Fifth Edition

PHARMACOTHERAPY

A Pathophysiologic Approach

Notice

Fifth Edition

PHARMACOTHERAPY

A Pathophysiologic Approach

Editors

Joseph T. DiPiro, PharmD, FCCP
Panoz Professor of Pharmacy, College of Pharmacy, University of Georgia;
Clinical Professor of Surgery, Medical College of Georgia, Augusta, Georgia

Robert L. Talbert, PharmD, FCCP, BCPS
Professor, College of Pharmacy, University of Texas at Austin;
Professor, Departments of Medicine and Pharmacology, University of Texas Health Science Center at San Antonio, San Antonio, Texas

Gary C. Yee, PharmD, FCCP
Professor and Chair, Department of Pharmacy Practice, College of Pharmacy,
University of Nebraska Medical Center, Omaha, Nebraska

Gary R. Matzke, PharmD, FCP, FCCP
Professor and Vice Chair, Department of Pharmacy and Therapeutics, School of Pharmacy;
Professor of Medicine, Renal-Electrolyte Division, School of Medicine,
University of Pittsburgh, Pittsburgh, Pennsylvania

Barbara G. Wells, PharmD, FASHP, FCCP, BCPP
Dean and Professor, School of Pharmacy, The University of Mississippi, University, Mississippi

L. Michael Posey, BS Pharm
President, PENS Pharmacy Editorial and News Services, Athens, Georgia

McGRAW-HILL
Medical Publishing Division

New York Chicago San Francisco Lisbon
London Madrid Mexico City Milan New Delhi
San Juan Seoul Singapore Sydney Toronto

McGraw-Hill
A Division of The McGraw-Hill Companies

Pharmacotherapy: A Pathophysiologic Approach, Fifth Edition

1 2 3 4 5 6 7 8 9 0 DOWDOW 0 9 8 7 6 5 4 3 2

ISBN 0-07-136361-0

This book was set in Times Roman by TechBooks, Inc.
The editors were Julie Scardiglia, Susan R. Noujaim, and Peter J. Boyle; the production supervisor was Richard Ruzycka; the text designer was Joan O'Connor; the cover designer was Elizabeth Pisacreta; Barbara Littlewood prepared the index.
R.R. Donnelley and Sons was printer and binder.

This book is printed on acid-free paper.

Cataloging-in-publication data is on file for this title at the Library of Congress.

INTERNATIONAL EDITION ISBN: 0-07-121264-7

Dedication

To those pharmacists who had the courage and perseverance to pioneer the development of the clinical practice of pharmacy.

To the contemporary pharmaceutical care practitioners who continue to expand their impact on patient outcomes and thereby serve as role models for their colleagues and students while clinging tenaciously to the highest standards of practice.

To our mentors, whose vision provided educational and training programs that encouraged our professional growth and challenged us to be innovators in our patient care, research, and educational endeavors.

To our faculty colleagues for their efforts and support for our mission to provide a comprehensive and challenging educational foundation for the clinical pharmacists of the future.

And finally to our families for the time that they have sacrificed so that this fifth edition would become a reality.

CONTENTS

Foreword

During the latter half of the twentieth century, clinical medicine enjoyed enormous progress. Many examples of success come to mind easily, and most of them involve two factors: better understanding of what goes wrong when disease occurs and new medications developed specifically to reverse these pathophysiologic aberrations. In the United States, more than 33,000 cases of polio were recorded in 1950. By 1998, a single case occurred, thanks to universal use of vaccines that have nearly eradicated this dreaded disease. Mortality from cardiovascular diseases decreased as treatment of hypertension, lipid disorders, and congestive heart failure improved. Histamine H_2-receptor antagonists, proton pump inhibitors, and antibiotics all reduced morbidity and mortality rate associated with peptic ulcer disease. Improved pharmacotherapy for benign prostatic hyperplasia led to a decline in the need for prostatectomies.

The United States offers the most advanced medical and surgical therapies. The rich and the famous from all over the world come to the United States for treatment of their most serious illnesses. However, a report from the Institute of Medicine in 2001 described a gap between the excellent care provided to some patients and the average care provided to a majority of Americans. This gap is too large to be ignored.

Further, the American health care system remains too fragmented and uncoordinated. Too many Americans do not receive proper health care, and more than 43 million Americans lack insurance to cover even the most basic health care services. Considering these problems, it is hardly surprising that the United States recently ranked 37th in the world in overall health care system performance, despite its first-place ranking in health care expenditures.

Within this respected but inefficient health care system, how is pharmacotherapy doing? Not entirely well. For example, one-third to two-thirds of patients with mental disorders do not receive optimal pharmacotherapy. Only 20 percent of the eligible patients receive a beta-blocker within 3 months after a myocardial infarction. Many studies have shown an overuse of antibiotics but an underuse of preventive vaccines.

This situation provides a perfect opportunity for pharmacists to show that we can solve pharmacotherapy-related problems in the most cost-effective fashion. We can take charge of providing the most rational pharmacotherapy to our patients, because we are the best educated and trained health professionals to do so.

How do we achieve this goal? The first step in achieving this goal is to offer a cutting-edge curriculum in our doctor of pharmacy (PharmD) programs. A strong sequence of courses in pathophysiology and pharmacotherapy that builds on the foundations of pharmaceutical sciences and extends to application in experiential education and training is critical to achieve this goal.

When I was in a PharmD program a quarter of a century ago, pathophysiology was covered only in a cursory fashion. This was even more true in baccalaureate pharmacy programs of that era. But how can one understand and optimize drug therapy without understanding the disease, its clinical features, associated laboratory abnormalities, and what and how to monitor in the patient to measure and document the therapeutic outcomes? This is why, at Ohio State University, we designed our PharmD program in 1980 for students to take pathophysiology with the medical students. We had no pharmacy textbook covering pathophysiology at that time.

When *Pharmacotherapy: A Pathophysiologic Approach* was originally published in the fall of 1988, it became the first pharmacy textbook to integrate the principles of pathophysiology and pharmacotherapy. It covers epidemiology, etiology, pathophysiology, clinical presentation, diagnosis and prognosis, patient evaluation, desired treatment outcome, general approach to treatment, supportive and pharmacologic treatment for the disease and its complications, pharmacotherapy recommendations while considering their advantages and disadvantages, evaluation of therapeutic outcomes, and key principles of pharmacotherapy. The text follows a consistent format and yet allows some flexibility to authors depending on the topic and style for their personal touch. The extensive use of figures and tables facilitate learning of content.

What is the future of pharmacotherapy, and where does this text fit in that picture? The process for drug discovery, design, and delivery will continue to be enhanced with new knowledge in science and technology. The prevention, diagnosis, and treatment of disease will also advance at a much faster pace than before, in part due to the burgeoning knowledge of pharmacogenetics, pharmacogenomics, proteomics, and bioinformatics. In the coming years, clinicians will likely know at the time of diagnosis which patients will respond best to which chemotherapeutic agents or antihypertensive drugs, avoiding the current somewhat arbitrary hit-or-miss, time-consuming approach. For certain diseases, gene therapy could provide definitive cures—although when and at what cost remain unknown.

The most important contribution pharmacists and other interested primary-care providers can make to patient care is to provide the most effective, safe, and economical pharmacotherapy, based on the best available evidence and documented by improved health outcomes and quality of life. For this purpose, *Pharmacotherapy: A Pathophysiologic Approach* provides excellent content, including information on which agents work best, what outcomes to monitor, and what key points to remember when treating patients. Further, thorough referencing to the original literature enables clinicians to consider the evidence for themselves and judge how it should be applied to the individual patient. Indeed, by going into detail on why recommendations are made, authors in *Pharmacotherapy* enable students and practitioners to understand their principles and thought processes in analyzing the evidence and making recommendations. "How to think" empowers the emerging clinician much more than does telling them "what to think." The available literature is out of date in a short few years, and the new evidence can render old evidence useless. Lifelong learning is required of all health care practitioners to remain current. Pharmacotherapists who study this text gain an understanding as to *why* the recommendations are made, and they are therefore ready to take on new information about drugs or disease and reach sound conclusions about ideas' impact on approaches to therapy.

To succeed in the twenty-first century, the new graduate must understand how to efficiently manage the dispensing function of pharmacy practice through use of technicians and technology; assess patients' conditions; evaluate, recommend, and monitor drug therapy; work and communicate with other health care practitioners; and educate and counsel patients so that they become involved with their own therapy. Our patients must know the desired outcomes to be achieved as well as possible adverse effects and drug–drug or drug–food interactions. They should know what to do when expected outcomes are not achieved or when unexpected adverse events occur with medicines. The patients should also understand the role of complementary or alternative medicines in the management of their illnesses. We are likely to achieve the desired goals only when our patients feel we care and take a genuine interest in their health and well-being.

Well-educated and well-trained pharmacists are not only finding satisfying careers in community pharmacies, medical centers, managed care, long-term care, clinics, academia, and industry, they are creating opportunities by offering the knowledge and skills no one else possesses about optimizing pharmacotherapy. Pharmacists have come a long way in the last three decades. It was a challenge for me to be the first pharmacist on rounds at Children's Hospital 23 years ago, and the attending physician wondered about the role of a pharmacist outside of a hospital pharmacy. The hospital now employs eight pharmacists with primary responsibility to provide patient care in a 170-bed facility. Practice models need to be developed now to offer patient focused care in the community pharmacies. I believe that pharmacists will continue to capture the opportunities to make unique contributions to health care of our society, and help elevate the profession to even greater heights.

Milap C. Nahata, MS, PharmD
Professor and Division Chairman
College of Pharmacy
Professor of Pediatrics
College of Medicine
The Ohio State University and Children's Hospital
Columbus, Ohio
July 2001

FOREWORD TO THE FIRST EDITION

Evidence of the maturity of a profession is not unlike that characterizing the maturity of an individual; a child's utterances and behavior typically reveal an unrealized potential for attainment, eventually, of those attributes characteristic of an appropriately confident, independently competent, socially responsible, sensitive, and productive member of society.

Within a period of perhaps 15 or 20 years, we have witnessed a profound maturation within the profession of pharmacy. The utterances of the profession, as projected in its literature, have evolved from mostly self-centered and self-serving issues of trade protection to a composite of expressed professional interests that prominently include responsible explorations of scientific/technological questions and ethical issues that promote the best interests of the clientele served by the profession. With the publication of *Pharmacotherapy: A Pathophysiologic Approach,* pharmacy's utterances bespeak a matured practitioner who is able to call upon unique knowledge and skills so as to function as an appropriately confident, independently competent pharmacotherapeutics expert.

In 1987, the Board of Pharmaceutical Specialties (BPS), in denying the petition filed by the American College of Clinical Pharmacy (ACCP) to recognize "clinical pharmacy" as a specialty, conceded nonetheless that the petitioning party had documented in its petition a specialist who does in fact exist within the practice of pharmacy and whose expertise clearly can be extricated from the performance characteristics of those in general practice. A refiled petition from ACCP requests recognition of "pharmacotherapy" as a Specialty Area of Pharmacy Practice. While the BPS had issued no decision when this book went to press it is difficult to comprehend the basis for a rejection of the second petition.

Within this book one will find the scientific foundation for the essential knowledge required of one who may aspire to specialty practice as a pharmacotherapist. As is the case with any such publication, its usefulness to the practitioner or the future practitioner is limited to providing such a foundation. To be socially and professionally responsible in practice, the pharmacotherapist's foundation must be continually supplemented and complemented by the flow of information appearing in the primary literature. Of course this is not unique to the general or specialty practice of pharmacy; it is essential to the fulfillment of obligations to clients in any occupation operating under the code of professional ethics.

Because of the growing complexity of pharmacotherapeutic agents, their dosing regimens, and techniques for delivery, pharmacy is obligated to produce, recognize, and remunerate specialty practitioners who can fulfill the profession's responsibilities to society for service expertise where the competence required in a particular case exceeds that of the general practitioner. It simply is a component of our covenant with society and is as important as any other facet of that relationship existing between a profession and those it serves.

The recognition by BPS of pharmacotherapy as an area of specialty practice in pharmacy will serve as an important statement by the profession that we have matured sufficiently to be competent and willing to take unprecedented responsibilities in the collaborative, pharmacotherapeutic management of patient-specific problems. It commits pharmacy to an intention that will not be uniformly or rapidly accepted within the established health care community. Nonetheless, this formal action places us on the road to an avowed goal, and acceptance will be gained as the pharmacotherapists proliferate and establish their importance in the provision of optimal, cost-effective drug therapy.

Suspecting that other professions in other times must have faced similar quests for recognition of their unique knowledge and skills I once searched the literature for an example that might parallel pharmacy's modern-day aspirations. Writing in the *Philadelphia Medical Journal,* May 27, 1899, D. H. Galloway, MD, reflected on the need for specialty training and practice in a field of medicine lacking such expertise at that time. In an article entitled "The Anesthetizer as a Speciality," Galloway commented:

> *The anesthetizer will have to make his own place in medicine: the profession will not make a place for him, and not until he has demonstrated the value of his services will it concede him the position which the importance of his duties entitles him to occupy. He will be obliged to define his own rights, duties and privileges, and he must not expect that his own estimate of the importance of his position will be conceded without opposition. There are many surgeons who are unwilling to share either the credit or the emoluments of their work with any one, and their opposition will be overcome only when they are shown that the importance of their work will not be lessened, but enhanced, by the increased safety and dispatch with which operations may be done. . . .*

It has been my experience that, given the opportunity for one-on-one, collaborative practice with physicians and other health professionals, pharmacy practitioners who have been educated and trained to perform at the level of pharmacotherapeutics specialists almost invariably have convinced the former that "the importance of their work will not be lessened, but enhanced, by the increased safety and dispatch with which" individualized problems of drug therapy could be managed in collaboration with clinical pharmacy practitioners.

It is fortuitous—the coinciding of the release of *Pharmacotherapy: A Pathophysiologic Approach* with ACCP's petitioning of BPS for recognition of the pharmacotherapy specialist. The utterances of a maturing profession as revealed in the contents of this book, and the intraprofessional recognition and acceptance of a higher level of responsibility in the safe, effective, and economical use of drugs and drug products, bode well for the future of the profession and for the improvement of patient care with drugs.

Charles A. Walton, PhD
San Antonio, Texas

Preface

Pharmacists, pharmacotherapists, and other health care professionals who rely each day on medications to treat diseases in people face many challenges in these early years of the 21st century. As we complete our work on this fifth edition of *Pharmacotherapy: A Pathophysiologic Approach,* we recognize just how much our tasks as editors have become equally complicated, trying to balance readers' needs for accurate, thorough, and unbiased information about drug treatment of diseases against the hard publishing realities of deadlines, word counts, and book length. We also keep foremost in our minds those precepts that first led us to compile this text:

- Advance the level of pharmaceutical care through understanding of pharmacotherapeutic principles.
- Stimulate the student to achieve higher levels of learning.
- Motivate the young practitioner to perform more advanced patient care.
- Challenge established pharmacists and other primary-care providers to learn concepts missed during years of practice.
- Inform the pharmacy profession as well as clinical medicine professionals more broadly about the standards of pharmaceutical care toward which we all should strive and which all patients will one day expect and, yes, demand.

Even more so than with previous updates, we have sought with this fifth edition to make certain that *Pharmacotherapy* remains on the cutting edge of clinical practice. Before soliciting chapters for this edition, we considered the dozens of new medications that became available in the late 1990s, and this process led us to create a new Urologic Disorders section and to add other new chapters, as detailed below. During editing, we reviewed each passage of text—and the references cited—for continued relevance and accuracy. We made deletions, asked authors to summarize concepts more succinctly or use tables to present details more concisely, included new medications as they came onto the U.S. market or emerged in other countries, and updated references. This process continued as the book entered production, and even during proofs, we continued to make sure that this book is as current and complete as any printed work of its size can be.

New chapters that long-time users of *Pharmacotherapy* will notice are the following:

- Evidence-Based Medicine
- Pharmacogenetics
- Disorders of Sodium, Water, Calcium, and Phosphorus Homeostasis (this chapter and the following one were covered in previous editions in a combined chapter, Electrolyte Homeostasis)
- Disorders of Potassium and Magnesium Homeostasis
- Endometriosis
- Erectile Dysfunction
- Benign Prostatic Hyperplasia
- Urinary Incontinence
- Superficial Fungal Infections

To incorporate these new chapters yet keep the book in only one volume, we have presented all text in the slightly smaller typeface used for the Treatment sections of the last edition. And as discussed above, the cooperation of many contributors in agreeing to make necessary deletions and summations was invaluable in this process.

The addition of more structure to disease-oriented chapters and the inclusion of more design elements, especially in the Treatment sections, were popular among readers of the fourth edition. These aspects have been retained, including sections on desired outcomes of treatment, improved flow diagrams that present standard elements, and the Principles of Pharmacotherapy section that concludes each chapter.

Standard formats have remained relatively unchanged since the very first edition of *Pharmacotherapy.* When seeking information in the disease-oriented chapters, users will find these sections: Epidemiology, Etiology, Pathophysiology, Clinical Presentation (including diagnostic considerations), Treatment (including desired outcomes, general approaches, nonpharmacologic therapy, pharmacologic therapy, and pharmacoeconomic considerations), Evaluation of Therapeutic Outcomes, and Principles of Pharmacotherapy.

As the world increasingly relies on electronic means of communication, we are committed to keeping *Pharmacotherapy* and its companion works, *Pharmacotherapy Casebook: A Patient-Focused Approach* and *Pharmacotherapy Handbook,* integral components of clinicians' toolboxes. Plans include a Web site with unique features that will benefit students, practitioners, and faculty. Watch the McGraw-Hill Web site (www.mcgraw-hill.com) for information about Pharmacotherapy Online.

In closing, we also stop once again to acknowledge the many hours that *Pharmacotherapy*'s 200 authors contribute to this labor of love. Without their devotion to the cause of improved pharmacotherapy and dedication in maintaining the accuracy, clarity, and relevance of their chapters, this text would unquestionably not be possible. In addition, we thank our colleagues at McGraw-Hill for their consistent support of the *Pharmacotherapy* family of resources, insights into trends in publishing and higher education, and the necessary and critical attention to detail so necessary in a book such as this one.

The Editors
January 2002

In Memoriam

Larry E. Boh (1953–2001) was a graduate of the University of Wisconsin School of Pharmacy and the University of Wisconsin Hospital pharmacy residency program. His career as a pharmacy educator began at the State University of New York at Buffalo. He returned to Wisconsin, where he rose to the rank of professor. He also served for many years as the chair of the Pharmacy Practice Division at the University of Wisconsin.

Professor Boh was widely known for his accomplishments in clerkship education. He was the editor of the *Clinical Clerkship Manual,* a text devoted to the clinical instruction of pharmacy students. Larry's skills and commitment were recognized by his peers and students in many ways, including being named a winner of the Rufus A. Lyman Award of the American Association of Colleges of Pharmacy, numerous "Teacher of the Year" awards at the University of Wisconsin School of Pharmacy, and the Distinguished Pharmacist of the Year Award from the Pharmacy Society of Wisconsin.

Contributors

Keith D. Aaronson, MD, MS
Assistant Professor of Internal Medicine, Medical Director, Cardiac Transplant Program, Division of Cardiology, Department of Medicine, University of Michigan Medical School, Ann Arbor, MI
Chapter 18

Betty J. Abate, PharmD, BCPS
Coordinator of Drug Information Services, Department of Pharmacy, Hurley Medical Center, Farmington Hills, MI
Chapter 104

Paul A. Abraham, MD
Associate Professor of Medicine, University of Minnesota; Chief of Nephrology, Regions Hospital, St. Paul, MN
Chapter 48

Val R. Adams, PharmD
Assistant Professor, Department of Pharmacy Practice, University of Kentucky, Lexington, KY
Chapter 129

Jeffrey R. Aeschlimann, PharmD
Assistant Professor of Pharmacy, University of Connecticut School of Pharmacy and St. Francis Hospital, Department of Research, Hartford, CT
Chapter 103

J. V. Anandan, PharmD, BCPS
Assistant Director of Pharmacy, Department of Pharmacy Services, Henry Ford Hospital; Adjunct Associate Professor, College of Pharmacy and Allied Health Professions, Wayne State University, Detroit, MI
Chapter 113

J. D. Anderson, PharmD
University of Minnesota Pharmaceutical Care Resident, Paynesville Area Health Care System, Paynesville, MN
Chapter 111

Edward P. Armstrong, PharmD, BCPS, FASHP
Associate Professor, Department of Pharmacy Practice and Science, University of Arizona, College of Pharmacy, Tucson, AZ
Chapter 116

Margaret Artz, RPh, PhD
Assistant Professor and Research Scientist, Institute for the Study of Geriatric Pharmacotherapy, College of Pharmacy, University of Minnesota, Minneapolis, MN
Chapter 7

George R. Bailie, MS, PharmD, PhD, FCCP
Professor of Pharmacy Practice, Albany College of Pharmacy, Albany, NY
Chapter 47

Jacquelyn L. Bainbridge, PharmD
Assistant Professor of Pharmacy Practice, School of Pharmacy, University of Colorado Health Sciences Center, Denver, CO
Chapter 55

Carol McManus Balmer, PharmD
Associate Professor, School of Pharmacy, University of Colorado Health Sciences Center, Denver, CO
Chapter 124

Jeffrey F. Barletta, PharmD
Clinical Specialist–Surgery/Critical Care, Adjunct Assistant Professor, Department of Pharmacy Services, Detroit Receiving Hospital and University Health Center, Wayne State University, Detroit, MI
Chapter 11

Steven L. Barriere, PharmD
Director, Medical Affairs, Gilead Sciences, Foster City, CA
Chapter 104

Larry A. Bauer, PharmD, FCP, FCCP
Professor of Pharmacy and Laboratory Medicine, University of Washington, Seattle, WA
Chapter 4

Jerry L. Bauman, PharmD, BCPS, FCCP, FACC
Professor, Departments of Pharmacy Practice and Medicine, University of Illinois, Chicago, IL
Chapter 16

Terry J. Baumann, PharmD, BCPS
Clinical Manager, Department of Pharmacy, Munson Medical Center, Traverse City, MI
Chapter 60

Eula D. Beasley, PharmD
Clinical Coordinator, Department of Pharmacy, The Washington Hospital Center, Washington, DC
Chapter 101

Brian E. Beckett, PharmD
Associate Professor of Pharmacy Practice, McWhorter School of Pharmacy, Samford University, Director of Pharmacy, Health South Metro West Hospital, Birmingham, AL
Chapter 61

Rosemary R. Berardi, PharmD, FASHP, FCCP
Professor of Pharmacy, College of Pharmacy, The University of Michigan; Clinical Pharmacist in Gastroenterology, Department of Pharmacy, the University of Michigan Health System, Ann Arbor, MI
Chapters 33, 39

Richard C. Berchou, PharmD
Assistant Professor, Department of Psychiatry and Behavioral Neurosciences, Wayne State University, Detroit, MI
Chapter 59

Joseph S. Bertino, Jr., PharmD
Section Chief Clinical Pharmacology, Bassett Healthcare, Clinical Pharmacology Research Center, Cooperstown, NY
Chapter 122

Betsy Bickert, PharmD
Oncology/BMT Specialist, Children's Hospital of Philadelphia, Philadelphia, PA
Chapter 100

Larry E. Boh, RPh, MS (1953–2001)
Professor and Former Chair of Pharmacy Practice, University of Wisconsin School of Pharmacy, Madison, WI
Chapter 92

John A. Bosso, PharmD, FCCP, BCPS
Professor, Colleges of Pharmacy and Medicine, Medical University of South Carolina, Charleston, SC
Chapter 30

Bradley A. Boucher, PharmD, BCPS, FCCP
Professor of Clinical Pharmacy and Associate Professor of Neurosurgery, Department of Clinical Pharmacy and Neurology, University of Tennessee Health Sciences Center, Memphis, TN
Chapters 57, 58

J. Chris Bradberry, PharmD, FASHP
Professor and Chair, Department of Pharmacy Practice and Pharmacoeconomics, College of Pharmacy, University of Tennessee Health Sciences Center, Memphis, TN
Chapter 20

Donald F. Brophy, PharmD, BCPS
Assistant Professor, Department of Pharmacy, School of Pharmacy, Virginia Commonwealth University, Richmond, VA
Chapter 52

Thomas E. R. Brown, BScPhm, PharmD
Clinical Coordinator–Women's Health, and Assistant Professor, University of Toronto, Pharmacy, Sunnybrook and Women's College Health Science Centre, Toronto, ON, Canada
Chapter 118

Kathryn K. Bucci, PharmD, FCCP, BCPP
Clinical Education Consultant, Pfizer, Inc., Southold, NY
Chapter 80

Karim Anton Calis, PharmD, MPH, BCPS, BCNSP, FASHP
Clinical Specialist, Endocrinology and Women's Health, Coordinator, Drug Information Service, Warren G. Magnuson Clinical Center, National Institutes of Health, Bethesda, MD; Clinical Associate Professor, University of Maryland, Baltimore, MD; Associate Clinical Professor, Medical College of Virginia, Virginia Commonwealth University, Richmond, VA; Clinical Associate Professor, Shenandoah University, Winchester, VA
Chapters 77, 83

Barry L. Carter, PharmD, FCCP, BCPS
Professor, The University of Iowa, College of Pharmacy and Department of Medicine, Iowa City, IA
Chapter 12

Peggy L. Carver, PharmD
Associate Professor of Pharmacy, University of Michigan College of Pharmacy; Clinical Pharmacist, Infectious Diseases, University of Michigan Health System, Ann Arbor, MI
Chapter 119

Nina Han Cheigh, PharmD
Clinical Assistant Professor and Coordinator of Academic Programs, University of Illinois College of Pharmacy, Chicago, IL
Chapters 96, 97

Kathleen Hammond Chessman, BS, PharmD, BCNSP, BCPS
Associate Professor of Pharmacy Practice, Clinical Pharmacy Specialist, Pediatrics/Pediatric Surgery, College of Pharmacy, Medical University of South Carolina, Charleston, SC
Chapters 135, 138

Thomas W. F. Chin, BScPhm, PharmD
Clinical Pharmacy Specialist, Pharmacy and Innercity Health Programme, St. Michael's Hospital; Assistant Professor, University of Toronto, Toronto, ON, Canada
Chapter 118

Elaine Chiquette, PharmD, BCPS
Scientific Medical Manager, Aventis, San Antonio, TX
Chapter 3

Marie A. Chisholm, PharmD
Associate Professor of Pharmacy and Clinical Associate Professor of Medicine, University of Georgia College of Pharmacy and the Medical College of Georgia, Augusta, GA
Chapter 31

Peter A. Chyka, FAACT, DABAT
Professor of Pharmacy Practice and Pharmacoeconomics, College of Pharmacy, University of Tennessee, Memphis, TN
Chapter 9

William R. Clark, PharmD, BCPP
Clinical Pharmacy Specialist, Psychiatry, Pharmacy Department, Central Texas Veterans Health Care System, Waco, TX
Chapter 65

Ann C. Collier, MD
Professor, University of Washington, AIDS Clinical Trials Unit, Harborview Medical Center, Seattle, WA
Chapter 123

Allan J. Collins, MD, FACP
Professor of Medicine, University of Minnesota; Director, United States Renal Data System, Minneapolis, MN
Chapter 45

Thomas J. Comstock, PharmD
Associate Professor, Department of Pharmacy, School of Pharmacy, Virginia Commonwealth University, Richmond, VA
Chapter 42

Stephen Joel Coons, PhD
Professor, University of Arizona College of Pharmacy, Tucson, AZ
Chapter 2

John R. Corboy, MD
Associate Professor, Director of the MS Center, University of Colorado Health Sciences Center, Department of Neurology, Denver, CO
Chapter 55

Elizabeth A. Coyle, PharmD
Assistant Professor, Department of Clinical Sciences, College of Pharmacy, University of Houston, Houston, TX
Chapter 114

M. Lynn Crismon, PharmD, FCCP, BCPP
Professor, Clinical Pharmacologist, University of Texas College of Pharmacy, Division of Pharmacy Practice, Pharmacy Administration and Pharmacotherapy and Center for Pharmacoeconomic Studies, Austin, TX
Chapters 65, 68

Michael A. Crouch, PharmD, BCPS
Assistant Professor, School of Pharmacy, Department of Pharmacy Practice, Virginia Commonwealth University, Richmond, VA
Chapter 109

Clarence E. Curry, Jr., PharmD
Associate Professor, School of Pharmacy, College of Pharmacy, Nursing and AHS, Howard University, Washington, DC
Chapter 101

Judy L. Curtis, PharmD, BCPP, FASHP
Assistant Professor, Pharmacy Practice and Science, School of Pharmacy, University of Maryland, Randallstown, MD
Chapter 73

Larry H. Danziger, PharmD
Professor of Pharmacy, Co-Director, Section of Infectious Disease Pharmacotherapy, Associate Vice-Chancellor for Research, College of Pharmacy, University of Illinois, Chicago, IL
Chapter 108

Joseph F. Dasta, MSc
Professor of Pharmacy, College of Pharmacy, Ohio State University, Columbus, Ohio
Chapter 23

Lisa E. Davis, PharmD, FCCP, BCPS, BCOP
Associate Professor of Clinical Pharmacy, Philadelphia College of Pharmacy, University of the Sciences in Philadelphia, Philadelphia, PA
Chapter 127

Susan R. Davis, PhD, MBBS, FRACP
Director of Research, Associate Professor, Monash University, Victoria, Australia
Chapter 83

Suzanne D. Day, PharmD, BCOP
BMT Clinical Specialist, Oncology and Hematology Associates, and Saint Luke's Hospital of Kansas City, Kansas City, MO
Chapter 131

Renee M. DeHart, PharmD, BCPS
Associate Professor, Clinical Pharmacy Specialist, Samford University, McWhorter School of Pharmacy, Birmingham, AL
Chapter 139

Jeffrey C. Delafuente, MS, FCCP
Professor and Director of Geriatric Programs, Department of Pharmacy, Virginia Commonwealth University, Richmond, VA
Chapter 88

Michel Deschênes, MD
Chargé d'enseignement, Médecine d'urgence, Université Laval, Faculté de médecine, Ste-Foy, PQ, Canada
Chapter 107

John W. Devlin, PharmD, BCPS
Clinical Specialist, Surgery/Critical Care, Detroit Receiving Hospital, Department of Pharmacy Services; Adjunct Assistant Professor of Pharmacy Practice, College of Pharmacy, Wayne State University, Detroit, MI
Chapter 121

Lori M. Dickerson, PharmD, BCPS
Director of Pharmacotherapy, Assistant Professor, Department of Family Medicine, Medical University of South Carolina, Charleston, SC
Chapter 80

Jennifer L. Difilippi, PharmD, BCPP
Clinical Pharmacy Specialist, Psychiatry, Pharmacy Department, Central Texas Veterans Health Care System, Temple, TX
Chapters 65

Joseph T. DiPiro, PharmD, FCCP
Panoz Professor of Pharmacy, College of Pharmacy, University of Georgia; Clinical Professor of Surgery, Medical College of Georgia, Augusta, GA
Chapters 34, 89, 112, 117

Paul L. Doering, MS
Distinguished Service Professor of Pharmacy Practice, College of Pharmacy, University of Florida, Gainesville, FL
Chapters 66, 67

Julie A. Dopheide, PharmD, BCPP
Assistant Professor of Clinical Pharmacy and Psychiatry and the Behavioral Sciences, Schools of Pharmacy and Medicine, University of Southern California, Los Angeles, CA
Chapter 63

Peter G. Dorson, PharmD, BCPP
Clinical Assistant Professor, University of Texas College of Pharmacy, Austin, TX
Chapter 68

Silvia S. Elias, PharmD
Pharmacist in Dermatology, Northwestern Medical Faculty Foundation, Chicago, IL
Chapters 96, 97

Mary E. Elliott, PharmD, PhD
Assistant Professor of Pharmacy Practice, University of Wisconsin School of Pharmacy, Madison, WI
Chapters 90, 92

Brian L. Erstad, PharmD
Associate Professor, Department of Pharmacy Practice and Sciences, College of Pharmacy, University of Arizona, Tucson, AZ
Chapter 24

Susan C. Fagan, PharmD, BCPS, FCCP
Professor of Pharmacy, University of Georgia, College of Pharmacy, Department of Neurology, Augusta, GA
Chapters 20, 54

Martha P. Fankhauser, MS Pharm, FASHP, BCPP
Clinical Associate Professor, Department of Pharmacy Practice and Science, University of Arizona, College of Pharmacy, Tucson, AZ
Chapters 70, 81

Sally A. Felton, PharmD, BCOP
Associate Clinical Oncology Manager, Aventis Clinical Oncology Programs, Nashville, TN
Chapter 126

Rebecca S. Finley, PharmD, MS, FASHP
Associate Professor and Chair, Department of Pharmacy Practice and Administration, University of the Sciences in Philadelphia, Philadelphia, PA
Chapter 126

Douglas N. Fish, PharmD, BCPS
Associate Professor of Pharmacy, School of Pharmacy, Department of Pharmacy Practice, University of Colorado Health Sciences Center, Denver, CO
Chapters 108, 120

Courtney V. Fletcher, PharmD
Professor, University of Colorado Health Sciences Center, School of Pharmacy, Department of Pharmacy Practice, Denver, CO
Chapter 123

Reginald F. Frye, PharmD, PhD
Assistant Professor, Department of Pharmaceutical Sciences, University of Pittsburgh, School of Pharmacy, Pittsburgh, PA
Chapter 50

Peter Gal, PharmD, BCPS, FCCP, FASHP
Director, Pharmacy Division, Greensboro Area Health Education Center, Greensboro, NC; Neonatal Pharmacotherapy Consultant, Women's Hospital of Greensboro, Moses Cone Health System, Greensboro, NC; Clinical Professor, Division of Pharmacotherapy, School of Pharmacy, University of North Carolina at Chapel Hill, Chapel Hill, NC
Chapter 28

William R. Garnett, PharmD, FCCP
Professor of Pharmacy and Pharmaceutics, Medical College of Virginia, College of Pharmacy, Richmond, VA
Chapter 56

Todd W. B. Gehr, MD
Professor of Medicine, Virginia Commonwealth University Medical College, Richmond, VA
Chapter 52

Barry E. Gidal, PharmD
Associate Professor, School of Pharmacy, University of Wisconsin, Madison, WI
Chapters 55, 56

Mark A. Gill, PharmD
Professor of Clinical Pharmacy, University of Southern California, Los Angeles, CA
Chapter 38

Mark L. Glover, PharmD
Assistant Professor, College of Pharmacy, Department of Pharmacy Practice, Nova Southeastern University, Ft. Lauderdale, FL
Chapter 106

Nina Graves, PharmD, FCCP
Epilepsy Program Manager, Staff Scientist, Medtronic, Inc., Minneapolis, MN
Chapter 56

David R. P. Guay, PharmD, CGP, FCP, FCCP, FASCP
Professor and Director of Education and Clinical Pharmacist Specialist in Geriatrics, University of Minnesota College of Pharmacy, Institute for the Study of Geriatric Pharmacotherapy, and Partnering Care Senior Services at Regions Hospital, Minneapolis and St. Paul, MN
Chapters 7, 86

John G. Gums, PharmD
Professor of Pharmacy and Medicine, Departments of Pharmacy Practice and Family Medicine, University of Florida, Gainesville, FL
Chapter 76

Brent W. Gunderson, PharmD
Infectious Disease Research Fellow, Experimental and Clinical Pharmacology, University of Minnesota College of Pharmacy, Minneapolis, MN
Chapter 105

Stuart T. Haines, PharmD, BCPS, CDE, CACP, FASHP
School Associate Professor, Clinical Instructor, Director, Antithrombosis Service, University of Maryland School of Pharmacy, Baltimore, MD
Chapter 19

Philip D. Hall, PharmD, FCCP, BCPS, BCOP
Associate Professor, Department of Pharmaceutical Sciences, Medical University of South Carolina, Charleston, SC
Chapter 87

Joseph T. Hanlon, PharmD, MS, BCPS, FASCP, FASHP
Professor, VFW Endowed Chair Pharmacotherapy for the Elderly, Director, and Clinical Pharmacist Specialist in Geriatrics, University of Minnesota College of Pharmacy, Institute for the Study of Geriatric Pharmacotherapy, and Minneapolis Veterans Affairs Medical Center, Minneapolis, MN
Chapter 7

J. William Harbilas, PharmD
Clinical Specialist, Ambulatory Care, Department of Pharmacy, Shands at the University of Florida, Gainesville, FL
Chapter 102

David W. Hawkins, PharmD
Professor of Pharmacy Practice and Senior Associate Dean, Mercer University Southern School of Pharmacy, Atlanta, GA
Chapter 93

Peggy E. Hayes, PharmD
Senior Strategic Consultant, Quintiles CNS Therapeutics, Medical and Regulatory Services, San Diego, CA
Chapters 69, 72

Mary S. Hayney, PharmD, BCPS
Assistant Professor of Pharmacy (CHS), University of Wisconsin School of Pharmacy, Madison, WI
Chapter 122

Thomas K. Hazlet, PharmD, DrPH
Assistant Professor, Department of Pharmacy, School of Pharmacy, University of Washington, Seattle, WA
Chapter 8

Amy M. Heck, PharmD
Clinical Assistant Professor of Pharmacy Practice, Purdue University School of Pharmacy and Pharmaceutical Sciences, Indianapolis, IN
Chapter 77

Karen L. Heim-Duthoy, PharmD, FCCP
Associate Professor, University of Minnesota, College of Pharmacy, Department of Pharmaceutical Care and Health Systems, Minneapolis, MN
Chapter 46

David W. Henry, MS, BCOP, FASHP
Associate Professor, Department of Pharmacy Practice, University of Kansas Medical Center, Kansas City, KS
Chapter 131

Katherine C. Herndon, PharmD, BCPS
Clinical Education Consultant, Pfizer, Inc., Birmingham, AL
Chapter 61

Gerald A. Hladik, MD
Clinical Assistant Professor, Division of Nephrology, School of Medicine, University of North Carolina, Chapel Hill, NC
Chapter 51

Collin A. Hovinga, PharmD
Neuropharmacology Research Specialist, Departments of Pharmacy and Neurology, Cleveland Clinics Foundation, Cleveland, OH
Chapter 57

Thomas R. Howdieshell, MD, FACS, FCCP
Associate Professor of Surgery, Medical College of Georgia, Department of Surgery, Augusta, GA
Chapter 112

Larisa M. Humma, PharmD, BCPS
Assistant Professor, Department of Pharmacy Practice, University of Illinois at Chicago, Chicago, IL
Chapter 5

Khalid H. Ibrahim, PharmD
Infectious Disease Research Fellow, Experimental and Clinical Pharmacology, University of Minnesota College of Pharmacy, Minneapolis, MN
Chapter 105

William L. Isley, MD
Associate Professor of Medicine, School of Medicine, University of Missouri, Kansas City, MO
Chapter 74

Mark W. Jackson, MD
Staff Physician, Baptist Hospital of East Tennessee and Fort Sanders Regional Medical Center, Knoxville, TN
Chapter 31

Stephen W. Janning, PharmD
Senior Regional Medical Scientist, North America Medical Affairs, Glaxo Smith Kline, Durham, NC
Chapter 121

Douglas D. Janson, PharmD, BCNSP
Assistant Professor, Department of Pharmacy and Therapeutics, University of Pittsburgh, School of Pharmacy, Pittsburgh, PA
Chapter 138

Donna M. Jermain, PharmD, BCPP
Senior Regional Medical Research Specialist, Pfizer, Inc., Georgetown, TX
Chapter 73

Thomas E. Johns, PharmD, BCPS
Manager, Clinical Practice Operations, Department of Pharmacy, Shands at the University of Florida, Gainesville, FL
Chapter 102

Heather J. Johnson, PharmD
Assistant Professor, Department of Pharmacy and Therapeutics, School of Pharmacy, University of Pittsburgh, Pittsburgh, PA
Chapter 46

Julie A. Johnson, PharmD, BCPS, FCCP
Professor of Pharmacy Practice and Medicine, University of Florida, College of Pharmacy and Medicine, Gainesville, FL
Chapter 13

Melanie S. Joy, PharmD
Clinical Assistant Professor, Director of Clinical Research, Division of Nephrology, School of Medicine, University of North Carolina, Chapel Hill, NC
Chapter 51

Laura L. Jung, PharmD
Research Fellow, Program of Molecular Therapeutics and Drug Development, University of Pittsburgh Cancer Institute, Pittsburgh, PA
Chapter 130

Thomas N. Kakuda, PharmD
Associate Clinical Research Scientist, Abbott Laboratories; Clinical Assistant Professor, University of Minnesota, Minneapolis, MN
Chapter 123

Sophia N. Kalantaridou, MD, PhD
Lecturer, Department of Obstetrics and Gynecology, University of Ioannina, School of Medicine, University Hospital, Ioannina, Greece
Chapter 83

Judith C. Kando, PharmD, BCPP
Director, Pharmacy Practice and Patient Safety, Assistant Clinical Professor of Psychiatry, Harvard Medical School, McKesson HBOC Medical Management, Tewksbury, MA
Chapter 69

S. Lena Kang-Birken, PharmD
Associate Professor, Department of Pharmacy Practice, University of the Pacific, Santa Barbara, CA
Chapter 117

Salmaan Kanji, PharmD
Critical Care Pharmacotherapy Fellow, Department of Pharmacy Practice, Wayne State University College of Pharmacy, Detroit, MI
Chapter 121

Janet L. Karlix, PharmD
Associate Professor, Department of Pharmacy Practice, College of Pharmacy, University of Florida, Gainesville, FL
Chapter 87

Bertram L. Kasiske, MD
Professor, School of Medicine, University of Minnesota; Director, Division of Nephrology, Hennepin County Medical Center, Minneapolis, MN
Chapter 44

H. William Kelly, PharmD, FCCP
Professor of Pharmacy and Pediatrics, The University of New Mexico, Children's Hospital of New Mexico, Department of Pediatrics, Albuquerque, NM
Chapters 26, 29

Mehmood Khan, MD, FACE
Senior Associate Consultant, Mayo Clinic, Division of Endocrinology, Rochester, MN
Chapter 140

William R. Kirchain, PharmD, CDE
Associate Professor of Community Pharmacy, College of Pharmacy, Medical University of South Carolina, Charleston, SC
Chapter 38

Cynthia K. Kirkwood, PharmD, BCPP
Associate Professor, Department of Pharmacy and Pharmaceutics, Virginia Commonwealth University, Richmond, VA
Chapter 71

Kenneth P. Klinker, PharmD, BCPS
Clinical Specialist, Critical Care, Department of Pharmacy, Shands at the University of Florida, Gainesville, FL
Chapter 102

Leroy C. Knodel, PharmD
Director of Drug Information Service and Associate Professor, Department of Pharmacology, University of Texas Health Sciences Center at San Antonio; Clinical Associate Professor, College of Pharmacy, University of Texas at Austin, San Antonio, TX
Chapter 115

Jill M. Kolesar, PharmD, BCPS
Assistant Professor, School of Pharmacy, University of Wisconsin-Madison, Madison, WI
Chapter 128

Sherri L. Konzem, PharmD
Clinical Assistant Professor of Pharmacy, Department of Clinical Sciences and Administration, College of Pharmacy, University of Houston and Memorial Family Practice Residency Program, Houston, TX
Chapter 27

Connie K. Kraus, PharmD, BCPS
Clinical Associate Professor of Pharmacy, University of Wisconsin-Madison School of Pharmacy, Madison, WI
Chapter 78

Janet L. Kwiatkowski, MD
Assistant Professor of Pediatrics, Children's Hospital of Philadelphia, Division of Hematology, Philadelphia, PA
Chapter 100

Thomas Lackner, PharmD
Professor, University of Minnesota College of Pharmacy and Institute for the Study of Geriatric Pharmacotherapy, Minneapolis, MN
Chapter 86

Kathleen D. Lake, PharmD, FCCP, BCPS
Director, Clinical Transplant Research and Therapeutics, Senior Associate Research Scientist, Departments of Medicine and Surgery, University of Michigan Medical School, Clinical Professor, University of Michigan College of Pharmacy, Ann Arbor, MI
Chapter 18

Y. W. Francis Lam, PharmD
Associate Professor, Departments of Pharmacology and Medicine, University of Texas Health Science Center at San Antonio, San Antonio, TX; Clinical Associate Professor and James O. Burke Endowed Centennial Fellow in Pharmacy, University of Texas, Austin, TX
Chapter 5

Tom A. Larson, PharmD, FCCP
Associate Professor of Pharmacy Practice, Department of Pharmacy Practice, University of Minnesota, Minneapolis, MN
Chapter 111

Alan H. Lau, PharmD, FCCP
Professor, Department of Pharmacy Practice, College of Pharmacy, University of Illinois at Chicago, Chicago, IL
Chapter 49

Mary W. L. Lee, PharmD, BCPS, FCCP
Dean and Professor of Pharmacy Practice, Midwestern University, Downers Grove, IL
Chapters 84, 85

Todd D. Lemke, PharmD
Clinical Pharmacist, Pharmacy/Family Practice, Paynesville Area Health Care System, Paynesville, MN
Chapter 111

Timothy S. Lesar, PharmD
Director of Pharmacy, Albany Medical Center, Albany, NY
Chapter 94

Stephanie M. Levine, MD
Associate Professor of Medicine, Department of Medicine, University of Texas Health Science Center, San Antonio, TX
Chapter 25

Matthew J. Lewis, PharmD, BCPS
Clinical Assistant Professor, Department of Pharmaceutical Care and Health Systems, College of Pharmacy, University of Minnesota; Clinical Pharmacy Specialist, Renal Division, Hennepin County Medical Center, Minneapolis, MN
Chapters 44, 45

Peter A. LeWitt, MD
Clinical Professor, Neurology and Psychiatry, Wayne State University, Detroit, MI, Sinai Clinical Neuroscience Center, Southfield, MI
Chapter 59

Cynthia L. Lieu, PharmD
Assistant Professor of Pharmacy Practice, School of Pharmacy, University of Southern California, Los Angeles, CA
Chapters 79, 82

Celeste Lindley, PharmD, MS, FCCP, BCPS
Associate Professor and Vice-Chair, School of Pharmacy, University of North Carolina, Chapel Hill, NC
Chapter 125

Gwynn D. Long, MD
Associate Clinical Professor, Department of Medicine, Duke University Medical Center, Durham, NC
Chapter 98

Larry M. Lopez, PharmD, FCCP
Professor of Pharmacy and Medicine, Chairman, Department of Pharmacy Practice, College of Pharmacy, University of Florida, Gainesville, FL
Chapter 15

Patricia A. Marken, BS Pharm, PharmD, BCPP
Chair, Associate Professor of Pharmacy Practice and Psychiatry, University of Missouri, Kansas City, MO
Chapter 62, 64

Patricia L. Marshik, PharmD
College of Pharmacy, Health Sciences Center, University of New Mexico, Albuquerque, NM
Chapter 29

Todd W. Mattox, PharmD, BCNSP
Nutrition Support Pharmacist, Department of Pharmacy, H. Lee Moffitt Cancer Center Hospital Inc., Lutz, FL
Chapter 137

Gary R. Matzke, PharmD, FCP, FCCP
Professor and Vice Chair, Department of Pharmacy and Therapeutics, School of Pharmacy; Professor of Medicine, Renal-Electrolyte Division, School of Medicine, University of Pittsburgh, Pittsburgh, PA
Chapters 47, 48, 50, 53

J. Russell May, PharmD
Director of Pharmacy, Medical College of Georgia Hospitals and Clinics; Adjunct Associate Professor, University of Georgia College of Pharmacy, Augusta, GA
Chapter 95

Margaret E. McGuinness, PharmD
Assistant Professor, Oregon State University, College of Pharmacy, Portland, OR
Chapter 10

Timothy R. McGuire, PharmD, FCCP
Associate Professor, Department of Pharmacy Practice, University of Nebraska Medical Center, Omaha, NE
Chapter 132

Sarah T. Melton, PharmD, BCPP
Consultant Pharmacist, Highlands Family Medicine, Lebanon, VA
Chapter 71

Gary Milavetz, PharmD
Associate Professor, College of Pharmacy, University of Iowa, Iowa City, IA
Chapter 30

Patricia A. Montgomery, PharmD
Clinical Pharmacy Specialist, Mercy General Hospital, Sacramento, CA
Chapter 39

Bruce A. Mueller, PharmD, FCCP, BCPS
Professor and Chair, Clinical Sciences Department, University of Michigan, College of Pharmacy, Ann Arbor, MI
Chapter 43

Milap C. Nahata, MS, PharmD
Professor and Chairman of Pharmacy Practice and Administration, and Professor of Pediatrics and Internal Medicine, Colleges of Pharmacy and Medicine, The Ohio State University, Columbus, OH
Chapter 6

Jean Nappi, PharmD, BCPS
Professor and Vice-Chair, Department of Pharmacy Practice, College of Pharmacy, Medical University of South Carolina, Charleston, SC
Chapter 17

Merlin V. Nelson, PharmD, MD
Neurologist, Department of Neurology, Affiliated Community Medical Center, Willmar, MN
Chapter 59

Fenwick T. Nichols, MD, FACP
Professor of Neurology, Medical College of Georgia, Augusta Veterans Administration Medical Center, Augusta, GA
Chapter 54

Thomas D. Nolin, MS, PharmD
PhD Candidate, University of Pittsburgh School of Pharmacy, Pittsburgh, PA
Chapter 48

Mary Beth O'Connell, PharmD, BCPS, FCCP, FSHP
Associate Professor of Experimental and Clinical Pharmacology, University of Minnesota College of Pharmacy, Minneapolis, MN
Chapter 90

Laura J. Odell, PharmD, CDE
Clinical Pharmacist, Pharmacy/Family Practice, Paynesville Area Health Care System, Paynesville, MN
Chapter 111

Julie C. Oki, PharmD, BCPS
Associate Professor, School of Medicine, University of Missouri, Kansas City, MO
Chapter 74

Dennis R. Ownby, MD
Professor of Pediatrics and Internal Medicine, Head, Section of Allergy and Immunology, Medical College of Georgia, Augusta, GA
Chapter 89

Paul M. Palevsky, MD
Chief Renal Section, Veterans Administration Pittsburgh Healthcare System; Professor of Medicine, Renal-Electrolyte Division, Department of Medicine, University of Pittsburgh School of Medicine, Pittsburgh, PA
Chapter 53

Robert B. Parker, PharmD, FCCP
Associate Professor of Clinical Pharmacy, University of Tennessee, College of Pharmacy, Department of Clinical Pharmacy, Memphis, TN
Chapter 13

Nital M. Patel, PharmD
Pharmacist in Dermatology, Northwestern Medical Faculty Foundation, Chicago, IL
Chapters 96, 97

J. Herbert Patterson, PharmD, FCCP, BCPS
Associate Professor of Pharmacy, School of Pharmacy, University of North Carolina at Chapel Hill, Chapel Hill, NC
Chapter 13

Steven Z. Pavletic, MD
Associate Professor, Department of Medicine, University of Nebraska Medical Center, Omaha, NE
Chapter 132

Charles A. Peloquin, PharmD
Director, Infectious Disease Pharmacokinetics Laboratory, National Jewish Medical and Research Center; Adjoint Associate Professor of Pharmacy and Medicine, University of Colorado, Denver, CO
Chapter 110

Susan L. Pendland, MS, PharmD
Assistant Professor, Department of Pharmacy, Director, Microbiology Research Laboratory, University of Illinois, Chicago, IL
Chapter 108

Janelle B. Perkins, PharmD, BCPS
Assistant Professor, Interdisciplinary Oncology Program and Manager, BMT Clinical Research, H. Lee Moffitt Cancer Center Hospital Inc., Tampa, FL
Chapter 134

Jay I. Peters, MD
Professor, Division of Pulmonary Medicine, Department of Medicine, University of Texas Health Science Center at San Antonio, San Antonio, TX
Chapter 25

William P. Petros, PharmD, FCCP
Associate Professor and Associate Director for Anticancer Drug Development, Mary Babb Randolph Cancer Center, West Virginia University, Morgantown, WV
Chapter 98

Stephanie J. Phelps, PharmD, FCCP
Professor of Clinical Pharmacy and Pediatrics, Department of Clinical Pharmacy and Neurology, University of Tennessee Health Science Center, Memphis, TN
Chapters 57, 58

Denise Walbrandt Pigarelli, PharmD
Clinical Assistant Professor of Pharmacy, Pharmacy Practice Division, University of Wisconsin-Madison School of Pharmacy, Madison, WI
Chapter 78

L. Michael Posey, BS Pharm
President, PENS Pharmacy Editorial & News Services, Athens, GA
Chapter 3

Randall A. Prince, PharmD
Professor, University of Houston, College of Pharmacy, Department of Clinical Sciences, Houston, TX
Chapter 114

Eric Racine, PharmD
Coordinator, Clinical Pharmacy Services, Harper Hospital, Detroit Medical Center, Clinical Assistant Professor, University of Michigan, Adjunct Assistant Professor, Wayne State University, Detroit, MI
Chapter 19

Marsha A. Raebel, PharmD, BCPS, FCCP
Pharmacotherapy Research Administrator, Kaiser Permanente of Colorado; Adjoint Associate Professor, University of Colorado School of Pharmacy, Clinical Research Unit, Denver, CO
Chapter 40

Daniel W. Rahn, MD
President and Professor of Medicine, Medical College of Georgia, Augusta, GA
Chapter 93

Hengameh H. Raissy, PharmD
The University of New Mexico, College of Pharmacy, Health Sciences Center, Albuquerque, NM
Chapter 29

Charles A. Reasner II, MD, FACE, FACP
Associate Professor, Department of Medicine, University of Texas Health Science Center, Austin; Medical Director, Texas Diabetes Institute, San Antonio, TX
Chapter 75

Michael D. Reed, PharmD, FCCP, FCP
Professor of Pediatrics and Director, Pediatric Clinical Pharmacology and Toxicology, School of Medicine, Case Western Reserve University and Rainbow Babies and Children's Hospital, Pediatric Pharmacology Division, Cleveland, OH
Chapter 106

Pamela D. Reiter, PharmD, BCPS
Clinical Pharmacy Specialist and Clinical Assistant Professor, Department of Pharmacy, University of Colorado Health Sciences Center, Denver, CO
Chapter 136

Monique Richer, PharmD, MA
Dean, Université Laval, Faculté de Pharmacie, Ste-Foy, PQ, Canada
Chapter 107

Gigi H. Ross, PharmD
Infectious Disease Specialist, Ican, Inc., Eden Prairie, MN
Chapter 105

John C. Rotschafer, PharmD
Professor, University of Minnesota College of Pharmacy, Experimental and Clinical Pharmacology, Minneapolis, MN
Chapter 105

Eric S. Rovner, MD
Assistant Professor of Urology, University of Pennsylvania School of Medicine and Hospital of the University of Pennsylvania, Philadelphia, PA
Chapter 86

Christine M. Ruby, PharmD, BCPS
Clinical Assistant Professor of Pharmacy, Senior Fellow, and Clinical Pharmacist Specialist in Geriatrics, University of North Carolina, Duke University Medical Center, and Durham Veterans Affairs Medical Center, Chapel Hill and Durham, NC
Chapter 7

Maria I. Rudis, PharmD, ABAT, BCPS
Assistant Professor of Clinical Pharmacy and Emergency Medicine, USC Schools of Pharmacy and Medicine, University of Southern California, Los Angeles, CA
Chapter 23

Michael J. Rybak, PharmD
Professor of Pharmacy and Medicine, Anti-Infective Research Laboratory, Detroit Receiving Hospital and Wayne State University College of Pharmacy and Allied Health Professions, Detroit, MI
Chapters 103, 121

Gordon S. Sacks, PharmD
Clinical Associate Professor, School of Pharmacy, University of Wisconsin, Madison, WI
Chapter 136

Lisa A. Sanchez, PharmD
President, PE Applications, Highlands Ranch, CO
Chapter 1

Joseph J. Saseen, PharmD, BCPS
Assistant Professor of Pharmacy and Family Medicine, Schools of Pharmacy and Medicine, University of Colorado Health Sciences Center, Denver, CO
Chapter 12

Robert R. Schade, MD
Professor, Department of Medicine, Chief, Section of Gastroenterology and Hepatology, Medical College of Georgia, Augusta, GA
Chapter 34

Lauren S. Schlesselman, PharmD
Clinical Pharmacy Specialist, Veterans Affairs Medical Center, Augusta, GA
Chapter 89

Mark E. Schneiderhan, BS Pharm, PharmD, BCPP
Clinical Assistant Professor, Pharmacotherapist, Psychiatry, University of Illinois at Chicago, Department of Pharmacy Practice, College of Pharmacy, Chicago, IL
Chapter 62

Marieka Dekker Schoen, PharmD, BCPS
Clinical Associate Professor, Departments of Pharmacy Practice and Medicine, University of Illinois, Chicago, IL
Chapter 16

Arthur A. Schuna, MS
Clinical Professor and Clinical Pharmacy Coordinator, University of Wisconsin School of Pharmacy and William S. Middleton Veterans Administration Medical Center, Madison, WI
Chapter 91

Rowena N. Schwartz, PharmD, BCOP
Associate Professor, Department of Pharmacy and Therapeutics, School of Pharmacy, University of Pittsburgh, Pittsburgh, PA
Chapter 133

Christopher L. Shaffer, PharmD, BCPS
Systems Manager, Department of Pharmacy Practice, Creighton University, Omaha, NE
Chapter 28

Alka Z. Somani, PharmD
Global Medical Affairs, Wyeth Pharmaceuticals, Radnor, PA
Chapter 41

Roger W. Sommi, Jr., BS Pharm, PharmD, BCPP
Associate Professor of Pharmacy Practice and Psychiatry, University of Missouri Kansas City, Department of Pharmacy, Kansas City, MO
Chapter 64

Christine A. Sorkness, PharmD
Professor of Pharmacy Practice, School of Pharmacy, University of Wisconsin-Madison, Madison, WI
Chapter 26

Thomas T. Sproat, PharmD, BCPS, PA-C
Product Manager, Infectious Diseases, Pharmacia Corporation, Peapack, NJ
Chapter 99

William J. Spruill, PharmD, FASHP
Associate Professor, University of Georgia, College of Pharmacy, Athens, GA
Chapter 36

John V. St. Peter, PharmD, BCPS
Clinical Associate Professor, College of Pharmacy, University of Minnesota; Division of Endocrinology, Hennepin County Medical Center, Minneapolis, MN
Chapter 140

Wendy L. St. Peter, PharmD, FCCP, BCPS
Associate Professor, College of Pharmacy, University of Minnesota, Director, Nephrology Pharmacy Associates, Minneapolis, MN
Chapters 44, 45

Andy Stergachis, PhD
Vice President, Drugstore.com and the Hope Heart Institute, Bellevue and Seattle, WA
Chapter 8

Jennifer A. Stoffel, PharmD, BCPS
Critical Care Specialist-Liver Transplant, Assistant Professor, Department of Pharmacy and Therapeutics, UPMC Health System and University of Pittsburgh School of Pharmacy, Pittsburgh, PA
Chapter 41

James J. Stragand, MD, PhD, FACP, FACG
Staff Gastroenterologist, Bend Memorial Clinic, Bend, OR
Chapter 37

Mark A. Stratton, PharmD, BCPS, FASHP
Professor, Department of Pharmacy Practice, University of Oklahoma, Oklahoma City, OK
Chapter 27

Kathleen A. Stringer, PharmD, FCCP
Associate Professor, School of Pharmacy, University of Colorado Health Sciences Center, Denver, CO
Chapter 15

Christopher J. Sullivan, MD
Assistant Professor of Medicine, University of Minnesota Medical School, St. Paul, MN
Chapter 105

Carol Taketomo, PharmD
Pharmacy Manager, Children's Hospital of Los Angeles, Los Angeles, CA
Chapter 6

Robert L. Talbert, PharmD, FCCP, BCPS
Professor, College of Pharmacy, University of Texas at Austin; Professor, Departments of Medicine and Pharmacology, University of Texas Health Science Center, San Antonio, TX
Chapters 10, 14, 21, 22, 75

A. Thomas Taylor, PharmD
Associate Professor, University of Georgia College of Pharmacy; Clinical Professor, Medical College of Georgia, Department of Family Medicine, Augusta, GA
Chapter 35

Kathleen M. Teasley-Strausburg, MS, BCNSP
Pharmacy/Nutrition Support Consultant, Denver, CO
Chapter 135

Chris M. Terpening, PhD, PharmD
Clinical Pharmacy Fellow, Department of Pharmacy Practice and Family Medicine, University of Florida College of Pharmacy and Medicine, Gainesville, FL
Chapter 76

Karen A. Theesen, PharmD, BCPP
Senior Regional Medical Scientist, North American Medical Affairs, Glaxo-Smithkline Inc, Research Triangle Park, NC
Chapter 63

Edward G. Timm, PharmD, MS
Senior Clinical Pharmacy Specialist, Critical Care, Albany Medical Center Hospital; Adjunct Assistant Professor, Albany College of Pharmacy, Albany, NY
Chapter 37

Margaret E. Tonda, PharmD
Associate Director of Clinical Research, Alza Pharmaceuticals, Mountain View, CA
Chapter 130

Amy Wells Valley, PharmD, BCOP
Oncology Pharmacy Specialist and Senior Consultant, Pharmacy Healthcare Solutions, Grapevine, TX; Clinical Assistant Professor, University of Texas College of Pharmacy, Austin, TX
Chapter 124

Thomas G. Vondracek, PharmD, BCPS
Clinical Pharmacy Specialist and Adjoint Assistant Professor, Exempla St. Joseph's Hospital and University of Colorado School of Pharmacy, Denver, CO
Chapter 40

Tracey A. Waddelow, PharmD
Program Director, Department of Leukemia, MD Anderson Cancer Center, Houston, TX
Chapter 99

William E. Wade, PharmD, FASHP, FCCP
Professor, College of Pharmacy, University of Georgia, Athens, GA
Chapter 36

Barbara G. Wells, PharmD, FASHP, FCCP, BCPP
Dean and Professor, School of Pharmacy, University of Mississippi, University, MS
Chapters 69, 72

Dianne B. Williams, PharmD, BCPS
Drug Information Specialist, Medical College of Georgia Hospitals and Clinics; Clinical Assistant Professor, University of Georgia College of Pharmacy, Augusta, GA
Chapter 32

Mary A. Worthington, PharmD
Assistant Professor, Clinical Pharmacy Specialist, Samford University, McWhorter School of Pharmacy, Birmingham, AL
Chapter 139

Jean F. Wyman, PhD, RN
Professor and Cora Meidl Siehl Chair in Nursing Research, University of Minnesota School of Nursing, Minneapolis, MN
Chapter 86

Jack A. Yanovski, MD, PhD
Head, Unit on Growth and Obesity, Developmental Endocrinology Branch, National Institute of Child Health and Human Development, National Institutes of Health, Bethesda, MD
Chapter 77

Gary C. Yee, PharmD, FCCP
Professor and Chair, Department of Pharmacy Practice, College of Pharmacy, University of Nebraska Medical Center, Omaha, NE
Chapters 129, 134

Tracey M. Yoshida, PharmD
Clinical Pharmacist, Share Ourselves Community Clinic, Costa Mesa, CA; Clinical Pharmacy Consultant, Women's Health, Redondo Beach, CA
Chapter 79

William C. Zamboni, PharmD
Assistant Professor, Program of Molecular Therapeutics and Drug Development, Departments of Pharmaceutical Sciences and Medicine, University of Pittsburgh Cancer Institute, Pittsburgh, PA
Chapter 130

Mario Zeolla, PharmD
Assistant Professor, Albany College of Pharmacy, Patient CAREPharmacist, Eckerd PatientCARE Center, Albany, NY
Chapter 19

Michael R. Zile, MD, FACC
Professor of Medicine, Cardiology Section, Department of Medicine, Gazes Cardiac Research Institute, University of South Carolina and the Veterans Administration Medical Center, Charleston, SC
Chapter 17

Guiding Principles of Pharmacotherapy

1. There should be a justifiable and documented indication for every medication that is used.
2. A medication should be used at the lowest dosage and for the shortest duration that is likely to achieve the desired outcome.
3. When a patient is adequately treated with a single drug, monotherapy is preferred.
4. Newly approved medications should be used only if there are clear advantages over older medications.
5. Whenever possible, the selection of a medication regimen should be based upon evidence obtained from controlled clinical trials.
6. The timing of drug administration should be considered as a possible influence on drug efficacy, adverse effects, and interactions with other drugs and food.
7. A medication regimen should be simplified as much as possible to enhance patient adherence.
8. A patient's perception of illness or the risks and benefits of therapy may affect adherence and treatment outcomes.
9. Careful observation of a patient's response to treatment is necessary to confirm efficacy, prevent, detect, or manage adverse effects, assess compliance, and determine the need for dosage adjustment or discontinuation of drug therapy.
10. A medication should not be given by injection when giving it by mouth would be just as effective and safe.
11. Before medications are used, lifestyle modifications should be made, when indicated, to obviate the need for drug therapy or to enhance pharmacotherapy outcomes.
12. Initiation of a drug regimen should be done with full recognition that a medication may cause a disease, sign, symptom, syndrome, or abnormal laboratory test.
13. When a variety of drugs are equally efficacious and equally safe, the drug that results in the lowest health care cost or is most convenient for the patient should be chosen.
14. When making a decision about drug therapy for individual patients, societal effects should be considered.
15. The possible reasons for failure of medication regimens include inappropriate drug selection, poor adherence, improper drug dose or interval, misdiagnosis, concurrent illness, interactions with foods or drugs, environmental factors, or genetic factors.

Joseph T. DiPiro, PharmD, FCCP
Barbara G. Wells, PharmD, FASHP, FCCP, BCPP
David W. Hawkins, PharmD
August 13, 2001

Fifth Edition

PHARMACOTHERAPY

A Pathophysiologic Approach

1
PHARMACOECONOMICS: PRINCIPLES

Lisa A. Sanchez

Today's cost-sensitive health care environment has created a competitive and challenging workplace for clinicians. Competition for diminishing resources has necessitated that the appraisal of health care goods and services extend beyond evaluations of safety and efficacy and consider the economic impact of these goods and services on the cost of health care. A challenge for health care professionals is to provide quality patient care with minimal resources.

An interest in defining the "value" of medicine is a common thread joining today's health care professionals, especially pharmacists. With serious concerns about rising medication costs and consistent pressure to decrease pharmacy expenditures and budgets, pharmacists must answer the question, "What is the value of the pharmaceutical goods and services I provide?" *Pharmacoeconomics,* or the discipline of placing a value on drug therapy,[1] has evolved to answer this question.

Challenged to provide high-quality patient care in the least expensive way, pharmacists have developed strategies aimed at containing costs. However, most of these strategies focus solely on determining the least expensive alternative rather than the alternative that represents the best value for the money. The "cheapest" alternative—with respect to drug acquisition cost—is not always the best value for patients, departments, institutions, and health care systems.

Quality patient care must not be compromised while attempting to contain costs. The products and services delivered by today's pharmacists should demonstrate "pharmacoeconomic value," that is, a balance of economic, humanistic, *and* clinical outcomes. Pharmacoeconomics can provide the systematic means for this quantification. This chapter discusses the principles and methods of pharmacoeconomics and how they can be applied to clinical pharmacy practice and thereby how they can assist in the valuation of pharmacotherapy and other modalities of treatment in clinical practice.

PRINCIPLES OF PHARMACOECONOMICS

Pharmacoeconomics has been defined as the description and the analysis of the cost of drug therapy to health care systems and society.[2] More specifically, pharmacoeconomic research is the process of identifying, measuring, and comparing the costs, risks, and benefits of programs, services, or therapies and determining which alternative produces the best health outcome for the resource invested.[3] For most pharmacists, this translates into weighing the cost of providing a pharmacy product or service against the consequences (outcomes) realized by using the product or service to determine which alternative yields the optimal outcome per dollar spent. This information can assist clinical decision makers in choosing the most cost-effective treatment options.[4]

There is a distinct relationship between pharmacoeconomics, outcomes research, and pharmaceutical care. Pharmacoeconomics is not synonymous with outcomes research. *Outcomes research* is defined more broadly as studies that attempt to identify, measure, and evaluate the results of health care services in general.[5] Outcomes research is discussed further in Chapter 2. Pharmacoeconomics is a division of outcomes research that can be used to quantify the value of pharmaceutical care products and services. *Pharmaceutical care* has been defined as the responsible provision of drug therapy for the purposes of achieving definite outcomes.[6] By accepting this as the paradigm or vision for our profession, pharmacy is accepting responsibility for managing drug therapy so that positive outcomes are produced.

Cost is defined as the value of the resources consumed by a program or drug therapy of interest. *Consequence* is defined as the effects, outputs, or outcomes of the program of drug therapy of interest. Consideration of both costs and consequences differentiates most pharmacoeconomic evaluation methods from traditional cost-containment strategies and drug-use evaluations.

Assessing costs and consequences—the value of a pharmaceutical product or service—depends heavily on the perspective of the evaluation. Common perspectives include those of the patient, provider (hospital, managed care organization), payer (government, insurer, employer), and society. A pharmacoeconomic evaluation can assess the value of a product or service from single or multiple perspectives. However, clarification of the perspective is critical because the results of a pharmacoeconomic evaluation depend heavily on the perspective taken. For example, if comparing the value of alteplase (tPA) with that of streptokinase from a patient or societal perspective, tPA may be the best-value alternative because a 1% reduction in mortality rates is observed in this large population. Yet, from a small community hospital's perspective, streptokinase may represent a better value because it provides similar outcomes for less money.

Once the perspective is clear, a full evaluation of the relevant costs and consequences can begin. Health care costs or economic outcomes can be grouped into several categories: direct medical, direct nonmedical, indirect nonmedical, and intangible costs.[7] *Direct medical costs* are those incurred for medical products and services used to prevent, detect, and/or treat a disease (e.g., drugs, laboratory tests, and hospitalizations).[7] *Direct nonmedical costs* are any costs for nonmedical services that are results of illness but do not involve purchasing medical services (e.g., costs of transportation and hotel rooms near a treatment center).[7] *Indirect nonmedical costs* are the costs of reduced productivity (e.g., morbidity and mortality costs).[7–9] *Intangible costs* are those costs incurred which represent other nonfinancial outcomes of disease and medical care and which are not appropriately expressed in a dollar value (e.g., pain, suffering, and grief).[7]

TABLE 1–1. Examples of Health Care Cost Categories

Cost Category	Costs
Direct medical costs	Drugs Supplies Laboratory tests Health care professionals' time Hospitalization
Direct nonmedical costs	Transportation Food Family care Home aides
Indirect costs	Lost wages (morbidity) Income forgone due to premature death (mortality)
Intangible costs	Pain Suffering Grief
Opportunity costs	Lost opportunity Revenue forgone

Costs also can be measured as opportunity costs. *Opportunity costs* represent the economic benefit forgone when using one therapy instead of the next best alternative therapy.[10] Therefore, if a resource has been used to purchase a program or treatment alternative, then the opportunity to use it for another purpose is lost. Table 1–1 contains examples of these costs. Again, the costs that are identified, measured, and ultimately compared will vary depending on the perspective. For example, from the patient perspective, costs are essentially what the patient pays for a product or service that is not covered by insurance, whereas from the provider perspective, costs are essentially the true expense of providing a product or service, regardless of the charge.

The consequences (or outcomes) of medical care also can be categorized. One way is to separate outcomes into three categories: economic, clinical, and humanistic. *Economic outcomes* are the direct, indirect, and intangible costs compared with the consequences of medical treatment alternatives.[11] *Clinical outcomes* are the medical events that occur as a result of disease or treatment (e.g., safety and efficacy end points).[11] *Humanistic outcomes* are the consequences of

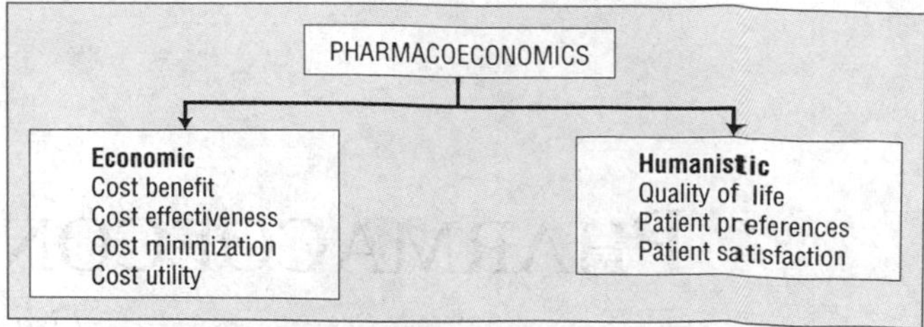

FIGURE 1–1. Components of pharmacoeconomics.

disease or treatment on patient functional status or quality of life along several dimensions (e.g., physical function, social function, general health and well-being, and life satisfaction).[11] These consequences (outcomes) also can be categorized as positive or negative. An example of a positive outcome is a desired effect of a drug, possibly manifested as an efficacy or effectiveness measure of the drug. A negative outcome is an undesired or adverse effect of a drug, possibly manifested as a treatment failure or an adverse drug reaction. Pharmacoeconomic evaluations should include assessments of both types of outcomes. Evaluating only positive outcomes may be misleading because of the potential detriment and expense associated with negative outcomes.

METHODS OF PHARMACOECONOMICS

The pharmacoeconomic methods of evaluation are listed in Figure 1–1. These methods or tools can be separated into two distinct categories: economic and humanistic evaluation techniques. These methods have been used in a variety of fields and are being applied increasingly to health care.[12] Those most commonly used by pharmacists are discussed in the next sections and briefly summarized in Table 1–2.

ECONOMIC EVALUATION METHODS

The basic task of economic evaluation is to identify, measure, value, and compare the costs and consequences of the alternatives being considered. The two distinguishing characteristics of economic evaluation are as follows: (1) is there a comparison of two or more

TABLE 1–2. Summary of Pharmacoeconomic Methodologies

Method	Description	Application	Cost Unit	Outcome Unit
COI	Estimates the cost of a disease on a defined population	Use to provide baseline to compare prevention/treatment options against	$$$	NA
CMA	Finds the least expensive cost alternative	Use when outcomes are the same	$$$	Assume to be equivalent
CBA	Measures benefit in monetary units and computes a net gain	Can compare programs with different objectives	$$$	$$$
CEA	Compares alternatives with therapeutic effects measured in physical units; computes a C/E ratio	Can compare drugs/programs that differ in clinical outcomes and use same unit of benefit	$$$	Natural units
CUA	Measures therapeutic consequences in utility units rather than physical units; computes a C/U ratio	Use to compare drugs/programs that are life extending with serious side effects or those producing reductions in morbidity	$$$	QALYs
QOL	Physical, social, and emotional aspects of patient's well-being that are relevant and important to the patient	Examines drug effects in areas not covered by laboratory or physiologic measurements	NA	QOL score

CBA = cost-benefit analysis; CEA = cost-effectiveness analysis; CMA = cost-minimization analysis; COI = cost-of-illness evaluation; CUA = cost-utility analysis; QOL = quality-of-life assessment; QALY = quality-adjusted life year gained.

alternatives? and (2) are both costs and consequences of the alternatives examined?[13] A full economic evaluation encompasses both characteristics, whereas a partial economic evaluation addresses only one.

Application of economic evaluation methods to health care products and services, especially pharmaceuticals, may increase their acceptance by health care professionals and society.[14] Popular economic evaluation methods include cost-of-illness evaluation and cost-minimization, cost-benefit, cost-effectiveness, and cost-utility analyses. Each method, except cost-of-illness evaluation, is used to compare competing programs or treatment alternatives. The methods are all similar in the way they measure cost (in dollars) and different in their measurement of outcomes. A brief discussion of each method is provided.

COST-OF-ILLNESS EVALUATION

A cost-of-illness (COI) evaluation identifies and estimates the overall cost of a particular disease for a defined population.[8] This evaluation method is often referred to as "burden of illness" and involves measuring the direct and indirect costs attributable to a specific disease. The costs of various diseases, including peptic ulcer disease, mental disorders, and cancer, in the United States have been estimated.

By successfully identifying the direct and indirect costs of an illness, one can determine the relative value of a treatment or prevention strategy. For example, by determining the cost of a particular disease to society, the cost of a prevention strategy could be subtracted from this to yield the benefit of implementing this strategy nationwide. COI evaluation is not used to compare competing treatment alternatives but to provide an estimation of the financial burden of a disease. Thus the value of prevention and treatment strategies can be measured against this illness cost.

COST-MINIMIZATION ANALYSIS

Cost-minimization analysis (CMA) involves the determination of the least costly alternative when comparing two or more treatment alternatives. With CMA, the alternatives must have an assumed or demonstrated equivalency in safety and efficacy (i.e., the two alternatives must be therapeutically equivalent). Once this equivalency in outcome is confirmed, the costs can be identified, measured, and compared in monetary units (dollars).

CMA is a relatively straightforward and simple method for comparing competing programs or treatment alternatives as long as the therapeutic equivalence of the alternatives being compared has been established. If no evidence exists to support this, then a more comprehensive method such as cost-effectiveness analysis should be employed. Remember, CMA shows only a "cost savings" of one program or treatment over another.[15]

Employing CMA is appropriate when comparing two or more therapeutically equivalent agents or alternate dosing regimens of the same agent.[15] For example, if drugs A and B are antiulcer agents, documented to be equal in efficacy and incidence of adverse drug reactions (ADRs), then the costs of using these drugs could be compared using CMA. These costs should extend beyond a comparison of drug acquisition costs and include costs of preparation, administration, and storage. The least expensive agent, considering all these costs, should be preferred.

COST-BENEFIT ANALYSIS

Cost-benefit analysis (CBA) is a method that allows for the identification, measurement, and comparison of the benefits and costs of a program or treatment alternative. The benefits realized from a program or treatment alternative are compared with the costs of providing it. Both the costs and the benefits are measured and converted into equivalent dollars in the year in which they will occur.[8,12] Future costs and benefits are discounted or reduced to their current value.

These costs and benefits are expressed as a ratio (a benefit-to-cost ratio), a net benefit, or a net cost. A clinical decision maker would choose the program or treatment alternative with the highest net benefit or the greatest benefit-to-cost (B/C) ratio.[9] Guidelines for the interpretation of this ratio are indicated.[12,15,16]

- If B/C ratio > 1, the program or treatment is of value. The benefits realized by the program or treatment alternative outweigh the cost of providing it.
- If B/C ratio = 1, the benefits equal the cost. The benefits realized by the program or treatment alternative are equivalent to the cost of providing it.
- If B/C ratio < 1, the program or treatment is not economically beneficial. The cost of providing the program or treatment alternative outweighs the benefits realized by it.

CBA should be employed when comparing treatment alternatives in which the costs and benefits do not occur simultaneously. CBA also may be used when comparing programs with different objectives, because all benefits are converted into dollars. CBA also can be used to evaluate a single program or compare multiple programs. However, valuing health benefits in monetary terms can be difficult and controversial. The expression of some health benefits as monetary units is neither appropriate nor widely accepted. Therefore, unless the benefits of a program or treatment alternative are appropriately expressed in dollars, CBA should not be employed.[15]

CBA may be an appropriate method to use in justifying and documenting the value of an existing health care service or the potential worth of a new one. For example, when competing for institutional resources, CBA can provide data to document that a clinical pharmacy service yields a high return on investment compared with other institutional services competing for the same resources. However, the relative magnitude of the costs and benefits for the service must be considered when making this resource allocation decision. If a service costs $100 to implement and results in a benefit to the hospital of $1000 and a service that costs $100,000 to implement results in a benefit of $1 million, both have a B/C ratio of 10.[15] Thus, caution should be exercised when using B/C ratios and CBA as a comparison tool.

COST-EFFECTIVENESS ANALYSIS

Cost-effectiveness analysis (CEA) is a way of summarizing the health benefits and resources used by competing health care programs so that policymakers can choose among them.[13] CEA involves comparing programs or treatment alternatives with different safety and efficacy profiles. Cost is measured in dollars, and outcomes are measured in terms of obtaining a specific therapeutic outcome. These outcomes are often expressed in physical units, natural units, or nondollar units (lives saved, cases cured, life expectancy, or mm Hg drop in blood pressure).[8,17,18]

The results of CEA are also expressed as a ratio—either as an average cost-effectiveness ratio (ACER) or as an incremental cost-effectiveness ratio (ICER). An ACER represents the total cost of a program or treatment alternative divided by its clinical outcome to yield a ratio representing the dollar cost per specific clinical outcome gained, independent of comparators. The ACER can be summarized as follows[7,15,18]:

$$\text{ACER} = \frac{\text{Health care costs (\$)}}{\text{Clinical outcome (not in \$)}}$$

This allows the costs and outcomes to be reduced to a single value to allow for comparison. Using this ratio, the clinician would choose the alternative with the least cost per outcome gained.[9] The most cost-effective alternative is not always the least costly alternative for obtaining a specific therapeutic objective. In this regard, cost-effectiveness need not be cost reduction but rather cost optimization.[19]

Often clinical effectiveness is gained at an increased cost. Is the increased benefit worth the increased cost? Incremental CEA may be used to determine the additional cost and effectiveness gained when one treatment alternative is compared with the next best treatment alternative.[7] Thus, instead of comparing the ACERs of each treatment alternative, the additional cost that a treatment alternative imposes over another treatment is compared with the additional effect, benefit, or outcome it provides. The ICER can be summarized as follows:

$$\text{ICER} = \frac{\text{cost (\$)}_A - \text{cost (\$)}_B}{\text{effect (\%)}_A - \text{effect (\%)}_B}$$

This formula yields the additional cost required to obtain the additional effect gained by switching from drug A to drug B.

CEA is particularly useful in balancing cost with patient outcome, determining which treatment alternatives represent the best health outcome per dollar spent, and when it is appropriate to measure outcome in terms of obtaining a specific therapeutic objective. In addition, CEA may provide valuable data to support drug policy, formulary management, and individual patient treatment decisions. Globally, CEA is being used to set public policies regarding the use of pharmaceutical products (national formularies) in countries such as Australia,[20] New Zealand, and Canada.[21]

When comparing antiemetic agents for development of a policy for the prevention of chemotherapy-induced emesis, CEA can be employed. Many of these agents differ with respect to effectiveness, safety, and cost. By performing a thorough CEA, these variables can be reduced to a single number (cost-effectiveness ratio), which will allow for a meaningful comparison. The treatment alternative with a better cost-effectiveness ratio than the others (i.e., lower cost per unit of outcome) would be selected and promoted for use.

COST-UTILITY ANALYSIS

Cost-utility analysis (CUA) is another method for comparing treatment alternatives. CUA integrates patient preferences and health-related quality of life (QOL). Cost is measured in dollars, and therapeutic outcome is measured in patient-weighted utilities rather than in physical units. Often the utility measure used is a quality-adjusted life year (QALY) gained. QALY is a common measure of health status used in CUA, combining morbidity and mortality data.

Results of CUA are also expressed in a ratio, a cost-utility ratio (C/U ratio). Most often, this ratio is translated as the cost per QALY gained.[8,12] The preferred treatment alternative is that with the lowest cost per QALY (or other health status utility).

CUA is the most appropriate method to use when comparing programs and treatment alternatives that are life extending with serious side effects (e.g., cancer chemotherapy), those which produce reductions in morbidity rather than mortality (e.g., medical treatment of arthritis),[19] and when QOL is the most important health outcome being examined. CUA is employed less frequently than other economic evaluation methods because of lack of agreement in measuring utilities, difficulty comparing QALYs across patients and populations, and difficulty quantifying patient preferences. Thus, CUA should be reserved for comparing treatment alternatives whose primary goal is improving QOL, and caution should be exercised when using this method.

HUMANISTIC EVALUATION METHODS

Pharmacoeconomic evaluations also may focus on humanistic concerns. Methods for evaluating the impact of disease and treatment of disease on a patient's health-related QOL, patient preferences, and patient satisfaction are all growing in popularity and application to pharmacotherapy decisions. These methods also can assist clinicians in quantifying the value of pharmaceuticals.

QOL has been defined as the assessment of the functional effects of illness and its consequent therapy as perceived by the patient.[22] These effects often are displayed as physical, emotional, and social effects on the patient.[14] Measurement of health-related QOL usually is achieved through the use of patient-completed questionnaires. Many questionnaires are available, and most are either disease-specific or generic measures of health status.[23,24] Various overviews on QOL and its application to pharmacy have been published.[24–27] For further discussion, refer to Chapter 2.

APPLICATIONS OF PHARMACOECONOMICS

Pharmacists, regardless of practice setting, can benefit from applying the principles and methods of pharmacoeconomics to their daily practice settings. *Applied pharmacoeconomics* is defined as putting pharmacoeconomic principles, methods, and theories into practice to quantify the "value" of pharmacy products and pharmaceutical care services used in "real world" environments. Today's pharmacy practitioners are increasingly required to justify the value of the products and services they provide. Applied pharmacoeconomics can provide the means or tools for this valuation.

One of the primary applications of pharmacoeconomics in clinical practice today is to aid clinical and policy decision making. Through the appropriate application of pharmacoeconomics, pharmacy practitioners and administrators can make better, more-informed decisions regarding the products and services they provide. Complete pharmacotherapy decisions should contain assessments of three basic outcome areas whenever appropriate: clinical, economic, and humanistic outcomes. Traditionally, most drug therapy decisions were based solely on the clinical outcomes (e.g., safety and efficacy) associated with a treatment alternative. Over the past 10 to 15 years, it has become quite popular to also include an assessment of the economic outcomes associated with a treatment alternative. The current trend is to also incorporate the humanistic outcomes associated with a treatment alternative, that is, to bring the patient back into this decision-making equation. In today's health care environment, it is no longer appropriate to make drug selection decisions based solely on acquisition costs. Thus, through the appropriate application of pharmacoeconomic principles and methods, incorporating these three critical components into clinical decisions can be accomplished.

Pharmacoeconomic data can be a powerful tool to support various clinical decisions, ranging from the level of the patient to the level of an entire health care system. Figure 1–2 shows various decisions that may be supported using pharmacoeconomics, including effective formulary management, individual patient treatment, medication policy, and resource allocation.[15,18] For discussion purposes, the application of pharmacoeconomics to decision making is divided

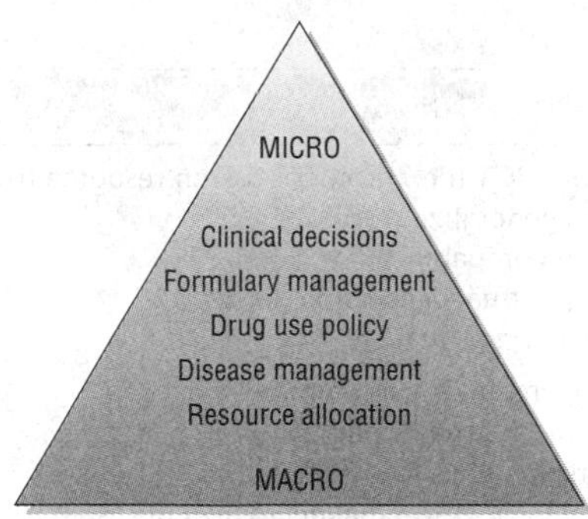

FIGURE 1–2. Decisions for pharmacoeconomic applications.

into two basic areas: drug therapy evaluation and clinical pharmacy service evaluation.

DRUG THERAPY EVALUATION

Historically, pharmacoeconomic principles and methods have been applied commonly to assist clinicians and practitioners in making more informed and complete decisions regarding drug therapy. For example, pharmacoeconomics can provide critical cost-effectiveness data to support the addition or deletion of a drug to or from a hospital formulary, with or without restriction. In fact, the pharmacoeconomic assessment of formulary actions is becoming a standardized part of many pharmacy and therapeutic (P&T) committees.

Selecting the most cost-effective drugs for an organizational formulary is important. However, it is equally important to determine the most appropriate way to use and prescribe these agents. Hence, developing and implementing appropriate use guidelines or policies, based on sound pharmacoeconomic data, can have a great impact on influencing prescribing patterns. Further, implementing sound drug use guidelines/policies will ensure the most appropriate and cost-effective use of pharmaceutical agents throughout the health care system.

The application of pharmacoeconomics also can be useful for making a decision about an individual patient's therapy. Evaluating the impact a drug has on a patient's health-related QOL can be useful when deciding between two agents for customizing a patient's pharmacotherapy. Although this can be one of the most difficult applications of pharmacoeconomics, it is also one of the most important.

CLINICAL PHARMACY SERVICE EVALUATION

The most recent application of pharmacoeconomic principles and methods has been for justifying the value of various health care services, particularly pharmacy services. When competing for hospital resources, pharmacoeconomics can provide the data necessary to justify that a specific service maximizes the resources allocated by health care system administrators. Pharmacoeconomics can be useful in determining the value of an existing service, estimating the potential worth of implementing a new service, or capturing the value of a "cognitive" clinical intervention. Practitioners and administrators can then use these data to make more informed resource-allocation decisions.

For example, suppose you want to implement a pharmacy-based therapeutic drug monitoring program. It is hypothesized that this service will improve quality of patient care and save money for the health care system. After negotiating with hospital administrators, the funding for this service is approved for a 1-year trial basis, after which you must document and justify the value of this practice. Theoretically, all the relevant costs and benefits of the program should be measured and, if appropriate, converted into dollars using CBA. Potential benefits may include decreased total drug costs and decreased incidence of ADRs. Potential program costs are primarily the salary and benefits for a pharmacist and additional laboratory tests to monitor patients. Data documenting that the benefit of this pharmacy service yields a high return on investment (ROI) should increase the probability of your program continuing to be funded by the health care system.

Unfortunately, previous reviews of the literature have revealed a disappointing number of rigorous economic evaluations of clinical pharmacy services published to date.[28–30] McGhan and colleagues evaluated 35 potential CBAs or CEAs of pharmacy services published before 1978 and concluded that only 5 of these studies were considered legitimate CBAs or CEAs.[28] MacKeigan and Bootman reviewed 22 CBAs or CEAs published between 1978 and 1987 and concluded that CBAs and CEAs have not been adopted extensively for the evaluation of clinical pharmacy services.[29] Most recently, Schumock and associates[30] reviewed economic evaluations of pharmacy services published between 1988 and 1995. Of the studies reviewed, only 19 were considered "full" or legitimate economic analyses, and the authors concluded that although the number of articles published has increased over the years, there is still a need for improvement in the quality or rigor of study design. Despite the relatively low number of methodologically sound studies, this review also revealed some results that demonstrate the potential value of clinical pharmacy services. Of the 109 studies evaluated, the various clinical services reviewed in this study yielded an average cost-benefit ratio of 16:1.

STRATEGIES TO INCORPORATE PHARMACOECONOMICS INTO PHARMACOTHERAPY

Various strategies are available to incorporate pharmacoeconomics into pharmacotherapy. Popular strategies for applying pharmacoeconomics to assess the value of pharmaceutical products and services include using the results of published pharmacoeconomic studies, building economic models, or conducting pharmacoeconomic research.[31] Advantages and disadvantages of these strategies are summarized in Table 1–3.

USE THE PHARMACOECONOMIC LITERATURE

Quantifying the value of pharmaceuticals through pharmacoeconomics has increased in popularity. Many pharmacoeconomic analyses are published in primary medical and pharmacy literature sources. However, the eagerness to conduct pharmacoeconomic evaluations of drugs often exceeds the quality of these evaluations. Variations in quality and indiscriminate use of pharmacoeconomic terminology are documented in medical and pharmacy literature sources.[4,28–30,32–34] To use this literature as an aid in clinical decision making, it must be (1) critically evaluated for quality and rigor and (2) interpreted correctly. Therefore, prior to using pharmacoeconomic data to make clinical and policy decisions, decision makers should recognize the potential limitations of those data.

A primary consideration when evaluating and interpreting a study is the ability to generalize or transfer the results to other health care settings and countries. It can be difficult to generalize and transfer the results of a published study primarily due to wide variations in practice patterns, patient populations, and costs among health care systems and countries. Further, differences in study perspectives, data sources, and analytical styles may present a challenge for practitioners

TABLE 1–3. Advantages and Disadvantages of Pharmacoeconomic Application Strategies

Strategy	Advantages	Disadvantages
Use published literature	Quick Inexpensive Subject to peer review Results may be from RCT Variety of results can be examined	Results from RCT (i.e., protocol-driven resource use) Difficult to generalize results May not be comparative Misuse of pharmacoeconomic terms Variations in rigor/quality
Build an economic model	Relatively quick Relatively inexpensive Yields organization-specific results Bridges efficacy and effectiveness Data collection is unobtrusive	Results dependent on assumptions Potential for researcher bias Controversial Reluctance of decision makers to accept results
Conduct a pharmacoeconomic evaluation	Flexible Usually comparative Yields organization-specific data Reflects "usual care" or effectiveness Data from multiple sources can be used	Expensive Time consuming Difficult to control and randomize Potential for patient selection bias Potential for small sample size

RCT = randomized controlled trial.

attempting to extrapolate or relate exact cost savings or cost ratios to their own practice setting. To enhance the ability to use pharmacoeconomic results published in the literature, consider the following points:

1. What is the technical merit of the study?
2. Are the results applicable to local decision making?
3. Do the results apply generally in different jurisdictions with different perspectives?[35]

Various guidelines, criteria, and consensus-based recommendations for evaluating, conducting, and reporting pharmacoeconomic literature have been published.[7,13,21,36–44] These guidelines and criteria have been combined and summarized into 11 categories most pertinent to pharmacotherapy.[39] A summary of these 11 criteria and pertinent questions for each category is given in Table 1–4. Each evaluation criterion is briefly discussed next.

STUDY OBJECTIVE

A clear statement of the purpose of the study should be given. This objective should be clear, concise, well defined, and measurable.

STUDY PERSPECTIVE

The researcher must select one or more perspectives (e.g., patient, provider, payer, or society) from which the analysis will be

TABLE 1–4. Basic Criteria for Evaluation of Pharmacoeconomic Literature

Objective
What is the question(s) being considered?
Is the question clear, defined, and measurable?
Perspective
What is the perspective(s) of the analysis?
Is it appropriate given the scope of the problem?
Pharmacoeconomic Method
What pharmacoeconomic tool was used?
Is it appropriate given the problem?
Is it actually what was conducted?
Study Design
What was the study design?
What were the data sources?
Is the evaluation suitable if carried out in a clinical trial?
Choice of Interventions
Were all appropriate alternatives considered and described?
Were any appropriate alternatives omitted?
Are the alternatives relevant to the perspective and clinical nature of the study?
Is there evidence that the alternatives' effectiveness has been established?
Costs and Consequences
What are the costs and consequences (outcomes) included?
Are the costs and outcomes relevant to the perspective chosen?
Do they include negative outcomes (failures, ADRs)?
How were they valued?
Were costs and consequences measured in the appropriate physical units?
Discounting
Was the study performed over time?
Were costs and consequences that occur in the future discounted to their present value?
Was any justification given for the discount rate used?
Results
Are the results accurate and practical for medical decision makers?
Were the appropriate statistical analyses performed?
Was an incremental analysis performed?
Are all the assumptions and limitations of the study discussed?
Sensitivity Analysis
Are cost ranges for significant variables tested for sensitivity?
Are the appropriate and relevant variables varied?
Do the findings follow the anticipated trend?
Conclusions
Are the conclusions of the study justified?
Is it possible to extrapolate the conclusions to daily clinical practice?
Sponsorship
Was there any bias due to the sponsorship of the study?

ADRs = adverse drug reactions.

conducted.[9] This perspective should be appropriate given the scope of the pharmacoeconomic problem identified. An evaluation may be conducted from single or multiple perspectives as long as the costs and consequences identified are relevant to the perspective(s) chosen.

PHARMACOECONOMIC METHOD

It should be clear which pharmacoeconomic method was employed (CEA, CMA, CBA, or CUA), and this method should be appropriate given the problem (e.g., CMA is appropriate if comparing two alternatives equivalent in therapeutic outcome but not if the alternatives differ in therapeutic outcome). Also, a researcher may claim a specific method was employed (e.g., CEA) but actually employ another method (e.g., CMA).

STUDY DESIGN

Pharmacoeconomic evaluations can be prospective or retrospective. Although prospective designs are usually preferred, retrospective evaluations can be rich with information and reflective of usual care. Many pharmacoeconomic evaluations today are conducted as a part of randomized, controlled clinical trials. Two cautions for interpreting pharmacoeconomic data collected in this manner include (1) costs can be protocol driven, not necessarily reflective of using a drug in common practice,[45] and (2) control of subjects and decreased complications may yield greater costs and benefits than those observed in common practice.[36]

CHOICE OF INTERVENTIONS

All relevant available treatment options should be described completely or mentioned. The treatment alternatives and dosages being compared should be those used in common practice, and evidence of their effectiveness should be established. Because pharmacoeconomic methods are tools to aid in choosing between treatment alternatives, assessing the cost of a single alternative is considered a partial economic evaluation.

COSTS AND CONSEQUENCES

All the important and relevant costs and consequences for each program or treatment alternative should be identified. The costs and consequences identified must be relevant to the study perspective(s) and measured in suitable terms using the appropriate physical units. Costs should include direct, indirect, and intangible costs. Consequences should include the positive and negative clinical and humanistic outcomes associated with the program or treatment alternative. All these costs and consequences must be valued credibly, with the data sources clearly identified.

DISCOUNTING

The comparison of programs or treatment alternatives should be made at one point in time; thus, any costs and consequences not occurring in the present must be addressed. *Discounting,* or adjusting for differential timing, is the process of reducing any costs and consequences that may occur in the future back to their present value. If a study is performed over time (more than 1 year), or if future cost savings are projected, discounting should be done using an appropriate discount rate. The rate used typically is 4% to 8%, representing annual inflation or bank interest rates. However, many researchers use a generally accepted discount rate of 5%.

STUDY RESULTS

A full discussion of the study assumptions and limitations and how to interpret the results in the context of different practice settings[13] should be provided. This discussion should include all relevant issues of concern to potential users of the study. The results should reflect that the appropriate statistical analyses were performed. Also, it may be appropriate to express the study results in terms of increases, that is, to use incremental cost analysis (additional cost of gaining an additional benefit by using one drug over another).

SENSITIVITY ANALYSIS

It is imperative that researchers test the sensitivity of study results using sensitivity analysis. *Sensitivity analysis* (SA) is the process of testing the robustness of an economic evaluation by examining changes in results. Specific variables such as percent effectiveness, incidence of ADRs, and dominant resources can be varied over a range of plausible values and the results recalculated. SA is of paramount importance because of the very common need for investigators to use assumptions and estimates for unknown variables.[34]

STUDY CONCLUSIONS

Researchers should assist the reader in extrapolating study conclusions to clinical practice. The conclusions drawn from the study results should be justified (internal validity) and able to be generalized (external validity).[39] Also, conclusions drawn from results that were "statistically" significant may or may not be "clinically" relevant, and vice versa.

SPONSORSHIP

Similar to evaluating the quality of a clinical trial, sponsorship of a pharmacoeconomic study should be considered when evaluating the quality and usefulness of that study.[37] Quality of studies conducted or funded by different companies or organizations will vary by sponsor, company, product, or evaluation, and the potential for bias should be neither ignored nor assumed. For example, many of the studies sponsored or conducted by the pharmaceutical industry to date have been academically rigorous as well as informative. A clear understanding of how to evaluate, critique, and use the pharmacoeconomic literature appropriately will minimize any potential effects of this criterion on clinical decision making.

BUILD AN ECONOMIC MODEL

Studies that "model" the economic impact of a pharmaceutical product or service on a defined population are increasing in popularity. Modeling studies use existing clinical and/or epidemiologic data to project future outcomes.[46] Use of economic models can provide support for various clinical decisions, especially those which are time-contingent.[31] Identifying assumptions regarding the treatment alternatives being compared, the patient outcomes under study, and the probability of those outcomes occurring can provide the basis for an economic simulation to assist in the medication decision-making process.

These studies can use data from various sources available within (internal) and from outside (external) a specific health care organization. Common approaches to modeling are to modify and adapt existing models or to develop a distinct model to answer a specific question.[47] Typically, economic modeling in today's practice settings employs *clinical decision analysis,* which has been defined as an explicit, quantitative, and prescriptive approach to choosing among alternative outcomes.[48,49] The tool used in decision analysis is a decision tree. A decision tree provides a framework to display graphically primary variables including treatment options, outcomes associated with those treatment options, and probabilities of the outcomes. The researcher can then algebraically reduce all these factors into a single value, allowing for comparison.

Building an economic model can help the clinician to forecast the impact of medication-use decisions on a patient, institution, or health care system. Also, as new drugs are marketed that can displace older agents, an economic model can expedite the reappraisal process for formulary management and drug-use policy decisions.[50] For building an economic model to assist in clinical decision making, various published examples can be considered.[51–56]

CONDUCT A PHARMACOECONOMIC EVALUATION

Clinicians may need to conduct a pharmacoeconomic evaluation if there is insufficient literature, if published results cannot be extrapolated to clinical practice, or if building a model is not appropriate. Before conducting a pharmacoeconomic evaluation, clinicians should be familiar with the similarities, differences, and appropriate application of pharmacoeconomic methods (discussed earlier in this chapter).

The decision to conduct a local pharmacoeconomic study is not without its own costs. Because both time and monetary resources are consumed by these evaluations, specific pharmacy products and services for pharmacoeconomic evaluation should be targeted. Thus, this strategy should be reserved for pharmacy decisions that may have a significant impact on cost or quality of care.

Conducting pharmacoeconomic research in a hospital or managed-care environment can be challenging. Lack of institutional resources, small sample sizes, difficulty randomizing, inability to compare with placebo, and difficulty generalizing results may all be limitations. For example, when asked to determine and recommend the most cost-effective antihypertensive agent for a formulary management decision, clinicians may lack monetary and time resources to conduct a scientifically rigorous study.

Conducting a pharmacoeconomic evaluation should be guided by the criteria for quality economic evaluations.[8,13,21,36–44] A 10-step process identified by Jolicoeur and associates[57] and 4 additional steps that I have added can provide readers with guidance for conducting a local pharmacoeconomic study.[58] This process contains 14 fundamental steps for conducting a pharmacoeconomic evaluation in a health care system and can be applied to virtually any therapeutic area or health care service. Although some of these steps are similar to those evaluation criteria detailed earlier in this chapter, they will now be discussed briefly in the context of conducting an evaluation.

STEP 1: DEFINE THE PHARMACOECONOMIC PROBLEM

A broad problem might be, "Which antiemetic regimen represents the best value for the prevention of chemotherapy-induced emesis (CIE)?" However, a more succinct and measurable problem would be, "Which regimen is the best value for preventing acute CIE in patients receiving highly emetogenic chemotherapy?"

STEP 2: ASSEMBLE A CROSS-FUNCTIONAL STUDY TEAM

The study team can provide early "buy-in" and additional resources for a pharmacoeconomic evaluation. Team members vary depending on the analysis but may include representatives from medicine, nursing, pharmacy, hospital administration, and information systems.

STEP 3: DEFINE THE APPROPRIATE STUDY PERSPECTIVE

Choose a study perspective(s) most relevant to the problem. For example, if the problem is as listed in step 1, then the perspective of the institution or health care system may be most appropriate.

STEP 4: IDENTIFY TREATMENT ALTERNATIVES AND OUTCOMES

Treatment alternatives can include pharmacologic and nonpharmacologic options but should include all clinically relevant alternatives. The outcomes identified should include both positive and negative clinical outcomes.

STEP 5: IDENTIFY THE APPROPRIATE PHARMACOECONOMIC METHOD TO EMPLOY

Pharmacoeconomic methods to choose from include CMA, CBA, CEA, and CUA. Employing the incorrect method can adversely affect medication decisions influencing both cost and quality of care.

STEP 6: PLACE A MONETARY VALUE ON TREATMENT ALTERNATIVES AND OUTCOMES

Placing a monetary value on treatment alternatives and outcomes includes not only drug administration and acquisition costs but also the cost of positive and negative clinical outcomes (e.g., determining the cost of ADRs and treatment failures). This can be measured prospectively or retrospectively or estimated using comprehensive databases or expert panels.

STEP 7: IDENTIFY RESOURCES TO CONDUCT STUDY IN AN EFFICIENT MANNER

Resources necessary will vary by study but may include access to medical or computerized records, average medical personnel wages, and specialty medical staff.

STEP 8: IDENTIFY PROBABILITIES THAT OUTCOMES MAY OCCUR IN STUDY POPULATION

What are the probabilities of the outcomes identified in step 4 actually occurring in clinical practice? Using primary literature and expert opinion, these probabilities can be obtained and may be manifested as efficacy rates and incidence of ADRs.

STEP 9: EMPLOY DECISION ANALYSIS

The use of decision analysis can assist in conducting various economic evaluations, including CEA. Although not necessary for all pharmacoeconomic evaluations, decision analysis and decision trees may provide a solid backbone or platform for the decision at hand. Using a decision tree, treatment alternatives, outcomes, and probabilities may be presented graphically and algebraically reduced to a single value for comparison (i.e., cost-effectiveness ratio).

STEP 10: DISCOUNT COSTS OR PERFORM A SENSITIVITY OR INCREMENTAL COST ANALYSIS

Costs and consequences that occur in the future must be discounted back to their present value. Sensitive variables must be tested over a clinically relevant range and results recalculated. If appropriate, an incremental analysis of the costs and consequences should be performed.

STEP 11: PRESENT STUDY RESULTS

Results should be presented to the cross-functional team and the appropriate committees. Presentation style and content may vary depending on the audience.

STEP 12: DEVELOP A POLICY OR AN INTERVENTION

Take the study results and develop a policy or an intervention that can improve or maintain quality of care, possibly at a cost savings.

STEP 13: IMPLEMENT POLICY AND EDUCATE PROFESSIONALS

Spend adequate time and resources strategically implementing the policy or intervention. Educate those health care professionals most likely to be affected by this policy, using various strategies, including verbal, written, and on-line communication.

STEP 14: FOLLOW-UP DOCUMENTATION

Once the intervention or policy has been implemented for a reasonable period of time, collect follow-up data. These data will provide feedback on the success and quality of the policy or intervention.

CONCLUSIONS

The principles and methods of pharmacoeconomics provide the means to quantify the value of pharmacotherapy through balancing costs and outcomes. Providing quality care with minimal resources is the future, and the future is here. By understanding the principles, methods, and application of pharmacoeconomics, pharmacists will be prepared to make better, more-informed decisions regarding the use of pharmaceutical products and services, that is, decisions that ultimately represent the best interests of the patient, the health care system, and society.

▶ PRINCIPLES OF PHARMACOTHERAPY

- Pharmacoeconomics seeks to describe and analyze the costs of drug therapy to the health care system and society.
- Values are placed on various economic, humanistic, and clinical outcomes using the methods of pharmacoeconomics.
- Health care costs can be categorized as direct medical, direct nonmedical, indirect nonmedical, intangible, and opportunity costs.
- To compare various health care choices, economic valuation methods are used, including cost-minimization, cost-benefit, cost-effectiveness, and cost-utility analyses. Comparisons may be expressed in monetary units, ratios, or mixed units (such as dollars per quality-adjusted life-year).
- Cost-of-illness evaluations identifies and estimates the overall cost of a particular disease for a defined population, but it is not used to compare alternative choices.
- In pharmacy practice, pharmacoeconomic methods can be used for effective formulary management, individual patient treatment, medication policy determination, and resource allocation.
- The following factors should be considered when evaluating published pharmacoeconomic studies: study objective, study perspective, pharmacoeconomic method, study design, choice of interventions, costs and consequences, discounting, study results, sensitivity analysis, study conclusions, and sponsorship.
- A standard method should be followed in performing pharmacoeconomic evaluations, as outlined in this chapter.

REFERENCES

1. Sanchez LA. Expanding the pharmacist's role in pharmacoeconomics: How and why? Pharmacoeconomics 1994;5:367–375.
2. Townsend RJ. Post-marketing drug research and development. Ann Pharmacother 1987;21:134–136.
3. Drummond M, Smith GT, Wells N. Economic Evaluation in the Development of Medicines. London, Office of Health Economics, 1988:33.
4. Lee JT, Sanchez LA. Interpretation of cost-effective and soundness of economic evaluations in the pharmacy literature. Am J Hosp Pharm 1991;48:2622–2627.
5. Bootman JL. Pharmacoeconomics and outcomes research. Am J Health System Pharm 1995;52(suppl 3):S16–S19.
6. Hepler CD, Strand LM. Opportunities and responsibilities in pharmaceutical care. Am J Hosp Pharm 1990;47:533–543.
7. Eisenberg JM. Clinical economics: A guide to economic analysis of clinical practices. JAMA 1989;262:2879–2886.
8. Bootman JL, Townsend RJ, McGhan WF. Principles of Pharmacoeconomics. Cincinnati, Harvey Whitney Books, 1991.
9. Freund DA, Dittus RS. Principles of pharmacoeconomic analysis of drug therapy. Pharmacoeconomics 1992;1:20–32.
10. Glossary of terms used in pharmacoeconomic and quality of life analysis. Pharmacoeconomics 1992;1:151.
11. Kozma CM, Reeder CE, Schulz RM. Economic, clinical, and humanistic outcomes: A planning model for pharmacoeconomic research. Clin Ther 1993;15:1121–1132.
12. Draugalis JR, Bootman LJ, Larson LN, McGhan WF. Current Concepts: Pharmacoeconomics. Kalamazoo, MI, Upjohn, 1989.
13. Drummond MF, Stoddart GL, Torrance GW. Methods for the Economic Evaluation of Health Care Programmes. Oxford, Oxford University Press, 1986:5–38, 74–111.
14. McGhan WF. Pharmacoeconomics and the evaluation of drugs and services. Hosp Formul 1993;28:365–378.
15. Sanchez LA, Lee JT. Use and misuse of pharmacoeconomic terms. Top Hosp Pharm Manage 1994;13:11–22.
16. Sanchez LA. Pharmacoeconomic principles and methods: An introduction for hospital pharmacists. Hosp Pharm 1994;29:1035–1040.
17. Bootman JL, Larson LN, McGhan WF, Townsend RJ. Pharmacoeconomic research and clinical trials: Concepts and issues. Ann Pharmacother 1989;23:693–697.
18. Detsky AS, Nagiie IG. A clinician's guide to cost-effectiveness analysis. Ann Intern Med 1990;113:147–154.

19. Bootman JL. The basics of pharmacoeconomic analysis. Pharm Rep 1993; 23:14–15.
20. Langley PC. The role of pharmacoeconomic guidelines for formulary approval: The Australian experience. Clin Ther 1993;15:1154–1176.
21. Detsky AS. Guidelines for economic analysis of pharmaceutical products: A draft document for Ontario and Canada. Pharmacoeconomics 1993;3: 354–361.
22. Schipper H, Clinch J, Powell V. Definitions and conceptual issues. In: Spilker B, ed. Quality of Life Assessments in Clinical Trials. New York, Raven, 1990.
23. Spilker B. Quality of Life Assessments in Clinical Trials. New York, Raven, 1990.
24. Spilker B, White WSA, Simpson RJ, Tilson HN. Quality of life bibliography and indexes—1990 update. Clin Pharmacoepidemiol 1992;6:157–158.
25. Coons SJ. Quality of life assessment: Understanding its use as an outcome measure. Hosp Formul 1993;28:486–498.
26. Jaeschke R, Guyatt GH, Cook D. Quality of life instruments in the evaluation of new drugs. Pharmacoeconomics 1992;1:84–94.
27. Mackeigan LD, Pathak DS. Overview of health-related quality-of-life measures. Am J Hosp Pharm 1992;49:2236–2245.
28. McGhan WF, Rowland CR, Bootman JL. Cost-benefit and cost-effectiveness: Methodologies for evaluating innovative pharmaceutical services. Am J Hosp Pharm 1978;35:133–140.
29. MacKeigan LD, Bootman JL. A review of cost-benefit and cost-effectiveness analyses of clinical pharmacy services. J Pharm Market Manage 1988;2:63–84.
30. Schumock GT, Meek PD, Ploetz PA, Vermeulen LC. Economic evaluations of clinical pharmacy services—1988–1995. Pharmacotherapy 1996; 16:1188–1208.
31. Sanchez LA. Pharmacoeconomic principles and methods: Including pharmacoeconomics into hospital pharmacy practice. Hosp Pharm 1994;29: 1035–1040.
32. Doubilet P, Weinstein MC, McNeil BJ. The use and misuse of the term "cost effective" in medicine. N Engl J Med 1986;314:253–256.
33. Bradley CA, Iskedjian M, Lanctot KL, et al. Quality assessment of economic evaluation in selected pharmacy, medical, and health economic journals. Ann Pharmacother 1995;29:681–689.
34. Udvarhelyi S, Colditz GA, Rai A, et al. Cost-effectiveness and cost-benefit analyses in the medical literature. Ann Intern Med 1992;116:238–244.
35. Mason J. The generalizability of pharmacoeconomic studies. Pharmacoeconomics 1997;11:503–514.
36. Sacristan JA, Soto J, Galende I. Evaluation of pharmacoeconomic studies: Utilization of a checklist. Ann Pharmacother 1993;27:1126–1133.
37. Hillman AL, Eisenberg JM, Pauly MV, et al. Avoiding bias in the conduct and reporting of cost-effectiveness research sponsored by pharmaceutical companies. N Engl J Med 1991;324:1362–1365.
38. McGhan WF, Lewis JV. Guidelines for pharmacoeconomic studies. Clin Ther 1992;14:486–494.
39. Sanchez LA. Pharmacoeconomic principles and methods: Evaluating the quality of published pharmacoeconomic evaluations. Hosp Pharm 1995; 30:146–152.
40. Clemans K, Townsend R, Luscombe F, et al. Methodological and conduct principles for pharmacoeconomic research. Pharmacoeconomics 1995; 8:169–174.
41. Task Force on Principles for Economic Analysis of Health Care Technology. Economic analysis of health care technology: A report on principles. Ann Intern Med 1995;122:61–70.
42. Russell LB, Gold MR, Siegel JE, et al. The role of cost-effectiveness analysis in health and medicine. JAMA 1996;276:1172–1177.
43. Weinstein MC, Siegel JE, Gold MR, et al. Recommendations of the panel on cost-effectiveness in health and medicine. JAMA 1996;276:1253–1258.
44. Siegel JE, Weinstein MC, Russell LB, et al. Recommendations for reporting cost-effectiveness analyses. JAMA 1996;276:1339–1341.
45. Eisenberg JM, Glick H, Koffer H. Pharmacoeconomics: Economic evaluation of pharmaceuticals. In: Strom BL, ed. Pharmacoepidemiology. New York, Churchill-Livingstone, 1989:325–350.
46. Milne RJ. Evaluation of the pharmacoeconomic literature. Pharmacoeconomics 1994;6:337–345.
47. Sanchez LA, Lee JT. Applied pharmacoeconomics: Modeling data from internal and external sources. Am J Health Syst Pharm 2000;57:146–158.
48. Sackett DL, Haynes RB, Tugwell P. Clinical Epidemiology: A Basic Science for Clinical Medicine. Boston, Little, Brown, 1985:126.
49. Barr JT, Schumacher GE. Applying decision analysis to pharmacy management and practice decisions. Top Hosp Pharm Manage 1994;13:60–71.
50. Schecter CB. Decision analysis in formulary decision making. Pharmacoeconomics 1993;3:454–461.
51. Bjornson DC, Hiner WO, Potyk RP, et al. Effect of pharmacists on health care outcomes in hospitalized patients. Am J Hosp Pharm. 1993;50:1875–1884.
52. Crane VS. Economic aspects of clinical decision making: Applications of clinical decision analysis. Am J Hosp Pharm 1988;45:548–553.
53. Harrison DL, Bootman JL, Cox ER. Cost-effectiveness of consultant pharmacists in managing drug-related morbidity and mortality at nursing facilities. Am J Health Syst Pharm 1998;55:1588–1594.
54. Kessler JM. Decision analysis in the formulary process. Am J Health Syst Pharm. 1997;54(suppl 1):S5–S8.
55. Mutnick AH, Szymusiak-Mutnick B, Schumacher GE, Barr JT. Using decision analysis in the evaluation of drug therapy. Pharm Times 1990;59–66.
56. Paladino JA. Cost-effectiveness comparison of cefepime and ceftazidime using decision analysis. Pharmacoeconomics 1994;5:505–512.
57. Jolicoeur LM, Jones-Grizzle AJ, Boyer JG. Guidelines for performing a pharmacoeconomic analysis. Am J Hosp Pharm 1992;49:1741–1747.
58. Sanchez LA. Pharmacoeconomic principles and methods: Conducting pharmacoeconomic evaluations in a hospital setting. Hosp Pharm 1995; 30:412–428.

2
HEALTH OUTCOMES AND QUALITY OF LIFE

Stephen Joel Coons

Over the past two decades, the medical care marketplace in the United States has undergone unprecedented change.[1] This change is evidenced by a variety of developments, including an increase in investor-owned organizations, heightened competition, numerous mergers and acquisitions, increasingly sophisticated clinical and administrative information systems, and new financing and organizational structures. In this dynamic and increasingly competitive environment, there is a concern that health care quality is being compromised in the rush to lower costs. As a consequence, there has been a growing movement to focus the evaluation of health care on the assessment of the end results, or *outcomes,* associated with medical care delivery systems as well as specific medical interventions. The primary objective of this effort is to maximize the net health benefit derived from the use of finite health care resources.[2] However, there is a serious lack of critical information as to what value is received for the tremendous amount of resources expended on medical care.[3] This lack of critical information as to the outcomes produced is an obstacle to optimal health care decision making at all levels.

HEALTH OUTCOMES

Although the implicit objective of medical care is to improve health outcomes, until recently, little attention was paid to the explicit measurement of them. An outcome is one of the three components of the conceptual framework articulated by Donabedian for assessing and ensuring the quality of health care: *structure, process,* and *outcome*.[4] Traditionally, the approach to evaluating health care has emphasized the structure and processes involved in medical care delivery rather than the outcomes. However, health care regulators, payers, providers, manufacturers, and patients are placing increasing emphasis on the outcomes that medical care products and services produce.[5] As stated by Ellwood, outcomes research is "designed to help patients, payers, and providers make rational medical care choices based on better insight into the effect of these choices on the patient's life."[6]

TYPES OF OUTCOMES

The types of outcomes that result from medical care interventions can be described in a number of ways. One classic list, called the *five D's,* although quite negatively worded, captures a wide range of outcomes used in assessing the quality of medical care.[7] The five D's are death, disease, disability, discomfort, and dissatisfaction.

A more comprehensive conceptual framework, the ECHO model, places outcomes into three categories: *e*conomic, *c*linical, and *h*umanistic *o*utcomes.[8] The model covers the five D's within the clinical and humanistic outcomes and provides an added economic outcomes dimension. As described by Kozma and associates, *clinical outcomes* are the medical events that occur as a result of the condition or its treatment. *Economic outcomes* are the direct, indirect, and intangible costs compared with the consequences of a medical intervention. Along with patient satisfaction, an essential humanistic or patient-reported outcome is self-assessed function and well-being, or *health-related quality of life*. This chapter focuses on health-related quality of life as an outcome of pharmacotherapeutic interventions.

QUALITY OF LIFE

DEFINITION

As mentioned, one of the essential elements of outcomes research is the assessment of patient *health-related quality of life*. However, there is no consensus on the definition of quality of life (QOL) or its overall conceptual framework.[9] In the literature, the term *quality of life* has been used in a variety of ways. It has been proposed that studies of health outcomes use the term *health-related quality of life* to distinguish health effects from the effects of job satisfaction, environment, and other factors on overall quality of life.[10] Only health outcomes are discussed in this chapter, so *quality of life* and *health-related quality of life* are used interchangeably, along with *health status*.

Quality of life, like other aspects of the human experience, is hard to define. In much of the empirical literature, explicit definitions of QOL are rare; readers must deduce the implicit definition of QOL from the manner in which it is measured. However, some authors have provided definitions. For example, Schron and Shumaker define QOL as "a multidimensional concept referring to a person's total well-being, including his or her psychological, social, and physical health status."[11] Patrick and Erickson propose that QOL is "the value assigned to duration of life as modified by the impairments, functional states, perceptions, and social opportunities that are influenced by disease, injury, treatment, or policy."[12] Although the two definitions differ in certain respects, a conceptual characteristic they share is the multidimensionality of quality of life. Although the terminology may vary with the author, commonly measured dimensions of health-related QOL include the following:

- Physical health and functioning
- Psychological health and functioning
- Social and role functioning
- Perceptions of general well-being

RELEVANCE OF QUALITY OF LIFE AS AN OUTCOME

For medical care providers, QOL increasingly is viewed as a therapeutic end point. An overriding factor leading to this has been the gradual shift in the focus of primary medical care from limiting mortality to limiting morbidity and the patient-reported impact of that morbidity. The pattern of illness in the United States has shifted from mostly acute disease to one in which chronic conditions predominate. In the early part of the twentieth century, many individuals died from infectious diseases for which cures (e.g., antibiotics) or effective preventive measures (e.g., increased sanitation, vaccines) were unavailable or underused. Today, although there are many diseases that may shorten life expectancy, it is more likely that a disease will have adverse health consequences leading to dysfunction and decreased well-being. For those conditions which shorten life expectancy and for which there are no cures, managing symptoms and maintaining function and well-being should be the primary objectives of medical care.

Because therapeutic interventions such as medications have the potential to increase or decrease QOL, medical care providers must strive to achieve enhanced QOL as an outcome of therapy. Although it must be assumed that QOL has always played an implicit role in the provision of health care, it has not always been viewed as equal in importance to the more clinical or physiologic outcome parameters (e.g., blood pressure). The subjective nature of QOL assessment has made many people uneasy with it as a measure of the patient outcomes produced by medical treatment.[13] However, there is growing awareness that in certain diseases, QOL may be the most important health outcome to consider in assessing treatment.[14] Physiologic measures may change without improving functioning and well-being. Likewise, patients may feel and function better without measurable change in physiologic values.

QUALITY OF LIFE AND PHARMACOTHERAPY

As described by Smith, there are four possible QOL outcomes associated with pharmacotherapy: (1) QOL is improved, (2) QOL is actively maintained, (3) QOL decreases, or (4) QOL remains unaffected.[15] To effectively assess these possible outcomes, moving beyond consideration of only the biologic or physical manifestations of a disease or its treatment is essential. The use of standardized measurement tools (e.g., self-reported QOL instruments) to collect information regarding the impact of pharmacotherapy on the quality of patients' lives is increasing.[16,17] However, the vast majority of QOL claims in prescription drug advertisements continue to be based on physiologic parameters and/or clinician-assessed physical function rather than patient-reported functioning and well-being.[18]

A study by Croog and colleagues[19] was one of the first in a growing body of literature reporting the QOL impact of pharmacotherapy, specifically the use of antihypertensive agents. Along with hypertension, examples of other therapeutic areas that are receiving increasing attention are arthritis, asthma, cancer, diabetes, and HIV/AIDS.[20–25] The type of condition and type of treatment dictate the importance of health-related QOL data in determining the value of pharmacotherapy. As discussed by Badia and Herdman,[26] in chronic conditions and palliative treatments (i.e., ameliorating symptoms but not curing the underlying disease), health-related QOL may be the primary measure of efficacy. However, with acute conditions and curative treatments, health-related QOL is likely to be secondary (although excluding it may underestimate the positive and negative impacts of the treatment).

Information about the impact of pharmacotherapy on QOL can provide additional data for making medication-use policy decisions.[27] Pharmacy and therapeutics committees should incorporate QOL data into the formulary and practice guideline decision-making process. QOL as an input to clinical decision making at the patient level is also very important. For example, alternative treatments may have equal efficacy based on traditional clinical parameters (e.g., blood pressure reduction) but produce very different effects on the patient's QOL. Thus a provider's selection among competing alternatives may hinge on documented differential impact on QOL. A perceived decrease in QOL attributed by the patient to an adverse effect of the drug may lead to a decrease in adherence to the medication regimen.[15]

TABLE 2–1. Taxonomy of Quality-of-Life Instruments

Generic Instruments
Health profiles
Preference-based measures
Specific Instruments
Disease specific (e.g., diabetes)
Population specific (e.g., frail older adults)
Function specific (e.g., sexual functioning)
Condition or problem specific (e.g., pain)

Adapted from Ref. 32.

MEASURING QUALITY OF LIFE

TYPES OF INSTRUMENTS

Hundreds of health-related QOL instruments are available.[28–30] Table 2–1 gives a taxonomy of the different types of instruments.[31] A primary distinction among QOL instruments is whether they are generic or specific.

GENERIC INSTRUMENTS

Generic, or general, QOL instruments are designed to be applicable across all diseases or conditions, across different medical interventions, and across a wide variety of populations.[32] Table 2–2 lists the dimensions or domains of five generic instruments. In choosing or evaluating the use of an instrument, the specific dimensions of functioning

TABLE 2–2. Domains Included in Selected Generic Instruments

EuroQol Group's EQ-5D[33]	
Mobility	Self-care
Usual activity	Pain/discomfort
Anxiety/depression	
Nottingham Health Profile (NHP)[34]	
Part I: Distress within the following domains	
Emotions	Energy
Sleep	Pain
Social isolation	Mobility
Part II: Health-related problems within the following domains	
Occupation	Sex life
Housework	Hobbies
Social life	Holidays
Home life	
Quality of Well-being Scale (QWB)[35]	
Symptoms/problems	Physical activity
Mobility	Social activity
Sickness Impact Profile (SIP)[36]	
Sleep and rest	Home management
Eating	Recreation and pastimes
Work	Body care and movement
Ambulation	Alertness behavior
Mobility	Emotional behavior
Communication	Social interaction
Health Utilities Index (HUI)—Mark III[37]	
Vision	Dexterity
Hearing	Cognition
Speech	Pain and discomfort
Ambulation	Emotion

TABLE 2–3. SF-36 Scales and Number of Items per Scale (SF-36/SF-12)

Physical functioning (10/2)
Role limitations attributed to physical problems (4/2)
Bodily pain (2/1)
General health (5/1)
Vitality (4/1)
Social functioning (2/1)
Role limitations attributed to emotional problems (3/2)
Mental health (5/2)
Health transition (1/0)

Compiled from Refs. 38 and 39.

and well-being covered must be considered. The instruments in Table 2–2 share common dimensions, but they also reflect the diversity and range of dimensions covered. The two main types of generic instruments are health profiles and utility- or preference-based measures.

Health Profiles

Health profiles provide an array of scores representing individual dimensions or domains of QOL or health status. An advantage of a health profile is that it provides multiple outcome scores that may be useful to clinicians and/or researchers attempting to measure differential effects of a condition or its treatment on various QOL domains.

A commonly used profile instrument is the Medical Outcomes Study 36-Item Short-Form Health Survey (SF-36).[38] The instrument includes nine health concepts or scales (Table 2–3). The SF-36 can be self-administered or administered by a trained interviewer (face to face or via telephone). This instrument has several advantages. For example, it is brief (it takes about 5 to 10 minutes to complete), and its reliability and validity have been documented in many clinical situations and disease states.[39,40] A means of aggregating the items into physical (PCS) and mental (MCS) component summary scores is available.[41] In addition, an abbreviated version of the SF-36, containing only 12 items (SF-12), has been introduced.[42] However, the scale scores and the mental and physical component summary scores derived from the SF-12 are based on fewer items and fewer defined levels of health and, as a result, are estimated with less precision and less reliability. The loss of precision and reliability in measurement can be a problem in small samples and/or with small expected effect sizes for an intervention.

Preference-Based Measures

QOL as measured by preference-based instruments is on a continuum from death (0.0) to perfect health (1.0). This approach incorporates the measurement of an individual's health status with an adjustment for the desirability, or preference, associated with that health state. The preferences are measured or assigned empirically through a variety of procedures. Although often called health state *utilities,* the term *preferences* will be used in this chapter as the broader term because it subsumes both *utilities* and *values.*[43]

Preference-based measures are useful in pharmacoeconomic research, specifically cost-utility analysis (CUA).[44] CUA, an economic technique discussed in Chapter 1, involves comparing the costs of an intervention (e.g., a medication) with its outcomes expressed in units such as quality-adjusted life years (QALYs) gained. QALYs gained is an outcome measure that incorporates both quantity and quality of life. This can be a key outcome measure, especially in diseases such as cancer, where the treatment itself can have a major impact on patient functioning and well-being. Numerous

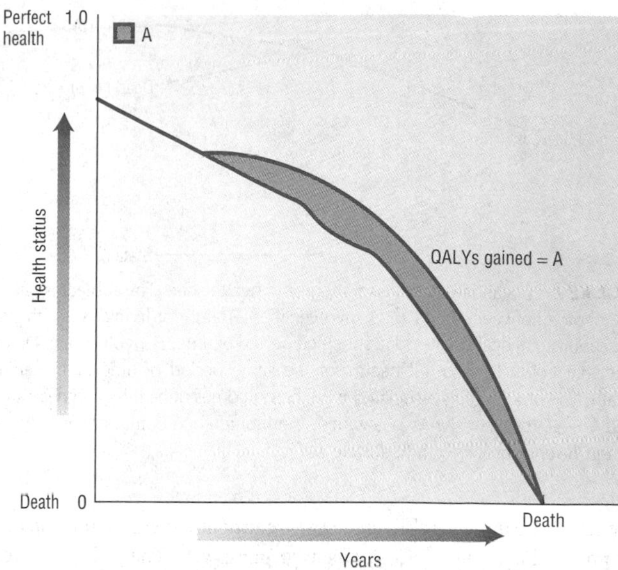

FIGURE 2–1. QALYs gained (i.e., area between the curves) as the outcome of a hypothetical health care intervention, such as a drug.

published studies have used CUA to evaluate the economic efficiency of health care interventions. A review of CUAs published from 1976–1997 by Neumann and colleagues[45] found that the number increased markedly during that time. Of the 228 articles reviewed, about one-third focused on pharmaceutical interventions. CUA data compiled during this extensive review can be accessed on the Web (at *www.hcra.harvard.edu/medical.html*).

QALYs can be produced by increases in QOL and/or length of life. Figure 2–1 represents a case in which QALYs were gained through an increase in QOL alone. The top curve represents the hypothetical life course of a cohort of individuals receiving a specific health care intervention compared with the life course of a cohort (i.e., lower curve) that did not receive the intervention. Average age at death did not differ between the two cohorts, but the intervention led to improvements in QOL in the treatment cohort. The area between the curves represents the QALYs gained through the intervention. This hypothetical case reflects a chronic disease, such as osteoarthritis, in which functioning and well-being are increased, but survival remains unchanged. Other hypothetical combinations of quality and quantity of life can be graphed in this manner. For example, an alternative scenario could reflect a temporary decrease in QOL but an increase in survival that may result from a chemotherapeutic regimen for cancer.

Direct Measures of Health State Values/Utilities. The most commonly used direct measurement techniques include visual analog scales, standard gamble, and time tradeoff.[46]

VISUAL ANALOG SCALES. The visual analog scale is a line, typically 10 cm in length, with the end points well defined (e.g., 0 = worst imaginable health state and 100 = best imaginable health state). The respondent is asked to mark the line where he or she would place one or more health states in relation to the two end points. If a subject rated his or her own health state or a health state described in a hypothetical scenario at the midpoint between 0 and 100 on the scale, the value for that health state would be 0.5.

STANDARD GAMBLE. The standard gamble offers a choice between two alternatives: choice A, living in health state *i* with certainty, or

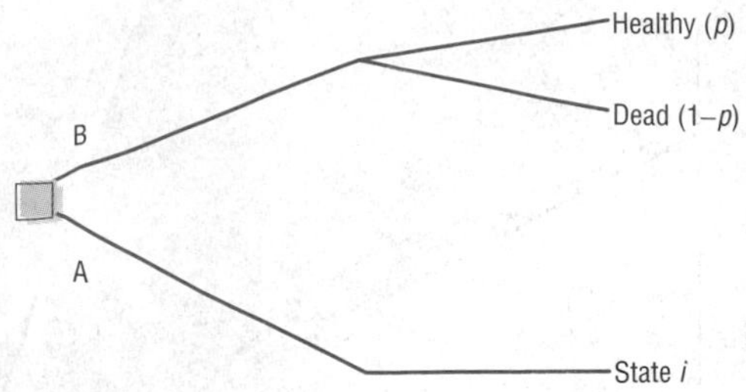

FIGURE 2–2. Standard gamble for a chronic health state. The subject is offered the choice between *A* and *B*. *A* involves the certainty of living in health state *i* (a suboptimal health state) for a specified period of time. *B* involves an intervention that could lead to full health for the same period of time or immediate death. The probabilities associated with the outcomes of healthy and dead are *p* and $1 - p$, respectively. As *p* is varied, the indifference point between choices *A* and *B* represents the utility of state *i*.

choice B, taking a gamble on a new treatment for which the outcome is uncertain. Figure 2–2 shows this gamble.[43] The subject is told that a hypothetical treatment will lead to perfect health, for a defined remaining lifetime, with a probability of p or immediate death with a probability of $1 - p$. The subject can choose between remaining, for the same defined lifetime, in state i, which is intermediate between healthy and dead, or taking the gamble and trying the new treatment. The probability p is varied until the subject is indifferent between choices A and B. For example, if a subject is indifferent between the choices A and B when $p = 0.75$, the utility of state i is 0.75.

TIME TRADEOFF. Figure 2–3 represents the time tradeoff technique for a chronic disease state.[47] Here, the subject is offered a choice of living for a variable amount of time x in perfect health or a defined amount of time t in a health state i that is less desirable. By reducing the time x of being healthy (at 1.0) and leaving the time t in the suboptimal health state fixed, an indifference point can be determined ($h_i = x/t$). For example, a subject may indicate that undergoing chronic hemodialysis for 2 years is equivalent to perfect health for 1 year. Therefore, the value of that health state would be 0.5 ($h_i = 1/2$).

Multiattribute Health Status Classification Systems. In addition to direct measures, instruments are available for which the health state utilities/values have been derived empirically through population studies. The instruments are administered to measure respondents' health status, which is then mapped onto a multiattribute health status classification system. Examples of such instruments include the Quality of Well-being Scale (QWB),[35] the Health Utilities Index (HUI),[37] and the EuroQol Group's EQ-5D.[33] Although each will be described briefly below, more thorough descriptions of these three instruments are provided elsewhere.[43,48]

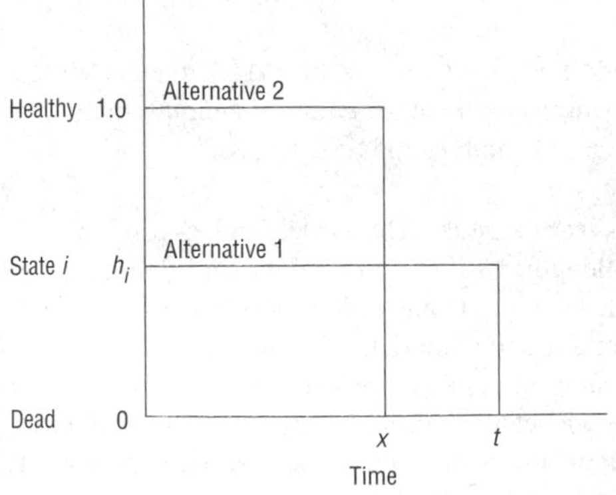

FIGURE 2–3. Time trade-off for a chronic health state. The subject chooses between living a varying amount of time in full-health (x) and living a specified amount of time (t) in state i. The length of time in full health is shortened until the subject is indifferent between the two choices. The value of health state i (h_i) is then calculated by dividing x/t.

The QWB is a generic QOL instrument that includes symptoms or problems plus three dimensions of functional health status (see Table 2–2). Standardized preference values for the health states represented by the QWB have been measured (via the category rating scale method, a technique related to visual analog scales) and validated on a general population sample.[35] The QWB was available originally only as an interviewer-administered version, but a self-administered version is now available.[49]

The HUI is another generic instrument that describes the health status of a person at a point in time in terms of his or her ability to function on a set of attributes or dimensions of health status. The HUI Mark III is a 15-item self-administered form. The measurements for the development of the health state preference system were made with visual analog scales and the standard gamble technique. The dimensions covered in the most recent version of the HUI (Mark III) are listed in Table 2–2.[37]

The EQ-5D was developed concurrently in five languages (Dutch, English, Finnish, Norwegian, and Swedish) by a multidisciplinary team of European researchers.[33] It was designed to be self-administered and short enough to be used in conjunction with other measures. The first of two parts classifies subjects into one of 243 health states within five dimensions. The health state preferences were estimated using the time tradeoff technique in a random sample of adults in the United Kingdom. The second part of the EQ-5D is a 20-cm visual analog scale (VAS) that has end points labeled "best imaginable health state" and "worst imaginable health state" anchored at 100 and 0, respectively. Respondents are asked to indicate how they rate their own health state by drawing a line from an anchor box to that point on the VAS that best represents their own health on that day.

SPECIFIC INSTRUMENTS

Specific instruments are intended to provide greater detail concerning particular outcomes, in terms of functioning and well-being, uniquely associated with a condition and/or its treatment. Several selected examples of disease-specific instruments are listed in Table 2–4. One of the instruments listed is the Asthma Quality of Life Questionnaire (AQLQ), a 32-item instrument developed to assess the impact of asthma on patients' everyday functioning and well-being.[51] Results from research in which the AQLQ was used have appeared in promotional materials for the GlaxoSmithKline salmeterol inhaler. As opposed to prior prescription drug advertisements that involved predominantly physiologic-based QOL claims,[18] this was one of the first times a pharmaceutical firm has promoted a product based on data from trials involving QOL as a primary outcome measure. This is likely to occur with increasing frequency as pharmaceutical firms

TABLE 2–4. Selected Disease-Specific Quality-of-Life Instruments

Arthritis Impact Measurement Scales (AIMS)[50]
Asthma Quality of Life Questionnaire (AQLQ)[51]
Diabetes Quality of Life (DQOL)[52]
Kidney Disease Quality of Life (KDQOL) Instrument[53]
Quality of Life in Epilepsy (QOLIE)[54]
Medical Outcomes Study HIV Health Survey (MOS-HIV)[55]

look for ways to demonstrate value and differentiate their products from those of the competition. Leidy and colleagues have provided useful recommendations for evaluating the validity of QOL claims for labeling and promotion of pharmaceuticals.[56] Disease- or condition-specific instruments may be more sensitive than a generic measure to particular changes in QOL secondary to the disease or its treatment. In addition, specific measures may appear to be more clinically relevant to patients and health care providers.[31]

However, a concern regarding the use of only specific instruments is that by focusing on the specific impact, the general or overall impact on functioning and well-being may be overlooked. In studies involving pharmacotherapy, the use of both a generic and a specific instrument may be the best approach. The generic instrument provides a more general outcome assessment and allows comparability across other disease states or conditions in which it has been used. An appropriately selected specific instrument should provide more detailed outcome information regarding expected changes in the particular patient population.

MEASUREMENT ISSUES

A number of issues must be considered when evaluating existing QOL research and/or choosing the appropriate instrument to use when designing a study involving QOL assessment. A thorough review of these issues is not within the scope of this chapter; more in-depth reviews of methodologic considerations are available in the literature.[12,57,58]

Of particular concern are the psychometric properties of a chosen instrument. *Psychometrics* refers to the measurement of psychological constructs, such as QOL. Instruments should be developed and tested such that one can place confidence in the measurement made. Psychometric properties of measures (e.g., reliability and validity) are considered in the review criteria developed by the Scientific Advisory Committee of the Medical Outcomes Trust (MOT).[59] The MOT is a depository and distributor of standardized health outcomes measurement instruments. Every instrument that is proposed for addition to the MOT list of approved instruments is reviewed against a rigorous set of eight attributes. These attributes provide a useful evaluative framework. The eight attributes of an instrument addressed by the review criteria are as follows: (1) conceptual and measurement model, (2) reliability, (3) validity, (4) responsiveness, (5) interpretability, (6) respondent and administrative burden, (7) alternative forms, and (8) cultural and language adaptations.

CONCEPTUAL AND MEASUREMENT MODELS

A *conceptual model* is the rationale for and description of the concepts that a measurement instrument is intended to assess and the interrelationships of those concepts. A *measurement model* is an instrument's scale and subscale structure and the procedures followed to create scale and subscale scores. An example is the well-defined conceptual and measurement models for the scales and scale structure of the SF-36.[38] The SF-36 contains 36 items that cover nine theory-based health concepts. Eight of these health concepts are measured by multi-item scales. There is a clearly defined means of creating the individual scale scores and the physical and mental component summary scales.[41]

RELIABILITY

Reliability refers to the extent to which measures give consistent or accurate results.[60] The purpose of evaluating the reliability of a QOL instrument is to estimate how much of the variation in a score is real as opposed to random. The two reliability assessment methods discussed most often in the QOL literature are internal consistency and test-retest reliability. *Internal consistency* is an assessment of the performance of items within a scale. It is a function of the number of items and their covariation.[61] Internal consistency is commonly measured using Cronbach's alpha coefficient. Alpha coefficients above 0.90 are recommended for making comparisons between individuals and above 0.70 for comparisons between groups.[62]

Test-retest reliability refers to the relationship between scores obtained from the same instrument on two or more separate occasions when all pertinent conditions remain relatively unchanged.[61] It is usually evaluated using a Pearson product-moment correlation coefficient. However, QOL is not assumed to be constant over the course of time. In fact, most clinical studies attempt to assess how QOL changes. Test-retest reliability estimates may have limited value in evaluating measures that are designed to assess a dynamic process.

Interrater reliability and *equivalent-forms reliability* are two other approaches to reliability assessment that are not used as commonly in QOL research. More in-depth discussions of these and the other reliability assessment methods are found elsewhere.[61,63]

VALIDITY

Reliability is necessary but not sufficient for valid measurement.[61] *Validity* is an estimation of the extent to which the instrument is measuring what it is supposed to be measuring. Validity is not an absolute property of an instrument. Hence a measurement instrument is not "valid," but empirical data can provide evidence to support its validity. Three types of validity commonly considered are criterion, content, and construct.

Criterion validity is demonstrated when a new measure corresponds to an established measure or observation that accurately reflects the phenomenon of interest. By definition, the criterion must be a superior measure of the phenomenon if it is to serve as a comparative norm. However, in QOL assessment, "gold standards" or criterion measures rarely exist against which a new measure can be compared.

Content validity, which is infrequently tested statistically, refers to how adequately the questions/items capture the relevant aspects of the domain or concept being measured.

Construct validity refers to the relationship between measures purporting to measure the same underlying theoretical construct (convergent evidence) or purporting to measure different constructs (discriminant evidence). For example, convergent evidence for the validity of a new measure of emotional well-being could be established by showing a strong association between the new scale and the mental health scale from the SF-36. Ware and colleagues[60] have provided a substantial amount of data supporting the validity of the SF 36. Evidence for the construct validity of other aspects of the measure might be established through comparisons with physiologic measures, organ pathology, or clinical signs.

RESPONSIVENESS

Responsiveness, or sensitivity to change, is the ability or power of the measure to detect clinically important change when it occurs.[64] Although some authors have suggested that responsiveness is a psychometric property of a measure distinct from validity,[65] others argue that responsiveness is an aspect of validity rather than a separate property.[61,66]

INTERPRETABILITY

Interpretability is the degree to which one can assign qualitative meaning to an instrument's quantitative scores. Interpretability is facilitated by comparison of a score or change in scores to a qualitative category that has clinical or commonly understood meaning. For example, it would be helpful to know how scale scores obtained in a specific patient sample compare with the scale scores of the general population. Again, Ware and colleagues have provided a substantial amount of normative data for the SF-36.[60]

RESPONDENT AND ADMINISTRATIVE BURDEN

Respondent burden refers to the time, energy, and other demands placed on those to whom the instrument is administered. *Administrative burden* refers to the demands placed on those who administer the instrument. A practical aspect of the measurement of QOL is length of the instrument or the administration time involved. Instruments should be as brief as possible without severely compromising the validity and reliability of the measurement. The longer an instrument, the greater is the respondent burden. This can lead to an individual's unwillingness or refusal to complete the instrument or to incomplete responses.

ALTERNATIVE FORMS

Alternative forms of an instrument include all modes of administration other than the original source instrument. Evidence should be provided that supports the comparability of the alternative mode of administration with that of the original instrument.[67] Many QOL measures can be administered in different ways. The primary modes of administration are (1) interviewer administered, either in person or over the telephone, or (2) self-administered.[31] Also used but not recommended are surrogate responders (i.e., using a health care provider, family member, or friend to respond for the subject when the subject is unable to complete the instrument). Because QOL is such a subjective concept, patients must have the opportunity to provide their perspective on the impact of medical care on their functioning and well-being. The patient's perspective has been shown to be quite different from that of outside observers, including physicians, family members, or significant others who are close to the patient.[68]

CULTURAL AND LANGUAGE ADAPTATIONS

Methods used to achieve conceptual and linguistic equivalence of cross-culturally adapted instruments should be explicitly stated.[69] Evidence should be provided that the measurement properties of the adaptation are comparable with those of the original instrument. It is obvious that this is an extremely important issue when planning cross-national QOL assessment projects. However, it is also very important within countries that are multicultural, such as the United States. Many of the English-language instruments have been developed for the dominant U.S. culture and may not be appropriate for all patients.

OTHER MEASUREMENT ISSUES

Selection of an Appropriate Instrument

It is essential that the purpose of the measurement be well-defined before selection of a QOL instrument. Is the purpose of the measurement to describe the health status or QOL of a patient population at a particular time or over time? Is it to document change in health outcomes associated with a particular intervention? These and other questions should be answered before QOL instruments are selected. Too many practitioner-researchers attempting to demonstrate improvements in outcomes resulting from a pharmaceutical product or service select a commonly used generic instrument, such as the SF-36, with the expectation that it will be sufficiently responsive to changes that may occur. The best approach may be to use the SF-36 or other generic instrument in conjunction with a more targeted, disease-specific instrument.

Availability of Instruments

Many QOL instruments are in the public domain. However, although they can be used for no or little cost, there may be a fee associated with the purchase of a user's guide or scoring manual. The MOT is a source of a wide array of instruments, including the SF-36, SF-12, QWB, MOS-HIV, AQLQ, and SIP (Sickness Impact Profile). For further information, the MOT home page is at *http://www.outcomes-trust.org*. Developers of particular instruments often can be contacted through addresses provided in other books referenced at the end of this chapter.[28–30,58]

CONCLUSIONS

The concept of QOL has gained increasing attention in the evaluation of the outcomes associated with medical care, including pharmacotherapy. In fact, in certain diseases, QOL may be the most important outcome to consider in assessing the effectiveness of health care interventions. Health care practitioners and policymakers must remember that efforts to increase QOL must not outstrip the ability to maintain or improve QOL.

Health-related QOL assessment is a relatively new field of endeavor, and a number of theoretical and methodological issues remain unresolved. However, some general concepts in the measurement of QOL outcomes should be considered carefully when designing a study, evaluating existing research, or evaluating new programs or services. This chapter has provided only a brief overview of the concepts in an effort to sensitize students and health care practitioners to the importance of the area as well as to provide insight as to how these concepts can and should be incorporated into their practices.

▶ PRINCIPLES OF PHARMACOTHERAPY

- The evaluation of health care is increasingly focused on the assessment of the end results, or *outcomes,* of medical interventions, including pharmacotherapy.
- Along with patient satisfaction, an essential humanistic or patient-reported outcome is self-assessed function and well-being, or health-related QOL.
- The patient's perspective has been shown to be quite different from that of outside observers, including clinicians and significant others.
- In certain chronic diseases and palliative conditions, QOL may be the most important health outcome to consider in assessing treatment.
- Information about the impact of pharmacotherapy on QOL can provide additional data for making medication-use decisions.
- A clinician's selection among competing therapeutic alternatives may hinge on documented differential impact on QOL.

- The assignment of numbers to psychosocial variables (e.g., attitudes, beliefs, well-being) according to predetermined rules makes it possible to quantify them in a uniform way.
- In QOL research, as with other areas of investigation, the quality of the data-collection tool is the major determinant of the overall quality of the results.
- Generic, or general, QOL instruments are designed to be applicable across all diseases or conditions, across different medical interventions, and across a wide variety of populations.
- Specific QOL instruments are intended to provide greater detail concerning particular outcomes, in terms of functioning and well-being, uniquely associated with a condition and/or its treatment.
- The use of QOL data in promotional activities is likely to occur with increasing frequency as pharmaceutical firms look for ways to demonstrate value and differentiate their products from those of the competition.

REFERENCES

1. Peterson MA, ed. Healthy Markets? The New Competition in Medical Care. Durham, NC: Duke University Press, 1999.
2. Gold MR, Siegel JE, Russell LB, Weinstein MC, eds. Cost-Effectiveness in Health and Medicine. New York, Oxford University Press, 1996.
3. Sloan FA, ed. Valuing Health Care: Costs, Benefits, and Effectiveness of Pharmaceuticals and Other Medical Technologies. New York, Cambridge University Press, 1996.
4. Donabedian A. Explorations in Quality Assessment and Monitoring, Vol. I: The Definition of Quality and Approaches to Its Assessment. Ann Arbor. MI, Health Administration Press, 1980.
5. Zitter M. Outcomes assessment: True customer focus comes to health care. Med Interface 1992;5:32–37.
6. Ellwood PM. Outcomes management: A technology of patient experience. N Engl J Med 1998;318:1551.
7. Lohr KN. Outcome measurement: Concepts and questions. Inquiry 1988;25:37–50.
8. Kozma CM, Reeder CE, Schulz RM. Economic, clinical, and humanistic outcomes: A planning model for pharmacoeconomic research. Clin Ther 1993;15:1121–1132.
9. Stewart AL. Conceptual and methodologic issues in defining quality of life: State of the art. Prog Cardiovasc Nurs 1992;7:3–11.
10. Kaplan RM, Bush JW. Health-related quality of life measurement for evaluation research and policy analysis. Health Psychol 1982;1:61–80.
11. Schron EB, Shumaker SA. The integration of health quality of life in clinical research: Experience from cardiovascular clinical trials. Prog Cardiovasc Nurs 1992;7(2):21.
12. Patrick DL, Erickson P. Health Status and Health Policy: Allocating Resources to Health Care. New York, Oxford University Press, 1993:22.
13. Schipper H, Clinch JJ, Olweny CLM. Quality of life studies: Definitions and conceptual issues. In: Spilker B, ed. Quality of Life and Pharmacoeconomics in Clinical Trials, 2d ed. Philadelphia, Lippincott-Raven, 1996:11–23.
14. Staquet M, Aaronson NK, Ahmedzai S, et al. Health-related quality of life research (Editorial). Qual Life Res 1992;1:3.
15. Smith M. Medication, quality of life and compliance: The role of the pharmacist. Pharmacoeconomics 1992;1:225–230.
16. Bungay KM, Boyer JG, Steinwald AB, Ware JE Jr. Health-related quality of life: An overview. In: Bootman JL, Townsend RJ, McGhan WF, eds. Principles of Pharmacoeconomics, 2d ed. Cincinnati, Harvey Whitney Books, 1996:126–148.
17. Revicki DA, Rothman M, Luce B. Health-related quality of life assessment and the pharmaceutical industry. Pharmacoeconomics 1992;1:394–408.
18. Rothermich EA, Pathak DS, Smeenk DA. Health-related quality of life claims in prescription drug advertisements. Am J Health Syst Pharm 1996;53:1565–1569.
19. Croog SH, Levine S, Testa MA, et al. The effects of antihypertensive therapy on quality of life. N Engl J Med 1986;319:1220–1221.
20. Côté I, Grégoire J-P, Moisan J. Health-related quality-of-life measurement in hypertension: A review of randomised controlled drug trials. Pharmacoeconomics 2000;18:435–450.
21. Juniper EF. Quality of life considerations in the treatment of asthma. Pharmacoeconomics 1995;8:123–138.
22. Fairclough DL, Fetting JH, Cella D, et al. Quality of life and quality adjusted survival for breast cancer patients receiving adjuvant therapy. Qual Life Res 1999;8:723–731.
23. Testa MA, Simonson DC. Health economic benefits and quality of life during improved glycemic control in patients with type 2 diabetes mellitus: A randomized, controlled, double-blind trial. JAMA 1998;280:1490–1496.
24. Briggs A, Scott E, Steele K. Impact of osteoarthritis and analgesic treatment on quality of life of an elderly population. Ann Pharmacother 1999;33:1154–1159.
25. Delate T, Coons SJ. The use of two health-related quality-of-life measures in a sample of persons infected with human immunodeficiency virus. Clin Infect Dis 2001;32(3):e47–e52.
26. Badia X, Herdman M. The importance of health-related quality-of-life data in determining the value of drug therapy. Clin Ther 2001;23:168–175.
27. Bukstein DA. Incorporating quality of life data into managed care formulary decisions: A case study with salmeterol. Am J Manag Care 1997;3:1701–1706.
28. Bowling A. Measuring Health: A Review of Quality of Life Measurement Scales, 2d ed. Buckingham, England, Open University Press, 1997.
29. Bowling A. Measuring Disease: A Review of Disease-Specific Quality of Life Measurement Scales, 2d ed. Buckingham, England, Open University Press, 1995.
30. McDowell I, Newell C. Measuring Health: A Guide to Rating Scales and Questionnaires, 2d ed. New York, Oxford University Press, 1996.
31. Guyatt GH, Feeny DH, Patrick DL. Measuring health-related quality of life. Ann Intern Med 1993;118:622–629.
32. Patrick DL, Deyo RA. Generic and disease-specific measures in assessing health status and quality of life. Med Care 1989;27:S217–S232.
33. Kind P. The EuroQol instrument: An index of health-related quality of life. In: Spilker B, ed. Quality of Life and Pharmacoeconomics in Clinical Trials, 2d ed. Philadelphia, Lippincott-Raven, 1996:191–201.
34. Hunt SM, McKewan J, McKenna SP. Measuring health status: A new tool for clinicians and epidemiologists. J R Coll Gen Prac 1985;35:185–188.
35. Kaplan RM, Anderson JP. The general health policy model: An integrated approach. In: Spilker B, ed. Quality of Life and Pharmacoeconomics in Clinical Trials, 2d ed. Philadelphia, Lippincott-Raven, 1996:309–322.
36. Bergner M, Bobbitt RA, Carter WB, Gilson BS. The sickness impact profile: Development and final revisions of a health status measure. Med Care 1976;14:57–67.
37. Feeny D, Furlong W, Boyle M, Torrance GW. Multiattribute health status classification systems: Health utilities index. Pharmacoeconomics 1995;7:490–502.
38. Ware JE Jr, Sherbourne CD. The MOS 36-item short-form health survey (SF-36): I. Conceptual framework and item selection. Med Care 1992;30:473–483.
39. McHorney CA, Ware JE Jr, Raczek AE. The MOS 36-item short-form health survey (SF-36): II. Psychometric and clinical tests of validity in measuring physical and mental health constructs. Med Care 1993;31:247–263.
40. McHorney CA, Ware JE Jr, Raczek AE. The MOS 36-item short-form health survey (SF-36): III. Tests of data quality, scaling assumptions, and reliability across diverse patient groups. Med Care 1994;32:40–66.
41. Ware JE Jr, Kosinski M, Keller SD. SF-36 Physical and Mental Health Summary Scales: A User's Manual. Boston, The Health Institute, 1994.
42. Ware JE Jr, Kosinski M, Keller SD. A 12-item short-form health survey: Construction of scales and preliminary test of reliability and validity. Med Care 1996;34:220.

43. Drummond MF, O'Brien B, Stoddart GL, Torrance GW. Methods for the Economic Evaluation of Health Care Programmes, 2d ed. Oxford, England, Oxford University Press, 1997.
44. Coons SJ, Kaplan RM. Cost-utility analysis. In: Bootman JL, Townsend RJ, McGhan WF, eds. Principles of Pharmacoeconomics, 2d ed. Cincinnati, Harvey Whitney Books, 1996:102–126.
45. Neumann PJ, Stone PW, Chapman RH, et al. The quality of reporting in published cost-utility analyses, 1976–1997. Ann Intern Med 2000;132:964–972.
46. Feeny DH, Torrance GW, Labelle R. Integrating economic evaluations and quality of life assessments. In: Spilker B, ed. Quality of Life and Pharmacoeconomics in Clinical Trials, 2d ed. Philadelphia, Lippincott-Raven, 1996:85–95.
47. Torrance GW, Thomas WH, Sackett DL. Utility maximization model for evaluation of health care programmes. Health Serv Res 1972;7:118–133.
48. Coons SJ, Rao S, Keininger DL, Hays RD. A comparative review of generic quality of life instruments. Pharmacoeconomics 2000;17:13–35.
49. Kaplan RM, Sieber WJ, Ganiats TG. The quality of well-being scale: Comparison of an interviewer-administered version with a self-administered questionnaire. Psychol Health 1997;12:783–791.
50. Meenan RF, Gertman PM, Mason JH. Measuring health status in arthritis: The arthritis impact measurement scales. Arthritis Rheum 1980;23: 146–152.
51. Juniper EF, Guyatt GH, Epstein RS, et al. Evaluation of impairment of health-related quality of life in asthma. Development of a questionnaire for use in clinical trials. Thorax 1992;47:76–83.
52. Parkerson GR, Connis RT, Broadhead WE, et al. Disease-specific versus generic measurement of health-related quality of life in insulin-dependent diabetic patients. Med Care 1993;7:629–639.
53. Hays RD, Kallich JD, Mapes DL, et al. Development of the kidney disease quality of life (KDQOL) instrument. Qual Life Res 1994;3:329–338.
54. Perrine KR. A new quality of life inventory for epilepsy patients: Interim results. Epilepsia 1993;34(Suppl 4):S28–S33.
55. Wu AW, Revicki DA, Jacobson D, Malitz FE. Evidence for reliability, validity and usefulness of the medical outcomes study HIV health survey (MOS-HIV). Qual Life Res 1997;6:481–493.
56. Leidy NK, Revicki DA, Geneste B. Recommendations for evaluating the validity of quality of life claims for labeling and promotion. Value Health 1999;2:113–127.
57. Staquet MJ, Hays RD, Fayers PM. Quality of Life Assessment in Clinical Trials: Methods and Practice. Oxford, England, Oxford University Press, 1998.
58. Fayers PM, Machin D. Quality of Life: Assessment, Analysis and Interpretation. Chichester, England, Wiley, 2000.
59. Lohr KN, Aaronson NK, Alonso J, et al. Evaluating quality of life and health status instruments: Development of scientific review criteria. Clin Ther 1996;18:979–992.
60. Ware JE Jr, Snow KK, Kosinski M, Gandek B. SF-36 Health Survey: Manual and Interpretation Guide. Boston, The Health Institute, 1993.
61. Hays RD, Anderson R, Revicki D. Psychometric considerations in evaluating health-related quality of life measures. Qual Life Res 1993;2: 441–449.
62. Nunnally J. Psychometric Theory, 2d ed. New York, McGraw-Hill, 1978.
63. Kaplan RM, Saccuzzo DP. Psychological Testing: Principles, Applications, and Issues, 3d ed. Pacific Grove, CA, Brooks/Cole, 1993.
64. Juniper EF, Guyatt GH, Jaeschke R. How to develop and validate a new health-related quality of life instrument. In: Spilker B, ed. Quality of Life and Pharmacoeconomics in Clinical Trials, 2d ed. Philadelphia, Lippincott-Raven, 1996:49–56.
65. Guyatt G, Walter S, Norman G. Measuring change over time: Assessing the usefulness of evaluative instruments. J Chron Dis 1987;40:171–178.
66. Hays RD, Hadorn D. Responsiveness to change: An aspect of validity, not a separate dimension. Qual Life Res 1992;1:73–75.
67. Cook DJ, Guyatt GH, Juniper E, et al. Interviewer versus self-administered questionnaires in developing a disease-specific, health-related quality of life instrument for asthma. J Clin Epidemiol 1993;46:529–534.
68. Jachuck SJ, Brierly H, Jachuck S, Wilcox PM. The effect of hypotensive drugs on the quality of life. J R Coll Gen Prac 1992;32:103–105.
69. Bullinger M, Power MJ, Aaronson NK, et al. Creating and evaluating cross-cultural instruments. In: Spilker B, ed. Quality of Life and Pharmacoeconomics in Clinical Trials, 2d ed. Philadelphia, Lippincott-Raven, 1996:659–668.

3
EVIDENCE-BASED MEDICINE

Elaine Chiquette and L. Michael Posey

In the information age, clinicians are presented with a daunting number of diseases and possible treatments to consider as they care for patients each day. As knowledge increases and as the technology for accessing information becomes widely available, health care professionals are expected to stay current in their fields of expertise and to remain competent throughout their careers. In addition, the number of information sources for the typical practitioner has ballooned, and clinicians must sort out information from many sources: college courses and continuing education (including seminars and journals), pharmaceutical representatives, colleagues, as well as guidelines from committees of health care facilities, governmental agencies, and expert committees and organizations.

How does the health care professional find valid information from such a cacophony? Increasingly, clinicians are turning to the principles of evidence-based medicine (EBM) to identify the best course of action for each patient. EBM strategies help health care professionals ferret out these gold nuggets, enabling them to integrate the best current evidence into their pharmacotherapeutic decision making. These strategies can help physicians, pharmacists, and other health care professionals reliably distinguish beneficial pharmacotherapies from those which are ineffective or harmful. Also, EBM approaches can be applied to keep up-to-date and to make an overwhelming task seem more manageable.

This chapter describes for the reader the principles of EBM, offers guidance for finding EBM sources on the World Wide Web, provides a model for applying EBM in patient care, and explains how EBM strategies can help a practitioner stay current.

WHAT IS EVIDENCE-BASED MEDICINE?

EBM is an approach to medical practice that uses the results of patient care research and other available objective evidence as a component of clinical decision making. Similarly, evidence-based pharmacotherapy, defined by Etminan and colleagues,[1] is an approach to decision making whereby clinicians appraise the scientific evidence and its strength in support of their therapeutic decisions.

While few would argue against the necessity for basing clinical decisions on the best possible evidence available, considerable controversy actually surrounds the practice of EBM. Critics note that not all questions relevant to the care of a patient are of a scientific nature and that EBM favors a cookbook approach. In fact, EBM integrates knowledge from research with other factors affecting clinical decision making. EBM does not replace clinical judgment. Rather, it informs clinical judgment with the current best evidence. The expertise and experience of the clinician who understands the disease are crucial in determining whether the external evidence applies to the patient and whether it should be integrated in the therapeutic plan. Also, nonmedical factors affect decision making, such as the patient's preferences and readiness and the health care delivery system's characteristics.

Other critics state that EBM considers randomized controlled trials (RCTs) as the only evidence to be used in clinical decision making. Actually, EBM seeks the best existing evidence from basic science to clinical research with which to inform clinical decision. For example, a decision about the accuracy of a diagnostic test is best informed by evidence from cross-sectional study, not an RCT. A cohort study, not an RCT, best answers a question about prognosis. However, in selecting a treatment, the randomized trial is the best study design to provide the most accurate estimate of treatment efficacy and safety.

EBM opponents note that RCTs usually are conducted in idealized environments or situations that are not sufficiently similar to the conditions of the "real world." In addition, errors can be made when results of an RCT of one drug are extrapolated to all members of that class of drugs.[2,3]

Regardless of one's view, RCTs have confirmed the value of many therapeutic options today and disproved or clarified the usefulness of others. For example, in 1970, observational studies had indicated a possible association between occurrence of premature ventricular contractions (PVCs) in patients after myocardial infarction (MI) and sudden death. As a result, the eighth edition of *Harrison's Principles of Internal Medicine* recommended the use of antiarrhythmic agents to eradicate post-MI PVCs and thereby minimize the risk of sudden death. However, an RCT tested the antiarrhythmic therapy in patients with frequent PVCs, and it showed that class 1 antiarrhythmic agents increased rather than decreased the risk of sudden death.[4,5] Today, guidelines discourage the use of antiarrhythmic agents to suppress PVCs in post-MI patients.[6]

More recently, the 1996 guidelines for the management of patients with acute MI concluded that observational studies "indicate that estrogen therapy does reduce mortality in women with moderate and severe coronary disease."[7] Subsequently, an RCT found no reduction in overall risk for nonfatal MI or coronary death with estrogen therapy. Rather, significantly more coronary events occurred during the first year of the trial among women receiving estrogen therapy compared with women taking placebo.[8] These results prompted revision of the guidelines to conclude: "On the basis of the finding of no overall cardiovascular benefit and a pattern of early increase in risk of coronary events, starting estrogen plus progestin is not recommended for the purpose of secondary prevention of coronary disease."[6]

In both these examples, conventional wisdom was wrong. Results from observational studies proved incorrect. Only through careful assessment using RCT methodology was the true estimate of the efficacy and safety of the therapeutic options discovered.

EBM ON THE WORLD WIDE WEB

For additional information and resources relevant to EBM, several comprehensive EBM sites exist on the World Wide Web. These sites include information on the history and development of EBM, glossaries of EBM terms, tutorials, training programs, software, links to EBM organizations and practice centers, guides to searching the medical literature, and results of evidence-based studies. For an excellent list of EBM links, access "Netting the Evidence: A ScHARR Introduction to Evidence Based Practice" (*http://www.shef.ac.uk/~scharr/ir/netting/*). A specialized EBM site dedicated to pharmacotherapy deserves special mention. It is provided by The Centre for Evidence-Based Pharmacotherapy (*http://www.aston.ac.uk/pharmacy/cebp/*). The mission of the center, created in 1995 by pharmacy professor Alain Li Wan Po, is to undertake research in the methodology of medicines assessment, pharmacoepidemiology, and pharmacoeconomics. In addition, the center offers postgraduate and distance learning in evidence-based pharmacotherapy.

INCORPORATING EBM INTO PHARMACOTHERAPEUTIC DECISION MAKING

The practice of EBM is to recognize an information need while caring for a patient, identify the best existing evidence to help resolve the problem, consider the evidence in light of the actual circumstances, and integrate the evidence into a medical plan. In this section, the four-step process of applying the EBM process to a pharmacotherapeutic decision is described[9]:

1. Recognize information needs and convert them into answerable questions.
2. Conduct efficient searches for the best evidence with which to answer these questions.
3. Critically appraise the evidence for its validity and usefulness.
4. Apply the results to patient situations to best assist clinical decision making.

BUILDING A FOCUSED QUESTION

Clinicians constantly balance the benefits and risks of various therapeutic choices. The questions they face are patient-specific:

- Should clopidogrel be prescribed to this 65-year-old man with unstable angina?
- Should hormone-replacement therapy be prescribed for this postmenopausal woman?
- Should amlodipine be discontinued in this patient with type 2 diabetes?

When searching for the best evidence to answer such questions, the questions must be rephrased with more precision and specificity. A well-formulated question includes the following elements: the patient or problem being addressed, the intervention being considered, the comparison intervention, and the outcome(s) of interest.[10] Using these four elements, the preceding questions can be reframed as follows:

- Would clopidogrel in addition to aspirin (*intervention*) prevent death or coronary events (*clinically relevant outcome*) in this patient with unstable angina (*patient with a problem*) who is currently on aspirin alone (*comparison intervention*)?
- Should we begin hormone-replacement therapy (*intervention compared with no intervention*) to prevent cardiovascular events (*outcome*) in this asymptomatic postmenopausal woman with a family history of coronary artery disease (*patient*)?
- Does amlodipine (*intervention*) compared with other antihypertensives (*comparison intervention*) increase the risk of death (*outcome*) in this patient with diabetes (*patient*)?

The acronym PICO can be helpful to remember the elements of a well-balanced question[11]:

P = patient
I = intervention
C = comparison
O = outcome

Focusing the question clarifies the target of the literature search and permits use of the appropriate guides for assessing external validity, that is, the applicability of the evidence found in the study to appropriate parts of the "real world."

CONDUCTING AN EFFICIENT SEARCH

Health care professionals have four options as they try to identify the best evidence available to answer a well-framed question:

1. Ask a colleague for his or her expert opinion.
2. Review practice guidelines (evidence-based or expert-opinion-based) or a textbook for appropriate disease management.
3. Consult electronic databases of systematic reviews and/or meta-analyses.
4. Conduct a literature search using an electronic database such as MEDLINE.

Each of these options has advantages and disadvantages, as described below.

Option 1. Asking an expert or colleague may provide a quick and easy answer to a clinical question. Exercise caution, however. These sources have become less reliable as the volume and complexity of medical information have grown exponentially. Colleagues may be out of date or biased by their own experiences.

Option 2. Online practice guidelines or current textbooks with evidence links are useful if the question relates to a common or well-established issue (e.g., *UpToDate, Harrison's Online,* and *Scientific American Medicine Online* electronic textbooks). As their names suggest, evidence-based clinical guidelines are guided by objective data and should be preferred over expert-opinion-based guidelines that refer loosely to evidence to support their opinions. Expert-opinion guidelines vary in their scientific validity and reproducibility.[12]

One Web site—the National Guideline Clearinghouse on the Web (*http://www.guideline.gov*)—provides links to many evidence-based clinical practice guidelines. For each guideline, this comprehensive database offers a short summary of the key attributes, including the bibliographic sources, guideline developers and endorsers, status of the guidelines, and major recommendations. In addition, the site provides the ability to generate side-by-side comparisons for any combination of two or more guidelines. Table 3–1 presents an annotated list of additional resources to find and access evidence-based clinical practice guidelines.

Option 3. Consulting electronic databases of systematic reviews and meta-analyses is attractive because of the limited amount of time health care professionals have to research and review the literature before they answer clinical questions or reach patient-care decisions. Busy health care professionals prefer summaries of information. Traditional narrative reviews are useful for broad overviews of particular therapies or diseases or for reports on the latest advances in a particular area where research may be limited.[13] However, information from narrative reviews is often gathered ad hoc, and the author's biases may enter into the process of gathering, analyzing, and reporting information.

TABLE 3–1. North American Sources of Evidence-Based Clinical Practice Guidelines

Resource/Web Address	Special Features
National Guideline Clearinghouse (NGC) (*www.guideline.gov*) NGC is a collaboration of U.S. Department of Health and Human Services and the Agency for Healthcare Research and Quality (AHRQ), in partnership with the American Medical Association (AMA) and the American Association of Health Plans (AAHP). NGC provides access to full text guidelines (when available) produced by a number of different professional medical associations and health care organizations. Each guideline is critically appraised using a standard instrument. The site permits side-by-side comparison of several guidelines.	• 966 guideline summaries • Weekly e-mail alerts • Advanced search queries based on guideline attributes • Annotated bibliography of resources relevant to guideline methodology
National Library of Medicine's Health Services/Technology Assessment Text (*http://text.nlm.nih.gov/ftrs/gateway*) This World Wide Web resource is a collection of AHRQ Supported Guidelines, AHRQ Technology Assessments and Reviews, ATIS (HIV/AIDS Technical Information), NIH Warren G. Magnuson Clinical Research Studies, NIH Consensus Development Program, Public Health Service (PHS) Guide to Clinical Preventive Services and the Substance Abuse, and Mental Health Services Administration's Center for Substance Abuse Treatment (SAMHSA/CSAT) Prevention Enhancement and Treatment Improvement Protocols.	1. 199 full-text guidelines 2. Metasearch capabilities to PubMed, Centers for Disease Control and Prevention (CDC) Prevention Guidelines Database, and National Guideline Clearinghouse 3. Access to quick-reference guides for clinicians and consumer brochures.
Primary Care Clinical Practice Guidelines (*http://medicine.ucsf.edu/resources/guidelines)* This Web resource offers a listing of online guidelines.	• Searchable by clinical content and organization
CDC Prevention Guidelines Database Home Page (*http://aepo-xdv-www.epo.cdc.gov/wonder/PrevGuid/prevquid.shtml)* The site is a comprehensive collection of all the official guidelines and recommendations published by the CDC about prevention of diseases, injuries, and disabilities.	• More than 500 prevention guidelines/documents • Searchable • Sort by date, by topic, or alphabetically
Cancer Care Ontario Practice Guidelines Initiative (CCOPGI) (*http://hiru.mcmaster.ca/ccopgi/guidelines.html*) This Web page includes published and unpublished guidelines related to cancer care. These guidelines are created by the CCOPGI and are available full text.	• 45 guidelines • When information is scarce, evidence summaries are created to review the best evidence available
Clinical Practice Guidelines Infobase (*http://www.cma.ca/cpgs/index.asp*) Guidelines in this collection were produce or endorsed in Canada by a national, provincial, or territorial medical/health organization, professional society, government agency, or expert panel. The database is searchable by category, title, or developer. Full text is available when possible.	• 255 guidelines • More than 2000 reviews, in French and English • Advanced search capabilities
Agency for Healthcare Research and Quality's Evidence-Based Practice Centers (AHRQ EPCs) (*http://www.ahcpr.gov/clinic/epcix.htm*) AHRQ has established 12 Evidence-Based Practice Centers to analyze and synthesize the scientific literature and develop evidence reports and technology assessments on clinical topics.	• 34 evidence reports • Full text available

In contrast, systematic reviews employ a comprehensive, reproducible data search and selection process to summarize all the best evidence. They follow a rigorous process to appraise and analyze the information, quantitatively (through the meta-analysis technique) or qualitatively, to best answer a defined clinical question. Systematic reviews are a useful means of assessing whether findings from multiple individual studies are consistent and can be generalized.[14]

The Cochrane Library represents one of the most comprehensive sources of systematic reviews summarizing the evidence about health care. More than 850 Cochrane reviews are currently available, and more than 750 additional reviews are in progress. As new reviews are added quarterly, eventually all areas of health care will be covered. The Cochrane Library includes the Database of Abstracts of Reviews of Effectiveness, which contains more than 2500 structured abstracts of good-quality published reviews about the effectiveness of health interventions. Table 3–2 lists accessible sources of systematic reviews and provides a search strategy developed by librarians at McMaster University to locate systematic reviews and meta-analyses in MEDLINE efficiently.[15]

Option 4. Consider conducting a literature search on an electronic database, such as MEDLINE, if the question relates to new developments in therapeutic options. In this case, health care professionals must consult primary literature. Dozens of electronic databases exist as primary sources of original research reports.

MEDLINE and PubMed, both produced by the National Library of Medicine (NLM), are the largest and best-known bibliographic databases of biomedical journal literature. PubMed's in-process records provide basic citation information and abstracts *before*

TABLE 3–2. Selected Resources for Systematic Reviews

Resources	Advantages	Disadvantages
Best Evidence Electronic version of both American College of Physicians (ACP) Journal Club and Evidence-Based Medicine (http://hiru.mcmaster.ca/acpjc/acpod.htm). Available on CD-ROM.	• All review articles are systematic reviews. • Updated every 6 months • Short title includes meta-analysis or review to facilitate identification	• Includes systematic reviews from only the journal scanned by ACP Journal Club and Evidence-Based Medicine
Medline Systematic review search strategy: (meta-analy$ or metanal$ or metaanal$).tw. or Meta-Analysis/ or meta-analysis (pt) or (quantitativ$ review$ or quantitativ$ overview$).tw. or (systematic$ review$ or systematic$ overview$).tw. or (methodologic$ review$ or methodologic$ overview$).tw. or medline.tw. or pooled.tw.) and eng.lg. and human/) not (letter or editorial or comment).pt	• Covers more than 4000 journals • Contains 11 million citations	• One-tenth of the citations are indexed as review articles. Even fewer are indexed as systematic reviews. • Requires search strategy to identify meta-analysis or systematic reviews.
Cochrane Library Electronic library of high-quality reviews (http://www.cochrane.org). Available on CD-ROM.	• Most comprehensive collection of systematic reviews. • Updated every 3 months • Abstracts of Cochrane Reviews are available free on the Internet at *http://www.cochrane.org.*	• Limited access; not all libraries subscribe to the Cochrane Library
United Kingdom National Health Services Centre for Reviews and Dissemination (*http://agatha.york.ac.uk/welcome.htm*) Includes the Database of Abstracts of Reviews of Effectiveness (DARE), NHS Economic evaluation database, and the Health Technology Assessment (HTA) database	• The DARE Web version, which is updated monthly, is more current than the Cochrane Library version.	• NHS economic evaluation, last update 1999
Effective Health Care Bulletins ***http://www.york.ac.uk/inst/crd/ehcb.htm***	• Reports of systematic reviews produced by NHS Centre for Reviews and Dissemination	• Limited number of reviews
National Institute for Clinical Excellence Part of the UK National Health Service (NHS). Provides guidelines and technology assessments to health care practitioners (http://nice.org.uk).	• Follows Cochrane methodology to develop technology assessments. Twenty-eight have been completed, and 38 are in progress.	• Limited number of guidelines and assessments available.

the citations are indexed with NLM's Medical Subject Headings (MeSH) Terms and added to MEDLINE. To optimize the efficiency of a clinical search, PubMed offers specialized searches using methodologic filters. These filters, based on work by Haynes and colleagues,[15] are validated search strategies to identify clinically relevant studies that answer questions about etiology, prognosis, diagnosis, or therapy of a disease.

To facilitate the searches of multiple Internet sources, metasearching is useful. Metasearch tools launch a single query across a set of Web-based health sites. One query returns a merged and often ranked list of hits, allowing the user to search several databases at once. Table 3–3 describes the specifics of new metasearch engines available to search for Internet-based health information.

Once the evidence is gathered, the clinician needs to determine whether the identified guideline, review article, or study report will help answer the clinical problem. This is accomplished by considering the validity and by judging the clinical relevance (usefulness) of the information.[16]

ASSESSING VALIDITY

The external validity refers to applicability and generazibility and is outlined in the section, "Applying the Results." The remainder of this section focuses on critically appraising the quality—that is, the internal validity—of individual trials. The internal validity is determined by how well the trial ensures that the known and unknown risk factors are equally distributed between the treatment and control groups. To ensure validity, the conduct of the trial should minimize systematic bias and random error as much as possible to provide results that are as accurate and close to the truth as possible. Four sources of bias are possible in trials of health care interventions: selection bias, performance bias, attrition bias, and detection bias. Bias can result in an overestimation or underestimation of the effectiveness of a drug therapy and mislead the reader. While it is beyond the scope of this chapter to present extensive details about critical appraisal, here are questions that must be answered in assessing the internal validity of an RCT:

TABLE 3–3. Metasearch Engines for Web-Based Health Information

Turning Research Into Practice (TRIP)
Web address: *www.tripdatabase.com*
Sources: Fifty-eight sites categorized as evidence-based, peer-reviewed journals, guidelines, or other. Sites include top 20 medical journals, EMB sites such as Bandolier, Critically Appraised Bank, Cochrane Database of Systematic Reviews, Journal Club on the Web, Evidence-Based Medicine series, guideline and systematic review sites such as SIGN, DARE, NICE, and National Guideline Clearinghouse.
Special features: Updated monthly. Searches use keywords in the title only. Results are displayed by categories: evidence-based, peer-reviewed journals, guidelines, or other.

SUMSearch
Web address: *http://SUMSearch.uthscsa.edu*
Sources: Three Internet sites: The National Library of Medicine, the Database of Abstracts of Reviews of Effectiveness, and the National Guideline Clearinghouse.
Special features: If the first search resulted in too many or not enough hits, SUMSearch uses metasearching and contingency search techniques to query the sites again.

Search.com
Web address: *http://www.search.com*
Sources: Twenty-two Internet sites containing health and medical information. Some of these sites are American College of Physicians Online, Centers for Disease Control and Prevention, *New England Journal of Medicine*, Agency for Healthcare Research and Quality, *Journal of the American Medical Association*, PubMed, Merck, Mayo Clinic, Food and Drug Administration, World Health Organization, WebMD, and Medical Subject Headings (MeSH).
Special features: The site allows customization in choosing search engines and how to display results.

Query Server
Web address: *http://queryserver.com*
Sources: Twelve sites containing health and medical information. These sites are American Health Consultants, American Heart Association, Centers for Disease Control and Prevention, Department of Health and Human Services, Food and Drug Administration, Johns Hopkins Infectious Diseases, Leukemia and Lymphoma Society, MEDLINE, Medscape Clinical Content, Medscape News, National Institutes of Health, National Library of Medicine.
Special features: Results are sorted according to content and/or source.

- *Was the subject's treatment allocation randomized?* To minimize selection bias, all participants should have an equal chance to be allocated to the treatment or control group. Randomization is the best method to create groups of similar known and unknown confounders. If important risk factors known to affect prognosis (such as disease severity or presence of comorbidities) are unevenly distributed between groups, then selection bias could falsely estimate the benefit of the intervention. Furthermore, recruiters should not know which assignment (treatment or control group) is next in line. Recruiters who assess eligibility criteria and are aware of the next random allocation may consciously or unconsciously select the healthiest patient to be enrolled in the control group or vice versa. Approaches to randomization that may allow the recruiters to manipulate the assignment include improper use of record numbers (e.g., if all odd numbers were assigned to control group), dates of birth, day of week, or open lists of random numbers. Examples of bias-free random allocations include centralized randomization (e.g., a central office unaware of subject characteristics allocates group assignments), pharmacy-controlled randomization (assuming the pharmacist is not recruiting the subjects), or opaque envelopes that are sequentially numbered and sealed.[17]
- *Was the study double-blinded?* To minimize performance bias (systematic differences in the care provided, apart from the intervention being evaluated), the subjects and the clinicians should be unaware of the therapy received. The double-blind method prevents subjects or clinicians from adding any additional treatments (or cointervention) to one of the groups. For example, clinicians who know that certain patients are receiving the therapy they perceive to be less effective (control group) may opt to check on those patients more often than is required in the study protocol. A third blind can be applied to the outcome assessor (e.g., a statistician or clinician whose role is to measure the outcome) to minimize detection bias (systematic differences in outcome assessment). The necessity for blinding outcome assessors is controversial at this time.
- *Was intention-to-treat analysis performed?* Intention-to-treat analysis means that the results from all subjects randomized in the study were accounted for and attributed to the group to which they were assigned. This strategy minimizes attrition bias and ensures that the known and unknown prognostic factors are kept equally distributed. For example, exclusion of subjects who withdrew early in treatment may bias the comparison because the reasons people withdraw early are often related to prognosis.[18] Excluding early withdrawals from the final analysis may select the subjects most likely to get the best outcome and thereby overestimate the benefit of the intervention.

For a more detailed description of the concepts in critical appraisal, a series of articles published in the *Journal of the American Medical Association (JAMA)* provides a useful tool for practitioners who are evaluating clinical trials.[19–50] These users' guides to the medical literature—developed by The Evidence-Based Medicine Working Group, a group of clinicians at Canada's McMaster University and colleagues across North America—can help assess the validity of primary studies as well as review articles.

TABLE 3–4. Checklist for Critical Appraisal of Articles Addressing Pharmacotherapeutic Decisions

Therapy

Internal validity
- Was subject's treatment allocation randomized?
- Was the study double-blinded?
- Was intention-to-treat analysis performed?
- Was the randomization successful?

Magnitude of the effect
- What was the impact of the treatment?
- How narrow is the 95% confidence interval range?
- Were clinically relevant outcomes considered?

Applicability
- Does this patient fulfill inclusion criteria for the trial?
- Do the treatment benefits outweigh the risks?

Harm

Internal validity
- Were the control subjects similar to the cases?
- Was bias minimized while measuring exposure and outcomes?
- Was length of follow-up appropriate?
- Does exposure precede the adverse outcome?
- Is there a dose-response relationship?

Magnitude of the effect
- How strong is the association between exposure and outcome?
- How precise is the estimate?
- How many patients must be exposed to the agent to cause an adverse event?

Applicability
- What is the likelihood of harm in my patient?
- What are the consequences of eliminating the agent from my patient's therapy?

Overview, Systematic Reviews, Meta-analysis

Internal validity
- Did the overview clearly state a well-formulated question?
- Were the criteria used to select articles for inclusion appropriate?
- Were all relevant studies included?
- Were included articles critically appraised for quality?
- Was bias minimized in the selection, data extraction, and analysis processes?
- Were all clinically important outcomes considered?
- Were the studies appropriately combined?

Magnitude of the effect
- What is the average effect?
- How precise are the results?

Applicability
- Are this patient's characteristics similar to the subjects included in the studies?
- Do the treatment benefits outweigh the risks?

Practice Guidelines

Internal validity
- Were the management options and outcomes clearly specified?
- Was all evidence relevant to each arm of the evidence model sought?
- Were systematic and explicit methods used to identify, select, and combine evidence?
- Were all clinically relevant outcomes evaluated?
- Is the guideline up-to-date?
- Does the guideline clearly present the evidence to support the benefit of following the recommendations?
- Has the guideline been peer-reviewed?

Magnitude of the effect
- How strong are the recommendations?
- What is the impact of uncertainty in the evidence on outcomes?

Applicability
- Are the guideline recommendations targeting my practice (e.g., family practice setting versus endocrinology setting)?
- Is my patient the intended target for this guideline?

Economic Analyses

Internal validity
- Were both costs and outcomes evaluated for all strategies considered?
- Were costs and outcomes measured and valued accurately?
- Was the potential impact of uncertainties in the analysis evaluated?
- Was the potential impact of different baseline risk in the treatment population estimated on costs and outcomes?

Magnitude of the effect
- What were the incremental costs and outcomes of each strategy considered?
- Do incremental costs and outcomes vary between selected groups of patients?
- What is the impact of sensitivity analyses on incremental cost?

Applicability
- Do the treatment benefits outweigh the treatment risk and cost?
- Are the results transferable to my practice setting (e.g., similar patient types, similar costs of resources)?

Adapted from Users' Guide Series (Refs. 19 to 50).

Online materials to support teaching of evidence-based health care, including the Users' Guides to Evidence-Based Practice, are now supported through the Centres for Health Evidence at *http://www.cche.net.* Table 3–4 summarizes the key elements to be addressed for each type of evidence to appraise internal validity and usefulness.[19–50]

CONSIDERING CLINICAL RELEVANCE

Once the clinician has gathered all relevant studies, eliminated those which addressed other questions, and identified those trials with the best methods, one question remains: So what? Also known as the "who cares" test,[51] applying this admittedly crude criterion begins the process of asking oneself, "Will these findings change the way I will treat or prevent this disease in my practice—and specifically for the patient sitting in front of me right now?"

The first step in making this decision is to consider the clinical value of the beneficial outcomes reported. Are the outcomes demonstrating improvements important to the patients? For example, a drug therapy that improves left ventricular ejection fraction (a surrogate end point) does not have the same clinical value as a drug that is shown to decrease mortality or improve functional status (primary end points) in an individual with heart failure.

The usefulness of an intervention depends not only on its efficacy but also on whether the magnitude of the benefit outweighs the risks, costs, and benefits of existing alternative interventions. In this context, the number needed to treat (NNT) and the number needed to harm (NNH) are clinically useful measures. NNT and NNH describe the number of patients who need to be treated and for how long to achieve one favorable or harmful outcome, respectively (Table 3–5 illustrates the value of NNT and NNH). The NNT strategy provides a way to estimate an intervention's impact and tradeoffs and to decide whether this therapy should be implemented.

TABLE 3–5. Number Needed to Treat and Number Needed to Harm

In this example, the clinical question is whether the addition of clopidogrel to the regimen of a 65-year-old man with unstable angina who is already taking aspirin would prevent death or coronary event? A search of published trials and presented papers at scientific meetings uncovered only one relevant study. It was presented in abstract form at the American College of Cardiology meeting on March 19, 2001.

In the trial:

- 12,562 subjects with coronary syndrome were randomized to aspirin alone or aspirin plus clopidogrel.
- On average, patients were followed for 9 months.
- The primary endpoint was to prevent cardiovascular (CV) death, myocardial infarction (MI), or stroke.

To calculate the number needed to treat (NNT), first calculate the absolute risk reduction (ARR). This is the absolute difference between the event rate in the control group (CER) minus the event rate in the experimental group (EER). The NNT is the inverse of the ARR.

The trial reports that 11.47% of the aspirin alone group (control group) had MI, stroke, or CV death. In contrast, 9.28% of the aspirin plus clopidogrel (experimental group) had these events.

Control Event Rate (Aspirin-Alone Group)	Experimental Event Rate (Aspirin Plus Clopidogrel)	RRR = (CER − EER)/CER	ARR = (CER − EER)	NNT = 1/ARR
11.47%	9.28%	19%	2.19%	46

Thus the NNT is 46. That is, treating 46 patients with unstable angina for 9 months with aspirin with clopidogrel should prevent MI, stroke, or CV death in 1 patient. To balance risks versus benefits of an intervention, we can generate a similar number needed to harm to express the risks associated to the intervention.

The trial reports that 2.7% of the aspirin-alone group had major nonfatal bleeding events compared with 3.6% in the intervention group (aspirin plus clopidogrel).

To calculate the number needed to harm (NNH), first calculate the absolute risk increase (ARI). This is the absolute difference between the event rate in the experimental group (EER) minus the event rate in the control group (CER). The NNH is the inverse of the ARI.

Control Event Rate	Experimental Event Rate	ARI (Absolute Risk Increase)	NNH
2.7%	3.6%	0.9%	111

The NNH is thus 111, meaning that treating 111 patients with both drugs for 9 months would result in 1 major nonfatal bleed. Combining the NNT and NNH and projecting the results to 1000 patients would lead to this conclusion: This randomized, controlled trial suggests that treating 1000 individuals with unstable angina with the combination of aspirin plus clopidogrel would prevent 21 patients from having a stroke, MI, or CV death at the cost of 9 major nonfatal bleeding events.

The relative risk reduction (RRR), as a measure of the magnitude of an intervention's effect, can be misleading. It does not discriminate between large and trivial absolute differences between the control and experimental groups. For example, an intervention may result in a 50% risk reduction for the adverse outcome, and this amount of decrease would sound impressive to most clinicians and patients. However, it might represent only a small difference in risk of rare event (e.g., 0.2% of patients in a placebo group died compared with 0.1% of patients on active drug). In contrast, a 50% risk reduction might reflect a much more meaningful difference, for instance, when 50% of placebo group died versus 25% of patients in the intervention group (an absolute difference 25%). The RRR is the same for both examples, but the magnitude of the impact of the intervention is drastically different. The information provided by RRR is incomplete because it does not take into account the baseline risk of subjects in the trial.

APPLYING THE RESULTS

For every health care professional, the ultimate test of which studies are important and which are not comes down to the decision of how to treat each patient. Thus, clinical judgment is crucial in assessing the importance of drug-therapy evidence.

Several patient-specific factors must be considered in the final analysis:

1. Compare the patient with those in the study (similar disease state and stage, similar baseline characteristics). This assessment should ensure that the population studied has a similar disease state and prognostic factors as the patient now being treated. For instance, the results of a trial assessing the mortality benefit of simvastatin in dyslipidemic men with known coronary artery disease would not likely apply to dyslipidemic women with no other coronary risk factors.
2. Consider the patient's baseline risk for the outcome of interest and other potential risks associated with the therapy. If this patient has a higher baseline risk for the outcome than the population studied, then treatment may yield an even higher benefit. In contrast, if the patient has a lower baseline risk than the population studied, then treatment-associated risks may outweigh the potential benefit. For example, premenopausal women, in general, have a lower cardiovascular mortality risk than do men. Therefore, an intervention shown to prevent cardiovascular mortality in men may result in a smaller benefit in women.

3. Consider the patient's values, beliefs, concerns, and readiness for the intervention. In addition, health care delivery characteristics (cost and accessibility) must be factored in. While not very long ago health care professionals were considered patriarchal figures who directed the patient's treatment, today patients are fully engaged partners in decisions about therapy. The evidence must be discussed and integrated with the specific patient's circumstances to result in successful outcomes.

KEEPING UP-TO-DATE BY USING EBM

The same combination of clinical experience and EBM skills that enables health care professionals to resolve patient-specific pharmacotherapeutic questions also aids health care professionals' continued efforts to keep up-to-date. The process is the same: (1) recognize information needs (the areas of one's practice), (2) identify literature relevant to clinical practice, (3) critically appraise the evidence for validity and utility, and (4) devise a mechanism to implement new evidence in daily practice.

Like human knowledge in general, medical information is growing exponentially. Clinicians have difficulty staying current; a few statistics explain why. The National Library of Medicine contains more than 11 million citations covering more than 4000 biomedical journals.[52] The number of citations *doubled* in just 6 years, from 1995 to 2001. Each year, 10,000 RCTs addressing the impact of health care interventions are published. Some influence how clinicians practice, others provide preliminary evidence that is too early to act on or is irrelevant to clinical practice, and others are seriously flawed and should not be implemented. Who has time to read it all and separate the good from the bad? A literature-sorting strategy, using the EBM approach, is one solution.

First, the clinician must recognize the areas important in his or her practice (e.g., internal medicine, cardiology, nuclear medicine, nutrition, psychiatry, or pharmacokinetics). Second, scan the literature for clinically relevant studies in that area of interest or practice. These are studies addressing clinical outcomes likely to be relevant to clinical practice and possibly change prescribing behaviors, such as those which report the effect of a pharmacotherapy on quality of life, cost-effectiveness, mortality, or morbidity. In contrast, trials addressing the impact of drug therapy on surrogate end points (e.g., biochemical markers) are most often irrelevant to current clinical practice and rarely would result in a change in practice. When in a "keeping up-to-date mode," choose the studies reporting clinically relevant outcomes over those with surrogate end points. Third, critically appraise the evidence for validity and usefulness. When addressing therapeutic efficacy, RCTs are considered the "gold standard" and should be preferred over observational studies for most clinical questions. Scan the abstracts of RCTs for obvious design flaws and size of the effect before appraising further. Shaughnessy and colleagues[53] have created a formula to help determine the usefulness of medical information (Fig. 3–1). Finally, integrate the new findings into one's daily practice.

$$\text{Usefulness of Medicine Information} = \frac{\text{Relevance} \times \text{Validity}}{\text{Work Factor}}$$

FIGURE 3–1. In this usefulness formula, *relevance* represents patient-oriented evidence that matters and affects health care, *validity* refers to a true estimate of the effect, and *work factor* describes the effort required to review the information.

If this process seems too labor-intensive for keeping pace with the medical literature, consider an evidence-based abstraction service. These services, which have grown tremendously in the past 10 years, claim to reduce by 98% the amount of clinical literature a clinician needs to read, enabling the busy health care professional to concentrate on the 2% that is most methodologically rigorous and useful to his or her practice.[54] In general, abstraction services consist of an editorial team that scans dozens of journals, usually organized by specialty. They identify articles of potential clinical relevance, critically appraise the studies, and provide commentary on the quality/validity and clinical significance of the results reported. Table 3–6 gathers a selected list of translation journals offering evidence-based abstracts of original research.

CONCLUSIONS

Is EBM realistic? The needed skills for practicing EBM may appear daunting, but once acquired, they can help health care professionals better use available resources and time by knowing how to focus a search and be more critical in what reading and information to integrate into their knowledge base. Several sites have demonstrated that EBM could be incorporated into practice successfully.[55–58]

Why practice EBM? Implementing EBM in a practice provides a framework and the skills to strengthen confidence in pharmacotherapeutic decisions and results in better communication with colleagues involved in the decision-making process. Furthermore, an evidence-based pharmaceutical care plan facilitates dialogue with patients about the rationale for the management decisions. Finally, using EBM principles enables practicing health care professionals to continuously update their knowledge.

This chapter provides tools for health care professionals to:

1. Identify rapidly evidence-based clinical practice guidelines.
2. Identify rapidly systematic reviews.
3. Conduct validated searches to identify studies answering pharmacotherapy questions.
4. Critically appraise the literature found.
5. Assess relevance and applicability of the evidence.
6. Develop strategies to triage the most useful literature and help keep pace with the evidence that makes a difference in one's practice.

▶ PRINCIPLES OF PHARMACOTHERAPY

- The best current evidence integrated into clinical expertise ensures optimal care for patients.
- The four-step process in applying EBM in practice are (1) formulate a clear question from a patient's problem, (2) identify relevant information, (3) critically appraise available evidence, and (4) implement the findings in clinical practice.
- The decision as whether to implement the results of a specific study, conclusions of a review article, or another piece of evidence in clinical practice depends on the quality (i.e., internal validity) of the evidence, its clinical importance, whether benefits outweigh risks and costs, and its relevance in the clinical setting and patient's circumstances.
- EBM strategies can be applied to help in keeping current.
- EBM is realistic.

TABLE 3–6. Evidence-Based Abstraction Services

ACP Journal Club (*http://www.acponline.org/journals/acpjc/jcmenu.htm*)
Audience: Internal medicine, primary care
Selection criteria: Original articles, systematic reviews, English, adult , clinically relevant with important outcomes, randomized controlled trials for treatment questions
Journals scanned: 26 journals

Bandolier (*http://www.jr2.ox.ac.uk/bandolier/*)
Audience: Internal medicine
Selection criteria: Those which look remotely interesting are read, and where they are both interesting and make sense, they are summarized
Journal scanned: Each month PubMed and the Cochrane Library are searched for systematic reviews and meta-analyses published in the recent past

Evidence-Based Cardiovascular Medicine (*http://www.harcourt-international.com/journals/ebcm/*)
Audience: Cardiology (adult and pediatric)
Selection criteria: Original articles, English, clinically relevant, adult or pediatric humans randomized controlled trials, double blinded
Journals scanned: 25 journals mostly cardiology specialty journals

Evidence-Based Health Care (*http://www.harcourt-international.com/journals/ebhc/*)
Audience: Managers
Selection criteria: Articles providing evidence for decision making; articles that are likely to be widely applicable
Journals scanned: More than 50 journals mostly with economics and public health focus

Evidence-Based Medicine (*http://www.evidence-basedmedicine.com*)
Audience: Internal medicine, general and family practice, surgery, psychiatry, pediatrics, and obstetrics and gynecologists
Selection criteria: Original articles, Cochrane Reviews, randomized controlled trial or therapeutic efficacy trial, clinically relevant outcomes, 80% follow-up
Journals scanned: More than 30 journals

Evidence-Based Mental Health (*http://www.ebmentalhealth.com/*)
Audience: Mental health clinicians
Selection criteria: Original articles, Cochrane Reviews, randomized controlled trial or therapeutic efficacy trial, clinically relevant outcomes, 80% follow-up
Journals scanned: Not available

Journal Watch series (*http://www.jwatch.org/*)
Audience: General medicine, dermatology, cardiology, psychiatry, women's health, emergency medicine, infectious disease, neurology, gastroenterology (specialty Journal Watch for each audience)
Selection criteria: Not given
Journals scanned: More than 50 journals

Journal of Family Practice (*http://www.jfp.msu.edu*)
Audience: Family practice, pharmacists
Selection criteria: High-quality articles with patient-oriented outcomes that have the greatest potential to change the way that primary care clinicians practice
Journals scanned: 80 journals

Journal Club on the Web (*http://www.Journalclub.org*)
Audience: Internal medicine
Selection criteria: Not given
Journals scanned: *New England Journal of Medicine, Annals of Internal Medicine, Journal of the American Medical Association, The Lancet*

REFERENCES

1. Etminan M, Wright JM, Carleton BC. Evidence-based pharmacotherapy: Review of basic concepts and applications in clinical practice. Ann Pharmacother 1998;32:1193–1200.
2. Swales JD. Evidence-based medicine and hypertension. J Hypertens 1999; 17:1511–1516.
3. Mancia G, Zanchetti A. Evidence-based medicine: An educational instrument or a standard for implementation (Editorial)? J Hypertens 1999; 17:1509–1510.
4. Echt DS, Liebson PR, Mitchell B, et al. Mortality and morbidity in patients receiving encainide, flecainide or placebo: The Cardiac Arrhythmia Suppression Trial. N Engl J Med. 1991,324.781–788.
5. Greene HL, Roden DM, Katz RJ, et al. The Cardiac Arrhythmia Suppression Trial: First CAST, then CAST II. J Am Coll Cardiol 1992;19:894–898.
6. Ryan TJ, Antman EM, Brooks NH, et al. 1999 Update: ACC/AHA guidelines for the management of patients with acute myocardial infarction: A report of the American College of Cardiology/American Heart Association Task Force on Practice Guidelines (Committee on Management of Acute Myocardial Infarction). J Am Coll Cardiol 1999;34:890–911.
7. Ryan TJ, Anderson JL, Antman EM, et al. ACC/AHA guidelines for the management of patients with acute myocardial infarction: A report of the American College of Cardiology/American Heart Association Task Force on Practice Guidelines (Committee on Management of Acute Myocardial Infarction). J Am Coll Cardiol 1996;28:1328–1428.

8. Hulley S, Grady D, Bush T, et al. Randomized trial of estrogen plus progestin for secondary prevention of coronary heart disease in postmenopausal women. Heart and Estrogen/progestin Replacement Study (HERS) Research Group. JAMA 1998;280:605–613.
9. Sackett DL, Richardson SW, Rosenberg W, Haynes BR. Evidence-Based Medicine: How to Practice and Teach EBM. New York, Churchill-Livingstone, 1997.
10. Richardson WS, Wilson MC, Nishikawa J, Hayward RSA. The well-built clinical question: A key to evidence-based decisions (editorial). ACP J Club 1995;123:A12–A13.
11. Ghosh AK, Ghosh K. Enhance your practice with evidence-based medicine. Patient Care. 2000;Feb:32–56.
12. Oxman A, Guyatt GH. The science of reviewing research. Ann NY Acad Sci 1993;703:125–134.
13. Mulrow CD. The medical review article: State of the science. Ann Intern Med 1987;106:485–488.
14. Mulrow CD. Rationale for systematic reviews. BMJ 1994;309:597–599.
15. Haynes RB, Wilczynski NL, McKibbon KA, et al. Developing optimal search strategies for detecting clinically sound studies in MEDLINE. J Am Med Inform Assoc 1994;1:447–458.
16. Huth EJ. How to Write and Publish Papers in the Medical Sciences, 2d ed. Philadelphia, ISI Press, 1990:56–57.
17. Chalmers TC, Smith H Jr, Blackburn B, et al. A method for assessing the quality of a randomized control trial. Control Clin Trials 1981;2: 31–49.
18. Horwitz RI, Viscoli CM, Berkman L, et al. Treatment adherence and risk of death after a myocardial infarction. Lancet 1990;336:542–545.
19. Oxman AD, Sackett DL, Guyatt GH. Users' guides to the medical literature: I. How to get started. The Evidence-Based Medicine Working Group. JAMA 1993;270:2093–2095.
20. Guyatt GH, Sackett DL, Cook DJ. Users' guides to the medical literature: II. How to use an article about therapy or prevention. A. Are the results of the study valid? Evidence-Based Medicine Working Group. JAMA 1993;270:2598–2601.
21. Guyatt GH, Sackett DL, Cook DJ. Users' guides to the medical literature: II. How to use an article about therapy or prevention. B. What were the results and will they help me in caring for my patients? Evidence-Based Medicine Working Group. JAMA 1994;271:59–63.
22. Jaeschke R, Guyatt G, Sackett DL. Users' guides to the medical literature: III. How to use an article about a diagnostic test. A. Are the results of the study valid? Evidence-Based Medicine Working Group. JAMA 1994;271:389–391.
23. Jaeschke R, Guyatt GH, Sackett DL. Users' guides to the medical literature: III. How to use an article about a diagnostic test. B. What are the results and will they help me in caring for my patients? The Evidence-Based Medicine Working Group. JAMA 1994;271:703–707.
24. Levine M, Walter S, Lee H, et al. Users' guides to the medical literature: IV. How to use an article about harm. Evidence-Based Medicine Working Group. JAMA 1994;271:1615–1619.
25. Laupacis A, Wells G, Richardson WS, Tugwell P. Users' guides to the medical literature: V. How to use an article about prognosis. Evidence-Based Medicine Working Group. JAMA 1994;272:234–237.
26. Oxman AD, Cook DJ, Guyatt GH. Users' guides to the medical literature: VI. How to use an overview. Evidence-Based Medicine Working Group. JAMA 1994;272:1367–1371.
27. Richardson WS, Detsky AS. Users' guides to the medical literature: VII. How to use a clinical decision analysis. A. Are the results of the study valid? Evidence-Based Medicine Working Group. JAMA 1995;273:1292–1295.
28. Richardson WS, Detsky AS. Users' guides to the medical literature: VII. How to use a clinical decision analysis. B. What are the results and will they help me in caring for my patients? Evidence Based Medicine Working Group. JAMA 1995;273:1610–1613.
29. Hayward RS, Wilson MC, Tunis SR, et al. Users' guides to the medical literature: VIII. How to use clinical practice guidelines. A. Are the recommendations valid? The Evidence-Based Medicine Working Group. JAMA 1995;274:570–574.
30. Wilson MC, Hayward RS, Tunis SR, et al. Users' guides to the medical literature: VIII. How to use clinical practice guidelines. B. What are the recommendations and will they help you in caring for your patients? The Evidence-Based Medicine Working Group. JAMA 1995;274:1630–1632.
31. Guyatt GH, Sackett DL, Sinclair JC, et al. Users' guides to the medical literature: IX. A method for grading health care recommendations. Evidence-Based Medicine Working Group. JAMA 1995;274:1800–1804.
32. Naylor CD, Guyatt GH. Users' guides to the medical literature: X. How to use an article reporting variations in the outcomes of health services. The Evidence-Based Medicine Working Group. JAMA 1996;275:554–558.
33. Naylor CD, Guyatt GH. Users' guides to the medical literature: XI. How to use an article about a clinical utilization review. Evidence-Based Medicine Working Group. JAMA 1996;275:1435–1439.
34. Guyatt GH, Naylor CD, Juniper E, et al. Users' guides to the medical literature: XII. How to use articles about health-related quality of life. Evidence-Based Medicine Working Group. JAMA 1997;277:1232–1237.
35. Drummond, M. F.; Richardson, W. S.; O'Brien, B. J.; Levine, M., and Heyland, D. Users' guides to the medical literature: XIII. How to use an article on economic analysis of clinical practice. A. Are the results of the study valid? Evidence-Based Medicine Working Group. JAMA 1997;277:1552–1557.
36. O'Brien BJ, Heyland D, Richardson WS, et al. Users' guides to the medical literature: XIII. How to use an article on economic analysis of clinical practice. B. What are the results and will they help me in caring for my patients? Evidence-Based Medicine Working Group. JAMA 1997;277:1802–1806.
37. Dans AL, Dans LF, Guyatt GH, Richardson S. Users' guides to the medical literature: XIV. How to decide on the applicability of clinical trial results to your patient. Evidence-Based Medicine Working Group. JAMA 1998;279:545–549.
38. Richardson WS, Wilson MC, Guyatt GH, et al. Users' guides to the medical literature: XV. How to use an article about disease probability for differential diagnosis. Evidence-Based Medicine Working Group. JAMA 1999;281:1214–1219.
39. Guyatt GH, Sinclair J, Cook DJ, Glasziou P. Users' guides to the medical literature: XVI. How to use a treatment recommendation. Evidence-Based Medicine Working Group and the Cochrane Applicability Methods Working Group. JAMA 1999;281:1836–1843.
40. Barratt A, Irwig L, Glasziou P, et al. Users' guides to the medical literature: XVII. How to use guidelines and recommendations about screening. Evidence-Based Medicine Working Group. JAMA 1999;281:2029–2034.
41. Randolph AG, Haynes RB, Wyatt JC, et al. Users' guides to the medical literature: XVIII. How to use an article evaluating the clinical impact of a computer-based clinical decision support system. JAMA 1999;282:67–74.
42. Bucher HC, Guyatt GH, Cook DJ, et al. Users' guides to the medical literature: XIX. Applying clinical trial results. A. How to use an article measuring the effect of an intervention on surrogate end points. Evidence-Based Medicine Working Group. JAMA 1999;282:771–778.
43. McAlister FA, Laupacis A, Wells GA, Sackett DL. Users' guides to the medical literature: XIX. Applying clinical trial results. B. Guidelines for determining whether a drug is exerting (more than) a class effect. JAMA 1999;282:1371–1377.
44. Hunt DL, Jaeschke R, McKibbon KA. Users' guides to the medical literature: XXI. Using electronic health information resources in evidence-based practice. Evidence-Based Medicine Working Group. JAMA 2000;283:1875–1879.
45. McAlister FA, Straus SE, Guyatt GH, Haynes RB. Users' guides to the medical literature: XX. Integrating research evidence with the care of the individual patient. Evidence-Based Medicine Working Group. JAMA 2000;283:2829–2836.
46. McGinn TG, Guyatt GH, Wyer PC, et al. Users' guides to the medical literature: XXII. How to use articles about clinical decision rules. Evidence-Based Medicine Working Group. JAMA 2000;284:79–84.

47. Giacomini MK, Cook DJ. Users' guides to the medical literature: XXIII. Qualitative research in health care. A. Are the results of the study valid? Evidence-Based Medicine Working Group. JAMA 2000;284:357–362.
48. Giacomini MK, Cook DJ. Users' guides to the medical literature: XXIII. Qualitative research in health care. B. What are the results and how do they help me care for my patients? Evidence-Based Medicine Working Group. JAMA 2000;284:478–482.
49. Richardson WS, Wilson MC, Williams JW Jr, et al. Users' guides to the medical literature: XXIV. How to use an article on the clinical manifestations of disease. Evidence-Based Medicine Working Group. JAMA 2000;284:869–875.
50. Guyatt GH, Haynes RB, Jaeschke RZ, et al. Users' guides to the medical literature: XXV. Evidence-based medicine: principles for applying the users' guides to patient care. Evidence-Based Medicine Working Group. JAMA 2000;284:1290–1296.
51. Huth EJ. Writing and Publishing in Medicine, 3d ed. Baltimore, Williams & Wilkins, 1999:10–12.
52. National Library of Medicine, Bethesda, MD, MEDLINE 2001.
53. Shaughnessy AF, Slawson DC, Bennet JH. Becoming an information master: A guidebook to the medical information jungle. J Fam Pract 1994;39:484–499.
54. Sackett DL, Haynes RB. 13 steps, 100 people, 1,000,000 thanks. Evidence Based Med 1997;2:101–102.
55. Ellis J, Mulligan I, Rower J, Sackett DL. Inpatient general medicine is evidence-based. Lancet 1995;346:407–410.
56. Geddes JR, Game D, Jenkins NE, Peterson LA, Pottinger GR, Sackett DL. What proportion of primary psychiatric interventions are based on randomised evidence? Qual Health Care 1996;5:215–217.
57. Gill P, Dowell AC, Neal RP, et al. Evidence based general practice: A retrospective study of interventions in our training practice. BMJ 1996;312:819–821.
58. Kenny SE, Shankar KR, Rentala R, et al. Evidence-based surgery: Interventions in a regional pediatric surgical unit. Arch Dis Child 1997;76: 50–53.

A

Evidence-Based Medicine Glossary

TERMS TO DESCRIBE THE BENEFIT OR HARM OF TREATMENT

		Outcome		
		Event	No Event	
Exposure	Treated (experimental group)	a	b	$a+b$
	Control (unexposed group)	c	d	$c+d$
		$a+c$	$b+d$	

Experimental event rate (EER) The proportion of patients in the treated group in whom an event is observed. Thus, if out of 100 treated patients ($a+b$), the event is observed in 27 (a), the event rate is 0.27 ($a/a+b$).

Control event rate (CER) The proportion of patients in the control group in whom an event is observed. CER = $c/c+d$.

Absolute risk The risk of having a disease at any point in time (incidence). For example, if the incidence of a disease is 1 in 100,000, then the absolute risk is 0.001%.

Absolute risk reduction (ARR) The difference in the event rate between control group (CER) and treated group (EER): ARR = CER − EER.

Number needed to treat (NNT) The inverse of the ARR (1/absolute risk reduction). NNT is the number of patients who need to be treated to prevent one bad outcome. If a drug reduced the risk of a bad outcome (e.g., stroke, myocardial infarction, death) from 40% to 20%, then

$$\text{ARR} = |0.2(\text{EER or the event rate in the experimental/treatment group}) - 0.4(\text{CER or event rate in the control group})|$$

$$\text{ARR} = |0.4 - 0.2| = 0.2\,(20\%)$$

Thus

$$\text{NNT} = 1/\text{ARR} = 1/0.2 = 5$$

Thus, 5 people would need to be treated with the drug to prevent one bad outcome.

Relative risk (RR) A ratio of two risks, the risk of the outcome/event in the treated group compared with the risk of the outcome in those not exposed (control group). Reported as a percentage, it is calculated as RR = EER/CER. A relative risk above 1 means that the treatment/exposure is associated with the outcome, and a value below 1 means that the treatment is negatively associated with the outcome. This is also referred to as *risk ratio*.

Relative risk reduction (RRR) The proportional reduction in events between control and treated groups. Reported as a percentage, it is calculated as (CER − EER)/CER or as 1 − RR.

Absolute risk increase (ARI) The risk difference in outcome rates between treated and control groups when the treatment harms more patients than the control. ARI is calculated as EER − CER.

Number needed to harm (NNH) The inverse of ARI (1/absolute risk increase). NNH is the number of patients who would need to be treated to cause one adverse outcome.

Odds ratio (OR) A ratio that describes the odds (probability) that a patient in an exposed or intervention group had an event (usually harmful event) relative to the odds that a patient in the control group had that event. When the outcome of interest is rare, the odds ratio approximates the relative risk. Odds ratio is used in case-control or retrospective trials. Odds ratio is calculated as OR = odds of being exposed in cases (a/c) divided by odds of being exposed in controls (b/d).

STUDY DESIGNS

Blinded study Study in which neither the study subject nor the study staff is aware of which group or intervention the subject has been assigned in a double-blinded study. In a single-blinded study, only the subject is not aware of his or her assignment. Blinding minimizes bias.

Case-control study Retrospective comparison of causal factors or exposures in a group of persons with disease (cases) and those of persons without the disease (controls). The purpose is to find the clinical finding that occurs more frequently in the cases than the control. The relative risk is estimated by odds ratio.

Case series Report on a series of patients with a specific disease. No control group is included.

Cohort study Retrospective or prospective follow-up study of exposed and nonexposed defined groups in which a variable of interest, usually disease rates, is measured. Exposure is measured before development of disease. Incidence, risk, and relative risk are measured.

Crossover study A trial comparing two or more treatments in which the participants, on completion of the course of one treatment, are switched to another. The therapies are administered in either a specified or random order to each participant.

Cross-sectional study A study that examines the presence or absence of a disease and other variable in a defined population and the potential risk factors at a particular point in time or time interval. Exposure and outcome are determined simultaneously. The temporal sequence of cause and effect cannot necessarily be determined.

Meta-analysis A systematic review that uses quantitative methods to summarize the results. The unit of analysis in the meta-analysis is the variable common to the studies being reviewed rather than the individual patient.

Open-label trial A study in which the investigators assign the interventions rather than using random allocation and both patients and investigators know which patients are receiving which therapies or interventions.

Randomized controlled trial (RCT) A comparative study in which the researchers randomly assign patients to treatment or control groups. Random allocation means that each participant has the same chance of receiving each of the possible groups under investigation.

Systematic review A comprehensive summary of best available evidence that addresses a defined question. The study uses systematic and explicit methods to identify, select, and critically appraise and collect data from relevant research. Systematic reviews may or may not include a quantitative analysis (such as that used in meta-analysis).

4

CLINICAL PHARMACOKINETICS AND PHARMACODYNAMICS

Larry A. Bauer

Pharmacokinetic concepts have been used successfully by pharmacists to individualize patient drug therapy for about a quarter of a century. Pharmacokinetic consultant services and individual clinicians routinely provide patient-specific drug dosing recommendations that increase the efficacy and decrease the toxicity of many medications. Laboratories routinely measure patient serum or plasma samples for many drugs, including antibiotics (aminoglycosides, vancomycin), theophylline, antiepileptics (phenytoin, carbamazepine, valproic acid, phenobarbital, ethosuximide), methotrexate, lithium, antiarrhythmics (lidocaine, procainamide, quinidine, digoxin), and immunosuppressants (cyclosporine, tacrolimus). Combined with a knowledge of the disease states and conditions that influence the disposition of a particular drug, kinetic concepts can be used to modify doses to produce serum drug concentrations that produce desirable pharmacologic effects without unwanted side effects. This narrow range of concentrations within which the pharmacologic response is produced and the adverse effects prevented in most patients is defined as the therapeutic range of the drug. Table 4–1 lists the therapeutic ranges for commonly used medications.

Although most individuals experience favorable effects with serum drug concentrations in the therapeutic range, the effects of a given serum concentration can vary widely among individuals. Clinicians should never assume that a serum concentration within the therapeutic range will be safe and effective for every patient. The response to the drug, such as number of seizures a patient experiences while taking an antiepileptic agent, always should be assessed when serum concentrations are measured.

Throughout this chapter, abbreviations for various pharmacokinetic parameters are used frequently. Commonly used abbreviations are listed in Table 4–2.

CLINICAL PHARMACOKINETIC CONCEPTS

Clinical pharmacokinetics is the discipline that describes the absorption, distribution, metabolism, and elimination of drugs in patients requiring drug therapy. When a drug is administered extravascularly to patients, it must be absorbed across biologic membranes to reach the systemic circulation. If the drug is given orally, the drug molecules must pass through the gastrointestinal tract wall into capillaries. For transdermal patches, the drug must penetrate the skin to enter the vascular system. In general, the pharmacologic effect of the drug is delayed when it is given extravascularly because time is required for the drug to be absorbed into the vascular system.

The vascular system generally provides the "transportation" for the drug molecule to its site of activity. After the drug reaches the systemic circulation, it can leave the vasculature and penetrate the various tissues or remain in the blood. If the drug remains in the blood, it may bind to endogenous proteins such as albumin or α_1-acid glycoprotein. This binding is usually reversible, and an equilibrium is created between protein-bound drug and unbound drug. Unbound drug in the blood provides the driving force for distribution of the agent to body tissues. If unbound drug leaves the bloodstream and distributes to tissue, it may become tissue-bound, it may remain unbound in the tissue, or if the tissue can metabolize or eliminate the drug, it may be rendered inactive and/or eliminated from the body. If the drug becomes tissue-bound, it may bind to the receptor that causes its pharmacologic or toxic effect or to a nonspecific binding site that causes no effect. Again, tissue binding is usually reversible so that the tissue-bound drug is in equilibrium with unbound drug in the tissue.

Certain organs—such as the liver, gastrointestinal tract wall, and lung—possess enzymes that metabolize drugs. The resulting metabolite may be inactive or have a pharmacologic effect of its own. The blood also contains esterases, which cleave ester bonds in drug molecules and generally render them inactive.

Drug metabolism usually occurs in the liver through one or both of two types of reactions. Phase I reactions generally make the drug molecule more polar and water soluble so that it is prone to elimination by the kidney. Phase I modifications include oxidation, hydrolysis, and reduction. Phase II reactions involve conjugation to form glucuronides, acetates, or sulfates. These reactions generally inactivate the pharmacologic activity of the drug and may make it more prone to elimination by the kidney.

Other organs have the ability to eliminate drugs or metabolites from the body. The kidney can excrete drugs by glomerular filtration or by such active processes as proximal tubular secretion. Drugs also can be eliminated via bile produced by the liver or air expired by the lungs.

LINEAR PHARMACOKINETICS

Most drugs follow linear pharmacokinetics: Serum drug concentrations change proportionally with long-term daily dosing. As an example, if the drug dose were doubled from 300 to 600 mg/d, the patient's serum drug concentration would double.

When a drug is given by continuous intravenous infusion, serum concentrations increase until an equilibrium is established between the drug dosage rate and the rate of drug elimination. At that point, the rate of drug administration equals the rate of drug elimination, and the serum concentrations therefore remain constant (Fig. 4–1). For example, if a patient were receiving a continuous intravenous infusion of theophylline at 40 mg/h, the theophylline serum concentration would increase until the patient's body was eliminating theophylline at 40 mg/h. When serum drug concentrations reach a constant value, steady state is achieved.

If the drug is given at intermittent dosage intervals, such as 250 mg every 6 hours, steady state is achieved when the serum-concentration-versus-time curves for each dosage interval are superimposable. The amount of drug eliminated during the dosage interval equals the dose.

TABLE 4–1. Selected Therapeutic Ranges

Drug	Therapeutic Range
Digoxin	0.5–2 ng/mL
Lidocaine	1.5–5 μg/mL
Procainamide/*N*-acetylprocainamide	10–30 μg/mL (total)
Quinidine	2–5 μg/mL
Amikacin[a]	20–30 μg/mL (peak) <5 μg/mL (trough)
Gentamicin, tobramycin, netilmicin[a]	5–10 μg/mL (peak) <2 μg/mL (trough)
Vancomycin	20–40 μg/mL (peak) 5–10 μg/mL (trough)
Chloramphenicol	10–20 μg/mL
Lithium	0.6–1.4 mEq/L
Carbamazepine	4–12 μg/mL
Ethosuximide	40–100 μg/mL
Phenobarbital	15–40 μg/mL
Phenytoin	10–20 μg/mL
Primidone	5–12 μg/mL
Valproic acid	50–100 μg/mL
Theophylline	10–20 μg/mL
Cyclosporine	150–400 ng/mL (blood)

[a]Using a multiple dose per day dosage schedule, single daily dose therapeutic concentrations not yet established.

BIOAVAILABILITY AND BIOEQUIVALENCE

When drugs are administered extravascularly, drug molecules must be released from the dosage form (dissolution) and pass through several biologic barriers before reaching the vascular system (absorption).

TABLE 4–2. Pharmacokinetic Abbreviations

Abbreviation	Definition
Cl	Clearance
k_0	Intravenous infusion rate
C_{ss}	Steady-state concentration
D	Dose
τ	Dosage interval
F	Fraction of drug absorbed into the systemic circulation
Q	Blood flow
E	Extraction ratio
f_b	Fraction of drug in the blood that is unbound
Cl_{int}	Intrinsic clearance
$C_{ss,u}$	Steady-state concentration of unbound drug
V_D	Volume of distribution
LD	Loading dose
MD	Maintenance dose
$t_{1/2}$	Half-life
k	Elimination rate constant
k_a	Absorption rate constant
α	Distribution rate constant
β	Terminal rate constant
t'	Postinfusion time
T	Duration of infusion
AUC	Area under serum or blood concentration-versus-time curve
V_{max}	Maximum rate of drug metabolism
K_m	Serum concentration at which the rate of metabolism equals $V_{max}/2$
C_{max}	Maximum serum or blood concentration
C_{min}	Minimum serum or blood concentration
DR	Dosage rate

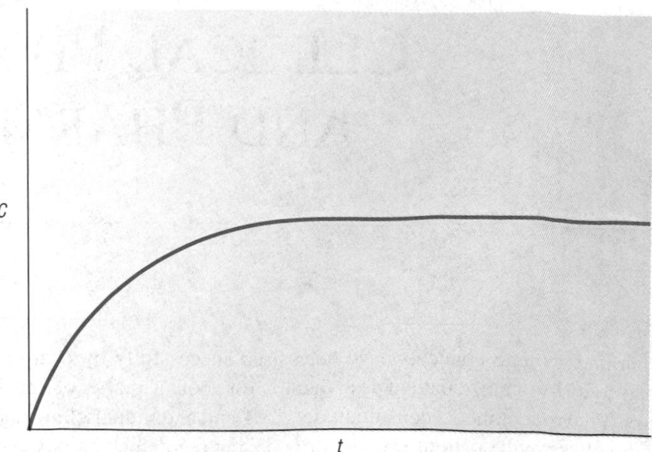

FIGURE 4–1. Normal serum concentration-time curve following a continuous intravenous infusion.

The fraction of drug absorbed into the systemic circulation (F) after extravascular administration is defined as its *bioavailability* and can be calculated after single intravenous and extravascular doses as[1]

$$F = D_{iv}(AUC_{0-\infty})/[D(AUC_{iv0-\infty})]$$

where D and D_{iv} are the extravascular and intravenous doses, respectively, and $AUC_{iv0-\infty}$ and $AUC_{0-\infty}$ are the intravenous and extravascular areas under the serum- or blood-concentration-versus-time curves, respectively, from time zero to infinity. The AUC represents the body's total exposure to the drug and is a function of the fraction of the drug dose that enters the systemic circulation via the administered route and clearance (Fig. 4–2). When F is less than 1 for a drug administered extravascularly, either the dosage form did not release all the drug contained in it or some of the drug was eliminated or destroyed (by stomach acid or other means) before it reached the systemic circulation.

When the extravascular dose is administered orally, part of the dose may be metabolized by enzymes contained in the liver or gastrointestinal tract wall before it reaches the systemic circulation.[2,3] This occurs commonly when drugs have a high liver extraction ratio

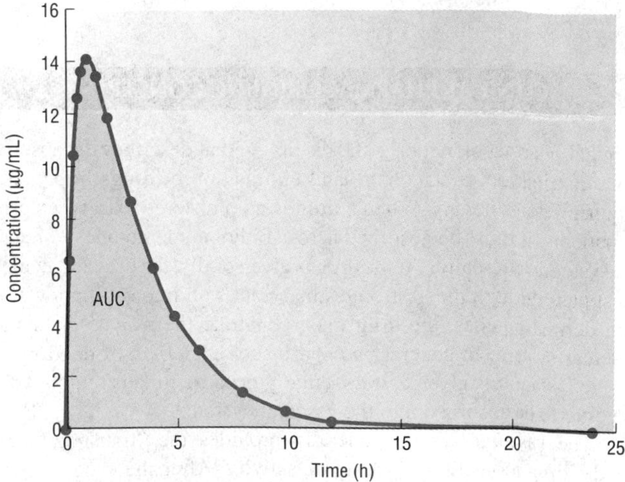

FIGURE 4–2. Area under the concentration-time curve (AUC) after the administration of an extravascular dose. The AUC is the function of the fraction of drug dose that enters the systemic circulation and clearance. AUCs measured after intravenous and extravascular doses can be used to determine bioavailability for the extravascular dose.

or are subject to gastrointestinal tract wall metabolism because, after oral administration, the drug must pass through the gastrointestinal tract wall and into the portal circulation of the liver. Transport proteins are also present in the gastrointestinal tract wall that can actively pump drug molecules that already have been absorbed back into the lumen of the gastrointestinal tract. P-Glycoprotein (PGP) is the primary transport protein that interferes with drug absorption by this mechanism. For example, if an orally administered drug is 100% absorbed from the gastrointestinal tract but has a hepatic extraction ratio of 0.75, only 25% of the original dose enters the systemic circulation. This first-pass effect through the liver and/or gastrointestinal tract wall is avoided when the drug is given by other routes of administration. The computation of F does not separate loss of oral drug metabolized by the first-pass effect and drug not absorbed by the gastrointestinal tract. Special techniques are needed to determine the fraction of drug absorbed orally for drugs with high liver extraction ratios or substantial gut wall metabolism.

Two different dosage forms of the same drug are considered to be bioequivalent when the $AUC_{0-\infty}$, maximum serum or blood concentrations (C_{max}), and the times that C_{max} occurs (t_{max}) are neither clinically nor statistically different. When this occurs, the serum-concentration-versus-time curves for the two dosage forms should be superimposable and therefore identical. Bioequivalence studies have become very important because many expensive drugs have become available recently in generic form. Most bioequivalence studies involve 18 to 25 healthy adults who are given the brand-name product and the generic product in a randomized, crossover study design.

CLEARANCE

Clearance (Cl) is the most important pharmacokinetic parameter because it determines the steady-state concentration for a given dosage rate. When a drug is given at a continuous intravenous infusion rate equal to k_0, the steady-state concentration (C_{ss}) is determined by the quotient of k_0 and Cl ($C_{ss} = k_0/\mathrm{Cl}$). If the drug is administered as individual doses (D) at a given dosage interval (τ), the average steady-state concentration (C_{ss}) over the dosage interval is given by the equation[4]

$$C_{ss} = [F(D/\tau)]/\mathrm{Cl}$$

where F is the fraction of dose absorbed into the systemic vascular system. The average steady-state concentration over the dosage interval is the steady-state concentration that would have occurred had the same dose been given as a continuous intravenous infusion (e.g., 300 mg every 6 hours would produce an average C_{ss} equivalent to the actual C_{ss} produced by a continuous infusion administered at a rate of 50 mg/h).

Physiologically, clearance is determined by (1) blood flow (Q) to the organ that metabolizes (liver) or eliminates (kidney) the drug and (2) the efficiency of the organ in extracting the drug from the bloodstream.[5] Efficiency is measured using an extraction ratio (E), calculated by subtracting the concentration in the blood leaving the extracting organ (C_{out}) from the concentration in the blood entering the organ (C_{in}) and then dividing the result by C_{in}:

$$E = (C_{in} - C_{out})/(C_{in})$$

Clearance for that organ is calculated by taking the product of Q and E: ($\mathrm{Cl} = QE$). For example, if liver blood flow equals 1.5 L/min and the drug's extraction ratio is 0.33, hepatic clearance equals 0.5 L/min. Total clearance is computed by summing all the individual organ clearance values. Clearance changes occur in patients when the blood flow to extracting organs changes or when the extraction ratio changes. Vasodilators such as hydralazine or nifedipine increase liver blood flow, whereas congestive heart failure and hypotension can decrease hepatic blood flow. Extraction ratios can increase when enzyme inducers increase the amount of drug-metabolizing enzyme. Extraction ratios may decrease if enzyme inhibitors inhibit drug-metabolizing enzymes or necrosis causes loss of parenchyma.

INTRINSIC CLEARANCE

The extraction ratio also can be thought of in terms of the unbound fraction of drug in the blood (f_b), the intrinsic ability of the extracting organ to clear unbound drug from the blood ($\mathrm{Cl_{int}}$), and blood flow to the organ (Q)[6,7]:

$$E = [f_b(\mathrm{Cl_{int}})]/\{Q + [f_b(\mathrm{Cl_{int}})]\}$$

By substituting this equation for E, the clearance equation becomes

$$\mathrm{Cl} = Q[f_b(\mathrm{Cl_{int}})]/\{Q + [f_b(\mathrm{Cl_{int}})]\}$$

Clearance changes will occur when blood flow to the clearing organ changes [in conditions where blood flow is reduced (shock, congestive heart failure) or when medications such as vasodilators increase blood flow], binding in the blood changes (if highly protein-bound drugs are displaced), or intrinsic clearance of unbound drug changes (when metabolizing enzymes are induced or inhibited by other drug therapy or functional organ tissue is destroyed by disease processes).

If $\mathrm{Cl_{int}}$ is large (enzymes have a high capacity to metabolize the drug), the product of f_b and $\mathrm{Cl_{int}}$ is much larger than Q. When $f_b(\mathrm{Cl_{int}})$ is much greater than Q, the sum of Q and $f_b(\mathrm{Cl_{int}})$ in the denominator of the clearance equation almost equals $f_b(\mathrm{Cl_{int}})$:

$$f_b(\mathrm{Cl_{int}}) \approx Q + f_b(\mathrm{Cl_{int}})$$

Substituting this expression in the denominator of the clearance equation and canceling common terms lead to the following expression for drugs with a large $\mathrm{Cl_{int}}$: $\mathrm{Cl} \approx Q$. In this case, the clearance of the drug is equal to blood flow to the organ; such drugs are called *high-clearance drugs* and have large extraction ratios. Propranolol, verapamil, morphine, and lidocaine are examples of high-clearance drugs. High-clearance drugs such as these typically exhibit high first-pass effects when administered orally.

If $\mathrm{Cl_{int}}$ is small (enzymes have a limited capacity to metabolize the drug), Q is much larger than the product of f_b and $\mathrm{Cl_{int}}$. When Q is much greater than $f_b(\mathrm{Cl_{int}})$, the sum of Q and $f_b(\mathrm{Cl_{int}})$ in the denominator of the clearance equation becomes almost equal to Q: $Q \approx Q + f_b(\mathrm{Cl_{int}})$. Substituting this expression in the denominator of the clearance equation and canceling common terms lead to the following expression for drugs with a small $\mathrm{Cl_{int}}$: $\mathrm{Cl} \approx f_b(\mathrm{Cl_{int}})$. In this case, clearance of the drug is equal to the product of the fraction unbound in the blood and the intrinsic ability of the organ to clear unbound drug from the blood; such drugs are known as *low-clearance drugs* and have small extraction ratios. Warfarin, theophylline, diazepam, and phenobarbital are examples of low-clearance drugs.

As mentioned previously, the concentration of unbound drug in the blood is probably more important pharmacologically than the total (bound plus unbound) concentration. The unbound drug in the blood is in equilibrium with the unbound drug in the tissues and reflects the concentration of drug at its site of action. Therefore, the pharmacologic effect of a drug is thought to be a function of the concentration of unbound drug in the blood. The unbound steady-state concentration ($C_{ss,u}$) can be calculated by multiplying C_{ss} and f_b: $C_{ss,u} = C_{ss} f_b$. The effect that changes in Q, f_b, and $\mathrm{Cl_{int}}$ have on $C_{ss,u}$ and therefore on the pharmacologic response of a drug depends on whether a high- or low-clearance drug is involved. Because $\mathrm{Cl} = Q$ for high-clearance drugs, a change in f_b or $\mathrm{Cl_{int}}$ does not change Cl or C_{ss} ($C_{ss} = k_0/\mathrm{Cl}$). However, a change in unbound drug fraction does alter $C_{ss,u}$ ($C_{ss,u} = f_b C_{ss}$), thereby affecting the pharmacologic response. Plasma-protein-binding displacement drug interactions are thus very important clinically, but they are also dangerous because the changes in $C_{ss,u}$ are not reflected in changes in C_{ss}. Since laboratories usually measure only total concentrations (concentrations of unbound drug are difficult to determine), the interaction is hard to detect. If Cl_{int} changes for high-clearance drugs, Cl, C_{ss}, $C_{ss,u}$, and pharmacologic responses do not change. Changes in Q cause a change in Cl; changes in C_{ss}, $C_{ss,u}$, and drug response are indirectly proportional to changes in Cl.

For low-clearance drugs, total clearance is determined by unbound drug fraction and intrinsic clearance: $Cl = f_b(Cl_{int})$. A change in Q does not change Cl, C_{ss}, $C_{ss,u}$, or pharmacologic response. However, a change in f_b or Cl_{int} does alter Cl and C_{ss} ($C_{ss} = k_0/Cl$). Changes in Cl_{int} will cause a proportional change in Cl. Changes in C_{ss}, $C_{ss,u}$, and drug response are indirectly proportional to changes in Cl. Altering f_b for low-clearance drugs produces interesting results. A change in f_b alters Cl and C_{ss} ($C_{ss} = k_0/Cl$). As Cl and C_{ss} change in opposite directions with changes in f_b, $C_{ss,u}$ ($C_{ss,u} = f_b C_{ss}$) and pharmacologic responses do not change with alterations in the fraction of unbound drug in the blood. For example, a low-clearance drug is administered to a patient until steady-state is achieved:

$$Cl = f_b(Cl_{int})$$

$$C_{ss} = k_0/CL$$

Suppose that another drug is administered to the patient that displaces the first drug from plasma protein binding sites and doubles f_b (f_b now equals $2f_b$). Cl doubles because of the protein-binding displacement [$2Cl = 2f_b(Cl_{int})$], and C_{ss} decreases by one-half because of the change in clearance [$\frac{1}{2}(C_{ss}) = k_0/(2Cl)$]. $C_{ss,u}$ does not change because even though f_b is doubled, C_{ss} decreased by one-half ($C_{ss,u} = f_b C_{ss}$). The potential for error in this situation is that clinicians may increase the dose of a low-clearance drug after a protein-binding displacement interaction because C_{ss} decreased. Since $C_{ss,u}$ and the pharmacologic effect do not change, the dose should remain unaltered. Plasma-protein-binding decreases occur commonly in patients taking phenytoin. Low albumin concentrations (as in trauma or pregnant patients) or plasma-protein-binding drug interactions (as with concomitant therapy with valproic acid) can result in subtherapeutic total phenytoin concentrations. Despite this fact, unbound phenytoin concentrations are usually within the therapeutic range, and often the patient is responding appropriately to treatment. Thus, in these situations, unbound rather than total phenytoin serum concentrations should be monitored and used to guide future therapeutic decisions.

CLEARANCES FOR DIFFERENT ROUTES OF ELIMINATION AND METABOLIC PATHWAYS

Clearances for individual organs can be computed if the excretion the organ produces can be obtained. For example, renal clearance can be calculated if urine is collected during a pharmacokinetic experiment. The patient empties his or her bladder immediately before the dose is given. Subsequent urine production is collected until the last serum concentration (C_{last}) is obtained. Renal clearance (Cl_R) is computed by dividing the amount of drug excreted in the urine by $AUC_{0-tlast}$. Biliary and other clearance values are computed in a similar fashion.

Clearances also can be calculated for each metabolite that is formed from the parent drug. This computation is particularly useful in drug interaction studies to determine which metabolic pathway is stimulated or inhibited. In the following metabolic scheme, the parent drug (D), is metabolized into two different metabolites (M_1, M_2) that subsequently are eliminated by the kidney (M_{1R}, M_{2R}):

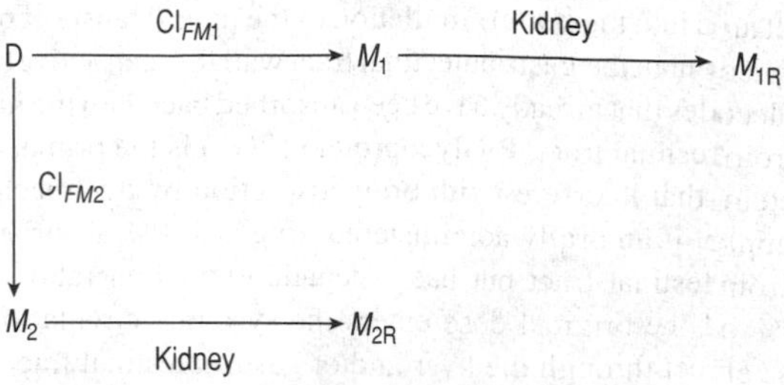

To compute the formation clearance of M_1 and M_2 (Cl_{FM1}, Cl_{FM2}), urine would be collected for five or more half-lives after a single dose or during a dosage interval at steady state. The amount of metabolite eliminated in the urine is then determined. The fraction of the dose (in moles, since the molecular weights of the parent drug and metabolites are not equal) eliminated by each metabolic pathway ($f_{M1} = M_{1R}/D$ and $f_{M2} = M_{2R}/D$) can then be computed. Formation clearance for each pathway can be calculated using the following equations: $Cl_{FM1} = f_{M1}Cl_M$ and $Cl_{FM2} = f_{M2}Cl_M$, where Cl_M is the metabolic clearance for the parent drug.

VOLUME OF DISTRIBUTION

The volume of distribution (V_D) is a proportionality constant that relates the amount of drug in the body to the serum concentration (amount in body $= CV_D$). V_D is used to calculate the loading dose (LD) of a drug that will immediately achieve a desired C_{ss} (LD $= C_{ss}V_D$). However, in practice, the patient's own V_D is not known at the time the loading dose is administered. In this case, an average V_D is assumed and used to calculate a loading dose. Because the patient's V_D is almost always different from the average V_D for the drug, a loading dose does not attain the calculated C_{ss}, but it hopefully achieves a therapeutic concentration. As usual, steady-state conditions are achieved in three to five half-lives for the drug.

The numeric value for the volume of distribution is determined by the physiologic volume of blood and tissues and how the drug binds in blood and tissues[8]:

$$V_D = V_b + (f_b/f_t)V_t$$

where V_b and V_t are the volumes of blood and tissues, respectively, and f_b and f_t are the fractions of unbound drug in blood and tissues, respectively.

HALF-LIFE

Half-life ($t_{1/2}$) is the time required for serum concentrations to decrease by one-half after absorption and distribution are complete. It takes the same amount of time for serum concentrations to drop from 200 to 100 mg/L as it does for concentrations to decline from 2 to 1 mg/L (Fig. 4–3).

Half-life is important because it determines the time required to reach steady state and the dosage interval. It takes approximately three to five half-lives to reach steady-state concentrations during continuous dosing. In three half-lives, serum concentrations are at about 90% of their ultimate steady-state values. Because most serum drug assays have about a 10% error, it is difficult to differentiate concentrations that are within 10% of each other. For this reason, many clinicians consider concentrations obtained after three half-lives to be C_{ss}.

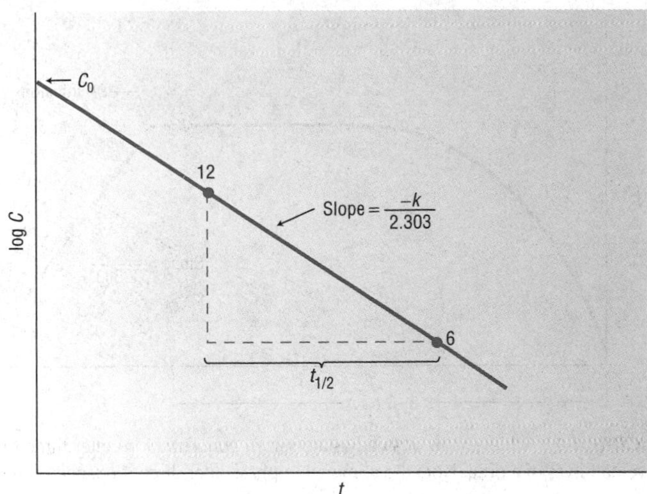

FIGURE 4–3. Calculation of the half-life of a drug following intravenous bolus dosing.

Half-life is also used to determine the dosage interval for a drug. For instance, it may be desirable to maintain maximum steady-state concentrations at 20 mg/L and minimum steady-state concentrations at 10 mg/L. In this case, it would be necessary to administer the drug every half-life because the minimum desirable concentration is one-half the maximum desirable concentration.

Half-life is a dependent kinetic variable because its value depends on the values of Cl and V_D.[8] The equation that describes the relationship among the three variables is $t_{1/2} = 0.693 V_D/\text{Cl}$. Changes in $t_{1/2}$ can result from a change in either V_D or Cl; a change in $t_{1/2}$ does not necessarily indicate that Cl has changed. Half-life can change solely because of changes in V_D. The elimination rate constant (k) is related to the half-life by the following equation: $k = 0.693/t_{1/2}$. Both the half-life and elimination rate constant describe how quickly serum concentrations decrease in the serum or blood.

NONLINEAR PHARMACOKINETICS

MICHAELIS-MENTEN KINETICS

Some drugs do not follow the rules of linear pharmacokinetics. Instead of C_{ss} and AUC increasing proportionally with dose, serum concentrations change more or less than expected (Fig. 4–4). One explanation for the greater than expected increase in C_{ss} and AUC after an increase in dose is that the enzymes responsible for the metabolism or elimination of the drug may start to become saturated. When this occurs, the maximum rate of metabolism (V_{max}) for the drug is approached. This is called *Michaelis-Menten kinetics*. The serum concentration at which the rate of metabolism equals $V_{max}/2$ is K_m. Practically speaking, K_m is the serum concentration at which nonproportional changes in C_{ss} and AUC start to occur when dose is increased. The Michaelis-Menten constants (V_{max} and K_m) determine the dosage rate (DR) needed to maintain a given C_{ss}: $\text{DR} = V_{max} C_{ss}/(K_m + C_{ss})$. Most drugs eliminated by the liver are metabolized by enzymes but still appear to follow linear kinetics. The reason for this disparity is that the therapeutic range for most drugs is well below the K_m of the enzyme system that metabolizes the agent. The therapeutic range is higher than K_m for some commonly used drugs. The average K_m for phenytoin is about 4 mg/L. The therapeutic range for phenytoin is usually 10–20 mg/L. Most patients experience Michaelis-Menten kinetics while taking phenytoin.

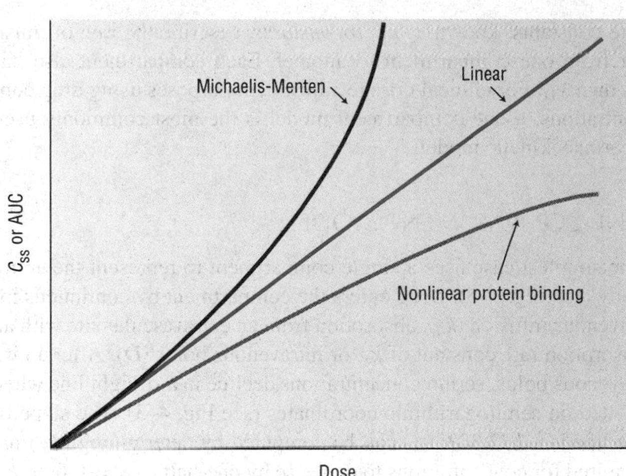

FIGURE 4–4. Relationship of dose and C_{ss} or AUC under linear and nonlinear conditions.

NONLINEAR PROTEIN BINDING

Another type of nonlinear kinetics can occur if C_{ss} and AUC increase less than expected after an increase in dose of a low-clearance drug. This usually indicates that plasma-protein-binding sites are starting to become saturated so that f_b increases with increases in dose (see Fig. 4–4). For a low-clearance drug, Cl depends on the values of f_b and Cl_{int} ($\text{Cl} = f_b \text{Cl}_{int}$). When a dosage increase takes place, f_b increases because nearly all plasma-protein-binding sites are occupied and no binding sites are available. If f_b increases, Cl increases and C_{ss} increases less than expected with the dosage change ($C_{ss} = k_0/\text{Cl}$). However, $C_{ss,u}$ increases proportionally with dose because $C_{ss,u}$ depends on Cl_{int} for low-clearance drugs ($C_{ss,u} = k_0/\text{Cl}_{int}$). Valproic acid[9] and disopyramide[10] both follow saturable-protein-binding pharmacokinetics.

PHARMACOKINETIC MODELS AND EQUATIONS

Pharmacokinetic models are useful to describe data sets, to predict serum concentrations after several doses or different routes of administration, and to calculate pharmacokinetic constants such as Cl, V_D, and $t_{1/2}$.[11] Compartmental models depict the body as one or more discrete compartments to which drug is distributed and/or from which drug is eliminated. The shape of the serum-concentration-versus-time curve determines the number of compartments in the pharmacokinetic model and the equation used in computations (Fig. 4–5). First-order

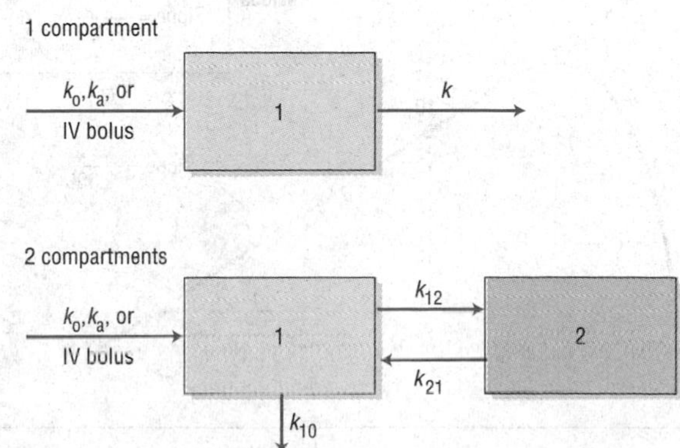

FIGURE 4–5. Visual representations of one- and two-compartment drug-distribution models.

rate constants, known as *microconstants,* describe the rate of transfer from one compartment to another. Each compartment also has its own V_D. For clinical dosage adjustment purposes using drug concentrations, a one-compartment model is the most commonly used pharmacokinetic model.

ONE-COMPARTMENT MODEL

The simplest case uses a single compartment to represent the entire body (see Fig. 4–5). Drug enters the compartment by continuous intravenous infusion (k_0), absorption from an extravascular site with an absorption rate constant of k_a, or intravenous bolus (D). After an intravenous bolus, serum concentrations decline in a straight line when plotted on semilogarithmic coordinates (see Fig. 4–3). The slope of the line is $-k/2.303$; $t_{1/2}$ can be computed by determining the time required for concentrations to decrease by one-half ($t_{1/2} = 0.693/k$). The equation that describes the data is $C = (D/V_D)e^{-kt}$. V_D is calculated by dividing the intravenous dose by the y intercept (the concentration at time zero, C_0) of the graph. CL is computed by taking the product of k and V_D. Once V_D and k are known, concentrations at any time after the dose can be computed [$C = (D/V_D)e^{-kt}$].

When an extravascular dose is given, one-compartment model serum concentrations rise during absorption, reach C_{max}, and then decrease in a straight line with a slope equal to $-k/2.303$. The equation that describes the data is $C = \{(FDk_a)/[V_D(k_a - k)]\}\ (e^{-kt} - e^{-k_a t})$, where F is the fraction of the dose absorbed into the systemic circulation. The absorption rate constant (k_a) is obtained using the method of residuals.

The method of residuals is used to obtain the individual rate constants (Fig. 4–6). A is determined by extrapolating the terminal slope to the y axis; k can be obtained by calculating the slope or $t_{1/2}$ and using the formulas given for the intravenous bolus case. At each time point in the absorption portion of the curve, the concentration value from the extrapolated line is noted and called the *extrapolated concentration.* For each point, the actual concentration is subtracted from the extrapolated concentration to compute the residual concentration. When the residual concentrations are plotted on semilogarithmic coordinates, a line with y intercept equal to A and slope equal to $-k_a/2.303$ is obtained. When these values are calculated, they can be placed into the equation ($C = Ae^{-kt} - Ae^{-k_a t}$, where $A = FDk_a/[V_D(k_a - k)]$) and used to compute the serum concentration at any time after the extravascular dose. The intercepts and rate constants also can be used to compute Cl and V_D: $\text{Cl} = FD/(A/k - A/k_a)$ and $V_D = \text{Cl}/k$, where F is the fraction of the dose absorbed into the systemic circulation.

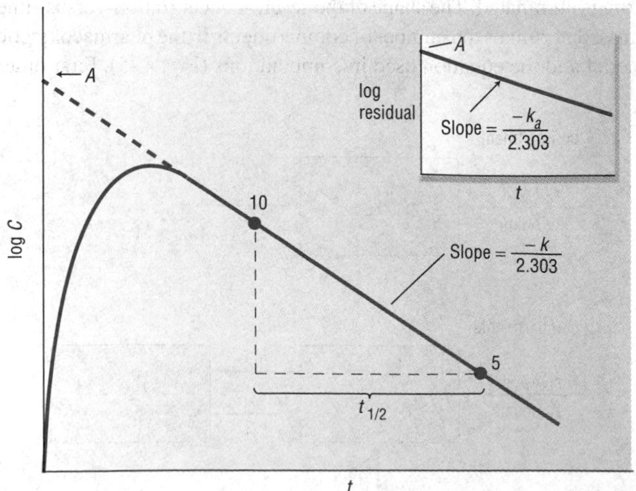

FIGURE 4–6. Calculation of the half-life of a drug following oral, intramuscular, or other extravascular dosing route.

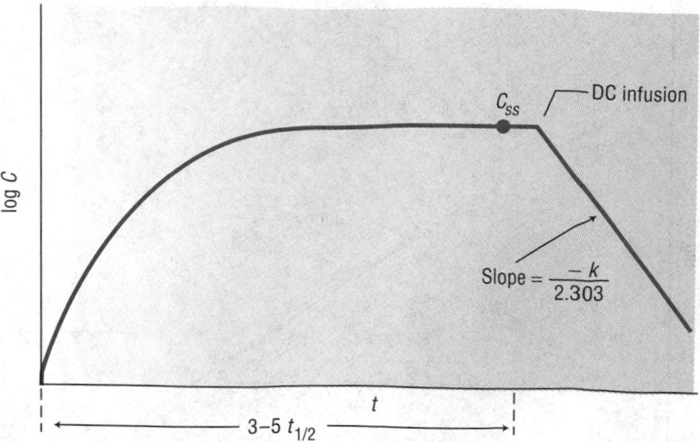

FIGURE 4–7. Achievement of steady-state serum concentrations after three to five half-lives of a drug. Note the elimination phase after discontinuance of the infusion.

During a continuous intravenous infusion, the serum concentrations in a one-compartment model change according to the following function: $C = (k_0/\text{Cl})(1 - e^{-kt})$. If the infusion has been running for more than three to five half-lives, the patient will be at steady state, and Cl can be calculated ($\text{Cl} = k_0/C_{ss}$). When the infusion is discontinued, serum concentrations appear to decline in a straight line when plotted on semilogarithmic paper with a slope of $-k/2.303$. V_D is computed by dividing Cl by k (Fig. 4–7).

MULTICOMPARTMENT MODEL

After an intravenous bolus dose, serum concentrations often decline in two or more phases. During the early phases, drug leaves the bloodstream by two mechanisms: (1) distribution into tissues and (2) metabolism and/or elimination. Because the drug is leaving the bloodstream through these two mechanisms, serum concentrations decline rapidly. After tissues and blood are in equilibrium, only metabolism and/or elimination remove drug from the blood. During this terminal phase, serum concentrations decline more slowly. The half-life is measured during the terminal phase by determining the time required for concentrations to decline by one-half.

After an intravenous bolus dose, serum concentrations decrease as if the drug were being injected into a central compartment that not only metabolizes and eliminates drug but also distributes drug to one or more other compartments. Of these multicompartment models, the two-compartment model is encountered most commonly (see Fig. 4–5). After an intravenous bolus injection, serum concentrations decrease in two distinct phases described by the equation:

$$C = D(\alpha - k_{21})/[V_{D1}(\alpha - \beta)]e^{-\alpha t} + D(k_{21} - \beta)/[V_{D1}(\alpha - \beta)]e^{-\beta t}$$

or $C = Ae^{-\alpha t} + Be^{-\beta t}$, where k_{21} is the first-order rate constant that reflects the transfer of drug from compartment 2 to compartment 1, V_{D1} is the V_D of compartment 1, $A = D(\alpha - k_{21})/[V_{D1}(\alpha - \beta)]$, and $B = D(k_{21} - \beta)/[V_{D1}(\alpha - \beta)]$. The rate constants α and β found in the exponents of the equations describe the distribution and elimination of the drug, respectively (Fig. 4–8). A and B are the y intercepts of the lines that describe drug distribution and elimination, respectively, on the log concentration-versus-time plot.

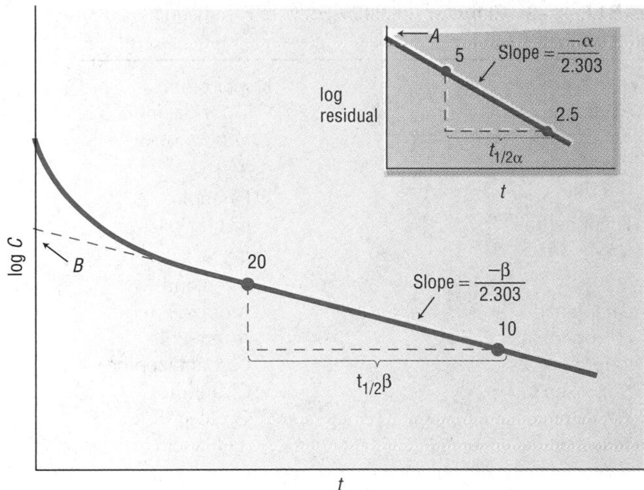

FIGURE 4–8. Calculation of α and β half-lives following intravenous dosing.

The residual line is calculated as before using the method of residuals. The terminal line is extrapolated to the y axis, and extrapolated concentrations are determined for each time point. Because actual concentrations are greater in this case, residual concentrations are calculated by subtracting the extrapolated concentrations from the actual concentrations. When plotted on semilogarithmic paper, the residual line has a y intercept equal to A. The slope of the residual line is used to compute α (slope $= -\alpha/2.303$). With the rate constants (α and β) and the intercepts (A and B), concentrations can be calculated for any time after the intravenous bolus dose ($C = Ae^{-\alpha t} + Be^{-\beta t}$) or pharmacokinetic constants can be computed: $\mathrm{Cl} = D/[(A/\alpha) + (B/\beta)]$, $V_{\mathrm{D},\beta} = \mathrm{Cl}/\beta$, $V_{\mathrm{D,ss}} = D[(A/\alpha^2) + (B/\beta^2)]/[(A/\alpha) + (B/\beta)]^2$.

If serum concentrations of a drug given as a continuous intravenous infusion decline in a biphasic manner after the infusion is discontinued, a two-compartment model describes the data set[12,13] (Fig. 4–9). In this instance, the postinfusion concentrations decrease according to the equation $C = Re^{-\alpha t'} + Se^{-\beta t'}$, where t' is the postinfusion time ($t' = 0$ when infusion is discontinued) and R, S, α, and β are determined from the postinfusion concentrations using the method of residuals with the y axis set at $t' = 0$. R and S are used to compute A and B. A and B are the y intercepts that would have occurred had the total dose given during the infusion ($D = k_0T$) been administered as an intravenous bolus dose:

$$A = RD\alpha/[k_0(1 - e^{-\alpha T})]$$
$$B = SD\beta/[k_0(1 - e^{-\beta T})]$$

where T is the duration of infusion. Once A, B, α, and β are known, the equations for an intravenous bolus are used to compute the pharmacokinetic constants. Often, when a drug is given as an intravenous bolus or continuous intravenous infusion, a two-compartment model is used to describe the data, but when the same agent is given extravascularly, a one-compartment model applies.[14] In this case, distribution occurs during the absorption phase, so a distribution phase is not observed.

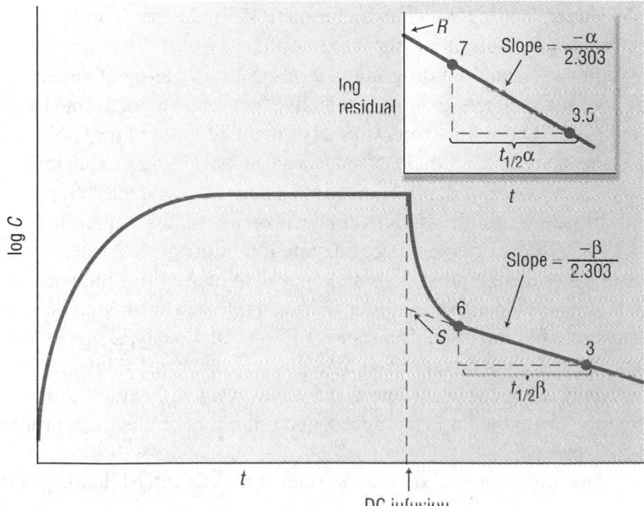

FIGURE 4–9. Calculation of α and β half-lives following a steady-state infusion.

VOLUMES OF DISTRIBUTION IN MULTICOMPARTMENT MODELS

Two different V_D values are needed as proportionality constants for drugs that require multicompartment models to describe the serum-concentration versus time curve. The V_D that is used to compute the amount of drug in the body during the terminal (β) portion of the curve is called $V_{\mathrm{D},\beta}$ (amount of drug in body $= V_{\mathrm{D},\beta}C$). During a continuous intravenous infusion at steady state, $V_{\mathrm{D,ss}}$ is used to compute the amount of drug in the body (amount of drug in body $= V_{\mathrm{D,ss}}C$). $V_{\mathrm{D,ss}}$ is also the V_D that can be computed using the physiologic volumes of blood and tissues and the ratio of unbound drug in blood to that in tissues [$V_{\mathrm{D,ss}} = V_\mathrm{b} + (f_\mathrm{b}/f_\mathrm{t})V_\mathrm{t}$]. Because the value of $V_{\mathrm{D},\beta}$ changes when Cl changes, $V_{\mathrm{D,ss}}$ should be used to indicate if drug distribution changes during pharmacokinetic or drug-interaction experiments.

MULTIPLE DOSING AND STEADY-STATE EQUATIONS

Any of these compartmental equations can be used to determine serum concentrations after multiple doses. The multiple-dosing factor $(1 - e^{-nK\tau})/(1 - e^{-K\tau})$, where n is the number of doses, K is the appropriate rate constant, and τ is the dosage interval, is simply multiplied by each exponential term in the equation, substituting the rate constant of each exponent for K. Time (t) is set at 0 at the beginning of each dosage interval. For example, a single-dose two-compartment intravenous bolus is calculated as follows: $C = Ae^{-\alpha t} + Be^{-\beta t}$. The equation for a multiple-dose two-compartment intravenous bolus is therefore

$$C = Ae^{-\alpha t}[(1 - e^{-n\alpha\tau})/(1 - e^{-\alpha\tau})] + Be^{-\beta t}[(1 - e^{-n\beta\tau})/(1 - e^{-\beta\tau})]$$

A single-dose one-compartment intravenous bolus is calculated as $C = (D/V_\mathrm{D})e^{-kt}$. For a multiple-dose one-compartment intravenous bolus the concentration is $C = (D/V_\mathrm{D})e^{-kt}[(1 - e^{-nk\tau})/(1 - e^{-k\tau})]$.

At steady state, the number of doses becomes large, $e^{-nk\tau}$ approaches zero, and the multiple-dosing factor equals $1/(1 - e^{-K\tau})$. Therefore, the steady-state versions of the equations are simpler than their multiple-dose counterparts:

$$C = [Ae^{-\alpha t}/(1 - e^{-\alpha\tau})] + [Be^{-\beta t}/(1 - e^{-\beta\tau})]$$

and

$$C = [(D/V_\mathrm{D})e^{-kt}]/(1 - e^{-k\tau})$$

for a steady-state two-compartment intravenous bolus and a steady-state one-compartment intravenous bolus, respectively.

USE OF PHARMACOKINETIC CONCEPTS FOR INDIVIDUALIZATION OF DRUG THERAPY

Many factors must be taken into consideration when deciding on the best drug dose for a patient. For example, the age of the patient is important because the dose (in milligrams per kilogram) for pediatric patients may be higher and for geriatric patients may be lower than the typically prescribed dose for young adults. Gender also can be a factor because males and females metabolize and eliminate some drugs differently. Patients who are significantly obese or cachectic also may require different drug doses because of clearance and volume-of-distribution changes. Other drug therapy that could cause drug interactions needs to be considered. Disease states and conditions may alter the drug-dosage regimen for a patient. Three disease states that deserve special mention are congestive heart failure, renal disease, and hepatic disease. Renal and hepatic diseases cause loss of organ function and decreased drug elimination and metabolism. Congestive heart failure causes decreased blood flow to organs that clear the drug from the body.

Many drug compounds are racemic mixtures of stereoisomers. In most cases, one of the isomers is more pharmacologically active than the other isomer, and each isomer may exhibit different pharmacokinetic properties. Warfarin, propranolol, verapamil, and ibuprofen are all racemic mixtures of stereoisomers. Some drug interactions inhibit or increase the elimination of only one stereoisomer. The importance of the drug interaction depends on which isomer is affected. Other drugs, such as dextromethorphan, levofloxacin, and diltiazem, are composed of just one stereoisomer.

Genetics also plays a role in drug metabolism. *Cytochrome P450* is a generic term for the group of enzymes that are responsible for most drug metabolism oxidation reactions. Several cytochrome P450 isozymes have been identified that are responsible for the metabolism of many important drugs (Table 4–3). CYP2C19 (P450IIC19, $P450_{mp}$; formerly included in CYP2C9) is responsible for aromatic hydroxylation of mephenytoin, and CYP2D6 (P450IID6, $P450_{db}$) oxidizes debrisoquine.[15] These subsets of the cytochrome P450 enzyme family are also responsible for the metabolism of several other drugs (CYP2D6: most tricyclic antidepressants, encainide, metoprolol). Both these isozymes appear to be under genetic control. As a consequence, there are "poor metabolizers" who lack the gene for the isozyme, cannot manufacture the isozyme, and therefore cannot metabolize the drug substrate very well. "Extensive metabolizers" have the gene for the isozyme and metabolize the drugs normally. Poor metabolizers usually are a minority of the general population. They may achieve toxic concentrations of drug when usual doses are prescribed for them or, if the active drug moiety is a metabolite, may fail to have any pharmacologic effect from the drug. The ethnic background of the patient can affect the likelihood that he or she will be a poor metabolizer.[15] For example, the incidence of poor metabolizers for CYP2D6 is about 5% to 10% for Caucasians and about 0% to 1% for Asians, whereas for CYP2C19 poor metabolizers make up about 3% to 6% of the Caucasian population and about 20% of the Asian population.

Other cytochrome P450 isozymes have been isolated.[15] CYP1A2 (P450IA2) is the enzyme that is responsible for the demethylation of caffeine and theophylline; CYP2C9 (P450IIC9) metabolizes phenytoin; tolbutamide, cyclosporine, and nifedipine are metabolized by CYP3A4 (P450IIIA4); and ethanol is a substrate for CYP2E1 (P450IIE1). It is important to recognize that a drug may be metabolized by more than one cytochrome P450 isozyme. While most tricyclic antidepressants are hydroxylated by CYP2D6, *N*-demethylation probably is mediated by a combination of CYP2C19, CYP1A2, and CYP3A4. Acetaminophen appears to be metabolized by both CYP1A2 and CYP2E1. The 4-hydroxy metabolite of propranolol is produced by CYP2D6, but side-chain oxidation of propranolol is probably a product of CYP2C19. The CYP3A enzyme family comprises approximately 90% of the drug-metabolizing enzyme present in the intestinal wall but only approximately 30% of the drug metabolizing enzyme found in the liver. The remainder of hepatic drug-metabolizing enzyme is approximately 20% for the CYP2C family, approximately 13% for CYP1A2, approximately 7% for CYP2E1, and approximately 2% for CYP2D6.

TABLE 4–3. Cytochrome P450 Enzyme Family and Selected Substrates

CYP1A2
- Acetaminophen
- Antipyrine
- Caffeine
- Tacrine
- Theophylline
- *R*-Warfarin

CYP2C9
- Diclofenac
- Hexobarbital
- Ibuprofen
- Naproxen
- Phenytoin
- Tolbutamide
- *S*-Warfarin

CYP2C19
- Diazepam
- Mephenytoin
- Omeprazole

CYP2D6
- Codeine
- Debrisoquine
- Dextromethorphan
- Encainide
- Fluoxetine
- Haloperidol
- Metoprolol
- Paroxetine
- Propafenone
- Risperidone
- Thioridazine
- Venlafaxine

CYP2E1
- Ethanol
- Isoniazid

CYP3A4
- Alfentanil
- Alprazolam
- Astemizole
- Carbamazepine
- Cisapride
- Cyclosporine
- Diltiazem
- Erythromycin
- Felodipine
- Fluconazole
- Itraconazole
- Ketoconazole
- Lidocaine
- Lovastatin
- Midazolam
- Nifedipine
- Quinidine
- Simvastatin
- Tacrolimus
- Terfenadine
- Verapamil

Understanding which cytochrome P450 isozyme is responsible for the metabolism of a drug is extraordinarily useful when predicting and understanding drug interactions. Some drug-metabolism inhibitors and inducers are highly selective for certain cytochrome P450 isozymes.[15] Quinidine is an extremely potent inhibitor of the CYP2D6 enzyme system[15]; a single 50-mg dose of quinidine can change a rapid metabolizer of debrisoquine into a poor metabolizer. Verapamil and diltiazem inhibit whereas tobacco or marijuana smoke induce CYP1A2. Some drugs that are enzyme inhibitors are also substrates for that same enzyme system and appear to cause drug interactions by being a competitive inhibitor. For example, erythromycin is both a substrate for and an inhibitor of CYP3A4. Obviously, if one knows that a new drug is metabolized by a given cytochrome P450 enzyme system, it is logical to assume that the new drug will exhibit drug interactions with the known inducers and inhibitors of that cytochrome P450 isozyme.

The importance of transport proteins in drug bioavailability and elimination is now better understood. The principal transport protein involved in the movement of drugs across biologic membranes is

P-glycoprotein (PGP). PGP is present in many organs, including the gastrointestinal tract, liver, and kidney. If a drug is a substrate for PGP, its oral absorption may be decreased when PGP transports drug molecules that have been absorbed back into the gastrointestinal tract lumen. In the liver, some drugs are transported by PGP from the blood into the bile, where the drug is eliminated by biliary secretion. Similarly, some drugs eliminated by the kidney are transported from the blood into the urine by PGP. Other possible mechanisms for drug interactions are when two drugs that are substrates for PGP compete for transport by the protein or when a drug is an inhibitor or inducer of PGP. Drug interactions involving inhibition of PGP decrease drug transportation in these organs and potentially can increase gastrointestinal absorption of orally administered drug, decrease biliary secretion of the drug, or decrease renal elimination of drug molecules. Many drugs that are metabolized by CYP3A4 are also substrates for PGP, and some of the drug interactions attributed to inhibition of CYP3A4 may be due to decreased drug transportation by PGP. Drug interactions involving induction of PGP have the opposite effect in these organs and may decrease gastrointestinal absorption of orally administered drug, increase biliary secretion of the drug, or increase renal elimination of drug molecules.

SELECTION OF INITIAL DRUG DOSES

When deciding on initial doses for drugs that are eliminated renally, the patient's renal function should be assessed. A common, useful way to do this is to measure the patient's serum creatinine concentration and convert this value into an estimated creatinine clearance ($CrCl_{est}$). Serum creatinine values alone should not be used to assess renal function because they do not include the effects of age, body weight, or gender. The Cockcroft-Gault equation[16] is probably the most widely used method to estimate creatinine clearance (in milliliters per minute) in adults (18 years or older) who are within about 30% of their ideal body weight and have stable renal function:

$$\text{Male}: CrCl_{est} = [(140 - \text{age})BW]/(S_{Cr} \cdot 72)$$
$$\text{Female}: CrCl_{est} = [0.85(140 - \text{age})BW]/(S_{Cr} \cdot 72)$$

where BW is body weight (in kilograms), age is the patient's age (in years), 0.85 is a correction factor to account for lower muscle mass in females, and S_{Cr} is serum creatinine (in milligrams per deciliter). For children, the following estimation equations are available according to the age of the child[17]: age 0 to 1 years: $CrCl_{est}$ (in mL/min/1.73 m^2) = $(0.45 \cdot Lt)/S_{Cr}$; age 1 to 20 years: $CrCl_{est}$ (in mL/min/1.73 m^2) = $(0.55 \cdot Lt)/S_{Cr}$, where Lt is patient length in centimeters. Other methods to determine $CrCl_{est}$ for obese adults[18] and patients with rapidly changing renal function[19] are available. Creatinine is a by-product of muscle breakdown in the body, so none of these estimation methods work well in patients with muscle disease, such as multiple sclerosis, or diseases that alter muscle mass, such as cachexia, malnutrition, cancer, or spinal cord injury. Nomograms that adjust initial doses according to a patient's renal function are available for several drugs, including digoxin,[20] vancomycin,[21] and the aminoglycoside antibiotics.[22] For many other drugs, William M. Bennett[23,24] occasionally updates his monograph of drug dosing in renal disease, which includes suggested dosage adjustments. For drugs that are eliminated primarily by the kidney (≥60% of the administered dose), some agents will need minor dosage adjustments for $CrCl_{est}$ between 30 and 60 mL/min, moderate dosage adjustments for $CrCl_{est}$ between 15 and 30 mL/min, and major dosage adjustments for $CrCl_{est}$ less than 15 mL/min. Postdialysis supplemental doses of some medications also may be needed for patients receiving hemodialysis if the drug is removed by the artificial kidney.

A similar assessment of liver function should be made for drugs that are metabolized hepatically. Unfortunately, there is no single test that can accurately estimate liver drug-metabolism capacity, and those which are used do not always prove accurate. High aminotransferase (AST or SGOT and ALT or SGPT) and alkaline phosphatase concentrations usually indicate acute hepatic cellular damage and do not reliably establish poor liver drug metabolism. Abnormal values for three tests that usually indicate that drugs will be metabolized poorly by the liver are high serum bilirubin, low serum albumin, and a prolonged prothrombin time. Bilirubin is metabolized by the liver, and albumin and clotting factors are manufactured by the liver, so aberrant values for all three of these tests are a more reliable indicator of abnormal liver drug metabolism. The Child-Pugh score,[25] a widely used clinical classification for liver disease that incorporates clinical signs and symptoms (ascites and hepatic encephalopathy) in addition to these three laboratory tests, can be used as an indicator of a patient's ability to metabolize drugs that are eliminated by the liver. A score in excess of 10 suggests very poor liver function. As a general rule, patients with cirrhosis have the most severe decreases in liver drug metabolism. Patients with acute or chronic hepatitis often retain relatively normal or slightly decreased hepatic drug-metabolism capacity. In the absence of specific pharmacokinetic dosing guidelines for a medication, a Child-Pugh score equal to 8 to 9 is grounds for a moderate decrease (approximately 25%) in initial daily drug dose for agents that are primarily (≥60%) hepatically metabolized, and a score of 10 or greater indicates that a significant decrease in initial daily dose (approximately 50%) is required for drugs that are mostly metabolized by the liver. As in any patient with or without liver dysfunction, initial doses are meant as starting points for dosage titration based on patient response and avoidance of adverse effects.

Since there are no good markers of liver function, clinicians have come to rely on pharmacokinetic parameters derived in various patient populations to compute initial doses of drugs that are eliminated hepatically. Table 4–4 contains average pharmacokinetic parameters

TABLE 4–4. Theophylline Pharmacokinetic Parameters for Selected Disease States/Conditions

Disease State/Condition	Mean Clearance (mL/min/kg)	Mean Dose (mg/kg/h)
Children 1–9 yr	1.4	0.8
Children 9–12 yr or adult smokers	1.25	0.7
Adolescents 12–16 yr or elderly smokers (>65 yr)	0.9	0.5
Adult nonsmokers	0.7	0.4
Elderly nonsmokers (>65 yr)	0.5	0.3
Decompensated CHF, cor pulmonale, cirrhosis	0.35	0.2

Mean volume of distribution = 0.5 L/kg.
Adapted from Ref. 49.

for theophylline in several disease states. Initial doses of many liver-metabolized drugs are computed by determining which disease states and/or conditions the patient has that are known to alter the kinetics of the drug and by using these average pharmacokinetic constants to calculate doses. The patient is then monitored for therapeutic and adverse effects, and drug serum concentrations are obtained to ensure that concentrations are appropriate and to adjust doses if necessary. The following computations illustrate the estimated intravenous loading and intravenous continuous infusion necessary to achieve a theophylline concentration of 10 mg/L for a 55-year-old, 70-kg male with liver cirrhosis (mean kinetic parameters obtained from Table 4–4):

$$V_D = (0.5\ \text{L/kg})(70\ \text{kg}) = 35\ \text{L}$$

$$\text{LD} = C_{ss}V_D = (10\ \text{mg/L})(35\ \text{L})$$

$$= 350\ \text{mg theophylline infused over } 20-30\ \text{min}$$

$$\text{Cl (in L/h)} = [(0.35\ \text{mL/min/kg})(70\ \text{kg})(60\ \text{min/h})]/1000\ \text{mL/L}$$

$$= 1.5\ \text{L/h}$$

$$k_0 = C_{ss}\text{Cl} = (10\ \text{mg/L})(1.5\ \text{L/h})$$

$$= 15\ \text{mg/h of theophylline to begin after loading dose given}$$

If theophylline is to be given as the aminophylline salt form, each dose would need to be changed to reflect the fact that aminophylline contains only 85% theophylline (LD = 350 mg of theophylline/0.85 = 410 mg of aminophylline infused over 20 to 30 minutes, k_0 = 15 mg/h of theophylline/0.85 = 18 mg/h of aminophylline to begin after loading dose given).

Heart failure is often overlooked as a disease state that can alter drug disposition. Severe heart failure decreases cardiac output and therefore reduces liver blood flow. Theophylline,[26] lidocaine,[27] and drugs with high extraction ratios are compounds whose clearance declines with decreased liver blood flow. Initial dosages of these drugs should be reduced in patients with moderate to severe heart failure by 25% to 50% until steady-state concentrations and response can be determined.

USE OF STEADY-STATE DRUG CONCENTRATIONS

Serum drug concentrations are readily available to clinicians to use as guides for the individualization of drug therapy. The therapeutic ranges for several drugs have been identified, and it is likely that new drugs also will be monitored using serum concentrations. Although several individualization methods have been advocated for specific drugs, one simple, reliable method is used commonly. For drugs that exhibit linear pharmacokinetics, C_{ss} changes proportionally with dose. To adjust a patient's drug therapy, a reasonable starting dose is administered for an estimated three to five half-lives. A serum concentration is obtained, assuming that it will reflect C_{ss}. Independent of the route of administration, the new dose (D_{new}) needed to attain the desired C_{ss} ($C_{ss,new}$) is calculated: $D_{new} = D_{old}\ (C_{ss,new}/C_{ss,old})$, where D_{old} and $C_{ss,old}$ are the old dose and old C_{ss}, respectively. To use this method, $C_{ss,old}$ must reflect steady-state conditions. Often patients are noncompliant with regard to their drug dosage and therefore are not at steady state. This occurs not only in outpatients but also in hospital inpatients. Inpatients can spit out oral doses or alter the infusion rates on intravenous pumps after the nurse leaves the hospital room. If $C_{ss,old}$ is much larger or smaller than expected for the D_{old} the patient is taking, one should suspect noncompliance and repeat the serum concentration after another three to five half-lives or change the patient's dose cautiously and monitor for signs of toxicity or lack of effect.

MEASUREMENT OF PHARMACOKINETIC PARAMETERS IN PATIENTS

If it is necessary to determine the kinetic constants for a patient to individualize his or her dose, a small kinetic evaluation is conducted in the individual. In these cases, the number of serum concentrations obtained from the patient is held to the minimum needed to calculate accurate pharmacokinetic parameters and doses. The reason for using fewer serum drug concentrations is to be as cost-effective as possible because these laboratory tests generally cost $20 to $50 each.

Although many drugs follow two-compartment model pharmacokinetics (especially after intravenous administration), a one-compartment model is used to compute kinetic parameters in patients because too many serum concentrations would be needed to accurately determine both the distribution and elimination phases found in the two-compartment model. Because of this, serum concentrations usually are not measured in patients during the distribution phase. Another important reason serum concentrations are not measured during the distribution phase for therapeutic drug monitoring purposes in patients is that drug in the blood and drug in the tissues are not in equilibrium during this time so that serum concentrations do not reflect tissue concentrations. When drug serum concentrations are obtained in patients for the purpose of assessing efficacy or toxicity, it is important that they be measured in the postdistribution phase when drug in the blood is in equilibrium with drug at the site of action.

In the case where the patient has received enough doses to be at steady state, pharmacokinetic parameters can be computed using a predose minimum concentration and a postdose maximum concentration. Under steady-state conditions, serum concentrations after each dose are identical, so the predose minimum concentration is the same before each dose (Fig. 4–10). This situation allows the predose concentration to be used to compute both the patient's $t_{1/2}$ and V. If the drug was given extravascularly or has a significant distribution phase, the postdose concentration should be collected after absorption or distribution is finished. To ensure that steady-state conditions have been achieved, the patient needs to receive the drug on schedule for at least three to five estimated half-lives. To make sure that this is the case, inpatients should have their medication administration

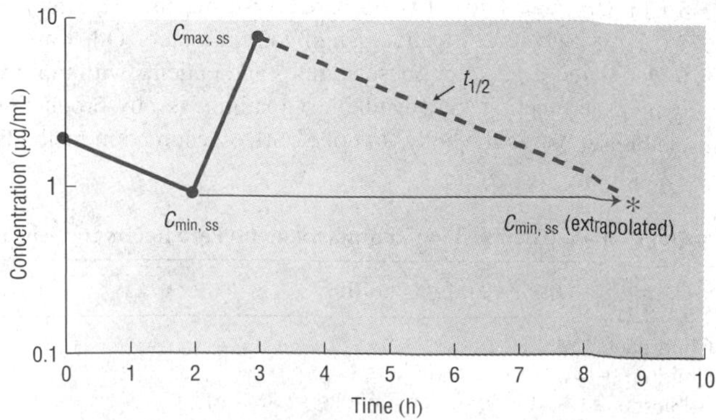

FIGURE 4–10. When a patient has received enough doses to be at steady state, steady-state maximum ($C_{max,ss}$) and minimum ($C_{min,ss}$) concentrations can be used to compute clearance, volume of distribution, and half-life. At steady state, consecutive $C_{min,ss}$ are equal, so the predose value can be extrapolated to the time before the next dose and be used to calculate half-life (dashed line).

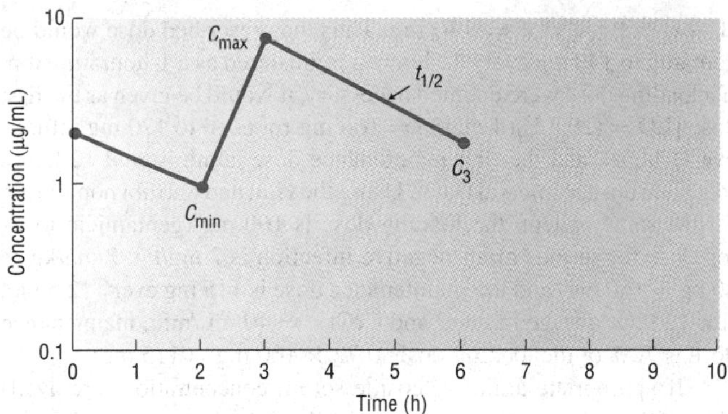

FIGURE 4–11. If a patient has not received enough doses to be at steady state, or doses have been given on an irregular schedule, the minimum concentration (C_{min}), maximum concentration (C_{max}), and an additional postdose concentration (C_3) can be used to compute clearance, volume of distribution, and half-life.

records checked, and the patient's nurse should be consulted regarding missed or late doses. Outpatients should be interviewed about compliance with the prescribed dosage regimen. When compliance with the dosage regimen has been verified, steady-state conditions can be reasonably assumed.

If the patient is not at steady state, an additional postdose serum concentration should be obtained to compute the patient's pharmacokinetic parameters. Ideally, the third concentration (C_3) should be acquired approximately one estimated half-life after the postdose maximum concentration. Getting serum concentrations too close together will hamper the drug assay's ability to measure differences between them, and getting the third sample too late could result in a concentration too low for the assay to detect. In this situation, the predose minimum and postdose maximum concentrations are used to compute V, and both postdose concentrations are used to calculate $t_{1/2}$ (Fig. 4–11).

After Cl, V, and $t_{1/2}$ have been computed for a patient, the dose and dosage interval necessary to achieve desired steady-state serum concentrations can be calculated using one-compartment model equations. Specific examples of these methods to calculate initial doses and individualized doses using serum concentrations are discussed later in this chapter for the aminoglycoside antibiotics, vancomycin, digoxin, theophylline, phenytoin, and cyclosporine.

COMPUTER PROGRAMS

Computer programs that aid in the individualization of therapy are available for many different drugs. The most sophisticated programs use nonlinear regression to fit Cl and V_D to actual serum concentrations obtained in a patient.[28] After drug doses and serum concentrations are entered into the computer, nonlinear least-squares regression programs adjust Cl and V_D until the sum of the squared error between actual (C_{act}) and computer-estimated concentrations (C_{est}) is at a minimum $[\Sigma(C_{est} - C_{act})^2]$. Once estimates of Cl and V_D are available, doses are calculated easily.

Many programs also take into account what the Cl and V_D should be on the basis of disease states and conditions present in the patient.[29] Incorporation of expected population-based parameters allows the computer to use a limited number of serum concentrations (one or two) to provide estimates of Cl and V_D. This type of computer program is called *Bayesian* because it incorporates portions of Bayes' theorem during the fitting routine.[30] Bayesian pharmacokinetic dosing programs are used widely to adjust the dose of a variety of drugs. In the case of renally eliminated drugs (aminoglycosides, vancomycin, digoxin), population estimates for kinetic parameters are generated by entering the patient's age, weight, height, gender, and serum creatinine concentration into the computer program. For hepatically eliminated drugs (theophylline, phenytoin), population estimates for kinetic parameters are computed using the patient's age, weight, and gender, as well as other factors that might change hepatic clearance, such as the presence or absence of disease states (cirrhosis, congestive heart failure) or other drug therapy that might cause a drug interaction. The Bayesian estimates of the pharmacokinetic parameters are then modified using nonlinear least-squares regression fits of serum concentrations to result in individualized parameters for the patient. The individualized parameters are used to compute doses for the patient that will result in desired steady-state concentrations of the drug.

AMINOGLYCOSIDES

Although aminoglycoside pharmacokinetics follow multicompartment models,[31] a one-compartment model appears sufficient to individualize doses in patients.[32] Aminoglycosides usually are given as short-term intermittent intravenous infusions and administered as a single daily dose or multiple doses per day. Initial doses for aminoglycosides can be computed using estimated kinetic parameters derived from population pharmacokinetic data. The elimination rate constant is estimated using the patient's creatinine clearance in the following formula: k (in h^{-1}) $= 0.00293$ (CrCl) $+ 0.014$, where CrCl is the measured or estimated creatinine clearance in milliliters per minute. The volume of distribution is estimated using the average population value for normal-weight (within 30% of ideal weight) individuals equal to 0.26 L/kg [$V = 0.26$(Wt), where Wt is patient weight] or for obese individuals (over 30% ideal weight)[33] by taking into account the patient's excess adipose tissue: $V = 0.26$ [IBW + 0.4(TBW – IBW)], where IBW is ideal body weight [IBW_{males} (in kilograms $= 50 + 2.3(\text{Ht} - 60)$ or $\text{IBW}_{females}$ (in kilograms) $= 45 + 2.3(\text{Ht} - 60)$, where Ht is patient height in inches]. Additional volume-of-distribution population estimates are available for other disease states and conditions such as cystic fibrosis,[34] ascites,[35] and neonates.[36]

Appropriate $C_{max,ss}$ and $C_{min,ss}$ values are selected for the patient based on the site and severity of the infection and the sensitivity of the known or suspected pathogen, as well as avoidance of adverse effects. For example, $C_{max,ss}$ values of 8 to 10 mg/L generally are selected for gram-negative pneumonia patients, whereas $C_{min,ss}$ values less than 2 mg/L usually are chosen to avoid aminoglycoside-induced nephrotoxicity when tobramycin and gentamicin are prescribed using conventional multiple-daily-dosing regimens. Once appropriate steady-state serum concentrations are selected, the dosage interval required to achieve those concentrations is calculated, and τ is rounded to a clinically acceptable value (e.g., 8, 12, 18, 24, 36, 48 hours): $\tau = [(\ln C_{max,ss} - \ln C_{min,ss})/k] + T$. Finally, a dose is computed for the patient using the one-compartment model intermittent intravenous infusion equation at steady state, and the dose is rounded off to the nearest 5 to 10 mg:

$$D = TkV_D C_{max,ss}[(1 - e^{-k\tau})/(1 - e^{-kT})]$$

The Hull and Sarrubi aminoglycoside dosage nomogram (Table 4–5) is based on this dosage calculation method and includes precalculated doses and dosage intervals for a variety of creatinine clearance values.[22] The nomogram assumes that $V_D = 0.26$ L/kg and should not be used to compute doses for disease states with altered V_D.

An example of this initial dosage scheme for a typical case is provided to illustrate the use of the various equations. Mr. JJ is a 65-year-old, 80-kg, 6-ft tall man with the diagnosis of gram-negative pneumonia. His serum creatinine equals 2.1 mg/dL and

TABLE 4–5. Aminoglycoside Dosage Chart

1. Compute patient's creatinine clearance (CrCl) using Cockcroft±Gault method: CrCl = [(140 − age)BW]/(Scr × 72). Multiply by 0.85 for females.
2. Use patient's weight if within 30% of IBW; otherwise use adjusted dosing weight = IBW + [0.40(TBW − IBW)].
3. Select loading dose in mg/kg to provide peak serum concentrations in range listed below for the desired aminoglycoside antibiotic:

Aminoglycoside	Usual Loading Doses	Expected Peak Serum Concentrations
Tobramycin Gentamicin Netilmicin	1.5 to 2.0 mg/kg	4 to 10 μg/mL
Amikacin Kanamycin	5.0 to 7.5 mg/kg	15 to 30 μg/mL

4. Select maintenance dose (as percentage of loading dose) to continue peak serum concentrations indicated above according to desired dosage interval and the patient's creatinine clearance. To maintain usual peak/trough ratio, use dosage intervals in clear areas.

CrCl (mL/min)	Est. Half-Life (h)	Percentage of Loading Dose Required for Dosage Interval Selected: 8 h (%)	12 h (%)	24 h (%)
>90	2–3	90	—	—
90	3.1	84	—	—
80	3.4	80	91	—
70	3.9	76	88	—
60	4.5	71	84	—
50	5.3	65	79	—
40	6.5	57	72	92
30	8.4	48	63	86
25	9.9	43	57	81
20	11.9	37	50	75
17	13.6	33	46	70
15	15.1	31	42	67
12	17.9	27	37	61
10[a]	20.4	24	34	56
7[a]	25.9	19	28	47
5[a]	31.5	16	23	41
2[a]	46.8	11	16	30
0[a]	69.3	8	11	21

[a]Note: Dosing for patients with CrCl ≤ 10 mL/min should be assisted by measuring serum concentrations.
Adapted from Ref. 22.

is stable. Compute a gentamicin dosage regimen (infused over 1 hour) that would provide approximate peak and trough concentrations of $C_{max,ss} = 8$ mg/L and $C_{min,ss} = 1.5$ mg/L, respectively. The patient is within 30% of his ideal body weight [$IBW_{male} = 50 + 2.3\,(72\text{ in} - 60) = 78$ kg] and has stable renal function, so the Cockcroft-Gault creatinine clearance estimation equation can be used: $CrCl_{est} = [(140 - 65\text{ yr})80\text{ kg}]/[72(2.1\text{ mg/dL})] = 40$ mL/ min. The patient's weight and estimated creatinine clearance are used to compute his V and k, respectively: $V = 0.26$ L/kg (80 kg) = 20.8 L, $k = 0.00293\,(40\text{ mL/min}) + 0.014 = 0.131\text{ h}^{-1}$ or $t_{1/2} = 0.693/0.131\text{ h}^{-1}) = 5.3$ h. The dosage interval and dose for the desired serum concentrations would then be calculated: $\tau = [(\ln 8\text{ mg/L} - \ln 1.5\text{ mg/L})/0.131\text{ h}^{-1}] + 1\text{ h} = 13.7$ h rounded to 12 h, $D = (1\text{ h})(0.131\text{ h}^{-1})(20.8\text{ L})(8\text{ mg/L})[(1 - e^{-(0.131\text{ h}^{-1})(12\text{ h})})/(1 - e^{-(0.131\text{ h}^{-1})(1\text{ h})})] = 140$ mg. Thus the prescribed dose would be gentamicin 140 mg every 12 hours administered as a 1-hour infusion. If a loading dose were deemed necessary, it would be given as the first dose [LD = (20.8 L)(8 mg/L) = 166 mg rounded to 170 mg infused over 1 hour], and the first maintenance dose administered 12 hours (e.g., one dosage interval) later. Using the Hull and Sarrubi nomogram for the same patient, the loading dose is 160 mg (gentamicin loading dose for serious gram-negative infection is 2 mg/kg: 2 mg/kg × 80 kg = 160 mg) and the maintenance dose is 115 mg every 12 hours (for 12 hour dosage interval and $CrCl_{est} = 40$ mL/min, maintenance dose is 72% of the loading dose: 0.72 × 160 mg = 115 mg).

If appropriate aminoglycoside serum concentrations are available, kinetic parameters can be calculated at any point in therapy. When the patient is not at steady state, serum aminoglycoside concentrations are obtained before a dose (C_{min}), after a dose administered as an intravenous infusion of about 1 hour, or as a ½-hour infusion followed by a ½-hour waiting period to allow for drug distribution (C_{max}), and at one additional postdose time (C_3) approximately one estimated half-life after C_{max}. The $t_{1/2}$ and k are computed using C_{max} and C_3: $k = (\ln C_{max} - \ln C_3)/\Delta t$ and $t_{1/2} = 0.693/k$, where Δt is the time that expired between the times C_{max} and C_3 were obtained. If the patient is at steady state, serum aminoglycoside concentrations are obtained before a dose ($C_{min,ss}$) and after a dose administered as an intravenous infusion of about 1 hour or as a ½-hour infusion followed by a ½-hour waiting period to allow for drug distribution ($C_{max,ss}$). The $t_{1/2}$ and k are computed using $C_{max,ss}$ and $C_{min,ss}$: $k = (\ln C_{max,ss} - \ln C_{min,ss})/(\tau - T)$ and $t_{1/2} = 0.693/k$, where τ is the dosage interval and T is the dose infusion time or dose infusion time plus waiting time.

Assuming a one-compartment model, the following equation is used to compute V_D[32]:

$$V_D = [(D/T)(1 - e^{-kT})]/\{k[C_{max} - (C_{min}e^{-kT})]\}$$

where D is dose and T is duration of infusion. Once these are known, the dose and dosage interval (τ) can be calculated for any desired maximum $C_{ss}(C_{max,ss})$ and minimum $C_{ss}(C_{min,ss})$:

$$\tau = [(\ln C_{max,ss} - \ln C_{min,ss})/k] + T$$

$$D = TkV_DC_{max,ss}[(1 - e^{-k\tau})/(1 - e^{-kT})]$$

The dose and dosage interval should be rounded to provide clinically accepted values (every 8, 12, 18, 24, 36, and 48 hours for dosage interval, nearest 5 to 10 mg for dose). This method also has been used to individualize intravenous theophylline dosage regimens.[37]

To provide an example of this technique, the problem given previously will be extended to include steady-state concentrations. Mr. JJ was prescribed gentamicin 140 mg every 12 hours (infused over 1 hour) for the treatment of gram-negative pneumonia. Steady-state trough ($C_{min,ss}$) and peak ($C_{max,ss}$) values were obtained before and after the fourth dose was given (more than three to five estimated half-lives), respectively, and equaled $C_{min,ss} = 2.8$ mg/L and $C_{max,ss} = 8.5$ mg/L. Clinically, the patient was improving with decreased white blood cell counts and body temperatures and a resolving chest x-ray. However, the serum creatinine value had increased to 2.5 mg/dL. Because of this, a new dosage regimen with a similar peak (to maintain high intrapulmonary levels) but lower trough (to decrease the risk of drug-induced nephrotoxicity) concentrations was suggested. The patient's elimination rate constant and half-life can be computed using the following formulas: $k = (\ln 8.5\text{ mg/L} - \ln 2.8\text{ mg/L})/(12\text{ h} - 1\text{ h}) = 0.101\text{ h}^{-1}$ and $t_{1/2} = 0.693/0.101\text{ h}^{-1} = 6.9$ h. The patient's volume of distribution can be calculated using the following equation:

$$V = \left[(140\ \text{mg/1 h})\left(1 - e^{-(0.101\ \text{h}^{-1})(1\ \text{h})}\right)\right] \Big/ \left(0.101\ \text{h}^{-1}\left\{8.5\ \text{mg/L} - \left[(2.8\ \text{mg/L})\, e^{-(0.101\ \text{h}^{-1})(1\ \text{h})}\right]\right\}\right) = 22.3\ \text{L}$$

Thus the patient's volume of distribution was larger and half-life was longer than originally estimated, and this led to higher serum concentrations than anticipated. To achieve the desired serum concentrations ($C_{\text{min,ss}} = 1.5$ mg/L and $C_{\text{max,ss}} = 8$ mg/L), the patient's actual kinetic parameters are used to compute a new dose and dosage interval: $\tau = [(\ln 8\ \text{mg/L} - \ln 1.5\ \text{mg/L})/0.101\ \text{h}^{-1}] + 1\ \text{h} = 17.6$ h, rounded to 18 h and

$$D = (1\ \text{h})(0.101\ \text{h}^{-1})(22.3\ \text{L})(8\ \text{mg/L})\left[\left(1 - e^{-(0.101\ \text{h}^{-1})(18\ \text{h})}\right) \Big/ \left(1 - e^{-(0.101\ \text{h}^{-1})(1\ \text{h})}\right)\right] = 157\ \text{mg, rounded to 160 mg}$$

Thus the new dose would be gentamicin 160 mg every 18 hours and infused over 1 hour; the first dose of the new dosage regimen would be given 18 hours (e.g., the new dosage interval) after the last dose of the old dosage regimen.

Because aminoglycoside antibiotics exhibit concentration-dependent bacterial killing and the postantibiotic effect is longer with higher concentrations, investigators studied the possibility of giving a higher dose of aminoglycoside once daily. Generally, these studies have shown comparable microbiologic and clinical cure rates for many infections and about the same rate of nephrotoxicity (approximately 5% to 10%) as with conventional dosing. Ototoxicity has not been monitored using audiometry in most of these investigations, but loss of hearing in the conversational range, as well as signs and symptoms of vestibular toxicity, usually has been assessed and found to be similar to that with aminoglycoside therapy dosed conventionally. Based on these data, clinicians have begun using extended-interval dosing in selected patients. For *Pseudomonas aeruginosa* infections where the organism has an expected MIC $\approx$ 2 mg/L, peak concentrations between 20 and 30 mg/L and trough concentrations of less than 1 mg/L for gentamicin or tobramycin have been suggested.[38] At the present time, there is not a consensus on how to approach concentration monitoring using this mode of administration. However, a nomogram that adjusts doses based on a single postdose concentration to achieve these steady-state concentration goals has been proposed (Fig. 4–12).

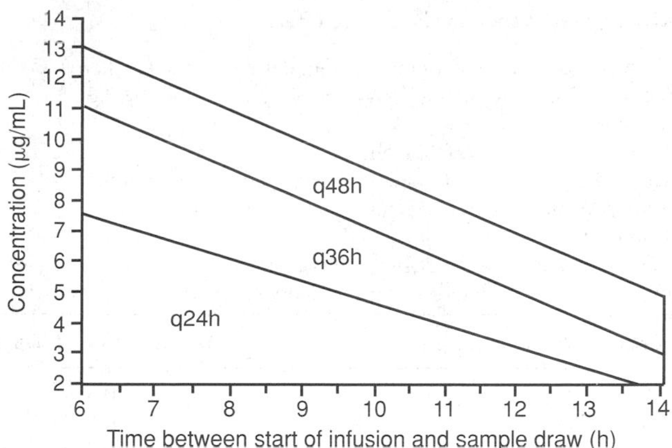

1. Administer 7 mg/kg gentamicin with initial dosage interval:

Estimated CrCl (mL/min)	Initial dosage interval
≥60 mL/min	q24h
40–59 mL/min	q36h
20–39 mL/min	q48h
<20 mL/min	Monitor serial concentrations and administer next dose when <1 μg/mL.

2. Obtain timed serum concentration 6 to 14 hours after dose (ideally first dose).
3. Alter dosage interval to that indicated by the nomogram zone (above q48h zone, monitor serial concentrations and administer next dose when <1 μg/mL)

FIGURE 4–12. Hartford nomogram for extended-interval aminoglycosides. (Adapted from Ref. 38.)

The dose is 7 mg/kg of gentamicin or tobramycin. The initial dosage interval is set according to the patient's creatinine clearance (see Fig. 4–12). The Hartford nomogram includes a method to adjust doses based on serum concentrations. This portion of the nomogram contains average serum concentration time lines for gentamicin or tobramycin in patients with creatinine clearances of 60, 40, and 20 mL/min. A serum concentration is measured 6 to 14 hours after the first dose is given, and this concentration/time point is plotted on the graph (see Fig. 4–12). The modified dosage interval is indicated by which zone the serum concentration/time point falls in. Because cystic fibrosis patients have a different volume of distribution (0.35 L/kg) than assumed by this dosing technique and extended-interval dosing has not been tested adequately in patients with endocarditis, the Hartford nomogram should not be used in these situations.

To illustrate how the nomogram is used, the same patient example used previously will be repeated for this dosage approach. Mr. JJ is an 80-kg man with a CrCl_{est} of 40 mL/min. Using the Hartford nomogram, the patient would receive gentamicin 560 mg every 36 hours (7 mg/kg $\times$ 80 kg = 560 mg, initial dosage interval for $\text{CrCl}_{\text{est}} =$ 40 mL/min is 36 hours). Ten hours after the first dose was given, the serum gentamicin concentration is 8.2 mg/L. According to the graph contained in the nomogram, the dosage interval should be changed to 48 hours. The new dose is 560 mg every 48 hours.

VANCOMYCIN

Vancomycin requires multicompartment models to completely describe its serum-concentration-versus-time curves. However, if peak serum concentrations are obtained after the distribution phase is completed (usually ½ to 1 hour after a 1-hour intravenous infusion), a one-compartment model can be used for patient dosage calculations. Also, since vancomycin has a relatively long half-life compared with the infusion time, only a small amount of drug is eliminated during infusion, and it is usually not necessary to use more complex intravenous infusion equations. Thus simple intravenous bolus equations can be used to calculate vancomycin doses for most patients. Although a recent review paper[39] questioned the clinical usefulness of measuring vancomycin concentrations on a routine basis, research articles[40,41] have shown potential benefits in obtaining vancomycin concentrations in selected patient populations. Some clinicians advocate monitoring only steady-state trough concentrations of vancomycin.[42] The

TABLE 4–6. Vancomycin Dosage Chart

1. Compute patient's creatinine clearance (CrCl) using Cockcroft–Gault method: CrCl = $[(140 - \text{age})\text{BW}]/(S_{cr} \times 72)$. Multiply by 0.85 for females.
2. Use patient's total body weight to compute doses.
3. Dosage chart designed to achieve peak serum concentrations of 30 μg/mL and trough concentrations of 7.5 μg/mL.
4. Compute loading dose of 25 mg/kg.
5. Compute maintenance dose of 19 mg/kg given at the dosage interval listed in the following chart for the patient's CrCl:

CrCl (mL/min)	Dosage Interval (Days)
≥120	0.5
100	0.6
80	0.75
60	1.0
40	1.5
30	2.0
20	2.5
10	4.0
5	6.0
0	12.0

Adapted from Ref. 45.

decision to conduct vancomycin concentration monitoring should be made on a patient-by-patient basis.

Initial doses of vancomycin can be computed for adult patients using estimated kinetic parameters derived from population pharmacokinetic data. Clearance is estimated using the patient's creatinine clearance in the following equation[41]: Cl (in mL/min/kg) = 0.695 (CrCl in mL/min/kg) + 0.05. The volume of distribution is computed assuming the standard value of 0.7 L/kg: $V_D = 0.7(\text{Wt})$, where Wt is patient weight. In the case of obese patients, actual or total body weight is used in the calculations.[44] The elimination rate constant is calculated using clearance and volume-of-distribution estimates, correcting for possible differences in units for these parameters: $k = \text{Cl}/V_D$. A nomogram that uses this type of approach for vancomycin therapy is available to rapidly determine initial doses for patients[45] (Table 4–6).

Steady-state peak and trough concentrations are chosen for the patient based on the site and severity of the infection as well as the known or suspected pathogen and avoidance of potential side effects. $C_{max,ss}$ values between 20 and 40 mg/L and $C_{min,ss}$ values between 5 and 10 mg/L typically are used for patients with moderate to severe methicillin-resistant *Staphylococcus aureus* infections. After appropriate steady-state concentrations are chosen, the dosage interval required to attain those concentrations is computed, and τ is rounded to a clinically acceptable value (12, 18, 24, 36, 48, and 72 hours): $\tau = (\ln C_{max,ss} - \ln C_{min,ss})/k$. Finally, the maintenance dose is computed for the patient using a one-compartment model intravenous bolus equation at steady state, and the dose is rounded off to the nearest 50 to 100 mg:

$$D = C_{max,ss} V_D(1 - e^{-k\tau})$$

If desired, a loading dose can be computed using the following equation:

$$\text{LD} = V_D C_{max,ss}$$

The following case will illustrate the use of this dosage methodology. Ms HJ is a 65-year-old, 68-kg, 5-ft 4-in tall coronary artery bypass graft surgery patient who has developed a surgical wound infection with *S. aureus* the suspected pathogen. Her serum creatinine is 1.8 mg/dL and stable. Compute a vancomycin dosage regimen that would provide approximate peak (obtained 1 hour after a 1-hour infusion) and trough concentrations of 30 and 7 mg/L, respectively. The patient is within 30% of her ideal body weight [$\text{IBW}_{female} = 45 + 2.3$ (64 in − 60) = 54 kg] and has stable renal function, so the Cockcroft-Gault creatinine clearance estimation formula can be used: $\text{CrCl}_{est} = 0.85[(140 - 65 \text{ yr})\ 68 \text{ kg}]/[72(1.8 \text{ mg/dL})] = 33$ mL/min. The patient's weight and estimated creatinine clearance are used to calculate her estimated Cl, V_D, and k, respectively: Cl = 0.695 (33 mL/min/68 kg) + 0.05 = 0.387 mL/min/kg, V_D = 0.7 L/kg (68 kg) = 48 L, and $k = [(0.387 \text{ mL/min/kg})(68 \text{ kg})(60 \text{ min/h})]/[(48 \text{ L})(1000 \text{ mL/L})] = 0.033 \text{ h}^{-1}$ or $t_{1/2} = 0.693/0.033 \text{ h}^{-1} = 21$ h. The dosage interval, maintenance dose, and loading dose for the desired serum concentrations can then be computed: $\tau = (\ln 30 \text{ mg/L} - \ln 7 \text{ mg/L})/0.033 \text{ h}^{-1} = 44$ h, rounded to 48 h, $D = (30 \text{ mg/L})\ (48 \text{ L})(1 - e^{-(0.033 \text{ h}^{-1})(48 \text{ h})}) = 1145$ mg, rounded to 1200 mg, LD = (48 L)(30 mg/L) = 1440 mg, rounded to 1450 mg. Therefore, the prescribed doses would be vancomycin 1200 mg every 48 hours administered as a 1-hour infusion. If a loading dose was used, it would be given as the first dose, and the first maintenance dose would be administered 48 hours (one dosage interval) later. Using the Matzke nomogram for the same patient, the loading dose would be 1700 mg (vancomycin loading dose is 25 mg/kg: 25 mg/kg × 68 kg = 1700 mg), followed by a maintenance dose of 1300 mg every 48 hours (for CrCl_{est} = 30 mL/min, maintenance dose is 19 mg/kg every 2 days: 19 mg/kg × 68 kg = 1292 mg, rounded to 1300 mg).

If appropriate vancomycin serum concentrations are available, kinetic parameters can be computed at any point in therapy. When the patient is not at steady state, serum vancomycin concentrations are obtained before a dose (C_{min}), after a dose administered as an intravenous infusion of 1 hour followed by a ½- to 1-hour waiting period to allow for drug distribution (C_{max}), and at one additional postdose time (C_3) approximately one estimated half-life after C_{max}. The $t_{1/2}$ and k are computed using C_{max} and C_3: $k = (\ln C_{max} - \ln C_3)/\Delta t$ and $t_{1/2} = 0.693/k$, where Δt is the time that expired between the times C_{max} and C_3 were obtained. If the patient is at steady state, serum vancomycin concentrations are obtained before a dose ($C_{min,ss}$) and after a dose administered as an intravenous infusion of about 1 hour followed by a ½- to 1-hour waiting period to allow for drug distribution ($C_{max,ss}$). The $t_{1/2}$ and k are computed using $C_{max,ss}$ and $C_{min,ss}$: $k = (\ln C_{max,ss} - \ln C_{min,ss})/(\tau - T_{max})$ and $t_{1/2} = 0.693/k$, where τ is the dosage interval and T_{max} is the dose infusion time plus waiting time. If only a steady-state trough concentration of vancomycin is available, the dose can be adjusted using linear pharmacokinetics: $D_{new} = D_{old}(C_{ss,new}/C_{ss,old})$.

Assuming a one-compartment model, the following equation is used to compute V_D:

$$V_D = D/(C_{max} - C_{min})$$

where D is dose and T_{max} is the dose infusion time plus waiting time. Once these are known, the dose and dosage interval (τ) can be calculated for any desired maximum $C_{ss}(C_{max,ss})$ and minimum $C_{ss}(C_{min,ss})$:

$$\tau = (\ln C_{max,ss} - \ln C_{min,ss})/k$$

$$D = C_{max,ss} V_D(1 - e^{-k\tau})$$

The dose and dosage interval should be rounded to provide clinically accepted values (every 12, 18, 24, 36, 48, and 72 hours for dosage interval, nearest 50 to 100 mg for dose).

To provide an example for this dosage-calculation method, the preceding problem will be extended to include steady-state concentrations. Ms HJ was prescribed vancomycin 1200 mg every 48 hours (infused over 1 hour) for the treatment of a surgical wound infection. Steady-state trough ($C_{min,ss}$) and peak ($C_{max,ss}$) values ($C_{max,ss}$ obtained 1 hour after end of infusion) were obtained before and after the third dose was given (more than three to five estimated half-lives), respectively, and equaled $C_{min,ss} = 2.5$ mg/L and $C_{max,ss} = 22.4$ mg/L. Clinically, the patient had improved somewhat, but the white blood cell count was still elevated, and the patient was still febrile. Because of this, a modified dosage regimen with a $C_{max,ss} = 30$ mg/L and $C_{min,ss} = 7$ mg/L was suggested to maintain trough concentrations three to five times above the minimal inhibitory concentration (MIC) for the suspected pathogen. The patient's actual elimination rate constant and half-life can be calculated using the following formulas: $k = (\ln 22.4\,\text{mg/L} - \ln 2.5\,\text{mg/L})/(48\,\text{h} - 2\,\text{h}) = 0.048\,\text{h}^{-1}$ and $t_{1/2} = 0.693/0.048\,\text{h}^{-1} = 14.4$ h. The patient's volume of distribution can be calculated using the following equation:

$$V_D = 1200\,\text{mg}/(22.4\,\text{mg/L} - 2.5\,\text{mg/L}) = 60\,\text{L}$$

Thus the patient's volume of distribution was larger and half-life shorter than originally estimated, and this led to lower serum concentrations than anticipated. To achieve the desired serum concentrations ($C_{max,ss} = 30$ mg/L and $C_{min,ss} = 7$ mg/L), the patient's actual kinetic parameters are used to calculate a new dose and dosage interval:

$$\begin{aligned}\tau &= (\ln 30\,\text{mg/L} - \ln 7\,\text{mg/L})/0.048\text{h}^{-1}\\ &= 30\,\text{h, rounded to } 36\,\text{h}\\ D &= (30\,\text{mg/L})(60\,\text{L})\left(1 - e^{-(0.048\,\text{h}^{-1})(36\text{h})}\right)\\ &= 1480\,\text{mg, rounded to } 1500\,\text{mg}\end{aligned}$$

The new dose would be vancomycin 1500 mg every 36 hours (infused over 1 hour); the first dose of the new dosage regimen would be given 36 hours (the new dosage interval) after the last dose of the old dosage regimen.

DIGOXIN

Digoxin pharmacokinetics are best described by a two-compartment model. However, because digoxin has a long half-life compared with its dosage interval and a very long distribution phase, simple pharmacokinetic equations can be used to individualize dosing when postdistribution serum concentrations are used. Digoxin can be given as an intravenous injection and orally as elixir ($F = 0.8$), tablets ($F = 0.7$), or capsules ($F = 0.9$). When given orally, the appropriate bioavailability fraction must be used to compute the correct dose. Initial doses of digoxin can be computed using population pharmacokinetic data obtained from published studies. Digoxin clearance is estimated using the patient's creatinine clearance in the following formula[20]: Cl (in milliliters per minute) = 1.303 (CrCl in milliliters per minute) + Cl_m, where Cl_m is metabolic clearance and equals 40 mL/min for patients with no or mild heart failure or 20 mL/min for patients with moderate to severe heart failure. The volume of distribution decreases with declining renal function and is estimated using the following equation[20]: V_D (in liters) = 226 + {[298 (CrCl in milliliters per minute)]/[29.1 + (CrCl in milliliters per minute)]}. The elimination rate constant can be computed by taking the product of Cl and V_D: $k = \text{Cl}/V_D$. For obese individuals, digoxin dosing should be based on ideal body weight.[46]

Appropriate C_{ss} values are chosen for the patient based on the disease state being treated, the goal of therapy, and the avoidance of adverse effects. The inotropic effects of digoxin occur at lower concentrations than do the chronotropic effects. Therefore, initial serum concentrations of digoxin for the treatment of heart failure generally are 1 ng/mL or less and for the treatment of atrial fibrillation are 1 to 1.5 ng/mL. Once the appropriate C_{ss} is selected, a dose is computed for the patient: $D/\tau = (C_{ss}\text{Cl})/F$.

An example of this initial dosage scheme is provided in the following case. Mr. PO is a 72-year-old, 83-kg, 5-ft 11-in man admitted to the hospital for the treatment of community-acquired pneumonia. While in the hospital, Mr. PO develops atrial fibrillation, and the decision is made to treat him with digoxin to provide ventricular rate control. His serum creatinine is 2.5 mg/dL and stable. Calculate an intravenous loading dose and oral maintenance dose that will achieve a C_{ss} of 1.5 ng/mL. The Cockcroft-Gault equation can be used to estimate the patient's creatinine clearance because his serum creatinine is stable and he is within 30% of his ideal weight [$\text{IBW}_{male} = 50 + 2.3(71\,\text{in} - 60) = 75$ kg]: CrCl = [(140 − 72 yr)83 kg]/[72(2.5 mg/dL)] = 31 mL/min. Using the estimated CrCl, both Cl and V_D can be computed:

$$\text{Cl} = 1.303(31\,\text{mL/min}) + 40 = 80\,\text{mL/min}$$

$$V_D = 226 + \{[298\,(31\,\text{mL/min})]/[29.1 + (31\,\text{mL/min})]\} = 380\,\text{L}$$

The maintenance dose will be given as digoxin tablets, so $F = 0.7$ in the dosing equation: $D/\tau = [(1.5\,\mu\text{g/L})\,(80\,\text{mL/min})\,(60\,\text{min/h})(24\,\text{h/d})]/[0.7(1000\,\text{mL/L})] = 247\,\mu\text{g/d}$, rounded to 250 μg/d. The loading dose will be given intravenously as digoxin injection: LD = (1.5 μg/L) (380 L) = 570 μg, rounded to 500 μg. The loading dose would be given 50% now (250 μg), 25% (125 μg) in 4 to 6 hours after monitoring the patient's heart rate and blood pressure and assessing the patient for digoxin adverse effects, and the final 25% (125 μg) 4 to 6 hours later after monitoring the same clinical parameters. The first maintenance dose would be given one dosage interval (in this case 24 hours) after the first part of the loading dose was given.

Adjustment of digoxin doses using steady-state concentrations is accomplished using linear pharmacokinetics and dosage ratios: $D_{new} = D_{old}(C_{ss,new}/C_{ss,old})$. For example, Mr. PO's atrial fibrillation responded to digoxin therapy, and he was discharged after resolution of his pneumonia. A month later he was followed up in the clinic with moderate nausea, possibly due to digoxin toxicity. His heart rate was 55 beats per minute. A steady-state digoxin concentration was obtained and reported by the clinic laboratory as 2.2 μg/L. Compute a new dose for the patient to achieve a C_{ss} of 1.5 μg/L. The digoxin C_{ss} and old dose would be used to calculate a new dose using the linear pharmacokinetic equation: $D_{new} = 250\,\mu\text{g/d}\,[(1.5\,\mu\text{g/L})/(2.2\,\mu\text{g/L})] = 170\,\mu\text{g/d}$. This approximate average daily dose could be achieved by having the patient alternate taking two 125-μg tablets (250 μg) and one 125 μg tablet daily giving an average dose equal to 187.5 μg/d ([250 μg + 125 μg]/2 = 187.5 μg/d).

THEOPHYLLINE

Theophylline disposition is described most accurately by nonlinear kinetics.[47,48] However, at the usual doses, theophylline acts as if it obeys linear kinetics in most patients. Initial theophylline doses are computed by taking a detailed medical history of the patient and noting disease states and conditions that are known to change theophylline disposition. Age, smoking of tobacco-containing products, heart failure, and liver disease are among the important factors that alter theophylline kinetic parameters and dosage requirements. Once the patient has been assessed, average theophylline kinetic parameters obtained from the literature for patients similar to the one being currently treated are used to compute either oral or intravenous doses. Dosage guidelines that take into account most common disease states and conditions that change theophylline kinetic parameters are available[49] (see Table 4–4). Once theophylline is administered, the patient is monitored for the therapeutic effect and potential adverse effects. Theophylline concentrations are then used to individualize the theophylline dose that the patient receives. An example of this approach was given previously for a patient case in the section on drug dosing in patients with liver disease.

Continuous intravenous infusions of theophylline (or its salt, aminophylline) can be individualized rapidly by determining the patient's Cl before steady state occurs.[50] Assuming that the patient receives theophylline only by continuous intravenous infusion (previous doses of sustained-release oral theophylline are completely absorbed), two serum theophylline concentrations are obtained 4 hours or more apart. The infusion rate (k_0) cannot be changed between the times the concentrations are drawn. With one-compartment model equations, the first (C_1) and second (C_2) theophylline concentrations are used to calculate theophylline Cl:

$$\mathrm{Cl} = 2k_0/(C_1 + C_2) + \{2V_D(C_1 - C_2)/[(C_1 + C_2)(t_2 - t_1)]\}$$

V_D is assumed to be 0.5 L/kg, and t_1 and t_2 are the times at which C_1 and C_2, respectively, are obtained. Once Cl is known, k_0 can be computed easily for any desired $C_{ss}(C_{ss} = k_0/\mathrm{Cl})$. This method probably can be applied to other drugs that are administered as continuous intravenous infusions, such as intravenous antiarrhythmics, when rapid individualization of drug dosage is desirable.

An example of this approach can be obtained by continuing the theophylline patient case from the section on drug dosing in liver disease. In this example, a 55-year-old, 70-kg man with liver cirrhosis was prescribed a loading dose of theophylline 350 mg intravenously over 20 to 30 minutes, followed by a maintenance dose of 15 mg/h of theophylline as a continuous infusion. The infusion began at 9 A.M., blood samples were obtained at 10 A.M. and 4 P.M., and the clinical laboratory reported the theophylline serum concentrations as 9.6 and 12.3 mg/L, respectively. The patient's theophylline clearance and revised continuous infusion to maintain a C_{ss} of 15 mg/L can be computed as follows (patient's V_D estimated at 0.5 L/kg):

$$\begin{aligned}\mathrm{Cl} &= 2(15\,\mathrm{mg/h})/(10.9\,\mathrm{mg/L} + 12.3\,\mathrm{mg/L})\\ &\quad + \{2(0.5\,\mathrm{L/kg} \times 70\,\mathrm{kg})(10.9\,\mathrm{mg/L} - 12.3\,\mathrm{mg/L})/\\ &\quad [(10.9\,\mathrm{mg/L} + 12.3\,\mathrm{mg/L})(16 - 10\,\mathrm{h})]\}\\ &= 0.59\,\mathrm{L/h}\\ k_0 &= C_{ss}\,\mathrm{Cl} = (15\,\mathrm{mg/L})(0.59\,\mathrm{L/h}) = 9\,\mathrm{mg/h\ theophylline}\end{aligned}$$

If theophylline is to be given as the aminophylline salt form, the doses would need to be changed to reflect the fact that aminophylline contains only 85% theophylline ($k_0 = 9$ mg/h theophylline/0.85 = 11 mg/h aminophylline).

If continuous intravenous infusions or oral dosage regimens are given long enough for steady state to occur (three to five estimated half-lives based on previous studies conducted in similar patients), linear pharmacokinetics can be used to adjust doses for either route of administration: $D_{new} = D_{old}(C_{ss,new}/C_{ss,old})$. For example, a patient receiving 200 mg of sustained-release oral theophylline every 12 hours with a theophylline steady-state serum concentration of 9.5 μg/mL can have the dose required to achieve a new steady-state concentration equal to 15 μg/mL computed by applying linear pharmacokinetics: $D_{new} = 200\,\mathrm{mg}[(15\,\mu\mathrm{g/mL})/(9.5\,\mu\mathrm{g/mL})] = 316\,\mathrm{mg}$, rounded to 300 mg. Thus the new theophylline dose would be 300 mg every 12 hours.

PHENYTOIN

Phenytoin doses are very difficult to individualize because the drug follows Michaelis-Menten kinetics and there is a large amount of interpatient variability in V_{max} and K_m. Initial maintenance doses of phenytoin in adults usually range between 4 and 7 mg/kg per day, yielding starting doses of 300–400 mg/d in most individuals. If needed, loading doses of phenytoin or fosphenytoin (a prodrug of phenytoin used intravenously) can be administered in adults at a dose of 15 mg/kg, which is approximately 1000 mg in many individuals. Loading doses of phenytoin can be given orally but need to be administered in divided doses separated by several hours in order to avoid decreased bioavailability (400 mg, 300 mg, and then 300 mg with each dose separated by 4 to 6 hours). Since phenytoin is metabolized hepatically, decreased doses may be needed in patients with liver disease. Because phenytoin follows dose-dependent pharmacokinetics, the half-life of phenytoin increases for a patient as the maintenance dose increases. Therefore, the time to steady-state phenytoin concentrations increases with dose. On average, at a phenytoin dose of 300 mg/d, it takes approximately 5 to 7 days to achieve steady state; at a dose of 400 mg/d, it takes approximately 10 to 14 days to achieve steady state; and at a dose of 500 mg/d, it takes approximately 21 to 28 days to achieve steady state. It should be noted that the injectable and capsule dosage forms of phenytoin are phenytoin sodium, and the labeled dosage amounts contain 92% of active phenytoin [300-mg phenytoin sodium capsules contain 276 mg (300 mg × 0.92 = 276 mg) of active phenytoin]. Unbound phenytoin concentrations are useful in patients with hypoalbuminemia (liver disease, nephrotic syndrome, pregnancy, cystic fibrosis, burns, trauma, malnourishment, elderly), in patients where displacement with endogenous compounds is possible (hyperbilirubinemia, liver disease, end-stage renal disease), or in patients receiving other drugs that may displace phenytoin from plasma-protein-binding sights (valproic acid, aspirin therapy > 2 g/d, warfarin, nonsteroidal anti-inflammatory drugs with high albumin binding).

After steady state has occurred, phenytoin serum concentrations can be obtained as an aid to dosage adjustment. A simple, easy way to approximate new serum concentrations after a dosage adjustment with phenytoin is to temporarily assume linear pharmacokinetics and then add 15% to 20% for a dosage increase or subtract 15% to 20% for a dosage decrease to account for Michaelis-Menten kinetics. For example, Ms PP is a 35-year-old, 65-kg patient with grand mal seizures who is receiving phenytoin capsules 300 mg orally at bedtime. A steady-state concentration of 9.2 μg/mL is measured. It is observed that her seizure frequency decreased by only about 15% and that she has no adverse effects due to phenytoin treatment. Because of this, her phenytoin dose is increased to 400 mg orally at bedtime. The expected phenytoin steady-state concentration would be estimated using linear pharmacokinetics [$C_{new} = (D_{new}/D_{old})C_{old} = (400\,\mathrm{mg}/300\,\mathrm{mg})/(9.2\,\mu\mathrm{g/mL}) = 12.3\,\mu\mathrm{g/mL}$] and then increased by 15% to 20% to account for nonlinear kinetics [$C_{new} = 1.15\,(12.3\,\mu\mathrm{g/mL}) = 14.1\,\mu\mathrm{g/mL}$]. (*Note:* A 15% increase was chosen for an estimated concentration of less than 15 μg/mL; a 20% increase would be used if the estimated concentration was 15 μg/mL or more.) Thus the patient would be expected to have a steady-state phenytoin concentration of approximately 14 μg/mL due to the dosage increase. An alternative approach would be to use a graphic Bayesian method that allows an estimate of V_{max} and K_m from one steady-state phenytoin concentration and the prediction of new steady-state concentrations when doses are changed.[51]

Other methods used to individualize phenytoin doses involve rearrangements of the Michaelis-Menten equation [$\mathrm{DR} = V_{max}C_{ss}/$

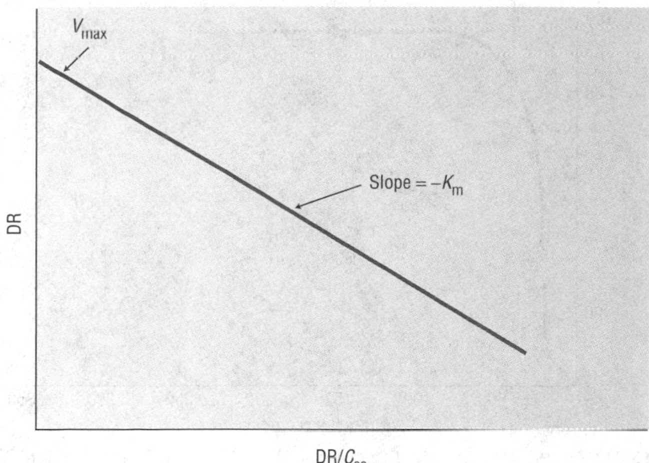

FIGURE 4–13. Relationship between dosage rate (DR) and steady state serum concentrations (C_{SS}).

$(K_m + C_{ss})$, in which DR is the dosage rate at steady state] so that two or more doses and C_{ss} values can be used to obtain graphic solutions for V_{max} and K_m. One rearrangement[52] is DR = $-K_m(\text{DR}/C_{ss}) + V_{max}$. When DR is plotted on the y axis and DR/C_{ss} is plotted on the x axis of Cartesian graph paper, a straight line with a y intercept of V_{max} and slope equal to $-K_m$ is found (Fig. 4–13). To use this method, patients are prescribed an initial phenytoin dose, and C_{ss} is obtained. The phenytoin dose is then changed, and a second C_{ss} from the new dose is obtained. Each dose is divided by its respective C_{ss} to derive DR/C_{ss} values. The DR/C_{ss} and C_{ss} values are plotted on the graph to calculate V_{max} (y intercept) and K_m (−slope). The steady-state Michaelis-Menten equation can be used to compute C_{ss} for a given DR or a DR for any C_{ss}.

CYCLOSPORINE

Because of the large amount of variability in cyclosporine pharmacokinetics, even when concurrent disease states and conditions are identified, many clinicians believe that the use of standard cyclosporine doses for various situations is warranted. Indeed, most transplant centers use doses that are determined using a cyclosporine dosage protocol. The original computations of these doses were based on the pharmacokinetic dosing methods described in preceding sections and subsequently modified based on clinical experience. In general, the expected cyclosporine steady-state concentration used to compute these doses depends on the type of transplanted tissue and the posttransplantation time line. Generally speaking, initial oral doses of 8–18 mg/kg per day or intravenous doses of 3–6 mg/kg per day (one-third the oral dose to account for approximately 30% oral bioavailability) are used and vary greatly from institution to institution. For obese individuals (more than 30% over ideal body weight), ideal body weight should be used to compute initial doses.

It is likely that doses computed using patient population characteristics will not always produce cyclosporine concentrations that are expected or desirable. Additionally, there is a very high amount of interday variation in cyclosporine concentrations. Because of pharmacokinetic variability, the narrow therapeutic index of cyclosporine, and the severity of cyclosporine adverse side effects, measurement of cyclosporine concentrations is mandatory for patients to ensure that therapeutic, nontoxic levels are present. When cyclosporine concentrations are measured in patients and a dosage change is necessary, clinicians should seek to use the simplest, most straightforward method available to determine a dose that will provide safe and effective treatment. In most cases, a simple dosage ratio can be used to change cyclosporine doses using steady-state concentrations and assuming that the drug follows linear pharmacokinetics:

$$D_{new} = D_{old}(C_{ss,new}/C_{ss,old}).$$

For example, LK is a 50-year-old, 75-kg, 5-ft 11-in male renal transplant recipient who is receiving oral cyclosporine 400 mg every 12 hours. The current steady-state blood cyclosporine concentration is 375 ng/mL. To compute a cyclosporine dose that will provide a steady-state concentration of 200 ng/mL, linear pharmacokinetic equations can be used. The new dose to attain the desired concentration should be proportional to the old dose that produced the measured concentration (total daily dose = 400 mg/dose × 2 doses/d = 800 mg/d):

$$D_{new} = (C_{ss,new}/C_{ss,old})D_{old} = (200\ \text{ng/mL}/375\ \text{ng/mL})$$
$$800\ \text{mg/d} = 427\ \text{mg/d, rounded to 400 mg/d}$$

The new suggested dose would be 400 mg/d or 200 mg every 12 hours of cyclosporine capsules to be started at the next scheduled dosing time.

CLINICAL PHARMACODYNAMICS

Pharmacodynamics is the study of the relationship between the concentration of a drug and the response obtained in a patient. Originally, investigators examined the dose-response relationship of drugs in humans but found that the same dose of a drug usually resulted in different concentrations in individuals because of pharmacokinetic differences in clearance and volume of distribution. Examples of quantifiable pharmacodynamic measurements include changes in blood pressure during antihypertensive drug therapy, decreases in heart rate during β-blocker treatment, and alterations in prothrombin time or international normalized ratio during warfarin therapy.

For drugs that exhibit a direct and reversible effect, the following diagram describes what occurs at the level of the drug receptor:

$$\text{Drug} + \text{receptor} \leftrightarrow \text{drug-receptor complex} \leftrightarrow \text{response}$$

According to this scheme, there is a drug receptor located within the target organ or tissue. When a drug molecule "finds" the receptor, it forms a complex that causes the pharmacologic response to occur. The drug and receptor are in dynamic equilibrium with the drug-receptor complex.

THE E_{max} AND SIGMOID E_{max} MODELS

The mathematical model that comes from the classic drug receptor theory shown previously is known as the E_{max} model:

$$E = \frac{E_{max} \times C}{EC_{50} + C}$$

where E is the pharmacologic effect elicited by the drug, E_{max} is the maximum effect the drug can cause, EC_{50} is the concentration causing one-half the maximum drug effect ($E_{max}/2$), and C is the concentration of drug at the receptor site. EC_{50} can be used as a measure of drug potency (a lower EC_{50} indicating a more potent drug), whereas E_{max} reflects the intrinsic efficacy of the drug (a higher E_{max} indicating greater efficacy). If pharmacologic effect is plotted versus concentration in the E_{max} equation, a hyperbola results with

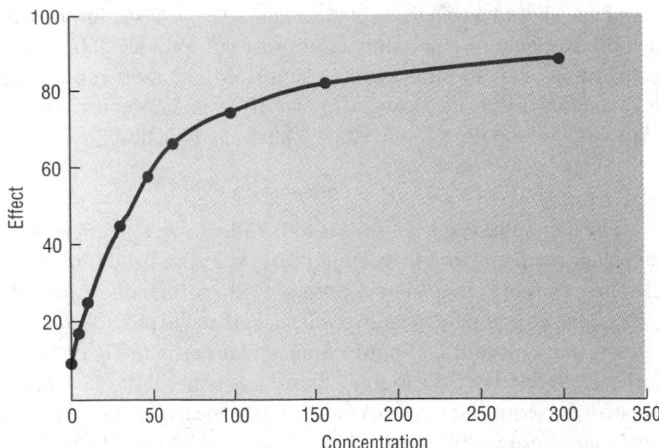

FIGURE 4–14. The E_{max} model [$E = (E_{max} \times C)/(EC_{50} + C)$] has the shape of a hyperbola with an asymptote equal to E_{max}. EC_{50} is the concentration where effect $= E_{max}/2$.

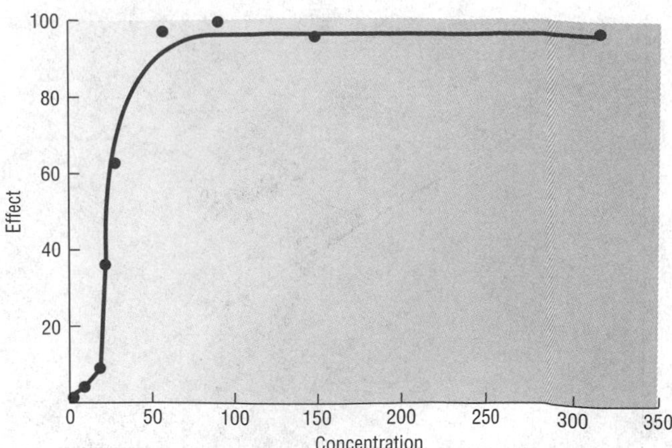

FIGURE 4–15. The sigmoid E_{max} model [$E = (E_{max} \times C^n)/(EC_{50}{}^n + C^n)$] has an S-shaped curve at lower concentrations. In this example, E_{max} and EC_{50} have the same values as in Fig. 4–14.

an asymptote equal to E_{max} (Fig. 4–14). At a concentration of zero, no measurable effect is present.

When dealing with human studies where a drug is administered to a patient and pharmacologic effect is measured, it is very difficult to determine the concentration of drug at the receptor site. Because of this, serum concentrations (total or unbound) usually are used as the concentration parameter in the E_{max} equation. Therefore, the values of E_{max} and EC_{50} are much different than if the drug were added to an isolated tissue contained in a laboratory beaker.

The result is that a much more empirical approach is used to describe the relationship between concentration and effect in clinical pharmacology studies. After a pharmacodynamic experiment has been conducted, concentration-effect plots are generated. The shape of the concentration-effect curve is used to determine which pharmacodynamic model will be used to describe the data. Because of this, the pharmacodynamic models used in a clinical pharmacology study are deterministic in the same way that the shape of the serum-concentration-versus-time curve determines which pharmacokinetic model is used in clinical pharmacokinetic studies.

Sometimes a hyperbolic function does not adequately describe the concentration-effect relationship at lower concentrations. When this is the case, the sigmoid E_{max} equation may be superior to the E_{max} model:

$$E = \frac{E_{max} \times C^n}{EC_{50}{}^n + C^n}$$

where n is an exponent that changes the shape of the concentration-effect curve. When $n > 1$, the concentration-effect curve is S- or sigmoid-shaped at lower serum concentrations. When $n < 1$, the concentration-effect curve has a steeper slope at lower concentrations (Fig. 4–15).

With both the E_{max} and sigmoid E_{max} models, the largest changes in drug effect occur at the lower end of the concentration scale. Small changes in low serum concentrations cause large changes in effect. As serum concentrations become larger, further increases in serum concentration result in smaller changes in effect. Using the E_{max} model as an example and setting $E_{max} = 100$ units and $EC_{50} =$ 20 mg/L, doubling the serum concentration from 5 to 10 mg/L increases the effect from 20 to 33 units (a 67% increase), whereas doubling the serum concentration from 40 to 80 mg/L only increases the effect from 67 to 80 units (a 19% increase). This is an important concept for clinicians to remember when doses are being titrated in patients.

LINEAR MODELS

When serum concentrations obtained during a pharmacodynamic experiment are between 20% and 80% of E_{max}, the concentration-effect curve may appear to be linear (Fig. 4–16). This occurs often because lower drug concentrations may not be detectable with the analytic technique used to assay serum samples, and higher drug concentrations may be avoided to prevent toxic side effects. The equation used is that of a simple line: $E = S \times C + I$, where E is the drug effect, C is the drug concentration, S is the slope of the line, and I is the y intercept. In this situation, the value of S can be used as a measure of drug potency (the larger the value of S, the more potent the drug). The linear model can be derived from the E_{max} model. When EC_{50} is much greater than C, $E = (E_{max}/EC_{50})C = S \times C$, where $S = E_{max}/EC_{50}$.

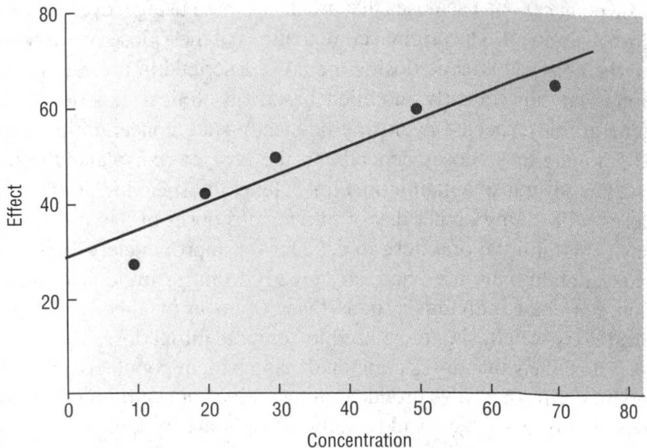

FIGURE 4–16. The linear model ($E = S \times C + 1$) is often used as a pharmacodynamic model when the measured pharmacologic effect is 20% to 80% of E_{max}. In this situation, the determination of E_{max} and EC_{50} is not possible. To illustrate this, effect measurements from Fig. 4–14 between 20% and 80% of E_{max} are graphed using the linear pharmacodynamic model.

The linear model allows a nonzero value for effect when the concentration equals zero. This may be a baseline value for the effect that is present without the drug, the result of measurement error when determining effect, or model misspecification. Also, this model does not allow the prediction of a maximum response.

Some investigators have used a log-linear model in pharmacodynamic experiments: $E = S \times (\log C) + I$, where the symbols have the same meaning as in the linear model. The advantages of this model are that the concentration scale is compressed on concentration-effect plots for experiments where wide concentration ranges were used, and the concentration values are transformed so that linear regression can be used to compute model parameters. The disadvantages are that the model cannot predict a maximum effect or an effect when the concentration equals zero. With the increased availability of nonlinear regression programs that can easily compute the parameters of nonlinear functions such as the E_{max} model, use of the log-linear model has been discouraged.[53]

BASELINE EFFECTS

At times, the effect measured during a pharmacodynamic study has a value before the drug is administered to the patient. In these cases, the drug changes the patient's baseline value. Examples of these types of measurements are heart rate or blood pressure. In addition, a given drug may increase or decrease the baseline value. Two basic techniques are used to incorporate baseline values into pharmacodynamic data. One way incorporates the baseline value into the pharmacodynamic model; the other way transforms the effect data to take baseline values into account.

Incorporation of the baseline value into the pharmacodynamic model involves the addition of a new term to the previous equations. E_0 is the symbol used to denote the baseline value of the effect that will be measured. The form that these equations takes depends on whether the drug increases or decreases the pharmacodynamic effect. When the drug increases the baseline value, E_0 is added to the equations:

$$E = E_0 + \frac{E_{max} \times C}{EC_{50} + C}$$

$$E = E_0 + \frac{E_{max} \times C^n}{EC_{50}{}^n + C^n}$$

$$E = S \times C + E_0$$

When E_0 is not known with any better certainty than any other effect measurement, it should be estimated as a model parameter similar to the way that one would estimate the values of E_{max}, EC_{50}, S, or n.[54,55] If the baseline effect is well known and has only a small amount of measurement error, it can be subtracted from the effect determined in the patient during the experiment and not estimated as a model parameter. This approach can lead to better estimates of the remaining model parameters.[55] Using the linear model as an example, the equation used would be $E - E_0 = S \times C$.

If the drug decreases the baseline value, the drug effect is subtracted from E_0 in the pharmacodynamic models:

$$E = E_0 - \frac{E_{max} \times C}{IC_{50} + C}$$

$$E = E_0 - \frac{E_{max} \times C^n}{IC_{50}{}^n + C^n}$$

$$E = E_0 - S \times C$$

where E_{max} represents the maximum reduction in effect caused by the drug, and IC_{50} is the concentration that produces a 50% inhibition of E_{max}. These forms of the equations have been called the *inhibitory* E_{max} and *inhibitory sigmoidal* E_{max} *equations*, respectively. In this arrangement of the pharmacodynamic model, E_0 is a model parameter and can be estimated. If the baseline effect is well known and has little measurement error, the effect in the presence of the drug can be subtracted from the baseline effect and not estimated as a model parameter. Using the inhibitory E_{max} model as an example, the formula would be $E_0 - E = (E_{max} \times C)/(IC_{50} + C)$.

When using the inhibitory E_{max} model, a special situation occurs if the baseline effect can be obliterated completely by the drug (decreased premature ventricular contractions during antiarrhythmic therapy). In this situation, $E_{max} = E_0$, and the equation simplifies to a rearrangement known as the *fractional* E_{max} *equation*:

$$E = E_0 \left(1 - \frac{C}{IC_{50} + C}\right)$$

This form of the model relates drug concentration to the fraction of the maximum effect.

An alternative approach to the pharmacodynamic modeling of drugs that alter baseline effects is to transform the effect data so that they represent a percentage increase or decrease from the baseline value.[55] For drugs that increase the effect, the following transformation equation would be used: percent effect$_t$ = [(treatment$_t$ − baseline)/baseline] × 100. For drugs that decrease the effect, the following formula would be applied to the data: percent inhibition$_t$ =[(baseline − treatment$_t$)/baseline] × 100. The subscript indicates the treatment, effect, or inhibition that occurred at time t during the experiment. If the study included a placebo control phase, baseline measurements made at the same time as treatment measurements (i.e., heart rate determined 2 hours after placebo and 2 hours after drug treatment) could be used in the appropriate transformation equation.[55] The appropriate model (excluding E_0) would then be used.

HYSTERESIS

Concentration-effect curves do not always follow the same pattern when serum concentrations increase as they do when serum concentrations decrease. In this situation, the concentration-effect curves form a loop that is known as *hysteresis*. With some drugs the effect is greater when serum concentrations are increasing, whereas with other drugs the effect is greater while serum concentrations are decreasing (Fig. 4–17). When individual concentration-effect pairs are joined in time sequence, this results in clockwise and counterclockwise hysteresis loops.

Clockwise hysteresis loops usually are caused by the development of tolerance to the drug. In this situation, the longer the patient is exposed to the drug, the smaller is the pharmacologic effect for a given concentration. Therefore, after an extravascular or short-term infusion dose of the drug, the effect is smaller when serum concentrations are decreasing compared with the time when serum concentrations are increasing during the infusion or absorption phase. Accumulation of a drug metabolite that acts as an antagonist also can cause clockwise hysteresis.

Counterclockwise hysteresis loops can be caused by the accumulation of an active metabolite, sensitization to the drug, or delay in time in equilibration between serum concentration and concentration of drug at the site of action. Combined pharmacokinetic-pharmacodynamic models have been devised that allow equilibration lag times to be taken into account.

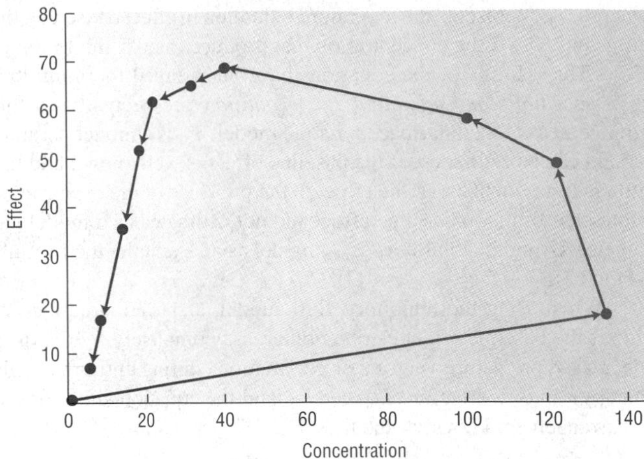

FIGURE 4–17. Hysteresis occurs when effect measurements are different at the same concentration. This is commonly seen after short-term intravenous infusions or extravascular doses where concentrations increase and subsequently decrease. Counterclockwise hysteresis loops are found when concentration-effect points are joined as time increases (shown by arrows) and effect is larger at the same concentration but at a later time. Clockwise hysteresis loops are similar, but the concentration-effect points are joined in clockwise order and the effect is smaller at a later time.

CONCLUSIONS

The availability of inexpensive, rapidly available serum drug concentrations has changed the way clinicians monitor drug therapy in patients. The therapeutic range for many drugs is known, and it is likely that more drugs will be monitored using serum concentrations in the future. Clinicians need to remember that the therapeutic range is merely an average guideline and to take into account interindividual pharmacodynamic variability when treating patients. Individual patients may respond to smaller concentrations or require concentrations that are much greater to obtain a therapeutic effect. Conversely, patients may show toxic effects at concentrations within or below the therapeutic range. Serum concentrations should never replace clinical judgment.

Three kinetic constants determine the dosage requirements of patients. Clearance determines the maintenance dose ($MD = ClC_{ss}$), volume of distribution determines the loading dose ($LD = V_D C_{ss}$), and half-life determines the time to steady state and the dosage interval. Several methods are available to compute these parameters.

Methods available to individualize drug therapy range from clinical pharmacokinetic techniques using simple mathematical relationships that hold for all drugs that obey linear pharmacokinetics to very complex computer programs that are specific to one drug. New techniques for monitoring serum drug concentrations are available on an experimental basis and may revolutionize clinical pharmacokinetics in the future.

▶ PRINCIPLES OF PHARMACOTHERAPY

- Clinical pharmacokinetics is the discipline that describes the absorption, distribution, metabolism, and elimination of drugs in patients requiring drug therapy.
- Clearance is the most important pharmacokinetic parameter because it determines the steady-state concentration for a given dosage rate. Physiologically, clearance is determined by blood flow to the organ that metabolizes or eliminates the drug and the efficiency of the organ in extracting the drug from the bloodstream.
- The volume of distribution is a proportionality constant that relates the amount of drug in the body to the serum concentration. The volume of distribution is used to calculate the loading dose of a drug that will immediately achieve a desired steady-state concentration. The value of the volume of distribution is determined by the physiologic volume of blood and tissues and how the drug binds in blood and tissues.
- Half-life is the time required for serum concentrations to decrease by one-half after absorption and distribution are complete. Half-life is important because it determines the time required to reach steady state and the dosage interval. Half-life is a dependent kinetic variable because its value depends on the values of clearance and volume of distribution.
- The fraction of drug absorbed into the systemic circulation after extravascular administration is defined as its bioavailability.
- Most drugs follow linear pharmacokinetics whereby steady-state serum drug concentrations change proportionally with long-term daily dosing.
- Some drugs do not follow the rules of linear pharmacokinetics. Instead of steady-state drug concentration changing proportionally with dose, serum concentrations change more or less than expected. These drugs follow nonlinear pharmacokinetics.
- Pharmacokinetic models are useful to describe data sets, to predict serum concentrations after several doses or different routes of administration, and to calculate pharmacokinetic constants such as clearance, volume of distribution, and half-life. The simplest case uses a single compartment to represent the entire body.
- Factors to be taken into consideration when deciding on the best drug dose for a patient include age, gender, weight, ethnic background, other concurrent disease states, and other drug therapy.
- Cytochrome P450 is a generic term for the group of enzymes that are responsible for most drug metabolism oxidation reactions. Several P450 isozymes have been identified, including CYP1A2, CYP2C9, CYP2C19, CYP2D6, CYP2E1, and CYP3A4.
- The importance of transport proteins in drug bioavailability and elimination is now better understood. The principal transport protein involved in the movement of drugs across biologic membranes is P-glycoprotein. P-glycoprotein is present in many organs including the gastrointestinal tract, liver, and kidney.
- When deciding on initial doses for drugs that are renally eliminated, the patient's renal function should be assessed. A common, useful way to do this is to measure the patient's serum creatinine concentration and convert this value into an estimated creatinine clearance ($CrCl_{est}$). For drugs that are eliminated primarily by the kidney ($\geq$ 60% of the administered dose), some agents will need minor dosage adjustments for $CrCl_{est}$ between 30 to 60 mL/min, moderate dosage adjustments for $CrCl_{est}$ between 15 to 30 mL/min, and major dosage adjustments for $CrCl_{est}$ < 15 mL/min. Postdialysis supplemental doses of some medications may also be needed for patients receiving hemodialysis if the drug is removed by the artificial kidney.
- When deciding on initial doses for drugs that are hepatically eliminated, the patient's liver function should be assessed. The Child–Pugh score can be used as an indicator of a patient's ability to metabolize drugs that are eliminated by the liver. In the absence of specific pharmacokinetic dosing guidelines for a medication, a

Child-Pugh score equal to 8 to 9 is grounds for a moderate decrease (~ 25%) in initial daily drug dose for agents that are primarily (≥ 60%) hepatically metabolized, and a score of 10 or greater indicates that a significant decrease in initial daily dose (~ 50%) is required for drugs that are mostly liver metabolized.

- For drugs that exhibit linear pharmacokinetics, steady-state drug concentration (C_{ss}) changes proportionally with dose (D). To adjust a patient's drug therapy, a reasonable starting dose is administered for an estimated three to five half-lives. A serum concentration is obtained assuming that it will reflect C_{ss}. Independent of the route of administration, the new dose (D_{new}) needed to attain the desired $C_{ss}(C_{ss,new})$ is calculated: $D_{new} = D_{old}$ $(C_{ss,new}/C_{ss,old})$, where D_{old} and $C_{ss,old}$ are the old dose and old C_{ss}, respectively.
- If it is necessary to determine the pharmacokinetic constants for a patient to individualize his or her dose, a small pharmacokinetic evaluation is conducted in the individual. Additionally, Bayesian computer programs that aid in the individualization of therapy are available for many different drugs.
- Pharmacodynamics is the study of the relationship between the concentration of a drug and the response obtained in a patient. If pharmacologic effect is plotted versus concentration for most drugs, a hyperbola results with an asymptote equal to maximum attainable effect.

REFERENCES

1. Koup JR, Gibaldi M. Some comments on the evaluation of bioavailability data. Drug Intell Clin Pharm 1980;14:327–330.
2. Gibaldi M, Boyes RN, Feldman S. Influence of first pass effect on availability of drugs on oral administration. J Pharm Sci 1971;60:1338–1340.
3. Wu C-Y, Benet LZ, Hebert MF, et al. Differentiation of absorption and first-pass gut and hepatic metabolism in humans: Studies with cyclosporine. Clin Pharmacol Ther 1995;58:492–497.
4. Wagner JG, Northam JI, Alway CD, et al. Blood levels of drug at the equilibrium state after multiple dosing. Nature 1965;207:1301–1302.
5. Rowland M, Benet LZ, Graham GG. Clearance concepts in pharmacokinetics. J Pharmacokinet Biopharm 1973;1:123–136.
6. Wilkinson GR, Shand DG. A physiological approach to hepatic drug clearance. Clin Pharmacol Ther 1975;18:377–390.
7. Nies AS, Shand DG, Wilkinson GR. Altered hepatic blood flow and drug disposition. Clin Pharmacokinet 1976;1:135–155.
8. Gibaldi M, Koup JR. Pharmacokinetic concepts: Drug binding, apparent volume of distribution and clearance. Eur J Clin Pharmacol 1981;20:299–305.
9. Bowdle TA, Patel IH, Levy RH, et al. Valproic acid dosage and plasma protein binding and clearance. Clin Pharmacol Ther 1980;28:486–492.
10. Lima JJ, Boudoulas H, Blanford M. Concentration-dependence of disopyramide binding to plasma protein and its influence on kinetics and dynamics. J Pharmacol Exp Ther 1981;219:741–747.
11. Gibaldi M, Perrier D. Pharmacokinetics, 2d ed. New York, Marcel Dekker, 1980.
12. Gibaldi M. Estimation of the pharmacokinetic parameters of the two-compartment open model from post-infusion plasma concentration data. J Pharm Sci 1969;58:1133–1135.
13. Loo JCK, Riegelman S. Assessment of pharmacokinetic constants from postinfusion blood curves obtained after IV infusion. J Pharm Sci 1970;59:53–55.
14. Wagner JG. Model-independent linear pharmacokinetics. Drug Intell Clin Pharm 1976;10:179–180.
15. Brosen K. Recent developments in hepatic drug oxidation: Implications for clinical pharmacokinetics. Clin Pharmacokinet 1990;18:220–239.
16. Cockcroft DW, Gault MH. Prediction of creatinine clearance from serum creatinine. Nephron 1976;16:31–41.
17. Traub SL, Johnson CE. Comparison of methods of estimating creatinine clearance in children. Am J Hosp Pharm 1980;37:195–201.
18. Salazar DE, Corcoran GB. Predicting creatinine clearance and renal drug clearance in obese patients from estimated fat-free body mass. Am J Med 1988;84:1053–1060.
19. Jelliffe RW, Jelliffe SM. A computer program for estimation of creatinine clearance from unstable serum creatinine levels, age, sex, and weight. Math Biosci 1972;14:17–24.
20. Koup JR, Jusko WJ, Elwood CM, Kohli RK. Digoxin pharmacokinetics: Role of renal failure in dosage regimen design. Clin Pharmacol Ther 1975;18:9–21.
21. Matzke GR, McGory RW, Halstenson CE, Keane WF. Pharmacokinetics of vancomycin in patients with various degrees of renal function. Antimicrob Agents Chemother 1984;25:433–437.
22. Sarubbi FA, Hull JH. Amikacin serum concentrations: Predictions of levels and dosage guidelines. Ann Intern Med 1978;89:612–618.
23. Sivan SK, Bennett WM. Drug dosing guidelines in patients with renal failure. West J Med 1992;156:633–638.
24. Aronoff GR, Berns JS, Brier ME, et al. Drug Prescribing in Renal Failure: Dosing Guidelines for Adults, 4th ed. Philadelphia, American College of Physicians, 1999.
25. Pugh RNH, Murray-Lyon IM, Dawson JL, et al. Transection of the oesophagus for bleeding oesophageal varices. Br J Surg 1973;60: 646–649.
26. Jusko WJ, Gardner MJ, Mangione A, et al. Factors affecting theophylline clearances: Age, tobacco, marijuana, cirrhosis, congestive heart failure, obesity, oral contraceptives, benzodiazepines, barbiturates, and ethanol. J Pharm Sci 1979;68:1358–1366.
27. Thomson PD, Melmon KL, Richardson JA, et al. Lidocaine pharmacokinetics in advanced heart failure, liver disease, and renal failure in humans. Ann Intern Med 1973;78:499–508.
28. Koup JR, Killen T, Bauer LA. Multiple-dose nonlinear regression analysis program: Aminoglycoside dose prediction. Clin Pharmacokinet 1983;8:456–462.
29. Sheiner LB, Beal S, Rosenberg B, et al. Forecasting individual pharmacokinetics. Clin Pharmacol Ther 1979;26:294–305.
30. Sheiner LB, Beal SL. Bayesian individualization of pharmacokinetics: Simple implementation and comparison with non-Bayesian methods. J Pharm Sci 1982;71:1344–1348.
31. Schentag JJ, Jusko WJ. Renal clearance and tissue accumulation of gentamicin. Clin Pharmacol Ther 1977;22:364–370.
32. Sawchuk RJ, Zaske DE, Cipolle RJ, et al. Kinetic model for gentamicin dosing with the use of individual patient parameters. Clin Pharmacol Ther 1977;21:362–369.
33. Bauer LA, Edwards WAD, Dellinger EP, Simonowitz DA. Influence of weight on aminoglycoside pharmacokinetics in normal weight and morbidly obese patients. Eur J Clin Pharmacol 1983;24:643–647.
34. Bauer LA, Piecoro JJ, Wilson HD, Blouin RA. Gentamicin and tobramycin pharmacokinetics in patients with cystic fibrosis. Clin Pharm 1983;2: 262–264.
35. Sampliner R, Perrier D, Powell R, Finley P. Influence of ascites on tobramycin pharmacokinetics. J Clin Pharmacol 1984;24:43–46.
36. Zank KE, Miwa L, Cohen JL, Waffarin F, Huxtable RF. Effect of body weight on gentamicin pharmacokinetics in neonates. Clin Pharm 1984;3:170–173.
37. Pancorbo S, Sawchuk RJ, Dashe C, et al. Use of a pharmacokinetic model for individual intravenous doses of aminophylline. Eur J Clin Pharmacol 1979;16:251–254.
38. Nicolau DP, Freeman CD, Belliveau PP, et al. Experience with a once-daily aminoglycoside program administered to 2184 adult patients. Antimicrob Agents Chemother 1995;39:650–655.
39. Cantu TG, Yamanaka-Yuen NA, Lietman PS. Serum vancomycin concentrations: Reappraisal of their clinical value. Clin Infect Dis 1994;18: 533–543.
40. Welty TE, Copa AK. Impact of vancomycin therapeutic drug monitoring on patient care. Ann Pharmacother 1994;28:1335–1339.
41. Zimmermann AE, Katona BG, Plaisance KI. Association of vancomycin serum concentrations with outcomes in patients with gram-positive bacteremia. Pharmacotherapy 1995;15:85–91.

42. Karam CM, McKinnon PS, Neuhauser MM, Rybak MJ. Outcome assessment of minimizing vancomycin monitoring and dosage adjustments. Pharmacotherapy 1999;19:257–266.
43. Moellering RC Jr, Krogstad DJ, Greenblatt DJ. Vancomycin therapy in patients with impaired renal function: A nomogram for dosage. Ann Intern Med 1981;94:343–346.
44. Blouin RA, Bauer LA, Miller DD, et al. Vancomycin pharmacokinetics in normal and morbidly obese subjects. Antimicrob Agents Chemother 1982;21:575–580.
45. Matzke GR, McGory RW, Halstenson CE, Keane WF. Pharmacokinetics of vancomycin in patients with various degrees of renal function. Antimicrob Agents Chemother 1984;25:433–437.
46. Abernethy DR, Greenblatt DJ, Smith TW. Digoxin disposition in obesity: Clinical pharmacokinetic investigations. Am Heart J 1981;102:740–744.
47. Sarrazin E, Hendeles L, Weinberger M, et al. Dose-dependent kinetics for theophylline: Observations among ambulatory asthmatic children. J Pediatr 1980;97:825–828.
48. Tang-Liu DDS, Williams RL, Riegelman S. Nonlinear theophylline elimination. Clin Pharmacol Ther 1982;31:358–369.
49. Edwards DJ, Zarowitz BJ, Slaughter RL. Theophylline In: Evans WE, Schentag JJ, Jusko WJ, eds. Applied Pharmacokinetics: Principles of Therapeutic Drug Monitoring. Vancouver, WA, Applied Therapeutics, 1992.
50. Vozeh S, Kewitz G, Wenk M, et al. Rapid prediction of steady-state serum theophylline concentrations in patients treated with intravenous aminophylline. Eur J Clin Pharmacol 1980;18:473–477.
51. Vozeh S, Muir KT, Sheiner LB, Follath F. Predicting individual phenytoin dosage. J Pharmacokinet Biopharm 1991;9:131–146.
52. Ludden TM, Allen JP, Valutsky WA, et al. Individualization of phenytoin dosage regimens. Clin Pharmacol Ther 1977;21:287–293.
53. Holford NHG, Sheiner LB. Understanding the dose-effect relationship: Clinical application of pharmacokinetic-pharmacodynamic models. Clin Pharmacokinet 1981;6:429–453.
54. Schwinghammer TL, Kroboth PD. Basic concepts in pharmacodynamic modeling. J Clin Pharmacol 1988;28:388–394.
55. Sheiner LB, Stanski DR, Vozeh S, et al. Simultaneous modeling of pharmacokinetics and pharmacodynamics: Application to D-tubocurarine. Clin Pharmacol Ther 1979;25:358.

5
PHARMACOGENETICS

Larisa M. Humma and Y. W. Francis Lam

Great variability exists among individuals in response to drug therapy, and it is often difficult to predict how effective or safe a medication will be for a particular patient. For example, when treating a patient with hypertension, it may be necessary to try several agents, or a combination of agents, before achieving adequate blood pressure control with acceptable tolerability. A number of factors may possibly influence drug response, including pharmacokinetics, age, ethnicity, and concomitant drug use. However, these alone do not sufficiently predict the likelihood of drug efficacy or safety for a given patient.

The observed interpatient variability in drug response may largely result from genetically determined differences in drug metabolism, drug distribution, and drug target proteins.[1] The influence of hereditary factors on drug response was demonstrated as early as 1956 with the discovery that an inherited deficiency of glucose-6-phosphate dehydrogenase was responsible for hemolytic reactions to the antimalarial drug primaquine.[2] Variations in the genetic makeup of cytochrome P450 (CYP) and other drug-metabolizing enzymes are now well recognized as causes of interindividual differences in plasma concentrations of certain drugs. These variations may have serious implications for narrow therapeutic index drugs such as warfarin, phenytoin, and mercaptopurine.[3–5] More recently, interest has been generated in the associations between drug response and genetic polymorphisms for drug transporters such as P-glycoprotein and drug targets such as receptors, enzymes, and proteins involved in intracellular signal transduction.

PHARMACOGENETICS: A DEFINITION

Pharmacogenetics involves the search for genetic variations that lead to interindividual differences in drug response. The term "*pharmacogenetics*" was first introduced by Vogel in 1959,[6] and is often used interchangeably with the term "*pharmacogenomics*." However, pharmacogenetics generally refers to monogenetic variants that affect drug response, whereas pharmacogenomics refers to the entire spectrum of genes that determine drug efficacy and safety. For simplicity, this review treats pharmacogenetics and pharmacogenomics as synonymous.

The goals of pharmacogenetics are to optimize drug therapy and to limit drug toxicity based on an individual's genetic profile. Thus, pharmacogenetics aims to use DNA information to deliver the right drug to the right patient at the right dose. The results of pharmacogenetic research may provide opportunities for clinicians to use genetic tests to predict individual responses to drug treatments, specifically select medications for patients based on DNA profiles, and develop novel strategies for disease treatment and prevention based on an understanding of genetic control of cellular functions.

HUMAN GENOME PROJECT

In 1988, Congress commissioned the Department of Energy and the National Institutes of Health to plan and implement the Human Genome Project. The goal of the Human Genome Project was to determine the entire sequence of the human genome by 2005. The mapping of the human genome, which officially began in 1990, has led to a better understanding of genetic contributions to disease susceptibility. To encourage research and ultimately maximize the societal benefits of the Human Genome Project, new sequence data are deposited into a freely accessible database, called GenBank, run by the National Center for Biotechnology Information (www.ncbi.nim.nih.gov).[7] As a consequence of these shared data, research efforts in the 1990s accelerated the process of discovery of genetic variations affecting treatment response and development of new treatments and preventive strategies for human diseases. Largely because of recent advances in biotechnology, the Human Genome Project completed its initial survey of the entire human genome in 2000, well ahead of schedule.

GENETIC CONCEPTS

The human genome contains approximately 3 billion base pairs, which codes for at least 30,000 genes. Two purine nucleotide bases, adenine (A) and guanine (G) and two pyrimidine nucleotide bases, cytosine (C) and thymine (T), are present in DNA, with purines and pyrimidines always pairing together to form base pairs. The majority of nucleotide base pairs are identical from person to person, with only 0.1% contributing to individual differences.

Three consecutive nucleotide base pairs form a codon, and codons specify amino acids, the basic constituents of protein. The code has substantial redundancy, in that two or more codons code for the same amino acid. For example, both GGA and GGC code for the amino acid glycine. Only 20 different amino acids, in various arrangements, form the basic units of all of the proteins in the human body.

A gene is a series of codons that specifies a particular protein. At each gene locus, an individual carries two alleles, one from each parent. Two identical alleles make up a homozygous genotype, and two different alleles make up a heterozygous genotype.

TYPES OF GENETIC VARIATIONS

Genetic variations occur as either rare defects or polymorphisms. Single nucleotide polymorphisms (abbreviated as SNPs and pronounced snips) are the most common genetic variations in human DNA, occurring on average at least once every 1,000 base pairs. Thus, there

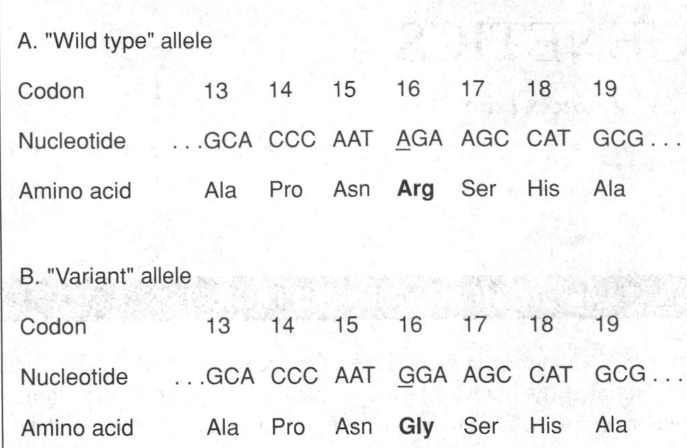

FIGURE 5–1. Nucleotide sequence of the β_2-adrenergic receptor gene from codons 13 through 19. **A**, Nucleotide sequence of the "wild type" allele with adenine (A) at nucleotide position 46 (underlined), located in codon 16 of the β_2-adrenergic receptor gene. The AGA codon designates the amino acid arginine (Arg), with an average frequency of 39% in the human population. **B**, Nucleotide sequence of the "variant" allele with guanine (G) at nucleotide position 46 (underlined), located in codon 16. The GGA codon designates the amino acid glycine (Gly), which occurs at an average frequency of 61%. Although the Arg16 polymorphism occurs less commonly than the Gly16 polymorphism, it is referred to as the wild-type because it was identified first.

are approximately 3 million SNPs distributed throughout the entire human genome. Polymorphisms are defined as those variations occurring at a frequency of at least 1% in the human population.[8] For example, the genes encoding the CYP enzymes 2A6, 2C9, 2C19, 2D6, and 3A4 are polymorphic with functional mutations of >1% in different ethnic groups. In contrast, rare mutations occur in <1% of the population and cause inherited diseases such as cystic fibrosis, hemophilia, and Huntington's disease.

SNPs occur when one nucleotide base pair replaces another, as illustrated in Fig. 5–1. Thus, SNPs are single base differences that exist between individuals. Nucleotide substitution results in two possible alleles. One allele, typically either the most commonly occurring allele or the allele originally sequenced, is considered the "wild-type," and the alternative allele is considered the "variant allele."

The nucleotide substitution may change the codon resulting in amino acid substitution, which may or may not alter gene expression. Many SNPs do not result in amino acid substitution, and are thus referred to as "silent." Referring to a previous example of redundancy in the genetic code, if adenine (A) replaces cytosine (C) in the codon GGC, the resulting amino acid is still glycine. If a SNP changes the expression of a protein that contributes to drug response, it may alter a patient's sensitivity to a drug or predispose a patient to adverse reactions from drug therapy.

Other examples of genetic variants include:

- *Insertion-deletion polymorphisms,* in which a nucleotide or nucleotide sequence is either added to or deleted from a DNA sequence
- *Tandem repeats,* in which a nucleotide sequence repeats in tandem (i.e., if "AG" is the nucleotide repeat unit, "AGAGAGAGAG" is a five-tandem repeat)
- *Defective splicing,* in which an internal polypeptide segment is abnormally removed and the ends of the remaining polypeptide chain are joined
- *Aberrant splice site,* in which processing of the protein occurs at an alternate site
- *Premature stop codon polymorphisms,* in which there is premature termination of the polypeptide chain by a stop codon (specific sequence of three nucleotides that do not code for an amino acid but rather specify polypeptide chain termination)

For more detailed information about genetic concepts, refer to the recommended genetics textbook.[9]

POLYMORPHISMS IN GENES FOR DRUG-METABOLIZING ENZYMES

Polymorphisms in the drug-metabolizing enzymes represent the first recognized, and, so far, the most documented examples of genetic variants with consequences in drug response and toxicity. The major phase I enzymes are the CYP superfamily of enzymes. *N*-Acetyltransferase, thiopurine *S*-methyltransferase, and glutathione *S*-transferase are examples of phase II metabolizing enzymes that exhibit genetic polymorphisms. Table 5–1 lists selected examples of polymorphic metabolizing enzymes, corresponding drug substrates, and the consequences of altered enzyme function as a result of gene mutation.

CYTOCHROME P450 ENZYMES

About 40 different CYP enzymes are present in humans. Of these, functional genetic polymorphism has been discovered for CYP2A6, CYP2C9, CYP2C19, and CYP2D6,[1] and, more recently, for CYP3A4.[10] A polymorphism in the regulatory region of the gene encoding for CYP1A2[11] has been identified, but its functional importance remains to be determined.

CYP2D6

Polymorphisms in the CYP2D6 gene are the best characterized of the CYP variants. Over the years, at least 48 gene variants and 53 alleles have been identified in the CYP2D6 gene.[12] Nevertheless, the CYP2D6 extensive metabolizer (EM) and poor metabolizer (PM) phenotypes (outward expression of genotypes) can be predicted with up to 99% confidence with six genotypic variants. *CYP2D6*1* is considered the wild-type variant and exhibits normal enzyme activity. *CYP2D6*2* has the same activity as *CYP2D6*1* but is capable of duplication or amplification. Both of these variants are present in EMs. The *CYP2D6*4* (defective splicing) and *CYP2D6*5* (gene deletion) variants are present in the PMs; these result in an inactive enzyme and absence of enzyme, respectively. The predominant variants in people of Asian and African descent are *CYP2D6*10* and *CYP2D6*17*, respectively, both resulting in single amino acid substitution and consequent reduction in enzyme activity.

CYP2D6 poor metabolizers carry two defective alleles, such as *CYP2D6*4* or *CYP2D6*5*, resulting in a total absence of active enzyme and an impaired ability to metabolize CYP2D6-dependent substrates. Examples of CYP2D6 substrates include neuroleptic medications, antidepressants such as tricyclic antidepressants and mianserin, antiarrhythmic drugs such as propafenone, and β-adrenergic receptor antagonists such as metoprolol (Table 5–1). Depending on the importance of the affected CYP2D6 pathway to overall drug metabolism and the drug's therapeutic index, clinically significant

TABLE 5–1. Selected Examples of Genetic Polymorphisms in Drug-Metabolizing Enzymes and Response to Drug Therapy

Gene	Drug	Drug Effect Associated with Polymorphism
CYP2D6	Perhexiline	Neuropathy in PMs[13]
	Codeine, Tramadol	Significant reduction in analgesic effect in PMs[17,18]
	Tricyclic antidepressants (e.g., desipramine, nortriptyline)	Inadequate antidepressant response in UMs[24,25]
	Antipsychotics (e.g., haloperidol)	Elevated plasma concentrations and exaggerated responses in IMs[27]
CYP2C9	Warfarin	Hemorrhage[3]
CYP2C9, CYP2C19	Phenytoin	Phenytoin toxicity[4]
CYP2C19	Omeprazole	Improved cure rates for *Helicobacter pylori* in PMs[34]
Glutathione *S*-transferase	Primaquine	Hemolytic reactions[2]
Thiopurine *S*-methyltransferase	Mercaptopurine	Bone marrow depression[5]
N-Acetyltransferase[2]	Isoniazid	More prone to peripheral neuropathy[98]
	Procainamide, Hydralazine	More prone to development of SLE-like syndrome[99,100]
	Sulfonamides	Increased hematologic and gastrointestinal adverse reactions[101]

PMs, poor metabolizers; IMs, intermediate metabolizers; UMs, ultrarapid metabolizers.

side effects may occur in PMs as a result of elevated parent drug concentrations. For example, as compared to EMs, PMs develop neuropathy after treatment with the antianginal agent perhexiline,[13] and experience more adverse effects with propafenone[14] and neuroleptic agents such as perphenazine.[15,16]

The therapeutic implication of CYP2D6 polymorphism is different if the substrate in question is a prodrug. In this case, PMs would be unable to convert the drug into the therapeutically active metabolite. Two examples of prodrugs dependent on CYP2D6-mediated conversion to active forms are codeine and tramadol. Codeine and tramadol are converted by CYP2D6 to morphine and *O*-desmethyltramadol, respectively; thus, CYP2D6 poor metabolizers would experience little or no analgesic relief after taking these drugs.[17,18]

Although PMs are at a disadvantage from the standpoint of drug toxicity and lack of efficacy for most CYP2D6 substrates and prodrugs, data suggest that they may be "protected" from abusing opiates such as codeine, oxycodone, and hydrocodone. This is primarily based on an observation that no PMs were found among opiate-dependent subjects, which likely reflects their inability to convert these drugs of abuse into their respective "pharmacologically active" moieties.[19] Given the reduced potential for opiate abuse among CYP2D6 PMs, investigators have used daily doses of fluoxetine 20 mg, a CYP2D6 inhibitor, as adjunctive therapy in the management of opiate abuse to "metabolically convert" drug abusers who are EMs to PMs.[20]

Furthermore, the potential and magnitude of drug interactions involving competitive inhibition of CYP2D6 is much greater in EMs than in PMs, who have either deficient or absent enzyme activity.[21,22] For example, Hamelin et al.[23] showed that in EMs, but not PMs, hemodynamic responses to metoprolol (a CYP2D6 substrate) were pronounced and prolonged during concomitant administration with diphenhydramine, a CYP2D6 inhibitor, administration. Thus, potent CYP2D6 inhibitors may significantly reduce the metabolic capacity of EMs, so that EMs phenotypically appear as PMs.[21,22]

Patients who are EMs have a wide range of CYP2D6 activity, with ultrarapid metabolizers (UMs) at one end of the spectrum and subjects with diminished activity at the other end. Both have clinical implications in terms of dosage adjustment for CYP2D6 substrates. UMs carry a duplicated or amplified mutant allele, resulting in two or multiple copies of the functional *CYP2D6*2*, and, therefore, very high CYP2D6 activity. Nontherapeutic plasma concentrations of nortriptyline, a CYP2D6 substrate, were observed in an UM given normal doses of the drug.[24] The CYP2D6 enzyme converts nortriptyline to 10-hydroxynortriptyline, and one study demonstrated a directly proportional relationship between the number of functional *CYP2D6* genes and the concentration of 10-hydroxynortriptyline after nortriptyline ingestion.[25] A patient with three copies of *CYP2D6*2* required nortriptyline doses three- to five-fold higher than normally recommended to achieve therapeutic plasma concentrations (50–150 μg/mL).[24,26] In the same report, another patient with duplicated *CYP2D6*2* required twice the usual recommended daily dose (300 mg vs 25–150 mg) to achieve adequate therapeutic response.[26]

The high prevalence of *CYP2D6*10* (associated with lower enzyme activity) in the Asian population provides a biologic and molecular explanation for the higher drug concentrations and/or lower dosage requirements of neuroleptic medications and mianserin in people of Asian descent.[27,28] The widespread presence of the *CYP2D6*17* variant among people of African descent suggests that native African populations metabolize CYP2D6 substrates at a slower rate than do other ethnic or racial groups.[29,30] However, there are no current genotype- and phenotype-based data to document the need of prescribing lower doses of psychotropics and other CYP2D6 substrates for the native African populations.

In addition to the therapeutic implications of genetic polymorphisms, a recent study showed that the CYP2D6 polymorphism also has an economic impact.[31] The annual cost of treating UMs and PMs (carriers of two nonfunctional CYP2D6 alleles) was $4,000 to $6,000 higher than the cost of treating EMs or intermediate metabolizers (carriers of one nonfunctional allele and one allele associated with diminished activity).

CYP2C19

The principal defective alleles for the CYP2C19 genetic polymorphism are *CYP2C19*2* (aberrant splice site) and *CYP2C19*3* (premature stop codon), which result in inactive CYP2C19 enzymes and the PM phenotype. The clinical implication of the CYP2C19 polymorphism has not been as extensively examined as that of the CYP2D6 polymorphism. However, PMs for the CYP2C19 polymorphism showed more than a 12-fold increase in the area-under-the-curve (AUC) of the CYP2C19 substrate omeprazole, as compared to EMs.[32] In a separate study, the steady-state AUC of omeprazole and other CYP2C19 substrate proton-pump inhibitors was five-fold higher in PMs than in EMs.[33]

The presence of a defective CYP2C19 allele has been associated with improved *Helicobacter pylori* cure rates after combination therapy with omeprazole and amoxicillin.[34] The cure rate was 100% in PMs, as compared to 60% and 29% in heterozygous and homozygous EMs, respectively. In another study, EMs had *H. pylori* eradication rates of 41% with dual therapy (omeprazole and amoxicillin) and 83% with triple therapy (omeprazole, amoxicillin, and clarithromycin).[35] In contrast, both dual- and triple-therapy regimens produced 100% cure rates in all 15 PMs included in this study. In a third study, EMs who failed initial therapy were retreated with high-dose lansoprazole (30 mg four times daily) and amoxicillin, resulting in 97% *H. pylori* eradication.[36]

Similar to the CYP2D6 polymorphism, people of Asian descent also metabolize most CYP2C19 substrates at a slower rate than do whites.[37] This is a reflection of a higher prevalence of both PMs and heterozygotes for the defective CYP2C19 allele in Asians.[38] This genotypic difference might explain the practice of prescribing lower diazepam dosages for patients of Chinese descent.[39]

CYP2C9

Warfarin, phenytoin, and tolbutamide are examples of narrow therapeutic index drugs that are metabolized by CYP2C9. Warfarin is a racemic mixture, and the S-isomer, which possesses about three times the anticoagulant effects of the R-isomer, is metabolized by CYP2C9. *CYP2C9*2* and *CYP2C9*3* are the two most common CYP2C9 variants, and both exhibit single amino acid substitutions at positions critical for enzyme activity.[40] This could have clinically important consequences in warfarin-treated patients. For example, a 90% reduction in S-warfarin clearance was reported in *CYP2C9*3* homozygotes, as compared to subjects homozygous for the wild-type variant.[41] In another study, an overrepresentation of *CYP2C9* mutant alleles was observed in 81% of patients requiring low-dose warfarin therapy (<1.5 mg/d).[3] The low-dose group was reported to have more difficulty with warfarin induction, requiring longer hospital stay to stabilize the warfarin regimen and experiencing a higher incidence of bleeding complications. In addition, a profound therapeutic response to usual doses of warfarin was observed in a patient homozygous for the *CYP2C9*3* allele, necessitating dose reduction to 0.5 mg/d.[42]

CYP2A6

A recent polymorphism was characterized for CYP2A6, with four variants identified: *CYP2A6*1* (wild type), *CYP2A6*2* (single amino-acid substitution), *CYP2A6*3* (gene conversion), and *CYP2A6del* (gene deletion).[43] Deletion of the CYP2A6 gene is very common in Asian patients.[43,44] Nicotine is metabolized by CYP2A6, and the clinical relevance of the CYP2A6 polymorphism lies in management of tobacco abuse.[45] Investigators reported that nonsmokers were more likely to carry the defective *CYP2A6* allele than were smokers. Smokers who had the defective *CYP2A6* allele smoked fewer cigarettes and were more likely to quit.[45] The inability to metabolize nicotine, secondary to the presence of a defective CYP2A6 allele, likely leads to enhanced nicotine exposure and increased adverse effects from nicotine. Based on these observations, CYP2A6 inhibition may have a role in the management of tobacco dependency.[46]

CYP3A4

Recently, CYP3A4 variants with amino acid substitutions in exons 7 and 12 have been associated with altered catalytic activity for a CYP3A4 substrate, nifedipine.[10] Ongoing studies in different laboratories will likely define the clinical importance of this finding, as well as identify consequences of this polymorphic variant for other CYP3A4 substrates.

PHASE II METABOLIZING ENZYMES

The clinical relevance of genetic polymorphisms in thiopurine *S*-methyltransferase (TPMT), dihydropyrimidine dehydrogenase (DPD), and UDP-glucuronosyl transferase (UGT) enzymes has been demonstrated in the treatment of cancer.[5,47,48] The TPMT gene has three mutant alleles: *TPMT*3A* (the most common), *TPMT*2*, and *TPMT*3C*. Patients who are homozygous or heterozygous for the *TPMT* mutant alleles are at higher risk for developing serious anemias during mercaptopurine treatment.[5] DPD mediates the metabolism of 5-fluorouracil; patients with a defective allele of the DPD gene cannot metabolize 5-fluorouracil and thus may experience enhanced drug-related neurotoxicity.[47] The camptothecin derivative irinotecan (CPT-11) is activated by carboxylesterase to SN-38, which is a potent topoisomerase I inhibitor. SN-38 is inactivated by glucuronidation via the polymorphic UDP-glucuronosyl transferase (UGT1A1) enzyme, which may play a role in CPT-11 related toxicity. A polymorphism in the promoter region of the UGT1A1 gene results in the $(TA)_7TAA$ allele, which possesses lower enzyme activity than the wild-type $(TA)_6TAA$ allele. A patient homozygous for the $(TA)_7TAA$ allele had impaired SN-38 glucuronidation.[48] As abnormally high SN-38 concentrations have been associated with diarrhea,[49] likely resulting from increased SN-38 excretion into the gut lumen, patients with the $(TA)_7TAA$ allele may be predisposed to developing diarrhea with usual CPT-11 doses.

POLYMORPHISMS IN DRUG TRANSPORTER GENES

Certain membrane proteins are responsible for drug transport across the gastrointestinal tract, drug excretion into the bile and urine, and drug distribution across the blood-brain barrier. Genetic variations in drug transport proteins may affect the distribution of drugs that serve as substrates for these proteins and alter drug concentration at their

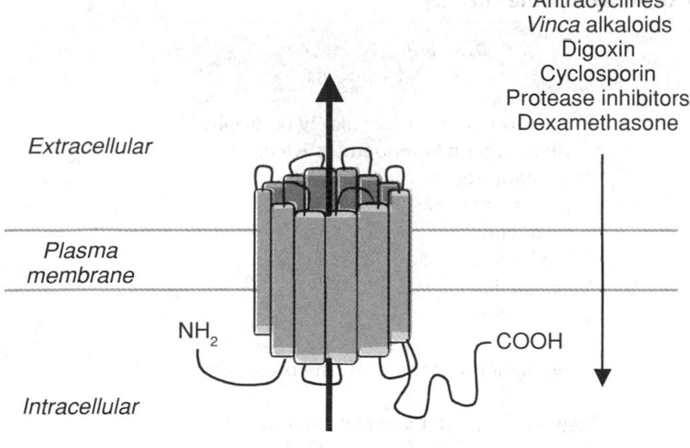

FIGURE 5–2. Active transport of drugs out of the cell by P-glycoprotein.

therapeutic sites of action. P-glycoprotein is an energy-dependent transmembrane efflux pump encoded by the multidrug-resistant (MDR-1) genes. Physiologically, P-glycoprotein serves a protective role by transporting toxic substances or metabolites out of cells. However, P-glycoprotein also affects the distribution of chemotherapeutic agents, digoxin, cyclosporine, HIV protease inhibitors, and other P-glycoprotein substrates (Fig. 5–2).[50] The expression of P-glycoprotein in cancer cells causes active cellular export of antineoplastics and can result in multidrug resistance to antineoplastic agents.[50]

P-glycoprotein is also widely distributed in normal cells including intestinal enterocytes, hepatocytes, renal proximal tubular cells, and capillary endothelial cells comprising the blood-brain barrier. Increased intestinal expression of P-glycoprotein can limit the absorption of drugs that are P-glycoprotein substrates, thus reducing their bioavailability and preventing attainment of therapeutic plasma concentrations. Conversely, decreased P-glycoprotein expression may result in supratherapeutic plasma concentrations and drug toxicity.

At least 15 polymorphisms occur in the MDR-1 gene that encodes for P-glycoprotein.[51] One common polymorphism in exon 26 of the MDR-1 influences P-glycoprotein expression *in vitro*.[51] In healthy volunteers, the homozygous form of this polymorphism resulted in significantly lower P-glycoprotein expression levels and in higher plasma digoxin concentrations.[51] The frequency of this polymorphism appears to be significantly lower among populations with African versus European ancestry.[52] Thus, the exon 26 polymorphism may serve as a useful marker for predicting plasma concentrations of P-glycoprotein substrates and may contribute to racial differences in the bioavailability of P-glycoprotein substrates.

Cyclosporine is an immunosuppressant commonly used in organ transplantation with highly variable oral absorption and a narrow therapeutic index. Subtherapeutic plasma cyclosporine concentrations increase the risk for organ rejection, and supratherapeutic levels predispose patients to drug-induced nephrotoxicity and neurotoxicity. Screening for the exon 26 polymorphism of the MDR-1 gene could aid in cyclosporine dosing and thus decrease the risks associated with nontherapeutic plasma levels.

Mutations in other drug transporters, such as those involved in neurotransmitter reuptake, are the focus of ongoing research.

POLYMORPHISMS IN DRUG TARGET GENES

Genetic variations at the drug target level may alter receptor function or sensitivity and influence responses to pharmacologic agonists and antagonists. Numerous studies demonstrate associations between genetic polymorphisms in receptors, enzymes, and other protein genes and the risk of disease development, severity, and prognosis. For example, the E4 allele of the apolipoprotein gene (ApoE4), which affects cholinergic function of the brain, has been strongly linked to familial late-onset Alzheimer's disease.[53] Several studies suggest associations between SNPs in the β_2-adrenergic receptor gene and hypertension.[54] Among patients with asthma, β_2-adrenergic receptor polymorphisms appear to be disease modifying in that they have been associated with steroid-dependent disease, airway reactivity, and nocturnal asthma.[55] In addition to contributing to disease pathophysiology, SNPs in drug target proteins appear to affect responses to drug therapy in a number of disease states. Table 5–2 lists examples of such genetic polymorphisms.

CARDIOVASCULAR DISEASE

Hypertension is the most common chronic disease in this country; it affects more than 50 million Americans.[56] The sympathetic nervous system and the renin-angiotensin-aldosterone system (RAAS) play major roles in the pathogenesis of hypertension. Thus, β-adrenergic receptor blockers and angiotensin-converting enzyme (ACE) inhibitors are commonly prescribed as antihypertensive agents. Substantial heterogeneity exists among hypertensive patients in their responses to drug treatment, with only about 50% of patients responding to β-blockers as monotherapy, and slightly fewer responding to ACE inhibitor monotherapy.[57] Because genetic factors are believed to contribute to the development of essential hypertension, genetic polymorphisms may contribute to the interindividual variability in response to antihypertensive therapy.

SNPs occur in genes encoding for components of the RAAS, including the ACE, angiotensinogen, and angiotensin II type 1-receptor genes. An insertion/deletion polymorphism occurs frequently in the ACE gene, and it has been correlated with transplant-free survival in heart failure patients and ACE inhibitor-induced regression of left ventricular hypertrophy in hypertensive patients.[58,59] Although data are conflicting, both the angiotensinogen and ACE genes have been linked with antihypertensive responses to ACE inhibitors.[60,61] In addition, several studies in patients with type 1 diabetes mellitus suggest that the ACE insertion/deletion polymorphism influences the magnitude of renoprotection by ACE inhibitors.[62–64] Despite similar reductions in blood pressure, those patients with diabetes who are homozygous for the insertion allele had greater reductions in albuminuria than those with other ACE genotypes. However, conflicting results were reported in patients with nondiabetic proteinuric nephropathies, with the homozygous deletion genotype predicting greater renoprotective effects from ACE inhibitors.[65]

To date, most studies examining the effects of genetic polymorphisms in the RAAS on ACE inhibitor response have focused on single polymorphic sites. Thus, one explanation for inconsistent and conflicting data is that the response to ACE inhibitors is influenced not by a single genetic polymorphism but rather by a combination of polymorphisms occurring in a number of genes involved in the RAAS pathway. This hypothesis is supported by the finding that four genes in the RAAS interact to determine hypertension risk.[66]

TABLE 5–2. Genetic Polymorphisms in Drug Targets and Response to Drug Therapy

Gene	Drug/Drug Class	Drug Effect Associated with Polymorphism
ACE	Enalapril, captopril	Regression of left ventricular hypertrophy,[58] BP reduction,[61] renoprotective effects[62–64]
	β-blockers	Transplant-free survival in heart failure patients[62]
Angiotensinogen	Captopril	BP reduction[60]
G_s protein α-subunit	β-blockers	BP reduction[68]
α-adducin	Hydrochlorothiazide	BP reduction[102]
G_i protein β_3-subunit	Hydrochlorothiazide	BP reduction[103]
Bradykinin	ACE inhibitors	Cough[67]
Cholesteryl ester transfer protein	Pravastatin	Slowing of progression of atherosclerosis[75]
LDL receptor	Fluvastatin	Reduction in total and LDL cholesterol[76]
Apolipoprotein E	Simvastatin	Reduction in postmyocardial infarction mortality risk[77]
Stromelysin-1 promoter	Pravastatin	Reduction in clinical events/coronary revascularization[78]
GP IIIa subunit of the platelet GP IIb/IIIa receptor	Aspirin, abciximab	Inhibition of platelet aggregation[104]
Combination of 5 long QT-syndrome genes	Antiarrhythmics	Sudden cardiac death[105]
5-lipoxygenase	Leukotriene modifier	Change in FEV_1[79]
β_2-Adrenergic receptor	Albuterol, salmeterol	Bronchodilatory response[81–84]
Combination of H_2, 5-HT_{2A}, 5-HT_{2C}, 5-HT transporter	Clozapine	Response in schizophrenia[85]
Dopamine D_2-receptor	Levodopa	Dyskinesia[87]
Dopamine D_3-receptor	Antipsychotics	Akathisia[86]
Dopamine transporter	Methylphenidate	Behavioral response in ADD[106]
5-HT transporter	Fluoxetine, paroxetine	Antidepressant effects[107]
Chemokine receptor	Combination of indinavir, zidovudine, lamivudine	HIV suppression[108]
Estrogen receptor-α	Estrogen	Increase in bone mineral density[109]

ACE, angiotensin-converting enzyme; ADD, attention-deficit disorder; BP, blood pressure; GP, glycoprotein; H, histamine; HIV, human immunodeficiency virus; LDL, low-density lipoprotein; FEV_1, forced expiratory volume in 1 second; 5-HT, serotonin.

Angiotensinogen and ACE are only two of many neurohormones involved in the RAAS (Fig. 5–3), and genetic polymorphisms are likely to occur for all RAAS components. Thus, future research may reveal that a combination of genetic variants in the RAAS best determines responses to ACE inhibitors and angiotensin II receptor blockers.

Genetic polymorphisms in the RAAS genes may also predict the likelihood of adverse reactions to ACE inhibitors. Approximately 10% of patients receiving ACE inhibitors develop a cough that persists for the duration of treatment.[67] It is believed that the accumulation of bradykinin during ACE inhibitor therapy causes this bothersome side effect. A SNP occurring in the core promoter region of the bradykinin B_2 gene (C or T) appears to be associated with the ACE inhibitor-induced cough.[67] Among hypertensive subjects, the frequencies of the homozygous TT genotype and the T allele were significantly greater among individuals who developed an ACE inhibitor-related cough versus cough-free patients.

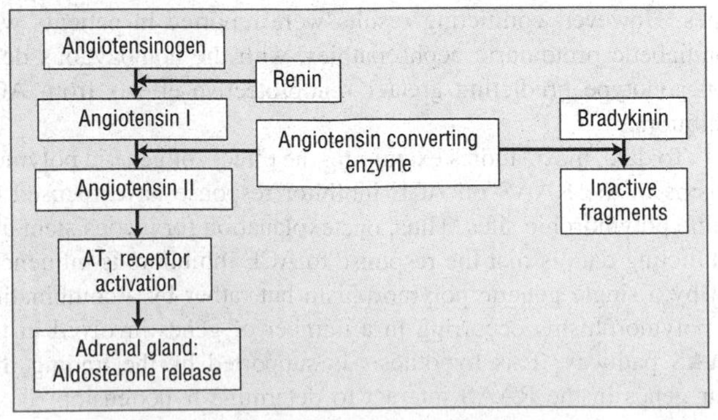

FIGURE 5–3. The renin-angiotensin-aldosterone system.

Angioedema is an infrequent but potentially life-threatening adverse effect of ACE inhibitor treatment. Gene polymorphisms in the RAAS may predispose patients to ACE inhibitor-induced angioedema. However, the associations between genetic polymorphisms and relatively rare adverse effects, such as angioedema, are difficult to examine unless data are available from a large number of patients. Investigators for many multicenter clinical drug trials are now asking study participants to provide consent for the collection of genetic samples, so that, in the future, genetic contributions to adverse drug effects may be examined in a large patient population.

Genetic polymorphisms also occur commonly in the β_1-adrenergic receptor and cell signaling proteins. Genetic polymorphisms in cell signaling proteins appear to influence the antihypertensive response to β_1-adrenergic receptor antagonists. The β_1 receptor is a G-protein coupled receptor in which a stimulatory G-protein (G_s-protein) couples the receptor to intracellular signaling mechanisms (Fig. 5–4). Receptor-coupled G_s-proteins contain α, β,

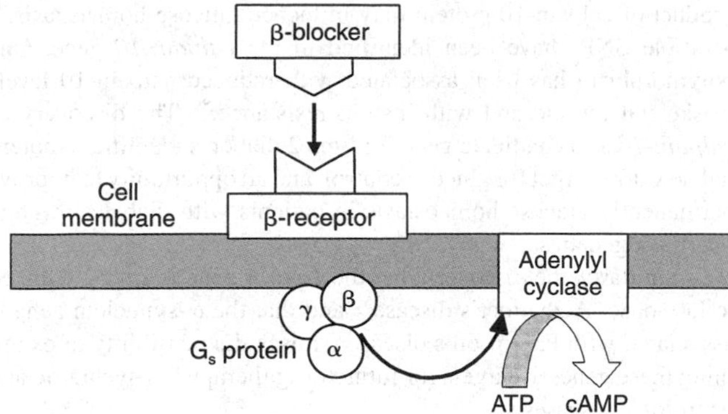

FIGURE 5–4. β_1-Adrenergic receptor coupled to intracellular signaling mechanisms by a stimulatory G-protein.

and γ subunits, which mediate the activation of adenylyl cyclase and generation of cyclic adenosine monophosphate (AMP) following receptor stimulation. A SNP occurring in the α-subunit of the G_s-protein has been linked to blood pressure response to β_1-adrenergic receptor blockers.[68]

Responses to cardiovascular drug therapy vary among racial groups. For example, African Americans in general have diminished antihypertensive responses to β-blockers and ACE inhibitors as compared to whites.[69] In addition, two recent clinical studies showed differences in ACE inhibitor efficacy between whites and African Americans with heart failure.[70,71] Specifically, in the second Vasodilator-Heart Failure Trial (V-HeFT II), enalapril, as compared to combination hydralazine and isosorbide dinitrate therapy, significantly reduced mortality among whites with left ventricular dysfunction, but not among African Americans with left ventricular dysfunction.[70] Similarly, treatment with enalapril versus placebo significantly reduced hospitalizations for worsening heart failure among whites but not among African Americans in the Studies of Left Ventricular Dysfunction (SOLVD).[71] SNPs in the β_1-adrenergic receptor and RAAS genes occur at different frequencies in African American versus white populations.[72,73] Thus, it is possible that racial differences in cardiovascular drug efficacy may be attributed to racial differences in the distribution of SNPs occurring in drug target genes, although this is yet to be determined. There are racial differences in the frequencies of nearly all drug target gene polymorphisms currently identified. The possibility that racial differences in drug target genotypes explain varying drug responses between racial groups is applicable to the treatment of a number of diseases.

Coronary artery disease is the leading cause of death in the United States.[56] Cholesterol-lowering treatment with HMG-CoA reductase inhibitors (the statins) slows the progression of coronary atherosclerosis and improves survival in patients with coronary artery disease.[74] Several SNPs appear to influence cholesterol lowering and clinical outcomes with statin therapy. A SNP in the cholesteryl ester transfer protein, which plays an important role in the metabolism of high-density lipoprotein cholesterol, was correlated with the ability of pravastatin to slow coronary atherosclerosis in men with coronary artery disease.[75] Two polymorphisms in the low-density lipoprotein (LDL) receptor gene were reported to predict the cholesterol-lowering response to fluvastatin.[76] The polymorphic apolipoprotein gene did not affect LDL levels in myocardial infarction survivors treated with simvastatin.[77] However, mortality risk reduction with simvastatin was greater among carriers of the ApoE4 allele than among non-ApoE4 carriers. Similarly, carriers of a common variant in the promoter region of the stromelysin 1 gene had greater reductions in coronary events and revascularization procedures with pravastatin therapy than homozygotes for the wild-type allele, despite similar reductions in cholesterol.[78]

PULMONARY DISEASE

Pharmacogenetic studies demonstrate relationships between drug target genotypes and responses to asthma mediations. In one asthma study, a polymorphism in the 5-lipoxygenase receptor gene affected bronchodilatory response to a 5-lipoxygenase inhibitor.[79] The 5-lipoxygenase pathway mediates bronchial inflammation through the production of leukotrienes. A polymorphism consisting of three to six tandem repeats of the GGGCGG nucleotide sequence occurs in the promoter region of the 5-lipoxygenase receptor gene. The five-tandem repeat polymorphism is considered the wild-type genotype because it occurs most commonly in the human population, with an average allele frequency of 77%.[79] After 12 weeks of treatment with a 5-lipoxygenase inhibitor, individuals with at least one wild-type allele had significantly greater improvement in forced expiratory volume in 1 second (FEV_1), as compared to those who were homozygous for the variant genotype (two variant alleles). Average change in FEV_1 was approximately 20% in carriers of the wild-type allele and −1% for those with two variant alleles.

β_2-Adrenergic receptors expressed on bronchial smooth-muscle cells mediate bronchodilation, and thus play a major role in the pathogenesis of asthma. Inhaled β_2-adrenergic receptor agonists are the most effective agents for acute reversal of bronchospasm. However, significant variability exists among individuals in their responses to inhaled bronchodilatory therapy.[80] More than 10 SNPs have been identified in the β_2 adrenergic receptor gene, and the consequences of these SNPs have been extensively studied in patients with asthma.[55] Three SNPs that result in amino acid changes commonly occur in the β_2-adrenergic receptor gene. Two are found in the gene's coding block at codons 16 and 27, and a third occurs upstream from the coding block at codon 19 of the gene's promoter region. This last polymorphism is located in a region believed to be important for overall receptor expression.

Several studies have demonstrated a correlation between the β_2-adrenergic receptor polymorphism at codon 16 and bronchodilatory response to inhaled β_2 agonists.[81–83] In a recent study, however, the combination of polymorphisms at codons 16 and 27 in the coding region and codon 19 in the promoter region—rather than individual SNPs—was found to be a better predictor of the bronchodilatory response to inhaled β_2-adrenergic receptor agonist treatment.[84]

These data suggest that future pharmacogenetic studies should focus on the combined effects of multiple SNPs on drug response rather than, or in addition to, evaluating the consequences of individual SNPs on treatment efficacy. Furthermore, these data may lead investigators to question whether the lack of apparent gene-drug response associations in previous studies may have been due to the examination of only a single genetic polymorphism.

PSYCHIATRIC DISORDERS

The idea that the interaction of multiple genes or multiple SNPs within a single gene may predict overall drug response has been applied to pharmacogenetic studies of psychiatric disorders. Genetic polymorphisms have been identified for a number of proteins believed to contribute to the development of depression, schizophrenia, and other psychiatric disorders. These polymorphisms include SNPs in the α-adrenergic receptor, dopamine D_2 and D_3 receptors, serotonin 2A,

2C, 3A, and 5A receptors, and histamine receptor genes. In addition, an insertion/deletion polymorphism occurs in the promoter region of the serotonin transporter gene.

Clozapine is an atypical antipsychotic indicated for severe schizophrenia in patients who fail to respond to adequate doses of standard antipsychotics. Overall, 30% to 60% of patients with refractory schizophrenia respond to clozapine.[85] Clozapine exerts its effects through the dopaminergic, serotonergic, adrenergic, and histaminergic receptors. In a retrospective study comparing clozapine responders versus nonresponders, a combination of six polymorphisms in the histamine and serotonin 2A and 2C receptor genes and the serotonin transporter gene were 77% predictive of response to clozapine.[85]

Genetic polymorphisms have been linked to adverse effects associated with medications used in the treatment of psychiatric and neurologic disorders. Movement disorders are the most common adverse effects of both neuroleptic agents and levodopa, and evidence suggests that genetic polymorphisms of dopamine receptors may contribute to their occurrence.[86,87] In one study, a short tandem repeat polymorphism in the dopamine D_2-receptor gene protected patients with Parkinson's disease against levodopa-induced dyskinesias.[87] A study involving schizophrenic patients demonstrated an association between a SNP in the dopamine D_3-receptor gene and neuroleptic-induced akathisia.[86]

REVIVAL OF OLDER DRUGS

The ability to predict the likelihood of adverse drug reactions by genetic analysis may revive the use of older drugs that are proven, effective treatments but seldom used because newer agents with less potential for toxicity were developed.

An example of this possibility is clozapine. Agranulocytosis occurs in 0.5% to 2% of clozapine-treated patients and limits the use of this agent as first-line therapy for schizophrenia, despite clozapine's proven superior efficacy as compared to typical antipsychotics. An association between polymorphisms in the human leukocyte antigen gene and clozapine-induced agranulocytosis has been reported.[88] Although confirmatory studies are necessary, screening for human leukocyte antigen gene polymorphisms may have clinical utility in predicting the risk of developing agranulocytosis with clozapine treatment. The results from this study are encouraging for future research of genetic variants linked to serious drug reactions that currently preclude the routine use of efficacious drugs.

NOVEL SITES FOR DRUG DEVELOPMENT

An improved understanding of the molecular mechanisms involved in disease pathophysiology has evolved from the discovery of genes that confer disease. Once associations between genes and diseases are discovered, scientists can elucidate the functions of the encoded proteins and more clearly define the consequences of genetic mutations. Insight into the genetic control of cellular functions may reveal new strategies for disease treatment and prevention.

For example, researchers recently identified a new gene that appears to confer susceptibility to type 2 diabetes.[89] It may serve as a new target for treatment intervention. The *calpain-10* gene, located on chromosome 2, encodes for calpain 10, a cysteine protease expressed in pancreatic islet cells, skeletal myocytes, and hepatocytes. These sites are important for controlling insulin secretion, peripheral insulin uptake, and hepatic glucose production, suggesting that the product of calpain-10 protein may influence glucose homeostasis.[90] Multiple SNPs have been identified in the *calpain-10* gene. One polymorphism has been associated with reduced calpain-10 levels in skeletal muscle and with insulin resistance.[89] The discovery of *calpain-10* as a candidate gene for type 2 diabetes identifies a potential new drug target for glucose control, and an opportunity to improve permanently glucose homeostasis in patients with diabetes through pharmacogenetics.

Similarly, the discovery that the ApoE4 gene is strongly linked to late-onset Alzheimer's disease[53] and that the α-synuclein gene is associated with Parkinson's disease[91] raises the possibility of examining these genes as targets for future drug therapy in psychiatric and neurologic diseases.

GENE THERAPY

Gene therapy has emerged as a possible approach to treating and curing disease by altering gene expression. The goal of gene therapy is to correct genetic defects permanently and thereby restore normal cellular function.

Most gene therapy techniques attempt to replace defective genes with normally functioning genes. Exogenous genes, called transgenes, can be transferred into either somatic (body) or germ-line (egg or sperm) cells of the recipient. In somatic cell gene transfer, genetic changes do not affect future generations. In contrast, germ-line cell transfer, which is currently prohibited by the Food and Drug Administration (FDA),[92] results in the passage of genetic alterations to offspring.

Initially, the focus of gene therapy was for the treatment of inherited disorders such as cystic fibrosis, sickle cell anemia, hemophilia, and adenosine deaminase deficiency.[93] Gene therapy trials were later expanded to include patients with acquired diseases such as cancer and heart disease.

The first clinical gene therapy trial began in 1990 for the treatment of adenosine deaminase deficiency.[92] B and T lymphocytes fail to develop in this autosomal recessive disease, resulting in a severe combined immunodeficiency syndrome. Adenosine deaminase deficiency was made famous by the "bubble boys" whose lives were confined to tents in an effort to keep them in a germ-free environment. Only two patients were included in this trial, and although both continued to demonstrate clinical improvement 10 years later, gene therapy did not cure the disease as investigators had hoped.

Since then, the FDA has approved more than 350 clinical gene-therapy trials.[93] The majority of these trials involve cancer patients; however, a number of studies also target inherited disorders. The results of gene therapy trials to date have been largely disappointing, with reports of serious toxicities and few therapeutic successes.

OBSTACLES TO SUCCESS

Reasons for limited success with gene therapy include inefficient gene delivery to target cells, inadequate gene expression, and unacceptable adverse effects.[92]

Sufficient amounts of the transgene must be inserted into a sufficient number of recipient cells to produce a therapeutic response. In addition, the transgene must be inserted into the correct chromosomal position of the correct cell nucleus so as not to disrupt normal gene function and expression. Incorrect chromosomal insertion of the transgene is a problem referred to as insertional mutagenesis. After the therapeutic gene is correctly integrated into host DNA, it must be expressed at adequate levels and at appropriate times to restore normal cell function. Finally, the delivery system and delivery technique should lack any potential to cause unwanted effects in the transgene recipient.

RETROVIRAL GENE DELIVERY

Because of their efficiency in integrating into human DNA, viruses are the most common vectors used to deliver therapeutic genes to recipient cell targets. Disease-causing genes are replaced with the desired therapeutic genes; the viral genes that control delivery mechanisms are retained.

The first viral vectors introduced were retroviruses, which are RNA viruses that integrate into the host cell genome and replicate during cell division. Thus, retroviral gene transfer is capable of permanently altering gene expression. Retroviruses may be used to deliver genes through either direct infusion into target organs or *ex vivo* manipulation of harvested cells followed by reinfusion into the recipient. The disadvantages of retroviral vectors are the limited size of the gene they can carry, relatively low efficiency, and the risk of insertional mutagenesis. Recently, scientists reported progress with retroviral-mediated gene therapy in the treatment of severe combined immunodeficiency.[93]

ADENOVIRAL GENE DELIVERY

Unlike retroviruses, adenoviruses do not integrate into the host genome, and thus, do not replicate. As a result, genes delivered by adenoviruses are only temporarily active. Adenoviral-mediated gene therapy is commonly employed in cancer patients because permanent gene expression is unnecessary in this patient population.

In a recent trial, adenoviral vectors carrying the herpes simplex virus-1 thymidine kinase gene were infused into tumor cells.[94] Subsequent treatment with ganciclovir, which is converted to its active, cytotoxic form by thymidine kinase, killed cancer cells expressing the thymidine kinase gene. Adenoviruses can be grown in high titers and do not carry the risk of insertional mutagenesis. The major disadvantage of adenoviruses is their immunogenic potential, which has resulted in one death and prompted federal oversight of gene therapy trials.[95]

OTHER MEANS OF GENE DELIVERY

Adeno-associated viruses are human DNA-containing viruses that appear neither to cause disease in humans nor to trigger immune responses upon injection. Similar to retroviruses, adeno-associated viruses are incapable of carrying a large amount of genetic material, and their use entails the risk of insertional mutagenesis. Investigators have had some success in treating hemophilia B using intramuscular injections of an adeno-associated virus vector that expresses the human coagulation factor IX gene.[96]

Scientists are also experimenting with nonviral delivery methods such as the use of direct DNA injection, cationic lipids, and electroporation.[92] Initial success was reported with intramuscular gene transfer of naked DNA into patients with severe, intractable angina.[97] Naked DNA—encoding for vascular endothelial growth factor—stimulated angiogenesis and improved myocardial perfusion in this patient population.

Scientists have enjoyed few successes with gene therapy in recent years, and it is unlikely that gene therapy will progress to have a lasting impact on medicine during the next decade. Improvements in gene delivery techniques and a better understanding of molecular processes controlling gene expression are necessary before gene therapy can successfully correct genetic defects and thus cure associated diseases without inducing adverse effects. Because of limited success with traditional approaches to gene therapy, scientists are exploring other strategies, such as repairing defected genes rather than replacing them. It is important that gene therapy eventually succeed so that diseases such as Huntington's disease, sickle cell anemia, and inherited immunodeficiency disorders may be cured and their associated morbidity and mortality alleviated.

ETHICAL CONSIDERATIONS

PHARMACOGENETICS

Traditionally, genetic testing refers to screening human genetic material to identify genotypes associated with disease susceptibility or carrier status for inherited diseases, such Huntington's disease, Alzheimer's disease, or breast cancer. This kind of testing can have profound legal, ethical, and social implications.[8] For example, knowledge that a patient is at risk for developing a genetic disorder could result in discrimination by employers and/or insurance companies. In addition, this information is likely to cause emotional distress for the individual at risk and his or her family members.

But within the context of pharmacogenetics, testing involves searching for genetic variations linked to drug efficacy or toxicity, rather than to disease susceptibility. Thus, this form of testing carries little to no risk for ethical, legal, and social concerns. To prevent public wariness and confusion, a term other than "genetic testing" should be used in reference to pharmacogenetics so that genotyping for polymorphisms associated with drug response can be distinguished from genotyping for mutations linked to increased susceptibility to inherited disorders.

GENE THERAPY

Many of the ethical concerns with gene therapy center on transgenic manipulation of somatic versus germ-line cells. Somatic gene therapy only affects the recipient. That is, genetic alterations introduced by gene therapy are not passed on to future generations. In contrast, with manipulation of germ-line cells, alterations are passed on to future children of the treated patient. Some argue that this is unethical because it violates the rights of future generations. Thus, it appears that most gene therapy in the foreseeable future will focus on somatic gene transfer.

ROLE OF PHARMACISTS

Although pharmacogenetics provides opportunities to improve drug therapy outcomes, it will likely increase the complexity of drug prescribing. In addition to considering factors such as age, concomitant drug therapy, and renal and hepatic function, prescribers will also have to interpret the results of genetic analyses when making drug therapy decisions. Further complicating the drug-prescribing process are many medications whose effects are not determined by single polymorphisms in single genes. Rather, pharmacologic effects for the majority of medications are likely determined by the interaction of several polymorphisms in multiple genes that encode proteins involved in the various pathways of drug metabolism, distribution, and effects.[1] For example, an individual who is prescribed metoprolol for hypertension may carry the CYP2D6 genotype that results in extensive metoprolol metabolism and the G_s-protein α subunit genotype that reduces receptor sensitivity to metoprolol. Thus, maximum therapeutic drug dosages may produce negligible pharmacologic effects because of low plasma concentrations and poor ability to respond to the drug. At the opposite extreme, if a patient carries the CYP2D6 genotype for poor metoprolol metabolism along with the G_s genotype with high sensitivity to β-blockade, low metoprolol doses may produce profound hypotension or heart block.

Pharmacists are broadly trained in a number of medication-related areas, including pharmacology, pharmacokinetics, and pharmacodynamics. This places pharmacists in an extremely valuable position in dealing with the complexities of the drug-decision process in the age of pharmacogenetics. Pharmacists will be in key positions to interpret the results of genetic tests, determine the ultimate effects of multiple genetic variations on drug response, and choose the most appropriate drug for a given patient based on the individual's DNA. Thus, it will be essential for pharmacists to stay abreast of significant discoveries in genotype-drug-response relationships.

FUTURE OF PHARMACOGENETICS

Pharmacogenetics may greatly influence the future practice of medicine. The application of pharmacogenetic principles to cancer treatment has already been realized. A biotechnology company has marketed a SNP test for thiopurine *S*-methyltransferase polymorphisms to identify patients at risk for toxicity from chemotherapeutic agents metabolized through this pathway. With SNP tests, clinicians will be able to predict the likelihood that an individual will respond to a particular medication based on the patient's genotype. Medications may be avoided or prescribed in lower doses with careful monitoring in patients genetically predisposed to their adverse effects. Thus, rather than using the trial and error approach of drug prescribing, clinicians will be able to use genetic information to match the right drug to the right patient at the right dose while minimizing adverse effects.

New drugs may be developed based on knowledge about genetic control of cellular functions. For example, the discovery that chronic myelogenous leukemia was caused by chromosome translocation and consequent production of an enzyme capable of producing life-threatening lymphocyte levels led to accelerated FDA approval of imatinib (Gleevec; also known as STI-571). Imatinib is an inhibitor of the translocation-created enzyme approved for chronic myelogenous leukemia. In addition, future drug development may focus on treating specific genetic subgroups instead of broadly treating all individuals with a particular disease. Ultimately, pharmacogenetics may improve the quality and reduce the overall costs of health care by decreasing the number of treatment failures and the number of adverse drug reactions and leading to the discovery of new genetic targets and therapeutic interventions for disease management.

▶ PRINCIPLES OF PHARMACOTHERAPY

- Genetic variations contribute to interpatient differences in drug response.
- Genetic variations occur for drug metabolism, drug transporter, and drug target proteins.
- Single nucleotide polymorphisms are the most common variations in the human genome.
- Genetic polymorphisms may be linked to drug efficacy and toxicity.
- Pharmacogenetics is the study of the impact of genetic polymorphisms on drug response.
- The goal of pharmacogenetics is to optimize drug efficacy and limit drug toxicity based on an individual's DNA.
- Gene therapy aims to cure disease caused by genetic defects by changing gene expression.
- Inadequate gene delivery and expression and serious adverse effects are obstacles to successful gene therapy.

REFERENCES

1. Evans WE, Relling MV. Pharmacogenomics: translating functional genomics into rational therapeutics. Science 1999;286:487–491.
2. Carson PE, Flanagan CL, Ickes CE, et al. Enzymatic deficiency in primaquine-sensitive erythrocytes. Science 1956;124:484–485.
3. Aithal GP, Day CP, Kesteven PJ, et al. Association of polymorphisms in the cytochrome P450 CYP2C9 with warfarin dose requirement and risk of bleeding complications. Lancet 1999;353:717–719.
4. Mamiya K, Ieiri I, Shimamoto J et al. The effects of genetic polymorphisms of CYP2C9 and CYP2C19 on phenytoin metabolism in Japanese adult patients with epilepsy: Studies in stereoselective hydroxylation and population pharmacokinetics. Epilepsia 1998;39:1317–1323.
5. Relling MV, Hancock ML, Rivera GK, et al. Mercaptopurine therapy intolerance and heterozygosity at the thiopurine *S*-methyltransferase gene locus. J Natl Cancer Inst 1999;91:2001–2008.
6. Vogel F. Moderne Probleme der Humangenetick. Ergebn Inn Med Kinderheilk 1959;12:52–125.
7. Collins F. Shattuck lecture-medical and societal consequences of the human genome project. N Engl J Med 1999;341:28–37.
8. Roses A. Pharmacogenetics and the practice of medicine. Nature 2000;405:857–865.
9. Mueller RF, Young ID. Emery's Elements of Medical Genetics, 10th ed. New York, Churchill Livingston, 1998.
10. Sata F, Sapone A, Elizondo G, et al. CYP3A4 allelic variants with amino acid substitutions in exons 7 and 12: Evidence for an allelic variant with altered catalytic activity. Clin Pharmacol Ther 2000;67:48–56.
11. Sachse C, Brockmoller J, Bauer S, et al. Functional significance of a C→A polymorphism in intron 1 of the cytochrome P450 CYP1A2 gene tested with caffeine. Br J Clin Pharmacol 1999;47:445–449.
12. Marez D, Legrand M, Sabbagh N, et al. Polymorphism of the cytochrome P450 CYP2D6 gene in a European population: characterization of 48 mutations and 53 alleles, their frequencies and evolution. Pharmacogenetics 1997;7:193–202.
13. Shah RR, Oates NS, Idle JR, et al. Impaired oxidation of debrisoquine in patients with perhexiline neuropathy. Br Med J 1982;284:295–299.
14. Lee JT, Kroemer HK, Silberstein DJ, et al. The role of genetically determined polymorphic drug metabolism in the beta-blockade produced by propafenone. N Engl J Med 1990;322:1764–1768.
15. Dahl-Puustinen ML, Liden A, Alm C, et al. Disposition of perphenazine is related to polymorphic debrisoquin hydroxylation in human beings. Clin Pharmacol Ther 1989;46:78–81.
16. Spina E, Ancione M, Di Rosa AE, et al. Polymorphic debrisoquine oxidation and acute neuroleptic-induced adverse effects. Eur J Clin Pharmacol 1992;42:347–348.
17. Poulsen L, Arendt-Nielsen L, Brosen K, et al. The hypoalgesic effect of tramadol in relation to CYP2D6. Clin Pharmacol Ther 1996;60: 636–644.
18. Sindrup SH, Brosen K, Bjerring P, et al. Codeine increases pain thresholds to copper vapor laser stimuli in extensive but not poor metabolizers of sparteine. Clin Pharmacol Ther 1990;48:686–693.
19. Tyndale RF, Droll KP, Sellers EM. Genetically deficient CYP2D6 metabolism provides protection against oral opiate dependence. Pharmacogenetics 1997;7:375–379.

20. Romach MK, Otton SV, Somer G, et al. Cytochrome P450 2D6 and treatment of codeine dependence. J Clin Psychopharmacol 2000;20: 43–45.
21. Alfaro CL, Lam YW, Simpson J, et al. CYP2D6 status of extensive metabolizers after multiple-dose fluoxetine, fluvoxamine, paroxetine, or sertraline. J Clin Psychopharmacol 1999;19:155–163.
22. Alfaro CL, Lam YW, Simpson J, et al. CYP2D6 inhibition by fluoxetine, paroxetine, sertraline, and venlafaxine in a crossover study: intraindividual variability and plasma concentration correlations. J Clin Pharmacol 2000;40:58–66.
23. Hamelin BA, Bouayad A, Methot J, et al. Significant interaction between the nonprescription antihistamine diphenhydramine and the CYP2D6 substrate metoprolol in healthy men with high or low CYP2D6 activity. Clin Pharmacol Ther 2000;67:466–477.
24. Bertilsson L, Aberg-Wistedt A, Gustafsson LL, et al. Extremely rapid hydroxylation of debrisoquine: A case report with implication for treatment with nortriptyline and other tricyclic antidepressants. Ther Drug Monit 1985;7:478–480.
25. Dalen P, Dahl ML, Ruiz ML, et al. 10-Hydroxylation of nortriptyline in white persons with 0, 1, 2, 3, and 13 functional CYP2D6 genes. Clin Pharmacol Ther 1998;63:444–452.
26. Bertilsson L, Dahl ML, Sjoqvist F, et al. Molecular basis for rational megaprescribing in ultrarapid hydroxylators of debrisoquine. Lancet 1993;341:63. Letter.
27. Lin KM, Finder E. Neuroleptic dosage for Asians. Am J Psychiatry 1983;140:490–491.
28. Mihara K, Otani K, Tybring G, et al. The CYP2D6 genotype and plasma concentrations of mianserin enantiomers in relation to therapeutic response to mianserin in depressed Japanese patients. J Clin Psychopharmacol 1997;17:467–471.
29. Masimirembwa C, Persson I, Bertilsson L, et al. A novel mutant variant of the CYP2D6 gene (CYP2D6*17) common in a black African population: Association with diminished debrisoquine hydroxylase activity. Br J Clin Pharmacol 1996;42:713–719.
30. Droll K, Bruce-Mensah K, Otton SV, et al. Comparison of three CYP2D6 probe substrates and genotype in Ghanaians, Chinese and Caucasians. Pharmacogenetics 1998;8:325–333.
31. Chou WH, Yan FX, de Leon J, et al. Extension of a pilot study: Impact from the cytochrome P450 2D6 polymorphism on outcome and costs associated with severe mental illness. J Clin Psychopharmacol 2000;20:246–251.
32. Andersson T, Regardh CG, Lou YC, et al. Polymorphic hydroxylation of *S*-mephenytoin and omeprazole metabolism in Caucasian and Chinese subjects. Pharmacogenetics 1992;2:25–31.
33. Andersson T, Holmberg J, Rohss K, et al. Pharmacokinetics and effect on caffeine metabolism of the proton pump inhibitors, omeprazole, lansoprazole, and pantoprazole. Br J Clin Pharmacol 1998;45:369–375.
34. Furuta T, Ohashi K, Kamata T, et al. Effect of genetic differences in omeprazole metabolism on cure rates for *Helicobacter pylori* infection and peptic ulcer. Ann Intern Med 1998;129:1027–1030.
35. Tanigawara Y, Aoyama N, Kita T, et al. CYP2C19 genotype-related efficacy of omeprazole for the treatment of infection caused by *Helicobacter pylori*. Clin Pharmacol Ther 1999;66:528–534.
36. Furuta T, Shirai N, Takashima M, et al. Effect of genotypic differences in CYP2C19 on cure rates for *Helicobacter pylori* infection by triple therapy with a proton pump inhibitor, amoxicillin, and clarithromycin. Clin Pharmacol Ther 2001;69:158–168.
37. Ghoneim MM, Korttila K, Chiang CK, et al. Diazepam effects and kinetics in Caucasians and Orientals. Clin Pharmacol Ther 1981;29:749–756.
38. Kalow W, Bertilsson L. Interethnic factors affecting drug response. Adv Drug Rev 1994;251:1–53.
39. Kumana CR, Lauder IJ, Chan M, et al. Differences in diazepam pharmacokinetics in Chinese and white Caucasians—Relation to body lipid stores. Eur J Clin Pharmacol 1987;32:211–215.
40. Stubbins MJ, Harries LW, Smith G, et al. Genetic analysis of the human cytochrome P450 CYP2C9 locus. Pharmacogenetics 1996;6:429–439.
41. Takahashi H, Kashima T, Nomoto S, et al. Comparisons between *in vitro* and *in vivo* metabolism of (S)-warfarin. Catalytic activities of cDNA-expressed CYP2C9, its Leu359 variant and their mixture versus unbound clearance in patients with the corresponding CYP2C9 genotypes. Pharmacogenetics 1998;8:365–373.
42. Steward DJ, Haining RL, Henne KR, et al. Genetic association between sensitivity to warfarin and expression of CYP2C9*3. Pharmacogenetics 1997;7:361–367.
43. Nunoya K, Yokoi T, Kimura K, et al. A new deleted allele in the human cytochrome P450 2A6 (CYP2A6) gene found in individuals showing poor metabolic capacity to coumarin and (+)-cis-3,5-dimethyl-2-(3-pyridyl)thiazolidin-4-one hydrochloride (SM-12502). Pharmacogenetics 1998;8:239–249.
44. Nunoya KI, Yokoi T, Kimura K, et al. A new CYP2A6 gene deletion responsible for the *in vivo* polymorphic metabolism of (+)-cis-3,5-dimethyl-2-(3-pyridyl)thiazolidin-4-one hydrochloride in humans. J Pharmacol Exp Ther 1999;289:437–442.
45. Pianezza ML, Sellers EM, Tyndale RF. Nicotine metabolism defect reduces smoking. Nature 1998;393:750. Letter.
46. Sellers EM, Tyndale RF. Mimicking gene defects to treat drug dependence. Ann N Y Acad Sci 2000;909:233–246.
47. Lu Z, Zhang R, Carpenter JT, et al. Decreased dihydropyrimidine dehydrogenase activity in a population of patients with breast cancer: Implication for 5-fluorouracil-based chemotherapy. Clin Cancer Res 1998;4:325–329.
48. Ando Y, Saka H, Asai G, et al. UGT1A1 genotypes and glucuronidation of SN-38, the active metabolite of irinotecan. Ann Oncol 1998;9: 845–847.
49. Wasserman E, Myara A, Lokiec F, et al. Severe CPT-11 toxicity in patients with Gilbert's syndrome: Two case reports. Ann Oncol 1997;8;1049–1051.
50. Wacher VJ, Silverman JA, Zhang Y, et al. Role of P-glycoprotein and cytochrome P450 3A in limiting oral absorption of peptides and peptidomimetics. J Pharm Sci 1998;87:1322–1330.
51. Hoffmeyer S, Burk O, von Richter O, et al. Functional polymorphisms of the human multidrug-resistance gene: Multiple sequence variations and correlation of one allele with P-glycoprotein expression and activity *in vivo*. Proc Natl Acad Sci U S A 2000;97:3473–3478.
52. Ameyaw MM, Regateiro F, Li T, et al. MDR1 pharmacogenetics: Frequency of the C3435T mutation in exon 26 is significantly influenced by ethnicity. Pharmacogenetics 2001;11:217–221.
53. Strittmatter WJ, Saunders AM, Schmechel D. Apolipoprotein E: High-avidity binding to B-amyloid and increased frequency of type 4 allele in late-onset familial Alzheimer disease. Proc Natl Acad Sci U S A 1993;90:1977–1981.
54. Nakagawa K, Ishizaki T. Therapeutic relevance of pharmacogenetic factors in cardiovascular medicine. Pharmacol Ther 2000;86:1–28.
55. Liggett S. Polymorphisms of the β_2-adrenergic receptor regulate receptor expression. J Clin Invest 1997;102:1927–1932.
56. American Heart Association. Heart and stroke statistical update 2000. Dallas, TX, American Heart Association, 1999.
57. Materson BJ, Reda DJ, Cushman WC, et al. Single-drug therapy for hypertension in men. A comparison of six antihypertensive agents with placebo. The Department of Veterans Affairs Cooperative Study Group on Antihypertensive Agents. N Engl J Med 1993;328:914–921.
58. Sasaki M, Oki T, Iuchi Aea. Relationship between the angiotensin converting enzyme gene polymorphism and the effects of enalapril on left ventricular hypertrophy and impaired diastolic filling in essential hypertension: M-mode and pulsed doppler echocardiographic studies. J Hypertens 1996;14:1403–1408.
59. McNamara DM, Holubkov R, Janosko K, et al. Pharmacogenetic interactions between beta-blocker therapy and the angiotensin-converting enzyme deletion polymorphism in patient with congestive heart failure. Circulation 2001;103:1644–1648.
60. Hingorani AD, Jia H, Stevens PA, et al. Renin-angiotensin system gene polymorphisms influence blood pressure and the response to angiotensin converting enzyme inhibition. J Hypertens 1995;13:1602–1609.
61. Dieguez-Lucena JL, Aranda Lara P, Ruiz-Galdon M, et al. Angiotensin I-converting enzyme genotypes and angiotensin II receptors. Response to therapy. Hypertension 1996;28:98–103.

62. Jacobsen P, Rossing K, Rossing P, et al. Angiotensin-converting enzyme gene polymorphism and ACE inhibition in diabetic nephropathy. Kidney Int 1998;53:1002–1006.
63. Penno G, Chaturvedi N, Talmud PJ, et al. Effect of angiotensin-converting enzyme (ACE) gene polymorphism on progression of renal disease and the influence of ACE inhibition in IDDM patients: Findings from the EUCLID Randomized Controlled Trial. EURODIAB Controlled Trial of Lisinopril in IDDM. Diabetes 1998;47:1507–1511.
64. Parving HH, Jacobsen P, Tarnow L, et al. Effect of deletion polymorphism of angiotensin converting enzyme gene on progression of diabetic nephropathy during inhibition of angiotensin converting enzyme: observational follow up study. BMJ 1996;313:591–594.
65. Perna A, Ruggenenti P, Testa A, et al. ACE genotype and ACE inhibitors induced renoprotection in chronic proteinuric nephropathies. Kidney Int 2000;57:274–281.
66. Williams SC, Addy JH, Phillips JA, et al. Combinations of variations in multiple genes are associated with hypertension. Hypertension 2000;36:2–6.
67. Mukae S, Aoki S, Itoh S. Bradykinin B_2 receptor gene polymorphism is associated with angiotensin-converting enzyme inhibitor-related cough. Hypertension 2000;36:127–131.
68. Jia H, Hingorani AD, Sharma P, et al. Association of the G(s)alpha gene with essential hypertension and response to beta-blockade. Hypertension 1999;34:8–14.
69. Joint National Committee on Prevention, Detection, Evaluation, and Treatment of High Blood Pressure. Sixth national report of the Joint National Committee on Prevention, Detection, Evaluation, and Treatment of High Blood Pressure (JNCVI). Arch Intern Med 1997;157:2413–2446.
70. Carson P, Ziesche S, Johnson G, Cohn JN. Racial differences in response to therapy for heart failure: analysis of the vasodilator-heart failure trials. J Card Fail 1999;5:178–187.
71. Exner DV, Dries DL, Domanski MJ, Cohn JN. Lesser response to angiotensin-converting-enzyme inhibitor therapy in black as compared with white patients with left ventricular dysfunction. N Engl J Med 2001;344:351–7.
72. Moore JD, Mason DA, Green SA, et al. Racial differences in the frequencies of cardiac β_1-adrenergic receptor polymorphisms: analysis of c145A>G and c1165G>C. Hum Mutat (online) 1999;14:271–273.
73. Stassen JA, Ginocchio G, Wang JG, et al. Genetic variability in the renin-angiotensin system: Prevalence of alleles and genotypes. J Cardiovasc Risk 1997;4:401–422.
74. Grundy S. Statin trials and goals of cholesterol-lowering therapy. Circulation 1998;97:1436–1439.
75. Kuivenhoven JA, Jukema JW, Zwinderman AH, et al. The role of a common variant of the cholesteryl ester transfer protein gene in the progression of coronary atherosclerosis. The Regression Growth Evaluation Statin Study Group. N Engl J Med 1998;338:86–93.
76. Salazar LA, Hirata MH, Qunitao EC, et al. Lipid-lowering response of the HMG-CoA reductase inhibitor fluvastatin is influenced by polymorphisms in the low-density lipoprotein receptor gene in Brazilian patients with primary hypercholesterolemia. J Clin Lab Anal 2000;14: 125–131.
77. Gerdes LU, Gerdes C, Kervinen K, et al. The apolipoprotein epsilon 4 allele determines prognosis and the effect on prognosis of simvastatin in survivors of myocardial infarction: A substudy of the Scandinavian Simvastatin Survival Study. Circulation 2000;101:1366–1371.
78. de Maat MP, Jukema JW, Ye S, et al. Effect of the stromelysin-1 promoter on efficacy of pravastatin in coronary atherosclerosis and restenosis. Am J Cardiol 1999;83:852–856.
79. Drazen JM, Yandava CN, Dube L, et al. Pharmacogenetic association between ALOX5 promoter genotype and the response to anti-asthma treatment. Nat Genet 1999;22:168–170.
80. Drazen JM, Israel E, Boushey HA, et al. Comparison of regularly scheduled with as-needed use of albuterol in mild asthma. Asthma Clinical Research Network. N Engl J Med 1996;335:841–847.
81. Kotani Y, Nishimura Y, Maeda H, et al. Beta-2-adrenergic receptor polymorphisms affect airway responsiveness to salbutamol in asthmatics. J Asthma 1999;36:583–590.
82. Lima JJ, Thomason DB, Mohamed MH, et al. Impact of genetic polymorphisms of the beta-2-adrenergic receptor on albuterol bronchodilator pharmacodynamics. Clin Pharmacol Ther 1999;65:519–525.
83. Martinez FD, Graves PE, Baldini M, et al. Association between genetic polymorphisms of the beta-2-adrenoceptor and response to albuterol in children with and without a history of wheezing. J Clin Invest 1997;100:3184–3188.
84. Drysdale CM, McGraw DW, Stack CB, et al. Complex promoter and coding region beta 2-adrenergic receptor haplotypes alter receptor expression and predict *in vivo* responsiveness. Proc Natl Acad Sci U S A 2000;97:10483–10488.
85. Arranz MJ, Munro J, Birkett J, et al. Pharmacogenetic prediction of clozapine response. Lancet 2000;355:1615–1616. Letter.
86. Eichhammer P, Albus M, Borrmann-Hassenbach M, et al. Association of dopamine D3-receptor gene variants with neuroleptic induced akathisia in schizophrenic patients: A generalization of Steen's study on DRD3 and tardive dyskinesia. Am J Med Genet 2000;96:187–191.
87. Oliveri RL, Annesi G, Zappia M, et al. Dopamine D2 receptor gene polymorphism and the risk of levodopa-induced dyskinesias in PD. Neurology 1999;53:1425–1430.
88. Lahdelma L, Ahokas A, Andersson L, et al. Human leukocyte antigen-A1 predicts a good therapeutic response to clozapine with a low risk of agranulocytosis in patients with schizophrenia. J Clin Psychopharmcol 2001;21:4–7.
89. Baier LJ, Permana PA, Yang X. A calpain-10 gene polymorphism is associated with reduced muscle mRNA levels and insulin resistance. J Clin Invest 2000;106:R69–73.
90. Horikawa Y, Oda N, Cox JH, et al. Genetic variation in the gene encoding calpain-10 is associated with type 2 diabetes mellitus. Nat Genet 2000;26:163–175.
91. Polymeropoulos MH, Lavedan C, Leroy E, et al. Mutation in the alpha-synuclein gene identified in families with Parkinson's disease. Science 1997;276:2045–2047.
92. Fibison W. Gene therapy. Nurs Clin North Am 2000;35:757–772.
93. Williams DA, Smith FO. Progress in the use of gene transfer methods to treat genetic blood diseases. Hum Gene Ther 2000;11:2059–2066.
94. Morris JC, Ramsey WJ, Wildner O, et al. A phase I study of intralesional administration of an adenovirus vector expressing the HSV-1 thymidine kinase gene (AdV.RSV-TK) in combination with escalating doses of ganciclovir in patients with cutaneous metastatic malignant melanoma. Hum Gene Ther 2000;11:487–503.
95. Marshall E. Gene therapy death prompts review of adenovirus vector. Science 1999;286:2244–2245.
96. Kay MA, Manno CS, Ragni MV, et al. Evidence for gene transfer and expression of factor IX in haemophilia B patients treated with an AAV vector. Nat Genet 2000;24:257–261.
97. Symes JF, Losordo DW, Vale PR, et al. Gene therapy with vascular endothelial growth factor for inoperable coronary artery disease. Ann Thorac Surg 1999;68:830–836.
98. Devadatta S, Gangadharam PRJ, Andrews RH, et al. Peripheral neuritis due to isoniazid. Bull World Health Organ 1960;23:587–598.
99. Henningsen NC, Cederberg A, Hanson A, et al. Effects of long-term treatment with procainamide. Acta Med Scand 1975;198:475–482.
100. Strandberg I, Bowan G, Hassler L, et al. Acetylator phenotype in patients with hydralazine-induced lupoid syndrome. Acta Med Scand 1976;200:367–371.
101. Pullar T, Hunter JA, Capell HA. Effect of acetylator phenotype on efficacy and toxicity of sulphasalazine in rheumatoid arthritis. Ann Rheum Dis 1985;44:831–837.
102. Cusi D, Barlassina C, Azzani T, et al. Polymorphisms of alpha-adducin and salt sensitivity in patients with essential hypertension. Lancet 1997;349:1353–1357.
103. Turner ST, Schwartz GL, Chapman AB, Boerwinkle E. C825T polymorphism of the G protein beta(3)-subunit and antihypertensive response to a thiazide diuretic. Hypertension 2001;37:739–743.

104. Michelson AD, Furman MI, Goldschmidt-Clermont P, et al. Platelet GP IIIa Pl(A) polymorphisms display different sensitivities to agonists. Circulation 2000;101:1013–1018.
105. Priori SG, Barhanin J, Hauer RN, et al. Genetic and molecular basis of cardiac arrhythmias: impact on clinical management parts I and II. Circulation 1999;99:518–528.
106. Winsberg B, Comings D. Association of the dopamine transporter gene (DAT1) with poor methylphenidate response. J Am Acad Child Adolesc Psychiatry 1999;38:1474–1477.
107. Kim DK, Lim SW, Lee S, et al. Serotonin transporter gene polymorphism and antidepressant response. Neuroreport 2000;11:215–219.
108. O'Brien TR, McDermott DH, Ioannidis JP, et al. Effect of chemokine receptor gene polymorphisms on the response to potent antiretroviral therapy. AIDS 2000;14:821–826.
109. Ongphiphadhanakul B, Chanprasertyothin S, Payatikul P, et al. Oestrogen-receptor-alpha gene polymorphism affects response in bone mineral density to oestrogen in post-menopausal women. Clin Endocrinol (Oxf) 2000;52:581–585.

6

PEDIATRICS

Milap C. Nahata and Carol Taketomo

Remarkable progress has been made in the clinical management of disease in pediatric patients. This chapter highlights important principles of pediatric pharmacotherapy that must be considered when the diseases discussed in other chapters of this book occur in pediatric patients, defined as those younger than 18 years of age. Newborn infants born before 37 weeks of gestational age are termed *premature;* those between 1 day and 1 month of age are *neonates;* 1 month to 1 year old, *infants;* 1 year to 12 years of age, *children;* and 12 to 16 years, *adolescents*. Covered are notable examples of problems in pediatrics, pharmacokinetic differences in pediatric patients, drug efficacy and toxicity in this patient group, and various factors affecting pediatric pharmacotherapy. Specific examples of problems and special considerations in pediatric patients are cited to enhance understanding.

Infant mortality had declined from 200 per 1000 births in the nineteenth century to 75 per 1000 births in 1925 to 7.2 per 1000 births in 1998.[1] This success has resulted largely from improvements in identification, prevention, and treatment of diseases once common during delivery and the period of infancy. Although most marketed drugs are used in pediatric patients, only one-fourth of the drugs approved by the Food and Drug Administration (FDA) have indications specific for use in the pediatric population. Data on the pharmacokinetics, pharmacodynamics, efficacy, and safety of drugs in infants and children are scarce. Lack of this type of information led to such disasters as gray baby syndrome from chloramphenicol, phocomelia from thalidomide, and kernicterus from sulfonamide therapy. Gray baby syndrome was first reported in two neonates who died after excessive chloramphenicol doses (100–300 mg/kg/d); the serum concentrations of chloramphenicol immediately before death were 75 and 100 μg/mL. Patients with gray baby syndrome usually have abdominal distention, vomiting, diarrhea, a characteristic gray color, respiratory distress, hypotension, and progressive shock.

Thalidomide is well known for its teratogenic effects. Clearly implicated as the cause of multiple congenital fetal abnormalities (particularly limb deformities), it also can cause polyneuritis, nerve damage, and mental retardation. Isotretinoin (Accutane) is another teratogen. Because it is used to treat acne vulgaris, common in teenage patients who may be sexually active but not willing to acknowledge that activity to authority figures such as health care professionals, isotretinoin has presented a difficult problem in patient education since its marketing in the 1980s.

Kernicterus was reported in infants receiving sulfonamides, which displaced bilirubin from protein-binding sites in the blood to cause a hyperbilirubinemia. This results in deposition of bilirubin in the brain and induces encephalopathy in infants.

Another area of concern in pediatrics is identifying an optimal dosage. Dosage regimens cannot be based simply on body weight or surface area of a pediatric patient extrapolated from adult data. Bioavailability, pharmacokinetics, pharmacodynamics, efficacy, and adverse-effect information can differ markedly between pediatric and adult patients, as well as among pediatric patients, because of differences in age, organ function, and disease state. Significant progress has been made in the area of pediatric pharmacokinetics during the last two decades, but few such studies have correlated pharmacokinetics with pharmacodynamics.

Several additional factors should be considered in optimizing pediatric drug therapy. Many drugs prescribed widely for infants and children are not available in suitable dosage forms. For example, extemporaneous liquid dosage forms of amiodarone, captopril, omeprazole, and spironolactone are prepared for infants and children who cannot swallow tablets or capsules, and injectable dosage forms of aminophylline, methylprednisolone, morphine, and phenobarbital are diluted to measure accurately small doses for infants. Alteration (dilution or reformulation) of dosage forms intended for adult patients raises questions about the stability and compatibility of these drugs. Because of low fluid volume requirements and limited access to intravenous sites, special methods must be used for the delivery of intravenous drugs to infants and children. As simple as it may seem, administration of oral drugs to young patients continues to be a difficult task for nurses and parents. Similarly, ensuring adherence to pharmacotherapy in pediatric patients poses a special challenge.

Finally, the need for additional pharmacologic or therapeutic research brings up the issue of ethical justification for conducting research. The investigators proposing studies and institutional review committees approving human studies must assess the risk-benefit ratio of each study to be fair to children who are not in a position to accept or reject the opportunity to participate in the research project.

Enormous progress has been made in pharmacokinetics in pediatric patients. Two factors have contributed to this progress: (1) the availability of sensitive and specific analytic methods to measure drugs and their metabolites in small volumes of biologic fluids and (2) awareness of the importance of clinical pharmacokinetics in optimization of drug therapy. Absorption, distribution, metabolism, and elimination of many drugs are different in premature infants, full-term infants, and older children, and this topic is discussed in detail in the next few sections.

ABSORPTION

GASTROINTESTINAL TRACT

Two factors affecting the absorption of drugs from the gastrointestinal tract are pH-dependent passive diffusion and gastric emptying time. Both processes are strikingly different in premature infants compared with older children and adults. In a full-term infant, gastric pH ranges from 6 to 8 at birth but declines to 1 to 3 within 24 hours.[2] In contrast, the gastric pH is elevated in premature infants because of immature acid secretion.[3]

In premature infants, higher serum concentrations of acid-labile drugs—such as penicillin,[4] ampicillin,[5] and nafcillin[6]—and lower serum concentrations of a weak acid such as phenobarbital[7] can be explained by higher gastric pH. Because of a lack of extensive data comparing serum concentration-time profiles after oral versus intravenous drug administration, differences in the bioavailability of drugs in premature infants are poorly understood. Studies also have shown that gastric emptying is slow in a premature infant.[8] Thus drugs with limited absorption in adults may be absorbed efficiently in a premature infant because of prolonged contact time with gastrointestinal mucosa.

INTRAMUSCULAR SITES

Drug absorption from an intramuscular site also may be altered in premature infants. Differences in relative muscle mass, poor perfusion to various muscles, peripheral vasomotor instability, and insufficient muscular contractions in premature infants compared with older children and adults can influence drug absorption from the intramuscular site. The net effect of these factors on drug absorption is impossible to predict; phenobarbital has been reported to be absorbed rapidly,[9] whereas diazepam absorption may be delayed.[10] Thus intramuscular dosing is used rarely in neonates except in emergency or when an intravenous site is inaccessible.

SKIN

Percutaneous absorption may be increased substantially in newborn infants because of an underdeveloped epidermal barrier (stratum corneum) and increased skin hydration. The increased permeability can produce toxic effects after the topical use of hexachlorophene soaps and powders,[11] salicylic acid ointment, and rubbing alcohol.[12] Interestingly, a study has shown that a therapeutic serum concentration of theophylline can be achieved to control apnea in premature infants of less than 30 weeks' gestation after a topical application of gel containing a standard dose of theophylline.[13] The use of this route of administration may minimize the unpredictability of oral and intramuscular absorption and complications of intravenous drug administration for certain drugs.

DISTRIBUTION

Drug distribution is determined by the physicochemical properties of the drug itself (pK_a, molecular weight, partition coefficient) and the physiologic factors specific to the patient. Although the physicochemical properties of the drug are constant, the physiologic functions often vary in different patient populations. Some important patient-specific factors include extracellular and total body water, protein binding by the drug in plasma, and the presence of pathologic conditions modifying physiologic function. Total body water, as a percentage of total body weight, has been estimated to be 94% in the fetus, 85% in premature infants, 78% in full-term infants, and 60% in adults.[14] Extracellular fluid volume is also markedly different in premature infants compared with older children and adults; the extracellular fluid volume may account for 50% of body weight in premature infants, 35% in 4- to 6-month-old infants, 25% in children 1 year of age, and 19% in adults.[14] This conforms to the observed gentamicin distribution volumes of 0.48 L/kg in neonates and 0.20 L/kg in adults.[15] Studies have shown that the distribution volume of tobramycin is largest in the most premature infants and decreases with increases in the gestational age and birth weight of the infant.[16]

Binding of drugs to plasma proteins is also decreased in newborn infants because of the decreased plasma protein concentration, lower binding capacity of protein, decreased affinity of proteins for drug binding, and competition for certain binding sites by endogenous compounds such as bilirubin. The plasma protein binding of many drugs—including phenobarbital, salicylates, and phenytoin—is significantly less in the neonate than in the adult.[17] The decrease in plasma protein binding of drugs can increase their apparent volumes of distribution. Therefore, premature infants require a larger loading dose than older children and adults to achieve a therapeutic serum concentration of such drugs as phenobarbital[18] and phenytoin.[19]

The consequences of increased concentrations of free or unbound drug in the serum and tissues must be considered. Pharmacologic and toxic effects are related directly to the concentration of free drug in the body. Increases in free drug concentrations may result directly from decreases in plasma protein binding or indirectly from, for example, drug displacement from binding sites. The increased mortality from the development of kernicterus secondary to displacement of bilirubin by sulfisoxazole in neonates has been well documented.[20] However, because drug bound to plasma proteins cannot be eliminated by the kidney, an increase in free drug concentration also may increase its clearance.[21]

The amount of body fat is substantially lower in neonates compared with adults, which may affect drug therapy. Certain highly lipid-soluble drugs are distributed less widely in infants than in adults. The apparent volume of distribution of diazepam has ranged from 1.4 to 1.8 L/kg in neonates and from 2.2 to 2.6 L/kg in adults.[22] In recent years, the numbers of mothers breast-feeding their infants has climbed. Thus certain drugs distributed in breast milk may pose problems for the infants. The American Academy of Pediatrics recommends that bromocriptine, cyclophosphamide, cyclosporine, doxorubicin, ergotamine, lithium, methotrexate, phenindione, and all drugs of abuse (e.g., amphetamine, cocaine, heroin, marijuana, and phencyclidine, or PCP) be contraindicated during breast feeding. Further, the use of nuclear medicines should be stopped temporarily during breast feeding.[23] Note that these recommendations are based on limited data; other drugs taken over a prolonged period by the mother also may be toxic to the infant. For example, acebutolol, aspirin, atenolol, clemastine, phenobarbital, primidone, sulfasalazine, and 5-aminosalicylic acid have been associated with adverse effects in some nursing infants.[23,24] Unless benefits outweigh the risks, the use of any drug should be avoided by the mother during pregnancy and while breast-feeding.

METABOLISM

Drug metabolism is substantially slower in infants compared with older children and adults. There are important differences in the maturation of various pathways of metabolism within a premature infant. For example, the sulfation pathway is well developed but the glucuronidation pathway is undeveloped in infants.[25] Although acetaminophen metabolism by glucuronidation is impaired in infants compared with adults, it is partly compensated for by the sulfation pathway. The cause of the tragic chloramphenicol-induced gray baby syndrome in newborn infants is a decreased metabolism of chloramphenicol by glucuronyl transferases to the inactive glucuronide metabolite.[26] This metabolic pathway appears to be age-related[27] and may take several months to a year to develop fully. Evidence for this is the increase in clearance with age up to 1 year.[28]

Interestingly, higher serum concentrations of morphine are required to achieve efficacy in premature infants than in adults because infants are not able to metabolize morphine adequately to its 6-glucuronide metabolite (20 times more active than morphine).[29]

Metabolism of drugs such as theophylline, phenobarbital, and phenytoin by oxidation is also impaired in newborn infants. The rate of metabolism, however, is more rapid with phenobarbital and phenytoin than with theophylline, perhaps due to the involvement of different cytochrome P450 isozymes. Total clearance of phenytoin surpasses adult values by 2 weeks of age, whereas theophylline clearance is not fully developed for several months.[17] Two additional observations should be noted about theophylline metabolism in pediatric patients. First, in premature infants receiving theophylline for the treatment of apnea, a significant amount of its active metabolite caffeine may be present, unlike in older children and adults.[17] Second, theophylline clearance in children 1 to 9 years of age exceeds the values in infants as well as adults. Thus a child with asthma often requires markedly higher doses on a weight basis of theophylline compared with an adult.[30] Because of decreased metabolism, doses of such drugs as theophylline, phenobarbital, phenytoin, and diazepam should be decreased in premature infants.

ELIMINATION

Drugs and their metabolites are often eliminated by the kidney. The processes of glomerular filtration, tubular secretion, and tubular reabsorption determine the efficiency of renal excretion. These processes may take several weeks to 1 year after birth to develop fully.

Studies in infants have shown that tobramycin clearance during the first postnatal week may increase with an increase in gestational age.[16] Netilmicin studies in infants up to 1 month after birth have suggested that postnatal age is also correlated directly with netilmicin clearance.[28] Thus premature infants require a lower daily dose of drugs eliminated by the kidney during the first week of life; the dosage requirement then increases with age.

Because of immature renal elimination, chloramphenicol succinate can accumulate in premature infants. Although chloramphenicol succinate is inactive, this accumulation may be the reason for an increased bioavailability of chloramphenicol in premature infants compared with older children.[27] These data indicate that dose-related toxicity may result from an underdeveloped glucuronidation pathway as well as increased bioavailability of chloramphenicol in premature infants.

DRUG EFFICACY AND TOXICITY

Besides the pharmacokinetic differences previously identified between pediatric and older patients, factors related to drug efficacy and toxicity also should be considered in planning pediatric pharmacotherapy. Unique pathophysiologic changes occur in pediatric patients with some disease states.

Examples of these pathophysiologic and pharmacodynamic differences are numerous. Clinical presentation of chronic asthma differs in children and adults.[31] Children present almost exclusively with a reversible extrinsic type of asthma, whereas adults have nonspecific, nonatopic bronchial irritability.[31] This explains the value of adjunctive hyposensitization therapy in the management of pediatric patients with extrinsic asthma.[32,33]

The maintenance dose of digoxin is substantially higher in infants than in adults. This is explained by a lower binding affinity of receptors in the myocardium for digoxin and increased digoxin-binding sites on neonatal erythrocytes compared with adult erythrocytes.[34] Insulin requirement is highest during adolescence because of the individual's rapid growth. Growth hormone therapy has allowed children with growth hormone deficiency to attain greater adult height. However, a recent study has shown that in "normal" short children (without growth hormone deficiency), early and rapid pubertal progression by growth hormone therapy may lead to a shorter final adult height than might have been attained naturally.[35] This emphasizes the need for identifying specific indications for the effective and safe use of drugs in pediatric patients.

Certain adverse effects of drugs are most common in the newborn period, whereas other toxic effects may continue to be important for many years of childhood. Chloramphenicol toxicity is increased in newborn infants because of immature metabolism and enhanced bioavailability. Similarly, propylene glycol—added to many injectable drugs, including phenytoin, phenobarbital, digoxin, diazepam, vitamin D, and hydralazine, to increase their stability—can cause hyperosmolality in infants.[36] Benzyl alcohol was a popular preservative in intravascular flush solutions until a syndrome of metabolic acidosis, seizures, neurologic deterioration, gasping respirations, hepatic and renal abnormalities, cardiovascular collapse, and death were described in premature infants. A decline in both mortality and the incidence of major intraventricular hemorrhage has been documented after the use of solutions containing benzyl alcohol was stopped in low-birth-weight infants.[37]

Tetracyclines are also contraindicated in pregnant women, nursing mothers, and children less than 8 years of age because they can cause dental staining and defects in enamelization of deciduous and permanent teeth, as well as a decrease in bone growth.[38]

The antibiotics of the fluoroquinolone class (e.g., ciprofloxacin) are not recommended for children or pregnant women because of an association between these drugs and development of permanent lesions of the cartilage of weight-bearing joints and other signs of arthropathy in immature animals of various species.[39] Reversible arthralgia, sometimes accompanied by synovial effusion, was associated with ciprofloxacin in 1.8% of pediatric patients with cystic fibrosis.[40] Although these drugs are used to treat certain infections in pediatric populations, further safety data are needed before they can be prescribed routinely in infants and children.

Some drugs may be less toxic in pediatric patients than in adults. Aminoglycosides appear to be less toxic in infants than in adults. In adults, aminoglycoside toxicity is related to both peripheral compartment accumulation and the individual patient's inherent sensitivity to these tissue concentrations.[41] Although neonatal peripheral tissue compartments for gentamicin have been reported to closely resemble those of adults with similar renal function,[15] gentamicin is rarely nephrotoxic in infants. This dissimilarity in the incidence of nephrotoxicity implies that newborn infants may have less inherent tissue sensitivity for toxicity than adults.

The differences in efficacy, toxicity, and protein binding of drugs in pediatric versus adult patients raise an important question about the acceptable therapeutic range in children. Therapeutic ranges for drugs are first established in adults and often are applied directly to pediatric patients, but specific studies should be conducted in pediatric patients to define optimal therapeutic ranges of drugs.

FACTORS AFFECTING PEDIATRIC THERAPY

DISEASE STATES

Because most drugs are either metabolized by the liver or eliminated by the kidney, hepatic and renal disease are expected to decrease the dosage requirements in patients. Nevertheless, not all diseases require lower doses of drugs; for instance, patients with cystic fibrosis require larger doses of certain drugs to achieve therapeutic concentrations.[42]

LIVER DISEASE

Because the liver is the main organ for drug metabolism, drug clearance usually is decreased in patients with hepatic disease; however, most studies on the influence of liver disease on dosage requirements have been carried out in adults, and these data may not be extrapolated uniformly to pediatric patients.

Drug metabolism by the liver depends on complex interactions among hepatic blood flow, ability of the liver to extract the drug from the blood, drug binding in the blood, and both type and severity of liver disease. Routine liver function tests—such as determination of serum aspartate transaminase, serum alanine transaminase, alkaline phosphatase, and bilirubin levels—have not correlated consistently with drug pharmacokinetics. Further, because of different pathologic changes in various types of liver diseases, patients with acute viral hepatitis may have different abilities to metabolize drugs compared with patients with alcoholic cirrhosis.[43]

On the basis of hepatic extraction characteristics, drugs can be divided into two categories. The first category consists of drugs with a high hepatic extraction ratio (>0.7; such drugs include morphine, meperidine, lidocaine, and propranolol). Clearance of these drugs is affected by hepatic blood flow. A decreased hepatic blood flow in the presence of such disease states as cirrhosis and congestive heart failure is expected to decrease the clearance of drugs with high extraction ratios. The second category comprises drugs with a low extraction ratio (<0.2) and a low affinity for plasma proteins. Metabolism of these drugs (e.g., theophylline, chloramphenicol, and acetaminophen) is influenced mainly by hepatocellular function and not as much by changes in hepatic blood flow or plasma protein binding. One report suggested that theophylline clearance may decrease by 45% in a child with acute viral hepatitis.[44] Because of a lack of specific data on dosage adjustment in liver disease, drug therapy should be monitored closely in pediatric patients to avoid potential toxicity from excessive doses, particularly for drugs with narrow therapeutic indices.

RENAL DISEASE

Renal failure decreases the dosage requirement of drugs eliminated by the kidney. Once again, because of limited studies, dosage adjustments in pediatric patients are based largely on data obtained in adults. For many important drugs—such as aminoglycoside antibiotics—renal clearance or rate of elimination is directly proportional to the glomerular filtration rate, as measured by endogenous renal creatinine clearance. Serum drug concentrations should be monitored for drugs with narrow therapeutic indices and eliminated largely by the kidney (e.g., aminoglycosides and vancomycin) to optimize therapy in pediatric patients with renal dysfunction. For drugs with wide therapeutic ranges (e.g., penicillins, cephalosporins), dosage adjustment may be necessary only in moderate to severe renal failure.

CYSTIC FIBROSIS

Drug therapy in pediatric patients with cystic fibrosis has been reviewed.[45] For unknown reasons, these patients require increased doses of certain drugs. Studies have reported higher clearance of such drugs as gentamicin, tobramycin, netilmicin, amikacin, dicloxacillin, cloxacillin, azlocillin, piperacillin, and theophylline in patients with cystic fibrosis compared with those without this disease; the apparent volume of distribution of certain drugs also may be altered in cystic fibrosis.[45] Severity of the illness may influence the change in dosage requirements, but this is not certain. Chapter 30 reviews these changes in detail.

OTHER DISEASES

Although specific dosage guidelines are not available, pediatric patients with gastrointestinal disease (e.g., celiac disease, gastroenteritis, and severe malabsorption) may require dosage adjustments.[42] Hypoxemia also has been shown to decrease the elimination of amikacin in low-birth-weight infants.[46] Critically ill adult and pediatric patients with severe head trauma require higher than normal doses of phenytoin in part because of increased intrinsic clearance.[47]

PAIN MANAGEMENT

For many years, the term *pain* could not be found in the index of any major pediatric medicine or pediatric surgical textbooks.[48] During the last years of the twentieth century, however, many research and clinical studies were performed in the areas of pain management and assessment in infants, children, and adolescents. Today, results of these discoveries have been incorporated into clinical practice, making effective pain therapy a standard of care and pain assessment the fifth vital sign in modern pediatric practice.[49]

The basic mechanisms of pain perception in infants and children are similar to those of adults except that pain impulse transmission in neonates occurs primarily along nonmyelinated C fibers rather than myelinated A-delta fibers. In addition, less precision in pain signal transmission exists in the spinal cord, and descending inhibitory neurotransmitters are lacking. The result is that young infants may perceive pain more intensely than older children or adults. It is now known that previous pain experience leads to long-term consequences such as alterations in response to a subsequent painful event.[50] Taddio and colleagues[51,52] reported that boys circumcised with the topical anesthetic EMLA had a lower pain response to subsequent immunizations than those who were circumcised without topical anesthesia. An inadequately treated initial painful procedure may decrease the effect of adequate analgesia in subsequent procedures due to altered pain response patterns.

Children consistently report that needles and shots are what they fear most. However, with the current immunization schedule that recommends 23 injections before adolescence, interventions to decrease injection pain need to be performed (Table 6–1).

Pharmacologic pain management for medical conditions and surgical and postoperative events has progressed considerably over the past decade with the use of continuous opioid infusions, epidural anesthesia, peripheral nerve blockade, local anesthetics, nonsteroidal anti-inflammatory drugs, use of different routes for traditional agents (i.e., transmucosal and transdermal), and nonopioid adjuvant drugs (Table 6–2).

DRUG ADMINISTRATION

Drugs often are given by the intravenous route to seriously ill patients. Flow rates and injection sites vary widely with pediatric intravenous drug delivery sets. Effective serum concentrations are expected to be achieved rapidly after drug infusion. Several studies demonstrated that the method of drug infusion has a profound influence on peak serum concentration and time to attain peak concentrations of chloramphenicol and tobramycin.[62,63] This has practical implications for routine therapeutic drug monitoring in that anticipated serum concentrations may be inaccurate, leading to unjustified, costly, and potentially harmful alterations in doses. Proper recommendations for obtaining patient specimens can be made only with the knowledge of drug characteristics and infusion method.

Intravenous drugs commonly are infused in an antegrade fashion. By this method, the doses injected at various sites of the intravenous set (e.g., a Y-site and a volumetric chamber such as Metriset Buretrol) are expected to move directly toward the patient (Fig. 6–1).

In vitro studies with gentamicin and aminophylline have shown that the delivery of these drugs may be delayed substantially depending on the flow rate and injection site.[64] These observations

TABLE 6–1. Techniques for Minimizing Pain Caused by Injections

Pharmacologic Methods	
EMLA[53] (eutectic mixture of lidocaine and prilocaine)	Penetrates the skin to provide anesthesia to a depth of 5 mm; effective in decreasing the pain of IM and subcutaneous injections, venipuncture, IV cannulation, lumbar puncture, circumcision, skin-graft harvesting, and laser dermal therapy; safe and effective in newborns ≥37 weeks' gestation. Disadvantages: Requires 1 hour before onset of adequate anesthesia, has a vasoconstrictive effect that may make starting IV catheters difficult, may induce methemoglobinemia.
Numby Stuff (lidocaine iontophoresis)[54]	Provides dermal anesthesia to a depth of 10 mm within 10–20 minutes; effective in decreasing the pain of IM injection, IV cannulation, venipuncture, lumbar puncture, skin biopsy, and bone marrow aspiration. Disadvantage: Tingling, itching or burning sensation from the electric current used to transport drug to the tissues.
Vapocoolant sprays (ethyl chloride or dichlorodifluoromethane)[55]	Vapocoolant is sprayed directly onto the skin or applied to a cotton ball that is held on the area to be anesthetized. Provides local anesthesia within 15 seconds; effective in reducing injection pain in children 4–6 years of age. Disadvantage: Brief duration of action so that procedure should be completed in 1 or 2 minutes; may not be effective in reducing injection pain in infants aged 2–6 months.
Local anesthetic (lidocaine)[56]	Use the smallest possible needle (30 gauge) for administration. Inject in the subcutaneous tissue first before raising the wheal. Neutralize the pH of the local anesthetic so that it will not sting (0.1 meq sodium bicarbonate is used for each 1 mL of 1% lidocaine). Warm the local anesthetic solution to body temperature to minimize the pain of lidocaine infiltration.
Other Techniques	
Site selection[57]	For children >18 months of age: Use of the deltoid muscle for IM injections; results in less pain than injections received in the thigh. For children >3 years of age: Use of the ventrogluteal area for injection is associated with less pain than the anterior thigh or dorsogluteal area.
Technique	Z-tract intramuscular injection technique is less painful (pull skin taut at the injection site, give injection, and then release the skin); use a higher-gauge needle when the injectable solution is not viscous.
Behavioral	Use of distraction methods such as blowing bubbles, providing music by headphones, relaxation, imagery, self-hypnosis, or having parents present for the procedure can be helpful.

TABLE 6–2. Opioid Administration for Acute and Severe Pain

Intermittent IV or PO Bolus Administration (not prn)

Weak opioids (e.g., codeine, hydrocodone, oxycodone) often are combined with acetaminophen or a nonsteroidal anti-inflammatory agent (NSAID) for moderate pain. With dose escalation of combination oral products, be aware that the dose does not exceed recommended daily amounts for acetaminophen or ibuprofen. IV administration of codeine has been associated with allergic reactions related to histamine release. Parenteral administration of codeine is not recommended.

Oxycodone and morphine are available in a sustained-release formulation for use with chronic pain (not acute pain). Disadvantage: tablet must be swallowed whole and cannot be administered to patients through gastric tubes.

Disadvantage: Wide fluctuation between peak and trough levels so that the patient alternates between peak blood levels associated with untoward effects and trough levels associated with inadequate pain relief when treating severe pain.

Intravenous Continuous Infusion[58,59]

Loading dose is administered to rapidly achieve a therapeutic blood level and pain relief (i.e., morphine loading dose of 0.05–0.15 mg/kg in children; 0.1 mg/kg infused over 90 minutes in neonates). Loading dose is followed by a maintenance continuous infusion. Doses that are considered safe in children can cause respiratory depression and seizures in neonates because neonates have decreased clearance, an immature blood-brain barrier at birth that is more permeable to morphine, and an increased unbound fraction of morphine that increases CNS sensitivity to the drug.

PCA (Patient-Controlled Analgesia)[60]

Gives patient some control over pain therapy. PCA allows the patient to self-administer small opioid doses. The PCA-Plus pump allows the patient to receive a continuous infusion together with a set number of self-administered doses per hour. PCA helps to eliminate wide peak and trough fluctuations so that blood levels remain in a therapeutic range. Children as young as 6 or 7 years of age can master the use of PCA.

Epidural and Intrathecal Analgesia[61]

Effective in the management of severe postoperative, chronic, or cancer pain. Spinal opioids can be administered by a single bolus injection into the epidural or subarachnoid space or by continuous infusion via an indwelling catheter. Dosage requirement by these routes is significantly less than with IV administration (epidural opioid doses: 10-fold lower than IV doses; intrathecal opioid doses: 100-fold lower than IV doses). Morphine, hydromorphone, fentanyl, and sufentanil are effective when administered intrathecally. The most commonly used local anesthetic in continuous epidural infusions is bupivacaine. Fentanyl, morphine, or hydromorphone usually is combined with bupivacaine for epidural infusions.

Transmucosal Administration

Fentanyl lozenge is absorbed transmucosally. It is useful for providing analgesia for breakthrough cancer pain. Advantages of this product include rapid onset of action (within 15 minutes), short duration of action (60–90 minutes), and painless administration because no IV access is needed. A common side effect is vomiting and mild to moderate oxygen desaturation. Doses of 10–15 μg/kg provide blood levels equivalent to 3–5 μg/kg IV.

New pain management techniques, education, research, and increasing awareness of pain management options have helped to improve the quality of life in children.

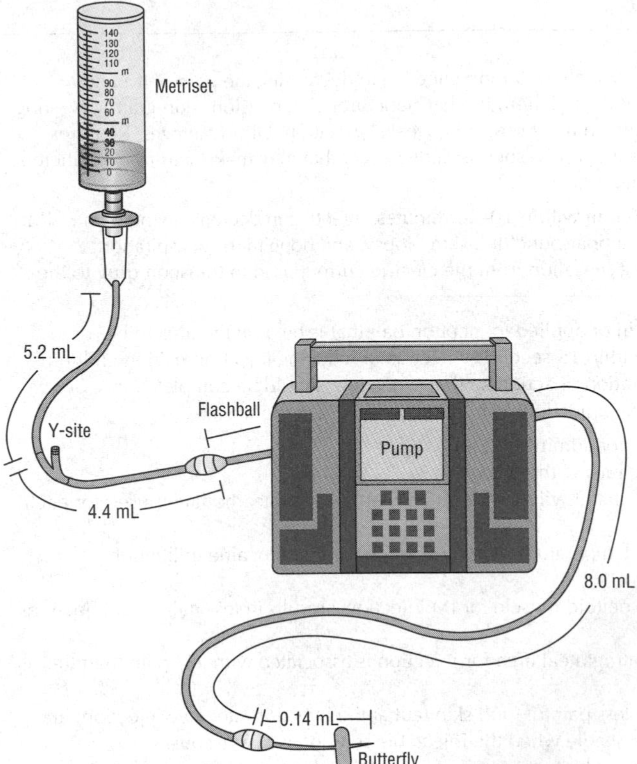

FIGURE 6–1. Schematic diagram of an intravenous set with a volumetric chamber (Metriset or Buretrol), Y-site, flashball, and butterfly. Values shown for the various components of the system are volume capacities. *(From Ref. 52, with permission.)*

were confirmed with infusion of chloramphenicol succinate[62] and tobramycin.[63] These studies clearly have demonstrated that the variables of intravenous drug infusion systems (e.g., flow rate, injection site, volume of drug, and fluid volume of the tubing) can markedly affect the serum concentrations of drugs after infusions into pediatric patients. For example, mean peak serum concentrations of chloramphenicol can be 5 μg/mL higher and occur 1 hour earlier after flashball injection compared with Buretrol injection in infants and children.[62] Similarly, the mean serum concentrations of tobramycin can be 2.3 to 2.5 μg/mL higher and occur 1 to 1.5 hours earlier after an infusion from a syringe pump compared with infusions from the Y-site of a system similar to that of Figure 6–1.[64] These differences can be important because of the narrow therapeutic indices of chloramphenicol and tobramycin. Furthermore, a lack of knowledge of these variables may result in inappropriate timing and interpretation of blood level data, leading to unnecessary dosage adjustments.

Specific gravity also can influence drug delivery at slow infusion rates.[65] For example, in vitro studies have indicated that drugs with a specific gravity lower than that of the maintenance fluid may layer at the top of the tubing, where delivery would be prolonged by laminar-flow characteristics.[65] Similarly, injections into a filter chamber, Y-site, or T-site with dead space also can prolong drug delivery.

No single infusion system is ideal for delivery of all drugs in all institutions for all patients. For example, a syringe pump with microbore tubing may be preferred for the infusion of vancomycin to neonates. Each facility must be cognizant of problems of drug delivery and develop specific guidelines for intravenous infusions. At our institution, specific guidelines are provided for administration of each drug. These guidelines take into account various infusion rates and provide consistency of delivery with each dose. As long as the time for actual delivery can be anticipated, times to obtain blood samples can be adjusted accordingly to generate meaningful data.

ALTERATION OF DOSAGE FORMS

Many drugs used in pediatric patients are not available in suitable dosage forms. This necessitates dilution of high concentrations of drugs intended for adult patients. Examples of these drugs include atropine, carbamazepine, diazepam, digoxin, epinephrine, hydralazine, insulin, morphine, phenobarbital, and phenytoin. Volumes ranging from 0.01 to 0.1 mL must be measured to dispense these drugs for use in infants. This obviously can be associated with large errors in measurements, and such errors have caused intoxication with digoxin[66] and morphine[67] in infants. One solution to this problem is to dilute these concentrated products, but such alterations can influence the stability or compatibility of these drugs. Because of limited data, pharmacists justifiably may be reluctant to alter dosage forms of certain drugs.

Selection of the appropriate vehicle to dilute the adult dosage forms for use in pediatric patients also can be difficult. Phenobarbital sodium contains propylene glycol in the original product to improve drug stability. Because propylene glycol can cause hyperosmolality in infants,[36] further addition of this vehicle may not be wise. Because of limited access to intravenous sites in pediatric patients, drugs must be administered through the same site; however, data on their compatibility often are missing. Newborn infants often require aminoglycosides for presumed or proven sepsis and calcium gluconate to correct hypocalcemia. Tobramycin and calcium gluconate have been found to be compatible at least during a 1-hour period of administration at the same site.[68]

Administration of oral drugs continues to challenge parents and nurses. Alteration of these drugs by crushing or mixing, refusal of patients to accept the medication, and loss of drug during administration are some factors that can affect pediatric therapy. A common practice is to mix medications in applesauce, syrup, ice cream, or other vehicles to make the drugs palatable.

A variety of extemporaneous formulations for oral, intravenous, and rectal administration are included in a compilation of products for use in pediatric patients.[69] A specific reference on the stability of many drugs of these formulations, however, is still lacking. This emphasizes the need for continued research in this area.

Drug administration into the middle ear, nose, or eye of a child requires special attention. Certain drugs (e.g., sodium valproate and morphine) can be administered rectally to infants who have limited access for intravenous drug administration or if oral drug administration cannot be accomplished.

Transdermal drug delivery can be used in pediatric patients (1) to avoid problems of drug absorption from the oral route and complications from the intravenous route and (2) to maximize duration of effect and minimize adverse effects of drugs. Unfortunately, the commercially available transdermal dosage forms (e.g., clonidine, scopolamine) are not intended for pediatric patients; these would deliver doses much higher than those needed for infants and children. Favorable results with percutaneous theophylline in infants with apnea[13] and with subcutaneous morphine in pediatric patients with cancer[70] form the basis for studies with additional drugs. Patients with asthma often receive drugs from various devices, and education should be offered to ensure complete delivery of doses.

MEDICATION ADHERENCE

The issue of medication adherence is more complex in pediatric patients than in adults. The parents must appreciate the importance of following the prescribing information. Among the factors that can negativly affect adherence are poor communication between the physician and patient or parent, insufficient prescribing information, lack of understanding about the severity of illness by the patient or parent, fear of side effects, failure of the patient or parent to remember to administer the drugs, inconvenient dosage forms or dosing schedules, and unpalatibility of drug products.[71] Studies in pediatric volunteers have been done to compare the palatability of antibiotics.[72] These data may have important implications for adherence in children.

MEDICATION SAFETY

The Institute of Medicine (IOM) reported that between 44,000 and 98,000 Americans die each year in hospitals from medical errors, with medication error being a leading cause.[73] According to this report, the vast majority of medical errors that cause harm to patients are preventable. Health care professionals have a responsibility for creating a safe medication environment and reducing risk to a vulnerable pediatric population.

Pediatric medication errors commonly occur at the medication-ordering step due to multiple calculations required with weight-based dosing and adjustments needed in providing therapy to the developing pediatric patient.[74–77] The medication-preparation step is also a high hazard point due to the need for dilution or manipulation of commercially available products only available in adult doses. Among drug administration–related errors, wrong dose, wrong technique, and wrong drug are the three most common errors and may be related to an inability to access pediatric drug information. Risk-reduction strategies include placement of a clinical pharmacist on pediatric wards in hospitals, simplifying the process, ordering standardized concentrations and doses, implementing computerized physician order-entry systems with dose range checking, dispensing pharmacy-prepared/ready-to-administer doses, standardizing infusion equipment, and using bar-coded medications and bar-coding systems that check the medication at the point of care.[77,78] Identifying and understanding the high-hazard areas or point of failure in the medication-use process will help us to design strategies to prevent problems before they arise.

CONCLUSIONS

Although tremendous progress has been made in the area of pediatric pharmacotherpy, many questions remain unanswered. The pharmacokinetics of many important drugs have been elucidated, but their pharmacodynamics has not been explored fully. Similarly, effect of disease states and patient characteristics such as genetic status have not been studied for most drugs. The effect of these factors on the development of cytochrome P450 isozymes (e.g., 3A4, 2D6, 1A2, and 2C19) and other enzymes needs to be studied (see Chaps. 4 and 5). Similarly, comparative efficacy and safety data for many therapies are unavailable. Influence of drug therapy on clinical and economic outcomes and on quality of life needs to be studied in pediatric patients.

The development of new drugs has contributed to improve patient care. The new FDA regulations can require the industry to conduct studies and seek labeling of important drugs for pediatric patients. As an incentive, a 6-month patent extension and waiver of supplemental new drug application fee are offered to the industry. This should encourage the industry to develop and market more drugs for the pediatric population. However, greater emphasis also should be placed on disease prevention. Millions of children die because of preventable diseases, particularly in developing countries of the world. Administration of vaccines and control of diarrhea alone could save millions of these lives annually. However, the developed countries face different problems. The infant mortality rate in the United States is nearly twice as high among blacks as whites. In some cities, more than 30% of the infants admitted to neonatal intensive care units were born to cocaine-abusing mothers.[79] Improved prenatal care, educational programs, and avoidance of alcohol, smoking, and drugs of abuse during pregnancy may decrease mortality as well as morbidity from illnesses, including acquired immunodeficiency syndrome.

Another exciting development is an identification of the genetic cause of common serious diseases such as cystic fibrosis. Nearly 70% of the gene mutations in cystic fibrosis are caused by the loss of a single trinucleotide codon, and the protein therefore lacks one amino acid, phenylalanine. One day it should be possible to offer gene therapy to correct the gene defects that cause a multitude of diseases.[80] Finally, certain procedures (e.g., extracorporeal membrane oxygenation, organ transplantation) and drugs (e.g., colony-stimulating factors, palivizumab, dornase alpha, epoetin alpha, immunoglobulins, surfactants, growth hormones) can improve quality of life or survival in patients.

Although much needs to be learned about the optimization of pediatric therapy, it is encouraging to witness the continued growth of knowledge in this area.

▶ PRINCIPLES OF PHARMACOTHERAPY

- Assess patients, medication history, and clinical/laboratory data.
- Document the need for drug therapy.
- Confirm the accuracy of patient's age, body weight, and dosage regimens of drugs.
- Select the most appropriate dosage form and regimen.
- Prepare a stable extemporaneous dosage form if one is not available commercially.
- Use the most effective, safe, palatable, and economical medicines based on comparative data.
- Establish therapeutic end points and measure health outcomes.
- Monitor for adverse effects and drug interactions.
- Implement changes in drug(s), dose(s), or dosage interval(s) as needed.
- Simplify regimens to improve adherence to and persistence with medication therapy.
- Counsel patients and caregivers.
- Periodically contact the patient and caregivers for continuity of care.

REFERENCES

1. Infant mortality statistics show variation by race, ethnicity, and state. National Vital Statistics Report, Vol. 48. Washington, U.S. Department of Health and Human Services, Centers for Disease Control, National Center for Health Statistics. 2000:15–16.
2. Avery GB, Randolph JG, Weaver T. Gastric acidity in the first day of life. Pediatrics 1966;37:1005–1007.
3. Agunod M, Yamaguchi N, Lopex R, et al. Correlative study of hydrochloric acid, pepsin, and intrinsic factor secretion in newborns and infants. Am J Dig Dis 1969;14:400–414.

4. Huang NN, High RN. Comparison of serum levels following the administration of oral and parenteral preparations of penicillin to infants and children of various age groups. J Pediatr 1953;42:657–668.
5. Silverio J, Poole JW. Serum concentrations of ampicillin in newborn infants after oral administration. Pediatrics 1973;51:578–580.
6. O'Connor WJ, Warren GH, Edrada LS, et al. Serum concentrations of sodium nafcillin in infants during the perinatal period. Antimicrob Agents Chemother 1965:220–222.
7. Jalling B. Plasma concentrations of phenobarbital in the treatment of seizures in newborns. Acta Paediatr Scand 1975;64:514–524.
8. Signer E, Fridrich R. Gastric emptying in newborns and young infants. Acta Paediatr Scand 1975;64:525–530.
9. Boreus IO. Plasma concentrations of phenobarbital in mother and child after combined prenatal and postnatal administration for prophylaxic of hyperbilirubinemia. J. Pediatr 1978;93:695.
10. Morselli PL. Serum levels and pharmacokinetics of anticonvulsants in the management of seizure disorders. In: Merkin B, ed. Clinical Pharmacology. Chicago, Year Book, 1978:89.
11. Tyrala FF, Hillman LS, Hillman RE, et al. Clinical pharmacology of hexachlorophene in newborn infants. J Pediatr 1977;91:481–486.
12. McFadden S, Haddow JE. Coma produced by topical application of isopropanol. Pediatrics 1969;43:622–623.
13. Evans NJ, Rutter N, Hadgraft J, et al. Percutaneous administration of theophylline in preterm infant. J Pediatr 1985;107:307–311.
14. Friis-Hansen B. Body water compartments in children: Changes during growth and related changes in body composition. Pediatrics 1961;28:169–181.
15. Haughey DB, Hilligoss DM, Grassi A, et al. Two-compartment gentamicin pharmacokinetics in premature neonates: A comparison to adults with decreased glomerular filtration rates. J Pediatr 1980;96:325–330.
16. Nahata MC, Powell DA, Durrell DE, et al. Effect of gestational age and birth weight on tobramycin kinetics in newborn infants. J Antimicrob Chemother 1984;14:59–65.
17. Roberts RJ. Pharmacologic principles in therapeutics in infants. In: Drug Therapy in Infants. Philadelphia, Saunders, 1984;3–12.
18. Pitlick W, Painter M, Pippenger C. Phenobarbital pharmacokinetics in neonates. Clin Pharmacol Ther 1978;23:346–350.
19. Painter MJ, Pippenger C, MacDonald H, et al. Phenobarbital and diphenylhydantoin levels in neonates with seizures. J Pediatr 1978;92:315–319.
20. Silverman WA, Anderson DH, Blanc WA, et al. A difference in mortality rate and incidence of kernicterus among premature infants allotted to two prophylactic antibacterial regimens. Pediatrics 1956;18: 614–624.
21. Odell GB. The dissociation of bilirubin from albumin and its clinical implications. J Pediatr 1959;55:268–279.
22. Morselli PL. Clinical pharmacokinetics in neonates. Clin Pharmacokinet 1976;1:81–98.
23. Committee on Drugs, American Academy of Pediatrics. The transfer of drugs and other chemicals into human milk. Pediatrics 1994;93:137–150.
24. Anderson PO. Drugs and breast milk. J Pediatr 1995;95:957.
25. Rane A. Basic principles of drug disposition and action in infants and children. In: Yaffe JF, ed. Pediatric Pharmacology: Therapeutic Principles in Practice. New York, Grune & Stratton, 1980:7–28.
26. Weiss CF, Glazko AJ, Weston JK. Chloramphenicol in the newborn infant: A physiologic explanation of its toxicity when given in excessive doses. N Engl J Med 1960;262:787–794.
27. Nahata MC, Powell DA. Comparative bioavailability and pharmacokinetics of chloramphenicol after intravenous chloramphenicol succinate in premature infants and older patients. Dev Pharmacol Ther 1983;6:23–32.
28. Kuhn R, Nahata MC, Powell DA, et al. Netilmicin pharmacokinetics in newborn infants. Eur J Clin Pharmacol 1986;29:635–637.
29. Chay PCW, Duffy BJ, Walker JS. Pharmacokinetic-pharmacodynamic relationships of morphine in neonates. Clin Pharmacol Ther 1992;51:334–342.
30. Edwards DJ, Zarowitz BJ, Slaughter RL. Theophylline. In: Evans WE, Schentag JJ, Jusko WJ, eds. Applied Pharmacokinetics, 3d ed. Vancouver, Applied Therapeutics, 1992;1–47.
31. Leffert FL. The management of chronic asthma. J Pediatr 1980;97:875–885.
32. Johnston DE. Immunotherapy in children: Past, present, and future, part I. Ann Allergy 1981;46:1–7.
33. Johnston DE. Immunotherapy in children: Past, present, and future, part II. Ann Allergy 1981;46:59–66.
34. Kearin M, Kelly JG, O'Malley K. Digoxin "receptors" in neonates: An explanation of less sensitivity to digoxin than in adults. Clin Pharmacol Ther 1980;28:346–349.
35. Kawai M, Momoi T, Yorifuji, T, et al. Unfavorable effects of growth hormone therapy on the final height of boys with short stature not caused by growth hormone deficiency. J Pediatr 1997;130:205–209.
36. Glasgow AM, Boeckx RL, Miller MK, et al. Hyperosmolality in small infants due to propylene glycol. Pediatrics 1983;72:353–355.
37. Hiller JL, Benda GI, Rahatzad M, et al. Benzyl alcohol toxicity: Impact of mortality and intraventricular hemorrhage among very low birth weight infants. Pediatrics 1986;77:500–506.
38. Grossman ER, Walchek A. Freedman H. Tetracyclines and permanent teeth: The relation between dose and tooth color. Pediatrics 1971;47:567–570.
39. Walker RC, Wright AJ. The quinolones. Mayo Clin Proc 1987;62:1007–1012.
40. Chysky V, Kapla M, Hullman R, et al. Safety of ciprofloxacin in children: Worldwide clinical experience based on compassionate usage. Infection 1991;19:289–296.
41. Schentag JJ, Plaut ME, Cerra FB, et al. Aminoglycoside nephrotoxicity in critically ill surgical patients. J Surg Res 1979;26:270–279.
42. Kauffman RE, Habersange R. Modification of dosage regimens in disease states of childhood. In: Mirking BL, ed. Clinical Pharmacology and Therapeutics: A Pediatric Perspective. Chicago, Year Book, 1978:73–88.
43. Roberts RJ. Special considerations in drug therapy in infants. In: Drug Therapy in Infants. Philadelphia, Saunders, 1984:25–35.
44. Feinstein RA, Miles MV. The effect of acute viral hepatitis on theophylline clearance. Clin Pediatr 1985;24:357–358.
45. Wallace CS, Hall M, Kuhn RJ. Pharmacologic management of cystic fibrosis. Clin Pharm 1993;12:657–674.
46. Myers MG, Roberts JF, Mirhig NJ. Effect of gestational age, birth weight, and hypoxemia on the pharmacokinetics of amikacin in serum of infants. Antimicrob Agents Chemother 1977;11:1027.
47. Bahal-O'Mara N, Jones R, Nahata MC, et al. Pharmacokinetics of phenytoin in children with acute neurotrauma. Crit Care Med 1995;23: 1418–1424.
48. Rana SR. Pain: a subject ignored (letter). Pediatrics 1987;79:309.
49. Franch LS, Greenberg CS, Stevens B. Pain assessment in infants and children. Pediatr Clin North Am 2000;47(3):487–512.
50. Fitzgerald M, Anand KJS. Development neuroanatomy and neurophysiology of pain. In: Schechter NL, Berde CB, Yaster M, eds. Pain in Infants, Children and Adolescents. Baltimore, Williams & Wilkins, 1993: 11–31.
51. Taddio A, Katz J, Ilersich Al, et al. Effect of neonatal circumcision on pain response during subsequent routine vaccination. Lancet 1997;349: 559–603.
52. Taddio A, Ohlsson A, Einarson T, et al. A systematic review of lidocaine-prilocaine cream for neonatal circumcision pain. N Engl J Med 1997;336:1197–1201.
53. Uhari M. Eutectic mixture of lidocaine and prilocaine for alleviating vaccination pain in infants. Pediatrics 1993;92:719–721.
54. Zempsky WT, Anand KS, Sullivan KM, et al. Lidocaine iontophoresis for topical anesthesia before intravenous line placement in children. J Pediatr 1998;132:1061–1063.
55. Reis EC, Holobukov R. Vapocoolant spray is equally effective as EMLA cream in reducing immunization pain in school-aged children. Pediatrics 1997;100:5.
56. Bartfield JM, Gennis P, Barbera J, et al. Buffered versus plain lidocaine as a local anesthetic for simple laceration repair. Ann Emerg Med 1990; 19:1387–1390.
57. Keen MF. Comparison of intramuscular injection techniques to reduce site discomfort and lesions. Nurs Res 1986;35:207–210.
58. Golianu B, Krane EJ, Galloway KS, et al. Pediatric acute pain management. Pediatr Clin North Am 2000;47(3):559–587.

59. Chay PCW, Duffy BJ, Walker JS. Pharmacokinetic-pharmacodynamic relationship of morphine in neonates. Clin Pharmacol Ther 1992;51:334–342.
60. Berde CB, Lehn BM, Yee JD, et al. Patient-controlled analgesia in children and adolescents: A randomized, prospective comparison with intramuscular administration of morphine for postoperative analgesia. J Pediatr 1991;118:460–466.
61. Nichols DG, Yaster M, Lynn AM, et al: Disposition and respiratory effects of intrathecal morphine in children. Anesthesiology 1993;79:733–738.
62. Nahata MC, Powell DA, Glazer JP, et al. Effect of intravenous flow rate and infection site on in vitro delivery of chloramphenicol succinate and in vivo kinetics. J Pediatr 1981;99:463–466.
63. Nahata MC, Powell DA, Durrell DE, et al. Effect of infusion methods on tobramycin serum concentrations in newborn infants. J Pediatr 1984;104:136–138.
64. Gould T, Robert RJ. Therapeutic problems arising from the use of intra venous route for drug administration. J Pediatr 1979;95:465–471.
65. Rajchgot P, Radde IC, MacLeod SM. Influence of specific gravity on intravenous drug delivery. J Pediatr 1981;99:658–661.
66. Berman W, Whitman V, Marks KH, et al. Inadvertent overadministration of digoxin to low birth weight infants. J Pediatr 1978;92:1024.
67. Zenk KE, Anderson S. Improving the accuracy of minivolume injections. Infusion 1982(Jan/Feb):7–11.
68. Nahata MC, Durrell DE. Stability of tobramycin sulfate in admixtures containing calcium gluconate. Am J Hosp Pharm 1985;42:1987–1988.
69. Nahata MC, Hipple TF. Pediatric Drug Formulations, 3d ed. Cincinnati, Harvey Whitney Books, 1997:1–118.
70. Nahata MC, Miser A, Miser J, et al. Analgesic plasma concentrations of morphine in children with terminal malignancy receiving a continuous subcutaneous infusion of morphine sulfate to control severe pain. Pain 1984;18:109–114.
71. Boreus LO. Drug compliance. In: Yaffe SJ, ed. Principles of Pediatric Pharmacology. New York, Churchill-Livingstone, 1982:176–192.
72. Matsui D, Barron A, Rieder MJ. Assessment of the palatability of antistaphylococcal antibiotics in pediatric volunteers. Ann Pharmacother 1996;30:586–588.
73. Institute of Medicine, Committee on Quality of Health Care in America. To Err Is Human: Building a Safer Health System. Washington, National Academy Press, 2000.
74. Wilson DG, McArtney RG, Newcombe RG, et al. Medication errors in paediatric practice: Insights from a continuous quality improvement approach. Eur J Pediatr 1998;157:769–774.
75. Raju TN, Kecskes S, Thornton JP, et al. Medication errors in neonatal and paediatric intensive-care units. Lancet 1989;2(8659):374–376.
76. Folli HL, Poole RL, Benitz WE, et al. Medication error prevention by clinical pharmacists in two children's hospitals. Pediatrics 1987;79:718–722.
77. Kaushal R, Bates DW, et al. Medication errors and adverse drug events in pediatric inpatients. JAMA 2001:285:2114–2120.
78. American Academy of Pediatrics Committee on Drugs and Committee on Hospital Care. Prevention of medication errors in pediatric inpatient setting. Pediatrics 1988;102:428–430.
79. Cherukuri R, Minkoff H, Feldman J, et al. A cohort study of alkaloidal cocaine (crack) in pregnancy. Obstet Gynecol 1988;72:147–151.
80. Nahata MC. Discovery of the gene defect in cystic fibrosis: implications for diagnosis and treatment. Clin Pharm 1990;9:716–717.

7

GERIATRICS

Joseph T. Hanlon, Christine M. Ruby, David Guay, and Margaret Artz

Pharmacotherapy for the elderly can cure or palliate disease as well as enhance health-related quality of life (HRQOL). HRQOL considerations for the elderly include focusing on improvement in physical functioning (e.g., activities of daily living), psychological functioning (e.g., cognition, depression), social functioning (e.g., social activities, support systems), and overall health (e.g., general health perception).[1–4] Despite the benefits of pharmacotherapy, HRQOL can be compromised by drug-related problems. The avoidance of drug-related adverse consequences in the elderly requires health care practitioners to become knowledgeable about a number of age-specific issues. To address these knowledge needs, this chapter will discuss the epidemiology of aging; physiologic changes associated with aging, with emphasis on those which can affect the pharmacokinetics and pharmacodynamics of drugs; common clinical conditions seen in geriatric patients; epidemiology of drug-related problems in the elderly; and an approach to reduce drug-related problems through the provision of comprehensive geriatric assessment.

EPIDEMIOLOGY OF AGING

In an era of limited resources and managed-care philosophy, it is important to assess the needs of both the community and the population in order to make clinical practice as effective as possible. In assessing these needs, a population's demographic and health characteristics provide the information necessary to allocate present resources. Using population projections, society can plan for the training, research, and resource needs necessary for future clinical practice and adequate health care.

In considering the entire older American population, the terms *diversity* and *heterogeneity* are applied frequently and appropriately. The demographics and health characteristics of persons aged 65 to 74 years are different from those 85 years of age and older, as are those who are institutionalized compared with those living in the community. It is teasing apart the various threads of wellness and illness, independence and dependence, and function and dysfunction that make the available demographic and health-status data relevant for clinical practice today and for planning for the future.

Currently, persons aged 65 or older account for 13% (35 million) of the total U.S. population. Women make up 58% of these 35 million and 70% of the segment that is aged 85 years and older.[5] The percentage of older persons in the United States is expected to increase only 1.3% per year over the next 10 years.[6] However, by 2030, one in five Americans will be over the age of 65 years, with 2.5% of the U.S. population aged 85 years and older. This 20% projection for persons aged 65 years and older will persist until 2050. However, the number of persons aged 85 years and older will further increase by 2050, to 5% (19 million) of the total U.S. population.[7]

The increase in the number of older persons is not just due to the post-World War II birth rate but also to a declining mortality rate and overall better health among elders.[8,9] The decline in early death and better elder health arise from a variety of reasons: (1) public health measures affecting all age groups (e.g., immunizations, prenatal care), (2) advances in medical procedures and drugs, (3) promotion of a healthy lifestyle, and (4) improvements in social living conditions.[10–14] Thus, while life expectancy at birth rose from 47 to 75 years through the first three-quarters of the twentieth century, projected estimates for 2050 range from 82 to 83 years.[6,15] More relevant to providers of care for older Americans is life expectancy at age 65. In 2000, white women 65 years of age can expect an average additional 19.7 years of life; black women, 17.8 years; white men, 16.2 years; and black men, 13.8 years.[6] Today, if a person survives to age 85, he can expect to live another 6 years and she another 7 years.[5] It is not surprising, then, that the number of centenarians nearly doubled during the 1990s to 70,000, with the Census Bureau projecting that this special population segment could number 834,000 by the middle of the next century.[16]

Along with changes in the life expectancy of future elders, there also will be changes in its racial composition. In 2000, an estimated 84% of persons age 65 years and older are non-Hispanic white, 8% were non-Hispanic black, and 6% were Hispanic. By 2050, the percentage of white elders will decline to 64%, and Hispanics and non-Hispanic blacks will account for 16% and 12% of the older population, respectively.[5]

Contrary to popular thinking, most older persons are self-sufficient and live in the community. However, as they age in the community, the likelihood of living alone increases, more so for women than for men. Only 4.3% of older persons reside in a long-term care facility, with the age distribution of nursing home residents being 13% for persons aged 65 to 74 years, 35% for persons aged 75 to 84 years, and 50% for persons aged 85+ years.[17]

Keeping persons independent for as long as possible is the primary goal in the clinical care of persons 65 years of age and older, a goal that ought to influence therapeutic decisions (e.g., prescribing). Similar to the distributions seen in living arrangement and nursing home status, disability is seen prominently in persons over 80 years of age, with almost three-fourths reporting at least one disability.[17] In contrast, recent data regarding older persons of all ages suggest that disability rates [measured as having one or more limitations performing activities of daily living (ADLs) for at least 90 days] declined from 1982 to 1994, from 24.0% in 1982 to 21.3% in 1994.[18] However, when considering only non-institutionalized persons who were aged 70 years and older, the disability rate was less (only 10%).[14,18] The picture is different for institutionalized older persons, where approximately 80% of them have some problems with mobility and 65% have difficulty controlling their bowels.[19] Nonetheless, whether disability rates will continue to decline at their present rate of 1.5% per year is debatable and depends on changes in the environment, changes in social roles, changes in the use of assistive devices, advancements in medicine and pharmacy, and changes in elders' education levels.[14]

A *chronic condition*, defined as an illness or impairment that cannot be cured, is often the cause of disability in the elderly.[20] The older population compared with younger persons is more affected by chronic conditions for several reasons: (1) the types of chronic conditions common among older persons tend to be more disabling (e.g., arthritis, heart disease), (2) the conditions become more severe with aging, and (3) several conditions are likely to be present.[8,21,22]

The most common chronic conditions of older Americans depend on their residence status. For noninstitutionalized older Americans, the list has changed little in the past decade.[23] These conditions, in rank order of prevalence, include arthritis (45%), high blood pressure (34%), hearing impairments (28%), heart disease (25%), cataracts (16%), orthopedic impairments (15%), sinusitis (11%), diabetes (9%), tinnitus (8%), and visual impairments (8%).[23,24] For elderly patients admitted to a nursing home, the common primary diagnoses are cardiovascular or cerebrovascular disease, mental disorders, nervous system or sensory impairment, or complications secondary to injuries.[25] A recent national report concerning hospital admissions notes that one-third of all elderly admissions are due to cardiovascular disease, 14% are due to respiratory problems, 6.5% are due to fractures, and 6.3% are due to cancer.[26]

Figure 7–1 illustrates the top 10 causes of death in elders. These causes have changed little in recent years. In 1980, heart diseases, cancers, or stroke accounted for 75% of deaths in those 65 years of age and older; in 1998, these diagnoses accounted for 64% of deaths.[19] The change in percentages is due, in part, to the gains made in the prevention and treatment of heart disease and stroke as well as increases in deaths due to respiratory diseases.

Elders are avid consumers of medical and prescription drug resources. With older persons accounting for 36% of all hospital stays and 49% of all days of care in hospitals, elders consume almost one-third of total U.S. health care expenditures.[17,27] By 2030, health

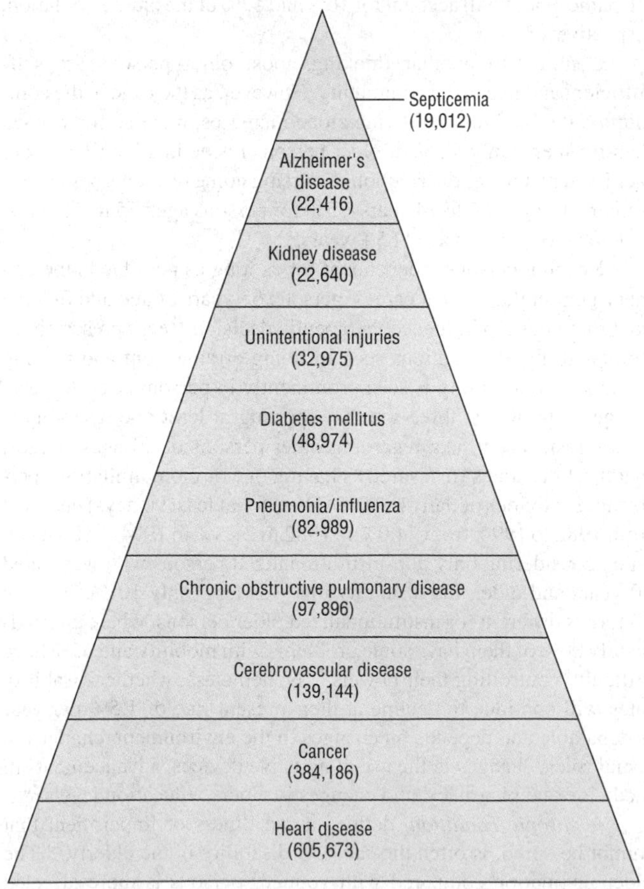

FIGURE 7–1. Leading causes of death in persons 65 years of age and older, 1998. (*Adapted from Ref. 19.*)

care spending by the U.S. population is projected to increase by 25%, simply because the average age of the population is increasing.[27] Although older persons comprise 13% of the U.S. population, they account for 34% of all prescription drug expenditures.[28] This was estimated at $25.1 to 26.7 billion per year in 1996.[29,30] Some 69% of elders (34 million Americans) have prescription drug coverage for at least part of any given year.[30] However, 17% to 40% of elders who are poor or near poor (but not eligible for Medicaid) have no prescription benefit.[28,30] The possible addition of a Medicare prescription drug benefit was a major point of discussion during the 2000 U.S. presidential campaign; hopefully, this important need of elders will be addressed by federal and/or state governments during the early years of the twenty-first century.

HUMAN AGING AND CHANGES IN DRUG PHARMACOKINETICS AND PHARMACODYNAMICS

There is a progressive functional decline in organ systems with advancing age. Table 7–1 reviews some common physiologic changes with an emphasis on those which can affect pharmacotherapy. For more detailed information, readers are referred to discussions in review articles.[31,32]

Age-associated physiologic changes may cause reductions in functional reserve capacity (or the ability to respond to physiologic challenges or stresses) and the homeostasis of the body.[33,34] To deal with physiologic challenges or stresses, an older individual may need 95% of his or her remaining reserve capacity.[31,32] However, physiologic aging slowly reduces functional reserve capacity and homeostatic control mechanisms, thus making an elder more susceptible to decompensation in a stressful situation. The cardiovascular, musculoskeletal, and central nervous systems may be most affected.[31,32] Examples of impaired homeostatic mechanisms include postural stability, orthostatic responses, thermoregulation, cognitive reserve, and bowel and bladder function. An event resulting in functional impairment may involve an insult for which the body cannot compensate, and relatively small stresses may result in major morbidity and mortality.[33]

A number of age-related physiologic changes occur that potentially could affect drug pharmacokinetics and pharmacodynamics (see Table 7–1). Unfortunately, limited data are available regarding the pharmacokinetics and pharmacodynamics of individual drugs commonly used in the elderly. This information gap may improve with the implementation of Food and Drug Administration (FDA) regulations establishing a "geriatric use" subsection in product labeling for all newly marketed drugs and all previously marketed drugs by 2003 and guidelines calling for pharmacokinetic studies by pharmaceutical companies for new molecular entities likely to have significant use in the elderly.[35,36]

ALTERED PHARMACOKINETICS

Table 7–2 and the following discussion summarize what is known about the effect of aging on each of the four major facets of pharmacokinetics.[37–39]

ABSORPTION

Most drugs are given orally, and thus a number of age-related changes in gastrointestinal physiology (see Table 7–1) potentially could affect the absorption of medications. Fortunately, most drugs are absorbed

TABLE 7–1. Physiologic Changes with Aging

Organ System	Manifestation
Body composition	↓ Total body water ↓ Lean body mass ↑ Body fat ↔ or ↓ Serum albumin ↔ or ↑ α_1-Acid glycoprotein (↑ by several disease states)
Cardiovascular system	↓ Myocardial sensitivity to β-adrenergic stimulation ↓ In baroreceptor activity ↓ Cardiac output ↑ Total peripheral resistance
Central nervous system	↓ In weight and volume of the brain Alterations in several aspects of cognition
Endocrine system	Thyroid gland atrophies with age Increase in incidence of diabetes mellitus, thyroid disease Menopause
Gastrointestinal system	↑ Gastric pH Delayed gastric emptying ↓ Gastrointestinal blood flow Slowed intestinal transit
Genitourinary system	Atrophy of the vagina secondary to decreased estrogen Prostatic hypertrophy secondary to androgenic hormonal changes Age-related changes may predispose to incontinence
Immune system	↓ Cell-mediated immunity
Liver	↓ Liver size ↓ Liver blood flow
Oral changes	Altered dentition ↓ Ability to taste sweetness, sourness, and bitterness
Pulmonary system	↓ Respiratory muscle strength ↓ In chest wall compliance ↓ Total alveolar surface ↓ Vital capacity ↓ Maximal breathing capacity
Renal system	↓ Glomerular filtration rate ↓ Renal blood flow ↑ Filtration fraction ↓ Tubular secretory function ↓ Renal mass
Sensory changes	↓ Accommodation of the lens of the eye, causing farsightedness Presbycusis (loss of auditory acuity) ↓ Conduction velocity
Skeletal system	Loss of skeletal bone mass (osteopenia)
Integument	Skin dryness, wrinkling, and changes in pigmentation, epithelial thinning, loss of dermal thickness ↓ In number of hair follicles ↓ In number of melanocytes in the hair bulbs

From Refs. 31 and 32.

TABLE 7–2. Age-Related Changes in Pharmacokinetics

Pharmacokinetic Phase	Pharmacokinetic Parameters
Gastrointestinal absorption	Unchanged passive diffusion and no change in bioavailability for most drugs ↓ Active transport and ↓ bioavailability for some drugs ↓ First-pass effect and ↑ bioavailability for some drugs
Distribution	↓ Volume of distribution and ↑ plasma concentration of water-soluble drugs ↑ Volume of distribution and ↑ terminal disposition half-life ($t_{1/2}$) for fat-soluble drugs ↑ or ↓ Free fraction of highly plasma protein bound drugs
Hepatic metabolism	↓ Clearance and ↑ $t_{1/2}$ for some oxidatively metabolized drugs ↓ Clearance and ↑ $t_{1/2}$ of drugs with high hepatic extraction ratio
Renal excretion	↓ Clearance and ↑ $t_{1/2}$ of renally eliminated drugs

From Refs. 37 to 39.

via passive diffusion, so age-related physiologic changes appear to have little influence on drug bioavailability.[40] A few drugs require active transport for their absorption, and thus their bioavailability may be reduced (e.g., calcium in the setting of hypochlorhydria). However, there is evidence for a decreased first-pass effect that results in increased bioavailability and higher plasma concentrations of drugs such as propranolol and morphine.[40] Increased drug bioavailability also may be seen with the concurrent ingestion of grapefruit juice; it inhibits the cytochrome P450 isoenzyme 3A4, thus decreasing first-pass metabolism and resulting in exaggerated pharmacologic effects.[41]

The effect of age-related changes in skin physiology on the bioavailability of drugs delivered transdermally is poorly understood. One study found that the bioavailability of transdermal fentanyl was enhanced in older individuals.[42] However, a study by Thompson and coworkers that compared the pharmacokinetics of transdermal fentanyl in 10 young and 8 elderly subjects found no significant differences in the mean maximum plasma concentration, time at which maximum plasma concentration occurred, terminal disposition half-life ($t_{1/2}$) after patch removal, or area under the plasma concentration-versus-time curve from time 0 to infinity.[43] However, the mean time for plasma concentrations to double after patch application was nearly three times longer in the elderly compared with the younger group. Whether these findings hold true for other drugs delivered transdermally remains to be determined.

DISTRIBUTION

The distribution of medications in the body depends on factors such as blood flow, plasma protein binding, and body composition, each of which may be altered with age (see Table 7–1). For example, the volume of distribution of water-soluble drugs is decreased, whereas lipophilic drugs will exhibit an increased volume of distribution.[37–39] Changes in the volume of distribution can have a direct impact on the amount of medication that needs to be given as a loading dose.

The two major plasma proteins to which medications can bind are albumin and α_1-acid glycoprotein (AAG), and concentrations of these proteins may change with concurrent pathologies seen with increasing age[44] (see Table 7–1). For acidic drugs such as naproxen, phenytoin, tolbutamide, and warfarin, decreased serum albumin may lead to an increase in free fraction. An increase in AAG induced by burns, cancer, inflammatory disease, or trauma may lead to a decreased free fraction of basic medications such as lidocaine, propranolol, quinidine, and imipramine. In the absence of compromise in excretory pathways, these potential changes are unlikely to have any deleterious clinical effect. However, they may be important to consider when interpreting serum concentrations for these drugs, since usually only total drug concentrations (sum of free and protein-bound drug) are reported.

METABOLISM

The liver is the major organ responsible for drug metabolism, including phase I (oxidative) and phase II (conjugative) reactions.[45] Recent data suggest that age-related declines in phase I metabolism are more likely the result of reduced liver volume rather than reduced hepatic enzymatic activity.[46] Decreased phase I metabolism (e.g., hydroxylation, dealkylation) producing decreased drug clearance and increased $t_{1/2}$ has been reported for medications such as diazepam, piroxicam, theophylline, and quinidine. Phase II metabolism (e.g., glucuronidation) of medications such as lorazepam and oxazepam appears to be relatively unaffected by age. Hepatic enzyme induction (e.g., by rifampin, phenytoin) or inhibition (e.g., by macrolides, ciprofloxicin, cimetidine) do not appear to be affected by the aging process.[47–50]

Age-related decreases in liver blood flow (see Table 7–1) also can significantly decrease the metabolism of high hepatic extraction ratio drugs such as imipramine, lidocaine, morphine, and propranolol.[45] The effect that age has on drugs that undergo polymorphic drug metabolism is less clear, although a recent study suggests that age has no biologically important effect on acetylator phenotype.[51] Moreover, a number of potential confounding factors, including race, sex, frailty, smoking, diet, and drug-drug interactions, may significantly affect hepatic metabolism in the elderly.[52]

ELIMINATION

Renal excretion is the primary route of elimination for many drugs. Although age-related reductions in glomerular filtration are well documented, as many as one-third of "normal" elderly subjects may have no decrease, as measured by creatinine clearance.[37–39] Moreover, emerging information suggests that tubular secretion may not decline in proportion to other renal processes.[53] The estimation of creatinine clearance, although not entirely accurate in all patients, can serve as a useful screening approximation.[54] One of the most commonly used equations for adults was created by Cockcroft and Gault[55]:

$$\text{Creatinine clearance (males)} = \frac{(140 - \text{age in years}) \times (\text{actual body weight in kg})}{(72) \times (\text{serum creatinine in mg/dL})}$$

For women, multiply this result by 0.85.

Medications whose excretion is primarily renal and for which there is evidence of age-related reduction in clearance include acetazolamide, amantadine, aminoglycosides, atenolol, captopril, cimetidine, digoxin, lithium, and vancomycin. Some hepatically metabolized medications can yield active, primarily renally excreted metabolites such as *N*-acetylprocainamide, normeperidine, and morphine-6-glucuronide, which can accumulate with advancing age due to reduced renal function.

ALTERED PHARMACODYNAMICS

There is some evidence in the elderly of enhanced drug response or "sensitivity." Four possible mechanisms have been suggested: (1) changes in receptor numbers, (2) changes in receptor affinity, (3) postreceptor alterations, and (4) age-related impairment of homeostatic mechanisms.[34,39,56] For example, muscarinic, parathyroid hormone, β-adrenergic, α_1-adrenergic and μ-opioid receptors exhibit reduced density with increasing age.[39] Evidence from epidemiologic and experimental studies suggest that, independent of pharmacokinetic alterations, the elderly are more sensitive to the central nervous system effects of benzodiazepines.[57] The elderly also exhibit a greater analgesic response to opioids when compared with their younger counterparts, even when pharmacokinetic parameters are similar between the groups.[58] In addition, the elderly demonstrate enhanced response to anticoagulants such as warfarin and heparin as well as thrombolytic therapy.[37] The elderly exhibit decreased pharmacodynamic sensitivity to certain drugs (e.g., β-agonists/antagonists).[59] In addition, reflex tachycardia, commonly seen with vasodilator therapy, is often blunted in the elderly, perhaps due to dampened baroreceptor function. Moreover, for some drugs (e.g., calcium-channel blockers), both enhanced pharmacodynamic sensitivity (as demonstrated by greater reduction in blood pressure) and decreased sensitivity (as demonstrated by reduced atrioventricular nodal blockade) occur simultaneously in elders.[57]

TABLE 7–3. The I's of Geriatrics: Common Problems in the Elderly

Immobility	Instability
Isolation	Intellectual impairment
Incontinence	Impotence
Infection	Immunodeficiency
Inanition (malnutrition)	Insomnia
Impaction	Iatrogenesis
Impaired senses	

From Ref. 31.

CLINICAL GERIATRICS

As mentioned previously, maintenance of independence and prevention of disability are primary goals in the clinical care of persons 65 years of age or older. To achieve these goals, it is necessary that pharmacists and other health care providers understand the concept of functional status because the elderly are not a homogeneous group. Typically, functional status can be determined by inquiring about an elderly person's ability to perform basic ADLs. Basic ADLs include activities such as feeding, dressing, ambulating, toileting, bathing, and grooming.[60] More complex activities are termed *instrumental activities of daily living* (IADLs). These include cooking, cleaning, shopping, using the telephone, managing money, and managing medications.[61] However, functional status depends not only on physical ailments but also on psychologic and social circumstances.[2]

One of the challenges of maintaining and improving functional status in geriatric individuals is diagnosing and managing conditions seen primarily in the elderly. Common problems found in older persons are sometimes referred to as the *I's of geriatrics*[31] (Table 7–3). Examples of diseases and syndromes that can present as these common problems include Parkinson's disease, falls, hip fractures, benign prostatic hypertrophy, dementia, glaucoma, postherpetic neuralgia, and tuberculosis.

Another factor that contributes to the challenge of clinical geriatrics is that approximately 50% of older patients present with atypical symptoms or complaints, making it difficult to use the classic medical model for diagnosis[62–65] (Table 7–4). For example, cardiac ischemia may present as syncope or weakness in an older person rather than the typical presentation of chest pain. Confusion may be the presenting symptom of an acute abdominal process rather than the expected severe pain, rigidity of the abdominal muscles, and leukocytosis. Serious adverse consequences may result if a diagnosis is delayed because of these atypical presentations. Such unusual presentations may result from factors associated with age-related physiologic changes, the presence of multiple comorbid illnesses, compromised functioning, and the presence of psychologic stressors.[62] Table 7–4 presents additional examples of medical illnesses that often present atypically in the elderly.[62–65] Other atypical symptoms also often are indicative of frailty and commonly include delirium, falls, and nonspecific functional decline.[62–64]

Multiple coexisting chronic illnesses are another common threat to independence that distinguishes the elderly from younger patients. It is not unusual for elderly patients to have multiple comorbidities such as osteoarthritis, heart disease, and diabetes. Although multiple comorbidities can have a substantial impact on a patient's functional status, the mere existence of multiple diseases alone does not determine functional impairment.

DRUG-RELATED PROBLEMS IN THE ELDERLY

Although medications used by the elderly can lead to improvement in HRQOL, negative outcomes due to drug-related problems are considerable.[66,67] Three important and potentially preventable negative outcomes due to drug-related problems that can occur in the elderly are adverse drug withdrawal events (ADWEs), which are clinically significant sets of symptoms or signs caused by the removal of a drug; therapeutic failure (inadequate drug therapy); and adverse drug reactions (ADRs).[68–70]

Limited data are available about the prevalence of ADWEs and related therapeutic failures in the elderly. Graves and colleagues reported ADWEs in 38 of 124 male outpatients who had 238 medications discontinued.[68] Grymonpre and coworkers reported that 19% of drug-associated hospital admissions in a group of older Canadians were related to therapeutic failure.[69] ADRs are thought to occur more commonly among elders compared with other age groups.[67] However, it is controversial whether age alone is a risk factor.[71] The reported rates of ADRs in the elderly range from 2.5% to 50.6%, depending on the study population and the methodology employed.[67] In the nursing home setting, a cost-of-illness study estimated that

TABLE 7–4. Atypical Disease Presentation in the Elderly[62–65]

Disease	Presentation
Acute myocardial infarction	Only about 50% present with chest pain, and diaphoresis and vomiting are uncommon in the absence of chest pain. In general, the elderly present with weakness, confusion, syncope, and abdominal pain; however, electrocardiographic findings are similar to younger patients.
Congestive heart failure	Instead of dyspnea, the patient may present with hypoxic symptoms, lethargy, restlessness, and confusion.
Gastrointestinal bleeding	Although the mortality rate is about 10%, the presenting symptoms are nonspecific, ranging from mental status change to syncope with hemodynamic collapse. Abdominal pain is often absent.
Upper respiratory infection	Older patients typically present with lethargy, confusion, anorexia, and decompensation of a preexisting medical condition. Fever, chills, and a productive cough may or may not be present.
Urinary tract infection	Dysuria, fever, and flank pain may be absent. More commonly, the elderly present with incontinence, confusion, abdominal pain, nausea/vomiting, and azotemia.

From Refs. 62 to 65.

drug-related problems (including ADRs and therapeutic failure) cost $4 billion per year.[72]

RISK FACTORS

A number of factors increase the risk of drug-related problems in the elderly, including suboptimal prescribing (e.g., overuse of medications or polypharmacy, inappropriate use, and underuse), medication errors (both dispensing and administration problems), and patient medication nonadherence (both intentional and unintentional). The following subsections address suboptimal prescribing and medication nonadherence, the most common problems.

OVERUSE

Polypharmacy can be defined as either the concomitant use of multiple drugs or the administration of more medications than are clinically indicated.[73,74] Polypharmacy is common in elderly persons; community-based surveys reveal that elders take an average of 2.7 to 4.2 prescription and nonprescription medications each day.[74–76] These studies also have shown that Caucasian patients, women, and those of advanced age are more likely to use greater numbers of prescription and nonprescription drugs.[77,78] The use of drugs increases to an average of 5 medications in elders who are hospitalized.[75] A recent nursing facility survey found that institutionalized elderly persons take an average of 6.69 routine medications, and 27.1% took 9 or more medications on a regular basis.[79] Drug-use studies that defined polypharmacy as use of one or more unnecessary medications showed that this occurs in 55% to 59% of elderly outpatients.[80,81] Multiple medication use has been strongly associated with ADRs.[67] The increase in ADR risk rises with increasing drug use. Polypharmacy is also problematic for elderly patients because it may increase the risk of geriatric syndromes, diminished functional status, and health care costs.[73,74]

INAPPROPRIATE PRESCRIBING

Inappropriate prescribing can be defined as prescribing of medications outside the bounds of accepted medical standards.[80,82,83] This phenomenon occurs commonly in elderly outpatients, as exemplified by one study in which 74% of drugs had at least one inappropriate rating based on clinical review applying explicit criteria.[80] Studies using explicit drug-use review criteria have found that between 7% and 53% of community-dwelling elders take one or more medications that have a dose, duration, duplication, or drug-interaction problem.[84–86]

Alternatively, *inappropriate prescribing* can be defined as those drugs whose use should be avoided because their risk outweighs potential benefit.[87,88] Applying explicit criteria developed by Beers and colleagues for medications or medication classes whose use should be avoided in the elderly, different investigators have found that 14% to 27% of persons 65 years of age and older living in the community take one or more such drugs.[88–90]

Inappropriate prescribing may pose important health risks. Limited retrospective data suggest that inappropriate prescribing is associated with drug-related hospital admissions and readmissions. A U.S. government report estimated that hospitalization due to inappropriate prescribing in the elderly costs $20 billion annually.[91] One study documented that 50% of ADRs causing hospital admissions in elderly patients resulted from inappropriate prescribing of drugs with contraindications or interactions.[92] Doucet and colleagues, in a prospective study of 1000 elderly people admitted to a hospital, found that 13% were related to a single type of inappropriate prescribing, drug-drug interactions.[93] Finally, Bero and associates found that 29% of drug-related hospital readmissions were due to medication inappropriateness.[94]

UNDERUSE

An important and increasingly recognized problem in elders is *underuse,* defined as the omission of drug therapy that is indicated for the treatment or prevention of a disease or condition.[95] One study found that 55% of 236 ambulatory elderly patients had one or more necessary drugs omitted because of lack of physician prescribing.[95] Another study of community-dwelling elders examined whether unrelated disorders are less likely to be treated in patients with chronic diseases.[96] They found that patients with diabetes mellitus were less likely to receive estrogen-replacement therapy, that patients with pulmonary emphysema were less likely to receive lipid-lowering medications, and that patients with psychotic syndromes were less likely to receive medications for arthritis.[96] Other investigators have focused on the omission of treatment of certain conditions such as hypertension, cancer chemotherapy, depression, underuse of angiotensin-converting enzyme (ACE) inhibitor medications in patients with congestive heart failure (CHF), underuse of anticoagulation in elderly patients with atrial fibrillation, and preventive therapy after myocardial infarction.[95,97,98] Underuse may have an important relationship with negative health outcomes in the elderly. For example, untreated depression has been associated with functional disability, health services use, and death.[99] Underuse of β-blockers in elderly survivors of acute myocardial infarction or underuse of ACE inhibitors in elders with CHF is associated with higher mortality.[100,101] The risk from underuse of medication in general due to limiting Medicaid patients' access to medications resulted in a more than doubling of the risk of admission to a nursing home.[102]

MEDICATION ADHERENCE

Medication nonadherence is a common problem in the elderly.[103] The prevalence rate ranges from 40% to 70% of patients (mean of approximately 50%).[104,105] Overall, these patients are adherent with about 75% of their medications.[106] It is commonly thought that the elderly have worse adherence than younger patients. However, this does not appear to be the case when the number of drugs taken by both groups is similar.[107] In fact, there is some evidence that adherence may be better in elders for some conditions.[108,109] What does seem to be different is that intentional nonadherence may be more common in the elderly.[110] Some have speculated that this may be related to the occurrence of ADRs and may represent intelligent nonadherence.[105] A recent study by Fincke and coworkers found that elders who perceived that they were overmedicated were more likely to have decreased adherence.[111]

Limited retrospective data suggest that nonadherence is associated with drug-related hospital admissions. A meta-analysis of studies published by Sullivan and associates that included patients of all ages determined that the rate of hospital admissions due to nonadherence was 5.5%.[112] A study by Col and coworkers evaluated 315 consecutive elderly patients admitted to a hospital and determined that 11.4% of admissions resulted from nonadherence.[113]

PROVISION OF COMPREHENSIVE GERIATRIC ASSESSMENT

Given that drug-related problems are common, costly, and clinically important, how can they be prevented? A solution may lie in comprehensive geriatric assessment. The term *comprehensive geriatric assessment* has been applied to geriatric evaluation and management (GEM), in which GEM clinicians manage the patient, and to consultative geriatric assessment, in which the geriatric multidisciplinary team makes recommendations to other clinicians for the management of the patient.[114–116] Comprehensive geriatric assessment has become a cornerstone in the care of the elderly; its effectiveness was summarized recently in a meta-analysis of 28 controlled trials.[117–119]

A number of published papers describe the role of pharmacists in optimizing pharmacotherapy for the elderly.[120–124] One has specifically documented the contribution of a clinical pharmacist to the effectiveness of interdisciplinary specialized geriatric care on drug-related problems.[124] The following subsections provide an approach to how pharmacists in any practice setting can optimize medication use through the provision of comprehensive geriatric assessment.

HISTORY TAKING

Several potential difficulties may occur while taking medication histories from the elderly. They include the following:

1. Communication problems (impaired hearing and vision)
2. Underreporting (health beliefs, cognitive impairment)
3. Vague or nonspecific symptoms (altered presentation)
4. Multiple diseases and medications
5. Reliance on a caregiver for the history
6. Lack of medical records to confirm findings

However, despite these potential difficulties, practitioners should find value in pursuing the collection of this vital medication history information. The importance of inquiry regarding nonprescription medication use in the elderly cannot be stressed enough, because one-third of all medications used by the ambulatory elderly are sold without a prescription, especially analgesics and laxatives.[76,125] Moreover, with the passage of the Dietary Supplement Health and Education Act of 1994, often referred to by its acronym, DSHEA, clinicians must probe for complementary and alternative medicines (e.g., dietary supplements, home or folk remedies, herbal medicines, homeopathic products, megavitamins).[126]

Asking elders and their caregivers about methods that they use to keep track of medicines is also important. This will allow one to design solutions to problems that are detected and prevent repeating ineffective and previously used methods.

Patients and caregivers also should be asked about risk factors for prescribing problems (e.g., multiple physicians and pharmacies) and for adherence problems (e.g., impaired hearing, vision, and cognition and ability to open safety caps, pay for medicines, and swallow medications).[127]

ASSESSING AND MONITORING DRUG THERAPY

The appropriateness of each prescribed medication should be assessed using a variety of methods.[83,88,128,129] One standardized measure that has demonstrated reliability and validity is the Medication Appropriateness Index (MAI).[129–132] It consists of 10 questions that should be asked about each medication (Table 7–5).

Several other factors that are not included in the MAI also should be assessed[128,133,134]:

- Suboptimal medication choice, based on effectiveness, safety, cost, and effects on health-related quality of life

TABLE 7–5. Medication Appropriateness Index[129–132]

Questions to Ask about Each Individual Medication
1. Is there an indication for the medication?
2. Is the medication effective for the condition?
3. Is the dosage correct?
4. Are the directions correct?
5. Are the directions practical?
6. Are there clinically significant drug-drug interactions?
7. Are there clinically significant drug-disease/condition interactions?
8. Is there unnecessary duplication with other drug(s)?
9. Is the duration of therapy acceptable?
10. Is this drug the least expensive alternative compared with others of equal utility?

From Refs. 129 to 132.

- Allergy (especially important with new prescriptions)
- Undertreatment (other medications that may be needed)
- Drug interactions with food or laboratory tests

Some additional factors to consider during drug-regimen review include adherence, medication storage problems, therapeutic end points, and ADRs.

DOCUMENTING PROBLEMS AND FORMULATING A THERAPEUTIC PLAN

The clinician must document the problems that have been detected, develop a therapeutic plan to resolve them, and establish reasonable therapeutic end points if these have not been set already. An important point to remember is that what may be a reasonable end point for a 40-year-old patient may not be as reasonable for an 80-year-old patient when comorbidities, functional status, and life expectancy are taken into consideration.

CONSULTING THE PHYSICIAN REGARDING PROBLEMS AND CONCERNS

In some cases, the pharmacist or other health professional must contact the patients' physician regarding problems and concerns that have been detected and documented. In discussing the patient in this context, the importance of optimizing the prescribing for elderly patients before implementing strategies to enhance their adherence cannot be over-stressed. Otherwise, the adherence intervention, if effective, may result in patient harm. Similarly in institutional settings, strategies to reduce medication administration errors may not improve patient outcomes if prescribing is not improved beforehand.

COUNSELING AND ADHERENCE AIDS

Some general factors to consider, before medication dispensing, to enhance adherence in the elderly include modifying medication schedules to fit patients' lifestyles, considering generic agents to reduce costs, using easy-to-open bottles and easy-to-swallow dosage forms, and using larger type on direction labels and auxiliary labels.[103,135,136] When dispensing medications (in particular, new medications or old ones that have changed in appearance or directions for use), both written and oral drug information should be provided to the patient and family.

To improve the likelihood of adherence, the health care professional also should recruit active patient and family involvement, stress the importance of adherence, and consider the use of adherence-enhancing aids (e.g., special packaging, medication record, drug calendar, medication boxes, magnification for insulin syringes, dose-measuring devices, and spacers for metered-dose inhalers).[137–139] In institutional settings, discussion of special considerations (medications that can be crushed and given via feeding tube) with health care professionals responsible for medication administration is also prudent.

DOCUMENTING INTERVENTIONS AND MONITORING PATIENT PROGRESS

All interventions must be documented, and the steps just outlined must be repeated over time with elderly patients. During follow-up contacts, minimum inquiry should include questions as to whether the patient has any questions or concerns regarding medicines and determining whether the therapeutic end points previously established have been achieved. Moreover, ask patients whether they are or have recently experienced any side effects, unwanted reactions, or other problems with their medications to assess potential ADRs.[140]

TARGETING HIGH-RISK ELDERLY

In busy practices, the approach outlined here may not be feasible for every patient. Therefore, practitioners may consider targeting these activities to patients at high risk for developing drug-related problems. Geriatric experts have identified 18 risk factors for drug-related problems in elderly nursing home patients.[141] These include the following medication-related factors:

- Polypharmacy (9 or more medications or 12 or more doses per day)
- Taking specific high-risk drugs (intermediate- and long-half-life benzodiazepines, sedative-hypnotic agents, antipsychotic drugs, anticholinergic medications, narcotic analgesics, chlorpropamide)
- Certain patient characteristics (low body weight, age 85 years or older, decreased renal function)
- Use of narrow-therapeutic-range drugs (e.g., lithium, digoxin, warfarin, anticonvulsants)
- History of a prior ADR
- Presence of six or more illnesses

The applicability of these criteria to elderly persons in other care settings and the relationship between identification of elderly patients with these potential risk factors and actual health outcomes remain to be determined.

CONCLUSIONS

The number of people above age 65 years is growing in the United States and around the world, and the fastest-growing segment of the American population is those over age 85. A number of physiologic changes with age affect pharmacokinetics and pharmacodynamics of drugs, especially hepatic metabolism and renal excretion. Improving and maintaining functional status and managing comorbidities are hallmarks of clinical geriatrics. Certain medical conditions are restricted to the elderly, and drug-related problems represent a major concern for this group. Innovative approaches, such as the provision of comprehensive geriatric assessment by pharmacists and other health care professionals, are needed to decrease the occurrence of these drug-related problems. Adherence to the principles outlined below also may result in more optimal pharmacotherapy for the elderly.

▶ PRINCIPLES OF PHARMACOTHERAPY

- Consider whether pharmacotherapy is absolutely necessary, but also check for untreated conditions or undertreatment of diseases.
- Streamline the number of medicines needed to treat common problems.
- Adjust doses and/or dosage intervals for medications based on patients' age, weight, renal and hepatic function, and concomitant diseases.
- Establish reasonable therapeutic end points for each medication, and monitor for these desired outcomes.
- Monitor for ADRs.
- Encourage adherence to medication and other therapies.
- Regularly review long-term medications.

REFERENCES

1. Applegate WB, Blass JP, Williams TF. Instruments for the functional assessment of older patients. N Engl J Med 1990;322:1207–1214.
2. Kane RA. Instruments to assess functional status. In: Cassel CK, Cohen HJ, Larson EB, et al., eds. Geriatric Medicine, 3d ed. New York, Springer-Verlag, 1997:169–179.
3. Ware JE, Sherbourne CD. The MOS 36-item short-form health survey (SF-36). Med Care 1992;30:473–483.
4. Weinberger M, Samsa GP, Hanlon JT, et al. Evaluation of a brief health status measure in elderly veterans. J Am Geriatr Soc 1991;39:691–694.
5. Federal Interagency Forum on Aging-Related Statistics. Older Americans 2000: Key indicators of well-being. *www.agingstats.gov;* August 2000.
6. U.S. Bureau of the Census. Current Population Reports. Population Projections of the United States by Age, Sex, Race, and Hispanic Origin: 1995 to 2050. Washington, U.S. Department of Commerce, Economics and Statistics Administration, 1996;25–113.
7. U.S. Bureau of the Census. Current Population Reports. Special Studies. Washington, U.S. Department of Commerce, Economics and Statistics Administration, 1997;23–193.
8. Applegate WB, Burns R. Geriatric medicine. JAMA 1996;275:1812–1813.
9. Horiuchi S. Demography: Greater lifetime expectations. Nature 2000; 405:744–745.
10. Davis MH, Burner ST. Three decades of Medicare: What the numbers tell us. Health Affairs 1995;14:231–243.
11. Fries JF, Green LW, Levine S. Health promotion and the compression of morbidity. Lancet 1989;1:481–483.
12. Verbrugge LM. The dynamics of population aging and health. In: Lewis SJ, ed. Connections '88: First International Symposium—Research and Public Policy on Aging and Health. Saskatoon, Saskatchewan, Canada, Lewis Publishers, 1988;23–40.
13. Kane RL, Ouslander JG, Abrass IB. The geriatric patient: Demography and epidemiology. In: Essentials of Clinical Geriatrics, 4th ed. New York, McGraw-Hill,1999:19–42.
14. National Center for Health Statistics. Annual Report on Nation's Health Spotlights Elderly Americans. Hyattsville, MD, U.S. Department of Health and Human Services, 1999.
15. Tuljapurkar S, Li N, Boe C. A universal pattern of mortality decline in the G7 countries. Nature 2000;405:789–792.
16. Velkoff, VA. New Census Report Shows Exponential Growth in Number of Centenarians. Washington, National Institutes of Health, National Institute of Aging, 1999.
17. Duncker A, Greenberg S. A Profile of Older Americans: 2000. Washington, Administration on Aging, 2001.

18. Manton KG, Corder L, Stallard E. Chronic disability trends in elderly United States: Populations—1982–1994. Proc Natl Acad Sci USA 1997;94:2593–2598.
19. National Center for Health Statistics. Health, United States, 2000. Hyattsville, MD, U.S. Department of Health and Human Services, 2000.
20. National Center for Chronic Disease Prevention and Health Promotion. Older Adults. Atlanta, GA, Centers for Disease Control and Prevention, 2000.
21. National Academy on an Aging Society. Challenges for the 21st Century: Chronic and Disabling Conditions. Washington, Gerontological Society of America, 1999.
22. Hoffman C, Rice D, Sung HY. Persons with chronic conditions: Their prevalence and costs. JAMA 1996;276:1473–1479.
23. National Center for Health Statistics. Current estimates from the National Health Interview Survey, 1994. Vital Health Stat 1995;10:81–82.
24. National Center for Health Statistics. Current estimates from the National Health Interview Survey, 1996. Vital Health Stat 1999;10:81–82.
25. National Center for Health Statistics. Characteristics of Elderly Nursing Home Residents: Data from the 1995 National Nursing Home Survey. Washington, U.S. Department of Health and Human Services, Centers for Disease Control and Prevention, Advance Data, 1997;289:1–9
26. National Center for Health Statistics. 1998 Summary: National Hospital Discharge Survey. Washington, U.S. Department of Health and Human Services, Centers for Disease Control and Prevention, Advance Data, 2000;316:1–8.
27. National Center for Chronic Disease Prevention and Health Promotion. Healthy Aging: Preventing Disease and Improving Quality of Life among Older Americans: At-a-glance 2000. Atlanta, GA, Centers for Disease Control and Prevention, 2000.
28. Soumerai SB, Ross-Degnan D. Inadequate prescription-drug coverage for Medicare enrollees: A call to action. N Engl J Med 1999;340:722–728.
29. Families USA. Cost Overdose: Growth in Drug Spending for the Elderly, 1992–2010. Families USA Foundation, Washington, DC, 2000.
30. Report to the President. Prescription Drug Coverage, Spending, Utilization, and Prices. Washington, U.S. Department of Health and Human Services, April 2000.
31. Kane RL, Ouslander JG, Abrass IB. Clinical implications of the aging process. In: Essentials of Clinical Geriatrics, 4th ed. New York, McGraw-Hill, 1999:3–18.
32. Taffet GE. Age-related physiologic changes. In: Cobbs EL, Duthie EH, Murphy JB, eds. Geriatrics Review Syllabus: A Core Curriculum in Geriatric Medicine, 4th ed. Dubuque, IA, Kendall/Hunt for the American Geriatrics Society, 1999:10–23.
33. Becker PM, Cohen HJ. The functional approach to the care of the elderly: A conceptual framework. J Am Geriatr Soc 1984;32:923–929.
34. Swift CG. Pharmacodynamics: changes in homeostatic mechanisms, receptor and target organ sensitivity in the elderly. Br Med Bull 1990; 46:36–52.
35. U.S. Food and Drug Administration. Guideline for Industry. Studies in Support of Special Populations: Geriatrics. ICH-E7, August 1994; available at *http://www.fda.gov/cder/guidance/iche7.pdf*.
36. U.S. Food and Drug Administration. Specific requirements on content and format of labeling for human prescription drugs: Addition of "geriatric use" subsection in the labeling. Fed Reg 1997;62:45313–45326.
37. Chapron DJ. Drug disposition and response. In: Delafuente JC, Stewart RB, eds. Therapeutics in the Elderly, 3d ed. Cincinnati, Harvey Whitney Books, 2000:257–288.
38. Kinross MT, Crone P. Clinical pharmacokinetic considerations in the elderly: An update. Clin Pharmacokinet 1997;33:302–312.
39. Hammerlein A, Derendorf H, Lowenthal DT. Pharmacokinetic and pharmacodynamic changes in the elderly: Clinical implications. Clin Pharmacokinet 1998;35:49–64.
40. Iber FL, Murphy PA, Connor ES. Age-related changes in the gastrointestinal system: Effects on drug therapy. Drugs Aging 1994;5:34–48.
41. Dresser GK, Bailey DG, Carruthers SG. Grapefruit juice–felodipine interaction in the elderly. Clin Pharmacol Ther 2000;68:28–34.
42. Holdsworth MT, Forman WB, Killilea TA, et al. Transdermal fentanyl disposition in elderly subjects. Gerontology 1994;40:32–37.
43. Thompson JP, Bower S, Liddle AM, et al. Perioperative pharmacokinetics of transdermal fentanyl in elderly and young adult patients. Br J Anaesthes 1998;81:152–154.
44. Grandison MK, Boudinot FD. Age-related changes in protein binding of drugs: Implications for therapy. Clin Pharmacokinet 2000;38:271–290.
45. Woodhouse K, Wynne HA. Age-related changes in hepatic function. Drugs Aging 1992;2:243–255.
46. Sotaniemi EA, Arranto AJ, Pelkonen O, Pasanen M. Age and cytochrome P450–linked drug metabolism in humans. Clin Pharmacol Ther 1997;61:331–339.
47. Guay DG. Quinolones. In: Piscitelli SC, Rodvold KA eds. Drug Interactions in Infectious Diseases. Totowa, NJ, Humana Press, 2000:121–150.
48. Crowley JJ, Cusack BJ, Jue SG, et al. Aging and drug interactions: II. Effect of phenytoin and smoking on the oxidation of theophylline and cortisol in healthy men. J Pharmacol Exp Ther 1988;245;513–523.
49. Loi CM, Parker BM, Cusack BJ, Vestal RE. Aging and drug interactions: III. Individual and combined effects of cimetidine and cimetidine and ciprofloxacin on theophylline metabolism in healthy male and female nonsmokers. J Pharmacol Exp Ther 1997;280:627–637.
50. Dilger K, Hofmann U, Klotz U. Enzyme induction in the elderly: Effect of rifampin on the pharmacokinetics and pharmacodynamics of propafenone. Clin Pharmacol Ther 2000;67:512–520.
51. Korrapati MR, Sorkin JD, Andres R, et al. Acetylator phenotype in relation to age and gender in the Baltimore Longitudinal Study of Aging. J Clin Pharmacol 1997;37:83–91.
52. O'Mahony MS, Woodhouse KW. Age, environmental factors and drug metabolism. Pharmacol Ther 1994;61:279–284.
53. Ujhelyi MR, Bottorff MB, Schur M, et al. Aging effects on the organic base transporter and stereoselective renal clearance. Clin Pharmacol Ther 1997;62:117–128.
54. Malmrose LC, Gray SL, Pieper CF, et al. Measured versus estimated creatinine clearance in a high-functioning elderly sample: MacArthur Foundation Study of Successful Aging. J Am Geriatr Soc 1993;41: 715–721.
55. Cockcroft DW, Gault MH. Prediction of creatinine clearance from serum creatinine. Nephron 1976;16:31–41.
56. Feely J, Coakley D. Altered pharmacodynamics in the elderly. Clin Geriatr Med 1990;6:269–283.
57. Klotz U. Effect of age on pharmacokinetics and pharmacodynamics in man. Int J Clin Pharmacol Ther 1998;36:581–585.
58. Scott JC, Stanski DR. Decreased fentanyl and alfentanil dose requirements with age: Simultaneous pharmacokinetic and pharmacodynamic evaluation. J Pharmacol Exp Ther 1987;240:159–165.
59. Turner MJ, Mier CM, Spina RJ, et al. Effects of age and gender on the cardiovascular responses to isoproterenol. J Gerontol 1999;54A: B393–B400.
60. Katz S, Akpom CA. A measure of primary sociobiologic functions. Int J Health Serv 1976;6:493–507.
61. Fillenbaum GG. Screening the elderly: A brief instrumental ADL measure. J Am Geriatr Soc 1985;33:698–706.
62. Fried LP, Storer DJ, King DE, et al. Diagnosis of illness presentation in the elderly. J Am Geriatr Soc 1991;39:117–123.
63. Jarrett PG, Rockwood K, Carver D, et al. Illness presentation in elderly patients. Arch Intern Med 1995;155:1060–1064.
64. Beers MH, Berkow R, eds. History and physical examination. In: Merck Manual of Geriatrics, 3d ed. Whitehouse Station, NJ, Merck, 2000: 24–40.
65. Johnson JC, Jayadevappa R, Baccash PD, Taylor L. Nonspecific presentation of pneumonia in hospitalized older people: Age effect or dementia. J Am Geriatr Soc 2000;48:1316–1320.
66. Atkin PA, Veitch PC, Veitch EM, Ogle SJ. The epidemiology of serious adverse drug reactions among the elderly. Drugs Aging 1999;14:141–152.
67. Hanlon JT, Schmader K, Gray SL. Adverse drug reactions. In: Delafuente JC, Stewart RB, eds. Therapeutics in the Elderly, 3d ed. Cincinnati, OH, Harvey Whitney Books, 2000;289–314.

68. Graves T, Hanlon JT, Schmader KE, et al. Adverse events after discontinuing medications in elderly outpatients. Arch Intern Med 1997; 157:2205–2210.
69. Grymonpre RE, Mitenko PA, Sitar DS, et al. Drug-associated hospital admissions in older medical patients. J Am Geriatr Soc 1988;36:1092–1098.
70. Karch FE, Lasagna L. Adverse drug reactions: A critical review. JAMA 1975;234:1236–1241.
71. Gurwitz JH, Avorn J. The ambiguous relation between aging and adverse drug reactions. Ann Intern Med 1991;114:956–966.
72. Bootman JL, Harrison DL, Cox E. The health care cost of drug-related morbidity and mortality in nursing facilities. Arch Intern Med 1997;157:2089–2096.
73. Montamat SC, Cusack B. Overcoming problems with polypharmacy and drug misuse in the elderly. Clin Geriatr Med 1992;8:143–158.
74. Stewart RB, Cooper JW. Polypharmacy in the aged: Practical solutions. Drugs Aging 1994;4:449–461.
75. Nolan L, O'Malley K. Prescribing for the elderly, part II. J Am Geriatr Soc 1988;36:245–254.
76. Hanlon JT, Fillenbaum GG, Burchett B, et al. Drug-use patterns among black and nonblack community dwelling elderly. Ann Pharmacother 1992;26:679–685.
77. Fillenbaum GG, Hanlon JT, Corder EH, et al. Prescription and nonprescription drug use among black and white community-residing elderly. Am J Public Health 1993;83:1577–1582.
78. Stewart RB, Marks RG, May FE, Hale WE. Factors which predict multiple drug use in the elderly. J Geriatr Drug Ther 1994;9:53–67.
79. Tobias DE, Sey M. General and psychotherapeutic medication use in 328 nursing facilities: A year 2000 national survey (Abstract). Consult Pharm 2000;15:964.
80. Schmader K, Hanlon JT, Weinberger M, et al. Appropriateness of medication prescribing in ambulatory elderly patients. J Am Geriatr Soc 1994;42:1241–1247.
81. Lipton HL, Bero LA, Bird JA, McPhee SJ. The impact of clinical pharmacists' consultations on physicians geriatric drug prescribing: A randomized controlled trial. Med Care 1992;30:646–658.
82. Murray MD. Medication Appropriateness Index: Putting a number on an old problem in older patients. Ann Pharmacother 1997;31:643–644.
83. Buetow SA, Sibbald B, Cantrill JA, Halliwell S. Appropriateness in health care: Application to prescribing. Soc Sci Med 1997;45:261–271.
84. Tamblyn RM, McLeod PJ, Abrahamowicz M, et al. Questionable prescribing for elderly patients in Quebec. Can Med Assoc J 1994; 150:1801–1809.
85. Briesacher BA, Stuart B, Peluso R. Drug use and prescribing problems in the community-dwelling elderly: A study of three state Medicaid programs. Clin Ther 1999;21:2156–2172.
86. Hanlon JT, Fillenbaum GG, Hu W, et al. Inappropriate drug prescribing for community dwelling elderly residents (Abstract). J Am Geriatr Soc 2000;48:S10.
87. Brook RH, Kamberg CJ, Mayer-Oakes A, et al. Appropriateness of acute medical care for the elderly: An analysis of the literature. Health Policy 1990;14:225–242.
88. Beers MH. Explicit criteria for determining potentially inappropriate medication use by the elderly: An update. Arch Intern Med 1997; 157:1531–1536.
89. Aparasu RR, Mort JR. Inapropriate prescribing for the elderly: Beers criteria-based review. Ann Pharmacother 2000;34:338–346.
90. Hanlon JT, Fillenbaum GG, Schmader KE, et al. Inappropriate drug use among community-dwelling elderly. Pharmacotherapy 2000;20:575–582.
91. Prescription Drugs and the Elderly: Many Still Receive Potentially Harmful Drugs Despite Recent Improvements. Washington, GAO Report (GAO/HEHS-95-152), July 1995:1–30.
92. Lindley CM, Tulley MP, Paramsothy V, Tallis RC. Inappropriate medication is a major cause of adverse drug reactions in elderly patients. Age Ageing 1992;21:294–300.
93. Doucet J, Chassagne P, Trivalle C, et al. Drug-drug interactions related to hospital admissions in older adults: A prospective study of 1000 patients. J Am Geriatr Soc 1996;44:944–948.
94. Bero LA, Lipton HL, Bird JA. Characterization of geriatric drug-related hospital readmissions. Med Care 1991;29:989–1003.
95. Lipton HL, Bero LA, Bird JA, McPhee SJ. Undermedication among geriatric outpatients: Results of a randomized controlled trial. Ann Rev Gerontol Geriatr 1992;12:95–108.
96. Redelmeier DA, Tan SH, Booth GL. The treatment of unrelated disorders in patients with chronic medical diseases. N Engl J Med 1998;338:1516–1520.
97. Rochon PA, Gurwitz JH. Prescribing for seniors: Neither too much nor too little. JAMA 1999;282:113–115.
98. Hanlon JT, Schmader KE, Ruby CM, Weinberger M. Suboptimal prescribing in elderly inpatients and outpatients. J Am Geriatr Soc 2001;49:200–209.
99. National Institute of Health consensus statement. Diagnosis and treatment of depression in late life: Consensus statement update. JAMA 1997;278:1186–1190.
100. Soumerai SB, McLaughlin TJ, Spieglelman D, et al. Adverse outcomes of underuse of beta-blockers in elderly survivors of acute myocardial infarction. JAMA 1997;277:115–121.
101. Havranek EP, Abrams F, Stevens E, Parker K. Determinants of mortality in elderly patients with heart failure: The role of angiotension-converting enzyme inhibitors. Arch Intern Med 1998;158:2024–2028.
102. Soumerai SB, Ross-Degnan D, Avorn J, et al. Effects of Medicaid drug-payment limits on admission to hospitals and nursing homes. N Engl J Med 1991;325:1072–1077.
103. Ryan AA. Medication compliance and older people: A review of the literature. Intern J Nur Stud 1999;36:153–162.
104. Stewart RB, Caranasos G. Medication compliance in the elderly. Med Clin North Am 1989;73:1551–1560.
105. Weintraub M. Compliance in the elderly. Clin Geriatr Med 1990;6:445–452.
106. Lipton HL, Bird JA. The impact of clinical pharmacists' consultations on geriatric patients' compliance and medical care use: A randomized controlled trial. Gerontologist 1994;34:307–315.
107. German PS, Klein LE, McPhee SJ, et al. Knowledge of and compliance with drug regimens in the elderly. J Am Geriatr Soc 1982;30:568–571.
108. Park DC, Hertzog C, Leventhal H, et al. Medication adherence in rheumatoid arthritis patients: Older is wiser. J Am Geriatr Soc 1999;47:172–183.
109. Buist DSM, LaCroix AZ, Black DM, et al. Inclusion of older women in randomized clinical trials: Factors associated with taking study medication in the Fracture Intervention Trial. J Am Geriatr Soc 2000;48:1126–1131.
110. Cooper JK, Love DW, Raffoul PR. International prescription nonadherence (noncompliance) by the elderly. J Am Geriatr Soc 1982;30:329–333.
111. Fincke BG, Miller DR, Spiro A 3d. The interaction of patient perception of overmedication with drug compliance and side effects. J Gen Intern Med 1998;13:182–185.
112. Sullivan SD, Kreling DH, Hazlet TK. Noncompliance with medication regimens and subsequent hospitalizations: Literature analysis and cost of hospitalization estimate. J Res Pharm Econ 1990;2:19–33.
113. Col N, Fanale JE, Kronholm P. The role of medication noncompliance and adverse drug reactions in hospitalizations in the elderly. Arch Intern Med 1990;150:841–845.
114. Rubenstein LZ. Geriatric assessment: An overview of its impact. Clin Geriatr Med 1987;3:1–16.
115. Becker PM, McVey LJ, Saltz CC, et al. Hospital acquired complications in a randomized controlled clinical trial of a geriatric consultation team. JAMA 1987;257:2313–2317.
116. Epstein AM, Hall JA, Besdine R, et al. The emergence of geriatric assessment units. Ann Intern Med 1987;106:299–303.
117. American College of Physicians. Comprehensive functional assessment of the elderly. Ann Intern Med 1988;109:70–72.

118. National Institute of Health Consensus Development Conference Statement. Geriatric assessment methods for clinical decision making. J Am Geriatr Soc 1988;36:342–347.
119. Stuck AE, Siu AL, Wieland GD, et al. Comprehensive geriatric assessment: A meta-analysis of controlled trials. Lancet 1993;342:1032–1036.
120. Adamcik BA, Rhodes RS. The pharmacist's role in rational drug therapy of the aged. Drugs Aging 1993;3:481–486.
121. Dyer CC, Oles KS, Davis SW. The role of the pharmacist in a geriatric nursing home: A literature review. Drug Intell Clin Pharm 1984;18:428–433.
122. Hanlon JT, Weinberger M, Samsa GP, et al. A randomized controlled trial of a clinical pharmacist intervention with elderly outpatients with polypharmacy. Am J Med 1996;100:428–437.
123. Owens NJ, Silliman RA, Fretwell MD. The relationship between comprehensive functional assessment and optimal pharmacotherapy in the older patient. Drug Intell Clin Pharm 1989;23:847–854.
124. Owens NJ, Sherburne NJ, Silliman RA, Fretwell MD. The Senior Care Study: The optimal use of medications in acutely ill older patients. J Am Geriatr Soc 1990;38:1082–1087.
125. Hanlon JT, Fillenbaum GG, Ruby CM, et al. Epidemiology of over-the-counter drug use in community dwelling elders. Drugs Aging 2001; 18:23–31.
126. Astin JA, Pelletier KR, Marie A, Haskell WL. Complementary and alternative medicine use among elderly persons: One-year analysis of a Blue Shield Medicare supplement. J Gerontol 2000;55:M4–9.
127. Ruscin JM, Semla TP. Assessment of medication management skills in older outpatients. Ann Pharmacother 1996;30:1083–1087.
128. Lipton HL, Bird JA, Bero LA, McPhee SJ. Assessing the appropriateness of physician prescribing for geriatric outpatients: Development and testing of an instrument. J Pharm Technol 1993;9:107–113.
129. Hanlon JT, Schmader KE, Samsa GP, et al. A method for assessing drug therapy appropriateness. J Clin Epidemiol 1992;45:1045–1051.
130. Samsa G, Hanlon JT, Schmader KE, et al. A summated score for the Medication Appropriateness Index: Development and assessment of clinimetric properties including content validity. J Clin Epidemiol 1994; 47:891–896.
131. Fitzgerald LS, Hanlon JT, Shelton PS, et al. Reliability of a modified Medication Appropriateness Index in ambulatory older persons. Ann Pharmacother 1997;31:543–548.
132. Schmader K, Hanlon JT, Landsman PM, et al. Inappropriate prescribing and health outcomes in the elderly in a pharmacist intervention trial. Ann Pharmacother 1997;31:529–533.
133. Cohen JS. Adverse drug effects, compliance, and initial doses of antihypertensive drugs recommended by the Joint National Committee vs the Physicians' Desk Reference. Arch Intern Med 2001;161:880–885.
134. Cohen JS. Dose discrepancies between the Physicians' Desk Reference and the medical literature, and their possible role in the high incidence of dose-related adverse drug events. Arch Intern Med. 2001;161:957–964.
135. Mallet L. Counseling in special populations: The elderly patient. Am Pharm 1992;NS32:71–81.
136. Opdycke RA, Ascione FJ, Shimp LA, Rosen RI. A systematic approach to educating elderly patients about their medications. Patient Educ Counsel 1992;19:43–60.
137. Murray MD, Birt JA, Manatunga AK, Darnell JC. Medication compliance in elderly outpatients using twice-daily dosing and unit-of-use packaging. Ann Pharmacother 1993;27:616–620.
138. Ascione FJ, Shrimp LA. The effectiveness of four education strategies in the elderly. Drug Intell Clin Pharm 1984;18:126–131.
139. Rivers PH. Compliance aids: Do they work? Drugs Aging 1992;2:103–111.
140. Hanlon JT, Schmader KE, Koronkowski MJ, et al. Adverse drug events in high risk elderly outpatients. J Am Geriatr Soc 1997;45:945–948.
141. Fouts MM, Hanlon JT, Pieper CF, et al. Identification of elderly nursing facility residents at high risk for drug-related problems. Consult Pharm 1997;12:1103–1111.

8

PHARMACOEPIDEMIOLOGY

Andy Stergachis and Thomas K. Hazlet

The practice of pharmacotherapy requires knowledge of the benefits and risks of pharmaceuticals as applied to human populations. Much of our understanding about the efficacy and safety of drugs arises from well-controlled studies conducted during the drug development and approval process. However, many additional risks and, to a lesser degree, additional benefits are only identified after the drug is used widely by the general population. Benefits and risks learned following a drug's approval may range from relatively minor to clinically important effects that seriously alter an individual drug's risk-benefit ratio. The association between certain appetite-suppressant drugs and primary pulmonary hypertension and valvular heart disease is an example where serious adverse effects were discovered only after these drugs had come into widespread use.[1,2] This example highlights both the inherent limitations of the drug development process and the need to study populations receiving medications obtained through usual clinical practice. The purpose of this chapter is to describe the role of pharmacoepidemiology in drug development and therapeutics and to characterize the primary methods and issues in this field.

Pharmacoepidemiology is a discipline that provides valuable information about the health and cost outcomes of drugs, devices, and biologics, particularly after their approval for clinical use. *Pharmacoepidemiology* is defined as the study of the use of and effects of drugs in large numbers of people.[3] The field as applied to the period after a drug enters the market is referred to as *postmarketing drug surveillance* (PMS). *Pharmacovigilance* refers to the continual monitoring for untwanted effects and other safety-related aspects of marketed drugs, primarily through the use of spontaneous reporting systems. One of the noteworthy developments in the field has been the use of automated, linked databases that permit efficient and rapid studies of drug effects, although recently heightened concerns about confidentiality of medical information may curtail future access to these data.

Epidemiologic study designs are essential for evaluating drug safety and effectiveness in situations where it is either infeasible or unethical to randomly assign patients to active treatment or placebo. While the randomized, controlled, blinded trial (RCT) is the standard against which other designs are measured, it is often not suitable for questions within the domain of pharmacoepidemiology. Randomized trials, for example, cannot contribute much to our understanding of the long-term or rare adverse effects associated with therapies. Clinical trials conducted prior to drug approval cannot uncover every important health effect of a pharmaceutical. For example, the adverse health effects of drugs on the human fetus can be estimated only through observational but not experimental methods. Epidemiologic studies of the patterns of drug prescribing and use are also essential to assess a drug's usefulness.[4] As a discipline, pharmacoepidemiology traditionally has concerned itself with the study of adverse drug effects. Epidemiologic study designs such as case-control and cohort studies are also used to identify beneficial effects of drugs in populations. For example, to determine the relationship between patterns of use of inhaled corticosteroids and the risk of fatal or near-fatal asthma, Suissa and colleagues conducted an epidemiologic study of 30,569 residents of Saskatchewan who were dispensed three or more asthma drugs in any 1 year from September 1975 through December 1991.[5] They found the death rate to be 21% lower among inhaled corticosteroid users for each additional canister used in the preceding year and an increased death rate in patients who had discontinued inhaled corticosteroid use. These findings support practice guidelines and quality performance measurements that recommend the use of inhaled anti-inflammatories in patients with moderate to severe asthma.

Whether or not a drug in fact achieves its desired effect in the real world, in contrast to RCTs, is referred to as its *effectiveness,* not efficacy. Studies of drug effectiveness generally are conducted using observational study designs, although RCTs also play a role in determining a drug's effectiveness.[6] It is widely recognized that results from an RCT offer the best evidence that a drug will perform under ideal conditions, and it is likely that the "well-controlled" design of RCTs will continue to be required for new drug applications (NDAs) to the Food and Drug Administration (FDA). As described in regulations governing NDAs, reports of adequate and well-controlled investigations provide the primary basis for determining whether there is "substantial evidence" to support the claims of effectiveness for new drugs.[7]

However, the rigorous circumstances surrounding design and implementation of an RCT do not necessarily extrapolate to the individual patient. Fletcher and associates draw a distinction between "efficacy"—Does the treatment work?—and "effectiveness"—Does the treatment's benefits outweigh its liabilities for those to whom it is offered in clinical practice?[8]

The tension between the conflicting goals of validity in efficacy trials and generalizability in effectiveness trials is shown in Figure 8–1. For example, in an efficacy trial, subjects are selected using narrowly defined eligibility criteria and are monitored closely to assure that they use or are exposed to the intervention in the manner defined in the trial's protocol and are cooperative with medical advice. In clinical practice, patients are not selected, and the manner in which the patient uses the intervention may vary widely from the intended use for which it was approved. For instance, in an effectiveness trial to compare stepped care beginning with niacin to the use of lovastatin in the treatment of elevated low-density lipoprotein cholesterol, Oster and coworkers found that insurance status and out-of-pocket expenses for drugs, issues that often would not surface in a clinical trial, had a major impact on adherence and therapeutic response.[9]

Clinical outcomes among RCT subjects often are better than in nontrial patients.[10] Trials to evaluate therapeutic effectiveness in clinical practice are difficult or expensive for researchers. If results from an effectiveness study are inconclusive, it could be due to a lack of the intervention's efficacy, patient behavior (such as lack of patient adherence), or both.

LIMITS OF KNOWLEDGE AT THE TIME OF NEW DRUG APPROVAL

The new drug approval process and the role of pharmacoepidemiology in the United States have evolved since the Federal Food, Drug, and Cosmetic (FD&C) Act of 1938 was enacted into law. The FD&C Act

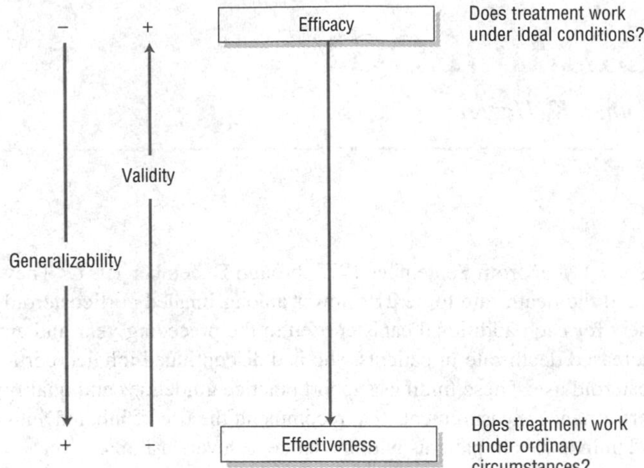

FIGURE 8–1. Schematic drawing showing the tension between conflicting goals of validity in efficacy trials and generalizability in effectiveness trials. *(Adapted from Ref. 8.)*

was adopted following the deaths of more than 100 patients of renal failure from sulfanilamide prepared in a diethylene glycol vehicle.[11] For the first time in U.S. history, the act required a drug to be proven safe under conditions of use intended by the manufacturer before marketing. The act also required manufacturers to conduct preclinical toxicity testing and gather and submit clinical data about drug safety to the FDA prior to drug marketing under an NDA. It also required new drugs to be labeled with adequate instructions and appropriate warnings for safe use. However, the FD&C Act required no proof of drug efficacy.

The FD&C Act was amended in 1962 following the epidemic of thalidomide-associated birth defects in Europe.[12] The Kefauver-Harris Amendments of 1962 strengthened the requirements for proof of drug safety and added a new requirement for demonstration of drug efficacy before marketing. Requiring "substantial evidence that the drug will have the effect it purports or is represented to have" resulted in the establishment of the RCT as the "gold standard" for proof of efficacy. The 1962 amendments also required manufacturers to report adverse drug events detected in the postmarketing setting to the FDA: Investigational new drug (IND) applications were required to be submitted to the FDA before clinical testing could begin. In 1985, requirements for manufacturers' adverse drug event (ADE) reporting were clarified, and specific regulations and guidelines were published to define the manufacturers' obligations in reviewing and reporting ADEs.

The Kefauver-Harris Amendments also identified explicit phases of preclinical animal testing followed by three phases of clinical testing (Fig. 8–2). In addition, a postapproval surveillance, phase 4 of drug development, is now common. Today we are witnessing even more regulatory changes to the drug approval process as it pertains to pharmacoepidemiology. The Food and Drug Administration Modernization Act (FDAMA) of 1997 resulted in new provisions stating that substantial evidence of drug effectiveness may consist of data from one adequate and well-controlled clinical investigation plus confirmatory evidence. This indicates that two or more well-controlled trials (the previous standard) are not always necessary and that the FDA should relate the number and type of trials to the specific product under development.

Phase 3 controlled clinical trials required by the FDA as part of the process of drug approval and labeling are the primary source of information about new drugs. Although these studies help ensure that a drug is efficacious and does not cause unacceptable harm, premarketing studies fail to provide much of the information needed to make therapeutic decisions.[13] Table 8–1 describes the major limitations of premarketing controlled clinical trials, which lend support to the need for further evaluation of drugs after their approval for marketing by the FDA. Briefly, clinical trials performed during drug development cannot be depended on to detect rare adverse drug events. In addition, they cannot be used directly to address the performance of drugs in the populations that will use the drug in ways not studied in clinical trials because clinical trials restrict the complexity of the patients tested. Thus often not included in drug testing are many persons who are likely to eventually receive new medicines—the chronically ill, women of childbearing age, and pregnant women. To improve the representativeness of populations included in clinical trials, the FDA has issued guidelines in support of inclusion of geriatric patients in phase 2 and phase 3 studies. Also, the FDA has issued guidelines and incentives to encourage manufacturers to provide efficacy, safety, pharmacokinetic, and pharmacodynamic information in support of the use of drugs and biologic products in pediatric populations.

Despite the rigorous process for drug approval and regulation, several important medications have been removed from the market because of serious ADEs over the past 30 years. Recent examples of serious but uncommon effects include acute flank syndrome associated with suprofen,[14] the gastrointestinal effects associated with nonsteroidal anti-inflammatory drugs (NSAIDs) in the elderly,[15] troglitazone and the risk of hepatotoxicity,[16] and the adverse effects of cisapride when used improperly.[17] Partially in response to concerns about ADEs, a number of epidemiology programs were developed beginning in the 1970s. An initial emphasis of early programs such as the Boston Collaborative Drug Surveillance Program was the estimation

	Early research preclinical testing		Clinical Trials: Phase I	Clinical Trials: Phase II	Clinical Trials: Phase III		FDA		Phase IV
Years	6.5	File IND at FDA	1.5	2	3.5	File NDA at FDA	1.5	15 Total	
Test population	Laboratory and animal studies		20–80 healthy volunteers	100–300 patient volunteers	1000–3000 patient volunteers		Review process/ approval		Additional post-marketing testing required by FDA
Purpose	Assess safety and biologic activity		Determine safety and dosage	Evaluate effectiveness, look for side effects	Confirm effectiveness, monitor adverse reactions from long-term use				
Success rate	5000 compounds evaluated		5 enter trials				1 approved		

FIGURE 8–2. The drug development and approval process in the United States.

TABLE 8–1. Limitations of Premarketing Clinical Trials

Short duration	Premarketing studies are limited in time Effects that develop following chronic use or those that have a long latency period cannot be detected
Small sample size	Few drugs are studied in more than 4000 subjects before FDA approval Effects that occur with a frequency of less than 1/1000 are difficult to detect
Narrowly defined population	Premarketing studies generally do not include special populations, such as children, women of childbearing age, or the elderly
Narrow set of indications	Manufacturers pursue specific indications for use during premarketing studies
Limited comparison groups	The comparison group is often limited to placebo

of drug use and adverse events among hospitalized patients.[18] The Drug Epidemiology Unit, now the Slone Epidemiology Unit, also was formed in the early 1970s to perform hospital-based case-control studies.[19] In the United Kingdom, the Drug Surveillance Research Unit established the Prescription Event Monitoring Program in 1980, now called the Drug Safety Research Trust.[20] Subsequent resources for pharmacoepidemiology evolved from the use of Medicaid data, followed by the use of databases from health maintenance organizations (HMOs) and other population-based data sources. Since the time of the 1980 report of the Joint Commission on Prescription Drug Use, there has been considerable interest in the use of HMO records for postmarketing drug surveillance.[21] Advantages to conducting PMS in an HMO setting include the availability of an identifiable population base for the estimation of rates, presence of a relatively stable population base, and access to medical records and computerized databases.[22]

ROLE OF FDA AND PHARMACOEPIDEMIOLOGY

Drug development should be viewed as a process that continues even after a drug is approved for marketing. As noted in the preceding section, it is not possible to detect all potential risks and benefits during premarketing studies. The FDA's postmarketing surveillance program provides important information on the clinical experience of medical products. The FDA's involvement in PMS includes monitoring approved drug use, monitoring the serious ADEs associated with the use of approved drugs, and the initiation of selected epidemiologic studies to estimate the risk or test specific hypotheses.[23] One of the primary uses of findings from PMS of drugs is modification of a drug's labeling or package insert. Other methods used to communicate the results of PMS efforts involve requiring the manufacturer to mail out a "Dear Doctor" letter, publishing an article in the *FDA Medical Bulletin*, presentation of findings at professional meetings, and publication of findings in peer-reviewed journals.

As a condition of approval for marketing, drug manufacturers are required to notify the FDA of all adverse events of which they are aware. It is important for clinicians to report ADEs either to the manufacturer or to the MedWatch program at the FDA. This program depends on health care professionals and the lay public to report serious ADEs observed in the course of their practice as part of their professional responsibility. The MedWatch form can be used to report ADEs or product problems related to any medical product, with the exception of those occurring with vaccines. Reports concerning vaccines should be sent to the Vaccine Adverse Event Reporting System (VAERS), a joint program of the FDA and the Centers for Disease Control and Prevention. Table 8–2 describes the FDA's MedWatch program.

The FDA provides limited funding for investigators to use large, automated databases to study the adverse effects of drugs marketed in the United States and its territories. Through its cooperative agreements program, the FDA has encouraged the use of large databases for use in pharmacoepidemiology. These agreements provide the FDA with access to data on the safety of pharmaceuticals. The objectives of these programs include the rapid and efficient conduct of pharmacoepidemiologic research designed to test hypotheses, particularly those arising from the MedWatch program. Current programs receiving funding for PMS from the FDA include Brigham and Women's Hospital and United HealthCare. Even though the FDA supports cooperative agreements for PMS, it lacks regulatory authority to require phase 4 studies for previously approved drugs. The FDAMA does require any sponsor of a drug that agreed to conduct a postmarketing study to report annually to the FDA on the progress of the study. To assist in translating information about the risks and benefits of drugs into action, the

TABLE 8–2. Characteristics of the FDA's MEDWATCH Program

Report experiences with:
- Medications (drugs or biologics)
- Medical devices (including in vitro diagnostics)
- Special nutritional products (dietary supplements, medical foods, infant formulas)
- Other products regulated by the FDA

Report SERIOUS adverse events. An event is serious when the patient outcome is:
- Death
- Life threatening (real risk of dying)
- Hospitalization (initial or prolonged)
- Disability (significant, persistent, or permanent)
- Congenital anomaly
- Required intervention to prevent permanent impairment or damage

Report even if:
- You're not certain that the product caused the event
- You don't have all the details

Report product problems—quality, performance, or safety concerns—such as:
- Suspected contamination
- Questionable stability
- Defective components
- Poor packaging or labeling
- Therapeutic failures

Important numbers:
- 1-899-FDA-0178 to Fax report
- 1-800-FDA-7737 to report by modem
- 1-800-FDA-1088 to report by phone, for more information, or to obtain software for reporting by modem
- 1-800-822-7967 for a VAERS form for vaccines
- FDA MedWatch Web site: http://www.fda.gov/medwatch/
  Download reporting forms (PDF format)
  MedWatch information

federal Agency for Healthcare Research and Quality (AHRQ) funds studies focused on patient outcomes associated with pharmaceutical therapy.

ADVERSE DRUG EVENTS

The field of pharmacoepidemiology concerns itself primarily with the study of adverse drug reactions. According to the World Health Organization, an *adverse drug reaction* (ADR) is any noxious, unintended, and undesired effect of a drug that occurs at doses used in humans for prophylaxis, diagnosis, or therapy.[24] The term *adverse drug event* (ADE) is used to describe an injury resulting from administration of a drug. Virtually any drug can have adverse effects. Between 3% and 11% of hospital admissions have been attributed to adverse effects.[25] The likelihood that a patient will experience an ADE during hospitalization ranges from 1% to 44% depending on the type of hospital, definition of an ADE, and study methodology.[26] The economic impact of ADEs is substantial and potentially avoidable.[27,28] Recently, the incidence of serious and fatal ADRs in hospital patients was reported to be as high as 6.7% and 0.32%, respectively.[29]

Although most ADEs can be anticipated, others are unpredictable, especially rare idiosyncratic reactions. ADRs have been separated into type A and B reactions.[30] Type A reactions are expected exaggerations of a drug's known pharmacologic effects. Therefore, they usually are dose-dependent, predictable, and preventable. Type A reactions are responsible for the majority of ADEs encountered. Examples include hypotension with antihypertensive agents and anticholinergic effects with tricyclic antidepressants. Type A reactions tend to occur in individuals who have one of three characteristics.[31] First, the individuals may have received more of a drug than is customarily required. Second, they may have received a conventional dose of the drug, but they may metabolize or excrete the drug unusually slowly, leading to drug levels that are too high, possibly due to concomitant disease or drug interactions. Third, they may have normal drug levels but for some reason are overly sensitive to them. Most type A reactions are identified prior to drug marketing and are listed in a product's labeling.

Type B reactions are idiosyncratic and tend to be unrelated to the known pharmacologic action of the drug. They are usually not related to dose, unpredictable, uncommon, and potentially more serious than type A reactions. They may be due to what are known as *hypersensitivity reactions* or *immunologic reactions*. Type B reactions may be the consequence of some other idiosyncratic reaction to the drug, such as an inherited susceptibility. These reactions may concentrate in certain body systems, including the liver, blood, skin, kidney, and nervous system.[32] Type B reactions represent a major focus of pharmacoepidemiologic studies of ADRs. Carcinogenic and teratogenic ADEs are considered type B reactions.

Because ADRs represent an important public health concern, institutions complying with the Joint Commission on Accreditation of Healthcare Organizations (JCAHO) are required to perform numerous steps pertaining to the surveillance and management of ADRs. They must define significant ADRs, initiate intensive assessments for ADRs meeting the institution's definition, and be able to provide evidence during accreditation surveys of sufficiently detailed follow-up on the causes of ADRs.[33] The JCAHO recently has instituted an additional requirement for reporting of sentinel events, which are those involving the occurrence of risk of death or serious physical or psychological injury. In situations where the sentinel event indicates an ongoing possibility of threat to life or safety, the JCAHO may conduct an unscheduled survey and require that the institution undertake extensive systems and process reviews and implement improvements to prevent recurrence of the sentinel event.

METHODOLOGIES FOR PHARMACOEPIDEMIOLOGIC STUDIES

A large number of study designs and methods are used to generate data on the uses and risks of new and older drugs. Epidemiologic methods, such as case-control, cohort, and cross-sectional studies, are used extensively. Large automated databases, meta-analyses, RCTs, and hybrid designs, such as nested case-control studies, also play an important role in pharmacoepidemiology. Epidemiologic studies typically do not use randomization to determine who will receive a particular drug exposure. Rather, associations between exposure(s) and disease(s) under study are determined through the use of observational study designs and statistical analyses. Observational methods are used in most situations because ethics and cost limit the use of experimentation. A number of methods are used to study health events associated with drug exposures. The usual approach to studying ADEs begins with the collection of spontaneous reports of drug-related morbidity or mortality.

There has been a growing interest in using computerized databases containing medical care information for pharmacoepidemiologic studies.[34] These databases usually consist of patient-level data from two or more separate files (e.g., billing files for pharmacy and medical services reimbursement) that were developed originally for clinical or administrative applications.[35] Through record linkage, it is possible to create person-based longitudinal files on an ad hoc basis. Multipurpose databases used for pharmacoepidemiologic studies include data from HMOs, the Medicaid program, the Medicare program, and geographically defined populations. In general, these databases include information on patient demographics, outpatient drugs, hospital discharge diagnoses, and ambulatory care encounters. The advantages and disadvantages of linked databases for pharmacoepidemiologic studies have been the subject of numerous publications.[36,37]

CASE REPORTS AND CASE SERIES

Case reports describe a single patient who was exposed to a drug and experienced a particular, usually adverse, outcome. For example, within the first 3 months of marketing, hemolytic anemia and acute renal failure following use of the antibiotic temafloxacin were reported to the Spontaneous Report System, the predecessor of the MedWatch system. Case reports are useful for raising hypotheses about drug effects to be tested with more rigorous study designs. It is uncommon for a case report or a series of case reports to be used to make a statement about causation. Case series are collections of patients, all of whom have a single exposure, whose clinical outcomes are then evaluated and described. They are useful for quantifying the incidence of an adverse reaction, particularly for a newly approved drug. Further, case series can be useful for being certain that the incidence rate of any particular adverse effects of concern does not occur in a population that is larger than that studied prior to drug's marketing.

If the event is rare and the exposure combination is very specific, the cause of the adverse health event may be inferred from a case-series study. In most situations, however, it is necessary to compare cases with a group of controls to identify risk factors. Thus the major disadvantage of a case-series study is the lack of a comparison group. However, recent methodologic advances in the analysis of case series data allow the estimation of relative incidence without the use of controls.[38]

CASE-CONTROL STUDIES

A case-control study assembles a group of cases (people who have the disease of interest) and controls (people who do not). The exposure histories of the cases and the controls are determined to establish the extent of association between exposure(s) of interest and disease. Case-control studies compare patients with a specific disease with a control group composed of similar people but without the disease. Case-control studies attempt to identify risk factors for a disease by examining differences in antecedent exposure variables between cases and controls. For example, one can select cases of women of childbearing age with ovarian cysts and compare them with controls, looking for differences in prior use of oral contraceptives. Such a study was performed to determine if the then newly introduced triphasic oral contraceptives were associated with functional ovarian cysts.[39]

Case-control studies have been used extensively to assess the safety of pharmaceuticals. There are many examples of case-control studies that have identified important associations between drugs and adverse health events: vaginal cancer and diethylstilbestrol (DES), Reye's syndrome and aspirin, peptic ulcer disease and NSAIDs, and venous thromboembolism and oral contraceptives. Data from case-control studies are used to calculate an odds ratio, which is the ratio of the odds of developing the disease for exposed patients to the odds of developing the disease for unexposed patients.

A classic example is a study of DES given during pregnancy and the risk of vaginal adenocarcinoma among female offspring nearly a generation later.[40] A study of hip fracture risk in relation to the prescription of benzodiazepines exemplifies a nested case-control design.[41] Hip fracture cases and controls were chosen from a large existing database on health care use among Saskatchewan residents. The use of a nested case-control design to efficiently assess the role of potential confounding factors is further illustrated in the previously cited study of inhaled corticosteroids and the risk of fatal and near-fatal asthma.[5] A nested case-control study is an efficient variation of a case-control and a cohort study. In a nested case-control study, all cases (or a sample of all cases) and only a random sample of all controls are chosen for study from the same defined population.

An advantage of the case-control design for the study of drug-outcome relationships is its efficiency for the study of rare or delayed outcomes. Compared with other strategies, the case-control study is relatively inexpensive. One potential problem with case-control studies is their susceptibility to certain types of bias, including selection bias and information bias. *Selection bias* refers to systematic differences between those selected for study and those who are not, whereas *information bias* is systematic differences in the quality of information gathered for study and comparison groups.

COHORT STUDIES

A cohort study assembles a group of persons without the disease(s) of interest at the onset of the study, ascertains the exposure status of each person, and then follows the cohort over time to determine the development of disease in exposed and nonexposed persons. Cohort studies involve the comparison of the incidence of one or more outcome events among those who received a drug or some other exposure of interest compared with the incidence of the event(s) for a comparison group. For example, much information about the risk of fatal cardiovascular diseases among oral contraceptive users has come from the Royal College of General Practitioners (RCGP) Oral Contraception Study, in which 23,000 oral contraceptive users were compared with 23,000 nonusers chosen from the same British general practices.[42] Death certificate records were used to ascertain instances of fatal events during the follow-up period.

Cohort studies can be prospective, as the RCGP study illustrates, or retrospective. Prospective cohort studies are one of the most valid types of observational study designs because exposure is measured and recorded prior to the development of the health outcome(s) of interest. Using a prospective cohort study design, Hooton and colleagues determined the association between contraceptive methods and symptomatic urinary tract infections in young women.[43] The investigators recruited sexually active young women who were starting a new method of contraception and followed them for 6 months to determine the incidence of symptomatic urinary tract infections by contraceptive method.

An alternative to the prospective cohort design is the retrospective cohort study. Retrospective cohort studies are useful when comparison cohorts of persons exposed and not exposed to drugs of interest can be identified at some time in the past from large preexisting databases and followed from that time to the present with regard to the incidence of a given outcome. Recently, Soumerai and associates used a retrospective cohort design to study the determinants and adverse health outcomes of β-blocker underuse in elderly patients with myocardial infarction.[44] Controlling for other predictors of survival, the mortality rate among β-blocker recipients was 43% less than that for the comparison group, suggesting that use of β-blockers reduces the risk of death among elderly patients with myocardial infarction.

Prospective cohort studies can provide strong evidence of associations between drugs and diseases because the exposure is assessed before the outcome occurs. However, because many cohort studies require large numbers of people followed for long periods of time, they can be expensive and, in some instances, infeasible. Retrospective or historical cohort studies can overcome these limitations if high-quality data have been collected already.

USE OF QUASI-EXPERIMENTAL DESIGNS IN PHARMACOEPIDEMIOLOGY

One of the opportunities that has emerged with increased computerization in health care is the use of large, linked databases for exploring pharmaceutical outcomes. The ability to use transaction or claims data from an insurance company or state Medicaid agency and link these data to files containing diagnosis and other patient-specific information has allowed researchers to explore outcomes questions at relatively low expense. Because these studies do not rely on random assignment of subjects, they have been described as *quasi experimental*.[45] The typical design includes a treatment (exposed) group, a control (unexposed) group, and some type of posttest assessment for both. Although efforts may be made to match treatment and control groups for important patient characteristics, the groups are not equivalent in the sense of an RCT. A refinement to this design is one where an analysis of underlying trends—factors that could influence study outcomes and progress independent of the study—is made using time-series methods. These studies often are used to evaluate the consequences of a change of policy, such as a prescription limit, or addition or removal of a drug from the marketplace. For instance, Soumerai and associates studied the effect of a prescription cap on the use of psychotropic drugs and emergency mental health services using claims data. They used pharmacy claims data collected over a 42-month period, including the 11 months that the prescription cap was in effect, and found that drug use decreased while costs to the state Medicaid program increased during the period of the cap.[46]

TABLE 8–3. Criteria for the Causal Nature of an Association

1. **The association makes biologic sense.** In other words, the proposed association is consistent with our knowledge of the mechanism of disease. You can use data from other human or animal studies, or data from in vitro studies.
2. **The suspected cause precedes the disease.** Even though this is self-evident, it can be overlooked when interpreting findings from certain observational studies.
3. **The association is strong.** Associations with a relative risk of less than 2.0 are considered to be weak. Risks of 2.0 to 4.0 are considered moderate, while those greater than 4.0 are strong. You also need to consider the 95% confidence interval.
4. **The association is found consistently when studied using different methods or populations.** An important characteristic of science is that a finding is reproducible.
5. **There is a dose–response relationship.** For example, there is a higher risk among persons with greater exposure to a risk factor.

INTERPRETATION OF PHARMACOEPIDEMIOLOGIC STUDIES

Not all associations represent a cause-effect relationship. Because most epidemiologic studies of drug effects do not employ random allocation, it is important to determine if a legitimate cause-effect relationship exists. A central methodologic concern in observational studies is *confounding*—that is, the possibility that the apparent effect of an exposure or intervention is due wholly or partly to other factors associated with it that have their own impact on the outcome of interest. Criteria have been proposed to help determine if an association is causal. The fewer criteria that are met, the less likely it is that an association is causal. Table 8–3 is adapted from the work of Hill and Stolly.[47,48] Practitioners should ask the series of questions listed in the table to interpret findings from studies to determine if an association is likely to be causal.

FUTURE DIRECTIONS

Pharmacoepidemiologic studies conducted during the postapproval period provide important information to assist in optimizing therapeutic responses to drugs. These studies can provide valuable information about the relationship between therapeutic agents and adverse and beneficial health outcomes. Information from pharmacoepidemiologic studies also contributes to population-based care and drug regulatory and reimbursement decisions. At the level of individual patient care, a combination of medical and epidemiologic knowledge leads to the choice to use a particular medication. Moreover, patient monitoring to optimize the therapeutic response to drugs also involves epidemiologic data and logic to balance likely benefits against potential risks. Epidemiologic information can provide vital information regarding safety, patterns of drug use, and effectiveness to assist in the provision of evidence-based health care. There is an inherent tradeoff between the need for more information about a drug's risks and the need to make a drug available for use. Because of limitations in the drug development process, more information emerges about a drug after its approval through PMS.

REFERENCES

1. Abenhaim L, Moride Y, Brenot F, et al. Appetite-suppressant drugs and the risk of primary pulmonary hypertension. N Engl J Med 1996;335:609–616.
2. Connolly HM, Crary JL, McGoon MD, et al. Valvular heart disease associated with fenfluramine-phentermine. N Engl J Med 1997;337:581–588.
3. Strom BL, ed. Pharmacoepidemiology. New York, Wiley, 1994.
4. Collett JP, Boissel JP. Pharmacoepidemiology: Epidemiologic approach to the study of drugs. Post Marketing Surveillance 1991;5:3–14.
5. Suissa S, Ernst P, Benayoun S, et al. Low-dose inhaled corticosteroids and the prevention of death from asthma. N Engl J Med 2000;343:332–336.
6. Strom BL, Melmon KL. The use of pharmacoepidemiology to study beneficial drug effects. In: Strom BL, ed. Pharmacoepidemiology. New York, Wiley, 1994.
7. 21 CFR Part 314.126, Adequate and well-controlled studies.
8. Fletcher RH, Fletcher SW, Wagner EH. Clinical Epidemiology, The Essentials, 3d ed. Baltimore, Williams & Wilkins, 1996.
9. Oster G, Borok GM, Menzin J, et al. Cholesterol-reduction intervention study (CRIS): A randomized trial to assess effectiveness and costs in clinical practice. Arch Intern Med 1996;156:731–739.
10. Fayers PM. Generalisation from phase III clinical trials: Survival, quality of life, and health economics. Lancet 1997;350:1025–1027.
11. Geiling EMK, Cannon PR. Pathogenic effects of elixir of sulfanilamide (diethylene glycol) poisoning. JAMA 1938;111:919–926.
12. Lenz W. Malformations caused by drugs in pregnancy. Am J Dis Child 1966;112:99–106.
13. Ray WA, Griffin MR, Avorn J. Evaluating drugs after their approval for clinical use. N Engl J Med 1993;329:2029–2032.
14. Rossi AC, Bosco L, Faich GA, et al. The importance of adverse reaction reporting by physicians: Suprofen and the flank pain syndrome. JAMA 1988;259:1203–1204.
15. Griffin MR, Piper JM, Daugherty JR, et al. Nonsteroidal anti-inflammatory drug use and increased risk for peptic ulcer disease in elderly persons. Ann Intern Med 1991;114:257–263.
16. Ault A. Troglitazone may cause irreversible liver damage. Lancet 1997; 350:1451.
17. Smalley W, Shatin D, Wysowski DK, et al. Contraindicated use of cisapride: Impact of Food and Drug Administration regulatory action. JAMA 2000;284:3036–3039.
18. Jick H, Miettinen OS, Shapiro S, et al. Comprehensive drug surveillance. JAMA 1970;213:1455–1460.
19. Shapiro S. Case-control surveillance. In: Strom BL, ed. Pharmacoepidemiology. New York, Wiley, 1994.
20. Inman WHW. Prescription event monitoring. Acta Med Scand Suppl 1984;683:119–126.
21. Joint Commission on Prescription Drug Use, 96th Congress. Washington, U.S. Government Printing Office, 1980.
22. Saunders KW, Stergachis A, Von Korff M. Group health cooperative. In: Strom BL, ed. Pharmacoepidemiology, 2d ed. New York, Wiley, 1994:171–185.
23. Arrowsmith-Lowe JB, Anello C. A view from a regulatory agency. In: Strom BL, ed. Pharmacoepidemiology, 2d ed. New York, Wiley, 1994: 87–97.
24. World Health Organization. International Drug Monitoring: The Role of the Hospital. Technical Report Series No. 425. Geneva, World Health Organization, 1966.
25. Beard K. Adverse reactions as a cause of hospital admission in the aged. Drugs Aging 1992;2:356–367.
26. Koch KE. Adverse drug reactions. In: Brown T, ed. Handbook of Institutional Pharmacy Practice, 3d ed. Bethesda, American Society of Hospital Pharmacists, 1992:279–291.
27. Johnson JA, Bootman JL. Drug-related morbidity and mortality: A cost-of-illness model. Arch Intern Med 1995;155:1949–1956.
28. Ernst FR, Grizzle AJ. Drug-related morbidity and mortality: Updating the cost-of-illness model. J Am Pharm Assoc. 2001;41:192–198.
29. Lazarou J, Pomeranz BH, Corey PN. Incidence of adverse drug reactions in hospitalized patients: A meta-analysis of prospective studies. JAMA 1998;279:1200–1205.
30. May JR. Adverse drug reactions and interactions. In: DiPiro JT, Talbert RL, Hayes PE, et al, eds. Pharmacotherapy: A Pathophysiologic Approach, 3d ed. Norwalk, CT, Appleton & Lange, 1995:101–116.
31. Strom BL. In: Strom BL, ed. Pharmacoepidemiology, 2d ed. New York: Wiley, 1994:3–14.

32. Park BK, Pirmohamed M, Kitteringham NNR. Idiosyncratic drug reactions: A mechanistic evaluation of risk factors. Br J Clin Pharmacol 1992;34:377–95.
33. Joint Commission on Accreditation of Healthcare Organizations. Comprehensive Accreditation Manual for Hospitals: The Official Handbook. Oakbrook Terrace, IL, JCAHO, 1996.
34. Strom BL, Carson JL. Use of automated databases for pharmacoepidemiology research. Epidemiol Rev 1990;12:87–107.
35. Stergachis A. Evaluating the quality of linked automated data sets for use in pharmacoepidemiology. In: Hartzema AG, Porta MS, Tilson HH, eds. Pharmacoepidemiology: An Introduction, 2d ed, Cincinnati, Harvey Whitney Books, 1991.
36. Shapiro S. The role of automated records linkage in the postmarketing surveillance of drug safety: A critique. Clin Pharmacol Ther 1989;46: 371–386.
37. Faich GA, Stadel BV. The future of automated record linkage for postmarketing surveillance: A response to Shapiro. Clin Pharmacol Ther 1989;46:387–389.
38. Farrington CP, Nash J, Miller E. Case series analysis of adverse reactions to vaccines: A comparative evaluation. Am J Epidemiol 1996;143:1165–1173.
39. Holt VL, Daling JR, Weiss NS, et al. Functional ovarian cyst risk associated with use of monophasic and triphasic oral contraceptives. Obstet Gynecol 1992;79:529–533.
40. Herbst AL, Ulfelder H, Poskanzer DC. Adenocarcinoma of the vagina: Association of maternal stilbestrol therapy with tumor appearance in young women. N Engl J Med 1971;284:878–881.
41. Ray WA, Griffin MR, Downey W. Benzodiazepines of long and short elimination half-life and the risk of hip fracture. JAMA 1989;262:3303–3307.
42. Royal College of General Practitioners. Oral Contraceptives and Health. London, Pitman, 1974.
43. Hooten TM, Scholes D, Hughs JP, et al. A prospective study of risk factors for symptomatic urinary tract infection in young women. N Engl J Med 1996;335:468–474.
44. Soumerai SB, McLaughlin TJ, Spiegelman D, et al. Adverse outcomes of underuse of beta-blockers in elderly survivors of acute myocardial infarction. JAMA 1997;277:115–121.
45. Cook TD, Campbell DT. Quasi-experimentation: Design and analysis issues for field settings. Boston, Houghton-Mifflin, 1979.
46. Soumerai SB, McLaughlin TJ, Ross-Degnan D, et al. Effects of limiting Medicaid drug-reimbursement benefits on the use of psychotropic agents and acute mental health services by patients with schizophrenia. N Engl J Med 1994;441:650–655.
47. Hill AB. The environment and disease: Association or causation? Proc R Soc Med 1965;58:295–300.
48. Stolly PD. How to interpret studies of adverse drug reactions. Clin Pharmacol Ther 1990;48:337–339.

9

CLINICAL TOXICOLOGY

Peter A. Chyka

Poisoning is an adverse effect from a chemical that has been taken in excessive amounts. The body is able to tolerate, and in some cases detoxify, a certain dose of a chemical, but once a critical threshold is exceeded, toxicity results. Poisoning can produce minor local effects that are treated readily in the outpatient setting or systemic life-threatening situations that require intensive medical intervention. This spectrum of toxicity is typical for many chemicals with which humans come in contact. Virtually any chemical can become a poison when taken in sufficient quantity, but the potency of some compounds leads to serious toxicity with small quantities[1] (Table 9–1). Poisoning by chemicals includes exposures to drugs, industrial chemicals, household products, plants, venomous animals, and agrochemicals. This chapter will describe some examples of this spectrum of toxicity, outline means to recognize poisoning risk, and present principles of treatment.

EPIDEMIOLOGY

Each year poisonings account for approximately 16,000 deaths, 225,000 hospitalizations, and 875,000 emergency department visits in the United States.[2,3] Young adults aged 25 to 44 years are at greatest risk of a poisoning death, and males have a twofold higher risk of death than females. Nearly one-half of all poisoning deaths of adults are due to suicide. Poisoning deaths in adults most commonly involve motor vehicle exhaust (carbon monoxide), other gases or vapors, antidepressants, tranquilizers, barbiturates, alcohol, opioids, and local anesthetics including cocaine.[4,5] Approximately 1% of poisoning deaths involve children under the age of 6 years. The elderly, those 75 years old and older, children under 5 years of age, and adolescents and young adults 15 to 24 years of age have the highest risk for nonfatal poisonings requiring hospitalization. The circumstances surrounding nearly one-half of hospitalized injuries are unrecorded; however, nearly two-thirds of those in which the intent is recorded are deemed to be intentional. Intentional[3] and unintentional[2] poisoning deaths (Fig. 9–1) have been increasing steadily during the last two decades. There are several databases in the United States that provide different levels of insight and documentation of the poisoning problem (Table 9–2). Poisonings documented by U.S. poison centers are compiled in the annual report of the American Association of Poison Control Centers Toxic Exposure Surveillance System (AAPCC-TESS).[6] Although it represents the largest database on poisoning, it is not complete because it relies on individuals contacting a poison control center and the center voluntarily reporting the incident. The AAPCC-TESS data set captures approximately 5% of the annual number of deaths from poisoning tabulated in death certificates.[3] Despite this shortcoming, AAPCC-TESS provides valuable insight into the characteristics and frequency of poisonings. In the 1999 AAPCC-TESS summary 2,201,156 poisoning exposures were reported by 64 participating poison centers that served a population of 261 million people.[6] Children younger than 6 years of age accounted for 53% of the cases. The site of exposure was the home in 92% of the cases, and a single substance was involved in 92% of the cases. An acute exposure accounted for 93% of the cases, 87% of which were unintentional or accidental exposures. Only 10% were intentional. Fatalities accounted for 873 (0.04%) cases, of which 3% were children younger than 6 years of age. The majority of fatalities (61%) occurred in 20- to 49-year old individuals. The distribution of substances most frequently involved in pediatric and adult exposures differed; however, medicines were the most frequently involved substance (Table 9–3). In summary, children account for the majority of reported poisonings with morbidity, but adults account for a greater proportion of mortality from poisoning.

ECONOMIC IMPACT OF POISONING

The economic impact of poisoning can be inferred from the role of poison control centers in cost avoidance. Poison control centers can optimize the use of health care resources by triaging patients to receive the appropriate level of medical care and thereby reduce overall health care costs. In one example, the cost for managing a case ranged from $23 for those managed at home by a poison control center to $635 when a call was placed to the 911 emergency service that resulted in ambulance transport to an emergency department.[7,8] Another economic analysis estimated that for every dollar spent on poison control center services, at least $6.50 in medical spending was saved, a value comparable with that obtained from immunizations.[9] This same analysis estimated that spending for poisoning treatment reached $3 billion in 1992.

Poisoning, which ranks fourth in cost of injury, accounted for 3% of the total injuries in this country and a total lifetime cost of $8.5 billion. The average lifetime cost per person for a fatal poisoning is $372,691, ranking second to the cost of a firearm fatality per person.[4] Estimates of the lifetime cost of injury include related health care costs and lost lifetime earnings of the victim; however, they do not include the costs of suffering, reduced productivity of caregivers, or legal costs. The average cost per person hospitalized for poisoning is $17,631 versus $171 for those not hospitalized.[4]

POISON PREVENTION STRATEGIES

The number of poisoning deaths in children has declined dramatically over the past three decades in part due to several poison prevention approaches.[10] These included the Poison Prevention Packaging Act of 1970, the evolution of regional poison control centers, the application of prompt first aid measures, improvements in overall critical care, development of less toxic product formulations, better clarity in the packaging and labeling of products, and public education on the risks and prevention of poisoning.[11] Although all these factors play a role in minimizing poisoning dangers, particularly in children, the Poison Prevention Packaging Act has perhaps had the most significant influence.[10] The intent of the act was to develop packaging that is difficult for children under 5 years of age to open or to obtain harmful amounts within a reasonable period of time. However, the

TABLE 9–1. Serious Toxicity Associated with Ingestion of One Mouthful or One Dosage Unit

Methanol[a]	Hydrocarbons[a]
Caustics or alkalis[a]	Acids[a]
Cationic detergents[a]	Selenous acid
Cyanide[a]	Anticholinesterase insecticides[a]
Phencyclidine or LSD	Clonidine
Colchicine	Chloroquine

[a]Concentrated or undiluted form.

packaging was not to be difficult for normal adults to use properly. There are a number of products and product categories for which safety packaging is required (Table 9–4). Child-resistant containers are not totally childproof and may be opened by children, which can result in poisoning. Despite the success of child-resistant containers, many adults disable the hardware or simply use no safety cap and thus place children at risk.[12] Fatigue of the packaging materials also can occur, which underscores the need for new prescription ware for refills, as required in the Act.[13]

Poison prevention requires constant vigilance because there are new generations of families where parents and grandparents need to be educated on poisoning risks and prevention strategies. New products and changes in product formulations also present different poisoning dangers and must be studied to provide optimal management. Strategies to prevent poisonings should consider the various psychosocial circumstances of poisoning (Table 9–5), prioritize risk groups and behaviors, and customize an intervention for specific situations.[14–16]

RECOGNITION AND ASSESSMENT

The clinician's initial responsibility is to determine whether a poisoning has occurred or if there is a potential for one to develop. Some patients provide a clear account of an exposure that has occurred with a known quantity of a specific agent. In other cases, the patient may appear with only an unexplained illness characterized by nonspecific signs and symptoms and no immediate history of ingestion. Exposure to folk remedies, herbal medicines, dietary supplements, and environmental toxins also should be considered. Patients with suicide gestures can deliberately give an unclear history, and poisoning should be suspected routinely. Poisoning and drug overdoses should be suspected in any patient with a sudden, unexplained illness or with a puzzling combination of signs and symptoms, particularly in high-risk age groups. Nearly any symptom can be seen with poisoning, but some signs and symptoms are suggestive of a particular toxin exposure.[17,18]

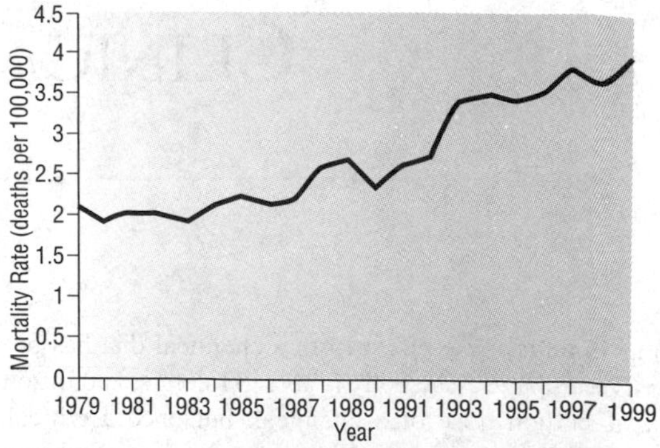

FIGURE 9–1. Unintentional poisoning mortality rates in the United States from 1979 to 1999. *(From Ref. 2.)*

Compounds that produce characteristic clinical pictures (toxidromes), such as organophosphate poisoning with pinpoint pupils, rales, bradycardia, central nervous system depression, sweating, excessive salivation, and diarrhea, are most readily recognizable.[19] Assessment of the patient may be aided by consultation with a poison control center. These centers can provide information on product composition, typical symptoms, the range of toxicity, laboratory analysis, treatment options, and bibliographic references. Furthermore, the center will have specially trained physicians, pharmacists, and toxicologists on staff or on file to assist with difficult cases. Contact with a poison control center also may identify changes in currently recommended therapy. A list of active poison control centers may be found in references such as *USP Drug Information*[20] and on the Internet (*http://www.aapcc.org*).

When the circumstances of a poison exposure indicate that it is minimally toxic, many poisonings can be managed successfully at the scene of the poisoning.[6] Poison control centers typically monitor the victim by telephone during the first 2 to 6 hours of the exposure to assess the patient's status and outcome of first aid. Once a poisoning is suspected and there is a need to confirm the diagnosis for medical or legal purposes, appropriate biologic material should be sent to the laboratory for analysis. Gastric contents may contain the greatest concentration of drug, but it is difficult to analyze. Blood or urine may be tested by qualitative screening in order to detect a drug's presence.[21,23] The results of a qualitative drug screen can be misleading due to interfering or low-level substances; it rarely guides therapy and thus has questionable value for nonspecific, general screening purposes.[19,21,22] Quantitative determination of serum concentrations may be important for the assessment of some poisonings, such as those with acetaminophen, ethanol, methanol, iron, theophylline, and digoxin.

TABLE 9–2. Strengths of Various Poisoning Databases

Database (abbreviation)	Strength
Death certificates from state health departments compiled by the National Center for Health Statistics (NCHS)	Compiles all U.S. death certificates where the cause of death was by disease or external forces, such as poisoning. Data typically verified by laboratory and clinical observations.
National Electronic Injury Surveillance System of U.S. Consumer Product Safety Commission (NEISS)	Surveys electronically all injuries, including poisonings, treated daily at a sample of U.S. emergency departments. Used to identify first-time and recurring product-related injuries.
Drug Abuse Warning Network (DAWN) of the Federal Substance Abuse and Mental Health Services Administration	Identifies drug-of-abuse–related episodes and deaths that are reported to 685 hospitals and 145 medical examiners in the United States.
Toxic Exposure Surveillance System of American Association of Poison Control Centers (AAPCC-TESS)	Represents largest database of poisonings with high representation of children based on voluntary reporting by poison control centers.

TABLE 9–3. Poison Exposures by Age Group and Fatal Outcome, Ranked in Decreasing Order

Pediatric	Adult	Fatal Outcome
Medicines	Medicines	Medicines
Cosmetics and personal care items	Cleaning substances	Alcohols
Cleaning substances	Bites or envenomations	Gases and fumes
Plants	Food products or food poisoning	Chemicals
Foreign bodies	Cosmetics and personal care items	Automotive products
Pesticides	Chemicals	Pesticides
Arts and crafts or office supplies	Alcohols	Hydrocarbons

From Ref. 6.

PHARMACOKINETICS OF OVERDOSE

The pharmacokinetic characteristics of drugs taken in overdose may differ from those observed following therapeutic doses[23,24] (Table 9–6). These differences are due to dose-dependent changes in absorption, distribution, metabolism, or elimination; pharmacologic effects of the drug; or pathophysiologic consequences of the overdose. Dose-dependent changes may decrease the rate and extent of absorption, whereas the bioavailability of the agent may be increased due to saturation of first-pass metabolism. The distribution of a compound may be altered due to saturation of protein-binding sites. Metabolism and elimination of a compound may be retarded due to saturated biotransformation pathways leading to nonlinear elimination kinetics. Delayed gastric emptying by anticholinergic drugs or as the result of general central nervous system (CNS) depression caused by many drugs may alter the rate and extent of absorption. The formation of concretions or bezoars of solid dosage forms may delay the onset, prolong the duration, or complicate the therapy of an acute overdose.[25] A combination of pharmacokinetic and pharmacodynamic factors may lead to the delayed onset of toxicity of several toxins, such as thyroid hormones, oral anticoagulants, acetaminophen, and drugs in sustained-release dosage forms.[26] Drug-induced hypoperfusion may affect drug distribution and result in reduced hepatic or renal clearance. Changes in blood pH may alter the distribution of weak acids and bases. Drug-induced renal or hepatic injury also can significantly decrease clearance. Implications of these changes for poisoning management include the delayed achievement of peak concentrations with a corresponding longer period of opportunity to remove drug from the gastrointestinal tract. The expected duration of effects may be much greater than those observed with therapeutic doses due to continued absorption and impaired clearance. The application of pharmacokinetic variables, such as percentage protein binding and volume of distribution, from therapeutic doses may not be appropriate in poisoning cases.[23] Data on toxicokinetics are often difficult to interpret and compare because the doses and times of ingestion are uncertain, the duration of sampling is often inadequate, active metabolites may not be measured, protein binding is typically not assessed, and the severity of toxicity may vary dramatically.

TABLE 9–4. Examples of Products Requiring Child-Resistant Closures

Aspirin	Acetaminophen
Ibuprofen	Diphenhydramine
Oral prescription drugs[a]	Iron pharmaceuticals
Turpentine	Kerosene
Ethylene glycol	Methanol
Sulfuric acid	Sodium hydroxide
Glue removers containing acetonitrile	Permanent hair wave neutralizers containing sodium bromate

[a]With certain exceptions such as nitroglycerin and oral contraceptives.

TABLE 9–5. Psychosocial Characteristics of Poisoning Patients

Children	Young Adults	Elderly
Act purposefully or are poisoned by caretaker or sibling	Intentional abuse or suicidal intent is possible	Suicidal intent or unintentional misuse
Act with developmentally appropriate curiosity	Disregard or cannot read directions	Confuse product identity and directions for use
Attracted by product appearance	Do not recognize poisoning risk	Do not recognize poisoning risk
Ingest substances that adults find unpleasant	Reluctant to seek assistance until ill	Comorbid conditions complicate toxicity
React to stressful and disrupted household	Exaggerate or misrepresent situation	Unable or unwilling to describe situation
Imitate adult behaviors (e.g., taking medicine)	Peer pressure to experiment with drugs	Multiple drugs may lead to adverse reactions

MECHANISMS OF TOXICITY

Characterization of the mechanism of toxicity of poisons is often limited by our understanding of the pharmacology and cellular mechanism of action of an agent. Although many toxic effects are an exag-

TABLE 9–6. Examples of the Influence of Drug Overdosage on Pharmacokinetic and Pharmacodynamic Characteristics

Effect of Overdosage[a]	Examples
Slowed absorption due to formation of poorly soluble concretions in the gastrointestinal tract	Aspirin, lithium, phenytoin, sustained-release theophylline
Slowed absorption due to slowed gastrointestinal motility	Benztropine, nortriptyline
Slowed absorption due to toxin-induced hypoperfusion	Procainamide
Decreased serum protein binding	Lidocaine, salicylates, valproic acid
Increased volume of distribution associated with toxin-induced acidemia	Salicylates
Slowed elimination due to saturation of biotransformation pathways	Ethanol, phenytoin, salicylates, theophylline
Slowed elimination due to toxin-induced hypothermia (<35°C)	Ethanol, propranolol
Prolonged toxicity due to formation of longer-acting metabolites	Carbamazepine, dapsone, glutethimide, meperidine

[a]Compared to characteristics following therapeutic doses or resolution of toxicity.
Adapted from Refs. 23 and 24.

geration of typical actions and effects, some chemicals produce toxic effects that are not observed with lower or therapeutic doses. Tricyclic antidepressants produce a characteristically widened QRS complex on electrocardiogram due to an exaggeration of their pharmacologic actions on the sodium channel of the myocardium. Overdoses of acetaminophen lead to accumulation of a hepatotoxic metabolite that typically is detoxified when taken in therapeutic doses. These and other examples will be described more fully later in this chapter.

Poisons may exhibit local effects on skin, eye, lung, gastrointestinal mucosa, or other tissue as the result of their pharmacologic, irritant, or corrosive action. Once a poison is absorbed, systemic effects may be immediate or delayed in onset. Local and systemic effects may set the stage for secondary effects that are a consequence of the initial injury, such as infection, metabolic acidosis, or reflex tachycardia. Finally, a single poisoning incident may result in permanent or disabling effects, such as blindness from methanol poisoning.

▶ TREATMENT: Clinical Toxicology

GENERAL APPROACHES TO TREATMENT OF THE POISONED PATIENT

PREHOSPITAL CARE

First Aid

The presence of adequate airway, breathing, and circulation should be assessed, and cardiopulmonary resuscitation should be started if needed. The most important step in preventing a minor exposure from progressing to a serious intoxication is early decontamination of the poison. Basic poisoning first-aid and decontamination measures (Table 9–7) should be instituted immediately at the scene of the poisoning.[28] If there is any question about the potential severity of the poison exposure, a poison control center should be consulted immediately. Recently a national toll-free phone service (1-800-222-1222) has been established that routes the caller to the local poison control center. While awaiting transport, placing the patient on the left side may afford easier clearing of the airway if emesis occurs and may slow absorption of drug from the gastrointestinal tract.[28]

Ipecac Syrup

Ipecac syrup induces emesis typically within 15 to 30 minutes by direct irritation of the stomach and stimulation of the CNS chemoreceptor trigger zone. Emesis typically occurs in one to six episodes lasting up to 1 hour.[29] The dose of ipecac syrup is 5 to 10 mL for a child 6 months to 1 year of age, 15 mL for children 1 to 12 years old, and 15 to 30 mL for patients over 12 years of age.[20] To aid gastric evacuation, 6 to 8 oz of water, fruit juice, or a carbonated drink should be administered with the ipecac syrup. The same dose is repeated in 30 minutes if no emesis occurs. Ipecac syrup produces emesis in 98% of individuals within 60 minutes.[29,30] The adverse effects of ipecac syrup when given in therapeutic doses include drowsiness (10% to 21%), diarrhea (5% to 26%), and protracted vomiting beyond 1 hour (13% to 17%). Rare complications include Mallory-Weiss tears, pneumomediastinum, and aspiration pneumonia.[30] Ipecac syrup should be considered for the prehospital care of poisonings of mild to moderate severity, when contraindications are not present, and it should be administered within 1 hour of the ingestion.[11,30]

TABLE 9–7. First Aid and Immediate Decontamination for Poison Exposures

Inhaled Poison
Immediately get the person to fresh air. Avoid breathing fumes. Open doors and windows. If victim is not breathing, start artificial respiration.

Poison on the Skin
Remove contaminated clothing and flood skin with water for 10 minutes. Wash gently with soap and water and rinse. Avoid further contamination of victim or first aid providers.

Poison in the Eye
Flood the eye with lukewarm or cool water poured from a glass 2 or 3 inches from the eye. Repeat for 10 to 15 continuous minutes. Keep eye open, but do not force the eyelid open.

Swallowed Poison
Unless the patient is unconscious, having convulsions, or cannot swallow, give 2 to 4 ounces of water immediately and then seek further help. Ipecac syrup should only be used on advice of a poison control center, emergency department, or physician.

There are several contraindications to its use.[30] If the patient is without a gag reflex; is lethargic, comatose, or convulsing; or is expected to become unresponsive within the next 30 minutes, emesis should not be induced. If a fruitful emesis has occurred spontaneously shortly after ingestion, ipecac syrup may not be necessary. Ingestions of caustics, corrosives, ammonia, and bleach are definite contraindications to ipecac-induced emesis. The ingestion of aliphatic hydrocarbons (e.g., gasoline, kerosene, and charcoal lighter fluid) typically does not require emesis. When the agent is definitely known to be nontoxic, induction of emesis is purposeless and potentially dangerous. The rapid onset of coma or seizures or the potential to exaggerate the toxic effects of the poison may preclude the use of ipecac syrup. Some examples include poisonings with diphenoxylate, propoxyphene, clonidine, tricyclic antidepressants, hypoglycemic agents, nicotine, strychnine, β-blocking agents, and calcium channel blockers. Debilitated, pregnant, and elderly patients may be further compromised by the induction of emesis. Ipecac syrup is not used routinely in emergency departments except for certain poisonings such as iron, where alternatives to ipecac syrup, such as activated charcoal, are not useful. If treatment at an emergency department is imminent, within an hour of ingestion, use of ipecac syrup should be withheld.

HOSPITAL TREATMENT

General Care

Supportive and symptomatic care is the mainstay of treatment of the poisoned patient. In the search for specific antidotes and methods to increase excretion of the drug, attention to vital signs and organ functions should not be neglected. Establishment of adequate oxygenation and maintenance of adequate circulation are the highest priority. Other components of the acute supportive care plan include the management of seizures, arrhythmias, hypotension, acid-base balance, fluid status, electrolyte balance, and hypoglycemia. Placement of an intravenous and urinary catheter is typical to ensure delivery of fluids and drugs when necessary and to monitor urine production, respectively.

Gastric Lavage

Gastric lavage involves the placement of an orogastric tube and washing out of the gastric contents through repetitive instillation and withdrawal of fluid. Gastric lavage should be considered only if a potentially toxic agent has been ingested within the past hour for most patients. If the patient is comatose or lacks a gag reflex, gastric lavage should be performed only after intubation with a cuffed or well-fitting endotracheal tube. The largest orogastric tube that can be passed (at least an external diameter of 12 mm in adults and 8 mm in children) should be used to ensure adequate evacuation, especially of undissolved tablets. Lavage should be performed with warm (37 to 38°C) normal saline or tap water until the gastric return is clear; this usually requires 2 to 4 L or more of fluid. Relative contraindications for gastric lavage include ingestion of a corrosive or hydrocarbon agent. Complications of gastric lavage include aspiration pneumonitis, laryngospasm, mechanical injury to the esophagus and stomach, hypothermia, and fluid and electrolyte imbalance.[31]

Single-Dose Activated Charcoal

Reduction of toxin absorption can be achieved by the administration of activated charcoal. It is a highly purified, adsorbent form of carbon that prevents the absorption of a drug from the gastrointestinal tract by chemically binding (adsorbing) it to the charcoal surface. There are no contraindications to its use, but it is generally ineffective for iron, lead, lithium, simple alcohols, and corrosives. It is not indicated for aliphatic hydrocarbons due to increased risk of emesis and pulmonary aspiration. Activated charcoal is most effective when given within the first few hours after ingestion, ideally within the first hour.[32] The recommended dose of activated charcoal for a child (1 to 12 years old) is 25 to 50 g; for an adolescent or adult it is 25 to 100 g. Children under 1 year of age may receive 1 g/kg.[4,20] Activated charcoal is mixed with water to make a slurry, shaken vigorously, and administered orally or by means of a nasogastric tube. Activated charcoal is contraindicated when the gastrointestinal tract is not intact. Activated charcoal is relatively nontoxic, but there are two identified risks: (1) emesis following administration and (2) pulmonary aspiration of charcoal and gastric contents leading to pneumonitis in patients with an unprotected airway or absent gag reflex.[32] Some activated charcoal products contain sorbitol, a cathartic that may be associated with an increased incidence of emesis following its use.[33]

Cathartics

Cathartics may decrease the rate of absorption by increasing gastrointestinal excretion of the poison and the poison-activated charcoal complex, but their value is unproven. Poisoned patients do not routinely require the administration of a cathartic, and it is rarely if ever given without concurrent activated charcoal administration.[34] If used, a cathartic should only be administered once and only if bowel sounds are present. The cathartics typically used are magnesium citrate, 4 mL/kg up to 300 mL per dose; 70% sorbitol, 1 to 2 mL/kg for adults; and 35% sorbitol, 4 mL/kg for children. Infants, the elderly, and patients with renal failure should be given saline cathartics cautiously, if at all.[11,34]

Whole-Bowel Irrigation

Polyethylene glycol electrolyte solutions, such as GoLytely and Colyte, are used routinely as whole bowel irrigants prior to colonoscopy and bowel surgery.[35] These solutions also can be used as a means to decontaminate the gastrointestinal tract of ingested toxins.[11,36] Large volumes of these osmotically balanced solutions are administered continuously through a nasogastric or duodenal tube for 4 to 12 hours or more. They quickly cause gastrointestinal evacuation and are continued until the rectal discharge is relatively clear. This procedure may be indicated for certain patients in whom the ingestion occurred several hours prior to hospitalization and the drug still is suspected to be in the gastrointestinal tract, such as cocaine smugglers who swallow condoms filled with cocaine.[37] In addition, patients who have ingested delayed-release or enteric-coated drug formulations or have ingested substances such as iron that are not well adsorbed by activated charcoal may benefit from whole-bowel irrigation.[36] It should not be used in patients with a bowel perforation or obstruction, gastrointestinal hemorrhage, ileus, or intractable emesis. Emesis, abdominal cramps, and intestinal bloating have been reported with whole-bowel irrigation.[36]

Perspectives on Gastric Decontamination

Although there are a variety of options for gastric decontamination, two clinical toxicology groups (the American Academy of Clinical Toxicology and the European Association of Poison Centers and Clinical Toxicologists) have concluded that no means of gastric decontamination should be used routinely for a poisoned patient without careful consideration.[30–32,34,36] They indicate that therapy is most effective within the first hour and that effectiveness beyond this time cannot be supported or refuted with the available data. A clinical policy statement by the American College of Emergency Physicians concludes that although no definitive recommendation can be made on the use of ipecac syrup, gastric lavage, cathartics, or whole-bowel irrigation, activated charcoal is advocated for most patients when appropriate.[38] The clinical policy also states that ipecac syrup is rarely of value in the emergency department and that the use of whole-bowel irrigation following ingestion of substances not well adsorbed by activated charcoal is not supported by evidence. Although gastric lavage can reduce drug absorption if performed within 1 hour of ingestion, its use is not recommended routinely.[31,38,39] In recent years, the use of ipecac syrup has declined (Fig. 9–2) in part because of its apparent lower efficacy compared with activated charcoal in minimizing drug absorption.[30,32] Recently, activated charcoal has been promoted for the treatment of poisonings at home, but issues of safety, patient compliance, and effectiveness have not been proven in the home setting.[40] Poison control centers may be a source of guidance on the contemporary application of gastric decontamination techniques for a specific patient.

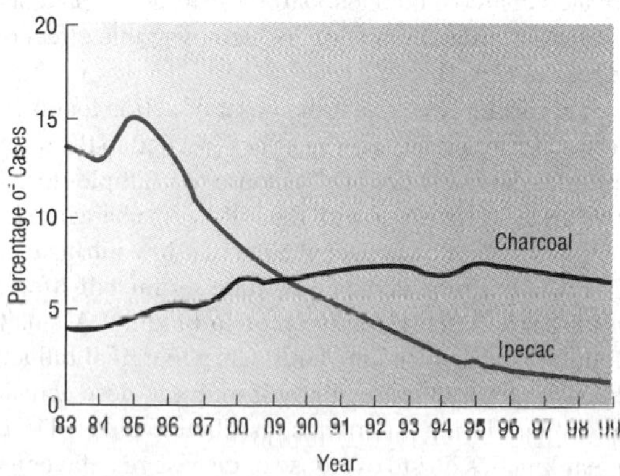

FIGURE 9–2. Trends in the use of ipecac syrup and activated charcoal based on cases reported by U.S. poison centers. *(From Ref. 6.)*

Enhanced Elimination

Numerous methods have been used to increase the rate of excretion of poisons from the body. Of these, only diuresis, multiple-dose activated charcoal, and hemodialysis are occasionally useful. These approaches should only be considered if the risks of the procedure are significantly outweighed by the expected benefits or if the recovery of the patient is seriously in doubt and the method has been shown to be helpful.

Diuresis. Diuresis may be used for poisons excreted predominantly by the renal route; however, most drugs and poisons are metabolized, and only a good urine flow, such as 2 to 3 mL/kg per hour, needs to be maintained for most patients. Fluid and electrolyte balance should be monitored closely. Ionized diuresis may increase excretion of certain chemicals that are weak acids or bases by trapping ionized drug in the renal tubule and minimizing reabsorption. Alkalinization of the urine to achieve a urine pH of 7.5 or greater for poisoning by weak acids such as salicylates or phenobarbital can be achieved by the intravenous administration of sodium bicarbonate, 1 to 2 mEq/kg over a 1- to 2-hour period. Complications of urinary alkalinization include alkalosis, fluid and electrolyte disturbances, and inability to achieve target urinary pH values.[41] Acid diuresis may enhance the excretion of weak bases, such as amphetamines, but it is rarely, if ever, used because it risks worsening rhadomyolysis commonly associated with amphetamine overdose.[42] Generally, ionized diuresis is rarely indicated for poisoned patients because it is inefficient relative to other methods of enhancing elimination, there is a risk of unacceptable adverse effects, and the renal elimination of most drugs is not enhanced dramatically.

Multiple-Dose Activated Charcoal. Multiple doses of activated charcoal can augment the body's clearance of certain drugs by enhanced passage from the bloodstream into the gastrointestinal tract and subsequent adsorption. This process, termed *charcoal intestinal dialysis* or *charcoal-enhanced intestinal exorption*, describes the attraction of drug molecules across the capillary bed of the intestine by activated charcoal in the intestinal lumen and subsequent adsorption of the drug to the charcoal.[43] Furthermore, it may interrupt the enterohepatic recirculation of certain drugs, such as tricylic antidepressants.[43,44] Once the drug is adsorbed to the charcoal, it is eliminated with the charcoal in the stool. The systemic clearance of several drugs has been shown to be enhanced by up to several-fold (Table 9–8). An international toxicology group's position statement on multiple-dose activated charcoal concluded that it should be considered only if a patient has ingested a life-threatening amount of carbamazepine, dapsone, phenobarbital, quinine, or theophylline.[45] Although a prospective, randomized study of the effects of multiple-dose activated charcoal on phenobarbital-overdosed patients demonstrated increased drug elimination, no demonstrable effect on patient outcome was observed.[46]

This approach provides a rapid onset of action that is limited by blood flow and a maximal "ceiling effect" related to the dose of charcoal present in the intestine. The response to multiple-dose activated charcoal is greatest for drugs with the following characteristics: good affinity for adsorption by activated charcoal, low intrinsic clearance, sufficient residence time in the body (long serum half-life), long distributive phase, and nonrestrictive protein binding. A small volume of distribution is also desirable, but it has a marginal influence as an isolated characteristic,[47] particularly if multiple-dose activated charcoal is instituted during the toxin's distributive phase. Development of nonlinear kinetics due to overdose or disease may favor a response for drugs otherwise shown to be unaffected with subtoxic doses in human volunteer studies.[48] A typical dosage schedule is 15 to 25 g of activated charcoal every 2 to 6 hours until serious symptoms abate or the serum concentration of the toxin is below the toxic range. This procedure has been used in premature and full-term infants in doses of 1 g/kg every 1 to 4 hours. Complications are the same as those for single-dose charcoal. The risks of aspiration pneumonitis in obtunded or uncooperative patients and of intestinal obstruction in patients prone to ileus following a period of bowel ischemia, for example, after cardiopulmonary arrest in the elderly may be higher.[44,49] Contraindications are the same as those for single-dose charcoal.

TABLE 9–8. Drugs Whose Elimination Half-Life Is Reduced by Multiple-Dose Activated Charcoal

Drug	Percent Reduction in Half-life[a]
Phenobarbital	62
Digitoxin	54
Dapsone	53
Piroxicam	51
Phenytoin	50
Theophylline	47
Carbamazepine	45
Quinine	45
Nortriptyline	35
Digoxin	33
Propoxyphene	32
Phenylbutazone	29
Amitriptyline	23

[a]Increased elimination in normal volunteers compared to a control group not receiving activated charcoal.
Adapted from Ref. 43.

Hemodialysis. Hemodialysis may be necessary for certain severe cases of poisoning. Dialysis should be considered when the duration of symptoms is expected to be prolonged, other pathways of excretion are unavailable, clinical deterioration is present, the drug is dialyzable, and appropriate personnel and equipment are available. Drugs that are effectively dialyzed possess a low molecular weight, are not highly or tightly protein bound, and are not highly distributed to tissues. The principles of hemodialysis for acutely ill individuals are described in Chapter 47. Hemodialysis and charcoal hemoperfusion are the most efficient methods of dialysis, but both pose serious risks related to anticoagulation, blood transfusions, loss of blood elements, fluid and electrolyte disturbances, and infection.[50] Hemodialysis may be lifesaving for methanol and ethylene glycol poisoning and quite effective for other poisons, such as lithium, salicylates, ethanol, and theophylline.[27,38] Charcoal hemoperfusion was popular in the 1970s and 1980s as a means to quickly remove toxins from the circulation, but this approach has fallen out of favor due to poor results, inappropriate use for drugs with large volumes of distribution, and limited commercial availability of charcoal hemoperfusion columns.

Antidotes

The search for and use of an antidote should never replace good supportive care.[38] Specific systemic antidotes are available for many common poisonings[51,52] (Table 9–9). Inadequate availability of antidotes at acute-care hospitals has been noted throughout the United States and can complicate the care of a poisoned patient. An evidenced-based consensus of experts has recommended minimum stocking requirements for 16 antidotes for acute-care hospitals.[53] These

TABLE 9–9. Systemic Antidotes Available in the United States

Antidote	Toxic Agent
Atropine	Anticholinesterase insecticides
Botulism antitoxin	Botulism
Calcium EDTA	Lead
Crotalidae polyvalent antivenin	Rattlesnakes, cottonmouth snakes, copperhead snakes
Crotalidae polyvalent immune Fab	Rattlesnakes, cottonmouth snakes, copperhead snakes
Cyanide antidote kit (Amyl nitrite, sodium nitrate, and sodium thiosulfate)	Cyanide
Deferoxamine	Iron
Digoxin immune Fab	Digoxin, digitoxin
Dimercaprol	Various heavy metals
Ethanol	Ethylene glycol, methanol
Flumazenil	Benzodiazepines
Fomepizole	Ethylene glycol, methanol
Lactrodectus mactans antivenin	Black widow spider
Methylene blue	Methemoglobinemia
Micrurus fulvius antivenin	Coral snake
N-acetylcysteine	Acetaminophen
Nalmefene	Opioids
Naloxone	Opioids
Oxygen	Carbon monoxide
Penicillamine	Various heavy metals
Phytonadione	Anticoagulants
Pralidoxime	Organophosphate insecticides
Succimer	Lead

recommendations may provide guidance to pharmacy and therapeutics committees in establishing a hospital's antidote needs. Drugs conventionally used for nonpoisoning situations may act as antidotes to reverse acute toxicity, such as glucagon for β-adrenergic blocker or calcium channel antagonist overdose and octreatide for sulfonylurea-induced hypoglycemia.[54] As our understanding of drug toxicity increases, antidotes may have applications beyond contemporary indications, such as *N*-acetylcysteine, which has shown promise for treating approximately 25 different poisonings and adverse drug reactions.[55] The use of toxin-specific antibodies (e.g., Fab antibody fragments for digoxin or crotalid snake venom[56,57]) has offered a new approach to the treatment of poisoning victims. With the development of other immunologic antidotes, such as those directed against antidepressants,[54] this approach may prove useful in the treatment of other intoxications.

ASSESSING THE EFFECTIVENESS OF THERAPIES

Our knowledge of poisoning treatment is derived from case reports, clinical studies, human volunteer studies, animal investigations, and in vitro tests. Each of these approaches has limited applicability to the care of humans who have been poisoned. Case reports often are difficult to assess because they are uncontrolled, the histories are uncertain, and multiple therapies are often used. They can, however, be useful to describe unique or new toxicities or characterize adverse effects associated with a therapy. Although clinical studies may describe tens to hundreds of patients, they can exhibit serious shortcomings, such as weak randomization procedures, no laboratory confirmation or correlation with history, insufficient number of severe cases, no control group, and no quantitative measure of outcome. Extrapolation of data from human volunteer studies to patients who overdose is difficult because of potential or unknown variations in pharmacokinetics (e.g., differing dissolution, gastric emptying, and absorption rates) seen with toxic as opposed to therapeutic doses,[23,24] differences in time to institute therapy in the emergency setting, and differences in absorption in fasted human volunteers compared with the full stomach of some patients who overdose. These studies, however, provide the most controlled and objective measures of the efficacy of a treatment. Experiences from animal studies cannot be applied directly to humans due to interspecies differences in toxicity and metabolism. In vitro tests serve to screen the efficacy of some approaches, such as activated charcoal adsorption, but they do not sufficiently mimic physiologic conditions to allow direct clinical application of the findings. Despite their limitations, these data comprise the basis for the therapy of poisoned patients and are tempered with the consideration of non-poisoning-related factors such as a particular patient's underlying medical condition, age, and need for concurrent supportive measures.

CLINICAL SPECTRUM OF POISONING

Poisoning and/or drug overdose with acetaminophen, anticholinesterase insecticides, calcium channel blockers, iron, theophylline, and tricyclic antidepressants are the focus of the remainder of this chapter because they represent commonly encountered poisonings for which pharmacotherapy is indicated. These agents also were chosen because they represent common examples with different mechanisms of toxicity, and they illustrate the application of general treatment approaches as well as some agent-specific interventions.

ACETAMINOPHEN

Signs and Symptoms. Acute acetaminophen poisoning characteristically results in hepatotoxicity.[58–61] Clinical presentation is determined by the time required for hepatic necrosis to occur, presence of risk factors, and the ingestion of other drugs. During the first 12 to 24 hours after ingestion, nausea, vomiting, anorexia, and diaphoresis may be observed; however, many patients are asymptomatic. During the next 1 to 3 days, a latent phase of lessened symptoms, patients often have an asymptomatic rise in liver enzymes and bilirubin. Signs and symptoms of hepatic injury become manifest 3 to 5 days after ingestion and include right upper quadrant abdominal tenderness, jaundice, hypoglycemia, and encephalopathy. Prolongation of the prothrombin time worsens as hepatic necrosis progresses and may lead to disseminated intravascular coagulapathy. By 7 to 8 days after ingestion, patients with hepatic damage may develop hepatic coma and hepatorenal syndrome. Death can occur,[59–61] but recovery is usually complete, even in patients with severe hepatotoxicity, with no residual functional or histologic abnormalities of the liver noted within 1 to 6 months of the incident.[60]

In many cases of severe hepatotoxicity, renal injury is also present and may range from oliguria to acute renal failure. The etiology of the renal injury may be a direct effect of a toxic metabolite of acetaminophen, *N*-acetyl-*p*-benzoquinone-imine (discussed in the next section), generated by renal cytochrome oxidase, or a consequence of hepatic injury resulting in hepatorenal syndrome.[62] Isolated cases of myocardial injury have been reported rarely.[63]

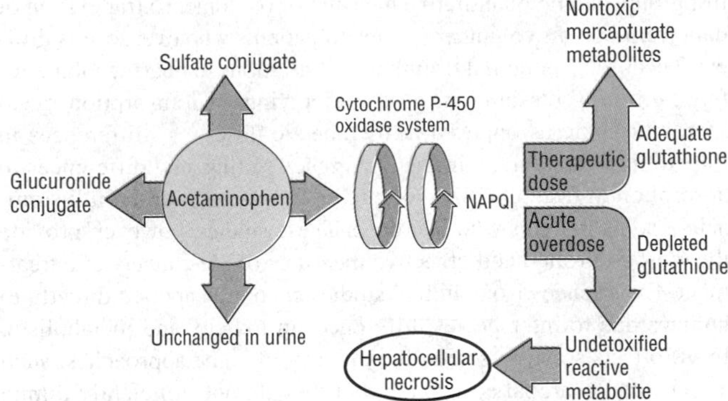

FIGURE 9–3. Pathway of acetaminophen metabolism and basis for hepatotoxicity. (NAPQI = *N*-acetyl-*p*-benzoquinone-imine, a reactive acetaminophen metabolite.)

Mechanism of Toxicity. Acetaminophen is metabolized in the liver primarily to glucuronide or sulfate conjugates, which are excreted into the urine with small amounts (less than 5%) of unchanged drug. Approximately 5% of a therapeutic dose is metabolized by the cytochrome P450 mixed-function oxygenase system, primarily CYP2E1, to a reactive metabolite, *N*-acetyl-*p*-benzoquinone-imine (NAPQI). This metabolite normally is conjugated with glutathione, a sulfhydryl-containing compound, in the hepatocyte and excreted in the urine as a mercapturate conjugate (Fig. 9–3).

In an acute overdose situation, sulfate stores are depleted, shifting more drug through the cytochrome system, thereby depleting the available glutathione used to detoxify the reactive metabolite. The reactive metabolite, NAPQI, then reacts with other hepatocellular sulfhydryl compounds such as those in the cytosol, cell wall, and endoplasmic reticulum. This results in centrilobular hepatic necrosis.[58]

Causative Agents. Acetaminophen, also known as paracetamol in other countries, is widely available without prescription as an analgesic and antipyretic. It is available in various oral dosage forms including an extended-release preparation. Acetaminophen may be combined with other drugs and marketed in cough and cold preparations, menstrual remedies, and allergy products.

Incidence. Acetaminophen is one of the most commonly ingested drugs by small children and is commonly used in suicide attempts by adolescents and adults. The 1999 AAPCC-TESS report documented 61,007 nonfatal exposures and 85 deaths from acetaminophen, with 53% of the exposures under 6 years of age.[6]

Age-based differences in the metabolism of acetaminophen appear to be responsible for major differences in the incidence of serious toxicity. Despite the common ingestion of acetaminophen by young children, few develop hepatotoxicity from acute overdosage.[58] In children under 9 to 12 years of age, acetaminophen undergoes more sulfation and less glucuronidation. The reduced fraction available for metabolism by the cytochrome system may explain the rare development of serious toxicity in young children who take large overdoses. Earlier treatment intervention and spontaneous emesis also may reduce the risk of toxicity in children.

Risk Assessment. There is a risk of developing hepatotoxicity when adolescents or adults acutely ingest more than 5 to 7.5 g of acetaminophen or when children acutely ingest greater than 150 mg/kg.[59] The least amount reported to produce death is 10 g in an adult; but others have survived much larger doses, particularly with early treatment. Initial symptoms, if present, do not predict how serious the toxicity eventually may become.

Chronic exposure to drugs that induce the cytochrome oxidase system—specifically isoenzyme CYP2E1, which is responsible for most of formation of NAPQI—may increase the risk of acetaminophen hepatotoxicity. Poorer outcomes have been noted in patients who chronically ingest alcohol and those receiving anticonvulsants, both known to induce CYP2E1.[60,61,64,65] Chronic, excessive acetaminophen consumption, defined as doses exceeding the recommended daily doses of 4 g for an adult and 90 mg/kg for a child for several days, has been associated with hepatotoxicity.[60,61] The incidence is unknown, and the basis of this association is not well understood. Patients who are fasting or have ingested alcohol in the preceding 5 days appear to be at greater risk.[66,67] Young children who receive acetaminophen in excess of the recommended total daily dose of 50 to 75 mg/kg have a risk of developing hepatotoxicity, particularly when they have been acutely fasting due to febrile illness or gastroenteritis.[68–70]

The risk of developing hepatotoxicity may be predicted from a nomogram (Fig. 9–4) comprised of a plot of the acetaminophen serum concentration and time after ingestion.[58,59] The treatment line of the nomogram (150 μg/mL at 4 hours), which allows a margin of error in laboratory analysis and time of ingestion, should be used to make treatment decisions. The other lines on the nomogram indicate differing levels of risk for hepatotoxicity based on a multicenter study of 11,195 patients.[59]

If the plasma concentration plotted on the nomogram falls above the nomogram treatment line, indicating that hepatic damage is possible, a full course of treatment with *N*-acetylcysteine is indicated. When the results of the acetaminophen determination will be available later than 8 hours after the ingestion, *N*-acetylcysteine therapy should be initiated based on the history and later discontinued if the results indicate nontoxic concentrations. The nomogram has not been evaluated and thus is not useful for assessing chronic exposure to acetaminophen.

Management of Toxicity. Therapy of an acute acetaminophen overdose depends on the amount ingested, time after ingestion, and the serum concentration of acetaminophen. When adolescents or adults ingest excessive amounts or when the history is unclear or suggests an

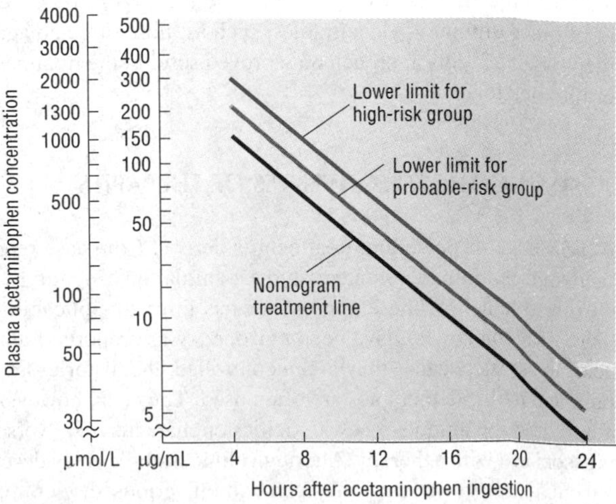

FIGURE 9–4. Nomogram for assessing hepatotoxic risk following acute ingestion of acetaminophen. *(Adapted from Ref. 59.)*

intentional ingestion, the patient must be evaluated at an emergency department and acetaminophen serum concentrations obtained. No prehospital care generally is indicated, and ipecac syrup typically is avoided because emesis may complicate later therapy.

If the patient presents to the emergency department within 4 hours of the ingestion or other drugs are suspected, one dose of activated charcoal should be administered. There has been concern that charcoal may minimize the effectiveness of subsequent orally administered therapy (i.e., *N*-acetylcysteine) by adsorbing it in the gastrointestinal tract. Recent evidence suggests that activated charcoal may not interfere with *N*-acetylcysteine to the extent previously thought, and it may be considered to be appropriate therapy.[32,58]

N-acetylcysteine, a sulfhydryl-containing compound, functionally replenishes the hepatic stores of glutathione by serving as a glutathione surrogate that combines directly with reactive metabolites or by serving as a source of sulfate, thus preventing hepatic damage.[58,59] It should be started within 10 hours of the ingestion to be most effective.[59] Initiation of therapy 24 to 36 hours after the ingestion may be of value in some patients, particularly those with measurable serum acetaminophen concentrations.[71,72] Patients with fulminant hepatic failure may benefit through other mechanisms by the administration or initiation of *N*-acetylcysteine several days after ingestion.[71] Therapy is initiated with a loading dose of 140 mg/kg orally followed in 4 hours by 70 mg/kg every 4 hours over a period of 68 hours (i.e., 17 maintenance doses). If the patient vomits a dose within an hour of administration, the dose should be repeated. *N*-acetylcysteine can be diluted with carbonated drinks, cola, juice, or water to a 5% solution and administered orally or through a nasogastric tube. Adverse effects of *N*-acetylcysteine therapy include nausea, vomiting, and rarely, hypersensitivity reactions.[58,59,73]

The unpleasant odor and associated emesis of *N*-acetylcysteine can limit the delivery of the full course of therapy. Aggressive antiemetic therapy with metoclopramide, ondansetron, or droperidol may enhance patient tolerability of *N*-acetylcysteine.[74] Other approaches include administration by a nasogastric or duodenal tube over 30 to 60 minutes or use of an investigational intravenous form of *N*-acetylcysteine.[73] A 52-hour course of intravenous *N*-acetylcysteine may be as effective as the 72-hour oral regimen.[75] Intravenous administration of the oral *N*-acetylcysteine product generally is not recommended because the product is not pyrogen-free. However, extemporaneous filtration with a 0.2-μm filter unit yields an intravenous product that has been associated with a limited number of adverse effects and potentially may be lifesaving when oral administration is not possible.[76] The local poison control center should be consulted for availability of the intravenous product.

When plasma concentrations are below the nomogram treatment line, there is little risk of toxicity, protective therapy with *N*-acetylcysteine is not necessary, and further medical therapy is unnecessary for the acetaminophen overdose.[59] The acetaminophen blood sample should be drawn no sooner than 4 hours after the ingestion to ensure that peak acetaminophen concentrations have been reached. If a concentration is obtained less than 4 hours after ingestion, it is uninterpretable, and a second determination should be done at least 4 hours after ingestion. Serial determinations of a serum concentration typically are unnecessary unless there is some evidence of slowed gastrointestinal motility from other ingested drugs (e.g., opioids or anticholinergic drugs) or unless an extended-release product is involved.

An extended-release formulation of acetaminophen was introduced in 1995 and raised significant issues in the management of overdose. One formulation (Tylenol-ER) delivers 325 mg in immediate release and another 325 mg in extended release. The pharmacokinetics of the extended-release preparation on overdose are unknown, but peak concentrations can occur approximately 16 hours after ingestion compared with the peak time of the standard-release preparation of 1 to 2 hours.[77] Concurrent ingestion of antihistamines (e.g., Tylenol PM) can delay the peak acetaminophen concentration to 10 hours after ingestion.[78] The validity of the toxic dose thresholds and the nomogram for extended-release formulation overdoses is untested to date. In 1994 a manufacturer, McNeil, suggested obtaining two serum acetaminophen concentrations 4 to 6 hours apart and continuing therapy with *N*-acetylcysteine if any concentration was above the treatment line of the nomogram and discontinuing therapy when both concentrations were below the treatment line.[58] Although young children have an inherently lower risk of acetaminophen-induced hepatotoxicity, these patients should be managed in the same manner as adults. When acetaminophen plasma concentrations predict that toxicity is probable, young children should receive *N*-acetylcysteine in the dosing regimen described previously.[58] If fulminant hepatic failure develops, the approaches described in Chapter 38 should be considered. In unresponsive cases, liver transplantation is a lifesaving option.[60]

Monitoring and Prevention. Baseline liver function tests (AST, ALT, bilirubin, prothrombin time), serum creatinine determination, and urinalysis should be obtained on admission and repeated at 24-hour intervals until at least 96 hours have elapsed for those at risk. Most patients with liver injury develop elevated transaminase concentrations within 24 hours of ingestion. Transaminase concentrations greater than 1000 IU/L commonly are associated with other signs of liver dysfunction and have been used as the threshold concentration in outcome studies to define severe liver toxicity.[59] The extent of transaminase elevation is not correlated directly with severity of the hepatic injury, with nonfatal cases demonstrating peak concentrations as high as 30,000 IU/L between 48 and 72 hours after ingestion.[60,61]

Prevention of acetaminophen poisoning is based on recognition of the maximum daily therapeutic doses, observance of general poison prevention practices, and early intervention in cases of suspected overdose.

ANTICHOLINESTERASE INSECTICIDES

Signs and Symptoms. The clinical manifestations of anticholinesterase insecticide poisoning include any or all of the following: pinpoint pupils, excessive lacrimation, excessive salivation, bronchorrhea, bronchospasm and expiratory wheezes, hyperperistalsis producing abdominal cramps and diarrhea, bradycardia, excessive sweating, fasciculations and weakness of skeletal muscles, paralysis of skeletal muscles (particularly those involved with respiration), convulsions, and coma.[79] Symptoms of anticholinesterase poisoning and their response to antidotal therapy depend on the action of excessive acetylcholinesterase at different receptor types (Table 9–10).

The time of onset and severity of symptoms depend on the route of exposure, potency of the agent, and total dose received. Toxic signs and symptoms develop most rapidly after inhalation or intravenous injection and slowest after skin contact. Anticholinesterase insecticides are absorbed through the skin, lungs, conjunctivae, and gastrointestinal tract. Severe symptoms can occur from absorption by any route. Within 6 hours, most patients are symptomatic, and without treatment, death may occur within 24 hours.[79] Death typically is

TABLE 9–10. Effects of Acetylcholinesterase Inhibition at Muscarinic, Nicotinic, and CNS Receptors

Muscarinic Receptors	**Nicotinic–Sympathetic Neurons**
Diarrhea	Increased blood pressure
Urination	Sweating and piloerection
Miosis[a]	Mydriasis[a]
Bronchorrhea	Hyperglycemia
Bradycardia[a]	Tachycardia[a]
Emesis	Priapism
Lacrimation	**Nicotinic–Neuromuscular Neurons**
Salivation	Muscular weakness
CNS Receptors (Mixed Type)	Cramps
	Fasciculations
Coma	Muscular paralysis
Seizures	

[a]Generally muscarinic effects predominate, but nicotinic effects can be observed.

caused by respiratory failure due to the combination of pulmonary and cardiovascular effects[79,80] (Fig. 9–5).

■ *Mechanism of Toxicity.* Anticholinesterase insecticides phosphorylate the active site of cholinesterase in all parts of the body. Inhibition of this enzyme leads to accumulation of acetylcholine at affected receptors and results in widespread toxicity. Acetylcholine is the neurohormone responsible for physiologic transmission of nerve impulses from preganglionic and postganglionic neurons of the cholinergic (parasympathetic) nervous system, preganglionic adrenergic (sympathetic) neurons, the neuromuscular junction in skeletal muscles, and multiple nerve endings in the CNS (Fig. 9–6).

■ *Causative Agents.* Anticholinesterase insecticides include organophosphate and carbamate insecticides. These insecticides are currently in widespread use throughout the world for eradication of insects in dwellings and crops. Carbamates typically are less potent and inactivate cholinesterase in a more reversible fashion through carbamylation compared with organophosphates.[79,80] The prototype anticholinesterase agent is the organophosphate, which will be the focus of this discussion. A large number of organophosphates are used as pesticides (Table 9–11), and several also have been used as potent chemical warfare agents (e.g., sarin, tabun, and VX, which are known as nerve gases). The chemical warfare agents act like organophosphate insecticides, but as a group they are highly potent, quickly absorbed, and deadly to humans.[81] An anticholinesterase insecticide typically is stored in a garage, a chemical storage area, or living areas. Anticholinesterase agents also can be found in occupational (e.g., pest exterminators) or agricultural (e.g., crop dusters or farm workers) settings. These agents also have been used as a means for suicide or homicide.

■ *Incidence.* Anticholinesterase insecticides are among the most poisonous substances commonly used for pest control and are a frequent source of serious poisoning in children and adults in rural and

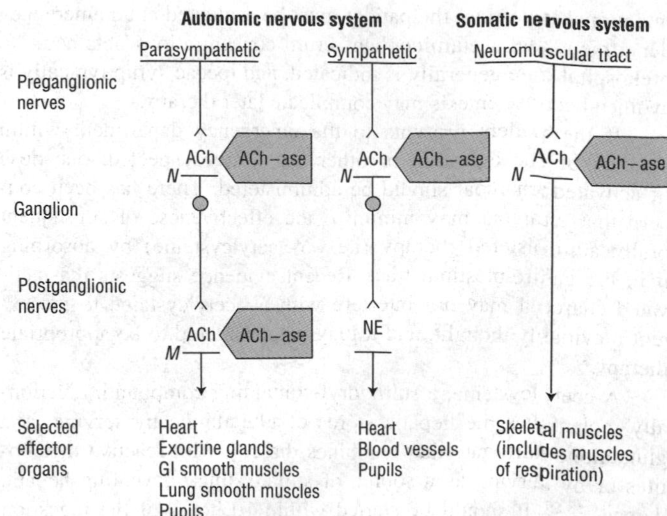

FIGURE 9–6. Organization of neurotransmitters of the peripheral nervous system and site of acetylcholinesterase action. (Ach = acetylcholine; Ach–ase = acetylcholinesterase; NE = norepinephrine; M = muscarinic receptor; N = nicotinic receptor.)

urban settings. The 1999 AAPCC-TESS report documented 14,306 nonfatal exposures and 5 deaths from anticholinesterase insecticides alone or in combination with other pesticides, with 31% of the exposures in children under 6 years of age.[6]

■ *Risk Assessment.* The triad of miosis, bronchial secretions, and muscle fasciculations should suggest the possibility of anticholinesterase insecticide poisoning and warrants a therapeutic trial of the antidote atropine. In cases of low-level exposure, failure to develop signs within 6 hours indicates a low likelihood of subsequent toxicity.[79]

Although the lethal dose for parathion is approximately 4 mg/kg, as little as 10 to 20 mg can be lethal to an adult and 2 mg (0.1 mg/kg) to a child. Small children may be more susceptible to toxicity because less pesticide is required per body weight to produce toxicity.[79,81] Estimation of an exact dose is impossible in most cases of acute poisoning, and tabulated "toxic" doses thus generally are not helpful in assessing risk of toxicity. Generally, ingestion of a small mouthful (5 mL or less) of the concentrated forms of an organophosphate intended to be diluted for commercial or agricultural use will produce serious toxicity, whereas a mouthful of an already diluted household product such as Raid or Black Flag typically does not produce serious toxic effects.[81] In 2000, the Environmental Protection Agency determined that the risk of chlorphyriphos, an organophosphate commonly used in homes, to humans, particularly young children, outweighed its benefits. This resulted in restrictions on its use in homes and agriculture.[82] The safety of other insecticides is now under review.

Measurement of acetylcholinesterase activity at the neuronal synapse is not feasible clinically. Cholinesterase activity can be

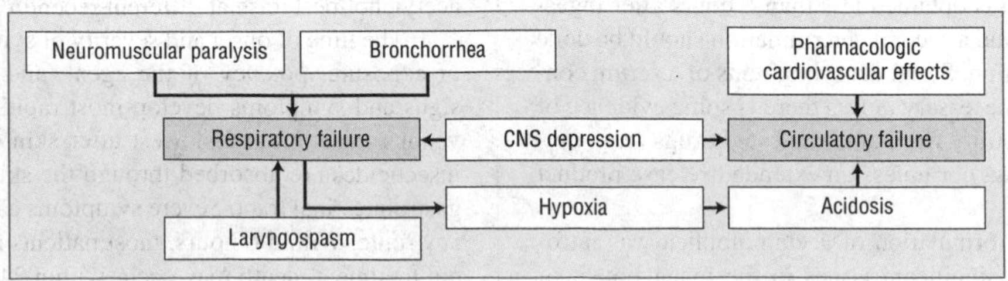

FIGURE 9–5. Pathogenesis of life-threatening effects of organophosphate poisoning.

TABLE 9–11. Commonly Used Organophosphate Insecticides

Chemical Name	Product Name Examples
Agricultural Use: High Potency	
Disulfoton	Di-syston
Mevinphos	Phosdrin
Parathion	Niagara Phos Kil Dust
Animal Use: Intermediate Potency	
Coumaphos	Co-Ral, Baymix
Dichlorphos	Agridip, Muscatox
Famphur	Brevinyl, DDVP, Vapona
Phosmet	Dovip, Warbex
Trichlorfon	Prolate, Smidan
Household Use: Low Potency	
Diazinon	Security Fire Ant Killer
Malathion	Ortho Malathion Insect Spray

measured in the blood as the pseudocholinesterase (butylcholinesterase) activity of the plasma and acetylcholinesterase activity in the erythrocyte. Both cholinesterases will be depressed with anticholinesterase insecticide poisoning.[79,80] Severity can be estimated roughly by the extent of depressed activity in relation to the low end of normal values. Because there are several methods to measure and report cholinesterase activity, each particular laboratory's normal range must be considered. Clinical toxicity usually is seen only after a 50% reduction in enzyme activity, and severe toxicity typically is observed with levels at 20% or less of the normal range. A clinical severity scoring system has been proposed as an alternative to cholinesterase activity determination.[79] The intrinsic activity of acetylcholinesterase may be depressed in some individuals, but the absence of any manifestations in most people does not permit the recognition of the relative deficiency in the general population. Therapy should not be delayed pending laboratory confirmation when the clinical suspicion of poisoning is present.

Management of Toxicity. People handling the patient should wear gloves and aprons to protect themselves against contaminated clothing, skin, or gastric fluid of the patient. Because many insecticides are dissolved in a hydrocarbon vehicle, there is an additional risk of pulmonary aspiration of the hydrocarbon leading to pneumonitis. The risks and benefits of prehospital ipecac-induced emesis should be considered carefully and should involve consultation with a poison control center or clinical toxicologist. Symptomatic cases of anticholinesterase insecticide exposure typically are referred to an emergency department for evaluation and treatment.

If the poison has been ingested, gastric lavage should be performed followed by the administration of activated charcoal. The patient with skin contamination should be washed with copious amounts of soap and water. An alcohol wash may be useful to remove residual insecticide due to its liphophillic nature. A surgical scrub kit for the hands, feet, and nails may be useful for exposure to those areas.

Supportive therapy should include maintenance of an airway, including bronchotracheal suctioning; provision of adequate ventilation; and establishment of an intravenous line. Based on a history of an exposure and presence of typical symptoms, the anticholinesterase syndrome should be recognized without difficulty.

The pharmacologic management of organophosphate intoxication relies on the administration of atropine and pralidoxime.[79,81] Atropine has no effect on inhibited cholinesterase, but it competitively blocks the actions of acetylcholine on cholinergic and some CNS receptors. It thereby alleviates bronchospasm and reduces bronchial secretions. Although atropine has little effect on the flaccid muscle paralysis or the central respiratory failure of severe poisoning, it is indicated in all symptomatic patients and can be used as a diagnostic aid. It should be given intravenously and in larger than conventional doses of 0.05 to 0.1 mg/kg in children under 12 years of age and 2 to 5 mg for adolescents and young adults.[81] It should be repeated at 5- to 10-minute intervals until bronchial secretions and pulmonary rales resolve. Therapy may require large doses over a period of several days until all absorbed organophosphate is metabolized and acetylcholinesterase activity is restored.

Restoration of enzyme activity is necessary for severe poisoning, characterized by reduction of cholinesterase activity to less than 20% of normal, profound weakness, and respiratory distress. Pralidoxime (Protopam), also called 2-PAM or pyridine aldoxamine methiodide, breaks the covalent bond between the cholinesterase and organophosphate and regenerates enzyme activity. Organophosphate-cholinesterase binding is initially reversible, but it gradually becomes irreversible. Therefore, therapy with pralidoxime should be initiated as soon as possible, preferably within 36 to 72 hours of exposure.[81] The drug should be given at a dose of 25 to 50 mg/kg up to 1 g intravenously over 5 to 20 minutes. If muscle weakness persists or recurs, the dose may be repeated after an hour and again if needed. A continuous infusion of pralidoxime has been shown to be effective in adults when administered at 3.2 mg/kg per hour preceded by a loading dose of 4 mg/kg[83] and in children at 10 to 20 mg/kg per hour with a loading dose of 15 to 50 mg/kg.[84] Both atropine and pralidoxime should be given together due to their complementary roles (Table 9–12). Carbamate insecticide poisonings typically do not require the administration of pralidoxime.

One of the pitfalls of therapy is the delay in administering sufficient doses of atropine or pralidoxime.[79,81] The adverse effects of atropine and pralidoxime, predictable extensions of anticholinergic actions, are minimally important compared with the life-threatening effects of severe anticholinesterase poisoning and can be minimized easily by decreasing the dose.

Monitoring and Prevention. Poisoned patients may require monitoring of vital signs, measurement of ventilatory adequacy such as blood gases and pulse oximetry, leukocyte count with differential to assess development of pneumonia, and chest radiographs to assess the degree of pulmonary edema or development of hydrocarbon

TABLE 9–12. Comparative Characteristics of Atropine and Pralidoxime for Anticholinesterase Poisoning

Characteristic	Atropine	Pralidoxime
Interaction	Synergy with pralidoxime	Reduces atropine dose requirement
Indication	Any anticholinesterase agent	Typically needed for organophosphates
Primary sites of action	Muscarinic, CNS	Nicotinic > muscarinic > CNS
Adverse effects	Coma, hallucinations, tachycardia	Dizziness, diplopia, tachycardia, headache
Daily dose[a]	2–1600 mg	1–12 g
Total dose[a]	2–11, 422 mg	1–92 g

[a]Range of some reported cases; higher doses may be required in rare cases.

pneumonitis. Workers involved in the formulation and application of pesticides should be monitored by periodic measurement of cholinesterase activity in their bloodstream. Untreated, anticholinesterase-depressed acetylcholinesterase activity returns to normal values in approximately 120 days.

Many anticholinesterase insecticide poisonings are unintentional due to misuse, improper storage, failure to follow instructions for mixing or application, or inability to read directions for use. Training and vigilant adherence to directions may minimize some poisonings. Storing pesticides in original or labeled containers can minimize the risk of unintentional ingestion. Keeping pesticides out of children's reach may decrease the risk of childhood poisoning.

CALCIUM CHANNEL BLOCKERS

Signs and Symptoms. Overdosage with calcium channel blockers typically results in bradycardia and hypotension (Fig. 9–7). Many patients become drowsy and may develop agitation and coma. If the degree of hypotension becomes severe or is prolonged, the secondary effects of seizures, coma, and metabolic acidosis usually develop. Pulmonary edema, nausea and vomiting, and hyperglycemia are frequent complications of calcium channel blocker overdoses. Paralytic ileus, mesenteric ischemia, and colonic infarction have been observed in patients with severe hypotension. Many symptoms become manifest within 1 to 2 hours of ingestion. If a sustained-release formulation is involved, the onset of overt toxicity may be delayed by 6 to 18 hours from the time of ingestion. Severe poisoning can result in refractory shock and cardiac arrest. Death can occur within 3 to 4 hours of ingestion.[85–88]

Mechanism of Toxicity. Most toxic effects of calcium channel blockers are produced by three basic actions on the cardiovascular system: vasodilation through relaxation of smooth muscles, decreased contractility by action on cardiac tissue, and decreased automaticity and conduction velocity through slow recovery of calcium channels. Calcium channel blockers interfere with calcium entry by inhibiting one or more of the several types of calcium channels and binding at one or more cellular binding sites.[89] Selectivity of these actions varies with the calcium channel blocker and provides some therapeutic distinctions (see Chap. 12), but these differences are less clear with overdosage.[88] Current experiences suggest that the signs and symptoms of calcium channel blocker toxicity are similar among the drugs in this class.

Causative Agents. There are approximately a dozen calcium channel antagonists marketed in the United States for the treatment of hypertension, certain dysrhythmias, and some forms of angina (see Chaps. 12, 14, and 16). The calcium channel blockers are classified by their chemical structure as phenylalkylamines (e.g., verapamil), benzothiapines (e.g., diltiazem), and dihydropyridines (e.g., amlodipine, felodipine, nicardipene, and nifedipine). Several of these agents, namely, diltiazem, nicardipine, nifedipine, and verapamil, are formulated as sustained-release oral dosage forms or have a slow onset of action and longer half-life (e.g., amlodipine[90]), allowing once-daily administration.

Incidence. In 1999, the AAPCC-TESS report documented 8844 people with a toxic exposure to a calcium channel blockers, with 243 patients exhibiting and surviving major toxic effects.[6] Sixty-one people died. Poison control center reports have shown a steady increase in the number of cases of morbidity and mortality following calcium channel blocker overdosage.

Risk Assessment. Ingestion of doses near or in excess of 1 gram of diltiazem, nifedipine, and verapamil may result in life-threatening symptoms or death in an adult.[85,91] Asymptomatic children who ingest less than 12 mg/kg of verapamil sustained release or 2.7 mg/kg of nifedipine sustained release may be monitored at home.[92] Doses associated with serious toxicity with the other agents have not been established. Patients on chronic therapy with these agents who acutely ingest an overdose may have a greater risk of serious toxicity. Elderly patients and those with underlying cardiac disease may not tolerate mild hypotension or bradycardia. Concurrent ingestion of β-adrenergic blocking drugs, digitalis, class I antiarrhythmics, and

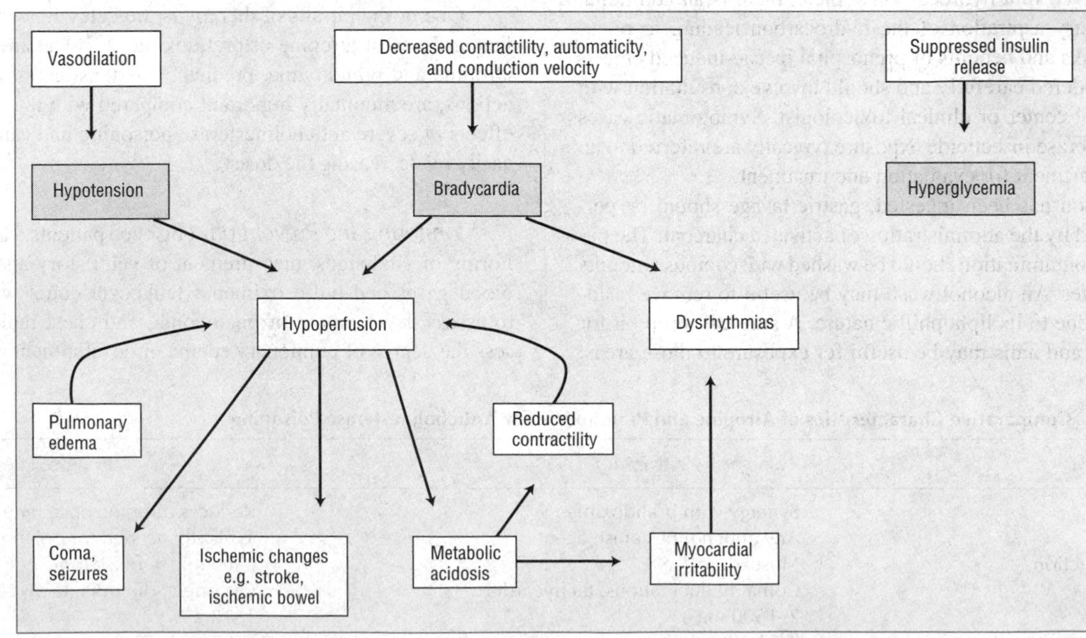

FIGURE 9–7. Pathophysiologic changes associated with calcium channel blocker poisoning.

other vasodilators may worsen the cardiovascular effects of calcium channel blockers.[86,88]

Management of Toxicity. There is no accepted specific prehospital care for calcium channel blocker poisoning except to summon an ambulance for symptomatic patients. Ipecac syrup should be avoided due to the risks of seizures and coma.[88,91] The therapeutic options for the management of calcium channel blocker poisoning include supportive care, gastric decontamination, and adjunctive therapy for the cardiovascular and metabolic effects. Supportive care consists of airway protection, ventilatory support, intravenous hydration to maintain adequate urine flow, and maintenance of electrolyte and acid-base balance. Maintaining vital organ perfusion is critical for successful therapy in order to allow time for calcium channel blocker toxicity to resolve.[87,88]

Gastric lavage and a single dose of activated charcoal should be administered if instituted within 1 to 2 hours of ingestion. Besides exhibiting a slower onset of symptoms, sustained-release formulations also can form concretions in the intestine.[88,91] Whole-bowel irrigation with polyethylene glycol electrolyte solution may accelerate rectal elimination of the sustained-release tablets and should be considered routinely for ingestion of sustained-release calcium channel antagonist formulations.[36,93]

Adjunctive therapy is focused on treating hypotension, bradycardia, and resulting shock. Hypotension is treated primarily by correction of coexisting dysrhythmias (e.g., bradycardia, heart block) and implementation of conventional measures to treat decreased blood pressure. Infusion of normal saline and placement of the patient in Trendelenberg position are initial therapy. Further fluid therapy should be guided by central venous pressure monitoring. Dopamine in conventional doses for cardiogenic shock should be considered next. If hypotension persists, dysrhythmias are present, or other signs of serious toxicity are present, calcium should be administered.[85,88]

A calcium chloride bolus test dose (10–20 mg/kg up to 1 to 3 g) is the preferred therapy for patients with serious toxicity. In adults, calcium chloride 10% can be diluted in 100 mL normal saline and infused over 5 minutes through a central venous line. If a positive cardiovascular response is achieved with this test dose, a continuous infusion of calcium chloride (20–50 mg/kg/h) should be started. Calcium gluconate is less desirable to use because it contains less elemental calcium per milligram of final dosage form. Intravenous calcium salts can produce vomiting and tissue necrosis on extravasation.[88,94] Atropine also may be considered for treatment of bradycardia, but it is seldom sufficient as a sole therapy.[87]

If the bradycardia and hypotension are refractory to the foregoing therapy, a bolus infusion of glucagon (0.05–0.20 mg/kg) should be considered. Benefit typically is observed within 5 minutes of administration and can be sustained with a continuous intravenous infusion (0.05–0.1 mg/kg/h) titrated to clinical response.[95] Glucagon possesses chronotropic and inotropic effects in part by stimulating adenyl cyclase and increasing cyclic AMP, which may promote intracellular entry of calcium through calcium channels. It thereby may improve hypotension and bradycardia.[54] Vomiting is not uncommon with these large doses of glucagon, and the airway should be protected to avoid pulmonary aspiration. Hyperglycemia may occur or be exacerbated in those patients receiving glucagon therapy. Hyperglycemia from calcium channel blocker toxicity or glucagon therapy typically does not require treatment with insulin. Intravenous sodium bicarbonate, however, may be necessary to establish acid-base balance and correct the metabolic acidosis that is common with serious calcium channel blocker overdoses.

Several life-saving options may be warranted for patients with cardiogenic shock that is refractory to conventional therapy. Electrical cardiac pacing may restore an acceptable heart rate in patients with severe bradycardia.[88] Intravenous infusion of regular insulin (0.5–1 units/kg bolus followed with a continuous infusion over one hour) with 50% dextrose (40 mL/hr) may improve myocardial contractility. Serum glucose and potassium concentrations should be closely monitored. The benefit of insulin therapy for calcium channel antagonist toxicity has been demonstrated in several cases,[54,97] but its effect on overall outcome is still being investigated.[94] Intra-aortic balloon counterpulsation or cardiopulmonary bypass may improve shock in patients unresponsive to other therapies.[88,94,96] Hypertonic sodium bicarbonate infusion has been shown to improve cardiac output and blood pressure in a swine model,[98] but it has not been demonstrated to be useful in humans to date.

Measures to enhance elimination from the bloodstream by hemodialysis or multiple-dose activated charcoal have not been shown to be effective and are not indicated for calcium channel blocker poisoning.[45,86,88,99]

Monitoring and Prevention. Regular monitoring of vital signs and electrocardiogram is essential in suspected calcium channel blocker poisoning. Determination of serum electrolytes, serum glucose, arterial blood gases, urine output, and renal function are indicated to assess and monitor symptomatic patients. If serious toxicity is likely to develop, overt symptoms will be manifest within 6 hours of ingestion.[87,88] For ingestions of sustained-release products in toxic doses, observation for 24 hours in a critical care unit may be prudent because the onset of symptoms may be slow and delayed up to 12 to 18 hours after ingestion.[93,99,100] Serum concentrations of these agents in overdose patients do not correlate well with the ingested dose, degree of toxicity, nor outcome.[88]

Poisonings due to these agents are likely to increase as their therapeutic indications and use increase. These poisonings may be the result of an intentional suicide or unintentional ingestion by young children. Prevention of calcium channel blocker poisonings in children rests with the education of patients receiving these agents, particularly of grandparents and those who infrequently have children visit their home, of their dangers on overdosage. Safe storage and use of child-resistant closures may reduce the opportunities for unintentional poisonings by children.[86]

IRON

Signs and Symptoms. In the first few hours of ingestion of toxic amounts of iron, symptoms of gastrointestinal irritation (e.g., nausea, vomiting, and diarrhea) are common. In certain severe cases, acidosis and shock can become manifest within 6 hours of ingestion. Some have observed a quiescent phase between 6 and 48 hours after ingestion where symptoms improve or abate, but this phenomenon is poorly characterized.[101] Continued gastrointestinal symptoms, poor perfusion, and oliguria should suggest the development of severe toxicity with other effects still to become manifest. Generally, within 24 to 36 hours after the ingestion, CNS involvement with coma and seizures; hepatic injury characterized by jaundice, increased prothrombin time, increased bilirubin, and hypoglycemia; cardiovascular shock; and acidosis also develop.[101] Adult respiratory distress syndrome (ARDS) may develop in patients with severe cardiovascular shock and further compromise recovery.[102] Coagulopathy with decreased thrombin formation is one of the early direct effects of excessive iron concentrations, and later disturbances of coagulation

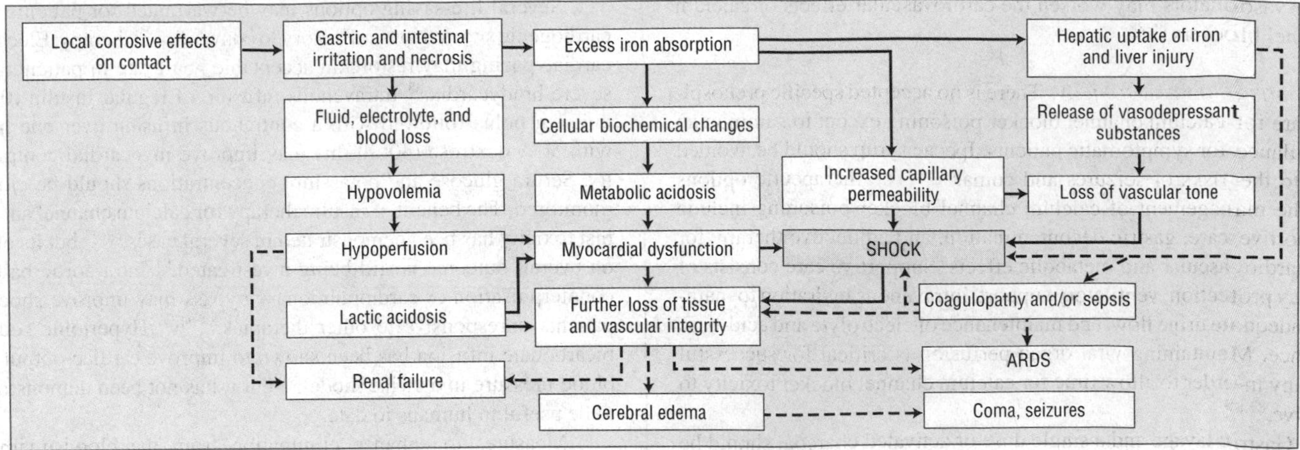

FIGURE 9–8. Pathophysiology of acute iron poisoning. Events indicated by dashed lines are not observed consistently in all serious poisonings. (ARDS = adult respiratory distress syndrome.)

(after 24 to 48 hours of ingestion) are a consequence of hepatotoxicity.[103] Mucosal injury, an iron-rich circulation, or deferoxamine therapy may promote septicemia with *Yersinia enterocolitica* during iron overdose; other bacteria or viruses also may cause septicemia.[101] The pathophysiologic relationships of acute iron toxicity are shown in Figure 9–8. Two to four weeks after the exposure some patients experience persistent vomiting from gastric outlet obstruction due to pyloric and duodenal stenosis from the earlier gastric mucosal necrosis. Autopsy findings in children indicate prominent iron deposition in intestinal mucosa and periportal necrosis of the liver that correlate with the primary symptoms of serious iron poisoning.[104]

Mechanism of Toxicity. The toxicity of acute iron poisoning includes local effects on the gastrointestinal mucosa and systemic effects induced by excessive iron in the body.[101,102] Iron is irritating to the gastric and duodenal mucosa, which may result in hemorrhage and occasional perforations. Once absorbed, iron is taken up by tissues, particularly the liver, and acts as a mitochondrial poison. It occasionally causes hepatic injury. Iron may significantly inhibit aerobic glycolysis and perturb the electron transport system. Further, iron may shunt electrons away from the electron transport system, thereby reducing the efficiency of oxidative phosphorylation. These biochemical factors, along with the cardiovascular effects of iron, lead to metabolic acidosis. The pathogenesis of shock is not well understood but may include development of hypovolemia and lactic acidosis, release of endogenous vasodilators, and direct vasodepressant effects of iron and ferritin on the circulation (see Fig. 9–8).

Causative Agents. Iron poisoning results from the ingestion and absorption of excessive amounts of iron from iron tablets, multiple vitamins with iron, and prenatal vitamins. Different iron salts and formulations contain varying amounts of elemental iron (see Chaps. 98 and 99). Generally, children's chewable vitamins are less likely to produce systemic iron poisoning due in part to lower iron content.

Incidence. Acute iron poisoning can produce death in children and adults.[104,105] An analysis by the Consumer Products Safety Commission concluded that iron poisoning remains a significant public health threat to young children based on injury and mortality data from 1980 through 1996.[105] The 1999 AAPCC-TESS report documented 28,809 nonfatal and 3 fatal cases, respectively, of iron poisoning, with 92% of the exposures in children under 6 years of age. In the majority of cases (87%), multiple vitamins with iron were the source of iron.[6]

Risk Assessment. The minimum lethal and toxic doses for acute iron poisoning are not well established. The ingestion of 10–20 mg/kg of elemental iron usually elicits mild gastrointestinal symptoms. The ingestion of 20–60 mg/kg is not likely to produce systemic toxicity, and typically these patients can be managed at home with observation and ipecac syrup, if indicated. Ingestions of greater than 60 mg/kg usually are associated with serious systemic toxicity and require medical attention. Immediate psychiatric and medical intervention is indicated for adults and adolescents who acutely ingest greater than 20 mg/kg of elemental iron because this suggests that the overdose was intentional.[101,102]

An abdominal radiograph (Fig. 9–9) may help confirm the ingestion of iron tablets and indicate the need for aggressive gastrointestinal evacuation. An abdominal radiograph is most useful within 2 hours of ingestion. The visualization of radio-opaque iron tablets is confounded by the presence of other hard-coated tablets and some extended-release tablets that are also radiopaque. Furthermore, the radio-opacity of iron tablets diminishes as the tablets disintegrate, and chewable and liquid formulations typically not are radiopaque.[106]

Most iron poisoning results in vomiting and diarrhea, but these symptoms are poor indicators of later serious toxicity. The presence of a combination of findings such as coma, radio-opacities, leukocytosis, and increased anion gap, however, is associated with dangerously high serum concentrations greater than 500 μg/dL. The presence of single signs and symptoms, such as vomiting, leukocytosis, or hyperglycemia, is not a reliable indicator of the severity of iron poisoning in adults or children.[107,108]

Once iron is absorbed, it is only eliminated by bleeding or sloughing of the intestinal and epidermal cells. Thus iron kinetics essentially represent a closed system with multiple compartments. The serum iron concentration represents a small fraction of the total-body content of iron and is at its greatest concentration in the postabsorptive and distributive phases, typically 2 to 10 hours after ingestion.[109] Serum iron concentrations in excess of 500 μg/dL have been associated with severe toxicity, whereas concentrations below 350 μg/dL typically are not associated with severe toxicity; however, exceptions have been reported for both thresholds. Serious toxicity is best determined by assessing the development of gross gastrointestinal bleeding, metabolic acidosis, shock, and coma regardless of the serum iron concentration.

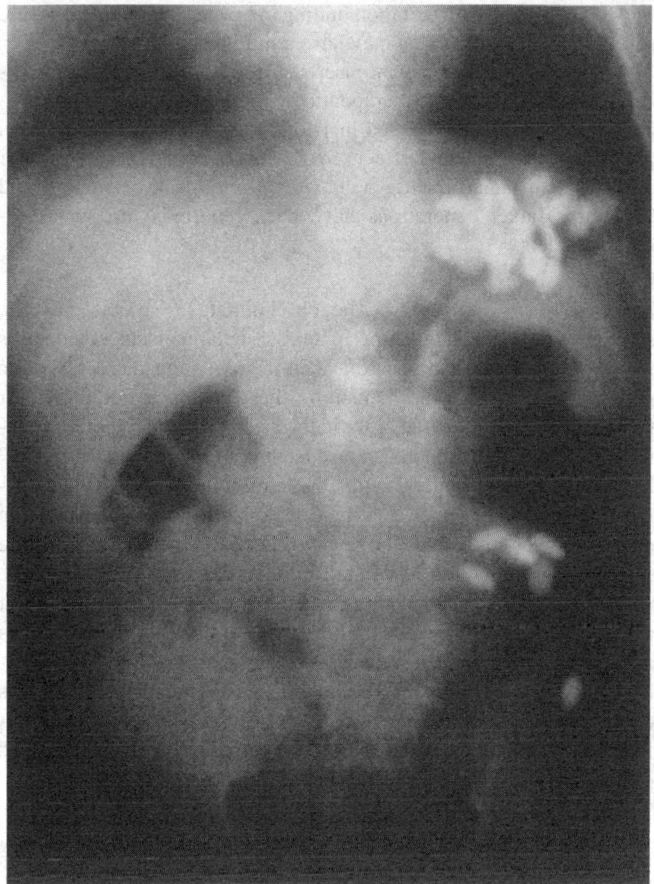

FIGURE 9–9. Abdominal radiograph of a 3-year-old boy who had ingested ferrous sulfate tablets.

The serum iron concentration serves as a guide for further assessment and treatment options. The ratio of the serum iron concentration to the total iron-binding capacity previously has been advocated to assess acute iron poisoning, but it is no longer used. This procedure is unreliable, insensitive, and has little relationship to toxicity.[108]

A deferoxamine challenge test has been proposed, on the basis that the presence of ferrioxamine as orange-red-colored urine would indicate that excess iron is present and able to be chelated. This approach is attractive in its simplicity and potential utility, but there has been no evaluation of its relationship to toxicity, there is no standardized protocol, and the color change may not be perceptible.

Management of Toxicity. Unless the patient has vomited spontaneously or contraindications to the use of ipecac are present, ipecac syrup should be considered for a recent ingestion of 10–60 mg/kg of elemental iron. The patient can be managed on the scene with follow-up contact to ascertain that emesis was induced. If symptoms such as persistent vomiting, bloody emesis, diarrhea, or unresponsiveness develop, if the patient ingested greater than 60 mg/kg, or if intentional overdosage is suspected, immediate referral to an emergency department is indicated.[101]

At the emergency department, ipecac syrup may be used if no more than 2 hours have elapsed since ingestion and spontaneous emesis is not evident. Gastric lavage with normal saline may be used to remove iron in unresponsive patients. Activated charcoal administration is not warranted routinely because it poorly adsorbs iron. Lavage with normal saline may remove iron tablet fragments and dissolved iron, but because the lumen of the tube is often smaller than some whole tablets, effective removal is unlikely.[101] If abdominal radiographs reveal a large number of iron tablets, whole-bowel irrigation with polyethylene glycol electrolyte solution is typically necessary.[36] Although removal by gastrostomy has been used in a few cases,[102] early and aggressive decontamination and evacuation of the gastrointestinal tract usually will be adequate to minimize iron absorption and thereby reduce the risk of systemic toxicity.

Patients with systemic symptoms (e.g., shock, coma, or gross gastrointestinal bleeding or metabolic acidosis) should receive deferoxamine as soon as possible. If the serum iron concentration exceeds 500 μg/dL, deferoxamine is also indicated because serious systemic toxicity is likely.[101,102] Its use is less clear in patients with serum iron concentrations in the range of 350–500 μg/dL because many of these patients do not develop systemic symptoms.

Deferoxamine is a highly selective chelator of iron that theoretically binds ferric (Fe^{3+}) iron in a 1:1 molar ratio (100 mg deferoxamine to 8.5 mg ferric iron) that is more stable than the binding of iron to transferrin. Deferoxamine removes excess iron from the circulation and some iron from transferrin by chelating ferric complexes in equilibrium with transferrin. The resulting iron-deferoxamine complex, ferrioxamine, is then excreted in the urine. Its action on intracellular iron is unclear, but it may have a protective intracellular effect or may chelate extramitochondrial iron.[102] The parenteral administration of deferoxamine produces an orange-red-colored urine within 3 to 6 hours due to the presence of ferrioxamine in the urine.[101] For mild to moderate cases of iron poisoning, where its use is unclear, the presence of discolored urine indicates the persistent presence of chelatable iron and the need to continue deferoxamine. The reliance on discolored urine as a therapeutic end point has been challenged because it is not sensitive and is difficult to detect.[110]

An initial intravenous infusion of 15 mg/kg per hour generally is indicated, although some have used up to 30 mg/kg per hour for life-threatening cases. In these situations, the dose must be titrated carefully to minimize deferoxamine-induced hypotension.[101,102,111] The rapid intravenous infusion of deferoxamine (>15 mg/kg/h) has been associated with tachycardia, hypotension, shock, generalized erythema, and urticaria.[101,113] Anaphylaxis has been reported rarely. The use of deferoxamine for greater than 24 hours at doses used for the treatment of acute poisoning has been associated with the exacerbation or development of adult respiratory distress syndrome.[112–114] Although the manufacturer states that the total dose in 24 hours should not exceed 6 g, the basis for this recommendation is unclear, and daily doses as high as 37.1 g have been administered without incident.[111,112] Good hydration and urine output may moderate some of the secondary physiologic effects of iron toxicity and ensure urinary elimination of ferrioxamine. In the patient who develops renal failure, hemodialysis or hemofiltration does not remove excess iron, but it will remove ferrioxamine.[101]

The desired endpoint for deferoxamine therapy is not clear. Some have suggested that deferoxamine therapy should cease when the serum iron concentration falls below 150 μg/dL.[102] The decline of serum iron concentrations, however, may not account for the potential cellular action of deferoxamine irrespective of its effect on iron elimination. The cessation of orange-red urine production that is indicative of ferrioxamine excretion is also not reliable because many individuals cannot distinguish its presence in the urine.[110] Considering these shortcomings, deferoxamine therapy should be continued for 12 hours after the patient is asymptomatic and the urine returns to normal color or until the serum iron concentration falls below 350 μg/dL and approaches 150 μg/dL.

Other Therapies. Lavage solutions of phosphate or deferoxamine have been proposed previously as a means to render iron insoluble, but they were found ineffective and dangerous.[102,115] Lavage with 1% to 2% sodium bicarbonate or administration of milk of magnesia may increase intragastric pH and precipitate iron, but the precipitate is reversibly soluble in the acidic pH of the stomach.[115] Administering deferoxamine orally with activated charcoal has been shown in volunteers to decrease iron absorption, but its application to the poisoned patient requires further evaluation.[108] Oral iron chelating agents, such as deferiprone,[117] are currently approved in Europe for the management of chronic iron overload states. Its role in the treatment of acute iron poisoning remains to be determined.

Monitoring and Prevention. Once a poisoning has occurred, acid-base balance (anion gap and arterial blood gases), fluid and electrolyte balance, and perfusion should be monitored. Other indicators of organ toxicity such as ALT, AST, bilirubin, prothrombin time, serum glucose, and creatinine and markers of physiologic stress or infection such as leukocytosis also should be monitored.

Iron poisoning often is not recognized as a potentially serious problem by parents or victims until symptoms develop, and thus valuable time to institute treatment is lost. Parents should be made aware of the potential risks and asked to observe basic poison prevention measures. Many chewable vitamins with iron are shaped like animal or cartoon characters that can be attractive to children and can lead to poisoning. Some hard-coated iron tablets resemble candy-coated chocolates and are easily confused by children. Based on these considerations and the frequency of this poisoning, iron tablets are packaged in child-resistant containers. In 1998, iron products were required to be sold in special packages, such as blister packs, which limit the total dose and present additional physical barriers for children.[105]

THEOPHYLLINE

Signs and Symptoms. Gastrointestinal, cardiovascular, neurologic, and metabolic effects have been observed following acute and chronic poisoning with theophylline.[118] Gastrointestinal symptoms include nausea and vomiting in 60% to 100% of cases, abdominal pain, diarrhea, and acute gastritis with gastrointestinal bleeding. Vomiting may be difficult to control despite antiemetic therapy. Supraventricular tachycardia is present in most cases. Peripheral vasodilation typically leads to hypotension in severe cases. Premature ventricular beats are also commonly observed. Ventricular tachycardia and fibrillation are associated with more severe intoxications and may be life-threatening. Atrial fibrillation is seen more frequently with chronic exposure.[119–121] Theophylline may produce tachypnea due to stimulation of CNS respiratory centers. Headache, hallucinations, disorientation, coma, ataxia, and tremor may be observed. Seizures are a common consequence of serious theophylline poisoning and are associated with increased mortality. The seizures typically are generalized, may occur without warning, and may be resistant to conventional anticonvulsant therapy. Irritability, vomiting, and headache may precede seizure activity. Neurologic complications of theophylline-induced seizure activity are more common with chronic toxicity and include amnesia, quadraplegia, persistent seizures, and intracerebral hemorrhage.[121,122] Theophylline poisoning typically produces marked hypokalemia, but its consequences are unclear. Blood glucose concentrations are elevated and in some cases may exceed 400 mg/dL. Hypercalcemia, hypophosphatemia, hypomagnesemia, and respiratory alkalosis also have been reported.[118–122] Metabolic acidosis is a common finding in cases of moderate to severe severity. Theophylline also may have a mild diuretic effect.

There are differences in onset and duration of toxic symptoms compared with effects at therapeutic doses. Peak effects from therapeutic doses may be observed in 1 to 2 hours, but with overdosage, peak concentrations and effects may occur from 2 to 8 hours after ingestion. Sustained-release preparations may peak between 6 and 24 hours. Tablet concretions have been reported with sustained-release tablets.[123]

Mechanism of Toxicity. Theophylline relaxes smooth muscles, stimulates the CNS, reduces peripheral vascular resistance, increases the rate and force of myocardial contractions, and increases urine production. The exact mechanism for these actions is not known for theophylline at therapeutic or toxic levels, but several hypotheses exist. Inhibition of phosphodiesterase leading to increased cyclic AMP has been proposed. General sympathetic stimulation may occur, as evidenced by increases in circulating catecholamines. The translocation of intracellular calcium as the result of increased permeability of the sarcoplasmic reticulum in striated muscles also has been observed. Another potential mechanism involves the competitive blockade of adenosine receptors thereby minimizing the effects of endogenous adenosine, a recognized bronchconstrictor, anticonvulsant, and regulator of cardiac rhythm.[118] Hypokalemia, one of the metabolic effects of theophylline toxicity, may result from cyclic AMP-mediated stimulation of the sodium-potassium-ATPase pump, resulting in decreased extracellular potassium.

Causative Agents. There are numerous theophylline-containing products on the market for the treatment of asthma and other pulmonary conditions (see Chaps. 26 and 27). No apparent difference in toxicity has been noted between products when equivalent doses of theophylline were ingested. Theophylline is available as a liquid and several solid dosage forms, including sustained-release formulations.

Incidence. The 1999 AAPCC-TESS report documented 1641 patients with an exposure to theophylline, of which 64% were greater than 19 years of age and 24% were intentional poisonings.[6] Sixty-five people experienced a major effect and 10 people died. As the therapy of asthma shifts away from the routine use of theophylline products, the availability of theophylline and the incidence of poisoning are likely to decline.[119]

Risk Assessment. The circumstances, symptoms, and toxic serum concentrations are different based on whether theophylline exposure is acute or chronic (Table 9–13). Theophylline toxicity is likely with the acute, single ingestion of 10 mg/kg or more of theophylline. Chronic theophylline toxicity typically results from overmedication, changes in metabolism of theophylline, or drug interactions[120–124] (see Chap. 26). Interpretation of serum theophylline concentrations should consider whether the exposure was acute or chronic. Ventricular tachycardia is associated with concentrations greater than 100 μg/mL, with acute exposures and concentrations of 40 μg/mL or greater following chronic exposures. Convulsions are seen in 50% of patients following acute exposures with serum concentrations over 120 μg/mL or chronic exposures with concentrations exceeding 40 μg/mL.[118–121] Patients with acute theophylline poisoning typically exhibit signs of minor toxicity at serum theophylline concentrations of 20–40 μg/mL, moderate toxicity in the range of 40–80 μg/mL, and severe toxicity with concentrations greater than 70–80 μg/mL. The serum theophylline concentration is less

TABLE 9–13. Comparison of Acute and Chronic Theophylline Toxicity

Characteristic	Acute	Chronic
Circumstance	Intentional overdose Unintentional ingestion	Patient increased dose Drug interaction Altered elimination Dosing/dispensing error
Symptoms	Vomiting, tremor, tachycardia, hypotension, hypokalemia, acidosis, seizures	Occasional vomiting Tachycardia, seizures
Life-threatening serum theophylline concentration (μg/mL)	>100	>40–60
Predictor of life-threatening events	Serum concentration (>100 μg/mL)	Extremes of age

predictive for chronic exposures[125,126]; patients have experienced seizures, arrhythmias, and death at serum concentrations as low as 20–30 μg/mL.[118,126]

With acute theophylline poisoning, few patient risk factors have been associated with the development of toxicity. The risk of toxicity from chronic exposure is increased by several factors, including drug interactions and saturable biotransformation. Because theophylline is metabolized by the cytochrome oxidase system, inhibitors of this enzyme system, such as erythromycin, oral contraceptives, allopurinol, cimetidine, and ciprofloxin (see Chap. 26), may lead to theophylline toxicity within several days of their concomitant use. Chronic toxicity is seen at lower serum concentrations than acute toxicity.[121,122,125] Possible explanations for chronic toxicity include CNS saturation or accumulation of 3-methylxanthine, an active metabolite of theophylline. Although seizures and serious dysrhythmias have been reported at concentrations of 15–20 μg/mL, they are seen more frequently with chronic serum theophylline concentrations of 35–70 μg/mL. Age rather than peak serum concentration is more predictive of major toxicity after chronic theophylline exposure, with the very young and the elderly at greatest risk.[120,121] Older patients with preexisting cardiopulmonary disease are more susceptible to the life-threatening complications of theophylline toxicity. Risk factors for life-threatening effects include the presence of seizures, hypotension, preexisting cardiac or hepatic disease, chronic exposure, and age over 50 years.[120,121,125,126]

Management of Toxicity. Routine supportive care and gastric decontamination procedures typically are indicated for theophylline poisoning. Due to the risk of theophylline-induced seizure activity, ipecac syrup is avoided. Activated charcoal adsorbs theophylline and may be useful for acute theophylline ingestions when the drug is still suspected to be present in the gastrointestinal tract. Vomiting is commonly associated with theophylline poisoning and may limit the ability to administer activated charcoal. Vomiting may be controlled by parenteral ranitidine, high-dose metoclopromide (0.5–1 mg/kg), ondansetron, or droperidol.[118,124] Whole-bowel irrigation has been used to evacuate the intestines following ingestion of sustained-release theophylline products.[36]

Because of the associated increase in mortality and resistance to anticonvulsant therapy, the anticipation and treatment of seizures are essential in the management of theophylline poisoning. Once seizures occur, they should be treated aggressively. Initially a benzodiazepine, such as diazepam or lorazepam, should be used and large doses may be required. Phenobarbital may be considered a second-line therapy, but phenytoin is avoided due to its ineffectiveness for theophylline-induced seizures.[119] If anticonvulsants are ineffective in terminating seizures, skeletal muscle paralysis and general anesthesia may be necessary.

Cardiac dysrhythmias, such as supraventricular tachycardia, may require no treatment. Hemodynamically significant supraventricular tachycardia may be treated with esmolol, adenosine, or verapamil,[118] but verapamil may exacerbate hypotension. Ventricular dysrhythmias may respond to lidocaine, β-blockers, or other antiarrhythmics depending on the cardiac disturbance. Hypotension, with an increased pulse pressure and diastolic hypotension, is often due to decreased vascular resistance and may respond to a modest intravenous fluid bolus followed by conventional vasopressors, such as dopamine, dobutamine, and norepinephrine, if needed.[124]

Hypokalemia, hyperglycemia, hypophosphatemia, hypercalcemia, and metabolic acidosis have been corrected by intravenous propranolol[124] and by specific replacement if indicated. Most metabolic disturbances do not require aggressive therapy. Propranolol or adenosine should be used cautiously in individuals susceptible to the risk of bronchoconstriction. Multiple-dose activated charcoal has proven to be effective at enhancing elimination of theophylline from the bloodstream even after intravenous overdose.[45,118] It has been shown to reduce theophylline half-life by 50%. Repeat-dose activated charcoal should be considered if serum concentrations in acute overdose are over 40 μg/mL, when patients are symptomatic (acute or chronic exposures), or in chronic intoxication with serum concentrations over 20 μg/mL.[119]

Charcoal hemoperfusion and hemodialysis are very effective in removal of theophylline from the bloodstream,[119,123] but they are frequently unnecessary when repeat-dose charcoal can be employed successfully.[45] Although hemoperfusion and hemodialysis are nearly similar in effectiveness, hemoperfusion is associated with more complications, whereas hemodialysis is more readily available.[127] Extracorporeal removal should be considered in acute overdose with serum concentrations over 100 μg/mL, for patients with seizure activity or hemodynamically significant dysrhythmias not responding to conventional therapy, or in chronic intoxication with serum concentrations over 40 μg/mL.[118,120]

Monitoring and Prevention. Theophylline may be detected reliably by enzyme-mediated immunoassays or high-performance liquid chromatography. Laboratory monitoring should include electrolytes, calcium, magnesium, phosphorus, arterial blood gases, and urine pH. Seizure activity should prompt the monitoring of serum creatine phosphokinase and myoglobinuria. When elevations occur, prophylactic treatment for rhabdomyolysis should be instituted, including alkaline diuresis to maintain a urine pH of 7.5 to 8 to minimize the risk of tubular deposition of myoglobin and resulting acute renal failure.

Theophylline poisoning may be prevented by recognition of its poisonous potential and institution of general poison prevention measures when young children are present. Monitoring of patients receiving theophylline for changes in health status (e.g., viral illness or cardiac disease, drug therapy leading to drug interactions, drug dosage by the patient or caregiver, and metabolism due to age-related changes in drug disposition) may identify patients at risk of developing chronic theophylline poisoning.[120,125]

TRICYCLIC ANTIDEPRESSANTS

Signs and Symptoms. Symptoms of tricyclic antidepressant poisoning typically occur within the first hour of ingestion and can progress rapidly to death in several hours. Patients may deteriorate rapidly and progress from no symptoms to life-threatening cardiotoxicity or seizures within 1 hour.[128,129] The principal effects of tricyclic antidepressant poisoning involve the cardiovascular system and the CNS and can result in arrhythmias, hypotension, coma, and seizures.

Prolongation of the QRS complex on electrocardiogram indicating nonspecific intraventricular conduction delay or bundle-branch block is the most distinctive feature of tricyclic antidepressant overdose.[129] Sinus tachycardia with rates typically under 160 beats per minute is common and does not cause serious hemodynamic changes in most patients. Ventricular tachycardia is a common ventricular arrhythmia, but it may be difficult to distinguish from sinus tachycardia in the presence of QRS prolongation and the apparent absence of P waves. It often occurs in patients with marked QRS prolongation or hypotension and may be precipitated by seizures.[129,130] High rates of mortality are associated with ventricular tachycardia; ventricular fibrillation is the terminal rhythm. Torsades de pointes is observed infrequently with tricyclic antidepressant poisoning. With massive tricyclic antidepressant overdose, slow ventricular rhythms may be observed. A few cases of sudden death from presumed fatal arrhythmias have been reported 2 to 5 days after ingestion, but these cases are isolated events that have an unclear causal relationship to tricyclic antidepressant overdose.[128] Hypotension is a significant factor in most cases of tricyclic antidepressant poisoning. Refractory hypotension leading to death is due to vasodilation and impaired cardiac contractility.[129] Other factors—such as extreme heart rates, intravascular volume depletion, hypoxia, hyperthermia, seizures, and acidosis—may contribute to refractory hypotension.

Coma usually is present in patients with tricyclic antidepressant poisoning and may or may not be associated with QRS prolongation. In severe cases, coma is sufficient to depress respirations. Delirium, manifest as agitation or disorientation, may occur early in the course of severe poisoning or with poisoning of moderate severity. Seizures often occur within 2 hours of ingestion and usually are generalized, single, and brief. Seizures may result in acidosis, hyperthermia, or rhabdomyolysis, and 10% to 20% of patients may abruptly develop cardiovascular deterioration.[129] Myoclonus also may be observed with tricyclic antidepressant overdose.

Hyperthermia often results from seizure and myoclonic activity in the presence of decreased sweating and is associated with a high incidence of neurologic sequelae and mortality. Anticholinergic symptoms, such as urinary retention, ileus, and dry mucous membranes, often are observed with tricyclic antidepressant overdose.[128,129] Pupil size is variable. Tricyclic antidepressant overdose can be staged based on the patient's symptoms and recovery time. In stage 1, patients are responsive to pain, have sinus tachycardia, and recover within 24 hours. In stage 2, seizures, coma, and cardiac conduction problems are evident; respiratory support typically is needed. Patients recover within 24 to 48 hours of ingestion. Stage 3 is characterized by the features of stage 2 with the addition of respiratory arrest, hypotension, ventricular dysrhythmias, and asystole, which may occur within 1 to 24 hours of ingestion.

Amoxipine, buproprion, and maprotiline are atypical antidepressants associated with a higher incidence of seizures on overdose; amoxipine produces minimal cardiotoxicity.[129,131] The selective serotonin reuptake inhibitors (SSRIs) generally produce a common toxicity profile on overdose despite their structural and pharmacologic distinctions.[132] The SSRIs inhibit the presynaptic neuronal uptake of serotonin, resulting in increased synaptic serotonin levels. When ingested in excess, SSRIs rarely cause death and typically produce nausea, vomiting, diarrhea, tremor, and decreased level of consciousness.[132] Tachycardia and seizures are infrequent.[129,131,133] Serotonin syndrome is associated with the coingestion of drugs increasing serotonin levels and develops within minutes to hours of the inciting action. It is characterized by a collection of neurobehavioral (e.g., confusion, agitation, coma, seizures), autonomic (e.g., hyperthermia, diaphoresis, tachycardia, hypertension), and neuromuscular (e.g., myoclonus, rigidity, tremor, ataxia, shivering, nystagmus) signs and symptoms.[134,135] Most cases are mild and resolve spontaneously within 24 to 72 hours. Cardiac arrest, coma, and multiple organ failure have been reported as consequences of serotonin syndrome.[134] Recognition of the syndrome is based on a high index of suspicion and identification of risk factors.

Mechanism of Toxicity. Many of the toxic effects of tricyclic antidepressants are associated with an exaggeration of their pharmacologic action. The tricyclic antidepressants, like type Ia antiarrhythmic drugs, inhibit the fast sodium channel so that phase zero depolarization of the myocardium is slowed.[129] This action leads to QRS prolongation, atrioventricular block, ventricular tachycardia, and decreased myocardial contractility. Tricyclic antidepressants also block vascular α-adrenergic receptors, resulting in vasodilation, which contributes to hypotension. Sinus tachycardia is related to the inhibition of norepinephrine reuptake and anticholinergic effects. Other anticholinergic effects include urinary retention, ileus, dry mucous membranes, and impaired sweating. Inhibition of norepinephrine reuptake also may account for the early, transient, and self-limiting elevation of blood pressure observed in some patients. The CNS toxicity of tricyclic antidepressants is not well understood.

Causative Agents. Tricylic antidepressants and SSRIs are used to treat a variety of behavioral conditions (see Chaps. 69 and 70). The tricyclic antidepressants include drugs such as amitriptyline, desipramine, doxepin, imipramine, and nortriptyline. Atypical agents include amoxapine, buproprion, and maprotilene. The SSRIs include fluoxetine, nefazadone, paroxetine, sertraline, trazadone, and venlafaxine. The tricyclic antidepressants are generally highly protein bound, exhibit a large volume of distribution, and possess elimination half-lives of 8 to 24 hours or more. Virtually none of the drug is eliminated unchanged in the urine. Metabolism of the parent drug produces active metabolites in most cases (e.g., amitriptyline to nortriptyline) which may contribute to toxicity after the first 12 to 24 hours.[129] Genetic polymorphism at CYP2D6 may lead to slower recovery in patients who are slow hydroxylators.[136]

Incidence. Tricyclic antidepressant poisoning is a common cause of death from drug overdose.[129,130] The 1999 AAPCC-TESS report documented 13,863 patients with exposures to tricyclic antidepressants, of whom 60% were intentional overdoses. A total of 1559 people experienced a major effect, and 101 people died.[6] The SSRIs accounted for 28,541 nonfatal exposures and 22 deaths.

Risk Assessment. Ingestion of greater that 1 g of a tricyclic antidepressant (greater than 10 mg/kg in children) typically results in life-threatening toxicity.[129] Because serious toxicity may occur within 1 to 2 hours of ingestion, prompt transport to an emergency department is crucial for overdoses. A QRS complex greater than 100 ms or progressive prolongation of the QRS are indicators of toxicity and often precede more serious symptoms.[129,130,137] Serum concentrations of tricyclic antidepressants in excess of 1000 ng/mL have been associated with a QRS complex of 100 ms or greater, but an electrocardiogram reading is more readily obtainable and serves as a more direct indicator of toxicity.[137] Although urine drug analyses routinely screen for tricyclic antidepressant, the qualitative result can only suggest or confirm a potential risk for the development of toxicity.

Patients with coexisting cardiovascular and pulmonary conditions (e.g., adult respiratory distress syndrome, pulmonary infection, pulmonary aspiration) may be more susceptible to the toxic effects or complications of tricyclic antidepressant poisoning. The influence of chronic exposure to tricyclic antidepressants on the risks of an acute overdose is unclear. Tricyclic antidepressants interact with other CNS depressant drugs, which together may lead to increased CNS and respiratory depression.

The risk of serotonin syndrome may be increased shortly after dosage increases of SSRIs or when drug interactions increase serotonin activity.[138] Concomitant or proximal use of SSRIs, tricyclic antidepressants, or monoamine oxidase inhibitors may cause serotonin syndrome. Further, the addition of certain drugs, such as tryptophan, dextromethorphan, cocaine, or sympathomimetics, to SSRI therapy may increase the risk of developing serotonin syndrome.[134,138]

Management of Toxicity. Once the ingestion of an overdose of tricyclic antidepressant is suspected, or for any intentional ingestion, medical evaluation and treatment should be sought promptly. If the patient is symptomatic, it may be prudent to call for an ambulance owing to the rapid progression of some cases. At the emergency department, the patient should be monitored carefully, have vital signs assessed regularly, and have an intravenous line started. Supportive and symptomatic care includes oxygen, intravenous fluids, and other treatments as indicated. Prompt administration of activated charcoal may decrease the absorption of any remaining tricyclic antidepressant. It also may be useful beyond the first hour of ingestion due to decreased gastrointestinal motility from the anticholinergic action of tricyclic antidepressants. Gastric lavage may be considered if the time of the ingestion is unknown or if it occurred within the past 1 to 2 hours. Some avoid gastric lavage altogether.[129] Ipecac syrup should be avoided in patients who ingest tricyclic antidepressants due to the rapid onset of toxicity. Multiple-dose activated charcoal has been shown to increase the elimination of some tricyclic antidepressants in human volunteers[45] and has been used in poisoned patients.[128,129] It may be most useful during the first 12 hours after ingestion, while the drug is distributing to tissue compartments. Because the tricyclic antidepressants possess such a large volume of distribution and so little of the drug is present in the bloodstream, hemodialysis is not useful for the extracorporeal removal of tricyclic antidepressants.

Intravenous sodium bicarbonate is part of the first-line treatment of QRS prolongation, ventricular arrhythmias, and hypotension caused by tricyclic antidepressant overdose[94,129,139] (Fig. 9–10). Typically 1–2 mEq/kg of sodium bicarbonate (1 mEq/mL) is administered as a bolus infusion (usually a 50-mEq ampule in an adult) and repeated as necessary to achieve an arterial blood pH of 7.50 to 7.55 or abatement of toxicity.[128,129] A therapeutic effect usually is observed within minutes. Excessive use of sodium bicarbonate may produce dangerous alkalemia, which is by itself associated with ventricular arrhythmias.[129] The mechanism of action of sodium bicarbonate is unclear. Although some have proposed that sodium bicarbonate increases protein binding of tricyclic antidepressants, this has been discounted. Sodium may play an important role by stabilizing tricyclic antidepressant-induced changes to the sodium gradient of the myocardium.[129,140] Regardless of its action, it is effective and generally safe. Hyperventilation to produce a mild state of respiratory alkalosis has been used to treat some dysrhythmias, but it is less widely used than sodium bicarbonate.[128,129]

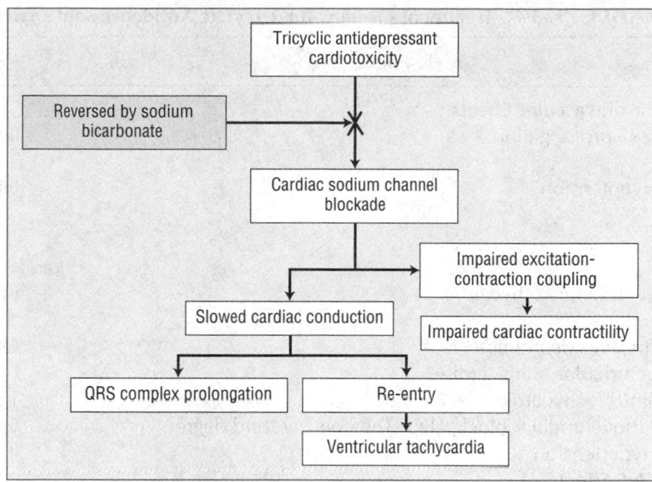

FIGURE 9–10. Role of sodium bicarbonate in limiting cardiotoxicity form tricyclic antidepressant poisoning. *(Adapted from Ref. 129.)*

Treatment of the complications of tricyclic antidepressant poisoning is outlined in Table 9–14 and includes pharmacologic and nonpharmacologic approaches.[129] Several agents generally should be avoided in the treatment of tricyclic antidepressant poisoning. Other drugs that inhibit the fast sodium channel, such as procainamide and quinidine, are contraindicated. Phenytoin has limited usefulness in treating tricyclic antidepressant seizures and has questionable efficacy in managing cardiotoxicity.[128] Physostigmine was used in the past as a treatment of tricyclic antidepressant cardiotoxicity and seizures because it antagonizes anticholinergic actions. However, physostigmine is otherwise ineffective, is associated bradycardia and asystole,[129,141] and has no role in the contemporary treatment of tricyclic antidepressant cardiovascular or CNS toxicity. Flumazemil is used to antagonize the effects of benzodiazepines, but its use in the presence of a tricyclic antidepressant has been associated with the development of seizures and should be avoided.[54,142]

Treatment of an overdose of the atypical antidepressants and SSRIs is directed primarily toward decontamination of the gastrointestinal tract with activated charcoal, symptomatic treatment, and general supportive care. Management of the serotonin syndrome involves discontinuation of the serotinergic agent and supportive therapy. Benzodiazepines, propranolol, and cyproheptadine, a serotonin antagonist, have been used successfully.[134]

Monitoring and Prevention. Measurement of vital signs, electrolytes, blood urea nitrogen, and a urinalysis are indicated for initial assessment. Patients should be continuously monitored by electrocardiogram, and a 12-lead electrocardiogram should be obtained if QRS prolongation is noted. If patients start to show signs of cardiotoxicity, arterial blood gases should be determined. Patients who show no signs of toxicity during 6 hours of observation and have promptly

TABLE 9–14. Treatment Options for Tricyclic Antidepressant Toxicity

Toxic Effect	Treatment
Cardiovascular Effects	
QRS prolongation	Intravenous sodium bicarbonate if QRS prolongation is marked or progressive (not clear if treatment is needed in the absence of hypotension or arrhythmias)
Hypotension	Intravascular volume expansion, intravenous sodium bicarbonate Vasopressors (norepinephrine) or inotropes (dopamine) Treat hyperthermia, acidosis, seizures Consider mechanical circulatory support
Ventricular tachycardia	Intravenous sodium bicarbonate, lidocaine, overdrive pacing Treat hypotension, hyperthermia, acidosis, seizures
Torsades de pointes	Overdrive cardiac pacing
Ventricular bradycardia	Chronotropes (epinephrine), cardiac pacemaker
Sinus tachycardia	Treatment rarely needed
Atrioventricular block—type II second or third degree	Cardiac pacemaker
Hypertension	If needed, rapidly titratable antihypertensive agent (nitroprusside)
CNS Effects	
Delirium and agitation	Physical restraints, benzodiazepines Neuromuscular blockade if hyperthermia or acidosis present
Seizures	Benzodiazepine Neuromuscular blockade if hyperthermia or acidosis present
Coma	Endotracheal intubation, mechanical ventilation if needed
Other Effects	
Hyperthermia	Treat seizures, agitation Cooling measures (cooling blanket, ice water lavage, cool water mist of body)
Acidosis	Intravenous sodium bicarbonate Treat hypotension, hypoventilation

Adapted from Ref. 129.

received activated charcoal require no further medical monitoring. Psychiatric evaluation is indicated for adolescents and adults. When signs of tricyclic antidepressant are present in a patient, cardiac monitoring generally is recommended for at least 24 hours after the patient is without findings.[129]

Prevention of tricyclic antidepressant poisoning poses unique challenges. Many of the dosage forms are small in size, and large numbers can be consumed easily by adults and children. In the course of treating depression, several antidepressant agents may be tried to achieve results. Instead of discarding unused medicines, a storehouse of potentially deadly drugs may be kept for children to discover or for the despondent patient to use to attempt suicide. Although patients take tricyclic antidepressants for therapeutic relief of depression, they are also a group likely to contemplate suicide with tricyclic antidepressants. Strategies that would limit the amount of tricyclic antidepressant prescribed at one time also would potentially impair adherence to a dosage regimen and thereby compromise the therapeutic potential of these agents.[129,139] Patients with a history of suicidal gestures may be candidates for the atypical antidepressants or SSRIs, which possess less cardiotoxicity. General poison prevention measures may limit childhood poisonings, and monitoring depressed patients for suicidal ideation may identify patients at risk.[143]

REFERENCES

1. Koren G. Medications which can kill a toddler with one tablet or teaspoonful. J Toxicol Clin Toxicol 1993;31:407–413.
2. Injury Facts, 2000 ed. Itasca, IL, National Safety Council. 2000:8–12, 18, 38–41, 126–129.
3. Hoppe-Roberts JH, Lloyd LM, Chyka PA. Poisoning mortality in the United States: Comparison of national mortality statistics and poison control center reports. Ann Emerg Med 2000;35:440–448.
4. Rice DJ, MacKenzie EJ. Cost of Injury in the United States: A Report to Congress. San Francisco, Institute for Health and Aging, University of California, and Injury Prevention Center, Johns Hopkins University, 1989:23–25, 37–85.
5. Fingerhut LA, Cox CS. Poisoning mortality. Public Health Rep 1998;113:218–233.
6. Litovitz TL, Klein-Schwartz E, White S, et al. 1999 annual report of the American Association of Poison Control Centers Toxic Surveillance System. Am J Emerg Med 2000;18:517–574.
7. Kearney TE, Olson KR, Bero LA, et al. Health care cost effects of public use of a regional poison control center. West J Med 1995;162:499–504.
8. Phillips KA, Homan RK, Hiatt PH, et al. The costs and outcomes of restricting public access to poison control centers: Results from a natural experiment. Med Care 1998;36:271–280.
9. Miller TR, Lestina DC. Cost of poisoning in the United States and savings from poison control centers: A benefit-cost analysis. Ann Emerg Med 1997;29:239–245.
10. Rodgers GB. The safety effects of child-resistant packaging for oral prescription drugs: Two decades of experience. JAMA 1996;275:1661–1665.
11. Shannon M. Ingestion of toxic substances by children. N Engl J Med 2000;342:186–191.
12. King WD, Palmisano PA. Ingestion of prescription drugs by children: An epidemiologic study. South Med J 1989;82:1468–1478.
13. Poison Prevention Packaging: A Textbook for Pharmacists and Physicians. Washington, U.S. Consumer Product Safety Commission, 1999. Publication number 384. Available at: *http://www.cpsc.gov/cpscpub/pubs/384.pdf.* Accessed September 7, 2001.
14. Rodgers GC, Tenenbien M. The role of aversive bittering agents in the prevention of pediatric poisonings. Pediatrics 1994;93:68–69.

15. Buckley NA, Whyte IM, Dawson AH, et al. Correlations between prescriptions and drugs taken in self-poisoning. Med J Aust 1995;162:194–197.
16. Haselberger MB, Kroner BA. Drug poisoning in older patients: Preventative and management strategies. Drugs Aging 1995;7:292–297.
17. Olson K, Pentel P, Kelley M. Physical assessment and differential diagnosis of the poisoned patient. Med Toxicol 1987;2:52–81.
18. Nice A, Leikin JB, Maturen A, et al. Toxidrome recognition to improve efficiency of emergency urine drug screens. Ann Emerg Med 1988;17:676–680.
19. Liang HK. Clinical evaluation of the poisoned patient and toxic syndromes. Clin Chem 1996;42:1350–1355.
20. USP Drug Information. Vol. I: Drug Information for the Health Care Professional, 20th ed. Englewood, CO, Micromedex, 2000.
21. Liu RH. Important considerations in the interpretation of forensic urine drug test results. Forens Sci Rev 1992;4:51–64.
22. Watson ID. Laboratory support for the poisoned patient. Ther Drug Monit 1998;20:490–497.
23. Rosenberg J, Benowitz NL, Pond S. Pharmacokinetics of drug overdose. Clin Pharmacokinet 1981;6:161–192.
24. Young-Jin S, Shannon M. Pharmacokinetics of drugs in overdose. Clin Pharmacokinet 1992;23:93–105.
25. Taylor JR, Streetman DS, Castle SS. Medication bezoars: A literature review and report of a case. Ann Pharmacother 1998;32:940–946.
26. Bosse GM, Matyunas NJ. Delayed toxidromes. J Emerg Med 1999;17:679–690.
27. Vernon DD, Gleich MC. Poisoning and drug overdose. Crit Care Clin 1997;13:647–667.
28. Vance MV, Selden BS, Clark RF. Optimal patient position for transport and initial management of toxic ingestions. Ann Emerg Med 1992;21:243–246.
29. Mowry JB, Sketris IS, Czajka PA. Ipecac syrup for poisoning at home: Availability, compliance, and response monitored by telephone. Am J Hosp Pharm 1981;38:1028–1030.
30. Krenzelok EP, McGuigan M, Lheur P. American Academy of Clinical Toxicology, European Association of Poison Centres and Clinical Toxicologists. Position statement: Ipecac syrup. J Toxicol Clin Toxicol 1997;35:699–709.
31. Vale JA. American Academy of Clinical Toxicology, European Association of Poison Centres and Clinical Toxicologists. Position statement: Gastric lavage. J Toxicol Clin Toxicol 1997;35:711–719.
32. Chyka PA, Seger D. American Academy of Clinical Toxicology, European Association of Poison Centres and Clinical Toxicologists. Position statement: Single-dose activated charcoal. J Toxicol Clin Toxicol 1997;35:721–741
33. McFarland AK III, Chyka PA. Selection of activated charcoal products for the treatment of poisonings. Ann Pharmacother 1993;27:358–361.
34. Barceloux D, McGuigan M, Hartigan-Go K. American Academy of Clinical Toxicology, European Association of Poisons Centres and Clinical Toxicologists. Position statement: Cathartics. J Toxicol Clin Toxicol 1997;35:743–752.
35. Oral electrolyte solutions for colonic lavage before colonoscopy or barium enema. Med Lett Drug Ther 1985;27:39–40.
36. Tenenbein M. American Academy of Clinical Toxicology, European Association of Poison Centres and Clinical Toxicologists. Position statement: Whole bowel irrigation. J Toxicol Clin Toxicol 1997;35:753–762.
37. Hoffman RS, Smilkstein MJ, Goldfrank LR. Whole bowel irrigation and the cocaine body-packer: A new approach to a common problem. Am J Emerg Med 1990;8:523–527.
38. American College of Emergency Physicians. Clinical policy for the initial approach to patients presenting with acute toxic ingestion or dermal or inhalation exposure. Ann Emerg Med 1999;33:735–761.
39. Grierson R, Green R, Sitar DS, Tenenbein M. Gastric lavage for liquid poisons. Ann Emerg Med 2000;35:435–439.
40. McGuigan MA. Activated charcoal in the home. Clin Pediatr Emerg Med 2000;1:191–194.
41. Elenbaas RM. Critical review of forced alkaline diuresis in acute salicylism. Crit Care Q 1982;4:89–95.
42. Scandling J, Spital A. Amphetamine-associated myoglobinuric renal failure. South Med J 1982;75:237–240.
43. Chyka PA. Multiple-dose activated charcoal and enhancement of systemic drug clearance: Summary of studies in animals and humans. J Toxicol Clin Toxicol 1995;33:399–405.
44. Neuvonen PJ, Olkkola KT. Oral activated charcoal in the treatment of intoxication: Role of single and repeated doses. Med Toxicol Adverse Drug Exp1988;3:33–58.
45. American Academy of Clinical Toxicology, European Association of Poison Centres and Clinical Toxicologists. Position statement and practice guidelines on the use of multidose activated charcoal in the treatment of acute poisoning. J Toxicol Clin Toxicol 1999;37:731–751.
46. Pond SM, Olson KR, Osterloh JD, et al. Randomized study of the treatment of phenobarbital overdose with repeated doses of activated charcoal. JAMA 1984;251:3104–3108.
47. Chyka PA, Holley JE, Mandrell TM, Sugathan P. Correlation of drug pharmacokinetics and effectiveness of multiple-dose activated charcoal therapy. Ann Emerg Med 1995;25:356–362.
48. Farrar HC, Herold DA, Reed MD. Acute valproic acid intoxication: Enhanced drug clearance with oral-activated charcoal. Crit Care Med 1993;21:299–301.
49. Tomaszewski C. Activated charcoal: Treatment or toxin? (Editorial). Clin Toxicol 1999;37:17–18.
50. Pond SM. Extracorporeal techniques in the treatment of poisoned patients. Med J Aust 1991;154:617–622.
51. Bowden CA, Krenzelok EP. Clinical applications of commonly used contemporary antidotes. Drug Saf 1997;16:9–47.
52. Trujillo MH, Guerrero J, Fragachan C, Fernandez MA. Pharmacologic antidotes in critical care medicine: A practical guide for drug administration. Crit Care Med 1998;26:377–391.
53. Dart RC, Goldfrank L, Chyka PA, et al. Combined evidence-based literature analysis and consensus guidelines for stocking of emergency antidotes in the United States. Ann Emerg Med 2000;36:126–132.
54. Liebelt EL. Newer antidotal therapies for pediatric poisonings. Clin Pediatr Emerg Med 2000;1:234–243.
55. Chyka PA, Butler AY, Holliman BJ, Herman MI. Utility of *N*-acetylcysteine in treating poisonings and adverse drug reactions. Drug Saf 2000;22:123–148.
56. Antman EM, Wenger TL, Butler VP, et al. Treatment of 150 cases of life-threatening digitalis intoxication with digoxin-specific Fab antibody fragments. Circulation 1990;81:1744–1752.
57. CroFab [Crotalidae Polyvalent Immune Fab (Ovine)] package insert. Nashville, TN, Protherics. Available at: *http://www.protherics.com/PRO0410000.html*. Accessed October 19, 2000.
58. Zed PJ, Krenzelok EP. Treatment of acetaminophen overdose. Am J Health Syst Pharm 1999;56:1081–1093.
59. Smilkstein MJ, Knapp GL, Kulig KW, Rumack BH. Efficacy of oral *N*-acetylcysteine in the treatment of acetaminophen overdose: Analysis of the national multicenter study (1976–1985). N Engl J Med 1988;319:1557–1562.
60. Makin AJ, Wendon J, Williams R. A 7-year experience of severe acetaminophen-induced hepatotoxicity (1987–1993). Gastroenterology 1995;109:1907–1916.
61. Schiodt FV, Rochling FA, Casey DL, Lee WM. Acetaminophen toxicity in an urban county hospital. N Engl J Med 1997;337:1112–1117.
62. Blantz RC. Acetaminophen: Acute and chronic effects on renal function. Am J Kid Dis 1996;28(Suppl 1):S3–S6.
63. Smilkstein MJ. APAP-induced heart injury? Maybe yes, maybe no. Next question. J Toxicol Clin Toxicol 1996;34:155–156.
64. Bray GP, Harrison PM, O'Grady JG, et al. Long-term anticonvulsant therapy worsens outcome in paracetamol-induced fulminant hepatic failure. Hum Exp Toxicol 1992;11:265–70.
65. Johnston SC, Pelletier LL Jr. Enhanced hepatotoxicity of acetaminophen in the alcoholic patient: Two case reports and a review of the literature. Medicine 1997;76:185–191.
66. Thummel KE, Slattery JT, Ro H, et al. Ethanol and production of the hepatotoxic metabolite of acetaminophen in healthy adults. Clin Pharmacol Ther 2000;67:591–599.

67. Draganov P, Durrence H, Cox C, Reuben A. Alcohol-acetaminophen syndrome: Even moderate social drinkers are at risk. Postgrad Med 2000;107:189–195.
68. Heubi JE, Barbacci MB, Zimmerman HJ. Therapeutic misadventures with acetaminophen: Hepatotoxicity after multiple doses in children. J Pediatr 1998;132:22–27.
69. Kearns GL, Leeder JS, Wasserman GS. Acetaminophen intoxication during treatment: What you don't know can hurt you. Clin Pediatr 2000;39(3):133–144.
70. Miles FK, Kamath R, Dorney SF, et al. Accidental paracetamol overdosing and fulminant hepatic failure in children. Med J Aust 1999;171:472–475.
71. Jones AL. Mechanism of action and value of *N*-acetylcysteine in the treatment of early and late acetaminophen poisoning: A critical review. J Toxicol Clin Toxicol 1998;36:277–285.
72. Tucker JR. Late-presenting acute acetaminophen toxicity and the role of *N*-acetylcysteine. Pediatr Emerg Care 1998;14:424–426.
73. Dhawan A, Sorrell MF. Acetaminophen overdose: Need to consider intravenous preparation of *N*-acetylcysteine in the United States. Am J Gastroenterol 1996;91:1476.
74. Clark RF, Chen R, Williams SR, et al. The use of ondansetron in the treatment of nausea and vomiting associated with acetaminophen poisoning. J Toxicol Clin Toxicol 1996;34:163–167.
75. Perry HE, Shannon MW. Efficacy of oral versus intravenous *N*-acetylcysteine in acetaminophen overdose: Results of an open-label clinical trial. J Pediatr 1998;132:149–152.
76. Yip L, Dart RC, Hurlbut KM. Intravenous administration of oral *N*-acetylcysteine. Crit Care Med 1998;26:40–43.
77. Bizovi KE, Aks SE, Paloucek F, et al. Late increase in acetaminophen concentration after overdose of Tylenol Extended Relief. Ann Emerg Med 1996;28:549–551.
78. Ho SY, Arellano M, Zolkowski-Wynne J. Delayed increase in acetaminophen concentration after Tylenol PM overdose (Letter). Am J Emerg Med 1999;17:315–317.
79. Bardin PG, van Eeden SF, Moolman JA, et al. Organophosphate and carbamate poisoning. Arch Intern Med 1994;154:1433–1441.
80. Goswamy R, Chaudhuri A, Hahashur AA. Study of respiratory failure in organophosphate and carbamate poisoning. Heart Lung 1994;23:466–472.
81. Organophosphates (management/treatment protocol). In: Toll LL, Hurlbut KM, eds. Poisindex System, Vol. 106. Englewood, CO, Micromedex, edition expires November 30, 2000.
82. Chlorpyriphos Revised Risk Assessment and Agreement with Registrants. Washington, Environmental Protection Agency (Prevention, Pesticides and Toxic Substance 7506C), June 2000. Available at *http://www.eps.gov/pesticides/op/chlorphyriphos/agreement.pdf.* Accessed on November 16, 2000.
83. Medicis JJ, Stork CM, Howland MA, et al. Pharmacokinetics following a loading dose plus a continuous infusion of pralidoxime compared with the traditional short infusion regimen in human volunteers. J Toxicol Clin Toxicol 1996;34:289–295.
84. Farrar HC, Wells TG, Kearns GL. Use of continuous infusion of pralidoxime for treatment of organophosphate poisoning in children. J Pediatr 1990;116:658–661.
85. Hofer CA, Smith JK, Tenholder MF. Verapamil intoxication: A literature review of overdoses and discussion of therapeutic options. Am J Med 1993;95:431–438.
86. Pearigen PD, Benowitz NL. Poisoning due to calcium antagonists: Experience with verapamil, diltiazem and nifedipine. Drug Saf 1991;6:408–430.
87. Ramoska EA, Spiller HA, Winter M, Borys D. A one-year evaluation of calcium channel blocker overdoses: Toxicity and treatment. Ann Emerg Med 1993;22:196–200.
88. Kline JA. Calcium channel antagonists. In: Ford M, Delaney K, Ling L, Erickson T, eds. Clinical Toxicology. Philadelphia, Saunders, 2001:370–378.
89. Michel T, Weinfled MS. Coronary artery disease. In: Carruthers SG, Hoffman BB, Melmon KI, Nierenberg DW, eds. Clinical Pharmacology: Basic Principles in Therapeutics, 4th ed. New York, McGraw-Hill, 1999:114–131.
90. Adams BD, Browne WT. Amlodipine overdose causes prolonged calcium channel blocker toxicity. Am J Emerg Med 1998;16:527–528.
91. Calcium antagonists managements. In: Toll LL, Hurlburt KM, eds. Poisindex system, Vol. 106. Greenwood Village, CO, Micromedex, edition expires November 2000.
92. Belson MG, Gorman SE, Sullivan K, Geller RJ. Calcium channel blocker ingestions in children. Am J Emerg Med 2000;18:581–586.
93. Buckley N, Dawson AH, Howarth D, Whyte IM. Slow-release verapamil poisoning: Use of polyethylene glycol whole-bowel lavage and high-dose calcium. Med J Aust 1993;158:202–204.
94. Albertson TE, Dawson A, de Latorre F, et al. Tox-ACLS: Toxicologic-oriented advanced cardiac life support. Ann Emerg Med 2001;37:S78–S90.
95. Papadopoulos J, O'Neil MG. Utilization of a glucagon infusion in the management of a massive nifedipine overdose. J Emerg Med 2000;18:453–455.
96. Holzer M, Sterz F, Schoerkhuber W, et al. Successful resuscitation of a verapamil-intoxicated patient with percutaneous cardiopulmonary bypass. Crit Care Med 1999;27:2818–2823.
97. Yuan TH, Kerns WP 2d, Tomaszewski CA, et al. Insulin-glucose as adjunctive therapy for severe calcium channel antagonist poisoning. J Toxicol Clin Toxicol 1999;37:463–474.
98. Tanen DA, Ruha AM, Cury SC, et al. Hypertonic sodium bicarbonate is effective in the acute management of verapamil toxicity in a swine model. Ann Emerg Med 2000;36:547–553.
99. Luomanmaki K, Tiula E, Kivisto KT, Neuvonen PJ. Pharmacokinetics of diltiazem in massive overdose. Ther Drug Monit 1997;19:240–242.
100. Morimoto S, Sasaki S, Kiyama M, et al. Sustained-release diltiazem overdose. J Hum Hypertens 1999;13:643–644.
101. Fine JS. Iron poisoning. Curr Probl Pediatr 2000;30(3):71–90.
102. Mills KC, Cury SC. Acute iron poisoning. Emerg Med Clin North Am 1994;12:397–413.
103. Tenenbein M, Israels SJ. Early coagulopathy in severe iron poisoning. J Pediatr 1988;113:695–697.
104. Pestaner JP, Ishak KG, Mullick FG, Centeno JA. Ferrous sulfate toxicity: A review of autopsy findings. Biol Trace Element Res 1999;69:191–198.
105. Morris CC. Pediatric iron poisonings in the United States. South Med J 2000;93:352–358.
106. Everson GW, Oukjhane K, Young LW, et al. Effectiveness of abdominal radiographs in visualizing chewable iron supplements following overdose. Am J Emerg Med 1989;7:459–463.
107. Palatnick W, Tenenbein M. Leukocytosis, hyperglycemia, vomiting, and positive x-rays are not indicators of severity of iron overdose in adults. Am J Emerg Med 1996;14:454–455.
108. Chyka PA, Butler AY. Assessment of acute iron poisoning by laboratory and clinical observations. Am J Emerg Med 1993;11:99–103.
109. Chyka PA, Butler AY, Holley JE. Serum iron concentrations and symptoms of acute iron poisoning in children. Pharmacotherapy 1996;16:1053–1058.
110. Eisen TF, Lacouture PG, Woolf A. Visual detection of ferrioxamine color changes in urine. Vet Hum Toxicol 1988;30:369–370.
111. Peck M, Rogers J, Riverbach J. Use of high doses of deferoxamine (Desferal) in an adult patient with acute iron overdosage. J Toxicol Clin Toxicol 1982;19:865–869.
112. Shannon M. Desferrioxamine in acute iron poisoning (Letter). Lancet 1992;339:1601.
113. Howland MA. Risks of parenteral deferoxamine for acute iron poisoning. J Toxicol Clin Toxicol 1996;34:491–497.
114. Tenenbein M, Kowalski S, Sienko A, et al. Pulmonary toxic effects of continuous desferrioxamine administration in acute iron poisoning. Lancet 1992;339:699–701.
115. Czajka PA, Konrad JD, Duffy JP. Iron poisoning: An in vitro comparison of bicarbonate and phosphate lavage solutions. J Pediatr 1981;98:491–494.

116. Gomez HF, McClafferty HH, Flory D, et al. Prevention of gastrointestinal iron absorption by chelation from an orally administered premixed deferoxamine/charcoal slurry. Ann Emerg Med 1997;30:587–592.
117. Berkovitch M, Livne A, Lushkov G, et al. The efficacy of oral deferiprone in acute iron poisoning. Am J Emerg Med 2000;18:36–40.
118. Stork CM, Howland MA, Goldfrank LR. Concepts and controversies of bronchodilator overdose. Emerg Med Clin North Am 1994; 12:415–436.
119. Shannon M. Theophylline: its rise, demise, and resurrection. Clin Pediatr Emerg Med 2000;1:217–221.
120. Shannon M. Life-threatening events after theophylline overdose: A 10-year prospective analysis. Arch Intern Med 1999;159:989–994.
121. Olson KR, Benowitz NL, Woo OF, Pond SM. Theophylline overdose: Acute single ingestion versus chronic repeated over medication. Am J Emerg Med 1985;3:386–394.
122. Shannon M, Lovejoy FH Jr. Effect of acute versus chronic intoxication on clinical features of theophylline poisoning in children. J Pediatr 1992;121:125–130.
123. American Academy of Pediatrics Committee on Drugs. Precautions concerning the use of theophylline. Pediatrics 1992;89:781–783.
124. Minton NA, Henry JA. Treatment of theophylline overdose. Am J Emerg Med 1996;14:606–612.
125. Shannon M, Lovejoy FH Jr. The influence of age versus peak serum concentration on life-threatening events after chronic theophylline intoxication. Arch Intern Med 1990;150:2045–2048.
126. Aitken ML, Martin TR. Life-threatening theophylline toxicity is not predictable by serum levels. Chest 1987;91:10–14.
127. Shannon MW. Comparative efficacy of hemodialysis and hemoperfusion in severe theophylline intoxication. Acad Emerg Med 1997;4:674–678.
128. Pimentel L, Trommer L. Cyclic antidepressant overdose: A review. Emerg Med Clin North Am 1994;12:533–547.
129. Pentel PR, Keyler DE, Haddad LM. Tricyclic antidepressants and selective serotonin reuptake inhibitors. In: Haddad LM, Shannon MW, Winchester JI, eds. Clinical Management of Poisoning and Drug Overdose, 3d ed. Philadelphia, Saunders, 1998:437–451.
130. James LP, Kearns GL. Cyclic antidepressant toxicity in children and adolescents. J Clin Pharmacol 1995;35:343–350.
131. Henry JA. Epidemiology and relative toxicity of antidepressant drugs in overdose. Drug Saf 1997;16:374–390.
132. Barbey JT, Roose SP. SSRI safety and overdose. J Clin Psychiatry 1998;59(Suppl 15):42–48.
133. Borys DJ, Setzer SC, Ling LJ, et al. Acute fluoxetine overdose: A report of 234 cases. Am J Emerg Med 1992;10:115–120.
134. Mills KC. Serotonin syndrome. Crit Care Clin 1997;13:763–783.
135. Corkeron MA. Serotonin syndrome: A potentially fatal complication of antidepressant therapy. Med J Aust 1995;163:481–482.
136. Spina E, Henthorn TK, Eleborg L, et al. Desmethylimipramine overdose: Nonlinear kinetics in a slow hydroxylator. Ther Drug Monit 1985;7:239–241.
137. Boehnert MT, Lovejoy FH. Value of QRS duration versus the serum drug level in predicting seizures and ventricular arrhthmias after an acute overdose of tricyclic antidepressants. N Engl J Med 1985;313:474–479.
138. Mitchell PB. Drug interactions of clinical significance with selective serotonin reuptake inhibitors. Drug Saf 1997;17:390–406.
139. Smilkstein MJ. Reviewing cyclic antidepressant cardiotoxicity: Wheat and chaff. J Emerg Med 1990;8:645–648.
140. McCabe JL, Cobaugh DJ, Mengazzi JJ, Fata J. Experimental tricyclic antidepressant toxicity: A randomized, controlled comparison of hypertonic saline solution, sodium bicarbonate, and hyperventilation. Ann Emerg Med 1998;32:329–333.
141. Shannon M. Toxicology reviews: physostigmine. Pediatr Emerg Care 1998;14:224–226.
142. Weinbroum AA, Flaishon R, Sorkine P. A risk-benefit assessment of flumazenil in the management of benzodiazepine overdose. Drug Saf 1997;17:181–196.
143. Jick SS, Dean AD, Jick H. Antidepressants and suicide. Br Med J 1995;310:215–218.

10
CARDIOVASCULAR TESTING

Margaret E. McGuinness and Robert L. Talbert

Cardiovascular (CVS) disease remains the leading cause of death in the United States. More than 50% of patients with ischemic heart disease (IHD) initially present with an acute myocardial infarction (AMI), and 50% of patients who suffer an AMI do not survive.[1] Although it may seem prudent to screen the population for CVS diseases such as IHD with the goal of reducing disease development, progression, and associated morbidities and mortality, currently there are no tests with adequate sensitivity or specificity or that have been shown to indeed have an impact disease outcomes. An awareness of symptoms of CVS disease and aggressive prevention and management of risk factors are more cost-effective than expensive diagnostic tests.

A plethora of tests exist to evaluate CVS disease. Four properties of the CVS system can be evaluated to provide diagnostic, prognostic, and therapeutic management information. These include (1) electrical conduction, (2) pump function, (3) myocardial perfusion and vasculature competence, and (4) anatomy.[2] Multiple test modalities are available to evaluate each of these functions. Selection of the most appropriate test is complex, due to overlap in available information from different tests, paucity of comparative data between tests, and "gold standards" that may not have been challenged by new technologies and drug therapies, making extrapolation of data difficult.[2,3] For example, myocardial perfusion can be evaluated using the gold standard angiography but also can be measured using echocardiography (ECHO), positron emission tomography (PET), computed tomographic (CT) scans, magnetic resonance imaging (MRI), and nuclear imaging, and it can be inferred from the exercise stress test (ET) and electrocardiogram (ECG). There is considerable debate as to how best to evaluate new tests, but for cost-effective use of tests, comparative head-to-head trials are essential. This chapter aims to outline each of the main groups of CVS testing modalities, highlight their advantages and disadvantages, give basic interpretation of results, and where possible, provide some comparative information. Tables 10–1 and 10–2 outline the use of different tests in CVS disease.

PATIENT INTERVIEW AND PHYSICAL EXAMINATION

In CVS disease, patient interview, history taking, and physical examination are the most important elements of patient assessment.[4–6] Technologically advanced tests can only be used effectively in conjunction with a complete physical examination and history.

The history and patient interview provide valuable insight into the patient's condition and help in the planning and interpreting of tests performed at a later date. History taking enables the examiner to establish a relationship with the patient and develop an awareness of the patient's perception of problems and quality of life and an assessment of problem acuity and severity. History taking covers elements such as chief complaint, present problems, past medical history, review of systems, and social and family history.

Primary signs and symptoms of CVS disease include chest pain, dyspnea with or without orthopnea, paroxysmal nocturnal dyspnea, cyanosis, fatigue, palpitations, cough, edema, and syncope.[4–6] During the interview and physical examination, identification and elucidation of characteristics and modulating factors for cardiac-related signs and symptoms are obtained.

PHYSICAL EXAMINATION

The CVS physical examination is divided into four categories:

1. Global examination of the patient for signs of CVS disease and a review of all body systems
2. Observation and assessment of physical findings (e.g., jugular venous pressure)
3. Measurement of parameters of CVS function (pulse, blood pressure)
4. Auscultation, percussion, and palpation of the chest and related cardiac structures.[4–6]

The initial part of the physical examination comprises inspection of the precordium for normal patterns of rise and fall and any abnormal markings or shape. The chest is then palpated for normal pulses, thrills (humming vibrations like the throat of a purring cat), and heaves (lifting of the chest wall). Thrills may indicate murmurs and heaves enlargement of one of the heart chambers or an abnormal vessel such as an aneurysm. The apical pulse [also known as the *point of maximum impulse* (PMI)] is helpful to estimate heart size and rotation. This is usually located in the fifth intercostal space, in the midsternal line, and radiates in an arc of 1 to 2 cm. Heightened intensity and/or displacement laterally suggests left or right ventricle enlargement, and reduced intensity may be a sign of fluid overload or pericardial effusion. Factors such as obesity, large breasts, muscularity, and pulmonary disease can interfere with determination of the apical pulse. The carotid pulse is examined for its intensity and, concurrently with the apical pulse, for concordance within the cardiac cycle. Decreased carotid pulsations may be due to reduced stroke volume or atherosclerotic narrowing of the carotid artery.

HEART SOUNDS

Auscultation with a stethoscope is used to characterize heart sounds. Auscultation is conducted in a systematic manner to ensure that all sites where normal and abnormal sounds are heard are reviewed

TABLE 10–1. Types of Tests Used to Evaluate the Cardiovascular System

	Cardiac Function[a]			
	Myocardial Perfusion	*Pump*	*Electrical Rhythm*	*Anatomy*
Type of test	Stress tests Nuclear imaging Angiography Echocardiography	Angiography MUGA Echocardiography	ECG Electrophysiologic studies Holter monitoring	Echocardiography Angiography Intravascular ultrasound Angioscopy
Parameters evaluated	Coronary anatomy and blood flow Myocardial perfusion	Cardiac output Ejection fraction Valvular function Shunts	Rhythm Rate Conduction pathways	Chamber size Wall motion Valve function Valve structure Pericardium Coronary anatomy

[a]Not all tests for any one cardiac function are used to evaluate all parameters listed.
MUGA = multigated acquisition; ECG = electrocardiogram.

(Fig. 10–1). Respiratory pattern, various maneuvers such as handgrip and the Valsalva maneuver, sitting versus standing, and pharmacologic agents (e.g., amyl nitrate) also may be used in the evaluation of heart sounds to accentuate or diminish the intensity of these sounds. Auscultation is an acquired art and requires considerable practice to become competent.

The normal heart sounds include S_1 (first heart sound) and S_2 (second heart sound) and occur with the closure of the mitral and tricuspid valves and the pulmonic and aortic valves, respectively. The sound of S_1 is thought to be generated by closure of the valvular leaflet. Other sounds, such as S_3 (third heart sound) and S_4 (fourth heart sound) and murmurs, are not considered normal but provide important diagnostic information.[4–6] Initially, the patient is examined lying partially on the left side to accentuate left-sided S_3 and S_4 and mitral murmurs, with the bell on the PMI. To identify S_1 and S_2, the patient can be examined lying or sitting. The other areas that are auscultated are the apex or base of the heart (mitral sounds), the lower left sternal border (tricuspid sounds), the second left interspace (pulmonic sounds), and the second right interspace (aortic sounds). At each of these locations, S_1 and S_2 should be heard.

Heart sounds are characterized by location, pitch, intensity, duration, and timing within the cardiac cycle. High-pitched sounds such as S_1 and S_2, murmurs of aortic and mitral regurgitation, and pericardial friction rubs are best heard with the diaphragm. The bell is preferred for low-pitched sounds such as S_3 and S_4. S_1 is heard as a click at the end of diastole and usually is synchronous with the apical pulse. The intensity of S_1 can be increased if systole begins prior to the mitral valve closing, which may occur in high output states (e.g., exercise, tachycardia, anemia, or hyperthyroidism) and mitral valve stenosis. S_1 intensity is decreased in first-degree heart block, mitral regurgitation, states of reduced myocardial contractility (such as heart failure or coronary artery disease), obesity (difficult to hear), and systemic or pulmonary hypertension. S_2 is heard at the end of systole and is best heard at the tricuspid and mitral areas. Most of the sound arises from aortic valve closure. Heart sounds may be "spilt" if the two valves do not close synchronously. Physiologic splitting of S_1 or S_2 is accentuated by inspiration and may disappear with expiration. Splitting of S_2 creates a pulmonic (P_2) and aortic (A_2) sound. S_2 frequently is heard as a split sound and is most predominant at the height of inspiration. Although S_1 also may be split, this is often difficult to hear.

Pathologic splitting of S_2 during expiration is described as *wide splitting, fixed splitting*, and *paradoxical splitting* and may be indicative of both stenosis and regurgitation. With right-sided heart failure, right bundle-branch block, pulmonic stenosis, or atrial septal defects, S_2 may be split due to delayed closure of the pulmonic valve. Fixed splitting of S_2 is associated with large atrial septal defects and right ventricular failure. Increased intensity of P_2 is seen in pulmonary

TABLE 10–2. Types of Tests for Various Cardiac Disorders or Features

Feature/Disorder	CXR	Echo	Angiography	Nuclear Scan	CT	MRI	ET	ECG	PET
Ischemic	—	+++	++++	+++	++/+++[a]	++	++	++	+++
Valvular	+	++++	+++	+	+++	+++	++	+	+
Congential	++	++++	+++	+	+++	++++	+	+	+
Anatomy	+	+++	++	+	+++	++++	—	+	+
Cardiomyopathy	+	++++	+++	++	+++	+++	—	—	++
Pericardial	+	++++	++	—	++++	++++	—	±	—
Endocarditis	—	++++[b]	+	—	++	+++	—	±	—
Masses	—	++++	+	—	+++	+++	—	—	+
Metabolism	—	—	—	+	—	—	—	—	++++
Graft patency	—	±	+++	++	+	++	++	+	+++
CA anatomy	—	—	++++	++	+	++	++	+	+
Ventricular function	—	++++	+++	++	+++	+++	+	—	++

CXR = chest x-ray; echo = echocardiography; CT = computed tomography; MRI = magnetic resonance imaging; ET = exercise testing; ECG = electrocardiogram; PET = positron emission tomography; CA = coronary artery.
[a]Ultrafast or cine-CT may be very useful in detecting ischemia based on calcium deposition.
[b]Transesophageal echocardiography is superior to transthoracic echocardiography.

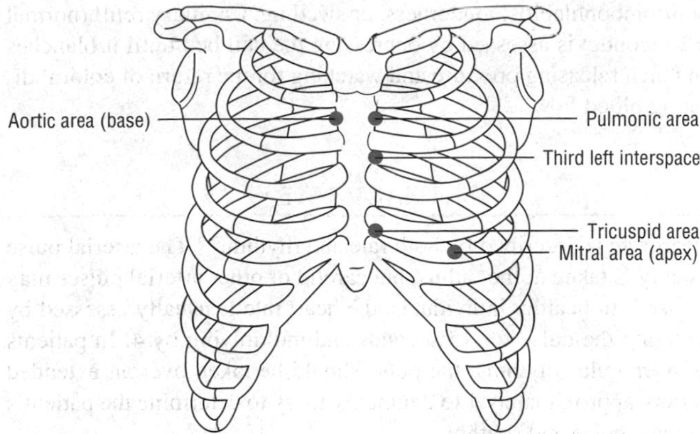

FIGURE 10–1. Schematic illustration of topographic areas on the precordium for cardiac auscultation. Auscultatory areas do not correspond to anatomic locations of the valves but to the sites at which particular valves are heard best. *(Redrawn from Kinney MR, Packa DR, eds. Andreoli's Comprehensive Cardiac Care, 8th ed. St. Louis: Mosby-Year Book, 1996, with permission.)*

hypertension and dilated pulmonary arteries and with atrial septal defects. Decreased or absent P_2 occurs with aging and in pulmonic stenosis. Extra heart sounds in systole include early systolic ejection sounds and clicks and midsystolic clicks. Early ejection sounds such as aortic or pulmonic ejection sounds are often associated with valvular disease. Midsystolic to late systolic clicks are usually due to mitral valve prolapse (MVP). MVP is best heard at or medial to the apex but also may be heard at the left lower sternal border.

The S_3 heart sound, or ventricular gallop, is an abnormal low-pitched sound, usually heard at the apex of the heart. It is thought to be due to rapid filling and stretching of the left ventricle when the left ventricle is somewhat noncompliant. This heart sound is characteristic of volume overloading such as in congestive heart failure (especially left-sided heart failure), tricuspid or mitral valve insufficiency, and atrial and/or ventricular septal defects. A physiologic S_3 is heard commonly in children and may persist into young adulthood. Localization of S_3 is helpful for determining heart rotation within the chest cavity.

The S_4 diastolic sound is a dull, low-pitched postsystolic atrial gallop (rapid blood flow), usually due to reduced ventricular compliance. It is best heard at the apex in the left lateral position. Like S_3, it occurs with reduced ventricular compliance and is present in conditions such as aortic stenosis, hypertension, hypertrophic cardiomyopathies, and coronary artery disease. It is less specific for congestive heart failure than S_3.

HEART MURMURS

Murmurs are auditory vibrations heard on auscultation, and they occur because of turbulent blood flow within the heart chambers or through the valves.[5,6] They are classified by timing and duration within the cardiac cycle (systolic, diastolic, and continuous), location, intensity, shape (configuration or pattern), pitch (frequency), quality, and radiation (Table 10–3).

Some murmurs are considered innocent or physiologic and result from rapid, turbulent flow of blood into the left ventricle during atrial systole and through the aorta during ventricular systole. Fever, anxiety, anemia, hyperthyroidism, and pregnancy exacerbate physiologic murmurs, and these murmurs need to be distinguished from those suggestive of valvular abnormalities.

As with heart sounds, accurate determination of murmurs requires practice. The intensity or loudness of a murmur is graded using a scale of grade I to VI. Grade I is so faint that it is heard only with special effort. Grade VI may be heard with the stethoscope just off the chest wall. Determinants of the grade include the amount of blood ejected across a valve, severity of the lesion, and chest anatomy.

Systolic murmurs begin with or after S_1 and end at or before S_2 depending on the origin of the murmur. They are classified based on time of onset and termination within systole: midsystolic, holosystolic (pansystolic), early, or late. Pathologic midsystolic murmurs are associated with pulmonic stenosis, aortic stenosis, and hypertrophic cardiomyopathy. Midsystolic murmurs include obstruction to ventricular outflow, dilatation of the aortic root or pulmonary trunk, an increased flow in the great arteries, anatomic changes in the semilunar valves, and some forms of regurgitation. Holosystolic murmurs occur when blood flows from a chamber of higher pressure to one of lower pressure, such as with mitral or tricuspid regurgitation and ventricular septal defects. Early systolic murmurs are decrescendo and may be associated with ventricular septal defects, mitral regurgitation, or tricuspid regurgitation. A late systolic murmur preceded by one or more midsystolic to late systolic clicks is the hallmark of MVP. Atherosclerotic obstruction of the carotid, subclavicular, or iliofemoral artery can give rise to a crescendo-decrescendo extracardiac systolic arterial murmur.

Early diastolic murmurs commonly are heard with aortic regurgitation. This murmur begins with A_2 and generally is decrescendo, reflecting the progressive decline in volume and rate of regurgitant flow during diastole. Aortic regurgitation is best heard by having the patient lean forward while holding his or her breath and listening with the diaphragm at the midleft sternal border. Pulmonary hypertension (Graham Steell's murmur) also may cause an early diastolic murmur. Middiastolic murmurs occur across the atrioventricular valves during rapid filling and are consistent with pure mitral stenosis or mitral

TABLE 10–3. Characteristics of Heart Sounds

Type of Murmur	Examples	Location	Pitch	Radiation	Quality
Midsystolic	Aortic stenosis	2nd RICS	Medium	Neck, left sternal border	Harsh
	Pulmonic stenosis	2nd and 3rd LICS	Medium	Left shoulder and neck	Harsh
	Hypertrophic cardiomyopathy	3rd and 4th LICS	Medium	Left sternal border to apex	Harsh
Pansystolic	Mitral regurgitation	Apex	Medium to high	Left axilla	Blowing
	Tricuspid regurgitation	Lower left sternal border	Medium	Right sternum, xiphoid	Blowing
	Ventricular septal defect	3rd, 4th, and 5th LICS	High		Often harsh
Diastolic	Aortic regurgitation	2nd to 4th LICS	High	Apex	Blowing
	Mitral stenosis	Apex	Low	Little or none	

RICS = right intercostal space; LICS = left intercostal space.

stenosis along with a ventricular septal defect or tricuspid regurgitation with an atrial septal defect. The Austin Flint murmur may be middiastolic or presystolic and results from antegrade flow across the mitral valve that is closing rapidly because of simultaneous left ventricular filling from aortic regurgitation. Continuous murmurs begin in systole and continue without interruption into all or part of diastole. Such murmurs are due mainly to aortopulmonary connections (e.g., patent ductus arteriosus), arteriovenous connections (e.g., arteriovenous fistula, coronary artery fistula), and disturbances of flow patterns in arteries or veins.

Anatomic correlation of murmurs may require cardiac catheterization or ECHO, where direct visualization of the blood flow abnormality and calculation of flow and chamber pressures can be obtained. PET and MRI are also possible options to evaluate flow patterns and gradients of murmurs across heart valves.

JUGULAR VENOUS PRESSURE

The jugular venous pressure (JVP) is used as a measure of right atrial pressure.[5,6] The JVP is measured in centimeters from the sternal angle and is best visualized with the patient's head rotated to the left. The JVP is described for its quality and character, effects of respiration, and patient position-induced changes. When reporting a JVP, both the measure and the patient position must be reported. The JVP can be reported as actual centimeters above the manubrium, or this value plus 5 to 7 cm to indicate the rise of the JVP above the right ventricle. For persons in whom the central venous pressure (CVP) is normal, JVP is observed in the right internal jugular vein with the patient supine at 30 degrees or less. In the presence of an elevated CVP, the JVP is measured at 60 to 90 degrees. In patients with poor myocardial function, the accuracy of the JVP as a measure of CVP is reduced, and is best measured directly by means of a Swan-Ganz catheter.

The normal JVP is a *v* wave 1 to 2 cm above the sternal ridge. If it is greater than halfway to the jaw angle, there is elevated CVP. Both the degree of elevation of the JVP and its wave flow in conjunction with the heart beat are noted. The first wave, or *a* wave, represents atrial contraction and occurs just prior to S_1, giving rise to an increased pressure. It is seen as an undulating pulsation in the internal jugular vein. The second and much larger wave, the *v* wave, represents the increased venous pressure that occurs during venous filling. To interpret the JVP accurately, the carotid pulse is palpated concurrently. The *a* wave occurs just before the pulse and the *v* wave just after.

PERIPHERAL CIRCULATION AND ARTERIAL PULSES

Arterial pulses are evaluated and characterized bilaterally by observation, palpation, and auscultation for presence, character, pattern, and rhythm.[4–6] Various arterial pulse patterns are described: pulsus alterans (variation in amplitude beat to beat), bisferans pulse (increased arterial pulse with a double systolic peak), bigeminal pulse (reduced amplitude associated with premature ventricular beats), and paradoxical pulse (decrease in amplitude with inspiration). Although each may be associated with certain disorders (e.g., bigeminal pulse in premature ventricular contractions), none is sensitive or specific enough to be diagnostic. The status of the patient's overall peripheral circulation is recorded, especially the presence and degree of edema or skin changes suggestive of venous or arterial insufficiency. Color, condition, and integrity of the skin are also recorded, including signs of thrombophlebitis, tenderness, or swelling. Capillary refill (normal <2 seconds) is assessed by depressing the nail bed until it blanches and then releasing pressure and watching for the return of color indicating blood flow.

HEART RATE

Heart rate is described by both rate and rhythm.[5,6] The arterial pulse usually is taken at the radius, but carotid or other arterial pulses may be used. In healthy individuals, the heart rate is usually assessed by counting the pulse for 15 seconds and multiplying by 4. In patients with irregular rhythms, the pulse should be taken over an extended period, approximately 1 to 2 minutes, to try to determine the patient's average pulse and rhythm.

Arterial pulses are an accurate measure of the ventricular rate in the healthy person with good ventricular function. In patients with a rapid ventricular rate—because of supraventricular tachyarrhythmias such as atrial flutter or fibrillation or rapid ventricular rates (e.g., ventricular tachycardia or premature ventricular beats)—extremity pulses (e.g., radial pulse) may be considerably slower than the true ventricular rate. A more accurate ventricular rate is determined by listening to the ventricles with the stethoscope (usually at the apex) or counting from an ECG. In patients with atrial fibrillation and a fast ventricular rate, a pulse deficit (measure of the difference in true ventricular rate and peripheral pulse rate) may exist. This may be as much as 10 to 20 beats per minute. Thus the location of the recorded pulse (radial or apical) should be recorded. The pulse deficit will be reduced as the ventricular rate is controlled with drug therapy or normal sinus rhythm is restored.

PRACTICE GUIDELINES FOR DIAGNOSTIC AND PROGNOSTIC TESTING IN CVS TESTING

The American Heart Association (AHA) and American College of Cardiology (ACC) task force on practice guidelines publishes guidelines as to the recommended uses for many diagnostic testing methods. Such guidelines were first developed in the 1980 and are updated as more information is available. These are evidence-based recommendations that rank the indications and uses of tests into three primary classes. Class I indications are those where there is evidence or agreement that the specific procedure is useful and effective. Class II indications are those situations where there is divergence of opinion as to the usefulness of the method. Class III indications are those where there is evidence or agreement that a diagnostic test is not useful. Each class (usually class II) may be broken down into two to three subcategories. Class IIa indications are those where there is evidence or opinion in favor of the test, whereas class IIb indications are those situations where there is less evidence. With each class of recommendation for a specific clinical scenario, the guidelines will indicate the level of evidence for the recommendation. Level A evidence is given if the recommendation is based on the availability of multiple randomized clinical trials Level B evidence is where only a single randomized trial or multiple nonrandomized trials exist. Level C evidence is awarded if the recommendation is afforded based on expert opinion only.

Each guideline provides a preamble to indicate how it was constructed and the peer review process. These documents provide the clinician with an extensive database on the testing methodologies and are endorsed by both organizations as acceptable standards of practice.

TESTING MODALITIES

CHEST X-RAY

The chest x-ray (CXR) provides supplemental information to the physical examination and is usually the first diagnostic test in a cardiac workup.[4–6] It does not provide details of internal cardiac structures but gives global information about position and size of the heart and chambers and surrounding anatomy. The standard CXRs for evaluation of lungs and heart are standing posteroanterior (PA) and lateral views taken at maximal inspiration. Portable CXRs usually are less satisfactory due to penetration difficulties, patient rotation, and poor inspiratory effort.

Initial assessment of the CXR evaluates the quality of the film for patient rotation, inspiratory effort, and penetration. Rotation is assessed by evaluating symmetry of the clavicles and central placement of the carina. Inspiratory effect is considered adequate if the diaphragms are pulled below the ninth rib. Lack of inspiratory effort and obesity lead to a poor-quality CXR. These make it more difficult to assess the presence of pleural effusions and fluid in the costophrenic angles. Where possible, comparison with previous or baseline films is done to determine the quality of film and comparison of structures.

The PA CXR outlines the superior vena cava, right atrium on the right and left sides, aortic knob, main pulmonary artery, left atrial appendage (especially if enlarged), and left ventricle. In the lateral view, the CXR visualizes the right ventricle, inferior vena cava, and left ventricle. These structures are visualized as shadows of differing density rather than discrete structures (Fig. 10–2).

The CXR is approached from two perspectives: (1) observation and (2) clinical correlation. Observation notes gross anatomic features such as size and placement of the cardiac silhouette, definition of the cardiac border, chamber enlargement, pulmonary vasculature, air-fluid levels, and diaphragm. Cardiac enlargement is determined by the cardiothoracic (CT) ratio, which is the maximal transverse diameter of the heart divided by the maximal transverse diameter of the thorax of a PA view. Normal averages 0.45, but it may be up to 0.55 in subjects with large stroke volumes (e.g., highly trained athletes). Heart conditions such as congestive heart failure or hypertension may enlarge the heart and so the CT ratio. Individual chamber enlargement can be seen on the CXR. Right ventricle enlargement is best seen on the lateral film, where the heart appears to occupy the retrosternal space. Left atrial enlargement is suspected if there is elevation of the left bronchus or an increase in the atrial appendage bulge. Left ventricular enlargement is the most common feature identified on CXR and is seen as an elongation and downward displacement of the apex of the heart. Sometimes a characteristic "boot" or "water bottle" outline is seen with left ventricular enlargement as in congestive heart failure (CHF).

The pulmonary vessels are examined for plumpness and definition of vessel walls. Decreased pulmonary flow (e.g., tetralogy of Fallot) causes central and peripheral vessels to be decreased in size. Increased pulmonary flow is associated with high output states such as hyperthyroidism and atrial septal defects. This may lead to enlargement and tortuosity of the central and peripheral vessels. Pulmonary arterial hypertension (increased pulmonary resistance) is identified by enlargement of the central vessels and diminished peripheral vessels. Pulmonary venous hypertension usually is due to mitral stenosis or left ventricular failure. This is characterized by larger than normal vessels in the upper lung zones due to recruitment of upper vessels from blood diverted from the lower constricted vessels (cephalization of flow).

Heart failure causes Kerley's B lines (edema of interlobular septa), which appear as thin, horizontal reticular lines in the costophrenic angles. At higher pressures, alveolar edema and pleural effusions appear in the pleural space or as blunting of the costophrenic angles. Pericardial effusions also may appear as a large heart, but because it usually occurs rapidly, there is no evidence of pulmonary venous congestion.

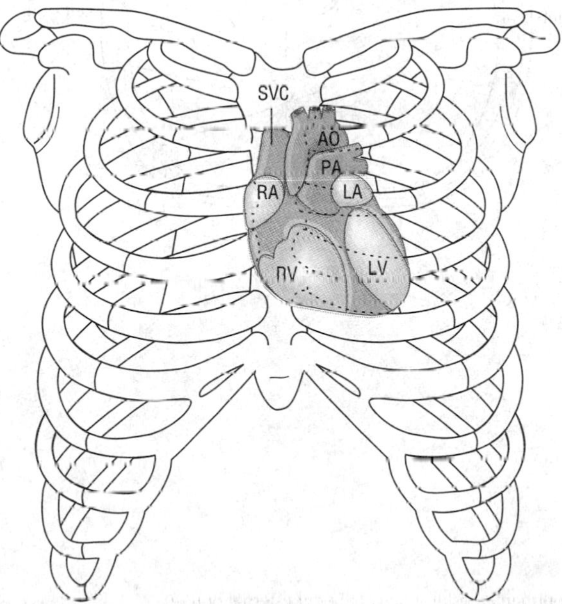

FIGURE 10–2. Schematic illustration of the parts of the heart. (AO = aorta; SVC = superior vena cava; RA = right atrium; PA = pulmonary artery; LA = left atrium; RV = right ventricle; LV = left ventricle.) *(Redrawn from Kinney MR, Packa DR, eds. Andreoli's Comprehensive Cardiac Care, 8th ed. St. Louis: Mosby Year Book, 1996, with permission.)*

ELECTROCARDIOGRAM (ECG)

Measurement of electrical activity in the heart, now known as the ECG, was introduced about 75 years ago by Willem Einthoven. The ECG is simple to perform and is the most frequently used, least invasive, and cheapest cardiovascular test.[7–10] It remains the procedure of first choice for evaluation of chest pain, dizziness, or syncope. In its simplest interpretation, the ECG characterizes rhythms and conduction abnormalities. However, the ECG also provides, by inference, information about the anatomy and structures of the heart, pathophysiologic changes, and hemodynamics of the CVS system.[3,8] ECG abnormalities are often the earliest sign of adverse drug effects, ischemia, and electolyte abnormalities.

Although few ECG recordings are highly specific or sensitive to a disease state, correlation of findings with clinical and pathologic states affords the ECG significant diagnostic and prognostic capabilities. Sensitivity and specificity of ECG changes depend primarily on the clinical setting, recording technique, and skill of interpreters. Sensitivity and specificity of findings are increased by interpretation in conjunction with patient information such as age, gender, medical history, and medications. Additionally, prior and/or serial ECGs should be obtained for comparison prior to identifying new findings on a current ECG as diagnostic. This is particularly important in patients with significant cardiac disease or on medications that alter the ECG (Table 10–4). The ECG is sensitive to detect rhythm abnormalities, but it does not record the actual activity of the conduction tissue.[7–9]

The AHA/ACC task force report from 1992 recommend ECGs as a tool for baseline and follow-up for responses to interventions in patients with known CVS disease. The ECG can be used to evaluate ischemia following angioplasty or other surgical interventions and to monitor responses to antiarrhythmic agents or in patients receiving drugs with potential cardiac effects. Refer to Table 10.5 for examples of conditions for which the ECG is a recommended evaluation tool.

Electrocardiography is based on the measurement of change in summated three-dimensional electrical vectors or forces that result from depolarization and repolarization of cells in the conduction system and heart muscle. The standard external 12-lead ECG uses two sets of leads: limb and chest (Fig. 10–3) The 6 limb leads look at the heart in a single frontal plane. Limb lead nomenclature is as follows: lead I, right arm/left arm; lead II, right arm/left leg; lead III, left arm/left leg. Altering resistances create the augmented limb leads, which are called aVR, aVL, and aVF. Unipolar chest leads are positioned across the chest and labeled V_1 to V_6. V_1 is positioned slightly to the right of the midline, and V_6 is positioned in the left midaxillary line (Fig. 10–4). Leads aVR and V_1 are considered right-sided leads, so they appear inverted, and leads aVL, I, II, and $V_{5,6}$ are left-sided leads, so they appear upright on the ECG. Leads II, III, and aVF are inferior leads. Leads V_1 to V_4 are anterior wall leads. Single-lead ECGs or ECG monitors frequently use lead II.

Recording of the ECG has several standard features. The paper is divided into squares of 1 mm; each 10 mm (10 small boxes) is equivalent to 1 mV. Paper speed is 25 mm/s. Each small box on the tracing paper equals 0.04 second (40 ms), and each big box is

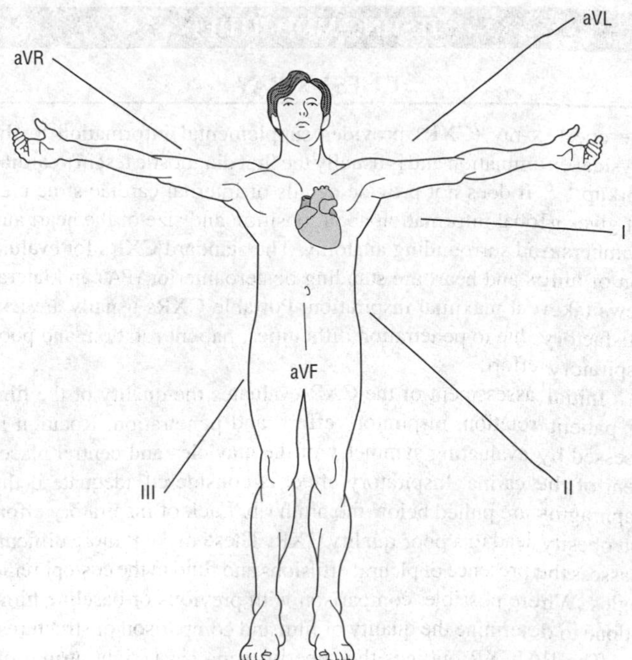

FIGURE 10–3. The torso with the 6 limb leads in a single frontal plane.

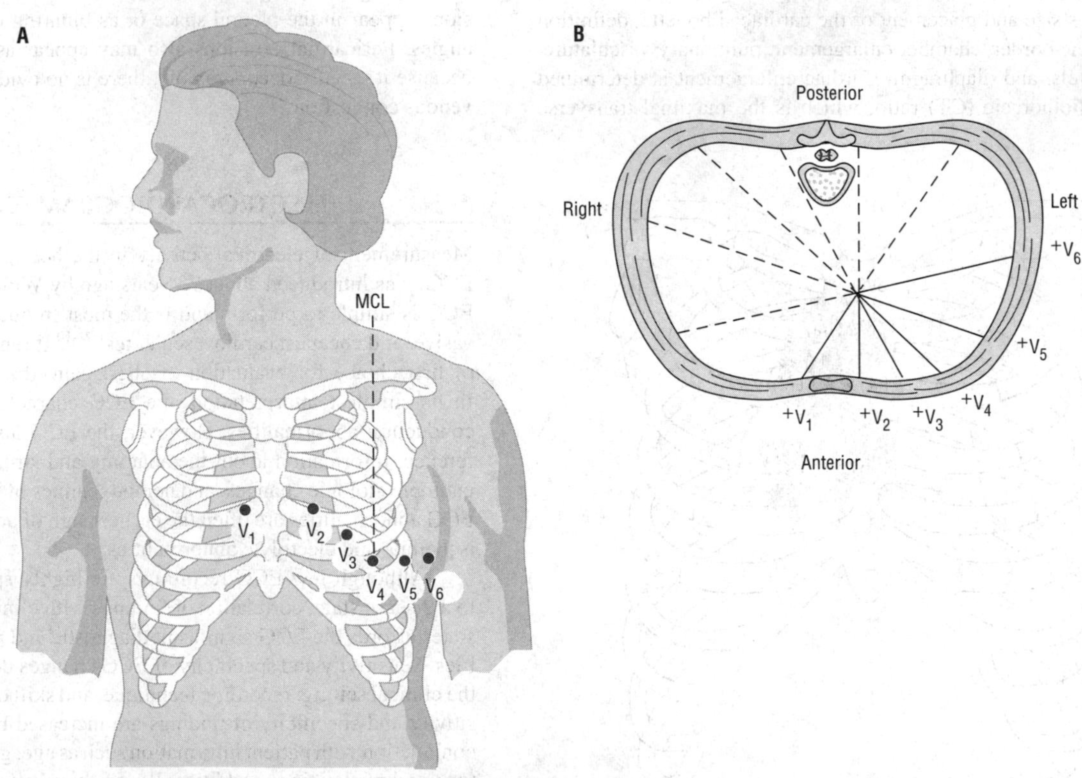

FIGURE 10–4. A. Electrode positions of the precordial leads (V_1 = fourth intercostal space at the right sternal border; V_2 = fourth intercostal space at the left sternal border; V_3 = halfway between V_2 and V_4; V_4 = fifth intercostal space at the midclavicular line; V_5 = anterior axillary line directly lateral to V_4; V_6 = anterior axillary space directly lateral to V_5.) **B.** The precordial reference figure. Leads V_1 and V_2 are called right-sided precordial leads; leads V_3 and V_4, midprecordial leads; and leads V_5 and V_6, left-sided precordial leads. *(Redrawn from Kinney MR, Packa DR, eds. Andreoli's Comprehensive Cardiac Care, 8th ed. St. Louis: Mosby-Year Book, 1996, with permission.)*

0.2 second. If there is one QRS complex per 6 big boxes (6 × 0.20 seconds), the patient has a heart rate of 50 beats per minute, whereas one QRS per big box indicates a heart rate of 300 beats per minute.

The ECG pattern is named alphabetically and is read from left to right, beginning with the P wave. Electrical activation (depolarization) of the right and then the left atrium due to discharge from the sinoatrial (SA) nodes causes an upward or positive deflection in lead II called the *P wave*. The normal duration of the P wave is up to 0.12 second, and it has an amplitude of 0.25 mV (i.e., 2.5 small boxes). The *PR segment* is created by passage of the impulse through the atrioventricular (AV) node and the bundle of His and its branches, and it has a duration of 0.12 to 0.21 second. The *QRS complex* primarily traces the electrical depolarization of the ventricles. Initially, there is a negative deflection, the *Q wave,* followed by a positive deflection, the *R wave,* and finally a negative deflection, the *S wave.* Q-wave duration is normally 0.4 second or less, and the amplitude is 25% or less of the overall height of the QRS complex. Normal duration of the QRS complex is 0.12 second. The QRS complex is positive in left-sided leads and negative in right-sided leads because the left ventricle is much thicker than the right, and the forces going left during depolarization dominate.

Following the QRS complex is a plateau phase called the *ST segment,* which extends from the end of the QRS complex (called the *J point*) to the beginning of the T wave. The ST segment is evaluated from its position relevant to the baseline, configuration, and leads where changes occur. The ST segment is normally on or slightly above the baseline. Configuration changes, convexity upward or downward, identify the presence of myocardial ischemia. Lead localization of ST-segment changes indicates the area of ischemia. The *QT interval* is measured from the start of the QRS complex to the end of the T wave. This varies with heart rate and is corrected (QTc) for heart rates greater than 60 beats per minute. The normal corrected QT is less than 0.42 seconds in men and 0.43 seconds in women.

Repolarization of the ventricle leads to the *T wave.* The T wave usually goes in the same direction as the QRS complex. The normal axis of the ECG is 30 degrees (above the horizontal) to +110 degrees (away from the horizontal (Fig. 10–5).

The ECG is evaluated in a systematic manner to avoid omission of important characteristics. All ECGs are interpreted for the following elements: rate, general rhythm, intervals, voltage, axis, waveforms, abnormal features (e.g., Q waves), and technical aspects such as adequacy of lead placement and calibration.[8] The number of P waves and QRS complexes (*RR interval*) is also used to determine rate. QRS complexes may be more useful if heart block exists. The rhythm from the ECG is identified by the following features:

1. The rate of the QRS (>100/min is tachycardia, and <60/min is bradycardia)
2. The regularity of the QRS [the presence or absence of the QRS complex with each P wave helps identify if the rhythm is atrial or ventricular in origin and if each atrial beat (P wave) is being conducted to the ventricles. The regularity of the QRS identifies conditions such as atrial fibrillation and extra beats]
3. Configuration of the QRS—wide or narrow—indicating if it is generated from electrical activity that arose in the atria or ventricles

Always reported are the RR, PR, QRS, and QT intervals and the duration, magnitude, and configuration of the P waves, QRS complexes, ST segments, T waves, and U waves. Computer interpretation of the ECG provides a standardized reading and records and calculates basic rhythm patterns, heart rate, and intervals but does not interpret arrhythmias. Independent review of the ECG is necessary for accurate translation of findings.[8]

In epidemiologic studies, the ECG is used to assess physical fitness, document the prevalence of IHD, and identify subclinical heart disease. The sensitivity and specificity of ECG changes are highly dependent on the pretest probability of heart disease. As the pretest probability of heart disease increases, the sensitivity and specificity of ECG findings increases. The use and value of the ECG as a screening tool are controversial. It is only used where the diagnosis of heart disease would preclude active employment, such as in airline pilots. The ECG frequently is used in conjunction with other diagnostic tests to provide additional data, to monitor the patient, and to identify if abnormalities detected during tests correlate with ECG changes.[7,8,10]

Gating, or linkage of and simultaneous recording of an ECG and other diagnostic tests, such as ECHO and CT scans, allows for

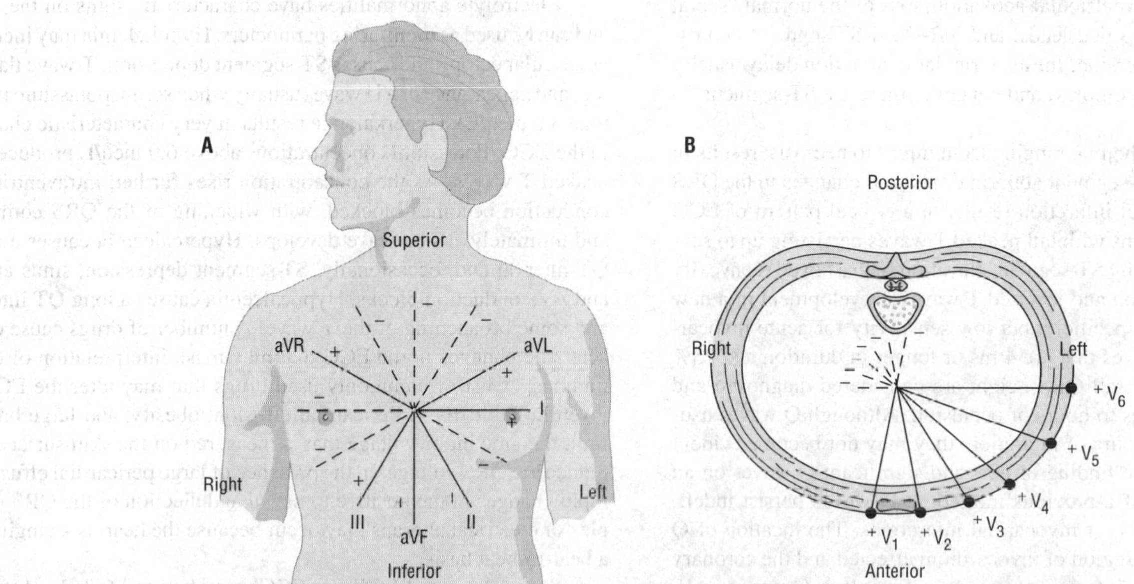

FIGURE 10–5. The 6 frontal plane (A) and the 6 horizontal plane (B) leads provide a three-dimensional representation of cardiac electrical activity. *(Redrawn from Ref. 7 with permission.)*

correlation of images with the cardiac cycle. Gating is either prospective, where a certain portion of the cardiac cycle is predetermined as the time during which the images are obtained, or retrospective, where the ECG and image are recorded simultaneously but independently and later matched for concurrent events. This allows multiple cardiac cycles to be overlayed, thus increasing the sensitivity to detect abnormalities.

Anomalies on the ECG include abnormal intervals, altered waveform configurations, and rate variability. Other findings give evidence for various forms of heart block, ischemia, infarction, atrial and ventricular enlargement and hypertrophy, atrial and ventricular rhythm disorders, pericarditis, metabolic abnormalities, drug-induced changes, and pacemaker-related changes. ECG patterns found on consecutive leads can help identify where a particular conduction defect or impulse generation is occurring or anatomic problem is located. For example, ST-segment elevation in V_2 to V_6 is indicative of anterior wall myocardial infarction from occlusion of the left anterior descending coronary artery. Single-lead abnormalities most frequently are attributed to poor lead placement, position of the patient, or recording artifacts.

Examples of some common findings will be briefly discussed.[7,8] Short PR intervals are associated with the Wolff-Parkinson-White and Lown-Ganong-Levine syndromes and reflect the presence of accessory pathways. Long PR intervals are measures of heart block. The presence of a Q wave is a marker for loss of electrically functioning myocardium and suggests a prior myocardial infarction. It also may be present in congenital heart disorders, hypertrophic cardiomyopathy, left ventricular hypertrophy, conduction defects such as Wolff-Parkinson-White syndrome, and intraventricular conduction defects. U waves are relatively nonspecific, the most common cause being hypertension. Bundle-branch blocks are frequent findings and indicate conduction defects in one of the bundles of His. Their presence confounds the interpretation of important ECG findings such as ischemia. Right bundle-branch block is associated with an R wave and the following abnormalities: QRS complex greater than or equal to 12 ms, delayed right ventricular forces resulting in terminal R waves in the right-sided leads and S wave in the left-sided lead, and right-sided ST-segment depression and T-wave inversion. Left bundle-branch block is characterized by the following: QRS complex greater than or equal to 12 ms, delayed left ventricular activation, loss of the normal "septal Q wave" in the left-sided leads, and left-sided ST-segment depression and T-wave inversion. Intraventricular conduction delay usually causes a wide QRS complex, and generally there are ST-segment–T-wave abnormalities.

Myocardial ischemia, ranging from injury to necrosis, results in T-wave changes, ST-segment abnormalities, and changes in the QRS complex. Myocardial infarction results in a typical pattern of ECG changes, which begins with tall peaked T waves persisting up to several hours, followed by ST-segment elevation with a coved (convexity upward) configuration and inverted T waves. Development of a new Q wave has a high specificity but low sensitivity for acute myocardial ischemia. Q waves that are 4 ms or longer in duration and 25% or greater of the overall QRS height are considered diagnostic and occur within minutes to hours of occlusion. Although Q waves usually evolve within hours of infarction, they may not become evident for several days. The finding of new and significant Q waves on an ECG is indicative of a previous infarction. Q waves persist indefinitely in 80% to 90% of myocardial infarctions. The location of Q waves identifies the region of myocardium affected and the coronary artery blocked (e.g., inferior infarction will result in Q waves in II, III, and aVF, associated with blockage in the right coronary artery). Non-Q-wave (subendocardial) myocardial infarction implies that the Q wave does not meet the diagnostic criteria for Q-wave infarction. ST-segment depression may be present.

ST-segment changes are very common and always should be compared with a previous ECG. ST-segment elevation may be seen in persons with no known coronary disease but is usually indicative of hyperacute ischemia. ST-segment depression is never considered a normal finding. ST-segment scooping (convexity downward) may be normal, but coving (convexity upward) is abnormal. Depression of the ST segment that does not return quickly to normal and changes in multiple leads suggest clinically significant heart disease. Diffuse ST-segment elevation in all leads except V_1 and aVR suggests the diagnosis of pericarditis. Exertion in normal individuals may cause J-point depression with a rapid rise of the ST segment, and this may be confused with ST-segment depression due to the configuration. Poor R-wave progression (usually increase in size moving from V_1 to V_6) suggests anterior myocardial infarction, but smaller R waves also can occur in diseases such as chronic obstructive pulmonary disease. T-wave changes are the most frequent and most sensitive abnormality on the ECG but are also the least specific and frequently are found in persons with no heart disease.

Left atrial enlargement is characterized by a P wave that is 12 mV in lead II, or the negative component of the biphasic P is 4 mV in duration and 0.1 mV in depth in lead V_1. In right atrial enlargement, the P wave in lead II can exceed 0.25 mV and usually has a vertical axis. Ventricular hypertrophy results in increased deflection of the QRS complex because of the increased muscle mass. Left ventricular hypertrophy (LVH) is diagnosed from the ECG using several different sets of criteria; none is considered highly sensitive or specific. LVH often is indicative of hypertension and resulting ventricular enlargement and strain. Voltage criteria indicating LVH commonly used are summation of the S wave in V_1 and the R wave in V_5 or the S wave in V_2 and the R wave in V_6, which exceeds 3.5 mV (35 small boxes), or the R wave in lead aVL, which exceeds 1.1 mV (11 small boxes). Right ventricular hypertrophy (RVH) is characterized by an R wave in V_1 that is equal to or greater than the S wave in that lead. In persons who are obese, increased voltage may not be apparent, making voltage criteria a less useful tool to identify hypertrophy. LVH also may be assessed using ECHO.

Electrolyte abnormalities have characteristic signs on the ECG and can be used as monitoring parameters. Hypokalemia may increase ventricular ectopy and causes ST-segment depression, T-wave flattening, and appearance of a U wave (usually when serum potassium is less than 3.0 meq/L). Hyperkalemia results in very characteristic changes in the ECG. Potassium concentrations above 6.0 meq/L produce tall, peaked T waves. As the concentration rises further, intraventricular conduction becomes blocked, with widening of the QRS complex, and ultimately, a sine wave develops. Hypercalcemia causes a short QT interval and, occasionally, ST-segment depression, sinus arrest, and AV conduction blocks. Hypocalcemia causes a long QT interval and some broadening of the T wave. A number of drugs cause characteristic changes in the ECG that may mask interpretation of other findings. A list of commonly used drugs that may alter the ECG is given in Table 10–4. Pericardial effusion, obesity, and large breasts limit the amount of voltage that is measured on the skin surface and reduce the QRS voltage. In the presence of large pericardial effusions, rapid changes in the positive to negative deflection of the QRS complex or electrical alterans may occur because the heart is swinging on a beat-to-beat basis.

Signal-averaged ECG (SAECG) may be used to help elucidate the presence of low-amplitude bioelectric potentials. Derangements

TABLE 10–4. Drugs That May Affect the Electrocardiogram

Digoxin	Pentamidine
Antiarrhythmics—classes I–IV	Lithium
Tricyclic antidepressants	Catecholamines (e.g., dopamine, albuterol)
H_1 antagonists (e.g., astemizole)	Diuretics (electrolyte abnormalities)
Methylxanthines	
Doxorubicin	

of ventricular activation and late potentials can be detected in the ECG after the QRS and ST segments and are thought to be associated with increased risk of ventricular arrhythmias. Traditional ECGs are unable to detect these potentials because they are "lost" in the noise of the ECG recording. SAECG improves the signal-to-noise ratio, enabling the low-amplitude potentials to be interpreted. SAECG can be used to identify patients at risk for developing sustained ventricular tachycardia after myocardial infarction. Patients with IHD and unexplained syncope who are at risk for sustained ventricular tachycardia also may be candidates for SAECG. Other potential uses of SAECG include patients with nonischemic cardiomyopathy with sustained ventricular tachycardia, detection of acute rejection of heart transplant, and assessing proarrthymia potential of antiarrhythmic drug therapy.

AMBULATORY ECG MONITORING

Ambulatory ECG monitoring (AEM), or Holter monitoring, named for its inventor, is an aid to detect, document, characterize, and evaluate arrhythmias and other ECG abnormalities over extended periods of time. AEM provides information regarding random abnormal cardiac electrical activity during daily activity and helps relate altered electrical activity to precipitating factors and patient symptomatology. Additionally, some findings on AEM have been used to confer prognostic implications.

Although controversial, AEM is used as a diagnostic and screening tool for asymptomatic ischemia. It is difficult to interpret changes in the ST segment recorded during AEM due to amplitude; and definitions of significant changes recorded with AEM are still in evolution. As a prognostic tool, it is used primarily to evaluate patients with known CVS disease who have symptoms that may be associated with an arrhythmia. It is also used in clinical trials to evaluate the efficacy of drug therapy.

Guidelines as to the recommended uses of AEM are available from AHA/ACC. The major class I indications for AEM include diagnosis in patients with symptoms suggestive of arrhythmias, prognostic delineation in patients with cardiac disease considered at risk for arrhythmia related events, and measurement of efficacy of interventions in patients with known and characterized arrhythmias. Examples of clinical indications are listed in Table 10–5.

A major limitation of AEM is the amount of data collected with ECG abnormalities that are of unknown clinical significance. High day-to-day variability of frequency and type of arrhythmias means that repeat AEM may demonstrate as much as a 90% difference in the number of premature ventricular contractions. Little correlation of arrhythmia suppression and clinical outcomes is available. No AEM study has shown a mortality advantage when used in conjunction with antiarrhythmic drugs or devices. Following an intervention (drugs or device), at least a 63% to 95% reduction in arrhythmia frequency is required for AEM to be considered as a valuable arrhythmia detection and evaluation tool. Compared with electrophysiology testing (EPS) in the Electrophysiologic Study Versus Electrocardiographic Monitoring (ESVEM) study, AEM was equivalent to but not superior in the ability to select initial drug therapy. The Asymptomatic Cardiac Ischemia Pilot (ACIP) study found that 75% of patients with asymptomatic evidence of ischemia on AEM had multivessel coronary artery disease on angiography.

TABLE 10–5. Clinical Uses of Ambulatory Electrocardiographic Monitoring (AHA/ACC Class I and II Recommendations)

Class I
Unexplained syncope or recurrent palpitations
Arrhythmias with characteristics suggestive of risk for sudden death
Antiarrhythmic drug therapy responses
Interrogation and setting of pacemakers and intracardiac defibrillators (ICDs)
Class II
Detection of arrhythmias for prognostic implications in patients with left ventricular dysfunction after myocardial infarction, congestive heart failure, or idiopathic hypertrophic cardiomyopathy
Detection of atrial flutter or fibrillation in patients with neurologic events
Evaluation of syncope or palpitations where a cause has been treated without full resolution of the condition
Detection of proarrhythmias and drug-induced arrhythmias

During AEM, the patient wears a portable ECG recorder that weighs about 8 to 16 oz. The recorder uses two to four chest leads (V_5 and V_3 most commonly). Additional leads do not improve the sensitivity of AEM significantly. If ST-segment changes are known to occur in certain leads, these can be used during AEM. Most AEM recordings are for 24 to 48 hours, but they can extend to weeks or months where the frequency of events related to ECG abnormalities is low. Implantable devices are used when long periods of monitoring are necessary. Currently used equipment is able to detect and analyze arrhythmias, ST-segment deviations, QRS complexes, RR intervals, and late potentials.

Three types of monitors are available: (1) continuous monitors, which record an ECG strip over the duration of the test, (2) event or intermittent recorders, which continuously monitor the ECG but only record preprogrammed abnormal ECG events or are patient-activated based on occurrence of symptoms, and (3) real-time analytical recorders, which record throughout the monitoring period and analyze each beat as it occurs. Monitors digitize, encode, and store the information in a solid-state memory or on magnetic tape. Event monitors are preprogrammed to record parameters such as the number of premature ventricular contractions and heart rate. During monitoring, the patient maintains a diary in which the occurrence, duration, and severity of symptoms (e.g., light-headedness, chest pain) are recorded, plus any specific activities undertaken, development of symptoms with the activity, and any interventions such as the taking of medication. A clocking device in the recorder allows later correlation of the patient's diary and the recorded ECG.

Evaluation and analysis of the ECG record is complex. Computer-assisted interpretation is used to scan the ECG and identify irregular rhythms, rates, and specific preprogramed changes. The main advantages of computer analysis are to reduce interpretation of artifact recordings. Each beat recorded during AEM is evaluated for its arrhythmia potential and classified as normal or abnormal. The morphology of each QRS-T section is examined for ischemia potential, although, as indicated previously, baseline ST-segment abnormalities and adjustments in amplitude of the recording may preclude

TABLE 10–6. Confounding Factors in Ambulatory ECG Monitoring

Patient Factors	Equipment Factors
Electrolyte abnormalities	Battery failure
Hyperventilation	Loose lead
Lead interference by patient	Mechanical failure of recorder
Medications	
Physiologic variations in waveforms	Motor failure
	Overrecording
Medications	Computer inability to detect arrhythmia
Patient activities (e.g., sudden exercise)	
Presence of atrial fibrillation	

interpretation of these segments. The new ACC/AHA guidelines provide detail as to the suitability of using ST segments for analysis of ischemia. Various drugs such as digoxin and the tricyclic antidepressants that cause baseline ECG abnormalities may preclude patients from being evaluated with AEM.

Sections identified by the computer as abnormal or those correlating with patient symptoms are then evaluated and characterized further (e.g., potentially pathologic rhythms) by technical personnel and physicians. Confounding factors when using AEM can arise from the patient and the device (Table 10–6). AEM is rapidly evolving, primarily related to improved technology with respect to data interpretation, signal quality, and improved understanding of the implications of ECG changes.

EXERCISE STRESS TESTING (ET)

ET is a noninvasive test used to evaluate clinical and cardiovascular responses to exercise. ET frequently is used as an initial test, in conjunction with physical examination and patient symptoms, to aid in the selection of additional testing modalities. It a simple test that can be conducted in a physician's office and is about 20 times less expensive than an angiogram and almost three times less expensive than stress ECHO. Almost two-thirds of ETs billed to Medicare in 1996 were conducted in physicians' offices, and one-third were conducted by noncardiologists.

The ET provides diagnostic information in patients with known or suspected IHD and prognostic information in patients after myocardial infarction or revascularization. However, there are no data that support its use as a screening tool for coronary artery disease (CAD) or for detection of early CAD in asymptomatic subjects.

The principle behind ET is to increase myocardial oxygen demand above myocardial oxygen supply and coronary reserve, thereby provoking ischemia (inadequate myocardial perfusion), using exercise as a stressor. Ischemia is detected by patient symptoms, ECG changes, and/or hemodynamic changes. The type of ECG changes, leads affected, and patient performance are used as an index of severity and location of disease. ET is a very practical test in that it can assess patients' functional capacity.

Some examples of class I, II, and III indications from the ACC/AHA guidelines on ET are presented here. The major class I indications are evaluation of males older than 40 years who have symptoms suggestive of CAD and risk factors for CAD or atypical symptoms suggestive of CAD. Another class I indication is to help assess prognosis and functional capacity in patients with confirmed CAD. Frequently, the ET is performed following an AMI for this purpose. Class II indications are patients with variant angina or women with a history of typical or atypical chest pain. Examples of class III indications are patients with simple premature ventricular contractions on a resting ECG with no other signs or symptoms of CAD. Additionally, ET is used to assess symptoms such as chest pain or breathlessness. The ET should only be used if the results are able to alter patient management or to assess patient function.

Guidelines for conducting and interpreting the tests and details of testing equipment and environment are outlined in the ACC/AHA guidelines on ET standards. ET is conducted on a treadmill or bicycle ergometer or by means of a handgrip. These dynamic methods are used to assess exercise tolerance because they induce both a volume and pressure load on the heart. Both modalities also allow the degree of stress to be delivered in a graded and calibrated manner. Treadmill walking is preferred over the ergometer because it involves more muscle mass and the VO_2max achieved with cycle ergometer is 10% to 15% lower than with the treadmill.

Many protocols have been designed and validated for use with ET, but the two most commonly used are the Bruce and Naughton protocols. Protocols help to decrease inter- and intrapatient variability and allow for standardization in the interpretation of the tests. Protocols may be customized for individual patients to ensure an exercise time of 6 to 12 minutes and a heart rate of 85% to 90% of maximum predicted (adjusted for age and gender). Protocols detail gradient, speed, and rates of change of these parameters during the test.

In preparation for ET, patients fast prior to the test for a minimum of 3 hours, may not exercise 12 hours prior to the test, and must dress suitably for exercise. Baseline evaluation consists of history and physical examination, blood pressure, heart rate, and ECG. The test begins with a 1-minute warmup period to orient the patient to the equipment. Each stage of the test is maintained for at least 3 minutes. Continuous blood pressure, heart rate, and ECG recordings are obtained, with definitive readings 2 minutes into each stage. Patients are questioned 2 to 3 minutes into each stage of the test about symptoms such as headache, dizziness, and chest pain. Clinical symptoms assessed include color of skin, level of perspiration, and evidence of peripheral cyanosis and light-headedness. Patients are encouraged to exercise as vigorously as they can to ensure an optimal test result. Onset, nature, and duration of all changes in symptoms, hemodynamics, and ECG are noted. Following the test there is a cool-down period during which the patient is seated or lying and is observed for changes as described earlier.

The ET requires considerable effort, with many patients requiring encouragement to perform to the best of their ability. Some patients use the test as a personal challenge, and perform better on repeated attempts. This is referred to as a *training effect* and may be a confounding factor in using ET to assess the effect of drug therapy or after interventions for IHD in clinical trials.

Interpretation of the ET requires correlation of clinical, ECG, and other parameters measured during the test with the patient's history (e.g., age, gender, concurrent risk factors, medical history) and concomitant therapy. Results of ET can be used as a guide to future patient management, including suitability for interventional cardiology and selection of pharmacotherapy. A positive ET is defined as 1 mm horizontal or downsloping depression or elevation of the ST segment for 60 to 80 ms after the QRS complex. For patients with baseline ST-segment depression, combinations of abnormal responses (e.g., 2-mm ST-segment depression with hemodynamic abnormalities) would be necessary to call a test positive. ST-segment depression of 2 mm or more, especially in conjunction with heart rates of less than 120 beats per minute, low levels of stress, or depression persisting for up to

6 minutes after the cessation of the ET, is associated with a poor prognosis. Depression of the ST segment in multiple leads is also significant. Other ECG changes include development of U waves and increased complexity and/or frequency of premature ventricular contactions or beats, especially if associated with bigeminy or periods of ventricular tachycardia.

Although ECG changes and heart rate responses are used as objective end points of an ET; patient and clinical end points are actually preferred. The use of the 85% to 90% maximally predicted heart rate is highly variable between patients and often is not achieved because of concomitant drug therapy and different levels of fitness. Symptom-limited or patient-directed tests are continued to the predetermined end point(s) unless the patient tires or certain characteristics are noted. Clinical symptoms, exhaustion, chest pain, and changes in blood pressure, heart rate, and the ECG (rhythm, configuration, and rate) are used as end points for such "open-ended tests." Also, patient performance, measured as exercise duration, time until symptoms, stress at which symptoms occur, and hemodynamic parameters are better indicators of an adequate test than heart rate response. "Close-ended testing" is the use of fixed end points such as time on the treadmill or maximal heart rate.

The product of blood pressure and heart rate (*double product*) is a measure of myocardial oxygen demand. In patients with stable angina, the double product is reproducible on repeat ETs; thus it is used as an objective parameter to follow an individual patient's disease. Inappropriate or inadequate responses in blood pressure and/or heart rate to exercise suggest heart disease. A reduction in heart rate or a flat response (failure to increase heart rate above 120 beats per minute) with increasing levels of stress has a poor prognosis. Likewise, failure to increase the systolic blood pressure or the finding of a sustained decrease of more than 10 mm Hg is also associated with a worse prognosis. Such responses indicate that the heart has an inadequate reserve to respond to stress. Patients who are unable to progress beyond stage II of the Bruce protocol have a poor prognosis and more severe IHD. Other rating scales (e.g., Borg, which measures perceived exertion) may be used in conjunction with the objective results from the ET to classify patients into high- and low-risk groups. Silent ischemia may confound the interpretation of ET because blood pressure and ECG changes may occur in the absence of symptoms.

To provide standardized comparability between tests and patients, metabolic equivalents (METs) are used as a measure of VO_2max. A MET is a measure of resting oxygen uptake. Activity energy demands can then be calculated in terms of METs. For example, 4 METs is equivalent to walking at 4 mi/h. The number of METs a patient can undertake without symptoms of ischemia correlates with prognosis and helps guide appropriate management strategies. Refer to Table 10–7 for examples of METs and activity correlations. Exercise capacities of less than 5 METs are associated with a poor prognosis; those greater than 13 METs have a good prognosis despite the presence of disease.

Metaanalysis of more than 24,000 patients in 147 studies showed a mean sensitivity of 68% and specificity of 77% for ET as a diagnostic test. The specificity of ET to detect the presence of CAD, compared with angiography, is 84%. Sensitivity ranges from 40% to 90% depending on the number of vessels affected, with a mean of 66%.

As a prognostic test, ET is very popular after myocardial infarction and can be conducted within 3 days of an acute event. It can be used to determine functional capacity, assess the degree of rehabilitation, and identify those patients at risk of further cardiovascular events. Immediately after myocardial infarction, a modified protocol is used; the test is terminated when a heart rate of 70% to 75% of age- and gender-predicted maximum is reached (e.g., 140 beats per minute for those under age 40 and 130 for those older than age 40) or a MET level of 5 for patients older than 40 or 7 for those younger than 40. Tests usually are done prior to discharge or within 6 weeks of infarction. In the peri-infarction period, mortality and reinfarction rates are 0.02% and 0.09%, respectively. Patients may be stratified into low-, intermediate-, and high-risk categories depending on the evidence for ischemia and the level of exercise tolerance.

TABLE 10–7. MET Relationship to Activity and Function

METs	Level of Activity	ET Result
1	Resting	<6 METs
2	Level walking at 2 mi/h	Symptom-limited lifestyle
4	Level walking at 4 mi/h	Sedentary lifestyle tolerated
13	Cycling 9–10 mi/h	Little or no activity limited lifestyle
20	Shoveling heavy snow	No limitations on lifestyle

ET is relatively safe, with an estimated risk of AMI or death of 10 per 10,000 tests overall. Most adverse effects are cardiac in nature, including arrhythmias (primarily bradyarrhythmias), sudden death, hypotension, and myocardial infarction. Patients in whom ET is contraindicated are those who are unable or who should not exercise because of physiologic or psychological limitations (Table 10–8). Unstable angina is usually a contraindication to ET because of the instability of the patient's disease state and because patients cannot exercise to a satisfactory level for the test to be considered adequate. However, once such a patient is stable, ET is excellent for prognostic evaluation. In patients with untreated life-threatening arrhythmias or CHF, ET is also contraindicated. Patients with comorbid diseases such as chronic obstructive pulmonary disease (COPD) or peripheral vascular disease (PVD) may be limited in their exercise capacity, whereas lower limb amputees are unable to perform the standard treadmill test. For patients with disabilities or other medical conditions that limit their exercise capacity independent of heart disease, pharmacologic stress testing with dipyridamole, adenosine, or dobutamine is an alternative (see "Pharmacologic Stress Testing" below).

Drug therapy rarely is discontinued for the test primarily because few data exist to support better test results off drug therapy. Patients on β-blockers or calcium channel blockers may not achieve maximal heart rates, but ET helps demonstrate patients' exercise capacity on drug therapy. Nitrates do not alter exercise capacity directly and

TABLE 10–8. Contraindications for Exercise Testing

Absolute	Relative
Unstable angina	Left main coronary artery disease
Syncope	Tachy or brady arrhythmias
<72 hours after AMI	Electrolyte abnormalities
Uncontrolled CHF	Hypertension (SBP >220 mm Hg)
Uncontrolled arrhythmias	High-degree AV block
Acute systemic illness	
Acute pulmonary embolism	
Acute myocarditis	
Thrombosis of lower extremity	

theoretically may improve patient response because they relieve or prevent symptoms of ischemia. Digoxin interferes with interpretation of ST-segment changes, and patients rarely achieve ST-segment changes greater than 1 mm even in the face of significant ischemia. Due to its long half-life, digoxin need not be discontinued prior to the test.

CARDIAC CATHETERIZATION AND ANGIOGRAPHY

The development of the cardiac catheterization technique was a major milestone in the diagnosis and management of CVS disease because it provided a physiologic and anatomic approach to assess patency of coronary vessels and hemodynamic parameters of cardiac function. Cardiac catheterization is the technique used to gain vascular access to the coronary arteries by intravsacular catheters and heart chambers. Once cardiac catheterization is complete, other diagnostic and therapeutic procedures, such as angiography, ventriculography, and percutaneous transluminal angioplasty (PTCA), and drug administration (e.g., thrombolytics) may be undertaken. Following interventional procedures such as PTCA, catheterization with angiography can be used to evaluate efficacy of the intervention. In recurrent clinical syndromes, following a procedure, catheterization is used to help delineate a new management strategy. Catheterization is also now used commonly with PTCA and/or drug therapy in the management of acute coronary syndromes.

Additionally, catheterization allows assessment of valvular function and computation of various cardiac performance parameters such as cardiac output, stroke volume, systemic vascular resistance, cardiac chamber pressures, and blood flow. It also allows for placement of cardiac pacemakers. Drug administration during cardiac catheterization is used primarily for assessment of end points in clinical trials (e.g., thrombolytics to assess coronary artery patency), for management of events (e.g., chest pain) during catheterization, or for diagnostic purposes (e.g., ergonovine to evaluate coronary spasm). Further applications of cardiac catheterization include aortic root angiography, pulmonary angiography, retrieval of foreign bodies, and atherectomy.

More than 1 million cardiac catheterizations are performed in the United States per year, making it the second most frequent in-hospital procedure. Images obtained during catheterization are stored on 35-mm cineradiographic film or are digitized, allowing comparison of studies at a later date. The ACC/AHA guidelines on angiography and PTCA describe the class I, II, and III indications for each of these procedures; examples are given in Table 10–9. The guidelines for angiography, PTCA, and catheterization also include recommendations regarding technique, procedures, facilities, personnel, and training.

The cardiac catheterization procedure requires vascular access, usually obtained percutaneously at brachial or femoral arteries or veins. Left-sided catheterization provides access to the aorta, left ventricle, and left atrium. Right-sided heart catheterization enables the right side of the heart, coronary sinus, pulmonary arteries, and pulmonary wedge position to be reached. Left-sided catheterization is used for coronary angiography and ventriculography, whereas right-sided catheterization is used for determination of cardiac performance parameters.

Prior to an elective procedure, the patient is given nothing by mouth (after midnight) except for oral medications. It is not necessary to stop any medications except warfarin prior to catheterization. Patients receiving warfarin may be transitioned to low-molecular-weight or unfractionated heparin or anticoagulation discontinued depending on the clinical scenario about 3 days prior to the procedure. Heparin products are stopped about 6 hours before the procedure to allow normalization of coagulation. There are no data to support low-molecular-weight heparin during catheterization procedures because its longer half-life may increase the risk of intra- and postprocedural bleeding. Patients who require anticoagulation prior to angiography (e.g., those with acute coronary syndromes) are usually treated with unfractionated heparin or low molecular heparin.

TABLE 10–9. Indications for Coronary Angiography

Class I
Patients with class III–IV angina or high risk for adverse outcomes not responding to medical therapy
Patients who have high-risk findings on noninvasive testing
Suspected abrupt closure or stent thrombosis following PTCA
Recurrent angina within 9 months of PTCA
Alternative to thrombolytic therapy in patients less than 12 hours from AMI
Class II
Patients with class III–IV angina who improve on medical therapy
Patients with CAD who fail to respond to medical therapy
Patients with CAD who cannot be risk stratified by other methodologies
Recurrent angina within 12 months of PTCA
Recurrent angina not controlled by medical therapy post PTCA
Class III
Patients after interventional procedure with no evidence of ischemia
Patients who are not candidates for or do not wish interventional procedures for revascularization
Assessment of atypical chest pain

Patients frequently develop chest pain and/or vasospasm during introduction and manipulation of catheters and injection of angiographic dyes. Nitroglycerin and/or morphine may be given for chest pain. Nitroglycerin also is used to prevent vasospasm and is given sublingually or by intravenous infusion. Sedatives, such as midazolam or other short-acting benzodiazepines, frequently are given to ensure patient comfort and safety, but the patient is awake and aware of the procedure. Patient cooperation is necessary to obtain the angiographic views and assess symptoms. The patient will be required to remain still for about 6 to 8 hours to reduce the risk of bleeding from the catheter entry site(s). Depending on the procedure, patients may be discharged the same day or within 24 hours if stable.

Heparin products are used during procedures such as angiography, left-sided heart catheterization, and PTCA to prevent thrombotic complications. Depending on the procedure undertaken, heparin is either discontinued almost immediately following the procedure or continued for 12 to 24 hours. Heparin administration during the procedure is measured with the activated clotting time (ACT) not the partial thromboplastin time (PTT). For patients undergoing PTCA, aspirin, clopidogrel or ticlopidine, and calcium channel blockers are used prior to and following the procedure. Despite the invasive nature of the procedure, there is no consensus as to the need for prophylactic antibiotics in patients at risk for bacterial endocarditis because of valvular prostheses or a prior history of rheumatic fever. With the advent of class IIb/IIIa receptor antagonists such as tirofiban, eptifibatide, and abciximab, which have been shown to improve short- and long-term coronary artery patency rates with PTCA, patients who receive a stent also will receive one of these agents prior to, during, and/or after the procedure.

During the procedure, hemodynamic parameters, blood pressure, and heart rate are monitored continuously. ECG monitoring and intermittent 12-lead ECGs are also maintained. Measurements taken during catheterization are obtained only after hemodynamic stabilization: at baseline, following catheter movement, or during pharmacologic intervention. Information obtained during catheterization is in

TABLE 10–10. Contraindications of Cardiac Catherization and Other Procedures[a]

Recent stroke	Patient noncompliance[b]
Advanced physiologic age	Digoxin intoxication
Severe anemia	Anaphylaxis to radiographic dyes
Severe hypertension	Active infection
Active gastrointestinal bleed	Severe electrolyte imbalances
Fever	Unstable condition
Other comorbid illnesses, e.g., COPD[c,d]	

[a]Primarily contraindications to procedures such as arteriography and PTCA.
[b]Patient not willing to undergo further treatment (e.g., surgery based on results of catherization).
[c]COPD = chronic obstructive pulmonary disease.
[d]Disease states that may prohibit or increase risk of other interventions (e.g., surgery).
[e]Patients in whom emergency cardiac surgery would pose a high risk (e.g., during acute asthma or acute exacerbation of COPD).

real time and is assumed to reflect the ongoing status of the coronary circulation. Procedurally related vasospasm may be misleading because the catheter itself is a powerful stimulus for spasm.

Complications associated with cardiac catheterization procedures and attending angiographic or interventional activites are related to the expertise and experience of the operator, with case load being a good indicator of the latter. The incidence of significant complications related to catheterization with angiography is reported to be less than 2%, with mortality about 0.11%. Patient factors such as hemodynamic stability and renal function increase risk. There are no absolute contraindications to coronary angiography, and the relative contraindications are not well substantiated (Table 10–10). Essentially, clinical stability of the patient and potential benefit of the procedure in terms of future patient management predicate the importance of relative contraindications. Complication rates, especially those of a thrombotic nature, increase with the dwell time of the catheters, duration of catheterization, catheter type, and operator technique. Bleeding complications can be reduced by ensuring that patients have normal coagulation studies prior to procedure and remain at bed rest for several hours after the procedure and that the nursing staff undertakes good care of the catheter entry and exit sites. In the event of bleeding complications, direct pressure is required with sandbags, followed by emergency surgery if there is no resolution, to prevent further complications. Heart perforation is an uncommon but potentially lethal complication requiring emergency surgical intervention. Other complications such as a vagal reflex with hypotension, bradycardia, and nausea can occur. These occur most frequently in conjunction with patient anxiety and can be prevented or treated with atropine. An increased predisposition to myocardial infarction during and after the procedure is seen in patients with unstable angina, recent subendocardial infarction, and Type 1 diabetes mellitus. After catheterization, patients may have elevated creatine phosphokinase and troponins due to tissue damage during the procedure. There is some controversy as to how to interpret these values with respect of what they indicate regarding myocardial damage. Acute closure of a cornary vessel or myocardial ischemia is managed by return to the catheterization laboratory or cardiac surgery. All facilities should be in close liaison with a cardiothoracic surgery unit.

Angiography, which accompanies most cardiac catheterization procedures, is defined as the "radiographic visualzation of coronary vessels after injection of radiopaque contrast medium." Despite the expanding role of cardiac catheterization, angiography is used most frequently to describe the presence and extent of CAD and to allow planning for medical or surgical intervention. Cardiac catheterization with angiography is the "gold standard" in the diagnosis and assessment of CAD, against which all new invasive and non invasive tests are measured. Unlike most other procedures, angiography determines the morphology of a stenotic lesion and the degree of luminal obstruction. However, this does not relate well to physiologic or functional significance of the lesion. For example, a 50% luminal occlusion not considered significant by radiologic standards may still be the lesion producing symptomatic chest pain, and a diabetic with significant microvascular CAD may appear to have unaffected larger arteries at angiography yet still be at risk of a cardiac event. Angiography also assess the presence of collateral circulation and dynamic abnormalities such as vasospasm.

The extent of disease by angiography is defined as the number of vessels, and the vessels affected are named. Angiography is able to detect lesions that occlude the vessel by as little as 20%. Occlusions of 75% or more are almost always seen on angiography. Significant narrowing is usually assumed to be 50% or more, although some studies use 70% narrowing as the cutoff point. The lesion can be measured in several ways. Considerable controversy exists as to the best methodology. During angiography, the lesion is compared visually to surrounding vessels. Inherent difficulties include individual evaluator variability and also the assumption that surrounding vessels are normal. Calipers can be used to document physical size, but generally, the degree of stenosis is reported as a percentage of narrowing. Various grading scales, such as the coronary artery score and myocardial jeopardy scores, are used, and these scores have been shown to predict long-term outcomes. Coronary artery lesions most prone to rupture and thrombosis are those with 40% to 60% narrowing, so lesions with less than 50% narrowing are not benign.

Multiple views are required to obtain a good image of the vessel; the right anterior oblique planes are most used commonly (two views at 90 degrees to each other). Lesions may be described as concentric and smooth (simple lesions) or eccentric and broad with a rough surface (complicated lesions). The number of lesions is also considered of importance to the severity and prognosis of IHD, although there is considerable variation in the accuracy of such predictions because angiographic and pathologic correlation of lesions is imperfect. The occurrence of spasm, variants in anatomy, and collateral filling also complicates interpretation of the angiogram.

Angiographic films are used to plan interventions, in particular coronary artery bypass grafting (CABG) and PTCA. They are also used during both surgery and PTCA to guide the procedure. Ventriculographic studies may be performed during cardiac catheterization to obtain information about the contours of the heart and to assess global and segmental function. Regional wall motion, filling defects, and the presence of mural thrombi also may be visualized. During this procedure, radiopaque dye is injected into the heart chambers, and serial films are taken to follow the dye passage. Left ventricular ventriculography is a routine part of left-sided catheterization unless ventricular function information is already available from other noninvasive studies or there are specific contraindications to the procedure.

Cardiac performance is also best assessed during catheterization procedures as direct visualization of performance along with calculated parameters that can be obtained simultaneously and represent real-time values. Measured and observed parameters obtained during catheterization are used to determine cardiac performance. Contractility, as judged by wall motion and ejection fraction, can be used to assess global cardiac performance and to plan and evaluate or assess therapy.

Invasive cardiology is growing rapidly not only in terms of the numbers of patients undergoing such procedures but also in terms of the diversity of procedures. The development of electrophysiologic studies for the assessment and treatment of arrhythmias was made possible because of catheterization. The diversity of techniques is "limited only by the imagination of the physician and inventiveness of the microtechnologist."

COMPUTED TOMOGRAPHY

CT scanning is rarely used as a primary diagnostic procedure in the evaluation of CVS disease and function because it provides similar information as other diagnostic procedures (e.g., ECHO) and is significantly more expensive. Enhanced definition and spatial resolution of structures are possible with CT scanning, which is useful in some specific indications such as to evaluate aortic and pericardial disease and assess paracardiac and cardiac masses. More accurate determination of chamber volume and size and mass calculations of myocardial wall thickness can be obtained from CT scanning than with other methods such as ECHO or angiography. Additionally, CT scanning acquires three-dimensional images.

New techniques such as ultrafast CT (cine-CT) scanning have resolved the problems of cardiac motion that distorted conventional CT images. With cine-CT scanning, complete tomograms are assembled within one cardiac cycle (50 ms), thus providing real-time images. For ultrafast CT scanners, a set event within the cardiac cycle (determined by ECG) usually is used as initiator for imaging to ensure standardization. Conventional CT scanning requires that images be correlated with the cardiac cycle by gating the CT to the ECG. Cine-CT scans examine the heart at 10 to 14 tomographic levels in 10-mm slices.

Although still in its infancy, cine-CT scanning has been proposed as a screening tool for evaluating the risk of developing obstructive CAD and as a diagnostic tool for CAD. Recent AHA/ACC guidelines address the current state of practice with this methodology. The CT scan will show localized areas of infarction and abnormal perfusion and allows quantifiation of the extent and density of coronary artery calcification. Cine-CT scanning is more sensitive and specific than fluoroscopy in identifying the extent and density of coronary artery calcification. The calcium score (calcium density and volume of calcium) in patients older than 30 to 70 years with known CAD is significantly higher than in subjects with no CAD and appears to correlate well with the degree of coronary artery occlusion.

CT scanning is more definitive and accurate in the diagnosis of aortic dissection and evaluation of the pericardium than ECHO. Diagnostic accuracy of aortic dissections with CT scanning is at least 90%. CT scanning affords definition of the edges of the intimal flap of the dissection, and true and false channels can be seen. It also demarcates the components of the myocardial wall from the inner endocardial wall through to the epicardial surface and pericardium, allowing visualization of abnormalities, such as aneurysms and thrombin. Detection of the presence of a thrombus on a CT scan is comparable in accuracy with two-dimensional ECHO. The pericardium appears as a distinct entity and can be evaluated for thickening and calcification. CT scanning is the most sensitive technique to differentiate types of pericarditis and estimate pericardial fluid volume. Compared with ECHO, CT scanning is equivocal to define loculated and hemorrhagic effusions.

In the evaluation of cardiac masses, CT scanning shows the mass as a distinct space-occupying entity. Tissue density differentiation as seen on a CT scan allows characterization of density, aiding in the determination of the nature of masses. Masses as small as 0.5 to 1 cm can be identified on CT scans.

Like radionuclide assessment, contrast angiography, and ECHO, CT scanning can be used to calculate ejection fraction, left ventricular volume, and stroke volume. The blood pool is defined with intravenous iodinated contrast material. Ventricular volumes, ejection fraction, and stroke volume are determined directly from the blood pool on each image. Values obtained with CT scanning are more accurate and reproducible than those obtained on angiography and ECHO. The three-dimensional image of a CT scan also allows determination of the extent and distribution of LVH in patients with hypertrophic or congestive cardiomyopathy.

CT scanning has proven to be an effective noninvasive method to visualize congenital heart disease, but its role is challenged by the higher-resolution capacity of MRI. For measuring parameters in some congenital disorders, such as evaluation of ventricular function and estimation of the volume of cardiac shunts, CT scanning still remains the evaluation method of choice.

In summary, CT scanning, especially cine-CT scanning, is a rapidly evolving technique for evaluation of CVS disease. It remains an expensive alternative to other methodologies in many instances, but the high resolution and spatial capabilities mean that CT scanning offers unique properties.

POSITRON EMISSION TOMOGRAPHY (PET)

PET is a relatively new modality for diagnostic imaging in CVS medicine.[48–54] PET has found a niche to characterize myocardial physiologic and metabolic activity, perfusion, and viability. PET can measure regional myocardial uptake of exogenous glucose and fatty acids, quantitate free fatty acid metabolism, define perfused myocardium energy source(s), and evaluate myocardial chemoreceptor sites.[50] Although many other techniques can be used similarly to evaluate myocardial function, PET images are superior in definition. The primary advantages of PET is its noninvasive nature; the ability to do repeat scans within a short period of time, such as before and after PTCA; and the reproducibility of images over time. PET is very expensive due to the need for on-site cyclotrons for many of the radiotracers, and there is limited availability of sites that offer the technique. Cheaper forms of PET-like scanning are in development, but image resolution is less.

PET uses positron-emitting isotopes such as oxgen-15, nitrogen-13, carbon-11, and fluoride-18. These are incoporated into substances such as water, glucose analogs, or fatty acids, the metabolic substrates for myocardial tissue. For myocardial perfusion studies, rubidium-82 (^{82}Rh), nitrogen-13 ammonia ($^{13}NH_3$), and $^{15}O_2$-labeled water are used. For myocardial substrate metabolism studies, [^{11}C]palmitate, [^{11}C]acetate, and [^{18}F]2-deoxyglucose (FDG) are used. All these substances have very short half lives, less than 10 minutes. In the fasted state, perfused myocardium primarily uses fatty acids as energy source. Postprandially, glucose is the preferred substrate. Ischemic myocardium primarily metabolizes glucose because mitochondial fatty acid oxidation is impaired. Hence, with PET using either a fatty acid or glucose substrate, ischemic versus nonischemic areas can be defined. Frequently, PET is used in conjunction with pharmacologic stress testing to provoke ischemia, with images obtained before and after stress application.

Uptake of ^{82}Rb occurs via the Na^+,K^+-ATPase pump and occurs preferentially in viable tissue. Net uptake into tissue resolving from an ischemic insult and infarcted tissue is reduced. With a half-life of 1.26 minutes, serial images of myocardial perfusion can be taken as frequently as every 5 minutes, and a dobutamine stress test is completed within 45 minutes. Comparative studies with ET, single-photon-emission computed tomography (SPECT), and stress ECHO show PET to be more accurate in the detection of IHD. The substrate $^{13}NH_3$ rapidly crosses capillary membranes and is trapped in the myocardium by glutamate-glutamine reactions. This product produces high-contrast images with a sensitivity of 88% to 97% and a specificity of 90% to 100% to detect IHD. Oxygen-15-labeled water has a high extraction ratio into myocardial tissue, which appears to be independent of blood flow or the metabolic state of the myocardium. Oxygen-15-labeled water studies are done in conjunction with [^{15}O]carbon monoxide (labels red blood cells in the vascular space) studies to help eliminate some of the background activity that occurs as a result of the high extraction ratio.[54]

Tracers used for assessment of myocardial metabolism are selected based on the type of metabolism of interest: FDG traces glucose metabolism, [^{11}C]palmitate traces mitochondrial fatty acid metabolism, and [^{11}C]acetate is an indirect marker for myocardial oxygen consumption, allowing assessment of ventricular performance. [^{11}C]Palmitate is a useful marker for normal myocardial oxygen consumption because baseline energy needs of the myocardium are met through fatty acid oxidation. Clearance of [^{11}C]palmitate is biexponential, and studies in animals and in healthy men have shown clearance to be proportional to cardiac workload and myocardial oxygen consumption. In acute ischemia, the first component of clearance is reduced and second is increased. The use of [^{11}C]palmitate to assess myocardial metabolism in ischemic tissue is limited because there is altered transport and storage of the compound and significant back-diffusion of the agent into the vascular space.

FDG accumulates in the heart proportional to glucose use by the myocardial cell and so is a marker of cell viability. FDG studies help identify the affected vascular bed and allow evaluation as to whether angioplasty or surgery might be used.[50] Detection of hibernating myocardium is possible because it predominantly uses glucose and can be seen readily on PET scans. Patients with a significant degree of jeopardized or hibernating myocardium identified on PET scanning could then be candidates for revascularization procedures. In contrast, a perfusion study would not show as good differentiation of infarcted versus hibernating tissue, and revascularization may not be considered. In studies of recovery of left ventricular function following revascularization, PET has a positive predictive value of 72% and a negative predictive of 83%. PET with FDG has been used in the assessment of cardiomyopathies. In ischemic cardiomyopathy, discrete regional ischemia is seen as a patchy, nonhomogeneous uptake of the tracers; dilated cardiomyopathies show global decreased uptake of tracers.

In coronary artery disease, PET is used to assess and follow the physiologic significance of stenotic lesions. After infarction, PET myocardial substrate metabolism studies are used to evaluate the amount and activity of viable tissue around the infarcted area and the site and extent of infarction. Myocardial perfusion studies with PET identify more accurately the viable and nonviable myocardium compared with technetium and thallium. PET also quantifies regional myocardial perfusion more accurately than other modalities. When linked with physiologic or pharmacologic stress tests, PET enables evaluation of the myocardium under stress conditions. Studies in patients with more than 50% stenosis on angiography suggest that dipyridamole–stress SPECT and [^{13}N]ammonia PET are comparable tests to assess coronary artery perfusion, with respective sensitivities of 98% and 96% and specificity of 88% and 81%.[51] SPECT analysis using FDG compared with PET with FDG shows comparable accuracy for the detection of CAD. Comparative studies with SPECT-thallium in conjunction with bicycle ergometer or dipyridamole versus PET perfusion scanning showed comparative sensitivities (76% to 79%) but improved specificity (90% versus 82%, $P < .005$).[53,54]

The future of PET appears promising. Improved tomographic scanners, development of new radiopharmaceuticals, and improved understanding of substrate metabolism and its relationship to myocardial tissue viability will provide new dimensions to assess and evaluate myocardial function. Research enterprises are developing agents to label receptors as a tool to determine cardiovascular physiology and how altered receptor function, biochemical abnormalities, substrate metabolism, or other as yet unrecognized abnormalities impair cardiac function.

ECHOCARDIOGRAM

ECHO is the use of ultrasound to visualize anatomic structures such as the valves within the heart and to describe wall motion. Clinically, ECHO is the most frequently used noninvasive cardiovascular test, aside from the ECG. It competes well with invasive techniques such as cardiac catheterization with angiography for the evaluation of ischemia and valvular abnormalities. ECHO is relatively cheap to perform and can be done at the bedside or in the physician's office. The major disadvantages of ECHO relate to technical limitations of operator-dependent images and competition from other noninvasive technologies such as MRI and CT scanning that provide similar information with superior tissue type resolution. ECHO is often used as an initial evaluative tool following auscultation detection of an abnormality, thus providing a baseline visual characterization. Serial determinations in a given patient, especially following a change in clinical condition or a procedure, allow evaluation of progression of disease over time.

ECHO remains the procedure of choice in the diagnosis and evaluation of a number of conditions such as valvular dysfunction (aortic and mitral stenosis and regurgitation, endocarditis), wall motion abnormalities associated with ischemia, and congenital abnormalities, such as ventricular or atrial septal defects. Images obtained from ECHO are used to estimate chamber wall thickness and left ventricle ejection fraction, assess ventricular function, and detect abnormalities of the pericardium such as effusions or thickening.

ECHO is based on the principle of differential acoustic impedance (or tissue density) and the laws of reflection and refraction. Sound waves directed across tissues from a transducer will reflect back sound waves of different frequencies. The ability of the ultrasonic beam to penetrate chest wall structures is inversely proportional to the frequency of the signal. With transthoracic ECHO, frequencies of 2.0 to 5.0 MHz are used commonly in adults, and 3.5 to 10.0 MHz are used in children. Serial determinations in a given patient using the same conditions and ECHO images (windows) provide the best form of internal control to allow comparisons of test results. In clinical trials, echocardiograms are read and interpreted independently by two or three clinicians to provide a means of control.

Two primary approaches to ECHO are used in clinical practice. Transthoracic echocardiography (TTE) is conducted with the transducer on the chest wall, whereas transesophageal echocardiography (TEE) is conducted with the transducer in the esophagus. In TTE, several modes of operation are possible, the most common being M-mode (motion) and two-dimensional (2D) imaging. Both M- mode and 2D ECHO provide visualization of heart structures and can indicate numerous structural abnormalities such as aneurysms, wall thickness abnormalities, chamber collapse (e.g., tamponade), and valvular stenosis. TEE is used primarily for assessment of valvular anatomy and function or to image intracardiac masses such as tumors or thrombi.

In M-mode ECHO, the transducer is placed at a single site on the chest (usually along the sternal border), and the ultrasound is directed posteriorly. M-mode ECHO records only static objects in one plane, producing a single picture of a small region of the heart or an "icepick" view. Results depend on the exact placement of the transducer with respect to the underlying structures. Conventional M-mode ECHO provides visualization of the right ventricle, left ventricle, and posterior left ventricular wall and pericardium. If the transducer is swept in an arc from the apex to the base of the heart, virtually the whole heart can be visualized, including the valves and left atrium. Images are displayed as "windows."

2D ECHO employs multiple windows of the heart; each view provides a wedge-shaped image. Windows most commonly used include parasternal long- and short-axis and apical two- and four-chamber views (Fig. 10–6). These views are processed onto a videotape to produce a motion picture of the heart. 2D ECHO renders increased accuracy in calculating ventricular volumes, wall thickness, and degree of valvular stenosis compared with M-mode ECHO. Patient-specific calculated parameters such as ejection fraction and wall thickness are compared with standardized values (population-based) or with previously obtained values from the patient. Although ejection fraction is still commonly obtained with ECHO, it is a derived number, so it is considered "subjective." Other tests to determine election fraction provide different numbers and highlight the difficulty of comparing results between tests. Ejection fraction from ECHO is also limited by the dimished views of total ventricular volume able to be viewed especially in persons with distorted ventricles. Despite these limitations, ECHO remains the most common modality for ejection fraction determination.

ECHO can be used for diagnosis and prognosis and as a serial evaluation tool to assessment of CAD. Areas of ischemic myocardium are seen on ECHO as aberrations in wall motion. Wall motion abnormalities are seen as altered thicknesses of various segments of the heart. Wall motion abnormalities are graded using descriptive terms such as *akinetic, hypokinetic, dyskinetic,* and *hyperkinetic*. It is possible to visualize the complete ventricle (in segments), allowing both global and regional left ventricular function to be assessed. Studies have shown that the location of segmental ventricular wall motion abnomalities correspond with areas of CAD. ECHO can be linked with the various stress tests (ET, dipyridamole) to assess stress-induced structural or functional abnormalities (e.g., changes in wall motion). As a serial monitoring test, ECHO is comparable with angiography as a prognostic tool and can be used as a treatment planning tool. After myocardial infarction, ECHO is a useful noninvasive diagnostic tool for detection of ventricular aneurysms, thrombi, and pericaridal effusions and can be used serially for diagnostic and prognostic information.

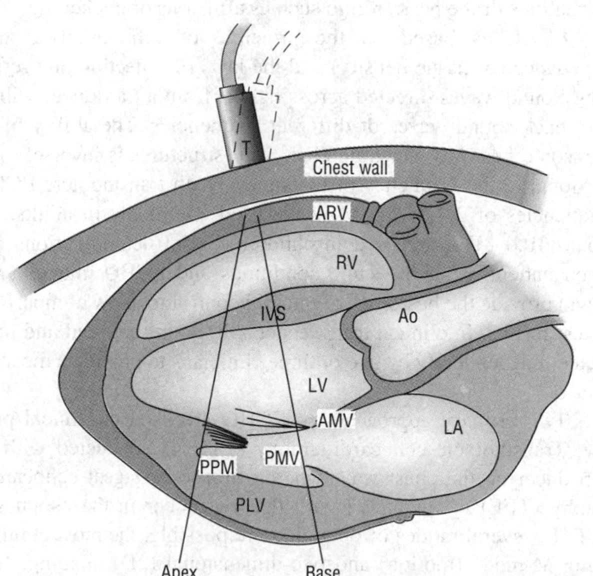

FIGURE 10–6. Schematic drawing of two-dimensional echocardiography to illustrate location of cardiac structures as "seen" by the transducer. The transducer is swept in an arc so several pictures of the heart are obtained to generate the final electrocardiogram. *(Redrawn from Corya BC et al. Applications of echocardiography in acute myocardial infarction. Cardiovasc Clin 1995; 2:113,1975, with permission.)*

In TEE, the transducer is advanced into the esophagus and rests just behind the heart. The transducer also can be passed into the fundus of the stomach to obtain better images of the ventricles. Images are obtained in either the horizontal or vertical plane.[58] This is a low-risk invasive procedure and does not require routine antibiotic prophylaxis for patients at risk of developing endocarditis. Complications such as esophageal tears or perforation, esophageal burns, transient ventricular tachycardia, minor throat irritation, and transient vocal cord paralysis have rarely been reported.[59] In one series of 10,218 studies, only 1 death (0.0098%) was reported, comparable with that with esophageal gastroduodenoscopy (0.004%).[58] TEE is contraindicated in patients with esophageal abnormalities, in whom passage of the transducer might be limited (e.g., esophageal strictures or varices).

TEE yields higher resolution and improved visualization of structures, especially pulmonary veins and valves, compared with TTE. Interference of ribs, lungs, and subcutaneous tissues is reduced, enabling TEE to be more useful in patients in whom TTE is limited because of pulmonary disease, mechanical ventilation, or obesity. A high-frequency transducer (5 MHz for adults) is used so producing better image resolution. TEE is used for the same indications as TTE. Visualization of the heart valves—in particular, the mitral valve—is superior, allowing more accurate evaluation of both native and prosthetic valves. Clinical studies have shown that it is posible to visualize valvular vegetations as small as 5 mm with TEE. The ACC/AHA guidelines do not recommend TEE as a first-line procedure for the evaluation of endocarditis or other valvular abnormalities. In a study comparing vegetation visualization, TEE detected vegetations in 90% of patients compared with 58% with TTE. It also can help define complications of endocarditis such as thrombosis or valve leakage. In aortic dissection, TEE is able to identify the initial flap and origin of dissection and has an overall sensitivity and specificity of 97% and 100%, respectively. CT remains the diagnostic method of choice for aortic dissection, but TEE offers a sensitive and fast test that can be conducted in the emergency room.

Other uses of TEE include identification of cardiac thrombus, especially those in the left atrium, and assessment of atrial dilation. After transient ischemic attacks or cerebrovascular accidents, TEE may enable identification of the site of cardiac emboli by providing excellent images of likely sources of such, namely, ventricular or atrial thrombus, valvular vegetation, cardiac shunts, cardiac tumors, or atrial and ventricular septal defects. In a study of almost 1500 patients with cerebral ischemia or nonvalvular atrial fibrillation, atrial thrombi were seen in 183 patients when evaluated by TEE versus only 2 patients using TTE. TEE can be used for intraoperative cardiac imaging to ascertain development of ischemia.

Another advance with ECHO has been the addition of Doppler and color-flow Doppler technology. The Doppler principle involves reflecting sound off a moving object—in the case of ECHO, the red blood cell. As the red cell moves in relation to the transducer, a frequency shift occurs in the reflected wave. Assessment with Doppler ECHO combines structural images and hemodynamic monitoring. Thus it is possible to evaluate the impact of structural disease on cardiac function and quantify the associated hemodynamics. Color enhancement allows flow direction to be visualized; different colors are used for antegrade and retrograde flow. These improve resolution of structures, identify patterns of blood flow, and allow calculation of flow gradients.

Doppler ECHO is used primarily in conjunction with traditional ECHO for analysis of valvular function or blood flow patterns. It allows measurement of transvalvular pressure gradients, valve area, and pressure changes on either side of the valve. Doppler ECHO is either continuous or pulsed; the former is used to assess pressure changes, whereas the latter is used to localize points of origin and creation of turbulent and high blood flow. Color Doppler is used to visualize blood flow (e.g., regurgitation). Turbulence associated with valvular and wall motion abnormalities can be visualized and quantified clearly. In aortic regurgitation, Doppler ECHO is the best noninvasive technique to assess the pressure and severity of regurgitation. Color-flow mapping allows tracing of the jet direction and an indication of its volume, point of wall contact, and width. Because Doppler ECHO distinguishes different types of turbulence, it can simultaneously identify more than one type of valvular abnormality (e.g., aortic regurgitation and mitral stenosis) and the source of concomitant heart murmur.

NUCLEAR CARDIOLOGY

Nuclear cardiology continues to be a major advance as a noninvasive testing methods. Radionuclides with short half-lives, which can be used either alone or combined with other substances to form agents with particular properties, such as technetium-99m pyrophosphate, have expanded the role for nuclear imaging in cardiology. Nuclear imaging techniques have demonstrated equal sensitivity and specificity to many of the invasive "gold standard" testing modalities. The major limitations of nuclear cardiology are the availability of suitable radionuclides and correlation of nuclear images with cardiovascular function.

Despite the availability of new radionuclides, technetium-99m (^{99m}Tc) and thallium-201 (^{201}Tl) remain the two most commonly used radionuclides. ^{99m}Tc is ideal for clinical imaging, with a half life of about 6 hours, a single 140-keV photon peak suitable for available imaging systems, primarily γ-ray emission, and ability to be combined with multiple pharmaceuticals. It is generated "in-house" by a benchtop generator that reduces transportation costs and provides immediate availability. The short half-life means high doses and repeat injections can be given to evaluate efficacy of interventional therapy over a relatively short period of time. ^{201}Th has a much longer half-life of 73 hours, which prevents the use of multiple doses close together but does mean that delayed imaging is possible following administration of the agent. Uptake into cells depends on blood flow. The energy from ^{201}Th is x-ray, with an energy level of 69 to 83 keV. Production of thallium requires a cyclotron. Images are obtained with a conventional gamma camera.

TECHNETIUM SCANNING

Technetium scanning is used for evaluation of blood pool and myocardial perfusion and as an infarct-avid agent to identify damaged myocardium. Analysis of the blood pool, as in a multigated angiography (MUGA), uses technetium either alone or as a red blood cell complex. The former obtains images following a bolus of technetium, and traces its passage from the venous system through the heart to the aorta and is known as *first-pass angiography*. Equilibrium tests where technetium is bound to red blood cells provide an imaging time of several hours, which allows serial images to be obtained. These tests are used to determine right and left ventricular ejection fractions, detect cardiac shunts, estimate ventricular volumes, and view wall motion.[64]

Infarct-avid radionuclides such as technetium-pyrophosphate (^{99m}Tc-PYP) are used to describe the presence and extent of damaged myocardium after myocardial infarction, in suspected myocardial contusion, and following chest wall injuries. Imaging with ^{99m}Tc-PYP is applicable when myocardial infarction is suspected clinically, but patient history, ECG changes, and laboratory evidence are not definitive. Uptake of ^{99m}Tc-PYP into infarcted tissue depends on regional blood flow, myocardial calcium concentration, the degree of irreversible myocardial injury, and time after infarction. ^{99m}Tc-PYP attaches to calcium deposited in the infarcted area, so the approach is known as "hot spot" scanning. False hot spots may occur where there is necrotic myocardial tissue as in myocarditis, myocardial abscesses, old infarctions, and myocardial trauma. Additionally, uptake has been seen during unstable angina and ventricular dyskinesia and at sites of ventricular aneursyms, suggesting that these are associated with transient low blood flow. In infarcted tissue, ^{99m}Tc-PYP levels can be as high as 18 to 20 times that of normal myocardium, which gives rise to very distinct borders between the infarcted and normal myocardium. Uptake of ^{99m}Tc-PYP into necrotic myocardium is delayed and not measurable until after about 4 hours of coronary occlusion. Scans prior to this time are usually negative and become positive about 12 hours after occlusion. Peak intensity of ^{99m}Tc-PYP is reached at 48 hours. Washout occurs over 5 to 7 days, so ^{99m}Tc-PYP is a useful late marker of infarction, especially in patients who present late or with a silent infarction. Images are viewed by comparing sternum and rib uptake to that seen in the myocardium. This type of imaging also can be used to assess graft patency after coronary artery bypass. Certain characteristics of the images obtained have been linked with various prognostic values but await confirmation in comparative and long-term prognostic trials.

Other technetium-labeled agents used include technetium-*t*-butyl isonitrile (^{99m}Tc-TIBI); technetium-carboxy isopropyl isonitrile (^{99m}Tc-CPI); technetium-sestamibi, also known as methoxy-isobutyl isonitrile (Tc-MIBI), and technetium-teboroxime. Technetium-sestamibi has a similar myocardial uptake pattern to thallium and produces similar results but with improved image quality because it generates a much higher photon yield. This is now popular as an alternative perfusion imaging agent to thallium. Technetium-teboroxime is still primarily an investigational agent. The main advantages of the newer technetium compounds is the lack of redistribution perfusion, allowing for delayed imaging. This is particularly useful in acute clinical settings; the radiopharmaceutical can be injected during the acute event and imaging undertaken when the patient is more stable.

THALLIUM SCANNING

Thallium is a potassium analog taken up into normal myocardium by passive diffusion and possibly by active transport via the Na^+, K^+-ATPase pump. Uptake depends on regional blood flow and in a linear fashion up to very high blood flow rates. It is used primarily for analysis of coronary and myocardial perfusion. High thallium uptake occurs in perfused myocardium; in ischemic myocardium, uptake is significantly reduced. Scans taken during acute ischemia or following infarction show areas of poor or nil distribution of thallium corresponding to the site of ischemia. A scan repeated 4 to 6 hours after the initial scan may show a redistribution of the thallium into areas that previously had little to no thallium uptake. These defects are referred to as *partial defects,* demonstrating areas hypoperfused during "stress" but viable myocardium at rest. Redistribution occurs because there is delayed washout of thallium from poorly perfused myocardium, resulting in less contrast between the density of thallium in different areas of the heart. This gives the appearance of "redistribution" of the radionuclide into the previously ischemic area. To enhance evaluation of potential partial defects, a second injection of thallium can be used. Areas of nil distribution are called *cold spots* or *fixed defects* and reflect infarcted myocardium.

Thallium scanning with the aid of computer analysis segregates the images into anatomic regions and specifically localizes areas of dead or necrotic myocardial tissue. In conjunction with ECHO or SPECT; thallium scans can correlate areas of abnormal wall motion with areas of poor perfusion. Sensitivity and specificity of thallium scanning to detect IHD disease are comparable with ET (75% and 80%, respectively). When used in conjunction with exercise ECG, sensitivity increases to about 80%. Thallium scanning also can be used in conjunction with ET to allow detection of lower levels of ischemia than may be determined from ECG abnormalities or patient symptoms. Thallium is injected at the peak of the ET, and exercise continues for another 30 to 60 seconds, when the initial images are taken. Repeat images are taken at 3 to 4 hours.

Thallium scanning is useful in patients with atypical chest pain and ambiguous or false-positive ET to determine if IHD is the cause of symptoms and the ET abnormalities. Thallium scanning is also used for postoperative evaluation of revascularization or angioplasty procedures and for preoperative evaluation for prognostic stratification for persons with IHD. A normal thallium scan heralds a benign outcome, even in patients who have angiographically evident CAD. The finding of redistribution is a marker of jeopardized but viable myocardium and has been shown to have important prognostic value. Major cardiac events such as myocardial infarction in patients with normal ^{201}Th studies average less than 1% per year. The best predictor of coronary events, which correlate thallium scans with clinical significance, are the number of myocardial segments with transient (redistribution) defects.

A number of other radiopharmaceuticals have found some use in cardiovascular testing, such as labeled antimyosin antibodies.[67] Theoretically, these antibodies should be more specific markers of myocyte necrosis. The currently used antibodies are a murine Fab fragment. Phase I, II, and III trials suggest that these are highly specific for irreversibly injured myocytes, but they have limitations in terms of pharmacokinetic properties. Uptake into myocardial tissues is very slow, with a prolonged blood pool activity seen for at least 24 hours. In clinical use, the antibody is given within 24 hours of the infarction, and planar or SPECT imaging is undertaken 24 to 48 hours later. Despite the supposed specificity of the antibody to myosin, localization is more dependent on blood flow than on myosin concentration, so measurement of infarction size is not as accurate as expected. Another investigational agent, [^{123}I]phenylpentadecanoic acid, is able to assess both myocardial perfusion and metabolism by virtue of its affinity for fatty acid metabolism.[67]

PHARMACOLOGIC STRESS TESTING

Pharmacologic stress testing is an alternative to ET and ET with thallium in patients who are unable or unwilling to undergo ET. Additionally, pharmacologic stress testing is now used more than 50% of the time to assess coronary perfusion. The pharmacologic agent produces stress by a hyperemic (vasodilator) response or by increasing myocardial oxygen demand (heart rate and myocardial contractility). Agents currently used include dipyridamole and adenosine (hyperemic stress) and dobutamine (myocardial stress). Pharmacologic stress tests can be linked to various imaging techniques such as thallium planar scanning, SPECT, MRI, and ECHO. Dobutamine is most frequently linked to ECHO, allowing quantification of wall motion abnormalities, which have been shown to correlate well with areas of ischemia.

The principle of dipyridamole and adenosine thallium imaging is related to their coronary arteriolar vasodilator properties. Dipyridamole inhibits adenosine cellular reuptake, resulting in increased concentrations of adenosine in the blood and tissues. Adenosine is a potent coronary artery vasodilator and can increase perfusion four to five times over baseline. Areas distal to a coronary artery obstruction will show a relative hypoperfusion compared with normal coronary arteries because there is reduced perfusion pressure due to preferential perfusion of normal segments over stenotic segments. Acutely, these areas will appear as cold spots, but on the redistribution scans, the defects will fill, indicating viable but jeopardized myocardium.

Dipyridamole is given intravenously in a dose of 0.142 mg/kg per minute over 4 minutes. This dose has been shown to increase baseline coronary blood flow in the normal tissues up to four to five times over control. Some studies have used doses up to 0.84 mg/kg to enhance the vasodilator response. At the higher dose, acute adverse effects such as chest pain are more common. Adenosine for stress testing is an unlabeled use of this drug. Adenosine is given over 6 minutes at a dose of 0.140 μg/kg per minute. At the end of infusion (dipyridamole) or after 3 minutes (adenosine), a 2.5- to 4-mCi dose of thallium is given. The maximum effect of dipyridamole occurs at 5 to 7 minutes and adenosine at about 30 seconds after the end of infusion. Imaging follows immediately and can be repeated at 24 hours (thallium scanning) to heighten the redistribution defects from fixed or partial defects.

Like exercise thallium scanning, dipyridamole and adenosine scanning or ECHO is used to detect IHD, evaluate the prognosis of patients with known disease, assess patients after myocardial infarction, and as a risk-stratification method prior to vascular, cardiac, and noncardiac surgery. Pharmacologic stress testing evaluates wall motion abnormalities and perfusion defects under stress and has been shown in numerous studies to have comparable sensitivity and specificity with the traditional ET. Using planar scanning and dipyridamole; sensitivity to detect IHD ranges from 67% to 95% with a 67% to 100% specificity. A summary of 13 studies in almost 900 patients gave a pooled sensitivity of 85% and specificity of 87%. SPECT scanning has at least comparable sensitivity and slightly lower specificity to planar imaging but produces higher-quality imaging, which may enhance quantitative interpretation.

Dipyridamole testing has been shown to be safe and effective in the elderly and in those with unstable angina immediately after myocardial infarction (within days). It also may be used to assess the status of revascularization procedures.[70] As a prognostic test, dipyridamole testing is very useful. In several studies, abnormal scans have shown about a 10-fold increase in event rates over 1 to 2 years of follow-up. Abnormal scans also have been shown to be an independent risk factor for myocardial infarction and death with a relative risk of 3.1. Reversible defects correlate best with events, with one study demonstrating a 4.41 relative risk for cardiac events.

Adverse effects with dipyridamole thallium testing are minimal, the main adverse effects being chest pain (with or without ischemic changes on the ECG), headache, dizziness, and nausea. Adverse effects are related to the increased adenosine activity and can be ameliorated by xanthine compounds because they are direct competitive antagonists of adenosine. Caffeine products must be avoided for about 24 hours prior to the test. Adenosine is associated with a higher incidence of adverse effects (80% versus 50%), but these are very transient, and some studies have shown that patients prefer it over dipyridamole. Both agents are relatively contraindicated in patients with a history of bronchospasm.

Dobutamine, a synthetic catecholamine, increases heart rate and cardiac output, resulting in an increase in myocardial oxygen demand. Ischemia develops in areas where stenosis prevents the increase in oxygen demand from being met with increased blood flow. Ischemia is detected by ECHO as regional wall motion abnormalities or with thallium scanning.

Dobutamine, when used as a stress test, is given in doses of 20–40 μg/kg per minute. The dose is titrated at 3-minute intervals in increments of 10 μ/kg per minute. If thallium is used, it is given 2 to 3 minutes before the end of infusion. Atropine 0.5–1 mg may be given to augment the heart rate response to 85% of the patient's calculated maximum. ECG and blood pressure are recorded continuously throughout the test, and ECHO recordings are made during the last minute of each dose level and during recovery.

β-Blocker and calcium channel blocker therapy may interfere with the heart rate response to dobutamine stress tests and is recommended to be discontinued prior to the test. Dobutamine stress testing is relatively well tolerated. Reasons to discontinue the test include development of severe chest pain, extensive new wall motion abnormalities, ST-segment elevation and depression suggestive of significant ischemia, tachyarrhythmias, and symptomatic reductions in blood pressure.[64,74] β-Blockers can be used to reverse most adverse effects if they persist. Dobutamine stress tests are contraindicated in patients with aortic stenosis, uncontrolled hypertension, and severe ventricular arrhythmias. Ventricular fibrillation and myocardial infarction occur at a rate of about 0.05%.

Dobutamine stress testing has been studied as a diagnostic, prognostic, and therapy assessment tool after myocardial infarction and for unstable and chronic angina. One study compared dobutamine, dipyridamole, and ET with coronary angiography for diagnostic accuracy in patients with IHD and showed an overall accuracy of 87% for ET, 82% for dobutamine, and 77% for dipyridamole. A recent review of 14 studies of 942 patients for the detection of IHD with dobutamine sttress testing calculated the sensitivity to be about 80% (70% to 100%) with a 75% (64% to 100%) specificity. Sensitivity is highest for detection of three-vessel disease (92%). Dobutamine-sestamibi stress testing seems to be less sensitive than thallium even for multivessel disease. Comparative studies with ET and dipyridamole ECHO show dobutamine to be more sensitive. After myocardial infarction, dobutamine stress testing identifies patients at high risk of subsequent cardiac events. For patients with suspected or known IHD, a positive dobutamine stress test is an independent predictor of cardiac events, and a negative test affords protection from cardiac death.

INTRAVASCULAR ULTRASOUND

Intravascular ultrasound (IVUS) combines braided polyethylene catheter technology with miniaturized ultrasound transducers that can be inserted into a variety of vascular beds within the body, including the coronary artery vasculature.[80,81] Catheter configuration varies and may include over-the-wire, monorail, and fixed-guidewire tip configurations, resulting in different torqueability, steerability, and pushability characteristics for each type of catheter. There are two basic types of transducers, the solid-state phased-array or a rotating mechanical transducer. In general, the phased-array transducers are smaller and may be mounted on more flexible catheters so that smaller vessels (such as coronary arteries) can be visualized, but they require a more complex system for image reconstruction and show more artifacts in imaging.

In contrast to angiography, IVUS provides quantitative information from within the vessel on diameter, circumference, luminal diameter, and percent stenosis. Qualitative information regarding the amount of plaque elevation, plaque composition (e.g., calcific, fibrous, or fatty plaque), and the presence of plaque versus thrombus, thrombus versus tumor, and aneurysm and hematoma can be provided with IVUS. IVUS is also used as a therapeutic adjunct with PTCA, atherectomy, stent or graft placement, and fibrinolysis. These combination procedures may be monitored in real time as the procedure (e.g., atherectomy) is being performed.

CORONARY ANGIOSCOPY

Percutaneous coronary angioscopy permits direct visualization of the luminal surface of coronary blood vessels.[82] The coronary angioscope is composed of a flexible catheter with a fiber-optic imaging bundle coupled with a video monitor and video recorder for live and archival viewing. Because a blood-free field is necessary for viewing, an occlusion catheter on the end of the catheter can be inflated for 45 to 90 seconds in a disease-free portion of the artery of interest and flushed with saline or lactated Ringer's solution to view diseased segments.

Although the role of angioscopy is still being developed, the recognized uses include guiding saphenous vein bypass graft interventions, postinterventional evaluation of lesions, identification of culprit and borderline lesions, stent deployment, and directing of procedures to achieve better outcomes with fewer complications. The limitations of angioscopy include lack of cross-sectional information, large fluid boluses to clear the field, large introducer size, and length of the procedure. Currently, this technology is not widely available, but it holds promise for future applications.

REFERENCES

1. Ryan TJ, Anderson JL, Rapaport E, et al. ACC/AHA guidelines for the management of patients with acute myocardial infarction: A report of the American College of Cardiology/American Heart Association task force on practice guidelines (committee on management of acute myocardial infarction.) J Am Coll Cardiol 1996;28:1328–1428.
2. American Heart Association. AHA medical/scientific statement: Classification of functional capacity and objective assessment of patients with diseases of the heart. Circulation 1994;90:644–645.
3. Bernstein SJ, Hilborne LH, Leape LL, et al. The appropriateness of use of cardiovascular procedures in women and men. Arch Intern Med 1994;1554:2759–2765.
4. Braunwald E. Physical examination. In: Braunwald E, ed. Heart Disease: A Textbook of Cardiovascular Medicine, 4th ed. Philadelphia, Saunders, 1992:13–42.
5. O'Rourke RA, Braunwald E. Physical examination of the cardiovascular system. In: Fauci AS, Braunwald E, Isselbacher KJ, et al., eds. Harrison's Principles of Internal Medicine, 14th ed. New York, McGraw-Hill, 1998:1231–1237.
6. Come PC, Lee RT, Braunwald E. Noninvasive methods of cardiac examination. In: Isselbacher KJ, Braunwald E, Wilson JD, et al., eds. Harrison's Principles of Internal Medicine, 13th ed. New York, McGraw-Hill, 1994:966–972.
7. Goldberger AL. Electrocardiography. In: Fauci AS, Braunwald E, Isselbacher KJ, et al., eds. Harrison's Principles of Internal Medicine, 14th ed. New York, McGraw-Hill, 1998:1237–1247.

8. Davis D. How to Quickly and Accurately Master ECG Interpretation, 2d ed. Philadelphia, Lippincott, 1992:89–95, 235–273.
9. Fisch C. Evolution of the clinical electrocardiogram. J Am Coll Cardiol 1989;14:1127–1138.
10. Garland JL, Wolfson AB. Routine admission electrocardiography in emergency department patients. Ann Emerg Med 1994;23:275–280.
11. ACC Expert Consensus Document. Signal averaged electrocardiography. J Am Coll Cardiol 1996;27:238–249.
12. Clinical competence in ambulatory electrocardiography: A statement for physicians from the ACP/ACC/AHA task force on clinical privileges in cardiolgoy. J Am Coll Cardiol 1993;22:331–335.
13. Fisch C, DeSanctis RW, Dodge HT, et al. Guidelines for ambulatory electrocardiography. J Am Coll Cardiol 1989;13:249–258.
14. DiMarco JP, Philbrick JT. Ambulatory electrocardiographic (Holter) monitoring. Ann Intern Med 1990;113:77–79.
15. Resch DD. Diagnostic and prognostic value of ambulatory electrocardiographic monitoring in older patients. J Am Geriatr Soc 1996;43:66–70.
16. Reiter MJ, Karagounis LA, Mann De, et al. Reproducibility of drug efficacy predictions by Holter monitoring in the electrophysiologic study versus electrocardiographic monitoring (ESVEM) trial. Am J Cardiol 1997;79:315–322.
17. Linzer M, Yang EH, Estes M, et al. Diagnosing syncope: 1. Value of history, physical examination and electrocardiography. Ann Intern Med 1997;126:989–996.
18. Sharaf BL, Williams DO, Miele RP, et al. A detailed angiographic analysis of patients with ambulatory electrocardiographic ischemia: Results from the Asymptomatic Cardiac Ischemia Pilot (ACIP) study of angiographic core laboratory. J Am Coll Cardiol 1997;29:78–84.
19. Chaitman B. Exercise stress testing. In: Braunwald E, ed. Heart Disease: A Textbook of Cardiovascular Medicine, 4th ed. Philadelphia, Saunders, 1992:161–179.
20. Gibbins RJ, Balady GJ, Beasley JW, et al. ACC/AHA guidelines for exercise testing: A report of the American College of Cardiology/American Heart Association task force on practice guidelines on exercise testing. J Am Coll Cardiol 1997;30:260–315.
21. Mark D. Prognostic value of a treadmill exercise score in outpatients with suspected coronary artery disease. N Engl J Med 1991;325:849–853.
22. Seceri S, Michelassi C. Prognostic impact of stress testing in coronary artery disease. Circulation 1991;83(Suppl 3):82–89.
23. Pina IL, Balady GJ, Hanson P, et al. Guidelines for clinical exercise testing laboratories: A statement for healthcare professionals from the committee on exercise and cardiac rehabilitation, American Heart Association. Circulation 1995;91:912–921.
24. Fletcher GF, Balady G, Froelicher VF, et al. Exercise standards: A statement for healthcare professionals from the American Heart Association. Circulation 1995;91:580–615.
25. Grossman W, Barry WH. Cardiac catheterization. In: Braunwald E, ed. Heart Disease: A Textbook of Cardiovascular Medicine, 4th ed. Philadelphia, Saunders, 1992:180–205.
26. Baim DS, Grossman W. Diagnostic cardiac catheterization and angiography. In: Fauci AS, Braunwald E, Isselbacher KJ, et al., eds, Harrison's Principles of Internal Medicine, 14th ed. New York, McGraw-Hill, 1998:1247–1253.
27. Levin DC, Gardiner GA. Cardiac arteriography. In: Braunwald E, ed. Heart Disease: A Textbook of Cardiovascular Medicine, 4th ed. Philadelphia, Saunders, 1992:235–275.
28. Report of the American College of Cardiology/American Heart Association Task Force on Assessment of Diagnostic and Therapeutic Cardiovascular Procedures (Subcommittee on Cardiac Catheterization). Guidelines for cardiac catheterization and cardiac catheterization laboratories. J Am Coll Cardiol 1991;18:1149–1182.
29. Report of the American College of Cardiology/American Heart Association Task Force on Assessment of Diagnostic and Therapeutic Cardiovascular Procedures (Subcommittee on Coronary Angiography). Guidelines for coronary angiography. J Am Coll Cardiol 1987;10:935–950.
30. Walder LA, Schaller FA. Diagnostic cardiac catheterization. When is it appropriate? Postgrad Med 1995;97:37–42.
31. Ryan TJ, Bauman WB, Kennedy JW, et al. Guidelines for percutaneous transluminal coronary 81 angioplasty: A report of the ACC/AHA Task Force on Assessment of Diagnostic and Therapeutic Cardiovascular Procedures (Committee on Percutaneous Transluminal Coronary Angioplasty). J Am Coll Cardiol 1993;22:2033–2054.
32. Foley DP, Escaned J, Strauss BH, et al. Quantitative coronary angiography (QCA) in interventional cardiology: Clinical application of QCA measurements. Prog Cardiovasc Dis 1994;36:363–384.
33. Reagan K, Boxt LM, Katz J. Introduction to coronary arteriography. Radiol Clin North Am 1994;32:419–433.
35. Gorlin R. Perspectives on invasive cardiology: The 24th Louis F. Bishop lecture. J Am Coll Cardiol 1994;23:525–532.
36. Topol EJ, Nissen SE. Our preoccupation with coronary luminology: The dissociation between clinical and angiographic findings on ischemic heart disease. Circulation 1995;92:2333–2342.
36. Landau C, Lange RA, Hillis LD. Percutaneous transluminal coronary angioplasty. New Engl J Med 1994;330:981–993.
37. Strauss BH, Escaned J, Foley DP, et al. Technological considerations and practical limitations in the use of quantitative angiography during percutaneous coronary recanalization. Prog Cardiovasc Dis 1994;36:343–362.
38. Higgins CB. Newer cardiac imaging techniques: CT, MRI. In:Braunwald E, ed. Heart Disease: A Textbook of Cardiovascular Medicine, 4th ed. Philadelphia, Saunders, 1992:312–341.
39. Higgins CB. New cardiac imaging techniques. In: Isselbacher KJ, Braunwald E, Wilson JD, et al., eds. Harrison's Principles of Internal Medicine, 13th ed. New York, McGraw-Hill, 1994:972–979.
40. Thompson BH, Stanford W. Evaluation of cardiac function with ultrafast computed tomography. Radiol Clin North Am 1995;32:537–554.
41. Lazem F, Barbir M, Banner N, et al. Coronary calcification detected by ultrafast computed tomography is a predictor of cardiac events in heart transplant recipients. Transplant Proc 1997;29:572–575.
42. Ganz W, Serafini A, Lerner D, et al. Cardiovascular magnetic resonance imaging goes beyond anatomy. Crit Rev Diagn Imaging 1995;36:479–503.
43. Hartiala J, Knuuti J. Imaging of the heart by MRI and PET. Ann Med 1995;27:35–45.
44. Hartiala J, Sakuma H, Higgins CB. Magnetic resonance imaging and spectroscopy of the human heart. Scand J Clin Lab Invest 1993;53:425–437.
45. McMillan RM. Cardiac magnetic resonance imaging. Cardiovasc Clin 1003;23:125–135.
46. De Roos A, van der Wall EE. Evaluation of ischemic heart disease by magnetic resonance imaging and spectroscopy. Radiol Clin North Am 1994;32:581–592.
47. Globits S, Higgins CB. Assessment of valvular heart disease by magnetic resonance imaging. Am Heart J 1995;129:369–381.
48. McGhie AI. Positron emission tomography. In: Raizner AE, ed. Topics in Cardiology: Indications for Diagnostic Procedures. New York, Igaku-Shoin, 1997:81–98.
49. Go RT, MacIntyre WJ, Chen EQ, et al. Current status of the clinical applications of cardiac positron emission tomography. Radiol Clin North Am 1995;32:501–520.
50. Schelbert HR. Metabolic imaging to assess myocardial viability. J Nucl Med 1994;35(Suppl):8s–14s.
51. Schwaiger M, Beanlands R, vom Dahl J. Metabolic tissue characterization in the failing heart by positron emission tomography. Eur Hear J 1994;15(Suppl D):14.
52. Canmici PG, Gropler RJ, Jones T, et al. The impact of myocardial blood flow quantification with PET on the understanding of heart diseases. Eur Heart J 1996;17:25–34.
53. Schwaiger M, Hutchins G. Quantification of regional myocardial perfusion by PET: Rationale and first clinical results. Eur Heart J 1995; 16(Suppl J):84–91.
54. Schwaiger M, Muzik O. Assessment of myocardial perfusion by perfusion emission tomography. Am J Cardiol 1991;67:35D–43D.
55. Feigenbaum H. Echocardiography. In: Braunwald E, ed. Heart Disease: A Textbook of Cardiovascular Medicine, 4th ed. Philadelphia, Saunders, 1992:64–115.
56. Popp RL. Echocardiography. In: Bennett JC, Plum F, Gill GN, et al., eds. Cecil's Textbook of Medicine, 20th ed. Philadelphia, Saunders 1996:194–199.

57. Cheitlin MD, Alpert JS, Armstrong WF, et al. ACC/AHA guidelines for the clinical application of echocardiography: A report of the American College of Cardiology/American Heart Association Task Force on Practice Guidelines (Committee on Clinical Application of Echocardiography). Circulation 1997;95:1686–1744.
58. Fisher EA, Stahl JA, Budd JH, et al. Transesophageal echocardiography: Procedures and clinical application. J Am Coll Cardiol 1991;18:1333–1348.
59. Seward JB, Khandheria BK, Oh JK, et al. Critical appraisal of transesophageal echocardiography: Limitations, pitfalls, and complications. J Am Soc Echocardiogr 1992;5:288–305.
60. Shively BK, Gurule FT, Roldan CA, et al. Diagnostic value of transesophageal compared with transthoracic echocardiography in infective endocarditis. J Am Coll Cardiol 1991;18:391–397.
61. Birmingham GD, Rahko PS, Ballantyne F III. Improved detection of infective endocarditis with transesophageal echocardiography. Am Heart J 1992;123:774–781.
62. Zaret BL, Wachers FJ, Soufer R. Nuclear cardiology. In: Braunwald E, ed. Heart Disease: A Textbook of Cardiovascular Medicine, 4th ed. Philadelphia, Saunders, 1992:276–311.
63. Taillefer R, Amyot R, Turpin S, Lambert R. Comparison between dipyridamole and adenosine as pharmacologic coronary vasodilators in detection of coronary artery disease with thallium 201 imaging. J Nucl Cardiol 1996;3:204–211.
64. Report of the American College of Cardiology/American Heart Association Task Force on Assessment of Diagnostic and Therapeutic Cardiovascular Procedures (Committee on Radionuclide Imaging, Developed in Collaboration with the American Society of Nuclear Cardiology). Guidelines for clinical use of cardiac radionuclide imaging. Circulation 1995;91:1278–1303.
65. Zaret BL, Wackers FJ. Nuclear imaging in cardiology, part I. N Engl J Med 1993;329:775–783.
66. Zaret BL, Wackers FJ. Nuclear imaging in cardiology, part II. N Engl J Med 1993;329:855–863.
67. Kahn JK, Pippin JJ, Corbett JR. New radionuclides for cardiac imaging: Descriptive applications. Cardiol Clin 1989;7:589–591.
68. Khan BA, Heber E. Imaging necrotic myocardium with 99m-technetium-pyrophosphate and radiolabeled antibodies. Cardiol Clin 1989;7:577–588.
69. Beller GA. Pharmacological stress testing. JAMA 1991;265:633–638.
70. Iskandrian AS, Heo J, Askenase A, et al. Dipyridamole cardiac imaging. Am Heart J 1988;115:432–443.
71. Stratmann HG, Kennedy HL. Evaluation of coronary artery disease in the patient unable to exercise: Alternatives to exercise stress testing. Am Heart J 1989;117:1344–1365.
72. Mahmarian JJ, Verani MS. Exercise thallium-201 perfusion scintigraphy in the assessment of coronary artery disease. Am J Cardiol 1991;67:2D–11D.
73. Verani MS. Adenosine thallium-201 myocardial perfusion scintigraphy. Am Heart J 1991;122:269–277.
74. Geleijnse ML, Fioretti PM, Roelandt JRTC. Methodology, feasibility, safety and diagnostic accuracy of dobutamine stress echocardiography. J Am Coll Cardiol 1997;30:595–606.
75. Sicari R, Picano E, Landi P, et al. Prognostic value of dobutamine-atropine stress echocardiography early after acute myocardial infarction. J Am Coll Cardiol 1997;29:254–260.
76. Greco CA, Salustri A, Seccareccia F, et al. Prognostic value of dobutamine echocardiography early after uncomplicated acute myocardial infarction: A comparison with exercise electrocardiography. J Am Coll Cardiol 1997;29:261–267.
77. Rallidis L, Cokkinos P, Tousoulis D, Nihoyannopoulos P. Comparison of dobutamine and treadmill exercise echocardiography in inducing ischemia in patients with coronary artery disease. J Am Coll Cardiol 1997;30:1660–1668.
78. Steinberg EH, Madmon L, Patel CP, et al. Long-term prognostic significance of dobutamine echocardiography in patients with suspected coronary artery disease: Results of a 5-year follow-up study. J Am Coll Cardiol 1997;29:969–973.
79. Beleslin BD, Ostojic M, Stepanovic J, et al. Stress echocardiography in the detection of myocardial ischemia: Head to toe comparison of exercise, dobutamine, and dipyridamole test. Circulation 1994;90:1168–1176.
80. Metz JA, Yock PG, Fitzgerald PJ. Intravascular ultrasound: Basic interpretation. Cardiol Clin 1997;15:1–16.
81. Benenati JF. Intravascular ultrasound: The role in diagnostic and therapeutic procedures. Cardiol Clin 1997;15:141–159.
82. Annex BH. Coronary angioscopy: Clinical applications. Cardiol Clin 1997;15:131–140.

11

CARDIOPULMONARY RESUSCITATION

Jeffrey F. Barletta

Cardiopulmonary arrest is the abrupt cessation of spontaneous and effective ventilation and circulation following a cardiac or respiratory event.[1] Cardiopulmonary resuscitation (CPR) provides artificial ventilation and circulation until it is possible to provide advanced cardiac life support (ACLS) and reestablish spontaneous circulation. In the United States, there are more than 300,000 victims of sudden cardiac arrest each year, with 60% to 70% occurring outside the hospital.[2]

Early attempts at resuscitation date back to the biblical era.[3] Modern day resuscitation began in the late 1950s when it was discovered that expired air delivered via a mouth-to-mouth technique can maintain adequate oxygenation of blood.[4] Later, in 1960, Kouwenhoven and colleagues described "closed chest cardiac massage," and together with mouth-to-mouth ventilation, modern day CPR was born.[5]

EPIDEMIOLOGY AND ETIOLOGY

In an adult patient, cardiopulmonary arrest usually results from the development of an arrhythmia.[1,2,6] Most cardiac arrests take place outside the hospital shortly after the onset of symptoms, and most victims have coronary artery disease.[7] The most common arrhythmia (80%) is either ventricular fibrillation (VF) or pulseless ventricular tachycardia (PVT).[8] The percentage of patients suffering out-of-hospital cardiac arrest actually found in VF or PVT is only 35% to 55%,[9] however, because of the time delay between the arrest and the arrival of a paramedic team with cardiac monitoring equipment. Hospital survival for VF or PVT is approximately 20% to 30%.[1,2,6]

Cardiopulmonary arrest is much less common in pediatric patients than in adults.[8] In pediatric patients, cardiopulmonary arrest is often the terminal event of progressive shock or respiratory failure.[8] The cause of cardiac arrest varies with age, the underlying health of the child, and the location of the event. Out-of-hospital arrests are frequently associated with events such as trauma, sudden infant death syndrome, drowning, poisoning, choking, and severe medical conditions (e.g., asthma, pneumonia). In-hospital arrests, on the other hand, are associated with sepsis, respiratory failure, drug toxicity, metabolic disorders, and arrhythmias. Pediatric out-of-hospital arrest generally presents with hypoxia and hypercarbia progressing to respiratory arrest, bradycardia, and finally to asystolic cardiac arrest. In contrast to adult patients, only 10% of pediatric patients present with VF or PVT as the initial rhythm.[8] Unfortunately, survival following pediatric out-of-hospital cardiopulmonary arrest ranges only from 3% to 17%, with most survivors having a poor neurologic status.[8]

PATHOPHYSIOLOGY

There are two proposed theories describing the mechanism of blood flow during CPR.[1,10,11] The first theory, known as the cardiac pump theory, states that the active compression of the heart between the sternum and the vertebrae creates an "artificial systole" in which intraventricular pressure increases, the atrioventricular valves close, the aortic valve opens, and blood is forced out of the ventricles. When ventricular compression ends, the decline in intraventricular pressure causes the mitral and tricuspid valves to open, and ventricular filling begins. The second, more recent theory is the thoracic pump theory. The basis for this theory is the belief that blood flow results from intrathoracic pressure alterations induced by chest compressions. During compression or systole, a pressure gradient develops between the intrathoracic arteries and extrathoracic veins, causing forward blood flow from the lungs into the systemic circulation. The heart merely acts as a passive conduit for flow. After compression ends, or diastole, intrathoracic pressure declines and blood flow returns to the lungs.

The concept of cough CPR supports the importance of changes in intrathoracic pressure as a means of generating forward blood flow.[10,11] During vigorous coughing, intrathoracic pressures increase secondary to contractions of the diaphragm, abdominal muscles, and intracostal muscles. These pressure changes occur without direct chest compression and are sufficient to maintain consciousness. The observation that cough alone can maintain consciousness led many investigators to question the cardiac pump theory and accept the thoracic pump theory. In reality, it is likely that both models apply to the mechanism of blood flow during CPR.[11]

▶ TREATMENT: Cardiopulmonary Resuscitation

DESIRED OUTCOME

The goal of cardiopulmonary resuscitation is to return effective ventilation and circulation as quickly as possible to minimize hypoxic damage to vital organs. It is not sufficient to restore spontaneous circulation if the patient is left neurologically devastated or incurs severe morbidity in the process. Factors proved to enhance prehospital survival include the presence of a witness at the arrest, rapid implementation of bystander CPR, presence of VF as the initial rhythm, and early defibrillation therapy for VF.[12] In one report, 43% of patients with out-of-hospital cardiac arrest due to VF survived to hospital discharge if CPR had been initiated by a bystander within 4 minutes and if definitive therapy had been delivered within 8 minutes.[13] This number decreased to less than 7% if CPR had not been initiated in the first 8 minutes after the arrest.

Considerable controversy surrounds the identification of patient-specific factors that affect resuscitation survival. Proposed risk factors are age, concomitant diseases, initial pH, duration of resuscitation, and end-tidal carbon dioxide. The accuracy of these predictors has not been consistent in clinical studies, however.[2]

GENERAL APPROACH TO TREATMENT

National conferences and organized committees have played a major role in encouraging widespread competency in CPR technique. The first national conference took place in 1966 and recommended the training of health care professionals in the techniques of CPR.[3] Since then, the American Heart Association (AHA) has organized six additional national conferences to update philosophies for providing CPR and emergency cardiovascular care (ECC) to the general population. The most recent conference was the Guidelines 2000 Conference, which provided the latest set of recommendations for CPR and ECC.[8] The resuscitation guidelines are now internationally developed, as well as evidence based, and a new intervention category has been added to the three categories originally established at the 1992 conference.[7] Class I interventions are considered to be appropriate and efficacious. Class II interventions are subdivided into those in Class IIa, meaning that they are probably beneficial and efficacious, and those in Class IIb, meaning that they are possibly beneficial without causing harm. Class III interventions are considered inappropriate and potentially harmful. The Guidelines 2000 Conference added Class Indeterminate, meaning that an intervention is acceptable, but not recommended.

In an effort to highlight the crucial components for successful CPR, the National Council on CPR and ECC has orchestrated a "chain of survival."[7] Based on the concept that "a chain is only as strong as its weakest link," each element in the chain is essential for a successful resuscitation outcome. If one of these critical actions is neglected or delayed, survival is unlikely. The four links of the chain of survival are

1. Early access, which encompasses the events initiated after the patient's collapse to arrival of paramedic personnel. Rapid emergency medical dispatch is a critical component of this link.
2. Early bystander basic life support and CPR. Basic life support is based on the assessment of the ABCs: airway, breathing, and circulation.
3. Early defibrillation. Because this is the link most likely to improve the survival rate, automatic external defibrillators (AEDs) have become more common in community settings. Public access defibrillation (PAD), which places AEDs in the hands of trained laypersons, has the potential to become the greatest advance in the treatment of cardiac arrest since the discovery of CPR.[8] Evidence supports the value of PAD programs in locations either where the frequency of cardiac arrests is greater than 1 arrest per 1,000 patient years or where conventional paramedic services cannot ensure a call-to-shock time of less than 5 minutes.[8]
4. Early ACLS, the final link in the "chain of survival."

The idea of a team approach toward cardiac resuscitation has existed since the early 1960s,[14] but it was not until the late 1960s that pharmacists began participating as cardiac resuscitation team members.[15] Defining roles for specific health care professionals, it is hoped, will make resuscitation attempts more efficient and, consequently, more effective. Team composition may vary among institutions, but a code team generally consists of a physician in charge, a surgeon, an anesthesiologist, a respiratory therapist, a nurse, and a pharmacist.[16] Table 11–1 lists the typical roles for each team member.[16]

VENTRICULAR FIBRILLATION AND PULSELESS VENTRICULAR TACHYCARDIA

NONPHARMACOLOGIC THERAPY

Because electrical defibrillation is the only effective method of restoring a perfusing cardiac rhythm,[17] early electrical defibrillation is the most crucial link in the "chain of survival." The probability of successful defibrillation is directly related to the time interval between the onset of VF and the delivery of the first shock.[8] With every minute, the chance of successful defibrillation decreases by 7% to 10%.[8] Persons in VF or PVT should receive electrical defibrillation with at least three shocks.[8] The initial defibrillation attempt should begin with 200 J. The second and third shock can be either the same or as high as 360 J. Repeated shocks, even at the same energy level, increase the probability of successful defibrillation. Following three unsuccessful attempts of defibrillation, the patient should receive roughly 1 minute of CPR. Endotracheal intubation and intravenous (IV) access

TABLE 11–1. Responsibilities for Cardiac Resuscitation Team Members

Team Member	Responsibilities
Physician–in–charge	Team leader; determines appropriate therapy; directs and oversees order implementation including provision of CPR, electrical therapy, endotracheal intubation, intravenous access, ECG monitoring, and drug administration; arranges postresuscitation care
Surgeon	Identifies surgically correctable causes for arrest
Anesthesiologist	Performs endotracheal intubation; provides adequate oxygenation; may assist with obtaining vascular access
Respiratory therapist	Maintains adequate oxygenation and ventilation
Nurse	Records timing and outcome of therapeutic interventions; may assist with chest compressions, obtaining peripheral venous access, administering fluids and medications, acquiring blood samples for laboratory determination
Pharmacist	Prepares medications for administration; provides drug information; documents medication administration and outcomes of interventions

CPR = cardiopulmonary resuscitation; ECG = electrocardiogram.
(Adapted from Ref. 16.)

obtained at this time. Once an airway is ensured, patients should be ventilated with 100% oxygen. Pharmacologic agents, such as sympathomimetics and antiarrhythmics, play a secondary role and are not recommended until an airway has been established and IV access attempted (Figure 11–1).

PHARMACOLOGIC THERAPY

SYMPATHOMIMETICS

The use of sympathomimetics is a major part of drug therapy in CPR. The goal of using these agents is to augment both coronary and cerebral perfusion pressures during the low-flow state seen with CPR. Coronary perfusion pressures of at least 15 mm Hg are associated with a higher rate of return of spontaneous circulation (ROSC).[18] Animal studies have shown that coronary perfusion pressure averages between 10 and 15 mm Hg with CPR alone following 10 minutes of ventricular fibrillation.[19] Sympathomimetics work primarily by increasing systemic arteriolar vasoconstriction, thus improving coronary and cerebral perfusion pressure. In addition, they also maintain vascular tone, decreasing arteriolar collapse, and shunt blood to the heart and brain.

Epinephrine continues to be a drug of first choice for the treatment of VF, PVT, asystole, and pulseless electrical activity (PEA). Epinephrine is both an α-receptor and a β-receptor agonist, although its effectiveness is thought to be due to its α effects. One study evaluated the importance of α-adrenergic, β-adrenergic, and any non-adrenergic activity mediated by epinephrine in dogs.[20] The first group received epinephrine along with phenoxybenzamine (an α-blocker) while a second group received epinephrine along with propranolol (a β-blocker). When α-receptors were blocked, epinephrine was not successful in restoring circulation. When β-receptors were blocked, epinephrine was successful in restoring circulation in six of eight animals ($P < .01$). It was concluded that the efficacy of epinephrine is due to the α-adrenergic receptor stimulation and that β stimulation is not important. It is unclear, however whether β effects are useful or harmful during CPR. It has been shown that β stimulation lowers the defibrillation threshold while β blockade increases it.[21] This would make epinephrine, a drug with both α and β properties, an ideal agent. Conversely, β stimulation increases myocardial oxygen demand and can increase the severity of postresuscitation myocardial dysfunction.[22,23]

Several studies have compared the effects of pure α_1-agonists, such as phenylephrine and methoxamine, with those of epinephrine to determine whether the β effects impact negatively on cardiac arrest outcome. These studies have shown the use of α_1-agonists to have no long-term survival advantage over the use of epinephrine.[24] One study found that both epinephrine (50 μg/kg) and phenylephrine (50 μg/kg) increased arterial blood pressure in dogs, but only epinephrine increased coronary and cerebral blood flows.[25] This study has been criticized, however, because doses were not equipotent. The primary reason that selective α_1-agonists are not superior to epinephrine is related to the α_2 effects. Agents that have potent α_2 effects (e.g., epinephrine, norepinephrine) may be more effective because the α_2-adrenergic receptors lie extrajunctionally in the intima of the blood vessels, making them more accessible to circulating catecholamines—even in low-flow states that occur during CPR.[24] Furthermore, during ischemia, the number of postsynaptic α_1-receptors decreases, which suggests a greater role for α_2-agonist activity during CPR.[26]

Another agent possessing α_2-agonist activity is norepinephrine (an α_1-, α_2-, β_1-agonist). Since it has been hypothesized that β_2-agonist–induced vasodilation may counteract the efficacy of α-agonist–induced vasoconstriction, investigators have compared the effects of the exogenous administration of epinephrine to those of norepinephrine in order to determine the impact of β_2-agonist activity during CPR. Callaham and associates conducted the only large-scale randomized, double-blind, prospective trial comparing the efficacy of norepinephrine to that of epinephrine in the prehospital cardiac arrest setting.[27] In this trial, 816 adults were randomized to receive standard-dose epinephrine (1 mg), high-dose epinephrine (15 mg), or high-dose norepinephrine (11 mg) after initial defibrillation attempts failed. Study end points were ROSC (i.e., measurable blood pressure or pulse for at least 5 minutes), hospital discharge rate, and neurologic status (cerebral performance criteria). Thirteen percent (35/260) of patients who received norepinephrine achieved ROSC prior to reaching the hospital. Thirteen percent (37/286) of patients who received 15 mg of epinephrine achieved ROSC, compared to 8% (22/270) of patients randomized to receive 1 mg of epinephrine ($P < .01$). Return of spontaneous circulation was not statistically different for either high-dose epinephrine or norepinephrine. Overall, only 1.8% (15/816) of all patients enrolled survived to hospital discharge. The percentages of patients discharged from the standard-dose epinephrine, high-dose epinephrine, and high-dose norepinephrine groups were not statistically different; they were 1.2%, 1.7%, and 2.6%, respectively. Neurologic survival was most favorable in the standard-dose epinephrine group; however, these differences were not statistically significant. The low number of surviving patients made it impossible to detect a meaningful difference in these two areas. Lindner and colleagues compared the efficacy of norepinephrine (1 mg) with repeated doses of epinephrine (1 mg) on the ROSC and hospital discharge rate in 50 patients.[28] In this study, there was an increase in ROSC with norepinephrine, but there was no difference in the hospital discharge rate.

A study using a swine model compared the effects of epinephrine (200 μg/kg) and norepinephrine (80, 120, and 160 μg/kg) on ventricular fibrillation.[19] Compared to epinephrine, there was a trend towards improved myocardial blood flow and successful defibrillation with the two highest doses of norepinephrine. A second study in a swine model examined the effects of epinephrine (45 μg/kg) and norepinephrine (45 μg/kg) on myocardial oxygen delivery and consumption.[29] In this trial, norepinephrine reduced myocardial oxygen consumption, thereby creating a more favorable profile between myocardial oxygen supply and demand than did epinephrine. Similarly, Brown and colleagues compared the effects of epinephrine (200 μg/kg) and three doses of norepinephrine (80, 120, and 160 μg/kg) on cerebral blood flow in a swine model.[30] Statistically significant increases in aortic diastolic pressure and coronary perfusion pressure occurred with epinephrine and the two highest doses of norepinephrine (120 and 160 μg/kg). Increased blood flow to the left cerebral cortex, midbrain, pons, medulla, and cervical spinal cord was also evident with the two highest doses of norepinephrine. Epinephrine, however, improved only flow to the medulla and cervical cord compared to 80 μg/kg of norepinephrine. Although norepinephrine has demonstrated beneficial effects over epinephrine on myocardial oxygen balance and ROSC, there is no difference in survival to hospital discharge. Consequently, epinephrine remains the first-line sympathomimetic for CPR until more definitive data become available.

Considerable controversy surrounds the optimal dose of epinephrine for CPR. The standard epinephrine dose is 1 mg administered by IV push every 3 to 5 minutes.[8] This epinephrine dose was derived from animal studies (0.1 mg/kg in a 10-kg dog) and equates to approximately 0.015 mg/kg for a 70-kg human.[31] Both animal and human studies have demonstrated a positive dose-response relationship with epinephrine.[32–35] Animal studies have suggested that

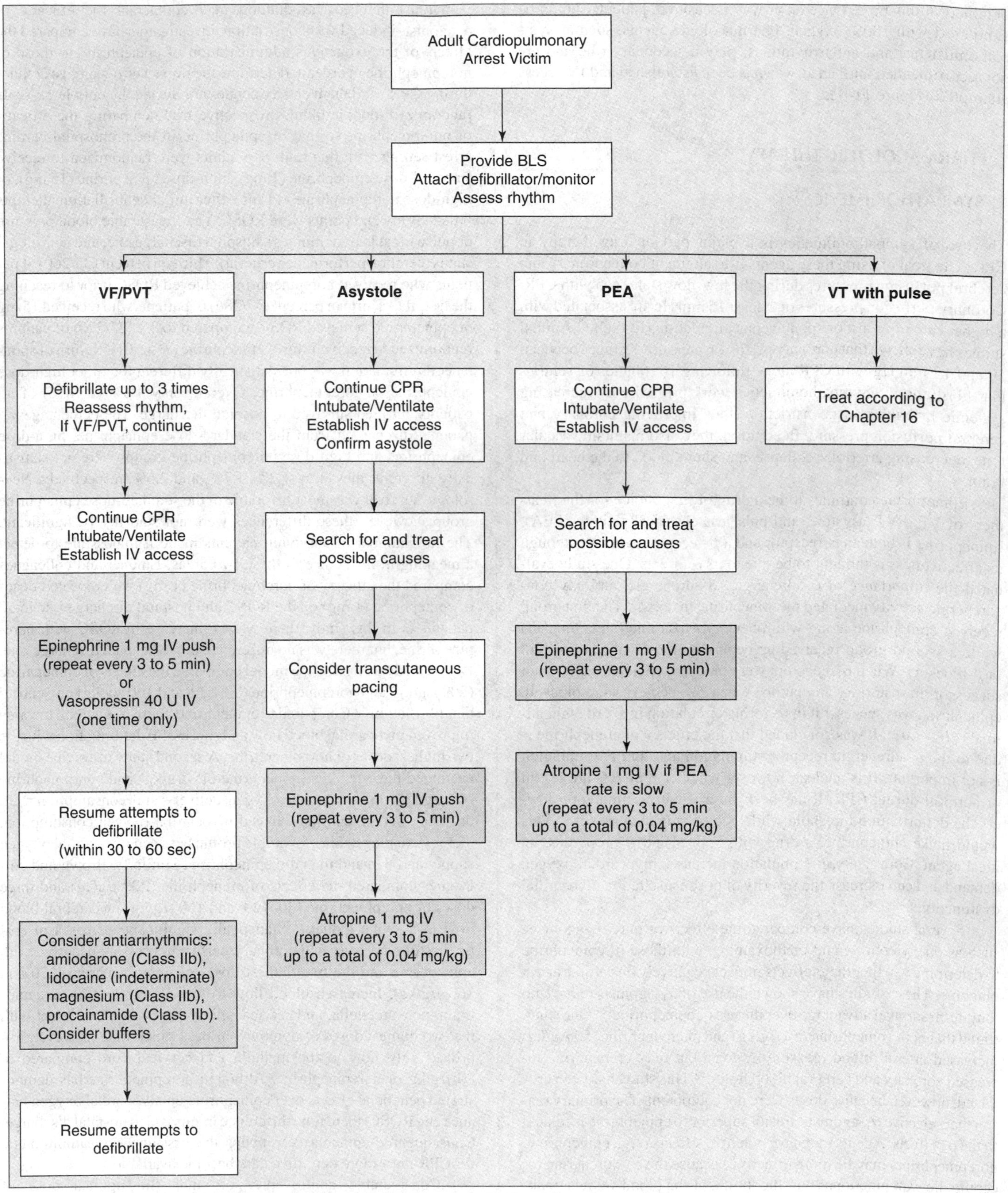

Adult Cardiopulmonary Arrest Victim

↓

Provide BLS
Attach defibrillator/monitor
Assess rhythm

VF/PVT

- Defibrillate up to 3 times
  Reassess rhythm,
  If VF/PVT, continue
- Continue CPR
  Intubate/Ventilate
  Establish IV access
- Epinephrine 1 mg IV push
  (repeat every 3 to 5 min)
  or
  Vasopressin 40 U IV
  (one time only)
- Resume attempts to defibrillate (within 30 to 60 sec)
- Consider antiarrhythmics:
  amiodarone (Class IIb),
  lidocaine (indeterminate)
  magnesium (Class IIb),
  procainamide (Class IIb).
  Consider buffers
- Resume attempts to defibrillate

Asystole

- Continue CPR
  Intubate/Ventilate
  Establish IV access
  Confirm asystole
- Search for and treat possible causes
- Consider transcutaneous pacing
- Epinephrine 1 mg IV push
  (repeat every 3 to 5 min)
- Atropine 1 mg IV
  (repeat every 3 to 5 min
  up to a total of 0.04 mg/kg)

PEA

- Continue CPR
  Intubate/Ventilate
  Establish IV access
- Search for and treat possible causes
- Epinephrine 1 mg IV push
  (repeat every 3 to 5 min)
- Atropine 1 mg IV if PEA rate is slow
  (repeat every 3 to 5 min
  up to a total of 0.04 mg/kg)

VT with pulse

- Treat according to Chapter 16

FIGURE 11–1. Treatment algorithm for adult cardiopulmonary arrest.

TABLE 11–2 Summary of Adult High–Dose Epinephrine Studies

Author (Date)	Design	Epinephrine Dosing SDE vs HDE	N	Initial Resuscitation SDE vs HDE		Hospital Discharge SDE vs HDE		Discharge Neurologic Status SDE vs HDE	
Gueugniaud et al.[36] (1998)	P, MC, R, DB	1 mg vs 5 mg up to 15 doses	3327	601/1650 (36.4%)	678/1677* (40.4%)	46/1650 (2.8%)	38/1677 (2.3%)	26/46 (56.5%)	26/38 (68.4%) Discharged without neurologic impairment
Sherman et al.[37] (1997)	P, MC, R, DB	0.01 mg/kg vs 0.1 mg/kg up to 4 doses	140	7/62 (11%)	15/78 (19%)	Not addressed		Not addressed	
Choux et al.[38] (1995)	P, R, DB	1 mg vs 5 mg up to 15 doses	536	85/265 (32%)	96/271 (35.5%)	20/54 (37%)	23/63□ (35.4%)	GCS ≥ 9 (at day 3): 4/20; EEG normal (at day 3): 1/20	3/23; 3/23
Lipman et al.[39] (1993)	P, R, DB	1 mg vs 10 mg up to 3 doses	35	11/16 (69%)	15/19 (79%)	1/16 (6.3%)	0/19 (0%)	Not addressed	
Stiell et al.[40] (1992)	P, R, DB	1 mg vs 7 mg up to 5 doses	650	76/333 (23%)	56/317 (18%)	16/333 (5%)	10/317 (3%)	94%	90% Remained in their best CPC upon discharge
Brown et al.[41] (1992)	P, MC, R, DB	0.02 mg/kg vs 0.2 mg/kg for the first dose	1280	190/632 (30%)	217/648 (33%)	26/632 (4%)	31/648 (5%)	92%	94% Conscious at discharge (CPC = 1–3)
Callaham et al.[27] (1992)	P, R, DB	1 mg vs 15 mg up to 3 doses	556	22/270 (8%)	37/286* (13%)	3/270 (1.2%)	5/286 (1.7%)	2.3	3.2 Mean CPC score
Lindner et al.[42] (1991)	P, R, DB	1 mg vs 5 mg for the first dose	68	6/40 (15%)	16/28* (57%)	2/40 (5%)	4/28 (14%)	Not addressed	
Callaham et al.[43] (1991)	Ret	HDE: ≥ 50 μg/kg or total dose > 2.8 μg/kg/min	68	Not addressed		11/35 (31%)	6/33 (18.2%)	Intact 8/11 vs 4/6; Impaired: 2/11 vs 2/6; Vegetative 1/11 vs 0/6	

* $P < .05$.
□ Number of patients admitted to the hospital alive on day 3.
SDE = standard–dose epinephrine; HDE = high–dose epinephrine; P = prospective; MC = multicenter; R = randomized; DB = double–blind; Ret = retrospective; GCS = Glasgow Coma Scale; EEG = electroencephalogram; CPC = cerebral performance category.

higher doses were necessary to improve hemodynamics and achieve successful resuscitation. These results, however, have not been replicated in human studies.[27,36–43] Collectively, these studies (Table 11–2) have shown that high-dose epinephrine may increase the initial resuscitation success rate, but overall survival is not significantly different. One study demonstrated an unfavorable neurologic outcome in patients treated with high-dose epinephrine.[44] Many of these patients would not have survived if given only standard-dose epinephrine, however, so this result wrongfully discredits high-dose epinephrine.

The discrepancy between animal and human studies may be due to the fact that most victims of cardiac arrest have coronary artery disease, a condition not present in an animal model. In a human model, however, atherosclerotic plaques can aggravate the balance between myocardial oxygen supply and demand. Moreover, the interval from arrest to treatment in animal studies is shorter than the interval frequently reported in human studies. As time to CPR and defibrillation are crucial variables for success, prolonging this time period can lower resuscitation rates. Because of the lack of evidence supporting high-dose epinephrine, the current guidelines recommend 1 mg IV push every 3 to 5 minutes or vasopressin as initial drug therapy for VF or PVT.[8] Tolerance to adrenergic stimulation can occur, especially when catecholamine levels are high. Therefore, if the standard dose of epinephrine is not successful, higher doses (up to 0.2 mg/kg) can be considered.

VASOPRESSIN

The algorithm for the treatment of VF/PVT now includes vasopressin. Also known as antidiuretic hormone, vasopressin is a potent vasoconstrictor that increases blood pressure and systemic vascular resistance. Although it acts on various receptors throughout the body, its vasoconstrictive properties are primarily due to its effects on the V_1 receptor.[45] Measurement of vasopressin levels in patients undergoing CPR has shown a high correlation between the levels of endogenous vasopressin released and the potential for ROSC.[46] Vasopressin may have several advantages over epinephrine. First, the metabolic acidosis that frequently accompanies cardiopulmonary arrest can blunt the vasoconstrictive effect of adrenergic agents like epinephrine. This effect does not occur with vasopressin. Second, the stimulation of β-receptors caused by epinephrine can increase myocardial oxygen demand and complicate the postresuscitative phase of CPR. Because vasopressin does not act on β-receptors, this effect does not occur with its use.

Several animal studies demonstrate the beneficial effect of vasopressin on coronary and cerebral blood flow.[47–49] Although vasopressin improves vital organ perfusion during ventricular fibrillation, myocardial oxygen consumption is lower with vasopressin than with epinephrine.[30] Vasopressin also may have a beneficial effect on renal blood flow by stimulating V_2 receptors in the kidney, causing

TABLE 11–3 Initial Doses of Drugs Used in Cardiac Arrest

Drug	Initial Dose	Comments
Epinephrine	1 mg IV every 3–5 min	If a 1–mg dose is not successful, then high–dose epinephrine (up to 0.2 mg/kg) is acceptable.
Vasopressin	40 U IV	A single dose of vasopressin may be used in place of epinephrine following the initial 3 unsuccessful defibrillation attempts. If there is no response to vasopressin after 5–10 min, epinephrine therapy may resume.
Amiodarone	VF or PVT: 300 mg diluted in a volume of 20–30 mL of saline or D_5W by rapid infusion	Supplementary doses of 150 mg may be administered by rapid infusion for recurrent or refractory VF/PVT, followed by an infusion of 1 mg/min for 6 h and then 0.5 mg/min, to a maximum daily dose of 2 g.
Lidocaine	VF or PVT: 1.5 mg/kg IV	A continuous infusion at 2–4 mg/min is reasonable if the drug was associated with the restoration of a stable rhythm. Reappearance of an arrhythmia during a constant infusion should be treated with a small bolus dose (0.5 mg/kg) of lidocaine and an increase in the infusion rate.
Magnesium	VF or PVT: 1–2 g diluted in 100 mL of D_5W administered over 1–2 min	For treatment of torsades de pointes, the patient should receive a loading dose of 1–2 g mixed in 50–100 mL of D_5W given over 5–60 min, followed by an infusion of 0.5–1 g/h.
Sodium bicarbonate	1 mEq/kg IV	Therapy should be guided by the bicarbonate concentration or calculated base deficit obtained from blood gas analysis or laboratory measurement. Complete correction of the base deficit should be avoided to minimize the risk of iatrogenically induced alkalosis.
Atropine	1 mg IV repeated as needed every 3–5 min	Maximum dose is 0.04 mg/kg. Doses less than 0.5 mg should be avoided to prevent paradoxical bradycardia.

IV = intravenous; VF = ventricular fibrillation; PVT = pulseless ventricular tachycardia; D_5W = dextrose in water.

vasodilation and increased water reabsorption. With regard to splanchnic blood flow, however, most studies have shown that vasopressin has a detrimental effect compared to epinephrine.[50,51]

Unfortunately, there are limited data on vasopressin in humans. Lindner and associates evaluated the use of vasopressin in 8 patients following in-hospital cardiac arrest.[52] After standard ACLS had failed, 40 U of vasopressin was administered intravenously. Spontaneous circulation returned in all 8 patients, but only 3 survived until hospital discharge. Following these results, Lindner and colleagues conducted the only prospective, randomized-controlled trial comparing vasopressin with epinephrine.[53] Forty patients who experienced out-of-hospital ventricular fibrillation resistant to electrical defibrillation were randomized to receive either 40 U of vasopressin or 1 mg of epinephrine as the initial drug for the treatment of cardiac arrest. In the vasopressin group, 16 patients (80%) achieved ROSC, compared to 11 patients (55%) in the epinephrine group ($P = .18$). Fourteen patients (70%) in the vasopressin group survived to hospital admission, and 12 patients (60%) survived more than 24 hours. Seven patients in the epinephrine group (35%) survived to hospital admission ($P = .06$), and 4 (20%) survived more than 24 hours ($P = .02$). There was no difference in hospital discharge rates between the groups: 8 patients (40%) in the vasopressin group and 3 patients (15%) in the epinephrine group ($P = .16$). Following administration of the study drug alone (i.e., no further ACLS), ROSC was achieved in 7 (35%) vasopressin patients compared to 2 (10%) epinephrine patients ($P < .001$). No adverse drug events secondary to vasopressin were observed. This trial showed a trend towards survival with vasopressin; however, statistical significance was evident only with survival longer than 24 hours and ROSC following use of the study drug alone.

There are concerns, however, about using vasopressin for cardiac arrest. Vasopressin has been reported to cause coronary artery constriction, with resultant myocardial ischemia at small doses.[45] In addition, vasopressin has a relatively long half-life (18 minutes) and may cause more persistent vasoconstriction in the postresuscitation phase than does epinephrine.[54] The doses for vasopressin and other agents used for cardiac arrest are listed in Table 11–3.

ANTIARRHYTHMICS

The primary reason for the use of antiarrhythmic agents following unsuccessful defibrillation and vasopressor administration is to prevent the development or recurrence of VF and PVT by raising the fibrillation threshold. There is, however, conflicting evidence and a divergence of opinion regarding the efficacy of these drugs and their place in CPR. These agents, therefore, receive either an indeterminate (meaning acceptable, but not recommended) or Class IIb intervention classification according to the 2000 guidelines for CPR and ECC.[8]

With drugs used as a secondary intervention, there is no recommendation for a specific antiarrhythmic. Many experts feel that amiodarone, the newest antiarrhythmic added to the VF/PVT algorithm (Class IIb), should be the agent of choice. Lidocaine remains on the algorithm, although its classification has been changed from a Class IIb to an indeterminate intervention. Bretylium, previously the second antiarrhythmic on the VF/PVT algorithm, is still acceptable for use, but has been dropped from the guidelines because of the difficulty in obtaining the raw materials necessary for production. Magnesium is a Class IIb intervention for polymorphic VT (torsades de pointes) and suspected hypomagnesemia. Procainamide is considered acceptable for refractory or recurrent VF/PVT (Class IIb); however, its usefulness is limited by the need for a prolonged administration time, which makes it unsuitable for cardiac arrest.

Amiodarone

Although officially classified as a Class III antiarrhythmic, amiodarone possesses electrophysiologic characteristics of all four Vaughn Williams classifications. Acutely, amiodarone administered IV displays mainly anti-adrenergic (Class II) and calcium channel–blocking (Class IV) properties. Consequently, hypotension, which occurs in roughly 20% of clinical trials, is a concern. This hypotension is more dependent on the rate of administration than on the amount of drug administered. A decrease in the infusion rate generally reverses hypotension induced by amiodarone.[55] The diluent used for the amiodarone solution, polysorbate 80, may also contribute to the hypotensive effect, since it is known to have vasodilatory actions.[56] Amiodarone has mild negative inotropic actions as well, but its vasodilatory action usually offsets this effect, resulting in a minimal change in cardiac output.[57] Other adverse effects noted acutely include fever, elevated values on liver function tests, confusion, nausea, and thrombocytopenia.

Kudenchuk and colleagues conducted the only randomized, double-blind, placebo-controlled study evaluating amiodarone for out-of-hospital cardiac arrest.[58] After receiving 1 mg of epinephrine, 504 patients with cardiac arrest secondary to VF or PVT were randomized to receive either 300 mg of amiodarone or placebo. Conventional ACLS was then followed. The primary end point was admission to the hospital with a spontaneously perfusing rhythm. Secondary end points included the number of precordial shocks required after the administration of amiodarone or placebo, the total duration of resuscitative efforts, and the need for additional antiarrhythmics. Survival to discharge and neurologic status at discharge were also evaluated, although the trial did not have sufficient statistical power to demonstrate differences in these outcomes. Recipients of amiodarone were more likely to be resuscitated and survive to hospital admission than were recipients of placebo (44% and 34%, respectively, $P = .03$) for a relative improvement of 29%. A subgroup analysis revealed that patients whose cardiac arrest was due to VF were more likely to survive to hospital admission than those with asystole or PEA (44% and 14%, respectively, $P < .001$). There were no significant differences in number of precordial shocks, total duration of resuscitative efforts, or need for additional antiarrhythmics. Based on these results, it was concluded that amiodarone resulted in a higher rate of hospital admission.

In 302 patients with refractory destabilizing PVT or VF,[56] high-dose amiodarone (1,000 mg/24 h) was equally as efficacious as bretylium (2,500 mg/24 h) in preventing PVT or VF. Bretylium, however, was associated with a higher rate of adverse effects, with hypotension being the most frequent, occurring in 32% of patients. Because of these findings and the lack of sufficient evidence supporting either lidocaine or bretylium, amiodarone is the preferred antiarrhythmic among many experts.[8]

Lidocaine

For many years, lidocaine has been used for treatment of ventricular arrhythmias in the setting of acute myocardial infarction (MI). The efficacy seen in cardiac arrest, however, has not mirrored that seen in acute MI. In the only published, case-control trial where patients were classified according to whether they received lidocaine, no significant difference was noted in ROSC, admission to the hospital, or survival to hospital discharge between groups.[59] Similarly, a prospective study comparing the effectiveness of lidocaine with that of standard-dose epinephrine showed not only a lack of benefit with lidocaine, but also a higher tendency to promote asystole.[60] In contrast, a retrospective analysis in patients with VF indicated that lidocaine was associated with a higher rate of ROSC and hospitalization ($P < .01$), but not an increase in the hospital discharge rate.[61]

Lidocaine has been shown to increase VF threshold in both the CPR and non–CPR setting.[62] Furthermore, it benefits the defibrillation threshold or the amount of energy required to convert VF to a more stable rhythm.[63] Although controversial, some studies show that lidocaine has a detrimental effect on defibrillation threshold.[64] These conflicting results may be related to drug interactions with lidocaine and the agents used for anesthesia.[64]

The antifibrillatory effects of lidocaine and bretylium were evaluated in the post–CPR setting in dogs.[65] A 2 mg/kg dose of lidocaine administered during CPR had a rapid effect (within 5 minutes) on VF threshold, but this effect was short-lived. The beneficial effect of lidocaine was associated with a plasma lidocaine level greater than 6 μg/mL. Furthermore, a 1 mg/kg dose was ineffective in this animal population. Bretylium, on the other hand, produced a delayed (within 10 minutes), but more persistent effect. Following these results, a similar animal model demonstrated that a combination of lidocaine (2 mg/kg) and bretylium (5 mg/kg) possessed both a rapid onset of action and prolonged duration of VF threshold elevation.[66]

There are two randomized, controlled trials evaluating the efficacy of lidocaine versus that of bretylium in adult prehospital cardiac arrest.[67,68] In the first trial, 60% of lidocaine-treated patients were successfully resuscitated compared to 58% of bretylium-treated patients ($P > .1$).[67] Hospital discharge rate was also similar between groups; 26% for those patients given lidocaine and 34% for those given bretylium ($P > .1$). In the second study, 56% of patients who received lidocaine converted to an organized rhythm compared to 35% of patients in the bretylium group ($P < .05$).[68] Hospital discharge rates were 10% for lidocaine-treated patients and 5% for bretylium-treated patients ($P =$ NS). Therefore, in the absence of any significant efficacy differences and the presence of a better adverse effect profile, lidocaine is preferred over bretylium.

Lidocaine pharmacokinetics have not been extensively studied during cardiac arrest. Lidocaine metabolism is dependent on hepatic blood flow. Because the reduction in cardiac output during cardiac arrest reduces hepatic blood flow, lidocaine clearance decreases.[69] The clinical significance of this has been questioned.[70] Although lidocaine levels may be variable and unpredictable during cardiac arrest,[71] they are nontoxic following ROSC and return of cardiac output.[70] Plasma concentrations should be monitored with prolonged maintenance infusions, and patients should be assessed for adverse effects, including slurred speech, altered consciousness, muscle twitching, and seizures.

THERAPEUTIC ALTERNATIVES FOR REFRACTORY VF OR PVT

Patients with persistent or recurrent VF or PVT following antiarrhythmic administration should be assessed for underlying electrolyte abnormalities as a cause for their refractory arrhythmia. The primary electrolyte abnormalities associated with refractory ventricular arrhythmias include hyperkalemia, hypokalemia, and hypomagnesemia.

In one study of prehospital cardiac arrests, 49% of resuscitated patients were found to be hypokalemic ($[K^+] < 3.6$ mEq/L) on hospital admission.[72] Although frequently debated, it is not yet known whether the hypokalemia most often precedes cardiac arrest or is a consequence of cardiac resuscitation.[72–74] Hypokalemia identified during cardiac arrest may also result from conditions that arise during resuscitation. For example, intracellular potassium shifts may occur secondarily to metabolic derangements or to elevated circulating catecholamine concentrations.[72–74] Similarly, hypomagnesemia has been associated with ventricular arrhythmias.[75] Investigators have found that in hospitalized patients, approximately 40% of hypokalemic patients have coexisting hypomagnesemia.[76] This is important because uncorrected hypomagnesemia may prevent successful potassium repletion.[76] The value of magnesium in cardiac arrest has not been demonstrated in randomized controlled trials, but anecdotal evidence is supportive. Therefore, the administration of magnesium is recommended only when a low level of magnesium is the suspected cause of an arrhythmia or when the patient experiences torsades de pointes.[8] Large doses of magnesium may produce hypotension, but do not compromise coronary perfusion pressure because of coronary artery dilatation.[7]

NON–VF/PVT RHYTHMS: PEA AND ASYSTOLE

NONPHARMACOLOGIC THERAPY

Pulseless electrical activity is defined as the absence of a detectable pulse and the presence of some type of electrical activity other than VF or PVT. Asystole is defined as the presence of a "flat line" on the ECG monitor. Although PEA is still classified as a "rhythm of survival," the success rate of treatment is much lower than the rates seen with VF/PVT.[6,77] The rate of survival among patients with asystole is a dismal 1% to 2%.[8] Successful treatment of both PEA and asystole depends almost entirely on diagnosis of the underlying cause (Table 11–4). The treatment of PEA is relatively similar to the treatment of asystole. Both conditions require CPR, intubation, and IV access. Emphasis, once again, should be placed on identifying a correctable cause. Asystole should be reconfirmed by checking a second lead on the cardiac monitor. Defibrillation should be avoided in patients with asystole, because the parasympathetic discharge that occurs with defibrillation may reduce the chance of ROSC and worsen the chance of survival. If available, transcutaneous pacing can be attempted. Asystole often represents confirmation of death rather than a rhythm to be treated; therefore, withdrawal of efforts must be strongly considered.

PHARMACOLOGIC THERAPY

The primary pharmacologic agents used in the treatment of asystole are epinephrine and atropine. The recommended epinephrine dose is identical to that used for the treatment of VF/PVT.

Atropine is an antimuscarinic agent that blocks the depressant effect of acetylcholine on both the sinus and atrioventricular nodes, thus decreasing parasympathetic tone. During asystole, parasympathetic tone may increase because of the vagal stimulation that occurs secondary to intubation, the effects of hypoxia and acidosis, or alterations in the balance of parasympathetic and sympathetic control.[78,79] Unfortunately, there are no large randomized trials showing benefit from atropine for the treatment of asystole. Evidence is limited to small case series or retrospective reviews.[80–85]

Gupta and colleagues demonstrated the beneficial effects of atropine in 4 patients with "cardiac standstill."[80] The response time for treatment in these patients was less than 22.5 seconds. Only 1 patient was actually in asystole when atropine was given, however. Iseri and colleagues reported a case series of 15 asystolic patients with 2 patients receiving atropine; none of these patients were successfully resuscitated.[81] Brown and coworkers reported results in 8 patients with asystole treated with atropine; 3 of the 8 patients survived to hospital discharge, but 2 of these surviving patients had developed asystole

TABLE 11–4 Potentially Reversible Causes of PEA and Asystole

Condition	Clues	Treatment
Hypovolemia	History, flat neck veins	Intravenous fluids
Hypoxia	Cyanosis, abnormal blood gases, airway problems	Ventilation, oxygen
Preexisting acidosis	History of bicarbonate–responsive preexisting acidosis	Sodium bicarbonate, hyperventilation
Hyperkalemia	History of renal failure, diabetes, recent dialysis, dialysis fistulas, medications	Calcium chloride, insulin, glucose, sodium bicarbonate, sodium polystyrene sulfonate, dialysis
Hypothermia	History of exposure to cold, low central body temperature	Rewarming, oxygen, intravenous fluids
Drug overdose	Bradycardia, history of ingestion, empty bottles at the scene, pupil size, neurologic examination	Drug screens, intubation, lavage, activated charcoal
Cardiac tamponade	History (trauma, renal failure, thoracic malignancy); no pulse with CPR; vein distention; impending tamponade–tachycardia; hypotension; low pulse pressure, changing to sudden bradycardia as terminal event	Pericardiocentesis
Tension pneumothorax	History (asthma, ventilator, chronic obstructive pulmonary disease, trauma), no pulse with CPR, neck vein distention, tracheal deviation	Needle decompression
Coronary thrombosis	History, ECG, elevated cardiac enzymes	Thrombolytics, oxygen, nitroglycerin, heparin, aspirin, morphine
Pulmonary thrombosis	History, no pulse with CPR, distended neck veins	Pulmonary arteriogram, surgical embolectomy, thrombolytics

CPR = cardiopulmonary resuscitation; ECG = electrocardiogram.
(Adapted from Ref. 7.)

secondary to cardiac catheterization.[79] Coon and associates published a prospective study of 21 patients with either asystole or pulseless idioventricular rhythm; although 10 patients received atropine, none survived to hospital discharge.[82] In a retrospective case-control study, Stueven and colleagues found a 14% (6/43) success rate with atropine compared to a 0% (0/41) rate with a control; as in previous trials, no patients survived to hospital discharge.[83] Ornato and associates published a retrospective study of 24 patients with asystole as the presenting rhythm; of the 22 patients who received atropine, asystole was abolished in 4.[84] Once again, none survived to hospital discharge. Finally, Tortolani and associates retrospectively reviewed the case histories of 123 patients with asystole.[85] Of the 101 patients who had received atropine, 24 were alive 24 hours postresuscitation. It is unclear how many survived to hospital discharge. These results show that although atropine may achieve ROSC in some instances, asystolic arrest is almost always fatal. Thus, the use of atropine for this indication is not harmful, but the beneficial effect is limited.

ACID–BASE MANAGEMENT DURING CPR

Acidosis seen during cardiac arrest results from decreased blood flow and inadequate ventilation. Chest compressions generate approximately 20% to 30% of normal cardiac output, leading to inadequate organ perfusion, tissue hypoxia, and metabolic acidosis. In addition, the lack of ventilation causes retention of carbon dioxide, leading to respiratory acidosis. This combined acidosis produces not only reduced myocardial contractility and negative inotropic effect, but also the appearance of arrhythmias because of a lower fibrillation threshold. In early cardiac arrest, adequate alveolar ventilation is the mainstay of control to limit the accumulation of carbon dioxide and control the acid-base imbalance.[8] With arrests of long duration, buffer therapy is often necessary.

Although sodium bicarbonate was once routinely given to reduce the detrimental effects associated with acidosis (e.g., reduced myocardial contractility), enhance the effect of epinephrine, and improve the rate of defibrillation, its use for cardiac arrest has become extremely controversial over the past several years. Unfortunately, there are few clinical data supporting sodium bicarbonate use.[86] Furthermore, sodium bicarbonate may have some detrimental effects.[86–88] The effect of sodium bicarbonate can be described by the following reaction:

$$[H^+] + [HCO_3^-] \rightleftharpoons H_2CO_3 \rightleftharpoons H_2O + CO_2$$

When sodium bicarbonate is added to an acidic environment, this reaction will shift to the right, thereby increasing tissue and venous hypercarbia. The carbon dioxide generated by this reaction will diffuse into the cell and decrease intracellular pH. The accumulation of intracellular carbon dioxide, specifically within the myocardium, is inversely correlated with coronary perfusion pressure produced by CPR. Intracellular acidosis will also decrease myocardial contractility, further complicating the low-flow state associated with CPR.[86] Furthermore, treatment with sodium bicarbonate often overcorrects extracellular pH, as sodium bicarbonate has a greater effect when the pH is closer to normal.[87] Alkalosis, created by overcorrection, causes an increase in the affinity of oxygen to hemoglobin, thus interfering with oxygen release into the tissues.

Recommendations for sodium bicarbonate vary (from Class I to Class III), depending on the clinical situation.[8] Sodium bicarbonate use is acceptable for patients with known, preexisting hyperkalemia (Class I); preexisting bicarbonate-responsive acidosis (Class IIa); overdoses of tricyclic antidepressants (Class IIa); to alkalinize the urine in aspirin and other drug overdoses (Class IIa). In addition, sodium bicarbonate may be of benefit in intubated and ventilated patients with a long arrest interval (Class IIb). Sodium bicarbonate may be harmful in hypercarbic acidosis, and patients with this condition should not receive it (Class III).

GUIDELINES FOR DRUG ADMINISTRATION DURING EMERGENCY SITUATIONS

Several routes of administration are available for drug delivery during CPR. The routes chosen represent a compromise between the practicality of access and their apparent efficacy in introducing the necessary drug into central circulation. The most efficacious method, obviously, is administration through a central venous catheter. Compared to peripheral administration, drug delivery via a central venous catheter results in a faster and higher peak concentration.[89] Central lines located above the diaphragm are preferable to those located below the diaphragm because of poor blood flow during CPR.[89,90] It is not practical, however, to interrupt CPR for an invasive procedure such as central line placement. Thus, if a central line is not already present, it is necessary to use a peripheral venous line. The antecubital vein is the first target for IV access.[7] Peripheral drug administration yields a peak concentration in the major systemic arteries in 1.5 to 3 minutes.[89] Circulation time is shortened by up to 40% if the drug is followed by a 20-mL fluid bolus with elevation of the extremity.[89]

In the event that neither central nor venous IV access is available, then a few drugs can be administered endotracheally. Those drugs are atropine, lidocaine, and epinephrine remembered by the AHA pneumonic A-L-E.[7] Animal studies have shown that endotracheal administration mimics the effects of IV administration.[78] Human studies, on the other hand, show that drugs administered endotracheally have a lower plasma concentration with a delayed peak, but a longer duration of action.[89] Therefore, it is recommended that the endotracheal dose be 2 to 2.5 times larger than the IV dose.[7]

The technique of endotracheal drug administration markedly influences the pattern of absorption.[78] The dose should first be diluted with 10 mL of sterile water or normal saline to permit distribution over the largest possible surface area. Cardiopulmonary resuscitation should be interrupted and the dose administered beyond the tip of the endotracheal tube. Immediately, three to five forceful insufflations should follow using a bag-valve device to aerosolize the drug and enhance bioavailability.

In pediatric patients, the intraosseous route can be used temporarily if no other route is available. Lastly, the intracardiac route is no longer recommended for patients of any age because of potential complications, such as myocardial laceration, coronary artery laceration, hemopericardium, and pneumopericardium.

ETHICAL AND ECONOMIC CONSIDERATIONS IN CPR

The primary objective of CPR is to obtain "neurologic survival." As this is often unobtainable, many health care professionals are attempting to identify patients unlikely to benefit from cardiac resuscitation. One difficulty in accomplishing this task is defining "medical futility." The two major determinants of medical futility are length of life and quality of life.[8] An intervention that cannot increase length or quality of life is considered futile. Key factors in CPR are the disease underlying the cardiac arrest and the expected state of health after resuscitation. One important question that is often debated is,

How low should the chance of survival be before medical therapy is considered futile? Should it be 0.1%, 1%, or 2%? Is the chance of one or two months of life for a patient an acceptable goal? These are important questions that must be addressed when determining resuscitation status.

Unfortunately, there is no scientific evidence or scoring system that can predict the outcome following CPR. Therefore, all patients in cardiac arrest should receive resuscitation unless the patient has a "do not resuscitate" order, signs of irreversible death, or vital organ function deterioration that makes it impossible to expect any benefit from CPR—despite maximum therapy.[8] Withholding CPR attempts in these futile cases would not only decrease the number of patients left in a vegetative state with poor neurologic status, but also improve the cost-effectiveness of CPR programs. Cardiopulmonary resuscitation is of minimal economic benefit if the only outcome following ROSC is a prolonged, expensive hospital stay.

EVALUATION OF THERAPEUTIC OUTCOMES

To gauge the success of resuscitation outcomes, therapeutic outcome monitoring should occur both during the resuscitation attempt and in the postresuscitation phase. The optimal outcome following CPR is an awake, responsive, spontaneously breathing patient. Patients must remain neurologically intact with minimal morbidity following the resuscitation if it is to be truly classified as a success. Heart rate, cardiac rhythm, and blood pressure should be assessed and documented throughout the resuscitation attempt and subsequent to each intervention. Determination of the presence or absence of a pulse is paramount to deciding which interventions may be appropriate. In addition, nonresponse to an array of suitable interventions may indicate that resuscitation is impossible.

The primary goal of resuscitation is the complete reestablishment of regional organ and tissue perfusion. Simple restoration of blood pressure and improvement in tissue gas exchange do not necessarily improve the patient's chance of survival.[8] Clinicians should consider the precipitating cause of the cardiac arrest, such as an acute MI, electrolyte imbalance, or primary arrhythmia. They should carefully review prearrest status, particularly if the patient was receiving drug therapy. Laboratory investigations, including a 12-lead ECG, portable chest x-ray film, measurement of arterial blood gases, and blood chemistry determinations are necessary. Altered cardiac, hepatic, and renal function resulting from ischemic damage during the cardiopulmonary arrest warrant special attention. Neurologic function should be assessed by means of the Glasgow Coma Scale and Cerebral Performance Category (Table 11–5).

TABLE 11–5 Assessment of Neurologic Function

A. Glasgow Coma Scale[90]

Eyes Opening	Spontaneous	4
	To command	3
	To pain	2
	No response	1
Best Motor Response	Obedience to verbal commands	6
	Localization of pain	5
	Withdrawal in response to pain	4
	Abnormal flexion (decorticate)	3
	Extensor response (decerebrate)	2
	Flaccidity	1
Verbal	Appropriate orientation	5
	Confused conversation	4
	Inappropriate words	3
	Incomprehensible sounds	2
	No response	1

B. Cerebral Performance Category[91]

Conscious and alert with normal function or only slight disability	1
Conscious and alert with moderate disability	2
Conscious with severe disability	3
Comatose or in a persistent vegetative state	4
Brain dead	5

▶ PRINCIPLES OF PHARMACOTHERAPY

- The goal of attempting cardiopulmonary resuscitation is to return effective ventilation and circulation as quickly as possible to minimize hypoxic damage to vital organs.
- For patients in VF/PVT, rapid defibrillation is the single most important intervention that affects survival.
- For VF or PVT, either epinephrine or vasopressin is the drug of first choice following electrical defibrillation, CPR, endotracheal intubation, and IV access.
- Amiodarone is the antiarrhythmic of first choice, according to many experts.
- For PEA, the primary focus should be diagnosis and identification of a reversible cause.

REFERENCES

1. Niemann JT. Cardiopulmonary resuscitation. N Engl J Med 1992; 327(15):1075–1080.
2. Thel MC, O'Connor CM. Cardiopulmonary resuscitation: historical perspective to recent investigations. Am Heart J 1999;137:39–48.
3. Paraskos JA. History of CPR and the role of the national conference. Ann Emerg Med 1993;22:275–280.
4. Safar P, Escarraga L, Elam JO. A comparison of the mouth-to-mouth and mouth-to-airway methods of artificial respiration with chest pressure arm-life method. N Engl J Med 1958;258:671–677.
5. Kouwenhoven WB, Jude JR, Knickerbocker GG. Closed-chest cardiac massage. JAMA 1960;173:1064–1067.
6. O'Nunain S, Ruskin J. Cardiac arrest. Lancet 1993;341:1641.
7. 1997–1999 Emergency Cardiovascular Care Programs, Advanced Cardiac Life Support. American Heart Association, 1997.
8. The American Heart Association in collaboration with the International Liaison Committee on Resuscitation. Guidelines 2000 for cardiopulmonary resuscitation and emergency cardiovascular care: an international consensus on science. Circulation 2000;102(Suppl 1):1–370.
9. Pepe PE, Levine RL, Fromm R. Cardiac arrest presenting with rhythms other than ventricular fibrillation: contribution of resuscitative efforts toward total survivorship. Crit Care Med 1993;21:1838–1843.
10. Chandra NS. Mechanisms of blood flow during CPR. Ann Emerg Med 1993;22:281–288.
11. Tucker KJ, Savitt MA, Idris A, Redberg RF. Cardiopulmonary resuscitation: historical perspectives, physiology, and future directions. Arch Intern Med 1994;154:2141–2150.
12. Becker LB, Berg RA, Pepe PE, et al. A reappraisal of mouth-to-mouth ventilation during bystander initiated cardiopulmonary resuscitation: a statement for healthcare professionals from the ventilation working group of the basic life support and pediatric life support subcommittees, American Heart Association. Ann Emerg Med 1997;30:654–666.
13. Eisenberg MS, Bergner L, Hallstrom A. Cardiac resuscitation in the community: Importance of rapid provision and implications for program planning. JAMA 1979;241:1905–1907.
14. Ayers SM. Preventing cardiac arrest. Crit Care Med 1994;22(2):189–191.
15. Edwards GA, Samuels TM. The role of the hospital pharmacist in emergency situations. Am J Hosp Pharm 1968;25:128–133.
16. Bardas SL. Demystifying the cardiopulmonary code team response. Pharm Technol 1992;8:151–154.
17. Bossaert LL. Fibrillation and defibrillation of the heart. Br J Anaesth 1997;79:203–213.
18. Paradis NA, Martin GB, Rivers EP, et al. Coronary perfusion pressure and the return of spontaneous circulation in human cardiopulmonary resuscitation. JAMA 1990;263:1106–1113.
19. Robinson LA, Brown CG, Jenkins J, et al. The effect of norepinephrine versus epinephrine on myocardial hemodynamics during CPR. Ann Emerg Med 1989;18:336–340.
20. Otto CW, Yakaitis RW, Blitt CD. Mechanism of action of epinephrine in resuscitation from asphyxial arrest. Crit Care Med 1981;9:321–324.
21. Paradis NA, Koscrove EM. Epinephrine in cardiac arrest: a critical review. Ann Emerg Med 1990;19:1288–1301.
22. Ditchey RV, Lindenfeld J. Failure of epinephrine to improve the balance between myocardial oxygen supply and demand during closed-chest resuscitation in dogs. Circulation 1988;78(2):382–389.
23. Tang W, Weil MH, Sun S, et al. Epinephrine increases the severity of postresuscitation myocardial dysfunction. Circulation 1995;92:3089–3093.
24. Ornato JP. Use of adrenergic agonists during CPR in adults. Ann Emerg Med 1993;22:411–416.
25. Holmes HR, Babbs CF, Voorhees WD, et al. Influence of adrenergic drugs upon vital organ perfusion during CPR. Crit Care Med 1980;8:137–140.
26. Brown C, Wiklund L, Bar-Joseph G, et al. Future directions for resuscitation research, IV: innovative advanced life support pharmacology. Resuscitation 1996;33:163–177.
27. Callaham M, Madsen CD, Barton CW, et al. A randomized clinical trial of high-dose epinephrine and norepinephrine vs standard-dose epinephrine in prehospital cardiac arrest. JAMA 1992;268:2667–2672.
28. Lindner KH, Ahnefeld FW, Grunert A. Epinephrine versus norepinephrine in prehospital ventricular fibrillation. Am J Cardiol 1991;67:427–428.
29. Lindner KH, Anhefeld FW, Schuermann W, et al. Epinephrine and norepinephrine in cardiopulmonary resuscitation: effects on myocardial oxygen delivery and consumption. Chest 1990;97:1458–1462.
30. Brown CG, Robinson LA, Jenkins J, et al. The effect of norepinephrine versus epinephrine on regional cerebral blood flow during cardiopulmonary resuscitation. Am J Emerg Med 1989;7(3):278–282.
31. Redding JS, Pearson JW. Evaluation of drugs for cardiac resuscitation. Anaesthesia 1963;24:203–207.
32. Kosnik J, Jackson R, Keats S, et al. Dose-related response of aortic diastolic pressure during closed-chest massage in dogs. Ann Emerg Med 1985;14:204–208.
33. Brown CG, Werman HA, Davis EA, et al. Comparative effect of graded doses of epinephrine on regional brain blood flow during CPR in a swine model. Ann Emerg Med 1986;15:1138–1144.
34. Brunette DD, Jameson SJ. Comparison of standard versus high-dose epinephrine in the resuscitation of cardiac arrest in dogs. Ann Emerg Med 1990;19:8–11.
35. Gonzalez ER, Ornato JP, Garnett AR, et al. Dose-dependent vasopressor response to epinephrine during CPR in human beings. Ann Emerg Med 1989;18:920–926.
36. Gueugniaud P, Mols P, Goldstein P, et al. A comparison of repeated high doses and repeated standard doses of epinephrine for cardiac arrest outside the hospital. N Engl J Med 1998;339:1595–1601.
37. Sherman BW, Munger MA, Foulke GE, et al. High-dose versus standard-dose epinephrine treatment of cardiac arrest after failure of standard therapy. Pharmacotherapy 1997;17(2):242–247.
38. Choux C, Gueugniaud P, Barbieux A, et al. Standard doses versus repeated high doses of epinephrine in cardiac arrest outside the hospital. Resuscitation 1995;29(1):3–9.
39. Lipman J, Wilson W, Kobilski S, et al. High-dose adrenaline in adult in-hospital asystolic cardiopulmonary resuscitation: a double-blind randomized trial. Anaesth Intensive Care 1993;21:192–196.
40. Stiell IG, Hebert PC, Weitzman BN, et al. High-dose epinephrine in adult cardiac arrest. N Engl J Med 1992;327:1045–1050.
41. Brown CG, Martin DR, Pepe PE, et al. A comparison of standard-dose and high-dose epinephrine in cardiac arrest outside the hospital. N Engl J Med 1992;327:1051–1055.
42. Lindner KH, Ahnefeld FW, Prengel AW. Comparison of standard and high-dose adrenaline in the resuscitation of asystole and electromechanical dissociation. Acta Anaesthesiol Scand 1991;35:253–256. al., 1992.
43. Callaham M, Barton CW, Kayser S. Potential complications of high-dose epinephrine therapy in patients resuscitated from cardiac arrest. JAMA 1991;265:1117–1122.

44. Behringer W, Kittler H, Sterz F, et al. Cumulative epinephrine dose during cardiopulmonary resuscitation and neurologic outcome. Ann Intern Med 1998;129:450–456.
45. Kelly CM, Ponzillo JJ. Vasopressin use in cardiopulmonary resuscitation. Ann Pharmacother 1997;31(12):1523–1525.
46. Lindner KH, Strohmenger HU, Ensinger H, et al. Stress hormone response during and after cardiopulmonary resuscitation. Anesthesiology 1992;77:662–668.
47. Wenzel V, Lindner KH, Prengel AW, et al. Vasopressin improves vital organ blood flow after prolonged cardiac arrest with postcountershock pulseless electrical activity in pigs. Crit Care Med 1999;27(3):486–492.
48. Wenzel V, Lindner KH, Krismer AC, et al. Repeated administration of vasopressin but not epinephrine maintains coronary perfusion pressure after early and late administration during prolonged cardiopulmonary resuscitation in pigs. Circulation 1999;99(10):1379–1384.
49. Wenzel V, Lindner KH, Krismer AC, et al. Survival with full neurologic recovery and no cerebral pathology after prolonged cardiopulmonary resuscitation with vasopressin in pigs. J Am Coll Cardiol 2000;35(2):527–533.
50. Lindner KH, Brinkmann A, Pfenninger EG, et al. Effect of vasopressin on hemodynamic variables, organ blood flow, and acid base status in a pig model of cardiopulmonary resuscitation. Anesth Analg 1993;77(3):427–435.
51. Voelckel WG, Lindner KH, Wenzel V, et al. Effects of vasopressin and epinephrine on splanchnic blood flow and renal function during and after cardiopulmonary resuscitation in pigs. Crit Care Med 2000;28(4):1083–1088.
52. Lindner KH, Prengel AW, Brinkmann A, et al. Vasopressin administration in refractory cardiac arrest. Ann Intern Med 1996;124(12):1061–1064.
53. Lindner KH, Dirks B, Strohmenger HU, et al. Randomized comparison of epinephrine and vasopressin in patients with out-of-hospital ventricular fibrillation. Lancet 1997;349:535–537.
54. Prengel AW, Lindner KH, Keller A, Lurie KG. Cardiovascular function during the postresuscitation phase after cardiac arrest in pigs: a comparison of epinephrine versus vasopressin. Crit Care Med 1996;24(12):2014–2019.
55. Gonzalez ER, Kannewurf BS, Ornato JP. Intravenous amiodarone for ventricular arrhythmias: overview and clinical use. Resuscitation 1998;39:33–42.
56. Kowey PR, Levine JH, Herre JM, et al. Randomized, double-blind comparison of intravenous amiodarone and bretylium in the treatment of patients with recurrent, hemodynamically destabilizing ventricular tachycardia or fibrillation. The Intravenous Amiodarone Multicenter Investigators Group. Circulation 1995;92(11):3255–3263.
57. Podrid PJ. Amiodarone: reevaluation of an old drug. Ann Intern Med 1995;122:689–700.
58. Kudenchuk PJ, Cobb LA, Copass MK, et al. Amiodarone for resuscitation after out-of-hospital cardiac arrest due to ventricular fibrillation. N Engl J Med 1999;341(12):871–878.
59. Harrison EE. Lidocaine in prehospital countershock refractory ventricular fibrillation. Ann Emerg Med 1981;10(8):420–423.
60. Weaver WD, Fahrenbruch CE, Johnson DD, et al. Effect of epinephrine and lidocaine therapy on outcome after cardiac arrest to ventricular fibrillation. Circulation 1990;82(6):2027–2034.
61. Herlitz J, Ekstrom L, Wennerblom B, et al. Lidocaine in out-of-hospital ventricular fibrillation: does it improve survival? Resuscitation 1997;33(3):199–205.
62. Chow MS. Advanced cardiac life support controversy: where do antiarrhythmic agents fit in? Pharmacotherapy 1997;17:84S–88S.
63. Kerber RE, Pandian NG, Jensen SR, et al. Effect of lidocaine and bretylium on energy requirements for transthoracic defibrillation: experimental studies. J Am Coll Cardiol 1986;7:397–405.
64. Jaffe AS. The use of antiarrhythmics in advanced cardiac life support. Ann Intern Med 1993;22:307–316.
65. Chow MS, Kluger J, DiPersio DM, et al. Antifibrillatory effects of lidocaine and bretylium immediately postcardiopulmonary resuscitation. Am Heart J 1985;110(5):938–943.
66. Hanyok JJ, Chow MS, Kluger J, Fieldman A. Antifibrillatory effects of high dose bretylium and a lidocaine-bretylium combination during cardiopulmonary resuscitation. Crit Care Med 1988;16(7):691–694.
67. Haynes RE, Chinn TL, Copass MK, Cobb LA. Comparison of bretylium tosylate and lidocaine in management of out of hospital ventricular fibrillation: a randomized clinical trial. Am J Cardiol 1981;48(2):353–356.
68. Olson DW, Thompson BM, Darin JC, Milbrath MH. A randomized comparison study of bretylium tosylate and lidocaine in resuscitation of patients from out-of-hospital ventricular fibrillation in a paramedic system. Ann Emerg Med 1984;13(9):807–810.
69. Pentel P, Benowitz N. Pharmacokinetic and pharmacodynamic considerations in drug therapy of cardiac emergencies. Clin Pharmacokinet 1984;9:273–308.
70. Hendrie J, O'Callaghan CJ. Lidocaine pharmacokinetics after cardiac arrest and external cardiopulmonary resuscitation. Am J Cardiol 1996;78(11):1322–1323.
71. Chow MS, Ronfeld RA, Ruggett D, Fieldman A. Lidocaine pharmacokinetics during cardiac arrest and external cardiopulmonary resuscitation. Am Heart J 1981;102(4):799–801.
72. Thompson RG, Cobb LA. Hypokalemia after resuscitation from out-of-hospital ventricular fibrillation. JAMA 1982;248:2860–2863.
73. Ornato JP, Gonzalez ER, Starke H, et al. Incidence and causes of hypokalemia associated with cardiac resuscitation. Am J Emerg Med 1985;3:503–506.
74. Higham PD, Adams PC, Murray A, Campbell RW. Plasma potassium, serum magnesium and ventricular fibrillation: a prospective study. Q J Med 1993;86:609–617.
75. Eisenberg MJ. Magnesium deficiency and sudden death. Am Heart J 1992;124:544–549.
76. Whang R, Flink EB, Dyckner T, et al. Magnesium depletion as a cause of refractory potassium repletion. Arch Intern Med 1985;145:1686–1689.
77. Herlitz J, Ekstrom L, Wennerblom B, et al. Survival among patients with out-of-hospital cardiac arrest found in electromechanical dissociation. Resuscitation 1995;29:97–106.
78. Gonzalez ER. Pharmacologic controversies in CPR. Ann Emerg Med 1993;22:317–323.
79. Brown DC, Lewis AJ, Criley JM. Asystole and its treatment: the possible role of the parasympathetic nervous system in cardiac arrest. JACEP 1979;8:448–452.
80. Gupta PK, Lichstein E, Chadda KD. Transient atrioventricular standstill: etiology and management. JAMA 1975;234:1038–1042.
81. Iseri LT, Humphrey SB, Siner EJ. Prehospital brady-asystolic cardiac arrest. Ann Intern Med 1978:88:741–745.
82. Coon GA, Clinton JE, Ruiz E. Use of atropine from bradyasystolic prehospital cardiac arrest. Ann Emerg Med 1981;10:462–467.
83. Stueven HA, Tonsfeldt DJ, Thompson BM, et al. Atropine in asystole: human studies. Ann Emerg Med 1984;13:815–817.
84. Ornato JP, Gonzalez ER, Morkunas AR, et al. Treatment of presumed asystole during prehospital cardiac arrest: superiority of electrical countershock. Am J Emerg Med 1985;3:395–399.
85. Tortolani AJ, Risucci DA, Powell SR, et al. In-hospital cardiopulmonary resuscitation during asystole: therapeutic factors associated with 24-hour survival. Chest 1989;96:622–626.
86. Levy MM. An evidence-based evaluation of the use of sodium bicarbonate during cardiac resuscitation. Crit Care Clin 1998;14(3):457–483.
87. Bjerneroth G. Tribonat: a comprehensive summary of its properties. Crit Care Med 1999;27(5):1009–1013.
88. Adgey AAJ. Adrenaline dosage and buffers in cardiac arrest. Heart 1998;80:412–414.
89. Vincent R. Drugs in modern resuscitation. Br J Anaesth 1997;79:188–197.
90. Jannett B, Teasdale G. Aspects of coma after severe head injury. Lancet 1977;1:878.
91. Jennett B, Bond M. Assessment of outcome after severe brain damage. Lancet 1975;1:480–484.

12

HYPERTENSION

Barry L. Carter and Joseph J. Saseen

Hypertension is a common disease that is simply defined by persistent elevation of arterial blood pressure. During the early and middle 1900s, elevated blood pressure was perceived to be necessary for adequate perfusion of essential organs. However, it is now identified as one of the most significant contributing factors to cardiovascular morbidity and mortality in the United States. Increased awareness has been placed on diagnosing and appropriately treating patients with hypertension in an attempt to reduce the risk of cardiovascular disease.

The Sixth Joint National Committee on the Detection, Evaluation, and Treatment of High Blood Pressure (JNC-VI) was developed to aid clinicians in the management of hypertension.[1] This chapter will review the relevant components of this evidence-based guideline, as well as the disease process and pharmacotherapy of hypertension. Data from 1991 to 1994 indicate that of the population of Americans with hypertension, 31.6% are not aware of their condition, only 27.4% have controlled blood pressure, and another 26.2% are on medication without control of blood pressure.[1] Therefore, there is ample opportunity for clinicians familiar with the management of this disease to improve the care of patients.

EPIDEMIOLOGY

It has been estimated that 50 million Americans have high blood pressure (≥140/90 mm Hg).[1,2] Specifically, the estimated prevalence of hypertension from the National Health and Nutrition Examination Survey III (Phases 1 and 2, 1988–1994) is 19.3% among white women, 24.4% among white men, 34.2% among black women, 35.0% among black men, 22.0% among Mexican-American women, and 25.2% among Mexican-American men.[2]

Blood pressure values continue to increase with age, and hypertension is very common in the elderly. However, most patients are diagnosed with hypertension during the third, fourth, and fifth decades of life. Up to the age of 55 years, more men than women have hypertension. From the ages of 55 to 74 years, slightly more women have hypertension than men, with this sex difference becoming quite clear in the very elderly (≥75 years). In the older population (age ≥60 years), the prevalence of hypertension is above 60%.

ETIOLOGY

Hypertension is a heterogeneous condition that can result from either an unknown pathophysiologic etiology (primary or essential hypertension) or a specific cause (secondary hypertension). The vast majority of individuals with high blood pressure have essential hypertension. Numerous mechanisms that may contribute to the pathogenesis of hypertension have been investigated to identify the underlying abnormality that results in high blood pressure. Hypertension often runs in families. This suggests that genetic factors may play an important pathogenic role in the development of essential hypertension. There is even some evidence that single genes might be responsible for specific subtypes of hypertension. These include genetic traits for high sodium-lithium countertransport, a low urinary kallikrein excretion, decreased nitric oxide, increased aldosterone and other adrenal steroids, and high angiotensinogen levels.[3–5] Identifying individuals with these traits could lead to more direct approaches to preventing or treating hypertension, but this is currently not recommended.

Fewer than 5% of people who suffer from high blood pressure have secondary hypertension. In most of these cases, renal dysfunction (either renovascular or renoparenchymal disease) is the cause of hypertension. Other conditions that are known to cause secondary hypertension include pheochromocytoma (adrenal tumor), Cushing's syndrome, hyperthyroidism, hyperparathyroidism, primary aldosteronism, pregnancy, increased intracranial pressure, and coarctation of the aorta. In some instances, drug-induced causes can be identified. The most common agents that potentially may increase blood pressure include adrenalcorticosteroids, alcohol (with chronic use), amphetamines, anorexiant agents, some antidepressants (monoamine oxidase inhibitors, venlafaxine), cyclosporine, estrogens, licorice, nonsteroidal anti-inflammatory agents, oral contraceptives, oral decongestants, and thyroid hormone products. When a secondary cause can be identified, treatment should be directed at removing the offending agent or treating the underlying condition.

ARTERIAL BLOOD PRESSURE

Arterial blood pressure is generated by the interplay between blood flow and the resistance to blood flow. Peak blood pressure values are achieved during cardiac contraction (systolic pressure) and nadir at the end of contraction (diastolic pressure). Arterial blood pressure conventionally is measured in millimeters of mercury and recorded as systolic pressure over diastolic pressure (e.g., 120/75 mm Hg). The difference between systolic blood pressure (SBP) and diastolic blood pressure (DBP) is called the *pulse pressure* and is an indicator of arterial wall tension. The mean arterial pressure (MAP) is the average pressure throughout the cardiac cycle of contraction. During a cardiac cycle, two-thirds of the time is spent in diastole and one-third in systole. Therefore, the MAP can be estimated by using the following equation:

$$\text{MAP} = (1/3\text{SBP}) + (2/3\text{DBP})$$

Under normal physiologic conditions, arterial blood pressure fluctuates only within a narrow range. It may increase to higher values during physical or emotional stress and typically is at its highest values during the midmorning. Arterial blood pressure usually falls to its lowest levels during sleep.

Arterial blood pressure (BP) can be defined hemodynamically as the product of cardiac output (CO) and total peripheral resistance (TPR): BP = CO × TPR. Cardiac output is the major determinant of SBP, whereas total peripheral resistance largely determines the level of DBP. In turn, cardiac output is a function of stroke volume, heart rate, and venous capacitance. Factors that increase stroke volume or heart rate may increase cardiac output and, consequently, can increase SBP. Venous capacitance affects the volume of blood (or preload) that is returned to the heart through the central venous circulation. Venous dilatation increases venous capacitance and decreases preload and systolic pressure. Constriction of peripheral veins conversely causes the opposite effect. Contraction and dilation of the arterioles regulate total peripheral resistance. Arteriolar constriction increases peripheral resistance and DBP. Other factors that affect intravascular resistance include the elasticity of aortic and arterial walls and blood viscosity.

Evidence from epidemiologic studies clearly indicates a strong correlation between blood pressure and cardiovascular morbidity and mortality.[6] The higher the pressure, the more likely it is that an individual will experience stroke, myocardial infarction, angina, heart failure, renal failure, or early death from a cardiovascular cause. Moreover, large-scale outcome trials have shown that the increased risks of cardiovascular events and death associated with elevated blood pressure are reduced substantially by interventions that lower blood pressure.[7–10]

The JNC-VI classifies hypertension in adults based on measured blood pressure values into various stages[1] (Table 12–1). Patients with DBP values of less than 90 mm Hg and SBP values of 140 mm Hg or higher have *isolated systolic hypertension.* Isolated systolic hypertension is believed to result from pathophysiologic changes in the arterial vasculature consistent with aging. These changes decrease the compliance of the arterial wall and portend an increased risk of cardiovascular morbidity and mortality. It is now believed that SBP is a much stronger marker for cardiovascular disease.[11] Additionally, pulse pressure may be an even better predictor of risk than SBP, but it is unlikely that it will be used to categorize patients clinically.[12] Pulse pressure is the difference between the SBP and the DBP. As pulse pressure widens or gets larger, it is a measure of increased arterial stiffness.

A marked or sharp increase in blood pressure (into the upper levels of stage 3) is considered a hypertensive crisis. Hypertensive crises can be either a hypertensive emergency or a hypertensive urgency. If the elevation in blood pressure is accompanied by acute target-organ injury, then a hypertensive emergency exists. Examples of acute target-organ injury include encephalopathy, intracranial hemorrhage, acute left ventricular failure with pulmonary edema, dissecting aortic aneurysm, unstable angina, and eclampsia or severe hypertension associated with pregnancy. Hypertensive emergencies require an immediate but gradual reduction in blood pressure over a period of several minutes to several hours. A reasonable goal is to lower the DBP gradually down to stage 2 values. Hypertensive urgencies signify severe hypertension (upper levels of stage 3) without signs or symptoms of acute target-organ complications. This situation requires a reduction in blood pressure generally down to stage 1 values over a period of several hours to several days.

TABLE 12–1. Classification of Blood Pressure for Adults Aged 18 Years and Older[a]

Category	Systolic, mm Hg	Diastolic, mm Hg	Percent of Population[b]
Optimal[c]	<120	<80	47%
Normal	<130	<85	21%
High normal	130–139	85–89	13%
Hypertension[d]			
Stage 1	140–159	90–99	14%
Stage 2	160–179	100–109	4%
Stage 3	≥180	≥110	1%

[a]Not taking antihypertensive drugs and not acutely ill. When systolic and diastolic pressures fall into different categories, the higher category should be selected to classify the individual's blood pressure status. For instance, 174/92 mm Hg should be classified as stage 2 hypertension, and 174/116 mm Hg should be classified as stage 3. Isolated systolic hypertension is defined as a systolic blood pressure of 140 mm Hg or greater and a diastolic blood pressure of less than 90 mm Hg and staged appropriately (e.g., 170/80 mm Hg is defined as stage 2 isolated systolic hypertension). In addition to classifying stages of hypertension on the basis of average blood pressure levels, clinicians should specify presence or absence of target-organ disease and additional risk factors. This specificity is important for risk classification and management.

[b]Percentage distribution of blood pressure levels in the U.S. adult population in each of the listed stages.[112]

[c]Optimal blood pressure with respect to cardiovascular risk is below 120/80 mm Hg. However, unusually low readings should be evaluated for clinical significance.

[d]Based on the average of two or more readings taken at each of two or more visits after an initial screening.

PATHOPHYSIOLOGY[5,13–20]

Multiple contributing factors have been identified as potential components involved in the development of primary hypertension. These include abnormal neuronal mechanisms, defects in peripheral autoregulation, malfunctions in either humoral or vasodepressor mechanisms, and disturbances in sodium, calcium, and natriuretic hormone. Although it is probable that none of these is solely responsible for essential hypertension, certain antihypertensive drug classes have been developed to specifically target these mechanisms.

NEURONAL MECHANISMS

Both the central and the autonomic nervous systems are intricately involved in the regulation of arterial blood pressure. A number of receptors that either enhance or inhibit norepinephrine release are located on the presynaptic surface of sympathetic terminals. The α and β presynaptic receptors play a role in negative and positive feedback to the norepinephrine-containing vesicles located near the neuronal ending. Stimulation of presynaptic α-receptors (α_2) exerts a negative inhibition on norepinephrine release. Stimulation of presynaptic β-receptors facilitates further release of norepinephrine.

Sympathetic neuronal fibers located on the surface of effector cells innervate the α- and β-receptors. Stimulation of postsynaptic α-receptors (α_1) on arterioles and venules results in vasoconstriction. There are two types of postsynaptic β-receptors, β_1 and β_2. Both types of β-adrenergic receptors are present in all tissue innervated by the sympathetic nervous system. However, the distribution of β-receptors is such that in some tissues β_1-receptors predominate and in other tissues β_2-receptors predominate. Stimulation of β_1-receptors in the heart results in an increase in heart rate and contractility, whereas stimulation of β_2-receptors in the arterioles and venules causes vasodilation.

The baroreceptor reflex system is the major negative-feedback mechanism controlling sympathetic activity. Baroreceptors are nerve endings lying in the walls of large arteries, especially in the carotid arteries and aortic arch. Changes in arterial pressure rapidly activate the baroreceptors, which then transmit impulses to the brain stem primarily through the ninth cranial nerve and vagus nerves. In this reflex system, an acute elevation in arterial pressure increases the rate of baroreceptor discharge. This will trigger vasodilation throughout the peripheral circulatory system and a decrease in heart rate and myocardial contractility. Conversely, a decrease in arterial pressure has the opposite effect on the baroreceptors, causing reflex vasoconstriction and an increase in heart rate and force of cardiac contraction. These baroreceptor reflex mechanisms may be blunted in elderly individuals.

Stimulation of certain areas within the central nervous system (nucleus tractus solitarius, vagal nuclei, vasomotor center, and the area postrema) can either increase or decrease blood pressure. For example, α_2-adrenergic stimulation within the central nervous system decreases blood pressure through an inhibitory effect on the vasomotor center. Increased angiotensin II, however, increases sympathetic outflow from the vasomotor center, which leads to an increase in blood pressure.

The primary purpose of these neuronal components is to maintain homeostatic blood pressure. However, pathologic disturbances in any of these neuronal components conceivably could lead to a sustained blood pressure elevation. It is reasonable to postulate that the primary defect can occur in any of the four major components: autonomic nerve fibers, adrenergic receptors, baroreceptors, or central nervous system. Considering that these systems are so physiologically interrelated, a defect in one component may disturb the normal function in another, and the combined abnormalities may then explain the development of hypertension.

PERIPHERAL AUTOREGULATORY COMPONENTS

Abnormalities in either the renal or tissue autoregulatory processes could cause hypertension. It is possible that individuals may first develop a renal defect for sodium excretion and then reset their tissue autoregulatory processes to a higher arterial blood pressure.

Under normal circumstances, the kidney maintains normal blood pressure through a volume-pressure adaptive mechanism. When blood pressure drops, the kidneys respond to this by increasing retention of sodium and water. This leads to plasma volume expansion, which increases blood pressure. Conversely, when blood pressure rises above normal, there is an increase in renal sodium and water excretion, which causes a decrease in plasma volume and cardiac output. This ultimately will result in blood pressure returning to normal.

Local autoregulatory processes maintain adequate tissue oxygenation. When oxygen demand is normal to low, the arteriolar bed remains in a relatively constricted state. However, increases in metabolic demand will trigger arteriolar vasodilation through autoregulation. This vasodilation will lower peripheral vascular resistance and increase blood flow and oxygen delivery.

Intrinsic defects in the renal adaptive mechanism could lead to plasma volume expansion and increased blood flow to peripheral tissues even when blood pressure is normal. Local tissue autoregulatory processes would then be needed to induce arteriolar constriction to offset increases in blood flow. This would raise the peripheral vascular resistance. If this is sustained, thickening of the arteriolar walls may occur, resulting in a sustained elevation in peripheral vascular resistance. An increase in total peripheral vascular resistance is a common underlying finding in patients with primary hypertension.

HUMORAL MECHANISMS

Humoral abnormalities may be involved in the development of essential hypertension. These include the renin-angiotensin-aldosterone system (RAS), the influence of natriuretic hormone that modulates sodium transport, and the presence of hyperinsulinemia.

THE RENIN-ANGIOTENSIN-ALDOSTERONE SYSTEM (RAS)

The primary purpose of the RAS is to regulate sodium, potassium, and fluid balance. Therefore, this system significantly influences vascular tone and sympathetic nervous system activity and ultimately contributes to the homeostatic regulation of blood pressure.

Renin is an enzyme that is synthesized and stored in the juxtaglomerular cells, which are located primarily in the media of the renal afferent arterioles. The release of renin is modulated by several factors. These can be categorized as intrarenal factors (e.g., renal perfusion pressure, catecholamines, angiotensin II) and extrarenal factors (e.g., sodium, chloride, and potassium).

The juxtaglomerular cells function as a baroreceptor-sensing device in the afferent arterioles. Decreased renal perfusion pressure stimulates the release of renin. The juxtaglomerular apparatus also contains a group of specialized distal tubule cells referred to collectively as the *macula densa*. The flux of sodium and chloride across the cells influences renin release. A decrease in the amount of sodium and chloride delivered in the distal tubule stimulates renin release.

Catecholamines increase renin release probably by directly stimulating the juxtaglomerular cells through an action involving the formation of cyclic AMP. Both potassium and calcium also may play a direct role in renin release. Decreased serum potassium or intracellular calcium stimulates renin release by the juxtaglomerular cells.

In blood, renin catalyzes the conversion of angiotensinogen to angiotensin I, which is then converted to angiotensin II by angiotensin-converting enzyme (ACE). After binding to specific receptors (classified as either AT_1 or AT_2 subtypes), angiotensin II exerts its biologic effects in several tissues. The AT_1 receptor is located in brain, renal, myocardial, vascular, and adrenal tissue. AT_1 receptors mediate the majority of responses critical to cardiovascular and renal function. The AT_2 receptor is located in adrenal medullary tissue, uterus, and brain. Stimulation of the AT_2 receptor does not directly influence blood pressure regulation.

Circulating angiotensin II can cause an elevation in blood pressure through both pressor and volume effects. The pressor effects of angiotensin II include direct vasoconstriction, stimulation of catecholamine release from the adrenal medulla, and a centrally mediated increase in sympathetic nervous system activity. Angiotensin II also stimulates the release of aldosterone from the adrenal gland. This leads to retention of both sodium and fluid, with a resulting increase in plasma volume and blood pressure. Clearly, any disturbance in the RAS that leads to an increase in any or all three components could produce hypertension.

Both the heart and brain contain a local RAS. In the heart, angiotensin II is also generated by a second enzyme, angiotensin I convertase (human chymase), which is not blocked by ACE inhibition. Activation of the myocardial RAS leads to increased cardiac contractility and stimulation of cardiac hypertrophy. The brain RAS has at least two functions. Angiotensin II modulates the production and release of hypothalamic and pituitary hormones. Angiotensin II also enhances sympathetic outflow from the medulla oblongata.

Local generation of biologically active angiotensin peptides in peripheral tissues may play an important role in the increased vascular resistance often observed in hypertensive individuals. Some evidence suggests that angiotensin produced by local tissue may interact with other humoral regulators and endothelium-derived growth factors to stimulate vascular smooth muscle growth and metabolism. This in situ generation of angiotensin peptides may, in fact, underlie the development of increased vascular resistance in forms of hypertension that are associated with low plasma renin activity. Components of tissue RAS may be responsible for long-term adaptation to hypertension (i.e., left ventricular hypertrophy, smooth muscle hypertrophy of blood vessels, and glomerular hypertrophy).

NATRIURETIC HORMONE

An increased concentration of circulating natriuretic hormone may be involved in the development of primary hypertension. Natriuretic hormone is believed to inhibit Na^+, K^+-ATPase and thus interfere with sodium transport across cell membranes. It has been suggested that an inherited defect in the kidney's ability to eliminate sodium would cause an increase in extracellular fluid and plasma volume, as discussed earlier. A compensatory increase in the concentration of circulating natriuretic hormone theoretically could increase urinary excretion of sodium and water. This same hormone, however, is also thought to block the active transport of sodium out of arteriolar smooth muscle cells. The increased intracellular concentration of sodium ultimately would increase vascular tone and blood pressure.

INSULIN RESISTANCE AND HYPERINSULINEMIA

Evidence has linked insulin resistance and hyperinsulinemia with the development of hypertension. Hypothetically, increased insulin concentrations may lead to hypertension because of increased renal sodium retention and enhanced sympathetic nervous system activity. Moreover, insulin has growth hormone–like actions that can induce hypertrophy of vascular smooth muscle cells. Insulin also may elevate blood pressure by increasing intracellular calcium concentration, which leads to increased vascular resistance. Truncal obesity and the development of dyslipidemia often accompany hyperinsulinemia, but even nonobese hypertensive individuals have been shown to be insulin-resistant, glucose-intolerant, and hyperinsulinemic. The exact mechanism by which insulin resistance and hyperinsulinemia occur in hypertension is unknown.

VASCULAR ENDOTHELIAL MECHANISMS

The vascular endothelium plays an important role in regulating blood vessel tone. These regulating functions are mediated through a variety of vasoactive substances synthesized by the endothelial cells. It has been postulated that a deficiency in the local synthesis of vasodilating substances such as prostacyclin and bradykinin or an increase in the production of vasoconstricting substances such as angiotensin II and endothelin I contribute to the pathogenesis of hypertension, atherosclerosis, and other diseases. Nitric oxide is a chemical that is produced in the endothelium and relaxes the vascular epithelium and is a very potent vasodilator. The nitric oxide system is an important regulator of arterial blood pressure. Hypertensive patients may have an intrinsic deficiency in nitric oxide release, resulting in inadequate vasodilation that may contribute to hypertension. Although the exact role of nitric oxide in hypertension is unclear, it is a focus of active research and may be a target for pharmacologic intervention in the future.

ELECTROLYTES AND OTHER CHEMICALS

Epidemiologic and clinical data have associated excess sodium intake with the development of hypertension. Population-based studies indicate that high salt intake is associated with a high prevalence of stroke and hypertension and that low salt intake is associated with a low prevalence of hypertension. Clinical studies consistently have shown that restriction of salt intake in the diet lowers blood pressure in many (but not all) subjects with elevated blood pressure. The exact mechanisms by which excess sodium leads to hypertension are not known, but they may be linked to an increase in circulating natriuretic hormone, as described previously. Natriuretic hormone inhibits intracellular sodium transport, which causes increased vascular reactivity and, consequently, a rise in blood pressure.

Altered calcium homeostasis also may play an important role in the pathogenesis of hypertension. A lack of dietary calcium hypothetically can disturb the balance between intracellular and extracellular calcium, resulting in an increased intracellular calcium concentration. This can alter vascular smooth muscle function and increase peripheral vascular resistance. Some studies have shown that supplementing the diet with calcium results in a modest reduction in the blood pressure of hypertensive subjects. More research is needed to confirm the role of altered calcium homeostasis in essential hypertension.

The role of potassium fluctuations is also inadequately understood. Potassium depletion may cause an increase in peripheral vascular resistance, but the clinical impact of small changes in the serum potassium concentration is not clearly defined. Furthermore, very limited data have suggested that potassium supplementation is associated with a reduced incidence of stroke, but this issue needs further study before supplementation can be endorsed.

The presence of hyperuricemia has been associated with cardiovascular events in hypertensive patients but remains controversial because of inconsistent data. Uric acid has no physiologic function and is considered a biologic waste product. Therefore, there is no rational explanation describing how uric acid would be harmful. However, it has been suggested that elevated uric acid be viewed as a supplemental marker of risk if present in hypertensive patients.

CLINICAL PRESENTATION

DIAGNOSIS

Hypertension has been termed the "silent killer" because patients with uncomplicated primary hypertension usually are asymptomatic. The most common physical finding is elevated blood pressure. It should be emphasized that the diagnosis of hypertension should not be based solely on one elevated blood pressure measurement. The average of two or more readings taken at each of two or more visits after an initial screening should be used to diagnose hypertension.[1] Thereafter, this blood pressure average can be used to initially confirm a diagnosis and classify the stage of hypertension present using Table 12–1.

BLOOD PRESSURE MEASUREMENT

Indirect measurement of blood pressure using a sphygmomanometer is a common routine medical screening tool that should be conducted at every health care encounter.[1] This procedure has been well described by the American Heart Association.[21] First, it is imperative that the equipment used for measurement (e.g., inflation cuff, stethoscope, manometer) meet certain certification criteria.[22] These criteria are used to ensure maximum quality and precision with measurement.

The following stepwise technique is recommended[1,21]:

- Patients should refrain from smoking or caffeine ingestion for 30 minutes and be seated in a position that provides support to the lower back with their bare arm resting near heart level. Measuring blood pressure in the supine or standing position may be required under special circumstances (i.e., if volume depletion is suspected). The environment ideally should be relatively free from excessively loud noise and should provide some level of privacy.
- Measurement should begin after at least a 5-minute period of rest.

- A properly sized cuff (pediatric, small, regular, large, or extra large) should be selected to avoid overestimating the actual pressure when the cuff is too small. The inflatable rubber bladder inside the cuff should encircle at least 80% of the arm, and the width of the cuff should be at least two-thirds the length of the upper arm.
- The palpatory method should be used to estimate the SBP. The cuff should be placed on the upper arm, attached to either a mercury or aneroid manometer, and the inflation valve should be closed and then inflated by pumping the inflation bulb with one hand while simultaneously palpating the radial pulse with the first and second fingers of the opposite hand. The point at which radial pulse disappears is the estimated SBP. Pressure can now be released from the cuff by turning the valve counterclockwise.
- A stethoscope should then be used with the earpieces inserted appropriately and with the bell of the stethoscope lying on the skin of the antecubital fossa over the brachial artery. The valve should be closed and the cuff inflated rapidly to about 30 mm Hg above the point at which the radial pulse disappeared. The value should be only slightly opened to release pressure at a rate of 2 to 3 mm Hg per second.
- The observer should listen for Korotkoff sounds that are heard through the stethoscope. The first phase of Korotkoff sounds consist of clear tapping sounds. The pressure that is noted at the first recognition of these sounds should be recorded. This is the SBP. As pressure continues to deflate, the pressure at the moment that all sounds disappear should be recorded (also known as the fifth Korotkoff phase). This is the DBP.
- Two or more readings should be measured separated by 2 minutes. The values should then be averaged. If the first two measurements differ by more than 5 mm Hg, additional readings should be collected and averaged.

Several additional factors, other than those mentioned previously, may result in erroneous blood pressure measurements. Pseudohypertension is a falsely high blood pressure that may be recorded in elderly patients with a rigid, calcified brachial artery.[12] In this situation, the true arterial blood pressure when measured directly with intraarterial measurement (the most accurate measurement of blood pressure) is much lower than that obtained by the indirect cuff method. The Osler's maneuver can be used to test for pseudohypertension. In this maneuver, the blood pressure cuff is inflated above peak SBP. If the radial artery remains palpable, the patient has rigid arteries. This is known as a *positive Osler's maneuver,* which indicates pseudohypertension.

Patients with an *auscultatory gap* may have blood pressure measurements that either underestimate systolic or overestimate diastolic pressures. In this situation, as the cuff pressure falls from the true systolic value, the Korotkoff sound may disappear sequentially (a false diastolic measurement), reappear (a false systolic measurement), and then disappear again at the true diastolic value. This may be identified by inflating the cuff an additional 30 mm Hg above the estimated SBP as determined by the palpatory method, as described above. If an auscultatory gap is present, Korotkoff sounds should be heard when pressure in the cuff is decreased initially after inflation. A third factor that may produce misleading values is an irregular ventricular rate because systolic and diastolic pressures may vary from one heartbeat to the next.

In all instances, it is recommended that the stethoscope bell, rather than the diaphragm, be used. Low-frequency Korotkoff sounds may not be heard clearly and accurately with the diaphragm, especially if the patient has faint or "distant" sounds.

Blood pressure varies with environmental temperature, the time of day and year, the timing of meals, physical activity, posture, smoking, and emotions.[23,24] Some individuals experience a rise in blood pressure in a medical setting that returns to normal outside the medical setting. This is known as *white coat hypertension* and appears to occur in approximately 20% of newly diagnosed hypertensive patients. Interestingly, such a rise in blood pressure dissipates gradually over several hours after leaving the office and may not be precipitated by other stresses in the patient's daily life. Aggressive treatment of white coat hypertension is controversial. However, patients with white coat hypertension may have increased cardiovascular risk compared with those without such blood pressure changes.[25]

Twenty-four-hour ambulatory blood pressure monitoring can document blood pressure at frequent time intervals throughout the day.[26,27] This may be warranted in patients with suspected white coat hypertension to delineate white coat hypertension from essential hypertension according to the National High Blood Pressure Education Program Coordinating Committee working group on ambulatory blood pressure monitoring.[28] It also appears that a patient's 24-hour blood pressure profile correlates better with end-organ damage than do casual office measurements. However, current limitations such as complexity of use, availability of devices, and costs prohibit routine use of such technology. Self-monitoring blood pressure at home is a less complicated alternative to evaluating blood pressure values outside a clinical setting, but these are not always reliable because patients may fail to record their values and then actually may add "ghost" values that were never measured.[29]

CLINICAL EVALUATION

Frequently, the only sign of primary hypertension is an elevated blood pressure. The rest of the physical examination may be completely normal. However, a complete medical evaluation is recommended after a diagnosis of hypertension. This includes a comprehensive medical history, physical examination, and laboratory and/or diagnostic tests. The purpose of this evaluation is to (1) identify known causes of hypertension, (2) identify other cardiovascular risk factors or comorbid conditions that may help define the prognosis and/or guide the choice of therapy, and (3) assess for the presence or absence of target-organ damage associated with elevated blood pressure.[1]

Basic tests that should be performed in all hypertensive patients prior to initiating drug therapy include urinalysis, complete blood cell count, serum chemistries (including sodium, potassium, creatinine, fasting glucose, total and high-density-lipoprotein cholesterol), and a 12-lead electrocardiogram. These are used to assess other risk factors and to develop baseline data for monitoring drug-induced metabolic changes.

SECONDARY CAUSES

The physical examination may provide clues for diagnosing secondary hypertension. For example, patients with coarctation of the aorta may have diminished or even absent femoral pulses, and patients with renal artery stenosis may have an abdominal systolic diastolic bruit. Of course, patients with Cushing's syndrome may have the classic physical features (i.e., moon face, buffalo hump, hirsutism, abdominal striae) that characterize individuals with this endocrine disorder.

Patients with secondary hypertension usually complain of symptoms suggestive of the underlying disorder. For example, many patients with pheochromocytoma have a history of paroxysmal headaches, sweating, tachycardia, and palpitations occurring singly or in combinations. More than half the patients with this form of secondary hypertension suffer episodes of orthostatic dizziness or syncope. In primary aldosteronism, hypokalemic symptoms usually include muscle cramps and muscle weakness. Patients who present with hypertension secondary to Cushing's syndrome may complain of weight gain, polyuria, edema, menstrual irregularities, recurrent acne, or muscular weakness.

Certain routine laboratory tests may help identify patients with secondary hypertension. A low serum potassium before antihypertensive therapy is begun may suggest mineralocorticoid-induced hypertension. The presence of protein, blood cells, and casts in the urine may indicate an underlying parenchymal kidney disease as the cause of hypertension. More specific laboratory tests are used to diagnose secondary hypertension. These include plasma norepinephrine and urinary metanephrine for pheochromocytoma, plasma and urinary aldosterone levels for primary aldosteronism, and plasma renin activity, captopril stimulation test, renal vein renins, and renal artery angiography for renovascular disease.

Certain medications and herbal products can result in drug-induced hypertension. The most common of these are adrenalcorticosteroids, amphetamines/anorexiants (e.g., phentermine, sibutramine), caffeine, cyclosporine, ethanol, ephedra, estrogens, monoamine oxidase inhibitors, nonsteroidal anti-inflammatory agents, oral contraceptives, oral decongestants (e.g., phenylpropanolamine, pseudoephedrine), thyroid hormone (in excess), tricyclic antidepressants, and venlafaxine. In some patients, the addition of these agents can be the cause of hypertension or they can exacerbate underlying hypertension. Identifying a temporal relationship between starting the suspected agent and observation of elevated blood pressure is most suggestive of drug-induced blood pressure elevation.

As hypertension progresses, signs of end-organ damage may appear. The primary organs involved are the eye, brain, heart, kidneys, and peripheral blood vessels. A comprehensive physical examination that includes a review of systems can identify pathologic changes in these organs that are consistent with organ involvement.

The funduscopic examination can detect hypertensive retinopathy, as evidenced by arteriolar narrowing, focal arteriolar constrictions, arteriovenous crossing changes, retinal hemorrhages and exudates, and disk edema. A neurologic assessment should be conducted to evaluate for the presence of either gross neurologic deficits in patients with previous cerebral infarcts or encephalopathy or a slight hemiparesis with some incoordination and hyperreflexia. Assessment of the systemic vasculature can detect evidence of atherosclerosis, which may present as bruits (in the aortic, abdominal, or peripheral arteries), distended veins, diminished or absent peripheral arterial pulses, or lower extremity edema. Lastly, cardiopulmonary abnormalities such as abnormal cardiac rate or rhythm, ventricular hypertrophy, precordial heave, heart clicks or murmurs, third and fourth heart sounds, and rales can be identified with a thorough cardiac and lung examination.

NATURAL COURSE OF DISEASE

Early in the course of primary hypertension, blood pressure may fluctuate between elevated and normal levels. This stage of the disease usually is referred to as *labile hypertension*. It may begin as early as the second decade of life. During this stage, many patients have a hyperdynamic circulation with increased cardiac output and normal or even low peripheral vascular resistance. As the disease progresses, peripheral vascular resistance increases, and blood pressure elevation is sustained. Most patients suffering from primary hypertension do not develop accelerated or severe hypertension (i.e., stage 3).

The main causes of death in hypertensive subjects are cerebrovascular accidents, cardiovascular events, and renal failure. The probability of premature death from any of these causes is correlated with the severity of blood pressure elevation.

Hypertension accelerates atherosclerosis and stimulates left ventricular and vascular hypertrophy. These pathologic changes are thought to be secondary to both a chronic pressure overload and a variety of nonhemodynamic stimuli. Some of the nonhemodynamic disturbances that have been implicated in the pathogenesis of cardiac and vascular hypertrophy include the adrenergic and renin-angiotensin systems, increased synthesis and secretion of endothelin I, and a decreased production of prostacyclin and endothelial-derived relaxing factor (also called *nitric oxide*). The mechanisms of accelerated atherogenesis in hypertension include proliferation of smooth muscle cells, lipid infiltration into the vascular endothelium, and an enhancement of vascular calcium accumulation.

Hypertension is a major risk factor for stroke. Stroke can result from lacunar infarcts caused by thrombotic occlusion of small vessels or intracerebral hemorrhage resulting from ruptured microaneurysms. Transient ischemic attacks secondary to atherosclerotic disease in the carotid arteries are common in hypertensive individuals.

A variety of retinopathies can occur in hypertension. Nonspecific changes include an increased light reflex, increased tortuosity of vessels, and arteriovenous nicking. These are all associated with the accelerated arteriosclerosis that accompanies hypertension. Focal arteriolar narrowing, retinal infarcts, and flame-shaped hemorrhages usually are pathognomonic of an accelerated or malignant phase of hypertension and are associated with increased arteriolar resistance and fibrinoid necrosis. Papilledema is a swelling of the optic disk and is caused by a breakdown in autoregulation of capillary blood flow in the presence of high pressure. Its presence is indicative of severe hypertension and hypertensive emergency.

Cardiac diseases are the most well-identified complications of hypertension. These include left ventricular hypertrophy, coronary heart disease, and congestive heart failure. The development of these complications may lead to cardiac arrhythmias, angina, myocardial infarction, and sudden death. Coronary heart disease and associated cardiac events are the most common causes of death in hypertensive patients.

The renal damage caused by hypertension is characterized pathologically by hyaline arteriosclerosis, hyperplastic arteriosclerosis, arteriolar hypertrophy, fibrinoid necrosis, and atheroma of the major renal arteries. Glomerular hyperfiltration and intraglomerular hypertension are early stages of hypertensive nephropathy. Microalbuminuria is followed by a gradual decline in renal function. The primary renal complication in hypertension is nephrosclerosis, which is secondary to accelerated arteriosclerosis. Atheromatous disease of a major renal artery may give rise to renal artery stenosis. Although renal failure is an uncommon complication of essential hypertension, it remains an important cause of end-stage renal disease, especially in African-Americans, Hispanics, and Native Americans. It is not completely understood why these ethnic groups are more at risk for end-stage renal disease. It may be due to genetic factors that cause more rapid acceleration of complications. It also may relate to other risk factors, such as the high rate of diabetes in Hispanics and Native Americans, which adds to the risk of end-stage renal disease.

▶ TREATMENT: Hypertension

DESIRED OUTCOMES

PRIMARY GOAL OF THERAPY

The overall goal of treating hypertension is to reduce morbidity and mortality by the least intrusive means possible.[1] Therefore, the purpose of controlling blood pressure in hypertension is to lower the risk of associated target-organ damage (i.e., cardiovascular events, cerebrovascular events, heart failure, etc.). This remains the primary goal of therapy and can influence the choice of drug therapy significantly.

SURROGATE GOAL OF THERAPY

Treating hypertensive patients aggressively enough to achieve a desired blood pressure reduction (i.e., achieving a goal blood pressure value) is simply a surrogate goal of therapy. Although reducing blood pressure to a target value does not guarantee that target-organ damage will not occur, it is well accepted that the closer a patient is to the normal blood pressure range, the lower is the risk. Targeting a goal blood pressure provides the clinician with a tool to easily evaluate response and is the primary method to titrate and modify therapy. Before hypertension is diagnosed, patients should receive blood pressure determinations on three separate occasions to confirm the diagnosis.

Most patients have a goal blood pressure value of less than 140/90 mm Hg. However, patients with renal impairment, heart failure, diabetes mellitus, severe renal disease who have more than 1 g/d of proteinuria, and isolated systolic hypertension have different goal values (Table 12–2). Recent recommendations from the National Kidney Foundation are to target a goal blood pressure of less than 130/80 mm Hg in patients with diabetes mellitus.[30] This is more aggressive than the JNC-VI goal of less than 130/85 mm Hg.

Some believe that achieving lower blood pressure values than those which are recommended may reduce cardiovascular risk even more. Contrary to this, a J-curve hypothesis in which lowering blood pressure too much might increase the risk of cardiovascular events has been described.[31] Lower goal blood pressure values have been evaluated prospectively in the Hypertension Optimal Treatment study (i.e., the HOT trial).[32] In this study, over 18,700 patients were randomized to target DBP values of 90 mm Hg or less, 85 mm Hg or less, or 80 mm Hg or less. Although the actual diastolic values achieved in these groups were 85.2, 83.2, and 81.1 mm Hg, respectively, the risk of major cardiovascular events was the lowest with a blood pressure of 139/83 mm Hg, and risk of stroke was lowest with a blood pressure of 142/80 mm Hg. Risk of events in subjects with either diabetes or ischemic heart disease were lowest at DBP values of less than 80 mm Hg. No J-curve relationship was seen. The results of the HOT study provide some validation of our present goal values but argue for more aggressive blood pressure lowering, especially in patients with diabetes.

TABLE 12–2. Goal Blood Pressure Values[1,30]

Population with Hypertension	Goal Value (mm Hg)
Uncomplicated hypertension	<140/90
Heart failure	<130/85
Renal impairment	<130/85
Diabetes mellitus	<130/85 (JNC-VI recommendation) <130/80 (National Kidney Foundation recommendation)
Severe renal disease with >1 g/d of proteinuria	<125/75
Isolated systolic hypertension	<160 mm Hg (systolic) initially, then <140 mm Hg eventually

GENERAL APPROACH TO TREATMENT

RISK STRATIFICATION

Cardiovascular risk stratification has been advocated as a method for evaluating an individual's risk of developing cardiovascular disease and complications releated to hypertension.[33] By implementing such an approach, patients with significant risk can be identified and treated accordingly. The JNC-VI has identified a risk stratification that incorporated individual risk factors and the presence of hypertension-related complications.[1]

After the diagnosis of hypertension, major risk factors for developing complications associated with hypertension should be noted, as described in Table 12–3. Although other factors such as sedentary lifestyle and obesity may increase the likelihood of hypertension and cardiovascular disease,[34] they are not included in this assessment. A complete medical examination and detailed history are needed in all patients suffering from hypertension to detect the presence of target-organ damage (TOD) and clinical cardiovascular disease (CCD), which are also presented in Table 12–3. With this patient-specific information, hypertensive individuals are further categorized into risk group A, B, or C. As noted in Table 12–4, patients with hypertension and no other major risk factors and no TOD/CCD are in risk group A. Those with either TOD/CCD or diabetes mellitus (independent of their number of major risk factors) are in risk group C.

The overall utility of risk stratification is to guide the implementation of therapy. Table 12–5 integrates recommended initial therapy with the risk group. Using these recommendations, patients who fall into risk group A with stage 1 hypertension can be managed with lifestyle modifications for up to 1 year. If after this time goal blood pressure is not achieved, drug therapy could be started. Moreover, high-risk patients such as those falling into risk group C would

TABLE 12–3. Assessment of Overall Risk of Hypertensive Patients[1]

Major Risk Factors
Smoking
Dyslipidemia
Diabetes mellitus
Patient age >60 years
Sex (men and postmenopausal women)
Family history of premature cardiovascular disease (age <65 years in women and <55 years in men)

Target Organ Damage/Clinical Cardiovascular Disease (TOD/CCD)
Heart disease (left ventricular hypertrophy, angina, prior myocardial infarction, prior coronary artery bypass graft or percutaneous transluminal coronary angioplasty, heart failure)
Cerebrovascular disease (stroke or transient ischemic attacks)
Nephropathy
Retinopathy
Peripheral arterial disease

TABLE 12–4. JNC-VI Risk Stratification[1]

Category	Major Risk Factors	TOD/CCD
Risk group A	None	None
Risk group B	≥1, but not diabetes mellitus	None
Risk group C	None to several	Present or none if diabetes mellitus

warrant drug therapy (in addition to lifestyle modification) initially after diagnosis when blood pressure is above the identified goal value. Of note, patients with at least one major risk factor (other than diabetes) but without TOD/CCD may be treated for up to 6 months with lifestyle modification if their blood pressure initially falls into stage 1. However, this population should be strongly considered for initial drug therapy if numerous risk factors are present.

NONPHARMACOLOGIC THERAPY

All treatment plans for hypertension should include lifestyle modifications. These are summarized in Table 12–6. Aside from lowering blood pressure, lifestyle modification can decrease the progression to hypertension in patients with high-normal blood pressure. Obesity, dyslipidemia, excessive salt intake, cigarette smoking, and alcohol consumption are important factors that should be addressed in formulating a rational antihypertensive treatment program.

A reasonable first step in the treatment of hypertension consists of a carefully constructed, aggressively promoted modification in lifestyle. Reasonable patient education, encouragement, and continued reinforcement are essential to the success of these modifications. A sensible dietary program is one that is designed to reduce weight gradually, if appropriate, and reduce dietary intake of saturated fat, cholesterol, and salt. The rationale for dietary treatment of hypertension is based on the following observations and facts:

1. Hypertension is two to three times more prevalent in overweight as compared with lean persons.
2. Sixty percent of hypertensive persons are overweight.
3. Weight loss, even as little as 10 pounds, can decrease blood pressure significantly in hypertensive, overweight individuals.[35]

TABLE 12–5. Recommended Initial Treatment Based on Risk Grouping[1]

Blood Pressure	Group A	Group B	Group C
High-normal	Lifestyle modification	Lifestyle modification	Drug therapy[b]
Stage 1	Lifestyle modification (up to 12 months)	Lifestyle modification (up to 6 months)[a]	Drug therapy
Stages 2 and 3	Drug therapy	Drug therapy	Drug therapy

Note: Lifestyle modification is adjunctive therapy for all patients recommended for drug therapy.

[a]For patients with multiple risk factors, initial drug therapy with lifestyle modification should be considered.

[b]For patients with diabetes, heart failure, or renal insufficiency.

TABLE 12–6. Lifestyle Modifications to Lower Blood Pressure in Hypertension[1]

Weight loss if overweight
Limiting alcohol intake to no more than 1 ounce of ethanol daily or less than 0.5 ounces per day for women and lighter people
Increasing aerobic physical activity (30 to 45 minutes most days of the week)
Reducing sodium intake to 2.4 g/d or less (or 6 g of sodium chloride)
Maintaining an adequate intake of dietary potassium
Maintaining an adequate intake of dietary calcium and magnesium for general health
Reducing daily intake of dietary saturated fat and cholesterol
Smoking cessation and reducing dietary intake of saturated fat and cholesterol for overall cardiovascular health

4. Upper body obesity is associated with insulin resistance and hyperinsulinemia. Hyperinsulinemia may be involved in the pathogenesis of hypertension as well as hyperlipidemia.
5. Diets rich in fruits and vegetables and low in saturated fat have been shown to lower blood pressure in hypertensive individuals.[36]
6. Although salt-sensitive hypertensives are most responsive to reducing dietary sodium intake, overall hypertensive and normotensive subjects experience some degree of systolic blood pressure reduction with sodium restriction.[37] Compared with the overall population, hypertensive patients with diabetes, African-Americans, and elderly persons respond best to sodium restriction.[38,39]

In addition to these dietary measures, it is important to moderate alcohol intake because excessive use of alcohol can either cause or worsen hypertension. Hypertensive patients who drink alcoholic beverages should restrict their intake to 1 ounce or less per day. One ounce of alcohol is contained in 2 ounces of 100 proof whiskey, 8 ounces of wine, or 24 ounces of beer.

Cigarette smoking is another major independent risk factor of coronary heart disease. Moreover, this is a modifiable risk factor. Patients with hypertension who smoke should be thoroughly counseled on the additional risks that smoking incurs as well as the potential benefits that cessation can provide. These patients must be encouraged to take advantage of available smoking-cessation programs and cessation aids.

Another useful lifestyle modification for hypertensive patients is a carefully designed program of regular aerobic physical exercise. Studies have shown that aerobic exercise, such as jogging, swimming, walking, and bicycling, can reduce blood pressure. These benefits can occur even in the absence of weight loss. Patients should consult their physicians before starting an exercise program, especially those with TOD/CCD.

PHARMACOLOGIC THERAPY

Antihypertensive drugs may be divided into nine classes: diuretics, β-blockers, ACE inhibitors, calcium channel blockers, angiotensin II receptor blockers, α-blockers, central α_2-agonists, adrenergic inhibitors, and vasodilators (Tables 12–7 and 12–8). Drug selection should be based on the scientific evidence for efficacy, safety, cost, and the presence of concomitant diseases and other risk factors. The

TABLE 12–7. Antihypertensive Agents

Class/Drug (Brand Name)	Usual Dose Range, mg/d (Maximum Dose)	Daily Frequency	Cost	Comments
Thiazide diuretics				
Chlorthalidone (Hygroton, generic)	12.5–25 (50)	1	$	Thiazides are more effective antihypertensives than loop diuretics except in patients with creatinine clearance <30 cc/min (serum creatinine >221 μmol/L or 2.5 mg/dL); lower doses and dietary measures should be used to avoid metabolic effects; hydrochlorothiazide or chlorthalidone are generally preferred.
Hydrochlorothiazide (HydroDIURIL, generic)	12.5–25 (50)	1	$	
Indapamide (Lozol, generic)	1.25–2.5 (5)	1	$$	
Metolazone (Mykrox)	0.5 (1)	1	$$$	
Metolazone (Zaroxolyn)	2.5 (5)	1	$$	
Loop diuretics				
Bumetanide (Bumex, generic)	0.5–2 (10)	2	$	Higher doses may be needed for patients with renal impairment or congestive heart failure. Bumetanide can be used in those allergic to furosemide.
Furosemide (Lasix, generic)	20–80 (320)	2	$	
Torsemide (Demadex)	2.5–5 (10)	1	$$	
Potassium-sparing diuretics				
Amiloride (Midamor, generic)	5 (10)	1 or 2	$$	Potassium-sparing agents are weak diuretics, used mainly in combination with other diuretics such as those listed here to reverse hypokalemia from other diuretics. Since hypokalemia from low-dose thiazides is uncommon, these agents should be reserved for treatment of hypokalemia (rather than prevention). Avoid in patients with creatinine clearance <30 cc/min (serum creatinine >221 μmol/L or 2.5 mg/dL). May cause hyperkalemia, and this may be exaggerated when combined with ACE inhibitors or potassium supplements.
Amiloride/HCTZ (Moduretic, generic)		1 or 2	$$	
Spironolactone (Aldactone, generic)	25–50 (100)	2 or 3	$$	
Spironolactone/HCTZ (Aldactazide, generic)		2 or 3	$	
Triamterene (Dyrenium)	50–100 (150)	1 or 2	$$	
Triamterene/HCTZ (Dyazide, generic)		1 or 2	$	
β-Blockers				
Atenolol (Tenormin, generic)	25–50 (100)+	1	$	Cardioselective agents also may inhibit β_2-receptors in higher doses; e.g., all may aggravate asthma.
Betaxolol (Kerlone)	5–20 (40)	1	$$$	
Bisoprolol (Zebeta)	2.5–10 (20)	1	$$$	
Metoprolol (Lopressor, generic)	50–100 (200)	1 or 2	$	
Metoprolol extended release (Toprol XL)	50–100 (200)	1	$$	
Nadolol (Corgard, generic)	40–80 (240)+	1		
Propranolol (Inderal, generic)	40–120 (240)	2	$$	
Propranolol long-acting (Inderal LA, generic)	60–120 (240)	1	$ $$$$	
Timolol (Blocadren, generic)	10–40 (60)	1	$$	
β-Blockers with ISA				
Acebutolol (Sectral, generic)	200–800 (1200)	2	$$	No clear advantage for agents with ISA except in those with bradycardia who must receive a β-blocker; they produce fewer or no metabolic side effects, but they may not be as cardioprotective as other β-blockers.
Carteolol (Cartrol)	2.5–5 (10)	1	$$$	
Penbutolol (Levatol)	20	1	$$$$	
Pindolol (Visken, generic)	10–40 (60)	2	$	
α/β Blockers				
Carvedilol (Coreg)	12.5–25 (50)	2	$$$$$	Similar properties as β-blockers but the α-blockade produces more orthostatic hypotension; carvedilol is indicated in congestive heart failure.
Labetalol (Normodyne, Trandate, generic)	200–800 (1200)	2	$$$$	
ACE Inhibitors				
Benazepril (Lotensin)	10–20 (40)+	1 or 2	$$$	Diuretic doses should be reduced or held for several days before starting ACE inhibitor whenever possible to prevent excessive hypotension. May cause hypokalemia in patients with renal impairment or in those receiving potassium-sparing diuretics. Can cause acute renal failure in patients with severe bilateral renal artery stenosis or severe stenosis in artery to solitary kidney.
Captopril (Capoten, generic)	12.5–100 (150)+	2	$	
Enalapril (Vasotec)	2.5–20 (40)+	1 or 2	$$$	
Fosinopril (Monopril)	10–20 (40)	1	$$$	
Lisinopril (Prinivil, Zestril)	5–20 (40)+	1	$$$	
Moexipril (Univasc)	7.5–30+	1	$$	
Quinapril (Accupril)	5–40 (80)+	1	$$$	
Ramipril (Altace)	1.25–10 (20)+	1	$$$	
Trandolapril (Mavik)	1–4+	1	$$	
Calcium antagonists, calcium channel blocking agents				
Diltiazem extended release (Cardizem CD, Dilator XR, generic)	180–240 (360)	1	$$$$	The FDA approved labeling lists three daily doses for short-acting verapamil, but studies have found twice-daily dosing to be effective especially in the elderly who have delayed elimination
Verapamil immediate release (Calan, Isoptin, generic)	80–360 (480)	2	$$	

TABLE 12–7. (Continued)

Class/Drug (Brand Name)	Usual Dose Range, mg/d (Maximum Dose)	Daily Frequency	Cost	Comments
Verapamil long acting (Calan SR, Isoptin SR, Generic)	120–360 (480)	1 or 2	$$$$	Short-acting diltiazem is not indicated for hypertension.
Verapamil controlled onset extended release (Covera-HS)	120–360 (480)	1++	$$$$	++ Coer verapamil is designed to be given at bedtime; it has a 4–5-hour delay in release and is designed to prevent the early morning surge in blood pressure; administer only at bedtime. These agents block slow channels in the heart and may reduce sinus rate and produce heart block.
Calcium antagonists, dihydropyridines				
Amlodipine (Norvasc)	2.5–5 (10)	1	$$$$	Short-acting dihydropyridines should be avoided, especially immediate-release nifedipine and nicardipine.
Felodipine (Plendil)	5–10 (20)	1	$$$	
Isradipine (DynaCirc)	2.5–5 (10)	2	$$$$	
Nicardipine sustained release (Cardene SR)	60–90 (120)	2	$$$$	Dihydropyridines are more potent peripheral vasodilators than diltiazem and verapamil and may cause more reflex sympathetic discharge (tachycardia), dizziness, headache, flushing, and peripheral edema.
Nifedipine long-acting (Adalat CC, Procardia XL)	30–60 (90)	1	$$$$	
Nisoldipine (Sular)	10–40 (60)	1	$$$	
α_1-Blockers				
Doxazosin (Cardura)	1–4 (8)	1	$$$	First dose should be given at bedtime; patients should be cautioned about rising rapidly.
Prazosin (Minipress, generic)	1–15 (20)	2 or 3	$	
Terazosin (Hytrin)	1–10 (20)	1 or 2	$$$$	All may cause postural effects, and titration should be based on standing blood pressure.
Angiotensin II antagonists				
Candesartan (Atacand)	8–32	1	$$$$	Only clear advantage for this class of drugs at this time is in patients with ACE inhibitor–induced cough.
Irbesartan (Avapro)	150–300	1	$$$$	
Losartan (Cozaar)	25–100	1–2	$$$$	
Telmisartan (Micardis)	40–80	1	$$$$	
Valsartan (Diovan)	80–320	1	$$$$	
Central α_2-agonists				
Clonidine (Catapres, generic)	0.1–0.8 (1.2)	2	$	Avoid abrupt withdrawal; avoid in nonadherent patients.
Clonidine patch (Catapres-TTS)	0.1–0.3	1 weekly	$$$	May be more effective if used with a diuretic
Methyldopa (Aldomet, generic)	250–1000 (2000)	2	$	The patch is replaced once per week.
Peripheral adrenergic antagonist				
Reserpine (generic)	0.05[a]–0.25		$	Reserpine is a very useful agent that has been used in many of the major clinical trials; should be used with a diuretic.
Direct vasodilators				
Minoxidil (Loniten, generic)	2.5–40 (80)	1 or 2	$$	Pretreat with β-blocker and diuretic to diminish fluid retention and reflex tachycardia.
Hydralazine (Apresoline, generic)	20–100 (200)	2–4	$	

Note: $ = <$10; $$ = $10.01–20; $$$ = $20.01–30; $$$$ = >$30. These costs are intended to be only estimates since many health systems and managed care organizations receive special prices for specific agents.
[a]A 0.1-mg dose may be given every other day to achieve this dosage.
+ = may require dosage reduction with renal impairment.
From Medical Letter 41:23–28, March 12, 1999.

TABLE 12–8. Less Commonly Used Antihypertensive Agents

Class/Drug (Brand Name)	Usual Dose Range, mg/d (Maximum Dose)	Daily Frequency	Cost	Comments
Peripheral adrenergic antagonists				
Guanabenz (Wytensin, generic)	4–32 (64)	2	$$	These agents should not be withdrawn abruptly; avoid in patients who do not adhere to treatment.
Guanfacine (Tenex, generic)	1 (3)	1	$$	
Methyldopa (Aldomet, generic)	250–1000 (2000)	2	$	

See notes for Table 12–7.

scientific evidence that should be used is not simply blood pressure reduction and tolerability but rather evidence that a given drug reduces morbidity and mortality in a hypertensive population. When considering these factors, the most useful agents are diuretics, β-blockers, ACE inhibitors, calcium channel blockers, and perhaps, angiotensin II receptor blockers.

UNCOMPLICATED HYPERTENSION

In the United States, the most recent guidelines for pharmacologic treatment of hypertension are the JNC-VI guidelines.[1] Figure 12–1 displays an algorithm for the treatment of hypertension. The guidelines suggest that patients with uncomplicated hypertension should receive a thiazide diuretic or a β-blocker. The vast majority of scientific evidence for reductions in stroke, congestive heart failure, myocardial infarction, and other cardiovascular events has been collected in clinical trials using these two drug classes.[1] The most impressive reductions have been obtained with thiazide diuretics, especially in elderly populations.[7] These trials have demonstrated reductions in stroke of 40% to 45%, congestive heart failure of 40% to 50%, and coronary artery disease of 16% to 25%.

Any given antihypertensive may control blood pressure to goal in approximately 40% of patients when control is defined as less than 140/90 mm Hg.[40,41] This finding means that many patients require two and perhaps three antihypertensives to control their blood pressure. The selection of the second drug must be rational, such that it has additive antihypertensive effects and is beneficial for any coexisting conditions that may be present. If a diuretic was not the first drug selected, it should be the second drug in the regimen if not contraindicated. The addition of a low dose of a thiazide diuretic often will provide blood pressure control in most patients (up to 75% of patients when it is part of a two-drug regimen).[42]

All antihypertensive medications are safe and generally well tolerated. Each agent has specific side effects for which the clinician must monitor. In the past it was always felt that hypertension was an asymptomatic condition, and medications frequently made patients feel worse. This was especially thought to be true for diuretics, β-blockers, and centrally acting agents. However, several studies have found that quality-of-life measures frequently are better on

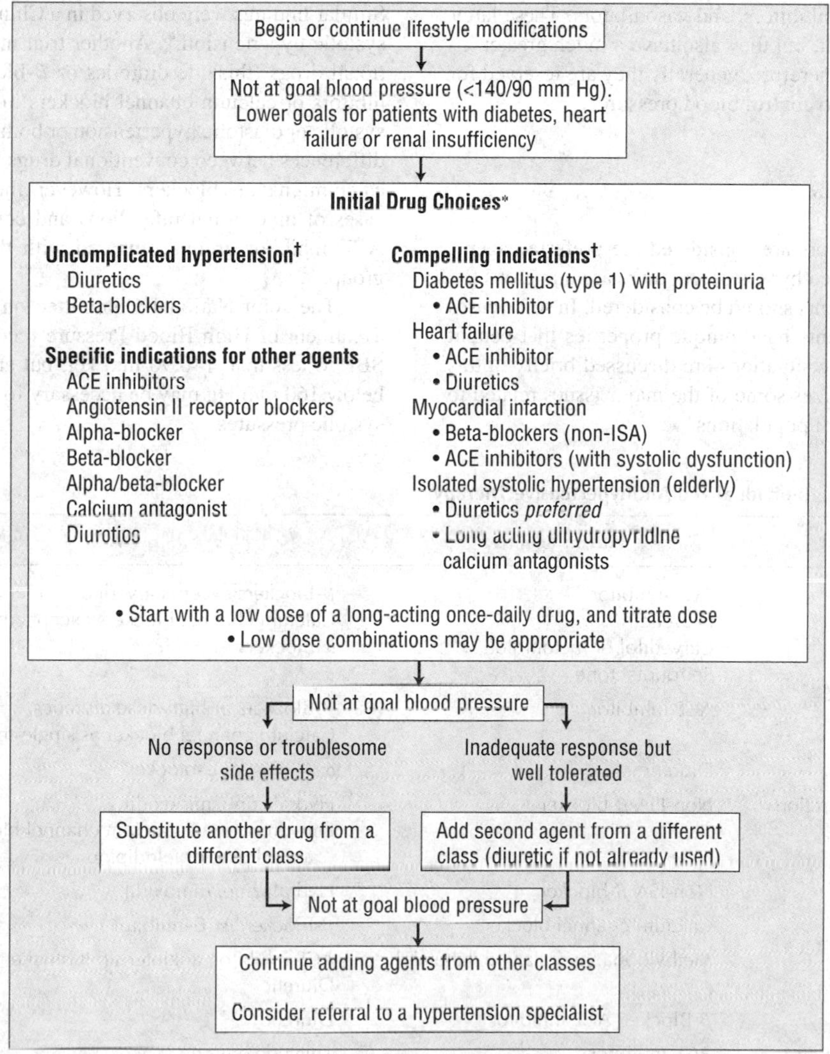

FIGURE 12–1. Algorithm for the treatment of hypertension.* Unless contraindicated. ACE = angiotensin converting enzyme; ISA = intrinsic sympathomimetic activity †Based on randomized controlled trials. *(From the Sixth Report of the Joint National Committee on Prevention, Detection, Evaluation, and Treatment of High Blood Pressure. Arch Intern Med, November 1997.)*

antihypertensive medications than with placebo.[40,43] Diuretics and β-blockers generally were tolerated, as well as ACE inhibitors and calcium channel blockers. Only central agents such as clonidine or the α-blocker prazosin clearly increased the rates of adverse effects.

New data also support slow dosage titration (doubling the dose every 6 weeks) rather than more rapid titration in patients with stage 1 or 2 hypertension.[44] The slower titration leads to equivalent blood pressure control and lower rates of adverse reactions.

ALTERNATIVE DRUG TREATMENTS

While thiazide diuretics and β-blockers are preferred for uncomplicated hypertension, patients frequently have coexisting conditions that must be considered in the treatment decision. For many patients, alternative drug treatments must be considered as either the first or second drug in the regimen. The most useful alternative drugs include the ACE inhibitors, calcium channel blockers, angiotensin II antagonists, and occasionally, the α-blockers. The role for these agents will be discussed within each section that discusses special populations. In some patients it becomes necessary to use other agents such as central α_2-agonists, adrenergic inhibitors, and vasodilators. These latter agents tend to be more potent, but they also have a much greater incidence of adverse effects. Therefore, generally they are reserved for patients with more difficult to control blood pressure.

SPECIAL POPULATIONS

While diuretics and β-blockers are considered the preferred agents in patients with uncomplicated hypertension, there are numerous examples where alternative agents should be considered. In some cases this is so because other agents have unique properties that benefit a coexisting condition. These situations are discussed briefly in this section. Table 12–9 summarizes some of the major issues related to drug selection in these special populations.

Hypertension in the Elderly[7,10,11,45,46]

The elderly may present with either isolated systolic hypertension or an elevation in both SBP and DBP. Epidemiologic data indicate that cardiovascular morbidity and mortality are more closely related to SBP than to DBP. The Coordinating Committee of the National High Blood Pressure Education Program recently issued a clinical advisory on the importance of systolic hypertension and its appropriate management.[11] Additionally, elevated pulse pressure (SBP − DBP) is an even better marker for cardiovascular risk.

In a double-blind, placebo-controlled trial, the Systolic Hypertension in the Elderly Program (SHEP), active treatment of isolated systolic hypertension resulted in a 36% reduction in the incidence of total stroke, a 27% reduction in coronary artery disease, and an impressive 55% reduction in congestive heart failure.[7] The SHEP trial initiated therapy with chlorthalidone, a thiazide diuretic, followed by atenolol or reserpine in those whose blood pressure was not controlled with the diuretic. Another placebo-controlled trial, the Systolic Hypertension–Europe (Syst-Eur) study, found a 42% reduction in stroke, a 26% reduction in coronary artery disease, and a 29% reduction in congestive heart failure when therapy was initiated with nitrendipine, a long-acting dihydropyridine calcium channel blocker.[10] Similar findings were observed in a Chinese population with isolated systolic hypertension.[47] Another trial in Sweden compared conventional drugs (thiazide diuretics or β-blockers) with either ACE inhibitors or calcium channel blockers in elderly patients with either systolic or diastolic hypertension or both.[48] There were no significant differences between conventional drugs and either ACE inhibitors or calcium channel blockers. However, there were significantly fewer cases of myocardial infarctions and congestive heart failure in the ACE inhibitor group compared with the calcium channel blocker group.

The Joint National Committee on Detection, Evaluation, and Treatment of High Blood Pressure recommends a reduction in the SBP to less than 140/90 mm Hg, but an interim goal of an SBP of below 160 mm Hg may be necessary for those with very high initial systolic pressures.

TABLE 12–9. Individualized Antihypertensive Therapy

Condition	Advantageous	Avoid
Heart failure	ACE inhibitor Diuretic Carvedilol or metoprolol Spironolactone	β-Blockers except carvedilol or metoprolol Calcium channel blockers except amlodipine α-Blockers
Diabetes	ACE inhibitor	β-Blockers or high-dose diuretics Calcium channel blocker as single-therapy
Elderly	Diuretic	α-Agonist or α-blocker
Myocardial infarction	Non-ISA β-blocker	Hydralazine, minoxidil Dihydropyridine calcium channel blocker except amlodipine or felodipine
Angina	Non-ISA β-blocker	Hydralazine, minoxidil
Bronchospasm	Calcium channel blocker	β-Blocker, ACE inhibitor
Pregnancy	Methyldopa, hydralazine, labetalol	ACE inhibitor, angiotensin II blocker Diuretic
Gout	β-Blocker, ACE inhibitor	Diuretic
Renal insufficiency	ACE inhibitor Loop diuretic Diltiazem Hydralazine Minoxidil	Thiazide diuretic Potassium-sparing diuretic

Elderly patients usually are more sensitive to volume depletion and sympathetic inhibition than younger individuals. This may lead to postural hypotension in the elderly. Therefore, antihypertensives that are frequently associated with dizziness and postural hypotension, such as the centrally acting agents and α-blockers, should be avoided. Treatment should be initiated with smaller-than-usual dosages. Most authorities agree that the initial drug should be a thiazide diuretic. The starting dose should be low (e.g., 12.5 mg hydrochlorothiazide) and increased gradually to no more than 25 mg/d. If diuretic therapy alone does not achieve the desired reduction in blood pressure, an ACE inhibitor can be added. Again, it is best to start with a low dose and increase the dose slowly, if necessary, but avoid excessive doses. While β-blockers frequently have been the second agent following a diuretic in many of the clinical trials, they typically have not been used alone for elderly patients. There is some concern that β-blockers may not be as effective as thiazide diuretics in older patients in their ability to reduce some cardiovascular events.[49] β-Blockers are the first drugs of choice, however, in elderly patients with hypertension and angina. ACE inhibitors are strongly preferred for hypertensive patients with diabetes or congestive heart failure.

Hypertension in Childhood[50–53]

Detecting hypertension in children requires special attention to measurement of the blood pressure, and detection is based on age-determined percentiles for excessive blood pressure.[50] Hypertensive children often have a family history of high blood pressure, and many are overweight. There is, however, one important distinction between hypertension in children and in adults: Secondary hypertension is much more common in children, and thus an appropriate workup for secondary causes is essential.

Renal disease is the most common cause of secondary hypertension in children. Pyelonephritis, glomerulonephritis, renal artery stenosis, pheochromocytoma, coarctation of the aorta, and renal cysts may all produce hypertension is children. Medical or surgical management of the underlying renal disorder usually restores blood pressure to normal.

Primary hypertension is much more common in children than was once thought. Nonpharmacologic treatment is the cornerstone of therapy, just as it is in adults. The goal of drug therapy is to reduce the blood pressure to below the 95th percentile for age. Diuretics and β-blockers are useful in treating hypertension in children and adolescents. ACE inhibitors are very effective in children and neonates but must be avoided in sexually active girls and in those who might have bilateral renal artery stenosis or unilateral stenosis in a solitary kidney. Long-acting nifedipine is the calcium channel blocker that has been used most successfully in children, but the safety of long-term use has not been determined.

Hypertension in Pregnancy[54–58]

The National High Blood Pressure Education Program Working Group Report on High Blood Pressure in Pregnancy was updated in 2000.[58] It is important to separate preeclampsia from chronic or transient hypertension of pregnancy because preeclampsia can lead rapidly to life-threatening complications for both mother and fetus. Whether treating chronic stage 1 or 2 hypertension is beneficial or not is controversial.

Preeclampsia usually presents after 20 weeks' gestation in primigravid women. The diagnosis of preeclampsia is based on the appearance of hypertension (>140/90 mm Hg) after 20 weeks' gestation with proteinuria. In the past, lower blood pressures also were considered diagnostic, but there is no evidence that pressures below 140/90 mm Hg cause adverse outcomes. Chronic hypertension, in contrast, is present before 20 weeks' gestation. Finally, preeclampsia can occur in women who were already hypertensive prior to pregnancy.

Definitive treatment of preeclampsia is delivery, and this is clearly indicated if pending or frank eclampsia (preeclampsia plus convulsions) is present. Otherwise, such measures as restriction of activity, bed rest, and close monitoring are in order. Salt restriction, or any other measures that may contract blood volume, should not be employed. Some experts would withhold treatment unless DBP is greater than 105 or 110 mm Hg. The most commonly used drug is intravenous hydralazine. Intravenous labetalol also has been effective. While immediate-release oral nifedipine has been used, it is important to note that it has never been approved by the Food and Drug Administration (FDA) for hypertension and that untoward fetal and maternal effects (hypotension with fetal distress) have been reported.

If drug treatment of hypertension is indicated for chronic hypertension, methyldopa is considered the drug of choice because most experience has been gathered with this agent. β-Blockers and the α/β-blocker labetalol appear safe and effective in simple hypertension of pregnancy. While there is some concern about effects on fetal heart rate, glucose intolerance, and growth retardation, β-blockers have not caused consistent ill effects. Calcium channel blockers have been used extensively in Europe and would seem to be a good choice. These agents also have been used successfully to treat preterm labor. ACE inhibitors are absolutely contraindicated because of reports of animal teratogenicity and acute renal failure in neonates. It is thought that this contraindication also applies to angiotensin II antagonists.

Several placebo-controlled studies have found that either 60 or 100 mg aspirin per day could reduce the risk of preeclampsia or gestational hypertension in pregnant women at risk for these conditions. Aspirin therapy usually was started at weeks 12 to 16 of gestation and continued until delivery. Pregnancy-induced hypertension, proteinuria, length of pregnancy, and fetal outcome were improved with aspirin therapy.[58] In another study, low-dose aspirin was shown to decrease the incidence of preeclampsia among nulliparous women, primarily through its effect in those who have elevated SBP initially. However, data from other studies have found conflicting results, and thus low-dose aspirin is not recommended for pregnant women.[58] Interestingly, these conflicting results may be related to the timing of administration of aspirin. A recent double-blind, randomized study found that giving aspirin at bedtime was much more effective at preventing increases in blood pressure than giving it on arising.[57] At this point, it is not clear what to recommend regarding the use of aspirin to prevent gestational hypertension or preeclampsia because the national guidelines recommend against its use. If aspirin is used, the dose should be 100 mg at bedtime.

African-Americans

Hypertension affects blacks at a disproportionately higher rate, and the consequences are more severe than in nonblacks. The reasons for the increased prevalence and severity of hypertension in blacks are not fully understood. Differences in electrolyte homeostasis, glomerular filtration rate, sodium excretion and transport mechanisms, plasma renin activity, and blood pressure response to plasma volume expansion have been noted. These differences may help explain the propensity for blacks to develop hypertension, but they do not account for the increased severity of hypertension in blacks as compared with whites.

Although dietary sodium intake is similar in blacks and whites, blacks ingest less potassium and calcium than whites. Supplemental potassium and calcium have both been shown to cause a modest reduction in blood pressure in some studies.

The lower plasma renin activity and increased blood pressure response to sodium and fluid loading observed in blacks suggest a more sodium- and volume-dependent hypertension than exists in nonblacks. Several clinical studies have shown that blacks are very responsive to diuretic therapy. These findings also point out the rationale of using diuretic therapy as the initial treatment of hypertension in blacks.

If diuretic therapy alone does not adequately control blood pressure in black patients with hypertension, then the addition of a β-blocker or ACE inhibitor is appropriate. Some clinicians have the misconception that β-blockers and ACE inhibitors are not effective in blacks, but 30% to 40% of blacks will have a good response to one of these agents. Although diuretics may be more effective as the initial treatment, diuretic therapy combined with β-blockers or ACE inhibitors is equally efficacious in hypertensive blacks and whites. The selection of the agent should be made based on coexisting conditions, if present. If patients tolerate a diuretic poorly, it might be added in very low doses (e.g., 12.5 mg hydrochlorothiazide) to one of these other agents.

Controlled clinical trials have shown that calcium channel antagonists are as effective at lowering blood pressure as diuretics in the initial pharmacologic treatment of hypertension in blacks. Thus an alternative to diuretic therapy might be a calcium channel blocker if a diuretic is contraindicated.

HYPERTENSION AND CONCOMITANT DISORDERS

Most patients with hypertension have some other coexisting conditions that must be considered in the overall treatment strategy for each patient. In some cases, an antihypertensive should be avoided because it may aggravate a concomitant disorder. In other cases, an antihypertensive can be used to treat both hypertension and another condition. Finally, there are some cases in which there is compelling evidence that a specific antihypertensive class may be preferred. These are outlined in Figure 12–1 and Table 12–9.

Asthma, COPD, and Peripheral Arterial Disease

β-Blockers, even those with β_1 selectivity, should be avoided in hypertensive patients with asthma, chronic obstructive pulmonary disease (COPD), and peripheral vascular disease. The α/β-blocker labetalol may not aggravate peripheral vascular disease as much as pure β-blockers, but it should be avoided in asthma and COPD. Since there are so many alternatives for hypertensive patients, it is usually not difficult to find acceptable alternatives. A β_1-selective β-blocker, however, is strongly indicated for a patient who has had a myocardial infarction.

Diabetes[30,59–67]

The blood pressure treatment goal in diabetic patients with hypertension is 130/85 mm Hg or less based on JNC-VI or less than 130/80 mm Hg based on the National Kidney Foundation guidelines.[1,30] No antihypertensive agent is specifically contraindicated for use in the diabetic population, but caution is needed with several drugs.

β-Blocker therapy may be problematic in patients with hypertension and tightly controlled diabetes. This is due to the effect β-adrenergic blockade produces during hypoglycemic episodes. Most of the symptoms of hypoglycemia (i.e., tremor, tachycardia, and palpitations) are mediated through the sympathetic nervous system, and these signs and symptoms are masked in the presence of β-adrenergic blockade. Sweating is a cholinergically mediated symptom of hypoglycemia that may still occur during a hypoglycemic episode with β-adrenergic blockade. Since recovery of hypoglycemia depends on various compensatory mechanisms, including those produced by catecholamine input, another consequence of β-adrenergic blockade is a delay in recovery time from hypoglycemia. Finally, hypertensive patients may experience marked elevations in blood pressure due to vasoconstriction caused by unopposed α-receptor stimulation during the hypoglycemic recovery phase due to epinephrine that is released in an effort to reverse the hypoglycemia. With these issues in mind, however, β-blockers have been shown in at least one study to be as effective as ACE inhibitors in protection against morbidity and mortality in patients with diabetes.[61] β-Blockers without intrinsic sympathomimetic activity are especially useful in diabetic patients with ischemic heart disease or in those who have had a myocardial infarction.

The α_1-antagonists may increase the risk of orthostatic hypotension, and the α_2-agonists may cause a paradoxical increase in blood pressure. Both these effects appear to be secondary to a more sensitive autonomic nervous system in patients with diabetic neuropathy.

Some evidence indicates that ACE inhibitors may increase insulin sensitivity, and there are a few case reports of hypoglycemia resulting from the combination of an ACE inhibitor and an oral hypoglycemic agent. While such interactions may occur and could be detrimental in some patients, the fact that ACE inhibitors improve insulin sensitivity is probably of limited clinical significance. Another potential benefit of ACE inhibitors in diabetic patients is their renal protective effects. In animal studies, ACE inhibitors and nondihydropyridine calcium channel antagonists have been shown to reduce intraglomerular hypertension. An increased glomerular pressure, hyperfiltration, and the accompanying microalbuminuria appear to be the earliest signs of diabetic nephropathy. Recent clinical studies support the renal protective effect of ACE inhibitors. Another study found, however, that atenolol was as effective as lisinopril in reducing urinary albumin excretion in patients with hypertension and diabetes.[68] Clearly, the most important strategy to protect the kidney is aggressive blood pressure control.

The most important outcome for patients with diabetes and hypertension is a reduction in cardiovascular events because these are the major causes of death. Three studies and a metaanalysis have been published that compared an ACE inhibitor with either a dihydropyridine calcium channel blocker or a β-blocker. In both studies that compared a dihydropyridine with an ACE inhibitor, the ACE inhibitor group had significantly lower rates of end points, including myocardial infarctions and all cardiovascular events.[59,60,66] The available evidence does not suggest that calcium channel blockers are harmful in diabetic patients, but it does suggest that they are not as protective as ACE inhibitors. While the data are limited, the nondihydropyridine calcium channel blockers (diltiazem and verapamil) appear to have more renal protective effects than the dihydropyridines.[30] In one trial that compared captopril with atenolol, there was no difference between the two drugs.[61] Based on the weight of this evidence, ACE inhibitors may be considered the preferred pharmacologic treatment of hypertension in the diabetic subject. If the ACE inhibitor does not control the blood pressure adequately, a low dose of a thiazide diuretic should be added.

Dyslipidemia[1,69]

Dyslipidemia significantly increases the risk of coronary artery disease attributed to hypertension. Therefore, every effort should be made not only to control high blood pressure but also to manage or prevent dyslipidemia effectively. While some antihypertensive agents may adversely affect serum lipids, namely, thiazide diuretics and β-blockers without intrinsic sympathomimetic activity (ISA), these effects generally are transient and of no clinical consequence. In addition, appropriate dietary modifications can reduce or eliminate these effects.[1] In the SHEP trial, patients with dyslipidemia were evaluated and found to have similar reductions in cardiovascular events as those who did not have dyslipidemia.[69] Therefore, diuretics and β-blockers are still useful agents in patients with dyslipidemia.

The α-adrenergic antagonists have been shown to decrease low-density lipoprotein cholesterol levels and increase high-density lipoprotein cholesterol levels. However, because they may not be as protective against cardiovascular end points as thiazide diuretics, they should not be specifically used therapeutically in patients with dyslipidemia.[70] ACE inhibitors and calcium channel antagonists have no effect on serum lipids.

Left Ventricular Hypertrophy

Left ventricular hypertrophy (LVH) is another independent risk factor for coronary artery disease. LVH is present in about 50% of hypertensive patients. With the exception of vasodilators, most classes of antihypertensive agents have been shown to prevent or regress LVH.[71] Prevention or regression of LVH should be considered an important objective in the overall management of hypertension. While ACE inhibitors are considered the most effective agents for regressing LVH, one study showed that the long-term use of diuretics led to the most regression.[43] Drug selections cannot be made based on a desire to prevent or cause a regression in LVH at this time.

Smoking

Smoking markedly increases cardiovascular risks associated with hypertension. Data from the Medical Research Council trial demonstrated that smoking eliminated any beneficial effect of propranolol in reducing cardiac events. Smoking induces catecholamine release, which, in the presence of β_2-receptor blockade, may lead to an increase in vascular resistance and therefore blood pressure and cardiac workload. It is also possible that smoking induced propranolol metabolism and lowered serum drug concentrations. All patients should be encouraged to stop smoking. The α-agonist clonidine has been shown to be useful in smoking cessation (particularly in women), and this antihypertensive agent may be considered in smokers who are trying quit. Otherwise, drug selection should be the same as for nonsmokers.

Coronary Artery Disease

β-Blockers and calcium channel antagonists offer the advantage of lowering blood pressure and reducing myocardial oxygen demand in patients with hypertension and ischemic heart disease. The cardiac stimulation that may occur with nifedipine or β-blockers with ISA, however, may make these agents less desirable in this clinical setting. Current guidelines suggest that non-ISA β-blockers are the agents of first choice in these patients. Calcium channel blockers should be reserved as second- or third-line therapy.

There has been concern that overtreating high blood pressure in patients with coronary artery disease may bring about more harm than good (the so called J-curve phenomenon). Since coronary blood flow occurs during diastole, the rate of flow is directly influenced by the DBP. Reducing the DBP excessively therefore may compromise coronary perfusion, especially in patients with fixed coronary artery stenosis, and lead to myocardial infarction. While this has been a theoretical concern based on retrospective analyses, prospective studies have not found a J-curve until DBPs were very low (e.g., <60 mm Hg).

For secondary prevention of infarction in hypertensive patients, calcium channel blockers do not afford the same degree of benefit as β-blockers. Diltiazem has been shown to reduce reinfarction in patients with non-Q-wave infarcts and may reduce cardiac events in post-myocardial infarction patients who do not have congestive heart failure. However, diltiazem was shown to be harmful if pulmonary congestion was present, where it increased the incidence of death. Similarly, verapamil offers some protection to post-myocardial infarction patients with normal left ventricular ejection fractions. Studies evaluating the use of calcium channel antagonists after myocardial infarction were not carried out in hypertensive patients.

Heart Failure

In patients with heart failure, ACE inhibitors have been shown to improve symptomatology and reduce hospitalizations and mortality. Although heart failure, not hypertension, was the focus of these studies, it seems logical to use ACE inhibitors to treat hypertension in the setting of concomitant heart failure. Because of the high renin and angiotensin II status of patients with heart failure, therapy with an ACE inhibitor should be initiated at low doses to avoid a profound drop in blood pressure. Low-dose β-blockers and spironolactone also have been found to reduce morbidity in patients with heart failure due to systolic dysfunction, but they must be titrated very carefully (see Chap. 11).

A β-blocker or nondihydropyridine calcium channel antagonist may improve left ventricular filling and cardiac output in patients with reduced cardiac output due to diastolic dysfunction. On the other hand, these agents may worsen heart failure in patients with systolic decompensation (see Chap. 11).

Renal Parenchymal and Renovascular Diseases[30,72]

Patients with hypertension and renal disease may have damage to either the renal tissue (parenchyma) or within the renal arteries. For patients with renal insufficiency due to renal damage, the most important strategy to slow the decline in renal function is strict blood pressure control (see Table 12–2). For patients with proteinuria in excess of 1 g/d, the goal blood pressure is less than 125/75 mm Hg. These blood pressures often will require two or more antihypertensive medications. In managing patients with hypertension and renal insufficiency, ACE inhibitors and angiotensin II receptor blockers may be particularly advantageous because they have been shown to reduce the intraglomerular pressures that result in further reductions in renal function. Diuretics may be a necessary addition to therapy, but thiazide diuretics may not be effective when creatinine clearances are below 20 to 30 mL/min. In these cases, a loop diuretic may be preferred.

An important caution, however, is that patients may experience a rapid and profound drop in blood pressure or acute renal failure when given ACE inhibitors. The potential for ACE inhibitors to produce acute renal failure is particularly noted in patients with bilateral renal artery stenosis or a solitary functioning kidney with stenosis. Patients with renal artery stenosis are usually older, and the condition is more common in patients with diabetes or those who smoke. Patients with renal artery stenosis do not necessarily have evidence of renal disease unless sophisticated tests are performed. Starting with low dosages and evaluating renal function shortly after starting the drug can minimize problems from ACE inhibitors.

Sexual Dysfunction[73,74,75]

Most antihypertensive agents have been associated with impotence or erectile dysfunction in males. It has been thought commonly that diuretics and β-blockers cause these side effects more often than newer antihypertensive agents such as ACE inhibitors and calcium channel blockers. In fact, several studies have borne this out.[74,75] However, hypertensive men frequently have arterial dysfunction, and this is even more prevalent if they also have diabetes. While specific drugs frequently are implicated, simply reducing blood pressure by any means can cause impotence in men. Thus drugs often are inappropriately implicated. Regardless, if a patient believes that a drug is the cause, it is likely that the dose will need to be reduced or the drug switched to an alternative agent. When a β-blocker is necessary, a cardioselective agent should be used. Other good alternatives include an ACE inhibitor or a calcium channel blocker. Centrally acting agents such as clonidine, methyldopa, and guanethidine should be avoided because they are associated with higher rates of sexual dysfunction. Unfortunately, little data are available concerning the effects of antihypertensives on sexual function in women. It is, however, believed that women may have difficulty achieving orgasm when blood pressure is reduced secondary to reduced blood flow to the vaginal tissues. This finding requires additional research.

INDIVIDUAL ANTIHYPERTENSIVE AGENTS

Diuretics[76]

There are four classes of diuretics: carbonic anhydrase inhibitors, thiazide and thiazide-like agents, loop diuretics, and potassium-sparing diuretics (see Table 12–7). In general, carbonic anhydrase inhibitors are weak antihypertensive agents and therefore are not used in the treatment of hypertension. The potassium-sparing diuretics are also weak antihypertensive agents when used alone but provide an additive hypotensive effect when used in combination with thiazide or loop diuretics. Moreover, they counteract the potassium- and magnesium-losing properties of other diuretic agents. Spironolactone actually may be a more potent antihypertensive than is usually thought in part due to its very slow onset of activity (up to 6 weeks). However, it has been shown to reduce mortality in heart failure.

In patients with adequate renal function (i.e., a glomerular filtration rate greater than 30 mL/min), thiazide diuretics are more effective hypotensive agents than loop diuretics such as furosemide. As renal function declines, however, sodium and fluid accumulate, and the use of a more potent diuretic is necessary to counter the effects that volume and sodium expansion have on arterial blood pressure. In this case, a loop diuretic should be considered.

All thiazide diuretics are equally effective in lowering blood pressure. The major differences between the various thiazides are the serum half-life and the duration of diuretic effect. These differences may not be relevant clinically, however, because the serum half-life of most antihypertensive agents does not correlate with the hypotensive duration of action. Moreover, diuretics may lower blood pressure primarily through extrarenal mechanisms. Until recently, all the major trials that evaluated morbidity and mortality outcomes started with a thiazide diuretic. The two most frequently used thiazide diuretics in clinical trials were hydrochlorothiazide and chlorthalidone.

The exact hypotensive mode of action of diuretics is not known. Acutely, diuretics lower blood pressure by causing a diuresis. The reduction in plasma volume and stroke volume associated with a diuresis decreases cardiac output and, consequently, blood pressure. The initial drop in cardiac output produced by the diuresis causes a compensatory increase in peripheral vascular resistance. With chronic diuretic therapy, the extracellular fluid volume and plasma volume return almost to pretreatment levels, and peripheral vascular resistance falls below its pretreatment baseline. The reduction in peripheral vascular resistance that occurs with chronic use of diuretics is responsible for their long-term antihypertensive effects.

The primary theory for the antihypertensive action of thiazide diuretics is that they mobilize sodium and water from arteriolar walls. This action would lessen the amount of physical encroachment on the lumen of the vessel created by excessive accumulation of intracellular fluid. As the diameter of the lumen increases, there is less resistance to the flow of blood through the vessel (i.e., peripheral vascular resistance drops). High dietary sodium intake can reverse and a low salt intake will potentiate the effect of diuretics on blood pressure.

Another postulated antihypertensive mode of action of the thiazide diuretics is direct relaxation of vascular smooth muscle. This theory is based on the known mechanism of action of diazoxide, a chemical closely related to the thiazide diuretics. Diazoxide is a direct vasodilator, and it has been proposed that the thiazide diuretics may exert a similar action.

Many patients require two or more antihypertensives to control blood pressure adequately. In these cases, one of the drugs should be a thiazide diuretic unless it is contraindicated. When diuretics are used in combination with other antihypertensive agents, an additive hypotensive effect usually is observed. This occurs as a result of two independent pharmacodynamic properties. First, it is a well-known pharmacologic principle that when two drugs cause the same effect through different mechanisms of action, their combined use results in an additive or synergistic response. This is especially useful when an agent such as a β-blocker or ACE inhibitor is necessary for an African-American, but it does not completely control the blood pressure. The addition of a diuretic frequently results in controlled blood pressure. Second, some alternative antihypertensive agents (e.g., clonidine, reserpine, hydralazine, minoxidil, and related agents) induce salt and water retention, which is counteracted by the concurrent use of a diuretic.

The side effects of thiazide diuretics include hypokalemia, hypomagnesemia, hypercalcemia, hyperuricemia, hyperglycemia, hyperlipidemia, and sexual dysfunction. Loop diuretics may cause the same side effects, although the effect on serum lipids and glucose is not as significant, and hypocalcemia may occur. Short-term studies indicate that indapamide does not adversely affect lipids or glucose tolerance or cause sexual dysfunction. Many of the preceding side effects were problematic with the thiazides when they were used in high doses (e.g., 100 mg/d) in the past. Current guidelines suggest limiting the dose of hydrochlorothiazide or chlorthalidone to 12.5 to 25 mg/d, which markedly reduces the risk for most metabolic side effects.

The hypokalemia and hypomagnesemia caused by diuretics may cause muscle fatigue or cramps. The most serious effects are cardiac arrhythmias in susceptible patients.[77] Patients at greatest risk are those receiving digitalis therapy, those with left ventricular hypertrophy, and those with ischemic heart disease. Low-dose diuretic therapy (i.e., 25 mg hydrochlorothiazide or chlorthalidone daily) seldom causes electrolyte disturbances in patients with uncomplicated hypertension. Every effort should be made to keep potassium in the therapeutic range by careful monitoring because hypokalemia also may negate the beneficial effects of the diuretic to reduce cardiovascular events.[78]

Diuretic-induced hyperuricemia may produce gouty arthritis or uric acid renal stones, especially in individuals who are predisposed to gout. In patients with no previous history of gout, acute gouty arthritis and nephrolithiasis are extremely unlikely consequences of diuretic-induced hyperuricemia. If some manifestation of gout does occur in a patient who requires diuretic therapy for effective treatment of hypertension, allopurinol can be given to prevent recurrent gouty attacks without compromising the antihypertensive effects of the diuretic. New information has appeared recently that suggests that an elevated uric acid value is a major risk factor for cardiovascular disease,[19,79] although this has not been found in all studies.[20] The evidence suggests that the benefit of thiazide diuretics can be negated if serum uric acid increases by more than 1 mg/dL over the patient's baseline. Thus serum uric acid should be monitored carefully.

At high doses, thiazide and loop diuretics may adversely affect glucose control and serum lipids. These effects, however, usually are transient and often inconsequential. Low-dose diuretic therapy is much less likely to produce these metabolic abnormalities.[69,80,81]

Potassium-sparing diuretics have the potential for causing hyperkalemia, especially in patients with renal insufficiency or diabetes and in patients receiving concurrent treatment with an ACE inhibitor, nonsteroidal anti-inflammatory drugs, or potassium supplements. The potassium-sparing drug spironolactone may cause gynecomastia.

β-Adrenoceptor Blockers[82,83]

The β-blockers are another category of antihypertensives that have been shown to reduce morbidity and mortality in patients with hypertension. In addition, numerous trials have shown a reduction in nonfatal reinfarction and death when using β-blockers following an acute myocardial infarction. Once considered contraindicated in congestive heart failure, carvedilol and metoprolol have been shown to reduce mortality in patients with heart failure who are receiving treatment with digoxin, diuretics, and an angiotensin-converting enzyme inhibitor (see Chap. 11).

Several mechanisms of action have been proposed for β-adrenoceptor blockers (β-blockers), but none of them has been shown to be consistently associated with a reduction in arterial blood pressure. β-Blockers reduce cardiac output because of their negative chronotropic and inotropic effects on the heart. Drugs that lower cardiac output lower blood pressure because blood pressure is the product of cardiac output and peripheral vascular resistance; however, cardiac output falls to the same degree in patients whose blood pressure is not lowered by β-blockers as in patients who respond with a fall in blood pressure. Finally, β-blockers with intrinsic sympathomimetic activity do not reduce cardiac output in the resting state, and yet they lower blood pressure and decrease peripheral resistance.

All β-blockers cross the blood-brain barrier, but the extent to which they enter the brain depends on their degree of lipophilicity. At one end of the spectrum is propranolol, a highly lipophilic drug; at the other end is atenolol, which is weakly lipophilic. One therefore would expect a much higher concentration of propranolol in the brain than atenolol after equivalent doses of the two drugs are given, and this indeed is the case. Despite differences in central nervous system concentration with various β-blockers, there is no difference in their hypotensive effectiveness. There is conflicting information concerning central nervous system side effects based on lipophilicity, with atenolol perhaps being better tolerated.

There are β-adrenoceptors located on the surface membranes of juxtaglomerular cells, and β-blockers inhibit the release of renin. However, there are conflicting studies as to the association between plasma renin levels and the ability of β-blocker therapy to lower blood pressure. In fact, some patients with low plasma renin levels do respond to β-blockers. Therefore, alternative or additional mechanisms need to be considered to account for the antihypertensive effect of β-adrenoceptor blocking agents. However, the ability of β-blockers to reduce plasma renin levels and thus angiotensin II concentrations may play a major role in their ability to reduce cardiovascular risk.

There are important pharmacodynamic and pharmacokinetic differences among the various β-blockers, but there is no difference in their clinical antihypertensive efficacy. Three pharmacodynamic properties of the β-blockers differentiate them to some extent. These are cardioselectivity, ISA, and membrane-stabilizing effects.

β-Blockers that possess a much greater affinity for β_1-receptors than β_2-receptors are called *cardioselective.* The β_1- and β_2-adrenoceptors are distributed throughout the body, but in certain organs and tissues, β_1-receptors predominate and in other organs and tissues β_2-receptors predominate. There is a preponderance of β_1-receptors in the heart and kidney, and a preponderance of β_2-receptors in the lungs, liver, pancreas, and arteriolar smooth muscle. Stimulation of β_1-receptors produces an increase in heart rate, contractility, and renin release. β_2-Receptor stimulation results in bronchodilation and vasodilation. β-Adrenergic blockers that bind more avidly to β_1-receptors than to β_2-receptors therefore are less likely to provoke bronchospasm and vasoconstriction. Also, because both insulin secretion and glycogenolysis are adrenergically mediated, blockade of β_2-receptors may reduce either process and cause hyperglycemia or blunt recovery from hypoglycemia, respectively.

At low doses, bisoprolol, metoprolol, atenolol, and acebutolol are cardioselective β-blockers. For this reason, they may be safer than nonselective β-blockers to use in patients with asthma, chronic obstructive pulmonary disease (COPD), peripheral vascular disease, and diabetes; however, it should be pointed out that cardioselectivity is a dose-dependent phenomenon. At higher doses, metoprolol, bisoprolol, atenolol, and acebutolol lose their relative selectivity for β_1-receptors and block β_2-receptors as effectively as they block β_1-receptors. The dose at which cardioselectivity is lost varies from patient to patient. Therefore, for patients with asthma, COPD, peripheral vascular disease, or diabetes, β-blockers should be avoided unless there is a compelling indication for their use. Compelling indications would include ischemic heart disease or prevention of a second myocardial infarction. In these latter cases, a cardioselective β-blocker would be preferred.

Another pharmacodynamic difference among the β-blockers is the *intrinsic sympathomimetic activity* (ISA). Pindolol, penbutolol, carteolol, and acebutolol are partial β-receptor agonists. This means that when they bind to the β-receptor, they stimulate it, but far less than a pure β-agonist. When sympathetic tone is low, as it is during resting states, β-receptors are partially stimulated by partial β-receptor agonists. Therefore, resting heart rate, cardiac output, and peripheral blood flow are not reduced when receptors are blocked. Theoretically, agents with ISA might have advantages over β-blockers in patients with borderline congestive heart failure, sinus bradycardia, or perhaps even peripheral vascular disease. Unfortunately, they do not appear to be as protective against cardiovascular events as other β-blockers and, in fact, actually may increase the risk of myocardial infarctions. Thus agents with ISA should not be used.

Finally, all β-blockers are capable of exerting a *membrane-stabilizing action* on cardiac cells if large enough doses are given. This activity is important for the antiarrhythmic properties of the β-blockers (see Chap. 14).

Pharmacokinetic differences among β-blockers can be found in first-pass metabolism, serum half-lives, degree of lipophilicity, and route of elimination. Propranolol and metoprolol undergo extensive first-pass metabolism. Therefore, the dose required to achieve β blockade with either drug is quite variable from patient to patient. Atenolol and nadolol, which have relatively long half-lives, are excreted renally, and the dosage of each may need to be adjusted in patients with renal insufficiency. Even though the half-lives of the other β-blockers are much shorter, once-daily administration still may be effective. As is the case with most other antihypertensive agents, the serum half-life does not correlate with the drug's hypotensive duration of action. β-Blockers also vary in terms of their lipophilic properties and thus central nervous system penetration.

Most of the side effects of β-blockers are due to their ability to antagonize β-adrenoceptors. β Blockade in the myocardium can be associated with bradycardia, atrioventricular conduction abnormalities, and the development of congestive heart failure. β-Blockers usually only produce heart failure if they are used in high initial doses in patients with preexisting left ventricular dysfunction. Blockade of β_2-receptors in the lung may cause acute exacerbations of bronchospasm in patients with asthma or chronic obstructive pulmonary disease. Blocking β_2-receptors in arteriolar smooth muscle may cause cold extremities and may aggravate intermittent claudication or Raynaud's phenomenon as a result of decreased peripheral blood flow. In addition, there is an increase of sympathetic tone during periods of hypoglycemia that may result in a significant increase in blood pressure because of unopposed α-receptor-mediated vasoconstriction.

Abrupt cessation of β-blocker therapy may produce unstable angina, myocardial infarction, or even death in patients predisposed to ischemic myocardial events. For this reason, it is always prudent to taper the dose of β-blocker gradually over 14 days before eventually discontinuing the drug. The acute withdrawal syndrome is believed to be secondary to a combination of factors, including progression of underlying coronary artery disease, hypersensitivity of β-adrenergic receptors, and failure to recognize the need to restrict physical activity on withdrawal of a drug that decreases myocardial oxygen requirements. In patients without coronary artery disease, abrupt discontinuation of β-blocker therapy may be associated with sinus tachycardia, increased sweating, and generalized malaise.

Like diuretics, β-blockers have been shown to increase serum lipids and glucose, but these effects generally appear to be transient and of little clinical importance. For instance, in patients with diabetes or hyperlipidemia, the reduction in cardiovascular events was as great with β-blockers as with an ACE inhibitor[61] and far superior to placebo.[69] β-Blockers increase serum triglyceride levels and decrease high-density lipoprotein cholesterol levels. β-Blockers with α-blocking properties (e.g., labetalol) produce no appreciable change in serum lipid concentration. Also, β-blockers with ISA do not adversely affect serum lipids and may even increase high-density lipoprotein cholesterol. The major concern in patients with diabetes is the fact that β-blockers blunt the symptoms of hypoglycemia and can prolong the duration of hypoglycemia. Therefore, they should be used very cautiously in tightly controlled diabetes, and a cardioselective β-blocker should be used.

Angiotensin-Converting Enzyme Inhibitors[44,48,59–61,84–88]

In recent years, several studies have helped clarify the role of ACE inhibitors. While they still are not recommended generally as first-line therapy in patients with uncomplicated hypertension, one study found that they were at least as effective in elderly patients when compared with diuretics and β-blockers,[48] and another study found captopril to be equivalent to atenolol except that more strokes were observed in the captopril group.[84] In addition, ACE inhibitors have many roles for patients with hypertension and coexisting conditions. Several studies have found that ACE inhibitors are superior to calcium channel blockers,[59,60] and another study found captopril equivalent to atenolol in preventing cardiovascular events in patients with diabetes.[61] ACE inhibitors are highly beneficial in reducing nonfatal and fatal events in patients with congestive heart failure, and they should be used in all these patients unless contraindicated. Finally, ACE inhibitors may be superior to other agents to reduce glomerular pressure and reduce the rate of decline in renal function in those with renal insufficiency.

Currently, there are nine ACE inhibitors on the U.S. market. Enalapril is metabolized to enalaprilat, which has a long half-life and duration of hypotensive action and therefore is given once daily in the treatment of hypertension. Lisinopril has an even longer duration of action but does not require metabolic conversion to exert its effect. Captopril, which has a much shorter half-life than enalapril, usually is administered two to three times daily. All three of these drugs are excreted in the urine, and therefore, an adjustment in dosage may be necessary in patients with renal dysfunction. The absorption of captopril, but not enalapril or lisinopril, is reduced by 30% to 40% by the presence of food in the stomach.

Benazepril, captopril, fosinopril, moexipril, quinapril, ramipril, and trandolapril can provide 24-hour blood pressure reduction with once- or twice-daily dosing depending on the agent. Benazepril, quinapril, and ramipril have the greatest effect on tissue ACE, but the significance of this effect has yet to be determined.

ACE is distributed widely in many tissues. It is present in several different cell types, but its principal location is in endothelial cells. Since the vascular endothelium covers a large surface area, the major site for angiotensin II production in the body is the blood vessels, not the kidney. ACE inhibitors block the conversion of angiotensin I to angiotensin II. This latter substance is a potent vasoconstrictor that also stimulates aldosterone secretion. ACE inhibitors also block the degradation of bradykinin and stimulate the synthesis of other vasodilating substances, including prostaglandin E_2 and prostacyclin. The observation that ACE inhibitors lower blood pressure in patients with normal plasma renin and ACE activity clearly indicates the importance of bradykinin and perhaps tissue production of ACE. Increased bradykinin has been shown to contribute to the blood pressure–lowering effects of ACE inhibitors.[85] ACE inhibitors effectively prevent or reverse (at least partially) left ventricular hypertrophy. ACE inhibitors also reduce the direct stimulation by angiotensin II on myocardial cells, which reverses left ventricular hypertrophy and prevents worsening heart failure.

Approximately 10% of patients who receive captopril develop a skin rash. In some cases, the rash is transient and disappears with lower doses and continued treatment with the drug. Another side effect of captopril is a reversible loss of taste or taste disturbance (dysgeusia), which has been reported in about 6% of patients who receive the drug. These side effects can occur with other ACE inhibitors, but the incidence is lower than with captopril. The higher incidence of skin rash, dysgeusia, and proteinuria with captopril has been attributed to its sulfhydryl group, which is not present on enalapril or lisinopril. Approximately 10% to 20% of patients will develop a persistent cough while on ACE inhibitors. While agents such as cromolyn and sulindac have been used to treat the cough, these options generally are not recommended.[87] Patients with cough may be switched to an angiotensin II receptor antagonist, which is less likely to produce cough, but it is not known if these drugs have the same cardiovascular and renal protective effects as ACE inhibitors.

Acute hypotension may occur at the onset on ACE inhibitor therapy, especially in patients who are severely sodium- or volume-depleted. It may be necessary to discontinue diuretics and reduce the dosage of other antihypertensive agents before initiating therapy with ACE inhibitors. It is also important to begin ACE inhibitors in very low doses with slow titration. A recent study initiated quinapril at 20 mg/d.[44] Patients were randomly assigned to a doubling of the dose at either 2- or 6-week intervals up to a maximum of 80 mg/d. Blood pressure control was essentially the same regardless of the titration scheme used, but serious adverse reactions occurred in 21% of patients in the fast-titration group and only 12% in the slow-titration group.

The most worrisome adverse effects of the ACE inhibitors are neutropenia and agranulocytosis, proteinuria, glomerulonephritis, acute renal failure, and angioedema. Fortunately, these serious adverse effects are rare, occurring in fewer than 1% of patients exposed. Patients with preexisting renal or connective tissue diseases appear to be most vulnerable to the renal and hematologic side effects. Patients with bilateral renal artery stenosis or unilateral stenosis of a solitary functioning kidney and patients dependent on the vasoconstrictive effect of angiotensin II on the efferent arteriole are particularly susceptible to developing acute renal failure on ACE inhibitors. Again, by slowly titrating the dose of ACE inhibitor and measuring renal function, adverse reductions in renal function can be detected early in those with renal artery stenosis.

Angioneurotic edema is a feared complication of ACE inhibitor therapy. It is more likely to occur in blacks than whites. Facial involvement is most common and only requires drug withdrawal. Laryngeal edema occasionally occurs and requires emergent medical care. Patients sensitive to one ACE inhibitor may be sensitive to another. There are reports of cross-reactivity between ACE inhibitors and angiotensin II antagonists.[88]

Hyperkalemia has been observed in patients treated with ACE inhibitors. Hyperkalemia is seen primarily in patients with renal disease or diabetes mellitus (especially with type IV renal tubular acidosis) or patients on concomitant nonsteroidal anti-inflammatory drugs, potassium supplements, or potassium-sparing diuretics.

ACE inhibitors are absolutely contraindicated in pregnancy because serious neonatal problems, including renal failure and death in the infant, have been reported when mothers took these agents during the second and third trimesters.

Angiotensin II Receptor Blockers[88–91]

Angiotensin II is generated by two enzymatic pathways: the renin-angiotensin pathway, which involves ACE, and an alternative pathway that uses other enzymes such as chymases. ACE inhibitors can block only the effects of angiotensin II produced by the renin-angiotensin system, whereas angiotensin II receptor blockers antagonize angiotensin II generated by either pathway. It is still not clear how these differences affect tissue concentrations of ACE. Because of these properties, ACE inhibitors do not completely block the effects of angiotensin. Angiotensin II receptor blockers directly block the angiotensin AT_1 receptor that mediates the known effects of angiotensin II in humans: vasoconstriction, aldosterone release, sympathetic activation, antidiuretic hormone release, and constriction of the efferent arterioles of the glomerulus. They do not block the AT_2 receptor, which means that the beneficial effects of angiotensin II mediated through stimulation of the AT_2 receptor are still intact, and these include vasodilation, tissue repair, and inhibition of cell growth.

Unlike ACE inhibitors, angiotensin II receptor blockers do not block the breakdown of bradykinin. This might have negative consequences in that some of the blood pressure–lowering effects of ACE inhibitors may be due to increased levels of bradykinin. The higher concentrations of bradykinin cause vasodilation and lower blood pressure. In addition, bradykinin has been shown to have important effects, including regression of myocyte hypertrophy, regression of fibrosis, and increased levels of tissue plasminogen activator (tPA).

Data from pooled analyses and direct comparisons have demonstrated that all the drugs in this class have similar antihypertensive efficacy, and they have a fairly flat dose-response curve. The latter finding suggests that increasing the dose above low or moderate doses is unlikely to result in additional blood pressure–lowering effects. The addition of low doses of a thiazide diuretic, however, can increase antihypertensive efficacy markedly.

While these drugs often have been considered to be "ACE inhibitors without the cough," the preceding differences highlight that they could have very different effects on vascular smooth muscle, myocardial tissue, and thus long-term cardiovascular effects when compared with ACE inhibitors. Whether their effects will lead to superior or inferior cardiovascular outcomes may be determined by the balance of these differences between effects on the AT_2 receptor and the bradykinin pathway. Unfortunately, there are no direct comparisons in hypertension. These drugs have been compared to ACE inhibitors in patients with congestive heart failure with mixed results. Because angiotensin II receptor blockers lack long-term cardiovascular outcome data, they should not be considered equivalent to ACE inhibitors at this time. Where they do appear to have a role is for patients who require an ACE inhibitor (e.g., congestive heart failure or diabetes) but cannot tolerate an ACE inhibitor (primarily due to cough) despite multiple attempts at lower doses or alternative ACE inhibitors.

Like ACE inhibitors, angiotensin II receptor blockers may cause renal insufficiency and hyperkalemia. Cough is very uncommon probably because these drugs do not block the breakdown of bradykinin. Angioneurotic edema is also less likely to occur than with ACE inhibitors, but cross-reactivity has been reported.[88] Angiotensin II blockers should be used cautiously in patients with a history of angioneurotic edema with ACE inhibitors.[88]

Currently, five angiotensin II receptor blockers are marketed for the treatment of hypertension: candesartan, irbesartan, losartan, telmisartan, and valsartan. Several others are under development, including eprosartan, tazosartan, and zolasartan.

Calcium Channel Antagonists[10,47,48,59,60,92–99]

Contraction of cardiac and smooth muscle cells requires an increase in the level of free intracellular calcium from the extracellular fluid. This is not the case for skeletal muscle cells. When cardiac or vascular smooth muscle is stimulated, voltage-sensitive channels in the cell membrane are opened, allowing calcium to enter the cells. The influx of extracellular calcium into the cell releases stored calcium from the sarcoplasmic reticulum. As the intracellular concentration of free calcium increases, it binds to a protein, calmodulin, which then activates myosin kinase. Activation of myosin kinase enables myosin to interact with actin to induce contraction. Calcium channel antagonists inhibit the influx of calcium across the cell membrane. There are two types of voltage-gated calcium channels: a high-voltage channel (L-type) and a low-voltage channel (T-type). Currently available calcium channel antagonists only block the L-type channel, which leads to coronary and peripheral vasodilation. Dihydropyridine calcium channel antagonists may cause reflex sympathetic activation, and all calcium channel antagonists (except amlodipine) may demonstrate negative inotropic effects.

Currently, there are eight calcium channel antagonists in use for the treatment of hypertension: verapamil, diltiazem, and six dihydropyridines: amlodipine, felodipine, isradipine, nicardipine, nifedipine, and nisoldipine. They are all similar in their antihypertensive effectiveness, but they differ somewhat in other pharmacodynamic effects. For example, verapamil decreases heart rate and slows atrioventricular nodal conduction. These properties make it an excellent drug for the treatment of supraventricular tachyarrhythmias. Verapamil also produces a negative inotropic effect that is responsible for its propensity to cause heart failure in subjects with borderline cardiac reserve. Diltiazem also decreases atrioventricular conduction and heart rate but to a lesser extent than verapamil. Nifedipine and, to a lesser extent, other dihydropyridine calcium channel antagonists cause a baroreceptor-mediated reflex increase in heart rate because of their potent peripheral vasodilating effects. Dihydropyridines usually do not alter conduction through the atrioventricular node and thus are not effective for supraventricular tachyarrhythmias. The reason that pharmacodynamic differences exist among the three major classes of calcium channel antagonists—verapamil, diltiazem, and the dihydropyridines—is that they all act at specific conformational sites on the calcium channel receptor on cell membranes. The density and distribution of specific types of calcium receptors vary from tissue to tissue.

Nifedipine rarely may cause an increase in the frequency, intensity, and duration of angina in association with acute hypotension. This effect is most likely due to the reflex sympathetic stimulation that occurs and may be obviated by using sustained-release formulations of nifedipine or other dihydropyridines. Immediate-release nifedipine has been associated with a greater incidence of adverse cardiovascular effects, it was never approved for treatment of hypertension, and it should not be used. Other side effects with dihydropyridines include dizziness, flushing, headache, gingival hyperplasia, peripheral edema, mood changes, and various gastrointestional complaints. The side effects due to vasodilation such as dizziness, flushing, headache, and peripheral edema occur more frequently with all dihydropyridines than with verapamil or diltiazem.

Diltiazem and verapamil rarely cause cardiac conduction abnormalities such as bradycardia, atrioventricular block, and congestive heart failure in otherwise healthy patients. These problems occur at increased frequency in those with preexisting abnormalities in the cardiac conduction system. Both can cause anorexia, nausea, peripheral edema, and hypotension. Verapamil causes constipation in about 7% of patients.

New randomized, controlled studies have demonstrated that calcium channel antagonists can reduce the risk of cardiovascular events markedly in both isolated systolic hypertension and combined diastolic/systolic hypertension. However, dihydropyridines may not provide as much protection against cardiac events such as myocardial infarction when compared with conventional therapy (diuretics and β-blockers)[96] or ACE inhibitors.[48] In addition, studies in patients with hypertension and diabetes demonstrate that ACE inhibitors are more protective against myocardial infarction and other cardiac events than dihydropyridines. Studies with diltiazem and verapamil are limited, but one study found diltiazem to be equivalent to diuretics and β-blockers in reducing cardiovascular events.[97] It is possible that these differences (beneficial with diltiazem and neutral with dihydropyridines) may relate to the sympathetic stimulation that can occur with dihydropyridines. Until research can better clarify the role of calcium channel antagonists, they should be reserved as alternative agents that may be the second or third drug in a therapeutic regimen.

Peripheral α_1-Receptor Blockers[70,100]

Prazosin, terazosin, and doxazosin are selective α_1-receptor blockers. These drugs do not cause the severe reflex tachycardia associated with the use of nonselective α-blockers. At higher doses and sometimes with chronic administration of low doses, fluid and sodium accumulate, and concurrent diuretic therapy is then required to maintain the hypotensive efficacy of the α-receptor blocker.

Even though the antihypertensive effect of these drugs is achieved through a peripheral mechanism of action, they do cross the blood-brain barrier and may cause central nervous system side effects such as lassitude, vivid dreams, and depression. A potentially severe side effect of selective α_1-blockers is the so-called first-dose phenomenon. This is characterized by transient dizziness or faintness, palpitations, and even syncope occurring within 1 to 3 hours of the first dose. This also may occur following later dosage increases. These episodes are accompanied by orthostatic hypotension and can be obviated by having the patient take the first dose and subsequent first increased dose at bedtime. Occasionally, orthostatic dizziness persists with chronic administration. For these reasons, these agents should be used very cautiously in elderly patients. α_1-Blockers also may cause priapism. One beneficial effect of α_1-blockers is that they provide symptomatic benefit to patients with benign prostatic hypertrophy.

Recently, the doxazosin arm of the Antihypertensive and Lipid-Lowering Treatment to Prevent Heart Attack Trial was stopped prematurely because of more cases of stokes, congestive heart failure, and all-cause cardiovascular events with doxazosin compared with the diuretic.[70] The other arms of the study (diuretic, ACE inhibitor, calcium channel antagonist) are continuing. These data suggest that doxazosin (and probably other α_1-receptor blockers) are not as protective against these cardiovascular events as other therapies. Therefore, α_1-receptor blockers in low doses should be reserved for unique cases such as males with benign prostatic hypertrophy if they are already receiving other standard therapy (e.g., diuretic, β-blocker, or ACE inhibitor). These agents block postsynaptic α_1-adrenergic receptors located on the prostate capsule, causing relaxation and decreased resistance to urinary outflow.

Central α_2-Receptor Agonists

Clonidine, guanabenz, guanfacine, and methyldopa all lower blood pressure primarily by stimulating α_2-adrenergic receptors in the brain. Such action leads to a reduction in sympathetic outflow from the vasomotor center in the brain and an associated increase in vagal tone. It is also possible that stimulation of presynaptic α_2-receptors peripherally may contribute to the reduction in sympathetic tone. As a consequence of reduced sympathetic activity, together with some enhancement of parasympathetic activity, heart rate is decreased, cardiac output decreases slightly, total peripheral resistance is lowered, plasma renin activity is reduced, and baroreceptor reflexes are blunted.

Chronic use of the centrally acting α-agonists results in sodium and fluid retention, which appears to be most prominent with methyldopa. Low doses of either clonidine, guanfacine, or guanabenz can be used to treat mild hypertension without the addition of a diuretic. Methyldopa, even at low doses, usually leads to enough sodium and fluid accumulation that tolerance to its hypotensive effect soon develops in the absence of concurrent diuretic therapy.

Sedation and dry mouth are common side effects of these antihypertensive agents. These symptoms may diminish or abate completely with chronic use of low doses. As with other centrally acting antihypertensive drugs, these agents may cause depression. Because they can cause orthostatic hypotension and dizziness more frequently than other antihypertensive agents, they should be used very cautiously in the elderly.

Abrupt cessation of a central α-receptor agonist may lead to rebound hypertension or overshoot hypertension. Rebound hypertension is characterized by a sudden increase in blood pressure to the pretreatment level, whereas overshoot implies an increase in excess of the pretreatment level. This is thought to occur secondary to a compensatory increase in norepinephrine release that follows a discontinuation of presynaptic α-receptor stimulation. The propensity for this is increased in patients receiving concurrent β-blocker and central α-receptor agonist therapy due to unopposed β-receptor stimulation.

In addition to the side effects already mentioned, methyldopa rarely may cause hepatitis or hemolytic anemia. A transient elevation in liver function tests is associated occasionally with methyldopa therapy and is clinically unimportant. However, a persistent increase in serum transaminases or alkaline phosphatase may herald the onset of a fulminant hepatitis, which can be fatal. A Coombs-positive hemolytic anemia occurs in less than 1% of patients receiving methyldopa, although 20% exhibit a positive direct Coombs test without anemia. For these reasons, methyldopa has limited usefulness.

One pharmaceutical formulation that may be associated with fewer side effects and increased adherence is the transdermal delivery system for clonidine. This patch is applied to the skin and left in place for 1 week before being replaced. It reduces blood pressure while avoiding the high peak serum drug concentrations seen with oral dosing and thought to contribute to the high incidence of adverse effects. The delivery system is ideal for patients who cannot take medication by mouth, such as the perioperative patient. However, most ambulatory patients will be taking other oral medications, so the advantage of adherence to this formulation may be limited. The disadvantages of this system are cost, a 20% incidence of local skin rash or irritation, and a 2- or 3-day delay of onset of effect so that oral medications should be overlapped for this period of time when patch therapy is first started. A similar delay in "offset" of action also may be seen when the patch is removed and the blood pressure returns to pretreatment values over a 2- or 3-day period.

Vasodilators

Hydralazine and minoxidil cause direct arteriolar smooth muscle relaxation through mechanisms that increase the intracellular concentration of cyclic GMP. They exert little effect, if any, on the venous side of the circulation and thus are considered afterload reducers. By decreasing the amount of systemic pressure in the arterial system, they reduce impedance to myocardial contractility.

These potent agents cause a reduction in perfusion pressure brought on by direct arteriolar vasodilation that activates the baroreceptor reflexes. This effect results in an increase in sympathetic outflow from the vasomotor center, which leads to an increase in heart rate, cardiac output, and renin release. Consequently, the hypotensive effectiveness of direct vasodilators diminishes in time unless the patient is also taking a sympathetic inhibitor and a diuretic to counteract the compensatory changes created by the baroreceptor reflexes. In older patients, however, baroreceptor mechanisms may be blunted enough that blood pressure may be lowered with vasodilatory therapy without causing sympathetic overactivity.

Patients who are candidates for these drugs generally should receive both a diuretic and a β-adrenergic blocker prior to using these agents. Direct vasodilator use can precipitate angina in patients with underlying coronary artery disease unless the baroreceptor reflex mechanism is completely blocked. This adverse effect can be minimized by using a β-adrenergic blocking agent, but another sympathetic inhibitor (e.g., clonidine) can be used in patients who have contraindications to β-blockers.

One side effect that is unique to hydralazine is a lupuslike syndrome that is dose-related. Hydralazine is eliminated by hepatic *N*-acetyltransferase. This enzyme displays genetic polymorphism, and "slow acetylators" are especially prone to develop a lupuslike reaction to hydralazine. The syndrome, which is more common in women, is reversible on discontinuation of the drug. By keeping the total daily dose below 200 mg, lupuslike reactions usually can be avoided. Other side effects associated with hydralazine include dermatitis, drug fever, peripheral neuropathy, hepatitis, and vascular headaches. For these reasons, hydralazine has limited usefulness in the treatment of hypertension. However, it is still used occasionally with isosorbide dinitrate in patients with congestive heart failure. Because sympathetic stimulation usually is maximal in patients with congestive heart failure, hydralazine rarely increases heart rate, and a β-adrenergic blocker is not necessary.

Because minoxidil is a more potent vasodilator, the compensatory increases in heart rate, cardiac output, renin release, and sodium retention are even more dramatic than those observed with hydralazine. Sodium and water retention can be so severe with minoxidil that congestive heart failure can be precipitated. It is even more important to coadminister a β-adrenergic blocker and a loop diuretic with minoxidil. Other sympathetic inhibitors and thiazide diuretics may prove inadequate in counteracting the minoxidil-induced baroreceptor reflex and intrarenal compensatory mechanisms.

A very troublesome side effect of minoxidil is hypertrichosis. Increased hair growth occurs on the face, arms, back, and chest. This drug induced hirsutism ceases with discontinuation of the drug. Other minoxidil side effects include pericardial effusion and a nonspecific T-wave change on the electrocardiogram. Minoxidil generally is reserved for very difficult to control hypertension.

Postganglionic Sympathetic Inhibitors

Guanethidine and guanadrel deplete norepinephrine from postganglionic sympathetic nerve terminals, and they inhibit the release of norepinephrine in response to sympathetic nerve stimulation. The fall in blood pressure produced by these agents is associated with a reduction in cardiac output and peripheral vascular resistance. Because reflex-mediated vasoconstriction is blocked by these drugs, a much greater hypotensive effect occurs in the upright posture, and postural hypotension is common. The use of postganglionic sympathetic inhibitors is associated with many other unwanted side effects, including impotence, diarrhea, and weight gain. The gastrointestinal side effects occur as a result of unopposed parasympathetic activity.

Long-term norepinephrine depletion leads to postsynaptic receptor supersensitivity. Therefore, the administration of drugs that compete with postganglionic inhibitors for uptake into the nerve terminals (such as tricyclic antidepressants and sympathomimetics) occasionally may provoke acute severe hypertensive episodes. Because of their potential to cause explosive diarrhea, impotence, orthostatic hypotension, and syncope, the postganglionic sympathetic inhibitors have little role in the current management of hypertension.

Reserpine[101]

Reserpine lowers blood pressure by depleting norepinephrine from sympathetic nerve endings, and it blocks the transport of norepinephrine into its storage granules. Reserpine reduces norepinephrine released into the synapse following nerve stimulation. This reduces sympathetic tone, peripheral vascular resistance, and blood pressure. Reserpine also depletes catecholamines from the brain and the myocardium, which may lead to sedation, depression, and decreased cardiac output.

Reserpine is a long-acting drug that can be given once daily, but it may take 2 to 6 weeks before the maximal effect of the drug is observed. Reserpine can cause significant sodium and fluid retention, and therefore, it should be administered in combination with a diuretic.

Reserpine's strong inhibition of sympathetic activity allows increased parasympathetic activity to occur, which is responsible for some of its side effects, including nasal stuffiness, increased gastric acid secretion, diarrhea, and bradycardia.

Reserpine has been implicated as a cause of mental depression, which is a consequence of central nervous system depletion of catecholamines and serotonin. Patients may complain of sadness, loss of appetite, loss of self-confidence, gradual loss of energy, impotence, and early morning awakening. The early reports of depression with reserpine from the 1950s are not consistent with current definitions of depression. Regardless, reserpine-induced depression may be dose-related because very high doses (e.g., in excess of 1.0 mg daily) frequently were used. The problem can be minimized by not exceeding a dose of 0.25 mg/d. At low doses, the rate of depression with reserpine is equivalent to that of β-blockers, diuretics, or placebo.[7,101]

It must be appreciated that reserpine was the sympathetic inhibitor in many of the major clinical trials that have documented the benefit in treating hypertension, including the VA Cooperative trials and the SHEP trial. Analysis of the SHEP data found that reserpine was very well tolerated. The combination of a diuretic and reserpine is a very effective, inexpensive antihypertensive regimen.

PHARMACOECONOMIC CONSIDERATIONS

While the cost of effectively treating hypertension is substantial, the cost is offset from the cost savings that would be realized by reducing the frequency of morbid events in hypertensive individuals, which can drive health care costs up substantially.[102] The cost per life-year saved from treating hypertension has been estimated to be $40,000 for younger adults and even less for older adults.[103] Treatments that cost less than $75,000 per life-year saved generally are considered favorable by health economists.

Drug costs can account for 70% to 80% of the total cost of hypertensive care. One model for calculating the cost-effectiveness of various initial monotherapies for mild to moderate hypertension found that the cost of life-year saved was $10,900 for propranolol, $16,400 for hydrochlorothiazide, $31,600 for nifedipine, $61,900 for prazosin, and $72,100 for captopril.[103] In a cost-minimization study that included the cost of drug acquisition, supplemental drugs, laboratory tests, clinic visits, and complications, the total costs of treating hypertension were $895 for β-blockers, $1043 for diuretics, $1165 for α-agonists, $1243 for ACE inhibitors, $1288 for α-blockers, and $1425 for calcium channel blockers.[104] Finally, another cost-minimization analysis found that 86 middle-aged patients or 29 elderly patients would need to be treated to prevent one myocardial infarction, stroke, or death.[105] The excess cost of preventing one event with a calcium channel blocker or ACE inhibitor instead of a diuretic or β-blocker was $89,000 to $341,000 for a middle-aged patient and $30,000 to $115,000 for an elderly patient. Depending on the agent chosen, the added cost would be $200 to $800 per year.

It therefore is crucial to identify ways to reduce the cost of care without increasing the morbidity and mortality associated with uncontrolled hypertension. The logical first step is to convince the patient of the need for lifestyle modification. A carefully designed program for smoking cessation, weight reduction, exercise, and moderation of dietary sodium and alcohol intake can be quite effective at preventing and treating hypertension at little cost.

If nonpharmacologic measures prove inadequate, either a diuretic or a β-blocker should be initiated if there are no compelling indications for another drug. Both of these are available in generic forms and as such are far less expensive than alternative antihypertensive agents. When a second-line antihypertensive agent that has been selected preferentially for initial treatment does not control blood pressure adequately, adding a low-dose diuretic should be considered. Adding a diuretic not only will keep the cost down but also likely will prove more effective than the addition of an alternative antihypertensive agent.

HYPERTENSIVE URGENCIES AND EMERGENCIES[1,92,106–111]

Elevated blood pressure alone, when not accompanied by symptoms or by new or progressive target-organ damage, rarely requires emergent therapy. A common error is that elevated blood pressures are treated too aggressively in the physician's office, nursing home, emergency department, and hospital. Hypertensive urgencies can be managed with oral medications and a gradual reduction in blood pressure, with a goal to achieve stage 1 levels after several days. For most cases of hypertensive urgencies, oral captopril is one of the agents of choice. Oral administration of captopril also has been used in doses of 25 to 50 mg orally at 1- to 2-hour intervals. The onset of action of oral captopril is 15 to 30 minutes, and a marked fall in blood pressure is unlikely to occur if no hypotensive response is observed within 30 to 60 minutes. Calcium channel blockers such as amlodipine 2.5 to 5 mg orally at 1- to 2-hour intervals are also useful for hypertensive urgencies.

Oral or sublingual nifedipine has been used in the office setting, in nursing home patients, in inpatients, and in postoperative patients whose blood pressure has risen to some specified level. This is a potentially dangerous practice, and rapid reduction in blood pressure is strongly discouraged due to reports of severe adverse events such as myocardial infarctions and strokes. There are no data confirming that the rapid reduction of blood pressure in patients with severe asymptomatic hypertension is more beneficial than the gradual reduction of blood pressure in these patients.[109] Since autoregulation of blood flow in chronically hypertensive patients occurs at a much higher range of pressure than in normotensive persons, there are some inherent risks in reducing blood pressure too precipitously, resulting in cerebrovascular accidents, myocardial infarction, and acute renal failure.

For patients with hypertensive rebound following withdrawal of clonidine, oral loading with the drug may be useful. With oral clonidine loading, 0.2 mg clonidine is given initially, followed by 0.2 mg hourly until the diastolic pressure falls below 110 mm Hg or a total of 0.7 mg clonidine has been administered. A single dose may be all that is necessary.

Hypertensive emergencies are those rare situations which require immediate blood pressure reduction to limit new or progressing target-organ damage (hypertensive encephalopathy, intracranial hemorrhage, unstable angina, acute myocardial infarction, dissecting aortic aneurysm, or eclampsia). Hypertensive emergencies generally require parenteral therapy, at least initially. The goal in hypertensive emergencies is not to lower blood pressure to normal (<140/90 mm Hg) but rather a reduction toward 160/100 mm Hg within 1 to 6 hours. Precipitous drops in blood pressure to the normotensive range or lower may lead to end-organ ischemia or infarction. After the goal DBP is reached, treatment should be designed to hold that level of pressure for several days to allow physiologic adjustments in autoregulatory function. Then the blood pressure can be reduced further to normotensive levels.

The treatment of hypertensive emergencies can be accomplished with any one of several antihypertensive agents depending on the clinical situation. Nitroprusside is widely considered the agent of choice for the minute-to-minute control in most cases of severe hypertension. It is a direct-acting vasodilator that decreases peripheral vascular resistance but does not increase cardiac output unless left ventricular failure is present. It is usually given as a continuous intravenous infusion at a rate of 0.25–8.0 μg/kg per minute. Its onset of hypotensive action is immediate, and its effect disappears within 2 to 5 minutes of discontinuation of the infusion. Nitroprusside can be given to treat any hypertensive emergency, but in aortic dissection, propranolol should be given first to prevent reflex sympathetic activation. Nitroprusside is metabolized to cyanide and then to thiocyanate and eliminated by the kidneys. When the infusion must be continued longer than 72 hours, serum thiocyanate levels should be measured, and the infusion should be discontinued if the level exceeds 12 mg/dL. The risk of thiocyanate toxicity is increased in patients with impaired renal function. Other side effects of nitroprusside include fatigue, nausea, anorexia, disorientation, psychotic behavior, muscle twitching, and rarely, hypothyroidism. Nitroprusside administration requires constant intraarterial pressure monitoring.

Intravenous nitroglycerin has many similar advantages as sodium nitroprusside. In large doses, nitroglycerin dilates both arterioles and venous capacitance vessels, thereby producing both afterload- and preload-reducing effects. By reducing end-diastolic volume and pressure, the drug decreases myocardial oxygen demand. It also dilates collateral coronary blood vessels and improves perfusion to ischemic myocardium. These properties make intravenous nitroglycerin particularly useful in the management of severe hypertension in the presence of myocardial ischemia. The dose of intravenous nitroglycerin is 5–100 μg/min. As is the case with other nitrates, intravenous nitroglycerin is associated with tolerance over 24 to 48 hours.

Intravenous nicardipine is administered at 5 15 mg/h, and it is adjusted by 1–2.5 mg/h after 15 minutes. Headaches, tachycardia, flushing, nausea, and vomiting are common side effects.

Labetalol has nonselective β-adrenergic and α-adrenergic blocking properties that has been used successfully in hypertensive emergencies. It reduces blood pressure by decreasing peripheral vascular resistance without significantly affecting heart rate or cardiac output. The initial dose is 20 mg by slow intravenous injection over a 2-minute period, followed by repeated injections of 40–80 mg at 10-minute intervals, up to a total dose of 300 mg. Alternatively, the drug can be administered by continuous infusion at an initial rate of 0.5–2 mg/min and adjusted according to blood pressure response. Because of its α-blocking effects, labetalol can cause orthostatic hypotension. Other side effects include nausea, vomiting, scalp tingling, sweating, dizziness, flushing, and headaches.

Hydralazine has an onset of action that ranges from 10 to 30 minutes, and its effects last 2 to 4 hours. When given intravenously, 10–20 mg is diluted in 20 mL of 5% dextrose in water (D_5W) and administered at a rate of 0.5–1.0 mL/min. Because the hypotensive response is less predictable than with other parenteral agents, its major role is in the treatment of eclampsia or hypertensive encephalopathy associated with renal insufficiency.

Diazoxide is now considered to be an obsolete agent when intensive monitoring is not available. The drug is a direct-acting arteriolar vasodilator that decreases peripheral resistance, increases cardiac output, and maintains or increases renal plasma flow. Because diazoxide increases plasma volume, it is common practice to give a diuretic concurrently unless the patient is volume-depleted. It has quick onset and a duration of action ranging from 4 to 12 hours. Diazoxide occasionally causes overshoot hypotension, which can be reversed by pressor agents. To avoid the precipitous fall in pressure that occurs when diazoxide is given as a 300-mg rapid bolus, smaller bolus doses (50–100 mg every 5 to 10 minutes) or slow infusion over 15 to 30 minutes should be used. Other side effects of diazoxide include nausea, vomiting, tachycardia, hyperglycemia, and hyperuricemia.

Two new dopamine-1 agonists also have been used in hypertensive emergencies, especially when accompanied by acute or chronic renal failure.[110,111] Fenoldopam is a parenteral agent that has been used as an alternative to nitroprusside for perioperative hypertension and hypertensive emergencies. The drug improves renal blood flow and is especially useful when renal function is impaired. It is given in a dose of 0.1–0.3 μg/kg per minute by intravenous infusion. This drug may cause tachycardia, flushing, and headache. Ibopamine is an orally active dopamine agonist that also has been used in hypertensive crisis. Additional research is required to identify their role in therapy compared with older, traditional agents used for hypertensive emergencies.

EVALUATION OF THERAPEUTIC OUTCOMES

The most important strategy to prevent cardiovascular morbidity and mortality is strict blood pressure control (<140/90 mm Hg). Additionally, other modifiable cardiovascular risk factors, such as smoking, hyperlipidemia, and diabetes mellitus, must be controlled. An attempt to lower blood pressure to the optimal range (approximately 130/80 mm Hg) should be pursued especially in patients with diabetes or renal insufficiency. This latter degree of blood pressure lowering should be done with caution in patients with coronary heart disease to avoid precipitation of ischemic myocardial events.

Patients should be monitored for any signs of progressive disease complications. A careful history for chest pain (or tightness), palpitations, dizziness, dyspnea, orthopnea, headache, sudden change in vision, one-sided weakness, slurred speech, and loss of balance should be taken to assess the likelihood of cardiovascular and cerebrovascular hypertensive complications.

Self-reported measurements of blood pressure or automatic ambulatory blood pressure monitoring should be performed to establish effective 24-hour control. The JNC-VI, however, recommends that ambulatory blood pressure monitoring only be used in select situations such as suspected white coat hypertension. Blood pressure control is especially important during the early morning hours when patients are particularly vulnerable to cardiac events.

Blood pressure readings should be taken after 2 to 4 weeks of initiating or making changes in therapy. Once the goal of therapy is achieved and the patient is asymptomatic, blood pressure readings need be evaluated only every 3 to 6 months. More frequent evaluations are required in patients with poor control, advancing target-organ damage, or symptoms of adverse drug effects.

Other clinical monitoring parameters that may be used to assess therapeutic efficacy include changes in funduscopic findings, left ventricular hypertrophy regression on electrocardiogram or echocardiogram, proteinuria, and changes in renal function. These should be monitored periodically because any sign of deterioration requires immediate assessment and follow-up.

Since hypertension is a relatively asymptomatic disease and the antihypertensive agents are not without adverse side effects, it is imperative to assess patient adherence with the therapeutic regimen on a regular basis. Detection of nonadherence should be followed up with appropriate patient education and counseling. Agents that can be given once daily are important for most patients, especially for those with documented difficulties with adherence. Another consideration is the impact aggressive treatment may have on various quality-of-life measures, although several studies have found that patients actually feel better once their blood pressure is reduced. Patients undergoing antihypertensive therapy should be questioned periodically about changes in their general health perception, energy level, physical functioning, and overall satisfaction with their treatment. At the present time, there is inadequate information to recommend any herbal therapy as a treatment strategy for hypertension.

Patients should be monitored routinely for adverse drug effects. The most common side effects that attend each class of antihypertensive agents are discussed in the treatment section of this chapter. The occurrence of an adverse drug event may require dosage reduction or substitution with an alternative antihypertensive agent. This will include laboratory monitoring for some agents (diuretics, ACE inhibitors). Typically, this would include assessments of potassium, uric acid, serum creatinine, and plasma glucose.

▶ PRINCIPLES OF PHARMACOTHERAPY

- Untreated or inadequately controlled hypertension is a major risk factor in the morbidity and mortality of cardiovascular, cerebrovascular, and renovascular diseases. Antihypertensive drug therapy should be individualized according to various patient characteristics and underlying pathophysiologic circumstances. Tables 12–7 and 12–8 provide a list of agents currently available for the treatment of hypertension in the United States.
- Carefully and accurately perform blood pressure measurements on three separate occasions to confirm the diagnosis of hypertension. A single elevated blood pressure does not necessarily mean that someone is hypertensive. Aggressive blood pressure control should be achieved in patients with diabetes, congestive heart failure, or renal insufficiency.
- Inquire as to self-medication as a cause of high blood pressure (e.g., nonsteroidal anti-inflammatory drugs, weight-reducing agents or sinus preparations containing phenylpropanolamine, herbal remedies, greater than 2 ounces of ethanol per day).
- Consider that heavy sodium intake may be a factor for hypertension.
- Implement lifestyle changes as the initial treatment for hypertension unless target-organ damage is present. This should include sodium restriction, weight reduction, ethanol abstinence or reduction, and increased physical activity.
- Evaluate the patient carefully in terms of target-organ damage (e.g., ischemic heart disease, heart failure, funduscopic changes, renal insufficiency), comorbid diseases (e.g., asthma, gout, diabetes, lipid disorder, benign prostatic hypertrophy), and lifestyle (e.g., athletic, restricted finances, heavy travel schedule).
- In patients with uncomplicated hypertension, diuretics and β-blockers should be considered as initial therapy. Other drug choices are dictated by target-organ damage, comorbid diseases, contraindications, and lifestyle issues.
- Use small doses of a single drug initially. Consider low-dose combinations if it is unlikely that a single drug will suffice. Wait 4 to 6 weeks to assess the response of the drug, but be sure to titrate to at least a moderate dose.
- Failure to control blood pressure after an additional titration should result in the addition of a second antihypertensive drug. Wait 4 to 6 weeks to assess the response of the combination.
- Failure to control blood pressure after an additional titration of the second drug should result in a reassessment of compliance, sodium intake, secondary causes of hypertension, alcohol abuse, drug-drug interactions, or the need to use a diuretic.
- If these issues are resolved, then add a diuretic. If the patient is already on a diuretic, switch to an alternative agent or add a rational third drug. Wait 4 to 6 weeks to assess the response of the new regimen.

REFERENCES

1. The Joint National Committee on Detection, Evaluation, and Treatment of High Blood Pressure. The Sixth Report of Joint National Committee on Detection, Evaluation, and Treatment of High Blood Pressure (JNC-VI). Arch Intern Med 1997;157:2413–2446.
2. American Heart Association. 1999 Heart and Stroke Statistical Update. Dallas, American Heart Association, 1998.
3. Williams R, Hunt SC, Hopkins PN, et al. Evidence for single gene contributions to hypertension and lipid disturbances: Definition, genetics, and clinical significance. Clin Genet 1994;46:80–87.
4. Caulfield M, Lavender P, Farrall M, et al. Linkage of the angiotensinogen gene to essential hypertension. New Engl J Med 1994;330:1629–1633.
5. Dominiczak AF, Bohr DF. Nitric oxide and its putative role in hypertension. Hypertension 1995;25:1202–1211.
6. MacMahon S, Petro R, Cutler J, et al. Blood pressure, stroke, and coronary heart disease. Lancet 1990;335:765–774.
7. SHEP Cooperative Research Group. Prevention of stroke by antihypertensive drug treatment in older persons with isolated systolic hypertension: Final results of the Systolic Hypertension in the Elderly Program (SHEP). JAMA 1991;265:3255–3264.
8. Dahlöf B, Lindholm LH, Hansson L, et al. Morbidity and mortality in the Swedish Trial in Old Patients with Hypertension (STOP-Hypertension). Lancet 1991;338:1281–1285.

9. MRC Working Party. Medical Research Council trial of treatment of hypertension in older adults: Principal results. Br Med J 1992;304:405.
10. Staessen JA, Fagard R, Thijs L, et al. Randomized double-blind comparison of placebo and active treatment for older patients with isolated systolic hypertension. Lancet 1997;350:757–764.
11. Izzo JL, Levy D, Black HR. Importance of systolic blood pressure in older Americans. Hypertension 2000;35:1021–1024.
12. Domanski MJ, Davis BR, Pfeffer MA, et al. Isolated systolic hypertension: Prognostic information provided by pulse pressure. Hypertension 1999;34:375–380.
13. Mancia G, Giannattasio C, Turrini D, et al. Structural cardiovascular alterations and blood pressure variability in human hypertension. J Hypertens 1995;13(Suppl 2):S7–S14.
14. Vane JR, Änggard EE, Botting RM. Regulatory functions of the vascular endothelium. New Engl J Med 1990;323:27–36.
15. Ferrario CM. Importance of the renin-angiotensin-aldosterone system (RAS) in the physiology and pathology of hypertension. Drugs 1990;39(Suppl 2):1–8.
16. Reaven GM. Role of insulin resistance in human disease. Diabetes 1988;37:1595–1607.
17. Reaven GM, Lithell H, Landsberg L. Hypertension and associated metabolic abnormalities—the role of insulin resistance and the sympathoadrenal system. New Engl J Med 1996;334:374–381.
18. Sowers JR. Insulin and insulin-like growth factor in normal and pathological cardiovascular physiology. Hypertension 1997;29:691–699.
19. Alderman MH, Cohen H, Madhavan S, Kivlighn S. Serum uric acid and cardiovascular events in successfully treated hypertensive patients. Hypertension 1999;34:144–150.
20. Culleton BF, Larson MG, Kannel WB, Levy D. Serum uric acid and risk for cardiovascular disease and death: The Framingham Heart Study. Ann Intern Med 1999;131:7–13.
21. Perloff D, Grim C, Flack J, et al. Human blood pressure determination by sphygmomanometry. Dallas, American Heart Association, 1994.
22. Prisant LM, Albert BS, Robbins CB, et al. American National Standard for nonautomated sphygmomanometers: Summary report. Am J Hypert 1995;8:210–213.
23. Smolensky MH. Chronobiology and chronotherapeutics: Applications to cardiovascular medicine. Am J Hypertens 1996;9:11S–21S.
24. Kristal-Boneh E, Harari G, Green MS. Seasonal change in 24-hour blood pressure and heart rate is greater among smokers than nonsmokers. Hypertension 1997;30:436–441.
25. Glen SK, Elliott HL, Curzio JL, et al. White coat hypertension as a cause of cardiovascular dysfunction. Lancet 1996;348:654–657.
26. Smolensky MH, Portaluppi F. Ambulatory blood pressure monitoring: Application to clinical medicine and antihypertensive medication trials. Ann NY Acad Sci 1996;783:278–294.
27. Prisant LM, Bottini PB, Carr AA. Ambulatory blood pressure monitoring: Methodological issues. Am J Nephrol 1996;16:190–201.
28. The National High Blood Pressure Education Program Coordinating Committee. The National High Blood Pressure Education Program Working Group Report on ambulatory blood pressure monitoring. Arch Intern Med 1990;150:2270–2280.
29. Pickering TG, for an American Society of Hypertension Ad Hoc Panel. Recommendations for the use of home (self) and ambulatory blood pressure monitoring. Am J Hypertens 1995;9:1–11.
30. Bakris GL, Williams M, Dworkin L, et al. Preserving renal function in adults with hypertension and diabetes: A consensus approach. Am J Kidney Dis 2000;36:646–661.
31. Farnett L, Mulrow CD, Linn WD, et al. The J-curve phenomenon and the treatment of hypertension: Is there a point beyond which pressure reduction is dangerous? JAMA 1991;265:489–495.
32. Hansson L, Zanchetti A, Carruthers SG, et al. Effects of intensive blood-pressure lowering and low-dose aspirin in patients with hypertension: Principal results of the Hypertension Optimal Treatment (HOT) randomised trial. Lancet 1998;351:1755–1762.
33. Black HR, Yi JY. A new classification scheme for hypertension based on relative and absolute risk with implications for treatment and reimbursement. Hypertension 1996;28:719–724.
34. Grundy SM, Pasternak R, Greenland P, et al. Assessment of cardiovascular risk by use of multiple-risk-factor assessment equations: A statement for health care professionals from the American Heart Association and the American College of Cardiology. Circulation 1999;100:1484–1492.
35. National Institutes of Health. National Heart, Lung, and Blood Institute. Clinical guidelines on the identification, evaluation, and treatment of overweight and obesity in adults: The evidence report. Obes Res 1998;6:51S–209S.
36. Appel LJ, Moore TJ, Obarzanek E, et al. A clinical trial of the effects of dietary patterns on blood pressure: DASH Collaborative Research Group. New Engl J Med 1997;336:1117–1124.
37. Midgley JP, Mathew AG, Greenwood AMT, et al. Effect of reduced dietary sodium on blood pressure: A metaanalysis of controlled trials. JAMA 1996;275:1590–1597.
38. Ergul A. Hypertension in black patients: An emerging role of the endothelin system in salt-sensitive hypertension. Hypertension 2000;36:62–67.
39. Grobbee DE. Methodology of sodium sensitivity assessment: The example of age and sex. Hypertension 1991;17(Suppl I):I109–I115.
40. Materson BJ, Reda DJ, Cushman WC, et al. Single-drug therapy for hypertension in men: A comparison of six antihypertensive agents with placebo. New Engl J Med 1993;328:914–921.
41. Materson BJ, Reda DJ. Correction: Single-drug therapy for hypertension in men. New Engl J Med 1994;330:1689–1691.
42. Materson BJ, Reda DJ, Preston RA, et al. Response to a second single antihypertensive agent used as monotherapy for hypertension after failure of the initial drug. JAMA 1995;155:1757–1762.
43. Neaton JD, Grimm RH, Prineas RJ, et al. Treatment of mild hypertension study: Final results. JAMA 1993;270:713–721.
44. Flack JM, Yunis C, Preisser J, et al. The rapidity of drug dose escalation influences blood pressure response and adverse effects burden in patients with hypertension: The Quinapril Titration Interval Management Evaluation (ATIME) study. Arch Intern Med 2000;160:1842–1847.
45. Insua JT, Sacks HS, Lau TS, et al. Drug treatment of hypertension in the elderly: A metaanalysis. Ann Intern Med 1994;121:355–362.
46. National High Blood Pressure Education Program. National High Blood Pressure Education Program working group report on hypertension in the elderly. Hypertension 1993;23:275.
47. Wang JG, Staessen JA, Gong L, Liu L. Chinese trial on isolated systolic hypertension in the elderly. Arch Intern Med 2000;160:211-220.
48. Hansson L, Lindholm LH, Tord E, et al. Randomized trial of old and new antihypertensive drugs in elderly patients: Cardiovascular mortality and morbidity the Swedish Trial in Old Patients with Hypertension-2 study. Lancet 1999;354:1751–1756.
49. Messerli FH, Grossman E, Goldbourt U. Are beta-blockers efficacious as first-line therapy for hypertension in the elderly? A systematic review. JAMA 1998;279:1903–1907.
50. National High Blood Pressure Education Program Working Group on Hypertension Control in Children and Adolescents. Update on the 1987 task force report on high blood pressure in children and adolescents: A working group report from the National High Blood Pressure Education Program. Pediatrics 1996;98:649–658.
51. Temple ME, Nahata MC. Treatment of pediatric hypertension. Pharmacotherapy 2000;20:140–150.
52. Sinaiko AR. Hypertension in children. New Engl J Med 1996;335:1968–1973.
53. Hohn AR. Diagnosis and management of hypertension in childhood. Pediatr Ann 1997;26:105–110.
54. Henriksen T. Hypertension in pregnancy: Use of antihypertensive drugs. Acta Obstet Gynaecol Scand 1997;76:96–106.
55. Sibai BM. Treatment of hypertension in pregnant women. New Engl J Med 1996;335:257–265.
56. Anonymous. CLASP: A randomized trial of low-dose aspirin for the prevention and treatment of preeclampsia among 9364 pregnant women. Lancet 1994;343:619–629.

57. Hermida RC, Ayala DE, Iglesias M, et al. Time-dependent effects of low-dose aspirin administration on blood pressure in pregnant women. Hypertension 1997;30:589–595.
58. National High Blood Pressure Education Program working group report on high blood pressure in pregnancy. Am J Obstet Gynecol 2000;183(Suppl 1):S1–S22.
59. Estacio RO, Jeffers BW, Hiatt WR, et al. The effect of nisoldipine as compared with enalapril on cardiovascular outcomes in patients with non-insulin-dependent diabetes and hypertension. New Engl J Med 1998;338: 645–652.
60. Tatti P, Pahor M, Byington RP, et al. Outcome results of the fosinopril versus amlodipine cardiovascular events randomized trial (FACET) in patients with hypertension and NIDDM. Diabetes Care 1998;21:597–603.
61. U.K. Prospective Diabetes Study Group. Efficacy of atenolol and captopril in reducing risk of macrovascular and microvascular complications in type 2 diabetes: UKPDS 39. Br Med J 1998;317:713–719.
62. U.K. Prospective Diabetes Study Group. Tight blood pressure control and the risk of microvascular complications in type 2 diabetes: UKPDS 38. Br Med J 1998;317:703–712.
63. National High Blood Pressure Education Program. National High Blood Pressure Education Program working group report on hypertension in diabetes. Hypertension 1994;23:145–158.
64. Arauz-Pacheco C, Raskin P. Hypertension in diabetes mellitus. Endocrinol Metab Clin North Am 1996;25:401–423.
65. Fatourechi V, Kennedy FP, Rizza RA, Hogan MJ. A practical guide for management of hypertension in patients with diabetes. Mayo Clin Proc 1996;71:53–58.
66. Pahor M, Psaty BM, Alderman MH, et al. Therapeutic benefits of ACE inhibitors and other antihypertensive drugs in patients with type 2 diabetes. Diabetes Care 2000;23:888–892.
67. Gress TW, Nieto FJ, Shahar E, et al. Hypertension and antihypertensive therapy as risk factors for type 2 diabetes mellitus. New Engl J Med 2000;342:905–912.
68. Nielsen FS, Rossing P, Gall MA, et al. Long-term effect of lisinopril and atenolol on kidney function in hypertensive NIDDM subjects with diabetic nephropathy. Diabetes 1997;46:1182–1188.
69. Savage PJ, Pressel SL, Curb JD, et al. Influence of long-term, low-dose, diuretic-based, antihypertensive therapy on glucose, lipid, uric acid, and potassium levels in older men and women with isolated systolic hypertension: The Systolic Hypertension in the Elderly Program. Arch Intern Med 1998;158:741–751.
70. The ALLHAT Officers and Coordinators for the ALLHAT Collaborative Research Group. Major cardiovascular events in hypertensive patients randomized to doxazosin versus chlorthalidone: The Antihypertensive and Lipid-Lowering Treatment to Prevent Heart Attack Trial (ALLHAT). JAMA 2000;283:1967–1975.
71. Eselin JA, Carter BL. Hypertension and left ventricular hypertrophy: Is drug therapy beneficial? Pharmacotherapy 1994;14:60–75.
72. National High Blood Pressure Education Program Working Group. 1995 update of the working group reports on chronic renal failure and renovascular hypertension. Arch Intern Med 1996;156:1938–1947.
73. Jensen J, Lendorf A, Stimpel H, et al. The prevalence and etiology of impotence in 101 male hypertensive outpatients. Am J Hypertens 1999;12:271–275.
74. Fogari R, Zoppi A, Carradi L, et al: Sexual dysfunction in hypertensive males treated with lisinopril and atenolol: A crossover study. Am J Hypertens 1998;11:1244–1247.
75. Barksdale JD, Gardner SF. The impact of first-line antihypertensive drugs on erectile dysfunction. Pharmcotherapy 1999;19:573–581.
76. Valvo E, D'Angelo G. Diuretics in hypertension. Kidney Int 1997; 59(Suppl): S36–S38.
77. Materson BJ. Diuretics, potassium, and ventricular ectopy. Am J Hypertens 1997;10:68S–72S.
78. Franse LV, Pahor M, DiBari M, et al. Hypokalemia associated with diuretic use and cardiovascular events in the systolic hypertension in the elderly program. Hypertension 2000;35:1025–1030.
79. Fang J, Alderman MH. Serum uric acid and cardiovascular mortality: The NHANES I epidemiologic follow-up study, 1971–1992. JAMA 2000;283:2404–2410.
80. Lakshman MR, Reda DJ, Materson BJ, et al. Diuretics and β-blockers do not have adverse effects at 1 year on plasma lipid and lipoprotein profiles in men with hypertension. Arch Intern Med 1999;159: 551–558.
81. Grimm RH, Flack JM, Grandits GA, et al. Long-term effects on plasma lipids of diet and drugs to treat hypertension. JAMA 1996;275:1549–1556.
82. Goldstein S. Beta-blockers in hypertensive and coronary heart disease. Arch Intern Med 1996;156:1267–1276.
83. Nadelmann J, Frishman WH. Clinical use of β-adrenoceptor blockade in systemic hypertension. Drugs 1990;39:862–876.
84. Hansson L, Lindholm LH, Niskanen L, et al. Effect of angiotensin-converting enzyme inhibition compared with conventional therapy on cardiovascular morbidity and mortality in hypertension: The Captopril Prevention Project (CAPPP) randomised trial. Lancet 1999;353: 611–616.
85. Gainer JV, Morrow JD, Loveland A, et al. Effect of bradykinin-receptor blockade on the response to angiotensin-converting enzyme inhibitor in normotensive and hypertensive subjects. New Engl J Med 1998;339:1285–1292.
86. White CM. Pharmacologic, pharmacokinetic, and therapeutic differences among ACE inhibitors. Pharmacotherapy 1998;18:588–599.
87. Luque CA, Ortiz MV. Treatment of ACE inhibitor-induced cough. Pharmacotherapy 1999;19:804–810.
88. Rivera JO. Losartan-induced angioedema. Ann Pharmacother 1999;33: 933–935.
89. Willenheimer R, Dohlöf B, Rydberg E, Erhardt L. AT_1-receptor blockers in hypertension and heart failure: Clinical experience and future directions. Eur Heart J 1999;20:997–1008.
90. Ellis ML, Patterson JH. A new class of antihypertensive therapy: Angiotensin II receptor antagonists. Pharmacotherapy 1996;16: 849–860.
91. Conlin PR, Spence JD, Williams B, et al. Angiotensin II antagonists for hypertension: Are there differences in efficacy? Am J Hypertens 2000;13:418–426.
92. Grossman E, Messerli FH, Grodzicki T, Kowey P. Should a moratorium be placed on sublingual nifedipine capsules given for hypertensive emergencies and pseudoemergencies? JAMA 1996;276:1328–1331.
93. Michalewicz L, Messerli FH. Cardiac effects of calcium antagonists in systemic hypertension. Am J Cardiol 1997;79:39–46.
94. Opie LH. Calcium channel blockers for hypertension: Dissecting the evidence for adverse effects. Am J Hypertens 1997;10:565–577.
95. van Zwieten PA. Clinical pharmacology of calcium antagonists as antihypertensive and anti-anginal drugs. J Hypertens 1996;14(Suppl): S3–S9.
96. Brown MJ, Palmer CR, Castaigne A, et al. Morbidity and mortality in patients randomized to double-blind treatment with a long-acting calcium-channel blocker or diuretic in the international nifedipine GITS study: Intervention as a Goal in Hypertension Treatment (INSIGHT). Lancet 2000;356:366–372.
97. Hansson LHT, Lund-Johansen P, Kjeldsen SE, et al. Randomized trial of effects of calcium antagonists compared with diuretics and β-blockers on cardiovascular morbidity and mortality in hypertension: The Nordic diltiazem (NORDIL) study. Lancet 2000;356:359–365.
98. Palma-Gamiz JL. High blood pressure and calcium antagonism. Cardiology 1997;88(Suppl 1):39–46.
99. Packer M, O'Connor CM, Ghali JK, et al. Effect of amlodipine on morbidity and mortality in severe chronic heart failure. New Engl J Med 1996;335:1107–1114.
100. Veelken R, Schmieder RE. Overview of alpha-1-adrenoceptor antagonism and recent advances in hypertensive therapy. Am J Hypertens 1996;9:139S–149S.
101. Prisant LM, Spruill WJ, Fincham J, et al. Depression associated with antihypertensive drugs. J Fam Pract 1991;33:481–485.

102. Moser M. Hypertension can be treated effectively without increasing the cost of care. J Hum Hypertens 1996;10(Suppl 2):533 538.
103. Edelson JT, Weinstein MC, Tosteson AN, et al. Long-term cost-effectiveness of various initial monotherapies for mild to moderate hypertension. JAMA 1990;263:407–413.
104. Hilleman DE, Mohjuddin SM, Lucas BD, et al. Cost-minimization analysis of initial antihypertensive therapy in patients with mild-to-moderate essential diastolic hypertension. Clin Ther 1994;16:88–102.
105. Pearce KA, Furberg CD, Psaty BM, et al. Cost-minimization and the number needed to treat in uncomplicated hypertension. Am J Hypertens 1998;11:618–629.
106. Rehman F, Mansoor GA, White WB. "Inappropriate" physician habits in prescribing oral nifedipine capsules in hospitalized patients. Am J Hypertens 1996;9:1035–1039.
107. Psaty BM, Heckbert SR, Koepsell TD, et al. The risk of myocardial infarction associated with antihypertensive therapy. JAMA 1995;274: 620–625.
108. Jick HJ, Derby LE, Gurewich V, et al. The risk of myocardial infarction associated with antihypertensive drug treatment in persons with essential hypertension. Pharmacotherapy 1996;16:321–326.
109. Zeller KR, Kuhnert LLV, Matthews C. Rapid reduction of severe asymptomatic hypertension. Arch Intern Med 1989;149:2186–2189.
110. Stefoni S, Mosconi G, La Manna G, et al. Low-dosage ibopamine treatment in progressive renal failure: A long-term multicentre trial. Am J Nephrol 1996;16:489–99.
111. Oparil S, Aronson S, Deeb GM, et al. Fenoldopam: A new parenteral antihypertensive. Consensus roundtable on the management of perioperative hypertension and hypertensive crisis. Am J Hypertens 1999;12: 653–64.
112. Burt VL, Whelton P, Roccella EJ, et al. Prevalence of hypertension in the U.S. adult population. Results from the third National Health and Nutrition Examination Survey, 1988–1991. Hypertension 1995;25:305–313.

13

HEART FAILURE

Julie A. Johnson, Robert B. Parker, and J. Herbert Patterson

Heart failure is a pathophysiologic state in which the heart is unable to pump blood at a rate sufficient to meet the metabolic needs of the body.[1] In the past it was commonly referred to as *congestive heart failure* (CHF); the preferred nomenclature is now *heart failure* because a patient can have the clinical syndrome of heart failure without having symptoms of congestion. Heart failure is not a classic disease entity, in that it may be caused by numerous cardiac disorders. However, once a patient develops the clinical syndrome of heart failure, there is a specific pathophysiologic process that seems to be independent of the initial cause, and in this sense heart failure then becomes a disease. The normal cardiac cycle is comprised of two main components: ventricular diastole and ventricular systole. Diseases that adversely affect either component may lead to heart failure. Filling of the ventricle occurs during ventricular diastole, whereas ventricular contraction and ejection of blood occur during ventricular systole. For many years it was believed that reduced myocardial contractility, or systolic dysfunction, was the sole disturbance in cardiac function responsible for heart failure. However, it is now recognized that disturbances in relaxation (lusitropic) properties of the heart, or diastolic dysfunction, account for symptoms of heart failure in approximately one-third of patients.[1] A diagnosis of isolated diastolic dysfunction is usually made in patients with symptoms of heart failure but normal systolic function. The remaining two-thirds of patients with heart failure symptoms have systolic dysfunction alone or systolic plus diastolic dysfunction.[1] This chapter will focus on treatment of patients with systolic dysfunction (with or without concurrent diastolic dysfunction), whereas Chapter 15 will focus on the treatment of heart failure with normal ejection fraction (isolated diastolic dysfunction).

EPIDEMIOLOGY

In 1996, it was estimated that approximately 4.8 million Americans carried a diagnosis of heart failure, with disease prevalence expected to reach 10 million by the year 2007.[2] It is estimated that 400,000 to 700,000 new diagnoses of heart failure are made each year. The incidence doubles with each decade of life, and heart failure is the most common hospital discharge diagnosis in individuals over age 65. Heart failure is more common in men than in women, which is thought to be due to the greater incidence of ischemic heart disease in men.[2] Unlike most other cardiovascular diseases, the incidence and morbidity/mortality from heart failure has not decreased over the last two decades, and the prevalence is expected to continue to increase over the next few decades. This is ascribed to the aging population, and the fact that more people are surviving early cardiovascular events (e.g., from myocardial infarction).

Heart failure hospitalizations increased fourfold in two decades, with over 2 million hospitalizations for heart failure as the primary or secondary diagnosis in 1991.[2] The economic impact of heart failure is tremendous, with this expected to increase markedly as the baby-boom generation ages. The annual expenditure for heart failure in 1991 (inpatient and outpatient) approached $38 billion, and based on additional recent data, it is estimated that the total cost for heart failure management in 1999 was $56 billion.[2] The relative economic burden of heart failure is highlighted in data from Health Care Financing Administration hospital expenditures for 1991, which showed that heart failure hospitalizations cost more than double that of the five most common cancers, and nearly double that for myocardial infarction.[2] Thus heart failure is a major medical problem, with substantial economic impact that is expected to become even more significant as the population ages.

The overall 5-year survival is 30% to 40% for all patients with a diagnosis of heart failure, with mortality increasing with symptom severity. For example, annual mortality in patients with mild, moderate, and severe heart failure is estimated at 10%, 20% to 30%, and 30% to 80%, respectively.[2,3] Death is classified as sudden in about 40% of patients,[2] implicating serious ventricular arrhythmias as the underlying cause of death in many patients with heart failure.

ETIOLOGY

Heart failure is a pathophysiologic state that can result from many cardiac diseases or disorders; common causes of heart failure are shown in Table 13–1.[1,4] The common cardiovascular diseases cause both systolic and diastolic dysfunction; thus many patients have heart failure as a result of abnormal ventricular filling and reduced myocardial contractility.

Systolic contractile dysfunction is a cardinal feature of dilated cardiomyopathies. Although the cause of reduced contractility frequently is unknown, abnormalities such as interstitial fibrosis, cellular infiltrates, cellular hypertrophy, and myocardial cell degeneration are seen commonly on histologic examination.[4]

Pressure or volume overload causes ventricular hypertrophy, which helps return contractility to a near-normal state. However, if the pressure or volume overload persists, the hypertrophied myocardial cells eventually become fibrotic, and contractility decreases. Ventricular hypertrophy also increases ventricular stiffness and slows relaxation, therefore impairing diastolic function.[1] Examples of pressure overload include systemic or pulmonary hypertension and aortic or pulmonic valve stenosis. Volume overload may occur in the presence of valvular regurgitation, shunts, or high-output states such as anemia or pregnancy.

Another cause of systolic dysfunction is reduction in muscle mass due to acute myocardial infarction (AMI). AMI leads to death of affected myocardial cells, and the degree to which contractility is decreased will depend on the size of the infarction. The surviving cells undergo a compensatory remodeling, which begins the negative process of heart failure. This is discussed in greater detail in the pathophysiology section. Myocardial ischemia and infarction also affect the diastolic properties of the heart by slowing ventricular relaxation and increasing ventricular stiffness. Thus, AMI frequently

TABLE 13–1. Causes of Heart Failure

Systolic Dysfunction (Decreased Contractility)
- Reduction in muscle mass (e.g., due to ischemia and myocardial infarction)
- Dilated cardiomyopathies (e.g., idiopathic, viral, alcoholic)
- Ventricular hypertrophy
  - Pressure overload (e.g., systemic or pulmonary hypertension, aortic or pulmonic valve stenosis)
  - Volume overload (e.g., valvular regurgitation, atrial and ventricular shunts, high-output states)

Diastolic Dysfunction (Restriction in Ventricular Filling)
- Increased ventricular stiffness
  - Ventricular hypertrophy (e.g., hypertrophic cardiomyopathy, other examples above)
  - Infiltrative myocardial diseases (e.g., amyloidosis, sarcoidosis, endomyocardial fibrosis)
  - Myocardial ischemia and infarction
- Mitral or tricuspid valve stenosis
- Pericardial disease (e.g., pericarditis, pericardial tamponade)

Compiled from Refs. 1 and 4.

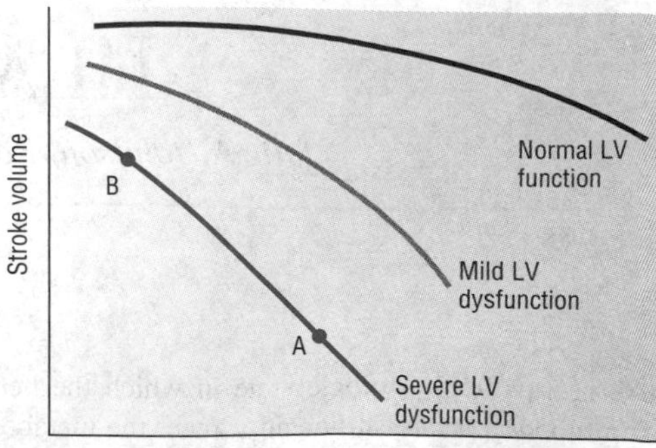

FIGURE 13–1. Relationship between stroke volume and systemic vascular resistance. In an individual with normal left ventricular (LV) function, increasing systemic vascular resistance has little effect on stroke volume. As the extent of LV dysfunction increases, the negative, inverse relationship between stroke volume and systemic vascular resistance becomes more important (*B* to *A*).

results in systolic and diastolic dysfunction. Less common causes of diastolic dysfunction are listed in Table 13–1 and include infiltrative myocardial diseases, mitral or tricuspid valve stenosis, and pericardial disease.

In the most recently published Framingham Study of patients with heart failure, ischemic heart disease alone was present in 19% of men and 7% of women with heart failure.[5] Hypertension alone was present in 30% of men and 37% of women, and hypertension plus ischemic heart disease was present in 40% of both genders. Thus, ischemic heart disease and/or hypertension contribute to development of heart failure in the majority of patients. Hypertension and ischemic heart disease were absent in 11% to 15% of patients,[5] suggesting that their heart failure was due to less common etiologies, including cardiomyopathies (idiopathic dilated, viral, alcoholic, hypertrophic) and valvular disease.[4,5] Many patients with pure diastolic dysfunction will have hypertension as their primary etiology, whereas in patients with any systolic dysfunction, ischemic heart disease is present in approximately 70%. The role of hypertension should not be underestimated based on this statistic, however, because hypertension is an important risk factor for ischemic heart disease and thus is also present in a high percentage of the patients with ischemic heart disease.

PATHOPHYSIOLOGY

NORMAL CARDIAC FUNCTION

To understand the pathophysiologic processes in heart failure, a basic understanding of normal cardiac function is necessary. *Cardiac output* (CO) is defined as the volume of blood ejected per unit time (L/min) and is the product of heart rate (HR) and stroke volume (SV):

$$CO = HR \times SV$$

The relationship between CO and mean arterial pressure (MAP) is:

$$MAP = CO \times \text{systemic vascular resistance (SVR)}$$

Heart rate is controlled by the autonomic nervous system. Stroke volume, or the volume of blood ejected during systole, depends on preload, afterload, and contractility.[1] As defined by the Frank-Starling mechanism, the ability of the heart to alter the force of contraction depends on changes in preload. As myocardial sarcomere length is stretched, the number of cross-bridges between thick and thin myofilaments increases, resulting in an increase in the force of contraction. The length of the sarcomere is determined primarily by the volume of blood in the ventricle; therefore, left ventricular end-diastolic volume (LVEDV) is the primary determinant of preload. In normal hearts, the preload response is the primary compensatory mechanism such that a small increase in end-diastolic volume results in a large increase in cardiac output. Because of the relationship between pressure and volume in the heart, left ventricular end-diastolic pressure (LVEDP) is often used in the clinical setting to estimate preload. The hemodynamic measurement used to estimate LVEDP is the pulmonary artery occlusion pressure (PAOP). Afterload is a more complex physiologic concept that can be viewed pragmatically as the sum of forces preventing active forward ejection of blood by the ventricle. Major components of global ventricular afterload are ejection impedance, wall tension, and regional wall geometry. In patients with left ventricular systolic dysfunction, an inverse relationship exists between afterload (or SVR) and stroke volume such that increasing afterload causes a decrease in stroke volume (Fig. 13–1). Contractility is the intrinsic property of cardiac muscle describing fiber shortening and tension development.

COMPENSATORY MECHANISMS IN HEART FAILURE

As cardiac function decreases secondary to one or more of the disorders described above, the heart relies on compensatory responses to maintain an adequate cardiac output. They are (1) tachycardia and increased contractility through sympathetic nervous system (SNS) activation, (2) the Frank-Starling mechanism, whereby an increase in preload results in an increase in stroke volume, (3) vasoconstriction, and (4) ventricular hypertrophy and remodeling. The benefits and detrimental consequences of these compensatory responses are described below and are summarized in Table 13–2.

TACHYCARDIA AND INCREASED CONTRACTILITY THROUGH SNS ACTIVATION

The change in heart rate and contractility that occurs in response to a drop in cardiac output is primarily due to release of norepinephrine from adrenergic nerve terminals. Because cardiac output equals the product of heart rate and stroke volume, one might expect cardiac output to change linearly with heart rate, but the relationship is much more complex. Because systolic time intervals change comparatively

TABLE 13–2. Beneficial and Detrimental Effects of the Compensatory Responses in Heart Failure

Compensatory Response	Beneficial Effects of Compensation	Detrimental Effects of Compensation
Increased preload (through Na^+ and water retention)	Optimize stroke volume via Frank-Starling mechanism	Pulmonary and systemic congestion and edema formation Increased MVO_2
Vasoconstriction	Maintain blood pressure in face of reduced cardiac output Shunt blood from nonessential organs to brain and heart	Increased MVO_2 Increased afterload decreases stroke volume and further activates the compensatory responses
Tachycardia and increased contractility (due to SNS activation)	Helps maintain cardiac output	Increased MVO_2 Shortened diastolic filling time B_1-receptor downregulation, decreased receptor sensitivity Precipitation of ventricular arrhythmias (?) Increased risk of myocardial cell death
Ventricular hypertrophy and remodelling	Helps maintain cardiac output Reduces myocardial wall stress Decreases MVO_2	Diastolic dysfunction Systolic dysfunction Increased risk of myocardial cell death Increased risk of myocardial ischemia Increased arrhythmia risk

Abbreviations: SNS = sympathetic nervous system; MVO_2 = myocardial oxygen demand.

little with changing heart rate, almost all cardiac cycle shortening occurs during diastole. Cardiac output continues to increase with heart rate until diastolic filling becomes compromised, which in the normal heart is at 170 to 200 beats per minute. When preexisting or acute diastolic dysfunction is present, however, the ventricle's need for more complete (longer) diastolic filling results in reduction of effective preload at significantly lower heart rates. Loss of atrial contribution to ventricular filling also can occur (atrial fibrillation, ventricular tachycardia), reducing ventricular performance even more. Because ionized calcium is sequestered into the sarcoplasmic reticulum and pumped out of the cell during diastole, shortened diastolic time also results in a higher average intracellular calcium concentration during diastole, increasing actin-myosin interaction, augmenting the active resistance to fibril stretch, and reducing lusitropy. Conversely, the higher average calcium concentration translates into greater filament interaction during systole, generating more tension.[6]

Increasing heart rate greatly increases myocardial oxygen demand. If ischemia is induced or worsened, both diastolic and systolic function may become impaired, and stroke volume can drop precipitously.

INCREASED PRELOAD

Augmentation of preload is another compensatory response that is rapidly activated in response to decreased cardiac output. Renal perfusion in heart failure is reduced due to both depressed cardiac output and redistribution of blood away from nonvital organs. The kidney interprets the reduced perfusion as an ineffective blood volume, thus stimulating sodium and water retention. Reduced renal perfusion and increased sympathetic tone also stimulate renin release from juxtaglomerular cells in the kidney. As shown in Figure 13–2, renin is responsible for conversion of angiotensinogen to angiotensin I.

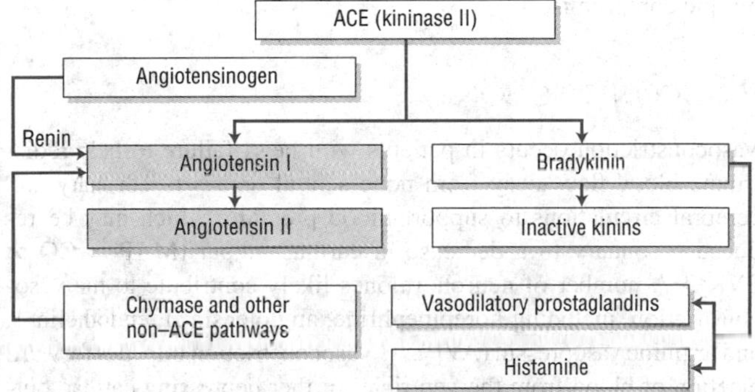

FIGURE 13–2. Activity of angiotensin-converting enzyme (ACE), which is identical to kininase II, on angiotensin and bradykinin.

Angiotensin I is converted to angiotensin II by angiotensin-converting enzyme (ACE). Angiotensin II feeds back on the adrenal gland to stimulate aldosterone release, thereby providing an additional mechanism for sodium and water retention in the kidney. As intravascular volume increases secondary to sodium and water retention, left ventricular volume and pressure (preload) increase, sarcomeres are stretched, and the force of contraction is enhanced.[1] While the preload response is the primary compensatory mechanism in normal hearts, the chronically failing heart usually has exhausted its preload reserve.[1] As can be seen in Figure 13–3, increases in preload will increase stroke volume only to a certain point. Once the flat portion of the curve is reached, further increases in preload will only lead to pulmonary or systemic congestion, a detrimental result.[1] Figure 13–3 also shows that the curve is flatter in patients with left ventricular dysfunction. Consequently, a given increase in preload in a patient with heart failure will produce a smaller increment in stroke volume than in an individual with normal ventricular function.

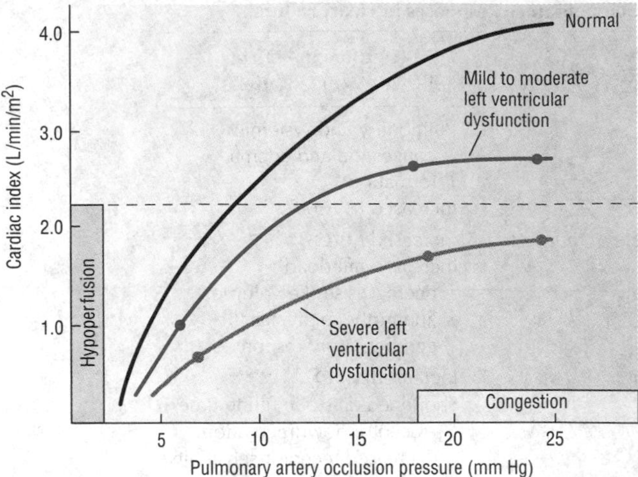

FIGURE 13–3. Relationship between cardiac output (shown as cardiac index, which is CO/BSA) and preload (shown as pulmonary artery occlusion pressure).

In addition to causing symptoms of congestion, augmentation of preload in the heart failure patient will increase afterload because increasing the radius of the ventricle elevates wall tension. Because the failing ventricle is highly afterload-dependent, increases in performance augmented by preload may at times be offset by the attendant increase in afterload. Additionally, the effects of increased preload on force of contraction and afterload will increase myocardial oxygen consumption. Thus an increase in preload can induce ischemia in the coronary patient, with subsequent lusitropic and inotropic compromise.[6]

VASOCONSTRICTION

Vasoconstriction occurs in patients with heart failure to help redistribute blood flow away from nonessential organs to coronary and cerebral circulations to support blood pressure, which may be reduced secondary to a decrease in cardiac output (MAP = CO × SVR).[1] A number of neurohormones likely contribute to the vasoconstriction, including norepinephrine, angiotensin II, endothelin-1, and arginine vasopressin (AVP).[1,6] Vasoconstriction impedes forward ejection of blood from the ventricle, further depressing cardiac output and heightening the compensatory responses. Because the failing ventricle usually has exhausted its preload reserve (unless the patient is intravascularly depleted), its performance is exquisitely sensitive to changes in afterload. Thus, increases in afterload often potentiate a vicious cycle of continued worsening and downward spiraling of the heart failure state.

VENTRICULAR HYPERTROPHY AND REMODELING[7,8]

While the ventricular hypertrophy or remodeling that occurs with heart failure does not cause signs and symptoms of heart failure as do the items described above, it is thought to be an important determinant of the long-term prognosis of patients with heart failure. *Ventricular hypertrophy* is a term used to describe an increase in ventricular muscle mass. *Cardiac remodeling* is a broader term describing changes in both myocardial cells and extracellular matrix that result in changes in the size, shape, and function of the heart. Ventricular hypertrophy and remodeling can be induced by a number of factors, including pressure or volume overload, loss of myocardial muscle mass due to AMI, inflammatory heart muscle disease (myocarditis), or decreases in contractility from a cardiomyopathy. It is well recognized that angiotensin II, norepinephrine, endothelin, aldosterone, and cytokines (especially tumor necrois factor alpha), as well as others under investigation, play an important role in initiating the signal-transduction cascade for ventricular remodeling. Pressure overload (and probably hormonal activation) associated with hypertension produces a concentric hypertrophy (increase in the ventricular wall thickness without chamber enlargement). Eccentric left ventricular hypertrophy (LVH; myocyte lengthening with increased chamber size and with minimal increase in wall thickness) characterizes the hypertrophy seen in patients with systolic dysfunction or previous myocardial infarction (MI). As the myocytes undergo changes, so do various components of the extracellular matrix. For example, there is evidence for collagen degradation, which may lead to slippage of myocytes, fibroblast proliferation, and increased fibrillar collagen synthesis, resulting in fibrosis and stiffening of the entire myocardium. Thus, a number of important ventricular changes that occur with remodeling include changes in the geometry of the heart from elliptical to spherical, increases in ventricular mass (from myocyte hypertrophy), and changes in ventricular composition (especially the extracellar matrix) and volumes, all of which likely contribute to the impairment of cardiac function. If the event that produces cardiac injury is acute (i.e., MI), the ventricular remodeling process begins immediately. However, it is the progressive nature of this process that results in continual worsening of the heart failure state, and thus is now the major focus of therapeutic targets. In fact, it is believed that all the heart failure therapies that have been associated with decreased mortality, and/or slowing of the disease, produce this effect largely through their ability to slow or reverse the ventricular remodeling process. Thus, while ventricular hypertrophy and remodeling may have some beneficial effects by helping maintain cardiac output, they also are believed to play an essential role in the progressive nature of heart failure.

THE NEUROHORMONAL MODEL OF HEART FAILURE AND THERAPEUTIC INSIGHTS IT PROVIDES[7]

Over the years, several different paradigms have guided the therapy of heart failure. The early paradigm is often called the *cardiorenal model,* where the problem was viewed as excess sodium and water retention, and diuretic therapy was the main therapeutic approach to combating the problem. The next paradigm was the *cardiocirculatory model,* which focused on impaired cardiac output (viewed as being due to both inadequate contractility and systemic vasoconstriction). This paradigm focused on positive inotropes and, later, vasodilators as the major mechanism by which to overcome the problems associated with heart failure. In fact, the first studies with ACE inhibitors were initiated with the thought that they might be effective due to their balanced (arterial and venous) vasodilation. While the therapeutic approaches associated with these paradigms provided some symptomatic benefits to patients with heart failure, they did little to slow progression of the disease (with the exception of ACE inhibitors). Subsequent realization that ACE inhibitors were providing benefit beyond their vasodilating effects, followed by the positive results with β-adrenergic receptor blockers and aldosterone antagonists has led to the current paradigm used to describe heart failure: the *neurohormonal model*. This model recognizes that there is an initiating event (e.g., AMI, longstanding hypertension) that leads to decreased cardiac output and begins the "heart failure state," but then the problems move beyond the heart, and it essentially becomes a systemic disease whose progression is mediated largely by neurohormones and autocrine/paracrine factors. While the former paradigms still guide us to some extent in the symptomatic management of the disease, it is the latter paradigm that helps us understand disease progression or, more important, the ways to slow disease progression. In the sections that follow, important neurohormones and autocrine/paracrine factors are described with respect to their role in heart failure and its progression. The benefits of current and investigational drug therapies can be better understood through a solid understanding of the neurohormones they regulate/affect.

ANGIOTENSIN II[1]

Of the neurohormones and autocrine/paracrine factors that play an important role in the pathophysiology of heart failure, angiotensin II is probably the best understood. The effects of angiotensin II are highlighted in Figure 13–4, and most of these contribute to its detrimental effects in heart failure. Angiotensin II increases systemic vascular resistance in heart failure through direct, potent vasoconstriction. Its ability to cause release of AVP and endothelin-1 also may contribute to vasoconstriction. Angiotensin II also facilitates release of norepinephrine from adrenergic nerve terminals, heightening SNS activation. It promotes sodium retention through direct effects on the renal tubules and by stimulating aldosterone release. Its vasoconstriction of the efferent glomerular arteriole helps to maintain perfusion pressure in patients with severe heart failure or impaired renal function. Thus, in patients dependent on angiotensin II for maintenance of perfusion pressure, initiation of an ACE inhibitor or angiotensin II type 1 (AT_1) receptor blocker causes efferent arteriole vasodilation, decreased perfusion pressure, and decreased glomerular filtration. This explains the risk of impairment in renal function associated with initiation of ACE inhibitor or AT_1 receptor blocker therapy. Finally, angiotensin II, and many of the neurohormones whose release/production is stimulated by angiotensin II, plays a central role in stimulating ventricular hypertrophy and remodeling. Clinical data suggest that blocking these effects contributes substantially to the prolonged survival of ACE inhibitor–treated heart failure patients.[8] The favorable effects of ACE inhibitors (and presumably angiotensin receptor blockers) on hemodynamics, symptoms, quality of life, and survival in heart failure highlight the importance of angiotensin II in the pathophysiology of heart failure.

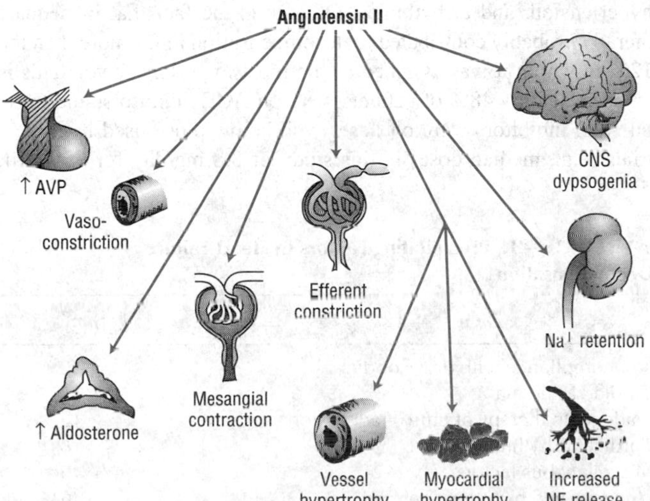

FIGURE 13–4. Biological effects of angiotensin II. See text for detailed explanation. Abbreviations: AVP = arginine vasopressin; NE = norepinephrine. *Reprinted from Am Heart J 1989;118:642, with permission.*

NOREPINEPHRINE[1,9,10]

Many of the detrimental effects of norepinephrine (NE) in heart failure are described above. It plays a central role in the tachycardia, vasoconstriction, and increased contractility observed in heart failure. Plasma NE concentrations are elevated in correlation with the degree of heart failure, and patients with the highest plasma NE concentrations have the poorest prognosis. In addition to the detrimental effects described, excessive SNS activation causes downregulation of β-receptors, with a subsequent loss of sensitivity to receptor stimulation. Excess catecholamines increase the risk of arrhythmias, and evidence suggests that NE can cause myocardial cell loss by stimulating both necrosis and apoptosis (programmed cell death). Finally, NE contributes to ventricular hypertrophy and remodeling. The detrimental effects of SNS activation are further highlighted by the clinical trials with chronic β-agonists, phosphodiesterase inhibitors, or other drugs that cause SNS activation, as since they have been shown uniformly to increase mortality in heart failure (discussed under "Other Drugs Studied in Heart Failure"). Additionally, β-blockers, ACE inhibitors, and digoxin all help to decrease SNS activation, through various mechanisms, and are beneficial in heart failure. Thus, it is clear that NE plays a critical role in the pathophysiology of the heart failure state.

ALDOSTERONE[11,12]

The effects of aldosterone on sodium retention, and thus a potential role in heart failure, have long been recognized. However, recent studies have revealed other direct effects of aldosterone on the heart that may be even more important in heart failure pathophysiology. Chief among these is the ability of aldosterone to produce interstitial cardiac fibrosis through increased collagen deposition in the extracellular matrix of the heart. This cardiac fibrosis may decrease systolic function, and also impair diastolic function by increasing the stiffness of the myocardium. Aldosterone also may increase the risk of ventricular arrhythmias through a number of mechanisms, including creation of reentrant circuits as a result of fibrosis, inhibition of cardiac NE reuptake, and impairment of parasympathetic traffic. In a recent study, low-dose spironolactone produced significant reductions in mortality in patients with moderate to severe heart failure, without appreciable effects on diuresis or hemodynamics,[13] providing substantial evidence that the direct cardiac effects of aldosterone play an important role in heart failure pathophysiology.

PROINFLAMMATORY CYTOKINES[14]

In addition to neurohormones, several proinflammatory cytokines are under extensive investigation for their role in the pathophysiology of heart failure. Tumor necrosis factor alpha (TNF-α), interleukin-6 (IL-6), and IL-1β have all been shown to be elevated in heart failure, with a direct relationship between the degree of elevation and the severity of heart failure. Of these cytokines, TNF-α is best studied for its pathophysiologic role in heart failure. Studies have demonstrated that TNF-α has negative inotropic effects, uncouples β-adrenergic receptors from adenylyl cyclase (thus reducing β-receptor-mediated responses), likely stimulates apoptosis of myocardial cells, and plays an important role in remodeling. With respect to remodeling, TNF-α promotes hypertrophy in cardiac myocytes, activates metalloproteinases, and inhibits expression of the inhibitors of metalloproteinases, thus activating extracellular matrix remodeling. These findings clearly implicate a role for TNF-α in the pathophysiology of heart failure. Based on this, anticytokine therapies are currently under investigation. Most promising in this regard is the study of the chimeric TNF-α-soluble receptor (etanercept). A phase II study of this drug, given to class III and IV heart failure patients for 3 months, showed improvements in left ventricular ejection fraction, and left ventricular remodeling, with trends toward improvements in functional status.[15] Thus, the long-term effects of etanercept are being tested in a large phase III trial. The results of this trial should further clarify the pathophysiologic role of TNF-α in heart failure and provide insight into the potential for anticytokine therapy in heart failure.

ENDOTHELIN[16]

There are three endothelin peptides, endothelin-1 (ET-1), endothelin-2 (ET-2), and endothelin-3 (ET-3), which bind to two distinct G-protein-coupled receptors, endothelin-A (ET_A) and endothelin B (ET_B). ET-1 is the most potent vasoconstrictor known (5 to 10 times as potent as angiotensin II) and may be involved in heart failure pathophysiology through a number of mechanisms. Its arterial and venous constrictive effects would increase preload and afterload, and its vasoconstriction of both efferent and afferent renal arterioles may decrease renal plasma flow and induce sodium retention. ET-1 has direct cardiotoxic effects, is a potent stimulator of cardiac myocyte hypertrophy, and has arrhythmogenic effects. It is also a positive inotrope and, like the β-agonists, over the long-term may be harmful due to the increased myocardial energy utilization. Finally, ET-1 also appears to modulate production of many other neurohormones involved in heart failure pathophysiology, including angiotensin II, aldosterone, and NE. Like other peptides and hormones described earlier, ET-1 plasma concentrations are elevated in heart failure and have been correlated directly with various findings in heart failure, including risk of death.

Both animal and clinical studies with endothelin-receptor antagonists also suggest that ET-1 may play an important role in the pathophysiology of heart failure. Clinical studies of the acute and short-term (2 weeks) hemodynamic effects of endothelin-receptor blockers have shown favorable effects on most hemodynamic parameters. Long-term endothelin therapy in animal models of heart failure have shown numerous beneficial effects, including beneficial modulation of left ventricular hypertrophy and survival benefits. The data to date seem to provide clear evidence for a role of ET-1 in heart failure pathophysiology. The challenge ahead is to try to translate this into beneficial effects for heart failure patients through endothelin-receptor blockade.

NATRIURETIC PEPTIDES AND NEUTRAL ENDOPEPTIDASE[17,18]

The natriuretic peptide family has three members, atrial natriuretic peptide (ANP), brain natriuretic peptide (BNP), and C-type natriuretic peptide (CNP). ANP is stored mainly in the right atrium, whereas BNP is found mainly in the ventricles. Both are released in response to pressure or volume overload. CNP is found mainly in the brain and has very low plasma concentrations. ANP and BNP are thought to balance the effects of the rennin-angiotensin-aldosterone (RAA) system by causing natriuresis, diuresis, vasodilation, decreased aldosterone release, decreased hypertrophy, decreased production of ET-1, and inhibition of the SNS and RAA system.

Numerous studies have found that plasma levels of ANP and BNP are good diagnostic markers. They are elevated in patients with heart failure in relation to the severity of the disease and can be followed to assess response to therapy. The elevation of ANP or BNP in heart failure appears to have no detrimental effects, but resistance to the natriuretic peptides' actions occurs in heart failure, possibly due to downregulation of the natriuretic peptide receptors, enhanced degradation by neutral endopeptidase (NEP), and the effects of the RAA system and other counter-regulatory systems overwhelming the beneficial effects of the natriuretic peptide family.

Based on the salutory effects of the natriuretic peptides in heart failure, research has focused on harnessing their therapeutic potential. Chronic natriuretic peptide therapy has been limited by the drug-delivery problems associated with peptides. However, the benefits of intravenous recombinant brain natriuretic peptide (nesiritide) for short-term management of acute heart failure has been documented recently.[19] It appears that the chronic benefits of the natriuretic peptides might be realized through inhibition of NEP, the ectoenzyme that catalyzes the breakdown of the natriuretic peptides, along with adrenomedullin and bradykinin. Studies have shown that NEP inhibition alone is largely ineffective because it results in increases in angiotensin II, and thus produces a pressor response. However, compounds that inhibit both ACE and NEP, called *vasopeptidase inhibitors,* show promise for the treatment of hypertension and heart failure.

PRECIPITATING FACTORS IN HEART FAILURE DECOMPENSATION

Patients may have a diagnosis of heart failure, yet appropriate therapy can maintain them in a "compensated" state, indicating that they are relatively symptom-free. However, there are many aggravating or precipitating factors that may cause a previously compensated patient to decompensate. Factors involved in precipitating a decompensation have been evaluated prospectively in patients admitted to the hospital with heart failure in several studies; with similar findings.[20] The results of one of the most recent studies are shown in Table 13–3. Consistently, the studies have shown that noncompliance with drugs or diet is the most common cause of heart failure decompensation. In this study, 43% of patients were assessed as having dietary sodium excess, 34% had excess fluid intake (defined as >2.5 L/day), and about 24% had drug noncompliance that may have contributed to their decompensation (although not necessarily defined as the primary cause of decompensation). Notably, drug noncompliance was fairly strictly defined as patients who had stopped their drugs or took them only intermittently, thus representing fairly extreme cases of noncompliance. The other common causes of decompensation included coronary ischemia, inadequate or inappropriate therapy, uncontrolled hypertension, and arrhythmias. Of note is the fact that inadequate therapy probably contributed to decompensation in far more than the 12% in whom it was assigned as the most important factor. This is so because only 48% of patients were on ACE inhibitors, and those on ACE inhibitors were on doses well below those used in clinical trials (e.g., median doses in this study of 8.8 mg/day for enalapril,

TABLE 13–3. Precipitating Factors in Heart Failure Decompensation

Factor	Patients (%)
Noncompliance with drugs or diet	42
Cardiac ischemia	13
Inadequate therapy at time of admission	12
Cardiac arrhythmias	6
Miscellaneous factors	6
Uncontrolled hypertension	6
No definite precipitant identified	15

Taken from Ref. 20, where prospective analysis was made to determine the single most important factor precipitating hospitalization of heart failure patients at the study hospital.

TABLE 13–4. Drugs That May Precipitate or Exacerbate Congestive Heart Failure

Negative Inotropic Effect
Antiarrhythmics (e.g., disopyramide, flecainide, and others)
β-Blockers (e.g., propranolol, metoprolol, atenolol, and others)
Calcium channel blockers (e.g., verapamil and others)
Itraconazole
Terbinafine
Rosiglitazone
Cardiotoxic
Doxorubicin
Daunomycin
Cyclophosphamide
Sodium and Water Retention
Nonsteroidal anti-inflammatory agents
COX-2 inhibitors
Glucocorticoids
Androgens
Estrogens
Salicylates (high dose)
Sodium-containing drugs (e.g., carbenicillin disodium, ticarcillin disodium)

25.6 mg/day for captopril; see Table 13–7 for recommended doses). Additionally, although inappropriate therapy was not a specific category in this study, calcium channel blockers and antiarrhythmics were used in 34% and 4% of patients, respectively. It is well recognized that many of the drugs in these categories can worsen heart failure through their negative inotropic effects.

What should be evident from careful examination of Table 13–3 is that many of the precipitating factors are preventable, particularly through appropriate pharmacist intervention. Specifically, patient education and counseling by a pharmacist should help to decrease the most common reason for heart failure exacerbation: noncompliance with dietary sodium and water restrictions, drug therapy, or both. Pharmacists also should be able to identify and address inadequate heart failure therapy, poorly controlled hypertension, and administration of drugs that may worsen heart failure due to their negative inotropic, cardiotoxic, or sodium-retaining properties. Specific examples of drugs that can worsen heart failure are given in Table 13–4. It should be noted that while the cyclooxygenase-2 (COX-2) inhibitors differ from the traditional nonsteroidal anti-inflammatory drugs (NSAIDs) in their gastric ulceration effects, their effects on renal function are similar to those of NSAIDs.[21] Thus, both NSAIDs and COX-2 inhibitors should be used judiciously in heart failure patients. It can be argued that heart failure exacerbations due to noncompliance, inadequate/inappropriate therapy, and poorly controlled hypertension are all preventable and amenable to pharmacist intervention. And based on the study highlighted in Table 13–3, this represents about 60% of all heart failure hospitilizations. Thus, the value of the pharmacist's role in careful and repeated education of patients, and monitoring of the drug regimen should not be underestimated.

CLINICAL PRESENTATION[22]

An understanding of the pathophysiologic and compensatory processes in heart failure makes it easy to understand the clinical signs and symptoms. The underlying pathophysiology in heart failure typically causes a reduction in cardiac output. In an attempt to compensate for reduced cardiac output, the SNS activates, as do mechanisms that increase preload. However, an overshoot of preload augmentation and an inability of the heart to efficiently accept or eject the increased

TABLE 13–5. Signs and Symptoms of Congestive Heart Failure

Symptoms	Signs
Right Ventricular Dysfunction	
Abdominal pain	Peripheral edema
Anorexia	Jugular venous distension
Nausea	Hepatojugular reflux
Bloating	Hepatomegaly
Constipation	
Ascites	
Left Ventricular Dysfunction	
Dyspnea on exertion	Bibasilar rales
Paroxysmal nocturnal dyspnea	Pulmonary edema
Orthopnea	S_3 gallop
Tachypnea	Pleural effusion
Cough	Cheyne-Stokes respiration
Hemoptysis	
Nonspecific Findings	
Exercise intolerance	Tachycardia
Fatigue	Pallor
Weakness	Cyanosis of digits
Nocturia	Cardiomegaly
CNS symptoms	

blood volume result in systemic and/or pulmonary congestion, the most common signs and symptoms in heart failure. Peripheral hypoperfusion and increased SNS activity are responsible for most of the remaining clinical findings in heart failure patients. Table 13–5 contains a summary of the signs and symptoms of congestive heart failure.

Congestion develops behind the failing ventricles, with left ventricular failure causing signs and symptoms of pulmonary congestion and right ventricular failure causing signs and symptoms of systemic congestion. Most patients initially have left ventricular failure. However, because the ventricles share a septal wall and left heart failure increases the workload of the right ventricle, both ventricles eventually fail. Many heart failure patients therefore present with symptoms of both right and left ventricular failure.

SIGNS AND SYMPTOMS OF LEFT VENTRICULAR FAILURE

When the left ventricle fails, it is unable to accept and eject the increased blood volume that is delivered to it. Consequently, pulmonary venous and capillary pressures rise, leading to interstitial and bronchial edema, increased airway resistance, and dyspnea. The associated signs and symptoms may include (1) dyspnea on exertion (DOE), (2) orthopnea, (3) paroxysmal nocturnal dyspnea (PND), (4) dyspnea at rest, and (5) pulmonary edema. Exertional dyspnea is a symptom of heart failure when there is a reduction in the level of exertion that causes breathlessness. This is typically described as more breathlessness than was associated previously with a specific activity (vacuuming, stair climbing). As heart failure progresses, many patients eventually have dyspnea at rest.

Orthopnea is dyspnea that occurs with assumption of the supine position. It occurs within minutes of recumbency and is due to reduced pooling of blood in the lower extremities and abdomen. Orthopnea is relieved almost immediately by sitting upright and typically is prevented by elevating the head with pillows. A change in the number of pillows required to prevent orthopnea (e.g., a change from "two-pillow" to "three pillow" orthopnea) suggests worsening heart failure. Pulmonary congestion also may cause a nonproductive cough, either with exertion or at night. Attacks of PND typically occur after 2 to 4 hours of sleep; the patient awakens from sleep with a sense of suffocation. The attacks are due to severe pulmonary and bronchial congestion, leading to shortness of breath and wheezing. Unlike orthopnea, the patient may have to sit upright for 30 minutes or more to obtain relief from an attack of PND. The reasons these attacks occur at night are unclear but may include (1) reduced pooling of blood in the lower extremities and abdomen (as in orthopnea), (2) slow resorption of interstitial fluid from sites of dependent edema, (3) normal reduction in sympathetic activity that occurs with sleep (e.g., less support for the failing ventricle), and (4) normal depression in respiratory drive that occurs with sleep.

Pulmonary edema is the most severe form of pulmonary congestion, and is caused by accumulation of fluid in the interstitial spaces and alveoli. In heart failure patients, it is the result of increased pulmonary venous pressure. The patient experiences extreme breathlessness and anxiety and may cough pink, frothy sputum. Pulmonary edema can be terrifying for the patient, causing a feeling of suffocation or drowning.

Rales (crackling sounds heard on auscultation) are present in the lung bases in patients with left-sided heart failure due to transudation of fluid into alveoli. The rales typically are bibasilar, but if heard unilaterally, they are usually right-sided. A third heart sound, or S_3 gallop, is heard frequently in patients with left ventricular failure and may be due to elevated atrial pressure and altered distensibility of the ventricle. Patients with very severe heart failure may have Cheyne-Stokes respiration, alternating between hyperventilation and apnea.

SIGNS AND SYMPTOMS OF RIGHT VENTRICULAR FAILURE

Signs and symptoms of right ventricular failure are the result of systemic venous congestion. Examination of the right internal jugular vein with the patient at a 45-degree angle is a simple method for assessing jugular venous pressure (JVP). Elevation of JVP more than 4 cm above the sternal angle suggests systemic venous congestion. In patients with mild right-sided heart failure, JVP may be normal at rest, but application of pressure to the abdomen will cause an elevation of JVP (hepatojugular reflux). Abdominal (especially hepatic) congestion and an inability of the right ventricle to accept or eject the increased blood volume cause this finding. Development of ascites and/or hepatomegaly uncommonly occurs in patients with longstanding systemic venous congestion.

Peripheral edema is a cardinal finding in right-sided heart failure. Edema usually occurs in dependent parts of the body, and thus is seen as ankle or pedal edema in ambulatory patients, although it may be manifested as sacral edema in bedridden patients. Adults typically have a 10-lb fluid weight gain before trace peripheral edema is evident; therefore, patients with acute heart failure may have no clinical evidence of systemic congestion except weight gain.

Symptoms associated with right-sided heart failure are less common than those of left-sided heart failure. These symptoms are related to hepatic and intestinal congestion and may include abdominal pain, anorexia, nausea, bloating, and constipation.

NONSPECIFIC FINDINGS IN HEART FAILURE

Physical examination and chest x-ray findings that suggest cardiomegaly are present in most patients with heart failure but are considered nonspecific. There are no specific electrocardiographic (ECG) findings associated with heart failure. Many patients will, however, have left ventricular hypertrophy by ECG. The remaining signs and symptoms of heart failure are primarily a result of reduced cardiac output or elevated SNS activity. Weakness, fatigue, and exercise intolerance are present in most patients with heart failure, related in part to inadequate oxygen delivery to skeletal muscles from reduced cardiac output. It must be kept in mind, however, that these symptoms also may be seen in many noncardiac disorders. Symptoms of central nervous system (CNS) hypoperfusion such as confusion, lethargy, hallucinations, nightmares, insomnia, and headache may occur in patients with severe heart failure, especially if they have underlying cerebral arteriosclerosis.

Increased SNS activity is responsible for the tachycardia often observed in heart failure. As described previously, numerous factors contribute to peripheral vasoconstriction, which manifests as pallor, cool extremities, or cyanosis of the digits. Vasoconstriction also serves to shunt blood away from nonvital organs such as the kidney. Nocturia is frequently noted in heart failure patients because of the reductions in sympathetic activation and cardiac output demands at night. Consequently, renal vasoconstriction diminishes, increasing renal blood flow and urine formation.

CLASSIFICATION OF HEART FAILURE PATIENTS

Systems that classify patients according to their level of disability are useful from several perspectives. They can be used to follow the progress of the patient longitudinally, to assess the impact of therapeutic maneuvers, or to provide a reference point for comparison with other patients. The most widely used classification system is the New York Heart Association (NYHA) Functional Classification System.[22] It divides patients into four categories (Table 13–6). There are obvious limitations to assigning a numerical score to subjective findings, but this system is fairly useful for monitoring patients and is widely used in heart failure studies.

TABLE 13–6. New York Heart Association Functional Classification

Functional Class	Description
I	Patients with cardiac disease but without limitations of physical activity. Ordinary physical activity does not cause undue fatigue, dyspnea, or palpitation.
II	Patients with cardiac disease that results in slight limitations of physical activity. Ordinary physical activity results in fatigue, palpitation, dyspnea, or angina.
III	Patients with cardiac disease that results in marked limitation of physical activity. Although patients are comfortable at rest, less than ordinary activity will lead to symptoms.
IV	Patients with cardiac disease that results in an inability to carry on physical activity without discomfort. Symptoms of congestive heart failure are present even at rest. With any physical activity, increased discomfort is experienced.

▶ TREATMENT: Chronic Heart Failure

DESIRED OUTCOMES

The goals of therapy in management of chronic heart failure are to improve the patient's quality of life, reduce symptoms, reduce hospitalizations, slow progression of the disease process, and prolong survival. A number of drug therapies have been clearly proven to affect one or more of these goals. Drugs that are currently recommended in consensus guidelines as standard therapy for treatment of systolic heart failure are described under the section entitled "Standard First-Line Therapies" and include ACE inhibitors, β-blockers, diuretics, and digoxin. Other drugs that also have certain proven benefits, and that may either be added to the standard therapy regimen or used as alternative therapy to a standard drug in the case of contraindications or poor tolerability are described under "Other Heart Failure Therapies" and include aldosterone antagonists (spironolactone), angiotensin II receptor blockers, and the hydralazine-nitrate combination. Finally, a number of drugs have been studied in heart failure and proven either ineffective or detrimental, and these are described briefly in a section entitled "Other Drugs Studied in Heart Failure."

HEART FAILURE TREATMENT GUIDELINES

In recent years, a number of clinical practice guidelines for the treatment of heart failure have been developed and published.[23–29] The philosophies behind the development of practice guidelines can vary.[30] Frequently, these documents are used to provide standards for the purpose of quality or process control, an application that has been controversial for many health care providers. In contrast, the philosophy of other guidelines is to provide insight into the actual treatment of heart failure patients that clinical trial data do not always provide. For example, when prescribing drug therapy, practitioners must write for a specific drug and dose given at a specific frequency for a designated period of time. They also must consider what impact the new medication will have on other agents (prescription drugs, over-the-counter drugs, herbal products) the patient may be taking. In many instances, clinical trial data do not provide information on these points. Thus, practice guidelines can help fill in these gaps and assist clinicians in actual treatment decisions for heart failure patients. Pharmacists are playing increasing roles in both guideline development[23,28] and management of heart failure patients.[31] The availability of treatment guidelines also provides pharmacists with an important mechanism for supporting their heart failure pharmacotherapy recommendations.

GENERAL APPROACH TO TREATMENT

The first step in management of chronic heart failure is to determine the etiology (see Table 13–1) and/or precipitating factors (see Table 13–3) of the syndrome. Treatment of underlying disorders such as anemia or hyperthyroidism may obviate the need for treatment of heart failure. Patients with valvular diseases may derive significant benefit from valve replacement or repair. Revascularization or anti-ischemic therapy in patients with coronary disease may reduce heart failure symptoms. Drugs that aggravate heart failure (see Table 13–4) should be discontinued if possible.

Restriction of physical activity reduces cardiac workload and is recommended for virtually all patients with acute congestive symptoms. However, once the patient's symptoms have stabilized and excess fluid is removed, restrictions on physical activity are discouraged. In fact, recent data suggest that low-intensity exercise training programs in stable heart failure patients improve exercise tolerance and functional capacity.[32]

Because a major compensatory response in heart failure is sodium and water retention, restriction of fluid intake and dietary sodium is an important nonpharmacologic intervention. Fluid intake typically is limited to a maximum of about 2 L/day from all sources. The typical American diet contains 3 to 6 g of sodium per day, and this should be reduced by about half (1.5 to 2 g of sodium per day). This can be accomplished by not adding salt to prepared foods and eliminating foods high in sodium (e.g., salt-cured meats, salted snack foods, pickles, soups, delicatessen meats, and processed foods). Further reductions in dietary sodium can be achieved by eliminating salt from cooking. However, this is not recommended for most heart failure patients because excessive sodium restriction produces an unpalatable diet, which leads to poor dietary compliance or compromised nutritional status. Additionally, the availability of potent diuretics makes excessive sodium restriction unnecessary in most cases. Although dietary sodium and water restriction should be instituted in all heart failure patients, pharmacologic therapy is required for slowing the disease progression and survival prolongation and is usually necessary for control of symptoms. Thus, all patients with systolic heart failure should be on pharmacologic therapy in addition to the nonpharmacologic therapies discussed earlier.

PHARMACOLOGIC THERAPY

STANDARD FIRST-LINE THERAPIES

A treatment algorithm for management of chronic heart failure is shown in Figure 13–5. It should be noted that most patients with symptomatic systolic heart failure should be on most or all of the drugs described in this section.

ACE Inhibitors

ACE inhibitors are the cornerstone of pharmacotherapy of patients with heart failure. These agents cause arterial and venous dilatation, reducing both preload and afterload. The vasodilation they produce appears to be due to both reduced formation of angiotensin II, a potent vasoconstrictor, and reduced breakdown of bradykinin, a vasodilator (see Figure 13–2). Bradykinin, which is inactivated by ACE (identical to kininase II), also enhances release of vasodilatory prostaglandins and histamine. The contribution of bradykinin effects to the efficacy of ACE inhibitors in heart failure is unknown, but will be clarified to some extent as angiotensin II receptor blockers (which lack bradykinin effects) are compared with ACE inhibitors in treatment of heart failure.

Numerous placebo-controlled trials have documented the favorable effects of ACE inhibitor therapy on hemodynamic variables, clinical status, and symptoms in heart failure.[33] Hemodynamic effects observed with long-term therapy include significant increases in

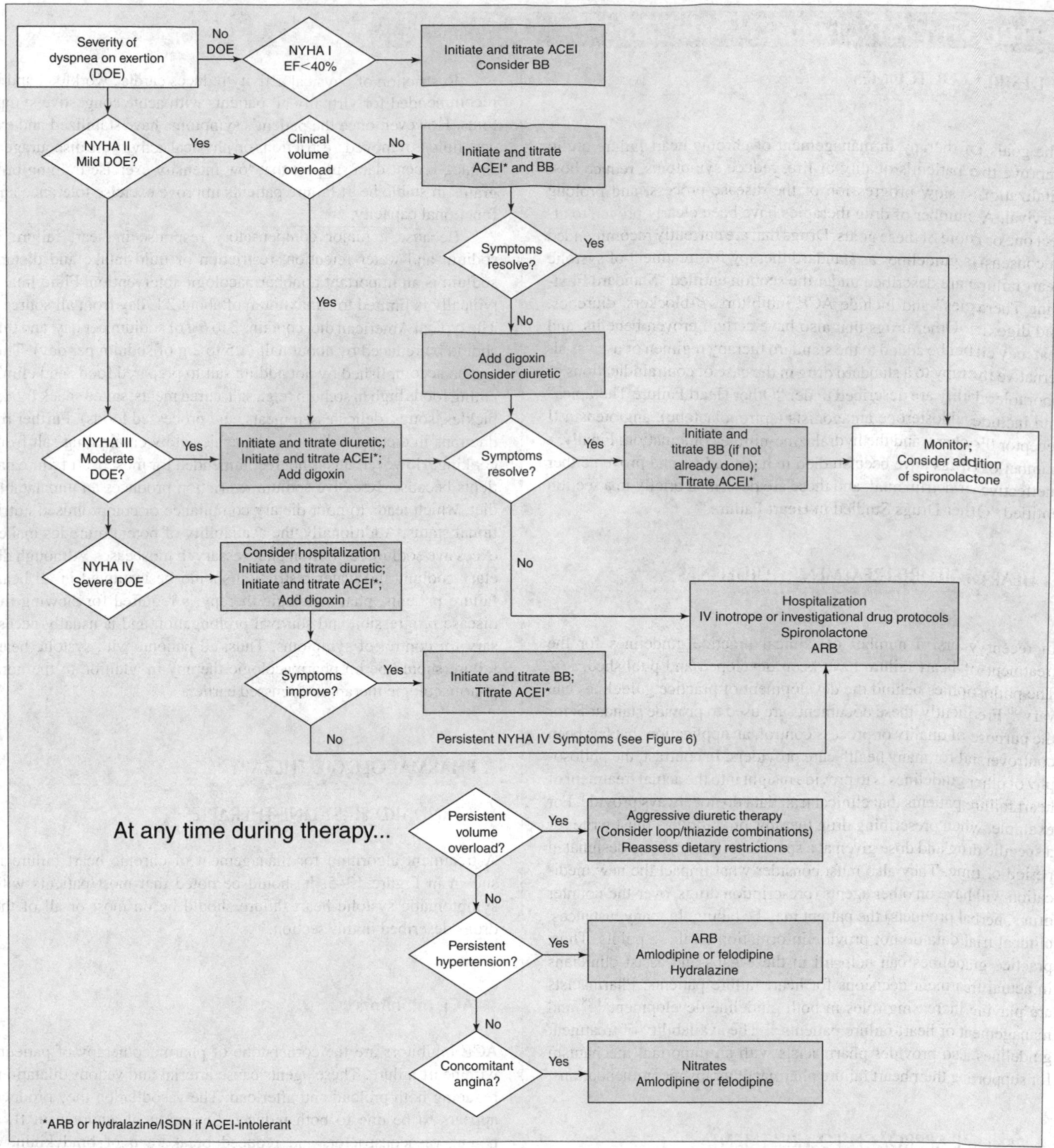

FIGURE 13–5. Treatment algorithm for patients with chronic heart failure. See text for details. Abbreviations: ACE = angiotensin converting enzyme; ACEI = ACE inhibitor; ARB = angiotensin II receptor blocker; BB = β-blocker; DOE = dyspnea on exertion; EF = ejection fraction; HF = heart failure; ISDN = isosorbide dinitrate; LV = left ventricular; NYHA = New York Heart Association. *Adapted from Ref. 23.*

cardiac index, stroke work index, and stroke volume index, as well as significant reductions in left ventricular filling pressure, SVR, mean arterial pressure, and heart rate. Significant improvements in clinical status, functional class, exercise tolerance, and left ventricular size are also well documented. When compared with placebo, patients treated with ACE inhibitors have fewer treatment failures, fewer hospitalizations, and fewer increases in diuretic dosages.[33,34] The acute response to ACE inhibitor therapy is greater in patients with high levels of plasma renin activity. However, long-term hemodynamic and clinical responses to ACE inhibition cannot be predicted from the plasma renin activity or from response to the initial dose of ACE inhibitor.

The beneficial effect of ACE inhibitors on mortality has been documented conclusively.[33,34] Since the publication of the first trial to show an improvement in heart failure survival with an ACE inhibitor (CONSENSUS),[35] numerous trials have documented a 20% to 30% relative reduction in mortality with ACE inhibitor therapy.[33,34] In addition to improving survival, ACE inhibitors also reduce the combined risk of death or hospitalization, slow the progression of heart failure, and reduce the rates of reinfarction.[33,34] The benefits of ACE inhibitor therapy are independent of the etiology of heart failure (ischemic versus non-ischemic) and are observed in patients with mild, moderate, or severe symptoms. ACE inhibitors are clearly superior to the other vasodilator regimen shown to reduce mortality in heart failure, specifically the hydralazine-nitrate combination.[36]

In addition to their benefits in patients with established heart failure, ACE inhibitors also are effective for prevention of heart failure. The SOLVD Prevention Trial showed that enalapril decreased the risk of hospitalization for worsening heart failure and reduced the composite end point of death and heart failure hospitalization in patients with asymptomatic left ventricular dysfunction.[37] The most common cause of heart failure is ischemic heart disease, where AMI results in loss of myocytes, followed by ventricular dilatation and remodeling. Since the SOLVD Prevention Trial, a number of studies therefore focused on the effects of ACE inhibitors in patients suffering an AMI. ACE inhibitors benefit post-MI patients whether they are initiated early (within 36 hours) and continued for 4 to 6 weeks[38] or started later and administered for several years.[34] Collectively, these studies indicate that ACE inhibitors after AMI improve overall survival, decrease development of severe heart failure, and reduce reinfarction and heart failure hospitalization rates. The benefit occurs within the first few days of therapy and persists during long-term treatment. The effects are most pronounced in higher-risk patients, such as those with symptomatic heart failure or reduced ejection fractions, with 20% to 30% reductions in mortality reported in these patients.[34,38] Post-MI patients without heart failure symptoms or decreases in ejection fraction also benefit from ACE inhibitors, but the magnitude of this effect is less pronounced, with all-cause mortality reduced by 7% to 11%.[38]

Despite the overwhelming benefit demonstrated with ACE inhibitors, there is substantial evidence that these agents are underused and underdosed in patients with heart failure.[39–41] These data indicate that significant numbers of heart failure patients do not receive ACE inhibitors and that, of those who are receiving these agents, up to 50% may be taking lower than recommended doses.[39–41] The most common reasons cited for underuse or underdosing are concerns about safety and adverse reactions to ACE inhibitors, especially in patients with underlying renal dysfunction or hypotension. However, recent evidence indicates that ACE inhibitors in post-MI patients with decreased left ventricular function may be more effective in those patients with renal insufficiency.[42] In this retrospective cohort study, nearly 21,000 Medicare patients with confirmed MIs and ejection fractions less than 40% on hospital discharge were studied. In patients receiving an ACE inhibitor at hospital discharge, those with a serum creatinine level greater than 3 mg/dL had a 37% increase in 1-year survival compared with only a 16% increase in patients with a serum creatinine level less than 3 mg/dL. The investigators also reported that aspirin attenuated the benefits of ACE inhibitors only in patients with renal insufficiency. These results suggest that renal dysfunction should not be a contraindication to ACE inhibitor use in patients with left ventricular dysfunction. The effect of using doses of ACE inhibitors that are lower than the target doses of large clinical trials was evaluated in the ATLAS Trial.[43] Over 3000 patients with NYHA class II–IV heart failure and an ejection fraction of 30% or less were randomized to receive either low-dose (2.5 to 5.0 mg/day) or high-dose (32.5 to 35 mg/day) lisinopril for a median of 45 months. Although the 8% relative reduction in mortality with high-dose lisinopril was not significant, the composite end point of death or hospitalization for any cause was significantly reduced by 12%, and heart failure hospitalizations decreased by 24% in the high-dose group. These results emphasize that for patients who can only tolerate low doses of ACE inhibitors, they are still apparently obtaining the benefit, although benefit is likely enhanced with higher doses.

In summary, the evidence that ACE inhibitors improve symptoms, slow disease progression, and decrease mortality in heart failure is unequivocal. As such, all patients with documented left ventricular dysfunction, irrespective of symptomatology, should receive ACE inhibitors, unless there are contraindications or intolerance is present.[25,28]

The mechanisms by which ACE inhibitors slow disease progression and decrease mortality are not entirely clear. Substantial evidence suggests these effects are due in part to inhibition of angiotensin II's growth-promoting effects on cardiac muscle and interstitium. Both clinical and animal studies provide compelling evidence that angiotensin II modulates left ventricular hypertrophy, dilatation, and remodeling.[44–46] Thus ACE inhibitor therapy appears to play an important role in preventing angiotensin II–mediated progressive worsening of myocardial function. Whether the ability of ACE inhibitors to impair breakdown of bradykinin also contributes to their beneficial effect in heart failure is unclear. Similarly, the contribution of the hemodynamic effects of ACE inhibitors to reducing disease progression and mortality is unknown. Hydralazine-nitrates lack the effects of ACE inhibitors on left ventricular hypertrophy yet have been shown to reduce mortality in heart failure. This would suggest that preload and afterload reduction contributes to some degree to the beneficial effects of ACE inhibitors on disease progression and mortality.

While ACE inhibitors improve morbidity and mortality in heart failure, the prognosis of these patients remains poor. Therefore, new therapies are needed to improve their outcome. One such new treatment that shows initial promise is vasopeptidase inhibition. Vasopeptidase inhibitors inhibit both ACE and NEP. Thus, in addition to reducing the vasoconstrictor peptide angiotensin II, inhibition of NEP results in increases in endogenous vasodilators such as natriuretic peptides and bradykinin and may more completely counter the hemodynamic derangements in heart failure. A recent report compared the effects of lisinopril with the vasopeptidase inhibitor omapatrilat in patients with NYHA class II–IV heart failure and an ejection fraction of 40% or less.[47] There was no difference in the primary end point of exercise tolerance between lisinopril and omapatrilat. The combined end point of death, hospital admission for heart failure, or withdrawal of study treatment for worsening heart failure was reduced by 48% by omapatrilat ($P = .035$). Serious adverse events involving the cardiovascular system were less common in patients receiving omapatrilat (7%) compared with lisinopril (12%; $P = .04$), as were increases in serum creatinine (1.8% with omapatrilat versus 6.1% with lisinopril ($P = .009$). However, effects on the gastrointestinal system (diarrhea, nausea/vomiting, and constipation) were more common with omapatrilat. An increased risk of angioedema with omapatrilat as compared with ACE inhibitors also has been raised as a concern.[48] Omapatrilat is currently being compared with ACE inhibitors in heart failure patients in trials sufficiently powered to detect differences in mortality and should provide important data on the efficacy and safety of this new drug class.

β-Blockers

It may seem paradoxical that, within this chapter, β-blockers are listed as drugs that may exacerbate or worsen heart failure (see Table 13–4) and as standard therapy for management of chronic heart failure, but both are true. Administration of normal doses of β-blockers to patients with heart failure has the potential to lead to symptomatic worsening or decompensation, due to their negative inotropic effect. However, there is now clear evidence that if stable patients are initiated on low doses of a β-blocker, with slow upward dose titration over several weeks, they should derive significant benefits. In fact, the Heart Failure Society of America (HFSA) Practice Guidelines recommend that β-blocker therapy should be considered in all clinically stable patients with systolic dysfunction (defined as left ventricular ejection fraction <40%) and mild to moderate symptoms (class II or III heart failure). These guidelines further recommend that β-blockers should be added to standard therapy, which typically includes ACE inhibitors, diuretics, and often, digoxin. The basis for this recommendation is the overwhelming data from clinical trials with carvedilol, metoprolol, and bisoprolol.

Carvedilol was the first β-blocker with data suggesting survival benefits in patients with heart failure. The U.S. Carvedilol Heart Failure Program was comprised of four different studies, none of which had mortality as an end point. However, these studies were stopped prematurely by the Data Safety Monitoring Board due to the significant reductions in mortality in patients treated with carvedilol (versus placebo).[49] Although combined data from these carvedilol studies showed a 65% reduction in mortality, many still questioned the benefits of β-blockers because this was not a prospectively designed mortality trial, and the duration of follow-up was short (about 6 months). However, subsequent, prospectively designed mortality studies with bisoprolol and metoprolol confirmed the benefits of these drugs in the heart failure population. CIBIS-II studied bisoprolol in over 2600 patients with class III or IV heart failure. The study was stopped prematurely (at an average follow-up of 1.3 years) due to the 34% reduction in mortality associated with bisoprolol.[50] Post hoc analyses showed a 44% reduction in sudden death and a 26% reduction in death due to worsening heart failure. The data from the largest β-blocker mortality trial to date, MERIT-HF, had data surprisingly similar to that with bisoprolol. In this study, nearly 4000 patients were randomized to metoprolol controlled-release/extended-release (CR/XL) or placebo.[51] Most of the patients had class II or III heart failure. Again, the study was halted prematurely at a mean follow-up of 1 year due to the impressive mortality reduction with metoprolol CR/XL. Specifically, there was a 34% reduction in total mortality, with a 41% reduction in sudden death and a 49% reduction in death from worsening heart failure. Multiple post hoc subgroup analyses suggested that all the subgroups analyzed benefited from the therapy. The subgroup within heart failure that has been less well studied with β-blockers is those with severe/advanced heart failure (class IIIb and IV), and this lack of data is the reason that the HFSA guidelines do not include class IV patients. However, the COPERNICUS study was designed to test carvedilol in the severe heart failure population and was stopped prematurely due the drug's significant survival benefit.[52] Specifically, carvedilol produced a 35% relative reduction in mortality, and an impressive 7.1% absolute reduction in mortality (from 18.5% to 11.4%). Thus, although not formally recommended in the HFSA guidelines, this more recent study suggests that patients with severe/advanced heart failure also derive significant benefit from β-blocker therapy.

As described in the pathophysiology section of this chapter, the current paradigm for heart failure suggests that compensatory neurohormal activation is responsible for progression of the disease. And the mortality data with β-blockers clearly support this paradi gm, suggesting that this therapy is interrupting the normal progression of the disease. Data on the effects of β-blockers on hospitalization further support the concept that these drugs interupt or slow the normal disease progression. For example, in the MERIT-HF trial, all-cause hospitalization was reduced by 18%, and hospitalizations for worsening heart failure were reduced by 35%. The positive effects of β-blockers on the left ventricle and systolic function also have be very consistent across studies. Following several weeks to months of therapy, β-blockers have been documented consistently to increase ejection fraction (EF) by 5 to 10 units (e.g., from an EF of 20% to 25% or 30%), decrease ventricular mass, improve the sphericity of the ventricle, and reduce systolic and diastolic volumes (left ventricular end-systolic volume and LVEDV).[53,54] These effects have been independent of the drug studied or the underlying cause of heart failure. Importantly, though, these changes, along with decreases in hospitalization and mortality, appear to depend on β-blocker dose, with greater benefit seen at higher doses.[54] Thus it seems important to make every effort to titrate patients to target doses when possible, although there are benefits over placebo of lower doses; thus the inability to titrate to the target dose is not a justification to discontinue therapy.

The positive effects of β-blockers on the left ventricle and disease progression have not always translated into symptomatic improvements. Many, but not all, studies have shown significant improvements in the NYHA functional class, patient symptom scores or quality-of-life assessments (such as the Minnesota Living with Heart Failure Questionnaire), and exercise performance, as assessed by the 6-minute walk test.[54–57] Thus it is important to inform patients that they may or may not notice dramatic symptomatic improvements with β-blocker therapy. However, even in the absence of noticeable symptomatic improvements, positive effects on disease progression and survival are still anticipated.

Since carvedilol, a nonselective β-blocker with α_1-receptor blockade and antioxidant effects, was the first to show clear benefits in heart failure, there has been much debate about whether ancillary properties contribute to the benefits of β-blockers in heart failure. The subsequent results of CIBIS-II and MERIT-HF, studies both conducted with β_1-selective blockers, would certainly suggest that the most important effect for β-blockers in heart failure is β_1-receptor blockade. However, whether carvedilol is superior to metoprolol and bisoprolol remains a subject of debate, and recent studies on this subject provide little additional insight.[57,58] In general, the data suggest that carvedilol may be superior in its effects on certain parameters, such as change in ejection fraction, and certain hemodynamic responses at peak exercise. However, it is not clear if these hemodynamic differences are significant clinically, and they did not translate into differences in symptom scores or exercise tolerance.[57,58] The ongoing COMET study is a mortality study directly comparing carvedilol and immediate-release metoprolol and should provide some insight into the question of superiority of certain β-blockers. Finally, a recent study of bucindolol in heart failure was stopped prematurely because of the low probability of showing any significant benefit over placebo.[58a] It appears that the lack of benefit with bucindolol is not attributable to the patient population studied but probably is related to the drug itself, most likely its instinsic sympathomimetic activity.[59] Thus it is not appropriate to assume that all β-blockers have the benefits in heart failure that have been documented with metoprolol, bisoprolol, and carvedilol. However, there are currently no data suggesting that one of these three is superior. Thus, selection of a drug from among these three is likely based on other factors, such as availability in starting doses, expected side effects/other effects, cost, and/or patient-compliance issues. These issues will be discussed in further detail in the section "Drug Class Information."

A number of potential mechanisms have been suggested to explain the beneficial effects of β-blockers in heart failure patients. Although not clearly elucidated, it seems likely that the mechanisms of benefit include antiarrhythmic effects, slowing or reversing the detrimental ventricular remodeling caused by sympathetic stimulation, decreased myocyte death from catecholamine-induced necrosis or apoptosis, prevention of fetal gene expression, and prevention of other detrimental effects of SNS activation described earlier.[52,53]

In summary, the data provide clear evidence that β-blockers slow the progression of heart failure, evidenced by reductions in mortality and hospitalizations. Many patients also will have improvements in quality of life associated with β-blocker therapy, although this is not a universal finding. Based on these data, β-blockers are recommended as standard therapy for all patients with systolic dysfunction and mild to moderate heart failure symptoms. More recent data suggest that they also should be considered in patients with severe heart failure symptoms (class IIIb and IV).

Diuretics[60–62]

The compensatory mechanisms in heart failure stimulate excessive sodium and water retention, often leading to signs and symptoms of systemic and pulmonary congestion. Consequently, diuretic therapy is recommended for all patients with clinical evidence of fluid retention. Although a majority of heart failure patients require chronic diuretic therapy, some may be well controlled without it. Therefore, diuretic therapy is a common component of a heart failure pharmacologic regimen, but should not be viewed as mandatory. The primary goal of diuretic therapy is to decrease edema and pulmonary congestion by reduction of preload. Although preload is a determinant of cardiac output, the Frank-Starling curve (see Figure 13–3) shows that patients with congestive symptoms have reached the flat portion of the curve. A reduction in filling pressure improves symptoms but has little effect on the patient's stroke volume or cardiac output until the steep portion of the curve is reached. Once diuretic therapy is initiated, dosage adjustments are based on symptomatic improvement and daily body weight. Change in body weight is a sensitive marker of fluid retention or loss, and it is recommended that patients monitor their status by taking daily, morning body weights. Patients who gain 1 lb/day for several consecutive days or 3 to 5 lb in a week should contact their health care provider for instructions (which often will be to temporarily increase the diuretic dose). Such action often will allow patients to prevent a full-blown decompensation.

Thiazide Diuretics. Thiazide diuretics such as hydrochlorothiazide block sodium and chloride reabsorption in the distal convoluted tubule (approximately 5% to 8% of filtered sodium). The thiazides therefore are relatively weak diuretics and are used alone infrequently in heart failure. However, as is reviewed in detail in the advanced/decompensated heart failure section under "Diuretic Resistance," thiazides or the thiazide-like diuretic metolazone can be used in combination with loop diuretics to promote a very effective diuresis.

Loop Diuretics. Loop diuretics are the most widely used diuretics in heart failure. They act in the thick ascending limb of the loop of Henle, where 20% to 25% of filtered sodium normally is reabsorbed. Because loop diuretics are highly bound to plasma proteins, they are not highly filtered at the glomerulus. They reach the tubular lumen by active transport via the organic acid transport pathway. Competitors for this pathway (probenecid or organic by-products of uremia) can inhibit delivery of loop diuretics to their site of action and decrease effectiveness. Loop diuretics also induce a prostaglandin-mediated increase in renal blood flow, which contributes to their natriuretic effect. Coadministration of NSAIDs blocks this prostaglandin-mediated effect and can diminish diuretic efficacy. Unlike thiazides, loop diuretics maintain their effectiveness in the presence of impaired renal function, although higher doses are necessary to obtain adequate delivery of the drug to the site of action.

Heart failure is one of the disease states in which the maximal response to loop diuretics is reduced, possibly due to increased proximal or distal tubule reabsorption of sodium. As a consequence, doses above the recommended "ceiling doses" do not produce additional effect. Thus, once these doses are reached, it is recommended to use more frequent dosing for additional effect, rather than give progressively higher doses. The appropriate chronic dose is that which maintains the patient at a stable weight without symptoms of dyspnea. (Ranges of doses of loop diuretics, and recommended ceiling doses are shown in Table 13–9.)

Digoxin

In 1785, William Withering was the first to report extensively on the use of foxglove, or *Digitalis purpurea,* for the treatment of dropsy (i.e., edema). Although digitalis glycosides have been in clinical use for more than 200 years, not until the 1920s were they clearly demonstrated to have a positive inotropic effect on the heart. Furthermore, it was not until the late 1980s that clinical trials were conducted to critically evaluate the role of digoxin in the therapy of chronic heart failure. The results of the Digitalis Investigation Group (DIG) trial helped clarify the role of digoxin in this setting.[63] This discussion focuses on digoxin because it is by far the most widely studied and frequently prescribed digitalis glycoside in the United States. The view of digoxin also has shifted over the past decade. While historically it was considered useful in heart failure because of its positive inotropic effects, it now seems clear that its real benefits in heart failure are related to its neurohormonal modulating effects.

Clinical Efficacy and Role in Therapy. The efficacy of digoxin in patients with heart failure and supraventricular tachyarrhythmias such as atrial fibrillation is well established and widely accepted.[64,65] Its role in heart failure patients with normal sinus rhythm has been considerably more controversial. Until the 1980s, most data supporting efficacy of digoxin in these patients came from anecdotal evidence and seriously flawed or uncontrolled studies. Since then, a number of clinical trials have shown that digoxin improves left ventricular ejection fraction, quality of life, exercise tolerance, and heart failure symptoms.[66–68] However, these studies involved small numbers of patients followed for short time periods, with many of the patients being withdrawn from preexisting digoxin treatment on entering the trial.[66,68] Although these trials demonstrated hemodynamic and symptomatic improvement in heart failure patients receiving digoxin, a more important question was the unknown effect of digoxin on mortality. This was of particular concern given the increased mortality seen with other positive inotropic drugs, and finally led to organization and performance of the DIG trial to determine the effects of digoxin on survival in patients with heart failure in sinus rhythm.[63]

The DIG trial was a double-blind, randomized, placebo-controlled trial with the primary end point of all-cause mortality. Patients ($n = 6800$) with heart failure symptoms and a left ventricular ejection fraction of 45% or less were eligible and were followed for a mean of 37 months.[63] Approximately 85% of patients were in NYHA functional class II or III, and ischemic cardiomyopathy was the primary cause of heart failure in 70% of patients. Most patients received background therapy with diuretics and ACE inhibitors. The mean serum digoxin concentration achieved was 0.80 ng/mL after 12 months of therapy. No significant difference in all-cause mortality was found between patients receiving digoxin and placebo (34.8% and 35.1%, respectively). A trend toward lower mortality due to worsening heart failure was observed in the digoxin group, although this was offset by a trend toward an increased mortality from other cardiovascular causes (presumably arrhythmias) in patients receiving digoxin. Hospitalizations for worsening heart failure were reduced 28% by digoxin compared with placebo ($P < .001$), whereas hospitalizations for other cardiovascular causes were increased in the digoxin group. In all, 64.3% of digoxin-treated patients were hospitalized compared with 67.1% of patients receiving placebo ($P = .006$). Therefore, DIG is the first trial to show that a positive inotropic agent does not increase mortality in patients with heart failure.

Although digoxin does not improve survival in heart failure patients, several recent analyses of data from the digoxin withdrawal studies, PROVED[68] and RADIANCE,[66] have helped clarify the role of digoxin use for patients in sinus rhythm and suggest that the drug produces important symptomatic benefits. In one study, worsening heart failure was less likely in patients receiving combined treatment with digoxin, diuretics, and ACE inhibitors (4.7%) than in patients treated with digoxin plus diuretics (19%), ACE inhibitor plus diuretics (25%), or diuretics alone (39%).[69] In another analysis, the effect of digoxin withdrawal in patients with mild to moderate heart failure (determined by heart failure score incorporating clinical signs and symptoms) was evaluated.[70] In patients with mild heart failure, digoxin withdrawal increased the risk of treatment failure and deterioration of exercise capacity and ejection fraction compared with patients continuing treatment with digoxin (23% versus 9%, respectively; $P < .01$). The effects were even more pronounced in patients with moderate symptoms, where 8.5% of patients continuing digoxin had treatment failures compared with 39% of patients randomized to digoxin withdrawal ($P = .011$). Finally, another retrospective evaluation of the PROVED and RADIANCE data indicated that the risk of symptomatic exacerbation of heart failure after digoxin discontinuation was highest in patients with the most severe symptoms.[71] Based on this evidence, digoxin is now recommended by current guidelines for use in patients with symptomatic heart failure (NYHA class II–IV).[28]

Digoxin's place in the pharmacotherapy of chronic heart failure therefore can be summarized for two patient groups. In patients with left ventricular systolic dysfunction and supraventricular tachyarrhythmias such as atrial fibrillation, it should be considered early in therapy to help control ventricular response rate. For patients in normal sinus rhythm, although digoxin does not improve survival, its positive inotropic effects, symptom reduction, and quality-of-life improvement are evident in patients with mild to severe heart failure. Therefore, it should be used together with other standard heart failure therapies, including diuretics, ACE inhibitors, and β-blockers, in patients with symptomatic heart failure. Clinicians may want to consider adding digoxin after instituting β-blocker therapy so that the potential bradycardic effect of digoxin does not preclude use of a β-blocker.

The appropriate dose or target plasma concentration for digoxin also has been clarified by recent trials. Two recent studies evaluated the dose-response to digoxin in heart failure patients receiving ACE inhibitors and diuretics.[72,73] One reported that an increase in the digoxin plasma concentration from a mean of 0.67 to 1.22 ng/mL resulted in a minor increase in left ventricular ejection fraction (23.7% to 27.1%), but no improvement in symptoms, exercise tolerance, or neurohormone levels.[72] The other study found that an increase in digoxin plasma concentration from 0.8 to 1.5 ng/mL produced no additional effect on ejection fraction and likewise did not improve other hemodynamic variables or indices of neurohormonal function.[73]

These results suggest that most of the benefit from digoxin is achieved at low plasma concentrations and that little additional effect is achieved with higher doses. Thus, for most patients, the target digoxin plasma concentration should be 0.5 to 1.0 ng/mL. This more conservative target also would be expected to decrease the risk of adverse effects from digoxin toxicity. In most patients with normal renal function, this plasma concentration can be achieved with a dose of 0.25 mg/day. Patients with decreased renal function, the elderly, or those receiving interacting drugs (e.g., amiodarone) should receive 0.125 mg or less daily. In patients with atrial fibrillation and a rapid ventricular response, the historic practice of increasing digoxin doses (and plasma concentrations) until rate control is achieved is no longer recommended.[28] Digoxin alone is often ineffective to control ventricular response in patients with atrial fibrillation, and increasing the dose only increases the risk of toxicity. Therefore, it should be dosed similarly irrespective of whether the patient is in sinus rhythm or atrial fibrillation. Adequate rate control can be achieved by adding a β-blocker or amiodarone. Several equations and nomograms have been proposed to estimate digoxin maintenance doses based on estimated renal function for a particular patient and population pharmacokinetic parameters. These methods are reviewed extensively elsewhere.[74] In the absence of tachyarrhythmias, a loading dose is not indicated because digoxin is a mild inotropic agent that will produce gradual effects over several hours, even after loading.

OTHER HEART FAILURE THERAPIES

Aldosterone Antagonists

Spironolactone has long been recognized as an inhibitor of aldosterone that produces a weak, potassium-sparing diuretic effect. However, only recently have the cardiovascular effects of aldosterone been described. As discussed in detail in the pathophysiology section of this chapter, aldosterone is now recognized as a neurohormone that plays an important role in ventricular remodeling, particularly by causing increased collagen deposition in the extracellular matrix and thus causing cardiac fibrosis. Based on these findings, a study was undertaken to determine the effects of aldosterone antagonism by spironolactone in patients with heart failure. The RALES study randomized over 1600 patients with class III and IV heart failure to 25 mg/day spironolactone or placebo, in addition to their standard heart failure regimen (however, only approximately 10% of patients were on a β-blocker).[13] Patients with a serum creatinine level above 2.5 mg/dL or a serum potassium level above 5.0 meq/L were excluded. The study was stopped prematurely after an average 24 months of follow-up due to the significant reduction in mortality associated with spironolactone. Specifically, spironolactone was associated with a 30% reduction in total mortality, a 36% reduction in death due to progressive heart failure, and a 29% reduction in sudden deaths. Spironolactone produced a significant 30% reduction in hospitalization for cardiac causes and a 35% reduction in hospitalization for heart failure. Spironolactone also was associated with significant improvements in symptoms, as assessed by changes in the patient's NYHA functional class.

The effects of spironolactone observed in this study are not likely related to any diuretic effect, since the dose-finding study for the RALES study found that 25 mg/day spironolactone produced no change in body weight, sodium-retention score, or urinary sodium excretion. This may not be surprising, given that the usual antihypertensive/diuretic dose ranges from 50 to 200 mg/day. The low dose of spironolactone in the RALES study also was extremely well tolerated. It produced statistically significant, although probably clinically unimportant, increases in serum creatinine and serum potassium of 0.05 to 0.10 mg/dL and 0.30 meq/L, respectively. Serious hyperkalemia was not different between groups, occurring in 1% on placebo and 2% on spironolactone. However, this was a highly selected patient population that was at low risk for developing hyperkalemia. The most common adverse effect associated with spironolactone was gynecomastia or breast pain, which occurred in 10% of men on spironolactone and 1% of men on placebo, although only 10 patients (1.7% of men) in the spironolactone group discontinued therapy due to the gynecomastia. Currently, a selective aldosterone antagonist that minimizes the occurrence of gynecomastia is under investigation.

In summary, spironolactone was associated with substantial benefits in patients with moderate to severe heart failure. At the doses used, it exhibited a very good safety profile. Given the potential benefits, the low risk, and the extremely low cost of spironolactone therapy, it seems reasonable to consider its use in all patients with symptomatic heart failure, even though it has not been studied in class II patients. Moreover, given the data from the RALES study, its use would be strongly recommended in all patients with class III and IV heart failure. However, the potential risk of hyperkalemia must be appreciated and serum potassium monitored routinely.

Angiotensin II Receptor Blockers

Although the beneficial effects of ACE inhibitors in heart failure are well established, chronic administration of ACE inhibitors can result in "ACE escape," with increased circulating angiotensin II, NE, and aldosterone.[75] In addition, angiotensin II can be formed in a number of tissues, including the heart, through non-ACE-dependent pathways.[76,77] Therefore, blockade of the detrimental effects of angiotensin II by ACE inhibition is incomplete. In addition, troublesome adverse effects of ACE inhibitors such as cough are linked to accumulation of bradykinin associated with these agents.[44] The angiotensin II receptor blockers (ARBs) block the angiotensin II receptor subtype, AT_1, preventing the deleterious effects of angiotensin II, regardless of its origin. They do not appear to affect bradykinin.[77] Thus these agents offer a theoretical advantage for the treatment of heart failure over ACE inhibitors by more complete blockade of the effects of angiotensin II without the ACE-associated effects on bradykinin. Also, by directly blocking AT_1 receptors, ARBs would allow unopposed stimulation of AT_2 receptors, causing vasodilation and inhibition of ventricular remodeling.[76,77] Whether ARBs are superior (or equivalent) to ACE inhibitors or more complete blockade of angiotensin II actions occurs with combination therapy is the subject of several ongoing studies.

Although ARBs are only approved for the treatment of hypertension, there is much interest in their use in heart failure. In patients with heart failure, ARBs and ACE inhibitors produce similar hemodynamic effects.[79] Losartan improves exercise capacity and NYHA functional class when added to maximally recommended or tolerated doses of ACE inhibitors in patients with class III-IV heart failure.[80] The RESOLVD study compared the effects of candesartan and enalapril alone and in combination on exercise capacity, ventricular function, quality of life, neurohormones, and tolerability in 768 patients with class II-IV heart failure. No important differences were found between treatments in most of the end points. Combination therapy was better at preventing increases in ventricular volumes than either drug given alone and also appeared to have favorable effects on neurohormones, with the greatest effect on angiotensin II and BNP levels. Combined candesartan and enalapril therapy also was well tolerated. Val-HEFT studied the addition of valsartan versus placebo to background heart failure therapy (which included an ACE inhibitor in 93% and a β-blocker in 35% of patients).[78] Valsartan had no effect on all-cause mortality but produced a 13% reduction in all-cause morbidity and mortality (principally due to reductions in heart failure hospitalizations). The benefits were greatest in those patients not receiving background ACE inhibitor therapy, and there appeared to be trends toward detrimental effects in those who had valsartan added to ACE inhibitor and β-blocker. Thus this study provides some insight into the benefits of combined ARB-ACE inhibitor therapy but does not provide clear support for use of the combination. Other ongoing trials, such as CHARM, and VALIANT, should help further clarify the role of combination ARB and ACE inhibitor therapy.

Two large trials have been performed to compare the effects of ARBs and ACE inhibitors in heart failure. In the ELITE study, losartan and captopril were compared in 722 patients with NYHA class II IV heart failure.[81] The primary end point of this trial, frequency of elevations in serum creatinine, was not different between the two groups. The secondary end point, all-cause mortality, was significantly reduced ($P = .035$) in patients receiving losartan compared with captopril (8.7% versus 4.8%, respectively; risk reduction 46%). However, this apparent mortality benefit was based on a small number of events. Therefore, these results served as the basis for a larger trial, ELITE II, to further compare the effects of these agents.

In ELITE II, over 3000 patients with NYHA class II–IV heart failure and an ejection fraction of less than 40% were randomly assigned to losartan titrated to a target dose of 50 mg once daily or captopril with a target dose of 50 mg three times daily.[82] The primary end point was all-cause mortality, and median follow-up was 555 days. In contrast to ELITE, there were no significant differences in mortality between the groups treated with losartan (17.7%) and captopril (15.9%). Thus the differences observed in ELITE are most likely due to chance. Significantly fewer patients taking losartan experienced drug-related adverse effects, including cough, than with captopril. Although losartan was better tolerated than captopril with equivalent mortality, these results should not be interpreted to mean ARBs and ACE inhibitors can be used interchangeably in heart failure. The overwhelming evidence favoring ACE inhibitors in heart failure, along with their documented efficacy after MI and in diabetes, indicates that they remain drugs of choice in heart failure.

At present, the role of ARBs in heart failure should be limited to those patients who are truly intolerant of ACE inhibitors, usually due to intractable cough or angioedema from an ACE inhibitor. However, patients experiencing cough with ACE inhibitors should be evaluated carefully before discontinuing treatment because in some cases cough is due to pulmonary congestion, rather than the drug. If congestion is present, the cough should improve with adjustment of diuretic therapy. Although initially believed to be safe in patients who have experienced angioedema from ACE inhibitors, this complication has been reported with ARB use, including reoccurrence of angioedema due to losartan after an earlier episode with an ACE inhibitor.[83] Therefore, ARBs should be used with caution in patients having angioedema from ACE inhibitors. In addition, ARBs are not a reasonable alternative in patients with hypotension, hyperkalemia, or renal insufficiency secondary to ACE inhibitors because they are as likely to cause these adverse effects.

Nitrates and Hydralazine

Nitrates and hydralazine were combined originally in the treatment of heart failure because of their complementary hemodynamic actions. Nitrates, by activating guanylate cyclase to increase cyclic guanosine monophosphate (cGMP) in vascular smooth muscle, are primarily venodilators, thus producing reductions in preload.[84] Hydralazine is a direct-acting vasodilator that acts predominantly on arterial smooth muscle to reduce SVR and increase stroke volume and cardiac output (see Figure 13–4); its effects on preload are minimal.[84] Recent evidence suggests these agents also may have beneficial effects in heart failure beyond their hemodynamic actions. Nitrates may inhibit the ventricular remodeling process,[85] whereas hydralazine prevents nitrate tolerance and may interfere with heart failure progression via an antioxidant effect.[86]

The combination of hydralazine and isosorbide dinitrate (ISDN) has been studied in two Veterans Affairs Cooperative studies (Vasodilators in Heart Failure Trial, V-HeFT-I and V-HeFT-II).[36,87] V-HeFT-I compared the effects of 75 mg hydralazine four times daily plus 40 mg ISDN four times daily, 5 mg prazosin four times daily, and placebo on mortality in patients already receiving standard heart failure therapy (diuretics and digoxin in most patients). Compared with placebo, mortality in the hydralazine-nitrate-treated patients was reduced by 38% after 1 year, 25% at 2 years, and 23% at 3 years.[87] V-HeFT-II compared the same hydralazine-nitrate regimen with enalapril, with enalapril producing superior mortality reduction (28% relative decrease in mortality).[36]

Adverse effects with both nitrates and hydralazine are common, limiting their use in many patients. In V-HeFT-I, one or both drugs were discontinued in 19% of patients due to side effects, and only 55% of patients could tolerate full doses of both drugs.[87] The ISDN-hydralazine combination was given four times daily in the V-HeFT studies, making patient compliance an important issue. Whether less frequent administration provides equivalent benefit is unknown.

Based on VHeFT-II data, the hydralazine-nitrate combination should not be used instead of ACE inhibitors as standard therapy in heart failure. Nevertheless, hydralazine and nitrates should be considered the most appropriate therapeutic option in patients who are unable to take ACE inhibitors because of renal insufficiency or possibly hypotension. For other patients with ACE intolerance, the hydralazine-nitrate combination or ARBs are considered appropriate alternatives. Although there are no controlled trials supporting this approach, some clinicians will add hydralazine and nitrates therapy to patients who remain symptomatic despite ACE inhibitor and/or β-blocker treatment.

OTHER DRUGS STUDIED IN HEART FAILURE

In addition to the drugs just described, which have been well documented to be appropriate therapy for management of patients with heart failure, there are a number of other drugs that have been studied, sometimes with negative results. They are described here briefly.

Given that up to 50% of heart failure deaths are sudden (and presumed arrhythmic), some investigations have focused on antiarrhythmics in heart failure. Based on data from the Cardiac Arrhythmia Suppression Trials, class I antiarrhythmics should be avoided in all patients with coronary disease and/or left ventricular dysfunction. More recent attention therefore has focused on alternative therapies, namely, class III antiarrhythmic drugs and implantable cardioverter defibrillators (ICDs). D-Sotalol was studied in heart failure, with a resulting increase in mortality in the D-sotalol arm. Clearly, the most favorable data for an antiarrhythmic in heart failure is with amiodarone, although some studies suggest that ICDs are superior to antiarrhythmic drugs.[88] Thus, in heart failure patients with ventricular arrhythmias, an ICD would be recommended, with amiodarone considered an appropriate alternative therapy. Many patients with ICDs implanted are also taking amiodarone to reduce the number of ICD firings. Antiarrhythmic strategies (either ICD or amiodarone) are currently not recommended for primary prevention of ventricular arrhythmias and death in patients with heart failure.

A number of previous studies demonstrate that calcium channel blockers worsen heart failure and may increase mortality, most likely due to their negative inotropic effects and SNS activation. However, the second-generation dihydropyridine agents amlodipine and felodipine were thought to offer theoretical advantages over other calcium antagonists for the treatment of heart failure. Studies undertaken to test the effect of these drugs in heart failure found no evidence of favorable clinical effects or mortality reduction.[89] However, the data from these studies do provide evidence that amlodipine and felodipine (particularly amlodipine) are safe in this setting and would be the calcium channel blockers of choice in patients with heart failure who need additional antianginal or antihypertensive therapy.

A number of other drugs have been studied in the treatment of chronic heart failure with unfavorable results, specifically increased mortality. These include amrinone, milrinone, enoximone, vesnarinone, xamoterol, dobutamine, ibopamine, flosequinan, and prostacyclin.[90] These drugs all share the common feature that they increase intracellular cyclic AMP, either directly through their pharmacologic actions or indirectly through reflex effects that activate the SNS. Given that β-blockers have now been well documented to have a positive impact on disease progression and survival in heart failure, it seems logical that drugs that have the opposite effect (i.e., increase intracellular cyclic AMP) would produce detrimental outcomes. Heart rate is a rather simple marker to detect a drug that might have negative outcomes in heart failure because drugs that have been shown to increase heart rate (even if only slightly) have been shown universally to increase mortality when used in the treatment of chronic heart failure. Thus the data from these trials provide further support for the neurohormonal paradigm of heart failure and for the concept that our goal is to block, not activate neurohormonal systems.

DRUG CLASS INFORMATION

ACE Inhibitors

A number of ACE inhibitors are available currently in the United States; those approved for use in heart failure are summarized in Table 13–7. The major differences in the ACE inhibitors are not in their pharmacologic properties but in their pharmacokinetic properties. Although it appears that mortality reduction with ACE inhibitors is probably a drug class effect, not all ACE inhibitors approved by the Food and Drug Administration (FDA) for treatment of heart failure have been tested for their effects on mortality in heart failure. Thus it seems most prudent to use those agents which have been documented to prolong survival because the dose required for this effect has been documented. Table 13–7 also contains a summary of the target doses for survival benefit.

Because of the high prevalence of coronary artery disease in patients with heart failure, aspirin is frequently coadministered with ACE inhibitors. Several retrospective cohort analyses suggest that aspirin may attenuate the hemodynamic and mortality benefits of ACE inhibitors.[91,92] The postulated mechanism of this

TABLE 13–7. ACE Inhibitors Approved for Use in Heart Failure

Generic Name	Brand Name	Usual Daily Dose (mg)	Dosing Frequency	Target Dosing Survival Benefit[a]	Prodrug	Elimination[b]	$t_{1/2}$ (h)
Captopril	Capoten	18.75–150	tid	50 mg tid	No	Renal	2
Enalapril	Vasotec	2.5–40	bid	10 mg bid	Yes	Renal	10[c]
Lisinopril	Zestril, Prinivil	5–40	qd	10 mg qd[d]	No	Renal	12[c]
Quinapril	Accupril	5–80	bid	No data	Yes	Renal	25[c]
Ramipril	Altace	1.25–20	qd or bid	5 mg bid	Yes	Renal	9–18[c]

Abbreviations: tid = three times daily; bid = twice daily; qd = once daily.
[a]Target doses associated with survival benefits in clinical trials.
[b]Primary route of elimination.
[c]Half-life of active metabolite.
[d]Note that in the ATLAS trial[43] no significant difference in mortality was found between low-dose (~5 mg/day) and high-dose (~35 mg/day) lisinopril therapy, although morbidity end points were significantly less frequent with the higher dose.

interaction involves opposing effects on synthesis of vasodilatory prostaglandins. The ACE inhibitor–mediated increase in bradykinin increases the synthesis of vasodilatory prostaglandins that have favorable hemodynamic benefits in heart failure. Because of aspirin's effect on prostaglandin synthesis, this potentially beneficial action of ACE inhibitors may be negated. However, in contrast with studies that showed an ACE inhibitor-aspirin interaction, other investigators have found no interaction[93,94] or that the effect of aspirin is dose-related.[95] Since there is no prospective evidence confirming an interaction between these agents, it is currently recommended that the decision to use each of these medications be made based on whether an individual patient has indications for each drug.

Adverse Effects of ACE Inhibitors. The primary adverse effects of ACE inhibitor therapy in heart failure are hypotension and functional renal insufficiency. Hypotension may be manifested as dizziness, lightheadedness, presyncope, or syncope. It occurs most commonly early in therapy or after an increase in dose, although it may occur at any time during treatment. Patients at increased risk of developing hypotension are those with hyponatremia (serum sodium < 130 meq/L) and recent increases in diuretic dose. The occurrence of hypotension may be minimized by initiating therapy with lower ACE inhibitor doses and/or temporarily withholding or reducing the dose of diuretic. Many patients who experience symptomatic hypotension early in therapy are still good candidates for long-term treatment if risk factors for low blood pressure are addressed.

Functional renal insufficiency is manifested as increases in serum creatinine and blood urea nitrogen. As cardiac output and renal blood flow decline, renal perfusion is maintained by the vasoconstrictor effect of angiotensin II on the efferent arteriole. Patients most dependent on this system for maintenance of renal perfusion (and therefore most likely to develop functional renal insufficiency with ACE inhibitors) are those with severe heart failure, hyponatremia, and dehydration.[96] Sodium depletion (usually secondary to diuretic therapy) is the most important factor in the development of functional renal insufficiency with ACE inhibitor therapy. Renal insufficiency therefore can be minimized in many cases by reduction in diuretic dosage or liberalization of sodium intake.

Careful dose titration can minimize the risks of hypotension and transient worsening of renal function. Thus usual initial doses should be about one-fourth the final target dose with slow upward dose titration over several days based on blood pressure and serum creatinine. In certain patients, especially those hospitalized patients who seem at high risk for hypotension or worsening of renal function, it also may be advisable to initiate therapy with a short-acting agent such as captopril. This will help minimize the duration of adverse effects should they occur. Once the patient is stabilized on ACE inhibitor therapy with captopril, he or she can then be switched to a longer-half-life drug.

Retention of potassium with ACE inhibitor therapy can occur and is due to the reduced feedback of angiotensin II to stimulate aldosterone release. Hyperkalemia rarely develops, although caution is necessary in patients with renal insufficiency and in patients taking concomitant potassium supplementation, potassium-containing salt substitutes, or potassium-sparing diuretic therapy.[44,96]

Rash and dysgeusia are troublesome side effects of ACE inhibitor therapy that appear to be more common with high doses; the rash may resolve with continued therapy. A dry, hacking cough occurs with a similar frequency (5% to 15% of patients) with all the agents and may be related to accumulation of tissue bradykinins. Cough occurs in up to 40% of patients with heart failure, independent of ACE inhibitor use, although ACE inhibitors significantly increase its incidence. However, in large clinical trials, only about 1% of participants discontinued ACE inhibitor therapy because of cough. Because cough is a bradykinin-mediated effect, replacement of ACE inhibitor therapy with an AT_1-receptor blocker or hydralazine-nitrates would be reasonable in those patients who discontinue ACE inhibitor therapy due to cough.

β-Blockers

Metoprolol, carvedilol, and bisoprolol have all been shown to reduce mortality in heart failure and are the β-blockers discussed here. Metoprolol is a lipophilic β_1-selective blocker, bisoprolol is a hydrophilic β_1-selective blocker, and carvedilol is a nonselective β-blocker with α_1-blocker and antioxidant effects. As was described earlier, there is currently no strong evidence that these pharmacologic differences have any important effects on the outcomes associated with β-blockers in heart failure. However, their pharmacologic differences may aid in selection of a specific agent. For example, the α_1 blockade of carvedilol causes more hypotension and dizziness than metoprolol or bisoprolol.[58] Thus metoprolol or bisoprolol may be preferred in patients with low blood pressure or in whom dizziness would be especially problematic. Conversely, carvedilol may be preferred in patients whose blood pressure is poorly controlled because it would be expected to have a greater antihypertensive effect than the others.

Bisoprolol is eliminated about 50% by the kidneys whereas metoprolol and carvedilol are essentially completely metabolized and undergo extensive hepatic first-pass metabolism. Both metoprolol and carvedilol are also substrates for the cytochrome P450-2D6, which is known to be polymorphic. Thus the 7% of the Caucasian population and 1% to 2% of the Asian and African descent populations who are

TABLE 13–8. Initial and Target Doses for β-Blockers Used in Treatment of Heart Failure

Drug	Initial Dose[a]	Target Dose
Bisoprolol[b]	1.25 mg qd	10 mg qd
Carvedilol[b]	3.125 mg bid	25 mg bid[c]
Metoprolol tartrate	6.25 mg bid	50–100 mg bid
Metoprolol succinate CR/XL[b]	12.5–25 mg qd[d]	200 mg qd

[a]Doses should be doubled approximately every 2 weeks or as tolerated by the patient until the highest tolerated or target dose is reached.
[b]Regimens proven in large trials to reduce mortality.
[c]Target dose for patients >85 kg is 50 mg bid.
[d]In MERIT-HF, the majority of class II patients were given 25 mg qd, while the majority of class III patients were given 12.5 mg qd as their starting dose.

CYP2D6 poor metabolizers would be expected to have more pronounced effects than anticipated at the usual doses of carvedilol and metoprolol.

An important aspect to the safe use of β-blockers in heart failure is initiation of therapy at a low dose with a slow, upward dose titration. Typically, starting doses have been one-tenth to one-twentieth the final dose. Doses typically are doubled no more frequently than every 2 weeks until the target dose is reached. The starting and target doses are described in Table 13–8. As shown in the table, the starting dose for bisoprolol is 1.25 mg/day. However, the smallest commercially available tablet of bisoprolol is a scored 5-mg tablet. Since the starting dosage of bisoprolol is not readily available, this drug is the least commonly used of the three in heart failure.

Another issue of debate is the clinical equivalency of metoprolol succinate CR/XL and immediate-release metoprolol (metoprolol tartrate). Due to differences in hepatic first-pass effects, the relative bioavailability of metoprolol controlled-release/extended-release (CR/XL) is only about 70% that of immediate-release metoprolol.[97] Thus, based on relative bioavailability, 200 mg/day of metoprolol CR/XL should produce approximately the same area under the curve as 150 mg/day of metoprolol tartrate. As might be expected, the plasma concentration-time profiles are also markedly different, with concentrations from the immediate-release preparation greatly exceeding those of CR/XL preparations for the first 8 to 10 hours but then dropping well below those of CR/XL preparations after 12 hours.[97] Consistent with the concentration-time profiles, metoprolol CR/XL produces a more consistent reduction in heart rate and blood pressure without the marked reductions that are observed at peak concentrations with the immediate-release preparations. Whether these pharmacokinetic differences translate into important differences in outcomes in heart failure is unclear. Given that immediate-release metoprolol has not been studied in a large mortality trial and is not readily available in the recommended starting doses, it seems prudent to use metoprolol CR/XL in those patients who can afford it. However, when cost considerations are a major factor, immediate-release metoprolol would appear to be a reasonable alternative.

Cost also may be an important factor in selection of carvedilol versus metoprolol CR/XL, since carvedilol is two to four times more expensive (depending on the target dose of 25 mg bid versus 50 mg bid) than the target dose of metoprolol CR/XL. Given that heart failure patients are typically on a large number of medications, cost can become an important differentiating factor when there is no evidence for differences in clinical outcomes, as is currently the case with the β-blockers.

Diuretics[60]

Loop diuretics, as described earlier, represent the typical diuretic therapy for patients with heart failure due to their potency and, as such, are the only diuretics discussed here. Currently, three loop diuretics are available that are used routinely: furosemide, bumetanide, and torsemide. They share many similarities in their pharmacodynamics, with their differences being largely pharmacokinetic in nature. Relevant information on the loop diuretics is shown in Table 13–9. Following oral administration, the peak effect with all the agents occurs in 30 to 90 minutes, with a duration of 2 to 3 hours (slightly longer for torsemide). Following intravenous administration, the diuretic effect begins within minutes. All three drugs are highly (>95%) bound to serum albumin and enter the nephron by active secretion in the proximal tubule. The biggest difference between the agents is bioavailability. Bioavailability of bumetanide and torsemide is essentially complete (80% to 100%), whereas furosemide bioavailability exhibits marked intra- and interpatient variability. Bioavailability for furosemide ranges from 10% to 100%, with an average of 50%. Thus, if bioequivalent intravenous and oral doses are desired, oral furosemide doses should be approximately double that of the intravenous dose, whereas intravenous and oral doses are the same for torsemide and bumetanide. Coadministration of furosemide and bumetanide with food can decrease bioavailability, whereas food has no effect on bioavailability of torsemide.

As noted in the preceding section on diuretics, the loop diuretics exhibit a ceiling effect in heart failure, meaning that once the ceiling dose is reached, no additional response is achieved by increasing the dose. Thus, when this dose is reached, additional diuresis is achieved by giving the drug more often or by giving combination diuretic therapy. The ceiling doses are listed in Table 13–9. While some heart failure patients take their diuretic once per day, many will take it twice per day and a small percentage three times per day. Multiple daily dosing is somewhat common in heart failure because of the ceiling dose effects and to achieve a more sustained diuresis throughout the day.

TABLE 13–9. Loop Diuretic Use in Heart Failure

	Furosemide	Bumetanide	Torsemide
Usual daily dose (PO)	20–160 mg/d	0.5–4 mg/d	10–80 mg/d
Ceiling dose[a]			
Normal renal function	80–160 mg	1–2 mg	20–40 mg
CL_{CR}: 20–50 mL/min	160 mg	2 mg	40 mg
CL_{CR} <20 mL/min	400 mg	8–10 mg	100 mg
Bioavailability	10–100% Average 50%	80–90%	80–100%
Affected by food	Yes	Yes	No
Half-life	0.3–3.4 h	0.3–1.5 h	3–4 h

[a]Ceiling dose: Single dose above which additional response is unlikely to be observed.
Adapted from Ref. 60.

When dosed two or three times daily, the first dose is usually given first thing in the morning and the final dose in late afternoon/early evening.

Diuretics cause a variety of metabolic abnormalities, with the severity related to the potency of the diuretic. The reader is referred to Chapter 12 for a detailed discussion on the adverse effects of diuretic therapy. The most common metabolic disturbances associated with both thiazide and loop diuretics is hypokalemia, which in heart failure patients may be exacerbated by hyperaldosteronism. Hypokalemia in these patients is also frequently accompanied by hypomagnesemia. And since adequate magenesium is necessary for entry of potassium into the cell, magnesium supplementation is also sometimes necessary to correct the hypokalemia. Hypokalemia is especially worrisome in the setting of heart failure because it can precipitate ventricular arrhythmias, a common mode of death for these patients. Digitalis-associated arrhythmias are also more common with concurrent hypokalemia. Concomitant ACE inhibitor therapy may help minimize diuretic-induced hypokalemia because these drugs tend to increase serum potassium through their effects on aldosterone. Nonetheless, serum potassium should be monitored closely in heart failure patients and supplemented appropriately when needed, either with potassium replacement or use of a potassium-sparing diuretic.

Digoxin

Pharmacology. Digoxin exerts its positive inotropic effect by binding to sodium- and potassium-activated adenosine triphosphatase (Na,K-ATPase or sodium pump).[65] Inhibition of Na,K-ATPase decreases outward transport of sodium and leads to increased intracellular sodium concentrations. Higher intracellular sodium concentrations favor calcium entry and reduce calcium extrusion from the cell through effects on the sodium-calcium exchanger.[65] The result is increased storage of intracellular calcium in the sarcoplasmic reticulum and, with each action potential, a greater release of calcium to activate contractile elements. Digoxin also has beneficial neurohumoral actions. These effects occur at low doses, where little inotropic effect is seen, and are independent of inotropic activity.[65,98] Unlike other positive inotropes that increase intracellular cyclic adenosine monophosphate (cAMP), digoxin blunts the excessive SNS activation present in heart failure patients.[65,98] Although the precise mechanism is unknown, a digoxin-mediated reduction in central sympathetic outflow and improvement in impaired baroreceptor function appear to play an important role.[65,98] Because mortality and progression of heart failure are linked to the extent of SNS activation, these sympathoinhibitory effects may be an important component of the clinical response to the drug. Chronic heart failure is also marked by autonomic dysfunction, most notably suppression of the parasympathetic (vagal) system.[65] Digoxin increases parasympathetic activity in heart failure patients and leads to a decrease in heart rate, thus enhancing diastolic filling.[65,99] The vagal effects also result in slowed conduction and prolongation of atrioventricular node refractoriness, thus slowing the ventricular response in patients with atrial fibrillation. Because atrial fibrillation is a common complication of heart failure, the combined positive inotropic, neurohormonal, and negative dromotropic effects of digoxin can be particularly beneficial for such patients. The overall response to digoxin is usually an increase in cardiac index, a decrease in SVR, PAOP, and plasma NE, but relatively little change in arterial blood pressure.[65]

Pharmacokinetics. Numerous studies of digoxin pharmacokinetics have been published and are summarized in Table 13–10.[74] Digoxin has a large volume of distribution and is extensively bound to various tissues, most notably to Na,K-ATPase in skeletal and cardiac muscles. Because it does not distribute appreciably to body fat, loading doses of digoxin (when necessary) should be calculated based on estimates of lean body weight. There is a long "distribution phase" after administration of oral or intravenous digoxin, resulting in a lag time before maximum pharmacologic response is observed (see Table 13–10). Transiently elevated serum digoxin concentrations (SDCs) during the distribution phase are not associated with increased therapeutic or adverse effects, although they can mislead the clinician who is unaware of the timing of blood sampling relative to the previous digoxin dose. Consequently, blood samples for measurement of SDCs should be collected at least 6 hours and preferably 12 hours or more after the last dose.

TABLE 13–10. Clinical Pharmacokinetics of Digoxin

Oral bioavailability	
Tablets	0.5–0.9 (0.65)[a]
Elixir	0.75–0.85 (0.80)
Capsules	0.9–1.0 (0.95)
Onset of action	
Oral	1.5–6 h
Intravenous	15–30 min
Peak effect	
Oral	4–6 h
Intravenous	1.5–4 h
Terminal half-life	
Normal renal function	36 h
Anuric patients	5 d
Volume of distribution at steady state	7.3 L/kg
Fraction unbound in plasma	0.75–0.80
Fraction excreted unchanged in urine	0.65–0.70

[a]Range and mean value in parenthesis.
Compiled from Ref. 74.

In patients with normal renal function, 60% to 80% of a dose of digoxin is eliminated unchanged in urine via glomerular filtration and tubular secretion. The terminal half-life of digoxin is approximately 1.5 days in subjects with normal renal function but approximately 5 days in anuric patients (see Table 13–10). It is important to emphasize that most studies of digoxin pharmacokinetics used immunoassays to measure digoxin concentrations in serum and urine. Lack of specificity with the immunoassays used in many studies of digoxin pharmacokinetics led to variable cross-reactivity with certain metabolites as well as endogenous digoxin-like immunoreactive substance(s) and probably affected the estimates of certain pharmacokinetic parameters.[74] Clinically important pharmacokinetic/pharmacodynamic drug interactions are summarized in Table 13–11. An extensive review of pharmacokinetics and pharmacodynamics of digoxin is available.[74]

Adverse Effects. Digoxin produces a variety of cardiac and noncardiac adverse effects (Table 13–12).[65] Noncardiac adverse effects frequently involve the CNS or gastrointestinal systems but also may be nonspecific (e.g., fatigue or weakness). Cardiac manifestations include numerous different arrhythmias caused by enhanced automaticity, slowed or accelerated conduction, or delayed afterdepolarizations (see Table 13–12). Cardiac arrhythmias may be the first evidence of toxicity in a patient (before any noncardiac symptoms occur). Rhythm disturbances are of particular concern because patients with chronic heart failure are already at increased risk for sudden cardiac death, presumably due to ventricular arrhythmias. Hypokalemia, hypercalcemia, and hypomagnesemia will predispose patients to cardiac manifestations of digoxin toxicity. Concomitant therapy with

TABLE 13–11. Digoxin Drug Interactions

Drugs	Mechanism/Effect	Suggested Clinical Management
Amiodarone	Inhibits P-glycoprotein resulting in decrease in renal and nonrenal clearance; can increase SDC by 70–100%	Monitor SDC and adverse effects; anticipate the need to reduce the dose by 50%
Antacids	Concurrent administration may decrease digoxin bioavailability by 20–35%	Space doses at least 2 h apart or avoid concurrent use if possible
Cholestrayramine, colestipol	Bind digoxin in gut and decrease bioavailability 20–35%; may also decrease enterohepatic recycling	Space doses at least 2 h apart or avoid concurrent use if possible
Diuretics	Thiazides or loop diuretics may cause hypokalemia and hypomagnesemia, thereby increasing the risk of digitalis toxicity	Monitor and replace electrolytes if necessary
Erthromycin, clarithromycin, tetracycline	Alter gut bacterial flora; bioavailability and SDC increase 40–100% in about 10% of patients who extensively metabolize digoxin in the gut, may also be due to inhibitian of P-glycoprotein by macrolides	Monitor SDC and anticipate the need to reduce the dose; avoid concurrent use if possible
Itraconazole	Decrease in renal and nonrenal clearance by inhibition of P-glycoprotein; SDC may increase by 50–100%	Monitor SDC and anticipate the need to reduce the dose by 50%
Kaolin-pectin	Large dose (30–60 mL) may decrease digoxin bioavailability by about 60%	Space doses at least 2 h apart or avoid concurrent use if possible
Metoclopramide	Increase in gut mobility may decrease bioavailability of slow dissolving tablets; unknown significance	Effect is minimized by administration of digoxin capsules
Neomycin, sulfasalazine	Decrease in bioavailability by 20–25%	Space doses at least 2 h apart or avoid concurrent use if possible
Propafenone	Decrease in renal clearance; SDC may increase 30–40%	Monitor SDC and anticipate the need to reduce the dose
Quinidine	Inhibits P-glycoprotein resulting in decrease in renal and nonrenal clearance; also displacement of digoxin from tissue binding sites with decrease in the volume of distribution; SDC generally increases about twofold.	Monitor SDC and adverse effects; anticipate the need to reduce dose by 50%
Spironolactone	Decrease in renal and nonrenal clearance; also interference with some digoxin assays thus increasing apparent SDC	Monitor SDC and anticipate the need to reduce dose; check assay for interference
Verapamil	Inhibits P-glycoprotein resulting in decrease in renal and nonrenal clearance, SDC may increase 70–100%	Monitor SDC and anticipate the need to reduce the dose by 50%; consider using another calcium channel blocker

Abbreviation: SDC = serum digoxin concentration.

TABLE 13–12. Signs and Symptoms of Digitalis Toxicity

Noncardiac (Mostly CNS) Adverse Effects
Anorexia, nausea, vomiting, abdominal pain
Visual disturbances
Halos, photophobia, problems with color perception (i.e., red-green or yellow-green vision), scotomata
Fatigue, weakness, dizziness, headache, neuralgia, confusion, delirium, psychosis

Cardiac Adverse Effects[a, b]
Ventricular arrhythmias
Premature ventricular depolarizations, bigeminy, trigeminy, ventricular tachycardia, ventricular fibrillation
Atrioventricular (A-V) block
First degree, second degree (Mobitz type I), third degree
A-V junctional escape rhythms, junctional tachycardia
Atrial arrhythmias with slowed A-V conduction or A-V block
Particularly paroxysmal atrial tachycardia with A-V block
Sinus bradycardia

[a]Some adverse effects may be difficult to distinguish from the signs/symptoms of heart failure.
[b]Digitalis toxicity has been associated with almost every known rhythm abnormality (only the more common manifestations are listed).
Compiled from Ref. 74.

diuretics may lead to electrolyte abnormalities and increase the likelihood of cardiac arrhythmias. Similarly, hypothyroidism, myocardial ischemia, and acidosis will increase the risk of cardiac adverse effects. Usual treatment of digoxin toxicity includes drug withdrawal or dose reduction and treatment of cardiac arrhythmias and electrolyte abnormalities. In patients with life-threatening digoxin toxicity, purified digoxin-specific Fab antibody fragments provide reversal of adverse effects within 1 hour in over 90% of cases.

Several retrospective analyses suggest that digoxin may increase mortality after MI, although it could not be determined if digoxin was the cause of death or was just a marker for patients with more severe heart disease.[100,101] One multivariate analysis that attempted to control for other confounding factors found a relative mortality risk of 1.8 for patients receiving digoxin after MI.[101] In a post hoc analysis of mortality in patients receiving digoxin in the Acute Infarction Ramipril Efficacy (AIRE) Study, treatment with digoxin was identified as an independent predictor of increased total mortality and sudden death.[100] These findings are supported by those of the DIG trial that reported an increased risk of cardiac death (defined as death from a cardiac cause other than worsening heart failure) in patients receiving digoxin.[63] Although not conclusive, the expected benefit of digoxin should be weighed carefully against the potential risk in a patient with recent MI.

▶ TREATMENT: Advanced/Decompensated Heart Failure

As discussed previously, the number of patients with heart failure is substantial and continues to increase. Although a large number of patients have the diagnosis of heart failure, most morbidity and mortality occurs in a relatively small group of patients with advanced disease.[102] Additionally, this group is responsible for the consumption of significant health care resources in a relatively short time period.[103]

A number of descriptive terms have been used to identify this group of patients including *advanced, severe, end-stage, complex, intractable,* and *refractory heart failure.* Irrespective of the term used, they are typically patients who require frequent hospitalization despite optimal therapy with ACE inhibitors, β-blockers, diuretics, and digoxin. Early identification and aggressive management of patients with advanced heart failure hopefully will reduce morbidity, mortality, and cost of care.

PATHOPHYSIOLOGY AND CLINICAL PRESENTATION

Patients requiring intensive therapy for advanced heart failure may present via several pathways. Patients with chronic progressive heart failure can become refractory to available oral therapy and decompensate following a relatively mild insult (e.g., dietary indiscretion), from medical noncompliance, from a noncardiac concurrent illness (e.g., infection), or simply from a progressive reduction in cardiac output ("low-output syndrome"). A new cardiac event, such as recurrent MI, myocarditis, or acute valvular insufficiency also can cause a stable patient to decompensate. A third group of patients consists of those with acute, massive MI whose initial presentation is severe heart failure. Regardless of their presentation, these patients represent the most advanced stage of heart failure.

The general pathophysiologic determinants of myocardial systolic (preload, afterload, inotropy) and diastolic function (ventricular compliance or lusitropic function) in these patients are essentially the same as described earlier in this chapter. However, the severity of their symptoms, lack of cardiopulmonary reserve, and potential for adverse responses to intervention make successful treatment of these patients a challenge.

HEMODYNAMIC MONITORING

Patients with severe heart failure typically have critically reduced cardiac output, usually with low arterial blood pressure and systemic hypoperfusion resulting in organ system dysfunction. They also may demonstrate pulmonary edema with hypoxemia, respiratory acidosis, and markedly increased work of breathing. Since cardiopulmonary support must be instituted and adjusted rapidly, immediate assessment of the results of an intervention limits risks and makes advances in therapy more prompt. ECG monitoring, continuous pulse oximetry, urine flow monitoring, and automated sphygmomanometric blood pressure recording are now the minimal noninvasive standard of care for critically ill patients with cardiopulmonary decompensation. Peripheral or femoral arterial catheters provide continuous and accurate assessment of arterial pressure.

Flow-directed pulmonary artery (PA) or Swan-Ganz catheters typically are placed percutaneously through a central vein,advanced through the right side of the heart and into the PA. Inflation of a balloon proximal to the end port allows the catheter to "wedge," yielding the PAOP, which estimates the pulmonary venous (left atrial) pressure and, in the absence of intracardiac shunt or mitral valve disease or pulmonary disease, LVEDP. Additionally, cardiac output may be measured and SVR calculated. Normal values for hemodynamic parameters are listed in Table 13–13. Although the routine use of PA catheters has come under scrutiny recently,[104] their efficacy and safety in individual patients with advanced heart failure seem well established. Hemodynamic monitoring often provides essential information necessary to achieve optimal drug therapy in patients with a confusing or complicated clinical picture and during dose titration of rapidly acting medications.

GENERAL APPROACH TO TREATMENT

Patients should be admitted to an intensive care unit (ICU) for decompensated heart failure when they show signs of significant systemic hypoperfusion (severe fatigue, shortness of breath at rest, hypotension, altered mental status, and depressed renal function), develop pulmonary vascular congestion requiring mechanical ventilation, manifest symptomatic sustained tachyarrhythmias, or require potent intravenous vasoactive or inotropic drugs or mechanical ventricular assistance. Reversible or treatable causes of the patient's decompensation such as a thyroid disorder or anemia should be addressed and corrected. The need for drugs that may aggravate heart failure (calcium channel blocking drugs, antiarrhythmics, NSAIDs) should be evaluated carefully and discontinued when possible.

The first step in the management of advanced heart failure is to ascertain that optimal treatment with oral medications has been achieved. If fluid retention is evident on physical examination, aggressive diuresis should be accomplished. Although increasing the dose of oral diuretic may be effective in some cases, the use of intravenous diuretics frequently is necessary. Most patients should be receiving digoxin at a low dose prescribed to achieve a trough serum concentration of 0.5 to 1.0 ng/mL. Additionally, every effort should be made to optimally treat the patient with an ACE inhibitor. Although β-blockers should not be started during this period of instability, it is desirable to continue their administration, if possible, in patients who are receiving them on a chronic basis. However, discontinuation occasionally may be necessary because some patients with advanced

TABLE 13–13. Hemodynamic Monitoring: Normal Values

Parameter	Normal value
Central venous (right atrial) pressure, mean	<5 mm Hg
Right ventricular pressure	25/0 mm Hg
Pulmonary artery pressure	25/10 mm Hg
PAP, mean	<18 mm Hg
Pulmonary artery occlusion pressure, mean	<12 mm Hg
Systemic arterial pressure	120/80 mm Hg
Mean arterial pressure	90–110 mm Hg
Cardiac index	2.8–4.2 L/min/m^2
Stroke volume index	30–65 mL/beat/m^2
Systemic vascular resistance	900–1400 dyn · s · m^{-5}
Pulmonary vascular resistance	150–250 dyn · s · m^{-5}
Arterial oxygen content	20 mL/dL
Mixed venous oxygen content	15 mL/dL
Arteriovenous oxygen content difference	3–5 mL/dL

heart failure may not be able to tolerate target doses of both ACE inhibitors and β-blockers.

There are two accepted approaches to maximize therapy in the advanced heart failure patient. One is to use simple clinical parameters (signs and symptoms, blood pressure, renal function) and the other is to use invasive hemodynamic monitoring. However, it is frequently necessary to combine the two approaches.

PRINCIPLES OF THERAPY BASED ON CLINICAL PRESENTATION

Appropriate medical management of the patient presenting with advanced heart failure is aided by determination of whether the patient has signs and symptoms of fluid overload ("wet" heart failure) or low cardiac output ("dry" heart failure).[102] Most patients present with congestion (or the "wet" profile). Symptoms of an elevated filling pressure include orthopnea and dyspnea with minimal exertion and can lead to systemic symptoms such as gastrointestinal discomfort, ascites, and peripheral edema. Patients with no or minimal fluid overload (or the "dry" category of advanced heart failure) may have symptoms that are more difficult to distinguish. This is a syndrome of low cardiac output and is characterized principally by fatigue and other symptoms not commonly attributed to cardiac causes such as poor appetite, nausea, and early satiety. Moreover, these patients frequently exhibit worsening renal function and a decline in serum sodium level. Many patients will present with signs and symptoms of both types of advanced heart failure. In these patients, low-output symptoms may not be obvious until congestion is treated. Based on the assessment of "wet" versus "dry" heart failure, the algorithm in Figure 13–6 may be considered.

PRINCIPLES OF THERAPY BASED ON HEMODYNAMIC SUBSETS

During the past 25 years, invasive hemodynamic monitoring has become a critically important tool in the management of patients with advanced/decompensated heart failure. In addition to the clinical presentation, invasive hemodynamic monitoring helps in the selection of appropriate medical therapy as well as in the classification of patients into specific subsets. These *hemodynamic subsets* were first proposed for patients with left ventricular dysfunction following an AMI but also are applicable to patients with acute or severe heart failure from other causes (Figure 13–7).[105] This hemodynamic classification has four subsets and is based on a cardiac index above or below 2.2 L/min/m^2 and a PAOP above or below 18 mm Hg. A treatment algorithm, based on hemodynamic subsets, is shown in Figure 13–8.

Subset I

Patients in hemodynamic subset I have a cardiac index and PAOP within generally acceptable ranges and have the lowest mortality of any subset. These patients do not need immediate specific interventions other than maximizing oral therapy and monitoring. It should be emphasized that patients with significant left ventricular dysfunction may still present in subset I because normal compensatory mechanisms and/or appropriate drug therapy may at least partially correct an otherwise abnormal hemodynamic profile.

Subset II

As shown in Figure 13–7, patients in subset II have an adequate cardiac index but a PAOP greater than 18 mm Hg. These patients are likely to have pulmonary congestion (i.e., "wet" heart failure) secondary to increased hydrostatic pressure in the pulmonary capillaries but no evidence of peripheral hypoperfusion. The primary goal of therapy in these patients is to reduce pulmonary congestion by lowering PAOP. However, it is critically important that PAOP not be decreased excessively so as to cause a significant decrease in cardiac index. Although the normal range of PAOP is 5 to 12 mm Hg for individuals without cardiac dysfunction, higher pressures of 15 to 18 mm Hg frequently are necessary for heart failure patients to optimize cardiac index while avoiding pulmonary congestion. Generally, the PAOP can be lowered to the range of 15 to 18 mm Hg with relatively little decrease in cardiac index because the Frank-Starling curve is flatter at higher PAOP values, particularly in patients with heart failure. Intravenous administration of agents that reduce preload (i.e., loop diuretics or nitroglycerin) is the most appropriate acute therapy to achieve the therapeutic goal for patients in subset II (see under specific drug classes that follow). These agents will produce a very rapid decrease in preload, although signs and symptoms of pulmonary congestion may take longer to resolve.

Subset III

Patients in hemodynamic subset III have a cardiac index of less than 2.2 L/min/m^2 but without an abnormally elevated PAOP (see Figure 13–7). These patients usually will present without evidence of pulmonary congestion, but the low cardiac index will result in signs and symptoms of peripheral hypoperfusion (i.e., decreased urine output, weakness, peripheral vasoconstriction, weak pulses). The mortality rate of subset III patients is reported to be four times higher than that of patients without hypoperfusion.[105] Although the treatment goal is to alleviate signs and symptoms of hypoperfusion by increasing cardiac index and perfusion to essential organs, therapy will differ among patients (see Figures 13–6 and 13–8). If the PAOP is significantly below 15 mm Hg, initial therapy will be to administer intravenous fluids to provide a more optimal left ventricular filling pressure of 15 to 18 mm Hg and consequently improve cardiac index. When there is only mild left ventricular dysfunction, intravenous fluid administration may be all that is necessary to achieve a cardiac index above 2.2 L/min/m^2. However, many patients will have significant left ventricular dysfunction and a depressed Frank-Starling relationship despite adequate preload (i.e., PAOP of 15 to 18 mm Hg). In these patients, intravenously administered positive inotropic agents (e.g., dobutamine, milrinone) and/or arterial vasodilators (e.g., nitroprusside, nitroglycerin) are often necessary to achieve an adequate cardiac index. It is noteworthy that many positive inotropic drugs also will have arterial vasodilating activity (see specific drug classes that follow).

Subset IV

Patients with a cardiac index of less than 2.2 L/min/m^2 and a PAOP higher than 18 mm Hg are in hemodynamic subset IV. These patients have the worst prognosis of any subset and illustrate the typical hemodynamic profile for the patient hospitalized for advanced heart failure.

Severe pump failure is evidenced by the fact that these patients cannot maintain an adequate cardiac index despite the elevated left

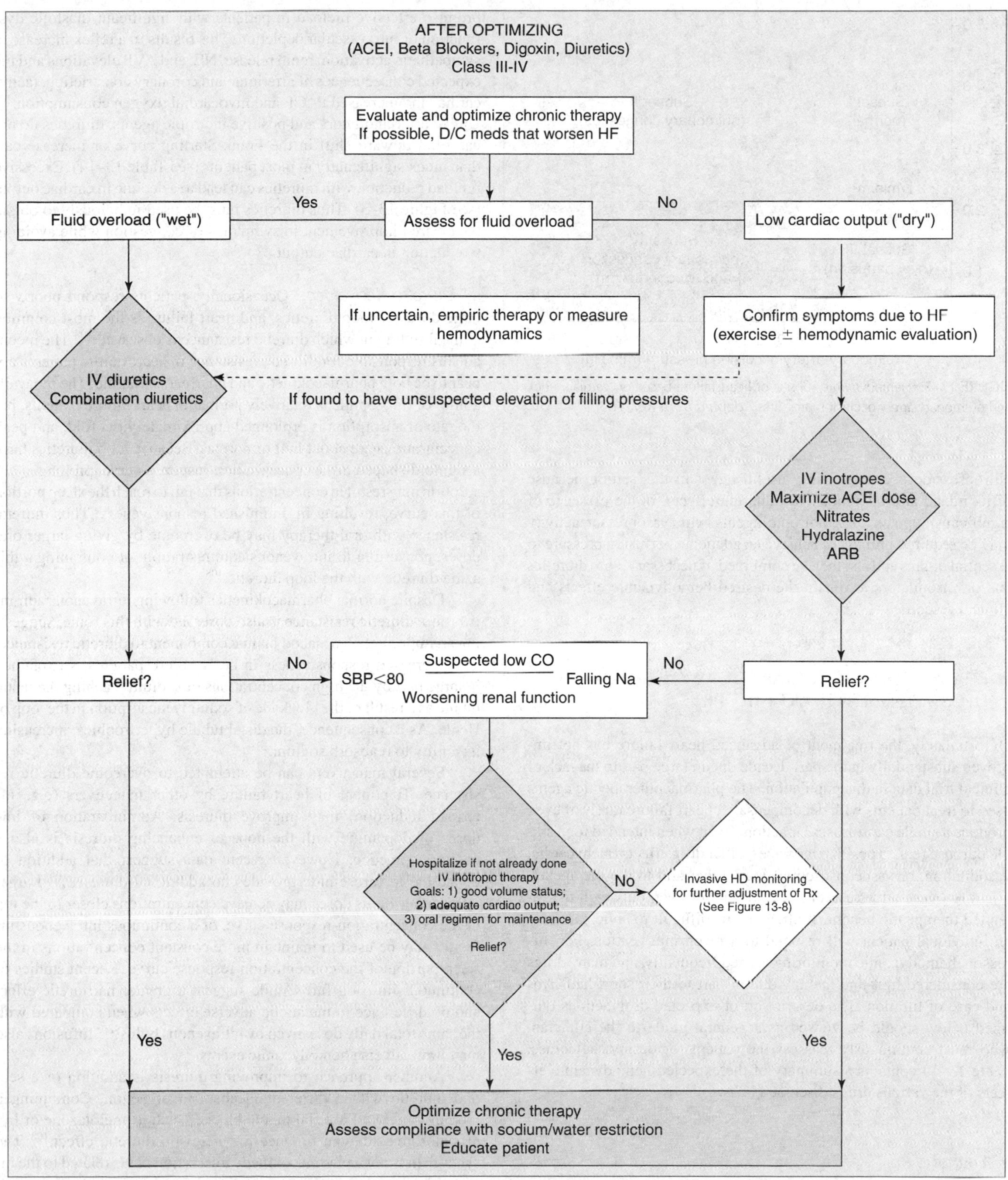

FIGURE 13–6. General treatment algorithm for advanced/decompensated heart failure based on clinical presentation. *Adapted from Ref. 102.*

ventricular filling pressure and increased myocardial fiber stretch. These patients will present with signs and symptoms of both "wet" and low-output ("dry") heart failure. The treatment goals are to alleviate these signs and symptoms by increasing cardiac index above 2.2 L/min/m^2 and reducing PAOP to 15 to 18 mm Hg while maintaining an adequate mean arterial pressure. Thus therapy will involve a combination of agents used for subset II and subset III patients to achieve these goals (i.e., combination of diuretic plus positive inotrope). These targets may be difficult to achieve and will necessitate careful monitoring and individualization of drug therapy.

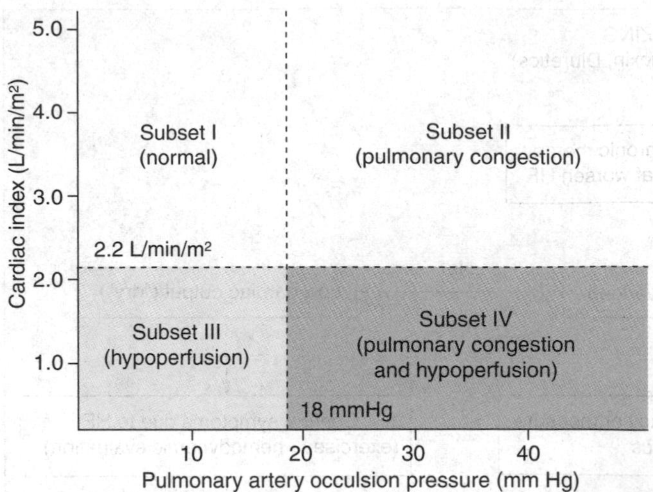

FIGURE 13–7. Hemodynamic subsets of heart failure based on cardiac index and pulmonary artery occlusion pressure. *Adapted from Ref. 105.*

Nitroprusside is a particularly useful agent in this setting because of its mixed arterial-venous vasodilating effects. In the presence of significant hypotension, inotropic agents with vasopressor activity may be required initially to achieve an adequate perfusion pressure to essential organs and can then be combined, if necessary, with diuretics and/or vasodilators to obtain the desired hemodynamic effects and clinical response.

PHARMACOLOGIC THERAPY OF ADVANCED OR DECOMPENSATED HEART FAILURE

Unfortunately, the treatment of advanced heart failure has not improved substantially in the past decade due in large part to the lack of clinical trial data in this population. The pharmacotherapeutic agents used to treat patients with decompensated heart failure rarely, if ever, produce a single cardiovascular action. Even when intended for a single purpose (e.g., a positive inotrope), other drug effects (tachycardia, vasodilation, or vasoconstriction) may either add to the therapeutic effect or cause adverse events that negate or even outweigh the intended therapeutic benefit. It often can be difficult to anticipate how an individual patient will respond to a given intervention. For this reason, hemodynamic monitoring is used frequently, and many drugs are considered first-line therapy due in part to their short half-lives and ease of titration. The description of expected drug actions outlined below should be viewed as a general guide to the clinician, who must continuously reassess the patient for desired outcomes. Table 13–14 contains a summary of the expected hemodynamic effects of the various drugs discussed below.

Diuretics

Intravenous loop diuretics, including furosemide, bumetanide, and torsemide, are used in the management of advanced heart failure, with furosemide the most widely studied and used agent in this setting. Bolus administration of diuretics decreases preload by functional venodilation within 5 to 15 minutes and later (>20 minutes) via sodium and water excretion, thereby improving pulmonary congestion.[106,107] However, the acute reduction in venous return may severely compromise effective preload in patients with significant diastolic dysfunction or intravascular depletion. This results in a reflex increase in sympathetic activation, renin release, NE, and AVP elevations and the expected consequences of arteriolar and coronary constriction, tachycardia, and increased PAOP and myocardial oxygen consumption.[107] Unlike arterial dilators and positive inotropic agents, diuretics do not cause an upward shift in the Frank-Starling curve or increase cardiac index significantly in most patients (see Table 13–14). Excessive preload reduction with diuretics can lead to a decline in cardiac output (see Figure 13–3). Thus diuretics must be used judiciously to obtain the desired improvement in symptoms of congestion while avoiding a reduction in cardiac output.

Diuretic Resistance. Occasionally, patients respond poorly to large doses of loop diuretics, and heart failure is the most common clinical setting in which diuretic resistance is observed.[108] The mechanisms responsible for diuretic resistance in heart failure patients appear to be both pharmacokinetic and pharmacodynamic. The bioavailability of furosemide is relatively normal in heart failure patients, but the rate of absorption is prolonged approximately twofold, and peak concentrations are about half of normal. Because loop diuretics have a sigmoid-shaped urine concentration-response curve, prolonged absorption may result in concentrations that fail to reach the steep portion of this curve, resulting in diminished responsiveness. Thus diuretic resistance with oral therapy may be overcome by giving larger oral doses, converting to intravenous administration, or combining a thiazide diuretic with the loop diuretic.[108]

Despite normal pharmacokinetics following intravenous administration, diuretic resistance is also observed with this route, suggesting an important pharmacodynamic component to diuretic resistance. The decreased responsiveness in heart failure patients is explained in large part by the high concentrations of sodium reaching the distal tubule as a result of the blockade of sodium reabsorption in the loop of Henle. As a consequence, the distal tubule hypertrophies, increasing its ability to reabsorb sodium.[108]

Several maneuvers can be attempted to overcome diuretic resistance. Treatment of heart failure by other maneuvers (e.g., afterload reduction) may improve diuresis. Administration of low doses of dopamine with the hope of enhancing diuresis is also a common practice. However, recent data suggest that addition of dopamine to furosemide provides no additional diuresis.[109] Larger intravenous bolus doses may achieve concentrations closer to the top of the concentration-response curve, or a continuous intravenous infusion may be used to maintain more constant concentrations in the steep portion of the concentration-response curve. Recent studies of continuous-infusion furosemide suggest a greater natriuretic effect and no difference in metabolic adverse effects when compared with the same total daily dose given by intravenous bolus.[110] Infusions also may limit adverse hemodynamic events.

Another approach to improving diuresis is addition of a second diuretic with a different mechanism of action. Combining a loop diuretic with a distal tubule blocker such as metolazone or hydrochlorothiazide can produce a synergistic diuretic effect.[108] The synergism is not a pharmacokinetic interaction but is related to the increased delivery of sodium to the distal convoluted tubule. Enhanced sodium delivery to (and reabsorption in) the distal tubule can then be blocked by the thiazide-type diuretic. Thus, when thiazide-type diuretics are added to a loop diuretic, they block more than their normal 5% to 8% of filtered sodium, and the combination results in synergistic natriuresis.[108]

The loop diuretic–thiazide combination generally should be reserved for the inpatient setting, where the patient can be monitored

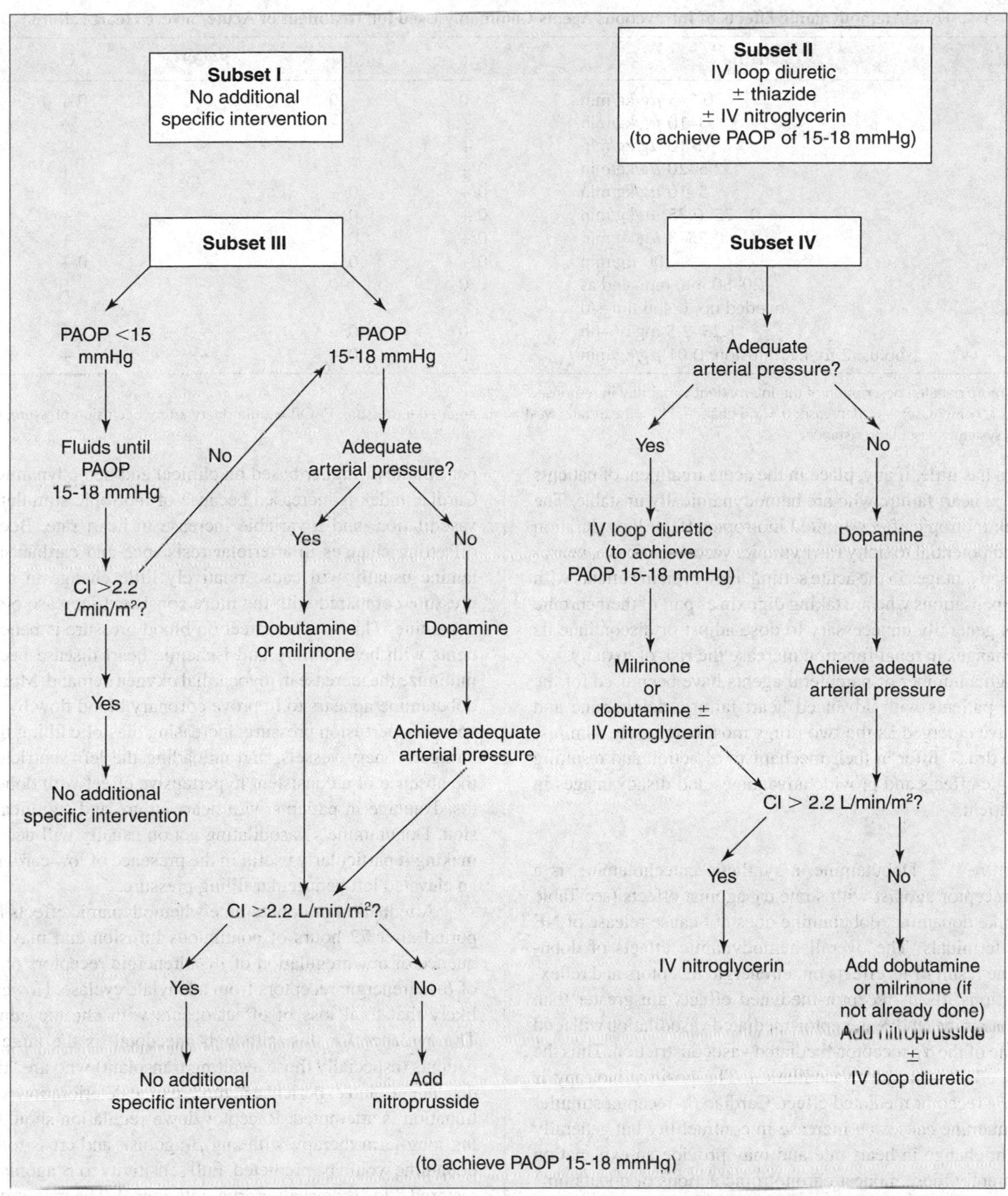

FIGURE 13–8. General treatment algorithm for patients with advanced/decompensated heart failure based on hemodynamic monitoring and hemodynamic subsets. See text for details. Abbreviations: CI = cardiac index; PAOP = pulmonary artery occlusion pressure.

closely, because it can induce a profound diuresis with severe sodium, potassium, and volume depletion. When used in the outpatient setting, very low doses or only occasional doses of the thiazide-type diuretic should be used along with close follow-up (weight, vital signs, dizziness) to avoid serious adverse events.

Positive Inotropic Agents

Drugs that increase intracellular cyclic adenosine monophosphate (cAMP) are the only positive inotropic agents currently approved for the treatment of acute heart failure. β-agonists activate adenylate cyclase through stimulation of β-adrenergic receptors, with the enzyme then catalyzing the conversion of ATP to cAMP. Phosphodiesterase inhibitors raise cAMP concentrations by reducing its degradation. Thus both drug classes increase intracellular cAMP, which enhances phospholipase (and subsequently phosphorylase) activity, increasing the rate and extent of calcium influx during systole and enhancing contractility. Additionally, cAMP enhances reuptake of calcium by the sarcoplasmic reticulum during diastole, improving active relaxation. The receptors on which the β-agonists work are summarized in Table 13–15. While rarely used in management of heart failure, the receptor effects of epinephrine, NE, and isoproterenol are provided for reference.

TABLE 13–14. Usual Hemodynamic Effects of Intravenous Agents Commonly Used for Treatment of Acute/Severe Heart Failure[a]

Drug	Dose	HR	MAP	PAOP	CO	SVR
Dopamine	0.5–3 μg/kg/min	0	0	0	0/+	–
Dopamine	3–10 μg/kg/min	+	+	0	+	0
Dopamine	>10 μg/kg/min	+	+	+	+	+
Dobutamine	2.5–20 μg/kg/min	0/+	0	–	+	–
Amrinone	5–10 μg/kg/min	0/+	0/–	–	+	–
Milrinone	0.375–0.75 μg/kg/min	0/+	0/–	–	+	–
Nitroprusside	0.25–3 μg/kg/min	0/+	0/–	–	+	–
Nitroglycerin	5–200 μg/min	0/+	0/–	–	0/+	0/–
Furosemide	20–80 mg, repeated as needed up to 4–6 times/d	0	0	–	0	0
Enalaprilat	1.25–2.5 mg q6–8h	0	0/–	–	+	+
Nesiritide	bolus: 2 μg/kg; infusion: 0.01 μg/kg/min	0	0/–	–	+	–

[a]See text for a more detailed description of the interpatient variability in response.
Abbreviations: + = increase; – = decrease; 0 = no change; HR = heart rate; MAP = mean arterial pressure; PAOP = pulmonary artery occlusion pressure; CO = cardiac output; SVR = systemic vascular resistance.

Digoxin has little, if any, place in the acute treatment of patients with advanced heart failure who are hemodynamically unstable. The delay in peak inotropic effect, limited inotropic effect, long duration of action, and potential toxicity (arrhythmic, vasoconstrictive, neurologic) are disadvantages in the acute setting. However, in patients with acute decompensations who are taking digoxin as part of their chronic therapy, it is generally unnecessary to dose adjust or discontinue its use unless changes in renal function increase the risk of toxicity.

Although a number of parenteral agents have been used for the treatment of patients with advanced heart failure, dobutamine and milrinone have emerged as the two drugs most commonly administered. These drugs differ in their mechanism of action and resulting pharmacologic effects and provide advantages and disadvantages in any given patient.

Dobutamine[111]. Dobutamine, a synthetic catecholamine, is a β_1- and β_2-receptor agonist with some α_1-agonist effects (see Table 13–15). Unlike dopamine, dobutamine does not cause release of NE from nerve terminals. The overall hemodynamic effects of dobutamine are the result of its effects on adrenergic receptors and reflex-mediated actions. Its β_2-receptor-mediated effects are greater than those with dopamine, and β_2-receptor-mediated vasodilation will tend to offset some of the α_1-receptor-mediated vasoconstriction. Thus the net vascular effect is usually vasodilation. The positive inotropy is primarily a β_1-receptor mediated effect. Cardiac β_1-receptor stimulation by dobutamine causes an increase in contractility but generally no significant change in heart rate and may provide an explanation for the apparently more modest chronotropic actions of dobutamine compared with dopamine.

The overall hemodynamic effects of dobutamine are those of a potent inotropic agent with vasodilating action. Initial doses of 2.5 to 5 μg/kg per minute can be increased progressively to 20 μg/kg per minute or higher based on clinical and hemodynamic responses. Cardiac index is increased because of inotropic stimulation, arterial vasodilation, and a variable increase in heart rate. Because of the offsetting changes in arteriolar resistance and cardiac index, dobutamine usually will cause relatively little change in mean arterial pressure compared with the more consistent increase observed with dopamine. This smaller effect on blood pressure is beneficial in patients with heart failure and ischemic heart disease because it will minimize the increase in myocardial oxygen demand. More important, dobutamine appears to improve coronary blood flow by augmenting coronary perfusion pressure, increasing diastolic filling time, vasodilating coronary vessels, and unloading the left ventricle. However, the absence of a consistent hypertensive effect with dobutamine is a disadvantage in patients with heart failure and significant hypotension. Dobutamine's vasodilating action usually will decrease PAOP, making it particularly useful in the presence of low cardiac index and an elevated left ventricular filling pressure.

Attenuation of dobutamine's hemodynamic effects has been reported after 72 hours of continuous infusion and may be a consequence of downregulation of β_1-adrenergic receptors or uncoupling of β_2-adrenergic receptors from adenylate cyclase. However, it is unlikely that total loss of effect occurs with chronic administration. The evidence for this, although anecdotal, is the large number of patients (especially those awaiting transplant) who are "dobutamine-dependent" and experience hemodynamic deterioration when discontinuation is attempted. Receptor down-regulation should occur during long-term therapy with any β-agonist, and cross-tolerance with dopamine would be predicted. Full sensitivity to β-agonists should be restored 7 to 10 days after drug withdrawal. The maximum inotropic effects of dobutamine are diminished in patients with severe heart failure compared with those without heart failure. The mechanism of this tolerance is decreased myocardial β-receptor density and uncoupling from G-protein, which is caused by chronically elevated circulating catecholamine concentrations in heart failure patients.

Despite the fact that dobutamine has a half-life of approximately 2.5 minutes, some patients may display sustained hemodynamic and symptomatic benefits for several days to months after a treatment course. These beneficial effects have been associated with widely different dobutamine dosage regimens used on a regular, intermittent basis (4- to 72-hour infusions every 3 to 7 days for 4 to 24 weeks). The mechanism of symptomatic benefit for these intermittent dobutamine infusions is unclear, but the drug may promote cardiovascular conditioning analogous to exercise training. However, a randomized, placebo-controlled multicenter trial in outpatients with chronic heart failure showed increased mortality in dobutamine-treated patients.[112]

TABLE 13–15. Relative Effects of Adrenergic Drugs on Receptors

Drug	α_1	β_1	β_2	$Dopamine_1$
Norepinephrine	++++	++++	0	0
Epinephrine	++++	++++	++	0
Dopamine[a]	++++	++++	++	++
Isoproterenol	0	++++	++++	0
Dobutamine[b]	+	++++	++	0

[a]See text for a more detailed description of the dose-dependent hemodynamic effects.
[b]Combined effects of the commercially available recemic mixture (see text).

Thus, despite symptomatic benefits, the potential for increased mortality should preclude the routine use of chronic scheduled administration of intermittent dobutamine infusions in most patients.

Milrinone and Amrinone.[111] Both milrinone and amrinone are bipyridine derivatives that work by inhibiting phosphodiesterase III and producing similar pharmacologic and hemodynamic effects during intravenous administration. Amrinone was the prototype drug in this group, but its use has been supplanted largely by milrinone due to the more frequent occurrence of thrombocytopenia with amrinone. Both positive inotropic and vasodilating effects contribute to the therapeutic response in heart failure patients; hence these drugs have been referred to as *inodilators*. The relative balance of these pharmacologic effects may vary in a particular patient with dose and underlying cardiovascular pathology.

During intravenous administration, there is an increase in stroke volume (and, therefore, cardiac output) with little change in heart rate (see Table 13–14). Despite the increase in cardiac index, mean arterial pressure generally remains constant because of the concomitant decrease in arteriolar resistance. However, the vasodilating effects may predominate in certain patients and lead to a decrease in blood pressure and a reflex tachycardia. The drugs lower PAOP by venodilation and thus are particularly useful in patients with a low cardiac index and an elevated left ventricular filling pressure. Such a reduction in preload, however, can be hazardous for patients without excessive filling pressure (especially those with symptoms of "dry" heart failure), leading to a decrease in cardiac index. Such an effect would blunt the improvement in cardiac output that would otherwise be produced by the positive inotropic and arterial dilating actions. These drugs should be used cautiously as single agents in severely hypotensive heart failure patients because they will not increase, and may even decrease, arterial blood pressure.

The results of controlled studies comparing dobutamine with amrinone or milrinone indicate that they produce generally similar hemodynamic effects to dobutamine. A clinically insignificant but greater increase in heart rate with dobutamine is the most consistent difference in these studies. The combination of dobutamine and a bipyridine produces additive effects on cardiac index and PAOP reduction, suggesting this regimen as an option in patients who have dose-limiting adverse effects with either class of drugs. It is unclear, however, if this combination provides a therapeutic advantage over the combination of a positive inotrope and a traditional pure vasodilator such as nitroprusside.

Milrinone and amrinone have longer terminal elimination half-lives than adrenergic agonists. The average half life in healthy subjects for milrinone is about 1 hour and for amrinone is 2 to 4 hours. This roughly doubles in patients with heart failure.[113] The long elimination half-lives of these drugs may be a disadvantage in this patient population because a loading dose may be necessary to obtain a prompt initial response, minute-to-minute titrations in dose cannot be made based on response, and adverse effects (arrhythmias or hypotension) will persist longer after drug discontinuation. The usual loading dose for milrinone is 50 μg/kg administered over 10 minutes and for amrinone is 0.75 mg/kg administered over 2 to 3 minutes. However, if rapid hemodynamic changes are not necessary, the loading dose should be eliminated due to the risk of hypotension and patients simply started on the maintenance infusion. The maintenance infusion for milrinone is 0.5 μg/kg per minute (range, 0.375 to 0.75 μg/kg/min) and for amrinone it is 5 to 10 μg/kg per minute. Over 80% of a dose of milrinone is excreted unchanged in urine, and unlike amrinone, its infusion rate should be decreased by 50% to 70% in patients with significant renal impairment.

In addition to undesirable hemodynamic effects, the most notable adverse events associated with inodilators are arrhythmias and thrombocytopenia. Thrombocytopenia is reported to occur in 2.4% of patients who have received intravenous amrinone, with decreased platelet survival from nonimmunologic platelet damage as the postulated mechanism. This adverse effect is dose-dependent and generally completely reversible within 5 to 7 days of drug discontinuation. The incidence of thrombocytopenia associated with milrinone therapy is very low (<0.5%). Milrinone therefore is preferable to amrinone because of its better side-effect profile. Patients who receive either drug should be monitored for signs of bleeding and have platelet counts determined before and during therapy.

Generally, milrinone should be considered for patients who are receiving chronic β-blocker therapy because its positive inotropic effect does not involve stimulation of β-receptors. Although it appears that β-agonists such as dobutamine still exert some beneficial effects in patients on β-blocker therapy, it is expected that higher than normal doses of these drugs would be needed to achieve the desired pharmacologic effect. Therefore, milrinone may provide a theoretical advantage in β-blocker-treated patients.

Dopamine.[111,114] Although dopamine generally should be avoided in the treatment of advanced heart failure, there are two clinical scenarios where its pharmacologic actions may be preferable to dobutamine or milrinone. The first is a patient with marked systemic hypotension or cardiogenic shock in the face of elevated ventricular filling pressures, where dopamine in doses greater than 5 μg/kg per minute may be necessary to raise central aortic pressure. The second use, although somewhat controversial, is to directly attempt to improve renal function in a patient with inadequate urine output despite volume overload and high ventricular filling pressures. Low doses (1 to 3 μg/kg/min) traditionally have been administered for this indication. As discussed earlier, however, there are no data to support this commonly employed practice.

Dopamine, the endogenous precursor of NE, exerts its effects by directly stimulating adrenergic receptors as well as causing release of NE from adrenergic nerve terminals. Dopamine produces dose-dependent hemodynamic effects because of its relative affinity for α_1-, β_1-, β_2-, and D_1- (vascular dopaminergic) receptors (see Table 13–15). The following dose-dependent actions are intended as a general guide to the clinician.

Positive inotropic effects mediated primarily by β_1-receptors become more prominent with dopamine doses of 3 to 10 μg/kg per minute. Cardiac index is increased because of an increase in stroke volume and a variable increase in heart rate, which is partially dose-dependent. There is usually little change in SVR, presumably because neither vasodilation (D_1- and β_2-receptor-mediated) nor vasoconstriction (α_1-receptor-mediated) predominates. Renal effects of dopamine may still be evident at these higher doses and are caused by a combination of D_1-mediated renovascular effects, increased cardiac index, and altered sodium tubular reabsorption. At doses above 10 μg/kg per minute, chronotropic and α_1 receptor mediated vasoconstricting effects become more prominent. Mean arterial pressure usually elevates because of an increase in both cardiac index and SVR (see Table 13–14). The vasoconstricting effects of higher doses could indirectly limit the increase in cardiac index by increasing afterload and PAOP, thus complicating the management of patients with preexisting high afterload. In such patients, alternative agents (dobutamine, milrinone) or the addition of diuretics and/or vasodilators may be necessary.

Dopamine, particularly at higher doses, may alter several parameters that increase myocardial oxygen demand (increased heart rate, contractility, and systolic pressure) and potentially decrease myocardial blood flow (coronary vasoconstriction and increased wall tension), worsening ischemia in some patients with coronary disease. Arrhythmogenesis is also more common at higher doses.

Vasodilators

Activation of the SNS, the RAA system, AVP, and endothelial and platelet-derived mediators all cause vasoconstriction and increased SVR. In patients with heart failure, stroke volume varies inversely with SVR such that an increase in peripheral resistance leads to a severe decline in stroke volume and cardiac output. (see Figure 13–1).

Vasodilators typically are described by their prominent site of action (arterial or venous). Arterial vasodilators act as impedance-reducing agents and typically cause an increase in cardiac output. Venodilators act as preload reducers by increasing venous capacitance, reducing symptoms of pulmonary congestion in patients with high cardiac filling pressures. Mixed vasodilators act on both resistance and capacitance vessels, reducing congestive symptoms while increasing cardiac output. Nitroprusside and nitroglycerin are the most widely studied and commonly used intravenous vasodilating agents in acute/severe heart failure. Other vasodilators have shown either tachyphylaxis, excessive reflex tachycardia, or refractory hypotension compromising coronary blood flow; they are rarely, if ever, used in this setting.

Nitroprusside.[113] Sodium nitroprusside, a mixed arterial-venous vasodilator, acts on vascular smooth muscle, increasing synthesis of nitric oxide to produce its balanced vasodilating action. As such, it both increases cardiac index and decreases venous pressure. Nitroprusside's effects on these parameters are qualitatively similar to those produced by dobutamine and phosphodiesterase inhibitors, despite the fact that it has no direct inotropic activity (see Table 13–14). However, nitroprusside generally causes a greater decrease in PAOP, SVR, and blood pressure than these agents. Mean arterial pressure may remain fairly constant but often decreases depending on the relative increase in cardiac output and reduction in arteriolar tone. Hypotension is an important dose-limiting adverse effect of nitroprusside and other vasodilators. Therefore, this drug is used primarily in patients who have a significantly elevated SVR.

Patients with normal left ventricular function will not have an increase in stroke volume when SVR falls because the normal ventricle is fairly insensitive to small changes in afterload. Consequently, these patients experience a significant decrease in blood pressure after administration of arterial vasodilators. This explains why nitroprusside is a potent antihypertensive agent in patients without heart failure but causes less hypotension and reflex tachycardia in patients with left ventricular dysfunction. Nonetheless, even a modest increase in heart rate could have adverse consequences in patients with underlying ischemic heart disease and/or resting tachycardia, and close monitoring is necessary during therapy.

Nitroprusside has been studied extensively and shown to be effective in the short-term management of patients with severe heart failure in a variety of settings (i.e., AMI, valvular regurgitation, after coronary bypass surgery, decompensated chronic heart failure). Generally, nitroprusside will not worsen, and may improve, the balance between myocardial oxygen demand and supply. This is mainly due to a decrease in oxygen demand caused by the lowering of left ventricular wall tension and a possible increase in subendocardial blood flow resulting from decreased LVEDP. However, an excessive decrease in systemic arterial pressure can reduce coronary perfusion and worsen ischemia, leading to increased risk of coronary steal.

Nitroprusside has a rapid onset of action and a duration of action of less than 10 minutes, necessitating its administration by continuous intravenous infusion. This allows for precise dose titration based on measured clinical and hemodynamic parameters. It, like other vasodilators used in heart failure, should be initiated at a low dose (0.1 to 0.25 μg/kg/min) to avoid excessive hypotension and then increased by small increments (0.1 to 0.2 μg/kg/min) every 5 to 10 minutes as needed and tolerated. Usually effective doses range from 0.5 to 3.0 μg/kg per minute. A rebound phenomenon has been reported after abrupt withdrawal of nitroprusside in patients with heart failure and is apparently due to reflex neurohumoral activation during therapy. If renal perfusion pressure is compromised by the drug, salt and water retention can contribute to volume expansion and tachyphylaxis; this is seen typically only in patients with chronic hypertension, baseline azotemia, or when therapeutic augmentation of cardiac output during therapy is minimal. When stopping nitroprusside and switching to oral drugs, it is usually advisable to taper doses slowly. Nitroprusside can cause cyanide and thiocyanate toxicity, but these are very unlikely when doses less than 3 μg/kg per minute are administered for less than 3 days, except in patients with a serum creatinine level greater than 3 mg/dL.

Nitroglycerin. Intravenous nitroglycerin is often considered the preferred agent for preload reduction in patients with severe heart failure. Because of its short half-life, intravenous nitroglycerin is administered by continuous infusion. Its major hemodynamic actions are reductions in preload and PAOP via functional venodilation and mild arterial vasodilation that is particularly evident in patients with heart failure and elevated SVR or when given in doses approaching 200 μg/min (see Table 13–14). Intravenous nitroglycerin is used primarily as a preload reducer for patients with pulmonary congestion and low-normal cardiac output or in combination with inotropic agents for patients with severely depressed systolic function and pulmonary edema. Combination therapy with nitroglycerin and dobutamine or dopamine produces complementary effects to increase cardiac index and decrease PAOP. As indicated previously, excessive PAOP reduction should be avoided to prevent suboptimal ventricular filling pressure and maintain cardiac index while relieving symptoms of pulmonary congestion. In higher doses, nitroglycerin displays potent coronary vasodilating properties and overall beneficial effects on myocardial oxygen demand and supply, making it the vasodilator of choice for patients with severe heart failure and ischemic heart disease.

Nitroglycerin should be initiated at a dose of 5 to 10 μg/min (0.1 μg/kg/min) and increased every 5 to 10 minutes as necessary and tolerated. Hypotension and an excessive decrease in PAOP are important dose-limiting side effects. Maintenance doses usually vary from 35 to 200 μg/min (0.5 to 3.0 μg/kg/min), although doses over 1000 μg/min (15 μg /kg/min) have been used in rare cases. Tolerance to the hemodynamic effects of nitroglycerin may develop over 12 to 72 hours of continuous administration, but some patients have a sustained response.[115] Neither nitroglycerin nor nitroprusside should be used in the presence of elevated intracranial pressure because either may worsen cerebral edema in this setting.

MECHANICAL CIRCULATORY SUPPORT

The intra-aortic balloon pump (IABP) is the most widely used form of mechanical circulatory assistance and typically is employed in patients with advanced heart failure who do not respond adequately to drug therapy or who have intractable myocardial ischemia as part of their presentation. The IABP is placed percutaneously into the high descending thoracic aorta. During counterpulsation, the balloon inflates during diastole, displacing aortic blood and thereby increasing aortic diastolic pressure and coronary perfusion. It deflates just prior to aortic valve opening and causes a sudden decrease in aortic pressure, allowing the left ventricle to pump against a reduced arterial impedance. IABP support results in increased cardiac index and coronary perfusion with decreased myocardial oxygen demand and is particularly useful for patients with decompensated heart failure in the setting of myocardial ischemia (evolving infarction, patients awaiting emergency coronary bypass surgery). It is also used as a bridge to cardiac transplantation when inotrpic drugs are no longer effective. Intravenous vasodilators and inotropic agents generally are used in conjunction with the IABP to maximize hemodynamic and clinical benefits.[116]

Several different ventricular assist devices and total artificial hearts are currently under investigation for the support of patients who cannot be sustained with pharmacologic therapy and IABP counterpulsation. These devices are approved for use as a temporary bridge to transplantation. Investigators also continue to study the use of assist devices for long-term management in selected patients.[116]

SURGICAL THERAPY

Orthotopic cardiac transplantation remains the best therapeutic option for patients with chronic, irreversible NYHA class IV heart failure, with a 5-year survival of approximately 60% to 70% in well-selected patients.[117] Unfortunately, the shortage of acceptable donor hearts has resulted in an average waiting time for transplant of more than 6 months, with only about one in five approved potential recipients receiving a heart before succumbing to their disease. Another large percentage of patients is rejected from consideration for transplant because of age, concurrent illnesses, psychosocial factors, and other reasons. See Chapter 18 for additional details on cardiac transplantation. The shortage of donor hearts has prompted development of new surgical techniques, including ventricular aneurysm resection, cardiomyoplasty, and partial left ventriculectomy (Batista procedure), which have shown variable degrees of symptomatic improvement.[117] Further development of these and other techniques may offer additional options in patients unable to receive transplantation.

EVALUATION OF THERAPEUTIC OUTCOMES

CHRONIC HEART FAILURE

Although mortality is an important end point, it does not give a complete measure of the overall effects of the disease on patient outcomes because many patients are hospitalized repeatedly for heart failure exacerbations and continue to survive. Thus some of the more important therapeutic outcomes in heart failure management, such as prolonged survival or prevention or slowing of the progression of heart failure, cannot be measured in an individual patient. However, symptomatic improvement is readily evaluated in the heart failure patient. This is most readily assessed by asking patients about the presence and severity of symptoms and how their symptoms affect their activities of daily living. The cardinal signs and symptoms of heart failure are caused by excess fluid retention, and symptomatic improvement can be documented by the disappearance of these signs and symptoms (see Table 13–5). Specifically, in a patient with pulmonary congestion, monitoring is indicated for resolution of rales and pulmonary edema and improvement or resolution of DOE, orthopnea, and PND. For patients with systemic congestion, a decrease or disappearance of peripheral edema, jugular venous distension, and hepatojugular reflux is sought. Other therapeutic outcomes include an improvement in exercise tolerance and fatigue, decreased nocturia, and a decrease in heart rate. Clinicians also will want to monitor blood pressure and ensure that the patient does not develop symptomatic hypotension as a result of drug therapy. Body weight is a sensitive marker of fluid loss or retention, and patients should be counseled to weigh themselves daily, reporting changes to their health care provider so that adjustments can be made in diuretic doses. It should be noted that, particularly with β- blocker therapy, symptoms may worsen initially and that it may take weeks to months of treatment before patients notice improvement in symptoms. Also, patients and health care providers should be aware that heart failure progression may be slowed even though symptoms have not resolved.

ADVANCED/DECOMPENSATED HEART FAILURE

Assessment of adequacy of therapy in the advanced heart failure patient can be separated into two general categories: initial improvement of physiologic parameters and safe discharge from the ICU following conversion to a chronic oral therapeutic regimen. Both goals must be achieved because hemodynamic improvement has not correlated with prolonged symptom improvement or enhanced survival.

Initial stabilization requires achievement of adequate arterial oxygen saturation and content. Cardiac index and blood pressure must be sufficient to ensure adequate organ perfusion, as assessed by alert mental status, creatinine clearance sufficient to prevent metabolic azotemic complications, hepatic function adequate to maintain synthetic and excretory functions, a stable heart rate (generally between 50 and 110 beats per minute) and rhythm (predominately sinus rhythm, rate-stabilized atrial fibrillation or flutter, or paced rhythm), absence of ongoing myocardial ischemia or infarction, skeletal muscle and skin blood flow sufficient to prevent ischemic injury, and normal arterial pH (7.34 to 7.47) with a normal serum lactate concentration. Although these goals are achieved most often with a cardiac index greater than 2.2 L/min/m^2, a mean arterial blood pressure greater than 60 mm Hg, and a PAOP of 25 mm Hg or greater, the absolute values are highly variable and depend on chronicity of illness, efficacy of chronic compensatory mechanisms, previous chronic therapy, and concurrent illness.

Discharge from the ICU requires maintenance of the preceding parameters in the absence of ongoing intravenous infusion therapy, mechanical circulatory support, or positive-pressure ventilation. Some patients may achieve this goal with markedly lower blood pressure or higher filling pressure than suggested earlier; hence numerical goals cannot always be substituted for clinical status. Nonpharmacologic treatments aimed at the precipitants of a patient's heart failure exacerbation include permanent pacing, coronary angioplasty or valvuloplasty, pericardial drainage, cardiac surgery (coronary bypass, valve replacement or reconstruction, closure of intracardiac shunts), or even cardiac transplantation to achieve initial stabilization, definitive therapy, or both.

PHARMACOECONOMIC CONSIDERATIONS

Heart failure imposes a tremendous economic burden on the health care system. In patients over age 65, it is the most common reason for hospitalization, with hospital admission rates for this disorder continuing to increase. Heart failure is also associated with 30% to 50% readmission rates during the 3 to 6 months after initial discharge. In 2000, the estimated costs of heart failure treatment in the United States were greater than $56 billion.[2] The prevalence of heart failure and the costs associated with patient care are expected to increase as the population ages and as survival from ischemic heart disease is improved. Thus approaches to improve the quality and cost-effectiveness of care for these patients may have a significant impact on health care costs.

Several studies have attempted to assess the cost-effectiveness of drug therapy for heart failure. Carvedilol reduced the number of heart failure-related hospital admissions compared with placebo, resulting in a significant savings in hospital costs. The cost per life-year saved with carvedilol was $12,799, which is similar to that of other medical therapies.[118] Similar results were reported with bisoprolol, in which the costs associated with bisoprolol treatment were offset by a reduction of inpatient treatment costs for heart failure.[119] In the DIG trial, patients treated with digoxin had fewer hospitalizations for heart failure, but digoxin produced an absolute decrease of only 2.8% in hospitalizations for any cause.[63] By slowing disease progression and reducing the number of heart failure-related hospitalizations, ACE inhibitors have been shown to be cost-effective.[120,121] Similarly, captopril therapy after MI in patients with an ejection fraction of 40% or lower also was shown to be cost-effective, with cost-effectiveness of therapy increasing with increasing age.[122] While not providing direct cost estimates, number needed to treat (NNT) is often a useful index that provides a sense of the cost-effectiveness of a given therapy. In the case of the ACE inhibitors and β-blockers, the NNT to prevent one death has ranged from 7 to 20 patients for the ACE inhibitor studies (including most of the post-MI studies) and from 14 to 26 patients for the β-blocker studies. These numbers compare favorably with, and in fact are superior to, most other cardiovascular therapies. In the case of both drug classes, the benefits are greater (NNT lower) for the patients with more severe heart failure.

Several studies recently have documented the benefits of multidisciplinary specialty care of heart failure patients over conventional care. In a comparison of heart failure patients receiving conventional care versus AHCPR guideline-guided care by a multidisciplinary team (consisting of nurses, dieticians, social services personnel, and cardiologists), overall hospital readmissions for heart failure were reduced by 56% in the multidisciplinary versus conventional care groups. Quality of life also improved significantly in treatment group patients. Cost of care was reduced by $460 per patient because of the reduction in hospital admissions.[123] Similar effects on health system resource use and reductions in hospitalizations have been reported using a home monitoring system (patient education, patient self-monitoring of weight, physician notification of weight gain, etc.) for heart failure patients.[124,125] The improvement in outcome in these studies may be related to better adherence to heart failure treatment guidelines by cardiologists compared with other physicians.[126,127] The impact of this specialty care on costs is unclear because some data suggest that there is no increase in costs with specialists,[126] whereas others report that cardiologist care increases costs.[128]

The impact of a pharmacist as a member of a multidisciplinary heart failure team was described recently.[31] The investigators randomly assigned 181 heart failure patients seen in an outpatient clinic to receive either conventional treatment (control group) or pharmacist intervention that included medication evaluation and therapeutic recommendations, patient education, and follow-up telephone monitoring. The primary end point, consisting of a composite of total mortality plus hospitalizations for heart failure, was reduced significantly in the pharmacist intervention group compared with the control group (4 versus 16 events, respectively; $P < .005$). This benefit was due primarily to a reduction in hospitalization for heart failure; mortality was not different between the groups. Target ACE inhibitor doses were achieved more frequently in patients in the intervention group, and in patients intolerant to ACE inhibitors, 75% in the intervention group received alternative vasodilators compared with 26% in the control group. These results suggest that pharmacists can play an important role in improving therapeutic outcomes in heart failure patients.

The cost of treatment of heart failure is due primarily to hospital admission charges because these are reported to account for 67% to 75% of the cost of treating patients.[129] Thus efforts aimed at reducing costs of heart failure should be aimed at reducing hospitalizations. This is probably accomplished most easily through appropriate drug therapy. However, it is well documented that many heart failure patients are not treated according to consensus guidelines[126,127] or fail to receive adequate doses of medications with documented beneficial effects.[31,39,43] The role and cost benefits of pharmacist involvement in the multidisciplinary care of heart failure patients are now apparent and should include optimizing doses of heart failure drug therapy, screening for drugs that exacerbate heart failure, monitoring for adverse drug effects and drug interactions, educating patients, and patient follow-up.

▶ PRINCIPLES OF PHARMACOTHERAPY

- Heart failure is a clinical syndrome caused by the inability of the heart to pump sufficient blood to meet the metabolic needs of the body. Heart failure can result from reduced ventricular filling (diastolic dysfunction) and/or reduced myocardial contractility (systolic dysfunction).
- In patients with heart failure, a number of compensatory responses are activated in an attempt to maintain adequate cardiac output, including the SNS, increased preload, vasoconstriction, and ventricular hypertrophy/remodeling. These compensatory mechanisms are responsible for the symptoms of heart failure and contribute to disease progression.
- All patients with symptomatic heart failure should receive ACE inhibitors or appropriate alternative therapy with the goals of improving survival, slowing disease progression, reducing hospitalizations, and improving quality of life. When ACE inhibitors are contraindicated or not tolerated, the combination of hydralazine and isosorbide dinitrate or an angiotensin II receptor blocker is a reasonable alternative. Doses for these drugs should be targeted at those shown in clinical trials to improve survival. Patients with asymptomatic left ventricular dysfunction also should be treated with ACE inhibitors, with the goal of preventing symptomatic heart failure and reducing mortality.
- β-Blockers are recommended for all patients with systolic dysfunction and mild to moderate heart failure. They also should be considered for patients with severe heart failure symptoms. They have been shown to prolong survival, decrease hospitalizations and need for transplantation, and cause "reverse remodeling" of the left ventricle. They must be instituted at low doses, with slow upward titration to the target dose.
- Although chronic diuretic therapy frequently is used in heart failure patients, it is not mandatory and is required only in those patients with peripheral edema and/or pulmonary congestion.
- Digoxin does not improve survival in patients with heart failure but does provide symptomatic benefits, particularly in patients with moderate and severe heart failure. Given its lack of effect on mortality, it should not be considered first-line therapy automatically in patients in normal sinus rhythm, particularly if

such use would preclude use of agents with mortality-reducing effects (e.g., β-blockers). Digoxin doses should be adjusted to achieve plasma concentrations of approximately 1 ng/mL; higher plasma concentrations are not associated with additional benefits but may be associated with increased risk of toxicity. Digoxin should be considered standard therapy in patients with heart failure and supraventricular tachyarrhythmias because it will help control the ventricular response rate.

- Aldosterone antagonism with low-dose spironolactone has been shown to reduce mortality in patients with class III and IV heart failure. Given its low cost and safety profile at the doses studied, it may be reasonable to consider in all patients with symptomatic heart failure and should be considered strongly in patients with severe heart failure.
- No therapy for advanced/decompensated heart failure studied to date has been shown conclusively to influence mortality. Treatment goals are directed toward restoration of systemic oxygen transport and tissue perfusion, relief of pulmonary edema, and limitation of further cardiac damage. Maximizing oral therapy and using combinations of short-acting intravenous medications with different cardiovascular actions are often needed to optimize cardiac output, relieve pulmonary edema, and limit myocardial ischemia. Invasive hemodynamic monitoring usually is required to provide immediate feedback on treatment efficacy and adverse effects.
- Pharmacists should play an important role as part of a multidisciplinary team to optimize therapy in heart failure. The pharmacist should be responsible for such activities as optimizing regimens for heart failure drug therapy (namely, ensuring that appropriate drugs at appropriate doses are used), educating patients about the importance of adherence to their heart failure regimen (including pharmacologic and dietary interventions), screening for drugs that may exacerbate or worsen heart failure, and monitoring for adverse drug effects and drug interactions.

REFERENCES

1. Colucci WS, Braunwald E. Pathophysiology of congestive heart failure. In: Braunwald E, ed. Heart Disease: A Textbook of Cardiovascular Medicine. Philadelphia: Saunders, 1997:394–420.
2. O'Connell JB. The economic burden of heart failure. Clin Cardiol 2000;23:III6–10.
3. Sharpe N, Doughty R. Epidemiology of heart failure and ventricular dysfunction. Lancet 1998;352(Suppl 1):SI3–7.
4. Wynne J, Braunwald E. The cardiomyopathies and myocarditides. In: Braunwald E, ed. Heart Disease: A Textbook of Cardiovascular Medicine. Philadelphia: Saunders; 1997:1404–1463.
5. Ho KK, Pinsky JL, Kannel WB, Levy D. The epidemiology of heart failure: The Framingham Study. J Am Coll Cardiol 1993;22:6A–13A.
6. Opie LH. Normal and abnormal contraction and relaxation. In: Braunwald E, ed. Heart Disease: A Textbook of Cardiovascular Medicine. Philadelphia: Saunders; 1997:360–393.
7. Mann DL. Mechanisms and models in heart failure: A combinatorial approach. Circulation 1999;100:999–1008.
8. Cohn JN, Ferrari R, Sharpe N. Cardiac remodeling—Concepts and clinical implications: A consensus paper from an international forum on cardiac remodeling. On behalf of an International Forum on Cardiac Remodeling. J Am Coll Cardiol 2000;35:569–582.
9. Colucci WS. The effects of norepinephrine on myocardial biology: Implications for the therapy of heart failure. Clin Cardiol 1998;21:120–124.
10. Colucci WS, Sawyer DB, Singh K, Communal C. Adrenergic overload and apoptosis in heart failure: Implications for therapy [In process citation]. J Card Fail 2000;6:1–7.
11. Richards AM, Nicholls MG. Aldosterone antagonism in heart failure. Lancet 1999;354:789–90.
12. Lijnen P, Petrov V. Induction of cardiac fibrosis by aldosterone. J Mol Cell Cardiol 2000;32:865–879.
13. Pitt B, Zannad F, Remme WJ, et al. The effect of spironolactone on morbidity and mortality in patients with severe heart failure. Randomized Aldactone Evaluation Study Investigators. N Engl J Med 1999;341: 709–717.
14. Feldman AM, Combes A, Wagner D, et al. The role of tumor necrosis factor in the pathophysiology of heart failure. J Am Coll Cardiol 2000;35:537–544.
15. Bozkurt B, Torre-Amione G, Warren MS, et al. Results of targeted anti-tumor necrosis factor therapy with etanercept (Enbrel) in patients with advanced heart failure. Circulation 2001;103:1044–1047.
16. Miyauchi T, Goto K. Heart failure and endothelin receptor antagonists. Trends Pharmacol Sci 1999;20:210–217.
17. Weber M. Emerging treatments for hypertension: potential role for vasopeptidase inhibition. Am J Hypertens 1999;12:139S–147S.
18. Chen HH, Burnett JC Jr. The natriuretic peptides in heart failure: Diagnostic and therapeutic potentials. Proc Assoc Am Phys 1999;111:406–416.
19. Colucci WS, Elkayam U, Horton DP, et al. Intravenous nesiritide, a natriuretic peptide, in the treatment of decompensated congestive heart failure. N Engl J Med 2000;343:246–253.
20. Michalsen A, Konig G, Thimme W. Preventable causative factors leading to hospital admission with decompensated heart failure. Heart 1998;80:437–441.
21. Swan SK, Rudy DW, Lasseter KC, et al. Effect of cyclooxygenase-2 inhibition on renal function in elderly persons receiving a low-salt diet: A randomized, controlled trial. Ann Intern Med 2000;133:1–9.
22. Braunwald E, Colucci WS, Grossman W. Clinical aspects of heart failure: High output heart failure—Pulmonary edema. In: Braunwald E, ed. Heart Disease: A Textbook of Cardiovascular Medicine. Philadelphia: Saunders; 1997:445–470.
23. Konstam MA, Dracup K, Baker DW, et al. Heart Failure: Evaluation and Care of Patients with Left-Ventricular Systolic Dysfunction. Rockville, MD: U.S. Department of Health and Human Services; 1994.
24. Vantrimpont P, Rouleau JL. Medical treatment of heart failure: The Canadian Cardiovascular Society's Consensus Conference revisited. Cardiovasc Drugs Ther 1997;10:711–716.
25. Packer M, Cohn JN. Consensus recommendations for the management of chronic heart failure. Am J Cardiol 1999;83:1A–38A.
26. American College of Cardiology/American Heart Association Task Force on Practice Guidelines. Guidelines for the evaluation and management of heart failure. Circulation 1995;92:2764–2784.
27. Task Force of the Working Group on Heart Failure of the European Society of Cardiology. The treatment of heart failure. Eur Heart J 1997;18:736–753.
28. Guideline Committee for the Heart Failure Society of America. HFSA guidelines for the management of patients with heart failure caused by left ventricular systolic dysfunction: Pharmacological approaches. J Card Fail 1999;5:357–382.
29. American College of Cardiology/American Heart Association Task Force on Practice Guidelines. ACC/AHA guidelines for the evaluation and management of chronic heart failure in the adult. Circulation 2001; 38:2101–2113.
30. Patterson JH, Adams KF Jr. Understanding the management of heart failure. Pharmacotherapy 2000;20:493–494.
31. Gattis WA, Hasselblad V, Whellan DJ, O'Connor CM. Reduction in heart failure events by the addition of a clinical pharmacist to the heart failure management team. Arch Intern Med 1999;159:1939–1945.
32. Braith RW. Exercise training in patients with CHF and heart transplant recipients. Med Sci Sports Exerc 1998;30:S367–S378.
33. Garg R, Yusuf S, for the Collaborative Group on ACE Inhibitor Trials. Overview of randomized trials of angiotensin-converting enzyme

inhibitors on mortality and morbidity in patients with heart failure. JAMA 1995;273:1450–1456.

34. Flather MD, Yusuf S, Kober L, et al., for the ACE-Inhibitor Myocardial Infarction Collaborative Group. Long-term ACE-inhibitor therapy in patients with heart failure or left-ventricular dysfunction: A systematic overview of data from individual patients. Lancet 2000;355:1575–1581.
35. The CONSENSUS Trial Study Group. Effects of enalapril on mortality in severe congestive heart failure: Results of the Cooperative North Scandinavian Enalapril Survival Study. N Engl J Med 1987;316:1429–1435.
36. Cohn JN, Johnson G, Ziesche S, et al. A comparison of enalapril with hydralazine-isosorbide dinitrate in the treatment of chronic congestive heart failure. N Engl J Med 1991;325:303–310.
37. The SOLVD Investigators. Effect of enalapril on mortality and the development of heart failure in asymptomatic patients with reduced left ventricular ejection fractions. N Engl J Med 1992;327:685–691.
38. ACE Inhibitor Myocardial Infarction Collaborative Group. Indications for ACE inhibitors in the early treatment of acute myocardial infarction: Systematic overview of individual data from 100,000 patients in randomized trials. Circulation 1998;97:2202–2212.
39. Stafford RS, Saglam D, Blumenthal D. National patterns of angiotensin-converting enzyme inhibitor use in congestive heart failure. Arch Intern Med 1997;157:2460–2464.
40. Echemann M, Zannad F, Briancon S, and the EPICAL Investigators. Determinants of angiotensin-converting enzyme inhibitor prescription in severe heart failure with left ventricular systolic dysfunction: The EPICAL Study. Am Heart J 2000;139:624–631.
41. Roe CM, Motheral BR, Teitelbaum F, Rich MW. Angiotensin-converting enzyme inhibitor compliance and dosing among patients with heart failure. Am Heart J 1999;138:818–825.
42. Frances CD, Noguchi H, Massie BM, et al. Are we inhibited? Renal insufficiency should not preclude the use of ACE inhibitors for patients with myocardial infarction and depressed left ventricular function. Arch Intern Med 2000;160:2645–2650.
43. Packer M, Poole-Wilson PA, Armstrong PW, et al. Comparative effects of low and high doses of the angiotensin-converting enzyme inhibitor, lisinopril, on morbidity and mortality in chronic heart failure. ATLAS Study Group. Circulation 1999;100:2312–2318.
44. Brown N, Vaughan D. Angiotensin-converting enzyme inhibitors. Circulation 1998;97:1411–1420.
45. Mann DL. Mechanisms and models in heart failure: A combinatorial approach. Circulation 1999;100:999–1008.
46. Sutton MSJ, Sharpe N. Left ventricular remodeling after myocardial infarction: Pathophysiology and therapy. Circulation 2000;101:2981–2988.
47. Rouleau JL, Pfeffer MA, Stewart DJ, et al., for the IMPRESS Investigators. Comparison of vasopeptidase inhibitor, omapatrilat, and lisinopril on exercise tolerance and morbidity in patients with heart failure: IMPRESS randomized trial. Lancet 2000;356:615–620.
48. Messerli FH, Nussberger J. Vasopeptidase inhibition and angio-oedema. Lancet 2000;356:608–609.
49. Packer M, Bristow MR, Cohn JN, et al. The effect of carvedilol on morbidity and mortality in patients with chronic heart failure. U.S. Carvedilol Heart Failure Study Group. N Engl J Med 1996;334:1349–1355.
50. The Cardiac Insufficiency Bisoprolol Study II (CIBIS-II): A randomised trial. Lancet 1999;353:9–13.
51. Effect of metoprolol CR/XL in chronic heart failure: Metoprolol CR/XL Randomised Intervention Trial in Congestive Heart Failure (MERIT-HF). Lancet 1999;353:2001–2007.
52. Packer M, Coats AJS, Fowler MB, et al. Effect of carvedilol on survival in severe chronic heart Failure. N Engl J Med 2001; 344:1651–1658.
53. Bristow MR. Mechanistic and clinical rationales for using beta-blockers in heart failure. J Card Fail 2000;6:8–14.
54. Bristow MR, Gilbert EM, Abraham WT, et al. Carvedilol produces dose-related improvements in left ventricular function and survival in subjects with chronic heart failure. MOCHA Investigators. Circulation 1996;94:2807–2816.
55. Hjalmarson A, Goldstein S, Fagerberg B, et al. Effects of controlled-release metoprolol on total mortality, hospitalizations, and well-being in patients with heart failure: The Metoprolol CR/XL Randomized Intervention Trial in congestive heart failure (MERIT-HF). MERIT-HF Study Group. JAMA 2000;283:1295–1302.
56. Krum H, Sackner-Bernstein JD, Goldsmith RL, et al. Double-blind, placebo-controlled study of the long-term efficacy of carvedilol in patients with severe chronic heart failure. Circulation 1995;92:1499–1506.
57. Kukin ML, Kalman J, Charney RH, et al. Prospective, randomized comparison of effect of long-term treatment with metoprolol or carvedilol on symptoms, exercise, ejection fraction, and oxidative stress in heart failure. Circulation 1999;99:2645–2651.
58. Metra M, Giubbini R, Nodari S, et al. Differential effects of beta-blockers in patients with heart failure: A prospective, randomized, double-blind comparison of the long-term effects of metoprolol versus carvedilol. Circulation 2000;102:546–551.
58a. The beta-blocker evaluation of survival trial investigators: A trial of the beta-blocker bucindolol in patients with advanced chronic heart failure. N Engl J Med 2001;344:1659–1667.
59. Willette RN, Aiyar N, Yue TL, et al. In vitro and in vivo characterization of intrinsic sympathomimetic activity in normal and heart failure rats. J Pharmacol Exp Ther 1999;289:48–53.
60. Brater DC. Pharmacology of diuretics. Am J Med Sci 2000;319:38–50.
61. Kramer BK, Schweda F, Riegger GA. Diuretic treatment and diuretic resistance in heart failure. Am J Med 1999;106:90–96.
62. Follath F. Do diuretics differ in terms of clinical outcome in congestive heart failure? Eur Heart J 1998;19(Suppl P):5–8.
63. The Digitalis Investigation Group. The effect of digoxin on mortality and morbidity in patients with heart failure. N Engl J Med 1997;336:525–533.
64. Smith T, Kelly R, Stevenson L, Braunwald E. The management of heart failure. In: Braunwald E, ed. Heart Disease: A Textbook of Cardiovascular Medicine. Philadelphia: Saunders; 1997:492–514.
65. Hauptman P, Kelly R. Digitalis. Circulation 1999;99:1265–1270.
66. Packer M, Gheorghiade M, Young J, et al. Withdrawal of digoxin from patients with chronic heart failure treated with angiotensin-converting enzyme inhibitors. N Engl J Med 1993;329:1–7.
67. The Captopril-Digoxin Multicenter Research Group. Comparative effects of therapy with captopril and digoxin in patients with mild to moderate heart failure. JAMA 1988;259:539–544.
68. Uretsky B, Young JB, Shahidi FE, et al. Randomized study assessing the effect of digoxin withdrawal in patients with mild to moderate chronic congestive heart failure: Results of the PROVED trial. J Am Coll Cardiol 1993;22:955–962.
69. Young J, Gheorghiade M, Uretsky B, et al. Superiority of "triple" drug therapy in heart failure: Insights from the PROVED and RADIANCE trials. J Am Coll Cardiol 1998;32:686–692.
70. Adams KF, Gheorghiade M, Uretsky BF, et al. Patients with mild heart failure worsen during withdrawal from digoxin therapy. J Am Coll Cardiol 1997;30:42–48.
71. Adams KF, Gheorghiade M, Uretsky BF, et al. Clinical predictors of worsening heart failure during withdrawal from digoxin therapy. Am Heart J 1998;135:389–397.
72. Gheorghiade M, Hall VB, Jacobsen G, et al. Effects of increasing maintenance doses of digoxin on left ventricular function and neurohormones in patients with chronic heart failure treated with diuretics and angiotensin-converting enzyme inhibitors. Circulation 1995;92:1801–1807.
73. Slatton ML, Irani WN, Hall SA, et al. Does digoxin provide additional hemodynamic and autonomic benefits in patients with mild to moderate heart failure and normal sinus rhythm? J Am Coll Cardiol 1997;29:1206–1213.
74. Reuning RH, Geraets DR, Rocci ML, Vlasses PH. Digoxin. In: Evans WE, Schentag JJ, Jusko WJ, eds. Applied Pharmacokinetics: Principles of Therapeutic Drug Monitoring. Spokane, WA: Applied Therapeutics, 1992:20–1–20–48.
75. Sutton MSJ, Pfeffer MA, Moye L, et al. Cardiovascular death and left ventricular remodeling two years after myocardial infarction: Baseline predictors and impact of long-term use of captopril. Information from the Survival and Ventricular Enlargement (SAVE) trial. Circulation 1997;96:3294–3299.

76. Goodfriend TL, Elliot ME, Catt KJ. Angiotensin receptors and their antagonists. N Engl J Med 1996;334:1649–1654.
77. Burnier M, Brunner HR. Angiotensin II receptor antagonists. Lancet 2000;355:637–645.
78. Presented Val-HEFT, American Heart Association, New Orleans, LA, 2000.
79. Dickstein K, Chang P, Willenheimer R, et al. Comparison of the effects of losartan and enalapril on clinical status and exercise performance in patients with moderate or severe heart failure. J Am Coll Cardiol 1995;26:438–445.
80. Hamroff G, Katz SD, Mancini D, et al. Addition of angiotensin II receptor blockade to maximal angiotensin-converting enzyme inhibition improves exercise capacity in patients with severe congestive heart failure. Circulation 1999;99:990–992.
81. Pitt B, Segal R, Martinez FA, et al. Randomised trial of losartan versus captopril in patients over 65 with heart failure (Evaluation of Losartan in The Elderly study, ELITE). Lancet 1997;349:747–752.
82. Pitt B, Poole-Wilson PA, Segal R, et al. Effect of losartan compared with captopril on mortality in patients with symptomatic heart failure: Randomised trial. The Losartan Heart Failure Survival Study ELITE II. Lancet 2000;355:1582–1587.
83. Rijnsoever EWv, Kwee-Zuiderwijk WJM, Feenstra J. Angioneurotic edema attributed to use of losartan. Arch Intern Med 1998;158:2063–2065.
84. Kelly RA, Smith TW. Pharmacologic treatment of heart failure. In: Hardman JG, Limbird LE, Molinoff PB, et al., eds. Goodman and Gilman's Pharmacological Basis of Therapeutics, 9th ed. New York: McGraw Hill; 1996:875–898.
85. Calderone A, Thaik CM, Takahashi N, et al. Nitric oxide, atrial natriuretic peptide, and cyclic GMP inhibit the growth-promoting effects of norepinephrine in cardiac myocytes and fibroblasts. J Clin Invest 1998;101:812–818.
86. Munzel T, Kurz S, Rajagopalan S, et al. Hydralazine prevents nitroglycerin tolerance by inhibiting activation of a membrane-bound NADH oxidase: A new action for an old drug. J Clin Invest 1996;98:1465–1470.
87. Cohn JN, Archibald DG, Ziesche S, et al. Effect of vasodilator therapy on mortality in chronic congestive heart failure: Results of the Veterans Administration Cooperative Study. N Engl J Med 1986;316:1547–1552.
88. Singh SN, Fletcher RD. Class III drugs and congestive heart failure: Focus on the congestive heart failure: Survival trial of antiarrhythmic therapy. Am J Cardiol 1999;84:103R–108R.
89. de Vries RJ, van Veldhuisen DJ, Dunselman PH. Efficacy and safety of calcium channel blockers in heart failure: Focus on recent trials with second-generation dihydropyridines. Am Heart J 2000;139:185–194.
90. Movsesian MA. Beta adrenergic receptor agonists and cyclic nucleotide phosphodiesterase inhibitors: Shifting the focus from inotropy to cyclic adenosine monophosphate. J Am Coll Cardiol 1999;34:318–324.
91. Al-Khadra AS, Salem DN, Rand WM, et al. Antiplatelet agents and survival: A cohort analysis from the Studies of Left Ventricular Dysfunction (SOLVD) trial. J Am Coll Cardiol 1998;31:419–425.
92. Nguyen KN, Aursnes I, Kjekshus J. Interaction between enalapril and aspirin on mortality after acute myocardial infarction: Subgroup analysis of the Cooperative New Scandinavian Enlaparil Survival Study II (CONSENSUS II). Am J Cardiol 1997;79:115–119.
93. Latini R, Tognoni G, Maggioni AP, Parker RB, on behalf of the Angiotensin-converting Enzyme Inhibitor Myocardial Infarction Collaborative Group. Clinical effects of early angiotensin-converting enzyme inhibitor treatment for acute myocardial infarction are similar in the presence and absence of aspirin. J Am Coll Cardiol 2000;35:1801 1807.
94. Leor J, Reicher-Reiss H, Goldbourt U, et al. Aspirin and mortality in patients treated with angiotensin-converting enzyme inhibitors. J Am Coll Cardiol 1999;33:1920–1925.
95. Nawarskas JJ, Spinler SA. Does aspirin interfere with therapeutic efficacy of angiotensin-converting enzyme inhibitors in hypertension or congestive heart failure? Pharmacotherapy 1998;18:1041 1052.
96. The SOLVD Investigators. Effect of enalapril on survival in patients with reduced left ventricular ejection fractions and congestive heart failure. N Engl J Med 1991;325:293–302.
97. Lundborg P, Abrahamsson B, Wieselgren I, Walter M. The pharmacokinetics and pharmacodynamics of metoprolol after conventional and controlled-release administration in combination with hydrochlorothiazide in healthy volunteers. Eur J Clin Pharmacol 1993;45:161–163.
98. vanVeldhuisen DJ, deGraeff PA, Remme WJ, Lie KI. Value of digoxin in heart failure and sinus rhythm: New features of an old drug? J Am Coll Cardiol 1996;28:813–819.
99. Krum H, Bigger JT, Goldsmith RL, Packer M. Effect of long-term digoxin therapy on autonomic function in patients with chronic heart failure. J Am Coll Cardiol 1995;25:289–294.
100. Spargias KS, Hall AS, Ball SG. Safety concerns about digoxin after acute myocardial infarction. Lancet 1999;354:391–392.
101. Kober L, Torp-Pedersen C, Gadsoll N, et al. Is digoxin an independent risk factor for long-term mortality after acute myocardial infarction? Eur Heart J 1994;15:382–388.
102. Stevenson LW, Massie BM, Francis GS. Optimizing therapy for complex or refractory heart failure: A management algorithm. Am Heart J 1998;135:S293–S309.
103. Schulman KA, Mark DB, Califf RM. Outcomes and costs within a disease management program for advanced congestive heart failure. Am Heart J 1998;135:S285–S292.
104. Connors AF, Jr., Speroff T, Dawson NV, et al. The effectiveness of right heart catheterization in the initial care of critically ill patients. SUPPORT Investigators. JAMA 1996;276:889–897.
105. Forrester JS, Diamond G, Chatterjee K, Swan HJC. Medical therapy of acute myocardial infarction by application of hemodynamic subsets. N Engl J Med 1976;295:1356–1362.
106. Francis GS, Siegel RM, Goldsmith SR, et al. Acute vasoconstrictor response to intravenous furosemide in patients with chronic congestive heart failure. Ann Intern Med 1985;103:1–6.
107. Kraus PA, Lipman J, Becker PJ. Acute preload effects of furosemide. Chest 1990;98:124–128.
108. Brater DC. Diuretic therapy in congestive heart failure. CHF 2000;6: 197–210.
109. Vargo DL, Brater DC, Rudy DW, Swan SK. Dopamine does not enhance furosemide-induced natriuresis in patients with congestive heart failure. J Am Soc Nephrol 1996;7:1032–1037.
110. Dorman TPJ, van Meyel JJM, Gerlag PGG, et al. Diuretic efficaccy of high dose furosemide in severe heart failure: bolus injection versus continuous infusion. J Am Coll Cardiol 1996;28:376–382.
111. Leier CV, Binkley PF. Parenteral inotropic support for advanced congestive heart failure. Prog Cardiovasc Dis 1998;41:207–224.
112. Dies F, Krell MJ, Whitlow P, et al. Intermittent dobutamine in ambulatory outpatients with chronic heart failure [Abstract]. Circulation 1986;74:II–138.
113. Kirsten R, Nelson K, Kirsten D, Heintz B. Clinical pharmacokinetics of vasodilators (part II). Clin Pharmacokinet 1998;35:9–36.
114. Bellomo R, Cole L, Ronco C. Hemodynamic support and the role of dopamine. Kidney Int 1998;53:S71–S74.
115. Elkayam U, Kulick D, McIntosh N, et al. Incidence of early tolerance to hemodynamic effects of continuous infusion of nitroglycerin in patients with coronary heart disease and heart failure. Circulation 1987;76:577–588.
116. Richenbacher WE, Pierce WS. Assisted circulation and mechanical heart. In: Braunwald E, ed. Heart Disease: A Textbook of Cardiovascular Medicine. Philadelphia: Saunders; 1997:534–547.
117. Uretsky BF, Pina I, Quigg RJ, et al. Beyond drug therapy: nonpharmacologic care of the patient with advanced heart failure. Am Heart J 1998;135:S264–S284.
118. Delea TE, Vera-Llonch M, Richner RE, et al. Cost-effectiveness of carvedilol for heart failure. Am J Cardiol 1999;83.890–896.
119. Malek M, Cunningham Davis J, Malek L, et al. A cost minimisation analysis of cardiac failure treatment in the UK using CIBIS Trial data. Int J Clin Pract 1999;53:19–23.
120. Szucs TD. Pharmacoeconomics of angiotensin converting enzyme inhibitors in heart failure. Am J Hypertens 1997;10(pt 2):272S–279S.
121. McMurray J, Davie A. The pharmacoeconomics of ACE inhibitors in chronic heart failure. Pharmacoeconomics 1996;3:188–197.

122. Tsevat J, Duke D, Goldman L, et al. Cost-effectiveness of captopril therapy after myocardial infarction. J Am Coll Cardiol 1995;26:914–919.
123. Rich MW, Beckham V, Wittenberg C, et al. A multidisciplinary intervention to prevent the readmission of elderly patients with congestive heart failure. N Engl J Med 1995;333:1190–1195.
124. Stewart S, Marley JE, Horowitz JD. Effects of a multidisciplinary, home-based intervention on planned readmissions and survival among patients with chronic congestive heart failure: A randomised controlled study. Lancet 1999;354:1077–1083.
125. Heidenreich PA, Ruggerio CM, Massie BM. Effect of a home monitoring system on hospitalization and resource use for patients with heart failure. Am Heart J 1999;138:633–640.
126. Philbin EF, Jenkins PL. Differences between patients with heart failure treated by cardiologists, internists, family physicians, and other physicians: Analysis of a large, statewide database. Am Heart J 2000;139:491–496.
127. Baker DW, Hayes RP, Massie BM, Craig CA. Variations in family physicians' and cardiologists' care for patients with heart failure. Am Heart J 1999;138:826–834.
128. Auerbach AD, Hamel MB, Davis RB, et al. Resource use and survival of patients hospitalized with congestive heart failure: Differences in care by specialty of the attending physician. Ann Intern Med 2000;132:191–200.
129. McMurray J, Hart W, Rhodes G. An evaluation of the cost of heart failure to the National Health Service in the UK. Br J Med Econ 1993;6:99–110.

14

ISCHEMIC HEART DISEASE

Robert L. Talbert

There is a disorder of the breast, marked with strong and peculiar symptoms, considerable for the kind of danger belonging to it, and not extremely rare, of which I do not recollect any mention among medical authors. The seat of it and sense of strangling and anxiety with which it is attended may make it not improper to be called angina pectoris.

Some Account of a Disorder of the Breast
William Heberden, 1768

Although Heberden did not understand the pathogenesis of ischemic heart disease (IHD), which is also known as coronary artery disease (CAD), it is now appreciated that atherosclerosis of the epicardial vessels is the main etiology of IHD. This process begins early in life, often not being clinically manifest until the middle-aged years and beyond. IHD may present as an acute coronary syndrome (which includes unstable angina and non-ST-segment-elevation myocardial infarction (NSTEMI) or ST-segment-elevation myocardial infarction and myocardial infarction (MI) diagnosed by biomarkers only), chronic stable exertional angina pectoris, and ischemia without clinical symptoms or due to coronary artery vasospasm (variant or Prinzmetal's angina). Other manifestations of atherosclerosis include heart failure, arrhythmias, cerebrovascular disease (stroke), and peripheral vascular disease. The American Heart Association (AHA) recently has published management guidelines for stable and unstable angina.[1,2]

EPIDEMIOLOGY

The syndrome of angina pectoris is reported to occur with an average annual incidence rate (number of new cases per time period divided by the total number of persons in the population for the same time period) of about 1.5% (range 0.1 to 5 per 1000) depending on the patient's age, gender, and risk factor profile.[3] The presenting manifestation in women is more commonly angina, whereas men more frequently have MI as the initial event. Estimates of the incidence and prevalence of angina are not entirely accurate owing to waxing and waning of symptoms; angina may disappear in up to 30% of patients with angina that is less severe and of recent onset.

Cardiovascular diseases (CVD) claimed 949,619 lives, or 1 of every 2.5 deaths, in the United States in 1998.[4] More than 2600 Americans die of CVD each day, or on average 1 death every 33 seconds. In 1998, the death rates from CVD were 532.0 (per 100,000) for black males, 419.3 for white males, 400.7 for black females, and 294.9 for white females.[4] CAD was responsible for 48% (459,841) of deaths from CVD. Men die earlier from IHD and acute MI than women, and aging of both sexes is associated with a higher incidence of these afflictions. The disparity in mortality from IHD between men and women decreases with aging, being about four to five times more common in men from the mid-30s to a preponderance of female deaths in the very elderly.

Data from the Framingham Study show that the prevalence was 5.9% for the 16-year period studied from earlier reports.[5] More recent data from the Framingham Study show that the prevalence in a 1970 cohort followed for 10 years was about 1.5% for women and 4.3% for men aged 50 to 59 years at inception.[3] The AHA estimates that the prevalence of angina was 6.4 million in 1998.[4] Other interesting trends noted included a 21% decline in the incidence of CVD in women but only a 6% decline in men over two cohorts from 1950 and 1970. CVD mortality was reduced by 59% in women and 53% in men from the same cohorts. The risk of developing IHD is not the same worldwide. Countries such as Japan and France are on the low end of the spectrum, whereas Finland, Northern Ireland, Scotland, and South Africa have very high rates of IHD.[6,7]

Angina may be classified according to symptom severity, disability induced, or a specific activity scale (Tables 14–1 and 14–2). The specific activity scale developed by Goldman and coworkers[8] may be preferable because it has been shown to be equal to or better than the New York Heart Association or Canadian Cardiovascular Society functional classifications for reproducibility and provides better agreement with treadmill testing.

An important determinate of outcome for the angina patient is the number of vessels obstructed. Twelve-year survival from the Coronary Artery Surgery Study (CASS) for patients with zero-, one-, two-, and three-vessel disease was 88%, 74%, 59%, and 40%, respectively.[9] Other factors that increase the risk of death in medically managed patients include the presence of heart failure (or markers such as poor ventricular wall motion and low ejection fraction), smoking, left main or left main equivalent CAD, diabetes, or prior MI. Twelve-year survival for patients with at least one diseased vessel and ejection fractions in the ranges of 50% to 100%, 35% to 49%, and 0% to 34% is 73%, 54%, and 21%, respectively. Of particular note, patients with left main CAD (or left main equivalent) are at extremely high risk and constitute a unique group for therapeutic consideration.[10] In the CASS, at 15 years of follow-up, 37% of the surgery group and 27% of the medical group are surviving; median survival is 13.3 versus 6.7 years, respectively ($P < .0001$). If systolic function was normal, then median survival and percentage surviving were not different between the surgery and medical groups (median survival of about 15 years). Patients screened but not randomized to CASS had similar survival rates, suggesting that results from randomized patients may be applicable to more generalized populations as a measure of external reliability. Other factors that predict outcome in acute coronary syndrome include age, heart rate, systolic blood pressure, ST-segment depression, signs of heart failure, and cardiac enzymes.[11]

PATHOPHYSIOLOGY

The pathophysiology that underlies this disease process is dynamic, evolutionary, and complex. An understanding of the determinants of myocardial oxygen demand (MVO_2), regulation of coronary blood flow, the effects of ischemia on the mechanical and metabolic function

TABLE 14–1. Criteria for Determination of the Specific Activity Scale Functional Class[a]

	Any Yes	No
1. Can you walk down a flight of steps without stopping (4.5–5.2 MET)?	Go to 2	Go to 4
2. Can you carry anything up a flight of 8 steps without stopping (5–5.5 MET)? Or can you:	Go to 3	Class III
a. Have sexual intercourse without stopping (5–5.5 MET)		
b. Garden, rake, weed (5.6 MET)		
c. Roller skate, dance fox trot (5–6 MET)		
d. Walk at a 4 mi/h rate on level ground (5–6 MET)		
3. Can you carry at least 24 lb up 8 steps (10 MET)? Or can you:	Class I	Class II
a. Carry objects that weigh at least 80 lb (18 MET)		
b. Do outdoor work, shovel snow, spade soil (7 MET)		
c. Do recreational activites such as skiing, basketball, touch football, squash, handball (7–10 MET)		
d. Jog/walk 5 mi/h (9 MET)		
4. Can you shower without stopping (3.6–4.2 MET)? Or can you:	Class III	Go to 5
a. Strip and make bed (3.9–5 MET)		
b. Mop floors (4.2 MET)		
c. Hang washed clothes (4.4 MET)		
d. Clean windows (3.7 MET)		
e. Walk 2.5 mi/h (3–3.5 MET)		
f. Bowl (3–4.4 MET)		
g. Play golf, walk and carry clubs (4.5 MET)		
h. Push power lawn mower (4 MET)		
5. Can you dress without stopping because of symptoms (2–2.3 MET)?	Class III	Class IV

[a]MET, metabolic equivalents of activity.

From Goldman L, Hashimoto B, Cook F, et al. Comparative reproducibility and validity of systems for assessing cardiovascular functional class: Advantages of a new specific activity scale. Circulation 1981;64:1228, with permission.

of the myocardium, and how ischemia is recognized is important to an understanding of the rationale for the selection and use of pharmacotherapy for IHD.

Ischemia may be defined as lack of oxygen and decreased or no blood flow to the myocardium. In contrast, *anoxia*, defined as the absence of oxygen to the myocardium, results in continued perfusion with washout of acid by-products of glycolysis, thereby preserving the mechanical and metabolic status of the heart to a greater extent than does ischemia for short periods of time.

TABLE 14–2. Grading of Angina Pectoris by the Canadian Cardiovascular Society Classification System

Class	Description of Stage
Class I	Ordinary physical activity does not cause angina, such as walking, climbing stairs. Angina occurs with strenuous, rapid, or prolonged exertion at work or recreation.
Class II	Slight limitation or ordinary activity. Angina occurs on walking or climbing stairs rapidly, walking uphill, walking or stair climbing after meals, or in cold, or in wind, or under emotional stress, or only during the few hours after wakening. Walking more than two blocks on the level and climbing more than one flight of ordinary stairs at a normal pace and in normal condition.
Class III	Marked limitations of ordinary physical activity. Angina occurs on walking one to two blocks on the level and climbing one flight of stairs in normal conditions and at a normal pace.
Class IV	Inability to carry on any physical activity without discomform-anginal symptoms may be present at rest.

From Campeau L. Grading of angina (letter). Circulation 1976;54:522–523, with permission.

DETERMINANTS OF OXYGEN DEMAND (MVO_2)

The major determinants of MVO_2 are (1) heart rate, (2) contractility, and (3) intramyocardial wall tension during systole. Overall, intramyocardial wall tension is thought to be the most important among these three factors. Since the consequences of IHD are a result of increased demand in the face of a fixed supply of oxygen in most situations, alterations in MVO_2 are critically important in producing ischemia and for interventions intended to alleviate ischemia. MVO_2 cannot be measured directly in patients; however, an indirect assessment that correlates reasonably well with MVO_2 as determined in experimental animal models is the tension-time index (TTI). This is a measure of the area under the curve of the left ventricular (LV) pressure curve. Tension in the ventricle wall is a function of the radius of the LV and intraventricular pressure. These factors are related through Laplace's law, which states that wall stress is related directly to the product of intraventricular pressure and internal radius and inversely to wall thickness multiplied by a factor of 2. Increasing systemic blood pressure or ventricular dilatation would increase wall tension and oxygen demand, whereas ventricular hypertrophy would tend to minimize increasing MVO_2. Clinical application of these principles has led to the use of the double product (DP), which is heart rate (HR) multiplied by systolic blood pressure (SBP) (that is, $DP = HR \times SBP$). Although this is a clinically useful indirect estimate of MVO_2, it does not consider changes in contractility (an independent variable), and because only changes in pressure are considered with the double product, volume loading of the LV and increased MVO_2 related to ventricular dilatation are underestimated.

REGULATION OF CORONARY BLOOD FLOW

Coronary blood flow is influenced by multiple factors; however, the caliber of the resistance vessels delivering blood to the myocardium and MVO_2 are the prime determinants in the occurrence of ischemia. The anatomy of the vascular bed will affect oxygen supply and, subsequently, myocardial metabolism and mechanical function.

ANATOMIC FACTORS

The normal coronary system (see Fig. 14–1 for normal anatomy) consists of large epicardial or surface vessels (R_1) that normally offer little intrinsic resistance to myocardial flow and intramyocardial arteries and arterioles (R_2), which branch into a dense capillary network (about 4000 capillaries per mm^2) to supply basal blood flow of 60 to 90 mL/min per 100 g of myocardium (Fig. 14–2). R_1 and R_2 are in series, and total resistance is the algebraic sum; however, under normal

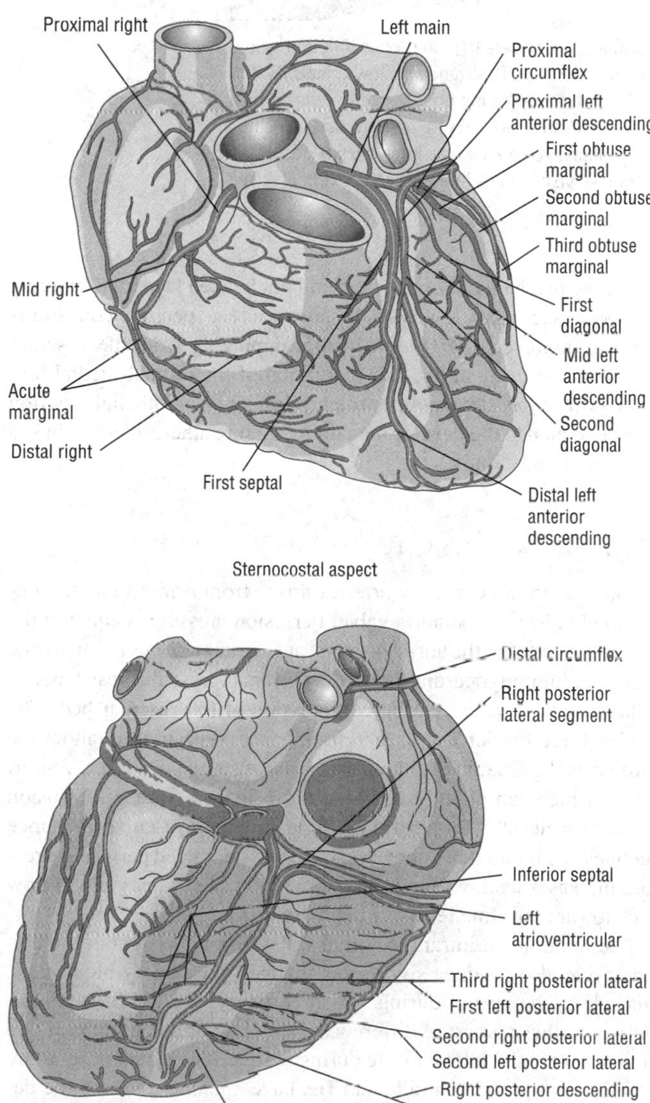

FIGURE 14–1. Coronary artery anatomy with sternocostal and diaphragmatic views.

circumstances, the resistance in R_2 is much greater. Myocardial blood flow is inversely related to arteriolar resistance and directly related to the coronary driving pressure. The arterioles dynamically alter their intrinsic tone in response to demands for oxygen and other factors, and as a result, myocardial oxygen delivery and myocardial oxygen demand are tightly coupled in a rapidly responsive system.

Atherosclerotic lesions encroaching on the luminal cross-sectional area of the larger epicardial vessels (R_1) transform the relationships among R_1, R_2, and blood flow. As resistance increases in R_1 owing to occlusion, R_2 can vasodilate to maintain coronary blood flow (see Fig. 14–2). This response is inadequate with greater degrees of obstruction, and the coronary flow reserve afforded by R_2 vasodilatation is insufficient to meet oxygen demand (also referred to as *autoregulation*). The extent of functional obstruction is important in the limitation of coronary blood flow, and the presence of relatively severe stenosis ($>70\%$) may provoke ischemia and symptoms at rest, whereas less severe stenosis may allow a reserve of coronary blood flow for exertion.[12]

The diameter of the lesion impeding blood flow through a vessel is important, but other factors such as length of the lesion and the influence of pressure drop across an area of stenosis also affect coronary blood flow and function of the collateral circulation. Resistance to flow in a vessel is directly related to length of the obstructing lesion, but resistance is inversely related to the diameter of the vessel to the fourth power. Diameter, therefore, is much more important. As blood flows across a stenotic lesion, the pressure drops (energy losses) owing to friction between blood and the lesion and owing to the abrupt turbulent expansion as blood emerges from the stenosis. This pressure drop is dynamic and directly related to flow, giving rise to a resistance that is not fixed but rather fluctuates as flow is changed. This relationship can affect collateral blood flow and its response to exercise dramatically, resulting in what has been called "coronary steal." A similar situation also may occur when the epicardial or subepicardial vessels "steal" blood flow from the endocardium in the presence of a stenotic lesion.

Large and small coronary arteries may undergo dynamic changes in coronary vascular resistance and coronary blood flow. Dynamic coronary obstruction can occur in normal vessels and vessels with stenosis in which vasomotion or spasm may be superimposed on a fixed stenosis. Although it is possible that these changes may be "active" in small coronary arteries, it is also possible that the observed changes may reflect collapse owing to poststenotic intraluminal pressure drop or increased intramyocardial compressive forces associated with inadequate ventricular relaxation.

Collateral blood flow exists to a certain extent from birth as native collaterals, but persisting ischemia may promote collateral growth as developed collaterals. These two types of collaterals differ in anatomy and in their ability to regulate coronary blood flow. Collateral development depends on the severity of obstruction, the presence of various growth factors [basic fibroblast growth factor (b-FGF) and vascular endothelial growth factor (VEGF)], endogenous vasodilators (e.g., nitrous oxide, prostacyclin), hormones such as estrogen, and potentially, exercise. Collateral development is highly species-dependent, and this should be considered when reading experimental literature.

METABOLIC REGULATION

Coronary blood flow is closely tied to oxygen needs of the heart. Changes in oxygen balance lead to very rapid changes in coronary blood flow. Although a number of mediators may contribute to these changes, the most important ones are likely to be adenosine, other nucleotides, nitric oxide, prostaglandins, CO_2, and H^+. Adenosine,

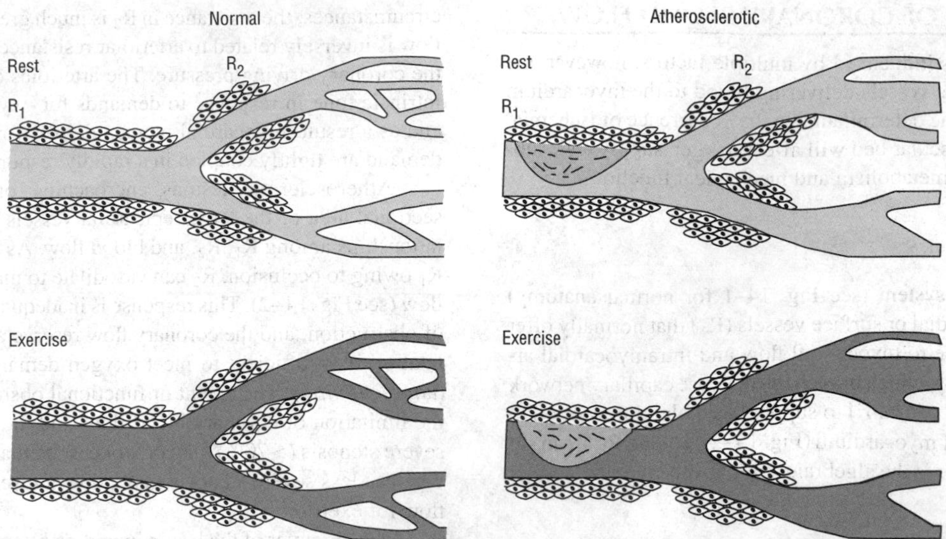

FIGURE 14–2. The coronary circulation with large epicardial conductance vessels (R_1) that offer little intrinsic resistance to myocardial blood flow and intramyocardial resistance arterioles (R_2). Resistance to flow equals $R_1 + R_2$ and R_2 resistance is normally much greater than R_1; hence flow is equal to the driving pressure across the coronary bed divided by the resistance in R_2. Dilatation in R_2 normally occurs in response to exercise or increased myocardial oxygen demand. When an atherosclerotic lesion narrows the conductance vessel, the arterioles dilate under resting conditions to prevent ischemia; however, with stress, the vasodilator reserve becomes limited. *(From Ref. 113, with permission.)*

which is formed from adenosine triphosphate (ATP) and adenosine monophosphate (AMP) under conditions of ischemia and stress, is a potent vasodilator that links decreased perfusion to metabolically induced vasodilation or "reactive hyperemia." The synthesis and release of adenosine into coronary sinus venous effluent occur within seconds after coronary artery occlusion, and about 30% of the hyperemic response can be blocked by metabolic blockers of adenosine.[13]

ENDOTHELIAL CONTROL OF CORONARY VASCULAR TONE[11]

The vascular endothelium, a single-cell tissue with an enormous surface area separating the blood from vascular smooth muscle of the artery wall, is capable of a broad range of metabolic functions. The endothelium functions as a protective surface for the artery wall, and as long as it remains intact and functional, it promotes vascular smooth muscle relaxation and inhibits thrombogenesis and atherosclerotic plaque formation; damaged endothelium reacts to numerous stimuli with vasoconstriction, thrombosis, and plaque formation. The vascular endothelium of the coronary arteries synthesizes large molecules such as fibronectin, interleukin-1, tissue plasminogen activator, and various growth factors. Small molecules that also are produced include prostacyclin, platelet-activating factor, endothelin-1, and endothelium-derived relaxing factor (EDRF) that is now characterized as nitric oxide. EDRF is synthesized from L-arginine via nitric oxide synthase and released by shear force on the endothelium as well as through interaction with many biochemical stimuli such as acetylcholine, histamine, arginine, catecholamines, arachidonic acid, adenosine diphosphate (ADP), endothelin-1, bradykinin, serotonin, and thrombin.[13] EDRF or nitric oxide then causes relaxation of the underlying smooth muscle and may be thought of as a paracrine homeopathic defense mechanism against noxious stimuli. Denudation or loss of the vascular endothelium results in loss of EDRF and this protective mechanism. Loss of the endothelial cell layer and function may occur secondary to physical disruption [e.g., percutaneous transluminal angioplasty (PTCA)], factors impinging from the vascular side (cyanide from smoke), or disruption of the intimal-medial layers (oxidized low-density lipoprotein). Impaired endothelial function may be related to the development of premature atherosclerosis based on recent family studies.[14]

FACTORS EXTRINSIC TO THE VASCULAR BED

Blood flow to the coronary arteries arises from orifices located immediately distal to the aorta valve. Perfusion pressure is equal to the difference between the aortic pressure at an instantaneous point in time minus the intramyocardial pressure. Coronary vascular resistance is influenced by phasic systolic compression of the vascular bed. The driving force for perfusion, therefore, is not constant throughout the cardiac cycle. Opening of the aortic valve also may lead to a Venturi effect, which can slightly decrease perfusion pressure. If perfusion pressure is elevated for a period of time, coronary vascular resistance declines and blood flow increases; however, continued perfusion pressure increases lead, within limits, to a return of coronary blood flow back toward baseline levels through autoregulation.

Alterations in intramyocardial wall tension throughout the cardiac cycle also produce significant changes in coronary blood flow. Diastole is the period during which coronary artery filling can occur due to these pressure differences, and little or no coronary blood flow occurs to the left ventricle during systole. The extent of pressure development in the ventricle and HR have a major effect on the development of wall tension, time for diastolic coronary artery filling, and myocardial oxygen demand.

Under normal conditions, the average global distribution of blood flow between the epicardial and endocardial layer is about 1:1 at rest and remains approximately even during exercise secondary to autoregulatory changes. Regional disparity of blood flow distribution does exist normally, and these disparities are magnified in the presence of diseased coronary arteries and with increased cardiac work as the vasodilator reserve in the resistance vessels of the subendocardium layers is exhausted. Factors that favor a reduction in subendocardial blood flow include decreased perfusion pressure due to decreased diastolic blood pressure or coronary artery obstruction by atherosclerotic plaques with or without vasomotion, abbreviation of diastole (increased HR), and increased intraventricular diastolic pressure (e.g., valvular obstruction to flow).

Extravascular resistance may decrease coronary blood flow, primarily during systole. This effect is much more pronounced in the left ventricle compared with the right ventricle. When the effect of increased contractility is separated from the effect of ventricular pressure, about 75% of extravascular resistance is accounted for by passive stretch in equilibrium with ventricular pressure, whereas only 25% results from active myocardial contraction.

FACTORS INTRINSIC TO THE VASCULAR BED

Metabolic factors, myogenic responses, neural reflexes, and humoral substances within the vascular bed of the coronary circulation function in an orchestrated fashion to maintain relative consistency in blood flow to the myocardium in the face of imposed changes in perfusion pressures. Autoregulation, mediated primarily through the effects of myogenic responses and metabolic factors, is thought to be responsible for maintaining regional blood flow in a narrow range while systemic pressure varies over a range of approximately 50 to 150 mm Hg.

Myogenic control (also known as the *Bayliss effect*) of coronary artery tone occurs when the vessel is stretched secondary to an increase in pressure and contracts to return blood flow to normal. It is thought that the myogenic response to stretching in coronary arteries is a modest one and that metabolic factors such as nitric oxide play a much larger role in autoregulation.

There are three well-studied metabolic factors that have the ability to modify coronary artery resistance and blood flow at the local level. Basal coronary blood flow meets oxygen demands of 8 to 10 mL/min per 100 g of myocardium with essentially complete extraction of oxygen from the blood. As cardiac output or mean arterial blood pressure increases, the increased demand for oxygen is met by increasing blood flow because little additional oxygen is available from hemoglobin. Decreased oxygen availability causes vasodilation of vascular smooth muscle and relaxation of precapillary sphincters, which increase tissue oxygen and help maintain blood flow on a regional basis.

At perfusion pressures below 60 mm Hg, as the coronary arteries are maximally dilated and the buffering effect of autoregulation has reached its capacity, further reduction in coronary blood flow will decrease perfusion pressure and tissue oxygenation. It is thought that autoregulation works more efficiently in the epicardial layers than in subendocardial layers, and this may contribute to coronary steal.

Neural components that participate in the regulation of coronary blood flow include the sympathetic nervous system, the parasympathetic nervous system, coronary reflexes, and possibly, central control of coronary blood flow. Within the sympathetic system, stimulation of the stellate ganglion elicits coronary vasodilation, which is associated with tachycardia and enhanced contractility. This indirect coronary vasodilation is secondary to increased MVO_2 related to increased HR, contractility, and aortic pressure and occurs following stellate stimulation. The direct effect of the sympathetic system is α_1-mediated vasoconstriction at rest and during exercise. Other receptor types, α_2 and β_1, have little influence on tone, whereas β_2 stimulation produces a modest vasodilatory effect. Although coronary atherosclerosis may decrease blood flow secondary to obstruction, severe coronary atherosclerosis and obstruction also may increase the sensitivity of coronary arteries to the effects of α_1 stimulation and vasoconstriction.

Vagal stimulation within the parasympathetic system produces a small to moderate increase in coronary blood flow, which involves the coronary efferent and afferent parasympathetic components (Bezold-Jarish reflex). Indirectly, vasoconstriction may result, with vagal stimulation as the result of bradycardia and decreased contractility reducing myocardial oxygen demand.

Coronary reflexes have an undetermined role in the regulation of coronary blood flow. Based on experimental data, coronary reflexes that may be important include the baroreceptor, the chemoreceptor, the Bezold-Jarish reflex, and the pulmonary inhalation reflex.

FACTORS LIMITING CORONARY PERFUSION

During exercise and pacing, as MVO_2 increases, coronary vascular resistance can be reduced to about 25% of basal values, which results in a four- to fivefold increase in coronary blood flow. The cross-sectional area can be reduced by about 80% prior to any mechanical or biochemical changes in the myocardium, reflecting a margin of safety for coronary blood flow. The extent of cross-sectional obstruction, the length of the lesion, lesion composition, and the geometry of the obstructing lesion can each affect flow across coronary arteries with atherosclerosis. Bernoulli's theorem states that the pressure drop across a lesion is directly related to the length of the lesion and inversely related to the radius of the lesion to the fourth power; critical stenosis occurs when the obstructing lesion encroaches on the luminal diameter and exceeds 70%. Lesions creating obstruction of 50% to 70% may reduce blood flow; however, these obstructions are not consistent, and vasospasm and thrombosis superimposed on a "noncritical" lesion may lead to clinical events such as myocardial infarction.[15] If the lesion enlarges from 80% to 90%, resistance in that vessel is tripled. Coronary reserve is diminished at about 85% obstruction owing to vasoconstriction. Exaggerated responsiveness can be seen when coronary stenosis reaches this critical level, and the role of vasoactive substances such as prostaglandins, thromboxanes, and serotonin may play more of a role in the regulation of coronary vascular tone and thrombosis.

Little reserve exists for coronary blood flow, and a relatively small reduction of 10% to 20% results in decreased myocardial fiber shortening as the first evidence for abnormal function. The subendocardial layers are affected to a greater extent than the epicardium by ischemia, considering changes in fiber shortening, arteriovenous (AV) difference in oxygen saturation, and lactate production. A reduction of 80% gives rise to akinesis, and a 95% reduction of coronary blood flow produces dyskinesis during contraction of the ventricles. Although these abnormalities of contraction are associated with transient impaired function, depletion of high-energy phosphate compounds and ultrastructural changes may last for days even after transient ischemia; this has been referred to as *stunned myocardium*. Chronic hypoperfusion may lead to *hibernation*, in which ventricular function is impaired over longer time intervals. Hibernating myocardium can be differentiated from necrosis with various techniques (see Chap. 10), and revascularization of hibernating myocardium is useful in improving ventricular function. Regional loss of contractility may impose a burden on the remaining myocardial tissue, resulting in heart failure, increased MVO_2, and rapid depletion of blood flow reserve. Consequently, zones of tissue with marginal blood flow may develop in a lateral or transmural fashion; such development puts this tissue at risk for more severe damage if the ischemic episode persists or becomes more severe. Nonischemic areas of myocardium may compensate for the severely ischemic and border zones of ischemia by developing more tension than usual in an attempt to maintain cardiac output. At the cellular level, ischemia and the attendant acidosis are thought to alter calcium release from storage sites such as the sarcolemma and the sarcoplasmic reticulum as well as inhibiting the binding of calcium to troponin, thereby impairing the association of actin and myosin. The clinical correlates of these cellular biochemical events leading to the development of left or right ventricular dysfunction include an S_3, dyspnea, orthopnea, tachycardia, fluctuating blood pressure, transient murmurs, and mitral or tricuspid regurgitation.

Calcium accumulation and overload secondary to ischemia impair ventricular relaxation as well as contraction. This is apparently a result of impaired calcium uptake after systole from the myofilaments, leading to a less negative decline in the pressure in the ventricle over time. Impaired relaxation is associated with enhanced diastolic stiffness, decreased rate of wall thinning, and slowed pressure decay, producing an upward shift in the ventricular pressure-volume relationship; put more simply, MVO_2 is likely to be increased secondary to increased wall tension. Impairment of both diastolic and systolic function leads to elevation of the filling pressure of the left ventricle.

CLINICAL PRESENTATION AND DIAGNOSIS

The classic symptoms associated with typical chest pain and angina caused by IHD appear in Table 14–3. Important aspects of the clinical history for chest pain for patients with angina include the nature or quality of the pain, precipitating factors, duration, pain radiation, and the response to nitroglycerin or rest. Because there can be considerable variation in the manifestations of angina, it is more accurate to refer to these symptoms as an *anginal syndrome*. For some patients with significant CAD, their presenting symptoms may differ from the classic symptoms, yet the symptoms are due to ischemic pain, and these are often referred to as *anginal equivalents*. Obtaining an accurate and detailed family history is useful in placing symptoms in perspective. Significant positive information includes premature coronary heart disease (<55 years of age in men and <65 years of age in women), manifested as fatal and nonfatal MI, stroke, or peripheral vascular disease, as well as other risk factors such as hypertension, smoking, familial lipid disorders, and diabetes mellitus. Typical pain radiation patterns include anterior chest pain (96%), left upper arm pain (83.7%), left lower arm pain (29.3%), and neck pain at some time (22%). Pain from other areas is less common. Ischemia detected by electrocardiographic (ECG) monitoring is more likely to be detected in the morning hours (6 AM to 12 noon) than other periods throughout the day. Patients suffering from variant or Prinzmetal's angina secondary to coronary spasm are more likely to experience pain at rest and in the early morning hours. Prinzmetal's anginal pain usually is not brought on by exertion or emotional stress nor relieved by rest, and the ECG pattern is that of current injury with ST-segment elevation rather than depression.

It is also important to differentiate the pattern of pain for stable angina from that of unstable angina. Unstable angina may be stratified into categories of risk ranging from high to low[2] (Table 14–4).

TABLE 14–3. Characteristics of Angina Pectoris

Quality
Sensation of pressure or heavy weight on the chest
Burning sensation
Feeling of tightness
Shortness of breath with feeling of constriction about the larynx or upper trachea
Visceral quality (deep, heavy, squeezing, aching)
Gradual increase in intensity followed by gradual fading away

Location
Over the sternum or very near to it
Anywhere between epigastrium and pharynx
Occasionally limited to left shoulder and left arm
Rarely limited to right arm
Limited to lower jaw
Lower cervical or upper thoracic spine
Left interscapular or suprascapular area

Duration
0.5–30 minutes

Precipitating factors
Relationship to exercise
Effort that involves use of arms above the head
Cold environment
Walking against the wind
Walking after a large meal
Emotional factors involved with physical exercise
Fright, anger
Coitus

Nitroglycerin relief
Relief of pain occurring within 45 s to 5 minutes of taking nitroglycerin

Radiation
Medical aspect of left arm
Left shoulder
Jaw
Occasionally right arm

From Helfant RH, Banka VS. A Clinical and Angiographic Approach to Coronary Heart Disease. Philadelphia, FA Davis, 1978:47, with permission.

Ischemia also may be painless or "silent" in 60% to 100% of patients depending on the series cited and the patient population.[16] In patients with myocardial ischemia, approximately 70% of the episodes of documented ischemia are painless, as determined by ambulatory ECG monitoring, and the ST-segment changes associated with these episodes can be ST-segment elevation or depression. The mechanism of silent ischemia is unclear, but studies have shown that patients not experiencing pain have altered pain perception, with the threshold and tolerance for pain being higher than that of patients who have pain more frequently. Although diabetics tend to have more extensive coronary disease than nondiabetics do and may suffer from autonomic neuropathy, asymptomatic ischemia is not more prevalent based on the Asymptomatic Cardiac Ischemia Pilot (ACIP) study.[17] Altered endorphin release is a plausible explanation, but investigations with naloxone to block endorphins do not consistently show altered pain thresholds to various stimuli compared with patients with symptomatic ischemia, and patients with asymptomatic ischemia do not necessarily have impaired somatic pain sensitivity.[18] Alternatively, adenosine and substance P release during ischemia and mechanical stretch on coronary arteries may play a role in the perception of pain.

Finally, it should be recognized that the threshold for pain owing to exertion is fixed in some patients and variable in others and that

TABLE 14–4. Short-Term Risk of Death or Nonfatal MI in Patients with Unstable Angina

Feature	High Risk (At least 1 of the following features must be present)	Intermediate Risk (No high-risk feature but must have 1 of the following)	Low Risk (No high- or intermediate-risk feature but may have any of the following)
History	Accelerating tempo of ischemic symptoms in preceding 48 h	Prior MI, peripheral or cerebrovascular disease, or CABG, prior aspirin use	
Character of pain	Prolonged ongoing (>20 min), rest pain	Prolonged (>20 min), rest angina, now resolved, with moderate or high likelihood of CAD	New-onset CCS class III or IV angina in the past 2 weeks without prolonged (>20 min) rest pain but with moderate or high likelihood of CAD
Clinical findings	Pulmonary edema, most likely due to ischemia New or worsening MR murmur S_3 or new/worsening rales Hypotension, bradycardia, tachycardia Age >75 yrs		
ECG	Angina at rest with transient ST-segment changes > 0.05 mV Bundle-branch block, new or presumed new	T-wave inversions > 0.2 mV Pathologic Q waves	Normal or unchanged ECG during an episode of chest discomfort
Cardiac markers	Markedly elevated (e.g., TnT or TnI > 0.1 ng/mL)	Slightly elevated (e.g., TnT > 0.01 but < 0.1 ng/mL)	Normal

Legend: MI = myocardial infarction; CABG = coronary artery bypass grafting; CAD = coronary artery disease; CCS = Canadian Cardiovascular Society; MR = mitral regurgitation; ECG = electrocardiogram; TnT = troponin T; TnI = troponin I

the amount of exercise or stress necessary to provoke symptoms can change over time. A fixed threshold for the induction of pain or ECG evidence of ischemia means that these indicators of ischemia occur at the same, or nearly so, double rate-pressure product. This is apparently owing to at least two factors. Over long periods of time, atherosclerosis may progress, leading to more severe stenosis, reduced oxygen supply, and less of an increase in demand to precipitate ischemic symptoms. Once stenotic lesions reach a critical level of about 80% or greater, vasomotion, vasospasm, and thrombotic occlusion become significant factors impairing blood flow to the myocardium. Consequently, anatomic considerations and vasoactive substances may interact to provide an environment amenable to changing thresholds for the production of angina.

There appears to be little relationship between the historical features of angina and the severity or extent of coronary artery vessel involvement. Therefore, one may speculate that severe symptoms might be associated with multivessel disease, but no predictive markers exist on a routine basis.

Chest pain may resemble pain arising from a variety of noncardiac sources, and the differential diagnosis of anginal pain from other etiologies may be quite difficult based on history alone. Table 14–5 outlines other common problems that may present with episodic chest pain. Although much less common, nonatherosclerotic etiologies of CAD do exist and should be excluded with appropriate tests. The clinical classification of chest pain encompasses typical angina, including (1) substernal chest pain with a characteristic quality and duration that is (2) provoked by exertion or emotional stress and (3) relieved by rest or nitroglycerin; atypical angina (meets two of the characteristics for typical angina); and non-cardiac chest pain (meets one or fewer of the typical angina characteristics).[1]

There are few signs apparent on physical examination to indicate the presence of CAD, and usually only the cardiovascular system reveals any useful information. Elevated HR or blood pressure can yield an increased DP and may be associated with angina, and it would be important to correct extreme tachycardia or hypertension if present. Other noncardiac physical findings that suggest that significant CVD may be associated with angina include abdominal aortic aneurysms or peripheral vascular disease. A controversial finding is that of a diagonal ear-lobe crease, which is said by some to be associated with significant CAD.[19] Cardiac examination findings in CAD are noted in Table 14–6. During an angina attack, these findings may appear or become more prominent, making them more valuable if present.

In addition to screening for CVD risk factors (see Table 21–7), other recommended tests include hemoglobin, fasting glucose, fasting lipoprotein panel, resting electrocardiogram, and chest x-ray in patients with signs or symptoms of heart failure, valvular heart disease, pericardial disease, or aortic dissection/aneurysm.[1] Hemoglobin is assessed to ensure adequate oxygen-carrying capacity. Fasting glucose determinations to exclude diabetes and glucose monitoring for concurrent diabetes should be performed routinely. Lipids assessed are total cholesterol, low-density lipoprotein–cholesterol, high-density lipoprotein–cholesterol, and triglycerides (see Chap. 21). Other risk factors that may be important for some patients include C-reactive protein, homocysteine level, evidence of *Chlamydia* infection, and elevations in lipoprotein-(a), fibrinogen, and plasminogen activator inhibitor.[20] Cardiac enzymes should all be normal in stable angina. Troponin T or I, myoglobin, or creatinine phosphokinase-MB isoform may be elevated in patients with unstable angina, and interventions such as anticoagulation or antiplatelet therapy have been

TABLE 14–5. Differential Diagnosis of Episodic Chest Pain Resembling Angina Pectoris

	Duration	Quality	Provocation	Relief	Location	Commet
Effort angina	5–15 min	Visceral (pressure)	During effort or emotion	Rest, NTG	Substernal, radiates	First episode vivid
Rest angina	5–15 min	Visceral (pressure)	Spontaneous (?with exercise)	NTG	Substernal, radiates	Often nocturnal
Mitral prolapse	Min–hours	Superficial (rarely visceral)	Spontaneous (no pattern)	Time	Left anterior	No pattern, variable
Esophageal reflux	10 min–1 h	Visceral	Spontaneous, cold liquids, exercise, lying down	Foods, antacids, H_2 blockers, proton pump inhibitors, NTG	Substernal, radiates	Mimics angina
Peptic ulcer	Hours	Visceral, burning	Lack of food, "acid" foods	Foods, antacids, H_2 blockers, proton pump inhibitors	Epigastric, substernal	
Biliary disease	Hours	Visceral (wax and wane)	Spontaneous, food	Time, analgesia	Epigastric, radiates	Colic
Cervical disc	Variable (gradually subsides)	Superficial	Head and neck, movement and palpation	Time, analgesia	Arm, neck	Not relieved by rest
Hyperventilation	2–3 min	Visceral	Emotion, tachypnea	Stimulus removed	Substernal	Facial paraesthesia
Musculoskeletal	Variable	Superficial	Movement, palpation	Time, analgesia	Multiple	Tenderness
Pulmonary	30 min	Visceral (pressure)	Often spontaneous	Rest, time bronchodilator	Subsernal	Dyspneic

TABLE 14–6. Cardiac Findings in Patients with Coronary Artery Disease

Sign	Clinical Significance	Frequency
Abnormal precordial systolic bulge	Left ventricular wall motion abnormality	Not usually present unless patient has sustained a prior MI (especially anterior wall) or is experiencing angina at time of examination
Decreased intensity of S_1	Decrease in left ventricular contractility	Difficult to evaluate in resting state, but can be commonly demonstrated during angina
Paradoxical splitting of S_2	Left ventricular wall motion abnormality	Very uncommon but occasionally noted during angina
S_3 (ventricular gallop)	Increased left ventricular diastolic pressure, with or without clinical CHF	Not usually present unless patient sustained extensive MI; may occasionally be present during angina
S_4 (atrial gallop)	Reduced ventricular compliance ("stiff heart")	Common; very common in patients who have sustained a prior MI as well as during angina
Apical systolic murmur (in absence of rheumatic mitral regurgitation or Barlow's syndome)	Papillary muscle dysfunction	Not usually present unless patient has sustained prior MI
Diastolic murmur (in absence of aortic regurgitation)	Coronary artery stenosis	Rare

Abbreviations: S = first heart sound; S_2 = second heart sound; S_3 = third heart sound; S_4 = fourth heart sound; MI = myocardial infarction.
From Cohn PF, ed. Diagnosis and Therapy of Coronary Artery Disease, 2d ed. Boston, Martinus Nijhoff, 1985:101, with permission.

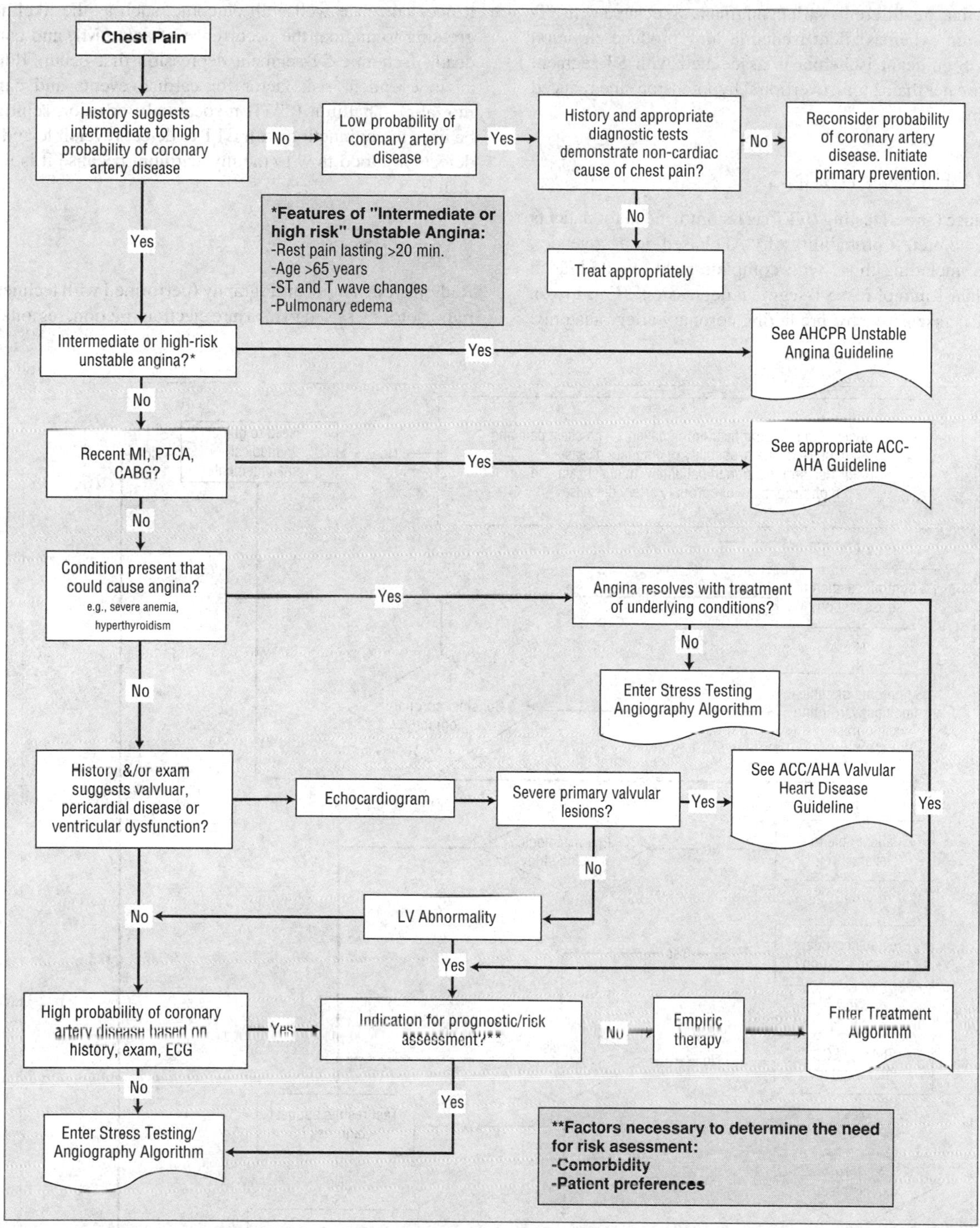

FIGURE 14–3. Clinical assessment. AHCPR indicates Agency for Health Care Policy and Research.

shown to reduce cardiac end points when these markers for injury are elevated[21] (see Table 14–4).

Patients presenting with chest pain are stratified into chronic stable angina or having features of intermediate or high-risk unstable angina (Fig. 14–3 and Table 14–4). These features include rest pain lasting more than 20 minutes, age greater than 65 years, ST-segment and T-wave changes, and pulmonary edema. Patients with acute coronary syndrome (e.g., unstable angina, NSTEMI, and ST-segment elevation MI) are managed differently than patients with chronic stable angina.

DIAGNOSTIC TESTS

See also Chapter 10.

ELECTROCARDIOGRAM

The electrocardiogram is normal in about one-half of patients with angina who are not experiencing an acute attack. Typical ST-T-wave changes include depression, T-wave inversion, and ST-segment elevation. Forms of ischemia other than exertional angina may have ECG manifestations that are different; variant angina is associated with ST-segment elevation, whereas silent ischemia may produce elevation or depression. Significant ischemia is associated with ST-segment depression of greater than 2 mm, exertional hypotension, and reduced exercise tolerance.

EXERCISE TOLERANCE TESTING

Exercise tolerance (stress) testing (ETT) is recommended for patients with intermediate pretest probability of CAD based on age, gender, and symptoms, including those with complete right bundle-branch block or less than 1 mm of rest ST-segment depression[1] (Fig. 14–4). Although ETT is insensitive for predicting coronary artery anatomy, it does correlate well with outcome, such as the likelihood of progressing to angina, the occurrence of acute MI, and cardiovascular death. Ischemic ST-segment depression that occurs during ETT is an independent risk factor for cardiac events and cardiovascular mortality. Thallium (^{201}Tl) myocardial perfusion scintigraphy may be used in conjunction with ETT to detect reversible and irreversible defects in blood flow to the myocardium because it is more sensitiv than ETT.

CARDIAC IMAGING

Radionuclide angiocardiography (performed with technetium-99m, a radioisotope) is used to measure ejection fraction, regional ventricular

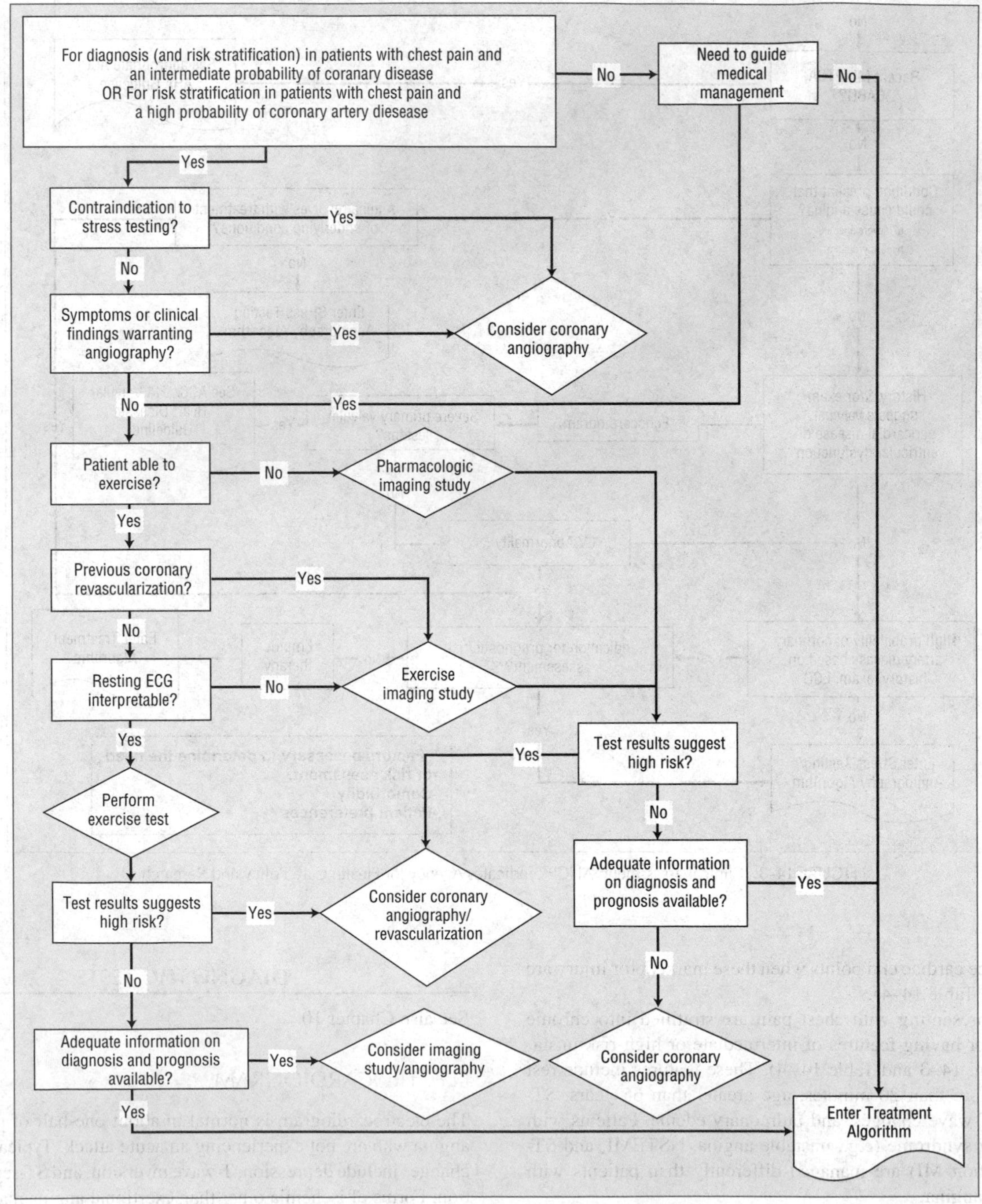

FIGURE 14–4. Stress testing/angiography.

performance, cardiac output, ventricular volumes, valvular regurgitation, asynchrony or wall motion abnormalities, and intracardiac shunts. Technetium pyrophosphate scans are used routinely for detection and quantification of acute MI (see Chap. 15). Positron emission tomography (PET) is useful for quantifying ischemia with metabolically important substrates such as oxygen, carbon, and nitrogen. Other metabolic probes use radiolabeled fatty acids and glucose to study metabolic processes that may be deranged during ischemia in animals and for investigative purposes in humans.

A new method using ultrarapid computed tomography (CT), also called spiral CT, ultrafast CT, or electron-beam CT, minimized artifact owing to motion of the heart during contraction and relaxation and provides a semiquantitative assessment of calcium content in coronary arteries.[22] Calcium scores greater than 150 provide a sensitivity of 74% and specificity of 89%, and this method may be cost-effective compared with ETT.

ECHOCARDIOGRAPHY

Echocardiography is useful if patients have a history or physical examination suggestive of valvular pericardial disease or ventricular dysfunction. For patients unable to exercise, pharmacologic stress echocardiography (e.g., dobutamine, dipyridamole, or adenosine) or pacing may be done to identify abnormalities during stress.

CARDIAC CATHETERIZATION AND CORONARY ARTERIOGRAPHY

Cardiac catheterization and angiography in patients with suspected CAD are used diagnostically to document the presence and severity of disease as well as for prognostic purposes. High-risk features during ETT suggesting the need for coronary angiography include early and significant (≥2 mm) changes on the electrocardiogram during ETT as well as multiple lead involvement, prolonged recovery from ischemia, low workload performance, abnormal blood pressure response (reduction in blood pressure), or ventricular arrhythmias. Multiple defects with thallium scans as well as lung uptake during exercise or post-exercise ventricular cavity dilatation are also high-risk indications for catheterization. Interventional catheterization is used for thrombolytic therapy in patients with acute MI and for the management of patients with significant CAD to relieve obstruction through PTCA, atherectomy, laser treatment, or stent placement. Catheterization and angiography may be done after coronary artery bypass grafting (CABG) to determine if the graft has closed or if CAD has progressed. Coronary artery intravascular ultrasound (IVUS) is useful for direct imaging of anatomy, calcified and fatty plaques, and thrombosis superimposed on plaque as well as determining patency following revascularization procedures. IVUS guidance of stent implantation may result in more effective stent expansion compared with angiographic guidance alone.[23]

▶ TREATMENT: Ischemic Heart Disease

MODIFICATION OF RISK FACTORS

Primary prevention of IHD through the identification and modification of risk factors prior to the initial morbid event would be the optimal management approach and should result in a significant impact on the prevalence of IHD. However, early recognition of some risk factors may not be possible in all cases, and in others, the patient may not be willing to undertake intervention until overt evidence of CAD is apparent. Secondary intervention continues to be pursued more commonly by both health care professionals and patients, and it is important to recognize this type of intervention as effective in reducing subsequent morbidity and mortality. The presence of risk factors in individual patients plays a major role in determining the occurrence and severity of IHD.[24] Risk factors are additive in nature and can be classified as alterable or unalterable. Unalterable risk factors include gender, age, family history or genetic composition, environmental influences (e.g., climate, air pollution, trace metal composition of drinking water), and to some extent, diabetes mellitus. Improved glycemic control reduces the microvascular complications of diabetes mellitus (see Chap. 74) and reduces coronary end points; however, based on the Diabetes Control and Complications study, the reduction was impressive (40 versus 23 major events) but not significant because the trial was underpowered to detect these changes.[25] Risk factors that can be altered include smoking, hypertension, hyperlipidemia, obesity, sedentary lifestyle, hyperuricemia, psychosocial factors such as stress and type A behavior patterns, and the use of certain drugs that may be detrimental, including progestins, corticosteroids, and cyclosporine.

Cigarette smoking is common; nearly 50 million people are regular smokers in this country, and the risk for IHD is increased by about 1.8 in active smokers and by about 1.3 for passive or environmental smoke exposure.[26] Approximately 430,700 Americans die each year from smoking-related illnesses, and 1 in 5 deaths due to CVD are attributable to smoking.[4] Risk due to smoking is related to the number of cigarettes smoked per day and the duration of smoking. Passive smoking in angina pectoris patients has been shown to decrease exercise time.[6] Pipe and cigar smokers are at increased risk compared with nonsmokers, but their risk is somewhat less than that of cigarette smokers.[27] The direct effects of cigarette smoke that are detrimental to patients with angina include (1) elevated HR and blood pressure from nicotine, which increase MVO_2, and impaired myocardial oxygen delivery owing to carboxyhemoglobin generation from carbon monoxide inhalation in smoke, (2) the negative inotropic effect of carboxyhemoglobin, (3) increased platelet adhesiveness and promotion of aggregation resulting in thrombotic tendencies owing to nicotine and carboxyhemoglobin, (4) lowered threshold for ventricular fibrillation during ischemia owing to carboxyhemoglobin, and (5) impaired endothelial function owing to smoking.[28] Similar changes have been noted for marihuana smoking as well. Smoking also accelerates the risk for MI, sudden death, cerebrovascular disease, peripheral vascular disease, and hypertension, and it reduces high-density lipoprotein concentrations. Clearly, primary prevention is needed for this risk factor, and much of the education effort to discourage initiation of smoking should be targeted to teenagers. Techniques for cessation of smoking that may be useful include aversive conditioning, group programs, self-help programs, hypnosis, "cold turkey," and the use of nicotine substitutes (lobeline) or other sources of nicotine (Nicorette chewing gum and transdermal nicotine systems) for short-term substitution during withdrawal syndrome. Cessation of smoking reduces the incidence of coronary events to about 15% to 25% of that associated with continued smoking, and these benefits are noted within 2 years of cessation.[29]

Hypertension, whether labile or fixed, borderline or definite, casual or basal, systolic or diastolic, at any age regardless of gender is the most common and a powerful contributor to atherosclerotic coronary vascular disease.[30] Morbidity and mortality increase progressively with the degree of blood pressure elevation of either systolic or diastolic pressure and pulse pressure, and no discernible critical value exists (see Chap. 12). Numerous trials have documented the reduction in risk associated with blood pressure lowering; however, most of these studies show that mortality and morbidity reduction is a result of fewer strokes and less renal failure and heart failure. The reduction in CAD end points is significant but not as dramatic. The reasons for this are unclear but perhaps relate to the multifactorial etiology of IHD.

Hypercholesterolemia is a significant cardiovascular risk factor, and risk is directly related to the degree of cholesterol elevation.[24] As with hypertension, there is no critical value that defines risk, but rather risk is incrementally related to the degree of elevation and the presence of other risk factors (see Chap. 21 for a detailed discussion). A fasting lipoprotein panel should be obtained in all patients with known CAD. The goals for total cholesterol, low-density lipoprotein–cholesterol, high-density lipoprotein–cholesterol, and triglycerides are discussed in Chapter 21. All patients should undertake therapeutic lifestyle changes. Reductions in low-density lipoprotein–cholesterol for primary prevention and secondary intervention have been shown to reduce total and CAD mortality and stroke as well as the need for such interventions as PTCA and CABG. Supplemental vitamin E or other antioxidants reduce the susceptibility of low-density lipoprotein–cholesterol to oxidation, but clinical trial data have failed to show any benefit with supplementation.[31]

The prevalence of obesity, defined as greater than 20% over ideal body weight, ranges from 7.4% to 17% in men and from 9.6% to 34.7% in women in this country. A body mass index [that is, weight (kg) divided by height (m) squared] greater than about 32 is associated with an increased mortality ratio compared with individuals of normal body weight, and the objective for patients with IHD is to maintain or reduce to a normal body weight. This may be accomplished through dietary modification, exercise, pharmacologic therapy, or surgical therapy. Frequently associated with obesity is a sedentary life-style, and inactivity may contribute to higher blood pressure, elevated blood lipid levels, and insulin resistance associated with glucose intolerance in diabetics (insulin resistance syndrome). Exercise to the level of about 300 kcal three times a week is useful in improving maximal oxygen uptake, improving cardiorespiratory efficiency, promoting collateral artery formation, and promoting potential alterations in the risk of ventricular fibrillation, coronary thrombosis, and improved tolerance to stress. Epidemiologic studies have found that mortality is directly related to resting HR and a low HR difference between resting and maximal exercise HR and inversely related to exercise HR.[32] Although a regular exercise program may not reduce CVD mortality, participants feel better, and their overall cardiovascular risk may be reduced.[33]

Competitiveness, intense striving for achievement, easily provoked hostility, a sense of urgency about doing things quickly and being punctual, impatience, abrupt and rapid speech and gestures, and concentration on self-selected goals to the point of not perceiving and attending to other aspects of the environment are traits that characterize the behavioral pattern known as the type A or coronary-prone personality. Although the issue is somewhat controversial, type A individuals may have increased cardiovascular risk, with risk ratios ranging from insignificant to three times that of a matched population. The mechanism by which personality affects the cardiovascular system is not understood but may reflect the activity of the sympathetic system and enhanced responsiveness of other stress hormones when compared with non-type A personalities.

Alcohol ingestion in small to moderate amounts (<40 g/d of pure ethanol) reduces the risk of CAD; however, consumption of large amounts (>50 g/d) or binge drinking of alcohol is associated with increased mortality from stroke, cancer, vehicular accidents, and cirrhosis. The mechanisms for the presumed protective effects of alcohol are not known, but the effects may be related to increased high-density lipoprotein levels, impaired platelet function, or associations between the amount of alcohol ingested and personality type. Whatever the relationship, it is well to remember that alcohol consumption is implicated in over 40% of all fatal automobile accidents and that consumption of alcohol predisposes to hepatic cirrhosis, the sixth to seventh most common cause of death in middle age in the United States. With this in mind, it seems illogical to suggest alcohol ingestion as a prophylactic measure for CAD but rather advise moderation of alcohol consumption, if it is the preference of the individual.

Thiazide diuretics have been shown to elevate serum cholesterol and triglyceride levels, whereas β-blockers tend to lower high-density lipoprotein and raise low-density lipoprotein slightly; however, a direct association between these drugs and cardiovascular risk is tenuous and based on aggregating results rather than on randomized clinical trials. Conjugated equine estrogen alone or in combination with progestin lowers low-density lipoprotein and raises high-density lipoprotein based on the Postmenopausal Estrogen/Progestin Interventions (PEPI) study.[34] Unfortunately, the Heart and Estrogen/Progestin Replacement Study (HERS) trial showed no benefit of hormone-replacement therapy for secondary intervention and increased risk for thromboembolism.[35] Unopposed estrogen is the optimal regimen for elevation of high-density lipoprotein, but the high rate of endometrial hyperplasia restricts use to women without a uterus. In women with a uterus, estrogen with cyclic medroxyprogesterone has the most favorable effect on high-density lipoprotein and no excess risk of endometrial hyperplasia. Use of oral contraceptives in women who smoke and are over the age of 35 years increases the risk of MI, stroke, and venous thromboembolism by threefold or higher. Alternative forms of contraception and cessation of smoking should be promoted in these patients. The risk for nonsmoking oral contraceptive users under the age of 35 is very small. Estrogen-replacement therapy (ERT) in the observational Nurses' Health Study reduced the risk of death in current or previous users of ERT compared with never users.[36] In women with a uterus, concurrent progestins (hormone-replacement therapy) should be used to offset the risk of endometrial carcinoma. The relative risk of breast cancer is increased, but in the absence of risk factors for breast cancer, the relative risk is approximately 1.3 (30% increase). Coffee consumption also has been linked to CAD, and caffeine does transiently elevate blood pressure; however, the overall risk, if any, appears to be low. Although thiazide diuretics and β-blockers (nonselective without intrinsic sympathomimetic activity) may elevate both cholesterol and triglycerides by some 10% to 20%, and these effects may be detrimental, no objective evidence exists from prospective, well-controlled studies to support avoiding these drugs at this time. This controversy is most pertinent in the treatment of mild hypertension, and it is discussed in greater detail in Chapter 12.

PHARMACOLOGIC THERAPY[37]

PLACEBO EFFECT

Historically, about 30% of anginal syndrome symptoms have responded regardless of which therapy was instituted. Examples of these placebo responses include drug therapies such as xanthines and khellin, as well as surgical procedures such as ligation of the internal mammary artery. These observations stem from two problems inherent in clinical trials undertaken to assess the efficacy of any therapy for angina: (1) adequate trial design incorporating appropriate controls and washout periods and (2) assessment of treatment effects using objective measures of efficacy including improvement in exercise performance, resting and ambulatory ECG improvement in ischemic changes, or other objective tests to address other aspects of myocardial function or metabolism. The use of pain episode frequency and nitroglycerin consumption is subjective, and their use as sole measures of efficacy should be avoided. Objective assessment using ETT has shown that placebo does not provide improvement in patients with exertional angina, substantiating this as a valid means to assess efficacy.

β-ADRENERGIC BLOCKING AGENTS[38]

Decreased HR, decreased contractility, and a slight to moderate decrease in blood pressure with β-adrenergic receptor antagonism reduce MVO_2. The predominant receptor type in the heart is the β_1-receptor, and competitive blockade minimizes the influence of endogenous catecholamines on the chronotropic and inotropic state of the myocardium. These beneficial effects may be countered to some degree with increased ventricular volume and ejection time seen with β blockade; however, the overall effect of β-blockers in patients with effort-induced angina is a reduction in oxygen demand (Table 14–7). The β-blockers do not improve oxygen supply, and in certain instances, unopposed α-adrenergic stimulation following the use of β-blockers may lead to coronary vasoconstriction. For patients with chronic exertional stable angina, β-blockers improve symptoms about 80% of the time, and objective measures of efficacy demonstrate improved exercise duration and delay in the time at which ST-segment changes and initial or limiting symptoms occur. β-Blockers do not alter the rate-pressure product (DP) for maximal exercise, therefore substantiating reduced demand rather than improved supply as the major consequence of their actions. Reflex tachycardia from nitrate therapy can be blunted with β-blocker therapy, making this a common and useful combination. Although β blockade may decrease exercise capacity in healthy individuals or in patients with hypertension, it may allow angina patients previously limited by symptoms to perform more exercise and ultimately improve overall cardiovascular performance through a training effect. Ideal candidates for β-blockers include patients in whom physical activity figures prominently in their anginal attacks, those who have coexisting hypertension, those with a history of supraventricular arrhythmias or post-MI angina, and those who have a component of anxiety associated with angina.[39] β-Blockers also may be used safely in angina and heart failure, as described in Chapter 13.

Pertinent pharmacokinetics for the β-blockers include half-life and route elimination, which are reviewed in Chapter 12. Drugs with longer half-lives need to be dosed less frequently than ones with shorter half-lives; however, disparity exists between half-life and duration of action for several β-blockers (e.g., metoprolol), and this may reflect attenuation of the central nervous system–mediated effects on the sympathetic nervous system as well as the direct effects of this category on HR and contractility. Renal and hepatic dysfunction can affect the disposition of β-blockers, but these agents are dosed to effect, either hemodynamic or symptomatic, and route of elimination is not a major consideration in drug selection.

Guidelines for the use of β-blockers in treating angina include the objective of lowering resting HR to 50 to 60 beats per minute and limiting maximal exercise HR to about 100 beats per minute or less. It also has been suggested that increases in exercise HR should be no more than about 20 beats per minute or a 10% increment over resting HR with modest exercise. Because β blockade is competitive and circulating catecholamine concentrations vary depending on the intensity of exercise and other factors and cholinergic tone may be important in controlling HR in some patients, these guidelines are general in nature. These effects generally are related to dose and plasma concentration, and for propranolol, plasma concentrations of 30 ng/mL are needed for a 25% reduction in anginal frequency. Initial doses of β-blockers should be at the lower end of the usual dosing range and titrated to response, as indicated above.

There is little evidence to suggest superiority of any β-blocker; however, the duration of β blockade depends in part on the half-life of the agent used, and those with longer half-lives may be dosed less frequently. Of note, propranolol may be dosed twice a day in most patients with angina, and the efficacy is similar to that seen with more frequent dosing. The ancillary property of membrane stabilizing activity is irrelevant in the treatment of angina, and intrinsic sympathomimetic activity appears to be detrimental in rest or severe angina because the reduction in HR would be minimized, therefore limiting a reduction in MVO_2. Cardioselective β-blockers may be used in some patients to minimize adverse effects such as bronchospasm in asthmatic or chronic obstructive pulmonary disease patients, intermittent claudication, and sexual dysfunction. It should be remembered that cardioselectivity is a relative property and that the use of larger doses (e.g., metoprolol 200 mg/d) is associated with the loss of selectivity and increased adverse effects. Patients with angina after acute MI are particularly good candidates for β blockade both because anginal symptoms may be treated as well as reducing the risk of post-MI reinfarction and because mortality has been demonstrated with timolol, propranolol, and metoprolol (see Chap. 15). Combined β (nonselective) and α blockade with labetolol may be useful in some patients with marginal LV reserve, and fewer deleterious effects on coronary blood flow are seen when compared with other β blockers.

Extension of pharmacologic effect is the underlying reason for many of the adverse effects seen with β blockade. Hypotension, heart failure, bradycardia and heart block, bronchospasm, peripheral vasoconstriction and intermittent claudication, and altered glucose metabolism are directly related to β-adrenoreceptor antagonism. Patients with preexisting LV dysfunction and the use of other negative inotropic agents are most prone to developing overt heart failure, and in the absence of these, heart failure is uncommon (less than 5%). Other drugs that depress conduction are additive to β blockade, and intrinsic conduction system disease predisposes the patient to conduction abnormalities. Altered glucose metabolism is most likely to be seen in insulin-dependent diabetics, and β blockade obscures the symptoms of hypoglycemia except for sweating. β-Blockers also may aggravate the lipid abnormalities seen in patients with diabetes; however, these changes are dose-related, are more common with normal baseline lipids than with dyslipidemia, and may be of short-term

TABLE 14–7. Effect of Drug Therapy on Myocardial Oxygen Demand[a]

			LV[b] Wall Tension	
	Heart Rate	Myocardial Contractility	Systolic Pressure	LV Volume
Nitrates	⇑	0	⇓	⇓⇓
β-Blockers	⇓⇓	⇓	⇓	⇑
Nifedipine	⇑	0 or ⇓	⇓⇓	0 or ⇓
Verapamil	⇓	⇓	⇓	0 or ⇓
Diltiazem	⇓⇓	0 or ⇓	⇓	0 or ⇓

[a]Calcium channel antagonists and nitrates also may increase myocardial oxygen supply through coronary vasodilation. Diastolic function also may be improved with verapamil, nifedipine, and perhaps, diltiazem. These effects may vary from those indicated in the table depending on individual patient baseline hemodynamics.
[b]LV = left ventricular.

significance only. One of the more common reasons for discontinuation of β-blocker therapy is related to central nervous system adverse effects of fatigue, malaise, and depression. Cognition changes seen with β-blockers are usually minimal and comparable with those of other categories of drugs based on studies done in hypertension.[40,41] Abrupt withdrawal of β-blocker therapy in patients with angina has been associated with increased severity and number of pain episodes and MI. The mechanism of this effect is unknown but may be related to increased receptor sensitivity or disease progression during therapy, which becomes apparent following discontinuation of β blockade. In any event, tapering of β-blocker therapy over about 2 days should minimize the risk of withdrawal reactions for those patients in whom therapy is being discontinued.

β-Adrenoreceptor blockade is effective in chronic exertional angina as monotherapy and in combination with nitrates and/or calcium channel antagonists. β-Blockers should be the first-line drug in chronic angina requiring daily maintenance therapy because β-blockers are more effective in reducing episodes of silent ischemia, reducing early morning peak of ischemic activity, and improving mortality after Q-wave MI than nitrates or calcium channel blockers[1,42] (Fig. 14–5). If β-blockers are ineffective or not tolerated, then monotherapy with a calcium channel blocker or combination therapy if monotherapy is ineffective for either alone may be instituted. Patients with severe angina, rest angina, or variant angina (i.e., a component of coronary artery spasm) may be better treated with calcium channel blockers or long-acting nitrates.

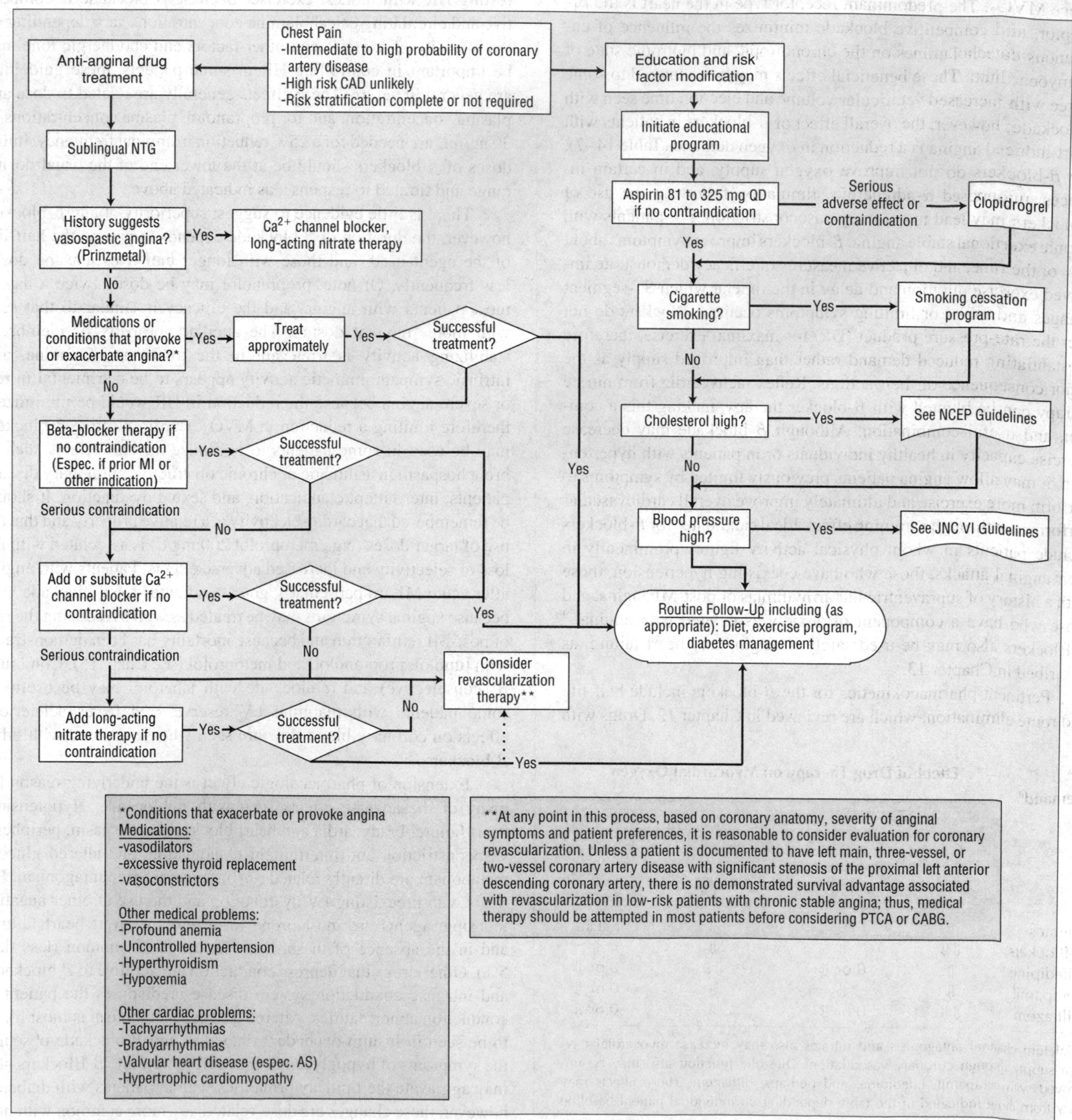

FIGURE 14–5. Treatment. NTG indicates nitroglycerin; NCEP, National Cholesterol Education Program; and JNC, Joint National Committee.

TABLE 14–8. Nitrate Products

Product	Onset (min)	Duration (min/h)	Initial Dose
Nitroglycerin			
IV	1–2	3–5	5 μg/min
Sublingual/lingual	1–3	30–60	0.3 mg
PO	40	3–6	2.5–9 mg tid
Ointment	20–60	2–8	1/2–1 in
Patch	40–60	>8	1 patch
Erythritol tetranitrate	5–30	4–6	5–10 mg tid
Penterythritol tetranitrate	30	4–8	10–20 mg tid
Isosorbide dinitrate			
Sublingual/chewable	2–5	1–2	2.5–5 mg tid
PO	20–40	4–6	5–20 mg tid
Isosorbide mononitrate	30–60	6–8	20 mg qd, bid[a]

[a]Product dependent.

NITRATES[43,44]

Nitroglycerin has a well-documented role in the alleviation of anginal attacks when used as rapidly absorbed and readily available preparations by the oral and intravenous routes (Table 14–8 and Fig. 14–5). Sublingual, buccal, or spray products are the products of choice for this indication. Prevention of symptoms may be accomplished by the prophylactic use of oral or transdermal products; however, recent concern has been expressed over the long-term efficacy of many of these preparations and the development of tolerance.

Nitrates have multiple potential mechanisms of action, and for a given patient, it is not always clear which of these is most important. In general, the major action appears to be indirectly mediated through a reduction of myocardial oxygen demand secondary to venodilation and arterial-arteriolar dilation, leading to a reduction in wall stress from reduced ventricular volume and pressure (see Table 14–7). Systemic venodilation also promotes increased flow to deep myocardial muscle by reducing the gradient between intraventricular pressure and coronary arteriolar (R^2) pressure. Direct actions on the coronary circulation include dilation of large and small intramural coronary arteries, collateral dilation, coronary artery stenosis dilation, abolition of normal tone in narrowed vessels, and relief of spasm; these actions occur even if the endothelium is denuded or dysfunctional. It is likely that depending on the underlying pathophysiology, different mechanisms become operative. For example, in the presence of a 60% to 70% stenosis, venodilation with MVO_2 reduction is most important; however, with higher-grade lesions, direct effects on the coronary circulation and vessel tone are the predominant effects. Although the cellular mechanism of vasodilation by nitrates is not entirely understood, organic nitrates are converted intracellularly to nitric oxide (EDRF) and 5-nitrosothiol via interaction with sulfhydryl groups. Nitric oxide, and perhaps 5-nitrosothiol, activates soluble guanylate cyclase to increase intracellular concentrations of cyclic GMP. Increased cyclic GMP induces a sequence of protein phosphorylation associated with reduced intracellular calcium release from the sarcoplasmic reticulum or reduced permeability to extracellular calcium and, consequently, smooth muscle relaxation.

Pharmacokinetic characteristics common to the organic nitrates used for angina include a large first-pass effect of hepatic metabolism, short to very short half-lives (except for isosorbide mononitrate), large volumes of distribution, high clearance rates, and large interindividual variations in plasma or blood concentrations. Pharmacodynamic-pharmacokinetic relationships for the entire class remain poorly defined, presumably owing to methodologic difficulty in characterizing the parent drug and metabolite concentrations at or within vascular smooth muscle and secondary to counterregulatory or adaptive mechanisms from the drug's effects as well as the occurrence of tolerance. Nitroglycerin is extracted by a variety of tissues and metabolized locally; differential extraction and metabolite generation occur depending on the tissue site. There are also numerous technical problems limiting the generation of reliable pharmacokinetic parameter estimates, including the following: assay sensitivity, arterial-venous extraction gradients and therefore extrahepatic metabolism, in vitro degradation, drug adsorption to polyvinyl chloride tubing and syringes, potentially saturable metabolism, accumulation of metabolites (some of which are active) with multiple doses, postural and exercise-induced changes in pharmacokinetics, and a variety of variables associated with transdermal delivery, including the delivery system (e.g., matrix, membrane-limited, ointment), vehicle used, the surface area and thickness of application, the site of application, and other skin variables (e.g., temperature, moisture content).

Nitroglycerin concentrations are affected by the route of administration, with the highest concentrations usually obtained with intravenous administration and the lowest seen with lower oral doses. Peak concentrations with sublingual nitroglycerin appear within 2 to 4 minutes, with the oral route producing peaks at about 15 to 30 minutes and the transdermal route at 1 to 2 hours. The half-life of nitroglycerin is 1 to 5 minutes regardless of route, hence the potential advantage of sustained-release and transdermal products. Transdermal nitroglycerin does produce sufficient concentrations for acute hemodynamic effects to occur, and these concentrations are maintained for long intervals; however, the hemodynamic and antianginal effects are minimal after 1 week or less with chronic, continuous (24 h/d) therapy.

Isosorbide dinitrate (ISDN) is metabolized to isosorbide 2-mono- and 5-mononitrate (isosorbide mononitrate). Isosorbide mononitrate is well absorbed, has a half-life of about 5 hours, and may be given once or twice daily depending on the product chosen. Multiple, larger doses of ISDN lead to disproportionate increases in the area under the plasma time profile, suggesting that metabolic pathways are being saturated or that metabolite accumulation may influence the disposition of ISDN. Little pharmacokinetic information is available for other nitrate compounds.

Nitrate therapy may be used to terminate an acute anginal attack, to prevent effort- or stress-induced attacks, or for long-term prophylaxis, usually in combination with β-blockers or calcium channel blockers. Sublingual nitroglycerin 0.3–0.4 mg will relieve pain in about 75% of patients within 3 minutes, with another 15% becoming pain-free in 5 to 15 minutes. Pain persisting beyond about 20 to 30 minutes following the use of two or three nitroglycerin tablets is suggestive of acute coronary syndrome, and the patient should be instructed to seek emergency aid. Patients should be instructed to keep nitroglycerin in the original, tightly closed glass container and to avoid mixing it with other medication because mixing may reduce nitroglycerin adsorption and vaporization. Additional counseling should include the facts that nitroglycerin is not an analgesic (rather, it partially corrects the underlying problem) and that repeated use is not harmful or addicting. Patients also should be aware that enhanced venous pooling in the sitting or standing position may improve the effect as well as the symptoms of postural hypotension and that inadequate saliva may slow or prevent tablet disintegration and dissolution. An acceptable, albeit expensive, alternative is lingual spray, which may be more convenient and has a shelf life of 3 years compared with 6 months or so for some forms of nitroglycerin tablets.

Chewable, oral, and transdermal products are acceptable for the long-term prophylaxis of angina; however, considerable controversy surrounds their use, and it appears that the development of tolerance or adaptive mechanisms limits the efficacy of all chronic nitrate therapies regardless of route. Dosing of the longer-acting preparations should be adjusted to provide a hemodynamic response, and as an example, this may require doses of oral ISDN ranging from 10 to 60 mg as often as every 3 to 4 hours owing to tolerance or first-pass metabolism, and similar large doses are required for other products. Nitroglycerin ointment has a duration of up to 6 hours, but it is difficult to apply in a cosmetically acceptable fashion over a consistent surface area, and response varies depending on the epidermal thickness, vascularity, and amount of hair. Percutaneous adsorption of nitroglycerin ointment may occur unintentionally if someone other than the patient applies the ointment, and limiting exposure through the use of gloves or some other means is advisable. Peripheral edema also may impair the response to nitroglycerin because venodilation cannot increase capacitance to a maximum and pooling may be reduced. Transdermal patch delivery systems were approved on the basis of sustained and equivalent plasma concentrations to other forms of therapy. Trials required by the Food and Drug Administration using transdermal patches as a continuous 24-hour delivery system revealed a lack of efficacy for improved exercise tolerance. Subsequently, large, randomized, double-blind, placebo-controlled trials of intermittent (10 to 12 hours on, 12 to 14 hours off) transdermal nitroglycerin therapy in chronic stable angina demonstrated modest but significant improvement in exercise time after 4 weeks for the highest doses at 8 to 12 hours after patch placement.[45] Subjective assessment methods for nitrate effects include reduction in the number of painful episodes and the amount of nitroglycerin consumed. Objective assessment includes the resolution of ECG changes at rest, during exercise, or with ambulatory ECG monitoring. Because nitrates work primarily through a reduction in MVO_2, the DP can be used to optimize the dose of sublingual and oral nitrate products. It is important to realize that reflex tachycardia may offset the beneficial reduction in systolic blood pressure and that calculation of the observed changes is necessary. The DP is best assessed in the sitting position and at intervals of 5 to 10 minutes and 30 to 60 minutes following sublingual and oral therapy, respectively. Owing to the placebo effect, unpredictable and variable course of angina, numerous pharmacologic effects of nitroglycerin, diurnal variation in pain patterns, stringent investigative protocols, and interindividual sensitivity to nitroglycerin, assessment with transdermal and sustained-release products is difficult. ETT provides valuable information concerning efficacy and mechanism of action for nitrates, but its use is usually reserved for clinical investigation rather than routine patient care. Most ETT studies have shown nitrates to delay the onset of ischemia (ST-segment changes or initial chest discomfort) at submaximal exercise, but the threshold for maximal exercise is unaltered, suggesting a reduction in oxygen demand rather than an improved oxygen supply. More sophisticated studies of myocardial function such as wall motion abnormalities and myocardial metabolism could be used to document efficacy; however, these studies are generally only for investigative purposes.

Adverse effects of nitrates are related most commonly to an extension of their pharmacologic effects and include postural hypotension with associated central nervous system symptoms, headaches and flushing secondary to vasodilatation, and occasional nausea from smooth muscle relaxation. If hypotension is excessive, coronary and cerebral filling may be compromised, leading to MI and stroke. While reflex tachycardia is most common, bradycardia with nitroglycerin has been reported. Other noncardiovascular adverse effects include rash with all products but particularly with transdermal nitroglycerin, the production of methemoglobinemia with high doses given for extended periods, and measurable concentrations of ethanol (intoxication has been reported) and propylene glycol (found in the diluent) with intravenous nitroglycerin.

Tolerance with nitrate therapy was first described in 1867 with the initial experience using amyl nitrate for angina and later widely recognized in munitions workers who underwent withdrawal reactions during periods of absence from exposure. Tolerance to nitrates is associated with a reduction in tissue cyclic GMP, which results from decreased production (guanylate cyclase) and increased breakdown via cyclic GMP phosphodiesterase and increased superoxide levels. One proposed mechanism for the lack of cyclic GMP is lack of conversion of organic nitrates to nitric oxide due to depletion of intracellular sulfhydryl cofactors (cysteine) in cells following chronic exposure to nitrates. This effect is more pronounced on the venous system than on the arterial system. Activation of neurohormonal systems following vasodilation with nitrates may result in vasoconstriction and sodium retention. The major systems thought to be involved in this second mechanism are the sympathoadrenal axis and the renin-angiotensin system. Concomitant use of captopril (25 mg tid) may attenuate increased sensitivity to phenylephrine and angiotensin II noted in patients with stable CAD.[46,47] Nitroglycerin administration is accompanied by a fall in hematocrit (caused by hemodilution rather than renal water conservation) and intravascular volume expansion, minimizing the ability of nitrates to decrease ventricular filling pressures, as a third mechanism of tolerance. Logically, a diuretic would minimize this mechanism; however, Parker and colleagues[48] found no effect on the development of tolerance to continuous transdermal nitroglycerin. Diuretic therapy itself has important antianginal effects and improves exercise capacity in patients with stable angina.[48] Supplemental vitamin E also has been studied to restore cyclic GMP production and the vasodilatory response to nitroglycerin.[49] Most of the published information from controlled trials examining nitrate tolerance have been done with either ISDN or transdermal nitroglycerin, and these studies demonstrate the development of tolerance within as little as 24 hours of therapy. While the onset of tolerance is rapid, the offset may be just as rapid, and one alternative dosing strategy to circumvent or minimize tolerance is to provide a daily nitrate-free interval of 6 to 8 hours. Studies with a variety of nitrate preparations and dosing schedules demonstrate that this approach is useful and that the nitrate-free interval should be a minimum of 8 hours and perhaps 12 hours for even better effects.[45] Another concern for intermittent transdermal nitrate therapy is the occurrence of rebound ischemia during the nitrate-free interval. Freedman and colleagues[50] found more silent ischemia during the patch-free interval during a randomized, double-blind, placebo-controlled trial than during the placebo patch phase, although others have not noted this effect. ISDN, for example, should not be used more often than three times per day if tolerance is to be avoided. Interestingly, hemodynamic tolerance does not always coincide with antianginal efficacy, but this is not well studied.[51]

Nitrates may be combined with other drugs for anginal therapy, including β-adrenergic blocking agents and calcium channel antagonists.[52] These combinations are usually instituted for chronic prophylactic therapy based on complementary or offsetting mechanisms of action (Table 14–7). Combination therapy generally is used in patients with more frequent or symptoms not responding to β-blockers alone (nitrates plus β-blockers or calcium blockers), in patients intolerant of β-blockers or calcium channel blockers, and in patients having an element of vasospasm leading to decreased supply (nitrates plus calcium blockers).[53]

CALCIUM CHANNEL ANTAGONISTS[51]

Modulation of calcium entry into vascular smooth muscle and myocardium as well as a variety of other tissues is the principal action of the calcium antagonists. The cellular mechanism of these drugs is not completely understood, and it differs among the available classes of the phenylalkylamines (verapamil-like), dihydropyridines (nifedipine-like), benzothiazepines (diltiazem-like), bepridil, and a recent class referred to as *T-channel blockers*. Receptor-operated channels stimulated by norepinephrine and other neurotransmittors and potential-dependent channels activated by membrane depolarization control the entry of calcium and consequently the cytosolic concentration of calcium responsible for activation of the actin-myosin complex leading to contraction of vascular smooth muscle and myocardium. In the myocardium, calcium entry triggers the release of intracellular stores of calcium to increase cytosolic calcium, whereas in smooth muscle, calcium derived from the extracellular fluid may do this directly. Binding proteins within the cell, calmodulin and troponin, after binding with calcium, participate in phosphorylation reactions leading to contraction. Decreased calcium availability, through the actions of calcium antagonists, inhibits these reactions.

Direct actions of the calcium antagonists include vasodilation of systemic arterioles and coronary arteries, leading to a reduction of arterial pressure and coronary vascular resistance as well as depression of the myocardial contractility and conduction velocity of the sinoatrial and atrioventricular nodes (see Chap. 16). Reflex β-adrenergic stimulation overcomes much of the negative inotropic effect, and depression of contractility becomes clinically apparent only in the presence of LV dysfunction and when other negative inotropic drugs are used concurrently. Verapamil and diltiazem cause less peripheral vasodilation than nifedipine, and consequently, the risk of myocardial depression is greater with these two agents. Conduction through the AV node is predictably depressed with verapamil and diltiazem, and they must be used with caution in patients with preexisting conduction abnormalities or in the presence of other drugs with negative chronotropic properties. Bepridil, in addition to having calcium channel blocking properties, also has class I and III antiarrhythmic activity. MVO_2 is reduced with all the calcium channel antagonists because of reduced wall tension secondary to reduced arterial pressure and, to a minor extent, depressed contractility (see Table 14–7). HR changes depend on the drug used and the state of the conduction system. Nifedipine generally increases HR or causes no change, whereas either no change or decreased HR is seen with verapamil and diltiazem because of the interaction of these direct and indirect effects. In contrast to the β-blockers, calcium channel antagonists have the potential to improve coronary blood flow through areas of fixed coronary obstruction and by inhibiting coronary artery vasomotion and vasospasm. Beneficial redistribution of blood flow from well-perfused myocardium to ischemic areas and from epicardium to endocardium also may contribute to improvement in ischemic symptoms. Overall, the benefit provided by calcium channel antagonists is related to reduced MVO_2 rather than improved oxygen supply based on lack of alteration in the rate-pressure product at maximal exercise in most studies performed to date. However, as CAD progresses and vasospasm becomes superimposed on critical stenotic lesions, improved oxygen supply through coronary vasodilation may become more important.

Absorption of the calcium channel antagonists is characterized by excellent absorption and large, variable first-pass metabolism resulting in oral bioavailability ranging from about 20% to 50% or greater for diltiazem, nicardipine, nifedipine, verapamil, felodipine, and isradipine. Amlodipine and bepridil have a range of bioavailability of approximately 60% to 80%. Saturation of this effect may occur with verapamil and diltiazem, resulting in greater amounts of drug being absorbed with chronic dosing. Nifedipine may have slow or fast absorption patterns, and the ingestion of food delays and impairs its absorption as well as potential enhanced absorption in elderly patients. This variability in absorption produces fluctuation in the hemodynamic response with nifedipine. Sublingual nifedipine is used frequently to provide a more rapid response; however, the rationale for this application is suspect because little nifedipine is absorbed from the buccal mucosa, and the swallowed drug is responsible for the observed plasma concentrations. Absorption of verapamil in sustained-release products may be influenced by food, and when used in the fasted state, dose dumping may occur, resulting in high peak concentrations with some products. The approved sustained-release products for nifedipine, verapamil, and diltiazem are approved primarily for the treatment of hypertension (see Chap. 12). The presence of severe liver disease (e.g., alcoholic liver disease with cirrhosis) has been shown to reduce the first-pass metabolism of verapamil, and this shunting of drug around the liver gives rise to higher plasma concentrations and lower dose requirements in these patients. Interestingly, this effect appears to be stereoselective for the more active isomer of verapamil. Verapamil also may reduce liver blood flow; however, evidence for this reduction is based primarily on animal experiments. Few data are available regarding the influence of liver disease on the kinetics of calcium blockers; however, these drugs undergo extensive hepatic metabolism, with little unchanged drug being renally excreted, and liver disease can be expected to alter the pharmacokinetics. Nifedipine has no active metabolites, whereas norverapamil possesses 20% or less activity of the parent compound. Desacetyldiltiazem has not been studied in humans, but canine studies suggest that its potency ranges from 100% to 40% of the parent compound for various cardiovascular effects; the clinical importance of these observations remains to be determined. With chronic dosing of verapamil and diltiazem, apparent saturation of metabolism occurs, producing higher plasma concentrations of each drug than those seen with single-dose administration. Consequently, the elimination half-life for verapamil is prolonged, and less frequent dosing intervals may be used in some patients. The elimination half-life for diltiazem is also somewhat prolonged and the half-life of desacetyldiltiazem is longer than that of the parent drug, but it is not clear if less frequent dosing may be used. Bepridil also undergoes hepatic elimination, and an active metabolite, 4-hydroxyphenyl bepridil, is produced; the parent compound has a long half-life of 30 to 40 hours. Nifedipine does not accumulate with chronic dosing; however, it is eliminated via oxidative pathways that may be polymorphic, and slow and fast metabolizers have been described for nifedipine. Most of the calcium channel blockers are eliminated via cytochrome P450 (CYP) isoenzyme 3A4 and other CYP isoenzymes, and many inhibit CYP 3A4 activity as well.[52] Renal insufficiency has little or no effect on the pharmacokinetics of these three drugs. Although disease alterations in kinetics have been described, the most important quantitative alteration is the influence of liver disease on bioavailability and elimination, which has been shown to reduce the clearance of verapamil and diltiazem; dosing in this population should be done with caution. Altered protein binding owing to renal disease, decreased protein concentration, or increased α_1-acid glycoprotein has been noted, but the clinical import of these changes is unknown.

Good candidates for calcium channel blockers in angina include patients with contraindications or intolerance of β-blockers, patients with coexisting conduction system disease (except for verapamil and diltiazem), patients with Prinzmetal's angina (vasospastic or variable threshold angina), patients with peripheral vascular disease or severe ventricular dysfunction (amlopidine is probably the calcium channel blocker of choice and others need to be used with caution if the ejection fraction is less than 40%), and patients with concurrent hypertension.

▶ TREATMENT: Stable Exertional Angina Pectoris[34,53–55]

After assessing and manipulating the alterable risk factors, as discussed previously, the next intervention that could be undertaken is the institution of a regular exercise program. Training is possible in many patients with angina, and the observed benefits include decreased HR and systolic blood pressure as well as increased ejection fraction and duration of exercise. Although the mechanism of these effects has been debated, improved overall cardiovascular and muscular condition is probably most important. Improved production of nitric oxide and coronary vasomotion may account partially for the beneficial effects of exercise. The intensity of exercise influences training, and more vigorous programs provide better overall results.[13,53] Obviously, an exercise program should be undertaken with caution and in a graded fashion with adequate supervision.

Chronic prophylactic therapy for patients with more than one angina episode per day also may be instituted with β-adrenergic blocking agents, and in many instances, β-blockers may be preferable because of less frequent dosing and other properties inherent in β blockade (e.g., potential cardioprotective effects, antiarrhythmic effects, lack of tolerance, and antihypertensive effects), as well as their antianginal effects and documented protective effects in patients after MI.[1] Patients who continue to smoke have reduced antianginal efficacy of β-blockers. This may be due to enhanced hepatic metabolism of drugs that are eliminated through this route or related to the effects of smoking on MVO_2 and oxygenation. The one characteristic that is relevant is the duration of effect on the DP. β-Blockers with longer half-lives (e.g., nadolol) are more likely to affect the DP for a longer period of time and require fewer doses per day. The choice of β-blocker for angina rests on choosing the appropriate dose to achieve the goals outlined for HR and DP, on choosing an agent that is well tolerated by individual patients, and on cost. Selective use may incorporate ancillary properties, but these are secondary considerations in overall drug product selection. Patients most likely to respond well to β blockade are those who have a high resting HR and those having a relatively fixed anginal threshold. In other words, their symptoms appear at the same level of exercise or work load on a consistent basis. Symptoms appearing with variable work loads suggest fluctuations in myocardial oxygen supply, perhaps due to coronary artery vasomotion, and these patients are more likely to respond to calcium channel antagonists.

Nitrate therapy should be the first step in managing acute attacks for patients with chronic stable angina if the attacks are infrequent (i.e., a few times per month) or for prophylaxis of symptoms when undertaking activities known to precipitate attacks. In general, if angina occurs no more often than once every few days, then sublingual nitroglycerin tablets or spray or buccal products may be sufficient to allow the patient to maintain an adequate life-style. For episodes of "first effort" angina occurring in a predictable fashion, nitroglycerin may be used in a prophylactic manner, with the patient taking 0.3–0.4 mg sublingually about 5 minutes prior to the anticipated time of activity. Nitroglycerin spray may be useful when inadequate saliva is produced to rapidly dissolve sublingual nitroglycerin or if a patient has difficulty opening the container. Most patients have a response that lasts about 30 minutes or so, but this is subject to interindividual variability. When angina occurs more frequently than once a day, a chronic prophylactic regimen using β-blockers as the first line of therapy should be considered (see Figure 14–5 for the stable angina algorithm). Chronic prophylactic therapy with long-acting forms of nitroglycerin (oral or transdermal), isosorbide dinitrate, 5-mononitrate, and pentaerythritol trinitrate may be effective; however, the development of tolerance is a major limiting step in their continued effectiveness. Since long-acting nitrates are not as effective as β-blockers and do not have beneficial effects, monotherapy with nitrates should not be first-line therapy unless β-blockers and calcium channel blockers are contraindicated or not tolerated. As described previously, providing a nitrate-free interval of 8 hours per day or longer appears to be the most promising approach to maintaining the efficacy of chronic nitrate therapy. Oral administration of nitrates is susceptible to a saturable first-pass effect; therefore, larger doses can produce a measurable hemodynamic effect and dose titration should be based on these changes in the double product. There are few well-controlled studies comparing oral or sublingual nitrate efficacy, and the choice among these products should be based on familiarity with the preparation, cost, and patient acceptance.

Calcium channel antagonists have the potential advantage of improving coronary blood flow through coronary artery vasodilation as well as decreasing MVO_2 and may be used instead of β-blockers for chronic prophylactic therapy; however, in chronic stable angina, comparative trials of long-acting calcium channel blockers with β-blockers do not show significant differences in response.[42,54] They are as effective as β-blockers and are most useful in patients who have a variable threshold for exertional angina. Calcium antagonists may provide better skeletal muscle oxygenation, resulting in decreased fatigue and better exercise tolerance. Additionally, if contraindications exist to β-blocker therapy, calcium antagonists can be used safely in many patients. The available calcium channel blockers appear to have similar efficacy in the management of chronic stable angina. Differences in their electrophysiology, peripheral and central hemodynamic effects, and adverse-effect profiles are useful in selecting the appropriate agent. Patients with conduction abnormalities and moderate to severe LV dysfunction (ejection fraction $< 35\%$) should not be treated with verapamil, whereas amlodipine may be used safely in many of these patients. Diltiazem has significant effects on the AV node and can produce heart block in patients with preexisting conduction disease or when other drugs, such as digoxin or β-blockers, with effects on conduction are used concurrently. Nifedipine may cause excessive HR elevation, especially if the patient is not receiving a β-blocker, and this may offset the beneficial effect it has on MVO_2. Gingival hyperplasia also has been reported with nifedipine, and some dental authorities say this may be seen in as many as 20% of patients on nifedipine. Bepridil prolongs the QT interval in patients with certain conditions (e.g., hypokalemia, advanced age, preexisting QT interval prolongation), and because of this potential proarrhythmic effect, it is indicated only in patients who have been inadequately controlled with other antianginal therapy. Case-control studies with calcium channel blockers suggest an increased risk for MI and cancer.[55,56] The relationship to cancer appears to be weak to nonexistent, whereas the risk for MI is probably real and related to the type of drug used and relationship to recent MI. Shorter-acting calcium blockers can activate the sympathetic nervous system and, in patients with recent MI or significant CAD, may induce ischemia. This effect has not been shown for longer-acting products. The hemodynamic effect of calcium antagonists is complementary to β blockade, and consequently, combination therapy is rational. However, clinical trial data do not support the notion that combination therapy is always more effective.[42,57]

▶ TREATMENT: Unstable Angina and NSTEMI[12,13,61,62]

Clinical and autopsy studies indicate that most patients who present with unstable angina and NSTEMI have significant underlying coronary atherosclerosis.[2] Precipitation of acute coronary syndromes is most often due to disruption of an atherosclerotic plaque and a subsequent cascade of platelet activation and aggregation, thrombosis, and coronary vasoconstriction leading to a decrease in coronary blood flow. The interrelationship of these mechanisms and potential therapeutic interventions are outlined in Figure 14–6. Patients at high risk of death or nonfatal MI are those presenting with a positive history, classic symptoms, clinical findings of heart failure, electrical instability, and positive biomarkers of cardiac injury (e.g., troponin T or I) found in Table 14–4.[2] Unstable angina differs from stable angina in that the initial event is thought to be a reduction in coronary blood flow rather than an increase in MVO_2, with corresponding ischemic changes in the ECG occurring prior to changes in HR and blood pressure.

Immediate management involves risk stratification that uses the history, physical examination, electrocardiogram (within 20 minutes), and initial cardiac biomarkers to assign patients into one of four categories: a noncardiac diagnosis, chronic stable angina, possible acute coronary syndrome, and definite acute coronary syndrome. Patients with definite or possible acute coronary syndrome should be transferred to a chest pain unit where an electrocardiogram and measurement of biomarkers should be repeated in 6 to 12 hours. If the follow-up 12-lead electrocardiogram and biomarkers are normal, then ETT may be used to further stratify the patient into low or intermediate risk. Low-risk patients may be discharged early. Patients with possible acute coronary syndrome and negative biomarkers and those who are unable to exercise or have an abnormal resting electrocardiogram should undergo a pharmacologic stress. Patients with definite acute coronary syndrome and ST-segment elevation should be evaluated for immediate reperfusion therapy (thrombolysis or primary coronary intervention).

Anti-ischemic therapy for unstable angina includes bed rest with continuous monitoring for ischemia and arrhythmia detection, supplemental oxygen if cyanotic or hypoxemic (maintain $SaO_2 > 90\%$), and immediate consideration of the use of sublingual nitroglycerin followed by intravenous nitroglycerin, aspirin, heparin, intravenous β-blockers followed by oral β-blockers, morphine sulfate 2 to 5 mg intravenously if pain is not relieved by nitrates, and an angiotensin-converting enzyme inhibitor if hypertension or LV dysfunction persists after nitroglycerin and β-blockers (see Fig. 14–7 for the unstable angina algorithm). Oral long-acting calcium channel blockers may be added or substituted for β-blockers if no contraindications exist and contraindications exist for β-blockers. If the history suggests vasospastic angina (Prinzmetal's angina) or chest pain or hypertension persists, calcium channel blockers would be appropriate. Immediate-release dihydropyridines calcium channel blockers should not be used in the absence of a β- blocker, and nitrates should not be given if sildenafil has been used within 24 hours. Use of antithrombotic therapy is based on the likelihood of acute coronary syndrome. If the patient is stratified as possible acute coronary syndrome, only aspirin is given. Likely or definite acute coronary syndrome should be treated initially with non-enteric-coated (chew and swallow) aspirin 160–325 mg followed by 75–160 mg/d of enteric- or non-enteric coated aspirin and subcutaneous low-molecular-weight heparin (LMWH) or intravenous unfractionated heparin (UFH). Definite acute coronary syndrome with continuing ischemia or other high-risk features (see Table 14–4) or planned percutaneous coronary intervention (PCI) should be treated with aspirin plus UFH or LMWH and an intravenous platelet glycoprotein IIb/IIIa receptor antagonist.

Platelet aggregation and thrombosis play a major role in acute coronary syndrome, and aspirin reduces the relative risk of recurrent acute MI and death by approximately 50% (12.5% versus 6.4%).[2] Alternative antiplatelet agents for patients intolerant of aspirin or who have failed aspirin are clopidogrel (75 mg/d) and ticlopidine (250 mg twice daily). If PCI is planned, combination therapy with aspirin plus clopidogrel or ticlopidine is now commonly used for 1 to 2 months after the procedure. Loading doses of clopidogrel (300–600 mg) or ticlopidine (500 mg) are also used for a rapid onset of inhibition of platelet aggregation.[58] Clopidogrel has become the preferred agent over ticlopidine for stent placement.[59,60] Monitoring of therapy is less complicated and less expensive (ticlopidine causes neutropenia in 2.4% of patients) and based on the Clopidogrel in Unstable angina to prevent Recurrent Events (CURE) trial, clopidogrel reduced cardiovascular death, nonfatal MI, or nonfatal stroke by 20% (9.28% versus 11.47%; $P = .00005$) compared with aspirin and placebo.[61] Major bleeding was slightly more common with clopidogrel (3.6% versus 2.7%; $P = .003$). Both ticlopidine (1 in 1600 to 5000 patients) and clopidogrel (less common) have been reported to cause thrombotic thrombocytopenic purpura.[62] Other drugs that have been tested in acute coronary syndrome but have shown no benefit include sulfinpyrazone, dipridamole, prostacyclin, prostacyclin analogs, and oral IIb/IIIa receptor antagonists (e.g., sibrafibin).[2] Intravenous abciximab was not useful for acute coronary syndrome without early coronary revascularization in the Global Use of Strategies To Open occluded Arteries (GUSTO-IV) trial and lead to slightly higher mortality at 30 days (9.1% for 48-hour infusion and 8.2% for 24-hour infusion versus 8.0% with placebo). Major bleeding was slightly more common with abciximab given for 48 hours than placebo (1% versus 0.3%).[63]

Historically, UFH has been the anticoagulant of choice for acute coronary syndrome, and compared with aspirin alone, the combination of UFH and aspirin reduces the risk of death or MI by 33% to 50% during short-term administration.[2,64] UFH is usually

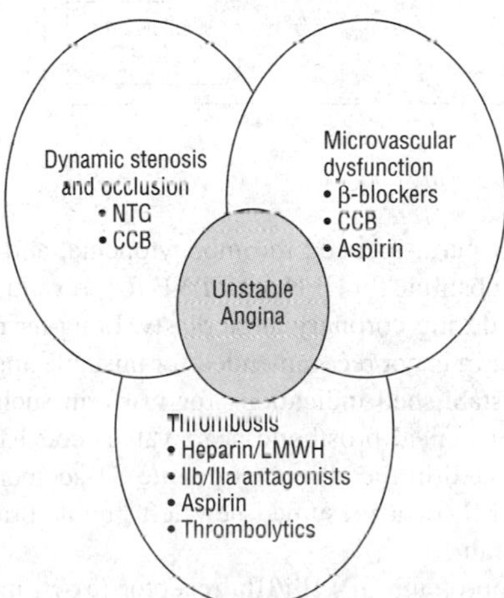

FIGURE 14–6. Pathophysiologic components of unstable angina and potentially useful therapeutic interventions. Dynamic stenosis or occlusion, microvascular dysfunction, and thrombosis interact equally to bring about unstable angina. NTG = nitroglycerin; CCB = calcium channel blocker; LMWH = low-molecular-weight heparin.

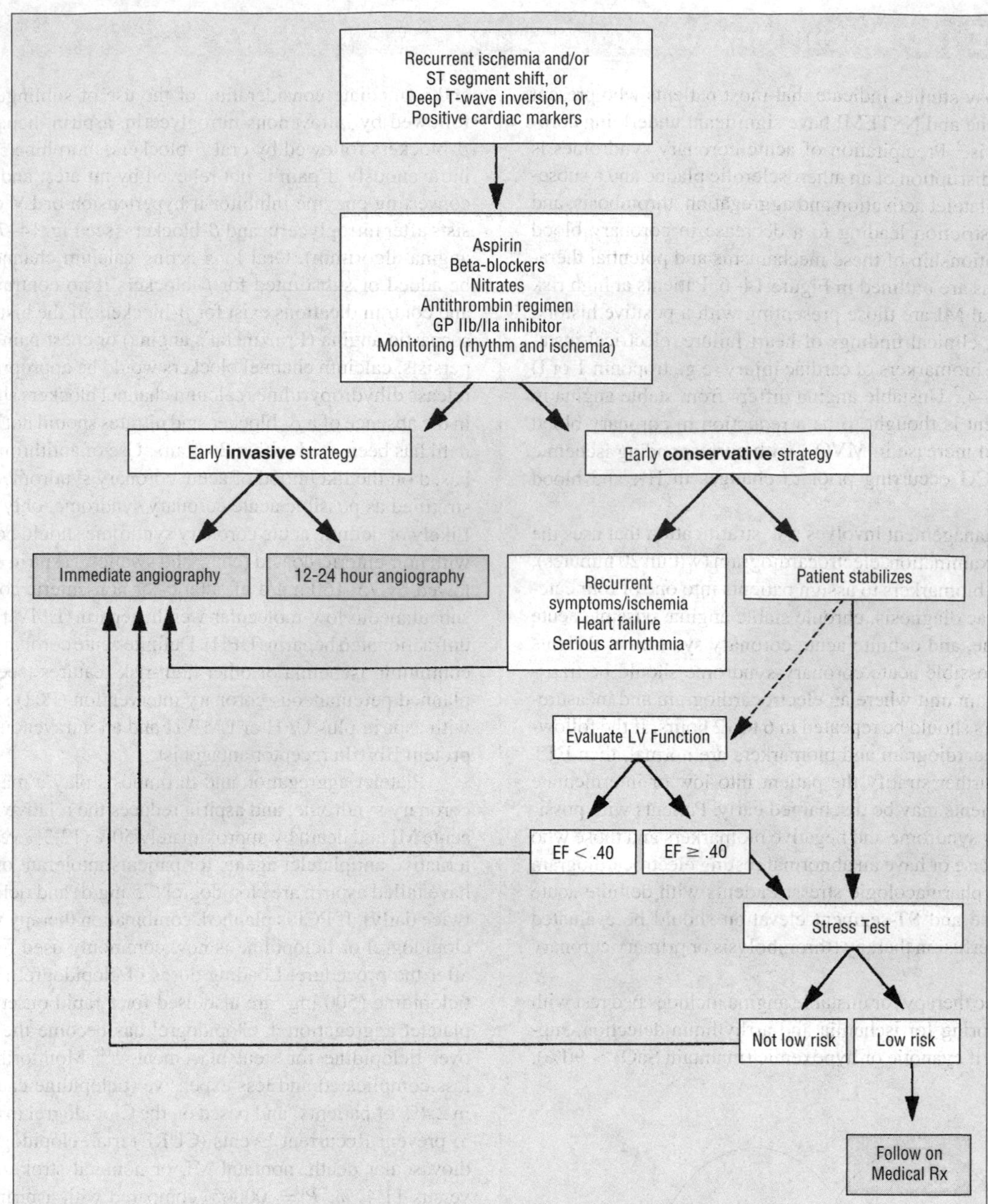

FIGURE 14–7. Unstable angina algorithm.

dosed by giving a loading dose of 60–70 units/kg, followed by an infusion of 12–15 units/kg per hour titrated to maintain an activated partial thromboplastin time of 1.5 to 2.5 times control. More recently, LMWH has been shown to provide comparable risk reduction to that seen with UFH (2.6% versus 5.5%). In the four trials comparing LMWH with UFH, mixed results have been seen with dalteparin or nadropain, but enoxaparin 1 mg/kg every 12 hours (ESSENCE and TIMI 11B trials) has consistently reduced death, MI, and recurrent ischemia with or without urgent revascularization to a greater extent than UFH.[65,66] More rigorous monitoring of anticoagulation therapy may be needed in patients who are obese or have renal insufficiency. Argatroban, lepirudin (Hirudin), and bivalirudin are direct thrombin inhibitors that have been used in unstable angina with some success but are not approved by the Food and Drug Administration for the treatment of acute coronary syndrome. Currently, argatroban and lepirudin are approved for heparin-induced thrombocytopenia, and bivalirudin is approved as a substitute for UFH or LMWH for prevention of ischemic complications during coronary angioplasty. Long-term anticoagulation with warfarin is not recommended for unstable angina/NSTEMI unless other established indications for warfarin such as atrial fibrillation or mechanical prosthetic heart valves coexist. Thrombolysis is not indicated in the absence of acute ST-segment elevation, a true posterior MI, or a presumed new left bundle-branch block on electrocardiogram.

The glycoprotein (GP) IIb/IIIa receptor ($\alpha_M\beta_3$ integrin) on the platelet surface undergoes a confirmation change when platelets are activated, increasing the affinity for binding of platelets to fibrinogen and other ligands. Binding of molecules of fibrinogen to receptors on different platelets results in platelet aggregation; binding of GP receptor antagonists prevents fibrinogen binding and thereby prevents platelet aggregation. Occupancy of 80% or more of the receptor population and inhibition of 80% or more of ADP-induced aggregation lead to potent antithrombotic effects. The pharmacokinetic and pharmacodynamic properties of abciximab, eptifibatide, and tirofiban differ, but the most important difference in the long duration of abciximab, which is due to strong affinity for the receptor. Abciximab antiplatelet activity persists for 24 to 48 hours after discontinuation, whereas the effects of eptifibatide and tirofiban are minimal 8 hours or so after discontinuation. The usual dosing regimens for these drugs are as follows: abciximab, 0.25 mg/kg bolus, followed by infusion of 0.125 μg/kg per minute (maximum 10 μg/kg per minute) for 12 to 24 hours; eptifibatide, 180 μg/kg bolus, followed by infusion of 2.0 μg/kg per minute for 72 to 96 hours; tirofiban, 0.4 μg/kg per minute for 30 minutes, followed by infusion of 0.1 μg/kg per minute for 48 to 96 hours. Approximately 12 large clinical trials (>1000 patients) have been conducted, and overall, there is a 20% reduction (9.1% versus 11.4%; $P < .001$) in the combined end point of death or recurrent MI with GP IIb/IIIa receptor antagonist use.[2] The effects of GP IIb/IIIa receptor antagonists are magnified in patients with acute coronary syndrome if a PCI is performed. PCI refers to a family of percutaneous techniques including PTCA, intracoronary stenting, and atheroablative technologies (e.g., atherectomy, thrombectory, laser). The majority of PCIs involve balloon dilatation and coronary stenting (~70%). In acute coronary syndrome trials where PCI is not performed, the absolute risk for death or MI is reduced by GP IIb/IIIa receptor antagonists from 13.2% to 11.7%, a 19% relative risk reduction. When PCI is performed, GP IIb/IIIa receptor antagonists reduce absolute risk for death or MI from 8.8% to 5.4%, a 38% relative risk reduction. Current guidelines recommend that a GP IIb/IIIa receptor antagonist be given along with aspirin and UFH or LMWH to patients with unstable angins/NSTEMI with active ischemia or with any of the high-risk features shown in Table 14–4.[2] The TARGET (do Tirofiban And ReoPro Give Similar Efficacy?) study was a direct comparison of abciximab 0.25 μg/kg bolus followed by 0.125 μg/kg per minute infusions for 12 hours versus tirofiban 10 μg/kg bolus followed by 0.15 μg/kg per minute infusion for up to 24 hours in patients undergoing stenting electively or for acute coronary syndrome.[67] The primary end point was the composite of death, MI, and urgent revascularization at 30 days. The primary end point was seen more commonly in the tirofiban group (7.55% versus 6.01%; $P = .037$), and the difference was greater in patients presenting with acute coronary syndrome. At this time, abciximab is considered the drug of choice for patients undergoing PCI with stenting, whereas tirofiban and eptifibatide generally are the preferred drugs for medical (pharmacologic) management of acute coronary syndrome.

If three doses of sublingual nitroglycerin 0.4 mg given 5 minutes apart do not relieve the patient's pain, then intravenous nitroglycerin provides a convenient method of titrating the dose and avoids uncertainty concerning drug delivery. Dosing should be started low (5–10 μg/kg per minute) and titrated upward by 10 μg/min every 3 to 5 minutes until symptoms are relieved or limiting adverse effects occur. A reduction in systolic blood pressure is expected and should be about a 25% reduction in mean arterial blood pressure or to a systolic pressure of 100 to 110 mm Hg. Caution is necessary in preload-dependent patients (with right ventricular infarct, hypovolemia, pericardial constriction, or effusion) to avoid hypotension and decreased coronary perfusion pressure as well as excessive HR elevation if the patient is not receiving β-blockers. After 24 hours free of symptoms, patients may be switched over to oral or topical nitrates.

Intravenous β-blockers are recommended for high-risk patients (oral for intermediate- and low-risk patients) in the absence of contraindications. Regimens are similar to those used in acute MI. Unstable patients with persisting or recurring pain while on nitrates and β-blockers should receive a calcium antagonist. β-Blockers in unstable angina reduces the risk of progression to MI slightly but have not been shown to reduce mortality. β-Blockers do have strong evidence supporting their use in acute MI and in post-MI patients, and this is sufficient evidence to recommend their routine use. In acute coronary syndrome, aggregated data suggest an approximate 13% reduction in progression to acute MI, β-Blocker therapy may prevent ischemia caused by tachycardia and reduce cardiac work. Patients should be screened for contraindications to therapy.

Several studies suggest efficacy of calcium channel blockers in unstable angina, and their effects are mediated via inhibition of increased coronary tone and through reduction in MVO_2. Calcium antagonists may be used to control ongoing or recurring ischemia-related symptoms for patients already on adequate doses of nitrates and β-blockers. Calcium channel antagonists also may be used if patients are intolerant of nitrates and/or β-blockers or for patients with variant angina. Verapamil and diltiazem should be avoided in patients with pulmonary edema or evidence of LV dysfunction. Amlodipine and felodipine may be tolerated in patients with heart failure. Nifedipine or short-acting calcium antagonists should not be used in the absence of concurrent β blockade. The largest randomized trial with nifedipine and metoprolol found metoprolol to be more effective than placebo, whereas nifedipine increased the risk of MI and recurrent angina compared with placebo; the combination was no better than metoprolol alone. Diltiazem may be more useful than other agents in the setting of unstable angina/NSTEMI because it has been shown to reduce reinfarction and refractory angina (see Chap. 15).

The need for conservative versus invasive strategies in management is based on risk stratification. Low-risk patients (see Table 14–4) who are free of ischemia at rest and heart failure may undergo noninvasive stress testing after 12 to 24 hours. Intermediate-risk patients who have been free of ischemia at rest or with low-level activity and free of heart failure for 2 or more days may undergo stress testing. Treadmill exercise is used most commonly, but the choice for testing depends on the resting electrocardiogram, ability to perform exercise, local expertise, and technologies available. An imaging modality is added in patients with resting ST-segment depression (≥0.10 mV), LV hypertrophy, bundle-branch block, intraventricular conduction defect, preexcitation, or digoxin who are able to exercise. Pharmacologic stress testing with adenosine or dobutamine is used when patients cannot exercise (e.g., arthritis, amputation, severe chronic obstructive pulmonary disease, peripheral arterial disease). Prompt angiography is recommended if patients with acute coronary syndrome who cannot be stabilized with medical therapy. Evaluation of LV function with an echocardiogram or radionuclide angiogram may be used in some patients not scheduled for angiography.[2,68] The Veterans Affairs Non-Q-Wave Infarction Strategies in Hospital (VANQWISH) study supports the concept that noninvasive testing correctly identifies high-risk patients who should be directed to angiography.[69] Coronary angiography should be considered in the following groups of patients: (1) patients with prior angioplasty, bypass surgery, or MI, (2) patients who fail to stabilize on medical therapy, (3) patients opting for early invasive strategy (CABG or PCI), (4) patients with high-risk clinical findings (described previously) or noninvasive test results (e.g., LV ejection fraction <0.35, high-risk treadmill score, stress-induced or multiple perfusion defects or wall motion abnormalities), or (5) patients with significant congestive heart failure or LV dysfunction.

An early invasive strategy for unstable angina/NSTEMI is recommended when patients have recurrent angina/ischemia at rest or with low-level activities (≤6.5 METs), develop heart failure symptoms or findings with ischemia despite intensive medical therapy, or have high-risk findings on stress testing, depressed LV function (ejection fraction <0.40), hemodynamic instability, sustained ventricular tachycardia, PCI in the past 6 months, and prior CABG. Invasive strategies also may be employed in patients with repeated presentations for acute coronary syndrome despite therapy and without evidence for ongoing ischemia or high risk and for patients over 65 years of age who present with ST-segment depression or elevated cardiac biomarkers and no contraindications to revascularization. The TACTICS (Treat Angina with Aggrastat and Determine Cost of Therapy with an Invasive or Conservative Strategy) study treated patients with aspirin 325 mg/d, a 5000-unit bolus of UFH followed by 1000 units/h for 48 hours, and a 0.4 mg/kg bolus of tirofiban followed by 0.1 mg/kg per minute for 48 hours until revascularization plus an additional 12 hours after revascularization and either an early invasive strategy (revascularization) or early conservative strategy (pharmacologic management).[70] At 6 months, the combined primary end point of death, nonfatal MI, and rehospitalization for acute coronary syndrome occurred in 15.9% of patients with the early invasive strategy versus 19.4% of patients with the conservative strategy (odds ratio 0.78, $P = .025$).

The decision to chose PCI or CABG for revascularization is based on the extent of CAD (number of vessels and location/amount of stenosis) and ventricular function. The recommended mode of coronary revascularization is outlined in Table 14–9.[2]

The largest randomized trial of PCI versus CABG is the Bypass Angioplasty Revascularization (BARI) trial conducted in 1829 patients with two- or three-vessel disease; 64% of these patients had an admitting diagnosis of unstable angins, and 19% were diabetic.[71] Seven-year survival for the total population was 84.4% for CABG and 80.9% for PTCA ($P = .043$). Patients with diabetes mellitus undergoing CABG had improved survival compared with nondiabetics (76.4% CABG and 55.7% PTCA; $P = .0011$). Among the remaining 1476 patients without treated diabetes, survival was virtually identical by assigned treatment (86.4% CABG and 86.8% PTCA; $P = .72$). The PTCA group had substantially higher subsequent revascularization rates than the CABG group (59.7% versus 13.1%; $P < .001$); however, the changes between the 5- and 7-year rates were similar for the two groups. Insulin-requiring diabetics seem to be at the highest risk, and CABG is the revascularization procedure of choice for this population.[72] In a large observational study by Hannan and colleagues, patients with proximal left anterior descending artery lesions and multivessel disease had higher survival rates with CABG than with PTCA.[73] High-risk patients who should be considered for CABG over PCI are those with LV systolic dysfunction, patients with diabetes, and those with two-vessel disease with severe proximal left anterior descending artery involvement or severe three-vessel or left main artery disease[2] (see Table 14–9). The AWESOME (Angina With Extremely Serious Operative Mortality) trial is large randomized trial comparing PTCA to CABG, and the results should further define which method of revascularization is best for patients with refractory ischemia and high risk of adverse outcomes.[74]

PCI has been used successfully in the management of unstable angina.[75–77] PTCA involves the insertion of a guidewire and inflatable balloon into the affected coronary artery and enlarging the lumen of the artery by stretching the vessel wall. This frequently causes atheroma plaque fracture by stretching inelastic components and denudation of the endothelium, resulting in loss of nitric oxide and other vasodilators and exposure of plaque contents to the vascular

TABLE 14–9. Recommended Mode of Coronary Revascularization

Extent of Disease	Treatment	Class/Level of Evidence
Left main disease,[a] candidate for CABG	CABG PCI	I/A III/C
Left main disease, not a candidate for CABG	PCI	IIb/C
Three-vessel disease with EF < 0.50	CABG	I/A
Multivessel disease including proximal LAD with EF < 0.50 or treated diabetes	CABG PCI	I/A IIb/B
Multivessel disease with EF > 0.50 and without diabetes	PCI	I/A
One- or two-vessel disease without proximal LAD but with large areas of myocardial ischemia or high-risk criteria on noninvasive testing (see text)	CABG or PCI	I/B
One-vessel disease with proximal LAD	CBAG or PCI	IIa/B
One- or two-vessel disease without proximal LAD with small area of ischemia or no ischemia on noninvasive testing	CABG or PCI	III/C
Insignificant coronary stenosis	CABG or PCI	III/C

[a] ≥50% diameter stenosis.

Abbreviations: CBAG = coronary artery bypass grafting; PCI = percutaneous coronary intervention; EF = ejection fraction; LAD = left anterior descending coronary artery. Class I evidence means conditions for which there is evidence and/or general agreement that a given procedure or treatment is useful and effective. Class IIa evidence means conditions for which there is conflicting evidence and/or divergence of opinion about usefulness/efficacy of a procedure or treatment. Class IIa indicates that the weight of evidence/opinion is in favor of usefulness/efficacy. Class IIb indicates that the usefulness/efficacy is less well established. Class III indicates that the evidence and/or general agreement that the procedure/treatment is not useful or effective and may be harmful. Level A evidence is derived from multiple randomized clinical trials with large numbers of patients. Level B evidence is derived from limited number of trials with small numbers of patients or from nonrandomized trials or observational studies. Level C evidence is based on expert opinion.

From Braunwald E, Antman EM, Beasley JW, et al. ACC/AHA guidelines for the management of patients with unstable angina and non-ST-segment elevation myocardial infarction: A report of the American College of Cardiology/American Heart Association Task Force on Practice Guidelines (Committee on the Management of Patients with Unstable Angina). J Am Coll Cardiol 2000;36:970–1062, with permission.

compartment. Consequently, immediate vascular recoil, platelet adhesion and aggregation, mural thrombus formation, smooth muscle proliferation, and synthesis of extracellular matrix may give rise to acute occlusion and early or late restenosis.[78,79] The presence of coronary artery spasm and intraluminal thrombus, common occurrences in unstable angina, increases the hazard of these complications. The advent of combination therapy with aspirin, UFH or LMWH, and glycoprotein IIb/IIIa receptor antagonists and coronary artery stents has reduced dramatically the occurrence of early reocclusion and late restenosis.[2,75] Patients best suited for PTCA are those with recent onset of worsening angina without a long history of symptoms. Angiographic characteristics associated with these clinical findings that allow the greatest probability of success for PTCA are severe, Patients with focal saphenous vein graft lesions who are poor candidates for reoperation have a class IIa recommendation for PCI. Class IIb indications include patients with one or more lesions to be dilated in vessels subtending a less than moderate area of viable myocardium and patients with multivessel disease and proximal left anterior descending artery lesions, diabetes, or abnormal LV function.[75] Candidates for PTCA also must be suited for CABG because a small percentage of procedures results in emergency CABG. Success of PCI may be defined as angiographic success (TIMI 3 flow and less than 20% residual stenosis), procedural success (lack of in-hospital clinical complications), and clinical success (anatomic and procedural success with relief of ischemic pain for at least 6 months). In trials of invasive versus conservative strategies (medical management) using PCI, death or MI is less frequent in some trials but not all.[69,76,80,81] Numerous studies support the use of glycoprotein IIb/IIIa receptor antagonists in addition to aspirin and UFH or LMWH, and as described previously, abciximab was superior to tirofiban in the only comparative study available.[2,67,75] The initial success rate for PTCA in unstable angina is approximately 80% to 90%, but these patients are at risk for more complications than are those with stable angina because of the underlying pathophysiology.

In the event of prolonged chest pain and ischemic ECG changes unrelieved by nitrate therapy or calcium channel antagonists, one may assume total occlusion of a coronary vessel, and steps should be taken to restore blood flow with either PCI or CABG.

▶ TREATMENT: Coronary Artery Spasm and Variant Angina (Prinzmetal's Angina)[54]

Prinzmetal, in his original description of variant angina pectoris, noted the waxing and waning course of this syndrome associated with ST-segment elevation that most commonly resolves without progression to MI. Patients who develop variant angina are usually younger and have fewer coronary risk factors but more commonly smoke than patients with chronic stable angina. Hyperventilation, exercise, and exposure to cold may precipitate variant angina attacks, or there may be no apparent precipitating cause. The onset of chest discomfort is usually in the early morning hours. The exact cause of variant angina is not well understood but may be an imbalance between endothelium-produced vasodilator factors (e.g., prostacyclin, nitric oxide) and vasoconstrictor factors (e.g., endothelin, angiotensin II) as well as an imbalance of autonomic control characterized by parasympathetic dominance.[82]

The diagnosis of variant angina is based on ST-segment elevation during transient chest discomfort (usually at rest) that resolves when the chest discomfort diminishes in patients who have a normal heart or nonobstructive coronary lesions. In the absence of ST-segment elevation, provocative test using ergonovine, acetylcholine, or methacholine may be used to precipitate coronary artery spasm, ST-segment elevation, and typical symptoms. Nitrates and calcium channel antagonists should be withdrawn prior to provocative testing. Provocative testing should not be used in patients with high-grade lesions. Hyperventilation also may be used to provoke spasm, and patients who have a positive hyperventilation test are more likely to have a higher frequency of attacks, multivessel disease, and a high degree of AV block or ventricular tachycardia.

Optimization of therapy includes dose titration using sufficiently high doses to obtain clinical efficacy without unacceptable adverse effects in individual patients. All patients should be treated for acute attacks and maintained on prophylactic treatment for 6 to 12 months following the initial episode. The occurrence of serious arrhythmias during attacks is associated with a greater risk of sudden death, and these patients should be treated more aggressively and for prolonged periods. In patients without arrhythmias who become asymptomatic and remain so for several months after treatment has been instituted, withdrawal of therapy may be safe after first ascertaining that disease activity is quiescent. Aggravating factors such as alcohol or cocaine use or cigarette smoking should be eliminated when instituting treatment.

Nitrates have been the mainstay of therapy for the acute attacks of variant angina and coronary artery spasm for many years. Most patients respond rapidly to sublingual nitroglycerin or isosorbide dinitrate; however, intravenous and intracoronary nitroglycerin may be very useful for patients not responding to sublingual preparations. In particular, vasospasm provoked by ergonovine may require intracoronary nitroglycerin. Although studies with nitrates generally show them to be efficacious, high doses often are required, and it is unclear if they reduce mortality. Because calcium channel antagonists may be more effective, have few serious adverse effects in effective doses, and can be given less frequently than nitrates, some consider them the agents of choice for variant angina.

Nifedipine, verapamil, and diltiazem are all equally effective as single agents for the initial management of variant angina and coronary artery spasm. Dose titration is important to maximize the response with calcium antagonists. Comparative trials, which are few in number, do not reveal significant differences among these three drugs for variant angina. Patients unresponsive to calcium antagonists alone may have nitrates added. Combination therapy with nifedipine-diltiazem or nifedipine-verapamil has been reported useful for patients unresponsive to single-drug regimens. This is probably rational because, at the cellular level, the drugs have different receptors, but the combination of verapamil-diltiazem should be used cautiously owing to their potential additive effects on contractility and conduction.

β-Adrenergic blockade has little or no role in the management of variant angina according to most authorities.[83] Although not all studies report increased painful episodes of variant angina with the addition of β-blockers, they may induce coronary vasoconstriction and prolong ischemia, as documented by continuous ECG monitoring. Other approaches to therapy attempting to modify sympathetic/parasympathetic tone include α-antagonists, anticholinergics, plexectomy, surgical interruption of the sympathetic innervation of the heart, thromboxane receptor antagonism, prostacyclin, lipoxygenase inhibition, and ticlopidine, but these drugs or procedures do not occupy a major place in therapy at the present time.

▶ TREATMENT: Silent Myocardial Ischemia[16]

The objective in the treatment of silent myocardial ischemia is to reduce the total number of ischemic episodes, both symptomatic and asymptomatic, regardless of the direction of ST-segment shift. The incidence of silent ischemia in the general, asymptomatic population is not known. Significant day-to-day variability in the number of episodes, the duration of ischemia, and the amount of ST-segment deviation complicates both the understanding of this process and the utility of various therapeutic interventions. Silent ischemia in patients with known CAD is common (80% of all ischemic episodes) and associated with the extent of disease as well as a high risk for MI and sudden death when compared with symptomatic episodes of ischemia. Although the underlying mechanisms for silent ischemia are continuing to be defined, increased physical activity, activation of the sympathetic nervous system, increased cortisol secretion, increased coronary artery tone, and enhanced platelet aggregation due to endothelia dysfunction leading to intermittent coronary obstruction may be additive in lowering the threshold for ischemia. Platelet aggregability is increased in the morning hours (7 to 11 AM), corresponding to circadian rhythms noted for the peak frequency of ischemia, acute MI, and sudden death. Silent ischemia is associated with ST-segment elevation or depression and frequently occurs without antecedent changes in HR or blood pressure, suggesting that this form of ischemia is a result of primary reduction in oxygen supply. Silent ischemia is classified into class I, patients who do not experience angina at any time, and class II, patients who have both asymptomatic and symptomatic ischemia. Patients with silent ischemia have a defective warning system for angina pain that may encourage excessive myocardial demand. Regardless of the exact mechanism, there is increasing concern that painless ischemia carries considerable risk for myocardial perfusion defects, detrimental hemodynamic changes, arrhythmogenesis, and sudden death. Silent ischemia is associated with reduced survival and increased need for PTCA and CABG as well as increased risk of acute MI.[84] Because it is apparently very common in some settings, major emphasis should be placed on its management. A consensus has not been reached for the most appropriate method of detecting and quantifying the magnitude of silent ischemia; however, ambulatory ECG monitoring is felt by many to be the most useful tool at the present time.

The initial step in management is to modify the major risk factors for IHD—hypertension, hypercholesterolemia, and smoking—and data from the Multiple Risk Factor Intervention Trial (MRFIT) show these interventions to be useful in patients with silent ischemia. In a subset of the study population who had abnormal baseline exercise ECG responses, the special intervention group had a 57% reduction in coronary heart disease death (22.2/1000 versus 51.8/1000) and a reduction in sudden death resulting from cessation of smoking and lowering of blood pressure and cholesterol when compared with the usual-care group.

The Asymptomatic Cardiac Ischemia Pilot (ACIP) study, a randomized trial of medical therapy versus revascularization (PTCA or CABG), at the 2-year follow-up demonstrates that total mortality was 6.6% in the angina-guided strategy (i.e., therapy based on symptoms), 4.4% in the ischemia-guided strategy (based on ECG changes), and 1.1% in the revascularization strategy ($P < .02$). The rate of death or MI was 12.1% in the angina-guided strategy group, 8.8% in the ischemia-guided strategy group, and 4.7% in the revascularization strategy group ($P < .04$).[85] The rate of death, MI, or recurrent cardiac hospitalization was 41.8% in the angina-guided strategy group, 38.5% in the ischemia-guided strategy group, and 23.1% in the revascularization strategy group ($P < .001$). Post-MI patients and those with a high levels of sympathetic nervous system activity are perhaps the best candidates for β-blocker therapy.

Calcium channel antagonists alone and in combination have been shown to be effective in reducing symptomatic and asymptomatic ischemia, but they do not interrupt the diurnal surge in ischemia observed on ambulatory monitoring, and in general, they are somewhat less effective than β-blockers for silent ischemia.[86,87] Nifedipine in particular seems to provide less protection and provides wide fluctuations in response, with approximate reductions in the number of episodes ranging from 0% to 93% and in duration from 23% to 65%, unless combined with β-blockers. Fewer studies are available with other calcium channel blockers, and comparative trials are uncommon. Earlier studies have shown that combination therapy with calcium channel blockers and β-blockers provides a better response than calcium channel blockers and nitrates or monotherapy.[88,89]

Surgical intervention using CABG does not appear warranted in asymptomatic patients *without* significant CAD. Based on the CASS 12-year follow-up results, survival following CABG was enhanced in men with three-vessel disease compared with medical therapy (61% versus 46%) but not for women (45% versus 50%) with silent ischemia.[90] The role for PTCA is promising in silent ischemia, and improvement in exercise tolerance and freedom from MI, CABG, and PTCA for new lesions or death may be seen in patients becoming asymptomatic after PTCA. However, exercise-induced silent myocardial ischemia frequently is seen early after successful PTCA and is more prevalent in patients undergoing multivessel angioplasty and incomplete revascularization. Both silent and symptomatic ischemia early after PTCA are predictors of an unfavorable prognosis.

▶ TREATMENT: Syndrome X[91]

Syndrome X refers to the occurrence of effort angina and exercise-induced ECG changes with a normal coronary arteriogram and no evidence of structural (stenosis) or functional (spasm) abnormalities. Although the basis for this syndrome is not yet established, it is thought that syndrome X may be a result of inducible myocardial ischemia caused by impaired functional coronary reserve at the microvascular level of intramural prearteriolar vessels.[92] It has been proposed that this defect is caused by defective prearteriolar regulation of blood flow into the arteriolar bed with subsequent focal, sustained, compensatory release of adenosine; excessive local concentrations of adenosine are then responsible for the pain seen in this syndrome. Cardiomyopathy and left bundle-branch block may result from ischemia in some patients. Follow-up studies have shown that the occurrence of left bundle-branch block in response to stress is associated with a greater likelihood of deterioration of LV performance, whereas stress-induced ST-segment depression does not predict a detrimental outcome in ventricular function. Esophageal abnormalities may be seen in these patients, and acid refluxing into the esophagus may reduce coronary blood flow.

β-Adrenergic blockers are much less effective in many studies in syndrome X than in exertional angina, and one characteristic, if present, that may predict a good response to β-blockers is increased sympathetic nervous system activity.[93] Angiotensin-converting enzyme (ACE) inhibitors have been shown to improve coronary reserve, exercise capacity, and exercise time in patients with microvascular angina.[94,95] ERT in postmenopausal women has been shown to restore endothelial responsiveness to acetylcholine, and this has potential in the management of syndrome X patients.[96]

▶ TREATMENT: Revascularization

CABG[97]

Following the introduction of saphenous vein graft replacement for severely occluded coronary arteries by Favorolo and Garrett in 1967, CABG became an accepted and commonly used approach for the management of IHD. The objectives in performing CABG are twofold: (1) reduce the number of symptomatic anginal attacks not controlled with medical management or PCI and improve the life-style of the patient and (2) reduce the mortality associated with CAD. Surgery is effective in providing pain relief in large numbers of patients, with about 70% to 95% being pain-free at 1 year and 46% to 55% being pain-free at 5 years. This compares favorably with medical management, with which only about 30% are free of symptoms at 5 years. Mortality at 10 years from the largest published studies is 26.4% with CABG and 30.5% with medical management ($P = .03$), but there are significant differences based on subgroup analysis (e.g., left main artery disease versus one-vessel without a proximal left anterior descending artery lesion).[97] The second objective is met in certain patients, and this has been addressed in three large, well-controlled trials of bypass surgery. These three studies, the Veterans Administration (VA) Study, the European Cooperative Surgery Study (ECSS), and CASS, are not directly comparable because the inclusion and exclusion criteria for entry into each study were different and patients were followed for different periods of time. They also have been criticized for not being representative of the population that may be candidates for surgery, lacking women or late-middle-aged or elderly patients, and for crossover of medically managed patients to the surgical group. A major change in medical practice that influences the interpretation of these older studies is the common procedure of stent placement at the time of angioplasty.[98] There are about 20 different types of stents available, and their use is associated with greater luminal diameter after angioplasty, fewer acute reocclusions, and less restenosis after stent placement. Consequently, the validity of generalizing the results from these studies to routine practice has been questioned, but these studies are useful for providing a basis for decisions concerning surgery. Current class I recommendations (Table 14–9) for CABG in asymptomatic or mild angina patient include significant (>50%) left main coronary artery stenosis, left main equivalent (≥70% stenosis of the proximal left anterior descending artery and the proximal left circumflex artery), and three-vessel disease, especially in patients with LV ejection fraction of less than 0.50.[97] Class IIa recommendations for CABG are proximal left anterior descending artery stenosis with one- or two-vessel disease, and Class IIb recommendations for CABG are one- or two-vessel disease not involving the proximal left anterior descending artery. In stable angina, class I recommendations are the same as for mild angina with the following additions: one- or two-vessel disease without significant proximal left anterior descending artery stenosis but with a large area of viable myocardium and high-risk criteria in noninvasive testing and disabling angina despite maximal medical therapy, when surgery can be performed with acceptable risk. Class IIb recommendations in stable angina include proximal left anterior descending artery stenosis with one-vessel disease and one- or two-vessel disease without significant proximal left anterior descending artery stenosis but with a moderate area of viable myocardium and ischemia on noninvasive testing. The indications for CABG in unstable angina/NSTEMI were described previously. In ST-segment MI, CABG is indicated for ongoing ischemia/infarction not responsive to maximal medical therapy (class IIb).

In patients with poor LV function, CABG is indicated for the same indications as in mild angina for class I. Class IIa recommendations include poor LV function with significant viable, noncontracting, revascularizable myocardium without any of the aforementioned anatomic patterns (e.g., left main artery disease). CABG is useful in patients with life-threatening ventricular arrhythmia in the presence of left main artery disease, three-vessel disease (class I), and bypassable one- or two-vessel disease causing life-threatening ventricular arrhythmias and proximal left anterior descending artery disease with one- or two-vessel disease (class IIa).

CABG also may be used for patients who have failed PTCA if there is ongoing ischemia or threatened occlusion with significant myocardium at risk and in patients with hemodynamic compromise (class I). Class IIa recommendations for failed PTCA include a foreign body in a crucial anatomic position and hemodynamic compromise in a patient with impairment of the coagulation system and without a previous sternotomy. CABG may be repeated in patients with a previous CABG if disabling angina exists despite maximal noninvasive therapy (class I) and if a large area of myocardium is threatened and is subtended by bypassable distal vessels (class IIa).

The need for nitrates and β-blockers is clearly reduced by surgery, with only 30% of CABG patients requiring chronic medication, whereas 70% of their medical counterparts received anginal drugs. Employment status after surgery has been shown in CASS to be more dependent on the pretreatment status than an effect induced by the treatment arm, and about 70% of patients are employed before and after surgery. Recent follow-up analyses of these studies suggest that patients who have diabetes or peripheral vascular disease, who are African-Americans, or who continue to smoke are at high risk for CAD events and that diabetics in particular are more likely to have a better outcome with CABG than PTCA.[71,99,100] The overall benefit noted after CABG is similar in men and women, and elderly patients appear to have outcomes similar to those of younger patients.

Operative mortality is reported to range from 1% to 3% and is related to the number of vessels involved and preoperative ventricular function. Patients in CASS with one-, two-, or three-vessel disease had operative mortalities of 1.4%, 2.1%, and 2.8%, respectively. The relationship to LV ejection fraction follows a similar trend, with ejection fractions of greater than 50%, 20% to 40%, and less than 20% having operative mortality rates of 1.9%, 4.4%, and 6.7%, respectively. Perioperative infarction averages 5% depending on the sensitivity of the method for assessment, and the occurrence of an infarct reduces long-term survival. Neurologic dysfunction is relatively common postoperatively in CABG patients (6%), but many of the deficits are clinically insignificant and resolve with time. Fatal brain damage occurs in 0.3% to 0.7%, stroke occurs in about 5%, and ophthalmologic defects occur in 25%, but only 3% have clinically apparent field defects. Peripheral nerve lesions (12%) and brachial plexopathy (7%) are also reported to occur. Other complications include constrictive pericarditis (0.2%), cellulitis at the site of the vein graft, and mediastinal infections (1% to 4%).

Graft patency influences the success of symptom control and survival, and the mechanism for early graft occlusion is probably different from that associated with late closure. Early occlusion is related to platelet adhesion and aggregation, whereas late occlusion may be related to endothelial proliferation and progression of atherosclerosis. Patency of grafts early on after the CABG is reported to range from 88% to 97% in at least one graft and 58% to 81% in all grafts at 1 year. Long-term patency based on the CASS Montreal Heart Institute experience suggests that 60% to 67% of all grafts remain patent at 5 to 11 years. Antiplatelet therapy has been demonstrated to improve early and late patency rates and probably should be used in all patients who do not have any contraindications. Aspirin with or without other antiplatelet agents (dipyridamole) reduces the late development of vein graft occlusions. Late graft closure is related to elevated lipid levels and the progression of atherosclerosis in the grafted vessels as well as the native circulation. Elevation of very low-density lipoprotein, low-density lipoprotein (LDL), and LDL–apolipoprotein B is correlated with disease progression and graft closure. Aggressive lipid lowering can stabilize the progression of CAD and may induce regression in selected coronary artery segments within a patient following CABG. Cessation of smoking is an important preoperative and postoperative objective, as well as in the management of other coronary risk factors (e.g., hypertension), and institution of a supervised, daily exercise program is recommended. Internal mammary artery grafts should be used for revascularizing the left anterior descending artery system when possible owing to better graft survival and clinical outcomes.

Valvular heart disease can coexist with CAD, although this is relatively uncommon with rheumatic valve disease, usually the mitral valve, and more common with aortic stenosis and regurgitation. Angina may occur in 35% to 65% of patients with aortic stenosis or regurgitation and, if severe, may be the cause of angina in the absence of CAD. Patients being evaluated for possible CABG also should be evaluated for valvular disease to determine if valve replacement needs to be performed along with bypass grafting.

PTCA[75]

Since the introduction into clinical cardiology of PTCA[101,102] by Gruentzig in 1977, this procedure has gained rapid acceptance as a safe and effective means of managing CAD. It is estimated that more than 750,000 PCI procedures are done each year in this country, and 525,000 of them are PTCAs. The proposed mechanisms of reduced stenosis with PTCA include (1) compression and redistribution of the atherosclerotic plaque, (2) embolization of plaque contents, (3) aneurysm formation, and (4) disruption of the plaque and arterial wall with distortion and tearing of the intima and media, which leads to denudation of the endothelium, platelet adhesion and aggregation, thrombus formation, and smooth muscle proliferation. Of these mechanisms, the last one is felt to be the most important, but the others may contribute to opening of the lesions in some situations.

The indications for PTCA have been provided by the American College of Cardiology and the AHA and now span single- or multivessel disease as well as asymptomatic and symptomatic patients[75] (Table 14–10). PTCA generally is *not* useful if only a small area of viable myocardium is at risk, when ischemia cannot be demonstrated, when borderline (<50%) stenosis or lesions are present that are difficult to dilate, or when patients are at high risk for morbidity or mortality or both (e.g., left main or equivalent disease or three-vessel disease). PTCA alone or when used in conjunction or sequentially with thrombolysis for acute MI is discussed in Chapter 15. Stent placement accompanies balloon angioplasty in about 70% of cases. The current recommendations for PCI are provided in Table 14–11 based on class of angina.

Assessment of outcome with PCI can be based on several angiographic, procedural, and clinical outcomes, as discussed previously. The success of PCI depends on the experience of the operator (high volume, better outcome), on complicating factors for the patient (including the number of vessels to be dilated), and on technical advances in the equipment used (e.g., steerable and low-profile catheters). The acute success rate for opening of uncomplicated stenotic lesions ranges from 96% to 99% with the combined balloon-device-pharmacologic approach in experienced hands, and angina is decreased or eliminated in about 80% of patients. The success rate for totally occluded lesions is somewhat less (65%). Mortality at 1 year is 1% and 2.5% for single-vessel disease and multiple-vessel involvement, respectively, reflecting the good prognosis associated with this degree of CAD. At 10 years, survival is 95% and 81% for single- and multivessel disease, respectively.[75] Most patients remain event-free (no death, MI, or CABG) for an extended period. Symptomatic status, as measured by the New York Heart Association (NYHA) classification, is improved in many patients. Restenosis is noted in 32% to 40% of patients after balloon angioplasty at 6 months, and half these patients will have symptoms associated with restenosis.[75] A few late restenotic events occur, but most restenosis occurs within the first 6 months. Anatomic factors that predict restenosis include lesions greater than 20 mm in length, excessive tortuosity of the proximal segment, extremely angulated segments (>90 degrees), total occlusions greater than 3 months old and/or bridging collaterals, inability to protect major side branches, and degenerated vein grafts with friable lesions. Clinical factors that predict worse outcome include diabetes, advanced age, female gender, unstable angina, heart failure, and multivessel disease. A four-variable scoring system that predicts cardiovascular collapse for failed PTCA includes percentage of myocardium at risk (e.g., >50% viable myocardium at risk and LV ejection fraction <25%), preangioplasty percentage diameter stenosis, multivessel CAD, and diffuse disease in the dilated segment or a high myocardial jeopardy score.[75] Strut thickness of the stent influences restenosis as well, and thicker struts are associated with angiographic and clinical restenosis.[103]

The overall complication rate ranges from 2% to 21% depending on the lesion type.[77] Coronary occlusion, dissection, or spasm occurs in 4% to 8% of patients, whereas Q-wave MI occurs in 1.6% to 4.8%.[75] Prolonged angina and ventricular tachycardia or fibrillation occurs in 6.9% and 2.3%, respectively. In-hospital mortality ranges from 0.7% to 2.5% overall, and high-risk events for mortality include ventricular arrhythmias and MI. The frequency of urgent CABG because of complications ranges from 0.4% to 5.8%.[75]

Antiplatelet therapy with aspirin 80–325 mg/d given at least 2 hours prior to angioplasty is currently recommended. If patients are sensitive to aspirin, clopidogrel and ticlopidine are acceptable alternatives. Most centers now use clopidogrel due to adverse effects (described under unstable angina) and prolonged time to onset of effect for ticlopidine. In elective settings, clopidogrel should be started at least 72 hours in advance of the procedure to allow for maximum antiplatelet effects. Alternatively, a loading dose of clopidogrel (300 mg)

TABLE 14–10. Recommendations for Primary Coronary Intervention Based on Angina Classification

Class I	Class IIa	Class IIb	Class III
Class I Angina			
Patients who not have treated diabetes with asymptomatic ischemia or mild angina with one or more significant lesions in one or two coronary arteries suitable for PCI with a high likelihood of success and a low risk of morbidity and mortality	The same clinical and anatomic requirements for class I, except the myocardial area at risk is of moderate size or the patient has treated diabetes	Patients with asymptomatic ischemia or mild angina with three or more coronary arteries suitable for PCI with a high likelihood of success and a low risk of morbidity	Patients with asymptomatic ischemia or mild angina who do not meet the criteria listed under class I or II and who have a. Only a small area of viable myocardium at risk b. No objective evidence of ischemia c. Lesions that have a low likelihood of successful dilation d. Mild symptoms that are unlikely to be due to myocardial ischemia e. Factors associated with increased risk of morbidity or mortality f. Left main disease g. Insignificant disease
The vessels to be dilated must subtend a large area of viable myocardium		The vessels to be dilated must subtend at least a moderate area of viable myocardium In the physician's judgment, there should be evidence of myocardial ischemia such as ECG exercise testing, stress nuclear imaging, stress echocardiography, ambulatory ECG monitoring, or intracoronary physiologic measurements	
Class II–IV Angina, UA/NSTEMI			
Patients with one or more significant lesions in one or more coronary arteries suitable for PCI with a high likelihood of success and a low risk of morbidity and mortality	Patients with focal saphenous vein graft lesions or multiple stenoses who are poor candidates for reoperative surgery	Patient has one or more lesions to be dilated with reduced likelihood of success or the vessel(s) subtend less than moderate area of viable myocardium	Patient has no evidence or myocardial injury or ischemia on objective testing and has not had a trial of medical therapy or has a. Only a small area of myocardium at risk b. All lesions or the culprit lesion to be dilated with morphology with a low likelihood of success c. A high risk of procedure-related morbidity or mortality
The vessel(s) to be dilated should subtend a moderate or large area of viable myocardium and have high risk		Patients with two- or three-vessel disease, with signficant proximal LAD CAD and treated diabetes or abnormal LV function	Patients with insignificant coronary stenosis (e.g., <50% diameter)
			Patients with left main CAD who are candidates for CABG

Note: See Table 14–9 for definitions for class I to III recommendations. *Abbreviations:* PCI = primary coronary intervention; ECG = electrocardiogram; LAD = left anterior descending coronary artery; CAD = coronary artery disease; CABG = coronary artery bypass grafting.
From ACC/AHA guidelines of percutaneous coronary interventions (revision of the 1993 PTCA guidelines): Executive summary. A report of the American College of Cardiology/American Heart Association Task Force on Practice Guidelines. J Am Coll Cardiol 2001;37:2239i–lxvi, with permission.

or ticlopidine (500 mg) may be given to achieve a more rapid antiplatelet effect.[60] The combination of aspirin plus clopidogrel is currently recommended for patients undergoing angioplasty and stenting, and this combination is safer and superior to antiplatelet therapy plus anticoagulation with warfarin-like drugs.[104] Follow-up for up to 4 years from the Intracoronary Stenting and Antithrombotic Regimen (ISAR) trial shows that the benefit of combined antiplatelet therapy evident afterx 30 days is maintained after 4 years.[105] Aspirin is an incomplete inhibitor of platelet aggregation, and combination therapy with aspirin plus a glycoprotein IIb/IIIa receptor antagonist for PCI has shown a relative risk reduction of 37.5% for death and nonfatal MI at 30 days, favoring glycoprotein IIb/IIIa receptor antagonists over placebo (absolute rates of 5.5% versus 8.9% based on PCI trials of EPIC, IMPACT-II, EPILOG, CAPTURE, RESTORE, and

TABLE 14–11. Recommendations for Pharmacologic Management of Patients Undergoing PCI

Drugs	Class I Angina	Class II–IV Angina, UA/NSTEMI	Transmural ML Acute-Phase MI	Hospital After Thrombolysis	Management Phase
Aspirin	I[a]	I	I	I	I
Clopidogrel[b]	I[e]	I	I	I	I[d]
Warfarin[c]	III	III	III	II	I[f]
GP blockers[g]	II	I	II	I	III
UFH/LMWH	I	I	I	II	III

[a]Roman numerals refer to ACC/AHA class recommendations for use. See Table 14–9 for definitions.
[b]In conjunction with stenting.
[c]To be given 24–48 hours before planned stenting, if possible.
[d]To be given 2–4 weeks after stent placement.
[e]In patients without atrial fibrillation or other preexisting clinical indications.
[f]Patients with anterior myocardial wall motion abnormalities or LV thrombus.
[g]Every indication may not apply to all available agents.
Abbreviations: PCI = primary coronary intervention; UA = unstable angina; NSTEMI = non-ST-segment myocardial infarction; MI = myocardial infarction; GP = glycoprotein receptor; UFH = unfractionated heparin; LMWH = low-molecular-weight heparin.
From ACC/AHA guidelines of percutaneous coronary interventions (revision of the 1993 PTCA guidelines): Executive summary. A report of the American College of Cardiology/American Heart Association Task Force on Practice Guidelines. J Am Coll Cardiol 2001;37:2239i–lxvi, with permission.

EPISTENT).[75] As discussed under unstable angina, high-risk patients and those having a stent placed are most likely to benefit from glycoprotein IIb/IIIa receptor antagonist use. Patients presenting with elevated cardiac biomarkers are also more likely to receive benefit from glycoprotein IIb/IIIa receptor antagonists than patients with normal levels of biomarkers.[106] In the only comparative trial (TARGET), abciximab was superior to tirofiban.[67]

During PTCA patients usually are heparinized to prevent immediate thrombus formation at the site of arterial injury and on coronary guidewires and catheters; anticoagulation is continued for up to 24 hours. The intensity of anticoagulation is monitored using the activated clotting time (ACT), and the targeted range for ACT is 250 to 300 seconds (HemoTec device) in the absence of glycoprotein IIb/IIIa receptor antagonist use.[75] When glycoprotein IIb/IIIa receptor antagonists are not used, UFH is given as an intravenous bolus of 70–100 IU/kg to achieve a target ACT of 200 seconds. The loading dose is lowered to 50–70 IU/kg when glycoprotein IIb/IIIa receptor antagonists are given. Target ACT for eptifibatide and tirofiban is less than 300 seconds during angioplasty; postprocedural UFH infusions are not recommended during glycoprotein IIb/IIIa receptor antagonist therapy. Some authors have advocated heparin alternatives such as hirudin or hirulog, but there is no apparent long-term advantage with these agents.[107–109]

Mechanisms that result in restenosis include acute lumen loss owing to "recoil," mural thrombosis formation, and smooth muscle cell proliferation with synthesis of extracellular matrix.[102] Approaches to prevent restenosis may be aimed at altering the underlying mechanisms. Recoil and loss of luminal diameter may be reduced by the use of stent placement; however, this beneficial effect is offset by an increased number of vascular complications. Cracking of the plaque leads to severe damage to the arterial wall, exposure of collagen, and endothelial dysfunction. These factors promote mural thrombi, and the propensity for thrombus formation is related, in part, to the composition of the plaque as well as the depth of injury. Combination therapy with aspirin, heparin, and glycoprotein IIb/IIIa receptor antagonists is recommended to minimize acute occlusion, and numerous clinical trials document the efficacy of this combined approach.[75] Unfortunately, antithrombotic therapy (e.g., warfarin, aspirin, dipyridamole, prostacyclin, UFH, hirudin, or antiplatelet combinations) has little effect on long-term restenosis rates.[110] Other pharmacologic interventions that have failed to alter restenosis include β-blockers, angiotensin-converting enzyme inhibitors, calcium channel blockers, and omega-3 fatty acids. Pharmacologic therapy for which some evidence exists that restenosis may be prevented include investigational antiproliferative agents (e.g., trapidil, angiopeptin, tranilast),[111–113] cilostanzol,[114] valsartan (angiotensin-receptor blocker),[115] enoxaparin,[116] and possibly ticlopidine.[117] One of the most promising approaches is the use of brachytherapy (local gamma or beta irradiation of stent and surrounding tissue).[78,118] Intracoronary irradiation with iridium-192 resulted in lower rates of clinical and angiographic restenosis and the need for revascularization (43.8% versus 28.2% assigned to iridium-192; $P = .02$), although it also was associated with a higher rate of late thrombosis, resulting in an increased risk of MI. If the problem of late thrombosis within the stent can be overcome, intracoronary irradiation with iridium-192 may become a useful approach to the treatment of in-stent restenosis.[119]

Alternatives to PTCA include directional coronary atherectomy (DCA), excimer laser, rotational atherectomy (rotablator), intracoronary stents, or some combination of these interventions.[120] Based on randomized trials, DCA produces greater initial luminal diameter but results in a higher rate of postprocedural complications such as non-Q-wave MI and death and is more expensive. Consequently, PTCA is considered to be superior to DCA for most patients. Tissue debulking with DCA is useful for in-stent restenosis, particularly for diabetic patients.[121] The use of abciximab may improve these results.[122] Excimer laser angioplasty followed by balloon angioplasty or rotational atherectomy provides no benefit over balloon angioplasty alone.[123]

When medical therapy, PTCA, and CABG have been compared, low-risk patients with single-vessel CAD and normal LV function had greater alleviation of symptoms with PTCA than with medical treatment; mortality rates and rates of MI were unchanged. In high-risk patients (risk was defined by severity of ischemia, number of diseased vessels, and presence of LV dysfunction), improvement of survival was greater with CABG than with medical therapy. In moderate-risk patients with multivessel CAD (most had two-vessel disease and normal LV function), PTCA and CABG produced equivalent mortality rates and rates of MI.[101] PTCA, DCA, and coronary stenting are considered to be cost-effective relative to medical therapy with a cost-effectiveness ratio of less than $20,000 per quality-adjusted life year.[75] In patients with one- or two-vessel CAD who are asymptomatic or have only mild angina, PCTA and CABG are not cost-effective compared with medical therapy. There is no cost-effectiveness difference for PCTA versus CABG.

Vascular gene transfer offers a promising new approach to prevention and treatment of atherosclerosis and its complications. Its potential has been shown in animal models and in the first human trials using VEGF, b-FGF, and E2F cell-cycle transcription factor decoy. However, further basic research on gene-transfer vectors, gene delivery techniques, and identification of effective treatment genes is needed to improve the efficacy and safety of human vascular gene therapy.[124]

▶ PRINCIPLES OF PHARMACOTHERAPY

- IHD is caused primarily by atherosclerosis and is very common in the U.S. population.
- Risk-factor identification and modification are important for individual patients with known or suspected IHD and as a population-based policy to reduce the impact of this disease.
- Major risk factors that can be altered include dyslipidemia (i.e., high total cholesterol, low-density lipoprotein–cholesterol, low high-density lipoprotein–cholesterol, and high triglycerides), smoking, glycemic control in diabetes mellitus, hypertension, and adoption of therapeutic lifestyle changes (e.g., exercise, weight reduction, and reduced cholesterol and fat in the diet).
- Nitroglycerin and other nitrate products are useful for prophylaxis of angina when patients are undertaking activities known to provoke angina; however, when angina is occurring on a regular, routine basis, chronic prophylactic therapy should be instituted.
- Chronic stable angina should be managed initially with β-blockers because they provide better symptomatic control, at least as effective as nitrates or calcium channel blockers, and decrease the risk of recurrent MI and CAD mortality.
- Although calcium channel blockers are effective as monotherapy, they generally are used in combination with β-blockers or as monotherapy if patients are intolerant of β-blockers; most patients with moderate to severe angina will require two drugs to control their symptoms.
- Pharmacologic management is as effective as revascularization (e.g., PTCA, CABG, etc.) if one or two vessels are involved and there are no differences in survival, recurrent MI, or other measures of effectiveness.
- Multivessel involvement, especially if the patient has left main coronary artery disease or left main equivalent disease or two- to three-vessel involvement with significant LV dysfunction, is best managed with revascularization.
- PTCA and CABG produce similar results overall, but certain patient subsets (e.g., diabetics) should have CABG done.

REFERENCES

1. Gibbons RJ, Chatterjee K, Daley J, et al. ACC/AHA/ACP-ASIM guidelines for the management of patients with chronic stable angina: Executive summary and recommendations. A Report of the American College of Cardiology/American Heart Association Task Force on Practice Guidelines (Committee on Management of Patients with Chronic Stable Angina). Circulation 1999;99:2829–2848.
2. Braunwald E, Antman EM, Beasley JW, et al. ACC/AHA guidelines for the management of patients with unstable angina and non-ST-segment elevation myocardial infarction: Executive summary and recommendations. A report of the American College of Cardiology/American Heart Association Task Force on Practice Guidelines (Committee on the Management of Patients with Unstable Angina). Circulation 2000;102:1193–1209.
3. Sytkowski PA, D'Agostino RB, Belanger A, Kannel WB. Sex and time trends in cardiovascular disease incidence and mortality: The Framingham Heart Study, 1950–1989. Am J Epidemiol 1996;143:338–350.
4. Association AH. 2001 Heart and Stroke Statistical Update. Dallas, TX: American Heart Association, 2000:1–33.
5. Kannel WB FM. Natural history of angina pectoris in the Framingham Study: Prognosis and survival. Am J Cardiol 1972;29:154–163.
6. Menotti A, Keys A, Blackburn H, et al. Comparison of multivariate predictive power of major risk factors for coronary heart diseases in different countries: Results from eight nations of the Seven Countries Study, 25-year follow-up. J Cardiovasc Risk 1996;3:69–75.
7. Keys A. Mediterranean diet and public health: Personal reflections. Am J Clin Nutr 1995;61:1321S–1323S.
8. Goldman L, Hashimoto B, Cook F, et al. Comparative reproducibility and validity of systems for assessing cardiovascular functional class: Advantages of a new specific activity scale. Circulation 1981;64:1227–1234.
9. Emond M, Mock MB, Davis KB, et al. Long-term survival of medically treated patients in the Coronary Artery Surgery Study (CASS) Registry. Circulation 1994;90:2645–2657.
10. Caracciolo EA, Davis KB, Sopko G, et al. Comparison of surgical and medical group survival in patients with left main coronary artery disease: Long-term CASS experience. Circulation 1995;91:2325–2334.
11. Boersma E, Pieper KS, Steyerberg EW, et al. Predictors of outcome in patients with acute coronary syndromes without persistent ST-segment elevation: Results from an international trial of 9461 patients. The PURSUIT Investigators. Circulation 2000;101:2557–2567.
12. Epstein SE CRI, Talbot TL. Hemodynamic principles in the control of coronary blood flow. Am J Cardiol 1985;56:4E–10E.
13. Gielen S, Schuler G, Hambrecht R. Exercise training in coronary artery disease and coronary vasomotion. Circulation 2001;103:E1–E6.
14. Hasdai D, Gibbons RJ, Holmes DR Jr, et al. Coronary endothelial dysfunction in humans is associated with myocardial perfusion defects (see comments). Circulation 1997;96:3390–3395.
15. Libby P. Coronary artery injury and the biology of atherosclerosis: Inflammation, thrombosis, and stabilization. Am J Cardiol 2000;86:3J–8J.
16. Cohn PF. Silent myocardial ischemia and infarction. In: Goldhaber SZ, Gounameaux H, eds. Fundamental and Clinical Cardiology. New York, Marcel Dekker, 2000:1–327.
17. Caracciolo EA, Chaitman BR, Forman SA, et al. Diabetics with coronary disease have a prevalence of asymptomatic ischemia during exercise treadmill testing and ambulatory ischemia monitoring similar to that of nondiabetic patients: An ACIP database study. Asymptomatic Cardiac Ischemia Pilot Investigators. Circulation 1996;93:2097–2105.
18. Glusman M, Coromilas J, Clark WC, et al. Pain sensitivity in silent myocardial ischemia. Pain 1996;64:477–483.
19. Elliott WJ, Powell LH. Diagonal earlobe creases and prognosis in patients with suspected coronary artery disease. Am J Med 1996;100:205–211.
20. Hoeg JM. Evaluating coronary heart disease risk: Tiles in the mosaic. JAMA 1997;277:1387–1390.
21. O'Rourke RA, Hochman JS, Cohen MC, et al. New approaches to diagnosis and management of unstable angina and non-ST-segment elevation myocardial infarction. Arch Intern Med 2001;161:674–682.
22. Raggi P, Callister TQ, Cooil B, et al. Evaluation of chest pain in patients with low to intermediate pretest probability of coronary artery disease by electron beam computed tomography. Am J Cardiol 2000;85:283–288.

23. Fitzgerald PJ, Oshima A, Hayase M, et al. Final results of the Can Routine Ultrasound Influence Stent Expansion (CRUISE) study. Circulation 2000;102:523–530.
24. Expert Panel on Detection, Evaluation, and Treatment of High Blood Cholesterol in Adults. Executive summary of the third report of the National Cholesterol Education Program (NCEP) Expert Panel on Detection, Evaluation, and Treatment of High Blood Cholesterol in Adults (ATP III). JAMA 2001;285:2486–2497.
25. Anonymous. Effect of intensive diabetes management on macrovascular events and risk factors in the Diabetes Control and Complications Trial. Am J Cardiol 1995;75:894–903.
26. Smith CJ, Fischer TH, Sears SB. Environmental tobacco smoke, cardiovascular disease, and the nonlinear dose-response hypothesis. Toxicologic Sci 2000;54:462–472.
27. Wald NJ, Watt HC. Prospective study of effect of switching from cigarettes to pipes or cigars on mortality from three smoking related diseases. Br Med J 1997;314:1860–1863.
28. Vogel RA. Coronary risk factors, endothelial function, and atherosclerosis: A review. Clin Cardiol 1997;20:426–432.
29. Russell LB, Carson JL, Taylor WC, et al. Modeling all-cause mortality: Projections of the impact of smoking cessation based on the NHEFS. NHANES I Epidemiologic Follow-up Study. Am J Public Health 1998;88:630–636.
30. Kannel WB. Blood pressure as a cardiovascular risk factor: Prevention and treatment. JAMA 1996;275:1571–1576.
31. Yusuf S, Dagenais G, Pogue J, et al. Vitamin E supplementation and cardiovascular events in high-risk patients. The Heart Outcomes Prevention Evaluation Study Investigators. N Engl J Med 2000;342:154–160.
32. Sandvik L, Erikssen J, Ellestad M, et al. Heart rate increase and maximal heart rate during exercise as predictors of cardiovascular mortality: A 16-year follow-up study of 1960 healthy men. Coronary Artery Dis 1995;6:667–679.
33. Dorn J, Naughton J, Imamura D, Trevisan M. Results of a multicenter randomized clinical trial of exercise and long-term survival in myocardial infarction patients: The National Exercise and Heart Disease Project (NEHDP). Circulation 1999;100:1764–1769.
34. Subbiah MT. Mechanisms of cardioprotection by estrogens. Proc Soc Exp Biol Med 1998;217:23–29.
35. Hulley S, Grady D, Bush T, et al. Randomized trial of estrogen plus progestin for secondary prevention of coronary heart disease in postmenopausal women. Heart and Estrogen/progestin Replacement Study (HERS) Research Group. JAMA 1998;280:605–613.
36. Grodstein F, Stampfer MJ, Colditz GA, et al. Postmenopausal hormone therapy and mortality. N Engl J Med 1997;336:1769–1775.
37. Gersh BJ, Rutherford JD. Chronic coronary artery disease. In: Brunwald E, ed. Heart Disease: A Textbook of Cardiovascular Medicine. Philadelphia, Saunders 1997:1289–1365.
38. Goldstein S. Beta-blocking drugs and coronary heart disease. Cardiovas Drugs Ther 1997;11:219–225.
39. Carbajal EV, Deedwania PC. Contemporary approaches in medical management of patients with stable coronary artery disease. Med Clin North Am 1995;79:1063–1084.
40. Prince MJ, Bird AS, Blizard RA, Mann AH. Is the cognitive function of older patients affected by antihypertensive treatment? Results from 54 months of the Medical Research Council's trial of hypertension in older adults. Br Med J 1996;312:801–805.
41. Rosenthal J, Bahrmann H, Benkert K, et al. Analysis of adverse effects among patients with essential hypertension receiving an ACE inhibitor or a beta-blocker. Cardiology 1996;87:409–414.
42. Pehrsson SK, Ringqvist I, Ekdahl S, et al. Monotherapy with amlodipine or atenolol versus their combination in stable angina pectoris. Clin Cardiol 2000;23:763–770.
43. Darius H. Role of nitrates for the therapy of coronary artery disease patients in the years beyond 2000. J Cardiovas Pharmacol 1999;34: S15–S20.
44. Thadani U. Oral nitrates: more than symptomatic therapy in coronary artery disease? Cardiovasc Drugs Ther 1997;11:213–218.
45. Parker JO, Amies MH, Hawkinson RW, et al. Intermittent transdermal nitroglycerin therapy in angina pectoris: Clinically effective without tolerance or rebound. Minitran Efficacy Study Group. Circulation 1995;91:1368–1374.
46. Pizzulli L, Hagendorff A, Zirbes M, et al. Influence of captopril on nitroglycerin-mediated vasodilation and development of nitrate tolerance in arterial and venous circulation. Am Heart J 1996;131:342–349.
47. Heitzer T, Just H, Brockhoff C, et al. Long-term nitroglycerin treatment is associated with supersensitivity to vasoconstrictors in men with stable coronary artery disease: Prevention by concomitant treatment with captopril. J Am Coll Cardiol 1998;31:83–88.
48. Parker JD, Parker AB, Farrell B, Parker JO. Effects of diuretic therapy on the development of tolerance to nitroglycerin and exercise capacity in patients with chronic stable angina. Circulation 1996;93:691–696.
49. Watanabe H, Kakihana M, Ohtsuka S, Sugishita Y. Randomized, double-blind, placebo-controlled study of supplemental vitamin E on attenuation of the development of nitrate tolerance. Circulation 1997;96:2545–2550.
50. Freedman SB, Daxini BV, Noyce D, Kelly DT. Intermittent transdermal nitrates do not improve ischemia in patients taking beta-blockers or calcium antagonists: Potential role of rebound ischemia during the nitrate-free period. J Am Coll Cardiol 1995;25:349–355.
51. Opie LH. First line drugs in chronic stable effort angina: The case for newer, longer-acting calcium channel blocking agents. J Am Coll Cardiol 2000;36:1967–1971.
52. Katoh M, Nakajima M, Shimada N, et al. Inhibition of human cytochrome P450 enzymes by 1,4-dihydropyridine calcium antagonists: Prediction of in vivo drug-drug interactions. Eur J Clin Pharmacol 2000;55:843–852.
53. Ades PA, Coello CE. Effects of exercise and cardiac rehabilitation on cardiovascular outcomes. Med Clin North Am 2000;84:251–265, x–xi.
54. Fox KM, Mulcahy D, Findlay I, et al. The Total Ischaemic Burden European Trial (TIBET). Effects of atenolol, nifedipine SR and their combination on the exercise test and the total ischaemic burden in 608 patients with stable angina. The TIBET Study Group. Eur Heart J 1996;17:96–103.
55. Howes LG, Edwards CT. Calcium antagonists and cancer: Is there really a link? Drug Safety 1998;18:1–7.
56. Opie LH, Yusuf S, Kubler W. Current status of safety and efficacy of calcium channel blockers in cardiovascular diseases: A critical analysis based on 100 studies. Prog Cardiovasc Dis 2000;43:171–196.
57. Knight CJ, Fox KM. Amlodipine versus diltiazem as additional antianginal treatment to atenolol. Centralised European Studies in Angina Research (CESAR) Investigators. Am J Cardiol 1998;81:133–136.
58. Muller I, Seyfarth M, Rudiger S, et al. Effect of a high loading dose of clopidogrel on platelet function in patients undergoing coronary stent placement. Heart 2001;85:92–93.
59. Muller C, Buttner HJ, Petersen J, Roskamm H. A randomized comparison of clopidogrel and aspirin versus ticlopidine and aspirin after the placement of coronary-artery stents. Circulation 2000;101:590–593.
60. Bertrand ME, Rupprecht HJ, Urban P, Gershlick AH. Double-blind study of the safety of clopidogrel with and without a loading dose in combination with aspirin compared with ticlopidine in combination with aspirin after coronary stenting : the clopidogrel aspirin stent international cooperative study (CLASSICS). Circulation 2000;102:624–629.
61. Mehta SR, Yusuf S. The clopidogrel in unstable angina to prevent recurrent events trial investigators. Effects of clopidogrel in addition to aspirin in patients with acute coronary syndromes without ST-segment elevation. N Engl J Med 2001;345:494–502.
62. Bennett CL, Connors JM, Carwile JM, et al. Thrombotic thrombocytopenic purpura associated with clopidogrel. N Engl J Med 2000; 342:1773–1777.
63. Investigators GI-A. Effect of glycoprotein IIb/IIIa receptor blocker abciximab on outcome in patients with acute coronary syndromes without early coronary revascularisation: The GUSTO IV-ACS randomised trial. Lancet 2001;357:1915–1924.

64. Hirsh J, Anand SS, Halperin JL, Fuster V. Guide to anticoagulant therapy: Heparin. A statement for healthcare professionals from the American Heart Association. Circulation 2001;103:2994–3018.
65. Cohen M, Demers C, Gurfinkel EP, et al. A comparison of low-molecular-weight heparin with unfractionated heparin for unstable coronary artery disease: Efficacy and Safety of Subcutaneous Enoxaparin in Non-Q-Wave Coronary Events Study Group. N Engl J Med 1997;337:447–452.
66. Antman EM, McCabe CH, Gurfinkel EP, et al. Enoxaparin prevents death and cardiac ischemic events in unstable angina/non-Q-wave myocardial infarction: Results of the thrombolysis in myocardial infarction (TIMI) 11B trial. Circulation 1999;100:1593–1601.
67. Topol EJ, Moliterno D, Herrmann HC, et al. Comparison of two platelet glycoprotein IIb/IIIa inhibitors, tirofiban and abciximab, for the prevention of ischemic events with percutaneous coronary revascularization. N Engl J Med 2001;344:1888–1894.
68. Gibbons RJ, Balady GJ, Beasley JW, et al. ACC/AHA guidelines for exercise testing: Executive summary. A report of the American College of Cardiology/American Heart Association Task Force on Practice Guidelines (Committee on Exercise Testing). Circulation 1997;96: 345–354.
69. Boden WE, O'Rourke RA, Crawford MH, et al. Outcomes in patients with acute non-Q-wave myocardial infarction randomly assigned to an invasive as compared with a conservative management strategy. Veterans Affairs Non-Q-Wave Infarction Strategies in Hospital (VANQWISH) Trial Investigators. N Engl J Med 1998;338:1785–1792.
70. Cannon CP, Weintraub W, Demopoulos L, et al. Comparison of early invasive and conservative strategies in patients with unstable coronary syndromes treated with the glycoprotein IIb/IIIa inhibitor tirofiban. N Engl J Med 2001;25:1879–1887.
71. Anonymous. Seven-year outcome in the Bypass Angioplasty Revascularization Investigation (BARI) by treatment and diabetic status. J Am Coll Cardiol 2000;35:1122–1129.
72. Weintraub WS, Stein B, Kosinski A, et al. Outcome of coronary bypass surgery versus coronary angioplasty in diabetic patients with multivessel coronary artery disease. J Am Coll Cardiol 1998;31:10–19.
73. Hannan EL, Racz MJ, McCallister BD, et al. A comparison of three-year survival after coronary artery bypass graft surgery and percutaneous transluminal coronary angioplasty. J Am Coll Cardiol 1999;33: 63–72.
74. Morrison DA, Sethi G, Sacks J, et al. A multicenter, randomized trial of percutaneous coronary intervention versus bypass surgery in high-risk unstable angina patients. The AWESOME (Veterans Affairs Cooperative Study 385, Angina with Extremely Serious Operative Mortality Evaluation) Investigators from the Cooperative Studies Program of the Department of Veterans Affairs. Controlled Clin Trials 1999;20:601–619.
75. Smith SC Jr, Dove JT, Jacobs AK, et al. ACC/AHA guidelines for percutaneous coronary intervention (revision of the 1993 PTCA guidelines): Executive summary. A report of the American College of Cardiology/American Heart Association Task Force on Practice Guidelines (Committee to Revise the 1993 Guidelines for Percutaneous Transluminal Coronary Angioplasty) endorsed by the Society for Cardiac Angiography and Interventions. Circulation 2001;103:3019–3041.
76. Williams DO, Braunwald E, Thompson B, et al. Results of percutaneous transluminal coronary angioplasty in unstable angina and non-Q-wave myocardial infarction: Observations from the TIMI IIIB trial. Circulation 1996;94:2749–2755.
77. Keelan ET, Nunez BD, Grill DE, et al. Comparison of immediate and long-term outcome of coronary angioplasty performed for unstable angina and rest pain in men and women. Mayo Clin Proc 1997;72:5–12.
78. Kaluza GL, Mazur W, Raizner AE. Basic science review: Radiotherapy for prevention of restenosis. Cathet Cardiovasc Intervent 2001;52: 518–529.
79. Cutlip DE. Stent thrombosis: Historical perspectives and current trends. J Thromb Thrombol 2000;10:89–101.
80. Pepine CJ. An ischemia-guided approach for risk stratification in patients with acute coronary syndromes. Am J Cardiol 2000;86:27M–35M.
81. Anonymous. Invasive compared with non-invasive treatment in unstable coronary-artery disease: FRISC II prospective randomised multicentre study. Fragmin and Fast Revascularisation during Instability in Coronary Artery Disease Investigators. Lancet 1999;354:708–715.
82. Sakata K, Miura F, Sugino H, et al. Assessment of regional sympathetic nerve activity in vasospastic angina: Analysis of iodine-123-labeled metaiodobenzylguanidine scintigraphy. Am Heart J 1997;133:484–489.
83. Lanza GA, Pedrotti P, Pasceri V, et al. Autonomic changes associated with spontaneous coronary spasm in patients with variant angina. J Am Coll Cardiol 1996;28:1249–1256.
84. Conti CR, Geller NL, Knatterud GL, et al. Anginal status and prediction of cardiac events in patients enrolled in the Asymptomatic Cardiac Ischemia Pilot (ACIP) study. ACIP investigators. Am J Cardiol 1997;79:889–892.
85. Davies RF, Goldberg AD, Forman S, et al. Asymptomatic Cardiac Ischemia Pilot (ACIP) study two-year follow-up: Outcomes of patients randomized to initial strategies of medical therapy versus revascularization (see comments). Circulation 1997;95:2037–2043.
86. Singh N, Mironov D, Goodman S, et al. Treatment of silent ischemia in unstable angina: A randomized comparison of sustained-release verapamil versus metoprolol. Clin Cardiol 1995;18:653–658.
87. Dwivedi SK, Saran RK, Mittal S, et al. Silent ischemic interval on exercise test is a predictor to drug therapy: A randomized crossover trial of metoprolol versus diltiazem in stable angina. Clin Cardiol 2001;24: 45–49.
88. Pratt CM, McMahon RP, Goldstein S, et al. Comparison of subgroups assigned to medical regimens used to suppress cardiac ischemia [the Asymptomatic Cardiac Ischemia Pilot (ACIP) Study]. Am J Cardiol 1996;77:1302–1309.
89. Davies RF, Habibi H, Klinke WP, et al. Effect of amlodipine, atenolol and their combination on myocardial ischemia during treadmill exercise and ambulatory monitoring. Canadian Amlodipine/Atenolol in Silent Ischemia Study (CASIS) Investigators. J Am Coll Cardiol 1995;25: 619–625.
90. Weiner DA, Ryan TJ, Parsons L, et al. Significance of silent myocardial ischemia during exercise testing in women: Report from the Coronary Artery Surgery Study. Am Heart J 1995;129:465–470.
91. Ali O, Smart FW, Nguyen T, Ventura H. Recent developments in microvascular angina. Curr Atherosclerosis Rep 2001;3:149–155.
92. Bellamy MF, Goodfellow J, Tweddel AC, et al. Syndrome X and endothelial dysfunction. Cardiovasc Res 1998;40:410–417.
93. Lanza GA, Colonna G, Pasceri V, Maseri A. Atenolol versus amlodipine versus isosorbide-5-mononitrate on anginal symptoms in syndrome X. Am J Cardiol 1999;84:854–856, A8.
94. Motz W, Strauer BE. Improvement of coronary flow reserve after long term therapy with enalapril. Hypertension 1996;27:1031–1038.
95. Nalbantgil I, Onder R, Altintig A, et al. Therapeutic benefits of cilazapril in patients with syndrome X. Cardiology 1998;89:130–133.
96. Roque M, Heras M, Roig E, et al. Short-term effects of transdermal estrogen replacement therapy on coronary vascular reactivity in postmenopausal women with angina pectoris and normal results on coronary angiograms. J Am Coll Cardiol 1998;31:139–143.
97. Eagle KA, Guyton RA, Davidoff R, et al. ACC/AHA guidelines for coronary artery bypass graft surgery: Executive summary and recommendations. A report of the American College of Cardiology/American Heart Association Task Force on Practice Guidelines (Committee to Revise the 1991 Guidelines for Coronary Artery Bypass Graft Surgery). Circulation 1999;100:1464–1480.
98. Colombo A, Tobis J. Techniques in Coronary Artery Stenting. London, Martin Dunitz, 2000:1–422.
99. Jacobs AK, Kelsey SF, Brooks MM, et al. Better outcome for women compared with men undergoing coronary revascularization: A report from the Bypass Angioplasty Revascularization Investigation (BARI). Circulation 1998;98:1279–1285.
100. Taylor HA Jr, Mickel MC, Chaitman BR, et al. Long-term survival of African Americans in the Coronary Artery Surgery Study (CASS). J Am Coll Cardiol 1997;29:358–364.

101. Solomon AJ, Gersh BJ. Management of chronic stable angina: Medical therapy, percutaneous transluminal coronary angioplasty, and coronary artery bypass graft surgery. Lessons from the randomized trials. Ann Intern Med 1998;128:216–223.
102. Landzberg BR, Frishman WH, Lerrick K. Pathophysiology and pharmacological approaches for prevention of coronary artery restenosis following coronary artery balloon angioplasty and related procedures. Prog Cardiovasc Dis 1997;39:361–398.
103. Kastrati A, Mehilli J, Dirschinger J, et al. Intracoronary stenting and angiographic results. Strut Thickness Effect on Restenosis Outcome (ISAR-STEREO) trial. Circulation 2001;103:2816–2821.
104. Schomig A, Neumann FJ, Walter H, et al. Coronary stent placement in patients with acute myocardial infarction: Comparison of clinical and angiographic outcome after randomization to antiplatelet or anticoagulant therapy. J Am Coll Cardiol 1997;29:28–34.
105. Schuhlen H, Kastrati A, Pache J, et al. Sustained benefit over four years from an initial combined antiplatelet regimen after coronary stent placement in the ISAR trial. Intracoronary Stenting and Antithrombotic Regimen. Am J Cardiol 2001;87:397–400.
106. Heeschen C, van Den Brand MJ, Hamm CW, Simoons ML. Angiographic findings in patients with refractory unstable angina according to troponin T status. Circulation 1999;100:1509–1514.
107. Shah PB, Ahmed WH, Ganz P, Bittl JA. Bivalirudin compared with heparin during coronary angioplasty for thrombus-containing lesions. J Am Coll Cardiol 1997;30:1264–1269.
108. Anonymous. A clinical trial comparing primary coronary angioplasty with tissue plasminogen activator for acute myocardial infarction. The Global Use of Strategies to Open Occluded Coronary Arteries in Acute Coronary Syndromes (GUSTO IIb) Angioplasty Substudy Investigators. N Engl J Med 1997;336:1621–1628.
109. Bittl JA, Strony J, Brinker JA, et al. Treatment with bivalirudin (Hirulog) as compared with heparin during coronary angioplasty for unstable or postinfarction angina. Hirulog Angioplasty Study Investigators. N Engl J Med 1995;333:764–769.
110. Lefkovits J, Topol EJ. Pharmacological approaches for the prevention of restenosis after percutaneous coronary intervention. Prog Cardiovasc Dis 1997;40:141–158.
111. Kosuga K, Tamai H, Ueda K, et al. Effectiveness of tranilast on restenosis after directional coronary atherectomy. Am Heart J 1997;134:712–718.
112. Emanuelsson H, Beatt KJ, Bagger JP, et al. Long-term effects of angiopeptin treatment in coronary angioplasty: Reduction of clinical events but not angiographic restenosis. European Angiopeptin Study Group. Circulation 1995;91:1689–1696.
113. Holmes D, Fitzgerald P, Goldberg S, et al. The PRESTO (Prevention of Restenosis with Tranilast and Its Outcomes) protocol: A double-blind, placebo-controlled trial. Am Heart J 2000;139:23–31.
114. Kozuma K, Hara K, Yamasaki M, et al. Effects of cilostazol on late lumen loss and repeat revascularization after Palmaz-Schatz coronary stent implantation. Am Heart J 2001;141:124–130.
115. Peters S, Gotting B, Trummel M, et al. Valsartan for prevention of restenosis after stenting of type B2/C lesions: The VAL-PREST trial. J Invas Cardiol 2001;13:93–97.
116. Kiesz RS, Buszman P, Martin JL, et al. Local delivery of enoxaparin to decrease restenosis after stenting: Results of initial multicenter trial. Polish-American Local Lovenox NIR Assessment (POLONIA) study. Circulation 2001;103:26–31.
117. Steinhubl SR, Ellis SG, Wolski K, et al. Ticlopidine pretreatment before coronary stenting is associated with sustained decrease in adverse cardiac events: Data from the Evaluation of Platelet IIb/IIIa Inhibitor for Stenting (EPISTENT) Trial. Circulation 2001;103:1403–1409.
118. Verin V, Popowski Y, de Bruyne B, et al. Endoluminal beta-radiation therapy for the prevention of coronary restenosis after balloon angioplasty. The Dose-Finding Study Group. N Engl J Med 2001;344:243–249.
119. Leon MB, Teirstein PS, Moses JW, et al. Localized intracoronary gamma-radiation therapy to inhibit the recurrence of restenosis after stenting. N Engl J Med 2001;344:250–256.
120. Ellis SG, Holmes DR Jr, eds. Strategic Approaches in Coronary Interventions. Philadelphia, Lippincott Williams & Wilkins, 1999.
121. Moustapha A, Assali AR, Sdringola S, et al. Percutaneous and surgical interventions for in-stent restenosis: Long-term outcomes and effect of diabetes mellitus. J Am Coll Cardiol 2001;37:1877–1882.
122. Ghaffari S, Kereiakes DJ, Lincoff AM, et al. Platelet glycoprotein IIb/IIIa receptor blockade with abciximab reduces ischemic complications in patients undergoing directional coronary atherectomy. EPILOG Investigators. Evaluation of PTCA to Improve Long-Term Outcome by c7E3 GP IIb/IIIa Receptor Blockade. Am J Cardiol 1998;82:7–12.
123. Appelman YE, Piek JJ, van der Wall EE, et al. Evaluation of the long-term functional outcome assessed by myocardial perfusion scintigraphy following excimer laser angioplasty compared to balloon angioplasty in longer coronary lesions. Int J Cardiac Imaging 2000;16:267–277.
124. Rutanen J, Rissanen TT, Kivela A, et al. Clinical applications of vascular gene therapy. Curr Cardiol Rep 2001;3:29–36.

15

UNCOMPLICATED MYOCARDIAL INFARCTION

Kathleen A. Stringer and Larry M. Lopez

Drug therapy and the management of patients who experience myocardial infarction (MI) have improved dramatically since the mid-1980s. Technological and therapeutic advances, as well as a greater understanding of the pathophysiology of acute coronary syndromes, have prompted the improvement of pharmacotherapy for MI. One of the most important advancements has been the introduction of fibrinolytic therapy. Though initially suggested as a potential therapeutic tool in the 1950s, fibrinolytic therapy was not evaluated in large clinical trials until the early 1980s. This delay was most likely due to the controversy that surrounded the etiology of MI, coupled with the negative results of small, underpowered trials of fibrinolytic therapy.[1,2] It was suggested as early as 1912 that thrombus formation played a critical role in the pathophysiology of MI, but it was not until 1980 that DeWood and associates definitively demonstrated that thrombus formation was the principal etiology of MI.[2] Once this pathology was established, a flurry of intracoronary fibrinolytic trials followed. Subsequently, the feasibility and usefulness of peripherally administered intravenous (IV) fibrinolytic therapy were demonstrated. Since that time, significant advances in reperfusion therapy, such as the use of intracoronary stents and the introduction of novel antithrombotic agents such as the low molecular weight heparins and the platelet glycoprotein IIb/IIIa inhibitors, have significantly improved the management of MI.

EPIDEMIOLOGY

Myocardial infarction is the number one killer of both men and women in the United States. Approximately 800,000 people experience acute MI each year.[3] Of these, nearly 213,000 die, at least half of these before they receive medical care.[3] In 1997, the mortality rate during hospitalization for acute MI was approximately 5% for patients between the ages of 45 and 64 years.[4] Older patients had a mortality rate of 15%. Patients with large anterior wall MIs, left ventricular dysfunction, and complex ventricular ectopy carry the highest 1-year mortality rate (22%).

The cost of coronary disease in the United States is high.[3,5] The estimated 2001 financial consequence of coronary artery disease (CAD) to the U.S. health care system is approximately $101 billion in direct and indirect costs.[3,4] Therefore, therapeutic interventions that reduce mortality and improve morbidity, as well as primary and secondary prevention strategies, will have a significant economic impact on the U.S. health care system.

ETIOLOGY

The formation of an atherosclerotic plaque in the coronary circulation is the underlying etiology of both CAD and MI.[6,7] The atherosclerotic process begins early in life, usually within the first decade. Fatty streaks appear on the coronary artery endothelium and may progress to form plaques, depending on whether risk factors are present. These risk factors include male gender, hypertension, diabetes mellitus, tobacco use, and hyperlipidemia. (See Chapter 14 for a detailed discussion of these risk factors.)

There is a growing body of evidence to suggest that an elevated plasma homocysteine concentration may be an independent risk factor for CAD,[8,9] although routine monitoring and treatment of elevated homocysteine levels remain controversial. It has also been suggested that there may be other risk factors, such as high plasma concentrations of C-reactive protein or fibrinogen, for the development of CAD. In fact, a recent review suggests that an elevated C-reactive protein level is an independent risk factor for CAD.[10] As with homocysteine, however, routine evaluation of C-reactive protein levels has not yet been adopted as a standard of care for the assessment of cardiovascular risk, although it appears that this procedure will soon move from the research arena into routine clinical practice. A number of studies have also attributed the development of CAD to an infectious etiology. The presence of antibodies to either *Chlamydia pneumoniae* or *Herpes simplex* type I (coupled with an elevated C-reactive protein level) has been shown to increase the risk of CAD. Although numerous studies have been published, an independent association between CAD, MI, and infection has not yet been established.[11]

Each CAD risk factor most likely has a discrete effect on the coronary vasculature (e.g., shear stress, oxygen radical production) that contributes to the development of atherosclerosis. It is now believed that the end result of these effects is endothelial injury.[7,12] The endothelium reacts to this injury with a variety of responses, rendering it dysfunctional. Ultimately, the dysfunction alters the endothelial surface from one that is antithrombotic to one that is prothrombotic. Furthermore, endothelial dysfunction appears to create a pro-inflammatory environment that propagates atherosclerotic lesion formation. In fact, atherosclerosis has been referred to as an inflammatory disorder, because its lesions represent a series of highly specific cellular and molecular responses–including increased cytokine release, infiltration of macrophages, enhanced growth factor activity, and the proliferation of smooth muscle cells–that collectively can be best described as an inflammatory process.[7] The early stages of plaque development (American Heart Association [AHA] types I–III) are eventually followed by the formation of fully developed complicated lesions (AHA type IV or type Va).[6] Regardless of its size, a complicated lesion, which has a large lipid core encapsulated by a thin fibrous cap, is more likely to rupture and to precipitate an acute coronary event than is an uncomplicated lesion.

PATHOPHYSIOLOGY

Thrombus formation precipitated by atherosclerotic plaque rupture or fissure is the cause of more than 85% of acute MIs.[2,6,7] Thrombosis over an atherosclerotic plaque occurs through one of two somewhat different processes.[6] The first, endothelial erosion, results from the endothelial denudation of so large an area that it exposes the surface of the subendothelial connective tissue of the plaque.[6] This exposure triggers activation of platelets and the coagulation cascade, and a thrombus forms, adhering to the plaque surface. The second mechanism is plaque rupture. In an unstable plaque, the lipid core is large and the fibrous cap is thin, enhancing the likelihood of plaque rupture. The occurrence of such a rupture exposes the highly thrombogenic lipid core, activating platelets and the coagulation cascade. In both scenarios, if thrombus formation is extensive and completely obstructs blood flow, myocardial cells die and infarction occurs. Subsequent to occlusive thrombus formation, platelet–thrombin microemboli can form. These microemboli may obstruct the microvasculature, which perpetuates inflammation, vasospasm, and endothelial dysfunction. It is now widely accepted that some degree of thrombus formation and platelet activation takes place in all acute coronary syndromes (i.e., unstable angina, MI). What most likely distinguishes MI from unstable angina, however, is the extent of thrombus formation and the magnitude of coronary vessel occlusion.

Although myocardial ischemia generally precedes MI, there are two distinct characteristics that differentiate the two. First, MI is precipitated by a sudden interruption of the blood supply to an area of the myocardium because of the complete, or near complete, occlusion of a coronary artery. Myocardial ischemia, on the other hand, is characterized by a temporary reduction in the blood supply or to an abrupt, but temporary, increase in myocardial oxygen demand in association with a fixed atherosclerotic obstruction. Second, the occlusion of MI persists long enough to compromise myocardial function and to lead to myocardial necrosis (i.e., nonviability). After the onset of ischemia, cell death is not immediate, but rather takes a finite period to develop. In some animal models, this time may be as little as 15 minutes, although it takes 6 hours before myocardial necrosis can be identified by post-mortem examination in humans.[13] Despite this rapid time course, it has been demonstrated that a significant percentage of myocardium "hibernates" in response to prolonged ischemia and is salvageable after as long as 12 to 24 hours of ischemia; this phenomenon may be due in part to the presence of collateral blood flow within the infarcted area.[13] Nevertheless, a process called myocardial "stunning" may delay full recovery of systolic function after complete restoration of blood flow.[14] These features of MI have important implications for the therapeutic management, prognosis, and outcome of patients with MI.

INFARCT LOCATION

The location of MI plays a very important role in determining the therapeutic management and the prognosis of the patient. Anterior wall MI involves the anterior wall of the left ventricle and most often represents occlusion of the left anterior descending (LAD) artery. Typically, anterior wall MI involves a much larger area of myocardium than does inferior wall MI; consequently, there is a risk of a greater loss of myocardium and myocardial function. Patients with anterior wall MI typically have the highest mortality rate of MI patients.

A right ventricular MI was not considered clinically important until recently. Although isolated right ventricular infarction accounts for fewer than 3% of all MIs, infarction of the right ventricle occurs in nearly 50% of patients with inferior wall MI.[15,16] In as many as 30% to 40% of the population, however, the right coronary artery is a large, dominant vessel that supplies not only the right ventricle, but also a significant portion of the inferior wall of the left ventricle. In these individuals, occlusion of the right coronary artery may result in an inferior wall MI or the combination of an inferior wall MI and a right ventricular MI, depending on where the occlusion in the right coronary artery occurs. Because approximately 50% of patients with an inferior wall MI may have right ventricular involvement, a right-sided electrocardiogram (ECG) should be obtained in all patients with inferior wall MI. The presence of ST-segment elevation in V_4R supports the diagnosis of right ventricular infarction, as does the presence of right bundle branch block or complete heart block.[15,16]

In addition to the ECG, patients with right ventricular MI may be differentiated from patients with left ventricular MI by their initial presentation and clinical course.[15,16] Hypotension, clear lung fields, and an elevated jugular venous pressure in a patient with an inferior wall MI is consistent with right ventricular infarction. Patients with right ventricular MI may present with or quickly develop hemodynamic compromise or cardiogenic shock due to dysfunction of the right ventricle and associated inadequate filling of the left ventricle. Therefore, patients with right ventricular MI usually require IV volume loading with normal saline to maintain right ventricular preload and cardiac output. If the administration of several liters of IV fluid does not improve the hemodynamic status of the patient, the use of inotropic and/or blood pressure support with dopamine may be necessary. Medications such as nitroglycerin, diuretics, and other drugs that reduce either preload or blood pressure should be avoided in patients with right ventricular MI. In patients with right ventricular MI accompanied by left ventricular dysfunction, the cautious IV use of nitroprusside may reduce afterload, and in severe cases where nitroprusside is not effective or tolerated, placement of an intra-aortic balloon pump may be necessary. Other than these exceptions, patients with right ventricular infarction should be managed in the same manner as patients with left ventricular infarction. Because right ventricular infarction accompanying inferior wall MI is associated with a substantial likelihood of mortality (25% to 30%),[15,16] these patients should be categorized as "high risk" and should be given high priority for reperfusion therapy.

TYPE OF INFARCTION

In addition to location, the type of MI has implications for therapeutic management. An ST-segment elevation MI, previously termed Q-wave or transmural MI, usually results in an injury that transects the entire thickness of the myocardial wall.[6,13] Subsequently, most of these patients develop pathologic Q waves on the ECG. Non–ST-segment elevation MI, previously termed non–Q-wave or nontransmural MI, involves only the subendocardial myocardium, and these patients do not develop a pathologic Q wave on the ECG. Essentially, a non–ST-segment elevation MI is smaller and less extensive than an ST-segment elevation MI.[6,13,17] Patients whose ECG does not show ST-segment elevation may have only subtle findings such as T-wave inversion, nonspecific ST-T–wave changes, or ST-segment depression. To confirm the diagnosis of MI an elevation in serum cardiac markers is necessary. Nevertheless, with the exception of fibrinolytic therapy, the therapeutic management of MI with and without ST-segment elevation is very similar.

PROGNOSIS

The most important prognostic indicator following MI is left ventricular function. The acute loss of myocardium following MI results in an abrupt increase in loading conditions that induces a unique pattern of *ventricular remodeling* in the infarcted border zone and remote noninfarcted myocardium.[18] This triggers a cascade of biochemical intracellular signaling events that initiates and propagates a complex response to injury. These responses include left ventricular dilatation, hypertrophy, and the formation of a discrete collagen scar.[18] The remodeling of the left ventricle is a reparative process by which mechanical, neurohormonal, and genetic factors regulate ventricular shape, size, and function.[18] Activation of the neurohumoral and renin-angiotensin systems, together with the release of vasopressin, ensue in response to increased left ventricular filling pressure. Sinus tachycardia, mediated by the activation of the adrenergic system, occurs first as a response to a drop in cardiac output; then, within hours of the MI, the infarcted area expands due to thinning and stretching of the infarcted region. Acute dilatation and hypertrophy of the noninfarcted myocardium follows this expansion. Ventricular remodeling may continue for weeks or months until the tensile strength of the collagen scar counterbalances the distending forces.[18] The size, location, and transmurality of the infarct, as well as the extent of myocardial stunning and the patency of the infarct-related artery, determine this balance.[18]

The initial ventricular remodeling process precipitates chronic changes in ventricular volume, leading to further ventricular dilation, hypertrophy, and eventually the development of heart failure–unfortunately, one of the most serious complications of MI. Patients who develop heart failure after MI have approximately a 50% 5-year mortality rate. Clinical trials evaluating the impact of early drug therapy intervention on this remodeling process and the subsequent development of heart failure have been completed and are reviewed later in this chapter.[19–22]

In addition to left ventricular function, several other factors have been implicated in predicting the outcome for patients with MI. Significant predictors of death within 30 days of MI include age greater than 70 years; hypertension, atrial fibrillation, and tachycardia; larger infarct size and anterior wall location; previous MI; and female gender.[23,24] Low-risk patients (a 2.5% 1-year cardiac mortality rate) are those younger than 71 years of age with a left ventricular ejection fraction greater than or equal to 40%.

Importantly, the highest risk of death from MI is early, generally within the first 48 hours, even in the patients who receive a fibrinolytic agent. Rapid identification of an MI patient and early risk stratification can reduce the likelihood of mortality, as well as the probability of long-term complications.[23] For the patient experiencing a first MI, the prognosis for survival is generally good. Those with a second or third MI have approximately a twofold higher risk of early mortality, and long term survival is substantially better in first-time MI patients than in those who have had more than one MI.

TABLE 15–1. Definitions of Thrombolysis in Myocardial Infarction (TIMI) Grade Flows

TIMI Grade	Definition
0	No perfusion; no antegrade flow beyond point of occlusion
1	Penetration without perfusion; failure of contrast medium to move out of area of obstruction and, thus, inability to opacify entire coronary bed distal to occlusion
2	Partial perfusion; passage of contrast medium through obstruction, but at slow rates of perfusion and clearance
3	Complete perfusion; prompt occurrence of antegrade flow distal to obstruction and clearance of contrast medium

Adapted from N Engl J Med 1985; 312:932–936.

TABLE 15–2. 90-minute Thrombolysis in Myocardial Infarction (TIMI) Grade Flow and the Corresponding Mortality Rate in Patients Enrolled in the GUSTO-I Study

TIMI Grade Flow	Mortality Rate (%)
0 or 1	8.9
2	7.4
3	4.4[a]

Difference between the mortality rate in patients with TIMI grade 3 flow versus TIMI grade 0 or 1 was significant ($P = .009$).
[a] $P = .08$ vs. TIMI grade 2.
Adapted from Ref. 25.

Both 30-day and 5-year mortality rates correlate with the patency of the infarct-related artery. Specifically, patients with thrombolysis in myocardial infarction (TIMI) grade 3 flow (Table 15–1) have a substantially lower mortality rate than do patients with TIMI grades 0 to 2 flow (Table 15–2), and TIMI grade flow has recently been confirmed as an independent predictor of survival.[25–27] Although there has been controversy about the importance of achieving TIMI grade 3 flow at *90 minutes* versus another time point (e.g., 24 hours), data now show that TIMI grade flow at *3 to 4 weeks* after fibrinolysis is an independent predictor of 5-year mortality.[28,29]

In addition to TIMI grade flow, troponin (I or T) concentration is a predictor of outcome for MI both with and without ST-segment elevation. The third Global Use of Strategies to Open Occluded Coronary Arteries study (GUSTO III) results demonstrated the predictive value of troponin T on 30-day mortality in MI patients whose ECG showed ST- segment elevation and who received treatment with fibrinolysis.[30] Similarly, in patients with non–ST-segment elevation MI, troponin I concentrations greater than or equal to 9 ng/mL were associated with a risk of death *nearly* eight times higher than that associated with a troponin I level of less than 0.4 ng/mL[17] Thus, the preferred biomarker for myocardial injury is now troponin.[13]

Historically, infarct type was believed to play a role in a patient's prognosis after MI, as patients with non–ST-segment elevation MI tend to be at higher risk for re-infarction and recurrent ischemia. With the advent of reperfusion therapy (specifically, percutaneous coronary intervention [PCI]) and new antithrombotic therapies, however, the incidence of these events is declining, and the usefulness of ST-segment elevation in predicting MI outcome may becoming less relevant. It has been proposed that categorization of MIs according to the presence or absence of ST-segment elevation on ECG should refer only to the extent of myocardial injury (as non–ST-segment elevation MI produces a smaller, less extensive injury) rather than to the potential outcome.[31] Regardless, assessment of prognosis involves the careful evaluation of *all* MI patients, including measurement of left ventricular function and evaluation of risk factors.

CLINICAL PRESENTATION

Chest pain is the predominant symptom that brings 70% to 80% of patients with MI to the emergency department.[32] Patients will, however, frequently describe their symptom as chest pressure or a squeezing sensation rather than pain. The pain or pressure may first be noticed in the epigastrum and be incorrectly interpreted as dyspepsia or indigestion. It may also develop in either or both arms, shoulders, or wrists, as well as the jaw or back. Movement, deep breathing, or a change in body position does not affect the pain. Unfortunately, the presence of such discomfort alone is not sufficient to make the diagnosis of MI, as it is a subjective symptom and is often difficult to distinguish from a variety of other cardiac and noncardiac events. Furthermore, absence of pain has been reported in as many as 15% to 25% of patients with MI, particularly in patients with diabetes mellitus.

Women who experience MI have a different clinical presentation and tend to have worse outcomes than men do. They tend to be older and to have a higher prevalence of diabetes, hypertension, and prior heart failure.[33] Fewer women than men have ST-segment elevation MI, and women also have a higher risk of death or re-infarction compared to men.

In addition to chest pain, patients may present with physical findings such as diaphoresis, nausea and vomiting, arm tingling/numbness, shortness of breath, weakness, light-headedness, or syncope. These symptoms are also not specific enough to confirm the diagnosis of MI; therefore, it is necessary to use objective criteria to confirm the diagnosis. These parameters include the 12-lead ECG and characteristic changes in concentrations of serum cardiac markers such as creatine kinase (CK) and its MB isoenzyme. Neither CK nor CK-MB, markers formerly used exclusively for the diagnosis of MI, are as sensitive as cardiac troponin I or T for the detection of myocardial necrosis.[13,32] Because troponin is not normally detectable in the blood of healthy individuals, it represents a much more sensitive measure of myocardial injury than does CK. Furthermore, because the amino acid sequences of the skeletal and cardiac isoforms of troponin are dissimilar, assays have been developed to detect the cardiac-specific isoform of both troponin T and I.[32] Another advantage associated with the use of troponin for the diagnosis of MI is the stoichiometric correlation to the magnitude of myocardial necrosis. This relationship translates to a correlation between an elevation in the troponin level and the prognosis (see Prognosis). Even though it is less cardiac-specific than troponin, however, measurement of CK-MB is still an acceptable alternative if troponin levels are not available.[13,32] The disadvantage of troponin is its inability to detect early MI and re-infarction.[13,32] Troponin levels are not detectable until approximately 2 to 4 hours from the onset of chest pain, although they persist for several days (I, 7 days; T,10 to 14 days; Fig. 15–1). Therefore, other cardiac markers such as the cardiac CK-MB isoform, $CK\text{-}MB_2$, or myoglobin may be more useful for early diagnosis.

In order to confirm the diagnosis of MI, elevated concentrations of troponin, either I or T, or CK-MB should appear in two or more successive blood samples collected several hours apart. For most patients, such sampling should occur upon admission, 6 to 8 hours later, and again at 12 to 24 hours. Neither measurement of the total concentration of CK, nor measurements of the concentrations of other proteins previously used (e.g., lactate dehydrogenase [LDH], aspartate aminotransferase [AST], alanine aminotransferase [ALT]) are recommended for diagnosis of MI.

An ECG should be obtained within 10 minutes of patient presentation.[16,32] The electrocardiographic diagnostic feature of MI with ST-segment elevation is the Q wave associated with a pattern of ST-segment changes.[16,32] It is critical not to base the diagnosis on a single ECG, but rather to obtain serial ECGs. This strategy significantly enhances the sensitivity of the ECG in making the diagnosis. The earliest change in the ECG in patients with ST-segment elevation MI is associated with the T wave; it may be prolonged, peaked, or inverted. T-wave alterations are soon followed by ST-segment elevation (Fig. 15–2). A pathologic Q wave may or may not be present on the initial ECG, or it may appear hours or sometimes days after an ST-segment elevation MI. Pathologic Q waves are those that are approximately one-third as deep as the size of the QRS complex and are at least 1 mm (0.04 s) wide. The ECG changes associated with non–ST-segment elevation MI may be less specific and can include ST-segment elevation or depression and/or T-wave inversion.

Ultimately, there are specific criteria to determine the diagnosis of MI.[13,16] There is a typical rise and gradual fall in troponin (I or T) or a more rapid rise and fall of biochemical markers (CK-MB) of myocardial necrosis with at least one of the following:

1. Ischemic symptoms.
2. Development of pathologic Q waves on the ECG (ST-segment elevation MI).
3. ECG changes indicative of ischemia (ST-segment elevation or depression) or new left bundle branch block.
4. Coronary artery intervention (e.g., coronary angioplasty). This criterion refers to patients who undergo percutaneous transluminal coronary angioplasty (PTCA) and experience an increase in cardiac biomarker levels following the procedure.

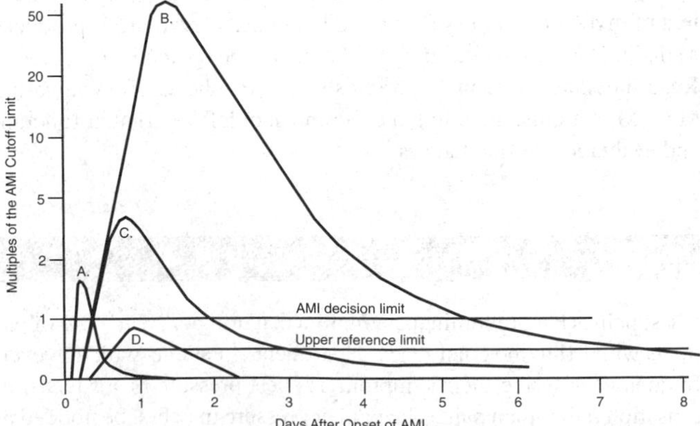

FIGURE 15–1. Timing of the release of various biomarkers following acute myocardial infarction (AMI). A = Early release of myoglobin or CK-MB after AMI. B = Cardiac troponin I level after AMI. C = CK-MB level after AMI. D = Cardiac troponin level after unstable angina. Data are plotted on a relative scale, where 1.0 is set at the AMI cutoff concentration. CK = creatine kinase. (*Adapted from Clin Chem 1999;45:1104–1121, with permission.*)

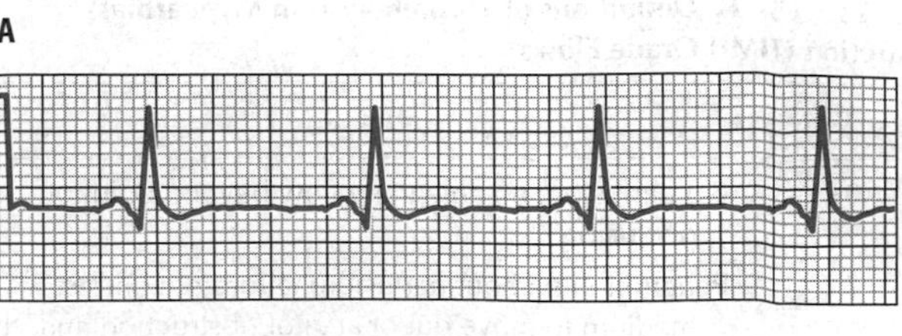

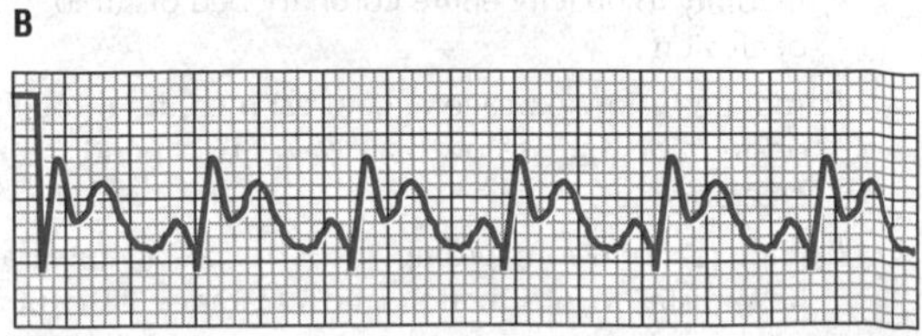

FIGURE 15–2. **(A)** Normal (isoelectric) ST segment with normal cardiac complexes and **(B)** ST-segment elevation with pathologic Q waves. Both rhythm strips are lead II.

▶ TREATMENT: Myocardial Infarction

DESIRED OUTCOMES

The foremost goals of therapy for patients with MI are (1) to minimize infarct size, (2) to salvage ischemic myocardium, (3) to prevent or minimize complications, and (4) to prevent mortality. The primary means of achieving these goals is the complete and timely restoration of coronary blood flow in the infarct-related artery.[34] Therapy has emphasized, and continues to emphasize, achievement and maintenance of the infarct-related artery's patency and preservation of left ventricular function. However, advancements in the understanding of the pathophysiology of MI, particularly the role of inflammation, are both changing the approach to treatment and expanding the knowledge of how certain drugs, some of which have been utilized in MI for some time, confer benefit.

GENERAL APPROACH

The highest incidence of MI complications and death is during the first 48 hours after the onset of symptoms.[16,23,32] Admission to an intensive care or coronary care unit is mandatory for the close observation and the acute care of MI patients with complications such as cardiogenic shock or those who may require such interventions as the insertion of an intra-aortic balloon pump.[16,32] Other patients may be admitted instead to an intermediate care unit where telemetry and defibrillation equipment are available and other forms of monitoring are not.[16,32] Close monitoring of vital signs, symptoms, and the ECG is recommended for the first 48 to 72 hours after uncomplicated MI. This approach is appropriate for patients who have been successfully treated with fibrinolytic therapy or primary PCI. Continued intensive monitoring is recommended beyond 72 hours if the patient is hemodynamically unstable, has persistent ischemia, or has hemodynamically significant cardiac arrhythmias.

A number of factors related to myocardial oxygen consumption require aggressive control. Activity should be restricted for the first 2 to 3 days and gradually increased as tolerated by the patient. Prolonged bed rest is not recommended other than for hemodynamically unstable patients, although a short period of bed rest of 12 hours is considered prudent.[16,32] The hospital diet should involve multiple small meals, sodium restriction, and reduced content of saturated fats and cholesterol. Dietary restrictions in the hospital need not include avoidance of caffeine, especially in routine caffeine drinkers.[16,32] To avoid the numerous potential problems associated with defecation-related Valsalva maneuver, the use of a stool softener, either docusate sodium (100 mg) or docusate calcium (240 mg) once or twice a day, is universally recommended.

Most interventions for MI are "acute" in nature and are frequently administered simultaneously or in close proximity to each other. Patients (both with and without ST-segment elevation MI) should be considered candidates for each therapy, based on a careful assessment of potential risks and benefits of each intervention.

NONPHARMACOLOGIC THERAPY

LABORATORY ASSESSMENTS

Patients with presumed acute MI should, if possible, have three large-bore (18-gauge) peripheral IV lines placed upon admission to the emergency department. Early establishment of IV access allows for the prompt administration of important drug therapy that will have an impact on the morbidity and mortality of the patient. In addition, IV access facilitates the collection of blood for tests that are imperative to the diagnosis and assessment of a patient's suitability for fibrinolytic therapy. One IV line should be reserved, if possible, for obtaining the frequent blood samples required. Pertinent laboratory tests on admission should include, but are not limited to, complete blood count (CBC) with platelet count; measurement of CK-MB and troponin I or T levels; and determination of activated partial thromboplastin time (aPTT), prothrombin time (PT), and international normalized ratio (INR). Serial measurements of CK-MB and/or troponin I or T should be obtained every 6 to 8 hours for 24 hours. In addition, it is recommended that all patients with acute MI have a lipid panel assessment within 24 hours of admission.[35] If the patient receives fibrinolytic and/or heparin therapy, a regular assessment of hemoglobin, hematocrit, and platelets is necessary. Details regarding appropriate laboratory monitoring of drug therapy are given in the following discussions of each agent when applicable.

PHARMACOLOGIC THERAPY

ADMINISTRATION OF OXYGEN

Patients may be moderately hypoxic even with an uncomplicated MI. This hypoxia may be due, in part, to a ventilation–perfusion mismatch.[16,32] Consequently, in the initial hours of therapy, supplemental oxygen (2–4 L/min by nasal cannula) should be administered. Although there appears to be little justification for its routine use beyond 2 to 3 hours, use of oxygen is especially important for patients with pulmonary edema or evidence of heart failure because hypoxia will be more severe in these patients. In some particularly severe cases, the administration of oxygen may not correct hypoxia, and the patient may require mechanical ventilation.

REPERFUSION THERAPY

Any intervention designed to re-open a partially or completely occluded coronary artery and, as a consequence, to reestablish normal or near normal blood flow can be called reperfusion therapy. All patients should be considered for reperfusion therapy, although non–ST-segment elevation MI patients are not considered eligible for fibrinolytic therapy. Available resources determine the most appropriate reperfusion strategy first and foremost. Fewer than 20% of hospitals in the United States have a cardiac catheterization laboratory, and only a fraction of these are capable of performing emergent PTCA.[16,32]

Fibrinolytic Therapy

An extremely important advancement in the treatment of ST-segment elevation MI, fibrinolytic therapy has had a huge impact on mortality reduction (up to 50%), and long-term (10 to 12 years) follow-up trials have demonstrated that this important benefit of fibrinolytic therapy is sustained.[29,36–38] Lately, the emphasis of clinical trials has been on achieving early patency of the infarct related artery and improving door-to-needle time. The development of bolus dose fibrinolytic agents such as reteplase (rPA; Retavase) and, more recently, tenecteplase (TNK-tPA; TNKase) has, in part, facilitated this improvement. The Food and Drug Administration (FDA) has approved these two medications, as well as streptokinase (Streptase/Kabikinase), recombinant tissue-type plasminogen activator (tPA; alteplase [Activase]), and anisoylated plasminogen streptokinase activator complex (APSAC; anistreplase [Eminase]), for use in patients with MI in the United States; additional agents are currently undergoing clinical evaluation.[38] None of these agents alter myocardial oxygen demand. Instead, they improve myocardial oxygen supply by dissolving the thrombus associated with acute MI and reestablishing blood flow to ischemic myocardium. Consequently, prompt fibrinolytic therapy limits the extent of myocardial necrosis and infarct size, thus significantly improving the likelihood of survival.[16,32]

Many clinical trials have established the efficacy, safety, and mortality benefit of fibrinolytic therapy in patients with ST-segment elevation MI. Controversy still exists regarding the superiority of one agent over any of the others, however, although there have been studies that have directly compared one agent to another.[39–44] The GUSTO-I (Global Utilization of Streptokinase and Tissue Plasminogen Activator for Occluded Coronary Arteries) trial tested the open artery hypothesis—i.e., *early and sustained infarct-related artery patency is associated with better survival in patients with MI*—and evaluated the efficacy of the accelerated administration of tPA (bolus of 15 mg, 0.75 mg/kg over 30 minutes, not to exceed 50 mg followed by 0.5 mg/kg over 60 minutes, not to exceed 35 mg), given in an open-label manner, compared to three other strategies: streptokinase, 1.5 million units over 1 hour with heparin given IV; streptokinase, 1.5 million units over 1 hour with heparin given subcutaneously; or the combination of streptokinase, 1.5 million units over 1 hour, and tPA (1 mg/kg over 1 hour not to exceed 90 mg with 10% given as a bolus).[42] Heparin was administered IV as a 5,000-U bolus, followed by a 1,000 U/h infusion, which was adjusted based on the aPTT. Subcutaneously, heparin was given as 12,500 U twice a day, starting 4 hours after the initiation of fibrinolytic therapy. All patients received aspirin, and patients without contraindications received 5 mg IV atenolol in two divided doses, followed by oral therapy of 50–100 mg/d. The primary end point of the study was the 30-day mortality rate. More than 41,000 patients were enrolled in GUSTO I, approximately 10,000 in each treatment arm. The 30-day mortality rate significantly favored the accelerated administration of tPA, and there was no significant difference between the two streptokinase regimens ($P = .731$). The benefit observed with the tPA regimen translates to approximately 9 lives saved per 1,000 patients, a risk reduction of 14%. However, there was a slightly higher incidence of stroke in patients who received tPA.

In addition to these findings, probably the most important observation made in the GUSTO-I trial was the relationship between TIMI grade flow and mortality (see Table 15–2). Other studies have also demonstrated that TIMI grade 3 flow is a strong predictor of mortality, and this premise served as the basis for the GUSTO-III trial, which compared the efficacy of rPA to that of tPA.[25,26,44] Because previous observations had revealed a higher incidence of TIMI grade 3 flow at 90 minutes with rPA than with front-loaded tPA, it was presumed that this would translate into a difference in mortality rates between the two agents.[43] This was not the case, however, and the importance of achieving TIMI grade 3 flow at 90 minutes (vs. a later time point) has been questioned.[28] Long-term follow-up from clinical trials of fibrinolysis demonstrate the importance of achieving and maintaining TIMI grade 3 flow, but not necessarily at 90 minutes.[26–29]

More recent studies of fibrinolysis have focused on improving the timely administration of fibrinolytic therapy. A door-to-needle time of less than 30 minutes is an important therapeutic goal for treating ST-segment elevation MI patients. Although the use of bolus dose fibrinolytics may facilitate achievement of this goal, there is little evidence to show that they improve TIMI grade flow or alter outcome. The infarct-related artery patency data from the TIMI 10B trial revealed that tenecteplase (40 mg), the newest fibrinolytic agent, and front-loaded tPA produced similar rates of 90-minute TIMI grade 3 flow (62.8% vs. 62.7%, respectively; $P =$ NS).[45] The results of the Second Assessment of Safety and Efficacy of a New Thrombolytic Agent (ASSENT-2) showed that tenecteplase and front-loaded tPA produced equivalent 30-day mortality rates.[46]

■ *Hemorrhagic Complications.* Stroke and intracranial hemorrhage are concerns with the administration of fibrinolytic therapy, although the overall incidences are low (<2% and <1%, respectively).[32] Notably, the cumulative 1-year medical costs are 60% higher in MI patients with stroke compared to MI patients without stroke.[47]

Intracranial hemorrhage is considered the greatest risk of fibrinolytic therapy. If it is going to occur, it usually occurs within the first 24 hours of therapy.[38] Although the risk of intracranial hemorrhage is similar for all of the fibrinolytic agents, there are severalpatient characteristics that may be associated with a higher risk of this event.[38] These include female gender, black ethnicity, age (>75 years), weight (<65 kg for females; <80 kg for males), known cerebral vascular disease or history of stroke, elevated diastolic blood pressure (>100 mm Hg), combined use of streptokinase and tPA, history of hypertension, and elevated systolic blood pressure (>140 mm Hg). In addition, front-loaded tPA or aggressive use of unfractionated heparin tend to put patients at greater risk for intracranial hemorrhage. Other bleeding (both major and minor) can occur during and following the administration of any fibrinolytic agent.

Major bleeding (i.e., events considered life-threatening) occur in approximately 1.1% of patients.[38] The most common cause of bleeding in patients who receive fibrinolytic therapy is the concomitant use of coronary revascularization procedures, although the most common site of these bleeding events is the insertion point of a peripheral IV catheter. As is the case with intracranial hemorrhage, there are risk factors that contribute to the probability of a major or severe bleeding event: advanced age, weight (lighter), and female gender.[38] Overall bleeding rates tend to be higher with streptokinase than with tPA and greater with tenecteplase than with tPA, although most of these differences are in the frequency of minor hemorrhagic events rather than major hemorrhages.[38]

■ *Patient Eligibility.* Patients with symptoms of ischemia and persistent ST-segment elevation on the ECG who present within 12 hours after the onset of chest pain should be evaluated as candidates for fibrinolytic therapy.[16,32] Patients who present between 12 and 24 hours are typically considered for fibrinolytic therapy only if they have signs and symptoms of ongoing ischemia, such as persistent ST-segment elevation and chest pain. Some of these patients may describe "stuttering" chest pain that has come and gone and come again in the last 6 to 12 hours. These patients represent a unique subgroup and require careful evaluation. It is essential to weigh the risks and benefits of fibrinolytic therapy before deciding to treat the patient with a lytic agent. Patients who present after 24 hours are considered ineligible for fibrinolytic therapy.

The decision to administer fibrinolytic therapy should be based on a timely assessment of risks and benefits. The sooner a patient is treated with fibrinolytic therapy, the better the outcome.[16,32] Outcome is optimal if eligible patients receive a fibrinolytic agent within 30 minutes of arrival at the emergency department.[16,32] Contraindications must be carefully considered when determining whether an

TABLE 15–3. Absolute and Relative Contraindications for Fibrinolytic Therapy in Patients with ST-segment Elevation Myocardial Infarction

Absolute Contraindications

- Previous hemorrhagic stroke at any time; other strokes or cerebrovascular events within 1 year
- Known intracranial neoplasm
- Active internal bleeding (does not include menses)
- Suspected aortic dissection

Cautions/Relative Contraindications

- Severe uncontrolled hypertension on presentation (blood pressure >180/110 mm Hg)
- History of prior cerebrovascular accident or known intracerebral pathology not covered in contraindications
- Current use of anticoagulants in therapeutic doses (INR ≥ 2–3)
- Known bleeding diathesis
- Recent trauma (within 2–4 weeks), including head trauma or traumatic or prolonged (>10 min) CPR or major surgery (<3 wk)
- Noncompressible vascular punctures
- Recent (within 2–4 weeks) internal bleeding
- For streptokinase and anistreplase: prior exposure (especially within 5 d–2 y) or prior allergic reaction; use rPA, tPA, or TNK
- Pregnancy
- Active peptic ulcer disease
- History of chronic severe hypertension

INR = international normalized ratio; CPR = cardiopulmonary resuscitation; rPA = reteplase; tPA = alteplase; TNK = tenecteplase.
From Ref. 16.

ST segment elevation MI patient should receive fibrinolytic therapy, however. So that therapy is not delayed, evaluation of potential contraindications must be made quickly.

Absolute and relative contraindications to fibrinolytic therapy are outlined in Table 15–3. The presence of more than one relative contraindication is considered an *absolute* contraindication to fibrinolytic therapy. Of considerable importance is the issue of the patient's age. Age is neither an absolute nor a relative contraindication. Although older individuals, particularly those over the age of 75 years, have a significantly higher rate of mortality from MI than their younger counterparts do, they still derive a benefit from fibrinolytic therapy. The risk of hemorrhagic stroke is higher, though, if a patient more than 75 years old is treated by the accelerated regimen of tPA.[38] Therefore, in the absence of an absolute contraindication, patients who are 75 years of age and older should not be excluded as candidates for fibrinolytic therapy; streptokinase may be the fibrinolytic agent of choice in these individuals.

The choice of fibrinolytic agent is another vital consideration in the decision-making process. A 1% mortality benefit of the accelerated regimen of tPA compared to a regimen of streptokinase was observed in the GUSTO I study, although *no* differences have been observed in subsequent comparative trials of rPA and tPA, and of tenecteplase and tPA.[42,44,46] In addition, a component of the decision-making process should include cost of the fibrinolytic agent. On average, tPA and rPA each cost approximately $2,400, tenecteplase (50 mg) $2,750, and streptokinase is about $220. Is the 1% mortality benefit observed with an accelerated regimen of tPA compared to a regimen of streptokinase worth the difference in cost between the two agents? The economic analysis of GUSTO-I determined the cost-effectiveness ratio of tPA to be approximately $33,000 per year of life saved.[48] This ratio varied considerably, depending on a number of different factors, such as patient age and infarct location. Patients with anterior wall MI had the lowest cost-effectiveness ratio (greatest cost-effectiveness).

These data, other cost-effectiveness data, and efficacy and adverse event data may guide clinicians in determining the most appropriate reperfusion strategy for their institution. As part of developing this strategy, clinicians should work together to facilitate the rapid identification of eligible MI patients and the timely administration of therapy. The availability of pharmacy services in the emergency department can facilitate the rapid administration of fibrinolytic therapy. Alternatively, pharmacists can assist in the development of fibrinolytic therapy "kits" that contain the agent, diluent, and instructions for preparation and administration. Pharmacists should also participate in the development of clinical pathways for the treatment of MI.

Dosing Guidelines. Patients with MI should be treated as soon as possible, but preferably within 30 minutes from the time they present to the emergency department, with one of the following regimens:

1. Tissue plasminogen activator (tPA, alteplase [Activase]), 15-mg bolus followed by 0.75 mg/kg infusion (not to exceed 50 mg) over 30 minutes followed by 0.5 mg/kg infusion (not to exceed 35 mg) over 1 hour
2. Streptokinase, 1.5 million units in 50 mL of normal saline or D_5W over 60 minutes
3. Anistreplase (APSAC, [Eminase]), 30 U by IV push over 2 minutes
4. Reteplase (rPA, [Retavase]), 10 U by IV push over 2 minutes followed 30 minutes later with another 10 U by IV push over 2 minutes
5. Tenecteplase (TNK [TNKase]), 30 mg in patients weighing less than 60 kg; 35 mg in patients weighing 60 to 69.9 kg; 40 mg in patients weighing 70 to 79.9 kg; 45 mg in patients weighing 80 to 89.9 kg; and 50 mg to patients 90 or more kg administered as a single IV bolus over 5 seconds.

Evaluation of Therapeutic Outcomes. Following fibrinolytic therapy administration, the patient should be carefully monitored for adverse events, as well as for signs and symptoms of reperfusion. A systemic lytic state develops rapidly after therapy begins and may persist for up to 24 hours, although it may be somewhat longer in patients who receive APSAC. Clinically, a fall in fibrinogen concentration, an increase in the concentration of fibrin degradation products, and prolongation of the aPTT characterize this systemic lytic state, and it is during this time that the risk of bleeding is the greatest.[38] If the patient begins to bleed during this period, timely management is essential. The algorithm outlined in Figure 15–3 for the management of bleeding that is not immediately life-threatening provides guidelines for intervention and assists in the decision-making process. Although intracranial hemorrhage is the most serious adverse effect associated with fibrinolysis, concern for this problem should not preclude administration of fibrinolytic therapy to an eligible patient.[38] Other adverse effects for which patients should be monitored include hypotension and allergic reactions, which occur more frequently with streptokinase and APSAC than with tPA , rPA, or tenecteplase.

Successful reperfusion with fibrinolytic therapy can be assessed by

1. Evaluation of the ECG. ST-segment elevation should normalize when reperfusion occurs.
2. Relief of chest pain. Initially, chest discomfort may actually become worse at the time of reperfusion, but it should ultimately be relieved.

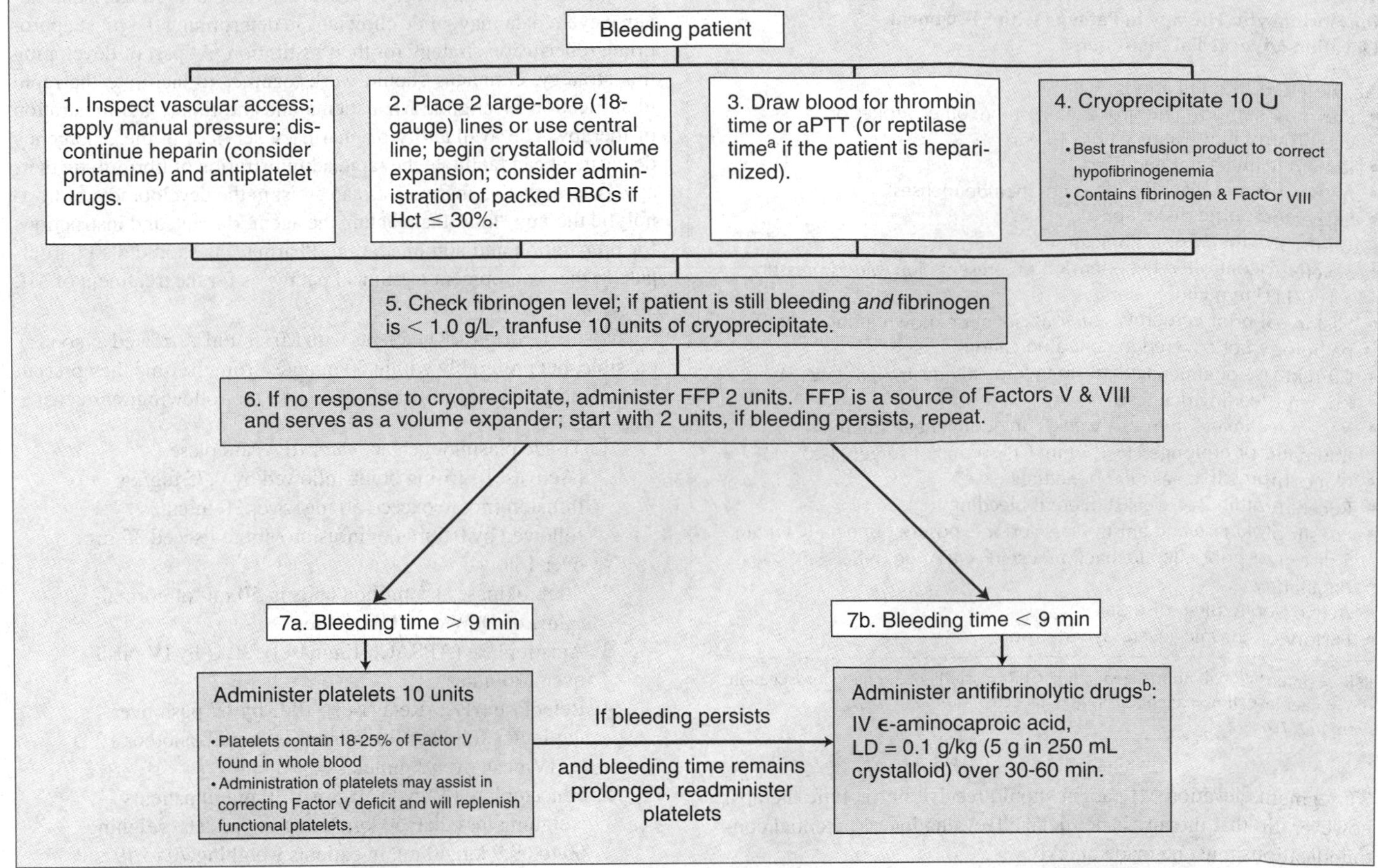

FIGURE 15–3. Sequential algorithm (steps 1–7) for the management of major bleeding associated with the administration of thrombolytic therapy. RBC = red blood cells; Hct = hematocrit; aPTT = activated partial thromboplastin time; FFP = fresh frozen plasma; LD = loading dose. [a]Will identify persistent lytic state in heparinized patients; [b]use with caution, consider as last line in actively bleeding patient. (*Adapted from Ann Intern Med 1989;111:1010–1022.*)

3. Abrupt onset of arrhythmias, usually ventricular in nature.[49]

Reperfusion arrhythmias are usually self-limiting or quite responsive to drug therapy (i.e., IV lidocaine) or direct current cardioversion, if necessary. Normalization of the ECG, relief of chest pain, and the appearance of reperfusion arrhythmias suggest that fibrinolysis has been successful. Unfortunately, presence or absence of these observations may not always be an accurate assessment of fibrinolytic success or failure, because fibrinolytic therapy is unsuccessful in approximately 22% to 30% of patients.[49] In addition, approximately 5% to 10% of patients will spontaneously reperfuse.

Combined Fibrinolytic and Platelet Glycoprotein IIb/IIIa Inhibitor Therapy

Strategies to improve the success of reperfusion therapy, particularly in regard to enhancing microvasculature patency, are continually being explored. In addition to the use of platelet glycoprotein IIb/IIIa inhibitors in PCI, the combined use of reduced-dose fibrinolytic agents and glycoprotein IIb/IIIa inhibitor therapy is being explored. The phase II, dose ranging TIMI 14 and Strategies for Patency Enhancement in the Emergency Department (SPEED) studies both showed that combination therapy is feasible and appears to be safe.[50,51] Larger outcome trials, the GUSTO-V and ASSENT-3, showed that the combination of either reteplase or tenecteplase and abciximab reduced cardiovascular events (versus rPA or TNK with unfractionated heparin), but resulted in more bleeding complications.[51a,51b]

Primary PTCA

Ever since the first report describing the use of primary PTCA as an alternative or adjunct to fibrinolysis, its role has been debated. In the GUSTO-IIb trial in which 1,138 patients with ST-segment elevation MI were randomized to either PTCA or fibrinolysis with tPA (100 mg over 90 minutes), the incidence of death, recurrent MI, or disabling stroke was significantly lower (9.6% vs. 13.6%, $P = .033$) in the PTCA-treated patients.[52] By 6 months, however, the differences between the two treatment groups were no longer significant (13.3% vs. 15.7%, $P =$ NS). Data from the Second National Registry of Myocardial Infarction (NRMI-2) also suggest that PTCA and fibrinolytic therapy offer similar efficacy.[53] In ST-segment elevation MI patients (without cardiogenic shock), the in-hospital mortality rate was 5.4% for tPA-treated patients and 5.2% for PTCA-treated patients. Importantly, this was also the case for higher risk patients, such as those more than 75 years of age and those with anterior wall MI. On the other hand, long-term (2-year) outcome data from the Primary Angioplasty in Myocardial Infarction (PAMI-I) trial showed that patients who underwent reperfusion with primary PTCA rather than fibrinolysis with tPA had less recurrent ischemia (36.4% vs. 48%, $P = .026$), lower re-intervention rates (27.2% vs. 46.5%, $P < .0001$), and reduced hospital re-admissions (58.5% vs. 69%, $P = .035$).[54] In addition, the combined end point of death or re-infarction was 14.9% for PTCA-treated patients and 23% for tPA-treated patients ($P = .034$).

Despite these promising results, primary PTCA should be offered as an alternative to fibrinolysis only (1) if it can be accomplished in a timely manner (within 90 minutes of admission) by skilled practitioners (those who perform more than 75 PTCAs/yr) in a high-volume center (where practitioners perform more than 200 PTCAs/yr) that specializes in the procedure or (2) in circumstances where fibrinolysis is otherwise contraindicated.[16,32] Obviously, the limitations of primary PTCA are that it is labor-intensive and not feasible for use on a routine basis in most institutions. In addition to these considerations, there have been advancements in adjunct PTCA therapy that clinicians should weigh. Improvement in the outcomes associated with primary PTCA in ST-segment elevation MI have been achieved, in part, by the addition of platelet glycoprotein IIb/IIIa inhibitor therapy.[55] For example, the use of abciximab (ReoPro, Eli Lilly, and Centocor) in primary PTCA was associated with a reduction (by treatment analysis) in death or re-infarction (4.7% vs. 1.4%, respectively, $P = .047$ at 7 days and 12% vs. 6.9%, respectively, $P = .07$ at 6 months) when compared to PTCA alone.[56] In addition, the need for "bail out" coronary stenting was reduced by 42% (20.4% vs. 11.9%, $P = .008$).

Patients with non–ST-segment elevation MI should also be considered for an "early invasive strategy" with PTCA if one or more markers of high risk for a poor outcome are present. Such markers include a decidedly elevated troponin level (e.g., >1.0 ng/mL), advanced age (>70 years), prior MI and/or revascularization, ST-segment depression on the ECG, heart failure, or depressed left ventricular function (i.e., left ventricular ejection fraction <40%). Consisting of coronary arteriography with PTCA, if necessary, the early invasive strategy should be reserved for high-risk non–ST-segment elevation MI patients (as described earlier). Patients without a high-risk factor should be managed pharmacologically.There may be system issues (e.g., timeliness of care) that make use of an early invasive strategy the preferred treatment at some centers, however.

PTCA Following Fibrinolytic Therapy

Although fibrinolysis is effective in the majority of patients with acute ST-segment elevation MI, approximately 75% to 90% of patients will have a residual stenosis following clot lysis, and PTCA has been shown to be very effective in reducing this residual stenosis.[57] Several studies have shown that PTCA immediately following full-dose fibrinolytic therapy is not beneficial and may actually contribute to morbidity and mortality, however.[16,32] Thus, PTCA *following* fibrinolytic therapy should be reserved for patients who have symptomatic or objective evidence of persistent or continuing ischemia. Clinical trials are ongoing to evaluate the utility of the use of low-dose fibrinolytic therapy in combination with PTCA (referred to as *facilitated* PTCA). The results of these trials are needed before this strategy can be recommended.

Coronary Artery Stenting

A coronary stent is a small, metal-mesh concentric scaffold that, when inserted into a coronary artery, maintains lumen patency (Fig. 15–4).

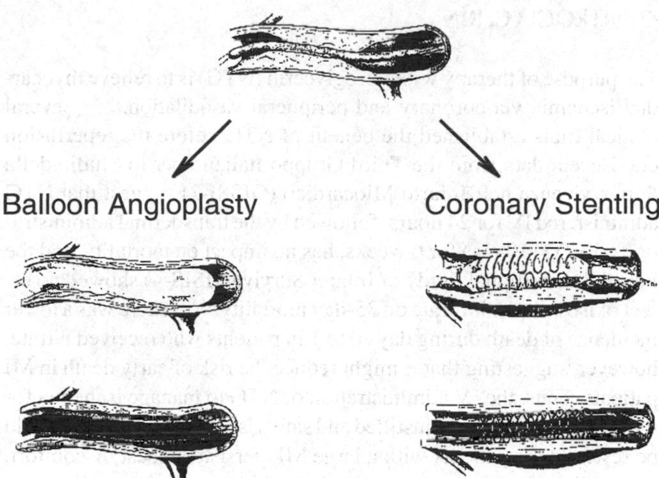

FIGURE 15–4. Percutaneous coronary intervention.

Stents are inserted angiographically and deployed using balloon angioplasty. Although still evolving as a reperfusion strategy for ST-segment elevation MI, current data suggest that stenting may improve outcomes over either fibrinolysis or PTCA alone.[58] When used in combination with a platelet glycoprotein IIb/IIIa inhibitor in ST-segment elevation MI patients ($n = 140$), stenting improved myocardial salvage and clinical outcomes compared to those achieved with fibrinolysis alone.[59]

Data also support the use of stents in non–ST-segment elevation MI, particularly in combination with a glycoprotein IIb/IIIa inhibitor.[60] The criteria for stenting in such patients are the same as those described earlier for primary PTCA.

ANALGESIA

Pain control and relief of anxiety are the most immediate objectives in the management of acute MI. Notably, recent experience with fibrinolytic agents strongly suggests that the pain associated with MI is due mainly to continuing ischemia of viable myocardium rather than to necrosis. Morphine sulfate, administered IV, is the drug of choice for acute management of pain associated with MI.[16,32] Morphine is particularly effective in the setting of acute MI because it blocks sympathetic efferent discharge from the central nervous system, resulting in peripheral arterial dilation. Overall, morphine reduces myocardial oxygen demand by decreasing systemic vascular resistance and afterload, and by decreasing circulating concentrations of catecholamines, which may, in turn, reduce the likelihood of ventricular arrhythmias.

Morphine should be administered slowly in small doses of 2–5 mg IV every 5 to 15 minutes as needed for pain. Blood pressure often guides dosage in that patients who are normotensive or hypertensive will tolerate higher morphine doses. A small number of patients whose pain persists may require as much as 25–30 mg before analgesia is adequate.

Morphine therapy should be continued until pain relief is achieved or an unacceptable end point, such as hypotension (systolic blood pressure <90 mm Hg), is reached. While receiving morphine, patients should be monitored closely for adverse effects such as hypotension, respiratory depression, and allergic reactions as well as the desired outcome, relief of pain

NITROGLYCERIN

The purpose of therapy with nitroglycerin (NTG) is to relieve myocardial ischemia via coronary and peripheral vasodilation.[16,32] Several clinical trials established the benefit of NTG before the reperfusion era. Recent data from the Third Gruppo Italiano per lo Studio della Sopravvivenza nell'Infarto Miocardico (GISSI-3) suggest that NTG administered IV for 24 hours, followed by the transdermal administration of NTG (10 mg) for 6 weeks, has no impact on mortality, and the Fourth International Study of Infarct Survival (ISIS-4) showed no effect of isosorbide dinitrate on 35-day mortality.[61,62] There was a lower incidence of death during days 0 to 1 in patients who received nitrate, however, suggesting that it might reduce the risk of early death in MI patients. Thus, the IV administration of NTG to manage ischemia for the first 24 to 48 hours is justified and safe. Use beyond 48 hours should be reserved for patients with a large MI, persistent chest discomfort, heart failure, hypertension, or persistent pulmonary congestion.

Dosing Guidelines

All patients with chest discomfort associated with ischemia and/or suspected MI should receive NTG sublingually unless blood pressure is less than 90 mm Hg and/or heart rate is less than 50 or more than 100 beats/min.[16,32] Nitroglycerin should be avoided in patients with right ventricular MI and used cautiously in patients with inferior wall MI. A sublingual dose of NTG should be given every 5 to 10 minutes or until such time that the IV administration of NTG can begin.

Nitroglycerin (0.4 mg) is often administered sublingually to determine whether chest pain is due to MI or ischemia. For this purpose, the sublingual administration of NTG may be repeated three times, once every 5 minutes, as long as heart rate and systolic blood pressure are more than 50 beats/min and more than 90 mm Hg, respectively. Following the administration of NTG, heart rate and blood pressure should be closely monitored and the ECG evaluated. It is possible that NTG administered sublingually will relieve some or all of the patient's initial chest pain, but ST-segment changes (elevation or depression) on the ECG may remain. The persistence of ST-segment changes despite pain relief supports (but does not confirm) the diagnosis of MI. If ischemic chest pain persists, the IV administration of NTG should begin.

The IV use of NTG is preferred over the use of long-acting oral or transdermal formulations in the management of MI because it is easily titrated and monitored.[16,32] However, topical or oral nitrates can be useful for patients with non–ST-segment elevation MI who respond favorably to β-blockers administered IV (see Early Administration of β-Adrenergic Blockers) or those without ongoing or continuing chest pain.[17] The administration of NTG may begin as an IV infusion at 10–20 μg/min via an infusion pump; a bolus dose is not necessary because of the very brief elimination half-life of NTG. The NTG infusion may be increased every 5 to 10 minutes by 5–10 μg/min until ischemic symptoms resolve or blood pressure declines by more than 10% in a normotensive patient or more than 30% in a hypertensive patient. If the patient develops hypotension while receiving NTG, the rate of the infusion should be reduced, or the infusion should be gradually discontinued. If upon discontinuation the patient remains hypotensive, fluids should be administered IV. An infusion of NTG should also be interrupted when the ECG normalizes or if heart rate exceeds 110 beats/min. Although there is no upper limit to the IV dose of NTG, a dose of more than 200 μg/min is associated with an increased risk for hypotension; therefore, this dose should not be exceeded.[16,32]

Evaluation of Therapeutic Outcomes

Use of NTG may lead to either tachycardia or bradycardia. If the patient develops either symptom, the NTG infusion rate should be decreased. It is necessary to monitor the ECG closely for recurrent ischemia, even if the patient does not experience chest pain. Management of bradycardia may also necessitate elevation of the legs or use of fluids and/or atropine. Nitroglycerin–associated headache is also common (>50%), and a small percentage of patients (<5%) may experience intolerable headache, which may require discontinuation of the drug. Decreasing the infusion rate and/or administering acetaminophen may relieve NTG-associated headache and should be attempted before discontinuation of the NTG infusion.

EARLY ADMINISTRATION OF β-ADRENERGIC BLOCKERS

For patients with either non–ST-segment elevation MI that is uncomplicated or ST-segment elevation MI, use of β-blockers is associated with an overall 40% reduction in mortality.[63] In the absence of contraindications, IV therapy with a β-blocker should be initiated early in these patients. Results of numerous clinical trials have established that early administration (within 12 hours of the onset of symptoms) of a β-blocker reduces the likelihood of ventricular arrhythmias, recurrent ischemia, re-infarction, and, most importantly, mortality in patients with acute MI.[16,32] It is thought that these benefits occur primarily as a result of β-blocker–induced reduction in myocardial workload secondary to reductions in heart rate, systemic blood pressure, and myocardial contractility. Also, prolonged diastole in association with the β-blocker–induced reduction in heart rate may improve perfusion to ischemic or injured areas of the myocardium. Use of a β-blocker, together with the IV administration of NTG, is theoretically appropriate because it would minimize the likelihood of tachycardia. Recent data also suggest that β-blockade may attenuate inflammatory cytokine expression, an effect that may mitigate the development of heart failure in the peri-infarction period.[64]

Dosing Guidelines

Administration of a β-blocker is recommended for MI patients without evidence of severe left ventricular dysfunction and other contraindications, whether or not a fibrinolytic agent has been administered.[16,17,32] A β-blocker may be especially beneficial for those patients with elevated blood pressure or a tachyarrhythmia. Notably, patients with signs of mild to moderate heart failure should still be considered candidates for β-blockade, as long as they can be monitored closely. Indeed, these patients are strong candidates for an oral β-blocker regimen following discharge.

Before therapy with a β-blocker begins, it is necessary to determine heart rate and blood pressure. Systolic blood pressure and heart rate should be greater than 100 mm Hg and greater than 55 beats/min, respectively.[16,17,32]

Evauation of Therapeutic Outcomes

After each IV dose, heart rate and blood pressure should be carefully reassessed and the ECG reviewed for bradycardia or advanced atrioventricular block. Additionally, the patient should be carefully observed for signs of worsening heart failure. A full assessment of these hemodynamic and ECG responses may require up to 5 to

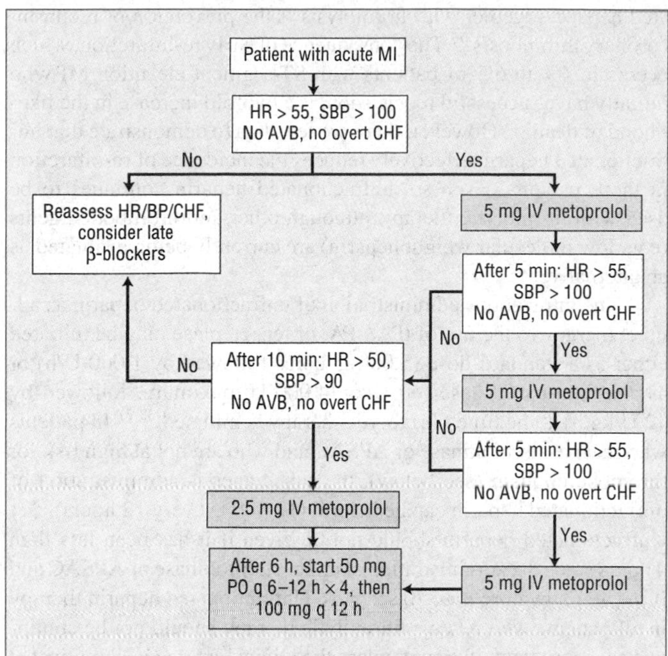

FIGURE 15–5. Algorithm for the early IV administration of metoprolol to patients with acute myocardial infarction (MI). HR = heart rate; SBP = systolic blood pressure; AVB = atrioventricular block; CHF = congestive heart failure.

10 minutes between doses. If the heart rate falls below 50 beats/min, the systolic blood pressure falls below 90 mm Hg, or the PR interval on the ECG becomes greater than 0.24 seconds, the IV administration of the β-blocker should cease–although hemodynamic and ECG monitoring continues. In some cases, bradycardia, hypotension, and atrioventricular block are transient and the IV regimen may resume once these problems resolve. If any of these problems persist, however, then the IV administration of the β-blocker should be terminated. Approximately 10% to 15% of patients will not tolerate the full IV regimen. This intolerance, however, does not preclude a patient from continuing with an oral regimen, which can be initiated 6 to 12 hours after the last IV dose. An algorithm outlining the decision-making process for acute β-blocker therapy is outlined in Figure 15–5.

LATE ADMINISTRATION OF β-ADRENERGIC BLOCKERS

The goal of the late administration of a β-blocker (at least 24 hours after MI) is prevention of recurrent MI and death. In addition, use of long-term β-blocker therapy improves left ventricular diastolic filling.[65] Patients who are not eligible for early IV β-blocker therapy may still be candidates for late administration. Such therapy, begun as early as 24 hours and as late as 28 days after MI, is associated with 23% and 32% reductions in occurrences of death and recurrent MI, respectively, for at least 2 to 3 years.[66]

In spite of these impressive results, β-blockers are underutilized, and it is estimated that 2,900 to 5,000 lives are lost in the first year following MI because of underprescribing.[67] The source of this apparent reluctance to use a β-blocker following MI is puzzling. The data supporting the use of long-term β-blockade following MI are so compelling that the use of a β-blocker is now advocated for patients with conditions that are considered relative contraindications to the use of β-blockers. Specifically, the β-blocker-associated rate of reduction in recurrent MI and mortality exceeds the risks in patients with asthma, insulin-dependent diabetes mellitus, chronic obstructive pulmonary disease (COPD), severe peripheral vascular disease, a PR interval of more than 0.24 seconds on the ECG, or moderate left ventricular failure.[16,17,32,63]

Dosing Guidelines

The β-blockers FDA-approved for use during and/or after MI are atenolol, metoprolol, propranolol, and timolol. Although other β-blockers, including carvedilol, may be used in selected patients, use of agents with intrinsic sympathomimetic activity (ISA) should be avoided.[16,17,68] Also, even a patient who cannot tolerate the maximum recommended dose can receive a β-blocker at a lower tolerable dose. Whenever possible, however, the β blocker dose should be maximized (Table 15–4). For secondary prevention of recurrent ischemia and re-infarction, β-blocker therapy should be continued indefinitely.[16,17,32]

Evaluation of Therapeutic Outcomes

Exercise heart rate is an important tool in assessing a patient's response to a β-blocker. The exercise heart rate goal for a post-MI patient who is taking a β-blocker is 60–70 beats/min. In addition, the patient should be followed closely for the development of congestive heart failure (CHF) and/or hypotension. Although patients who leave the hospital with some degree of left ventricular compromise (e.g., an ejection fraction < 40%) derive the greatest mortality benefit from the use of a β-blocker, they also may be more prone to the drug's adverse effects. If such effects occur, either the β-blocker dose should be decreased or therapy discontinued. Patients should also be monitored for symptomatic bradycardia and for long-term adverse reactions such as impotence, depression, and claudication. Similarly, a patient with asthma, COPD, insulin-dependent diabetes mellitus, or severe peripheral vascular disease should be monitored for exacerbation of any of these conditions. If such exacerbation occurs, dose reduction of the β-blocker should be attempted first, followed by discontinuation, if necessary.

ANTITHROMBOTIC THERAPY

Antithrombotic therapy plays an important role in the management of patients with acute MI. This therapeutic category is rapidly

TABLE 15–4. Early (IV) and Late (Oral) Dosing Regimens of β-Blockers for Patients with ST-segment or Non–ST-segment Elevation Myocardial Infarction)

Early Dosing Regimens	
IV Doses	
Propranolol	0.1 mg/kg two to three divided doses every 10 min
Metoprolol	15 mg in three divided doses every 5 min
Atenolol	5–10 mg in two divided doses every 5–10 min
Late Dosing Regimens	
Oral Doses	
Propranolol	180–240 mg/day in four divided doses
Metoprolol	200 mg/day in two divided doses
Atenolol	100 mg/day as a single dose
Timolol	20 mg/day in two divided doses

expanding: Over the past few years, aspirin and unfractionated heparin have been joined by clopidogrel, low molecular weight heparins, and platelet glycoprotein (GP) IIb/IIIa intibitors.

Aspirin

Due in no small part to observations from the Second International Study of Infarct Survival (ISIS-2) trial,[69] aspirin has become a critical component of acute MI therapy. In this study, 17,187 patients with suspected MI were assigned in a randomized, double-blind fashion to receive either streptokinase (1.5 million units IV over 1 hour), aspirin (160 mg daily for 1 month), both aspirin and streptokinase, or placebo. Compared with the placebo, aspirin was associated with a highly significant 23% reduction ($P < .00001$) in mortality. Furthermore, for patients assigned to receive both aspirin and streptokinase, the mortality rate was 39% lower than that observed in the placebo group ($P < .00001$). These observations clearly established the beneficial contribution of early aspirin administration with concomitant fibrinolysis in patients with acute MI.

Although the inhibition of cyclooxygenase-dependent platelet activation is the most likely mechanism responsible for these beneficial effects, the anti-inflammatory activity of aspirin may play a role. Furthermore, there is no evidence that other platelet inhibitors, such as dipyridamole, ticlopidine, or clopidogrel, have any advantage over aspirin in reducing the mortality risk.[70,71] In aspirin-sensitive patients, however, clopidogrel should be considered as an alternative.[32,72] Notably, there is also no evidence that aspirin has differential effects on any particular subgroup of patients, nor is there a time-dependent effect on early mortality similar to that observed with fibrinolysis.

Current recommendations for aspirin therapy in patients with suspected MI call for the immediate initiation of non–enteric-coated aspirin, 160–325 mg, that the patient should chew and swallow to achieve a rapid antiplatelet effect.[16,71] Patients who present to the emergency department with suspected MI should also receive aspirin, regardless of the reperfusion strategy being considered. The only exceptions to this recommendation are for patients who have an allergy to aspirin or an intolerance because of gastrointestinal problems. Patients scheduled for PTCA should be pretreated with (if not already receiving) aspirin (80–325 mg).

Clopidogrel/Ticlopidine

For patients undergoing PTCA who cannot tolerate aspirin, pretreatment with clopidogrel (300 mg given orally as a loading dose, followed by 75 mg daily) is recommended,[55] even though evidence to support the use of a loading dose is lacking. Alternatively, ticlopidine can be useful, but it has a less favorable side effect profile than does clopidogrel. For those patients who are tolerant of aspirin, however, the combination of aspirin and clopidogrel is recommended and may be preferable to the combination of aspirin and ticlopidine because of clopidogrel's more favorable side effect profile.

Unfractionated Heparin

Unfractionated Heparin in Combination with Fibrinolytic Therapy. Despite a paucity of data to support its use,[34] unfractionated heparin has long been considered routine adjunct therapy to fibrinolysis. The primary justification for the use of unfractionated heparin together with fibrinolysis is the prevention of recurrent coronary thrombosis.[72] The consequence of early re-infarction, which occurs in 4% to 6% of patients with ST-segment elevation MI who initially have successful reperfusion, is a twofold increase in the likelihood of death.[73] However, there are few data to demonstrate that unfractionated heparin effectively reduces the incidence of re-infarction in these patients. Even so, unfractionated heparin continues to be used with fibrinolytic therapy, although other antithrombotic agents (e.g., low molecular weight heparin) are currently being evaluated as an alternative.

The intravenous administration of unfractionated heparin as adjunct therapy to the use of tPA, rPA, or tenecteplase may be initiated either as a standard-dose (5,000-U bolus followed by 1,000 U/h) or as a weight-based dose (60 U/kg, 4,000 U maximum, followed by 12 U/kg/h) at the time fibrinolytic therapy is initiated.[38,71] In patients who receive streptokinase or APSAC and who are not at high risk for thromboembolism (see below), the subcutaneous administration of unfractionated heparin can be helpful (12,500 U every 12 hours).[38,71] Unfractionated heparin should not be given if it has been less than 4 hours since the administration of either streptokinase or APSAC and if the aPTT is more than 70 seconds. Unfractionated heparin therapy in all patients who receive fibrinolytic therapy should not be continued for more than 48 hours unless the clinical course is complicated by refractory or recurrent chest pain.

Despite these recommendations, optimal unfractionated heparin dosing should reflect institution-specific determinations of the therapeutic unfractionated heparin concentration and aPTT range.[74] These criteria should also serve as the basis for unfractionated heparin infusion titrations. The aPTT is the coagulation test most commonly used to assess the level of unfractionated heparin anticoagulation. So-called "therapeutic" aPTTs vary substantially between institutions because of the number and variety of aPTT reagents and instruments available. Practitioners should contact the clinical laboratory to determine the aPTT range that corresponds to therapeutic heparin levels (0.2–0.4 U/mL by protamine neutralization or 0.35–0.7 U/mL by anti-Xa activity).[74] On average, the aPTT range is 60 to 80 seconds, but it can be as low as 50 seconds to as high as 110 seconds. In the absence of local laboratory information, the current recommendation is an aPTT range of 50 to 70 seconds.[38,71] The aPTT should be measured 6 hours after the initiation of an unfractionated heparin infusion or a change in its rate and, because of the delayed distribution of unfractionated heparin (full dose) administered subcutaneously, 12 hours after a subcutaneous dose. Once an appropriate infusion rate is established, the aPTT should be checked once a day. In addition to the aPTT, patients receiving unfractionated heparin should have routine assessment of their CBC and platelet count, particularly if the unfractionated heparin infusion is to be continued beyond 48 hours.

During continuous IV or full-dose subcutaneous unfractionated heparin therapy, each patient should be monitored closely for signs and symptoms of bleeding, recurrent ischemia, and thromboembolism. Recurrent MI can occur even in a patient receiving adequate anticoagulation.

Unfractionated Heparin for Prevention of Thromboembolism. Patients who do not receive either IV unfractionated heparin or full-dose subcutaneous unfractionated heparin therapy, should receive unfractionated heparin subcutaneously (at least 7,500 U twice daily) within 4 hours of the onset of chest pain to prevent thromboembolic complications of MI. This regimen should be continued until the patient is ambulatory; follow-up therapy with warfarin is not necessary in these patients.[32] Although there is no need to monitor the aPTT, patients receiving low-dose subcutaneous unfractionated heparin still require monitoring for signs and symptoms of bleeding. In addition, the potential for heparin-induced thrombocytopenia remains despite the use of a lower heparin dosage.

Patients who are at high risk for thromboembolism (e.g., those who have anterior wall MI, severe left ventricular dysfunction, a history of systemic or pulmonary embolism or documented left ventricular thrombus) and who do not receive fibrinolysis should receive unfractionated heparin given IV (approximately 75 U/kg then 1,000–2,000 U/h) followed by warfarin (target INR 2.5, range 2.5 to 3.5) for up to 3 months.[71] Furthermore, patients at high risk of thromboembolism who receive either streptokinase or APSAC should also receive unfractionated heparin (60 U/kg then 12 U/kg/h) given IV provided that at least 4 hours have passed since the administration of fibrinolytic therapy and the aPTT is less than 70 seconds.[38,71]

Low Molecular Weight Heparins

In 1993, low molecular weight heparins were introduced into clinical practice, and in 1995, clinical data became available for their use in unstable angina and non–ST-segment elevation MI. Data from the Efficacy and Safety of Subcutaneous Enoxaparin in Non-Q wave Coronary Events (ESSENCE) and the TIMI 11B study showed that the use of enoxaparin (1 mg/kg administered subcutaneously every 12 hours) was superior to the use of unfractionated heparin (administered IV and titrated to an aPTT of 55 to 85 seconds) in reducing the incidence of the composite end point of death, MI, or recurrent angina at 14 days.[75–77] Importantly, the magnitude of the benefit derived from enoxaparin was proportional to the number of risk factors present (e.g., age $\geq$ 65 years, ST-segment deviation on the ECG, elevated serum cardiac markers).[78] Data on the other low molecular weight heparins are not as compelling.

Enoxaparin, dalteparin, and nadroparin have also been evaluated in ST-segment elevation MI for use in combination with fibrinolysis or PCI. Administration of dalteparin (vs. placebo) in combination with streptokinase resulted in improved patency of the infarct-related artery at 24 hours (as assessed by myoglobin levels) and less recurrent ischemia. Dalteparin (100 IU/kg administered subcutaneously) was given just prior to streptokinase administration and a second injection (120 IU/kg administered subcutaneously) was given 12 hours later.[79] Nadroparin combined with tPA in an open-labeled feasibility study resulted in 80% patency rates at 3 to 5 days with no major bleeding complications.[80] A comparison of enoxaparin with unfractionated heparin in combination with tPA for the purpose of assessing the stability of their anticoagulant effects showed that enoxaparin produced stable therapeutic anti-Xa levels while unfractionated heparin produced wide swings in the aPTT.[81] Also, the recent data from the National Investigators Collaborating on Enoxaparin-3 (NICE 3) study suggest that enoxaparin can be given safely with the glycoprotein IIb/IIIa inhibitor, tirofiban.[82] This study also demonstrated that it is feasible and safe to transition patients to the cardiac catheterization laboratory on the combination. Recently the ASSENT-3 study showed that the addition of enoxaparin to tenecteplase resulted in fewer cardiovascular end points (e.g., refractory ischemia) compared with the combination of unfractionated heparin and tenecteplase.[51b] Although bleeding rates were higher in enoxaparin treated patients, the difference was not statistically significant.

Although data are still emerging it is anticipated that low molecular weight heparins will replace unfractionated heparin as the anticoagulant of choice in MI. Data presently support their use, particularly that of enoxaparin, in high-risk patients with non–ST-segment elevation MI.[78] For this indication, enoxaparin should be administered subcutaneously, 1 mg/kg every 12 hours. Therapy should be continued through hospitalization as the patient's clinical course warrants or until the patient has undergone PCI or a coronary artery bypass graft (CABG). As with unfractionated heparin, patients should still be monitored for signs and symptoms of bleeding, including the routine CBC and platelet count, and for recurrent ischemia. Monitoring of the aPTT is not needed, however, and routine monitoring of anti-Xa levels is currently not recommended. Anti-Xa levels may be useful in special populations (e.g., those who are obese, those who have renal dysfunction) where dosage adjustments may be necessary. Use of a low molecular weight heparin can also be considered as an alternative to the subcutaneous administration of unfractionated heparin for prophylaxis of thromboembolism.[71]

Platelet Glycoprotein IIb/IIIa Inhibitors

Like the role of the low molecular weight heparins, the role of platelet glycoprotein IIb/IIIa inhibitors is rapidly evolving. They have been extensively evaluated in patients undergoing PCI and those with unstable angina or non–ST-segment elevation MI. More recent studies have evaluated them in combination with fibrinolytic therapy for the treatment of ST-segment elevation MI.[51a,51b]

The platelet glycoprotein IIb/IIIa receptor antagonists represent the newest and most potent antiplatelet agents available.[83,84] Presently, three agents, abciximab [Reopro], tirofiban [Aggrastat], and eptifibatide [Integrilin]), are approved for IV use. In combination with heparin and aspirin, eptifibatide and abciximab reduce the incidence of the combined end point of death, MI, and recurrent ischemia in patients with either unstable angina or non–ST-segment elevation MI who undergo PCI.[84] For abciximab, this is also true if the patient has ST-segment elevation MI. Tirofiban and eptifibatide also reduce the incidence of this combined end point in patients with unstable angina or non–ST-segment elevation MI who do not undergo intervention. The greatest benefit of these agents, however, is for those patients who are at high risk and those who undergo PCI.[17] Risk stratification of patients with unstable angina and non–ST-segment elevation MI is important for determining who should receive a glycoprotein IIb/IIIa inhibitor as part of their medical management. Indicators of high risk for early death in patients with unstable angina or non–ST-segment elevation MI include a markedly elevated level of troponin (>0.1 ng/mL), prolonged (>20 minutes) ongoing rest pain, age more than 75 years, or angina at rest with ST-segment changes of more than 0.05 mV.[17]

The role of glycoprotein IIb/IIIa inhibitors in patients with ST-segment elevation MI who do not undergo PCI is still evolving. The quest for the reperfusion strategy that results in more complete and expedient infarct-related artery patency with less risk of reocclusion or re-infarction has perpetuated the evaluation of the efficacy and safety of glycoprotein IIb/IIIa inhibitors in ST-segment elevation MI.[34,85] Trials to date evaluating glycoprotein IIb/IIIa inhibitors as adjunct therapy to full-dose fibrinolysis have collectively shown that this combination results in more rapid and complete reperfusion of the infarct-related artery.[34] A higher rate of bleeding complications accompanies this benefit, however. Therefore, more recent studies have evaluated the combination of reduced-dose fibrinolytic therapy with glycoprotein IIb/IIIa inhibition.[51a,51b] Data from these trials, however, suggest some improvement in efficacy but at the expense of more bleeding events. (Additional information regarding the use of glycoprotein IIb/IIIa inhibitors appears in Reperfusion Therapy.)

OTHER DRUGS

Angiotensin-Converting Enzyme Inhibitors (ACEI)

Over 120,000 ST segment elevation MI patients have been studied in clinical trials of ACEIs.[22] Collectively, these studies have shown that administration of an ACEI is associated with a number of favorable outcomes.[19] Notably, two of these were large trials of patients who received a fibrinolytic agent as part of their routine care for ST-segment elevation MI and, as a consequence, observations from these trials are directly applicable to the current care of patients with ST-segment elevation MI.

In the first of these clinical trials, 19,394 patients with acute ST-segment elevation MI received, in addition to standard care, either placebo or lisinopril, 5–10 mg daily, begun within 24 hours of admission.[61] After 42 days of therapy, a 12% reduction in mortality rate was observed in patients receiving lisinopril as compared with those receiving placebo ($P = .03$). In the second study, patients ($n = 58,050$) with acute MI, also within 24 hours of onset of symptoms, were randomly assigned to receive either placebo or captopril, 6.25–50 mg twice daily.[62] All patients received standard care as well and were followed for 35 days. Use of captopril in this study was associated with a modest, but significant 7% reduction in mortality compared with placebo ($P = .02$).

Experience from these trials also suggests that therapy should be initiated within 24 hours of onset of symptoms of MI, preferably after completion of fibrinolytic therapy and subsequent stabilization of blood pressure. Subsequent studies involving other ACEIs have confirmed these results and have illustrated the importance of blood pressure stabilization before the initiation of therapy.[16,19–22,32]

The use of angiotensin II (AT II) receptor inhibitors, either alone or in combination with an ACEI, may also benefit patients with ST-segment elevation MI, although data from large clinical trials are not yet available.[86]

Current recommendations call for the use of an ACEI within the first 24 hours of a suspected anterior wall MI or ST-segment elevation MI associated with clinical heart failure in patients when there are no contraindications to ACEI therapy.[16,32] The use of an ACEI is also recommended for patients with ST-segment elevation MI and asymptomatic heart failure (left ventricular ejection fraction <40%), as well as for those without evidence of left ventricular dysfunction, provided that there are no contraindications to ACEI and hypotension is not a problem.

To achieve maximal benefit and minimize adverse effects, dosing strategies and dosages of individual agents should be restricted to those used in the clinical trials described earlier. Specifically, ACEI therapy should be withheld until fibrinolytic therapy has been completed and the patient's blood pressure has stabilized, preferably with a systolic blood pressure higher than 100 mm Hg. Additionally, initial doses of lisinopril, captopril, or trandolapril should not exceed 5 mg, 6.25 mg, and 1.0 mg, respectively. The goal of therapy should be to provide the maximum dosage used in these trials, that is, 10 mg daily, 50 mg two or three times daily, and 4 mg once daily, respectively. Notably, although an appreciable number of patients will not be able to tolerate these maximal dosages, therapy with the chosen ACEI should continue at the maximally tolerated dosage.

When ACEI therapy is initiated, blood pressure should be monitored closely. Usually, if a hypotensive response to an ACEI is going to occur, it will do so following the initial dose. Patients who are hyponatremic and/or hypertensive tend to be at greater risk for a hypotensive response to ACEI. Blood pressure should be monitored regularly on an outpatient basis throughout therapy. Other monitoring parameters for ACEI therapy include signs and symptoms of worsening heart failure, renal function, and serum potassium level, particularly if the patient is concomitantly taking a diuretic and potassium supplementation. Common side effects of ACEIs that practitioners should question patients about are altered taste, dizziness, cough, and diarrhea.

Calcium Channel Antagonists

Verapamil or diltiazem should be considered for use only in patients who have either ST-segment elevation MI or non–ST-segment elevation MI and have continuing or frequently recurring ischemia when β-blockers are contraindicated or when β-blockers and nitrates are at fully tolerated doses.[16,17,32] Neither verapamil nor diltiazem should be used for MI in the presence of severe left ventricular dysfunction or other contraindications (e.g., atrioventricular block, bradycardia).[17]

Lidocaine

Ventricular fibrillation accounts for the majority of early deaths during acute ST-segment elevation MI. The incidence of ventricular fibrillation is highest (3% to 5%) during the first 4 hours after MI and then declines sharply thereafter.[87] The incidence of ventricular tachycardia follows a similar time course. Because the incidence of ventricular fibrillation is approximately 5% with a mortality rate of nearly 50%, it would seem reasonable to administer prophylactic lidocaine to these patients. Although such use of lidocaine is associated with a 33% reduction in the frequency of ventricular fibrillation, the benefit is offset by a corresponding increase in all-cause mortality.[87] Consequently, the prophylactic use of lidocaine in the early management of ST-segment elevation MI is not recommended.[17,32] Lidocaine should be reserved for patients who experience ventricular fibrillation and/or hemodynamically compromising ventricular tachycardia.[87] (In light of the recently published revised advanced cardiovascular life support [ACLS] guidelines, the reader is referred to Chapter 16 for details regarding the management of ventricular rhythm disturbances.)

Amiodarone

Patients who continue to manifest frequent premature ventricular contractions (PVCs) and/or ventricular arrhythmias following MI represent a subgroup of patients at high risk for sudden cardiac death.[16,23,32] Amiodarone, a Class III antiarrhythmic drug, possesses unique characteristics, such as mild calcium channel–blocking and β-blocking properties, that may make it useful in post-MI patients at high risk for sudden cardiac death. Results of clinical trials have confirmed some of these assumptions. The Canadian Amiodarone Myocardial Infarction Arrhythmia Trial (CAMIAT) and the European Myocardial Infarction Amiodarone Trial (EMIAT) both showed that the use of amiodarone was associated with a significant reduction in risk of ventricular fibrillation and arrhythmic death, but no reduction in the overall mortality rate. Importantly, neither of these trials had sufficient numbers of patients to detect less than a 33% reduction in total mortality.[88,89] However, a recently completed study that evaluated the effect of amiodarone on morbidity and mortality when it was administered first by the IV route and then orally to patients with ST-segment elevation MI and symptoms of heart failure showed that amiodarone, even in low doses, should be reserved for MI patients who manifest life-threatening ventricular arrhythmias.[90] Thus, the use of amiodarone should not preclude the use of a β-blocker. Data from both the CAMIAT and EMIAT databases now show that the adjunct of amiodarone to β-blockers is not hazardous, and β-blocker therapy should be continued if possible in patients for whom amiodarone is indicated.[91]

Magnesium

Although magnesium was used as an antiarrhythmic in the management of MI in the 1960s, only small studies were conducted. With the attention of most clinical trials focused on fibrinolytic and antithrombotic therapy, the potential role of magnesium was not aggressively pursued until recently.

The Fourth International Study of Infarct Survival (ISIS-4) is the largest trial to date evaluating the usefulness of magnesium in the management of MI.[62] In this study of 58,050 patients with suspected MI, 29,011 received an IV dose of magnesium, and 29,039 made up a control group. The mortality rate of patients who received magnesium did not differ significantly from that observed in patients who did not receive magnesium (7.28% vs. 6.92%, respectively; P = NS). So, despite a large difference in mortality in early studies, the results of ISIS-4 do not support the routine use of magnesium in patients with MI. However, there are sources of heterogeneity between ISIS-4 and previous trials that may explain the lack of benefit observed in association with magnesium in ISIS-4. First, magnesium was administered late in the ISIS-4 trial relative to the administration of fibrinolytic therapy. This delay is relevant because one of the presumed benefits of magnesium is a reduction in myocardial reperfusion injury following fibrinolysis. Second, the mortality rate in the control group was lower than anticipated; a slightly higher mortality rate in the control group would have produced a significant benefit of magnesium.

Recent data from a small study (n = 150) of ST-segment elevation MI patients evaluating the ability of magnesium to preserve left ventricular function in conjunction with PTCA showed that whether given before, during, or after reperfusion, magnesium did not decrease myocardial damage (as determined by peak CK level and the incidence of ventricular tachycardia/ventricular fibrillation).[92] In support of these results, recent NRMI-2 data show that although magnesium is used infrequently, its use is associated with worse outcomes.[93] The ongoing Magnesium in Coronary Disease (MAGIC) study is designed to further evaluate the role of magnesium in high-risk ST-segment elevation MI patients, specifically the effect of its early administration prior to fibrinolytic therapy.[94] Until the results of this trial are known, the routine use of magnesium is not recommended. Its use should be reserved for those patients who have documented hypomagnesemia.

Glucose-Insulin-Potassium Infusions

The rationale for the administration of glucose-insulin-potassium infusions is based on observational data suggesting that hypokalemia occurs in 9% to 25% of patients with ST-segment elevation MI and that there is an association between hypokalemia and poor outcome.[95] Furthermore, there is some evidence that glucose-insulin-potassium infusion may improve regional myocardial perfusion and function.[96] Presently, insufficient evidence exists to recommend the routine use of glucose-insulin-potassium infusion. Clinical trials are ongoing to evaluate its clinical utility, however.

SECONDARY PREVENTION

Aspirin

Results of numerous studies have revealed that aspirin is useful for prevention of recurrent cardiovascular events following acute MI. Aspirin, when started within 7 days to 7 years of MI, significantly reduces the frequency of recurrent events. The Antiplatelet Trialists' Collaboration has shown that the use of aspirin following MI reduces the risk of death from cardiovascular causes (including MI and stroke) by one-sixth, while it reduces the risk of a second nonfatal MI by one-third.[97]

Collectively, studies involving more than 16,000 MI patients have demonstrated that aspirin (75–1,500 mg/day) decreases the risk of recurrent MI by 30% to 49%.[71] These observations also suggest that a low dose of aspirin may be effective, which would diminish the likelihood of aspirin-related adverse effects as well. Despite the introduction of new, novel antiplatelet agents, the clinical evidence still supports the use of aspirin for secondary prevention.[71]

It is recommended that aspirin, originally given for the management of the acute phase of MI, be continued indefinitely in patients following either ST-segment elevation MI or non–ST- segment elevation MI.[35] Aspirin dosage for such long-term therapy may be as low as 75 mg (75–325 mg) daily. In patients with true aspirin sensitivity, clopidogrel (75 mg/day) or warfarin (INR 2.0–3.0) may be used as an alternative.[16,35,71] Patients should be followed on a regular basis and examined for signs and symptoms of recurrent ischemia. Though aspirin is very effective in preventing recurrent ischemia, as many as 30% to 40% of patients will experience recurrent ischemia or reinfarction despite aspirin therapy.

Bleeding and gastrointestinal side effects of aspirin are the most common adverse events, although the risk of these events is dose-dependent. The incidence of such events associated with a daily dose of aspirin that is less than 325 mg is indistinguishable from that associated with placebo. The incidence of gastrointestinal complications such as stomach pain, heartburn, and nausea is as high as 40% to 60% in patients receiving 900 to 1,300 mg/day of aspirin, while the incidence of these side effects is 4% to 13% in patients receiving 75 mg/day. The use of enteric-coated aspirin also reduces the incidence of gastrointestinal side effects. The overall incidence of intracranial hemorrhage with low-dose aspirin is 0.3%, which increases as the dose of aspirin increases.

Warfarin

Whether or not anticoagulant therapy with warfarin should be continued following either non–ST-segment elevation MI or ST-segment elevation MI to prevent recurrent ischemia or re-infarction remains controversial. Although more data are available, including results from two recently completed clinical trials, the role of warfarin in secondary prevention remains unclear.

In the Anticoagulants in the Secondary Prevention of Events in Coronary Thrombosis-2 (ASPECT-2) study, 993 patients were randomized to either aspirin alone (80 mg), aspirin (80 mg) in combination with warfarin (dosed to an INR of 2 to 2.5), or warfarin alone (dosed to an INR of 3 to 4).[98] The composite end point of death, MI, and stroke occurred in 9.2% of patients on aspirin, 5.1% of patients on combination therapy, and 5.2% of patients on warfarin. The mortality rates were 4.5% for aspirin, 2.7% for combination therapy, and 1.2% for warfarin. Major bleeding events occurred more frequently in patients on combination therapy (0.9% for aspirin vs. 2.1% for combination therapy vs. 0.9% for warfarin alone), but the differences were not statistically significant. Importantly, this study was halted prematurely because of slow enrollment. Therefore, the reliability of the study's assessment of the effect of warfarin on mortality should be questioned.

Results of the Antithrombotics in Prevention of Reocclusion in Coronary Thrombolysis-2 (APRICOT-2) study were similar.[99] This trial assessed the 3-month angiographic rate of reocclusion in ST-segment elevation MI patients ($n = 308$) treated with fibrinolysis and then randomized to either aspirin alone (80 mg) or the combination of aspirin (80 mg) plus warfarin (dosed to an INR of 2 to 3). Reocclusion occurred in 30% of patients treated with aspirin compared with 18% of patients receiving combination therapy ($P < .05$). There was no significant difference in the incidence of major bleeding events, although the incidence of minor bleeding was higher (3% vs. 6%) in the combination-treated patients. This study was too small to make conclusions regarding mortality.

Observations from an earlier, larger clinical trial of combination therapy (aspirin, 80 mg, plus 1 or 3 mg of warfarin) did not show a reduction in subsequent events following MI compared with aspirin alone (160 mg).[100] Furthermore, the likelihood of spontaneous major hemorrhage was nearly twofold higher in patients receiving aspirin and warfarin as compared with those receiving aspirin alone (1.4% vs. 0.74%, respectively; $P < .014$).

As a consequence of these observations, warfarin alone is currently recommended as an alternative to clopidogrel for secondary prevention of recurrent ischemia and re-infarction in MI patients who are intolerant or allergic to aspirin.[16,71] The routine use of the combination of aspirin and warfarin is presently not recommended, although it may be useful in patients with recurrent ischemic episodes following MI.[71] Warfarin therapy should be used, however, in patients with persistent or paroxysmal atrial fibrillation, extensive left ventricular wall motion abnormalities, severe left ventricular dysfunction (left ventricular ejection fraction <35%), or a documented left ventricular thrombus for prevention of thromboembolism.[71,101] Patients should be monitored closely for signs and symptoms of bleeding, as well as for recurrent ischemia. (The reader is referred to Chapter 19 for detailed guidelines for appropriate follow-up of these patients.)

Angiotensin Converting Enzyme Inhibitors

Results of a number of studies have shown that the long-term use of an ACEI following MI can reduce the incidence of recurrent MI and congestive heart failure.[19] In the Survival and Ventricular Enlargement (SAVE) trial, for example, the use of captopril (6.25 to 50 mg three times daily, initiated 3 to 16 days following MI and continued for 42 months) for patients with a left ventricular ejection fraction of less than 40% was associated with a 25% reduction in risk of recurrent MI compared with placebo ($P = .015$).[102] A 19% reduction in all-cause mortality ($P = .019$) and a 21% reduction in risk of death from cardiovascular causes ($P = .014$) were also observed. A number of other clinical trials using an array of ACEIs have confirmed these observations, collectively showing up to a 30% reduction in cardiovascular mortality.[19] Secondary analyses of some of these results revealed that the benefit of therapy from an ACEI following MI occurs primarily in patients with anterior wall MI or those with an ejection fraction equal to or less than 40%.[19,22] Recent evidence, however, from a study evaluating the efficacy of an ACEI in high-risk patients, only half of whom had had an MI, supports the use of an ACEI in all MI patients and high-risk patients with cardiovascular disease.[20,35] Post-MI patients should be treated indefinately.[16,32] (For a more detailed discussion of use of ACEIs in heart failure, the reader is referred to Chapter 13.)

Antihyperlipidemic Drugs

A history of CAD that includes previous MI is a major risk factor for recurrent MI. Further, recurrent MI is four to seven times more likely to occur in a patient with clinically apparent CAD than in an individual without such evidence. Given the intimate association between elevated concentrations of lipids and CAD, it would seem logical to assume that aggressive management of hyperlipidemia would benefit patients who have experienced MI. A summary of secondary prevention trials provided by the last report of the National Cholesterol Education Program (NCEP) revealed that management of cholesterol through both drugs and diet was associated with an overall 25% reduction in recurrent nonfatal MI and a 14% reduction in fatal MI.[103] Notably, none of the studies included in this overview evaluated the effects of an HMG-CoA reductase inhibitor on recurrent MI.

Since publication of that report, several studies on the role of cholesterol in recurrent MI have been completed. For example, the Cholesterol and Recurrent Events (CARE) trial included patients ($n = 4{,}159$) who adhered to a step I/II diet and took either placebo or pravastatin, 40 mg, every evening beginning 3 to 20 months after MI.[104] After 5 years of therapy, those taking pravastatin had a 24% reduction in the primary end point of fatal CAD and nonfatal MI compared with those taking placebo. Notably, the beneficial effects of cholesterol reduction observed were in patients with only mild to moderate elevations in serum cholesterol level. Average baseline total and low-density lipoprotein (LDL)-cholesterol values were 209 mg/ dL and 139 mg/dL, respectively. Similar studies that used simvastatin, lovastatin, or fluvastatin have supported these observations.

Furthermore, results from the recent Reduction of Cholesterol in Ischemia and Function of the Endothelium (RECIFE) trial showed that pravastatin (40 mg) initiated at the time of hospital discharge in ST-segment elevation MI patients and continued for 6 weeks reduced total and LDL-cholesterol by 23% and 33%, respectively, compared with placebo ($P < .05$ and $P < .01$, respectively).[105] In addition, the effects of pravastatin on endothelial function were examined by using brachial ultrasound to measure endothelial-dependent flow-mediated dilatation. Compared with placebo, pravastatin increased flow-mediated dilatation by 42% ($P = .02$). These data, as well as other long-term (1 year) data, suggest that early statin treatment in patients with MI results in a significant lowering of LDL-cholesterol levels, a possible benefit on endothelial function, and a reduction in mortality.[106] Unfortunately, despite this convincing evidence, lipid-lowering medications are underutilized in patients following MI, particularly those at high risk.[107] These trials establish the benefit of such therapy following MI—even in patients without profound elevations in total and LDL-cholesterol concentrations.

An assessment of the patient's LDL-cholesterol level should be made within the first 24 hours of acute MI.[35] All patients whose LDL-cholesterol level is equal to or greater than 100 mg/dL should be started on a statin as soon as possible, but no later than at hospital discharge. Total and LDL-cholesterol levels should be re-assessed at 3 months and every 6 months thereafter. The use of either niacin or gemfibrozil is currently recommended in patients whose triglyceride concentrations exceed 200 mg/dL.[32] (The reader is referred to Chapter 21 for details regarding dosing guidelines and evaluation of therapeutic outcomes for these agents.) The AHA step II diet and lipid-lowering drug therapy are integral components of treatment designed to prevent the recurrence of MI in patients with an LDL-cholesterol level higher than 100 mg/dL. In patients with normal cholesterol levels, but with high-density lipoprotein (HDL)-cholesterol levels less than 35 mg/dL, the combined use of nonpharmacologic approaches (e.g., smoking cessation, exercise) and pharmacologic therapies (e.g., gemfibrozil) to raise the HDL level is recommended.[108] In addition to the aforementioned therapies, post-MI patients should receive a β-blocker indefinitely and smoking cessation, blood pressure control, and an exercise/weight control program should be part of secondary prevention.[35] In diabetic patients, maintaining a hemoglobin AI_c (H_bAI_c) <7% is also part of secondary prevention.[35]

RISK STRATIFICATION FOLLOWING MI

Patients with uncomplicated MI should be discharged from the hospital within 1 week. Notably, recent cost effectiveness data suggest that it is economically unattractive to hospitalize uncomplicated MI patients beyond 3 days.[109] As a consequence, patients are sometimes discharged after an uncomplicated MI within 3 to 4 days.

In-hospital management plays a critical role in the outcome for MI patients, as approximately 25% of deaths during the first year post-MI occur within the first 48 hours of hospitalization.[23] What happens after hospital discharge is also important, however. Risk stratification of MI patients should begin at the time of admission and continue through hospital discharge.[23,24] Because patients after their first MI have a very good prognosis, it is essential to ensure that they understand all aspects of their post-MI care. Prior to discharge, there should be a frank and open discussion among clinicians, the patient, and the patient's family regarding strategies for prevention of recurrent MI. Topics covered should include risk factor modification such as tobacco use, hyperlipidemia, and hypertension. Other important topics are the rationale and appropriate use of medications, as well as the role of diet and exercise. Guidelines for safe resumption of customary activities, such as returning to work or recreational activities, should also be discussed in detail. All questions should be answered to the patient's satisfaction.

In addition to counseling following MI, clinicians should make an objective assessment of a patient's prognosis and stratification for risk of recurrent cardiovascular events. This assessment should include a determination of left ventricular function and the presence or absence of other risk factors that have been shown to be predictive of outcome, such as diabetes (Fig. 15–6). In addition, it may include an evaluation of the patency of the infarct-related artery (i.e., TIMI grade flow).[24] Assessment of left ventricular function is important, because it is a primary determinant of long-term mortality following MI (Fig. 15–7).[23,24] These parameters will help to guide further evaluation and treatment. A multitude of procedures and tests are available to assist in the stratification of patients after MI. However, many have limited utility and are extremely expensive. It is important to select a procedure/test that is cost-effective and will provide useful and prognostic information about the patient.

Probably the most common noninvasive test that is performed after MI is the exercise tolerance test.[23] This test is typically performed using a treadmill or bicycle and continuous ECG and blood pressure monitoring. This procedure determines what the patient's overall exercise capacity is; how the patient's blood pressure responds to exercise; if ischemia develops, at what point during exercise it occurs; and whether activity precipitates arrhythmias. Exercise testing can be safely performed as early as 3 days post-MI in low-risk patients.[110]

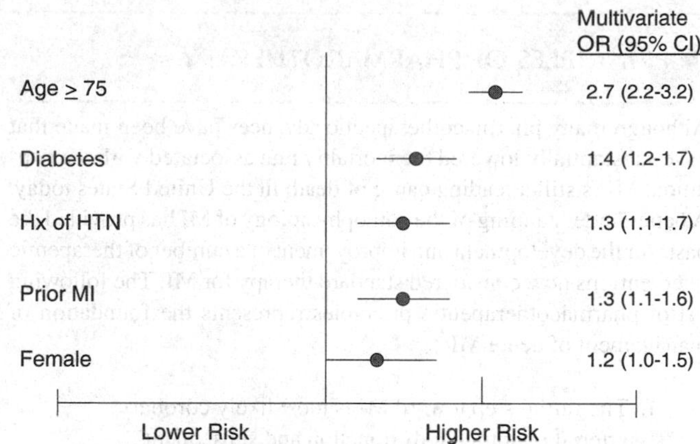

FIGURE 15–6. Odds of death by 30 days following myocardial infarction (MI): examples of independent predictors of 30-day mortality. OR = odds ratio; CI = confidence interval; HX = history; HTN = hypertension. (*Adapted from Circulation 2000;102:2031–2037.*)

Patients with a high risk of recurrent MI are easily identified by their low exercise capability, failure of the systolic blood pressure to rise above the resting value during exercise (frequently referred to as an inadequate blood pressure response to exercise), and chest pain associated with ischemic changes on the ECG.[24,110] In some cases, patients may experience ventricular ectopy during or shortly after exercise. These patients require further evaluation by invasive means (i.e., coronary angiography) to assess coronary anatomy. In patients without these findings, no further diagnostic evaluation is necessary, and the risk of a subsequent cardiac event is very low.

Many procedures exist to evaluate left ventricular function. No one test is considered the "gold standard;" the type of test used depends on the expertise that exists at the given institution. Echocardiography, coronary angiography, and radionuclear ventriculograms are a few examples of methods that may be available to assess left ventricular function.

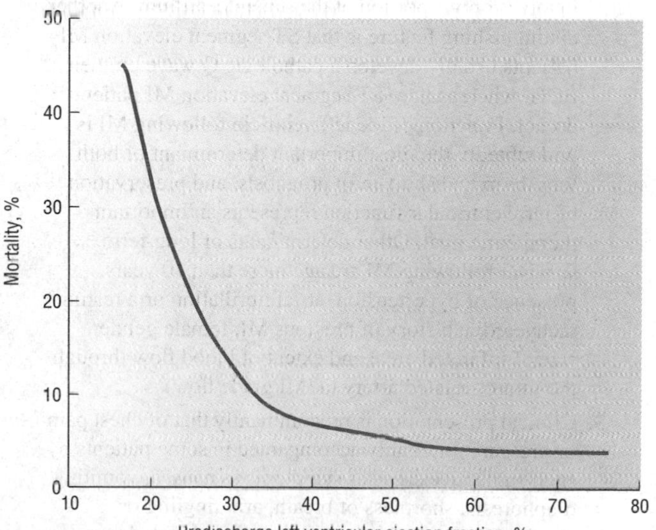

FIGURE 15–7. Relationship between left ventricular ejection fraction (%) at hospital discharge and mortality in patients following an acute myocardial infarction. (*Adapted from Ref. 23.*)

▶ PRINCIPLES OF PHARMACOTHERAPY

Although many pharmacotherapeutic advances have been made that have substantially lowered the mortality rate associated with the condition, MI is still a leading cause of death in the United States today. A better understanding of the pathophysiology of MI has provided the basis for the development and improvement of a number of therapeutic interventions now considered standard therapy for MI. The following list of pharmacotherapeutic principles represents the foundation of management of acute MI:

1. The initial step toward MI is most likely coronary arterial endothelial dysfunction and subsequent development of atherosclerosis and clinically evident CAD in association with one or more risk factors. Myocardial infarction occurs when an unstable atherosclerotic lesion in a coronary artery either fissures or ruptures, releasing its highly thrombogenic core of contents into the coronary circulation and subsequently causing the formation of a thrombus that completely occludes blood flow and leads to myocardial cell death.
2. The most important determinants of prognosis following MI include type and location of MI, and resulting left ventricular function. An anterior wall MI usually involves a larger area of myocardium than does an inferior wall MI; as a consequence, the risk of complications, including mortality, are greater with an anterior wall MI than with an inferior wall MI. A right ventricular MI occurs less frequently, but may also involve the inferior wall. Although the management of right ventricular MI is similar to that of either an anterior wall MI or an inferior wall MI, the IV administration of fluids and stabilization of blood pressure usually precedes other interventions. An ST-segment elevation MI results in an injury that transects the entire thickness of the myocardial wall, whereas a non–ST-segment elevation MI usually involves only a portion of the subendocardium. Another distinguishing feature is that ST-segment elevation MI patients usually develop a pathologic Q wave on their ECG, whereas non–ST-segment elevation MI patients do not. Function of the left ventricle following MI is undoubtedly the most important determinant of both long-term and short-term prognosis, and preservation of left ventricular function represents an important therapeutic goal. Other determinants of long-term survival following MI are age more than 70 years, presence of hypertension, atrial fibrillation or a resting tachycardia, history of previous MI, female gender, size of infarcted area, and extent of blood flow through the infarct-related artery (TIMI grade flow).
3. Clinical presentation is predominantly that of chest pain or pressure unreliably accompanied in some patients by such subjective signs or symptoms as nausea, vomiting, diaphoresis, shortness of breath, arm tingling or numbness, generalized weakness, light-headedness, or syncope. Objective signs include characteristic ECG changes such as T-wave abnormalities, ST-segment changes, formation of a pathologic Q wave, and/or new left bundle branch block. Other objective signs include an increase and subsequent fall in the concentrations of troponin I or T and/or CK-MB.
4. Goals of therapy include immediate relief of presenting symptoms, preservation or salvage of ischemic myocardium, prevention or minimization of both short-term and long-term complications, and prevention of mortality. A patient with an MI is managed initially in an emergency department and is subsequently admitted to a coronary care unit or an intensive care unit. Management frequently involves aggressive and sometimes simultaneous administration of a number of different therapeutic agents.
5. The cornerstone of therapy for MI is reperfusion, either mechanically or pharmacologically. Following diagnosis, a fibrinolytic agent should be administered as soon as possible (within 30 minutes of arrival in the emergency department) to patients who have no contraindications and who have arrived within 12 hours of the onset of symptoms. Patients receiving a fibrinolytic agent should be monitored for signs and/or symptoms of hemorrhage (especially intracranial hemorrhage), hypotension, and severe allergic reactions. Signs of successful reperfusion include normalization of the ECG (except for the Q wave), relief of chest discomfort (possibly preceded by an increase), and abrupt onset of ventricular arrhythmias. If it can be accomplished within 90 minutes of admission, emergent PTCA should be offered as an alternative to patients for whom a fibrinolytic agent is contraindicated.
6. Other important pharmacotherapeutic agents include the following:

   Morphine sulfate for relief of pain.
   Nitroglycerin given IV for relief of ischemia and preservation of ischemic myocardium.
   β-blocker given IV for prevention of ventricular arrhythmias and for the same reasons as nitroglycerin given IV.
   Aspirin for synergy with the fibrinolytic agent (although it should also be used in patients who do not receive a fibrinolytic agent).
   Unfractionated heparin (full dose given IV) for prevention of re-occlusion simultaneously with tPA, rPA, or tenecteplase. Following the administration of streptokinase or APSAC, it should be held until 4 hours after the administration of the fibrinolytic agent and then used subcutaneously in patients at low risk for a thromboembolic event. For prevention of thromboembolism, unfractionated heparin should be given subcutaneously until the patient is fully ambulatory. The role of the low molecular weight heparins is still evolving for patients with ST-segment elevation MI, but it should be used in patients with non–ST-segment elevation MI.
   ACEIs in the first 24 hours after admission in patients whose blood pressure has been stabilized and preferably after administration of the fibrinolytic agent.

7. Secondary prevention of MI should include all of the following:

Aspirin indefinitely unless contraindicated; alternatively, clopidogrel.

Warfarin in patients otherwise intolerant of aspirin or clopidogrel and those with other risk factors for thromboembolism, such as atrial fibrillation, severe left ventricular dysfunction, or documented left ventricular thrombus.

β-blocker even if the patient was considered ineligible for use during the acute period. Use of a β-blocker for secondary prevention of MI is *not* contraindicated in patients with asthma, insulin-dependent diabetes, COPD, severe peripheral vascular disease, first degree atrioventricular block, or moderate left ventricular failure. Use of a β-blocker should continue indefinitely.

Angiotensin-converting enzyme inhibitors should be continued indefinately.

Pravastatin, fluvastatin, simvastatin, or lovastatin started as soon as possible given in a dose designed to achieve an LDL-cholesterol concentration of less than 100 mg/dL.

8. The following agents should be used only in limited clinical circumstances:

Verapamil or diltiazem if a β-blocker is contraindicated or ischemia persists in a patient receiving maximally tolerated doses of β-blocker and nitroglycerin given IV.

Lidocaine for acute management of ventricular arrhythmias. It should not be used prophylactically.

Amiodarone for the long-term management of ventricular arrhythmias.

Magnesium only for management of documented hypomagnesemia.

Glucose-insulin-potassium infusion has no place in the management of MI because of the absence of sufficient documentation of benefits.

REFERENCES

1. Collins R, MacMahon S. Reliable assessment of the effects of treatment on mortality and major morbidity, I: clinical trials. Lancet 2001;357:373–380.
2. DeWood MA, Spores J, Notske R, et al. Prevalence of total coronary occlusion during the early hours of transmural myocardial infarction. N Engl J Med 1980;303:897–902.
3. http://www.americanheart.org (accessed February 8th, 2001).
4. National Heart, Lung and Blood Institute Morbidity and Mortality Chart book, 2000. http://www.nhlbi.gov/resources/docs/oochtbk.pdf (accessed February 8th, 2001).
5. Sloan FA, Rankin PJ, Whellan DJ, Conover CJ. Medicaid, managed care, and the care of patients hospitalized for acute myocardial infarction. Am Heart J 2000;139:567–576.
6. Davies MJ. The pathophysiology of acute coronary syndromes. Heart 2000;83:361–366.
7. Ross R. Atherosclerosis—an inflammatory disease. N Engl J Med 1999;340:115–126.
8. Nygard O, Nordrehaug JE, Refsium H, et al. Plasma homocysteine levels and mortality in patients with coronary artery disease. N Engl J Med 1997;337:230–236.
9. Aronow WS, Ahn C. Increased plasma homocysteine is an independent predictor of new coronary events in older persons. Am J Cardiol 2000;86:346–347.
10. Lagrand WK, Visser CA, Hermens WT, et al. C-reactive protein as a cardiovascular risk factor. More than epiphenomenon? Circulation 1999; 100:96–102.
11. Wald NJ, Law MR, Morris JK, et al. *Chlamydia pneumoniae* infection and mortality from ischaemic heart disease: large prospective study. BMJ 2000;321:204–207.
12. Abrams J. Role of endothelial dysfunction in coronary artery disease. Am J Cardiol 1997;79(12B):2–9.
13. The Joint European Society of Cardiology/American College of Cardiology Committee. Myocardial infarction redefined—a consensus document of the Joint European Society of Cardiology/American College of Cardiology for the redefinition of myocardial infarction. J Am Coll Cardiol 2000;36;959–969.
14. Redwood SR, Ferrari R, Marber MS. Myocardial hibernation and stunning: from physiological principles to clinical practice. Heart 1998;80:218–222.
15. Kinch JW, Ryan TJ. Right ventricular infarction. N Engl J Med 1994; 330:1211–1217.
16. Ryan TJ, Anderson JL, Antman EM, et al. ACC/AHA guidelines for the management of patients with acute myocardial infarction: a report of the American College of Cardiology/American Heart Association Task Force on Practice Guidelines (Committee on Management of Acute Myocardial Infarction). J Am Coll Cardiol 1996;28:1328–1428.
17. Braunwald E, Antman EM, Beasley JW, et al. ACC/AHA guidelines for the management of patients with unstable angina and non–ST-segment elevation myocardial infarction: executive summary and recommendations. Circulation 2000;102:1193–1209.
18. St. John Sutton MG, Sharpe N. Left ventricular remodeling after myocardial infarction: pathophysiology and therapy. Circulation 2000;101: 2981–2988.
19. ACE Inhibitor Myocardial Infarction Collaborative Group. Indications for ACE inhibitors in the early treatment of acute myocardial infarction. Circulation 1998;97:2202–2212.
20. The Heart Outcomes Prevention Evaluation Study Investigators. Effects of an angiotensin-converting enzyme, inhibitor, ramipril, on cardiovascular events in high-risk patients. N Engl J Med 2000;342:145–153.
21. Torp-Pedersen C, Kober L, Trandolapril Cardiac Evaluation (TRACE) Study Group. Effect of ACE inhibitor trandolapril on life expectancy of patients with reduced left-ventricular function after acute myocardial infarction. Lancet 1999;354:9–12.
22. O'Keete JH, Wetzel M, Moe RR, et al. Should an angiotensin-converting enzyme inhibitor be standard therapy for patients with atherosclerotic disease? J Am Coll Cardiol 2001;37:1–8.
23. Peterson ED, Shaw LJ, Califf RM. Risk stratification after myocardial infarction. Ann Intern Med 1997;126:561–582.
24. Michaels AD, Goldschlager N. Risk stratification after acute myocardial infarction in the reperfusion era. Prog Cardiovasc Dis 2000;42:273–309.
25. The GUSTO Angiographic Investigators. The effect of tissue plasminogen activator, streptokinase, or both on coronary-artery patency, ventricular function, and survival after acute myocardial infarction. N Engl J Med 1993;329:1615–1622.
26. Lenderink T, Simoons ML, Van Es G-A, et al. Benefit of fibrinolytic therapy is sustained throughout five years and is related to TIMI perfusion grade 3 but not grade 2 flow at discharge. Circulation 1995;92:1110–1116.
27. Puma JA, Sketch MH, Thompson TD, et al. Support of the open-artery hypothesis in survivors of acute myocardial infarction: analysis of 11,228 patients treated with thrombolytic therapy. Am J Cardiol 1999;83:482-7.
28. Stringer KA. TIMI grade flow, mortality and the GUSTO III trial. Pharmacotherapy 1998;18:699–705.
29. French JK, Hyde TA, Patel H, et al. Survival 12 years after randomization to streptokinase: the influence of thrombolysis in myocardial infarction flow at three to four weeks. J Am Coll Cardiol 1999;34:62–69.
30. Ohman EM, Armstrong PW, White HD. Global Use of Strategies to Open Occluded Coronary Arteries (GUSTO III) Investigators. Risk stratification with a point-of-care cardiac troponin T test in acute myocardial infarction. Am J Cardiol 1999;84:1281–1286.

31. Phibbs B, Marcus F, Marriott HJ, et al. Q-wave versus non-Q wave myocardial infarction: a meaningless distinction. J Am Coll Cardiol 1999;33:576–582.
32. Ryan TJ, Antman EM, Rapaport E, et al. 1999 Update: ACC/AHA guidelines for the management of patients with acute myocardial infarction. A report of the American College of Cardiology/American Heart Association Task Force on Practice Guidelines (Committee on Management of Acute Myocardial Infarction). J Am Coll Cardiol 1999;34:890–911.
33. Hochman JS, Tamis JE, Thompson TD, et al. Sex, clinical presentation, and outcome in patients with acute coronary syndromes. N Engl J Med 1999;341:226–232.
34. Campbell KR, Ohman EM, Cantor W, et al. The use of glycoprotein IIb/IIIa inhibitor therapy in acute ST-segment elevation myocardial infarction: current practice and future trends. Am J Cardiol 2000;85:32C–38C.
35. Smith SC, Blair SN, Bonow RO, et al. AHA/ACC guidelines for preventing heart attack and death in patients with atherosclerotic cardiovascular desease: 2001 update. Circulation 2001;104:1577–1579.
36. Franzosi MG, Santoro E, DeVita C. Gruppo Italiano per lo Studio della Sopravvivenza nell'Infarto (GISSI) Investigators. Ten-year follow-up of the first megatrial testing thrombolytic therapy in patients with acute myocardial infarction: results of the Gruppo Italiano per lo Studio della Sopravvivenza nell'Infarto-1 study. Circulation 1998;98:2659–2665.
37. Topol EJ. Acute myocardial infarction: thrombolysis. Heart 2000; 83:122–126.
38. Ohman EM, Harrington RA, Cannon CP, et al. Intravenous thrombolysis in acute myocardial infarction. Chest 2001;119:253S–277S.
39. Gruppo Italiano per lo Studio della Sopravvivenza nell'Infarto Miocardico (GISSI-2). A factorial randomised trial of alteplase versus streptokinase and heparin versus no heparin among 12,490 patients with acute myocardial infarction. Lancet 1990;336:65–71.
40. The International Study Group. In-hospital mortality and clinical course of 20,891 patients with suspected acute myocardial infarction randomised between alteplase and streptokinase with or without heparin. Lancet 1990;336:71–75.
41. Third International Study of Infarct Survival (ISIS-3) Collaborative Group. A randomised comparison of streptokinase vs tissue plasminogen activator vs anistreplase and of aspirin plus heparin vs aspirin alone among 41,299 cases of suspected acute myocardial infarction. Lancet 1992;339:753–770.
42. The Global Utilization of Streptokinase and Tissue Plasminogen Activator for Occluded Coronary Arteries (GUSTO) Investigators. An international randomized trial comparing four fibrinolytic strategies for acute myocardial infarction. N Engl J Med 1993;329:673–682.
43. Bode C, Smalling RW, Berg G, et al. Randomized comparison of coronary fibrinolysis achieved with double bolus reteplase (rPA) and front-loaded "accelerated" alteplase (tPA) in patients with acute myocardial infarction. Circulation 1996;94:891–898.
44. The Global Use of Strategies to Open Occluded Coronary Arteries (GUSTO III) Investigators. A comparison of reteplase with alteplase for acute myocardial infarction. N Engl J Med 1997;337:1118–1123.
45. Cannon CP, Gibson CM, McCabe CH, et al. TNK-tissue plasminogen activator compared with front-loaded alteplase in acute myocardial infarction: results of the TIMI 10B trial. Circulation 1998;98:2805–2814.
46. Anonymous. Single-bolus tenecteplase compared with front-loaded alteplase in acute myocardial infarction: the ASSENT-2 double-blind randomised trial. Lancet 1999;354:716-22.
47. Tung CY, Granger CB, Sloan MA. Global Utilization of Streptokinase and Tissue Plasminogen Activator for Occluded Coronary Arteries (GUSTO I) Investigators. Effects of stroke on medical resource use and costs in acute myocardial infarction. Circulation 1999;99:370–376.
48. Mark DB, Hlatky MA, Califf RM, et al. Cost effectiveness of fibrinolytic therapy with tissue plasminogen activator as compared with streptokinase for acute myocardial infarction. N Engl J Med 1995;332:1418–1424.
49. Stringer KA. Clinical trials in fibrinolytic therapy, part 1: outcome markers that go beyond mortality reduction. Am J Health Syst Pharm 1997;54(suppl 1):S23–S26.
50. Antman EM, Giugliano RP, Gibson CM, et al. Abciximab facilitates the rate and extent of thrombolysis: results of Thrombolysis in Myocardial Infarction (TIMI) 14 trial. Circulation 1999;99:2720–2732.
51. Strategies for Patency Enhancement in the Emergency Department (SPEED) Group. Trial of abciximab with and without low-dose reteplase for acute myocardial infarction. Circulation 2000;101:2788–2794.
51a. The GUSTO-V Investigators. Reperfusion therapy for acute myocardial infarction with fibrinolytic therapy or combination reduced fibrinolytic therapy and platelet glycoprotein IIb/IIIa inhibition: the GUSIO V randomised trial. Lancet 2001;357:1905–1914.
51b. The Assessment of the Safety and Efficacy of a New Thrombolytic Regimen (ASSENT)-3 Investigators. Efficacy and safety of tenecteplase in combination with enoxaparin, abciximab, or unfractionated heparin: the ASSENT-3 randomised trial in acute myocardial infarction. Lancet 2001;358:605–613.
52. Anonymous. A clinical trial comparing percutaneous transluminal coronary angioplasty with tissue plasminogen activator for acute myocardial infarction. The Global Use of Strategies to Open Occluded Coronary Arteries in Acute Coronary Syndromes (GUSTO IIb). N Engl J Med 1997;336:1621–1628.
53. Tiefenbrunn AJ, Chandra NC, French WJ, et al. Clinical experience with primary percutaneous transluminal coronary angioplasty compared with alteplase (recombinant tissue-type plasminogen activator) in patients with acute myocardial infarction: a report from the Second National Registry of Myocardial Infarction (NRMI-2). J Am Coll Cardiol 1998;31:1240–1245.
54. Nunn CM, O'Neill WW, Rothbaum D, et al. Long-term outcome after primary angioplasty: report from the primary angioplasty in myocardial infarction (PAMI-I) trial. J Am Coll Cardiol 1999;33:640–646.
55. Popma JJ, Ohman EM, Weitz J, et al. Antithrombotic therapy in patients undergoing percutaneous coronary intervention. Chest 2001;119:321S–336S.
56. Brener SJ, Barr LA, Burchenal JEB, et al. Randomized, placebo-controlled trial of platelet glycoprotein IIb/IIIa blockade with primary angioplasty for acute myocardial infarction. Circulation 1998;98:734–741.
57. Vaitkus PT, Laskey WK. Efficacy of adjunctive fibrinolytic therapy in percutaneous transluminal coronary angioplasty. J Am Coll Cardiol 1994;24:1415–1423.
58. Yhip PJ, Smalling RW. Primary stenting for acute myocardial infarction. Thromb Haemost 1999;82(suppl 1):160–163.
59. Schomig A, Kastrati A, Dirschinger J, et al. Coronary stenting plus platelet glycoprotein IIb/IIIa blockade compared with tissue plasminogen activator in acute myocardial infarction. N Engl J Med 2000:343;385–391.
60. Evaluation of Platelet IIB/IIIa Inhibitor for Stenting (EPISTENT) Investigators. Randomised placebo-controlled and balloon-angioplasty–controlled trial to assess safety of coronary stenting with use of platelet glycoprotein IIb/IIIa blockade. Lancet 1998;352:87–92.
61. Gruppo Italiano per lo Studio della Sopravvivenza nell'Infarto Miocardico (GISSI-3): Effects of lisinopril and transdermal glyceryl trinitrate singly and together on 6-week mortality and ventricular function after acute myocardial infarction. Lancet 1994;343: 1115–1122.
62. The Fourth International Study of Infarct Survival (ISIS-4) Collaborative Group. A randomised factorial trial assessing early oral captopril, oral mononitrate, and intravenous magnesium sulfate in 58,050 patients with suspected acute myocardial infarction. Lancet 1995; 345:669–685.
63. Gottlieb SS, McCarter RJ, Vogel RA. Effect of beta-blockade on mortality among high-risk and low-risk patients after myocardial infarction. N Engl J Med 1998;339:489–497.
64. Prabhu SD, Chandrasekar B, Murray DR, Freeman GL. β-adrenergic blockade in developing heart failure: effects on myocardial inflammatory cytokines, nitric oxide, and remodeling. Circulation 2000;101:2103–2109.
65. Poulsen SH, Jensen SE, Egstrup K. Effects of long-term adrenergic beta-blockade on left ventricular diastolic filling in patients with acute myocardial infarction. Am Heart J 1999;138:710–720.
66. Hennekens CH, Albert CM, Godfried SL, et al. Adjunctive drug therapy of acute myocardial infarction—evidence from clinical trials. N Engl J Med 1996;335:1660–1667.

67. Bradford WD, Chen J, Krumholz HM. Under-utilisation of β-blockers after acute myocardial infarction: pharmacoeconomic implications. Pharmacoeconomics 1999;15:257–268.
68. Senior R, Basu S, Kinsey C, et al. Carvedilol prevents remodeling in patients with left ventricular dysfunction after acute myocardial infarction. Am Heart J 1999;137:646–652.
69. Second International Study of Infarct Survival (ISIS-2). Randomised trial of intravenous streptokinase, oral aspirin, both, or neither among 17,187 cases of suspected acute myocardial infarction. Lancet 1988;ii:349–360.
70. CAPRIE Steering Committee. A randomised, blinded, trial of clopidogrel versus aspirin in patients at risk of ischaemic events (CAPRIE). Lancet 1996;348:1329–1339.
71. Cairns JA, Theroux P, Lewis HD, et al. Antithrombotic agents in coronary artery disease. Chest 2001;119:228S–252S.
72. Wood AJJ. Aspirin, heparin and fibrinolytic therapy in suspected acute myocardial infarction. N Engl J Med 1997;336:847–860.
73. Gersh BJ. Current issues in reperfusion therapy. Am J Cardiol 1998; 82:3P 11P.
74. Olson JD, Arkin CF, Brandt JT, et al. College of American Pathologists Conference XXXI on laboratory monitoring of anticoagulant therapy. Laboratory monitoring of unfractionated heparin therapy. Arch Pathol Lab Med 1998;122:782–798.
75. Cohen M, Demers C, Gurfinkel EP, et al. A comparison of low-molecular-weight heparin with unfractionated heparin for unstable coronary artery disease. N Engl J Med 1997;33;7:447–452.
76. Antman EM, McCabe CH, Gurfinkel EP, et al. Enoxaparin prevents death and cardiac ischemic events in unstable angina/non–Q-wave MI. Circulation 1999;100:1593–1601.
77. Monrad ES. Role of low molecular weight heparins in the management of patients with unstable angina and non-Q wave acute myocardial infarction. Am J Cardiol 2000;85:2C–9C.
78. Antman EM, Cohen M, Bernink PJLM, et al. The TIMI risk score for unstable angina/non-ST elevation MI. JAMA 2000;284:835–842.
79. Frostfeldt G, Ahlberg G, Gustafsson G, et al. Low molecular weight heparin (dalteparin) as adjuvant treatment of thrombolysis in acute myocardial infarction—a pilot study: biochemical markers in acute coronary syndromes (BIOMACS II). J Am Coll Cardiol 1999;33:627–633.
80. Chamuleau SAJ, de Winter RJ, Levi M, et al. Low molecular weight heparin as an adjunct to thrombolysis for acute myocardial infarction: the FATIMA study. Heart 1998;80:35–39.
81. Ross AM, Coyne K, Hammond M, Lundergan CF. Low-molecular-weight heparins in acute myocardial infarction: rationale and results of a pilot study. Clin Cardiol 2000;23:483–485.
82. Ferguson JJ. Combining low-molecular-weight heparin and glycoprotein IIb/IIIa antagonists for the treatment of acute coronary syndromes: the NICE3 story. J. Invasive Cardiol 2000;Suppl E:E10–E13.
83. Lefkovits J, Plow EF, Topol EJ. Platelet glycoprotein IIb/IIIa receptors in cardiovascular medicine. N Engl J Med 1995;332:1553–1559.
84. Stringer KA. The evolving role of platelet glycoprotein IIb/IIIa inhibitors in the management of acute coronary syndromes. Ann Pharmacotherapy 1999;33:712–722.
85. Mukherjee D, Moliterno DJ. Achieving tissue-level perfusion in the setting of acute myocardial infarction. Am J Cardiol 2000;85:39C–46C.
86. Yousef ZR, Redwood SR, Marber MS. Postinfarction left ventricular remodelling: where are the theories and trials leading us? Heart 2000;83:76–80.
87. Anonymous. Part 7: The era of reperfusion. Section 1: Acute coronary syndromes (acute myocardial infarction). Advanced cardiovascular life support. Circulation 2000;102:1–172.
88. Cairns JA, Connolly SJ, Roberts RS, CAMIAT Investigators. Randomised trial of outcome after myocardial infarction in patients with frequent or repetitive ventricular premature depolarisations: CAMIAT. Lancet 1997;349:675–682.
89. Julian DG, Camm AJ, Frangin G, et al. Randomised trial of effect of amiodarone on mortality in patients with left ventricular dysfunction after recent myocardial infarction. EMIAT. Lancet 1997;349:667–674.
90. Elizari MV, Martinez JM, Belziti C, Grupo de Estudios Multicentricos en Argentina (GEMICA). Morbidity and mortality following early administration of amiodarone in acute myocardial infarction. Eur Heart J 2000;21:198–205.
91. Boutitie F, Boissel J-P, Connolly SJ, et al. Amiodarone interaction with β-blockers: analysis of the merged EMIAT and CAMIAT databases. Circulation 1999;99:2268–2275.
92. Santoro GM, Antoniucci D, Bolognese L, et al. A randomized study of intravenous magnesium in acute myocardial infarction treated with direct coronary angioplasty. Am Heart J 2000;140:891–897.
93. Ziegelstein RC, Hilbe JM, French WJ, et al. Magnesium use in the treatment of acute myocardial infarction in the United States (observations from the Second National Registry of Myocardial Infarction). Am J Cardiol 2001:87:7–10.
94. The MAGIC Steering Committee. Rationale and design of the magnesium in coronaries (MAGIC) study: a clinical trial to reevaluate the efficacy of early administration of magnesium in acute myocardial infarction. Am Heart J 2000;139:10–14.
95. Madias JE, Shah B, Chintalapally G, et al. Admission serum potassium in patients with acute myocardial infarction: its correlates and value as a determinant of in-hospital outcome. Chest 2000;118:904–913.
96. Marano L, Bestetti A, Lomuscio A, et al. Effects of infusion of glucose-insulin-potassium on myocardial function after a recent myocardial infarction. Acta Cardiol 2000;55:9–15.
97. Antiplatelet Trialists' Collaboration. Collaborative overview of randomised trials of antiplatelet therapy—I: prevention of death, myocardial infarction, and stroke by prolonged antiplatelet therapy in various categories of patients. BMJ 1994;308:81–106.
98. Anticoagulants in the Secondary Prevention of Events in Coronary Thrombosis-2 (ASPECT-2) study. Presented at the European Society of Cardiology meeting, 2000.
99. Antithrombotics in Prevention of Reocclusion in Coronary Thrombolysis-2 (APRICOT-2) study. Presented at the European Society of Cardiology meeting, 2000.
100. Coumadin Aspirin Reinfarction Study [CARS] Investigators. Randomised double-blind trial of fixed low-dose warfarin with aspirin after myocardial infarction. Lancet 1997;350:389–396.
101. Loh E, St. John Sutton M, Wun C-CC, et al. Ventricular dysfunction and the risk of stroke after myocardial infarction. N Engl J Med 1997;336:251–257.
102. Pfeffer MA, Braunwald E, Moye LA, et al. Effect of captopril on mortality and morbidity in patients with left ventricular dysfunction after myocardial infarction. N Engl J Med 1992;327:669–677.
103. National Cholesterol Education Program. Second Report of the Expert Panelon Detection, Evaluation, and Treatment of High Blood Cholesterol in Adults (Adult Treatment Panel II). Circulation 1994;89: 1333–1345.
104. Sacks FM, Pfeffer MA, Braunwald E, et al. for the CARE Investigators. Effect of pravastatin on coronary events after myocardial infarction in patients with average cholesterol levels. N Engl J Med 1996;335:1001–1009.
105. Dupuis J, Tardif J-C, Cernacek P, Theroux P. Cholesterol reduction rapidly improves endothelial function after acute coronary syndromes: the RECIFE (Reduction of Cholesterol in Ischemia and Function of the Endothelium) trial. Circulation 1999;99:3227–3233.
106. Stenestrand U, Wallentin L. Early statin treatment following acute myocardial infarction and 1-year survival. JAMA 2001;285:430–436.
107. Fonarow GC, French WJ, Parsons LS, et al. Use of lipid-lowering medications at discharge in patients with acute myocardial infarction: data from the National Registry of Myocardial Infarction 3. Circulation 2001;103:38–44.
108. Boden WE, Pearson TA. Raising low levels of high-density lipoprotein cholesterol is a target of therapy. Am J Cardiol 2000;85:645–650.
109. Newby KL, Eisenstein EL, Califf RM, et al. Cost effectiveness of early discharge after uncomplicated acute myocardial infarction. N Engl J Med 2000;342:749–755.
110. Senaratne MP, Smith G, Gulamhusein SS. Feasibility and safety of early exercise testing using the Bruce protocol after acute myocardial infarction. J Am Coll Cardiol 2000;35:1212–1220.

16

ARRHYTHMIAS

Jerry L. Bauman and Marieke Dekker Schoen

The heart has two basic properties, namely an electrical property and a mechanical property. The synchronous interaction between these two properties is complex, precise, and relatively enduring. The study of the electrical properties of the heart has grown at a slow steady rate, interrupted by periodic salvos of scientific breakthroughs. Einthoven's pioneering work allowed graphic electrical tracings of cardiac rhythm and probably represents the first of these breakthroughs. This discovery (of the surface electrocardiogram [ECG]) has remained the cornerstone of diagnostic tools for cardiac rhythm disturbances. Intracardiac recordings and programmed cardiac stimulation have further advanced our understanding of arrhythmias, while microelectrode, voltage clamp, and patch clamping techniques have allowed considerable insight into the electrophysiologic actions and mechanisms of antiarrhythmic drugs. Certainly, the new era of molecular biology and mapping of the human genome promises even greater insights into mechanisms (and potential therapies) of arrhythmias. Noteworthy in this regard is the discovery of genetic abnormalities in the ion channels that control electrical repolarization in patients with the heritable long QT syndromes.

The clinical use of drug therapy started with the use of digitalis, followed by quinidine, followed in turn by a surge of new agents. The theme of drug discovery was initially to find orally absorbed lidocaine-congeners (e.g., mexilitene and tocainide). Later, the emphasis was on drugs with extremely potent effects on conduction (i.e., flecainide-like agents). The current focus of investigational antiarrhythmic drugs is on the potassium channel blockers, with dofetilide being the most recently approved in the United States.

Previously, there had been some expectation that advances in antiarrhythmic drug discovery would lead to a highly effective and nontoxic agent that would be effective for a majority of patients. Instead, significant problems with drug toxicity and proarrhythmia have resulted in a decline in the overall volume of antiarrhythmic drug usage in the United States over the past decade. The development of very effective non-drug therapies has also significantly contributed to the decline in drug usage. Technical advances have made it possible to interrupt reentry circuits with radiofrequency ablation, which renders long-term antiarrhythmic drug use obsolete in certain arrhythmias. Further refinement of internal cardioverter/defibrillators continues to advance at an impressive rate, and this, combined with the now known hazards of drugs, have led most clinicians to choose this form of therapy as the first-line treatment of serious, recurrent ventricular arrhythmias. What does the future hold for the use of antiarrhythmic drugs? Certainly new knowledge and technologic advances have forced investigators and clinicians to rethink the concept of traditional membrane-active drugs. Although considerable enthusiasm exists for some of the newer agents, the overall impact of these drugs has yet to be determined.

ARRHYTHMOGENESIS

NORMAL CONDUCTION

Electrical activity moves through cardiac tissue by a tree-like conduction network. Under normal circumstances, the sinoatrial node initiates cardiac rhythm, because this tissue possesses the highest degree of automaticity or rate of spontaneous impulse generation. The autonomic nervous system influences the degree of automaticity of the sinoatrial node in that both cholinergic and sympathetic innervation control sinus rate. Most tissues within the conduction system also possess varying degrees of inherent automatic properties. However, the rates of spontaneous impulse generation of these tissues are less than that of the sinoatrial node. Thus, these latent automatic pacemakers are continuously excited, but they are overdriven by impulses arising from the sinoatrial node (primary pacemaker) and, therefore, do not become clinically apparent.

From the sinoatrial node, electrical activity moves in a wavefront through an atrial specialized conducting system and eventually gains entrance to the ventricle via an atrioventricular node and a large bundle of conducting tissue referred to as the bundle of His. Aside from this atrioventricular nodal-Hisian pathway, a fibrous atrioventricular ring that will not permit electrical stimulation separates the atria and the ventricles. The conducting tissues bridging the atria and ventricles are referred to as the junctional areas. Again, this area of tissue (junction) is under the significant influence of autonomic input and possesses a relatively high degree of inherent automaticity (but still less than that of the sinoatrial node). From the bundle of His, the cardiac conduction system bifurcates into several (usually three) bundle branches: one right bundle and two left bundles. These bundle branches further arborize into a conduction network referred to as the Purkinje system. The conduction system as a whole innervates the mechanical myocardium and serves to initiate excitation-contraction coupling and the contractile process. After the electrical stimulation of a cell or group of cells within the heart, a brief period of time follows in which those cells cannot again be excited. This time period is referred to as the refractory period. As the electrical wavefront moves down the conduction system, the impulse eventually encounters tissue refractory to stimulation (recently excited) and subsequently dies out. Then the sinoatrial node recovers, fires spontaneously, and begins the process again.

Prior to cellular excitation, an electrical gradient exists between the inside and the outside of the cell membrane. At this time, the cell is said to be polarized. In atrial and ventricular conducting tissue, the intracellular space is about 80–90 mV negative with respect to the extracellular environment. The electrical gradient just prior to excitation is referred to as the resting membrane potential (RMP) and is

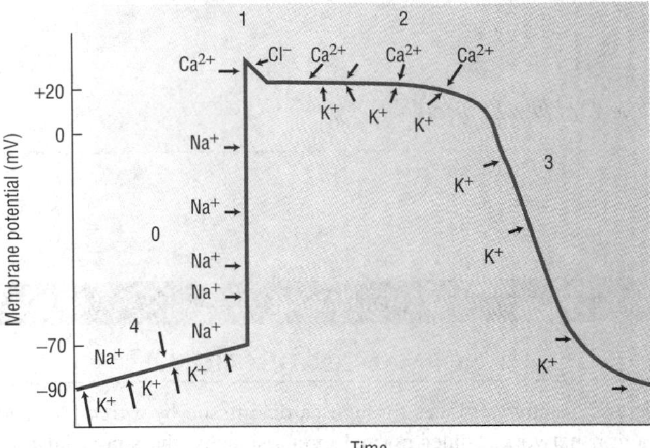

FIGURE 16–1. Purkinje fiber action potential showing specific ionflux responsible for the change in membrane potential.

the result of differences in ion concentrations between the inside and the outside of the cell. At the RMP, the cell is polarized primarily by the action of active membrane ion pumps, the most notable of these being the sodium-potassium pump. For example, this specific pump (in addition to other systems) attempts to maintain the intracellular sodium concentration at 5–15 mEq/L and the extracellular sodium at 135–142 mEq/L; the intracellular potassium concentration at 135–140 mEq/L and the extracellular potassium concentration at 3–5 mEq/L. The RMP can be calculated by using the Nernst equation:

$$\text{RMP} = -61.5 \log \frac{[\text{ion outside}]}{[\text{ion inside}]}$$

Electrical stimulation (or depolarization) of the cell will result in changes in membrane potential over time or a characteristic action potential curve (Fig. 16–1). Resulting from the transmembrane movement of specific ions, the action potential curve is divided into different phases. The initial, rapid depolarization of atrial and ventricular tissues, or phase 0, is due to an abrupt increase in the permeability of the membrane to sodium influx. This rapid depolarization more than equilibrates (overshoots) the electrical potential, leading to a brief initial repolarization, or phase 1. Phase 1 is due to a transient and active potassium efflux. Calcium begins to move into the intracellular space at about −60 mV (during phase 0), causing a slower depolarization. Calcium influx continues throughout the plateau phase of the action potential, or phase 2, and is balanced to some degree by potassium efflux. Calcium entrance (only through L channels in myocardial tissue) distinguishes cardiac conducting cells from nerve tissue and provides the critical ionic link to excitation-contraction coupling and the mechanical properties of the heart as a pump (see Chapter 13, Heart Failure). The membrane remains permeable to potassium efflux during phase 3, resulting in cellular repolarization. Phase 4 of the action potential is the gradual depolarization of the cell and is related to a constant sodium leak into the intracellular space balanced by a decreasing (over time) efflux of potassium. The slope of phase 4 depolarization determines, in large part, the automatic properties of the cell. As the cell is slowly depolarized during phase 4, an abrupt increase in sodium permeability occurs, allowing the rapid cellular depolarization of phase 0. The juncture of phase 4 and phase 0 where rapid sodium influx is initiated is referred to the threshold potential of the cell. The level of threshold potential also regulates the degree of cellular automaticity.

Not all cells in the cardiac conduction system rely on sodium influx for initial depolarization. Some tissues depolarize in response to a slower inward ionic current caused by calcium influx. These "calcium-dependent" tissues are found primarily in the sinoatrial and atrioventricular nodes (both L and T channels) and possess distinct conduction properties in comparison to "sodium-dependent" fibers. Calcium-dependent cells generally have a less negative RMP (−40 to −60 mV) and a slower conduction velocity. Furthermore, in calcium-dependent tissues, recovery of excitability outlasts full repolarization, whereas in sodium-dependent tissue, recovery is prompt after repolarization. These two types of electrical fibers also differ dramatically in the way that drugs modify their conduction properties.

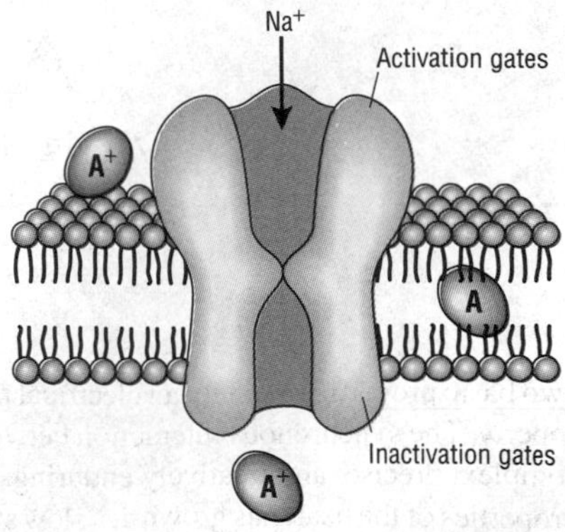

FIGURE 16–2. Lipid bilayer, sodium channel, and possible sites of action of the type I agents (A). Type I antiarrhythmic drugs may theoretically inhibit sodium influx at an extracellular, intramembrane, or intracellular receptor site. However, all approved agents appear to block sodium conductance at a single receptor site by gaining entrance to the interior of the channel from an intracellular route. Active ionized drugs block the channel predominantly during the activated or inactivated state and bind and unbind with specific time constants (described as fast on-off, slow on-off, and intermediate).

Ion conductance across the lipid bilayer of the cell membrane occurs via the formation of membrane pores or "channels" (Fig. 16–2). Selective ion channels probably form in response to specific electrical potential differences between the inside and the outside of the cell (voltage dependence). The membrane itself is composed of both organized and disorganized lipids and phospholipids in a dynamic sol-gel matrix. During ion flux and electrical excitation, changes in this sol-gel equilibrium permit the formation of activated ion channels. Intrachannel proteins or phospholipids, referred to as gates, also help to regulate the transmembrane movement of ions. These gates are believed to be positioned strategically within the channel to modulate ion flow (see Fig. 16–2). Each ion channel conceptually has two types of gates: an activation gate and an inactivation gate. The activation gate opens during depolarization to allow the ion current to enter or exit from the cell, and the inactivation gate closes to stop ion movement. When the cell is in a rested state, the activation gates are closed, and the inactivation gates are open. The activation gates then open to allow ion movement through the channel, and the inactivation gates later close to stop ion conductance. Therefore, the cell cycles between three states: resting, activation, and inactivation. Activation of sinoatrial and atrioventricular nodal tissue is dependent on a slow depolarizing current through calcium channels and gates, whereas the activation of atrial and ventricular tissue is dependent on a rapid depolarizing current through sodium channels and gates.

ABNORMAL CONDUCTION

The mechanisms of tachyarrhythmias have been classically divided into two general categories: those resulting from an abnormality in impulse generation or "automatic" tachycardias and those resulting from an abnormality in impulse conduction or "reentrant" tachycardias.

Automatic tachycardias depend on spontaneous impulse generation in latent pacemakers and may be due to several different mechanisms. Experimentally, chemicals such as digitalis glycosides or catecholamines and conditions such as hypoxemia, electrolyte abnormalities (e.g., hypokalemia), or fiber stretch (cardiac dilatation) may lead to an increased slope of phase 4 depolarization in cardiac tissues other than the sinoatrial node. These factors, which experimentally lead to abnormal automaticity, are also known to be arrhythmogenic in clinical situations. The increased slope of phase 4 causes heightened automaticity of these tissues and competition with the sinoatrial node for dominance of cardiac rhythm. If the rate of spontaneous impulse generation of the abnormally automatic tissue exceeds that of the sinoatrial node, then an automatic tachycardia may result. Automatic tachycardias have the following characteristics: (1) the onset of the tachycardia is not related to an initiating event, such as a premature beat; (2) the initiating beat is usually identical to subsequent beats of the tachycardia; (3) the tachycardia cannot be initiated by programmed cardiac stimulation; (4) the tachycardia often occurs in association with digitalis toxicity, high degrees of sympathetic tone, hypokalemia, and/or severe pulmonary disease; and (5) the onset of the tachycardia is usually preceded by a gradual acceleration in rate and termination by a deceleration in rate.

Triggered automaticity is also a possible mechanism for abnormal impulse generation. Briefly, transient membrane depolarizations that occur during repolarization (early after-depolarizations) or after repolarization (delayed after-depolarizations), but prior to phase 4 of the action potential, may "trigger" abnormal repetitive impulses. After-depolarizations may be related to abnormal calcium and sodium influx during or just after full cellular repolarization. Experimentally, early after-depolarizations may be precipitated by hypokalemia, type III and Ia antiarrhythmic drugs, or slow stimulation rates, and they have been implicated as a cause of torsades de pointes. Late after-depolarizations may be precipitated by digitalis or catecholamines and suppressed by calcium channel inhibitors; furthermore, they have been suggested as the mechanism for multifocal atrial tachycardia and exercise-provoked ventricular tachycardia. Triggered automatic rhythms possess some of the characteristics of automatic tachycardias and some of the characteristics of reentrant tachycardias.

As previously mentioned, the impulse originating from the sinoatrial node in an individual with sinus rhythm eventually meets previously excited and thus refractory tissue. Reentry is a concept that involves indefinite propagation of the impulse and continued activation of previously refractory tissue. There are three conduction requirements for the formation of a viable reentrant focus: two pathways for impulse conduction, an area of unidirectional block (prolonged refractoriness) in one of these pathways, and slow conduction in the other pathway (Fig. 16–3). Usually, a critically timed premature beat initiates reentry. This premature impulse enters both conduction pathways, but encounters refractory tissue in one of the pathways at the area of unidirectional block. The impulse dies out because it is still refractory from the previous (sinus) impulse. Although it fails to propagate in one pathway, the impulse may still proceed in a forward direction (antegrade) through the other pathway because of this pathway's relatively shorter refractory period. The impulse may then proceed through a loop of tissue and "reenter" the area of unidirectional block in a backward direction (retrograde). Because the antegrade pathway has slow conduction characteristics, the area of unidirectional block has time to recover its excitability. The impulse can proceed retrogradely through this (previously refractory) tissue and continue around the loop of tissue in a circular fashion. Thus, the

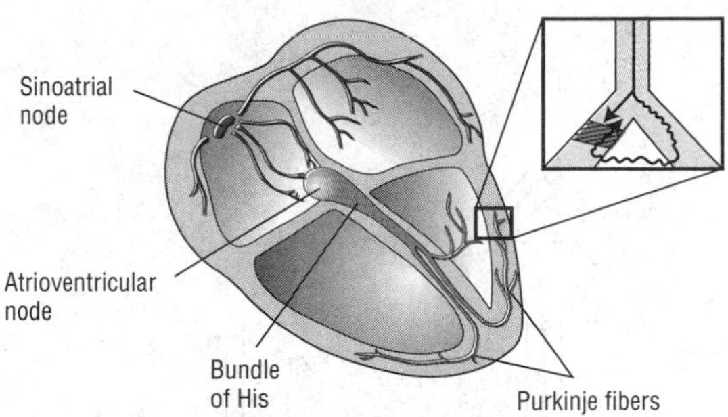

FIGURE 16–3. Conduction system of the heart. The magnified portion shows a bifurcation of a Purkinje fiber traditionally explained as the etiology of reentrant ventricular tachycardia. A premature impulse travels to the fiber, damaged by heart disease or ischemia. It encounters a zone of prolonged refractoriness (area of unidirectional block—hatched area), but fails to propagate because it remains refractory to stimulation from the previous impulse. However, the impulse may slowly travel (squiggly line) through the other portion of the Purkinje twig and will "reenter" the cross-hatched area if the refractory period is over and it is now excitable. Thus, the premature impulse never meets refractory tissue; circus movement ensues. If this site stimulates the surrounding ventricle repetitively, clinical reentrant ventricular tachycardia results.

key to the formation of a reentrant focus is the presence of crucial conduction discrepancies in the electrophysiologic characteristics of the two pathways. The reentrant focus may excite surrounding tissue at a rate greater than that of the sinoatrial node, and a clinical tachycardia results. The model described is anatomically determined in that there is only one pathway for impulse conduction with a fixed circuit length.

Another model of reentry, referred to as a functional reentrant loop or leading circle model, may also occur (Fig. 16–4).[1] In a functional reentrant focus, the length of the circuit may vary, depending on the conduction velocity and recovery characteristics of the impulse. The area in the middle of the loop is continually kept refractory by the inwardly moving impulse. The length of the circuit is not fixed, but is the smallest circle possible, such that the leading edge of the wavefront is continuously exciting tissue just as it recovers; the head of the impulse chases its tail. It differs from the anatomic model in that the leading edge of the impulse is not preceded by an excitable gap of tissue, it does not have an obstacle in the middle, and it does not have a fixed anatomic circuit.

Clinically, many reentrant foci probably have both anatomic and functional characteristics. In the figure 8 model, there is a zone of unidirectional block, which allows for two impulse loops that join and reenter the area of block in a retrograde fashion, forming a pretzel-shaped reentrant circuit. This model combines functional characteristics with an excitable gap. All of these theoretical models require a critical balance of refractoriness and conduction velocity within the circuit, and each has helped to explain the effects of drugs on terminating, modifying, and causing cardiac rhythm disturbances.

What causes reentry to become clinically manifest? Reentrant foci may occur at any level of the conduction system: within the branches of the specialized atrial conduction system, the Purkinje network, and even within portions of the sinoatrial and atrioventricular nodes. The anatomy of the Purkinje system is felt to provide a suitable substrate for the formation of microreentrant loops and is often used as a model to facilitate the understanding of reentry concepts (see Fig. 16–4). Of course, reentry does not usually occur in normal, healthy conduction tissue, and therefore, various forms of heart disease or conduction abnormalities must usually be present before reentry becomes manifest. In other words, the various forms of heart disease can alter conduction in the pathways of a suitable

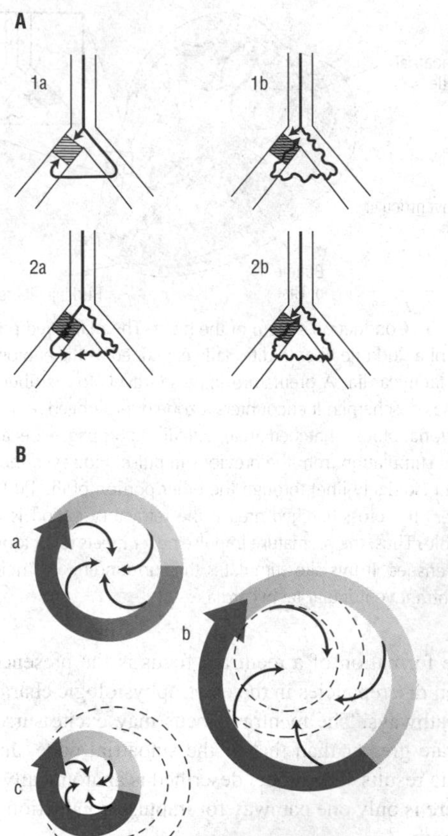

FIGURE 16–4. A. Possible mechanism of proarrhythmia in the anatomic model of reentry. (1a) Nonviable reentrant loop due to bidirectional block (shaded area). (1b) Instance where a drug slows conduction velocity without significantly prolonging the refractory period. The impulse is now able to reenter the area of unidirectional block (shaded area), because slowed conduction through the contralateral limb allows recovery of the block. A new reentrant tachycardia may result. (2a) Nonviable reentrant loop due to a lack of a unidirectional block. (2b) Instance where a drug prolongs the refractory period without significantly slowing conduction velocity. The impulse moving antegrade meets refractory tissue (shaded area), allowing for unidirectional block. A new reentrant tachycardia may result. **B.** Mechanism of reentry and proarrhythmia. (a) Functionally determined (leading circle) reentrant circuit. This model should be contrasted with anatomic reentry: here the circuit is not fixed (it does not necessarily move around an anatomic obstacle), and there is no excitable gap. All tissue inside is held continuously refractory. (b) Instance where a drug prolongs the refractory period without significantly slowing conduction velocity. The tachycardia may terminate or slow in rate as shown because of a greater circuit length. The dashed lines represent the original reentrant circuit prior to drug treatment. (c) Instance where a drug slows conduction velocity without significantly prolonging the refractory period (i.e., type Ic agents) and accelerates the tachycardia. The tachycardia rate may increase (proarrhythmia) as shown because of a shorter circuit length. The dashed lines represent the original reentrant circuit prior to drug treatment. *(From Ref. 8, with permission.)*

reentrant substrate. An often used example is reentry occurring as a consequence of ischemic or hypoxic damage: with inadequate cellular oxygen, cardiac tissue resorts to anaerobic glycolysis for adenosine triphosphate (ATP) production. As the high-energy phosphate concentration diminishes, the activity of the transmembrane ion pumps declines, and the RMP rises. This increase in the RMP inactivates the voltage-dependent sodium channel, and the tissue begins to assume slow conduction characteristics. If changes in conduction parameters occur in a discordant manner because of varying degrees of ischemia or hypoxia, then a reentry circuit may become manifest. Furthermore, an ischemic, dying cell liberates intracellular potassium, which also causes a rise in the RMP. In other cases, reentry may occur due to anatomic or functional variants in the normal conduction system. For instance, patients may possess two (instead of one) conduction pathways near or within the atrioventricular node, or they may have an anomalous, extranodal atrioventricular pathway that possesses different electrophysiologic characteristics from the normal atrioventricular nodal pathway. Reentry in these cases may occur within the atrioventricular node or encompass both atrial and ventricular tissue. Reentrant tachycardias have the following characteristics: (1) the onset of the tachycardia is usually related to an initiating event (i.e., premature beat); (2) the initiating beat is usually different in morphology from subsequent beats of the tachycardia; (3) the initiation of the tachycardia is usually possible with programmed cardiac stimulation; and (4) the initiation and termination of the tachycardia usually occurs abruptly, without an acceleration or deceleration phase.

ANTIARRHYTHMIC DRUGS

In a theoretical sense, drugs may have antiarrhythmic activity by directly altering conduction in several ways. First, a drug may depress the automatic properties of abnormal pacemaker cells. An agent may do this by decreasing the slope of phase 4 depolarization and/or by elevating threshold potential. If the rate of spontaneous impulse generation of the abnormally automatic foci becomes less than that of the sinoatrial node, normal cardiac rhythm can be restored. Second, drugs may alter the conduction characteristics of the pathways of a reentrant loop.[1,2] An agent may facilitate conduction (shorten refractoriness) in the area of unidirectional block, allowing antegrade conduction to proceed. On the other hand, an antiarrhythmic may further depress conduction (prolong refractoriness) either in the area of unidirectional block or in the pathway with slowed conduction and a relatively shorter refractory period. Prolongation of refractoriness in the area of unidirectional block makes it impossible for retrograde propagation of the impulse to occur, causing a "bidirectional" block. In the anatomic model, prolongation of refractoriness in the pathway with slow conduction prevents antegrade conduction of the impulse through this route. In either case, drugs that reduce the discordance and cause uniformity in conduction properties of the two pathways may suppress the reentrant substrate. In the functionally determined model, if refractoriness is prolonged without significantly slowing conduction velocity, the tachycardia may terminate or slow in rate due to a greater circuit length (see Fig. 16–4). There are other possible ways to stop reentry; a drug may eliminate the critically timed premature impulse that triggers reentry, for example, or a drug may slow conduction velocity to such an extent that conduction is extinguished.

CATEGORIZATION OF ANTIARRHYTHMIC DRUGS

In patients with or without heart disease, antiarrhythmic drugs have specific electrophysiologic actions that alter cardiac conduction. These actions form the basis of grouping antiarrhythmics into specific categories based on their electrophysiologic actions *in vitro*. Vaughan Williams first proposed the most frequently used classification system. (Table 16–1).[2] This classification has been criticized because (1) it is incomplete and does not allow for the classification of agents such as digoxin or adenosine; (2) it is not pure, and many agents have properties of more than one class of drugs; (3) it does not incorporate drug characteristics such as mechanisms of tachycardia termination/prevention, clinical indications, or side effects; and (4) agents become "labeled" within a class, although they may be distinct in many regards.[3] These criticisms became the rationale for an attempt to reclassify antiarrhythmic agents according

TABLE 16–1. Classification of Antiarrhythmic Drugs

Type	Drug	Conduction Velocity[a]	Refractory Period	Automaticity	Ion Block
Ia	Quinidine Procainamide Disopyramide	↓	↑	↓	Sodium (intermediate)
Ib	Lidocaine Mexiletine Tocainide	0/↓	↓	↓	Sodium (fast on-off)
Ic	Flecainide Propafenone[c] Moricizine[d]	↓↓	0	↓	Sodium (slow on-off)
II[b]	β-Blockers	↓	↑	↓	Calcium (indirect)
III	Amiodarone[c,e] Bretylium[c] Dofetilide Sotalol[c] Ibutilide	0	↑↑	0	Potassium
IV[b]	Verapamil Diltiazem	↓	↑	↓	Calcium

[a]Variables for normal tissue models in ventricular tissue.
[b]Variables for sinoatrial and atrioventricular nodal tissue only.
[c]Also has type II, β-blocking actions.
[d]Classification controversial.
[e]Amiodarone also blocks calcium and sodium channels (fast on-off).

to a variety of basic and clinical characteristics (called the Sicilian Gambit[3]). Nonetheless, the Vaughan Williams classification remains the most frequently used, despite many proposed modifications and alternative systems.

TYPE I ANTIARRHYTHMIC AGENTS

The type Ia drugs such as quinidine, procainamide, and disopyramide slow conduction velocity, prolong refractoriness, and decrease the automatic properties of sodium-dependent (normal and diseased) conduction tissue. Therefore, the type Ia agents can be effective in automatic tachycardias, decreasing the rate of spontaneous impulse generation of atrial or ventricular foci. In reentrant tachycardias, these drugs generally depress conduction and prolong refractoriness, theoretically transforming the area of unidirectional block into a bidirectional block. Clinically, type Ia drugs are broad-spectrum antiarrhythmics, as they are effective for both supraventricular and ventricular arrhythmias.

Historically, lidocaine and phenytoin were categorized separately from quinidine-like drugs. Early work demonstrated that lidocaine had distinctly different electrophysiologic actions. It was found that in normal tissue models, lidocaine generally facilitates actions on cardiac conduction by shortening refractoriness and having little effect on conduction velocity. Thus, it was postulated that these agents could improve antegrade conduction, eliminating the area of unidirectional block. Of course, arrhythmias do not usually arise from normal tissue, leading investigators to study the actions of lidocaine and phenytoin in ischemic and hypoxic tissue models. Interestingly, studies have shown these drugs to possess quinidine-like properties in diseased tissues. Therefore, it is probable that lidocaine acts in clinical tachycardias in a similar fashion to the type Ia drugs (i.e., accentuated effects in diseased tissues leading to bidirectional block in a reentrant circuit). Lidocaine and similar agents have accentuated effects in ischemic tissue because of the local acidosis and potassium shifts that occur during cellular hypoxia. Changes in pH alter the time that local anesthetics occupy the sodium channel receptor and, therefore, affect the agent's electrophysiologic actions. The type Ib agents such as lidocaine (and structural analogs such as tocainide or mexiletine) are considerably more effective in ventricular arrhythmias than in supraventricular arrhythmias.

The third group of type I drugs, type Ic agents, includes flecainide, propafenone, and moricizine. These agents profoundly slow conduction velocity while leaving refractoriness relatively unaltered. Type Ic agents theoretically eliminate reentry by slowing conduction to a point where the impulse is extinguished and cannot propagate further. Although effective for both ventricular and supraventricular arrhythmias, their use for ventricular arrhythmias has been limited by the risk of proarrhythmia.

Type I drugs exert their effects on a subcellular basis by inhibiting the transmembrane influx of sodium. In essence, type I agents can be referred to as sodium channel blockers. The receptor site for the antiarrhythmics is probably inside the sodium channel so that, in effect, the drug plugs the pore. The agent may gain access to the receptor either via the intracellular space through the membrane lipid bilayer or directly through the channel. There are several principles inherent in antiarrhythmic–sodium channel receptor theories:[4]

1. Type I antiarrhythmics have predominant affinity for a particular state of the channel (e.g., during activation or inactivation). For example, lidocaine and flecainide block sodium current primarily when the cell is in the inactivated state, whereas quinidine is predominantly an open (or activated)-channel blocker.
2. Type I antiarrhythmics have specific binding and unbinding characteristics to the receptor. For example, lidocaine binds to and dissociates from the channel receptor quickly (termed fast on-off), but flecainide has very "slow on-off" properties. This explains why flecainide has such potent effects on slowing ventricular conduction, but lidocaine has little effect on normal tissue. In general, the type Ic agents are slow

on-off; the type Ib agents, fast on-off; and the type Ia agents, intermediate in their binding kinetics.
3. Type I antiarrhythmics possess rate dependence (i.e., sodium channel blockade and slowed conduction are greatest at fast heart rates and least during bradycardia). For slow on-off drugs, sodium channel blockade is evident at normal rates (60–100 beats/min) but for fast on-off agents, slowed conduction is apparent only at rapid rates of stimulation.
4. Type I antiarrhythmics (except phenytoin) are weak bases with a pKa more than 7 and block the sodium channel in their ionized form. Therefore, pH will alter these actions: acidosis accentuates and alkalosis diminishes sodium channel blockade.
5. Type I antiarrhythmics appear to share a single receptor site in the sodium channel.

These principles are important in understanding additive drug combinations (e.g., quinidine and mexiletine), antagonistic combinations (e.g., flecainide and lidocaine), and potential antidotes to excess sodium channel blockade (e.g., sodium bicarbonate or propranolol).

TYPE II ANTIARRHYTHMIC AGENTS

The β-adrenergic antagonists are classified as type II antiarrhythmic drugs. For the most part, the clinically relevant antiarrhythmic mechanisms of the β-blockers result from their antiadrenergic actions. Because adrenergic innervation strongly influences the sinoatrial and atrioventricular nodes, β-blockers are most useful in tachycardias in which these nodal tissues are abnormally automatic or are a portion of a reentrant loop. These agents are also helpful in slowing ventricular response in atrial tachycardias (e.g., atrial fibrillation) because of their effects on the atrioventricular node. Furthermore, β-blockers may be useful for those tachycardias that are exercise-related or precipitated by states of high sympathetic tone (perhaps through triggered activity). β-Adrenergic stimulation results in increased conduction velocity, shortened refractoriness, and increased automaticity of the nodal tissues; β-adrenergic blockers will antagonize these effects. Propranolol is often noted to have "local anesthetic" or quinidine-like activity; however, suprapharmacologic concentrations are usually required to elicit this action. In the nodal tissues, β-blockers interfere with calcium entry into the cell by altering catecholamine-dependent channel integrity and gating kinetics. In sodium-dependent atrial and ventricular tissue, β-blockers shorten repolarization somewhat, but otherwise have little direct effect. The antiarrhythmic properties of β-blockers observed with long-term, chronic therapy in patients with heart disease are less well understood. Although it is clear that β-blockers decrease the likelihood of sudden death (presumably arrhythmic death) after myocardial infarction, the reason remains unclear, but may relate to the complex interplay of changes in sympathetic tone, damaged myocardium, and ventricular conduction.

TYPE III ANTIARRHYTHMIC AGENTS

Type III antiarrhythmics include those agents that specifically prolong refractoriness in atrial and ventricular fibers. This class includes very different drugs: bretylium, amiodarone, sotalol, ibutilide, and recently dofetilide; they share the common effect of delaying repolarization by blocking potassium channels. The electrophysiologic actions of bretylium are related to its multifaceted pharmacology. Bretylium is structurally similar to guanethidine and can, likewise, cause an initial increase in catecholamine release from the adrenergic neuron. This action may potentially affect arrhythmogenesis by an indirect mechanism: an increase in coronary blood flow and myocardial perfusion, which reverses ischemia-related arrhythmias (similar to epinephrine's action in a patient with ventricular fibrillation). After causing catecholamine release, bretylium then causes an uncoupling of autonomic nerve stimulation from the release step, resulting in antiadrenergic effects. Theoretically, bretylium may also be antiarrhythmic by these sympatholytic actions. Nonetheless, bretylium prolongs repolarization due to blockade of potassium conductance, independent of the sympathetic nervous system, and many researchers feel that these direct actions account for its clinical effectiveness. Importantly, bretylium increases the ventricular fibrillation threshold and seems to have selective antifibrillatory, but not antitachycardic, effects. In other words, bretylium can be effective in ventricular fibrillation, whereas it is often ineffective in ventricular tachycardia.

In contrast, amiodarone and sotalol are effective in most tachycardias. Amiodarone displays electrophysiologic characteristics consistent with each class within the Vaughan Williams scheme; it is a sodium channel blocker with relatively fast on-off kinetics, has nonselective β-blocking actions, blocks potassium channels, and also has a small degree of calcium antagonist activity. At normal heart rates and with chronic use, its primary effect is to prolong repolarization. Upon intravenous (IV) administration, it begins to act relatively quickly (unlike the oral form), and β-blockade predominates initially. Theoretically, amiodarone, like type I agents, may interrupt the reentrant substrate by transforming an area of unidirectional block into an area of bidirectional block. However, electrophysiologic studies utilizing programmed cardiac stimulation imply that amiodarone may leave the reentrant loop intact. Rather, it is possible that amiodarone abolishes the premature impulse that usually triggers the reentry process. In addition, the potent β-blocking properties of amiodarone may contribute significantly to its acute and chronic efficacy. The impressive effectiveness of amiodarone, coupled with its low proarrhythmic potential, has challenged the notion that selective ion channel blockade by antiarrhythmic agents is preferable. Sotalol is a potent inhibitor of outward potassium movement during repolarization and also possesses β-blocking actions. Indeed, it was first synthesized as a nonselective β-antagonist, but now has evolved into the prototype type III agent on which most investigational agents are based. Ibutilide and, more recently, dofetilide have been approved for the conversion and prevention of atrial fibrillation, respectively; these agents are structurally similar to sotalol. Both possess type III activity, blocking the rapid component of the delayed potassium rectifier current (I_{Kr}).

There are a number of different potassium channels that function during normal conduction, but the most relevant in terms of approved and investigational antiarrhythmic drugs is the delayed rectifier current (I_K) responsible for phase 2 and phase 3 repolarization. Subcurrents make up I_K: an ultrarapid component, I_{Kur}; a rapid component, I_{Kr}; and the slow component, I_{Ks}. *N*-acetylprocainamide (NAPA) and dofetilide selectively block I_{Kr} whereas amiodarone and azimilide (investigational) block both I_{Kr} and I_{Ks}. The clinical relevance of selectively blocking components of the delayed rectifier current remains to be determined. Potassium current blockers (particularly those with selective I_{Kr} blocking properties) display "reverse use-dependence," (i.e., their effects on repolarization are greatest at low heart rates). Sotalol and like drugs also appear to be much more effective in preventing ventricular fibrillation (in dog models) than the traditional sodium blockers. They also decrease the defibrillation threshold, in contrast to type I agents, which tend to increase this parameter. Thus, patients with automatic internal defibrillators as concurrent therapy with type I agents may require more energy for successful cardioversion, or worse, these devices may become ineffective in terminating tachycardia. Although the current focus of antiarrhythmic drug therapy centers around sotalol-like, type III agents, all of these drugs may cause proarrhythmia in the form of torsades de pointes; more long-term data regarding safety and efficacy are necessary in order to ascertain their true place in therapy.

TYPE IV ANTIARRHYTHMIC AGENTS

The calcium channel antagonists comprise the type IV antiarrhythmic category. At least two types of calcium channels are operative in sinoatrial and atrioventricular nodal tissues: an L-type channel and a T-type channel. Therefore, both L-channel blockers (verapamil and diltiazem) and selective T-channel blockers (mibefradil) will slow conduction, prolong refractoriness, and decrease automaticity of the calcium-dependent tissue in the sinoatrial and atrioventricular nodes. These agents are effective in automatic or reentrant tachycardias that arise from or utilize the sinoatrial or atrioventricular nodes. In atrial tachycardias, these drugs can slow ventricular response (e.g., atrial fibrillation) by slowing atrioventricular nodal conduction. Furthermore, because calcium entry seems to be integral to tachycardias related to exercise and/or tachycardias due to some forms of triggered automaticity, preliminary evidence shows effectiveness in these types of arrhythmias. In all likelihood, verapamil and diltiazem work at different receptor sites because of their dissimilar chemical structures and pharmacologic actions. Nifedipine (or any of the dihydropyridine calcium antagonists) does not have significant antiarrhythmic activity because a reflex increase in sympathetic tone due to vasodilation counteracts this agent's direct negative dromotropic action. Calcium antagonists can slightly shorten repolarization in normal sodium-dependent tissue, but otherwise have little effect.

SIDE EFFECTS OF ANTIARRHYTHMIC DRUGS

All antiarrhythmic agents currently available have an impressive side effect profile (Table 16–2). A considerable percentage of patients cannot tolerate long-term therapy with these drugs, and chances are good that it will be necessary to discontinue an agent because of side effects. In one trial,[5] more than 50% of patients had to discontinue the long-term use of procainamide (mostly because they developed a lupus-like syndrome) after myocardial infarction. In another study,[6] disopyramide caused anticholinergic side effects in approximately 70% of patients. Flecainide and disopyramide may precipitate congestive heart failure in a significant number of patients with underlying left ventricular dysfunction.[7] The type Ib agents, such as tocainide and mexiletine, cause neurologic and/or gastrointestinal toxicity in a high percentage of patients. Tocainide, specifically, has been reported to cause both pulmonary fibrosis and leukopenia, the significance of which came to light only after the Food and Drug Administration (FDA) had approved the use of the drug. Clearly, the most frightening adverse effects related to antiarrhythmic drugs are the aggravation of underlying ventricular arrhythmias and the precipitation of new (and life-threatening) ventricular arrhythmias.[8]

Amiodarone has taken a prominent place in the treatment of both chronic and acute arrhythmias and is now the most commonly prescribed antiarrhythmic drug. Once considered a drug of last resort, it is now the first drug considered in many symptomatic tachycardias. Yet amiodarone is a peculiar and complex drug, displaying unusual pharmacologic effects, pharmacokinetics, dosing schemes, and multisystem side effects. Amiodarone has an extremely long elimination phase and large volume of distribution; therefore, the onset of action with the oral form is delayed (days to weeks) despite a loading regimen, and its effects persist long (months) after discontinuation. Amiodarone inhibits most CYP enzymes (including p-glycoprotein), resulting in many common drug interactions; for example, it causes digoxin levels to approximately double and makes it necessary to reduce the maintenance dose of warfarin by one third to one-half. Patients can usually tolerate the acute administration well, but severe toxicities may result with chronic use. Severe bradycardia (sometimes requiring pacing to allow the patient to remain on amiodarone), hyper- and hypothyroidism, photosensitivity, and a blue-gray skin discoloration on exposed areas are common. Hepatitis and pulmonary fibrosis have caused death.[9,10] These side effects mandate close and continued monitoring (i.e., liver enzyme measurements, thyroid function tests, eye examinations, chest x-rays, pulmonary function tests)

TABLE 16–2. Side Effects of Antiarrhythmic Drugs

Drug	Side Effects
Quinidine	Cinchonism, diarrhea, GI, hypotension, torsades de pointes, aggravation of underlying heart failure, conduction disturbances or ventricular arrhythmias, hepatitis, thrombocytopenia, hemolytic anemia
Procainamide	Systemic lupus erythematosus, GI, torsades de pointes, aggravation of underlying heart failure, conduction disturbances or ventricular arrhythmias, agranulocytosis
Disopyramide	Anticholinergic symptoms, GI, torsades de pointes, heart failure, aggravation of underlying conduction disturbances and/or ventricular arrhythmias, hypoglycemia, hepatic cholestasis
Lidocaine	CNS, seizures, psychosis, sinus arrest, aggravation of underlying conduction disturbances
Mexiletine	CNS, psychosis, GI, aggravation of underlying conduction disturbances or ventricular arrhythmias
Tocainide	CNS, psychosis, GI, aggravation of underlying conduction disturbances or ventricular arrhythmias, rash/arthralgias, pulmonary infiltrates, agranulocytosis, thrombocytopenia
Moricizine	Dizziness, headache, GI, aggravation of underlying conduction disturbances or ventricular arrhythmias
Flecainide or Propafenone	Blurred vision, dizziness, headache, GI, bronchospasm[a], aggravation of underlying heart failure, conduction disturbances or ventricular arrhythmias
Amiodarone	CNS, corneal microdeposits/blurred vision, optic neuropathy/neuritis, GI, aggravation of underlying ventricular arrhythmias, torsades de pointes, bradycardia or atrioventricular block, bruising without thrombocytopenia, pulmonary fibrosis, hepatitis, hypothyroidism, hyperthyroidism, photosensitivity, blue-gray skin discoloration, myopathy, hypotension, phlebitis (IV use)
Dofetilide	Torsades de pointes
Ibutilide	Torsades de pointes, hypotension
Sotalol	Fatigue, GI, depression, torsades de pointes, bronchospasm, aggravation of underlying heart failure, conduction disturbances or ventricular arrhythmias
Bretylium	Hypotension, GI

GI = gastrointestinal effects (e.g., nausea, anorexia); CNS = central nervous system effects (e.g., confusion, paresthesias, tremor, ataxia).
[a]Propafenone only

and have led to a proliferation of "amiodarone clinics" designed just for patients receiving this agent on a chronic basis.

The pharmacokinetics of the antiarrhythmic agents are summarized in Table 16–3, and a nomogram for estimating initial effective dosages of the oral forms (except amiodarone and dofetilide) is shown in Figure 16–5. Dosing recommendations for the IV forms are shown in Table 16–4. When dosing oral amiodarone, clinicians usually employ a loading dose, then sometimes an intermediate priming dose before maintenance treatment, although there is no standardized regimen. Oral loading doses range from 800–1600 mg/day (in divided daily doses) for 5–7 days then maintenance therapy at 200–400 mg/day (given once daily). For those with supraventricular tachycardias or ventricular arrhythmias with an implantable cardioverter-defibrillator, one usually tries to reach a chronic maintenance dose of 200 mg/day. When dosing dofetilide, clinicians must pay particular attention to the patient's renal function. High dosages in patients with renal dysfunction will lead to drug accumulation and a high risk of proarrhythmia (see later). Per the manufacturer's recommendations, patients with creatinine clearances of > 60 mL/min should receive an initial dofetilide dose of 500 μg bid, for 40–60 mL/min 125 μg bid and for 20–40 mL/min 125 μg once daily. Dofetilide is contraindicated at estimated creatinine clearances < 20 mL/min. Initial dosages will require adjustment based upon the QTc prolongation.

SUPRAVENTRICULAR ARRHYTHMIAS

The common supraventricular tachycardias that often require drug treatment are (1) atrial fibrillation or atrial flutter, (2) paroxysmal supraventricular tachycardia, and (3) automatic atrial tachycardias. Other common supraventricular arrhythmias that usually do not require drug therapy include premature atrial complexes (PACs), wandering atrial pacemaker, sinus arrhythmia, and sinus tachycardia. Because PACs rarely cause symptoms and never cause hemodynamic compromise, drug therapy is usually not indicated for this condition. Likewise, sinus tachycardia is usually the result of underlying metabolic or hemodynamic disorders (e.g., infection, dehydration, hypotension), and the underlying cause, not the tachycardia per se, should be the focus of therapy. Of course, there are exceptions to these suggestions. For example, sinus tachycardia may be deleterious in patients after cardiac surgery or myocardial infarction. In another unusual tachycardia termed nonparoxysmal sinus tachycardia, chronically elevated heart rates may cause alterations in left ventricular function. In these instances, antiarrhythmic drugs such as β-blockers may indeed be indicated. Stated in another way, although many arrhythmias generally do not require therapy, clinical judgment and patient-specific variables play an important role in this decision.

Supraventricular tachycardias may cause a variety of symptoms. Some patients may be totally asymptomatic or complain only of minor palpitations or irregular pulse. In contrast, severe and even life-threatening symptoms can sometimes occur in association with supraventricular tachycardia. Patients may experience dizziness or acute syncopal episodes with the onset of their tachycardia because of an abrupt drop in cardiac output, blood pressure, and cerebral perfusion. This drop in forward cardiac output results from the rapid ventricular rate with resultant poor ventricular filling and asynchronous atrioventricular contraction. Heart failure symptoms may also develop, and patients with preexisting left ventricular dysfunction

TABLE 16–3. Pharmacokinetics of Antiarrhythmic Drugs

Drug	Bioavailability (%)	Primary Route of Elimination	Substrate	Inhibitor	$V_{D,ss}$ (L/Kg)	Protein Binding (%)	$t_{1/2}$	Therapeutic Range (mg/L)
Quinidine	70–80	H	CYP3A4	CYP2D6 P-GP	2.0–3.5	80–90	5–9 h	2–6
Procainamide	75–95	H/R	NAT		1.5–3.0	10–20	2.5–5.0 h	4–15
Disopyramide	70–95	H/R	CYP3A4		0.8–2.0	50–80	4–8 h	2–6
Lidocaine	20–40	H	CYP3A4 CYP2D6		1–2	65–75	60–180 min	1.5–5.0
Mexiletine	80–95	H	CYP2D6 CYP1A2		5–12	60–75	6–12 h	0.8–2.0
Tocainide	90–95	H			1.5–3.0	10–30	12–15 h	4–10
Moricizine	34–38	H			6–11	92–95	1–6 h	—
Flecainide	90–95	H/R	CYP2D6		8–10	35–45	13–20 h	0.3–2.5
Propafenone[a]			CYP2D6					
Poor	11–39	H			2.5–4.0	85–95	12–32 h	—
Extensive							2–10 h	
Amiodarone	22–28	H	CYP3A4	CYP1A2 CYP2C9 CYP2D6 CYP3A4 P-GP	70–150	95–99	15–100 d	1.0–2.5
Sotalol	90–95	R			1.2–2.4	30–40	12–20 h	—
Dofetilide	85–95	R	CYP3A4		2.5–3.5	60–70	6–10 h	—
Ibutilide	—	H			6–12	40–50	3–6 h	—
Bretylium	15–20	R			4–8	Negligible	5–10 h	0.5–2.0
Verapamil	20–40	H	CYP3A4 CYP1A2	CYP3A4 P-GP	1.5–5.0	95–99	4–12 h	>0.05
Diltiazem	35–50	H	CYP3A4	CYP3A4 P-GP	3–5	70–85	4–10 h	>0.05

H = hepatic; R = renal; CYP = cytochrome P450 isoenzyme; NAT = N-acetyltransferase; P-GP = P-glycoprotein.
[a]Variables for parent compound (not 5-OH, propafenone).

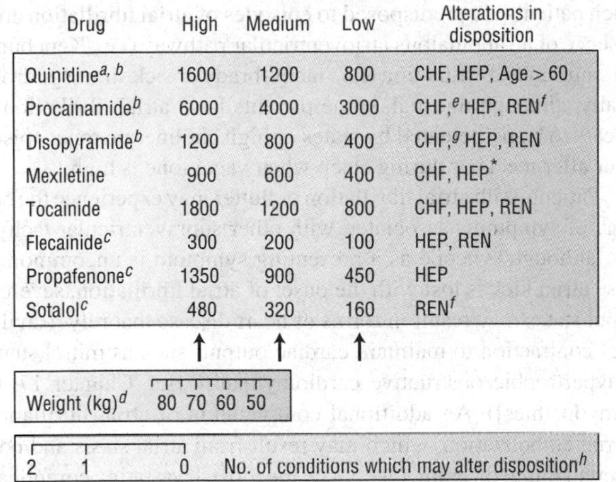

Drug	High	Medium	Low	Alterations in disposition
Quinidine[a, b]	1600	1200	800	CHF, HEP, Age > 60
Procainamide[b]	6000	4000	3000	CHF,[e] HEP, REN[f]
Disopyramide[b]	1200	800	400	CHF,[g] HEP, REN
Mexiletine	900	600	400	CHF, HEP*
Tocainide	1800	1200	800	CHF, HEP, REN
Flecainide[c]	300	200	100	HEP, REN
Propafenone[c]	1350	900	450	HEP
Sotalol[c]	480	320	160	REN[f]

FIGURE 16–5. Nomogram for estimating effective oral dosages of commonly used antiarrhythmic drugs for acute efficacy testing. The dosages are grouped into high, medium, and low categories based on commonly used regimens and commercially available dosage forms. The dosages for each drug are listed as milligrams per day and are expected to result in the average steady-state concentrations shown in Table 16–3. CHF = congestive heart failure; HEP = hepatic disease; REN = renal insufficiency (creatinine clearance < 50 mL/min).

[a]Sulfate salt equivalents.

[b]Sustained release forms may allow less fluctuation in concentrations.

[c]Best to initiate low-dose regimens in all patients and slowly escalate.

[d]Ideal body weight

[e]Conflicting data regarding alteration in disposition.

[f]Significant accumulation of active metabolites or patent in renal disease limit use.

[g]Disopyramide not recommended in congestive heart failure.

[h]Use 1 for each suspected alteration, but 2 where indicated (*).

Use of nomogram:

Step 1. Connect a straight line from the bar indicating the number of alterations in disposition, through the patient's weight to the base of the box.

Step 2. Approximate daily dosage is shown directly above the arrow. When the line connects between the arrows, use the crossbars between the arrows to choose high, medium, or low dosages or estimate an intermediate amount. Exercise caution when choosing dosages in the high range.

Example: A 70-kg patient with poor left ventricular function (i.e., CHF) and frequent paroxysmal episodes of atrial fibrillation is to be treated with oral quinidine. A straight line drawn between 1 on the conditions bar and 70 kg on the weight bar will intersect near the center arrow on the box. Directly above the point of intersection are the medium dosage ranges; quinidine sulfate can be initiated at 1,200 mg/day or 300 mg every 6 hours in this patient. *(From Ref. 62, with permission.)*

TABLE 16–4. Intravenous Antiarrhythmic Dosing

Drug	Clinical Situation	Dosage
Amiodarone	Recurrent VT/VF	150 mg/10 min IV push 1 mg/min for 6 h, then 0.5 mg/min infusion
	Cardiac arrest	300 mg IV push
Bretylium	Acute VF	5 mg/min IV push (May repeat to total dose 30 mg/kg) 1–2 mg/min infusion if needed
Diltiazem	PSVT; rate control AF	0.25 mg/kg IV push (May repeat with 0.35 mg/kg) 5–15 mg/h infusion
Ibutilide	Termination AF	1 mg/10 min IV push (May repeat if needed)
Lidocaine	VT/VF	100 mg IV push (May repeat up to total dose 300 mg) (limit total to 200 mg if CHF present) 2–4 mg/min infusion (1–2 mg/min if liver disease or CHF)
Procainamide	AF, VT	15–18 mg/kg at 20–50 mg/min load 1–6 mg/min infusion
Verapamil	PSVT; rate control AF	5 mg IV push (May repeat up to 20 mg) 5–15 mg/h infusion

VT = Ventricular tachycardia; VF = ventricular fibrillation; PSVT = paroxysmal supraventricular tachycardia; AF = atrial fibrillation; CHF = congestive heart failure.

tolerate the tachycardia particularly poorly. Furthermore, patients with underlying coronary obstruction may experience anginal chest pain because of altered coronary perfusion (low cardiac output) and elevated myocardial oxygen demand (rapid heart rate). More often, patients complain of a choking or pressure sensation during the tachycardia episode, which can be confused with angina pectoris. Symptoms such as palpitations and even syncope correlate rather poorly with documented recurrences of the tachycardia.

ATRIAL FIBRILLATION AND ATRIAL FLUTTER

Among the more common supraventricular tachycardias are atrial fibrillation and atrial flutter. These tachycardias occur more often in men and in those who are elderly. The overall incidence of atrial fibrillation is about 1% to 2% (independent of gender and age), and this approximately doubles in elderly men.[11] These arrhythmias may present as acute atrial fibrillation (first appeared within previous 48 hours); paroxysmal atrial fibrillation (terminates spontaneously); persistent atrial fibrillation (has continued for more than 48 hours and does not terminate spontaneously); and permanent atrial fibrillation (does not terminate with attempts at pharmacologic or electrical cardioversion).

Atrial fibrillation is characterized as an extremely rapid (400–600 atrial beats/min) and disorganized atrial activation. With this disorganized atrial activity, there is a loss of the contribution of atrial contraction (atrial kick) to forward cardiac output. Supraventricular impulses penetrate the atrioventricular conduction system in variable degrees, resulting in an irregular activation of the ventricles and an irregularly irregular pulse. Because the atrioventricular junction will not conduct most of the supraventricular impulses, the ventricular response is considerably slower (120–180 beats/min) than the atrial rate.

Atrial flutter occurs less frequently than atrial fibrillation, but is similar in its precipitating factors, consequences, and drug therapy approach (with some exceptions noted in the following). This arrhythmia is characterized by rapid (270–330 atrial beats/min), but regular atrial activation. The slower and regular electrical activity results in a regular ventricular response and pulse that is in approximate multiples of 300 beats/min (i.e., 1:1 atrioventricular conduction = ventricular rate of 300 beats/min; 2:1 atrioventricular conduction = ventricular rate of 150 beats/min; 3:1 atrioventricular conduction = ventricular rate of 100 beats/min). Atrial flutter may occur in two distinct forms (type I and type II). Type I flutter is the more common, classic form with atrial rates of approximately 300 beats/min and the typical "sawtooth" pattern of atrial activation as shown by the surface ECG. Type II flutter tends to be faster, being somewhat of a hybrid between classic atrial flutter and atrial fibrillation. Although the ventricular response usually has a regular pattern, atrial flutter that occurs with varying degrees of atrioventricular block or with episodes of atrial fibrillation ("fib-flutter") can cause an irregular ventricular rate and pulse.

It is generally accepted that the predominant mechanism of atrial fibrillation and atrial flutter is reentry. Atrial fibrillation appears to result from multiple atrial reentrant loops (or wavelets), and atrial flutter is due to a single, dominant reentrant substrate. Atrial fibrillation or flutter usually occurs in association with forms of organic heart disease that cause atrial distention. Conditions that commonly lead to atrial stretch and precipitate atrial fibrillation or flutter include ischemia or infarction, hypertensive heart disease, valvular disorders such as mitral stenosis, mitral insufficiency, congenital abnormalities such as septal defects, and primary myocardial disease such as dilated or hypertrophic cardiomyopathy. Disorders that cause right atrial stretch and have a known association with atrial fibrillation or flutter include acute pulmonary embolus and chronic lung disease resulting in pulmonary hypertension and cor pulmonale. It is sometimes said, "Atrial fibrillation begets atrial fibrillation." That is, the arrhythmia tends to perpetuate itself; long episodes are more difficult to terminate, perhaps because of tachycardia-induced changes in atrial function (mechanical and electrical "remodeling"). Atrial fibrillation may also occur in association with states of high adrenergic tone, such as thyrotoxicosis, alcohol withdrawal, sepsis, or excessive physical exertion. Established or paroxysmal atrial fibrillation occurring without identifiable heart disease or known precipitating factors is termed "lone" atrial fibrillation. Other states in which patients are predisposed to episodes of atrial fibrillation are the presence of an anomalous atrioventricular pathway (i.e., Kent bundle) and sinus node dysfunction (i.e., tachy-brady or sick sinus syndrome). Finally, although unusual, some patients have atrial fibrillation that appears to be perpetuated by states of high cholinergic tone; episodes occur after meals or during sleep when vagal tone is high.

Patients with atrial fibrillation or flutter may experience the entire range of symptoms associated with other supraventricular tachycardias, although syncope as a presenting symptom is uncommon. Because atrial kick is lost with the onset of atrial fibrillation, severe low output states may result in forms of heart disease that rely heavily on atrial contraction to maintain cardiac output (such as mitral stenosis or hypertrophic obstructive cardiomyopathy [see Chapter 17, Cardiomyopathies]). An additional complication of atrial fibrillation is arterial embolization, which may result from atrial stasis and poorly adherent mural thrombi. Of course, the most devastating complication in this regard is the occurrence of an embolic stroke. The overall incidence of stroke in patients with atrial fibrillation who do not receive antithrombotic therapy is about 3% to 6%.[12,13] Patients with atrial fibrillation and concurrent mitral stenosis or severe systolic heart failure are at a particularly high risk for cerebral embolism. Other risk factors for stroke identified from recent trials are increasing age, history of hypertension, previous transient ischemic event or stroke, and diabetes.[12] Stroke can precede the onset of documented atrial fibrillation, probably because paroxysms were undetected prior to the onset of established atrial fibrillation. In contrast, patients with atrial fibrillation in whom precipitating factors cannot be identified (i.e., lone atrial fibrillation) and those with only atrial flutter have a low risk of embolic stroke.[13]

▶ TREATMENT: Atrial Fibrillation and Atrial Flutter

The ultimate treatment goals of atrial fibrillation or flutter are the restoration of sinus rhythm, the prevention of thromboembolic complications, and the prevention of further recurrences (Fig. 16–6). However, the methods by which to attain these goals vary, depending on the patient's symptom severity. If presenting symptoms are severe, patients with new onset atrial fibrillation or flutter may need direct-current cardioversion (DCC) to immediately restore sinus rhythm. Atrial flutter often requires relatively low energy levels of countershock (i.e., 25–50 W/s), whereas atrial fibrillation often requires higher energy levels (i.e., >200 W/s). On the other hand, if symptoms are tolerable, no such emergency measures are necessary.

CONTROL OF RAPID VENTRICULAR RESPONSE

Type Ia and III antiarrhythmic agents may restore sinus rhythm, but should not be administered initially. These agents may paradoxically increase ventricular response in the absence of drugs that slow atrioventricular nodal conduction. Traditionally, this observation has been attributed to the vagolytic action of these drugs, despite the fact that only disopyramide displays significant anticholinergic side effects. It seems more likely that all of these agents slow atrial conduction, decreasing the number of impulses that reach the atrioventricular node; as a result, the atrioventricular node paradoxically allows more impulses to gain entrance to the ventricular conduction system (increasing ventricular rate). Because of this phenomenon and the lack of any need for the immediate restoration of sinus rhythm, drugs that slow conduction and increase refractoriness in the atrioventricular node should be used as initial therapy. Loading dosages of digoxin have generally been used because of its time-proved effectiveness and the prevalence of concurrent heart failure in these patients. Questions have arisen, however, about the place of digoxin in therapy in both acute and chronic settings.[14,15] Digoxin is sometimes ineffective and often slow in onset; although an initial decrease in ventricular response can sometimes be observed within 1 hour of IV administration, full control (i.e., heart rate less than 100 beats/min) is usually not achieved for 24 to 48 hours. Digoxin will not restore sinus rhythm, but atrial fibrillation may end spontaneously in some patients during the loading procedure.

As mentioned previously, patients can present with a wide variety of symptoms. Consequently, clinical judgment is necessary in choosing the proper treatment strategy. For example, the IV administration of calcium antagonists (diltiazem or verapamil) provides an alternative approach, allowing for a rapid decrease in ventricular rate and symptomatic relief without the need for DCC.[16,17] Because control of ventricular response can be transient, diltiazem or verapamil can be given as an initial IV bolus followed by a continuous infusion titrated to heart rate. Digoxin has in the past been considered the drug of first choice to slow ventricular rate, but many now choose calcium antagonists for most patients with atrial fibrillation or flutter. Further, atrial fibrillation or flutter precipitated by states of high adrenergic tone, such as thyrotoxicosis, is often resistant to digoxin therapy, as digoxin slows atrioventricular nodal conduction primarily through vagotonic mechanisms. In these cases, the IV administration of β-blockers (e.g., propranolol, esmolol) can be highly effective and should be considered first.

Although calcium blockers and β-blockers have taken a more prominent role in controlling rate in patients with rapid atrial fibrillation or flutter, most patients with these tachycardias have concomitant symptoms of heart failure, and these two forms of drug therapy may initially worsen the situation. Usually, a prompt decline in rate and an

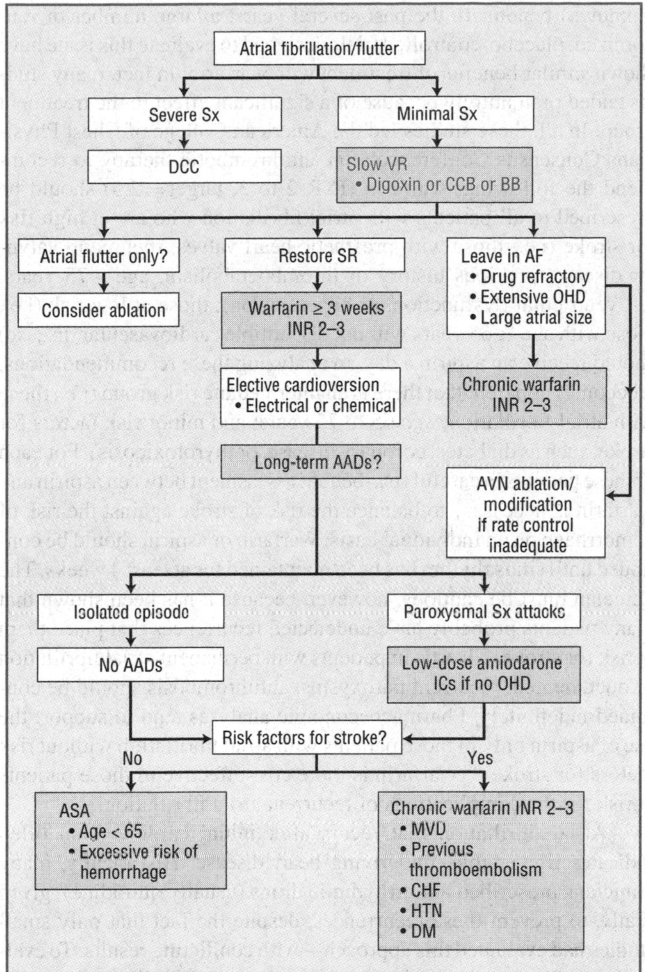

FIGURE 16–6. Algorithm for the treatment of atrial fibrillation and atrial flutter. Sx = symptoms; DCC = direct-current cardioversion; VR = ventricular rate; AVN = atrioventricular node; CCB = calcium channel antagonist (verapamil or diltiazem); BB = β-blocker; SR = sinus rhythm; AF = atrial fibrillation/flutter; OHD = organic heart disease; INR = international normalized ratio; AADs = antiarrhythmic drugs; IC = type IC antiarrhythmic drugs; ASA = aspirin; MVD = mitral valve disease, CHF = congestive heart failure, HTN = hypertension, DM = diabetes mellitus. AADs = antiarrhythmic drugs

increase in stroke volume balance the decrease in contractility seen with β-blockers or calcium blockers such that heart failure symptoms remain unchanged. Occasionally, however, severe reactions and hypotension occur; preliminary information implies that diltiazem may be safer than verapamil.[17]

Patients may present with a slow ventricular response (in the absence of atrioventricular nodal-blocking drugs) and, thus, do not require therapy with digoxin, verapamil, or esmolol. This type of presentation should alert the clinician to the possibility of preexisting sinoatrial or atrioventricular nodal conduction disease, such as sick sinus syndrome. Direct-current cardioversion should not be attempted in these patients without a temporary pacemaker in place.

RESTORATION OF SINUS RHYTHM

After treatment with atrioventricular node-blocking agents and a subsequent decrease in ventricular response, the patient should undergo an evaluation for the possible restoration of sinus rhythm. This evaluation should include consideration of several factors. For example, maintenance of sinus rhythm for a significant length of time is not feasible in some patients, such as those with a history of chronic (more than 1 year) established atrial fibrillation or those with large atrial size (greater than 45 mm determined by echocardiography). Therefore, cardioversion may not be attempted, and these patients can remain in atrial fibrillation, chronically treated with atrioventricular node-blocking agents to control ventricular response (e.g., resting rate ≈ 80 beats/min). Often, long-term therapy with digoxin alone will not control exercise-related increases in ventricular response and tachycardia symptoms. It may be necessary to add small doses of calcium antagonists or β-blockers; treadmill exercise testing or simple ambulation can easily determine the need for these ancillary agents. Occasionally, patients have a condition that is highly refractory to atrioventricular node-blocking agents (including combination drug therapy), and ventricular response remains rapid. Aggressive attempts to lower rate are necessary; chronic tachycardias can result in a progressive decline in left ventricular function, causing so-called tachycardia cardiomyopathy. Hence, in drug-refractory conditions, ablation or modification of the atrioventricular node by a transvenous catheter that delivers radiofrequency current is indicated.[18] This procedure often completely blocks conduction from the atrium to the ventricle, requiring the concurrent implantation of a permanent pacemaker with a ventricular lead.

Restoration of sinus rhythm itself (by either pharmacologic or electrical means) is associated with an increased risk of thromboembolism. The return of sinus rhythm restores an effective contraction, which may dislodge poorly adherent thrombi. Anticoagulation prior to cardioversion prevents clot growth, keeps new thrombi from forming, and allows existing clots to become organized and well adherent to the atrial wall. This form of preventive therapy has been shown to prevent stroke associated with cardioversion, but a regimen of several weeks of anticoagulation is necessary. Therefore, current recommendations are to institute warfarin treatment (international normalized ratio [INR] 2 to 3) for at least 3 weeks prior to cardioversion. The common clinical scenario is to discharge the patient from the hospital, monitor him or her on an ambulatory basis, and readmit for elective cardioversion after this time period.[13] After restoration of sinus rhythm, full atrial contraction does not occur immediately. Rather, it returns gradually to a maximum contractile force over a 3- to 4-week period. Therefore, warfarin should be continued for at least 1 month after effective cardioversion and return of sinus rhythm.

There are several exceptions to this recommended process of anticoagulation. In patients with atrial fibrillation of less than 48 hours' duration, anticoagulation prior to cardioversion is probably not necessary because there has not been sufficient time for atrial thrombi to form. The exact time of onset is unclear in most presentations of atrial fibrillation, however. Because the risk of thromboembolism appears lower in general, some clinicians do not routinely anticoagulate patients with only atrial flutter. But current consensus recommendations give strong consideration to treating atrial flutter in the same way as atrial fibrillation (i.e., generally, at least 3 weeks of anticoagulation prior to elective cardioversion).[18a]

Transesophageal echocardiography (TEE) is also serving as a tool to differentiate patients who may require anticoagulation prior to DCC from those who may not. If there is no indication of atrial thrombus or severe stasis ("smoke") on TEE, then perhaps these patients do not require the 3 weeks of warfarin pretreatment before cardioversion. Initial data are promising; the approach seems cost-effective, as it obviates the need for more than 3 weeks of prior warfarin treatment and subsequent readmission to the hospital. Recently, the use of TEE in this manner was compared to the use of the conventional 3 weeks of anticoagulation before cardioversion in patients with atrial fibrillation.[19] In this large multicenter randomized trial, the incidence of thromboembolic events was not different between the two strategies, but bleeding episodes occurred more frequently in the group that received 3 weeks of treatment with warfarin. Patients in the TEE strategy group were more likely to revert to sinus rhythm, probably because the longer a patient remains in atrial fibrillation (i.e., "atrial fibrillation begets atrial fibrillation"), the more difficult it is to terminate it. These impressive data will more than likely place the use of TEE in patients with atrial fibrillation in a much more prominent role.

After prior anticoagulation or TEE, there are two methods of restoring sinus rhythm in patients with atrial fibrillation or flutter: pharmacologic cardioversion and DCC. Which of these is the method of choice is generally a matter of clinical preference. Recently, in its updated International Consensus Guidelines, the American Heart Association[41] recommended that elective cardioversion be considered first. Indeed, one recent economic analysis determined that DCC as first-line therapy was less costly than the strategy of first trying a drug (such as ibutilide), then proceeding to DCC in the event of drug failure.[20] Nonetheless, some clinicians elect to use antiarrhythmic drugs first, then resort to electrical cardioversion in the event that these agents fail.

Nearly all types Ia, Ic, and III agents have been demonstrated to be effective, and because of the risk of proarrhythmia, their administration should be initiated in an inpatient, monitored setting. In a recent meta-analysis supported by the Agency for Healthcare Research and Quality (AHRQ), there was strong evidence for efficacy only for the type Ic agents (e.g., flecainide, propafenone) and the type III pure I_K blockers (e.g., ibutilide, dofetilide).[21] Oral loading doses of the type Ic antiarrhythmic propafenone (600 mg as a single dose) have been demonstrated effective compared to placebo and provide a simple regimen.[22] Ibutilide given IV or dofetilide given orally appears to be more effective than sotalol and procainamide, albeit with a significant risk of proarrhythmia in the form of torsades de pointes.[23,24] There is inconclusive evidence that the IV administration of amiodarone is effective in terminating atrial fibrillation, although it is being used more frequently for this (non-FDA-approved) indication.

The disadvantages of pharmacologic cardioversion are the risk of significant side effects, such as drug-induced torsades de pointes,[25] the inconvenience of drug-drug interactions (e.g., digoxin-quinidine), and the fact that drugs are generally less effective when compared to DCC. The advantages of DCC are that it is quick and more often successful. The disadvantages of DCC are the need for prior sedation/anesthesia and a risk (albeit small) of serious complications such as sinus arrest or ventricular arrhythmias. Contrary to past beliefs, DCC carries very little risk in patients who are receiving digoxin and have no evidence of digitalis toxicity.

PREVENTION OF COMPLICATIONS: THROMBOEMBOLISM AND RECURRENCE OF ATRIAL FIBRILLATION/FLUTTER

After sinus rhythm is restored, what chronic medications should the patient receive? In many cases, maintenance digoxin therapy is continued simply because of underlying ventricular dysfunction. In a patient with normal left ventricular function, there is no need to continue digoxin. There are two other forms of therapy that the clinician must consider in each patient: (1) long-term antithrombotic therapy to prevent stroke and (2) long-term antiarrhythmic drugs to prevent recurrences of atrial fibrillation. In the past, patients with atrial fibrillation did not routinely receive anticoagulant therapy (unless there was a history of stroke or concurrent mitral valve disease), because it was felt that the risk of warfarin exceeded its potential (though unknown) benefit. In the past several years, a large number of randomized, placebo-controlled trials designed to evaluate this issue have shown similar benefits of treatment with warfarin; in fact, many studies ended prematurely because of a significant effect in the treatment group. In all, these studies led the American College of Chest Physicians Consensus Conference[13] on antithrombotic therapy to recommend the following: warfarin (INR 2 to 3, target = 2.5) should be prescribed to all patients with atrial fibrillation who are at high risk for stroke (i.e., those with prosthetic heart valves, rheumatic valvular disease, previous history of thromboembolism, age > 75 years, left ventricular dysfunction, or hypertension); those at low risk (i.e., those with age < 65 years without discernible cardiovascular disease) should receive an aspirin a day. In analyzing these recommendations, it becomes apparent that there is an intermediate risk group (i.e., those with atrial fibrillation; age 65 to 75 years; and minor risk factors for stroke, such as diabetes, coronary disease, or thyrotoxicosis). For each of these patients, a careful risk-benefit assessment between aspirin and warfarin is necessary to balance the risk of stroke against the risk of hemorrhage on an individual basis. Warfarin or aspirin should be continued until sinus rhythm has been maintained for at least 4 weeks. The clinician must be cautious, however, because it has been shown that many patients probably have undetected recurrences that place them at risk for stroke. Clearly, in patients with permanent atrial fibrillation or documented, recurrent paroxysms, antithrombosis should be continued indefinitely. Pharmacoeconomic analyses tend to support the use of aspirin only in those patients with atrial fibrillation without risk factors for stroke.[26] Warfarin is more cost-effective in those patients at risk for the complications of recurrent atrial fibrillation.

Atrial fibrillation that recurs after initial cardioversion often indicates irreversible, underlying heart disease. Historically, many clinicians prescribed antiarrhythmic drugs (usually quinidine), given orally, to prevent these recurrences, despite the fact that only small studies had evaluated this approach—with conflicting results. To evaluate the efficacy of quinidine in preventing atrial fibrillation, a meta-analysis of the existing literature was completed.[27] This meta-analysis demonstrated that, indeed, more patients remain in sinus rhythm with quinidine therapy (compared to placebo), although about 50% have recurrences of atrial fibrillation within a year despite quinidine. This reported effectiveness was at the cost of an associated increase in mortality (presumably due, in part, to proarrhythmia) in the quinidine-treated patients, however. These disturbing results (published soon after the Cardiac Arrhythmia Suppression Trial [CAST][28]) became widely quoted and highly visible, making clinicians question the wisdom of the long-term prevention of recurrences of atrial fibrillation with antiarrhythmic drugs. Although the results were questioned because some of the reported causes of death in the treated patients could not be directly attributed to quinidine, a subsequent study tended to support the findings of the meta-analysis.[29]

It is possible that the type Ic and the type III agents provide alternatives to quinidine. Flecainide and propafenone tend to be better tolerated than the type Ia agents, and they have been shown to be highly effective in the termination and prevention of atrial fibrillation. With the type Ic agents, however, there is the risk of ventricular proarrhythmia. The CAST[28] and other studies have demonstrated that patients being treated for ventricular arrhythmias with coexisting ischemic heart disease and poor left ventricular function are at increased risk of proarrhythmia. Patients with atrial fibrillation often fall into this category. For that reason, type Ic agents, although effective, should be reserved for patients with lone atrial fibrillation (i.e., young patients without evidence of heart disease).

Another alternative, sotalol, has been shown to be at least as effective as quinidine in preventing recurrences of atrial fibrillation.[30] Treatment with sotalol is associated with an incidence of torsades de pointes much like that of quinidine, however. Because this form of proarrhythmia occurs primarily with higher doses of sotalol (quinidine causes torsades de pointes at low to therapeutic concentrations), it may be more easily predicted and therefore avoided with sotalol. Nonetheless, sotalol may increase mortality in patients with atrial fibrillation as quinidine does, and this requires further study.[31]

The newest type III agent, dofetilide, also appears to be effective in preventing recurrences of atrial fibrillation. Preliminary evidence suggests that dofetilide is at least as effective as sotalol when used for this purpose. Like sotalol, dofetilide has significant potential to cause torsades de pointes (in a dose-related fashion); therefore, it appears that dofetilide should not be first-line therapy for recurrent atrial fibrillation at this time. Uncontrolled studies indicate that low doses of amiodarone (100–200 mg/d) are highly effective in preventing the recurrence of atrial fibrillation, perhaps at a lower risk of serious toxicity than that associated with higher doses (400 mg/d).[32] In one of the few comparative trials with amiodarone,[33] it was shown to be more effective than either sotalol or propafenone in maintaining sinus rhythm. These data, coupled with a low incidence of proarrhythmia associated with amiodarone, have prompted many now to choose amiodarone first in patients with recurrent atrial fibrillation (and organic heart disease), despite the risk of other toxicities.

In view of the studies implying that mortality increases in association with the time-honored approach of prescribing long-term quinidine and other agents, the following approach is suggested. That is, chronic antiarrhythmic drugs should be reserved for those patients with documented symptomatic recurrences or symptomatic paroxysmal atrial fibrillation. Those with an isolated episode should not receive chronic preventive therapy. In terms of drug choice, low-dose amiodarone is the preferred agent for most patients. After appropriate oral loading doses, patients should receive 200 mg/d on a continuing basis. If this dosage has successfully prevented recurrences, the clinician may attempt to reduce it to 100 mg/d, but more data are required on this practice. Although the oral methods of loading amiodarone vary considerably, it is appropriate to use 800 mg/d for 1 week, followed by 400 mg/d for 1 month before initiation of the 200 mg/d maintenance dose for patients with recurrent atrial fibrillation. For those patients with symptomatic recurrences of atrial fibrillation, but no evidence of organic heart disease (e.g., recurrent lone atrial fibrillation), type Ic agents such as flecainide or propafenone are highly effective and safe as first-line drugs.

Studies are currently under way to compare the long-term use of antiarrhythmic drugs to prevent atrial fibrillation/flutter with the use of drugs that simply control ventricular rate (e.g., digoxin and/or calcium antagonists) with mortality as the primary end point. These studies should more clearly define the best long-term approach to these arrhythmias. One such study, the Atrial Fibrillation Follow-up Investigation of Rhythm Management (AFFIRM), began in 1996 and will randomize patients to an arm with strategies to maintain sinus rhythm (e.g., antiarrhythmic drugs) or an arm with strategies to control ventricular response (e.g., atrioventricular node-blocking drugs). It is possible that, in the future, most patients can be managed by strategies to control rate only (drugs, atrioventricular nodal ablation) without chronic antiarrhythmic drug therapy.

Non-drug forms of therapy designed to maintain sinus rhythm are either currently in use or under active investigation. For patients who have "pure" (i.e., not associated with concurrent atrial fibrillation) type I atrial flutter, ablation of the reentrant substrate with radiofrequency current is highly effective (80%).[34] This form of therapy is rapidly becoming an attractive alternative to chronic drug treatment. For patients with atrial fibrillation, an innovative surgical procedure referred to as the "maze" operation has been used for more than a decade.[35] Because of its highly complex nature, the maze should be reserved for highly drug-refractory patients. Some have attempted to replicate the ideas of the maze procedure by using catheter ablation technologies, but success has been varied; complications have included recurrences of atrial fibrillation (and flutter) and thromboembolism. Interestingly, in a subset (often those with lone atrial fibrillation) of patients with paroxysmal atrial fibrillation, premature beats that arise in the pulmonary veins appear to initiate the episodes. In these cases, ablation of the pulmonary venous foci can prevent recurrences in a high percentage of patients.[36]

PAROXYSMAL SUPRAVENTRICULAR TACHYCARDIA CAUSED BY REENTRY

Reentrant mechanisms such as atrioventricular node reentry, atrioventricular reentry incorporating an anomalous atrioventricular pathway, sinoatrial node reentry, and intra-atrial reentry can all give rise to paroxysmal supraventricular tachycardia (PSVT). Sinus node reentry or intra atrial reentry occur less commonly and are not as well described as atrioventricular node or atrioventricular reentry. Aside from a characteristic abrupt onset and termination coupled with subtle changes in P-wave morphology, these tachycardias can be difficult to diagnose. Electrophysiologic studies may be necessary to determine the ultimate mechanism of the PSVT. Atrioventricular node reentry and atrioventricular reentry are by far the most common of these tachycardias, and inasmuch are discussed in detail below.

The underlying substrate of atrioventricular node reentry is the functional division of the atrioventricular node into two (or more) longitudinal conduction pathways or "dual" atrioventricular nodal pathways.[37] Although there is some disagreement, most electrophysiologists now believe that there are not two distinct, anatomic pathways inside the atrioventricular node itself. Rather, it is likely that a fan-like network of perinodal fibers inserts into the atrioventricular node and represents the second pathway. The two pathways possess key differences in conduction characteristics: one is a fast conducting pathway with a relatively long refractory period (fast pathway), and the other is a slower conducting pathway with a shorter refractory period (slow pathway). The presence of dual pathways does not necessarily imply that the patient will have clinical PSVT. In fact, it is estimated that from 10% to nearly 50% of the general population have discernible dual pathways, but the incidence of PSVT is considerably lower.[37] Sustenance of the tachycardia depends on the critical electrophysiologic discrepancies, the ability of one pathway (usually the slow) to allow repetitive antegrade conduction, and the ability of the other pathway (usually the fast) to allow repetitive retrograde conduction. During sinus rhythm, a patient with dual pathways conducts supraventricular impulses in an antegrade direction through both pathways. Electrical activity reaches the distal common pathway at the level of or above the His bundle and continues to depolarize the ventricles in an antegrade direction. Conduction proceeds via the two pathways but reaches the distal common pathway first through the fast atrioventricular node route (Fig. 16–7). For this reason, a short PR interval is sometimes observed during sinus rhythm.

Paroxysmal supraventricular tachycardia caused by atrioventricular node reentry may occur by the following sequence of events. An appropriately timed premature impulse penetrates the atrioventricular node, but is blocked in the fast pathway, which is still refractory from the previous beat. However, the slow pathway, which has a shorter refractory period, permits antegrade conduction of the premature impulse. By the time the impulse has reached the distal common pathway, the fast pathway has recovered its excitability and permits

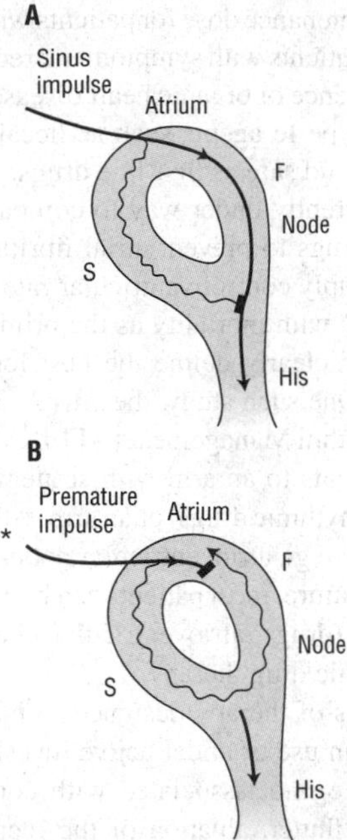

FIGURE 16–7. Reentry mechanism of dual atrioventricular nodal pathway paroxysmal supraventricular tachycardia (PSVT). **(A)** Sinus rhythm: the impulse travels from the atrium through the fast pathway (F) and then to the His-Purkinje system. The impulse also travels through the slow pathway (S), but is stopped when refractory tissue is encountered. **(B)** Dual atrioventricular nodal reentry: a critically timed premature impulse (*) is stopped in the fast pathway (because of prolonged refractoriness), but is able to travel antegrade down the slow pathway and retrograde through the fast pathway.

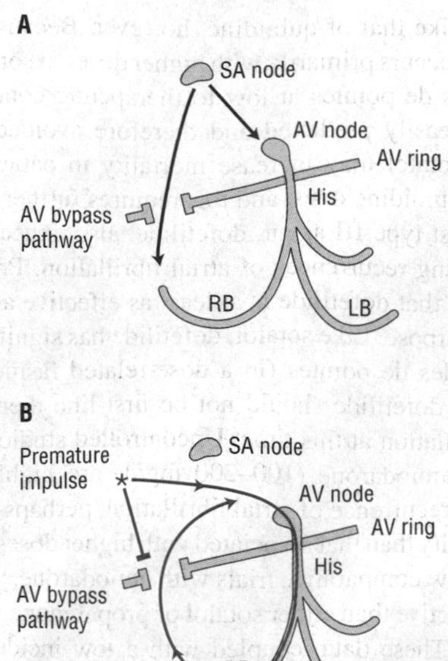

FIGURE 16–8. Reentry mechanism for atrioventricular (AV) accessory pathway paroxysmal supraventricular tachycardia (PSVT) in Wolff-Parkinson-White syndrome. (**A**) Sinus rhythm: the impulse travels from the atrium to the ventricle by two pathways—the atrioventricular node and an accessory bypass pathway. (**B**) Atrioventricular reentry: a critically timed premature impulse (*) is stopped in the Kent bundle (because of prolonged refractoriness), but travels antegrade through the atrioventricular node and retrograde through the Kent bundle. SA = sinoatrial; RB = right bundle; LB = left bundle.

retrograde conduction. The impulse reaches the common proximal pathway, preceded by an excitable gap of tissue, and reenters the slow pathway. A reentrant circuit that does not require atrial or ventricular tissue is completed within (or nearly so) the atrioventricular node, and a tachycardia is thereby initiated (see Fig. 16–7). The common form of this tachycardia uses the slow pathway for antegrade conduction and the fast pathway for retrograde conduction; an uncommon form exists in which the reentrant impulse travels in the opposite direction.

Atrioventricular reentrant tachycardia depends on the presence of an anomalous, or accessory, extranodal pathway that bypasses the normal atrioventricular conduction pathway. Several different types of accessory pathways have been described, depending on the specific anatomic areas that they connect (e.g., atrioventricular bundles, nodoventricular tracts). Some are also referred to by eponyms; the Kent bundle, for example, is an extranodal atrioventricular connection that is associated with the Wolff-Parkinson-White syndrome. During sinus rhythm (Fig. 16–8), patients with this syndrome depolarize the ventricles simultaneously through both atrioventricular pathways (atrioventricular node pathway and the Kent bundle), creating a fusion pattern on the early portion of the QRS complex (Δ wave). The degree of ventricular "preexcitation" depends on the contribution of antegrade ventricular activation through the accessory pathway. Patients may have an accessory pathway that is not evident on surface ECGs, or they may have a "concealed" Kent bundle. These concealed accessory pathways are often incapable of antegrade conduction and can accept electrical stimulation only in a retrograde fashion. The ECG expression of preexcitation (Δ wave) depends on the location of the accessory pathway, the distance from the wavefront of sinus activation, and the conduction characteristics of the various structures involved. Like patients with dual atrioventricular nodal pathways, not all patients with preexcitation with an accessory atrioventricular pathway are capable of having clinical PSVT.

Patients with an accessory atrioventricular pathway may have three forms of supraventricular tachycardia: orthodromic reentry, antidromic reentry, and/or atrial fibrillation or flutter. Analogous to atrioventricular node reentry, atrioventricular reentrant PSVT usually involves two pathways (the normal atrioventricular node pathway and the accessory atrioventricular pathway), which have different electrophysiologic characteristics. The atrioventricular node pathway generally has a relatively slower conduction velocity and a shorter refractory period, and the accessory pathway has a faster conduction velocity and a longer refractory period. A critically timed premature impulse may block the accessory pathway, because it is still refractory from the previous sinus beat. However, the atrioventricular node pathway, with a relatively shorter refractory period, may accept antegrade conduction of the premature impulse. Meanwhile, the accessory pathway may recover its excitability and allow retrograde conduction. These circumstances initiate a macroreentrant tachycardia in which the antegrade pathway is the atrioventricular node pathway; the distal common pathway is the ventricle; the retrograde pathway the accessory pathway; and the proximal common pathway is the atrium (see Fig. 16–8).

This sequence of events (down node, up Kent bundle), termed orthodromic PSVT, is the common variety of reentry in patients with an accessory atrioventricular pathway, resulting in a narrow QRS complex tachycardia. In the uncommon variety of reentry (down Kent bundle, up node), conduction proceeds in the opposite direction, resulting in a wide QRS complex tachycardia, termed antidromic PSVT.

Patients with Wolff-Parkinson-White syndrome can have a third type of tachycardia, namely, atrial fibrillation. The mechanism for its occurrence is unknown, but the occurrence of this arrhythmia can be very serious and may lead to sudden death. As atrial fibrillation is an extremely rapid atrial tachycardia, conduction can proceed down the accessory atrioventricular pathway, producing a very fast ventricular response or even ventricular fibrillation. Unlike the atrioventricular nodal pathway, the refractory period of the accessory bundle shortens in response to rapid stimulation rates.

▶ TREATMENT: Paroxysmal Supraventricular Tachycardia

Both pharmacologic and nonpharmacologic methods have been used to treat patients with PSVT. Drugs used in the treatment of PSVT can be divided into three broad categories: (1) those that directly or indirectly increase vagal tone to the atrioventricular node, such as digoxin; (2) those that depress conduction through slow, calcium-dependent tissue, such as adenosine, β-blockers, and calcium channel blockers; and (3) those that depress conduction through fast, sodium-dependent tissue, such as quinidine, procainamide, disopyramide, and flecainide. Drugs within these categories alter the electrophysiologic characteristics of the reentrant substrate so that PSVT cannot be sustained.[38,39] In PSVT caused by atrioventricular node reentry, type I antiarrhythmic drugs, such as procainamide, act primarily on the fast, retrograde pathway. Digoxin and propranolol may work on either the fast, retrograde or the slow, antegrade limb. Verapamil, diltiazem, and adenosine prolong conduction time and increase refractoriness primarily in the slow, antegrade pathway of the reentrant loop. In PSVT caused by atrioventricular reentry incorporating an extranodal pathway, type I drugs increase refractoriness in the fast accessory pathway or within the His Purkinje system. Propranolol, digoxin, adenosine, and verapamil all act by their effects on the atrioventricular nodal (slow, antegrade) portion of the reentrant circuit. Regardless of the mechanism, treatment measures are directed at first terminating an acute episode of PSVT and then preventing symptomatic recurrences.

As in any rapid reentrant tachycardia resulting in severe symptoms (i.e., syncope, near syncope, anginal chest pain, and severe heart failure), synchronized DCC is the treatment of choice. Even at low energy levels (such as 25 W/s), DCC is almost always effective in quickly restoring sinus rhythm and correcting symptomatic hypotension in patients with PSVT. Patients with only mild to moderate symptoms usually do not require DCC, and non-drug measures that increase vagal tone to the atrioventricular node can be used initially. Unilateral carotid sinus massage, Valsalva maneuver, ice water facial immersion, induced retching, and other more elaborate vagomimetic measures are often successful in terminating PSVT, although carotid massage and Valsalva maneuver are the simplest, least obtrusive, and most frequently used of these techniques.

In the event that these methods fail, drug therapy is the next option. A therapeutic approach to the acute therapy of the different forms of reentrant PSVT is presented in Figure 16–9. This approach is based on analysis of the ECG characteristics of the rhythm, because PSVT is not always discernible from other arrhythmias, and some forms of PSVT require different treatment. In patients with a narrow QRS complex, regular arrhythmia (atrioventricular node reentry or orthodromic atrioventricular reentry), verapamil (5–10 mg given IV), diltiazem (15–25 mg given IV), or adenosine (6–12 mg) are all equally efficacious; any may be the agent of first choice. About 80% to 90% of PSVT episodes will revert to sinus rhythm within 5 minutes of IV therapy with verapamil, diltiazem, or adenosine.[40] Verapamil has the advantage in terms of cost, being available in generic formulations; whereas adenosine (although it has a higher frequency of side effects) may be safer because of its ultrashort duration of action. The most recent guidelines for emergency care from the American Heart Association promote adenosine as the drug of first choice in patients with PSVT.[41] These recommendations are particularly important when treating a patient who presents with a wide QRS complex, regular tachycardia that may be ventricular tachycardia, or PSVT (caused by

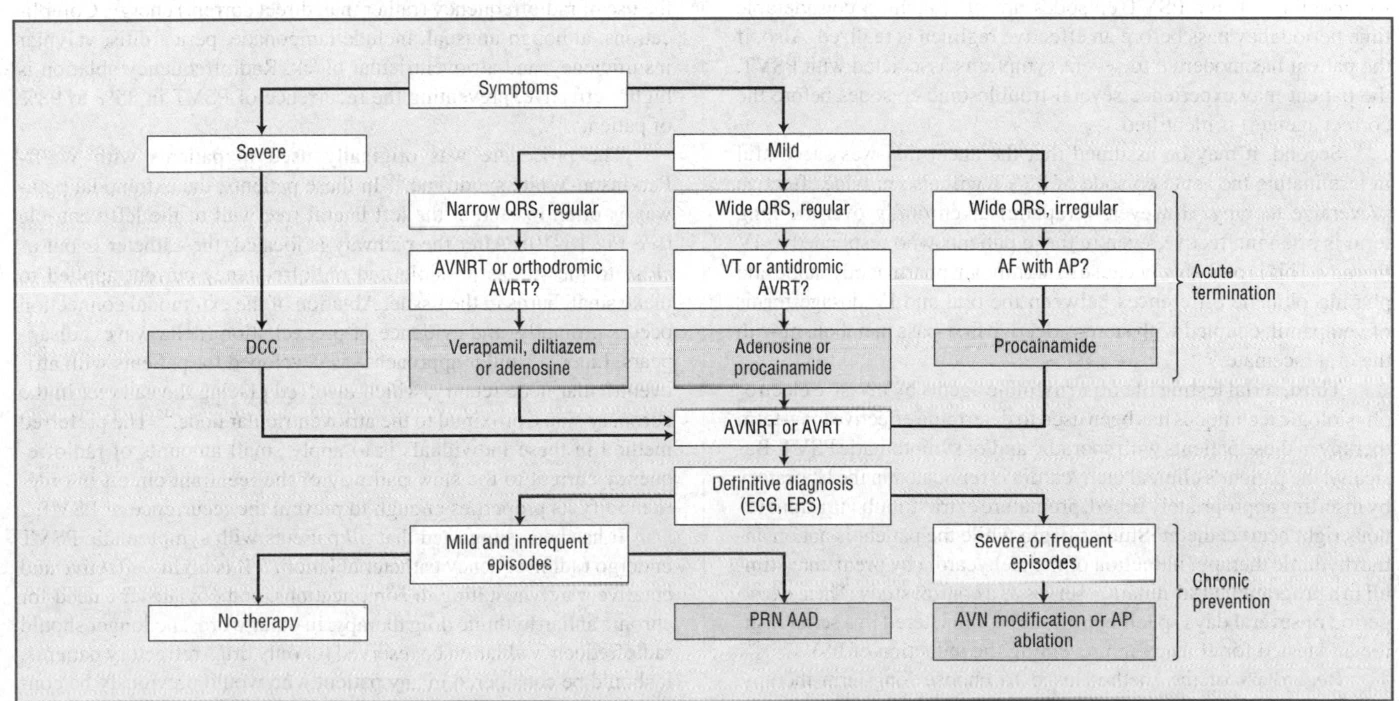

FIGURE 16–9. Algorithm for the treatment of acute (top portion) PSVT and chronic prevention of recurrences (bottom portion). DCC = direct-current cardioversion; AVN = atrioventricular node; AVNRT = atrioventricular node reentrant tachycardia; AVRT = atrioventricular reentrant tachycardia; VT = ventricular tachycardia; AF = atrial fibrillation; AP = accessory pathway; ECG = electrocardiographic monitoring, EPS = electrophysiologic studies, PRN = as needed, AAD = antiarrhythmic drugs. Note: For empiric bridge therapy prior to radiofrequency ablation procedures, calcium antagonists (or other atrioventricular node blockers) should not be used if the patient has atrioventricular reentry with an accessory pathway.

antidromic atrioventricular reentry or aberrancy). Because of its short duration of action (i.e., seconds), adenosine will not cause the severe and prolonged hemodynamic compromise seen in patients with ventricular tachycardia who were mistakenly treated with verapamil and suffer from its negative inotropic effects and vasodilator properties.[42] If, in fact, the arrhythmia is PSVT, adenosine will likely terminate it.

An alternative treatment for this type of patient is the IV administration of procainamide, which may terminate antidromic PSVT (by increasing refractoriness in the sodium-dependent extranodal pathway) as well as ventricular tachycardia. Procainamide given IV or perhaps IV amiodarone should be used for the patient who presents with a wide QRS complex and an irregular arrhythmia that is hemodynamically stable. This rhythm could represent atrial fibrillation with ventricular activation through an extranodal pathway. The IV administration of verapamil or adenosine to these patients could result in a paradoxical increase in ventricular response, causing severe symptoms and requiring cardioversion. These agents (particularly long-acting atrioventricular node blockers such as verapamil, diltiazem, and digoxin) are contraindicated in this specific setting.

Once the acute episode of PSVT is terminated, a decision on long-term preventive therapy must follow. Some patients may require long-term therapy; preventive treatment is indicated if (1) frequent episodes occur that necessitate therapeutic intervention (i.e., emergency department visits or interference with the patient's lifestyle); or (2) infrequent, but severe, symptoms occur. For those patients who need preventive treatment, there are three traditional strategies. First, clinicians may use a trial-and-error approach on an ambulatory basis for those patients with frequently recurrent, mildly symptomatic PSVT. Ambulatory ECG recordings (Holter) or telephonic transmissions of cardiac rhythm (event monitors) can be used to objectively document the efficacy or failure of drug therapy. The trial-and-error methods for determining drug effectiveness have inherent shortcomings. If the PSVT episodes are infrequent, a considerable time period may pass before an effective regimen is realized. Also, if the patient has moderate to severe symptoms associated with PSVT, the patient may experience several troublesome episodes before the correct agent(s) is identified.

Second, it may be assumed that the agent that was successful in terminating the acute episode of PSVT will also provide effective preventive therapy. However, verapamil taken orally over the long term is often ineffective, even in those patients who responded to IV therapy. This is probably because of significant pharmacodynamic and pharmacokinetic differences between the oral and IV dosage forms of verapamil, coupled with stereoselective first-pass metabolism with the oral racemate.[43]

Third, serial testing of antiarrhythmic agents by invasive electrophysiologic techniques has been used to determine effective long-term therapy in those patients with sporadic and/or symptomatic PSVT. Basically, the patient's clinical tachycardia is replicated in the laboratory by inserting appropriately timed, premature extra stimuli via a transvenous right heart catheter. Studies begin while the patient is not on antiarrhythmic therapy; induction of the tachycardia by premature stimuli in a programmed stimulation serves as a control study. Then, over a period of several days specific drugs are administered in a serial fashion and tested for efficacy in preventing the induction of PSVT.[38,39]

Regardless of the method used to choose long-term therapy, chronic antiarrhythmic drug treatment in these often young, otherwise healthy patients is problematic. Besides the necessity of taking daily medication, possibly for life, antiarrhythmic drugs are not well tolerated, sometimes precipitate severe side effects, and are commonly ineffective. For these reasons, non-drug therapies have been receiving attention. One such procedure, namely, transcutaneous

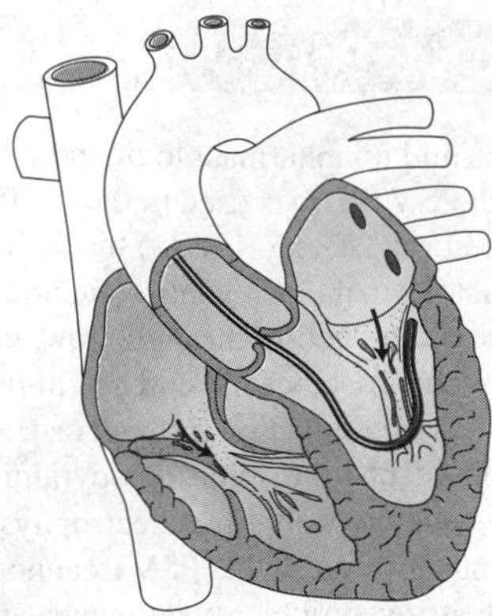

FIGURE 16–10. Catheter placement for radiofrequency ablation of left free wall accessory pathway. Here, the retrograde arterial approach is taken, although a venous (atrial) transseptal puncture has also been used. *(From M.M. Scheinman. Catheter ablation: Present role and projected impact on health care for patients with cardiac arrhythmias. Circulation 1991;83:1489–1498, with permission.)*

catheter ablation using radiofrequency current on the PSVT substrate has dramatically altered the traditional treatment of these patients (Fig.16–10). Radiofrequency energy delivered through a transvenous or arterial catheter causes small, discrete lesions through thermal energy. During invasive electrophysiologic studies, portions of the reentrant circuit can be located (or "mapped") by the use of a number of catheters. Once this is completed, radiofrequency energy is applied to kill or damage the tissue necessary for reentry. The destruction of the substrate for reentry "cures" the patient of recurrent episodes of PSVT and obviates the need for chronic drug therapy. Historically, ablation procedures were reserved for drug-refractory patients, because they necessitated open-heart surgery; however, breakthroughs in technology have allowed, first, transvenous catheter approaches and, then, the use of radiofrequency (rather than direct current) energy. Complications, although unusual, include tamponade, pericarditis, valvular insufficiency, and atrioventricular block. Radiofrequency ablation is highly effective, preventing the recurrence of PSVT in 85% to 98% of patients.[44,45]

The procedure was originally used in patients with Wolff-Parkinson-White syndrome.[44] In these patients, the extranodal pathway is often located at the left lateral free wall of the left ventricle (see Fig.16–10). After the pathway is located, the catheter is put as close to the site as possible and radiofrequency current applied to make small burns in the tissue. Ablation of the extranodal connection occurs promptly, and evidence of preexcitation (delta waves) disappears. Later, a similar approach was developed for patients with atrioventricular node reentry, which involved placing the catheter in the coronary sinus, proximal to the atrioventricular node.[45] The preferred method in these individuals is to apply small amounts of radiofrequency current to the slow pathway of the reentrant circuit in order to modify its properties enough to prevent the recurrence of PSVT.

It has been suggested that *all* patients with symptomatic PSVT undergo radiofrequency catheter ablation.[46] It is highly effective and curative, rarely resulting in complications, and obviates the need for chronic antiarrhythmic drug therapy. In other words, no longer should radiofrequency ablation be reserved for only drug-refractory patients; it should be considered in any patient who would previously be considered for chronic antiarrhythmic drug treatment. Radiofrequency ablation is also a cost-effective approach (in the long term) because, if effective, it eliminates the costs of drugs and repeated hospital visits. In one cost-effectiveness analysis, radiofrequency ablation improved quality of life and reduced lifetime medical expenditures by nearly $30,000 compared to chronic drug treatment.[47]

AUTOMATIC ATRIAL TACHYCARDIAS

Supraventricular foci with enhanced automatic properties appear to be the source of automatic atrial tachycardias, such as multifocal atrial tachycardia.[48] It is presumed that multifocal atrial tachycardia (sometimes referred to as chaotic atrial tachycardia) is the result of multiple ectopic atrial pacemakers, which accounts for the variable and differing P-wave morphology. In unifocal atrial tachycardia (sometimes referred to as ectopic atrial tachycardia) a single P-wave morphology different from that of sinus rhythm is recorded. In either case, the underlying, precipitating disorder present in the majority (60% to 80%) of these patients is severe pulmonary disease. Other disease states associated with these arrhythmias include acute infection (pneumonia and sepsis) and dilated congestive cardiomyopathy. Rarely, young patients without associated precipitating factors may present with rapid atrial tachycardias from unknown causes. In these cases, long-standing tachycardias cause the cardiomyopathic state. Effective treatment of the tachycardia may reverse the left ventricular dysfunction. Traditionally, many factors (i.e., electrolyte disturbances, hypoxia, catecholamines, tissue stretch) may cause an elevated slope of phase 4 depolarization and theoretically result in abnormal heightened automaticity. Many of these factors are oftentimes clinically present in patients with concurrent pulmonary disease and automatic atrial tachycardia. However, recent information[48,49] implies that triggered activity is a more likely mechanism in the genesis of these tachycardias. Atrial tachycardias with atrioventricular block or a slow ventricular response should alert the clinician to the possibility of digitalis toxicity.

▶ TREATMENT: Automatic Atrial Tachycardia

The first step in the treatment of automatic atrial tachycardia is to correct the underlying, precipitating factors.[48] The clinician should ensure proper oxygenation and ventilation, and correct acid-base or electrolyte disturbances. These measures alone may result in the return of sinus rhythm, but in some cases, the tachycardia will persist. Patients with an asymptomatic atrial tachycardia and a relatively slow ventricular response usually require no drug therapy. In symptomatic patients, medical therapy can be tailored either to control ventricular response or to restore sinus rhythm. Type I antiarrhythmic drugs such as procainamide or quinidine are occasionally effective in restoring sinus rhythm, presumably by their ability to decrease the automatic properties of latent pacemakers, but these agents are usually not considered first-line therapy. Direct-current cardioversion is ineffective in restoring sinus rhythm; serial drug testing is of no value, as programmed stimulation will not replicate the clinical tachycardia. To slow ventricular response, β-blockers are usually contraindicated because of the frequent coexistence of severe pulmonary disease or heart failure. Digoxin has been used, but is controversial because of its ability to increase the automatic properties of atrial tissue. Further, the high sympathetic state of these patients frequently overrides the vagotonic effects of digoxin, rendering it ineffective. Calcium antagonists such as verapamil are most effective and may now be considered first-line drug therapy.[49] Surprisingly, verapamil seems to decrease ventricular response by altering atrial automaticity, not by slowing atrioventricular node conduction.[49] Magnesium given IV (independent of serum magnesium) can also be effective, but the high doses necessary and transient duration render it impractical.[48] Both verapamil and magnesium given parenterally probably act by suppressing calcium-mediated triggered activity.

VENTRICULAR ARRHYTHMIAS

The common ventricular arrhythmias include (1) ventricular premature beats (VPBs), (2) ventricular tachycardia, and (3) ventricular fibrillation. Again, these arrhythmias may result in a wide variety of symptoms. Often, VPBs cause no symptoms or only mild palpitations. The presentation of ventricular tachycardia may range from a life-threatening situation associated with hemodynamic collapse to a totally asymptomatic one. Ventricular fibrillation, by definition, is an acute medical emergency necessitating cardiopulmonary resuscitation.

VENTRICULAR PREMATURE BEATS

Very common ventricular rhythm disturbances, VPBs occur in patients with or without heart disease. Experimental models have shown that abnormal automaticity, triggered activity, or reentrant mechanisms may elicit premature ventricular depolarizations. It has become well-known that VPBs often occur in apparently healthy individuals, although they occur more frequently and in more complex forms in patients with detectable heart disease. In overtly normal subjects without discernible heart disease, VPBs seem to have little, if any, prognostic significance. In patients with myocardial infarction (acute or remote), however, those with some forms of VPBs are at higher risk for "sudden death" than are those without these minor rhythm disturbances. Sudden cardiac death can be defined as unexpected death occurring in a patient within 1 hour of experiencing symptoms. Studies of patients who experienced sudden cardiac death (and happened to be wearing an ECG monitor at the time) often demonstrate the cause to be ventricular fibrillation preceded by a short run of ventricular tachycardia and frequent VPBs.[50] Therein lies the basis of the so-called VPB hypothesis: preventing more minor arrhythmias, such as VPBs, may prevent the occurrence of sudden death.

Historically, investigators promoted the concept that patients in the acute phase of myocardial infarction may have certain types of VPBs that are predictive of ventricular fibrillation and sudden cardiac death. Referred to as "warning arrhythmias," these types of VPBs include frequent ectopy (more than 5 beats per minute), multiform configuration (different morphology), couplets (two in a row), and R-on-T phenomenon (VPBs occurring during the repolarization phase of the preceding sinus beat in the vulnerable period of ventricular recovery). Through the use of sophisticated monitoring techniques, however, it has become apparent that almost all patients have warning arrhythmias in the acute infarction setting. In those patients who experience ventricular fibrillation, warning arrhythmias are no more common than in those without ventricular fibrillation. Therefore, warning arrhythmias observed during acute myocardial infarction are neither sensitive nor specific in predicting which patients will have ventricular fibrillation. Therefore, in patients with acute myocardial infarction, there is little need to direct drug therapy (usually lidocaine) specifically at VPB suppression. Studies have shown that effective prevention of ventricular fibrillation in the acute infarction setting may be achieved without the abolition of VPBs. The inability of VPBs (warning arrhythmias) to predict the occurrence of ventricular fibrillation, coupled with the lack of correlation between a drug's effectiveness in preventing ventricular fibrillation and suppressing VPBs, form the rationale for suggesting antiarrhythmic drug prophylaxis (e.g., with lidocaine, magnesium) for all patients with an uncomplicated acute myocardial infarction.

On the other hand, data strongly imply that VPBs documented in the convalescence period of myocardial infarction do carry important long-term prognostic significance.[51] Those VPBs that occur after a myocardial infarction seem to be a risk factor for patient death that is independent of the degree of left ventricular dysfunction or the extent of coronary atherosclerosis. Lown and Wolf have developed a grading scale for classifying different types of VPBs:[52] grade 0, no ectopy; grade I, less than 30 VPBs/h of uniform morphology; grade II, more than 30 VPBs/h of uniform morphology; grade III, multiform VPBs; grade IVa, couplets; grade IVb, 3 or more consecutive VPBs (nonsustained ventricular tachycardia); grade V, R-on-T phenomenon. It is a common assumption that the higher grades of VPBs within this classification system imply a higher risk of subsequent arrhythmogenic death. This assumption has never been proved.

Ruberman and co-workers devised a simple alternative classification based on the significance of simple or benign (infrequent and monomorphic) versus "complex" (all other types in the Lown classification) forms of VPBs.[51] These investigators found that the presence of complex ventricular ectopy in the setting of ischemic heart disease was associated with a higher incidence of cardiac death (but not necessarily arrhythmogenic death). Within the controversy about the significance of VPBs, there is clearly a basic question: are complex forms of VPBs simply an unimportant marker of underlying structural heart disease, or are VPBs an important electrical disorder that should be addressed independently?

▶ TREATMENT: Ventricular Premature Beats

Because VPBs without associated heart disease in apparently healthy individuals carry little or no risk, drug therapy is unnecessary. The prognostic significance of complex VPBs in patients with heart disease has made the use of antiarrhythmic drug therapy to suppress them controversial in these patients, however. Traditionally, many have supported aggressive drug therapy designed to suppress a high percentage of VPBs, based on the Lown grading system. The underlying reason for this approach is to attempt to eliminate a risk factor for cardiac death in patients with coronary disease, namely, the presence of complex VPBs.Others have favored a more conservative approach and disregarded drug therapy in the absence of significant symptoms. The release of the initial CAST results[28] clearly supports the later, conservative approach.

The National Institutes of Health (NIH) initiated the CAST[28,53] in 1987 to determine if suppression of ventricular ectopy with encainide, flecainide, or moricizine could decrease the incidence of death from arrhythmia in patients who had suffered a myocardial infarction. Entrance criteria included documented myocardial infarction between 6 days and 2 years prior to enrollment, and 6 or more VPBs/h without runs of ventricular tachycardia greater than 15 beats in length. Also, patients were required to have an ejection fraction equal to or less than 55% if recruited within 90 days of myocardial infarction or equal to or less than 40% if recruited 90 days or more after infarction. Patients with an ejection fraction less than 30% were randomized only to a regimen of encainide or moricizine. Patients were randomized to receive drug therapy or placebo after demonstrating VPB suppression with one of the agents. The drug and dose were determined during an open-label dose titration phase that preceded randomization.

In April of 1989, a routine, preliminary review of the study by the Safety and Monitoring Board revealed alarming results, and the study was interrupted. The results showed that compared to treatment with placebo, treatment with encainide or flecainide was associated with a significantly higher rate of total mortality and death due to arrhythmia, presumably due to proarrhythmia (Fig. 16–11). Analysis of the moricizine arm indicated neither harm nor benefit from this therapy; therefore, only this portion of the study was allowed to continue as CAST II. Later (July 1991), however, CAST II was also prematurely stopped, when a trend toward an increase in mortality was observed in moricizine-treated patients. This was particularly true during the dose titration phase, but not during the chronic treatment phase. The overall results of the two CASTs conclusively prove that patients with VPBs after myocardial infarction do not benefit from chronic antiarrhythmic drug therapy (beyond the general use of β-blocking agents), and, in fact, most drugs are detrimental. The study also puts into perspective the risk associated with the use of antiarrhythmic therapy and the need to administer antiarrhythmic drugs only to those patients with a defined therapeutic benefit.

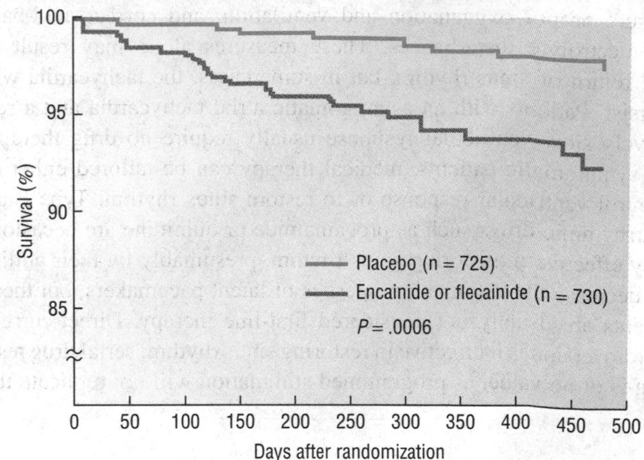

FIGURE 16–11. Life table curves from the CAST, specifically for patients receiving encainide or flecainide (lighter line) and matching placebo (darker line). Note the divergent slopes of each line, implying sustained risk of death (presumed proarrhythmia). *(From N Engl J Med 1989;321:406–412, with permission.)*

The CAST is one of the most important trials ever undertaken by the NIH and has had a tremendous influence on the overall approach to the treatment of tachycardias; in addition, it has had a far-reaching impact on new drug development. The results have colored the long-term use of all antiarrhythmics, causing a broad skepticism toward the risk-benefit profile of this class of drugs. Pharmaceutical companies, as a result, have shifted their drug discovery and investigative efforts away from potent sodium channel blockers. As immediate fallout, the pharmaceutical company pulled encainide from the market, and another pharmaceutical manufacturer decided not to market the type Ic agent indecainide despite Food and Drug Administration (FDA) approval. The CAST findings also provided additional fuel for the pursuit of non-drug therapies for tachycardias, such as ablation and implantable devices.

Post-myocardial infarction patients with complex ventricular ectopy remain at risk for death. Therefore, other drugs besides the type Ic agents have been studied. One of these, sotalol, is marketed as a racemic mixture of a *d* and *l* isomer: both are type III potassium blockers, but the *l* isomer has β-blocking actions. Chronic therapy with *d*-sotalol was studied in patients with remote myocardial infarction complicated by complex ectopy in the Survival With Oral *d*-Sotalol (SWORD) trial.[54] Unlike the CAST, *d*-sotalol treatment was not designed to suppress VPBs, yet like the CAST, the trial was halted prematurely because of excessive mortality in the treatment arm. Again, the presumed reason for this happening was *d*-sotalol-related proarrhythmia.

Currently, only two antiarrhythmic drugs have been shown *not* to increase mortality with long-term use: amiodarone and dofetilide. A number of trials have shown amiodarone to decrease the incidence of sudden (or arrhythmic) death, but not total mortality in post-myocardial infarction patients with complex ventricular ectopy.[55,56] A meta-analysis of all trials (6,553 combined patients) demonstrated a reduction in total mortality (by 13%) with long-term amiodarone therapy.[57] It is unclear if this finding can be attributed to one property (e.g., β-blocking) or a combination of amiodarone's complex pharmacologic effects on conduction. In two major studies, patients treated with amiodarone *and* a β-blocker generally did better than those who did not receive a β-blocker.[55,56] Clearly, because of its impressive adverse effect profile and its inability to improve survival, amiodarone cannot routinely be recommended in patients with heart disease such as remote myocardial infarction and complex VPBs. Two randomized, controlled trials have shown chronic therapy with dofetilide to have no effect on overall mortality in patients who have suffered myocardial infarction with left ventricular dysfunction.[58,59] Dofetilide (not approved for prevention of sudden death) caused torsades de pointes in about 5% of patients, necessitating a protocol amendment with dosage adjustments during both trials (particularly in those with renal disease, because the primary route of elimination is through the kidney).

How should the clinician approach the patient at risk for sudden cardiac death? Clearly, VPBs should not be suppressed with antiarrhythmic drugs. Indeed, those with risk factors for arrhythmic death (recent myocardial infarction, left ventricular dysfunction, complex VPBs) should not be routinely given *any* type I or III antiarrhythmic agent.[60] Only β-blockers have been conclusively proved to prevent overall mortality in these patients; therefore, chronic drug therapy should be restricted to these agents.

VENTRICULAR TACHYCARDIA

A wide QRS tachycardia, ventricular tachycardia may acutely occur as a result of metabolic abnormalities, ischemia, or drug toxicity; it may chronically recur as a paroxysmal form. On ECG inspection, ventricular tachycardia may appear as either repetitive monomorphic or polymorphic ventricular complexes. The definition of ventricular tachycardia is 3 or more repetitive VPBs, occurring at a rate greater than 100 beats/min. Severe electrolyte abnormalities (e.g., hypokalemia), hypoxemia, or digitalis toxicity may precipitate an acute episode of ventricular tachycardia; most commonly, it occurs during an acute myocardial infarction. In these cases, correction of the underlying precipitating factors will usually prevent further recurrences of ventricular tachycardia. For example, if ventricular tachycardia occurs during the first 24 hours of an acute myocardial infarction and treatment is effective, it will probably not reappear on a chronic basis after the infarcted area has healed or ischemia resolved. This form of acute ventricular tachycardia may result either from enhanced automatic properties of a ventricular focus or from reentrant mechanisms within the ischemic ventricle.

In contrast, some patients have a chronic, recurrent form of ventricular tachycardia that is almost always associated with some type of underlying organic heart disease. Common examples are paroxysmal ventricular tachycardia associated with idiopathic dilated cardiomyopathy or remote myocardial infarction with a left ventricular aneurysm. Indeed, left ventricular dysfunction and aneurysm formation are risk factors for the development of recurrent ventricular tachycardia after myocardial infarction. In chronic, recurrent ventricular tachycardia, microreentry within the distal Purkinje network is presumed to be responsible for the underlying substrate in a large majority of patients (see Fig. 16–3). Theoretically, electrophysiologic discrepancies occur as a result of structural damage and heart disease within the ventricular conducting system. The reentrant circuit may possess both anatomically determined and functional properties, coursing through normal tissue, damaged (but not dead) tissue, and islands of necrosed tissue. In a minority of patients, macroreentrant circuits may be responsible for recurrent ventricular tachycardia, including reentry that incorporates the bundle branches.

▶ TREATMENT: Ventricular Tachycardia

Patients with acute ventricular tachycardia associated with a precipitating factor often suffer severe symptoms requiring immediate treatment measures. Chronic, recurrent ventricular tachycardia may also cause severe hemodynamic compromise, but sometimes only mild, generally well tolerated symptoms result. There are different varieties of ventricular tachycardia. Sustained ventricular tachycardia is that which requires therapeutic intervention to restore a stable rhythm or lasts a relatively long time (usually > 30 seconds). Nonsustained ventricular tachycardia is that which self-terminates after a brief duration (usually < 30 seconds). If the patient has ventricular tachycardia more frequently than sinus rhythm (i.e., if ventricular tachycardia is the dominant rhythm), the condition is referred to as incessant ventricular tachycardia. Exercise-induced ventricular tachycardia is that which occurs during times of high sympathetic tone, such as physical exertion. Monomorphic ventricular tachycardia has a consistent QRS configuration, whereas polymorphic ventricular tachycardia has varying QRS complexes. A characteristic type of polymorphic ventricular tachycardia, in which the QRS complexes appear to undulate around a central axis and is associated with evidence of delayed ventricular repolarization (long QT interval or prominent U waves), is referred to as torsades de pointes.

Like other rapid tachycardias, the initial management of an acute episode of ventricular tachycardia requires a quick assessment of the patient's status and symptoms. If symptoms are severe, then DCC should be instituted to restore sinus rhythm immediately. An investigation should be made into possible precipitating factors, and these should be corrected if possible. The diagnosis of acute myocardial infarction should be entertained. If the episode of ventricular tachycardia is felt to be an isolated electrical event associated with a transient initiating factor (e.g., acute myocardial ischemia, digitalis toxicity), there is no need for long-term antiarrhythmic therapy once the precipitating factors are corrected (e.g., an infarct has healed, the patient is stable). Nevertheless, the patient should be monitored closely for possible recurrences of ventricular tachycardia.

Patients with mild or no symptoms during an acute episode of ventricular tachycardia can be initially treated with antiarrhythmic drugs, but DCC should be readily available. (See the most recent Guidelines for Cardiopulmonary Resuscitation and Emergency Cardiac Care put forth by the American Heart Association.[41]) The IV administration of amiodarone is now usually the first step in this situation. Procainamide or lidocaine given IV are suitable alternatives, although one small study comparing these two agents showed procainamide to be superior in terminating ventricular tachycardia.[61] If the patient's status deteriorates, ventricular tachycardia degenerates to ventricular fibrillation, or drug therapy fails, DCC should be instituted. As an alternative to DCC, a transvenous pacing wire can be inserted and ventricular tachycardia terminated by overdrive pacing methods.

Once an acute episode of sustained ventricular tachycardia has been successfully terminated by electrical or pharmacologic means and an acute myocardial infarction ruled out, the possibility of paroxysmal ventricular tachycardia recurring should be considered. The use of invasive electrophysiologic study using programmed ventricular stimulation can often confirm this possibility. The management of the patient with chronic, recurrent sustained ventricular tachycardia deserves considerable attention because these patients are at extremely high risk for death; trial-and-error attempts to find effective therapy are unwarranted. Two methods of identifying effective drug therapy, using surrogate end points have been used: (1) inability to induce sustained ventricular tachycardia with programmed extrastimuli by invasive electrophysiologic studies and (2) suppression of ventricular ectopy by serial 24-hour continuous ECG (Holter) monitoring.

Electrophysiologic studies based on programmed stimulation incorporate the concepts of reentry in order to replicate the patient's clinical tachycardia in a controlled laboratory setting. The patient is admitted to the hospital (often in an intensive care setting), and ECG strips of the clinical tachycardia are carefully analyzed. All antiarrhythmic drugs are discontinued. After the systemic elimination of these drugs, the patient is brought to the electrophysiology laboratory unsedated. Here transvenous multipolar catheters, which can both pace the heart and record electrical activity, are inserted into the right heart. Next, attempts are made to replicate the clinical tachycardia by the insertion of early beats and/or pacing methods via programmed stimulation. If the clinical tachycardia is replicated, this initial study (done without drug therapy) serves as a control that can be compared to subsequent studies on drug therapy. Once ventricular tachycardia has been induced by programmed stimulation, it can be terminated by programmed stimulation, overdrive pacing, or DCC, depending on the patient's status. Antiarrhythmic drugs can then be serially administered, and the electrophysiologic study is repeated (at presumed drug steady state). If the control study induces sustained ventricular tachycardia, then the inability to reproduce ventricular tachycardia or the induction of only brief, self-terminating episodes of ventricular tachycardia (usually less than 15 beats) upon repeat testing during drug treatment generally predicts that that drug will be effective in preventing recurrent episodes on a long-term basis. When drug therapy renders ventricular tachycardia noninducible, a serum drug level should be obtained immediately. This serum level then serves as the patient's target level for chronic oral therapy (Fig. 16–12). Efforts should be directed to keep the serum level at or above this target to prevent recurrence of the arrhythmia.[62]

Although this method can be efficacious in determining effective antiarrhythmic drug therapy in patients with recurrent ventricular tachycardia, it has several drawbacks besides its invasive nature. Foremost is the fact that the yield for finding an effective drug is low. Sustained monomorphic ventricular tachycardia can be rendered noninducible or nonsustained in only 20% to 25% of patients. Therefore, the clinician frequently must search for other therapeutic options or settle for other treatment end points, such as slower and more tolerable inducible ventricular tachycardia. Amiodarone is clearly the most effective (about 50% effective after 2 years) agent in patients with recurrent ventricular tachycardia; however, electrophysiologic drug testing does not necessarily predict the clinical efficacy of amiodarone. Patients may have continued inducibility of ventricular tachycardia on amiodarone despite the success of long-term therapy. Indeed, empiric amiodarone has been compared to therapy with other agents guided by electrophysiologic testing in patients at high risk for recurrent ventricular tachycardia.[63] In this trial, amiodarone therapy without invasive testing was superior in preventing cardiac death and recurrences of severe ventricular arrhythmias at all time points.

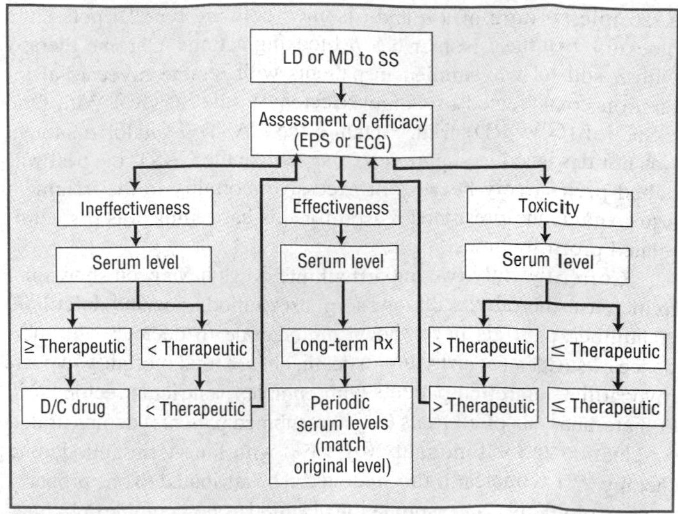

FIGURE 16–12. Algorithm for the clinical approach to therapeutic drug monitoring of antiarrhythmic drugs. LD = loading dose; MD = maintenance dose; SS = steady-state; EPS = electrophysiologic study; ECG = continuous electrocardiographic monitoring; D/C = discontinue drug.

Older trials that seemingly demonstrated the usefulness of serial drug testing in identifying effective chronic agents always lack a control group (i.e., a group of patients whose ventricular tachycardia was rendered noninducible after treatment with an antiarrhythmic drug and who are not treated chronically with that agent). This was obviously done because of ethical concerns, but raises the possibility that noninducibility simply identifies low-risk patients, independent of drug treatment.

As noted earlier, the second method used to determine therapy for patients with chronic, recurrent sustained ventricular tachycardia is the use of serial Holter monitors with drug testing. The surrogate end point in this case is the suppression of ventricular ectopy and total abolition of nonsustained ventricular tachycardia compared to control (drug-free) recordings. Clinicians in the United States did not use this method routinely; initial small studies[64] demonstrated a superiority of invasive electrophysiologic testing over serial Holter recordings.[64] Nonetheless, there was enough controversy to initiate a large study to compare the two methods of drug testing. The Electrophysiologic Study Versus Electrocardiographic Monitoring (ESVEM) Trial enrolled patients with documented clinical ventricular tachycardia/ventricular fibrillation, inducible ventricular tachycardia, and frequent ventricular ectopy.[65,66] These patients were randomized to electrophysiologic studies or serial Holter recordings to test up to seven antiarrhythmic drugs (imipramine, mexiletine, pirmenol, procainamide, quinidine, propafenone, or sotalol). Holter testing identified effective agents in more patients, and there was no statistical difference between this method and electrophysiologic testing in terms of ventricular tachycardia recurrence or sudden death. Although patients with poor left ventricular systolic function could not receive it in the ESVEM Trial, sotalol proved to be the most effective drug in the trial. The relatively impressive results in the ESVEM Trial with racemic sotalol, in contrast to the poor results of its *d*-isomer in the SWORD Study (which admittedly involved a different population), speak strongly for the importance of chronic treatment with β-blockers in patients with serious ventricular arrhythmias. Regardless of the methods of drug testing, recurrence rate of ventricular tachycardia in the ESVEM Trial was high (20% to 50% per year depending on the drug chosen). These findings and the impressive side effect profiles of antiarrhythmic agents have led investigators to study non-drug approaches to the treatment of recurrent ventricular tachycardia/ventricular fibrillation.[67]

Some centers have had excellent results with the surgical excision of the ventricular tachycardia focus in appropriate candidates for this extensive procedure. With the aid of endocardial mapping techniques, procedures such as ventricular aneurysectomy, encircling ventriculotomy, and cryoablation or laser ablation can successfully abolish the arrhythmogenic substrate. However, the introduction and advances in the automatic implantable cardioverter-defibrillator (ICD), coupled with its demonstrated effectiveness, has obviated the need for serial drug testing (by invasive or noninvasive methods) and many risky surgical procedures (Fig. 16–13). Early ICDs required a thoracotomy for placement and were programmed to tachycardia rate. Once the patient's rate rose to a certain level, a series of internal defibrillations were delivered. Although effective in terminating ventricular tachycardia/ventricular fibrillation, inappropriate shocks were sometimes delivered for either sustained ventricular tachycardia episodes or nonsustained ventricular tachycardia. Further, the pulse generator that was placed in the abdomen had a relatively short battery life in these early models. ICD technology is rapidly expanding so that the newer devices employ a "tiered therapy approach;" they provide, sequentially, programmed stimulation, overdrive pacing, and then low energy cardioversion before internal defibrillation is employed as a last step. In addition, backup bradycardia pacing and extended battery lives have made these devices much more attractive. Importantly, most institutions are now routinely using transvenous insertion techniques that do not require a thoracotomy, and the pulse generator is now small enough to implant in the pectoral region of the chest (see Fig. 16–13).

Most would agree that the ICD is the most highly effective method in preventing sudden death due to recurrent ventricular tachycardia or ventricular fibrillation,[68] although several problems remain.

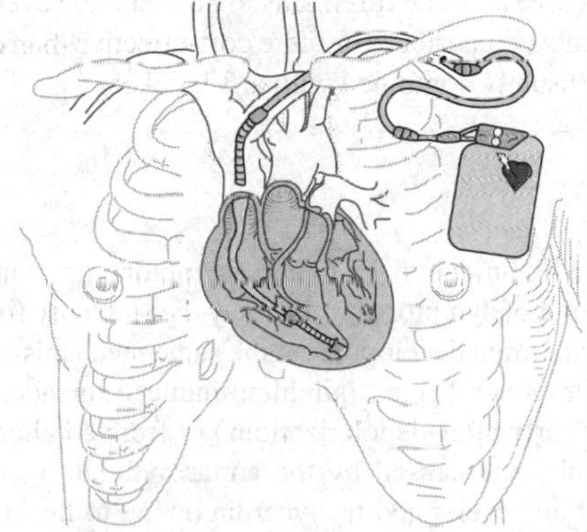

FIGURE 16–13. Automatic implantable cardioverter-defibrillators with newer methods of device placement. There is an endocardial lead system in which the leads are placed transvenously without the need for a thoracotomy. The generator is now small enough to be placed in the pectoral region of the chest. *(From Cardiac Pacemakers, Inc. St. Paul, MN, with permission.)*

First, the device and its implantation are expensive. Total cost for the device, implantation procedure, electrophysiologic studies, hospitalization, and physician fees may be as much as $50,000. Second, many patients (as high as 50%) end up receiving antiarrhythmic drugs (usually amiodarone) as well. Here, the end point of drug therapy is different from that of therapy without the ICD, in that the drugs do not necessarily need to prevent all sustained recurrences. Antiarrhythmic drugs are prescribed in this instance to decrease the frequency of ventricular tachycardia/ventricular fibrillation episodes and nonsustained ventricular tachycardia, minimize patient discomfort, and save battery life. The management of each patient should be individualized and antiarrhythmic drugs administered in those with frequent ventricular tachycardia and shocks. Because many agents alter defibrillation thresholds, the addition of antiarrhythmic drugs to ICD therapy necessitates reprogramming of the device.[69]

Which is better: antiarrhythmic drugs or the ICD? The use of the ICD in patients with remote myocardial infarction, left ventricular dysfunction, and nonsustained ventricular tachycardia who had inducible sustained ventricular tachycardia during programmed stimulation was compared to the chronic administration of antiarrhythmic drug (>90% empiric amiodarone) therapy in the Antiarrhythmic drug Versus Internal Defibrillator (AVID) Trial.[70] The trial was stopped early because of a demonstrated superiority of the ICD: patients in the ICD group had a better overall survival (75% vs. 64% at 3 years). In other words, in this important study, the benefit of the ICD was superior to that of the most effective drug known, namely, amiodarone. Despite the high costs, these results provide strong support for the aggressive use of the ICD in patients at high risk for recurrent life-threatening ventricular arrhythmias. Further, in patients who have inducible sustained ventricular tachycardia (after out-of-hospital cardiac arrest), early ICD implantation has been shown to be more cost-effective than antiarrhythmic drug therapy guided by electrophysiologic studies.[71] Although nearly all clinicians now consider implantation of the ICD as first-line treatment in patients with recurrent sustained ventricular tachycardia/ventricular fibrillation, there is one patient group that may possibly do as well with drug therapy alone. In the AVID trial, patients with only mild left ventricular dysfunction (i.e., ejection fraction > 35%) treated with amiodarone (especially with a β-blocker) did just as well as if they had been treated with an ICD. It is possible that this specific subgroup of patients could be treated without an ICD. The results of several ongoing trials may aid in this decision and help stratify which patients should receive the ICD and which should not. For instance, the Sudden Cardiac Death in Heart Failure Trial (SCD-Heft) will evaluate survival in patients with left ventricular dysfunction who are at risk for sudden death and are treated with amiodarone or an ICD.[72]

At this time, it is clear that patients with complex ventricular ectopy should not receive type I or type III antiarrhythmic drugs and that those with recurrent, sustained ventricular tachycardia definitely require some form of preventive treatment, generally an ICD with or without amiodarone, but the approach to nonsustained ventricular tachycardia remains an area of controversy. Obviously, those patients with long, symptomatic episodes require drug therapy, but most have no symptoms. Epidemiologic data indicate that patients with nonsustained ventricular tachycardia and coronary disease are at increased risk for sudden death.[73] However, partly because of the results of the CAST and similar trials with antiarrhythmic drugs, clinicians have sought more clear risk stratification before initiating drug therapy.

Traditionally, there are three strategies to approach the treatment of nonsustained ventricular tachycardia: (1) conservative (no antiarrhythmic drug treatment beyond β-blockers); (2) empiric amiodarone, and (3) aggressive (i.e., electrophysiologic) studies with possible insertion of an ICD. A number of early studies have

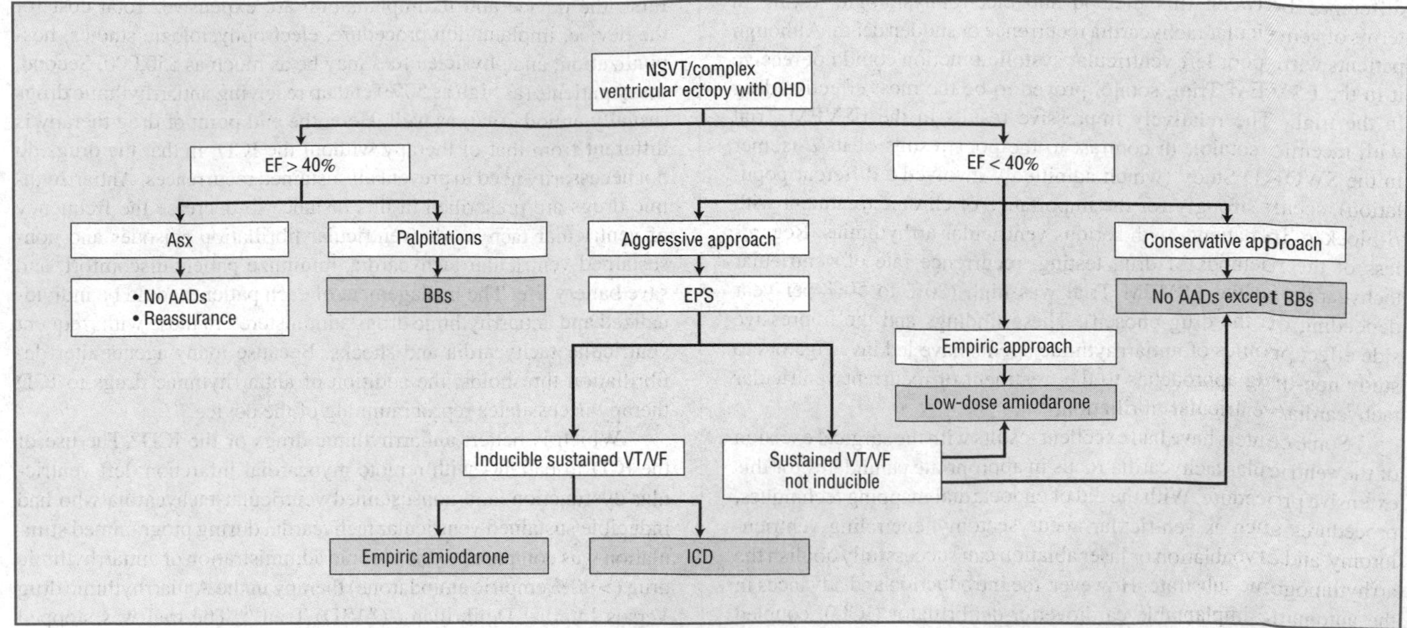

FIGURE 16–14. Algorithm for the management of patients with ventricular ectopy or nonsustained ventricular tachycardia (NSVT) in patients with organic heart disease (OHD, usually after myocardial infarction). EF = ejection fraction; Asx = asymptomatic; AADs = antiarrhythmic drugs; BBs = β-blockers; EPS = electrophysiologic studies; VT/VF = ventricular tachycardia/ventricular fibrillation; ICD = implantable cardioverter-defibrillator.

suggested that tests such as electrophysiologic studies could be used to determine long-term risk in patients with nonsustained ventricular tachycardia.[74,75] For instance, Wilber and associates demonstrated that post-myocardial infarction patients with nonsustained ventricular tachycardia and inducible, sustained ventricular tachycardia after programmed stimulation were at increased risk for subsequent ventricular tachycardia/ventricular fibrillation or sudden death compared to those in whom sustained ventricular tachycardia could not be induced.[74] These data provide the basis for the Multicenter Unsustained Tachycardia Trial (MUST).[76] In the MUST, patients with asymptomatic clinical nonsustained ventricular tachycardia (more than 3 beats), inducible sustained ventricular tachycardia, or left ventricular dysfunction were randomized to the conservative approach (no antiarrhythmic drug therapy beyond β-blockers) or electrophysiologic guided therapy (antiarrhythmic drugs and/or ICD). The results showed that the conservative approach had a significantly higher rate of events (cardiac arrest or death). When the results of the electrophysiologically guided group were further stratified, however, the outcomes of those receiving only antiarrhythmic drugs (no ICD) were no different from the outcomes of those who received no treatment. In other words, only those treated with an ICD had a significantly lower event rate and greater survival. One problem with the MUST is that because of the time frame in which the trial was initiated (1989), nearly 50% of patients received type I antiarrhythmic drugs or drugs that are now known not to improve survival in patients with coronary disease and ventricular arrhythmias; only 10% received the most effective agent in this setting, amiodarone.

In summary, at this time, patients with coronary disease, left ventricular dysfunction, or nonsustained ventricular tachycardia should undergo electrophysiologic studies. If these patients do not have inducible sustained ventricular tachycardia/ventricular fibrillation, they need no antiarrhythmic drug therapy targeted specifically to the arrhythmia on a chronic basis. On the other hand, if sustained ventricular tachycardia/ventricular fibrillation is inducible, chronic preventive therapy is warranted (Fig. 16–14). Because of the result of the MUST, many will receive an ICD. It remains to be seen, however, if the ICD in these patients is superior to or more cost-effective than empiric oral amiodarone (usually combined with a β-blocker).

PROARRHYTHMIA

All antiarrhythmic agents have the potential to aggravate existing arrhythmias or to cause new arrhythmias. It is believed that antiarrhythmic drugs may cause proarrhythmia in 5% to 20% of patients.[10] Although drug-induced arrhythmias have been recognized for several years, only recently has this adverse effect gained widespread attention. Many definitions for proarrhythmia have been proposed; in simplest terms, it indicates the development of a significant new arrhythmia (e.g., ventricular tachycardia, ventricular fibrillation, or torsades de pointes) or an exacerbation of an existing arrhythmia (longer, faster, or more frequent episodes). As with all arrhythmias, the consequences of proarrhythmia are varied. Some patients who develop proarrhythmia may be totally asymptomatic; others may notice a worsening of symptoms; some may die suddenly from this side effect. Proarrhythmia develops from the same mechanisms that cause arrhythmias in general (e.g., quinidine-induced torsades de pointes as a result of early after-depolarizations) or from an alteration in the underlying substrate caused by the antiarrhythmic agent (e.g., development of an accelerated tachycardia owing to flecainide, which decreases conduction velocity without significantly altering the refractory period).[10] (See Fig. 16–4.) The diagnosis of proarrhythmia is sometimes difficult to make because of the variable nature of the underlying arrhythmias. However, in all cases, the agent should be discontinued if proarrhythmia is detected or suspected.

Associated with type Ic antiarrhythmia agents, the prototypical form of proarrhythmia is a rapid, sustained, monomorphic ventricular tachycardia with a characteristic sinusoidal QRS pattern that is often resistant to resuscitation with cardioversion or overdrive pacing. Sometimes referred to as sinusoidal or incessant ventricular tachycardia, it is the result of excessive sodium channel blockade and slowed conduction. A rare heritable form of this tachycardia (Brugada's syndrome) has been described and linked to genetic abnormalities in the fast sodium channel. Sinusoidal ventricular tachycardia caused by type Ic agents was thought to occur within the first several days of drug initiation; however, the results of the CAST indicate that the risk may exist as long as the agent is continued. Factors that definitely predispose patients to this form of proarrhythmia are (1) the presence of underlying ventricular arrhythmias, (2) ischemic heart disease, and (3) poor left ventricular function. Provocation of proarrhythmia owing to the type Ic agents is sometimes reported during exercise; this is more than likely because of augmented slowed conduction at rapid heart rates (i.e., rate-dependent sodium blockade). The incidence of proarrhythmia is greatest in patients with all three risk factors (approximately 10% to 20%) and considerably less (<5%) in those without risks, such as patients with good left ventricular function and supraventricular tachycardias. Interestingly, in one study of risk factors, the incidence of death from proarrhythmia associated with the use of encainide and flecainide was approximately the same as the chance of long-term effectiveness.[77] Other factors that have a less defined association with proarrhythmia are elevated serum concentrations of the antiarrhythmic agent and rapid escalation of dosage. It has been proposed that the presence of underlying ventricular conduction delays may also pose a risk. As mentioned earlier, this arrhythmia is resistant to resuscitation; however, some have had success with the IV administration of lidocaine (which competes for sodium channel receptor) or the administration of sodium bicarbonate (which reverses the excessive sodium channel blockade).

TORSADES DE POINTES

With torsades de pointes, a rapid form of polymorphic ventricular tachycardia, there is evidence of delayed ventricular repolarization (long QT interval or prominent U waves) on surface ECGs (Fig. 16–15). Polymorphic ventricular tachycardia, occurring in the setting of a normal QT interval, is similar to monomorphic ventricular tachycardia in terms of etiology and treatment strategies. Torsades de pointes may occur in association with hereditary syndromes or in an acquired form. The underlying cause in both cases is delayed ventricular repolarization because of blockade of potassium conductance. Two well described heritable forms are Romano and Ward's syndrome (long QT interval, torsades de pointes, and high incidence of sudden death) and Jervell and Lange-Neilson's syndrome (long QT interval, torsades de pointes, high incidence of sudden death, and congenital deaf-mutism). These relatively unusual syndromes originate in genetic abnormalities in the function of the cardiac potassium or sodium channels that govern repolarization. Recent breakthroughs in the understanding of the exact genetic abnormalities of these disorders have been made.[78] It is possible, however, that many individuals have a partially expressed form of these congenital syndromes, but never suffer torsades de pointes unless some other external factor (drugs, diseases) further delay ventricular repolarization.

Acquired forms of torsades de pointes are associated with electrolyte disturbances (hypokalemia or hypomagnesemia), subarachnoid hemorrhage, myocarditis, liquid protein diets, arsenic poisoning, hypothyroidism, or drug therapy (notably, therapy with phenothiazines, antihistamines, antidepressants, and antiarrhythmics; Table 16–5). The type Ia (especially quinidine) and type III I_{Kr} blockers are most notorious for precipitating torsades de pointes; type Ib and Ic agents rarely, if ever, cause it. The syndrome often referred to as "quinidine syncope" is, in most cases, a drug-induced torsades de pointes. Quinidine syncope occurs in 4% to 8% of patients treated with this agent. Associated features, most of which are shared with other forms of drug-induced torsades de pointes, are as follows[25]: (1) low to "therapeutic" quinidine serum concentrations without other evidence of quinidine-related toxicity, such as prolonged QRS intervals; (2) concurrent organic heart disease, commonly ischemic; (3) evidence of mild delayed repolarization prior to quinidine therapy; (4) documentation, usually within 1 week of initiating therapy; (5) high incidence of cross-sensitivity (recurrence of torsades de pointes) with other type Ia antiarrhythmic agents, but not type Ib and Ic agents, or amiodarone; (6) frequent coexisting electrolyte disturbances, such as hypokalemia or hypomagnesemia; and (7) a characteristic long-short initiating sequence ("pause" dependence) of the episode of torsades de pointes (see Fig. 16–15); and (8) female gender. However, none of these associations are absolute prerequisites to the occurrence of quinidine syncope and torsades de pointes. Although more frequently documented early in the course of therapy, patients may suffer torsades de pointes during chronic quinidine treatment.[79] Other drug-related causes of torsades de pointes occur with high concentrations and doses of such agents as sotalol, dofetilide, and *N*-acetylprocainamide. Amiodarone is an infrequent cause of torsades de pointes; the incidence is estimated at 1% or less.[79a] The potent potassium channel blockers cisapride and terfenadine were recently withdrawn from the market because of their association with torsades de pointes. Both of these agents are rapidly metabolized to active moieties that are not proarrhythmic by cytochrome (CYP) P450 3A4.

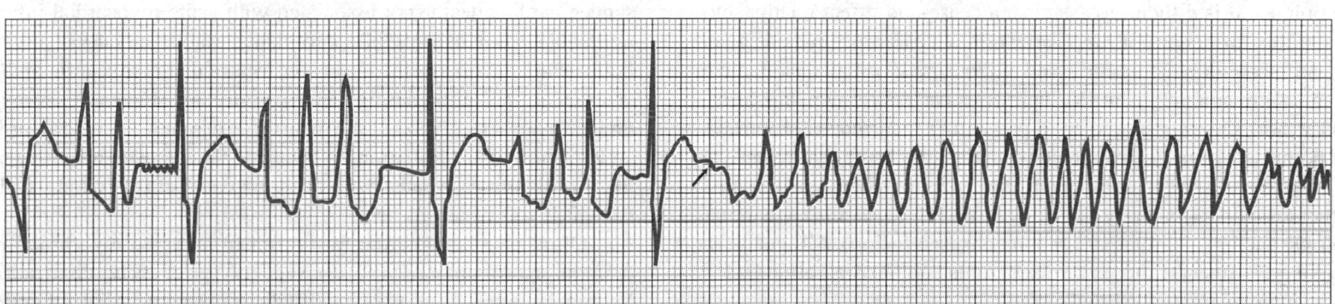

FIGURE 16–15. Torsades de pointes as a result of quinidine. A couplet and two triplets follow each extra systolic pause. The pause grows progressively longer until it is long enough to result in an episode of sustained torsades de pointes. Also, as the pause lengthens, discernible U waves (labeled ↑) (EADs?) begin to appear. The amplitude of the U wave is somewhat greater with the longest pause. *(From Hosp Med 1995;31:24, with permission.)*

TABLE 16–5. Reported Causes of QT Prolongation and Torsades de Pointes

Conditions	Drugs (continue)
Congenital long QT syndromes	—haloperidol/droperidol
Myocarditis	—pimozide
Myocardial ischemia/infarction	—thioridazine
Severe bradycardia owing to atrioventricular block; <50 beats/min	Toxins
Hypokalemia	—organophosphate insecticides
Severe hypothermia	—arsenic
Hypomagnesemia	Antihistamines
Hypothyroidism	—terfenadine[a]
Cardiomyopathy	—astemizole[a]
Subarachnoid hemorrhage	Antibiotics
Drugs	—pentamidine
Antiarrhythmic/vasodilating drugs	—clarithromycin
—quinidine	—erythromycin
—procainamide	—trimethoprim-sulfamethoxazole
—*N*-acetylprocainamide	—grepafloxacin[a]/sparfloxacin
—disopyramide	Miscellaneous
—amiodarone	—liquid protein diets[b]
—dofetilide	—corticosteroids[b]
—sotalol	—diuretics[b]
—ibutilide	—vasopressin
—bepridil[a]	—quinine
Psychotropics	—chloroquine
—phenothiazines	—chloral hydrate
—tricyclic and tetracyclic antidepressants	—cisipride[a]
	—sumitriptan
	—tacrolimus
	—tamoxifen

[a]Withdrawn from market because of torsades de pointes.
[b]Due, more than likely, to severe electrolyte imbalance.

In the presence of drugs that block the CYP3A4 isozyme (e.g., ketoconazole, erythromycin, diltiazem), however, the parent compounds (which are potent I_K blockers) may accumulate—torsades de pointes and death may follow.

It has been suggested that torsades de pointes may be due to discrepancies in ventricular repolarization and inhomogeneous ventricular recovery, allowing the formation of multiple reentrant circuits. In addition, recent investigations have suggested that torsades de pointes is likely the result of triggered activity (early after-depolarizations) caused by a delay in ventricular repolarization. For an acute episode of torsades de pointes, most patients will require and respond to DCC. Torsades de pointes tends to be paroxysmal in nature, however, and often will rapidly recur after countershock. Therefore, after the initial restoration of a stable rhythm, therapy designed to prevent recurrences of torsades de pointes should be instituted. Almost all antiarrhythmics have been reported to be successful in isolated case reports, but because of the unpredictable and self-terminating nature of torsades de pointes, it is difficult to establish a cause-and-effect relationship. Drugs that further prolong repolarization, such as procainamide given IV, are absolutely contraindicated. Lidocaine is usually ineffective. Magnesium sulfate, given IV, suppresses early after-depolarizations and is now the drug of choice in preventing recurrences of torsades de pointes.[80] If ineffective, treatment strategies designed to increase heart rate and shorten ventricular repolarization should be initiated: either temporary transvenous pacing (105–120 beats/min) or pharmacologic pacing (isoproterenol or epinephrine infusion). All agents that prolong QT interval should be discontinued and exacerbating factors (e.g., hypokalemia) corrected.

In heritable long QT interval syndromes, propranolol has been shown to prevent recurrences of torsades de pointes and prevent sudden death.[81] Although effective, β-blockers may not prevent all episodes; therefore, they are commonly employed with an ICD. In acquired long QT interval syndromes, correction of the underlying cause is the key to long-term preventive therapy. No drug agents are necessary on a chronic basis. In the case of quinidine-induced torsades de pointes, type Ia agents should be strictly avoided for the future treatment of the patient's underlying arrhythmias.

VENTRICULAR FIBRILLATION

Because ventricular fibrillation is electrical anarchy of the ventricle that results in no cardiac output and cardiovascular collapse, death will ensue rapidly without effective treatment measures. Sudden cardiac death accounts for about 400,000 deaths per year or 1,000 deaths per day in the United States. It occurs most commonly in patients with ischemic heart disease or primary myocardial disease associated with left ventricular dysfunction, less commonly in patients with Wolff-Parkinson-White syndrome or mitral valve prolapse, and occasionally in those without associated heart disease. Patients who have sudden cardiac death (not associated with acute myocardial infarction), but survive because of appropriate cardiopulmonary resuscitation usually have inducible sustained ventricular tachycardia and/or ventricular fibrillation during electrophysiologic studies.[82] These individuals are at high risk for the recurrence of ventricular tachycardia and/or ventricular fibrillation. In contrast, patients who have ventricular fibrillation associated with acute myocardial infarction usually have little risk of recurrence.

Of all patients who die as a result of an acute myocardial infarction, approximately 50% die suddenly prior to hospitalization. Ventricular fibrillation associated with acute myocardial infarction can be subdivided into two types: (1) primary and (2) complicated or secondary. Primary ventricular fibrillation occurs in an uncomplicated myocardial infarction not associated with heart failure; secondary ventricular fibrillation occurs in a myocardial infarction complicated by heart failure. The time course, incidence, mechanisms, treatment, and complications of these two forms of ventricular fibrillation are different. For example, about 2% to 6% patients with acute myocardial infarction suffer primary ventricular fibrillation within 24 hours of chest pain, but the risk of ventricular fibrillation declines rapidly over time and is nearly zero after the initial 24-hour period. Complicated ventricular fibrillation does not follow such a predictable time course and may occur in the late infarction period. The rationale behind the prophylactic administration of antiarrhythmic drugs to all patients with uncomplicated myocardial infarction is based on (1) the inability to predict which patients are at risk for primary ventricular fibrillation and (2) the predictable time course of primary ventricular fibrillation (in contrast to the complicated form).

Of the prophylactic therapies used, lidocaine has been the most widely debated and studied. Lie and co-workers performed the classic study showing the effectiveness of lidocaine in preventing primary ventricular fibrillation.[83] Although lidocaine significantly reduced the incidence of ventricular fibrillation compared with placebo, there was no difference between the groups in the rate of overall mortality. This fact and the effectiveness of rapidly instituted DCC in modern coronary care units with sophisticated monitoring techniques have caused most to reject the notion of prophylactic lidocaine administration for all patients with uncomplicated myocardial infarction. In support of this, two meta-analyses indicated that the use of prophylactic lidocaine should not be routine because of a possible increase in mortality in lidocaine-treated patients[84] and the declining incidence of primary ventricular fibrillation documented in recent years (in the acute coronary intervention era that provides rapid treatment with β-blockade and thrombolytics).[85]

The IV use of magnesium sulfate has also been under consideration for the prevention of ventricular fibrillation during the acute infarction period. A meta-analysis of small trials that had suggested the effectiveness of magnesium therapy showed a decrease in the incidence of ventricular tachycardia/ventricular fibrillation and a reduction in total mortality with this approach.[86] A subsequent large multicenter trial produced similar results, although most of the decrease in mortality was (surprisingly) attributed to deaths caused by heart failure rather than deaths caused by ventricular arrhythmias.[87] These results would lead to the conclusion that magnesium sulfate should be routinely administered to patients with suspected myocardial infarction because of its ease of administration and safety. However, data from the Fourth International Study of Infarct Survival (ISIS-4) apparently have verified no such effectiveness of magnesium therapy in this setting.[88] Hence, the prophylactic use of magnesium also cannot be recommended. Indeed, no therapies (lidocaine, magnesium, or other antiarrhythmic drugs) have shown a conclusive benefit to prevent ventricular fibrillation in the acute infarction period, and this form of therapy cannot be recommended at this time.

A patient with ventricular fibrillation (with or without associated myocardial ischemia) should be managed according to the American Heart Association's recommendations for advanced cardiac life support.[41] Prior to the initiation of drug therapy, DCC should be instituted and repeated twice (if unsuccessful). If DCC does not restore a stable rhythm, epinephrine (administered IV or intratracheally if a line is not established) should be given prior to the next DCC. It has been debated whether the standard dose of epinephrine (i.e., 1 mg) is sufficient (see Chapter 11, Cardiopulmonary Resuscitation). A large multicenter trial found that "high-dose" epinephrine (0.2 mg/kg) had no greater effect on the success or survival of patients with cardiac arrest (including ventricular fibrillation) than did the standard dose (0.02 mg/kg).[89] New in the American Heart Association's 2000 guidelines is that vasopressin (40 U given IV one time only) is a recommended alternative to epinephrine. Nevertheless, if the use of epinephrine or vasopressin (coupled with DCC) is unsuccessful, an antiarrhythmic drug should be selected and administered, then DCC repeated as necessary.

It appears clear from the new guidelines that amiodarone given IV is now the antiarrhythmic drug of first choice for most patients with ventricular fibrillation. When administered IV, as opposed to orally, amiodarone has a quick onset of action and may be effective in 40% to 60% of patients with ventricular tachycardia or ventricular fibrillation refractory to lidocaine therapy. In one trial,[90] amiodarone was shown to be as effective as bretylium, but caused less post-conversion hypotension. The promotion of amiodarone given IV to be the preferred first antiarrhythmic drug used during ventricular fibrillation (and the corresponding demotion of lidocaine) is the result of (1) a lack of data demonstrating the effectiveness of other agents and (2) the Amiodarone for Resuscitation after Out-of-Hospital Cardiac Arrest due to Ventricular Fibrillation Study.[91] In this multicenter randomized trial, significantly more patients in a group receiving 300 mg IV of amiodarone survived to hospital admission than did those in a corresponding placebo group. Survival to hospital *discharge* was no different (although the study was not powered to determine this end point). Nonetheless, this study has encouraged the recent change (away from lidocaine and toward amiodarone) in the treatment of acute ventricular fibrillation. Indeed, amiodarone may be the only drug used in this situation because the new guidelines suggest that only one antiarrhythmic agent be given to patients with ventricular fibrillation. This is in contrast to the tradition of adding drugs if the first fails.

Once the patient is successfully resuscitated, antiarrhythmics should be continued until the patient's rhythm and overall status are stable. If the episode of ventricular fibrillation was associated with acute ischemia, the long-term use of antiarrhythmic drugs is probably unnecessary, but the patient needs close monitoring for recurrence of ventricular tachycardia and/or ventricular fibrillation. If, on the other hand, ventricular fibrillation was not associated with acute myocardial infarction (or a known precipitating factor), the patient should undergo invasive electrophysiologic studies and (depending on the results) probably ICD implantation (Fig. 16–16).

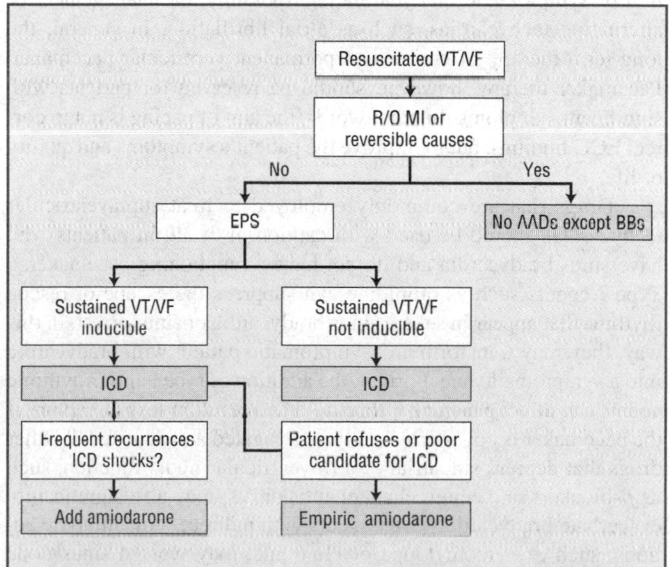

FIGURE 16–16. One approach to the management of survivors of cardiac arrest (resuscitated ventricular tachycardia/ventricular fibrillation [VT/VF]). Reversible causes of cardiac arrest (e.g., electrolyte abnormalities, acute phase of myocardial infarction [MI]) should be treated with specific therapy. AADs = antiarrhythmic drugs; BBs = β-blockers; EPS = electrophysiologic studies; ICD = implantable cardioverter-defibrillator.

BRADYARRHYTHMIAS

For the most part, the symptoms of bradyarrhythmias result from a decline in cardiac output. Because cardiac output decreases as heart rate decreases (to a point), patients experience symptoms in association with hypotension such as dizziness, syncope, fatigue, and confusion. If left ventricular dysfunction exists, patients may have an exacerbation of congestive heart failure symptoms. Except in the case of recurrent syncope, these symptoms are often subtle and nonspecific.

SINUS BRADYCARDIA

It is common to find sinus bradyarrhythmias (heart rate less than 60 beats/min), especially in young, athletically active individuals. It usually neither produces symptoms nor requires therapeutic intervention. On the other hand, some patients, particularly the elderly, have sinus node dysfunction. This is usually reflective of diffuse conduction disease and may be the result of underlying organic heart disease and the normal aging process which, over time, attenuate sinoatrial nodal function. Referred to as sick sinus syndrome, this process results in symptomatic sinus bradycardia and/or periods of sinus arrest.[92] Accompanying atrioventricular block is not uncommon.

In the "tachy-brady syndrome," alternating periods of tachycardias, such as atrial fibrillation, may accompany symptomatic bradyarrhythmias. In this instance, atrial fibrillation sometimes presents with a rather slow ventricular response (in the absence of atrioventricular node-blocking drugs) because of the diffuse conduction disease. The occurrence of paroxysmal atrial fibrillation in a patient with sinus node dysfunction may be due to underlying heart disease with atrial dysfunction or to atrial escape in response to reduced sinus node automaticity. In fact, because the rate of impulse generation by the sinus node is generally depressed or may fail altogether, other automatic pacemakers within the conduction system may "rescue" the sinus node. These rescue rhythms often occur as paroxysmal atrial rhythms (e.g., atrial fibrillation) or as a junctional escape rhythm.

The treatment of sinus node dysfunction involves the elimination of symptomatic bradycardia and, possibly, the management of alternating tachycardias, such as atrial fibrillation. In general, the long-term therapy of choice is a permanent ventricular pacemaker. Pacemaker therapy, however, should be reserved for patients with significant symptoms. In other words, the aim of pacing is not to correct ECG findings, but to improve the patient's symptoms and quality of life.

Drugs that are commonly employed to treat supraventricular tachycardias should be used with caution, if at all, in patients who have sinus bradycardia and do not have a functioning pacemaker.[92] Type I agents such as quinidine can suppress the escape or rescue rhythms that appear in severe sinus bradycardia or sinus arrest. In this way, they may transform an asymptomatic patient with bradycardia into a symptomatic one. Further, the addition of type I antiarrhythmic agents can affect pacemaker threshold and result in loss of capture if the pacemaker is not appropriately interrogated and adjusted.[69] Other drugs that depress sinoatrial or atrioventricular nodal function, such as β-blockers or calcium channel antagonists, may also significantly exacerbate bradycardia. Even agents with indirect sympatholytic actions, such as α-methyldopa or clonidine, may worsen sinus node dysfunction. Digitalis use in these patients is controversial, but in most cases, it can be used safely.

Another reason for paroxysmal bradycardia and sinus arrest that is not due directly to sinus node dysfunction is carotid sinus hypersensitivity.[93,94] Again, this syndrome occurs commonly in the aged who have underlying heart disease. Symptoms occur when stimulation of the carotid sinus results in an accentuated baroreceptor reflex. Thus, the patient may experience paroxysmal episodes of dizziness or syncope because of sinus arrest due to increased vagal tone and sympathetic withdrawal (cardioinhibitory type), a drop in systemic blood pressure due to sympathetic withdrawal (vasodepressor type), or both (mixed cardioinhibitory and vasodepressor types). Performing carotid sinus massage with ECG and blood pressure monitoring in controlled conditions makes it possible to confirm the diagnosis.

The treatment of symptomatic carotid sinus hypersensitivity should include permanent pacemaker therapy.[93] However, some patients, particularly those patients whose condition has a significant vasodepressor component, still experience syncope or dizziness. In these cases, α-adrenergic stimulants such as midodrine, sometimes in combination with β-blockers to achieve maximal α-sympathetic stimulation, can be tried in addition to the pacemaker.[94]

Still another syndrome, vasovagal syncope, is believed to be the cause of syncope in many patients who develop recurrent syncope of unknown origin.[95,96] This reaction is presumed to be a neurally mediated, paradoxical reaction involving stimulation of cardiac mechanoreceptors (i.e., Bezold-Jarisch reflex). Forceful contractions of the ventricle (e.g., as with adrenergic stimulation), coupled with low ventricular volumes (e.g., with upright posture or dehydration), provide a powerful stimulus for cardiac mechanoreceptors. Syncope results from the spontaneous development of transient hypotension (sympathetic withdrawal) and bradycardia (vagotonia).The true mechanism of vasovagal syncope remains to be definitively determined, however. For instance, the observation that patients with denervated hearts (e.g., heart transplant recipients) can still experience this form of syncope has led some to question the ultimate role of the Bezold-Jarisch reflex in these patients.[97] Despite concerns about the sensitivity and reproducibility of the test, the condition of patients believed to have frequent episodes of vasovagal syncope has commonly been diagnosed by means of the upright body tilt test, a potent stimulus for the development of vasovagal symptoms.

Vasovagal syncope can usually be successfully treated with the oral administration of β-blockers. Although these agents may seem peculiar choices to treat a syndrome resulting from vasodilation and bradycardia, their purpose is to block an inappropriate vasovagal reaction. β-Blockers act by inhibiting the sympathetic surge that causes forceful ventricular contraction that precedes the onset of hypotension and bradycardia. Drug testing with esmolol or metoprolol, given IV, during repeat head-up tilt tests has been used to predict a patient's long-term response to the oral use of β-blockers.[98] Other drugs that have been used successfully (with or without β-blockers) include anticholinergic agents (scopolamine patches, disopyramide), α-adrenergic agonists (midodrine), adenosine analogs (theophylline, dipyridamole), and selective serotonin receptor reuptake inhibitors (sertraline, fluoxetine). More research is necessary, particularly comparative trials with effective agents, before it will be possible to draw definitive conclusions regarding the place of these alternatives to β-blockers in this disorder. Chronic pacing has been used with some success, but should be reserved for drug-refractory patients.[99]

ATRIOVENTRICULAR BLOCK

Conduction delay or block may occur in any area of the atrioventricular conduction system: the node, the His bundle, or the bundle branches. Atrioventricular block is usually categorized into three different types, based on surface ECG findings (Table 16–6).

TABLE 16–6. Forms of Atrioventricular (AV) Block

Type	Criteria
First-degree block	Prolonged PR interval (>0.2 s), 1:1 AV conduction
Second-degree block	
Mobitz I	Progressive PR prolongation until QRS complex is dropped, <1:1 AV conduction
Mobitz II	Random nonconducted beats (absence of QRS complex), <1:1 AV conduction
Third-degree block	AV dissociation Absence of AV conduction

First-degree atrioventricular block is 1:1 atrioventricular conduction with a prolonged PR interval. Second-degree atrioventricular block is divided into two forms: Mobitz I atrioventricular block (Wenkebach periodicity) is less than 1:1 atrioventricular conduction with progressively lengthening PR intervals until a ventricular complex is dropped; Mobitz II atrioventricular block is intermittently dropped ventricular beats in a random fashion without progressive PR lengthening. Third-degree atrioventricular block is complete heart block where atrioventricular conduction is totally absent (atrioventricular dissociation).

By using intracardiac His bundle ECGs, the clinician can determine the actual site of conduction delay/block and the exact diagnosis. First-degree atrioventricular block usually represents prolonged conduction in the atrioventricular node. Second-degree Mobitz I atrioventricular block is also usually due to prolonged conduction in the atrioventricular node. Indeed, Wenkebach periodicity is a normal atrioventricular node response to rapid supraventricular stimulation or high vagal tone. In contrast, second-degree Mobitz II atrioventricular block is usually due to conduction disease below the node (i.e., at the His bundle). Third-degree atrioventricular block may be due to disease at any level of the atrioventricular conduction system: complete atrioventricular node block, His bundle block, or trifascicular block. The ventricle will beat independently of the atria (atrioventricular dissociation), and the site of the atrioventricular block will determine the rate of ventricular activation and QRS configuration. The usual degree of automaticity of ventricular pacemakers progressively declines as impulses move down the conduction system. Therefore, the ventricular escape rate in cases of trifascicular block will be significantly less than complete atrioventricular node block.

Atrioventricular block may occur without underlying heart disease (e.g., in trained athletes) or during sleep when vagal tone is high. It may be transient when the underlying cause is reversible, as in myocarditis or myocardial ischemia; when it follows cardiovascular surgery; or when it develops during drug therapy. β-Blockers, digitalis, or calcium antagonists may cause atrioventricular block, primarily in the atrioventricular nodal area. Type I antiarrhythmic agents may exacerbate conduction delays below the level of the atrioventricular node (sodium-dependent tissue). In other cases, atrioventricular block may be irreversible, such as that due to acute myocardial infarction, rare degenerative diseases, primary myocardial disease, or congenital conditions.

The cornerstone of treatment for acute, symptomatic bradycardia or atrioventricular block is temporary pacing, either through a transvenous wire or, in the event of an emergency, by transcutaneous leads.[41] Atropine (0.5–1 mg) should be given IV as the leads for pacing are being placed. Drugs such as atropine will facilitate the effectiveness of transcutaneous pacing. In the past, isoproterenol infusion was frequently chosen for this purpose, but it is no longer recommended because of its vasodilating properties and its ability to increase myocardial oxygen consumption (particularly during acute infarction). Sympathomimetic infusions such as epinephrine or dopamine can be useful in the event of atropine failure, and they are particularly effective in sinus bradycardia/arrest and atrioventricular node block. These agents will usually not help when the site of atrioventricular block is below the atrioventricular node (e.g., Mobitz II or trifascicular atrioventricular block).

Chronic symptomatic atrioventricular block warrants the insertion of a permanent pacemaker. It is sometimes enough to follow patients without symptoms closely, without inserting a pacemaker at first. Because symptoms often correlate with the ventricular rate and the ventricular rate corresponds to the site of the block, pacemaker therapy is usually necessary in distal atrioventricular blocks, such as those occurring in the His bundle or the bundle branches. Patients with acute myocardial infarction and evidence of new atrioventricular block or conduction disturbances often require the insertion of a temporary transvenous pacemaker. Atrioventricular block more commonly occurs as a complication of inferior wall infarcts because of the high vagal innervation at this site, and the coronary blood flow to the nodal areas usually supplies the inferior wall. However, the atrioventricular block may be only transient, obviating the need for permanent pacing. In patients with chronic atrioventricular conduction disturbances, intracardiac recordings (His bundle ECGs) are sometimes used to document the actual site of block and define the potential need for and specific type of pacemaker therapy.

EVALUATION OF THERAPEUTIC AND ECONOMIC OUTCOMES

Generally, monitoring can show one or several possible outcomes of therapy for tachyarrhythmias. Obviously, it is possible to document the presence or recurrence of any arrhythmia by ECG means (e.g., surface ECG, Holter monitor, event monitor). Further, patients may experience a decrease in blood pressure that may result in symptoms from light-headedness to abrupt syncope, depending on the rate of the arrhythmia and the status of the underlying heart disease. For some patients, the potential alteration in hemodynamics may lead to death if the arrhythmia is not detected and treated immediately. Besides these clinical outcomes, many patients with arrhythmias experience alterations in quality of life—either because of recurrent symptoms of the arrhythmia or because of side effects of therapy. Finally, there are the economic considerations of medical or surgical intervention, continued medical care, and chronic drug or non-drug treatment.

Compared to the treatment of other forms of cardiovascular disease, there are relatively few pharmacoeconomic analyses of the treatment of arrhythmias available.[100,101] Most of the studies are limited to the use of non-drug therapies, such as the ICD or radiofrequency ablation. As technology is evolving rapidly, what is not cost-effective now may indeed become cost-effective in the next several years. For example, original cost-effectiveness analysis of the ICD showed it to be highly sensitive to the life of the generator, yet newer devices have made significant advances not only in the size of the device, but also in the life of the battery. More recent data on the effect of the ICD on mortality, coupled with the declining costs of an ICD, imply that the device is indeed cost-effective in certain subsets of patients.

Some therapeutic outcomes are unique to certain arrhythmias. For instance, patients with atrial fibrillation or flutter need to be monitored for thromboembolism and for complications of anticoagulation therapy (e.g., bleeding, drug interactions) prescribed to prevent it. However, the most important monitoring parameters for most patients fall into the following categories:

- Mortality
  - —Total, all-cause
  - —Arrhythmic death (i.e., sudden)
- Recurrences documented by ECG
  - —Time to recurrence
  - —Frequency of recurrences
- Tolerance
  - —Symptoms
  - —Blood pressure
  - —Rate of tachycardia
- Necessity of non-drug interventions (e.g., ICD)
- ICD shocks
- Side effects of drugs/treatment complications
- Quality of life
- Economics
- Outcomes specific to tachycardia (e.g., ventricular rate, systemic embolism in atrial fibrillation)

When evaluating the arrhythmia literature, clinicians should take care to consider real outcomes. For example, total mortality is more meaningful than only sudden death rates; it is possible that an intervention prevents arrhythmic death, but patients die from other causes, leaving all cause mortality unaltered. Likewise, surrogate markers of drug efficacy (e.g., noninducible tachycardia, suppression of minor arrhythmias) should be judged with a degree of skepticism. One should ask, Did the treatment make patients live longer (reduce mortality)? Did it make them feel better (improve humanistic outcomes or quality of life)? Was it economically worth it (cost-effective)?

▶ PRINCIPLES OF PHARMACOTHERAPY

- Clinical tachycardias most often result from reentry, and available drugs used in these disorders work by altering transmembrane ion movement, which affects electrical conduction within the reentrant circuit.
- The use of antiarrhythmic drugs in the United States is declining because of major trials that show increased mortality with their use in several clinical situations, the recognition of proarrhythmia as a significant side effect, and the advancing technology of non-drug therapies such as ablation and the implantable cardioverter-defibrillator.
- Antiarrhythmic drugs are complex in their pharmacokinetic characteristics and frequently cause side effects. The therapeutic range of these agents provides only a rough guide to modifying treatment; it is preferable to attempt to define an individual's effective (or target) concentration and match that during long-term therapy.
- In patients with atrial fibrillation, therapy is aimed at controlling ventricular response (e.g., with digoxin, calcium antagonists, β-blockers), preventing thromboembolic complications (e.g., with warfarin, aspirin), and restoring and maintaining sinus rhythm (e.g., with antiarrhythmic drugs, direct-current cardioversion).
- Paroxysmal supraventricular tachycardia is usually due to reentry in or proximal to the atrioventricular node or atrioventricular reentry incorporating an extranodal pathway; common tachycardias can be terminated acutely with atrioventricular node-blocking agents such as adenosine, and recurrences can be prevented by ablation with radiofrequency current.
- Patients with Wolff-Parkinson-White syndrome may have several different tachycardias that are treated by different strategies in their acute phase: orthodromic reentry (adenosine), antidromic reentry (adenosine or procainamide), and atrial fibrillation (procainamide or amiodarone). Atrioventricular node-blocking drugs are contraindicated with Wolff-Parkinson-White syndrome and atrial fibrillation.
- Because of the results of the Cardiac Arrhythmia Suppression Trial (CAST) and other trials, antiarrhythmic drugs (excepting β-blockers) should not be routinely used in patients with prior myocardial infarction or left ventricular dysfunction.
- Life-threatening proarrhythmia generally takes two forms: sinusoidal or incessant monomorphic ventricular tachycardia (treated with type Ic agents) and torsades de pointes (treated with type Ia or type III agents and others, such as select antihistamines).
- The clinical approach to patients with left ventricular dysfunction and nonsustained ventricular tachycardia is a major remaining controversy with three divergent strategies: (1) invasive electrophysiologic studies with possible internal cardioverter-defibrillator implantation, (2) empiric amiodarone therapy, and (3) conservative management (i.e., no treatment beyond β-blockers). Invasive electrophysiologic studies can aid in deciding among these strategies.
- Patients with hemodynamically significant ventricular tachycardia or ventricular fibrillation *not* associated with an acute myocardial infarction who are successfully resuscitated (e.g., by means of electrical cardioversion, vasopressors, amiodarone) are at high risk for death and should have an implantable cardioverter-defibrillator.

REFERENCES

1. Alice MA, Bonke FIM, Schopman FJG. Circus movement in rabbit atrial muscle as a mechanism of tachycardia III. The "leading circle" concept: a new model of circus movement in cardiac tissue without the involvement of an anatomic obstacle. Circ Res 1977;41:9–18.
2. Vaughan Williams EM. A classification of antiarrhythmic actions reassessed after a decade of new drugs. J Clin Pharmacol 1984;24:129–147.
3. Working Group on Arrhythmias of the European Society of Cardiology. The Sicilian Gambit: a new approach to the classification of antiarrhythmic drugs based upon their actions on arrhythmogenic mechanisms. Circulation 1991;84:1831–1851.
4. Hondeghem LM, Katzung BG. Antiarrhythmic agents: the modulated receptor mechanism of action of sodium and calcium channel-blocking drugs. Ann Rev Pharmacol Toxicol 1984;24:387–423.
5. Kosowsky BD, Taylor J, Lown B, et al. Long-term procaine amide following acute myocardial infarction. Circulation 1973;47:1204–1210.
6. Bauman JL, Gallastegui J, Strasberg B, et al. Long-term therapy with disopyramide phosphate: side effects and effectiveness. Am Heart J 1986;111:654–660.
7. Podrid PJ, Schoeneburger A, Lown B. Congestive heart failure caused by oral disopyramide. N Engl J Med 1980;302:614–617.
8. McCollam PL, Parker RB, Beckman KJ, et al. Proarrhythmia: a paradoxic response to antiarrhythmic agents. Pharmacotherapy 1989;9:144–153.
9. Dusman RE, Stanton MS, Miles WM, et al. Clinical features of amiodarone-induced pulmonary toxicity. Circulation 1990;82:51–59.
10. Podrid PJ. Amiodarone: reevaluation of an old drug. Ann Intern Med 1995;122:689–700.

11. Prystowsky EN, Benson W, Fuster V, et al. Management of patients with atrial fibrillation: a statement for healthcare professionals from the Subcommittee in Electrocardiography and Electrophysiology, American Heart Association. Circulation 1996;93:1262–1277.
12. Atrial Fibrillation Investigators. Risk factors for stroke and efficacy of antithrombotic therapy in atrial fibrillation: analysis of pooled data from five randomized controlled trials. Arch Intern Med 1994;154:1449–1457.
13. Albers GW, Dalen J, Laupacis A, et al. Antithrombotic therapy in atrial fibrillation. Chest 2001;119:194S–206S.
14. Falk RH, Leavitt JI. Digoxin for atrial fibrillation: a drug whose time has gone? Ann Intern Med 1991;114:573–575.
15. Roberts SA, Diaz C, Nolan PE, et al. Effectiveness and costs of digoxin treatment for atrial fibrillation and flutter. Am J Cardiol 1993;72:567–573.
16. Ellenbogen KA, Dias VC, Plumb VJ, et al. A placebo-controlled trial of continuous intravenous diltiazem infusion for 24-hour heart rate control during atrial fibrillation and atrial flutter: a multicenter study. J Am Coll Cardiol 1991;18:891–897.
17. Phillips BG, Gandhi AJ, Sanoski CA, et al. Comparison of intravenous diltiazem and verapamil for the acute treatment of atrial fibrillation and flutter. Pharmacotherapy 1997;17:1238–1245.
18. Feld GK, Fleck P, Fujimura O, et al. Control of rapid ventricular response by radiofrequency catheter modification of the atrioventricular node in patients with medically refractory atrial fibrillation. Circulation 1994;90:2299–2307.
18a. American College of Cardiology/American Heart Association Task Force on Practice Guideline's and the European Society of Cardiology Committee for Practice Guidelines and Policy Conferences. ACC/AHA/ESC guidelines for the management of patients with atrial fibrillation Executive Summary. J Am Coll Cardiol 2001;38:1231–1265.
19. Klein AL, Grimm RA, Murray D, et al. Use of transesophageal echocardiography to guide cardioversion in patients with atrial fibrillation. N Engl J Med 2001;344:1411–1420.
20. Murdock DK, Schumock GT, Kaliebe J, et al. Clinical and case comparison of ibutilide and direct-current cardioversion for atrial fibrillation and flutter. Am J Cardiol 2000;85:503–506.
21. Management of New Onset Atrial Fibrillation. Summary, Evidence Report/Technology Assessment: Number 12. Rockville, MD: Agency for Healthcare Research and Quality; May 2000. AHQR Publication No. 00–E006.
22. Boriani G, Biffi M, Alessandro C, et al. Oral propafenone to convert recent-onset atrial fibrillation in patients with and without underlying heart disease: a randomized, controlled trial. Ann Intern Med 1997;126:621–625.
23. Murray KT. Ibutilide. Circulation 1998;97:493–497.
24. Cropp JS, Antal EG, Talbert RL. Ibutilide: a new class III antiarrhythmic agent. Pharmacotherapy 1997;17(1):1–9.
25. Bauman JL, Bauernfeind RA, Hoff JV, et al. Torsades de pointes due to quinidine: observations in 31 patients. Am Heart J 1984;107:425–430.
26. Gage BF, Cardinally AB, Abers GW, Owens DR. Cost-effectiveness of warfarin and aspirin for prophylaxis of stroke in patients with nonvalvular atrial fibrillation. JAMA 1995;274:1839–1845.
27. Coplen SE, Antman EM, Berlin JA, et al. Efficacy and safety of quinidine therapy for maintenance of sinus rhythm after cardioversion: a meta-analysis of randomized control trials. Circulation 1990;82:1106–1116.
28. Echt DS, Liebson PR, Mitchell B, et al. Mortality and morbidity in patients receiving encainide, flecainide, or placebo: the Cardiac Arrhythmia Suppression Trial. N Engl J Med 1991;324:781–788.
29. Flaker GC, Blackshear JL, McBride R, et al. Antiarrhythmic drug therapy and cardiac mortality in atrial fibrillation. J Am Coll Cardiol 1992;20:527–532.
30. Juul-Moller S, Edvardsson N, Rehnqvist-Ahlberg N. Sotalol versus quinidine for the maintenance of sinus rhythm after direct current conversion of atrial fibrillation. Circulation 1990;82:1932–1939.
31. Southworth MR, Zarembski D, Viana M, Bauman JL. Comparison of sotalol versus quinidine for maintenance of normal sinus rhythm in patients with chronic atrial fibrillation. Am J Cardiol 1999;83:1629–1632.
32. Gosselink ATM, Crijns HJM, VanGelder IC, et al. Low-dose amiodarone for maintenance of sinus rhythm after cardioversion of atrial fibrillation or flutter. JAMA 1992;267:3289–3292.
33. Roy D, Talajic M, Dorian P, et al. Amiodarone to prevent recurrence of atrial fibrillation: Canadian Trial of Atrial Fibrillation. N Engl J Med 2000;324:913–920.
34. Fischer B, Haissaguerre M, Garrigues S, et al. Radiofrequency catheter ablation of common atrial flutter in 80 patients. J Am Coll Cardiol 1995; 225:1365–1372.
35. Cox JL, Schuessler RB, Loppas DG, Boineau JP. An 8 1/2 year clinical experience with surgery for atrial fibrillation. Ann Surg 1996;224: 267–275.
36. Chen SA, Hsieh MH, Tai CT, et al. Initiation of atrial fibrillation by ectopic beats originating from the pulmonary veins: electrophysiologic characteristics, pharmacologic responses and the effects of radiofrequency ablation. Circulation 1999;80:1527–1535.
37. Sung RJ, Lauer MR, Chun H. Atrioventricular node reentry: current concepts and new perspectives. PACE 1994;17:1413–1430.
38. Bauernfeind RA, Wyndham CR, Dhingra RC, et al. Serial electrophysiologic testing of multiple drugs in patients with atrioventricular nodal reentrant paroxysmal tachycardia. Circulation 1980;62:1341–1349.
39. Wu D, Amat-Y-Leon F, Simpson R, et al. Electrophysiological studies with multiple drugs in patients with atrioventricular reentrant tachycardias utilizing an extra nodal pathway. Circulation 1977;56:727–736.
40. DiMarco JP, Miles W, Akhtar M, et al. Adenosine for paroxysmal supraventricular tachycardia: dose ranging and comparison with verapamil. Assessment in placebo-controlled, multicenter trials. Ann Intern Med 1990;1113:104–110.
41. American Heart Association in collaboration with the International Liaison Committee on Resuscitation. Guidelines 2000 for cardiopulmonary resuscitation and emergency cardiovascular care. Circulation 2000;102(8):I-1–I-384.
42. Rankin AC, McGovern BA. Adenosine or verapamil for the acute treatment of supraventricular tachycardia? Ann Intern Med 1991;114:513–515.
43. Hoon TJ, Bauman JL, Rodvold KA, et al. The pharmacodynamic and pharmacokinetic differences of the *d*- and *l*-isomers of verapamil: implications in the treatment of PSVT. Am Heart J 1986;112:396–403.
44. Jackman WM, Wang Z, Friday KJ, et al. Catheter ablation of accessory atrioventricular pathways (Wolff-Parkinson-White syndrome) by radiofrequency current. N Engl J Med 1991;324:1605–1611.
45. Jackman WM, Beckman KJ, McClelland JH, et al. Treatment of supraventricular tachycardia due to atrioventricular nodal reentry by radiofrequency catheter ablation of slow pathway conduction. N Engl J Med 1992;327:313–318.
46. Scheinman MM. Radiofrequency catheter ablation for patients with supraventricular tachycardia. PACE 1993;16:671–679.
47. Cheng CH, Sanders GD, Hlatky MA, et al. Cost effectiveness of radiofrequency ablation for supraventricular tachycardia. Ann Intern Med 2000;133:864–876.
48. McCord J, Borzak S. Multifocal atrial tachycardia. Chest 1998;113:203–209.
49. Levine JH, Michael JR, Guarnier T. Treatment of multifocal atrial tachycardia with verapamil. N Engl J Med 1985;312:21–25.
50. Bayes deLuna A, Coumel P, LeClercq IF. Ambulatory sudden cardiac death: mechanisms of production of fatal arrhythmia on the basis of data from 157 cases. Am Heart J 1989;117:151–159.
51. Ruberman W, Weinblatt E, Goldberg JD, et al. Ventricular premature beats and mortality after myocardial infarction. N Engl J Med 1977;297:750–757.
52. Lown B, Wolf M. Approaches to sudden death from coronary heart disease. Circulation 1971;44:130–142.
53. The Cardiac Arrhythmia Suppression Trial II Investigators. Effect of the antiarrhythmic agent moricizine on survival after myocardial infarction. N Engl J Med 1992;327:227–233.

54. Waldo AL, Camm AJ, deRuyter H, et al. Effect of *d*-sotalol on mortality in patients with left ventricular dysfunction and remote myocardial infarction. Lancet 1996;348:7–12.
55. Julian DG, Camm AJ, Frangin G, et al. Randomised trial of effect of amiodarone on mortality in patients with left ventricular dysfunction after recent myocardial infarction: EMIAT. Lancet 1997;349:667–674.
56. Cairns JA, Connolly SJ, Roberts R, et al. Randomised trial of outcome after myocardial infarction in patients with frequent or repetitive ventricular premature depolarisations; CAMIAT. Lancet 1997;349:675–682.
57. Amiodarone Trials Meta-Analysis Investigators. Effect of prophylactic amiodarone on mortality after acute myocardial infarction and in congestive heart failure: meta-analysis of individual data from 6,500 patients in randomized trials. Lancet 1997;350:1417–1424.
58. Torp-Pederson C, Moller M, Bloch-Thomsen PE, et al. Dofetilide in patients with congestive heart failure and left ventricular dysfunction. N Engl J Med 1999;341:857–865.
59. Kober L, Bloch-Thomsen PE, Moller M, et al. Effect of dofetilide in patients with recent myocardial infarction and left ventricular dysfunction: a randomized trial. Lancet 2000;356:2052–2058.
60. Hilleman DE, Bauman JL. Role of antiarrhythmic therapy in patients at risk for sudden cardiac death: an evidence-based review. Pharmacotherapy 2001;21:556–575.
61. Gorgels A, van den Dool A, Hofs A, et al. Comparison of procainamide and lidocaine in terminating sustained monomorphic ventricular tachycardia. Am J Cardiol 1996;78:43–46.
62. Bauman JL, Schoen MD, Hoon TJ. Practical optimization of antiarrhythmic drug therapy using pharmacokinetic principles. Clin Pharmacokinet 1991;20:151–166.
63. The CASCADE Investigators. Randomized antiarrhythmic drug therapy in survivors of cardiac arrest (the CASCADE Study). Am J Cardiol 1993;72:280–287.
64. Mitchell LB, Duff HJ, Manyari DE, et al. A randomized clinical trial of the noninvasive and invasive approaches to drug therapy of ventricular tachycardia. N Engl J Med 1987;317:1681–1687.
65. Mason JW and the Electrophysiologic Study versus Electrocardiographic Monitoring Investigators. A comparison of electrophysiologic testing with Holter monitoring to predict antiarrhythmic drug efficacy for ventricular tachyarrhythmias. N Engl J Med 1993;329:445–451.
66. Mason JW and the Electrophysiologic Study versus Electrocardiographic Monitoring Investigators. A comparison of seven antiarrhythmic drugs in patients with ventricular tachyarrhythmias. N Engl J Med 1993;329:452–458.
67. Zipes DP. Cardiac electrophysiology: Promises and contributions. J Am Coll Cardiol 1989;13:1329–1352.
68. Powell AC, Fuchs T, Finklestein DM, et al. Influence of implantable cardioverter-defibrillators on long-term prognosis of survivors of out-of-hospital cardiac arrest. Circulation 1993;88:1083–1092.
69. Tworek DA, Nazari J, Ezri M, Bauman JL. Interference by antiarrhythmic agents with the function of electrical cardiac devices. Clin Pharm 1992;11:48–56.
70. Moss AJ, Hall WJ, Cannom DS, et al. Improved survival with an implanted defibrillator in patients with coronary disease at high risk for ventricular arrhythmia. N Engl J Med 1996;335:1933–1940.
71. Wever EFD, Hauer RNW, Schrijvers G, et al. Cost-effectiveness of implantable defibrillator as first-choice therapy versus electrophysiologically guided tiered strategy in post infarct sudden death survivors: a randomized study. Circulation 1996;93:489–496.
72. Klein H, Auricchio A, Reek S, Geller C. New primary prevention trials of sudden death in patients with left ventricular dysfunction: SCD-Heft and Madit II. Am J Cardiol 1999;83:91D–97D.
73. Mitra Rl, Buxton AE. The clinical significance of nonsustained ventricular tachycardia. J Cardiovasc Electrophys 1993;4:490–496.
74. Wilber DJ, Olshansky B, Moran JF, et al. Electrophysiological testing and nonsustained ventricular tachycardia: use and limitations in patients with coronary artery disease and impaired ventricular function. Circulation 1990;82:350–358.
75. Buxton AE, Leek KL, DiCarlo L, et al. Electrophysiologic testing to identify patients with coronary artery disease who are at risk for sudden death: Multicenter Unsustained Tachycardia Trial. N Engl J Med 2000;342:1937–1945.
76. Gomes JA, Winters SL, Stewart D, et al. A new noninvasive index to predict sustained ventricular tachycardia and sudden death in the first year after myocardial infarction: Based on signal-averaged electrocardiogram, radionuclide ejection fraction and Holter monitoring. J Am Coll Cardiol 1987;10:349–357.
77. Herre JM, Titus C, Oeff M, et al. Inefficacy and proarrhythmic effects of flecainide and encainide for sustained ventricular tachycardia and ventricular fibrillation. Ann Intern Med 1990;113:671–676.
78. Ackerman MJ, Clapham DE. Ion channels—Basic science and clinical disease. N Engl J Med 1997;336(22):1575–1586.
79. Oberg KC, O'Toole MF, Gallastegui JL, Bauman JL. "Late" proarrhythmia due to quinidine. Am J Cardiol 1994;74:192–194.
79a. Hohnloser SH, Klingenheben T, Singh BN. Amiodarone-associated proarrhythmic effects. A review with special reference to torsade de pointes tachycardia. Ann Intern Med 1994;121:529–535.
80. Tzivoni D, Banai S, Schuger C, et al. Treatment of torsades de pointes with magnesium sulfate. Circulation 1987;77:392–397.
81. Moss AJ, Zareba W, Hall WJ, et al. Effectiveness and limitations of beta-blocker therapy in congenital long-QT syndrome. Circulation 2000;101:616–623.
82. Ruskin JN, DiMarco JP, Garan H. Out-of-hospital cardiac arrest: electrophysiologic observation and selection of long-term antiarrhythmic therapy. N Engl J Med 1980;303:607–613.
83. Lie KI, Wellens HJJ, Van Capelle FJ. Lidocaine in the prevention of primary ventricular fibrillation. N Engl J Med 1974;291:1324–1326.
84. MacMahon S, Collin R, Peto R, et al. Effects of prophylactic lidocaine in suspected acute myocardial infarction: an overview of results from the randomized controlled trials. JAMA 1988;260:1910–1916.
85. Antman EM, Berlin JA. Declining incidence of ventricular fibrillation in myocardial infarction: implications for the prophylactic use of lidocaine. Circulation 1992;86:764–773.
86. Horner SM. Efficacy of intravenous magnesium in acute myocardial infarction in reducing arrhythmias and mortality: meta-analysis of magnesium in acute myocardial infarction. Circulation 1992;86:774–779.
87. Woods KL, Fletcher S, Roffe C, Haider Y. A randomized trial of intravenous magnesium sulfate in suspected acute myocardial infarction: Results of the Second Leicester Intravenous Magnesium Intervention Trial (LIMIT-2). Lancet 1992;339:1553–1558.
88. Sleight P. Vasodilators after myocardial infarction—ISIS IV. Am J Hypertens 1994;7:1025–1055.
89. Brown CG, Martin DR, Pepe PE, et al. A comparison of standard-dose and high-dose epinephrine in cardiac arrest outside the hospital. N Engl J Med 1992;327:1051–1055.
90. Kowey PR, Levine JH, Herre JM, et al. Randomized, double-blind comparison of intravenous amiodarone and bretylium in the treatment of patients with recurrent, hemodynamically destabilizing ventricular tachycardia or fibrillation. Circulation 1995;92:3255–3263.
91. Kudenchuk PJ, Cobb LA, Copass MK, et al. Amiodarone for resuscitation after out-of-hospital cardiac arrest due to ventricular fibrillation. N Engl J Med 1999;341:871–878.
92. Talano JV, Euler D, Randall WC, et al. Sinus node dysfunction: an overview with emphasis on autonomic and pharmacologic considerations. Am J Med 1978;64:773–781.
93. Sugrue DD, Gersh BJ, Holmes DR, et al. Symptomatic "isolated" carotid sinus hypersensitivity: natural history and results of treatment with anticholinergic drugs or pacemaker. J Am Coll Cardiol 1986;7:158–162.
94. Strasberg B, Sagie A, Erdman S, et al. Carotid sinus hypersensitivity and the carotid sinus syndrome. Prog Cardiovasc Dis 1989;31:379–391.
95. Milstein S, Reyes WJ, Benditt DG. Upright body tilt for evaluation of patients with recurrent, unexplained syncope. PACE 1989;12:117–124.
96. Almquist A, Goldenberg I, Milstein S. Provocation of bradycardia and hypotension by isoproterenol and upright posture in patients with unexplained syncope. N Engl J Med 1990;320:346–351.
97. Somers VK, Abboud FM. Neurocardiogenic syncope. Adv Intern Med 1996;41:399–435.

98. Sra JS, Vishnubhakta S, Murthy S, et al. Use of intravenous esmolol to predict efficacy of oral beta-adrenergic blocker therapy in patients with neurocardiogenic syncope. J Am Coll Cardiol 1992;19:402–408.
99. Zagga M, Massumi A. Neurally mediated syncope. Tex Heart Inst J 2000;27:268–272.
100. Kupersmith J, Holmes-Novner M, Hogan A, et al. Cost-effectiveness analysis in heart disease, Part I: general principles. Prog Cardiovasc Dis 1994;37:161–184.
101. Kupersmith J, Holmes-Novner M, Hogan A, et al. Cost-effectiveness analysis in heart disease, Part III: ischemia, congestive heart failure, and arrhythmias. Prog Cardiovasc Dis 1995;37:307–346.

17

ISOLATED DIASTOLIC HEART FAILURE AND THE CARDIOMYOPATHIES

Jean Nappi and Michael R. Zile

Heart failure may be the result of a primary abnormality in systolic function, in diastolic function, or in both. Making the distinction is important, because the prevalence, prognosis, and treatment of heart failure are quite different, depending on whether the predominant mechanism is systolic or diastolic dysfunction. Some clinical studies have reported as many as 30% to 50% of patients with congestive heart failure (CHF) have preserved left ventricular function, making isolated diastolic heart failure (DHF) very common.[1] In addition, abnormalities in diastolic function can play an important role in the development of symptoms in patients with cardiomyopathy and systolic heart failure.

DIASTOLIC HEART FAILURE

Patients with DHF have impaired myocardial relaxation and incomplete filling. The ventricle is unable to accept an adequate volume of blood from the venous system, does not fill at low pressure, and is unable to maintain normal stroke volume. In its most severe form, DHF results in overt symptoms of CHF. In modest DHF, symptoms of dyspnea and fatigue occur only during stress or activity, when heart rate and/or end diastolic volume increase. In its mildest form, DHF can be manifested as a slow or delayed pattern of relaxation and filling with little or no elevation in diastolic pressure and few or no cardiac symptoms. The congestive symptoms that occur with DHF are a manifestation of increased pulmonary venous pressures. DHF is caused by impaired myocardial relaxation and/or increased diastolic stiffness. When an isolated abnormality in diastolic function causes CHF, the ventricular chamber is not enlarged, and the ejection fraction is normal.[2–5] Figure 17–1 demonstrates the pressure-volume relationship in a patient with normal versus abnormal diastolic function. Changes in the myocardium are associated with a shift upward and to the left of the pressure-volume curve. Thus, for any increase in left ventricular volume, diastolic pressure rises to a much greater level than would normally occur. Clinically, patients with elevated left ventricular diastolic pressures present with reduced exercise tolerance and dyspnea.

EPIDEMIOLOGY

The prevalence of mild diastolic dysfunction with no clinical symptoms and moderate diastolic CHF limited to exercise-induced symptoms is not known. Studies performed in the 1980s suggested that the prevalence of DHF in patients with overt CHF vary over a wide range, that as many as one-third of patients presenting with overt CHF have a normal ejection fraction; and that these patients have clinically significant diastolic dysfunction and isolated DHF.[6–11] However, it has also become clear that the prevalence of DHF depends on a number of determinants: patient age, patient gender, study design, the particular population under consideration, and ejection fraction.[8] It is important to recognize that these determinants are not independent, but interdependent. The most important determinant appears to be patient age. Diastolic heart failure is relatively uncommon in young and middle-aged patients, especially those preselected for clinical research or cared for at tertiary care centers. The prevalence of DHF increases with age, approximating 15% in patients less than 60 years, 35% in patients between 60 and 70 years, and 50% in patients more than 70 years of age.[9–11]

ETIOLOGY

Several disorders can impair ventricular function and play a role in the development of isolated DHF. Primary DHF often appears in patients with hypertension, coronary artery disease, valvular heart disease, and hypertrophic cardiomyopathies. Hypertension is the most common underlying cardiovascular disorder in patients with isolated DHF.[1] There are several proposed mechanisms by which hypertension may impair diastolic function. Hypertension can alter diastolic function by affecting (1) intramyocardial wall tension, (2) myocardial hypertrophy and fibrosis, or (3) small vessel structure and function, or by predisposing the patient to epicardial coronary artery disease. An association between impaired left ventricular filling and subnormal high-energy phosphate metabolism has been shown in hypertensive patients, even in the absence of left ventricular hypertrophy.[12]

Left ventricular hypertrophy plays a central role in the adaptation of the myocardium to pressure overload. Severe and long-standing pressure overload has been associated with phenotypic alterations at the myocyte level, which differs from the physiologic hypertrophy seen in athletes.[13] Long-term, chronic pressure overload stimulates cardiac growth and collagen production, which lead to an increase in myocardial mass and structural remodeling. The results of these changes are an increase in myocardial stiffness and a decrease in diastolic filling.

Diastolic dysfunction has been reported to be present in 90% of patients with coronary artery disease.[13] For example, patients with exercise-induced ischemia, but normal function at rest; patients with myocardial stunning; and patients with previous myocardial infarction may all exhibit signs of diastolic dysfunction.

In patients with valvular heart disease, the chronic pressure or volume overload leads to either concentric or eccentric hypertrophy. Mitral or aortic regurgitation may lead to volume overload, which is associated with increased diastolic wall stress and eccentric hypertrophy. Severe pressure overload, seen with aortic stenosis, is associated with an increase in systolic wall stress and concentric hypertrophy. Both types of hypertrophy are accompanied by impaired relaxation. Most patients with aortic stenosis and systolic dysfunction also have diastolic dysfunction.[13]

Hypertrophic cardiomyopathy is the prototype for DHF. The grossly thickened myocardium, structural changes, and interstitial fibrosis severely alter the passive elastic properties of the myocardium.

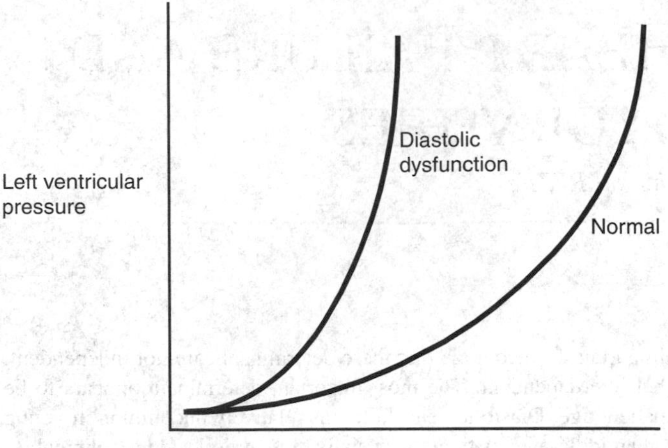

FIGURE 17–1. Diastolic pressure–volume relationship in a normal patient (right side) and a patient with diastolic dysfunction (left side).

Patients with hypertrophic obstructive cardiomyopathy are so sensitive to small changes in volume that small decreases in filling pressure and left ventricular end diastolic volume can lead to a dramatic fall in stroke volume and cardiac output.

PATHOPHYSIOLOGY

The pathologic disease processes that cause DHF include myocardial ischemia with or without epicardial coronary artery disease, pressure overload hypertrophy, genetic hypertrophy, and constrictive pericarditis. Hypertrophy consequent to a woman's physiologic adaptation to pregnancy, hypertrophy that occurs in athletes, and volume overload hypertrophy do not cause abnormalities in diastolic function and do not cause the development of DHF.

The basic mechanisms by which pressure overload hypertrophy and genetic hypertrophy cause diastolic CHF include both myocardial and extramyocardial factors, such as changes in the cardiac muscle cell and in the extracellular matrix that surrounds the cardiomyocyte (Table 17–1).[2–5,14–19] Intracellular processes such as changes in calcium homeostasis, contractile and noncontractile proteins, energetics, and the cytoskeleton contribute to abnormalities in myocardial relaxation and stiffness. Changes in the extracellular matrix, particularly changes in fibrillar collagen, alter relaxation and stiffness. In addition to the cardiomyocyte and the extracellular matrix, local myocardial neuroendocrine activation can impair relaxation and increase stiffness. Activation of neurohormones such as the renin-angiotensin-aldosterone system may act directly to alter diastolic properties or act indirectly by altering calcium homeostasis. Finally, extramyocardial changes in loading conditions and changes in myocardial synchrony and synergy occur in hypertrophied ventricles and contribute to changes in relaxation and stiffness so that, even when the myocardium itself is normal, changes in these extramyocardial factors can cause abnormalities in diastolic function.

Myocardial ischemia, particularly in the subendocardial region, is common in the presence of ventricular hypertrophy. Slow or delayed myocardial relaxation and perivascular fibrosis can adversely affect coronary blood flow and coronary blood flow reserve. This may contribute to the development of myocardial ischemia.[20,21] Therefore, myocardial ischemia may be part of the clinical syndrome of DHF—even if there is no epicardial coronary artery disease.

Both in its acute manifestations of myocardial ischemia and in its chronic consequences of myocardial fibrosis, epicardial coronary artery disease is frequently the underlying pathologic cause of DHF.[22–24] Myocardial ischemia, caused either by an acute decrease in supply (because of coronary artery spasm, but not occlusion) or an increase in demand (because of exercise and tachycardia), impairs relaxation and leads to an acute increase in myocardial stiffness.[24] An acute coronary artery occlusion actually can initially lower myocardial stiffness by the hydraulic effect.[20] Chronic coronary artery occlusions, however, result in myocardial fibrosis, remodeling, and DHF. It is clear that the same basic mechanisms—myocardial and extramyocardial, cellular and extracellular—that cause diastolic dysfunction in the presence of pressure overload hypertrophy underlie the changes that coronary artery disease produces.

TABLE 17–1. Potential Pathologic Mechanisms of Diastolic Heart Failure

A. Mechanisms directly affecting myocardial tissue
  1. Cardiomyocyte
    a. Increase in intracellular Ca^{2+}
      1. Increased Ca^{2+} influx into cells, producing Ca^{2+} overload
      2. Decreased sarcoplasmic reticulum function, resulting in inability to resequester Ca^{2+}
    b. Myofilaments
      1. Increased troponin-C Ca^{2+} binding
      2. Increased myofilament Ca^{2+} sensitivity
    c. Cytoskeleton: Decrease in ATP availability, leading to a decreased rate or extent of actomyosin dissociation
  2. Extracellular matrix
    a. Increased content of fibrillar collagen
    b. Thickening of existing fibrillar collagen
    c. Increased MMP and/or decreased TIMP
  3. Neurohormones
    a. Increased renin-angiotensin-aldosterone
    b. Increased endothelin
B. Extramyocardial mechanisms
  1. Increased hemodynamic load: preload or afterload
  2. Increased heterogeneity
  3. Systemic neurohormones: increased levels of angiotensin II
  4. Pericardium: possible constraining effect as LV filling pressure and end diastolic volume increase

ATP = adenosine triphosphate; MMP = matrix metalloproteinase; TIMP = tissue inhibitor of MMP; Ca^{2+} = calcium; LV = left ventricular.

CLINICAL PRESENTATION

Patients with DHF have a marked limitation in exercise tolerance. There are a number of mechanisms responsible for this limitation. Exercise in a healthy patient is accompanied by an increase in the myocardial relaxation rate, an increase in the rate of left ventricular pressure decline, a decrease in the left ventricular minimum pressure, and an increase in the early left ventricle to left atrium transmitral pressure gradient—all of which together result in an increased filling rate during diastole. In addition, there is an increase in the left ventricular end diastolic volume, allowing the ventricle to use the Frank-Starling mechanism to augment stroke volume and ejection fraction. In patients with DHF, the ability to use the Frank-Starling mechanism is limited despite the increased filling pressures, because increased diastolic stiffness prevents the increase in left ventricular end diastolic volume that normally accompanies exercise (see Fig. 17–1).[25–27] As a result, the ejection fraction and stroke volume fail to rise, and patients experience dyspnea and fatigue.

Frequently, patients with DHF experience an exaggerated rise in blood pressure and heart rate in response to exercise. The exaggerated increase in blood pressure increases the left ventricular load, which in turn impairs left ventricular emptying as well as myocardial relaxation and filling.[19] In addition, the abnormal relaxation rate versus frequency relationship that exists in patients with DHF prevents augmentation of relaxation rate as heart rate increases during exercise.[28–30] These changes in load and heart rate result in an increase in diastolic filling pressures. Elevated diastolic pressures cause a reduction in lung compliance, increase the work of breathing, and evoke the symptom of dyspnea. Increased left ventricular diastolic pressure during exercise may also limit subendocardial blood flow during a period of increased myocardial oxygen demand, further worsening diastolic function. An inadequate cardiac output during exercise contributes to anaerobic metabolism of skeletal muscles, lactate accumulation, and, consequently, fatigue of the legs and the accessory muscles of respiration.

DIAGNOSIS

Making the diagnosis of DHF is difficult, as the requisite features to make the diagnosis remain controversial. However, making the diagnosis accurately is extremely important. Guidelines from the European Study Group on Diastolic Heart Failure propose three requirements for the diagnosis of DHF: (1) symptoms or signs of CHF, (2) normal systolic function, and (3) abnormal diastolic function (abnormal relaxation, filling, diastolic distensibility or diastolic stiffness).[31] Some of these three requirements appear to be well justified; others may not be.

With few exceptions, DHF cannot be distinguished from systolic CHF on the basis of the history, physical examination, chest radiograph, and electrocardiogram (ECG) alone.[5] Echeverria and colleagues showed that the frequency with which patients had symptoms of CHF, signs of CHF on physical examination, or indications of CHF on chest radiograph was not dependent on whether they had systolic or diastolic CHF.[6] But, there are exceptions. Pulsus alternans, a PMI displaced into the axilla, or cor bovinum on chest radiograph indicate that an abnormality in systolic function is causing CHF.

The data from a number of studies demonstrate that signs and symptoms of CHF do not predict ejection fraction. In contrast, they do predict the presence of increased left ventricular diastolic pressure. The question then becomes whether the increase in left ventricular diastolic pressure occurs in association with normal left ventricular volume and ejection fraction, as would occur in DHF, or whether the increase in left ventricular diastolic pressure occurs in association with an increased left ventricular volume and decreased ejection fraction, as would occur with systolic heart failure. Therefore, determining whether CHF is the result of diastolic or systolic dysfunction requires some estimate of left ventricular size and ejection fraction. These measurements can be made by means of echocardiography, radionuclide ventriculography, or contrast ventriculography. Measuring indices of left ventricular diastolic function can supplement this clinical approach; however, acquisition of these data may not be essential to establish the diagnosis of DHF. When a patient presents with dyspnea, pulmonary rales, and radiographic evidence of pulmonary venous hypertension, the detection of normal left ventricular end diastolic volume and normal ejection fraction supports the diagnosis of isolated DHF. Conditions such as mitral stenosis, noncardiogenic pulmonary edema, and chronic obstructive pulmonary disease (COPD) must be ruled out because they can cause similar symptoms.

Although some guidelines for the diagnosis of DHF require only the presence of symptoms of CHF, there are a number of clinical situations in which the presence of symptoms alone may lead to a misdiagnosis. This is especially true in older patients in whom symptoms of dyspnea on exertion may reflect deconditioning or noncardiac problems like COPD. To avoid this diagnostic problem, guidelines should require the presence of *both* symptoms and signs of CHF. Thus, the diagnosis of DHF is functionally a diagnosis of exclusion in which patients have symptoms and signs of CHF, but have normal left ventricular volume and have a preserved ejection fraction.

It has been argued that this clinical description characterizes patients with "CHF and normal EF" [ejection fraction]—certainly a narrow and precise description. Some clinicians are reluctant to use the term *diastolic heart failure,* arguing that (1) these patients do not have diastolic dysfunction; (2) the left ventricular ejection fraction may change episodically (e.g., decreased when symptoms are present, but normal at the time of the left ventricle study, thus obscuring the link between CHF and decreased ejection fraction, and preventing the diagnosis of systolic CHF); (3) it is often easy to misinterpret the left ventricular ejection fraction, because mitral regurgitation can maintain a normal ejection fraction even when contractility is abnormal and high blood pressure can suppress ejection fraction even when contractility is normal so that loading conditions can mask the ability of the ejection fraction to reflect the contractile state; and (4) the presence of an arrhythmia-like atrial fibrillation can make measurement of the left ventricular ejection fraction inaccurate.

There appear to be straightforward clinical approaches to deal with these concerns about the use of the term *diastolic heart failure*. If the accuracy of the volume or ejection fraction determination is in question, two diagnostic techniques can be helpful. Significant mitral regurgitation can be ruled out with echo-Doppler. Blood pressure should be assessed at the time the studies are performed. If there is a question of episodic mitral regurgitation or ischemia, an echocardiogram should be done while the symptoms of CHF are present. Although many clinicians believe that patients with symptoms and signs of CHF who have normal volume and ejection fraction, in fact, have abnormal diastolic function, no prospective controlled trials have yet addressed this point. However, a study by Soufer and associates supports this conclusion.[7] For a 12-month period, these researchers screened by means of nuclear medicine consecutive patients with symptoms and signs of CHF and ejection fractions of more than 45%. Of these patients, 65% had abnormal filling patterns by radionuclide ventriculography. Of the remaining 35%, one-third had left heart catheterizations (10% of total patients). The average left ventricular end-diastolic pressure was more than 20 mm Hg, and all patients had a pressure greater than 15 mm Hg. Thus, at least 75% of these patients had demonstrable abnormalities in diastolic function. It is suspected that if diastolic function was measured in patients with symptoms and signs of CHF, normal ejection fraction, and normal end-diastolic volume, then virtually 100% would have measurable abnormalities in diastolic function.

The major limitation in quantifying diastolic function is that the majority of the measurements of isovolumic and auxotonic relaxation and passive diastolic stiffness depend on the use of invasive techniques that are not always applicable to routine clinical diagnosis. Thus, clinicians have come to rely largely on noninvasive techniques to screen patients for diastolic dysfunction. All of these noninvasive techniques use parameters that reflect the process of filling. For example, filling dynamics can be assessed using echo-Doppler techniques in which the E wave represents early rapid filling and the A wave represents late filling produced by atrial contraction. Diastolic filling can be quantified by measuring the peak velocity, the area within the velocity versus time integral, the rate of deceleration, and the E:A velocity ratio. When diastolic dysfunction is present, the E-wave velocity is markedly reduced, the A-wave velocity is increased, the velocity versus time integral is decreased, the deceleration time is prolonged, and the E:A velocity ratio is decreased.

Like all of the proposed measurements of diastolic function, however, filling dynamics are influenced by changes in loading conditions, heterogeneity, and patient age.[2–5] Above the age of 60 to 65 years, a decreased E wave and an increased A wave may represent a normal pattern, rather than the presence of diastolic dysfunction or disease.[32] When left atrial pressure increases, a pseudonormalization of the pattern may occur and mask the presence of diastolic dysfunction.

PROGNOSIS

The prognosis of patients with DHF, although less ominous than that of patients with systolic CHF, does exceed the prognosis of age-matched control patients.[8,22,23,33] The annual mortality rate for patients with DHF approximates 5% to 8%. In comparison, the annual mortality rate for patients with systolic CHF approximates 10% to 15%, while that of age-matched control patients approaches 1%. In patients with DHF, the clinical pathologic cause of the disease also affects the prognosis. When patients with coronary artery disease are excluded, the annual mortality rate for those with isolated DHF approximates 2% to 3%;[22,23] most of the remaining patients are those with pressure overload left ventricular hypertrophy. In addition to the clinical pathologic cause of CHF, age and ejection fraction are determinants of mortality. Like prevalence, these are interactive, with the most important determinant being age. The 5-year mortality rate in patients with DHF is 25%. In patients 60 to 70 years of age, however, it is 35%; in patients more than 70 years of age, 50%.

The mode of death is similar in patients with systolic versus diastolic heart failure. Sudden death and death from progressive pump failure occurred with equal frequency in systolic versus diastolic CHF patients. The morbidity rate from DHF is quite high, requiring frequent outpatient visits, hospital admissions, and the expenditure of significant health care resources. The 1-year readmission rate approaches 50% in patients with DHF. Surprisingly, this morbidity rate is nearly identical to that of patients with systolic CHF.[34]

▶ TREATMENT: Diastolic Heart Failure

The general principles used to guide the treatment of systolic CHF are based on randomized, double-blind, placebo-controlled, multicenter trials. Unfortunately, no such randomized trials have been performed in patients with diastolic CHF. Consequently, the guidelines for the management of DHF are based on clinical investigations in relatively small groups of patients, clinical experience, and an understanding of the pathophysiology of the disease process.[2–4,35–37] The treatment regimen outlined in Table 17–2 applies to those patients with DHF who have clear manifestations of congestion, either at rest or with exertion. Whether treatment of asymptomatic diastolic dysfunction confers any benefit has not been examined.

DESIRED OUTCOMES

Treatment should be targeted at reducing symptoms, principally those of increased pulmonary venous pressure. For example, treatment should include decreasing diastolic pressure by decreasing left ventricular volume, maintaining atrial contraction, and reducing heart rate. Second, treatment should be targeted at the pathologic disease that is causing diastolic CHF. For example, coronary artery disease, hypertensive heart disease, and aortic stenosis provide relatively specific therapeutic goals, such as lowering blood pressure, inducing left ventricular hypertrophy (LVH) regression, performing aortic valve replacement, and countering ischemia by increasing myocardial blood flow and reducing myocardial oxygen demand. Third, treatment should be targeted at the underlying mechanisms that the disease processes mentioned are altering.

NONPHARMACOLOGIC THERAPY

DIET AND LIFESTYLE

The initial effort in the treatment of DHF is aimed at decreasing symptoms. The first step in this effort is to decrease pulmonary congestion by decreasing left ventricular volume through sodium and fluid restriction. A low sodium diet (<2 g daily) will help to prevent volume overload. Judicious fluid restriction will also help to prevent volume overload. Both sodium and fluid restriction must be done with care, however. Excessive restriction can lead to hypotension, low output, and/or renal insufficiency. Monitoring the patient's daily weight may help evaluate excess volume. It is important for the

TABLE 17–2. General Approach to Treatment of Diastolic Heart Failure

Type of Treatment	Strategy	Drug
Symptom-targeted treatment	Decrease pulmonary venous pressure	
	Reduce left ventricular volume	Diuretics, salt restriction
	Maintain atrial contraction	Cardioversion of atrial fibrillation
	Reduce heart rate	β-Blockers, diltiazem, verapamil
	Improve exercise tolerance	As above
	Use positive inotropic agents with caution	
Disease-targeted treatment	Prevent/treat myocardial ischemia	β-Blockers, diltiazem, verapamil, nitrates
	Prevent/regress ventricular hypertrophy	Antihypertensive therapy
Mechanism-targeted treatment	Modify myocardial and extramyocardial mechanisms	Possibly ACE inhibitors or angiotensin receptor blockers, diuretics, spironolactone
	Modify intracellular and extracellular mechanisms	Possibly ACE inhibitors or angiotensin receptor blockers, spironolactone

ACE = angiotensin-converting enzyme.

patient to avoid dietary and lifestyle factors that increase the risk of epicardial coronary artery disease and high blood pressure. Moderate aerobic exercise to improve cardiovascular conditioning is beneficial to maintain a slower heart rate, improve cardiac reserve, and maintain skeletal muscle function. Isometric exercise should be avoided.

INTERVENTIONAL/SURGICAL PROCEDURES

An important step in symptom-targeted therapy that acts to decrease pulmonary venous pressures is to maintain atrial contraction and atrioventricular synchrony. These factors are important both in preserving normal cardiac output and keeping left ventricular diastolic pressure low. Chemical or electrical cardioversion of persistent atrial tachyarrhythmias will decrease diastolic pressure, increase cardiac output, and resolve pulmonary edema. An atrioventricular sequential pacemaker should be used to treat bradyarrhythmias in patients who require pacing.

Therapy should also be aimed at preventing or treating the underlying pathologic cause of DHF. Symptomatic patients with pressure overload hypertrophy caused by aortic stenosis should undergo aortic valve replacement. Selected patients with DHF caused by coronary artery disease-induced myocardial ischemia need revascularization. In addition, myocardial oxygen consumption and myocardial blood flow should be increased by means of medical treatment, including the administration of nitrates, β-blockers, and calcium channel blockers.

INDICATIONS FOR HOSPITALIZATION

Patients with DHF may present with an acute onset of pulmonary edema. There are a number of potential causes for the acute decompensation of these patients, including volume overload, uncontrolled hypertension, acute myocardial ischemia, progressive valvular disease (aortic stenosis), progressive constrictive pericardial disease, and new-onset or uncontrolled tachyarrhythmias. Treatment strategies for these patients may include surgery, in the case of valvular disease, or the intravenous (IV) use of diuretic agents, in the case of volume overload. Caution must be exercised to avoid overdiuresis, which can lead to hypotension.

A recent study involving patients who required emergency treatment for pulmonary edema focused on the association of clinical findings with prognosis or outcome.[38] In this study of 186 patients, 40% had no recognized precipitating factor identified for their hospitalization. Patients who responded to diuretic therapy with a good urine output had a better outcome than did patients who did not respond as well. This study did not examine whether prognosis was related to the presence of systolic or diastolic heart failure. Based on this information, diuretics are first-line therapy for acute decompensation and pulmonary edema.

PHARMACOLOGIC THERAPY

With a few notable exceptions, many of the drugs used to treat systolic heart failure are also used to treat DHF. However, the rationale for their use, the pathophysiologic process that the drug is altering, and the dosing regimen may be entirely different, depending on whether the patient has systolic or diastolic CHF. For example, β-blockers are recommended for the treatment of both systolic and diastolic CHF. In systolic CHF, β-blockers are used over the long term to increase inotropic state and modify left ventricular remodeling. In diastolic CHF, β-blockers are used to decrease heart rate, increase diastolic duration, and modify the hemodynamic response to exercise. Similarly, diuretics are used in the treatment of both systolic and diastolic heart failure; however, the doses of diuretics used to treat DHF are, in general, much smaller than the doses used in systolic CHF. Some drugs are used to treat either systolic or diastolic CHF, but not both. Calcium channel blockers such as diltiazem, nifedipine, and verapamil have little utility in the treatment of systolic CHF. In contrast, each of these has been proposed as useful in the treatment of DHF.

DIURETICS

By acting to decrease systemic and left ventricular volume, diuretics can provide symptom-targeted therapy. When left ventricular diastolic volumes decrease, left ventricular pressures slide down the curvilinear diastolic pressure-volume relationship toward a lower, less steep portion of this curve (see Fig. 17–1). As pressure throughout diastole falls, mean diastolic pressure, pulmonary capillary wedge pressure, and pulmonary venous pressures also fall. Diuretic agents effectively reduce the central blood volume, lower diastolic pressures, and thus alleviate the symptoms of the congestive state. They can provide disease-targeted therapy by decreasing blood pressure and favorably affecting the myocardial oxygen supply versus demand ratio. Lower left ventricular diastolic pressures may increase subendocardial blood flow, preventing or alleviating the imbalance between myocardial oxygen supply and demand. Diuretics alone and especially in combination with other antihypertensive drugs are an effective approach to therapy.

Treatment with diuretics should begin at low doses in order to avoid hypotension and fatigue. Hypotension can be a significant problem in the treatment of DHF because these patients have a very steep left ventricular diastolic pressure-volume curve such that a small change in volume causes a large change in filling pressure and cardiac output. After the completion of the acute treatment of DHF, long-term treatment should include small to moderate doses of diuretics (furosemide, 20–40 mg/d administered orally, or hydrochlorothiazide, 25 mg/d administered orally). If prompt and sustained diuresis is not achieved, the dosage of a single diuretic should be increased, or a loop and thiazide or thiazide-like diuretic should be used in combination. Aldosterone antagonists such as spironolactone may be especially effective in long-term use because they have potassium-sparing effects and because their antagonism of renin-angiotensin-aldosterone system activation may alter the intra- and extramyocardial mechanisms that cause abnormalities in diastolic function. Thiazide diuretics are generally ineffective in patients with a creatinine clearance of less than 30 mL/min.

Excessive diuresis may result in hypotension, low-output syndrome, and worsening renal insufficiency. Electrolyte imbalances, including hypokalemia and hypomagnesemia, are common with thiazide diuretics. Carbohydrate intolerance and hyperuricemia are dose-related adverse drug reactions seen with thiazide diuretics. Spironolactone can cause hyperkalemia and gynecomastia. However, diuretic agents are very cost-effective agents in the management of DHF.

NITRATES

Similar to diuretics, nitrates can provide symptom-targeted therapy by acting to decrease left ventricular volume, by increasing venous capacitance. In addition, nitrates can provide disease-targeted therapy through their anti-ischemic effects in patients with coronary artery disease-induced DHF.

Like therapy with diuretics, therapy with nitrates should be initiated at low doses in order to avoid hypotension. Isosorbide dinitrate (10 mg three or four times each day), isosorbide mononitrate (Imdur; 30 mg/d), nitroglycerin paste (0.5–1 inch every 4 to 6 hours), or nitroglycerin patch (0.1–0.2 mg/h applied each day) are common initial dosages. Doses can be increased during long-term therapy and titrated against symptoms. Nitrate tolerance has not been studied in this patient population, but probably does occur. Just as diuretics can, nitrates can cause hypotension and low-output syndrome. Headaches are common, but may become less frequent with continued use.

Patients who develop shortness of breath with mild exercise may find the sublingual use of nitroglycerin tablets or a nitroglycerin spray beneficial. They should use these medications in much the same way that the patient with ischemic symptoms uses them. Nitroglycerin will decrease left ventricular end-diastolic volume, resulting in relief of breathlessness.

β-ADRENERGIC BLOCKERS

Not only can β-blockers provide symptom-targeted therapy by decreasing heart rate, but also they can provide disease-targeted therapy by treating high blood pressure and coronary artery disease. By decreasing heart rate and increasing the duration of diastole, β-blockers can help to reduce pulmonary venous pressure and maintain it at a lower level.

Tachycardia is poorly tolerated by patients with DHF for several reasons. First, rapid heart rates increase myocardial oxygen demand and decrease coronary perfusion time. This rapid rate can promote ischemic diastolic dysfunction, even in the absence of epicardial coronary disease, especially in patients with left ventricular hypertrophy. Second, relaxation between cardiac cycles may be incomplete, resulting in an increase in diastolic pressure relative to volume. Thus, left ventricular distensibility is reduced. Third, a rapid rate reduces diastolic filling time and ventricular filling. Fourth, hearts with diastolic dysfunction exhibit a flat or even negative relaxation rate versus frequency relationship.[28–30] Thus, as heart rate increases in these hearts, relaxation does not become augmented, so that relaxation may become slow and incomplete, causing diastolic pressures, especially early in diastole, to increase. For these and other reasons, most clinicians use β-blockers (and calcium channel blockers) to prevent excessive tachycardia and produce a relative bradycardia in patients with diastolic dysfunction. However, excessive bradycardia can result in a fall of cardiac output, despite an increase in left ventricular filling.[28,39] Such considerations underscore the need for individualizing therapeutic interventions that affect heart rate. Although it is necessary to determine the optimal heart rate on an individual basis, an initial goal may be a resting heart rate of approximately 60 beats/min with a blunted exercise-induced increase in heart rate not to exceed 110 beats/min.[40]

β-Blockers (and calcium channel blockers) directly reduce relaxation rate by their actions on intracellular processes. On the other hand, they normalize loading conditions, decrease heart rate, prevent ischemia, and cause the regression of hypertrophy. The indirect effects of these mechanisms are to speed relaxation and to increase filling. Taken together, these effects result in symptomatic improvement in patients with DHF. However, it is an oversimplification to suggest that β-blockers (and calcium channel blockers), in and of themselves, speed relaxation by a direct effect on the cardiac muscle cell.

There is no evidence to suggest that one β-blocker has a specific therapeutic advantage over others. Selective and nonselective β-blockers appear equally effective in DHF, although β-blockers with intrinsic sympathomimetic activity may be less effective because they slow the heart rate less. In general, it is not necessary to start the chosen drug at an extremely low dose and titrate the β-blocker in a slow progressive fashion in DHF as it is in systolic heart failure. As the population is older, it is prudent to start with a moderate dose of metoprolol (25 mg two times a day), or atenolol (25 mg/d), and titrate to a higher dose with the treatment target of a heart rate of approximately 60 beats/min.

Prinzmetal's vasospastic angina, bronchospastic COPD, asthma, occlusive peripheral vascular disease, type I diabetes mellitus that is prone to hypoglycemia, heart block, and excessive bradycardia are contraindications to the use of β-blockers. The main side effects are depression, fatigue, bradycardia, bronchospasm, and impotence. Many of the β-blockers are eliminated via hepatic metabolism, which may be affected by other drugs that either inhibit (e.g., cimetidine, verapamil) or enhance (e.g., barbiturates) the hepatic enzymes. Because the doses are titrated to patient response, these interactions are easily managed. Several β-blockers (i.e., propranolol, metoprolol, atenolol, nadolol, timolol) are available as generic formulations, making them very cost-effective.

CALCIUM CHANNEL BLOCKERS

The symptom-targeted treatment provided by calcium channel blockers comes from the ability of these drugs to decrease heart rate and increase exercise tolerance. They can provide disease-targeted treatment by treating high blood pressure and coronary artery disease. Although the beneficial effect of these agents on exercise tolerance does not always parallel improved left ventricular diastolic function or increased relaxation rate, a number of small clinical trials have shown that the use of these agents results in both short-term and long-term improvement of exercise capacity in patients with DHF.[21,41]

Of the calcium channel blockers, the nondihydropyridines (i.e., verapamil and diltiazem) are the most effective, because they lower both heart rate and blood pressure. Nifedipine, because of its strong vasodilator properties, tends to cause hypotension and reflex tachycardia. In addition, nifedipine causes peripheral edema. These characteristics make it less useful in DHF. Amlodipine is also effective, because it reduces blood pressure. Initial dosages are verapamil, 120–240 mg/d; diltiazem, 90–120 mg/d; and amlodipine, 2.5 mg/d.

The most common side effects of the nondihydropyridine calcium channel blockers are bradycardia and heart block. Peripheral edema and headache are also common. Heart block is a contraindication for the use of nondihydropyridines. Further, these drugs exacerbate the bradycardic effects of β-blockers, and verapamil raises digoxin serum concentrations by 70%. Diltiazem raises cyclosporine serum concentrations. Calcium salts given IV inhibit the pharmacologic effect of calcium channel blockers. Generic formulations or similar products, but not necessarily generic equivalents to the original brand names, are available for verapamil, diltiazem, and nifedipine.

NEUROHUMORAL ANTAGONISTS

Both basic and clinical studies suggest that DHF is associated with activation of systemic and local cardiac neuroendocrine systems, such as the renin-angiotensin-aldosterone system.[15,16] Activation of these neuroendocrine systems contribute to the fluid retention and the increases in central and systemic volume that occur in patients with DHF. Therefore, treatment for DHF should include agents such as angiotensin-converting enzyme inhibitors (ACEIs), angiotensin receptor antagonists, and aldosterone antagonists, which attenuate the fluid retention caused by neuroendocrine activation.

In addition to promoting fluid retention, neuroendocrine activation can have direct effects on cellular and extracellular mechanisms that contribute to the development of DHF. Modulation of neuroendocrine activation may provide mechanism-targeted treatment by decreasing fibroblast activity and interstitial fibrosis, improving intracellular calcium handling, and decreasing myocardial stiffness. Finally, renin-angiotensin-aldosterone system antagonists provide disease-targeted treatment by treating hypertension.

The mechanisms that evoke the activation of the neuroendocrine system in patients with diastolic CHF remain incompletely understood. A number of factors have been suggested. Myocardial ischemia, uncontrolled hypertension, and excessive dietary sodium may contribute to neuroendocrine activation. Limited distensibility of the atria may attenuate the secretion of atrial natriuretic factor and thereby reduce its diuretic effect.[42] In others, low systemic vascular resistance and/or low arterial pressure may contribute to an increase in renin-angiotensin-aldosterone system activation, as well as to salt and water retention.[43] Elevated venous pressure may directly cause renal sodium retention.[44] The reduction in blood volume that follows the use of diuretics triggers an increase in sympathetic tone and further activates the renin-angiotensin-aldosterone system. Such neurohormonal activation can lead to vasoconstriction and a worsening of the congestive state. Some vasodilators, particularly nitrates and pure arteriolar vasodilators, evoke a similar response. By contrast, ACEIs (and β-blockers) blunt neurohormonal activation and decrease the salt and water retention that complicates the treatment of CHF.

ANGIOTENSIN-CONVERTING ENZYME INHIBITORS

By decreasing left ventricular volume and directly improving relaxation, ACEIs can provide symptom-targeted treatment. They can provide disease-targeted treatment by treating high blood pressure, preventing LVH, promoting regression, and preventing fibrosis. Treatment of high blood pressure with ACEIs has been shown to normalize load, prevent left ventricular hypertrophy and/or cause it to regress, correct the abnormality in intracellular processes, and modify the extracellular matrix response.[45] Recently, a small, prospective, double-blind, randomized trial compared the effectiveness of lisinopril to that of hydrochlorothiazide in 35 patients with primary hypertension, left ventricular hypertrophy, and left ventricular diastolic dysfunction.[46] After 6 months of therapy, lisinopril had caused regression of myocardial fibrosis and improved left ventricular diastolic function, although left ventricular hypertrophy was unchanged.

At this time, there is no evidence to suggest an advantage of one ACEI over another. Their effects appear to be a class effect. Initial doses should be to small to moderate in order to avoid hypotension, especially if volume status indicates dehydration. A single daily dose improves compliance. Examples of initial starting dosages are captopril, 6.25 mg administered orally three times a day; enalapril, 2.5 mg/d administered orally; or lisinopril, 2.5 mg/d administered orally.

Severe renal failure, a history of angioedema, and pregnancy are contraindications to ACEIs. Hyperkalemia, persistent cough, hypotension, taste disturbances, and worsening renal function are common side effects.

ANGIOTENSIN RECEPTOR BLOCKERS

To treat symptoms, angiotensin receptor blockers decrease left ventricular pressure, decrease left ventricular volume, and increase exercise tolerance. They can provide disease-targeted treatment by lowering blood pressure.

In a randomized, double-blind, placebo-controlled trial in 20 patients with diastolic dysfunction, losartan or placebo was added to the existing medical regimen for a 2-week period.[47] Patients enrolled in the study had a marked hypertensive response to exercise, an ejection fraction greater than 50%, and no evidence of ischemia on stress echocardiogram. Their blood pressure at rest was well controlled (143/79 mm Hg); however, the mean peak systolic blood pressure after 11 minutes of exercise was 226 mm Hg. Although the resting systolic and diastolic blood pressure did not change with the administration of either losartan or placebo, the peak systolic blood pressure in those given losartan declined to 193 mm Hg, compared to placebo (217 mm Hg) and baseline (226 mm Hg). Losartan increased the exercise time, and improved New York Heart Association class and quality of life as assessed by the modified Minnesota Living With Heart Failure survey.

The specific mechanism of the losartan-induced improvement is not known. Angiotensin II slows the rate of left ventricular relaxation and increases left ventricular diastolic pressures. In a 2-week period of time, there was no evidence of improved diastolic function. Losartan did slow the increase in systolic blood pressure during exercise and decreased the peak systolic blood pressure by a mean of 33 mm Hg. Although the patients had no evidence of myocardial ischemia, losartan may have improved endothelial function and coronary perfusion.

No angiotensin receptor blocker has yet been shown to have any major advantages over another. Initial doses of candesartan start at 8 mg/d; irbesartan, 150 mg/d; losartan, 25 mg/d; telmisartan, 40 mg/d; and valsartan, 80 mg/d. As with the ACEIs, angiotensin receptor blockers are contraindicated in pregnancy. The side effects of these drugs are similar to those of the ACEIs, but they are not associated with persistent cough.

ALDOSTERONE ANTAGONISTS

The symptom-targeted treatment provided by aldosterone antagonists comes from their ability to decrease left ventricular volume; the disease-targeted treatment, from their ability to decrease the fibrosis that accompanies LVH. In a subgroup of the RALES (Randomized Aldactone Evaluation Study) study, spironolactone significantly decreased the levels of three different serum markers for cardiac collagen turnover. The benefit from spironolactone occurred in patients with the highest baseline levels of the three markers for extracellular matrix turnover.[48] This was the first study to show that high serum levels of markers of cardiac collagen synthesis were associated with a poor clinical outcome and that spironolactone could decrease those levels. This property distinguishes spironolactone from other diuretics that have no effect on myocardial necrosis or collagen turnover.

Like other diuretics, spironolactone should be initiated at a low dose and increased to treat symptoms. It may be initiated at doses of 12.5–25 mg/d. Spironolactone should be avoided in severe renal failure. Hyperkalemia and gynecomastia are the most common side effects.

β-ADRENERGIC AGONISTS

Positive inotropic agents like β-agonists are generally not used in the treatment of patients with isolated DHF because this condition preserves the left ventricular ejection fraction and there appears to be little potential for a beneficial effect. Moreover, positive inotropic agents sometimes worsen the pathophysiologic processes that cause diastolic CHF. Despite the doubts regarding their long-term use, positive inotropic drugs may be beneficial in the short-term treatment of pulmonary edema associated with diastolic CHF. Positive inotropes such as β-adrenergic agonists (and phosphodiesterase inhibitors) can enhance sarcoplasmic reticular function, promote more rapid complete relaxation, increase splanchnic blood flow, increase venous capacitance, and facilitate diuresis.[37,49–51] However, even short-term treatment with these agents may adversely affect energetics, induce ischemia, raise heart rate, and induce arrhythmias.[37] Therefore, these agents should be used with caution in patients with DHF, if they are used at all.

DIGITALIS DERIVATIVES

Digoxin, by inhibiting the sodium–potassium–adenosine triphosphatase (ATPase) pump, augments intracellular calcium and thereby augments the contractile state. In this manner, digoxin increases systolic energy demands while adding to a relative calcium overload in diastole. These effects may not be clinically apparent under many circumstances, but during hemodynamic stress or ischemia, digoxin may promote or contribute to diastolic dysfunction.[48] Therefore, until recently, digoxin was not used in the treatment of DHF—except to slow ventricular rate in patients with chronic atrial fibrillation. However, results of the DIG trial suggest that even patients with a normal ejection fraction may have fewer symptoms and fewer hospitalizations if they are treated with digoxin.[34] This salutary effect is not likely to result from digoxin's effect on inotropy, but rather from its blunting of neuroendocrine activation.

THE CARDIOMYOPATHIES

Diastolic dysfunction plays a role in the presentation of some cardiomyopathies, a variety of diseases that affect the myocardium in either a diffuse or multifocal manner and that frequently result in heart failure. The terminology and classification used for the cardiomyopathies are confusing because of overlap among the diseases and/or classification schemes. Cardiomyopathies are sometimes defined according to their cause. Primary cardiomyopathies are disorders that affect either the structure or function of the myocardium in the *absence* of other known causes of heart disease or systemic diseases known to affect the heart. Secondary forms of cardiomyopathy are conditions in which a recognized factor is causing the myocardial abnormality. Infectious agents, inflammation, metabolic disorders, infiltrative diseases, and toxins are a few of the causative factors of secondary cardiomyopathy.[52,53]

Many times, a specific cause is not evident. Therefore, another commonly used categorization of the cardiomyopathies is based on the structural and/or functional abnormalities present. The three groups of cardiomyopathies are usually described as: dilated (congestive), hypertrophic, and restrictive (Table 17–3). The distinction among the cardiomyopathies is not absolute, and there is some overlap in the functional abnormalities. An understanding of the pathophysiologic basis for each type of cardiomyopathy leads to a rational selection of drug therapy or other treatment modality, however.

In dilated cardiomyopathy (DCM), the cardinal feature is dilatation of the ventricles. Systolic function is abnormal, leading to a decreased cardiac output. (For a thorough discussion of the pathophysiology and treatment of dilated cardiomyopathy, see Chapter 13, Heart Failure.) In those patients with hypertrophic cardiomyopathy (HCM), the ventricular muscle mass is increased. Ventricular cavity size is normal or decreased, and systolic function is often preserved. Patients with HCM may have an obstructive or nonobstructive form. Patients with restrictive cardiomyopathy have inadequate ventricular compliance, causing diastolic dysfunction as a result of endocardial and/or myocardial disease. The clinical presentation is similar to that of constrictive pericarditis.

Other terms are frequently encountered in discussions of patients with cardiomyopathy. *Familial cardiomyopathy* denotes a condition found in more than one family member. *Genetic predisposition* may occur in all three functional types. Patients with occlusive atherosclerotic coronary artery disease and left ventricular dysfunction are said

TABLE 17–3. Characteristics of the Cardiomyopathies

	Dilated	Hypertrophic	Restrictive
Myocardial mass	↑→↑↑	↑↑↑	nl →↑
Ventricular cavity size	↑↑→↑↑↑↑	↓↓→ nl	nl →↓
Contractile function	↓↓↓	↑↑→↓	nl →↓
LV filling pressure	↑↑	nl →↑	↑
Chest radiograph	Moderate to marked cardiac enlargement	Mild to moderate cardiac enlargement	Mild cardiac enlargement
Electrocardiogram	ST and T-wave abnormalities	ST and T-wave abnormalities, LV hypertrophy	Low voltage, conduction defects
Echocardiogram	LV dilatation and dysfunction	Asymmetric septal hypertrophy systolic anterior motion of the mitral valve	Increased LV wall thickness possible
Radionuclide studies	LV dilatation and dysfunction	Vigorous systolic function	Normal systolic function

↑ = increased; ↓ = decreased; nl = normal; LV = left ventricular.

to have *ischemic cardiomyopathy*—although this is not a true cardiomyopathy because there is an identifiable cause of the ventricular muscle dysfunction.

Myocardial hypertrophy is one of the most important adaptive measures that the failing heart uses to compensate for pressure and volume overload conditions. However, these hypertrophied cells are not normal, and this "cardiomyopathy of overload" may eventually lead to myocardial cell deterioration and death.[54] The role of altered gene expression in the hypertrophied myocardium is an area of extensive research. It appears that the phenotype of the hypertrophied heart differs from that of the normal heart. The expression of genes that encode the proteins responsible for contraction (myosin and actin) and relaxation (calcium-ATPase and phospholamban) appear to be of primary importance.[55]

HYPERTROPHIC CARDIOMYOPATHY

A primary myocardial disorder, HCM is characterized by a hypertrophied and nondilated left ventricle with no apparent cause. The distribution of the hypertrophy is usually asymmetric, meaning segments of the left ventricle are thickened to varying degrees. There may also be enlargement of the atria, thickening of the mitral valve leaflets, and fibrotic areas within the ventricular wall. In the past, HCM has been termed idiopathic hypertrophic subaortic stenosis (IHSS) and hypertrophic obstructive cardiomyopathy (HOCM). These latter terms are used less frequently now, because they overemphasize the obstructive component of the disease, which is present in only a minority of patients.[56] Treatment strategies are aimed at improving symptoms and preventing sudden cardiac death.

PATHOPHYSIOLOGY

The genetic predisposition to HCM is thought to be an autosomal dominant trait with variable penetrance. Because of the wide variability of presentation, not all cases in a family may be detected. Usually, HCM is the result of mutations in the genes for β-myosin heavy chain, α-tropomyosin, myosin-binding protein C, or cardiac troponin T.[57,58] It appears that HCM has several different pathophysiologic mechanisms leading to similar clinical manifestations, although the prognoses for patients will vary. Overall, HCM has an estimated prevalence in the United States of 1 in 500.

The pathophysiology of HCM is a complex relationship among several factors, including (1) asymmetric left ventricular hypertrophy, (2) diastolic dysfunction, (3) dynamic obstruction of the outflow tract, and (4) myocardial ischemia. Each of these components contributes to the overall presentation of the patient to a varying degree.

Left Ventricular Hypertrophy

The hypertrophy seen in HCM is usually diffuse, and it involves the septum and left ventricular anterolateral free wall to a greater degree than the posterior segment. Asymmetric septal hypertrophy is a sensitive marker for HCM, but is not specific for this disorder. In patients with outflow obstruction, the basal septum is usually markedly thickened at the level of the mitral valve. In patients with nonobstructive HCM, the outflow tract is larger, and the septal hypertrophy that occurs has a more distal or apical distribution.

Cellular disorganization is a common histologic finding of HCM. Morphologic abnormalities occur at the gross, microscopic, and ultrastructural levels. The disarray of myocytes may contribute to diastolic and systolic dysfunction and may serve as a nidus for ventricular arrhythmias. The greater the degree of left ventricular hypertrophy, the worse the clinical course. Patients with severe and diffuse hypertrophy are predisposed to symptoms of heart failure, lethal arrhythmias, and sudden death.

Diastolic Dysfunction

The most common abnormality found in patients with HCM is diastolic dysfunction. Approximately 80% of patients will exhibit symptoms associated with this finding. Examination of the left ventricle led to the realization that diastolic dysfunction is the result of abnormalities in relaxation, distensibility (compliance), and filling. These abnormalities can be both regional and global, and they lead to an incoordination of contraction and relaxation. Abnormal relaxation is manifested by a prolonged isovolumic relaxation period and a reduced rate of decline in left ventricular pressure. Filling of the left ventricle is prolonged in most patients. The presence of mitral regurgitation tends to normalize these abnormalities. β-Adrenergic stimulation can aggravate these abnormalities, whereas β-blockade may diminish them.[56,59]

Myocardial relaxation is an energy-dependent process that is sensitive to episodes of ischemia. Diastolic resequestration of calcium ions by the sarcoplasmic reticulum is also an energy-dependent process. In the event of ischemia, the sequestration of calcium is inhibited, allowing the calcium to continue its interaction with the myofibrillar contractile proteins. Calcium channel–blocking drugs have been used with some success in patients with diastolic dysfunction.[56]

Abnormalities in filling are also associated with the changes in chamber stiffness that occur in HCM. This stiffness may be the result of myocardial fibrosis, cellular disorganization, or the increase in myocardial mass. The decreased distensibility leads to an abnormally steep slope of the diastolic pressure-volume curve (see Fig. 17–1), such that an increase in left ventricular volume results in a disproportionate increase in diastolic pressure.[56]

Systolic Function and Outflow Tract Obstruction

Abnormalities of systolic function also occur in patients with HCM. The hypertrophied left ventricle may cause a powerful, but sometimes uncoordinated contraction, presumably because of the abnormal architecture of the myocardium. The increase seen in the left ventricular wall thickness results in decreased wall stress during systole. Therefore, the left ventricle contracts against a decreased afterload so that the left ventricle is described as being hyperdynamic rather than hypercontractile.[56] Ejection fraction is often increased.

Considerable controversy has surrounded the issue of the importance of outflow tract obstruction in conjunction with HCM. The presence of a gradient (the systolic pressure difference between the body and outflow tract of the left ventricle) is indicative of a dynamic obstruction of the left ventricular outflow tract. Outflow tract gradients occur in about 25% of patients with HCM. The obstruction that occurs usually shows spontaneous variability, and interventions that decrease myocardial contractility may reduce it. Factors that increase contractility can augment the gradient (Table 17–4).[56]

Enhanced contraction, apposition of the anterior mitral leaflet to the hypertrophied septum impeding aortic flow, large papillary muscles, and reduced left ventricular cavity size are factors that may contribute to a systolic pressure gradient. The importance of the pressure gradient remains controversial because there is a poor correlation between the presence of a gradient and the clinical symptoms or prognosis of a patient.

Myocardial Ischemia

Chest pain in the absence of coronary artery disease is a common symptom of patients with HCM. There are several mechanisms

TABLE 17–4. Factors Known to Affect Gradients

- Factors That Diminish Gradients
  - Decreasing myocardial contractility
    - β-Blocking drugs
    - Verapamil
  - Increasing ventricular volume
  - Increasing arterial pressure
- Factors That Enhance Gradients
  - Increasing myocardial contractility
    - Exercise
    - Inotropic agents
  - Decreasing ventricular volume
  - Decreasing arterial pressure

proposed for the myocardial ischemia that occurs in this patient population. Capillary density may be inadequate in relation to the increased left ventricular muscle mass. The small intramural coronary arteries may be abnormally narrowed or excessively compressed during systole. Impaired relaxation during diastole may inhibit blood flow to the subendocardium. Once myocardial ischemia develops, left ventricular filling pressure may increase further, which in turns leads to more ischemia. Repeated episodes of ischemia may be responsible for progressive myocyte loss and fibrosis. The subendocardium is at greatest risk for ischemic damage due to the lower capillary density and higher oxygen demand secondary to wall tension.[59]

CLINICAL PRESENTATION

The natural history of HCM is quite variable, and its form ranges from an asymptomatic illness to a severe, life-threatening illness. There is no relation between the presence or absence of an outflow tract gradient and clinical presentation or prognosis. However, the presence of hypertrophy does correlate directly with myocardial infarction, heart failure, stroke, and ventricular arrhythmias.[60]

The clinical presentation varies widely, ranging from no symptoms to severe symptoms of angina and heart failure, to sudden cardiac death. The most common symptoms are chest pain, dyspnea, fatigue, palpitations, presyncope, and syncope. In general, the severity of symptoms corresponds to the degree of left ventricular hypertrophy, but this relationship is not absolute. Some patients with mild or localized hypertrophy have severe symptoms, whereas other patients with marked hypertrophy have minimal symptoms. Furthermore, the presence or absence of a dynamic obstruction does not seem to play a role in the patient's presentation. The symptoms of fatigue, orthopnea, and dyspnea are usually due to the elevated pulmonary pressures secondary to diastolic dysfunction. Some patients may develop dyspnea as a result of systolic dysfunction secondary to myocardial ischemia and fibrosis. Chest pain occurs in as many as 75% of patients, even though the incidence of atherosclerotic coronary artery disease is much less. The chest pain may have atypical features, such as a prolonged duration, occurrence at rest, and limited relief from nitrates.[59]

DIAGNOSIS

It may be difficult to make the diagnosis of HCM, as the disorder may be confused with coronary artery disease, mitral regurgitation, and aortic stenosis. Patients with HCM are often physically active. The physical signs of the cardiac examination depend on the presence of a systolic pressure gradient within the left ventricle. If a gradient is present, a late-onset systolic murmur is often heard. The murmur is intensified by standing and the Valsalva maneuver and lessened with squatting or handgrip. Very rarely, some patients develop an end-stage left ventricular dilatation and a declining left ventricular ejection fraction that is often confused with idiopathic DCM.[59]

Echocardiography is used to confirm the diagnosis. Findings consistent with HCM include a low normal or decreased end-diastolic dimension, a septal wall thickness equal to or greater than 15 mm, and a septal to posterior wall thickness ratio equal to or greater than 1.3:1. The presence of a hyperdynamic left ventricle and systolic anterior motion of the anterior mitral leaflet increased the likelihood of the diagnosis. Recently, the classic echocardiographic criteria have been called into question, because there is overlap between the genetically affected and unaffected persons of left ventricular wall thickness.[61]

PROGNOSIS

The development or increase of a murmur in a patient with HCM suggests progression of disease, but the disappearance of a murmur does not imply improvement. In fact, the disappearance of a murmur may herald further impairment of systolic function. Some patients progress to CHF as a result of atrial fibrillation, mitral regurgitation, or myocardial infarction. If heart failure develops, the patient has a poor prognosis.

Of major concern is the incidence of sudden cardiac death among patients with HCM. Sometimes, the first manifestation of HCM is sudden death. The mechanisms responsible for sudden cardiac death are ill defined. Younger age, marked left ventricular hypertrophy, family history of sudden death, and the presence of nonsustained ventricular tachycardia on ambulatory ECGs have been identified as risk factors for sudden death in patients with HCM.[56]

In one long-term study of 314 patients with HCM and 82 patients with DCM, 68% of the deaths that occurred in the HCM patients were sudden.[62] Age less than 30 years, fractional shortening less than 35%, and left ventricular end-diastolic pressures greater than 20 mm Hg were factors associated with sudden cardiac death. Patients who were less than 30 years of age rarely (5%) had ventricular tachycardia on Holter monitoring. It was suggested that young patients with hypertrophic cardiomyopathy may die suddenly as a result of exercise-induced ischemia rather than ventricular arrhythmias.

A variety of other rhythm abnormalities may accompany HCM, including supraventricular and ventricular tachyarrhythmias, bradyarrhythmias, aberrant atrioventricular nodal pathways and complete heart block. In 25 children with HCM, 6 (24%) were found to have a prolonged QT interval.[63] Either DCM or HCM may be a cause of QT prolongation.

Less often, sudden death may be the result of hemodynamic changes. The onset of atrial fibrillation in the face of severe left ventricular diastolic dysfunction may result in a significant decrease in stroke volume. This decrease in cardiac output could lead to acute left ventricular failure, myocardial infarction, or sudden death.

Quantification of the risk of sudden death for patients with HCM remains elusive. However, the magnitude of hypertrophy appears to be a strong predictor. Recently, Spirito and colleagues found that the magnitude of hypertrophy is directly related to the risk of sudden cardiac death, with the cumulative risk nearly zero for patients with a wall thickness of 19 mm or less.[64] Young patients with severe hypertrophy (wall thickness >30 mm) are at a high risk for sudden death, even if they are asymptomatic. It is recommended that young patients with HCM refrain from competitive athletics. A high left ventricular outflow tract pressure gradient (>30 mm Hg) is a strong predictor of sudden death in older patients.[65]

Development of HCM in the latter decades of life is common. In general, the prognosis of patients who present with HCM at an advanced age (>65 years) is no different from that of age- and gender-matched controls.[66] It is not clear whether this elderly patient subgroup has a better prognosis than do patients presenting at a younger age with HCM as a result of a different pathophysiologic process. Elderly patients presenting with New York Heart Association functional class III dyspnea had a higher mortality rate than did a control group. Increased left atrial size was associated with reduced survival.

▶ TREATMENT: Hypertrophic Cardiomyopathy

Because there are no known means available to prevent HCM, the focus must be on methods to minimize the consequences of the disorder. The treatment of HCM is designed to reduce symptoms, to improve exercise tolerance, to retard disease progression, and to improve prognosis. Agents that decrease contractility, improve diastolic function, reduce ischemia, and suppress arrhythmias have been used with some success.

NONPHARMACOLOGIC THERAPY

Surgical treatment is generally reserved for the patients whose condition is refractory to medical management and who have an outflow gradient of 50 mm Hg or more, a very thick ventricular septum, and high left ventricular pressures. The purpose of surgical intervention is to relieve the outflow obstruction and the elevated left ventricular pressures. The surgeon accomplishes this by performing a partial septal resection and/or incision (ventricular myotomy-myectomy). There is likely to be an overall early mortality rate following surgery of approximately 5%. Complications may include septal perforation and late occurrence of CHF. However, significant improvement can be expected in patients with symptoms of dyspnea, angina, near-syncope and syncope.[67]

Mitral valve replacement has been used to abolish the subaortic gradient that results from the anterior motion of the mitral leaflets during systole. This procedure is generally reserved for patients with severe mitral regurgitation or those with mild ventricular septal hypertrophy such that myotomy-myectomy may cause perforation.[56,57,59] Dual chamber pacing has been helpful to some patients with obstructive cardiomyopathy that pharmacologic approaches has failed to resolve.[68] Ablation of the myocardium with alcohol is another approach in selected centers.

PHARMACOLOGIC THERAPY

β-BLOCKING AGENTS

Since the 1960s, β-blocking agents have been used in obstructive and nonobstructive forms of HCM. Approximately one-third to one-half of patients with angina, dyspnea, light-headedness, or syncope will have a favorable response to these agents. Patients should receive maximally tolerated doses; most patients require doses of 320 mg/d of propranolol or its equivalent.[59] Standing heart rate should be 60 beats/min, and the maximum exercise heart rate should be less than 130 beats/min. The benefits of β-blockade come from the inhibition of sympathetic stimulation of the heart. Myocardial oxygen demand is reduced by decreasing heart rate, left ventricular contractility, and myocardial wall stress during systole. Outflow tract obstruction may be minimized with β-blockade, especially under conditions of stress or exercise, when sympathetic stimulation is high. Furthermore, consequences of a decreased resting and exercise heart rate include an increase in left ventricular diastolic filling time, reduction of the abnormally prolonged isovolumic relaxation period, and lengthening of early rapid filling. Cardioselective β-blocking drugs are thought to be less desirable, because their effect on outflow tract gradient is less. It has been suggested that they should be reserved for those patients with COPD. Furthermore, β-blocking agents with intrinsic sympathomimetic activity may not reduce resting heart rate sufficiently.[59]

CALCIUM CHANNEL–BLOCKING AGENTS

Patients who have no response to β-blockade may respond to verapamil.[57] There are several reasons that calcium channel–blocking agents may be of benefit to patients with HCM. Increased calcium concentrations play a role in prolonging the ventricular action potential, as well as the duration of isometric contraction and relaxation. Patients with HCM have a hyperdynamic ventricle in systole with delayed relaxation and decreased compliance during diastole. Calcium channel–blocking drugs decrease the myocardial oxygen demand, thus improving the balance between oxygen supply and demand; therefore, diastolic function may also improve.

In one study of 101 patients, 85% of previously symptomatic patients reported improvement or complete relief of symptoms when treated with a calcium channel blocker.[69] Most patients with HCM who have been treated with a calcium channel blocker have received verapamil, although other drugs have also been used. The IV administration of verapamil reduces the outflow tract gradient in those patients with obstructive HCM. The mechanism may be a decrease in systolic function, as well as an increase in left ventricular volumes due to enhanced left ventricular diastolic filling.

The adverse effects associated with the use of verapamil include sinus node blockade, prolongation of the PR interval, atrioventricular dissociation, hypotension, and pulmonary congestion.[61] The risks may outweigh the benefits in those patients with (1) a pulmonary capillary wedge pressure or pulmonary artery occlusion pressure greater than 20 mm Hg, (2) a history of paroxysmal nocturnal dyspnea or orthopnea, (3) sick sinus syndrome or significant atrioventricular nodal disease in the absence of a permanent pacemaker, (4) low systolic blood pressure, and (5) a substantial outflow gradient.[56] Verapamil should be avoided in patients with heart failure caused by systolic dysfunction.

Studies using other calcium channel blockers are limited. Although they may improve diastolic function, the dihydropyridines may cause a reflex increase in heart rate, cause hypotension, or worsen the outflow tract gradient. It has been suggested that a combination of a β-blocker with a calcium channel blocker may be useful. In that situation, a β-blocker should be initiated before a dihydropyridine is started.[59] If verapamil has been used first, additional benefit has been reported with the addition of pindolol.[70] Trials using combination therapy are extremely limited.

There is no evidence that either β-blockade or verapamil protects the patient from sudden cardiac death.

ANTIARRHYTHMIC AGENTS

The incidence of sudden cardiac death in patients with HCM is a cause of great concern. Sudden death is thought to be related to ventricular arrhythmias as a primary event or secondary to myocardial ischemia, diastolic dysfunction, outflow obstruction, systemic hypotension, or supraventricular tachyarrhythmias.[57] Patients who are identified to be at high risk for sudden death should receive aggressive treatment. Such patients include survivors of cardiac arrest with documented ventricular fibrillation, those with episodes of recurrent sustained ventricular tachycardia, and young patients with a family history (two or more family members) of sudden death. It is less clear whether other patients with nonsustained ventricular tachycardia benefit from antiarrhythmic agents. Unfortunately, electrophysiologic testing has not been shown to be helpful in identifying patients at high risk. Patients with characteristics known to be associated with a low risk of sudden death should be reassured that their condition does not warrant therapy with antiarrhythmic agents nor restriction of activities.

Patients with HCM at high risk for sudden death should be considered eligible for treatment with amiodarone or an implantable cardioverter-defibrillator (ICD). Amiodarone is a complex agent with α, β, and calcium blocking effects. As a result, it has negative chronotropic, inotropic, and coronary vasodilating properties. Amiodarone may relieve symptoms and prolong exercise duration in some patients, independent of its antiarrhythmic actions.[71] Disopyramide has been used in treating both the supraventricular and ventricular arrhythmias that may occur in patients with HCM. In addition, disopyramide's negative inotropic effect and ability to increase peripheral vascular resistance has been used to reduce outflow tract obstruction.[69] The number of patients receiving disopyramide is small, however, and there are few controlled trials available. The anticholinergic side effects (blurred vision, dry mouth, and urinary retention) make disopyramide a less desirable agent for long-term therapy.

A significant portion of patients with HCM develop atrial fibrillation. Amiodarone is one of the most effective agents available to maintain normal sinus rhythm for these patients. For those patients requiring rate control, β-blockade or verapamil is beneficial. Anticoagulation therapy should be considered, as these patients are at a risk for systemic embolization and stroke. If amiodarone is added to the regimen of a patient already receiving warfarin, the prothrombin time or international normalized ratio (INR) should be closely monitored.[57]

NEW TYPES OF PHARMACOLOGIC THERAPY

Because growth factors have been shown to be associated with primary HCM, researchers are now investigating approaches to treatment through interruption of growth stimulation. Octreotide is a somatostatin analog that can prevent the stimulating effect of growth factors. It has been given to small numbers of patients with HCM and has demonstrated a positive hemodynamic effect.[72] This type of therapy may hold promise for the future.

RESTRICTIVE CARDIOMYOPATHY

Defined as heart muscle disease that results in impaired filling, with normal or decreased diastolic volume, restrictive cardiomyopathy is the least common cardiomyopathy. Systolic function is normal early in the course of the disease, but deteriorates later in the disease process. Restrictive cardiomyopathy is one type of diastolic dysfunction; it results from an increased stiffness of the myocardium that causes ventricular pressure to rise dramatically with only small increases in volume.[73] Either one or both of the ventricles may be affected; therefore, restrictive cardiomyopathy may present as either left- or right-sided heart failure.

EPIDEMIOLOGY AND ETIOLOGY

Because of the rare occurrence of restrictive cardiomyopathy, the natural course of the disease is not well characterized, and reports on its prognosis have been highly variable. Restrictive cardiomyopathies may be classified as either myocardial or endomyocardial. The myocardial types may be noninfiltrative, infiltrative, or storage diseases. The endomyocardial types may be due to endomyocardial fibrosis, hypereosinophilic syndrome, carcinoid heart disease, metastatic cancers, radiation, anthracycline toxicity, or they may be secondary to drugs known to cause fibrosis.[73]

The most common cause in the industrialized world is amyloidosis, whereas endomyocardial fibrosis is a common cause in tropical areas of the world. There is a genetic predisposition to idiopathic restrictive cardiomyopathy.[73]

The cause of the disease, the severity of heart failure symptoms, and the presence of cardiac thrombi and arrhythmias are factors that affect long-term survival. Children with restrictive cardiomyopathy have a worse prognosis than do adults and should be considered for early cardiac transplantation.[74]

PATHOPHYSIOLOGY

The major hemodynamic abnormality in restrictive cardiomyopathy is a limitation of ventricular filling that leads to increased filling pressures. Thrombi are frequently found in the cardiac chambers. Patients have signs and symptoms consistent with CHF. The abnormality is similar to that observed in pericardial disease causing constriction or tamponade. Atrial dimensions are often increased.

Restrictive myocardial disease may result from several local or systemic disorders. Amyloidosis, hemochromatosis, scleroderma, carcinoid sarcoidosis, pseudoxanthoma elasticum, and endomyocardial fibrosis have been known to cause restrictive cardiomyopathy.[75]

CLINICAL PRESENTATION

Patients who have restrictive cardiomyopathy present with dyspnea, orthopnea, fatigue, edema, ascites, and at times chest pain. The heart is either normal in size or has atrial enlargement. Significant jugular venous distention is quite common. Mitral and/or tricuspid regurgitant murmurs may be audible. The ECG may show atrial arrhythmias, tachy-brady syndrome, or conduction abnormalities. An accurate diagnosis can be made only by means of standard catheterization techniques.

The diagnosis of restrictive cardiomyopathy should be considered in the patient who presents with signs and symptoms of CHF, but has only mild cardiomegaly. It is important to differentiate restrictive cardiomyopathy from constrictive pericarditis since pericardectomy is an effective form of treatment for constrictive pericarditis.

▶ TREATMENT: Restrictive Cardiomyopathy

The treatment of restrictive cardiomyopathy is complex because of the heterogeneity of the pathophysiologic abnormalities. Diuretics and vasodilators are used for the symptoms of CHF in the presence of restrictive cardiomyopathy; caution is advisable, however, because these patients require high filling pressures to maintain an adequate stroke volume and cardiac output. Hypotension and hypoperfusion may occur as a result of the use of diuretics. Because systolic function is often normal, digoxin is of no benefit. Amiodarone is used to maintain normal sinus rhythm in patients who have atrial fibrillation. Anticoagulation therapy is necessary to decrease the risk of systemic embolization, particularly in those patients with atrial fibrillation, valvular regurgitation, and low cardiac output. In the case of hemachromatosis, chelation therapy and/or repeated phlebotomy may be of benefit. Treatment with corticosteroids and cytotoxic drugs has been successful in the early phase of endomyocardial fibrosis and eosinophilic cardiomyopathy.[73]

EVALUATION OF THERAPEUTIC OUTCOMES

The goal of treatment for patients with DHF and HCM is primarily to reduce their symptoms of dyspnea and exercise intolerance. In DHF, symptom relief may be accomplished by management of the patient's volume through dietary restriction of sodium and careful use of diuretics. Long-acting nitrates are also helpful in relieving symptoms of pulmonary congestion. Other strategies include maintaining normal sinus rhythm and controlling blood pressure. β-blockers or calcium channel blockers that lower heart rate play an important role in patient care. Neurohumoral antagonists, such as angiotensin-converting enzyme inhibitors (ACEIs), angiotensin receptor blockers and spironolactone are used to lower left ventricular pressures and thereby provide symptom relief. There is some evidence to suggest that spironolactone may also affect collagen turnover which could inhibit the underlying disease process.

Most patients with HCM also have diastolic dysfunction. Either β-blockers or calcium channel blockers may be used to reduce their symptoms of dyspnea and exercise intolerance. If a β-blocker is the agent chosen, it is best to use one that does not have intrinsic sympathomimetic activity. The dose should be maximized. If the patient cannot tolerate a β-blocker or has a contraindication to the use of a β-blocker, then a rate-lowering calcium channel blocker may be effective. The most commonly used calcium channel blocker is verapamil. Patients should be monitored for resolution of symptoms (although they may not be resolved for months) and an increase in exercise tolerance. In addition, both β-blockers and calcium channel blockers may cause hypotension and conduction abnormalities. β-Blockers may worsen pulmonary function. Combination therapy with a β-blocker and a calcium channel blocker may be tried if the desired therapeutic response is not achieved with either agent alone. If dyspnea continues with maximal doses of a β-blocker and a calcium channel blocker, a diuretic agent or a nitrate may be added with caution. Those patients who are at high risk for sudden cardiac death should be considered candidates for amiodarone or an ICD.

Those patients who have a significant obstruction to left ventricular outflow and do not respond to medical management may require a surgical approach. Septal myotomy-myectomy has been employed. Surgical therapy is generally reserved for those patients who have an outflow gradient of more than 50 mm Hg and/or severe symptoms and who have failed an adequate trial of medical therapy.

The first step in assessing and treating a patient with restrictive cardiomyopathy is to rule out constrictive pericarditis, because the two conditions have a similar presentation. Constrictive pericarditis is easily treatable with surgery, whereas the treatment of restrictive cardiomyopathy varies according to the cause of the disorder. The treatment for restrictive cardiomyopathy is aimed at relieving the symptoms associated with high filling pressures, generally through the use of diuretics. Therapy with diuretics should be initiated with low doses. Normalization of filling pressures is not possible or desirable. Patients' symptoms should be monitored for improvement. Overdiuresis will result in an inadequate cardiac output. Chelation therapy has been advocated for patients with hemochromatosis. Prednisone has been suggested for patients with sarcoidosis. There is no curative treatment for restrictive cardiomyopathy.

▶ PRINCIPLES OF PHARMACOTHERAPY

- Patients with diastolic dysfunction are treated differently from those with systolic dysfunction.
- The diagnosis of diastolic heart failure can be made when a patient has (1) both symptoms and signs on physical examination of congestive heart failure (CHF), and (2) normal left ventricular volume and ejection fraction. Documentation of abnormal diastolic function is confirmatory, but not mandatory.
- Diastolic heart failure is a frequent cause of CHF (prevalence of 35% to 50%) and has a significant effect on mortality (5-year mortality rate of 25% to 35%) and morbidity (1-year readmission rate of 50%).
- Treatment should be targeted at symptom reduction, causal clinical disease, and underlying basic mechanisms.
- Pharmacologic therapy is aimed at symptoms. Decrease pulmonary venous pressure by using diuretics and long-acting nitrates; maintain atrial contraction and atrioventricular synchrony; reduce heart rate by using β-adrenergic blockers and calcium channel blockers. Increase exercise tolerance by reducing exercise-induced increases in blood pressure and heart rate, using angiotensin-converting enzyme inhibitors (ACEIs), angiotensin receptor blockers, and calcium channel blockers.
- Disease-targeted therapy includes preventing or treating myocardial ischemia, and preventing or regressing left ventricular hypertrophy.
- Future approaches may include modifying neurohumoral activation by using renin-angiotensin-aldosterone system antagonists (ACEIs, angiotensin receptor blockers, aldosterone, and renin antagonist), endothelin antagonists, nitric oxide agonists, and atrial natriuretic peptide agonists, as well as altering intracellular mechanisms and extracellular matrix structures.
- Patients with HCM who are at high risk for sudden cardiac death should receive amiodarone or an ICD.
- Patients with HCM who are symptomatic may benefit from β-blockade or verapamil.

REFERENCES

1. Yamamoto K, Wilson DJ, Canzanello VJ, Redfield MM. Left ventricular diastolic dysfunction in patients with hypertension and preserved systolic dysfunction. Mayo Clin Proc 2000;75:148–155.
2. Gaasch WH, Schick EC, Zile MR. Management of left ventricular diastolic dysfunction. In: Smith TW, ed. Cardiovascular Therapeutics: A Companion to Braunwald's Heart Disease. Philadelphia, WB Saunders, 1996:237–242.
3. Zile MR: Diastolic dysfunction and heart failure in hypertrophied hearts. Congestive Heart Failure 1998;4:32–42.
4. Gaasch WH, Blaustein AS, LeWinter MM. Heart failure and clinical disorders of left ventricular diastolic dysfunction. In: Gaasch WH, LeWinter MM, eds. Left Ventricular Diastolic Dysfunction and Heart Failure. Philadelphia, Lea & Febiger, 1994:245.
5. Gaasch WH. Diagnosis and treatment of heart failure based on left ventricular systolic or diastolic dysfunction. JAMA 1994;271:1276–1280.
6. Echeverria HH, Bilisker MS, Myerburg RJ, Kessler KM. Congestive heart failure: echocardiographic insights. Am J Med 1983;75:750–755.
7. Soufer R, Wohlgelemter D, Vita NA, et al. Intact systolic left ventricular function in clinical congestive heart failure. Am J Cardiol 1985;55:1032–1036.
8. Cohn JN, Johnson G, and the Veterans Administration Cooperative Study Group. Heart failure with normal ejection fraction: the V-HeFT study. Circulation 1980;81(suppl III):48–53.
9. Luchi RJ, Snow E, Luchi JM, et al. Left ventricular function in hospitalized geriatric patients. J Am Geriatr Soc 1982;30:700–705.
10. Forman DE, Coletta D, Kenny D, et al. Clinical issues related to discontinuing digoxin therapy in elderly nursing home patients. Arch Intern Med 1991;151:2194–2198.
11. Wong WF, Gold S, Fukuyama O, Blanchette PL. Diastolic dysfunction in elderly patients with congestive heart failure. Am J Cardiol 1989;63:1526–1528.
12. Lamb HJ, Beyerbacht HP, van der Laarse A, et al. Diastolic dysfunction in hypertensive heart disease. Circulation 1999;99:2261–2267.
13. Mandinov L, Eberli FR, Seiler C, Hess OM. Diastolic heart failure. Cardiovasc Res 2000:45;813–825.
14. Apstein CS, Morgan JP. Cellular mechanisms underlying left ventricular diastolic dysfunction. In: Gaasch WH, LeWinter MM, eds. Left Ventricular Diastolic Dysfunction and Heart Failure. Philadelphia, Lea & Febiger, 1994:3.
15. Weber KT, Brilla CG. Pathological hypertrophy and cardiac interstitium: fibrosis and renin-angiotensin-aldosterone system. Circulation 1991;83:1849–1865.
16. Weber KT, Sun Y, Guarda E. Structural remodeling in hypertensive heart disease and the role of hormones. Hypertension 1994;23:869–887.
17. Zile MR, Richardson K, Cowles MK, et al. Constitutive properties of adult mammalian cardiac muscle cells. Circulation 1998;98:567–579.
18. Tian R, Nascimben L, Ingwall JS, Lorell BH. Failure to maintain a low ADP concentration impairs diastolic function in hypertrophied rat hearts. Circulation 1997;96:1313–1319.
19. Zile MR, Nishimura RA, Gaasch WH. Hemodynamic loads and left ventricular diastolic function: factors affecting the indices of isovolumetric and auxotonic relaxation. In: Gaasch WH, LeWinter MM, eds. Left Ventricular Diastolic Dysfunction and Heart Failure. Philadelphia, Lea & Febiger, 1994:219.
20. Watanabe J, Levine MJ, Bellotto F, et al. Left ventricular diastolic chamber stiffness and intramyocardial coronary capacitance in isolated dog hearts. Circulation 1993;88:2929–2940.
21. Udelson JE, Bonow RO, O'Gara PT, et al. Verapamil prevents silent myocardial perfusion abnormalities during exercise in asymptomatic patients with hypertrophic cardiomyopathy. Circulation 1989;79:1052–1060.
22. Judge KW, Pawitan Y, Caldwell J, et al. Congestive heart failure in patients with preserved left ventricular systolic function: analysis of the CASS registry. J Am Coll Cardiol 1991;18:377–382.
23. Brogen WC, Hillis LD, Flores ED, et al. The natural history of isolated left ventricular diastolic dysfunction. Am J Med 1992;92:627–630.
24. Paulus WJ, Bronzwaer JGF, de Bruyne B, Grossman W. Different effects of "supply" and "demand" ischemia on left ventricular diastolic function in humans. In: Gaasch WH, LeWinter MM, eds. Left Ventricular Diastolic Dysfunction and Heart Failure. Philadelphia, Lea & Febiger, 1994:286.
25. Kitzman DW, Higginbotham MB, Cobb FR, et al. Exercise intolerance in patients with heart failure and preserved left ventricular systolic function: failure of the Frank-Starling mechanism. J Am Coll Cardiol 1991;17:1065–1072.
26. Packer M. Abnormalities of diastolic function as a potential cause of exercise intolerance in chronic heart failure. Circulation 1990;81(suppl 3):78–86.
27. Chikamori T, Counihan PJ, Doi YL, et al. Mechanisms of exercise limitation in hypertrophic cardiomyopathy. J Am Coll Cardiol 1992;19:507–512.
28. Liu CP, Ting CT, Lawrence W, et al. Diminished contractile response to increased heart rate in intact human left ventricular hypertrophy: systolic versus diastolic determinants. Circulation 1993;88:1893–1906.
29. Mulieri LA, Hasenfuss G, Leavitt B, et al. Altered myocardial force-frequency relation in human heart failure. Circulation 1992;85:1743–1750.
30. Gwathmey JK, Warren SE, Briggs M, et al. Diastolic dysfunction in hypertrophic cardiomyopathy: effect on active force generation during systole. J Clin Invest 1991;87:1023–1031.
31. European Study Group on Diastolic Heart Failure. How to diagnose diastolic heart failure. Eur Heart J 1998;19:990–1003.
32. Warren SE, Cohn LH, Schoen FJ, et al. Advanced diastolic heart failure in familial hypertrophic cardiomyopathy managed with cardiac transplantation. J Appl Cardiol 1988;3:415–419.
33. Setaro JF, Soufer R, Remetz MS, et al. Long-term outcome in patients with congestive heart failure and intact systolic left ventricular performance. Am J Cardiol 1992;69:1212–1216.
34. The Digitalis Investigation Group. The effect of digoxin on mortality and morbidity in patients with heart failure. N Engl J Med 1997;336:525–533.
35. Topol EJ, Traill TA, Fortuin NJ: Hypertensive hypertrophic cardiomyopathy of the elderly. N Engl J Med 1985;312;277–283.
36. Bonow RO, Dilsizian V, Rosing DR, et al. Verapamil-induced improvement in left ventricular filling and increased exercise tolerance in patients with hypertrophic cardiomyopathy: short and long term results. Circulation 1985;72:853–863.
37. Setaro JF, Zaret BL, Schulman DS, et al. Usefulness of verapamil for congestive heart failure associated with abnormal left ventricular diastolic filling and normal left ventricular systolic performance. Am J Cardiol 1990;66;981–986.
38. LeConte P, Countant V, N'Guyen JM, et al. Prognostic factors in acute cardiogenic pulmonary edema. Am J Emerg Med 1999;17:329–332.
39. Udelson JE, Cannon RO, Bacharach SL, et al. Beta adrenergic stimulation with isoproterenol enhances left ventricular diastolic performance in hypertrophic cardiomyopathy despite potentiation of myocardial ischemia: comparison to rapid atrial pacing. Circulation 1989;79:371–382.
40. Levine HJ. Optimum heart rate of large failing hearts. Am J Cardiol 1988;61:633–636.
41. Udelson JE, Bonow RO. Left ventricular diastolic function and calcium channel blockers in hypertrophic cardiomyopathy. In: Gaasch WH, LeWinter MM, eds. Left Ventricular Diastolic Dysfunction and Heart Failure. Philadelphia, Lea & Febiger, 1994:465.
42. Anand IS, Ferrari R, Kalra GS, et al. Pathogenesis of edema in constrictive pericarditis: studies of body water and sodium, renal function, hemodynamics, and plasma hormones before and after pericardectomy. Circulation 1991;83:1880–1887.
43. Anand IS, Chandrashekhar Y, Ferrari R, et al. Pathogenesis of congestive state in chronic obstructive pulmonary disease: studies of body water and sodium, renal function, hemodynamics, and plasma hormones during edema and after recovery. Circulation 1992;86:12–21.
44. Firth JD, Raine AEG, Ledingham JGG. Raised venous pressure: a direct cause of renal sodium retention in oedema. Lancet 1988;1:1033–1035.
45. Hoit BD, Walsh RA. Diastolic function in hypertensive heart disease. In: Gaasch WH, LeWinter MM, eds. Left Ventricular Diastolic Dysfunction and Heart Failure. Philadelphia, Lea & Febiger, 1994:354.

46. Brilla CG, Funck RC, Rupp H. Lisinopril-mediated regression of myocardial fibrosis in patients with hypertensive heart disease. Circulation 2000;102:1388–1393.
47. Warner JG, Metzger C, Kitzman DW, et al. Losartan improves exercise tolerance in patients with diastolic dysfunction and a hypertensive response to exercise. J Am Coll Cardiol 1999;33:1567–1572.
48. Zannad F. The survival benefit of spironolactone therapy in patients with congestive heart failure could be explained by the limitation of the excessive cardiac fibrosis; insights from the RALES trial. http://www.escardio.org/pubinfo/mediaservices/APR/Zannad.htm (accessed 9/8/00).
49. Lorell BH, Isoyama S, Grice WN, et al. Effects of ouabain and isoproterenol on left ventricular diastolic function during low-flow ischemia in isolated, blood-perfused rabbit hearts. Circ Res 1988;63:457–467.
50. Lang RM, Carroll JD, Nakamura S, et al. Role of adrenoceptors and dopamine receptors in modulating left ventricular diastolic function. Circ Res 1988;63:126–134.
51. Monrad ES, McKay R, Baim DS, et al. Improvement in indexes of diastolic performance in patients with congestive heart failure treated with milrinone. Circulation 1984;70:1030–1037.
52. Wynne J, Braunwald E. The cardiomyopathies and myocarditides. In: Braunwald E, ed. Heart Disease: A Textbook of Cardiovascular Medicine, 5th ed. Philadelphia, WB Saunders, 1997:1404–1463.
53. Mason JW. Classification of cardiomyopathy. In: Schlant RC, Alexander RW, eds. Hurst's The Heart, 8th ed. New York, McGraw-Hill, 1994:1585–1590.
54. Katz AM. Cardiomyopathy of overload: an unnatural growth response in the hypertrophied heart. Ann Intern Med 1994;121:363–371.
55. Schwartz K, Chassagne C, Boheler K. The molecular biology of heart failure. J Am Coll Cardiol 1993;22(Supplement A):30A–33A.
56. Maron BJ, Roberts WC. Hypertrophic cardiomyopathy. In: Schlant RC, Alexander RW, eds. Hurst's The Heart, 8th ed. New York, McGraw-Hill, 1994:1621–1635.
57. Spirito P, Seidman CE, McKenna WJ, Maron BJ. The management of hypertrophic cardiomyopathy. N Engl J Med 1997;336:775–785.
58. Watkins H, McKenna WJ, Thierfelder L, et al. Mutations in the genes for cardiac troponin T and α tropomyosin in hypertrophic cardiomyopathy. N Engl J Med 1995;332:1058–1064.
59. von Dohlen TW, Frank MJ. Current perspectives in hypertrophic cardiomyopathy: diagnosis, clinical management and prevention of disability and sudden cardiac death. Clin Cardiol 1990;13:247–252.
60. St. John Sutton M, Epstein JA. Hypertrophic cardiomyopathy—beyond the sarcomere. N Engl J Med 1998;338:1303–1304.
61. Posma JL, van der Wall EE, Blanksma PK, et al. New diagnostic options in hypertrophic cardiomyopathy. Am Heart J 1996;132:1031–1041.
62. Koga Y, Ogata M, Kihara K, et al. Sudden death in hypertrophic and dilated cardiomyopathy. Jpn Circ J 1989;53:1546–1556.
63. Martin AB, Garson A, Perry JC. Prolonged QT interval in hypertrophic and dilated cardiomyopathy in children. Am Heart J 1994;127:64–70.
64. Spirito P, Bellone P, Harris KM, et al. Magnitude of left ventricular hypertrophy and risk of sudden death in hypertrophic cardiomyopathy. N Engl J Med 2000;342:1778–1785.
65. Maki S, Ikeda H, Muro A, et al. Predictors of sudden cardiac death in hypertrophic cardiomyopathy. Am J Cardiol 1998;82:774–778.
66. Fay WP, Talierco CP, Ilstrup DM, et al. Natural history of hypertrophic cardiomyopathy in the elderly. J Am Coll Cardiol 1990;16:821–826.
67. McCully RB, Nishimura RA, Tajik AJ, et al. Extent of clinical improvement after surgical treatment of hypertrophic obstructive cardiomyopathy. Circulation 1996;94:467–471.
68. Nishimura RA, Symanski JD, Hurrell DG, et al. Dual chamber pacing for cardiomyopathies: a 1996 clinical perspective. Mayo Clin Proc 1996;71:1077–1087.
69. Hopf R, Kaltenbach M. Management of hypertrophic cardiomyopathy. Annu Rev Med 1990;41:75–83.
70. Dimitrow PP, Dubiel JS. Effects on left ventricular function of pindolol added to verapamil in hypertrophic cardiomyopathy. Am J Cardiol 1993;71:313–316.
71. Fananapazir L, Leon MB, Bonow RO, et al. Sudden death during empiric amiodarone therapy in symptomatic hypertrophic cardiomyopathy. Am J Cardiol 1991;67:169–174.
72. Gunal AI, Isik A, Celiker H, et al. Short-term reduction of left ventricular mass in primary hypertrophic cardiomyopathy by octreotide injections. Heart 1996;76:418–421.
73. Kushwaha S, Fallon JT, Fuster V. Restrictive cardiomyopathy. N Engl J Med 1997;336:267–276.
74. Lewis AB. Clinical profile and outcome of restrictive cardiomyopathy in children. Am Heart J 1992;123:1589–1593.
75. Hoit BD. Restrictive, obliterative and infiltrative cardiomyopathies. In: Fuster V, Alexander RW, O'Rourke RA, Roberts R, King SB, Wellens HJJ eds. Hurst's The Heart, 10th ed. New York, McGraw-Hill 2001:1989–2000.

18

CARDIAC TRANSPLANTATION

Kathleen D. Lake and Keith D. Aaronson

Despite advances in heart failure management, cardiac transplantation remains the most successful treatment option for appropriately selected patients with end-stage cardiac disease. The use of refined donor and recipient selection criteria, improved donor organ preservation techniques, endomyocardial biopsy surveillance for acute rejection, advances in the diagnosis and treatment of infectious and malignant complications of long-term immunosuppression, and the introduction of new immunosuppressive agents have all contributed to the dramatic improvements in survival following transplantation. Recent actuarial survival rates in the era 1996–1999 are in excess of 85% and 79% at 1 and 3 years, respectively.[1] Long-term survival is now limited primarily by the development of late-stage problems, including cardiac allograft vasculopathy (CAV), also known as *transplant coronary artery disease* or *accelerated graft atherosclerosis* and analogous to chronic rejection processes seen with the other solid-organ transplants, and complications related to chronic maintenance immunosuppression (e.g., infections, malignancy, and nephrotoxicity).[2–9]

The number of patients transplanted annually in the United States increased progressively over time until 1994, when, due to a shortage of donors, the number of transplants plateaued at approximately 2,350 per year.[10] In 1999, 2,185 heart transplants were performed in the United States and 3,646 worldwide. More than 58,000 heart and heart-lung transplants have been performed worldwide to date.[1]

Heart failure affects an estimated 4.9 million Americans, and approximately 400,000 new case are diagnosed each year.[11,12] It is estimated that there are 15,000 to 25,000 patients 55 years of age and younger with end-stage cardiac disease for whom survival and quality of life could be improved through cardiac transplantation.[13] This number could increase to 40,000 if patients up to age 65 are included and if the current progression rate to end-stage heart failure were to remain unchanged. In the United States, an estimated $20.2 billion is spent annually for care of patients with heart failure. Heart transplantation improves the quality of life for these patients and has been reported to be cost-effective.[14,15]

Although demand for cardiac donors continues to grow, the number of potential organ donors, according to current brain death criteria, remains relatively fixed at 14,000 per year. Of these 14,000 patients, only 4,500 become organ donors, and of these, only slightly more than 2,300 are suitable cardiac donors. Currently, there are more than 4,100 patients on the national organ network waiting list for cardiothoracic transplantation.[16] Procurement of donor hearts with longer ischemic times, in addition to the use of older donors, those with borderline left ventricular function, and even those with mild coronary artery disease amenable to bypass grafting have been considered in an effort to increase donor supply.[17,18] Due to the progressive reduction in survival when cold ischemic preservation time is greater than 3 hours, donor hearts rarely are transported more than 1,000 miles to a waiting recipient.

CONDITIONS LEADING TO THE NEED FOR CARDIAC TRANSPLANTATION

RECIPIENT SELECTION

Cardiac transplant candidates typically are patients with end-stage heart failure who have New York Heart Association (NYHA) class III or IV symptoms despite maximal medical management and have an expected 1-year mortality risk of 25% or greater without a transplant. The majority of recipients are white males (78%) between 50 and 64 years of age.[10] The major etiologies of heart failure in potential heart transplant recipients include idiopathic cardiomyopathy in 43.7% and ischemic heart disease in 44.3%.[1] Other less common etiologies include valvular disease (4%), retransplantation for graft atherosclerosis or dysfunction (2%), and congenital heart disease (1.5%). Implantable defibrillators and improved surgical and catheter-based techniques have reduced substantially the need for transplantation as a treatment for recurrent malignant ventricular arrhythmias and refractory angina, respectively.

Based on the large number of patients who currently meet the NYHA end-stage heart failure classification, more objective methods of identifying patients with the poorest prognosis as candidates for cardiac transplantation are needed[19] (Table 18–1). Two national consensus conferences have been held during the past decade to identify uniform criteria for listing patients for heart transplantation. The American College of Cardiology Bethesda Conference met in 1992 and the United Network for Organ Sharing (UNOS) developed guidelines in 1996 that emphasize optimizing medical therapy and objectively assessing the patient's functional status. Oxygen consumption measured during maximal exercise (peak V_{O_2}) provides an objective assessment of functional capacity, an indirect assessment of cardiovascular reserve, and a valuable estimation of prognosis.[20] However, a number of factors, including age, gender, conditioning status, muscle mass, and angina, can limit peak V_{O_2}, and adjustment for these factors may be useful in certain circumstances.[21] Other predictors of poor survival include lower resting blood pressure, higher resting heart rate, presence of sustained ventricular arrhythmias, right ventricular failure, hyponatremia, and elevated serum catecholamines. A prospectively validated index of survival, the Heart Failure Survival Score, combines multiple, easily measured prognostic characteristics to estimate survival prognosis.[22]

Absolute contraindications to orthotopic cardiac transplantation include the presence of an active infection (except in the case of an infected ventricular assist device, which is an indication for urgent transplantation) or the presence of other diseases (i.e., malignancy) that may limit survival and/or rehabilitation. Severe, irreversible pulmonary hypertension [defined as a fixed pulmonary vascular resistance (PVR) greater than 3 Wood units or a transpulmonary gradient (difference in mean pulmonary artery pressure and capillary wedge

TABLE 18–1. Criteria for Transplantation

I. Accepted Indications for Transplantation
1. Maximal V_{O_2} < 10 mL/kg/min with achievement of anaerobic metabolism
2. Severe ischemia consistently limiting routine activity not amenable to bypass surgery or angioplasty
3. Recurrent symptomatic ventricular arrhythmias refractory to all accepted therapeutic modalities, including ICD

II. Probable Indications for Cardiac Transplantation
1. Maximal V_{O_2} < 14 mL/kg/min and major limitation of patient's daily activities
2. Recurrent unstable ischemia not amenable to bypass surgery or angioplasty
3. Instability of fluid balance/renal function not owing to patient noncompliance with regimen of weight monitoring, flexible use of diuretic drugs, and salt restriction

III. Inadequate Indications for Transplantation
1. Ejection fraction < 20% in an asymptomatic or mildly symptomatic patient
2. History of Class III or IV symptoms of heart failure
3. Previous ventricular arrhythmias
4. Maximal V_{O_2} > 15 mL/kg/min without other indications

pressure greater than 15 mm Hg)] is also a contraindication because it could cause posttransplantation right ventricular failure. Candidates with elevations in pulmonary resistance should be assessed to determine reversibility of pulmonary hypertension with vasodilatory agents such as nitroprusside, prostaglandin E_1 (PGE_1), prostacyclin, or nitric oxide.[23] A patient with reversible pulmonary hypertension may be an acceptable candidate if the pulmonary hypertension does not progress. The patient needs to be reassessed periodically to ensure suitability for transplantation. Patients with elevated pulmonary artery resistances who do not respond to hemodynamic maneuvers may be candidates for heterotopic heart transplantation or heart-lung transplantation depending on the transplant center's policy and expertise. Some centers are placing these patients on a left ventricular assist device to more fully unload the left ventricle in hopes that a large reversible component of pulmonary hypertension was present despite failure of vasodilators.

Other exclusion criteria are listed in Table 18–2. Reversible renal and hepatic dysfunction may be the sequelae of chronic heart failure and do not necessarily disqualify the candidate.[19]

TABLE 18–2. Secondary Exclusion Criteria for Heart Transplantation

Pulmonary hypertension with irreversibly high pulmonary vascular resistance
Coexistent systemic illness with poor prognosis
Irreversible pulmonary parenchymal disease
Irreversible renal dysfunction with serum creatinine > 2 mg/dL or creatinine clearance < 50 mL/min
Irreversible hepatic dysfunction
Severe peripheral and cerebrovascular obstructive disease
Insulin-dependent diabetes with end-organ damage
Active infection
Coexisting or recent neoplasm
Acute pulmonary embolism or infarction
Active diverticulosis or diverticulitis
Active peptic ulcer disease
Myocardial infiltrative and inflammatory diseases (e.g., amyloidosis)
Severe obesity
Severe osteoporosis
Psychosocial instability or substance abuse, or both

Once it is determined that the patient is a candidate for heart transplantation, the patient's name is placed on the UNOS waiting list. UNOS maintains a national registry of all candidates waiting for donor organs. Patients are matched initially with available organs based on blood type and body weight, and then the organ is given to the patient who has accrued the longest waiting time. Critically ill status 1 patients (e.g., those in intensive care units requiring intravenous inotropes or mechanical assistance) receive priority for the available organs. Individual waiting times vary considerably based on recipient blood type (e.g., type O patients wait the longest at 352 days versus type AB patients at 82 days), body size, clinical condition (e.g., status 1 patients wait 58 days versus 351 days for status 2), and geographic location. As a result of this prolonged waiting time, 1 of every 10 patients accepted for transplantation dies while waiting for a donor organ.[24,25]

PRETRANSPLANT MANAGEMENT

Optimal recipient management in the pretransplantation period has been shown to reduce the morbidity and mortality associated with end-stage heart failure. Urgent transplantation is the obvious choice for patients with irreversible cardiogenic shock and no significant contraindications. Most of these patients will require intravenous inotropic agents (e.g., dobutamine, milrinone, or dopamine) to maintain effective end-organ function while awaiting a suitable donor organ. When these measures are ineffective, some form of mechanical circulatory assist device is required. Insertion of an intraaortic balloon pump (IABP) may be helpful temporarily (particularly in patients with unstable angina), but the modest improvement in cardiac output (i.e., 10% to 15%) and the inevitable development of vascular complications with long-term use limit its application in this setting. Implantable left ventricular assist devices (LVADs) are now used commonly, with successful "bridging" to transplantation in 70% of patients.[26] Extracorporeal life support [also known as extracorporeal membrane oxygenation (ECMO)] has been instituted when death would otherwise occur within minutes, allowing subsequent safe and successful LVAD implantation.[27]

Medical therapy for the ambulatory advanced heart failure patient includes the use of angiotensin-converting enzyme (ACE) inhibitors, spironolactone, β-blockers, digoxin, diuretics, and potassium supplements.[28–30] Intermittent inotropic infusion therapy (e.g., dopamine, dobutamine, or milrinone) has been used by some centers, but there are no randomized clinical trials to support this practice; an American College of Cardiology/American Heart Association. Consensus statement advises against it.[30a] Frequent patient follow-up with careful attention to weight gain, nutrition, and electrolyte surveillance appears to reduce morbidity and the need for hospital admission.[31]

DONOR SELECTION

Patients with irreversible neurologic damage become candidates for organ donation following a declaration of brain death. Conventional cardiac donor criteria (Table 18–3), such as age, have been expanded considerably over the past several years in response to the continuing imbalance between donor supply and recipient demand. The use of donors older than 45 years of age is associated with a higher risk for 1-year mortality, but this must be viewed in the context of the higher risk of death with longer time on the waiting list if only younger donors are used.[1] Several principles remain standard in donor selection. There should be ABO blood group compatibility with the prospective heart recipient because mismatching in this system will result in hyperacute

TABLE 18–3. Criteria for Cardiac Donation

ABO blood type compatibility
Negative T-cell crossmatch if PRA[a] ≥ 10% to 20%
Age ≤ 60 years (older organs may be used in older recipients)
Size within 30% of recipient
Negative cardiac history
Normal electrocardiogram
Normal echocardiogram
Minimal pressor support (e.g., <10 μg/kg/min dopamine or equivalent)
Central venous pressure ≤ 12 mm Hg

[a]PRA = panel reactive antibody.

rejection. Human leukocyte antigen (HLA) tissue matching of the donor organ and recipient is not performed routinely before heart transplantation. However, if the potential recipient is reactive against a panel of random donor antigens (i.e., patient has a positive panel reactive antibody [PRA] > 10% to 20%) then a negative T-cell crossmatch is required prior to transplantation. The donor should be hemodynamically stable, requiring only mild to moderate vasopressor support following volume replacement, and have a normal echocardiogram. Some centers will accept donors with mild left ventricular dysfunction, particularly if the myocardial wall motion abnormalities are not in an anatomic pattern suggestive of coronary artery disease. These abnormalities may be a consequence of brain death, in which case they may reverse after transplantation. Hearts with severe left ventricular hypertrophy should be excluded due to the increased risk of ischemic injury (i.e., inadequate myocardial preservation) during the harvest procedure. Ideally, the donor should have no active infection or history of behavior placing the recipient at risk for transmissible infections (Table 18–4). Recent studies have shown, however, that use of organs from donors with gram-positive bacteremia who are treated with antibiotics poses little, if any, risk of transmission; donors with gram-negative bacteremia should be excluded.[32,33]

TABLE 18–4. Absolute and Relative Contraindications to Cardiac Donation

Absolute contraindications include:

1. Death from carbon monoxide poisoning, with blood carboxyhemoglobin level >20%
2. Intractable ventricular arrhythmia
3. Inadequate oxygenation, with arterial saturation < 80% on ventilatory support
4. Documented previous myocardial infarction
5. Clinically significant structural heart disease, intracardiac tumor, or severe global hypokinesia with ejection fraction < 30% as determined by echocardiogram
6. Severe occlusive coronary artery disease on arteriography

Relative contraindications include:

1. Hepatitis B surface antigen positivity (? except in cases of surface-antigen-positive recipients)
2. Bacterial sepsis
3. Hepatitis C positivity
4. History of metastatic cancer
5. Extensive chest wall trauma with evidence of cardiac contusion by ECG or echocardiography
6. Prolonged hypotension, defined as a systolic blood pressure < 60 mm Hg for > 6 h
7. Recurrent supraventricular and ventricular arrhythmias
8. Prolonged need for inotropic support, defined as a dopamine dosage > 20 μg/kg/min for > 24 h or comparable dosage of other β-agonist or epinephrine, norepinephrine, or dobutamine for the same period
9. Prolonged resuscitation time after cardiopulmonary arrest, defined as attempted cardiopulmonary resuscitation for > 30 min performed within 24 h of organ harvest or multiple episodes of attempted cardiopulmonary resuscitation
10. Severe left ventricular hypertrophy on electrocardiogram or echocardiogram
11. Echocardiogram revealing moderate hypokinesia
12. Noncritical coronary disease on arteriogram
13. History of carbon monoxide inhalation, with blood carboxyhemoglobin < 20%
14. History of intravenous drug abuse

PHYSIOLOGIC CONSEQUENCES OF CARDIAC TRANSPLANTATION

The heart reimplanted into the orthotopic position is surgically denervated and no longer responds to physiologic stimuli in a normal manner. The most clinically significant consequence of denervation is that these patients do not experience classic angina. In situations requiring an increased heart rate (e.g., exercise or hypotension), the denervated heart is unable to acutely increase heart rate but instead relies on the Frank-Starling mechanism by increasing the stroke volume. The heart remains sensitive to circulating catecholamines and is able to increase heart rate later in the course of exercise or hypotension. The overall maximum exercise capacity of heart transplant recipients is subnormal and most likely related to the denervated state. Most patients are able to resume normal lifestyles and reasonably vigorous activity levels. Studies have documented that partial reinnervation may occur over time, thereby facilitating more normal physiologic (e.g., presence of classic angina), pharmacologic responses, and better exercise capacity.[34–39]

The physiologic performance of the transplanted heart is a result of a complex interaction between parasympathetic and sympathetic denervation, intrinsic myocardial autoregulatory reflexes, catecholamine responsiveness, anatomic factors (donor recipient size match, atrial anastomosis characteristics), skeletal muscle conditioning, and chronic complications.[40] For purposes of therapeutic consideration, it is perhaps useful to divide a discussion of physiology with its implications for management into the acute postoperative phase (0–6 weeks) and a chronic phase.

Immediately following transplantation, a number of autoregulatory, anatomic, and physiologic responses present in the normal heart are interrupted or blunted. In the acutely denervated heart (absence of tonic vagal and sympathetic influence), the changes in cardiac output (heart rate × stroke volume) largely depend on heart rate changes engendered by circulating catecholamines. The donor sinus node function may be impaired by preservation injury, direct surgical trauma at excision, the presence of long-acting antiarrhythmics (e.g., amiodarone) taken prior to transplant by the recipient,[41] and a lack of "conditioning" responsiveness to catecholamines. Therefore, the transplanted heart generally requires chronotropic support with either milrinone or pacing in the early posttransplant period to maintain a heart rate of 90 to 110 beats per minute and satisfactory hemodynamics (i.e., blood pressure, urine output, and tissue perfusion). Approximately 10% to 20% of transplant patients will have persistent chronotropic incompetence requiring either cardiac pacing or pharmacologic manipulation of the heart with theophylline, or terbutaline after hospital discharge however, only about 4% of patients who receive a pacemaker use it permanently.[42] Transplant with the bicaval anastamosis instead of the classical Shumway's donor-recipient atrial anastamosis has been reported to decrease the incidence of sinus node dysfunction and permanent pacer requirements and to improve right-sided heart hemodynamics.[43] In the early posttransplant period, anatomic variables may further compromise optimal hemodynamic function and complicate hemodynamic assessment of the patient. Right ventricular function frequently is impaired, presumably as a result of preservation injury and elevated pulmonary vascular resistance. A "restrictive" hemodynamic pattern may be present initially, but it usually improves over the 6 weeks following transplantation. Also, donor-recipient size mismatch may contribute to early post-transplantation hemodynamic abnormalities characterized by higher right and left ventricular end-diastolic pressures. Supraventricular arrhythmias are not uncommon in the early posttransplant period but usually are transient. In the immediate perioperative period, they may result from overvigorous use of catecholamines or milrinone; later, they should raise suspicion for acute rejection.

The transplanted heart has been studied extensively both at rest and in response to exercise, which may unmask physiologic abnormalities not seen in the resting state.[44] Persistent abnormalities of diastolic function are noted in the transplanted heart such that intracardiac pressures increase in an exaggerated fashion with response to exercise and/or volume infusion. These abnormalities of diastolic function are due, at least in part, to denervation, but also to acute rejection or to the scarring secondary to previously treated rejection episodes, hypertension or cardiac allograft vasculopathy.

The peculiar physiology of the transplanted heart has several implications for pharmacologic therapy. Drugs such as digoxin and atropine, whose mechanism of action is mediated by the parasympathetic nervous system, will have no effect on the atrioventricular (AV) node; but digoxin's inotropic effect remains intact. Augmentation of cardiac output usually is mediated by heart rate increases and, to a lesser extent, inotropic responses. Thus drugs such as epinephrine with its marked β-adrenergic effect are particularly useful in increasing cardiac output in transplant patients, whereas β-blocking agents may impair the heart rate response and should be used very cautiously. The sinus node of the denervated heart is particularly sensitive to the negative chronotropic effects of acetylcholine or adenosine, and caution must be used if these agents are given. Life-threatening asystole for 0.5 minute or longer may occur if adenosine is administered to treat a supraventricular arrhythmia or if it is used as the pharmacologic "stress" for nuclear perfusion imaging.[45]

QUALITY OF LIFE AFTER TRANSPLANTATION

Most heart transplant patients return to NYHA functional class I following transplantation. In fact, 89.9% of patients consider themselves to have no limitations on activity at 1-year follow-up; however, not all have returned to work.[46] Many transplant patients are retired or disabled and chose not to work, whereas younger recipients may find it difficult to return to work because of insurance limitations.

CARE OF THE CARDIAC TRANSPLANT PATIENT

POSTOPERATIVE MANAGEMENT

Immediate postoperative care is similar to that provided for other patients undergoing cardiac surgery. Patients are generally extubated on the first postoperative day. Early ambulation, vigorous pulmonary toilet, and removal of all central lines, catheters, and chest tubes are of considerable importance in minimizing infectious complications. The uncomplicated patient is transferred out of the intensive care unit within 48–72 hours and discharged from the hospital after 10–14 days.

Many early postoperative complications in the heart transplant recipient can be avoided by carefully screening donors (see Tables 18–3 and 18–4) and recipients prior to transplantation (see Tables 18–1 and 18–2). Myocardial depression resulting from a combination of poor preservation, myocardial ischemia, catecholamines, and high-energy phosphate depletion frequently occurs and generally requires inotropic support and occasionally transient mechanical support. Commonly used inotropic agents include dobutamine, milrinone, and epinephrine. Cardiac output in the transplanted heart is largely rate-dependent; therefore, milrinone may be required to maintain the heart rate in the range of 90–110 beats per minute to optimize cardiac output. Some centers prefer to pace the heart using the epicardial pacing wires that are placed routinely during surgery. The incidence of right ventricular failure secondary to high pulmonary vascular resistances can be decreased by carefully screening recipients.[23,47] On occasion, intra- or postoperative administration of vasodilators, including nitric oxide, and inotropic agents may be necessary to treat right-sided failure in the transplant patient; milrinone and isoproterenol are the preferred inodilators in this setting. Cardiac function generally returns to "normal" within 3–4 days, during which time most patients can be weaned from chronotropic and inotropic support. Fortunately, irreversible ventricular dysfunction (primary graft failure) is infrequent.

Hypertension often occurs following surgery. Endogenous catecholamine levels and systemic vascular resistance are severely elevated in patients with end-stage heart failure. When a healthy new "pump" should be placed in this milieu, hypertension results. Systolic blood pressure is maintained at 110–120 mm Hg enhance cardiac function. Initial treatment may include nitroprusside or nitroglycerin; hydralazine or amlodipine are used later.

Because the incidence of acute rejection is highest during the first 6 months following transplantation, routine surveillance endomyocardial biopsies are performed at regularly scheduled intervals following transplantation.

IMMUNOSUPPRESSION PROTOCOLS

Triple-drug regimens remain the cornerstone of most heart transplant protocols in use today; however, new drugs and regimen modifications (e.g., early withdrawal of corticosteroids, calcineurin-sparing regimens) have been introduced to decrease complication rates and improve long-term results. Current maintenance immunosuppressive regimens consist of combinations of immunosuppressive agents that are used for the lifetime of the graft, such as cyclosporine modified solution (Neoral or its multiple generics) or tacrolimus (Prograf), mycophenolate mofetil (Cellcept) or azathioprine (Imuran or generic), corticosteroids, and most recently, sirolimus (Rapamune).

Current preoperative regimens consist primarily of mycophenolate mofetil (3.0 g orally) and varying dosages of cyclosporine modified solution (CsA) (0–10 mg/kg) or tacrolimus (0–0.05 mg/kg) administered orally 2–6 hours prior to surgery. All patients receive methylprednisolone 500 mg intravenously immediately after discontinuation of cardiopulmonary bypass and 125 mg intravenously every 8 hours for the first 24 hours after surgery. The administration of lower doses of CsA (e.g., 1–3 mg/kg/day) or tacrolimus (0.05 mg/kg/day) is often employed until day 3 or 4 to decrease potential nephrotoxicity in the immediate postoperative period. CsA is usually titrated to achieve whole-blood levels as assayed by high-performance liquid chromatography in the range of 200–300 ng/mL. Intravenous cyclosporine or tacrolimus may be used in patients who have difficulty absorbing these agents. Due to the poor oral bioavailability of both drugs, the intravenous dose of tacrolimus and cyclosporine should be reduced to 25% to 33% of the oral dose and titrated to achieve similar trough concentrations.

Cyclosporine was introduced in the 1980s and became incorporated in to most triple-drug regimens shortly thereafter. It is credited with the success seen with solid-organ transplantation. Initially, much higher doses of CsA were used (e.g., 15–25 mg/kg); however, because of the concentration-related side effects, dosages have decreased through the years. Cyclosporine has numerous unwanted side effects, most of which result from calcineurin inhibition.[48] The most serious adverse drug effects include renal dysfunction (decreased glomerular filtration rate, hyperkalemia, and hypermagnesemia), hypertension, hyperlipidemia, gout, osteoporosis, posttransplant diabetes, and cholelithiasis.[3,4,7,8] Other side effects include neurotoxicity (e.g., tremors, peripheral neuropathy), gingival hyperplasia, and hirsutism.

Drug interactions occur commonly with cyclosporine and tacrolimus and require very close monitoring. Cyclosporine is metabolized by the cytochrome P-450 3A4 system in both the gut and the liver, which accounts for both its poor bioavailability and numerous drug interactions. Cyclosporine is also a substrate for *p*-glycoprotein, which contributes to its drug interactions.[49,50]

Tacrolimus (formerly FK506) was approved in 1994 and has been used as an alternative agent for cyclosporine in double- and triple-drug regimens.[51] It has gained widespread acceptance in kidney, liver, and lung transplantation but is still used less frequently than cyclosporine in hearts. It has similar mechanisms of action, pharmacokinetic profiles, and analytical difficulties.

The majority of experience with tacrolimus in cardiac transplant recipients comes from four trials, one nonrandomized and three randomized, comparing tacrolimus- and cyclosporine-based protocols.[52–55] The overall incidence of rejection during the first year appears similar to that with CsA; however, the incidence of side effects such as hyperlipidemia and hypertension is lower with tacrolimus. Other advantages of tacrolimus compared with CsA is that it does not cause gingival hyperplasia and hirsutism. The incidence of neurotoxicity and nephrotoxicity appears similar to that for cyclosporine and most likely is concentration-related.[56] Other side effects include alopecia and a higher incidence of posttransplant diabetes, which also appears to be concentration-related. In a recent renal study targeting lower tacrolimus concentrations, the incidence of posttransplant diabetes in patients receiving tacrolimus and mycophenolate was identical to that of those receiving cyclosporine and mycophenolate, suggesting that other factors (e.g., steroid usage) may play a more significant role.[57] Tacrolimus also has been used as a "rescue" agent in patients with recalcitrant rejection on maintenance cyclosporine.[58]

The usual starting dosage of tacrolimus for cardiac transplant patients is 0.1 mg/kg per day administered orally as a twice-daily dosage or 0.025–0.05 mg/kg per day as a continuous intravenous infusion. Initially, tacrolimus concentrations are titrated to achieve whole-blood levels of 12–15 ng/mL or plasma levels of 0.5–2 ng/mL; lower concentrations (5–10 ng/mL) are used after 6 months if there are no rejection episodes.[52 55,59] Since tacrolimus is a substrate for cytochrome P-450 3A4 and *p*-glycoprotein, the propensity for drug interactions with tacrolimus appears to be similar to that reported with CsA. Drug concentrations need to be monitored whenever the patient's condition changes, toxicity is suspected, or other drugs metabolized by cytochrome P-450 3A4 are administered concomitantly (Table 18–5). Until clinical data document the contrary, drugs known to interact with CsA should be assumed to interact with tacrolimus[49,50] (Table 18–6).

Most heart transplant centers currently use mycophenolate mofetil (MMF) (formerly RS61443) as their preferred antiproliferative agent; however, many previously transplanted patients are still maintained on azathioprine. Mycophenolate mofetil was approved for use in renal transplant patients in 1995, heart transplant patients in 1998, and liver transplant patients in 2000 as an alternative to azathioprine. This drug is a prodrug that is hydrolyzed rapidly to the active ingredient mycophenolic acid, which is an anti-T- and B-cell agent that has less bone marrow toxicity than azathioprine.[60,61] It has demonstrated efficacy both as maintenance immunosuppression and "rescue" therapy for rejection episodes.[62–64] An international multicenter, randomized, blinded 3-year comparison of MMF (3 g/d) versus azathioprine (1.5–3.0 mg/kg/d) in combination with cyclosporine and oral corticosteroids of 650 primary heart transplant recipients was published recently.[65] In treated patients (MMF, $n = 289$; azathioprine, $n = 289$), MMF treatment was associated with significant reduction in mortality at 1 year (6.2% vs 11.4%; $P = .031$) and a significant reduction in the requirement for rejection treatment (65.7% vs 73.7%; $P = .026$). Opportunistic infections, mostly herpes simplex, were more common in the MMF group (53.3% vs 43.6%; $P = .025$). A recent analysis of 5599 patients in the joint International Society for Heart and Lung Transplantation (ISHLT) and UNOS Thoracic Registry showed an actuarial survival advantage for MMF when comparing MMF with azathioprine (1 year, 96% vs 93%; 3 years, 91% vs 86%; $P = .0012$).[66] This study focused on patients who were actually discharged from the hospital, whereas the original MMF trial was an intent-to-treat analysis, which included all patients randomized prior to transplantation, some of whom received only a few or no doses of the study medication.[65] Since mycophenolate is more expensive than azathioprine, some centers have suggested switching patients to azathioprine after the first year; however, one study reported a higher incidence of late rejection following conversion from MMF to azathioprine.[67] The cost of treating and diagnosing one rejection episode typically nullifies any cost savings incurred by the switch.[68]

Mycophenolic acid (MPA) is eliminated primarily by the kidneys and is also highly protein bound to albumin, The drug is largely metabolized in the liver to an inactive glucuronide metabolite (MPAG), most of which is eliminated by the kidneys, but a small portion is eliminated through the bile and undergoes enterohepatic recycling. Therapeutic drug monitoring may prove useful in optimizing efficacy and/or minimizing toxicity for this agent.[69,70] Drug interactions have resulted in decreased absorption of MMF in combination with cholestyramine, iron, or antacids containing magnesium and aluminum. Competition for renal tubular secretion may result in increased acyclovir and MPAG metabolite concentrations.[60] Decreased MPA trough concentrations have been reported when MMF is administered with CsA as compared with those achieved with similar MMF doses in patients receiving tacrolimus or sirolimus.[71–73] This interaction was thought originally to be caused by a drug interaction with tacrolimus that resulted in increased MPA levels but, in fact, is most likely due to CsA interfering with the enterohepatic recycling of the MPAG, which results in decreased MPA concentrations.[74] To achieve equivalent MPA and MPAG concentrations, it is necessary to administer MMF 3.0 g/day with CsA as compared with MMF 2.0 g/day with concomitant tacrolimus, making MMF-tacrolimus a less costly regimen.

As an alternative to MMF, azathioprine (AZA) is initiated at 2 mg/kg per day, and the dose is adjusted to maintain a peripheral white blood cell count of 3,500 to 6,000 cells/mm^3. AZA is a prodrug that is hydrolyzed rapidly to 6-mercaptopurine, which is then metabolized via xanthine oxidase to its active metabolites. Major side effects include bone marrow suppression and gastrointestinal

TABLE 18–5. Substrates, Inducers, and Inhibitors of Cytochrome P450 Enzymes

	CYP1A	CYP2C	CYP2D6	CYP3A
Substrates	Acetaminophen Amitriptyline Antipyrine Caffeine Chlorotrianisene Chlorzoxazone Clarithromycin Clomipramine Clozapine Dantrolene Diethylstilbestrol Estradiol Flutamide Fluvoxamine Haloperidol Imipramine Lidocaine Methadone Ondansetron Paracetamol Paraxathine Phenacetin Procarbazine Propafenone Prostaglandins R-warfarin Ritonavir Tacrine Tamoxifen Theobromine Theophylline Toltrazuril Verapamil	Amitriptyline Benzphetamine Clomipramine Cyclophosphamide Dapsone Diazepam Diclofenac Ethosuximide Hexobaribital Ibuprofen Lansoprazole Mephenytoin Naproxen Nelfinavir Nifedipine Omeprazole Phenylbutazone Phenytoin Piroxicam Progesterone Proguanil Propranolol Ritonavir S,R-warfarin Sulfinpyrazone Sulfaphenazole Sulfonamides Tamoxifen Taxol Tenoxicam Testosterone Tetrahydrocannabinol Tolbutamide Tricyclics Trimethadione Valproic acid	Amitripyline Bufuralol Captopril Citalopram Chlorpromazine Clomipramine Clozapine Codeine Debrisoquine Desipramine Dextromethorphan Doxepin Encainide Ethylmorphine Flecainide Fluoxetine (40%) Fluphenazine Haloperidol (small %) Imipramine Indoramin Labetolol Lidocaine Maprotiline (R)-methadone (active isomer) Metoprolol Mexiletine Morphine Nelfinavir Nortriptyline Omeprazole Ondansetron Phenformin Propafenone Propranolol Quinidine Retinoic acid Risperidone Ritonavir RU486 Sparteine Tamoxifen Taxol Teniposide Testosterone Thioridazine Timolol Tramadol Trazadone Triazolam Trifluperidol Trimipramine Venlafaxine Vinblastine Zonisamide	ABT-378 Alfentanil Alprazolam Amiodarone Amiodipine Antipyrine Astemizole Benzphetamine Carbamazepine Cisapride Chlorpromazine Clarithromycin Cocaine Cortisol Cyclophosphamide Cyclosporine Dantrolene Dapsone Delavirdine Dextromethorphan (min %) Diazepam Digitoxin Diltiazem Disopyramide Enalapril Erythromycin Estradiol Estrogen Ethosuximide Ethylmorphine Etoposide Felodipine FK506 Flutamide Indinavir Itraconazole Ketoconazole Lidocaine Loratadine Lovastatin Mephenytoin Miconazole Midazolam Nefazodone Melfinavir Nevirapine Nicardipine Nifedipine Omeprazole Paclitaxel Paracetamol Prednisone Propafenone Progasterone Quindine R-warfarin (minor) Ritonavir Saquinavir Sertraline Tacrolimus Tamoxifen Taxol Terfenadine Testosterone Triazolam Verapamil Vinblastine
Inducers	Charbroiled food Cigarette smoke Cruciferous vegetables Omeprazole Phenobarbital Phenytoin	For CYP2C9/10: rifampicin dexamethasone phenobarbital For CYP2C19: none identified	None identified	Carbamazepine Dexamethasone DMP-266 Isoniazid Nevirapine Phenobarbital Phenytoin Prednisone Rifabutin/rifampicin
Inhibitors	Cimetidine Ciprofloxacin Enoxacin Fluvoxamine Nalidixic acid Norfloxacin	Amiodarone (2C9/10) Cimetidine Disulfiram Fluconazole Fluoxetine Fluvoxamine Ketoconazole (2C9/10) Omeprazole (2C9/10) Ritonavir Sertraline	Cimetidine Clomipramine Desipramine Fluoxetine Fluvoxamine (weak) Haloperidol Methadone Moclobemide Norfluoxetine Paroxetine Perphenazine Quinidine Ritonavir Sertraline Thioridazine	Cimetidine Clarithromycin Clotrimazole Delavirdine Diltiazem Erythromycin Fluoxetine Fluvoxamine Grapefruit juice (6′, 7′-dihydroxybergamottin) Indinavir Itra/flu/ketoconazole Miconazole Nefazodone Nelfinavir Nifedipine Norfloxacin Omeprazole Paroxetine Propoxyphene Ritonavir Saquinavir Sertraline Verapamil

TABLE 18–6. Drug Interactions of CsA and Tacrolimus

CsA Levels		Tacrolimus Levels	
Increase	***Decrease***	***Increase***	***Decrease***
Ketoconazole	Rifampicin	Ketoconazole	Rifampin
Fluconazole	Phenytoin	Fluconazole	Dexamethasone
Itraconazole	Phenobarbital	Itraconazole	Phenytoin
Erythromycin	Carbamazepine	Erythromycin	
Diltiazem	Sulfadimidine	Diltiazem	
Verapamil	Trimethoprim	Verapamil	
Danazol		Danazol	
Nicardipine		Cimetidine	
Metoclopramide		Clotrimazole	
Methylprednisolone		CsA	
Norethisterone			
Sirolimus			
Tacrolimus			

From Ref. 49.

toxicity. Clinically significant interactions include other bone marrow toxins (e.g., ganciclovir, trimethoprim-sulfamethoxazole, and sirolimus), other gastrointestinal irritants, and allopurinol, which inhibits xanthine oxidase. Allopurinol blocks the metabolism of AZA, resulting in increased bioavailability and a fourfold increase in 6-mercaptopurine concentrations, which may result in life threatening pancytopenia if not managed appropriately.[75] If it is necessary to administer allopurinol concomitantly with AZA, it is recommended that the dosage of AZA be reduced to 25% of the previous dosage. Many practitioners preferentially would switch the patient to MMF because it does not interact with allopurinol. Since CsA can cause hyperuricemia, another option is to switch the patients to tacrolimus, thereby minimizing the complication rather than adding another medication to treat the drug-induced hyperuricemia.

Prednisone is tapered from an initial dose of 1 to 1.5 to 0.3 mg/kg per day on day 30 and 0.1 mg/kg per day on day 90 after transplantation. Many programs attempt to gradually withdraw prednisone 6 months after transplantation in patients who are thought to be at low risk (e.g., no or infrequent prior rejection, older patients, males) or in patients at risk for steroid-related complications (e.g., females, children who are still growing).[76,77] Potential benefits of steroid with drawal include a lower incidence of osteoporosis, hypertension, hyperlipidemia, obesity, and diabetes. However, no multicenter studies have been conducted to assess the full impact of early steroid withdrawal on the incidence of CAV and long-term survival. One observational study suggested a higher rate of "late" rejection occurring months to years after steroid weaning.[78]

In addition to maintenance therapy, a number of centers use either monoclonal or polyclonal induction agents including the interleukin-2 receptor blockers (e.g., basiliximab or daclizumab), OKT3, or the antithymocyte globulins (e.g., Thymoglobulin or Atgam) for short periods of time immediately after transplantation in high risk patients (e.g., high Panel reactive antibody, retransplants) or to spare the kidney from exposure to nephrotoxicity of CsA or tacrolimus.[79,80] To date, pooled data series show no clear-cut survival advantages with induction therapy, although it appears that a higher percentage of patients may be weaned from prednisone, thereby reducing the incidence of steroid-associated complications.[79,81] Controversy exists as to whether prophylactic therapy with these cytolytic agents confers any added benefit other than delaying the onset of the first rejection episode.[79,81] In addition, cytolytic therapy is very expensive, is inconvenient to administer, possibly alters the incidence and character of infectious complications, and may result in a higher incidence of malignancy, but this more likely related to the cumulative immunosuppressive load rather than one specific agent.[82]

Daclizumab, the first humanized monoclonal antibody, was approved in 1997 by the Food and Drug Administration (FDA) for prophylaxis of acute organ rejection in renal transplant recipients.[83] In a single-center experience, induction with daclizumab produced favorable results with a lower incidence of acute rejection (defined as ISHLT grade of 2 or higher): 18% in the daclizumab-treated patients as compared with 63% in the group receiving CsA, MMF, and prednisone with no induction therapy ($P = .04$). The time to occurrence of the first rejection episode also was signifantly longer in the daclizumab-treated patients.[84] There were no adverse reactions to daclizumab and no significant differences between the groups in the incidence of infection or cancer during follow-up. A large multicenter randomized, prospective, placebo-controlled trial evaluating daclizumab is currently underway at 32 centers in the United States, Canada, and Europe. Daclizumab 1 mg/kg is given within 12 hours of transplant and on days 8, 22, 36, and 50. Maintenance immunosuppression includes CsA, MMF, and prednisone.

Simulect is a chimeric interleukin 2 receptor blocker that was approved by the FDA in 1998 for induction therapy in renal transplant patients but has not been studied in heart transplant recipients.[85] All these medications are reviewed in greater detail in Chapter 46.

MORTALITY

Mortality in the early posttransplant period (first 3 months) occurs as a result of early graft failure usually owing to poor graft preservation, right ventricular failure caused by pulmonary hypertension, or acute rejection or infection. Risk factors for death within the first postoperative year include prior transplantation, very young or old recipient (< 5 or > 60 years of age), older donor, ischemia time, patient being in the intensive care unit prior to transplantation, patient requiring mechanical ventilation, and patient having received an LVAD or IABP.[10] However, some programs have showed improved survival in patients receiving mechanical assist devices because the patient is no longer in congestive heart failure at the time of transplantation.[86] Considerable progress has been made over the last two decades, with 1- and 3-year heart transplant survival rates increasing from 51.2% and 28.1% in 1968–1979 to 83.2% and 70% in 1998, respectively.[10]

The mortality rate is approximately 3% to 4% per year beyond the first posttransplant year. In addition to infection and acute graft rejection, late mortality (>12 months) occurs as a result of CAV, malignancy, cerebrovascular accident, and renal or hepatic failure.[2–9] The overall median survival time is 9.8 years, and for patients surviving the first year after transplantation, the median survival is 12 years.[16]

IMMUNOSUPPRESSION-RELATED COMPLICATIONS

ACUTE REJECTION

Despite advances in immunosuppression and refinement of postoperative care, acute cardiac allograft rejection remains a major determinant of survival following cardiac transplantation. Acute rejection continues to account for approximately 17% of all deaths.[87] The incidence of rejection is substantially higher during the early months following transplantation, with 90% of all rejections occurring within the first 6 months. In addition, the severity of rejection tends to be greater when it occurs early in the postoperative period. Although a minority of patients (37%) remains rejection-free, most will experience at least one episode of rejection during the first year (the cumulative number of rejection episodes is 1.3 ± 0.7 per patient).[87]

Rejection of the cardiac allograft is not necessarily accompanied by overt clinical signs or symptoms. Nonspecific findings may include low-grade fever, malaise, and mild reduction in exercise capacity, whereas heart failure or atrial arrhythmias may reflect more severe rejection. The "gold standard" for detection of rejection is histologic confirmation using endomyocardial specimens obtained by transvenous biopsy of the right ventricle. Since most patients remain asymptomatic, regularly scheduled surveillance biopsies are performed on all patients, with extra biopsies performed whenever rejection is suspected. A typical schedule would be to perform weekly biopsies for the first postoperative month, biweekly biopsies for the next 2 months, monthly biopsies for the next 4 to 6 months, and bimonthly biopsies for the next 7 to 12 months. Biopsy frequency subsequently decreases to every 3 to 12 months. To assess cardiac function, either echocardiography or measurement of right-sided heart and pulmonary wedge pressures and cardiac output by pulmonary artery catheterization is performed with each biopsy. Biopsy specimens are examined for evidence of rejection and are graded, based on histologic severity of the rejection, as ISHLT grade 0 (none) to grade 4 (severe).[88] Because an endomyocardial biopsy is an invasive, expensive, and labor-intensive procedure, great efforts have been expended to identify an accurate and reproducible noninvasive method/marker to detect or predict acute rejection.[89] Unfortunately, none of the methods studied thus far has the reliability of the endomyocardial biopsy. The treatment of rejection is based on a number of factors, including type, histologic grade, clinical symptoms, hemodynamic changes, noninvasive findings, and duration of time after transplantation.

Mild degrees of acute cellular rejection (ISHLT grades 1A and 1B) usually are not treated unless the patient is symptomatic, whereas the presence of moderate to severe rejection (grades 3A, 3B, and 4) with or without necrosis mandates treatment.[90] Treatment of grade 2 rejection is still a subject of debate. Winters and colleagues reported that approximately 40% to 45% of grade 2 rejections occurring in the first 6 months progress to grade 3A on the next biopsy, whereas only about 15% of grade 2 biopsies occurring later progress to grade 3A.[91] Early acute rejection occurring during the first 3 months usually is treated with daily "pulses" of methylprednisolone 500–1,000 mg administered intravenously for 3 days. Lower doses (250 mg) may be equally effective. Unless the rejection is recurrent or hemodynamically compromising, an oral prednisone regimen (1–1.5 mg/kg/day for 3 days) is administered and then tapered to the baseline dose over 5–10 additional days.[92] An endomyocardial biopsy usually is repeated within 7–14 days. If there is evidence of continuing or worsening rejection, the steroid therapy may be repeated and/or cytolytic therapy (Thymoglobulin or OKT3 Atgam) may be employed. Cytolytic therapy is used when there is hemodynamic compromise; Atgam or thymoglobulin is preferred over OKT3 when the wedge pressure is markedly elevated due to concern that development of a capillary leak syndrome (e.g., noncardiogenic pulmonary edema) associated with OKT3's cytokine release syndrome could be catastrophic in this setting. Other innovative forms of therapy for persistent or intractable rejection have been investigated, including mycophenolate mofetil,[62,64] tacrolimus,[58] low-dose methotrexate,[93,94] sirolimus (formerly rapamycin),[95–98] total lymphoid irradiation,[94] and photopheresis (e.g., immune-modulating therapy, which involves apheresis with isolation of peripheral blood leukocytes, treatment of the leukocytes ex vivo with 8-methoxypsoralen and ultraviolet light, and subsequent reinfusion into the patient).[99]

The majority of rejection episodes (i.e., cellular rejection) are characterized histologically by lymphocytic infiltrates with or without myocyte degeneration; however, in approximately 20% of those episodes associated with hemodynamic compromise, myocyte damage and lymphocytic infiltrates are absent. In contrast, extensive vascular damage is present and characterized by endothelial cell swelling, hemorrhages, interstitial edema, and occlusion of small capillaries. Immunofluorescence staining has shown deposition of immunoglobulins (IgG), complement, and fibrinogen at the level of the capillaries. This form of rejection is called *humoral* or *vascular rejection* and usually is preceded by the appearance of circulating immune complexes and the deposition of immunoglobulins.[100,101] Humoral rejection is an antibody-mediated process directed against HLA class II antigens present on the donor vascular endothelium. The diagnosis is suspected when a recipient develops ventricular dysfunction in the absence of cellular rejection and is confirmed by immunoflourescence staining of biopsy specimens showing deposition of IgG, C3, and C4 on coronary endothelium. This form of rejection generally occurs in the first 3 months after transplantation, appears to be more common when antilymphocyte antibodies are used for rejection prophylaxis, and is associated with an increased fatality rate and a higher incidence of CAV. Affected individuals are treated with high-dose intravenous glucocorticoids, antithymocyte globulin, cyclophosphamide, mycophenolate mofetil plasmapheresis, and heparin.

INFECTION

Both the severity and incidence of infections and deaths due to infections have decreased dramatically since the introduction of CsA and the use of lower steroid dosages. Nonetheless, infection and rejection remain the most frequently encountered complications associated with immunosuppression in the first year after transplantation.[102] The major cause of hospitalization remains infection, with 15.8% of readmissions in the first year and 7.8% in the fourth year attributed to infections.[10] The risk of infection is directly related to the overall level of immunosuppression and is greatest during the first 3 postoperative months, as well as following treatment of rejection episodes.[103] Laboratory or clinical evidence of an evolving infectious process necessitates the institution of aggressive diagnostic and frequently empirical therapeutic strategies. Infections in the transplant recipient can be categorized as nosocomial (catheter- or wound-related or pneumonia with *Staphylococcus* or gram-negative bacteria), donor-related [toxoplasmosis, hepatitis, cytomegalovirus (CMV)], or opportunistic

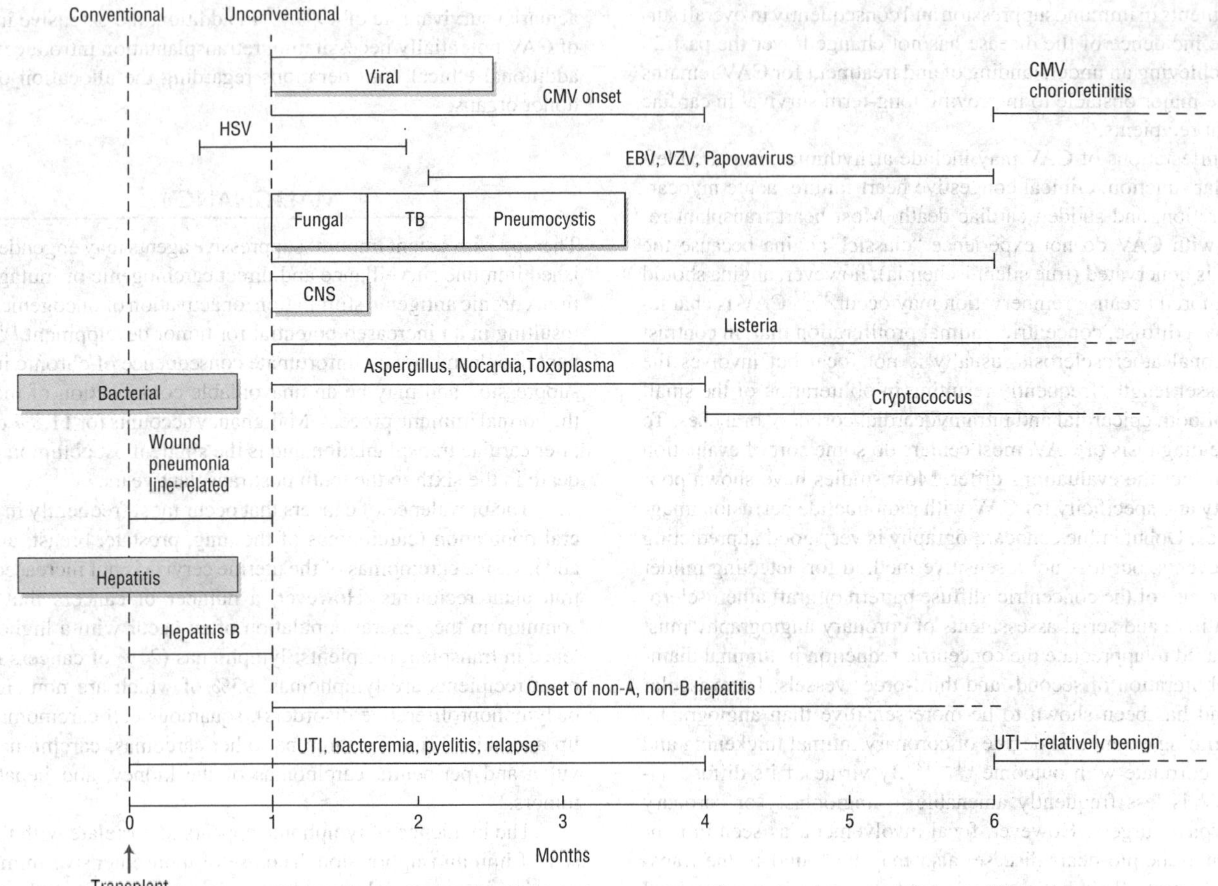

FIGURE 18–1. Timetable of infection for organ transplantation.

(CMV, *Pneumocystis, Nocardia,* fungal).[103,104] The infections usually present in a characteristic time course (Fig. 18–1) following transplantation. The most common sites of infection include lung, blood, urine, gastrointestinal tract, and sternal wound. The latter accounts for only 7% of infections but represents 25% of the deaths; therefore, mediastinitis in an immunosuppressed thoracic transplant recipient can be devastating.[102] A number of preventive strategies are employed routinely in the transplant recipient and include trimethoprim-sulfamethoxazole (*Pneumocystis, Toxoplasma,* and *Nocardia* prophylaxis), miconazole (*Candida*), and antiviral agents (acyclovir, ganciclovir, immune globulin, CMV hyperimmune globulin) for CMV, herpes simplex virus (HSV), and Epstein-Barr virus (EBV).[104–107] Pyrimethamine–folinic acid for 6 weeks has been used as an alternative for *Toxoplasma* prophylaxis in high-risk patients (e.g., negative recipients of positive organs). Other infections that may occur in heart transplant recipients and should be included in the differential diagnosis are *Legionella* pneumonia and *Listeria* meningitis, and bacteremia.

CMV can cause direct damage (infection) or indirect damage such as stimulating antigen expression, enhancing immune responses resulting in rejection, or allowing opportunistic infections and possibly chronic rejection.[104] Based on the premise that preventing CMV infection is preferable to treating CMV disease, most centers have adopted some type of preventive regimen.[107] The major limitation is that the anti-CMV agents appear to be most efficacious in preventing reactivation (secondary infection) but have had little impact on the incidence of primary infection in the highest-risk group (CMV-negative recipients of CMV-positive allografts).[105,106] The added benefit of ganciclovir prophylaxis is that it has significant activity against the other herpes viruses, including EBV, which may provide a protective effect against posttransplant lymphoproliferative disease. Based on the current literature, there is no ideal regimen for CMV prevention. More aggressive strategies including intravenous ganciclovir plus or minus CMV hyperimmune globulin followed by oral ganciclovir may be most appropriate for the highest-risk patients (CMV-negative recipients of CMV-positive organs or those receiving antilymphocyte therapy with OKT3, Atgam, or Thymoglobulin), whereas selective preemptive therapy with ganciclovir (treating the infection once it manifests itself rather than administering prophylaxis to all patients) may be used in CMV-positive recipients at risk for reactivation.[104]

CARDIAC ALLOGRAFT VASCULOPATHY (CAV)

CAV, also referred to as *transplant coronary artery disease* or *chronic rejection,* has been defined as the occurrence of an accelerated atherosclerosis in the coronary arteries of the graft. This is the single most common cause of death in patients who survive the first year after cardiac transplantation. Numerous reports have suggested that the average incidence of CAV is approximately 10% per year such that 40% to 50% of recipients have angiographically defined CAV by year 5 following transplantation. More recently, it has been reported to be present in 80% to 100% of patients at 5 years when intravascular ultrasound is used as the diagnostic tool.[108] This entity is thought to be similar to the chronic rejection processes also seen in renal (chronic allograft nephropathy), lung (obliterative bronchiolitis), and liver (vanishing bile duct syndrome) allografts. Despite improvements in immunosuppression and consequently in overall survival, the incidence of the disease has not changed over the past 20 years. Achieving an understanding of and treatment for CAV remains the single major obstacle to improving long-term survival in cardiac transplant recipients.[109]

Manifestations of CAV may include arrhythmias, impaired left ventricular function, clinical congestive heart failure, acute myocardial infarction, and sudden cardiac death. Most heart transplant recipients with CAV do not experience "classic" angina because the allograft is denervated (true silent ischemia); however, angina should not be ignored because reinnervation may occur.[36,37] CAV is characterized by a diffuse, concentric, intimal proliferation that, in contrast to traditional atherosclerosis, usually is not focal but involves the entire vessel length, frequently resulting in obliteration of the small vessels of both epicardial and intramyocardial coronary branches. To aid in the diagnosis of CAV, most centers do some sort of evaluation each year, but the evaluations differ. Most studies have shown poor sensitivity and specificity for CAV with radionuclide perfusion imaging studies. Dobutamine echocardiography is very good at predicting adverse events, but it is not a sensitive method for detecting milder CAV. Because of the concentric, diffuse pattern of graft atherosclerosis, quantitive and serial assessments of coronary angiography must be compared to appreciate the concentric reduction in luminal diameter or obliteration of second- and third-order vessels. Intravascular ultrasound has been shown to be more sensitive than angiography in determining extent and degree of coronary intimal thickening and to better correlate with outcome.[110–112] By virtue of its diffuse nature, CAV is less frequently amenable to angioplasty or coronary artery bypass surgery. However, focal involvement, as seen in nontransplant ischemic heart disease, also may be found in the transplanted allograft. This latter process tends to occur in the proximal portions of the extramural coronary vessels and may be amenable to percutaneous balloon dilation. However, this is only palliative at best.[113]

The pathogenesis of CAV has not yet been delineated, but the frequent observation of intimal thickening and a mononuclear cell inflammatory reaction within the intima suggests that it may in part be caused by rejection, possibly as a result of a reaction to immunologic markers carried on vascular endothelial cells. Traditional risk factors, including hypercholesterolemia, hypertriglyceridemia, obesity, glucose intolerance, and smoking, most likely contribute to the adverse milieu. It has been reported that CMV infection and subsequent rejection episodes are associated with the development of atherosclerosis in the transplanted heart.[114] It is possible that the CMV contributes to an initial injury to the coronary endothelium, perhaps on an immunologic basis, that progresses to coronary artery disease. The potential long-term benefit of ganciclovir prophylaxis and treatment of CMV infections and its association with CAV remain to be assessed.

Conventional preventive measures used to decrease the incidence of CAV in the transplant recipient include maintenance of ideal body weight, control of blood pressure (goal blood pressure around 130/80 mm Hg), and implementation of dietary and drug therapy for lipid disorders (goal low-density lipoprotein level of 100 mg/dL or less). Studies with pravastatin and simvastatin show decreased coronary artery disease and prolongation of survival.[115,116]

As mentioned previously, percutaneous transluminal coronary angioplasty and coronary bypass surgery are not usual options for treatment of diffuse graft atherosclerosis, even if both have been used, leaving retransplantation as the only potential therapy. The prognosis following retransplantation is suboptimal, as reflected by a 1-year actuarial survival rate of 49%.[117] In addition, the extensive incidence of CAV potentially necessitating retransplantation introduces several additional ethical considerations regarding the allocation of scarce donor organs.

MALIGNANCY

Therapy with potent immunosuppressive agents may engender diminished immune surveillance and direct carcinogenic or mutagenic action, chronic antigenic stimulation, or activation of oncogenic viruses, resulting in an increased potential for tumor development.[118] Malignant neoplasms are an unfortunate consequence of chronic immunosuppression and may be an unavoidable complication of modifying the normal immune process. Malignancy accounts for 11.8% of deaths after cardiac transplantation and is the single most common cause of death in the sixth to the tenth posttransplant years.

The prevalence of cancers that occur most frequently in the general population (carcinomas of the lung, prostate, breast, and colon and invasive carcinomas of the uterine cervix) is not increased among transplant recipients. However, a number of cancers that are uncommon in the general population often occur with a higher prevalence in transplant recipients: lymphomas (21% of cancers in transplant recipients are lymphomas, 93% of which are non-Hodgkin's or lymphoproliferative disorders), squamous cell carcinomas of the lip and skin, Kaposi's sarcoma, other sarcomas, carcinomas of the vulva and perineum, carcinomas of the kidney, and hepatobiliary tumors.

The incidence of lymphoma appears to correlate with the intensity of immunosuppression. The use of more intensive immunosuppression in extrarenal transplant recipients is particularly common and is reflected in the higher incidence of lymphomas seen in cardiac recipients when compared with renal recipients.[119]

The incidence, time to occurrence, and features of the tumors appear to vary with use of various immunosuppressive agents. AZA-based immunosuppressive regimens have been associated with a high incidence (40% of all malignancies) of cutaneous malignancies. One possible mechanism to explain this unusually high incidence of skin cancer involves AZA's metabolite, nitroimidazole, which causes significant photosensitivity, resulting in subsequent skin cancer.[120] AZA therapy is associated with a 2:1 predominance of squamous over basal cell carcinomas, whereas basal cell carcinoma occurs more frequently in the general population. AZA-induced cutaneous squamous cell carcinoma is also associated with more metastatic disease and accounts for 6% of all deaths in comparison with less than 1% with CsA. Patients must be encouraged to use effective techniques to reduce sun exposure.

With the introduction of CsA, the relative frequency of non-Hodgkin's lymphoma or posttransplant lymphoproliferative disorder (PTLD) increased to 29% as compared to 11% with regimens based on AZA or cyclophosphamide. The tumors tended to occur earlier (15 months after transplantation in the CsA group vs 48 months in the AZA or cyclophosphamide group), and 32% occurred within 4 months postoperatively in the CsA group versus 11% for older non-CsA-based regimens. Among patients treated with OKT3 and other monoclonal antibodies, lymphomas account for 64% of all tumors. These lymphomas frequently develop soon after transplantation (average 7 months).[119] In one report, PTLD developed in 1.3% of patients receiving triple-drug immunosuppression as compared with 11.4% in patients receiving the monoclonal antibody OKT3. A statistically significant increase in incidence was noted in patients receiving a cumulative OKT3 dose of greater than 75 mg.[82] This report demonstrates the contribution of overall immunosuppressive load in comparison with centers using lower doses. Similarly, the use of Atgam was found to increase the risk of PTLD.[119] T-cell-specific agents (CsA, OKT3, Atgam) that directly impair T-cell function may produce a reduction in host response to viral infections, particularly EBV and CMV. EBV has been shown to have infectious as well as oncogenic properties and may play a causal role in the development of mononucleosis, Burkitt's lymphoma, and nasopharyngeal carcinoma.

The clinical presentation of PTLD may vary from a flu-like syndrome to multisystem organ failure. A higher proportion of patients receiving conventional immunosuppression have extranodal involvement as compared with CsA-based regimens. Extranodal involvement, with tumors present in the gastrointestinal tract, lung, and central nervous system, occurs in 69% of cases in transplant recipients versus 24% to 48% in the general population. Central nervous system involvement occurs more frequently in patients with conventional immunosuppression (39%) as compared with CsA-based regimens (14%).

The diagnosis of PTLD is made by a tissue biopsy. The histologic types of PTLD are described in Chapter 14. Treatment depends on symptoms, presentation, and extent of involvement. In general, reduction of immunosuppression and concomitant therapy with acyclovir often have been associated with resolution and remission of PTLD.[121] Radiotherapy, chemotherapy, and surgical excision may be necessary in certain situations as palliative therapy but are rarely curative. Optimal preventive therapy is to avoid overimmunosuppression in transplant recipients. A 5-year mortality rate of 37% has been reported in patients with PTLD.[119]

IMMUNOSUPPRESSION-RELATED ADVERSE EFFECTS

HYPERTENSION

Arterial hypertension is the most common posttransplantation medical problem, which, despite intensive investigation, remains poorly understood. The incidence of posttransplantation hypertension in cardiac recipients has increased from less than 20% in the conventional immunosuppression era to greater than 90% in the current era using CsA-based regimens.[122] In the conventional era, hypertension was felt to be a result of mineralocorticoid excess engendered by immunosuppressive regimens based heavily on prednisone. Paradoxically, with the introduction of CsA-based regimens allowing for steroid dosage reduction or discontinuation, hypertension has become more prevalent.[122]

The primary mechanism of CsA-associated hypertension in heart transplant recipients may be related to the CsA-induced stimulation of intact renal sympathetic nerves and the absence of reflex cardiac inhibition of the sympathetic nervous system,[122] but a number of other mechanisms, including decreased prostacyclin and nitric oxide production, also have been proposed.[123,124] In addition to CsA's propensity to cause peripheral vasoconstriction, it promotes sodium retention by increasing proximal tubular sodium retention, resulting in extracellular fluid volume expansion. Thus diuretics and dietary sodium restriction are used routinely in heart transplant recipients. Because CsA and diuretics also induce renal magnesium wasting, hypomagnesemia may contribute to the hypertension because magnesium is purported to be a vasorelaxant. Magnesium supplementation is usually necessary in CsA-treated patients unless they have renal insufficiency.

No single antihypertensive agent has been found to be uniformly effective in controlling CsA-associated hypertension. Currently, the use of calcium channel antagonists (e.g., diltiazem) and ACE inhibitors has been found to be effective in the treatment of this form of hypertension.[125] Calcium channel blockers, particularly diltiazem, often are considered drugs of choice because they have other purported benefits on the development of graft atherosclerosis and also may be protective of the kidneys.[126] It is important to remember that a number of the calcium channel blockers (e.g., diltiazem, nicardipine, verapamil, and amlodipine) interact with CsA, tacrolimus, and sirolimus, resulting in increased immunosuppressant concentrations. Drug concentrations of the immunosuppressants must be monitored as doses of the antihypertensive agents are adjusted or therapy is switched. Polydrug antihypertensive regimens often are necessary. β-Blockers usually are avoided because a decrease in heart rate is not desirable in heart transplant patients. α-Blockers tend not to be well tolerated because of the propensity to exacerbate orthostatic hypotension. Compared with CsA, a lower incidence of hypertension has been reported with tacrolimus-based immunosuppressive regimens[52] and with regimens that eliminate prednisone after transplantation.

NEPHROTOXICITY

One of the most common side effects observed in heart transplant recipients receiving maintenance CsA or tacrolimus therapy is nephrotoxicity. Two types of toxicity occur. Acute nephrotoxicity often is seen early and is dose-dependent and reversible, but chronic nephropathy is more common. Clinical manifestations of CsA nephrotoxicity include elevated serum creatinine and blood urea nitrogen, hyperkalemia, hyperuricemia, mild proteinuria, and a decreased fractional excretion of sodium.

The predominant mechanism for CsA nephrotoxicity is renal vasoconstriction, primarily of the afferent arteriole, resulting in increased renal vascular resistance, decreased renal blood flow by up to 40%, reduced glomerular filtration rate by up to 30%, and increased proximal tubular sodium reabsorption with a reduction in urinary sodium and potassium excretion.[124] A number of other mechanisms have been implicated, including changes in the rennin-angiotensin-aldosterone system, prostaglandin synthesis, nitrous oxide production, sympathetic nervous system activation, and calcium handling.[124]

Measures to reduce CsA nephrotoxicity include delaying its administration immediately postoperatively in patients at high risk for nephrotoxicity (using alternative induction protocols including OKT3, Atgam, or Thymoglobulin), monitoring CsA trough blood levels and reducing the CsA dosage if the vasoconstrictive effects are problematic, and avoiding other nephrotoxins (e.g., aminoglycosides, amphotericin B, nonsteroidal anti-inflammatory agents) when possible. When using these agents, drug concentrations of CsA and those of the other drugs, if available, should be monitored closely. In addition, the concomitant administration of drugs [e.g., azole antifungals, especially ketoconazole and to a lesser extent fluconazole and itraconazole; the macrolide antibiotics (erythromycin, clarithromycin but not azithromycin); the calcium antagonists (diltiazem, nicardipine, verapamil); and antidepressants (nefazadone, fluvoxamine)] known to elevate CsA levels requires intentional dosage reductions to avoid unnecessary renal and other toxicity.[49] Similar management strategies are useful when dealing with tacrolimus because it is at least as nephrotoxic as CsA.[58] Other drugs also may increase CsA and tacrolimus concentrations (see Table 18–6). Some centers take advantage of these interactions by routinely using CsA-sparing agents to reduce the dosage and cost of therapy while maintaining the same therapeutic concentrations.[127]

Currently, no proven therapies consistently prevent or reverse the nephrotoxic effects of CsA; however, a number of agents have been studied, including prostaglandin analogs, pentoxyphylline, fish oils, and so on.[126]

HYPERLIPIDEMIA

Although hypercholesterolemia is a known risk factor for the development of coronary artery disease and reduction of serum cholesterol levels decreases cardiac morbidity and mortality in the general population, conflicting evidence exists regarding the relationship between the hyperlipidemia commonly seen in heart recipients and the development of CAV.[128] A progressive rise in serum cholesterol and triglycerides occurs in a time-dependent fashion following cardiac transplantation. Steroids, CsA, and sirolimus are known to increase serum cholesterol and triglyceride levels. Other drugs, including diuretics, β-blockers, and ethanol, may aggravate hyperlipidemia in transplant patients. Drug therapy to reduce cholesterol and triglycerides may be used, but dosage reduction of lovastatin and monitoring for myositis are necessary to avoid rhabdomyolysis if it is used concomitantly with CsA.[129] Pravastatin is preferred as a result of its lower interactive potential with CsA because it is not metabolized by cytochrome P-450 3A4, and it may have a salutory immunosuppressive effect as well.[116,128,130] Atorvastatin may substantially reduce LDL cholesterol in patients with persistently elevated levels despite pravastatin therapy.[131] Management of hyperlipidemia in the heart transplant recipient is reviewed elsewhere.[115,116,129,130]

SUMMARY

A number of factors, including refined selection criteria, improvements in immunosuppressive regimens and diagnostic techniques for rejection, donor organ preservation, and treatment of infectious complications, have contributed to the overall success of cardiothoracic transplantation. The majority of patients return to NYHA functional class I and are able to achieve a desirable quality of life following transplantation. Despite the tremendous progress made in cardiothoracic transplantation over the last decade, much remains to be done.

The therapeutic-to-toxic ratio of currently used immunosuppressive agents remains narrow, mandating lifelong monitoring of patients. The identification of more specific immunosuppressive agents, with a higher therapeutic-to-toxic index or one capable of inducing tolerance to the grafted organ, remains a desirable although elusive goal at this time. Similarly, the development of noninvasive techniques for the diagnosis of graft rejection would reduce the inconvenience, cost, and morbidity associated with long-term surveillance substantially.

Chronic graft atherosclerosis remains to be understood, and until the pathogenesis and appropriate treatment are defined, graft dysfunction secondary to this form of atherosclerosis will remain the leading impediment to long-term survival.

Although, ideally, legislative and public awareness programs will have an impact on resolving the chronic shortage of suitable donors, the rapidly increasing number of patients afflicted with congestive heart failure will necessitate developing alternative options for patients with end-stage disease. The roles of long-term mechanical circulatory assistance and xenotransplantation remain to be defined. It is likely that the coming decade will witness enhanced therapeutic and laboratory research designed to evaluate and refine the clinical, immunologic, and socioeconomic impact of using these alternative options.

▶ PRINCIPLES OF PHARMACOTHERAPY

- Survival and quality of life after heart transplantation are limited by posttransplant events, such as infection and acute and chronic rejection.
- Patients require lifelong immunosuppression to maintain the stability of their grafts.
- Overimmunosuppression predisposes patients to infection, malignancy, and drug toxicity, whereas underimmunosuppression increases the risk of rejection.
- Combinations of two or three immunosuppressants are usually necessary to maximize immunosuppressive efficacy while minimizing the toxicity of the individual agents.
- Immunosuppressant-induced side effects, including nephrotoxicity, hypertension, hyperlipidemia, and diabetes, occur frequently and usually require additional drug therapy.
- Antimicrobial prophylaxis is necessary to decrease the risk of bacterial, viral (e.g., CMV, HSV, EBV), fungal (e.g., *Candida, Aspergillus*), and other opportunistic infections (e.g., *Pneumocystis, Nocardia*).
- Heart transplant patients receive multiple medications, and both pharmacokinetic and pharmacodynamic interactions are very common.
- The consequences of drug interactions (e.g., over- or underimmunosuppression) can be life-threatening, and heart transplant patients must be monitored closely whenever new drugs are added or existing medications are discontinued from their drug therapy regimens.
- As more immunosuppressive agents are introduced to the marketplace, drug therapy regimens in heart transplant patients need to be individualized based on each patient's immunologic status and toxicity-risk profile.
- CAV remains the number one cause of long-term morbidity and mortality, and the incidence has been minimally affected by the advent of new immunosuppressants.

REFERENCES

1. Hosenpud JD, Bennett LE, Keck BM, et al. The Registry of the International Society for Heart and Lung Transplantation: Eighteenth official report—2001. J Heart Lung Transplant 2001;20:805–815.
2. Brann WM, Bennett LE, Keck BM, Hosenpud JD. Morbidity, functional status, and immunosuppressive therapy after heart transplantation: An analysis of the joint International Society for Heart and Lung Transplantation/United Network for Organ Sharing Thoracic Registry. J Heart Lung Transplant 1998;17:374–382.
3. Bennett WM. Renal complications after heart transplantation. Transplant Proc 1999;31:88.
4. de Mattos AM, Olyaei AJ, Bennett WM. Nephrotoxicity of immunosuppressive drugs: Long-term consequences and challenges for the future (Editorial). Am J Kidney Dis 2000;35:333–346.
5. Gallo P, Agozzino L, Angelini A, et al. Causes of late failure after heart transplantation: A ten-year survey. J Heart Lung Transplant 1997; 16:1113–1121.

6. Esposito S, Renzulli A, Agozzino L, et al. Late complications of heart transplantation: An 11-year experience. Heart Vessels 1999;14: 272–276.
7. Esposito C, Semeraro L, Bellotti N, et al. Risk factors for chronic renal dysfunction in cardiac allograft recipients. Nephron 2000;84:21–28.
8. Frimat L, Villemot JP, Cormier L, et al. Treatment of end-stage renal failure after heart transplantation. Nephrol Dial Transplant 1998;13:2905–2908.
9. Yamani MH, Starling RC. Long-term medical complications of heart transplantation: Information for the primary care physician. Cleve Clin J Med 2000;67:673–680.
10. Keck BM, Bennett LE, Rosendale J, et al. Worldwide Thoracic Organ Transplantation: A report from the UNOS/ISHLT International Registry for Thoracic Organ Transplantation. In: JM Cecka, PI Terasaki, eds. Clinical Transplants 1999. Los Angeles: UCLA Immunogenetics Center, 1999:35–49.
11. American Heart Association. 1998 Heart and Stroke Statistical Update. Dallas: AHA, 1998.
12. National Heart, Lung & Blood Institute. Congestive Heart Failure in the United States: A New Epidemic. Bethesda, MD: National Heart, Lung & Blood Institute, 1996.
13. O'Connell JB, Bristow MR. Economic impact of heart failure in the United States: Time for a different approach. J Heart Lung Transplant 1994;13:S107–S112.
14. Grady KL, Jalowiec A, White-Williams C. Improvement in quality of life in patients with heart failure who undergo transplantation. J Heart Lung Transplant 1996;15:749–757.
15. Starling R. Economics of heart transplantation. In: Norman DJ, Suki WN, eds. Primer on Transplantation. Thorofare, NJ: American Society of Transplant Physicians, 1998:405–408.
16. UNOS 1999 Annual Report: The U.S. Scientific Registry of Transplant Recipients and the Organ Procurement and Transplantation Network. UNOS Web site; available at *http://www.unos.org*.
17. Young JB. Age before beauty: The use of "older" donor hearts for cardiac transplantation. J Heart Lung Transplant 1999;18:488–491.
18. Bennett LE, Edwards EB, Hosenpud JD. Transplantation with older donor hearts for presumed "stable" recipients: An analysis of the Joint International Society for Heart and Lung Transplantation/United Network for Organ Sharing Thoracic Registry [published erratum appears in J Heart Lung Transplant 1998;17(11):1138]. J Heart Lung Transplant 1998;17:901–905.
19. Costanzo MR, Augustine S, Bourge R, et al. Selection and treatment of candidates for heart transplantation: A statement for health professionals from the Committee on Heart Failure and Cardiac Transplantation of the Council on Clinical Cardiology, American Heart Association. Circulation 1995;92:3593–3612.
20. Mancini DM, Eisen H, Kussmaul W, et al. Value of peak exercise oxygen consumption for optimal timing of cardiac transplantation in ambulatory patients with heart failure. Circulation 1991;83:778–786.
21. Aaronson KD, Mancini DM. Is percentage of predicted maximal exercise oxygen consumption a better predictor of survival than peak exercise oxygen consumption for patients with severe heart failure? [published erratum appears in J Heart Lung Transplant 1996;15(1 Pt 1):106–107]. J Heart Lung Transplant 1995;14:981–989.
22. Aaronson KD, Schwartz JS, Chen TM, et al. Development and prospective validation of a clinical index to predict survival in ambulatory patients referred for cardiac transplant evaluation. Circulation 1997;95:2660–2667.
23. Costard-Jackle A, Fowler MB. Influence of preoperative pulmonary artery pressure on mortality after heart transplantation: Testing of potential reversibility of pulmonary hypertension with nitroprusside is useful in defining a high risk group. J Am Coll Cardiol 1992;19:48–54.
24. Kauffman HM, McBride MA, Shield CF, et al. Determinants of waiting time for heart transplants in the United States [published erratum appears in J Heart Lung Transplant 19991;18(7):733]. J Heart Lung Transplant 1999;18:414–419.
25. Harper AM, Rosendale JD, McBride MA, et al. The UNOS OPTN waiting list and donor registry. Clin Transplant 1998;73–90.
26. Hunt SA, Frazier OH. Mechanical circulatory support and cardiac transplantation. Circulation 1998;97:2079–2090.
27. Pagani FD, Lynch W, Swaniker F, et al. Extracorporeal life support to left ventricular assist device bridge to heart transplant: A strategy to optimize survival and resource utilization. Circulation 1999;100:II206–II210.
28. Packer M, Bristow MR, Cohn JN, et al. The effect of carvedilol on morbidity and mortality in patients with chronic heart failure. U.S. Carvedilol Heart Failure Study Group. N Engl J Med 1996;334:1349–1355.
29. Stevenson LW. Selection and management of candidates for heart transplantation. Curr Opin Cardiol 1996;11:166–173.
30. Pitt B, Zannad F, Remme WJ, et al. The effect of spironolactone on morbidity and mortality in patients with severe heart failure. Randomized Aldactone Evaluation Study Investigators. N Engl J Med 1999;341:709–717.
30a. Hunt SA, Baker DW, Chin MH, et al. ACC/AHA guidelines for the evaluation and management of chronic heart failure in the adult: Executive summary: A report of the American College of Cardiology/American Heart Association Task Force on Practice Guidelines (Committee to Revise the 1995 Guidelines for the Evaluation and Management of Heart Failure). J Am Coll Cardiol 2001;38:2101–2113.
31. Fonarow GC, Stevenson LW, Walden JA. Impact of a comprehensive heart failure management program on hospital readmissions and functional status of patients with advanced heart failure. J Am Coll Cardiol 1997;30:725–732.
32. Rubin RH, Fishman JA. A consideration of potential donors with active infection: Is this a way to expand the donor pool? Transplant Int 1998;11:333–335.
33. Lopez-Navidad A, Domingo P, Caballero F, et al. Successful transplantation of organs retrieved from donors with bacterial meningitis. Transplantation 1997;64:365–368.
34. Givertz MM, Harley H, Colucci WS. Long-term sequential changes in exercise capacity and chronotropic responsiveness after cardiac transplantation. Circulation 1997;96:232–237.
35. Mancini D. Surgically denervated cardiac transplant: Rewired or permanently unplugged? Circulation 1997;96:6–8.
36. Wilson RF. Reinnervation reexamination (Editorial). J Heart Lung Transplant 1998;17:137–139.
37. Bengel FM, Ueberfuhr P, Schiepel N, et al. Effect of sympathetic reinnervation on cardiac performance after heart transplantation. N Engl J Med 2001;345:731–738.
38. Burke MN, McGinn AL, Homans DC, et al. Evidence for functional sympathetic reinnervation of left ventricle and coronary arteries after orthotopic cardiac transplantation in humans. Circulation 1995;91: 72–78.
39. Stark RP, McGinn AL, Wilson RF. Chest pain in cardiac transplant recipients: Evidence of sensory reinnervation after cardiac transplantation. N Engl J Med 1991;324:1791–1794.
40. Young JB, Winters WL Jr, Bourge R, Uretsky BF. 24th Bethesda conference: Cardiac transplantation. Task Force 4: Function of the heart transplant recipient. J Am Coll Cardiol 1993;22:31–41.
41. Chelimsky-Fallick C, Middlekauff HR, Stevenson WG, et al. Amiodarone therapy does not compromise subsequent heart transplantation. J Am Coll Cardiol 1992;20:1556–1561.
42. Redmond JM, Zehr KJ, Gillinov MA, et al. Use of theophylline for treatment of prolonged sinus node dysfunction in human orthotopic heart transplantation. J Heart Lung Transplant 1993;12:133–138; discussion, 138–139.
43. Traversi E, Pozzoli M, Grande A, et al. The bicaval anastomosis technique for orthotopic heart transplantation yields better atrial function than the standard technique: An echocardiographic automatic boundary detection study. J Heart Lung Transplant 1998;17:1065–1074.
44. Kao AC, Van Trigt P 3d, Shaeffer-McCall GS, et al. Central and peripheral limitations to upright exercise in untrained cardiac transplant recipients. Circulation 1994;89:2605–2615.
45. McCollam PL, Uber WE, Van Bakel AB. Adenosine-related ventricular asystole. Ann Intern Med 1993;118:315–316.

46. Hosenpud JD, Bennett LE, Keck BM, et al. The Registry of the International Society for Heart and Lung Transplantation: Fifteenth official report—1998. J Heart Lung Transplant 1998;17:656–668.
47. Chen JM, Levin HR, Michler RE, et al. Reevaluating the significance of pulmonary hypertension before cardiac transplantation: Determination of optimal thresholds and quantification of the effect of reversibility on perioperative mortality. J Thorac Cardiovasc Surg 1997;114:627–634.
48. Kahan BD. Cyclosporine. N Engl J Med 1989;321:1725–1738.
49. Lake KD, Canafax DM. Important interactions of drugs with immunosuppressive agents used in transplant recipients. J Antimicrob Chemother 1995;36:11–22.
50. Mignat C. Clinically significant drug interactions with new immunosuppressive agents. Drug Saf 1997;16:267–278.
51. Shapiro R. Tacrolimus in solid organ transplantation: An update. Transplant Proc 1999;31:2203–2205.
52. Taylor DO, Barr ML, Radovancevic B, et al. A randomized, multicenter comparison of tacrolimus and cyclosporine immunosuppressive regimens in cardiac transplantation: Decreased hyperlipidemia and hypertension with tacrolimus. J Heart Lung Transplant 1999;18:336–345.
53. Reichart B, Meiser B, Vigano M, et al. European Multicenter Tacrolimus (FK506) Heart Pilot Study: One-year results. European Tacrolimus Multicenter Heart Study Group. J Heart Lung Transplant 1998;17:775–781.
54. Meiser BM, Uberfuhr P, Fuchs A, et al. Single-center randomized trial comparing tacrolimus (FK506) and cyclosporine in the prevention of acute myocardial rejection. J Heart Lung Transplant 1998;17:782–788.
55. Pham SM, Kormos RL, Hattler BG, et al. A prospective trial of tacrolimus (FK 506) in clinical heart transplantation: Intermediate-term results. J Thorac Cardiovasc Surg 1996;111:764–772.
56. Bennett WM. The nephrotoxicity of immunosuppressive drugs. Clin Nephrol 1995;43(Suppl 1):S3–S7.
57. Johnson C, Ahsan N, Gonwa T. Randomized trial of tacrolimus (Prograf) in combination with azathioprine or mycophenolate mofetil versus cyclosporine (Neoral) with mycophenolate mofetil after kidney transplantation. Transplantation 2000;69:834–841.
58. Meiser BM, Uberfuhr P, Fuchs A, et al. Tacrolimus: A superior agent to OKT3 for treating cases of persistent rejection after intrathoracic transplantation. J Heart Lung Transplant 1997;16:795–800.
59. Taylor DO, Barr ML, Meiser BM, et al. Suggested guidelines for the use of tacrolimus in cardiac transplant recipients. Heart Lung Transplant 2001;20:734–738.
60. Sievers TM, Rossi SJ, Ghobrial RM, et al. Mycophenolate mofetil. Pharmacotherapy 1997;17:1178–1197.
61. Fulton B, Markham A. Mycophenolate mofetil: A review of its pharmacodynamic and pharmacokinetic properties and clinical efficacy in renal transplantation. Drugs 1996;51:278–298.
62. Renlund DG, Gopinathan SK, Kfoury AG, Taylor DO. Mycophenolate mofetil (MMF) in heart transplantation: Rejection prevention and treatment. Clin Transplant 1996;10:136–139.
63. Taylor DO, Ensley RD, Olsen SL, et al. Mycophenolate mofetil (RS-61443): Preclinical, clinical, and three-year experience in heart transplantation. J Heart Lung Transplant 1994;13:571–582.
64. Kirklin JK, Bourge RC, Naftel DC, et al. Treatment of recurrent heart rejection with mycophenolate mofetil (RS-61443): Initial clinical experience. J Heart Lung Transplant 1994;13:444–450.
65. Kobashigawa J, Miller L, Renlund D, et al. A randomized active-controlled trial of mycophenolate mofetil in heart transplant recipients. Mycophenolate Mofetil Investigators. Transplantation 1998;66:507–515.
66. Hosenpud JD, Bennett LE. Mycophenolate mofetil compared to azathioprine improves survival in patients surviving the initial cardiac transplant hospitalization: An analysis of the joint ISHLT /UNOS Thoracic Registry. J Heart Lung Transplant 2000;19:72.
67. Taylor DO, Sharma RC, Kfoury AG, Renlund DG. Increased incidence of allograft rejection in stable heart transplant recipients after late conversion from mycophenolate mofetil to azathioprine. Clin Transplant 1999;13:296–299.
68. Sullivan SD, Garrison LP, Best JH. The cost-effectiveness of mycophenolate mofetil in the first year after primary cadaveric transplant. U.S. Renal Transplant Mycophenolate Mofetil Study Group. J Am Soc Nephrol 1997;8:1592–1598.
69. DeNofrio D, Goldberg LR, Loh E, et al. Reduced mycophenolic acid concentrations are associated with an increased risk of rejection following heart transplantation. Circulation 1999;100:I-526.
70. Meiser BM, Pfeiffer M, Schmidt D, et al. Combination therapy with tacrolimus and mycophenolate mofetil following cardiac transplantation: Importance of mycophenolic acid therapeutic drug monitoring. J Heart Lung Transplant 1999;18:143–149.
71. Smak Gregoor PJH, de Sevaux RGL, Hene RJ. Effect of cyclosporine on mycophenolic acid trough levels in kidney transplant recipients. Transplantation 1999;68:1603–1606.
72. Glanemann M, Klupp J, Langrehr JM, et al. Higher immunosuppressive efficacy of mycophenolate mofetil in combination with FK 506 than in combination with cyclosporine A. Transplant Proc 2000;32:522–523.
73. Smak Gregoor PJ, van Gelder T, van Besouw NM, et al. Mycophenolic acid trough levels after kidney transplantation in a cyclosporine-free protocol. Transplant Int 2000;13(Suppl 1):S333–S335.
74. Zucker K, Rosen A, Tsaroucha A, et al. Unexpected augmentation of mycophenolic acid pharmacokinetics in renal transplant patients receiving tacrolimus and mycophenolate mofetil in combination therapy and analogous in vitro findings. Transplant Immunol 1997;5:225–232.
75. Kennedy DT, Hayney MS, Lake KD. Azathioprine and allopurinol: The price of an avoidable drug interaction. Ann Pharmacother 1996;30:951–954.
76. Olivari MT, Jessen ME, Baldwin BJ, et al. Triple-drug immunosuppression with steroid discontinuation by six months after heart transplantation. J Heart Lung Transplant 1995;14:127–135.
77. Taylor DO, Bristow MR, O'Connell JB, et al. Improved long-term survival after heart transplantation predicted by successful early withdrawal from maintenance corticosteroid therapy. J Heart Lung Transplant 1996;15:1039–1046.
78. Kobashigawa JA, Lin P, Moriguchi JD, et al. Do heart transplant patients on corticosteroid-free immunosuppression have less rejection? Circulation 1999;100:I-525.
79. Prieto M, Lake KD, Pritzker MR, et al. OKT3 induction and steroid-free maintenance immunosuppression for treatment of high-risk heart transplant recipients. J Heart Lung Transplant 1991;10:901–911.
80. Costanzo-Nordin MR, O'Sullivan EJ, Johnson MR, et al. Prospective randomized trial of OKT3-versus horse antithymocyte globulin-based immunosuppressive prophylaxis in heart transplantation. J Heart Transplant 1990;9:306–315.
81. Wilde MI, Goa KL. Muromonab CD3: A reappraisal of its pharmacology and use as prophylaxis of solid organ transplant rejection. Drugs 1996;51:865–894.
82. Swinnen LJ, Costanzo-Nordin MR, Fisher SG, et al. Increased incidence of lymphoproliferative disorder after immunosuppression with the monoclonal antibody OKT3 in cardiac-transplant recipients (See comments). N Engl J Med 1990;323:1723–1728.
83. Wiseman LR, Faulds D. Daclizumab: A review of its use in the prevention of acute rejection in renal transplant recipients [published erratum appears in Drugs 2000;59(3):476]. Drugs 1999;58:1029–1042.
84. Beniaminovitz A, Itescu S, Lietz K, et al. Prevention of rejection in cardiac transplantation by blockade of the interleukin-2 receptor with a monoclonal antibody (See comments). N Engl J Med 2000;342:613–619.
85. Onrust SV, Wiseman LR. Basiliximab. Drugs 1999;57:207–213; discussion, 214.
86. Aaronson KD, Eppinger MJ, Dyke DB, et al. LVAD therapy improves utilization of donor hearts. J Am Coll Cardiol. In press.
87. Kobashigawa JA, Kirklin JK, Naftel DC, et al. Pretransplantation risk factors for acute rejection after heart transplantation: A multiinstitutional study. The Transplant Cardiologists Research Database Group. J Heart Lung Transplant 1993;12:355–366.
88. Billingham ME, Cary NR, Hammond ME, et al. A working formulation for the standardization of nomenclature in the diagnosis of heart and lung rejection. Heart Rejection Study Group, The International Society for Heart Transplantation. J Heart Transplant 1990;9:587–593.

89. Tugulea S, Ciubotariu R, Colovai AI, et al. New strategies for early diagnosis of heart allograft rejection. Transplantation 1997;64:842–847.
90. Winters GL, Marboe CC, Billingham ME. The International Society for Heart and Lung Transplantation grading system for heart transplant biopsy specimens: Clarification and commentary. J Heart Lung Transplant 1998;17:754–760.
91. Winters GL, Loh E, Schoen FJ. Natural history of focal moderate cardiac allograft rejection: Is treatment warranted? Circulation 1995;91:1975–1980.
92. Hosenpud JD, Norman DJ, Pantely GA. Low-dose oral prednisone in the treatment of acute cardiac allograft rejection not associated with hemodynamic compromise. J Heart Transplant 1990;9:292–296.
93. Costanzo MR, Koch DM, Fisher SG, et al. Effects of methotrexate on acute rejection and cardiac allograft vasculopathy in heart transplant recipients. J Heart Lung Transplant 1997;16:169–178.
94. Ross HJ, Gullestad L, Pak J, et al. Methotrexate or total lymphoid radiation for treatment of persistent or recurrent allograft cellular rejection: A comparative study. J Heart Lung Transplant 1997;16:179–189.
95. Miller L, Bozena S, Valantine H. Treatment of acute cardiac allograft rejection with rapamycin: A multicenter dose-ranging study. J Heart Lung Transplant 1997;16:44.
96. Kelly PA, Gruber SA, Behbod F, Kahan BD. Sirolimus, a new, potent immunosuppressive agent. Pharmacotherapy 1997;17:1148–1156.
97. Straatman LP, Coles JG. Pediatric utilization of rapamycin for severe cardiac allograft rejection. Transplantation 2000;70:541–543.
98. Haddad H, MacNeil DM, Howlett J, O'Neill B. Sirolimus, a new potent immunosuppressant agent for refractory cardiac transplantation rejection: Two case reports. Can J Cardiol 2000;16:221–224.
99. Barr ML. Immunomodulation in transplantation with photopheresis. Artif Organs 1996;20:971–973.
100. Olivari MT, May CB, Johnson NA, et al. Treatment of acute vascular rejection with immunoadsorption. Circulation 1994;90:II70–II73.
101. Hammond EH, Yowell RL, Nunoda S, et al. Vascular (humoral) rejection in heart transplantation: Pathologic observations and clinical implications. J Heart Transplant 1989;8:430–443.
102. Miller LW, Naftel DC, Bourge RC, et al. Infection after heart transplantation: A multiinstitutional study. Cardiac Transplant Research Database Group. J Heart Lung Transplant 1994;13:381–392; discussion, 393.
103. Thaler SJ, Rubin RH. Opportunistic infections in the cardiac transplant patient. Curr Opin Cardiol 1996;11:191–203.
104. Rubin RH. Prevention and treatment of cytomegalovirus disease in heart transplant patients. J Heart Lung Transplant 2000;19:731–735.
105. Merigan TC, Renlund DG, Keay S, et al. A controlled trial of ganciclovir to prevent cytomegalovirus disease after heart transplantation. N Engl J Med 1992;326:1182–1186.
106. Griffiths PD. Prophylaxis against CMV infection in transplant patients. J Antimicrob Chemother 1997;39:299–301.
107. Couchoud C, Cucherat M, Haugh M, Pouteil-Noble C. Cytomegalovirus prophylaxis with antiviral agents in solid organ transplantation: A meta-analysis. Transplantation 1998;65:641–647.
108. Weis M, von Scheidt W. Cardiac allograft vasculopathy: A review. Circulation 1997;96:2069–2077.
109. Libby P, Tanaka H. The pathogenesis of coronary arteriosclerosis ("chronic rejection") in transplanted hearts. Clin Transplant 1994;8:313–318.
110. Buszman P, Zembala M, Wojarski J, et al. Comparison of intravascular ultrasound and quantitative angiography for evaluation of coronary artery disease in the transplanted heart. Transplant Proc 1996;28:3535–3537.
111. Liang DH, Gao SZ, Botas J, et al. Prediction of angiographic disease by intracoronary ultrasonographic findings in heart transplant recipients. J Heart Lung Transplant 1996;15:980–987.
112. Mehra MR, Ventura HO, Jain SP, et al. Heterogeneity of cardiac allograft vasculopathy: Clinical insights from coronary angioscopy. J Am Coll Cardiol 1997;29:1339–1344.
113. Halle AA 3d, DiSciascio G, Massin EK, et al. Coronary angioplasty, atherectomy and bypass surgery in cardiac transplant recipients. J Am Coll Cardiol 1995;26:120–128.
114. McDonald K, Rector TS, Braulin EA, et al. Association of coronary artery disease in cardiac transplant recipients with cytomegalovirus infection. Am J Cardiol 1989;64:359–362.
115. Kobashigawa JA, Katznelson S, Laks H, et al. Effect of pravastatin on outcomes after cardiac transplantation. N Engl J Med 1995;333:621–627.
116. Wenke K, Mesiser B, Thiery J, et al. Simvastatin reduces graft vessel disease and mortality after heart transplantation: A four-year randomized trial. Circulation 1997;96:1398 1402.
117. Srivastava R, Keck BM, Bennett LE, Hosenpud JD. The results of cardiac retransplantation: An analysis of the Joint International Society for Heart and Lung Transplantation/United Network for Organ Sharing Thoracic Registry. Transplantation 2000;70:606–612.
118. Penn I. Post-transplant malignancy. The role of immunosuppression. Drug Safety 2000;23:101–113.
119. Aull MJ, Troge J, Alloway RR, et al. Experience with 274 cardiac transplant recipients with post-transplant lymphoproliferative disorder: A report from the Israel Penn International Transplant Tumor Registry. Am J Transplant 2001;1(Suppl 1):283. Abstract 585.
120. Buell JF, Trofe J, Hanaway MJ, et al. Transmission of donor cancer into cardiothoracic tansplant recipients. Surgery 2001;130:660–668.
121. Walker RC, Paya CV, Marshall WF, et al. Pretransplantation seronegative Epstein-Barr virus status is the primary risk factor for posttransplantation lymphoproliferative disorder in adult heart, lung, and other solid organ transplantations. J Heart Lung Transplant 1995;14:214–221.
122. Textor SC, Taler SJ, Canzanello VJ, Schwartz L. Cyclosporine, blood pressure and atherosclerosis. Cardiol Rev 1997;5:141–151.
123. Ventura HO, Malik FS, Mehra MR, et al. Mechanisms of hypertension in cardiac transplantation and the role of cyclosporine. Curr Opin Cardiol 1997;12:375–381.
124. Sturrock ND, Struthers AD. Hormonal and other mechanisms involved in the pathogenesis of cyclosporin-induced nephrotoxicity and hypertension in man (Editorial). Clin Sci 1994;86:1–9.
125. Brozena SC, Johnson MR, Ventura H, et al. Effectiveness and safety of diltiazem or lisinopril in treatment of hypertension after heart transplantation: Results of a prospective, randomized multicenter trial. J Am Coll Cardiol 1996;27:1707–1712.
126. Epstein M. Calcium antagonists and the kidney: Implications for renal protection. Am J Hypertens 1993;6:251S–259S.
127. Jones TE. The use of other drugs to allow a lower dosage of cyclosporine to be used: Therapeutic and pharmacoeconomic considerations. Clin Pharmacokinet 1997;32:357–367.
128. Kobashigawa JA, Kasiske BL. Hyperlipidemia in solid organ transplantation. Transplantation 1997;63:331–338.
129. Lake KD. Management of post-transplant obesity and hyperlipidemia. In: Emery RW, Miller L, eds. Handbook of Cardiac Transplantation. Philadelphia: Hanley & Belfus, 1995:147–164.
130. Keogh A, Macdonald P, Kaan A, et al. Efficacy and safety of pravastatin vs simvastatin after cardiac transplantation. J Heart Lung Transplant 2000;19:529–537.
131. Patel DN, Pagani F, Koelling T, et al. Safety and efficacy of atorvastatin in heart transplant recipients. J Heart Lung Transplant. In press.

19

VENOUS THROMBOEMBOLISM

Stuart T. Haines, Eric Racine, and Mario Zeolla

Venous thromboembolism (VTE) is a potentially fatal disorder and a significant national health problem in our aging society.[1–3] Although it can strike young, otherwise healthy adults, it most frequently occurs in patients who sustain multiple trauma, undergo major surgery, are immobile for a lengthy period of time, or have a hypercoagulable disorder. Resulting from clot formation within the venous circulation (Fig. 19–1), VTE is manifested as deep vein thrombosis (DVT) and pulmonary embolism (PE). Death from pulmonary embolism can occur within minutes after the onset of symptoms, before effective treatment can be given.

Unfortunately, the disease is often clinically silent, and the first manifestation may be sudden death. In some case series, 80% of patients who died suddenly had some evidence of pulmonary embolism at the time of autopsy.[4] Beyond the symptoms produced by the acute event, the long-term sequelae of VTE, such as the post-thrombotic syndrome and recurrent thromboembolic events, also cause substantial pain and suffering.[1]

The treatment of VTE is fraught with substantial risks.[5] Antithrombotic drugs require precise dosing and meticulous monitoring.[6–9] Systematic approaches to drug therapy management substantially reduce the risks, but bleeding remains an all too common and serious complication of administering antithrombotic drugs.[9] Therefore, the prevention of VTE in at-risk patients is paramount to improving outcomes. When there is a suspicion of VTE, the rapid and accurate diagnosis of the disorder is critical to making appropriate treatment decisions.[10] The optimal use of antithrombotic drugs requires not only an in-depth knowledge of their pharmacology and pharmacokinetic properties, but also a comprehensive approach to patient management.[7,11]

EPIDEMIOLOGY

The true incidence of VTE in the general population is unknown, because a substantial portion of patients, perhaps greater than 50%, have clinically silent disease. An estimated 2 million people in the United States develop VTE each year; 600,000 are hospitalized, and 60,000 die.[12] The estimated annual direct medical costs of managing the disease are well over $1 billion and growing. The best available data indicate the age-adjusted annual incidence of symptomatic VTE in Caucasians to be 117/100,000.[13] The incidence of VTE nearly doubles in each decade of life over the age of 50 and is slightly higher in men (Table 19–1). The age-adjusted incidence of pulmonary embolism has declined slightly in recent years, presumably because of heightened awareness of VTE, effective prevention strategies, early diagnosis, and prompt treatment. However, as the population ages, the total number of cases of DVT and pulmonary embolism continues to climb.

Relatively little is known about the risk of VTE in ethnic populations. African Americans appear to be at somewhat higher risk of VTE than are Americans of predominantly European ancestry, while Hispanic Americans may be somewhat protected.[14] Asian Americans and Pacific Islanders appear to have a striking lower incidence of VTE.

The incidence of VTE in specific high-risk patient populations has been extensively studied.[15] Patients who sustain multiple trauma or undergo an orthopedic procedure involving a lower extremity are at particularly high risk, with the incidence of VTE often exceeding 50% in the absence of effective prophylaxis.[15,16] Among those undergoing major surgeries other than procedures involving the lower extremities, the incidence of VTE is 20% to 40% when one or more other risk factors are present, such as age over 60 years. The long-term incidence of VTE among patients who have a prior history of VTE and who have metastatic cancer is extremely high.[17–19] Likewise, the incidence of VTE after a myocardial infarction, stroke, and spinal cord injury is high. Several disorders of hypercoagulability have also been linked to a high lifetime incidence of VTE.[20–22]

PATHOPHYSIOLOGY AND RISK FACTORS

The arrest of bleeding following vascular injury, or hemostasis, is essential to life.[23,24] Within the vascular system, blood remains in a fluid state, transporting oxygen, nutrients, plasma proteins, and waste. With vascular injury, a dynamic series of reactions involving a complex interplay of thrombogenic and antithrombotic stimuli result in the local formation of a hemostatic plug that seals the vessel wall and prevents further blood loss (Table 19–2; Figs. 19–2, 19–3, and 19–4). A disruption of this delicate system of checks and balances may lead to inappropriate clot formation within the blood vessel that subsequently obstructs blood flow or embolizes to a distant vascular bed. In the late 1800s, Dr. Rudolf Virchow, a German pathologist, recognized the role played by blood vessels, circulating elements in the blood, and the speed of blood flow in the regulation of clot formation.[25] Alterations in any one of these elements, known today as Virchow's triad, may lead to pathologic clot formation. Numerous risk factors for such alterations and, thus, VTE have been identified (Table 19–3).

Under normal circumstances, the endothelial cells that form the intima of vessels maintain blood flow by producing a number of substances that inhibit platelet adherence, prevent the activation of the coagulation cascade, and facilitate fibrinolysis.[23] Vascular injury can expose the subendothelium (see Fig. 19–3). Platelets readily adhere to the subendothelium, using glycoprotein Ib receptors found on their surfaces and facilitated by von Willebrand factor. This causes platelets to become activated, releasing a number of procoagulant substances into the local circulation that stimulate platelets to expose glycoprotein IIb-IIIa receptors. These receptors allow the platelets to adhere to one another, resulting in platelet aggregation. In addition, the damaged vascular tissue releases tissue factor, also known as tissue thromboplastin, which activates the extrinsic pathway of the coagulation cascade (see Fig. 19–4).

The coagulation cascade is a stepwise series of enzymatic reactions that result in the formation of a fibrin mesh.[23,24] Clotting factors circulate in the blood in inactive forms. Specific stimuli convert an

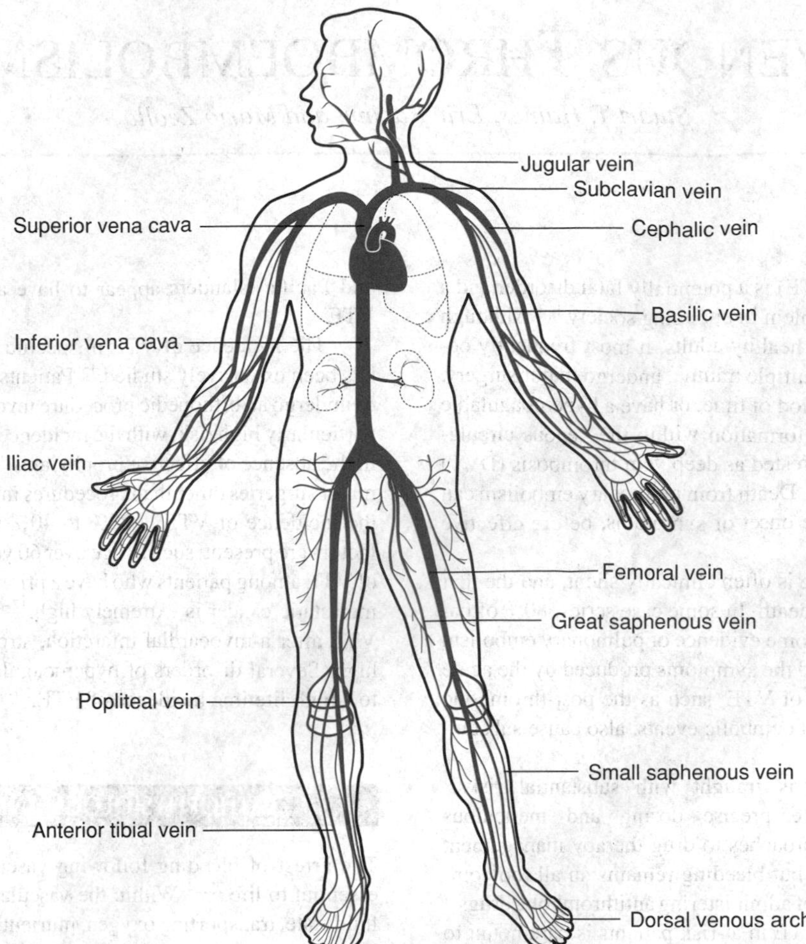

FIGURE 19–1. Venous circulation.

inactive precursor into an active form that, in turn, converts the next precursor in the sequence. It was once believed that all clotting factors were proteolytic enzymes, known as zymogens. It is now known that factors V and VIII have no enzymatic activity themselves, but rather serve as cofactors that greatly accelerate the enzymatic activity of their respective partners. The final steps in the cascade are the conversion of prothrombin to thrombin and fibrinogen to fibrin. Thrombin plays a key role in the coagulation cascade; it is responsible not only for the production of fibrin, but also for the conversion of factors V and VIII, creating a positive feedback loop that greatly accelerates the production of more thrombin. Additionally, thrombin enhances platelet aggregation through its interactions with the glycoprotein IIb-IIIa receptor.

TABLE 19–1. Annual Incidence of Diagnosed Venous Thromboembolism in Olmsted County, Minnesota (1966–1990)

Gender and Age (Years)	Rate/100,000 Residents
Females	
<19	6
20–29	63
30–39	74
40–49	90
50–59	122
60–69	227
70–79	424
>80	830
Males	
<19	3
20–29	27
30–39	42
40–49	84
50–59	146
60–69	337
70–79	673
>80	1054

Adapted with permission from Ref. 13.

Traditionally, the coagulation cascade has been divided into three distinct parts: the intrinsic, extrinsic, and common pathways (see Fig. 19–4).[23,24] This artificial division is somewhat misleading, as there are numerous interactions between the three pathways. The extrinsic pathway, sometimes referred to as the tissue factor pathway, appears to be the principal mechanism that triggers the coagulation cascade. Tissue factor, released from the subendothelium, forms a complex with factor VIIa. The factor VIIa-tissue factor complex activates factor X in the common pathway and factor IX in the intrinsic pathway. The intrinsic pathway may begin in several ways. Negatively charged surfaces in contact with the blood will activate factor XII, and activated platelets can convert factor XI. Both the intrinsic and extrinsic pathways meet at a common point with the activation of factor X. With its partner, factor Va, factor Xa converts prothrombin (II) to thrombin (IIa), which then cleaves fibrinogen to form fibrin monomers. Finally, as the fibrin monomers reach a critical concentration, they begin to precipitate and polymerize to

TABLE 19–2. Factors Regulating Hemostasis and Thrombosis

	Thrombogenic	Antithrombotic
Vessel wall	Exposed subendothelium Tissue factor Plasminogen activator inhibitor–1	Heparan sulfate Dermatan sulfate Thrombomodulin Tissue plasminogen activator (t-PA) Urokinase plasminogen activator (u-PA)
Circulating elements	Platelets Platelet activating factor (PAF) Clotting factors Prothrombin (Factor II) Fibrinogen (Factor I) Von Willebrand factor (vWF) α_2-Antiplasmin	Antithrombin (AT) Heparin cofactor II Protein C Protein S Plasminogen Tissue factor pathway inhibitor Proteolytic enzymes
Blood flow	Slow rate of flow Turbulent flow	Fast rate of flow Laminar flow

From Ref. 23.

form fibrin strands. Factor XIIIa covalently bonds these strands to one another.

Normally, a number of tempering mechanisms control coagulation (see Table 19–2 and Fig. 19–2).[23,24] Without effective self-regulation, the coagulation cascade would proceed unabated until all the clotting factors and platelets were consumed. Thus, the intact endothelium adjacent to the damaged tissue actively secretes several antithrombotic substances. As its name implies, thrombomodulin modulates thrombin activity by converting protein C to its active form. When joined with its cofactor protein S, protein C enzymatically inactivates factors Va and VIIIa. Activated protein C also stimulates the release of tissue plasminogen activator (t-PA). Antithrombin is a circulating protein that inhibits thrombin and factor Xa. Heparan sulfate, a heparin-like compound secreted by endothelial cells, exponentially accelerates antithrombin activity. By a similar mechanism, heparin cofactor II also inhibits thrombin. Tissue factor pathway inhibitor (TFPI) plays an important role by regulating the initiation of the coagulation cascade. When these self-regulatory mechanisms are intact, the formation of the fibrin clot is limited to the zone of tissue

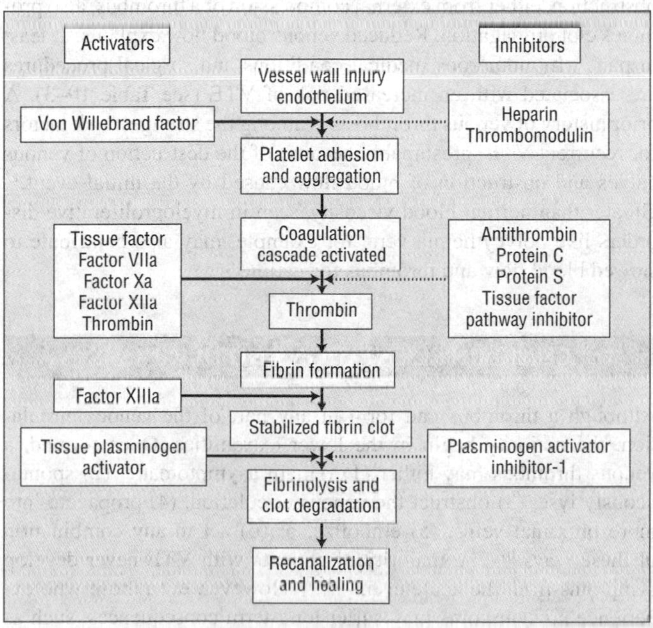

FIGURE 19–2. Hemostasis and thrombosis.

injury. However, disruptions in the system, so-called hypercoagulable states, often result in thrombosis.[22,26]

A growing list of hereditary deficiencies, gene mutations, and acquired diseases have been linked to hypercoagulability (see Table 19–3).[17,20–22,27,28] Activated protein C resistance is the most common genetic disorder of hypercoagulability, with a prevalence rate approaching 5% among community-dwelling Caucasians and a rate as high as 40% among those who suffer an idiopathic DVT or who have a strong family history of VTE. Although these patients have normal plasma concentrations of protein C, they often have a mutation on factor V that renders it resistant to degradation by activated protein C. This mutation is known as factor V Leiden, named after the city of Leiden, Holland where the defect was initially reported. The prothrombin 20210A mutation also appears to be a relatively common defect, occurring in as many as 3% of healthy individuals of Southern European descent and 16% of those with an idiopathic DVT. Although less common, inherited deficiencies of the natural anticoagulants protein C, protein S, and antithrombin place patients at a high lifetime risk for VTE. Conversely, excessively high concentrations of factors VIII, IX, and XI also increase the risk of VTE. Given the prevalence of these inherited abnormalities in the general population, some patients have multiple genetic defects that have additive effects in terms of increasing the lifetime thrombotic risk.

Acquired disorders of hypercoagulability may result from malignancy, the presence of antiphospholipid antibodies, and estrogen use. The strong link between cancer and thrombosis has been recognized since the late 1800s.[27] Tumor cells secrete a number of procoagulant substances that activate the coagulation cascade. Further, patients with cancer often have suppressed levels of protein C, protein S, and antithrombin. It has been postulated that cancer cells use thrombotic mechanisms to recruit a blood supply (angiogenesis), metastasize, and create a barrier against host defense mechanisms. Antiphospholipid antibodies, most commonly found in patients with autoimmune disorders such as systemic lupus erythematosus (SLE) and inflammatory bowel disease, can cause venous and arterial thrombosis. These antibodies are also associated with repeated pregnancy loss because of placental thrombosis. The precise mechanism by which the antiphospholipid antibodies provoke thrombosis is unclear, but they appear to activate the coagulation cascade and platelets, as well as to inhibit the anticoagulant activity of proteins C and S.[29] Estrogren-containing oral contraceptive pills, estrogren replacement therapy, and the selective estrogren receptor modulators (SERMs) have all been linked to venous thrombosis. Again, the mechanisms are not clearly

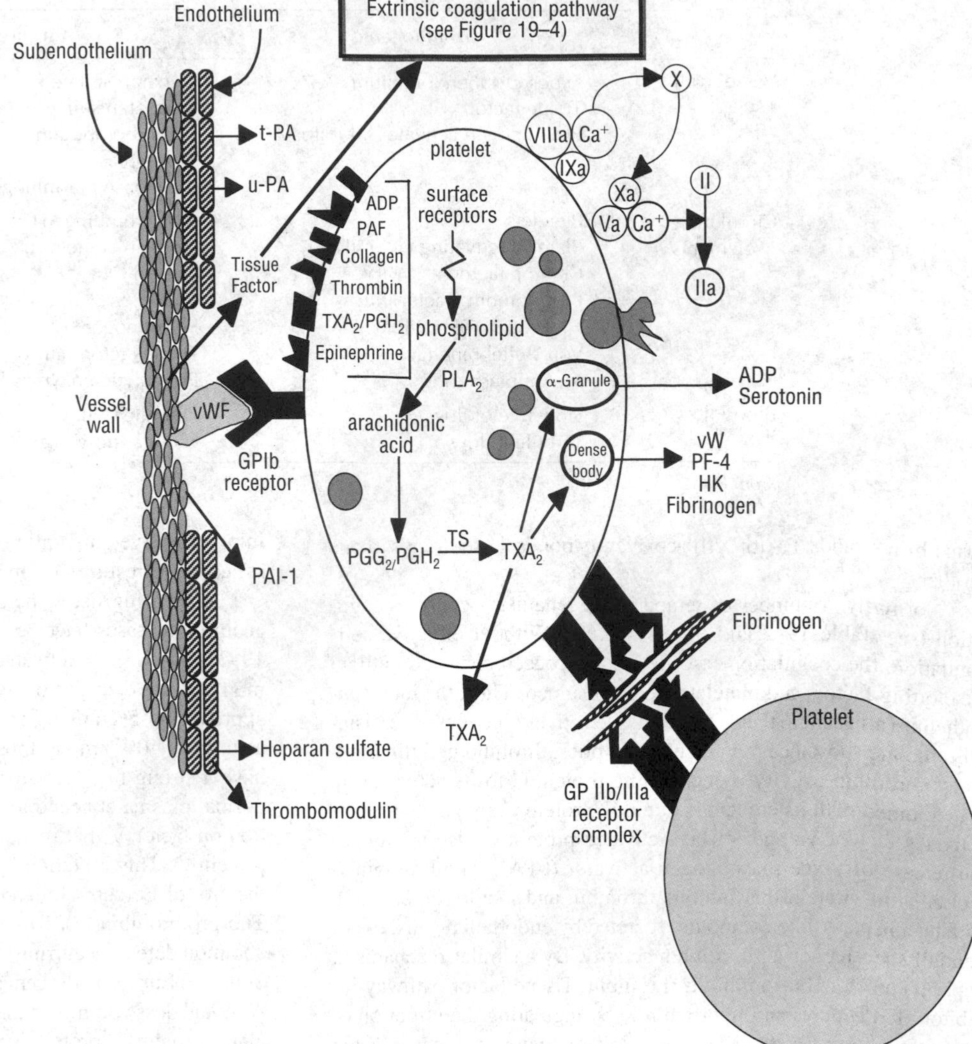

FIGURE 19–3. Vascular injury and thrombosis. ADP = adenosine diphosphate; CO = cyclo-oxygenase; GP Ib = glycoprotein Ib; GP IIb/IIIa = glycoprotein IIb/IIIa; HK = high-molecular-weight kininogen; PAF = platelet activating factor; PAI-1 = plasminogen activator inhibitor-1; PF-4 = platelet factor-4; PGG/PGH = prostaglandins; PGI = prostacyclin; PLA = phospholipase A; TS = thromboxane synthetase; TXA_2 = thromboxane A_2; t-PA = tissue plasminogen activator; u-PA = urokinase plasminogen activator; vWF = von Willebrand factor.

understood, but estrogens increase serum clotting factor concentrations and induce activated protein C resistance.[3,30] Increased serum estrogen concentrations may explain, in part, the increased risk of VTE observed during pregnancy and the immediate postpartum period.[30,31]

The fibrinolytic protein plasmin degrades the fibrin mesh into soluble end products collectively known as fibrin split products or fibrin degradation products.[23,24] The fibrinolytic system is also under the control of a series of stimulatory and inhibitory substances. Tissue plasminogen activator (t-PA) and urokinase plasminogen activator (u-PA) convert plasminogen to plasmin. Plasminogen activator inhibitor-1 (PAI-1) inhibits the plasminogen activators, and α_2-antiplasmin inhibits plasmin activity. Aberrations in the fibrinolytic system have also been linked to hypercoagulability.

Rapid blood flow has an inhibitory effect on thrombus formation, but a slow rate of flow reduces the clearance and dilution of activated clotting factors in the zone of injury and slows the influx of regulatory substances.[23] Stasis tips the delicate balance of procoagulation and anticoagulation in favor of thrombogenesis. The rate of blood flow in the venous circulation, particularly in the deep veins of the lower extremities, is relatively slow. Valves in the deep veins of the legs, as well as contraction of the calf and thigh muscles, facilitate the flow of blood back to the heart and lungs. Damage to the venous valves and prolonged periods of immobility result in venous stasis. Vessel obstruction, either from external compression or a thrombus, also promotes clot propagation. Reduced venous blood flow explains, at least in part, why numerous medical conditions and surgical procedures are associated with an increased risk of VTE (see Table 19–3). A prior history of venous thrombosis is among the strongest risk factors for recurrent VTE, presumably because of the destruction of venous valves and obstruction of blood flow caused by the initial event.[17] Greater than normal blood viscosity, seen in myeloproliferative disorders like polycythemia vera, for example, may also contribute to slowed blood flow and thrombus formation.

CLINICAL PRESENTATION AND DIAGNOSIS

Although a thrombus can form in any part of the venous circulation, the majority begin in the lower extremities. Once formed, a venous thrombus may either (1) remain asymptomatic, (2) spontaneously lyse, (3) obstruct the venous circulation, (4) propagate into more proximal veins, (5) embolize, or (6) act in any combination of these ways.[10] The majority of patients with VTE never develop symptoms from the acute event.[1,15,32] However, even those who experience no symptoms may suffer long-term consequences, such as the post-thrombotic syndrome and recurrent VTE.[33]

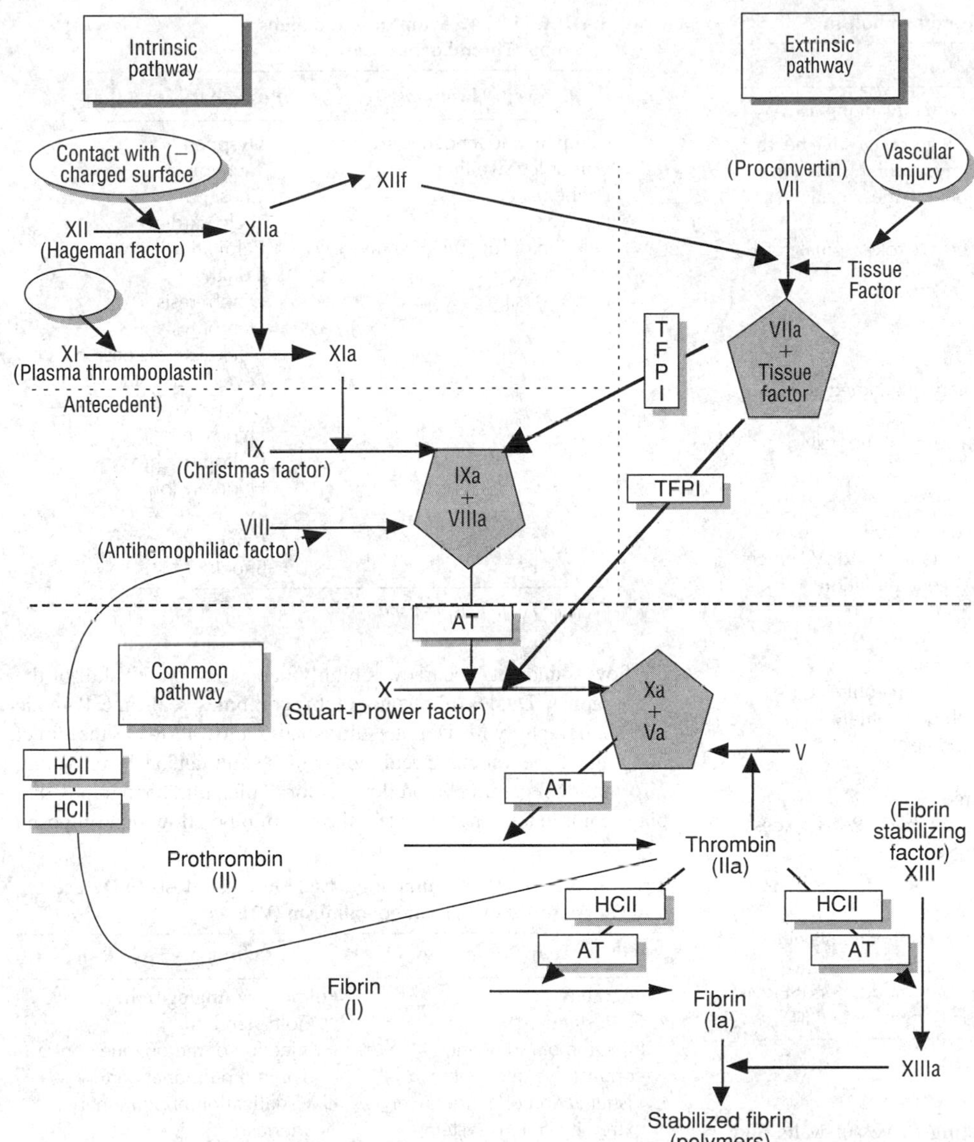

FIGURE 19–4. Coagulation cascade. AT = antithrombin; HCII = heparin cofactor II; TFPI = tissue factor pathway inhibitor.

Even when symptoms of DVT or pulmonary embolism are present (Table 19–4), they are nonspecific.[10,11,34] It is extremely difficult to distinguish VTE from other disorders, and additional objective tests are required to confirm or exclude the diagnosis (Table 19–5). The classic symptoms associated with DVT include unilateral leg swelling, pain, tenderness, erythema, and warmth. During physical examination of the patient, dorsiflexion of the foot may elicit pain behind the knee (Homans' sign), and the affected vein may feel like a rope deep under the skin in the calf or thigh (palpable cord). The post-thrombotic syndrome, a long-term complication of DVT caused by damage to the venous valves, can produce symptoms very similar to those of an acute thrombotic event. The symptoms of the post-thrombotic syndrome include chronic lower extremity swelling, pain, tenderness, skin discoloration, and ulceration. Symptomatic pulmonary embolism often produces dyspnea, tachypnea, and tachycardia. Pleuritic chest pain occurs in the majority of patients with symptomatic pulmonary embolism. Hemoptysis, while distressing, occurs in less than one-third of patients. Cardiovascular collapse, characterized by cyanosis, shock, and oliguria, is an ominous sign.

Given that VTE can be debilitating or fatal, it is important to treat it quickly and aggressively.[1,3,10,34] On the other hand, because major bleeding with antithrombotic therapy can be equally harmful, it is important to avoid treatment when the diagnosis is not a reasonable certainty. Assessment of the patient's status should focus on the search for risk factors in the patient's medical history (see Table 19–3; Table 19–6).[35] Venous thrombosis is uncommon in the absence of risk factors, and the effects of these risks are additive. Conversely, even in the absence of symptoms, VTE should be strongly suspected in those with multiple risk factors.

Because radiographic contrast studies are the most accurate and reliable methods for the diagnosis of VTE, they are considered the gold standards in clinical trials.[3,10,11,34] Contrast venography allows visualization of the entire venous system in the lower extremity and abdomen. Pulmonary angiography allows the visualization of the pulmonary arteries. The patient is placed on a fluoroscopy table, radiopaque contrast media is injected, and a series of x-ray films are subsequently taken. The diagnosis of VTE can be made if there is a persistent intraluminal filling defect observed on multiple x-ray films. Although they can provide a definitive diagnosis, contrast studies are expensive, invasive procedures that are technically difficult to perform and evaluate. Severely ill patients often are unable to tolerate the procedure, and many develop hypotension and cardiac arrhythmias.

TABLE 19–3. Risk Factors for Venous Thromboembolism

Risk Factor	Example
Age	Exponential increase with advancing age
Venous stasis	Major medical illness (e.g., congestive heart failure, status post; myocardial infarction) Major surgery (e.g., general anesthesia >30 minutes) Paralysis (e.g., status post; stroke, spinal cord injury) Polycythemia vera Obesity Varicose veins
Vascular injury	Major orthopedic surgery (e.g., knee and hip replacement) Trauma (especially fractures of the pelvis, hip, or leg) In-dwelling venous catheters
Hypercoagulable states	Malignancy, diagnosed or occult Activated protein C resistance/factor V Leiden Prothrombin (20210A) gene mutation Protein C deficiency Protein S deficiency Antithrombin (AT) deficiency Factor VIII excess (>90th percentile) Factor XI excess (>90th percentile) Antiphospholipid antibodies Dysfibrinogenemia Hyperhomocysteinemia Plasminogen activator inhibitor (PAI-1) excess Inflammatory bowel disease Nephrotic syndrome Pregnancy/postpartum
Drug therapy	Estrogen-containing oral contraceptive pills Estrogen replacement therapy Selective estrogen receptor modulators (SERMs) Heparin-induced thrombocytopenia (HIT)

Compiled from Refs. 15, 20, and 21.

Furthermore, the contrast medium is irritating to vessel walls and toxic to the kidneys. For these reasons, noninvasive tests, such as ultrasonography and the ventilation/perfusion (VQ) scan, are frequently used in clinical practice for the initial evaluation of patients with suspected VTE.[10,36]

Several ultrasonography technologies are available and can be performed at the bedside.[10,37,38] Real-time B-mode ultrasonography allows the visualization of leg veins by means of a transducer that emits high-frequency sound waves that are reflected off soft tissues. The sonographer begins the examination by placing the transducer at the patient's groin to locate the common femoral vein and then proceeds distally, using light compression to look for intraluminal thrombi. Vein incompressibility is considered diagnostic for DVT. Doppler ultrasonography is used to determine the rate of blood flow through reflections of sound waves off red blood cells. The change in sound frequency, the so-called Doppler effect, is proportional to the velocity of blood flow. Venous blood flow typically produces a low-pitched sound. If there is no blood flow, there is no sound. Doppler ultrasonography is also useful in the assessment of venous valve competence. If the venous valves are severely damaged, retrograde blood flow may be heard. Doppler ultrasonography can sensitively detect large thrombi that occlude the proximal veins, but is relatively insensitive to smaller nonocclusive thrombi and calf vein thrombi. As the Doppler test requires a subjective interpretation of the flow sounds, its accuracy is highly dependent on the skill of the sonographer. Duplex ultrasonography combines real-time B-mode ultrasonography with Doppler ultrasonography, allowing the direct imaging of the venous circulation while simultaneously providing information regarding blood flow. Color duplex ultrasonography displays color images that represent the rate of blood flow superimposed

TABLE 19–4. Symptoms and Signs of Venous Thromboembolism

Deep Vein Thrombosis	Pulmonary Embolism
Calf pain and tenderness Calf or leg swelling Erythema Leg warmth Dilation of superficial veins Palpable cord Homans' sign	Dyspnea Tachypnea Chest pain Tachycardia Palpitations Cough Diaphoresis Hemoptysis Neck vein distension Fever (low-grade) Cyanosis Hypoxemia Gallop rhythm Hypotension Syncope Oliguria Shock

Compiled from Refs. 1–3 and 10.

TABLE 19–5. Most Commonly Used Objective Tests to Detect and Diagnose Venous Thromboembolism (VTE)

Deep Vein Thrombosis	Pulmonary Embolism
Venography • Gold standard • Injection of radiopaque contrast dye into foot vein • Visualization of entire lower extremity venous system • High cost • Nephrotoxicity of contrast medium • Possible induction of VTE • Expertise required to interpret • Invasive procedure	**Pulmonary Angiography** • Gold standard • Injection of radiopaque contrast dye into pulmonary artery • Visualization of pulmonary arteries • High cost • High risk of adverse effects in acutely ill • Expertise required to interpret • Invasive procedure
Ultrasonography • Emission of high-pitched sound waves through a transducer • Several technologies available (Doppler, B-Mode, Duplex, Color Duplex) • Visualization of soft tissues and large vessels (B-Mode) • Production of sound waves proportional to rate of blood flow (Doppler) • Detection of retrograde flow (Doppler) • Insensitivity for small thrombi and most distal DVTs • Noninvasive procedure	**Ventilation/Perfusion (VQ) Scan** • Inhalation of radiolabeled particles and administration of radiolabeled albumin • Distribution of blood and air flow in the lungs recorded by a gammacamera • High probability of pulmonary embolism if a large mismatch • Expertise required to interpret • More testing required after intermediate probability scans • Less invasive procedure than pulmonary angiography

DVTs = deep vein thromboses.
Compiled from Refs. 3, 10, 38, and 39.

TABLE 19–6. Clinical Assessment Model for Deep Vein Thrombosis (DVT)

Major Points	Minor Points
Active cancer (treatment ongoing or within 6 months) Paralysis, paresis, immobilization of leg(s) Bedridden >3 days (within 4 weeks) Major surgery (within 4 weeks) Localized tenderness along deep veins Thigh and calf swelling Calf swelling 3 cm > than symptomless side Strong family history of DVT (≥2 first-degree relatives)	Recent trauma to leg Unilateral leg swelling Dilated superficial leg veins Hospitalized within 6 months Erythema
	Clinical Probability of DVT
High	≥3 major points and no alternative diagnosis ≥2 major points + ≥2 minor points and no alternative diagnosis
Moderate	Any combination that does not satisfy the HIGH or LOW probability criteria
Low	1 major point + ≥2 minor points and has alternative diagnosis 1 major point + ≥1 minor point and no alternative diagnosis 0 major points + ≥3 minor points and has alternative diagnosis 0 major points + ≥1 minor point and no alternative diagnosis

Adapted with permission from Ref. 35.

over anatomic images. Although color duplex ultrasonography is not superior to other ultrasonograpic techniques in the hands of an experienced sonographer, it is widely used because the results are easier to interpret.

The ventilation/perfusion (VQ) scan is the principal screening test for pulmonary embolism.[11,39] Perfusion to the lung tissue is determined by giving the patient radiolabeled, macroaggregated human albumin that becomes trapped in the pulmonary capillary beds. A gammacamera records the distribution of blood flow. Perfusion defects as small as 2 cm in diameter can be detected, but such defects do not specifically indicate that a pulmonary embolus is present. To determine ventilation to the lung tissue, the patient inhales aerosolized radiolabeled particles. An x-ray image of the air flow distribution in the alveoli is taken. If a large section of lung tissue is ventilated, but not perfused—a so-called VQ mismatch—there is a high probability of a pulmonary embolism. The results of the VQ scan must be read by an experienced radiologist, who interprets the scan as either high probability, intermediate probability, or low probability of a pulmonary embolism, or normal. Although a normal scan reasonably excludes the diagnosis of pulmonary embolism, abnormal readings in the absence of a clinical assessment have relatively poor diagnostic accuracy.[3] Because most patients with a pulmonary embolism will have an antecedent DVT (with or without symptoms), ultrasonography of the lower extremities should be used to supplement the diagnostic workup of a patient with an intermediate probability VQ scan.

Despite its pitfalls, clinical assessment improves the diagnostic accuracy of an objective, noninvasive test.[10,11,35] A simple assessment checklist can be used to stratify patients into high, moderate, and low probability of VTE (see Table 19–6). Patients with a high pretest probability of VTE have a greater than 80% chance of having VTE compared with only 5% in the low pretest probability group. Clinical assessment can rule in or rule out the diagnosis of VTE with reasonable certainty when its results are concordant with those of a noninvasive test.[35,40] In those patients with a moderate pretest probability of VTE and an abnormal lower extremity ultrasonogram, the diagnosis of VTE can be reasonably concluded. If the results of the clinical assessment and the ultrasonogram are discordant, venography or angiography should be performed to make the definitive diagnosis.

▶ TREATMENT: Venous Thromboembolism

PHARMACOLOGIC AGENTS USED IN THE MANAGEMENT OF VTE

UNFRACTIONATED HEPARIN

Since the 1930s, clinicians have used unfractionated heparin (UFH) for the prevention and treatment of thrombosis.[8,41] McLean discovered UFH in 1916 when he found that an extract of liver inhibits coagulation. It has been known since 1939 that UFH requires a "heparin cofactor" to produce an anticoagulant effect, but it was not until 1968 that antithrombin (previously known at antithrombin III) was identified and isolated. Soon thereafter, it was recognized that UFH greatly accelerates the activity of antithrombin. Commercially available UFH preparations are derived from bovine lung or porcine intestinal mucosa. Although some differences exist between those two preparations, no differences in antithrombotic activity have been demonstrated. Today, UFH and the low molecular weight heparins (LMWHs) are the mainstays for the acute treatment of arterial and venous thrombosis.

Pharmacology/Pharmacokinetics

A heterogeneous mixture, UFH is composed of sulfated glycosaminoglycans of variable lengths and pharmacologic properties.[8,41–43] Each heparin molecule is composed of repetitive units of D-glycosamine and uronic acid. The molecular weight of these molecules ranges from 5,000 to 30,000 daltons with a mean of 15,000 daltons. The anticoagulant profile and clearance of each UFH molecule varies based on its length. The smaller chains are cleared less rapidly than their longer counterparts.

The anticoagulant effect of UFH is mediated through a specific pentasaccharide sequence on the heparin molecule that binds to antithrombin, provoking a conformational change (Fig. 19–5).[8,41] Only one-third of the UFH molecules possess the unique pentasaccharide sequence with affinity for antithrombin. The UFH-antithrombin complex is 100 to 1,000 times more potent as an anticoagulant compared to antithrombin alone. Antithrombin inhibits the activity of factors IXa, Xa, XIIa, and thrombin (IIa). Through its action on thrombin, the UFH-antithrombin complex also inhibits the thrombin induced

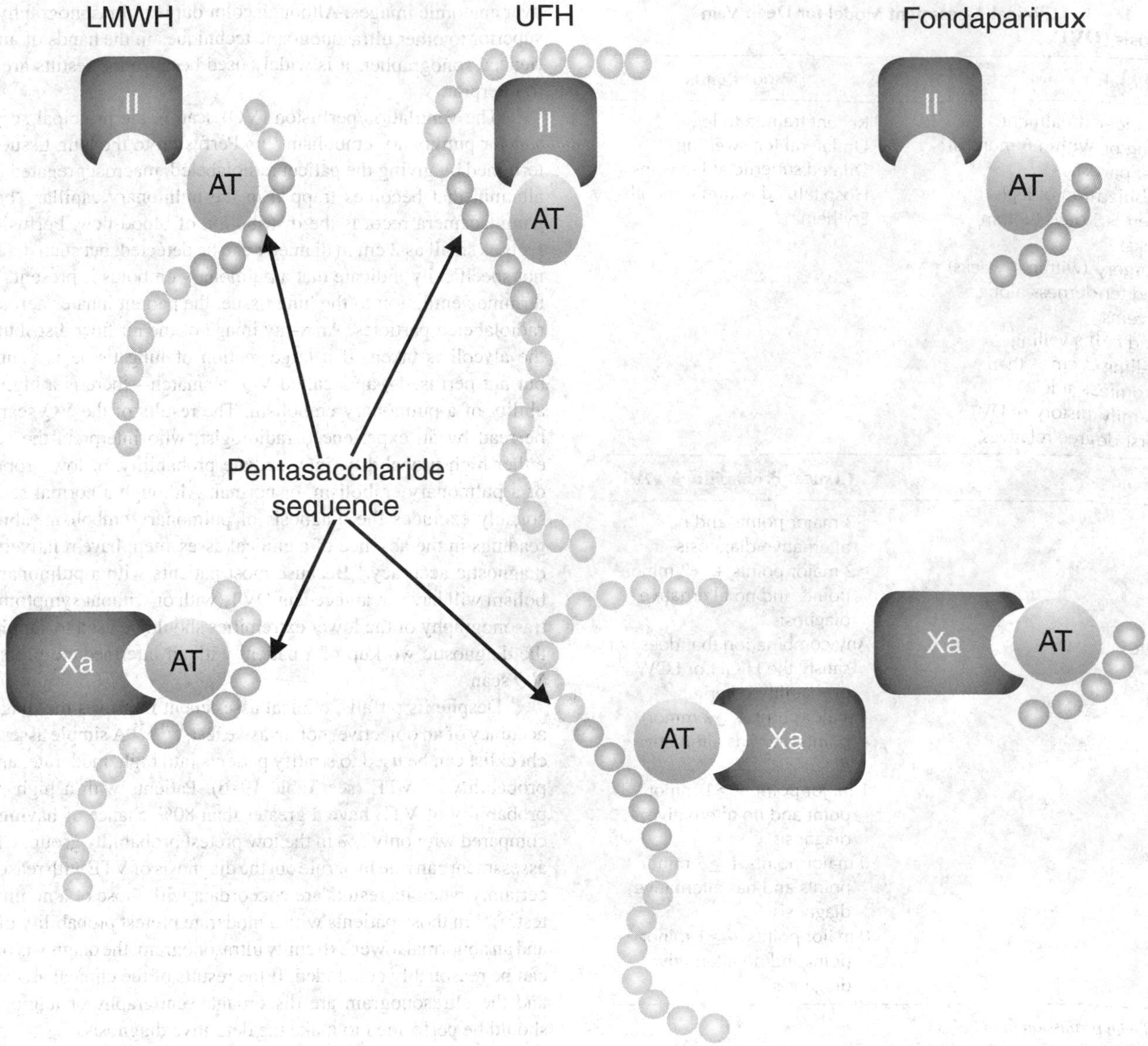

FIGURE 19–5. Pharmacologic activity of unfractionated heparin, low–molecular weight heparin, and fondaparinux. AT = antithrombin.

activation of factors V and VIII. Not only does UFH prevent the growth and propagation of a formed thrombus, but it also allows the patient's own thrombolytic system to degrade the clot. Further, UFH may have some direct effects on thrombolysis.

Factors IIa and Xa are the most sensitive to inhibition by the UFH-antithrombin complex. In order to inactivate thrombin, the heparin molecule must form a ternary complex as a bridge between antithrombin and thrombin (see Fig. 19–5).[8] Only molecules that contain more than 18 saccharide units are able to bind both antithrombin and thrombin simultaneously. Smaller heparin molecules cannot facilitate the interaction between antithrombin and thrombin. In contrast, the inactivation of factor Xa does not require UFH to form a bridge with antithrombin. It requires only that UFH bind to antithrombin, using the specific pentasaccharide sequence. Heparin molecules with as few as 5 saccharide units are able to catalyze the inhibition of factor Xa. Heparin uncouples from antithrombin after it has produced its effect and quickly re-couples with another antithrombin molecule. Because of its relatively large size, the UFH-antithrombin complex is incapable of inactivating thrombin or factor Xa that is within a formed clot or is bound to surfaces. At high doses, UFH also binds to heparin cofactor II, further inhibiting the activity of thrombin. In addition, UFH increases the release of TFPI from endothelium, augmenting its inhibitory effect on factor Xa. UFH also modulates vessel wall permeability, prevents the proliferation of vascular smooth muscle cells, and inhibits platelet aggregation.

The absorption of UFH is not reliable when patients take it orally because of its large molecular size and anionic structure.[8] Recently, lipophilic vehicles have been developed to facilitate the transport of heparin across the intestinal lumen into the systemic circulation. One such vehicle, sodium N-(8-[2-hydroxybenzoyl]) amino caprylate (SNAC) markedly improves the gastrointestinal absorption of UFH.[44] Unfortunately, when given in high doses, the SNAC vehicle has been associated with considerable nausea and vomiting. Further, the bioavailability of heparin in the SNAC vehicle is rather variable, limiting its usefulness. Until a reliable and well tolerated vehicle for oral delivery is available, UFH must be given parenterally, preferably by the intravenous (IV) or subcutaneous route. Intramuscular administration is discouraged because the absorption is erratic and it may result in large hematomas.

Its propensity to bind to plasma proteins, platelet factor-4 (PF-4), macrophages, and endothelial cells limits the bioavailability and biologic activity of UFH.[8,41,45] This may explain the substantial inter- and intrapatient variability observed in the anticoagulation response to UFH. Patients who are acutely ill or have active thrombosis have rapid changes in the circulating levels of these heparin-binding proteins. These patients often appear to have "heparin resistance," requiring relatively high doses of UFH to achieve a therapeutic response.[8,46]

The subcutaneous bioavailability of UFH is dose-dependent and ranges from 30% at low doses to as much as 70% at high doses. Higher doses presumably saturate protein-binding sites, thereby permitting a larger proportion to reach the systemic circulation. The onset of anticoagulation activity is usually evident 1 to 2 hours after subcutaneous injection. Because of its unpredictable absorption and delayed onset when administered subcutaneously, heparin should be administered IV when the patient requires rapid anticoagulation. A continuous IV infusion is preferable. Intermittent intravenous boluses produce relatively high peaks in anticoagulation activity and have been associated with a greater risk of major bleeding.

The volume of distribution (V_D) of UFH is similar to blood volume ($V_D = 60$ mL/kg). The dose required to achieve a therapeutic anticoagulation response is correlated to weight. Obese patients do not have a proportional increase in blood volume relative to body weight, however, so it is unclear if the ideal, adjusted, or total body weight should be used when calculating heparin doses.

UFH has a dose-dependent half-life of approximately 30 to 90 minutes, but it may be prolonged to as much as 150 minutes when given in high doses to some patients. There are two primary mechanisms for the elimination of UFH.[8,42,43] The relative contribution of each mechanism to the total clearance of heparin is related to the dose and size of the UFH molecules. One mechanism is a rapid, but saturable zero-order process. Heparinases and desulfatases enzymatically inactivate heparin molecules bound to endothelial cells and macrophages, reducing them to smaller and less sulfated molecules. Heparin is also eliminated renally. This first-order process is slower and nonsaturable. Low doses of UFH are cleared principally by the saturable, rapid zero-order mechanism, while the renal route predominates at very high doses. With typical regimens, a combination of the two mechanisms are used to eliminate UFH. Renal and hepatic dysfunction reduces the rate of clearance of UFH. Patients with active thrombosis may eliminate UFH more rapidly, possibly because of increased binding to acute phase reactants.

Laboratory Monitoring

Administration of UFH requires close monitoring owing to the unpredictable anticoagulant response among patients.[8,47] Several tests are available to monitor UFH therapy, including determinations of whole blood clotting time, activated partial thromboplastin time (aPTT), activated clotting time (ACT), anti-factor Xa activity, and plasma heparin concentrations. Although UFH monitoring with anti-factor Xa heparin activity is commonly used in some European countries, the aPTT is the most widely used test in North America to determine the degree of anticoagulation (Table 19–7). The therapeutic range of the aPTT is considered to be 1.5 to 2.5 times the mean normal control value. Different commercial aPTT reagents vary in their responsiveness to heparin.[48] Many currently available aPTT reagents do not accurately measure the response to heparin within this fixed therapeutic range. Furthermore, there is no standard definition for the term *control value,* which may be interpreted to be either the average aPTT in healthy volunteers or the patient's baseline prior to treatment.

Recognizing the substantial variability in the aPTT, the College of American Pathologists recommends monitoring UFH therapy by establishing an institution-specific aPTT therapeutic range that correlates with a plasma heparin concentration of 0.2–0.4 units/mL by protamine titration assay or 0.3–0.7 units/mL by the chromogenic anti-factor Xa assay.[47] Ideally, aPTT measurements should be compared with heparin levels or anti-factor Xa activity in plasma samples obtained from patients treated with heparin. Alternatively, but considered a less reliable method, the aPTT reagent can be calibrated by using known samples created by adding heparin at several clinically relevant concentrations *in vitro* to several plasma samples.

The use of the aPTT has several limitations.[8] First, the aPTT does not reliably correlate with heparin concentrations, because factors such as reagent sensitivity, temperature, collection methods, and hemodilution produce variability. Second, the turnaround time in most institutions is relatively slow owing to the time required to collect and process the sample in a central laboratory. Substantial delays are undesirable because adjustments in heparin dosing must be made in a timely manner to provide optimal care. Third, while the aPTT can

TABLE 19–7. Tests to Monitor Anticoagulation Response to Unfractionated Heparin

Laboratory Test	Specimen	Advantages	Limitations
Activated partial thromboplastin time (aPTT)	Plasma specimen	▪ Performed in central laboratory in batches ▪ Measures activity of thrombin and factor Xa	▪ Slow turnaround time ▪ Results affected by several variables: reagent sensitivity, anticoagulant used in the blood collection tube, time between obtaining sample and performing the assay, storage conditions for sample, centrifugation parameters, concurrent warfarin use ▪ Has lower and upper limit of heparin detection
Activated clotting time (ACT)	Whole blood	▪ Bedside measurement ▪ Rapid turnaround time (5–10 min) ▪ Accurate measurement of heparin concentration between 1–5 units/mL ▪ Measures the activity of factors VII, VIII, IX, X, XI	▪ Insensitive to factor VII deficiency ▪ Low sensitivity at low heparin concentrations ▪ Results affected by several variables: sample volume, anticoagulant used in blood collection tube storage conditions for sample, centrifugation parameters

TABLE 19–8. Weight-based Dosing[a] for Unfractionated Heparin Administered by Continuous Intravenous Infusion

Indication	Initial Loading Dose	Initial Infusion Rate
Deep vein thrombosis, pulmonary embolism	80–100 units/kg Maximum = 10,000 units	17–20 units/kg/h Maximum = 2,300 units/h
Acute coronary syndromes (with aspirin and thrombolytic agent or glycoprotein IIb/IIIa receptor antagonist)	60–70 units/kg Maximum = 5,000 units bolus	12–15 units/kg/h Maximum = 1,000 units/h

[a]Use actual body weight for all calculations. Adjusted body weight may be used for obese patients (>130% of ideal body weight).
Compiled from Refs. 8 and 49.

measure the intensity of anticoagulation when the heparin concentration is 0.1–1.0 units/mL, it is prolonged beyond measurable limits when the concentration exceeds 1 unit/mL. Consequently, the aPTT is not suitable to monitor heparin therapy in patients requiring high doses of heparin.

Dosing and Administration

The indication, the therapeutic goals, and the patient's individual response to therapy determine the appropriate dose and route of administration for UFH.[8] The dose is expressed in units of activity. The number of units per milligram is variable and depends on the manufacturing process. For the prevention of VTE, UFH can be given by subcutaneous injection in the abdominal fat layer over the iliac crest. The typical dose for prophylaxis is 5,000 units every 8 to 12 hours. When immediate and full anticoagulation is required, a weight-based IV bolus dose followed by a continuous IV infusion is preferred (Tables 19–8 and 19–9).[8,49] Although some clinicians continue to use the time-honored "standard" dosing regimen of a 5,000 unit bolus followed by an infusion rate of 1,000–1,200 units/h, a weight-based approach to UFH dosing is clearly superior. In clinical trials, weight-based dosing protocols substantially increased the proportion of patients who achieved a therapeutic response in the first 24 hours of therapy and decreased the number of recurrent thromboembolic events.[49] Specialized inpatient anticoagulation management services that actively monitor patients receiving UFH and warfarin therapy not only improve the quality of care, but also reduce the overall cost of care.[50]

TABLE 19–9. Adjusted Heparin Dose Based on Activated Partial Thromboplastin Time (aPTT) Measurements

aPTT (sec)	Dose Adjustment
<37 (or >12 sec below institution-specific therapeutic range)	80 units/kg bolus then increase infusion by 4 units/kg/h
37–47 (or 1–12 sec below institution-specific therapeutic range)	40 units/kg bolus then increase infusion by 2 units/kg/h
48–71 (within institution-specific therapeutic range)	No change
72–93 (or 1–22 sec above institution-specific therapeutic range)	Decrease infusion by 2 units/kg/h
>93 (or >22 sec above institution-specific therapeutic range)	Hold infusion for 1 hour then decrease by 3 units/kg/h

Compiled from Refs. 8 and 49.

Therapeutic Monitoring

When used in full therapeutic doses, UFH must be monitored to determine the appropriate dose.[8,47] The choice of assay, which includes aPTT, ACT, or anti-factor Xa heparin activity, is based on clinician preference and institutional availability. If the aPTT is used, it should be measured prior to the initiation of therapy to determine the patient's baseline. When UFH is administered by IV infusion, the response to therapy should be measured 6 hours after the initiation of therapy or a dose change. This is the time required for heparin to reach steady state. The dose of heparin should be promptly adjusted based on the patient's response and the institution-specific therapeutic range (see Table 19–9). The ACT is the most suitable assay when high doses of heparin are given, especially during coronary angioplasty or coronary bypass surgery.[47] Although either the aPTT or ACT may be used to monitor heparin therapy, they should not be used interchangeably because there is a poor correlation between the two tests.

Many patients with acute VTE and myocardial infarction have a diminished response to heparin, presumably because of variations in the plasma concentrations of heparin-binding proteins. Some patients have been reported to have acute elevations in factor VIII, preventing the prolongation of the aPTT by UFH. In some cases, antithrombin deficiency may be the culprit. The recommended management of patients with "heparin resistance" is to adjust the UFH dose based on anti-factor Xa concentrations. Approximately 50% of patients with this "heparin resistance" have dissociation between aPTT and heparin concentration as a result of elevated factor VIII. If anti-factor Xa concentrations cannot be readily measured, the dose of UFH should be increased until a therapeutic aPTT is achieved.

Adverse Effects

Bleeding is the primary adverse effect associated with UFH.[5,51] The rate of major bleeding for patients receiving full therapeutic doses of UFH is estimated to be 0.8%/d, and the rate of minor bleeding is approximately 2%/d. Low-dose UFH administered subcutaneously is associated with a minimal risk of major bleeding. The risk of bleeding increases with age. Elderly women appear to be at particularly high risk, with an incidence of major bleeding twice that of men. There are several contraindications to anticoagulation therapy (Table 19–10). In addition, recent surgery, hemostatic defects, heavy alcohol

TABLE 19–10. Contraindications to Anticoagulation Therapy

Type	Contraindication
General	
	Active bleeding
	Hemophilia or other hemorrhagic tendencies
	Severe liver disease with elevated baseline prothrombin time (PT)
	Severe thrombocytopenia (platelet count <20,000)
	Malignant hypertension
	Inability to meticulously supervise and monitor treatment
Product-Specific Contraindications	
Unfractionated Heparin (UFH)	
	Hypersensitivity to UFH
	History of heparin-induced thrombocytopenia (HIT)
Low–Molecular Weight Heparins (LMWHs)	
	Hypersensitivity to LMWH, UFH, pork products, methylparaben, or propylparaben
	History of HIT or suspected HIT
Danaparoid	
	Hypersensitivity to danaparoid
	Positive *in vitro* platelet aggregation test in presence of danaparoid in patients with HIT
Lepirudin	
	Hypersensitivity to hirudins
Argatroban	
	Hypersensitivity to argatroban
Warfarin	
	Hypersensitivity to warfarin
	Pregnancy
	History of warfarin-induced skin necrosis
	Inability to obtain follow-up PT/INR measurements
	Inappropriate medication use or lifestyle behaviors

INR = international normalized ratio.

TABLE 19–11. Risk Factors for Major Bleeding While Taking Anticoagulation Therapy

Anticoagulation intensity (e.g., INR > 4.0)
Initiation of therapy (first few days and weeks)
Unstable anticoagulation response
Age > 65 years
Concurrent antiplatelet drug use
Concurrent NSAID use
History of gastrointestinal bleeding
Recent surgery or trauma
High risk for fall/trauma
Heavy alcohol use
Renal failure
Cerebrovascular disease
Malignant cancer

INR = international normalized ratio; NSAID = nonsteroidal anti-inflammatory drug.

consumption, renal failure, peptic ulcers, and neoplasms increase the risk of major bleeding in patients who are receiving UFH (Table 19–11).[51]

The most common sites for bleeding are the gastrointestinal and urinary tracts, as well as soft tissues. Bruising at the site of injection is also common. Local irritation, mild pain, erythema, histamine-like reactions, and hematoma can occur. The calcium UFH preparation has been reported to cause hematoma less frequently than the sodium preparation.

Thrombocytopenia, defined as a platelet count less than 150,000, is common with UFH therapy.[52–55] Up to 30% of patients have some appreciable decline in their platelet count. Thrombocytopenia occurs more frequently with UFH preparations derived from bovine lung tissue than with those from porcine gut. Two distinct clinical presentations of the disorder can occur during heparin therapy. Heparin-associated thrombocytopenia (HAT) is a benign, transient, and mild phenomenon that generally occurs within the first 5 days of treatment. Platelet counts rarely drop below 100,000 in patients with HAT, and they rebound with continued therapy. On the other hand, heparin-induced thrombocytopenia (HIT) is a serious drug-induced problem that requires immediate intervention (see Heparin-Induced Thrombocytopenia). Platelet counts must be monitored every 2 to 3 days, and the patient's condition should be rigorously evaluated for HIT if the platelet count drops by more than 50% or to a point below 100,000.

Hypersensitivity reactions involving chills, fever, urticaria, and rarely bronchospasm, nausea, vomiting, and shock have been reported to occur in patients with HIT. Cutaneous necrosis is a rare, but serious complication of UFH therapy that can occur in the setting of HIT. Long-term UFH has been reported to cause alopecia, priapism, and suppressed aldosterone synthesis with subsequent hyperkalemia. Bone loss and osteoporosis are also well recognized complications of long-term UFH administration.[31]

Few drug interactions have been reported in association with UFH. Concurrent use with other antithrombotic drugs, thrombolytics, and antiplatelet agents will increase the risk of bleeding, however.

Management of Bleeding and Excessive Anticoagulation

Hemorrhage can occur at any site in patients receiving UFH, and close monitoring for signs and symptoms of bleeding is crucial.[3,8,31] In addition to an appropriate coagulation study to measure the response to UFH, it is necessary to monitor hemoglobin, hematocrit, and blood pressure regularly. Bleeding can produce a wide variety of symptoms, depending on the site of hemorrhage. Symptoms may include severe headache, joint pain, chest pain, abdominal pain, swelling, tarry stools, frank hematuria, or the passage of bright red blood through the rectum. Life-threatening bleeding, due either to a significant volume loss or to the location (e.g., bleeding into a critical space), must be recognized swiftly and treated immediately. Critical areas include intracranial, pericardial, and intraocular sites, as well as the adrenal gland.

When major bleeding occurs, UFH should be immediately discontinued, and IV protamine sulfate, 1 mg per 100 units of UFH up to a maximum of 50 mg, should be administered. Protamine sulfate has intrinsic anticoagulation activity, but when administered with UFH, it forms a stable salt that results in the loss of anticoagulation activity of both drugs. Protamine sulfate neutralizes UFH in 5 minutes, and its activity persists for 2 hours. It should be given by slow IV infusion over 10 minutes. In cases of large heparin overdoses, a "rebound" effect may occur with a return of some anticoagulant activity several hours after the administration of protamine sulfate. Therefore, the patient's coagulation status should be closely monitored. Multiple doses of protamine sulfate may be necessary if hemorrhage continues.

Use in Special Populations

Classified by the Food and Drug Administration (FDA) as a pregnancy category C agent, UFH is the anticoagulant of choice during pregnancy.[8,56] Although UFH appears to be safer for pregnant women than warfarin, it is not without risks. Its use has been associated with stillbirths and premature births. UFH should be used cautiously during the last trimester of pregnancy and the peripartum period because of the risk of maternal hemorrhage. As UFH is not excreted in breast milk, it is considered safe to use by women who are breastfeeding.

For the treatment of acute thrombosis in children, the dosage of UFH is 50 units/kg bolus, followed by a continuous infusion at 20,000 units/m^2/24 hours.[57] Alternatively, an initial loading dose of 75 units/kg over 10 minutes, followed by a maintenance dose of 28 units/kg/h for infants up to 12 months and 20 units/kg/h for children 1 year old or greater may be used.

LOW-MOLECULAR WEIGHT HEPARINS

Produced by either chemical or enzymatic depolymerization (Table 19–12), LMWHs are fragments of UFH.[8,45,58] They are heterogeneous mixtures of sulfated glycosaminoglycans with approximately one-third the molecular weight of UFH. Although all the LMWHs share similarities in their mechanisms of action with UFH, their molecular weight distributions vary, resulting in differences in their activity against factor Xa and thrombin, affinity for plasma proteins, propensity to release TFPI, and duration of activity. The mean molecular weight of the LMWHs is product-specific. These agents have several advantages over UFH, including (1) predictable anticoagulation dose response, (2) improved subcutaneous bioavailability, (3) dose-independent clearance, (4) longer biologic half-life, (5) lower incidence of thrombocytopenia, and (6) a reduced need for routine laboratory monitoring.

Currently, there are three LMWH products available in the United States. The usefulness of LMWHs has been extensively evaluated for a wide array of indications, including the treatment of acute coronary syndromes, DVT, and pulmonary embolism, as well as the

TABLE 19–12. Chemical and Pharmacokinetic Properties of Antithrombotic Drugs Used for Venous Thromboembolism

Agent (Trade Name)	FDA-Approved (2001)	Method of Preparation	Mean Molecular Weight (Daltons)	Plasma Half-Life	Anti-Xa: Anti-IIa Activity	Bioavailability
Unfractionated heparin	Yes	Extracted from porcine gut mucosa or beef lung	15,000	30–90 min (dose-dependent)	1:1	SC: 30%–70% (dose-dependent)
Low–Molecular Weight Heparins						
Ardeparin (Normiflo)	Yes (no longer marketed in U.S.)	Peroxidative depolymerization	6,000	200 min	1.9:1	SC: 90%
Dalteparin (Fragmin)	Yes	Nitrous acid depolymerization	6,000	119–139 min	2.7:1	SC: 87%
Enoxaparin (Lovenox)	Yes	Benzylation and alkaline depolymerization	4,200	129–180 min	3.8:1	SC: 92%
Nadroparin (Fraxiparine)	No (available in Canada and Mexico)	Nitrous acid depolymerization	4,500	132–162 min	3.6:1	SC: 99%
Tinzaparin (Innohep)	Yes	Heparinase digestion	4,500	111–234 min	2.8:1	SC: 90%
Heparinoid						
Danaparoid (Orgaran)	Yes	Extracted from porcine gut mucosa	6,500	22–24 h	20:1	SC: 95%
Anti–factor Xa Inhibitors						
Fondaparinux (Arixtra)	Yes	Synthetic	1,728	15–18 h	100% anti-Xa	SC: 100%
Direct Thrombin Inhibitors						
Argatroban (Argatroban)	Yes	Synthetic	509	30–50 min	100% anti-IIa	
Lepirudin (Refludan)	Yes	Recombinant DNA technology	6,980	80 min	100% anti-IIa	SC: 70%
Ximelagatran (Exanta)	No	Synthetic	474	3 h	100% anti-IIa	Oral: 40%–45%
Vitamin K Antagonists						
Warfarin (Coumadin)	Yes	Synthetic	330	40 h	1:1	Oral: 100%

FDA = Food and Drug Administration; SC = subcutaneous.

Compiled from Refs. 23, 45, 69, 78, 79.

TABLE 19–13. Indications and Doses for the Low-Molecular Weight Heparins (LMWHs)

Indication	Enoxaparin	Dalteparin	Tinzaparin
Hip replacement surgery (prophylaxis)	30 mg SC q 12 h initiated 12–24 h after surgery[a] OR 40 mg SC q 24 h initiated 12 h prior to surgery.[a] Extended prophylaxis may be given for up to 3 weeks.[a]	2,500 U SC given 2 h prior to surgery, followed by 2,500 IU the evening after surgery and at least 6 h after first dose, then 5,000 IU SC q 24 h[a] OR 5,000 IU SC q 24 h initiated the evening prior to surgery.[a]	750 units/kg SC q 24 h initiated the evening prior to surgery or 12 h after surgery OR 4,500 units SC q 24 h initiated 12 h prior to surgery.
Knee replacement surgery (prophylaxis)	30 mg SC q 12 h initiated 12–24 h prior to surgery.[a]		75 units/kg SC q 24 h initiated the evening prior to surgery or 12 h after surgery.
Abdominal surgery (prophylaxis)	40 mg SC q 24 h initiated 2 h prior to surgery.[a]	2,500 units SC q 24 h initiated 1–2 h prior to surgery.[a] Patients with malignancy: 5,000 units SC the evening prior to surgery, then 5,000 units SC q 24 h[a] OR 2,500 units SC 1–2 h prior to surgery, then 2,500 units 12 h after surgery followed by 5,000 units SC q 24 h.[a]	3500 U SC Q 24 hrs initiated 1–2 hrs prior to surgery.
Acute medical illness (prophylaxis)	40 mg SC q 24 h.[a]	2,500 units SC q 24 h.	
Trauma (prophylaxis)	30 mg SC q 12 h starting 12–36 hours after injury.		
DVT treatment (with or without PE)	1 mg/kg SC q 12 h[a] OR 1.5 mg/kg SC q 24 h.[a]	100 units/kg SC q 12 h OR 200 units/kg SC q 24 h.	175 units/kg SC q 24 h.
Unstable angina or non-Q-wave MI	1 mg/kg SC q 12 h.	120 units/kg SC q 12 h.	

[a]Dose approved by the Food and Drug Administration for indication.
SC = subcutaneous; DVT = deep vein thrombosis; PE = pulmonary embolism; MI = myocardial infarction.
From Ref. 15.

prevention of VTE in several high-risk populations. The FDA-approved indications and doses for the LMWHs are product-specific (Table 19–13). Some authorities have advocated that the LMWHs should replace UFH for the prevention and treatment of VTE. Institutional resources and individual patient needs should determine their precise role in the management of VTE.

Pharmacology/Pharmacokinetics

The LMWHs prevent the growth and propagation of formed thrombi.[8,58–60] Like UFH, the LMWHs enhance and accelerate the activity of antithrombin by binding to a specific pentasaccharide sequence. Approximately 20% of the LMWH molecules contain the specific sequence necessary to interact with antithrombin, compared with nearly 30% for UFH. The principal difference in the pharmacologic activity of the LMWHs and UFH is their relative inhibition of factor Xa and thrombin (IIa). Because of their smaller chain length, the LMWHs have limited activity against thrombin (see Fig. 19–5). Fewer than 50% of the LMWH molecules have the requisite chain length to simultaneously bind antithrombin and thrombin. For this reason, the LMWHs have proportionally greater anti-factor Xa activity. The ratio of anti-factor Xa:IIa activity is product-specific. Like UFH, the LMWHs cause the endothelium to release TFPI, which is believed to enhance the inhibition of factor Xa and to inactivate factor VIIa.

Compared with UFH, the LMWHs have a more predictable anticoagulation response. The improved pharmacokinetic profile of the LMWHs is the result of reduced binding to proteins and cells (Table 19–14). The bioavailability of the LMWHs varies between 85% and 99% when administered subcutaneously, while the absorption of UFH is relatively poor and erratic. The subcutaneous bioavailability of the available LMWH products differs only slightly. The peak anticoagulation effect is seen in 3 to 5 hours.

The renal route is the predominant mode of elimination for the LMWHs.[8,58] Consequently, their biologic half-life may be prolonged in patients with renal impairment. Longer heparin chains bind to macrophages and are rapidly degraded. Therefore, anti-factor Xa activity, which is mediated by smaller heparin molecules, persists longer than antithrombin activity. The plasma half-life of the LMWH preparations is two to four times longer than that of UFH. The clearance of the LMWHs is independent of dose.

Dosing and Administration

The LMWHs are given in fixed or weight-based doses based on the product and indication (see Table 19–13).[8,58–60] The dose for enoxaparin is expressed in milligrams, while those for dalteparin, tinzaparin, and ardeparin are expressed in units of anti-factor Xa activity. Although they can be given by continuous IV infusion, the LMWHs are generally given by subcutaneous injection in the abdominal area while the patient is in a supine position. The clinician or patient pinches a layer of skin between the thumb and forefinger, and then introduces the entire length of the needle into a skin fold at a 90° angle. Following

TABLE 19–14. Biologic and Clinical Consequences of Reduced Binding of LMWHs to Proteins and Cells

Binding Target	Biologic Effects	Clinical Consequence
Thrombin	Reduced anti-IIa activity	None known
Proteins	Improved bioavailability; predictable anticoagulant response	Effective when given by subcutaneous injection, but monitoring of anticoagulant effect usually unnecessary
Macrophages	Renally cleared	Longer plasma half-life; once daily administration effective
Platelets	Reduced incidence of heparin-induced antibodies	Reduced incidence of HIT
Osteoblasts	Reduced activation of osteoblasts	Reduced incidence of osteopenia and osteoporosis

LMWHs = low-molecular weight heparins; HIT = heparin-induced thrombocytopenia.

subcutaneous administration, the drug is absorbed slowly, resulting in sustained antithrombotic activity over several hours.

The dosing interval for the LMWHs is every 12 or 24 hours, depending on the indication and product. Larger doses are given for once daily administration and produce significantly higher peak plasma concentrations. Given that the elimination half-life of the LMWHs is prolonged in patients with severe renal impairment (e.g., serum creatinine <30 mL/min), high doses may lead to a significant accumulation in these patients. Few data are available to guide the dosing of LMWHs in the setting of renal insufficiency, but monitoring anti-factor Xa activity is considered prudent until more studies are completed.

For the prevention of VTE, the LMWHs have been studied in a variety of high-risk circumstances, including orthopedic surgery, abdominal surgery, acute spinal cord injury, neurosurgery, multiple trauma, and critical illnesses. The effectiveness of the LMWHs has been extensively evaluated for the treatment of VTE in hospitalized patients and in the outpatient management of DVT. They are also a reasonable alternative to warfarin therapy in circumstances when monitoring by prothrombin time or international normalized ratio (INR) is unavailable. The LMWHs have also been demonstrated to be safe and effective for the treatment of unstable angina and non-ST-segment elevation myocardial infarction.

Therapeutic Monitoring

The LMWHs achieve predictable anticoagulant response when given subcutaneously. Therefore, routine laboratory monitoring is unnecessary to guide the dosing of these agents. The prothrombin time, the ACT, and the aPTT are minimally affected by LMWH heparin. Prior to the initiation of the LMWH, a baseline prothrombin time/INR, aPTT, complete blood cell (CBC) with platelet count, and serum creatinine level should be obtained. Periodic monitoring of the CBC, including platelet count, and occult fecal blood is recommended during LMWH therapy.

Several methods have been used to monitor the LMWHs: the Heptest, thrombin time (TT), chromogenic anti-factor Xa activity assay, anti-IIa activity assay, thrombin generation, and release of TFPI. The Heptest appears to be the most useful marker for LMWH activity. However, this test is not readily available at most commercial laboratories. Measurement of anti-factor Xa activity has been the most widely used method to monitor LMWH therapy in clinical practice. Routine anti-factor Xa activity measurement is not necessary in patients whose condition is stable and uncomplicated. Although very limited data support the use of laboratory monitoring to guide LMWH therapy, measuring anti-factor Xa activity may be helpful in patients who have significant renal impairment (e.g., creatinine clearance <30 mL/min), weigh less than 50 kg, are morbidly obese, or require prolonged therapy (e.g., longer than 14 days). Periodic anti-factor Xa activity monitoring may also be useful in women treated with an LMWH during pregnancy because of changing pharmacokinetic variables (e.g., volume of distribution and renal function). Patients who are at very high risk of bleeding or thrombotic recurrence may also benefit from anti-factor Xa monitoring to avoid periods of over- or under-anticoagulation. Newborns have unpredictable pharmacokinetic profiles; therefore, they may require monitoring to ensure adequate therapy.

When anti-factor Xa activity is used to monitor LMWH therapy, the sample should be drawn approximately 4 hours after the subcutaneous injection, during the peak period of anti-factor Xa activity.[8] A calibrated LMWH should be used to establish the standard curve for the assay. The therapeutic range for anti-factor Xa activity is not well defined. For the treatment of VTE, an acceptable therapeutic target range is 0.5–1.0 units/mL. In one small study, bleeding was associated with peak anti-factor Xa activity greater than 0.8 units/mL. Specific algorithms for dosing adjustments based on anti-factor Xa activity are not available at the present time.

Adverse Effects

As with UFH, bleeding is the most common adverse effect of the LMWHs.[5,8] Although not consistently demonstrated in clinical trials, the frequency of major bleeding has been purported to be less with the LMWHs than with UFH.[8,61,62] This difference may be due in part to their reduced effects on platelet function, endothelial cells, and microvascular permeability. The incidence of major bleeding reported in clinical trials is less than 3% and varies among the LMWH preparations, their indication for use, patient population, and dose administered. Minor bleeding, particularly at the site of injection, occurs frequently with LMWH use. Several cases of epidural and spinal hematoma resulting in long-term or permanent paralysis have been reported with the use of enoxaparin during spinal and epidural anesthesia or spinal puncture. The risk of these events is higher with the use of in-dwelling epidural catheters and concomitant use of drugs that affect hemostasis. Epidural catheters should be removed only after a minimum of 12 hours has elapsed after the last dose of the LMWH, and any subsequent dose should be given at least 2 hours later.

If major bleeding occurs in a patient receiving an LMWH, it is recommended that protamine sulfate be administered IV.[8] However, because of its limited binding to the shorter LMWH chains, protamine sulfate cannot completely neutralize their anticoagulant effects. When given in equimolar concentrations, protamine sulfate neutralizes an estimated 60% to 75% of their antithrombotic activity. The recommended dose of protamine sulfate is 1 mg/100 anti-factor Xa units of the LMWH dose administered in the previous 8 hours. If the LMWH dose was given in the previous 8 to 12 hours, a 0.5-mg dose of protamine should be given for every 100 anti-factor Xa units. The use of protamine sulfate is not recommended if the LMWH was administered more than 12 hours earlier.

Although thrombocytopenia can occur, the incidence of HIT with the use of an LMWH is substantially lower than that observed with the use of UFH.[8,63] The explanation may lie in the reduced propensity of the LMWHs to bind to platelets and PF-4. The LMWHs exhibit 70% to 100% cross-reactivity with heparin antibodies *in vitro*.[52,64] Therefore, the LMWHs should be avoided in patients with an established diagnosis or history of HIT. Platelet counts must be periodically monitored in all patients receiving an LMWH, and thrombocytopenia of any degree should be promptly evaluated.

The use of UFH for longer than 1 month has been associated with significant bone loss.[8,58] The risk of osteoporosis appears to be substantially lower with the LMWHs, and they have not caused appreciable changes in bone mineral density after several months of use.[30,56] They have been used in a limited number of patients with established heparin-induced osteoporosis. Although these reports are promising, it cannot be concluded that the LMWHs have no effect on bone formation until well designed clinical trials are available.

Use in Special Populations

There is growing experience with the use of LMWHs during pregnancy.[30,56] The LMWHs do not cross the placenta. According to the results of a few large case series, the LMWHs appear to be relatively safe to use during pregnancy and are an attractive alternative to UFH when long-term anticoagulation therapy is required. Furthermore, the LMWHs do not appear to affect bone formation. Ardeparin has been classified as FDA pregnancy category C. Dalteparin, enoxaparin, and tinzaparin are classified as FDA pregnancy category B. The safety and effectiveness of the LMWHs to treat VTE in children and infants has not been extensively studied.[57] Limited data exist for enoxaparin. The recommended treatment dosage for enoxaparin in patients less than 1 year old is 1.5 mg/kg every 12 hours and 1 mg/kg every 12 hours in children 1 year of age or older. Until more data are available, it is prudent to periodically monitor anti-factor Xa activity in these special populations during long-term use.

HEPARINOIDS

Danaparoid sodium is the only heparinoid available in North America.[8,65,66] It is derived from porcine gut mucosa (see Table 19–12). It is a mixture of three sulfated glycosaminoglycans: heparan (84%), dermatan (12%), and chondroitin (4%). Although related to UFH and the LMWHs, danaparoid does not contain heparin. It is FDA-approved for VTE prophylaxis in patients undergoing elective hip replacement surgery, and it has been used for a number of other indications, including the treatment of VTE and ischemic stroke. It has also served as an alternative anticoagulant in patients with HIT.[66,67]

Danaparoid binds to antithrombin and heparin cofactor II and greatly accelerates their activity.[66] It inhibits factor Xa and to a lesser extent thrombin (factor IIa). Danaparoid's Xa to IIa ratio (20:1) is substantially greater than that of the LMWHs. Danaparoid also inhibits the formation of factor IXa, further contributing to its antithrombotic activity. It does not bind to or activate platelets and has minimal cross-reactivity with heparin-induced antibodies.

Subcutaneously administered, danaparoid has excellent bioavailability.[66] Although the pharmacokinetic properties of danaparoid have been evaluated in healthy volunteers, they are difficult to characterize because the agent is a mixture of different naturally occurring molecules. Plasma anti-factor Xa activity is directly related to the administered dose, and the peak effect is seen with 5 hours. Peak anti-IIa activity usually occurs slightly sooner. Danaparoid's anticoagulation effect is relatively durable, with a terminal anti-factor Xa activity half-life of approximately 22 hours. Full anticoagulation activity requires 4 to 5 days to reach steady state. Because the elimination of danaparoid takes place primarily by renal excretion, significantly impaired renal function may result in accumulation; however, specific dosing recommendations in this setting are not available. There are few known clinically important drug interactions associated with danaparoid. It does not cross the placenta, and the FDA has designated it a pregnancy category B agent. Even so, its use in pregnant women has not been systematically evaluated, and it should be used only when UFH or the LMWHs are contraindicated.

Bleeding is the most common adverse effect associated with danaparoid use.[65,66] The reported incidence of major bleeding in clinical trials varies from 3% to 7%. Minor bleeding or bruising at the site of injection is common. Nonhemorrhagic complications associated with danaparoid use, such as fever, nausea, constipation, and skin rash, are uncommon. The contraindications and precautions for danaparoid are similar to those for other anticoagulant drugs.

Like the LMWHs, danaparoid does not require routine therapeutic laboratory monitoring.[68] Although poorly correlated with efficacy, determination of its anti-factor Xa activity may be useful when there is doubt regarding the appropriate dose of danaparoid, such as in patients who have significant renal impairment or who are morbidly obese. Because danaparoid has little anti-IIa activity, it does not appreciably affect the aPTT or prothrombin time, and these tests are not useful in monitoring therapy. A CBC should be obtained at baseline and periodically thereafter to monitor for thrombocytopenia and blood loss. In patients with a history of HIT, danaparoid therapy should be discontinued when the presence of cross-reactive heparin-induced antibodies is confirmed. No known antidote is available to reverse the effect of danaparoid, and major bleeding must be treated with supportive measures.[66,67]

FACTOR Xa INHIBITORS

A number of direct and indirect factor Xa inhibitors are currently under development.[69] The direct factor Xa inhibitors thwart thrombin generation by binding directly to circulating and clot-bound factor Xa. They are not dependent on antithrombin to produce their antithrombotic effects. Discovered in nature, a number of direct factor Xa inhibitors, including tick anticoagulation peptide (TAP) as well as antistasin and lefaxin from leeches, are currently under investigation in early clinical trials.

Similar to UFH and the LMWHs, the indirect factor Xa inhibitors bind to antithrombin, greatly accelerating its activity.[69,70] However, because of their small molecular size, they do not enhance the enzymatic activity of antithrombin against factor IIa (thrombin).

Fondaparinux, also known as a pentasaccharide, is a synthetic molecule (molecular weight = 1,728 daltons) consisting of the five critical saccharide units that bind specifically, but reversibly to antithrombin (see Fig. 19–5 and Table 19–12). Because of its high specificity for antithrombin, it does not bind to other plasma proteins. Furthermore, it demonstrates excellent bioavailability after subcutaneous injection and a long half-life. Fondaparinux circulates in the plasma bound to antithrombin and passes unchanged out of the body in the urine. It does not bind to PF-4 and does not cross-react with heparin-induced antibodies in patients with HIT. Data from phase II and III clinical trials indicate that fondaparinux is highly effective in the prevention of VTE among high-risk patients and in the treatment of VTE.[70,70a,70b] Fondaparinux has also been evaluated for the treatment of DVT.[71] Fondaparinux has been approved initially for the prevention of VTE following lower extremity orthopedic procedures and is given 2.5 mg subcutaneously every 24 hours.

DIRECT THROMBIN INHIBITORS

A relatively new class of very potent anticoagulant agents, the direct thrombin inhibitors, includes lepirudin, bivalirudin, argatroban, and ximelagatran. These agents have been studied for a number of indications, such as the prophylaxis and treatment of VTE, acute coronary syndromes, and HIT.[69,72] The oral administration of direct thrombin inhibitors, such as ximelagatran, is currently under intense clinical investigation.

Direct thrombin inhibitors, as their name implies, interact directly with the thrombin molecule (Fig. 19–6).[72,73] Unlike the heparins, danaparoid, or fondaparinux, direct thrombin inhibitors do not require antithrombin or heparin cofactor II to have antithrombotic activity. They are capable of inhibiting both circulating and clot-bound thrombin, a potential advantage over UFH and the LMWHs.[74] Further, they do not induce immune-mediated thrombocytopenia.

Hirudin, the prototype of this class, was isolated from the salivary secretions of the medicinal leech (*Hirudo medicinalis*).[23,72] Mass production of several synthetic hirudin analogs with the potential for

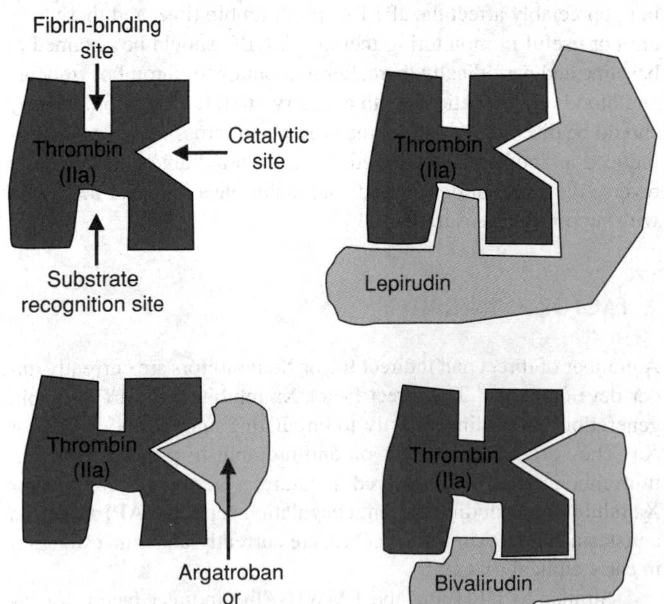

FIGURE 19–6. Pharmacologic activity of lepirudin, bivalirudin, argatroban, and ximelagatran.

wide clinical application became possible only with the advent of recombinant DNA technology. Lepirudin, a recombinant analog of hirudin, is a 65-amino acid polypeptide that irreversibly binds with high specificity to thrombin. The hirudins form a noncovalent bond in a 1:1 ratio to the catalytic and substrate recognition sites on the thrombin molecule. Hirudins must be administered parenterally and are usually given by continuous IV infusion. The primary route of elimination for lepirudin is through renal excretion, and systemic clearance is directly proportional to the glomerular filtration rate. Many patients develop antibodies to lepirudin.[72] Although these complexes do not appear to appreciably alter the pharmacologic activity of lepirudin, they do reduce its renal clearance rate. The probability that the patient will develop lepirudin antibodies increases with the duration of therapy. Up to 40% of patients treated with lepirudin for 10 days or more will develop antibodies. Lepirudin has an elimination half-life of approximately 90 minutes.

Bivalirudin, formerly known as hirulog, is a semisynthetic 20-amino acid polypeptide analog of recombinant hirudin.[69,72] Unlike lepirudin, bivalirudin is a reversible inhibitor of thrombin and provides transient antithrombotic activity with an estimated half-life of 20 to 30 minutes. This difference may reduce the risk of bleeding and antibody production.[75] Although only 20% of an IV dose of bivalirudin is eliminated in the urine, the manufacturer recommends specific dose reductions in patients with renal impairment.

Argatroban is a small synthetic molecule derived from arginine that reversibly binds to the catalytic site of thrombin.[76] It is primarily eliminated by hydroxylation and aromatization in the liver to inactive metabolites. A small percentage is excreted unchanged in the bile. The terminal elimination half-life of argatroban is 30 to 50 minutes.

Ximelagatran is a pro-drug converted by hydrolysis and reduction in the liver to melagatran, the active moiety.[69,72] Bioavailability following oral administration is good, and food does not appear to affect it. Peak plasma concentrations are evident within 120 minutes following an oral dose, so melagatran's antithrombotic activity is relatively rapid. The elimination half-life is approximately 3 hours, making twice daily administration necessary. Melagatran is primarily eliminated in the urine. Based on early clinical trials, ximelagatran appears to produce a predictable antithrombotic response in fixed doses and has a relatively large therapeutic window. Therefore, this agent may not require routine laboratory monitoring in clinical practice.

Contraindications for the use of direct thrombin inhibitors are similar to those for the use of other antithrombotic drugs. Hemorrhage is the most serious and common adverse effect related to the direct thrombin inhibitors.[67,72] In studies evaluating the use of lepirudin for the treatment of patients with HIT, the incidence of major bleeding was relatively high (13% to 17%).[78] However, no fatal or intracranial bleeding events occurred. A slightly lower rate of major hemorrhage was reported in HIT trials using argatroban (approximately 5%), and similarly, there were no reports of fatal or intracranial bleeding.[79] Minor bleeding and small reductions in red blood cell counts occurred relatively frequently, but typically did not require drug discontinuation. There are no known agents that reverse the activity of the direct thrombin inhibitors. Given their relatively short half-lives, the intensity of their anticoagulation activity declines rapidly after drug discontinuation. Nonhemorrhagic effects such as fever, nausea, vomiting, and allergic reactions occur infrequently.

Although the direct thrombin inhibitors produce changes in the prothrombin time/INR, the aPTT is used to monitor the patient's response to lepirudin and argatroban therapy.[67] After baseline coagulation studies have been obtained, the dose should be titrated to achieve the institution-specific therapeutic range or an aPTT 1.5 to 3.0 times the mean normal control. The eccarin clotting time is a potentially more suitable test to measure the antithrombotic activity of the direct thrombin inhibitors, but it is not readily available in the United States.[73] A CBC should be obtained at baseline and periodically thereafter to detect potential bleeding.

The concurrent use of direct thrombin inhibitors and thrombolytic agents substantially increases the bleeding risk, particularly the risk of intracranial hemorrhage, and should be done with great caution. Warfarin and antiplatelet agents can be concurrently initiated with these agents. Few pharmacokinetic drug interactions with this class of agents are known. Drugs that alter renal function could prolong lepirudin activity. Although drugs that inhibit liver enzymes have the potential to interact with argatroban, erythromycin did not appreciably alter argatroban pharmacokinetics in healthy volunteers in one small study.[77]

The FDA has classified lepirudin and argatroban as pregnancy category B drugs, but they should be used cautiously in women of childbearing age because experience is very limited.[78,79] Lepirudin has been evaluated in a small number of children. Further study is required to develop dosing guidelines for patients with renal and hepatic insufficiency.

The direct thrombin inhibitors appear to offer great promise for a number of indications, but the relatively high incidence of bleeding observed in early clinical trials and their relatively high cost have limited their use to date. Currently, lepirudin and argatroban are most frequently used in the management of patients with HIT, while bivalirudin is indicated for use with aspirin in patients who have unstable angina and are to undergo percutaneous transluminal coronary angioplasty (PCTA). There are only very limited data available regarding the use of bivalirudin for the treatment or prevention of VTE. Given its immediate onset of action, the good bioavailability when it is taken orally, wide therapeutic window, fixed dosing, and promising results from early clinical trails, ximelagatran (and other direct thrombin inhibitors that can be administered orally) could revolutionize the treatment of VTE in the next 5 years.

WARFARIN

The most widely prescribed anticoagulant in North America is warfarin (Coumadin®). It was serendipitously discovered in the early 1940s at the University of Wisconsin after hemorrhagic deaths occurred in cattle eating spoiled sweet clover.[80] Warfarin is FDA-approved for the prevention and treatment of VTE, as well as for the prevention of thromboembolic complications associated with atrial fibrillation, heart valve replacement, and myocardial infarction. Because of its narrow therapeutic index, predisposition to drug and food interactions, and propensity to cause hemorrhage, warfarin requires continuous patient monitoring and education in order to achieve optimal outcomes.[6]

Pharmacology/Pharmacokinetics

Warfarin exerts its anticoagulation effect by inhibiting the enzymes responsible for the cyclic interconversion of vitamin K (Fig. 19–7). Reduced vitamin K is a cofactor required for the carboxylation of the vitamin K-dependent coagulation proteins—namely, prothrombin (factor II); factors VII, IX, and X; as well as the endogenous anticoagulant proteins C and S. Carboxylation of the N-terminal region of these proteins in the liver is required for biologic activity. By inhibiting the supply of vitamin K that is available to serve as a cofactor in the production of these proteins, warfarin indirectly slows their rate

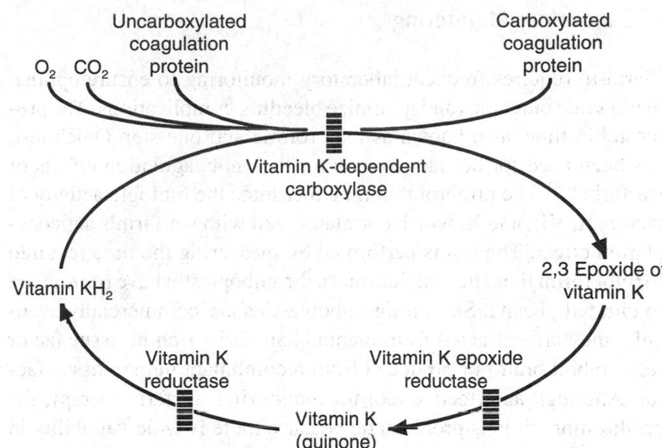

FIGURE 19–7. Vitamin K recycling and warfarin. Thrombin; factors VII, IX, and X; as well as proteins C and S are carboxylated to their circulating forms by a vitamin K–dependent enzyme. Recycling is necessary to maintain sufficient intracellular concentrations of vitamin K to serve as a cofactor in this reaction. Warfarin and other coumarin derivatives inhibit the reductase enzymes responsible for vitamin K recycling.

of synthesis. Warfarin has no direct effect on previously circulating clotting factors or previously formed thrombi. The time required for warfarin to achieve its pharmacologic effect depends on the elimination half-lives of the coagulation proteins (Table 19–15).[81] Given that prothrombin has a 2- to 4-day half-life, warfarin's full antithrombotic effect is not achieved for 8 to 16 days after the initiation of therapy. By suppressing the production of clotting factors, warfarin prevents the initial formation and propagation of thrombi.

Commercially available warfarin is a racemic mixture of R and S isomers.[6,7,80] The S isomer is two to five times more potent that the R isomer. Rapidly and extensively absorbed from the gastrointestinal tract, warfarin reaches its peak plasma concentration in approximately 90 minutes with a bioavailability of more than 90% following oral administration. In plasma, both the R and S isomers are extensively (97% to 99%) bound to albumin. The R isomer has a slightly higher affinity for albumin and is bound at a ratio of 1.6:1 relative to the S isomer. Warfarin is hepatically metabolized via the cytochrome P450 enzyme system, including the isoenzymes CYP1A2, 2C9, 2C19, 2C18, and 3A4. Warfarin's metabolism is isomer-specific. The CYP2C enzymes metabolize the S isomer, whereas the CYP1A2 and 3A4 isoenzymes degrade the R isomer. Given the relatively greater potency of the S isomer, drugs that induce or inhibit the CYP2C isoenzymes are more likely to produce a clinically significant effect. The pharmacokinetic parameters of warfarin, particularly hepatic metabolism, varies substantially among individuals. These variations likely explain the large differences in interpatient dose-response seen with warfarin in clinical practice.

TABLE 19–15. Biologic Half-Life of Vitamin K–Dependent Coagulation Proteins

Protein	Half-life (Hours)
Prothrombin (factor II)	60–100
Factor VII	4–6
Factor IX	20–30
Factor X	24–40
Protein C	8–10
Protein S	40–60

From Ref. 6.

Laboratory Monitoring

Warfarin requires frequent laboratory monitoring to ensure optimal therapeutic outcomes and minimize bleeding complications. The prothrombin time, also known as the protime and one-step Quick test, has been used for decades to monitor the anticoagulation effects of warfarin.[6,82] The prothrombin time measures the biologic activity of factors II, VII, and X, which correlates well with warfarin's anticoagulation effect. The test is performed by measuring the time required for clot formation after calcium and a thromboplastin have been added to citrated plasma. Several thromboplastins are commercially available; they are extracted from mammalian tissue rich in tissue factor (e.g., rabbit brain) or produced from recombinant human tissue factor. Although an effective tool for monitoring warfarin therapy, the prothrombin time is problematic because there is wide variability in the sensitivity of the thromboplastin reagents. Given the same blood sample, different thromboplastins will produce substantially different results that may prompt clinicians to make potentially inappropriate dosing decisions. The World Health Organization (WHO) addressed the need for standardization in the late 1970s when it developed a reference thromboplastin and recommended the use of the INR to monitor warfarin therapy. The INR corrects for differences in the thromboplastin reagents through the following formula:

$$\mathrm{INR} = \left(\frac{\mathrm{PT}^{\mathrm{Patient}}}{\mathrm{PT}^{\mathrm{Control}}}\right)^{\mathrm{ISI}}$$

The International Sensitivity Index (ISI) is a measure of the thromboplastin's responsiveness compared with the WHO reference standard. Each thromboplastin reagent manufactured has an ISI value that should be used to calculate the INR. Although the INR system has a number of potential problems, it is currently the best means available to interpret the prothrombin time and the preferred method for monitoring oral anticoagulation therapy.

Dosing and Administration

The dosing of warfarin is patient-specific.[6,7,80] The appropriate dose is based not only on the indication for therapy (Table 19–16), but also on the patient's individual response. There is tremendous interpatient variability with regard to the pharmacodynamic response and pharmacokinetic handling of warfarin. Furthermore, there is substantial intrapatient variability over time. Therefore, the dose of warfarin must be based on continual clinical and laboratory monitoring. At the initiation of therapy, it is difficult to predict the specific dose that an individual patient will require.

Although the average weekly dose of warfarin is between 30 and 40 mg, some patient-related variables suggest the need for a lower than usual dose: advanced age (>65 years old), elevated baseline INR, poor nutritional status, liver disease, and concomitant use of medications known to enhance the effects of warfarin (Table 19–17). Prior to initiating therapy, the clinician should screen the patient for the presence of contraindications to anticoagulation therapy and risk factors for major bleeding (see Tables 19–10 and 19–11). It is essential to collect a

TABLE 19–16. Recommended Target INR and Goal Range for Warfarin Therapy Based on Indication

Indication	Target INR (Goal Range)
Prophylaxis for venous thromboembolism	2.5 (2.0–3.0)
Treatment for venous thromboembolism	2.5 (2.0–3.0)
Arterial thrombosis and stroke prevention	
Atrial fibrillation	2.5 (2.0–3.0)
Acute myocardial infarction[a]	2.5 (2.0–3.0)
Valvular heart disease	2.5 (2.0–3.0)
Prosthetic tissue heart valve	2.5 (2.0–3.0)
Prosthetic mechanical heart valve[b]	3.0 (2.5–3.5)

INR = international normalized ratio.
[a]A target INR of 3.0 (2.5–3.5) is appropriate for patients following an acute myocardial infarction to prevent recurrent cardiac events.
[b]A target INR of 2.5 (2.0–3.0) is appropriate for patients who have a mechanical bileaflet valve in the aortic position, normal cardiac chamber size, and no other risk factors for stroke.
From Ref. 6.

TABLE 19–17. Clinically Important Warfarin Drug Interactions

Increased Anticoagulation Effect (⇑ INR)	Decreased Anticoagulation Effect (⇓ INR)	Increased Bleeding Risk
Acetaminophen	Amobarbital	Argatroban
Alcohol binge	Butabarbital	Aspirin
Allopurinol	Carbamazepine	Clopidogrel
Amiodarone	Cholestyramine	Danaparoid
Cefamandol	Dicloxacillin	Dipyridamole
Chloral hydrate	Griseofulvin	NSAIDs
Chloramphenicol	Nafcillin	Ticlopidine
Cimetidine	Phenobarbital	UFH/LMWHs
Ciprofloxacin	Phenytoin	
Clofibrate	Primidone	
Danazol	Rifabutin	
Disulfiram	Rifampin	
Doxycycline	Secobarbital	
Erythromycin	Sucralfate	
Fenofibrate	Vitamin K	
Fluconazole		
Fluorouracil		
Fluoxetine		
Fluvoxamine		
Gemfibrozil		
Influenza vaccine		
Isoniazid		
Itraconazole		
Lovastatin		
Metronidazole		
Miconazole		
Moxalactam		
Neomycin		
Norfloxacin		
Ofloxacin		
Omeprazole		
Phenylbutazone		
Piroxicam		
Propafenone		
Propoxyphene		
Quinidine		
Sertraline		
Sulfamethoxazole		
Sulfinpyrazone		
Tamoxifen		
Testosterone		
Vitamin E		
Zafirlukast		

INR = international normalized ratio; UFH = unfractionated heparin; LMWHs = low-molecular weight heparins; NSAIDs = nonsteroidal anti-inflammatory drugs.
Compiled from Refs. 6 and 98.

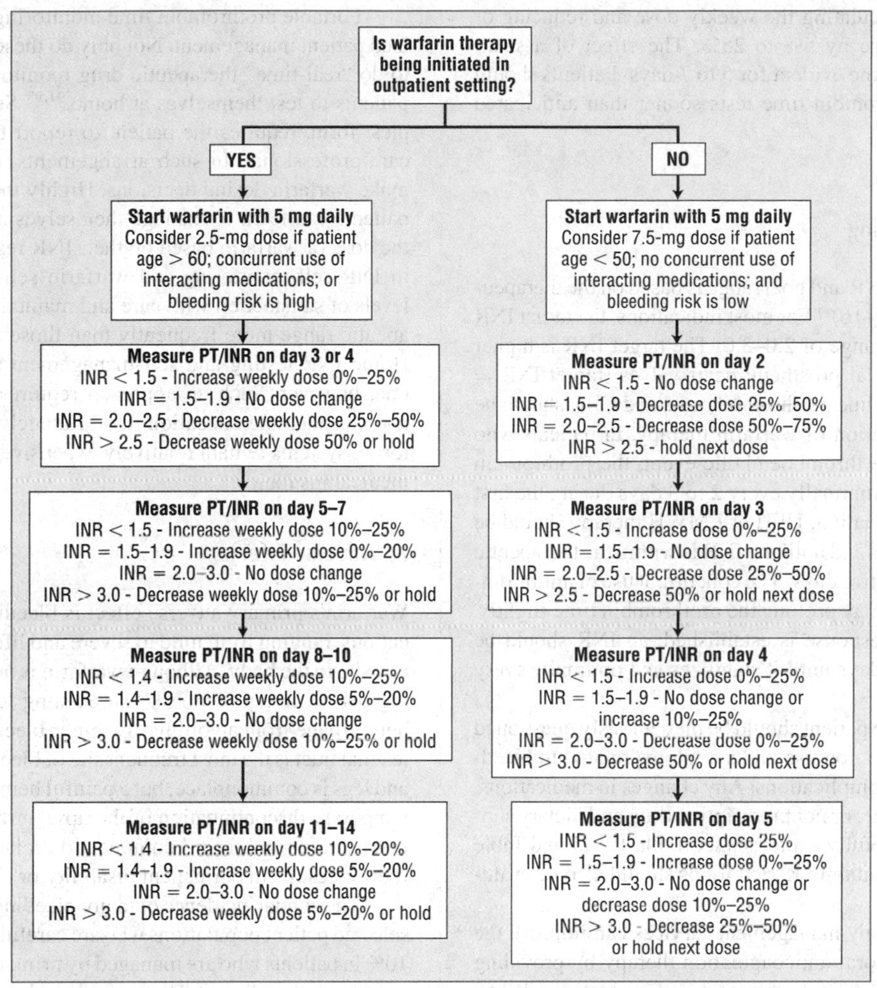

FIGURE 19–8. Initiation of warfarin therapy. PT = prothrombin time; INR = international normalized ratio.

complete medication history. Absolute contraindications to warfarin include active bleeding, hemorrhagic tendencies, pregnancy, and a history of warfarin-induced skin necrosis. Warfarin should be used with great caution in patients who have a history of gastrointestinal bleeding, recent neurosurgery, alcoholic liver disease, or severe renal impairment, and those who are unable or unlikely to keep follow-up appointments for monitoring.

There is some controversy regarding the optimal method for initiating warfarin therapy (Fig. 19–8).[7] To achieve a therapeutic INR in the least amount of time, many clinicians have used relatively high doses (10 mg) for the first few days of therapy and then adjusted the dose based on the patient's response. Recent data suggest that a 5-mg initial dose is preferable to a 10-mg dose, calling into the question the practice of giving a dose larger than the anticipated maintenance dose during the initiation of therapy.[83,84] Unless there is a clear reason to do so, initial dosing greater than 10 mg should be avoided. Although a 10-mg dose appears to produce a more rapid response in the INR, many patients given such a dose become excessively anticoagulated. A 10-mg dose may also increase the theoretical risk for early thrombotic complications, such as warfarin-induced skin necrosis.

After the initiation of warfarin therapy, the level of protein C, which has a relatively short half-life, declines rapidly, but prothrombin concentrations remain near normal for several days. If protein C concentrations are severely suppressed relative to prothrombin, there is a potential for inducing a hypercoagulable state. It is known that patients with hereditary protein C deficiency are at greater risk for developing warfarin-induced skin necrosis.[85]

A 10-mg dose results in a more severe depression in factor VII concentrations. This early response to therapy may make it appear that a therapeutic INR has been achieved after only 2 or 3 days. Patients are not truly anticoagulated at this point, however, because a significant reduction in prothrombin concentrations requires at least 5 days to occur. The achievement of a full antithrombotic effect requires up to 16 days. Several dosing nomograms have been developed and prospectively evaluated.[83,84,86–89] For patients with acute venous thrombosis, heparin and warfarin therapy should be overlapped for at least 5 days, regardless of whether the target INR has been achieved earlier.[7,90]

Warfarin therapy can begin safely on an outpatient basis, provided that there is no urgent need for anticoagulation (e.g., prevention of venous thrombosis, atrial fibrillation). Given that laboratory monitoring is performed less frequently in the outpatient setting, warfarin therapy should be undertaken a bit more cautiously. In most circumstances, the initial dose should not exceed the anticipated maintenance dose. Older patients (age > 65 years) and those taking potentially interacting medications should be started on a 2-mg or 2.5-mg dose. The response to therapy should be measured every 3 to 5 days until it stabilizes.

When adjusting the dose of warfarin, the clinician should allow sufficient time for changes in the INR to occur.[7] In general, dose changes should not be made more frequently than every 3 days. Doses should be adjusted by calculating the weekly dose and reducing or increasing the weekly dose by 5% to 25%. The effect of a small dose change may not become evident for 5 to 7 days. Patients should not have follow-up prothrombin time tests sooner than anticipated changes are likely to occur.

Therapeutic Monitoring

The recommended target INR and goal range is based on the therapeutic indication (see Table 19–16).[6] For most indications, the target INR is 2.5 with an acceptable range of 2.0–3.0. The target INR is higher for patients with mechanical prosthetic heart valves (target INR = 3.0, range 2.5–3.5). A baseline prothrombin time and CBC should be obtained prior to the initiation of warfarin therapy. In patients who have experienced an acute thromboembolic event, the prothrombin time should be measured minimally every 2 to 3 days during the first week of therapy. In this situation, UFH or LMWH therapy should be continued for at least 5 days and until the INR is within the therapeutic range for at least 2 consecutive days. The concurrent use of antithrombotic drugs with warfarin may prolong the prothrombin time slightly. Once the patient's dose response is established, an INR should be determined every 7 to 14 days until it stabilizes and optimally every 4 weeks thereafter.

At each encounter, the patient should be meticulously questioned regarding his or her medication use and symptoms related to bleeding and thromboembolic complications. Any changes in medications, including changes in dosage, or nonprescription drug and dietary supplement use should be carefully explored (see Table 19–17 and Table 19–18). Dietary intake of vitamin K-rich foods should also be evaluated (see Table 19–19).

Anticoagulation therapy management services can improve the care of patients who take oral anticoagulation therapy by providing structured, comprehensive patient education and evaluation.[7] When staffed by experienced and knowledgeable practitioners, anticoagulation management services improve the safety and effectiveness of warfarin therapy.[9,91] Data also suggest that these specialized patient management services reduce the overall cost of care by reducing the frequency of major bleeding and recurrent thromboembolic events.[9,92]

Portable prothrombin time monitoring devices have revolutionized patient management. Not only do these devices permit clinicians to do "real-time" therapeutic drug monitoring, but also they enable patients to test themselves at home.[91,93] Self-monitoring, in its simplest form, requires the patient to report the test results to a health care professional. In such arrangements, the clinician continues to make warfarin dosing decisions. Highly motivated and sophisticated patients can learn to manage themselves and to independently alter the dose of warfarin based on their INR results. Patients who engage in INR self-monitoring and warfarin self-management report high levels of satisfaction with care and maintain the INR within the therapeutic range more frequently than those managed by "usual care." Home INR testing and self-management are clearly not for everyone, however. Such an approach requires careful patient selection and considerable education. Unfortunately, prothrombin time monitoring systems remain relatively expensive and are rarely covered by medical insurance.

Adverse Effects

Warfarin's primary adverse effect is bleeding. Hemorrhagic complications, ranging from mild to severe and life-threatening, can occur at any site in the body. Although warfarin is not believed to cause bleeding per se, it can "unmask" an existing lesion or enable a massive hemorrhage from an ordinarily minor bleeding source. The gastrointestinal tract is the most frequent site of bleeding. Bruising on the arms and legs is commonplace, but a painful hematoma may necessitate the temporary discontinuation of therapy. Intracranial hemorrhage is the most serious and feared complication related to warfarin therapy, as it often results in permanent disability or death.

The annual incidence of major bleeding ranges from 1% in highly selected patient populations who are carefully managed to greater than 10% in patients who are managed by primary care physicians, according to some studies.[7,9] There are no universally accepted criteria for defining a bleeding event as major or minor. Most studies have defined major bleeding as any bleeding event that warrants hospitalization, requires transfusion of 2 units of whole blood or plasma, or leads to a greater than 2 percentage point drop in hematocrit. Bleeding that does not meet the criteria for a major hemorrhage is considered to be a

TABLE 19–18. Potential Warfarin Interactions with Herbal and Nutritional Products

Increased Anticoagulation Effect (⇑ INR)	Decreased Anticoagulation Effect (⇓ INR)	Possible Increase in Bleeding Risk	
Danshen	Coenzyme Q_{10}	Angelica root	Ginkgo
Devil's claw	Ginseng	Amica flower	Horse chestnut
Dong quai	Green tea	Anise	Licorice root
Papain		Asafoetida	Lovage root
Vitamin E		Bogbean	Meadowsweet
		Borage seed oil	Onion
		Bromelain	Parsley
		Capsicum	Passionflower herb
		Celery	Poplar
		Chamomile	Quassia
		Clove	Red clover
		Fenugreek	Rue
		Feverfew	Sweet clover
		Garlic	Tumeric
		Ginger	Willow bark

INR = international normalized ratio.
From Ref. 101.

TABLE 19–19. Vitamin K Content of Select Foods[a]

Very High (>200 μg)	High (100–200 μg)	Medium (50–100 μg)	Low (<50 μg)
Brussels sprouts	Basil	Apple, green	Apple, red
Chick pea	Broccoli	Asparagus	Avocado
Collard greens	Canola oil	Cabbage	Beans
Coriander	Chive	Cauliflower	Breads, grains
Endive	Coleslaw	Mayonnaise	Carrot
Kale	Cucumber (w/peel)	Nuts, pistachio	Celery
Lettuce, red leaf	Green onion/scallion	Squash, summer	Cereal
Liver	Lettuce, butterhead		Coffee
Parsley	Mustard greens		Corn
Spinach	Soybean oil		Cucumber (w/o peel)
Swiss chard			Dairy products
Tea, black			Eggs
Tea, green			Fruit (varies)
Turnip greens			Lettuce, iceberg
Watercress			Meats, fish, poultry
			Pasta
			Peanuts
			Peas
			Potato
			Rice
			Tomato

[a]Approximate amount of vitamin K per 100 g (3.5-oz.) serving.
From Ref. 99.

minor bleeding episode. Minor bleeding is very common. Few studies have prospectively evaluated the incidence of minor bleeding, but it is likely to be greater than 15% annually even in the most expertly managed patients.

Several risk factors for bleeding among patients receiving anticoagulation therapy have been identified (see Table 19–11).[5,94] The intensity of anticoagulation therapy appears to be the most powerful risk factor. Patients whose target INR is greater than 3.0 have twice the incidence of major bleeding than do those with a goal range of 2.0–3.0. The risk of intracranial hemorrhage increases significantly when the INR is greater than 4.0. Patients given very low intensity warfarin therapy (goal INR, 1.3–1.9) have a negligible risk of bleeding. Wide variability in the anticoagulation response, as seen in patients with very unstable INR values, also appears to be associated with an increased risk of bleeding. The risk of hemorrhage is greatest during the first few weeks of therapy; however, bleeding can occur at any time, and the cumulative incidence steadily increases over time.

Nonhemorrhagic adverse effects associated with warfarin are uncommon, but can be serious when they do occur.[95] The "purple toe syndrome," manifested as a purplish discoloration of the toes, is an extremely rare event reported in only a handful of patients who have taken warfarin. The etiology of this unusual phenomenon is unknown, but it is thought to be the result of cholesterol microembolization into the arterial circulation of the toe. Warfarin-induced skin necrosis is an uncommon, but very serious dermatologic reaction that is manifested by a painful maculopapular rash and ecchymosis or purpura that subsequently progresses to necrotic gangrene. It appears most frequently in areas of the body rich in subcutaneous fat, such as the breasts, thighs, buttocks, and abdomen. The incidence of warfarin-induced skin necrosis is less than 0.1%. It occurs most commonly in middle-aged women who are being treated for acute venous thrombosis. Although symptoms generally appear during the first week of therapy, it has been reported in a small number of patients who had taken warfarin for months and even years.

The pathogenesis of warfarin-induced skin necrosis is not clearly understood. Many believe that imbalances between procoagulant and anticoagulant proteins early in the course of warfarin therapy result in capillary thrombosis and secondary hemorrhages. The observation that patients with a deficiency in either protein C or protein S appear to be at greater risk for warfarin-induced skin necrosis further supports this theory. Warfarin-induced necrosis has also been reported in patients with other disorders of hypercoagulability, such as antithrombin deficiency and those with antiphospholipid antibodies. Patients who receive large "loading" doses of warfarin may also be at greater risk. It is strongly recommended that heparin therapy be overlapped for a minimum of 7 days when warfarin therapy is initiated in any patient who may have a hypercoagulable state or who has a strong family history of venous thrombosis. If the diagnosis of skin necrosis is suspected, warfarin therapy should be immediately discontinued, vitamin K administered, and full-dose UFH or LMWH therapy initiated. Warfarin therapy should be restarted with extreme caution in patients with a history of skin necrosis, if at all.

Gastrointestinal side effects of warfarin therapy are uncommon and usually self-limited. Because warfarin interferes with vitamin K metabolism, there has been some theoretical concern that it may adversely affect bone formation and cause osteoporosis with long-term use.[96] To date, the association between warfarin and osteoporosis is inconclusive, and the risk of fracture appears to be negligible.

Management of Bleeding and Excessive Anticoagulation

Specific recommendations for the management of patients with an elevated INR are published by the American College of Chest Physicians (ACCP) Consensus Conference on Antithrombotic Therapy (Fig. 19–9).[7] Patients with a mildly elevated INR (3.5–5.0) should be examined for signs and symptoms of bleeding, as well as for risk factors that increase bleeding risk. In this circumstance, either reducing the dose of warfarin or holding one dose will safely manage most

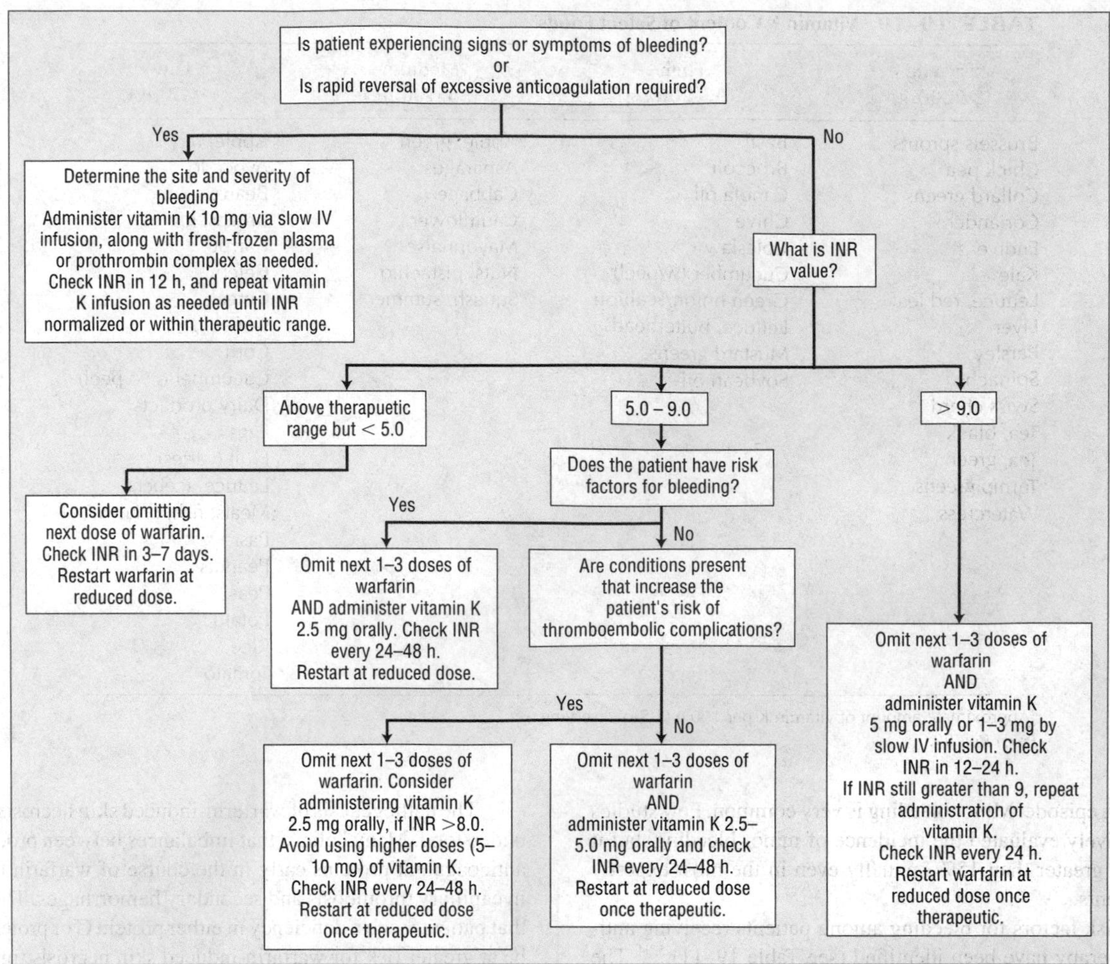

FIGURE 19–9. Management of an elevated international normalized ratio (INR). Dose reductions should be made by determining the weekly warfarin dose and reducing the weekly dose by 10% to 25% based on degree of INR elevation. See Table 19–11 for risk factors for major bleeding. Conditions that increase the risk of thromboembolic complications include history of hypercoagulability disorders (e.g., protein C or S deficiency, presence of antiphospholipid antibodies, antithrombin deficiency, Activated Protein C resistance); arterial or venous thrombosis within the previous month; thromboembolism associated with malignancy; mechanical mitral valve in conjunction with atrial fibrillation, previous stroke, poor ventricular function, or coexisting mechanical aortic valve.

patients. When a swift reduction in an elevated INR is required, the oral or parenteral administration of vitamin K_1 (phytonadione) can be given.[7,97] In the absence of major bleeding, the oral route of administration is preferred. Although the IV route produces the most rapid reversal of anticoagulation, it has been associated with anaphylactoid reactions. If the INR is 5–9, a low dose of oral vitamin K (2.5 mg) should be given. If the INR is greater than 9, a 5-mg oral dose is usually sufficient. Low doses of vitamin K consistently reduce the INR within 12 to 24 hours without making the patient's INR subtherapeutic. If needed, additional doses can be given. High doses of vitamin K (e.g., 10 mg) administered IV have been associated with prolonged resistance to warfarin therapy. In the event of serious or life-threatening bleeding, vitamin K should be administered IV, together with fresh-frozen plasma or clotting factor concentrates.

Drug and Food Interactions

The pharmacokinetic and pharmacodynamic properties of warfarin, coupled with its narrow therapeutic index, predispose this agent to numerous clinically important food and drug interactions (see Tables 19–17, 19–18, and 19–19).[6,98,99] Vitamin K can reverse warfarin's pharmacologic activity, and many foods contain sufficient vitamin K to reduce the anticoagulation effect of warfarin if a patient consumes them in large portions or repetitively in a short period of time.[99] Patients should be given a list of vitamin K-rich foods and instructed to maintain a relatively consistent intake. It is important to stress consistency and moderation rather than absolute abstinence. Abrupt changes in vitamin K intake should always be suspected when unexplained changes in the INR occur. Alternative sources of vitamin K, such as multivitamins and nutritional supplements (e.g., Sustical, Ensure), should also be considered. Patients who require parenteral nutrition should not receive a weekly bolus dose of vitamin K if they are taking warfarin therapy.

Pharmacokinetic drug interactions with warfarin are due primarily to alterations in its hepatic metabolism or binding to plasma proteins.[100] As noted earlier (see Pharmacology/Pharmacokinetics), commercially available warfarin is a racemic mixture of R and S isomers. Drugs that inhibit or induce the isoenzymes that metabolize these isomers have the greatest potential to significantly alter the response to warfarin therapy. Protein-binding displacement interactions can also occur. However, in the absence of hepatic disease or a diminished capacity to metabolize warfarin, changes in protein binding result in only transient changes in the INR. Drugs that alter hemostasis, platelet function, or the production of clotting factors can alter the response to warfarin therapy or increase the risk of bleeding by pharmacodynamic mechanisms.

The explosive increase in the use of herbal and alternative therapies in North America has raised concern regarding their potential to affect warfarin therapy.[101] Although there are a growing number of case reports and some *in vivo* data, the clinical importance of specific warfarin-herbal interactions remains unclear. All patients on warfarin therapy should be questioned regarding the use of herbal drugs and dietary supplements. Clinicians should advise patients on warfarin therapy to seek information about potential interactions with warfarin whenever they start to take a new drug product, whether it is prescribed or purchased over the counter. If there is a known drug interaction or doubt about its potential to alter the response to warfarin, more frequent prothrombin time testing following the initiation of the new agent is prudent.

Use in Special Populations

In the absence of a clear and compelling indication, warfarin should not be used during pregnancy because of the potential for fetal hemorrhage and teratogenic complications.[56] Warfarin crosses the placenta and has been associated with several embryopathies, particularly CNS abnormalities, which have occurred throughout gestation. The FDA has designated warfarin a pregnancy category X agent. As they are large molecules that do not cross the placental barrier, UFH and the LMWHs are considered the drugs of choice for anticoagulation therapy during pregnancy. Warfarin is excreted into the breast milk in very low concentrations and is generally considered safe for use by women who are breastfeeding.

Warfarin use among elderly patients is increasingly common. Although the drug has been extensively studied in this population, some debate still remains regarding the relative risks of warfarin therapy in the elderly.[5,94] Data supporting the notion that older age increases hemorrhagic risk are somewhat conflicting. Age greater than 75 years has been associated with an increased risk of intracranial hemorrhage, but the overall incidence of major bleeding is similar to that among younger users. Elderly patients may be more likely to be excessively anticoagulated because of nutritional deficiencies, comorbidities, and multiple drug interactions. Furthermore, they are often at greater risk of falls. Although they often derive the greatest benefit from anticoagulation therapy, elderly patients should be monitored with greater vigilance, and warfarin dosing changes should be made more cautiously.

PREVENTION OF VTE

Given that VTE is often clinically silent and potentially fatal, strategies to prevent DVT in at-risk populations will have the greatest impact on patient outcomes.[15,102] To rely on the early diagnosis and treatment of VTE is unacceptable, because many patients will die before treatment can be initiated. Furthermore, even clinically silent disease may lead to long-term morbidity from the post-thrombotic syndrome and predisposes the patient to future thromboembolic events.[33] Despite an immense body of literature that overwhelmingly supports the widespread use of pharmacologic and nonpharmacologic strategies to prevent VTE, prophylaxis is underused in most hospitals.[15,103] Even when prophylaxis is given, it is less than optimal for many patients who receive it. Educational programs and clinical decision support systems have been shown to improve the appropriate use of VTE prevention methods.[15,104]

The goal of an effective VTE prophylaxis program is to identify all patients at risk, determine each patient's level of risk, select and implement regimens that provide sufficient protection for the level of risk, and avoid or limit complications from the selected regimens. As hospitalized patients are frequently at high risk for VTE, screening all patients prior to or at the time of admission to determine their level of risk is the first step in an effective prophylaxis program. The risk classification criteria and recommended prophylaxis strategies promulgated by the ACCP Consensus Conference on Antithrombotic Therapy are widely used in North America (Table 19–20).[15] Several pharmacologic and nonpharmacologic methods are highly effective for preventing VTE (Table 19–21), and these can be used alone or in combination. Nonpharmacologic methods improve venous blood flow by mechanical means, while drug therapy counteracts the propensity for thrombosis formation by dampening the coagulation cascade.

Resumption of ambulation as soon as possible following surgery has been shown to reduce the incidence of VTE in low-risk patients.[15] Walking increases venous blood flow and promotes the flow of natural antithrombotic factors into the lower extremities.[105] During prolonged surgeries, electrical calf muscle stimulation devices that mimic the pumping action produced during ambulation can be beneficial.[15] Although these devices can reduce the risk of DVT by more than 50%, their use is painful, and they can be used only when the patient is under general anesthesia. Continuous passive motion devices and plantar compression systems are also available, but their effectiveness is not certain.[106]

Graduated compression stockings reduce the incidence of VTE by approximately 60% following general surgery, neurosurgery, and stroke.[107–109] Compression stockings work by increasing the velocity of venous blood flow. They apply a graded amount of pressure, with the greatest amount of pressure applied at the ankle. Inexpensive and safe, they are an excellent choice when pharmacologic interventions are either contraindicated or difficult to monitor adequately. When combined with pharmacologic interventions, graduated compression stockings have an additive effect.[15] Some patients are unable to wear compression stockings because of the size or shape of their legs, however.

Like graduated compression stockings, intermittent pneumatic compression (IPC) devices increase the velocity of blood flow in the lower extremities.[15,110,111] The technique involves the sequential inflation of a series of cuffs wrapped around the patient's legs. Using graded pressure, the cuffs inflate in 1- to 2-minute cycles continually throughout the day from the ankles to the thighs. IPC has been shown to reduce the risk of VTE by more than 60% following general surgery, neurosurgery, and orthopedic surgery.[15] There is some theoretical concern that external compression may dislodge a previously formed clot.[112] If a patient has been immobile for several days prior to the initiation of IPC, it is recommended that an objective noninvasive test be performed to rule out the presence of a large proximal vein thrombus. Although IPC is well tolerated and safe to use in patients who have contraindications to pharmacologic therapies, it does have a few drawbacks. It is more expensive than the use of graduated compression stockings, it is a relatively cumbersome technique, and some patients may have difficulty sleeping while using it.[15] Like graduated compression hose, IPC can increase the effectiveness of pharmacologic prophylaxis.

Inferior vena cava (IVC) filters, also known as Greenfield filters, provide short-term protection against pulmonary embolism

TABLE 19–20. Venous Thromboembolism (VTE) Risk Classification and Recommended Prophylaxis Strategies

Level of Risk	Calf Vein Thrombosis (%)	Symptomatic PE (%)	Fatal PE (%)	Effective Prevention Strategies
Low				
Minor surgery, age <40 years, and no clinical risk factors	2	0.2	0.002	Ambulation
Moderate				
Major or minor surgery, age 40–60 years, and no clinical risk factors Major surgery, age <40 years, and no clinical risk factors Minor surgery, with clinical risk factor(s) Acutely ill (e.g., MI, ischemic stroke, CHF exacerbation), and no clinical risk factors	10–20	1–2	0.1–0.4	LDUFH (5,000 units q 12 hours) LMWH IPC Graduated compression stockings
High				
Major surgery, age >60 years, and no clinical risk factors Major surgery, age 40–60 years, with clinical risk factor(s) Acutely ill (e.g., MI, ischemic stroke, CHF exacerbation), with risk factor(s)	20–40	2–4	0.4–1.0	LDUFH (5,000 units q 8 hours) LMWH IPC
Highest				
Major lower extremity, orthopedic surgery Hip fracture Multiple trauma Major surgery, age >40 years, and prior history of VTE Major surgery, age >40 years, and malignancy Major surgery, age >40 years, and hypercoagulable state Spinal cord injury or stroke with limb paralysis	40–80	4–10	0.2–5	LMWH Fondaparinux Warfarin IPC with LDUFH or LMWH ADUFH

PE = pulmonary embolism; LDUFH = low-dose unfractionated heparin; LMWH = low–molecular weight heparin; IPC = intermittent pneumatic compression; MI = myocardial infarction; CHF = congestive heart failure; ADUFH = Adjusted dose unfractionated heparin.
From Ref. 15.

in very high risk patients by preventing the embolization of a thrombus formed in the lower extremities into the pulmonary circulation.[15,113,114] Percutaneous insertion of a filter into the IVC is a minimally invasive procedure performed via fluoroscopy. Despite the widespread use of IVC filters, there are very limited data regarding their effectiveness and long-term safety. The evidence suggests that IVC filters, particularly in the absence of effective antithrombotic therapy, increase the long-term risk of recurrent DVT. In the

TABLE 19–21. Comparative Efficacy of Pharmacologic Strategies to Prevent Venous Thromboembolism: Reduction in Relative Risk of Deep Vein Thrombosis

Drug	General Surgery	Post–MI	Ischemic Stroke	Hip Replacement	Knee Replacement
Aspirin	20%			26%	13%
LDUFH	68%	71%	56%	45%	33%
Warfarin				59%	27%
LMWHs	76%		58%	70%	52%
Danaparoid			82%	71%	
ADUFH		86%		74%	

MI = myocardial infarction; LDUFH = low-dose unfractionated heparin; LMWHs = low–molecular weight heparins; ADUFH = adjusted-dose unfractionated heparin, subcutaneous or intravenous.
From Ref. 15.

only randomized clinical trial examining the short- and long-term effectiveness of the filters in patients with a documented proximal DVT, treatment with IVC filters in combination with anticoagulation therapy reduced the risk of pulmonary embolism by more than 75% during the first 12 days following insertion.[114] However, this benefit was not sustained during 2 years of follow-up, and the long-term risk of recurrent DVT was nearly twofold higher in those who received a filter. Although IVC filters can reduce the short-term risk of pulmonary embolism in patients at highest risk, they should be reserved for patients in whom other prophylactic strategies are not feasible. Further, to reduce the long-term risk of VTE in association with IVC filters, pharmacologic prophylaxis is necessary, and warfarin therapy should begin as soon as the patient is able to tolerate it.

Several pharmacologic interventions to prevent VTE have been extensively evaluated in numerous randomized clinical trials.[15] Appropriately selected drug therapies can dramatically reduce the incidence of VTE following hip replacement, knee replacement, general surgery, myocardial infarction, and ischemic stroke (Table 19–22). The choice of agent and dose to use for VTE prevention must be based on the patient's level of risk for thrombosis and bleeding complications, as well as on the cost and the availability of an adequate drug therapy monitoring system.

Although a meta-analysis by the Antiplatelet Trialists' Collaboration challenges this view, most randomized controlled trials fail to show a significant benefit from aspirin therapy in the prevention of VTE.[15,115] The ACCP Consensus Conference continues to recommend against the use of aspirin as the primary method of VTE prophylaxis. Antiplatelet drugs clearly reduce the risk of coronary artery and cerebrovascular events in patients with arterial disease, but aspirin produces a very modest reduction in VTE following orthopedic surgeries of the lower extremities. The relative contribution of platelets in the pathogenesis of venous thrombosis compared with that of arterial thrombosis can explain the reason for this difference. Venous thrombosis results primarily from venous stasis, while arterial thrombosis is most often the result of vascular wall injury.

Previously in wide use, dextran has been largely abandoned for the prevention of VTE because of perceptions that it is only modestly effective and has a high potential for adverse effects.[15] Dextrans are large molecules with a molecular weight of 40,000 to 70,000 daltons that are believed to produce an antithrombotic effect by interfering with platelet aggregation and fibrin polymerization. In clinical trials, dextran 70 reduced the risk of DVT following hip replacement by approximately 40%. Although less effective for the prevention of DVT when compared with other pharmacologic choices, dextran 70 appears to have a more favorable impact on the incidence of pulmonary embolism. Unfortunately, dextran is costly, requires IV administration, may cause volume overload and pulmonary congestion in patients with renal insufficiency and poor cardiac reserve, and may provoke allergic reactions, including anaphylaxis. For these reasons, dextran is no longer considered the best choice for most patients who require VTE prophylaxis.

The most extensively studied agents for the prevention of VTE are UFH, the LMWHs, and fondaparinux.[15,70a,70b] Danaparoid has also been studied in several high-risk populations. The LMWHs, fondaparinux, and danaparoid provide superior protection against VTE when compared with low dose UFH.[15,116,117] Their more predictable

TABLE 19–22. Dosing of Antithrombotic Drugs for the Prevention of Venous Thromboembolism

Drug	Level of Risk/Indication	Dose, Route, and Initiation Time
LDUFH	Moderate risk—general surgery or medical conditions	5,000 units q 12 h, SC, started 1–2 before surgery or as soon as possible
	High risk—general surgery or medical conditions	5,000 units q 8 h, SC, started 1–2 h before surgery or as soon as possible
ADUFH	Highest risk—total hip replacement	3,500 units q 8 h, SC, started 1–2 h before surgery and adjusted by +/−500 units/dose to maintain a high-normal aPTT drawn 4–6 h post dose
Dalteparin	Moderate risk—general surgery or medical conditions	2,500 units q 24 h, SC, started before surgery or as soon as possible
	High and highest risk—general or orthopedic surgery	5,000 units q 24 h, SC, started before surgery or 12–24 h after surgery
Enoxaparin	Moderate risk—general surgery or medical conditions	20–40 mg q 24 h, SC, started before surgery or as soon as possible
	High risk—general surgery or medical conditions	40 mg q 24 h, SC, started before surgery or 12–24 h after surgery
	Highest risk—orthopedic surgery, multiple trauma, spinal cord injury	30 mg q 12 h, SC, started before surgery or 12–24 h after surgery or 12–36 h after injury
Tinzaparin	Moderate risk—general surgery or medical conditions	3,500 units q 24 h, SC, started 1–2 h before surgery or as soon as possible
	High and highest risk—general surgery, orthopedic surgery	75 units/kg q 24 h, SC, started 1–2 h before surgery or 12–24 h after surgery
Danaparoid	High and highest risk—general surgery, orthopedic surgery, or medical conditions	750 units q 12 h, SC, started 1–2 h before surgery or as soon as possible
Fondaparinux	Highest risk—orthopedic surgery	2.5 mg q 12 h, SC, started 6 h after surgery
Warfarin	Highest risk—orthopedic surgery	5 mg q 24 h, orally, started on the day of or after surgery and adjusted to maintain an INR = 2.0–3.0

LDUFH = low dose unfractionated heparin; SC = subcutaneous; ADUFH = adjusted-dose unfractionated heparin; aPTT = activated partial thromboplastin time; INR = international normalized ratio.

absorption when given by subcutaneous injection may be the explanation. Even so, UFH remains a highly effective, cost-conscious choice for many patient populations, provided that it is given in the appropriate dose (Table 19–22). Low-dose UFH (5,000 units every 12 hours or every 8 hours) given subcutaneously has been shown to reduce the risk of VTE by 55% to 70% in patients undergoing a wide range of general surgical procedures and following a myocardial infarction or stroke. For the prevention of VTE following hip and knee replacement surgery, the effectiveness of low-dose UFH is considerably lower.[15,118] Adjusted-dose heparin therapy provided subcutaneously, which requires dose adjustments to maintain the aPTT at the high end of the normal range, appears to be substantially more effective in the highest risk patient populations.[119] However, adjusted-dose heparin has been studied in only a few relatively small clinical trials and requires frequent laboratory monitoring.[15] The LMWHs and danaparoid appear to provide a high degree of protection against VTE in most high-risk populations. The appropriate prophylactic dose for each LMWH product is indication-specific. There is no evidence that one LMWH is superior to another for the prevention of VTE. Fondaparinux was significantly more effective than enoxaparin in several clinical trials that enrolled patients undergoing high risk orthopedic procedures but has not been shown to reduce the incidence of symptomatic pulmonary embolism or mortality.[70a,70b] To provide optimal protection, some experts believe that LMWHs should be initiated prior to surgery.[15,120]

Warfarin is a commonly used option for the prevention of VTE following orthopedic surgeries of the lower extremities.[15,121] The evidence is equivocal regarding the relative effectiveness of warfarin compared with that of the LMWHs for the prevention of clinically important VTE events in the highest risk populations.[15,122] When used to prevent VTE, the dose of warfarin must be adjusted to maintain an INR between 2.0 and 3.0. Oral administration and low drug cost give warfarin some advantages over the LMWHs and fondaparinux. However, warfarin does not achieve its full antithrombotic effect for several days, requires frequent monitoring and periodic dosage adjustments, and carries a substantial risk of major bleeding. For these reasons, warfarin is reserved for the highest risk patients. Furthermore, warfarin should be recommended only when a well developed monitoring system is available.[7,123]

The optimal duration for VTE prophylaxis is not well established.[15] Prophylaxis should be given throughout the period of risk. For general surgical procedures and medical conditions, once the patient is able to ambulate regularly and other risk factors are no longer present, prophylaxis can be discontinued. Because of the relatively high incidence of VTE in the first month following hospital discharge among patients who have undergone a lower extremity orthopedic procedure, extended prophylaxis following hospital discharge with either an LMWH or warfarin appears to be beneficial. Most, but not all, clinical trials support the use of antithrombotic therapy for 21 to 35 days following total hip and knee replacement surgeries.[124–126]

Only a handful of studies have formally evaluated the cost-effectiveness of VTE prevention strategies. The acquisition costs of graduated compression stockings, heparin, and warfarin are considerably less than those of the LMWHs, danaparoid, and fondaparinux. However, the acquisition cost for drug therapy is relatively small when compared with the overall cost of care. Economic analyses must take into account the efficacy of the strategy, treatment complications, and monitoring costs.

The determination of the cost-effectiveness of VTE prophylaxis is based on the premise that a reduction in future VTE events will reduce future costs.[127] Furthermore, the incremental cost per patient will decrease proportionally with an increase in the frequency of VTE in the population. Stated another way, the cost of providing prophylaxis to 1,000 patients will decline as the incidence of VTE in the given population increases. More expensive and effective strategies, therefore, become more cost-effective in higher risk populations. In populations at low risk for VTE, early ambulation appears to be the most cost-effective strategy. In populations at moderate risk, the use of graduated compression stockings, the least expensive intervention, results in a lower overall cost of care when compared with no prophylaxis.[127] The administration of low-dose UFH, together with IPC, slightly increases the overall cost, but these prophylactic strategies result in fewer VTE events and deaths. The use of low-dose heparin in moderate VTE risk populations is estimated to cost an additional $50,000 (US$ 1990) per 1,000 patients when compared with no prophylaxis.[127,128] This compares favorably with the incremental costs associated with other routinely employed preventive measures. Although the LMWHs provide slightly greater reductions in the risk of VTE, the additional cost per 1,000 patients who are at moderate risk of VTE is estimated to be $107,000 (US$ 1999) when compared with the cost of low-dose UFH.[129] Whether universal use of LMWHs in moderate-risk patients is a cost-effective strategy remains controversial.

In high-risk patients, the cost-effectiveness of prevention is far greater because the incidence of VTE is higher. Following hip replacement surgery, regardless of the strategy selected, prophylaxis saves money when compared with no prophylaxis.[130] The LMWHs slightly increase the total mean cost of care after total hip and knee replacement when compared with low-dose UFH and warfarin.[131] However, because of their superior effectiveness, the LMWHs have a significantly lower cost per DVT and pulmonary embolism avoided.[118,131–133] As determined by typical drug acquisition costs, the LMWHs appear to be a cost-effective choice in the highest risk patient populations. To date, no formal pharmacoeconomic analysis has been performed comparing fondaparinux to other pharmacological strategies.

GENERAL APPROACH TO THE TREATMENT OF VTE

Anticoagulation therapy remains the mainstay of treatment for VTE. Full "therapeutic" doses of antithrombotic drugs not only prevent thrombus extension and embolization, but also reduce the risk of long-term sequelae such as the post-thrombotic syndrome and recurrent thromboembolism.[90,134] The standard approach is to initiate therapy with UFH by continuous IV infusion or an LMWH by subcutaneous injection and to make the transition to an oral anticoagulant for maintenance therapy (Fig. 19–10). In some circumstances, elimination of the obstructing thrombus is warranted, and venous thrombectomy or thrombolysis can be considered.[3,39,90,135,136] Interruption of the IVC with a filter is also an option in some patients who have contraindications to anticoagulation therapy.

The parenteral administration of UFH followed by warfarin has been the conventional treatment of patients with VTE for more than 40 years.[90,134] Although UFH can be given by either subcutaneous or IV injection, continuous IV infusion is preferable because of improved dosing precision and a lower risk of major bleeding. The aPTT or a suitable coagulation study should be used to monitor the effect of UFH. The infusion rate should be adjusted to maintain an appropriate therapy range corresponding to a heparin concentration of 0.2–0.4 units/mL or an anti-factor Xa level of 0.3–0.7 units/mL. Weight-based dosing of UFH achieves a therapeutic aPTT in the vast majority of patients in the first 24 hours (see Table 19–9). Failure to achieve a therapeutic aPTT in the first 24 hours increases the risk of thromboembolic recurrence.[49,90]

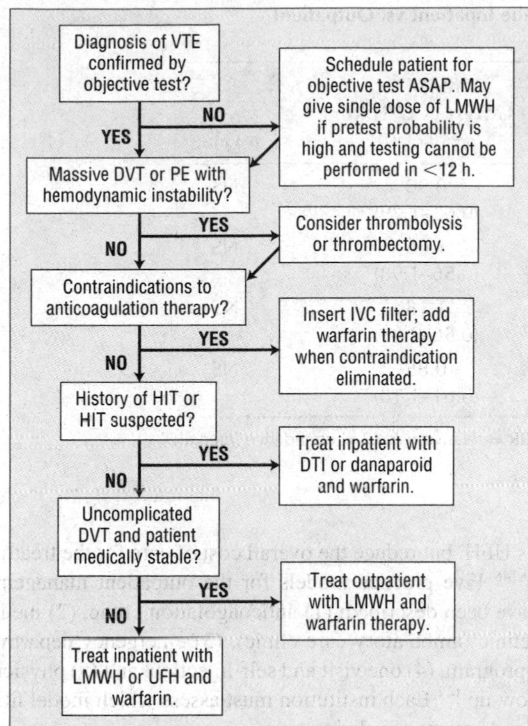

FIGURE 19–10. Treatment of venous thromboembolism (VTE). ASAP = as soon as possible; LMWH = low-molecular weight heparin; DVT = deep vein thrombosis; PE = pulmonary embolism; IVC = inferior vena cava; HIT = heparin-induced thrombocytopenia; DTI = direct thrombin inhibitor; UFH = unfractionated heparin.

Because of their improved pharmacokinetic profile and ease of use, the LMWHs have incrementally replaced UFH in the treatment of VTE in many institutions. Warfarin is an unacceptable choice for the acute treatment of VTE because it does not produce a rapid anticoagulation effect and is associated with a high incidence of recurrent thromboembolism.[134] However, warfarin is very effective in the long-term management of VTE and should begin concurrently with UFH or LMWH therapy. The LMWH or UFH should overlap with warfarin therapy for at least 5 days and until a therapeutic INR has been achieved.[90] The initial dose of warfarin should be 5–10 mg, and the dose should be periodically adjusted to achieve an INR of 2.0–3.0. Warfarin should be continued for at least 3 months. However, the optimal duration of treatment for patients with VTE remains unclear.[1,90] A shorter duration (e.g., 6 weeks) may be adequate for some patients who suffer a postoperative DVT and who have no other risk factors for VTE. Patients with an idiopathic first episode VTE should be treated for at least 6 months. A longer duration (e.g., greater than 1 year) is recommended in those patients who have persistent risk factors, a hypercoagulability disorder, or who suffer a recurrent VTE event.

The LMWHs have now become widely accepted alternatives to UFH for the treatment of DVT with or without pulmonary embolism. The LMWHs given subcutaneously are at least as effective as UFH given IV in the treatment of VTE.[61,90] For the treatment of DVT, the efficacy and safety of ardeparin, dalteparin, enoxaparin, nadroparin, reviparin, and tinzaparin have been well established in numerous clinical trials. Their efficacy and safety in pulmonary embolism has also been well studied.[137–139]

A number of meta-analyses comparing LMWHs to UFH in the treatment of VTE have demonstrated no differences in clinically important end points, including recurrent VTE, pulmonary embolism, major or minor bleeding, and thrombocytopenia.[61,62,140] Surprisingly, patients who received a LMWH have a significantly lower mortality rate (Table 19–23).[61,62] The reduction in mortality was seen primarily in patients with cancer.[61,141] The explanation for this survival advantage in unknown, but studies are under way to further examine this finding.[27,28,90] There appears to be no difference in the risk of recurrent VTE between patients who are treated on an inpatient basis and those treated on an outpatient basis with an LMWH for DVT.[62] However, inpatient treatment was associated with a lower risk of major bleeding (Table 19–24). There appears to be no difference in the efficacy or safety of once-daily versus twice-daily dosing regimens (Table 19–25).[62,142]

OUTPATIENT MANAGEMENT OF DVT WITH LMWHs

Given the predictable response and the reduced need for laboratory monitoring with the LMWHs, selected patients with lower extremity DVT who have no other comorbid conditions requiring hospitalization can be discharged early from the hospital or treated entirely on an outpatient basis (Table 19–26).[143,144] The efficacy and safety of

TABLE 19–23. Meta-Analysis Comparing LMWHs to UFH in the Acute Treatment of Venous Thromboembolism (VTE)

Outcome	LMWH Events (%)	UFH Events (%)	RR (95% CI)	p Value
Recurrent VTE	4.3	5.1	0.85 (0.65–1.12)	NS
Pulmonary embolism	1.9	1.8	1.02 (0.64–1.62)	NS
Total mortality	4.9	6.5	0.76 (0.59–0.98)	NS
Major bleeding	1.5	2.6	0.63 (0.37–1.05)	NS
Minor bleeding	5.6	4.7	1.18 (0.87–1.61)	NS
Thrombocytopenia	1.0	1.3	0.85 (0.45–1.62)	NS

LMWH = low-molecular weight heparin; UFH = unfractionated heparin; RR = relative risk; CI = confidence interval; p value = probability; NS = not significant.
From Ref. 62.

TABLE 19–24. Meta-Analysis Comparing LMWHs to UFH in the Inpatient vs. Outpatient Management of Venous Thromboembolism (VTE)

Outcome	Inpatient LMWH vs UFH RR (95% CI)	p Value	Outpatient LMWH vs UFH RR (95% CI)	p Value
Recurrent VTE	0.80 (0.53–1.19)	NS	0.90 (0.63–1.29)	NS
Pulmonary embolism	0.97 (0.49–1.94)	NS	1.06 (0.56–1.98)	NS
Major bleeding	0.40 (0.21–0.76)	<0.01	1.18 (0.56–2.49)	NS
Total mortality	0.63 (0.42–0.95)	NS	0.85 (0.61–1.18)	NS

LMWH = low-molecular weight heparin; UFH = unfractionated heparin; RR = relative risk; CI = confidence interval; p value = probability; NS = not significant.
From Ref. 62.

the LMWHs in the home-based treatment of proximal DVT were initially established in two large clinical studies.[145,146] The Tasman Study was a multicenter, randomized trial comparing nadroparin administered subcutaneously at home to UFH administered IV in hospital for the treatment of proximal DVT.[145] The rate of recurrent thromboembolism was similar in each group: 6.9% in the nadroparin-treated patients and 8.6% in the UFH-treated patients ($p > 0.05$). The rate of major bleeding was slightly higher in the UFH group (2%) compared with those treated with nadroparin (0.5%). Likewise, in a similarly designed home treatment trial comparing enoxaparin to UFH, Levine and colleagues found no differences in the rate of recurrent thromboembolism (5.3% vs. 6.7%) and major bleeding (2% vs. 1.2%) between the two groups ($p > 0.05$).[146] However, the mean length of hospital stay was 1.1 days for the enoxaparin group, compared with 6.5 days for the UFH group. Additional studies have confirmed that outpatient treatment of DVT with the LMWHs is effective, well tolerated, and convenient. Patient self-administration has been shown to be as effective as nurse-administered therapy.[8,144]

A number of cost-effectiveness analyses using decision modeling suggest that the treatment of DVT with an LMWH is more cost-effective than is the treatment with UFH.[140,147] According to these decision models, the LMWHs will reduce overall health care cost if as few as 8% of patients are treated entirely on an outpatient basis or if 13% of patients are discharged from hospital early. Evidence from prospective clinical trials confirms that the LMWHs are as effective and safe as UFH, but reduce the overall cost of care for the treatment of VTE.[90,148] Five practice models for the outpatient management of DVT have been described: (1) anticoagulation clinic, (2) medical day care clinic (ambulatory care clinic), (3) emergency department fast-track program, (4) one visit and self-injection, and (5) physician-office follow-up.[149] Each institution must assess which model fits its resources and patient population best.

THROMBOLYSIS AND THROMBECTOMY

Most cases of VTE require only anticoagulation therapy. In some cases, however, removal of the occluding thrombus by either pharmacologic or surgical means may be warranted.[90,150] There is a relative paucity of data supporting either thrombolysis or thrombectomy in the management of VTE, and more study is clearly needed to clarify their precise role.[151]

Thrombolytic agents are proteolytic enzymes that enhance the conversion of plasminogen to plasmin, which subsequently degrades the fibrin matrix. Alteplase and streptokinase have been the most widely used agents in the treatment of VTE, but studies comparing their relative effectiveness and safety have not been conducted (Table 19–27). During the infusion of the thrombolytic agent, UFH or LMWH therapy should be temporarily withheld. Continuous infusion with UFH should be restarted without a bolus dose following

TABLE 19–25. Meta-Analysis Comparing Twice-Daily or Once-Daily LMWH to UFH for the Treatment of Venous Thromboembolism (VTE)

Outcome	Twice-Daily LMWH vs. UFH RR (95% CI)	p Value	Once-Daily LMWH vs. UFH RR (95% CI)	p Value
Recurrent VTE	0.84 (0.62–1.14)	NS	0.98 (0.49–1.93)	NS
PE	1.01 (0.60–1.70)	NS	1.06 (0.38–2.92)	NS
Major bleeding	0.70 (0.36–1.37)	NS	0.46 (0.20–1.07)	NS
Total mortality	0.82 (0.61–1.11)	NS	0.61 (0.37–0.99)	NS

LMWH = low-molecular weight heparin; UFH = unfractionated heparin; RR = relative risk; CI = confidence interval; p value = probability; NS = not significant.
From Ref. 62.

TABLE 19–26. Outpatient Treatment Protocol for Deep Venous Thrombosis

Eligibility (All of the following criteria must be met)

- Acute DVT is documented by ultrasonography or venography.
- Patient is otherwise healthy with no comorbid condition requiring admission or continued hospitalization.
- Patient or caregiver (or both) have the skill to inject LMWH subcutaneously at home.
- Patient has access to emergency care.
- Patient's creatinine clearance is >30 mL/min.
- Patient understands benefits and risks and agrees to outpatient therapy.

Exclusion Criteria

- Symptomatic pulmonary embolism
- Active bleeding
- Recent head trauma
- Intracranial neoplasm
- History of hemorrhagic CVA
- Arterio-venous malformation
- Uncontrolled hypertension: SBP ≥ 180 or DBP ≥ 110
- Major surgery or trauma within the past two weeks
- History of heparin-induced thrombocytopenia (HIT)
- Platelet count <100,000 per cubic milliliter (unless physician waives exclusion)
- Hypersensitivity to LMWH
- Hepatic failure
- Pregnancy
- Likelihood of poor adherence to treatment plan (e.g., substance abuse, psychiatric disorder)

Drug Dosing

- LMWH dosed by ACTUAL BODY WEIGHT every 12 hours or 24 hours (product-specific). If patient previously on intravenous UFH, infusion should be discontinued 1 hour before first injection of LMWH.
- Initiate warfarin therapy with 5 mg PO on day 1; target INR = 2.5 (range 2.0 to 3.0). Patient-specific factors favoring a lower initial dosage will be evaluated and dosage adjusted accordingly. First dose to be given no sooner than 3 hours after the first dose of LMWH. Subsequent warfarin doses to be adjusted according to INR results.
- LMWH and warfarin must overlap for a minimum of 5 days and until the patient has had 2 consecutive therapeutic INRs.

Laboratory Monitoring

- Baseline data—aPTT, PT/INR, CBC, BUN, creatinine, weight, height, and pregnancy test, if applicable—should be obtained.
- Platelet counts should be measured on the first day of LMWH treatment and on day 5. If therapy is continued beyond 7 days, platelet count should be done every other day.
- PT/INR should be obtained every 2 to 3 days after initiation of warfarin therapy until target levels of anticoagulation have been achieved, then as indicated.

Patient Activity

- The physician is to document on the order sheet the activity for the patient.

Compression Stockings

- The use of compression stockings is at the discretion of the physician.

Pain Management

- Pain medication is prescribed at the discretion of the physician (aspirin and NSAIDs are not recommended for pain management).

Patient Education

- Deep vein thrombosis (DVT) and its complications
- Treatment regimen of LMWH and warfarin (mechanism of action; dosing schedule; side effects; emergency instructions; drug/drug, drug/food interactions; over-the-counter products to avoid while on LMWH and warfarin).
- Explanation of laboratory tests and need for dose adjustment
- Demonstrated ability to correctly administer LMWH, including injection site selection, injection technique, and syringe disposal
- Activity (elevation of affected extremity, no standing or sitting for prolonged periods of time, no crossing of legs, no restrictive clothing)
- How to reduce the chance of bleeding, and how to monitor for signs and symptoms of bleeding
- Phone numbers—anticoagulation clinic, primary care physician

Patients Follow-up Visits

- Interview patient to determine medication use behavior and symptoms (e.g., improvement in DVT symptoms and absence of bleeding).
- Reinforce patient education on disease process, medications, and potential complications.
- Instruct the patients to avoid anti-inflammatory drugs or antiplatelet agents unless otherwise prescribed by the physician.
- Coordinate lab draws, interpret INR results, and write orders for warfarin dose adjustments.
- Notify the physician if signs and symptoms of recurrent DVT, PE, bleeding, or pain uncontrolled by prescribed analgesia.
- If the patient is being followed by home nursing agency, the pharmacist will work directly with the home nursing agency as needed

DVT = deep vein thrombosis; LMWH = low-molecular weight heparin; CVA = cerebrovascular accident; SBP = systolic blood pressure; DBP = diastolic blood pressure; UFH = unfractionated heparin; PO = by mouth; INR = international normalized ratio; aPTT = activated partial thromboplastin time; PT = prothrombin time; CBC = complete blood count; BUN = blood urea nitrogen [level]; NSAIDs = nonsteroidal anti-inflammatory drugs; PE = pulmonary embolism.

From Harper Hospital, Detroit Medical Center.

TABLE 19–27. Thrombolytic Regimens for the Treatment of Venous Thromboembolism

Thrombolytic	PE Treatment Dose	DVT Treatment Dose
Alteplase (t-PA)	100 mg infusion over 2 h	0.05 mg/kg/h continuous infusion over 24 h (maximum = 150 mg) or 80–100 mg infusion over 2 h
Reteplase	10 units IV bolus followed 30 min later by a second 10 units IV bolus	
Streptokinase	250,000 units bolus infusion over 30 min followed by a 100,000 units/h continuous infusion for 24 h	250,000 units bolus infusion over 30 min followed by a 100,000 units/h continuous infusion for 24–72 hours
Urokinase[a]	4,400 units/kg bolus over 10 min followed by 4,400 units/kg/h infusion for 12 h	2,000–4,400 units/kg over 10 min followed by infusion of 2,000–4,400 units/kg/h for 12–72 hours

[a]Urokinase currently unavailable in the United States.
PE = pulmonary embolism; DVT = deep vein thrombosis.

the administration of the thrombolytic when the aPTT returns to less than twice normal. UFH may be administered immediately following the completion of alteplase infusion.

Thrombolytic therapy for DVT was once believed to improve long-term outcomes by preventing the post-thrombotic syndrome.[90,150] Indeed, thrombolytic therapy has been shown to improve venous patency.[150] However, clinical trials have failed to demonstrate a substantial benefit from the routine use of thrombolytic therapy.[151] Patients with massive DVT and limb gangrene despite anticoagulation therapy are candidates for thrombolysis. Some authorities recommend thrombolytic treatment for patients with iliofemoral venous thromboembolism who present with leg pain and discoloration at rest.[150]

In the management of pulmonary embolism, alteplase, streptokinase, and urokinase have all been shown to more rapidly restore pulmonary artery patency when compared to UFH alone.[3,39,90,150] However, this early benefit does not improve long-term patient outcomes. One week following acute treatment, clot lysis and vessel patency are similar with or without thrombolytic therapy.[152] Thrombolytic therapy has never been shown to improve morbidity or mortality, but has been associated with a substantial risk of hemorrhage. Admittedly, clinical trials to date have been underpowered to detect a benefit from thrombolytic therapy. Given the relative lack of data to support their routine use, thrombolytic agents should be reserved for those patients with pulmonary embolism who are most likely to benefit. Patients who had thrombus in the right atrium or ventricle or who have hemodynamic compromise as evidenced by significant hypotension or severe right ventricular strain may benefit from thrombolytic therapy.[3,90,152]

Although it is an uncommon choice, venous thrombectomy is a reasonable approach to remove a massive obstructive thrombus in a patient with significant iliofemoral venous thrombosis, particularly if the patient is either not a candidate for or has not responded to thrombolysis.[90,135] The surgical technique has been refined over the past 20 years. The procedure uses a balloon catheter to extract the thrombus while the patient is under general anesthesia. Fluoroscopy and venography guide the procedure. Balloon angioplasty, with or without stent placement, can be used if a focal iliac vein stenosis is discovered. Full-dose anticoagulation therapy is essential during the entire operative and postoperative period. These patients still need chronic anticoagulation therapy given orally for the usual recommended duration of treatment.

TREATMENT OF DVT AND PULMONARY EMBOLISM IN SPECIAL POPULATIONS

Pediatric Patients

Anticoagulation with UFH and warfarin remains the most frequently used approach for the treatment of VTE in pediatric patients.[57] The recommended target aPTT and INR ranges, as well as the duration of therapy, are extrapolated from clinical trials in adults. The recommended initial bolus dose of UFH is 75–100 units/kg given IV over 10 minutes, followed by a maintenance infusion of 28 units/kg/h for infants 2 to 12 months of age and 20 units/kg/h for children 1 year or older. Subsequent adjustments should be made every 4 to 6 hours to maintain the aPTT within the institution-specific therapeutic range.

The usual warfarin starting dose is 0.2 mg/kg with a maximum of 10 mg.[57,153] The INR target range is 2.0–3.0. Because the LMWHs require less frequent laboratory testing, they are an attractive alternative in pediatric patients.[57] The recommended dose of enoxaparin in patients less than 1 year old is 1.5 mg/kg every 12 hours and 1 mg/kg every 12 hours in children 1 year of age or older. It is also recommended that anti-Xa activity be monitored and the dosing adjusted to maintain anti-factor Xa levels of 0.5–1.0 units/mL. Warfarin can be initiated concurrently with UFH or LMWH therapy. Therapy should be overlapped for a minimum of 5 days and until the INR is therapeutic. Warfarin should be continued for at least 3 months. Thrombolysis and thrombectomy have been successfully employed in pediatric patients, but published data are very limited.

Patients with Cancer

Several meta-analyses and one randomized clinical trial comparing LMWH with UFH for treatment of VTE have shown improved survival rates for patients with cancer who received a LMWH.[61,62,141] Although the reduction in mortality may be attributable to a decline in fatal pulmonary embolism, several other mechanisms have been postulated, including alterations in tumor angiogenesis and metastasis.[27,28] *In vitro* data suggest that small to mid-sized heparin molecules have anti-angiogenic properties. It is premature to recommend the use of LMWHs as the treatment of choice in all cancer patients with VTE because there are no published prospective, randomized trials. Several trials controlling for tumor type and stage, as well as baseline performance status, are now under way to assess this promising observation.[8]

NONPHARMACOLOGIC STRATEGIES

For patients who have contraindications to anticoagulation therapy, IVC interruption with a filter can protect against embolization of the thrombus into the pulmonary bed.[90,154] Placement of an IVC filter is also an attractive option when used concomitantly with warfarin therapy in those patients with recurrent embolism despite therapeutic anticoagulation or with a free-floating iliac vein or IVC thrombus. Another group of patients who would likely benefit from IVC interruption are patients with limited cardiorespiratory reserve for whom even a small pulmonary embolus carries a high risk of mortality. The most common reason for placing an IVC filter is a contraindication to anticoagulation therapy, such as active bleeding, recent hemorrhagic cerebrovascular accident, or an underlying bleeding diathesis. Because IVC interruption does not reduce the long-term recurrence of DVT, routine re-evaluation of the contraindications is warranted to determine when anticoagulation can be initiated.

Following the acute management of DVT, graduated compression stockings are recommended and appear to prevent the development of the post-thrombotic syndrome.[155] Fearing that a poorly adherent thrombus may embolize, some practitioners have recommended strict bedrest in the first few days following an acute event. However, there is no evidence that ambulation increases the risk of pulmonary embolism. Patients should be encouraged to ambulate as soon as they are able.

HEPARIN-INDUCED THROMBOCYTOPENIA

An uncommon, but extremely serious adverse effect associated with heparin use is HIT.[52,55] The immune-mediated platelet activation and thrombin generation seen during HIT can lead to severe and unusual thrombotic complications. Morbidity and mortality associated with HIT is disturbingly high—up to 50% of patients who develop the disorder will suffer a thrombotic complication or die within 30 days in the absence of treatment. The diagnosis of HIT is based on clinical and laboratory findings that confirm heparin-induced antibody formation and platelet activation. To prevent the thrombotic complications associated with HIT, prompt discontinuation of heparin and initiation of an alternative anticoagulant therapy is imperative.

PATHOPHYSIOLOGY OF HIT

Two types of thrombocytopenia associated with heparin use have been described.[8,55,64] As many as 25% of patients receiving heparin therapy develop a benign, mild reduction in platelet counts referred to as non-immune-mediated heparin-associated thrombocytopenia (HAT), previously called HIT type 1. Early in the course of therapy, typically between days 2 and 4, HAT produces a transient fall in platelet count. The degree of thrombocytopenia is usually mild, with platelet counts rarely going below 100,000. It is not necessary to discontinue heparin therapy in these patients, as platelet counts generally rebound to baseline values despite continued therapy. The exact mechanism of HAT is unknown; however, it may be the result of platelet aggregation, a dilutional effect, or the diminished platelet production often seen in acutely ill patients. No clinical sequelae are associated with this benign phenomenon.

The second type of thrombocytopenia associated with heparin use, known as heparin-induced thrombocytopenia (HIT), is immune-mediated.[8,52,55,64] A severe pathologic adverse effect of heparin, HIT has a significant potential to cause thrombotic complications. The time course and magnitude of thrombocytopenia associated with HIT differs from that of HAT. Platelet counts typically begin to fall after 5 or more days of continuous heparin use, most often between days 7 and 14 of therapy. The development of thrombocytopenia can be delayed up to 20 days in patients naive to heparin therapy, but can occur rapidly (24 to 48 hours) in patients with recent exposure to heparin (i.e., the past 3 months).[156] Platelet counts commonly fall below 120,000 and can nadir as low as 20,000. In some cases, overt thrombocytopenia may not occur, but a drop in platelet count greater than 50% from baseline is considered indicative of HIT.[54]

The frequency of immune-mediated HIT is most powerfully related to the duration and type of heparin used and, to a lesser extent, the dose and route of administration.[54,55] The incidence of HIT associated with full-dose UFH given IV for prolonged periods is significantly higher than that of low-dose heparin or the LMWHs given subcutaneously. The estimated overall incidence of HIT after 5 days of UFH use is 1% to 3%, but the cumulative incidence may be as high as 6% after 14 days of continuous IV use. The LMWHs are associated with a significantly lower risk of HIT (<1%).[8,63]

The pathogenesis of HIT involves an immunoglobulin-mediated response to the heparin molecule, leading to platelet activation and thrombin generation (Fig. 19–11).[52,55] With platelet activation, there is release of platelet factor-4 (PF-4) from platelet granules (see Figure 19–3). Heparin binds to PF-4, forming a negatively charged polysaccharide molecule that is highly antigenic and stimulates the production of IgG antibodies. Although heparin-induced antibody formation occurs in 10% to 20% of patients treated with heparin, the vast majority of these patients never develop HIT. In patients who develop HIT, the heparin–PF-4–IgG complexes bind to the Fc receptor on platelets, leading to further platelet activation and the release of PF-4 and procoagulant microparticles from platelet granules. In addition, PF-4 and heparin-like molecules bind to the surface of endothelial cells, resulting in antibody-induced endothelial cell damage and the release of tissue factor. The net result of this cascade of events is an increased risk of thrombotic events secondary to platelet activation, endothelial damage, and thrombin generation despite moderate to severe thrombocytopenia.

CLINICAL PRESENTATION AND DIAGNOSIS OF HIT

Thrombotic complications are the most common clinical sequelae of HIT.[53] The incidence of thrombosis is as high as 50% in those patients with laboratory-confirmed immune-mediated thrombocytopenia. Thrombosis may occur in patients with seemingly mild thrombocytopenia, but their platelet counts invariably have dropped more than 50% from baseline. This syndrome is poorly recognized, and many, perhaps most, patients diagnosed with HIT initially presented with thrombosis. Even among those who are diagnosed prior to the development of thrombosis, the prognosis is poor. In one case series of patients who were diagnosed with HIT without thrombosis, the cumulative incidence of thrombosis over the next 30 days was greater than 50% despite the discontinuation of heparin therapy.[157]

Venous thrombosis is the most common thrombotic complication associated with HIT, and the majority of patients develop

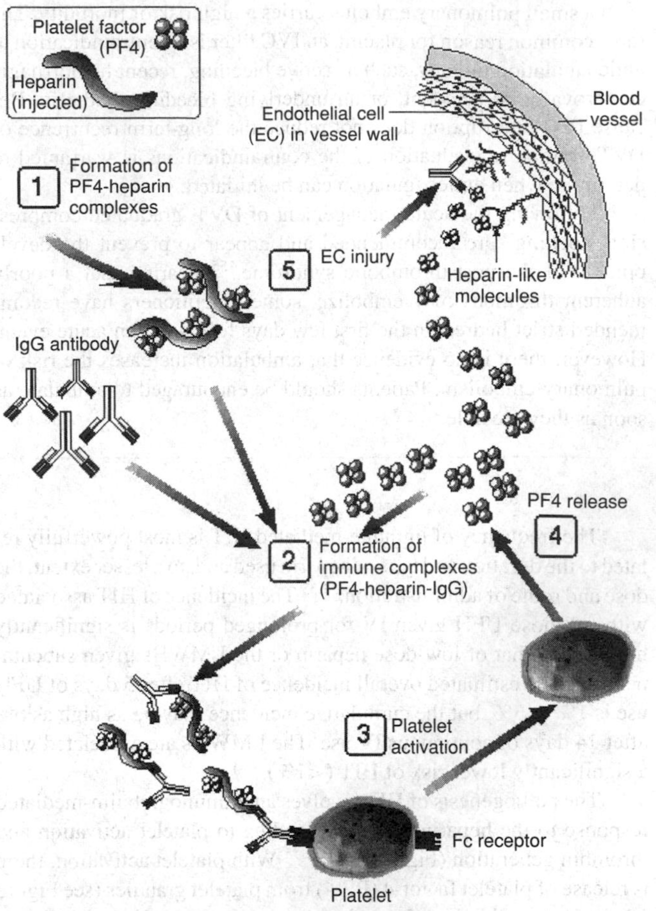

FIGURE 19–11. Pathogenesis of heparin-induced thrombocytopenia. (1) The formation of heparin–PF-4 complexes leads to the development of IgG antibodies. (2) Antibodies bind to the heparin–PF-4 complex and lead to platelet activation (3) and release of additional PF-4. (4) Excess PF-4 binds to heparin-like molecules on endothelial cell surfaces. (5) Endothelial cell injury and expression of tissue factor further promote thrombin generation. *Republished with permission from Aventis Pharmaceuticals.*

proximal DVT.[53,157] A large percentage of patients develop asymptomatic VTE. Pulmonary embolism occurs in 25% of patients with thrombotic complications and contributes significantly to the mortality rate. Arterial thrombosis occurs less commonly. Limb artery occlusion, stroke, and myocardial infarction are the most commonly reported arterial events. Heparin-induced skin lesions occur in 10% to 20% of patients with HIT. Lesions range from painful, localized erythematous plaques to widespread dermal necrosis that frequently requires amputation. Mortality from HIT may be as high as 36% in patients with acute thrombosis. Because of the relatively high frequency of thrombotic complications and poor outcomes associated with HIT, prompt recognition and diagnosis are critical.

The diagnosis of immune-mediated HIT is based on clinical findings supplemented by laboratory tests that confirm the presence of antibodies to heparin or platelet activation induced by heparin.[54,55,64] Although thrombocytopenia is the most common initial event to suggest the diagnosis of HIT, clinicians should evaluate all the potential causes. The time course and magnitude of thrombocytopenia are the features distinguishing immune-mediated HIT from HAT. Acute thrombosis and skin lesions may occur prior to the development of overt thrombocytopenia. Clinicians should immediately suspect HIT when these events occur in any patient on UFH or LMWH therapy.

Laboratory testing must be performed to confirm the diagnosis of HIT.[55,157,158] This testing is particularly helpful in patients with only mild to moderate thrombocytopenia in whom HIT is suspected. Two types of assays are available to detect the presence of heparin-induced antibodies. Platelet activation assays, also known as functional assays, confirm *in vitro* platelet activation in the presence of therapeutic heparin levels. Functional assays include the heparin-induced platelet activation (HIPA) assay, the serotonin release assay (SRA), and the platelet aggregation assay (PAA). The HIPA and SRA tests have higher sensitivity and specificity than the PAA assay, but are technically more difficult to perform. Antigen assays that detect the presence of specific antibodies against the heparin–PF-4 complex using enzyme-linked immunosorbent assays (ELISA) are also available. These tests have reasonably high sensitivity and specificity. The optimal test for laboratory confirmation of immune-mediated HIT is unclear. The most readily available test with the greatest sensitivity and specificity should be used. The combined use of functional and ELISA assays may reduce false-negative results. When the results of one test are negative or indeterminate in a patient with suspected HIT, another test should be considered.

▶ TREATMENT: Heparin-Induced Thrombocytopenia

Once the diagnosis of HIT is established or strongly suspected, *all* sources of heparin, including heparin flushes, should be discontinued and an alternative anticoagulant agent initiated (Table 19–28; Fig. 19–12).[8,54,55,64] Even in the absence of thrombosis, patients with HIT are at extremely high risk for serious thrombotic complications over the next 30 days without treatment. The time required for laboratory results to be reported can be prolonged, a factor that requires consideration in the management of HIT. It is crucial that patients receive anticoagulation therapy by some other means to prevent new thrombosis. The goal of therapy is not only to treat existing thrombosis, but also to prevent new thrombotic events and to return platelet counts to near baseline levels.

Anticoagulant agents that rapidly inhibit thrombin activity are the drugs of choice for the management of HIT. The LMWHs are not recommended for use in HIT because they have nearly 100% cross-reactivity with heparin antibodies by *in vitro* testing.[63,64,159] Lepirudin and argatroban are FDA-approved for the treatment of HIT. Although it is not FDA-approved for this indication, danaparoid has been formally evaluated in clinical trials and used in many institutions for the treatment of HIT. The comparative efficacy of these agents has not been examined, and all three are considered suitable for the initial treatment of HIT. Many clinicians consider argatroban the best alternative because of its shorter half-life, modest bleeding risk, and lower cost compared with that of lepirudin and danaparoid. Fondaparinux is also a potential alternative auticoagulant because it does not cross-react with heparin-induced antibodies *in vitro*. However, to date, fondaparinux has not been formally evaluated for the management of patients with HIT.

For the treatment of HIT, lepirudin, argatroban, and danaparoid are administered by IV infusion.[8,64,67] Lepirudin and argatroban should be titrated based on aPTT testing with a target of 1.5 to 3 times the normal control or the institution-specific therapeutic range. Danaparoid does not require routine laboratory monitoring to determine the response to therapy. In morbidly obese patients and those

TABLE 19–28. Recommended Dose and Monitoring Parameters for Direct Thrombin Inhibitors

Agent	Dose	Monitoring Parameters	Clinical Considerations
Lepirudin	0.4 mg/kg slow IV bolus, followed by 0.15 mg/kg/h IV infusion	Obtain baseline PT, aPTT, CBC, SCr. Check aPTT 4 h after initiation and adjust dose to achieve aPTT 1.5–3 times control. Once stable, monitor aPTT q 12 h.	Initial dose must be reduced in patients with renal impairment. Antihirudin antibodies can occur in up to 40% of patients and can lead to reduced clearance. Concomitant warfarin requires dose adjustment.
Argatroban	2 μg/kg/min continuous IV infusion	Obtain baseline PT, aPTT. Monitor aPTT 2 h after initiation and adjust dose to achieve therapeutic aPTT.	Initial dose must be reduced to 0.5 μg/kg/min for those with hepatic impairment. Agent will cause significant elevation in PT/INR; concurrent warfarin therapy requires special management.
Danaparoid	1,500–3,750 units bolus based on weight, followed by 400 units/h for 4 h, then 300 units/h for 4 h and 150–200 units/h thereafter	Routine monitoring of anticoagulation response is not recommended. Anti-factor Xa can be measured (target 0.5–0.8 units/mL).	*In vitro* cross-reactivity with heparin antibodies is seen in 10% of cases. Dose should be reduced in patients with renal impairment.

PT = prothrombin time; aPTT = activated partial thromboplastin time; CBC = complete blood count; SCr = Serum creatinine; INR = international normalized ratio.

with renal insufficiency, the dose of danaparoid can be adjusted based on anti-factor Xa activity, with a target range of 0.5–1 units/mL.

The use of warfarin during the initial treatment of HIT is potentially dangerous.[64,160] The rapid reduction in protein C concentrations induced early in the course of warfarin therapy further increases the risk of thrombosis in patients with HIT. The observation that several patients with HIT have developed venous limb gangrene when treated with warfarin supports this concern. These patients had relatively high INRs after the initiation of warfarin therapy and presumably had a rapid depletion of protein C. One case series found a low incidence of venous limb gangrene among HIT patients treated with low to moderate doses of warfarin.[161] As a result of conflicting data, warfarin is not recommended for the initial treatment of patients diagnosed with HIT.[8,64,67,161] However, it is safe for patients requiring long-term anticoagulation for the management of HIT. Warfarin can be concomitantly initiated with lepirudin, argatroban, or danaparoid. Therapy should be overlapped until the thrombocytopenia has resolved and the full anticoagulant effect of warfarin has been achieved. Initial doses of warfarin greater than 5 mg should be strictly avoided in these patients.

The appropriate duration of therapy for HIT is unknown.[8,64,67] In patients with HIT without thrombosis, treatment should be continued until the platelet counts have normalized. Patients with thrombosis, either at the time of presentation or following the diagnosis of HIT, should be given warfarin therapy for at least 6 months. The anticoagulant used initially should be continued until the INR is persistently greater than 2.0.

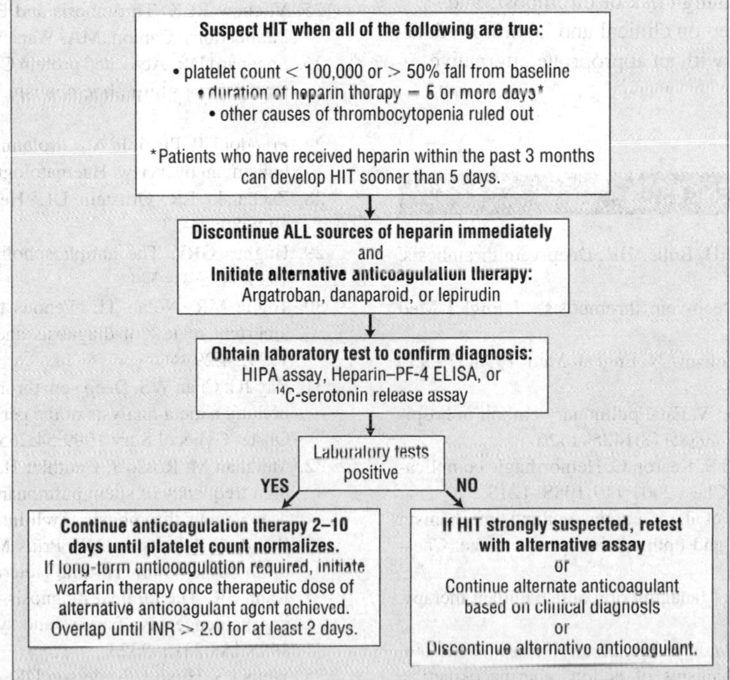

FIGURE 19–12. Treatment of heparin-induced thrombocytopenia (HIT). HIPA assay = heparin-induced platelet activation assay; ELISA = enzyme linked immunosorbent assay, INR = international normalized ratio.

▶ PRINCIPLES OF PHARMACOTHERAPY

- The risk of venous thromboembolism (VTE) is related to several easily identifiable factors, including age, major surgery (particularly orthopedic procedures of the lower extremities), previous VTE, trauma, malignancy, and hypercoagulable states. These risks are additive.
- At the time of hospital admission, all patients should receive prophylaxis against VTE that corresponds to their level of risk. Prophylaxis should be continued throughout the period of risk.
- The diagnosis of VTE must be confirmed by an objective test.
- In the absence of contraindications, the treatment of VTE should initially include a rapid-acting anticoagulant (e.g., unfractionated heparin [UFH], a low-molecular weight heparin [LMWH], fondaparinux) overlapped with warfarin for 5 days and until the patient's international normalized ratio (INR) is therapeutic on 2 consecutive days. The oral administration of anticoagulation therapy should be continued for a minimum of 3 months. The duration of anticoagulation therapy should be based on the patient's risk of VTE recurrence and major bleeding.
- Antithrombotic therapies require meticulous and systematic monitoring, as well as ongoing patient education. Well organized anticoagulation management services improve the quality of patient care and reduce overall cost.
- Many patients with a proximal deep vein thrombosis (DVT) can be managed on an outpatient basis with a LMWH and warfarin.
- Bleeding is the most frequent complication related to antithrombotic therapy. The patient's risk of major hemorrhage is related to the intensity and stability of therapy, concurrent drug use, history of gastrointestinal bleeding, risk of fall/trauma, and age.
- Warfarin is prone to numerous clinically important food and drug interactions.
- Heparin-induced thrombocytopenia (HIT) is frequently unrecognized. Associated with a high risk of thrombosis and mortality, HIT is diagnosed based on clinical and laboratory data. It requires aggressive treatment with an appropriate alternative antithrombotic drug.

REFERENCES

1. Lensing AW, Prandoni P, Prins MH, Buller HR. Deep-vein thrombosis. Lancet 1999;353:479–485.
2. Weinmann EE, Salzman EW. Deep-vein thrombosis. N Engl J Med 1994;331:1630–1641.
3. Goldhaber SZ. Pulmonary embolism. N Engl J Med 1998;339:93–104.
4. Rubinstein I, Murray D, Hoffstein V. Fatal pulmonary emboli in hospitalized patients. Arch Intern Med 1988;148:1425–1426.
5. Levine M, Raskob GE, Landefeld S, Kearon C. Hemorrhagic complications of anticoagulant treatment. Chest 2001;119:108S–121S.
6. Hirsh J, Dalen JE, Anderson DR, et al. Oral anticoagulants: mechanism of action, clinical effectiveness, and optimal therapeutic range. Chest 2001;119:8S–21S.
7. Ansell J, Hirsh J, Dalen JE, et al. Managing oral anticoagulant therapy. Chest 2001;119:22S–38S.
8. Hirsh J, Warkentin TE, Shaughnessy SG, et al. Heparin and low-molecular-weight heparin: mechanisms of action, pharmacokinetics, dosing, monitoring, efficacy, and safety. Chest 2001;119:64S–94S.
9. Chiquette E, Amato MG, Bussey HI. Comparison of an anticoagulation clinic with usual medical care: anticoagulation control, patient outcomes, and health care costs. Arch Intern Med 1998;158:1641–1647.
10. Haines ST, Bussey HI. Diagnosis of deep vein thrombosis. Am J Health Syst Pharm 1997;54:66–74.
11. Ginsberg JS. Management of venous thromboembolism. N Engl J Med 1996;335:1816–1828.
12. Hirsh J, Hoak J. Management of deep vein thrombosis and pulmonary embolism: a statement from the Council on Thrombosis (in consultation with the Council on Cardiovascular Radiology), American Heart Association. Circulation 1996;93:2212–2245.
13. Silverstein MD, Heit JA, Mohr DN, et al. Trends in the incidence of deep vein thrombosis and pulmonary embolism: a 25-year population-based study. Arch Intern Med 1998;158:585–593.
14. White RH, Zhou H, Romano PS. Incidence of idiopathic deep venous thrombosis and secondary thromboembolism among ethnic groups in California. Ann Intern Med 1998;128:737–740.
15. Geerts WH, Heit JA, Clagett GP, et al. Prevention of venous thromboembolism. Chest 2001;119:132S–175S.
16. Geerts WH, Code KI, Jay RM, et al. A prospective study of venous thromboembolism after major trauma. N Engl J Med 1994;331:1601–1606.
17. Hansson PO, Sorbo J, Eriksson H. Recurrent venous thromboembolism after deep vein thrombosis: incidence and risk factors. Arch Intern Med 2000;160:769–774.
18. Heit JA, Mohr DN, Silverstein MD, et al. Predictors of recurrence after deep vein thrombosis and pulmonary embolism: a population-based cohort study. Arch Intern Med 2000;160:761–768.
19. Levitan N, Dowlati A, Remick SC, et al. Rates of initial and recurrent thromboembolic disease among patients with malignancy versus those without malignancy: risk analysis using Medicare claims data. Medicine 1999;78:285–291.
20. Federman DG, Kirsner RS. An update on hypercoagulable disorders. Arch Intern Med 2001;161:1051–1056.
21. Seligsohn U, Lubetsky A. Genetic susceptibility to venous thrombosis. N Engl J Med 2001;344:1222–1231.
22. Thomas DP, Roberts HR. Hypercoagulability in venous and arterial thrombosis. Ann Intern Med 1997;126:638–644.
23. Haines ST, Bussey HI. Thrombosis and the pharmacology of antithrombotic agents. Ann Pharmacother 1995;29:892–905.
24. Dahlback B. Blood coagulation. Lancet 2000;355:1627–1632.
25. Virchow RLK. Thrombosis and Emboli (1846–1856). Science History Publications. Canton, MA, Watson Publishing International, 1998.
26. Sheppard DR. Activated protein C resistance: the most common risk factor for venous thromboembolism. J Am Board Fam Pract 2000;13:111–115.
27. Prandoni P, Piccioli A, Girolami A. Cancer and venous thromboembolism: an overview. Haematologica 1999;84:437–445.
28. Zacharski LR, Ornstein DL. Heparin and cancer. Thromb Haemost 1998;80:10–23.
29. Hughes GRV. The antiphospholipid syndrome: ten years on. Lancet 1993;342:341–344.
30. Toglia MR, Nolan TE. Venous thromboembolism during pregnancy: a current review of diagnosis and management. Obstet Gynecol Surv 1999;54:29–41.
31. Ray JG, Chan WS. Deep vein thrombosis during pregnancy and the puerperium: a meta-analysis of the period of risk and the leg of presentation. Obstet Gynecol Surv 1999;54:265–271.
32. Meignan M, Rosso J, Gauthier H, et al. Systematic lung scans reveal a high frequency of silent pulmonary embolism in patients with proximal deep venous thrombosis. Arch Intern Med 2000;160:159–164.
33. Prandoni P, Lensing AW, Prins MR. The natural history of deep-vein thrombosis. Semin Thromb Hemost 1997;23:185–188.
34. Kahn SR. The clinical diagnosis of deep venous thrombosis: integrating incidence, risk factors, and symptoms and signs. Arch Intern Med 1998;158:2315–2323.
35. Wells PS, Hirsh J, Anderson DR, et al. Accuracy of clinical assessment of deep-vein thrombosis. Lancet 1995;345:1326–1330.

36. Perrier A, Desmarais S, Miron MJ, et al. Non-invasive diagnosis of venous thromboembolism in outpatients. Lancet 1999;353:190–195.
37. Kearon C, Ginsberg JS, Hirsh J. The role of venous ultrasonography in the diagnosis of suspected deep venous thrombosis and pulmonary embolism. Ann Intern Med 1998;129:1044–1049.
38. Kearon C, Julian JA, Math M, et al. Noninvasive diagnosis of deep venous thrombosis. Ann Intern Med 1998;128:663–677.
39. Tai NRM, Atwal AS, Hamilton G. Modern management of pulmonary embolism. Br J Surg 1999;86:853–868.
40. Rosenow EC, 3rd. Venous and pulmonary thromboembolism: an algorithmic approach to diagnosis and management. Mayo Clin Proc 1995;70:45–49.
41. Hirsh J. Heparin. N Engl J Med 1991;324:1565–1574.
42. Ambrosioni E, Strocchi E. Pharmacokinetics of heparin and low molecular weight heparins. Haemostasis 1990;20 (Suppl 1):94–97.
43. Boneu B, Caranobe C, Sie P. Pharmacokinetics of heparin and low molecular weight heparin. Baillieres Clin Haematol 1990;3:531–544.
44. Baughman RA, Kapoor SC, Agarwal RK, et al. Oral delivery of anticoagulant doses of heparin: a randomized, double-blind, controlled study in humans. Circulation 1998;98:1610–1615.
45. Hirsh J, Levine MN. Low molecular weight heparin. Blood 1992;79: 1–17.
46. Brill-Edwards P. Heparin resistance. In: Ginsberg JS, Kearon C, Hirsh J, eds. Clinical Decisions in Thrombosis and Hemostasis. Hamilton, Ontario, Canada. B.C. Decker, 1998:117–122.
47. Olson JD, Arkin CF, Brandt JT, et al. College of American Pathologists Conference XXXI on laboratory monitoring of anticoagulation therapy: laboratory monitoring of unfractionated heparin therapy. Arch Pathol Lab Med 1998;122:782–788.
48. Volles DF, Ancell CJ, Michael KA, et al. Establishing an institution-specific therapeutic range. Am J Health Syst Pharm 1998;55:2002–2006.
49. Raschke RA, Reilly BM, Guidry JR, et al. The weight-based heparin dosing nomogram compared with a "standard care" nomogram. Ann Intern Med 1993;119:874–881.
50. Mamdani MM, Racine E, McCreadie S, et al. Clinical and economic effectiveness of an inpatient anticoagulation service. Pharmacotherapy 1999;19:1064–1074.
51. Ibrahim SA, Landefeld CS. Bleeding and unfractionated heparin. In: Ginsberg JS, Kearon C, Hirsh J, eds. Clinical Decisions in Thrombosis and Hemostasis. Hamilton, Ontario, Canada. B.C. Decker, 1998:154–160.
52. Greinacher A. Heparin-induced thrombocytopenia—pathogenesis and treatment. Thromb Haemost 1999;82(Suppl 1):148–156.
53. Warkentin TE, Kelton JG. A 14-year study of heparin-induced thrombocytopenia. Am J Med 1996;101:502–507.
54. Warkentin TE, Chong BH, Greinacher A. Heparin-induced thrombocytopenia: towards consensus. Thromb Haemost 1998;79:1–7.
55. Warkentin TE. Heparin-induced thrombocytopenia: a clinicopathologic syndrome. Thromb Haemost 1999;82:439–447.
56. Ginsberg JS, Greer IA, Hirsh J. Use of antithrombotic agents during pregnancy. Chest 2001;119:122S–131S.
57. Monagle P, Michelson AD, Bovill E, Andrew M. Antithrombotic therapy in children. Chest 2001;119:344S–370S.
58. Weitz JI. Low-molecular-weight heparins. N Engl J Med 1997;337:688–698.
59. Turpie AG. Pharmacology of the low-molecular-weight heparins. Am Heart J 1998;135:S329–S335.
60. Hirsh J. Low-molecular-weight heparin for the treatment of venous thromboembolism. Am Heart J 1998;135:S336–S342.
61. Gould MK, Dembitzer AD, Doyle RL, et al. Low-molecular-weight heparins compared with unfractionated heparin for treatment of acute deep venous thrombosis: a meta-analysis of randomized, controlled trials. Ann Intern Med 1999;130:800–809.
62. Dolovich L, Ginsberg JS, Douketis J, et al. A meta-analysis comparing low-molecular-weight heparins with unfractionated heparin in the treatment of venous thromboembolism. Arch Intern Med 2000;160: 181–188.
63. Warkentin TE, Levine MN, Hirsh J, et al. Heparin-induced thrombocytopenia in patients treated with low-molecular-weight heparin or unfractionated heparin. N Engl J Med 1995;332:1330–1335.
64. Warkentin TE, Barkin RL. Newer strategies for the treatment of heparin-induced thrombocytopenia. Pharmacotherapy 1999;19:181–195.
65. Tardy-Poncet B, Tardy B, Reynaud J, et al. Efficacy and safety of danaparoid sodium (ORG 10172) in critically ill patients with heparin-associated thrombocytopenia. Chest 1999;115:1616–1620.
66. Wilde MI, Markham A. Danaparoid: a review of its pharmacology and clinical use in the management of heparin-induced thrombocytopenia. Drugs 1997;54:903–924.
67. Greinacher A. Treatment of heparin-induced thrombocytopenia. Thromb Haemost 1999;82:457–467.
68. Laposata M, Green D, Van Cott EM, et al. College of American Pathologists Conference XXXI on laboratory monitoring of anticoagulant therapy: the clinical use and laboratory monitoring of low-molecular-weight heparin, danaparoid, hirudin and related compounds, and argatroban. Arch Pathol Lab Med 1998;122:799–807.
69. Weitz JI, Hirsh J. New anticoagulant drugs. Chest 2001;119:95S–109S.
70. Turpie AG, Gallus AS, Hoek JA. A synthetic pentasaccharide for the prevention of deep-vein thrombosis after total hip replacement. N Engl J Med 2001;344:619–625.
70a. Eriksson BI, Baner KA, Lassen MR, et al. Fondaparinux compared with enoxaparin for the prevention of venous thromboembolism after hip-fracture surgery. N Engl J Med 2001;345:1298–1304.
70b. Baner KA, Eriksson BI, Lassen MR, et al. Fondaparinux compared with enoxaparin for the prevention of venous thromboembolism after elective major knee surgery. N Engl J Med 2001;345:1305–1310.
71. Rembrandt-Investigators. Treatment of proximal deep vein thrombosis with a novel synthetic compound (SR90107A/ORG31540) with pure anti-factor Xa activity: a phase II evaluation. Circulation 2000;102:2726–2731.
72. Agnelli G, Sonaglia F. Clinical status of direct thrombin inhibitors. Crit Rev Oncol Hematol 1999;31:97–117.
73. Fareed J, Callas D, Hoppensteadt DA, et al. Antithrombin agents as anticoagulants and antithrombotics: implications in drug development. Med Clin North Am 1998;82:569–586.
74. Harker LA. Therapeutic inhibition of thrombin activities, receptors, and production. Hematol Oncol Clin North Am 1998;12:1211–1230.
75. Bates SM, Weitz JI. Direct thrombin inhibitors for treatment of arterial thrombosis: potential differences between bivalirudin and hirudin. Am J Cardiol 1998;82:12P–18P.
76. Swan SK, Hursting MJ. The pharmacokinetics and pharmacodynamics of argatroban: effects of age, gender, and hepatic or renal dysfunction. Pharmacotherapy 2000;20:318–329.
77. Swan SK, St. Peter JV, Lambrecht LJ, Hursting MJ. Comparison of anticoagulant effects and safety of argatroban and heparin in healthy subjects. Pharmacotherapy 2000;20:756–770.
78. Refludan Product Labeling. Aventis Pharmaceuticals, Inc., 1998.
79. Argatroban Product Labeling. SmithKline Beecham, 2000.
80. Ansell JE. Oral anticoagulant therapy—50 years later. Arch Intern Med 1993;153:586–596.
81. Stirling Y. Warfarin-induced changes in procoagulant and anticoagulant proteins. Blood Coagul Fibrinolysis 1995;6:361–373.
82. Fairweather RB, Ansell J, van den Besselaar AM, et al. College of American Pathologists Conference XXXI on laboratory monitoring of anticoagulant therapy: laboratory monitoring of oral anticoagulant therapy. Arch Pathol Lab Med 1998;122:768–781.
83. Crowther MA, Ginsberg JB, Kearon C, et al. A randomized trial comparing 5-mg and 10-mg warfarin loading doses. Arch Intern Med 1999;159:46–48.
84. Harrison L, Johnston M, Massicotte MP, et al. Comparison of 5-mg and 10-mg loading doses in initiation of warfarin therapy. Ann Intern Med 1997;126:133–136.
85. Chan YC, Valenti D, Mansfield AO, Stansby G. Warfarin induced skin necrosis. Br J Surg 2000;87:266–272.
86. Erban S. Initiation of warfarin therapy: recommendations and clinical pearls. J Thromb Thrombolysis 1999;7:145–148.

87. Crowther MA, Harrison L, Hirsh J. Warfarin: less may be better. Ann Intern Med 1997;124:332–333.
88. Roberts GW, Druskeit T, Jorgensen LE, et al. Comparison of an age adjusted warfarin loading protocol with empirical dosing and Fennerty's protocol. Aust N Z J Med 1999;29:731–736.
89. Kovacs MJ, Cruickshank M, Wells PS, et al. Randomized assessment of a warfarin nomogram for initial oral anticoagulation after venous thromboembolic disease. Haemostasis 1998;28:62–69.
90. Hyers TM, Agnelli G, Hull RD, et al. Antithrombotic therapy for venous thromboembolic disease. Chest 2001;119:176S–193S.
91. Ansell JE, Hughes R. Evolving models of warfarin management: anticoagulation clinics, patient self-monitoring, and patient self-management. Am Heart J 1996;132:1095–1100.
92. Holden J, Holden K. Comparative effectiveness of general practitioner versus pharmacist dosing of patients requiring anticoagulation in the community. J Clin Pharm Ther 2000;25:49–54.
93. Ansell JE. Empowering patients to monitor and manage oral anticoagulation therapy. JAMA 1999;281:182–183.
94. Landefeld CS, Beyth RJ. Anticoagulant-related bleeding: clinical epidemiology, prediction, and prevention. Am J Med 1993;95:315–328.
95. Gallerani M, Manfredini R, Moratelli S. Non-haemorrhagic adverse reactions of oral anticoagulant therapy. Int J Cardiol 1995;49:1–7.
96. Booth SL, Mayer J. Warfarin use and fracture risk. Nutr Rev 2000;58: 20–22.
97. Taylor CT, Chester EA, Byrd DC, Stephens MA. Vitamin K to reverse excessive anticoagulation: a review of the literature. Pharmacotherapy 1999;19:1415–1425.
98. Wells PS, Holbrook AM, Crowther NR, Hirsh J. Interactions of warfarin with drugs and food. Ann Intern Med 1994;121:676–683.
99. Booth SL, Centurelli MA. Vitamin K: a practical guide to the dietary management of patients on warfarin. Nutr Rev 1999;57:288–296.
100. Porter RS, Sawyer WT. Wafarin. In: Evans WE, Schentag JJ, Jusko WJ, eds. Applied Pharmacokinetics: Principles of Therapeutic Drug Monitoring. Vancouver, WA, Applied Therapeutics, 1992:31.1–31.46.
101. Heck AM, DeWitt BA, Lukes AL. Potential interactions between alternative therapies and warfarin. Am J Health Syst Pharm 2000;57:1221–1227.
102. Verstraete M. Fortnightly review: prophylaxis of venous thromboembolism. BMJ 1997;314:123–125.
103. Stratton MA, Anderson FA, Bussey HI, et al. Prevention of venous thromboembolism: adherence to the 1995 American College of Chest Physicians consensus guidelines for surgical patients. Arch Intern Med 2000;160:334–340.
104. Durieux PMDMPH, Nizard RMD, Ravaud PMDP, et al. A clinical decision support system for prevention of venous thromboembolism: effect on physician behavior. JAMA 2000;283:2816–2821.
105. Sochart DH, Hardinge K. The relationship of foot and ankle movements to venous return in the lower limb. J Bone Joint Surg Br 1999;81:700–704.
106. Blanchard J, Meuwly JY, Leyvraz PF, et al. Prevention of deep-vein thrombosis after total knee replacement: randomised comparison between a low-molecular-weight heparin (nadroparin) and mechanical prophylaxis with a foot-pump system. J Bone Joint Surg Br 1999;81:654–659.
107. Muir KW, Watt A, Baxter G, et al. Randomized trial of graded compression stockings for prevention of deep-vein thrombosis after acute stroke. QJM 2000;93:359–364.
108. Best AJ, Williams S, Crozier A, et al. Graded compression stockings in elective orthopaedic surgery: an assessment of the in vivo performance of commercially available stockings in patients having hip and knee arthroplasty. J Bone Joint Surg 2000;82:116–118.
109. Agu O, Hamilton G, Baker D. Graduated compression stockings in the prevention of venous thromboembolism. Br J Surg 1999;86:992–1004.
110. Elliott CG, Dudney TM, Egger M, et al. Calf-thigh sequential pneumatic compression compared with plantar venous pneumatic compression to prevent deep-vein thrombosis after non-lower extremity trauma. J Trauma 1999;47:25–32.
111. Hooker JA, Lachiewicz PF, Kelley SS. Efficacy of prophylaxis against thromboembolism with intermittent pneumatic compression after primary and revision total hip arthroplasty. J Bone Joint Surg 1999;81: 690–696.
112. Siddiqui AU, Buchman TG, Hotchkiss RS. Pulmonary embolism as a consequence of applying sequential compression device on legs in a patient asymptomatic of deep vein thrombosis. Anesthesiology 2000;92:880–882.
113. Velmahos GC, Kern J, Chan LS, et al. Prevention of venous thromboembolism after injury: an evidence-based report—part II: analysis of risk factors and evaluation of the role of vena caval filters. J Trauma 2000;49:140–144.
114. Decousus H, Leizorovicz A, Parent F, et al. A clinical trial of vena caval filters in the prevention of pulmonary embolism in patients with proximal deep-vein thrombosis. N Engl J Med 1998;409–415.
115. Collaborative overview of randomised trials of antiplatelet therapy—III: reduction in venous thrombosis and pulmonary embolism by antiplatelet prophylaxis among surgical and medical patients. Antiplatelet Trialists' Collaboration. BMJ 1994;308:235–246.
116. Koch A, Bouges S, Ziegler S, et al. Low molecular weight heparin and unfractionated heparin in thrombosis prophylaxis after major surgical intervention: update of previous meta-analyses. Br J Surg 1997;84:750–759.
117. Mismetti P, Laporte-Simitsidis S, Tardy B, et al. Prevention of venous thromboembolism in internal medicine with unfractionated or low-molecular-weight heparins: a meta-analysis of randomised clinical trials. Thromb Haemost 2000;83:14–19.
118. Anderson DR, O'Brien BJ, Levine MN, et al. Efficacy and cost of low-molecular-weight heparin compared with standard heparin for the prevention of deep vein thrombosis after total hip arthroplasty. Ann Intern Med 1993;119:1105–1112.
119. Leyvraz PF, Richard J, Bachmann F, et al. Adjusted versus fixed-dose subcutaneous heparin in the prevention of deep-vein thrombosis after total hip replacement. N Engl J Med 1983;309:954–958.
120. Hull RD, Brant RF, Pineo GF, et al. Preoperative vs postoperative initiation of low-molecular-weight heparin prophylaxis against venous thromboembolism in patients undergoing elective hip replacement. Arch Intern Med 1999;159:137–141.
121. Leclerc JR, Geerts WH, Desjardins L, et al. Prevention of venous thromboembolism after knee arthroplasty: a randomized, double-blind trial comparing enoxaparin with warfarin. Ann Intern Med 1996;124:619–626.
122. Hull RD, Pineo GF, Francis C, et al. Low-molecular-weight heparin prophylaxis using dalteparin in close proximity to surgery vs warfarin in hip arthroplasty patients: a double-blind, randomized comparison. The North American Fragmin Trial Investigators. Arch Intern Med 2000;160:2199–2207.
123. McIntyre K. Medicolegal implications of the consensus conference. Chest 2001;199:337S–343S.
124. Hull RD, Pineo GF, Francis C, et al. Low-molecular-weight heparin prophylaxis using dalteparin extended out-of-hospital vs in-hospital warfarin/out-of-hospital placebo in hip arthroplasty patients: a double-blind, randomized comparison. The North American Fragmin Trial Investigators. Arch Intern Med 2000;160:2208–2215.
125. Heit JA, Elliott CG, Trowbridge AA, et al. Ardeparin sodium for extended out-of-hospital prophylaxis against venous thromboembolism after total hip or knee replacement: a randomized, double-blind, placebo-controlled trial. Ann Intern Med 2000;132:853–861.
126. Bergqvist D, Benoni G, Björgell O, et al. Low–molecular-weight heparin (enoxaparin) as prophylaxis against venous thromboembolism after total hip replacement. N Engl J Med 1996;335:696–700.
127. Corditz GA. Cost-effectiveness of prevention. In: Bergqvist D, Comerota A, Nicolaides AN, Scurr JH, eds. Prevention of Venous Thromboembolism. London, Med-Orion Publishing Company, 1994:403–420.
128. Oster G, Tuden RL, Colditz GA. Prevention of venous thromboembolism after general surgery: cost-effectiveness analysis of alternative approaches to prophylaxis. Am J Med 1987;82:889–899.

129. Etchells E, McLeod RS, Geerts W, et al. Economic analysis of low-dose heparin vs the low–molecular-weight heparin enoxaparin for prevention of venous thromboembolism after colorectal surgery. Arch Intern Med 1999;159:1221–1228.
130. Oster G, Tuden RL, Colditz GA. A cost-effectiveness analysis of prophylaxis against deep-vein thrombosis in major orthopedic surgery. JAMA 1987;257:203–208.
131. Hawkins DW, Langley PC, Krueger KP. Pharmacoeconomic model of enoxaparin versus heparin for prevention of deep vein thrombosis after total hip replacement. Am J Health Syst Pharm 1997;54:1185–1190.
132. Hawkins DW, Langley PC, Krueger KP. A pharmacoeconomic assessment of enoxaparin and warfarin as prophylaxis for deep vein thrombosis in patients undergoing knee replacement surgery. Clin Ther 1998;20:182–195.
133. Menzin J, Richner R, Huse D, et al. Prevention of deep-vein thrombosis following total hip replacement surgery with enoxaparin versus unfractionated heparin: a pharmacoeconomic evaluation. Ann Pharmacother 1994;28:271–275.
134. Hirsh J, Bates SM. Clinical trials that have influenced the treatment of venous thromboembolism: a historical perspective. Ann Intern Med 2001;134:409–417.
135. Comerota AJ. Venous thrombectomy. In: Ginsberg JS, Kearon C, Hirsh J, eds. Clinical Decisions in Thrombosis and Hemostasis. Hamilton, Ontario, Canada. B.C. Decker, 1998:72–77.
136. Ng CM, Rivera JO. Meta-analysis of streptokinase and heparin in deep vein thrombosis. Am J Health Syst Pharm 1998;55:1995–2001.
137. Hull RD, Raskob GE, Brant R, et al. Low–molecular-weight heparin vs heparin in the treatment of patients with pulmonary embolism. Arch Intern Med 2000;160:229–236.
138. Simmoneau G, Sors J, Charbonnier B, et al. A comparison of low–molecular-weight heparin with unfractionated heparin for acute pulmonary embolism. N Engl J Med 1997;337:663–669.
139. The Columbus Investigators. Low–molecular-weight heparin in the treatment of patients with venous thromboembolism. N Engl J Med 1997;337:657–662.
140. Gould MK, Dembitzer AD, Sanders GD, Garber AM. Low–molecular-weight heparins compared with unfractionated heparin for treatment of acute deep venous thrombosis: a cost-effectiveness analysis. Ann Intern Med 1999;130:789–799.
141. Hull RD, Raskob GE, Pineo G, et al. Subcutaneous low–molecular-weight heparin compared with continuous intravenous heparin in the treatment of proximal-vein thrombosis. N Engl J Med 1992;326:975–982.
142. Merli GJ, Spiro TE, Olson C, et al. Subcutaneous enoxaparin once or twice daily compared with intravenous unfractionated heparin for treatment of venous thromboembolic disease. Ann Intern Med 2001;134:191–202.
143. Yusen RD, Haraden BM, Gage BF, et al. Criteria for outpatient management of proximal lower extremity deep venous thrombosis. Chest 1999;115:972–979.
144. Yeager BF, Matheny SC. Low–molecular-weight heparin in outpatient treatment of DVT. Am Fam Physician 1999;59:945–952.
145. Koopman M, Prandoni P, Piovella F, et al. Treatment of venous thrombosis with intravenous unfractionated heparin administered in the hospital as compared with subcutaneous low–molecular-weight heparin administered at home. The Tasman Study Group. N Engl J Med 1996;334:682–687.
146. Levine MN, Gent M, Hirsh J, et al. A comparison of low–molecular-weight heparin administered primarily at home with unfractionated heparin administered in the hospital for proximal deep-vein thrombosis. N Engl J Med 1996;334:677–681.
147. Rodger M, Bredeson C, Wells PS, et al. Cost-effectiveness of low–molecular-weight heparin and unfractionated heparin in treatment of deep vein thrombosis. CMAJ 1998;159:931–938.
148. Tillman DJ, Charland SL, Witt DM. Effectiveness and economic impact associated with a program for outpatient management of acute deep vein thrombosis in a group model health maintenance organization. Arch Intern Med 2000;160:2926–2932.
149. Leong WA. Outpatient deep vein thrombosis treatment models. Pharmacotherapy 1998;18:170S–174S.
150. Anderson DR. Thrombolytic therapy for pulmonary embolism and deep vein thrombosis. In: Ginsberg JS, Kearon C, Hirsh J, eds. Clinical Decisions in Thrombosis and Hemostasis. Hamilton, Ontario, Canada, B.C. Decker, 1998:61–66.
151. Horne MK, 3rd, Chang R. Thrombolytic therapy for deep venous thrombosis? JAMA 1999;282:2164–2166.
152. Dalen JE, Alpert JS, Hirsh J. Thrombolytic therapy for pulmonary embolism: Is it effective? Is it safe? When is it indicated? Arch Intern Med 1997;157:2550–2556.
153. Buck ML. Anticoagulation with warfarin in infants and children. Ann Pharmacother 1996;30:1316–1322.
154. Cisek PL, Malone MD, Comerota AJ. Inferior vena cava interruption. In: Ginsberg JS, Kearon C, Hirsh J, eds. Clinical Decisions in Thrombosis and Hemostasis. Hamilton, Ontario, Canada, B.C. Decker, 1998:67–71.
155. Brandjes DP, Büller HR, Heijboer H, et al. Randomised trial of effect of compression stockings in patients with symptomatic proximal-vein thrombosis. Lancet 1997;349:759–762.
156. Warkentin TE, Kelton JG. Temporal aspects of heparin-induced thrombocytopenia. N Engl J Med 2001;344:1286–1292.
157. Januzzi JL, Jr, Jang IK. Heparin induced thrombocytopenia: diagnosis and contemporary antithrombin management. J Thromb Thrombolysis 1999;7:259–264.
158. Bauters A, Zawadzki C, Trillot N, et al. Laboratory diagnosis of heparin-induced thrombocytopenia: comparison of the diagnosis value of platelet aggregation test and platelet-factor 4/heparin complexes ELISA. Br J Haematol 1998;102:262, Abstract p–1049.
159. Horellou MH, Conard J, Lecrubier C, et al. Persistent heparin induced thrombocytopenia despite therapy with low molecular weight heparin. Thromb Haemost 1984;51:134.
160. Warkentin TE, Elavathil LJ, Hayward CP, et al. The pathogenesis of venous limb gangrene associated with heparin-induced thrombocytopenia. Ann Intern Med 1997;127:804–812.
161. Wallis DE, Quintos R, Wehrmacher W, Messmore H. Safety of warfarin anticoagulation in patients with heparin-induced thrombocytopenia. Chest 1999;116:1333–1338.

20
STROKE

J. Chris Bradberry and Susan C. Fagan

Stroke, or brain attack, is a syndrome and is a major manifestation of cerebrovascular disease. *Stroke* refers to the sudden onset of a focal neurologic deficit. *Cerebrovascular disease* refers to any type of pathophysiologic vascular disease of the brain. This vascular pathology can include any abnormality of the vessel, blood flow, or quality of the blood. Abnormalities of the vessel include many processes such as developmental defects, arteritis, aneurysm, hypertensive disease, vasoconstriction, and atherosclerosis. Blood flow can be affected by disease of the vessels as well as by thrombotic or embolic processes. The changes in the brain that these abnormalities can produce are either a decrease in blood flow, sometimes leading to ischemia, or bleeding. Ischemia can be present with or without brain tissue infarction. When a stroke occurs, the neurologic manifestations produced are the result of the location of insult in the brain and the extent of ischemia, infarct, or hemorrhage. A stroke may show varied manifestations, reversible and irreversible, ranging from hemiplegia to sensory deficits. Hemiplegia may or may not be accompanied by other manifestations. It is a challenge for the clinician to accurately diagnose a particular lesion because of these variations in presentation; however, a good neurologic examination can aid in locating a lesion. The advent of imaging studies such as computed tomographic (CT) scanning and magnetic resonance imaging (MRI) has been of tremendous importance in the diagnosis and assessment of neurologic disorders, particularly stroke. Results of the CT scan must be known prior to therapy of certain stroke syndromes with anticoagulants, thrombolytics, or platelet antiaggregating agents.

EPIDEMIOLOGY AND ETIOLOGY

Figure 20–1 outlines the classification by mechanism of stroke. Since the 1940s, stroke death rates have declined in the United States.[1] In fact, during the mid-1970s, the rate of decline in mortality from cerebrovascular disease was far greater than that from cardiovascular disease and probably is related to the effective treatment of hypertension. In 1993, stroke mortality increased for the first time since the 1950s, and death rates from heart disease and cancer have been declining consistently.[1]

General population studies show that atherothrombotic infarction is the most common type of stroke, representing almost 65% of the reported cases of the 85% caused by ischemia. Therefore, the majority of strokes are caused by ischemia and infarction secondary to disease of the large, small, and medium-sized arteries supplying the brain. Cerebral embolism causes stroke about 20% of the time. Hemorrhage into the brain tissue (cerebral or intraparenchymal hemorrhage) and subarachnoid hemorrhages account for about 15% of all strokes. In 1997, the American Heart Association (AHA) estimated that in the United States more than 159,000 (1 of every 15 deaths) people died from a stroke and that there were 4.4 million stroke survivors nationwide.[2] Stroke remains the third leading cause of death in the United States, even though mortality has declined. It is estimated in aggregate that 600,000 people per year have a new or recurrent stroke.

One of the major impacts of stroke is the resulting disability in more than 50% of patients hospitalized for stroke. The overall direct and indirect economic impact is estimated to be as high as $40.9 billion annually and expected to increase further.[2,3] Obviously, with this impact, both economically and emotionally, stroke is one of the most devastating diseases in this country. Prevention is of primary importance, and proper prevention requires management of risk factors in persons at highest risk.[4] As noted earlier, there is good evidence to show that improved treatment, specifically of hypertension, may decrease death from stroke. The risk factors for stroke are shown in Table 20–1 and are divided into groups on the basis of their relationship to stroke.[2,3]

SINGLE RISK FACTORS

It is clear that stroke incidence is related to increasing age, with doubling of stroke rates each decade after 55.[2] Approximately 72% of stroke victims are 65 years of age or older.[2] Stroke generally has a 19% higher incidence in men than in women. There is a higher death rate in blacks, Asian Pacific Islanders, and Hispanics than whites. In blacks, this may be a result of the increased incidence of hypertension and environmental factors. Diabetes mellitus contributes independently to atherothrombotic brain infarction, and the risk is greater in women than in men. An individual with a prior stroke has a high risk of developing a recurrent stroke. Carotid bruits are associated with increased risk of stroke; however, asymptomatic carotid bruits have been a controversial topic with regard to treatment. In asymptomatic individuals, a carotid bruit reflects underlying generalized atherosclerotic disease and does not necessarily indicate that a cerebral infarction will occur in the cerebral territory supplied by the affected carotid.

Of the single risk factors identified, hypertension (HTN) is the major predisposing factor for stroke and is strongly related to atherothrombotic brain infarction as well as cerebral hemorrhage. HTN is a factor in almost 70% of all strokes. The Framingham Study indicated that there is a direct relationship between elevation of blood pressure and stroke risk.[5] Elevated pulse pressure may indicate stronger evidence of increased cardiovascular risk than either systolic or diastolic pressure.[6] There does not seem to be a gender difference in the risk for hypertensive patients, and elevated blood pressure appears to be closely associated with stroke. The risk does not decrease with age; however, with effective treatment, the elderly have a reduction in stroke as great as or greater than that of the younger population. Heart disease is the next most important single treatable risk factor for stroke. Individuals with cardiac diseases such as coronary heart disease, congestive heart failure, left ventricular hypertrophy, arrhythmias, and specifically atrial fibrillation have more than twice the stroke risk compared with those with no manifest heart disease. Cardiovascular risk reduction must be implemented to reduce the risk of coronary heart disease (CHD) and, in turn, stroke risk. Atrial fibrillation is strongly correlated with embolic stroke, and patients with nonrheumatic atrial fibrillation have a sixfold increase in stroke frequency over those without fibrillation.[7–9]

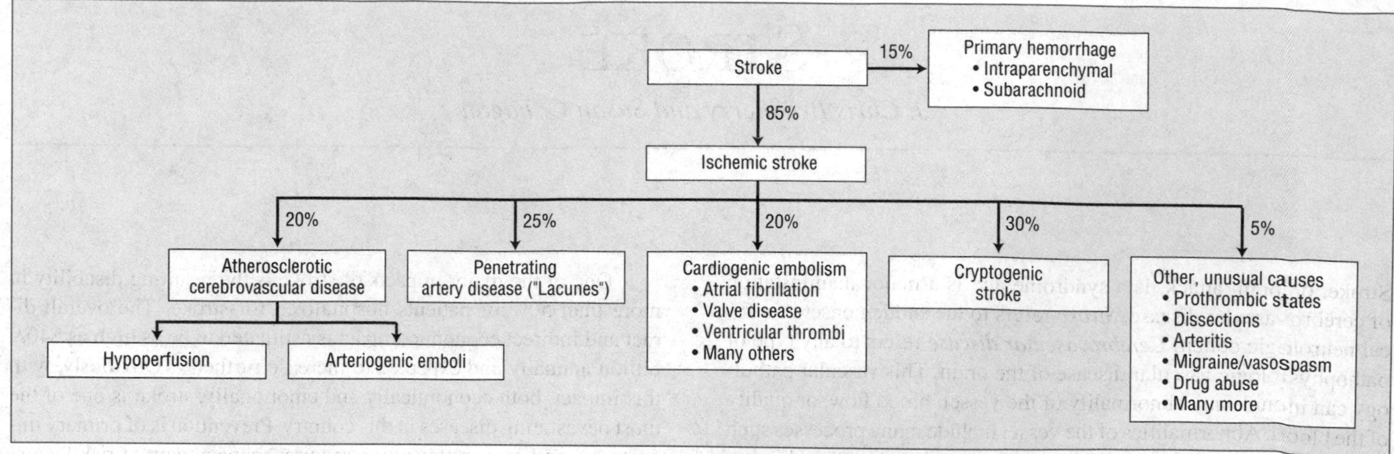

FIGURE 20–1. A classification of stroke by mechanism with estimates of the frequency of various categories of abnormalities. About 30% of ischemic strokes are cryptogenic. *(From Fourth ACCP Consensus Conference on Anti-thrombotic Therapy.)*

Transient ischemic attacks (TIAs) are defined as episodes of focal ischemic neurologic deficit lasting less than 24 hours. The neurologic deficit depends on the thrombotic or embolic activity in the particular arterial supply to the brain. TIAs precede an ischemic stroke in about 60% of cases, and 35% of untreated patients will develop a stroke within 5 years of a TIA. TIAs precede 10% of strokes from all causes. The greatest risk for stroke is early, within the first few weeks of the TIA, with about 20% occurring within the first month after the TIA and 50% within the first year after the TIA. The more frequently TIAs occur, the higher is the probability of stroke, and a previous stroke is a greater risk factor for subsequent stroke than a TIA alone.[9] TIAs as risk factors are also influenced by other stroke risk factors; therefore, treatment of other risk factors may influence the occurrence of stroke in patients with TIAs. Another risk factor is elevated hematocrit. Stroke in patients with elevated hematocrits has been attributed to decreased collateral flow caused by increased blood viscosity. Sickle cell disease also increases the risk of stroke. Stroke in middle-age men has been shown to correlate significantly with a maternal history of stroke.

Dyslipidemia is a risk factor for atherosclerosis in both the coronary and cerebral vascular beds, and hypercholesterolemia is a modest risk factor for stroke. It has been clearly established that lipoproteins play a primary role in atherogenesis and that lowering plasma cholesterol concentration reduces arterial cholesterol accumulation.[10] A recent review of published studies involving 29,000 patients treated with 3-hydroxy-3-methylglutaryl coenzyme A reductase inhibitors (statins) showed that lowering cholesterol for primary and secondary prevention of CHD reduced the risk of stroke 29% and total mortality

TABLE 20–1. Risk Factors in Ischemic Stroke

Single Risk Factors
- Nonmodifiable risk factors or risk markers
  - Age
  - Gender
  - Race
  - Ethnicity
  - Heredity
- Potentially modifiable
  - Hypertension—single most important risk factor for ischemic stroke
  - Cardiac disease
    - Atrial fibrillation—most important and treatable cardiac cause of stroke
    - Mitral stenosis
    - Mitral annular calcification
    - Left atrial enlargement
    - Structural abnormalities such as atrial-septal aneurysm
    - Myocardial disease
      - 1% to 6% of myocardial infarction patients develop a stroke
  - Transient ischemic attacks—major independent risk factor
  - Diabetes—independent risk factor
  - Hypercholesterolemia—positive risk factor for extracranial atherosclerosis but link still under study for ischemic stroke
  - Cigarette smoking
  - Alcohol
  - Illicit drug use—cocaine, heroin, amphetamines, LSD, PCP and others linked with stroke
  - Life-style factors—associated with stroke risk
    - Obesity
    - Physical inactivity
    - Diet
    - Acute triggers—emotional stress
  - Oral contraceptives—positive only with estrogen content >50 μg
  - Migraine—risk not clear
  - Hemostatic and inflammatory factors—fibrinogen linked to increased risk; elevated hematocrit and sickle cell disease are positive risk factors
  - Homocysteine—still under study, but hyperhomocysteinemia may be related to increased stroke risk
  - Asymptomatic carotid stenosis
  - Subclinical disease—aortic arch atheromas

Multiple Risk Factors—Stroke is Increased by the Presence of Multiple Risk Factors
- Framingham profile
  - Elevated systolic blood pressure
  - Elevated serum cholesterol
  - Glucose intolerance
  - Cigarette smoking
  - Left ventricular hypertrophy

22%, thus clearly emphasizing the importance of elevated cholesterol as a risk factor for stroke.[11–14]

Cigarette smoking is a major risk factor for ischemic and hemorrhagic strokes. Smoking causes increased concentration of fibrinogen, increased hematocrit and platelet aggregation, and reduction in high-density lipoprotein–cholesterol (HDL-C); all these factors may impair endothelial cell function. Smokers had two to three times the risk of stroke compared with nonsmokers and a fourfold to sixfold increase in stroke risk compared with those who had never smoked.[15] Cessation of smoking significantly reduces stroke risk. The risk of stroke for women smokers is higher than that for men smokers, but the risk for all smokers decreases to that of nonsmokers 2 to 5 years after cessation.

Low levels of alcohol consumption and ischemic stroke are inversely related, and risk in men increases with heavy consumption (≥300 g/week). Alcohol should not be construed as a preventative measure for stroke.

The association between oral contraceptives as an independent risk factor and the incidence of stroke is not certain. Higher-dose formulations have been shown to increase stroke risk in subgroups of women, such as those greater than 35 years of age, smokers, hypertensives, those with hyperlipidemia, and those with histories of migraine. Newer products contain much lower doses of estrogen and progestogen, and more recent studies have not shown an association between oral contraceptive use and stroke. Caution is recommended in the use of oral contraceptives in women at high risk for stroke.

MULTIPLE RISK FACTORS

The Framingham Study determined five factors for stroke: elevated systolic blood pressure, elevated serum cholesterol, glucose intolerance, cigarette smoking, and left ventricular hypertrophy by electrocardiogram (ECG). These factors, if present, can be used to identify the 10% of the population who will have one-third of the strokes. Interestingly, various combinations of factors have been studied, including low ponderal index (height in inches divided by the cube root of weight in pounds), and risk can vary four- to eightfold depending on the number of multiple risk factors present. The most important single factor, however, was found to be elevated blood pressure. Table 20–1 summarizes the nonmodifiable and modifiable risk factors for ischemic stroke. In addition, certain risk factors have been identified that can help to determine those at high risk for ischemic stroke. Table 20–2 shows these high risk factors and stroke rates.

The treatable single risk factors should be addressed vigorously, and when risk factors occur in combination, therapy should be initiated aggressively, with particular emphasis on hypertension and lifestyle changes.

TABLE 20–2. High-Risk Factors for Ischemic Stroke

High-Risk Factor	Ischemic Stroke Rate per Year (%)
Asymptomatic bruit	1.5
Prior myocardial infarction	1.5
Asymptomatic carotid stenosis	2.0
NVAF	5.0
TIA (varies with territory involved)	6
Prior ischemic stroke	10

Stroke rate for the general population 70 years of age = 0.6%.
NVAF, nonvalvular atrial fibrillation.

PATHOPHYSIOLOGY OF ACUTE STROKE

The vascular anatomy of the brain with blood flow from the heart is shown in Fig. 20–2. The reader also may refer to the diagrams of the brain territory supplied by the middle cerebral artery (Fig. 20–3), and the vertebral-basilar system (see Fig. 20–4).

The large majority of acute strokes result either from ischemic infarction or from inadequate blood flow, whereas only 15% result from primary intracranial hemorrhage. Exact pathophysiologic mechanisms remain controversial. Figure 20–5 describes the anatomy of stroke syndromes.

CEREBROVASCULAR DISEASE

ATHEROTHROMBOTIC DISEASE

Atherosclerosis of brain arteries is a process similar to that found in other extracranial vessels. It is generally held that the atherosclerotic process occurs in parallel fashion throughout the body, although the severity may be slightly less in arteries of the brain than in such arteries as the aorta, the arteries of the extremities, and the coronary

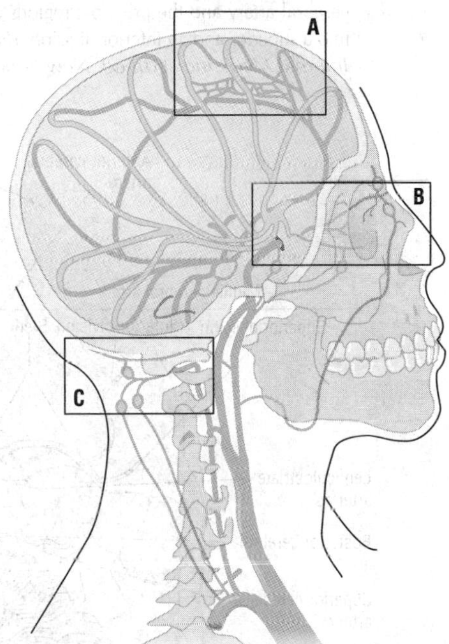

FIGURE 20–2. Arrangement of the major arteries of the right side carrying blood from the heart to the brain. Also shown are vessels of collateral circulation that may modify the effects of cerebral ischemia (*A–C*). Not shown is the circle of Willis, which also provides a source for collateral circulation. (*A*) The anastomotic channels between the distal branches of the anterior and middle cerebral artery, termed *borderzone* or *watershed anastomotic channels*. Note that they also occur between the posterior and middle cerebral arteries and the anterior and posterior cerebral arteries. (*B*) Anastomotic channels occurring through the orbit between branches of the external carotid artery and the ophthalmic branch of the internal carotid artery. (*C*) Wholly extracranial anastomotic channels between the muscular branches of the ascending cervical arteries and the muscular branches of the occipital artery that anastomose with the distal vertebral artery. Note that the occipital artery arises from the external carotid artery, thereby allowing reconstitution of flow in the vertebral artery from the carotid circulation. *(From Braunwald E. Isselbacher KJ, et al., eds. Harrison's Principles of Internal Medicine, 11th ed. New York, McGraw-Hill, 1987:1931, with permission.)*

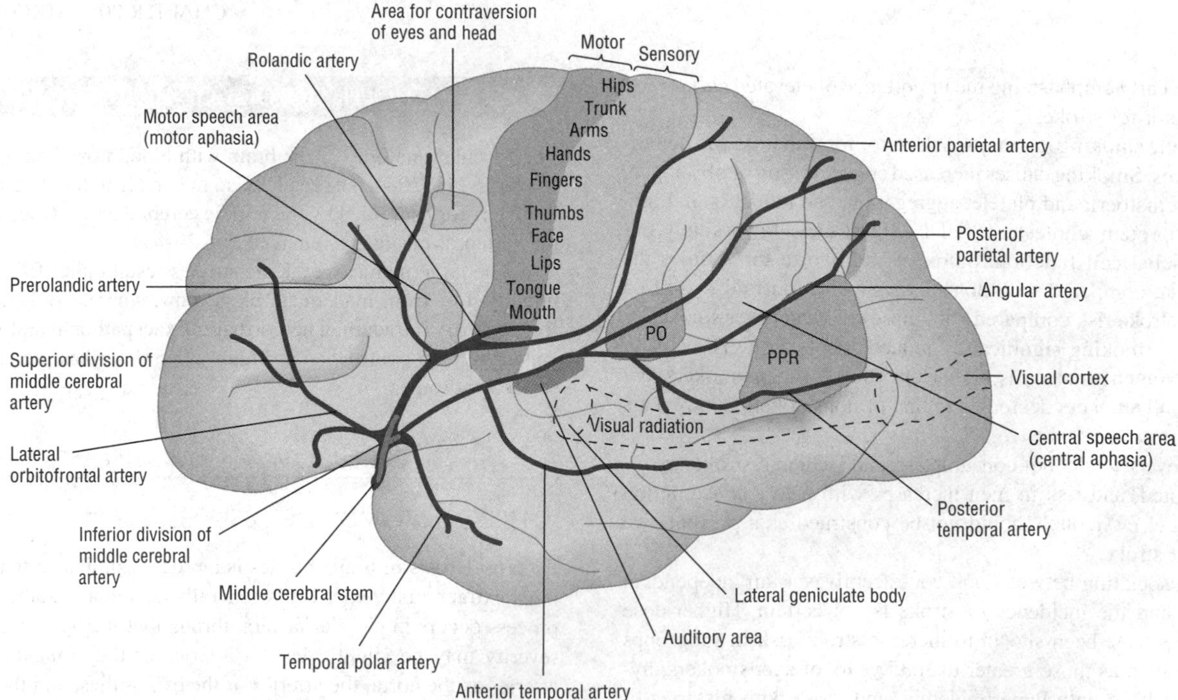

FIGURE 20–3. Diagram of a cerebral hemisphere, lateral aspect, showing the branches and distribution of the middle cerebral artery and the principal regions of cerebral localization. Note the bifurcation of the middle cerebral artery into a superior and an inferior division. *(From Braunwald E, Isselbacher KJ, et al., eds. Harrison's Principles of Internal Medicine, 11th ed. New York, McGraw-Hill, 1987:1936, with permission.)*

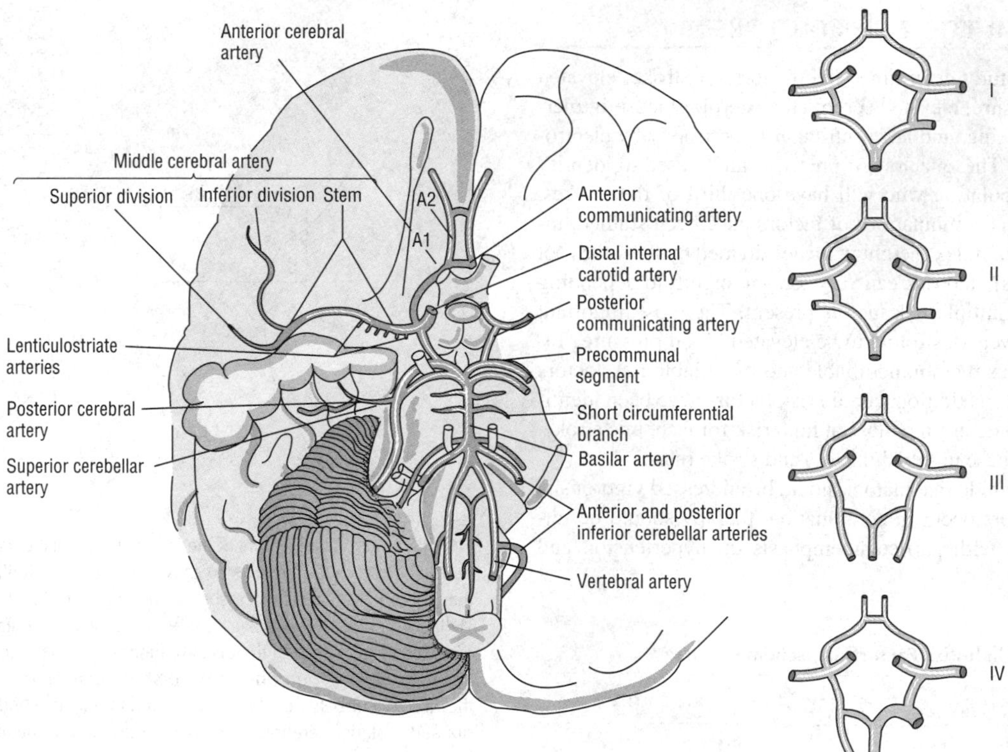

FIGURE 20–4. Diagram of the brain stem, cerebellum, inferior right frontal lobe, and temporal lobe transected. Principal branches of the vertebrobasilar arterial system are pictured. Small branches of the vertebral and basilar arteries that penetrate the medulla and pons are not pictured. The stem of the middle cerebral artery with its small, deep penetrating lenticulostriate arteries and the circle of Willis with its small, deep penetrating branches are pictured. Roman numerals I, II, III, and IV represent some of the possible variations of the circle of Willis resulting from atresia of one or more of its arterial components. Great variability in infarct size and location occurs when the basilar or vertebral arteries, or one of their penetrating branches, occlude because of variation in arterial anatomic location and available collateral circulation. Thus the stroke syndromes produced are often atypical or incomplete, or merge with one another. *(From Braunwald E, Isselbacher KJ, et al., eds. Harrison's Principles of Internal Medicine, 11th ed. New York, McGraw-Hill, 1987:1932, with permission.)*

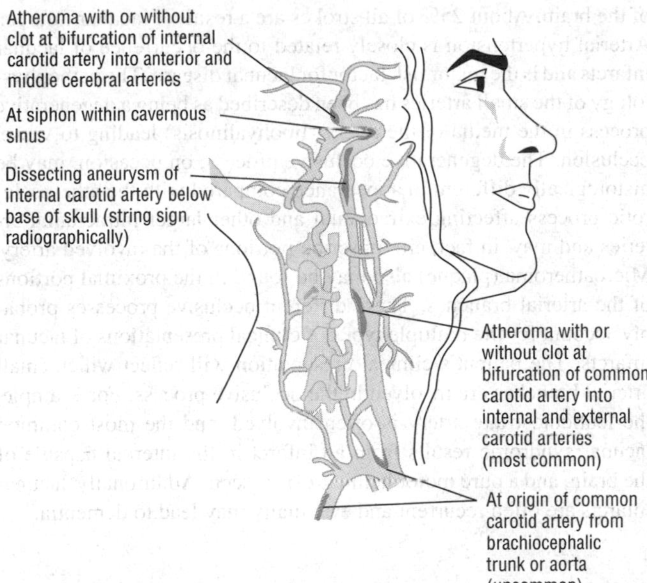

FIGURE 20–5. Common sites of atherosclerotic disease in the aortocranial circulation. *(From Ciba Collection of Medical Illustrations. Ciba Foundation, 1982, vol I pt II, p 55, with permission.)*

arteries. Atherosclerosis and subsequent plaque formation result in arterial narrowing or occlusion and constitute the most common cause of aortacranial stenosis. Atherosclerosis is seen initially as a fatty streak on the vascular wall. This fatty streak starts as a deposition of lipids in the endothelial cells of the vessel wall. This process may regress, remain stable, or progress. If the process continues, yellow fatty, fibrous plaques are formed. Again, if there is progression, an atheromatous lesion may form secondary to the interaction of a number of atherogenic substances including low-density lipoprotein–cholesterol (LDL-C) and others and hemorrhage into the plaque, and subintimal necrosis, loss of intimal integrity, ulcer formation, or calcification may occur.[16,17] The process of atherosclerosis results in plaque formation, which enhances platelet aggregation. Thrombosis may be more likely to occur in areas where plaque has caused the greatest narrowing of the vessel. Formation of a blood clot superimposed on an atherosclerotic plaque may cause significant stenosis of large extracranial arteries of the deep penetrating intracerebral arteries. Additional factors such as blood hypercoagulability and increased platelet counts and hematocrit also may contribute to clotting and sludging of blood flow.

Embolism can produce a stroke when a clot, plaque, or platelet aggregate breaks off into the circulation and blocks an artery. When atherosclerotic plaque ulcerates and is embolized distally, the emboli are called *artery-to-artery emboli*. Other embolic phenomena are discussed in the section "Cerebral Embolism and Cardiogenic Embolism" under "Clinical Presentation and Diagnosis" later in this chapter. Platelets play an important role in thrombosis and loss of integrity of the endothelial surface of the arterial wall, even if the defect is minor, and the resulting platelet activation can lead to formation of a thrombus. This endothelial damage can result from trauma or from diseases such as atherosclerosis, and when this occurs, vessel collagen can be exposed to the blood. This exposed collagen acts as a trigger mechanism to activate the platelets. This activation results in release of adenosine diphosphate (ADP) from the platelets, which in turn causes platelets to aggregate. Aggregation is consolidated by coagulation factors, red blood cells, and formation of a fibrin network. Other factors are also produced, including thromboxane A_2, which promotes platelet aggregation and vasoconstriction. This is balanced by the production of prostacyclin (PGI_2) by the vessel endothelium. The atherosclerotic process is variable, and the ischemic consequences resulting from this process depend on (1) the adequacy of blood flow and collateral circulation and (2) embolism. These factors determine the outcome of any individual ischemic event. To produce a low-blood-flow state leading to ischemia, the blood pressure must be reduced distal to the stenosis or occlusion and, usually, the carotid lumen must be reduced 75% in diameter. Impaired collateral circulation to the affected area is also critical. The collateral circulation is composed of a network of arteries on the surface of the brain and those of the circle of Willis.

The most common sites for the atherosclerotic process to occur are at the bifurcation of the common carotid siphon, the origin of the common carotid artery from the aorta, and less commonly in the aortic arch; at the bifurcation of the internal carotid artery into the anterior and middle cerebral arteries; and in the circle of Willis at the proximal segments of the anterior, middle, and posterior cerebral arteries (Fig. 20–4).

The process of atherogenesis also may be stimulated by vascular endothelial damage caused by the increased expression of cell adhesion molecules in patients with dyslipidemia. Adhesion molecules such as vascular cell adhesion molecule (VCAM-1), which is specific for monocytes, promote atherogenesis by binding monocytes on the endothelium and increasing their numbers in the atherosclerotic lesion. Additionally, intracellular adhesion molecules (ICAM-1) can contribute to neutrophil adhesion and movement into endothelial cells.[18–21] Refer to Chapter 21 for additional details.

CEREBRAL ISCHEMIA

Cerebral ischemia can be divided into focal and general (or global) ischemia. Global ischemia is associated with lack of collateral blood flow, and irreversible brain damage occurs in a short period of time (4–8 minutes). In focal ischemia, however, there remains some degree of collateral circulation; therefore, this may allow for survival of brain cells and reversal of neuronal damage after periods of ischemia. Because of this potential for recovery, focal ischemia is considered treatable in some cases. The pathophysiologic characteristics of focal ischemia may be reviewed in terms of cerebral ischemia thresholds, metabolic derangements, and microcirculatory changes.[18]

CEREBRAL ISCHEMIA THRESHOLDS

Normal cerebral blood flow (CBF) in humans is about 53 mL per 100 g of brain tissue per minute. Reductions in CBF to the range 15–18 mL/100 g/min result in abnormal brain electrical activity. At a flow of 10 mL/100 g/min, alterations in intracellular calcium and extracellular potassium homeostasis occur. Also, free fatty acids are released, and adenosine triphosphate (ATP) is depleted. A severe intracellular acidosis ensues in cells in the ischemic area. A CBF of 10 mL/100 g/min results in failure of ionic regulation and is thought to result in rapid irreversible damage to neurons. The CBF range between electrical failure and ionic failure is thought to be enough to maintain cell function for a time, possibly up to 4 hours, and recovery might be possible in acute focal ischemia, provided adequate collateral flow could supply basic energy requirements. Clinical outcome, as noted earlier, depends on the severity and duration of the decreased CBF.

METABOLIC DERANGEMENTS

When the CBF decreases to 10 mL/100 g/min, accumulation of lactic acid, depletion of ATP, and an increase in intracellular calcium may be seen. Extracellular potassium increases because of a failure of the ATP-dependent sodium-potassium pump. This rise in extracellular K^+ and sodium depolarizes the neuronal membrane, which in turn stimulates opening of the voltage-dependent calcium channels, and an influx of calcium into the intracellular space occurs. Calcium cannot be pumped out normally because of the failure of the ATP-dependent calcium transport system, and in addition, calcium is not taken up normally by the endoplasmic reticulum. This unbalanced intracellular increase in calcium is thought to result in production of free fatty acids from membrane phospholipids. This loss of phospholipid decreases the integrity of the cell, and the permeability of the cell membranes increases and further impairs calcium homeostasis.

Excitatory substances, such as amino acids, glutamate, and aspartate, are released from the neuron as a result of depolarization. Glutamate activates the *N*-methyl-D-asparate (NMDA) receptor as well as other receptors, allowing further influxes of calcium and sodium into the cell and thereby enhancing depolarization.

Accumulation of free fatty acids, including arachidonic acid, results in oxidation via cyclooxygenase and lipoxygenase pathways, producing prostaglandins, leukotrienes, and free radicals. Thromboxane A_2 is a potent vasoconstrictor, leukotrienes affect membrane permeability, and free radicals can attack cell membranes. Free radical production during ischemia overwhelms the endogenous methods for scavenging, and these free radicals can further disrupt cell membranes and produce vasoconstriction. All these actions can lead to further intracellular acidosis and increasingly impair cell function. Ischemia and the subsequent production of intracellular acidosis can have devastating effects on the brain cell. These effects include glial edema and denaturation of proteins. Focal ischemia is associated with preserved but marginal CBF, and continued glucose delivery in the face of ischemia promotes anaerobic glycolysis with production of lactic acidosis. This continues to worsen the intracellular acidosis.

ISCHEMIC EDEMA

Swelling is one of the primary responses of brain tissue to acute injury. An early or intracellular phase and a late or extracellular phase occur. The early phase involves primarily the glial cells surrounding the vessel itself, suggesting a defect in vascular permeability, possibly enhanced by lactic acidosis. The primary difficulty caused by the glial edema is that collateral flow is decreased as a result of the "squeezing down" on the collateral circulation. The late or extracellular phase occurs hours to days after vessel occlusion and probably is a result of ischemic damage to vessel endothelial tissue. Movement of plasma into the extracellular space results in increased intracranial pressure. Brain herniation can result from the increased pressure. In animals, there are regional differences in brain tissue vulnerability to ischemia, and some tissues may be more or less resistant to ischemic damage than other tissues. Some investigators postulate that these differences may result from the greater number of calcium channels in those tissues which are most vulnerable.

LACUNAR INFARCTS

Occlusion of the small arterial branches of the circle of Willis and of the anterior, middle, and posterior cerebral and basilar arteries can result in infarcts deep in the cerebral hemispheres (subcortical) and brain stem. These are small arteries with diameters in the range of 100–400 μm, and their occlusion results in small infarcts 2–15 μm in diameter. The term *lacunar* or *lacune* refers to the small cavity left after necrotic tissue has been removed. The pathophysiology of these infarcts is somewhat different from that of infarcts closer to the surface of the brain. About 25% of all strokes are a result of lacunar infarcts. Arterial hypertension is closely related to the occurrence of lacunar infarcts and is the major risk factor for lacunar disease. The pathophysiology of the small arteries has been described as being a degenerative process in the media of the artery (lipohyalinosis) leading to vessel occlusion. The degenerative occlusive process, on occasion, may be histologically different in appearance compared with the atherosclerotic process affecting extracranial and other larger intracranial arteries and may, in fact, circumscribe portions of the involved artery. Microatheroma (plaque) also may be found in the proximal portions of the arterial branches. These different occlusive processes probably account for the multiple types of clinical presentations of lacunar infarcts. The patient's clinical presentation will reflect which small arterial branches are involved in the occlusive process. For example, the lenticulostriate artery is often involved, and the most common lacunar syndrome results from an infarct in the internal capsule of the brain, and a pure motor hemiparesis is seen. Additionally, lacunar infarcts are often recurrent and eventually may lead to dementia.

TRANSIENT ISCHEMIC ATTACKS

TIAs are episodes of temporary focal cerebral dysfunction of vascular origin in which the onset is rapid, is of variable duration, and lasts from a few seconds up to 24 hours. The most common duration is a few seconds up to 5 to 10 minutes depending on the territory of the brain where the event occurs. Between attacks, there may be no neurologic abnormality. The clinical manifestation reflects the territory of the artery involved and usually occurs in the carotid system or in the vertebrobasilar system or both. TIAs have great significance in that they herald an impending stroke. *Threatened stroke* is a term used to describe any prestroke syndrome, such as TIAs, or patients who have had small or minor strokes or progressing or evolving stroke and are at further risk for a major stroke.

The pathophysiology of TIAs involves the atherosclerotic process of thrombus formation in cerebrovascular arteries and low CBF. It is from the cerebral thrombus that small microemboli, in the form of platelet aggregates and cholesterol crystals, break off and travel to distal areas and lodge, producing the ischemic attack. Cerebral or cerebellar artery thrombosis is most commonly responsible for TIAs. Low flow also will result in a TIA when the CBF is sufficiently reduced in stenosed arteries. Other causes include emboli from the heart caused by valvular disease or endocardial damage and increased blood viscosity from conditions such as polycythemia. Polycythemia is an uncommon cause of TIA. Transient monocular blindness (amaurosis fugax), although not a TIA, is a focal retinal deficit caused by localized retinal ischemia.

CEREBRAL EMBOLISM

Any region of the brain can be affected by embolism, but the area or territory of the middle cerebral artery is commonly involved. Embolism may result from pieces or fragments of an arterial thrombus that have broken off or from a heart valve vegetation. Occasionally, an embolus may form from an ulcerated atheromatous plaque. Other forms of embolism such as air, fat, or tumor cells occur only rarely. Cerebral embolism from bacterial sepsis occurs frequently, but bacterial emboli large enough to produce a stroke are infrequent. After breaking off from a thrombus or heart valve vegetation, an embolism usually circulates until it is too large to traverse the arterial lumen. The point of occlusion may be at a bifurcation or other narrowed area. Both hemispheres of the brain appear to be equally affected. Hemorrhagic

TABLE 20–3. Major Causes of Cardiogenic Cerebral Embolism

Nonvalvular atrial fibrillation	50%
Coronary heart disease	20%
Myocardial infarction	
Rheumatic heart disease	15%
Mitral stenosis ± atrial fibrillation	
Prosthetic cardiac valves	10%
Other	5%
Cardiomyopathy	
Cardiac tumors	
Septic endocarditis	
Nonbacterial thrombotic endocarditis (marantic)	
Congenital heart disease	
Venous clots/intracardiac shunt (paradoxic emboli)	
Mitral annulus calcification	
Calcific aortic stenosis	
Mitral valve prolapse	

From Easton JD, Hart RG, Sherman DG, et al. Diagnosis and management of ischemic stroke. Part 1. Threatened stroke and its management. Curr Prob Cardiol 1983;8:20.

infarction frequently occurs in the embolic process because of reperfusion of blood into the ischemic tissue, causing hemorrhage, and the area of the middle cerebral artery is often the involved site. This usually develops in 1 to 2 days after the infarct. The size of the embolus may vary from large to very small; in fact, the embolus may be so small that it produces no infarct or produces an infarct so small that it cannot be detected.

Cerebral embolism secondary to thrombotic disease usually has a rapid onset, and it is not preceded by a TIA. This rapid onset is problematic because there is less time for collateral circulation to develop as in cerebral thrombosis. As a result, embolic strokes often are functionally devastating. Cerebral embolism may result from heart disease. It is currently recognized that cardiogenic embolism accounts for 20% of all ischemic strokes. Embolism has been associated with many types of heart disease, and the following discussion focuses on the most common types (Table 20–3).

CARDIOGENIC EMBOLISM AND ATRIAL FIBRILLATION

Chronic atrial fibrillation (AF) is the most common cause of cardiogenic embolism and is the most common sustained dysrhythmia. The incidence of AF increases with age such that 2% to 5% of patients older than 60 years of age have AF, and more than half of AF-associated strokes occur in individuals older than 75 years.[22]

Patients with nonvalvular AF have about the same stroke risk as patients who experience a TIA. AF enhances the development of left atrial thrombi and arterial embolism. The most common site (75%) in which left atrial thrombi form in patients with nonvalvular AF (NVAF) is the atrial appendage rather than the atrial wall. Patients with AF and valvular disease have thrombi both on the atrial wall and on the appendage in equal incidence. Factors involved in the pathogenesis of atrial thrombus formation in patients with AF include increased left atrial pressure and outflow obstruction. Mitral valve obstruction can enhance left atrial stasis similar to that seen in AF alone. Enlargement of the left atrium occurs in AF, and the incidence of thrombus formation increases with left atrial enlargement. Damage to the endothelial surface also could induce thrombus formation and initiate AF. Such disorders as rheumatic heart disease, myocardial infarction, and pericarditis also can initiate AF by involvement of the sinoatrial node and change the atrial endothelial surface such that thrombus formation is enhanced. The risk of stroke in patients with AF is high, and 20% to 35% of all patients with AF will have an embolic stroke of clinical significance.[22] The risk of stroke in those with AF is five to six times that of the general population and averages about 5% per year. Those at greatest risk are patients with AF and rheumatic valvular disease. The risk for development of systemic embolism for these individuals is 17 times that of the general population. The largest group of patients comprises those with NVAF; their rate of systemic embolism is around 35%, and their stroke risk is six times that of the general population.[22] Predictors of stroke risk in AF include history of hypertension, prior stroke or transient ischemic attack, diabetes, and recent (within 3 months) heart failure. Risk factors have been identified by various authors and groups and are summarized in the literature.[23] The clinical utility of this risk stratification will be discussed under treatment. Even patients with idiopathic AF have an increased rate of embolism of 7% in the first year and up to 14% at 5 years. The presence of carotid stenosis also may help to identify a subgroup with NVAF who are at higher risk of stroke.[24] Patients who develop AF have a high rate of embolus formation soon after the onset of AF. Recurrence of embolism is frequent. Up to 50% of patients who develop one embolus develop another. In addition, changing the rhythm by cardioversion increases the rate of embolus occurrence, and about 2% of these patients may develop an embolus the first few days after cardioversion of AF to normal sinus rhythm. Generally, anticoagulation should be used 3 weeks before conversion and continued for 4 weeks after conversion.[25,26] Reversion to normal sinus rhythm versus ventricular rate control in AF in a recent report in a small number of patients has shown that neither approach is superior.[27] Results of the large trial Atrial Fibrillation Follow-up Investigation of Rhythm Management (AFFIRM) is awaited.[28]

Ischemic heart disease and ischemic stroke share the same risk factors, and most younger patients with TIAs and stroke die from myocardial infarction. In myocardial infarction, the primary cause of emboli is mural thrombus formation in the left ventricle. Thrombus formation is thought to be started by platelet adherence to and deposition on the damaged (infarcted) akinetic or dyskinetic endocardial surface. There is also an inflammatory white cell response in the damaged area secondary to the tissue infarction. Additionally, the infarcted area may develop into an aneurysmal region where fibrin accumulation can occur. Mural thrombus formation depends on the size and location of the infarct. Thrombus formation and the presence of apical akinesis or dyskinesis are seen almost exclusively in anterior myocardial infarctions. Aneurysms occur most frequently in the apex region of the heart. About 50% to 60% of patients with aneurysm formation in the left ventricle develop a mural thrombus. Most of these mural thrombi develop within the first week of the acute myocardial infarction, and patients who have mural thrombi, as evidenced by echocardiography after acute myocardial infarction, are most probably those patients at risk for eventual embolization. The overall incidence of systemic emboli in patients who suffer an anterior acute myocardial infarction is around 5% to 6% and is similar to the incidence in those patients who develop a left ventricular aneurysm. Therefore, of the 50% to 60% of patients with an aneurysm who develop a mural thrombus, only 5% to 6% develop a systemic embolus. In patients surviving acute myocardial infarction who develop congestive heart failure, the risk of stroke is approximately 2% per year, and it is increased during the first three months after acute myocardial infarction.[29,30] Risk factors for stroke in patients surviving acute myocardial infarction are advanced age, presence of AF, prior stroke, previous myocardial infarction, and left ventricular dysfunction as shown by echocardiography. Therefore, cardiogenic embolism may be likely if there is severe impairment of left ventricular function or if there is a left ventricular thrombus that is mobile or protruding.

VALVULAR HEART DISEASE

Thromboembolism is commonly found in patients with valvular heart disease, such as rheumatic mitral disease, and in those with prosthetic heart valves. Thrombus formation in patients with valvular disease or prosthetic valves most often occurs in the left ventricle or on the prosthetic valve. Thrombi also can form, but with a lower incidence, in the left atrium.

In valvular heart disease, patients with mitral stenosis and those with mitral stenosis combined with incompetence of the mitral valve have a thromboembolic event rate of 15% to 20%. Up to 16% of these events may be fatal. Patients with only mitral incompetence are at less risk than those with mitral stenosis, and the embolic rate is approximately 3%, although this rate may be higher in patients with a severe form of mitral incompetence. Prolapse of the mitral valve appears to carry a very low risk of embolism. The risk of embolism also appears to be low in patients with aortic valve disease. Additional factors that increase risk for systemic embolism in patients with valvular disease are atrial fibrillation, increased left atrial size, increased age, and history of a previous embolic event. AF is the most important single risk factor, and as noted previously, thrombus formation is rare in patients with a normal sinus rhythm. AF is closely associated with mitral valve disease, and emboli may develop shortly after fibrillation develops. Enlargement of the left atrium usually occurs with mitral valve disease, and left atrial enlargement predisposes to AF; therefore, there is an indirect relationship between left atrial enlargement and embolism. Recurrent embolic events can occur in up to 20% of mitral stenosis patients with previous embolic history. The mortality rate is high in this group of patients and may reach 42%.

PROSTHETIC CARDIAC VALVES

Thrombus formation on prosthetic cardiac valves (PCVs), whether aortic or mitral valves, is related to the production of turbulence in blood flow by the valve and the thrombogenic potential of the valve material. Patients who have had PCV replacement are at long-term risk of arterial thrombolism. Examples of mechanical valves currently used are the Starr-Edwards ball valve, the Bjork-Shiley disk valve, the St. Jude Medical valve, and others. The early Starr-Edwards valve, used in the 1960s, may have a higher embolic rate than those used in recent years. This may be a result of improved operative procedures and valve factors, as well as less severe disease and better atrial and ventricular function. The embolism rate with the Bjork-Shiley valve is similar to that with the Starr-Edwards valve; however, a newer material, pyrolytic carbon, in the disk of the valve is less thrombogenic, and the embolism rate is lower. The bioprosthetic valves, such as the Hancock, Carpentier-Edwards, and Lonescu-Shiley valves, have a different design—a central flow design. This design produces less turbulence in blood flow, the biologic material (porcine valve) is less thrombogenic, and thus thromboembolism occurs less frequently than with the other valves. Other risk factors include AF, large left atrium, valve placement in the mitral position, inadequate anticoagulation, multiple PCVs, and a previous embolic event.

The overall risk of neurologic deficit with mechanical prosthetic valve-induced embolism is high. For instance, data from follow-up of the older Starr-Edwards ball valve show that 85% of systemic emboli entered the cerebral circulation and 50% of these emboli resulted in a neurologic deficit, with 10% of all embolic events being fatal. Overall, the rate of embolism in anticoagulated patients with mechanical PCVs averages 3% per year for mitral valves and 1.5% per year for aortic valves.[31] Embolic rates for nonanticoagulated patients with bioprosthetic valves are 2% to 4% per year. A new stentless porcine tissue aortic valve from St. Jude Medical has been approved recently by the Food and Drug Administration (FDA). This valve does not have the plastic or metal support structure that other tissue valves have, and it may be more similar to the natural heart valve. Postmarketing follow-up is necessary to determine the place in treatment of this valve. There is general agreement that all adults with any type of mechanical valve should be on long-term anticoagulation and that bioprosthetic valves also require treatment with short-term anticoagulation and optional long-term antiplatelet therapy.[31]

INFECTIVE ENDOCARDITIS

Emboli may result from bacterial vegetations that can form in infective endocarditis. Arterial emboli are one of the most frequent complications of this disease. Major cerebral emboli have been observed in nearly one-third of patients with endocarditis, with the middle cerebral artery and its branches being involved most frequently. The highest frequency of major embolic events occurs in association with infections on the left side of the heart that produce large, mobile vegetations from *Hemophilus parainfluenzae* or slow-growing fastidious gram-negative bacilli, fungi *(Aspergillus)*, and *Streptococcus viridans*. Emboli from the right side of the heart, as seen in intravenous drug abusers, often are caused by staphylococcal organisms and can produce clinical manifestations of pulmonary emboli. Cerebral emboli from right-sided endocarditis also can occur if the patient has a patent foramen ovale (PFO). About 15% of adults have PFO. There is another type of endocarditis, called *nonbacterial thrombotic endocarditis* (NBTE), in which sterile thrombi are present on the valves. This condition is seen most often in patients with mucin-secreting adenocarcinomas and other debilitating diseases, and the vegetations are composed mainly of platelets and fibrin.[32]

UNUSUAL AND OTHER CAUSES OF INFARCTION

Other causes of cerebral infarction are listed in Table 20–4.

TABLE 20–4. Unusual Causes of Infarction

Venous thrombosis	Contraceptive steroid use
Systemic hypotension	Polycythemia
Arteriography	Idiopathic thrombocytosis
Carotid occlusion	Dissecting aortic aneurysm
Arteritis	Hypercoagulable states
Moyamoya disease	

INTRACRANIAL HEMORRHAGE

Approximately 15% of cases of stroke are due to intracranial hemorrhage. The more frequent causes of stroke from intracranial hemorrhage are hypertensive intracerebral hemorrhage, ruptured saccular aneurysms, hemorrhage associated with bleeding disorders, and arteriovenous malformations (AVMs).

Hypertensive intracerebral hemorrhage occurs generally when the blood pressure is elevated significantly. The bleeding occurs in the brain tissue as a result of rupture of an artery. This allows for an extravasation of blood into the brain tissue, which forms a mass. This mass damages the tissue and continues to enlarge as bleeding

TABLE 20–5. Causes of Intracranial Hemorrhage

Hypertensive intracerebral hemorrhage
Lobar hemorrhage of undetermined cause and intracerebral hemorrhage associated with congophilic angiopathy (analyzed)
Ruptured saccular aneurysm, giant aneurysm, or mycotic aneurysm
Ruptured angioma
Hemorrhagic disorders: leukemia, aplastic anemia, thrombocytopenic purpura, liver disease, complication of anticoagulant therapy, hyperfibrinolysis, hypofibrinogenemia, hemophilia, Christmas disease
Trauma, including posttraumatic apoplexy
Hemorrhage into primary and secondary brain tissue
Hemorrhagic infarction, arterial or venous
Inflammatory disease of the arteries and veins
Miscellaneous rare types: after vasopressor drugs, upon exertion, during arteriography, during painful urologic examination, as a late complication of early-life carotid occlusion, complication of carotid–cavernous arteriovenous fistula, with anoxemia, migraine, teratomatous malformations (acute inclusion body encephalitis produces xanthochromia and up to 2000 red blood cells or more in the cerebrospinal fluid; acute necrotizing hemorrhagic encephalopathy may be associated with up to 100 red blood cells in the cerebrospinal fluid; tularemia and snake venom poisoning may cause bloody cerebrospinal fluid)

From Braunwald F, Isselbacher KJ, et al, eds. Harrison's Principles of Internal Medicine, 11th ed. New York, McGraw-Hill, 1987:1952, with permission.

continues. Brain tissue is pushed, displaced, and compressed, and brain functions may be impaired. The larger the hemorrhage, the greater is the displacement of tissue. Escape of blood into the ventricles of the brain can occur, and when this happens, the spinal fluid becomes bloody. The cerebrospinal fluid may remain clear if the hemorrhage is small or at a distance from the ventricular system. The extravascular blood undergoes changes such as phagocytosis, and the mass shrinks gradually; after 2 to 6 months, only discoloration is left at the site. Hemorrhagic infarcts, discussed earlier, are due primarily to the reflow or reperfusion of ischemic tissue, with resulting bleeding into the tissue. In hypertensive hemorrhage, the vessels most often involved are the penetrating arteries in the putamen and internal capsule and parts of the white matter, including the frontal lobe, thalamus, pons, and cerebellar hemisphere. Causes of intracranial hemorrhage are listed in Table 20–5.

CLINICAL PRESENTATION AND DIAGNOSIS

ATHEROTHROMBOTIC DISEASE

Thrombosis of cerebral vessels produces variable clinical manifestations as compared with embolic disease or intracranial hemorrhage. In a large percentage of cases (≥50%), the stroke is preceded by one or more TIAs. If the evolving thrombosis involves the internal carotid and middle cerebral arteries, then such focal symptoms as mono- or hemiplegia, mono- or hemiparesthesia, blindness in one eye, and speech disturbance may occur. If the vertebrobasilar system is involved, such symptoms as dizziness, diplopia, numbness, impaired vision, and dysarthria may occur. Usually these attacks are short-lived and resolve in less than 10 minutes. The stroke itself most often develops suddenly as a single attack, or it may show an intermittent or stuttering progression pattern over hours to days. Additionally, a patient may suffer a partial stroke, improve for several hours, and then develop full paralysis of one or more parts of the body; other parts become paralyzed in a stepwise manner until the stroke is completed. When the thrombosis produces a developing involvement over hours, days, or weeks, it is called *stroke in evolution* or *progressing stroke.* Interestingly, the majority of cerebral thrombotic strokes occur at rest while sleeping or after arising. Headache may occur but is often absent; when present, it may occur several days prior to the other symptoms of the stroke.

Diagnosis consists of evaluation of the clinical presentation and laboratory findings. In addition to the clinical presentation just discussed, laboratory evaluation can include tests such as cerebral arteriography, imaging studies such as CT scan (with or without contrast enhancement), MRI, radioactive brain scan study (such as a technetium scan), x-rays of the head, electroencephalogram, ECG, transcranial Doppler studies, digital subtraction angiogram, and lumbar puncture (LP). The definitive test for arterial occlusion or narrowing is the arteriogram; however, the procedure carries a neurologic risk itself and should only be used if the diagnosis of vascular disease is not clear or if vascular surgery is a possibility, such as in carotid TIA patients. Complications from cerebral angiography occur in 2% to 12% of patients and consist primarily of aortic or carotid dissection and embolic stroke. Hydration may reduce these risks. Because of the risks of arteriography, brain imaging is the most important test after a stroke has occurred. When it is performed, transfemoral angiography is usually the procedure of choice as compared with the direct carotid puncture procedure. The CT scan in cerebral thrombosis usually shows an area of decreased attenuation or hypodense lesion in the infarcted area. The CT scan is often normal, however, during the first 48 hours after the thrombotic infarction. The CT scan is extremely useful in excluding tumors and identifying intracranial hemorrhage, both of which dictate different treatment modalities. CT scans, however, may not show small ischemic strokes, especially on the cortical surface, and bone may cause difficulty in interpretation. MRI can adequately detect small infarcts in the cortical surface and elsewhere usually within 1 hour of occurrence. MRI is a noninvasive imaging technique that, unlike CT and positron-emission tomography (PET), does not require x-rays or isotopes. MRI uses magnetic fields to generate images, and it takes longer to perform than a CT scan, although recent advances in MRI (ultrafast and echoplanar imaging) has made it as fast as CT.

Radioisotopic brain scans can be helpful and show infarcts earlier than CT scans. Skull x-rays usually are not helpful, and the electroencephalogram and LP are of limited value because they are usually normal. Noninvasive techniques such as Doppler flow studies and Doppler scanning have been developed but have some disadvantages with consistent differentiation of stenosis from occlusion and detection of distal atherosclerosis. Transcranial Doppler studies recently have been shown to detect circulating microemboli that cannot be detected by other imaging techniques. This technique may be useful in patient risk assessment and risk stratification.

Digital subtraction angiography (DSA) is a recent addition, and it holds promise as a diagnostic tool. Arterial injection of contrast medium in DSA currently provides better imaging of the cerebral vasculature than does intravenous administration, which gives imperfect detail. Other new diagnostic imaging techniques aimed at measuring cerebral blood flow and/or metabolism include xenon-CT blood flow; PET assessment of glucose and oxygen metabolism; single-photon-emission computed tomography (SPECT), which can give an image of dynamic physiology after injection of positron-emitting isotopes; and MRI angiography (MRA). MRA allows noninvasive visualization of the cerebral vasculature as well as extracerebral vessels and may become the most used of the techniques because it does not require arterial access and can be done in the course of a routine MRI study.

Recommendations for imaging of the brain in suspected hemispheric TIA are as follows[33]:

1. CT scan, without contrast, should be done to exclude other lesions that may produce TIA-like manifestations such as a tumor.
2. MRI is not routinely recommended over CT scanning unless the CT scan is a failure or inadequate.
3. Routine use of MRI in vertebrobasilar TIA is not recommended.

Recommendations for imaging of the brain in acute stroke are as follows[33]:

1. CT scan of the head, without contrast, can detect rapidly almost 100% of hemorrhages in the first 12 to 24 hours.
2. Follow-up CT scan, without contrast, is done 2 to 7 days after the acute event if the initial CT scan was negative in order to document potential hemorrhagic transformation or to determine the location of the infarction; MRI can be used after 12 to 24 hours (diffusion-weighted and perfusion-weighted MRI adds to clinical findings as early as 8 hours) to detect the exact location and size of the infarction. MRI (diffusion-weighted and perfusion-weighted) is superior to CT scanning in detecting brain edema.
3. MRI is not recommended for routine evaluation in acute stroke at this time.

LACUNAR INFARCTS

The clinical presentation varies depending on the perforating cerebral arteries involved. The most frequently occurring lacunar syndrome is pure motor hemiparesis, which is due to an infarct in the posterior portion of the internal capsule. This infarct results from occlusion of a middle or posterior cerebral perforating artery. The manifestations of the pure motor hemiparesis syndrome are hemiparesis or hemiplegia of the arm, leg, face, and trunk. In addition, a mild dysarthria occurs without sensory or consciousness alterations or visual field defects. The different parts of the body involved in the stroke display the same degree of weakness. This is in contrast to a stroke in the cortical region involving the middle or anterior cerebral artery, where there is usually an unequal degree of weakness of the affected parts of the body.

Diagnosis usually is based on clinical evaluation of the patient after careful neurologic examination. A CT scan or MRI scan can provide evidence of the infarction if performed within about 7 to 10 days of the event; however, infarcts smaller than 2 mm may be missed. Treatment after lacunar stroke requires control of hypertension to help in the prevention of progression of the degenerative occlusive process.

TRANSIENT ISCHEMIC ATTACKS

Most TIAs last 5 to 10 minutes, and those lasting one or more hours may be a result of embolism rather than ischemia or atherosclerosis. A TIA resulting from a carotid system lesion and anterior cerebral artery involvement manifests as weakness in the opposite leg and shoulder. Refer to Fig. 20–3 for anatomic correlation. If the anterior cortical branches of the middle cerebral artery are involved, a sensory and motor loss results in the contralateral face, arm, and hand. If the ischemia is in the dominant hemisphere, a nonfluent (Broca's) aphasia usually is present. Ischemia occurring in the posterior portions of the middle cerebral artery often produces contralateral sensory loss and homonymous hemianopia (defective vision or blindness affecting the right halves or the left halves of the visual fields of the two eyes). If there is posterior middle cerebral artery involvement in the dominant hemisphere, a fluent aphasia is likely to occur. Ischemia of the lenticulostriate arteries may result in findings that involve motor and sensory defects in the arms, legs, face, and trunk, as noted in the discussion of lacunar infarcts. Clinical manifestations of TIAs arising from ischemia in the vertebrobasilar circulation are numerous. Vertigo and ataxia are seen in ischemia affecting cerebellar and vestibular areas. Bilateral weakness of the extremities indicates that the corticospinal nerve tracts are involved as they cross the brain stem. TIAs occurring with an increasing frequency, longer duration, and of greater severity are termed *crescendo TIAs*. These should be treated urgently because they usually represent an unstable internal carotid artery stenosis or ulceration or both or possibly extracranial arterial aneurysm.

Diagnosis of a TIA is difficult because the episode is usually over before the patient can be examined. Therefore, the diagnosis is really made on the basis of the patient's recollection of the symptoms. Table 20–6 shows the symptoms of TIAs. There are many singular symptoms or events that can be confused with TIAs and usually are not TIAs. Some of these events are fainting, convulsions, loss of consciousness, dizziness, spots before the eyes, dysarthria, imbalance and falling, and headache. Diagnostic studies may indicate the presence of vascular disease; however, history is a key to the diagnosis of a TIA. Proper attention to the history is important because treatment of TIAs is important in stroke prevention.

Laboratory studies in the diagnosis of TIA should rule out blood or other disorders that may produce decreased cerebral blood flow. Routine studies include erythrocyte sedimentation rate, complete

TABLE 20–6. Symptoms of Transient Ischemic Attacks

Carotid system TIAs	
Unilateral weakness—usually hemiparesis	
Unilateral sensory complaints—numbness, paresthesia	
Aphasia—language comprehension, output, or both	
Monocular visual loss (amaurosis fugax)	
Vertebrobasilar system TIAs	
Motor deficit—especially if bilateral	
Sensory complaints—especially if bilateral	
Simultaneous, bilateral visual complaints	
Diplopia	Only in combination, not as isolated symptoms
Vertigo	
Dysarthria[a]	
Ataxia without weakness	
Dysphagia	
Either carotid or vertebral TIAs	
Severe dysarthria[a]	
Homonymous visual complaints	
Isolated symptoms rarely resulting from TIAs	
Vertigo, dizziness	
Diplopia	
Loss of consciousness	
Confusion	
Bilateral leg weakness, falling spells	

[a]Often difficult to distinguish from nonfluent dysphasia on the basis of history.
From Easton JD, Hart RG, Sherman DG, et al. Diagnosis and management of ischemic stroke. Part 1. Threatened stroke and its management. Curr Prob Cardiol 1983;8:13, with permission.

blood count, platelet count, blood chemistry, urinalysis, coagulation profile, and syphilis (serology). To reveal systemic disease in selected patients, serum protein electrophoresis, antinuclear antibody titers, blood and plasma viscosities, plasma fibrinogen, and cerebrospinal fluid examination may be performed. Embolism of cardiac origin should be a consideration in every patient with a single TIA. In these cases, a 12-lead ECG should be performed to test for recent myocardial infarction and/or dysrhythmias such as atrial fibrillation. Other laboratory tests include a chest x-ray to exclude heart enlargement or disease of the valves. In patients suspected of having TIAs of embolic origin, echocardiography is an important diagnostic tool.[34] Two-dimensional echocardiography is indicated in patients with cerebral ischemia who have evidence of cardiac disease such as AF, enlarged heart, and mitral valve prolapse. The yield of thrombus detection in the hearts of these patients is 10% to 20%. The lower limit of clot size that is detected accurately by echocardiography is 2 to 3 mm. In addition, results from the Stroke Prevention in Atrial Fibrillation Investigators (SPAF) studies indicate that echocardiography in NVAF can serve as a clinical predictor of thromboembolism by detecting increased left atrial size and left ventricular dysfunction.[23,29] Left atrial size and left ventricular size are strong independent predictors of later thromboembolism. Therefore, the echocardiogram can add to the clinical variables for risk stratification. If transthoracic echocardiography (TTE) detects an embolic source, transesophageal echocardiography (TEE) generally is not necessary. As mentioned earlier, cerebral angiography should be performed only in selected patients, and patients who have had a carotid TIA should be studied with angiography as soon as reasonably possible because of the high risk of cerebral infarction in these patients.

CEREBRAL EMBOLISM AND CARDIOGENIC EMBOLISM

Cardiogenic brain embolism is the major cause of cerebral embolism. The brain is involved in approximately 70% of all emboli from the heart, whereas systemic or noncerebral nervous system emboli often go unrecognized. Cardiogenic brain embolism accounts for 20% of all ischemic strokes. The clinical diagnosis is based on a variety of findings, as shown in Table 20–7. The onset is characteristically abrupt, often occurring in an awake patient.

A stuttering course may be seen in about 10% of patients. This represents a distal lodging of emboli. Most cardiogenic emboli that go to the brain lodge in the middle cerebral artery (MCA) or one of its branches. Vertebrobasilar or anterior cerebral artery emboli occur less frequently (<10%) than MCA emboli. Cardiogenic embolism may be suspected when there are multifocal neurologic findings. Seizure or headache at the onset of the stroke is not as useful an indicator as once thought. Cardiogenic embolism should be considered when the following conditions are present: age over 60, sudden onset of maximal neurologic deficit, prior cortical infarct, past history of valvular heart disease or left ventricular myocardial infarct, and atrial fibrillation or congestive heart failure. Laboratory studies in those with suspected cardiogenic brain embolism may include two-dimensional (2D) TTE to assess the presence of left ventricular thrombi and mitral valve dysfunction and M-mode echocardiography for the presence of left ventricular dysfunction.[34] TTE does not reliably indicate atrial thrombi, although TEE may be better at detection than TTE. The ECG may indicate a dysrhythmia such as AF. MRI and CT scanning are currently being evaluated for their clinical usefulness in detecting cardiogenic emboli.

TABLE 20–7. Clinical Features Suggestive of Cardiogenic Brain Embolism

Primary Features
Abrupt onset of maximal deficit
Presence of a potential embolic source
Infarct involving the cerebral cortex or cerebellum
Previous ischemic events in other vascular territories

Secondary Evidence
Hemorrhagic infarct by CAT
Absence of occlusive cerebrovascular disease by cerebral angiography or reliable noninvasive imaging
Angiographic evidence of vanishing occlusions
Evidence of embolism to other organs
Cardiac thrombi demonstrated by echocardiography, catheterization, cardiac CAT, or MRI

From Sherman DG, Dyken ML, Fisher M, et al. Cerebral embolism. Chest 1986;89(suppl 2):845, Table 2, with permission.

INTRACRANIAL HEMORRHAGE

Usually the clinical manifestations of intracranial hemorrhage have an abrupt onset, and changes generally occur over minutes to hours (up to 24 hours). This gradual evolution depends primarily on the bleeding rate and accounts for the time range for the neurologic deficit to become maximal. The neurologic physical findings vary with the site of bleeding and the size of the bleed. The majority of patients lose consciousness, and many die without recovering awareness.

Typically, the patient with spontaneous intracerebral hemorrhage may experience head pain and dizziness prior to losing consciousness. In the case of hypertension-related external capsule (putaminal) hemorrhage, the patient quickly develops signs of hemiplegia and loss of consciousness. Hypertensive intracerebral hemorrhages are associated most often with prolonged and sustained hypertension and occur frequently while the patient is awake.

Conjugate deviation of the eyes to the side opposite of the affected limbs is seen commonly. If the lesion becomes larger, compression of the upper brain stem produces deepening coma, and the patient has dilated and fixed pupils, Babinski signs, bilateral motor hypertonus, and irregular respirations.

In the case of internal capsule (thalamic) hemorrhage, the onset is similar to that for putaminal hemorrhage; however, if the patient is still alert, homonymous hemianopia may be seen because of optic nerve involvement in the internal capsule. The location of this hemorrhage produces a variety of gaze disturbances, including defective vertical and lateral gaze, fixed downward deviation of the eyes, and unequal pupils.

In the diagnosis of hypertensive intracerebral hemorrhage, the sudden onset and quick evolution of the physical findings are important. Headache occurs at the onset in approximately 50% of the cases, whereas the occurrence of headache in thromboembolism is less than 25%. Neck rigidity is common, and the funduscopic examination of the eye may reveal periarteriolar hemorrhages and decreased arteriolar size. Ocular signs are very helpful in localizing hemorrhages of putaminal and thalamic origin. Convulsions are common, as is vomiting, and a history of hypertension is an important clue. Generally, the immediate prognosis for intracerebral hemorrhage is extremely poor, with up to 70% of patients dying in a few days.

Important laboratory findings include evidence of bleeding on the CT scan. CT scanning, without contrast, is the diagnostic procedure of choice in assessing intracranial and subarachnoid hemorrhage. It is extremely sensitive in detection of blood in very small amounts, as noted earlier, and is extremely useful in the differential diagnosis of hemorrhage versus infarction.

▶ TREATMENT: Stroke

GENERAL THERAPEUTIC CONSIDERATIONS

The therapeutic approach to patients with cerebrovascular disease involves multiple phases, including preventive measures against stroke and vascular disease in general, supportive and medical management during the acute phase of a stroke, measures necessary to mitigate the pathologic or atherothrombotic process, and appropriate rehabilitative and physical therapy programs during the poststroke period. Importantly, significant public attention has been focused on stroke (brain attack). The development of practice guidelines, stroke teams, and stroke care units in hospitals has greatly improved the awareness and care of patients with acute stroke.

Prevention of cerebrovascular disease is the most important aspect of therapeutic management, and elimination and/or management of the risk factors discussed earlier under epidemiology and etiology are required. Control of hypertension, hyperlipidemia, obesity, cigarette smoking, alcohol use, and other tobacco use as well as other risk factors for atherothrombotic disease is essential to the overall care of the patient with cerebrovascular disease. In the patient with hypertension who has atherosclerotic cerebrovascular disease or who has developed an ischemic infarction, care must be taken to avoid drug-induced or other hypotensive episodes. In general, preservation of the systemic circulation in acute stroke and avoidance of orthostatic changes are also advised. Management of blood pressure after stroke is controversial. Elevated pressure after a stroke usually is not considered an emergency. Elevated pressure usually will go down when other problems such as pain, agitation, and increased intracranial pressure are addressed. Recommendations for treatment differ depending on the type of stroke and if the patient is to receive thrombolytic therapy. If thrombolytic therapy is indicated, strict control of blood pressure is necessary to decrease the possibility of bleeding. Consensus recommendations for antihypertensive therapy in those not eligible for thrombolytic therapy are shown in Table 20–8.[35]

ISCHEMIC CEREBROVASCULAR DISEASE

The major goals of treatment for patients with acute ischemic stroke are (1) to remove or limit the obstruction to flow in the vessel and (2) to protect brain cells distal to the obstruction or blockage from suffering hypoxic changes. It is currently possible to attain the first goal with thrombolytic and anticoagulation therapy, thus reducing mortality and improving functional outcome; however, neuroprotective therapy is still under study.

TABLE 20–8. Antihypertensive Therapy in Acute Stroke

Blood Pressure (mm Hg)	Treatment
Diastolic blood pressure >140	Sodium nitroprusside—target is 10% to 20% reduction in diastolic blood pressure
Systolic blood pressure >220, diastolic blood pressure 121 to 140 or mean arterial pressure >130	Labetalol IV 10 to 20 mg over 1 to 2 minutes; may repeat every 20 minutes to dose of 150 mg
Systolic blood pressure <220, diastolic blood pressure ≤120 or MAP <130	Defer treatment unless presence of AMI, severe CHF, or hypertensive encephalopathy

THROMBOLYTIC THERAPY

Thrombolytic therapy for acute ischemic stroke was first proposed in the 1950s; however, intracranial hemorrhage was such a limiting factor that use of thrombolysis as a therapy became dormant until just recently, when better understanding about brain hemorrhage, use of plasminogen activators, and better imaging techniques have shed new light on this type of therapy in acute ischemic stroke.[36] The therapeutic effect of tissue plasminogen activators is to activate plasmin and thereby lyse fresh thromboemboli. Agents include streptokinase, anisoylated plasminogen streptokinase activator complex (APSAC), and tissue plasminogen activator (t-PA) single chain (alteplase). Results of major clinical trials using streptokinase have been reported recently.[37,38] In all these trials, treatment with streptokinase (SK) resulted in increased mortality and morbidity from intracranial hemorrhage, and thus SK cannot be recommended in stroke therapy. Recently, two major trials have been reported using alteplase in acute ischemic stroke: the European Cooperative Acute Stroke Study (ECASS) and the National Institute of Neurological Disorders and Stroke t-PA Trial (NINDS).[39,40] The ECASS trial was established to assess the safety and efficacy of alteplase in acute ischemic stroke. The study was a double-blind, placebo-controlled, randomized, prospective multicenter trial. A total of 620 patients were randomized to alteplase or placebo 6 hours or less following the onset of ischemic stroke symptoms and after hemorrhagic stroke had been excluded by CT scanning. Alteplase was infused at a rate of 1.1 mg/kg over 60 minutes, after a bolus of 10% of total dose. Primary end points measured were the Barthel Index and modified Rankin Scale at 30 and 90 days, 30-day mortality, and the Scandinavian Stroke Scale at 30 days. These stroke scales quantify neurologic functioning and overall functional disability. Because of protocol violations (intravenous heparin) and difficulty in interpreting the results, the conclusion reached was that alteplase improves some functional measures and neurologic outcomes in patients but that t-PA should not be used in the general stroke population.

The NINDS trial had the same objective as ECASS, but the design of the study was quite different in that it was in two parts. The study consisted of two sequential randomized trials comparing t-PA with placebo in which 624 patients were randomized to one of two treatment groups within 3 hours of stroke. Alteplase was infused at a rate of 0.9 mg/kg (maximum 90 mg) over 1 hour after a bolus of 10% of the total dose over 1 minute. Careful review of the CT scan before treatment for evidence of hemorrhage, exclusion of patients with hypertension, good blood pressure control, and no heparin or aspirin use in the first 24 hours were significant parameters used to select the most appropriate patients. Part 1 evaluated 291 patients and showed that a favorable clinical improvement at 24 hours was evident: 47% improvement with alteplase versus 39% with placebo ($P = .18$). Part 2 of the study was the same as part 1 except that it evaluated outcomes of 333 randomly assigned patients on four stroke scales at 3 months. Part 2 is considered to be a pivotal study, and the

TABLE 20–9. NINDS Combined Results of Part 1 and Part 2

End Points	TPA	Placebo	RR (95% CI)	*P* Value
NIHSS at 24 h (% with improvement)	47	39	1.2 (1.0–1.4)	.06
0–90 min (% with favorable outcome)				
Global test			1.9 (1.2–2.9)	.005
Barthel index	53	38	1.8 (1.2–2.9)	.010
Modified Rankin scale	40	28	1.7 (1.0–2.6)	.035
Glasgow outcome scale	43	32	1.6 (1.0–2.5)	.057
NIHSS	34	20	2.0 (1.2–3.4)	.008
91–180 min (% with favorable outcome)				
Global test			1.9 (1.3–2.9)	.002
Barthel index	51	38	1.6 (1.1–2.5)	.026
Modified Rankin scale	45	25	2.4 (1.5–3.7)	<.001
Glasgow outcome scale	47	30	2.0 (1.3–3.2)	.002
NIHSS	34	21	2.0 (1.2–3.2)	.008
Mortality at 90 days (%)	17	21		NS

investigators were blinded to the outcomes of part 1. Results of part 2 show sustained clinical benefit that was statistically significant on all four stroke scales (Barthel Index, modified Rankin Scale, Glasgow outcome, and NIHSS). The global statistic for improvement on all four stroke scales was significant, thereby denoting the clinical improvement seen in these study patients. A subgroup analysis of the study showed that the benefit was across all subtypes of stroke and patient groups. There was, however, a significant increase in the occurrence of cerebral hemorrhage (6.4% of all t-PA patients versus 1% in placebo group) within 36 hours of treatment. Most of these hemorrhages were in patients with large strokes. Even with the increased rate of hemorrhage, t-PA did not cause a significant increase in early or late mortality. The conclusion is that alteplase, when administered within 3 hours of acute ischemic stroke onset, improves 3-month clinical outcome. These findings represent a most significant advance in the acute treatment of ischemic stroke. Table 20–9 shows the combined results of parts 1 and 2. Additionally, it has been shown recently that the NIHSS score is strongly predictive of patient recovery after stroke.[41] The TOAST trial reported that early intravenous use (within 24 hours) of the heparinoid danaparoid produced favorable outcomes in patients with ipsilateral occlusion of the internal carotid artery identified by carotid duplex imaging. This was a small study of 119 patients. The NIHSS score was shown to predict recovery in this trial if the score was less than or equal to 6. A score greater than or equal to 16 predicts a high probability of death or severe disability.

RECOMMENDATIONS AND MONITORING

The development of t-PA therapy is indeed an exciting advance in the treatment of acute ischemic stroke, but caution must be exercised in using this mode of therapy, and adherence to clinical protocol is a necessity.[42] Summary of the recommended alteplase treatment protocol is (1) stroke team activation, (2) onset of symptoms within 3 hours, (3) a cranial CT scan to rule out hemorrhage, (4) intravenous administration of alteplase at 0.9 mg/kg (maximum of 90 mg) over 1 hour after a bolus of 10% of the total dose given over 1 minute, and (5) monitoring of patient for response and hemorrhage. Table 20–10 summarizes the inclusion and exclusion criteria for use of alteplase in acute ischemic stroke.

ANTICOAGULATION THERAPY

This mode of therapy was the first to gain acceptance in ischemic cerebrovascular disease, and because this therapy has been used for some time, some conclusions can be drawn about the usefulness of anticoagulation in various types of ischemic cerebrovascular disease.

TABLE 20–10. Inclusion and Exclusion Criteria for Alteplase Use in Acute Ischemic Stroke

Inclusion Criteria (all YES boxes must be checked before treatment)

YES

☐ Age 18 years or older
☐ Clinical diagnosis of ischemic stroke causing a measurable neurological deficit
☐ Time of symptom onset well established to be less than 180 minutes before treatment would begin

Exclusion Criteria (all NO boxes must be checked before treatment)

NO

☐ Evidence of intracranial hemorrhage on noncontrast head CT
☐ Only minor or rapidly improving stroke symptoms
☐ High clinical suspicion of subarachnoid hemorrhage even with normal CT
☐ Active internal bleeding (e.g., GI/GU bleeding within 21 days)
☐ Known bleeding diathesis, including but not limited to platelet count <100,000/mm^3
☐ Patient has received heparin within 48 hours and had an elevated APTT
☐ Recent use of anticoagulant (e.g., warfarin) and elevated PT (>15 sec)/INR
☐ Intracranial surgery, serious head trauma, or previous stroke within 3 months
☐ Major surgery or serious trauma within 14 days
☐ Recent arterial puncture at noncompressible site
☐ Lumbar puncture within 7 days
☐ History of intracranial hemorrhage, arteriovenous malformation, or aneurysm
☐ Witnessed seizure at stroke onset
☐ Recent acute myocardial infarction
☐ SBP >185 mm Hg or DBP >110 mm Hg at time of treatment

A number of studies have been performed with heparin and coumarin derivatives since the 1970s; however, criticisms of poor design, wrong diagnoses, and inadequate numbers of patients for comparative purposes have limited the acceptance of these studies.

The following is a brief review of anticoagulation therapy in TIA, progressing stroke, and completed stroke.

TRANSIENT ISCHEMIC ATTACKS/PROGRESSING STROKE (STROKE IN EVOLUTION)

No randomized clinical trial evidence exists to support the use of anticoagulation in patients with either TIA or progressing stroke. Some clinicians opt to use anticoagulation in patients while they are being urgently evaluated for either crescendo TIAs or neurologic deterioration (progressing stroke) after intracranial hemorrhage has been ruled out. There is no evidence to support these practices.

COMPLETED STROKE

Seven randomized studies have addressed anticoagulation therapy in completed stroke. These studies showed no difference between treatment and control groups in the incidence of recurrent stroke or death. There is also a risk of major bleeding in patients treated for several months with anticoagulation therapy. Therefore, the risk of anticoagulation therapy in completed stroke outweighs any benefits obtained, and based on the best studies to date, anticoagulation generally should not be used.

The risk of hemorrhage is highest in patients with ischemic cerebrovascular disease when anticoagulation therapy lasts longer than 4 weeks. Compared with other indications for anticoagulation, anticoagulation for stroke is associated with a greater risk of hemorrhagic complications. Although intensity of therapy and type of reagents used in laboratory testing were the source of some of the differences in European and North American studies, hemorrhagic complications are still the major risk in anticoagulated patients with ischemic cerebrovascular disease.

RECOMMENDATIONS AND MONITORING

It is recommended that anticoagulation not be used routinely in patients with TIAs or progressing stroke and not be used at all in patients with completed stroke. Prophylaxis of recurrent cerebral thromboembolism is important in patients with completed stroke, however, because prior stroke is a risk factor for another stroke. Aspirin 50 to 325 mg/d, clopidogrel, or an aspirin-dipyridamole combination product can be recommended. Patients who remain symptomatic with TIAs on optimal antiplatelet therapy who do not have surgical disease may be candidates for anticoagulation. Some would use a combination of aspirin and clopidogrel if aspirin alone fails, and this is currently under study. In general, if warfarin is to be used for chronic anticoagulation, it should overlap with heparin for approximately 5 days to obtain warfarin antithrombotic activity. By maintaining an international normalized ratio of 2.0 to 3.0, a slightly less intensive anticoagulation effect is obtained with a decreased incidence of bleeding without a decrease in efficacy. Continuous monitoring for minor and major bleeding is required. The use of special anticoagulation services can be of significant assistance in the therapy and monitoring of patients on warfarin therapy and is recommended whenever possible.

ANTIPLATELET THERAPY

Antiplatelet agents have been studied for use in ischemic cerebrovascular disease for a number of years; the proposed mechanism of action is an alteration in blood platelet aggregation, thus inhibiting the formation of thrombi in arterial vessels. The antiplatelet agents currently available include aspirin, clopidogrel, extended-release dipyridamole-aspirin combination, and ticlopidine. Cilostazol is under investigation and shows promise.

ASPIRIN

The antiplatelet effects of aspirin are theoretically responsible for aspirin's beneficial antithrombotic effects in TIAs. Aspirin inhibits platelet aggregation by irreversible inactivation of the enzyme cyclooxygenase, which, in platelets, prevents conversion of arachidonic acid to thromboxane A_2 (TXA_2), which is a powerful vasoconstrictor and stimulator of platelet aggregation. Platelets remain impaired for their life span (5–7 days) after exposure to aspirin. Aspirin also inhibits prostacyclin activity in the smooth muscle of vascular walls. PGI_2 inhibits platelet aggregation, and the vascular endothelium can synthesize prostacyclin such that the platelet antiaggregating effect is maintained. The suppression of PGI_2 production by aspirin has been found to be related to dose and duration; the higher the dose, the longer the cyclooxygenase production is suppressed. Therefore, the lower the aspirin dose, the less effect there is on prostacyclin. The optimal dose of aspirin is still under study, but it should be the dose that inhibits TXA_2 with the least amount of prostacyclin inhibition. It has been shown that an aspirin dose of 325 mg/d will inhibit TXA_2 but will not significantly inhibit PGI_2 production. There is probably a point at which lower doses of aspirin do not completely block TXA_2, and recent studies indicate that the lowest effective dose may be in the range of 30–50 mg/d.

Aspirin (acetylsalicylic acid) was found in the early 1970s to prevent amaurosis fugax (monocular visual loss) and to decrease the number of TIAs without affecting the death rate. The Canadian Cooperative Study Group study was published in 1978.[43] This study involved treatment of 585 patients with one or more cerebral or retinal ischemic attacks. These patients were randomized to aspirin, sulfinpyrazone, and placebo. The average follow-up was 26 months, and the aspirin dose was 325 mg four times daily and sulfinpyrazone 200 mg four times daily. For the overall study group, aspirin reduced the risk of TIA, stroke, or death by 19% ($P < .05$). If only stroke or death was considered, aspirin reduced the risk of these by 31% ($P < .05$). Interestingly, no significant benefit was shown for women in this study, but this sex difference was not confirmed in later studies.[44] Sulfinpyrazone did not show any risk reduction for TIA. Other randomized trials have been done, and all show statistically significant differences between aspirin and placebo for some ischemic events.

The doses of aspirin used in ischemic cerebrovascular disease studies have ranged from 30 mg/d to 1.5 g/d. A controversy still exists over the appropriate dose of aspirin. Although low doses of aspirin (325 mg/d) have been shown to be effective in other conditions such as protection against myocardial infarction in unstable angina patients, prevention of coronary bypass shunt thrombosis, and prevention of thrombosis in arteriovenous shunts of chronic hemodialysis patients, the effectiveness of low doses in preventing stroke is still controversial. One of the recent studies to address the low-dose issue is the United Kingdom Transient Ischemic Attack/Aspirin Trial (UKTIA).[45] This is the first large study to evaluate low-dose versus high-dose aspirin (300 versus 1200 mg/d). Between July 1979 and September 1985, 2435 patients were enrolled in the study. All patients had experienced at least one TIA or mild ischemic stroke within 3 months of entry. The mean age was 60, and 75% of patients were male. Patients were randomly assigned to three groups. One group received 600 mg aspirin twice daily, the second group received 300 mg daily, and the third group received placebo. The dose ranges were selected somewhat arbitrarily, and patients were followed an average of 4 years. Reported results indicate that the incidence of stroke, myocardial infarction, or sudden death was the same in both aspirin-treated groups and 20% lower (statistically significant) than the incidence in the placebo-treated groups. The risk of cerebral infarction alone was 11% higher in the placebo group, although this was not statistically significant. When women were considered separately in the study, no significant differences were found between aspirin and placebo in risk for cerebral infarction or other major vascular event. The investigators note, however, that the number of women in the study was small. Side effects were less frequent with the lower dose of aspirin (29%) as compared with the 1200 mg dose (39%) and were least frequent in the placebo group (24%). Therefore, the lower dose of aspirin in this study was just as effective as the higher dose and had fewer side effects. Although this study showed that aspirin had less effect on fatal events than on nonfatal events, antiplatelet treatment conclusively reduces the risk of nonfatal vascular events.

Another recent study to address the low-dose aspirin issue is the Dutch TIA Trial.[46] This study was a double-blind trial in patients with TIAs or nondisabling stroke. This study had a different twist in that two main hypotheses were tested; first is the question of the effectiveness of 30 mg aspirin per day versus 300 mg/d in preventing vascular death and disability, and second was the question of whether 50 mg atenolol is more effective than placebo in preventing vascular death and disability. A double randomization technique was used to compare these two different therapeutic modalities. A total of 3131 patients were enrolled, and follow-up was 2.6 years. It was found that 30 mg/d of aspirin is no less effective than 300 mg/d in the prevention of the composite outcome event of death from vascular causes, nonfatal stroke, or nonfatal myocardial infarction. There also were fewer adverse effects in the 30 mg/d group. Therefore, a dose of 30 mg/d of aspirin was effective in TIA prevention.

Meta-analysis of 29,000 patients with histories of TIAs, minor strokes, unstable angina, or myocardial infarction was reported by the Antiplatelet Trialists' Collaboration. This analysis represented 25 trials. All antiplatelet agents and regimens were evaluated. Results of the analysis showed an overall 25% odds reduction (similar to relative risk reduction) for vascular events (i.e., stroke, myocardial infarction, or death from a vascular cause) and a 27% odds reduction in nonfatal stroke. A second meta-analysis from this group evaluated more than 100,000 patients in 145 trials.[47] A 25% overall odds reduction was shown for vascular events and 22% for patients with previous minor stroke or TIAs.

Pharmacodynamically, aspirin is converted to salicylate among four other metabolites during the normal metabolic process, and the ratio of salicylate to aspirin may be important because salicylate may prevent aspirin inhibition of PGI_2. Excessive salicylate concentrations may displace or prevent aspirin from binding to platelets, thereby potentially minimizing the antiplatelet effect of aspirin. Whether or not this proves to be clinically relevant remains to be shown in clinical studies. The interaction can be minimized by using low doses and sustained-release preparations. There is also some suggestion that a specific dose of aspirin in a specific patient may work at one point in time but at a later time may be ineffective.

The effectiveness of doses lower than 50 mg/d for TIAs or minor strokes of arterial origin is still not resolved, and additional study is required to adequately answer the dose questions. Other potential mechanisms of antithrombotic action of aspirin are currently under investigation. Aspirin also has been evaluated for treatment of acute ischemia stroke, and two large trials have found that use of aspirin 50 to 300 mg/d within 48 hours of stroke onset reduces stroke recurrence and mortality.[48,49]

CLOPIDOGREL

This agent has unique platelet antiaggregatory effects in that it is an inhibitor of the ADP pathway of platelet aggregation and inhibits known stimuli to platelet aggregation. This effect causes an alteration of the platelet membrane and interference with the membrane-fibrinogenic interaction leading to a blockage of the platelet glycoprotein IIb/IIIa receptor. A time lag of 3 to 7 days before the antiplatelet effect is maximal should be expected. Clinical effectiveness and tolerability appear similar to those of aspirin in preliminary studies using a dose of 75 mg/d. A large international trial (CAPRIE) comparing 75 mg/d of clopidogrel with 325 mg/d of aspirin in secondary prevention of ischemic disease in 19,000 patients with atherosclerotic disease has been published.[50] The atherosclerotic processes evaluated were ischemic stroke, myocardial infarction, and vascular death. Patients were followed for 1 to 3 years, and intention-to-treat analysis on the first events showed that clopidogrel had an annual 5.32% risk of ischemic stroke, myocardial infarction, or vascular death compared with 5.83% for aspirin. This represents a relative risk reduction of 8.7% ($P = .043$) in favor of clopidogrel. On-treatment analysis showed a relative risk reduction of 9.4%. Importantly, the safety profile was at least as good as that of aspirin with regard to bleeding, with no difference as compared with aspirin in neutrophil reduction. CAPRIE concluded that long-term administration of clopidogrel in patients with the atherosclerotic diseases studied is more effective than aspirin and at least as safe. In clinical use, however, there have been rare cases of thrombotic thrombocytopenic purpura (TTP) reportedly associated with the drug. This rare adverse effect occurs more frequently in patients treated with ticlopidine, however. In the published case series, all but 1 of 11 cases occurred within the first 2 weeks of therapy. Clopidogrel has evolved as an effective, safe treatment in patients who have had a TIA or stroke.

EXTENDED-RELEASE DIPYRIDAMOLE-ASPIRIN (ERDP-ASA)

Early studies of the role of dipyridamole in stroke prevention failed to show a benefit over that realized by aspirin alone. The European Stroke Prevention Study (ESPS) 2, published in 1996, demonstrated the efficacy of high-dose, extended-release dipyridamole (ERDP) alone and in combination with aspirin in secondary stroke prevention.[51] ESPS-2 was a randomized, double-blind evaluation of aspirin 25 mg bid, ERDP 200 mg bid, a combination of the two, or placebo in 6602 patients. Patients were followed for 2 years for stroke recurrence. All three of the treatment groups experienced significantly lower rates of stroke than the placebo group: aspirin alone, 18.1% reduction ($P = .013$); ERDP alone, 16.3% reduction ($P = .039$); and the ERDP-aspirin (ASA) combination product, 37% reduction ($P < .001$) compared with placebo. In addition, this was the first study to demonstrate the benefits of combination antiplatelet therapy (the combination was significantly more effective than either agent alone). More than 15% of the patients who received dipyridamole (alone or in combination) discontinued the therapy early, and this was twice as common as in the aspirin alone group. The main reasons were gastrointestinal problems or headache.

ERDP-ASA (ERDP 200 mg + ASA 25 mg) one capsule twice daily has been recommended as a first-line therapy (along with ASA and clopidogrel) in patients who have experienced a TIA or minor stroke. Due to the fact that 50 mg/d of ASA has never been shown to protect against recurrent myocardial infarction, some clinicians may opt to add an additional dose of ASA in these patients.

TICLOPIDINE

Ticlopidine, another thienopyridine, has been evaluated in two large clinical trials, and the results in stroke prevention have been beneficial in both men and women. In the TASS trial, the relative risk reduction for fatal or nonfatal stroke at 3 years was 21% greater with ticlopidine as compared to ASA.[52] The CATS trial showed a 30% relative risk reduction as compared with placebo.[53] Ticlopidine does possess a significant side-effect profile and is costly. Side effects include suppression of bone marrow, rash, diarrhea, and elevation of serum cholesterol. Neutropenia may occur in up to 2% of patients but is reversible on discontinuation of therapy. Monitoring is required because of these side effects, and it is recommended that patients have complete blood counts with differential every 2 weeks for 3 months. More than 50% of patients report at least one side effect, with gastrointestinal complaints being the most common. Drug interactions may occur with digoxin, theophylline, and antacids, and these efforts should be monitored. Ticlopidine was relegated to third-line status in stroke prevention due to its adverse-events profile. Ticlopidine 250 mg twice daily can be recommended as an alternative antiplatelet therapy in patients who fail or are intolerant of other strategies.

RECOMMENDATIONS AND MONITORING

Clinical trials have shown the beneficial effects of ASA in prevention of secondary TIAs as well as in producing a decrease in major vascular events. Currently, a dose of 50–325 mg/d can be recommended in the secondary prevention of TIAs and stroke. An enteric-coated product may be better tolerated by some individuals and may be used if needed. Patients should be monitored for gastrointestinal bleeding because the risk for bleeding is slightly increased. Clopidogrel, ticlopidine, and ERDP-ASA have all been shown to be superior to ASA in secondary stroke prevention, but the side-effect profiles and the increased cost of the newer agents have allowed ASA to maintain its status as a first-line drug in this category. Clopidogrel (75 mg/d) should be used if aspirin has failed to decrease or eliminate TIAs or stroke or if the patient cannot tolerate or has an allergy to aspirin. ERDP (200 mg) and ASA (25 mg) twice daily also can be used in patients who fail aspirin, but this combination should not be used in patients with coronary artery disease. Ticlopidine (250 mg bid) has been relegated to third-line status. Patients require careful monitoring while on ticlopidine, as noted previously, particularly during the first 3 months of therapy.

SURGICAL THERAPY

The purpose of surgery in ischemic cerebrovascular disease is to prevent the occurrence of cerebral infarctions and TIAs. Generally, the goal of a surgical procedure is to remove the source of occlusion and/or embolus and, hopefully, to increase cerebral blood flow to an ischemic area.

Carotid endarterectomy (CEA) is the most common surgical procedure used for occlusive cerebrovascular disease. This procedure has been popular since its introduction over 30 years ago. CEA involves exposing the carotid artery in the neck and removing the occlusive atheromatous plaque usually at the carotid bifurcation. The indications generally have been considered to be TIAs and mild completed stroke in the presence of ulcerated or highly stenotic (≥75%) plaque. Two recent multicenter studies of CEA in symptomatic carotid artery disease have been reported: the North American Symptomatic Carotid Endarterectomy Trial Collaborators (NASCET) study (still ongoing) and the European Carotid Surgery Trial (ECST).[54–56] In both of these trials, analysis showed that for symptomatic patients with stenosis of 70% or greater, CEA was superior to medical treatment alone at 2 to 3 years. In the NASCET study, surgery was not beneficial in patients with less than 50% stenosis and less than 70% stenosis in ECST. Patients with lesser degrees of stenosis were harmed by surgery. The rate of complications such as stroke or death due to CEA for an institution should be equal to or better than the NASCET figure (<5%) in order to have an acceptable risk-benefit ratio. Additionally, in symptomatic carotid artery stenosis, the number-needed-to-treat analysis indicates that six CEAs would need to be performed to prevent one stroke over a 2-year span. Other indications such as asymptomatic bruits and progressing stroke are controversial; however, results from the Asymptomatic Cartoid Atherosclerosis Study (ACAS) show that symptom-free patients with 60% to 99% carotid artery stenosis had a 55% relative risk reduction for ipsilateral stroke or any stroke or death after CEA compared with medical therapy.[57] Number-needed-to-treat analysis has shown that in patients with asymptomatic carotid artery stenosis, 67 CEAs would have to be performed to prevent one stroke over a 2-year period. CEA is not indicated in patients with permanent deficits from moderate to severe completed strokes.

INVESTIGATIONAL THERAPY

Therapy to improve or reverse the effects of an acute ischemic stroke is being actively pursued. As knowledge of the pathophysiologic processes involved has increased, the number of potential targets for therapy have multiplied. Strategies aimed at restoring blood flow to the ischemic brain have been most promising. Ancrod, a defibrinogenating agent, has been shown to improve 90-day outcome when initiated within 3 hours of onset of symptoms.[58] Prourokinase, when administered intraarterially to patients with large strokes within 6 hours of symptom onset, also has been shown to improve stroke outcome at 90 days.[59] Intraarterial thrombolysis may be more effective than intravenous therapy in patients with large clots. Other nonpharmacologic strategies under investigation to open the artery include laser embolectomy, intracranial angioplasty, and suction embolectomy.

Neuroprotective therapy has shown less promise. Although many compounds have been neuroprotective in animal models of stroke, success in human clinical trials has been elusive. Some reasons for the lack of success may be an inability to give the drug early enough, incomplete delivery of the drug to the site of action due to reduced blood flow, and selection of patients less likely to benefit from the therapy.[60] Dozens of compounds that interfere at various time points in the ischemic cascade are being studied. Compounds under study include glutamate antagonists, gamma-aminobutyric acid (GABA) agonists, ion channel modulators, and free radical scavengers. An area

TABLE 20–11. Antithrombotic Therapy in Patients with AF

Study	Type[a]	*n*	Target INR or Aspirin Dosage	Relative Risk Reduction % (*P*)[b]	Absolute Risk Reduction (%/yr)	NNT
Warfarin Versus Placebo						
AFASAK	1°	671	2.8–4.2	58 (<.05)	2.6	39
SPAF I	1°	421	2.0–4.58[c]	65 (.01)	4.7	22
BAATAF	1°	420	1.5–3.0[c]	86 (.002)	2.6	39
CAFA	1°	378	2.0–3.0	33 (>.05)	2.5	40
SPINAF	1°	571	1.5–3.0[c]	79 (.001)	3.4	30
EAFT	2°	439	2.5–4.0	66 (.001)	8.4	12
Aggregate[d]				68 (<.001)		
Aspirin Versus Placebo						
AFASAK	1°	672	75 mg/d	18 (>.05)	0.7	143
SPAF 1	1°	1120	325 mg/d	44 (.01)	2.5	40
EAFT	2°	782	300 mg/d	15 (>.05)	1.3	77
Aggregate				21 (<.05)		
Warfarin Versus Aspirin						
SPAF II	1°	1100	325 mg/d	31 (<.05)	0.8	125
AFASAK	1°	671	2.8–4.2, 75 mg/d	50 (.05)	1.9	53
SPAF III	1°	1044	325 mg/d[e]	76 (.001)	6.0	17
EAFT	2°	455	2.5–4.0, 300 mg/d	62 (.001)	6.4	16
Aggregate				55 (<.01)		

INR = International Normalized Ratio; NNT = number needed to treat to prevent one ischemic stroke per year; AFASAK = Atrial Fibrillation Aspirin Study of Anticoagulation from Kocenhaven; SPAF = Stroke Prevention in Atrial Fibrillation; BAATAF = Boston Area Anticoagulation Trial for Atrial Fibrillation; CAFA = Canadian Atrial Fibrillation Anticoagulation; SPINAF = Stroke Prevention in Nonrheumatic Atrial Fibrillation; EAFT = European Atrial Fibrillation Trial.

[a]1° = Primary prevention (in several studies, 5% to 10% of patients had remote thromboembolism); 2° = secondary intervention (previous transient ischemic attack or stroke).

[b]Reduction compared with control (active treatment or placebo) by intention-to-treat analysis.

[c]INR estimated for BAATAF, SPAF 1, and SPINAF, which used prothrombin time ratios.

[d]Average of all studies cited.

[e]Aspirin 325 mg/day plus warfarin given to achieve an INR in the range of 1.2–1.5.

Adapted from Ref. 26.

of intense interest is recovery enhancement. Stroke patients generally continue to improve for months after their acute event. Investigators are interested in facilitating this recovery, enhancing it, and making it available to all stroke victims regardless of how long it has been. An early study of the feasibility of injecting cultured human neuronal cells (transplantation) into stroke patients was published recently, giving additional hope to the stroke community.[61]

CEREBRAL EMBOLISM OF CARDIAC ORIGIN

In patients with cardiogenic brain embolism, immediate anticoagulation should be considered because approximately 12% of such patients have a second embolic stroke within 2 weeks. In nonhypertensive patients with small to moderate stroke, heparin should be given 24 hours after stroke onset without a loading dose so that a less intensive anticoagulation effect is obtained. The partial thromboplastin time (PTT) should be no greater than 1.5 times the control value using rabbit brain thromboplastin. Before heparin is started, however, a CT scan should document the absence of spontaneous hemorrhagic transformation. Anticoagulation should be maintained with warfarin at an INR of 2.0 to 3.0. In patients who develop hemorrhagic transformation shortly after embolic stroke, anticoagulation should be postponed 8 to 10 days.

The role of platelet antiaggregating agents in this situation is not clear, but antiplatelet agents generally are not recognized to have therapeutic value in those instances where red thrombi can develop, as in patients with cardiac mural thrombi, venous thrombosis, or large thrombi in any artery. In general, anticoagulation with warfarin is recommended in these situations. Obviously, prevention of the embolic event is the best therapy, and patients at high risk for cardiogenic embolism, such as those with AF or mechanical or prosthetic valves, should be treated with prophylactic chronic anticoagulation with warfarin. Six recent studies looking at preventative therapy in patients with NVAF have been completed. Five were primary intervention trials, and one (European Atrial Fibrillation Trial) was for secondary intervention. Table 20–11 summarizes the studies of antithrombotic therapy in patients with AF.[25]

In summary, these studies indicate that patients with NVAF can be treated effectively and safely with either warfain or ASA. The overall reduction of the relative risk of stroke in AF patients treated with warfarin was 68% compared with placebo, and the reduction with ASA was 21% compared with placebo. In all studies, the aggregate relative risk reduction is about 1.5% per year. Therefore, in order to gain maximum therapeutic benefit, the risk of intracranial bleeding must be less than the benefit of stroke prevention. In addition, warfarin may be the agent of choice in the stasis-related thromboembolism seen in patients with NVAF and heart failure.

RECOMMENDATIONS

Because of the potential for intracerebral hemorrhage in elderly patients and the probability of lifetime treatment with warfarin, identification of subgroups of AF patients with high and low rates of stroke has been studied in two large trials (SPAF I and SPAF II).[23,29] The new consensus recommendations for AF require risk stratification into high risk, moderate risk, and those with no high or moderate risk factors.[62] High risk factors are prior stroke or TIA or systemic embolism, history of hypertension, poor left ventricular function, age greater than 75 years, rheumatic mitral valve disease, and prosthetic heart valve. Moderate risk factors are age 65 to 75 years, diabetes mellitus, and coronary artery disease with preserved left ventricular systolic function. High-risk AF patients require anticoagulation with warfarin to a target INR of 2.5 (range 2.0–3.0). Patients with more than one moderate risk factor should be anticoagulated like high-risk patients. In patients with one moderate risk factor, warfarin (INR 2.0–3.0) or ASA (325 mg/d) may be used. Patients with AF who are younger than 65 years with no clinical or echocardiographic evidence of cardiovascular disease should be treated with ASA (325 mg/d). In AF patients who have had an ischemic stroke or TIA, anticoagulation with warfarin is usually recommended.

Patients who have had prosthetic cardiac valve replacement have a clinically significant and long-term risk of thromboembolism. The pathophysiologic events that precede arterial thromboembolism actually begin as soon as the device is sewn in place and blood flows across the PCV. Generally, patients who have undergone aortic valve replacement are at a lower risk of thromboembolism than those with mitral PCVs. Patients with both aortic and mitral valve replacement are usually considered to have the highest risk of thromboembolism. Other risk factors for thromboembolism include presence of AF, a large left atrium, previous thromboembolism, left ventricular dysfunction, and valve type and design.

Treatment recommendations for patients with mechanical PCVs are based on prospective, randomized trials of anticoagulant therapy with and without a platelet inhibitor. Thromboembolism is less frequent after bioprosthetic valve replacement. Even though the thrombogenicity of bioprosthetic valves is lower than that of mechanical valves, specific therapy is still required. The current recommendations for antithrombotic therapy for PCV replacement are presented for mechanical and bioprosthetic valves.

MECHANICAL PCVs

Therapy should begin with intravenous heparin or low-molecular-weight heparin (LMWH) 6 hours after surgery and warfarin as soon as possible after operation and dosed to maintain the INR in the therapeutic range for 2 consecutive days before discontinuing heparin or LMWH. A target INR of 2.5 (range 2.0–3.0) is recommended for St. Jude Medical bileaflet, Carbomedics bileaflet, and Medtronic-Hall tilting-disk valves in the aortic position if the left atrium is normal and the patient is in sinus rhythm.[31] Patients who have these valves in the mitral position require an INR target of 3.0 (range 2.5–3.5). If AF is present in patients with these valves in the aortic position, a target INR of 3.0 (range 2.5–3.5) is recommended. In patients with older caged-ball or caged-disk valves, a target INR of 3.0 (range 2.5–3.5) is recommended. In patients with mechanical valves and additional risk factors, a target INR of 3.0 (range 2.5–3.5) plus low-dose ASA (80–100 mg/d) is recommended. Patients who develop systemic embolism in the face of recommended therapy should receive ASA (80–100 mg/d) and have a target INR of 3.0 (range 2.5–3.5).

BIOPROSTHETIC PCVs

Initial therapy with unfractionated heparin or LMWH described for mechanical valves followed by warfarin overlap can be considered. Valves in the mitral position require warfarin for 3 months at an INR target of 2.5 (range 2.0–3.0). Long-term therapy with ASA (80 mg/d) is recommended after 3 months of warfarin. Patients who have a history of systemic embolism should receive warfarin at an INR target of 2.5 (range 2.0–3.0) for 3 to 12 months. Finally, long-term ASA (80 mg/d) is recommended for patients in sinus rhythm.

INTRACRANIAL HEMORRHAGE

General medical management and supportive therapy are indicated in the patient with this condition. This condition, as noted earlier, generally has a poor prognosis. Preventive therapy of intracranial bleeding is possible in the case of hypertension, where blood pressure can be controlled by diet and/or medication. Surgical management in the acute or early stage of the event is removal of the clot by aspiration or evacuation; this treatment usually is beneficial only in those patients whose hemorrhage is near the surface of the brain and who are not comatose. Cerebellar hemorrhage, on the other hand, often is amenable to surgery within the first 2 days of onset.

Corticosteroids and, more recently, dexamethasone have been used in the treatment of cerebral edema resulting from primary intracerebral hemorrhage. However, the use of steroids in this condition is not recommended.[62] The use of mannitol and other osmotic agents to reduce edema around the hemorrhage is appropriate, provided systemic hypotensive and hypertensive episodes are avoided. The use of mannitol is well established and is guided by maintaining the serum osmolality and arterial pressure. Generally, 0.25–2 g/kg mannitol can be administered intravenously every 4 to 8 hours until the serum osmolality is raised between 300 and 310 mosm/L. Cerebral edema is rarely a problem in ischemic stroke unless a very large MCA territory infarction occurs. Treatment is the same as noted for intracranial hemorrhage. Cerebral vasospasm in subarachnoid hemorrhage can be severe, and therapeutic efforts to prevent or treat the vasospasm have been disappointing. Reserpine, kanamycin, isoproterenol, aminophylline, and nitroprusside have all failed in this condition. Dopamine (3–6 μg/kg/min) has been used, but there is a risk of rebleeding. Percutaneous intra-arterial angioplasty, although not recommended, may be considered when vasospasm persists despite optimal medical treatment. However, data from well-designed trials are lacking. Barbiturate coma has been used to reduce intracranial pressure resulting from intracerebral hemorrhage when pressure reduction with dopamine or mannitol has not been successful. Further research is needed in the treatment of cerebral vasospasm and the resulting increased intracranial pressure.

PHARMACOECONOMIC CONSIDERATIONS

Cost-effectiveness of therapy in acute ischemic stroke has been examined in only a few studies. In antithrombotic prophylaxis for atrial fibrillation, warfarin therapy was evaluated using quality-adjusted life-years (QALY) saved.[63] It was found that in patients with AF and one additional risk factor, warfarin therapy cost \$8000 per QALY saved. In high-risk patients, those with AF and two or more risk factors, warfarin use was estimated to save \$6200 in costs from stroke and TIAs. Costs of monitoring and hemorrhages from warfarin were estimated to be \$5500, thus showing a positive savings from warfarin use. Those without risk factors were much more costly to treat at an estimated $370,000 per QALY saved when compared with ASA treatment. Warfarin is cost-effective in high-risk patients, particularly if the hemorrhagic side effects are lower relative to the stroke risk. For comparison purposes, hypertension screening is estimated to cost $10,000 to $50,000 per QALY saved. A Swedish study reported the cost-effectiveness of primary stroke prevention in AF patients with oral anticoagulants or ASA based on four published clinical trials.[64] The authors found that the total cost per stroke prevented was a $16 savings if the intracerebral bleeding was 0.3% and a $43 savings if the bleeding rate was 2%. At a bleeding complication rate of 1.3%, warfarin would prevent 1000 strokes per year and save about $29 million. Cost-analysis data on the NINDS trial with t-PA estimates that total health care costs (including acute and long-term costs) could be reduced by almost $5 million for every 1000 patients treated with t-PA.[65] Although t-PA is expensive, when the total health care costs are factored in, savings can accrue to the health care system as a direct result of appropriate t-PA therapy. Primary prevention strategies that address the risk factors for ischemic stroke can be powerful in reducing the costs of stroke. Many of the stroke risk factors can be modified and some eliminated at very low costs (lifestyle changes); therefore, developing risk-factor reduction strategies may be the most cost-effective measure of all. More research is needed to identify the cost-effectiveness of other forms of acute stroke treatment.

▶ PRINCIPLES OF PHARMACOTHERAPY

- Prevention of cerebrovascular disease is most important. Heart and brain healthy lifestyle changes and control of modifiable risk factors are key steps in prevention of ischemic stroke.
- Anticoagulation for TIA is not recommended routinely.
- Antiplatelet therapy is the therapy of choice for secondary prevention of TIA; 50–325 mg/d ASA is recommended.
- ASA 50 to 325 mg/d is recommended for secondary stroke prevention if the stroke is not due to AF.
- Clopidogrel 75 mg/d orally and the combination of ASA 25 mg and ERDP 200 mg twice daily are also acceptable for initial therapy in those who fail aspirin.
- AF patients should be stratified according to risk prior to oral anticoagulation. High risk factors are prior stroke/TIA or systemic embolism, history of hypertension, poor left ventricular systolic function, age greater than 75 years, rheumatic mitral valve disease, and PCVs. Moderate risk factors are age 65 to 75 years, diabetes mellitus, and coronary artery disease with good left ventricular function.
- High-risk AF patients should receive warfarin with an INR target of 2.5 (range 2.0–3.0).
- AF patients with one moderate risk factor should receive either warfarin (INR target 2.5) or ASA (325 mg/d). AF patients with more than one moderate risk factor should be treated as high-risk patients.
- AF patients younger than 65 years of age with no clinical or echocardiographic evidence of cardiovascular disease should be treated with ASA (325 mg/d).
- Mechanical PCVs require warfarin therapy indefinitely, dosed to an INR of 2.5–3.5. Bioprosthetic PCVs in the mitral position require warfarin dosed to an INR of 2.0–3.0 for the first 3 months after placement followed by long-term ASA (80 mg/d).
- Ateplase 0.9 mg/kg infused over 1 hour after a bolus of 10% of total dose is recommended as emergency therapy in acute ischemic stroke if a CT scan is negative for intracranial hemorrhage and if therapy can be initiated within 3 hours of the acute event. Patient selection is critical, and strict adherence to the AHA guidelines is mandatory to avoid bleeding complications. Monitor patients closely for bleeding.[42]

REFERENCES

1. Gorelick PB, Sacco RL, Smith DB, et al. Prevention of a first stroke: A review of guidelines and a multidisciplinary consensus statement from the National Stroke Association. JAMA 1999;281:1112–1120.
2. Heart and Stroke Facts: 2001 Statistical Supplement. Dallas, American Heart Association, 2000.
3. Taylor TN, Davis PH, Torner JC, et al. Lifetime cost of stroke in the United States. Stroke 1996;27:1459–1466.
4. Helgason CM, Wolf PA. American Heart Association Prevention Conference IV: Prevention and rehabilitation of stroke. Circulation 1997;96:701–707.
5. Bronner LL, Kanter DS, Manson JE. Primary prevention of stroke. New Engl J Med 1995;333:1392–1400.
6. Circulation 2000;102(Suppl 1):I204–216.
7. Albers GW, Dalen JE, Laupacis A, et al. Antithrombotic therapy in atrial fibrillation. Chest 2001;119(Suppl):194S–206S.
8. Allessie MA, Royden PA, Camm J, et al; Pathophysiology and prevention of atrial fibrillation. Circulation 2001;103:769–777.
9. WHO Task Force on Stroke and Other Cerebrovascular Disorders. Recommendations on stroke prevention, diagnosis, and therapy. Stroke 1989;20:1407–1431.
10. Adult Treatment Panel II. National Cholesterol Education Program: Second report of the Expert Panel on Detection, Evaluation, and Treatment of High Blood Cholesterol in Adults. Circulation 1994;89;1333–1445.
11. Hebert PR, Gaziano JM, Chan KS, Hennekens CH. Cholesterol lowering with statin drugs, risk of stroke, and total mortality: An over view of randomized trials. JAMA 1997;278:313–321.
12. Scandinavian Simvastatin Survival Study Group. Randomized trial of cholesterol lowering in 4444 patients with coronary heart disease: The Scandinavian Simvastatin Survival Study (4S). Lancet 1994;344:1383–1389.
13. Byrington RP, Davis BR, Plehn JF, et al., for the PPP Investigators. Reduction of stroke events with pravastatin: The Prospective Pravastatin Pooling (PPP) Project. Circulation 2001;103:387–392.
14. Long-Term Intervention with Pravastatin in Ischemic Disease (LIPID) Study Group. Prevention of cardiovascular events and death with pravastatin in patients with coronary heart disease and a broad range of initial cholesterol levels. N Engl J Med 1998;339:1349–1357.
15. Bonita R, Duncan J, Trualson T, et al. Passive smoking as well as active smoking increases the risk of acute stroke. Tob Control 1998;8:156–160.
16. O'Brien KD, Chait A. The biology of the artery wall in atherogenesis. Med Clin North Am 1994;78:41–67.
17. Ross R. The pathogenesis of atherosclerosis: An update. N Engl J Med 1986;314:488–500.
18. Fisher M, Garcia JH. Evolving stroke and the ischemic penumbra. Neurology 1996;47:884–888.
19. Schiter W, Pietersma A, Lamers JM, Koster JT. Leukocyte adhesion molecules on the vascular endothelium: Their role in the pathogenesis of cardiovascular disease and the mechanisms underlying their expression. J Cardiovasc Pharmacol 1993;22(Suppl 4):S37–S44.
20. Hackman A, Abe Y, Insull W, et al. Levels of soluble cell adhesion molecules in patients with dyslipidemia. Circulation 1996;93:1334–1338.
21. Libby P, Sukhova G, Lee RT, Galis ZS. Cytokines regulate vascular function related to stability of the atherosclerotic plaque. J Cardiovasc Pharmacol 1995;25(Suppl 2):S9–S12.
22. Feinberg WM, Blackshear JL, Laupacis A, et al. Prevalence, age distribution and gender of patients with atrial fibrillation. Arch Intern Med 1995;155:469–473.

23. Stroke Prevention in Atrial Fibrillation Investigators. Predictors of thromboembolism in atrial fibrillation: I. Clinical features of patients at risk. Ann Intern Med 1992;116:1–5.
24. Tegeler C. Carotid stenosis in atrial fibrillation (abstract). Neurology 1989;39(Suppl):159.
25. Nelson KM, Talbert RL. Preventing stroke in patients with nonrheumatic atrial fibrillation. Am J Hosp Pharm 1994;51:1175–1183.
26. American Society of Health-System Pharmacists. ASHP therapeutics position statement on antithrombotic therapy in chronic atrial fibrillation. Am J Health Syst Pharm 1998;55:376–381.
27. Hohnloser SH, Kuck KH, Lilienthal J. Rhythm or rate control in atrial fibrillation: Pharmacologic Intervention in Atrial Fibrillation (PIAF): A randomized trial. Lancet 2000;356:1789–1794.
28. National Heart, Lung, and Blood Institute (NHLBI) AFFIRM Investigators. Atrial fibrillation follow-up investigation of rhythm management: The AFFIRM study design. The planning and steering committee of the AFFIRM study for the NHLBI AFFIRM investigators. Am J Cardiol 1997;79:1198–2202.
29. Stroke Prevention in Atrial Fibrillation Investigators. Predictors of thromboembolism in atrial fibrillation: II. Echocardiographic features of patients at risk. Ann Intern Med 1992;116:6–12.
30. Tanne D, Goldbourt U, Zion M, et al. Frequency and prognosis of stroke/TIA among 4808 survivors of acute myocardial infarction. Stroke 1993;24:1490–1495.
31. Stein PD, Alpert JS, Bussey HI, et al. Antithrombotic therapy in patients with mechanical and biologic prosthetic heart valves. Chest 2001;119:220S–227S.
32. Lopez JA, Ross RS, Fishbein MC, et al. Nonbacterial thrombotic endocarditis: A review. Am Heart J 1987;113:773–784.
33. Culebras A, Kase CS, Masdeu JC, et al. Practice guidelines for the use of imaging in transient ischemic attacks and acute stroke. Stroke 1997;28:148–149.
34. Cheitlin MD, Alpert JJ, Armstrong WF, et al. ACC/AHA guidelines for the clinical application of echocardiography: Executive summary. A report of the American College of Cardiology/American Heart Association Task Force on Practice Guidelines. J Am Coll Cardiol 1997;29:862–879.
35. Adams HS, Brott T, Crowell R, et al. Guidelines for the management of patients with acute ischemic stroke: A statement for healthcare professionals from a special writing group of the Stroke Council American Heart Association. Stroke 1994;25:1901–1914.
36. Dumo P, Fagan SL, Carhuapoma J. Thrombolysis in acute ischemic stroke. Am J Health Syst Pharm 1997;54:2213–2217.
37. Multicentre Acute Stroke Trial, Italy. Randomised controlled trial of streptokinase, aspirin, and combination of both in treatment of acute ischemic stroke. Lancet 1995;346:1509–1514.
38. Multicentre Acute Stroke Trial, Europe Study Group. Thrombolytic therapy recombinant tissue plasminogen activator for acute hemispheric stroke. N Engl J Med 1996;335:145–150.
39. Hacke W, Kaste M, Fieschi C, et al. Intravenous thrombolysis with recombinant tissue plasminogen activator for acute hemispheric stroke: The European Cooperative Acute Stroke Study (ECASS). JAMA 1995;274:1017–1025.
40. The National Institute of Neurological Disorders and Stroke rt-PA Stroke Study Group. Tissue plasminogen activator for acute ischemic stroke. N Engl J Med 1995;333:1581–1587.
41. Adams HP, Davis PH, Leira EC, et al. Baseline NIH Stroke Scale score strongly predicts outcomes after stroke: A report of the Trial of Org10172 in Acute Stroke Treatment (TOAST). Neurology 1999;53:126–131.
42. Adams HP Jr, Brott TG, Furla AJ, et al. Guidelines for thrombolytic therapy for acute stroke: A supplement to the guidelines for the management of patients with acute ischemic stroke. A statement for healthcare professionals from a special writing group of the Stroke Council, American Heart Association. Circulation 1996;94:1167–1174.
43. Canadian Cooperative Study Group. A randomized trial of aspirin and sulfinpyrazone in threatened stroke. New Engl J Med 1978;299: 53–59.
44. Kelton JG, Hirsh J, Carter CJ, et al. Sex differences in the antithrombotic effects of aspirin. Blood 1978;52:1073–1076.
45. UK-TIA Study Group. United Kingdom transient ischemic attack (UK-TIA) aspirin trial: Interim results. Br Med J 1988;296:316–320.
46. Dutch TIA Study Group. The Dutch TIA trial: Protective effects of low-dose aspirin and atenolol in patients with transient ischemic attacks or nondisabling stroke. Stroke 1988;19:512–517.
47. Antiplatelet Trialists'collaboration. Collaborative overview of randomized trials of antiplatelet therapy: I. Prevention of death, myocardial infarction, and stroke by prolonged antiplatelet therapy in various categories of patients. Br Med J 1994;308:81–106.
48. Chinese Acute Stroke Trial (CAST) Collaboration Group. A randomized, placebo-controlled trial of early aspirin use in 20,000 patients with acute ischemia stroke. Lancet 1997;349:1641–1649.
49. The International Stroke Trial (IST). A randomized trial of aspirin, subcutaneous heparin, both, or neither among 19,435 patients with acute ischemic stroke. Lancet 1997;349:1569–1581.
50. CAPRIE Steering Committee. A randomized, blinded trial of clopidogrel versus aspirin in patients at risk of ischaemic events (CAPRIE). Lancet 1995;348:1329–1339.
51. Diener HC, Cunha L, Forbes C, et al. European Stroke Prevention Study 2: Dipyridamole and acetylsalicylic acid in the secondary prevention of stroke. J Neurol Sci 1996;143:1–13.
52. Hass WT, Easton JD, Adams HP, et al. A randomized trial comparing ticlopidine hydrochloride with aspirin for the prevention of stroke in high-risk patients. N Engl J Med 1989;321:501–507.
53. Gent M, Blabely JA, Easton JD. The Canadian American Ticlopidine Study (CATS) in thromboemboli stroke. Lancet 1989;1:1215–1220.
54. North American Symptomatic Carotid Endarterectomy Trial Collaborators. Beneficial effect of carotid endartecrectomy in symptomatic patients with high-grade carotid stenosis. New Engl J Med 1991;325:445–453.
55. North American Symptomatic Carotid Endarterectomy Trial (NASCET) Group. Long-term progressive and effect of endarectomy in patients with symptomatic severe carotid stenosis and contralateral carotid stenosis or occlusion: Results from NASCET. Neurosurgery 1995;83:778–782.
56. Rothwell PM, Gibson RJ, Slattery J, et al. Risk of stroke in the distribution of an asymtomatic carotid artery. The European Carotid Surgery Trialists' Collaborative Group. Lancet 1995;345:209–212.
57. Executive Committee for the Asymptomatic Carotid Atherosclerosis Study. Endarterectomy for asymptomatic carotid artery stenosis. JAMA 1995;273:1421–1428.
58. Sherman DG, Atkinson RP, Chippendale T, et al., for the STAT participants. Intravenous Ancrod for treatment of acute ischemic stroke. The STAT Study: A randomized controlled trial. JAMA 2000;283:2395–2403.
59. Furlan A, Higashida R, Wechsler L, et al., for the PROACT investigators. Intra-aterial prourokinase for acute ischemic stroke. The PROACT II study: A randomized controlled trial. JAMA 1999;282:2003–2011.
60. Brott T, Bogousslavsky J. Treatment of acute ischemic stroke. New Engl J Med 2000;343:710–722.
61. Kondziolka D, Wechsler L, Goldstein S, et al. Transplantation of cultured human neuronal cells for patients with stroke. Neurology 2000;55:565–569.
62. Broderich JP, Adams HP, Barran W, et al. Guidelines for the management of spontaneous intracerebral hemorrhage: A statement for healthcare professionals from a special writing group of the Stroke Council, American Heart Association. Stroke 1999;30:905–915.
63. Gage BF, Cardinalli AB, Albers GW, Owens DK. Cost-effectiveness of warfarin and aspirin for prophylaxis of stroke in patients with nonvalvular artrial fibrillation. JAMA 1995;274:1839–1845.
64. Gustafsson C, Asplund K, Britton M, et al. Cost-effectiveness of stroke prevention in atrial fibrillation. Br Med J 1992;305:1457–1460.
65. Fagan SC, Morgenstein LB, Peitta A, et al. and the NINDDS rt-PA Stroke Study Group. Cost-effectiveness of tissue plasminogen activator for acute ischemic stroke. Neurology 1998;50:883–890.
66. Albers GW, Amarenco P, Eastin JD, et al. Antithrombotic and thrombolytic therapy for ischemic stroke. Chest 2001;119:300S–320S.

21

HYPERLIPIDEMIA

Robert L. Talbert

Cholesterol, triglycerides, and phospholipids are the major lipids in the body and they are transported as complexes of lipid and specialized proteins (apolipoproteins) known as lipoproteins. Plasma lipoproteins are spherical particles with surfaces that consist largely of phospholipid, free cholesterol, and protein, and cores that consist mostly of triglyceride and cholesterol ester (Fig. 21–1). Abnormalities of plasma lipoproteins can result in a predisposition to coronary, cerebrovascular and peripheral vascular arterial disease. Accumulating evidence over the last decades had linked elevated total and low-density lipoprotein cholesterol (LDL-C) and reduced high-density lipoprotein cholesterol (HDL-C) to the development of coronary heart disease (CHD). Premature coronary atherosclerosis, leading to the manifestations of ischemic heart disease (see Chap. 14), is the most common and significant consequence of hyperlipidemia. In 2001, the National Cholesterol Education Program (NCEP) adult treatment panel III (ATP III) published its third report summarizing these data and giving recommendations for the management of hypercholesterolemia in adults.[1] This report modifies earlier recommendations and provides a new way of risk-stratifying patients.[2] The American Heart Association also provides guidelines for primary and secondary prevention of CHD.[3–5]

Total cholesterol and LDL-C increase throughout life in men and women, representing an atherogenic pattern characteristic of Westernized society diets (Fig. 21–2). Based on the National Health and Nutrition Examination Survey (NHANES 1988 to 1994) and ATP III guidelines, an estimated 100,870,000 American adults have total cholesterol levels of 200 mg/dL or higher. Assuming that dietary intervention would reduce LDL-C by about 10%, then about 7% (approximately 12.7 million Americans) might be candidates for lipid-lowering drugs. This reflects about 4 million Americans with known CHD and about 8.7 million adults without established CHD. Of the latter group, as many as 3.1 million are aged 65 years and older.[6] Although these numbers seem staggering in their enormity, substantial progress has been made, and the number of Americans with a desirable blood cholesterol level (<200 mg/dL) has risen to 49% from 45% from the earlier survey (1976 to 1980), while the average total cholesterol in this country has fallen from 220 mg/dL in 1960 to 1962, to 203 mg/dL in 1988 to 1994.[7] Patients who are at risk but who have not yet experienced their first cardiovascular or cerebrovascular event [e.g., myocardial infarction (MI)] are termed primary prevention, whereas those with manifest vascular disease are termed secondary intervention.

Data from the Framingham study and from other studies demonstrate that the risk for developing cardiovascular disease is related to the degree of total cholesterol and LDL-C elevation in a graded, continuous fashion.[8,9] Hypercholesterolemia is additive to the other nonlipid risk factors for CHD, including cigarette smoking, hypertension, diabetes, low HDL-C levels, and electrocardiographic abnormalities. The presence of established CHD or prior MI increases the risk of MI five to seven times that seen in men or women without CHD, and LDL-C is a significant predictor of subsequent morbidity and mortality.[10] About 50% of all MIs and at least 70% of CHD deaths occur in patients with known CHD, and these patients should therefore be a target for screening, identification, and treatment. Unfortunately, the identification of patients at high risk because of hypercholesterolemia or other lipid disorders is too frequently overlooked, because blood lipid levels are not always evaluated in this population even after an event such as MI.[10,11]

A comparison of the United States to other countries shows similar relationships between total cholesterol, LDL-C, and an inverse relationship with HDL-C to coronary artery disease (CAD) mortality.[8,12] On a positive note, the U.S. mortality rate is midway among the countries studied, and this country has had the greatest decline in CAD mortality (35% to 40%) in men and women over the last 10 years as compared to other countries. A decline in the prevalence of hypercholesterolemia in certain segments of the U.S. population parallels these trends in mortality.[13] LDL-C and the ratio of LDL-C to HDL-C have also been used to assess risk, but their use adds little information to total cholesterol alone unless HDL-C is abnormally high or low. HDL-C has been shown to be protective for the occurrence of CHD, and an inverse relationship exists between CHD and HDL-C levels.[14]

Two fractions of HDL-C occur, HDL_2-C and HDL_3-C, and it is thought that HDL_2 is more important for prevention of cardiovascular disease.[12] HDL transports cholesterol from lipid-laden foam cells to the liver. In general, for every 1 mg/dL decline in HDL, CHD risk is increased by 2% to 3%. Elevated triglycerides may cause pancreatitis, but their relationship to CHD is much weaker than cholesterol, and studies of unselected patients have not found a significant relationship between triglycerides and the prevalence of CHD. Very-low-density lipoprotein (VLDL), which is enriched with cholesterol esters, is smaller, denser, and more atherogenic than less-dense VLDL. Routine measurement of triglycerides cannot distinguish between the types of VLDL present in plasma. Elevation of triglyceride-rich lipoproteins is associated with low HDL, and this ratio predicts increased risk. The 8-year follow-up of the Copenhagen male study found a clear gradient of risk of ischemic heart disease (IHD) with increasing triglyceride levels within each level of HDL cholesterol. When compared to the lowest tertile of triglyceride concentrations; the highest tertile had 2.2 relative risk for IHD and the relationship extended across all concentrations of HDL-C.[15] The Helsinki heart study shows that hypertriglyceridemia and low HDL-C are associated with obesity (body mass index [BMI] >26 kg/m^2), smoking, sedentary life-style, blood pressure of $\geq$140/90 mm Hg, and blood glucose above 4.4 mmol/L, and that the benefit of gemfibrozil (risk reduction 68%, $P < 0.03$) was largely confined to overweight subjects. The Stockholm IHD study using niacin and clofibrate found the greatest reduction in CHD in patients with elevated triglycerides.[16] Hypertriglyceridemia in certain instances—for example, diabetes mellitus, nephrotic syndrome, and chronic renal disease, and perhaps in women—is associated with increased cardiovascular risk. This is thought to be a consequence of the presence of atherogenic lipoproteins and of hypertriglyceridemia being a marker for them, as triglycerides are usually not independently predictive for CHD.

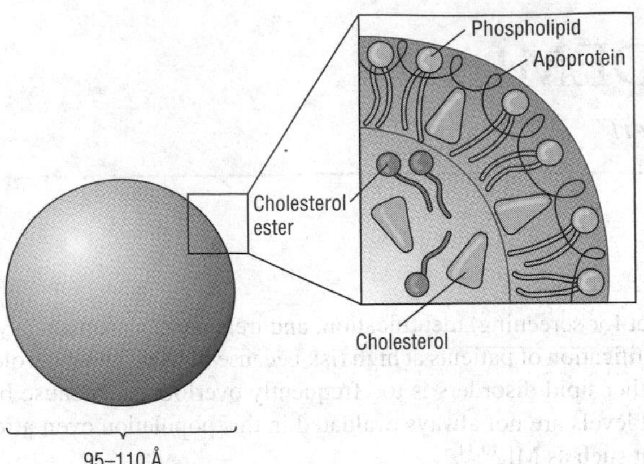

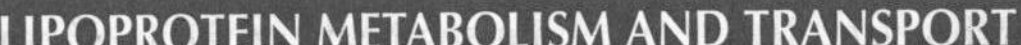

FIGURE 21–1. A high-density-lipoprotein particle. The protein is represented as having a helical structure and forming the outer 110-Å shell of the particle. The polar head groups of phospholipids are shown interacting with the helices of the protein. Cholesteryl esters are drawn such that the cholesterol moiety interacts with the fatty acyl chains of the phospholipids.

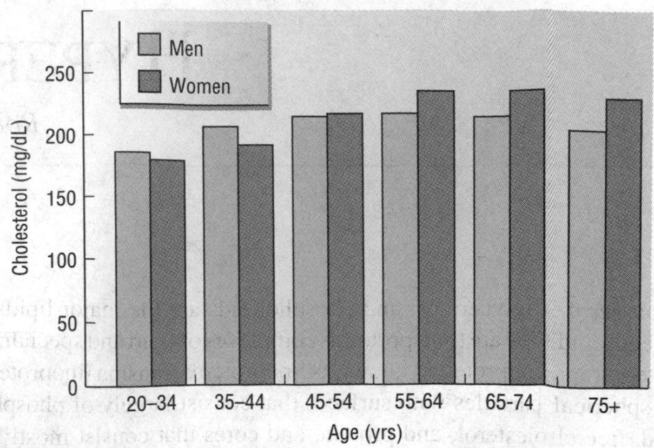

FIGURE 21–2. Serum cholesterol levels in men and women 20 years of age and over from 1988 to 1994. *(Based on data from the Third National Health and Nutrition Examination survey. Health, United States, 1996–1997. Hyattsville, MD, National Center for Health Statistics, 1997:1–345.)*

LIPOPROTEIN METABOLISM AND TRANSPORT

Cholesterol and triglycerides, as the major plasma lipids, are essential substrates for cell membrane formation and hormone synthesis, and provide a source of free fatty acids.[17,18] Hyperlipidemia is defined as an elevation of one or more of cholesterol, cholesterol esters, phospholipids, or triglycerides. Lipids, being water immiscible, are not present in free form in the plasma, but rather circulate as lipoproteins. Hyperlipoproteinemia describes an increased concentration of the lipoprotein macromolecules that transport lipids in the plasma. The density of plasma lipoproteins is determined by their relative content of protein and lipid. Density, composition, size, and electrophoretic mobility divide lipoproteins into four classes (Table 21–1).

LDL has been further divided into LDL_1, or intermediate-density lipoprotein (density 1.006–1.019 g/mL), and LDL_2 (1.019–1.063 g/mL). LDL_2 is the major LDL component in plasma and it carries 60% to 70% of the total serum cholesterol. HDL has been subfractionated into HDL_2 (density 1.063–1.125 g/mL) and HDL_3 (1.125–1.21 g/mL). Fluctuations in HDL are usually caused by alterations in the levels of HDL_2. HDL normally carries about 20% to 30% of the total cholesterol. VLDL has also been subdivided into three classes, and it carries about 10% to 15% of serum cholesterol and most of the triglyceride in the fasting state. VLDL is the precursor for LDL, and VLDL remnants may also be atherogenic. Table 21–2 shows the characteristics of the protein constituent of lipoproteins known as apolipoproteins.

Chylomicrons, large triglyceride-rich particles containing apolipoprotein B-48, B-100, and E, are formed from dietary fat solubilized by bile salts in intestinal mucosal cells (Fig. 21–3). Chylomicrons are normally not present in the plasma after a fast of 12 to 14 hours and are catabolized by lipoprotein lipase (LPL), which is activated by apolipoprotein C-II and in the vascular endothelium and hepatic lipase to form chylomicron remnants. The remnants that contain apolipoprotein E (Fig. 21–3) are taken up by the "remnant receptor," which may be an LDL receptor-related protein, in the liver. Free cholesterol is liberated intracellularly after attachment to the remnant receptor. Chylomicrons also function to deliver dietary triglyceride to skeletal muscle and adipose tissue. During the catabolism of nascent chylomicrons to remnants, triglyceride is converted to free fatty acids and apolipoproteins A-I, A-II, A-IV (free in plasma), C-I, C-II, and C-III, and phospholipids are transferred to HDL. Apolipoprotein E and apolipoprotein C-II are transferred to chylomicrons from HDL and eventually back through these metabolic events. Hepatic VLDL synthesis is regulated in part by diet and hormones, and is inhibited by uptake of chylomicron remnants in the liver. VLDL is secreted from the liver and serially converted via LPL to intermediate-density lipoprotein (IDL), and, finally, to LDL. VLDL receptors are found in adipose tissue and muscle, and bear close homology to the structure of LDL receptors.

LDL, the major cholesterol transport lipoprotein and having virtually only apolipoprotein B-100, is mostly derived from VLDL catabolism and cellular synthesis. When fasting and on low-fat intake in normal subjects, most cholesterol is synthesized and used in the extrahepatic organs, while most of the cholesterol carried by LDL is taken up by the liver for catabolism.[17] In patients with homozygous familial hypercholesterolemia, enhanced synthesis of LDL may occur,

TABLE 21–1. Composition of Lipoprotein Isolated from Normal Subjects

			Composition (Weight %)				
					Cholesterol		
Lipoprotein Class	Density Range (g/mL)	Diameter (nm)	*Protein*	*Triglyceride*	*Free*	*Ester*	*Phospholipid*
Chylomicrons	<0.94	75–1200	1–2	80–95	1–3	2–4	3–9
VLDL	0.94–1.006	30–80	6–10	55–80	4–8	16–22	10–20
LDL	1.006–1.063	18–25	18–22	5–15	6–8	45–50	18–24
HDL	1.063–1.21	5–12	45–55	5–10	3–5	15–20	20–30

HDL, high-density lipoprotein; LDL, low-density lipoprotein; VLDL, very-low-density lipoprotein.

TABLE 21–2. Characteristics and Functions of Apolipoproteins

Apolipoprotein	Lipoprotein Density Class	Approximate Plasma Concentration (mg/dL)	Approximate Molecular Weight (kDa)	Reported Functions	Major Site of Synthesis
A-I	Chylomicrons, HDL	120	28	Cofactor with LCAT, structural protein on HDL, ligand for HDL receptor	Liver, intestine
A-II	Chylomicrons, HDL	35	17	Structural protein for HDL, ligand for HDL receptor	LIver
A-IV	Chylomicrons, 1.21B	15	46	Possibly facilitates transfer of other apos between HDL and chylomicrons	Intestine
ApoLp(a)	LDL, HDL	10	500±	Bound to B-100, high homology with plasminogen, may prevent LDL uptake by B, E receptors	Liver
B-100	VLDL, LDL, IDL	100	540	Necessary for assembly and secretion of VLDL from the liver, structural protein of VLDL, IDL, LDL, ligand for LDL receptor	Liver
B-48	Chylomicrons	Trace	264	Necessary for assembly and secretion of chylomicrons from the small intestine	Intestine
C-I	Chylomicrons, VLDL, HDL	7	6.6	Cofactor with LCAT; may inhibit hepatic uptake of chylomicron and VLDL remnants	Liver
C-II	Chylomicrons, VLDL, HDL	4	8.9	Activator of LPL	Liver
C-III	Chylomicrons, VLDL, HDL	13	8.8	Inhibitor with LPL; may inhibit hepatic uptake of chylomicron and VLDL remnants	LIver
D	HDL	6	32	?	?
E2–E4	Chylomicrons, VLDL, HDL	5	34	Ligand for several lipoproteins to LDL receptor, LRP and possibly to a separate hepatic apoE receptor	Liver

HDL, high-density lipoprotein; HL, hepatic lipase; IDL, intermediate-density lipoprotein; LCAT, lecithin-cholesterol acyltransferase; LDL, low-density lipoprotein; LRP, LDL receptor-related protein; VLDL, very-low-density lipoprotein.

because LDL clearance is reduced as a consequence of the lack of LDL receptors. LDL is catabolized through interaction of cell surface receptors found on liver, adrenal, and peripheral cells (including fibroblasts and smooth-muscle cells). These cells recognize apolipoprotein B-100 on LDL, and after binding to a receptor on the cell membrane, LDL is internalized and degraded. In the normal fasting state, approximately 70% of LDL is cleared through receptor-dependent mechanism, although this is highly dependent on the availability and type of saturated and mono- or polyunsaturated fat from dietary sources. Ingestion of cholesterol and saturated fatty acids such as C12:0, C14:0, and C16:0 are associated with reduction in LDL receptor activity, increased LDL production rate, and elevation in LDL plasma concentration. Receptor-independent mechanisms are also involved to a lesser extent in the catabolism of LDL, and these receptors are present in many tissues but are most active in animals in the adrenals and ovary.[17] Increased intracellular cholesterol resulting from LDL catabolism inhibits the activity of 3-hydroxy-3-methylglutaryl coenzyme A reductase (HMG-CoA reductase), the rate-limiting enzyme for intracellular cholesterol biosynthesis (Fig. 21–4). Additional consequences of increased intracellular cholesterol include reduced synthesis of LDL receptors, which limits subsequent cholesterol uptake from the plasma, and accelerated activity of acyl coenzyme-A:cholesterol acyltransferase to facilitate cholesterol storage within cells. LDL cholesterol may also be excreted into bile and become part of the enterohepatic pool or may be lost in the stool. Lp(a) is a cholesterol-rich lipoprotein similar to LDL in composition and density and with close homology to fibrinogen; it is reported to be an important independent risk factor for the development of premature cardiovascular disease.

Nascent HDL is derived from liver and gut synthesis primarily in the form of apolipoprotein A-I phospholipid discs. Esterification of free cholesterol in nascent HDL and from peripheral tissues to cholesteryl esters by lecithin-cholesterol acyltransferase (LCAT) results in the production of HDL_3. Further addition of tissue cholesterol to HDL_3 results in the formation of HDL_2. HDL_2 can also be formed from remodeling of chylomicrons and VLDL catabolism. HDL_2 may be converted back to HDL_3 by the action of hepatic lipase and by the transfer of cholesteryl esters to the liver, LDL, and VLDL. Apolipoprotein A-I production is increased by estrogens, leading to higher HDL levels in women and in individuals receiving estrogen. Transfer of excess cholesterol from peripheral tissues by HDL is called *reverse cholesterol transport.* Putative HDL receptors in peripheral cells facilitate the uptake of cholesterol by HDL, which transfers cholesterol to either VLDL and LDL or to the liver for secretion into bile or conversion into bile acids. These processes serve to rid peripheral tissue (e.g., coronary arteries) of excessive amounts of cholesterol, and account for some of the protective effects noted with increasing HDL in women and other factors that elevate HDL levels. HDL has been further separated into subtypes HDL_{2a}, HDL_{2b}, HDL_{3a}, HDL_{3c}. The importance of each subtype is being investigated. Variants of the cholesterol ester transfer protein (CETP) have been demonstrated in humans, and the B1B1 genotype is associated with lower HDL and progression of coronary atherosclerosis.

The "response-to-injury" hypothesis states that risk factors such as oxidized LDL, mechanical injury to the endothelium (e.g., percutaneous transluminal angioplasty), excessive homocysteine, immunologic attack, or infection-induced (e.g., *Chlamydia,* herpes simplex virus-1) changes in endothelial and intimal function lead to endothelial dysfunction and a series of cellular interactions that culminate in atherosclerosis.[19,20] C-reactive protein (CRP) is an acute phase reactant and a marker for inflammation; it may be useful in

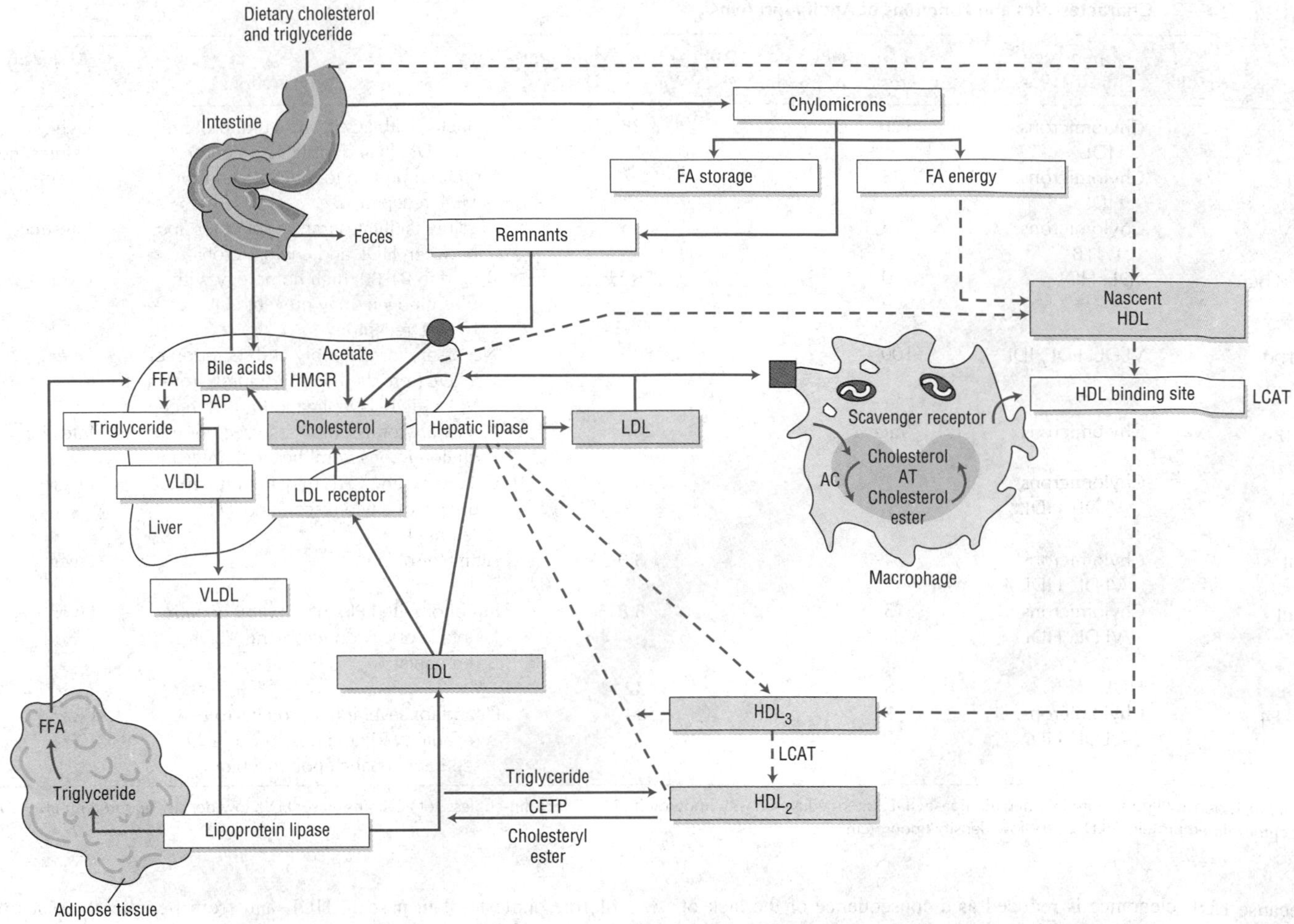

FIGURE 21–3. Overview of lipoprotein metabolism. (ACAT, acyl CoA:cholesterol acyltransferase; CETP, cholesteryl ester transfer protein; FFA, free fatty acid; HMGR, HMG CoA reductase; LCAT, lecithin:cholesterol acyltransferase; PAP, phosphatidic acid phosphatase). *(From Ref. 12, with permission.)*

identifying patients at risk for developing CAD.[21] The eventual outcomes of this cascade are clinical events such as angina, MI, arrhythmias, stroke, peripheral arterial disease, abdominal aortic aneurysm, and sudden death. Atherosclerotic lesions are thought to arise from transport and retention of plasma LDL-cholesterol through the endothelial cell layer into the extracellular matrix of the subendothelial space. Once in the artery wall, LDL is chemically modified through oxidation and non-enzymatic glycation. Mildly oxidized LDL then recruits monocytes into the artery wall, which become transformed into macrophages. Macrophages have tremendous potential for accelerating LDL oxidation and apolipoprotein B accumulation, and altering the receptor-mediated uptake of LDL into the artery wall from the usual LDL-receptor to a "scavenger receptor" not regulated by cell content of cholesterol. Oxidized LDL increases plasminogen inhibitor levels (promotion of coagulation), induces the expression of endothelin (vasoconstrictive substance), inhibits the expression of nitric oxide (a vasodilator and platelet inhibitor), and is toxic to macrophages if highly oxidized. As oxidation of biologically active lipids proceeds, other lipids such as lysophosphatidylcholine, hydroperoxides, aldehydic breakdown products of fatty acids and oxysterol are formed, which continue the reaction within the tissue. These events lead to a massive accumulation of cholesterol. The cholesterol-laden cells are called foam cells; foam cells are the earliest recognized cells of the arterial fatty streak.

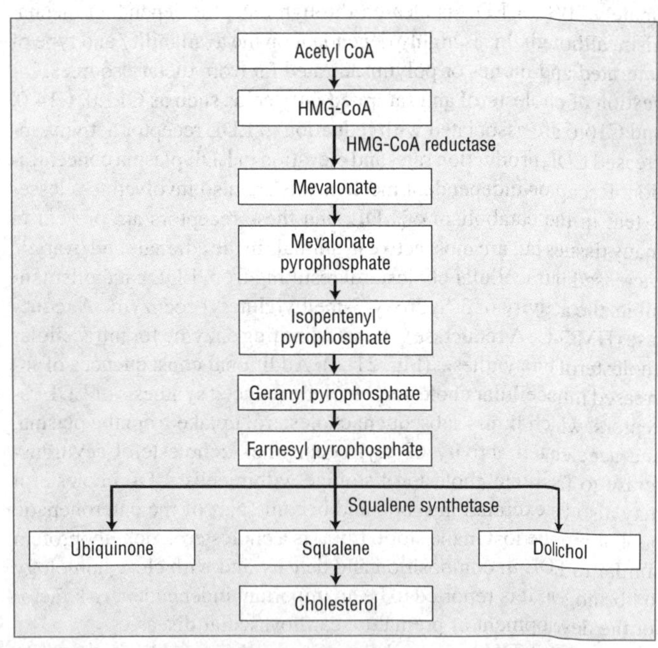

FIGURE 21–4. Biosynthetic pathway for cholesterol. The rate-limiting enzyme in this pathway is 3-hydroxy-3-methylglutaryl coenzyme A reductase (HMG-CoA reductase).

Oxidized LDL provokes an inflammatory response, which is mediated by a number of chemoattractants and cytokines. Examples of each that appear to be involved at different stages of lesion development include monocyte chemoattractant protein 1 (MCP-1); monocyte colony stimulating factor (M-CSF); *gro;* vascular cell adhesion molecule (VCAM-1); E-selectin (ELAM-1); intercellular adhesion molecule (ICAM-1); platelet-derived growth factor (PDGF); vascular endothelial growth factor (VEGF); transforming growth factors (TGFα and TGFβ); interleukin-1 and interleukin-6 (IL-1, IL-6); and the ratio of interleukin-10 and interleukin-12 (IL-10, IL-12). It appears that some of these factors (e.g., MCP-1 and M-CSF) participate early in the process of monocyte-macrophage attachment and transmigration across the endothelium, whereas others (PDGF and VCAM-1) promote later lesion growth.[22] The extent of oxidation and the inflammatory response is under genetic control of a major gene termed *Ath*-1 based on murine model studies. The process of aging may lead to lipoproteins that are more susceptible to oxidation and have longer resident time in the vascular compartment.[23] Two proteins associated with HDL—apolipoprotein J (apoJ) and paraxonase (PON)—appear to play an important role to minimize the oxidation of LDL-C.[24,25] Increased recognition of the role of these growth-regulatory molecules provides the possibility of future directions for antagonists to regulatory molecules such as PDGF, TGFβ, and the interleukins. Repeated injury and repair within an atherosclerotic plaque eventually leads to a fibrous cap protecting the underlying core of lipids, collagen, calcium and inflammatory cells such as T-lymphocytes. Maintenance of the fibrous plaque is critical to prevent plaque rupture and subsequent coronary thrombosis. An imbalance between plaque synthesis and degradation may lead to a weakened or vulnerable plaque prone to rupture. The fibrous cap may become weakened through decreased synthesis of the extracellular matrix or increased degradation of the matrix. The cytokine interferon-γ, produced by T-lymphocytes, inhibits the ability of smooth-muscle cells to synthesize collagen, a structurally important component of the fibrous cap. A family of enzymes known as matrix metalloproteinases can degrade all major constituents of the vascular extracellular matrix: collagen, elastin, and proteoglycans.[22]

TABLE 21–3. Fredrickson-Levy-Lees Classification of Hyperlipoproteinemia

Type	Lipoprotein Elevation
I	Chylomicrons
IIa	LDL
IIb	LDL + VLDL
III	IDL (LDL_1)
IV	VLDL
V	VLDL + Chylomicrons

IDL, intermediate-density lipoprotein; LDL, low-density lipoprotein; VLDL, very-low-density lipoprotein.

Lipoprotein disorders are classified into six categories, which are commonly used for phenotypical description of hyperlipidemia (Table 21–3). Specific genetic defects with disrupted protein, cell, and organ function give rise to several disorders within each family of lipoproteins (Table 21–4). In other words, an elevated cholesterol

TABLE 21–4. Lipoprotein Disorders

Lipid Phenotype	Plasma Lipid Levels, mmol/L (mg/dL)L	Lipoproteins *Elevated*	Lipoproteins *Phenotype*	Clinical Signs
Isolated Hypercholesterolemia				
Familial hypercholesterolemia	Heterozygotes TC = 7–13 (275–500)	LDL	IIa	Usually develop xanthomas in adulthood and vascular disease at 30–50 years of age
	Homozygotes TC >13 (>500)	LDL	IIa	Usually develop xanthomas in adulthood and vascular disease in childhood
Familial defective apo B100	Heterozygotes TC = 7–13 (275–500)	LDL	IIa	
Polygenic hypercholesterolemia	TC = 6.5–9 (250–350)	LDL	IIa	Usually asymptomatic until vascular disease develops; no xanthomas
Isolated Hypertriglyceridemia				
Familial hypertriglyceridemia	TG = 2.8–8.5 (250–750)	VLDL	IV	Asymptomatic; may be associated with increased risk of vascular disease
Familial LPL deficiency	TG > 8.5 (750)	Chylomicrons, VLDL	I, V	May be asymptomatic; may be associated with pancreatitis, abdominal pain, hepatosplenomegaly
Familial apo CII deficiency	TG > 8.5 (>750)	Chylomicrons, VLDL	I, V	As above
Hypertriglyceridemia and Hypercholesterolemia				
Combined hyperlipidemia	TG = 2.8–8.5 (250–750); TC = 6.5–13 (250–500)	VLDL, LDL	IIb	Usually asymptomatic until vascular disease develops; familial form may also present as isolated high TG or an isolated high LDL cholesterol
Dysbetalipoproteinemia	TG = 2.8–8.5 (250–750); TC = 6.5–13 (250–500)	VLDL, IDL; LDL normal	III	Usually asymptomatic until vascular disease develops; may have palmar or tuboeruptive xanthomas

IDL, intermediate-density lipoprotein; LDL, low-density lipoprotein; LPL, lipoprotein lipase; TC, total cholesterol; TG, triglycerides; VLDL, very low density lipoprotein.

TABLE 21–5. Secondary Causes of Lipoprotein Abnormalities

Hypercholesterolemia	Hypothyroidism Obstructive liver disease Nephrotic syndrome Anorexia nervosa Acute intermittent porphyria Drugs: progestins; thiazide diuretics; glucocorticoids; β-blockers; isotretinoin; protease inhibitors; cyclosporine; mirtazapine; sirolimus
Hypertriglyceridemia	Obesity Diabetes mellitus Lipodystrophy Glycogen storage disease Ileal bypass surgery Sepsis Pregnancy Acute hepatitis Systemic lupus erythematosus Monoclonal gammopathy: multiple myeloma, lymphoma Drugs: alcohol; estrogens; isotretinoin; β-blockers; glucocorticoids; bile-acid resins; thiazides; asparaginase; interferons; azole antifungals; mirtazapine; anabolic steroids; sirolimus; bexarotene
Hypocholesterolemia	Malnutrition Malabsorption Myeloproliferative diseases Chronic infectious diseases: AIDS, tuberculosis Monoclonal gammopathy Chronic liver disease
Low HDL	Malnutrition Obesity Drugs: non-ISA β-blockers; anabolic steroids; probucol; isotretinoin; progestins

level does not necessarily equate with familial hypercholesterolemia or type IIa, as cholesterol may also be elevated in other lipoprotein disorders and the lipoprotein pattern does not describe the underlying genetic defect. The preceding discussion has focused on primary or genetic hyperlipoproteinemia; it should be remembered that secondary forms exist and that several drugs may also elevate lipid levels (Table 21–5). These secondary forms of hyperlipidemia should be initially managed by correcting the underlying abnormality, including modification of drug therapy when appropriate.

Familial hypercholesterolemia is characterized by (a) a selective elevation in the plasma level of LDL; (b) deposition of LDL-derived cholesterol in tendons (xanthomas) and arteries (atheromas); and (c) inheritance as an autosomal dominant trait with homozygotes more severely affected than heterozygotes. Homozygotes (prevalence 1 in 1,000,000) have severe hypercholesterolemia (650–1000 mg/dL), with the early appearance of cutaneous xanthomas and fatal CHD generally before the age of 20. The primary defect in familial hypercholesterolemia is the inability to bind LDL to the LDL receptor (LDL-R) or, rarely, a defect of internalizing the LDL-R complex into the cell after normal binding. Homozygotes have essentially no functional LDL receptors. This leads to lack of LDL degradation by cells and unregulated biosynthesis of cholesterol, with total cholesterol and LDL-C being inversely proportional to the deficit in LDL receptors. Heterozygotes have only about one-half of the normal number of LDL receptors, total cholesterol levels in the range of 300–600 mg/dL and cardiovascular events beginning in the third and fourth decades of life.

Familial LPL deficiency is a rare, autosomal recessive trait characterized by a massive accumulation of chylomicrons and corresponding increase in plasma triglycerides or a type I lipoprotein pattern. VLDL concentration is normal. The presenting manifestations include repeated attacks of pancreatitis and abdominal pain, eruptive cutaneous xanthomatosis, and hepatosplenomegaly beginning in childhood. Symptom severity is proportional to dietary fat intake, and consequently to the elevation of chylomicrons. LPL is normally released from vascular endothelium or by heparin and hydrolyzes chylomicrons and VLDL (see Fig. 21–3). Diagnosis is based on low or absent enzyme activity with normal human plasma or apolipoprotein C-II, a cofactor of the enzyme.[26] Accelerated atherosclerosis is not associated with this disease. Abdominal pain, pancreatitis, eruptive xanthomas, and peripheral polyneuropathy characterize type V (VLDL and chylomicrons). Symptoms may occur in childhood, but usually the disorder is expressed at a later age. The risk of atherosclerosis is increased with this disorder. These patients are commonly obese, hyperuricemic, and diabetic, and alcohol intake, exogenous estrogens, and renal insufficiency tend to be exacerbating factors.

Patients with familial type III hyperlipoproteinemia (also called dysbetalipoproteinemia, broad-band or β-VLDL) develop these clinical features after 20 years of age: xanthoma striata palmaris (yellow discolorations of the palmar and digital creases); tuberous or tuberoeruptive xanthomas (bulbous cutaneous xanthomas); and severe atherosclerosis involving the coronary arteries, internal carotids, and abdominal aorta. A defective structure of apolipoprotein E does not allow normal hepatic surface receptor binding of remnant particles derived from chylomicrons and VLDL (known as IDL); aggravating factors such as obesity, diabetes, or pregnancy may promote overproduction of apo-B-containing lipoproteins. Although homozygosity for the defective allele (E_2/E_2) is common (1 in 100), only 1 in 10,000 express the full-blown picture, and interaction with other genetic or environmental factors, or both, is needed to produce clinical disease.

Type IV hyperlipoproteinemia is common and occurs in adulthood primarily in patients who are obese, diabetic, and hyperuricemic and do not have xanthomas. It may be secondary to alcohol ingestion and can be aggravated by stress, progestins, oral contraceptives, thiazides, or β-blockers. Two genetic patterns occur in type IV hyperlipoproteinemia: familial hypertriglyceridemia, which does not carry a great risk for premature CAD, and familial combined hyperlipidemia, which is associated with increased risk of cardiovascular disease.

Rare forms of lipoprotein disorders may include hypobetalipoproteinemia, abetalipoproteinemia, Tangier disease, LCAT deficiency (fish-eye disease), cerebrotendinous xanthomatosis, and sitosterolemia. Most of these rare lipoprotein disorders do not result in premature atherosclerosis, with the exceptions of familial LCAT deficiency, cerebrotendinous xanthomatosis (CTX), and sitosterolemia with xanthomatosis. Their treatment consists of dietary restriction of plant sterols (sitosterolemia with xanthomatosis), chenodeoxycholic acid (CTX), or, potentially, blood transfusion (LCAT deficiency).

PATIENT EVALUATION

A fasting lipoprotein profile including total cholesterol, LDL-C, HDL-C, and triglycerides should be measured in all adults 20 years of age or older at least once every 5 years.[1] If the profile is obtained in the nonfasted state, only total cholesterol and HDL-C will be usable because LDL-C is usually a calculated value; if total cholesterol is ≥200 mg/dL, or if HDL-C is <40 mg/dL, a followup fasting lipoprotein profile should be obtained. After a lipid abnormality is confirmed (Table 21–6), major components of the evaluation are the history (including age, gender, and, if female, menstrual and estrogen replacement status), physical examination, and laboratory investigations. A complete history and physical exam should assess (a) presence or absence of cardiovascular risk factors (Table 21–7) or definite cardiovascular disease in the individual; (b) family history of premature cardiovascular disease or lipid disorders; (c) presence or absence of secondary causes of lipid abnormalities, including concurrent medications (see Table 21–5); and (d) presence or absence of xanthomas or abdominal pain, or history of pancreatitis, renal or liver disease, peripheral vascular disease, abdominal aortic aneurysm, or cerebral vascular disease (carotid bruits, stroke, or transient ischemic attack). An important change in the ATP III guidelines is that diabetes mellitus is regarded as a CHD risk equivalent. The presence of diabetes in patients without known CHD is associated with the same level of risk as patients without diabetes but having confirmed CHD.[27] ATP III identifies three categories of risk that modify the goals and modalities of LDL-lowering therapy (Table 21–8). The highest category is known CHD or CHD risk equivalents, which is defined as the risk for major coronary events equal to or greater than established CHD; that is, >20% per 10 years (2% per year). The next category consists of patients with multiple (2+) risk factors in which 10-year risk for CHD is ≤20%. The lowest risk category is persons with 0 to 1 risk factor, which is usually associated with a 10-year risk of CHD of <10%. Risk is estimated from Framingham risk scores.[14] Risk is estimated based on the patient's age, LDL-C or total cholesterol level, blood pressure, the presence of diabetes, and smoking status (Table 21–7). This approach for a single patient is referred to as case finding or patient-based; whereas large-scale screening and recommendations for the general populace, health care providers, and the food industry are called a population-based approach.

Measurement of plasma cholesterol (which is about 3% lower than serum determinations), triglyceride, and HDL-C levels after a 12-hour or longer fast is important, as triglycerides may be elevated in nonfasted individuals; total cholesterol is only modestly affected by fasting. Analytic and biologic variability can have a major impact on the measurement and interpretation of cholesterol (or any other laboratory test). Analytic variability can be minimized through the use of adequate quality-control procedures, including internal training, routine calibration and monitoring, and external proficiency testing. Even with these measures, the coefficient of variability in the best procedures can acceptably be up to 5%, and when combined with average biologic variability, total variability may be as high as about 22%. Analytic variability with desktop equipment generally is greater in the fingerstick capillary blood methods, usually yielding measurements less than those from a clinical laboratory, and this technology should be considered for use only as a screening method. Reliance on desktop methods can result in misclassification of 7% to 14% of patients if capillary blood is used. Two determinations, 1 to 8 weeks apart, with the patient on a stable diet and weight, and in the absence of acute illness, are recommended to minimize variability and to obtain a reliable baseline.[1] If the total cholesterol is greater than 200 mg/dL, a second determination is recommended, and if the values are more than 30 mg/dL apart, the average of three values should be used. Familiarity with the method and quality control procedures employed by local laboratories is essential for interpretation of reported values. If the physical examination and history are insufficient to diagnose a familial disorder, then agarose-gel lipoprotein electrophoresis is useful to determine which class of lipoproteins is affected. If the triglyceride levels are below 400 mg/dL and neither type III hyperlipidemia nor chylomicrons are detected by electrophoresis, then one can calculate VLDL-C and LDL-C concentrations: VLDL-C = triglyceride/5; LDL-C = total cholesterol − (VLDL-C + HDL-C).

Because total cholesterol is comprised of cholesterol derived from LDL, VLDL, and HDL, determination of HDL-C is useful when total plasma cholesterol is elevated. HDL-C may be elevated by moderate alcohol ingestion (less than two drinks per day), physical exercise, smoking cessation, weight loss, oral contraceptives, phenytoin, and terbutaline. Smoking, obesity, a sedentary lifestyle and drugs such as β-blockers lower HDL. Only exercise and smoking cessation could be recommended as interventions for low HDL-C concentrations. Niacin and gemfibrozil also increase HDL concentrations.

The range of lipid concentrations represents a population mean plus or minus two standard deviations and does not define the risk of disease. Reference values for plasma total, LDL, and HDL cholesterol concentrations for men and women, as well as various ethnic groups, are available from the NHANES III.[7] Cholesterol and triglycerides

TABLE 21–6. Classification of Total, LDL, HDL Cholesterol and Triglycerides

Total cholesterol	
<200 mg/dL	Desirable
200–239 mg/dL	Borderline high
≥240 mg/dL	High
LDL cholesterol	
<100 mg/dL	Optimal
100–129 mg/dL	Near or above optimal
130–159 mg/dL	Borderline high
160–189 mg/dL	High
≥190 mg/dL	Very high
HDL cholesterol	
<40 mg/dL	Low
≥60 mg/dL	High
Triglycerides	
<150 mg/dL	Normal
150–199 mg/dL	Borderline high
200–499 mg/dL	High
≥500 mg/dL	Very high

HDL, high-density lipoproteins; LDL, low-density lipoproteins.

TABLE 21–7. Major Risk Factors (Exclusive of LDL Cholesterol) That Modify LDL Goals[a]

Age
- Men: ≥45 years
- Women: ≥55 years or premature menopause without estrogen replacement therapy

Family history of premature CHD (definite myocardial infarction or sudden death before 55 years of age in father or other male first-degree relative, or before 65 years of age in mother or other female first-degree relative)

Cigarette smoking

Hypertension (≥140/90 mm Hg or on antihypertensive medication)

Low HDL cholesterol (<40 mg/dL)[b]

[a]Diabetes is regarded as a coronary heart disease (CHD) risk equivalent; LDL, low-density lipoprotein; HDL, high-density lipoprotein.
[b]HDL cholesterol (≥60 mg/dL) counts as a "negative" risk factor; its presence removes 1 risk factor from the total count.

increase throughout life until about the seventh decade for both men and women. At that point, total cholesterol and LDL plateau and fall slightly in men, but continue to rise in women. HDL tends to fall slightly with time and more rapidly after menopause in women. Institution of a population-based approach for cholesterol reduction should shift the entire curve to the left, and the potential reduction in cardiovascular mortality would be proportional to mean reductions at any cholesterol concentration.

TREATMENT RECOMMENDATIONS

Based on a careful review of the experimental pathologic, genetic, and epidemiologic evidence relating to the relationship between blood cholesterol levels and CHD, the adult treatment panel III of the NCEP recommends that a fasting lipoprotein profile and risk factor assessment be used in the initial classification of adults.[1] If total cholesterol is less than 200 mg/dL, then the patient has a *desirable blood cholesterol level* (Table 21–6). Cholesterol levels between 200 and 239 mg/dL are classified as *borderline-high blood cholesterol levels,* and assessment of risk factors (Table 21–7) is needed to more clearly define disease risk. Blood cholesterol levels of 240 mg/dL and above are classified as *high blood cholesterol levels.* If the total cholesterol is below 200 mg/dL and the HDL is above 40 mg/dL, no further follow-up is recommended for patients without known CHD and who have fewer than two risk factors. In patients with evidence of CHD or other clinical atherosclerotic disease, the LDL goal is less than 100 mg/dL and most patients will require diet and/or drug intervention. Decisions regarding classification and management are based on the LDL-C levels as outlined in Table 21–8. An increasing number of persons have the metabolic syndrome (previously termed syndrome X) which is characterized by abdominal obesity, atherogenic dyslipidemia (elevated triglycerides, small LDL particles, low HDL-C), raised blood pressure, insulin resistance (with or without glucose intolerance), and prothrombotic and proinflammatory states. ATP III recognizes the metabolic syndrome as a secondary target of risk-reduction therapy after LDL-C has been addressed.

The Expert Panel on Children and Adolescents of the NCEP recommends screening in higher-risk children (positive family history or parental high blood cholesterol, ≥240 mg/dL).[28] The rationale, in part, for this approach is based on the recognition that atherosclerosis begins in the childhood and adolescent years as documented in the pathobiologic determinants of atherosclerosis in youth (PDAY) and the Bogalusa studies.[29] Similarly, if children with high blood lipids or lipoprotein levels are identified, and the levels in the parents are unknown, the parents should be screened as well, as they are likely to be at high risk. Racial and gender differences do exist in the determination of lipoprotein fractions, and these factors should be considered in screening. Use of the serum cholesterol level alone may be of insufficient specificity or sensitivity, depending on the cut points used in screening, and other discretionary factors, such as hypertension, smoking, obesity, high-fat diet, and use of cholesterol-raising medication, may be needed to correctly identify children at risk. Table 21–9 presents these recommendations. Presently, children over the age of 10 years are candidates for drug therapy if a trial of diet (6 months to 1 year) proves to be inadequate and LDL-C remains above 190 mg/dL, or above 160 mg/dL if two or more risk factors or CHD are present in the child or adolescent, or if there is a history of premature CHD. The Dietary Intervention Study in Children (DISC) in pubertal children found that a fat restricted diet modestly lowered LDL-C and maintained psychologic well-being.[30] Bile acid sequestrants are the recommended drugs for this population.[31] The long-term consequences of drug therapy in this population are unknown. In special instances, familial hypercholesterolemia (particularly the homozygous form), or the existence of CHD or two or more risk factors in the child, would prompt the earlier institution of drug therapy after a trial of dietary intervention.[32]

The goals of therapy expressed as LDL-C levels and the level of initiation of diet and drug therapy are provided in Tables 21–8 and 21–9 for adults and children, respectively. Ideally, therapeutic life-style changes including reduced intake of saturated fats and cholesterol, increased stanol/sterol and fiber intake, weight reduction, and increased physical activity should be used to attain lower LDL-C and to achieve reductions in CHD risk. Based on angiographic studies, aggressive reduction in total and LDL cholesterol is beneficial to prevent the development of atheromatous lesions in vascular beds and to induce the regression of existing lesions. Furthermore, data from trials of secondary and primary intervention also provide evidence that CHD morbidity and mortality as well as total mortality can be reduced with diet and drug therapy. The extent of lipid reduction is related to CHD risk reduction, and the goals outlined in the tables should be considered as *minimal* goals. Hypertriglyceridemia is classified as normal, borderline, high, or very high, as outlined in Table 21–6.

TABLE 21–8. LDL Cholesterol Goals and Cutpoints for Therapeutic Life-style Changes (TLC) and Drug Therapy in Different Risk Categories[a]

Risk Category	LDL Goal (mg/dL)	LDL Level at Which to Initiate TLC (mg/dL)	LDL Level at Which to Consider Drug Therapy (mg/dL)
CHD or CHD risk equivalents (10-year risk >20%)	<100	≥100	≥130 (100–129: drug optional)[b]
2+ Risk factors (10-year risk ≤20%)	<130	≥130	10-year risk 10–20%; ≥130 10-year risk <10%; ≥160
0–1 Risk factor[c]	<160	≥160	≥190 (160–189: LDL-lowering drug optional)

[a]CHD, coronary heart disease; LDL, low-density lipoprotein.

[b]Some authorities recommend use of LDL-lowering drugs in this category if an LDL cholesterol level of <100 mg/dL cannot be achieved by TLC. Others prefer use of drugs that primarily modify triglycerides and HDL; e.g., nicotinic acid or fibrates. Clinical judgment also may call for deferring drug therapy in this subcategory.

[c]Almost all people with 0–1 risk factor have a 10-year risk <10%; thus, 10-year risk assessment in people with 0–1 risk factor is not necessary.

TABLE 21–9. Classification of Total and Low-Density Lipoprotein Cholesterol Levels in Children and Adolescents from Families with Hypercholesterolemia or Premature Cardiovascular Disease*

Category	Total Cholesterol (mg/dL)	LDL Cholesterol (mg/dL)	Dietary Intervention
Acceptable	<170	<110	Recommended population eating pattern
Borderline	170–199	110–129	Step 1 diet prescribed and other risk factor intervention
High	≥200	≥130	Step 1 diet prescribed and then Step 2 diet if necessary

*For use in children with a definite family history of premature (<50 y in females; <60 y in males) coronary heart disease including diagnostic coronary arteriography, angioplasty, coronary artery bypass grafting, myocardial infarction, angina pectoris, peripheral vascular disease, or cerebrovascular disease before age 55 years. Screening should also be done in the offspring of a parent or sibling with blood cholesterol of ≥240 mg/dL, or, in the absence of family history, in the presence of other risk factors (corticosteroid use, juvenile diabetes mellitus, hypothyroidism or other renal, endocrine, or hepatic disease known to affect cholesterol level).
(From Expert Panel. National Cholesterol Education Program. Report of the Expert Panel on blood cholesterol levels in children and adolescents. Pediatrics 1998;101:141–147.)

▶ TREATMENT: Hyperlipidemia

NONPHARMACOLOGIC THERAPY

Results from numerous epidemiologic studies suggested that elevated blood cholesterol levels increased the risk for CHD. However, proof of the lipid hypothesis (that reduction of elevated cholesterol would reduce risk) was lacking until the publication of the Lipid Research Clinics Coronary Primary Prevention Trial (LRC-CPPT) in the early 1980s, which unequivocally demonstrated a reduction in CHD death and nonfatal MI in a large number of asymptomatic men with primary hypercholesterolemia.[33,34] The investigators found that for every 1% reduction in cholesterol, approximately a 2% reduction in CHD was seen; in more recent trials, however, the relationship has been 1:1. More recently, the Scandinavian simvastatin survival study (4S), a secondary intervention trial, demonstrated that intervention with diet and simvastatin reduces CHD mortality and total mortality as compared to diet and placebo treatment.[35] Results from angiographic studies demonstrate halting of progression of established lesions, prevention of new lesion formation, and, to a lesser extent, regression of existing atherosclerotic plaques in coronary arteries. This has been shown in native vessels or venous bypass grafts in patients who have undergone coronary artery bypass grafting. Of interest, these angiographic trials, which typically cause small changes in luminal diameter (e.g., about a 0.04-mm difference in change between placebo and active treatment), result in fewer clinical events such as MI or the need for revascularization.[36] This unexpected finding suggests that plaque size and luminal encroachment by plaque may be less important than the effects that cholesterol lowering may have on the activity in the plaque and endothelial dysfunction. These studies provide a strong rationale for attempting to lower plasma cholesterol and LDL in patients with hypercholesterolemia. Present evidence clearly demonstrates the benefit of cholesterol lowering in patients with known CHD and in patients with multiple risk factors. Many more patients without established CHD or risk factors must be treated to show a reduction in cardiovascular end points; however, the LRC-CPPT[33,34] and the West of Scotland[37] trials provide convincing evidence that primary intervention is also effective.

DIETARY THERAPY

The objectives of dietary therapy are to progressively decrease the intake of total fat, saturated fatty acids (i.e., saturated fat), and cholesterol, and to achieve a desirable body weight. Typical American diets now include 13% to 20% of total calories from saturated fat and a cholesterol intake of 350–450 mg/d, both in excess of a "heart healthy" diet for normal Americans, let alone patients with a lipid disorder. The targeted saturated fatty acids have carbon chain lengths of 12 (lauric acid), 14 (myristic acid), and 16 (palmitic acid). The rationale for using a nutritionally balanced low-fat, low-cholesterol diet for the treatment of hypercholesterolemia is based on these principles: (a) it represents a reasonable extension of the diet recommended for the general public; (b) it progressively decreases the major cholesterol-raising constituent of the diet; (c) it precludes large intakes of polyunsaturated fats; and (d) it facilitates weight reduction by removing foods of high caloric density.[2] Dietary modification, weight control, and increased physical activity are essential first steps in the treatment of most lipid disorders. Table 21–10 outlines the therapeutic life-style changes diet recommended by the NCEP ATP III for treating high blood cholesterol.

Many patients with hyperlipidemia may be managed with dietary therapy alone, obviating the need for drugs. Diet is a cost-effective form of intervention.[1,2] Diet is the cornerstone for most forms of

TABLE 21–10. Nutrient Composition of the TLC Diet

Nutrient	Recommended Intake
Total fat	25%–35% of total calories
Saturated fatty acids	<7% of total calories
Polyunsaturated fatty acids	Up to 10% of total calories
Monounsaturated fatty acids	Up to 20% of total calories
Carbohydrates	50%–60% of total calories
Protein	~15% of total calories
Fiber	20–30 g/d
Cholesterol	<200 mg/d
Total calories	To achieve and maintain desirable body weight

hyperlipidemia, and the use of a dietitian for patient counseling is recommended. Several cookbooks with recipes generally suitable for implementing an alternate diet as part of the stepped diet approach have been published (contact the American Heart Association). The basic rationale for reducing dietary cholesterol, saturated fat, and excessive calories is based on the overproduction of VLDL and, subsequently, LDL. Excessive dietary intake of cholesterol and saturated fatty acids leads to decreased hepatic clearance of LDL and deposition of LDL and oxidized LDL in peripheral tissues.[17] The predicted reduction in total serum cholesterol following institution of the therapeutic life-style changes diet is 8% to 14%.[2] Considering the baseline LDL-C concentration, the percentage of patients who were prescribed diet was 26%, 30%, and 40% for patients with less than two risk factors, two or more risk factors, and known CHD, respectively, based on the NHANES III survey data.[7] Some individuals are more responsive to dietary therapy than others and deviation from the predictions can be expected. Assessment of response to dietary therapy can be done with a dietary assessment instrument as described in the ATP III report. Life-style therapies are begun on visit 1 including reducing saturated fat and cholesterol, encouraging moderate physical activity, and possible referral to a dietitian. Visit 2 should be 6 weeks later with reinforcement of the changes instituted on visit 1 and consider adding stanols/sterols, increasing fiber intake, and additional dietary counseling. Six weeks later at visit 3, drug therapy may be considered if the LDL-C goal is not achieved. At that time, therapy for the metabolic syndrome should be initiated, weight management and exercise should be intensified, and referral to a dietitian if this has not been done previously. In general, drug therapy should not be instituted until the trial of diet has continued for 12 weeks. Exceptions to these suggestions include patients with severe forms of hyperlipidemia, or the presence of two or more risk factors, or definite CHD, or risk equivalents. Long-term counseling of the patient and family to encourage diet compliance, and education about the risks and benefits that can be derived from diet modification and life-style changes, are important. Overall, reduction of cholesterol and saturated fat intake provides a reduction of coronary heart risk. This seems to be true regardless of the time of intervention (primary versus secondary), and diet modification works adjunctively with other risk-factor interventions, such as cessation of smoking and treating hypertension. Continuation of diet therapy is imperative if drug therapy is to be optimal. After the LDL-C goal is achieved, monitoring of adherence to therapeutic life-style changes should occur at 4 to 6 months.

Adherence to diet therapy may be improved by presenting the changes in diet in a positive perspective and by making changes over a reasonable time frame. The entire family, including the preparer of meals, should be included in diet counseling. Realistic goals should be set, and monitoring of response to diet intervention with feedback to the patient and family will improve compliance. A registered dietitian is an important member of the team. Dietary expertise in providing a wide range of options and suggestions in preparation of food can make the difference between a good or an inadequate response to diet. Information concerning eating out in a healthy fashion and advice for shopping are also important factors for success in diet therapy. An example is being aware of products with misleading labels such as coffee creamers that state they contain "no cholesterol," when they may contain hydrogenated (saturated) fats or oils (e.g., palmitic acid, palm kernel oil, or coconut oil), which makes them undesirable because of their saturated fat content. Variations in polyunsaturated and saturated fat and cholesterol intake influence the LDL concentration, but the amount of cholesterol has been found to have a greater effect than the proportion of polyunsaturated or saturated fat. There were also racial differences in elevation of LDL with high saturated fat diets being greater in whites than in other racial groups. The isomeric form of fatty acids is also important. Fatty acids with the *cis* configuration are the preferred substrate for the ACAT reaction and significantly increase hepatic LDL receptor clearance while reducing LDL cholesterol production rate. The *trans* isomeric form cannot be used by ACAT and is biologically inactive with no effect on LDL concentration.[17] In addition to the commercial publications mentioned earlier, the NCEP also has publications available that assist in diet therapy.

Other dietary interventions or diet supplements may be useful in certain patients with lipid disorders. Increased intake of soluble fiber in the form of oat bran, pectins, certain gums, and psyllium products can result in useful adjunctive reductions in total and LDL cholesterol, but these dietary alterations or supplements should not be substituted for more active forms of treatment. Total daily fiber intake should be about 20–30 g/d, with about 25% or 6 g/d, being soluble fiber.[2] Studies with psyllium seed in doses of 10–15 g/d show reductions in total and LDL cholesterol ranging from about 5% to 20%.[38] They have little or no effect on HDL-C or triglyceride concentrations. These products may also be useful in managing constipation associated with the bile acid sequestrants. Psyllium binds cholesterol in the gut but also reduces hepatic production and clearance.[39] Fish oil supplementation provides an increased amount of the omega-3 polyunsaturated fatty acids such as eicosapentaenoic acid and docosahexaenoic acid. In epidemiologic studies from Scandinavia, ingestion of large amounts of cold water fish is associated with a reduction in CHD risk, but it is unclear whether the same advantage is conferred with commercially prepared fish oil products. Fish oil supplementation has a fairly large effect in reducing triglycerides and VLDL-C, but it either has no effect on total and LDL cholesterol or may cause elevations in these fractions. Other actions of fish oil may account for their protective effects. These effects include quantitative and qualitative alterations in the synthesis of prostanoid substances, changes in immune function and cellular proliferation, and potential antioxidative actions.[40] Responses noted with fish oil are further discussed under drug therapy.

Fat substitutes such as Olestra (Olean, sucrose polyester, Procter and Gamble), a mixture of hexa-, hepta-, and octa-esters formed from the reaction of sucrose with long-chain fatty acids, are approved by the FDA as a nondigestible, nonabsorable, noncaloric fat substitute for snack foods. Olestra is heat stable, an advantage over several other fat substitutes, enabling it to be used in the preparation of fried and baked foods. It is similar in composition to triglycerides, but Olestra is not hydrolyzed in the gastrointestinal tract by pancreatic lipase, and, consequently, is not taken up by the intestinal mucosa. The principal adverse effects associated with Olestra use are bloating, flatulence, diarrhea, and "anal leakage." Because of the ability of Olestra to solubilize lipophilic substances, there has been concern over potential drug interactions in which lipophilic drugs (e.g., digitoxin, cyclosporin, or colchicine) or vitamins (vitamins A, D, E, and K) are solubilized in Olestra and excreted in the feces. Drug therapy is indicated following an adequate trial of therapeutic life-style changes as outlined in Tables 21–8 and 21–9.

PHARMACOLOGIC THERAPY

Several excellent reviews on the treatment of hyperlipidemia and the adverse effects of the drugs used have been published.[41–44] Although many efficacious lipid-lowering drugs exist, none is effective

TABLE 21–11. Effects of Drug Therapy on Lipids and Lipoproteins

Drug	Mechanism of Action	Effects on Lipids	Effects on Lipoproteins	Comment
Cholestyramine, colestipol and colesevelam	↑ LDL catabolism ↓ Cholesterol absorption	↓ Cholesterol	↓ LDL ↑ VLDL	Problem with compliance; binds many coadministered drugs
Niacin	↓ LDL and VLDL synthesis	↓ Triglyceride and ↓ cholesterol	↓ VLDL; ↓ LDL; ↑ HDL	Problems with patient acceptance; good in combination with bile acid resins
Probucol	↑ LDL clearance	↓ Cholesterol	↓ LDL and HDL	Lowers HDL; modest efficacy but inhibits LDL oxidation and facilitates reverse cholesterol transport
Gemfibrozil, fenofibrate, clofibrite	↑ VLDL clearance ↓ VLDH synthesis	↓ Triglyercide and cholesterol	↓ VLDL; ↑↓ LDL; ↑ HDL	Possible long-term toxicity; raises HDL
Lovastatin, pravastatin, simvastatin, fluvastatin, atorvastatin, rosuvastatin	↑ LDL catabolism; inhibit LDL synthesis	↓ Cholesterol	↓ LDL	Highly effective in heterozygous familial hypercholesterolemia and in combination with other agents

in all lipoprotein disorders, and all such agents are associated with some adverse effects.[45] Lipid-lowering drugs can be broadly divided into agents that decrease the synthesis of VLDL and LDL, agents that enhance VLDL clearance, agents that enhance LDL catabolism, agents that decrease cholesterol absorption, agents that elevate HDL, or some combination of these characteristics (Table 21–11). Table 21–12 lists recommended drugs of choice for each lipoprotein phenotype and alternate agents. Table 21–13 lists available products and their doses.

Treatment of type I hyperlipoproteinemia is directed toward reduction of chylomicrons derived from dietary fat with the subsequent reduction in plasma triglycerides. Total daily fat intake should be no more than 10–25 g/d, or approximately 15% of total calories. Secondary causes of hypertriglyceridemia (see Table 21–5) should be excluded or, if present, the underlying disorder should be treated appropriately. Type V hyperlipoproteinemia also requires a stringent restriction of the fat component of dietary intake; in addition, drug therapy is indicated, as outlined in Table 21–12, if the response to diet alone is inadequate. Medium-chain triglycerides, which are absorbed without chylomicron formation, may be used as a dietary supplement for caloric intake if needed for types I and V. Hepatic fibrosis has been reported with medium-chain triglycerides. Omega-3 fatty acids may be useful in lipoprotein lipase deficiency in some patients. In patients with apolipoprotein C-II deficiency, infusion of plasma may normalize plasma triglyceride levels.

TABLE 21–12. Lipoprotein Phenotype and Recommended Drug Treatment

Lipoprotein Type	Drug of Choice	Combination Therapy
I	Not Indicated	—
IIa	HMG Co-ARI (statins)	Niacin or BAR
	Cholestyramine or colestipol	Statins or niacin
	Niacin	Statins or BAR ERT/HRT[a]
IIb	Statins	BAR or fibrates or niacin
	Fibrates	Statins or niacin or BAR[b]
	Niacin	Statins or fibrates
III	Fibrates	Statins or niacin
	Niacin	Statins or fibrates
IV	Fibrates	Niacin
	Niacin	Fibrates
V	Fibrates	Niacin
	Niacin	Fish oils

BAR, bile acid resins; ERT/HRT, estrogen replacement therapy or hormone replacement therapy; fibrates includes gemfibrozil or fenofibrate; HMG Co-ARI, hydroxymethylglutaryl coenzyme-A reductase inhibitors.

[a]In selected women, ERT may be first-line therapy and may be adequate to reach LDL C and HDL-C targets.

[b]BAR are not used as first-line therapy if triglycerides are elevated at baseline because hypertriglyceridemia may worsen with BAR alone.

Primary hypercholesterolemia (familial hypercholesterolemia, familial combined hyperlipidemia, type IIa hyperlipoproteinemia) is treated with the bile acid resins or sequestrants (BAR, colestipol, cholestyramine, and colesevelam), HMG Co-A reductase inhibitors (statins), or niacin. The primary action of BAR is to bind bile acids in the intestinal lumen, with a concurrent interruption of enterohepatic circulation of bile acids and a markedly increased excretion of acidic steroids in the feces. This decreases the bile acid pool size and stimulates hepatic synthesis of bile acids from cholesterol. Depletion of the hepatic pool of cholesterol results in an increase in cholesterol biosynthesis and an increase in the number of LDL receptors on the hepatocyte membrane. The increased number of receptors stimulates an enhanced rate of catabolism from plasma and lowers LDL levels. CETP, which is correlated with total and LDL cholesterol concentrations, is also reduced by BAR, perhaps by interfering with hepatic microsomal cholesterol content.[46] Patients with homozygous familial hypercholesterolemia genetically lack the ability to increase synthesis of LDL receptors and bile acid resins are generally ineffective. The increase in hepatic cholesterol biosynthesis may be paralleled by increased hepatic VLDL production and, consequently, bile acid resins may aggravate hypertriglyceridemia in patients with combined hyperlipidemia. Gastrointestinal complaints of constipation, bloating, epigastric fullness, nausea, and flatulence are most commonly reported.[45] With intensive education, patients can learn to tolerate resins on a long term basis as evidenced by adherence in clinical trials to active drug regimens but in routine clinical practice 40% or more of patients will discontinue therapy within 1 year.[47–49] These

TABLE 21–13. Comparison of Drugs Used in the Treatment of Hyperlipidemia

Drug	Manufacturer	Dosage Forms	Usual Daily Dose	Maximum Daily Dose
Cholestyramine (Questran)	Bristol	Bulk powder/4-g packets	8 g tid	32 g
Cholestyramine (Questran Light)	Bristol	Bulk powder/4-g packets		
Cholestyramine (Cholybar)	Parke-Davis	4-g resin per bar		
Colestipol hydrochloride (Colestid)	Upjohn	Bulk powder/1- and 5-g packets	8 g bid	16 g
Colesevelam (Welchol)	Sankyo	625 mg tablets	1,875 mg bid	4,375 mg
Niacin	Various	50-, 100-, 250-, and 500-mg tablets; 125-, 250-, and 500-mg capsules	2 g tid	9 g
Probucol (Lorelco)	Merrell Dow	250-mg tablets	500 mg bid	1 g
Clofibrate (Atromid-S)	Ayerst	500-mg capsules	1 g bid	2 g
Fenofibrate (Tricor)	Abbott	54, 160-mg tablets	160 mg	160 mg
Gemfibrozil (Lopid)	Parke-Davis	600-mg tablets	600 mg bid	1200 mg
Lovastatin (Mevacor)	MSD	10-, 20-, and 40-mg tablets	20–40 mg	80 mg
Pravastatin (Pravachol)	Bristol-Myers Squibb	10-, 20-, and 40-mg tablets	10–20 mg	40 mg
Simvastatin (Zocor)	MSD	5-, 10-, 20-, 40-, and 80-mg tablets	10–20 mg	80 mg
Atorvastatin (Lipitor)	Parke-Davis	10-, 20-, 40, and 80-mg tablets	10 mg	80 mg
Rosuvastatin (Crestor)	Astra-Zeneca	5- and 10-mg tablets	5 mg	10 mg

Probucol is no longer on the market in the United States; gemfibrozil and lovastatin are available as generic products.

adverse effects can be managed by increasing the fluid intake, modifying the diet to increase bulk, and using stool softeners. The other major limiting complaint is the gritty texture and bulk; these problems may be minimized by mixing the powder with orange drink or juice. Tablet forms of bile acid sequestrants should help in improving compliance with this form of therapy, whereas the bar does not improve compliance.[31] Other potential adverse effects include impaired absorption of fat-soluble vitamins A, D, E, and K; hypernatremia and hyperchloremia; gastrointestinal obstruction; and reduced bioavailability of acidic drugs such as coumarin anticoagulants, digitoxin, nicotinic acid, thyroxine, acetaminophen, hydrocortisone, hydrochlorothiazide, loperamide, and possibly iron.[45] Hyperchloremic metabolic acidosis, hypernatremia, and gastrointestinal obstruction have been reported almost exclusively in children, and malabsorption of fat-soluble vitamins is probably most common with high doses (e.g., 30 g/d of cholestyramine) of the bile acid resins. Drug interactions may be avoided by alternating administration times with an interval of 6 hours or greater between the bile acid resin and other drugs. Colestipol and cholestyramine have comparable side effects; however, colestipol may have better palatability because it is odorless and tasteless. Colesevelam is the newest BAR and total and LDL-C reduction is dose related. The adverse effects are qualitatively similar to the older BAR but may occur less often. Because of adverse effects occurring commonly with BAR at higher doses, BARs are increasingly used in combination with other drugs, as low doses are tolerated well and they work in a complementary fashion with other agents.

Niacin (nicotinic acid) may also be used in primary hypercholesterolemia in combination with bile acid sequestrants or as monotherapy for this disorder and others (Table 21–12). Niacin reduces the hepatic synthesis of VLDL, which, in turn, leads to a reduction in the synthesis of LDL. Factors responsible for decreased production of VLDL include inhibition of lipolysis with a decrease in free fatty acids in plasma, decreased hepatic esterification of triglycerides, and a possible direct effect on the hepatic production of apolipoprotein B. The complementary action of niacin and bile acid sequestrants to increase catabolism and decrease synthesis of LDL may account for the additive effects of this combination in hyperlipidemia. Niacin also increases HDL by reducing its catabolism. Niacin selectively decreases hepatic removal of HDL apoA-I but not removal of cholesterol esters, thereby increasing the capacity of retained apoA-I to augment reverse cholesterol transport in isolated hepatic cells. The principal use of niacin is for mixed hyperlipemia or as a second-line agent in combination therapy for hypercholesterolemia. It is also considered to be the first-line agent or an alternative for the treatment of hypertriglyceridemia.[50] There are numerous smaller trials suggesting that lower doses of niacin may be combined with statins or gemfibrozil to minimize adverse effects and maximize response. These combinations require careful monitoring because interactions do occur.

Niacin has many adverse drug reactions that occur commonly; fortunately, most of the symptoms and biochemical abnormalities seen do not require discontinuation of therapy. Cutaneous flushing and itching appear to be prostaglandin mediated and can be reduced by aspirin 325 mg given shortly before niacin ingestion.[51] Flushing seems to be related to rising plasma concentrations of niacin; taking the dose with meals and slowly titrating the dose upward may minimize these effects. Gastrointestinal intolerance and flushing are common problems. Acanthosis nigricans, a darkening of the skin in skinfold areas and an external marker of insulin resistance, may be seen with high doses of niacin. Sustained-release products may minimize these complaints in some patients, but controlled trials with regular-release products do not demonstrate much of a difference between sustained- and regular-release products. One possible exception is a newer product, Niaspan. In controlled trials, it is reported to have fewer dermatologic reactions.[52,53] Potentially important laboratory abnormalities occurring with niacin therapy include elevated liver function tests, hyperuricemia, and hyperglycemia. Recent experience with niacin in diabetes suggests that some diabetic patients do not have worsened glycemic control with dose-titration and sustained-release products.[54] With less than 3 g/d, the degree of liver function test elevation is generally not marked and often transient, and a temporary reduction in dosage frequently corrects the problem. Niacin-associated hepatitis is more common with sustained-release preparations, and their use should be restricted to patients intolerant of regular-release

TABLE 21–14. Pharmacokinetics of the Statins

Parameter	Lovastatin	Simvastatin	Pravastatin	Fluvastatin	Atorvastatin	Rosuvastatin	Cerivastatin
Isoenzyme	3A4	3A4	None	2C9	3A4	2C9/2C19	3A4
Lipophilic	Yes	Yes	No	Yes	Yes	No	Yes
Protein binding (%)	>95	95–98	~50	>90	96	NA	>99
Active metabolites	Yes	Yes	No	No	Yes	No	Yes
Elimination half-life (h)	3	2	1.8	1.2	14	20	2

Isoenzyme refers to the specific isoenzyme in the cytochrome P450 system that is responsible for the metabolism of each drug. Pharmacokinetic parameters in this table are based on studies and reviews presented in the literature. NA, not available.

products.[55] Sustained-release products are often more expensive and given the lack of data for reduced adverse effects and increased incidence of hepatitis, regular-release products should always be used first. Preexisting gout and diabetes may be exacerbated by niacin; these patients should be monitored more closely and their medication titrated appropriately. Niacin is contraindicated in patients with active liver disease. Dry eyes and other ophthalmologic complaints are also occasionally noted. Concomitant alcohol and hot drinks may magnify flushing and pruritus with niacin and they should be avoided at the time of ingestion. Nicotinamide should not be used in the treatment of hyperlipidemia, as it does not effectively lower cholesterol or triglyceride levels.

Statins interrupt the conversion of HMG-CoA to mevalonate, the rate-limiting step in de novo cholesterol biosynthesis, by inhibiting HMG-CoA reductase (see Fig. 21–4). Currently available products include lovastatin, pravastatin, simvastatin, fluvastatin, and atorvastatin. Rosuvastatin should become available in 2002 and will likely be the most potent statin on the market. Table 21–14 lists the pharmacokinetic properties of the statins.[56] The plasma half-lives for all the statins are reported to be short except for atorvastatin and rosuvastatin, and this may account for their potency.[57] In CURVES, the largest head-to-head comparison of statins, atorvastatin was found to be the most potent drug for lowering total cholesterol and LDL-C, with reductions in LDL-C of 38%, 46%, 51%, and 54% for the 10-, 20-, 40-, and 80-mg doses, respectively.[58] Metabolic studies with statins in normal volunteers and patients with hypercholesterolemia suggest reduced synthesis of LDL-C, as well as enhanced catabolism of LDL mediated through LDL receptors, as the principal mechanisms for lipid-lowering effects.[2] Total and LDL cholesterol are reduced in a dose-related fashion by 30% or more on average when added to dietary therapy, with the effects being more pronounced in nonfamilial than in familial hypercholesterolemia. Combination therapy with bile acid sequestrants and lovastatin is rational as LDL receptor numbers are increased, leading to greater degradation of LDL-C; intracellular synthesis of cholesterol is inhibited, and enterohepatic recycling of bile acids is interrupted. In the expanded clinical evaluation of lovastatin (EXCEL) study of more than 8000 patients, lovastatin reduced LDL-C by 24% to 40% when given in doses ranging from 20 mg once daily to 40 mg twice daily.[59] Constipation in placebo-treated patients occurred in 4.7% of patients, while lovastatin was associated with constipation in 4.2% to 7.7% of patients (20 mg twice a day). Elevation of serum transaminase levels (primarily alanine aminotransferase) to greater than three times the upper limit of normal and associated muscle symptoms (myopathy) were most common at higher doses (40 mg given twice a day)—1.5% as compared to placebo of 0.1%. Creatine kinase (CK) greater than 10 times the upper limit of normal and muscle symptoms occurred in 0% of the placebo group versus 0.2% of the lovastatin group, and any elevation of CK was highest at 40 mg given twice a day, 3.5% versus 1.6% for placebo. Lens opacities have been reported with lovastatin; however, in the age groups studied, these abnormalities are common and tend to wax and wane with time irrespective of drug therapy, and no statistical association is known to exist. As a category of monotherapy, the HMG-CoA reductase inhibitors are the most potent total and LDL cholesterol-lowering agents and among the best tolerated.[35,37,60–63] Recently, a potential mechanism for poor response to statin therapy was described.[64] Poor responders had a low basal rate of cholesterol synthesis that may be secondary to a genetically determined increase in cholesterol absorption, possibly mediated by apolipoprotein E4.

Combined hyperlipoproteinemia (type IIb) may be treated with statins, niacin, or gemfibrozil to lower LDL cholesterol without elevating VLDL and triglycerides. Niacin is the most effective agent and may be combined with a bile acid sequestrant. Bile acid resins alone in this disorder may elevate VLDL and triglycerides, and their use as single agents for treating combined hyperlipoproteinemia should be avoided. Fibric acid (gemfibrozil, fenofibrate, clofibrate) monotherapy is effective in reducing VLDL, but a reciprocal rise in LDL may occur, and total cholesterol values may remain relatively unchanged. Gemfibrozil reduces the synthesis of VLDL and, to a lesser extent, apolipoprotein B, with a concurrent increase in the rate of removal of triglyceride-rich lipoproteins from plasma. Plasma HDL concentrations may rise 10% to 15% or more with fibrates. Early studies with clofibrate were associated with a number of unacceptable adverse effects (see below); however, evidence from the Helsinki Heart Study shows no significant differences between gemfibrozil and placebo.[65] Gastrointestinal complaints occur in 3% to 5% of patients; rash in 2% of patients; dizziness in 2.4% of patients; and transient elevations in transaminase levels and alkaline phosphatase in 4.5% and 1.3% of patients, respectively. Similar to clofibrate, gemfibrozil may enhance the formation of gallstones associated with an increase in the lithogenic index; however, the rate is low (0.6%) and similar to that seen with placebo in the Helsinki heart study. Other studies have found the relative risk for gallstones to be 1.7.[66] Fibric acid derivatives may potentiate the effects of oral anticoagulants and the prothrombin time and international normalized ratio should be monitored very closely with this combination.

Type III hyperlipoproteinemia may be treated with fibric acid derivatives or niacin. Although clofibrate has been suggested as the drug of choice for this disorder, given the lack of data supporting its efficacy in altering cardiovascular mortality in the major studies on hypercholesterolemia, and its numerous, well-documented, and serious adverse effects, it is reasonable to consider niacin, gemfibrozil or fenofibrate prior to the use of clofibrate. Clofibrate increases the activity of lipoprotein lipase and reduces to a lesser extent the synthesis or secretion of VLDL from the liver into the plasma. Clofibrate is less effective than gemfibrozil or niacin in reducing VLDL production. The most disturbing aspects of clofibrate's adverse effects are its potential to induce gallstones (4.7%, clofibrate; 0.54%, placebo), promote ventricular ectopy, and potentially cause gastrointestinal malignancy, causing a greater overall mortality than placebo alone.[67]

A myositis syndrome of myalgia, weakness, stiffness, malaise, and elevations in creatinine phosphokinase and aspartate aminotransaminase is seen with the fibric acid derivatives, and it seems to be more common in patients with renal insufficiency. Enhanced hypoglycemic effects are reported to occur when fibric acid derivative are given to patients on sulfonylurea compounds, but the mechanisms for these interactions are not well understood. Rifampin, an hepatic enzyme inducer of oxidative pathways, may induce the metabolism of clofibrate but the long-term consequences are unknown.

Three fibric acid derivatives (clofibrate, gemfibrozil, and fenofibrate) are approved in the United States; however, several others are under development or are being used in Europe, including bezafibrate and ciprofibrate. All reduce LDL-C by 20% to 25% in heterozygous familial hypercholesterolemia. The response of LDL-C, HDL-C, and triglycerides to this category of drug is very dependent on the specific lipoprotein type (e.g., type IIa versus IIb) and the baseline triglyceride concentration.[68]

As a potential alternative therapy, for this phenotype, numerous epidemiologic and normal volunteer studies have found that diets high in omega-3 polyunsaturated fatty acids (from fish oil), mostly commonly eicosapentaenoic acid, reduce cholesterol, triglycerides, LDL-C, and VLDL-C, and may elevate HDL-C.[17,69] The effects of fish oil on lipoprotein metabolism are mediated through a reduction in VLDL production and suppression of VLDL apolipoprotein B. In patients with hypertriglyceridemia, either phenotypes type IIb or type V, a diet high in omega-3 fatty acids given for 4 weeks reduced cholesterol 27% and 45%, and triglyceride 64% and 79%, in the type IIb and type V patients, respectively.[70] A diet high in eicosapentaenoic acid given to hyperlipidemic hemodialysis patients resulted in significant decreases in cholesterol and triglycerides for as long as 13 weeks. Fish oil supplementation may be most useful in patients with hypertriglyceridemia; however, its role in treatment is not well defined. Potential complications of fish oil supplementation, such as thrombocytopenia and bleeding disorders, have been noted, especially with high doses (eicosapentaenoic acid 15–30 g/d); and well-controlled trials are needed to determine if fish oils are safe and effective before their use may be broadly recommended.

Combination drug therapy may be considered after adequate trials of monotherapy and for patients documented compliant to the prescribed regimen. Two or three lipoprotein profiles at 6-week intervals should confirm lack of response prior to initiation of combination therapy. Cholestyramine may be added in patients with fasting hypertriglyceridemia, but it should not be used as the initial drug, because triglycerides are likely to increase. Contraindications to and drug interactions with combined therapy should be carefully screened, as well as consideration of the extra cost of drug product and monitoring that may be required. In general, a statin and a BAR or niacin with a BAR provide the greatest reduction in total and LDL cholesterol. Regimens intended to increase HDL levels should include either gemfibrozil or niacin, and it should be remembered that statins combined with either of these drugs may result in a greater incidence of hepatotoxicity or myositis. Familial combined hyperlipidemia may respond better to a fibric acid and a statin than to a fibric acid and a BAR.[71,72]

Severe forms of hypercholesterolemia—such as familial hypercholesterolemia, familial defective apolipoprotein B-100, severe polygenic hypercholesterolemia, familial combined hyperlipidemia, and familial dysbetalipoproteinemia (type III)—may require more intensive therapy. In particular, familial hypercholesterolemia patients often require combination therapy (two or three drugs) and are managed with surgical therapy (partial ileal bypass), plasmapheresis (LDL-apheresis), and liver transplantation (to replace LDL receptors).

HYPERTRIGLYCERIDEMIA

It is important to remember that lipoprotein pattern types I, III, IV, and V are associated with hypertriglyceridemia, and that these primary lipoprotein disorders and underlying diseases should be excluded prior to implementing therapy (see Table 21–5). A positive family history of CHD is important in identifying patients at risk for premature atherosclerosis.[73,74] If a patient with CHD has elevated triglycerides, the associated abnormality is probably a contributing factor to CHD and should be treated.[50]

High serum triglycerides (see Tables 21–6 and 21–12) should be treated by achieving desirable body weight, consumption of a low saturated fat and cholesterol diet, regular exercise, smoking cessation, and restriction of alcohol (in selected patients). ATP III identifies the sum of LDL-C + VLDL-C (termed *non-HDL-C* [total cholesterol − HDL-C]) as a secondary target of therapy in persons with high triglycerides (≥200 mg/dL). The goal for non-HDL-C in persons with high serum triglycerides can be set at 30 mg/dL higher than that for LDL-C on the premise that a VLDL-C level ≤30 mg/dL is normal. In patients with borderline-high triglycerides but with accompanying risk factors of established CHD disease, family history of premature CHD, concomitant LDL elevation or low HDL, and genetic forms of hypertriglyceridemia associated with CHD (familial dysbetalipoproteinemia, familial combined hyperlipidemia), drug therapy with niacin should be considered. Niacin (crystalline immediate release, Niacor) may be used cautiously in diabetics based on the results of the ADMIT trial, which found triglycerides were reduced by 23%, HDL-C increased by 29%, only a slight increase in glucose (mean 8.7 mg/dL), and no change in hemoglobin A_{1c}.[75] Alternative therapies include gemfibrozil, statins, and fish oil.[76–78] Fibrates may increase LDL, and their use in borderline-high triglyceridemia requires careful monitoring to detect this deleterious change in lipid profile. Statins may also be used, because they provide modest reductions in triglycerides and modest elevations in HDL.[78,79] Atorvastatin, in the currently approved doses, has the greatest triglyceride-lowering effects of the available statins. Higher doses of atorvastatin and fluvastatin may reduce HDL-C as well as LDL-C and triglycerides.[80] The goal of therapy in this situation is to lower triglycerides and VLDL particles that may be atherogenic, increase HDL, and reduce LDL.

Very high triglycerides are associated with pancreatitis and other consequences of the chylomicron syndrome. At this level of elevation of triglycerides, a genetic form of hypertriglyceridemia often coexists with other causes of elevated triglycerides such as diabetes. Dietary fat restriction (10% to 20% of calories as fat), weight loss, alcohol restriction, and treatment of the coexisting disorder are the basic elements of management. Drugs useful in hypertriglyceridemia include gemfibrozil, niacin, and certain statins (atorvastatin and simvastatin). Gemfibrozil is the preferred drug in diabetics because of the effect of niacin on glycemic control unless the newer sustained-release forms are used. Success in treatment is defined as a reduction in triglycerides below 500 mg/dL.[1,2]

LOW HDL CHOLESTEROL

Low HDL-C is a strong independent risk predictor of CHD. ATP III redefined low HDL-C as <40 mg/dL, but specified no goal for HDL-C raising.[1] Low HDL-C may be a consequence of insulin resistance, physical inactivity, Type 2 diabetes, cigarette smoking, very high carbohydrate intake, and certain drugs (see Table 21–5). In low HDL-C the primary target remains LDL-C according to ATP III, but emphasis shifts to weight reduction, increased physical activity, and smoking cessation, and if drug therapy is required, to fibric acid derivatives and niacin. Niacin has the potential for the greatest increase in HDL-C and the effect is more pronounced with regular or immediate-release forms than with sustained-release forms.[55]

DIABETIC DYSLIPIDEMIA

Diabetic dyslipidemia is characterized by hypertriglyceridemia, low HDL-C, and LDL-C that is minimally elevated. Small, dense LDL-C (pattern B) in diabetes is more atherogenic than larger, more buoyant forms of LDL-C (pattern A); routine lipoprotein profiles do not differentiate between pattern A and pattern B.[81] Diabetes in ATP III is a CHD risk equivalent and the primary target is LDL-C with a goal of treatment being to lower LDL-C <100 mg/dL.[82] When LDL-C is >130 mg/dL, most patients will require simultaneous therapeutic lifestyle changes and drug therapy. When LDL-C is between 100 and 129 mg/dL, intensifying glycemic control, adding drugs for the atherogenic dyslipidemia (fibric acid derivatives, niacin) and intensifying LDL-C-lowering therapy are options. Because the primary target is LDL-C in diabetic dyslipidemia, statins are considered by many to be initial drugs of choice.[83] The relative risk reduction for CHD in diabetics versus nondiabetics is greater in the West of Scotland (37% versus 20%),[37] AFCAPS/TexCAPS (43% versus 36%),[61] CARE (25% versus 23%),[62,64] and 4S (55% versus 32%) trials.[35] All statins are fairly comparable in triglyceride lowering and because statins differ in potency for LDL-C reduction, a ratio of LDL-C reduction to triglyceride reduction can be applied. Statin therapy may protect against the development of diabetes but the observations from the West of Scotland study with pravastatin needs to be confirmed in a prospective trial.[84]

Fenofibrate, according to the DIAS trial, reduced the angiographic progression of CAD in type 2 diabetes.[85] Fewer CHD events were seen with fenofibrate compared with placebo but the difference was not significant. Fibric acids principally lower VLDL and triglycerides while increasing HDL with only modest lowering of total and LDL cholesterol; on occasion, fibric acid derivatives may increase LDL levels. Fibric acid derivatives tend to improve glucose tolerance, in contrast to niacin; the greatest effect has been seen with bezafibrate. The Helsinki Heart Study found gemfibrozil to be most effective in diabetic dyslipidemia.[65] Although the effect of statins on triglycerides and HDL-C abnormalities commonly seen in diabetes is less than with fibric acids, the subgroup analyses cited earlier suggest that they reduce CHD risk significantly. Cholestyramine in diabetic patients may result in lower LDL levels, but VLDL and triglyceride levels, which are commonly elevated in diabetes, may be further increased in this population. Resins may aggravate constipation, which is common in diabetics. Niacin is very effective in lowering total and LDL cholesterol and raising HDL concentrations, but it may be associated with worsened glycemic control.[86–88]

SPECIAL CONSIDERATIONS

ELDERLY

Hypercholesterolemia is an independent risk factor for CHD in the elderly (>65 years old), as it is in the younger patient. The attributable risk, which is the difference in absolute rates of CHD between segments of the population with higher or lower serum cholesterol levels, increases with age. Older patients potentially benefit to a greater extent from cholesterol lowering than younger populations. Data from studies of elderly men in a variety of settings are consistent with a relative risk of at least 1.5 in the highest compared to the lowest quartile of cholesterol levels.[89] Treatment of hypercholesterolemia in the elderly may bring about a comparable reduction in absolute risk to that obtained in younger persons.[2] Subgroup analyses of the West of Scotland (primary) and 4S (secondary) intervention studies show that elderly patients have lower CHD risk reduction (relative risk reduction of 27% and 29%, respectively) as compared to younger patients (relative risk reduction of 40% and 39%, respectively).[35,37] The Framingham study suggests that elderly women are at higher risk because of high blood cholesterol levels, but no other large studies included women; and their risks or benefits from cholesterol reduction are not well defined. Primary prevention in younger patients requires about 2 years before reduction in CHD risk is apparent, and this lag time should be taken into consideration in patient selection for therapy. Non-lipid CHD risk factors do not decline in relative risk with aging, and aggressive management of the modifiable non-lipid risk factors is important in the older patient. Because most women with CHD are elderly and also at risk for osteoporosis, they are logical candidates for diet therapy with consideration of calcium intake consistent with osteoporosis prevention, exercise, and perhaps estrogen replacement therapy. Recent evidence suggests that statins may reduce the risk of osteoporosis; however, there are conflicting data from various studies.[90,91]

Drug therapy in principle differs little from younger patients, and older patients respond to lipid-lowering drugs as well as younger patients based on the 4S trial and smaller studies.[37,92,93] Predicted reductions in CHD morbidity and mortality suggest that elderly patients with hypercholesterolemia should benefit from treatment; however, the gain in life expectancy may be small depending on the age at the start of treatment and the magnitude of cholesterol reduction.[94] Changes in body composition, renal function, and other physiologic changes of aging may make older patients more susceptible to adverse effects of lipid-lowering drug therapy. In particular, older patients are more likely to have constipation (bile acid resins), skin and eye changes (niacin), gout (niacin), gallstones (fibric acid derivatives), and bone/joint disorders (fibric acid derivatives, statins). Therapy should be started with lower doses and titrated up slowly to minimize adverse effects.

WOMEN

Cholesterol is an important determinant of CHD in women, but the relationship is not as strong as that seen in men. HDL may be a more important predictor of disease in women.[95] LDL and HDL genetic regulation in women and men does not appear to be different. Based on the Nurses' Health Study, obesity is an important determinant of CHD in women, with the relative risk being 3.3 in the highest Quetelet index (weight in kilograms divided by the square of the height in meters) as compared to the lowest category (i.e., <21 vs ≥29); low HDL levels usually accompany obesity.[96] No major differences exist in the influence of exercise, alcohol ingestion, and smoking on lipid levels between men and women. Women in the highest tertile of cholesterol appear to be more responsive to dietary therapy than those in the lower tertiles, and more responsive than formulas based on men predict. Oral contraceptives adversely influence LDL and HDL, and the products containing the lowest estrogen dose and the strongest antiestrogenic progestin produce the largest changes. Unopposed estrogen replacement for menopausal therapy increases HDL by 9% to 13% and decreases LDL by 4% to 10%, which is enough to influence CHD risk. Cyclic therapy with estrogen-progestin therapy may offset the beneficial effect of estrogen alone, depending on the particular estrogen-progestin combination and the doses used. The relative risk reduction of CHD in women was greater than in men in AFCAPS/TexCAPS (54% versus 34%),[61] CARE (46% versus 20%),[62] and 4S (35% versus 34%),[35] but less in LIPID (7% versus 25%). Regression of coronary atherosclerosis in women can be induced with aggressive therapy and, based on one study, the mean percent change in area of stenosis was greater in women than in men when LDL was reduced by about 38% and HDL was increased by 28%.[97]

Cholesterol and triglyceride levels rise progressively throughout pregnancy, with an average increment in cholesterol of 30–40 mg/dL occurring around the 36th to 39th weeks. Triglyceride levels may go up by as much as 150 mg/dL. Drug therapy is not instituted nor is it usually continued during pregnancy. Dietary therapy is the mainstay of treatment, with emphasis on maintaining a nutritionally balanced diet as per the needs of pregnancy.

CHILDREN

Drug therapy in children is not recommended until the age of 10 years or older, and the guidelines for institution of therapy and the goals of therapy are different from those in adults (see Table 21–9).[28] Younger children are generally managed with therapeutic life-style changes until after the age of 2 years.[98–100] Bile acid sequestrants are used in children because they minimize the risks of systemic toxicity.[31,101] Some literature does exist suggesting that resins are safe and effective in children.[32,102] Severe forms of hypercholesterolemia (e.g., familial hypercholesterolemia) may require more aggressive treatment.

CONCURRENT DISEASE STATES

Nephrotic syndrome, end-stage renal disease and nephrotic syndrome, and hypertension compound the risk of dyslipidemia and may present difficult-to-treat lipid abnormalities. Abnormalities of lipoprotein metabolism in the nephrotic syndrome include elevated total and LDL cholesterol, Lp(a), VLDL, and triglycerides. The apolipoprotein C-III to C-II ratio is elevated, consistent with greater lipoprotein lipase inhibitor activity, and the extent of hypoalbuminemia is correlated with dyslipidemia. The basic abnormality appears to be one of overproduction of LDL-apoB from VLDL, rather than reduced clearance of LDL-C and related proteins.[103,104] Protein restriction and a "vegan" diet corrects lipid abnormalities to some extent.[104] Statins have been shown to be effective in reducing elevated total and LDL cholesterol in the nephrotic syndrome, although the levels do not usually return to normal.[105,106] Clofibrate should not be used if renal insufficiency exists, whereas the pharmacokinetics of gemfibrozil are apparently not altered by renal insufficiency and it is effective in lowering total cholesterol by about 15% for this disorder.[107,108] Fenofibrate but not cerivastatin reduces remnant lipoproteins. Fibric acid derivatives and statins reduce small, dense LDL-C by different mechanisms, suggesting a potential role for combination therapy to optimize lowering of small, dense LDL-C and remnant lipoproteins.[78]

Renal insufficiency without proteinuria leads to hypertriglyceridemia, slightly elevated total and LDL cholesterol (particularly with chronic ambulatory peritoneal dialysis), and low HDL levels (especially during hemodialysis). These abnormalities are thought to be caused by a deficiency in apolipoprotein C-II, perhaps as a result of sustained use of heparin during hemodialysis and depletion of lipoprotein lipase, carbohydrate-induced obesity and hypertriglyceridemia, loss of carnitine during hemodialysis, use of acetate buffer (acetate is a precursor to fatty acid synthesis) during hemodialysis, and decreased LCAT activity during hemodialysis. Dialysis does not correct the lipid abnormalities. Renal transplantation may correct lipid abnormalities in some patients; however, in others, the use of transplantation-related medications such as corticosteroids, cyclosporine, and certain antihypertensive agents (see Chaps. 12 and 46) may aggravate the lipid abnormalities. Cyclosporine interferes with the metabolism of reductase inhibitors, and patients need to be observed closely for myositis and worsening renal function. Of interest, correction of lipid abnormalities may improve renal hemodynamics.[109] Small, short-term studies suggest that fluvastatin may be safer than other reductase inhibitors, but this needs to be validated in larger, long-term trials.[110] Diet will modify lipoprotein levels and polyunsaturated fatty acids may have a role in impeding the progression of renal disease as well as the cardiovascular complications. Bile acid sequestrants do not correct the lipid abnormalities seen in renal insufficiency. Lovastatin or its active metabolite may accumulate in renal insufficiency, and lower doses of reductase inhibitors should be used to avoid adverse effects. Gemfibrozil may be used with caution as its pharmacokinetics are unchanged and it lowers triglycerides and increases HDL.[108] Statins and fibric acid derivatives may increase the risk of severe myopathy, and attention to symptoms of myositis is needed. Niacin may also be useful in nondiabetic patients with renal insufficiency.

Hypertensive patients have a greater-than-expected prevalence of high blood-cholesterol levels and, conversely, patients with hypercholesterolemia have a higher than expected prevalence of hypertension caused by the metabolic syndrome. Recommendations for the management of hypertension in patients with hypercholesterolemia include avoiding the use of drugs that elevate cholesterol such as diuretics and β-blockers and using agents that are either lipid-neutral or that may reduce cholesterol slightly (see Chap. 12).[2] Bile acid sequestrants may bind to thiazide diuretics and some β-blockers, and may interfere with their absorption; reaction may be avoided by giving the antihypertensive 1 hour before or 4 hours after the resin. Niacin may magnify the hypotensive effects of vasodilators.

COST-EFFECTIVENESS OF ANTIHYPERLIPIDEMIC THERAPY

The clinical benefits of lipid-lowering therapy for primary and secondary intervention are now well established based on the results of the AFCAPS/TexCAPS, 4S, and other studies showing a reduction in CHD morbidity and mortality. The balance of benefits and costs has been examined in a few studies.[94,111,112] The cost per year of life saved has been estimated to range from less than $10,000 to over $1 million dollars depending on the presence or absence of CHD, age of the patient, baseline total or LDL-C level and reduction in cholesterol, and number of risk factors present. In general, intervention in patients with known CHD, those who have CHD risk equivalents or those with a 10-year risk of 10% to 20% are cost-effective with statin therapy, while other types of therapy may be cost-effective if certain assumptions concerning compliance, efficacy, and so forth, are met. The range for secondary intervention based on the 4S study is $3,800 for a 70-year-old man with a high cholesterol level to $27,400 per year of life gained for a middle-aged woman with an average cholesterol level.[94] In contrast, primary prevention in men based on the West of Scotland trial averages about $35,000 per year of life gained.[111] These studies demonstrate that primary and secondary intervention are well within the accepted boundary of less than $50,000 for a medical intervention to be considered cost-effective. Based on the specific lipoprotein phenotype, fibric acid derivatives, niacin, or combination therapy of statins plus BAR may be cost-effective.[113] Cost-effectiveness is maximized by treating high-risk patients and those with established CHD.

Specialty lipid clinics have become increasingly popular and many use pharmacists to provide direct patient care in this setting. An interesting recent analysis shows that a specialty clinic may be more expensive ($659 ± $43 versus $477 ± $42 per patient, $P < .001$) than usual care. However, the overall cost-effectiveness is improved when expressed as program costs per unit (mmol/L) reduction in the LDL-C, a measure of cost-effectiveness that was significantly lower for specialized care ($758 ± $58 versus $1,058 ± $70, $P = .002$) because more patients achieve their targeted goal.[114]

OTHER THERAPIES

Partial ileal bypass has been used in severe heterozygous and homozygous familial hypercholesterolemia; however, it is ineffective in the latter case. Ileal bypass removes the site of bile acid reabsorption, depleting the bile acid pool and increasing the catabolism of cholesterol. A randomized trial of diet versus surgery, program on the surgical control of the hyperlipidemias (POSCH), reported that total and LDL cholesterol were decreased (23.3% and 37.7%, respectively) and HDL increased (4.3%) in patients who had undergone ileal bypass for hypercholesterolemia.[115,116] Overall death was delayed by nearly 3 years ($P = .032$) and CHD mortality was delayed by nearly 4 years ($P = .046$) by surgery, as compared to the control group. Revascularization procedures were delayed by an average of 7 years ($P < .001$). Post-surgery diarrhea was more common in the surgical group, as was the rate of kidney stones (4% versus 0.4%), gallstones (10% versus 2%), and bowel obstruction (13.5% versus 3.6%).

Portacaval shunts have been used to decrease the formation of LDL-C and reductions of 10% to 20% have been reported.[117] Plasma exchange combined with niacin was found to reduce plasma cholesterol levels by about 50% in homozygous familial hypercholesterolemia over 5 years, and coronary atherosclerosis did not progress as documented by angiography. LDL-apheresis, selective removal of LDL-C via a filtering system, plus statin therapy is effective in LDL-C and appears to affect the progression of vascular disease.[118,119] LDL-apheresis may be combined with statin therapy for greater effect.[120] Combined liver and heart transplantation in homozygous familial hypercholesterolemia reduces total and LDL cholesterol concentrations from about 1100 and 900 mg/dL to about 300 and 185 mg/dL, prior to and after surgery, respectively. Liver transplantation replaced the missing LDL receptors, enhanced catabolism, and reduced lipoprotein synthesis in this patient.[117]

SUMMARY OF MAJOR STUDIES

Primary and secondary prevention diet and drug trials have been performed to determine whether lowering of cholesterol will prevent CHD; Tables 21–15 and 21–16 summarize these trials. A number of angiographic studies have also been performed that demonstrate that cholesterol reduction leads to regression of atherosclerosis. Most of the primary and secondary studies were double blinded, randomized, and placebo controlled, lasting for 5 years or longer, and most had sufficient patient numbers to be meaningful. Exceptions to these qualifications were seen in the early studies such as the Newcastle and Edinburgh trials, which were small; and the Coronary Drug Project (CDP) using dextrothyroxine, which was terminated early due to adverse effects on CHD mortality.[121–124] In the Edinburgh study, 180 patients were also given warfarin, and the patients remained blinded although the physicians were aware of the treatment group allocation. The Helsinki heart study, using gemfibrozil, resulted in a reduction in nonfatal MI, which was the primary contributor to reduced CHD incidence (Table 21–15).[65,125]

Total and LDL cholesterol were reduced an average of 13.4% and 20.3%, respectively, by cholestyramine in the LRC-CPPT, and the reduction of lipid levels was related to the amount of drug ingested[33,34] (e.g., 1 to 2 packets, 5.4% reduction in total cholesterol, versus 5 or more packets, 19.0% reduction). The prescribed dose of cholestyramine was 24 g, or 6 packets, per day. The cholestyramine group experienced a 19% reduction in risk ($P < .05$) of the primary end point—definite CHD death and/or definite nonfatal MI—reflecting a 24% reduction in definite CHD death and a 19% reduction in nonfatal MI. Other end points were reduced by 25%, 20%, and 21% for new positive exercise tests, angina, and coronary bypass surgery, respectively. Death from all causes was not significantly reduced by cholestyramine secondary to more accidents and violence in this group. The mean falls in total and LDL cholesterol in the cholestyramine group were 8% and 12% relative to levels in placebo-treated men, providing evidence that for every 1% reduction in cholesterol, a 2% decline in CHD mortality can be realized.

The cooperative trial sponsored by WHO used clofibrate 1.6 g/d in high-risk males (upper one-third of cholesterol distribution) and compared that group to a similar high-risk group given placebo and to a low-risk group (lower one-third of cholesterol distribution).[126] Cholesterol was reduced an average of 9%, but ranged from 7% to 11% from the three study centers in the clofibrate-treated group. Clofibrate reduced nonfatal myocardial infarcts by 25% and CHD was reduced by 20%, primarily caused by nonfatal MI reductions. Fatal MI was similar in the two high-cholesterol groups, and all-cause mortality was higher ($P < .05$) in the clofibrate-treated group. Mortality from gastrointestinal malignancy was seen more commonly with clofibrate, and the cholecystectomy rate for gallstones was also significantly higher. AFCAPS/TexCAPS is the most recent primary prevention trial. In this study, conducted in 6605 men and women aged 57 to 63 years with average total cholesterol and LDL (<221 mg/dL and <150 mg/dL, respectively) who were treated with lovastatin 20–40 mg/d for 5.2 years, a 37% reduction ($P < .001$) was shown in the risk for first acute major coronary event (fatal or nonfatal MI, unstable angina, or sudden cardiac death).[61] The need for revascularization procedures was also reduced by 33% ($P < .001$). The implications of this trial are enormous; potentially millions of "normal" people could benefit from lipid-lowering with statins based on these results. The number of patients that need to be treated (NNT, Table 21–15) for primary prevention ranges from 43 in the West of Scotland trial to 71 in the Helsinki Heart Study. This range is within the typical boundary used for treatment decisions and described previously; cost-effectiveness is achieved routinely in patients with moderate to high risk.

In the secondary intervention trials, clofibrate (1.5 g/d) in the Newcastle study significantly reduced mortality (11.1% versus 19.0%) from sudden deaths (9 versus 21 patients in clofibrate and placebo groups, respectively) but not from MI or congestive heart failure.[124] Nonfatal infarcts were 11.9% with clofibrate versus 18.2% in the placebo group ($P < .055$). Clofibrate (1.6–2 g/d) in the Edinburgh trial was less impressive, with no significant effect on the occurrence of fatal or nonfatal MI or overall mortality seen.[123]

Niacin in the CDP significantly reduced definite, nonfatal MI as compared to placebo (10.1% versus 13.9%), whereas clofibrate did not reduce death from any cause or nonfatal or fatal MI at the 5-year followup period.[122] Clofibrate did increase the rate of definite or suspected fatal or nonfatal pulmonary embolism or thrombophlebitis compared to placebo (5.8% versus 3.6%) after adjusting for baseline characteristics for total follow-up.[121] Other findings with clofibrate that occurred more frequently than with placebo included intermittent claudication, arrhythmias, palpable spleen, cholelithiasis (including cholecystectomy), and more frequent use of anticoagulants. Skin reactions, gastrointestinal complaints, and the use of gout medication were more common with niacin than with placebo. The 5-year total mortalities were 20.0% for clofibrate and 20.9% for placebo. The 5-year total mortality for niacin was 21.2%. Long-term follow-up of the CDP has shown a reduction in total mortality with niacin which occurred 9 years after the drug had been stopped.[122] The mechanism for this effect is unclear.

One of the most important studies published in the last few years is the 4S trial, a secondary intervention trial in a large number of patients.[35] Simvastatin, 20–40 mg/d, reduced LDL cholesterol by 35% and reduced the risk of death from any cause by 30%. Coronary deaths were also reduced with simvastatin (relative risk, 0.58; confidence interval, 0.46–0.73). Therapy was also shown to be effective in women (18% to 19% of patients enrolled) and in the elderly (≥60 years). Indeed, the relative risk of death or major coronary event was reduced to a greater extent in the elderly than in younger patients. Death from noncardiovascular causes was similar for simvastatin and placebo (2.1% and 2.2%, respectively). The survival curves for simvastatin and placebo began to separate at 1 year and became more divergent with additional follow-up. The 4S study clearly demonstrates the benefit in cholesterol lowering and placates long-held fears of death from non-CHD causes. The long-term intervention with pravastatin in ischemic disease (LIPID) study ($N = 7498$ men and 1516 women) has investigated the effect of pravastatin on CHD mortality in patients with prior MI or unstable angina and mean cholesterol level of 219 mg/dL over 6 years.[127] Pravastatin reduced the risk of CHD mortality by 24% (8.3% versus 6.4%, $P = .0004$) and total mortality by 23% (14.1% versus 11.0%, $P = .00002$); stroke was also reduced by 20% (4.3% versus 3.5%, $P = .22$) as well as reduction in the need for coronary artery bypass graft (11.3% versus 8.9%, $P = .0001$) or percutaneous transluminal coronary angioplasty (5.3% versus 4.4%, $P = .04$).

The Veterans Administration High-Density Lipoprotein intervention trial (VA-HIT) was a double-blind trial that compared gemfibrozil (1200 mg/d) with placebo in 2531 men with CHD, an HDL cholesterol level of ≤40 mg/dL, and an LDL cholesterol level of ≤140 mg/dL.[128] The primary study outcome was nonfatal MI or death from coronary causes. The median follow-up was 5.1 years. At 1 year, the mean HDL cholesterol level was 6% higher, the mean triglyceride level was 31% lower, and the mean total cholesterol level was 4% lower in the gemfibrozil group than in the placebo group. LDL cholesterol levels did not differ significantly between the groups. A primary event occurred in 21.7% of the patients assigned to placebo and in 17.3% of the patients assigned to gemfibrozil. The overall reduction in the risk of an event was 4.4 percentage points, and the reduction in relative risk was 22% ($P = 0.006$). This trial presents the strongest evidence to date that raising HDL-C and lowering triglycerides reduces risk for CHD.

The Heart and Estrogen/Progestin Replacement Study (HERS) was undertaken to determine whether estrogen plus progestin therapy alters the risk for CHD events in postmenopausal women with established coronary disease.[129] A total of 2763 women (mean age, 66.7 years) with coronary disease, who were younger than 80 years and postmenopausal with an intact uterus, were randomized to receive either 0.625 mg of conjugated equine estrogens plus 2.5 mg of medroxyprogesterone acetate in 1 tablet daily (n = 1380) or a placebo of identical appearance (n = 1383). Follow-up averaged 4.1 years. The primary outcome was the occurrence of nonfatal MI or CHD death. There were no significant differences between groups in the primary outcome or in any of the secondary cardiovascular outcomes. More women in the hormone group than in the placebo group experienced venous thromboembolic events and gallbladder disease. Based on the finding of no overall cardiovascular benefit and a pattern of early increase in risk of CHD events, the authors did not recommend starting this treatment for the purpose of secondary prevention of CHD. In this study of secondary intervention of relatively elderly postmenopausal women, there was no evidence of benefit from hormone replacement therapy (HRT) and only an increase for thromboembolism was seen. If women are on HRT at the time of event, then they should be given a choice to continue. The role of HRT in primary prevention will be clarified with the publication of results from the Women's Health Initiative (Table 21–15).

The Atorvastatin Versus Revascularization Treatments (AVERT) study compared atorvastatin 80 mg/d with percutaneous transluminal coronary angioplasty.[130] The follow-up period was 18 months. Of the patients who received aggressive lipid-lowering treatment with atorvastatin, 13% had ischemic events, as compared to 21% of the patients who underwent angioplasty. The incidence of ischemic events was thus 36 % lower in the atorvastatin group over an 18-month period ($P = 0.048$, which was not statistically significant after adjustment for interim analyses). This reduction in events was because of a smaller number of angioplasty procedures, coronary-artery bypass operations, and hospitalizations for worsening angina (the most common end point). As compared to the patients who were

TABLE 21–15. Primary Prevention Trials with Lipid-Lowering Drugs

Trial	F/U (y)	N	Treatment	Control Events	Treatment Events	p Value	RRR	ARR	NNT
AFCAPS/TexCAPS	5	6,605	Lovastatin 20–40 mg	5.5%	3.5%	<0.001	36.4%	2.0%	50
Helsinki	5	4,081	Gemfibrozil 1200 mg	4.1%	2.7%	<0.02	34.0%	1.4%	71
LRC-CPPT	7.4	3,806	Cholestyramine 24 g	9.8%	8.1%	<0.05	17.3%	1.7%	59
Oslo	5	1,232	Diet + smoking cessation	4.2%	2.5%	0.03	40.5%	1.7%	59
WOSCOPS	4.9	6,595	Pravastatin 40 mg	7.8%	5.5%	<0.001	29.5%	2.3%	43
ALLHAT		40,000+	Usual care Pravastatin	NA					
WHI		27,500	Usual care Diet, HRT	NA					

AFCAPS/TexCAPS, Air Force/Texas Coronary Atherosclerosis Prevention Study (Downs et al., 1998).
Helsinki, The Helsinki Heart Study (Frick et al., 1987); LRC-CPPT, The Lipid Research Clinics Coronary Primary Prevention Trial (Insull et al., 1984); Oslo, The Oslo Study (Hjermann et al., 1988).
WOSCOPS, The West of Scotland Coronary Prevention Study (Shepherd et al., 1995); ALLHAT, Antihypertensive and Lipid-Lowering Treatment to Prevent Heart Attack Trial; WHI, Women's Health Initiative; RRR, relative risk reduction; ARR, absolute risk reduction; NNT, number needed to treat; NA, not available.

TABLE 21–16. Secondary Prevention Trials with Lipid-Lowering Drugs

Trial	F/U (y)	N	Treatment	Control Events	Treatment Events	p Value	RRR	ARR	NNT
VA-HIT	5.1	2531	Gemfibrozil 1200 mg	21.7%	17.3%	0.006	22%	4.4%	23
AVERT	1.5	341	Atorvastatin 80 mg	21%	13%	0.048	38%	8%	12
CARE	5	4,159	Pravastatin 40 mg	13.2%	10.2%	0.003	22.7%	3.0%	33
CDP	5	8,341	Niacin 3 g + Clofibrate 1.8 g	20.9%	20.6%	NS	1.4%	0.3%	333
HERS	4.1	2,673	Estrogen 0.625 mg + Progestin 2.5 mg	12.7%	12.5%	0.91	1.6%	0.2%	500
LIPID	7.4	3,806	Pravastatin 40 mg	9.8%	8.1%	<0.05	17.3%	1.7%	59
4S	5	4,444	Simvastatin 20 mg	11.5%	8.2%	0.0003	28.7%	3.3%	30
WHO	5.3	15,745	Clofibrate 1.6 g	3.9%	3.1%	<0.005	20.5%	0.8%	125
BIP	6.2	3,090	Placebo Bezafibrate 400 mg	15.0%	13.6%	0.26	9.3%	1.4%	72

VA-HIT, Veterans Administration-High-Density Lipoprotein Cholesterol (HDL-C) Intervention Trial; AVERT, The Atorvastatin Versus Revascularization Treatments; CARE, Cholesterol and Recurrent Events (Melendez et al., 1996); CDP, Coronary Drug Project (Berge et al., 1975); HERS, Heart and Estrogen Replacement Study (Hulley et al., 1998); LIPID, Long-Term Intervention with Pravastatin in Ischaemic Disease Study (MacMahon et al., 1995); 4S, Scandinavian Simvastatin Survival Study (Pederson et al., 1994); WHO, World Health Organization (Committee of Principal Investigators, 1978); BIP, Bezafibrate Infarction Prevention; RRR, relative risk reduction; ARR, absolute risk reduction; NNT, number needed to treat; NA, not available.

treated with angioplasty and usual care, the patients who received atorvastatin had a significantly longer time to the first ischemic event ($P = 0.03$). In low-risk patients with stable CAD, aggressive lipid-lowering therapy is at least as effective as angioplasty and usual care in reducing the incidence of ischemic events.

The Bezafibrate Infarction Prevention (BIP) study was a double-blind trial of 3090 patients with a previous MI or stable angina, a total cholesterol of 180–250 mg/dL, HDL-C ≤45 mg/dL, triglycerides ≤300 mg/dL, and low-density lipoprotein cholesterol ≤180 mg/dL, who were randomized to receive either 400 mg of bezafibrate per day or a placebo; they were followed for a mean of 6.2 years. The primary end point was fatal or nonfatal MI or sudden death. Bezafibrate increased HDL-C by 18% and reduced triglycerides by 21%. The frequency of the primary end point was 13.6% on bezafibrate versus 15.0% on placebo ($P = 0.26$). In a post hoc analysis of the subgroup with high baseline triglycerides (≥200 mg/dL), the reduction in the cumulative probability of the primary end point by bezafibrate was 39.5% (12.0% versus 19.7%, $P = 0.02$). Total and noncardiac mortality rates were similar, and adverse events and cancer were equally distributed. Bezafibrate was safe and effective in elevating HDL-C levels and in lowering triglycerides. An overall trend in a reduction of the incidence of primary end points was observed. The reduction in the primary end point in patients with high baseline triglycerides (≥200 mg/dL) requires further confirmation. The overall baseline HDL C was higher and triglycerides lower in BIP than VA-HIT and this may explain the disparate outcomes of these two trials.

Numerous studies demonstrate regression of atherosclerosis and atheromatous plaques in various arterial systems. Intensive dietary and drug therapy was used in these trials, and the duration of therapy required for regression to be seen is about 2 years. Regression was noted in native vessels, as well as in grafted vessels in coronary artery bypass grafts. Regression was seen in the carotid, as well as in the coronary system. Presumably, regression can also be induced in other vascular beds, and these effects appear to be independent of the drug therapy used to induce regression. Based on meta-analysis and pooling project analysis of angiographic trial data, clinical outcomes such as MI and the need for interventions are reduced in a time frame not consistent with regression of plaque.[131–133] This interesting observation suggests that alteration in plaque activity, so-called plaque stabilization, may play an important role favoring aggressive lipid lowering that has not been previously recognized.

EVALUATION OF THERAPEUTIC OUTCOMES

Short-term evaluation of therapy for hyperlipidemia is based on response to diet and drug treatment as measured in the clinical laboratory by total cholesterol, LDL cholesterol, HDL cholesterol, and triglycerides for patients being treated for primary intervention, as well as on response to secondary intervention. The interval for follow-up is dependent on the severity of illness, and patients with known CAD or multiple risk factors should be monitored more closely. Less commonly used laboratory measurements include C-reactive protein, homocysteine, apolipoprotein B, and Lp(a) levels. Because many patients being treated for primary hyperlipidemia have no symptoms and may not have any clinical manifestations of a genetic lipid disorder such as xanthomas or eruptions, monitoring and outcome are solely laboratory based. In patients treated for secondary intervention, symptoms of atherosclerotic cardiovascular disease, such as angina or intermittent claudication, may improve over months to years. If patients have xanthomas or other external manifestations of hyperlipidemia, these lesions should regress with therapy. Lipid measurements should be obtained in the fasted state to minimize interference from chylomicrons, and once the patient is stable, monitoring is needed at intervals of 6 months to 1 year. The goals for LDL and HDL cholesterol are provided in Tables 21–8 and 21–9.

Patients with multiple risk factors and established CHD should also be monitored and evaluated for progress in managing their other risk factors such as hypertension, smoking cessation, exercise and weight control, and glycemic control if diabetic. The goals are to maintain a blood pressure of below 140/90 mm Hg or less (presence of diabetes or renal insufficiency), stop smoking, maintain an ideal body weight, exercise for at least 20 minutes three or more times per week, and keep plasma glucose below 126 mg/dL. Invasive evaluation, such as cardiac catheterization, is useful in patients with established CHD and is typically used for planning revascularization rather than monitoring of lipid-lowering therapy.

Evaluation of dietary therapy is part of the outcome evaluation for treating hyperlipidemia and the assistance of a dietitian is recommended. Use of diet diaries and recall survey instruments enable information about diet to be collected in a systematic fashion and may improve patient adherence to dietary recommendations.

▶ PRINCIPLES OF PHARMACOTHERAPY

- Hypercholesterolemia, elevated LDL-C, and low HDL-C are unequivocally linked to increased risk for CHD and cerebrovascular morbidity and mortality.
- Reductions in elevated total cholesterol and LDL-C reduce CHD mortality and total mortality. Aggressive treatment of hypercholesterolemia results in fewer patients progressing to myocardial infarction, angina, and stroke, and reduces the need for interventions such as coronary artery bypass graft and percutaneous transluminal coronary angioplasty.
- Initial therapy for any lipoprotein disorder is therapeutic life-style changes with restricted intake of total and saturated fat and cholesterol and a modest increase in polyunsaturated fat intake along with a program of regular exercise and weight reduction if needed.
- Recent clinical trials in primary and secondary intervention with the statins show a 25% to 35% reduction in CHD risk, and patients with high to moderate LDL-C concentrations benefit from treatment.
- Considering compliance, adverse effects and effectiveness, statins are the drugs of choice for patients with hypercholesterolemia because they are the most potent form of monotherapy and are cost-effective in patients with known CAD or multiple risk factors and in high-risk primary prevention patients.
- Gemfibrozil, cholestyramine, and niacin reduce nonfatal MI and niacin may also reduce total mortality.
- Patients not responding to statin monotherapy may be treated with combination therapy for hypercholesterolemia, but should be monitored closely because of an increased risk for adverse effects and drug interactions.
- Hypertriglyceridemia usually responds well to niacin, gemfibrozil, or high-dose/potency statins (atorvastatin, simvastatin); niacin should be used cautiously in diabetics because of worsening glycemic control.
- Low HDL-C is addressed with life-style modifications such as smoking cessation and increased exercise; niacin and gemfibrozil can significantly increase HDL-C as well.

REFERENCES

1. Expert Panel on Detection E, and Treatment of High Blood Cholesterol in Adults. Executive summary of the third report of the National Cholesterol Education Program (NCEP) Expert Panel on Detection, Evaluation and Treatment of High Blood Cholesterol in Adults (Adult Treatment Panel III). JAMA 2001;285:2486–2497.
2. National, Cholesterol, Education, Program. Second report of the National Cholesterol Education Program (NCEP) Expert Panel on detection, evaluation, and treatment of high blood cholesterol in adults (Adult Treatment Panel II). Circulation 1994;89:1329–1445.
3. Grundy SM, Balady GJ, Criqui MH, et al. Primary prevention of coronary heart disease: Guidance from Framingham: A statement for healthcare professionals from the AHA Task Force on Risk Reduction. American Heart Association. Circulation 1998;97:1876–1887.
4. Grundy SM. Cholesterol management in patients with heart disease. Emphasizing secondary prevention to increase longevity. Postgrad Med 1997;102:81–84, 87–90.
5. Grundy SM, Bazzarre T, Cleeman J, et al. Prevention Conference V: Beyond secondary prevention: Identifying the high-risk patient for primary prevention: Medical office assessment: Writing Group I. Circulation (Online) 2000;101:E3–E11.
6. Sempos CT, Cleeman JI, Carroll MD, Johnson CL, et al. Prevalence of high blood cholesterol among US adults. An update based on guidelines from the second report of the National Cholesterol Education Program Adult Treatment Panel. JAMA 1993;269:3009–3014.
7. Fingerhut LA, Warner M. Health, United States, 1996–97 and Injury Chartbook. Hyattsville, MD, National Center for Health Statistics, 1997:1–345.
8. Menotti A, Keys A, Blackburn H, et al. Comparison of multivariate predictive power of major risk factors for coronary heart diseases in different countries: Results from eight nations of the Seven Countries Study, 25-year follow-up. J Cardiovasc Risk 1996;3:69–75.
9. Kannel WB, Wilson PW. Comparison of risk profiles for cardiovascular events: Implications for prevention. Adv Intern Med 1997;42:39–66.
10. Kannel WB. Range of serum cholesterol values in the population developing coronary artery disease. Am J Cardiol 1995;76:69C–77C.
11. Menotti A, Seccareccia F, Blackburn H, Keys A. Coronary mortality and its prediction in samples of US and Italian railroad employees in 25 years within the Seven Countries Study of cardiovascular diseases. Int J Epidemiol 1995;24:515–21.
12. Gotto AMJ. Low high-density lipoprotein cholesterol as a risk factor in coronary heart disease. Circulation 2001;103:2213–2218.
13. Sytkowski PA, D'Agostino RB, Belanger A, Kannel WB. Sex and time trends in cardiovascular disease incidence and mortality: the Framingham Heart Study, 1950–1989. Am J Epidemiol 1996; 143:338–350.
14. Wilson PW, D'Agostino RB, Levy D, Belanger AM, Silbershatz H, Kannel WB. Prediction of coronary heart disease using risk factor categories. Circulation 1998;97:1837–1847.
15. Jeppesen J, Hein HO, Suadicani P, Gyntelberg F. Triglyceride concentration and ischemic heart disease: An eight-year follow-up in the Copenhagen Male Study. Circulation 1998;97:1029–1036.
16. Carlson LA, Rosenhamer G. Reduction of mortality in the Stockholm Ischaemic Heart Disease Secondary Prevention Study by combined treatment with clofibrate and nicotinic acid. Acta Medica Scandinavica 1988;223:405–418.
17. Dietschy JM. Dietary fatty acids and the regulation of plasma low-density lipoprotein cholesterol concentrations. J Nutr 1998;128:444S–448S.
18. Shepherd J. Lipoprotein metabolism. Drugs 1994;47:1–10.
19. Ross R. Cellular and molecular studies of atherogenesis. Atherosclerosis 1997;131:S3–S4.
20. Wierzbicki WB, Hagmeyer KO. *Helicobacter pylori, Chlamydia pneumoniae,* and cytomegalovirus: Chronic infections and coronary heart disease. Pharmacotherapy 2000;20:52–63.
21. Ridker PM, Stampfer MJ, Rifa IN. Novel risk factors for systemic atherosclerosis. A comparison of C-reactive protein, fibrinogen, homocysteine, lipoprotein (a), and standard cholesterol screening predictors of peripheral arterial disease. JAMA 2001;285:2481–2485.
22. Libby P, Schoenbeck U, Mach F, Selwyn AP, Ganz P. Current concepts in cardiovascular pathology: The role of LDL cholesterol in plaque rupture and stabilization. Am J Med 1998;104:14S–18S.
23. Reaven PD, Napoli C, Merat S, Witztumc JL. Lipoprotein modification and atherosclerosis in aging. Exp Gerontol 1999;34:527–37.
24. Turban S, Fuentes F, Ferlic L, et al. A prospective study of paraxonase gene Q/R192 polymorphism and severity, progression and regression of coronary atherosclerosis, plasma lipid levels, clinical events and response to fluvastatin. Atherosclerosis 2001;154:633–640.
25. Navab M, Hama-Levy S, Van Lenten BJ, et al. Mildly oxidized LDL induces an increased apolipoprotein J/paraxonase ratio. J Clin Invest 1997;99:2005–19.
26. Jukema JW, van Boven AJ, Groenemeijer B, et al. The Asp9 Asn mutation in the lipoprotein lipase gene is associated with increased progression of coronary atherosclerosis. REGRESS Study Group, Interuniversity

Cardiology Institute, Utrecht, The Netherlands. Regression Growth Evaluation Statin Study. Circulation 1996;94:1913–8.
27. Haffner SM, Miettinen H. Insulin resistance implications for type II diabetes mellitus and coronary heart disease. Am J Med 1997;103:152–162.
28. American Academy of Pediatrics, Committee on N. American Academy of Pediatrics, Committee on Nutrition. Cholesterol in childhood. Pediatrics 1998;101:141–147.
29. Strong JP, Malcom GT, Oalmann MC, Wissler RW. The PDAY Study: Natural history, risk factors, and pathobiology. Pathobiological determinants of atherosclerosis in youth. Ann N Y Acad Sci 1997;811:226–235; discussion 235–237.
30. The Writing Group for the DISC. Efficacy and safety of lowering dietary intake of fat and cholesterol in children with elevated low-density lipoprotein cholesterol: The Dietary Intervention Study in Children (DISC). JAMA 1995;273:1429–1435.
31. McCrindle BW, O'Neill MB, Cullen-Dean G, Helden E. Acceptability and compliance with two forms of cholestyramine in the treatment of hypercholesterolemia in children: A randomized, crossover trial. J Pediatr 1997;130:266–73.
32. Lambert M, Lupien PJ, Gagne C, et al. Treatment of familial hypercholesterolemia in children and adolescents: effect of lovastatin. Canadian Lovastatin in Children Study Group. Pediatrics 1996;97:619–28.
33. Anonymous. The Lipid Research Clinics Coronary Primary Prevention Trial results. II. The relationship of reduction in incidence of coronary heart disease to cholesterol lowering. JAMA 1984;251:365–374.
34. Anonymous. The Lipid Research Clinics Coronary Primary Prevention Trial results. I. Reduction in incidence of coronary heart disease. JAMA 1984;251:351–364.
35. Anonymous. Randomised trial of cholesterol lowering in 4444 patients with coronary heart disease: The Scandinavian Simvastatin Survival Study (4S). Lancet 1994;344:1383–1389.
36. Blankenhorn DH, Azen SP, Crawford DW, et al. Effects of colestipol-niacin therapy on human femoral atherosclerosis. Circulation 1991;83:438–447.
37. Shepherd J, Cobbe SM, Ford I, et al. Prevention of coronary heart disease with pravastatin in men with hypercholesterolemia. West of Scotland Coronary Prevention Study Group. N Engl J Med 1995;333:1301–1307.
38. Spence JD, Huff MW, Heidenheim P, et al. Combination therapy with colestipol and psyllium mucilloid in patients with hyperlipidemia. Ann Intern Med 1995;123:493–9.
39. Turley SD, Dietschy JM. Mechanisms of LDL-cholesterol lowering action of psyllium hydrophilic mucilloid in the hamster. Biochim Biophys Acta 1995;1255:177–84.
40. Harris WS. N-3 fatty acids and human lipoprotein metabolism: An update. Lipids 1999;34:S257–S258.
41. Maron DJ, Fazio S, Linton MF. Current perspectives on statins. Circulation 2000;101:207–213.
42. Vaughan CJ, Gotto AM Jr, Basson CT. The evolving role of statins in the management of atherosclerosis. J Am Coll Cardiol 2000;35:1–10.
43. Duplaga BA. Treatment of childhood hypercholesterolemia with HMG-CoA reductase inhibitors. Ann Pharmacother 1999; 33:1224–1227.
44. Gotto AMJ. Cholesterol management in theory and practice. Circulation 1997;96:4424–4430.
45. Steiner A, Weisser B, Vetter W. A comparative review of the adverse effects of treatments for hyperlipidaemia. Drug Saf 1991;6:118–130.
46. Carrilho AJ, Medina WL, Nakandakare ER, Quintao EC. Plasma cholesteryl ester transfer protein is lowered by treatment of hypercholesterolemia with cholestyramine. Clin Pharmacol Ther 1997;62:82–88.
47. Andrade SE, Walker AM, Gottlieb LK, et al. Discontinuation of antihyperlipidemic drugs—do rates reported in clinical trials reflect rates in primary care settings? N Engl J Med 1995;332:1125–1131.
48. Konzem SL, Gray DR, Kashyap ML. Effect of pharmaceutical care on optimum colestipol treatment in elderly hypercholesterolemic veterans. Pharmacotherapy 1997;17:576–583.
49. Tsuyuki RT, Bungard RJ. Poor adherence with hypolipidemic drugs: A lost opportunity. Pharmacotherapy 2001;21:627–635.
50. Grundy SM. Consensus statement: Role of therapy with "statins" in patients with hypertriglyceridemia. Am J Cardiol 1998;81:1B–6B.
51. Whelan AM, Price SO, Fowler SF, Hainer BL. The effect of aspirin on niacin-induced cutaneous reactions. J Fam Pract 1992;34:165–168.
52. Guyton JR, Blazing MA, Hagar J, et al. Extended-release niacin vs gemfibrozil for the treatment of low levels of high-density lipoprotein cholesterol. Niaspan-Gemfibrozil Study Group. Arch Intern Med 2000;160:1177–1184.
53. Goldberg A, Alagona P Jr, Capuzzi DM, et al. Multiple-dose efficacy and safety of an extended-release form of niacin in the management of hyperlipidemia. Am J Cardiol 2000;85:1100–1105.
54. Garg R, Elam MB, Crouse JR 3rd, et al. Effective and safe modification of multiple atherosclerotic risk factors in patients with peripheral arterial disease. Am Heart J 2000;140:792–803.
55. McKenney JM, Proctor JD, Harris S, Chinchili VM. A comparison of the efficacy and toxic effects of sustained- vs immediate-release niacin in hypercholesterolemic patients. JAMA 1994;271:672–677.
56. Bottorff M, Hansten P. Long-term safety of hepatic hydroxymethyl glutaryl coenzyme A reductase inhibitors: The role of metabolism-monograph for physicians. Arch Intern Med 2000;160:2273–2280.
57. Naoumova RP, Dunn S, Rallidis L, et al. Prolonged inhibition of cholesterol synthesis explains the efficacy of atorvastatin. J Lipid Res 1997;38:1496–1500.
58. Jones P, Kafonek S, Laurora I, Hunninghake D. Comparative dose efficacy study of atorvastatin versus simvastatin, pravastatin, lovastatin, and fluvastatin in patients with hypercholesterolemia (the CURVES study). Am J Cardiol 1998;81:582–587.
59. Bradford RH, Shear CL, Chremos AN, et al. Expanded Clinical Evaluation of Lovastatin (EXCEL) study results: Two-year efficacy and safety follow-up. Am J Cardiol 1994;74:667–673.
60. Pedersen TR, Berg K, Cook TJ, et al. Safety and tolerability of cholesterol lowering with simvastatin during 5 years in the Scandinavian Simvastatin Survival Study. Arch Intern Med 1996;156:2085–2092.
61. Downs JR, Clearfield M, Weis S, et al. Primary prevention of acute coronary events with lovastatin in men and women with average cholesterol levels. JAMA 1998;279:1615–1622.
62. Sacks FM, Pfeffer MA, Moye LA, et al. The effect of pravastatin on coronary events after myocardial infarction in patients with average cholesterol levels. Cholesterol and Recurrent Events Trial investigators. N Engl J Med 1996;335:1001–1009.
63. Anonymous. The effect of aggressive lowering of low-density lipoprotein cholesterol levels and low-dose anticoagulation on obstructive changes in saphenous-vein coronary-artery bypass grafts. The Post Coronary Artery Bypass Graft Trial Investigators. N Engl J Med 1997;336:153–162.
64. O'Neill FH, Patel DD, Knight BL, Clare KY. Determinants of variable response to statin treatment in patients with refractory familial hypercholesterolemia. Arterioscler Thromb Vasc Biol 2001;21:832–837.
65. Frick MH, Elo O, Haapa K, et al. Helsinki Heart Study: Primary-prevention trial with gemfibrozil in middle-aged men with dyslipidemia. Safety of treatment, changes in risk factors, and incidence of coronary heart disease. N Engl J Med 1987;317:1237–1245.
66. Caroli-Bosc FX, Le Gall P, Pugliese P, et al. Role of fibrates and HMG CoA reductase inhibitors in gallstone formation: Epidemiological study in an unselected population. Dig Dis Sci 2001;46:540–544.
67. Anonymous. A co-operative trial in the primary prevention of ischaemic heart disease using clofibrate. Report from the Committee of Principal Investigators. Br Heart J 1978;40:1069–1118.
68. Steinmetz A, Schwartz T, Hehnke U, Kaffarnik H. Multicenter comparison of micronized fenofibrate and simvastatin in patients with primary type IIA or IIB hyperlipoproteinemia. J Cardiovasc Pharmacol 1996;27:563–570.
69. Nestel PJ. Fish oil and cardiovascular disease: Lipids and arterial function. Am J Clin Nutr 2000;71:228S–231S.
70. Connor WE, DeFrancesco CA, Connor SL. N-3 fatty acids from fish oil. Effects on plasma lipoproteins and hypertriglyceridemic patients. Ann N Y Acad Sci 1993;683:16–34.
71. Athyros VG, Papageorgiou AA, Hatzikonstandinou HA, et al. Safety and efficacy of long-term statin-fibrate combinations in patients with

refractory familial combined hyperlipidemia. Am J Cardiol 1997;80: 608–613.
72. Guerin M, Bruckert E, Dolphin PJ, Turpin G, Chapman MJ. Fenofibrate reduces plasma cholesteryl ester transfer from HDL to VLDL and normalizes the atherogenic, dense LDL profile in combined hyperlipidemia. Arterioscler Thromb Vasc Biol 1996;16:763–772.
73. Austin MA, McKnight B, Edwards KL, et al. Cardiovascular disease mortality in familial forms of hypertriglyceridemia: A 20–year prospective study. Circulation 2000;101:2777–82.
74. Sveger T, Flodmark CE, Nordborg K, Nilsson-Ehle P, Borgfors N. Hereditary dyslipidaemias and combined risk factors in children with a family history of premature coronary artery disease. Arch Dis Child 2000;82:292–296.
75. Elam MB, Hunninghake DB, Davis KB, et al. Effect of niacin on lipid and lipoprotein levels and glycemic control in patients with diabetes and peripheral arterial disease: The ADMIT study: A randomized trial. Arterial Disease Multiple Intervention Trial. JAMA 2000;284:1263–1270.
76. Yang CY, Gu ZW, Xie YH, et al. Effects of gemfibrozil on very-low-density lipoprotein composition and low-density lipoprotein size in patients with hypertriglyceridemia or combined hyperlipidemia. Atherosclerosis 1996;126:105–116.
77. Sheu WH, Jeng CY, Lee WJ, Lin SY, Pei D, Chen YT. Simvastatin treatment on postprandial hypertriglyceridemia in type 2 diabetes mellitus patients with combined hyperlipidemia. Metabolism 2001;50:355–359.
78. Deighan CJ, Caslake MJ, McConnell M, Boulton-Jones JM, Packard CJ. Comparative effects of cerivastatin and fenofibrate on the atherogenic lipoprotein phenotype in proteinuric renal disease. J Am Soc Nephrol 2001;12:341–8.
79. Zambon D, Ros E, Rodriguez-Villar C, et al. Randomized crossover study of gemfibrozil versus lovastatin in familial combined hyperlipidemia: Additive effects of combination treatment on lipid regulation. Metabolism 1999;48:47–54.
80. Bakker-Arkema RG, Davidson MH, Goldstein RJ, et al. Efficacy and safety of a new HMG-CoA reductase inhibitor, atorvastatin, in patients with hypertriglyceridemia. JAMA 1996;275:128–133.
81. Krauss RM. Atherogenic lipoprotein phenotype and diet-gene interactions. J Nutr 2001;131:340S–343S.
82. Howard BV, Robbins DC, Sievers ML, et al. LDL cholesterol as a strong predictor of coronary heart disease in diabetic individuals with insulin resistance and low LDL: The Strong Heart Study. Arterioscler Thromb Vasc Biol 2000;20:830–835.
83. Insull W, Kafonek S, Goldner D, Zieve F. Comparison of efficacy and safety of atorvastatin (10 mg) with simvastatin (10 mg) at six weeks. ASSET Investigators. Am J Cardiol 2001;87:554–559.
84. Freeman DJ, Norrie J, Sattar N, et al. Pravastatin and the development of diabetes mellitus: Evidence for a protective treatment effect in the West of Scotland Coronary Prevention Study. Circulation (Online) 2001;103:357–362.
85. Anonymous. Effect of fenofibrate on progression of coronary-artery disease in type 2 diabetes: The Diabetes Atherosclerosis Intervention Study, a randomised study. Lancet 2001;357:905–910.
86. Crouse JR 3rd. New developments in the use of niacin for treatment of hyperlipidemia: New considerations in the use of an old drug. Coron Artery Dis 1996;7:321–326.
87. Garg A, Grundy SM. Nicotinic acid as therapy for dyslipidemia in non-insulin-dependent diabetes mellitus. JAMA 1990;264:723–726.
88. Gray DR, Morgan T, Chretien SD, Kashyap ML. Efficacy and safety of controlled-release niacin in dyslipoproteinemic veterans. Ann Intern Med 1994;121:252–258.
89. Kannel WB. Cardiovascular risk factors in the elderly. Coron Artery Dis 1997;8:565–575.
90. Mundy G, Garrett R, Harris S, et al. Stimulation of bone formation in vitro and in rodents by statins. Science 1999;286:1946–1949.
91. Reid IR, Hague W, Emberson J, et al. Effect of pravastatin on frequency of fracture in the LIPID study: Secondary analysis of a randomised controlled trial. Long-term intervention with pravastatin in ischaemic disease. Lancet 2001;357:509–512.
92. Grundy SM, Cleeman JI, Rifkind BM, Kuller LH. Cholesterol lowering in the elderly population. Coordinating Committee of the National Cholesterol Education Program. Arch Intern Med 1999;159:1670–1678.
93. Campeau LMD, Hunninghake DBMD, Knatterud GLP, et al. Aggressive cholesterol lowering delays saphenous vein graft atherosclerosis in women, the elderly, and patients with associated risk factors: NHLBI Post Coronary Artery Bypass Graft Clinical Trial. Circulation 1999;99:3241–3247.
94. Johannesson M, Jonsson B, Kjekshus J, Olsson AG, Pedersen TR, Wedel H. Cost effectiveness of simvastatin treatment to lower cholesterol levels in patients with coronary heart disease. Scandinavian Simvastatin Survival Study Group. N Engl J Med 1997;336:332–336.
95. Welty FK. Cardiovascular disease and dyslipidemia in women. Arch Intern Med 2001;161:514–522.
96. Abate N. Obesity and cardiovascular disease. Pathogenetic role of the metabolic syndrome and therapeutic implications. J Diabetes Complications 2000;14:154–174.
97. Kane JP, Malloy MJ, Ports TA, Phillips NR, Diehl JC, Havel RJ. Regression of coronary atherosclerosis during treatment of familial hypercholesterolemia with combined drug regimens. JAMA 1990;264:3007–3012.
98. Salo P, Seppanen-Laakso T, Laakso I, et al. Low-saturated fat, low-cholesterol diet in 3year-old children: Effect on intake and composition of trans fatty acids and other fatty acids in serum phospholipid fraction—The STRIP study. Special Turku coronary Risk factor Intervention Project for children. J Pediatr 2000;136:46–52.
99. Dixon LB, McKenzie J, Shannon BM, Mitchell DCMS, Smiciklas-Wright H, Tershakovec A. The effect of changes in dietary fat on the food group and nutrient intake of 4- to 10-year-old children. Pediatrics 1997;100:863–872.
100. Nader PR, Stone EJ, Lytle LA, et al. Three-year maintenance of improved diet and physical activity: The CATCH cohort. Child and Adolescent Trial for Cardiovascular Health. Arch Pediatr Adolesc Med 1999;153:695–704.
101. Tonstad S. A rational approach to treating hypercholesterolaemia in children. Weighing the risks and benefits. Drug Saf 1997;16:330–341.
102. Knipscheer HC, Boelen CC, Kastelein JJ, et al. Short-term efficacy and safety of pravastatin in 72 children with familial hypercholesterolemia [published erratum appears at Pediatr Res 1996;40(6):866]. Pediatr Res 1996;39:867–871.
103. Aguilar-Salinas CA, Barrett PH, Kelber J, Delmez J, Schonfeld G. Physiologic mechanisms of action of lovastatin in nephrotic syndrome. J Lipid Res 1995;36:188–199.
104. Gentile MG, Fellin G, Cofano F, et al. Treatment of proteinuric patients with a vegetarian soy diet and fish oil. Clin Nephrol 1993;40:315–320.
105. Toto RD, Grundy SM, Vega GL. Pravastatin treatment of very-low-density, intermediate-density and low-density lipoproteins in hypercholesterolemia and combined hyperlipidemia secondary to the nephrotic syndrome. Am J Nephrol 2000;20:12–17.
106. Thomas ME, Harris KP, Ramaswamy C, et al. Simvastatin therapy for hypercholesterolemic patients with nephrotic syndrome or significant proteinuria. Kidney Int 1993;44:1124–1129.
107. Spencer CM, Barradell LB. Gemfibrozil. A reappraisal of its pharmacological properties and place in the management of dyslipidaemia. Drugs 1996;51:982–1018.
108. Samuelsson O, Attman PO, Knight-Gibson C, et al. Effect of gemfibrozil on lipoprotein abnormalities in chronic renal insufficiency: A controlled study in human chronic renal disease. Nephron 1997;75:286–294.
109. Fuiano G, Esposito C, Sepe V, et al. Effects of hypercholesterolemia of renal hemodynamics: Study in patients with nephrotic syndrome. Nephron 1996;73:430–435.
110. Lintott CJ, Scott RS, Bremer JM, Shand BI. Fluvastatin for dyslipoproteinemia, with or without concomitant chronic renal insufficiency. Am J Cardiol 1995;76:97A–101A.
111. Caro J, Klittich W, McGuire A, et al. The West of Scotland coronary prevention study: Economic benefit analysis of primary prevention with pravastatin. BMJ 1997;315:1577–1582.

112. Hilleman DE, Wurdeman RL, Lenz TL. Therapeutic change of HMG-CoA reductase inhibitors in patients with coronary artery disease. Pharmacotherapy 2001;21:410–415.
113. Perreault S, Hamilton VH, Lavoie F, Grover S. A head-to-head comparison of the cost effectiveness of HMG-CoA reductase inhibitors and fibrates in different types of primary hyperlipidemia. Cardiovasc Drugs Ther 1997;10:787–794.
114. Schectman G, Wolff N, Byrd JC, Hiatt JG, Hartz A. Physician extenders for cost-effective management of hypercholesterolemia. J Gen Intern Med 1996;11:277–286.
115. Buchwald H, Campos CT, Boen JR, Nguyen PA, Williams SE. Disease-free intervals after partial ileal bypass in patients with coronary heart disease and hypercholesterolemia: Report from the Program on the Surgical Control of the Hyperlipidemias (POSCH). J Am Coll Cardiol 1995;26:351–357.
116. Matts JP, Buchwald H, Fitch LL, et al. Subgroup analyses of the major clinical endpoints in the Program on the Surgical Control of the Hyperlipidemias (POSCH): Overall mortality, atherosclerotic coronary heart disease (ACHD) mortality, and ACHD mortality or myocardial infarction. J Clin Epidemiol 1995;48:389–405.
117. Hoeg JM. Pharmacologic and surgical treatment of dyslipidemic children and adolescents. Ann N Y Acad Sci 1991;623:275–284.
118. Kroon AA, Aengevaeren WR, van der Werf T, et al. LDL-Apheresis Atherosclerosis Regression Study (LAARS). Effect of aggressive versus conventional lipid lowering treatment on coronary atherosclerosis. Circulation 1996;93:1826–1835.
119. Donner MG, Richter WO, Schwandt P. Long-term effect of LDL apheresis on coronary heart disease. Eur J Med Res 1997;2:270–274.
120. Kroon AA, van't Hof MA, Demacker PN, Stalenhoef AF. The rebound of lipoproteins after LDL-apheresis. Kinetics and estimation of mean lipoprotein levels. Atherosclerosis 2000;152:519–526.
121. Anonymous. Coronary Drug Project report on clofibrate and niacin. Atherosclerosis 1978;30:239–240.
122. Canner PL, Berge KG, Wenger NK, et al. Fifteen-year mortality in Coronary Drug Project patients: Long-term benefit with niacin. J Am Coll Cardiol 1986;8:1245–1255.
123. Dewar HA, Oliver MF. Secondary prevention trials using clofibrate: A joint commentary on the Newcastle and Scottish trials. Br Med J 1971;790:784–786.
124. Anonymous. Trial of clofibrate in the treatment of ischaemic heart disease. Five-year study by a group of physicians of the Newcastle upon Tyne region. Br Med J 1971;790:767–775.
125. Huttunen JK, Manninen V, Manttari M, et al. The Helsinki Heart Study: Central findings and clinical implications. Ann Med 1991;23:155–159.
126. (WHO) CoPI. A co-operative trial in the primary prevention of ischaemic heart disease using clofibrate. Br Heart J 1978;40:1069–1118.
127. Anonymous. Prevention of cardiovascular events and death with pravastatin in patients with coronary heart disease and a broad range of initial cholesterol levels. The Long-Term Intervention with Pravastatin in Ischaemic Disease (LIPID) Study Group. N Engl J Med 1998;339:1349–1357.
128. Rubins HB, Robins SJ, Collins D, et al. Gemfibrozil for the secondary prevention of coronary heart disease in men with low levels of high-density lipoprotein cholesterol. Veterans Affairs High-Density Lipoprotein Cholesterol Intervention Trial Study Group. N Engl J Med 1999;341:410–418.
129. Hulley S, Grady D, Bush T, et al. Randomized trial of estrogen plus progestin for secondary prevention of coronary heart disease in postmenopausal women. Heart and Estrogen/progestin Replacement Study (HERS) Research Group. JAMA 1998;280:605–613.
130. Pitt B, Waters D, Brown WV, et al. Aggressive lipid-lowering therapy compared with angioplasty in stable coronary artery disease. Atorvastatin versus Revascularization Treatment Investigators. N Engl J Med 1999;341:70–76.
131. Byington RP, Jukema JW, Salonen JT, et al. Reduction in cardiovascular events during pravastatin therapy. Pooled analysis of clinical events of the Pravastatin Atherosclerosis Intervention Program. Circulation 1995;92:2419–2425.
132. Watts GF, Burke V. Lipid-lowering trials in the primary and secondary prevention of coronary heart disease: new evidence, implications and outstanding issues. Curr Opin Lipidol 1996;7:341–355.
133. Sacks FM, Pasternak RC, Gibson CM, Rosner B, Stone PH. Effect on coronary atherosclerosis of decrease in plasma cholesterol concentrations in normocholesterolaemic patients. Harvard Atherosclerosis Reversibility Project (HARP) Group. Lancet 1994;344:1182–1186.

22

PERIPHERAL VASCULAR DISEASE

Robert L. Talbert

The term *peripheral vascular disease* (PVD), in its broadest sense, applies to disease of any of the blood vessels outside the heart and thoracic aorta and to disease of the lymph vessels. Although this term includes cerebrovascular and hypertensive vascular disease, these two topics are discussed in Chapters 12 and 20. The other major area included in this term is PVD of the extremities, which can be divided into two distinct systems: (1) venous disorders such as acute deep vein thrombosis and its complications of pulmonary embolism and postthrombotic syndrome (see Chapter 21), and (2) peripheral arterial disease resulting from occlusion and arterial vasospasm.[1,2] This chapter will focus on peripheral arterial disease. Because there are several distinct peripheral arterial diseases, epidemiology, pathophysiology, clinical presentation, and treatment are oriented to the particular disease. A general review of the structure and function of the normal vascular system and its reactive changes is presented first to aid in the understanding of the specific peripheral vascular disorders.[3–6]

STRUCTURE/FUNCTION OF THE NORMAL VASCULAR SYSTEM

The vascular system consists of varying histologic portions of five component parts: endothelium, basement membrane, elastic tissue, collagen, and smooth muscle[5,7] (Fig. 22–1). The endothelium is the monolayer lining of the luminal surface of the entire vascular system and functions to regulate the flow of blood in and out of the vessel lumen. Endothelial cells have several important functions including the active transport of circulating substances through their cytoplasm. Endothelium-derived relaxing factor (EDRF), which is nitric oxide or a mixture of *S*-nitrosothiol and nitric oxide, is synthesized through three pathways by the endothelium from L-arginine in response to a host of neurochemical and mechanical stimuli including wall and shear stress, endothelin-1, platelet activation, thrombin, serotonin, adenosine diphosphate (ADP), arachidonic acid, catecholamines, vasopressin, histamine, and acetylcholine.[8–10] EDRF diffuses from endothelial cells to adjacent smooth muscle cells and relaxes vascular smooth muscle and counteracts the action of numerous vasoconstrictor substances on smooth muscle as well as inhibiting platelet aggregation. The effects of EDRF seem to be most pronounced in the basal state and contribute to dilator tone of the skin and extremities, but less of an effect is seen during reflex sympathetic vasoconstriction.[11] Vasorelaxation and inhibition of platelet aggregation derived from the actions of EDRF stem from stimulation of the formation of cyclic guanosine monophosphate (cGMP) from guanosine triphosphate (GTP) and elevated cytosolic concentrations of cGMP, which stimulates intracellular binding of free calcium. Endothelin-1, the arachidonic acid metabolites prostacyclin H_2 and thromboxane A_2, and angiotensin II are vasoconstricting substances derived from the endothelium that are counterbalanced by the vasodilating properties of nitric oxide when endothelial function is normal.[3,12] Downregulation of the endothelin receptor (ETA) may reflect overactivity of this system.[9] Loss of endothelium from atherosclerotic plaque formation, percutaneous transluminal angioplasty, or other means of disruption of this monolayer of cells such as smoking reduces synthesis of EDRF and the protective homeostatic function of this paracrine substance (Fig. 22–2). Disease states that facilitate this process or are worsened because of it include hypertension, diabetes mellitus, dyslipemia (hypercholesterolemia and hypertriglyceridemia, and low high-density lipoprotein cholesterol), atherosclerosis, coronary artery disease, and others.[13,14]

Basement membrane is a dense sheath adjacent to the external surface of endothelial cells that serves as a transport barrier and support structure. The basement membrane contains a ground substance that is a mixture of mucopolysaccharides, protein-polysaccharide complexes, and glycoproteins, which retain large amounts of water and provide a gelatinous medium for transport of materials. Elastic tissue encircles the wall just outside the endothelium and basement membrane. It is also found in the media and adventitia of all vessels except the terminal arterioles, capillaries, and small venules and allows for expansion of the vessel. The internal elastic lamella is prominently affected by nearly all pathologic changes that involve the vascular system.

Another important component of vessel walls is collagen. In normal vessels it is present in the media and adventitia and is involved in all reactions of vessels to injury.[5] Collagen is highly resistant to stretching and functions to prevent overdistension of the vessels. The fifth component is smooth muscle, which is the actively contracting element of the vascular system. Arterial metabolism depends mainly on smooth muscle cells. These are the major connective tissue–forming cells of the vascular wall, producing elastic tissue, collagen, mucopolysaccharides, and myosin. Smooth muscle cells can metabolize glucose; synthesize fatty acids, cholesterol, phospholipids, and triglycerides; and facilitate the entry of lipoproteins into the cell. Several catabolic enzymes such as mixed-function oxidases, fibrinolysins, and lysosomal hydrolases are also present. This function and proliferative nature of smooth muscle cells are important factors in the reaction of arterial walls to injury and atherogenesis. In contrast to the differentiated, contractile type of smooth muscle cell usually seen in adults, smooth muscle cells lose their contractility and instead gain the ability to secrete extracellular matrix components and divide, which is thought to be an early step in the development of atherogenesis.

The structural organization of the vessel wall consists of three well-defined layers: the intima, the media, and the adventitia (see Fig. 22–1). The intima is a single continuous layer of endothelial cells and associated basement membrane. It is delineated on its outer surface by a perforated tube of elastic tissue, the internal elastic lamella. This structure is especially prominent in large elastic arteries and medium-caliber muscular arteries but is not seen in capillaries. The media consists of only one cell type, the smooth muscle cell. These cells are surrounded by small amounts of collagen and elastic tissue. The media is delineated on the luminal side by internal elastic lamina and on the abluminal side by a less continuous sheet of elastic tissue, the external elastic lamella. The outer portion is nourished by small blood vessels (vasa vasorum) in the adventitia, and the inner layers

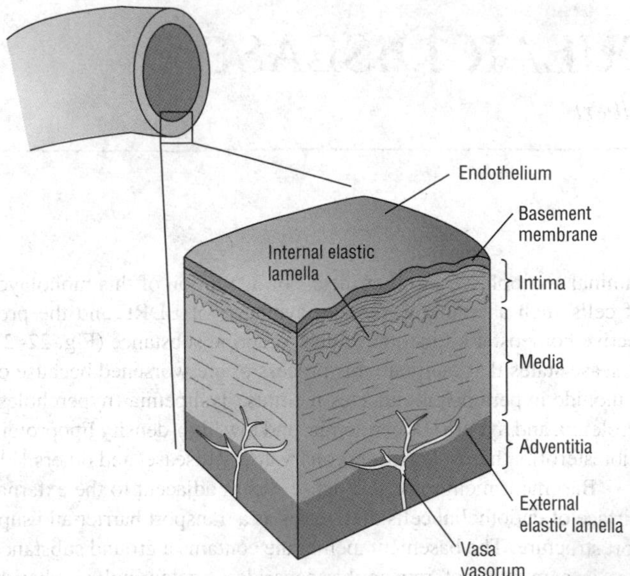

FIGURE 22–1. Schematic drawing of structural organization of the vascular wall. *(From Lie JR. The structure of the normal vascular system and its reactive changes. In: Juergens JL, Spittell JA, Fairbairn JF, eds. Peripheral Vascular Diseases. Philadelphia, Saunders, 1980:57, with permission.)*

receive nutrients from the lumen. The outer layer of the vascular wall is the adventitia. This layer contains a mixture of collagen, elastic fibers, smooth muscle fibers, and fibroblasts. This outer layer also contains nerve fibers, the vasa vasorum, and lymphatics that nourish the vessel wall and remove metabolic waste products.

The vascular system can be divided into elastic arteries, muscular arteries, arterioles, capillaries, veins, and lymphatics. Elastic arteries, such as the aorta and major pulmonary arteries, contain large amounts of elastic tissue. The walls of these arteries distend and increase their elastic tension with systole. During diastole, the elastic fibers recoil, which helps propel the blood distally and maintain flow (see Chapter 12).

Smooth muscle cells predominate in muscular arteries such as the renal, superior mesenteric, and femoral arteries. These arteries regulate peripheral flow and supply organs that require a specific blood supply based on the amount of work they are performing. These arteries can vary their caliber by contracting (vasoconstriction) and relaxing (vasodilation) so that a given cardiac output can be allocated to various tissues depending on their current needs. Thus muscular arteries function as resistance vessels and are major regulators of systemic blood pressure.

Arterioles are branches of the muscular arteries that differ structurally and functionally from small arteries only by their size. Because of their large number, arterioles form the most important class of resistance channels in the vascular system. Capillaries are blood vessels that have a diameter similar to that of a red blood cell.

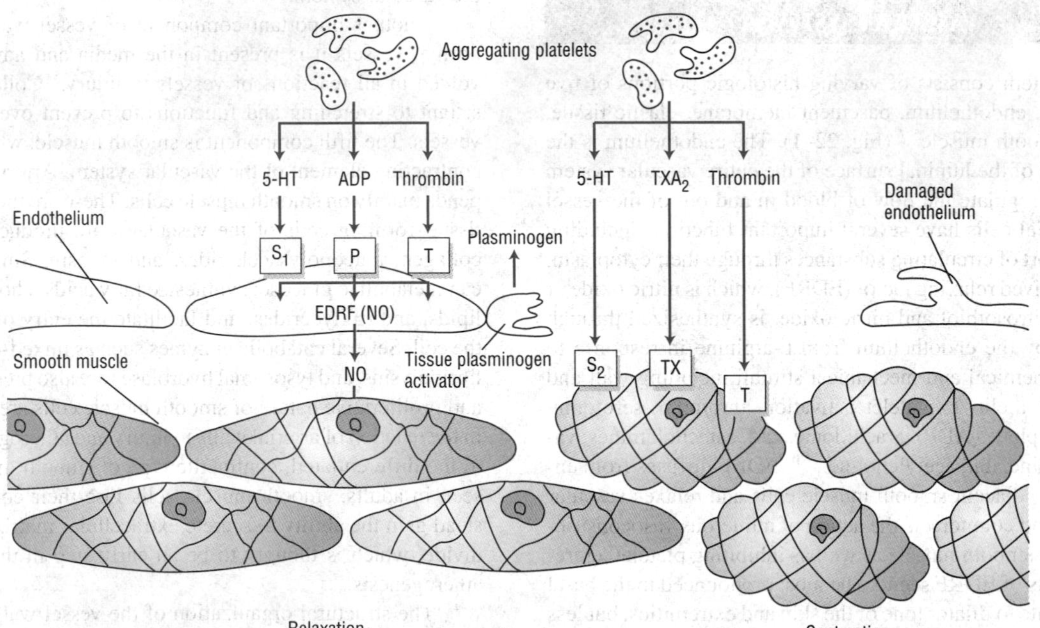

FIGURE 22–2. Mechanisms of vasospasm in atherosclerotic arteries. *Left:* Normal endothelium. If platelets were to aggegate and release 5-hydroxytryptamine (5-HT; serotonin) and adenosine diphosphate (ADP), these would act on specific receptors on the endothelial cells (S_1, serotoninergic receptor; P, purinergic receptor) to release endothelium-derived relaxing factor (EDRF). EDRF is nitric oxide (NO) or a nitrosothiol. Also, if any thrombin were formed, this would act on a specific receptor (T) to enhance the release of relaxing factor. Also, tissue plasminogen activator would be stimulated to form plasminogen. *Right:* If the endothelium is damaged, platelets aggregate because of the loss of the inhibitory action of NO and prostacyclin. The resulting release of 5-HT and thromboxane A_2 (TXA_2) and the formation of thrombin cause vasoconstriction or vasospasm by acting directly on receptors on the smooth muscle cells. Not shown is the fact that some of the 5-HT can be taken up by the sympathetic nerve endings and released again as a false transmitter to enhance the contraction. Also, the resulting tissue hypoxia-anoxia releases a contracting factor from the vessel wall, which further aggravates and prolongs the vasospasm. *(From Shepherd JT, Katusic ZS. Endothelium-derived vasoactive factors: I. Endothelium dependent relaxation. Hypertension 1991;18(Suppl 3):76–85, by permission of the American Heart Association, Inc.)*

Veins are considerably larger than their associated arteries. Their structure reflects both the low pressure of this system and their reservoir function. The walls of the veins are thinner, and the media contains fewer smooth muscle cells, collagen, and elastic fibers. Smooth muscle cells are responsible largely for the vasoconstrictive activity of the veins that is seen mainly in the small peripheral veins in the skin. The larger veins can actively constrict during acute changes in pressure, but they passively dilate with slow increases in pressure. The lymphatic channels are the simplest parts of the vascular system. The intima consists of endothelial cells and a few collagen and muscle fibers.

REACTIVE CHANGES OF THE VASCULAR SYSTEM

The arteries are not static structures, but rather they change in response to various physical and chemical stimuli, react to injury, and undergo structural alterations throughout growth and aging.[7] The major change that occurs with normal aging is a slow, continuous, and symmetric increase in the intimal thickness, especially in the large elastic arteries. This process results from a gradual accumulation of smooth muscle cells (which presumably migrate from the media) and diffuse connective tissue and an accumulation of sphingomyelin and cholesterol. This diffuse age-related thickening is to be distinguished from discrete, raised fibromuscular plaques, a characteristic feature of atherosclerosis. After the sixth decade, the intima also becomes more collagenized, and there is a loss of cellular constituents and granular degranulation of elastic fibers. The rate of aortic intimal thickening is more prominent in men and accelerated in patients with hypertension. Structural changes in small arteries and arterioles differ somewhat from that in systemic vessels in that there is progressive fibrotic thickening of the adventitia and media with little intimal change. These changes are closely linked to hypertension and diabetes mellitus.

In the normal arterial wall, lipid content, mainly cholesterol and phospholipid (especially sphingomyelin), also increase progressively with age. Phospholipid synthesis rises with age, followed by a compensatory increase in all phospholipases except sphingomyelinase. Accumulations of cholesterol and low-density lipoprotein (LDL) appear to be derived from plasma. Functionally, these changes result in increased rigidity of arteries and loss of endothelial function. Endothelial dysfunction leads to vasoconstriction, thrombosis, and greater involvement of the inflammatory response, promoting atherosclerosis. The larger arteries may become dilated, elongated, and tortuous, and aneurysms may form in areas of degenerating arteriosclerotic plaques.

The veins also undergo age-related changes. *Phlebosclerosis,* also called *hyperplastic phlebitis,* refers to thickening of the veins. It appears to be age related and is particularly prominent in veins of the lower extremity that are subject to stasis and increased luminal pressure.

PHYSIOLOGY OF LIMB BLOOD FLOW

Arterial blood pressure and resistance to flow, which is provided by the physical characteristics of blood vessels and of the blood itself, control blood flow to the limbs. There are two major components to resistance: the viscosity of the blood and the tube factor or hindrance, based on size, shape, smoothness, branching, and other physical aspects of the wall. Poiseuille's law governs the flow of fluids through cylindrical tubes, and it states that resistance to flow is proportional to the fourth power of the radius. Viscosity is usually fairly constant, but exceptions to this would be the presence of abnormal or abnormally high numbers of red or white blood cells such as in chronic obstructive airways disease, sickle cell disease, high circulating levels of fibrinogen, or certain types of leukemia. Active changes in the radius of the resistance vessels in the limbs are caused by local and neurogenic mechanisms.[7]

LOCAL CONTROL

Local control of limb blood flow includes intrinsic, metabolic, humoral, and physical factors. The relative importance of each of these varies for different tissues and for different vessels within the same tissue. Intrinsic smooth muscle tone appears to be influenced directly by changes in wall tension, which in turn is determined by intravascular pressure. A decrease in intravascular pressure and wall tension would result in spontaneous activity of the smooth muscle cells, and an increase in intravascular pressure would have the opposite effect.

The intrinsic myogenic activity is modified by chemical changes in the resistance vessels, which adjust blood flow to the limbs (active hyperemia). Similar increases are seen after temporary arrest of circulation to the limbs (reactive hyperemia). Metabolic factors play an important role in controlling blood flow to skeletal muscles. The accumulation of metabolic products such as carbon dioxide, potassium, phosphate, and adenosine during exercise, an increase in the osmolality of venous effluent, or a change in pH causes direct vasodilation of peripheral vessels (Fig. 22–3). The humoral factors that cause dilation of skeletal muscle vessels include epinephrine, acetylcholine, histamine, prostaglandins, and serotonin. As described previously, many of the effects of these substances are mediated via the endothelial release of EDRF. Norepinephrine, angiotensin, and vasopressin cause vasoconstriction. In skin, epinephrine causes vasoconstriction because there is a preponderance of α-adrenergic receptors in cutaneous vessels, in contrast to skeletal muscle vessels, which have both α- and β-receptors. Epinephrine has a greater affinity for β_2-receptors in skeletal muscle resistance vessels and thus causes vasodilation.

Such physical factors as local temperature also control blood flow to extremities. Low temperatures can cause vasoconstriction or vasodilation depending on the thermal state of the body. Application of heat to an extremity dilates the blood vessels. This vasodilation is enhanced by increasing the temperature of the body as a whole.

NEURAL CONTROL

The skin of the hands and feet is innervated by sympathetic fibers that mediate reflex changes in vessel tone. Alterations in activity of these fibers under central control cause large fluctuations in the flow to all fingers simultaneously. Skin vasoconstrictive sympathetic reflex is preserved in chronically ischemic limbs with PVD, suggesting that sympathetic nerve fibers are relatively resistant to chronic ischemia; however, diabetics do not have preserved sympathetic reflexes.[15] Temperature changes alter the sympathetic outflow to the skin. Exposure of the body to cold augments the vasoconstrictor tone, whereas an increase in body temperature decreases tone. The circulation in the skin also plays an essential role in thermal homeostasis. Arteriovenous anastomoses, which are numerous in fingers and toes, favor heat dissipation. Sweat glands cause local production of bradykinin, and consequently vasodilation, when stimulated by sympathetic cholinergic nerves.

Changes in the diameter of resistance vessels in skeletal muscle are influenced by sympathetic adrenergic nerves, which are abundant in small arteries and arterioles. Sympathetic nerve fibers to muscle are of two types: vasoconstrictor fibers, whose activity is mediated by

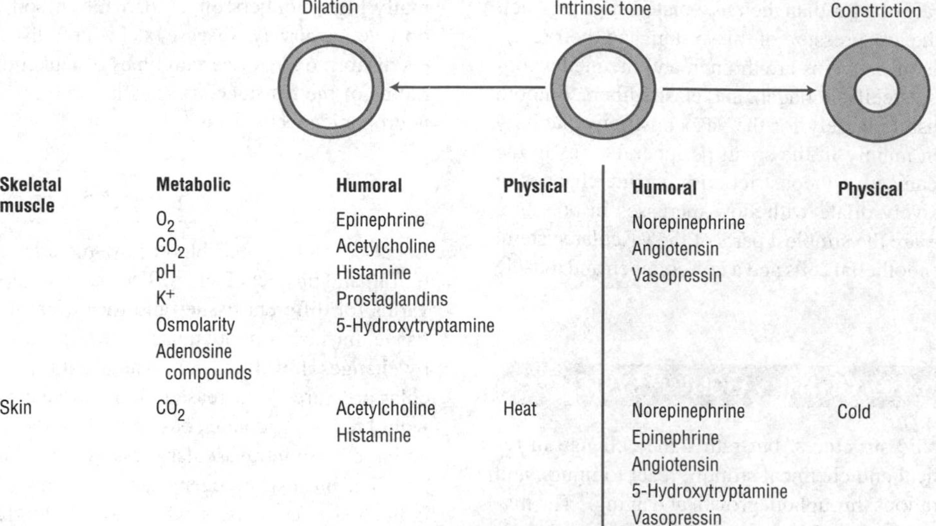

FIGURE 22–3. Active changes in vascular diameter are caused by local and nervous mechanisms. Local control includes intrinsic, metabolic, humoral, and physical factors, and the relative importance of each of these varies for different tissues and for different vessels within the same tissue. This figure identifies actions of local factors that can alter arterial diameter in skeletal muscle and skin. *(From McGrath MA, Verhaeghe RH, Shepherd JT. The physiology of limb blood flow. In: Juergens JL, Spittell JA, Fairbairn JF, eds. Peripheral Vascular Diseases. Philadelphia, Saunders, 1980:84, with permission.)*

the release of norepinephrine, and vasodilator fibers, whose activity is mediated through the release acetylcholine. Although vessels in both the skin and muscles are innervated by sympathetic fibers, the vasomotor centers controlling these vessels can function independently. In reflex control of body temperature, only the vessels to the skin are involved, whereas with alterations in position, the reflex changes are confined to the vessels in the muscles.

PERIPHERAL ARTERIAL DISORDERS

PVD of the arteries generally can be classified as obstructive and vasospastic. Examples of an obstructive abnormality include arteriosclerosis obliterans and thromboangiitis obliterans (Buerger's disease). Raynaud's disease is the most common example of a vasospastic disorder.

ARTERIOSCLEROSIS OBLITERANS

Arteriosclerosis obliterans, also called *atherosclerosis obliterans* (ASO), is a chronic occlusive arterial disease of the aorta, particularly the terminal portion of the abdominal aorta and its major branches to the extremities. It is one of several types of chronic arterial occlusive disease (Table 22–1). This disease also involves the large and medium-sized arteries of the extremities, especially the iliofemoral and popliteal arteries and, in the lower leg, the posterior tibial artery at the ankle and the anterior tibial artery at its origin. ASO is considered a segmental disease, with significant variation in its extent. The clinical classification of the severity of PVD is based on exercise limitation and symptoms and is referred to as the *Fontaine classification* (Table 22–2).

EPIDEMIOLOGY

Arteriosclerosis obliterans occurs primarily in men between the ages of 50 and 70 years, and the reported prevalence of symptomatic disease ranges from 1% to 6%; however, the prevalence is age-related.[2,16] In men aged 40 to 44 years, 50 to 54 years, and 60 to 64 years, the reported incidence is 0.9%, 3.6%, and 7.5%, respectively. The disease affects women less commonly (about 0.07%), usually after age 60 years, perhaps in part because of a menopausal loss of the protective effect of estrogens and an increased incidence of diabetes in women of this age.[17] If noninvasive testing is performed, the prevalence of large leg artery disease is 11.7% and small artery disease is 16%, although only 10% or fewer report symptoms.[18] Asymptomatic arterial insufficiency may be detected using the ankle-brachial index (ABI), and the incidence is about 10% when the ABI is less than 0.9.[19] As in the case of atherosclerosis, hypercholesterolemia plays an important role in the development of this disease. Arteriosclerotic lesions

TABLE 22–1. Causes of Chronic Arterial Occlusive Disease

Arteriosclerosis obliterans
Thromboangiitis obliterans (Buerger's disease)
Arteritis
Trauma
Congenital arterial narrowing

TABLE 22–2. Fontaine Classification for Claudication

Stage	Symptoms
I	Asymptomatic
II	Intermittent claudication
IIa	Pain-free, claudication walking >200 m
IIb	Pain-free, claudication walking <200 m
III	Rest/nocturnal pain
IV	Necrosis/gangrene

in the lower extremities are commonly associated with coronary and cerebrovascular disease, as noted in the Coronary Artery Surgery Study (CASS) and others.[20] Patients undergoing revascularization procedures who have PVD have worse outcomes than those who do not have PVD. Diabetes mellitus significantly increases the prevalence (11-fold) and severity of ASO (10 years earlier than if diabetes is not present). Other risk factors important for the pathogenesis of ASO include age, hypertension, hypercholesterolemia, and smoking.[21,22] Patients with PVD have greater relative risk for death from all causes (range 1.6–3.3) and cardiovascular disease (range 2.0–5.1) compared with that of control patients.[2]

PATHOPHYSIOLOGY

The primary lesion in ASO is an intimal plaque that narrows progressively and, in many cases, leads to complete occlusion of these arteries. The histopathologic changes are essentially identical to those of arteriosclerotic occlusive disease of the visceral and cerebral arteries. The primary physiologic disturbance is obstruction of blood flow through large arteries and, therefore, ischemia of those tissues of the extremity supplied by these arteries. The degree of ischemia is proportional to (1) the proximal limit of the occluding process, (2) the patency of collateral blood vessels, and (3) the rapidity of occlusion development. The ischemia produced by the obstruction may be increased by arteriolar constriction from any cause. If the occlusion is not too extensive, dilation may improve circulation. Obstruction of the large arteries decreases pressure and blood flow in smaller arteries distal to the obstruction, and thrombosis and gangrene may result. Peripheral occlusive arterial disease is often associated with increased blood viscosity, hyperfibrinogenemia, and a relatively high hematocrit.

CLINICAL PRESENTATION

Unless there is acute arterial occlusion due to thrombosis, the signs and symptoms of ASO have a gradual onset. The most common presentation is intermittent claudication, which is described as pain, cramping, numbness, or weakness in certain muscles that develops only during exercise. Distress is quickly relieved by rest without change in position. About one-third of patients with PVD will have typical symptoms of intermittent claudication. Intermittent claudication is caused by inadequate blood supply to muscles(s) stressed by exercise. The distance a person is able to walk before the pain develops varies with the extent and severity of arterial occlusion. It is usually unilateral at first, may become bilateral with time, and often is worse in one of the extremities if both are involved. The location of the involved muscle group may predict the most proximal level of occlusion. For example, claudication of the calf muscles suggests occlusion of the popliteal artery or higher; claudication of the hip indicates disease low in the aorta or in the iliac artery. Edema of disuse and dependency may occur if a limb is kept in the dependent position for long periods of time in the attempt to relieve symptoms.

Another important group of symptoms includes pain at rest, paresthesias, and numbness. These symptoms are usually the result of more severe ischemia of tissues and a more advanced form of the disease resulting from multiple levels of occlusion or obstruction of collateral vessels. It is usually felt in the digits but may be noted in the foot and lower leg as well. Ulceration and gangrene are common when the disease reaches this stage. Pain caused by ischemic neuropathy is another clinical feature of ASO, especially in diabetic patients. Peripheral nervous tissue has a low metabolism and requires very little blood to keep it healthy; this ischemic neuropathy, regardless of symptoms, is consistent with advanced disease. This pain may be continuous or paroxysmal and may be described as a series of sharp pains or the sensation of electrical shocks. A sensation of numbness, coldness, or burning also may occur. When diabetics with a neuropathy develop ulcers, the lesions are often painless.

The physical findings in arteriosclerosis of the extremities are for the most part indistinguishable from those seen in other occlusive arterial diseases. Impairment of arterial pulsations, often noted by palpation, is the most important and consistent finding. Others include systolic bruits over the involved arteries, color (i.e., waxy, pale, and dry appearance) and temperature changes in the skin of the extremity, edema, and hypoesthesia and hyporeflexia in patients with severe neuropathy.

DIAGNOSIS

The diagnosis of ASO often is made on the basis of a good history and physical examination. Sophisticated laboratory studies and diagnostic tests rarely are necessary to establish the diagnosis; however, routine laboratory tests such as blood chemistry, electrocardiogram, and x-ray studies may be needed to determine the extent of associated disease as well as prognosis and therapy. The magnitude of arterial occlusion can be assessed simply by measuring the extremity blood pressure at rest and after exercise to the point of claudication. Another easily obtained measure of disease severity is the ABI.[2] This is done using a Doppler ultrasonography to measure systolic blood pressure. The ABI (sometimes called the *arm-ankle index,* or AAI) is abnormal if the ratio of the arm (right or left) to dorsalis pedis (DP) or posterior tibial (PT) blood pressure is 0.9 or less. If both DP and PT pressures are abnormal, the extent of disease is more severe, and atherosclerosis is likely to be widespread. An ABI between 0.41 to 0.90 is consistent with mild to moderate PVD; an ABI between 0.00 to 0.40 is consistent with severe PVD. ABI is inversely related to cardiovascular risk factors as well as subclinical and clinical cardiovascular disease in older adults. The lower the ABI, the greater is the increase in cardiovascular disease risk. Even those with asymptomatic reductions in the ABI (0.8 to 1.0) appear to be at increased risk of cardiovascular disease.[23] The 6-minute walk or accelerometer and pedometer also may be used as reproducible measures of disability due to occlusive arterial disease, and they correlate fairly well with the ABI and rating scales of physical activity.[24] Arteriography is rarely necessary to establish the diagnosis but usually is used prior to surgery to precisely locate the disease. Traditional or digital subtraction arteriography is considered to be the "gold standard" diagnostic tests for PVD. Other techniques include vascular songraphy (standard and color Doppler ultrasound), magnetic resonance imaging, computed axial tomography, and angioscopy that uses a thin, flexible fiberoptic scope to directly visualize the vessel lumen. A triple-lumen probe to detect skin surface Po_2 has been developed and correlates well with laser-Doppler flowmetry (LDF). If the ABI is 0.91 to 1.30, the patient undergoes treadmill exercise and repeat ABI. If the ABI is greater than 1.30, then duplex ultrasonography or other pressure-volume measures are employed.[25] After physical examination and ABI determination, the next diagnostic test is usually ultrasonography. The sensitivity and specificity of duplex ultrasonography are greater than 80% unless adjacent segments have stenoses of greater than 50%; color duplex sonongraphy improves the sensitivity and specificity.[26] The clinical differentiation of ASO from other types of occlusive peripheral arterial diseases is given in Table 22–3.

▶ TREATMENT: Arteriosclerosis Obliterans

The goals of therapy in patients with ASO are to arrest progression of the disease, improve blood flow, relieve exertional pain, improve walking and quality of life, and prevent and treat ulceration and gangrene. Progression of the disease may be prevented by control of hyperlipoproteinemia, control of any associated diseases such as diabetes and hypertension, and tobacco abstinence.[2,27] Regression of atherosclerosis with lipid lowering is described in Chapter 21. Normalizing serum cholesterol levels through diet and drug therapy and LDL-apheresis in patients with peripheral atherosclerosis improve both endothelium-dependent and -independent relaxation in human peripheral small arteries.[28] For patients who have severe ischemia manifested by rest pain, ulceration, and gangrene, rest of the extremity is an important adjunct of treatment. If the pain is severe, narcotics and other pain medications may be necessary as well as either angioplasty or surgery. It is important to take meticulous care of the extremities and avoid even minor trauma because it may lead to ulceration. In these patients, ulceration usually is treated with local care, medical management (including antibiotics if necessary), and surgical amputation if required.

Another effective method of improving blood flow to the extremities is to increase collateral flow. This can be accomplished by a warm environmental temperature; avoidance of vasoconstriction caused by drugs, cold, and tobacco; elevation of the head of the bed 12 to 16 inches; and exercise. A daily exercise training program is very effective in patients with mild to moderate intermittent claudication. Important features of a successful program are (1) repetitive daily walks to 75% of the claudication distance with intermittent periods of rest (1–2 minutes), (2) weekly increases in walking time and distance, and (3) continuation of this program, because cessation results in loss of improvement. In general, the exercise program needs to be 20 minutes per session or more three times per week for at least 6 months.[29] Controlled studies have shown a 25% to 30% increase in walking distance with an average of about 1000 feet, although 40% of patients may show increases of nearly a mile even though the ABI may not be increased significantly.[30] Compared with strength training, treadmill training provides more improvement in exercise time and maximum oxygen uptake. A consistent exercise training program will prevent abrupt deterioration and the need for amputation and may reduce mortality compared with patients with claudication not on an exercise program.[31] The mechanism by which exercise improves functionality and symptoms is not clear.[32]

Cigarette smoking is one of the most important risk factors for chronic PVD, and continued smoking is associated with a greater risk for disabling claudication, limb-threatening ischemia, amputation, and the need for intervention. Although smoking cessation is universally recommended in patients with PVD, there are few data suggesting improvement in PVD with cessation other than that smoking cessation improved postoperative graft patency rates and reduced the complications of peripheral arterial disease.[33] Smoking cessation should be attempted to improve coronary artery disease end points, and this alone justifies this intervention.

Various vasodilating drugs (e.g., tolazoline, nylidrin, isoxsuprine, niacin derivatives, cyclandelate, and papaverine) have been used in ASO, but none has been shown to be consistently effective. Ischemia is one of the most potent stimuli for vasodilation, and drug therapy does not augment the physiologic response to ischemia. Vasodilators are of no value in treating ASO.[1,2]

Controversy surrounds the use of β-adrenergic blocking agents in PVD patients with concurrent coronary artery disease or hypertension. A number of case reports have been published indicating that these agents can cause or worsen intermittent claudication. By reducing systemic blood pressure, these agents could decrease blood flow through stenotic arteries or collateral vessels. A nonselective β-blocker may attenuate epinephrine-induced vasodilation during exercise by blocking β_2-receptors in peripheral vessels. Controlled trials using both selective and nonselective agents have produced mixed results in patients with PVD. A few studies have demonstrated an increase in muscle blood flow and symptomatic improvement when β-blockers were withdrawn or no effect on either blood flow or claudication. A metaanalysis of six trials found that β-blockers do not adversely affect walking capacity or symptoms of intermittent claudication in patients with mild to moderate peripheral arterial disease.[34] β-Adrenergic blocking agents, if used, probably should be cardioselective agents; however, because other drugs are available for hypertension and angina, β-blocker use should be minimized.

Pentoxifylline (Trental) has been shown to be of benefit in patients with chronic occlusive arterial disease; however, the results have been small improvement in walking distance (20–40 m) and inconsistent due, in part, to placebo responses.[35,36] Pentoxifylline increases red blood cell deformability and decreases platelet adhesiveness, blood fibrinogen, and neutrophil elastase/α_1-proteinase inhibitor complex levels, which are thought to lead to a reduction in blood viscosity and improved blood flow.[37] The average increase in walking distance was about one-half of a city block, and pentoxifylline has been shown to be effective in moderately severe chronic obstructive arterial disease if the resting ABI is less than 0.8 and if symptoms of intermittent claudication have been present for longer than 1 year.[38] Patients more likely to improve with pentoxifylline are those with moderately severe ischemia and without rest pain, ischemic ulcers, or severe claudication.[39] In contrast to the unpredictable and less than impressive effects with oral pentoxifylline for chronic therapy, intravenous pentoxifylline (400 mg twice daily) given for 21 days improved the symptoms of critical limb ischemia.[40] Pentoxifylline has been used to prevent postoperative rethrombosis after vascular surgery for arterial occlusive disease, but worldwide, aspirin and anticoagulation are used more commonly to prevent graft occulsion depending on the graft site.[41] Pentoxifylline has been evaluated in various diabetic complications including PVD; the effects are inconsistent and only marginally better than placebo. A cost-effectiveness analysis suggests that pentoxifylline may reduce the risk of vascular surgery while not increasing the total cost of PVD care.[42] Modification of risk factors such as hypertension, tobacco use, and hyperlipidemia is also considered to be cost-effective.[43,44]

Antiplatelet therapy with aspirin (325 mg daily) in the U.S. Physicians' Health Study reduced the relative risk of peripheral artery surgery in the aspirin group to 0.54 (95% confidence intervals 0.30–0.95; $P = .03$).[45] Aspirin (81–325 mg/d) or clopidogrel (75 mg/d) is recommended by the American College of Chest Physicians Consensus Conference because patients with PVD are at high risk for myocardial infarction and stroke.[46] Several small studies have used dipyridamole in combination with aspirin, but the effects of dipyridamole alone are unclear. The Swedish Ticlopidine Multicenter Study, a large randomized, placebo-controlled trial with ticlopidine found no significant improvement in walking distance or ABI with ticlopidine.[47] EMATAP, a randomized, stratified, placebo-controlled, double-blind multicenter trial with ticlopidine did find a significant reduction in first events (i.e., sudden deaths, myocardial infarctions, and strokes) compared with placebo.[48] Aspirin

(81–325 mg/d) is also recommended for patients undergoing saphenous vein or prosthetic femoropopliteal bypass operation.[46] More recently, a French trial assessed the utility of ticlopidine 250 mg twice daily in patients with femoropopliteal or femorotibial saphenous vein bypass grafts for 2 years. Cumulative graft patency with ticlopidine was 82%, whereas 63% of the grafts in the placebo group were patent.[49] A randomized, blinded trial of clopidogrel versus aspirin (CAPRIE) found that clopidogrel use had an annual 5.32% risk of ischemic stroke, myocardial infarction, or vascular death compared with 5.83% for aspirin, a small but significant difference (relative risk reduction of 8.7%) between the two drugs. Most of the benefit from clopidogrel was restricted to patients entering the study with peripheral arterial disease.[50,51] Recent large, randomized, double-blinded trials of iloprost, an oral prostaglandin analog, have shown that short-term (4 weeks, $N = 178$) improvement in the proportion of patients who survived without major amputation, ulcers, or gangrene and had no rest pain was 11% in the placebo group, 19% in the low-dose iloprost (50–100 μg) group, and 28% in the high-dose iloprost (150–200 μg) group ($P = .04$).[52] In a long-term study (1 year, $N = 624$), there was no treatment benefit in terms of a primary end point of amputation and death. The secondary combined end point of patients who survived without a major amputation, ulcers, or gangrene and had no rest pain, nor a need for regular analgesia, was favorable for iloprost, with 18% of patients in the placebo group reaching this optimal secondary end point compared with 23% in the low-dose iloprost group and 26% in the higher-dose iloprost group ($P < 0.05$). The main limitation for iloprost use is tolerability; fewer than half the patients started on therapy were maintained at the end of the trial. Cilostazol was approved in 1999 by the Food and Drug Administration (FDA) for the treatment of claudication.[2,53] It works by inhibiting phosphodiesterase type 3, which increases intracellular concentrations of cyclic adenosine monophosphate (cAMP) in platelets and vascular smooth muscle cells and therefore is a potent antiplatelet agent and vasodilator that reduces vascular proliferation and has lipid-lowering effects in vivo. Cilostazol is metabolized by cytochrome P-450 3A4 (CYP3A4) and to a lesser extent via CYP2C19 and CYP1A2. Consequently, drugs that inhibit CYP3A4 (e.g., ketoconazole) are likely to impair the clearance of cilostazol. The half-life is approximately 11 hours, and steady-state concentrations are reached in approximately 4 days.[54] Several clinical trials with cilostazol 200 mg/d for 3 to 6 months have shown a 30% to 80% improvement in maximal treadmill walking distance and improved quality of life compared with placebo.[2] Compared with pentoxifylline, cilostazol improved maximal walking distance by 54% versus 30% ($P < 0.001$) and with similar withdrawal rates due to adverse effects (16% to 19%).[55]

Short-term studies with calcium channel blocker also have shown some promise; however, interest has focused recently on the potential for antiatherosclerosis effects of calcium blockers.[56] In the PREVENT trial, amlodipine did not delay the progression of atherosclerosis in the coronary circulation, but intimal-medial thickness (IMT) was improved in the carotid arteries, with amlodipine producing a 0.0126-mm decrease in IMT compared with a 0.033 mm increase with placebo ($P = .007$).[57] The reasons for these disparate effects are not obvious, and the role for calcium antagonists remains uncertain. Defibrotide, an investigational agent, has been shown to improve walking time in about 50% of treated patients.[58] Defibrotide increases tissue plasminogen activator production and release and prostaglandin I_2 formation and inhibits platelet activation.

Based on results from the Prevention of Atherosclerosis Complications with Ketanserin (PACK) trial, ketanserin has no significant effect in reducing the symptoms of intermittent claudication.[59] Another approach, based on improved muscle metabolism with L-carnitine (1 g twice a day for 12 months), improved walking distance by 62% compared with 45% for placebo, and it was more effective in patients unable to walk 250 m at baseline.[60] Carnitine skeletal muscle stores are reduced in animal models, and when they are replenished, muscle performance is improved. At this point, an appropriate reminder would be that many trials in the treatment of PVD and intermittent claudication are either poorly controlled or have significant design flaws and that an inverse correlation exists between the sample size and the number of studies reporting positive results.[36]

Intraarterial thrombolysis should be considered (1) in an attempt, time permitting, to convert an emergent surgical procedure into an elective one, (2) to convert a major surgical procedure into a less extensive one, (3) to restore the patency of any acutely occluded vessel that is inaccessible to mechanical thrombectomy, (4) to identify the underlying cause of thrombosis so that it can be corrected with salvage of native artery or a bypass graft, (5) to prevent arterial intimal damage from balloon thrombectomy, and (6) to reduce the level of ampuation when clot retrivial is incomplete.[1] The success rate for acute native arterial occlusion ranges from 58% to 100%, and the need for adjunctive revascularization procedures is comparable with bypass grafting, thrombectomy, or percutaneous transluminal angioplasty (PTA). Ouriel and colleagues, in a randomized, multicenter trial [Thrombolysis or Peripheral Arterial Surgery (TOPAS)], compared intraarterial urokinase (4000 IU/h for 4 hours and then 2000 IU/h until lysis was complete) with vascular surgery in patients ($N = 272$ in each group) with acute occlusion of native or bypass grafts (45% and 55%, respectively) and found that the amputation-free survival was similar (65.0% and 69.6%; $P = .23$), whereas the need for open operative procedures was greater in the surgery group.[61] Patients with thrombi less than 30 cm in length did better with urokinase than with longer occlusions.[62] Major hemorrhage was more significantly common with urokinase (12.5% versus 5.5%). Tissue plasminogen activator (TPA), urokinase, and streptokinase all have been used for acute arterial occlusion, and none is clearly superior. Passage of a guidewire through the thrombus predicts success and is the most common method of thrombolytic delivery; however, the extact method of delivering thrombolytics (e.g., pulse-spray, slow infusion), the relative efficacy among available agents, optimal patients to be treated, and duration of response remain to be determined.[1] Based on the results of the TOPAS study, the projected life expectancy for patients who underwent initial surgery was 5.04 years versus 4.75 years for initial thrombolysis. The lifetime costs were $57,429 for surgery and $76,326 for thrombolysis. In performing sensitivity analyses, a threshold cost-effectiveness ratio of $60,000 was considered what society would pay for accepted medical interventions.[63] Thrombolysis became cost-effective if the 1-year mortality rate for lysis was lowered from 20% to 10.7%, if the amputation rate for lysis diminished from 15% to 3.9%, or if the 1-year cost of lysis could be reduced to a level below $13,000. In chronic native arterial thrombosis, the duration of occlusion (<7 days versus >6 months) has a large effect on the success of clot lysis (72% versus 24%, respectively).

When medical management with exercise, control of risk factors, and vasodilator or antithrombotic therapy is inadequate, interventional therapeutic technology is useful. The indication for revascularization is true incapacitation by exercise limitations or critical limb ischemia. The types of technology used include atherectomy, atheroablation, PTA and endovascular stents, angioscopy, and laser angioplasty; direct open arterial surgery using endarterectomy, prosthetic bypass grafts, or vein-patch arterioplasty may be effective in bypassing or removing areas of stenosis but should be reserved for patients with severe and disabling symptoms (Fontaine class IIb and above). Indications for surgery include relief of symptoms of limb-threatening ischemia, including ischemic pain at rest, ischemic ulcers, and gangrene. Intermittent claudication is only a relative indication for surgery and only after an adequate trial of nonsurgical therapy.[1] Patients most likely to have complete relief of symptoms and normalization of pressure gradients are those with smaller, more focal segments involved (2 to 5 cm or so depending on the vascular bed), those without calcification, and those with less than total occlusion. Revascularization through angioplasty or surgery has been shown to be more cost-effective than amputation of a limb because of high rehabilitation costs and the fact that angioplasty is more cost-effective than surgery if the 5-year patency rate with angioplasty is 30% or greater.[64,65] Intravascular stents (e.g., Palmaz stents) may be combined with thrombolysis for critical ischemia, and initial technical success was achieved in 65 of 77 limbs (84%) with thrombolysis alone versus 76 of 77 (99%) limbs in the stent group ($P = .009$).[66] Major complications were similar in the two groups. There was no difference between treatment groups. Hemodynamic/clinical success at 1 and 2 years in the PTA group was 72% and 65% versus 77% and 65% in the stent group. The cumulative 1- and 2-year angiographic primary patency rates were 63% and 53%, respectively, for both groups. The secondary 1- and 2-year angiographic patency rates were 86% and 74% in the PTA group versus 79% and 73% in the stent group ($P = .5$). Endovascular brachytherapy may reduce restenosis after revascularization procedures.[67] Vein grafts are preferred for infrainguinal bypass because of a lower incidence of thrombosis and occlusion compared with synthetic materials (e.g., 68% versus 38%). An aortic bifurcation prosthesis appears to provide the same outcome as aortofemoral bypass for aortoiliac disease.[1] For patients with venous insufficiency, sclerotherapy with hypertonic saline or dextrose of sodium morrhuate, sodium tetradecyl sulfate, or polidocanol and others may be useful in controlling telangiectasias and varicosities.

As with atherectomy, atheroablation, and angioplasty procedures for coronary revascularization, these revascularization procedures for peripheral artery occlusion are associated with primary failure and restenosis, hematomas at the site of device insertion, dissection, and pseudoaneurysms at the site of catheter entry.[68,69] Acute closure occurs in 1% to 4% of peripheral angioplasties, and antithrombotic therapy with urokinase or other thrombolytics and heparin may be used to reopen a vessel occluded with thrombus. Spasm after the procedure is managed with nitroglycerin and calcium channel blockers. Longer-term antithrombotic therapy may be continued with aspirin. Aspirin alone or in combination with glycoprotein IIb/IIIa receptor antagonists may lower the rate of acute closure.[70,71] Neither antiplatelet agents nor anticoagulation with warfarin has been shown to be very effective in preventing long-term restenosis; however, omega-3 polyunsaturated fatty acid supplementation with fish oil shows some promise.[69] Longer-term patency rates following angioplasy typically have ranged from about 60% to 75% at 1 year depending on the site of intervention, and this compares favorably with surgery. Human gene therapy is being attempted in PVD to prevent restenosis by percutaneous catheter-based delivery of a plasmid carrying the gene encoding vascular endothelial growth factor (VEGF) to promote therapeutic angiogenesis.[72]

Percutaneous lumbar neurolytic sympathetic blockade (NSB) using 1.5 mL ethanol 95% has been shown to improve walking distance and muscle metabolic activity in a small trial.[73] Lumbar sympathectomy may be useful in patients with mild ischemic rest pain, but temporary sympathectomy with local anesthetics should be performed first to ensure benefit from the procedure. Sympathectomy does alter the long-term course of ASO.

THROMBOANGIITIS OBLITERANS (BUERGER'S OR VON WINIWERTER DISEASE)[74]

Thromboangiitis obliterans (TAO) is a disease involving segmental inflammatory and proliferative nonatheromatous lesions of the medium and small arteries, veins, and nerves that usually occurs in young males and frequently leads to nonhealing ulcers and gangrene (see Table 22–3). The cause of TOA is unknown, but virtually all patients are heavy smokers of cigarettes or use other forms of tobacco. Many patients show cutaneous sensitivity to tobacco, and there is a high prevalence of the human leukocyte antigens (HLA) A9 and B5 in affected persons, which suggests a genetic basis for the disease. Lymphocyte sensitivity to type I and III collagens has been shown for 77% of patients, and about 50% have anticollagen antibodies.

Common presenting complaints include a superficial, migratory, nodular phlebitis associated with cutaneous erythema and tenderness. TAO may present with intermittent claudication, most commonly in the arch of the foot (relieved by rest) or less commonly in the calf and occasionally on both sides. Rest pain may present as a severe ache or numb, gnawing pain that may worsen by elevation of the limb. Cold sensitivity of the hands occurs in about 50% of TAO patients. Pulsations in the DP and PT arteries may be impaired or absent, and affected extremities may be abnormally red. Segmental thrombophlebitis occurs in about 40% of the patients.

Goals of therapy in TAO include arresting progression of the disease, producing vasodilation, relieving pain, and treating ulcers and gangrene. All patients with TAO should abstain completely and permanently from tobacco of any type. Failure to abstain from tobacco results in disease progression, severe rest pain, ulceration, and amputation. Other measures that have been suggested but do not work well include anticoagulants, sympathectomy, vascular surgery, and vasodilating drugs. Oral iloprost (100 μg twice daily) improves pain control in TAO but has no effect on healing of skin lesions.[75] None of these measures can be recommended at the present time. Patients should be advised to avoid cold exposure and vasoconstricting drugs.

RAYNAUD'S DISEASE[76–79]

In 1862, Maurice Raynaud described episodes of discoloration of the skin of the digits on exposure to cold, and he thought that this was due to increased sensitivity of the sympathetic nervous system. This condition, which is limited to the skin, usually accompanied by cyanosis, rubor, pain, or parethesias and associated gangrene, came to be termed *Raynaud's disease*. More than a century later, the pathogenesis, diagnosis, and treatment are still unclear. Raynaud's disease may be classified as primary, in which the cause is unknown, or secondary, in which an associated condition exists (Table 22–4).

EPIDEMIOLOGY

The prevalence of Raynaud's disease in the general population is unknown, but the gender ratio is 4 or 5 to 1 female to male, and most

TABLE 22–3. Factors in Differential Diagnosis of Peripheral Vascular Disease

Factor	Arteriosclerosis Obliterans	Thromboangiitis Obliterans	Raynaud's Phenomenon
Gender distribution	Predominantly male	98% male	90% female
Age at onset of symptoms	Usually over 50 yr Earlier in diabetes	<35 yr	Usually 11–45 yr
Symmetry	Often asymmetrical	Generally asymmetrical	Symmetrical
Onset	Insidious	Acute and preceded by migratory phlebitis (30–70%)	Often in cold climate and after stress
Intermittent claudication	Common	Common	Absent
Vasospasm	Not remarkable	Almost invariable in involved limb	Invariably symmetrical
Absent pulses	Infrequent in upper and common in lower extremities	Common in upper and lower extremities	Occurs only in late and extreme cases
Skin (if involved)	Thin, often hairless	Thin, atrophic, and red or cyanotic	Normal except during spasm
Ulcers (if any)	Dry and usually superficial	Moist, deep, inflamed, and invasive	Dry, fingertip
Plain radiograms	Calcification of artery	Normal	Often atrophy of phalanges
Cholesterol	High	Borderline	Normal
Presence of coronary or cerebral disease	Common	Rare early in disease	Coincidental

Modified from McCombs PR, Horwitz O. Diseases of the arteries of extremities. In: Horwitz O, McCombs PR, Roberts B, eds. Diseases of Blood Vessels. Philadelphia, Lea & Febiger, 1985:210–211.

cases occur prior to age 40 years (Table 22–3). Men with Raynaud's disease generally present at an older age and have a much higher incidence of associated atherosclerosis, which accounts for their symptoms when compared with women.

TABLE 22–4. Classification of Raynaud's Phenomenon

I. Primary Raynaud's syndrome or phenomenon—no known association or contributing condition
  A. Raynaud's disease
II. Secondary Raynaud's phenomenon
  A. After trauma—pneumatic hammer, pianists, typists
  B. Neurogenic lesions—carpal tunnel syndrome, thoracic outlet syndrome
  C. Occlusive arterial disease—ASO, TAO, thrombotic arterial occlusion
  D. Miscellaneous diseases and conditions
    1. Common causes—connective tissue diseases
    2. Uncommon causes—cryoproteinemias, polycythemia, vinyl chloride, hepatitis B antigenemia, hypothyroidism, renal disease
  E. Drugs
    1. β-Andrenergic receptor blocking drugs
    2. Ergot preparations
    3. Methysergide
    4. Vinblastine and bleomycin
    5. Amphetamines (?cocaine)
    6. Imipramine
    7. Bromocriptine
    8. Clonidine
    9. Cyclosporin

Modified from Coffman JD. Raynaud's phenomenon: An update. Hypertension 1991;17:593–602; and Spittell JA Jr. Raynaud's phenomenon and allied vasospastic disorders. In: Juergens JL, Spittell JA, Fairbairn F, eds. Peripheral Vascular Diseases. Philadelphia, Saunders, 1980:554–583.

One interesting group of patients with Raynaud's symptoms comprises those whose occupations involve routine use of vibratory equipment or frequent exposure to cold temperature. Between 40% and 90% of loggers and 50% of miners using vibratory equipment have been diagnosed with Raynaud's disease. Heredity also may play a role in the development of this disease.[80]

PATHOPHYSIOLOGY

The two theories of the cause of digital artery vasospasm in primary Raynaud's disease are an increased activity of the sympathetic nervous system and a local fault in the digital arteries.[76] Although several lines of evidence favoring increased sympathetic activity exist, evidence against this mechanism includes the facts that there is lack of increased cutaneous nervous system activity, that local cooling of one hand does not lead to reflex vasoconstriction in the opposite hand, and that normal plasma and urinary catecholamine concentrations are seen in primary Raynaud's disease. In contrast, the local fault theory is supported by the induction of vasospastic attacks in sympathetically denervated fingers, the induction of attacks in single fingers, an enhancement of reflex sympathetic vasoconstriction by local hand cooling, and a loss of digital systolic blood pressure with a local ischemia and cold stimulus. One of the mechanisms to explain these observations focuses on the activity of α_2-adrenergic receptors in patients with primary Raynaud's disease and the sensitivity of the receptor to cold exposure. Patients with primary Raynaud's disease have a greater sensitivity of the α_2-receptor with exposure to cold, and specific agonists and antagonists for α_1- and α_2-receptors point to altered α_2 activity as one of the defects in this syndrome. Reflex sympathetic stimulation also leads to greater S_2-sertonergic receptor activity even in the presence of α_1 and α_2 blockade, suggesting a pathophysiologic role for serotonin (5-hydroxytryptamine) in vasospasm of Raynaud's disease. Coffman has studied Raynaud's patients and could not document a role for sertontin in these patients.[81] It is still possible that serotonin is produced at the local level and contributes to the disease, but this remains to be further clarified. Young women with primary Raynaud's disease usually exhibit the purest form of vasospasm. These patients have lower digital, artery, and arteriolar systolic blood pressures than normal subjects.[82] Older male patients usually have secondary Raynaud's disease involving both a vasospastic and obstructive disease. In these patients, a normal vasoconstrictive stimulus acting on an arterial bed with reduced intraluminal pressure is sufficient to cause arterial closure. Initially these patients may demonstrate pure vasospasm, but later they develop obstruction as underlying autoimmune processes cause damage to the arterial wall.

Additional factors that may contribute to the pathogenetic mechanisms of Raynaud's disease include increased blood viscosity, platelet abnormalities, low systemic blood pressure, abnormal secretion of prostacyclin and thromboxane B_2, and abnormal endothelial function. Evidence does exist for increased factor VIII/von Willebrand factor antigen and factor activity along with elevated fibrinogen levels that promote hyperviscosity (especially in connective tissue disorders) and thrombosis, but the importance of these factors as well as the others described remains to be determined. An imbalance between endothelin-1 and calcitonin gene–related peptide may be responsible for the vasospastic phenomenon.[83]

CLINICAL PRESENTATION

Digital color changes are a common manifestation of this disease. A classic attack begins with a sudden loss of arterial blood flow, causing blanching. Next, a small quantity of blood enters the capillary and venous system and desaturates, and the digits become cyanotic. The third phase of the attack involves vasodilation, causing rubor. Not all patients exhibit a triphasic color change; many demonstrate only pallor or cyanosis, during which the digits turn absolutely white. At first, only the tips of the fingers of both hands are involved; later, the more proximal parts of the fingers are affected. In the late stage, the color change may extend back to involve the rest of the hands. Symptoms are worse in the cold season and less severe in warm weather. Pain is not a prominent symptom during the attack or in the interval between attacks. Paresthesias are common during the attack and consist of numbness, tingling, burning, or a feeling of tightness. Slight swelling of the involved fingers may occur, but only during attacks.

DIAGNOSIS

Primary Raynaud's disease usually includes the following features:

1. Vasospastic attack induced by cold exposure
2. Bilateral involvement of the extremities
3. Absence of gangrene or involvement of only the skin of the fingertips
4. History of symptoms for at least 2 years
5. No evidence of underlying disease, including absence of antinuclear antibodies, a normal erythrocyte sedimentation rate, and normal nailfold capillaroscopy and esophageal motility studies[82]

All patients should have a complete history and physical examination, with special emphasis on signs and symptoms of connective tissue disease. Routine laboratory tests should include a complete blood count; erythrocyte sedimentation rate; chemistry profile; determinations of antinuclear antibody, rheumatoid factor, and cryoglobulins; urinalysis; and hand radiography. Digital plethysmography (pulse volume recordings) often is used to follow the course of the disease or to evaluate the response to therapy. Digital systolic blood pressure and its response to cold stress and ischemia also have been used to aid in diagnosis. Hand arteriography sometimes may be used in assessing the relative roles of vasospastic and occlusive disease but is used rarely to establish a diagnosis.

▶ TREATMENT: Raynaud's Disease[76,78,84]

Conservative measures will suffice for the majority of patients with primary or secondary Raynaud's disease. General considerations for treatment include avoidance of cold temperatures, tobacco, emotional situations, and certain drugs (Table 22–4). These patients should dress warmly, wear lined gloves, and use Styrofoam coasters when handling iced drinks. Large meals and long periods of standing should be avoided because they both reduce peripheral circulation.

Therapy for Raynaud's disease is aimed at increasing digital blood flow and consists of behavioral therapy or biofeedback and drug therapy. Temperature biofeedback was not better than its control treatment and was inferior to sustained-release nifedipine for treating primary Raynaud's phenomenon in one large trial.[85] The goal with these techniques is to self-regulate the nervous system and reduce vasoconstrictive autonomic tone. When attacks interfere with a patient's ability to function normally, drug therapy should be tried. Drug therapy is associated with significant adverse effects, and objective changes in blood flow do not always correlate with symptom improvement. In addition, only about two-thirds of patients can be expected to respond to drug therapy.

Drug therapy for Raynaud's disease is directed toward vasodilation and involves several classes of drugs toward this end, including sympatholytics, α-adrenergic antagonists, direct-acting vasodilators, calcium channel antagonists, serotonin receptor antagonists, angiotensin-converting enzyme inhibitors, prostaglandins, and thyroid hormones.

SYMPATHOLYTIC AGENTS[86]

Reserpine and other drugs have been used for years in the treatment of Raynaud's disease; unfortunately, there are few controlled trials with these agents to suggest that any benefit is derived from their use. Reserpine in oral doses of 0.25–0.75 mg daily may increase capillary blood flow in short-term studies, but long-term improvement is doubtful. Reserpine in higher doses causes several unpleasant adverse effects, including nasal congestion, bradycardia, postural hypotension, dyspepsia, fluid retention, lethargy, and depression. Intraarterial reserpine has been shown to be no better than placebo. Guanethidine in doses of 10–50 mg daily produces postural hypotension, explosive diarrhea, fatigue, and impotence and generally is not well tolerated. It may increase capillary blood flow during cooling in patients with Raynaud's disease resulting from scleroderma. Methyldopa has been shown to offer subjective improvement in uncontrolled studies, but no objective benefit has been observed in comparisons with other drugs. Adverse effects seen with methyldopa include drowsiness, headache, dry mouth, postural hypotension, nasal congestion, edema, and diarrhea.

α-ADRENERGIC ANTAGONISTS[87]

Prazosin and terazosin have been studied in Raynaud's disease, but the trials have mixed results. Although prazosin produces about a 60% response rate, larger doses of prazosin lead to an unacceptable number of adverse effects, and a dose of 1 mg three times a day is best tolerated and improves symptoms, finger skin blood flow, and temperature. The early response to prazosin may dissipate in a few weeks, and increasing to maximum tolerated doses leads to multiple adverse effects such as headache, dizziness, fatigue, edema, dyspnea, rash, or diarrhea.

Other nonselective α-adrenergic antagonists such as phentolamine and phenoxybenzamine provide inconsistent improvement in blood flow and symptoms. Their use is further limited by difficulties in oral dosing as well as frequent and bothersome adverse effects. Intraarterial phentolamine infused at 50 150 g/min or as a single brachial artery injection of 0.05–10 mg improves finger blood flow, digital pulse volume amplitude, and forearm blood flow, and this route is useful for unrelenting vasospasm and ischemia when the sympathetic nervous system is the cause.[88]

DIRECT-ACTING VASODILATORS

Nitroglycerin, nitroprusside, niacin and its derivatives, papaverine, isoxsuprine, griseofulvin, cyclandelate, and hydralazine fall into this category. With the exception of nitroglycerin, none of these agents can be recommended because of the lack of controlled studies to support their use and the frequency of adverse effects. Nitroglycerin ointment usually improves the symptoms, and at times, objective measures of effectiveness have been shown in patients with primary and secondary Raynaud's disease. Nitroglycerin transdermal patches reduced the number and severity of attacks, but headache symptoms limited patient acceptance.[89] Headaches, dizziness, and postural hypotension are the most frequent reasons for failure with nitroglycerin.

CALCIUM CHANNEL ANTAGONISTS

Numerous studies with calcium channel antagonists, particularly nifedipine, have been performed in patients with Raynaud's disease. As the name implies, these drugs block the entry of calcium ions through the slow channel that reduces the availability of cytosolic calcium and decreases smooth muscle contractility. Additionally, they may inhibit vascular responses evoked by α_2-adrenergic receptors, which are activated predominantly during reflex sympathetic stimulation of body cooling. Subjective and objective improvements have been demonstrated with drugs in this category. Table 22–5 summarizes clinical trials of calcium channel antagonists for Raynaud's disease. Nifedipine is more effective in primary Raynaud's disease, and its effects are more pronounced early in therapy. Chronic therapy may result in loss of response, as determined by objective measures and reported by Gush and Wollersheim (see Table 22–5). Nifedipine also may be used as prophylactic therapy prior to cold exposure.

Newer calcium blockers such as nicardipine, isradipine, and nisoldipine also have been used with varying degrees of success for Raynaud's disease. Nicardipine provides subjective improvement in about half of patients receiving it, and the frequency and severity of attacks are reduced significantly with its use. It is more effective in primary Raynaud's disease than in secondary disease, and subjective symptomatic improvement is seen more often than objective improvement. Other studies (also see Table 22–5) have shown no benefit, either subjective or objective, from nicardipine, even though the drug was shown to inhibit platelet aggregation. Nifedipine was compared with misoprostol 200 μg every 12 hours for 10 days, and both drugs caused similar effects on attack severity and blood flow[90] (see Table 22–5).

SEROTONIN RECEPTOR ANTAGONISTS

Serotonin (5-hydroxytryptamine, or 5-HT) has been shown to induce vasospasm and platelet aggregation in animals and humans through the 5-HT_2 receptor. Ketanserin is a selective antagonist of the 5-HT_2 receptor, and it also may have some α_1-adrenoreceptor blocking activity. It increases finger blood flow with intraarterial and intravenous injection during sympathetic vasoconstriction induced by body cooling, and its effects are evident in the presence of α blockade.[91] The largest study ($N = 222$) with oral use found that ketanserin (40 mg three times a day) decreased the duration and frequency of attacks (34% reduction versus 18%) and was preferred by both patients and investigators over placebo.[92,93] About 50% to 70% of the patients experienced subjective mild to moderate improvement. Ketanserin had no effect on total finger blood flow in warm or cold environments. There was no difference in response between primary and secondary Raynaud's disease. Headache, asthenia, dizziness, and gastrointestinal complaints were the most common symptoms seen with ketanserin; respiratory infections also were more common with ketanserin than with placebo. Ketanserin also may prolong the QT interval, and it should be used cautiously in patients with hypokalemia, second- or third-degree heart block, ventricular arrhythmias, and prolonged QT interval at baseline or in combination with potassium-losing diuretics or antiarrhythmics.[59] Part of the variability in response to ketanserin may be due to the frequency in dosing, since some evidence exists that its effects on platelet aggregation are minimal at 12 hours after dosing.

ANGIOTENSIN-CONVERTING ENZYME INHIBITORS/ANGIOTENSIN RECEPTOR BLOCKADE[94]

The proposed mechanism for improvement of Raynaud's disease with angiotensin-converting enzyme (ACE) inhibitors is the inhibition of the breakdown of bradykinin and vasodilation resulting from its accumulation. Early studies showed improved blood flow and some improvement in symptoms. Double-blinded, placebo-controlled trials have not documented any improvement with enalapril 20 mg/d, and since up to one-third of patients with PVD have renal artery stenosis, ACE inhibitors would be a logical choice.[95] Losartan (50 mg/d), an angiotensin receptor blocker, has been compared with nifedipine (40 mg/d) in primary and secondary Raynaud's phenomenon, and

TABLE 22–5. Effect of Calcium Channel Antagonists in the Treatment of Raynaud's Disease

Reference	No. Patients	Study Duration (wk)	Additional Assessment	Results
Nifedipine				
Aldoori et al. Cardiovasc Res 1986;20:446	30p + 10s	3	Digital blood flow	9/13 patients had improved clinical symptoms
Belcaro et al. Panminerva Med 1987;29:223	34p	3	Digital blood flow	N improved digital blood flow
Challenor et al. Angiology 1989;40:122	22	3	Vibrotactile thresholds	40% reduction in mean number of attacks; better response at lower thresholds
Corbin et al. Eur Heart J 1986;7:165	23p	4	Digital blood pressure	N significantly reduced the number of attacks
Finch et al. Clin Rheum 1986;5:493	16s	4	Digital blood pressure	N produced "better" clinical results than placebo
Fisher et al. Zeit Kardiol 1985;74:298	6 PAH		Hemodynamic testing	Raynaud's patients more responsive to nifedipine than other PAH patients
Gjorup et al. Am Heart J 1986;3:742	19p	4		N significantly reduced frequency of attacks and attack severity
Gush et al. J Cardiovasc Pharmocol 1987;9:628	9p	5 d	Peripheral blood flow	Tendency for N to offer some protection against reductions in blood flow
Hawkins et al. Rheum Int 1986;6:85	20p + 37s	3	Mitogenic activity	Overall, N reduced both frequency and severity of attacks, but large individual variations in response. N inhibited mitogen-induced lymphocyte proliferation but only in patients who responded to the drug clinically
Kallenberg et al. J Rheum 1987;14:284	8p + 8s	4	Digital blood flow	N reduced frequency and severity of attacks and improved digital blood flow
Lewis et al. Eur Heart J 1987;8 (suppl): 83	20	OD	Radial artery blood flow	N prevented reduction in blood flow by cooling
Meyrick et al. Br J Derm 1987;117:237	10	6	Digital blood flow	Reduction in number and severity of attacks but no change in blood flow or red blood cell deformability or white blood cell CL
Nilsson et al. Acta Med Scand 1987;221:53	28p	2	Digital blood pressure	17 patients showed symptomatic improvement with N versus 5 with placebo; digital blood pressure improved significantly with N
Riccio et al. Clin Ther 1987;9:232	6p + 7s	5 d	Thermography	More marked increases of hand tissue temperature in patients with secondary disease (progressive systemic sclerosis) than primary disease
Sarkozi et al. J Rheum 1986;13:331	39p	10		N significantly reduced frequency and severity of attacks compared with placebo
Waller et al. Br J Clin Pharm 1986;22:449	34p	4	Rheology	N produced a 25% reduction in mean number of attacks; no difference versus placebo in red cell deformability
White et al. Am J Med 1986;80:623	6p + 5s	1	Digital skin temperature recovery time	9/11 patients reported symptomatic improvement; N significantly improved skin temperature recovery time
Wollersheim. J Clin Pharmacol 1987;27:907	16	4	Digital blood flow	Open label, no correlation between sublingual acute use and oral long term; lack of objective long-term benefit
Dompeling and Smit. Vasa Suppl 1992;34:34–37	14p	1d	Photoelectric plethysmography	Single-dose study; N better than placebo and a potassium channel opener, pinacidil
Varela-Aguila. Rev Clin Esp 1997;197:77	20s	10d	Doppler duplex	
Diltiazem				
Da Costa et al. J Rheumatol 1987;14:858–859	1p + 14s	4	Digital rheology	No difference in vasospastic attacks or rheology
Nicardipine				
French Cooperative Multicenter Group. Am Heart J 1991;122:352–355	69p		Symptomatic	Double-blind, placebo-controlled study; 21% symptomatic improvement; no improvement in cold-reactive hyperemia test
Ferri et al. Clin Rheumatol 1992; 11(1):76–80	21p + s	3	Peak flow after postischemic reactive hyperanemia	18/21 completed study; subjective improvement noted with fewer episodes and improved hand disability score

TABLE 22–5. Effect of Calcium Channel Antagonists in the Treatment of Raynaud's Disease (*cont.*)

Reference	No. Patients	Study Duration (wk)	Additional Assessment	Results
Wollersheim et al. J Cardiovasc Pharmacol 1991;18:813–818	16p + 9s	3	Finger skin temperature and laser Doppler flux	Double-blind, placebo-controlled study; NS between nicardipine and placebo for number, duration, or severity of vasospastic attacks or for any of the microcirculatory parameters
Felodipine				
Kallenberg et al. Eur J Clin Pharmacol 1991;40:313–315	10p	6	Symptomatic and finger plethysmography	Single blind; subjective improvement in the number and intensity of attacks; blood flow improved only at certain temperatures
Flunarizine				
Centonze et al. Clin Ter 1991;137:77–82	28	4	Symptomatic	Flunarizine caused NS clinical improvement; adverse effects were common

p = primary Raynaud's disease; s = secondary Raynaud's disease; N = nifedipine; PAH = pulmonary arterial hypertension; CL = clearance; OD = one dose; NS = not significant.

losartan provided a greater reduction in number and severity of episodes.[96]

PROSTANOIDS

Prostacyclin, iloprost, and prostaglandins E_1 and E_2 have been studied in Raynaud's disease because of their properties of vasodilation and inhibition of platelet aggregation. Intravenous prostacyclin analogs and oral analogs such as beraprost and iloprost improve blood flow and walking distance acutely but do not seem to have benefit long term.[97–99] An intravenous prodrug of prostaglandin E_1 (AS-013) incorporated into lipid microspheres provides modest improvement (24–28 m) in walking distance for up to 8 weeks in early trials.[100]

THYROID HORMONES

Triiodothyronine (T_3) 80 μg/d has been shown in one small ($N = 18$) double-blind, controlled crossover trial to reduce the frequency, duration, and severity of attacks as well as increase skin temperatures and promote ulcer healing.[101] The proposed mechanisms for this effect are activation of heat-dissipating mechanisms and enhanced β_2-adrenoreceptor activity in vascular smooth muscle. T_3 significantly elevated T_3 and T_4 concentrations and reduced thyroid-stimulating hormone concentrations to less than 0.1 mIU/L in 14 of 18 patients. Palpitations, headaches, and weight loss were reported by about one-third of patients. The overall attack rate reduction was approximately 75%, somewhat higher than that reported for other types of treatment. The authors suggest follow-up studies using a lower dose of 60 μg/d of T_3 to minimize adverse effects and chemical hyperthyroidism. Other case reports suggest similar findings.[102]

Other approaches to therapy have included β-adrenergic blocking agents and pentoxiphylline. Atenolol and/or nifedipine had no effect on walking distance or foot temperature.[103] Pentoxifylline, in a study of 11 patients, was reported to improve symptoms in 7 patients and to improve red cell filtration.[104] Improved skin temperatures to cold challenge have been noted with pentoxiphylline as well.[78]

Calcitonin gene-related peptide is an endogenous vasodilator that seems to be specific for skin blood flow, and it may be deficient in Raynaud's disease.[105] Trials giving this substance intravenously for up to 5 days have shown improved hand warming and skin temperature, improved hand and digital blood flow, and ulcer healing in small groups of patients, and it seems to be better tolerated than prostacyclin. Another drug with some promise is piracetam, an antiplatelet agent that also increases the synthesis of prostaglandin I_2.[106]

EVALUATION OF THERAPEUTIC OUTCOMES

Drug therapy responses in peripheral vascular disease may be evaluated using patient symptoms, presence or absence of peripheral pulses at various sites, the ABI, exercise capacity, angiographic documentation of improved flow, and the need for subsequent procedures and surgery. Using the Fontaine classification system (see Table 22–2) or other rating scales that are available,[1,69] semiquantitative assessments of symptomatic clinical improvement can be obtained, and for example, a patient might move from class IIb to class IIa or I as a measure of improvement following pharmacotherapeutic or interventional therapy. The ABI provides an estimate of the restoration of blood flow to an extremity, and this index can be obtained easily by measuring blood pressures at different points of the circulatory system. Exercise capacity can be evaluated using the Fontaine classification or through other estimates made by the patient or clinician of exercise duration or effort. This could be expressed as the time to cover a set distance (e.g., one block) or the total amount of distance covered without a time restriction. Angiographic studies to document improved blood flow usually are not necessary and are used more often for research purposes to objectively assess outcome of some intervention. The need for a revascularization procedure as primary or secondary intervention or the need for vascular surgery after pharmacotherapy or interventional technologies also could be used as an outcome measure. This would be more important for groups of patients than for individual patients, but the need for revascularization certainly would suggest failure of the primary mode of therapy.

Symptom remission is the primary method of evaluating therapy for Raynaud's disease. Digital plethysmography and finger blood pressure would be used for a more objective method of assessment or for research purposes. Patients with TAO should be evaluated for symptom response, but smoking cessation is important as well. This may be evaluated through history, but more a objective means would be serum cotinine concentrations.

▶ PRINCIPLES OF PHARMACOTHERAPY

- All patients 55 years of age and older should have pedal pulses evaluated, and if they are nonpalpable, the ABI or other examination should be used to evaluate the patient for arterial insufficiency.
- The cornerstone of therapy for arterial insufficiency is risk-factor modification, including an exercise program, smoking cessation, and diabetic, hypertension, and dyslipidemia management.
- Aspirin 80–325 mg/d should be given to most patients with PVD to reduce the risk of future cardiovascular events (i.e., stroke, myocardial infarction, or vascular death); aspirin does not affect the development of atherosclerosis.
- Pentoxifylline is not recommended for intermittent claudication because the trial results are inconsistent and show only marginal benefit over exercise alone. Cilostazol has been shown to provide mild to moderate symptomatic improvement.
- PTA and surgery are effective treatments for intermittent claudication and are recommended after an adequate trial of nonoperative therapy.
- Intraarterial thrombolytic therapy is recommended for acute thrombotic or embolic occlusion of a native artery or prosthetic graft and may delay or prevent vascular surgery. No particular agent has documented superiority.
- Conservative management of Raynaud's disease, including avoidance of cold, emotion stress, tobacco and certain drugs, should be tried before trials of drug therapy.
- Calcium channnel blockers, in particular nifedipine, are the best-studied form of pharmacotherapy for Raynaud's disease, and they provide at least symptomatic relief; evidence for efficacy with other vasodilating drugs (e.g., nitroglycerin) is available in a limited number of studies.
- Although still under investigation, ketanserin, a serotonin antagonist, improves the symptoms of Raynaud's disease.
- Other approaches for Raynaud's disease such as prostacyclin and its analogues, thyroid hormones, and calcitonin gene-related protein are under development.

REFERENCES

1. Weitz JI, Byrne J, Clagett GP, et al. Diagnosis and treatment of chronic arterial insufficiency of the lower extremities: A critical review. Circulation 1996;94:3026–3049.
2. Hiatt WR. Medical treatment of peripheral arterial disease and claudication. N Engl J Med 2001;344:1608–1621.
3. Clement DL, Shepherd JT. Vascular Diseases in the Limbs: Mechanisms and Principles of Treatment. St. Louis, Mosby–Year Book, 1993:1–219.
4. Young JR, Olin JW, Bartholomew JR. Peripheral Vascular Disease. St. Louis, Mosby–Year Book, 1996:1–752.
5. Loscalzo J, Creager MA, Dzau VJ. Vascular Medicine: A Textbook of Vascular Biology and Diseases. Boston, Little, Brown, 1996:1–1312.
6. Anonymous. Management of peripheral arterial disease (PAD). Trans-Atlantic Inter-Society Consensus (TASC). Section B: Intermittent claudication. Eur J Vasc Endovasc Surg 2000;19:S47–S114.
7. Lie JR. The structure of the normal vascular system and its reactive changes. In: Juergens JL, Spittell JA, Fairbairn JF, eds. Peripheral Vascular Diseases. Philadelphia, Saunders, 1980:51–81.
8. Bell DM, Johns TE, Lopez LM. Endothelial dysfunction: Implications for therapy of cardiovascular diseases. Ann Pharmacother 1998;32: 459–470.
9. Newby DE, Flint LL, Fox KA, et al. Reduced responsiveness to endothelin-1 in peripheral resistance vessels of patients with syndrome X. J Am Coll Cardiol 1998;31:1585–1590.
10. Schellong SM, Boger RH, Burchert W, et al. Dose-related effect of intravenous L-arginine on muscular blood flow of the calf in patients with peripheral vascular disease: A H215O positron emission tomography study. Clin Sci 1997;93:159–165.
11. Coffman JD. Effects of endothelium-derived nitric oxide on skin and digital blood flow in humans. Am J Physiol 1994;267:H2087–H2090.
12. Berkenboom G, Crasset V, Giot C, et al. Endothelial function of internal mammary artery in patients with coronary artery disease and in cardiac transplant recipients. Am Heart J 1998;135:488–494.
13. Curb JD, Masaki K, Rodriguez BL, et al. Peripheral artery disease and cardiovascular risk factors in the elderly. The Honolulu Heart Program. Arterioscler Thromb Vasc Biol 1996;16:1495–1500.
14. Violi F, Criqui M, Longoni A, Castiglioni C. Relation between risk factors and cardiovascular complications in patients with peripheral vascular disease: Results from the ADEP study. Atherosclerosis 1996;120: 25–35.
15. Nukada H, van Rij AM, Packer SG, Patterson A. Preservation of skin vasoconstrictor responses in chronic atherosclerotic peripheral vascular disease. Angiology 1998;49:181–188.
16. Ouriel KE. Lower Extremity Vascular Disease. Philadelphia, Saunders, 1995:1–440.
17. Gerhard M, Baum P, Raby KE. Peripheral arterial-vascular disease in women: Prevalence, prognosis, and treatment. Cardiology 1995;86: 349–355.
18. Shepherd JT, Bergan JJ, Cohen RA, et al. Report of the Task Force on Vascular Medicine. Circulation 1994;89:532–535.
19. Fowkes FG, Housley E, Cawood EH, et al. Edinburgh Artery Study: Prevalence of asymptomatic and symptomatic peripheral arterial disease in the general population. Int J Epidemiol 1991;20:384–392.
20. Rihal CS, Eagle KA, Mickel MC, et al. Surgical therapy for coronary artery disease among patients with combined coronary artery and peripheral vascular disease. Circulation 1995;91:46–53.
21. Criqui MH, Denenberg JO, Langer RD, Fronek A. The epidemiology of peripheral arterial disease: Importance of identifying the population at risk. Vasc Med 1997;2:221–226.
22. Newman AB, Naydeck BL, Sutton–Tyrrell K, et al., Cardiovascular Health Study Research Group. The role of comorbidity in the assessment of intermittent claudication in older adults. J Clin Epidemiol 2001;54:294–300.
23. Newman AB, Tyrrell KS, Kuller LH. Mortality over four years in SHEP participants with a low ankle-arm index. J Am Geriatr Soc 1997;45:1472–1478.
24. Montgomery PS, Gardner AW. The clinical utility of a six-minute walk test in peripheral arterial occlusive disease patients. J Am Geriatr Soc 1998;46:706–711.
25. Androulakis AE, Giannoukas AD, Labropoulos N, et al. The impact of duplex scanning on vascular practice. Int Angiol 1996;15:283–290.
26. de Vries SO, Hunink MG, Polak JF. Summary receiver operating characteristic curves as a technique for meta-analysis of the diagnostic performance of duplex ultrasonography in peripheral arterial disease. Acad Radiol 1996;3:361–369.
27. Dormandy JA, Rutherford RB. Management of peripheral arterial disease (PAD). TASC Working Group, Trans-Atlantic Inter-Society Concensus (TASC). J Vasc Surg 2000;31:S1–S296.

28. Kroon AA, van Asten WN, Stalenhoef AF. Effect of apheresis of low-density lipoprotein on peripheral vascular disease in hypercholesterolemic patients with coronary artery disease. Ann Intern Med 1996;125:945–954.
29. Gardner AW, Katzel LI, Sorkin JD, et al. Improved functional outcomes following exercise rehabilitation in patients with intermittent claudication. J Gerontol [A] 2000;55:M570–M577.
30. Regensteiner JG, Gardner A, Hiatt WR. Exercise testing and exercise rehabilitation for patients with peripheral arterial disease: Status in 1997. Vasc Med 1997;2:147–155.
31. Tan KH, De Cossart L, Edwards PR. Exercise training and peripheral vascular disease. Br J Surg 2000;87:553–562.
32. Tan KH, Cotterrell D, Sykes K, et al. Exercise training for claudicants: Changes in blood flow, cardiorespiratory status, metabolic functions, blood rheology and lipid profile. Eur J Vasc Endovasc Surg 2000;20: 72–78.
33. Smith I, Franks PJ, Greenhalgh RM, et al. The influence of smoking cessation and hypertriglyceridaemia on the progression of peripheral arterial disease and the onset of critical ischaemia. Eur J Vasc Endovasc Surg 1996;11:402–408.
34. Radack K, Deck C. Beta-adrenergic blocker therapy does not worsen intermittent claudication in subjects with peripheral arterial disease: A meta-analysis of randomized controlled trials. Arch Intern Med 1991, 151:1769–1776.
35. Girolami B, Bernardi E, Prins MH, et al. Treatment of intermittent claudication with physical training, smoking cessation, pentoxifylline, or nafronyl: A meta-analysis. Arch Intern Med 1999;159:337–345.
36. Moher D, Pham B, Ausejo M, et al. Pharmacological management of intermittent claudication: A meta-analysis of randomised trials. Drugs 2000;59:1057–1070.
37. Currie MS, Simel DL, Christenson RH, et al. Anti-inflammatory effects of pentoxifylline in claudication. Am J Med Sci 1991;301:85–90.
38. Lindgarde F, Labs KH, Rossner M. The pentoxifylline experience: Exercise testing reconsidered. Vasc Med 1996;1:145–154.
39. AbuRahma AF, Woodruff BA. Effects and limitations of pentoxifylline therapy in various stages of peripheral vascular disease of the lower extremity. Am J Surg 1990;160:266–270.
40. Anonymous. Intravenous pentoxifylline for the treatment of chronic critical limb ischaemia. The European Study Group. Eur J Vasc Endovasc Surg 1995;9:426–436.
41. Lindblad B, Wakefield TW, Stanley TJ, et al. Pharmacological prophylaxis against postoperative graft occlusion after peripheral vascular surgery: A world-wide survey. Eur J Vasc Endovasc Surg 1995;9: 267–271.
42. Stergachis D, Sheingold S, Luce BR, et al. Medical care and cost outcomes after pentoxifylline for peripheral arterial disease. Arch Intern Med 1992;152:1220–1224.
43. West JA. Cost-effective strategies for the management of vascular disease. Vasc Med 1997;2:25–29.
44. Hirsch AT, Treat-Jacobson D, Lando HA, Hatsukami DK. The role of tobacco cessation, antiplatelet and lipid-lowering therapies in the treatment of peripheral arterial disease. Vasc Med 1997;2:243–251.
45. Goldhaber SZ, Manson JE, Stampfer MJ, et al. Low-dose aspirin and subsequent peripheral arterial surgery in the Physicians' Health Study. Lancet 1992;340:143–145.
46. Jackson MR, Clagett GP. Antithrombotic therapy in peripheral arterial occulsive disease. Chest 2001;119:283S–299S.
47. Fagher B. Long-term effects of ticlopidine on lower limb blood flow, ankle/brachial index and symptoms in peripheral arteriosclerosis: A double-blind study. The STIMS Group in Lund, Swedish Ticlopidine Multicenter Study. Angiology 1994;45:777–788.
48. Blanchard J, Carreras LO, Kindermans M. Results of EMATAP: A double-blind placebo-controlled multicentre trial of ticlopidine in patients with peripheral arterial disease. Nouv Rev Franc Hematol 1994;35:523–528.
49. Becquemin JP. Effect of ticlopidine on the long-term patency of saphenous-vein bypass grafts in the legs. Etude de la Ticlopidine apres Pontage Femoro-Poplite and the Association Universitaire de Recherche en Chirurgie. N Engl J Med 1997;337:1726–1731.
50. Anonymous. A randomised, blinded trial of clopidogrel versus aspirin in patients at risk of ischaemic events (CAPRIE). CAPRIE Steering Committee. Lancet 1996;348:1329–1339.
51. Harker LA, Boissel JP, Pilgrim AJ, Gent M. Comparative safety and tolerability of clopidogrel and aspirin: Results from CAPRIE. CAPRIE Steering Committee and Investigators (Clopidogrel versus Aspirin in Patients at Risk of Ischaemic Events). Drug Saf 1999;21:325–335.
52. Anonymous. Two randomised and placebo-controlled studies of an oral prostacyclin analogue (Iloprost) in severe leg ischaemia. The Oral Iloprost in severe Leg Ischaemia Study Group. Eur J Vasc Endovasc Surg 2000;20:358–362.
53. Reilly MP, Mohler ER 3d. Cilostazol: treatment of intermittent claudication. Ann Pharmacother 2001;35:48–56.
54. Bramer SL, Forbes WP, Mallikaarjun S. Cilostazol pharmacokinetics after single and multiple oral doses in healthy males and patients with intermittent claudication resulting from peripheral arterial disease. Clin Pharmacokinet 1999;37:1–11.
55. Dawson DL, Cutler BS, Hiatt WR, et al. A comparison of cilostazol and pentoxifylline for treating intermittent claudication. Am J Med 2000;109:523–530.
56. Schachter M. Calcium antagonists and atherosclerosis. Int J Cardiol 1997;62:S9–S15.
57. Pitt B, Byington RP, Furberg CD, et al. Effect of amlodipine on the progression of atherosclerosis and the occurrence of clinical events. PREVENT Investigators. Circulation 2000;102:1503–1510.
58. Violi F, Marubini E, Coccheri S, Nenci GG. Improvement of walking distance by defibrotide in patients with intermittent claudication: Results of a randomized, placebo-controlled study (the DICLIS Study). Thromb Haemost 2000;83:672–677.
59. Verstraete M. The PACK trial: Morbidity and mortality effects of ketanserin (Prevention of Atherosclerotic Complications). Vas Med 1996;1:135–140.
60. Brevetti G, Diehm C, Lambert D. European multicenter study on propionyl-L-carnitine in intermittent claudication. J Am Coll Cardiol 1999;34:1618–1624.
61. Ouriel K, Veith FJ, Sasahara AA. A comparison of recombinant urokinase with vascular surgery as initial treatment for acute arterial occlusion of the legs. Thrombolysis or Peripheral Arterial Surgery (TOPAS) Investigators. N Engl J Med 1998;338:1105–1111.
62. Ouriel K, Veith FJ. Acute lower limb ischemia: Determinants of outcome. Surgery 1998;124:336–341; discussion, 341–342.
63. Patel ST, Haser PB, Bush HL Jr, Kent KC. Is thrombolysis of lower extremity acute arterial occlusion cost-effective? J Surg Res 1999;83: 106–112.
64. Hunink MG, Wong JB, Donaldson MC, et al. Revascularization for femoropopliteal disease: A decision and cost-effectiveness analysis. JAMA 1995;274:165–171.
65. Singh S, Evans L, Datta D, et al. The costs of managing lower limb-threatening ischaemia. Eur J Vasc Endovas Surg 1996;12:359–362.
66. Cejna M, Thurnher S, Illiasch H, et al. PTA versus Palmaz stent placement in femoropopliteal artery obstructions: A multicenter prospective randomized study. J Vasc Intervent Radiol 2001;12:23–31.
67. Minar E, Pokrajac B, Maca T, et al. Endovascular brachytherapy for prophylaxis of restenosis after femoropopliteal angioplasty: Results of a prospective, randomized study. Circulation 2000;102:2694–2699.
68. Rosenfield K, Schainfeld R, Isner JM. Percutaneous revascularization in peripheral arterial disease. Curr Prob Cardiol 1996;21:7–93.
69. Pentecost MJ, Criqui MH, Dorros G, et al. Guidelines for peripheral percutaneous transluminal angioplasty of the abdominal aorta and lower extremity vessels: A statement for health professionals from a special writing group of the Councils on Cardiovascular Radiology, Arteriosclerosis, Cardio-Thoracic and Vascular Surgery, Clinical Cardiology, and Epidemiology and Prevention, the American Heart Association. Circulation 1994;89:511–531.
70. Schweizer J, Kirch W, Koch R, et al. Short- and long-term results of abciximab versus aspirin in conjunction with thrombolysis for patients with

peripheral occlusive arterial disease and arterial thrombosis. Angiology 2000;51:913–923.

71. Minar E, Ahmadi A, Koppensteiner R, et al. Comparison of effects of high-dose and low-dose aspirin on restenosis after femoropopliteal percutaneous transluminal angioplasty. Circulation 1995;91:2167–2173.
72. Isner JM, Walsh K, Symes J, et al. Arterial gene therapy for therapeutic angiogenesis in patients with peripheral artery disease. Circulation 1995;91:2687–2692.
73. Gleim M, Maier C, Melchert U. Lumbar neurolytic sympathetic blockades provide immediate and long-lasting improvement of painless walking distance and muscle metabolism in patients with severe peripheral vascular disease. J Pain Sympt Manage 1995;10:98–104.
74. Olin JW. Thromboangiitis obliterans (Buerger's disease). N Engl J Med 2000;343:864–869.
75. Anonymous. Oral iloprost in the treatment of thromboangiitis obliterans (Buerger's disease): A double-blind, randomised, placebo-controlled trial. The European TAO Study Group. Eur J Vasc Endovasc Surg 1998;15:300–307.
76. Cerinic MM, Generini S, Pignone A. New approaches to the treatment of Raynaud's phenomenon. Curr Opin Rheumatol 1997;9:544–556.
77. Ho M, Belch JJ. Raynaud's phenomenon: State of the art 1998. Scand J Rheumatol 1998;27:319–322.
78. Belch JJ, Ho M. Pharmacotherapy of Raynaud's phenomenon. Drugs 1996;52:682–695.
79. Belch J. Raynaud's phenomenon. Cardiovasc Res 1997;33:25–30.
80. Chetter IC, Kent PJ, Kester RC. The hand arm vibration syndrome: A review. Cardiovasc Surg 1998;6:1–9.
81. Coffman JD, Cohen RA. Plasma levels of 5-hydroxytryptamine during sympathetic stimulation and in Raynaud's phenomenon. Clin Sci 1994;86:269–273.
82. Coffman JD. Raynaud's phenomenon: An update. Hypertension 1991;17:593–602.
83. Noel B. Pathophysiology and classification of the vibration white finger. Int Arch Occup Environ Health 2000;73:150–155.
84. Wigley FM, Flavahan NA. Raynaud's phenomenon. Rheum Dis Clin North Am 1996;22:765–781.
85. Anonymous. Comparison of sustained-release nifedipine and temperature biofeedback for treatment of primary Raynaud phenomenon: Results from a randomized clinical trial with 1-year follow-up. Arch Int Med 2000;160:1101–1108.
86. Coffman JD. Pathogenesis and treatment of Raynaud's phenomenon. Cardiovasc Drugs Ther 1990;4:45–51.
87. Pope J, Fenlon D, Thompson A, et al. Prazosin for Raynaud's phenomenon in progressive systemic sclerosis. Cochrane Database of Systematic Reviews (computer file) 2000:CD000956.
88. Sylaidis P, Logan A. Local injection of phentolamine to treat digital ischaemic necrosis in Raynaud's syndrome. J Wound Care 1997;6: 356–357.
89. Teh LS, Manning J, Moore T, et al. Sustained-release transdermal glyceryl trinitrate patches as a treatment for primary and secondary Raynaud's phenomenon. Br J Rheumatol 1995;34:636–641.
90. Varela-Aguilar JM, Sanchez-Roman J, Talegon Melendez A, Castillo Palma MJ. Comparative study of misoprostol and nifedipine in the treatment of Raynaud's phenomenon secondary to systemic diseases: Hemodynamic assessment with Doppler duplex. Rev Clin Espanola 1997;197:77–83.
91. Frishman WH, Huberfeld S, Okin S, et al. Serotonin and serotonin antagonism in cardiovascular and noncardiovascular disease. J Clin Pharmacol 1995;35:541–572.
92. Coffman JD, Clement DL, Creager MA, et al. International study of ketanserin in Raynaud's phenomenon. Am J Med 1989;87:264–268.
93. Pope J, Fenlon D, Thompson A, et al. Ketanserin for Raynaud's phenomenon in progressive systemic sclerosis. Cochrane Database of Systematic Reviews (computer file) 2000:CD000954.
94. Challenor VF. Angiotensin converting enzyme inhibitors in Raynaud's phenomenon. Drugs 1994;48:864–867.
95. Wachtell K, Ibsen H, Olsen MH, et al. Prevalence of renal artery stenosis in patients with peripheral vascular disease and hypertension. J Hum Hypertens 1996;10:83–85.
96. Dziadzio M, Denton CP, Smith R, et al. Losartan therapy for Raynaud's phenomenon and scleroderma: Clinical and biochemical findings in a fifteen-week, randomized, parallel-group, controlled trial. Arthritis Rheum 1999;42:2646–2655.
97. Belch JJ, Capell HA, Cooke ED, et al. Oral iloprost as a treatment for Raynaud's syndrome: A double-blind multicentre placebo controlled study. Ann Rheum Dis 1995;54:197–200.
98. Vayssairat M. Controlled multicenter double blind trial of an oral analog of prostacyclin in the treatment of primary Raynaud's phenomenon. French Microcirculation Society Multicentre Group for the Study of Vascular Acrosyndromes. J Rheumatol 1996;23:1917–1920.
99. Pope J, Fenlon D, Thompson A, et al. Iloprost and cisaprost for Raynaud's phenomenon in progressive systemic sclerosis. Cochrane Database of Systematic Reviews (computer file) 2000:CD000953.
100. Belch JJ, Bell PR, Creissen D, et al. Randomized, double-blind, placebo-controlled study evaluating the efficacy and safety of AS-013, a prostaglandin E_1 prodrug, in patients with intermittent claudication. Circulation 1997;95:2298–2302.
101. Dessein PH, Morrison RC, Lamparelli RD, van der Merwe CA. Triiodothyronine treatment for Raynaud's phenomenon: A controlled trial. J Rheumatol 1990;17:1025–1028.
102. Gledhill RF, Dessein PH, Van der Merwe CA. Treatment of Raynaud's phenomenon with triiodothyronine corrects coexistent autonomic dysfunction: preliminary findings. Postgrad Med J 1992;68:263–267.
103. Solomon SA, Ramsay LE, Yeo WW, et al. β-Blockade and intermittent claudication: Placebo-controlled trial of atenolol and nifedipine and their combination. Br Med J 1991;303:1100–1104.
104. Neirotti M, Longo F, Molaschi M, et al. Functional vascular disorders: Treatment with pentoxifylline. Angiology 1987;38:575–580.
105. Bunker CB, Goldsmith PC, Leslie TA, et al. Calcitonin gene-related peptide, endothelin-1, the cutaneous microvasculature and Raynaud's phenomenon. Br J Dermatol 1996;134:399–406.
106. Moriau M, Lavenne-Pardonge E, Crasborn L, et al. Treatment of the Raynaud's phenomenon with piracetam. Arzneimittel Forsch 1993;43: 526–535.

23

Vasopressors and Inotropes in Shock

Maria I. Rudis and Joseph F. Dasta

Shock is an acute, generalized state of inadequate perfusion of critical organs that can produce serious pathophysiologic consequences, including death. Thirty years ago, mortality from septic or cardiogenic shock exceeded 70%. Currently, approximately 10% of patients admitted to hospitals have a diagnosis of severe sepsis or septic shock. Mortality in septic shock remains approximately 50%–70% despite enhanced treatment modalities and sophisticated monitoring techniques.[1,2]

Hemodynamic and perfusion monitoring can be categorized into two broad areas: global and regional monitoring. Global parameters, such as systemic blood pressure and pulse oximetry, assess perfusion and oxygen use by the entire body. Regional monitoring techniques, such as gastrointestinal tonometry, focus on flow and subsequent changes in metabolism of individual organs and tissues. Normal values for commonly monitored parameters are listed in Table 23–1.

GLOBAL PERFUSION MONITORING

ARTERIAL BLOOD PRESSURE MEASUREMENT

Arterial blood pressure is the product of cardiac output and systemic vascular resistance. Conditions that may lower blood pressure in the critically ill include cardiac failure or hypovolemia (by a reduction of cardiac output) and vasodilation (by sepsis, drugs, or neurotrauma). Arterial blood pressure determinations can be either noninvasive or invasive. All noninvasive blood pressure monitoring techniques depend on the use of an occluding cuff. Systolic and diastolic blood pressure are further measurable by auscultation, palpation (systolic pressure only), oscillometry, or Doppler technique (most reliable for systolic pressures). Auscultation is the most commonly used method outside the intensive care unit (ICU), although its usefulness is limited in patients with hypovolemia, hypothermia, or cardiogenic shock when pulses or Korotkoff sounds may be difficult to hear. Similar constraints exist for the palpation and oscillometric methods. However, oscillometry is preferred in edematous patients. Oscillometry measures blood pressure by sensing arterial blood pressure changes, or oscillations, against an inflated cuff. Rapid changes in oscillation amplitude correspond to systolic and diastolic pressure. It is the only noninvasive method to measure mean arterial pressure even in low-flow states, and it lends itself to automatic cycling and serial measurements (every 1 to 3 minutes) that do not require operator intervention, a key component in ICU monitoring. The use of narrow cuffs or cuffs applied too loosely can result in falsely high readings, whereas wide cuffs may produce falsely low readings.[3] Fingertip devices offer another avenue for continuous indirect blood pressure measurement, but their accuracy in ICU patients may be significantly diminished by the concurrent administration of vasoactive drugs.[4]

The use of invasive arterial catheters makes it possible to measure arterial blood pressures continuously, as well as to obtain blood samples for blood gas monitoring. The radial artery is the most commonly used vessel, but the dorsalis pedis, femoral, brachial, and axillary arteries (and the umbilical artery in the newborn) are also accessible. This method of blood pressure monitoring is a standard technique against which all other methods are compared. Major complications of peripheral artery catheterization include infection and distal ischemia. Catheter-related bacteremia and acute distal ischemia occur in less than 1% of catheter insertions. Ischemia is most common in patients with multiple or prolonged arterial cannulations, hypertension, or vasopressor therapy.[3] Invasive techniques are labor-intensive, require aseptic techniques, and offer potential sources of equipment errors, such as length and quality of tubing, air bubbles, stopcocks, thrombus formation, tube kinking, and placement of transducer. Hypertension, advanced age, and atherosclerosis may also affect the accuracy of invasive blood pressure readings.[5]

CENTRAL VENOUS CATHETER

Through a central venous catheter, clinicians can measure the central venous pressure (CVP), obtain venous blood gas samples, and administer drugs or fluids directly to the central circulation. A triple-lumen catheter makes it possible to administer drugs with known incompatibility. Blood volume, venous wall compliance, right cardiac function, intra-abdominal and intrathoracic pressure, and vasopressor therapy affect the CVP. Although not a reliable estimate of blood volume, the CVP can be used to qualitatively assess blood volume changes in patients during the early phases of fluid resuscitation. Sustained elevated pressures are indicative of fluid overloading.[6] There are few data supporting the use of CVP monitoring in the ICU. However, initial reports involving patients with sepsis suggest that CVP monitoring of fluid therapy during shock was associated with a reduction in the mortality rate of more than 50%.

PULMONARY ARTERY CATHETER

Introduced in 1970, pulmonary artery catheterization is a routinely performed bedside procedure in many ICUs. With the pulmonary artery catheter, also known as the Swan-Ganz catheter, the practitioner can obtain multiple cardiovascular parameters, including central venous, pulmonary artery, and pulmonary artery occlusive pressures, and cardiac output. Mixed venous blood samples from the pulmonary artery may also be obtained. In an effort to reduce blood loss from samples, many clinicians are using special pulmonary artery catheters called SvO_2 catheters that measure mixed venous oxygen saturation continuously by fiberoptic technology. Hence, trends in the venous oxygen saturation can be observed, and any necessary action can be taken.

Most important, inflation of the balloon at the catheter tip occludes the pulmonary artery, isolates the distal catheter tip from the right side of the heart, and allows the user to measure the pulmonary artery occlusion pressure (PAOP), an approximate measure of the left ventricular end-diastolic volume and a major determinant of left ventricular preload. Ideally, the pulmonary artery catheter should be fluoroscopically positioned; however, satisfactory placement may also be obtained by observing pulmonary artery pressure readings during

TABLE 23–1. Hemodynamic and Oxygen Transport Monitoring Parameters

Parameter	Normal Value
Blood pressure (systolic/diastolic)	100–130/70–85 mm Hg
Mean arterial pressure (MAP)	80–100 mm Hg
Pulmonary artery pressure (PAP)	25/10 mm Hg
Mean pulmonary artery pressure (MPAP)	12–15 mm Hg
Central venous pressure (CVP)	2–6 mm Hg
Pulmonary artery occlusion pressure (PAOP)	8–12 mm Hg (normal), 15–18 (ICU) mm Hg
Heart rate (HR)	60–80 beats/min
Cardiac output (CO)	4–7 L/min
Cardiac index (CI)	2.8–3.6 L/min/m^2
Stroke volume index (SVI)	30–50 ml/m^2
Systemic vascular resistance index (SVRI)	1300–2100 dyne·sec/m^{2}cm^5
Pulmonary vascular resistance index (PVRI)	45–225 dyne·sec/m^{2}cm^5
Arterial oxygen saturation (Sao_2)	97% (range, 95%–100%)
Mixed venous oxygen saturation (Svo_2)	75% (range, 60%–80%)
Arterial oxygen content (Cao_2)	20.1 vol % (range, 19–21)
Venous oxygen content (Cvo_2)	15.5 vol % (range, 11.5–16.5)
Oxygen content difference ($C(a\text{-}v)o_2$)	5 vol % (range, 4–6)
Oxygen consumption index (Vo_2)	131 mL/min/m^2 (range, 100–180)
Oxygen delivery index (Do_2)	578 mL/min/m^2 (range, 370–730)
Oxygen extraction ratio (O_2 ER)	25% (range, 22%–30%)
Intragastric mucosal pH	7.40 (range, 7.35–7.45)
Index	Parameter indexed to body surface area

catheter advancement. Proper positioning in the lower lung (zone 3) is essential to measure the PAOP and to prevent distal pulmonary artery collapse. Catheter migration, patient movement, mechanical ventilation, or eccentric balloon inflation may cause poor positioning.

Pulmonary artery catheters equipped with a distal thermistor also allow measurement of cardiac output by thermodilution. Rapid injection of saline solutions via the right atrial port permits complete mixing of blood with injectate, and the resultant change in blood temperature is measured in the pulmonary artery. From the temperature change, the patient's cardiac output can be calculated. Newer pulmonary artery catheters contain a temperature coil that intermittently warms the blood in the right ventricle for near-continuous cardiac output measurement.[7] Significant tricuspid regurgitation, an intracardiac shunt, and significant positive end-expiratory pressure (PEEP) decrease the validity of cardiac output measurements.

Despite its ubiquitous use, much controversy surrounds the safety and utility of the pulmonary artery catheter. The most common complications of pulmonary artery catheterization include mural thrombus formation (14% to 91%), transient ventricular tachydysrhythmias (11% to 63%), pulmonary infarction (1% to 7%), pulmonary artery rupture (0.06% to 2.0%), and sepsis (0.3% to 0.5%).[8] Tuman and colleagues found that pulmonary artery catheterization did not affect outcome in 1,094 patients who underwent coronary artery surgery.[9] In fact, Connors and associates observed in a multicenter, retrospective, matched-case study of 5,735 critically ill patients that pulmonary artery catheter use was associated with an increase in mortality and resource utilization.[10] In a subsequent consensus statement, a panel of experts found few studies investigating the device's impact on patient outcome. The catheter was, however, found useful in the diagnosis of cardiovascular alterations and in guidance of cardiovascular drug therapy, especially in patients who are undergoing high-risk procedures or who are severely ill.[11]

Studies in both Europe and the United States have found that one of two physicians incorrectly interpreted a tracing from the right heart catheter.[12] These findings could explain some of the results of studies concluding that right heart catheterization has no benefit. As such, a recently convened task force recommended standardizing and monitoring physician and nurse education on the proper use of the catheter, conducting clinical trials to assess the safety and efficacy of the catheter, and evaluating new device technology on patient outcome.[8]

OXYGEN PRESSURE AND SATURATION MONITORING

Arterial oxygen pressure (Pao_2) and saturation (Sao_2) may be measured invasively by obtaining an arterial blood sample. Arterial blood gases measured by conventional arterial sampling are standard, but poor sampling techniques, transportation and analysis delays, questionable analyzer accuracy, sample cellular metabolism, and inability to trend results affect their accuracy and usefulness. In-dwelling fiberoptic and electrochemical systems allow continuous monitoring and trend analysis of blood pH, Pao_2, and $Paco_2$ while decreasing the patient blood loss that results from frequent sampling. Unfortunately, studies evaluating the *in vitro* accuracy of these devices may not apply to the ICU environment. The in-dwelling sensors may exhibit lower Pao_2, higher $Paco_2$, and lower pH levels than central arterial blood measurements when peripheral flow is diminished. Furthermore, sensor contact with the blood vessel wall and vigorous arterial line flushing will also diminish sensor accuracy.[13]

Mixed venous oxygen saturation (Svo_2) is dependent on cardiac output, oxygen demand, hemoglobin concentration, and arterial oxygen saturation. It may be measured in patients with a Swan-Ganz catheter. In critically ill patients with sepsis, the values are likely to be more elevated (Svo_2, 70%–75%) than in those without sepsis. This occurs because of a maldistribution of blood flow and a lack of extraction of oxygen in the arteriolar beds. A low Svo_2 in patients with sepsis and other conditions should prompt rapid intervention to increase oxygen delivery to tissues.[14]

Subcutaneous tissue oxygenation ($Psqo_2$) is linked to tissue perfusion and, by extension, to total body hemodynamic status. The main limitation to subcutaneous tissue oximetry is its sensitivity to peripheral flow changes induced by catecholamines. Transcutaneous oximetry, a similar noninvasive method, is currently used in some neonatal ICUs. Unlike invasive subcutaneous tissue oximetry, this method may artificially elevate tissue oxygen values and is less sensitive to changes in perfusion. Both methods, however, provide continuous measurement of $Psqo_2$.[15]

Pulse oximetry is based on the principles of the Lambert-Beer law, which states that light transmission is inversely proportional to the density of a substance (hemoglobin). Thus, the concentrations of different types of hemoglobin (oxygenated, deoxygenated, carboxy, and methemoglobin) can be measured at different wavelengths. Pulse oximeters measure oxygen saturation by determining the ratio of oxygenated hemoglobin to total hemoglobin in a finger or toe.

Increased concentrations of carboxyhemoglobin (resulting from carbon monoxide toxicity) may elevate $Sa{O_2}$ readings. In contrast, increased levels of methemoglobin (methemoglobinemia) and methylene blue (a methemoglobinemia antidote) may decrease $Sa{O_2}$ readings. Nail polish, onychomycosis, dark skin pigmentation, strong light sources, patient motion, and peripheral vasoconstriction may also affect $Sa{O_2}$ readings. These effects are more pronounced when saturations are decreased. The incidence of equipment malfunction is approximately 1% to 2%.[16]

The use of pulse oximetry is very common in the perioperative arena or ICU. Despite this, few studies have addressed its usefulness. The false-positive alarm rate for pulse oximeters used in the ICU may be in excess of 80%.[17] In a large study of 20,802 patients, pulse oximetry was not shown to alter outcome following general surgery.[18] In a retrospective review of 17,093 surgical patients, however, Cullen and coworkers concluded that pulse oximetry reduced the rate of unintended ICU admissions from the recovery area.[19] A recent advance in pulse oximetry is the development of signal extraction technology. One device that uses this technology eliminates motion artifact and provides more accurate readings in states of low perfusion.

OXYGEN DELIVERY AND CONSUMPTION

The concept of tissue oxygen debt as a determinant of organ damage in critical illness arose more than 10 years ago. In normal individuals, oxygen consumption ($V{O_2}$) is dependent on oxygen delivery ($D{O_2}$) up to a certain critical level ($V{O_2}$ flow dependency). At this point, tissue oxygen requirements have apparently been satisfied and further increases in $D{O_2}$ will not alter consumption ($V{O_2}$ flow independency; Fig. 23–1). Although animal models of sepsis have substantiated this relationship, studies in critically ill humans show a continuous, pathologic dependence relationship of $V{O_2}$ on $D{O_2}$. Furthermore, ICU survivors exhibited higher $D{O_2}$ and $V{O_2}$ levels than did nonsurvivors. This became the rationale for targeting supranormal levels of $D{O_2}$ and $V{O_2}$ in the treatment of ICU patients.[20] However, a recent meta-analysis of randomized clinical trials involving 1,016 adult ICU patients failed to show that achieving this goal improved patient mortality.[21] This may, in part, have been due to the heterogeneous nature of the ICU patients studied, the lack of study blinding, crossover patients (i.e., control patients who achieve supranormal $D{O_2}$ and $V{O_2}$ levels by themselves), or a lack of adequate control of co-interventions.

The debate continues in more homogeneous patient populations. In high-risk surgical patients, supranormal $D{O_2}$ values correlate with a decrease in mortality. Two recent randomized studies further evaluated the effect of increasing $D{O_2}$ values to more than 600 mL/min/m^2 in a homogeneous population of elderly surgical patients with systemic inflammatory response syndrome, sepsis, severe sepsis, or septic shock-with conflicting results. Yu and associates demonstrated that the intervention group had a significant increase in survival at 24 hours

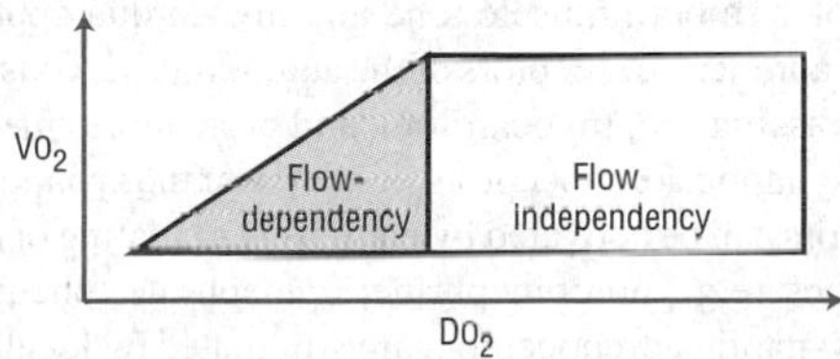

FIGURE 23–1. Relationship between oxygen consumption ($V{O_2}$) and oxygen delivery ($D{O_2}$).

(21% vs. 52%, $P = .01$) compared to the control group of patients between 50 and 75 years of age.[22] This benefit was not evident in those older than 75 years of age. The authors suggested that the combination of increasing $D{O_2}$ and maintaining the $V{O_2}$:$D{O_2}$ ratio (oxygen extraction ratio, or O_2ER) below 0.25 without a changing $V{O_2}$ may be helpful in maintaining or improving the reserve of the body to meet the oxygen demands. This may be true, particularly in older patients who have a lower baseline $V{O_2}$. In the second study, the same intervention revealed a significant reduction in the 60-day survival rate in high-risk elderly surgical patients randomized to have their $D{O_2}$ increased to the same level (i.e., more than 600 mL/min/m^2).[23] Thus, it is not yet certain that the benefits of supranormal $D{O_2}$ in these patients originate in the prevention and reversal of tissue hypoxia.

A recent review on alternative potential mechanisms for the beneficial effect of supranormal $D{O_2}$ suggests that catecholamines exert anti-inflammatory actions by modulating cytokine response.[24] In general, catecholamines inhibit pro-inflammatory cytokine (e.g., tumor necrosis factor [TNF]-α) production and may enhance anti-inflammatory cytokine (e.g., interleukin [IL]-6 and IL-10) production.[24] Further evidence to support these actions comes from studies which show that the actions of epinephrine on these cytokines are blocked by propranolol and thus are mediated by β-adrenergic receptors. These data must be interpreted with caution, because most investigators have used animal or cell models of sepsis, have pretreated patients with vasopressors prior to endotoxin infusion, and have used doses that may not always be clinically relevant.

Further problems with therapy directed to supranormal oxygen transport values arise from the fact that the apparent linear relationship between $D{O_2}$ and $V{O_2}$ has been questioned. The equations share variables; this so-called mathematical coupling can produce artifactual relationships between the two. The $D{O_2}$ and $V{O_2}$ indexed parameters are calculated as follows:

$$D{O_2} = CI \times Ca{O_2}$$

$$V{O_2} = CI \times (Ca{O_2} - Cv{O_2}),$$

where CI = cardiac index, $Ca{O_2}$ = arterial oxygen content, and $Cv{O_2}$ = mixed venous oxygen content.

Variable relationships between $D{O_2}$ and $V{O_2}$ have been observed when $V{O_2}$ is measured independently by indirect calorimetry. A linear relationship between $D{O_2}$ and $V{O_2}$ may, therefore, be the result of mathematical coupling or flow-dependent $V{O_2}$. Currently available data do not support the concept that treatment measures directed to achieve supranormal levels of $D{O_2}$ and $V{O_2}$ may alter patient outcome or survival.[21] In fact, a recent consensus conference concluded that although pulmonary artery catheterization is useful to guide therapy, routinely increasing the cardiac index to predetermined supranormal values has not been shown to improve outcome.[25] Furthermore, achievement of a supranormal value for $D{O_2}$ does not ensure parallel improvements in regional organ blood flow and oxygenation.[26] The O_2ER can be used to assess adequacy of perfusion and metabolic response. Patients who are able to increase $V{O_2}$ when $D{O_2}$ is increased are more likely to survive. However, low $V{O_2}$ and O_2ER values are indicative of poor oxygen utilization and lead to greater mortality.[27] Another approach that may decrease the effect of mathematical coupling and provide individualized therapy may lie in titrated therapy, with sequential measurements of $D{O_2}$ and $V{O_2}$ to achieve $V{O_2}$ flow independency, along with normalization of blood lactate and hemodynamic parameters.[28,29]

SERUM LACTATE

The use of serum lactate concentrations may be an alternate or complementary measure of tissue oxygenation and function, as DO_2 and VO_2 may change independently of blood lactate levels.[20] In some patients, lactate concentrations may show better correlation with outcome than do oxygen transport parameters,[29] and they may be superior to hemodynamic markers in determining the adequacy of systemic oxygenation restoration.[30]

Lactate is a metabolic product of pyruvate, and its production increases under anaerobic conditions, as may occur during shock. However, lactate may also accumulate in patients with significant liver dysfunction who are not in shock and in patients with the acute respiratory distress syndrome and endotoxin-inactivated pyruvate dehydrogenase.[31] Interestingly, the intestines and kidneys may take up lactate during near-zero flow states.[32] Furthermore, because both well perfused and poorly perfused tissues contribute to arterial and mixed venous lactate concentrations, these levels are not reflective of regional perfusion.

Increased lactate concentrations have been correlated with increased mortality,[33] but the utility of blood lactate measurements in guiding therapy has not been clearly demonstrated. Serial blood lactate measurements are more useful than single isolated measurements. Blood lactate levels also have a greater prognostic value than oxygen-derived variables in predicting outcome in septic shock.[14]

REGIONAL PERFUSION MONITORING

Blood pressures, cardiac output, serum lactate, and global oxygen homeostasis parameters do not offer information about individual organ perfusion and oxygenation. The measurement of regional perfusion to detect inadequate tissue oxygenation has focused on the splanchnic circulation, because it is sensitive to changes in blood flow and oxygenation. There are several reasons for this sensitivity. First, most of the normally large amount of blood that flows to the gut mucosa is redistributed toward the serosa and muscularis. Second, the gut may have a higher critical DO_2 threshold than do other organs. Third, the tip of the villus has a countercurrent oxygen exchange mechanism, rendering it very sensitive to reduction in regional blood flow and oxygenation.[14]

Gastric tonometry measures gut luminal PCO_2 at equilibrium by placing a saline- or air-filled gas-permeable balloon in the gastric lumen. Assuming that CO_2 permeates freely among tissues and that the arterial bicarbonate (HCO_3^-) concentration is equal to that of the gut mucosa, the intramucosal pH (pHi) may be calculated using the Henderson-Hasselbach equation:

$$\text{pHi} = 6.1 + \log(\text{HCO}_3^-)0.03 \times P\text{CO}_2$$

Increases in mucosal PCO_2 and calculated decreases in pHi are associated with mucosal hypoperfusion and perhaps increased mortality.[34] Increases in luminal PCO_2, as may occur when patients use buffering antacids, can confound the calculation of pHi. Patients may use histamine-2-receptor antagonists instead. The presence of respiratory acid-base disorders, systemic bicarbonate administration, arterial blood gas measurement errors, enteral feeding solutions, blood or stool in the gut may also confound pHi determinations.[35]

The time delay associated with this measurement (30 minutes) makes this method inconvenient for routine bedside monitoring. Recent investigations suggest that an air-filled balloon may require a shorter equilibrium time, be simpler to use, and be equally accurate.[36]

A randomized, prospective, multicenter trial of pHi-directed therapy was not able to show that the use of pHi reduced mortality in critically ill patients.[37] However, patients who had a normal pHi (>7.35) upon admission and subsequently received pHi-guided treatment to increase DO_2 experienced a 38% reduction in mortality. In a smaller trial of 57 patients, Ivatury and associates compared pHi-directed therapy (end point pHi > 7.3) to DO_2-directed therapy (end point DO_2 > 600 mL/min/m^2).[38] The incidence of multiple organ failure and the rate of mortality were not statistically different between the groups, although this may have been due to a small sample size. Many clinicians believe that measurements of gastric mucosal PCO_2 may be more accurate than calculations of pHi. Furthermore, because the arterial PCO_2 influences the mucosal PCO_2, consensus is that the mucosal–arterial PCO_2 difference (PCO_2 gap) may be the optimum measurement.[34] Although promising, gastric tonometry is not yet ready for routine clinical use.

A subsequent technology to gastric tonometry is sublingual capnometry. One device has recently gained the approval of the Food and Drug Administration (FDA) and consists of a catheter placed sublingually for the determination of sublingual PCO_2 ($P_{sl}CO_2$). In a study evaluating the feasibility of using sublingual capnometry to diagnose and quantify the severity of circulatory shock, Weil and colleagues found that the capnographer reliably detected the physical signs of shock, particularly when the $P_{sl}CO_2$ exceeded 70 mm Hg (positive predictive value [PPV] = 1.00). This study was controlled for the presence of circulatory shock, as defined by physical symptoms and arterial blood lactate levels greater than 2.5 mmol/L, and for the presence of acute illness through the use of healthy controls.[39] Initial clinical results look promising, and sublingual capnometry may represent a convenient way to assess the adequacy of regional perfusion.

VASOPRESSORS AND INOTROPES

In septic shock, when volume resuscitation fails to maintain adequate blood pressure (mean arterial pressure [MAP] $\geq$ 65 mm Hg), and organ and tissue perfusion, it is necessary to use vasopressors and inotropes. The clinician must decide on the choice of agent, therapeutic end points, and the safe and effective doses of vasopressors and inotropes to be used.

Although agents other than catecholamines (e.g., phosphodiesterase III inhibitors, naloxone, nitric oxide synthase inhibitors, vasopressin) have been used as inotropes and vasopressors in shock states, the focus of this chapter is on catecholamines.

RECEPTOR PHARMACOLOGY

The comparative receptor activity of endogenous and exogenously administered catecholamines are summarized in Table 23–2. Endogenous catecholamines are responsible for regulation of vascular and bronchiolar smooth muscle tone and myocardial contractility.[40] Sympathetic adrenergic receptors of the autonomic nervous system located in the vasculature, myocardium, and bronchioles mediate these effects. Postsynaptic adrenoceptors lie at or near the synaptic junction. These receptors can be activated by naturally circulating or exogenous catecholamines (e.g., norepinephrine, epinephrine, phenylephrine), whereas presynaptic adrenoceptors are stimulated by locally released neurotransmitters (e.g., norepinephrine) and are controlled by a negative feedback mechanism.

TABLE 23–2. Adrenergic and Dopaminergic Receptor Pharmacology and Organ Distribution

Effector Organ	Receptor Subtype	Physiologic Response
Heart		
SA Node	β_1, β_2	Increased heart rate
Atria	β_1, β_2	Increased contractility Increased conduction velocity
AV Node	β_1, β_2	Increased automaticity Increased conduction velocity
His-Purkinje system	β_1, β_2	Increased automaticity Increased conduction velocity
Ventricles	β_1, β_2, α_1	Increased contractility Increased conduction velocity Increased automaticity Increased rate idioventricular pacemaker cells
Arterioles		
Coronary	α_1, α_2, β_2, DA_1	Constriction; dilatation
Skin and mucosa	α_1, α_2	Constriction
Skeletal muscle	α_1, β_2	Constriction, dilatation
Cerebral	α_1	Constriction (slight)
Pulmonary	α_1, β_2	Constriction, dilatation
Abdominal viscera (mesentery)	α_1, β_2, DA_1	Constriction, dilatation
Renal	α_1, α_2, β_1, β_2, DA_1	Constriction, dilatation
Veins (systemic)	α_1, α_2, β_2	Constriction, dilatation
Lungs		
Trachial/bronchial smooth muscle	β_2	Relaxation
Bronchial glands	α_1, β_2	Decreased, increased secretion
Stomach		
Motility and tone	α_1, α_2, β_2	Decrease (usually)
Sphincter	α_1	Contraction (usually)
Intestine		
Motility and tone	α_1, α_2, β_1, β_2	Decrease
Sphincters	α_1	Contraction
Secretions	α_2	Inhibition (?)
Kidney		
Renin secretion	α_1	Decrease
Skeletal muscle	β_2	Increased contractility, glyconeogenesis, K^+ uptake
Liver	α_1, β_2	Glycogenolysis and gluconeogenesis

SA = sinoatrial; AV = atrioventricular; DA = dopamine.
Compiled from Refs. 40 and 127.

Figure 23–2 depicts adrenoceptor–G protein interaction. Once activated by the β- and dopamine $(DA)_1$-adrenoceptor agonists, the stimulatory G protein, Gs, dissociates from the receptor and activates membrane-bound adenyl cyclase. The α_2- and DA_2-agonists activate the inhibitory G protein, Gi, which dissociates from the receptor and blocks adenyl cyclase. Because adenyl cyclase converts adenosine triphosphate (ATP) to cyclic adenosine monophosphate (cAMP), which stimulates protein kinases, blocking it alters cellular functions.

The heart contains primarily postsynaptic β_1-receptors, which increase the rate and the force of contraction when stimulated. This

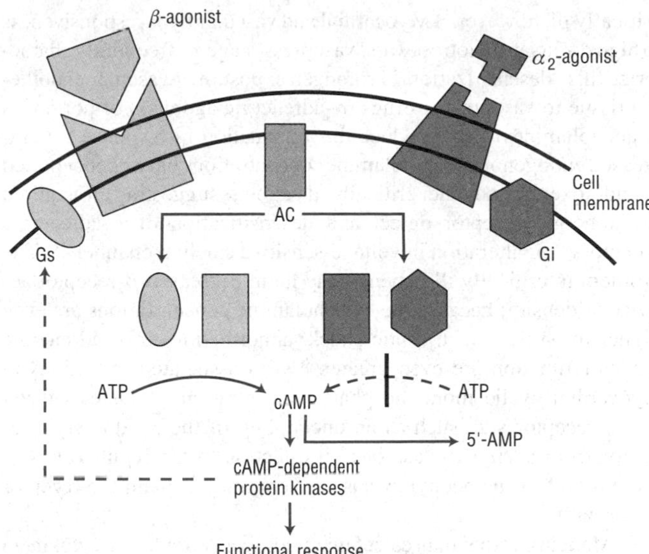

FIGURE 23–2. Adrenoceptor–G protein interaction. AC = adenyl cyclase; α_2-agonist = α_2-adrenergic receptor agonist; AMP = adenosine monophosphate; ATP = adenosine triphosphate; β_1-agonist = β-adrenergic receptor agonist; cAMP = cyclic adenosine monophosphate; Gs = G stimulatory protein; Gi = G inhibitory protein. *(Adapted with permission from Ref. 43.)*

effect appears to result from the activation of adenyl cyclase and the subsequent generation and accumulation of cAMP. Stimulation of postsynaptic cardiac α_1-receptors causes a significant increase in contractility without an increase in rate, an effect apparently not mediated by cAMP. The increased contractility is more pronounced at lower heart rates, and it has a slower onset and longer duration in comparison with β_1-mediated inotropic responses. Presynaptic α_2-adrenoceptors are also found in the heart and appear to be activated by norepinephrine released by the sympathetic nerve itself. Their activation inhibits further norepinephrine release from the nerve terminal.

Both postsynaptic and presynaptic adrenoceptors are present in the vasculature. Postsynaptic α_1- and α_2-receptors mediate vasoconstriction, whereas postsynaptic β_2-receptors induce vasodilation. Presynaptic α_2-receptors inhibit norepinephrine release in the vasculature as well. Presynaptic β_1-adrenoceptors promote neurotransmitter release. Stimulation of peripheral DA_1-receptors produces renal, coronary, and mesenteric vasodilation and a natriuretic response. Stimulation of DA_2-receptors inhibits norepinephrine release from sympathetic nerve endings, as well as prolactin release, and it may induce nausea and vomiting.[41] In addition, DA_1- and DA_2-receptor stimulation also suppresses peristalsis and may precipitate ileus.[41] Cloning techniques have identified novel DA_1- and DA_2-like receptors, but their function beyond positive and negative adenyl cyclase coupling to the α-subunit of the G proteins has yet to be determined.[42]

ALTERED ADRENOCEPTOR FUNCTION: IMPLICATIONS FOR THE CRITICALLY ILL

The majority of the work describing receptor function and associated clinical pharmacology has been done either in animal models or human volunteers and not in critically ill patients with sepsis or septic shock. Derangements in adrenergic receptor activity may result in resistance to exogenous catecholamine administration in the critically ill, however.[43] Myocardial and vascular hyporesponsiveness to high dosages of inotropes and vasopressor agents frequently characterize this "desensitization." Prolonged exposure of vascular endothelial tissue to vasopressor drugs (α-adrenergic agonists) or hormones (catecholamines) may produce this attenuation in response.[44,45] Increased endogenous catecholamine concentrations have been reported in endotoxemic and other critically ill patients, suggesting an acquired β-adrenergic receptor defect and desensitization of β-adrenergic receptors[46] or alteration in voltage-sensitive calcium channels.[47] The problem in critically ill patients may lie in decreased β-receptor activity or density; because the catecholamine concentrations are even higher in patients with septic shock, abnormalities in β-adrenergic receptor function are even greater,[46] with associated reductions in myocardial cyclic monophosphate concentrations.[47] Defects distal to the receptor site, such as an uncoupling of the β-adrenergic receptor from adenyl cyclase or a dysfunction in the regulatory (G)-protein unit of the adenyl cyclase system, may explain the receptor abnormality.[47]

Mediators other than catecholamines (e.g., circulating cytokines) may be responsible for these distal alterations. Macrophage-derived IL-1 and TNF-α impair the coupling of β-adrenergic receptors to adenyl cyclase in rat cardiac myocytes.[45] Septic shock patients have exhibited impaired β-adrenergic receptor stimulation of cAMP associated with myocardial hyporesponsiveness to dobutamine and reduced myocardial performance when compared to normal volunteers, nonbacteremic critically ill, and patients who have sepsis, but are not in shock.[45] However, increased chronotropic sensitivity to β-adrenergic stimulation with hypersensitivity of the adenyl cyclase system to isoproterenol stimulation has also been reported in animal models of bacteremia and endotoxemia.[45] In the presence of intrinsic myocardial dysfunction and increased metabolic demands, this dysfunctional adrenergic system is incapable of mobilizing functional cardiac reserve to maintain adequate myocardial performance.[45] These conflicting findings were observed in the early stages of sepsis, and thus adrenergic receptor sensitivity may be time-dependent. In fact, in an *in vivo* rodent model of sustained endotoxemia (48 hours) and continuous parenteral nutrition that simulated advanced critical illness, Dickerson and colleagues showed no difference in α_1-adrenergic maximal responsiveness (in MAP) to phenylephrine.[44] Time-dependent alterations in the production of endothelium-derived nitric oxide, a potent vasodilator, may explain the apparent differences in vascular reactivity to phenylephrine during the phases of endotoxemia.[44] These findings suggest that the clinical response to vasopressor and inotropic agents is variable during the stages of the hemodynamic, myocardial, and peripheral vascular derangements of septic shock. These derangements vary among patients and during each bacteremic insult; therefore, the appropriate doses of catecholamines vary from patient to patient and during the insult. For these reasons, these drugs should be dosed to clinical end points, not to arbitrary maximal doses.

CLINICAL PHARMACOLOGY OF CATECHOLAMINES

The receptor selectivity of clinically used vasopressors and inotropes, and their hemodynamic effects are listed in Table 23–3. In general, these drugs act rapidly with short durations of action. As such, these drugs are given as continuous infusions. Care in monitoring and calculating infusion rates is advised because dosing adjustments are made frequently and more concentrated solutions are used in volume-restricted patients.

Dopamine is often recommended as the initial catecholamine in sepsis because it increases blood pressure by increasing myocardial contractility and vasoconstriction. Dopamine has dose-related receptor activity at DA_1-, β_1-, and α_1-receptors. Unfortunately, this dose-response relationship has not been confirmed in critically ill patients. In patients with septic shock, there is a great overlap of hemodynamic effects, even at doses as low as 3 μg/kg/min.[48] Tachydysrhythmias are common because of the release of endogenous norepinephrine by dopamine entering the sympathetic nerve terminal. Dopamine may increase the PAOP through pulmonary vasoconstriction.[49] Furthermore, this drug may depress ventilation and worsen hypoxemia in patients dependent on the hypoxic ventilatory drive.

Dobutamine, a synthetic catecholamine, is primarily a selective β_1-agonist with mild β_2- and vascular α_1-activity, resulting in strong positive inotropic activity without concomitant vasoconstriction. In comparison with dopamine, dobutamine produces a larger increase in cardiac output and is less arrhythmogenic.[43] Ruffolo showed that α_1-adrenoceptors in the heart are directly stimulated by the (−)

TABLE 23–3. Receptor Pharmacology of Selected Inotropic and Vasopressor Agents Used in Septic Shock[a]

Agent	α_1	α_2	β_1	β_2	DA[b]
Dobutamine (500 mg/250 mL D_5W or NS)					
2–10 μg/kg/min	+	0	++++	++	0
>10–20 μg/kg/min	++	0	++++	+++	0
Dopamine (800 mg/250 mL D_5W or NS)					
1–3 μg/kg/min	0	0	+	0	++++
3–10 μg/kg/min	0/+	0	++++	++	++++
>10–20 μg/kg/min	+++	0	++++	+	0
Dopexamine (investigational)					
0.5–4.0 μg/kg/min	0	0	++[c]	+++	++++
Epinephrine (2 mg/250 mL D_5W or NS)					
0.01–0.05 μg/kg/min	++	++	++++	+++	0
>0.05 μg/kg/min	++++	++++	+++	+	
Norepinephrine (4 mg/250 mL D_5W or NS)					
0.02–3.0 μg/kg/min (2–20 μg/min)	+++	+++	+++	+/++	0
Phenylephrine (50 mg/250 mL D_5W or NS)					
0.5–9 μg/kg/min	+++	+	?	0	0

[a]activity ranges from no activity (0) to maximal (++++) activity or ? when activity is not known.
[b]DA = Dopaminergic.
[c]Dopexamine inhibits neuronal reuptake of norepinephrine (see text).
Compiled from Refs. 53 and 55.

isomer of dobutamine, and the β_1- and β_2-agonist activity resides in the (+) isomer.[41] This suggests that the strong inotropic action of dobutamine is a function of its structure, the additive effect of the cardiac α_1- and β_1-agonist activity, and a relatively weak chronotropic effect limited to the (+) isomer action on the β-receptors. Clinically, the increased myocardial contractility and subsequent reflex reduction in sympathetic tone leads to a decrease in systemic vascular resistance (SVR).[40,50,51] Even though dobutamine is optimally used for low cardiac output states with high filling pressures, or in cardiogenic shock, vasopressors may be needed to counteract arterial vasodilation.

Norepinephrine is a combined α- and β-agonist, but mainly produces vasoconstriction. It acts primarily via its more prominent α-effects on all vascular beds, thus increasing SVR.[40,50,51] Norepinephrine administration generally produces either no change or a slight decrease in cardiac output.

Phenylephrine is a pure α_1-agonist and is believed to increase blood pressure through vasoconstriction. This may result in a reflexive bradycardia. However, given the presence of cardiac α_1-receptors, phenylephrine may also increase contractility and cardiac output.[52]

Epinephrine exerts combined α- and β-agonist effects and has traditionally been reserved as the vasopressor of last resort because of reports of peripheral vasoconstriction, particularly in the splanchnic and renal beds. At the high epinephrine infusion rates used in septic shock, predominantly α-adrenergic effects are seen, and SVR and MAP are increased.[53]

Dopexamine is an investigational synthetic catecholamine with marked intrinsic agonist activity at β_2-receptors and less activity at dopaminergic (DA_1 and DA_2) receptors. Direct stimulation of cardiac β_2-receptors may result in a reflex baroceptor stimulation and mild inotropic activity. Dopexamine has no clinically significant direct β_1-agonist activity and no α- effects. Cardiac β_1-receptors are indirectly stimulated through inhibition of neuronal reuptake of catecholamines.[54,55]

CLINICAL USE OF VASOPRESSORS AND INOTROPES

Optimizing MAP as the goal of vasopressor therapy does not uniformly correlate with a decrease in mortality in septic shock.[56] Historically, significant concerns about the adverse effects of the vasopressors limited their use. Goal-directed therapy, with optimization of oxygen transport variables to supranormal values, has also yielded poor results in patients with septic shock.[21,56] In fact, normalization of systemic Do_2 and Vo_2, whether spontaneously or by design, is associated with improved outcome and is not dependent on the administration of vasopressor agents. Part of our inability to detect an improvement with vasopressor or inotrope therapy may result from our limited ability to quantify regional tissue perfusion.

ADVERSE EFFECTS

Catecholamine vasopressors may result in adverse peripheral vasoconstrictive, metabolic, and dysrhythmogenic effects that limit or outweigh their positive effects on the central circulation.[57] Norepinephrine, phenylephrine, and epinephrine can produce a lactic acidosis secondary to excessive constriction in peripheral arterioles or enhanced glycogenolysis, or as a result of mobilization of lactate from peripheral tissues through improved oxygenation.[57,58] Additionally, excessive peripheral vasoconstriction may cause ischemia or necrosis of already poorly perfused areas, such as the skin, mesenteric, and splanchnic circulations.[43,59] The use of epinephrine and phenylephrine in septic shock patients, who are significantly hypovolemic, increases the profound vasoconstrictive effects. These agents are used in the context of late septic shock, where hypotension is refractory to less selective vasoconstrictors (e.g., norepinephrine, dopamine) such that very large doses of epinephrine or phenylephrine are required. Myocardial ischemia and dysrhythmias may occur in patients with coronary artery disease, atherosclerosis, cardiomyopathies, left ventricular hypertrophy, congestive heart failure, and underlying dysrhythmias resulting from their inability to tolerate β_1-cardiac stimulation that mediates increases in cardiac output. The effect is usually the opposite, however, in young patients with healthy myocardium. These patients tolerate β_1-cardiac stimulation well, their ventricular filling pressures decrease, and their cardiac output and Do_2 increase, with a resulting increase in peripheral perfusion. An extensive review of the dysrhythmogenic potential of the catecholamine vasopressors reveals a variety of resulting atrial and ventricular arrhythmias.[60]

Sympathomimetic vasopressors have also been found to occupy neutrophil β_2-receptors (e.g., epinephrine) and directly scavenge oxygen free radicals (e.g., dopamine, dobutamine).[61] These effects may be either beneficial (e.g., dampening the harmful effects of oxygen free radical–mediated tissue injury, or deleterious (e.g., reducing neutrophilic defense against bacteria). At clinically relevant concentrations, dopamine inhibits *in vitro* endothelial adhesion molecule expression of E-selectin.[62] This and other adhesion molecules mediate leukocyte interaction with and adherence to endothelial cells, which is implicated in enhancing sepsis-induced multiple organ failure and lung injury in many animal models.[61,62] Epinephrine, dopamine, and other β-adrenergic agonists can inhibit production of TNF-α by neutrophils or expression of cellular adhesion molecules such as E-selectin by increasing cAMP, but the mechanism is more complex than previously thought.[62,63]

Vasopressor catecholamines have the potential to cause extravasation-associated tissue damage if infusions infiltrate during peripheral administration. In the event of infiltration, an α-receptor antagonist such as phentolamine (10 mg in 10 mL of saline) should be injected intradermally to reverse local vasoconstriction. Administering vasopressor drugs into a large central vein can help to avoid this problem.

HEMODYNAMIC OXYGEN TRANSPORT AND CLINICAL OUTCOMES: EFFECT OF VASOPRESSORS AND INOTROPES

Traditionally, there have been few vasopressors and inotropes used for hemodynamic support in shock: dopamine, norepinephrine, dobutamine, phenylephrine, and epinephrine.

Dopamine

The initial vasopressor used in septic shock is frequently dopamine. Doses of 5–10 μg/kg/min are given to improve MAP. Most studies in patients with septic shock have shown that at these doses, dopamine increases cardiac index by improving ventricular contractility and heart rate, resulting primarily from its β_1-effects. It increases arterial pressure and SVR both as a result of the increased cardiac output and, at higher doses (> 10 μg/kg/min), as a result of the α_1-effects.

Oxygen transport variables parallel the hemodynamic effects. Dopamine improves global Do_2 in patients with sepsis, but compromises tissue oxygen extraction in the splanchnic and mesenteric circulation by α_1-mediated vasoconstriction. Indeed, despite increasing systemic Do_2 and Vo_2, large doses of dopamine worsen gastric pHi and ΔpCO_2. This is reflected by a decrease or lack of change in regional VO_2 and a decrease in the tissue O_2ER.

The clinical utility of dopamine in the setting of septic shock is limited, because large doses are frequently necessary to maintain cardiac output and blood pressure. At doses exceeding 20 μg/kg/min, further improvement in cardiac performance and regional hemodynamics is unlikely to be significant. Tachycardia and tachydysrhythmias frequently hamper the clinical use of dopamine. Although the tachydysrhythmias should theoretically not occur until 5–10 μg/kg/min of dopamine, these β_1-effects may be evident with doses as low as 3 μg/kg/min. They seem to be more prevalent in patients who are elderly, who have preexisting or concurrent cardiac ischemia or dysrhythmias, or who are currently receiving other dysrhythmogenic agents, including vasopressors and inotropes. In the instance of high filling pressures, tachycardia or tachydysrhythmias in the presence of refractory hypotension, dopamine should be replaced by another vasopressor or inotrope, such as norepinephrine, dobutamine, phenylephrine, or epinephrine, depending on the desired effect.

Other adverse effects that may limit the use of dopamine in septic shock are increases in PAOP and pulmonary shunt, and decreases in PaO_2.[49] The increase in PAOP may be the result of changes in diastolic volumes from decreased cardiac compliance or increased venous return to the heart by α-adrenergic receptor–mediated venoconstriction. This may affect gas exchange and decrease PaO_2. The increase in pulmonary shunt may also result from acute enhancement of pulmonary blood flow to nonhomogeneous lung regions. Thus, dopamine should be used with caution in patients with elevated preload, as the drug may exacerbate pulmonary edema.

In the critical care setting, low doses (1–3 μg/kg/min) of dopamine are frequently used in septic shock patients who are receiving vasopressors with or without oliguria. The goal of therapy is to prevent or reverse renal vasoconstriction caused by other pressors, to prevent oliguric renal failure, or to convert it to nonoliguric renal failure. Dopamine has been shown to increase renal blood flow and increase urine output, either because of its dopaminergic effect at low doses, natriuretic effects (inhibition of Na^+/K^+ adenosine triphosphate in renal tubular cells), or because of an increase in cardiac index.[64,65] In normal volunteers, the addition of dopamine to incremental doses of norepinephrine may blunt norepinephrine-induced renal vasoconstriction, thereby maintaining renal blood flow, natriuresis, urine output,[48,66] and, in one study, glomerular filtration.[66] In oliguric patients, dopamine may increase fractional excretion of sodium and increase urine output. These effects have also been observed during the course of dopamine administration in oliguric patients without septic shock,[67] as well as in oliguric[68,69] and nonoliguric[64,70,71] patients with septic shock.

Dopamine is often added in low doses to other vasopressors or inotropes (e.g., norepinephrine). More commonly, however, pressor doses of dopamine are found to be ineffective (or are not tolerated), and an additional agent is given. At this point, the dopamine is titrated to a low dose. Despite the frequent use of low-dose dopamine, there is no evidence to support its utility in preserving kidney function in oliguria, with or without septic shock, or in reversing vasopressor-induced vasoconstriction in septic shock.[64,65,68,71,72] Studies in septic shock patients stabilized with norepinephrine and then given low-dose dopamine as an additional agent have shown disappointing results. An increase in urine output is most often associated with an increase in cardiac index and a natriuretic effect rather than a sustained increase in glomerular filtration rate. Low-dose dopamine did not reduce the incidence of acute renal failure, the need for dialysis, or the 28-day mortality rate in patients with oliguria due to septic shock in a retrospective analysis of a randomized trial.[73] Lherm and coworkers demonstrated a different response to low-dose dopamine in septic shock patients on catecholamines compared with nonoliguric patients with sepsis syndrome.[74] The latter group showed an increase in creatinine clearance and diuresis, but the former did not. Furthermore, tolerance to the vasodilatory effects of dopamine after 24 to 48 hours was evident in the nonoliguric patients with sepsis syndrome and has been reported in others.[74,75] The lack of response to dopamine in septic shock patients on vasopressors and the tolerance that develops in responders to low-dose dopamine may be partly explained by time- and disease-dependent desensitization of dopamine receptors;[74,75] this may not occur in those with sepsis syndrome or normal volunteers.[48,74] Furthermore, differences in the extent of preexisting vasodilation and in the pathophysiology of renal dysfunction in oliguric and septic shock may also contribute to the inconsistent responses to the administration of low doses of dopamine.

Undesirable effects of low-dose dopamine on regional hemodynamics are now being recognized. Inappropriate use of dopamine, together with hypovolemia, may induce tachycardia with myocardial ischemia. The fact that dopamine blocks tubuloglomerular feedback, an important mechanism in decreasing the oxygen demand of renal tubular cells in ischemic states, may override its benefits of reducing tubular cell oxygen consumption by inhibiting sodium resorption. Dopamine at low or pressor doses impairs gastric motility in critical illness and may aggravate gut ischemia in septic shock.[76–79]

Although splanchnic blood flow and DO_2 may increase, there is no preferential increase in the splanchnic perfusion as a fraction of cardiac output and systemic increases in DO_2.[69,70] One study found an inverse relationship between fractional splanchnic flow at baseline and the change in fractional splanchnic blood flow; that is, dopamine was effective in increasing the fractional splanchnic blood flow in those patients with normal flow, but worsened it in those patients with high baseline values, such as occurs with redistribution of regional blood flow in septic shock.[69] Clinically, it is difficult to prospectively distinguish either subset of patients. Lastly, immune suppression of T-cell proliferation, pituitary hormone secretion, blunting of growth, and thyroid hormones and prolactin secretion are also potentially clinically significant unwanted neuroendocrine effects.

Currently, there is insufficient evidence to promote the use of low-dose dopamine because it does not improve regional hemodynamics, oxygen transport variables, and functional parameters of organ perfusion in a sustained manner and may even impair them. These findings are raising a controversy about consideration of dopamine as the first-line vasopressor agent in severe sepsis or septic shock.[78,80]

Norepinephrine

Three decades ago, prior to the development of the newer synthetic catecholamines dopamine and dobutamine, norepinephrine was first used for the treatment of hypotensive states. Traditionally, norepinephrine was believed to cause significant peripheral tissue vasoconstriction, which could selectively impair regional flow and thus DO_2 to the renal and splanchnic beds. However, recent clinical studies of norepinephrine support the primary use of norepinephrine to restore blood pressure in septic shock.[47,50,56,81] In fact, in a retrospective study of 100 ICU patients treated with norepinephrine for severe hypotension and evidence of end- organ hypoperfusion unresponsive to both fluid resuscitation and dopamine treatment, the early administration of norepinephrine was associated with the lowest mortality rate.[82] In patients with higher Sequential Organ Failure Assessment (SOFA) scores and associated multiorgan failure, treatment with norepinephrine no longer offered an advantage. Early, aggressive vasopressor support may be the key to a positive outcome in septic shock.

In clinical practice, norepinephrine is initiated after vasopressor doses of dopamine (4–20 μg/kg/min) alone or in combination with dobutamine (2–40 μg/kg/min) fail to achieve the desired goals.[50,51,56,83] Doses of dopamine and dobutamine may be kept constant or stopped altogether; in some instances, dopamine is kept at low doses for its purported renal protection.[56,59,84] It may be wiser to use norepinephrine, with its combined α_1- and β-agonist effects, because of the diminished sensitivity of cardiac β-receptors and the diminished myocardial contractility in septic shock.[85] Norepinephrine infusions may be titrated to preset goals of MAP (usually > 70 mm Hg), improvement in peripheral perfusion (to restored urine output or decreased blood lactate concentration), and/or achievement of desired oxygen transport variables, while not compromising cardiac index. Norepinephrine, 0.01–2 μg/kg/min, reliably and predictably improves hemodynamic parameters to "normal" or "supranormal" values in the majority of patients with septic shock. Doses that exceed those recommended by the manufacturer are necessary in critically ill patients with septic shock to achieve predetermined goals. An increase in the SVR generally accompanies a significant increase in MAP. Heart rate either decreases or remains unchanged, although insignificant increases have been reported.[56] Cardiac index either increases or does not change with few exceptions,[47,50,56] and there is no change in the PAOP.[50,51,56,86]

Whereas the effects on MAP, SVR, cardiac index, and heart rate appear to be desirable and more predictable, the effect of norepinephrine on urine output is variable and may depend on concurrently administered vasoactive agents.[48,56,51] Concurrent inotropic support with dobutamine and dopamine, or low doses of dopamine, preclude attributing any beneficial effects to norepinephrine alone.[56] An increase in urine output may be due to increased renal perfusion pressure secondary to the increases in MAP and SVRI, especially given that norepinephrine has a greater vasoconstrictive effect on the efferent arteriole of the kidney than on the afferent arteriole.[50]

The effect of norepinephrine on oxygen transport parameters is variable and depends on baseline values and concurrently administered vasoactive agents. The majority of the studies have shown either an increase or no change in Do_2 with no change in O_2ER, particularly when mean Do_2 values were "supranormal" prior to therapy.[56,84,87] In all but one study,[88] patients had received dobutamine and/or dopamine prior to the initiation of goal-directed therapy with norepinephrine. Martin and associates found norepinephrine alone to be superior to dopamine in achieving and maintaining for at least 6 hours preset levels for hemodynamic and oxygen transport variables (93% vs. 31% of patients, $P < .001$).[88] These investigators suggested that differences between the two agents resulted from norepinephrine's combined increase in Vo_2 and decrease in lactate concentrations through correction of splanchnic ischemia and efficient hepatic clearance of lactate, or through a preferential increase in Do_2 to areas of greatest oxygen demand, thus optimizing O_2ER.

Recently, Martin and colleagues, in a prospective, observational, cohort study of 97 adult patients with septic shock, determined that the use of norepinephrine to provide hemodynamic support was associated with a significant decrease in hospital mortality.[81] Martin also showed that the addition of norepinephrine in patients with dobutamine-resistant septic shock resulted in significant improvements (40%) in cardiac index and stroke volume index during a 4-hour study period.[47] This occurred despite an increase in left ventricular afterload, suggesting that either a positive inotropic effect or the correction of systemic hypotension was responsible. The authors further speculated that older patients may benefit from a combined α- and β-vasopressor versus a pure β-agonist (i.e., dobutamine), given the higher incidence of coronary disease and compromised ventricles in these patients. By virtue of restored MAP and, hence, coronary perfusion, norepinephrine increases cardiac index in older patients, whereas in younger patients, who have less coronary artery disease and a higher cardiac index at baseline, norepinephrine acts primarily as a vasopressor. In younger patients in this study, norepinephrine did not significantly increase cardiac index or stroke volume index.

Taken together, these recent data suggest that norepinephrine should potentially be repositioned as the vasopressor of choice in septic shock because of its multiple benefits: (1) it attenuates inappropriate vasodilation and low global oxygen extraction; (2) it attenuates myocardial depression, at unchanged or increased cardiac output and increased coronary blood flow; (3) it improves renal perfusion pressure and renal filtration; and (4) it improves splanchnic perfusion.[86]

Dobutamine

An inotrope with vasodilatory properties (so-called "inodilator"), dobutamine is used in the treatment of septic and cardiogenic shock to increase cardiac index. In septic shock, the left ventricular ejection fraction and right ventricular function are depressed, despite a high cardiac index, while ventricular volumes and compliance are increased. Stroke index is maintained by an increased heart rate and ventricular dilatation. In survivors, the myocardial depression is reversible and normalizes at 5 to 10 days after the onset of sepsis.[89] Dobutamine has been shown to increase stroke index, left ventricular stroke work index, and thus cardiac index and Do_2 without increasing the PAOP in septic shock in animals, human volunteers, or in controlled studies of human septic shock.[56,90–92]

Most prospective, randomized, controlled studies of goal-directed therapy with dobutamine were performed in surgical and medical critically ill patients with septic shock refractory to concurrently administered vasopressors (dopamine and/or norepinephrine).[56,90,93–95] The oxygen transport effects of dobutamine may not be significant, or may be transient, particularly during prolonged infusions. It appears that the achievement of supranormal oxygen transport values with dobutamine in hyperdynamic septic shock refractory to fluid resuscitation and vasopressors is of little benefit as compared to treatment to achieve normal values. In addition, the administration of dobutamine to achieve these high values has resulted in an unchanged or an increased mortality and a greater incidence of adverse effects,[95] with the exception of a study in older high-risk surgical patients without sepsis.[23] Results in medical and surgical patients may differ because of differences in the time when the dobutamine infusion began, the duration of the infusion, and the dosages administered. Subgroups of patients with septic shock (6% to 34%) among critically ill, high-risk, trauma, and surgical patients have small and insignificant changes in Do_2, Vo_2, O_2ER, and cardiac index.[56,94] The lack of response may be related to late treatment (>72 hours after surgery), resulting in irreversible changes caused by hypoperfusion and hypoxia. In the group of medical patients, the lack of sustained effect may have been attributed to the fact that very large doses were needed to achieve the desired effects over a longer treatment period (72 hours).[96] The requirement for vasopressor support with dopamine may have decreased the O_2ER and negated the beneficial effects of increased delivery. The O_2ER, mixed venous oxygen tension, and relative changes in SVR were not reported.

In populations of medical[93] and surgical patients,[90,95] dobutamine did not increase the likelihood of patients achieving supranormal oxygen transport values. Continuation of dobutamine until death or resolution of acute illness resulted in an increased mortality rate, despite an increase in the mean area under the Do_2 curve. The fact that no change in Vo_2 was evident, and thus O_2ER decreased, partially explains the higher mortality rate. Also, patients received much higher doses of dobutamine in this study.[95] Of the 50 patients in the experimental group, 17 received 50 μg/kg/min or more of dobutamine at some time during the study. Despite these high doses, 35 of 50 patients (70%) were unable to achieve the predetermined goals. In fact, despite the absence of preexisting cardiac abnormalities, complications (e.g., tachycardia, ischemic changes on ECG, hypertension, and tachydysrhythmias) limited dose increments of dobutamine in half of the dobutamine patients in the treatment group.

Recent studies have focused on the effects of dobutamine on gastric mucosal flow and the splanchnic circulation. Duranteau and associates found that the addition of dobutamine (5 μg/kg/min) to norepinephrine improved gastric mucosal perfusion without increasing cardiac index.[96] This result is consistent with findings in clinical studies indicating that dobutamine may improve pHi and mucosal perfusion in septic patients.[97,98] The addition of dobutamine to epinephrine regimens has been shown to improve gastric mucosal perfusion, as measured by improvements in pHi, arterial lactate concentrations, and $P\text{CO}_2$ gap.[99] The findings of Duranteau and associates were likely related to a blood flow redistribution toward gastric mucosa. This effect may result from either an increase in the fraction of the cardiac output that was distributed to the global hepatosplanchnic blood flow or a redistribution of blood flow within gastric wall layers toward mucosa by 'stealing' blood away from the muscularis, potentially owing to the greater β_2-mediated vasodilation. Other investigations support this hypothesis.[97,100,101]

Dobutamine should be started with doses ranging from 2.5 to 5.0 μg/kg/min. Although there is generally a dose response, recent evidence suggests that doses in excess of 5 μg/kg/min not only may provide limited beneficial effects on oxygen transport values and hemodynamics, but also may increase adverse cardiac effects.[102] If given to patients who are intravascularly depleted, dobutamine will result in hypotension and a reflexive tachycardia. Klem and associates found significant inter- and intrapatient variability in the pharmacokinetics of dobutamine in unstable critically ill patients.[103] Pathophysiologic factors influence dosing requirements and pharmacokinetic parameters over the time course of the illness and the duration of the infusion. Thus, infusion rates should be guided by clinical end points. Decreases in $Pa\text{O}_2$ and increases in $P\bar{v}\text{O}_2$, as well as myocardial adverse effects such as tachycardia, ischemic changes on ECG, tachydysrhythmias, and hypotension, may occur.[95] Dobutamine, like other inotropes, is usually given until there is an improvement in myocardial function with resolution of the septic episode or when dose-limiting side effects appear.[90,93]

Phenylephrine

Despite its purported use in refractory septic shock, very little information is published regarding the clinical efficacy of phenylephrine. Nevertheless, it is an attractive agent for use in sepsis because of its selective α-agonism and primarily vascular effects, its rapid onset, and its short duration of action. It is generally initiated at dosages of 0.5 μg/kg/min and may be titrated quickly to desired effect.

Three clinical trials involving 38 patients have evaluated the use of phenylephrine in septic shock. Phenylephrine (0.5–9 μg/kg/min), when used alone or in combination with dobutamine or low doses of dopamine, improves blood pressure and myocardial performance in fluid-resuscitated patients with sepsis.[104] Incremental doses of phenylephrine over 3 hours result in linear dose-related increases in MAP, SVR, heart rate, and stroke index when administered as a single agent in stable, nonhypotensive, but hyperdynamic, volume-resuscitated surgical ICU patients. In septic shock, phenylephrine does not impair cardiac index, PAOP, or peripheral perfusion.[52,86] Yamazaki and associates showed that although its administration improved myocardial performance in hyperdynamic, normotensive patients with sepsis, phenylephrine worsened it in cardiac controls.[104] At a dosage of 70 μg/min, phenylephrine improved cardiac index and MAP by increasing venous return to the heart (increase in CVP and stroke index) and by acting as a positive inotrope because SVR did not change. There was a clinically insignificant decrease in heart rate (3 beats/min). However, in cardiac patients, myocardial performance worsened as a result of an increase in MAP and SVR, and a decrease in cardiac index with no change in heart rate. Although these results suggest caution, it is noteworthy that the cardiac indices of the two groups were not comparable at baseline.

In septic shock, phenylephrine appears to increase global tissue oxygen use, although there is conflicting information regarding the relationship of the oxygen transport variables with increases in MAP and cardiac index.[52,86] Increases in $V\text{O}_2$ appear to be dissociated from $D\text{O}_2$, representing an increase in O_2ER because cardiac index remains unchanged. Increases in $V\text{O}_2$ may result from the redistribution of blood flow to previously underperfused areas, thus improving oxygen use due to changes in MAP and SVRI. With phenylephrine administration, no organ dysfunction was documented, and evidence of globally improved peripheral tissue perfusion was seen as the lactic acid level fell or remained unchanged and urine output increased significantly at increased or maximal $V\text{O}_2$. An increased O_2ER may contribute to improved tissue use of oxygen.[52,86]

In one small study, measured $D\text{O}_2$ and $V\text{O}_2$ values paralleled MAP in most patients.[86] As with epinephrine, phenylephrine doses required to achieve the goals of therapy were significantly higher (1.3–3.7 μg/kg/min) than those traditionally recommended for use. When phenylephrine (0.5 μg/kg/min) was titrated to a plateau in $V\text{O}_2$ or the appearance of adverse cardiac effects, there was a greater than 15% increase in $D\text{O}_2$ and $V\text{O}_2$. When combined with dobutamine, phenylephrine resulted in a more consistent and statistically significant increase in both $D\text{O}_2$ and $V\text{O}_2$. However, these observations may be biased, because baseline $D\text{O}_2$ and $V\text{O}_2$ values were somewhat higher in patients who did not require dobutamine (5 of 11).

In a second study, Flancbaum and colleagues evaluated the use of phenylephrine as a single agent, without another cardiotonic agent, in 10 septic, hyperdynamic surgical ICU patients.[52] Of the 10 patients, 8 had a clinically significant increase ($>15\%$) in $V\text{O}_2$ with variable doses of phenylephrine, while $D\text{O}_2$ increased in only 3 patients. Phenylephrine predictably increased MAP, but not $V\text{O}_2$ in a dose-dependent fashion in the surgical patient population.

There are very few data regarding the effect of phenylephrine on regional hemodynamics and oxygen transport variables. When phenylephrine replaced norepinephrine in patients with septic shock, it selectively reduced splanchnic blood flow, and thus the splanchnic $D\text{O}_2$ and the splanchnic lactate uptake rate, without changing the overall splanchnic $V\text{O}_2$.[105] Because all these parameters normalized when norepinephrine was reinstated, these data suggest that exogenous β-adrenergic stimulation (norepinephrine) may determine hepatosplanchnic perfusion and oxygen availability, but not utilization, in septic shock. This study also demonstrated that while the phenylephrine-induced reduction in splanchnic DO_2 also reduced the *de novo* synthesis of glucose (a highly oxygen-dependent pathway in the periportal region), it did not affect the formation of monoethylglycylxylide (MEGX), an active metabolite of lidocaine (a cytochrome P450–dependent pathway in the perivenous region). This finding suggests that the latter metabolic activity is not so dependent on oxygen, is retained in septic shock, and reflects the heterogeneity of metabolic function in different areas of the liver.[105]

The available data on hemodynamics, oxygen transport variables, and mortality associated with the use of phenylephrine in septic shock may not be generalizable because of the small numbers of patients involved in the studies. Adverse effects such as tachydysrhythmias are notably infrequent with phenylephrine, particularly when used as a single agent or with higher doses. It is unclear, however, what the optimal duration of therapy with phenylephrine is in septic shock and how sustained the beneficial effects may be with longer administration.[52] In an experimental animal model, sustained endotoxemia (48 hours) did not result in desensitization of α_1-adrenergic responsiveness when phenylephrine was used.[44] Other mechanisms may be responsible for the ineffectiveness of vasopressors during advanced sepsis. Phenylephrine may be an appropriate choice when β-adrenergic receptor desensitization becomes a clinical problem. Like other vasopressors, phenylephrine is continued until resolution of the hemodynamic instability associated with the septic episode and stopped when patients are clinically stable.

Epinephrine

By convention, epinephrine has been reserved as a last-line agent in hemodynamic support of sepsis. There are very few objective data evaluating its comparative efficacy in early sepsis; most studies examine the effects of epinephrine in refractory septic shock.[56] Despite this, epinephrine is an acceptable choice as a single agent because of its combined vasoconstrictor and inotropic effects. Epinephrine infusion rates of 0.04–1 μg/kg/min alone increase hemodynamic and oxygen transport variables to "supranormal" values without adverse effects in patients who do not have coronary artery disease. In 69 patients evaluated in five studies, epinephrine alone or combined with either dobutamine or low doses of dopamine, achieved the desired outcomes.[44,58,106–108] Large doses (0.5–1 μg/kg/min) are required when epinephrine is added to other agents.[58] Smaller doses (0.10–0.50 μg/kg/min) are effective if dobutamine and dopamine infusions are kept constant, possibly because of exposure to less β-receptor stimulation and thus less receptor desensitization.[108]

The same holds true when epinephrine is used as a first-line agent and when it is used in younger patients.[45,106,107] A linear dose-response curve is seen, with a rapid improvement of hemodynamic variables and Do_2. Although Do_2 increases mainly as a function of consistent increases in cardiac index and a more variable increase in SVR, Vo_2 may not increase, and O_2ER may fall. A transient fall in pHi may occur during the epinephrine administration, but dobutamine can counteract this impairment in gastric mucosal perfusion. The lactate concentration may rise during the first few hours of epinephrine therapy; however, it normalizes over the ensuing 24 hours in survivors.[58,109] The increase in the lactate concentration may be due to a worsened Do_2 to the liver (and subsequent anaerobic metabolism) or to the hepatosplanchnic circulation, or, alternately, due to a direct increase by epinephrine in calorigenesis and breakdown of glcyogen and lactate production.

There is recent evidence to suggest that epinephrine, unlike dopamine, may increase the proportion of total cardiac output delivered to the splanchnic circulation, although Vo_2 is not increased sufficiently to increase O_2ER.[110] In contrast, when epinephrine is compared to a combination of norepinephrine and dobutamine, a short infusion (2 hours) of it preferentially decreases splanchnic Do_2, worsens pHi, and increases systemic lactate concentration without increasing Vo_2.[26] Methodologic limitations preclude drawing significant conclusions from this study, however. For example, the crossover period was not randomized and had confounding factors, including pharmacologic carryover, failure of patients to achieve a steady state before crossover, and the use of time-dependent response measures. It is also unclear whether patients were comparable at baseline, whether they had received the same or other vasoactive agents before the study period, and if so, how long they had received them.[111]

Another crossover study in dopamine-resistant volume-replete patients with septic shock was designed to compare the gastric mucosal perfusion obtained with epinephrine and that obtained with norepinephrine.[96] For the same level of MAP, epinephrine induced a greater increase in mucosal perfusion. Because similar ratios between gastric mucosal perfusion and Do_2 were observed with both epinephrine and norepinephrine, it is likely that the greater increase in mucosal perfusion by epinephrine was secondary to a larger increase in Do_2 by this agent (increase in cardiac index via an increase in heart rate).[96]

Despite the large doses used in all of the studies discussed, no clinically important ventricular or supraventricular dysrhythmias were reported in the young patients, in older patients, or in those with long-standing underlying cardiac disease states.[45,106,107] Nevertheless, caution must be exercised before using epinephrine in managing hypoperfusion in hypodynamic patients with coronary artery disease where ischemia, chest pain, and myocardial infarction may result. Factors that may influence successful therapy with epinephrine may include the time from the onset of septic shock to effective therapy, its use as a primary or initial agent, and the age of the population.

EXPERIMENTAL THERAPIES

DOPEXAMINE

An investigational synthetic catecholamine, dopexamine is used in low cardiac output states with coexisting elevated systemic or pulmonary vascular resistance. Dopexamine has been used in acute heart failure, impaired left ventricular function after surgery, and in septic shock. As is the case with dobutamine in septic shock, dopexamine is most frequently administered in combination with a vasopressor agent such as norepinephrine or dopamine because of coexisting refractory hypotension.

Dopexamine improves cardiac performance by a marked vasodilation and a mild inotropic activity. In two studies of septic shock in predominantly surgical patients ($n = 39$), dopexamine produced a dose-related (range, 2–6 μg/kg/min) increase in cardiac index, stroke volume, and heart rate, as well as a decrease in SVR, over the course of the infusion (0.5–1 hour).[54,55] Epinephrine[55] or norepinephrine and dobutamine[54] dosages were kept constant during the study period. There appears to be a smaller increase in myocardial oxygen demand than with dopamine, although tachycardia and tachydysrhythmias may lead to myocardial ischemia, particularly in patients with ischemic heart disease.[54,55]

Global oxygen transport variables are similar to those of dopamine. Oxygen delivery increases significantly, but Vo_2 increases insufficiently and thus O_2ER decreases. Dopexamine's combined β_2-adrenergic and DA_1-agonist activities theoretically should be advantageous in improving distribution of blood flow in septic shock. Only one study has evaluated the regional effects of dopexamine.[56] During dopexamine infusion, pHi increased ($n = 7/10$) and remained high an hour after discontinuation of the drug. The improvements in pHi, however, did not parallel changes in cardiac output and Do_2. The authors suggested that this may represent a preferential effect on gastric mucosal blood flow. When administered before and during major abdominal surgery, low doses of dopexamine increased small bowel serosal tissue oxygen content ($p_{tiss}O_2$) but decreased gastric ΔpCO_2, indicating an improvement of blood flow in the small bowel at the expense of shunting blood away from the gastric mucosa.[112]

The same results were found with escalating doses of dopexamine to dobutamine-resistant septic shock patients.[113] Initial data do not appear to support a significant role for dopexamine in improving regional hemodynamics and blood flow in the supportive management of septic shock.

NITRIC OXIDE SYNTHASE INHIBITORS

Nitric oxide is a short-acting, potent vasodilator derived from the enzymatic oxidation of arginine. Its production is under the control of nitric oxide synthase (NOS). This enzyme is present (expressed) in two forms: a constitutive form (ecNOS) and an inducible form (iNOS). The vascular endothelium normally produces small amounts of nitric oxide under the control of ecNOS for the physiologic control of vascular tone and blood flow distribution. Under pathophysiologic conditions such as stimulation by lipopolysaccharide or cytokines, iNOS becomes diffusely expressed, producing large amounts of nitric oxide. The latter has been implicated in the cardiovascular failure of septic shock.[114,115]

Pharmacologic inhibition of nitric oxide production has been investigated as an adjunct to standard therapies of septic shock. L-arginine analogs such as monomethyl-L-arginine (L-NMMA) or L-arginine-methylester (L-NAME) are competitive inhibitors of NOS and have been shown to increase blood pressure and partially restore vascular reactivity in experimental and human septic shock.[116] However, because these arginine analogs nonselectively block ecNOS and iNOS, their use has been associated with extensive vasoconstriction, decreased cardiac output, and regional hypoperfusion, thus promoting organ failure and mortality. Currently, there is increased focus on identification of selective inhibitors of iNOS.[114,115] Some S-substituted thiourea derivatives have demonstrated both *in vitro* and *in vivo* (rodent) dose-dependent selectivity for iNOS inhibition. Recently, Rosselet and associates demonstrated that low doses (0.1 mg/kg/h) of S-methyl-isothiourea (SMT) were superior to norepinephrine in the treatment of rat endotoxic shock. These doses of SMT prevented hypotension by maintaining cardiac index, without increasing SVRI as did norepinephrine. However, only low doses of SMT limited the development of lactic acidosis.[114]

CORTICOSTEROIDS

The use of corticosteroids in the treatment of septic shock has been a topic of controversy for many years. The renewed interest in the use of corticosteroids in the treatment of sepsis has emerged because of the recent focus on adrenocortical insufficiency in critically ill patients, including those with septic shock.[117] Relative adrenal insufficiency has been defined as a poor adrenal response (9 μg/dL) irrespective of the initial serum cortisol level) to a dose of synthetic corticotropin, indicating a low functional reserve of the adrenal cortex.[117] Although absolute insufficiency is rare, relative adrenal insufficiency in the presence of normal or high cortisol levels at baseline is present in 30% to 50% of patients with septic shock, and is associated with a poor outcome.[118]

Two studies have shown that the administration of moderate "supraphysiologic" doses (200–300 mg/day) of hydrocortisone may reverse septic shock.[119,120] The corticosteroid improves hemodynamics and reduces the length of time that the patient needs vasopressor support. One of the studies showed a trend toward an improvement in survival at 28 days.[119] In two other studies, the responsiveness to norepinephrine was the greatest and fastest in patients with inadequate endogenous production of cortisol in comparison with those with adequate endogenous production.[121,122] All these studies differ from earlier studies of steroids in septic shock in that the steroids were administered late in the septic shock, for longer than 5 days, and at lower doses—all in patients receiving relatively high doses of catecholamine vasopressors.

In order to understand further the interaction between vasopressors and corticosteroids, Bellissant and colleagues evaluated the hydrocortisone-phenylephrine MAP dose-response relationship in 12 septic shock patients within 3 hours of ICU admission and in normal controls.[123] The patients with septic shock were severely ill (Acute Physiology And Chronic Health Evaluation [APACHE II] 61 $\pm$ 22), received fluids to achieve a PAOP of 14–18 mm Hg, and began treatment with incremental doses of phenylephrine only at first with the subsequent addition of hydrocortisone. An E_{max} model was developed in both groups of patients before and after the addition of hydrocortisone. In septic shock patients, hydrocortisone reversed the blunted response to phenylephrine to that of controls. The hyporesponsiveness to phenylephrine was related to its vascular, rather than its central (no alteration in baroreflex sensitivity), effects. The corticosteroid effects were deemed not to be related to activation of the sympathetic or renin-angiotensin systems nor to nitric oxide pathways, because no significant relationship was found between pharmacodynamic parameters and circulating catecholamines, renin, aldosterone, or nitrite/nitrate levels. The methods used by these investigators made it impossible to exclude more indirect mechanisms of effect on adrenergic receptor activity.

Current proposed mechanisms of the vasoconstrictor effect of corticosteroids may include increasing the number and stimulating the function of α_1- and β-adrenergic receptors. In addition, corticosteroids may attenuate the production of mediators responsible in part for the vasodilation and hyperdynamic state of sepsis (perhaps indirectly through i NOS inhibition or through improved binding affinity of the cortisol receptor).[117,118]

Given the current data, corticosteroids may be administered to patients with septic shock on high doses of vasopressors for prolonged periods of time if (1) reversible causes of hypotension are eliminated; (2) absolute corticosteroid deficiency is checked with corticotropin stimulation testing; and (3) corticosteroids are used for at least 5 to 7 days and progressively reduced.[117] Issues that remain unclear include which patients may benefit from corticosteroids, whether corticosteroids improve survival, and what the optimal dosing regimen is (i.e., the lowest minimum dose, the timing and duration of administration).

VASOPRESSIN

Recently, vasopressin has been used anecdotally in a series of patients with vasodilatory septic shock who remained hypotensive on vasopressors.[124,125] Arginine vasopressin has little pressor activity in normal subjects, but markedly increases blood pressure when sympathetic nerve function is impaired, including in an experimental animal model of septic shock. When administered in low doses (0.01–0.05 U/min) to patients with vasodilatory septic shock who were receiving high doses and long courses of norepinephrine, vasopressin successfully increased arterial blood pressure and SVRI; cardiac output remained stable.

In a case series, urine flow rates increased significantly in three of five patients, most likely because of increased renal perfusion and arterial pressure. In four of five patients, norepinephrine therapy was successfully tapered and discontinued within 15 minutes. No clinical or laboratory signs of cardiac or mesenteric ischemia were observed, nor was PAOP or oxygenation adversely affected.[124] In a double-blind, placebo-controlled trial involving trauma patients who required vasopressors for vasodilatory shock, a vasopressin infusion (0.04 U/min) significantly improved arterial pressure resulting from peripheral vasoconstriction and permitted the withdrawal of catecholamine vasopressors (norepinephrine, phenylephrine, or dopamine).[126] All patients receiving vasopressin survived the 24-hour study period and had all other catecholamine vasopressors withdrawn and blood pressure maintained solely with a low-dose vasopressin infusion. Although vasopressin may be a useful agent in the treatment of refractory septic shock, it should not be used in patients with hypovolemia, cardiogenic shock, or septic shock with myocardial depression, as it may decrease cardiac output and cause profound cutaneous vasoconstriction and necrosis.[125]

GENERAL CONCLUSIONS AND RECOMMENDATIONS

The choice of vasopressor or inotropic agent in septic shock should be made according to the needs of the patient (Figure 23–3). The traditional algorithm suggests a stepwise approach first using dopamine, then norepinephrine; dobutamine is added for low cardiac output states, and occasionally epinephrine and phenylephrine are necessary. Although this approach is empirical, it is broadly used in clinical practice and has been justified by a desire to avoid strong vasoconstriction and by the sense of safety that graded doses of dopamine provide. This dose-response relationship, however, has never been established in the critically ill. Furthermore, recent observations of improved outcomes with norepinephrine and decreased regional perfusion with dopamine are calling into question the use of dopamine as a first-line agent.

For all catecholamine vasopressors, larger doses than those traditionally recommended are required for goal-directed therapy to the desired MAP and for normalization of oxygen transport variables, DO_2 and VO_2. Attainment of supranormal DO_2 and VO_2 values is difficult in the majority of patients, even if large doses are used. Patients who develop supranormal DO_2 and VO_2 have a lower mortality rate, but

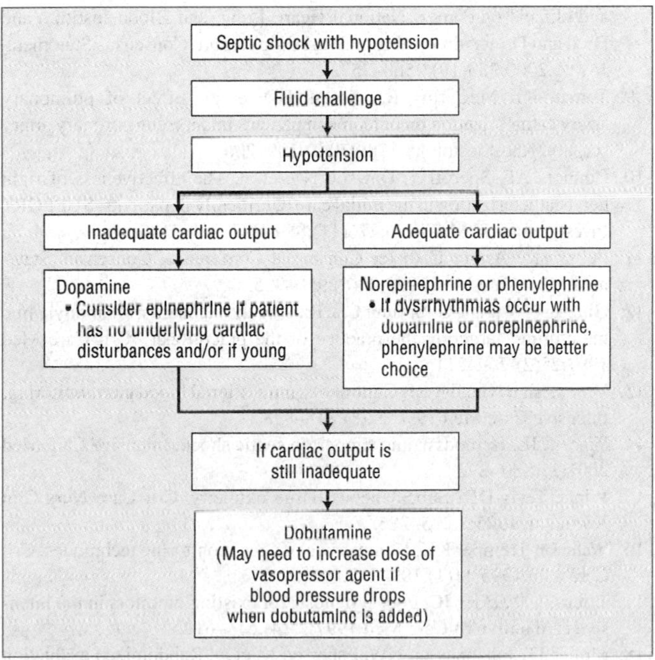

FIGURE 23–3. Algorithmic approach to the use of vasopressors and inotropes in septic shock. Approach is intended to be used in conjunction with clinical judgment, hemodynamic monitoring parameters, and therapy end points. *(Modified from Ref. 25.)*

whether this is achieved intrinsically or with exogenous administration of vasopressors/inotropes appears inconsequential. Goal-directed therapy to supranormal oxygen transport values cannot therefore be recommended, as little or no benefit of this approach has been demonstrated to date. Further work is required to better elucidate the differential effects of vasopressors on regional hemodynamic and oxygen transport values, as measures of local tissue perfusion.

Although difficult to demonstrate, there may be true differences in the pharmacologic activity of vasopressors and inotropes. For example, recent evidence suggests that when used appropriately with fluid replenishment, norepinephrine is safe and effective in decreasing mortality, particularly when initiated early. It is effective in optimizing hemodynamic variables and improving systemic and regional (e.g., renal, gastric mucosal, splanchnic) perfusion, probably because of its β_2 vasodilatory effects. Epinephrine causes a greater increase in cardiac index and DO_2 than does norepinephrine, and it increases gastric mucosal flow; however, it may not adequately preserve splanchnic circulation because of its predominant vasoconstrictive α effects. Epinephrine may cause a short-lived increase in the concentration of lactic acid. This resolves in 24 hours, and no difference in clinical outcome has been documented. Epinephrine may be particularly useful when used earlier in the course of septic shock in young patients and those who do not have any known cardiac abnormalities. Unlike epinephrine, dopamine does not preferentially increase the proportion of cardiac output that preferentially goes to the splanchnic circulation. The inability of dopamine to increase cardiac output by more than 35% and the associated tachycardia or tachydysrhythmias limit its utility. Dopamine, as opposed to norepinephrine, has been shown to worsen splanchnic VO_2 and O_2ER. Low-dose dopamine has not been shown to consistently increase the glomerular filtration rate, does not prevent renal failure, and indeed worsens splanchnic tissue oxygen utilization. Routine use of concurrently administered dopamine with vasopressors is not recommended. Phenylephrine should be used when a pure vasoconstrictor is desired in patients who may not require or cannot tolerate the β effects of dopamine or norepinephrine with or without dobutamine. In patients with high filling pressure and hypotension, the combination of phenylephrine and dobutamine may be useful.

The methodologic shortcomings of the studies that have been done prevent definitive conclusions. Short infusions (not exceeding 2 hours) during studies may show differences that are not clinically significant at 24 hours or more, as demonstrated for epinephrine and dobutamine. Clinically, vasopressors and inotropes are used for hours to days. Also, variable stages of sepsis or septic shock when a study is initiated, the inherent differences in circulating catecholamine levels, and changes in receptor activity all may be confounding factors, as may be the prestudy duration and type of exogenous catecholamine administration.

Recent data with moderate doses of corticosteroids (200–300 mg/day) infused over 5 to 7 days may reverse septic shock and dependency on vasopressor agents, particularly in patients with relative adrenal insufficiency. Data are still needed regarding optimal dosing and the effect on outcomes such as mortality. Initial uncontrolled studies with vasopressin suggest that it has a potential role in the management of vasopressor-refractory septic shock, although additional data are needed.

Further pharmacotherapeutic and outcome studies are still required to elucidate the place in therapy that individual vasopressors and inotropes or their combinations occupy in the supportive care of patients with bacteremia or septic shock. Once this is accomplished, it will be necessary to direct our efforts to the pharmacoeconomics and cost-effectiveness of these therapies.

▶ PRINCIPLES OF PHARMACOTHERAPY

- Continuous and invasive hemodynamic monitoring with an arterial catheter and a pulmonary artery catheter should be used early and throughout the course of septic shock to assess intravascular fluid status and ventricular filling pressures, to determine cardiac output, and to monitor arterial and venous oxygenation. They should also be used to monitor the response to drug therapy and to guide dosage titration.
- Derangements in adrenergic receptor sensitivity or activity frequently result in resistance to vasopressor and inotropic therapy in critically ill patients. These changes may be a function of endogenous catecholamine concentrations, dose/duration of exposure to and type of exogenously administered vasopressors, stage of septic shock, preexisting illness, as well as other factors.
- In refractory septic shock, the use of vasopressor or inotropic agents should be guided by receptor activity, pharmacologic characteristics, and regional and systemic hemodynamic effects of the drug; treatment should be tailored to the patient's physiologic needs. Pharmacologically sound combinations of agents should be initiated early to optimize response.
- Goals of therapy with vasopressors and inotropes should be predetermined and should optimize regional perfusion to tissues (e.g., cardiac, renal, mesenteric, periphery). Goal-directed therapy with vasopressors and inotropes to supranormal global oxygen transport values cannot be recommended, as there is no clear benefit and morbidity may increase. However, achievement of supranormal values for oxygen delivery (DO_2) and oxygen consumption (VO_2), whether intrinsically or pharmacologically, is associated with decreased mortality in septic shock.
- Much higher dosages of all vasopressors and inotropes than traditionally recommended are required in order to improve the hemodynamic and oxygen transport variables in patients with septic shock.
- The "best clinical response" should guide dose titration and monitoring of vasopressor and inotropic therapy. It is important to watch for and minimize the effect of any evidence of myocardial ischemia (e.g., tachydysrhythmias, electrocardiogram [ECG] changes), renal difficulties (e.g., decreased glomerular filtration rate and/or urine output), splanchnic/gastric problems (e.g., low intramucosal pH, bowel ischemia), or peripheral (cold extremities) hypoperfusion; and worsening of PaO_2, the pulmonary artery occlusion pressure (PAOP); and other hemodynamic variables.
- Dopamine is typically used as an initial vasopressor agent for hemodynamic support, but is limited by its ability to increase cardiac output (35%). Its use is frequently complicated by tachycardia and tachydysrhythmias, and occasionally by an increase in the PAOP. In contrast to norepinephrine, it decreases splanchnic oxygen use. Although commonly used, low-dose dopamine either with norepinephrine or other agents has not been proved to be of any benefit in oliguric patients in septic shock.
- Phenylephrine may be a particularly useful alternative in those who cannot tolerate tachycardia or tachydysrhythmias with dopamine or norepinephrine, or those patients with known underlying myocardial dysfunction.
- Epinephrine appears to be safe and effective as a single agent and as an add-on agent. It is particularly useful in the young, in patients with otherwise healthy myocardia, and early in the course of treatment. It causes a significant increase in the lactate level, which gradually resolves, and it appears to cause little cardiac disturbance in patients with no known cardiac abnormalities. It should be used cautiously in patients with a history of coronary artery disease or underlying cardiac disturbances.
- Therapy with vasopressors and inotropes is continued until the myocardial depression and vascular hyporesponsiveness of septic shock improves, usually measured in hours to days. Discontinuation of vasopressor or inotropic therapy should take place slowly; "weaning" from therapy helps to avoid a precipitous worsening in regional and systemic hemodynamics.

REFERENCES

1. Balk RA. Severe sepsis and septic shock: definitions, epidemiology, and clinical manifestations. Crit Care Clin 2000;16(2):179–192.
2. Hollenberg SM, Kavinsky CJ, Parrillo JE. Cardiogenic shock. Ann Intern Med 1999;131(1):47–59.
3. Ahrens T. Hemodynamic monitoring. Crit Care Nurs Clin North Am 1999;11(1):19–31.
4. Lal SK, Henderson RJ, Cejnar M, et al. Physiological influences on continuous finger and simultaneous intra-arterial blood pressure. Hypertension 1995;26(2):307–314.
5. Headley JM. Invasive hemodynamic monitoring: applying advanced technologies. Crit Care Nurs Q 1998;21(3):73–84.
6. Ayres SM, Grenvik A, Holbrook PR, et al. Invasive and noninvasive physiologic monitoring. In: Shoemaker WC, Parsa MH, eds. Textbook of Critical Care. Philadelphia, Saunders, 1995:252–266.
7. Burchell SA, Yu M, Takiguchi SA, et al. Evaluation of a continuous cardiac output and mixed venous oxygen saturation catheter in critically ill surgical patients. Crit Care Med 1997;25(3):388–391.
8. Bernard GR, Sopko G, Cerra F, et al. Pulmonary artery catheterization and clinical outcomes: National Heart, Lung, and Blood Institute and Food and Drug Administration Workshop Report. Consensus Statement. JAMA 2000;283(19):2568–2572.
9. Tuman KJ, McCarthy RJ, Spiess BD, et al. Effect of pulmonary artery catheterization on outcome in patients undergoing coronary artery surgery. Anesthesiology 1989;70(2):199–206.
10. Connors AF, Speroff T, Dawson NV, et al. The effectiveness of right heart catheterization in the initial care of critically ill patients. SUPPORT Investigators. JAMA 1996;276(11):889–897.
11. Pulmonary Artery Catheter Consensus Conference. Consensus Statement. Crit Care Med 1997;25(6):910–925.
12. Ginosar Y, Thijs LG, Sprung CL. Raising the standard of hemodynamic monitoring: targeting the practice or the practitioner? Crit Care Med 1997;25(2):209–211.
13. Venkatesh B, Hendry SP. Continuous intra-arterial blood gas monitoring. Intensive Care Med 1996;22(8):818–828.
14. Vincent JL. Hemodynamic support in septic shock. Intensive Care Med 2001;27:S80–S92.
15. Wipke-Tevis DD. Subcutaneous tissue oximetry. Crit Care Nurs Clin North Am 1995;7:275–285.
16. Wahr JA, Tremper KK. Noninvasive oxygen monitoring techniques. Crit Care Clin 1995;11(1):199–217.
17. Tsien CL, Fackler JC. Poor prognosis for existing monitors in the intensive care unit. Crit Care Med 1997;25(4):614–619.
18. Moller JT, Johannessen NW, Espersen K, et al. Randomized evaluation of pulse oximetry in 20,802 patients: II. Perioperative events and postoperative complications. Anesthesiology 1993;78(3):445–453.
19. Cullen DJ, Nemeskal AR, Cooper JB, et al. Effect of pulse oximetry, age, and ASA physical status on the frequency of patients admitted un-

expectedly to a postoperative intensive care unit and the severity of their anesthesia-related complications. Anesth Analg 1992;74(2):181–188.
20. Yu M. Oxygen transport optimization. New Horizons 1999;7:46–53.
21. Heyland DK, Cook DJ, King D, et al. Maximizing oxygen delivery in critically ill patients: a methodologic appraisal of the evidence. Crit Care Med 1996;24(3):517–524.
22. Yu M, Burchell S, Hasaniya NW, et al. Relationship of mortality to increasing oxygen delivery in patients > or = 50 years of age: a prospective, randomized trial. Crit Care Med 1998;26(6):1011–1019.
23. Lobo SM, Salgado PF, Castillo VG, et al. Effects of maximizing oxygen delivery on morbidity and mortality in high-risk surgical patients. Crit Care Med 2000;28(10):3396–3404.
24. Uusaro A, Russell JA. Could anti-inflammatory actions of catecholamines explain the possible beneficial effects of supranormal oxygen delivery in critically ill surgical patients? Intensive Care Med 2000;26(3):299–304.
25. Task Force of the American College of Critical Care Medicine, Society of Critical Care Medicine. Practice parameters for hemodynamic support of sepsis in adult patients. Crit Care Med 1999;27(3): 639–660.
26. Meier-Hellmann A, Reinhart K, Bredle DL, et al. Epinephrine impairs splanchnic perfusion in septic shock. Crit Care Med 1997;25(3): 399–404.
27. Kelly KM. Does increasing oxygen delivery improve outcome? Yes. Crit Care Clin 1996;12(3):635–644.
28. Dasta JF, Brackett CC. Defining and achieving optimum therapeutic goals in critically ill patients. Pharmacotherapy 1994;14(6):678–688.
29. Tuchschmidt JA, Mecher CE. Predictors of outcome from critical illness: shock and cardiopulmonary resuscitation. Crit Care Clin 1994;10(1): 179–195.
30. Rady MY, Rivers EP, Nowak RM. Resuscitation of the critically ill in the ED: responses of blood pressure, heart rate, shock index, central venous oxygen saturation, and lactate. Am J Emerg Med 1996;14(2):218–225.
31. Brown SD, Clark C, Gutierrez G. Pulmonary lactate release in patients with sepsis and the adult respiratory distress syndrome. J Crit Care 1996;11(1):2–8.
32. Schlichtig R, Tonnessen TI, Nemoto EM. Detecting dysoxia in "silent" organs. Critical Care State of the Art, Society of Critical Care Medicine. 1993;14:239–273.
33. Bakker J, Coffernils M, Leon M, et al. Blood lactate levels are superior to oxygen-derived variables in predicting outcome in human septic shock. Chest 1991;99(4):956–962.
34. Chapman MV, Mythen MG, Webb AR, Vincent JL. Report from the meeting: Gastrointestinal tonometry: state of the art. 22nd-23rd May 1998, London, UK. Intensive Care Med 2000;26(5):613–622.
35. Temmesfeld-Wollbrück B, Mayer K, Grimminger F. Assessment of intestinal tissue oxygenation: the canary sings-but what does the twitter tell us? Intensive Care Med 2000;26(8):1025–1027.
36. Creteur J, De Backer D, Vincent JL. Monitoring gastric mucosal carbon dioxide pressure using gas tonometry: in vitro and in vivo validation studies. Anesthesiology 1997;87(3):504–510.
37. Gutierrez G, Palizas F, Doglio G, et al. Gastric intramucosal pH as a therapeutic index of tissue oxygenation in critically ill patients. Lancet 1992;339(8787):195–199.
38. Ivatury RR, Simon RJ, Islam S, et al. A prospective randomized study of end points of resuscitation after major trauma: global oxygen transport indices versus organ-specific gastric mucosal pH. J Am Coll Surg 1996;183(2):145–154.
39. Weil MH, Nakagawa Y, Tang W, et al. Sublingual capnometry: a new noninvasive measurement for diagnosis and quantitation of severity of circulatory shock. Crit Care Med 1999;27(7):1225–1229.
40. Hardman JG, Gilman AG, Limbird LE, et al. The autonomic and somatic motor nervous system. In: Lefkovitz RJ, Hoffman BB, Taylor P, eds. Goodman & Gilman's The Pharmacological Basis of Therapeutics. New York: McGraw-Hill; 1996:110–111.
41. Ruffolo R. Cardiovascular adrenoceptors: physiology and critical care implications. In: Chernow B, Brater DC, Holaday JW, et al., eds. The Pharmacological Approach to the Critically Ill Patient. Baltimore: Williams & Wilkins; 1994:167–181.
42. Sokoloff P, Schwartz JC. Novel dopamine receptors half a decade later. Trends Pharmacol Sci 1995;16(8):270–275.
43. Zaritsky AL. Catecholamines, inotropic medications, and vasopressor agents. In: Chernow B, Brater DC, Holaday JW, et al., eds. The Pharmacological Approach to the Critically Ill Patient. Baltimore: Williams & Wilkins; 1994:387–404.
44. Dickerson RN, Lima JJ, Kuhl DA, et al. Effect of sustained endotoxemia on alpha1-adrenergic responsiveness in parenterally fed rats. Pharmacotherapy 1998;18(1):170–174.
45. Silverman HJ, Penaranda R, Orens JB, Lee NH. Impaired beta-adrenergic receptor stimulation of cyclic adenosine monophosphate in human septic shock: association with myocardial hyporesponsiveness to catecholamines. Crit Care Med 1993;21(1):31–39.
46. Hahn PY, Wang P, Tait SM, et al. Sustained elevation in circulating catecholamine levels during polymicrobial sepsis. Shock 1995;4(4): 269–273.
47. Martin C, Viviand X, Arnaud S, et al. Effects of norepinephrine plus dobutamine or norepinephrine alone on left ventricular performance of septic shock patients. Crit Care Med 1999;27(9):1708–1713.
48. Richer M, Robert S, Lebel M. Renal hemodynamics during norepinephrine and low-dose dopamine infusions in man. Crit Care Med 1996;24(7):1150–1156.
49. Jindal N, Hollenberg SM, Dellinger RP. Pharmacologic issues in the management of septic shock. Crit Care Clin 2000;16(2):233–249.
50. Dasta JF. Norepinephrine in septic shock: renewed interest in an old drug. Drug Intell Clin Pharm 1990;24(2):153–156.
51. Redl-Wenzl EM, Armbruster C, Edelmann G, et al. The effects of norepinephrine on hemodynamics and renal function in severe septic shock states. Intensive Care Med 1993;19(3):151–14.
52. Flancbaum L, Dick M, Dasta J, et al. A dose-response study of phenylephrine in critically ill, septic surgical patients. Eur J Clin Pharmacol 1997;51(6):461–465.
53. Wilson W, Lipman J, Scribante J, et al. Septic shock: does adrenaline have a role as a first-line inotropic agent? Anaesth Intensive Care 1992;20(4):470–474.
54. Hannemann L, Reinhart K, Meier-Hellmann A, et al. Dopexamine hydrochloride in septic shock. Chest 1996;109(3):756–760.
55. Smithies M, Yee TH, Jackson L, et al. Protecting the gut and the liver in the critically ill: effects of dopexamine. Crit Care Med 1994;22(5):789–795.
56. Rudis MI, Basha MA, Zarowitz BJ. Is it time to reposition vasopressors and inotropes in sepsis? Crit Care Med 1996;24(3):525–537.
57. Marino PL. Oxygen transport. In: Marino PL, ed. The ICU Book. Philadelphia: Lea & Febiger; 1991:14–24.
58. Bollaert PE, Bauer P, Audibert G, et al. Effects of epinephrine on hemodynamics and oxygen metabolism in dopamine-resistant septic shock. Chest 1990;98(4):949–953.
59. Hayes MA, Yau EH, Hinds CJ, Watson JD. Symmetrical peripheral gangrene: association with noradrenaline administration. Intensive Care Med 1992;18(7):433–436.
60. Tisdale JE, Patel R, Webb CR, et al. Electrophysiologic and proarrhythmic effects of intravenous inotropic agents. Prog Cardiovasc Dis 1995;38(2):167–180.
61. Weiss M, Schneider EM, Tarnow J, et al. Is inhibition of oxygen radical production of neutrophils by sympathomimetics mediated via beta-2 adrenoceptors? J Pharmacol Exp Ther 1996;278(3):1105–1113.
62. Fortenberry JD, Huber AR, Owens ML. Inotropes inhibit endothelial cell surface adhesion molecules induced by interleukin-1beta. Crit Care Med 1997;25(2):303–308.
63. van der Poll T, Calvano SE, Kumar A, et al. Epinephrine attenuates down-regulation of monocyte tumor necrosis factor receptors during human endotoxemia. J Leukoc Biol 1997;61(2):156–160.
64. Girbes AR, Patten MT, McCloskey BV, et al. The renal and neurohumoral effects of the addition of low-dose dopamine in septic critically ill patients. Intensive Care Med 2000;26(11):1685–1689.
65. Ichai C, Soubielle J, Carles M, et al. Comparison of the renal effects of low to high doses of dopamine and dobutamine in critically ill patients: a single-blind randomized study. Crit Care Med 2000;28(4):921–928.

66. Hoogenberg K, Smit AJ, Girbes AR. Effects of low-dose dopamine on renal and systemic hemodynamics during incremental norepinephrine infusion in healthy volunteers. Crit Care Med 1998;26(2):260–265.
67. Rudis MI, Zarowitz BJ. Low-dose dopamine in acute oliguric renal failure. Am J Med 1997;102(3):320–322.
68. Bellomo R, Chapman M, Finfer S, et al. Low-dose dopamine in patients with early renal dysfunction: a placebo-controlled randomised trial. Australian and New Zealand Intensive Care Society (ANZICS) Clinical Trials Group. Lancet 2000;356(9248):2139–2143.
69. Meier-Hellmann A, Bredle DL, Specht M, et al. The effects of low-dose dopamine on splanchnic blood flow and oxygen uptake in patients with septic shock. Intensive Care Med 1997;23(1):31–37.
70. Olson D, Pohlman A, Hall JB. Administration of low-dose dopamine to nonoliguric patients with sepsis syndrome does not raise intramucosal gastric pH nor improve creatinine clearance. Am J Respir Crit Care Med 1996;154(6 Pt 1):1664–1670.
71. Day NP, Phu NH, Mai NT, et al. Effects of dopamine and epinephrine infusions on renal hemodynamics in severe malaria and severe sepsis. Crit Care Med 2000;28(5):1353–1362.
72. Klahr S, Miller SB. Acute oliguria. N Engl J Med 1998;338(10): 671–675.
73. Marik PE, Iglesias J. Low-dose dopamine does not prevent acute renal failure in patients with septic shock and oliguria. NORASEPT II Study Investigators. Am J Med 1999;107(4):387–390.
74. Lherm T, Troche G, Rossignol M, et al. Renal effects of low-dose dopamine in patients with sepsis syndrome or septic shock treated with catecholamines. Intensive Care Med 1996;22(3):213–219.
75. Ichai C, Passeron C, Carles M, et al. Prolonged low-dose dopamine infusion induces a transient improvement in renal function in hemodynamically stable, critically ill patients: a single-blind, prospective, controlled study. Crit Care Med 2000;28(5):1329–1335.
76. Dive A, Foret F, Jamart J, et al. Effect of dopamine on gastrointestinal motility during critical illness. Intensive Care Med 2000;26(7):901–907.
77. Meier-Hellmann A, Sakka S, Reinhart K. Aspects in monitoring and treatment of gastrointestinal underperfusion in sepsis: diagnosis and therapy of gastrointestinal underperfusion in sepsis. Anasthesiol Intensivmed Notfallmed Schmerzther 1998;33(Suppl 2):S60–S69.
78. Meier-Hellmann A, Sakka SG, Reinhart K. Catecholamines and splanchnic perfusion. Schweiz Med Wochenschr 2000;130(50):1942–1947.
79. Yu M. A peek at renal blood flow, renal function, and oxygen consumption with epinephrine and dopamine therapy. Crit Care Med 2000;28(5):1661–1663.
80. Reinhart K, Sakka SG, Meier-Hellmann A. Haemodynamic management of a patient with septic shock. Eur J Anaesthesiol 2000;17(1): 6–17.
81. Martin C, Viviand X, Leone M, Thirion X. Effect of norepinephrine on the outcome of septic shock. Crit Care Med 2000;28(8):2758–2765.
82. Abid O, Akca S, Haji-Michael PL, Vincent JL. Strong vasopressor support may be futile in the intensive care unit patient with multiple organ failure. Crit Care Med 2000;28(4):947–949.
83. Marik PE, Mohedin M. The contrasting effects of dopamine and norepinephrine on systemic and splanchnic oxygen utilization in hyperdynamic sepsis. JAMA 1994;272(17):1354–1357.
84. Lucas CE. A new look at dopamine and norepinephrine for hyperdynamic septic shock. Chest 1994;105(1):7–8.
85. Groeneveld AB, Girbes AR, Thijs LG. Treating septic shock with norepinephrine. Crit Care Med 1999;27(9):2022–2023.
86. Gregory JS, Bonfiglio MF, Dasta JF, et al. Experience with phenylephrine as a component of the pharmacologic support of septic shock. Crit Care Med 1991;19(11):1395–1400.
87. Ruokonen E, Takala J, Kari A, et al. Regional blood flow and oxygen transport in septic shock. Crit Care Med 1993;21(9):1296–1303.
88. Martin C, Papazian L, Perrin G, et al. Norepinephrine or dopamine for the treatment of hyperdynamic septic shock? Chest 1993;103(6):1826–1831.
89. Parrillo JE. Myocardial depression during septic shock in humans. Crit Care Med 1990;18(10):1183–1184.
90. Yu M, Levy MM, Smith P, et al. Effect of maximizing oxygen delivery on morbidity and mortality rates in critically ill patients: a prospective, randomized, controlled study. Crit Care Med 1993;21(6):830–838.
91. Bhatt SB, Hutchinson RC, Tomlinson B, et al. Effect of dobutamine on oxygen supply and uptake in healthy volunteers. Br J Anaesth 1992;69(3):298–303.
92. Haywood GA, Tighe D, Moss R, et al. Goal-directed therapy with dobutamine in a porcine model of septic shock: effects on systemic and renal oxygen transport. Postgrad Med J 1991;67(Suppl 1):S36–S39.
93. Tuchschmidt J, Fried J, Astiz M, Rackow E. Elevation of cardiac output and oxygen delivery improves outcome in septic shock. Chest 1992;102(1):216–220.
94. Shoemaker WC, Appel PL, Kram HB. Oxygen transport measurements to evaluate tissue perfusion and titrate therapy: dobutamine and dopamine effects. Crit Care Med 1991;19(5):672–688.
95. Hayes MA, Timmins AC, Yau EH, et al. Elevation of systemic oxygen delivery in the treatment of critically ill patients. N Engl J Med 1994;330(24):1717–1722.
96. Duranteau J, Sitbon P, Teboul JL, et al. Effects of epinephrine, norepinephrine, or the combination of norepinephrine and dobutamine on gastric mucosa in septic shock. Crit Care Med 1999;27(5):893–900.
97. Gutierrez G, Clark C, Brown SD, et al. Effect of dobutamine on oxygen consumption and gastric mucosal pH in septic patients. Am J Respir Crit Care Med 1994;150(2):324–329.
98. Neviere R, Mathieu D, Chagnon JL, et al. The contrasting effects of dobutamine and dopamine on gastric mucosal perfusion in septic patients. Am J Respir Crit Care Med 1996;154(6 Pt 1):1684–1688.
99. Reinelt H, Radermacher P, Fischer G, et al. Effects of a dobutamine-induced increase in splanchnic blood flow on hepatic metabolic activity in patients with septic shock. Anesthesiology 1997;86(4):818–824.
100. Parviainen I, Ruokonen E, Takala J. Dobutamine-induced dissociation between changes in splanchnic blood flow and gastric intramucosal pH after cardiac surgery. Br J Anaesth 1995;74(3):277–282.
101. Levy B, Bollaert PE, Lucchelli JP, et al. Dobutamine improves the adequacy of gastric mucosal perfusion in epinephrine-treated septic shock. Crit Care Med 1997;25(10):1649–1654.
102. De Backer D, Moraine JJ, Berre J, et al. Effects of dobutamine on oxygen consumption in septic patients: direct versus indirect determinations. Am J Respir Crit Care Med 1994;150(1):95–100.
103. Klem C, Dasta JF, Reilley TE, Flancbaum LJ. Variability in dobutamine pharmacokinetics in unstable critically ill surgical patients. Crit Care Med 1994;22(12):1926–1932.
104. Yamazaki T, Shimada Y, Taenaka N, et al. Circulatory responses to afterloading with phenylephrine in hyperdynamic sepsis. Crit Care Med 1982;10(7):432–435.
105. Reinelt H, Radermacher P, Kiefer P, et al. Impact of exogenous beta-adrenergic receptor stimulation on hepatosplanchnic oxygen kinetics and metabolic activity in septic shock. Crit Care Med 1999;27(2):325–331.
106. Mackenzie SJ, Kapadia F, Nimmo GR, et al. Adrenaline in treatment of septic shock: effects on haemodynamics and oxygen transport. Intensive Care Med 1991;17(1):36–39.
107. Moran JL, O'Fathartaigh MS, Peisach AR, et al. Epinephrine as an inotropic agent in septic shock: a dose-profile analysis. Crit Care Med 1993;21(1):70–77.
108. Lipman J, Roux A, Kraus P. Vasoconstrictor effects of adrenaline in human septic shock. Anaesth Intensive Care 1991;19(1):61–65.
109. Levy B, Bollaert PE, Charpentier C, et al. Comparison of norepinephrine and dobutamine to epinephrine for hemodynamics, lactate metabolism, and gastric tonometric variables in septic shock: a prospective, randomized study. Intensive Care Med 1997;23(3):282–287.
110. Day NP, Phu NH, Bethell DP, et al. The effects of dopamine and adrenaline infusions on acid-base balance and systemic haemodynamics in severe infection. Lancet 1996;348(9022):219–223.
111. Uusaro A, Takala J. Vasoactive drugs and splanchnic perfusion in septic shock. Crit Care Med 1998;26(8):1458–1460.

112. Muller M, Boldt J, Schindler E, et al. Effects of low-dose dopexamine on splanchnic oxygenation during major abdominal surgery. Crit Care Med 1999;27(11):2389–2393.
113. Meier-Hellmann A, Bredle DL, Specht M, et al. Dopexamine increases splanchnic blood flow but decreases gastric mucosal pH in severe septic patients treated with dobutamine. Crit Care Med 1999;27(10): 2166–2171.
114. Rosselet A, Feihl F, Markert M, et al. Selective iNOS inhibition is superior to norepinephrine in the treatment of rat endotoxic shock. Am J Respir Crit Care Med 1998;157(1):162–170.
115. Griffiths MJ, Messent M, Curzen NP, Evans TW. Aminoguanidine selectively decreases cyclic GMP levels produced by inducible nitric oxide synthase. Am J Respir Crit Care Med 1995;152(5 Pt 1):1599–1604.
116. Grover R, Zaccardelli D, Colice G, et al. An open-label dose escalation study of the nitric oxide synthase inhibitor, N(G)-methyl-L-arginine hydrochloride (546C88), in patients with septic shock. Glaxo Wellcome International Septic Shock Study Group. Crit Care Med 1999;27(5): 913–922.
117. Bollaert PE. Stress doses of glucocorticoids in catecholamine dependency: a new therapy for a new syndrome? Intensive Care Med 2000;26(1):3–5.
118. Spijkstra JJ, Girbes AR. The continuing story of corticosteroids in the treatment of septic shock. Intensive Care Med 2000;26(5):496–500.
119. Bollaert PE, Charpentier C, Levy B, et al. Reversal of late septic shock with supraphysiologic doses of hydrocortisone. Crit Care Med 1998;26(4):645–650.
120. Briegel J, Forst H, Haller M, et al. Stress doses of hydrocortisone reverse hyperdynamic septic shock: a prospective, randomized, double-blind, single-center study. Crit Care Med 1999;27(4):723–732.
121. Annane D, Bellissant E, Sebille V, et al. Impaired pressor sensitivity to noradrenaline in septic shock patients with and without impaired adrenal function reserve. Br J Clin Pharmacol 1998;46(6):589–597.
122. Oppert M, Reinicke A, Graf KJ, et al. Plasma cortisol levels before and during "low-dose" hydrocortisone therapy and their relationship to hemodynamic improvement in patients with septic shock. Intensive Care Med 2000;26:1747–1755.
123. Bellissant E, Annane D. Effect of hydrocortisone on phenylephrine—mean arterial pressure dose-response relationship in septic shock. Clin Pharmacol Ther 2000;68(3):293–303.
124. Landry DW, Levin HR, Gallant EM, et al. Vasopressin deficiency contributes to the vasodilation of septic shock. Circulation 1997;95(5):1122–1125.
125. Landry DW, Levin HR, Gallant EM, et al. Vasopressin pressor hypersensitivity in vasodilatory septic shock. Crit Care Med 1997;25(8): 1279–1282.
126. Malay MB, Ashton RC Jr, Landry DW, Townsend RN. Low-dose vasopressin in the treatment of vasodilatory septic shock. J Trauma 1999;47(4):699–703.
127. Hardman JG, Gilman AG, Limbird LE, et al. Catecholamines, sympathomimetic drugs and adrenergic receptor antagonists. In: Hoffman BB, Lefkovitz RJ, eds. Goodman & Gilman's The Pharmacological Basis of Therapeutics. New York: McGraw-Hill;1996:199–248.

24

HYPOVOLEMIC SHOCK

Brian L. Erstad

This chapter discusses the assessment and management of hypovolemic shock. Depending on the classification scheme being used for shock, spinal and anaphylactic shock may be considered separately from hypovolemic shock because fluid loss from the body is not necessary for their occurrence. For example, there are distributive forms of shock, such as spinal shock resulting from loss of sympathetic, and anaphylactic shock, resulting from increased vascular permeability of immunologic origin.[1] Although these forms of shock are not discussed in detail, it is important to note that the initial therapy for both is the same as for hypovolemic shock (i.e., adequate volume replacement) because circulating volume is decreased. In this regard, adequate fluid resuscitation to maintain circulating blood volume is a common principle in managing all forms of shock.

EPIDEMIOLOGY

It is estimated that approximately one million deaths a year in the United States occur in patients with shock.[2] The number is much higher when one considers that all causes of death ultimately result in circulatory failure (i.e., the last stage of shock). It is much more difficult to estimate the number of patients with reversible organ dysfunction or patients with end-organ damage who survived an episode of hypovolemic shock. Part of the problem is defining when progressive circulatory insufficiency results in the loss of normal compensatory responses by the body, which could reverse the processes leading to irreversible organ dysfunction. This loss of appropriate compensation varies from patient to patient and is not always readily apparent during the initial patient presentation.

ETIOLOGY

Hypovolemic shock may result from a number problems including plasma loss, sequestered fluid within a compartment in the body (e.g., third-spacing), thermal injury, and various forms of dehydration. Plasma loss may occur from hemorrhage, or from sustained gastrointestinal or urinary losses that are insufficiently replaced. In some cases, such as in postoperative patients, a number of these problems may occur at the same time. For example, a patient may have had blood loss secondary to trauma or surgery with additional fluid being third-spaced postoperatively. The third-spaced fluid may occur as tissue edema in the gastrointestinal tract with a concomitant ileus. As the example of third-spaced fluid indicates, fluid (i.e., plasma) does not have to be lost from the body for a person to develop hypovolemic shock.

Dehydration may result from primary water deficiency, usually because of decreased intake, but in some instances (e.g., diabetes insipidus), it may result from increased losses of water. In general, the term *dehydration* implies intracellular and interstitial fluid depletion, in contrast to *volume depletion,* which implies extracellular, and particularly intravascular, sodium and water. In the case of a primary water deficit, cell dehydration occurs, with delayed circulatory failure from decreased circulatory volume with ongoing losses.[3] Initially, the patient may be thirsty and possibly have some mental status changes, such as confusion. If the cellular dehydration occurs slowly, intracellular substances, referred to as *idiogenic osmols,* develop, which limit progressive complications (e.g., cerebral edema, coma). With combined water and salt deficiencies as might occur with gastrointestinal losses (e.g., diarrhea), interstitial and intravascular depletion are an early occurrence. Fortunately, dehydration is relatively easy to prevent with routine vigilance and water replacement compared to some of the other causes of shock.

PATHOPHYSIOLOGY

Hypovolemic shock is often described in terms of monitoring parameters such as lowered blood pressure, but patients with shock may die despite normal surrogate markers of circulatory insufficiency. Therefore, an appropriate definition should mention the underlying problem, which is inadequate tissue perfusion resulting from circulatory failure. In the case of hypovolemic shock, the cause of the altered perfusion is fluid (or volume) depletion resulting from trauma, surgery, thermal injury, or some form of dehydration. Figure 24–1 provides a simplified version of the pathophysiology of circulatory insufficiency. Cell damage and death may occur from the primary insult or from reperfusion injury.[4] The latter problem is most frequently associated with trauma and blood loss that cause the release of a multitude of mediators of inflammation and injury that have complex interactions.[5] Cells have varying responses to hypoxia, ranging from astrocytes that quit functioning almost immediately to hepatic cells that may function for several hours postinjury.[3] Left unmitigated, cell death occurs.

The body attempts to compensate for volume depletion, beginning with autoregulatory changes involving smaller blood vessels. When the cause of circulatory insufficiency continues unabated, local mechanisms eventually fail to provide adequate compensation and macrocirculatory changes ensue. Approximately 75% of blood volume is contained in venous capacitance vessels, with gravity being the major impedance of flow back to the heart.[3] With increasing volume depletion, blood flow to the heart (preload) is decreased, with subsequent activation of baroreceptors and chemoreceptors leading to sympathetic discharge. Also, fluid shifting from the interstitial space to the intravascular space occurs through a phenomenon known as transcapillary refill, and hormones (adrenocorticotrophic hormone, angiotensin, catecholamines, vasopressin) that cause sodium and water retention by the kidneys are released. The phenomenon of transcapillary refill means that the body can have fluid losses exceeding normal plasma volume. These responses cause alterations in stroke volume, heart rate, and peripheral vascular resistance so that blood pressure and hence tissue perfusion can be maintained.

The microcirculatory changes associated with shock are complex and difficult to study. Although some mediators such as endothelin-1 cause vasoconstriction, other mediators, such as adenosine and nitric oxide, yield vasodilation.[6] These changes result in hypoperfusion

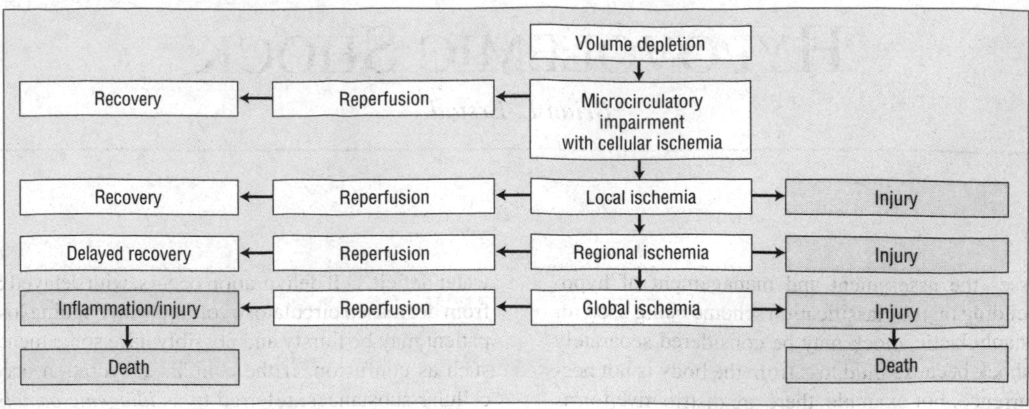

FIGURE 24–1. Pathophysiology of circulatory insufficiency.

or hyperperfusion depending on the area. As these microcirculatory changes fail to maintain adequate organ perfusion, more widespread sympathetic nervous system activation and vasoconstriction ensue.

The factors involved in fluid shifting between the intravascular and interstitial spaces are described by the modified Starling equation:

$$J_V = K_{f,c}\,[(P_c - P_t) - \sigma(\pi_c - \pi_t)]$$

where

J_V = net transvascular flow rate; cannot be measured in clinical setting

$K_{f,c}$ = capillary filtration coefficient for fluids; cannot be measured in clinical setting

P_c = capillary hydrostatic pressure; indirectly estimated in clinical setting (e.g., pulmonary artery occlusive pressure)

P_t = tissue hydrostatic pressure; cannot be measured in clinical setting

σ = reflection coefficient for proteins; cannot be measured in clinical setting

π_c = plasma colloid osmotic pressure; not usually measured in clinical setting, but technology is available

π_t = tissue colloid osmotic pressure; cannot be measured in clinical setting

Proteins act as osmotic (or oncotic) agents in each of these spaces to attract fluid, while hydrostatic forces push fluid into or out of the vessels. The equation has distinct permeability values for water and protein, because each crosses the vascular membrane at a different rate. Although the Starling equation is useful to the practitioner in terms of understanding the factors involved in fluid shifting between compartments, the rate and direction of transvascular flow cannot be accurately calculated in the clinical setting because the majority of factors cannot be measured directly.

The body's compensatory mechanisms may have beneficial and harmful consequences. For example, if preload is not substantially decreased, cardiac output can be increased approximately fivefold by increases in stroke volume or heart rate.[1] Although this may be useful for providing blood flow to inadequately perfused tissues, it may cause large (e.g., fourfold) increases in oxygen consumption by the heart that could aggravate preexisting ischemia in patients with underlying coronary artery disease. Another example is the sympathetic-nervous-system-mediated vasoconstriction that causes blood to shift from the skin, skeletal muscle, and some internal organs such as the kidneys and gastrointestinal tract to organs (e.g., heart, brain) that are less tolerant of inadequate flow. If the vasoconstriction continues unabated, the hypoperfused organs eventually become damaged. Figure 24–2

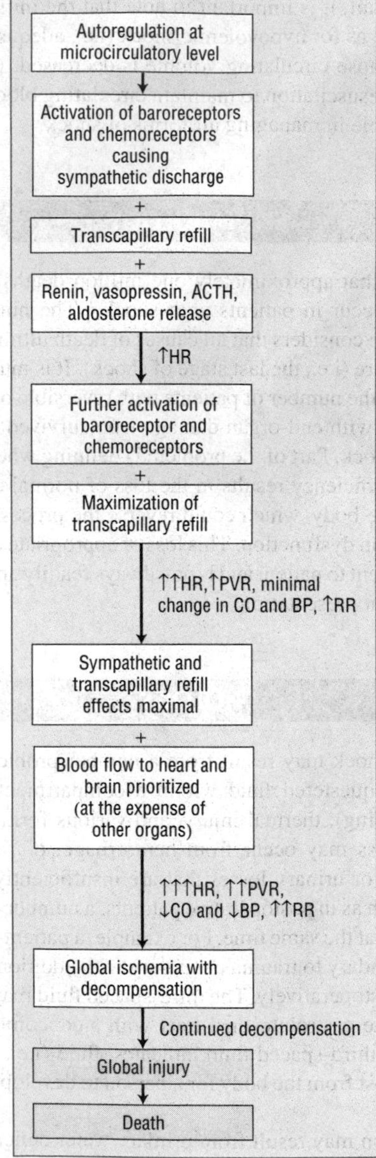

FIGURE 24–2. Activation of compensatory mechanisms with loss of circulatory volume. Certain stages may be absent depending on a number of factors such as age, preexisting disease states, and cause of circulatory insufficiency. BP, blood pressure; CO, cardiac output; HR, heart rate; PVR, peripheral vascular resistance; RR, respiratory rate.

provides an overview of the compensatory changes that occur with a loss of circulating blood volume.

In addition to the more acute implications of hypovolemia and attendant complications, reperfusion damage is likely to occur particularly after prolonged resuscitation attempts. In addition to oxygen free-radical damage of cell membranes, a number of cellular (e.g., white blood cells, platelets) and humoral (e.g., procoagulants, anticoagulants, complement, kinins) components are activated, causing the release of other inflammatory mediators.[6] The resulting reperfusion injury may range from readily reversible organ dysfunction to multiple organ failure and death.

Although the basic pathophysiology is similar for the various causes of hypovolemic shock, there are unique considerations relative to each. For example, whereas isolated head injuries associated with trauma typically do not result in substantial blood loss or shock, pelvic fractures may sequester several liters of blood as hematoma formation.[7] Patients with traumatic or thermal injuries, as well as postoperative patients, may have substantial fluid accumulation in sites where it cannot be readily transferred back into blood vessels (i.e., third-spaced fluid) for maintaining pressure. With these types of injuries, prompt control of compressible bleeding sources with rapid patient transfer to the hospital for definitive treatment may preclude the cascade of events leading to shock. Indeed, with trauma patients, a "scoop and run" approach is used in most urban hospitals, which places a priority on rapid transport to a hospital.[8]

In the case of hemorrhagic shock, prompt attention must be given to cell, as well as plasma, losses. Red blood cells lost during the bleeding episode may lead to ischemic damage in vital organs. Packed red blood cell transfusions may be needed to increase the oxygen-carrying capacity of the blood, because oxygen transport is a function not only of cardiac output, but also of hemoglobin concentration and saturation and of hemoglobin affinity for oxygen.

Clotting factors and platelets are also lost in hemorrhage. The resulting bleeding problems may be aggravated by the dilutional effect of fluid resuscitation on clotting factor activity. Fresh-frozen plasma that contains necessary clotting factors and platelets is often needed in massive blood loss to restore adequate coagulation. On the other hand, trauma patients are at increased risk for deep venous thrombosis and pulmonary embolism caused by multiple factors, including vessel damage, abnormal blood flow patterns, and the hypercoagulable state associated with injury. Therefore, some form of venous thromboembolism prophylaxis is usually indicated in multiple-trauma patients or patients with severe single-system injuries (e.g., spinal cord damage).

The pathophysiology becomes more complicated if the severity of shock is sufficient to require admission to the intensive care unit (ICU) after initial resuscitation or surgery. The majority of patients admitted to the ICU have a systemic inflammatory response syndrome (SIRS), which is the body's response to injury. This syndrome is defined by a number of hypermetabolic changes reflected in the patient's temperature, white blood cell count and differential, and respiratory and heart rates. The stress response involves complex interactions between the nervous system and immunomodulating substances and has similar (if not the same) harmful and helpful consequences described with reperfusion following shock.[9] If the underlying problems are left untreated, the patient with SIRS may develop multiple organ dysfunction syndrome (MODS) during the final stages of illness.

CLINICAL PRESENTATION

The initial presentation of patients with suspected volume depletion can vary markedly depending on factors such as age, concomitant disease states and medications, and the etiology and rapidity of depletion. Intravascular depletion as a consequence of blood loss is signified by postural vital sign changes, and such measurements should be performed unless the diagnosis is obvious as in the case of bleeding associated with trauma.[10] Early signs and symptoms of dehydration and intravascular depletion caused by gastrointestinal or urinary losses are often relatively nonspecific. Plasma volume losses of less than 10 mL/kg of body weight are usually associated with minor signs and symptoms of distress. For example, in most patients greater than 12 years of age the heart and respiratory rates would be less than 100 beats per minute and 20 breaths per minute, respectively, and the blood pressure and urine output would be normal, but the person would appear somewhat anxious. Larger losses are not likely to be well tolerated (Table 24–1), particularly in patients greater than 65 years of age. Such patients would have marked increases in heart rate (e.g., >120 beats/min) and respiratory rate (e.g., >30 breaths/min) assuming no concurrent diseases or drugs that alter these rates, and substantial decreases in blood pressure (e.g., systolic blood pressure <90 mm Hg) and urine output (e.g., <0.5 mL/kg/h). An 18-year-old athlete and a 65-year-old sedentary individual are likely to have much different responses to a similar amount of fluid loss. The young patient may lose one-fourth of his or her circulating blood volume with minimal changes in arterial blood pressure and a relatively low heart rate. However, the elderly patient may have orthostatic changes in blood pressure that are not well tolerated by organs such as the kidneys.[3] Unfortunately, this same elderly patient may not have common signs and symptoms of volume depletion such as skin turgor changes or thirst, but, instead, may have more subtle changes (e.g., mental status alterations).[11] Regardless of patient age or preexisting

TABLE 24–1. Acute Circulatory Insufficiency: Initial Presentation and Therapy*

	Mild	Severe
Plasma/blood loss	10 mL/kg adult 20 mL/kg child	30 mL/kg adult 35 mL/kg child
Mental status/level of consciousness	None—small changes (e.g., anxious, irritable)	Marked changes (e.g., confusion to unconscious)
Vital signs/orthostatic changes	Minor changes	Marked changes
Therapy	20 mL/kg lactated Ringer's IV* over 10–15 min Unlikely to need blood cell replacement even if hemorrhagic loss	Lactated Ringer's IV as rapidly as possible until response in adult, then decrease rate of infusion 20 mL/kg lactated Ringer's IV in child (repeat quickly if minimal response); likely to need blood cell replacement and surgery if hemorrhagic

*Patients may have intermediate degrees of volume loss in addition to those listed, but the amount of loss is often difficult to quantify. The presentations may also vary greatly in patients with similar amounts of loss (young athlete vs sedentary, elderly person). Refer to text for a more in-depth discussion of some of the guidelines in this table.

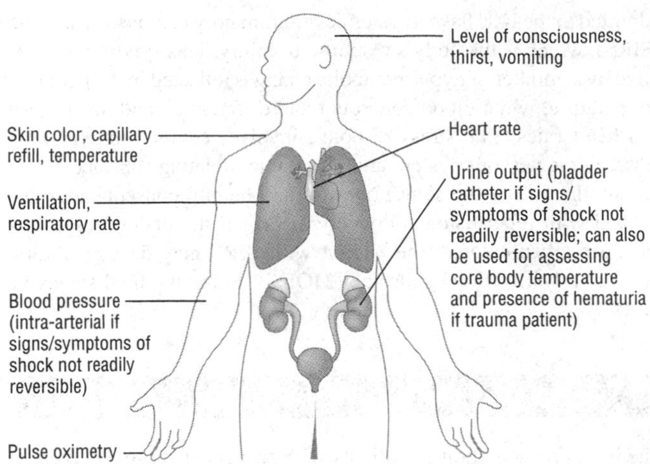

FIGURE 24–3. Noninvasive assessment of circulatory insufficiency.

conditions, the initial monitoring of a patient with suspected volume depletion should include the following noninvasive parameters: vital signs, urine output, mental status, and physical examination (Fig. 24–3).

While the presenting signs and symptoms of circulatory insufficiency are variable, patients will usually have decreased blood pressure, increased heart and respiratory rates, and a normal or low-normal temperature (e.g., 36–37°C [96.8–98.6°F]) in the absence of infection or exposure to extremes of temperature. As mentioned earlier, blood pressure and heart rate recordings must be interpreted in light of known or suspected baseline conditions. For example, medications such as β-blockers and calcium channel blockers may alter resting blood pressure and heart rate, as well as the subsequent response to therapeutic interventions. Similarly, although a blood pressure reading of 110/70 mm Hg (systolic/diastolic) may be acceptable in many patients, it may be inadequate for a patient with preexisting hypertension who normally has a blood pressure of 170/105 mm Hg. At the other extreme, patients with very low blood pressure may have inaudible or inaccurate determinations with cuff (sphygmomanometric) measurements. Chapter 12 details blood pressure measurement (e.g., cuff size, position). In this case, intra-arterial monitoring is indicated. As a noninvasive tool, the respiratory rate may correlate better than the heart rate with volume loss, but respiratory rate is often not used.[3] The respiratory rate may be elevated because of anxiety or as a compensatory mechanism for the metabolic acidosis caused by lactic acidosis associated with poor tissue perfusion.

Although the kidneys continually produce urine, the bladder stores the urine for intermittent elimination. For the initial diagnosis and management of acute circulatory insufficiency, a catheter can be inserted into the bladder for measuring urine output. In contrast to thirst, which is a relatively insensitive indicator of volume depletion, urine output is generally diminished with inadequate fluid administration and increases with appropriate resuscitation. This presumes, of course, that acute renal failure or medications, such as diuretics, are not altering the expected response. Adults should produce at least 0.5–1 mL/kg/h of urine, whereas children up to 12 years of age should produce at least 1 mL/kg/h (2 mL/kg/h if younger than 1 year of age).[7]

Mental status changes associated with volume depletion, if present, may range from subtle fluctuations in mood to unconsciousness. Although the latter finding is typically indicative of more severe depletion, less dramatic findings should not be interpreted as indicating mild fluid deficits. Losses of 4 L of plasma volume may be associated only with lassitude in an otherwise healthy adult patient.[3] Similar interpretation difficulties must be considered when performing the initial physical examination. An orderly progression from warm, reddish skin with appropriate capillary refill (rapid return of blood flow to extremity after removal of compression) to cold, cyanotic discoloration with impaired refill may not occur. Also, dry mucous membranes in elderly patients may be caused by mouth breathing or anticholinergic medications, and not by fluid depletion.[11]

▶ TREATMENT: Hypovolemic Shock

DESIRED OUTCOME

The desired outcomes of therapy for circulatory insufficiency that has led to hypovolemic shock are to prevent further progression of the disease with subsequent organ damage and, to the extent possible, to reverse organ dysfunction that has already taken place.

GENERAL APPROACH TO TREATMENT

Milder forms of volume depletion may be managed in outpatient settings. For example, supplemental fluids can be added to the usual estimated daily requirements of 30–35 mL/kg in patients greater than 12 years of age with dehydration. Commercially available carbohydrate/electrolyte drinks are generally more palatable than water and may promote earlier recovery.[11] When the dehydration involves substantial losses of salt, as well as water, additional sodium may need to be added to these drinks because they usually contain ≤50 mEq/L of sodium. This is less than the amounts of sodium (e.g., 90–120 mEq/L) generally recommended for rehydration.[12] The additional sodium will increase osmolarity, but this does not appear to delay gastric emptying.[13] Also, guidelines for oral rehydration of children with acute diarrhea are available, which, if used appropriately, may prevent future hospitalization.[14] Intravenous rehydration of children in outpatient settings has been accomplished, but patients must be carefully selected.[15,16] Outpatient rehydration of children generally should be limited to those with uncomplicated (e.g., vomiting <48 hours) acute gastroenteritis and relatively mild dehydration, after the exclusion of more severe illnesses such as bowel obstruction.

Hospitalization is indicated in more severe forms of circulatory insufficiency. If access to the circulatory system for fluids and medication administration was not obtained prior to hospitalization, this should be a priority. Venous access is generally obtained during the preliminary examination process that includes the ABCs of life support (i.e., airway, breathing, and circulation), assessment of vital signs and mental status, and urine output after catheterization. Whenever large-volume fluid resuscitation is expected, as in hemorrhagic shock, it is desirable to have at least two IV catheters. Because flow is a function of tubing length and catheter diameter, large-bore peripheral IVs are preferred over longer central lines. Unfortunately, vascular access in some patients may be problematic and other routes (e.g., intraosseous infusion in children) may be necessary.[7] One interesting method of fluid administration that has been investigated in elderly patients is subcutaneous infusion or hypodermoclysis. This route of administration is not commonly used probably because of concerns of adverse effects that were found in early studies that used

TABLE 24–2. Fluid Distribution and Major Indications[a]

Fluid	Intracellular	Interstitial	Intravascular	Major Indication
Normal saline or lactated Ringer's	None	750 mL	250 mL	Intravascular repletion in symptomatic patients
3% sodium chloride	→	750 mL+	250 mL+	Small amounts (e.g., 250 mL) have been used in conjunction with normal saline or lactated Ringer's for severe intravascular depletion in adults
5% dextrose/0.45% sodium chloride	333 mL	500 mL	167 mL	Maintenance fluid in euvolemic or dehydrated (sodium and water loss) patients with mild signs/symptoms of volume depletion
5% dextrose	667 mL	250 mL	83 mL	Dehydration (primarily water loss) in patients with mild signs/ symptoms of volume depletion
5% albumin	None	None	1000 mL[b]	Intravascular repletion in symptomatic patients
25% albumin	→	→	1000 mL+[b]	Smaller amounts (e.g., 50–100 mL or by continuous infusion in adults) titrated to response in hypovolemic patients with excess total body water

[a]Based on the administration of 1 L of each solution (*which may not be an appropriate amount for clinical use*); numbers are approximations; arrows indicate direction of fluid shift and plus signs indicate fluid retention in that compartment.
[b]After distribution, 60% of albumin (and associated fluid) is in interstitial compartment and 40% is in intravascular compartment.

excessively hypotonic or hypertonic solutions. Although alternative methods of fluid administration, such as hypodermoclysis are desirable, there is a need for well-conducted trials before such methods can be recommended for routine use.

PHARMACOLOGIC THERAPY

Dextrose-in-water solutions may be appropriate for uncomplicated dehydration caused by water deprivation, but crystalloid (sodium-containing) solutions should be used for forms of circulatory insufficiency that are associated with hemodynamic instability. In the latter situation, IV solutions with sodium concentrations approximating normal serum sodium values are usually indicated because they cause more expansion of the intravascular and interstitial spaces compared to dextrose solutions (Table 24–2). Lactated Ringer's and normal saline solutions are examples of such crystalloid solutions, although lactated Ringer's is the preferred solution according to some published guidelines (see *Advanced Trauma Life Support Guidelines*) because it is unlikely to cause the hyperchloremic metabolic acidosis that is seen with infusion of large amounts of normal saline (Table 24–3).[7] A "large" amount of fluid does not mean the typical bolus volumes used as fluid challenges in critically ill patients. Isolated boluses (e.g., 500 mL in patients greater than 18 years of age) are unlikely to cause substantial changes in blood pressure or acid-base balance.[17]

Although lactated Ringer's solution does contain lactate, it does not cause substantial elevations in circulating lactate concentrations when used as a resuscitation solution.[18] However, blood samples for lactate determinations drawn through catheters (arterial and venous) that have not been cleared appropriately may have spurious increases or decreases in lactate concentrations because of retained lactated Ringer's and nonlactated solutions (e.g., varying concentrations of dextrose-in-water or sodium chloride), respectively.[19] Therefore, blood samples for lactate concentrations should be drawn from a catheter that has been adequately cleared (e.g., 5 mL) of infusate after temporarily stopping the fluid infusion.

While a number of pharmacologic therapies show promise in animal models of shock, few demonstrate success in subsequent trials involving patients with shock. In large part this is a result of the lack of acceptable animal models of shock that mimic the pathophysiology of patients.[20] In cases in which a relevant animal model is available, care must be taken in extrapolating the information to forms of shock other than the one under study. This may be the problem with naloxone, which has been shown to raise blood pressure in some studies of shock but not in others.[21] In light of the lack of other demonstrated pharmaceutical interventions, fluids remain the mainstay of therapy, although their use is not devoid of controversy.

Larger-molecular-weight solutions (i.e., >30,000) known as colloids have been recommended in conjunction with, or as replacements for, crystalloid solutions. Examples of colloids used as plasma expanders include albumin, hetastarch, and dextran. Albumin is known as a monodisperse colloid because all of its molecules are of the same molecular weight (approximately 67,000), whereas hetastarch and dextran solutions are polydisperse compounds with molecules of varying molecular weights (*average* molecular weights of 450,000 [range, 10,000–1,000,000] for hetastarch and 40,000 [range, 10,000–90,000] or 70,000–75,000 [range, 20,000–200,000] for dextran 40 or dextran 70 or 75, respectively). This has important implications for

TABLE 24–3. Adverse Effects of Plasma Expanders: Crystalloids

Normal saline
- Primarily extensions of pharmacologic actions (e.g., fluid overload, dilutional coagulopathy)
- Hyperchloremic metabolic acidosis (has 154 mEq/L of chloride)
- Hypernatremia (has 154 mEq/L of sodium)

Lactated Ringer's
- Primarily extensions of pharmacologic actions (e.g., fluid overload, dilutional coagulopathy)
- Hyponatremia (has 130 mEq/L of sodium)
- Aggravation of preexisting hyperkalemia (has 4 mEq/L potassium)

Hypertonic saline
- Primarily extensions of pharmacologic actions (e.g., fluid overload; dilutional coagulopathy; intracellular volume depletion)
- Hypernatremia (has 513 mEq/L of sodium)
- Hyperchloremia (has 513 mEq/L of chloride)

the distribution of the products, because lower-molecular-weight substances are retained in the intravascular space for a shorter period of time because of more rapid leakage across the vessel membrane. The theoretical usefulness of colloids is based on their increased molecular weight (average molecular weight in the case of hetastarch and dextran) that corresponds to increased intravascular retention time in the absence of increased capillary permeability compared with crystalloids. Even in patients with intact capillary permeability, the colloid molecules will eventually leak through the membrane. In the case of albumin, approximately 60% of the albumin molecules (and associated fluid) are contained in the interstitial space within 5 days of exogenous administration. In patients with altered permeability (e.g., acute respiratory distress syndrome), the leakage of albumin from the intravascular to the interstitial space may occur within hours, not days.

Albumin is available in 5% and 25% concentrations. Plasma protein fraction has oncotic actions similar to a 5% albumin solution, which is not surprising as albumin is the predominant protein in this product. It takes approximately four times as much lactated Ringer's or normal saline solution to yield the same volume expansion as 5% albumin solution, but when given in equipotent amounts, albumin is much more costly than crystalloid solutions. Additionally, the 5% and 25% albumin solutions are typically priced in such a way that there is no cost savings associated with dilution of the 25% product to make a 5% concentration. The 5% albumin solution is relatively iso-oncotic, which means that it does not pull fluid into the compartment in which it is contained. In contrast, 25% albumin is referred to as hyperoncotic albumin because it tends to pull fluid into the compartment containing the albumin molecules. In general, the 5% albumin solution is used for hypovolemic states. The 25% solution should not be used for acute circulatory insufficiency unless it is used in combination with other fluids, or unless it is being used in patients with excess total body water but intravascular depletion, as a means of pulling fluid into the intravascular space. An example of the latter condition would be cirrhosis with ascites in which total body water is substantially increased but the patient is hypotensive as a consequence of lack of intravascular volume. This use of hyperoncotic albumin presumes that there is evidence of adverse effects associated with this excess water such as interstitial fluid accumulation in the lungs. Although theoretically appealing, improved outcomes related to the fluid shifting associated with hyperoncotic albumin have not been documented in randomized controlled trials. Additionally, the effect is temporary because the albumin crosses the vascular membrane over time.

Hetastarch 6% has comparable plasma expansion to a 5% albumin solution but is usually less expensive, which accounts for much of its use. The majority of trials comparing albumin to hetastarch for volume expansion have found no significant differences in clinically important outcomes (e.g., mortality). Few trials have directly compared hetastarch to crystalloid solutions for intravascular expansion. Although hetastarch is often stated as being contraindicated in bleeding disorders, it has been most-studied in patients with blood loss (e.g., trauma and perioperative patients). Although the definition of severe bleeding is somewhat nebulous, hetastarch should be avoided in conditions such as intracranial bleeding; it may aggravate bleeding through mechanisms specific to this colloid (e.g., decreased factor VIII activity). These mechanisms have not been well elucidated and are often difficult to distinguish from the dilutional effects on clotting factors caused by all plasma expanders. Hetastarch may cause elevations in serum amylase concentrations but does not cause pancreatitis.

Dextran 40, dextran 70, and dextran 75 are available for use as plasma expanders in the United States. The numbers refer to the average molecular weight of the solutions. In general, dextran solutions are not used as often as albumin or hetastarch solutions for plasma expansion, possibly because of concerns related to aggravation of bleeding (i.e., anticoagulant actions related to inhibiting stasis of microcirculation) and anaphylaxis that is more likely to occur with the higher-molecular-weight solutions. However, both of these concerns can be reduced if proper attention is paid to patient selection and, in the case of bleeding, published dosing guidelines with regards to the amounts of these products that should be infused. There are few comparative trials involving the dextran solutions, but the intravascular expansion within hours after infusion is approximately equal to the amount of dextran infused.

The crystalloid versus colloid debate was intensified when a meta-analysis by a well-respected group (Cochrane) found an overall increase in mortality associated with albumin using pooled results of randomized investigations.[22] The meta-analysis involved 30 randomized trials with 1,419 patients (relative risk of death with albumin vs no administration or crystalloid administration 1.68, 95% confidence interval = 1.26–2.23).[68] For hypovolemia (caused by blood loss in the majority of studies), the risk of death associated with albumin administration was not quite statistically significant (relative risk 1.46, 95% confidence interval 0.97–2.22). However, the most comprehensive meta-analysis to date did not find increased mortality attributable to albumin when looking at overall mortality (relative risk of death 1.11, 95% confidence interval = 0.95 to 1.28) or for any category of indications.[23] The presumed comparability of studies needed to perform such analyses does raise questions concerning extrapolation of the results to specific patient populations. With this caution in mind, these trials provide additional evidence that crystalloid solutions should be considered first-line therapy in patients with hypovolemic shock.

SPECIAL POPULATIONS

Trauma/Perioperative Patients

The immediate treatment of hemorrhagic circulatory insufficiency with plasma expanders (i.e., crystalloids or colloids) seems obvious and has widespread acceptance, but no large, well-controlled trials in humans have been conducted that support this practice.[24] To the contrary, there is evidence to suggest that fluid resuscitation beyond minimal levels (i.e., mean arterial pressure >40–60 mm Hg) is harmful. One prospective study involving 598 adult patients with gunshot or stab wound injuries to the torso and systolic blood pressure measurements ≤90 mm Hg found that delayed fluid resuscitation until operation was associated with increased survival and discharge from the hospital ($P = .04$).[25] However, concerns were expressed about comparability of the immediate and delayed resuscitation groups, particularly because true randomization did not take place.[26] Additionally, the study was conducted in a populated urban area with approximately 2 hours from time of injury to operation. Therefore, the results may not be applicable to rural areas with extended transport times. While the applicability of this study to other populations and settings is debatable, the *presumption* of benefits from immediate plasma expansion in all perioperative patients with circulatory insufficiency caused by hemorrhage is no longer valid. Instead, the initial priority should be surgical control of the bleeding source.

The latter study has dampened interest in other solutions being investigated primarily for prehospital use.[27] For example, hypertonic solutions have several characteristics that make them attractive for acute resuscitation. The intravascular and interstitial expansion resulting from the administration of these solutions is much greater than the volume infused by emergency personnel. By causing redistribution (i.e., pulling fluid) from the intracellular space, hypertonic solutions cause rapid expansion of the intravascular compartment, which is essential for vital organ perfusion. In head-injured patients, this redistribution should decrease intracranial pressure because the vessels of the brain are more impermeable to sodium ions than vessels in other areas of the body.[27] Additionally, hypertonic saline solutions have beneficial immunomodulating actions when compared to more isotonic solutions in experiments with animals.[28,29]

Potential adverse effects associated with hypertonic fluid administration for circulatory insufficiency include cellular crenation and damage caused by the dramatic fluid shifts, as well as peripheral vein destruction from their high osmolality. Also, in the case of hypertonic sodium chloride solutions, there are the possibilities of neurologic damage from hypernatremia and hyperchloremic metabolic acidosis from hyperchloremia. In the limited number of studies conducted in humans to date, such adverse effects have been uncommon and apparently of little clinical importance.[30,31]

Unfortunately, beneficial outcome data attributable to administration of these hypertonic solutions have also been lacking.[32] Most of these studies were conducted in prehospital and emergency department settings using 250 mL of 7.5% sodium chloride with or without 6% dextran 70. A meta-analysis of randomized controlled trials found no statistical difference between the survival rates of patients receiving the hypertonic saline solutions and those receiving standard isotonic crystalloid solutions.[33] Part of the explanation for this finding may be related to supplemental crystalloid fluids that were routinely given to patients in both the treatment and control groups, which would probably increase the number of patients needed to demonstrate a statistically significant difference in mortality. Until the concerns regarding efficacy and toxicity of these solutions have been resolved, normal saline could be considered as an alternative for head-injured patients when a hypertonic solution is desirable because it contains 154 mmol/L of both sodium and chloride. Given their relatively poor intravascular expansion and association with poor outcome in animal models of closed head injury, hypotonic solutions should be avoided in this population.[34]

In addition to crystalloid solutions, colloids have been used for plasma expansion in patients with hemorrhagic circulatory insufficiency. In the United States, albumin and starch (i.e., hetastarch) derivatives are most commonly used, although dextran solutions are also commercially available. The theoretical advantage to these compounds is their prolonged intravascular retention time compared to crystalloid solutions. In contrast to isotonic crystalloid solutions that have substantial interstitial distribution within minutes of intravenous administration, colloids remain in the intravascular space for hours or days depending on factors such as capillary permeability.

The colloids, in particular albumin, are expensive solutions. Therefore, it is difficult to justify the additional cost of colloidal products unless the benefit-to-risk ratio is substantially greater than that associated with inexpensive crystalloid solutions. This does not appear to be the case based on four randomized controlled studies comparing colloid and crystalloid solutions for acute circulatory insufficiency. In one study involving 94 patients being resuscitated by an emergency surgical service, albumin administration was titrated based on albumin levels.[35] All patients were given crystalloids and blood products in addition to the supplemental albumin. There were statistically significant increases in length of stay and pulmonary shunting in patients randomized to receive albumin, albeit the clinical significance of the calculated shunting differences is questionable. Pulmonary shunting refers to blood that is diverted through the lungs without being oxygenated. It is an indirect indicator of impaired oxygenation and is estimated by calculations that use various measured arterial and venous respiratory parameters (and hemoglobin concentration). Values greater than 20% are usually considered substantial impairment. Three additional studies titrated albumin to achieve hemodynamic stabilization. In the two larger studies (141 and 36 patients) involving patients undergoing exploratory laparotomy, there were no significant differences in ventilatory support, pulmonary shunting, or alveolar-arterial oxygen difference between groups receiving crystalloids or albumin.[36,37] The third study randomized 26 elderly patients (mean age, 79 years) to receive albumin, hetastarch, or normal saline for hypovolemic shock.[38] Despite the small number of patients in each group, the incidence of pulmonary edema was 22% in patients receiving the colloids, but 87.5% in the patients receiving the saline ($P < .05$). In addition to the small number of patients enrolled in this investigation, another concern was the radiographic definition of pulmonary edema at 24 hours postresuscitation without supporting clinical data. In summary, of the four randomized studies comparing colloids to crystalloids for acute circulatory insufficiency, there is no obvious benefit to using colloid products for resuscitation with the possible exception of elderly patients in shock based on one short-term study involving a small number of patients.

Because other colloids, such as hetastarch, have almost always been compared to albumin and not to crystalloid solutions in published clinical studies (with no clinically important differences being found), there is no reason to suspect these other colloids have any unique advantages as volume expanders. Adverse effects associated with colloids appear to be uncommon and are generally extensions of their pharmacologic activity (Table 24–4), but this is also true of crystalloids. The benefit-to-risk ratio appears to be similar for colloids and crystalloids; thus, based on cost, crystalloids are preferred for initial treatment of circulatory insufficiency.

Another consideration in the patient with injuries or surgery is the potential need for blood-product administration (Table 24–5) to replace oxygen-carrying and clotting functions. Although a small group of trauma patients respond to the initial fluid bolus and remain stable, most patients respond initially and then deteriorate.[7] The latter patients, as well as patients undergoing blood loss associated with surgery, frequently need blood components such as packed red blood cells. In the case of the latter component, red blood cells contain hemoglobin that delivers oxygen to tissues. Neither crystalloids nor colloids perform this function.

Blood products are not risk free. For example, there is the rare, but important, risk of virus transmission (e.g., HIV, hepatitis). The administration of blood products has its own risks. For example, citrate that is added to stored blood to prevent coagulation may bind to calcium, resulting in hypocalcemia. In contrast, potassium and phosphate concentrations are often elevated in stored blood, particularly when hemolysis has occurred during storage. Additionally, administration of excessive blood products may be counterproductive. In the case of red blood cells, attempts to raise the hematocrit to high normal or supranormal concentrations may decrease oxygen delivery by increasing blood viscosity.[3] Although there is no optimal hematocrit value for all patients, a minimum hematocrit concentration of 30% is usually indicated in patients at particular risk for ischemia, such as those with coronary artery disease. Other issues that must be considered with blood-product administration include monitoring for transfusion-related reactions and attention to appropriate warming, particularly when large volumes are given to pediatric patients, because hypothermia is associated with increased fluid requirements and mortality.[39]

Patients with Thermal Injuries

There are a wide variety of formulas for estimating fluid requirements in thermally injured patients, but there is little reason to choose one over another based on well-controlled studies. In general, the amount

TABLE 24–4. Adverse Effects of Plasma Expanders: Colloids

Albumin
- Primarily extensions of pharmacologic actions (e.g., fluid overload; dilutional coagulopathy; crystalloids are usually needed with 25% albumin in hypovolemic states to prevent intracellular volume depletion and renal failure)
- Amino acid profile and catabolism alterations (clinical significance?); potential protein overload if given with exogenous protein (e.g., parenteral nutrition)
- Anaphylactoid/anaphylaxis (life-threatening reactions rare; higher in patients with IgA deficiency)
- Infectous complications (all reported cases have been associated with improper handling by manufacturer or institution; no reported cases of HIV or hepatitis transmission)
- Interactions with medications and nutrients (clinical significance varies)
- Metal loading, particularly aluminum (long-term administration in patients with renal failure)
- Negative inotropic effect, reductions in ionized calcium concentrations?
- Pyrogenic reactions?

Hetastarch
- Primarily extensions of pharmacologic actions (e.g., fluid overload; dilutional coagulopathy)
- Bleeding (decreases factor VIII/C activity; not recommended in patients with severe bleeding conditions such as subarachnoid hemorrhage)
- Macroamylase formation may cause elevation in blood amylase that leads to inaccurate diagnosis of pancreatitis

Dextrans
- Primarily extensions of pharmacologic actions (e.g., fluid overload; dilutional coagulopathy)
- Anaphylaxis (increased incidence with increased molecular weight)
- Bleeding (sometimes used for anticoagulant activity so not recommended in patients with severe bleeding)

of loss corresponds to the size of the thermal injury.[3] Approximately 3 mL/kg of isotonic fluid (lactated Ringer's) for each percent burn can be used for calculating the expected fluid requirements for the first 24 hours postburn. For example, a 60-kg person with 30% body-surface-area burns is expected to require 5,400 mL of fluid over the initial 24 hours. Regardless of the calculated deficit, fluids should be administered until adequate tissue perfusion has been documented or adverse effects (e.g., pulmonary edema) occur. While the choice of plasma expander is based primarily on cost considerations for blood loss as a consequence of trauma or surgery, crystalloids are preferred as initial therapy for burn victims because they are less likely to cause interstitial fluid accumulation. Only one randomized trial has been conducted in which patients were given either albumin or lactated Ringer's solution to maintain urine output and vital signs during the first 24 hours after occurrence of the burn.[40] Lung water accumulation was significantly higher ($P < .0001$) in the albumin-treated patients, and there were trends toward increased pulmonary edema and death in the albumin group. In another study conducted immediately after the first 24-hour resuscitation period, infusion of albumin reduced glomerular filtration rate ($P < .05$) despite increasing plasma volume by 37%.[41]

TABLE 24–5. General Indications for Blood Products in Acute Circulatory Insufficiency Due to Hemorrhage*

Packed red blood cells
- Increase oxygen-carrying capacity of blood—usually indicated in patients with continued deterioration after volume replacement or obvious exsanguination; needs to be warmed, particularly when used in children

Fresh-frozen plasma
- Replacement of clotting factors—generally overused; indicated if ongoing hemorrhage in patients with PT/PTT > 1.5 times normal, severe hepatic disease, or other bleeding diathesis

Platelets
- Used for bleeding due to severe thrombocytopenia (i.e., platelet count < 10,000 μL) or rapidly dropping platelet counts as would occur with massive bleeding

Other products
- Components such as cryoprecipitate and factor VIII are generally not indicated in acute hemorrhage, but rather are used after specific deficiencies are identified

*Although whole blood could be used for large-volume blood loss, most hospitals use component therapy, and use crystalloids or colloids for plasma expansion. PT, prothrombin time; PTT, partial thromboplastin time.

In a more recent randomized trial involving 70 patients younger than 19 years of age with more than 20% body-surface-area thermal injuries, patients were given albumin based on albumin concentrations.[42] Both groups received conventional resuscitation with crystalloid solutions. In one group, albumin was given if the concentration decreased to less than 2.5 g/dL, whereas patients in the other group were given albumin only if the concentration was less than 1.5 g/dL. No statistically significant differences were found in any of the resuscitation or nutritional parameters.

Some novel therapies for thermal resuscitation are currently under study. For example, in guinea pigs with 70% body-surface-area burns, antioxidant therapy with high-dose vitamin C (340 mg/kg/24 h) has been shown to decrease the amount of resuscitation fluid needed for maintaining cardiac output.[43] The proposed mechanism is reduction in free-radical-induced increases in capillary permeability.

ONGOING MONITORING

Although the monitoring of patients in the emergency department is relatively straightforward, it becomes much more controversial in other settings such as the ICU. This is particularly true as regards the value of right-heart catheterization (aka pulmonary artery or Swan-Ganz catheter). However, most clinicians would agree that certain forms of monitoring are important, because patients in the postresuscitation phase of management are at risk for various complications secondary to ischemia. A more complete discussion of invasive and noninvasive hemodynamic monitoring is found in Chap. 23.

One form of monitoring that may take place in the emergency and operating rooms, as well as in the intensive care unit, requires placement of a central venous pressure (CVP) line. Monitoring of CVP provides the clinician with an indirect and insensitive, yet useful estimate of the relationship between increased right atrial pressure and cardiac output.[7]

A number of laboratory tests are indicated for the subacute monitoring of shock. These include a renal battery for assessing possible electrolyte alterations and kidney perfusion (blood urea nitrogen, creatinine). Among other things, a complete blood count will enable assessment of possible infection (white blood cell count), oxygen-carrying capacity of the blood (hemoglobin, hematocrit), and ongoing bleeding (hemoglobin, hematocrit, platelet count). The prothrombin time (PT) and partial thromboplastin time (PTT) will give an indication of the ability of the blood to clot because, in the case of hemorrhagic shock, clotting factors are lost and diluted. An increasing lactate concentration (arterial, mixed venous, or central venous)[44] and base deficit are consistent with inadequate perfusion, leading to anaerobic metabolism with accumulation of lactic acid. These tests are often considered the optimal end points of resuscitation in certain populations such as trauma patients.[45] Other tests may be indicated if organ dysfunction is likely. For example, when blood flow to the liver is interrupted because of sustained hypotension, a condition known as shock liver may occur. In this condition, the transaminases on a liver panel may be markedly elevated in the first couple of days after marked hypotension, although the concentrations should decrease over time.[3] Along with laboratory testing, a more extensive history can be obtained during the subacute monitoring period.

The value of pulmonary artery catheters has been hotly debated since their introduction. Such catheters are placed to obtain various oxygen transport variables, some of which cannot be reliably determined from peripheral or other central vessels.[46] The debate was intensified when early studies suggested improved outcomes when cardiac output and other oxygen transport variables were raised to supranormal levels, the monitoring of which required placement of a pulmonary artery catheter. Subsequent studies using similar monitoring parameters associated with pulmonary artery catheterization gave conflicting results.[47]

A resolution to this controversy involving oxygen transport therapeutic goals seemed possible with a study involving the largest number of patients to date.[48] This study randomized 762 patients to a control group in which traditional therapies were titrated to normal physiologic values, a treatment group in which therapies were titrated to achieve a supranormal cardiac index of >4.5 L/min/m^2, and a treatment group in which therapies were titrated to achieve a normal mixed venous oxygen saturation of ≥70%. Morbidity, mortality, and length of stay were similar for all three groups. This study did not prove that supranormal goals are undesirable in any patient, however, because it included a heterogeneous group of patients most of whom were studied postoperatively. In contrast, the studies that show value in titrating therapies to supranormal goals were conducted in high-risk surgery or trauma patients with early (preoperative or intraoperative) initiation of monitoring by pulmonary artery catheterization.[49] It would be expected that most of these patients would have a hypovolemic form of shock. It is important to realize that most clinicians would agree that *conservative* management of patients with circulatory insufficiency is inappropriate.[50]

The titration of therapies to supranormal therapeutic goals requires placement of a pulmonary artery catheter, but the controversy surrounding this type of catheterization extends beyond this particular issue. A large observational study involving 5,735 critically ill patients found that placement of a pulmonary artery catheter for a variety of reasons resulted in increased mortality, as well as increased costs.[51] An editorial accompanying the published study was more controversial than the study itself because the authors recommended a moratorium on pulmonary artery catheter placement *if* a multicenter, randomized trial was not initiated.[52] At least one organization condemned the suggestion of a moratorium on catheter placement and made plans for a consensus conference to address the issue of pulmonary artery catheterization. Results of the consensus conference, which was endorsed by five major health professional organizations, were subsequently published.[53] The consensus participants concluded that while a randomized controlled trial would be ethical, a moratorium on pulmonary artery catheter placement should not be enacted pending such a trial. The debate between catheter proponents and opponents has continued with the publication of a meta-analysis that found a statistically significant reduction in *morbidity* using pulmonary artery catheters to guide therapy.[54]

Part of the concern regarding pulmonary artery catheterization relates to the interpretation of its results by inexperienced practitioners. Studies in both Europe and the United States found that one of two physicians incorrectly interpreted a tracing from a pulmonary artery catheter.[55] This could explain some of the results of studies finding no benefits to pulmonary artery catheterization or, in some cases, worse outcomes in the pulmonary artery catheterization group by actions taken as a result of inaccurate measurements or misinterpretation of information obtained from the monitoring process. In light of these and other concerns, the National Heart, Lung, and Blood Institute and the Food and Drug Administration conducted a workshop to develop recommendations for pulmonary artery catheter use. The problems in conducting trials in trauma patients were discussed and no specific recommendations for a future, well-designed trial were made. However, trials were recommended for problems such as septic shock and the acute respiratory distress syndrome, and it was acknowledged that the results of these trials could have important implications for the management of trauma patients.[56]

Complications related to pulmonary artery catheter insertion, maintenance, and removal include damage to vessels and organs during insertion, arrhythmias, infections, and thromboembolic damage.[57] To avoid the complications associated with pulmonary artery catheterization, other less-invasive tools were developed to obtain similar information. For example, cardiac output determinations have been made by Doppler, bioimpedance, dye, and ionic dilution techniques, although such measurements would not provide other data that are routinely obtained with pulmonary artery catheters (e.g., left-heart-filling pressure).[58] Additionally, advances in pulmonary artery catheter technology that expand the information obtained from such monitoring (e.g., mixed venous oxyhemoglobin) are under investigation.[59] However, given the lack of well-defined outcome data associated with pulmonary artery catheterization, its use is best reserved for complicated cases of shock not responding to conventional fluid and medication therapies.

Commonly measured and calculated hemodynamic and oxygen transport indices associated with invasive monitoring are primarily global indicators of tissue perfusion. There have been attempts to find regional and local indicators of hypoperfusion so that circulatory insufficiency can be treated before overt shock occurs. One focus of recent research has been monitoring modalities involving the gastrointestinal tract.

It has been demonstrated that intramucosal stomach pH (pHi) determinations <7.35 are associated with very high mortality (>65%), which may not be altered by standard interventions. For example, one study used a protocol (normal saline boluses followed by a dobutamine infusion if the pHi remained <7.35) aimed at increasing oxygen transport and reducing oxygen demand in patients with initial pHi determinations <7.35 or ≥7.35 after "conventional" therapy had been used to stabilize all patients.[60] Survival in the protocol group was not improved when compared to a control group for patients with pHi values <7.35 on admission. However, mortality was significantly decreased in the protocol, as compared to the control group, in patients with relatively normal pHi values (i.e., initial pHi values ≥7.35) on admission. Interestingly, pulmonary artery catheterization was not used in this study, but there were limits placed on the dose of dobutamine (e.g., no more than 10 μg/kg/min) to try to decrease the incidence of drug toxicity. Although the literature is fairly consistent concerning low pHi values being predictive of death,[61] pHi-guided therapy to decrease mortality has not been demonstrated.[62] Additionally, there are a number of technical considerations that remain to be resolved when using pHi, or more recently capnometry (luminal PCO_2 tonometry), for monitoring and therapy.[63] Despite these concerns, measures of regional tissue oxygenation continued to be investigated through a variety of novel monitoring techniques.[64]

In addition to regional monitoring of tissue perfusion, local methods of monitoring are also being studied. For example, subcutaneous measurement of tissue oxygen pressure shows promise in preliminary investigations. It is unlikely that regional and local measurements will replace more global indicators of perfusion, but rather that the methods will complement each other.

ONGOING MANAGEMENT

Proper attention to plasma expansion must be continued into the intraoperative and postoperative periods. A number of neurohormonal changes take place that affect urine output and patients may have substantial third-spacing of fluid depending on the operation and the preexisting condition of the patient. Furthermore, postoperative patients are prone to hyponatremia from renal generation of electrolyte-free water and from antidiuretic hormone release.[65] As in acute resuscitation, the administration of hypotonic solutions in the perioperative period does not prevent the decrease in extracellular volume that often occurs. Therefore, although excess fluid administration is to be avoided in the perioperative setting, isotonic crystalloid solutions should be used when fluids are indicated to prevent intravascular depletion and circulatory insufficiency.

Of the randomized studies comparing albumin to crystalloid solutions in the perioperative period, the majority found no statistically significant differences between groups.[66] The significant differences that have been found have involved isolated hemodynamic or respiratory variables with no obvious clinical correlates (e.g., duration of mechanical ventilation). Therefore, albumin (and other colloids) cannot be recommended for the prevention or initial treatment of circulatory insufficiency, although their use may be appropriate in patients who are not responding to crystalloids and are developing problems such as interstitial fluid accumulation. Practice guidelines published by a consortium of academic medical centers reflect this recommendation, but colloids continue to be widely used.[67]

In general, medications are not indicated in the initial therapy of hypovolemic shock. With hypovolemia, the body's natural response is to increase cardiac output and to constrict blood vessels to maintain blood pressure. There is no reason why most patients should need inotropic or vasoactive agents assuming fluid therapy is adequate. For that matter, there is no evidence that these medications improve outcome in patients with hypovolemic shock. However, once the cause of acute circulatory insufficiency has been stopped or treated and fluids have been optimized, some patients continue to have signs and symptoms of inadequate tissue perfusion. This may be caused by reperfusion injury. Although the search for a cryptogenic source (e.g., intra-abdominal bleeding in a trauma patient) should continue, the clinician may need to administer medications to improve perfusion.

Pressor agents such as norepinephrine and high-dose dopamine are to be avoided, if possible, because they may increase blood pressure at the expense of peripheral tissue ischemia. Some sources use stronger language and state that vasopressors are contraindicated in certain forms of shock (e.g., hemorrhagic).[7] This does not help the clinician who is treating a patient with unstable blood pressure despite massive fluid replacement and increasing interstitial fluid accumulation. In such situations, inotropic agents such as dobutamine are preferred if blood pressure is adequate (e.g., systolic blood pressure ≥90 mm Hg), because they should not aggravate the existing vasoconstriction. The inotropic agents are justified by presumed inadequate cardiac output for the specific situation, although the measured values may be in the normal range.[3]

When pressure cannot be maintained with inotropic agents, or when inotropic agents with vasodilatory properties cannot be used because of inadequate blood pressure concerns, pressors may be required as a last resort. In general, the need for pressors is predictive of the development of MODS and increased length of stay.[68] Although the response to pressor agents may be variable in hypovolemic shock, there does not appear to be resistance as a consequence of altered receptor response as is sometimes seen in patients with septic shock.[3] Potent vasoconstrictors such as norepinephrine and phenylephrine should be given through central veins because of the possibility of extravasation and necrosis with peripheral administration.

A number of interesting treatments for shock are under investigation, including autotransfusion for removing harmful cytokines from the body. Various alternatives to conventional blood components are also being studied, such as stroma-free hemoglobin and perfluorocarbon compounds, as virus-free alternatives to red blood cell transfusion. Hopefully these will be useful adjuncts to adequate volume replacement, which is the primary therapeutic intervention in managing acute circulatory insufficiency due to volume depletion.

PHARMACOECONOMIC CONSIDERATIONS

The primary therapy for hypovolemic shock is fluid replacement. The institutional cost of 1 L of most crystalloid solutions is less than $1. Assuming such fluids are used, it is the associated costs of personnel and equipment that become the primary economic considerations in the resuscitation of patients with hypovolemic shock. However, as mentioned, many clinicians recommend that colloid plasma expanders (e.g., albumin, hetastarch, dextrans) be used to replace some or all of the standard crystalloid solutions. Although the costs of these solutions vary, depending on contractual arrangements as might occur with purchasing groups, in general, albumin solutions are more expensive than hetastarch and dextran products. All of these are markedly more costly than crystalloid solutions; in some cases, there are 50- to 100-fold differences, even when used in equipotent amounts.

The only recent trial that investigated albumin use on a large-scale basis was an observational study involving 15 academic medical centers in the United States. Based on previously published guidelines, 62% of albumin use was defined as inappropriate at a cost of $124,939.[69] Presuming equal efficacy and toxicity (as available studies indicate) between crystalloid and colloid solutions, cost minimization analysis clearly indicates the economic advantages of the crystalloids.

Because medications are not simply alternatives to crystalloids, but rather are used when crystalloid therapy has been optimized, there is little reason to compare medication and fluid therapies from an economic perspective. Furthermore, there are no economic comparisons of the various inotropic and vasopressor medications used in the treatment of hypovolemic shock.

CONCLUSIONS

Figure 24–4 is an algorithm that summarizes many of the treatment principles discussed in this chapter. The algorithm is an example of one approach to the adult patient presenting with hypovolemic shock. It presumes that initial rehydration attempts (i.e., outpatient or prehospital) were unsuccessful in restoring circulation. Obviously, modifications may be needed for patient-specific forms of hypovolemic shock. Other limitations of the algorithm should be recognized, particularly the decisions to add or to substitute colloid or medication therapies when crystalloid solutions are not yielding desired results and when to perform pulmonary artery catheterization for more invasive monitoring. Medications become more important for the ongoing management of hypovolemic shock, particularly when the patient is unresponsive to fluids (see Fig. 24–5). Additionally, it is hoped that the options for more complicated cases of hypovolemic shock do not detract from the primary effective resuscitative measure for most patients: fluid.

▶ PRINCIPLES OF PHARMACOTHERAPY

Restoring circulating blood volume is a common goal in managing all forms of shock.

Tissue injury and death may result from inadequate tissue perfusion during the primary shock event or from reperfusion injury associated with subsequent compensatory changes.

The presentation of patients with acute circulatory insufficiency can vary markedly depending on the cause, as well as patient-specific considerations, such as age, concomitant disease states, and medications.

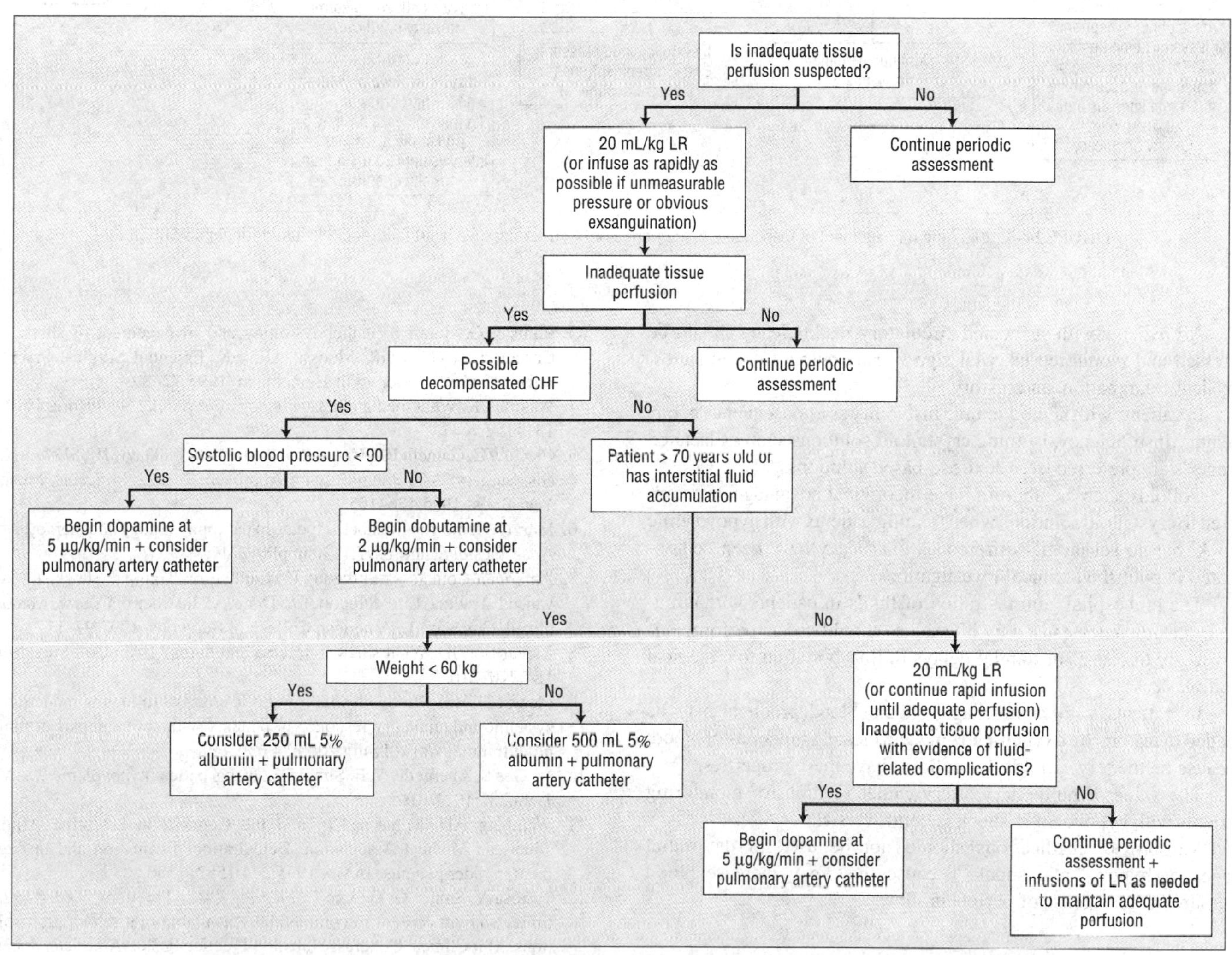

FIGURE 24–4. Hypovolemia protocol for adults. This protocol is not intended to replace or delay therapies such as surgical intervention or blood products for restoring oxygen-carrying capacity or hemostasis. If available, some measurements may be used in addition to those listed in the algorithm, such as mean arterial pressure or pulmonary artery catheter recordings. The latter may be used to assist in medication choices (e.g., agents with primary pressor effects may be desirable in patients with normal cardiac outputs, whereas dopamine or dobutamine may be indicated in patients with suboptimal cardiac outputs). Lower maximal doses of the medications in this algorithm should be considered when pulmonary artery catheterization is not available. CHF, congestive heart failure; LR, lactated Ringer's solution. Colloids that may be substituted for albumin are hetastarch 6% and dextran 40. See text for an in-depth discussion of these and other issues involved in this protocol.

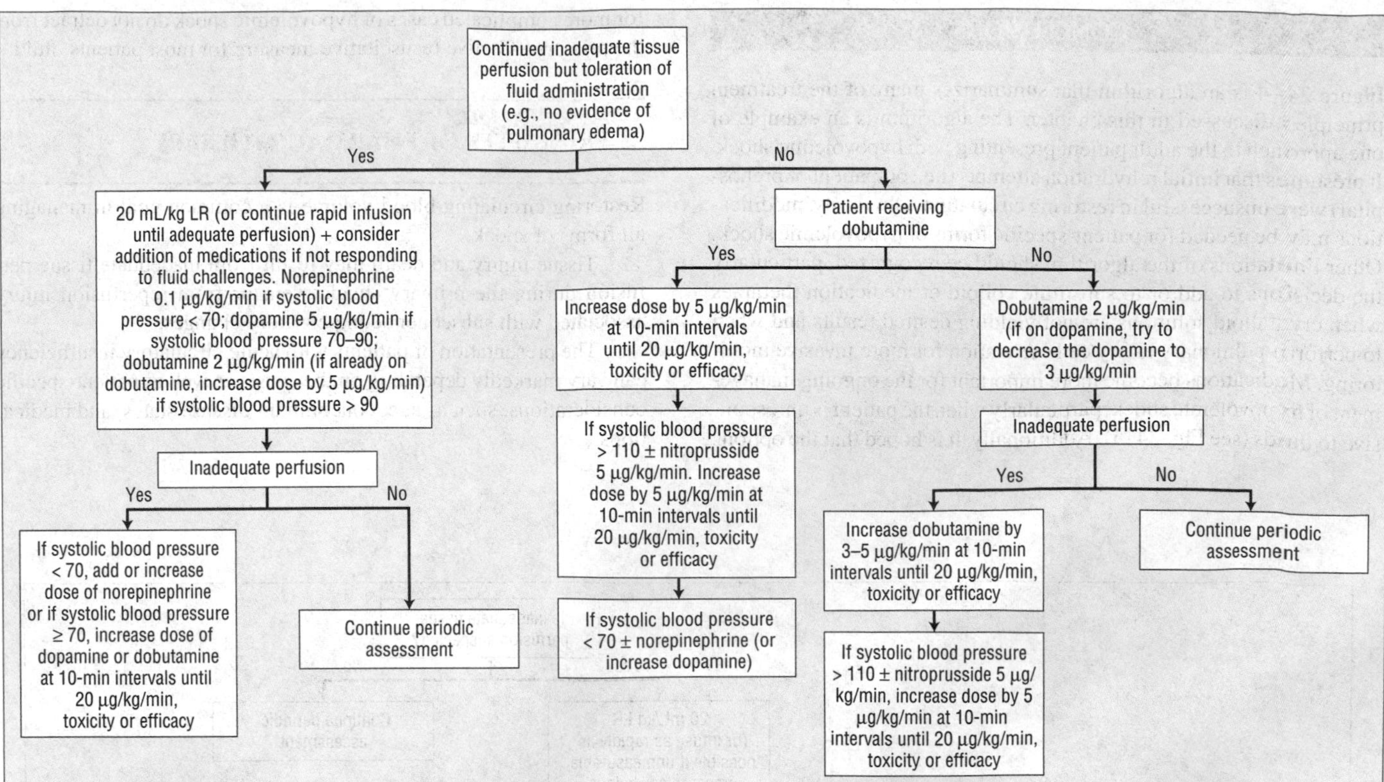

FIGURE 24–5. Ongoing management of inadequate tissue perfusion. CHF, congestive heart failure; LR, lactated Ringer's solution.

All patients with suspected circulatory insufficiency should be assessed and monitored by vital signs, urine output, mental status, physical examination, and history.

In patients with hemodynamic instability as a consequence of circulatory insufficiency, isotonic crystalloid solutions such as lactated Ringer's are preferred over dextrose-based solutions.

Colloids such as albumin have theoretical advantages as compared to crystalloid solutions when treating patients with hypovolemic shock, but no substantial differences in efficacy have been demonstrated in published clinical investigations.

The prehospital administration of fluids in patients with circulatory insufficiency caused by blood loss should not be performed if it is likely to cause substantial delays in transportation to a medical facility.

In patients with hemorrhagic shock, blood products may be needed to restore the oxygen-carrying and clotting functions of blood, because neither crystalloids nor colloids have these properties.

The value of pulmonary artery catheterization for monitoring patients with hypovolemic shock is controversial.

Vasopressor medications should not be used in the initial stages of hypovolemic shock, because they may increase blood pressure at the expense of peripheral flow.

REFERENCES

1. Jimenez EJ. Shock. In: Civetta JM, Taylor RW, Kirby RR, eds. Critical Care, 3rd ed. Philadelphia, PA, Lippincott-Raven, 1997:359–387.
2. Shoemaker WC. Temporal physiologic patterns of shock and circulatory dysfunction based on early descriptions by invasive and noninvasive monitoring. New Horiz 1996;4:300–318.
3. Ramsay G, Boom S. Pathophysiology and management of shock. In: Cuschieri A, Giles GR, Moossa AR, eds. Essential Surgical Practice, 3rd ed. Oxford, Butterworth-Heinemann, 1995:72–89.
4. Waxman K. What mediates tissue injury after shock? New Horiz 1996;4: 151–152.
5. Cioffi WG, Gamelli RL. Circulation and shock. In: Davis JH, Sheldon GF, eds. Surgery: A Problem-Solving Approach, 2nd ed. St. Louis, Mosby-Year Book, 1995:126–165.
6. Marzi I. Hemorrhagic shock: Update in pathophysiology and therapy. Acta Anaesthesiol Scand 1997;111(suppl):42–44.
7. American College of Surgeons Committee on Trauma. Shock. In: Advanced Trauma Life Support for Doctors: Instructor Course Manual, 6th ed. Chicago, IL, American College of Surgeons, 1997:97–117.
8. Richardson JD. What's new in trauma and burns? J Am Coll Surg 1997; 184:210–216.
9. Plank LD, Hill GL. Sequential metabolic changes following induction of systemic inflammatory response in patients with severe sepsis or major blunt trauma. World J Surg 2000;24:630–638.
10. McGee S, Abernethy WB, Simel DL. Is this patient hypovolemic? JAMA 1999;281:1022–1029.
11. Weinberg AD, Minaker KL, and the Council on Scientific Affairs, American Medical Association. Dehydration: Evaluation and management in older patients. JAMA 1995;274:1552–1556.
12. Tarrosa V, Stoner G, George L, Fleming CR. Alterations needed to optimize sodium content in commercially available oral rehydration solutions. 21st Clinical Congress Nutrition Practice Poster. American Society of Parenteral and Enteral Nutrition. San Francisco, California, January 1997.
13. Brouns F, Senden J, Beckers EJ, Saris WHM. Osmolarity does not affect the gastric emptying rate of oral rehydration solutions. J Parenter Enteral Nutr 1995;19:403–406.
14. Duggan C, Santosham M, Glass RI. The management of acute diarrhea in children: Oral rehydration, maintenance, and nutritional therapy. MMWR Morb Mortal Wkly Rep 1992;41:1–20.

15. Reid SR, Bonadio WA. Outpatient rapid intravenous rehydration to correct dehydration and resolve vomiting in children with acute gastroenteritis. Ann Emerg Med 1996;28:318–323.
16. Luten RC. Rapid rehydration of pediatric patients. Ann Emerg Med 1996; 28:353–355.
17. Axler OA, Tousiganant C, Thompson CR, et al. Small hemodynamic effect of typical rapid volume infusions in critically ill patients. Crit Care Med 1997;25:965–970.
18. Didwania A, Miller J, Kassel D, et al. Effect of intravenous lactated Ringer's solution infusion on the circulating lactate concentration: Results of a prospective, randomized, double-blind, placebo-controlled trial. Crit Care Med 1997;25:1851–1854.
19. Jackson EV, Wiese J, Sigal B, et al. Effects of crystalloid solutions on circulating lactate concentrations: Part 1. Implications for the proper handling of blood specimens obtained in critically ill patients. Crit Care Med 1996;24:1840–1846.
20. Deitch EA. Animal models of sepsis and shock: A review and lessons learned. Shock 1998;9:1–11.
21. Napolitano LM. Naloxone therapy in shock: The controversy continues. Crit Care Med 2000;28:887–888.
22. Cochrane Injuries Group Albumin Reviewers. Human albumin administration in critically ill patients: Systematic review of randomized controlled trials. BMJ 1998;317:235–240.
23. Wilkes MM, Navickis RJ. Patient survival after human albumin administration: A meta-analysis of randomized, controlled trials. Ann Intern Med 2001;135:149–164.
24. Mattox KL, Brundage SL, Hirshberg A. Initial resuscitation. New Horiz 1999;7:4–9.
25. Bickell WH, Wall MJ, Pepe PE, et al. Immediate versus delayed fluid resuscitation for hypotensive patients with penetrating torso injuries. N Engl J Med 1994;331:1105–1109.
26. Jacobs LM. Timing of fluid resuscitation in trauma. N Engl J Med 1994; 331:1153–1154.
27. Prough DS, Zornow MH. Solutions in search of problems. Crit Care Med 1996;24:1104–1105.
28. Saetzler RK, Badellino MM, Buckman RF, et al. Hypertonic saline attenuates leukocyte/endothelium and leukocyte/platelet interactions following hemorrhagic shock. Surg Forum 1996;47:41–43.
29. Angle N, Coimbra R, Hoyt DB, et al. Hypertonic saline resuscitation prevents lung injury following hemorrhagic shock. Surg Forum 1996;47: 43–45.
30. Vassar MJ, Fischer RP, O'Brien PE, et al. A multicenter trial for resuscitation of injured patients with 7.5% sodium chloride: The effect of added dextran 70. Arch Surg 1993;128:1003–1013.
31. Suarez JI, Qureshi AI, Bhardwa A, et al. Treatment of refractory intracranial hypertension with 23.4% saline. Crit Care Med 1998;26:1118–1122.
32. Valadka AB, Robertson CS. Should we be using hypertonic saline to treat intracranial hypertension? Crit Care Med 2000;28:1245–1246.
33. Wade CE, Kramer GC, Grady JJ, et al. Efficacy of hypertonic 7.5% saline and 6% dextran-70 in treating trauma: A meta-analysis of controlled studies. Surgery 1997;122:609–616.
34. Gurevich B, Talmore D, Artru AA, et al. Brain edema, hemorrhagic necrosis volume, and neurological status with rapid infusion of 0.45% saline or 5% dextrose in 0.9% saline after closed head trauma in rats. Anesth Analg 1997;84:554–559.
35. Lucas CE, Ledgerwood AM, Higgins RF, Weaver DW. Impaired pulmonary function after albumin resuscitation from shock. J Trauma 1980; 20:446–451.
36. Lowe RJ, Moss GS, Jilek J, Levine HD. Crystalloid vs colloid in the etiology of pulmonary failure after trauma: A randomized trial in man. Surgery 1977;81:676–683.
37. Moss GS, Lowe RJ, Jilek J, Levine HD. Colloid or crystalloid in the resuscitation of hemorrhagic shock: A controlled clinical trial. Surgery 1981; 89:434–438.
38. Rackow EC, Falk JL, Fein A, et al. Fluid resuscitation in circulatory shock: A comparison of the cardiorespiratory effects of albumin, hetastarch, and saline solutions in patients with hypovolemia and septic shock. Crit Care Med 1983;11:839–850.
39. Gentileilo LM, Jurkovich GJ, Stark MS, et al. Is hypothermia in the victim of major trauma protective or harmful: A randomized, prospective study. Ann Surg 1997;226:439–449.
40. Goodwin CW, Dorethy J, Lam V, Pruitt BA. Randomized trial of efficacy of crystalloid and colloid resuscitation on hemodynamic response and lung water following thermal injury. Ann Surg 1983;197:520–531.
41. Gore DC, Dalton JM, Gehr TWB. Colloid infusions reduce glomerular filtration in resuscitated burn victims. J Trauma 1996;40:356–360.
42. Greenhalgh DG, Housinger TA, Kagan RJ, et al. Maintenance of serum albumin levels in pediatric burn patients: A prospective, randomized trial. J Trauma 1995;39:67–74.
43. Tanaka H, Matsuda H, Shimazaki S, et al. Reduced resuscitation fluid volume for second-degree burns with delayed initiation of ascorbic acid therapy. Arch Surg 1997;132:158–161.
44. Gallagher EJ, Rodriguez K, Touger M. Agreement between peripheral venous and arterial lactate levels. Ann Emerg Med 1997;29:479–483.
45. Porter JM, Ivatury RR. In search of the optimal end points of resuscitation in trauma patients: A review. J Trauma Inj Infect Crit Care 1998;44:908–914.
46. Edwards JD, Mayall RM. Importance of the sampling site for measurement of mixed venous oxygen saturation in shock. Crit Care Med 1998; 26:1356–1360.
47. Yu. Oxygen transport optimization. New Horiz 1999;7:46–53.
48. Gattinoni L, Brazzi L, Pelosi P, et al. A trial of goal-oriented hemodynamic therapy in critically ill patients. N Engl J Med 1995;333:1025–1032.
49. Wilson J, Woods I, Fawcett J, et al. Reducing the risk of major elective surgery: Randomised controlled trial of preoperative optimisation of oxygen delivery. BMJ 1999;318:1099–1103.
50. Hinds C, Watson D. Manipulating hemodynamics and oxygen transport in critically ill patients. N Engl J Med 1995;333:1074–1075.
51. Connors AF, Speroff T, Dawson NV, et al. The effectiveness of right heart catheterization in the initial care of critically ill patients. JAMA 1996; 276:889–897.
52. Dalen JE, Bone RC. Is it time to pull the pulmonary artery catheter? JAMA 1996;276:916–918.
53. Taylor RW, Ahrens T, Beilin Y, et al. Pulmonary artery consensus conference: Consensus statement. Crit Care Med 1997;25:190–200.
54. Ivanov R, Allen J, Calvin JE. The incidence of major morbidity in critically ill patients managed with pulmonary artery catheters: A meta-analysis. Crit Care Med 2000;28:615–619.
55. Ginosar Y, Thijs LG, Sprung CL. Raising the standard of hemodynamic monitoring: Targeting the practice or the practitioner? Crit Care Med 1997; 25:209–211.
56. Bernard GR, Sopko G, Cerra F, et al. Pulmonary artery catheterization and clinical outcomes. JAMA 2000;283:2568–2572.
57. Connors AF. Right-heart catheterization: Is it effective? New Horiz 1997; 5:195–200.
58. Peruzzi WT. Hemodynamic monitoring: Does the end justify the means? Crit Care Med 1997;25:1767–1768.
59. Burchell SA, Yu M, Takiguchi SA, Ohta RM. Evaluation of a continuous cardiac output and mixed venous oxygen saturation catheter in critically ill surgery patients. Crit Care Med 1997;2:388–391.
60. Gutierrez G, Palizas F, Doglio G, et al. Gastric intramucosal pH as a therapeutic index of tissue oxygenation in critically ill patients. Lancet 1992; 339:195–199.
61. Ivatury RR, Simon RJ, Islam S, et al. A prospective randomized study of end points of resuscitation after major trauma: Global oxygen transport indices versus organ-specific gastric mucosal pH. J Am Coll Surg 1996; 183:145–154.
62. Gomersall CD, Joynt GM, Freebairn RC, et al. Resuscitation of critically ill patients based on the results of gastric tonometry: A prospective, randomized, controlled trial. Crit Care Med 2000;28:607–614.

63. Groeneveld ABJ, Kolkman JJ. Factors affecting gastrointestinal luminal P_{CO_2} tonometry. Intensive Care Med 1999;25:249–251.
64. Siegemund M, van Bommel J, Ince C. Assessment of regional tissue oxygenation. Intensive Care Med 1999;25:1044–1060.
65. Steele A, Gowrishankar M, Abrahamson S, et al. Postoperative hyponatremia despite near-isotonic saline infusion: A phenomenon of desalination. Ann Intern Med 1997;126:20–25.
66. Erstad BL. Concerns with defining appropriate uses of albumin by meta-analysis. Am J Health Syst Pharm 1999;56:1451–1454.
67. Fox DL, Vermeulen LC. UHC Technology Assessment: Albumin, Nonprotein Colloid, and Crystalloid Solutions. University Health System Consortium, Oak Brook, IL, May 2000.
68. Goncalves JA, Hydo LJ, Barie PS. Factors influencing outcome of prolonged norepinephrine therapy for shock in critical surgical illness. Shock 1998;10:231–236.
69. Yim JM, Vermeulen LC, Erstad BL, et al. Albumin and nonprotein colloid solution use in US academic health centers. Arch Intern Med 1995; 155:2450–2455.

25
INTRODUCTION TO PULMONARY FUNCTION TESTING

Jay I. Peters and Stephanie M. Levine

GENERAL CONCEPTS

The primary function of the respiratory system is to maintain Pa_{O_2} and Pa_{CO_2} (the arterial pressure of oxygen and carbon dioxide) within the normal range. To accomplish this task, several processes must be accomplished, including alveolar ventilation, pulmonary perfusion, ventilation-perfusion matching, and gas transfer across the alveolar-capillary membrane.

Alveolar ventilation is achieved by the cyclic process of air movement in and out of the lung. During inspiration, the inspiratory muscle contracts and generates negative pressure in the pleural space. This pressure gradient between the mouth and the alveoli draws fresh air (tidal volume) into the lung. Approximately, one-third of the inspired gas stays in the conducting airways (dead space) while two-thirds reaches the alveoli.

The human lung contains a series of branching, progressively tapering airways that originate at the glottis and terminate in a matrix of thin-walled alveoli. Coursing through this matrix of alveoli is a rich network of capillaries that originate from the pulmonary arterioles and terminate in the pulmonary venules. The adequacy of respiration in each gas exchange unit depends on the opposition of a thin film of mixed venous blood with just the right amount of fresh alveolar gas. During "ideal" gas exchange, there is uniform blood flow and uniform ventilation; accordingly, there is no alveolar-arterial P_{O_2} difference (P_{A-aO_2} gradient, sometimes called the A-a gradient). Gas exchange is not perfect, however, even in the normal lung. Normally, there is less alveolar ventilation than pulmonary blood flow, and the overall ventilation-to-perfusion ratio is 0.8 (not 1.0).

Normal expiration is a passive process and when the inspiratory muscles end their contraction, the elastic recoil of the lung pulls the lung back to its original size and shape. This process makes the alveolar pressure positive relative to the pressure at the mouth and air flows out of the lung. During inspiration, the respiratory muscles must overcome the elastic properties of the lung (elastic recoil) and the resistance to airflow by the airways. During expiration, the flow of air is primarily determined by the elastic recoil and airway resistance.

Different pulmonary function tests are used to evaluate the physiologic process of the respiratory system. Physiologic abnormalities that can be measured by pulmonary function testing include obstruction to airflow, restriction of lung size, and decrease in the transfer of gas across the alveolar-capillary membrane. Abnormal values on pulmonary function tests are those outside the range of values obtained from a group of normal individuals matched according to age, height, sex, and race. A pulmonary function test is labeled abnormal when the results fall outside the range in which 95% of people the same age, height, and sex would be found (95% confidence interval). This definition is arbitrary and may misclassify a small percentage of normals as having lung dysfunction. Therefore, clinical correlation and serial pulmonary function testing (PFT) may be necessary for optimal interpretation of PFTs.

Potential uses of pulmonary function testing include the evaluation of patients with known or suspected lung disease; the evaluation of symptoms such as chronic cough, dyspnea, or chest tightness; monitoring the effects of exposure to dust, chemicals, or pulmonary toxic drugs; risk stratification prior to surgery; monitoring the effectiveness of therapeutic interventions; and objective assessment of impairment or disability.[1]

DEFINITIONS OF LUNG VOLUMES AND EXPIRATORY FLOWS

The air within the lung at the end of a forced inspiration can be divided into four compartments or lung volumes (Fig. 25–1). The volume of air exhaled during normal quiet breathing is termed "tidal volume" (V_T). The maximal volume of air inhaled above tidal volume is called the inspiratory reserve volume (IRV) and the maximal air exhaled below tidal volume is called the expiratory reserve volume (ERV). The residual volume (RV) is the amount of air remaining in the lungs after a maximal exhalation.

The combinations or sums of two or more lung volumes are termed capacities (Fig. 25–1). Vital capacity (VC) is the maximal amount of air that can be exhaled after a maximal inspiration. It is equal to the sum of the IRV, TV, and ERV. When measured on a forced expiration, it is called the forced vital capacity (FVC). When measured over an exhalation of at least 30 seconds, it is called the slow vital capacity (SVC, VC). The VC is approximately 75% of the total lung capacity (TLC) and when the SVC is within the normal range, a significant restrictive disorder is unlikely. Normally, the value for SVC and FVC are very similar unless airway obstruction is present.

The TLC is the volume of air in the lung after the maximal inspiration and is the sum of the four primary lung volumes (IRV, V_T, ERV, and RV). Its measurement is difficult because the amount of air remaining in the chest after maximal exhalation (RV) must be measured by indirect methods. The definition of restrictive lung disease is based on a reduction in TLC (i.e., inability to get air into the lung or restriction to air movement on inhalation).

The functional residual capacity (FRC) is the volume of air remaining in the lungs at the end of a quiet expiration. FRC is the

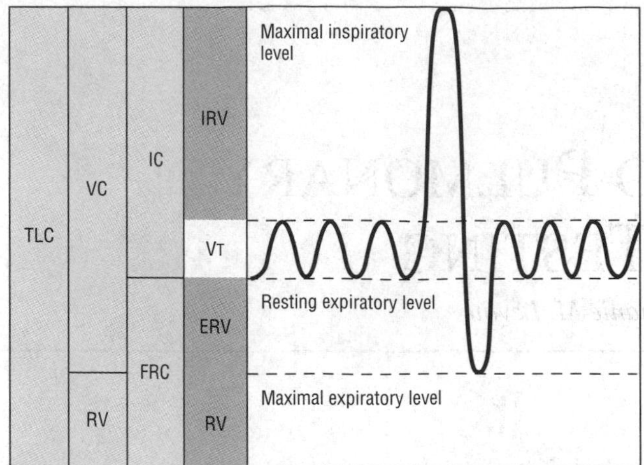

FIGURE 25–1. Lung volumes and capacities. ERV, expiratory reserve volume; FRC, functional residual capacity; IC, inspiratory capacity; IRV, inspiratory pressure volume; RV, residual volume; TLC, total lung capacity; VC, vital capacity; V_T, tidal volume.

normal resting position of the lung and occurs when there is no contraction of either inspiratory or expiratory muscles and is normally 40% of TLC. Inspiratory capacity (IC) is the maximal volume of air that can be inhaled from the end of a quiet expiration and represents the sum of V_T and IRV.

The FVC, which represents the total amount of air than can be exhaled can be expressed as a series of timed volumes. The forced expiratory volume in 1 second (FEV_1) is the volume of air exhaled during the first second of the FVC maneuver. Although the FEV_1 is a volume, it conveys information on obstruction because it is measured over a known time interval. The FEV_1 is dependent upon the volume of air within the lung and the effort during exhalation; therefore, it can be diminished by a decrease in TLC, or by a lack of effort. A more sensitive way to measure obstruction is to express the FEV_1 as a ratio of FVC. This ratio is independent of the patient's size or the TLC; therefore, the FEV_1/FVC is a specific measure of airway obstruction with or without restriction. Normally, this ratio is 75% or greater and any value below 70% to 75% suggests obstruction.

Because flow is defined as the change in volume with time, forced expiratory flow may be determined graphically by dividing the volume change by the time change. The forced expiratory flow (FEF) during 25% to 75% of FVC ($FEF_{25\%-75\%}$) represents the mean flow during the middle half of the FVC. The $FEF_{25\%-75\%}$, formerly called the maximal midexpiratory flow (MMEF), is frequently reported to assess small airways. The 95% confidence limit is so wide that the $FEF_{25\%-75\%}$ has limited utility in the early diagnosis of small airways disease in an individual subject. The peak expiratory flow (PEF), also called maximum forced expiratory flow (FEF_{max}) is the maximum flow obtained during the FVC. This measurement is often used in the outpatient management of asthma because it can be measured with inexpensive peak flow meters.

SPIROMETRY/FLOW-VOLUME LOOP

Spirometry is the most widely available and useful PFT. It takes only 15 to 20 minutes, carries no risks, and provides information about obstructive and restrictive disease. Spirometry allows for the measurement of all lung volumes and capacities except RV, FRC, and TLC, and allows the assessment of FEV_1 and $FEF_{25\%-75\%}$. Spirometry measurements can be reported in two different formats—standard

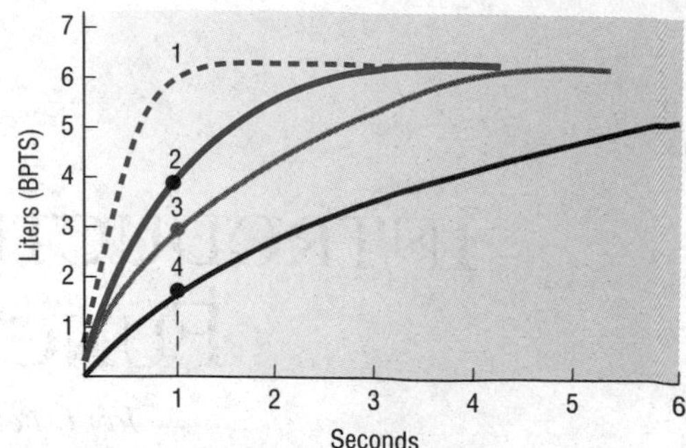

FIGURE 25–2. Standard spirometry. Curve (1) is a normal subject with a normal FEV_1; (2) FEV_1 in a patient with mild airways obstruction; (3) a patient with moderate airways obstruction; (4) a patient with severe airways obstruction. BPTS, body temperature saturated with water vapor.

spirometry (Fig. 25–2) and the flow-volume loop (Fig. 25–3). In standard spirometry, the volumes are recorded on the vertical (y) axis and the time on the horizontal (x) axis. In flow-volume loops, volume is plotted on the horizontal (x) axis and flow (derived from volume/time) is plotted on the vertical (y) axis. The shape of the flow-volume loop can be helpful in differentiating obstructive and restrictive defects and in the diagnosis of upper airway obstruction (Fig. 25–4). This curve gives a visual representation of obstruction because the expiratory descent becomes more concave with worsening obstruction.

LUNG VOLUMES

Spirometry measures three of the four basic lung volumes but cannot measure RV (residual volume). Residual volume must be measured to determine the TLC. TLC should be measured anytime there is a reduced vital capacity. In the setting of chronic obstructive pulmonary disease (COPD) with a low VC, measurement of TLC can help to determine whether there is a superimposed restrictive disorder. There are four methods to measure TLC: helium dilution, nitrogen washout, body plethysmography, and chest x-ray measurement (planimetry). The first two methods are called dilution techniques and only measure lung volumes in communication with the upper airway. In patients with airway obstruction who have trapped air, dilution techniques will underestimate the actual volume of the lungs. Planimetry measures the circumference of the lungs on the posterior-anterior

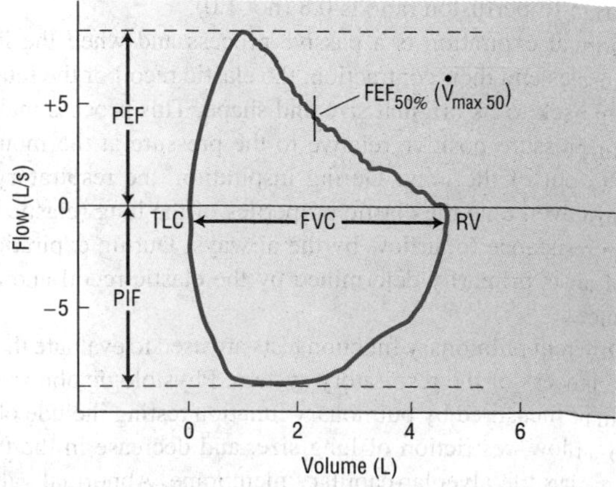

FIGURE 25–3. Normal flow volume loop. Flows measured on the vertical (y) axis and lung volumes measured on the horizontal (x) axis. FVC can be read from the tracing as the maximal horizontal deflection. Instantaneous flow (V_{max}) at any point in FVC can also be measured directly. FVC, forced vital capacity.

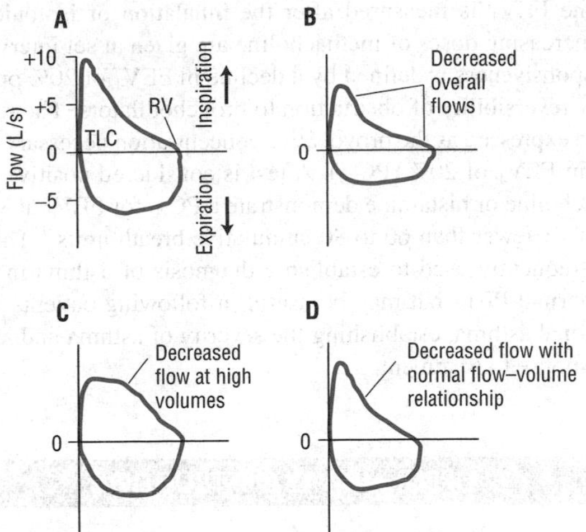

FIGURE 25–4. Flow-volume loop depicting **(A)** mild obstruction characterized by decrease flow at low lung volumes. **B,** Moderate airflow obstruction characterized by a more concave curve. **C,** Variable intrathoracic obstruction in which peak flow is decreased at higher lung volume with normalization of curve at lower lung volumes. **D,** Restrictive lung disease with a curve that is decreased in width but with a normal shape.

view and lateral view of a chest x-ray and estimates the total lung volume.

Body plethysmography or body box is the most accurate technique for lung volume determinations. It measures all the air in the lungs, including trapped air. The principle of the measurement of the body box is Boyle's gas law ($P_1V_1 = P_2V_2$): a volume of gas in a closed system varies inversely with the pressure applied to it. The changes in alveolar pressure are measured at the mouth as well as pressure changes in the body box. The volume of the body box is known. Lung volumes can be determined measuring the changes in pressures caused by panting against a closed shutter.[2] The measurement of lung volumes provides useful information about elastic recoil of the lungs. If elastic recoil is increased (as in interstitial lung disease), the lung volumes (TLC) are reduced. When the elastic recoil is reduced (as in emphysema), the lung volumes are increased.

CARBON MONOXIDE DIFFUSING CAPACITY

The diffusing capacity of the lungs (D_L) is a measurement of the ability of a gas to diffuse across the alveolar-capillary membrane. Carbon monoxide is the usual test gas because it is not normally present in the lungs and is much more soluble in blood than lung tissue. When the diffusing capacity is determined with carbon monoxide, the test is called the carbon monoxide diffusing capacity (D_{LCO}). Because the D_{LCO} is directly related to the alveolar volume (V_A), it is frequently normalized to this value (D_L/V_A), which allows for its interpretation in the presence of abnormal lung volumes (e.g., after surgical lung resection).

The diffusing capacity will be reduced in all clinical situations in which there is impairment of gas transfer from the alveoli to capillary blood.[2,3] Common conditions that reduce the D_{LCO} include lung resection, emphysema (loss of functioning alveolar-capillary units), and interstitial lung disease (thickening of the alveolar-capillary membrane). Normal PFTs with a reduced D_{LCO} should suggest the possibility of pulmonary vascular disease (e.g., pulmonary embolus) but can also be seen with anemia, early interstitial lung disease, and mild Pneumocystis carinii (PCP) infection in AIDS patients.

OBSTRUCTIVE LUNG DISEASE

Obstructive lung disease implies a reduced capacity to get air through the conducting airways and out of the lungs. This reduction in airflow may be caused by a decrease in the diameter of the airways (bronchospasm), a loss of their integrity (bronchomalacia), or from a reduction in the elastic recoil (emphysema) with a resultant decrease in the driving pressure. The most common diseases associated with obstructive pulmonary functions are asthma, emphysema, and chronic bronchitis; however, bronchiectasis, infiltration of the bronchial wall by tumor or granuloma, aspiration of a foreign body, and bronchiolitis also cause obstructive pulmonary function tests. The standard test used to evaluate airway obstruction is the forced expiratory spirogram.

Standard spirometry and flow-volume loop measurements include many variables; however, according to the American Thoracic Society Guidelines, the diagnosis of obstructive and restrictive ventilatory defects should be made using the basic measurements of spirometry.[3] A reduction in FEV_1 (with a normal FVC) establishes the diagnosis of obstruction. When both the FEV_1 and FVC are reduced, the FEV_1 cannot be used to assess airway obstruction because such patients may have either obstruction or restriction. In restrictive lung disease, the patient has an inability to get air into the lung, which results in a reduction of all expiratory volumes (FEV_1, FVC, SVC). In obstructive patients a better measurement is the ratio of the FEV_1 to FVC. Patients with restrictive lung disease have a reduced FEV_1 and a reduced FVC, but the FEV_1/FVC ratio remains normal. Although a normal FEV_1/FVC % is above 70% to 75%, the ratio is age-dependent and slightly lower values may be normal in older patients. Caution should be used in interpreting obstruction when the ratio of FEV_1/FVC is below normal but the FEV_1 and FVC are both within the normal range, because this pattern can be seen with healthy, athletic subjects. The measurement of $FEF_{25\%-75\%}$ is also abnormal in patients with obstructive airways disease. In general, this test has so much variability that it adds little to the measurement of FEV_1 and FEV_1/FVC ratio. The $FEF_{25\%-75\%}$ has been of value in monitoring lung transplant patients for graft rejection[4] and a reduced value may be an early indicator of acute rejection.

Although there is no standardization for interpretation of severity of obstruction, most pulmonary laboratories state than an FEV_1/FVC ratio of less than 75% of the predicted value is mild obstruction, less than 60% of the predicted value is moderate obstruction, and less than 40% of the predicted value is severe obstruction. In patients with obstruction, a dose of a bronchodilator (e.g., isoproterenol) by metered dose inhaler is given during the initial exam. If patients have angina or a history of cardiac arrhythmias, a β_2 selective drug (e.g., albuterol) is used. An increase in the FEV_1 of more than 12% and greater than 0.2 L suggest an acute bronchodilator response.[3] Because bronchodilator responsiveness is variable over time, the lack of an acute bronchodilator response should not preclude a 6- to 8-week trial of bronchodilators and/or corticosteroids.

Although all patients with obstructive lung disease of any etiology will have reduced flow rates on forced exhalation, the pattern on pulmonary function tests may be helpful in differentiating among the various etiologies (see Table 25–1). Asthma is characterized by variable obstruction that often improves or resolves with appropriate therapy. Since asthma is an inflammatory disorder of the airways (predominately large airways), the diffusing capacity of carbon monoxide (D_{LCO}) is normal. Most patients with acute asthma have a bronchodilator response of over 15–20%; however, this response is also seen in 20% of patients with COPD. These patients are said to have asthmatic bronchitis. Chronic bronchitis may be limited to

TABLE 25–1. Specific Patterns of Pulmonary Function in Patients with Chronic Obstructive Pulmonary Disease (COPD)

		COPD	
	Asthma	*Chronic Bronchitis*	*Emphysema*
Decreased FEV_1	++++	++++	++++
Decreased FEV_1/FVC	++++	++++	++++
Increased airway resistance	++++	++++	+
Decreased D_{LCO}	—	—/++[a]	++++
Response to bronchodilators	++++	+[b]	—[b]

D_{LCO} = diffusing capacity of carbon monoxide; FEV_1 = forced expiratory volume after 1 second; FVC = forced vital capacity.
[a]Most smokers with chronic bronchitis have reduced D_{LCO}.
[b]Twenty percent of patients with COPD have large (++++) bronchodilator response.

the airways but the vast majority of patients with chronic bronchitis and airway obstruction have a mixture of bronchitis and emphysema and have a reduction in D_{LCO}. Therefore, D_{LCO} is the best pulmonary function test in separating asthma from COPD.

After the diagnosis of obstructive airways disease is established, the course and response to therapy is best followed by serial spirometry. The multicenter Lung Health Study demonstrated an abnormally rapid decline (90–150 mL/y) in patients with COPD who continue to smoke.[5]

Smoking cessation often resulted in an increase in FEV_1 during the first year and a near normal rate of decline (30–50 mL/y) in subsequent years.

AIRWAY HYPERREACTIVITY

Airway hyperreactivity or hyperresponsiveness is defined as an exaggerated bronchoconstrictor response to physical, chemical, or pharmacologic stimuli. Individuals with asthma by definition have hyperresponsive airways. Recently, the Lung Health Study Group[6] observed nonspecific hyperresponsiveness in a significant number of patients with COPD. This group of patients with airway hyperreactivity appears to have a worse prognosis and an accelerated rate of decline in FEV_1.

Some patients with asthma (especially cough-variant asthma) present with no history of wheezing and normal pulmonary function tests. The diagnosis of asthma can still be established by demonstrating hyperresponsiveness to provocative agents. The two agents most widely used in clinical practice are methacholine and histamine. Other agents used for bronchial provocation include distilled water, cold air, and exercise. During a typical bronchoprovocation test, a baseline FEV_1 is measured after the inhalation of isotonic saline, then increasing doses of methacholine are given at set intervals. Hyperresponsiveness is defined by a decline in FEV_1 of 20% or greater, and by reversibility of obstruction to bronchodilators. The result can best be expressed as the provocative concentration necessary to cause a fall in FEV_1 of 20% (PC_{20}). A test is considered positive if either methacholine or histamine demonstrate a PC_{20} for FEV_1 at 8 mg/mL or less, or fewer than 60 to 80 cumulative breath units.[7] This test is most frequently used to establish a diagnosis of asthma in patients with normal PFTs but may be useful in following patients with occupational asthma, establishing the severity of asthma and assessing the response to treatment.

UPPER AIRWAY OBSTRUCTION

Obstruction of airflow by abnormalities in the upper airway often go undiagnosed or misdiagnosed because of improper interpretation of the pulmonary function tests. The patients have obstructive physiology and often are misclassified as asthma or COPD. The shape of the flow-volume loop, which includes inspiratory and expiratory flow-volume curves, and ratio of the expiratory and inspiratory flow at 50% of vital capacity ($FEF_{50\%}/FIF_{50\%}$) may be useful in the diagnosis of upper airway obstruction.[8]

The shape of the flow-volume curve differs depending on whether the obstruction is fixed or variable (Fig. 25–5). Fixed lesions, as in strictures from previous intubation or tracheostomy, cause a uniform caliber of the airway during inspiration and expiration. With variable lesions, however, the airway caliber changes with changes in intrathoracic pressure. Variable lesions are subclassified into variable intrathoracic and variable extrathoracic. If the lesion is intrathoracic, as with tumors of the trachea, the negative pressure generated during inspiration opens the obstruction while the positive pressure during expiration worsens the obstruction. If there is variable extrathoracic obstruction, as with vocal cord dysfunction, the negative pressure within the airways will pull the vocal cord toward the midline and potentiate the obstruction. In this case, there will be a plateau on the inspiratory limb on the flow-volume loop and the $FEF_{50\%}/FIF_{50\%}$ will be greater than 1. Typical flow-volume curves from upper airway obstruction are shown in Fig. 25–4.

Another test used to distinguish upper airway obstruction from COPD and asthma is the $FEV_1/FEV_{0.5}$ (FEV at 1 second/FEV at 0.5 seconds). This ratio is usually greater than 1.5 in patients with upper airway obstruction.[9] This is because the $FEV_{0.5}$ is proportionately more reduced in upper airway obstruction because forced expiration measured at 0.5 seconds better reflects obstruction at high lung volumes. The abnormality seen on the flow-volume loop has been referred to as "straightening" of the curve during early expiration.

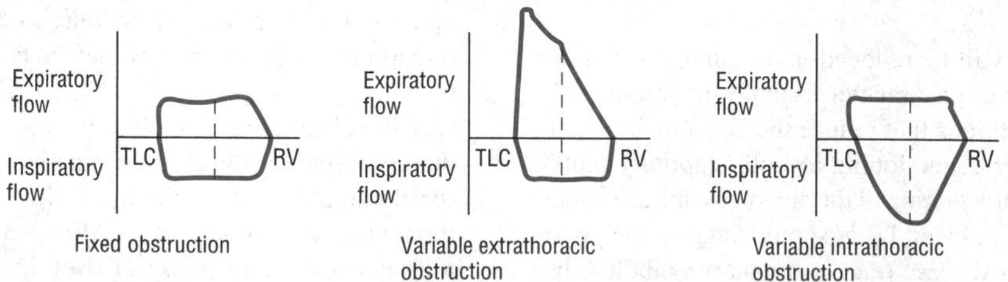

FIGURE 25–5. Maximum expiratory flow volume curves from patients with fixed obstruction, variable extrathoracic obstruction, and variable intrathoracic obstruction. RV, residual volume; TLC, total lung capacity.

RESTRICTIVE LUNG DISEASE

Restrictive lung disease is defined as an inability to get air into the lungs and to maintain normal lung volumes. Restrictive lung disease reduces all the subdivisions of lung volumes (IRV, VT, ERV, RV) without reduction in airflow. These patients have normal airway resistance and their FEV_1/FVC ratio is greater than 75%.

Although restriction could be defined as a reduction in vital capacity (VC or FVC) with a normal FEV_1/FVC ratio, poor effort will also reduce FVC with a normal FEV_1/FVC ratio. A reduction in the TLC is the most accurate measurement of restrictive lung function. As mentioned previously, TLC can be measured by various techniques. The gas dilution methods (helium dilution, nitrogen washout) are unable to measure gas trapped in cysts or bullae and may underestimate the true lung volume. Therefore, TLC is best measured by plethysmography. Most restrictive lung disease is associated with impairment or destruction of the alveolar capillary membrane and therefore, the D_{LCO} is reduced in most patients with restrictive lung disease. The reduction of D_{LCO} may occur prior to reduction in lung volumes and is used as a marker of early interstitial (restrictive) lung disease. The D_{LCO} may be abnormal even with a normal chest x-ray and thin-cut computed tomography (CT) scans of the chest may be required to diagnose early interstitial lung disease. Because peribronchiolar inflammation and fibrosis occurs in patients with restrictive parenchymal lung disease, the $FEF_{25\%-75\%}$ may be reduced and fail to respond to bronchodilators.

The severity of restrictive disease has not been standardized; however, many laboratories classify patients with a reduced TLC into mild (TLC $\leq$ 80%), moderate (TLC $\leq$ 65%), and severe (TLC $\leq$ 50%). These definitions are completely arbitrary because a patient with obstructive lung disease may start with a TLC of 120% and subsequently develop a moderately severe restrictive lung disease while maintaining a TLC within the normal range. On flow-volume loop, patients with restrictive disease have normal-shaped curves with a reduction in the height and width of the curve because the peak expiratory flow rate (PEFR) and VC are both dependent upon the amount of air within the lung prior to performing expiratory maneuvers (Fig. 25–3).

Restrictive lung function can be produced by increased elastic recoil of the lung parenchymal (interstitial lung disease), respiratory muscle weakness, mechanical restrictions (chest wall deformities) and/or poor effort. Table 25–2 lists common causes of restrictive lung disease.

Restrictive lung function from parenchymal lung disease can usually be differentiated from processes causing mechanical restriction as a result of chest bellows malfunction (Table 25–3). Restrictive parenchymal diseases are associated with a reduction in alveolar volume and an increase in lung elastic recoil. All lung volumes, as well as the D_{LCO}, are reduced. The RV/TLC ratio (normal $\leq$ 30%) and measurements of maximal inspiratory pressure (MIP; normal = negative 75 cm H_2O males, negative 50 cm H_2O females) remain normal. In addition, these patients exhibit mild resting hypoxemia that worsens with exercise. Monitoring gas exchange during exercise may be the most sensitive test for detecting progression of interstitial lung disease.[10]

Mechanical restriction caused by chest bellows malfunction may result from chest wall or skeletal deformity, loss of neuromuscular function, fibrosis of the pleural space, and abdominal overdistention causing upward displacement of the diaphragm, as well as decreased diaphragm movement. The most common pulmonary function pattern seen in these patients is a decrease in TLC and VC with only a slight decrease in RV. The RV is maintained in these diseases because lung compliance remains normal. The D_{LCO} is normal or only minimally reduced and the D_{LCO}/V_A (corrected for alveolar volume) is normal. The RV/TLC ratio is often increased in patients with restrictive chest bellows disease. Patients with neuromuscular disease also have reduced respiratory muscle function with a reduction in their MIP.

TABLE 25–2. Causes of Restrictive Lung Disease

Interstitial lung diseases
- Idiopathic pulmonary fibrosis
- Sarcoidosis
- Collagen vascular disease
- Pneumoconiosis
- Drug-induced lung disease
- Pulmonary edema

Infiltrative lung diseases
- Granulomatosis
- Tumor

Pleural diseases
- Pleural effusion
- Fibrothorax
- Pneumothorax

Chest wall diseases
- Kyphoscolioisis
- Ankylosing spondilitis
- Neuromuscular disease

Miscellaneous causes
- Obesity
- Pregnancy
- Ascites
- Paralyzed diaphragm

Lung resection

TABLE 25–3. Patterns of Pulmonary Function

	Obstructive Lung Disease		Restrictive Lung Disease	
	Asthma	*COPD*	*Parenchymal Disease*	*Chest Bellows Disease*
FVC	Nl or I	Nl or I	D	D
FEV_1	D	D	D	D
FEV_1/FVC	<75%	<75%	≥75%	≥75%
TLC	Nl or I	Nl or I	D	D
RV/TLC	Nl or I	Nl or I	Nl	I
Airway resistance	I	I	Nl	Nl
D_{LCO}	Nl	D	D	Nl

D = decreased; I = increased; Nl = normal.

PULMONARY GAS EXCHANGE

The essential function of the lungs is to maintain blood gas homeostasis. Arterial blood gas measurement plays an important role in the diagnosis and management of patients with pulmonary disease and should be ordered whenever hypoxemia, hypercapnia (CO_2 retention), and/or acid-base disorders are clinically suspected. Every time arterial blood gases are ordered, the A-a gradient (the difference between the partial pressure of oxygen in the alveolus minus the partial pressure of oxygen in arterial blood) should be calculated. This is done by computer on all automated blood gas machines and a normal $P(A\text{-}a)O_2$ can be approximated for sea level breathing room air by multiplying the age by 0.3. The presence of hypoxemia with a normal A-a gradient usually implies alveolar hypoventilation (e.g., sedative overdose). Most patients develop hypoxemia secondary to mismatching of ventilation and perfusion and the $P(A\text{-}a)O_2$ will be significantly elevated.

Pulse oximetry is widely used in clinical practice to monitor arterial saturation (SpO_2). A pulse oximeter is a small battery-operated device that is placed on the finger or the earlobe. This device emits and reads the reflected light from capillary blood, estimating the saturation. Although very useful clinically, SpO_2 is only an estimate of the arterial saturation and the actual arterial oxygen saturation (SaO_2) can be $\pm 4\%$ of the oximetry reading. The error may be even greater with a saturation of less than 88%. Pulse oximeters do not measure carboxyhemoglobin and the SpO_2 may be significantly overestimated in patients with smoke inhalation or recent smokers. An initial validation of pulse oximetry with direct measurement of SaO_2 is recommended in any critically ill patient.

EXERCISE TESTING

The major indications for exercise testing are dyspnea upon exertion, evaluation of exercise-induced bronchospasm, and suspected arterial desaturation during exercise.[11–12] Exercise testing can also be useful in the evaluation of ventilatory or cardiovascular limitations to work; assessment of general fitness or conditioning; evaluation of disability; establishment of safe levels for exercise; evaluation of drug therapy; determining the need and liter flow for supplemental oxygen therapy during exercise; assessment of the effects of a rehabilitation program; and as a preoperative assessment before lung resection.[11–13]

Tests for general fitness include the 6-minute walking distance and the Harvard step test.[11,13] For the 6-minute walking distance, the subject simply walks a predetermined route or circuit as fast as possible for 6 minutes. The greater the distance covered, the better the patient's general fitness and exercise tolerance. For the Harvard step test, the subject steps up and down on a 20-inch step at a set rate for 5 minutes. A 1-minute rest period is followed by measurement of the subject's recovery heart rate. The lower the recovery heart rate, the better the subject's general fitness.

Exercise testing is sometimes done to determine if exercise results in arterial oxygen desaturation ($SaO_2 < 90\%$).[12,13] This may be useful to quantify the level of exertion the patient can perform during the activities of daily living, as well as determining appropriate levels of supplemental oxygen therapy. Typically, this test is done using a treadmill or cycle ergometer. A baseline measurement of arterial blood gas values or pulse oximetry is followed by up to 6 minutes of exercise, during which time the patient is monitored for oxygen desaturation using pulse oximetry. If significant desaturation occurs (saturation $\leq$ 88–90%), the test is terminated. In the event of oxygen desaturation, the test may be repeated to determine the level of supplemental oxygen therapy needed to compensate for the desaturation that would otherwise occur.

Exercise tolerance tests or cardiopulmonary stress testing may include the measurement of oxygen consumption ($\dot{V}O_2$), carbon dioxide production ($\dot{V}CO_2$), minute volume ($\dot{V}E$), oxygen saturation via pulse oximeter (SpO_2), heart rate, blood pressure, and recording or monitoring the subject's electrocardiogram (ECG). During exercise, oxygen consumption ($\dot{V}O_2$) increases with work load in a linear fashion, until a maximum oxygen consumption level is reached ($\dot{V}O_{2max}$). Consequently, $\dot{V}O_{2max}$ is a measure of an individual's muscular work capacity.[11–13] Normal $\dot{V}O_{2max}$ is about 1,700 mL/min for a sedentary person and up to 5,800 mL/min in a trained athelete.[13] This compares to a resting $\dot{V}O_2$ of about 250 mL/min. Ventilatory equivalents for oxygen and carbon dioxide and O_2 pulse are often calculated. Ventilatory equivalent for oxygen is a measure of the efficiency of the ventilatory pump at various workloads[11,13] and is calculated as follows:

$$\text{Ventilatory equivalent for } O_2 = \dot{V}E/\dot{V}O_2$$

A normal ventilatory equivalent for oxygen is 20 to 30.[11,13]

O_2 pulse is an estimate of oxygen consumption per cardiac cycle and may be decreased with cardiac problems. O_2 pulse can be calculated as follows:

$$O_2 \text{ pulse} = (\dot{V}O_2 \times 1{,}000)/\text{heart rate}$$

TABLE 25–4. Indications and Contraindications for Exercise Testing

Indications
Dyspnea upon exertion
Exercise induced bronchospasm
Suspected arterial desaturation with exercise
Evaluation of ventilatory limitations to exercise
Evaluation of cardiac limitations to exercise
Assessment of general fitness or conditioning
Evaluation of cardiopulmonary disability
Establishment of safe levels for exercise
Evaluation of drug therapy
Determining appropriate use of supplemental oxygen therapy
Assessment of the effect of a rehabilitation program
Evaluation of specific disease states or conditions (e.g., asthma; COPD; interstitial lung disease; pulmonary vascular disorders; coronary artery disease; other vascular disorders; neuromuscular disorders; obesity; anxiety-induced hyperventilation)
Assessment before resection

Contraindications
PaO_2 less than 40 mm Hg on room air
$PaCO_2$ greater than 70 mm Hg
FEV_1 less than 30% of predicted
Recent (within 4 weeks) myocardial infarction
Unstable angina pectoris
Second- or third-degree heart block
Rapid ventricular/atrial arrhythmias
Orthopedic impairment
Severe aortic stenosis
Congestive heart failure
Uncontrolled hypertension
Limiting neurologic disorders
Dissecting/ventricular aneurysms
Severe pulmonary hypertension
Thrombophlebitis or intracardiac thrombi
Recent systemic or pulmonary embolus
Acute pericarditis

TABLE 25–5. Typical Findings During Maximum Exercise with Poor Conditioning, Pulmonary Limitations to Exercise, and Cardiac Limitations to Exercise

Test Parameter	Poor Conditioning	Pulmonary Limitation	Cardiac Limitation
$\dot{V}O_{2max}$	↓	↓	↓
SpO_2	N	↓	N
O_2 pulse	N	N or ↓	↓
Anaerobic threshold	↓ or N	↓ or N	↓
Ventilatory reserve* ($MVV-V_{Emax}$)	N	↓	N or ↑

*Ventilatory reserve = Maximum voluntary ventilation (MVV) – minute volume during maximum exercise (V_{Emax}).
N = normal.
(Adapted from Madama VE. Pulmonary function testing and cardiopulmonary stress testing. Albany, NY, Delmar, 1993.)

A normal O_2 pulse is 2.5–4.0 mL/beat at rest increasing to 10–15 mL/beat during strenuous exercise.[11,13]

The anaerobic threshold is the point during strenuous exercise at which anaerobic metabolism and lactic acid production begins.[11,13] Carbon dioxide production ($\dot{V}CO_2$) increases with exercise at about the same rate as $\dot{V}O_2$, until the subjects anaerobic threshold is reached. From that point on, $\dot{V}CO_2$ increases faster than $\dot{V}O_2$ and this change can be used to estimate the anaerobic threshold. A breath by breath plot of the ventilatory equivalents for O_2 and CO_2 can also be used to determine the anaerobic threshold. Anaerobic threshold is a measure of fitness in normal subjects and aerobic training can delay the anaerobic threshold.[11,13]

For exercise-tolerance testing, the subject is typically subjected to either a constant work load (steady-state tests) or to an increasing work load (progressive multistage tests) using a cycle ergometer or treadmill.[11,13] With the progressive multistage tests, the subject is exercised until exhaustion or the occurrence of an adverse reaction, at which point the test is stopped. Safety during exercise testing is of major importance and rigorous guidelines for the termination of the test should be followed. Both types of tests can be used to determine $\dot{V}O_{2max}$. A limit to exercise, as indicated by a decrease in $\dot{V}O_{2max}$, can be as a result of (a) poor conditioning, (b) a pulmonary limitation, (c) a cardiac limitation, or (d) poor effort. In the case of poor conditioning, SpO_2 and O_2 pulse will be normal. With a pulmonary limitation to exercise, SpO_2 will be reduced and O_2 pulse will be normal. With a cardiac limitation to exercise, SpO_2 will be normal and O_2 pulse reduced. Table 25–4 summarizes the indications and contraindications and indications for exercise testing. Table 25–5 summarizes the findings during maximum exercise associated with poor conditioning, pulmonary limitations to exercise, and cardiac limitations to exercise.

REFERENCES

1. American College of Physicians Consensus Statement. Preoperative pulmonary function testing. Ann Intern Med 1990;112:793–794.
2. Crapo RO. Pulmonary function testing. N Engl J Med 1994;331:25–30.
3. Crapo RO, Hankinson JL, Irvin C, et al. American Thoracic Society statement: Standardization of spirometry. 1994 update. Am J Respir Crit Care Med 1995;152:1107–1136.
4. Peters JI, Levine SM. Lung transplantation. In: George RB, Light RW, Matthaw MA, eds. Chest Medicine: Essentials of Pulmonary and Critical Care Medicine, 3rd ed. Baltimore, MD, Williams & Wilkins, 1995: 540–563.
5. Anthonisen NR, Connett JE, Kiley JP, et al. Effects of smoking intervention and the use of an inhaled anticholinergic bronchodilator on the rate of decline of FEV_1: The Lung Health Study. JAMA 1994;272:1497–1505.
6. Tashkin DP, Altose MD, Bleeker ER, et al. The Lung Health Study: Airway responsiveness to inhaled methacholine in smokers with mild to moderate airflow limitation. Am Rev Respir Dis 1992;145:301–310.
7. Crapo RO, Casaburi R, coates AL, et al. American Thoracic Society statement: Guidelines for methacholine and exercise challenge testing—1999. Am J Respir Crit Care Med 2000;161:309–329.
8. Acres JC, Kryger MH. Upper airway obstruction. Chest 1981;80:207–211.
9. Bright P, Miller MR, Franklyn JA, et al. The use of a neural network to detect upper airway obstruction caused by goiter. Am J Respir Crit Care Med 1998;157:1885–1891.
10. Leith DE, Brown R. ERS/ATS Workshop Series: Human lung volumes and the mechanisms that set them. Eur Respir J 1999;13:468–472.
11. Wasserman K, Hansen JE, Sue DY, Whipp BJ. Principles of Exercise Testing and Interpretation: Including Pathophysiology and Clinical Applications, 3rd ed. Philadelphia, Lippincott Williams & Wilkins, 1999.
12. Ruppel GE. Manual of Pulmonary Function Testing. St. Louis, Mosby, 1994.
13. Madama VC. Pulmonary Function Testing and Cardiopulmonary Stress Testing. Albany, NY, Delmar, 1993.

26

ASTHMA

H. William Kelly and Christine A. Sorkness

Asthma has been known since antiquity, yet it is a disease that still defies precise definition. The word *asthma* is of Greek origin and means "panting." More than 2000 years ago, Hippocrates used the word *asthma* to describe episodic shortness of breath; however, the first detailed clinical description of the asthmatic patient was made by Aretaeus in the second century.[1] Since that time, asthma has been used to describe any disorder with episodic shortness of breath or dyspnea. However, asthma now refers to a disorder of the respiratory system characterized by episodes of difficulty in breathing. An expert panel of the National Institutes of Health, the National Asthma Education and Prevention Program (NAEPP), has provided the following working definition of asthma[2]:

> Asthma is a chronic inflammatory disorder of the airways in which many cells and cellular elements play a role, in particular, mast cells, eosinophils, T-lymphocytes, macrophages, neutrophils, and epithelial cells. In susceptible individuals, this inflammation causes recurrent episodes of wheezing, breathlessness, chest tightness, and coughing, particularly at night or in the early morning. These episodes are usually associated with widespread but variable airflow obstruction that is often reversible either spontaneously or with treatment. The inflammation also causes an associated increase in the existing bronchial hyperresponsiveness to a variety of stimuli.

Although the precise pathogenic defect of asthma remains elusive, the current descriptive definition does allow for the important heterogeneity of the clinical presentation of asthma. Molecular and genetic technologies have added substantially to our understanding of the pathogenesis of asthma, and ongoing research continues to define genetic influences. However, the preceding definition adequately describes the scientific and clinically accepted characteristics of asthma.

EPIDEMIOLOGY

An estimated 14 to 15 million persons in the United States have asthma (about 5% of the population). The reported prevalence has increased 75% from 1980 to 1994 to 54 per 1000 population.[2] The prevalence of asthma has been increasing worldwide primarily in Westernized urban populations. Asthma accounts for 1.6% of all ambulatory care visits (13.7 million) according to the National Ambulatory Medical Care Survey and results in more than 470,000 hospitalizations per year.[3] It is the third leading cause of preventable hospitalization in the United States. Children have the highest prevalence of asthma, with the 1996 estimate at 68.6 per 1000 population less than 18 years old.[4] Asthma is the most common chronic disease in children, affecting 4.8 million and accounting for more than 10 million missed school days per year. Although recent estimates have suggested a possible decreasing prevalence in children for the years 1997 and 1998, this is most likely a result of a change in the National Health Interview Survey question that asked whether or not the child had physician-diagnosed asthma.[4] In young children (0–10 years of age), the risk of asthma is greater in boys than in girls, becomes about equal during puberty, and then is significantly greater in women than in men [relative risk (RR) = 1.38–5.91).[5] This gender reversal of the cumulative incidence of asthma with age suggests that airway caliber and/or hormonal factors influence the development of asthma.

Ethnic minorities continue to share the burden of asthma disproportionately. African-Americans and Hispanics have higher prevalences than whites, and African-Americans are twice as likely to be hospitalized.[2] In middle-class populations, African-American children have twice the lifetime prevalence of asthma (12% versus 6%) than white children.[4] The lifetime prevalence of probable undiagnosed asthma is also higher in African-American children (16.6% versus 10.8%). While this indicates a true prevalence difference in asthma between African-American and white children, recent analyses suggest that this difference is attributable primarily to urban living and not a result of race or socioeconomic differences.[6] This is consistent with previous findings of a similar prevalence of asthma in whites and Hispanics in rural communities.[7]

The estimated cost of asthma in the United States in 1998 was \$12.6 billion, and this is expected to be \$14.5 billion in 2000.[8] The average societal burden of asthma (including both direct and indirect medical expenditures) in the United States averages \$640 per patient per year, with direct medical expenditures accounting for 40% to 50% of total costs.[8] In 1997 an estimated cost of \$1 billion dollars per year in lost productivity accrued from parents staying home to care for their children.[8]

NATURAL HISTORY

The natural history of asthma is still not well defined. Between 30% and 70% of children with asthma will improve markedly or become symptom-free by early adulthood; chronic disease persists in about 30% to 40% of patients, and generally 20% or less develop severe chronic disease.[9] Risk factors for early (less than 3 years of age) recurring wheezing include low birth weight, male gender, and parental smoking, all of which is due to small airways, but children who continue to wheeze up to age 6 years are more likely to have a family history of asthma and an elevated immunoglobulin E (IgE) level.[9] Data from the large longitudinal Tucson Children's Respiratory Study have been used to develop two indices for the prediction of asthma.[10] A *stringent* index includes frequent wheezing during the first 3 years of life and either one major risk factor (e.g., parental history of asthma or eczema) or two of three minor risk factors (e.g., eosinophilia, wheezing without colds, and allergic rhinitis). A *loose* index requires any wheezing during the first 3 years of life plus the same combination of risk factors just described. Children with a positive loose index were 2.6 to 5.5 times more likely to have active asthma between the ages of 6 and 13 than children with a negative loose index. When a stringent index was used, the risk of having subsequent asthma increased to

4.3 to 9.8 times. Over 95% of children with a negative stringent index never had active asthma between the ages of 6 and 13.

Atopic status is the strongest indicator of a poor prognosis, although initial severity also markedly predicts severity as an adult. Some early epidemiologic studies have suggested that children with persistent asthma may not attain normal lung growth; however, a recent 4- to 6-year longitudinal clinical trial failed to detect diminished lung growth in children with mild to moderate persistent asthma.[11] Diminished lung growth may occur only in children with uncontrolled severe asthma. Low lung function and increased bronchial hyperresponsiveness (BHR) are independent risk factors for low lung function in early adulthood.[12]

In adults, the majority of longitudinal studies have suggested a more rapid rate of decline in lung function, primarily forced expiratory volume in 1 second (FEV_1), in asthmatics than in normal volunteers.[9] However, the annual decline is less than in smokers or those patients with a diagnosis of emphysema. In general, subjects with less frequent attacks and normal pulmonary function on initial assessment have higher remission rates, whereas smokers have the lowest remission and highest relapse rates. The level of BHR tends to predict rate of decline in FEV_1, with a greater decline with high levels of BHR.[9,12] These studies suggest that airways obstruction in asthma not only may become irreversible but also may worsen over time due to airway remodeling. To what degree airway remodeling occurs and whether or not therapy can alter the course of this chronic deterioration are the subject of intensive ongoing research and debate.

Evidence exists that both the morbidity and mortality from asthma are increasing. Although death from asthma is still relatively uncommon, only 5000 deaths per year, the annual death rate rose 118% from 1980 to 1993; however, from 1994 to 1997 the death rates stabilized.[13] African-Americans have two to three times the death rate from asthma as whites. This discrepancy is even more evident in children, where the death rate for African-Americans was six times higher than for whites in children 0 to 4 years old.[2] Hospitalization rates from the National Hospital Discharge Survey also vindicate that asthma morbidity is increasing.[3] Hospitalizations for asthma among children 0 to 17 years of age increased 4.5% per annum, whereas total hospitalizations for all causes actually decreased.

Despite the relatively low number of asthma deaths, 80% to 90% are preventable.[2] Most deaths from asthma occur outside the hospital, and death is rare after hospitalization. The most common cause of death from asthma is inadequate assessment of the severity of airways obstruction by the patient or physician and inadequate therapy. Studies of the cause and prevention of death from asthma are disturbing in that they indicate that 80% to 90% of the deaths are preventable.[2] Since inner-city populations have a disproportionate share of deaths from asthma, inadequate access to the health care system may play a significant role.[3,7] The most common cause of death in the hospitalized patient is also inadequate or inappropriate therapy. Thus the key to prevention of death from asthma, as advocated by the NAEPP, is education.[2] This includes education of the patients as well as the clinicians caring for them. Recently, the use of inhaled corticosteroids (ICSs) has been associated with a significant reduction in the risk of death from asthma.[14]

ETIOLOGY

The heterogeneity of asthma appears most obvious when listing the diverse triggers of bronchospasm in asthmatic subjects (Table 26–1). In the past, a good deal of the confusion concerning the definition and etiology of asthma centered on the inclusion of the various triggering

TABLE 26–1. List of Agents and Events Triggering Asthma

Respiratory infection
- Respiratory syncytial virus (RSV), rhinovirus, influenza, parainfluenza, *Mycoplasma pneumonia*

Allergens
- Airborne pollens (grass, trees, weeds), house-dust mites, animal danders, cockroaches, fungal spores

Environment
- Cold air, fog, ozone, sulfur dioxide, nitrogen dioxide, tobacco smoke, wood smoke

Emotions
- Anxiety, stress, laughter

Exercise
- Particularly in cold, dry climate

Drugs/preservatives
- Aspirin, NSAIDs (cyclooxygenase inhibitors), sulfites, benzalkonium chloride, β-blockers

Occupational stimuli
- Bakers (flour dust); farmers (hay mold); spice and enzyme workers; printers (arabic gum); chemical workers (azo dyes, anthraqui none, ethylenediamine, toluene diisocyanates, polyvinyl chloride); plastics, rubber, and wood workers (formaldehyde, western cedar, dimethylethanolamine, anhydrides)

events as the etiology. Thus asthma has been variously defined as an allergic or atopic, emotional, and infectious disease. However, it has become clear that asthma is first a lung disease and that specific triggering events have relative degrees of importance from patient to patient. Asthma is a complex syndrome with many clinical phenotypes in children and adults.

Epidemiologic studies strongly support the concept of a genetic predisposition to the development of asthma. Twin studies suggest that genetic factors account for 50% of the susceptibility.[15] Asthma represents a complex genetic disorder in that the asthma phenotype is likely a result of polygenic inheritance or different combinations of genes. Currently, genome-wide searches to establish links between atopy (genetically determined state of hypersensitivity to environmental allergens) or BHR[15] are being carried out. BHR is uniformly increased responsiveness to challenge with a variety of stimuli, including methacholine, histamine, and exercise, and often is used to define and diagnose asthma.

Studies of occupational asthma and the induction of BHR in healthy individuals emphasize the effect of environment on the development of asthma. Early exposure of infants to house dust mites and tobacco smoke is associated with increased incidence of asthma in children.[2] Atopy or a family history of atopy is strongly associated with continuing asthma in those infants who have wheezing with viral infections.[2] Thus genetic predisposition to atopy is a significant risk factor for developing asthma, although not all atopic individuals develop asthma, nor do all asthmatics exhibit atopy.

PATHOPHYSIOLOGY

The major characteristics of asthma include a variable degree of airflow obstruction (related to bronchospasm, edema, and hypersecretion), BHR, and airways inflammation (Fig. 26–1). Evidence of inflammation arose from the studies of nonspecific BHR, bronchoalveolar lavage (BAL), bronchial biopsies, and induced sputum, as well as from postmortem observations of patients with asthma who

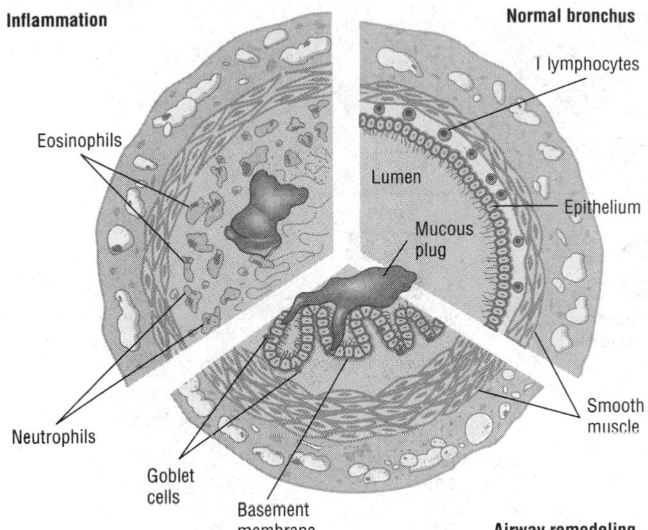

FIGURE 26–1. Representative illustration of the pathology found in the asthmatic bronchus compared with a normal bronchus (upper right). Each section demonstrates how the lumen is narrowed. Hypertrophy of the basement membrane, mucous plugging, smooth muscle hypertrophy, and constriction contribute (lower section). Inflammatory cells infiltrate, producing submucosal edema, and epithelial desquammation fills the airway lumen with cellular debris and exposes the airway smooth muscle to other mediators (upper left).

died from an attack of asthma or from other causes. To understand the pathogenetic mechanisms that underlie the many variants of asthma, it is critical to identify factors that initiate, intensify, and modulate the inflammatory response of the airways and to determine how these immunologic and biologic processes produce the characteristic airways abnormalities. Immune responses mediated by IgE antibodies are of foremost importance.

ACUTE INFLAMMATION AND ASSOCIATED SYMPTOMS

Sudden symptomatic attacks of asthma are caused by both unknown and known factors such as exposure to allergens, viruses, or indoor and outdoor pollutants, and each may induce an acute inflammatory response. Inhaled allergen challenge models contribute most to our understanding of acute inflammation in asthma.[16]

Inhaled allergen challenge in allergic patients leads to an early-phase allergic reaction that, in some cases, may be followed by a late-phase reaction. The activation of cells bearing allergen-specific IgE initiates the early-phase reaction. It is characterized primarily by the rapid activation of airway mast cells and macrophages. The activated cells rapidly release proinflammatory mediators such as histamine, eicosanoids, and reactive oxygen species that induce contraction of airway smooth muscle, mucus secretion, and vasodilatation.[17] The bronchial microcirculation has an essential role in this inflammatory process. Inflammatory mediators induce microvascular leakage with exudation of plasma in the airways.[16] Acute plasma protein leakage induces a thickened, engorged, and edematous airway wall and a consequent narrowing of the airway lumen. Plasma exudation may compromise epithelial integrity, and its presence in the lumen may reduce mucus clearance.[18] Plasma proteins also may promote the formation of exudative plugs mixed with mucus and inflammatory and epithelial cells. Together these effects contribute to airflow obstruction (Fig. 26–1).

The late-phase inflammatory reaction occurs 6 to 9 hours after allergen provocation and involves the recruitment and activation of eosinophils, $CD4^+$ T cells, basophils, neutrophils, and macrophages.[16] There is selective retention of airway T cells, the expression of adhesion molecules, and the release of selected proinflammatory mediators and cytokines involved in the recruitment and activation of inflammatory cells.[19,20] The activation of T cells after allergen challenge leads to the release of T-helper cell type 2 (Th2)–like cytokines that may be a key mechanism of the late-phase response.[21] The release of preformed cytokines by mast cells is the likely initial trigger for the early recruitment of cells. This cell type may recruit and induce the more persistent involvement by T cells.[16] The enhancement of nonspecific BHR usually can be demonstrated after the late-phase reaction but not after the early-phase reaction following allergen or occupational challenge.

This bronchoconstrictive response associated with acute inflammation results in brief symptoms that include wheezing, dyspnea, and shortness of breath that last for a day or so. Treatment and/or prevention of these brief symptoms is best achieved by short- or long-acting β_2-agonists.

CHRONIC INFLAMMATION SITE AND CELL SURVIVAL

Airways inflammation has been demonstrated in all forms of asthma, and an association between the extent of inflammation and the clinical severity of asthma has been demonstrated in selected studies.[16] It is accepted that both central and peripheral airways are inflamed. Eosinophilic apoptosis limits inflammatory tissue injury and promotes resolution rather than progression of inflammation.[22] The persistence of inflammation may be due to changes in the regulation of cell apoptosis leading to a chronic and self-perpetuating inflammatory cell survival and accumulation. Once at the site of airways inflammation, the survival of eosinophils as activated cells is increased as a consequence of reduced apoptosis and increased expression of adhesion molecules on epithelial cells.[16] Increased eosinophil survival in asthma is associated with reduced apoptosis.[22] Several cytokines and chemokines that are overexpressed in asthmatic airways may promote cell survival; these include granulocycte–macrophage–colony–stimulating factor (GM-CSF), interleukin (IL) 3 (IL-3), IL-5, and RANTES (a member of the interleukin 8 superfamily).[23] Antiasthmatic treatments may resolve inflammation by causing apoptosis.

CHARACTERISTICS OF CHRONIC INFLAMMATION

In asthma, all cells of the airways are involved and become activated (Fig. 26–2). Included are eosinophils, T cells, mast cells, macrophages, epithelial cells, fibroblasts, and bronchial smooth muscle cells. These cells also regulate airway inflammation and initiate the process of remodeling by the release of cytokines and growth factors.[23]

EPITHELIAL CELLS

Bronchial epithelial cells traditionally have been considered as a barrier, participating in mucociliary clearance and removal of noxious agents. However, epithelial cells also participate in inflammation by the release of eicosanoids, peptidases, matrix proteins, cytokines, and nitric oxide (NO). Epithelial cells can be activated by IgE-dependent mechanisms, viruses, pollutants, or histamines. Further, epithelial cells perform an immune function by their capacity to express human leukocyte–associated antigen DR (HLA-DR) and present antigen.[16]

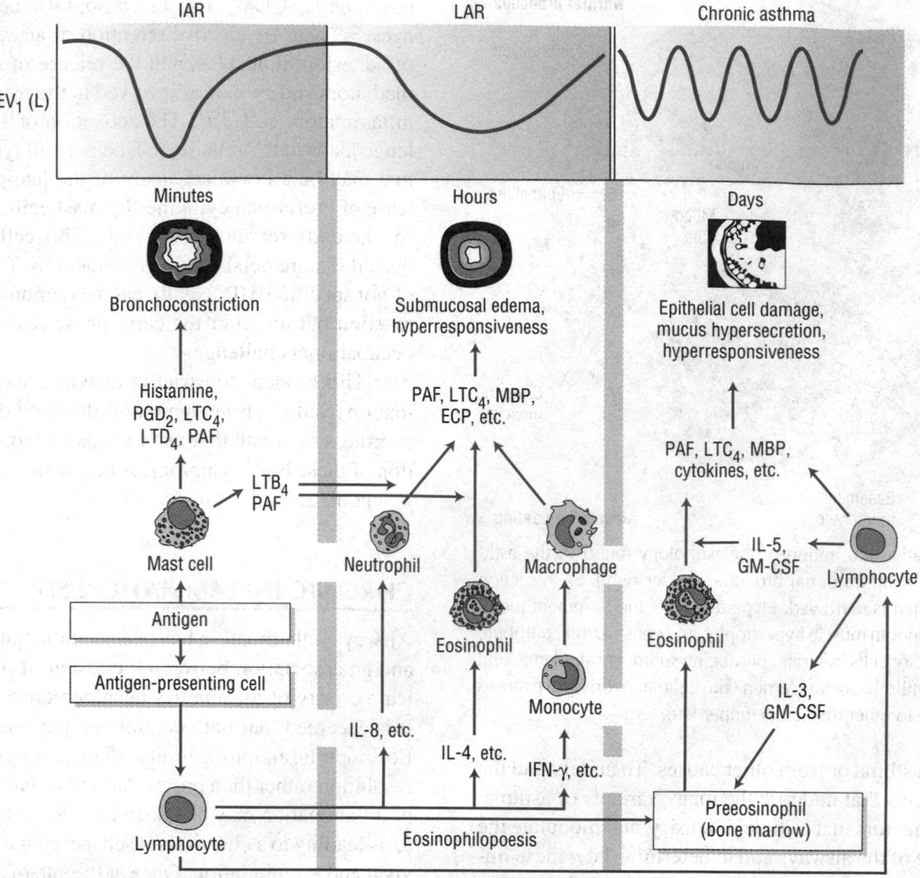

FIGURE 26–2. Diagrammatic presentation of the relationship between inflammatory cells, lipid and preformed mediators, inflammatory cytokines, and proposed pathogenesis and clinical presentation in asthma. See text for details. PG = prostaglandin; LT = leukotriene; PAF = platelet-activating factor; IL = interleukin; MBP = major basis protein; GM-CSF = granulocyte-macrophage colony-stimulating factor.

In asthma, especially fatal asthma, extensive epithelial shedding occurs. Contributors to epithelial shedding include plasma exudation, toxic inflammatory mediators, oxygen free radicals, tumor necrosis factor alpha (TNF-α), mast cell proteolytic enzymes, and metalloproteases from epithelial cells or macrophages.[16] The functional consequences of epithelial shedding may include heightened airways responsiveness, altered permeability of the airway mucosa, depletion of epithelial-derived relaxant factors, and loss of enzymes responsible for degrading proinflammatory neuropeptides. The integrity of airway epithelium may influence the sensitivity of the airways to various provocative stimuli. Epithelial cells also may be important in the regulation of airway remodeling and fibrosis.

EOSINOPHILS

Eosinophils play an effector role in asthma by release of proinflammatory mediators, cytotoxic mediators, and cytokines.[16,23] Circulating eosinophils migrate to the airways by cell rolling, through interactions with selectins, and eventually adhere to the endothelium through the binding of integrins to adhesion proteins [vascular cell adhesion molecule 1 (VCAM–1) and intercellular adhesion molecule 1 (ICAM–1)]. As eosinophils enter the matrix of the membrane, their survival is prolonged by interleukin 5 and GM-CSF. On activation, eosinophils release inflammatory mediators such as leukotrienes and granule proteins to injure airway tissue.[23]

LYMPHOCYTES

Mucosal biopsy specimens from patients with asthma contain lymphocytes, many of which express surface markers of inflammation. There are two types of T-helper CD4$^+$ cells. Type 1 T-helper (Th1) cells produce interleukin 2 and interferon γ, both essential for cellular defense mechanisms. Th2 cells produce cytokines (IL-4, -5, -6, -9, and -13) that mediate allergic inflammation. It is known that Th1 cytokines inhibit the production of Th2 cytokines, and vice versa. It is hypothesized that allergic asthmatic inflammation results from a Th2-mediated mechanism (an imbalance between Th1 and Th2 cells).[23]

TH1 AND TH2 CELL IMBALANCE

It has been postulated that the Th1/Th2 imbalance contributes to the cause and evolution of atopic diseases, including asthma. The T-cell population in the cord blood of newborn infants is skewed toward a Th2 phenotype.[24] The extent of the imbalance between Th1 and Th2 cells (as indicated by diminished interferon γ production) during the neonatal phase may predict the subsequent development of allergic disease, asthma, or both.[23] It has been suggested that infants at high risk of asthma and allergies should be exposed to stimuli that upregulate Th1-mediated responses in order to restore the balance during a critical time in the development of the immune system and the lung.

The *hygiene hypothesis* has been articulated as a means to explain the increasing prevalence of asthma in Western countries.[25,26]

The basic premise of this hypothesis is that the newborn's immune system is skewed toward Th2 cells and needs timely and appropriate environmental stimuli to create a balanced immune response. Factors have been identified that enhance Th1-mediated responses and that are associated with a reduced incidence of allergy, asthma, or both.[23] These factors include infection with *Mycobacterium tuberculosis,* measles virus, and hepatitis A virus; increased exposure to infections through contact with older siblings; attendance at day care during the first 6 months of life; and a reduction in the production of interferon γ. Restoration of the balance between Thl and Th2 cells may be impeded by frequent administration of oral antibiotics, with concomitant alterations in gastrointestinal flora.

Other factors favoring the Th2 phenotype include Western lifestyle, urban environment, diet, and sensitization to house dust mites and cockroaches. Immune "imprinting" may begin in utero by transplacental transfer of allergens and cytokines.[27] The validity of the hygiene hypothesis has been challenged and will continue to generate intense debate.[28]

MAST CELLS

Mast cell degranulation is important in the initiation of immediate responses following exposure to allergens.[2] Mast cells are found throughout the walls of the respiratory tract, and increased numbers of these cells (three- to fivefold) have been described in the airways of asthmatics with an allergic component. Once binding of allergen to cell-bound IgE occurs, mediators such as histamine, eosinophil and neutrophil chemotactic factors, leukotrienes C_4, D_4, and E_4, prostaglandins, platelet-activating factor, and others are released from mast cells (see Fig. 26–2). Histologic examination has revealed decreased numbers of granulated mast cells in the airways of patients who have died from acute asthma attacks, suggesting that mast cell degranulation is a contributing factor in the progression of the disease. Mast cell degranulation is believed to be an integral cause of exercise-induced bronchospasm (EIB) following either drying or cooling of the airways.[29]

ALVEOLAR MACROPHAGES

The primary function of alveolar macrophages in the normal airway is to serve as "scavengers," engulfing and digesting bacteria and other foreign materials. They are found in large and small airways, ideally located for affecting the asthmatic response. A number of mediators produced and released by macrophages have been identified, and their roles in initiating and amplifying inflammation in allergic asthma have been determined. A partial list of mediators produced by these cells includes platelet-activating factor, leukotriene B_4, leukotriene C_4, and leukotriene D_4.[16] Additionally, alveolar macrophages are able to produce neutrophil chemotactic factor and eosinophil chemotactic factor, which in turn further the inflammatory process.

NEUTROPHILS

The role of neutrophils in the pathogenesis of asthma remains somewhat unclear because they normally may be present in the airways and usually do not infiltrate tissues showing chronic allergic inflammation despite the potential to participate in late-phase inflammatory reactions. However, high numbers of neutrophils have been reported to be present in the airways of patients who died from sudden-onset fatal asthma.[30] This suggests that neutrophils may play a pivotal role in the disease process, at least in the sudden onset fatal cases and in some patients with long-standing or corticosteroid dependent asthma. The neutrophil also can be a source for a variety of mediators, including platelet-activating factor, prostaglandins, thromboxanes, and leukotrienes, that contribute to BHR and airway inflammation.

FIBROBLASTS AND MYOFIBROBLASTS

Fibroblasts are found frequently in connective tissue. Human lung fibroblasts may behave as inflammatory cells on activation by IL-4 and IL-13. The myofibroblast may contribute to the regulation of inflammation via the release of cytokines and to tissue remodeling. In asthma, myofibroblasts are increased in numbers beneath the reticular basement membrane, and there is an association between their numbers and the thickness of reticular basement membrane.[16]

INFLAMMATORY MEDIATORS

Associated with asthma for many years, histamine is capable of inducing smooth muscle constriction and bronchospasm and is thought to play a role in mucosal edema and mucus secretion.[2] Lung mast cells are an important source of histamine. The release of histamine can be stimulated by exposure of the airways to a variety of factors, including physical stimuli (such as exercise) and relevant allergens.[2,29] Histamine is involved in acute bronchospasm following allergen exposure; however, other mediators such as leukotrienes are also involved. Antihistamines have only a small benefit in asthma.

Besides histamine release, mast cell degranulation releases interleukins, proteases, and other enzymes that activate the production of other mediators of inflammation. Several classes of important mediators, including arachidonic acid and its metabolites (i.e., prostaglandins, leukotrienes, and platelet-activating factor), are derived from cell membrane phospholipids.

Once arachidonic acid is released, it can be broken down by the enzyme cyclooxygenase to form the prostaglandins. A further breakdown product, prostaglandin D_2, has been well characterized and is a potent bronchoconstricting agent. It is unlikely that prostaglandin D_2 can produce sustained effects on airway function or inflammation; however, its role in asthma remains to be determined. Similarly, prostaglandin $F_{2\alpha}$ is a potent bronchoconstrictor in patients with asthma and can enhance the effects of histamine.[2] However, its pathophysiologic role in asthma is unclear. Another cyclooxygenase product, prostacyclin (prostaglandin I_2), is known to be produced in the lung. It is unclear whether prostaglandin I_2 is important as a bronchoconstricting agent in humans; however, it may contribute to inflammation and edema owing to its effects as a vasodilator.

Thromboxane A_2 is produced by alveolar macrophages, fibroblasts, epithelial cells, neutrophils, and platelets within the lung.[31] Indirect evidence from animal models suggests that thromboxane A_2 may have several effects, including bronchoconstriction, involvement in the late asthmatic response, and involvement in the development of airway inflammation and BHR. Potent and specific thromboxane synthetase inhibitors will be crucial tools for understanding the role of thromboxanes in asthma.

The 5-lipoxygenase pathway of arachidonic acid breakdown is responsible for production of the class of compounds called *cysteinyl leukotrienes* (LTs).[16] Leukotrienes C_4, D_4, and E_4 (cysteinyl LTs) constitute the slow-reacting substance of anaphylaxis (SRS-A). These leukotrienes are liberated during inflammatory processes in the lung. LTs D_4 and E_4 share a common receptor (LTD_4 receptor) that, when stimulated, produces bronchospasm, mucus secretion, microvascular permeability, and airway edema. Potent LTD_4 receptor antagonists can produce improvement in symptoms and lung function in patients with chronic asthma. Specific LTD_4 receptor antagonists and

5-lipoxygenase inhibitors have Food and Drug Administration (FDA) approval for the treatment of asthma.[32]

Thought to be produced by macrophages, eosinophils, and neutrophils within the lung, platelet-activating factor (PAF) is involved in the mediation of bronchospasm, sustained induction of BHR, edema formation, and chemotaxis of eosinophils.[16] Selective and potent PAF receptor antagonists have been developed but have so far been disappointing in clinical trials of asthma.

ADHESION MOLECULES

An important step in the inflammatory process is the adhesion of the various cells to each other and the tissue matrix to facilitate infiltration and migration of these cells to the site of inflammation. To promote this, cell membranes express a number of glycoproteins, or adhesion molecules. Adhesion molecules have additional functions involved in the inflammatory process aside from promoting cell adhesion, including activation of cells and cell-cell communication, and promoting cellular migration and infiltration.[2] The many adhesion molecules are divided into families on the basis of their chemical structure. These families are the integrins, cadherins, immunoglobulin supergene family, selectins, vascular adressins, and carbohydrate ligands.[33] Those thought to be important in inflammation include the integrins, immunoglobulin supergene family, selectins, and carbohydrate ligands including ICAM-1 and VCAM-1.[23]

Adhesion molecules are found on a variety of cells, such as neutrophils, monocytes, lymphocytes, basophils, eosinophils, granulocytes, platelets, endothelial cells, and epithelial cells, and can be expressed or activated by the many inflammatory mediators present in asthma.[23] Thus complex interactions occur whereby mediators affect expression of adhesion molecules and adhesion molecules can produce mediators. In addition to these interactions, a major role of adhesion molecules is in the recruitment of leukocytes from the vascular lumen to tissues. The initial step involved in this leukocyte–endothelial cell adhesion cascade is transient and reversible binding of the adhesion molecule to specific ligands on endothelial cells, which results in slowing or rolling of the circulating leukocyte along the surface of the vasculature. Activation of the leukocytes or endothelial cells follows in response to a mediator or the initial adhesion event. Finally, firm adhesion (anchoring) of the leukocytes to endothelial cell surfaces allows for diapedesis between endothelial cells and migration of leukocytes into the extracellular matrix. For instance, ICAM-1 and VCAM-1 are involved in the migration of lymphocytes and eosinophils.[23]

Although the role of adhesion molecules in the pathogenesis of asthma remains undefined, studies have begun to address the mechanisms of leukocyte infiltration into the airways. The availability of monoclonal antibodies to the functional epitopes of adhesion molecules will facilitate our understanding of their role in inflammation. In addition, specific blocking of adhesion molecules by monoclonal antibodies appears promising as a novel therapeutic approach or complement to existing anti-inflammatory therapy.

CLINICAL CONSEQUENCES OF CHRONIC INFLAMMATION

Chronic inflammation is associated with nonspecific BHR and induces asthma exacerbations. Exacerbations are characterized by symptoms or worsening of asthma over a period of days or even weeks. Although the inflammatory nature of chronic asthma is not completely understood, corticosteroids remain the most potent anti-inflammatory drugs for use in the treatment of asthma. The treatment of exacerbations is based on the use of long-term control medications.

Hyperresponsiveness of the airways to physical, chemical, and pharmacologic stimuli is a hallmark of asthma.[2] BHR also occurs in some patients with chronic bronchitis and allergic rhinitis.[2] Normal healthy subjects also may develop a transient BHR after viral respiratory infections or exposure to ozone. However, the degree of BHR is quantitatively greater in asthmatic patients than in other groups. Bronchial responsiveness of the general population fits a unimodal distribution that is skewed toward increased reactivity. Patients with clinical asthma represent the extreme end of the distribution. The degree of BHR within asthmatics correlates with the clinical course of their disease and medication requirement necessary to control symptoms.[2] Patients with mild symptoms or in remission demonstrate lower levels of responsiveness, although still greater than the normal population.

Our current understanding recognizes that the increased BHR seen in asthma is at least in part owing to an inflammatory response within the airways.[16] Early investigations found correlations with inflammatory cells in BAL fluids and degree of BHR.[2] Newer evidence suggests that airways remodeling, subepithelial fibrosis, or collagen deposition correlates with BHR.[34] Although the precise link is not known, BHR is in part related to the extent of inflammation in the airways.

REMODELING OF THE AIRWAYS

Acute inflammation is a beneficial, nonspecific response of tissues to injury and generally leads to repair and restoration of the normal structure and function. In contrast, asthma represents a chronic inflammatory process of the airways followed by healing. The end result may be an altered structure referred to as a *remodeling of the airways*.[35] Repair involves replacement of injured tissue by parenchymal cells of the same type and replacement by connective tissue and its maturation into scar tissue. In asthma, the repair process can be followed by complete or altered restitution of airways structure and function, presenting as fibrosis and an increase in smooth muscle and mucus gland mass.[16]

The precise mechanisms of remodeling of the airways are under intense study. Airway remodeling is of concern because it may represent an irreversible process that can have more serious sequelae such as the development of chronic obstructive pulmonary disease.[2] Recent observations in children with asthma (ages 5–12 years) suggest that prevention of the progressive loss of lung function in childhood may require recognition and treatment of the disease during the first 5 years of life.[36] Whether there is a mechanistic link between this loss of airway function and structural remodeling of the airway in early life is unknown.[23]

MUCUS PRODUCTION

The mucociliary system is the lung's primary defense mechanism against irritants and infectious agents. Mucus, composed of 95% water and 5% glycoproteins, is produced by bronchial epithelial glands and goblet cells.[37] The lining of the airway consists of a continuous aqueous layer controlled by active ion transport across the epithelium where water moves toward the lumen along the concentration gradient. Catecholamines and vagal stimulation enhance the ion transport and fluid movement.[22] Mucus transport depends on the viscoelastic properties of the mucus. Mucus that is either too watery or too viscous will not be transported optimally. The exudative inflammatory process and sloughing of epithelial cells into the airway lumen impair mucociliary transport. The bronchial glands are increased in size and the goblet cells are increased in size and number in asthma. Expectorated mucus from patients with asthma tends to have a high viscosity. The mucus plugs in the airways of patients who died in status asthmaticus are tenacious and tend to be connected by mucous strands to the goblet cells.[37] Asthmatic airways also may become plugged with casts consisting of epithelial and inflammatory cells. Although it is tempting to speculate that death from asthma attacks is a result of the mucus plugging resulting in irreversible obstruction, there is no direct evidence for this. Autopsies of asthmatics who died from other causes have shown similar pathology. In addition, some subjects who have died of sudden severe asthma did not show the characteristic mucus plugging on necropsy.[37]

AIRWAY SMOOTH MUSCLE

The smooth muscle of the airways does not form a uniform coat around the airways but is wrapped around in a connecting network best described as a spiral arrangement.[37] The muscle contraction displays a sphincteric action that is capable of completely occluding the airway lumen. The airway smooth muscle extends from the trachea through the respiratory bronchioles. When expressed as percentage of wall thickness, the smooth muscle represents 5% of the large central airways and up to 20% of the wall thickness in the bronchioles.[37] Total smooth muscle mass decreases rapidly past the terminal bronchioles to the alveoli, so the contribution of smooth muscle tone to airway diameter in this region is relatively small. In the large airways of asthmatics, smooth muscle may account for 11% of the wall thickness.[37] Airway smooth muscle contraction in vivo is measured indirectly by determining the flow of air into and out of the patient. The difficulties in using changes in airflow as a measurement of smooth muscle contraction have been delineated elsewhere.[37] The relationship between airway diameter and flow is dictated by Poiseuille's law:

$$P = 8nl/r^4$$

where n is the viscosity of the air, l is the length of the tube, r is the radius of the tube, and P is the drop in pressure. Because resistance is equal to P divided by airflow, a 2-fold change in airway diameter would produce a 16-fold change in airflow resistance. It is possible that the increased smooth muscle mass of the asthmatic airways is important in magnifying and maintaining BHR in chronic asthma.[37] However, it appears that the hypertrophy and hyperplasia are secondary processes caused by chronic inflammation and are not the primary cause of BHR.[37]

NEURAL CONTROL/NEUROGENIC INFLAMMATION

The airway is innervated by parasympathetic, sympathetic, and nonadrenergic inhibitory nerves.[2] Parasympathetic innervation of the smooth muscle consists of efferent motor fibers contained in the vagus nerves and sensory afferent fibers in the vagus and other nerves.[37] The normal resting tone of human airway smooth muscle is maintained by vagal efferent activity.[37] Maximum bronchoconstriction mediated by vagal stimulation occurs in the small bronchi and is absent in the small bronchioles. The nonmyelinated C fibers of the afferent system lie immediately beneath the tight junctions between epithelial cells lining the airway lumen.[37] These endings probably represent the irritant receptors of the airways. Stimulation of these irritant receptors by mechanical stimulation, chemical and particulate irritants, and pharmacologic agents such as histamine produces reflex bronchoconstriction.[37]

The sympathetic innervation of the airway smooth muscle is sparse and does not directly control airway smooth muscle tone.[37] All airway smooth muscle contains noninnervated β_2-adrenergic receptors that produce bronchodilation.[37] Circulating catecholamines play an important role in regulating bronchial tone. The major resistance airways contain α-adrenergic receptors whose stimulation produces bronchoconstriction that is enhanced by pretreatment with histamine.[37] The importance of these receptors in asthma is unknown; however, specific α-adrenergic blockers have minimal effect on asthma. One theory on the pathogenesis of BHR is that asthma represents a relative β-adrenergic blockade. The demonstration of a β-adrenergic defect in asthmatic patients has been inconsistent, and the production of β blockade in normal subjects is insufficient, by itself, to cause bronchial hyperreactivity.

The nonadrenergic, noncholinergic (NANC) nervous system has been described in the trachea and bronchi. Substance P, neurokinin A, neurokinin B, and vasoactive intestinal peptide (VIP) are the best characterized neurotransmitters in the NANC nervous system.[38] VIP is an inhibitory neurotransmitter in the system. Inflammatory cells in asthma can release peptidases that can degrade VIP, producing exaggerated reflex cholinergic bronchoconstriction.38 NANC excitatory neuropeptides such as substance P and neurokinin A are released by stimulation of C-fiber sensory nerve endings.[38] The NANC system may play an important role in amplifying inflammation in asthma by releasing NO.

NITRIC OXIDE

NO is produced by cells within the respiratory tract. It has been thought to be a neurotransmitter of the NANC nervous system.[38] Endogenous NO is generated from the amino acid L-arginine by the enzyme NO synthase.[39] There are three isoforms of NO synthase. One isoform is induced in response to proinflammatory cytokines, inducible NO synthase (iNOS), in airway epithelial cells and inflammatory cells of asthmatic airways.[39] NO produces smooth muscle relaxation in the vasculature and bronchials; however, it appears to amplify the inflammatory process and is unlikely to be of therapeutic benefit. Recent investigations measuring exhaled NO concentrations have suggested that it may be a useful measure of ongoing lower airways inflammation in patients with asthma and for measuring effectiveness of therapy.[40]

CLINICAL PRESENTATION

CHRONIC ASTHMA

Classic asthma is characterized by episodic dyspnea associated with wheezing; however, the clinical presentation of asthma is as diverse as the number of triggering events. Although wheezing is the characteristic symptom of asthma, the medical literature is replete with the warning that "not all that wheezes is asthma." A wheeze is a high-pitched, whistling sound created by turbulent airflow through an obstructed airway, so any condition that produces significant obstruction can result in wheezing as a symptom. In addition, "all of asthma does not wheeze" is an equally justifiable warning. Patients may present with a chronic persistent cough as their only symptom.[2]

The diagnosis of asthma is based primarily on a good history of recurrent episodes of dyspnea and/or wheezing[2] (Table 26–2). The patient may complain of a feeling of tightness in the chest or sometimes a burning sensation. The patient may have a family history of allergy or asthma or have symptoms of allergic rhinitis.[2] A history

TABLE 26–2. Sample Questions[a] for the Diagnosis and Initial Assessment of Asthma

A "yes" answer to any question suggests that asthma diagnosis is likely. In the past 12 months, . . .

- Have you had a sudden severe episode or recurrent episodes of coughing, wheezing (high-pitched whistling sounds when breathing out), or shortness of breath?
- Have you had colds that "go to the chest" or take more than 10 days to get over?
- Have you had coughing, wheezing, or shortness of breath during a particular season or time of the year?
- Have you had coughing, wheezing, or shortness of breath in certain places or when exposed to certain things (e.g., animals, tobacco smoke, perfumes)?
- Have you used any medications that help you breathe better? How often?
- Are the symptoms relieved when the medications are used?

In the past 4 weeks, have you had coughing, wheezing, or shortness of breath . . .

- At night that has awakened you?
- In the early morning?
- After running, moderate exercise, or other physical activity?

[a] *These questions are recommended by the NAEPP but have not been formally validated.*

of exercise or cold air precipitating the dyspnea or an association of increased symptoms during specific allergen seasons also would point to asthma.

Asthma has a widely variable presentation from chronic daily symptoms to only intermittent symptoms. The intervals between symptoms could be weeks, months, or years. It is a disease characterized by recurrent exacerbations and remissions. The next variable is severity. The NAEPP has provided a means of classifying asthma that is presented in Table 26–3.[2] The intermittent and/or chronic nature of symptoms does not necessarily determine the severity of symptoms during exacerbations. The severity is by lung function and symptoms prior to therapy, as well as by the amount of medication required to control the patient's symptoms adequately. Patients can present with a range from mild intermittent symptoms that require no medications or only occasional use of inhaled bronchodilators to severe chronic asthma symptoms despite receiving multiple medications.

ACUTE SEVERE ASTHMA

Uncontrolled asthma, with its inherent variability, can progress to an acute state where inflammation, airways edema, excessive accumulation of mucus, and severe bronchospasm result in a profound airways narrowing that is poorly responsive to usual bronchodilator therapy.[2,41] Although this progression is the most common scenario, some patients experience rapid onset or hyperacute attacks.[2,41] Hyperacute attacks are associated with neutrophilic as opposed to eosinophilic infiltration and resolve rapidly with bronchodilator therapy, suggesting that smooth muscle spasm is the major pathogenic mechanism.[30,42] In most cases, emergency department visits for acute severe asthma represent the failure of an adequate therapeutic regimen for chronic asthma. Underutilization of anti-inflammatory drugs and excessive reliance on short-acting inhaled β_2-agonists are the major risk factors for severe exacerbations.[2] A blunted perception of airway obstruction may predispose certain asthmatics to fatal attacks.[2] This may occur more commonly in patients who have labile asthma (fluctuation of daily peak flows of 50% or greater). Patients present with severe dyspnea, inspiratory as well as expiratory wheezing, anxiety, tachypnea, tachycardia, and in severe cases, cyanosis. They exhibit supraclavicular and intercostal retractions, a hyperinflated chest, and coughing. In severe obstruction, air movement in and out of the lungs is substantially decreased so that wheezing actually may decrease.[2]

ALLERGIC ASTHMA

An allergic component can be demonstrated in 35% to 55% of asthmatic patients, and this may be higher in childhood asthma.[2] The allergens (see Table 26–1) that provoke asthma are airborne and evoke an asthmatic response through the classic allergic pathway. Although the allergic reaction plays an important role in the atopic asthmatic patient, atopy is not necessary for the development of asthma, and not all atopic individuals develop asthma.[2] Many patients with hay fever

TABLE 26–3. Classification of Asthma Severity: Clinical Features Before Treatment

	Symptoms	Lung Function[a]
Step 1 Mild Intermittent	Daytime ≤ 2 times/wk Asymptomatic between exacerbations Exacerbations brief (from a few hours to a few days); intensity may vary Nocturnal ≤ 2 times/mo	FEV_1 or PEF ≥ 80% PEF variability < 20%
Step 2 Mild Persistent	Daytime > 2 times/wk but < 1 time/day Exacerbations may affect activity Nocturnal > 2 times/mo	FEV_1 or PEF ≥ 80% PEF variability 20% to 30%
Step 3 Moderate Persistent	Daily symptoms Daily use of inhaled, short-acting β_2-agonists Exacerbations affect activity Exacerbations ≥ 2 times/wk; may last days Nocturnal > 1 time/wk	FEV_1 or PEF > 60% to < 80% PEF variability > 30%
Step 4 Severe Persistent	Continual symptoms Limited physical activity Frequent exacerbations Nocturnal frequent	FEV_1 or PEF ≤ 60% PEF variability > 30%

[a] The presence of one of the features of severity is sufficient to place a patient in that category. An individual should be assigned to the most severe grade in which any feature occurs. The characteristics noted are general and may overlap because asthma is highly variable. Furthermore, an individual's classification may change overtime. Patients at any level of severity can have mild, moderate, or severe exacerbations. Some patients with intermittent asthma experience severe and life threatening exacerbations separated by long periods of normal lung function and no symptoms.

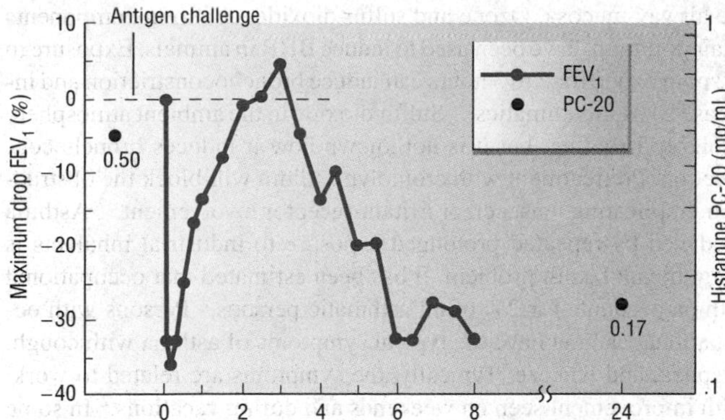

FIGURE 26–3. Biphasic response to allergen exposure in a sensitive patient with asthma. The immediate response occurs within 10 to 30 minutes following exposure and may revert to baseline without intervention. The late asthmatic response occurs within 2 to 8 hours following exposure. The provocative concentration of inhaled histamine, which produces a 20% decrease in forced expiratory volume in 1 second (FEV_1) (PC-20), an index of airways reactivity, also shows a marked decrease following development of a late asthmatic response. This is suggestive of an increase in the propensity of the airways to constrict to nonspecific stimuli.

will develop some BHR (although less than asthmatics) during their allergen season. However, the study of the response to allergens has improved our understanding of the role of inflammation in asthma.

When allergic asthmatics are given an inhalational challenge with an allergen to which they are sensitized, the patients demonstrate an early-phase asthmatic reaction (EAR) (Fig. 26–3). The reaction is characterized by a drop in pulmonary function that reaches maximum intensity in 10 to 20 minutes and reverses spontaneously by 60 to 120 minutes.[29] In addition, many subjects experience a late-phase asthmatic reaction that begins 4 hours after the challenge, reaches maximum intensity in 6 to 9 hours, is often more severe than the EAR, and may last as long as 24 hours. The late asthmatic reaction (LAR) may be the pathogenic mechanism for inducing and maintaining BHR in atopic asthmatics.[16] Patients who experience an LAR demonstrate increased BHR that may last up to 6 weeks, whereas subjects who experience only the EAR demonstrate no increased BHR. The degree of BHR and its duration correlate with the intensity of the LAR. The LAR is associated with greater degrees of obstruction in small airways and air trapping than occur with the EAR.

The measurement of BHR is made by having the patient breathe increasing log concentrations or doubling doses of histamine or methacholine. Following each increment, the patient performs spirometric measurement until the FEV_1 drops at least 20% from the baseline value. Then either a provocative dose (PD) or provocative concentration (PC) that produces the 20% drop is calculated (the PC20 in Fig. 26–3).[26] Most patients with asthma will have a PC20FEV_1 of $\leq$ 8 mg/L methacholine. The usual variation over time without change in therapy does not exceed one dose step or one doubling dose, so a clinically significant change is considered to be at least 1.5 to 2 doubling doses.[43] The NAEPP considers drugs to be anti-inflammatory if they reduce markers of airway inflammation and decrease BHR.[2]

The EAR is easily blocked or reversed with inhaled β_2-agonists.[2,44] Theophylline, anticholinergics, and oral β_2-agonists blunt the response but are inconsistently effective.[2] The LAR is not prevented by treatment with any of these bronchodilators, although the bronchospastic component may be attenuated if therapeutic doses are administered at the time of the LAR.[43] Glucocorticoid pretreatment does not alter the EAR but prevents the LAR, whereas pretreatment with cromolyn sodium or nedocromil blocks both responses.[2] Long-term treatment with glucocorticoids can attenuate the immediate response by decreasing overall BHR.[2]

Clinically, allergic asthmatics develop increased BHR with increased exposure to allergens during a pollen season.[45] Avoidance of the pollen or prophylaxis with cromolyn sodium prevents the increased bronchial hyperreactivity.[43,45] Studies have shown that long-term therapy with cromolyn, nedocromil, and glucocorticoids reduces BHR.[43,45] In contrast, long-term therapy with β_2-agonists and theophylline has not been associated with similar decreases in bronchial hyperreactivity.[2,44] The LT modifiers have not demonstrated a reduction in BHR.

EXERCISE-INDUCED BRONCHOSPASM

During vigorous exercise, pulmonary function in asthmatic patients (as measured by forced expiratory maneuvers) increases during the first few minutes but then begins to decrease after 6 to 8 minutes[29] (Fig. 26–4). EIB is defined as a drop in FEV_1 of greater than 15% to 20% of baseline (preexercise value).[2,29] Most studies suggest that 70% to 90% of asthmatics experience EIB.[2] The exact pathogenesis of EIB is unknown; however, heat loss and/or water loss from the central airways appears to play an important role.[29] EIB is more easily provoked in cold, dry air, and warm, humid air can blunt or block it.[29]

Studies using isocapnic hyperventilation of cold air and inhalation of hypertonic saline have demonstrated similar degrees of bronchospasm as seen in EIB.[29] A number of studies have demonstrated increased plasma histamine and tryptase concentrations during EIB, suggesting a role for mast cell degranulation. In addition, pretreatment with cromolyn sodium, a drug that stabilizes mast cells, inhibits EIB and inhibits the associated rise in neutrophil chemotactic factor.[29] A small number of patients with EIB will have a late response similar to the LAR and associated with a secondary rise in neutrophil chemotactic factor.

A refractory period following EIB lasts up to 3 hours after exercise. During this period, repeat exercise of the same intensity produces either no decrease in pulmonary function or a drop of less than 50% of the initial response.[29] The refractory period is thought to be caused by an acute depletion of mast cell mediators and time required for their repletion. Patients with known refractoriness to exercise will still

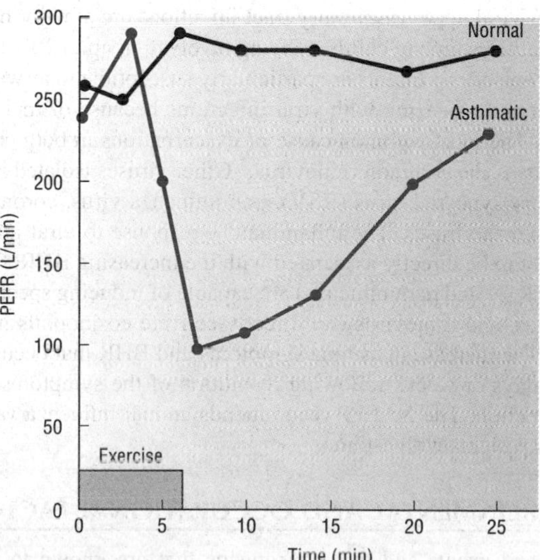

FIGURE 26–4. Typical responses to exercise in a normal subject and an asthmatic subject. Note the initial bronchodilation. PEFR = peak expiratory flow rate.

respond to histamine, so acute hyporesponsiveness of airway smooth muscle does not appear to be a factor.[29]

EIB is believed to be a reflection of the increased BHR of asthmatics. A correlation, though not perfect, exists between EIB and reactivity to histamine and methacholine.[43] Other patient groups with BHR (e.g., after viral infection, cystic fibrosis, or hay fever) show bronchoconstriction after exercise to a lesser degree (5% to 10%) than asthmatics (20% to 40%).[29] Asthmatics will not always demonstrate the same sensitivity. During periods of remission, they often have a decreased sensitivity to the same degree of exercise. Finally, a number of children and adults with EIB are otherwise normal, without symptoms or abnormal pulmonary function.

NOCTURNAL ASTHMA

Worsening of asthma during sleep is referred to as *nocturnal asthma.* Patients with nocturnal asthma exhibit significant falls in pulmonary function between bedtime and awakening.[2,46] Although the pathogenesis of this phenomenon is unknown, it has been associated with diurnal patterns of endogenous cortisol secretion and circulating epinephrine.[46] Direct evidence for an inflammatory component to nocturnal asthma includes increased circulating histamine and activated eosinophils at night associated with increased hyperresponsiveness to methacholine.[46] It has been postulated that the decrease in endogenous hormones results in enhanced pulmonary T-cell release of proinflammatory cytokines, which then activate the airway inflammatory cells at night. Increased urinary LT excretion has been found in patients with nocturnal asthma.

Numerous other factors that may affect nocturnal worsening of asthma, including allergies and improper environmental control, gastroesophageal reflux, and sinusitis, also must be considered when evaluating these patients.[2,37] Although nocturnal asthma often can be controlled with long-acting bronchodilators, most experts consider it a symptom of inadequately treated persistent asthma and advocate increased anti-inflammatory therapy.[2]

FACTORS CONTRIBUTING TO ASTHMA SEVERITY

VIRAL INFECTIONS

Viral infections are primarily responsible for exacerbations of asthma.[2] Viral upper respiratory tract infections are a major precipitant of acute asthma in children, being involved in up to 20% to 40% of acute episodes.[2] Infants are particularly susceptible to airways obstruction and wheezing with viral infections because of their small airways. The most common cause of exacerbations in both children and adults is the common rhinovirus.[2] Other viruses isolated include respiratory syncytial virus (RSV), parainfluenza virus, coronavirus, and influenza viruses. The inflammatory response to viral infection is thought to be directly associated with the increasing BHR. Certain viruses (RSV and parainfluenza) are capable of inducing specific IgE antibodies, and rhinovirus can directly activate eosinophils in asthmatics. The increase in asthma symptoms and BHR that occurs may last for days or weeks following resolution of the symptoms of the viral infection. The NAEPP recommends annual influenza vaccinations for patients with asthma.[2]

ENVIRONMENTAL AND OCCUPATIONAL FACTORS

Agents and events and the mechanisms that are known to trigger asthma are listed in Table 26–1. The general mechanisms are unknown but are presumably the result of epithelial damage and inflammation in the airway mucosa. Ozone and sulfur dioxide, common components of air pollution, have been used to induce BHR in animals. Exposure to 0.2 ppm ozone for 2 to 3 hours can induce bronchoconstriction and increase BHR in asthmatics.[37] Sulfur dioxide in the ambient atmosphere is highly irritating, but it is not known how it induces bronchoconstriction. Pretreatment with cromolyn sodium will block the obstruction, implicating mast cell or irritant-receptor involvement.[37] Asthma produced by repeated prolonged exposure to industrial inhalants is a significant health problem. It has been estimated that occupational asthma accounts for 2% of all asthmatic persons.[2] Persons with occupational asthma have the typical symptoms of asthma with cough, dyspnea, and wheeze. Typically, the symptoms are related to work, with improvement seen on weekends and during vacations.[2] In some instances, symptoms may persist even after termination of exposure.[2]

PSYCHOLOGICAL FACTORS

Emotions and stress rarely can precipitate attacks of asthma but more commonly worsen an attack in progress.[2] Bronchoconstriction from psychological factors appear to be mediated primarily through excess parasympathetic input.[37] Atropine has been shown to block experimental psychogenic bronchoconstriction.[37] It is most important to emphasize to patients and to parents of asthmatic children that asthma is not an emotional disease; however, calming influences and relaxation techniques may benefit the patient who becomes severely emotionally distraught during an asthma attack.

SINUSITIS AND RHINITIS

Disorders of the upper respiratory tract, particularly sinusitis and rhinitis, have been linked with asthma for many years. As many as 40% to 50% of asthmatics have abnormal sinus radiographs.[37] However, chronic sinusitis may just represent a nonbacterial coexisting condition with allergic asthmatics because the histologic changes in the paranasal sinuses are similar to those seen in the lung and nose.[2] Some studies have shown that asthma symptoms improve with treatment of sinusitis. The mechanism by which sinusitis aggravates asthma is unknown. The treatment of allergic rhinitis with inhaled corticosteroids and cromolyn but not antihistamines will reduce BHR in asthmatic patients.[2] It has been postulated that transport of mucus chemotactic factors and inflammatory mediators from nasal passages during allergic rhinitis into the lung may accentuate BHR.

GASTROESOPHAGEAL REFLUX

Gastroesophageal reflux has been associated with asthma for many years.[2,37] Nocturnal asthma may be associated with nighttime reflux.[46] Reflux of acidic gastric contents into the esophagus is thought to initiate a vagally mediated reflex bronchoconstriction.[37] Also of concern is that most medications that decrease airways smooth muscle tone have a relaxant effect on gastroesophageal sphincter tone as well. The therapeutic approach most commonly taken for patients with gastroesophageal reflux and asthma is to initiate standard antireflux therapy and observe the asthma symptoms.

MENSTRUATION-RELATED ASTHMA

Premenstrual worsening of asthma has been reported in as many as 30% to 40% of women in some studies, whereas worsening of pulmonary functions has been reported even in women not aware of worsening of symptoms.[47] The pathophysiology is uncertain because estrogen replacement in postmenopausal women has been shown to worsen asthma, whereas estradiol and progesterone administration is reported to improve asthma in women with premenstrual asthma.[47,48] Studies would indicate that, in general, BHR and symptoms improve in asthmatics during pregnancy.[2] An abnormal regulation of β_2-adrenergic receptors has been demonstrated in women who experience premenstrual asthma.[48] The clinical significance of menstruation-related asthma is still unclear because some studies have reported up to 50% of emergency department visits by women were premenstrual, whereas others have reported no association with menstrual phase.[47,49]

FOODS, DRUGS, AND ADDITIVES

Documentation in the literature of food allergens as triggers for asthma is not available.[37] However, additives, specifically sulfites used as preservatives, can trigger life-threatening asthma exacerbations. Beer, wine, dried fruit, and open salad bars in particular have high concentrations of metabisulfites.[2] Severe oral corticosteroid-dependent patients should be warned about ingesting foods processed with sulfites. Another additive producing bronchospasm is benzalkonium chloride, which is found as a preservative in some nebulizer solutions of antiasthmatic drugs.

Aspirin and other nonsteroidal anti-inflammatory drugs can precipitate an attack in up to 20% of adults with asthma.[37] The mechanism is related to cyclooxygenase inhibition, and 5-lipoxygenase inhibition can prevent the symptoms.[19] The prevalence increases with age. The greatest frequency occurs in severe corticosteroid-dependent asthmatics in their fourth and fifth decades who also have perennial rhinitis and nasal polyposis (presence of several polyps).[37] Other drugs that do not precipitate bronchospasm but which prevent its reversal are the β-blocking agents.[2]

▶ TREATMENT: Asthma

AEROSOL THERAPY FOR ASTHMA

Aerosol delivery of drugs for asthma has the advantages of being site-specific and thus enhancing the therapeutic ratio.[2,50] Inhalation of short-acting β_2-agonists provides more rapid bronchodilation than either parenteral or oral administration as well as the greatest degree of protection against EIB and other challenges.[44] ICSs appear to have a greater effect on BHR than corticosteroids administered systemically.[51] Other agents (e.g., cromolyn, nedocromil, formoterol, salmeterol, and ipratropium) are only effective by inhalation.[2,52] Due to the international ban on the production and use of chlorofluorocarbons (CFCs), the manufacturers of CFC-propelled metered-dose inhalers (MDIs) are developing new devices for delivering topically active medication.[2,53] Therefore, an understanding of aerosol drug delivery is essential to optimal asthma therapy. Table 26–4 lists the factors determining lung deposition of therapeutic aerosols.

LUNG DEPOSITION

Devices used to generate therapeutic aerosols include jet nebulizers (JNs), ultrasonic nebulizers, MDIs, and dry-powder inhalers (DPIs). The single most important device factor determining the site of aerosol deposition is particle size.[50] Devices for delivering therapeutic aerosols generate particles with aerodynamic diameters from 0.5 to 35 μm in diameter.[50] Particles larger than 10 μm deposit in the oropharynx, particles between 5 and 10 μm deposit in the trachea and large bronchi,

TABLE 26–4. Factors Determining Lung Deposition of Aerosols

Device	Device Factors	Patient Factors
Metered-dose inhaler (MDI)	Canister held inverted Formulation (CFC, HFA, solution, suspension) Actuator cleanliness Addition of a spacer device	Inspiratory flow (slow, deep) Breath-holding Coordinating actuation with inhalation Priming and shaking the device
Dry-powder inhaler (DPI)	Device cleanliness Resistance to inhalation Humidity	Inspiratory flow (deep, forceful) Tilting head back Maintaining parallel to ground once activated
Jet nebulizer (small volume)	Volume fill (3–6 mL) Gas flow (6–12 L/min) Dead-space volume Open versus closed system Thumb-activating valve Mouthpiece versus facemask	Inspiratory flow (slow, deep) Breath-holding Tapping nebulizer
Ultrasonic nebulizer	Volume fill Not effective for suspensions Mouthpiece versus facemask	Inspiratory flow (slow, deep) Breath-holding Tapping nebulizer
Spacer device	Volume (≥650 mL) One-way valves Holding chamber versus opened-ended Metal versus plastic Mouthpiece versus facemask	Inspiratory flow (slow, deep) Time between actuation and inhalation (<5 s) Cleaning with detergent to reduce static Multiple actuations decreases delivery Coordination of actuation and inhalation for the simple open-tube spacers

particles 1 to 5 μm reach the lower airways, and particles smaller than 0.5 μm act as a gas and are exhaled. In asthma, the airways, not the alveoli, are the target for delivery. Respirable particles are deposited in the airways by three mechanisms: (1) inertial impaction, (2) gravitational sedimentation, and (3) Brownian diffusion.[50] The first two are the most important for therapeutic aerosols and probably are the only factors that can be manipulated by patients.

The most important patient factor determining aerosol deposition is inspiratory flow.[2,50] High inspiratory flows increase the degree of deposition due to impaction of particles of any size, thereby increasing deposition centrally (i.e., large airways) and decreasing peripheral deposition.

Besides the two major factors, a number of other factors can be altered to improve delivery and efficacy of clinical aerosols. Most of these factors tend to be device-specific and will be discussed along with the individual devices. Patient factors that cannot be controlled include interpatient variability in airway geometry (particularly the differences between children and adults),[52] the effect of bronchospasm, edema, and mucus hypersecretion. Mild obstruction increases aerosol deposition; however, severe obstruction probably leads to increased central deposition from impaction.[50]

In general, a delivery device should be easy to use and deliver a consistent amount of drug to the lungs across a wide age range of patients while avoiding oropharyngeal deposition, which can lead to increased systemic activity.[54] The absolute delivery to the lung is not as important as consistency of delivery, provided a sufficient dose to produce the desired therapeutic effect is achieved. Variability in patient response should not be a result of inconsistent delivery. However, no device is the best for all patients. The ideal device would deliver an effective dose with the patient placing the device in the mouth and breathing in through the mouth at a normal rate. Table 26–5 lists the differing characteristics of inhalation devices.

TABLE 26–5. Characteristics of Various Inhalation Devices

Device	Drugs	Breath-Activated	Dose Counter	Other Excipients	Disadvantages
CFC MDI	All classes	No	No	Propellants, surfactants	Requires coordination of actuation and inhalation Large pharyngeal deposition Difficult to teach
HFA-MDI	Albuterol	No	No	Propellants, surfactants, cosolvents	Same as CFC MDI
	Beclomethasone	No	No		
Autohaler MDI	Pirbuterol	Yes	No	CFC propellant, surfactant	Requires rapid inhalation to activate
MDI plus holding chamber	All classes	No	No		More expensive than MDI alone; less portable; some payers will not pay; inconsistent effect on delivery
Jet nebulizers	All classes except long-acting β_2-agonists	No	—	Preservatives in some solutions	Significant interbrand variability; expensive and time-consuming; less efficient than MDIs; contamination possible; preparations may be light- and temperature-sensitive (short shelf-life)
Ulrasonic nebulizer	Cromolyn solution short acting β_2-agonist solutions	No	—	Preservatives in some solutions	Sames as for jet nebulizers plus cannot be used for suspensions
Rotahaler	Albuterol	Yes	—	Lactose filler	Single-dose capsule; requires high inspiratory flow
Turbuhaler	Budesonide	Yes	Indicator for last 20 doses	No	Requires high inspiratory flow (60 L/min). Pharyngeal deposition. Not approved for <6 years of age
Diskhaler	Fluticasone	Yes	Yes	Lactose filler	Rotadisk contains 4 doses Needs assembly and cleaning
Diskus	Fluticasone Salmeterol Fluticasone/salmeterol	Yes	Yes	Lactose filler	Not approved for <4 years of age
Aerolizer	Formoterol	Yes	—	Lactose filler	Single-dose capsules. Not approved for <5 years of age Requires high inspiratory flow (≥60L/min)
Twisthaler	Mometasone	Yes	Yes	Lactose filler	Not approved for <12 years of age

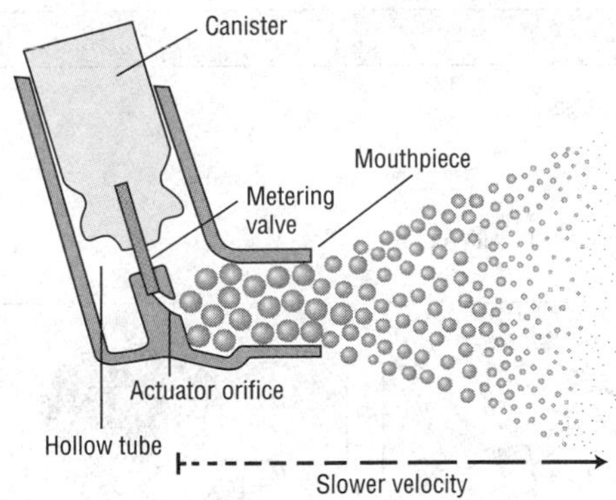

FIGURE 26–5. Illustration of a metered-dose inhaler demonstrating the particle size difference as the aerosol cloud extends outward.

METERED-DOSE INHALERS

MDIs are still the most popular form of aerosol delivery because of their convenience (easy portability) and efficacy (Fig. 26–5). They consist of a pressurized canister with a metering valve containing active drug, low-vapor-pressure propellants such as chlorofluorocarbon (CFC) or hydrofluoroalkane (HFA), cosolvents, and/or surfactants.[50] With any change of these components, the FDA considers it to be a new drug that requires stability, safety, and efficacy studies for approval prior to marketing. The drug is either in solution or a suspended micronized powder. In order to disperse the suspension for accurate delivery, the canister must be shaken. The metering chamber measures a liquid volume, and therefore, the device must be held with the valve stem downward so that the chamber is covered with liquid.[50] The canister is placed inverted in an actuator, and when pressed, the device releases the propellant and drug in a forceful spray whose particles are large [mass median aerodynamic diameter (MMAD) = 45 μm], with the exception of HFA-propelled MDIs, whose spray is less forceful and particles are smaller.[50] As evaporation occurs, the particle size is reduced to a final MMAD of 2.8 to 5.5 μm, depending on the MDI. The aerosol cloud of a CFC-propelled MDI extends at least 10 in beyond the MDI at the lowest MMAD and that of an HFA-propelled MDI about 6 in.[50] Although CFCs can produce cardiac arrhythmias at high doses, investigations have failed to detect adverse effects from the dose delivered via MDIs in recommended dosages. Surfactants, particularly oleates, can produce lung irritation and coughing at excessive doses.[50]

The patient needs to be aware of a number of practical issues for optimal use of CFC propelled MDIs. Prior to initial use and after the device has not been used for several days, it should be primed (actuated once) before use, or the initial dose will contain a lower and variable amount of drug.[50] The CFC-propelled MDIs have a tailing off of drug delivered despite appearing to work at the end of the labeled number of doses due to CFC excess in the canister. In extreme cold, CFC inhalers may malfunction. Many of these characteristics have been improved with the HFA-propelled MDIs.[50]

Appropriate technique is required to achieve optimal drug delivery and therapeutic effect from an MDI[50,52] (Fig. 26–6). With optimal technique, about 10% to 30% of the metered dose is deposited in the lung depending on the device.[50,54] Approximately 70% to 80% impacts on the oropharynx due to the initial high velocity, and this portion is then swallowed; the rest is either left in the actuator or exhaled.[54] The newer HFA-propelled beclomethasone dipropionate MDI is a marked exception, delivering 50% to 60% of its actuated dose to the lungs with optimal technique.[50] It is important that actuation occurs during inhalation, although the time during inspiration is unimportant provided the inspiratory flow is slow (30 L/min or 5 to 10 seconds for the entire inspiration).[2,52] Although studies using radiolabeling indicate improved delivery by holding the actuator 2 to 3 cm in front of an open mouth to allow more evaporation and less impaction, physiologic studies with bronchodilators have failed to document an advantage for this method.[50] Numerous studies have shown that many patients do not use their MDIs optimally and also that patient instruction with demonstration is the most effective means of improving inhaler technique.[2,50,52] Even with instruction, up to 30% of patients, particularly young children and the elderly, cannot master the use of an MDI. For these patients, the attachment of auxiliary devices or spacers to the MDI or use of a breath-activated MDI can improve efficacy significantly.[2,50]

HOLDING-CHAMBER/SPACER DEVICES

Advantages to the use of spacers with an MDI are decreased oropharyngeal deposition and enhanced lung delivery.[2,52] However, not all spacer devices produce similar effects. The design of spacers varies from simple open-ended tubes that maintain the MDI away from the mouth to holding chambers with one-way valves that open during inhalation. The purpose of a spacer is to allow evaporation of the propellant prior to inhalation. This allows inhalation after actuation of the device, obviating the need for good hand-lung coordination, and permits a greater number of drug particles to achieve a respirable droplet size.[52,54] Additionally, most of the large particles that normally would deposit in the oropharynx rain out in the spacer.[52] All the available spacers significantly reduce oropharyngeal deposition of CFC-propelled aerosols, with the holding-chamber devices superior to the open-ended tubes.[52] This is an important factor in reducing local adverse effects (i.e., hoarseness, thrush), may decrease hypothalamic-pituitary-adrenal axis suppression from orally bioavailable inhaled glucocorticoids,[55] and may have clinical importance for bronchodilators delivered by MDI in acute severe asthma.[56] The use of spacers significantly enhances the clinical effect from bronchodilators in ambulatory patients with poor hand-lung coordination but offers no advantage in those patients who can optimally use an MDI alone, despite the fact that radiolabeling studies show an increased lung deposition.[54] Either the increased amount of bronchodilator drug deposited in the lung is clinically insignificant, or these patients reside at the top of the dose-response curve. The inconsistent result also would be due to the use of different spacers. The lung delivery depends on both the MDI and the drug, where one device may enhance delivery with one MDI preparation and decrease delivery with others.[51] In general, the larger-volume holding chambers (>600 mL) consistently enhance delivery.[54] The new HFA-propelled MDIs have not been studied adequately with spacers.

BREATH-ACTUATED MDIs

The breath-actuated MDI Autohaler is cocked with a lever to "load" the dose of medication, a baffle is opened by inspiratory pressure, and the dose is expelled from the canister metering chamber.[50] While the need for hand lung coordination for proper actuation is reduced significantly with breath-actuated MDIs, these devices do not allow the use of a spacer. Also, use of these devices improve pulmonary drug deposition only in patients unable to coordinate the use of conventional MDIs adequately.[50] These devices may be particularly helpful in the elderly, who have difficulty actuating conventional MDIs.[50]

Steps for Using Your Inhaler

Please demonstrate your inhaler technique at every visit.

1. Remove the cap and hold inhaler upright.
2. Shake the inhaler.
3. Tilt your head back slightly and breathe out slowly.
4. Position the inhaler in one of the following ways (A or B is optimal, but C is acceptable for those who have difficulty with A or B. C is required for breath-activated inhalers):

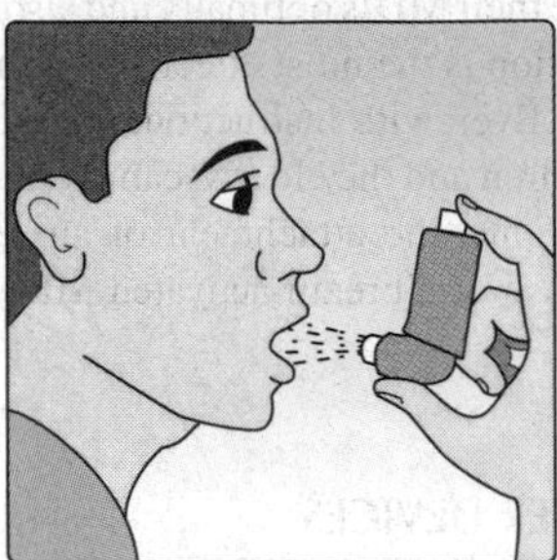

A Open mouth with inhaler 1 to 2 inches away.

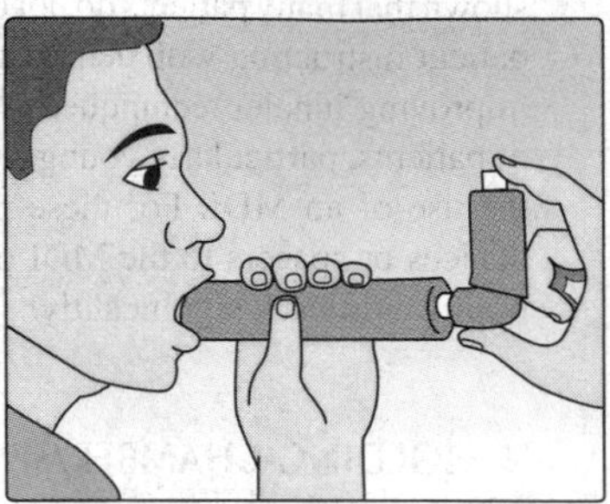

B Use spacer/holding chamber (that is recommended especially for young children and for people using corticosteroids).

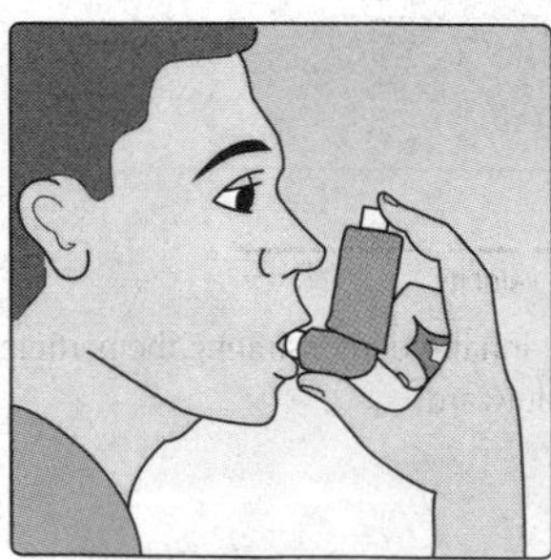

C In the mouth. Do not use for corticosteroids.

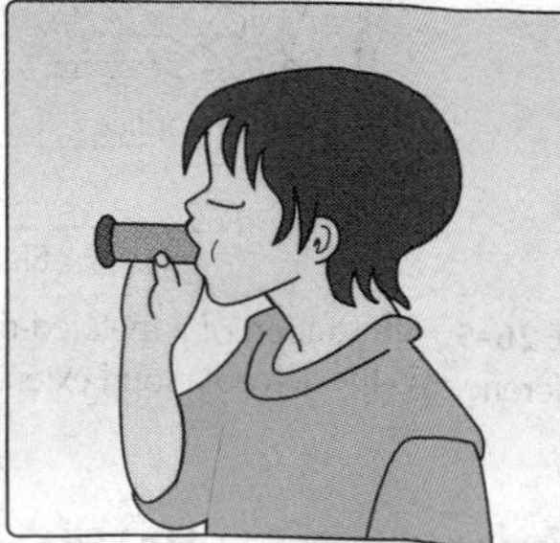

D NOTE: Inhaled dry powder capsules require a different inhalation technique. To use a dry powder inhaler, it is important to close the mouth tightly around the mouthpiece of the inhaler and to inhale rapidly.

5. Press down on the inhaler to release medication as you start to breathe in slowly.
6. Breathe in slowly (3 to 5 seconds).
7. Hold your breath for 10 seconds to allow the medicine to reach deeply into your lungs.
8. Repeat puff as directed. Waiting 1 minute between puffs may permit second puff to penetrate your lungs better.
9. Spacers/holding chambers are useful for all patients. They are particularly recommended for young children and older adults and for use with corticosteroids.

Avoid common inhaler mistakes. Follow these inhaler tips:

- Breathe out *before* pressing your inhaler.
- Inhale *slowly*.
- Breathe in through your mouth, not your nose.
- Press down on your inhaler at the *start* of inhalation (or within the first second of inhalation).
- Keep inhaling as you press down on inhaler.
- Press your inhaler only *once* while you are inhaling (one breath for each puff).
- Make sure you breathe in evenly and deeply.

NOTE: Other inhalers are becoming available in addition to those illustrated above. Different types of inhalers require different techniques.

FIGURE 26–6. Instructions for inhaler use from the NAEPP Expert Panel Report 2.[2]

NEBULIZERS

Nebulizers come in two basic forms, the jet nebulizer and the ultrasonic nebulizer. JNs produce an aerosol from a liquid solution or suspension placed in a cup. A tube connected to a stream of compressed air or oxygen flows up through the bottom and draws the liquid up an adjacent open-ended tube.[50] The air and liquid strike a baffle, creating a droplet cloud that is then inhaled.[50] Ultrasonic nebulizers produce an aerosol by vibrating liquid lying above a transducer at speeds of about 1 mHz.[50] Both produce similar degrees of lung deposition, with the exception that ultrasonic nebulizers are ineffective for nebulizing micronized suspensions.[54] Large droplets adhere to the sides of the nebulizer and baffles, coalesce, and drip to the bottom to be renebulized. The aerosol output and lung delivery vary between the commercially available JNs even when operated in the same manner.[50] This is due to differing dead-space volumes, output characteristics, and baffle systems.[50] Altering the operating parameters also can affect lung delivery significantly. Because dead space (i.e., the volume left behind after nebulization stops) remains constant, increasing fill volume will increase the total amount of drug delivered; however, it also will take longer to nebulize the dose.[50] A total fill volume of 4 to 6 mL is considered optimal but will take 10 to 15 minutes to complete.[50] Tapping the side of the nebulizer during operation induces the droplets on the sides to fall back into the reservoir, minimizing loss. The MMAD of the droplets is directly related to the gas flow, with flows of 5 to 12 L/min providing an aerosol cloud with an MMAD of 4 to 8 μm for most nebulizers.[54] Putting a hole in the gas supply tube so that nebulization will occur only during inhalation when the patient closes his or her thumb over the hole also decreases aerosol loss. Quiet tidal breathing through a mouthpiece or facemask is the usual method of aerosol delivery from a nebulizer; however, slow, deep inhalation and breathholding also will improve delivery from this device as well as from an MDI. JNs are used primarily to deliver aerosols to hospitalized patients or patients with acute asthma exacerbations presenting to the clinic or emergency department, although they are also used to deliver long-term controller medications for patients with difficulty operating MDIs plus holding chambers (e.g., infants and elderly patients).[2,50,56] They have the advantage of not requiring significant patient coordination or cooperation other than tidal breathing.

Approximately 10% (5% to 15%) of the dose placed in a nebulizer is delivered to the patient's lung, with 60% to 80% lost in the apparatus, up to 20% exhaled, and 2% deposited in the mouth under usual operating conditions.[50,54] Nebulizers generally are less efficient at delivering drug to the lung than MDIs plus holding chambers.[50] Numerous studies in acute severe asthma have shown that bronchodilators delivered by an MDI plus holding chamber are equally effective as the same drug nebulized.[56] However, the dose ratios have varied from 1:2.5 to 1:10 (i.e., requires 10 times the dose delivered by nebulizer). Use of a facemask versus a mouthpiece significantly reduces lung delivery by either method due to nasal filtering.[54] Adults receive about one-half the dose to the lung when using a facemask versus a mouthpiece.[52,54]

DRY-POWDER INHALERS

Dry micronized powders can be inhaled directly into the lung. Five DPIs are available for use in the United States (i.e., Diskhaler, Diskus, Rotahaler, Turbuhaler, and Aerolyzer), with the Twisthaler expected to receive approval soon and other DPI devices under development.[50] The Rotahaler requires that a capsule of medication be placed in the back of the device, and then the device is twisted to break open the capsule and release the medication for inhalation. The Aerolyzer also requires that a capsule be inserted into the device prior to inhalation. The Diskhaler allows the patient to place a four-dose disk into the device and then requires "loading" a dose prior to inhalation by puncturing a blister of medication in the disk.[50] The Diskus, Turbuhaler, and Twisthaler are all self-contained with at least a month of therapy (depending on the dosing schedule). Each device has specific characteristics that are compared in Table 26–5.

An advantage of DPIs is that they are breath-actuated and require minimal hand-lung coordination.[50,54] In general, DPIs require higher inspiratory flows (>60 L/min) and a change in inhalation technique (i.e., deep, forceful inspiration) for optimal actuation as compared with MDIs, which in turn increase the amount of drug delivered to the larger central airways.[50,54] However, this difference in delivery has not been shown to produce clinically significant differences.[50] Some DPIs are more flow-dependent than others.[50,54] Thus, similar to MDIs and spacers, delivery data from one DPI cannot be extrapolated to another. Mouth rinsing following treatment with DPI-inhaled corticosteroids is important to minimize local effects and oral absorption.[52,54] The higher inspiratory flows required and inherent inhaler resistance of DPIs have raised concern that patients in acute distress will be unable to actuate the devices adequately for symptomatic relief. Another concern is that the powder may be irritating and may produce cough, but this has not been reported widely.[52,54]

The Turbuhaler device has the highest mean lung deposition at the optimal inspiratory flow of 60 L/min, and its flow rate is approximately twice that of its corresponding MDI for both budesonide and terbutaline.[52,54] However, it has a greater flow dependency and higher variability than the Diskhaler and Diskus.[50,54] Children 6 to 12 years of age received approximately one-half the dose of radio-labeled budesonide than those greater than 12 years of age, whereas children less than 6 years of age received one-quarter of the dose.[54] The Diskhaler and Diskus deliver about 15% of the dose to the airways, and this appears to be similar at both 30 and 60 L/min inspiratory flows; both have been approved for children down to 4 years of age.[50,54]

ACUTE SEVERE ASTHMA

Environmental exposures are the most important precipitants of asthma exacerbations. Environmental tobacco smoke exposure and exposure to smoke from fireplaces and wood-burning stoves are associated with asthma exacerbations.[2] The role of air pollution in cities is still unclear; some studies report an increase in hospital use associated with increased atmospheric ozone and sulfate levels, whereas others have reported increasing death rates despite decreasing concentrations of major pollutants.[57] Epidemics of severe asthma in cities have followed exposures to high concentrations of aeroallergens.[2] Viral respiratory tract infections remain the single most significant precipitant of severe asthma in children.[2] The risk of severe life-threatening asthma may be reduced by ICS therapy,[14] teaching age-appropriate self-management, and providing clearly written crisis plans for the family.[2] Excessive use of inhaled β_2-agonists (>2 canisters per month), particularly a pattern of increasing use, is a marker of worsening asthma and an increased risk of life-threatening exacerbations.[58,59] The primary cause of death during acute asthma exacerbations is respiratory failure and is not cardiac-related.[2] The primary goal is prevention of life- threatening asthma by early recognition of signs of deterioration and early intervention (Figs. 26–7 and 26–8).

ASSESSMENT

The NAEPP suggests that objective measures of oxygenation and lung function are the most important factors for determining severity of an exacerbation of asthma.[2] Early response to treatment as measured by the improvement in FEV_1 at 30 minutes following inhaled β_2-agonists is the best predictor of outcome.[57] The introduction of peak expiratory flow (PEF) guidelines in the emergency department has resulted in a decrease in the number of children hospitalized with asthma.[57]

Gas exchange at the alveoli-capillary interface depends on ventilation ($\dot{V}_a$), or the mechanical properties of the lung, perfusion ($\dot{Q}$), the flow of blood, and diffusion of the gases across the membrane. In acute severe asthma, diffusion capacity is slightly increased or unchanged.[57] Arterial hypoxemia is common during acute asthma attacks and is caused by $\dot{V}_a/\dot{Q}$ mismatch.[2,57] When lungs initially become obstructed, patients demonstrate a marked respiratory drive thought to be caused by stimulation of the irritant receptors because it is not obliterated by correcting the hypoxemia.[2] As a result, the asthmatic tends to "blow off" carbon dioxide (CO_2), and the arterial CO_2 concentration decreases.[2] Unfortunately, the patient is forced to breathe at higher lung volumes because of air trapping. This requires the use of accessory respiratory muscles. When obstruction worsens ($FEV_1 < 20\%$ of predicted) and the accessory respiratory muscles begin to fatigue, the patient will begin to retain CO_2, signaling impending respiratory failure.[2,57] Thus more severely obstructed patients may have "normal" or elevated $PaCO_2$ values.

Most patients who present with severe asthma in an urgent-care setting will present with a mild metabolic acidosis (lactic acidosis from hypoxic metabolism in accessory respiratory muscles) and a low PaO_2 and $PaCO_2$. The measurement of oxygen saturation (SaO_2) of hemoglobin by pulse oximetry is a less invasive means to evaluate oxygenation.[2] To assess ventilation, arterial $PaCO_2$, is necessary for assessing the risk of respiratory failure in those patients presenting with severe obstruction (FEV_1 or PEF < 30% of predicted).[57] Capillary gases for assessing $PaCO_2$ may be particularly useful in infants.[2] Generally accepted criteria for impending respiratory failure and the need to intubate and mechanically ventilate a patient include hypoxia unresponsive to O_2 ($PaO_2 < 60$ mm Hg or $FiO_2 > 60$ percent), $PaCO_2 > 65$ mm Hg or increasing more than 5 mm Hg per hour despite adequate therapy, and significant metabolic acidosis.[2] In infants and young children less than 6 years of age, lung function measures are difficult to obtain and are less reliable indicators of asthma severity. Thus a combination of objective and subjective measures may be used to assess severity in young patients.[2]

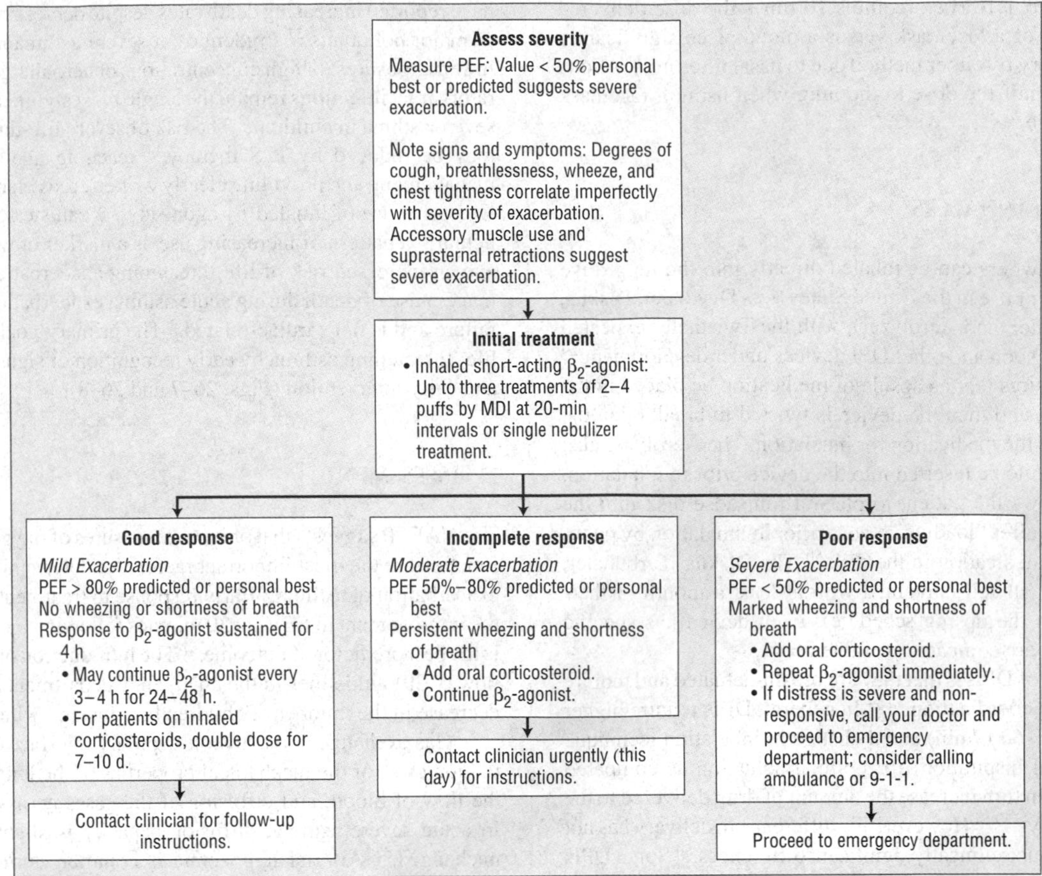

FIGURE 26–7. Home management of acute asthma exacerbation. Patients at risk of asthma-related death should receive immediate clinical attention after initial treatment. Additional therapy may be required. *(From Ref. 2.)*

A brief history and physical examination are essential to the appropriate assessment and management of an acute asthma exacerbation. However, it is important that initial therapy not be delayed, and it is recommended that the history and physical examination be obtained while initial therapy is being provided. A history of the severity of previous asthma exacerbations (e.g., hospitalizations, intubations, or hypoxic seizures) as well as potentially complicating illnesses (e.g., cardiac disease, diabetes, or psychosis) should be obtained.[2]

The physical examination helps to assess severity as well as general patient health status, such as hydration and the presence of cyanosis. The patient should be examined for the presence of pneumonia, pneumothorax, pneumomediastinum, and upper airway obstruction. The use of accessory muscles of respiration, particularly supraclavicular retractions, indicates an FEV_1 of less than 50% of normal predicted value. Mild dehydration occurs commonly in small children due to increased insensible losses.

A complete blood count may be appropriate for patients with fever or purulent sputum, but many patients will have a leukocytosis from a viral infection or secondarily to corticosteroid administration. Routine chest radiographs have not been shown to be of value unless physical findings suggestive of consolidations or pneumothoraces are present.[2] Serum electrolytes should be monitored if high-dose continuous inhaled or systemic β_2-agonists are to be used because they can produce transient decreases in potassium, magnesium, and phosphate.[60] The combination of high-dose β_2-agonists and systemic corticosteroids occasionally may result in excessive elevations of glucose.[57]

THERAPY

The goals of treatment for acute asthma are (1) rapid reversal of airflow obstruction, (2) correction of significant hypoxemia, (3) restoration of lung function to normal as soon as possible, (4) reduction of the rate of recurrent of severe asthma symptoms, and (5) development of a written action plan in case of a further exacerbation.[2]

The first goal should be achieved within minutes, and most patients experience significant improvement within the first 30 to 60 minutes of therapy, with most patients doubling their FEV_1 or PEF. In patients ultimately admitted to the hospital, only a 10% to 20% predicted improvement is seen within the first 2 hours. Hypoxemia is immediately correctable by low-flow O_2. While reversal into the normal range may take 12 to 24 hours, complete restoration to normal lung function takes much longer, up to 3 to 7 days. A strategy to prevent recurrence such as systemic corticosteroids and peak-flow monitoring should be used. It is essential to provide the patient with a self-management plan that includes a written action plan for dealing with exacerbations. Patients at risk for severe exacerbations should be taught how to use a peak-flow meter and monitor morning peak flows at home. In young children, an increased respiratory rate, increased heart rate, and inability to speak more that one or two words between breaths are signs of severe obstruction.[2] Oxygen saturations by pulse oximetry and peak flows should be measured in all patients not completely responding to initial intensive inhaled β_2-agonist therapy. Initially, on admission, the peak flows or clinical symptoms should be monitored every 2 to 4 hours. Prior to discharge from the

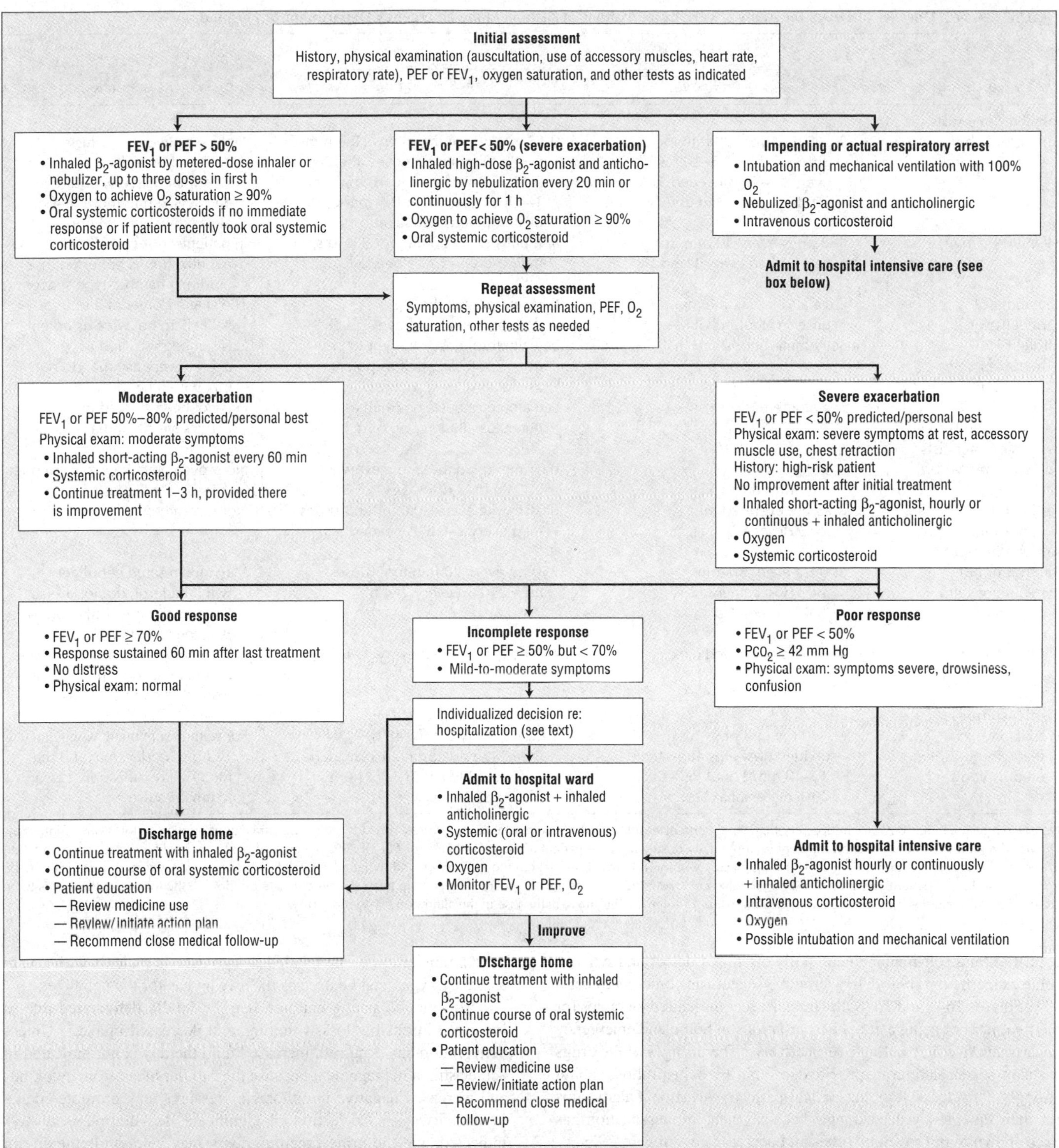

FIGURE 26–8. Emergency department and hospital care of acute asthma exacerbations. *(From Ref. 2.)*

emergency department or hospital, the patient should be given sufficient prednisone to finish his or her course, taught the purpose of the medications and how to use inhalers correctly, and given an appointment for a follow-up visit.

The key points for the management of acute asthma are early recognition of deterioration and aggressive treatment. For both to occur, there must be patient and/or parent education and written action plans for early institution of therapy for acute exacerbations. For more moderate to severe patients, this therapeutic plan also may include the availability of oral prednisone to begin at home.[2] Easy access by telephone to health care providers is also needed. Because of the rapid progression to severe asthma that can occur, patients and parents should be encouraged to communicate promptly with their primary care provider during an exacerbation. Systemic corticosteroids and aggressive use of inhaled β_2-agonists continue to be the cornerstone of therapy for acute severe asthma exacerbations.[3] Families given adequate

TABLE 26–6. Dosages of Drugs for Acute Severe Exacerbations of Asthma in the Emergency Department or Hospital

Medications	Dosages: >6 Years Old	Dosages: ≤6 Years Old	Comments
Inhaled β-agonists			
Albuterol nebulizer soln. (5 mg/mL)	2.5–5 mg every 20 min for 3 doses, then 2.5–10 mg every 1–4 h as needed, or 10–15 mg/h continuously	0.15 mg/kg (minimum dose 2.5 mg) every 20 min for 3 doses, then 0.15–0.3 mg/kg up to 10 mg every 1–4 h as needed, or 0.5 mg/kg/h by continuous nebulization	Only selective β_2-agonists are recommended For optimal delivery, dilute aerosols to minimum of 4 mL at gas flow of 6–8 L/min
MDI (90 μg/puff)	4–8 puffs every 30 min up to 4 h, then every 1–4 h as needed	4–8 puffs every 20 min for 3 doses, then every 1–4 h as needed	In patients in severe distress, nebulization is preferred; use holding-chamber-type spacer
Levalbuterol nebulizer soln.	Give at one-half the mg dose of albuterol above	Give at one-half the mg dose of albuterol above	The single isomer of albuterol is likely to be twice as potent
Bitolterol nebulizer soln. (2 mg/mL)	See albuterol dose	See albuterol dose; thought to be as potent to one-half as potent as albuterol on a μg basis	Has not been studied in acute severe asthma; do not mix with other drugs
Pirbuterol MDI (200 μg/puff)	See albuterol dose	See albuterol dose; one-half as potent as albuterol on a μg basis	Has not been studied in acute severe asthma
Systemic β-agonists			
Epinephrine 1:1000 (1 mg/mL)	0.3–0.5 mg every 20 min for 3 doses SQ	0.01 mg/kg up to 0.5 mg every 20 min for 3 doses SQ	No proven advantage of systemic therapy over aerosol
Terbutaline (1 mg/mL)	0.25 mg every 20 min for 3 doses SQ	0.01 mg/kg every 20 min for 3 doses, then every 2–6 h as needed SQ	Not recommended
Anticholinergics			
Ipratropium Br. nebulizer soln. (0.25 mg/mL)	500 μg every 30 min for 3 doses, then every 2–4 h as needed	250 μg every 20 min for 3 doses, then 250 μg every 2–4 h	May mix in same nebulizer with albuterol; do not use as first-line therapy; only add to β_2-agonist therapy
MDI (18 μg/puff)	4–8 puffs as needed every 2–4 h	4–8 puffs as needed every 2–4 h	Not recommended because dose in inhaler is low and has not been studied in acute asthma
Corticosteroids			
Prednisone, methylprednisolone, prednisolone	60–80 mg in 3 or 4 divided doses for 48 h, then 30–40 mg/d until PEF reaches 70% of personal best	1 mg/kg every 6 h for 48 h, then 1–2 mg/kg/day in 2 divided doses until PEF is 70% of normal predicted	For outpatient "burst" use 1–2 mg/kg/day, max. 60 mg, for 3–7 days; it is unnecessary to taper course

Note: No advantage has been found for very-high-dose corticosteroids in acute severe asthma, nor is there any advantage for intravenous administration over oral therapy. The usual regimen is to continue the frequent multiple daily dosing until the patient achieves and FEV_1 or PEF of 50% of personal best or normal predicted value and then lower the dose to twice-daily dosing. This usually occurs within 48 hours. The final duration of therapy following a hospitalization or emergency department visit may be from 7 to 14 days. If patients are then started on inhaled corticosteroids, studies indicate there is no need to taper the systemic steroid dose. If the follow-up therapy is to be given once daily, studies indicate there may be an advantage to giving the single daily dose in the afternoon at around 3:00 P.M.

education and self-management skills often can detect and manage acute exacerbations before they progress to requiring emergency care.

Figures 26–7 and 26–8 illustrate the recommended therapies for the treatment of acute asthma exacerbations in home and emergency department/hospital settings, respectively.[2] The dosages of the drugs for acute severe asthma are provided in Table 26–6. Institutions should strongly consider developing critical-pathways/treatment algorithms for their emergency departments because their implementation has been shown to improve outcomes and decrease cost of care.[61]

GENERAL SUPPORTIVE THERAPY

Supplemental oxygen therapy by mask or nasal cannulae should be titrated to maintain SaO_2 normal for altitude (>95% at sea level). Inhaled β_2-agonists can transiently decrease SaO_2 through worsening $\dot{V}/\dot{Q}$ mismatch due to vasodilation.[61] However, this is a mild effect that is easily overcome by oxygen administration and should not delay the administration of the inhaled β_2-agonists. In patients with severe asthma, oxygen can be used as the driving gas for the nebulizer.

Infants and young children may be mildly dehydrated due to increased insensible loss, vomiting, and decreased intake.[57] Unless dehydration has occurred, increased fluid therapy is not indicated in acute asthma management because the capillary leak from cytokines and increased negative intrathoracic pressures may promote edema in the airways.[2] Correction of significant dehydration is always indicated, and the urine specific gravity may help guide therapy in young children, in whom the state of hydration may be difficult to determine.[57]

Chest physical therapy and mucolytics are not indicated in the therapy of acute asthma.[2] Sedatives should not be given because anxiety may be a sign of hypoxemia, which could be worsened by central nervous system depressants. Antibiotics are also not indicated routinely because viral respiratory tract infections are the primary cause of asthma exacerbations.[2] Antibiotics should be reserved for patients who have signs and symptoms of pneumonia (e.g., fever, pulmonary consolidation, and purulent sputum from polymorphonuclear leukocytes). *Mycoplasma* and *Chlamydia* are infrequent causes of severe asthma exacerbations but should be considered in those patients with high oxygen requirements.

All patients who have an exacerbation of asthma requiring emergency department care or hospitalization should receive asthma education (including intensification of usual chronic medication), instruction in self- assessment, and a follow-up appointment.[2] Written instructions that include an action plan for managing any recurrence should be given prior to discharge. Sufficient medication (i.e., prednisone) should be prescribed to continue the treatment plan. Consideration should be given to issuing a peak-flow meter with instruction for its use. For hospitalized patients or those who have visited the emergency department twice within a year, referral to an asthma specialist should be considered because specialist care for these patients has been shown to reduce subsequent emergency department use.[2]

PHARMACOTHERAPY

β_2-AGONISTS

Aerosol versus Systemic Administration

The short-acting inhaled β_2-agonists are the most effective bronchodilators and the treatment of first choice for the management of acute severe asthma.[2] Most well-controlled clinical trials have demonstrated equal to greater efficacy and greater safety of aerosolized β_2-agonists over systemic administration.[60] Even in severely obstructed hypercapnic adults, twice as many patients respond successfully to nebulized albuterol than to intravenous albuterol (86% versus 48%).[62] Hypokalemia is more pronounced in patients receiving intravenous albuterol, whereas heart rate decreases in those receiving nebulized therapy versus intravenous therapy. A controlled trial in children reported more rapid improvement with a single intravenous dose of albuterol added to every-20-minute nebulized albuterol than with nebulized therapy alone.[63] However, the study design does not allow differentiation between greater improvement as a result of systemic administration of albuterol or just a higher overall dose. Considering the potential for increased toxicity, it is unclear why the practice of using intravenous β_2-agonists persists. Even children younger than 2 years of age achieve clinically significant responses from nebulized albuterol.[2,57] Effective doses of aerosolized β_2-agonists even can be delivered through mechanical ventilator circuits to infants, children, and adults in respiratory failure from severe airways obstruction.[50]

Continuous Nebulization

Frequent administration of inhaled β_2-agonists has been found to be superior to the same dosage administered at 1-hour intervals.[60] Numerous trials of continuously nebulized albuterol (CNA) have had mixed results. This is likely a result of the heterogeneity of patients enrolled in the trials. For instance, CNA at 10 or 15 mg/h offered no benefit over intermittent hourly therapy in less severely obstructed patients (initial FEV_1 > 50% of predicted or PEF >200 L/min).[57] However, in the subset of more severely obstructed patients, CNA decreased the hospital admission rate and provided greater improvement in the FEV_1 and PEF when compared with intermittent nebulized albuterol in the same total dose. In a four-way comparison of 2.5 and 7.5 mg of albuterol nebulized continuously or intermittently every 1 hour, the two high-dose regimens and the low-dose continuous regimen produced a greater improvement in FEV_1 than the lower-dose intermittent regimen.[64]

In children admitted to an intensive care unit with severe asthma, CNA at a dose of 0.3 mg/kg per hour produced more rapid improvement and shorter hospital stays than the same dose given on an hourly basis.[57] Thus, in this severely obstructed population, CNA provided a more cost-effective therapy than standard intermittent administration. Thus CNA is recommended for patients having an unsatisfactory response (achieving less than 50% of normal FEV_1 or PEF) following the initial three doses (every 20 minutes) of aerosolized β_2-agonists and possibly patients presenting initially with PEF or FEV_1 less than 30% of predicted normal.[57] Up to 66% of adults presenting to an emergency department require only three doses of 2.5 mg nebulized albuterol to be discharged.[57]

The dose of inhaled β_2-agonists for acute severe asthma has been derived empirically as a result of the difficulty in determining dose-response curves in acutely ill patients. The β_2-agonists follow a log-linear dose-response curve.[44,60] In addition, the dose-response curve is shifted to the right by more severe bronchospasm or by increased concentrations of bronchospastic mediators, which is characteristic of functional antagonists.[60] The ability to increase the dose of the short-acting aerosolized β_2-agonists by as much as five- to tenfold over doses producing adequate bronchodilation in chronic stable asthmatics is what contributes to their efficacy in reversing the bronchospasm of acute severe asthma.[60] In children with severe asthma, greater improvement in FEV_1 has been documented as dosing has increased from 0.15 to 0.45 mg/kg per hour.[60] The nebulizer dose of inhaled β_2-agonists for children is often listed on a weight basis (mg/kg). However, the use of a minimum fixed dose of 2.5 mg albuterol or equivalent in children 4 to 12 years of age was as safe and effective as a dose of 0.1 mg/kg.[57] We use a fixed minimum dose of 10 mg/h albuterol for any patient requiring CNA. A fixed minimal dose as opposed to a weight-adjusted dose is more appropriate in younger children because children younger than 5 years of age receive a lower lung dose.[54] In addition, adults dosed on a weight basis demonstrate excessive cardiac stimulation.[57]

High-dose nebulized albuterol has been associated with a 20% decrease in serum potassium concentration, a 16% increase in heart rate,[60] and a 54% increase in serum glucose, with a mean level of 180 mg/dL, respectively.[57] In children prospectively monitored, no cardiac toxicity other than sinus tachycardia was found at doses up to 3 mg/kg per hour of CNA, which is six times the recommended starting dose of 0.5 mg/kg per hour.[57] In adults, a dose of 0.4 mg/kg per hour CNA for 4 hours (or approximately 28 mg/h) produced a mean increase in heart rate of 16.3%, with one patient developing supraventricular tachycardia.[57] The heart rate increased greater in those on theophylline (22 versus 7 beats per minute). On the other hand, CNA at 15 mg/h in adults provided a significant improvement in FEV_1 and a decrease in heart rate.[57]

Delivery by MDI versus Nebulizer

A recent systematic review from the Cochrane Library found no evidence for a difference in efficacy between delivery of β_2-agonists by nebulizer versus MDI plus spacer, with most studies suggesting greater efficiency of delivery with the MDI plus spacer.[65] However, the dose ratios of MDI plus spacer to nebulizer have ranged from 1:1 to 1:10. The explanations for this large range include the intrinsic variability between various small-volume JNs and the spacers used in the trials.[50] In the setting of more severe asthma, where continuous nebulization has been shown to be more effective than intermittent nebulization, MDI plus holding chamber has not been tested. In the emergency department studies, trained personnel, either nurses or respiratory therapists, assist the patient with either mode of administration so that the cost savings must derive primarily from the difference in cost between the drug, nebulizer, and spacer devices.[50]

DPIs generally are not indicated for the treatment of acute severe asthma exacerbations. In adults presenting to an emergency department, administration of albuterol by a DPI (Rotahaler) was equivalent to administration by nebulizer or MDI plus spacer (Aerochamber).[57] However, children younger than 6 years old hospitalized for acute wheezing could not empty a Rotahaler capsule.[57]

Systemic Corticosteroids

Systemic corticosteroids are indicated in all patients with acute severe asthma not responding completely to initial inhaled β_2-agonist administration.[2] Intravenous therapy offers no therapeutic advantage over oral administration.[66] This therapy is usually continued until hospital discharge. Tapering the dose in acute asthma following discharge from the hospital appears unnecessary.[2] Most patients achieve 70% predicted normal FEV_1 within 48 hours and 80% of predicted by 6 days after plateauing by day 3.[66] This indicates that maintaining patients on systemic corticosteroid courses for 10 to 14 days may be unnecessarily long in some patients. Indeed, many patients respond to 3- to 5-day courses of systemic corticosteroids. It is recommended that a full dose of the corticosteroid be continued until the patient's peak flow reaches 80% of predicted normal or personal best.[2] Although clinical trials have not confirmed that this is necessary, it seems a reasonable target.

Multiple daily dosing of systemic corticosteroids for the initial therapy of acute asthma exacerbations appears warranted. The binding affinities of lung steroid receptors are decreased in the face of airway inflammation.[67] Pharmacodynamic studies suggest that the decreased binding affinity would be best overcome by maintaining the concentration of corticosteroids at the receptor site as opposed to giving higher single doses of corticosteroids.[57] Indeed, high-dose and very-high-pulse-dose corticosteroid regimens have not been shown to enhance the outcomes in acute severe asthma but are associated with a higher likelihood of developing myopathy and other side effects.[66]

Short courses of oral prednisone (3–10 days) have been effective in preventing hospitalizations in infants and young children.[2] Following the institution of systemic corticosteroids in acute severe asthma, a lag of 6 to 8 hours occurs prior to improvement in pulmonary function.[66] Thus early institution of systemic corticosteroids would appear to provide an advantage. The current recommendation is to reserve the use of corticosteroids to patients who are incompletely responsive to aggressive inhaled β_2-agonists (every 20 minutes for three to four doses).[2]

A common practice is to increase or double the dose of ICSs in patients who are experiencing a deterioration of their asthma control to prevent an exacerbation that requires emergency care. However, studies of ICSs in acute exacerbations of asthma have provided conflicting results.[68,69] Currently, there is insufficient evidence supporting efficacy. However, it seems like a reasonable recommendation because inflammation is the underlying cause of deterioration in most cases.

ANTICHOLINERGICS

Inhaled ipratropium bromide generally produces a further improvement in lung function of 10% to 15% over inhaled β_2-agonists alone. Randomized trials in children of multiple-dose ipratropium bromide added to initial therapy produced a greater improvement in FEV_1 than β_2-agonists alone, and more important, in the subset of patients with an FEV_1 of less than 30% predicted at baseline, ipratropium reduced hospitalization rate.[70,71] A systematic review recommends the additive use of ipratropium bromide.[72]

Unlike atropine sulfate, which is a tertiary amine and is well absorbed, ipratropium, a quaternary amine, is poorly absorbed and produces minimal to no systemic effects. Care should be used when administering ipratropium by nebulizer. If a tight mask or mouthpiece is not used, the ipratropium that deposits in the eye may produce pupillary dilatation and difficulty in accomodation. Ipratropium is not a vasodilator, so unlike β_2-agonists it will not worsen $\dot{V}/\dot{Q}$ mismatch.[2]

AMINOPHYLLINE

The emergency department use of aminophylline for acute asthma has not been recommended for a number of years.[2] Several clinical trials of aminophylline in children hospitalized with acute asthma have reported a lack of clinical improvement and an increased risk of adverse effects.[57] Similar results, though less consistent, have been reported in controlled clinical trials in adults hospitalized for acute asthma. Every study that has added aminophylline to regular administration of inhaled β_2-agonists as the primary therapy has failed to show an added benefit.[57] However, a recent study of aminophylline in children with severe disease requiring intensive care suggested a possible benefit.[73] However, study design flaws raise concerns about this conclusion.

EXPERIMENTAL THERAPIES

MAGNESIUM SULFATE

Magnesium, an abundant intracellular cation, is involved in the regulation of a number of enzymatic and cellular activities in the body. Magnesium produces relaxation of smooth muscle and central nervous system depression.[74] The mechanism for producing bronchodilation possibly may be by competing with Ca^{2+} ion for binding sites. A systematic review stated that the routine administration of intravenous $MgSO_4$ to patients presenting to the emergency department was not justified.[74] However, the review also stated that a subset of the most severe patients who responded poorly to β_2-agonists benefited from $MgSO_4$. Unfortunately, the subset analysis consisted of very few patients of unequal numbers, and it was not always clear what happened with the standard therapy of inhaled β_2-agonists from study to study.[74] The lack of adequate control of baseline therapy was not considered by the systematic review. For instance, a newly published study in children administered 40 mg/kg $MgSO_4$ intravenously up to 2 g following the initial three doses of albuterol, which may or may not have been combined with ipratropium.[75] The doses of albuterol and ipratropium were not provided by the authors. After beginning the $MgSO_4$, patients received on average 1.6 nebulization treatments over the next 110 minutes, whereas recommended therapy would be to continue to administer 1 treatment every 20 minutes (5 treatments) or a minimum of 1 treatment per hour (at least 2 to 3 treatments). Thus the baseline therapy could not be considered adequately controlled to determine if $MgSO_4$ added significantly or whether it was just better than inadequate baseline therapy. Magnesium sulfate produces moderate degrees of bronchodilation in acute severe asthma when inhaled β_2-agonists are withheld.[74] The administration of magnesium has not consistently produced added bronchodilation or improved therapeutic outcomes when patients have continued to receive standard recommended inhaled β_2-agonist therapy for acute severe asthma.

The adverse effects of magnesium sulfate include hypotension, facial flushing, sweating, nausea, loss of deep tendon reflexes, and respiratory depression.[57] Patients have required dopamine to treat the hypotension.[57] Until well-controlled trials that rigorously address the issue of adequacy of standard therapy are performed, the use of $MgSO_4$ should still be considered experimental.

HELIOX

Helium is an inert gas of low density with no pharmacologic properties that can lower resistance to gas flow and increase ventilation because the low density decreases the pressure gradient needed to achieve a given level of turbulent flow, converting turbulent flow to laminar flow.[57] Helium is given as a mixture of helium and oxygen (heliox) usually 60% to 70% percent helium with 30% to 40% oxygen.[57] Heliox has been reported to improve $PaCO_2$ when given to adults in an emergency department as well as to patients receiving mechanical ventilation and to decrease pulsus paradoxus and dyspnea score and improve pulmonary function tests in children.[76] However, not all studies demonstrate a consistent effect.

The use of heliox is limited to patients who do not require high inspired oxygen concentrations because the decrease in density generally is considered clinically insignificant with less than 60% helium.[57] In general, an 80:20 mixture of helium and oxygen is blended with pure oxygen to deliver the desired concentrations of oxygen and helium. Heliox can be administered with either a facemask or a tent, and it appears to be free of side effects. For patients receiving continuous nebulization of β_2-agonists, the heliox blend can be used as the carrier gas. When heliox is used in patients receiving mechanical ventilation, a separate oxygen analyzer is needed because ventilator blenders are calibrated for air/oxygen.[57] More important, most ventilators use pneumotachs that rely on a pressure drop to calculate flow and tidal volumes. These will be falsely low when using helium because of the lower density of the gas.[57] Either the ventilator pneumotach should be recalibrated or conversion factors should be calculated to overcome this problem.

ANESTHETICS

The inhalational anesthetics halothane, isoflurane, and enflurane have all been reported to have a positive effect in children and adults with severe asthma unresponsive to standard medical therapy.[57] The proposed mechanisms for halothane, a bronchodilator, include direct action on bronchial smooth muscle, inhibition of airway reflexes, attenuation of histamine-induced bronchospasm, and interaction with β_2-adrenergic receptors.[57] Isoflurane and enflurane presumably act through similar mechanisms.

Concerns regarding the use of inhalational anesthetics for severe acute asthma include myocardial depression, vasodilation, potential for arrhythmias, and depression of mucociliary function. In addition, the practical problem of delivery and scavenging these agents in the intensive-care environment as opposed to the operating room is a concern. The use of volatile anesthetics should be reserved for mechanically ventilated patients in whom maximal bronchodilator therapy is failing and where the appropriate equipment is available to deliver anesthetic gases.

Ketamine has been recommended for rapid induction of anesthesia in patients with asthma. It is thought to produce bronchodilation from a combination of an increase in circulating catecholamines, direct smooth muscle relaxation, and inhibition of vagal flow.[57] While anecdotal reports have suggested that ketamine is useful as short-term adjunct in acute severe asthma, the only controlled trial using 0.5 mg/kg per hour in spontaneously breathing adults with severe asthma reported no additional bronchodilation with standard therapy.[77]

Ketamine has several significant adverse effects, including the anesthesia emergence reaction, which can alter mood and cause delirium. These emergence phenomena occur in at least 25% of patients over 16 years of age; the incidence seems to be much lower in younger patients.[57] Other risks include an increase in heart rate, arterial blood pressure, and cerebral blood flow because of its sympathetic effects.[57]

PHARMACOECONOMICS

The number of emergency department visits for asthma exceeds the number of hospitalizations by approximately four times, yet the annual expenditures for emergency department visits ($478.6 million) is significantly less than the estimated $1.8 billion spent on inpatient hospital services for patients with acute severe asthma.[78] Thus, reducing the number of patients requiring hospitalizations is a primary goal of therapy. Inpatient services have declined as a percentage of total medical expenditures primarily as a result of decreasing duration of hospitalizations.[78] Few of the therapies used in the management of acute severe asthma have been formally evaluated for their pharmacoeconomic impact. One evaluation based on a metaanalysis of inhaled anticholinergics added to inhaled β_2-agonists in children with acute severe asthma suggested that this approach was cost-effective and would reduce overall costs by reducing hospitalizations.[79] In children with acute severe asthma admitted to an intensive-care unit, the use of continuously nebulized albuterol resulted in a decreased cost of care compared with intermittent nebulization.[80] A number of studies have suggested that conversion from small-volume nebulizers to MDIs with spacers in stable hospitalized patients, as well as use in the emergency department, can reduce the cost of aerosol therapy.[50] However, this strategy may require careful selection of patients, and the reduced costs must come from the cost of drugs and devices because personnel time is a fixed expense.[50]

CHRONIC ASTHMA

DIAGNOSIS

The diagnosis of asthma is made primarily by history and confirmatory spirometry.[2,37] The NAEPP has provided a list of questions that would lead to the diagnosis of asthma (see Table 26–2). In the older child and adult patient in whom spirometric evaluations can be performed, abnormal pulmonary functions that improve 15% or more following bronchodilator administration help confirm the diagnosis.[2] Failure of pulmonary functions to improve acutely does not necessarily rule out asthma. Patients with long-standing disease or substantial inflammation may require an intensive, prolonged course of bronchodilators and glucocorticoids before reversibility is detected.[2,37] If baseline spirometry is normal, challenge testing with exercise, histamine, or methacholine can be used to elicit BHR.[2] Patients with significant symptoms and/or an FEV_1 of less than 65% of predicted normal should not be challenged. Spirometry and bronchoprovocation have been shown to be more reliable indicators of BHR than a history of wheezing and physical examination.[37] Studies for atopy such as serum IgE and sputum and blood eosinophil determinations are not necessary to make the diagnosis of asthma, but they may help differentiate asthma from chronic bronchitis in adults. Clinically, this distinction is often difficult to make. Some patients with chronic bronchitis may have a reversible component, and some patients with long-standing severe chronic asthma may have significant irreversible damage and obstruction. Very high peripheral blood eosinophil counts may point to the diagnosis of aspergillosis or other hypereosinophilic syndromes.[37] Skin testing is of no value in diagnosing asthma but may be useful in identifying triggers.[2] In small infants unable to perform spirometry, the diagnosis is more difficult. They may demonstrate hyperinflation on the chest roentgenogram.[2] Radiologic examination is helpful in ruling out other causes of wheezing (e.g., foreign-body aspiration, parenchymal lung disease, cardiac disease, and congenital anomalies).[2] In place of pulmonary functions, the parents should be given a diary card to record symptoms and precipitating events.

GOALS OF MANAGEMENT

The NAEPP has provided the following goals for asthma management[2]:

1. Maintain normal activity levels (including exercise and other physical activity).
2. Maintain (near) normal pulmonary functions.
3. Prevent chronic and troublesome symptoms (e.g., coughing or breathlessness in the night, in the early morning, or after exertion).
4. Prevent recurrent exacerbations of asthma and minimize the need for emergency department visits or hospitalizations.
5. Provide optimal pharmacotherapy with minimal or no adverse effects.
6. Meet patients' and families' expectations of satisfaction with asthma care.[2]

Toward these goals, every effort should be made to decrease the patient's baseline BHR and prevent it from increasing.

NONPHARMACOLOGIC THERAPY

Although the mainstay of the management of asthma is pharmacologic therapy, it is likely to fail without attending to the nonpharmacologic therapy issues. Figure 26–9 depicts the stepwise approach to asthma therapy recommended by the NAEPP.[2] It is important to see that the nonpharmacologic aspects of therapy are incorporated into the steps. The guidelines were designed to give primary health care providers a framework from which to develop the proper approach to the individualized therapy of patients. The heterogeneity of asthma demands an individualized approach to therapy with the basic goals of therapy as primary outcome measures.[2]

The knowledge that inflammation plays a primary role in the pathogenesis of asthma has led to the conviction that the focus of therapy is the prevention and suppression of the underlying inflammation.[2] Thus current therapeutic options in asthma consist of acute reliever medications used for acute exacerbations and long-term control medications used for the prevention of symptoms and the suppression of inflammation.[2] The currently accepted approach is to use drugs that suppress the inflammatory response as primary long-term control therapy, thereby reducing the degree of BHR and improving long-term control and outcomes in asthma by preventing airway remodeling.[2]

The development of a partnership in care through patient education and the teaching of patient self- management skills should be the cornerstone of any treatment program.[2] There are a number of published self-management programs for children and adults available through local American Lung Association chapters as well as asthma treatment centers and nationally through the NAEPP and the Asthma and Allergy Foundation of America.[2] Asthma self-management programs have been shown to improve patient adherence to medication regimens, improve self-management skills, and improve use of health care services.[2] The object of these programs is to develop a partnership relationship between the patient and the health care provider. Table 26–7 lists the key educational messages recommended by the NAEPP.[2]

Self-management programs instruct patients in the pathogenesis of asthma and the appropriate use of their medications but focus principally on teaching patients to recognize triggers for their asthma and how to recognize early signs of deterioration. Use of objective measurement of airflow obstruction with a home peak-flow meter is integral to many of the programs.[2] However, following a review of the literature, the NAEPP suggests that routine peak-flow monitoring in and of itself does not improve patient outcomes.[2]

The NAEPP now advocates the routine use of peak-flow meters for only those patients with moderate and severe persistent asthma.[2] The NAEPP also has recommended a system based on a traffic light scenario (based on percentage of normal predicted values or personal best values): Green zone is equal to 80% to 100%; yellow zone is equal to 50% to 79%; red zone is less than 50%. The yellow zone is cautionary and requires increasing as needed bronchodilator use and either increasing the anti-inflammatory dose or beginning prednisone if not improved, whereas the red zone warrants contacting the patient's health care provider.[2] This approach can assist the patient and health professional in determining the next level of therapy.

Patient education is essential before monitoring can be effective. Patient education has proven successful regardless of the health professional who provided the information (physician, nurse, or pharmacist). The NAEPP advocates significant involvement of the primary health care provider in the educational process. The provision of written treatment plans enhances the success of education and peak-flow monitoring and is considered an essential component of care.[2] Samples of clinically tested written action plans are available from the NAEPP Expert Panel Report 2.[2]

In patients with known allergic triggers for their asthma, allergen avoidance has resulted in an improvement in symptoms, a reduction in medication use, and a decrease in BHR.[2,37] Relatively simple environmental controls for patients with house dust mite allergy such as removing carpeting from bedrooms, washing sheets in hot water (>130°F), and using plastic pillow and mattress covers can reduce symptoms and need for medications.[2,37] Obvious environmental triggers (i.e., warm-blooded animals, cockroaches), if the patient is sensitive, should be avoided; however, there is very little evidence that extensive environmental controls (i.e., home air-filtering systems and chemicals for killing house dust mites) are of any value.[2] Patients who smoke should be encouraged to stop. Parents of children with asthma should stop or at least not smoke around their children.[81]

The role of immunotherapy (allergy shots) in asthma, although a proven and accepted therapy for allergic rhinitis, is still controversial.[2] Some studies have shown that immunotherapy of patients with a very specific allergy reduces the number of late asthmatic responses and decreases BHR to the allergen, whereas others have shown no effect. A recent metaanalysis of immuotherapy trials suggested a positive

Treatment			Preferred treatments are in bold print.
	Long-term control	Quick relief	Education
STEP 4 Severe Persistent	Daily medications: • **Anti-inflammatory: inhaled corticosteroid (high dose)** AND • Long-acting bronchodilator: either **long-acting inhaled β_2-agonist,** sustained-release theophylline, or long-acting β_2-agonist tablets AND • Corticosteroid tablets or syrup long term (2 mg/kg/d, generally do not exceed 60 mg/d/).	• Short-acting bronchodilator: **inhaled β_2-agonists** as needed for symptoms. • Intensity of treatment will depend on severity of exacerbation; see component 3–Managing Exacerbations. • Use of short-acting inhaled β_2-agonists on a daily basis, or increasing use, indicates the need for additional long-term–control therapy.	Steps 2 and 3 actions plus: • Refer to individual education/counseling
STEP 3 Moderate Persistent	Daily medication: • Either **Anti-inflammatory: inhaled corticosteroid (medium dose)** OR **Inhaled corticosteroid (low-medium dose)** and add a long-acting bronchodilator, especially for nighttime symptoms: either **long-acting inhaled β_2-agonist,** sustained-release theophylline, or long-acting β_2-agonist tablets. • If needed Anti-inflammatory: **inhaled corticosteroids (medium-high dose)** AND **Long-acting bronchodilator**, especially for nighttime symptoms; either **long-acting inhaled β_2-agonist,** sustained-release theophylline, or long-acting β_2-agonist tablets.	• Short-acting bronchodilator: **inhaled β_2-agonists** as needed for symptoms. • Intensity of treatment will depend on severity of exacerbation; see component 3—Managing Exacerbations. • Use of short-acting inhaled β_2-agonists on a daily basis, or increasing use, indicates the need for additional long-term–control therapy.	Step 1 actions plus: • Teach self-monitoring • Refer to group education if available • Review and update self-management plan
STEP 2 Mild Persistent	One daily medication: • **Anti-inflammatory:** either **inhaled corticosteroid** (low doses) or **cromolyn or nedocromil** (children usually begin with a trial of cromolyn or nedocromil). • Sustained-release theophylline to serum concentration of 5–15 μg/mL is an alternative, but not preferred, therapy. Zafirlukast or zileuton may also be considered for patients ≥ 12 years of age, although their position in therapy is not fully established.	• Short-acting bronchodilator: **inhaled β_2-agonists** as needed for symptoms. • Intensity of treatment will depend on severity of exacerbation; see component 3—Managing Exacerbations. • Use of short-acting inhaled β_2-agonists on a daily basis, or increasing use, indicates the need for additional long-term–control therapy.	
STEP 1 Mild Intermittent	• No daily medication needed.	• Short-acting bronchodilator: **inhaled β_2-agonists** as needed for symptoms. • Intensity of treatment will depend on severity of exacerbation; see component 3–Managing Exacerbations. • Use of short-acting inhaled β_2-agonists more than 2 times a week may indicate the need to initiate long-term–control therapy.	• Teach basic facts about asthma • Teach inhaler/spacer/holding chamber technique • Discuss roles of medications • Develop self-management plan • Develop action plan for when and how to take rescue actions, especially for patients with a history of severe exacerbations • Discuss appropriate environmental control measures to avoid exposure to known allergens and irritants (See component 4.)

↓ Step down
Review treatment every 1–6 months; a gradual stepwise reduction in treatment may be possible.

↑ Step up
If control is not maintained, consider step up. First, review patient medication technique, adherence, and environmental control (avoidance of allergens or other factors that contribute to asthma severity).

Note:
- **The stepwise approach presents general guidelines to assist clinical decision making; it is not intended to be a specific prescription. Asthma is highly variable; clinicians should tailor specific medication plans to the needs and circumstances of individual patients.**
- Gain control as quickly as possible; then decrease treatment to the least medication necessary to maintain control. Gaining control may be accomplished by either starting treatment at the step most appropriate to the initial severity of the condition or starting at higher level of therapy (e.g., a course of systemic corticosteroids or higher dose of inhaled corticosteroids).
- A rescue course of systemic corticosteroids may be needed at any time and at any step.
- Some patients with intermittent asthma experience severe and life-threatening exacerbations separated by long periods of normal lung function and no symptoms. This may be especially common with exacerbations provoked by respiratory infections. A short course of systemic corticosteroids is recommended.
- At each step, patients should control their environment to avoid or control factors that make their asthma worse (e.g., allergens, irritants); this requires specific diagnosis and education.
- Referral to an asthma specialist for consultation or comanagement is *recommended* if there are difficulties achieving or maintaining control of asthma or if the patient requires step 4 care. Referral may be *considered* if the patient requires step 3 care.

FIGURE 26–9. Stepwise approach for managing asthma in adults and children older than 5 years of age. *(From Ref. 2.)*

benefit for specific immunotherapy against known allergens; however, the benefit was small in comparison with placebo.[82] A recent trial demonstrating an initial response to immunotherapy in the first year failed to find a continued effect in the second year.[83] Studies comparing immunotherapy with pharmacotherapy are warranted to determine the role for immunotherapy in asthma treatment.

PHARMACOLOGIC THERAPY

The current NAEPP recommendations for therapy of chronic asthma and acute exacerbations are illustrated in Fig. 26–11. Regardless of the long-term control therapy, all patients need to have quick relief medication available for acute symptoms.

TABLE 26–7. Key Educational Messages for Patients

Basic Facts About Asthma
- The contrast between asthmatic and normal airways
- What happens to the airways in an asthma attack

Roles of Medications
- How medications work
  Long-term control: medications that prevent symptoms, often by reducing inflammation
  Quick relief: short-acting bronchodilator relaxes muscles around airways
- Stress importance of long-term-control medications and not to expect quick relief from them

Skills
- Inhaler use (patient demonstrate)
- Spacer and holding chamber use
- Symptom monitoring, peak flow monitoring, and recognizing early signs of deterioration

Environmental Control Measures
- Identifying and avoiding environmental precipitants or exposures

When and How to Take Rescue Actions
- Responding to changes in asthma severity (daily self-management plan and action plan)

TABLE 26–8. Pharmacologic Responses to Sympathomimetic Agonists

Tissue	Receptor Type	Response
Airways	β_2	Smooth muscle relaxation (bronchodilation), increased ciliary beat, increased serous secretion, and inhibition of mast cell degranulation
	α	Smooth muscle contraction (bronchoconstriction?)
Heart	β_1	Inotropic and chronotropic
	β_2	Chronotropic
Vasculature	β_2	Vasodilation, decrease microvascular leakage
	α	Vasoconstriction
Skeletal	β_2	Increased neuromuscular transmission (tremor and increased strength of contraction)
Uterus	β_2	Relaxation (tocolysis)
Metabolic	α, β_1	Glycogenolysis, lipolysis
	β_2	Gluconeogenesis, hypokalemia, increased lactate production

β_2-Agonists

The β_2-agonists are the most effective bronchodilators available. The β_2-adrenergic receptors (β_2-ARs) are transmembrane proteins consisting of clusters of seven helices of amino acids that form the ligand-binding core.[84,85] Interestingly, the human β_2-ARs are polymorphic in their structure, with the most common polymorphisms in the amino terminus of the receptor at amino acid positions 16 [encoding either arginine (Arg) or glycine (Gly)] and 27 [encoding either glutamine (Gln) or glutamic acid (Glu)].[86] Some of the polymorphisms determine responsiveness to β_2-agonists, whereas others may act as disease modifiers (see below).[86] Stimulation of β_2-ARs activates cytoplasmic G proteins, which in turn activates adenylyl cyclase to produce cyclic adenosine monophosphate (cAMP), generally thought to be responsible for the bulk of activity through activation of various proteins by cAMP-dependent protein kinase (PKA).[86] This in turn decreases unbound intracellular calcium, producing smooth muscle relaxation, mast cell membrane stabilization, and skeletal muscle stimulation.[44] Despite the fact that β_2-agonists are potent inhibitors of mast cell degranulation in vitro, they do not inhibit the late asthmatic response to allergen challenge or the subsequent bronchial hyperresponsiveness.[2,44] Long-term administration of β_2-agonists does not reduce BHR, confirming a lack of significant anti-inflammatory activity.[44] β_2-Adrenergic stimulation also activates Na^+,K^+-ATPase, produces gluconeogenesis, and enhances insulin secretion, producing a mild to moderate decrease in serum potassium concentration by driving potassium intracellularly.[44] The chronotropic response to β_2-agonists is mediated in part by baroreceptor reflex mechanisms as a result of the drop in blood pressure from vascular smooth muscle relaxation, as well as by direct stimulation of cardiac β_2 receptors and some β_1 stimulation at high concentrations.[44] Table 26–8 lists the pharmacologic effects of adrenergic receptor stimulation. Because β_1-receptor stimulation produces excessive cardiac stimulation resulting in cardiac arrhythmias and the inotropic effect enhancing myocardial oxygen consumption leads to myocardial necrosis, there is no rationale for using non-β_2-selective agonists in the treatment of asthma.[44]

Table 26–9 compares the various β-adrenergic agonists in terms of selectivity, potency, oral activity, and duration of action. The β_2-agonists are functional or physiologic antagonists in that they

TABLE 26–9. Relative Selectivity, Potency, and Duration of Action of the β-Adrenergic Agonists

	Selectivity			Duration of Action[b]		
Agent	β_1	β_2	Potency, β_2[a]	*Bronchodilation (h)*	*Protection (h)*[c]	Oral activity
Isoproterenol	++++	++++	1	0.5–2	0.5–1	No
Metaproterenol	+++	+++	15	3–4	1–2	Yes
Isoetharine	++	+++	6	0.5–2	0.5–1	No
Albuterol	+	++++	2	4–8	2–4	Yes
Bitolterol	+	++++	5	4–8	2–4	No
Pirbuterol	+	++++	5	4–8	2–4	Yes
Terbutaline	+	++++	4	4–8	2–4	Yes
Formoterol	+	++++	0.24	≥12	6–12	Yes
Salmeterol	+	++++	0.5	≥12	6–>12	No

[a]Relative molar potency to isoproterenol: 15 = lowest potency.
[b]Median durations with the highest value after a single dose and lowest after chronic administration.
[c]Protection refers to the prevention of bronchoconstriction induced by exercise or nonspecific bronchial challenges.

relax airway smooth muscle regardless of the mechanism for constriction.[84,85] When administered in equipotent doses, all the short-acting drugs produce the same intensity of response; the only differences are in duration of action and cardiac toxicity.[2,85] The catecholamine derivatives all have the disadvantage of rapid inactivation of their 3,4 hydroxyl (OH) catechol group from catechol-*O*-methyltransferase found in the gastrointestinal tract, rendering them orally inactive. In addition, catecholamines are rapidly taken up into tissues by secondary uptake mechanisms that limit their receptor occupancy and thus have a shorter duration of action.[44,85] All the β_2-agonists are more bronchoselective when administered by the aerosol route.[44] Differences in myocardial effects are discernible between selective and nonselective agents even when administered as aerosols, particularly at the higher doses used for acute severe asthma. The β_2-agonists also differ in efficacy or ability to activate the β_2-ARs. Full agonists include the catecholamines, metaproterenol, and formoterol. Partial agonists include albuterol, terbutaline, pirbuterol, and salmeterol.[84] The principal differences between full and partial agonists is that full agonists require a lower fraction of receptor occupancy to produce their maximum effect and more easily produce receptor desensitization.[84]

All synthetic β_2-agonists are 1:1 racemic mixtures of two mirror images (enantiomers) due to an asymmetric or chiral carbon.[87] As most, physiologic functions (receptor occupancy and activation and enzymatic metabolism) are stereoselective; the (*R*) enantiomers of the β_2-agonists are the most pharmacologically active isomer.[87] While it was felt initially that the (*S*) enantiomers were essentially inactive due to the 1000-fold potency difference between the enantiomers, studies in animal models and isolated in vitro tissue preparations have suggested that the (*S*) enantiomers may be proinflammatory and could induce BHR.[87] However, evidence that this occurs consistently in humans or is clinically relevant is lacking (see below).[85,87] The pharmacokinetics are stereoselective as well, although not as predictable. (*R*)-Albuterol is more rapidly metabolized than (*S*)-albuterol, which could lead to accumulation of the (*S*)-albuterol with continued dosing. This is more exaggerated with oral dosing, as would be expected from a drug with a high first-pass effect.[84] On the other hand, (*S*)-terbutaline is eliminated more rapidly than (*R*)-terbutaline.[84]

Besides enhancing bronchoselectivity, the aerosol administration of β_2-agonists provides greater protection against provocations that induce bronchospasm such as exercise and allergen challenges than does systemic administration.[44] Currently, the only disadvantage to aerosol administration of β_2-agonists is the relative complexity of administration. The two long-acting β_2-agonists formoterol and salmeterol provide long-lasting bronchodilation (12 or more hours) when administered as aerosols.[44,84] Unlike the more water-soluble short-acting β_2-agonists, the long-acting agents are lipid-soluble, readily partitioning into the outer phospholipid layer of the cell membrane.[85] Salmeterol is more β_2-selective than albuterol and more bronchoselective by virtue of its property of remaining in the lung tissue cell membrane, which produces its longer duration.[84] However, both formoterol and salmeterol will produce dose-dependent systemic β_2-agonist effects.[85]

For the short-acting β_2-agonists, both the intensity and duration of response are dose-dependent, and more important, the dose-response relationship is dynamic.[44] At increasing levels of baseline bronchoconstriction (irrespective of the stimulus), the dose-response curve is shifted to the right, and the duration of bronchodilation is decreased.[60] This is reflected in the need for higher, more frequent doses in acute asthma exacerbations, and this is why the duration of protection against significant provocation is much less than the duration of bronchodilation in chronic stable asthma[44] (see Table 26–9).

Tolerance. Chronic administration of β_2-agonists can lead to a downregulation (decreased number of β_2 receptors) and a decreased binding affinity for these receptors.[44,84] Systemic corticosteroid therapy can both prevent and partially reverse this phenomenon.[2,44] However, the ability of ICSs to prevent tolerance to β_2-agonists has been inconsistent.[84] The glycine substitution at codon 16 (GLY-16) form of the receptor downregulates to a much greater extent compared with the arginine form (ARG-16) of the receptor after exposure to a β_2-agonist.[86] The heterozygous ARG-16/GLY-16 is intermediately desensitized compared with the homozygous GLY-16. On the other hand, glutamate substitution at codon 27 (GLU-27) protects against downregulation compared with the glutamine form (GLN-27) of the receptor.[86] However, the GLY-16 overcomes any protective effect of GLU-27.[86] Tolerance primarily reduces duration of bronchodilation as opposed to peak response. A significantly greater tolerance develops in other tissues (e.g., lymphocytes and cardiac and skeletal muscle) compared with the lung primarily as a result of the surplus β_2 receptors found in respiratory smooth muscle.[44] Tolerance to the extrapulmonary effects (cardiac stimulation and hypokalemia) may account for a lack of significant cardiac effects with retention of the bronchodilator response despite chronic inhaled β_2-agonist therapy, whereas tolerance to mast cell stabilization may be a drawback to chronic use.[44] Thus chronic β_2-agonist administration produces a tolerance of minimal clinical significance that is easily overcome by increasing the dose or by administering corticosteroids.[2,44] Most of the tolerance occurs within a week of regular administration and does not worsen with continued administration.

As would be expected from a receptor phenomenon, tolerance also develops to the long-acting β_2-agonists.[44] Long-term trials have shown no diminution in bronchodilator response but a significant reduction in protection against bronchoprovocation. In particular, the duration of protection against EIB following a single dose of salmeterol is up to 9 hours but is reduced to less than 4 hours following regular treatment.[85] Following regular treatment with salmeterol, decreased protection against nonspecific bronchoprovocation with methacholine also occurs, although it provides greater protection than placebo.[84] Responsiveness to short-acting β_2-agonists has been reported to be slightly decreased (although easily overcome by increasing the dose) or not affected by chronic therapy with long-acting β_2-agonists.[85]

The β_2-Agonist Controversy. The potential for chronic use of inhaled β_2-agonists to worsen asthma and for excessive use to increase the risk of dying from asthma has been a concern for over 30 years. A complete review is beyond the scope of this chapter. A number of short-term trials suggest an increased responsiveness to allergen and a rebound increase in BHR following regular treatment with short-acting inhaled β_2-agonists.[84] However, two multicenter double-blind, placebo-controlled trials in large numbers of patients with both mild and moderate persistent asthma have not confirmed that regular administration short-acting inhaled β_2-agonists worsens asthma.[88,89] A recent retrospective genotyping of patients from the U.S. study suggests that the homozygous ARG-16 predisposes to worsening asthma as measured by lower morning PEFs but not increasing BHR during regular use of short-acting β_2-agonists.[90] This needs confirmation with a prospective trial because the number of patients homozygous for ARG-16 was small (16% of patients). Morning PEFs did not fall in any other group, suggesting that the potential for worsening asthma is unrelated to β_2 receptor downregulation. Long-term studies with the long-acting inhaled β_2-agonists have not demonstrated a rebound increase in BHR after discontinuation or a worsening of asthma.[84]

Numerous epidemiologic studies have suggested an increased risk of asthma death and near-death episodes associated with excessive use of β_2-agonists by MDI. However, case-control studies are confounded by disease severity affecting therapy. The increased risk appeared primarily if the increased use of the β_2-agonists occurred in the 2 months prior to the event, suggesting that the increased use was a marker for asthma deterioration as opposed to a causative factor.[14] No evidence exists for an increased risk of death from regular use of the long-acting inhaled β_2-agonists.[2,44]

Clinical Use. Inhaled short-acting selective β_2-agonists are indicated for the treatment of intermittent episodes of bronchospasm and are the bronchodilator as well as the first treatment of choice for acute severe asthma.[2,44,60] The inhaled selective β_2-agonists are the treatment of choice for EIB.[2,44] They inhibit EIB in a dose-dependent fashion and provide complete protection for a 2-hour period following inhalation with varying levels of patient-dependent protection over 4 hours.[44] The new long-acting agents provide significant protection for 8 to 12 hours after a single dose but are likely not superior to the short-acting agents with regular use as the duration diminishes.[84] Although the regular administration of β_2-agonists slightly decreases the effect on EIB, two inhalations prior to exercise still essentially blocks EIB completely (1% versus 5% drop in FEV_1).[91]

Since the use of short-acting inhaled β_2-agonists does not improve control of symptoms, their use can be used to measure asthma control, so it is recommended that they only be used as needed for symptoms.[2] Although the long-acting inhaled β_2-agonists are preferred over oral sustained-release β_2-agonists or sustained-release theophylline for nocturnal asthma, nocturnal asthma may be an indicator of inadequate anti-inflammatory treatment, and the introduction of or dosage adjustment of these agents should be considered.[92] Long-acting inhaled β_2-agonists are indicated as adjunctive long-term control for patients with symptoms who are already on low to medium doses of ICSs prior to advancing to medium- or high-dose ICSs (see below).[2] Patients should be warned that salmeterol is ineffective for acute severe asthma because it can take up to 20 minutes for onset and 1 to 4 hours for maximum bronchodilation following inhalation.[2,44] Patients need to be counseled to continue to use their short-acting inhaled β_2-agonists for acute exacerbations.

Methylxanthines

Methylxanthines have been used for asthma therapy for over 50 years. Theophylline is the primary methylxanthine of interest, although others such as caffeine, dyphylline, and enprophylline also produce bronchodilation.[2,93,94] Like the β_2-agonists, the methylxanthines are functional antagonists of bronchospasm; however, their clinical potency is limited by their low therapeutic index.[2] Theophylline as a sustained-release product is the preferred oral preparation, whereas its complex with ethylenediamine (aminophylline) is the preferred injectable product due to increased solubility.[94]

The mechanism by which theophylline produces bronchodilation appears to be through phosphodiesterase (PDE) inhibition.[93] Inhibition of PDE results in increased cAMP and cyclic GMP concentrations. The PDE isoenzymes currently thought to be important in asthma are PDE III, predominant in airway smooth muscle, and PDE IV, important in inflammatory cell regulation such as mast cells, eosinophils, and T-lymphocytes.[93] PDE inhibition is consistent with various nonbronchodilator activities that may be relevant to asthma, including decreased mast cell mediator release, decreased eosinophil basic protein release, decreased T-lymphocyte proliferation, decreased T-cell cytokine release, and decreased plasma exudation. Selective PDE isoenzyme inhibitors are currently being evaluated for possible treatment of asthma. Theophylline is a nonselective PDE inhibitor.[93] Some clinical trials indicate that theophylline may provide anti-inflammatory activity in asthma.[93] However, studies have failed to demonstrate an effect on BHR except when the drug is present as a functional antagonist to the provocative agent.[2] Theophylline is a competitive antagonist of adenosine and stimulates endogenous catecholamine release.[93] These latter two effects are important determinants of toxic symptoms of excess theophylline.[2,93]

Both bronchodilation and protection against bronchoprovocation challenges are concentration-dependent. Theophylline produces linear increases in bronchodilation with logarithmic increments in serum drug concentrations.[94] The majority of chronic stable asthmatics will obtain significant bronchodilation when the serum theophylline concentration reaches 5 μg/mL, and most patients will have no toxic symptoms with serum concentrations of less than 15 μg/mL.[2,95] The percentage of patients experiencing adverse effects is approximately 18% at serum concentrations between 15 and 20 μg/mL.[95] This increases sharply to 60% at concentrations between 20 and 30 μg/mL and to 80% at concentrations greater than 30 μg/mL. As with the β_2-agonists, the dose-response curves for smooth muscle relaxation by theophylline are dynamic and shifted to the right in the face of increasing contractile stimuli.[95] This probably explains theophylline's relative lack of bronchodilatory effect in acute severe asthma.[2,57] The severity of theophylline's toxicity precludes even doubling the usual dosage.

Other effects that may be important to theophylline's antiasthmatic action include decreasing vascular permeability, enhancing mucociliary clearance, and strengthening of contractions of a fatigued diaphragm.[93] In vitro theophylline inhibits the release of histamine in sensitized human lung fragments but has provided an inconsistent protection against the early asthmatic response to allergen.[95] When present in therapeutic concentrations, theophylline attenuates the bronchospasm of the late asthmatic response but has no apparent effect on the subsequent increase in BHR.[2,95]

Other Effects. Theophylline stimulates the central nervous system through its adenosine antagonism and produces cerebral vasoconstriction, potentiating seizures.[95] Theophylline acts as a respiratory stimulant by enhancing the hypoxic ventilatory drive, it decreases the lower esophageal sphincter pressure and increases gastric acid secretion, and it has both inotropic and chronotropic cardiac effects.[95] Acutely, theophylline acts as a diuretic, but tolerance develops rapidly.

Pharmacokinetics. Routine monitoring of serum concentrations is essential for the safe and effective use of theophylline.[94,95] Theophylline is eliminated primarily by metabolism via the hepatic cytochrome P-450 mixed-function oxidase microsomal enzymes (primarily the CYP1A2 and CYP3A3 isozymes), with 10% or less excreted unchanged in the kidney.[94] The major metabolic pathways for theophylline are saturable within the usual therapeutic concentration, so theophylline frequently, though not always, exhibits nonlinear pharmacokinetics.[94] This may explain in part the relatively large intrapatient variability in theophylline clearance (often as great as 30%) over time.[94] Theophylline clearance is age-dependent, with 1- to 9-year-olds having the greatest clearances and therefore requiring the largest dosages (on a weight basis). However, even within the same age groups theophylline clearance can vary two- to threefold.[94] Figure 26–10 gives a dosing and monitoring schedule for theophylline.

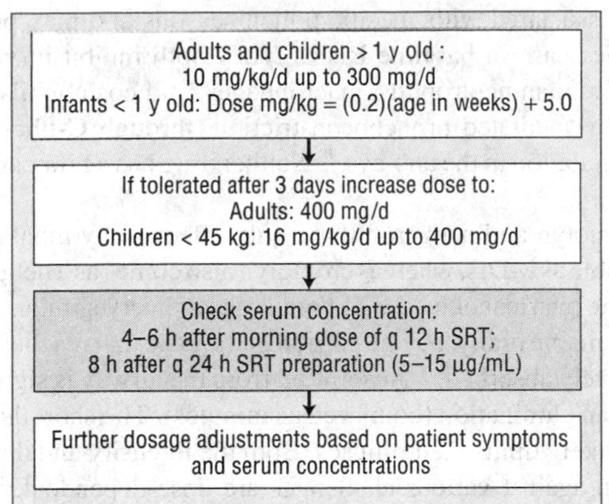

Adults and children > 1 y old :
10 mg/kg/d up to 300 mg/d
Infants < 1 y old: Dose mg/kg = (0.2)(age in weeks) + 5.0
If tolerated after 3 days increase dose to:
Adults: 400 mg/d
Children < 45 kg: 16 mg/kg/d up to 400 mg/d
Check serum concentration:
4–6 h after morning dose of q 12 h SRT;
8 h after q 24 h SRT preparation (5–15 μg/mL)
Further dosage adjustments based on patient symptoms
and serum concentrations

FIGURE 26–10. Algorithm for slow titration of theophylline dosage and guide for final dosage adjusment based on serum theophylline concentration measurement. For infants <1 year of age, the initial daily dosage can be calculated by the following regression equation: Dose (mg/kg) = (0.2) (age in weeks) + 5.0. *Whenever side effects occur, dosage should be reduced to a previously tolerated lower dose.*

The hepatic cytochrome P-450 enzymes are susceptible to induction and inhibition by various environmental factors and drugs. These are listed in Table 26–10. Only those drugs or diseases which produce a 20% or greater inhibition or 50% or greater induction of theophylline metabolism are likely to result in clinically significant interactions.[94,95]

Due to the relatively short elimination half-life of theophylline (3–5 hours in children and 6–12 hours in adults), sustained-release oral preparations are favored for outpatient therapy.[2] These preparations can be administered every 8 to 24 hours in patients and maintain relatively constant therapeutic serum concentrations.[93,94] The degree of serum theophylline concentration fluctuation over the dosing interval depends on the release characteristics of the products, as well as on the elimination-rate characteristics of the patients.[93] Thus patients with rapid clearances for theophylline will experience greater fluctuations than patients with slow clearances, given the same product over the same dosing interval. Neither an optimal nor an acceptable maximum fluctuation has been established absolutely for theophylline serum concentration, but it seems reasonable that it should not exceed the usual therapeutic range. That is, it should not exceed 100% for twice-daily dosing or 150% for once-daily dosing, where percent fluctuation $= Cp_{max} - Cp_{min}/Cp_{min}$. Each of the sustained-release theophylline products has different release characteristics, and the products are variably susceptible to altered absorption from food or gastric pH changes.[94,95] Preparations with slower release characteristically exhibit a significant diurnal variation in absorption, with the rate significantly slower at night in the recumbent patient.[94] As a result of these differences, it is best not to consider the sustained-release preparations interchangeable. In general, preparations unaffected by food that can be administered a minimum of every 12 hours in most patients are preferable.

Clinical Use. Regular theophylline administration can reduce asthma symptoms, reduce the amount of as-needed inhaled β_2-agonists used, and reduce the oral steroid requirement in steroid-dependent asthmatics.[93] Sustained-release theophylline once nightly is effective for nocturnal asthma.[93] Comparative studies between sustained-release theophylline and oral sustained-release β_2-agonists have not shown any advantage for theophylline.[2] Comparisons of cromolyn and theophylline as first-line therapy for chronic asthma have failed to demonstrate an advantage for theophylline over cromolyn.[95] Although the addition of theophylline to ICSs reduces the number of asthma exacerbations, it is overall less effective than the long-acting inhaled β_2-agonists as adjunctive therapy.[96] Significant disadvantages to chronic theophylline therapy are the dangers inherent in giving a drug that can produce severe cardiac arrhythmias and neurologic toxicity, including seizures, permanent neurologic deficit, and death at serum concentrations only twofold greater than optimal therapeutic concentrations. Death has occurred in children receiving their usual doses of theophylline during acute systemic viral illnesses.[95]

The therapeutic range for theophylline of 5–15 μg/mL is not an absolute but a statistical concept.[94] This therapeutic range has been recommended by the NAEPP as an effective and safe range of steady-state concentrations for most patients.[2] Due to the log-linear nature of the concentration-response curve, there is little bronchodilation to gain by going from 15 to 20 μg/mL. Patients whose theophylline concentrations are maintained near 20 μg/mL are more susceptible to developing serious adverse effects when confronted with an environmental exposure that inhibits theophylline metabolism. Due to its high risk-benefit ratio, theophylline is considered a second- or third line drug in the therapy of asthma.[2]

TABLE 26–10. Factors Affecting Theophylline Clearance

Decreased Clearance	% Decrease	Increased clearance	% Increase
Cimetidine	−25 to −60	Rifampin	+53
Macrolides:	−25 to −50	Carbamazepine	+50
Erythromycin, TAO, clarithromycin		Phenobarbital	+34
		Phenytoin	+70
Allopurinol	−20	Charcoal-broiled meat	+30
Propranolol	−30		
Quinolones:	−20 to −50	High-protein diet	+25
Ciprofloxacin, enoxacin, pefloxacin		Smoking	+40
Interferon	−50	Sulfinpyrazone	+22
Thiabendazole	−65	Moricizine	+50
Ticlopidine	−25	Aminoglutethimide	+50
Zileuton	−35		
Systemic viral illness	−10 to −50		

Anticholinergics

The anticholinergic agents have been used for centuries in the form of stramonium herbal treatments for asthma.[1,2] However, their systemic effects, particularly involving the central nervous system, limited their usefulness. Anticholinergics are competitive inhibitors of muscarinic receptors.[97] Unlike β_2-agonists and theophylline, they are not functional antagonists; they only produce bronchodilation in cholinergic-mediated bronchoconstriction.[72] Normal bronchial tone is maintained through parasympathetic innervation of the airways via the vagus nerve. A number of the triggers and mediators of asthma (i.e., histamine, prostaglandins, sulfur dioxide, exercise, and allergens) produce bronchoconstriction in part through vagal reflex mechanisms.[2] Studies of asthmatics consistently demonstrate that anticholinergics are effective bronchodilators, although not as potent as β_2-agonists. Anticholinergics attenuate but do not block allergen- or exercise-induced asthma in a dose-dependent fashion and have no effect on the LAR or BHR.[2]

Currently available anticholinergics are nonselective muscarinic receptor blockers, and blockade of inhibitory muscarinic receptors theoretically could result in an increased release of acetylcholine and overcome the block on the smooth muscle receptors (M_3).[97] This mechanism may explain why some patients have experienced paradoxical bronchoconstriction from nebulized anticholinergics. Only the quaternary ammonium derivatives (ipratropium bromide) should be used because they have the advantage of poor absorption across mucosae and the blood-brain barrier. This results in negligible systemic effects with a prolonged local effect (i.e., bronchodilation). In addition, the quaternary compounds do not appear to produce a decrease in mucociliary clearance.[97] Ipratropium bromide has a duration of action of 4 to 8 hours. Both intensity and duration of action are dose-dependent. Time to reach maximum bronchodilation is considerably slower than from aerosolized short-acting β_2-agonists (2 hours versus 30 minutes). However, this is of little clinical consequence because some bronchodilation is seen within 30 seconds, 50% of maximum response occurs within 3 minutes, and 80% of maximum is reached within 30 minutes.[97]

Clinical Use. The role of anticholinergics in the treatment of asthma is limited. Unfortunately, the addition of ipratropium bromide has not improved outcomes in chronic asthma over β_2-agonists alone, so asthma is not an approved indication.[2] Ipratropium bromide is only indicated as adjunctive therapy in acute severe asthma not completely responsive to β_2-agonists alone.[2,72]

Cromolyn Sodium and Nedocromil Sodium

Cromolyn sodium has been available for the prophylactic treatment of asthma for over 30 years, whereas nedocromil sodium, a pyranoquinoline dicarboxylic acid that is pharmacologically similar, is a more recent addition.[2] Although they are classified as mast cell stabilizers, the exact mechanism of action for these agents is still unknown. While minor differences in activity do exist, the principal difference appears to be potency, with 4 mg nedocromil by MDI equivalent to 10 mg cromolyn assessed by bronchoprovocation.[98] However, there is no apparent difference in the clinical efficacy between these two drugs.[2] They produce mast cell membrane stabilization, inhibiting the EAR to allergen challenge as well as EIB.[2,98] Cromolyn and nedocromil also inhibit the LAR and prevent the subsequent increased BHR.[98] Long-term treatment with cromolyn prevents the usual rise in BHR associated with specific pollen seasons and may produce a modest decrease in baseline BHR.[2] They both inhibit in vitro activation of human neutrophils, macrophages, and eosinophils, as well as neurally mediated bronchoconstriction, through C-fiber sensory nerve stimulation in the airways.[98] Neither drug has a bronchodilatory effect.

Cromolyn and nedocromil are only effective by inhalation and are available as MDIs, whereas cromolyn also comes as a nebulizer solution. The pharmacokinetics of both drugs are very similar. They are not bioavailable orally, but the portion of the dose that reaches the lung is completely absorbed.[98] Absorption from the airway is significantly slower than elimination (hours versus minutes). The short duration in the lung likely limits their efficacy. Both the intensity and duration of protection against various challenges are dose-dependent.[98] Higher doses produce greater and more prolonged protection.

Both drugs are remarkably nontoxic. No evidence of mutagenesis or teratogenesis has been found for cromolyn. Cough and wheeze have been reported following inhalation of each and bad taste and headache following nedocromil.[2] The taste from nedocromil is sufficiently bad in some patients (approximately 20%) to preclude them from taking the drug. Cromolyn is undoubtedly the least toxic drug used to treat asthma, with significant adverse effects occurring in less than 1 in 10,000 patients.[99] Tolerance to cromolyn or nedocromil has not been demonstrated. Short-term clinical trials suggest that approximately 60% to 75% of patients (adults and children) with mild persistent asthma will receive a positive benefit from cromolyn.[2] Nedocromil but not cromolyn may be able to produce a decrease in inhaled steroid dosage.[2,98]

Comparative studies between cromolyn and theophylline do not demonstrate a significant advantage for either agent in controlling symptoms of asthma or improving baseline pulmonary functions.[99] Comparisons with the LT antagonists also suggest equivalent efficacy.[100] Neither cromolyn nor nedocromil is as effective as the ICSs for controlling persistent asthma.[10,99]

Clinical Use. Cromolyn and nedocromil are indicated for the prophylaxis of mild persistent asthma in both children and adults regardless of etiology. They may be particularly effective for allergic asthmatics on a seasonal basis or just prior to an acute exposure (i.e., animals or mowing the lawn).[2] Cromolyn is the second drug of choice for the prevention of EIB and may be used in conjunction with a β_2-agonist in more severe cases not completely responding to either agent alone.[2] Most patients will experience an improvement in 1 to 2 weeks, but it may take longer to achieve maximum benefit. Patients initially should receive cromolyn or nedocromil four times daily, and then only after stabilization of symptoms may the frequency be reduced to two times daily for nedocromil and three times daily for cromolyn. The NAEPP and the more recently released "Pediatric Asthma: Promoting Best Practice" have suggested that cromolyn and nedocromil should be the anti-inflammatories of first choice for childhood asthma due to their efficacy and safety.[2,101] However, the results from two large, well-controlled clinical trials have questioned the validity of these recommendations. In 1- to 4-year-olds ($N = 218$) with moderate asthma, cromolyn 10 mg three times daily by MDI plus spacer was no better than placebo over 22 weeks of therapy.[102] In 5- to 12-year-olds ($N = 730$) with mild to moderate persistent asthma, nedocromil 8 mg twice daily by MDI plus spacer device reduced only urgent care visits and prednisone usage over a 4- to 6-year span.[11] All other measures of asthma control including BHR, baseline lung function, use of as-needed albuterol, hospitalizations, episode-free

TABLE 26–11. Pharmacodynamic/Pharmacokinetic Comparison of the Corticosteroids

Systemic	Anti-inflammatory Potency	Mineralcorticoid Potency	Duration of Biologic Activity (h)	Elimination Half-Life (h)
Hydrocortisone	1	1.0	8–12	1.5–2.0
Prednisone	4	0.8	12–36	2.5–3.5
Methylprednisolone	5	0.5	12–36	3.3
Dexamethasone	25	0	36–54	3.4–4.0
ICS	**Receptor Binding Affinity**	**Topical Skin Blanching**	**Oral Bioavailability (%)**	**Systemic Clearance (L/h)**	**Half-Life (h) IV/Inhaled**
BDP/BMP	0.4/13.5	600/400	15–20	UK	0.5/1.5–6.5
BUD	9.4	980	11	55–84	2.8/2.0
FLU	1.8	330	20	58	1.6/1.6
FP	18	1200	≤1	66	7.8/14.4
MF	27[a]	UK	<1	53	5.8/UK
TAA	3.6	330	23	45–69	2.0/3.6

Note: Receptor binding affinities and topical skin blanching are relative to dexamethasone equal to 1. UK = unknown.
[a]MF studied in a different receptor system. Value estimated from relative values of BDP, TAA, and FP in that system.

days, and symptom scores were not different from placebo. In addition, a recent metaanalysis of 24 placebo controlled trials in children suggested that there was insufficient evidence that cromolyn was beneficial as maintenance treatment for chronic asthma.[103] Thus their status as first-line agents would seem to be diminishing.

Corticosteroids

The corticosteroids are the most effective anti-inflammatories available to treat asthma.[2,51] The mechanism of action and use of corticosteroids in asthma have been reviewed extensively.[51,104–108] Actions useful in treating asthma include (1) increasing the number of β_2-ARs and improving the receptor responsiveness to β_2-adrenergic stimulation, (2) reducing mucus production and hypersecretion, (3) reducing BHR, and (4) preventing and reversing airway remodeling.[51,105] The glucocorticosteroid receptor is found in the cytoplasm of most cells throughout the body, explaining the multiple effects of systemic corticosteroids. The corticosteroids are highly lipophilic, readily cross the cell membrane, and combine with the glucocorticoid receptor. The activated complex then enters the nucleus, where it acts as a transcription factor leading to gene activation or suppression.[105] This leads to specific mRNA production, resulting in increased production of anti-inflammatory mediators such as lipocortin-1, β_2-ARs, neutral endopeptidase, and endonucleases.[104,105] Other mRNA is suppressed decreasing the synthesis and release of several proinflammatory cytokines such as IL 1, GM CSF, IL-3, IL-4, IL-5, IL-6, and IL-8; reducing inflammatory cell activation, recruitment, and infiltration; and decreasing vascular permeability.[104,105] In addition, the activated glucocorticosteroid receptor complex can act directly with cytoplasmic transcription factors, nuclear factor kappa B, and activating protein 1 to prevent the action of proinflammatory cytokines on the cell.[105]

Time Course of Response. Due to the mechanism to modify gene expression, the time required to see the particular effect depends on the time required for new protein synthesis, decreased formation of the particular mediator, and resolution of the response.[106] Generally, the cellular and biochemical effects are immediate, but varying amounts of time are required to produce a clinical response. β_2-Receptor density increases within 4 hours of corticosteroid administration.[105] Improved responsiveness to β_2-agonists occurs within 2 hours.[66] In acute severe asthma, 4 to 12 hours may be required before any clinical response is noted.[66] Reversal of seasonal increased BHR requires at least 1 week of therapy.[105] Sensitivity to EIB decreases after 4 weeks of therapy with ICSs.[104] Although single doses do not inhibit the immediate asthmatic response to antigen challenge, continued therapy for 1 week partially suppresses the response. These two latter effects are likely due to a reduction in mucosal mast cells.[51,105]

The response to ICSs is somewhat more delayed. Most patients' symptoms will improve in the first 1 to 2 weeks of therapy and reach maximum improvement in 4 to 8 weeks. Improvement in baseline FEV_1 and PEFs may require 3 to 6 weeks for maximum improvement,[104,106] whereas improvement in BHR requires 1 to 3 months and may continue to improve over 1 year.[106] No evidence indicates that the use of corticosteroids in the persistent asthmatic will induce a state of steroid dependence. In fact, most of the evidence demonstrating a decrease in BHR and cellular infiltration with corticosteroid therapy implies just the opposite.

Systemic Corticosteroid Therapy. The corticosteroids used in asthma are compared in Table 26–11. Besides acute severe asthma, systemic corticosteroids are also recommended for the treatment of impending episodes of severe asthma unresponsive to bronchodilator therapy.[2,66] The effects of corticosteroids in asthma are dose- and duration-dependent. This is true for the adverse effects as well (Table 26–12). The clinician is continually forced to balance the toxicity

TABLE 26–12. Adverse Effects of Chronic Systemic Glucocorticoid Administration

Hypothalamic–pitutitary-adrenal suppression	Hypertension
Growth retardation	Skin striae
Skeletal muscle myopathy	Impaired wound healing
Osteoporosis/fractures	Inhibition of leukocyte and monocyte function
Aseptic necrosis of bone	Subcutaneous tissue atrophy
Pancreatitis	Glaucoma
Pseudotumor cerebri	Posterior subcapsular cataracts
Psychiatric disturbances	Moon facies
Sodium and water retention	Central redistribution of fat
Hypokalemia/hyperglycemia	

of chronic systemic corticosteroid therapy with control of asthma symptoms. Because short-term (1–2 weeks) high-dose corticosteroids (1–2 mg/kg/d prednisone) do not produce serious toxicities, the ideal use is to administer the systemic corticosteroids in a short "burst" and then maintain the patient on appropriate long-term control therapy with long periods between systemic corticosteroid treatment.[2] In general, therapy for more than 5 days at doses that exceed the usual physiologic endogenous cortisol production will cause temporary aberration in adrenal cortisol release.[66] However, in studies, this hypothalamic-pituitary-adrenal (HPA) axis suppression is short-lived (1–3 days) and readily reversible following short bursts (10 days or less) of pharmacologic doses.[66] A maximum number of short bursts that a patient can receive probably exists, after which chronic corticosteroid side effects occur. Patients receiving at least eight bursts (of at least 10 days each) were shown to have a similar decrease in trabecular bone density as patients on daily or alternate-day steroids over 1 year.[66] Children who received four or more bursts of prednisone exhibited a subnormal response to hypoglycemic stress or adrenocorticotropic hormone (ACTH) administration.[66] Very short courses of (3–5 days) have been effective in reducing hospitalization from acute exacerbations.[2,66]

In patients who require chronic systemic corticosteroids for control of asthma, the lowest possible dose required to control symptoms should be used. Physicians often will sacrifice complete control of the patient's symptoms to avoid toxicity. Two methods of decreasing the toxicity are to use alternate-day therapy or high-dose ICSs. Studies have suggested that administering a single daily dose at 3:00 to 5:00 P.M. provides increased efficacy without increasing toxicity.[2,92] Once control is achieved, the prednisone dose is tapered and replaced by ICSs if possible.

Inhaled Corticosteroids. The ICSs beclomethasone dipropionate (BDP), budesonide (BUD), flunisolide (FLU), fluticasone propionate (FP), mometasone furoate (MF), and triamcinolone acetonide (TAA) that are currently available for use are compared and listed in Table 26–13. The ICSs differ significantly in topical potency and have pharmacokinetic differences that result in different topical/systemic activity.[104,107] Most evidence is consistent with log-linear dose-response curves for both indirect and direct responses.[107] The log-linear nature of the dose-response curve for corticosteroid activity raises the issue of how much of a difference in dose (or lung delivery) or potency is detectable. The dose-response curves for the ICSs are relatively flat, primarily because all the measures used to assess efficacy (lung function, BHR, symptoms, and as- needed β_2-agonist use) are downstream events from the anti-inflammatory activity.[104] However, clinical trials of sufficient power have been able to detect twofold differences in potency.[104] The NAEPP provides clinically comparable doses to be used by clinicians.[2] However, the comparisons are primarily based on in vitro potency differences, limited pharmacokinetic studies, and a small number of clinical comparative trials. There have now been over 35 direct comparative ICS clinical trials in over 6000 patients.[108] The table of comparative doses (see Table 26–13) is based on this recent information as well as some of the newer formulations that have become available. Clinical comparative doses

TABLE 26–13. Available Inhaled Corticosteroid Products, Lung Delivery, and Comparative Doses

ICS	Product	Lung Delivery[a]
Beclomethasone dipropionate (BDP)	42 μg/actuation CFC MDI, 200 actuations	4–10%
	40 and 80 μg/actuation HFA MDI, 120 actuations	55–60%
Budesonide (BUD)	200 μg/dose DPI, Turbuhaler, 200 doses	32% (16–59%)
	200 and 500-μg ampules, 2 mL each	6%
Flunisolide (FLU)	250 μg/actuation CFC MDI, 100 actuations	32%
Fluticasone propionate (FP)	44, 110, and 220 μg/actuation CFC MDI, 120 actuations	26–30%
	50, 100, and 250 μg/dose DPI, Rotadisk, 4 doses	15% (13–18%)
	50, 100, and 250 μg/dose DPI, Diskus, 60 doses	15%
Mometasone furoate (MF)	200 and 400 μg/dose DPI, Twisthaler, 14, 30, 60, and 120 doses	Unknown
Triamcinolone acetonide (TAA)	100 μg/actuation CFC MDI, 240 actuations with spacer	22%

	Comparable Daily doses (μg)		
	Low Dose, Child/Adult	*Medium Dose, Child/Adult*	*High Dose, Child/Adult*
BDP			
CFC MDI	84–336/168–504	336–672/504–840	>672/>840
HFA MDI	40–160/80–240	160–320/240–400	>320/>400
BUD			
DPI	100–200/200–400	200–400/400–800	>400/>800
Nebules	250–500/UK	500–1000/UK	>1000/UK
FLU, CFC MDI	500–750/500–1000	750–1250/1000–2000	>1250/>2000
FP			
CFC MDI	88–176/88–264	176–440/264–660	>440/>660
DPIs	100–200/100–300	200–400/300–600	>400/>600
MF, DPI	UK/200–400	UK/400–800	UK />800
TAA, CFC MDI	400–800/400–1000	800–1200/1000–2000	>1200/>2000

[a]Lung delivery from in vivo radiolabel scintigraphy or pharmacokinetic studies.

take into consideration potency differences as well as lung delivery differences.

The ICSs have high anti-inflammatory potency, approximately 1000-fold greater than endogenous cortisol, and differ from each other by as much as 4- to 6-fold.[104] However, potency differences, which are simply a measure of binding affinity to the receptor, can be overcome simply by giving different microgram dosages of drug. For example, the CFC-propelled MDIs of BDP and TAA are equivalent on a per-puff basis because of the difference in microgram per puff in each inhaler.[107] Aerosol delivery of the preparations is remarkably variable, ranging from 10% to 60% of the nominal dose (i.e., that dose which leaves an actuator for an MDI or in the case of a DPI that which is released on activation of the inhaler).[50,108] Different devices for the same chemical entity may result in 2-fold differences in delivery, such as with fluticasone propionate and budesonide, or as much as 8-fold with BDP preparations.[108] Thus the delivery method can make a significant difference in the relative comparable dose.[2,108]

Differences in the pharmacokinetic profile are required to produce differences in the topical-systemic effect ratio.[107] Pharmacokinetic properties that enhance improved topical selectivity include rapid systemic clearance, poor oral bioavailability, and long residence time in the lung.[107] Due to their high lipophilicity, systemic clearance of the available ICSs is very rapid, approaching the rate of liver blood flow.[107] However, the ICSs differ markedly in their oral bioavailability, although they all undergo rather extensive first-pass metabolism to less active substances when absorbed[55] (see Table 26–11). The ICSs produce dose-dependent systemic effects from a combination of the orally absorbed fraction and the fraction absorbed from the lung[55,106] (Table 26–14). Essentially all the drug that reaches the lung is systemically absorbed; thus a slow absorption from the lung results in an apparent long elimination $t_{1/2}$ and will enhance topical selectivity by lowering the systemic concentration.[107] The potential advantage of the drugs with low orally bioavailability is obviated by using a spacer device with the MDI for the drugs with higher oral bioavailability because appropriate spacers reduce the oral dose by 80%.[106] The ability of spacer devices to enhance lung delivery is inconsistent and should not be relied on. Mouth rinsing and spitting also will reduce the oral availability and is particularly useful for DPI devices.[2]

TABLE 26–14. Effects of Inhaled Corticosteroids

Beneficial Effects	Potential Adverse Effects
Decrease eosinophil numbers	Growth retardation, skeletal muscle myopathy
Decrease mast cell numbers	Osteoporosis, fractures and aseptic necrosis of hip
Decrease T-lymphocyte cytokine production	Posterior subcapsular cataract formation and glaucoma
Inhibit transcription of inflammatory genes in airway epithelium	Adrenal axis suppression, immunosuppression
Reduce endothelial cell leak	Impaired wound healing, easy bruising, skin striae
Upregulate β_2 receptor production	Hyperglycemia/hypokalemia, hypertension
Reduce airway epithelial subbasement membrane thickening	Psychiatric disturbances

Local adverse effects of ICSs include oropharyngeal candidiasis and dysphonia that are dose-dependent. The dysphonia appears to be due to a local corticosteroid-induced myopathy of the vocal chords.[51] The use of a spacer device can decrease oropharyngeal deposition and decrease the incidence and severity of local side effects.[50,55] In infants who require delivery through a facemask, the parent should clean their nasal-perioral area with a damp cloth following each treatment.

Optimal dosing of inhaled steroids has not been investigated thoroughly. Most patients with moderate disease can be controlled with twice-daily dosing.[2,106] Twice-daily dosing produces less thrush than three- to four-times-daily dosing regimens. In milder asthma, once-daily dosing is often sufficient to maintain control.[107,109] Some of the newer products have gained once-daily dosing indications.[109] Chronobiologic dosing studies have demonstrated that dosing at 3:00 to 5:00 P.M. improves efficacy and may decrease adverse effects; however, this is a very difficult time to achieve for working adults and school children.[110] There does not appear to be any specific pharmacologic or pharmacokinetic aspect of the ICSs that allows for once-daily dosing because all those agents studied (both the older low-potency and newer high-potency ICSs) have been effective provided the patients had relatively mild to moderate asthma.[107] More severe patients require multiple daily dosing. The inflammatory response of asthma has been shown to inhibit steroid receptor binding.[67] This provides strong theoretical evidence for initially beginning patients on higher and more frequent doses and then tapering down once control has been achieved. Many specialists have used this approach, and it is now advocated by the NAEPP.[2]

Clinical Use. The early ongoing intervention with ICSs has been advocated as a means of preventing irreversible loss of lung function in patients with persistent asthma secondary to airway remodeling.[104,111] This has been tempered by concerns of potential for long-term adverse effects including growth suppression in children, osteoporosis in the elderly, and glaucoma and cataracts.[112] These contravening issues have led to explorations of combinations with adjunctive therapy that would enhance efficacy and decrease the potential for toxicity (see below). Despite these concerns, the ICSs have been proven to be the most effective long-term control therapy for persistent asthma, regardless of the severity, and the only therapy to reduce the risk of death from asthma even in relatively low doses.

LT Modifiers

Two clinically distinct cysteinyl LT receptor antagonists (zafirlukast and montelukast) and one inhibitor of LT synthesis (zileuton) have been available in the United States since 1996 for both children and adults with persistent asthma.[113] In challenge studies, they reduce allergen-, exercise-, cold-air hyperventilation-, irritant-, and aspirin-induced asthma.[113] Clinical use of zileuton is limited due to the need for four-times-daily dosing, the potential for elevated liver enzymes (especially in the first 3 months of therapy), and the potential inhibition of drugs metabolized by the CYP3A4 isoenzymes.[100]

In clinical trials, the LTD_4 receptor antagonists (zafirlukast and montelukast) have demonstrated efficacy in adults and children with persistent asthma. These drugs improve pulmonary function tests (FEV_1 or PEF), decrease nocturnal awakenings and β_2-agonist use, and improve asthma symptoms.[32,113] A major advantage is that they are effective orally, administered once or twice a day, and contribute to patient adherence and satisfaction with therapy.[32] However, they are less effective in asthma than low doses of ICSs, although some patients (even those with severe disease) may have useful clinical improvement.[114–116] For example, in 533 patients (>15 years old) with persistent asthma, treatment with fluticasone 176 μg by MDI twice daily improved mean morning FEV_1 at end point by 22.9% versus montelukast 10 mg daily improvements of 14.5% ($P < .001$).[116] All other asthma outcomes were improved to a greater extent by fluticasone therapy. It is not yet possible to predict which patients respond best to LT modifiers, although there is some evidence that patients with aspirin- sensitive asthma do well, as predicted by studies showing increased cysteinyl LT production in these patients.[113] It is possible that genetic polymorphisms in the 5-LO or LTC_4 synthase pathways or in cys-LT_1 receptors might predict better responders in the future.[32] Antileukotrienes also may have modest efficacy in allergic rhinitis.

In general, the LTD_4 receptor antagonists are well tolerated and do not appear to have serious class-specific effects. In the early 6-month zafirlukast trials, nonrespiratory or laboratory abnormalities did not occur with greater frequency in the treatment group than in the placebo groups. However, postmarketing surveillance reports include elevations in serum aminotranferase concentrations and clinical hepatitis (thought to be rare).[113] An idiosyncratic syndrome similar to the Churg-Strauss syndrome, with marked circulating eosinophilia, heart failure, and associated eosinophilic vasculitis, has been reported in a small number of patients treated with zafirlukast or montelukast.[113] The majority of these patients had been receiving high-dose inhaled or oral corticosteroids and were able to reduce the dose as a consequence of the LTD_4 receptor antagonists. It is unclear whether the increased reports are due to increased case finding among patients with asthma prescribed a new drug or whether the syndrome is related to glucocorticoid dose reduction or an idiosyncratic effect of LT modifiers in general. Whatever the cause, it appears to be a rare syndrome, with an estimated incidence of less than 1 case per 15,000 to 20,000 patient-years of treatment.[113] Montelukast has been prescribed widely worldwide, due to its approval for children as young as 2 years of age. Churg-Strauss syndrome has not been reported in children, and the drug has been very well tolerated and palatable (4- and 5-mg chewable cherry tablets).[117]

Combination Controller Therapy: ICS/LABA versus ICS/LT Receptor Agonists

Whereas ICS therapy is considered the most effective anti-inflammatory treatment, in cases of moderate to severe persistent asthma, the addition of a second long-term control medication to ICS therapy is one recommended treatment option. A combination-product inhaler (Advair) was developed to treat both the inflammatory and bronchoconstrictive components of asthma by delivering a dose of fluticasone (100, 250, or 500 μg) with a fixed dose of salmeterol (50 μg). Advair, in a variety of clinical trials in persistent asthma, was superior to the individual components at the same doses, comparable with concurrent therapy at the same doses, had a rapid onset of effect (within 1 week), and demonstrated clinical benefits that improved over the duration of the studies. Importantly, salmeterol therapy allows reduction in ICS dosage by 50% in patients with persistent asthma.[118,119] Further, salmeterol plus low-dose fluticasone has been found to be more effective than higher-dose fluticasone alone in reducing asthma exacerbations in patients with persistent asthma.[118] The ability to detect deteriorating asthma and the severity of exacerbation was similar between groups.

LT receptor agonists also have been found to be successful as additive therapy in patients inadequately controlled on ICS alone and as inhaled corticosteroid-sparing therapy.[32] However, the magnitude of these benefits is less than those reported with the addition of long-acting beta agonists (LABA).[118]

MISCELLANEOUS THERAPIES

Methotrexate

Low-dose methotrexate (15 mg/wk) used for inflammatory diseases, psoriatic and rheumatoid arthritis, and polymyositis has been used to reduce the systemic steroid dose in patients with severe steroid-dependent asthma.[100] Double-blind, placebo-controlled trials have given decidely mixed results, with half the studies showing no effect.[100] A metaanalysis determined that a statistically significant reduction (mean 4.37 mg/d prednisone or 23% of original dose) can be achieved.[100] The mechanism of action is unknown but may be anti-inflammatory or immunomodulatory effects. Methotrexate inhibits chemotaxis of neutrophils, inhibits leukotriene B_4–induced adherence to endothelium, and inhibits the proinflammatory activity of IL-1. Low-dose weekly methotrexate is not without hazard. Both hepatotoxicity and pulmonary fibrosis have been reported in patients receiving similar therapy for psoriasis and rheumatoid arthritis.[100] No evidence for induction of asthma remission exists because patients' corticosteroid requirement returns on discontinuation of the methotrexate. Methotrexate should still be considered experimental and reserved for only severe steroid-dependent asthmatics under the care of specialties. Patients require careful monitoring, including periodic liver biopsies. Owing to the marginal effect of methotrexate, the risk-benefit should be evaluated carefully prior to institution.

Other Agents

As a result of the inflammatory nature of asthma and the risk of toxicities from corticosteroids, a number of the drugs with anti-inflammatory or immunomodulatory activity such as hydroxychloroquine, dapsone, gold, intravenous γ–globulin, cyclosporine, and colchicine have been studied in severe steroid-dependent asthma with mixed results.[2,100]

Future Therapies

Agents that are now in development for asthma focus on the treatment of allergic inflammation.[120,121] Examples include inhibitors of eosinophilic inflammation, drugs that may inhibit allergen presentation, and inhibitors of Th2 cells. Multiple cytokines have been implicated in allergic inflammation, and several possible inhibiting approaches are being explored. These range from drugs that inhibit cytokine synthesis (cyclosporin A and tacrolimus), humanized blocking blocking antibodies to cytokines or their receptors, soluble receptors to mop up secreted cytokines, receptor antagonists, or drugs that block the signal-transduction pathways activated by cytokines.[120] Specifically, humanized monoclonal antibodies to IL-5 and nebulized soluble IL-4 receptors have been tested but have been disappointing to date.[120,121]

Clinical studies with a humanized murine monoclonal antibody (E25) directed to the high-affinity IgE receptor show reduction in early and late responses to inhaled allergen and eosinophil counts in induced sputum. RhuMab-E25 forms complex with free IgE and block its interaction with mast cells and basophils. Some steroid-sparing effects have been demonstrated in patients with moderate to severe asthma. Therapy with anti-IgE antibodies requires intravenous or subcutaneous administration and is likely to be expensive.

PHARMACOECONOMIC CONSIDERATIONS

Of the estimated $12.6 billion cost of asthma in the United States in 1998, direct medical expenditure accounted for 58% of the total, with emergency care (emergency department and inpatient hospital care) reaching $2.5 billion and prescription medications ($3.2 billion) as the single largest direct medical expenditure.[8,78] A cost-of-illness approach takes in all measurable costs; both indirect costs or costs to society and direct medical costs are considered.[113] Using this approach, the costs per patient per year in 1994 in the United States was $756, a slight decrease in inflation-adjusted expenditures over the past 10 years.[8] Two–thirds of this was indirect costs such as lost work and death.

The medication cost increase over the past 10 years resulted from a doubling of prescribed medications as well as a 169%t increase in unit cost per medication, presumably due to a shift to more expensive anti-inflammatory drugs consistent with the recommendations of the NAEPP guidelines.[2] Asthma severity obviously has an impact on cost of care. Studies from health-maintenance organizations suggest that up to 45% of the cost of asthma is accrued by 10% of the patients, primarily as a result of emergency care.[122]

Numerous studies have demonstrated the cost-effectiveness of patient education programs for asthma, particularly those providing guided self-management.[122] Several studies have reported positive results from pharmacist interventions reducing overall cost of care.[122] Similar studies have demonstrated the cost-effectiveness of specialist care compared with generalist care. However, the results of these trials may be confounded by changes in prescribing as part of the overall program. Indeed, ICS therapy has been shown to reduce both morbidity, particularly hospitalizations, and mortality in asthma patients.[11,14,123]

However, the NAEPP recommendations provide numerous alternatives for long-term controllers in mild to moderate persistent asthma, and few studies have compared their relative cost-effectiveness. This is important because outside the realm of randomized clinical trials that evaluate efficacy, other factors such as concern about adverse effects and adherence to therapy may alter the overall clinical effectiveness. ICSs in children have produced a cost of $9.45 per symptom-free day gained.[122] In a mixed group of adults with asthma and chronic obstructive pulmonary disease, the addition of ICSs to β_2-agonists provided an incremental cost-effectiveness ratio of $5.00 per symptom-free day.[122] More recently, retrospective analyses of large managed-care-linked pharmacy claims and health care utilization databases has allowed direct comparisons of the various long-term controllers in a general population to assess clinical effectiveness and cost-effectiveness. These studies primarily have confirmed comparative randomized clinical trials showing ICSs to be significantly more cost-effective than LT modifiers despite slightly better compliance with the LT modifiers.[124] When administered in equipotent doses, the newer ICSs budesonide and fluticasone propionate are comparable with less expensive (based on average wholesale price), older preparations.[103] In addition, preliminary studies have suggested that from the payer perspective, the more potent ICS fluticasone propionate is more cost-effective than the older less potent ICSs (beclomethasone dipropionate, triamcinolone acetonide, and flunisolide).[125] Obviously, many more studies are needed to confirm these early findings.

EVALUATION OF THERAPEUTIC OUTCOMES

The desired outcomes have been described previously. *Control of asthma* is defined as achieving a minimal need for "rescue" short-acting β_2-agonists (ideally none), no acute episodes, no limitations on activity, no emergency care visits, no nocturnal symptoms, normal pulmonary functions (FEV_1 and PEF), minimal to no medication side effects, and satisfaction of the patient and family with their asthma care. Depending on the severity of the patient's asthma, compromises from the ideal control are made, and the best possible outcome balancing disease control and possible adverse effects from the drugs is attempted.

Monitoring consists of quantitating the use of inhaled short-acting β_2-agonists, days of limited activity, and number of symptoms (especially nocturnal). The NAEPP recommends yearly spirometric studies. In moderate to severe persistent asthma, once-daily (on awakening) peak-flow monitoring is recommended. Patients also should be asked about exercise tolerance. All patients on inhaled drugs should have their inhalation delivery technique evaluated periodically–monthly initially and then every 3 to 6 months.

Following initiation of anti-inflammatory therapy or an increase in dosage, most patients should begin experiencing a decrease in symptoms in 1 to 2 weeks and achieve maximum symptomatic improvement within 4 to 8 weeks. The use of higher doses or more potent agents may accelerate the process. Improvement in FEV_1 and PEF should follow a similar time frame; however, a decrease in BHR, as measured by morning PEF, PEF variability, and exercise tolerance, may take longer and improve over 1 to 3 months.[2] Patients should be informed that following a viral respiratory infection they may experience increased exercise intolerance for up to 4 weeks.

Initial visits with the patient should focus on the patient's concerns, expectations, and goals of treatment. Basic education should focus on asthma as a chronic lung disease, the types of medications, and how they are to be used. Inhaler technique is taught, as is when to seek medical advice. Written action plans should be provided. The first follow-up visit should be in 2 to 4 weeks. At this time the educational messages of the first visit should be repeated as well as questions about the patient's current medications and any difficulties related to the therapy.

CONCLUSION

Asthma is a complicated disease with a multitude of clinical presentations. The exact defect in asthma has not been defined, and it may be that asthma is a common presentation of a heterogeneous group of diseases. Asthma is defined and characterized by excessive reactivity of the bronchial tree to a wide variety of noxious stimuli. The reaction is characterized by bronchospasm, excessive mucus production, and inflammation. The central role of inflammation in inducing and maintaining BHR is now becoming widely appreciated and studied. The goal of asthma therapy is to normalize, as much as possible, the patient's life and prevent chronic irreversible lung changes. Drugs are the mainstay of asthma therapy. The goal of drug therapy is to use the minimum amount possible to completely control the disease. In chronic asthma, therapy should be aimed at both bronchospasm and inflammation in order to produce the best results. Patients should be followed and monitored diligently for toxicities. Although death from asthma is an uncommon event, the most common cause of death is underassessment of the severity of obstruction either by the patient or by the clinician; the next common cause is undertreatment. A cornerstone of any therapy is education and the realization that most asthma deaths are avoidable.

▶ PRINCIPLES OF PHARMACOTHERAPY

- Asthma is a chronic inflammatory disease of the lung characterized by intermittent symptoms of airway obstruction and reactivity to numerous stimuli that also may progress to irreversible changes.
- Therapeutic agents are classified by how they are used as either quick-relief or long-term control medication.
- Drugs with anti-inflammatory activity (especially the ICSs) are preferred for long-term control therapy.
- A stepwise approach to asthma therapy is preferred, but it is recommended that patients be started at a higher step initially to gain control and then step down.
- The preferred quick-relief medication for asthma is short-acting inhaled β_2-agonists.
- Regular use of β_2-agonists does not worsen asthma, but short-acting agents should be used as needed so that the frequency of use can be used to assess the appropriateness of long-term controller therapy.
- Education and development of a partnership in care are essential to the success of any pharmacotherapy plan.
- Written action plans are considered essential for all patients to assist in self-management.

REFERENCES

1. Rosenblatt MB. History of bronchial asthma. In: Weiss EB, Segal MS, Stein M, eds. Bronchial Asthma: Mechanisms and Therapeutics, 2d ed. Boston, Little, Brown, 1976: 5–17.
2. NHLBI, National Asthma Education and Prevention Program, Expert Panel Report 2. Guidelines for the Diagnosis and Management of Asthma. NIH Publication No. 97-4051. Bethesda, MD, U.S. Department of Health and Human Services, 1997.
3. CDC. Surveillance for asthma–United States 1960–1995. MMWR 1998; 47(SS–1).
4. CDC. Measuring childhood asthma prevalence before and after the 1997 redesign of the National Health Interview Survey–United States. MMWR 2000;49:908–911.
5. De Marco R, Locatelli F, Sunyer J, Burney P, and the European Community Respiratory Health Survey Study Group. Differences in incidence of reported asthma related to age in men and women. Am J Respir Crit Care Med 2000;162:68–74.
6. Aligne CA, Auinger P, Byrd RS, Weitzman M. Risk factors for pediatric asthma; Contributions of poverty, race, and urban residence. Am J Respir Crit Care Med 2000;162:873–877.
7. Coultas DB, Gong H Jr, Grad R, et al. Respiratory diseases in minorities of the United States. Am J Respir Crit Care Med 1993;149:S93–S131.
8. Weiss KB, Sullivan SD. The health economics of asthma and rhinitis: I. Assessing the economic impact. J Allergy Clin Immunol 2001;107:3–8.
9. Ahmed IH, Sarnet JM. The natural history of asthma. In: Murphy S, Kelly HW, eds. Pediatric Asthma. New York, Marcel Dekker, 1999: 41–69.
10. Castro-Rodriquez JA, Holberg CJ, Wright AL, Martinez FD. A clinical index to define risk of asthma in young children with recurrent wheezing. Am J Resp Crit Care Med 2000;162:1403–1406.
11. The Childhood Asthma Management Program Research Group. Long-term effects of budesonide or nedocromil in children with asthma. New Engl J Med 2000;343:1054–1063.
12. Grol MH, Gerritsen J, Vonk JM, et al. Risk factors for growth and decline of lung function in asthmatic individuals up to age 42 years: A 30-year follow-up study. Am J Respir Crit Care Med 1999;160:1830–1837.
13. Sly RM. Decreases in asthma mortality in the United States. Ann Allergy Asthma Immunol 2000;85:121–127.
14. Suissa S, Ernst P, Benayoun S, et al. Low-dose inhaled corticosteroids and the prevention of death from asthma. New Engl J Med 2000;343: 332–336.
15. Sandford A, Weir T, Pare P. The genetics of asthma. Am J Respir Crit Care Med 1996;153:1749–1765.
16. Bousquet J, Jeffery PK, Busse WW, et al. Asthma: From bronchoconstriction to airways inflammation and remodelling. Am J Respir Crit Care Med 2000;161:1720–1745.
17. Jarjour N, Calhoun W, Becky-Wells E, et al. The immediate and late-phase allergic response to segmental bronchopulmonary provocation in asthma. Am J Respir Crit Care Med 1997;155:1515–1521.
18. Wanner A, Salathe M, O'Riordan TG. Mucociliary clearances in the airways. Am J Respir Crit Care Med 1996;154:1868–1902.
19. Gratziou C, Carroll M, Montefort S, et al. Inflammatory and T-cell profile of asthmatic airways 6 hours after local allergen provocation. Am J Respir Crit Care Med 1996;153:515–520.
20. Smith HR, Larsen GL, Cherniack RM, et al. Inflammatory cells and eicosanoid mediators in subjects with late asthmatic responses and increases in airway responsiveness. J Allergy Clin Immunol 1992;89: 1076–1084.
21. Kay AB. "Helper" (CD4$^+$) T cells and eosinophils in allergy and asthma. Am Rev Respir Dis 1992;145:S22–S26.
22. Woolley KL, Gibson PG, Carty K, et al. Eosinophil apoptosis and the resolution of airway inflammation in asthma. Am J Respir Crit Care Med 1996;154:237–243.
23. Busse WW and Lemanske RF Jr. Asthma. New Engl J Med 2001;344: 350–362.
24. Prescott SL, Macaubus C, Holt BJ, et al. Transplacental priming of the human immune system to environmental allergens: Universal skewing of initial T cell responses toward the Th2 cytokine profile. J Immunol 1998;160:4730–4737.
25. Strachan DP. Hay fever, hygiene, and household size. Br Med J 1989;299: 1259–1260.
26. Mattes J, Karmaus W. The use of antibiotics in the first year of life and development of asthma: Which comes first? Clin Exp Allergy 1999;29: 729–732.
27. Warner JA, Jones CA, Williams TJ, et al. Maternal programming in asthma and allergy. Clin Exp Allergy 1998;28:35–38.
28. Bodner C, Godden D, Seaton A. Family size, childhood infections and atopic diseases. Thorax 1998;53:28–32.
29. McFadden ER, Gilbert IA. Exercise-induced asthma. New Engl J Med 1994;330:1362–1367.
30. Sur S, Crotly TB, Kephart GM, et al. Sudden-onset fatal asthma: A distinct entity with few eosinophils and relatively more neutrophils in the airway submucosa? Am Rev Respir Dis 1993;148:713–719.
31. Kay AB. Asthma and inflammation. J Allergy Clin Immunol 1991;87: 893–910.
32. Sorkness CA. Leukotriene receptor antagonists in the treatment of asthma. Pharmacotherapy 2001;21(2 Pt 3):34S–37S.
33. Calderon E, Lockey RF. A possible role for adhesion molecules in asthma. J Allergy Clin Immunol 1992;90:852–865.
34. Boulet L-P, Laviolette M, Turcotte H, et al. Bronchial subepithelial fibrosis correlates with airway responsiveness to methacholine. Chest 1997;112:45–52.

35. Rennard SI. Repair mechanisms in asthma. J Allergy Clin Immunol 1996; 98:S278–S286.
36. Martinez FD, Wright AL, Taussig CM, et al. Asthma and wheezing in the first six years of life. New Engl J Med 1995;332:133–138.
37. Weiss EB, Stein M, eds. Bronchial Asthma: Mechanism and Therapeutics, 3d ed. Boston, Little Brown, 1993.
38. Global Initiative for Asthma. Global strategy for asthma management and prevention NHLBI/WHO workshop report. National Institutes of Health, National Heart, Lung and Blood Institute Publication No. 95–3659. Washington, 1995.
39. Barnes PJ. NO or no NO in asthma? Thorax 1996;51:218–220.
40. Barnes PJ, Kharitonov SA. Exhaled nitric oxide: A new lung function test. Thorax 1996;51:233.
41. Strunk RC. Death due to asthma: New insights into sudden unexpected deaths, but the focus remains on prevention. Am Rev Respir Dis 1993;148:550–552.
42. Kallenbach JM, Frankel AH, Lapinsky SE, et al. Determinants of near fatality in acute severe asthma. Am J Med. 1993;95:265–272.
43. Kelly HW, Murphy S. Assessment of inflammation and its suppression in lung disease. J Biopharm Sci 1992;3:155–161.
44. Nelson HS. β-Adrenergic bronchodilators. New Engl J Med 1995;333: 499–506.
45. Duff AL, Platts-Mills TAE. Allergens and asthma. Pediatr Clin North Am 1992;39:1277–1291.
46. Martin RJ. Nocturnal asthma: Circadian rhythms and therapeutic interventions. Am Rev Respir Dis 1993;147(suppl):S25–S28.
47. Alberts WM. "Circa menstrual" rhythmicity and asthma. Chest 1997; 111:840–842.
48. Chandler MH, Schuldheisz HS, Phillips BA, Muse KN. Premenstrual asthma: The effect of estrogen on symptoms, pulmonary function, and β_2-receptors. Pharmacotherapy 1997;17:224–34.
49. Zimmerman JL, Woodruff PG, Clark S, Camargo CA Jr, MARC Investigators. Relation between phase of menstrual cycle and emergency department visits for acute asthma. Am J Respir Crit Care Med 2000;162: 512–515.
50. Dolovich MA, MacIntyre NR, Dhand R, et al. Consensus conference on aerosols and delivery devices. Respir Care 2000;45:588–776.
51. Barnes PJ. Inhaled glucocorticoids for asthma. New Engl J Med 1995; 332:868–875.
52. Bisgaard H. Delivery of inhaled medication to children. J Asthma 1997; 34:443–67.
53. Department of Health and Human Services, Food and Drug Administration. Chlororofluorocarbon propellants in self-pressurized containers: Determinations that uses are no longer essential–Request for comments. Fed Reg 1997;62:10242–10247.
54. Kelly HW. Aerosol delivery. In: Murphy S, Kelly HW, eds. Pediatric Asthma. Lung Biology in Health and Disease Series 126. New York, Marcel Dekker, 1999: 463–487.
55. Lipworth BJ. Airway and systemic effects of inhaled corticosteroids in asthma: Dose response relationship. Pulm Pharmacol 1996;9:19–27.
56. Cates C. Comparison of holding chambers and nebulisers for β agonists in acute asthma (Cochrane Review). In: Cochrane Library Issue 1. Oxford, United Kingdom, Update Software, 1998.
57. Kelly HW, Murphy SJ. The management of acute severe asthma in children. In: Busse WW, Holgate S, eds. Asthma and Rhinitis. Boston, Blackwell Science, 2001.
58. Spitzer WO, Suissa S, Ernst P, et al. The use of β-agonists and the risk of death and near death from asthma. New Engl J Med 1992;326:501–506.
59. Suissa S, Blais L, Ernst P. Patterns of increasing β-agonist use and the risk of fatal or near-fatal asthma. Eur Respir J 1994;7:162–169.
60. Kelly HW, Murphy S. β-Adrenergic agonists for acute, severe asthma. Ann Pharmacother 1992;26:81–91.
61. McFadden ER Jr, Elsanadi N, Dixon L, et al. Protocol therapy for acute asthma: Therapeutic benefits and cost savings. Am J Med 1995;99:651–661.
62. Salmeron S, Brochard L, Mal H, et al. Nebulized versus intravenous albuterol in hypercapnic acute asthma: A multicenter, double-blind, randomized study. Am J Respir Crit Care Med 1994;149:1466–1470.
63. Browne GJ, Penna AS, Phung X, Soo M. Randomised trial of intravenous salbutamol in early management of acute severe asthma in children. Lancet 1997;349:301–305.
64. Shrestha M, Bidadi K, Gourlay S, Hayes J. Continuous versus intermittent albuterol, at high and low doses, in the treatment of severe acute asthma in adults. Chest 1996;110:42–47.
65. Cates C. Comparison of holding chambers and nebulisers for β-agonists in acute asthma (Cochrane Review). In: Cochrane Library Issue 1. Oxford, United Kingdom, Update Software, 1998.
66. Kelly HW, Murphy S. Corticosteroids for acute severe asthma. DICP Ann Pharmacother 1991;25:72–79.
67. Spahn JD, Leung DYM, Surs W, et al. Reduced glucocorticoid binding affinity in asthma is related to ongoing allergic inflammation. Am J Respir Crit Care Med 1995;151:1709–1714.
68. Rodrigo G, Rodrigo C. Inhaled flunisolide for acute severe asthma. Am J Respir Crit Care Med 1998;157:698–703.
69. Schuh S, Reisman J, Alshehri M, et al. A comparison of inhaled fluticasone and oral prednisone for children with severe acute asthma. New Engl J Med 2000;343:689–694.
70. Schuh S, Johnson DW, Callahan S, et al. Efficacy of frequent nebulized ipratropium bromide added to frequent high-dose albuterol therapy in severe childhood asthma. J Pediatr 1995;126:639–645.
71. Qureshi D, Pestian J, Davis P, Zaritsky A. Effect of nebulized ipratropium on the hospitalization rates of children with asthma. New Engl J Med 1998;339:1030–1035.
72. Plotnick LH, Ducharme FM. Should inhaled anticholinergics be added to β_2-agonists for treating acute childhood and adolescent asthma? A systematic review. Br Med J 1998;317:971–977.
73. Yung M, South M. Randomised controlled trial of aminophylline for severe acute asthma. Arch Dis Child 1998;79:405–410.
74. Rowe BH, Bretzlaff JA, Bourdon C, et al. Intravenous magnesium sulfate treatment for acute asthma in the emergency department: A systematic review of the literature. Ann Emerg Med 2000;36:181–190.
75. Ciarallo L, Brousseau D, Reinert S. Higher-dose intravenous magnesium therapy for children with moderate to severe asthma. Arch Pediatr Adolesc Med 2000;154:979–983.
76. Kudukis T, Manthous CA, Schmidt GA. Effect of inhaled helium:oxygen (heliox) during the treatment of status asthmaticus in children. J Pediatr 1997;130:217–224.
77. Howton JC, Rose J, Duffy S, et al. Randomized, double-blind, placebo-controlled trial of intravenous ketamine in acute asthma. Ann Emerg Med 1996;27:170–175.
78. Weiss KB, Sullivan SD, Lyttle S. Trends in the cost of illness for asthma in the United States, 1985–1994. J Allergy Clin Immunol 2000;106: 493–499.
79. Lord J, Ducharme FM, Stamp RJ, et al. Cost-effectiveness analysis of inhaled anticholinergics for acute childhood and adolescent asthma. Br Med J 1999;319:1470–1471.
80. Papo MC, Frank J, Thompson AE. A prospective, randomized study of continuous versus intermittent nebulized albuterol for severe status asthmaticus in children. Crit Care Med 1993;21:1479–1486.
81. Murray AB, Morrison BJ. The decrease in severity of asthma in children of parents who smoke since the parents have been exposing them to less cigarette smoke. J Allergy Clin Immunol 1993;91:102–110.
82. Abramson MJ, Puy RM, Weiner JM. Is allergen immunotherapy effective in asthma? A meta-analysis of randomized controlled trials. Am J Respir Crit Care Med 1995;151:969–974.
83. Creticos PS, Reed CE, Norman PS, et al. Ragweed immunotherapy in adult asthma. New Engl J Med 1996;334:501–506.
84. Jenne JW, Kelly HW. β_2-agonists. In: Murphy S, Kelly HW, eds. Pediatric Asthma. New York, Marcel Dekker, 1999: 279–326.
85. Anderson GP. Interactions between corticosteroids and β-adrenergic agonists in asthma disease induction, progression, and exacerbation. Am J Respir Crit Care Med 2000;161:S188–S196.
86. Liggett SB. β_2-Adrenergic receptor pharmacogenetics. Am J Respir Crit Care Med 2000;161:S197–S201.
87. Waldeck B. Enantiomers of bronchodilating β_2-adrenoceptor agonists: Is there a cause for concern? J Allergy Clin Immunol 1999;103:742–748.

88. Drazen JM, Israel E, Boushey HA, et al. Comparison of regularly scheduled with as needed use of albuterol in mild asthma. New Engl J Med 1996;335:841–847.
89. Dennis SM, Sharp SJ, Vickers MR, et al. Regular inhaled salbutamol an asthma control: the TRUST randomised trial. Lancet 2000;355: 1675–1679.
90. Israel E, Drazen JM, Liggett SB, et al. The effect of polymorphisms of the β_2-adrenergic receptor on the response to regular use of albuterol in asthma. Am J Respir Crit Care Med 2000;162:75–80.
91. Inman MD, O'Byrne PM. The effect of regular inhaled albuterol on exercise-induced bronchoconstriction. Am J Respir Crit Care Med 1996;153: 65–69.
92. Martin RJ. Nocturnal asthma: circadian rhythms and therapeutic interventions. Am Rev Respir Dis 1993;147(Suppl):S25–S28.
93. Weinberger M, Hendeles L. Theophylline in asthma. New Engl J Med 1996;334:1380–1388.
94. Edwards D, Zarowitz BJ, Slaughter RL. Theophylline. In: Evans WE, Schentag JJ, Jusko WJ, eds. Applied Pharmacokinetics: Principles of Therapeutic Drug Monitoring, 3d ed. Vancouver, Applied Therapeutics, 1992: 13- 1–13-38.
95. Blake K. Theophylline. In: Murphy SA, Kelly HW, eds. Pediatric Asthma. New York, Marcel Dekker, 1999: 363–431.
96. Evans DJ, Taylor DA, Zetterstrom O, et al. A comparison of low-dose inhaled budesonide plus theophylline and high-dose inhaled budesonide for moderate asthma. New Engl J Med 1997;337:1412–1418.
97. Campbell SC. Clinical aspects of inhaled anticholinergic therapy. Respir Care. 2000;45:864–867.
98. Wasserman SI, ed. Nedocromil sodium: A pyranoquinoline antiinflammatory agent for the treatment of asthma. J Allergy Clin Immunol 1993; 92(Suppl):143–216.
99. Murphy S, Kelly HW. Cromolyn sodium: A review of mechanisms and clinical use in asthma. Drug Intell Clin Pharm l987;21:22–35.
100. Sorkness CA. Cromolyn, nedocromil, leukotriene modifiers, and alternative anti-inflammatory agents in the treatment of pediatric asthma. In: Murphy SA, Kelly HW, eds. Pediatric Asthma. New York, Marcel Dekker, 1999: 433–462.
101. American Academy of Allergy, Asthma and Immnology. Pediatric Asthma: Promoting Best Practice. Guide for Managing Asthma in Children. Milwaukee, WI, American Academy of Allergy, Asthma and Immnology, 1999.
102. Tasche MJ, van der Wouden JC, Uijen JH, et al. Randomised placebo-controlled trial of inhaled sodium cromoglycate in 1–4-year-old children with moderate asthma. Lancet. 1997;350:1060–1064.
103. Tasche MJ, Uijen JH, Bernsen R, et al. Inhaled disodium cromoglycate (DSCG) as maintenance therapy in children with asthma: A systematic review. Thorax. 2000;55(11):913–920.
104. Pederson S, O'Byrne P. A comparison of the efficacy and safety of inhaled corticosteroids in asthma. Allergy 1997;52(Suppl 39):1–34.
105. Lee TH, Brattsand R, Leung D, eds. Corticosteroid action and resistance in asthma. Am J Respir Crit Care Med 1996;154(Suppl):S1–S79.
106. Kamada A, Szefler SJ, Martin RJ, et al. Issues in the use of inhaled glucocorticoids. Am J Respir Crit Care Med 1996;153:1739–1748.
107. Kelly HW. Comparison of inhaled corticosteroids. Ann Pharmacother 1998;32:220–232.
108. Kelly HW. Pharmacology of inhaled glucocorticoids: Comparative properties. Immunol Allergy Clin North Am 1999;19:725–738.
109. McFadden ER, Casale TB, Edwards TB, et al. Administration of budesonide once daily by means of turbuhaler to subjects with stable asthma. J Allergy Clin Immunol 1999;104:46–52.
110. Pincus DJ, Szefler SJ, Ackerson LM, Martin RJ. Chronotherapy of asthma with inhaled steroids: The effect of dosage timing on drug efficacy. J Allergy Clin Immunol 1995;95:1172–1178.
111. Olivieri D, Chetta A, Del Dono M, et al. Effect of short-term treatment with low-dose inhaled fluticasone propionate on airway inflammation and remodeling in mild asthma: A placebo-controlled study. Am J Respir Crit Care Med 1997;155:1864–1871.
112. Sorkness CA. Comparison of systemic activity and safety among different inhaled corticosteroids. J Allergy Clin Immunol 1998;102:S52–S64.
113. Drazen JM, Israel E, O'Byrne PM. Treatment of asthma with drugs modifying the leukotriene pathway. New Engl J Med 1999;340: 197–206.
114. Malmstrom K, Rodriguez-Gomez G, Guerra J, et al. Oral montelukast, inhaled beclomethasone, and placebo for chronic asthma. Ann Intern Med 1999;130:487–495.
115. Bleeker ER, Welch MJ, Weinstein SF, et al. Low-dose inhaled fluticasone propionate versus oral zafirlukast in the treatment of persistent asthma. J Allergy Clin Immunol 2000;105:1123–1129.
116. Busse W, Raphael GD, Galant S, et al. Low-dose fluticasone propionate compared with montelukast for first- line treatment of persistent asthma: a randomized clinical trial. J Allergy Clin Immunol 2001;107:461–468.
117. Price D. Tolerability of montelukast. Drugs 2000;59(Suppl 1):35–42.
118. Nelson HS. Advair: Combination treatment with fluticasone propionate/salmeterol in the treatment of asthma. J Allergy Clin Immunol 2001; 107:397–416.
119. Lemanske RF Jr, Sorkness CA, Mauger EA, et al. Inhaled corticosteroid reduction and elimination in patients with persistent asthma receiving salmeterol: A randomized controlled trial. JAMA 2001;285:2594–2603.
120. Barnes PJ. New directions in allergic diseases: Mechanism based anti-inflammatory therapies. J Allergy Clin Immunol 2000;106:5–16.
121. Sterling RG, Chung KF. New immunological approaches and cytokine targets in asthma and allergy. Eur Respir J 2000;16:1158–1174.
122. National Asthma Education and Prevention Program Task Force report on the cost effectiveness, quality of care, and financing of asthma care. Am J Respir Crit Care Med 1996;154(Suppl):S81–S130.
123. Donahue JG, Weiss ST, Livingston JM, et al. Inhaled steroids and the risk of hospitalization for asthma. JAMA 1997;277:887–891.
124. Stempel DA, Meyer JW, Stanford RH, Yancey SW. One-year claims analysis comparing inhaled fluticasone propionate with zafirlukast for the treatment of asthma. J Allergy Clin Immunol 2001;107: 94–98.
125. Stempel DA, Kelly HW, Clous J, et al. One-year claims analysis comparing inhaled fluticasone propionate with triamcinolone, beclomethasone dipropionate and flunisolide for the treatment of asthma. Respir Med (submitted).

27

CHRONIC OBSTRUCTIVE LUNG DISEASE

Sherri L. Konzem and Mark A. Stratton

Chronic obstructive lung disease (COLD) is defined as a disease state characterized by the presence of airflow obstruction owing to chronic bronchitis or emphysema; the airflow obstruction generally is progressive, may be accompanied by airway hyperreactivity, and may be partially reversible. The definition provided here is the one adopted by the American Thoracic Society in the 1995 statement of the Standards for the Diagnosis and Care of Patients with Chronic Obstructive Pulmonary Disease and serves to distinguish COLD from asthma or other potentially reversible causes of lung dysfunction such as tuberculosis or tumors.[1] More recently, the National Heart, Lung and Blood Institute and the World Health Organization have launched the Global Initiative for Chronic Obstructive Lung Diseases (GOLD) and have proposed a new definition of COLD as a disease characterized by a progressive airflow limitation caused by an abnormal inflammatory reaction to the chronic inhalation of particles.[2] The newer definition captures the prevailing opinion that the dominant pathology seen in chronic bronchitis and emphysema is as a result of inflammation due to inhalation of particles, of which particles from cigarette smoking are the most prevalent. This initiative is to jointly develop guidelines that will present evidence-based recommendations for the management of COLD. Currently, eleven different societies have proposed their own guidelines for COLD management, often based on insufficient evidence and clinical experience. The GOLD initiative is designed to standardize care of the COLD patient similar to the asthma model, which has been shown to improve care for patients. The terms *chronic obstructive airway disease* (COAD) and *chronic obstructive pulmonary disease* (COPD) are synonymous with COLD.

COLD conventionally has included the subsets of chronic bronchitis and emphysema, although one should note that COLD may exist before evidence of airflow obstruction is demonstrated. Although the pathology and clinical characteristics of these subsets differ, most patients with COLD show characteristics of both these subsets. Peripheral airway disease contributes significantly to the airway obstruction in both conditions and is further worsened by mucous plugging.[3]

Chronic bronchitis is a condition with chronic or recurrent excess mucus secretion into the bronchial tree with cough that occurs on most days during a period of at least 3 months of the year for at least 2 consecutive years in a patient in whom other causes of chronic cough have been excluded.[1] Bronchitis is defined in clinical terms, but emphysema is defined in terms of anatomic pathology. Emphysema classically was defined on histologic examination at autopsy. Because this definition is of no clinical value, emphysema has been defined as a condition of the lung characterized by abnormal, permanent enlargement of the airspaces distal to the terminal bronchioles, accompanied by destruction of their walls, yet without obvious fibrosis.[1] Peripheral airway disease is a condition that includes inflammation of the terminal and respiratory bronchioles, fibrosis with narrowing of airway walls, and goblet cell metaplasia of the bronchiolar epithelium. These changes appear before clinically detectable emphysema is present and are consistent with the pathology traditionally associated with chronic bronchitis.

EPIDEMIOLOGY

In 1996, over 16 million Americans suffered from COLD—about 14.2 million from chronic bronchitis and about 2 million from emphysema.[4] It is the fourth most common cause of death in the United States. This is notable because COLD is the only leading cause of death that is increasing in prevalence.[5,6] Data from the National Center for Health Statistics indicate that in the 17-year period from 1980 to 1997, the age-adjusted mortality from COLD remained stable in men (26.1 per 100,000 in 1980 and 26.1 per 100,000 in 1997), whereas in women the rate increased nearly 100% (8.9 per 100,000 in 1980 and 17.5 per 100,000 in 1997).[7] Rates of death from COLD increase with age, and in 1998, rates for males and females were nearly equal, with a total of 112,584 people dying from COLD and allied conditions, including 5438 deaths from asthma.[6] This represented a 45.9% increase in COLD mortality since 1979, even though the prevalence of smoking has decreased since 1965 but still remains at 24% in the United States.[6,8] This probably reflects the long latency period between smoking exposure and death from COLD. The prevalence rate of chronic bronchitis has increased from 1982 to 1999, whereas that of emphysema has remained stable during this period.[7,9]

Although the mortality associated with COLD is impressive, the disability associated with it is also of concern. COLD is the second leading cause of disability in the United States. Assessing the use of medical resources can provide an estimate of the impact of COLD on society. From 1979 to 1985, physician office visits for COLD increased 15% for men and 8% for women. In addition, individuals with COLD have approximately double the number of hospital stays, days of restricted activity, and days of being confined to bed than do individuals without COLD.[10] In 1997, there were over 13 million physician office visits made for COLD and 634,000 hospitalizations with an average length of stay of 5.4 days.[9] The economic impact is estimated at greater than $23 billion annually.[11]

Of the numerous risk factors (Table 27–1) associated with the development of chronic bronchitis and emphysema, clearly cigarette smoking is the most common. The median risk ratio for smokers versus nonsmokers to develop chronic bronchitis is 5.3 for men and 4.2 for women. Eighty-five percent of COLD mortality is a result of smoking in men and 69.4% in women.[1] Although the risk is lower in pipe and cigar smokers, it is still higher than for nonsmokers. Age of starting, total pack-years, and current smoking status are predictive of COLD mortality. However, only 15% of smokers go on to develop COLD, and not all smokers who have equivalent smoking histories develop the same degree of pulmonary impairment, suggesting that other physiologic and environmental factors contribute to the degree of lung dysfunction in smokers. As the field of molecular genetics continues to unfold, we may be better able to identify those at greatest risk of developing COLD through various genetic markers.[3] Nevertheless, the rate of loss of lung function is above all determined by smoking status and history.[1] Children and spouses of smokers are also at increased risk of developing significant pulmonary dysfunction

TABLE 27–1. Risk Factors for the Development of COLD

Major	Minor
Smoking	Air pollution
Age	Race
Male gender	Nutritional status
Existing impaired lung function	Family history
Occupation	Socioeconomic status
α_1-Antitrypsin deficiency	Respiratory tract infection
	Bronchial reactivity

by passive smoking, also known as *environmental tobacco smoke* or *secondhand smoke.*

Increasing age, male gender, and existing impaired lung function also have been identified as risk factors for the development of COLD. Individuals with existing impairment experience a greater decline in lung function over time than their counterparts with normal pulmonary function. Other increasingly identified familial factors are genetic and environmental.

Occupational hazards are difficult to identify because they primarily affect blue-collar workers, who also have a higher incidence of cigarette smoking and may live in areas of higher air pollution. Reduced lung function and deaths from COLD are higher for individuals who work in gold and coal mining, in the glass or ceramic industries with exposure to silica dust, and in jobs that expose them to cotton dust or grain dust, toluene diisocyanate, or asbestos. Cigarette smokers have a higher incidence of pulmonary dysfunction than their nonsmoking counterparts in jobs with these types of exposures. Numerous other possible occupational risk factors also exist.

It is unclear whether or not air pollution alone is a significant risk factor for the development of COLD. However, in individuals with existing pulmonary dysfunction, significant air pollution worsens symptoms. Studies have shown an association between intensity of air pollution and number of emergency room admissions for COLD.[12] There are as yet insufficient data to suggest that air pollution contributes to the development of COLD in smokers and nonsmokers with normal pulmonary function.

α_1-Antitrypsin (AAT) deficiency clearly has been defined as a genetic disorder that contributes to the risk of developing COLD, specifically emphysema. True AAT deficiency accounts for less than 1% of COLD cases.[1] AAT is a protease inhibitor that normally inhibits trypsin and other proteases from destroying normal lung tissue. The protease inhibitor (Pi) phenotypes with the highest incidence of COLD are the homozygous PiZZ (because they have the lowest level of AAT) and, to a lesser extent, PiSZ and Pi-null phenotypes.[1] PiMZ heterozygotes have lower levels of AAT than normal, but there is as yet an unclear association with an increased risk of COLD from smoking.

PATHOLOGY/PATHOPHYSIOLOGY

The prevailing opinion regarding the pathology of COLD revolves around the dominant role of inflammation in the pathology of chronic bronchitis and emphysema. In COLD, there are chronic inflammatory processes that are distinctly different than those seen in asthma.[3] The site of inflammation is in the peripheral airways and the lung parenchyma. Patients with COLD have increased numbers of macrophages, CD8+ (cytotoxic) T cells, and neutrophils. Eosinophils are not present during exacerbations of COLD, as seen in asthma. Exactly which inflammatory mediators are involved has not been fully defined. There is probably a complex interaction between these inflammatory mediators and cells that result in progressive changes in small airways and parenchyma that contribute to obstruction. At the site of destruction, there are large numbers of macrophages that can be activated by cigarette smoke and other irritants to release neutrophil chemotactic factors (e.g., leukotriene B_4 and interleukin-8). When neutrophils and macrophages are activated, they release proteinases that break down connective tissue in the lung parenchyma, leading to emphysema and mucus production. Cytotoxic T cells may further contribute to the destruction of alveolor walls through the release of porphyrins and tumor necrosis factor-α (TNF-α). Pathology and pathophysiology of COLD can best be understood by examining chronic bronchitis and emphysema separately. Peripheral airway disease is a major component of both conditions, contributing to obstruction. In the majority of patients, evidence of each condition is present. Figure 27–1 provides a graphic depiction of the mechanisms of airflow limitation in COLD that characterizes the role of both conditions along with mucus plugging.[3]

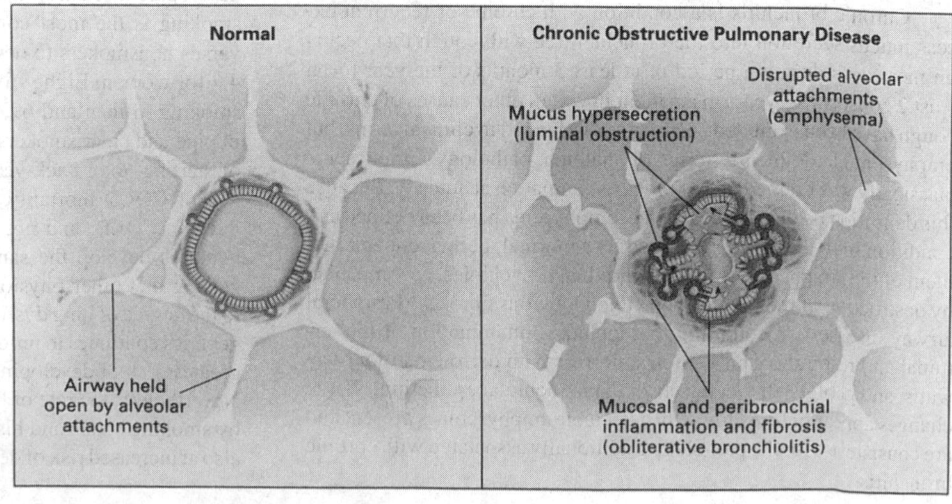

FIGURE 27–1. Mechanisms of airflow limitation in chronic obstructive pulmonary disease. In the peripheral airways of patients with chronic obstructive pulmonary disease, as compared with normal peripheral airways, there is airflow limitation due to a variable mixture of loss of alveolar attachments, inflammatory obstruction of the airway, and luminal obstruction with mucus. *(From Ref. 3.)*

CHRONIC BRONCHITIS

As described earlier, chronic bronchitis is characterized by excessive tracheobronchial mucus secretion with cough. This excessive production of mucus results from hyperplasia and hypertrophy of mucus-producing glands and goblet cells owing to continued bronchial irritation. Additional morphologic changes occur in the bronchi, including increased smooth muscle, cartilage atrophy, inflammation characterized by neutrophil and lymphocyte infiltration, and loss of cilia. These bronchial changes do not contribute significantly to obstruction.

In the COLD patient with predominant chronic bronchitis, changes in the peripheral airways contribute most to obstruction. Inflammation exists with mucus production and narrowing of the lumen in the more distal noncartilagenous or membranous bronchioles. In addition, there is fibrosis, tortuosity, and irregularity of these smaller airways. Autopsies have shown that individuals with chronic bronchitis have more airways smaller than 0.4 mm in diameter when compared with nonbronchitic patients.

Many chronic bronchitis patients will show minimal improvement with bronchodilators. Some display much more improvement in obstruction after bronchodilator therapy and would be more appropriately referred to as patients with chronic asthmatic bronchitis. There may be a component of atopy in these patients.[13] Ventilatory impairment is unrelated to atopic status in individuals without a history of asthma, further supporting the theory that nonallergic inflammation is important in the pathogenesis of chronic airflow obstruction.

The lung damage produced by smoking or exposure to other chronic irritants has long been considered to begin in the small airways. These small airways (i.e., those less than 2 mm in diameter) contribute to only 10% to 20% of normal resistance to airflow. However, their total cross-sectional diameter is much greater than that of larger airways; thus, by the time obstruction is detected by pulmonary function tests, extensive damage has occurred. The best predictor of moderate disease has been suggested to be the presence of diminished breath sounds on physical examination, especially when combined with a clinical history consistent with COLD. As chronic bronchitis progresses over several years, the changes in small airways begin to impair ventilation (V), whereas perfusion (Q) remains fairly adequate, resulting in a V/Q imbalance and hypoxemia. This can be assessed by measuring the alveolar-arterial Po_2 difference.[13] Hypoxemia leads to pulmonary hypertension with subsequent right ventricular failure (cor pulmonale). Autopsy data indicate that patients with pulmonary hypertension have markedly increased intima and media in the musculature of the pulmonary arteries, specifically the larger vessels. These alterations do not, however, correlate with either the severity or the ability of the vasculature to respond to oxygen.[14] The persistent hypoxemia stimulates erythropoiesis with resulting secondary polycythemia and increased blood viscosity, with its attendant complications of mental confusion and thrombotic stroke. Why some patients with predominant chronic bronchitis suffer more severe hypoxemia and hypercarbia than others with equal degrees of obstruction is not clear but probably is best explained simply by individual differences in ventilatory drive in response to decreased oxygen or elevated carbon dioxide.[13]

An additional component of chronic bronchitis is repeated respiratory infections. Patients are predisposed to repeated infections owing to excessive mucus production, mucus stagnation and plugging, as well as lack of cilia or ciliary movement to clear mucus. The signs of infection usually consist of sputum changes, such as an increase in volume, thickening, and a change in color. Fever or other objective evidence of infection need not be present. Repeated respiratory infections in the patient with chronic bronchitis can cause severe acute exacerbations in pulmonary status and can contribute significantly to accelerating the decline in pulmonary function tests resulting from the inflammation-induced fibrosis of bronchi and bronchioles. The most frequent respiratory pathogens are viral, although bacterial infection may follow a viral infection. The respiratory syncytial virus is considered the most common overall pathogen, whereas *Streptococcus pneumoniae* and *Hemophilus influenzae* are the most common bacterial pathogens. Because these are not the only bacteria that act as pathogens, the host's condition and environment must be considered when searching for a pathogen in a patient with chronic bronchitis with a suspected respiratory infection.

EMPHYSEMA

Emphysema refers specifically to involvement of the acinus, which is the unit of the lung responsible for gas exchange. It consists of three levels proceeding distally—respiratory bronchioles, alveolar ducts, and alveolar sacs. In a simplistic sense, emphysema is a condition in which there is destruction of walls within the acinus such that the surface area for gas exchange is diminished.

Several types of emphysema have been described and deserve comment:

1. *Proximal acinar emphysema.* This type includes the centrilobular emphysema (i.e., central lobes of the acinus) characteristically seen in cigarette smokers, especially in the upper lobes, and simple pneumoconiosis of coal workers. This type of emphysema is confined largely to the proximal portion of the acinus, with the respiratory bronchioles being particularly affected.
2. *Panacinar emphysema.* The entire acinus is involved in this type. It is found in those genetically susceptible individuals who possess the homozygous PiZZ phenotype. These patients have a deficiency of protease inhibitors (AAT) such that proteases are allowed to destroy the alveolar walls of the acinus. This type usually involves the entire lung field.
3. *Distal (paraseptal) emphysema.* As the term suggests, this type of emphysema is associated with the distal portion of the acinus. It is seen as a consequence of spontaneous pneumothorax in young adults.
4. *Irregular emphysema.* This type of emphysema is produced as a consequence of trauma to lung tissue.

Our understanding of the pathogenesis of centrilobular emphysema (the most common type) extends from an understanding of the panacinar emphysema associated with protease inhibitor deficiency states. In centrilobular emphysema specifically caused by smoking, an imbalance develops between the protective protein inhibitors and proteases from activated neutrophils and macrophages. Women are less likely to experience this imbalance, possibly because of a protective effect of estrogens that may stimulate synthesis of protease inhibitors. Damage occurs because cigarette smoke causes a macrophage alveolitis and a respiratory bronchiolitis. These macrophages are chemotactic for neutrophils. Both the macrophages and neutrophils release a greater amount of elastase (which breaks down elastin, a protein integral to the structural integrity of alveolar walls) in response to smoke in smokers than in nonsmokers. Cigarette smoke is also thought to impair the synthesis of elastin.[15] Alveolar inflammatory cells in smokers with emphysema have been shown to spontaneously inactivate α_1-proteinase inhibitor, suggesting that the progressive lung damage is related to an ongoing inflammation in peripheral airways.[3]

The destruction of the surface area for gas exchange within the acinus results in a loss of elastic recoil. This loss permits compression of distal airways during expiration, contributing to the significant obstructive pattern seen in pulmonary function tests. The exact changes in pulmonary function are described later in this chapter. In cigarette smokers with centrilobular emphysema, the respiratory bronchiolitis leads to narrowing of the terminal bronchioles.[16] In addition to a reduction in elastic recoil, loss of alveolar walls results in a loss of the capillary network essential to adequate perfusion. This results in not only a decrease in ventilation (V) but also a loss in perfusion (Q); thus the V/Q ratio is maintained better than in chronic bronchitis.[16] Therefore, although predominant emphysematous patients experience greater dyspnea than predominant chronic bronchitis patients, the former are better able to preserve gas exchange because they have better ventilatory response to hypoxia.[13] The net result of this on other physiologic systems is less cor pulmonale and less polycythemia than seen in the predominant chronic bronchitic.

CLINICAL PRESENTATION

Patients with COLD typically present with a smoking history of at least 20 cigarettes per day for 20 or more years before symptoms develop. They commonly present with symptomatic shortness of breath, a productive cough, or an acute chest illness in the fifth decade.[1] By the time a patient presents with obstructive airway disease, the diagnosis can be made rapidly often simply by observing the patient's breathing pattern. Early in the disease, chest examination reveals only slowed expiration and wheezing on forced exhalation. As the disease progresses, breath sounds become decreased, hyperinflation is evident, exhalation is further prolonged, and wheezes are more frequent along with coarse crackles in the lung bases.[1] The clinical features are presented in Table 27–2. As described previously, although the majority of patients with COLD will have components of both chronic bronchitis and emphysema, it is best to describe the physical examination of each predominant constituent condition separately.

CHRONIC BRONCHITIS

The patient presenting with predominant chronic bronchitis often is overweight and has an impressive history of productive cough and increasing dyspnea on exertion. By history, the cough has been increasing in frequency and duration. Predominant chronic bronchitis patients are classically referred to as "blue bloaters" (type B) because they tend to retain carbon dioxide because of a decreased ventilatory response. Commonly they will have peripheral edema from cor pulmonale and usually a normal or only slightly increased respiratory rate at rest. With advanced disease, the anteroposterior diameter of the chest often is increased, resulting in the classical "barrel chest" appearance. This does not always indicate advanced disease because it is also a normal part of the aging process. Percussion of the chest is resonant, and the breath sounds are distant on auscultation. Rhonchi and wheezes are heard frequently and change in location as the patient breathes deeply or coughs. A rapid assessment of obstruction can be done by placing the stethoscope over the trachea and instructing the patient to forcefully expire. Forced expiration lasting greater than 4 seconds correlates with obstruction in pulmonary function tests. Use of the scalene or sternocleidomastoid muscles of the neck to assist respiration may not be apparent unless severe obstruction is present.

As the degree of obstruction worsens and the arterial oxygen tension (PaO_2) continues to drop, pulmonary hypertension from vasoconstriction ensues. This leads to right ventricular strain and ultimately cor pulmonale. On physical examination, this is manifested by jugular venous distension, hepatomegaly, hepatojugular reflux, and peripheral edema. Conventional cardiac examination may be difficult if a barrel chest is present; however, by palpating the epigastric area, a heave may be felt or even seen in thin patients, and auscultation of the area may reveal a gallop rhythm suggestive of right ventricular hypertrophy.

In the face of chronic hypoxemia, cyanosis of the lips, mucous membranes, or extremities may be seen. The cyanosis worsens during the night, frequently because of chronic oxygen desaturation secondary to sleep apnea. Clubbing of the fingers is seen rarely in chronic bronchitis. Sleep apnea recently has become an area of increasing study in patients with COLD and may play a much greater role than previously understood in the pathophysiology of COLD, especially with respect to cor pulmonale and polycythemia. Individuals with sleep apnea are at greater risk for developing respiratory insufficiency. These consequences are more likely in the obese COLD patient.[17]

TABLE 27–2. Clinical Features of COLD

	Predominant Emphysema	Predominant Chronic Bronchitis
Age	60±	50±
Dyspnea	Severe	Mild
Cough	After dyspnea starts	Before dyspnea starts
Sputum	Scanty, mucoid	Copius, purulent
Bronchial infection	Less frequent	More frequent
Respiratory insufficiency episodes	Often terminal	Repeated
$PaCO_2$ (mm Hg)	35–40	50–60
PaO_2 (mm Hg)	65–75	45–60
Hematocrit (%)	35–45	50–60
Cor pulmonale	Rare	Common

Adapted from Ref. 13.

EMPHYSEMA

The patient presenting with predominant emphysema characteristically is older than the chronic bronchitis patient. The chief complaint is often increasing dyspnea, even at rest, with minimal cough. These patients classically have been termed "pink puffers" (type A) because of their obvious tachypnea and flushed appearance, which is a result of greater ventilatory responsiveness to hypoxemia.[13]

These patients frequently are thin in physical stature and will present with "pursed lip" breathing. This maneuver compensates for loss of elastic recoil so that exhalation of a larger volume of air is possible. They also are tachypneic at rest and often sit with their chests forward and hands resting on their knees; this position requires the least energy for breathing. Frequently, the patient uses accessory muscles of the chest and neck to assist in the work of breathing. Percussion of the chest is hyperresonant, and auscultation reveals diminished breath sounds with rhonchi and minimal wheezes. Excursion of the diaphragm is limited because of persistent hyperinflation of the lungs.

Hypoxemia is not a significant problem in the predominant emphysema patient until late in the disease state. As a result, cor pulmonale is not as common a problem as seen in the predominant chronic bronchitic until the terminal stages.

DIAGNOSTIC TESTS

PULMONARY FUNCTION TESTS

Measurements of pulmonary function by objective means are considered essential in any patient with COLD to determine the severity of the disease, responsiveness to therapeutic agents, and prognosis. Several tests of small airway function are available, including the single-breath nitrogen test and mid- and end-expiratory flows from spirometry. Spirometry has been used extensively and is preferred owing to its cost, technical ease, and clinical applicability.

In patients with chronic bronchitis and/or emphysema leading to COLD, there are reductions in forced expiratory volume after 1 second (FEV_1), forced vital capacity (FVC), FEV_1/FVC ratio, and forced expiratory flow ($FEF_{25\%-75\%}$). The FEV_1/FVC ratio, expressed as a percentage, is helpful in determining the degree of obstruction. If it is less than 80%, obstruction is present. The FEF over the middle 50% of the expiratory curve [maximum midexpiratory flow rate (MMFR), $FEF_{25\%-75\%}$, or $FEF_{50\%}$] is helpful specifically in the predominant emphysema patient because it represents the elastic recoil of the lung. It is now understood that in addition to loss of elastic recoil (i.e., elasticity of the lung parenchyma) in the emphysema patient, there is also a significant component of peripheral airway disease, also referred to as *bronchiolitis,* that also contributes to the obstructive picture.

The majority of patients with mixed disease usually will experience exertional dyspnea when the FEV_1 is less than 50% of predicted and will have dyspnea at rest when the FEV_1 is less than 25% of predicted. Patients with predominant chronic bronchitis experience carbon dioxide retention and cor pulmonale when the FEV_1 is greater than 25% of predicted values, but the predominantly emphysematous patient does not experience these complications until the FEV_1 is less than 25% of predicted.

In both chronic bronchitis and emphysema, the vital capacity (VC) is decreased, the residual volume (RV) is increased, and the total lung capacity (TLC) often is normal in chronic bronchitis and increased in emphysema.[13] Measurement of diffusion capacity using carbon monoxide (DCO) can help distinguish predominant bronchitis from emphysema. In emphysema, the diffusion capacity is diminished because of loss of surface area available for gas diffusion. In bronchitis, the diffusion capacity is normal or only slightly decreased, although this test and the lung volume tests rarely are necessary in clinical practice.

The American Thoracic Society has proposed a staging system for COLD based on pulmonary function tests. The purpose of this system would be to aid in standardization of clinical trials, epidemiologic studies, health resource planning, and application of clinical recommendations. The society has proposed the following: Stage I is $FEV_1 \geq 50\%$ of predicted; stage II is $FEV_1 \geq 35\%$ to 49% of predicted; and stage III is $FEV_1 < 35\%$ of predicted.[1]

ARTERIAL BLOOD GASES

While arterial blood gas measurements are important, they do not carry the prognostic value of pulmonary function tests. Patients with COLD in stage I do not warrant arterial blood gas determination, but for those with stage II or III disease, arterial blood gas determinations are considered essential.[1] Arterial blood gases should be determined at rest and after exercise for those patients in stage II and III. The predominant chronic bronchitis patient is characterized as having a low arterial oxygen tension ($Pa{O_2}$ = 45 to 60 mm Hg) and an elevated arterial carbon dioxide tension ($Pa{CO_2}$ = 50 to 60 mm Hg). The predominantly emphysematous patient has, by comparison, a higher $Pa{O_2}$ and usually normal $Pa{CO_2}$ with similar degrees of pulmonary dysfunction. In the predominant chronic bronchitis patient, the initial abnormality is a decrease in the $Pa{O_2}$. The major cause of this hypoxemia is an underventilation (V) of acini relative to perfusion (Q) of the area. This low V/Q ratio will progress over a period of several years, resulting in a consistent decline in the $Pa{O_2}$. For reasons that are not entirely understood, the predominant chronic bronchitic loses the ability to increase the rate or depth of respiration in response to persistent hypoxemia. This decreased ventilatory drive may have its origin in either abnormal peripheral or central respiratory receptors. This relative hypoventilation subsequently leads to hypercapnia. The respiratory centers again do not respond to the persistently increasing $Pa{CO_2}$. These changes in $Pa{O_2}$ and $Pa{CO_2}$ are subtle and progress over a period of many years; as a result, the pH usually is nearly normal because the kidneys compensate by retaining bicarbonate. If an acute change occurs, such as might be seen in an acute pneumonia with impending respiratory failure, the $Pa{CO_2}$ may rise sharply, temporarily resulting in a primary respiratory acidosis until the kidneys can compensate (24 to 72 hours later) or the acid-base defect is corrected by mechanical ventilation.

The persistent hypoxemia leads to pulmonary vascular constriction and cor pulmonale. The hypoxemia and hypercarbia lead to an increase in 2,3-diphosphoglyceric acid (2,3-DPG) and a shift of the oxyhemoglobin dissociation curve to the right. This results in a decrease in the affinity of hemoglobin for oxygen, allowing more oxygen to be released to tissues in which the $Pa{O_2}$ is lowest. Hypoxemia also stimulates erythropoiesis, which leads to the secondary polycythemia common in the predominant chronic bronchitic. Patients with predominant chronic bronchitis who are also obese have more severe nocturnal hypoxemia associated with episodes of sleep apnea. As a result, these particular patients tend to have more severe cor pulmonale and secondary polycythemia.[13]

Compared with the predominant chronic bronchitic, the predominant emphysematous patient can maintain a near-normal $Pa{O_2}$ in the face of declining pulmonary function until the terminal stages because ventilation and perfusion decrease proportionately. These individuals have normal or excess responsiveness of peripheral and central respiratory receptors to hypoxemia or hypercarbia. This explains why the predominant emphysematous patient does not develop cor pulmonale, cyanosis, or polycythemia until the end stages of the disease process but does have more noticeable tachypnea.

CHEST ROENTGENOGRAM AND COMPUTED TOMOGRAPHY

A chest roentgenogram (posteroanterior and lateral views) is most useful in the diagnosis of the predominant emphysema patient. Characteristic findings include flattened diaphragms that move less than 3 cm between inspiration and expiration, loss of peripheral vascular markings, bullous lesions (i.e., an empty space greater than 1 cm in diameter usually in the lower lung field), and increased retrosternal airspace. All these findings indicate extensive air trapping consistent with severe emphysema. Whether or not the dimensions of the thoracic cage itself are truly increased is a matter of controversy; it may be that the cage appears large because of the loss of physical mass in the rest of the body. Unfortunately, these changes are more reflective of severe disease and are not as consistently present in mild to moderate emphysema. High-resolution computed tomography (CT) is more specific and sensitive than chest radiography but is of limited clinical value because results from CT do not change therapy except in the instances where surgical resection of portions of the lung is being considered for some emphysema patients.[13]

In the predominant chronic bronchitic, the only changes on chest x-ray are increased bronchovascular markings in the lower lung field and an increased cardiac silhouette in the presence of right ventricular failure with prominent pulmonary arteries.

ELECTROCARDIOGRAM

The electrocardiogram is helpful in COLD patients only when cor pulmonale develops. Common findings are right-axis deviation, prominent R waves in V_1 and V_2, S wave in V_5 or V_6 that are 7 mm or greater, and tall peaked P waves in lead II.

OTHER LABORATORY TESTS

HEMATOLOGY

In the predominant chronic bronchitic patient, the hemoglobin and hematocrit will be elevated secondary to erythropoiesis caused by hypoxemia. In exacerbations of chronic bronchitis, the white cell count may or may not rise, and a left shift may or may not be present.

SPUTUM

Examination of sputum (e.g., Gram stain) is helpful in exacerbations of chronic bronchitis to identify potential bacterial pathogens that may have precipitated the exacerbation and aid in the selection of antimicrobial therapy. It is important to ensure that what is examined microscopically is truly sputum and not saliva. Sputum is identified by the presence of alveolar macrophages; saliva is identified by squamous epithelial cells. Many laboratories have developed scoring systems to help clinicians assess the adequacy of the sputum sample being examined. Sputum also should be examined for eosinophils to rule out an allergic component that would be consistent with asthmatic bronchitis.

α_1-ANTITRYPSIN ASSAY

This test is particularly useful in patients younger than 40 years of age who present with emphysema and obstructive lung disease. Markedly low levels may indicate a PiZZ phenotype. Moderately low levels may indicate other Pi phenotypes who may be more predisposed to emphysema caused by smoking than the general population.

COURSE AND PROGNOSIS

The clinical course and prognosis of patients having chronic bronchitis and/or emphysema with obstructive pulmonary disease are marked by variable morbidity and mortality. Little is known of the early natural history of COLD, but it is probably characterized by slowly deteriorating pulmonary function for several years before clinical illness is appreciated by the patient. Much more is known of the prognosis and clinical course once symptomatology has become evident. Delay in recognition of the true impact of COLD may occur because the disease develops at a time of life when people generally begin to modify activities to less stressful pursuits. There also may be a process of physical detraining that obscures the fact that dyspnea is the underlying cause of their reduced exercise tolerance. This may result in a loss of cardiopulmonary fitness and some disuse atrophy of leg muscles. This is of interest and importance because patients with lung disease may cease exercise because of leg fatigue rather than dyspnea, and patients with COLD have relatively poor work efficiency.

The predominant emphysema patient's pattern is characterized by progressive dyspnea without exacerbations precipitated by increased sputum production, as is characteristic of the predominant chronic bronchitic patient. The predominant emphysema patient's terminal event often is characterized by rapidly progressive cor pulmonale and intractable hypercapnia leading to respiratory arrest. The usual course of a patient with predominant bronchitis is characterized by increasing frequency of exacerbations of acute pulmonary insufficiency precipitated by bronchitis. This is accompanied by progressive decline in pulmonary function, with the chronic complications (previously described) of cor pulmonale, hypercapnia, and polycythemia. Exacerbations of bronchitis are characterized by increased mucopurulent sputum and frequently lead to acute respiratory failure from which the patient recovers rapidly with appropriate antibiotics and other therapies. These episodes tend to increase in severity and frequency until intractable cor pulmonale and hypercapnia occur.

Mean rate of decline of FEV_1 appears to be a useful objective tool to assess the course of COLD. The rate of decline in FEV_1 for normal patients from age alone is 25 to 30 mL per year. The rate of decline for smokers is steeper. It is also steeper for heavy smokers than for light smokers. The decline in pulmonary function is a steady curvilinear path. The more severely diminished the FEV_1 at diagnosis, the steeper is the rate of decline. Greater numbers of years of smoking and number of cigarettes smoked also correlate with a steeper decline in pulmonary function.[18] The rate of decline of blood gases has not been shown to be a useful parameter to assess progression of the disease.

In terms of functional capacity, the predominant chronic bronchitic patient will show more physical impairment at a higher FEV_1 than the predominant emphysema patient because of the comparatively worse arterial blood gases. Most people with mixed disease are not able to perform extremely vigorous activity once the FEV_1 falls below 1.5 L, but they can work. Once the FEV_1 falls below 1.0 L, their ability to perform usual daily activities becomes impaired.

The survival rate of patients with COLD is related to the initial level of impairment in the FEV_1 and age. Other less important factors include degree of reversibility with bronchodilators, resting pulse, perceived physical disability, diffusing capacity, cor pulmonale, and blood gas abnormalities. A rapid decline in pulmonary function tests indicates a poor prognosis. People living at high altitudes also have a reduced survival rate. Median survival is approximately 10 years when the FEV_1 is 1.4 L, 4 years when the FEV_1 is 1.0 L, and about 2 years when the FEV_1 is 0.5 L.

As yet it is not clear that treatment with pharmacologic agents improves survival; however, they do improve the quality of life, probably reduce hospitalizations, and may prevent some premature deaths. In recent years, several disease-specific quality-of-life measures have been developed to assess the overall efficacies of therapies for COLD, including the Chronic Respiratory Questionnaire (CRQ) and the St. George's Respiratory Questionnaire (SGRQ).[19] These questionnaires measure the impact of various therapies on disease variables such as severity of dyspnea and level of activity; they do not measure impact of therapies on survival. Currently, they have been used only to a limited degree to quantify short-term health gain obtained from bronchodilators; however, there appears to be a trend toward greater use of these disease-specific quality-of-life measures. The only intervention shown to improve survival rate is oxygen therapy. Smoking cessation leads to decreased symptomatology and slows the rate of decline of pulmonary function even after significant abnormality in pulmonary function tests have been detected ($FEV_1/FVC < 60\%$).[18]

ACUTE RESPIRATORY FAILURE IN COLD

The diagnosis of acute respiratory failure in COLD is made on the basis of an acute change in the arterial blood gases. Defining acute respiratory failure as a PaO_2 of less than 50 mm Hg or a $PaCO_2$ of greater than 50 mm Hg often may be incorrect and inadequate because these values may not represent a significant change from a patient's baseline values. A more precise definition is an acute drop in PaO_2 of 10 to 15 mm Hg or any acute increase in $PaCO_2$ that decreases the serum pH to 7.3 or less.[13] Additional acute clinical manifestations of respiratory failure include restlessness, confusion, tachycardia, diaphoresis, cyanosis, hypotension, irregular breathing, miosis, and unconsciousness.

The most common cause of acute respiratory failure in COLD is acute exacerbation of bronchitis with an increase in the volume and viscosity of sputum. This serves to worsen obstruction and further impair alveolar ventilation, resulting in worsening hypoxemia and hypercapnia. Additional causes of acute respiratory failure in COLD are pneumonia, pulmonary embolism, left ventricular failure, pneumothorax, and use of central nervous system depressants.

▶ TREATMENT: Chronic Obstructive Lung Disease

DESIRED OUTCOMES, SMOKING CESSATION, AND NONPHARMACOLOGIC THERAPY

Therapy of the patient with COLD is multifaceted. Goals of therapy include smoking cessation, improvement in chronic obstructive status, treatment and prevention of acute exacerbations, reduction in the rate of progression of disease, improvement in physical and psychological well-being, and reduction in mortality, hospitalizations, and days lost from work. The importance of smoking cessation cannot be overemphasized—it is the obvious and first step in the secondary prevention plan. As confirmed by the Lung Health Study, smoking cessation is the only intervention proven at this time to affect long-term decline in FEV_1 and slow the progression of COLD.[20] In this 5-year prospective trial, smokers with early COLD were randomly assigned to smoking-cessation intervention or usual care groups. Smokers who underwent smoking-cessation intervention had fewer respiratory symptoms and a lesser decline in FEV_1 compared with smokers who received usual care. Nicotine replacement therapy (e.g., gum, patch, or inhaler), bupropion, and clonidine may be helpful in assisting the smoker to quit. Bupropion appears to be the most promising treatment available to aid with smoking cessation. Nicotine patch, buproprion, and the combination of bupropion and the nicotine patch were compared with placebo in a controlled trial.[21] The treatment groups that received bupropion had higher rates of smoking cessation than the groups that received placebo or the nicotine patch. The addition of the nicotine patch to bupropion slightly improved the smoking-cessation rate compared with bupropion monotherapy. Behavioral modification techniques or other forms of psychotherapy also may be helpful in assisting in smoking cessation. Programs that address the many issues associated with smoking (i.e., learned behaviors, environmental influences, chemical dependence) using a team approach are more likely to be successful. The role of alternative medicine therapies in smoking cessation is controversial. Hypnosis may aid in improving abstinence rates when added to a smoking-cessation program but appears to give little benefit when used alone. Acupuncture has not been shown to contribute to smoking cessation and is not recommended.[1]

Pulmonary rehabilitation programs are an integral component in the management of COLD and should include exercise training along with smoking cessation, breathing exercises, optimal medical treatment, psychosocial support, and health education. High-intensity training (70% maximal workload) is possible even in advanced COLD patients, and the level of intensity improves peripheral muscle and ventilatory function. Studies have demonstrated that pulmonary rehabilitation with exercise three to seven times per week can produce long-term improvement in activities of daily living, quality of life, and exercise tolerance in patients with moderate to severe COLD.[22] Programs using less intensive exercise regimens (two times per week) have not been shown to be of benefit.[23]

Adjunctive therapies to consider as part of a pulmonary rehabiliation program are psychoeducational care, nutritional support, and the use of supplemental oxygen. Psychoeducational care (such as relaxation) has been associated with improving the functioning and well-being of adults with COLD.[24] The role of nutritional support in patients with COLD is controversial. Several studies have shown an association between malnutrition, low body mass index (BMI), and impaired pulmonary status among patients with COLD. However, in a recent metaanalysis, the effect of nutritional support on outcomes in COLD was small and was not associated with improved anthropometric measures, lung function, or functional exercise capacity.[25]

PHARMACOLOGIC THERAPY

There was a long-standing opinion that COLD was associated with irreversible obstruction. This reasoning allowed pharmacotherapy to be chosen empirically. However, studies now suggest that many individuals with COLD do obtain some degree of improvement in their obstruction from bronchodilators. This group may include many patients who would now be described as having an asthmatic component to their disease. In addition, COLD patients with the greatest bronchodilatory response have the lowest annual decline in FEV_1 and the greatest 5-year survival. It also appears that a single test of reversibility using an inhaled sympathomimetic followed by pulmonary function tests is not adequate to assess whether patients with COLD will benefit from bronchodilators. Even if a positive response is not detected, these patients deserve an adequate therapeutic trial of pharmacologic agents for the following reasons: (1) although objective tests may not reveal a response, possibly because of sensitivity of equipment, a subjective improvement may occur, (2) some patients may respond to inhaled sympathomimetics on one occasion and not on another, (3) the response to bronchodilators may require prolonged administration, (4) patients may respond to pharmacologic agents via mechanisms besides bronchodilation, (5) patients not responding in initial tests with sympathomimetics may respond to anticholinergics or methylxanthines, and (6) some parameters may be improved (e.g., exercise capacity) while others are not (e.g., FEV_1).[10,26] Patients whose disease is caused primarily by bronchial wall inflammation accompanied by bronchospasm, as seen in the chronic bronchitic, respond better to bronchodilator therapy than patients suffering primarily from irreversible emphysematous damage. The decision of drug therapy selection should be based on patient compliance, individual response, and side effects. For the purposes of this chapter, agents will be presented in the sequence indicated by current trends in therapy and are divided into two tiers. Tier one therapy includes anticholinergics and sympathomimetics; tier two therapy is represented by methylxanthines and corticosteroids.

ANTICHOLINERGICS

In the past decade, anticholinergic agents have emerged as first-line therapy for the stable COLD patient. The only anticholinergic agents currently available in the United States are atropine and ipratropium bromide. When given by inhalation, anticholinergics produce bronchodilation by competitively inhibiting cholinergic receptors in bronchial smooth muscle. This activity blocks acetylcholine, with the net effect being a reduction in cyclic guanosine monophosphate (GMP), which normally acts to constrict bronchial smooth muscle. These agents maintain their effectiveness during years of regular continuous use.[26–28] Ipratropium bromide has been shown to decrease the effectiveness of voluntary cough on clearing mucus from the airways, which may affect its role in the treatment of patients who have excessive mucus production.[29] The clinical significance of this effect is unknown.

The inhaled anticholinergics have been well demonstrated in the literature to be effective bronchodilators in COLD.[26–29] However, data from the Lung Health Study demonstrate that the rate of decline of lung function in smokers with mild to moderate COPD can be slowed significantly by smoking cessation but not by ipratropium.[30] Anticholinergic agents have been compared with inhaled sympathomimetic agents and have been found to produce greater improvement in pulmonary function tests than the sympathomimetic agents with fewer systemic side effects such as tachycardia.[31–33] This is likely so because patients with COLD do not exhibit dramatic responsiveness to adrenergic compounds, unlike patients with asthma. Moreover, with aging, the sensitivity of the adrenergic system decreases, making the cholinergic system the more readily manipulated for purposes of achieving bronchodilation. Ipratropium has a slower onset of action and a more prolonged bronchodilator effect compared with standard β-agonists and has been considered to be less suitable for use on an "as needed" basis for immediate relief of bronchospasm.[1,34] However, it has been demonstrated that in acute exacerbations of COLD in the critically ill patient, anticholinergics may be valuable as additive agents or as single agents for patients intolerant to β-agonist side effects.[35]

Ipratropium is considered the anticholinergic agent of choice for COLD. Atropine has a tertiary structure and is absorbed readily across the oral and respiratory mucosae, whereas ipratropium has a quaternary structure that is absorbed poorly. The lack of systemic absorption of ipratropium greatly diminishes the anticholinergic side effects such as blurred vision, urinary retention, nausea, and tachycardia associated with atropine. Ipratropium bromide is available as a metered-dose inhaler (MDI) and a solution for inhalation. It provides a peak effect in 1.5 to 2 hours and has a duration of effect of 4 to 6 hours. Although the recommended dose is 2 puffs four times a day, many clinicians prescribe two to three times this dose to produce maximal bronchodilation. Ipratropium has been shown to increase maximum exercise performance in stable COLD patients with doses of 8 to 12 puffs prior to exercise but not with doses of 4 puffs or less.[36,37] During sleep, ipratropium also has been shown to improve arterial oxygen saturation and sleep quality.[38] Side effects of ipratropium appear to be limited to dry mouth and an occasional metallic taste.

Tiotropium bromide, not yet available in the United States, is a long-acting quarternary anticholinergic agent. Binding studies of tiotropium in the human lung show that it is approximately 10-fold more potent than ipratropium and protects against cholinergic bronchoconstriction for greater than 24 hours.[39] Recently, the efficacy and safety of tiotropium, administered via a dry-powder inhaler, were compared with ipratropium, administered by MDI, in a multicenter, double-blind 13-week study.[40] Patients who received once-daily tiotropium demonstrated significantly greater improvements in trough, average, and peak lung function compared with patients who received ipratropium four times daily. The safety profile of tiotropium was similar to that of ipratropium. Tiotropium has a long onset of action and likely would not be of benefit for the treatment of rescue or acute exacerbations.

SYMPATHOMIMETICS

Sympathomimetics are considered tier one therapy for chronic maintenance of COLD. However, most authorities recommend that sympathomimetics be used after an adequate trial of anticholinergics, either to supplement or to replace ipratropium for patients who do not obtain satisfactory clinical benefit from ipratropium alone.[34] However, in acute exacerbations and for rescue, sympathomimetics remain the initial treatment of choice owing to their rapid onset of action. The clinical situations in which sympathomimetics are used other than acute exacerbations include (1) as-needed use for monotherapy for mild, episodic symptomatic COLD, (2) as-needed use for chronically stable, symptomatic COLD in combination with other agents (i.e., anticholinergics), and (3) as a fixed-schedule plus as-needed agent for chronically stable symptomatic COLD.

Numerous sympathomimetics currently are available in the U.S. market; however, it is more desirable to use the newer agents with greater β_2 selectivity and longer duration of action. These agents include albuterol, levalbuterol, bitolterol, pirbuterol, salmeterol, and terbutaline. β_2-Selective sympathomimetics cause bronchodilation by stimulating the enzyme adenyl cyclase to increase the formation of adenosine-3',5'-monophosphate (3',5'-cAMP).[28] In addition, they are thought to improve mucociliary clearance. Although shorter-acting and less selective β-agonists are still used widely (e.g., metaproterenol, isoetharine, isoproterenol, and epinephrine), it is difficult to advocate their continued use because of the shorter duration of action and increased cardiostimulatory effects. Note that salmeterol, which has the longest onset and duration of action of the inhaled β-agonists, is used for chronic, not acute, therapy.

β-Agonists cause only a small improvement in FEV_1 acutely but may improve respiratory symptoms and exercise tolerance despite the small improvement in spirometric measurements.[41–43] In contrast to asthma, there is little evidence to suggest that the regular use of a β-agonist is deleterious in COLD. However, some studies suggest that use of β-agonists may result in a greater rate of decline of FEV_1 than that which is related to normal COLD deterioration.[31,44] At the present time, there is no evidence to suggest that prolonged use of β-agonists increases or decreases survival in patients with COLD. The peak response tends to be preserved over the course of long-term therapy with a β-agonist, but a slight decline in duration of the bronchodilation may develop. The reader is referred to Chapter 26 for a comparative table of these agents.

In a recent randomized, double-blind, placebo-controlled trial, the efficacy and safety of salmeterol were compared with ipratropium in patients with symptomatic COLD. Patients received salmeterol 42 μg (2 puffs) twice daily, ipratropium 36 μg (2 puffs) four times daily, or inhaled placebo twice daily. Both salmeterol and ipratropium resulted in greater improvements in respiratory symptoms compared with placebo.[45] However, salmeterol was significantly better at improving lung function than ipratropium. Clinical evidence suggests that higher doses of ipratropium are more effective than the lower doses that were used in this trial.[46] An additional potential benefit of long-acting β-agonists in COLD is a potential for a decrease in infectious exacerbations. Salmeterol has been shown to reduce adherence of bacteria such as *H. influenzae* to airway epithelial cells.[47]

Sympathomimetics are available in inhaled, oral, and parenteral dosage forms. The preferred route of administration is by inhalation. The use of oral and parenteral β-agonists in COLD is discouraged because they are no more effective than a properly used MDI or dry-powder inhaler (DPI) and the incidence of systemic adverse effects (tachycardia and hand tremor) is greater.[34] The inhalation route minimizes the intracellular shift of potassium and resulting hypokalemia, which is augmented by theophylline.[28] Administration of β-agonists in the outpatient and emergency room settings via inhalers (MDI or DPI) is at least as effective as nebulization therapy and usually favored for reasons of cost and convenience.[48–50] The reader is referred to Chapter 26 for a complete description of the devices used for delivering aerosolized medication.

If response to ipratropium alone is unsatisfactory, all patients with COLD should receive a trial of an inhaled β_2-selective agonist even if their FEV_1 is not changed because mechanisms other than bronchodilation may be helpful (e.g., increase in mucociliary clearance). An individual's perceived benefit from these agents may affect their usefulness significantly. The dose of the β-agonist can be increased in an acute exacerbation, although the limiting factor is an excessive increase in heart rate. In patients whot exhibit cardiotoxicity to traditional sympathomimetics, levalbuterol is a possible alternative. Albuterol, in all marketed forms, is a racemic mixture of (R)-albuterol that is responsible for the bronchodilator effect and (S)-albuterol that has no therapeutic effect and may be responsible for many of the side effects associated with the drug.[51] Levalbuterol is the (R)-isomer of albuterol. Levalbuterol has not yet been evaluated for the treatment of COLD, is only available as an inhalation solution for nebulization, and is considerably more costly than albuterol.[52]

COMBINATION ANTICHOLINERGICS AND SYMPATHOMIMETICS

The body of evidence indicates that combination inhaled anticholinergic and β_2-agonist regimens are more effective than either as monotherapy.[53–55] Before the combination is used, the dose of the anticholinergic first should be titrated. A combination of albuterol and ipratropium (Combivent) is available as an MDI in the United States for chronic maintenance therapy of COLD. When ipratropium and β-agonists (e.g., albuterol) are used in combination, often a greater number of inhalations (puffs) of ipratropium are required compared with the β_2-agonist. This disparity in number of inhalations makes use of the combination product difficult in many patients.

METHYLXANTHINES

Methylxanthines have been available for the treatment of COLD for at least five decades and at one time were considered first-line therapy. However, in the past 20 years, with the advent of long-acting inhaled β-agonists and inhaled anticholinergics, they have been relegated to second-tier status in terms of preference. Theophylline, the most common methylxanthine used in clinical practice, can be an effective bronchodilator in many patients with chronic, stable disease.[1] The methylxanthines may produce bronchodilation through numerous mechanisms, including (1) inhibition of phosphodiesterase, thereby increasing cyclic adenosine monophosphate levels, (2) inhibition of calcium ion influx into smooth muscle, (3) prostaglandin antagonism, (4) stimulation of endogenous catecholamines, (5) adenosine receptor antagonism, and (6) inhibition of release of mediators from mast cells and leukocytes.[28] However, there is no certainty about these mechanisms. Long-term theophylline use in patients with COLD has been demonstrated to exert improvements in lung function, including VC, FEV_1, minute ventilation, and gas exchange.[56] Subjectively, theophylline has been shown to lessen dyspnea, enhance exercise tolerance, and improve respiratory drive in COLD patients.[37,57–59] Other nonpulmonary effects of theophylline that may contribute to improved overall functional capacity in patients with COLD include improved cardiac function and decreased pulmonary artery pressure.[56]

Numerous reliably absorbed sustained-release theophylline (1,3-dimethylxanthine) preparations are available currently. These have the advantages of improving patient compliance and achieving more consistent serum concentrations over rapid-release theophylline and aminophylline preparations; however, caution must be used in switching from one sustained-release preparation to another because there are considerable variations in sustained-release characteristics.[57] Aside from aminophylline, there is no need to use any of the various other theophylline complexes. There is no indication for rectal suppositories of theophylline or aminophylline or intramuscular administration of these drugs. Dissolution from rectal suppositories is inconsistent, absorption from intramuscular injections is unreliable, and the injections are painful. Aminophylline and theophylline with 5% dextrose are available as intravenous preparations. Oral and intravenous theophylline are equivalent in terms of dosage strength. Aminophylline is 80% anhydrous theophylline. Aminophylline can be converted to intravenous or oral theophylline by using 80% of the aminophylline dose.

Theophylline has been shown to be of value in exacerbations of COLD.[60] In acute exacerbations, loading doses of theophylline or aminophylline should be administered to achieve therapeutic serum concentrations rapidly. Without a loading dose, COLD patients would require 40 to 60 hours (five half-lives, using the usual elimination half-life of 8 to 12 hours) before steady-state serum concentrations would be reached with maintenance dosing only. Loading doses may be administered orally or intravenously. Oral theophylline is well absorbed from the intestines and is effective for loading when gastrointestinal function is thought to be intact. Intravenous therapy should be reserved for severe acute decompensation in patients unable to take oral medication. The loading dose is based on actual body weight.[60] Recommended loading doses are 5 mg/kg (theophylline) and 6 mg/kg (aminophylline) for patients who have not taken any theophylline in the previous 24 hours. Each 0.5 mg/kg (theophylline) or 0.6 mg/kg (aminophylline) will raise the serum theophylline concentration by approximately 1 μg/mL. Ideally, for patients currently taking theophylline, the loading dose should be deferred until a theophylline concentration can be obtained rapidly. However, if this is not possible, then it is recommended to administer a partial loading dose of 2.5 mg/kg (theophylline) or 3 mg/kg (aminophylline) if the patient has taken sustained release theophylline within the past 24 hours or immediate-release theophylline within the past 12 hours.

The intravenous administration rate of aminophylline and theophylline with dextrose should not exceed 25 mg/min to avoid cardiac arrhythmias or cardiovascular collapse. A controlling device is recommended when infusing aminophylline or theophylline.

TABLE 27–3. Maintenance Doses of Intravenous Aminophylline in Exacerbations of COLD

Usual loading dose, mg/kg	6
Maintenance dose, mg/kg/h	
Smokers	0.8
Nonsmokers	0.5
Elderly	0.3
Cor pulmonale	0.3
Congestive heart failure	0.1–0.2
Liver disease	0.1–0.2

Traditionally, the desired therapeutic range of theophylline is 10 to 20 μg/mL; however, the literature is absent of studies to support any particular theophylline concentration range. Because of the high incidence of theophylline-associated toxicity, many practitioners advocate a more conservative therapeutic range of 10–15 or 8–12 μg/mL. This latter lower concentration range is preferable in the elderly, who are especially prone to theophylline-associated side effects. Factors in COLD patients that decrease theophylline clearance leading to reduced maintenance-dose requirements include advanced age, bacterial or viral pneumonia, left or right ventricular failure, liver dysfunction, hypoxemia from the acute decompensation, and use of drugs such as cimetidine, macrolide, and fluoroquinolone antibiotics. Factors that may enhance theophylline clearance, resulting in the need for higher maintenance doses, include tobacco and marijuana smoking, hyperthyroidism, and the use of such drugs as phenytoin, phenobarbital, and rifampin. Maintenance-dose recommendations for intravenous aminophylline for these conditions have been proposed and are summarized in Table 27–3. Again, when using oral or intravenous theophylline, 80% of the aminophylline dose should be used. These recommendations should be considered as starting points because serum theophylline concentrations must be obtained to guide and individualize therapy. The conditions described are dynamic, and as they fluctuate, so will the clearance of theophylline.

Oral therapy should be substituted for intravenous therapy once the patient is stabilized, serum concentrations are reasonably consistent, and the patient is able to take oral medications. The oral sustained-release preparation can be initiated at the time the intravenous solution is stopped. The oral dose is calculated from the 24-hour intravenous theophylline dose. The total 24-hour dose may then be divided in thirds or halves depending on the desired interval and strength of preparation available. Another regimen used clinically is to administer long-acting theophylline preparations at bedtime. This has been demonstrated to reduce overnight declines in FEV_1 and morning respiratory symptoms.[61]

In the severely decompensated patient, serum concentrations should be obtained 12 to 24 hours after administration of the loading dose and every 24 hours thereafter until the patient is stable. The reason for evaluating concentrations early is that should the patient have a clearance much lower than anticipated, the dose can be reduced before the patient becomes toxic, and should the clearance be much higher than anticipated, modest elevations in dose can be made. Maintenance therapy in the non-acutely ill patient can be initiated at 400–900 mg/d of the sustained-release preparation. Trough serum levels should be evaluated 1 to 2 weeks after initiation of therapy or with any dose adjustment. Once a dose is established, it should not be necessary to monitor serum concentrations routinely unless the patient's disease worsens or toxicity is suspected.

Attempting to make adjustments in dose to attain a desired concentration using first-order pharmacokinetic equations is fraught with error. Theophylline is metabolized by microsomal enzymes to three major metabolites: 1,3-dimethyluric acid, 1-methyluric acid, and 3-methylxanthine. Each metabolic pathway is potentially saturable. This results in nonlinear kinetics of theophylline that are witnessed in acute overdoses. Apparent nonlinearity may occur because of physiologic changes that happen during therapy of acute exacerbations. Diminished hemodynamics due to either right or left ventricular failure may result in hepatic congestion, which affects theophylline clearance. Acutely ill and hypoalbuminemic patients may have increased free (as opposed to protein-bound) theophylline concentrations while their total serum theophylline concentrations are in the "therapeutic range."[62] This perhaps explains why toxicity develops at low serum concentrations in some patients. Because there are other pharmacologic interventions for COLD, it is unnecessary to push the theophylline dose to toxicity.

Serum theophylline concentrations above 20 μg/mL are associated with nausea and vomiting, and those above 35–40 μg/mL are associated with arrhythmias and seizures. In the elderly, these values should not be used to judge the likelihood of toxicity because this population exhibits these catastrophic side effects at lower serum concentrations. Nausea is a common complication in elderly patients with concentrations greater than 15 μg/mL, and seizures and atrial tachyarrhythmias have been reported with serum concentrations of 20–30 μg/mL. Theophylline-induced seizures and arrhythmias are quite refractory to conventional treatment.

There has been considerable debate as to the relative risk-benefit ratio of methylxanthines in COLD patients.[10] Regular use of methylxanthines has not been shown to have either a beneficial or a detrimental effect on the course of COLD. Because of the uncertainty regarding their role, they are now considered second-tier therapy, placed after anticholinergics and sympathomimetics. Methylxanthines may be added to the treatment plan of patients who have not achieved an optimal clinical response to ipratropium and an inhaled β-agonist. Studies suggest that adding theophylline to the combination of albuterol and ipratropium can result in maximum benefit in stable COLD patients, supporting the hypothesis that there is a synergistic bronchodilatory effect.[61,63,64] When methylxanthines are used to treat COLD patients, parameters other than objective measurements, such as FEV_1, should be monitored to assess efficacy. Subjective parameters, such as perceived exercise tolerance, become increasingly important in assessing the acceptability of methylxanthines for COLD patients. Note that although objective improvement may be minimal, clinical benefit to the individual may be meaningful.[61,63,64]

CORTICOSTEROIDS

Therapeutic trials evaluating the use of corticosteroids in COLD have been going on for more than 40 years.[65] Because of the potential role of inflammation in the pathogenesis of the disease, corticosteroids theoretically should be useful agents in COLD management. However, their use continues to be debated, especially in the management of stable COLD. The anti-inflammatory mechanisms whereby corticosteroids exert their beneficial effect in COLD include (1) reduction in capillary permeability to decrease mucus, (2) inhibition of release of proteolytic enzymes from leukocytes, and (3) inhibition of prostaglandins. These desired effects occur because of the ability of steroids to be transported into the nucleus of the cell and stimulate RNA synthesis. Corticosteroids may be used in COLD in many different clinical scenarios, including (1) systemic use for acute exacerbations, (2) systemic use for chronic stable COLD, and (3) inhalation for chronic stable COLD.

Until recently, the literature supporting the use of corticosteroids in acute exacerbations of COLD was sparse and debatable. However, since 1996, three randomized, placebo-controlled studies have been performed that advocate corticosteroid use for exacetrbations.[66–68] The Systemic Corticosteroids in Chronic Obstructive Pulmonary Disease Exacerbations (SCCOPE) trial evaluated three groups of patients hospitalized for exacerbations of COLD.[66] The first group received an 8-week course of corticosteroids given as methylprednisolone 125 mg intravenously every 6 hours for 72 hours, followed by once-daily oral prednisone (60 mg on days 4 through 7, 40 mg on days 8 through 11, 20 mg on days 12 through 43, 10 mg on days 44 through 50, and 5 mg on days 51 through 57). The second group received a 2-week course given as methylprednisolone 125 mg intravenously every 6 hours for 72 hours, followed by oral prednisone (60 mg on days 5 through 7, 40 mg on days 8 through 11, and 20 mg on days 12 through 15) and placebo on days 16 through 57. The third group received placebo for all 57 days of study. Rates of treatment failure and hospital stay were significantly higher in the placebo group than in either treatment group at 30 and 90 days. Groups randomized to corticosteroid treatment also had a significantly shorter length of hospital stay compared with the placebo group. The 8-week regimen was not found to be superior to the 2-week regimen. Significant treatment benefits were no longer evident at 6 months. Davies and colleagues evaluated the oral use of corticosteroids in hospitalized patients with acute exacerbations of COLD.[67] Patients received either 30 mg daily of oral prednisolone or placebo for 14 days. Patients who were treated with corticosteroids had a significantly more rapid improvement in FEV_1 and a shorter hospital stay than did patients who received placebo. There was no significant difference between groups at 6-week follow up. Thompson and colleagues found oral prednisone to be more effective than placebo in outpatients with acute exacerbations of COLD using a 9-day tapering dose (60 mg on days 1 through 3, 40 mg on days 4 through 6, and 20 mg on days 7 through 9) that resulted in a more rapid improvement in PaO_2, alveolar-arterial oxygen gradient, FEV_1, and peak expiratory flow.[68] Prednisone also resulted in fewer treatment failures compared with placebo. Based on these trials, patients with acute exacerbations of COLD should receive a short course of intravenous or oral corticosteroids. If intravenous steroids are used, they should be converted to oral steroids after improvement in pulmonary status is noted and the patient has a functioning gastrointestinal tract. If steroid treatment is continued for greater than 2 weeks, a tapering oral schedule should be employed to avoid hypothalamic-pituitary-adrenal (HPA) axis suppression.

Oral steroid use in chronic stable COLD patients was evaluated in a review by Callahan and associates.[69] In this metaanalysis, 33 original studies of oral steroids in COLD published since 1951 were evaluated. The authors concluded that COLD patients treated with steroids showed clinically significant improvement in baseline FEV_1 (increase of 20%) 10% more often than similar patients who received placebo. It therefore appears that the number of stable COLD patients who will benefit from steroids is modest at best. Attempts to determine patient characteristics that may be helpful in assessing which patients would most likely benefit from steroid administration appear to show that an increased proportion of eosinophils on sputum examination ($\geq$3%) and a significant response on pulmonary function tests to sympathomimetics are the best predictors.[70] A 25% or greater response of the FEV_1 has been reported to be the best predictor of responsiveness.[2]

The role of inhaled corticosteroids in COLD continues to be debated in the literature, unlike asthma, where their use is clearly advocated. Numerous trials have been performed that have evaluated the use of inhaled corticosteroids in this population.[71–78] Evaluating the effect of steroids based on these trials is difficult because treatment durations and doses of steroids used differ between trials, as do end points of efficacy and interpretation of these end points.[2,3,77,78] Two of the most recent larger and well-designed studies, European Respiratory Society on Chronic Obstructive Pulmonary Disease (EUROSCOP) and Inhaled Steroids in Obstructive Lung Disease in Europe (ISOLDE), found that inhaled corticosteroids improve post-bronchodilator FEV_1 acutely, but they found no evidence that long-term treatment reduced the progression of COLD.[71,73] An added potential benefit of inhaled corticosteroids is a reduction in the incidence of acute exacerbations.[75,76]

Based on the lack of consensus of the efficacy of oral and inhaled corticosteroids for the management of chronic stable COLD, they are considered second-tier therapy after an adequate trial of inhaled anticholinergics, sympathomimetics, and possibly theophylline. A common finding among many trials that have evaluated oral and inhaled steroids in COLD is that there are two types of patients with COLD: those who do respond to steroids (steroid responders) and those who do not. It is suggested that many steroid responders with COLD have an asthmatic component in their disease. Regardless, current COLD guidelines recommend that steroids only should be used for the management of stable COLD in patients who show objective benefit during a steroid trial.[1,79]

Systemic corticosteroids produce significant side effects; therefore, many clinicians follow the axiom that as small a dose as possible should be used for as short a duration as possible. Objective parameters should be followed to substantiate drug use. A short- to intermediate-acting corticosteroid is preferred to minimize suppression of the HPA axis. In prolonged therapy, the ideal is to achieve the lowest possible effective dose with a minimal likelihood of HPA axis suppression (e.g., prednisone 7.5 mg/d). The dose should be given once per day in the morning to mimic the normal diurnal variation of endogenous cortisol secretion. If possible, the patient should be moved to an alternate-day schedule. This is accomplished by raising one day's dose while decreasing the alternate day's dose. Side effects of inhaled corticosteroids seen in COLD trials are relatively mild and include hoarseness, sore throat, oral candidiasis, and skin bruising. More severe side effects associated with prolonged use of inhaled corticosteroids, such as HPA axis suppression, osteoporosis, and cataract formation, have been reported.[80]

LONG-TERM OXYGEN

Although long-term oxygen has been used for many years in patients with advanced COLD, it was not until 1980 that data became available documenting its benefits. At that time, the Nocturnal Oxygen Therapy Trial Group published its data comparing nocturnal oxygen therapy (NOT) (12 h/d) with continuous oxygen therapy (COT) (average of 20 h/d).[81] The patients were followed for at least 12 months. The results revealed a mortality rate in the NOT group nearly double that of the COT group, 41 in 80 versus 23 in 87. Statistical estimates of the COT group suggest that COT may have added 3.25 years to a COLD patient's life. The decline in mortality with oxygen therapy was further substantiated in 1981 in a study by the British Medical Research Council that compared 15 h/d of oxygen versus no supplemental oxygen in COLD patients.[82] Additional data from the Nocturnal Oxygen Therapy Trial Group revealed that COT patients had fewer (but statistically insignificant) hospitalizations, improved quality of life and neuropsychological function, reduced hematocrits, and decreased pulmonary vascular resistance. Recent analyses have shown that long-term oxygen therapy provides even more benefit in terms of survival after at least 5 years of use, and it improves the quality of life of these patients by increasing walking distance and neuropsychological condition and reducing time spent in the hospital.[83,84] Once stable on oxygen for 6 months, patients do not need to be reevaluated more often than every 6 months. Whether oxygen therapy consistently improves exercise tolerance or sleep remains controversial.

Before patients are considered for long-term oxygen therapy, they should be stabilized in the outpatient setting for 1 month, and pharmacotherapy should be optimized. Once this is accomplished, long-term oxygen therapy should be instituted if either of two conditions exists:

1. A resting PaO_2 of less than 55 mm Hg
2. Evidence of right-sided heart failure, polycythemia, or impaired neuropsychiatric function with a PaO_2 of less than 60 mm Hg

The most practical means of administering long-term oxygen is with the nasal cannula, which provides 24% to 28% oxygen. The goal is to raise the PaO_2 above 60 mm Hg. Patients known to retain carbon dioxide should be cautioned to not raise the PaO_2 so high that they depress their respiratory drive. Patient education about flow rates and avoidance of flames is of the utmost importance.

There are three different ways to deliver oxygen, including (1) in liquid reservoirs, (2) compressed into a cylinder, and (3) via an oxygen concentrator. Although the conventional liquid oxygen and compressed oxygen are quite bulky, smaller, portable tanks are available to permit the patient more mobility. Oxygen concentrator devices separate the nitrogen from room air and concentrate the oxygen. These are the most convenient and the least expensive method of oxygen delivery. Oxygen-conservation devices are available that allow oxygen to flow only during inspiration, making the supply last longer. These may be particularly useful to prolong the oxygen supply for mobile patients using portable cylinders. However, the devices are bulky and subject to failure.Controversy exists concerning the efficacy and tolerability of nasal nocturnal positive-pressure ventilation for COLD, and many patients may be unwilling to accept this form of oxygen therapy.[83]

ANTIBIOTICS

Acute bacterial exacerbations in COLD can cause considerable morbidity and mortality, particularly in the elderly. Although the majority of infections are viral, bacterial infection may follow the initial viral infection. Effective antibiotic therapy results in fewer hospitalizations and better resolution of symptoms. Saint and colleagues performed a metaanalysis of six studies evaluating the effectiveness of antibiotics in treating exacerbations of COLD.[85] They summarized that patients receiving antibiotics had a greater improvement in peak expiratory flow rate than those who did not. This metaanalysis concluded that antibiotics are of most benefit and should be initiated if at least two of the following three symptoms are present: increased dyspnea, increased sputum volume, and increased sputum purulence. The utility of sputum Gram stain and culture is questionable because some patients have chronic bacterial colonization of the bronchial tree between exacerbations.[86]

The emergence of drug-resistant organisms has mandated that antibiotic regimens be chosen judiciously. Selection of empirical antimicrobial therapy should be based on the most likely organism(s) thought to be responsible for the infection based on the individual patient profile. The most common organisms for any acute exacerbation of COLD are *H. influenzae*, *M. catarrhalis*, *S. pneumoniae*, and *H. parainfluenzae*. More virulent bacteria may be present in patients with more complicated acute exacerbations of COLD, including drug-resistant pneumococci, β-lactamase producing *H. influenzae* and *M. cattarhalis,* as well as enteric gram-negative organisms including *Pseudomonas aeruginosa*. Table 27–4 summarizes recommended antimicrobial therapy for exacerbations of COLD and the most common organisms based on patient presentation.[87]

Therapy should be initiated within 24 hours of symptoms to prevent unnecessary hospitalization. It is also important to prevent an accelerated rate of decline in pulmonary function from irritation and mucus plugging owing to the infectious process. Therapy generally should be continued for at least 7 to 10 days. Studies evaluating shorter treatment courses (usually 5 days) with the fluoroquinolones, second- and third-generation cephalosporins, and macrolide antimicrobials have demonstrated comparable efficacy with the longer treatment regimens.[88–93] If the patient deteriorates or does not improve as anticipated, hospitalization may be necessary, and more aggressive attempts should be made to identify potential pathogens responsible for the exacerbation. Parenteral antibiotics may be required.

IMMUNOTHERAPY

Because influenza is a common complication in COLD that can lead to respiratory failure, an annual influenza vaccine is recommended to protect those individuals who are not allergic to eggs. Amantadine can be considered for patients with COLD who have not received the vaccination and who are at risk for influenza A or for patients with early influenza A infection. The dose should be decreased from 100 mg twice daily to 100 mg once daily in those older than 65 years of age owing to reduced renal clearance. Newer antivirals such as rimantadine, zanamivir inhalant, and oseltamivir may be reasonable alternatives, although zanamivir may be less than ideal in the COLD patient due to potential irritant properties exhibited when this powder formulation is inhaled.

The polyvalent pneumococcal vaccination, administered one time, is widely recommended for people from 2 to 64 years of age who have chronic lung disease. Although the recommendation of the pneumococcal vaccine has been questioned, the argument for continued use is that the current vaccine has 23 antigens and now provides coverage for 85% of pneumococcal disease. Currently, administering the vaccine remains the standard of practice and is recommended by the Centers for Disease Control and Prevention and the American Lung Association.[94] Repeated vaccination with the 23-valent product is not recommended for patients aged 2 to 64 years with chronic lung disease; however, revaccination is recommended for patients over 65 years of age if the first vaccination was more than 5 years earlier and the patient was younger than age 65. Individuals who received the original 18-valent product should receive the 23-valent vaccine.

RESPIRATORY STIMULANTS

The role of respiratory stimulants in COLD patients is controversial. There is no role for respiratory stimulants in the long-term management of COLD.[95] Agents that have shown some utility in the acute setting include amiltrine and doxapram. However, amiltrine is available only in Europe, and its usefulness is limited by neurotoxicity.[96] Doxapram is available for intravenous use only and may be no better than nasal intermittent positive-pressure ventilation.

TABLE 27–4. Recommended Antimicrobial Therapy in Acute Exacerbations of COLD

Patient Characteristics	Likely Pathogens	Recommended Therapy
Uncomplicated exacerbations < 4 exacerbations per year No comorbid illness FEV_1 > 50% of predicted	*S. pneumoniae* *H. influenzae* *M. catarrhalis* *H. parainfluenzae* Resistance uncommon	Macrolide (azithromycin, clarithromycin) Second- or third-generation cephalosporin Doxycycline Therapies not recommended[a]: TMP/SMX, amoxicillin, first-generation cephalosporins, and erythromycin
Complicated exacerbations Age ≥ 65 > 4 exacerbations per year FEV_1 < 50% but > 35% of predicted	As above plus drug-resistant pneumococci, β-lactamase–producing *H. influenzae* and *M. catarrhalis* Some enteric gram-negatives	Amoxicillin/clavulanate Fluoroquinolone with enhanced pneumococcal activity (levofloxacin, gatifloxacin, moxifloxacin)
Complicated exacerbations with risk of *P. aeruginosa* Chronic bronchial sepsis[b] Need for chronic Corticosteroid therapy Resident of nursing home > 4 exacerbations per year FEV_1 > 35% of predicted	As above plus *P. aeruginosa*	Fluoroquinolone with enhanced pneumococcal and *P. aeruginosa* activity (levofloxacin, gatifloxacin, moxifloxacin) IV therapy if required: β-lactamase resistant penicillin with antipseudomonal activity Third- or fourth-generation cephalosporin with antipseudomonal activity

[a]TMP/SMX should not be used due to increasing pneumococcal resistance; amoxicillin and first-generation cephalosporins are not recommended due to β-lactamase susceptibility; and erythromycin is not recommended due to insufficient activity against *H. influenzae.*
[b]In sepsis, double antipseudomonal coverage should be considered (e.g., addition of aminoglycoside).
Adapted from Ref. 87.

CHOICE OF THERAPY

An algorithm to provide guidance in the choice of therapy for a patient with chronic stable COLD is given in Figure 27–2. Therapeutic options for acute exacerbations of COLD are summarized in Table 27–5. It cannot be stressed enough that individualized treatment regimens are necessary to optimize outcome because patients differ in their compliance with medication, technique in using inhalers and equipment, and values in terms of quality of life.

COMPLICATIONS

COR PULMONALE

Long-term oxygen therapy and diuretics have been the mainstays of therapy for cor pulmonale. Increasing the PaO_2 above 60 mm Hg with supplemental oxygen therapy decreases pulmonary hypertension and thus decreases the force against which the right ventricle has to work. While diuretics decrease preload and in this manner improve right-sided heart failure, the greatest concern with using diuretics is hypokalemic metabolic alkalosis. The hypokalemia may be exacerbated by concomitant use of β-agonists or corticosteroids. Therefore, the decision to use diuretics must be based on a risk-benefit ratio. If only peripheral edema exists without hepatic congestion, the risk of diuretics may exceed potential benefit. If hepatic congestion is evident, judicious use of diuretics is certainly indicated because other modes of therapy may be compromised by the congestion. Digitalis glycosides have no role in the treatment of cor pulmonale.

Other pharmacologic agents that have been investigated to treat cor pulmonale include hydralazine, calcium channel blockers, angiotensin-converting enzyme inhibitors, and angiotensin II antagonists.[97,98] Data are currently insufficient to offer guidelines for the role of these agents in COLD patients with cor pulmonale.

POLYCYTHEMIA

Polycythemia secondary to chronic hypoxemia in COLD patients can be improved by either oxygen therapy or periodic phlebotomy if oxygen is not sufficient. COT was shown by the Nocturnal Oxygen Therapy Trial Group to reduce hematocrits.[81] Acute phlebotomy is indicated if the hematocrit is above 55% to 60% and the patient is experiencing central nervous system effects suggestive of sludging from high blood viscosity. Long-term oxygen can then be used to maintain a lower hematocrit.

α_1-PROTEINASE INHIBITOR (α_1-ANTITRYPSIN)

This genetically engineered compound is indicated for patients with panacinar emphysema who have the PiZZ and Pi-null phenotypes. Its use should not be considered in patients with emphysema who have other Pi phenotypes. The therapeutic objective is to maintain ATT serum concentrations higher than 80 mg/dL to have sufficient antielastase activity in the lung epithelial lining fluid. The recommended

TABLE 27–5. COLD Therapy Recommendations in Acute Exacerbations

Disorder	Therapy	Comments
Bacterial infection of airways	Antibiotics	Recommended if two or more of the following are present: Increased dyspnea; Increased sputum volume; Increased sputum purulence
Airway inflammation	Corticosteroids	Oral or intravenous therapy may be used If intravenous is used, it should be changed to oral after improvement in pulmonary status If continued longer than 14 days, then the dose should be tapered to avoid HPA axis suppression
Bronchoconstriction	β_2-Agonist Ipratropium β_2-Agonist + ipratropium Theophylline + other bronchodilator	MDIs and DPIs equal in efficacy to nebulization β-Agonists also may increase mucociliary clearance
Secretions	Stop smoking	Other therapies such as expectorants, iodides, chest physiotherapy have no proven therapy in acute setting
Impaired gas exchange and acute ventilatory failure	Supplemental oxygen Treat comorbid conditions that impair gas exchange and muscle function Doxapram Noninvasive assisted ventilation or intubation and mechanical intubation	Titrate supplemental oxygen by response

Adapted from Ref. 86.

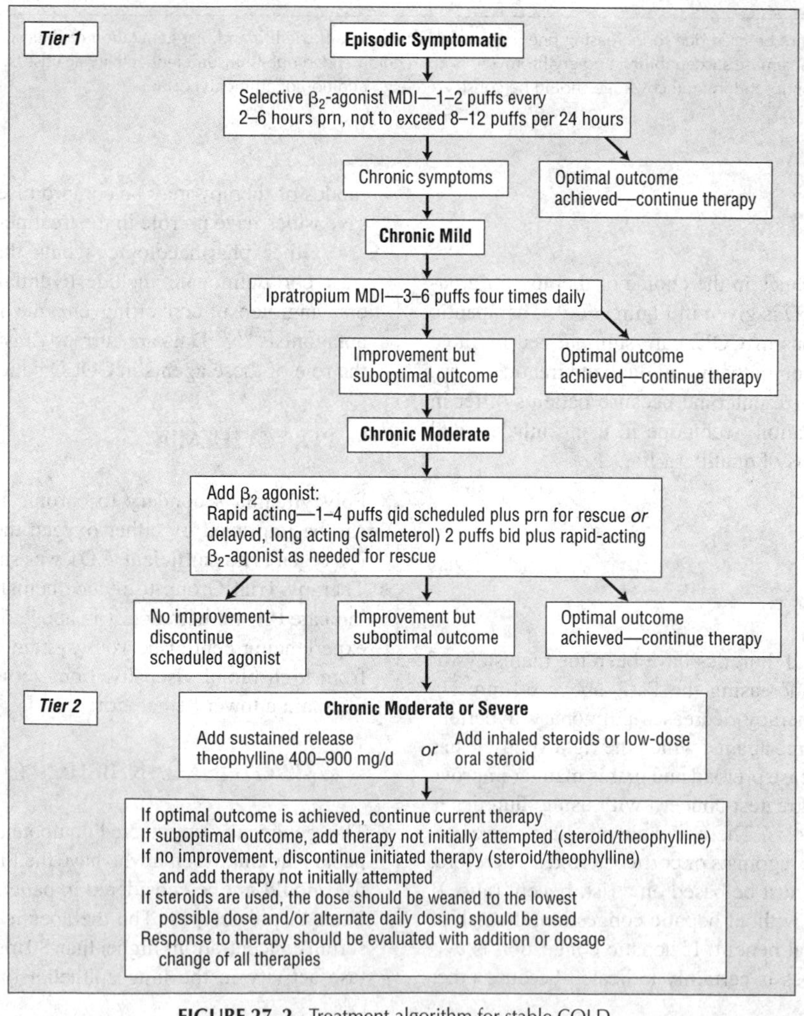

FIGURE 27–2. Treatment algorithm for stable COLD.

dosing regimen is 60 mg/kg administered intravenously once a week at a rate of 0.08 mL/kg per minute (adjusted to patient tolerance). It has been estimated that this form of augmentation therapy will have an annual cost of $20,000 to $30,000 per patient.[99]

ACUTE RESPIRATORY FAILURE

Acute respiratory failure is an emergency situation. When it occurs in a patient with COLD, all pharmacologic maneuvers should be optimized initially and low-flow oxygen delivered. If these agents fail to stabilize or improve the patient's condition, intubation and mechanical ventilation must be considered. This is an extremely difficult decision. Ideally, all severe COLD patients should be involved in the decision to intubate. Preferably, this decision should be made before an acute event occurs. If a decision is made to mechanically ventilate because of impending respiratory failure, it is important that ventilator settings not be adjusted to return the patient to normal values; rather, settings should be adjusted to achieve the patient's baseline values in a stable state. This will facilitate weaning from the ventilator. Maintaining the physical strength and nutritional status of the patient is vital in aiding the weaning procedure. Data indicate that a systematic multiparameter approach to assessing nutritional status is critical for COLD patients requiring mechanical ventilation because malnutrition is common and has a deleterious effect on the weaning process.[100] Physical therapy and a nutritional intake of 3000 kcal/d with a relatively high proportion of protein are advised. Unfortunately, most patients remain in negative nitrogen balance, and muscle wasting is strongly correlated with the dose of corticosteroid used. If mechanical ventilation persists beyond 5 to 7 days, the patient should be switched to a tracheostomy to prevent tracheal erosion and to facilitate feeding.

Many patients requiring mechanical ventilation for COLD are able to undergo extubation without weaning. However, some require gradual weaning. The most important factors that determine the ability of patients to wean from prolonged mechanical ventilation are neuromuscular reserve capacity relative to respiratory load, cardiovascular performance, oxygenation, and psychologic factors.[1] A number of objective indices (e.g., maximum inspiratory pressure, VC, respiratory frequency/tidal volume) are designed to evaluate patients for extubation. Weaning values are institution-specific, and no clear physiologic indices assist the selection of patients for weaning, determination of the rapidity of weaning, or identification of the ideal weaning method. For example, for patients with an FiO_2 of 40% or less and a tidal volume of 400 mL or less, extubation can be considered. Methods that can assist in weaning include T-piece trials, intermittent mandatory ventilation (IMV), and pressure-support ventilation (PSV).[101] IMV and PSV are preferred because they provide partial support when the patient is connected to the ventilator and they provide less opportunity for barotrauma.[1]

CONTROVERSIES AND NEW TREATMENTS

EXPECTORANTS AND MUCOLYTICS

Water has been, and continues to be, the expectorant of choice in COLD patients. Adequate hydration is safe and effective when compared with saturated solutions of potassium iodide, ammonium chloride, or guaifenesin. Although these agents may promote expectoration, the doses required are so large that they are frequently associated with undesirable side effects.

Use of the mucolytic agent acetylcysteine to aid clearance of mucus has been a matter of controversy for some time. There is no question that it is effective as a mucolytic. However, it causes irritation when administered via nebulization, which may cause further narrowing of the airways. For this reason, use of inhaled acetylcysteine has fallen into disfavor. It should always be preceded by an inhaled sympathomimetic if this route is chosen. Another mucolytic, iodinated glycerol, was compared with placebo at a dose of 60 mg four times a day and was found to be superior in terms of cough frequency, cough severity, and chest discomfort, but no improvement in blood oxygenation or pulmonary function was reported.[102] However, objective evidence of benefit was deemed insufficient, and the Food and Drug Administration required that marketing of the drug be discontinued.

DIETARY SUPPLEMENTS

In the past decade, use of nonenzymatic antioxidants, including vitamins E and C and β-carotene, has increased dramatically. They have been used for a variety of disease states, including lung and heart disease. It is postulated that they may be beneficial in COLD as a result of an imbalance between oxidants and antioxidants that has been considered in the pathogenesis of smoking-induced lung disease.[103] A recent study evaluated the effect of vitamin E on exhaled ethane in cigarette smokers.[104] This trial failed to find a significant change in ethane values and demonstrated a negative trend between vitamin E administration and lung function.[104] Rautalahti and colleagues evaluated the effect of β-carotene and vitamin E on COLD symptoms.[105] They found that neither antioxidant improved COLD symptoms. Based on the results of these trials, the use of vitamin E or β-carotene to improve lung function in COLD cannot be advocated.

Lack of sleep is associated with low melatonin secretion. The use of melatonin has been evaluated in a double-blind, placebo-controlled trial in intensive care COLD patients suffering from lack of sleep.[106] Patients who received controlled-release melatonin had an improved duration of sleep and quality of sleep.

INVESTIGATIONAL THERAPIES

Several classes of drugs are currently being investigated for the treatment of COLD.[3] Leukotriene antagonists that inhibit mediators of inflammation have been shown to have a beneficial effect in the treatment of asthma. Leukotriene B_4 antagonists and 5'-lipooxygenase inhibitors (which prevent the synthesis of leukotriene B_4) are currently being evaluated for the treatment of COLD. Neutrophil elastase is implicated in the induction of bronchial disease causing structural changes in lungs, impairment of mucociliary clearance, and impairment of host defenses. Protease inhibitors, namely, inhibitors of neutrophil elastase, are being investigated currently for the treatment of COLD. As discussed previously, inflammation is thought to play a key role in the pathogenesis of COLD. New anti-inflammatory treatments currently are being investigated, the most promising of which are the phosphodiesterase 4 inhibitors. The phosphodiesterase 4 inhibitor SB207499 has been evaluated and has been shown to improve symptoms, quality of life, and lung function in COLD patients.[107]

SURGICAL INTERVENTION

Recent trials have evaluated the effect of bilateral lung volume reduction surgery (LVRS) for management of severe COLD. Short-term trials have compared the effects of pulmonary rehabilitation plus LVRS with pulmonary rehabilitation alone.[108,109] In these studies, patients who received LVRS plus pulmonary rehabilitation were noted to have greater improvements in lung function, gas exchange, and quality of life at 3 months after LVRS compared with patients who received only pulmonary rehabilitation. Long-term trials evaluating the effect of LVRS compared with pulmonary rehabilitation are lacking. However, in a nonrandomized, noncontrolled trial, Gelb and investigators did note improvement in lung function after more than 3 years in 9 of 26 patients who received LVRS.[110] The National Emphysema Treatment Trial (NETT), a prospective, randomized trial to evaluate the long-term effects of LVRS plus pulmonary rehabilitation compared with pulmonary rehabilitation alone, has been terminated due to high mortality rates in high-risk patients.[111]

OTHER ASPECTS OF MANAGEMENT

The standard of practice for many years was to avoid administering narcotics and benzodiazepines to patients with COLD. These drugs can further depress respiration, especially when given parenterally. Recent work in this area suggests that this issue is not yet settled. The current debate is over the risk of loss of sleep versus the risk of sedatives. As yet, there is no clear resolution to this issue. Zolpidem, an imidazopyridine with a hypnotic action close to that of benzodiazepines, has been evaluated in patients with stable COLD in a single-blind, placebo-controlled study.[112] Patients who received zolpidem did not show impairments in nocturnal respiratory and sleep architecture parameters or in diurnal pulmonary function tests, central control of breathing, and physical performance compared with patients receiving placebo. Some have found diphenhydramine useful as an anxiolytic or sedative, but there has not been an objective analysis of its effectiveness or safety in patients with COLD. Opiates alone or with phenothiazines have been used to increase exercise tolerance in individuals in whom dyspnea is severely disabling; however, the various trials do not show consistent results.[113,114] Inhaled morphine does not appear to be effective in decreasing exercise-induced breathlessness in patients with COLD.[115]

PHARMACOECONOMIC CONSIDERATIONS

The overall cost of therapy is an important consideration in contemporary medical practice. Meaningful cost analysis goes beyond the cost of the medication itself and incorporates the impact of a given therapeutic agent on overall health care cost. Pharmacoeconomic analyses in COLD, although limited, are available regarding antibiotic use in acute exacerbations and some therapies for management of chronic stable COLD.

Grossman and colleagues conducted a trial investigating the use of aggressive antimicrobial therapy (ciprofloxacin) compared with usual antibiotic therapy (defined as any nonquinolone) in the treatment of acute exacerbations of COLD.[116] The overall results indicated no preference for either treatment arm. However, in patients who were categorized as high risk (severe underlying lung disease, more than four exacerbations per year, duration of bronchitis greater than 10 years, elderly, significant comorbid illness), the use of aggressive antibiotic therapy was associated with improved clinical outcome, higher quality of life, and fewer costs. The results of this study are consistent with Table 27–4, which suggests that higher-risk patients are likely to have more resistant strains of organisms and thus require more aggressive antimicrobial treatment.

Jubran and associates performed a Markov analysis comparing the strategies of treatment with theophylline or ipratropium and found that ipratropium was only marginally better than theophylline in terms of efficacy.[117] However, the total cost per year (e.g., hospitalization for toxic events, monitoring of blood levels) was significantly higher for patients using theophylline despite the fact that ipratropium costs more on formularies. This study reinforces the concept that the total cost of therapy and not simply the cost of a drug must be taken into account when determining the cost-effectiveness of a given therapeutic regimen.

Friedman and colleagues conducted a post hoc pharmacoeconomic evaluation of two multicenter, randomized trials comparing the combination of ipratropium and albuterol with both drugs used as monotherapy.[118] Patients who received a combination of ipratropium and albuterol had lower rates of exacerbations, lower overall treatment costs, and improved cost-effectiveness compared with either drug used alone.

EVALUATION OF THERAPEUTIC OUTCOMES

To effectively evaluate therapeutic outcomes of COLD, the practitioner must first delineate between chronic stable COLD and acute exacerbations. In chronic stable COLD pulmonary function tests, namely, FEV_1, should be assessed with any therapy addition, change in dose, or deletion of therapy and periodically throughout the course of the disease. In acute exacerbations of COLD, pulmonary function tests, white blood cell count, vital signs, chest x-ray, and changes in frequency of dyspnea, sputum volume, and sputum purulence should be assessed at the onset and throughout treatment of an exacerbation. In more severe exacerbations, arterial blood gases and oxygen saturation also should be monitored. As with any drug therapy, patient compliance to therapeutic regimens, side effects, potential drug interactions, and subjective measures of quality of life also must be evaluated.

ADDENDUM

The reader is referred to the U.S. National Heart, Lung and Blood Institute and the World Health Organization workshop summary on a strategy for the diagnosis, management, and prevention of chronic obstructive pulmonary disease.[119] This workshop summary was published after the text of this chapter was approved and finalized. This summary has been endorsed by the American Thoracic Society and represents the most up-to-date information.

▶ PRINCIPLES OF PHARMACOTHERAPY

- COLD includes the terms *chronic bronchitis* and *emphysema*. Bronchitis is defined in clinical terms, whereas emphysema is defined in terms of anatomic pathology. Most patients have a combination of chronic bronchitis and emphysema.
- The most common cause of COLD is cigarette smoking. The first and most important step in the treatment of COLD is smoking cessation.
- The main classes of drug treatment for COLD include anticholinergics, sympathomimetics, methylxanthines, and

corticosteroids. Anticholinergics and sympathomimetics are considered tier-one therapies, whereas methylxanthines and corticosteroids are relegated to second-line or tier-two therapies.

- The foregoing therapies have demonstrated improvement in subjective and objective symptoms. However, it is unknown whether morbidity and mortality associated with COLD are decreased. The only treatment shown to increase survival is oxygen administered for most of the hours of the day.
- The treatment of COLD is not an exact science and is very patient-dependent. For instance, some patients may respond better to one bronchodilator than another or may respond to pharmacologic agents via mechanisms other than bronchodilation.
- Many agents, particularly corticosteroids and methylxanthines, are not without considerable potential toxicity. Therefore, embarking on a pharmacologic plan for the treatment of a COLD patient requires weighing the risk-benefit ratio carefully and having a comprehensive plan to assess subjectively and objectively the efficacy and toxicity of the chosen therapy.
- Antibiotics should be used during acute exacerbations if the patient exhibits at least two of the following: increased dyspnea, increased sputum volume, and increased sputum purulence. Selection of an antimicrobial agent should be based on the most likely causative pathogens based on individual patient characteristics.

REFERENCES

1. American Thoracic Society. Standards for the diagnosis and care of patients with chronic obstructive pulmonary disease. Am J Respir Crit Care Med 1995;152:S77–S120.
2. Pauwels RA. National and international guidelines for COPD: The need for evidence. Chest 2000;117:20S–22S.
3. Barnes PJ. Chronic obstructive pulmonary disease. N Engl J Med 2000;343:269–280.
4. National Center for Health Statistics. FA Stats 2000. Washington, 2000.
5. Hurd S. The impact of COPD on lung health worldwide: Epidemiology and incidence. Chest 2000;117:1S–4S.
6. National Vital Statistics Report 2000. Washington, 2000.
7. National Vital Statistics Report 1999. Washington, 1999.
8. Health, United States, 2000. Washington, 2000.
9. NHLBI Morbidity and Mortality Chartbook 2000. Washington, 2000.
10. Edelman NH, Kaplan RM, Buist AS, et al. Chronic obstructive pulmonary disease. Chest 1992;102(Suppl):243–256.
11. Sullivan SD, Ramsey SD, Lee TA. The economic burden of COPD. Chest 2000;117:5S–9S.
12. Sunyer J, Saez M, Murillo C, et al. Air pollution and emergency room admissions for chronic obstructive pulmonary disease: A 5-year study. Am J Epidemiol 1993;137:701–705.
13. Honig EG, Ingram RH. Chronic bronchitis, emphysema, and airways obstruction. In: Fauci AS, Braunwald E, Isselbacher KJ, et al, eds. Harrison's Textbook of Internal Medicine, 14th ed. N York, McGraw-Hill, 1998:1451–1460.
14. Wright JL, Petty T, Thurlbeck WM. Analysis of the structure of the muscular pulmonary arteries in patients with pulmonary hypertension and COPD: National Institutes of Health Nocturnal Oxygen Therapy Trial. Lung 1992;170:109–124.
15. Shapiro SD. The pathogenesis of emphysema: The elastase:antielastase hypothesis 30 years later. Proc Assoc Am Physicians 1995;107:346–352.
16. Lamb D. Chronic bronchitis, emphysema, and the pathological basis of chronic obstructive pulmonary disease. In: Hasleton PS, ed. Spencer's Pathology of the Lung, 5th ed. N York, McGraw-Hill, 1996:597–629.
17. Jokic R, Fitzpatrick MF. Obstructive lung disease and sleep. Med Clin North Am 1996;80:821–850.
18. Celli BR. The importance of spirometry in COPD and asthma. Chest 2000;117:15S–19S.
19. Jones PW. Issues concerning health-related quality of life in COPD. Chest 1995;107:187S–193S.
20. Kanner RE, Connett JE, Williams DE, Buist AS. Effects of randomized assignment to a smoking cessation intervention and changes in smoking habits on respiratory symptoms in smokers with early chronic obstructive pulmonary disease: The Lung Health Study. Am J Med 1999;106: 410–416.
21. Jorenby DE, Leischow SJ, Nides MA, et al. A controlled trial of sustained-release bupropion, a nicotine patch or both for smoking cessation. N Engl J Med 1999;340:685–691.
22. Bredstrup KE, Ingemann Jensen J, Holm S, Bengtsson B. Out-patient rehabilitation improves activities of daily living, quality of life and exercise tolerance in chronic obstructive pulmonary disease. Eur Respir J 1997;10:2801–2806.
23. Ringbaek TJ, Broendum L, Hemmingsen K, et al. Rehabilitation of patients with chronic obstructive pulmonary disease: Exercise twice a week is not sufficient! Respir Med 2000;94:150–154.
24. Devine EC, Pearcy J. Meta-analysis of the effects of psychoeducational care in adults with chronic obstructive pulmonary disease. Patient Educ Couns 1996;29:167–178.
25. Ferreira IM, Brooks D, Lacasse Y, et al. Nutritional support for individuals with COPD: A meta analysis. Chest 2000;117:672–678.
26. Anthonisen NR, Wright EC, IPPB Trial Group. Response to inhaled bronchodilators in COPD. Chest 1987;91:36S–39S.
27. Gross NJ. Ipratropium bromide. N Engl J Med 1989;319:486–494.
28. Skorodin MS. Pharmacotherapy for asthma and chronic obstructive pulmonary disease. Arch Intern Med 1993;153:814–828.
29. Bennett WD, Chapman WF, Mascarella JM. The acute effect of ipratropium bromide bronchodilator therapy on cough clearance in COPD. Chest 1993;103:488–495.
30. Anthonisen NR, Connett JE, Kiley JP, et al. Effects of smoking intervention and the use of an inhaled anticholinergic bronchodilator on the rate of decline of FEV_1: The Lung Health Study. JAMA 1994;272:1497–1505.
31. Friedman M. A multicenter study of nebulized bronchodilator solutions in chronic obstructive pulmonary disease. Am J Med 1996;100 (Suppl 1A):30S–39S.
32. Wiggins J. The role of anticholinergics in "stable" chronic obstructive pulmonary disease: Unanswered questions. Respiration 1994;61: 303–304.
33. Colice GL. Nebulized bronchodilators for outpatient management of stable chronic obstructive pulmonary disease. Am J Med 1996;100(Suppl 1A):11S–18S.
34. Schapira RM, Reinke LF. The outpatient diagnosis and management of chronic obstructive pulmonary disease: Pharmacotherapy, administration of supplemental oxygen, and smoking cessation techniques. J Gen Intern Med 1995;10:40–55.
35. Siefkin AD. Optimal pharmacologic treatment of the critically ill patient with obstructive airways disease. Am J Med 1996;100(Suppl 1A):54S–61S.
36. Ikeda A, Nishimura K, Koyama H, et al. Dose-response study of ipratropium bromide aerosol on maximum exercise performance in stable patients with chronic obstructive pulmonary disease. Thorax 1996;51: 48–53.
37. Tsukino M, Nishimura K, Ikeda A, et al. Effects of theophylline and ipratropium bromide on exercise performance in patients with stable chronic obstructive pulmonary disease. Thorax 1998;53:269–273.
38. Martin RJ, Bartelson BL, Smith P, et al. Effect of ipratropium bromide treatment on oxygen saturation and sleep quality in COPD. Chest 1999;115:1338–1345.
39. Barnes PJ. The pharmacological properties of tiotropium. Chest 2000; 117:63S–66S.
40. van Noord JA, Bantje TA, Eland ME, et al. A randomized, controlled comparison of tiotropium and ipratropium in the treatment of chronic obstructive pulmonary disease. The Dutch tiotropium study. Thorax 2000;55:289–294.

41. O'Donnel DE, Lam M, Webb KA. Measurement of symptoms, lung hyperinflation, and endurance during exercise in chronic obstructive pulmonary disease. Am J Respir Crit Care Med 1998;158:1557–1565.
42. Boyd G, Morice AH, Pounsford JC, et al. An evaluation of salmeterol in the treatment of chronic obstructive pulmonary disease (COPD). Eur Respir J 1997;10:815–821.
43. Grove A, Lipworth BJ, Reid P, et al. Effects of regular salmeterol on lung function and exercise capacity in patients with chronic obstructive airways disease. Thorax 1996;51:689–693.
44. Van Schayck CP, Dompeling E, van Herwaarden LA, et al. Bronchodilator treatment in moderate asthma or chronic bronchitis: Continuous or on demand? A randomized controlled study. Br Med J 1991;303(6815):1426–1431.
45. Mahler DA, Donohue JF, Barbee RA, et al. Efficacy of salmeterol xinafoate in the treatment of COPD. Chest 1999;115:957–965.
46. Ferguson GT, Cherniack RM. Management of chronic obstructive pulmonary disease. N Engl J Med 1993;328:1017–1022.
47. Dowling RB, Johnson M, Cole PJ, Wilson R. Effect of salmeterol on *Haemophilus influenzae* infection of respiratory mucosa in vitro. Eur Respir J 1998;11:86–90.
48. Mandelberg A, Chen E, Noviski N, Priel IE. Nebulized wet aerosol treatment in emergency department: Is it essential? Comparison with large spacer device for metered-dose inhaler. Chest 1997;112:1501–1505.
49. Ikeda A, Nishimura K, Koyama H, et al. Comparison of the bronchodilator effects of salbutamol delivered via a metered-dose inhaler with spacer, a dry-powder inhaler, and a jet nebulizer in patients with chronic obstructive pulmonary disease. Respiration 1999;66:119–123.
50. Turner MO, Patel A, Ginsburg S, FitzGerald JM. Bronchodilator delivery in acute airflow obstruction. Arch Intern Med 1997;157:1736–1744.
51. Nelson HS. Clinical experience with levalbuterol. J Allergy Clin Immunol 1999;104:S77–S84.
52. Asmus MJ, Hendeles L. Levalbuterol nebulizer solution: Is it worth five times the cost of albuterol? Pharmacotherapy 2000;20:123–129.
53. Combivent Inhalation Aerosol Study Group. In chronic obstructive pulmonary disease, a combination of ipratropium and albuterol is more effective than either agent alone. Chest 1994;105:1411–1419.
54. Campbell S. For COPD a combination of ipratropium bromide and albuterol sulfate is more effective than albuterol base. Arch Intern Med 1999;159:156–160.
55. Dorinsky PM, Reisner C, Ferguson GT, et al. The combination of ipratropium and albuterol optimized pulmonary function reversibility testing in patients with COPD. Chest 1999;115:966–971.
56. Vaz Fragoso CA, Miller MA. Review of the clinical efficacy of theophylline in the treatment of chronic obstructive pulmonary disease. Am Rev Respir Dis 1993;147:S40–S47.
57. Ramsdell J. Use of theophylline in the treatment of COPD. Chest 1995;107:206S–209S.
58. Fink G, Kaye C, Sulkes J, et al. Effect of theophylline on exercise performance in patients with severe chronic obstructive pulmonary disease. Thorax 1994;49:332–334.
59. Ashutosh K, Sedat M, Fragale-Jackson J. Effects of theophylline on respiratory drive in patients with chronic obstructive pulmonary disease. J Clin Pharmacol 1997;37:1100–1107.
60. McKay SE, Howie CA, Thomson AH, et al. Value of theophylline treatment in patients handicapped by chronic obstructive lung disease. Thorax 1993;48:227–232.
61. Man GC, Chapman KR, Ali SH, Darke AC. Sleep quality and nocturnal respiratory function with once-daily theophylline (Uniphyl) and inhaled salbutamol in patients with COPD. Chest 1996;110:648–653.
62. Zarowitz B, Shlom J, Eichenhorn MS, Popovich J. Alterations in therapy protein binding in acutely ill patients with COPD. Chest 1985;87: 766–769.
63. Nishimura K, Koyama H, Ikeda A, et al. The additive effect of theophylline on a high-dose combination of inhaled salbutamol and ipratropium bromide in stable COPD. Chest 1995;107:718–723.
64. Karpel JP, Kotch A, Zinny M, et al. A comparison of inhaled ipratropium, oral theophylline plus inhaled beta agonist, and the combination of all three in patients with COPD. Chest 1994;105:1089–1094.
65. Franklin W, Michaelson AL, Lowell FC, et al. Bronchodilators and corticosteroids in the treatment of obstructive pulmonary emphysema. N Engl J Med 1958;278:774–778.
66. Niewoehner DE, Erbland ML, Deupree RH, et al. Effect of systemic glucocorticoids on exacerbations of chronic obstructive pulmonary disease. Department of Veterans Affairs Cooperative Study Group. N Engl J Med 1999;340:1941–1947.
67. Davies L, Angus RM, Calverley PMA. Oral corticosteroids in patients admitted to hospital with exacerbations of chronic obstructive pulmonary disease: A prospective, randomised controlled trial. Lancet 1999; 354:456–460.
68. Thompson WH, Nielson CP, Carvalho P, et al. Controlled trial of oral prednisone in outpatients with acute COPD exacerbation. Am J Respir Crit Care Med 1996;154:407–412.
69. Callahan CM, Dittus RS, Katz BP. Oral corticosteroid therapy for patients with stable chronic obstructive pulmonary disease: A meta-analysis. Ann Intern Med 1991;114:216–223.
70. Pizzichini E, Pizzichini MM, Gibson P, et al. Sputum eosinophilia predicts benefit from prednisone in smokers with chronic obstructive bronchitis. Am J Respir Crit Care Med 1998;158:1511–1517.
71. Pauwels RA, Claes-Goran L, Latinen LA, et al. Long-term treatment with inhaled budesonide in persons with mild chronic obstructive pulmonary disease who continue smoking. N Engl J Med 1999;340:1948–1953.
72. Vestbo J, Sorenson T, Lange P, et al. Long-term effect of inhaled budesonide in mild and moderate chronic obstructive pulmonary disease: A randomized, controlled trial. Lancet 1999;353:1819–1823.
73. Burge PS, Calverley PM, Jones PW, et al. Randomised, double-blind, placebo-controlled study of fluticasone propionate in patients with moderate to severe chronic obstructive pulmonary disease: The ISOLDE trial. Br Med J 2000;320:1297–1303.
74. Nishimura K, Koyama H, Ikeda A, et al. The effect of high-dose inhaled beclomethasone dipropionate in patients with stable COPD. Chest 1999;115:31–37.
75. Weir DC, Bale GA, Bright P, Sherwood Burge P. A double-blind placebo-controlled study of the effect of inhaled beclomethasone dipropionate for 2 years in patients with nonasthmatic chronic obstructive pulmonary disease. Clin Exp Allergy 1999;29(Suppl 2):125–128.
76. Paggiaro PL, Dahle R, Bakran I, et al. Multicentre, randomized, placebo-controlled trial of inhaled fluticasone propionate in patients with chronic obstructive pulmonary disease. International COPD Study Group. Lancet 1998;351:773–780.
77. Postma DS, Kerstjens HAM. Are inhaled glucocorticosteroids effective in chronic obstructive pulmonary disease? Am J Respir Crit Care Med 1999;160:S66–S71.
78. van Grunsven PM, van Schayck CP, Derenne JP, et al. Long-term effects of inhaled corticosteroids in chronic obstructive pulmonary disease: A meta-analysis. Thorax 1999;54:7–14.
79. Ferguson GT. Recommendations for the management of COPD. Chest 2000;117:23S–28S.
80. Lipworth BJ. Systemic adverse effects of inhaled corticosteroid therapy: A systematic review and meta-analysis. Arch Intern Med 1999;159:941–955.
81. Nocturnal Oxygen Therapy Trial Group. Continuous or nocturnal oxygen therapy in hypoxemic chronic obstructive lung disease. Ann Intern Med 1980;93:391–398.
82. Medical Research Council Working Party. Long-term domiciliary oxygen therapy in chronic hypoxic cor pulmonale complicating chronic bronchitis and emphysema. Lancet 1981;1:681–685.
83. O'Donohue WJ. Home oxygen therapy. Med Clin North Am 1996; 80:611–622.
84. Weitzenblum E, Apprill M, Oswald M. Benefit from long-term O_2 therapy in chronic obstructive pulmonary disease patients. Respiration 1992:59(Suppl 2):14–17.
85. Saint S, Bent S, Vittinghoff E, Grady D. Antibiotics in chronic obstructive pulmonary disease exacerbations: A meta-analysis. JAMA 1995;273:957–960.
86. Madison JM, Irwin RS. Chronic obstructive pulmonary disease. Lancet 1998;352:467–473.

87. Niederman MS. Antibiotic therapy of exacerbations of chronic bronchitis. Semin Respir Infect 2000;15:59–70.
88. Wilson R, Kubin R, Ballin I, et al. Five-day moxifloxacin therapy compared with 7-day clarithromycin therapy for the treatment of acute exacerbations of chronic bronchitis. J Antimicrob Chemother 1999;44:501–513.
89. Chodosh S, DeAbate C, Haverstock D, et al. Short-course moxifloxacin therapy for treatment of acute bacterial exacerbations of chronic bronchitis. Respir Med 2000;94:18–27.
90. Langan C, Clecner B, Cazzola CM, et al. Short-course cefuroxime axetil therapy in the treatment of acute exacerbations of chronic bronchitis. Int J Clin Pract 1998;52:289–297.
91. Guest N, Langan C. Comparison of the efficacy and safety of a short course of ceftibuten with that of amoxycillin/clavulanate in the treatment of acute exacerbations of chronic bronchitis. Int J Antimicrob Agents 1998;10:49–54.
92. Wasilewski MM, Johns D, Sides GD. Five-day dirithromycin therapy is as effective as seven-day erythromycin therapy for acute exacerbations of chronic bronchitis. J Antimicrob Chemother 1999;43:541–548.
93. Cazzola M, Vinciguerra A, Di Perna F, et al. Comparative study of dirithromycin and azithromycin in the treatment of acute bacterial exacerbations of chronic bronchitis. J Chemother 1999;11:119–125.
94. Nuorti, PJ, Butler JC, Breiman RF. Prevention of pneumococcal disease. *MMWR* 1997;46(RR8):1–24.
95. Barnes PJ. Nonantimicrobial aspects of therapy. Semin Respir Infect 2000;15:52–58.
96. Winkelmann BR, Kullmer TH, Kneissl DG, et al. Low-dose almitrine bismesylate in the treatment of hypoxemia due to chronic obstructive pulmonary disease. Chest 1994;105:1383–1391.
97. Sajkov D, Wang T, Frith PA, et al. A comparison of two long-acting vasoselective calcium antagonists in pulmonary hypertension secondary to COPD. Chest 1997;111:1622–1630.
98. Kiely DG, Cargill RI, Wheeldon NM, et al. Haemodynamic and endocrine effects of type 1 antiotensin II receptor blockade in patients with hypoxaemic cor pulmonale. Cardiovas Res 1997;33:201–208.
99. MacDonald JL, Johnson CE. Pathophysiology and treatment of α_1-antitrypsin deficiency. Am J Health Syst Pharm 1995;52:481–489.
100. Laaban JP, Kouchakji B, Dor MF, et al. Nutritional status of patients with chronic obstructive pulmonary disease acute respiratory failure. Chest 1993;103:1362–1368.
101. Curtis JR, Hudson LD. Emergent assessment and management of acute respiratory failure in COPD. Clin Chest Med 1994;15:481–500.
102. Morgan EJ, Petty TL. Summary of the national mucolytic study. Chest 1990;97:24S–27S.
103. Rahman I, MacNee W. Role of oxidants/antioxidants in smoking induced lung diseases. Free Radic Biol Med 1996;21:669–681.
104. Habib MP, Tank LJ, Lane LC, Garewal HS. Effect of vitamin E on exhaled ethane in cigarette smokers. Chest 1999;115:684–690.
105. Rautalahti M, Virtamo J, Haukka J, et al. The effect of alpha-tocopherol and beta-carotene supplementation on COPD. Am J Respir Crit Care Med 1997;156:1447–1452.
106. Shilo L, Dagan Y, Smorjik Y, et al. Effect of melatonin on sleep quality of COPD intensive care patients: A pilot study. Chronobiol Int 2000;17:71–76.
107. Torphy TJ, Barnette MS, Underwood DC, et al. Ariflo (SB 207499), a second-generation phosphodiesterase 4 inhibitor for the treatment of asthma and COPD: From concept to clinic. Pulm Pharmacol Ther 1999;12:131–135.
108. Criner GJ, Cordova FC, Furukawa S, et al. Prospective, randomized trial comparing bilateral lung volume reduction surgery to pulmonary rehabilitation in severe chronic obstructive pulmonary disease. Am J Respir Crit Care Med 1999;160:2018–2027.
109. Leyenson V, Furukawa S, Kuzma AM, et al. Correlation of changes in quality of life after lung volume reduction surgery with changes in lung function, exercise, and gas exchange. Chest 2000;118:728–735.
110. Gelb AF, McKenna RJ, Brenner M. Lung function 4 years after lung volume reduction surgery for emphysema. Chest 1999;116:1608–1615.
111. The National Emphysema Treatment Trial Research Group. Rationale and design of the National Emphysema Treatment Trial: A prospective, randomized trial of lung volume reduction surgery. Chest 1999;116:1750–1761.
112. Girault C, Muir JF, Mihaltan F, et al. Effects of repeated administration of zolpidem on sleep, diurnal and nocturnal respiratory function, vigilance and physical performance in patients with COPD. Chest 1996;110:1203–1211.
113. Light RW, Stansbury DW, Webster JS. Effect of 30 mg of morphine alone or with promethazine or prochlorperazine on the exercise capacity of patients with COPD. Chest 1996;109:975–981.
114. Poole PJ, Veale AG, Black PN. The effect of sustained-release morphine on breathlessness and quality of life in severe chronic obstructive pulmonary disease. Am J Respir Crit Care Med 1998;157:1877–1880.
115. Leung R, Hill P, Burdon J. Effect of inhaled morphine on the development of breathlessness during exercise in patients with chronic lung disease. Thorax 1996;51:596–600.
116. Grossman RF, Mukerjee J, Vaughan D, et al. A one-year community-based health economic study of ciprofloxacin versus usual antibiotic treatment in acute exacerbations of chronic bronchitis. Chest 1998;113:131–141.
117. Jubran A, Gross N, Ramsdell J, et al. Comparative cost-effectiveness analysis of theophylline and ipratropium bromide in chronic obstructive pulmonary disease three-center study. Chest 1993;103:678–684.
118. Friedman M, Serby CW, Menjoge SS, et al. Pharmacoeconomic evaluation of a combination of ipratropium plus albuterol compared with ipratropium alone and albuterol alone in COPD. Chest 1999;115:635–641.
119. Pauwells RA, Buist AS, Calverly PMA, et al. Global strategy for the diagnoses management, and prevention of chronic obstruction pulmonary disease. Am J. Respir Crit Care Med. 2001;163:1256–1276.

28

ACUTE RESPIRATORY DISTRESS SYNDROME

Peter Gal and Christopher L. Shaffer

This chapter addresses the problems of acute respiratory distress syndromes in neonates and adults. Abbreviations are used throughout the text, and a glossary for physiology, diseases, and drugs is presented in Table 28–1. Descriptions of ventilator-related terms are provided in Tables 28–2 and 28–3. Because the physiology of neonatal respiratory distress syndrome (RDS) and acute respiratory distress syndrome (ARDS) have some differences, these diseases will be discussed separately.

NEONATAL RESPIRATORY DISTRESS SYNDROME

RDS, historically known as *hyaline membrane disease* (HMD), is more appropriately termed *surfactant-deficiency RDS.* RDS is associated with considerable morbidity and mortality. Before 35 weeks' gestation, the risk of RDS and the severity of disease increase with greater degree of prematurity and, in the absence of antenatal interventions, occurs in over 50% of newborns of 30 weeks or less gestation.[1] The Vermont Oxford Network experience for 1999 describes over 27,000 neonates below 1500 g from 325 neonatal intensive care unit (NICU) sites. The annual report noted that RDS occurred in over 80% of premature infants below 1000 g and that there was a gradual decline to about 42% of neonates with birth weights between 1400 and 1500 g.

RDS is attributed primarily to insufficient formation and differentiation of type II pneumocytes with consequent impaired production and release of surfactant. Pulmonary surfactant contains phospholipids that function at the air-liquid interface in the alveolus to lower surface tension, thus preventing alveolar collapse. In the face of surfactant deficiency, atelectasis and impaired gas exchange occur. Additionally, alveolar transudation of protein-rich fluid forms a hyaline membrane, giving rise to the term *hyaline membrane disease.*[1]

Epithelial sodium channel (ENaC) maturation also appears important in RDS. In utero, fluid is actively secreted into lungs via chloride channels. At birth, the ENaC takes over, and fluid is actively reabsorbed from the lungs. In premature infants, immaturity of the ENaC results in failure to reabsorb lung fluid, with consequent pulmonary edema.[2] In term infants, this conversion occurs at birth in response to circulating catecholamines. Failure of the conversion to occur in preterm infants results in an inability to clear alveolar fluid and consequent pulmonary edema.[3]

Measurement of lung maturation in amniotic fluid using biochemical markers of surfactant deficiency is an important consideration in preventive and therapeutic interventions, as well as in predicting the likelihood of developing RDS. Measurement of surfactant components in amniotic fluid using either the ratio of lecithin to sphingomyelin (L/S ratio), or phosphatidylglycerol (PG) have been particularly useful for confirming lung maturity. PG is the better test because, unlike the L/S ratio, it is reliable in the presence of blood, meconium, or maternal diabetes. Also, turnaround time for PG is more rapid.[4] A positive PG test or L/S ratio is associated with a sensitivity of 95% to 99% and a positive predictive value of 97% to 98%. Both tests suffer from limited specificity (30% to 70%) and limited negative predictive value (54% to 56%). Thus a test result indicating immaturity does not ensure development of RDS, but a test indicating maturity makes RDS very unlikely.[4] RDS severity and risk are made worse by a variety of perinatal factors including perinatal hypoxia or asphyxia, acidosis, cold stress, patent ductus arteriosus, and maternal diabetes mellitus. These factors may further compromise pulmonary blood supply, consequently causing death of an already limited number of type II alveolar cells and limiting surfactant production.

Chronic intrauterine stress, on the contrary, lowers the risk of RDS by promoting lung maturation, perhaps by increasing endogenous glucocorticoid concentrations.[1]

CLINICAL PRESENTATION

A premature infant with RDS may appear normal at birth, although evidence of intrapartum depression or asphyxia often is present. During the first few hours after birth, these newborns develop early signs of respiratory failure (e.g., forceful intercostal retractions, the use of accessory neck muscles, expiratory grunting, paradoxical seesaw respirations, gradual increase in oxygen requirements, and tachycardia). Pallor or cyanosis also may develop. Fluid retention, edema, and oliguria are common in the first 48 hours.

A characteristic chest x-ray film (Fig. 28–1) shows a reticulogranular (ground-glass) pattern to the peripheral lung fields, along with clearly defined large airways (air bronchograms) resulting from the presence of air in the large airways and the collapse of small air-spaces around the large airways.[1]

A number of neonatal disorders may mimic and be indistinguishable from RDS, the most important being sepsis caused by group B β-hemolytic *Streptococcus*, pneumococcus, or gram-negative bacilli. Sepsis accounted for 8% of consecutively admitted infants with RDS during a 1-year study.[5] All neonates with suspected RDS should be evaluated for sepsis. Antibiotics should be used until sepsis can be ruled out or a full therapeutic course is completed. Other etiologies for RDS include transient tachypnea of the newborn, spontaneous pneumothorax, congenital cyanotic heart disease, and diaphragmatic hernia.

PREVENTION

Several perinatal/antenatal interventions can be adopted to prevent or minimize the severity of RDS. These include optimizing care at labor and delivery and control of maternal diseases to avoid factors known to predispose to RDS. Additionally, drug therapy to delay premature delivery (tocolytics) or to assist with lung maturation (steroids) can be instituted (Fig. 28–2). Early initiation of antibiotics to treat bacterial vaginosis and trichomoniasis also has been associated with significant reduction in preterm births.[6]

Delaying delivery with tocolysis (usually a β-sympathomimetic) is feasible for only a few days in most cases. However, this may provide sufficient time to resolve a reversible etiology or promote fetal lung maturation. Tocolysis generally is started when frequent

TABLE 28–1. Glossary of Terms and Abbreviations

ABG	Arterial blood gas
ALI	Acute lung injury
ARDS	Acute respiratory distress syndrome
BPD	Bronchopulmonary dysplasia
CO	Cardiac output
CXR	Chest x-ray
ECMO	Extracorporeal membrane oxygenation
ENaC	Epithelial sodium channel
HMD	Hyaline membrane disease
IVH	Intraventricular hemorrhage
L/S ratio	Lecithin/sphingomyelin ratio
MODS	Multiple organ dysfunction syndrome
Mvo_2	Mixed venous saturation
NEC	Necrotizing enterocolitis
NO	Nitric oxide
$Paco_2$	Arterial blood gas carbon dioxide
Pao_2	Arterial blood gas oxygen
PCWP	Pulmonary capillary wedge pressure
PDA	Patent ductus arteriosus
PFC	Perfluorocarbon
PG	Phosphatidylglycerol
PIE	Pulmonary interstitial emphysema
PVL	Periventricular leukomalacia
RDS	Neonatal respiratory distress syndrome
Sao_2	Oxygen saturation
SRT	Surfactant replacement therapy
TRH	Thyrotropin releasing hormone
VILI	Ventilator-induced lung injury

TABLE 28–2. Glossary of Terms for Ventilator Settings and Management

Et	Expiratory time; in the ventilatory cycle, the amount of time devoted to exhalation.
It	Inspiratory time; in the ventilatory cycle, the amount of time devoted to inspiration.
I:E	Ratio of inspiratory time to expiratory time; in a normal, spontaneously breathing patient this is 1:1.5.
Pao_2	Partial pressure of oxygen present in arterial blood; normal level for adults is 80–100 mm Hg; normal level for premature babies is 50–70 mm Hg.
$Paco_2$	Partial pressure of carbon dioxide present in arterial blood; normal is 35–45 mm Hg, but higher levels are acceptable to minimize ventilator support.
PEEP	Positive end-expiratory pressure; positive pressure at the end of exhalation designed to prevent alveoli from collapsing during expiration.
PIP	Peak inspiratory pressure; the maximum level of pressure achieved by the ventilator during inspiration.
IMV	Intermittent mandatory ventilation; a mode of ventilation designed to deliver a preset inspiratory rate; continuous flow of gas is available for patient's spontaneous breaths.
Fio_2	Fraction (percentage) of inspired oxygen.
TV	Tidal volume; volume of gas delivered during a single inspiration.
MAP	Mean airway pressure; a constant distending pressure.
Hz	Hertz; normally described as cycles per second, this is the number of breaths per minute.
FRC	Functional residual capacity; the volume of air remaining in the lung after normal expiration.
Amp	Amplitude; a wavelike change in pressure centered around a mean airway pressure.
Sigh	A breath that recruits and maintains alveolar patency, used in HFJV. Similar to pressure provided with PIP.
CWF	Chest wiggle factor; a clinical observation ensuring appropriate chest wall movement with HFOV.
BPM	Breaths per minute.

contractions are noted. Although preterm labor may be overdiagnosed in up to 70% of cases using this approach, waiting for cervical changes will reduce the likelihood of successful inhibition of labor.[7] The contribution of tocolysis should not be underestimated. For example, around 25 weeks' gestation, even a 2-day increase in the length of gestation could increase survival by 15% to 25%.[3] Contraindications to tocolytic therapy include fetal death or lethal abnormality, eclampsia, abruptio placentae, and proven chorioamnionitis. Relative contraindications are preeclampsia, severe chronic hypertension, renal disease, heart disease, fetal distress, and fetal growth retardation.

Fetal lung maturation can be accelerated with antenatal corticosteroids. Contrary to previous beliefs, glucocorticoid benefits are seen at all gestational ages below 35 weeks' gestation.[8–10] The mechanisms by which corticosteroids enhance lung maturation include acceleration of the normal rise in the antioxidant enzymes—for example, superoxide dismutase, catalase, and glutathione peroxidase—that protect lungs against damage from O_2 free radicals,[9] increased production of surfactant,[9] and upregulation of ENaC to promote alveolar

TABLE 28–3. Mechanical Ventilator Types and Modes of Ventilation

CMV	Controlled mechanical ventilation; a ventilator mode in which RR + TV are under machine rather than patient control.
AC	Assist control; mode in which patient receives a full TV if the patient breathes over the ventilator.
PC	Pressure control; ventilator delivers a TV until a certain pressure is achieved.
SIMV	Synchronized intermittent mandatory ventilation; a ventilator breath "synchronized" with patient's inspiratory effort.
PS	Pressure support; pressure on inspiration designed to assist generation of tidal volume.
IRV	Inverse ratio ventilation; ventilator mode in which inspiratory time is prolonged in comparison to expiration time. Used to decrease plateau pressure and improve oxygenation.
HFOV	High frequency oscillatory ventilation; a mechanical diaphragm produces oscillations superimposed on a constant gas flow. Can provide from 180 to 900 breaths per minute. Both inpiration and expiration are actively promoted.
HFJV	High-frequency jet ventilation; small volumes of air are released in a pulsating fashion through a jet nozzle and directed down the airway in a patient simultaneously receiving conventional ventilation. Can provide from 240 to 660 breaths per minute. Inspiration is active but expiration is passive, predisposing to air trapping.
HFFI	High-frequency flow interruption; similar to HFJV, but air pulses are delivered at lower pressures and volumes.
HFPPV	High-frequency positive-pressure ventilation; conventional mechanical ventilation at faster-than-usual rates.
PPAV	Patient proportional assist ventilation; a collective term describing ventilators using patient controlled rates and tidal volumes.
OH	Oxygen hood; a clear plastic enclosure placed over a nonintubated infant to allow humidification of room air (21% Fio_2 or increased Fio_2).

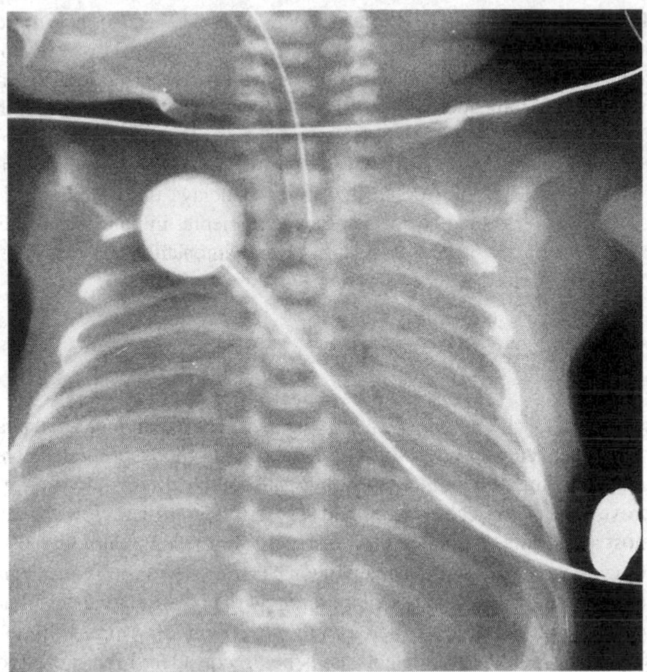

FIGURE 28–1. Chest x-ray demonstrating hyaline membrane disease with ground-glass appearance and air bronchograms.

fluid absorption.[3] The National Institutes of Health (NIH) consensus conference published in 1995 concluded that all fetuses between 24 and 34 weeks' gestation at risk for preterm delivery should receive corticosteroids regardless of gender, race, maternal infection, and availability of surfactant.[9] Failure to treat all appropriate candidates is common, as noted by the observation that in the early 1990s corticosteroids were given to 12% to 18% of women delivering infants weighing 500 to 1500 g.[9] Progress has been made in this area, and the 1999 experience from the Vermont Oxford Network reported that 60% to 70% of neonates below 1500 g received antenatal steroids.[1] Many women who are appropriate candidates are still untreated. Treatment with three or more courses of antenatal steroids is discouraged because of concerns for impaired fetal growth and long-term neurodevelopmental delays.[10] Use of one or two courses of antenatal steroid therapy is relatively devoid of toxicity and markedly improves neonatal morbidity and mortality. Betamethasone appears to provide superior benefits to dexamethasone.[9] The odds ratio [95% confidence interval (CI)] for developing RDS is reduced to 0.49 (CI 0.41 to 0.6) if steroids are started 24 hours to 7 days before delivery. Even if treatment is started less than 24 hours or more than 7 days from delivery, risk is still reduced (odds ratio 0.69, CI 0.50 to 0.94).[9] Antenatal steroids also reduced the risk of intraventricular hemorrhage (odds ratio 0.5, CI 0.3 to 0.9), necrotizing enterocolitis (odds ratio 0.35, CI 0.18 to 0.68), and neonatal mortality (odds ratio 0.6, CI 0.5 to 0.8).[8,9] An estimated number of patients needed to treat (NNT)

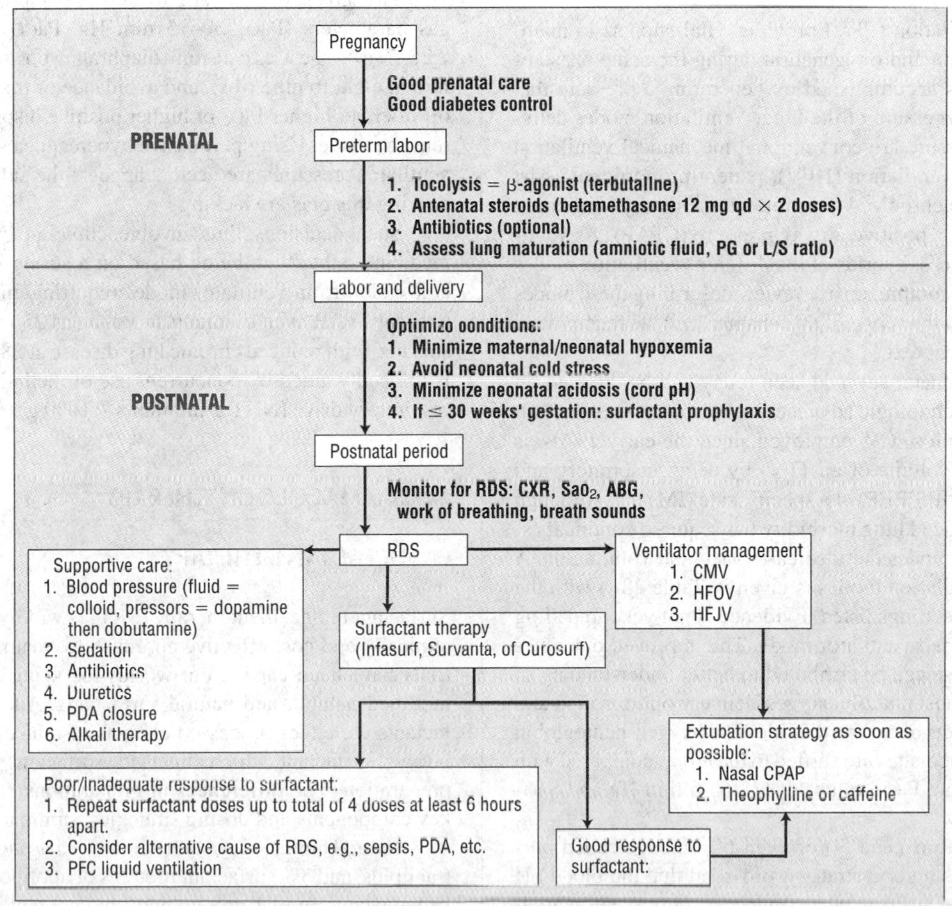

FIGURE 28–2. Algorithm for prevention and treatment of neonatal RDS.

to prevent RDS in one preterm infant less than 30 weeks' gestation, where RDS occurs in 50% of untreated cases, is six patients.[9] One report estimated that over $3000 was saved per treated neonate and that if treatment rates increased to 60%, annual savings in health care costs from initial hospitalization alone would exceed $157 million.[9]

Use of thyrotropin-releasing hormone (TRH) as an adjunct to antenatal corticosteroids was thought to further accelerate fetal lung maturation.[9] However, the Australian Collaborative Trial of Antenatal Thyrotropin-Releasing Hormone (ACTOBAT) study failed to show additional benefits from TRH 200 μg every 12 hours. The frequencies of RDS (relative risk 1.17, CI 1.00 to 1.36) and need for ventilation (relative risk 1.15, CI 1.01 to 1.31) were not reduced, and treatment was associated with maternal nausea, vomiting, and lightheadedness.[10] Of more concern was the 12-month follow-up report in which TRH treatment was associated with motor delays (odds ratio 1.51, CI 1.11 to 2.05), sensory impairment (odds ratio 2.00, CI 1.06 to 3.74), social delays (odds ratio 1.41, CI 1.01 to 1.95), and severe neurodevelopmental impairment (odds ratio 1.75, CI 1.07 to 2.87).[11] At this point, antenatal TRH treatment cannot be advised.

▶ TREATMENT: Neonatal Respiratory Distress Syndrome

GENERAL APPROACH TO TREATMENT

Recently, treatment options for RDS have significantly advanced. Effective drug therapies include surfactant, and perfluorocarbons (PFCs). Extracorporeal membrane oxygenation (ECMO) has been used as a final resort. Supportive therapies such as mechanical ventilation, management of acidosis, and diuresis are also important. An algorithm for prevention and treatment of neonatal RDS is presented in Figure 28–2.

NONPHARMACOLOGIC THERAPY

VENTILATOR THERAPY

Positive-pressure ventilation (PPV) provides vital support to maintain adequate ventilation and oxygenation during the acute phase of RDS. Effective PPV is accomplished by generating a pressure that exceeds the "closing" pressure of the lung. Ventilation modes delivering this positive pressure are conventional mechanical ventilation (CV), high-frequency ventilation (HFV), patient proportional assist ventilation (PPAV), synchronized intermittent mandatory ventilation (SIMV), and continuous positive airway pressure (CPAP). As ventilator technology advances, hybrids of the different ventilation modes also have been tried. A comprehensive review describing these modes of ventilation is beyond the scope of this chapter, and we recommend the reader to an excellent text.[12]

The increased neonatal survival seen today can be credited, in part, to the extensive technologic advances in respiratory care, including mechanical ventilation. CV, employed since the early 1970s, is based on delivering a volume of air (TV) by using inspiratory and expiratory pressures (PIP/PEEP) at a specific rate (IMV).[13] Although successful, the CV-induced lung morbidity has required continual assessment of ventilator modes that decrease baro- and volutrauma. A summary of these ventilation modes is given in Table 28–4 with the range of typical initial settings listed. Evidence is not yet compelling to recommend a preferred ventilator mode. The improved outcomes in premature infants also can be attributed to better understanding of neonatal physiology, most notably oxygen delivery optimization and cerebral protective effects of carbon dioxide. The oxygen-hemoglobin dissociation curves in neonates are shifted to the left as compared with adults, resulting in target Pa_{O_2} values of 50 to 75 mm Hg and Sa_{O_2} values greater than 90%.

Allowing Pa_{CO_2} to exceed 50 or even 60 mmHg (called *permissive hypercapnia*) is a good strategy, provided that the blood pH remains acceptable, because it means that less aggressive ventilator pressures are needed. Too aggressive ventilation can result in hypocarbia, which is associated with periventricular leukomalacia and consequent neurodevelopmental delays. The more comprehensive understanding of neonatal physiology allows the clinician to use improved ventilator technologies and select strategies that allow for the most appropriate fit for the circumstance. For example, although CV remains a good choice for many neonates, those with pulmonary air leaks probably are managed more safely with high-frequency oscillatory ventilation (HFOV). Increasingly, HFOV using a "high volume" strategy, which avoids atelectasis, is being considered the preferred first-line ventilator therapy. This must be tempered by an inability of studies to show differences in outcomes between CV and HFOV. Since rapid and early ventilator weaning is becoming popular and the optimal approach to weaning from HFOV is unknown, the pendulum may shift back to CV when prophylactic surfactant is used and rapid advancement to extubation is anticipated.

The goals of CV are to achieve appropriate arterial blood gas parameters (Pa_{O_2} 50–75 mm Hg, Pa_{CO_2} 40–60 mm Hg, pH 7.28–7.40), chest expansion (diaphragm position on an inspiratory film at eight to nine ribs), and avoidance of toxicities. Often a trade-off of either higher F_{IO_2} or higher positive inspiratory pressure (PIP) must be made. Using permissive hypercapnea so that less aggressive ventilator pressures are needed appears the safer approach, but data proving this bias are lacking.

Such decisions thus involve clinician bias and the "art" of medicine rather than being based on a strong scientific basis. Early conversion from ventilator modes requiring endotracheal intubation to nasal CPAP, even in infants as young as 25 weeks' gestation, is associated with reduced chronic lung disease at 28 days (NNT 6).[14] This is markedly aided by concurrent use of methylxanthines to increase respiratory drive (NNT 2 in infants $<$1000 g).[13]

PHARMACOLOGIC THERAPY

SURFACTANT THERAPY

Surfactant replacement therapy (SRT) is widely accepted as the most clinically and cost-effective approach to treatment of RDS. Clinical trials have been carried out worldwide using an array of artificial, modified natural, and natural surfactants. Additionally, natural surfactants are either processed extracts of minced lungs or extracts of lavaged surfactant, which affects the surfactant protein makeup of the preparation. The differences in preparations can be discerned from key components and dosing strategies, summarized in Table 28–5.

Natural human surfactant contains 85% phospholipids, 10% neutral lipids, and 5% surfactant proteins or apolipoproteins. Animal surfactants have similar protein and lipid content. Surfactant is synthesized in type II pneumocytes in the alveoli. After secretion, the major

TABLE 28–4. Ventilator Management and Considerations in RDS

Ventilator Type	Setting	Normal Initial Settings <1500 g	>1500 g	Advantages	Disadvantages
CMV	PIP (cm H_2O)	18–20	20–22	High inspiratory pressures allow "popping open" of alveoli	Larger tidal volumes and inspiratory pressures causing lung injury
	Target TV (mL/kg)	4–6	6–8		
	PEEP (cm H_2O)	4	4–5		
	IMV (bpm)	40–60	40–60		
CPAP	(cm H_2O)	5–7	6–8	Little barotrauma/volutrauma	Lack of tidal volume
HFOV	MAP (cm H_2O)	7–10	8–12	Less risk volutrauma/barotrauma Increased alveolar recruitment Approved for air-leak syndromes Simple to operate	Risk for IVH/PVL? Unable to give aerosolized respiratory medications Hypotension, increased mucostasis?
	Amplitude	*To appropriate CWF*			
	Hz	15	15		
HFJV	PIP (cm H_2O)	18–20	20–22	Increased CO_2 removal	Risk for IVH/PVL? Two machines Increased gas trapping Unable to give respiratory medicines
	PEEP (cm H_2O)	4–5	4–5		
	Sigh rate (bpm)	5–10	5–10		
	Rate (bpm)	420	420		
PPAV SIMV	Rate (bpm)	20–30	10–20	Less barotrauma due to "synchronizing" with patient's own breath Patient sensitive Reduced need for sedation	Lack of clinical experience
	Volume (mL/kg)	8–15	10–15		

Assistance provided by Andrew Davey, M.D., neonatologist, The Women's Hospital of Greensboro, Moses Cone Health System, Greensboro, North Carolina.

route of clearance is via reuptake by type II cells. Small quantities are removed by absorption into the lymphatics and clearance by alveolar macrophages. After reuptake into the type II cells, the phospholipids are either recycled for secretion or degraded and reused to synthesize new phospholipids.[15]

Most exogenous surfactants incorporate dipalmitoyl phosphatidylcholine (DPPC), which constitutes 45% to 70% of endogenous lung surfactant and is the major phospholipid causing the low surface tension of surfactant. Other phospholipids, mainly phosphatidyl ethanolamine, phosphatidyl glycerol, phosphatidylinositol, and

TABLE 28–5. Exogeneous Surfactants Used for the Treatment of Neonates with RDS

Surfactant Type	Dose (mg/kg)/Volume (mL/kg)	Source	Components
Artificial Surfactants			
Pulmactant (ALEC)	100/1.2	Synthetic	DPPC, unsaturated phosphatidylglycerol
Colfosceril palmitate (Exosurf)	67.5/5.0	Synthetic	DPPC, hexadecanol, tyloxapol
Human Surfactants			
Human	60/3.0	Aminotic fluid whole surfactant	Surfactant lipids, SP-A, SP-B (2.0–5.0%), SP-C, SP-D
Animal Surfactants			
Calfactant (Infasurf)	100/3.0	Calf lung lavage	Surfactant lipids, SP-B (1.7%), SP-C
CLSF	100/3.0	Calf lung lavage	Surfactant lipids, SP-B (1.7%), SP-C
SFRI 1 (Alveofact)	50/1.2	Cow lung lavage	Surfactant lipids, SP-B (1.7%), SP-C
Poractant alfa (Curosurf)	(Dose 1) 200/2.5 (Doses 2–4) 100/1.25	Minced pig lung extract purified by chromatography	Lung phospholipids, SP-B (0.2%), SP-C
Surfacten (Surfactant-TA)	100/4.0	Minced cow lung extract + synthetic lipids	Lung lipids + DPPC, tripalmitin, palmitic acid
Beractant (Survanta)	100/4.0	Minced cow lung extract + synthetic lipids	Lung lipids + DPPC, tripalmitin, palmitic acid, SP-B (<0.1%), SP-C

ALEC-artificial lung expanding compound; CLSE-calf lung surfactant extract; DPPC-dipalmitoyl phosphatidylcholine; SP-A-surfactant protein A; SP-B-surfactant protein B; SP-C-surfactant protein C. Doses reported per milligram of phospholipid and milliliter of surfactant product.

sphingomyelin, are responsible for adsorbing to the air-liquid interface. Four surfactant proteins (SP-A, SP-B, SP-C, and SP-D) comprise 2% to 5% of the weight of natural surfactant.[15,16] SP-A appears to regulate pulmonary surfactant turnover, formation of tubular myelin, and immune regulation. Since natural surfactant products undergo an organic solvent extraction procedure, no substantial quantities of SP-A are present in these products. SP-B appears to be involved in the formation of tubular myelin. It is also the most active hydrophobic protein in improving the surface activity of surfactant, perhaps by increasing the lateral stability of the phospholipid layer. Increasing SP-B content of surfactant preparations is associated with increased activity and resistance to inactivation by various endogenous substances. Genetic deficiency of SP-B in full-term infants results in death from respiratory failure. SP-C is speculated to be involved in the spreadability and surface activity of surfactant by increasing the adsorption of DPPC and other phospholipids to the air-liquid interface. SP-D function is unknown, but it has the structure of lectins and proteins responsible for bacterial opsonization.[15]

When given in the delivery room as prophylaxis, natural surfactant can be given as a single bolus down the endotracheal tube, although the manufacturers still recommend divided doses using the same procedure as for treatment.[16] For neonates with established RDS who are stabilized on the ventilator, surfactant is best administered via a sideport in the endotracheal adapter in two bolus fractional doses at a 45-degree upward tilt angled to the right and then left.[17] Animal studies confirm that the bolus technique delivers and distributes surfactant evenly. Use of the slow infusion technique delivered surfactant primarily to the upper lobes,[18] and nebulized surfactant concentrated in select pockets of each lobe, resulting in areas of hypo- and hyperinflation.[19] Bolus administration of natural surfactants may require extra attention if the neonate is on HFOV. Anecdotal experience with HFOV is that patients actually may suffer sudden loss of oxygenation, which appears to be from airway obstruction. When neonates are suctioned in these circumstances, the surfactant appears to be removed from the endotracheal tube. One theory for this occurring is that the linear flow of air pulses is both into and out of the lungs during HFOV, and the surfactant, instead of being pushed down into the lungs, essentially percolates back up and blocks the bronchi or endotracheal tube. Suctioning in this case probably does remove the surfactant, depriving the neonate of the dose. An apparent solution, which probably should be used routinely for surfactant delivery, is to hand-bag the surfactant in for about 5 minutes before reconnecting the HFOV mode. The optimal dose of exogenous surfactant remains uncertain. Controlled trials comparing single and multiple doses of surfactant have shown multiple doses to significantly reduce the incidence of pneumothorax and neonatal mortality.[20] This makes physiologic sense because animal studies suggest that much of the initial surfactant dose is inhibited by soluble proteins and other factors in the small airways and alveoli. Multiple doses may overcome this initial inactivation. Many clinicians use up to four doses of natural surfactant based on clinical need. A typical strategy is repeating surfactant doses if after 6 hours or more from the previous dose the patient continues to require mechanical ventilation and the FIO_2 exceeds 30% or 40%, depending on the clinician's preference. A summary of trials[21–27] comparing surfactant doses is shown in Table 28–6. A requirement of four doses of Survanta to treat RDS may be a valuable predictor of increasing oxygen requirements around day 10, with the subsequent development of bronchopulmonary dysplasia (BPD).[28]

SRT can be initiated as prophylaxis in the delivery room, prior to the first breath, or as rescue therapy after clinical signs of RDS appear. The proposed advantages for prophylaxis involve more even distribution of surfactant after delivery and preventing the onset of respiratory deficiency, thus avoiding excess ventilatory support and associated barotrauma.[29,30] On the downside, this may result in unnecessary treatment and costs. In reports of recent trials using surfactant rescue[31,32] in newborns weighing 501 to 1500 g in over 5000 patients, only 45% actually required treatment. Alternatively, over 80% of neonates with birth weights below 1000 g had RDS in the 1999 Vermont Oxford Network experience reporting on over 27,000 neonates with birth weights below 1500 g. Any surfactant treatment approach provides multiple outcome benefits (Table 28–7). A recent systematic review and metaanalysis makes a strong argument for prophylaxis rather than treatment when using a natural surfactant in neonates less than 30 weeks' gestation.[30] Relative risk (RR) for prophylaxis versus treatment was reduced for pneumothorax (RR 0.62, CI 0.42, 0.89), pulmonary interstitial emphysema (RR 0.54, CI 0.36, 0.82), and mortality (RR 0.75, CI 0.59, 0.96). For every 100 infants treated with prophylactic surfactant, 2 fewer pneumothoraces and 5 fewer deaths can be expected.

The only known consequence of exposing some infants unnecessarily to surfactant is the cost. This should be somewhat offset by decreased need for additional surfactant doses, the decreased morbidity and mortality, and ultimately the cost savings from facilitation of initiating strategies to switch neonates to early nasal CPAP rather

TABLE 28–6. Dosing Comparison Studies for Different Surfactants

			Effects of Higher Doses Compared to Lower Doses	
Ref.	Surfactant	Doses	*Short Term*	*Long Term*
21	Exosurf	5 mL/kg ≤4 versus ≤2 doses	Not stated	28 days; no differences
22	Exosurf	2.5 versus 5 mL	⇓ FIO_2, ⇓ vent (MAP)	14 days; no differences
		2.5 versus 7.5 mL	⇓ FIO_2, ⇓ vent (MAP)	
		5 versus 7.5 mL	No difference	
23	Infasurf	100 mg /kg 1 versus ≤4 doses	⇓ FIO_2, ⇓ vent (PIP × IMV)	28 days; ⇓ O_2 suppl (0 versus 8.3%) ⇓ pneumothorax (11.1% versus 16.7%)
24	Surfactant TA	30 mg/mL 2 versus 4 mL/kg	⇓ FIO_2	30 days; ⇓ O_2 suppl (13% versus 43.5%) ⇓ vent (4.3% versus 30.4%)
25	Curosurf	200 mg/kg × 1 versus 200 mg/kg × 1 + 100 mg/kg (× ≤2)	⇓ FIO_2, ⇓ vent (MAP)	28 days; ⇓ death (13% versus 21%) ⇓ pneumothorax (9% versus 18%)
26	Curosurf	100 mg/kg × ≤3 versus 200 mg/kg + 100 mg/kg (× ≤4)	⇓ FIO_2	28 days; no differences
27	Alveofact	100 mg/kg versus 50 mg /kg (repeat doses to max 200 mg /kg)	⇓ FIO_2	28 days; ⇓ pulmonary air leak (14% versus 33%)

TABLE 28–7. Relative Risks for Potential Beneficial and Adverse Effects of Synthetic and Natural Surfactants

	Synthetic Surfactant				Natural Surfactant			
Outcome	*No.*	*Prophylaxis*	*No.*	*Rescue*	*No.*	*Prophylaxis*	*No.*	*Rescue*
Pneumothorax	5	0.64 (0.49–0.89)	3	0.52 (0.42–0.65)	9	0.31 (0.22–0.44)	12	0.34 (0.27–0.44)
BPD	5	1.09 (0.80–1.47)	3	0.68 (0.46–0.99)	7	0.88 (0.67–1.17)	10	1.01 (0.81–1.27)
Death	7	0.67 (0.52–0.88)	3	0.47 (0.30–0.74)	9	0.60 (0.42–0.85)	11	0.59 (0.47–0.74)
Death + BPD	3	0.82 (0.63–1.08)	2	0.65 (0.50–0.82)	7	0.64 (0.49–0.84)	10	0.66 (0.53–0.82)
All IVH	4	0.94 (0.73–1.21)	2	0.77 (0.62–0.97)	8	0.95 (0.73–1.24)	10	0.94 (0.76–1.15)
Severe IVH						1.05 (0.86–1.18)		0.91 (0.72–1.14)
PDA	5	1.27 (1.03–1.57)	3	0.73 (0.60–0.88)	9	1.16 (0.89–1.50)	12	0.96 (0.79–1.18)
Pulmonary bleed	4	3.12 (1.54–6.32)	3	1.49 (0.57–3.79)	2	0.73 (0.31–1.69)	2	1.25 (0.74–2.13)

than prolonged mechanical ventilation and its attendant chronic lung problems.[33]

Outcome measures examined during surfactant trials include oxygen and ventilator requirements, severity of RDS, RDS mortality, total mortality, pneumothorax and other air-leak syndromes, pulmonary interstitial emphysema (PIE), BPD, and complications some investigators associate with surfactant therapy, such as intraventricular hemorrhage (IVH), pulmonary hemorrhage, and patent ductus arteriosus (PDA) (Table 28–8). In general, the primary benefits are more rapid resolution and milder course of RDS and lower risk of pneumothorax, death, or chronic lung disease. These benefits are seen with natural and synthetic surfactants and are enhanced markedly when antenatal glucocorticoids also are used.[9] Despite the high success rates, 20% of neonates fail to respond to treatment. Factors associated with poor response include sepsis, pneumonia, PDA, congenital heart disease, and pulmonary hypoplasia.[15] Whether retreatment of RDS with surfactant after resolution of these factors is useful is currently unknown.

Although surfactant appears to be generally well tolerated, some possible toxicities and associated problems include bradycardia, airway obstruction, and oxygen desaturation during administration; pulmonary hemorrhage; IVH; and the theoretical risk of allergy to natural surfactants,[31] although antibodies were absent in over 1400 Survanta-treated neonates.[32]

Problems during administration appear to be related to the volume of surfactant delivered, so surfactants using lower administration volumes may be better tolerated. Surfactant treatment is also associated with higher likelihood of clinically significant PDA. Pulmonary edema is associated with PDA. The pink respiratory secretions are thought to represent hemorrhagic pulmonary edema due to capillary leakage of blood rather than the serious pulmonary hemorrhage seen in 10% to 45% of neonates with RDS in the presurfactant era.[15] Furthermore, this pulmonary hemorrhage seems primarily to be a risk for prophylaxis with Exosurf[34] (see Table 28–8). Early closure of the PDA may minimize the risk of hemorrhagic pulmonary edema as well as optimize surfactant response. While the relationship of IVH to surfactant use is controversial, cerebral blood flow velocity has been shown to be altered in some studies.[20] The risks of surfactants causing periventricular leukomalacia (PVL), a marker of hypoxic-ischemic brain injury, is poorly understood, but two recent trials[29,35] comparing Infasurf and Exosurf found increased risk with Infasurf (odds ratio 2.03, CI 1.09 to 3.80).[29] A theoretical basis for this is the more rapid and greater pulmonary beneficial effects with Infasurf, resulting in overventilation and hypocarbia, since this is associated with decreased cerebral blood flow. If this is the correct cause, a more intense respiratory monitoring approach and aggressive ventilator weaning can avoid the problem. This trend needs to be assessed for all surfactants in additional studies that better measure this important prognostic marker for neurodevelopment.

Selection of surfactant products will require measuring positive and adverse outcomes in direct comparisons and meta-analyses with sufficient study numbers to document small differences in clinically important end points because sample sizes cannot be achieved readily in individual clinical trials. Studies comparing Exosurf with natural

TABLE 28–8. Comparison of Rescue SRT on Outcomes in Neonates <1750 g

	Adverse Outcomes			
% Events	*Air Leaks*	*PIE*	*Died from RDS*	*Died and/or BPD*
Controls, mean (range)	23 (15–31)	38 (33–44)	24 (18–29)	57 (44–67)
NNT				
Exosurf versus control[a]	+11 (6, 100)*	+4 (3, 5)*	+14 (8, 100)*	+5 (3, 14)*
Survanta versus control[a]	+8 (6, 20)*	+4 (3, 5)*	+10 (7, 25)*	+5 (3, 14)*
Infasurf versus control[a]	+8 (6, 20)*	+3 (3, 4)*	+9 (6, 20)*	+4 (3, 9)*
Survanta versus Exosurf[b]	+17*	NA	+50	+33
Infasurf versus Exosurf[b]	+20*	+17*	+25	I=E
Infasurf versus Survanta[b]	+33	+25	−20*	+25

*Statistically significant difference ($P < .05$)

NA = information not available; NNT = the number of neonates needed to be treated with the test surfactant (listed first) compared with second listed treatment to avoid (+) or cause (−) one adverse outcome in one patient

[a]Compared to data from separate studies.

[b]Direct comparison of treatments.

Untreated controls data from Refs. 31 and 32; SRT data from Refs. 29, 36, and 38.

surfactants (Survanta[36,37] and Infasurf[29,35]) found that the natural surfactant groups have a more rapid onset and lower requirements for oxygen supplementation and PPV. Natural surfactant treatment resulted in fewer air leaks (e.g., pneumothorax).[29,35–37] Although survival trends favored natural surfactants (2% to 4% lower mortality rates), a statistically significant reduction in death was not shown and would require a study of at least 9000 patients to demonstrate statistical significance.[38] Typically, mortality rates are below 20% and often below 10%, depending on the gestational ages of the patients included in the study.

Comparisons of currently marketed natural surfactants show that Infasurf[39] and Curosurf[40] have a more rapid onset of pulmonary benefits (decreased oxygen supplementation and ventilator pressures) and longer duration of action[37] than the modified natural surfactant (Survanta). This can be resolved by adding surfactant protein B supplement to Survanta so that the SP-B content increases to 2% to 3%.[41] However, in clinical trials comparing Infasurf and Survanta, no clinically significant outcomes (e.g., incidence of chronic lung disease or days on a ventilator) were statistically different, except the counterintuitive finding that fewer RDS-related deaths occurred with Survanta prophylaxis than with Infasurf prophylaxis.

Curosurf trials have been in relatively small study populations and cannot be used to make conclusive statements about its relative effectiveness, other than that preliminary experiences are very positive.[16,33]

Because studies are limited, natural surfactants should be considered equivalent at this time, although the problems of hypocarbia and PVL documented with Infasurf[29,35] must be studied for all surfactants for the true risk to be clarified. If problems with increased PVL risk are unique to Infasurf (which seems unlikely), it would place this surfactant product at a disadvantage. Most likely, this problem can be avoided by more aggressive ventilator weaning strategies with the newer surfactants that have more rapid onset and possibly greater pharmacologic effect on lung dynamics. In fact, rapid extubation to nasal CPAP is feasible, even in neonates with birth weights below 1000 g. This was accomplished with prophylactic Curosurf.[33] Whether prophylactic use of the current formulation of Survanta with relatively low SP-B has similar benefits is an important issue because Survanta remains in widespread use. Comparative trials of natural surfactants using this prophylaxis strategy with early extubation are needed.

Pharmacoeconomics of SRT

The pharmacoeconomic impact of SRT is examined in several reports.[42–44] SRT has lowered RDS mortality by at least 30%. From 1989 to 1990 (when Exosurf was introduced), 80% of the decline in infant mortality nationwide was attributable directly to SRT.[42] The reduction in resource use resulted in projected savings (using 1991 dollars) of $5800 in survivors and $4400 in infants who died.[42] Survanta use was projected to save $3300 in hospital resources for infants surviving to 28 days.[43] Savings as high as $18,000 in total hospital charges per surviving infant were projected in one analysis.[44] Each RDS- or treatment-related adverse outcome confers cost to health care.

Although data are limited, the number of neonates with RDS needed to treat with SRT to avoid selected RDS-related complications is estimated in Table 28–8. Use of prophylactic surfactant in combination with new respiratory strategies to rapidly extubate neonates to nasal CPAP is not measured in these economic analyses, and it is likely that the economic savings are larger than reported in these studies if this strategy is applied to neonates born at 30 weeks or less of gestation. Also, as newer surfactants have entered the market, the price for surfactants had fallen, making the benefits even greater.

LIQUID VENTILATION WITH PERFLUOROCHEMICALS

An investigational but highly promising approach to treating refractory RDS is the use of partial liquid ventilation, also called *perfluorocarbon-associated gas exchange* (PAGE).[45] Studies with perflubron, a PFC, have reported a dramatic increase in partial pressure of oxygen in arterial blood (PaO_2) and dynamic lung compliance within 1 hour of starting therapy, and treatment resulted in prevention of RDS-associated deaths.[46] PFCs are inert liquids in which oxygen and carbon dioxide are highly soluble. PFCs have low surface tension and are distributed evenly throughout the lung at low inflation pressures. The surface tension with PFCs at the alveolar air-liquid interface is markedly lower than seen with air ventilation, allowing for markedly lower ventilator pressures and a reduced risk of barotrauma.[45] Clinically, PFCs have been dosed by instillation into the endotracheal tube through the sideport at a rate of 1 mL/kg per minute without interrupting mechanical gas ventilation until a column of fluid is welled up in the endotracheal tube. This volume of PFC is felt to represent the infant's liquid functional residual capacity (FRC). Fluid that evaporates is replaced hourly to maintain this liquid FRC.[46]

In animal studies, PFCs also offered a vehicle for improved drug delivery via the lungs.[46] Addition of exogenous surfactant to PFC ventilation appears to improve surfactant delivery and enhance response to PFCs and surfactant in animals,[47,48] although studies in humans are unavailable. Adverse events associated with PFC use are mild and manageable, although long-term studies are lacking. Problems include endotracheal tube obstruction, hypoxic episodes, pneumothorax or fluorothorax (i.e., PFC leakage into the pleural space), and pulmonary hemorrhage.[46] These are not necessarily causal relationships, and overall, PFCs have been remarkably toxicity-free. The limited experience with PFCs and PAGE requires that this therapy be viewed as a promising but investigational option in RDS unresponsive to surfactant.

NITRIC OXIDE

Nitric oxide (NO) is a natural endothelium-derived relaxing factor that is important in regulating vascular tone, especially the pulmonary vasculature.[49] Under normal physiologic conditions, NO is synthesized in endothelial cells and released into the vascular smooth muscle, where it stimulates cyclic GMP for vascular dilatation. At birth, NO helps in the transition from the markedly elevated pulmonary pressures in utero to normal pulmonary pressures and respiratory function.[49] Clinical studies have demonstrated the benefits of NO in persistent pulmonary hypertension of the newborn, meconium aspiration syndrome, and RDS. An exogenous NO product and delivery system was approved by the Food and Drug Administration (INOmax and INOvent, INO Therapeutics, Inc.). Dosages of 5–80 parts per million (ppm) usually are targeted. While inhaled NO therapy was effective in term and near-term infants with respiratory failure, it has not appeared beneficial in preterm neonates, although further studies are justified.[50] Potential toxicities are few but include methemoglobinemia, inhibited platelet aggregation, and severe acute pulmonary edema secondary to the NO_2 oxidant metabolite. Further studies are needed to examine the clinical impact of this adjunctive therapy and the cost-benefit ratio as well.

SUPPORTIVE PHARMACOTHERAPY

Supportive pharmacotherapy in RDS is aimed at alleviating pain and discomfort, minimizing ventilator complications, and correcting any metabolic and/or fluid imbalance.

Narcotics/Benzodiazepines

Appropriate pharmacologic treatment is effective in alleviating pain and discomfort in neonates. Many ventilator-induced complications are secondary to asynchrony between ventilator rates and patient-driven respirations, resulting in pneumothorax and increased cerebral pressures that may promote IVH. Avoidance of these serious adverse effects can be accomplished by nonpharmacologic methods (e.g., PPAV) or through the use of sedative and paralytic agents. A comprehensive review of sedation in neonates is available[51]; therefore, the following discussion will be limited. The most commonly used analgesics and sedative agents are morphine, fentanyl, and lorazepam. Studies have shown a significantly greater percentage of ventilator time in synchrony and a decrease in catecholamine levels in neonates who routinely receive narcotics. A recent comparison of morphine and fentanyl in this patient population showed fentanyl to have a better side-effect profile at equivalent efficacy.[52] One concern is that studies examining fentanyl have shown an increase in ventilator support, tolerance, and physiologic dependence effects with long-term use.[53]

All narcotics are expected to have this problem. The most common side effects demonstrated with narcotics include decreased gastrointestinal motility and risk of hypotension. Lorazepam is the preferred sedative agent in the absence of pain owing to its fast onset of action, its lack of hemodynamic toxicities, and its low risk of metabolite accumulation in comparison with diazepam. Midazolam continuous infusion is a reasonable alternative, although more costly and requiring additional fluid, which may be detrimental in a patient predisposed to PDA. Muscle paralysis has been used to reduce ventilator fighting and the consequent complications. However, its role in RDS has diminished owing to adverse effects (i.e., edema, hypoventilation). If paralysis is induced, assessment of sedation and seizures is confounded. Consequently, concurrent phenobarbital serum concentrations of 40 mg/L are recommended. Independent of agent use, it is imperative to establish target sedation and pain scores to guide the clinical team in optimizing drug dosage. The use of sedation scores provides a mechanism to titrate drug to effect, which maximizes effectiveness while limiting complications.

Acidosis

Acidosis is associated with a number of physiologic effects that increase the severity of RDS, including increased pulmonary vascular resistance, impaired synthesis of surfactant, reduced cardiac output, and depressed ventilation. Consequently, measures that reduce the risk of acidosis, such as prevention of hypoxemia, hypotension, and excessive blood loss through venipuncture and minimizing oxygen consumption through careful temperature control, are critical. Correction of metabolic acidosis with sodium bicarbonate or 0.3 *M* tromethamine (THAM) is recommended when blood pH falls below 7.25 and base excess is 5 or less. Patients should not receive sodium bicarbonate in congestive heart failure or any other conditions where sodium administration worsens the clinical condition. Patients receiving THAM should be monitored for episodes of apnea and bradycardia, which may worsen following administration. THAM should be avoided in uremic or anuric patients and should not be given via umbilical artery catheter.

Diuretics

Pulmonary edema is a prominent feature of RDS. The severity of RDS is correlated with the presence of factors that cause pulmonary edema. This is not unexpected because excess fluid in the alveolar and interstitial spaces impairs pulmonary gas exchange, lowers lung compliance, and reduces FRC. Prevention of fluid overload and pulmonary edema is critical to minimize the risk of opening the ductus arteriosus and the need for high ventilatory pressures. Pulmonary edema can benefit from positive end-expiratory pressure (PEEP) because of redistribution of fluid from airspaces to interstitial tissue and improvement in gas exchange. Oliguria is well recognized during the early stages of RDS. The routine use of a diuretic, furosemide, to correct this oliguria was not shown to improve markers of ventilation, oxygenation, or mortality.[54] The potential benefits of furosemide must be weighed against its risks, especially electrolyte imbalance. Furosemide also promotes prostaglandin synthesis, which dilates the ductus arteriosus and may increase the risk of developing a PDA. The intermittent use of furosemide 1–2 mg/kg when pulmonary edema is thought to play a clinical role is justified and often beneficial clinically.

CONCLUSIONS

Advances in prevention and reversal of RDS have had considerable impact on morbidity and mortality from RDS. Nevertheless, chronic lung disease, although less severe, continues to occur in 10% to 45% of neonates depending on the institution studied. The challenge for the future is to manage effectively the 20% of neonates with RDS responding poorly to surfactant. Also, institutions need to use multidisciplinary committees that enhance proficiency with therapies that will further reduce long-term pulmonary sequelae associated with RDS. A good example is ensuring surfactant availability at all preterm deliveries so that prophylactic surfactant treatment can be used when appropriate. Also, rapid extubation to nasal CPAP and use of methylxanthines to facilitate this are useful NICU policies. Finally, if more than one surfactant is used in an institution, the pharmacodynamic differences between surfactants must be understood to optimize timing of arterial blood gas measurements to guide ventilator weaning and thus avoid serious sequelae from under- or overventilation.

ACUTE RESPIRATORY DISTRESS SYNDROME (ARDS)

Acute respiratory distress syndrome (formerly known as *adult respiratory distress syndrome*) was first described in 1967 in 12 patients presenting with acute respiratory distress, cyanosis refractory to oxygen therapy, decreased lung compliance, and diffuse infiltrates seen on chest x-ray.[55,56] Although the clinical description is similar to neonatal RDS, the underlying pathophysiology and ultimate morbidity and mortality differ considerably. A proper diagnostic definition of ARDS and acute lung injury (ALI) is necessary in order for clinical trials to include appropriate patients. Efforts to arrive at a standard definition were initially made in 1971, modified in 1988, and revised again in 1994. Establishing epidemiologic data is influenced by the definition used. Comparing results across clinical trials has been confounded by the lack of a standardized definition. Designing a controlled, prospective study is difficult because of so many variables and possible measures of response, although pulmonary morbidity and death are frequent end points. Limited patient numbers in clinical trials have resulted in insufficient power to detect potentially important but modest benefits of therapies. Recently, attention has focused on the systemic inflammatory response syndrome (SIRS) and the ablation of such response in limiting lung dysfunction, with mixed results.[55–62] In this situation, biochemical markers of the disease process also may prove useful for comparisons of clinical and therapeutic interventions. Management of ARDS is still primarily supportive, with general focus on ventilator management, prevention or limiting pulmonary tissue damage, hemodynamic support, and prevention of multiorgan dysfunction syndrome (MODS).

EPIDEMIOLOGY AND ETIOLOGY

Accurate estimation of the incidence of ARDS has been confounded historically by variation in definition parameters. In an effort to standardize definitions, the 1994 American-European Consensus Conference (AECC) provided the clinical definition of ARDS by the following: (1) acute onset of arterial hypoxemia with a PaO_2/FIO_2 ratio of less than 200 mm Hg, (2) bilateral infiltrates on frontal chest radiograph consistent with pulmonary edema, and (3) pulmonary wedge pressure of 18 mm Hg or less without clinical evidence of left atrial hypertension.[63] A broader term attempting to encompass patients with milder gas exchange abnormalities ($PaO_2/FIO_2 < 300$ mm Hg) is ALI. The 1994 consensus definitions were designed to develop homogeneity for epidemiologic and clinical research aspects; however, it is now recognized that these definitions are a temporary solution for a complex disease state.[64] While this definition has the advantages that it is easy to use and recognizes the spectrum of the clinical disorder, it fails to recognize the cause or the presence or absence of multiorgan dysfunction.[55]

The most recent data using the AECC criteria demonstrates an incidence of ARDS at 4.8 to 8.3 cases per 100,000 individuals.[65] These data are extrapolated from one state, with national projections of 13,000 to 22,000 cases annually. Alternatively, the incidence may be as high as 75 per 100,000.[55] Certain groups are predisposed to developing ARDS, and the risks vary within these groups. Patients with aspiration pneumonia or sepsis are at the highest risk for developing ARDS.[65,66] Other causes of ARDS include pneumonia, pulmonary contusion, fat emboli, inhalational injury, near-drowning, severe trauma with shock, multiple transfusions of blood products, acute pancreatitis, cardiopulmonary bypass, and drug overdose.[55,65]

Mortality associated with ARDS typically has been 40% to 60% in most studies but appears to be declining in more recent reports.[55,67] The explanation for this is unclear.[67] Subgroup analysis suggests that patients with trauma-induced ARDS are more likely to survive than those with an infectious etiology.[67] The constellation of underlying pathophysiologic conditions and the individual response to the inflammatory cascade appears to place the underlying subgroups at higher or lower risks for mortality.[68]

PATHOPHYSIOLOGY

Damage to the alveolar epithelium and the microvascular endothelium compromises the alveolar-capillary barrier and results in influx of protein-rich edema fluid during the acute phase of ALI and ARDS. The extent of alveolar epithelial injury is predictive of outcome. Epithelial injury is thought to predispose to progression of the disease process in five ways: (1) increased fluid permeability resulting in alveolar flooding, (2) type II pneumocyte damage impairing removal of edema fluid from alveoli, (3) type II pneumocyte injury reducing surfactant production, (4) damaged epithelial barrier predisposing to systemic infection, and (5) disorganized or insufficient epithelial repair possibly leading to fibrosis.[55] After the acute phase of ALI or ARDS, there may be rapid resolution of the disorder, or it may progress to a fibrosing alveolitis. This fibrotic process may begin early in the disease course and be detectable histologically as early as 5 days after onset of the disease. Proinflammatory cell mediators, especially interleukin-1, are thought to stimulate this cascade of events.[69] The inflammatory process is thought to reflect a balance between proinflammatory cytokines and anti-inflammatory mediators.[55] Neutrophils predominate in the pulmonary edema fluid and bronchoalveolar fluid obtained from affected patients. Neutrophils release oxidants, proteases, leukotrienes, platelet-activating factor, and other proinflammatory molecules that may play a role in causing lung injury. However, the importance of neutrophils in this cascade of lung damage was called into question recently because ALI and ARDS also occur in neutropenic patients and do not occur more frequently in patients with pneumonia who are treated with therapies to increase the number of circulating neutrophils.[55] Cytokine-mediated proinflammatory response appears to be further enhanced in association with ventilator-induced lung injury (VILI). The cascade of proinflammatory cytokine release is thought to be stimulated by alveolar overdistension and possibly by cyclic opening and closing of atelectatic alveoli.[55,70] This can result not only in local pulmonary effects but also in a systemic inflammatory response with multiple systemic organ failure.[71] No single mediator or clinical feature adequately predicts which patient will develop ARDS.[56] One postulate is that a genetic predisposition for lung injury when combined with inflammatory mediators may contribute to this lack of predictive value.[71] Nonetheless, inflammatory mediators compromise the pulmonary endothelium, resulting in increased protein permeability across endothelial and epithelial cells. This results in arterial hypoxemia and bilateral radiographic infiltrates from a protein-rich edema that is a chemotactant for further inflammatory mediators. The "leakage" of fluid into the pulmonary interstitium results in three physiologic alterations: (1) an impairment of tissue integrity that compromises normal expansion of alveolar tissue, (2) a physical impairment of oxygen-carbon dioxide exchange on an alveolar level, and (3) inactivation of endogenous surfactant resulting in alveolar collapse and development of pulmonary ventilation-perfusion mismatch. Not all areas of the lung are equally affected. Fluid-filled alveoli, atelectasis, and consolidation occur primarily in dependent lung zones, whereas other areas may be relatively spared.[55,56] This creates problems with mechanical ventilation because positive pressure can overdistend normal alveoli while trying to open other atelectatic alveoli.

CLINICAL PRESENTATION

The clinical presentation of ARDS is associated most often with concomitant factors that can complicate the differential diagnosis. As such, ARDS presents clinically as refractory hypoxemia (blood oxygen saturation <90%) with bilateral pulmonary infiltrates on chest radiography. However, chest radiographs may be interpreted differently for diagnosis of ARDS even among experienced intensivists.[72] In addition, since the failure is not cardiogenic, the pulmonary artery obstruction pressure should be normal (<18 mm Hg), and left ventricular function is also normal. To assist with the diagnosis of ARDS, computed tomography (CT) is being used with increased regularity to detect underlying conditions such as abscesses, surgical emphysema, and pneumothorax. Further, CT has been used to evaluate pulmonary response to ventilatory and positioning maneuvers.[73]

▶ TREATMENT: Acute Respiratory Distress Syndrome

DESIRED OUTCOME

No effective therapy is available to treat the underlying pathophysiology of ARDS. Thus initial therapy is focused on maintaining adequate oxygenation and tissue perfusion. Identifying and appropriately managing the precipitating factors and minimizing nosocomial complications related to infection, ventilator management, and other interventions also play prominent roles. Prevention of MODS is important because studies have shown that mortality is linked to a variety of factors, including nonpulmonary organ dysfunction.[55,74] Finally, investigational pharmacologic therapies to attenuate the inflammatory response may be a part of the clinician's approach to the ARDS patient. Treatment options are outlined in Figure 28–3.

VENTILATOR MANAGEMENT

The cornerstone for the treatment of ARDS is mechanical ventilation. This area of management is evolving rapidly due to newer ventilator technologies and improved understanding of lung physiology and VILI. Traditionally, ventilator management has focused on giving patients a tidal volume sufficient to maintain normal arterial blood gas values for $PaCO_2$ or pH. Typically, this has required supraphysiologic tidal volumes of 10–15 mL/kg of predicted ideal body weight (normal physiologic volume is 7–8 mL/kg). It has become apparent that this high-volume approach causes excessive distension of normally aerated portions of affected lungs with consequent release of inflammatory mediators. This is one mechanism thought to perpetuate ALI as well as nonpulmonary organ damage. Several investigators have tried a "low volume" strategy and administered tidal volumes of 6 mL/kg.[55,74–77] The Acute Respiratory Distress Syndrome Network compared ventilator strategies using a traditional tidal volume approach, i.e., initial tidal volume of 12 mL/kg, and adjusted to give a plateau pressure (measured after a 0.5-s pause at the end of inspiration) of 45–50 cm H_2O, with a low volume strategy, i.e., initial tidal volume 6 mL/kg, and adjusted to give a plateau pressure of 25–30 cm H_2O.[74] Both groups used a volume-assist-control ventilator mode until the patient was weaned from the ventilator or until day 28 of the study. The ratio for the duration of inspiration to the duration of expiration (I:E ratio) was set at 1.1 to 1.3. Ventilator settings were adjusted overall to achieve target goals for arterial blood pH of 7.3–7.45 and PaO_2 of 55–80 mm Hg or oxygen saturation of 88% to 95%. This study, which included over 400 patients in each treatment group, showed that the "low volume" strategy significantly reduced mortality (31.0% versus 39.8%), increased the percentage breathing without assistance by day 28 (65.7% versus 55.0%), reduced the number of days without ventilator use during the first 28 days (12 ± 11 versus 10 ± 11), and reduced days without failure of nonpulmonary organs (15 ± 11 versus 12 ± 11). Day 3 interleukin-6 plasma concentrations were lower in the low-volume strategy group, supporting the clinical findings.[74] This approach using gentler ventilation with adjunctive therapies to maintain acceptable arterial blood oxygenation and pH also was embraced in the accompanying editorial.[77] The risk with using a low-volume strategy is that it may result in lung derecruitment, atelectasis, and promotion of inflammatory response. Also, this approach of using higher PEEP and lower tidal volumes with conventional ventilation may lead to hypoventilation and respiratory acidosis. This could lead to increased need for sedation or neuromuscular blockade. Myopathy and neuropathy are recognized increasingly as a concern with prolonged neuromuscular blocker use, especially when systemic steroids are used concurrently. Since ventilator management is as much of an art as a science, only individuals experienced with ventilator modes and options should oversee selection of ventilator strategy and changes in ventilator settings in such a life-threatening situation.

Clinicians caring for critically ill patients must have a rudimentary understanding of the technical aspects of mechanical ventilation to optimize therapy. Therefore, the following section simply provides an overview of ventilator technology and issues. Mechanical ventilation management is based on evaluations of respiratory and hemodynamic measurements. Arterial blood gas (ABG) determination is a key component to the respiratory management of ARDS because it describes perfusion (pH), oxygenation (PaO_2), and degree of ventilation ($PaCO_2$). In addition, the ABG determination allows assessment of the acid-base balance of a patient to differentiate whether acidosis or alkalosis is from metabolic, respiratory, or mixed etiologies so that the appropriate management can be implemented. Acid-base disorders are discussed extensively in Chapter 53.

Appropriate lung distension is evaluated by clinical observation of chest wall expansion and radiography, notably the chest x-ray. Chest x-rays also provide important information, including endotracheal tube placement, severity of lung disease, markers of pulmonary toxicity, presence of air leaks, and an estimation of heart size.

The goal of mechanical ventilation is to provide adequate oxygen delivery while promoting the removal of CO_2. The target SaO_2 traditionally has been greater than 90% on the lowest possible FIO_2. In light of the recent study using low-tidal-volume ventilator strategy, slightly lower oxygen saturation, and more liberal use of the FIO_2 to avoid increased ventilator pressures should be tolerated. The use of ventilatory maneuvers that achieve these end points while minimally disrupting the anatomic and physiologic aspects of respiratory and hemodynamic function is another goal. For the purpose of this discussion, there are six main types of ventilator management. A brief explanation of each follows. In reality, a number of hybrids between different ventilator modes also exist.

CONTROL-MODE VENTILATION (CMV)

CMV administers a breath independent of the patient's efforts. Ventilator settings determine the end of inspiration and the beginning of expiration (the I:E ratio, normally 1:2). PEEP is used to prevent alveolar collapse at the end of expiration. The "best PEEP" is determined clinically by monitoring the patient's oxygenation and most often is between 10 to 15 cm H_2O. PEEP rarely should exceed 20 cm H_2O. The tidal volume associated with the breath is independent of the patient and is set between 6 and 15 mL/kg ideal weight. However, if highly compliant endotracheal tubing is used, higher volumes may be

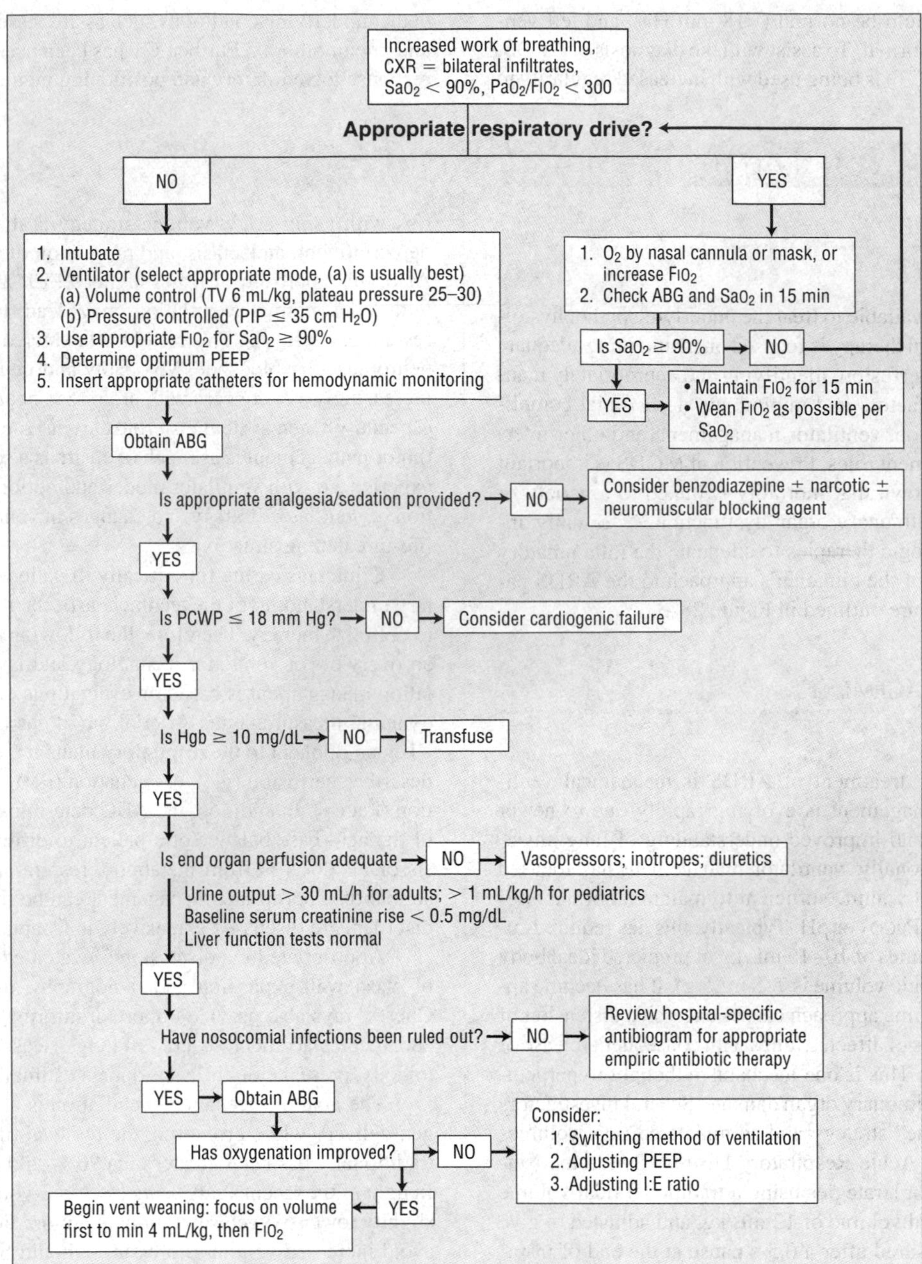

FIGURE 28–3. Algorithm for treatment of ARDS and ALI.

warranted. Risk associated with this form of ventilation is overdistension with possible pneumothorax. Some clinicians advocate an I:E ratio of 1:1, which purportedly allows use of more PEEP without pushing up peak inspiratory pressure or plateau pressure. This is reasonable in patients unless they have chronic obstructive pulmonary disease.

ASSIST-CONTROL VENTILATION (ACV)

ACV uses a mechanically set rate for breaths per minute but does allow patient-initiated breaths. The ventilator senses a patient's "trigger" of an inspiratory phase by noting a change in pressure within the endotracheal tubing. After such a trigger, the patient receives a full-tidal-volume inspiration. In the absence of a patient's inspiratory effort, the machine will deliver a programmed number of breaths per minute. Disadvantages of ACV include discomfort in "conforming" to predetermined tidal volumes while being alert enough to generate an inspiratory effort. Another disadvantage associated with the delivery of a complete-tidal-volume breath is the increased likelihood of developing respiratory alkalosis.

INTERMITTENT MANDATORY VENTILATION/SYNCHRONIZED INTERMITTENT MANDATORY VENTILATION

Intermittent mandatory ventilation (IMV) is a form of mechanical ventilation that not only delivers a preset number of breaths per minute but also allows the patient to breathe spontaneously between mechanical breaths. Thus, as the patient begins to initiate an increasing number of breaths, the preset mechanical IMV number can be dialed down. This form of ventilation allows the patient to increase his or her work of breathing; thus it is ideal for patients who are weaning from mechanical ventilation. An evolution of IMV is SIMV, which allows for the mechanical breaths to coincide with the inspiratory effort generated by the patient. Although functionally similar, SIMV prevents the "stacking" of breaths that may lead to higher peak airway pressures and higher intrathoracic pressures. The use of SIMV for the initial phase of ARDS is not indicated because patients generally are unable to initiate an inspiratory effort nor maintain such effort for a prolonged period of time.

PRESSURE-CONTROL VENTILATION (PCV)

PCV is a time-cycled ventilation that limits inspiratory pressures, thereby maximizing alveolar pressure. Ventilation is independent of the patient's effort but depends on pulmonary compliance. Thus there is a reduced likelihood of overdistension and pulmonary tissue damage because inspiration is limited once the predetermined peak pressure is obtained. Thus it is assumed that VILI is reduced.

PRESSURE-SUPPORT VENTILATION (PSV)

PSV is a type of mechanical ventilation that uses a patient's inspiratory effort and supplements to a select level of positive airway pressure. The patient controls the ventilatory rate and inspiratory assist time while the PSV supplements inspiratory flow and tidal volume. Because PSV is heavily reliant on the patient's effort, this form of ventilation may not be optimal in patients unable to generate sufficient effort. However, it is the modality of choice in patients who are unable to synchronize with other modes of support.

HIGH-FREQUENCY VENTILATION (HFV)

HFV has been mentioned as a ventilator option for neonatal RDS (see Table 28–2). The basic concept for its use in ARDS is that the pressure-volume curve in ARDS creates a narrow window of safety for PPV. If staying between the points of low inflection (where atelectasis occurs) and high inflection (where overdistension occurs) are the goals, then theoretically HFV, which delivers small, frequent tidal volumes, should be an optimal ventilator strategy. However, initial clinical trials of HFV for patients with ARDS have failed to demonstrate superior outcomes, giving little incentive at this time for clinicians to switch from control-mode ventilation.[55,78] Advocates for HFV have noted several problems in the studies failing to find HFV superior to control-mode ventilation. The most serious flaw cited is that the studies lacked sufficient statistical power to recognize modest benefits. One recent editorial[78] noted that only 447 patients had thus far been included in all HFV studies combined. The authors point out that about 500 patients would be needed for each arm of the study (total 1000 patients) to detect a 10% reduction in mortality. Only the recent low-volume strategy study with control-mode ventilation published by the ARDS Network[74] approaches this. Another criticism is that early studies used a low-pressure/low-volume strategy that permitted pressures below the lower inflection point, allowing for the shear stress associated with repeated collapse and opening of terminal airways. This strategy would promote inflammatory mediator release and would be unlikely to improve outcomes. Ventilation using sufficient PEEP to recruit alveoli above the lower inflection point combined with HFV to deliver small tidal volumes warrants an appropriately designed and powered clinical trial.[78] Finally, ventilator technology for HFV has been insufficient to support proper use of this ventilator mode. HFOV seems most appropriate because it promotes expiration as well as inspiration and avoids air trapping. A newer high-frequency oscillatory ventilator (3100B Ventilator, SensorMedics) purportedly is able to provide the extended levels of continuous distending pressures needed to follow a high-volume strategy necessary for HFOV to succeed in adults with ARDS. Theoretically, this strategy would provide the most physiologic ventilator approach because both airway collapse and overdistension can be avoided while gradually recruiting and opening atelectatic alveoli. Clinical trials testing this ventilator are in progress.

VILI AND OTHER COMPLICATIONS

Irreversible loss of disease control or serious ventilator-related toxicities through oxygen toxicity, barotrauma, and volutrauma can occur if ventilatory management is not monitored and optimized continuously. These ventilator-related toxicities may occur even with appropriate ventilator management, and minimizing these toxicities is one of the major goals of ventilator management.

Despite increasing evidence that pressure is more damaging to lungs than oxygen toxicity, oxygen supplementation remains a serious concern in ARDS as well as RDS. Toxicity occurs as the result of oxygen-derived free radicals. The combination of high O_2 concentrations with the underlying lung damage may create a proinflammatory condition that further worsens underlying lung damage. There does not appear to be a universally accepted duration of exposure or O_2 concentration that correlates with lung damage, thereby suggesting that disease severity and individual susceptibility are the most important factors.[57] However, with the increasing attention to pressure-related lung damage, oxygen toxicity may be the lesser evil if compromises must be made to achieve adequate oxygenation.

ARDS does not uniformly affect the lung; there are consolidated and necrotic areas not available for gas exchange, areas of collapse that may be recruited, and normal alveolar components. It has been reported that in severe cases of ARDS, the inflation capacity of the lungs may be less that one-third normal.[56] Although traditional ventilator management has described tidal volumes of 10–15 mL/kg, consolidated or collapsed areas of the lung volume will "shunt" to areas of least resistance, i.e., alveoli that are not collapsed. Thus areas of hyperinflation can be located next to hypoinflation within the lung field. Furthermore, these areas of altered ventilation may not be evident in gross examination of mean airway pressure because this parameter is calculated under passive inflation.[56] The volutrauma of ARDS is a result of regional overdistension of alveolar components and generally occurs in patients with a static pressure greater than 30 mm Hg. The risk of volutrauma occurs later in the course of ARDS, presumably because of the uneven degradation of the lung structure creating areas of weakened tissue and increased risk for alveolar disruption.[79] As mentioned earlier, a low-tidal-volume strategy appears to be the safer course.

In addition to the damage incurred with tidal volume, barotrauma can ensue. The shearing force of a tidal volume associated with alveolar collapse and reinflation is an important aspect of VILI.[56] Thus the employment of PEEP can limit this barotrauma. In addition, PEEP can limit the FIO_2 needed for adequate oxygen saturation. PEEP is a pressure applied by the ventilator that prevents complete lung emptying at end expiration, increasing lung volume. This improved gas exchange redistributes (but does not decrease) lung water. The concept behind the ability of PEEP to reduce lung injury stems from the prevention of continued alveolar collapse and reopening with consequent inflammation and worsening ARDS.[55] However, finding the "best PEEP" can be challenging because too much volume remaining in the alveoli can cause overdistension and damage, with possible hemodynamic effects. One additional adverse consequence of a ventilator strategy that uses a large tidal volume is the translocation of bacteria and endotoxins with subsequent systemic sequelae.[80,81]

PERFUSION MANAGEMENT

Tissue perfusion is a critical component of ARDS. In order to optimize oxygen dissociation on a cellular level, appropriate tissue perfusion is required. In addition, adequate perfusion supplies glucose and electrolytes while eliminating metabolic by-products. Clinical monitoring of the ARDS patient requires assessment of perfusion in two capacities: hemodynamic/fluid support and end-organ function.

HEMODYNAMIC AND FLUID MANAGEMENT

Theoretically, improving oxygen supply should improve oxygen delivery to the tissues. Although the validity of this direct relationship has been scrutinized, most clinicians optimize cardiac output in ARDS patients to ensure adequate perfusion by using fluids, blood transfusions, inotropic agents, and afterload-reducing agents. In addition to the ABG and hemoglobin determinations, hemodynamic parameters such as cardiac output, pulmonary artery obstruction pressure, and mean arterial pressure are monitored to determine which agent is most appropriate to improve perfusion. These parameters, combined with evaluation of tissue hypoxia, contribute extensively to the fluid management decisions of ARDS (Table 28–9). The importance of appropriate fluid management cannot be overstated. Sufficient intravascular volume is needed for adequate perfusion. Avoiding a persistent positive fluid balance is important to reduce the likelihood of pulmonary edema, which is associated with a poorer prognosis.[80] A randomized trial of restricted versus liberal fluid management is planned by the National Institutes of Health ARDS Network.[54]

PERFUSION AND PREVENTION OF END-ORGAN DAMAGE

Another marker of sufficient tissue perfusion can be clinical assessment of end-organ function. As mentioned previously, prevention of MODS is an important factor in reducing ARDS-associated mortality. Clinically, assessment of urine output and serum electrolytes is an important aspect of renal function monitoring, whereas liver function tests (aminotransferases AST and ALT) are important laboratory parameters for monitoring hepatic function. Central nervous system assessment can be difficult in the ARDS patient and is confounded by concurrent drug therapies (e.g., sedatives, narcotics, etc.) that alter neurologic status.

Stress-induced gastrointestinal bleeding is another complication of ARDS. Mechanical ventilation, altered gastric blood flow, and coagulopathy are indications for stress ulcer prophylaxis.[55] However, considerable controversy exists as to the role of pH-altering drugs for stress prophylaxis and the relationship with nosocomial pneumonia. Due to the considerable risk of mortality with gastrointestinal bleeding in patients with ARDS, it is our opinion that prophylactic agents be used. There does not appear to be a uniform clinical advantage of either histamine antagonists or proton pump inhibitors; therefore, selection should be based on costs.

Nosocomial Pneumonia

Nosocomial pneumonia in ARDS patients causes mortality in 67% of patients, versus 23% of patients without pneumonia. Prevention and early treatment are critical to decreasing ARDS mortality. Ventilator-associated pneumonia correlates directly with length of mechanical ventilation.[82] Diagnosis of ventilator-associated pneumonia is difficult because no diagnostic method, even protected specimen brush, correlates with microbiologic results on autopsy or affects mortality.[83] Mechanically ventilated patients are always colonized with pathogenic organisms. When clinical findings suggest ventilator-associated pneumonia, the causative organism correlates with the organism colonizing the upper airway and should be the target of antimicrobial therapy.[84]

Gastric colonization does not correlate with ventilator-associated pneumonia and mortality differences. Attempts to decontaminate the gastrointestinal tract have not become established norms.[84] Antibiotic use carries the risk of acquiring multiresistant organisms, which can adversely affect hospital and community antibiograms. Based on the epidemiologic and financial costs of resistant organisms generated with such a procedure, its routine practice cannot be advocated.

Catheter-Related Infection

ARDS patients are also at risk for the development of catheter-related infections, especially bacteremia, which is life-threatening. Appropriate hospital hygiene and the standard use of sterile technique are of extreme importance in preventing infections. Catheter-related infections are dealt with elsewhere in this text (see Chapter 137). Diagnosis of catheter-related infections can be difficult, although most clinicians agree that semiquantitative cultures of the removed catheters

TABLE 28–9. Hemodynamic and Fluid Support Decisions in ARDS

PAOP	MAP	CO	Tissue Hypoxia	Therapeutic Manuever
Decreased	Decreased	Decreased	Yes	Fluid bolus
Decreased	Decreased	Increased	Yes	Vasopressor ± fluid bolus
Decreased	Decreased	Increased	No	Vasopressor
Decreased	Increased	Increased	No	Diuresis and negative fluid balance
Decreased	Increased	Decreased	Yes	After-load reduction
Decreased	Increased	Decreased	No	After-load reduction and negative fluid balance

PAOP, pulmonary artery occlusion pressure; MAP, mean arterial pressure; CO, cardiac output.

are helpful. Catheter-associated organisms usually are gram-positive bacteria, namely, *Staphylococcus* species. Catheter removal and antimicrobial therapy are cornerstones of treatment.

Nutritional Support

Nutritional support does not affect the outcome of intensive care unit patients, but most clinicians nonetheless initiate this therapy.[85] Parenteral nutrition is often necessary in seriously ill ARDS patients because blood flow to the gastrointestinal tract is limited. Enteral nutrition is preferred if tolerable, even in small amounts. The advantages of enteral feedings include decreased need for central catheter access, increased gastrointestinal access, increased gastrointestinal blood flow decreasing the risk of gut contamination, and decreased risk for ulceration. It is important for the clinician to remember that using a high amount of intravenous carbohydrates as the major source of caloric intake increases the production of carbon dioxide, which can further complicate management of the ARDS patient. Interest has increased in the potential benefits of selected enteral nutritional approaches. Use of an enteral formula containing eicosapentaenoic acid (EPA, fish oil), gamma-linolenic acid (GLA, borage oil), and antioxidants was compared recently with a standard ready-to-feed high-fat, low-carbohydrate (corn oil base) formula.[86] This preliminary trial reported that both formulas were well tolerated by most patients and resulted in fewer days on the ventilator and in the intensive care unit and fewer instances of new organ failures. The authors speculate that the benefits are due to the anti-inflammatory effects of the EPA + GLA formulation. This formula contained polyunsaturated long-chain fatty acids (PUFAs) with an N-6:N-3 ratio of 1:1 (compared with 54:1 for the standard formulation). For patients who can tolerate enteral feedings, formulas with lipid content high in N-3 PUFAs are worth considering.

INVESTIGATIONAL THERAPIES

Various therapies have been evaluated to reverse or limit the pulmonary damage associated with ARDS. These entities range from inhibiting the underlying etiology (i.e., antiendotoxin immunotherapy) to altering inflammatory mediators (i.e., cyclooxygenase inhibitors) to directly improving oxygenation (i.e., NO and surfactant). To date, no single therapy has uniformly demonstrated benefits in clinical trials. These trials have been summarized in a recent comprehensive review.[54] The failure to prove clinical benefits to the various therapies should not discourage further research of any approach. A recent editorial challenges the negative findings in these large trials and tries to reconcile the promising experimental evidence with the trial outcomes.[87] The author questions the definitions used for ARDS and the end point of death as perhaps issues to resolve. Most studies also suffer from problems with insufficient patient numbers to ensure the validity of negative findings, inappropriate selection of drug-delivery technique (as in the case of surfactant[89]), and uncertainty about optimal dosing. Nevertheless, some recent studies performed by the National Institutes of Health ARDS Network and other multicenter groups involved large patient numbers and placebo-controlled trials. These studies failed to show improved outcomes for mortality, pulmonary and nonpulmonary organ morbidity, and measures of interleukins or other markers of inflammation.

At this juncture, despite laboratory experiments raising expectations of benefits and in some cases experiential reports favorable to the therapy, studies to date have failed to demonstrate benefits with systemic glucocorticoids, liposomal prostaglandin E1, inhaled NO, ketoconazole, procysteine, and lisofylline.[54] Synthetic surfactant (Exosurf) was studied in a placebo-controlled trial of patients with ARDS.[88] While this therapy also failed to show benefits, the drug was aerosolized over 5 days to administer 240 mL of Exosurf. Since aerosolized surfactant is poorly delivered and was shown recently to be ineffective in neonates with RDS, this trial cannot be considered of value in gauging the efficacy of surfactant for ARDS. Systemic glucocorticoids, while apparently ineffective during the acute phase of ARDS, may have a role in patients with ARDS who remain unimproved for 7 days. Therapy at this point is targeting the fibrosing-alveolitis phase of the disease.[89] In a small trial, methylprednisolone was started at 2 mg/kg per day and tapered gradually over 32 days.[57] Treatment was associated with significant reduction in mortality, lung injury score, and multiorgan dysfunction. The prolonged high-dose methylprednisolone course differs from studies of glucocorticoids during the acute phase of ARDS. The study investigators challenge the negative findings for early steroid use on the basis of their findings. Ultimately, steroid use remains controversial but probably should be considered investigational during the acute phase of ARDS.

A large number of additional therapies have been or are under review. These therapies include nonsteroidal anti-inflammatory agents, proinflammatory agents (GM-CSF), antiadhesion molecules, gene therapy, antiendotoxin therapy, and antioxidants (i.e., superoxide dismutase).[56] Therapies will continue to focus on the early interventions to prevent the progressive downward spiral of lung injury, inflammation, and hypoxemia.

EVALUATION OF OUTCOMES AND MONITORING PLANS

Mortality, intensive care unit stay, and duration of mechanical ventilation are common outcome measures used in ARDS studies. However, there is considerable debate not only on the definition of ARDS but also on the usefulness of these markers or other surrogate markers in determining efficacy of ARDS therapies.

Monitoring ventilatory parameters, ABGs, and oxygen saturation assists in determination of illness severity and provides rudimentary end points of perfusion. For example, most clinicians agree that maintaining an oxygen saturation more than 90% is important. Effects of inotropic agents, blood products, and vasopressors must be measured to optimize oxygenation. Thus appropriate monitoring of invasive hemodynamic parameters (i.e., pulmonary artery obstruction pressure) through a pulmonary artery catheter is critical in appropriate management of the ARDS patient. Radiographically, ARDS cannot be distinguished from cardiogenic pulmonary edema; therefore, a pulmonary artery catheter is almost essential. In addition, because ventilatory maneuvers can reduce cardiac output (excessive PEEP), appropriate hemodynamic monitoring can be essential for establishing appropriate ventilator settings. A summary of monitoring parameters for patients with ARDS can be found in Table 28–10.

CONCLUSIONS

ARDS-related mortality plagues the modern intensive care unit. Therapy is primarily supportive but requires extensive comprehension of

TABLE 28–10. Monitoring Parameters in ARDS

Hemodynamic	Ventilator Status	Infection	End-Organ Damage
PCWP	FiO_2	White blood cells/differential	BUN
Cardiac output/index	PaO_2	Chest x-ray findings	Creatine
Oxygen saturation (SaO_2)	SaO_2	Temperature	Urine output
Mixed venous oxygenation (MvO_2)	MvO_2	Cultures	Liver function tests
Hemoglobin/hematocrit	Plateau pressure	Changes in color/quality sputum	PT/PTT
Urine output	Respiratory effort/rate	New onset hypotension	
		Abdominal examination	
		Number of central catheter days	

the underlying pathophysiology to ensure optimal pharmacotherapy. Vigilance in monitoring ventilatory and hemodynamic end points to prevent MODS is the priority, with prevention of secondary complications such as pneumonia and catheter-related infections very significant. Research is ongoing for pharmacologic therapies directed at the underlying disease process.

▶ PRINCIPLES OF PHARMACOTHERAPY

- Neonatal RDS is predominantly a disease of surfactant deficiency.
- Surfactant availability can be affected antenatally with maternal glucocorticoids to promote production and postnatally with surfactant replacement therapy.
- Surfactant replacement therapy markedly reduces neonatal pulmonary morbidity and mortality.
- Modified natural and natural surfactants appear superior to synthetic surfactant in these effects.
- Early extubation of preterm infants is feasible and is aided by methylxanthine use.
- ARDS is a syndrome characterized by bilateral pulmonary infiltrates, high oxygen requirements, and noncardiogenic pulmonary edema that occurs secondary to an inflammatory insult such as sepsis.
- No drug therapy modality has adequate evidence-based documentation to confidently claim improved outcome in ARDS. Supportive therapy is necessary while the lung injury heals.
- Infection and end-organ failure are the usual causes of ARDS mortality.
- Mechanical ventilation is essential to manage the respiratory failure associated with RDS and ARDS.
- Selection of ventilator maneuvers is based on a combination of clinical experience and scientific merits.
- Low-volume ventilator strategies are preferred for managing adults with ARDS.
- Mechanical ventilation has serious toxicities; therefore, every effort should be made to limit duration of ventilation.
- Positive-pressure ventilation can reduce cardiac output, resulting in diminished organ perfusion and drug elimination. It also may cause systemic inflammatory response if atalectasis or lung overdistension occurs.
- Anti-inflammatory therapies (drugs and nutrition) are expected to help ARDS and ALI, but studies confirming the theoretical benefits have yet to be done.

REFERENCES

1. Vermont Oxford Network Annual Database Summary, 1999. Burlington, VT, Vermont Oxford Network, 2000.
2. Barker PM, Gowen CW, Lawson EE, Knowles MR. Decreased sodium ion absorption across nasal epithelium of very premature infants with respiratory distress syndrome. J Pediatr 1997;130:373–377.
3. O'Bradovich HM. The role of active Na^+ transport by lung epithelium in the clearance of airspace fluid. New Horiz 1995;3:240–247; Gerdes JS. Assessment of lung maturity. In: Spitzer AR, ed. Intensive Care of the Fetus and Newborn. St. Louis, Mosby-Year Book, 1996:130–134.
4. Boyle RJ, Oh W. Respiratory distress syndrome. Clin Perinatol 1978;5:287–297.
5. Novy MJ, McGregor JA, Iams JD. New perspectives on the prevention of extreme prematurity. Clin Obstet Gynecol 1995;38:790–808.
6. Leonardi MR, Hankins GDV. What's new in tocolytics. Clin Perinatol 1992;19:367–384.
7. Kierse MJ. New perspectives for the effective treatment of preterm labor. Am J Obstet Gynecol 1995;173:618–628.
8. Ballard PL, Ballard RA. Scientific basis and therapeutic regimens for use of antenatal glucocorticoids. Am J Obstet Gynecol 1995;173:254–262.
9. French NP, Hagan RH, Evans SE, et al. Repeated antenatal steroids: Size at birth and subsequent development. Am J Obstet Gynecol 1999;180: 114–121.
10. ACTOBAT Study Group. Australian Collaborative Trial of Antenatal Thyrotropin-Releasing Hormone (ACTOBAT) for prevention of neonatal respiratory disease. Lancet 1995;345:877–882.
11. Crowther CA, Hiller JE, Studs DS, et al. Australian Collaborative Trial of Antenatal Thyrotropin-Releasing Hormone: Adverse effects at 12-month follow-up. Pediatrics 1997;99:311–317.
12. Goldsmith JP, Karotkin EH. Assisted Ventilation of the Neonate, 3d ed. Philadelphia, Saunders, 1996.
13. Halliday HL. Towards earlier neonatal extubation. Lancet 2000;355: 2091–2092.
14. Curosurf. Med Lett Drugs Ther 2000;42:27–28.
15. Zola EM, Gunkel JH, Chan RK, et al. Comparison of three dosing procedures for administration of bovine surfactant to neonates with respiratory distress syndrome. J Pediatr 1993;122:453–459.
16. Veda T, Ikegami M, Rider ED, Jobe AH. Distribution of surfactant and ventilation in surfactant-treated preterm lambs. J Appl Physiol 1994;76: 45–55.
17. Lewis JF, Tabor B, Ikegami M, et al. Lung function and surfactant distribution in saline-lavaged sheep given instilled versus nebulized surfactant. J Appl Physiol 1993;74:1256–1264.
18. Lewis JF, Ikegami M, Jobe AH, Tabor B. Aerosolized surfactant treatment of preterm lambs. J Appl Physiol 1991;70:869–876.
19. Soll RF. Multiple- versus single-dose natural surfactant extract for severe respiratory distress syndrome. (Systematic review). Cochran Neonatal Review Group. Cochrane Database Syst Rev 2000;3.
20. OSIRIS. Early versus delayed neonatal administration of a synthetic surfactant the judgment of OSIRIS. Lancet 1992;340:1363–1369.

21. Berry DD, Pramanik AK, Phillips JB, et al. Comparison of the effect of three doses of a synthetic surfactant on the alveolar-arterial oxygen gradient in infants weighing <1250 grams with respiratory distress syndrome. J Pediatr 1994;124:294–301.
22. Dunn MS, Shennan AT, Possmayer F. Single- versus multiple-dose surfactant replacement therapy in neonates of 30 to 36 weeks gestation with respiratory distress syndrome. Pediatrics 1990;86:564–570.
23. Konishi M, Fujiwara T, Naito T, et al. Surfactant replacement therapy in neonatal respiratory distress syndrome: A multicenter, randomized clinical trial. Comparison of high- versus low-dose of surfactant-TA. Eur J Pediatr 1988;147:20–25.
24. Speer CP, Robertson B, Curstedt T, et al. Randomized European Multicenter Trial of Surfactant Replacement Therapy for Severe Neonatal Respiratory Distress Syndrome: Single versus multiple doses of Curosurf. Pediatrics 1992;89:13–20.
25. Halliday HL, Tarnow-Mardi WO, Corcoran JD, Patterson CC. Multicenter randomized trial comparing high and low surfactant regimens for the treatment of respiratory distress syndrome (The Curosurf 4 Trial). Arch Dis Child 1993;69:276–280.
26. Gotner L, Pohlandt F, Bartmann P, et al. High-dose versus low-dose bovine surfactant treatment in very premature infants. Acta Paediatr 1994;83:135–141.
27. Sobel DB, Carroll A. Postsurfactant slump: Early prediction of neonatal chronic lung disease? J Perinatol 1994;14:268–271.
28. Hudak ML, Martin DJ, Egan EA, et al. A multicenter, randomized, masked comparison trial of natural versus synthetic surfactant for the treatment of respiratory distress syndrome. Pediatrics 1997;100:39–50.
29. Soll RF, Morley CJ. Prophylactic versus selective use of surfactant for preventing morbidity and mortality in preterm infants (Systematic review). Cochrane Neonatal Review Group. Cochrane Database Syst Rev 2000;3.
30. Survanta (beractant) Package Insert. Ross Products Division, Abbott Laboratories, April 1995.
31. Spafford PS, Kendig JW, Maniscalco WM. Use of natural surfactants to prevent and treat respiratory distress syndrome. Semin Perinatol 1993;17:285–294.
32. Verder H, Robertson B, Greisen G, et al. Surfactant therapy and nasal continuous positive airway pressure for newborns with respiratory distress syndrome. New Engl J Med 1994;331:1051–1055.
33. Rajo TNK, Langenberg P. Pulmonary hemorrhage and exogenous surfactant therapy: A meta-analysis. J Pediatr 1995;123:603–610.
34. Hudak ML, Martin DJ, Egan EA, et al. A multicenter randomized masked comparison trial of synthetic surfactant versus calf lung surfactant extract in the prevention of neonatal respiratory distress syndrome. J Pediatr 1996;128:396–406.
35. Harbor JD, Wright LL, Soll RF, et al. A multicenter randomized trial comparing two surfactants for the treatment of neonatal respiratory distress syndrome. J Pediatr 1993;123:757–766.
36. Vermont-Oxford Neonatal Network. A multicenter, randomized trial comparing synthetic surfactant with modified bovine surfactant extract in the treatment of neonatal respiratory distress syndrome. Pediatrics 1996;97: 1–6.
37. Tarnow-Mardi WO, Soll RF. Artificial versus natural surfactant: Can we base clinical practice on a firm scientific footing? Eur J Pediatr 1994;153(Suppl):17–21.
38. Bloom BT, Kattwinkel J, Hall RT, et al. Comparison of Infasurf (calf lung surfactant extract) to Survanta (beractant) in the treatment of respiratory distress syndrome. Pediatrics 1997;100:31–38.
39. Speer CP, Gofeller O, Groneck P, et al. Randomized clinical trial of two treatment regimens of natural surfactant preparations in neonatal respiratory distress syndrome. Arch Dis Child 1995;72:8–13; Mizuno K, Ikegami M, Chen C, et al. Surfactant protein-B supplementation improves in vivo function of a modified natural surfactant. Pediatr Res 1995;37: 271–276.
40. Schwartz RM, Luby AM, Scalon JW, et al. Effect of surfactant on morbidity, mortality, and resource use in newborn infants weighing 500 to 1500 g. N Engl J Med 1994;330:913–936.
41. Soll RF, Jacobs J, Pashko S, Thomas R. Cost-effectiveness of beractant in the prevention of respiratory distress syndrome. Pharmacoeconomics 1993;4:278–286.
42. Maniscalco WM, Kendig JW, Shapiro DL. Surfactant replacement therapy: Impact on hospital charges for premature infants with respiratory distress syndrome. Pediatrics 1989;83:1–6.
43. Gal P, Reed MD, Nahata MC. Recent advances in pediatrics. Ann Pharmacother 1995;29:66–70.
44. Leach CL, Greenspan JS, Rubenstein SD. Partial liquid ventilation with perflubron in premature infants with severe respiratory distress syndrome. New Engl J Med 1996;335:761–767.
45. Wolfson MR, Greenspan JS, Shaffer TH. Pulmonary administration of vasoactive substances by perfluorochemical ventilation. Pediatrics 1996;97:449–455.
46. Tarczy-Hornoch P, Hildebrandt J, Mates EA. Effects of exogenous surfactant on lung pressure-volume characteristics during liquid ventilation. J Appl Physiol 1996;80:1764–1771.
47. Anderson TJ, Meredith IT, Ganz P, et al. Nitric oxide and nitrovasodilators: Similarities, differences and potential interactions. J Am Coll Cardiol 1994;24:555–566.
48. Kinsella JP, Walsh WF, Bose CL, et al. Inhaled nitric oxide in premature neonates with severe hypoxaemic respiratory failure: A randomised, controlled trial. Lancet 1999;354:1061–1065.
49. Jacqz-Aigrain E, Burtin P. Clinical pharmacokinetics of sedatives in neonates. Clin Pharmacokinet 1996;31:423–443.
50. Saarenmaa E, Huttunen P, Leppaluoto J, et al. Advantages of fentanyl over morphine in analgesia for ventilated newborn infants after birth: A randomized trial. J Pediatr 1999;134:144–150.
51. Orsini AJ, Leef KH, Costarino A, et al. Routine use of fentanyl infusions for pain and stress reduction in infants with respiratory distress syndrome. J Pediatr 1996;129:140–145.
52. Brion LP, Soll RF. Diuretics for respiratory distress syndrome in preterm infants (Systematic review). Cochrane Neonatal Review Group. Cochrane Database Syst Rev 2000;3.
53. Ware LB, Matthay MA. The acute respiratory distress syndrome. New Engl J Med 2000;342:1334–1349.
54. Artigas A, Bernard GR, Carlet J, et al., and the Consensus Committee. The American-European consensus on ARDS: 2. Ventilatory, pharmacologic, supportive therapy, study design strategies, and issues related to recovery and remodeling. Am J Respir Crit Care Med 1998;157:1332–1347.
55. Meduri GU, Headley AS, Golden E, et al. Effect of prolonged methylprednisolone therapy in unresolving acute respiratory distress syndrome: A randomized, controlled trial. JAMA 1998;280:159–165.
56. Bernard G, Luce JM, Sprung CL, et al. High dose corticosteroids in patients with adult respiratory distress syndrome. New Engl J Med 1987;317:1565–1570.
57. NIH ARDS Network. Ketoconazole does not reduce mortality in patients with the acute respiratory distress syndrome. JAMA 2000;283:1995–2002.
58. Yu M, Tomasa GA. A double-blind, prospective, randomized trial of ketoconazole, a thromboxane synthetase inhibitor, in the prophylaxis of the adult respiratory distress syndrome. Crit Care Med 1993;21:1635–1642.
59. Bernard GR, Artigas A, Brigham KL, et al., and the Consensus Committee. Report of the American-European consensus conference on acute respiratory distress syndrome: 1. Definitions, mechanisms, relevant outcomes, and clinical trial coordination. Am J Respir Crit Care Med 1994; 149:818–824.
60. Abraham E, Matthay MA, Dinarello CA, et al. Consensus conference definitions for sepsis, septic shock, acute lung injury and acute respiratory distress syndrome: time for a reevaluation. Crit Care Med 2000;28:232–235.
61. American Lung Association. Acute respiratory distress syndrome. Lung Disease Data, 1998–1999. New York, American Lung Association. 1998: 45–46.
62. Hudson LD, Millberg JA Anardi D, Maunder RJ. Clinical risks for development of the acute respiratory distress syndrome. Am J Respir Crit Care Med 1995;29:1002–1009.

63. Milbergh JA, Daris DR, Steinberg KP, Hudson LD. Improved survival of patients with acute respiratory distress syndrome (ARDS): 1983–1993. JAMA 1995;273:306–309.
64. Fein AM. Acute lung injury and acute respiratory distress syndrome in sepsis and septic shock. Crit Care Clin 2000;16(2):289–317.
65. Sloan PJ, Gee MH, Gottlieb JE, et al. A multicenter registry of patients with acute respiratory distress syndrome: Physiology and outcome. Am Rev Respir Dis 1992;146:419–426.
66. Pugin J, Verghese G, Widmer M, Matthay MA. The alveolar space is the site of intense inflammatory and profibrotic reactions in the early phase of acute respiratory distress syndrome. Crit Care Med 1999;27: 304–312.
67. Ranieri VM, Suter PM, Tortorella C, et al. Effect of mechanical ventilation on inflammatory mediators in patients with acute respiratory distress syndrome: A randomized, controlled trial. JAMA 1999;282:54–61.
68. Slutsky AS, Tremblay LN. Multiple system organ failure: Is mechanical ventilation a contributing factor? Am J Respir Crit Care Med 1998;157:1721–1725.
69. Donnelly SC, Strieter RM, Kunkel SL, et al. Interleukin-8 and development of adult respiratory distress syndrome in at-risk patient groups. Lancet 1993;341:643–647.
70. Bohn, D. Lung salvage and protection ventilatory techniques. Pediatr Clin North Am 2001;48:553–572.
71. Meade MO, Cook RJ, Guyatt GH, et al. Interobserver variation in interpreting chest radiographs for the diagnosis of acute respiratory distress syndrome. Am J Respir Crit Care Med 2000;161:85–90.
72. Desai SR, Hansell DM. Lung imaging in the adult respiratory distress syndrome: Current practice and new insights. Intensive Care Med 1997; 23:7–15.
73. Knaus WA, Wagner DP. Multiple systems organ failure: Epidemiology and prognosis. Crit Care Clin 1989;5:221–232.
74. The Acute Respiratory Distress Syndrome Network. Ventilation with lower tidal volumes as compared with traditional volumes for acute lung injury and the acute respiratory distress syndrome. N Engl J Med 2000;342:1301–1308.
75. Amato MBP, Barbas CSV, Medeiros DM, et al. Effect of a protective ventilation strategy on mortality in the acute respiratory distress syndrome. N Engl J Med 1998;338:347–354.
76. Tobin MJ. Culmination of an era in research on the acute respiratory distress syndrome. N Engl J Med 2000;342:1360–1361.
77. Herridge MS, Slutsky AS, Colditz GA. Has high-frequency ventilation been inappropriately discarded in adult acute respiratory distress syndome? Crit Care Med 1998;26:2073–2077.
78. Gammon RB, Shin MS, Groves RH, et al. Clinical risk factors for pulmonary barotrauma: A multivariate analysis. Am J Respir Crit Care Med 1995;152:1235–1240.
79. Murphy DB, Cregg N, Tremblay L, et al. Adverse ventilatory strategy causes pulmonary-to-systemic translocation of endotoxin. Am J Respir Crit Care Med 2000;162:27–33.
80. Schuster DP. Fluid management in ARDS: "Keep them dry" or does it matter? Intensive Care Med 1995;21:101–103.
81. Bonten MJ, Bergmans DC, Ambergen AW, et al. Risk factors for pneumonia and colonization of respiratory tract and stomach in mechanically ventilated ICU patients. Am J Respir Crit Care Med 1996;154:1339–1346.
82. Torres A, El-Ebiary M, Padro L, et al. Validation of different techniques for the diagnosis of ventilator-associated pneumonia. Am J Crit Care Med 1994;149:324–331.
83. DeLatorre FL, Pont T, Ferrer A, et al. Patterns of tracheal colonization during mechanical ventilation. Am J Respir Crit Care Med 1995; 152:1028–1033.
84. D'Amico R, Pifferi S, Leonetti C, et al. Effectiveness of antibiotic prophylaxis in critically ill adult patients: Systematic review of randomized controlled trials. Br Med J 1998;316:1275–1285.
85. Koretz RL. Nutritional supplementation in the ICU. Am J Respir Crit Care Med 1995;151:570–573.
86. Gadek JE, DeMichele SJ, Karlstad MD, et al. Effect of enteral feeding with eicosapentaenoic acid, linolenic acid, and antioxidants in patients with acute respiratory distress syndrome. Crit Care Med 1999;27:1409–1420.
87. Brochard L, Brun-Buisson C. Clinical trials in acute respiratory distress syndrome: What is ARDS? Crit Care Med 1999;27:1657–1658.
88. Anzueto A, Baughman RP, Guntupalli KK, et al. Aerosolized surfactant in adults with sepsis-induced acute respiratory distress syndrome. New Engl J Med 1996;334:1417–1421.
89. Brun-Buisson C, Brochard L. Corticosteroid therapy in acute respiratory distress syndrome. Better late than never? JAMA 1998;280:182–183.

29

DRUG-INDUCED PULMONARY DISEASES

Hengameh H. Raissy, Patricia L. Marshik, and H. William Kelly

The manifestations of drug-induced pulmonary diseases span the entire spectrum of pathophysiologic conditions of the respiratory tract. As with most drug-induced diseases, the pathologic changes are nonspecific. Therefore, the diagnosis often is difficult and, in most cases, is based on exclusion of all other possible causes. In addition, the true incidence of drug-induced pulmonary disease is difficult to assess as a result of the pathologic nonspecificity and the interaction between the underlying disease state and the drugs.

Considering the physiologic and metabolic capacity of the lung, it is surprising that drug-induced pulmonary disease is not more common. The lung is the only organ of the body that receives the entire circulation. In addition, the lung contains a heterogeneous population of cells capable of various metabolic functions, including *N*-alkylation, *N*-dialkylation, *N*-oxidation, reduction of *N*-oxides, and *C*-hydroxylation.

Evaluation of epidemiologic studies on adverse drug reactions provides a perspective on the importance of drug-induced pulmonary disease. In a 2-year prospective survey of a community-based general practice, 41% of 817 patients experienced adverse drug reactions.[1] Four patients, or 0.5% of the total respondents, experienced adverse respiratory symptoms. Respiratory symptoms occurred in 1.2% of patients experiencing adverse drug reactions. A surveillance study of 3181 general pediatric outpatients receiving 4244 courses of drug therapy reported adverse reactions in 473 (11.1%) of the courses.[2] Of these, only 200 were considered definite or probably related to the drug. Gastrointestinal symptoms, skin reactions, and central nervous system (CNS) symptoms made up 96.5% of the reactions, with respiratory symptoms included with all other reactions.

Adverse pulmonary reactions are uncommon in the general population but are among the most serious reactions, often requiring intervention. In a study of 270 adverse reactions leading to hospitalization from two populations, 3.0% were respiratory in nature.[3] Of the reactions considered to be life-threatening, 12.3% were respiratory. An early report on death caused by drug reactions from the Boston Collaborative Drug Surveillance Program indicated that 7 of 27 drug-induced deaths were respiratory in nature.[4] This was confirmed in a follow-up study in which 6 of 24 drug-induced deaths were respiratory in nature.[5]

DRUG-INDUCED APNEA

Apnea may be induced by CNS depression or respiratory neuromuscular blockade (Table 29–1). Patients with chronic obstructive airway disease, alveolar hypoventilation, and chronic carbon dioxide retention have an exaggerated respiratory depressant response to narcotic analgesics and sedatives. In addition, the injudicious administration of oxygen in patients with carbon dioxide retention can remove their hypoxic ventilatory drive, producing apnea.[6] Although the benzodiazepines are touted as causing less respiratory depression than barbiturates, they may produce a profound additive or synergistic effect when taken in combination with other respiratory depressants. Combining intravenous diazepam with phenobarbital to stop seizures in an emergency department frequently results in admission to an intensive care unit (ICU) for a short period of assisted mechanical ventilation regardless of the drug administration rate. Too rapid intravenous administration of any of the benzodiazepines, even without coadministration of other respiratory depressants, will result in apnea. The risk appears to be the same for the various available agents (i.e., diazepam, lorazepam, midazolam). Respiratory depression and arrest resulting in death and hypoxic encephalopathy have occurred following rapid intravenous administration of midazolam for conscious sedation prior to medical procedures. This has been reported more commonly in the elderly and the chronically debilitated or in combination with opioid analgesics.

Prolonged apnea may follow administration of any of the neuromuscular blocking agents for surgery, particularly in patients with hepatic or renal dysfunction. In addition, persistent neuromuscular blockade and muscle weakness have been reported in critically ill patients receiving neuromuscular blockers continuously for more than 2 days to facilitate mechanical ventilation.[7] This has resulted in delayed weaning from mechanical ventilation and prolonged ICU stays. The prolonged neuromuscular blockade has been confined principally to pancuronium and vecuronium in patients with renal disease. Both agents have pharmacologic active metabolites that are excreted renally. The persistent muscular weakness is less well defined but appears to represent an acute myopathy.[7] High-dose corticosteroids appear to produce a synergistic effect, supported by animal studies showing that corticosteroids at dosages greater than or equal to 2 mg/kg per day of prednisone produce atrophy in denervated muscle.[8] The fluorinated corticosteroids (e.g., triamcinolone) appear to be more myopathic.[9] Dose-dependent respiratory muscle weakness has been reported in chronic obstructive pulmonary disease (COPD) and asthma patients receiving repeated short courses of oral prednisone in the previous 6 months.[10]

Respiratory failure has been known to occur following local spinal anesthesia. Apnea from respiratory paralysis and rapid respiratory muscle fatigue has followed the administration of polymyxin and aminoglycoside antibiotics.[6] The mechanism appears to be related to the complexation of calcium and its depletion at the myoneural junction. Intravenous calcium chloride has been variably effective in reversing the paralysis.[6] The aminoglycosides competitively block neuromuscular junctions. This has resulted in life-threatening apnea when neomycin, gentamicin, streptomycin, or bacitracin has been administered into the peritoneal and pleural cavities.[6] The aminoglycosides will produce an additive blockade and ventilatory paralysis with curare or succinylcholine and in patients with myasthenia gravis or myasthenic syndromes.[6] Intravenous administration of aminoglycosides has resulted in respiratory failure in babies with infantile botulism. The treatment consists of ventilatory support and administration of an anticholinesterase agent (neostigmine or edrophonium).[6]

TABLE 29–1. Drugs That Induce Apnea

Central Nervous System Depression	
Narcotic analgesics	F[a]
Barbiturates	F
Benzodiazepines	F
Other sedative and hypnotics	I
Tricyclic antidepressants	R
Phenothiazines	R
Ketamine	R
Promazine	R
Anesthetics	R
Antihistamines	R
Alcohol	I
Fenfluramine	R
L-Dopa	R
Oxygen	R
Respiratory Muscle Dysfunction	
Aminoglycoside antibiotics	I
Polymyxin antibiotics	I
Neuromuscular blockers	I
Quinine	R
Digitalis	R
Myopathy	
Corticosteroids	F
Diuretics	I
Aminocaproic acid	R
Clofibrate	R

[a]Relative frequency of reactions: F = frequent; I = infrequent; R = rare.

TABLE 29–2. Drugs That Induce Bronchospasm

Anaphylaxis (IgE-Mediated)		**Anaphylactoid Mast-Cell Degranulation**	
Penicillins	F[a]	Narcotic analgesics	I
Sulfonamides	F	Ethylenediamine	R
Serum	F	Iodinated-radiocontrast media	F
Cephalosporins	F	Platinum	R
Bromelin	R	Local anesthetics	I
Cimetidine	R	Steroidal anesthetics	I
Papain	F	Iron–dextran complex	I
Pancreatic extract	I	Pancuronium bromide	R
Psyllium	I	Benzalkonium chloride	I
Subtilase	I	**Pharmacologic Effect**	
Tetracyclines	I	β-Adrenergic receptor blockers	I–F
Allergen extracts	I	Cholinergic stimulants	I
L-Asparaginase	F	Anticholinesterases	R
Pyrazolone analgesics	I	α-Adrenergic agonists	R
Direct Airway Irritation		Ethylenediamine tetraacetic acid (EDTA)	R
Acetate	R	**Unknown Mechanisms**	
Bisulfite	F	ACE inhibitors	I
Cromolyn	R	Anticholinergics	R
Smoke	F	Hydrocortisone	R
N-Acetylcysteine	F	Isoproterenol	R
Inhaled steroids	I	Monosodium glutamate	I
Precipitating IgG Antibodies		Piperazine	R
α-Methyldopa	R	Tartrazine	R
Carbamazepine	R	Sulfinpyrazone	R
Spiramycin	R	Zinostatin	R
Cyclooxygenase Inhibition		Losartan	R
Aspirin/NSAIDs	F		
Phenylbutazone	I		
Acetaminophen	R		

[a]Relative frequency of reactions: F = frequent; I = infrequent; R = rare.

DRUG-INDUCED BRONCHOSPASM

Bronchoconstriction is the most common drug-induced respiratory problem. Bronchospasm can be induced by a wide variety of drugs through a number of disparate pathophysiologic mechanisms (Table 29–2). Regardless of the pathophysiologic mechanism, drug-induced bronchospasm is almost exclusively a problem of patients with preexisting bronchial hyperreactivity (e.g., asthma, COPD).[11] By definition, all patients with nonspecific bronchial hyperreactivity will experience bronchospasm if given sufficiently high doses of cholinergic or anticholinesterase agents. Severe asthmatics with a high degree of bronchial reactivity may wheeze following the inhalation of a number of particulate substances, such as the lactose in dry-powder inhalers (DPIs) and inhaled corticosteroids, presumably through direct stimulation of the central airway irritant receptors. Other pharmacologic mechanisms for inducing bronchospasm include β_2-receptor blockade and nonimmunologic histamine release from mast cells and basophils.[11] A great number of agents are capable of producing bronchospasm through reactions mediated by immunoglobulin E (IgE).[11] These drugs can become a significant occupational hazard for pharmacists, nurses, and pharmaceutical industry workers.[11]

ASPIRIN-INDUCED BRONCHOSPASM

Aspirin sensitivity or intolerance occurs in 4% to 20% of all asthmatics.[12] The frequency of aspirin-induced bronchospasm increases with age. Patients older than 40 years have a frequency approximately four times that of patients younger than 20 years.[12] The frequency increases to 14% to 23% in patients with nasal polyps.[12] Women predominate over men, and there is no evidence for a genetic or familial predisposition.[13]

The classic description of the aspirin-intolerant asthmatic includes the triad of severe asthma, nasal polyps, and aspirin intolerance. The typical patient experiences intense vasomotor rhinitis, which may or may not be associated with aspirin exposure, beginning during the third or fourth decade of life.[14] Over a period of months, nasal polyps begin to appear, followed by severe asthma exacerbated by aspirin. Bronchospasm typically begins within minutes to hours following ingestion of aspirin and is associated with rhinorrhea, flushing of the head and neck, and conjunctivitis.[14] The reactions are severe and often life-threatening.

All aspirin-sensitive asthmatics do not fit the classic "aspirin triad" picture, and not all patients with asthma and nasal polyps develop sensitivity to aspirin.[13] In most cases, aspirin-sensitive asthmatics are clinically indistinguishable from the general population of asthmatics except for their intolerance to aspirin and other nonsteroidal anti-inflammatory drugs (NSAIDs). Aspirin-induced asthmatics are not at higher risk of having fatal asthma if aspirin and other NSAIDs are avoided.[15]

Diagnosis of aspirin-induced asthma requires a detailed medical history. The definitive diagnosis is made by oral provocation with aspirin.[13] Although there is no in vitro laboratory test to diagnose aspirin-intolerant asthma, bronchial provocation with lysine-aspirin has been used as a diagnostic tool to identify these patients.[16,17] When lysine-aspirin bronchoprovocation was compared with oral aspirin provocation, both methods were equally sensitive.[18]

TABLE 29–3. Tolerance of Anti-Inflammatory and Analgesic Drugs in Aspirin-Induced Asthma

Cross-Reactive Drugs	Drugs With No Cross-Reactivity
Diclofenac	Acetaminophen[a]
Diflunisal	Benzydamine
Fenoprofen	Chloroquine
Flufenamic acid	Choline salicylate
Flurbiprofen	Corticosteroids
Hydrocortisone hemisuccinate	Dextropropoxyphene
Ibuprofen	Phenacetin[a]
Indomethacin	Salicylamide
Ketoprofen	Sodium salicylate
Mefenamic acid	
Naproxen	
Noramidopyrine	
Oxyphenbutazone	
Phenylbutazone	
Piroxicam	
Sulindac	
Sulfinpyrazone	
Tartrazine	
Tolmetin	

[a]A very small percentage (5%) of aspirin-sensitive patients react to acetaminophen and phenacetin.

PATHOGENESIS

Aspirin-induced asthma is classified correctly as an idiosyncratic reaction in that the pathogenesis is still unknown. Patients with aspirin intolerance have increased plasma histamine concentrations after ingestion of aspirin and elevated peripheral eosinophil counts.[13,14] All attempts to define an immunologic mechanism have been unsuccessful. Chemically similar drugs such as salicylamide and choline salicylate do not cross-react, whereas a large number of chemically dissimilar NSAIDs do produce reactions.[13,14] Table 29–3 lists the analgesics that do and do not cross-react with aspirin.

The currently accepted hypothesis of aspirin-induced asthma is that aspirin intolerance is integrally related to inhibition of cyclooxygenase. This is supported by the following evidence: (1) All NSAIDs that inhibit cyclooxygenase produce reactions, (2) the degree of cross reactivity is proportional to the potency of cyclooxygenase inhibition, and (3) each patient with aspirin sensitivity has a threshold dose for precipitating bronchospasm that is specific for the degree of cyclooxygenase inhibition produced, and once established, the dose of another cyclooxygenase inhibitor needed to induce bronchospasm can be estimated.[14]

The mechanism by which cyclooxygenase inhibition produces bronchospasm in susceptible individuals is unknown. Arachidonic acid metabolism through the 5-lipoxygenase pathway may lead to the excess production of leukotrienes (LTs) C_4 and D_4.[15] LTC_4, LTD_4, and LTE_4 produce bronchospasm and promote histamine release from mast cells,[14] whereas the administration of leukotriene receptor antagonists and 5-lipoxygenase inhibitors ablates the pulmonary and nonpulmonary responses to aspirin in aspirin-sensitive asthmatics.[19] The precise mechanism by which augmented leukotriene production occurs is unknown, and available hypotheses do not explain why only a small number of asthmatic patients react to aspirin and NSAIDs.

DESENSITIZATION

Patients with aspirin sensitivity can be desensitized. The ease of desensitization correlates with the sensitivity of the patient.[14] Highly sensitive patients who initially react to less than 100 mg of aspirin require multiple rechallenges to produce desensitization.[13] Desensitization usually persists for 2 to 5 days following discontinuance, with full sensitivity reestablished within 7 days.[13] Cross-desensitization has been established between aspirin and all NSAIDs tested to date. Because patients may experience life-threatening reactions, desensitization should be attempted only in a controlled environment by personnel with expertise in handling these patients. In addition, there have been reports of patients who have failed to maintain a desensitized state despite continued aspirin administration.[13] The chronic asthma symptoms have improved markedly in a number of aspirin-sensitive asthmatics who have undergone desensitization.[13]

CROSS-SENSITIVITY WITH FOOD AND DRUG ADDITIVES

Up to 80% of aspirin-sensitive asthmatics will have an adverse reaction to the yellow azo dye tartrazine (FD&C Yellow No. 5), which is widely used for coloring foods, drinks, drugs, and cosmetics.[12] However, those studies reporting high cross-reactivity were poorly controlled and often used only subjective criteria.[12,20] In double-blind, placebo-controlled trials using pulmonary function testing, sensitivity to tartrazine has proven to be a rare event.[20] Tartrazine sensitivity appears to occur only in aspirin-intolerant patients at a prevalence of 2%.[20] Although rare, due to severity of reaction and widespread use of tartrazine, the Food and Drug Administration (FDA) has required labeling for the products containing this dye.[21] The likely mechanism is dose-related histamine release, and the clinical presentation is the same as reaction to aspirin in aspirin-sensitive patients.[21]

Reactions to other azo dyes, monosodium glutamate (MSG), parabens, and non–azo dyes have been reported much less frequently than reactions to tartrazine and have been equally difficult to confirm with controlled challenges.[20] Positive reactions to sodium benzoate, a food preservative, have been reported in as many as 23% of aspirin-sensitive individuals.[12] Acetaminophen is a weak inhibitor of cyclooxygenase. As such, approximately 5% of aspirin-sensitive asthmatics will experience reactions to acetaminophen.[12] Most aspirin-sensitive asthmatics can use acetaminophen as a safe alternative to aspirin. Sporadic cases of worsening bronchospasm and anaphylaxis have been reported in aspirin-sensitive asthmatics receiving intravenous hydrocortisone succinate but have not been reported with the use of other corticosteroids.[13] It is not known whether it is the hydrocortisone or the succinate that is the problem.

▶ TREATMENT: Aspirin-Sensitive Asthma

Therapy of aspirin-sensitive asthmatics takes one of two general approaches: desensitization or avoidance. Avoidance of triggering substances seldom alters the clinical course of the patients' asthma. The therapy of asthma has been nonspecific; however, in theory, 5 lipoxygenase inhibitors such as zileuton or LT antagonists should provide specific therapy. A few studies have investigated use of LT modifiers to prevent aspirin-induced bronchospasm in aspirin-sensitive asthmatic patients.[22–24] Pretreatment with zileuton in eight aspirin-sensitive asthmatic patients protected them from the same threshold-provoking doses of aspirin.[22] However, larger escalating doses of aspirin above the threshold challenge doses were not examined in this study. Furthermore, in a recent study, when doses of aspirin were escalated above the threshold-provoking doses, zileuton did not prevent formation of LTs.[23] In a similar study, pretreatment with 10 mg daily of montelukast did not protect the patients when aspirin doses were increased above their threshold doses.[24] Although initial studies suggested that LT modifiers blocked aspirin-induced reactions, it is now apparent that they merely shift the dose-response curve to the right, leaving the patient at risk at higher doses. Thus even patients who might benefit from LT modifiers should avoid aspirin and all NSAIDs. A case of ibuprofen-induced (400 mg) asthma was reported in an asthmatic patient on 20 mg zafirlukast twice daily.[25] Furthermore, most of the challenge studies are based on incremental doses of aspirin or NSAIDs, and exposure of patients to full clinical doses of aspirin or NSAIDs can overcome the antagonistic effect of LT modifiers. Many of these patients require chronic steroid therapy to control the asthma. No placebo-controlled clinical trials comparing LT modifiers and other controller medications in this subgroup of asthmatic patients has been published. The respiratory symptoms can be decreased but not prevented by pretreatment with antihistamines, cromolyn, and nedocromil.[13,26]

β-BLOCKERS

β-Adrenergic receptor blockers comprise the other large class of drugs that can be hazardous to asthmatics. Even the more cardioselective agents, such as acebutolol, atenolol, and metoprolol, have been reported to cause asthma attacks.[11] Asthmatics may take nonselective and β_1-selective blockers without incident for long periods; however, the occasional reports of fatal asthma attacks resistant to therapy with β-agonists should provide ample warning of the dangers inherent in β-blocker therapy.[11]

If a patient with bronchial hyperreactivity requires β-blocker therapy, one of the relatively selective β_1-blockers (i.e., acebutolol, atenolol, metoprolol, or pindolol) should be used at the lowest possible dose. Celiprolol and betaxolol appear to possess greater cardioselectivity than currently marketed drugs.[27,28] Fatal status asthmaticus has occurred with the topical administration of the nonselective timolol maleate ophthalmic solution for the treatment of open-angle glaucoma.[29] Early investigations with ophthalmic betaxolol suggest that it is well tolerated even in timolol-sensitive asthmatics.[30]

SULFITES

Severe, life-threatening asthmatic reactions following the ingestion of restaurant meals and wine have occurred secondary to ingestion of the food preservative potassium metabisulfite.[20] Sulfites have been used for centuries as preservatives in wine and food. As antioxidants, they prevent fermentation of wine and discoloration of fruits and vegetables caused by contaminating bacteria.[32] Previously, sulfites had been given generally-recognized-as-safe (GRAS) status by the FDA. Sensitive patients react to concentrations ranging from 5 to 100 mg, amounts that are consumed routinely by anyone eating in restaurants. Consumption of sulfites in U.S. diets is estimated to be 2 to 3 mg/d in the home, with 5 to 10 mg per 30 mL of beer or wine consumed.[20] Anaphylactic or anaphylactoid reactions to sulfites in nonasthmatics are extremely rare. In the general asthmatic population, reactions to sulfites are uncommon. Approximately 5% of steroid-dependent asthmatics demonstrate sensitivity to sulfiting agents, but the prevalence is only around 1% in non-steroid-dependent asthmatic patients.[32]

MECHANISM

Three different mechanisms have been proposed to explain the reaction to sulfites in asthmatic patients.[32] The first is explained by the inhalation of sulfur dioxide, which produces bronchoconstriction in all asthmatics through direct stimulation of afferent parasympathetic irritant receptors. Furthermore, inhalation of atropine or the ingestion of doxepin protected sulfite-sensitive patients from reaction to ingestion of sulfites. The second theory, IgE-mediated reaction, is supported by reported cases of sulfite-sensitive anaphylactic reactions in patients with a positive sulfite skin test. Finally, a reduced concentration of sulfite oxidase enzyme (the enzyme that catalyzes oxidation of sulfites to sulfates) as compared with normal individuals has been demonstrated in a group of sulfite-sensitive asthmatics.

A number of pharmacologic agents contain sulfites as preservatives and antioxidants. The FDA now requires warning labels on drugs containing sulfites. Most manufacturers of drugs for the treatment of asthma have discontinued the use of sulfites. In addition, labeling is required on packaged foods that contain sulfites at 10 ppm or more, and sulfiting agents are no longer allowed on fresh fruits and vegetables (excluding potatoes) intended for sale.

Pretreatment with cromolyn, anticholinergics, and cyanocobalamine has protected sulfite-sensitive patients.[32,33] Presumably, pharmacologic doses of vitamin B_{12} catalyze the nonenzymatic oxidation of sulfite to sulfate.

OTHER PRESERVATIVES

Both ethylenediamine tetraacetic acid (EDTA) and benzalkonium chloride used as stabilizing agents and bacteriostatics, respectively, can produce bronchoconstriction.[34] In addition to producing bronchoconstriction, EDTA potentiates the bronchial responsiveness to histamine.[34] These effects presumably are mediated through calcium chelation by EDTA. Benzalkonium chloride is more potent than EDTA, and its mechanism appears to be a result of mast cell degranulation and stimulation of irritant C fibers in the airways.[34]

The bronchoconstriction from benzalkonium chloride can be blocked by cromolyn but not the anticholinergic ipratropium bromide.[35] Benzalkonium chloride is found in the commercial multiple-dose nebulizer preparations of ipratropium bromide and beclomethasone diproprionate marketed in the United Kingdom and Europe and is presumed to be in part responsible for paradoxical wheezing following administration of these agents.[34–36] Benzalkonium chloride is also found in albuterol nebulizer solutions marketed in the United States and has been implicated as a possible cause of paradoxical wheezing in infants receiving this preparation.[34] In a recent study, subjects with stable asthma were assigned randomly to inhale up to four 600-μg nebulized doses of EDTA and benzalkonium chloride and normal saline in order to evaluate the effect of these agents on FEV_1 when used in the amount administered for treatment of acute asthma.[37] Change in FEV_1 was not different between the EDTA and placebo groups, but benzalkonium chloride was associated with a statistically significant decrease in FEV_1 compared with placebo. It is important to consider that these agents are always used in combination with bronchodilators, that β_2-agonists are potent mast cell stabilizers, and that the anecdotal reports have not yet been confirmed with controlled investigations.[34,35]

CONTRAST MEDIA

Iodinated radiocontrast materials are the most common cause of anaphylactoid reactions producing bronchospasm.[38] The reader is referred to Chapter 89 for a discussion of this topic.

NATURAL RUBBER LATEX ALLERGY

Allergy to natural rubber latex, first reported in 1989 in the United States, is a common cause of occupational allergy for health care workers.[39] Natural rubber is a processed plant product from the commercial rubber tree, *Hevea brasiliensis.*[40] Latex allergens are proteins found in both raw latex and the extracts present in finished rubber products. Latex gloves are the largest single source of exposure to the protein allergens.[40]

The reported prevalence of latex allergy depends on the sample population. In the general population, latex allergy is less than 1%, but the prevalence increases in health care workers to 5% to 15%.[40] Risk factors for latex allergy include frequent exposure to rubber gloves, history of atopic disease, and presence or history of hand dermatitis. Patients with spina bifida are at increased risk of latex allergy, with an incidence of 24% to 60% due to early and repeated exposure to rubber devices during the surgical procedures required for correction.[40]

Clinical manifestations of latex allergy range from contact dermatitis to urticaria, rhinitis, and asthma and reported cases of anaphylaxis.[39,40] The early manifestation of rubber allergy is contact urticaria, which is an IgE-mediated reaction to rubber proteins following direct contact with the medical devices, mainly rubber gloves.[40] Contact dermatitis may occur within 1 to 2 days. Contact dermatitis is a cell-mediated delayed-type hypersensitivity reaction to additive chemical components of rubber products.[40] Rhinitis and asthma may follow inhalation of allergens by means of the cornstarch powder used to coat the latex gloves. Asthma caused by occupational exposure is seen mostly in atopic patients with histories of seasonal and perennial allergies and asthma.[40] There are also isolated cases of wheezing due to latex exposure in patients without a history of asthma.[40]

The diagnosis of latex allergy is based on the presence of latex-specific IgE as well as symptoms consistent with IgE-mediated reactions.[41] The mainstay of therapy for latex allergy is avoidance. The FDA requires appropriate labeling for all medical devices containing natural rubber latex to ensure avoidance and a latex-free environment. The role of pretreatment with antihistamine and corticosteroids and allergen immunotherapy remains to be determined and supported by controlled clinical trials.[40,41]

ANGIOTENSIN-CONVERTING ENZYME INHIBITOR–INDUCED COUGH

Cough has become a well-recognized side effect of angiotensin-converting enzyme (ACE) inhibitor therapy. According to spontaneous reporting by patients, cough occurs in 1% to 10% of patients receiving ACE inhibitors, with a preponderance of females. In a retrospective analysis, 14.6% of women had cough compared with 6.0% of the men on ACE inhibitors. It is suggested that women have a lower cough threshold, resulting in reporting of this adverse effect more commonly than by men.[42] Studies specifically evaluating cough caused by ACE inhibitors have reported a prevalence of 19% to 25%.[43,44] Patients receiving ACE inhibitors had a 2.3 times greater likelihood of developing cough than a similar group of patients receiving diuretics.[43] Patients with hyperreactive airways do not appear to be at greater risk.[45] African-Americans and the Chinese have a higher incidence of cough.[42] When different disease states were compared, 26% of patients with heart failure had ACE inhibitor–induced cough compared with 14% of those with hypertension.[42] Cough occurs with all ACE inhibitors.[45]

The cough typically is dry and nonproductive, persistent, and not paroxysmal.[45] The severity of cough varies from a "tickle" to a debilitating cough with insomnia and vomiting. Sixty percent of patients who discontinued their ACE inhibitor therapy reported cough as the main reason.[40] The cough can begin within 3 days or have a delayed onset of up to 12 months following initiation of ACE inhibitor therapy.[45] The cough remits within 1 to 4 days of discontinuing therapy but, rarely, can last up to 4 weeks and recur with rechallenge.[45] Patients should be given a 4-day withdrawal to determine if the cough is indeed induced by the ACE inhibitor. The chest x-ray is normal, as are pulmonary function tests (spirometry and diffusing capacity). Bronchial hyperreactivity, as measured by histamine and methacholine provocation, may be worsened in patients with underlying bronchial hyperreactivity such as asthma and chronic bronchitis. However, bronchial hyperreactivity is not induced in others.[45,47] The cough reflex to capsaicin is enhanced but not to nebulized distilled water or citric acid.[45]

The mechanism of ACE inhibitor–induced cough is still unknown. ACE is a nonspecific enzyme that also catalyzes the hydrolysis of bradykinin and substance P (see Chapter 25) that produce or facilitate inflammation and stimulate lung irritant receptors.[45] ACE inhibitors also may induce cyclooxygenase to cause the production of prostaglandins. NSAIDs, benzonatate, inhaled bupivacaine, theophylline, beclofen, thromboxane A_2 synthase inhibitor,[42,48] and cromolyn sodium all have been used to suppress or inhibit ACE inhibitor–induced cough.[45,49] The cough is generally not responsive to cough suppressants or bronchodilator therapy. No long-term trials evaluating different treatment options for ACE inhibitor–induced cough exist. Cromolyn sodium may be considered first because it is the most studied agent and has minimal toxicity.[42] The preferred therapy is withdrawal of the ACE inhibitor and replacement with an alternative antihypertensive agent. Owing to their fewer side effects than ACE inhibitors, angiotensin II (AT2) receptor antagonists are often recommended in place of an ACE inhibitor, but there are rare reports of this agent inducing bronchospasm.[50] Clinical trials suggest that AT2 receptor antagonists have the same incidence of cough as placebo. Furthermore, when AT2 receptor antagonists were compared with ACE inhibitors, cough occurred much less frequently. Reduction in incidence of cough with AT2 receptor antagonists is likely due to the lack of effect on clearance of bradykinin and substance P.[46] The use of alternative therapies to treat ACE inhibitor–induced cough generally is not recommended.[45]

PULMONARY EDEMA

Pulmonary edema may result from the failure of any of a number of homeostatic mechanisms. The most common cause of pulmonary edema is an increase in capillary hydrostatic pressure because of left ventricular failure. Excessive fluid administration in compensated and decompensated heart failure patients is the most frequent cause of iatrogenic pulmonary edema. Besides hydrostatic forces, other homeostatic mechanisms that may be disrupted include the osmotic and oncotic pressures in the vasculature, the integrity of the alveolar epithelium, interstitial pulmonary pressure, and interstitial lymph flow.[6] The edema fluid in cardiogenic pulmonary edema contains a low amount of protein, whereas noncardiogenic pulmonary edema fluid has a high protein concentration.[6] This indicates that noncardiogenic pulmonary edema results primarily from disruption of the alveolar epithelium. The reader is referred to Chapter 28 for a detailed discussion of this topic.

The clinical presentation of pulmonary edema includes persistent cough, tachypnea, dyspnea, tachycardia, rales on auscultation, hypoxemia from ventilation-perfusion imbalance and intrapulmonary shunting, widespread fluffy infiltrates on chest roentgenogram, and decreased lung compliance (stiff lungs). Noncardiogenic pulmonary edema may progress to hemorrhage; cellular debris collects in the alveoli, followed by hyperplasia and fibrosis with a residual restrictive mechanical defect.[6]

NARCOTIC-INDUCED PULMONARY EDEMA

The most common drug-induced noncardiogenic pulmonary edema is produced by the narcotic analgesics[6] (Table 29–4). Narcotic-induced pulmonary edema is associated most commonly with intravenous heroin use but also has occurred with morphine, methadone, meperidine, and propoxyphene use.[6,51] There also have been a few reported cases associated with the use of the opiate antagonist naloxone and nalmefene, a long-acting opioid antagonist.[52,53] The mechanism is unknown but may be related to hypoxemia similar to the neurogenic pulmonary edema associated with cerebral tumors or trauma or a direct toxic effect on the alveolar capillary membrane.[51] Initially thought to occur only with overdoses, most evidence now supports the theory that narcotic-induced pulmonary edema is an idiosyncratic reaction to moderate as well as high narcotic doses.[51]

TABLE 29–4. Drugs That Induce Pulmonary Edema

Cardiogenic Pulmonary Edema	
Excessive intravenous fluids	F[a]
Blood and plasma transfusions	F
Corticosteroids	F
Phenylbutazone	R
Sodium diatrizoate	R
Hypertonic intrathecal saline	R
β_2-Adrenergic agonists	I
Noncardiogenic Pulmonary Edema	
Heroin	F
Methadone	I
Morphine	I
Oxygen	I
Propoxyphene	R
Ethchlorvynol	R
Chlordiazepoxide	R
Salicylate	R
Hydrochlorothiazide	R
Triamterene + hydrochlorothiazide	R
Leukoagglutinin reactions	R
Iron–dextran complex	R
Methotrexate	R
Cytosine arabinoside	R
Nitrofurantoin	R
Dextran 40	R
Fluorescein	R
Amitriptyline	R
Colchicine	R
Nitrogen mustard	R
Epinephrine	R
Metaraminol	R
Bleomycin	R
Iodide	R
Cyclophosphamide	R
VM-26	R

[a]Relative frequency of reactions: F = frequent; I = infrequent; R = rare.

Patients with pulmonary edema may be comatose with depressed respirations or dyspnea and tachypnea. They may or may not have other signs of narcotic overdose. Symptomology varies from cough and mild crepitations on auscultation with characteristic radiologic findings to severe cyanosis and hypoxemia even with supplemental oxygen. Symptoms may appear within minutes of intravenous administration but may take up to 2 hours to occur, particularly following oral methadone administration.[51] Hemodynamic studies in the first 24 hours have demonstrated normal pulmonary capillary wedge pressures in the presence of pulmonary edema.

Clinical symptoms generally improve within 24 to 48 hours, and radiologic clearing occurs in 2 to 5 days. However, the abnormalities in pulmonary function tests may persist for 10 to 12 weeks. Therapy consists of naloxone administration, supplemental oxygen, and ventilatory support if required. Mortality is less than 1%.[51]

OTHER DRUGS THAT CAUSE PULMONARY EDEMA

Noncardiogenic pulmonary edema also has been associated with the oral and intravenous administration of ethchlorvynol.[51] A parodoxical pulmonary edema has been reported in a few patients following hydrochlorothiazide ingestion but not any other benzothiazide diuretic.[6] Acute pulmonary edema rarely has followed the injection of high concentrations of contrast medium into the pulmonary circulation during angiocardiography.[6] Rare occurrences of pulmonary edema have followed the intravenous administration of bleomycin, cyclophosphamide, and vinblastine.[6]

The selective β_2-adrenergic agonists terbutaline and ritodrine have been reported to induce pulmonary edema when used as tocolytics.[6] This disorder commonly occurs 48 to 72 hours after tocolytic therapy.[53] This has never occurred with their use in asthma patients, even in inadvertent overdosage. This reaction may result from excess fluid administration used to prevent the hypotension from β_2-mediated vasodilation or the particular hemodynamics of pregnancy. In a review of 330 patients who received tocolytic therapy and were monitored closely for their fluid status, no episode of pulmonary edema was reported.[53]

Inteleukin-2, a cytokine used alone or in combination with cytotoxic drugs, has been reported to induce pulmonary edema. Although other cytokines have been associated with pulmonary edema, the problem is most significant with interleukin-2. A weight gain of 2 kg has been reported after treatment with interleukin-2.[53]

Pulmonary edema has occurred occasionally with salicylate overdoses. The serum salicylate concentrations are often greater than 45 mg/dL, and the patients have other signs of toxicity, although some cases have been associated with concentrations in the usual therapeutic range.[51]

PULMONARY EOSINOPHILIA

Pulmonary infiltrates with eosinophilia (Loeffler's syndrome) have been associated with nitrofurantoin, *para*-aminosalicylic acid,

TABLE 29–5. Drugs That Induce Pulmonary Infiltrates with Eosinophilia (Loeffler's Syndrome)

Nitrofurantoin	F[a]2	Tetracycline	R
para-Aminosalicylic acid	F	Procarbazine	R
Sulfonamides	I	Cromolyn	R
Penicillins	I	Niridazole	R
Methotrexate	I	Gold salts	R
Imipramine	I	Chlorpromazine	R
Chlorpropamide	R	Naproxen	R
Carbamazepine	R	Sulindac	R
Phenytoin	R	Ibuprofen	R
Mephenesin	R		

[a]Relative frequency of reactions: F = frequent; I = infrequent; R = rare.

methotrexate, sulfonamides, tetracycline, chlorpropamide, phenytoin, NSAIDs, and imipramine[6,54] (Table 29–5). The disorder is characterized by fever, nonproductive cough, dyspnea, cyanosis, bilateral pulmonary infiltrates, and eosinophilia in the blood.[6] Lung biopsy has revealed perivasculitis with infiltration of eosinophils, macrophages, and proteinaceous edema fluid in the alveoli. The symptoms and eosinophilia generally respond rapidly to withdrawal of the offending drug.

Sulfonamides were first reported as causative agents in users of sulfanilamide vaginal cream.[6] *para*-Aminosalicylic acid frequently produced the syndrome in tuberculosis patients being treated with this agent.[6] There have been nine reported cases associated with sulfasalazine use in inflammatory bowel disease.[54] The drug most frequently associated with this syndrome is nitrofurantoin.[6,51] Nitrofurantoin-induced lung disorders appear to be more common in postmenopausal women.[51] Lung reactions made up 43% of 921 adverse reactions to nitrofurantoin reported to the Swedish Adverse Drug Reaction Committee between 1966 and 1976.[54] No apparent correlation exists between duration of drug exposure and severity or reversibility of the reaction.[54] Most cases occur within 1 month of therapy. Typical symptoms include fever, tachypnea, dyspnea, dry cough, and less commonly, pleuritic chest pain. Radiographic findings include bilateral interstitial infiltrates, predominant in the bases and pleural effusions 25% of the time. Although there are anecdotal reports that steroids are beneficial, the usual rapid improvement following discontinuation of the drugs brings their utility into question. Complete recovery usually occurs within 15 days of withdrawal.

A few cases of pulmonary eosinophilia have been reported in asthmatics treated with cromolyn.[6,54] The significance of this is unknown in light of the occasional spontaneous occurrence of pulmonary eosinophilia in asthmatic patients. Cases of acute pneumonitis and eosinophilia have been reported to occur with phenytoin and carbamazepine therapy.[54] Patients have had other symptoms of hypersensitivity, including fever and rashes. The symptoms of dyspnea and cough subside following discontinuation of the drug.

OXYGEN TOXICITY

Because of the similarity to pulmonary fibrosis, oxygen-induced lung toxicity is reviewed briefly. More extensive reviews on this topic have been published.[55,56]

The earliest manifestation of oxygen toxicity is substernal pleuritic pain from tracheobronchitis.[56] The onset of toxicity follows an asymptomatic period and presents as cough, chest pain, and dyspnea. Early symptoms usually are masked in ventilator-dependent patients. The first noted physiologic change is a decrease in pulmonary compliance caused by reversible atelectasis. Then decreases in vital capacity occur, followed by progressive abnormalities in carbon monoxide diffusing capacity (DLCO).[56] Decreased inspiratory flow rates, reflected in the need for high inspiratory pressures in ventilator-dependent patients, occur as the fractional concentration of inspired oxygen (FiO_2) requirement increases. The lungs become progressively stiffer as the ability to oxygenate becomes more compromised.

The FiO_2 and duration of exposure are both important determinants of the severity of lung damage. Normal human volunteers can tolerate 100% oxygen at sea level for 24 to 48 hours with minimal to no damage.[55] Oxygen concentrations of less than 50% are well tolerated even for extended periods. Inspired oxygen concentrations between 50% and 100% carry a substantial risk of lung damage, and the duration required is inversely proportional to the FiO_2.[54] Underlying disease states may alter this relationship.

Oxygen-induced lung damage generally is separated into the acute exudative phase and the subacute or chronic proliferative phase. The acute phase consists of perivascular, peribronchiolar, interstitial, and alveolar edema with alveolar hemorrhage and necrosis of pulmonary endothelium and type I epithelial cells.[55] The proliferative phase consists of resorption of the exudates and hyperplasia of interstitial and type II alveolar lining cells. Collagen and elastin deposition in the interstitium of alveolar walls then leads to thickening of the gas-exchange area and the fibrosis.[55]

The biochemical mechanism of the tissue damage during hyperoxia is the increased production of highly reactive, partially reduced oxygen metabolites[56] (Fig. 29–1). These oxidants normally are produced in small quantities during cellular respiration and include the superoxide anion (O_2), hydrogen peroxide (H_2O_2), the hydroxyl radical (OH^-), singlet oxygen ($^1O_2$), and hypochlorous acid (HOCl).[56] Oxygen free radicals normally are formed in phagocytic cells to kill invading microorganisms, but they are also toxic to normal cell components. The oxidants produce toxicity through destructive redox reactions with protein sulfhydryl groups, membrane lipids, and nucleic acids.[56]

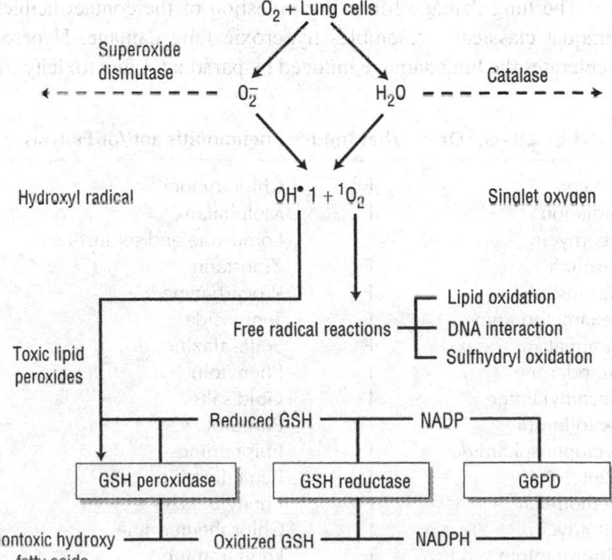

FIGURE 29–1. Schematic of the interaction of oxygen radicals and the antioxidant system. GSH = glutathione; G6PD = glucose-6-phosphate dehydrogenase; NADP = nicotinamide-adenine dinucleotide phosphate; NADPH = reduced NADP.

The oxidants are products of normal cellular respiration that are normally counterbalanced by an antioxidant defense system that prevents tissue destruction. The antioxidants include superoxide dismutase, catalase, glutathione peroxidase, ceruloplasmin, and α-tocopherol (vitamin E). Antioxidants are ubiquitous in the body. Hyperoxia produces toxicity by overwhelming the antioxidant system. There is experimental evidence that a number of drugs and chemicals produce lung toxicity through increasing production of oxidants (e.g., bleomycin, cyclophosphamide, nitrofurantoin, and paraquat) and/or by inhibiting the antioxidant system (e.g., carmustine, cyclophosphamide, and nitrofurantoin).[57,58]

PULMONARY FIBROSIS

A great number of drugs have been associated with chronic pulmonary fibrosis with or without a preceding acute pneumonitis (Table 29–6). The cancer chemotherapeutic agents make up the largest group and have been the subject of numerous reviews.[57,58] Although the mechanisms by which all the drugs produce pneumonitis and/or fibrosis are not known, the clinical syndrome, pulmonary function abnormalities, and histopathology present a relatively homogeneous pattern.[57] The histopathologic picture closely resembles oxidant lung damage, and in some experimental cases, oxygen enhances the pulmonary injury.[51] Although the terms *pulmonary fibrosis* or *interstitial pneumonitis* have been used widely to describe pneumonia after bone marrow transplantation, in 1991 a National Institutes of Health workshop recommended that the term *idiopathic pneumonia syndrome* (IPS) should be used to avoid histopathologic terms and to define the inherent heterogeneity of this disorder.[59] IPS accounts for more than 40% of deaths related to bone marrow transplantation.[59] Suggested causes of IPS include radiation or chemotherapy regimens prior to transplantation, graft versus host disease, unrecognized infections, and other inflammation-related lung injuries.[60,61] IPS is characterized by dyspnea, hypoxemia, nonproductive cough, diffuse alveolar damage, and interstitial pneumonitis in the absence of lower respiratory infection. IPS has been reported early and late, up to 24 months after bone marrow transplantation.[61]

The lung damage following ingestion of the contact herbicide paraquat classically resembles hyperoxic lung damage. Hyperoxia accelerates the lung damage induced by paraquat. Lung toxicity from paraquat occurs following oral administration in humans and aerosol administration and inhalation in experimental animals.[58] The pulmonary specificity of paraquat results in part from its active uptake into lung tissue. Paraquat readily accepts an electron from reduced nicotinamide-adenine dinucleotide phosphate (NADPH) and is then rapidly reoxidized, forming superoxide and other oxygen radicals.[58] The toxicity may be a result of NADPH depletion (see Fig. 29–1) and/or excess oxygen free-radical generation with lipid peroxidation. Treatment with exogenous superoxide dismutase has had limited and conflicting results.[58]

TABLE 29–6. Drugs That Induce Pneumonitis and/or Fibrosis

Drug	Frequency	Drug	Frequency
Oxygen	F[a]	Chlorambucil	R
Radiation	F	Melphalan	R
Bleomycin	F	Lomustine and semustine	R
Busulfan	F	Zinostatin	R
Carmustine	F	Procarbazine	R
Hexamethonium	F	Teniposide	R
Paraquat	F	Sulfasalazine	R
Amiodarone	F	Phenytoin	R
Mecamylamine	I	Gold salts	R
Pentolinium	I	Pindolol	R
Cyclophosphamide	I	Imipramine	R
Practolol	I	Penicillamine	R
Methotrexate	I	Phenylbutazone	R
Mitomycin	I	Chlorphentermine	R
Nitrofurantoin	I	Fenfluramine	R
Methysergide	I		
Azathioprine, 6-mercaptopurine	R		

[a]Relative frequency of reactions: F = frequent; I = infrequent; R = rare.

TABLE 29–7. Possible Causes of Pulmonary Fibrosis

Idiopathic pulmonary fibrosis (fibrosing alveolitis)
Pneumoconiosis (asbestosis, silicosis, coal dust, talc berylliosis)
Hypersensitivity pneumonitis (molds, bacteria, animal proteins, toluene diisocyanate, epoxy resins)
Smoking
Sarcoidosis
Tuberculosis
Lipoid pneumonia
Systemic lupus erythematosus
Rheumatoid arthritis
Systemic sclerosis
Polymyositis/dermatomyositis
Sjögren's syndrome
Polyarteritis nodosa
Wegener's granuloma
Byssinosis (cotton workers)
Siderosis (arc welders' lung)
Radiation
Oxygen
Chemicals (thioureas, trialkylphosphorothioates, furans)
Drugs (see Tables 29–5, 29–6, and 29–8)

A number of furans have been shown to produce oxidant injury to lungs.[58] Occasionally, patients with acute nitrofurantoin lung toxicity will progress to a chronic reaction leading to fibrosis, and rarely, a patient may develop chronic toxicity without an antecedent acute reaction. Like paraquat, nitrofurantoin undergoes cyclic reduction and reoxidation that may produce superoxide radicals or deplete NADPH. In addition, nitrofurantoin inhibits glutathione reductase, an enzyme involved in the glutathione antioxidant system (see Fig. 29–1). Table 29–7 provides a list of possible nondrug causes of pulmonary fibrosis.

DRUGS ASSOCIATED WITH PULMONARY FIBROSIS

ANTINEOPLASTICS

A number of cancer chemotherapeutic agents produce pulmonary fibrosis. In an excellent review,[57] six predisposing factors for the development of cytotoxic drug-induced pulmonary disease were described: (1) cumulative dose, (2) increased age, (3) concurrent or previous radiotherapy, (4) oxygen therapy, (5) other cytotoxic drug therapy, and (6) preexisting pulmonary disease. Drugs that are directly toxic to the lung would be expected to show a dose-response relationship. Dose-response relationships have been established for bleomycin, busulfan, and carmustine (BCNU).[57] Bleomycin and busulfan exhibit threshold cumulative doses below which a very small percentage of patients exhibit toxicity, but carmustine shows a more linear relationship.[58] Older patients appear to be more susceptible, possibly as a result of a decrease in the antioxidant defense system.

Excessive irradiation produces a pneumonitis and fibrosis thought to be caused by oxygen free-radical formation.[57] Evidence for synergistic toxicity with radiation exists for bleomycin, busulfan, and mitomycin.[57] Hyperoxia has shown synergistic toxicity with bleomycin, cyclophosphamide, and mitomycin.[57] Carmustine, mitomycin, cyclophosphamide, bleomycin, and methotrexate all appear to show increased lung toxicity when they are part of multidrug regimens.

NITROSOUREAS

BCNU is associated with the highest incidence of pulmonary toxicity (20% to 30%).[57] The lung pathology generally resembles that produced by bleomycin and busulfan. Unique to BCNU is the finding of fibrosis in the absence of inflammatory infiltrates. BCNU preferentially inhibits glutathione reductase, the enzyme required to regenerate glutathione, thus reducing glutathione tissue stores.[57,58] The patients present with dyspnea, tachypnea, and nonproductive cough that may begin within a month of initiation of therapy but may not develop for as long as 3 years.[57] A more recent report suggested that most patients receiving BCNU develop fibrosis that may remain asymptomatic or become symptomatic any time up to 17 years after therapy.[62] The cumulative dose has ranged from 580 to 2100 mg/m^2.[55] The disease usually is slowly progressive, with a mortality rate from 15% to greater than 90% depending on the study and period of follow-up. In a retrospective study, the risk factors for development of IPS and prognostic factors for outcomes were evaluated in 94 patients with relapsed Hodgkin's disease treated with BCNU containing high-dose chemotherapy and hematopoietic support. The risk factors for pulmonary fibrosis and mortality were female sex and dose of BCNU, with all deaths reported in those who received BCNU at doses of more than 475 mg/m^2.[63] Rapid progression and death within a few days occur in a small percentage of patients.[57] Corticosteroids do not appear to be effective in reducing damage.[57] Other nitrosoureas, lomustine, and semustine also have been reported to produce lung damage in patients receiving unusually high doses.[57]

BLEOMYCIN

Bleomycin is the best-studied cytotoxic pulmonary toxin. Because of its lack of bone marrow suppression, pulmonary toxicity is the dose-limiting toxicity of bleomycin therapy. The incidence of bleomycin lung toxicity is about 4%, which may be affected by the following risk factors: bleomycin cumulative dose, age, high concentration of inspired oxygen, radiation therapy, and multidrug regimens, particularly those with cyclophosphamide.[53] Age at the time of treatment with bleomycin may be a risk factor as well; patients younger than 7 years at the time of bleomycin therapy are more likely to develop pulmonary toxicity compared with older subjects.[53] The cumulative dose above which the incidence of toxicity significantly increases is 450 to 500 units.[57] However, rapidly fatal pulmonary toxicity has occurred with doses as low as 100 units.[57]

Experimentally, bleomycin generates superoxide anions, and the lung toxicity is increased by radiation and hyperoxia.[57] Pretreatment with superoxide dismutase and catalase reduces toxicity in experimental animals.[57] Bleomycin also oxidizes arachidonic acid, which may account for the marked inflammation. Bleomycin also may affect collagen deposition by its stimulation of fibroblast growth.[57] Combination of bleomycin with other cytotoxic agents, particularly regimens containing cyclophosphamide, may predispose patients to pulmonary damage.

There are two distinct clinical patterns of bleomycin pulmonary toxicity. Chronic progressive fibrosis is the most common; acute hypersensitivity reactions occur infrequently. Patients present with cough and dyspnea. The first physiologic abnormality seen is a decreased DLCO.[57] Chest radiographs show a bibasilar reticular pattern, and gallium scans show marked uptake in the involved lung.[57] Chest radiographic changes lag behind pulmonary function abnormalities. Spirometry tests before each bleomycin dose are not predictive of toxicity. The single-breath DLCO is the most sensitive indicator of bleomycin-induced lung disease. Although it is not absolutely predictive, a drop of 20% or greater in the DLCO is an indication for using alternative therapies.[57] The prognosis of bleomycin lung toxicity has improved due to early detection, but the mortality rate is approximately 25%. Mild cases respond to discontinuation of bleomycin therapy.[53] Corticosteroid therapy appears to be helpful in patients with acute pneumonitis, although there have been no controlled trials. Patients with chronic fibrosis would be less likely to respond. Although corticosteroids have been used for a number of drug-induced pulmonary problems, a study in mice showing a potential for worsening of lung damage when administered early during the repair stage should sound a word of caution against their indiscriminate use.[64]

MITOMYCIN

Mitomycin is an alkylating antibiotic that produces pulmonary fibrosis at a frequency of 3% to 12%.[57] The mechanism is unknown, but oxygen and radiation therapy appear to enhance the development of toxicity.[57] The clinical presentation and symptoms are the same as for bleomycin. The mortality rate is about 50%. Early withdrawal of the drug and administration of corticosteroids appear to significantly improve the outcome.

ALKYLATING AGENTS

A number of alkylating agents have been associated with pulmonary fibrosis (see Table 29–5). The incidence of clinical toxicity is around 4%, although subclinical damage is apparent in up to 46% of patients at autopsy. The mechanism of toxicity is unknown, but epithelial cell damage that triggers the arachidonic acid inflammatory cascade may be the initiating event.[57] The clinical presentation is insidious, with 4 years being the average duration of therapy before the onset of symptoms.[57] Patients present with low-grade fever, weight loss, weakness, dyspnea, cough, and rales.[57] Pulmonary function tests initially show abnormal diffusion capacity followed by a restrictive pattern (low vital capacity). The histopathologic findings are nonspecific. The prognosis is one of slow progression, with a mean survival of 5 months following diagnosis.[57] Although there is no direct dose-dependent correlation, patients receiving less than 500 mg of busulfan do not develop the syndrome without concomitant radiation or use of other pulmonary-toxic chemotherapeutic agents.[57] There are anecdotal reports of beneficial responses to corticosteroids, but no controlled studies have been done.

Cyclophosphamide infrequently produces pulmonary toxicity. More than 20 well-documented cases have been reported to date. In animal models, cyclophosphamide produces reactive oxygen radicals. High oxygen concentrations produce synergistic toxicity with cyclophosphamide. The duration of therapy before the onset of symptoms is highly variable, and there may be a delay of several months between the onset of symptoms and discontinuation of the drug.[57] Cyclophosphamide may potentiate carmustine lung toxicity.[57] Clinical symptoms usually consist of dyspnea on exertion, cough, and fever.

Inspiratory crackles and the bibasilar reticular pattern typical of cytotoxic drug–induced radiographic changes are present. Histopathologic changes are also nonspecific. Approximately 60% of patients recover. Corticosteroid therapy has been reported to be beneficial, but death despite corticosteroid administration also has been reported.

Chlorambucil, melphalan, and uracil mustard also have been associated with pulmonary fibrosis. Of the alkylating agents, only nitrogen mustard and thiotepa have not been reported to cause fibrotic pulmonary toxicity.[57]

ANTIMETABOLITES

Methotrexate was first reported to induce pulmonary toxicity in 1969.[57] The pulmonary toxicity to methotrexate is unique in that discontinuation is not always necessary, and reinstitution of the drug may not produce recurrence of symptoms.[6] Methotrexate pulmonary toxicity most commonly appears to result from hypersensitivity,[54] and it can occur 3 or more years following methotrexate therapy.[65] Age, sex, underlying pulmonary disease, duration of therapy, or smoking is not associated with an increased risk of pneumonitis with methotrexate.[65] Serial pulmonary function tests did not help identify pneumonitis in patients receiving methotrexate before the onset of clinical symptoms.[65] Reductions in DLCO and lung volumes are the most common manifestations of methotrexate lung toxicity.[53] Pulmonary edema and eosinophilia are common, and fibrosis occurs in only 10% of the patients who develop acute pneumonitis.[57] Systemic symptoms of chills, fever, and malaise are common before the onset of dyspnea, cough, and acute pleuritic chest pain. Methotrexate also has been associated with granuloma formation.[57]

The prognosis of methotrexate-induced pulmonary toxicity is good, with a 1% or less mortality rate.[54] Pulmonary toxicity has followed intrathecal as well as oral administration and has occurred after single doses as well as long-term daily and intermittent administration.[57] Pneumonitis has been reported to occur up to 4 weeks following discontinuation of therapy.[57] Numerous anecdotal reports have claimed dramatic benefit from corticosteroid therapy. It is unknown whether intermittent (weekly) dosing as is done for rheumatoid arthritis decreases the risk of methotrexate-induced pulmonary toxicity, and pneumonitis has occurred with this form of dosing.

Rarely, azathioprine and its major metabolite, 6-mercaptopurine, have been reported to produce an acute restrictive lung disease. Procarbazine, a methylhydrazine more commonly associated with Loeffler's syndrome, rarely has been associated with pulmonary fibrosis.[54] The *Vinca* alkaloids vinblastine and vindesine have been reported to produce severe respiratory toxicity in association with mitomycin. The incidence with the combination is 39% and may represent a true synergistic effect between these agents.[57]

NONCYTOTOXIC DRUGS

Pulmonary fibrosis associated with the ganglionic-blocking agent hexamethonium was first reported in 1954[6] (see Table 29–6). Patients developed extreme dyspnea after several months on the drug. Pathologic findings were consistent with bronchiectasis, bronchiolectasis, and fibrosis.[6] This phenomenon occasionally has occurred with use of the other ganglionic blockers mecamylamine and pentolinium.[6]

In 1959, radiographic changes characteristic of diffuse pulmonary fibrosis were reported in 87% of 31 patients who had taken phenytoin for 2 years or more.[51] Since then, studies have been conflicting. If phenytoin does produce chronic fibrosis, it would appear to be a relatively rare event.

Gold salts (sodium aurothiomalate) used in the treatment of rheumatoid arthritis have produced pulmonary fibrosis with cough, dyspnea, and pleuritic pain 5 to 16 weeks following institution of therapy.[51] Pulmonary function tests show a restrictive defect, and patients generally have an eosinophilia. The reactions improve on discontinuation of the gold therapy and promptly recur on reexposure. The pulmonary deficit may not improve completely.

AMIODARONE

Amiodarone, a benzofuran derivative, produces pulmonary fibrosis when used for supraventricular and ventricular arrhythmias[66] (see Table 29–6). The duration of amiodarone therapy before the onset of symptoms has ranged from 4 weeks to 6 years.[51,66] The estimated incidence is 1 in 1000 to 2000 treated patients per year. The clinical course is variable, ranging from acute onset of dyspnea with rapid progression into severe respiratory failure to death caused by slowly developing exertional dyspnea over a few months. Patients generally improve on discontinuation of the drug.[66] The majority of patients develop reactions while taking maintenance doses greater than 400 mg daily for more than 2 months or smaller doses for more than 2 years.[60,61] The risk of amiodarone pulmonary toxicity is higher during the first 12 months of therapy even at a low dosage.[67] Other risk factors include cardiopulmonary surgery combined with the administration of high concentrations of oxygen.[67] Routine spirometry does not appear to be predictive of patients at risk.[68] Carbon monoxide diffusing capacity studies are sensitive indicators of amiodarone pulmonary toxicity but have only a 21% positive predictive value.[68] Clinical findings include exertional dyspnea, nonproductive cough, weight loss, and occasionally low-grade fever.[51,68] Radiographic changes are nondiagnostic and include diffuse bilateral interstitial changes consistent with a pneumonitis. Pulmonary function abnormalities include hypoxia, restrictive changes, and diffusion abnormalities.

The mechanism of amiodarone-induced pulmonary toxicity is multifactorial. Amiodarone and its metabolite can damage lung tissue directly by a cytotoxic process or indirectly by immunologic reactions.[67] Amiodarone is an amphiphilic molecule that contains both a highly apolar aromatic ring system and a polar side chain with a positively charged nitrogen atom.[66] Amphiphilic drugs characteristically produce a phospholipid storage disorder in the lungs of experimental animals and humans.[58] Chlorphentermine, an anorectic, is the prototypical amphiphilic compound. The mechanism is currently believed to be the inhibition of lysosomal phospholipases.[58] The inflammation and fibrosis are thought to be a late finding resulting from nonspecific inflammation following the breakdown of phospholipid-laden macrophages.[66]

In a review of 39 cases, 9 patients died, and the remaining 30 patients had resolution of abnormalities after withdrawal of the drug.[66] Some patients have had resolution with lowering of the dosage, and therapy has been reinstituted at lower doses without problems in others. Of the patients who died, one-half received corticosteroids. There have been reports of a protective effect with prophylactic corticosteroids and other reports of patients developing amiodarone lung toxicity while on corticosteroids.[66] At this time, any benefit of corticosteroids is unclear because most patients improve on stopping the drug.

PULMONARY HYPERTENSION

Primary pulmonary hypertension (PPH) is a rare disorder occurring with an approximate incidence of 1 to 2 cases per 1 million persons in the general population.[69] With progression of the disease, right ventricular afterload increases, and the ability to increase cardiac output with activity decreases. This progresses to right-sided heart failure and death.[70]

Patients with PPH often complain of exertional dyspnea, chest pain, and syncope. Owing to the nonspecific nature of these symptoms and lack of a noninvasive diagnostic test for detecting PPH, there are often delays in the diagnosis of the disease, many times up to a year after the onset of symptoms.[70]

The factors leading to the development of PPH are unclear, although associations with portal hypertension and pregnancy have been detected. Obesity by itself may double the risk of PPH.[71] Additionally, the use of cocaine, oral contraceptives, infection with human immunodeficiency virus (HIV), the use of anorexic agents,[72] hepatic cirrhosis, genetic susceptibility, and female sex in the third to fourth decades of life also have been implicated as predisposing factors.[71] Exposure of patients to fenfluramine or dexfenfluramine has been associated with 20% of all diagnosed cases of PPH.[71]

The first reports of the association between PPH and the use of anorexic agents occurred in the late 1960s and early 1970s in western Europe when the drug aminorex was used for weight reduction.[73] The incidence of PPH returned to baseline after the drug was removed from the market. In the early 1990s, an association between fenfluramine use and PPH was established.[74] Shortly thereafter, the International Primary Pulmonary Hypertension Study Group investigated the potential role of anorexic agents in causing PPH.[72] Included in this multinational case-control study were 95 patients with pulmonary hypertension and 355 controls from general practices, matched for gender and age. The use of anorexic agents, primarily fenfluramine and dexfenfluramine, within the last year was associated with an increased risk of PPH with an odds ratio of 10:1. When anorexic drugs were used for a total of more than 3 months, the odds ratio increased to 23:1.

In a 12-year observational study, 62 patients with fenfluramine associated PPH were compared with 125 sex-matched patients with PPH unrelated to the use of fenfluramine derivatives. In most of the cases (81%), fenfluramine derivatives were used for at least 3 months. The time frame between the initiation of the therapy and the onset of dyspnea ranged from 27 days to 23 years. Both patients with fenfluramine-associated PPH and the control group had similar levels of New York Heart Association functional class and symptoms as well as an overall survival rate of 50% in 3 years.[75]

The mechanism by which anorexic agents cause PPH is unknown. Studies have shown that fenfluramine, dexfenfluramine, and aminorex inhibit potassium channels in isolated pulmonary artery smooth muscle cells in rats, which results in vasoconstriction. Potassium channel activity is altered in pulmonary artery smooth muscle cells obtained from patients with PPH, leading to speculation that anorexic agents may cause vasoconstriction followed by vascular growth and remodeling.[70] Another potential mechanism involves serotonin, which has been found in increased levels in patients with PPH.[70] Serotonin can be stored in platelets when serotonin plasma concentration is high. Serotonin acts as a pulmonary vasoconstrictor when it is released from the platelets.[71]

Patients with PPH associated with anorexic use may experience a considerable improvement in their condition or possibly even remission within 1 to 3 months following discontinuation of the drug.[71,76] Pharmacologic agents used in the treatment of PPH include high-dose calcium channel blockers and anticoagulants.[69] Epoprostenol, also known as *prostacyclin*, a strong vasodilator of all vascular beds, was approved for the long-term therapy of PPH in 1995.[77] Additionally, lung and heart-lung transplantations have played a role in the treatment of PPH. However, the 4-year survival rate is less than 60% in PPH patients receiving any transplant.[77]

In September 1997, the FDA requested the manufacturers of fenfluramine and dexfenfluramine to voluntarily withdraw their products from the market. This was done following case reports of valvular heart disease in patients taking either medication as monotherapy or in combination with another anorexic agent, phentermine. Because no association has been found between phentermine alone and valvular heart disease, it is still available. Isolated case reports of PPH and phentermine monotherapy have been published,[78,79] but present data do not support an association. Although fenfluramine and phentermine were both approved by FDA to be used as anorectic agents, the combination therapy, "fen-phen," was never approved.

MISCELLANEOUS PULMONARY TOXICITY

Drugs may produce serious pulmonary toxicity as part of a more generalized disorder. The pleural thickening, effusions, and fibrosis that occur as an extension of the retroperitoneal fibrotic reactions of methysergide and practolol or as part of a drug-induced lupus syndrome are the most common examples (Table 29–8).

Methysergide therapy for prophylaxis of poorly controlled migraine headache occasionally results in pulmonary toxicity associated with pleural effusions. The patients develop pleural pain, dyspnea, and fever. Chest radiography reveals a uniform hazy shadowing over the lower lung fields, and a loud pleural rub is heard on auscultation.[6] The mechanism is unknown, and most patients improve with discontinuation of the drug. Pleural and pulmonary fibrosis has been reported in one patient taking pindolol, a β-blocker structurally similar to practolol, an agent known to produce fibrosis.[51] Acute pleuritis with pleural effusions and fibrosis is a prominent manifestation of drug-induced lupus syndrome. Procainamide is associated with the largest number of pulmonary reactions, with 46% of patients with the lupus syndrome developing pulmonary complications.[6] Symptoms include pleuritic pain and fever with muscle and joint pain. Chest radiographs show bilateral pleural effusions

TABLE 29–8. Drugs That May Induce Pleural Effusions and Fibrosis

Idiopathic	
Methysergide	F[a]
Practolol	F
Pindolol	R
Methotrexate	R
Nitrofurantoin	R
Owing to Drug-Induced Lupus Syndrome	
Procainamide	F
Hydralazine	F
Isoniazid	R
Phenytoin	R
Mephenytoin	R
Griseofulvin	R
Trimethadione	R
Sulfonamides	R
Phenylbutazone	R
Streptomycin	R
Ethosuximide	R
Tetracycline	R
Pseudolymphoma Syndrome	
Cyclosporine	R
Phenytoin	R

[a]Relative frequency of reactions: F = frequent; I = infrequent; R = rare.

and linear atelectasis. Patients have a positive antinuclear antibody (ANA) test. Symptoms usually resolve within 6 weeks of drug withdrawal.[6]

Hydralazine is the next most common cause of lupus syndrome. Most patients who develop pleuropulmonary manifestations have antecedent symptoms of generalized lupus.[6] Other drugs that produce the lupus syndrome include isoniazid and phenytoin. Phenytoin also can produce hilar lymphadenopathy as part of a generalized pseudolymphoma or lymphadenopathy syndrome.[6]

MONITORING THERAPEUTIC OUTCOMES

Monitoring for drug-induced pulmonary diseases consists primarily of having a high index of suspicion that a particular syndrome may be drug-induced. Most hypersensitivity or allergic reactions (bronchospasm) occur rapidly, within the first 2 weeks of therapy with the offending agent and reverse rapidly with appropriate therapy (e.g., withdrawal of the offending agent, administration of corticosteroids and bronchodilators). Loeffler's syndrome and acute pulmonary edema syndromes also improve rapidly in 1 to 2 days for the dyspnea. However, some residual defect in diffusion capacity and roentgenogram may persist for a few weeks. It is probably unnecessary to do follow-up spirometry or diffusion capacity in these patients unless there is some concern that the syndrome will progress to pulmonary fibrosis (through use of bleomycin or nitrofurantoin).

The routine monitoring of patients receiving known pulmonary toxins with dose-dependent toxicity such as amiodarone, bleomycin, or carmustine is still controversial. For chronic fibrosis, the DLCO is the most sensitive test and may be useful in patients receiving bleomycin for detecting and preventing further deterioration of lung function with continued administration. Carmustine lung toxicity may be delayed up to 10 years following administration, and routine monitoring has not proven preventive. Monitoring patients receiving amiodarone in doses greater than 400 mg daily every 4 to 6 months may prove useful in detecting early disease that requires lowering the amiodarone dose or stopping the drug. Because there is no evidence of a cumulative dose effect, once it has been established that a patient can tolerate the elevated dose, continued routine monitoring past the first year is unnecessary.

REFERENCES

1. Martys CR. Adverse reactions to drugs in general practice. Br Med J 1979;2:1194–1197.
2. Kramer MS, Hutchinson TA, Flegel KM, et al. Adverse drug reactions in general pediatric outpatients. J Pediatr 1985;106:305–310.
3. Levy M, Kewitz H, Altwein W, et al. Hospital admissions due to adverse drug reactions: A comparative study from Jerusalem and Berlin. Eur J Clin Pharmacol 1980;17:25–31.
4. Shapiro S, Slone D, Lewis GP, et al. Fatal drug reactions among medical inpatients. JAMA 1971;216:467–472.
5. Porter J, Jick H. Drug-related deaths among medical inpatients. JAMA 1977;237:879–881.
6. Brewis RAL. Respiratory disorders. In: Davies DM, ed. Textbook of Adverse Drug Reactions, 2d ed. New York, Oxford University Press, 1981:154–178.
7. Hansen-Flaschen J, Cowen J, Raps EC. Neuromuscular blockade in the intensive care unit: More than we bargained for. Am Rev Respir Dis 1993;147:234–236.
8. Lieu F, Powers SK, Herb RA, et al. Exercise and glucocorticoid-induced diaphragmatic myopathy. J Appl Physiol 1993;75:763–771.
9. Dekhuijzen PNR, Gayan-Ramirez G, de Bock V, et al. Triamcinolone and prednisolone affect contractile properties and histopathology of rat diaphragm differently. J Clin Invest 1993;92:1534–1542.
10. Decramer M, Lacquet LM, Fagard R, et al. Corticosteroids contribute to muscle weakness in chronic airflow obstruction. Am J Respir Crit Care Med 1994;150:11–16.
11. Fisher HK. Drug-induced asthma syndromes. In: Weiss EB, Segal MS, Stein M, eds. Bronchial Asthma: Mechanisms and Therapeutics, 3d ed. Boston, Little, Brown, 1993:1154–1179.
12. Settipane GA. Aspirin and allergic diseases: A review. Am J Med 1983;74(Suppl 6a):102–109.
13. Stevenson DD. Diagnosis, prevention, and treatment of adverse reactions to aspirin and nonsteroidal anti-inflammatory drugs. J Allergy Clin Immunol 1984;74:617–622.
14. Szczeklik A, Gryglewski RJ. Asthma and anti-inflammatory drugs: Mechanisms and clinical patterns. Drugs 1983;25:533–543.
15. Matsuse H, Shimoda T, Matsua N, et al. Aspirin-induced asthma as a risk factor for asthma mortality. J Asthma 1997;34:314–317.
16. Dahlen B, Melillo G. Inhalation challenge in ASA-induced asthma. Respir Med 1998;92:378–384.
17. Milewski M, Mastalerz L, Nizankowska E, et al. Nasal provocation test with lysine-aspirin for diagnosis of aspirin-sensitive asthma. J Allergy Clin Immunol 1998;101:581–586.
18. Dahlen B, Zetterstrom O. Comparison of bronchial and per oral provocation with aspirin in aspirin-sensitive asthmatics. Eur Respir J 1990;3:527–534.
19. Lee TH. Mechanism of bronchospasm in aspirin-sensitive asthma. Am Rev Respir Dis 1993;148:1442–1443.
20. Mathison DA, Stevenson DD, Simon RA. Precipitating factors in asthma: Aspirin, sulfites, and other drugs and chemicals. Chest 1985; 87(Suppl):50–54.
21. American Academy of Pediatrics, Committee on Drugs. "Inactive" ingredients in pharmaceutical products: Update. Pediatrics 1997;99:268–278.
22. Israel E, Fischer A, Rosenberg M, et al. The pivotal role of 5-lipoxygenase products in the reaction of aspirin-sensitive asthmatics to aspirin. Am Rev Respir Dis 1993;148:1447–1451.
23. Paul JD, Simon RA, Daffern PJ, et al. Lack of effect of the 5-lipoxygenase inhibitor zileuton in blocking oral aspirin challenges in aspirin-sensitive asthmatics. Ann Allergy Asthma Immunol 2000;85:40–45.
24. Stevenson DD, Simon RA, Mathison DA, Christiansen SC. Montelukast is only partially effective in inhibiting aspirin response in aspirin-sensitive asthmatics. Ann Allergy Asthma Immunol 2000;85:477–482.
25. Menendez R, Venzor J, Ortiz G. Failure of zafirlukast to prevent ibuprofen-induced anaphylaxis. Ann Allergy Asthma Immunol 1998;80:225–226.
26. Robuschi M, Gambaro G, Setini P, et al. Attenuation of aspirin-induced bronchoconstriction by sodium cromoglycate and nedocromil sodium. Am J Respir Crit Care Med 1997;155:1461–1464.
27. Riddell JG, Shanks RG. Effects of betaxolol, propranolol, and atenolol on isoproterenol-induced β-adrenoceptor responses. Clin Pharmacol Ther 1985;38:554–559.
28. Hauck RW, Schulz CH, Emslander HP, Bohm M. Pharmacological actions of the selective and non-selective β-adrenoeceptor antagonists celiprolol, bisoprolol and propranolol on human bronchi. Br J Pharmacol 1994;113:1043–1049.
29. Fraunfeder FT, Barker AF. Respiratory effects of timolol. N Engl J Med 1984;311:1441.
30. Dunn TL, Gerber MJ, Shen AS, et al. The effect of topical ophthalmic instillation of timolol and betaxolol on lung function in asthmatic subjects. Am Rev Respir Dis 1986;133:264–268.
31. ADRAC. Systemic adverse reactions with betaxolol eye drops. Med J Aust 1995;162:84.
32. Simon RA. Update on sulfite sensitivity. Allergy 1998;53:78–79.
33. Anibarro B, Caballero T, Garcia-Ara C, et al. Asthma with sulfite intolerance in children: A blocking study with cyanocobalamine. J Allergy Clin Immunol 1992;90:103–109.
34. Beasley R, Rafferty P, Holgate ST. Adverse reactions to the nondrug constituents of nebulizer solutions. Br J Clin Pharmacol 1988;25:283–287.

35. Zhang YG, Wright WJ, Tam WK, et al. Effect of inhaled preservatives on asthmatic subjects: II. Benzalkonium chloride. Am Rev Respir Dis 1990;141:1405–1408.
36. Beasley R, Fishwick, D, Miles JF, et al. Preservatives in nebulizer solutions: Risks without benefit. Pharmacotherapy 1998;18:130–139.
37. Asmus MJ, Barros MD, Liang J, et al. Pulmonary function response to EDTA, an additive in nebulized bronchodilators. J Allergy Clin Immunol 2001;107:68–72.
38. Greenberger PA. Contrast media reactions. J Allergy Clin Immunol 1984;74:600–605.
39. Tilles SA. Occupational latex allergy: Controversies in diagnosis and prognosis. Ann Allergy Asthma Immunol 1999;83;640–644.
40. Yunginger JW. Natural rubber latex allergy. In: Middleton E Jr, Reed CE, Ellis EF, et al., eds. Allergy Principles and Practice, 5th ed. St. Louis, Mosby, 1998;1073–1078.
41. Poley GE, Slater JE. Latex allergy. J Allergy Clin Immunol 2000;105:1054–1162.
42. Luque CA, Ortiz MV. Treatment of ACE inhibitor-induced cough. Pharmacotherapy 1999;19:804–810.
43. Sebastian JL, McKinney WP, Kaufman J, et al. Angiotensin-converting enzyme inhibitors and cough: Prevalence in an outpatient medical clinic population. Chest 1991;99:36–39.
44. Simon SR, Black HR, Moser M, Berland WE. Cough and ACE inhibitors. Arch Intern Med 1992;152:1698–1700.
45. Israili ZH, Hall WD. Cough and angioneurotic edema associated with angiotensin-converting enzyme inhibitor therapy: A review of the literature and pathophysiology. Ann Intern Med 1992;117:234–242.
46. Pylypchuk GB. ACE inhibitor-versus angiotensin II blocker-induced cough and angioedema. Ann Pharmacother 1998;32:1060–1066.
47. Kaufman J, Casanova JE, Riendl P, et al. Bronchial hyperreactivity and cough due to angiotensin-converting enzyme inhibitors. Chest 1989;95:544–548.
48. Malini PL, Strocchi E, Zanardi M, et al. Thromboxane antagonism and cough induced by angiotensin-converting-enzyme inhibitor. Lancet 1997;350:15–18.
49. Allen TL, Gora-Harper ML. Cromolyn sodium for ACE inhibitor–induced cough. Ann Pharmacother 1997;31:773–775.
50. Dicpinigaitis PV, Thomas SA, Sherman MB, et al. Losartan-induced bronchospasm. J Allergy Clin Immunol 1996;98:1128–1130.
51. Cooper JAD, White DA, Matthay RA. Drug-induced pulmonary disease: 2. Noncytotoxic drugs. Am Rev Respir Dis 1986;133:488–505.
52. Henderson CA, Reynolds, JE. Acute pulmonary edema in a young male after intravenous nalmefene. Anesth Analg 1997;84:218–219.
53. Copper JA Jr. Drug-induced lung disease. Adv Intern Med 1997;42:231–268.
54. Obermiller T, Lakshminarayan S. Drug-induced hypersensitivity reactions in the lung. Immunol Allergy Clin North Am 1991;11:575–594.
55. Frank L, Massaro D. Oxygen toxicity. Am J Med 1980;69:117–126.
56. Jackson RM. Pulmonary oxygen toxicity. Chest 1985;88:900–905.
57. Cooper JAD, White DA, Matthay RA. State of the art: Drug-induced pulmonary disease: 1. Cytotoxic drugs. Am Rev Respir Dis 1986;133:321–340.
58. Kehrer JP, Kacew S. Systematically applied chemicals that damage lung tissue. Toxicology 1985;35:251–293.
59. Clark JG, Hansen JA, Hertz MI, et al. Idiopathic pneumonia syndrome after bone marrow transplantation. Am Rev Respir Dis 1993;147:1601–1606.
60. Wiedemann HP. Toward an understanding of idiopathic pneumonia syndrome after bone marrow transplantation. Crit Care Med 1999;27:2040–2041.
61. Quabeck K. The lung as a critical organ in marrow transplantation. Bone Marrow Transplant 1994;14:S19–S28.
62. O'Driscoll BR, Hasleton PS, Taylor PM, et al. Active lung fibrosis up to 17 years after chemotherapy with carmustine (BCNU) in childhood. N Engl J Med 1990;323:378–382.
63. Rubio C, Hill ME, Milan S, et al. Idiopathic pneumonia syndrome after high-dose chemotherapy for relapsed Hodgkin's disease. Br J Cancer 1997;75:1044–1048.
64. Jantz MA, Sahn SA. Corticosteroids in acute respiratory failure. Am J Respir Crit Care Med 1999;160:1079–1100.
65. Lynch JP, McCune WJ. Immunosuppressive and cytotoxic pharmacotherapy for pulmonary disorders. Am J Crit Care Med 1997;155:395–420.
66. Rakita L, Sobol SM, Mostow N, et al. Amiodarone pulmonary toxicity. Am Heart J 1983;106:906–914.
67. Jessurun GAJ, Boersma WG, Crijns HJGM. Amiodarone-induced pulmonary toxicity: Predisposing factors, clinical symptoms and treatment. Drug Safety 1998;18:339–344.
68. Gleadhill IC, Wise RA, Schonfeld SA, et al. Serial lung-function testing in patients treated with amiodarone: A prospective study. Am J Med 1989;86:4–10.
69. Rubin LJ. Primary pulmonary hypertension. N Engl J Med 1997; 336:111–117.
70. McCann UD, Seiden LS, Rubin LJ, Ricaurte GA. Brain serotonin neurotoxicity and primary pulmonary hypertension from fenfluramine and dexfenfluramine: A systematic review of the evidence. JAMA 1997;278;666–672.
71. Vivero LE, Anderson PO, Clark RF. Pharmacology in emergency medicine: A close look at fenfluramine and dexfenfluramine. J Emerg Med 1998;16:197–295.
72. Abenhaim L, Moride Y, Brenot F, et al. Appetite-suppressant drugs and the risk of primary pulmonary hypertension. N Engl J Med 1996;335:609–616.
73. Gurtner HP. Aminorex and pulmonary hypertension: A review. Cor Vasa 1985;27:160–171.
74. Brenot F, Herve P, Petitpretz P, et al. Primary pulmonary hypertension and fenfluramine use. Br Heart J 1993;70:537–541.
75. Simonneau G, Fartoukh M, Sitbon O, et al. Primary pulmonary hypertension associated with the use of fenfluramine derivatives. Chest 1998;114:195S–199S.
76. Nall KC, Rubin LJ, Lipskind S, Sennesh JD. Reversible pulmonary hypertension associated with anorexigen use. Am J Med 1991;91:97–99.
77. Bever KA, Perry PJ. Dexfenfluramine hydrochloride: An anorexigenic agent. Am J Health Syst Pharm 1997;54:2059–2072.
78. Heuer L, Benoit W, Heydrich D. Diagnostic error: Pulmonary hypertension caused by an appetite suppressant (Mirapront). Chir Praxis 1978;23:497–504.
79. Schnabel KF, Schultz V, Busch S, Just H. Drug-induced primary vascular pulmonary hypertension. Med Welt (Stuttgart) 1976;27:1300–1303.

30

Cystic Fibrosis

John A. Bosso and Gary Milavetz

Cystic fibrosis is the most common lethal, genetically inherited disease affecting the Caucasian population. It is a disease mainly involving the exocrine glands and thus affects a number of organs or organ systems (Table 30–1). The more common manifestations of the disease involve the gastrointestinal and pulmonary systems, with most of the observed morbidity and mortality associated with the latter. Most pathology is a result of production of viscous secretions. The underlying disorder leading to this pathophysiology is a chloride transport channel defect at the secretory epithelial cell level. The protean nature of the disease dictates that care be multidisciplinary with a wide variety of therapeutic interventions.

EPIDEMIOLOGY

Cystic fibrosis is inherited through an autosomal (Mendelian) recessive genetic mode. This implies that each parent must be at least a carrier (heterozygous) for the trait, and with such a couple, each child would have a one-in-four chance of having the disease, a one-in-two chance of being a carrier, and a one-in-four chance of being normal (having neither the disease nor the trait). The incidence of cystic fibrosis is greatest in the Caucasian population, with a rate of 1 in 2000 live births in the United States.[1] The incidence of the trait (carrier state) in this group is about 5%. The frequency of the disease is considerably less in other races, occurring in 1 in 17,000 blacks and about 1 in 90,000 Asians.[2]

After years of intensive research, the cystic fibrosis gene was discovered and cloned.[3–5] The protein [cystic fibrosis transmembrane regulator (CFTR)] encoded by this gene, which is on the long arm of chromosome 7, is a membrane protein that represents a channel involved in the transport of electrolytes and water. The most common genetic mutation associated with cystic fibrosis involves a 3-base-pair deletion at position 508,[3–5] but over 700 cystic fibrosis–associated mutations within the gene have been described. The common mutation is referred to as the ΔF_{508} allele and is present in about 70% of patients. The possible mutations have been divided into four classes: I—defective protein production; II—defective protein processing; III—defective regulation; and IV—defective conduction.[6] Patients who are homozygous for the ΔF_{508} mutation, which falls into class II, tend to be diagnosed at an earlier age, owing to earlier onset of airway disease, and have a greater frequency of pancreatic insufficiency (99% versus 72% in heterozygotes and 36% in patients with other genotypes).[7,8]

PATHOPHYSIOLOGY

Cystic fibrosis is a disease of secretory epithelial cells or tissues involved with the transport of chloride, sodium, and water into and out of the blood. In the normal state, there is a net chloride transport out of blood with sodium and water following this flux. This net secretion is activated or affected by hormones or neurotransmitters such as protein kinases and further involves intracellular second messengers such as cyclic adenosine 3′,5′-monophosphate (cAMP) or calcium.[9] It is an apical membrane cAMP-stimulated chloride channel where activity is apparently affected in cystic fibrosis, leading to a decrease in secretion of chloride and water and increased absorption of sodium (Fig. 30–1). ΔF_{508}-homozygous individuals have this abnormal chloride channel in the cells of several exocrine organs, including pancreatic and hepatobiliary ducts, microvilli of the gastrointestinal tract, and the lungs. In pulmonary epithelial cells, there also appears to be excessive absorption of sodium. These phenomena then lead to the thick, dehydrated secretions or mucus, depending on the organ. These secretions can block pancreatic and hepatobiliary exocrine outflow and also accumulate in and obstruct the airways.

GASTROINTESTINAL TRACT

Involvement of the gastrointestinal tract in cystic fibrosis is a result of both the increased viscosity of mucus secretions and a relative deficiency of pancreatic digestive enzymes. In 10% to 16% of cystic fibrosis patients, the first gastrointestinal manifestation of the disease is an intestinal obstruction evident shortly after birth and is known as *meconium ileus.* Again, the basic electrolyte transport defect is involved, and this complication is caused by an inability of these patients to evacuate the abnormally viscid meconium. A similar condition, known as *distal intestinal obstruction syndrome* or *meconium ileus equivalent,* occurs in older cystic fibrosis patients; it is also thought to result from abnormally viscous gastrointestinal secretions and fecal impaction often following ingestion of fatty meals or nonadherence with pancreatic enzyme therapy. Other intestinal complications include intussusception, volvulus, gastroesophageal reflux, atresia, perforation, giant cystic meconium peritonitis, and rectal prolapse.

A deficiency of pancreatic digestive enzymes (pancreatic achylia) is present with most genotypes and thus is present in 85% of patients. Pancreatic lesions including fibrosis, fatty replacement, and cyst formation are secondary to obstruction of small pancreatic ducts by thickened secretions and cellular debris. Inspissated eosinophilic material is also present in acini and ductules. As a result, pancreatic secretions are viscous and low in volume and in concentrations of pancreatic enzymes and bicarbonate. Affected enzyme concentrations include trypsin, chymotrypsin, carboxypeptidase, amylase, and lipase. This leads to a maldigestion of ingested nutrients, including fats and protein. Increased fecal loss of bile acids (binding to undigested fecal fat decreases enterohepatic recycling) also contributes to fat maldigestion.

Because of the lipase deficiency, fat-soluble vitamin (A, D, E, and K) deficiencies sometimes occur. Whether lipase is involved in fat soluble vitamin absorption directly (e.g., in micelle formation) or indirectly, with continuing steatorrhea resulting in abnormally high losses of these nutrients in the feces, is unclear. Vitamin B_{12} and zinc deficiencies also can occur as a result of the pancreatic enzyme deficiency. Although pancreatic involvement is predominantly exocrine in nature, insulin deficiency/glucose intolerance occurs in many older

TABLE 30–1. Organ Involvement in Cystic Fibrosis

Organ System/Organ	Abnormality	Consequence
Gastrointestinal		
Pancreas	Digestive enzyme deficiency	Maldigestion
		Malnutrition
	Insulin deficiency	Glucose intolerance
Intestines	Viscous secretions	Obstruction
Liver	Biliary cirrhosis/fatty infiltration	Portal hypertension/ esophageal varices
Pulmonary	Viscous secretions	Chronic obstruction
	Infection	Endobronchial infection
Sweat glands	Failure to reabsorb sodium	Hyponatremia
Reproductive	Obstruction of epididymis, vas deferens, and seminal vesicles	Aspermia
	Viscous cervical mucus	Decreased fertility
Hematologic	Chronic disease?	Anemia
Bone and joint	Unknown	Arthritis, osteopenia

cystic fibrosis patients. The carbohydrate intolerance observed is characterized by low insulin concentrations and enhanced peripheral sensitivity to insulin but not the presence of islet cell or anti-insulin antibodies nor by ketosis common to type 1 diabetes. This complication involves an increase in the number of insulin receptors with decreased affinity for insulin. Despite a concomitantly increased tissue affinity for insulin, 8% of cystic fibrosis children over 12 years of age require insulin therapy.

The liver is sometimes involved in cystic fibrosis. Biliary cirrhosis secondary to bile duct obstruction occurs in as many as 18% of patients, whereas fatty infiltration occurs in about 30% of patients in a pattern unrelated to nutritional status. Bile duct obstruction occurs with inspissated mucus and may lead to focal or multilobar cirrhosis.[10] Such hepatic involvement, which can occur at any age, is more common as the cystic fibrosis life span increases and can lead to portal hypertension and thus bleeding esophageal varices and hypersplenism. The most common laboratory abnormality associated with hepatic involvement is elevated serum alkaline phosphatase (hepatic isoenzyme).

PULMONARY SYSTEM

Manifestations within this organ system result from the accumulation of viscous mucus in the small airways. There are two important consequences of this pulmonary condition: obstruction and infection/inflammation. Obstruction of both small and large airways by thick mucus results in air trapping, bronchiectasis, and atelectasis, resulting in a chronic obstructive pulmonary disease–like phenomenon. Thus a progression of lung disease from small airways obstruction to large airways or generalized obstruction and finally to a restrictive lung disease component is evident. Hyperinflation or dilation of the airspaces is the common lesion. Further, the persistent mucus is an excellent growth medium for microorganisms, and pulmonary infections are commonplace. Although systemic host defenses appear normal in cystic fibrosis, recent evidence suggests that local defenses in the airways (i.e., human β-defensin) are inhibited by the high salt concentrations present in respiratory secretions of affected patients[11] and that abnormal CFTR itself may contribute to susceptibility to infection with *Pseudomonas aeruginosa.*[12] Although bacterial infection is thought to be the major factor in this aspect of the respiratory disease, it is clear that viruses and other nonbacterial pathogens play an important pathologic role as well.[13–15] Environmental factors, such as exposure to tobacco smoke, also contribute.[16] The three most common bacterial pathogens isolated from the respiratory secretions (sputum) of cystic fibrosis patients are *Staphylococcus aureus, P. aeruginosa,* and *Hemophilus influenzae,* with *P. aeruginosa* predominating throughout life. *Proteus* and *Klebsiella* species and *Stenotrophomonas maltophilia* are observed much less frequently. Mucoid strains (alginate producers) of *P. aeruginosa* commonly observed in cystic fibrosis may be particularly resistant to antibiotics,[17] as are nonmotile forms. The isolation of *Burkholderia cepacia* from the sputum of cystic fibrosis patients has become more common at some cystic fibrosis centers. The significance of the presence of this highly contagious organism varies from one patient to the next. Three fairly distinct syndromes associated with this *B. cepacia* have been described, these being asymptomatic colonization, chronic deterioration with intermittent fever and weight loss, and rapid, usually fatal deterioration.[18] The nature of the initially cultured oropharyngeal flora in patients less than 2 years of age has prognostic significance. The finding of *P. aeruginosa* or *P. aeruginosa* plus *S. aureus* in initial cultures appears related to increased morbidity and mortality, respectively.[19]

The presence of the preceding bacteria is responsible for a portion of the destructive changes to the lungs in cystic fibrosis owing to both direct damage from bacterial toxins and the body's immune reaction to the presence of these same bacteria. For example, *P. aeruginosa,* which elaborates a number of extracellular toxins, proteases, hemolysins, and exopolysaccharides, may be responsible for direct or indirect pulmonary damage, increases mucin production in respiratory epithelium, and stimulates the production of immune complexes (IgG and IgM), which also may contribute to local damage. Elevated levels of such mediators as granulocyte elastase, tumor necrosis factor-α, interleukin-1 and -2, and related complexes with associated inhibitors have been well documented in cystic fibrosis patients. One inflammatory mediator that clearly contributes to pulmonary pathophysiology is neutrophil elastase. Present in excess, it overwhelms and neutralizes native antiproteases [α_1-antitrypsin and secretory leukocyte protease inhibitor (SLPI)], destroys structural fibers, and inhibits complement-mediated phagocytosis and antipseudomonal antibodies. Combined with other inflammatory mediators, a self-sustaining, vicious cycle leading to progressive and often permanent tissue damage is established. The neutrophil influx that is part of this cycle results in release of neutrophil-derived DNA, which is thought to contribute to sputum viscosity. The occasional presence of *Aspergillus fumagatus* in the sputum of these patients also may contribute to the pulmonary pathology because it can induce a steroid-responsive allergic reaction.

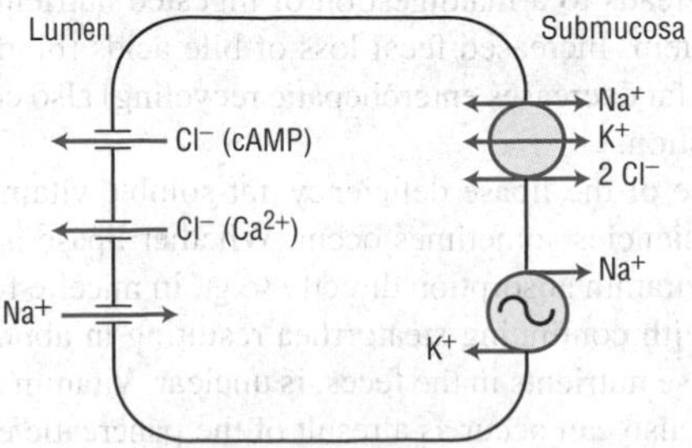

FIGURE 30–1. Electrolyte transport in the airway epithelial cell. CFTR is the cyclic-3′,5′-AMP (cAMP)-dependent chloride channel.

The major consequence of these pulmonary processes is a decrease in gas exchange by the lungs. The challenge of moving air into and out of such congested airways often requires the use of accessory muscles, resulting in an increased anteroposterior chest diameter (also referred to as *barrel chest*), a flattened diaphragm, and pulmonary hypertension. The increased work of breathing in these patients produces a relative exercise intolerance and increased resting energy expenditure. Hemoptysis secondary to bronchiectasis occurs but is seldom massive. Other respiratory complications include gastroesophageal reflux, pneumothorax, and right-sided heart failure (cor pulmonale) secondary to the pulmonary hypertension. Although seldom overt clinically, findings such as right ventricular hypertrophy, increased heart weight, and right atrial and right ventricular chamber dilatation are usually present at autopsy. Digital clubbing, a common finding in cystic fibrosis as well as other chronic pulmonary conditions, may be related to chronic hypoxia.

The upper respiratory tract is also involved, and chronic rhinitis is common. Sinusitis and nasal polyposis occur in 90% and 50% of patients, respectively.[20] Sinusitis is chronic in character, and acute symptoms are unusual. Although its etiology is not entirely clear, sinusitis may result from obstruction of the sinus ducts, thus preventing drainage. The bacteria generally isolated in these cases include *P. aeruginosa, H. influenzae,* streptococci, and anaerobes. Usually, the same strain of *P. aeruginosa* found in the lungs is present in the upper airways (nasopharynx, sinuses), which may represent a reservoir for the pathogen. Symptomatic patients are often treated medically or surgically.

SWEAT GLANDS

The abnormally high concentrations of both sodium and chloride in the sweat of cystic fibrosis patients owing to defective salt reabsorption can result in the need for supplementary dietary intake of these electrolytes and forms the basis for the diagnosis of the disease. Sodium and chloride are not excreted in abnormally high concentrations by the sweat glands. Instead, there is a failure of the sweat ducts to reabsorb these electrolytes in a normal fashion, again owing to the chloride impermeability in the epithelial cells of the sweat ducts. Similar abnormalities are seen in the excretions of the salivary glands.

REPRODUCTIVE SYSTEM

Of males with cystic fibrosis, 95% are sterile because of obstruction of the epididymis, vas deferens, and seminal vesicles with resulting aspermia. There is late maturation of the reproductive system with delayed onset of puberty in both sexes. Females also have less than normal fertility owing to the production of abnormal cervical mucus. Menstrual irregularity and oligomenorrhea are also common. Nonetheless, owing to greater life expectancy in these patients, increasing numbers are becoming mothers. In these individuals, the course and tolerance of pregnancy are related to pregravid nutritional and pulmonary status.

HEMATOLOGIC SYSTEM

Anemia is observed in some cystic fibrosis patients despite chronic hypoxia. The apparent deficient erythroid response occurs, at least in part, from disturbances in erythropoietin regulation and iron availability (impaired gastrointestinal absorption). Despite the chronic hypoxia characteristic of cystic fibrosis, erythropoietin concentrations are normal or low. The condition is characterized by decreased hematocrit and serum ferritin, increased carboxyhemoglobin, and normal or low hemoglobin. Many patients have documented iron deficiency, the causes of which appear to include decreased dietary intake, malabsorption, and blood loss.

BONE AND JOINT

Arthritis occurs in cystic fibrosis patients and can take one of several forms.[21] This arthritis may be either mono- or polyarticular and usually is nondestructive. An episodic form is most common and may be due to immune complexes formed in response to the chronic pulmonary infections. Hypertrophic osteoarthropathy occurs in cystic fibrosis, as it does in association with other pulmonary diseases. The incidence of arthritis may be increasing as median survival age increases. Osteopenia and osteoporosis also occur with abnormally high frequency in adult cystic fibrosis patients. The causes of the resulting bone demineralization are multifactorial and include vitamin D malabsorption and decreased vitamin conversion (via sunlight), delayed puberty and endocrine development, poor nutrition, limited physical activity, and chronic acidosis.

CLINICAL PRESENTATION

The clinical findings of cystic fibrosis occur as direct consequences of the pathophysiologic processes described earlier. Thus the clinical findings can be subdivided conveniently by organ system.

GASTROINTESTINAL SYSTEM

Intestinal symptomatology is secondary to obstruction and maldigestion of nutrients. Obstruction, manifested as meconium ileus or distal intestinal obstruction syndrome, causes symptoms such as vomiting of bile-stained material, abdominal distension, and pain. Pain may be an especially prominent feature when obstruction results in intussusception.

The more frequent gastrointestinal clinical presentation is caused by maldigestion of ingested food, resulting in steatorrhea and malnutrition. Stools are characterized by their foul smell, bulk, greasy nature, and abnormally high number per day; they may precipitate rectal prolapse. The stool's high fat content results from the relative lipase deficiency. Perhaps the most significant consequence of maldigestion is malnutrition; cystic fibrosis children characteristically fall below age-related norms for both weight and height.

PULMONARY SYSTEM

The respiratory symptoms of cystic fibrosis are those of obstructive disease and pneumonia. Hypoxia with resulting cyanosis and digital clubbing are common. Likewise, labored breathing with retractions and resulting increased anteroposterior chest diameter, flattened diaphragm, and overaeration observed on chest roentgenogram are frequent findings.

A patient's respiratory status follows a cyclic pattern from a state of relative well-being to one of acute pulmonary deterioration, theoretically paralleling the course of the infectious process. Marked declines in pulmonary status (presumably secondary to infection) are referred to as *acute respiratory exacerbations* and generally are associated with symptoms of acute bacterial endobronchial infection. Thus fever, increased coughing, increased sputum production, change in sputum character (e.g., thicker, change in color), increased respiratory rate, dyspnea on exertion, increased oxygen requirements, and decreased exercise tolerance are commonly described. Symptoms of chronic sinusitis and nasal polyposis may include rhinorrhea, nasal obstruction, pain over affected sinuses, and disturbances of smell.

Concomitantly, laboratory tests of peripheral blood reveal an increased white blood cell count with increased polymorphonuclear leukocytes and immature forms consistent with acute infection. Tests of pulmonary function often demonstrate both acute and long-term changes in forced vital capacity (FVC), forced expiratory volume (FEV), and residual volume. Tests reflective of small airways function are more markedly affected as the pulmonary disease progresses. Arterial blood gases typically reveal hypoxia and hypercapnia.

OTHER SIGNS AND SYMPTOMS

The relative insulin deficiency observed in older cystic fibrosis patients is often asymptomatic and only detected on laboratory analysis of serum performed for other reasons. Symptomatic patients present as untreated cases of diabetes mellitus type 2. Cases of cor pulmonale usually are not evident clinically until signs of left-sided heart failure ensue. An enlargement of cardiac size often is noted on routine chest roentgenogram prior to that time, however. Signs and symptoms of anemia and arthritis with cystic fibrosis patients do not differ from those in other patients.

Although the abnormal loss of sodium and chloride in the sweat of cystic fibrosis patients seldom results in profound symptoms such as those of heat prostration, this phenomenon has formed the basis of some large-scale public awareness/screening programs owing to the resulting "salty" taste on the skin of affected patients.

DIAGNOSIS

Cystic fibrosis normally is diagnosed on the basis of an abnormal sweat test. Although diagnosis through chromosomal analysis is now possible, this test as well as others such as nasal cell potential difference are currently reserved for patients in whom results of sweat testing are unclear.[22] With the former, a sample of sweat is collected (usually with the use of pilocarpine iontophoresis), and the concentration of chloride is determined. A chloride concentration of 60 mEq/L or more is considered diagnostic, although values up to 80 mEq/L may be observed in non-cystic fibrosis adults. A number of other disorders, such as adrenal insufficiency and hypothyroidism, may be inconsistently associated with elevated sweat chloride concentrations but generally do not present a problem in the differential diagnosis of cystic fibrosis. Ninety-eight percent of cystic fibrosis patients will have a sweat chloride concentration of 60 mEq/L or greater. The remaining 2% will have sweat chloride concentrations between 50 and 60 mEq/L, and the test may have to be repeated one or more times to obtain definitive results. Nonetheless, the results of a sweat test are not necessarily proof positive of the presence or absence of cystic fibrosis. The presence of chronic obstructive respiratory disease, exocrine pancreatic insufficiency, and/or a positive family history of the disease help to confirm the diagnosis. The diagnosis is established in most patients by 7 months of age. Genetic (DNA) analysis may be used to diagnose the disease in utero or to detect heterozygotes (carriers) with obvious implications for genetic counseling. Although newborn screening is possible, more study of its potential benefits on long-term outcomes is needed before it receives an unqualified recommendation.[23]

COURSE

Cystic fibrosis is a heterogeneous disease in terms of initial presentation, organ involvement, and clinical course. Most patients are not diagnosed at birth. Only 16% of affected patients have meconium ileus, the value of neonatal screening programs have not been proven, and prenatal diagnosis is early in its implementation. Therefore, the average patient is diagnosed later in life based on a history of recurrent respiratory infections, steatorrhea, and/or failure to thrive. The median age at diagnosis is 7 months, and most patients are diagnosed by 12 years of age.[24]

The course of the disease after diagnosis varies markedly from one patient to the next. Some patients have a rapid downhill course based on early pulmonary involvement, whereas others suffer only from gastrointestinal complaints for many years. Although the expected life span of cystic fibrosis patients has increased to 25 to 30 years of age in the last two decades, some patients still die early in life secondary to a fulminant pulmonary process. Others, owing to minimal involvement and mild course, are not diagnosed until their second decade of life. The increased longevity now realized with early diagnosis and aggressive treatment has led to an increase in formerly unusual complications such as diabetes and hepatic disease. Two-year mortality rates above 50% are associated with a forced expiratory volume in 1 second (FEV_1) of less than 30% of predicted, Pa_{O_2} less than 50 mm Hg, or P_{CO_2} greater than 50 mm Hg.[25]

▶ TREATMENT: Cystic Fibrosis

DESIRED OUTCOME

The desired pharmacotherapeutic outcomes for cystic fibrosis are both long and short term. In the long term, one obviously wants to slow or halt the progression of the disease to allow normal growth and development. In the short term, acute problems must be dealt with. The ultimate goal of pharmacotherapy for the gastrointestinal involvement of cystic fibrosis is optimal nutrition. On a day-to-day basis, normal bowel habits and continued weight gain are desirable. Acute goals of therapy for the pulmonary component center around air movement and gas exchange. Thus antibiotic and bronchodilator/mucolytic therapy are geared toward treating the complications that compromise these functions. For an acute pulmonary exacerbation, return of pulmonary function to preexacerbation status is the central goal of therapy.

GENERAL APPROACH TO TREATMENT

The Cystic Fibrosis Foundation has published clinical guidelines for the diagnosis and care of cystic fibrosis patients, including applicable pharmacotherapy.[26] The following information is generally in agreement with those guidelines except that it may contain more current information. The interested reader is referred to that publication for more detail on the drug treatment of cystic fibrosis and its various complications.

GASTROINTESTINAL SYSTEM

The treatment of gastrointestinal involvement ultimately is aimed at correcting the nutritional deficit present in so many patients.[27] In addition to the pancreatic enzyme replacement and other drug therapy described below, nutritional supplementation is employed frequently. Nutritional interventions range from behavioral modification to nocturnal feedings via gastrostomies.[28]

Pancreatic Enzyme Supplementation

The backbone of gastrointestinal therapy in cystic fibrosis is pancreatic enzyme replacement or supplementation. The preferred products are microencapsulated pancreatic enzymes, although powders are marketed and are useful in patients unable to swallow capsules or to otherwise use the microencapsulated beads they contain. Microencapsulated products protect the contained enzymes from destruction by gastric acid and may be given in much lower doses than their predecessors, which were susceptible to acid breakdown. Most contemporary enzyme-replacement products vary mainly in enzyme content per capsule, with lipase content being the chief variable. Representative products and their contents are presented in Table 30–2. Infants normally are given 2000 to 4000 lipase units per 120 mL of formula or breast milk, which provides 450 to 900 lipase units per gram of ingested fat. In general, patients require 500 to 4000 lipase units per gram of ingested fat, with the average pediatric or adult patient requiring 1800 units per gram of fat. Enzymes also may be dosed based on weight, with an initial dose of 1000 lipase units being administered per kilogram of body weight per meal. One-half this amount is administered with snacks.

Before the introduction of microencapsulated enzyme products, various maneuvers were used to circumvent or overcome the problem of acid breakdown. The most obvious of these was to administer large quantities of enzyme product. Enteric-coated (microencapsulated) pancreatic enzymes have largely solved this problem. The occasional patient may yet require large quantities of even the microencapsulated enzyme product. Whether such difficulties are caused by residual acid breakdown or perhaps low pH in the upper small intestine (secondary to deficient bicarbonate excretion by the pancreas) resulting in a failure to dissolve the coating of the microencapsulated beads is unknown. Defective enteric coating on some generic brands also has been described and led to Food and Drug Administration (FDA) reclassification of these products, requiring biocquivalence data. Histamine H_2-receptor antagonists and omeprazole have been used to reduce the enzyme dose when residual acid breakdown of enzymes is suspected. Another possible maneuver is to administer both microencapulated and non-enteric-coated enzyme products (e.g., powder) concomitantly.

For patients who are unable to swallow capsules, the contents may be emptied into applesauce, jelly, or some other nonalkaline vehicle, provided that the patient does not chew the microencapsulated beads. Side effects of pancreatic enzyme products are uncommon. Perianal irritation resembling diaper rash may occur in infants fed excess quantities of enzyme powders. Hyperuricosuria also has been reported to occur secondary to pancreatic enzyme use, apparently related to their high purine content. Proximal colonic stricture (fibrosing colonopathy) is a dose-related side effect associated with lipase doses in excess of 24,000 units per kilogram per day.[29]

Vitamin Supplementation

Patients should receive two multivitamin tablets per day, which will provide adequate water-soluble vitamins along with reasonable amounts of vitamins D and K. While clinically evident fat-soluble vitamin deficiencies are unusual in patients taking adequate pancreatic enzymes and receiving a balanced diet, obvious vitamin K deficiency, manifested as bleeding diathesis, can occur. Demineralization of bone also has been described, and vitamin E deficiency has been related to neurologic dysfunction. Further, appropriate laboratory tests (serum carotene, vitamin E, and cholecalciferol concentrations) often will help document other deficiencies, leading to recommendations for additional supplementation of these vitamins. Water-miscibilized vitamin A, 4000 international units (IU) per day, and vitamin E, 100 to 400 IU/d, also should be administered either singly or in the form of a water-miscibilized combination product (containing vitamins A, D, E, and K). Vitamin K, in a dose of 5 mg twice weekly, should be given to patients with prolonged prothrombin times. It also should be noted that appropriately adjusted doses of fat-soluble preparations may be more

TABLE 30–2. Pancreatic Enzyme Products

		Enzyme Content (Units)			
Trade Name	Manufacturer	*Lipase*	*Protease*	*Amylase*	*Form*[a]
Cotazym	Organon	8000	30,000	30,000	C
Cotazym-S		5000	20,000	20,000	ECM
Creon	Reid-Rowell	8000	13,000	30,000	ECM
Ilozyme	Adria	11,000	30,000	30,000	T
Ku-Zyme	Schwarz Pharma	8000	30,000	30,000	C
Pancrease	McNeil	4000	25,000	20,000	ECM
Pancrease MT4		4000	12,000	12,000	ECM
Pancrease MT10		10,000	30,000	30,000	ECM
Pancrease MT16		16,000	48,000	48,000	ECM
Pancrelipase	Geneva	4000	25,000	20,000	ECM
Protilase	Rugby	4000	25,000	20,000	ECM
Ultrase MT12	Scandipharm	12,000	39,000	39,000	ECM
Ultrase MT20		20,000	65,000	65,000	ECM
Ultrase MT24		24,000	78,000	78,000	ECM
Viokase	Robins	8000	30,000	30,000	T
Viokase		16,800	70,000	70,000	P[b]
Zymase	Organon	12,000	24,000	24,000	ECM

[a]Dosage form: C = capsule; ECM = enteric-coated microspheres or beads; T = tablet; P = powder.
[b]Viokase powder, units of enzymes per 700 mg.

cost-effective than their water-miscible counterparts (e.g., 800 IU fat-soluble vitamin E versus 200 IU water-miscible vitamin E).[30]

Treating Meconium Ileus and Distal Intestinal Obstruction Syndrome

The treatment of meconium ileus or distal intestinal obstruction syndrome sometimes can be limited to the use of enemas with isoosmolar contrast material. Unfortunately, surgery (bowel resection and primary anastomosis) is sometimes necessary to treat this condition and prevent its complications. Distal intestinal obstruction syndrome usually responds to management by oral administration of electrolyte lavage solutions. The adequacy of enzyme dosage should be reassessed in the face of distal intestinal obstruction.

Prevention and Treatment of Cirrhosis

Ursodeoxycholic acid, a bile acid with choleretic properties, has been shown to produce morphologic and functional improvement in affected patients with long-term treatment. The effects are dose-related and 15–20 mg/kg per day has been used, sometimes in combination with taurine supplementation.[31,32]

CARDIOVASCULAR SYSTEM

Various modalities have been used in attempts to treat the pulmonary hypertension and secondary cor pulmonale of cystic fibrosis. These treatments, which include the use of vasodilators, inotropic agents, and diuretics, have all resulted in limited and transient effects. This is most likely due to the fact that none of these modes of therapy addresses the underlying cause of the cor pulmonale, namely, hypoxia. Likewise, supplemental (often nocturnal) oxygen treatment also has failed to affect mortality rates or disease progression, although it does appear to prevent exercise-induced oxygen desaturation as well as that occurring with sleep. Thus the most beneficial approach may be to attempt to improve oxygenation with aggressive pulmonary therapy.

PULMONARY SYSTEM

Management of the pulmonary component of cystic fibrosis can be broken down into two areas: respiratory therapy, including anti-inflammatory therapy, and anti-infective therapy.[33]

Respiratory Therapy

The cornerstone of pulmonary therapy is percussion and postural drainage, which aids in the clearance of pulmonary mucus and is performed once or twice daily in "healthy" patients and as often as five times daily or more during an acute pulmonary exacerbation. New flutter devices also appear to be useful adjuncts in this regard. Percussion often is preceded by nebulizer therapy during which nebulized sterile water or 0.9% sodium chloride solution is breathed to liquefy pulmonary secretions. Bronchodilators and/or mucolytic agents (e.g., *N*-acetylcysteine; Mucomyst, Mead Johnson) may be added to the nebulizer solution to prevent bronchospasm and further liquefy pulmonary secretions, respectively. Although the effects of bronchodilators administered by inhalation are readily demonstrated with pulmonary function tests, those of mucolytic agents are not as obvious, and a number of attempts to demonstrate the effects of inhaled *N*-acetylcysteine have been unsuccessful. Moreover, many patients prefer not to use *N*-acetylcysteine because of its unpleasant taste and odor and because it often induces bronchospasm. Normal saline and sodium bicarbonate solution also are administered commonly by aerosol as aids to sputum expectoration, but again, documentation of efficacy is elusive.

Recombinant human DNase has been approved for use in cystic fibrosis. When given by inhalation (2.5 mg once or twice daily), rhDNase reduces the viscosity of cystic fibrosis sputum and leads to statistically significant, though modest, improvement in indices of pulmonary function.[34] Importantly, rhDNase use may lower the incidence (or lengthen the time between) respiratory exacerbations and thus improve quality of life and may indirectly decrease the overall costs of care in patients with mild to moderate disease. Should these outcomes be borne out in further long-term studies, the cost of this therapy may well be justified for some patients.

In attempts to block the consequences of the inflammatory component of the disease, corticosteroid therapy has been evaluated. Although results of preliminary trials were encouraging, a large, multicenter, placebo-controlled trial found alternate-day prednisone treatment at 2 mg/kg to have positive effects on pulmonary function but negative consequences on growth and glucose metabolism.[35] Reanalysis of the data from this same study suggested that the benefits of a 1 mg/kg dose might outweigh the risks.[36] The efficacy of short-term systemic corticosteroid use, as well as inhalation of these agents, will continue to be evaluated. Although data concerning inhaled corticosteroids are scant, a long-term trial of oral ibuprofen indicates a positive effect in slowing pulmonary deterioration.[37] Unfortunately, therapeutic drug monitoring (periodic determination of ibuprofen serum concentrations) is required.

Because many cystic fibrosis patients have a reactive airways component to their pulmonary disease, systemic bronchodilators such as theophylline and β-agonists may be of benefit. Wheezing and responsiveness to bronchodilators represent legitimate indications. Responsiveness to such agents (>15% improvement in FEV_1) should be documented, however, before a protracted course is begun. Normal antiasthmatic doses of most bronchodilators should be appropriate for cystic fibrosis patients. However, theophylline clearance may be different in cystic fibrosis patients, and bioavailability of some products may be decreased, sometimes necessitating the use of higher than usual doses.[38] Because of the necessity of pharmacokinetic monitoring and its involvement in a number of common drug interactions, theophylline should be considered second-line bronchodilator therapy at most in these patients. Because cystic fibrosis patients are at high risk to develop the complications of influenza, influenza vaccine should be administered on a yearly basis, and amantadine prophylaxis or treatment may be indicated as well.

Antibiotic Therapy

Antibiotics are used for two purposes in cystic fibrosis: for chronic suppressive therapy and for treatment of acute exacerbations. The use of antibiotics in cystic fibrosis patients is somewhat controversial and certainly challenging. Controversy exists because of the observation that during treatment for an acute pulmonary exacerbation, clinical improvement occurs despite failure to eradicate bacterial pathogens from the sputum. This suggests to some practitioners that the bacteria present are colonizers rather than pathogens, which would argue against the use of antibiotics. The results of one published study comparing antibiotic therapy with placebo indicated that antibiotics may not always contribute to recovery from an acute exacerbation.[39] However, this small study only evaluated patients with mild to moderate disease and therefore is not convincing. At the same time, these results do emphasize the fact that not all exacerbations of pulmonary disease in cystic fibrosis are caused by bacteria. It is logical that other factors such as viral infection and air pollutants could at least contribute to such episodes. Clearly, bacteria such as *P. aeruginosa* are pathogenic by virtue of both inherent properties such as exotoxin release and the body's immune response to their presence and products. Moreover, it is apparent that sublethal effects of antibiotics on *P. aeruginosa* (e.g., decreased exoenzyme production) contribute to clinical improvement.[40] Therefore, the routine presence of known bacterial pathogens dictates antibiotic use, and most, if not all, clinicians caring for cystic fibrosis patients regularly employ antibiotic therapy. Suppressive or prophylactic therapy is given with the intention of prolonging the time between acute exacerbations. Although intuitively attractive, the practice is not supported by well-designed clinical trials.[41] Moreover, the practice of routine quarterly administration of intravenous courses of antibiotics used at some European centers is also lacking in proof of efficacy.[42]

Once one is committed to antibiotic therapy, a number of other important, and sometimes perplexing, issues emerge. These include the selection of the best antibiotic(s) for the individual patient, the best dosage and dosage regimen given altered pharmacokinetics, the optimal route of administration, emergence of antibiotic-resistant bacteria, and identification of appropriate end points of therapy.

Selection of Antibiotic. Suppressive therapy usually is accomplished with the use of common orally administered antibiotics such as trimethoprim-sulfamethoxazole, amoxicillin–clavulanic acid, or one of the many oral cephalosporins. Specific therapy for acute exacerbations is directed at proven or likely pathogens such as *P. aeruginosa* and *S. aureus* and usually includes an aminoglycoside and an extended-spectrum penicillin. Since most *S. aureus* encountered are β-lactamase producers, use of an extended-spectrum penicillin–β-lactamase inhibitor combination (e.g., ticarcillin-clavulanate) will help avoid the necessity of triple-drug therapy. Single-agent therapy with newer antibiotics, especially on an outpatient basis, frequently is employed at some centers where significant resistance to these agents has not yet emerged. Such agents would include ceftazidime, aztreonam, and ciprofloxacin. However, the evidence supporting the clinical superiority of two-drug combinations over single-agent therapy leads many clinicians to treat only with combinations.[43–46] The fact that such combinations are sometimes synergistic in vitro and the possibility that they may act to suppress or delay the emergence of resistance provide attractive rationales for their use. Further, in vitro synergism has been reported to persist even in the face of resistance to one of the single agents in a given combination.[47] Last, monodrug therapy has been met with rapid emergence of resistance.[48]

Unlike other cases of lower respiratory tract infection, organism-specific drug treatment may be based on results from sputum cultures in cystic fibrosis patients because good agreement between sputum and thoracotomy cultures has been demonstrated.[49] Typically, such results will lead one to prescribe or recommend aminoglycoside–extended-spectrum penicillin combinations, although other antibiotics such as ciprofloxacin and older agents such as colistin also may play a role. While the complete eradication of *S. aureus* and *H. influenzae* are practical goals or end points of antibiotic therapy, the total eradication of *Pseudomonas* species is infrequent and transient. Thus, once a patient has been colonized/infected with *P. aeruginosa*, it is prudent to assume that it is always present regardless of culture

TABLE 30–3. Changes in Pharmacokinetics in Cystic Fibrosis[38,50]

Agent	$\beta t_{1/2}$	V_d	Cl_B	Cl_R
Antibiotics				
Methicillin	NC	I	I	I
Cloxacillin	D	I	I	I
Dicloxacillin	I	NR	NR	I
Azlocillin	D	I	I	NR
Piperacillin	D	I	I	NR
Ticarcillin	D	NC	I	I
Aztreonam	D	I	I	I
Ceftazidime	D	I	I	I
Imipenem	NC	I	I	NR
Trimethoprim-sulfamethoxazole	D/D	NC/NC	I/I	I/NC
Gentamicin	NC	I	I	NR
Tobramycin	NC	I	I	NC
Amikacin	NC	I	I	I
Netilmicin	NC	I	I	NR
Fleroxacin	D	D	I	D
Other				
Theophylline	D	I	I	I
Furosemide	NC	NC	I	NC
Acetaminophen	NC	NR	I	NR

$\beta t_{1/2}$ = elimination half-life; V_d = apparent volume of distribution; Cl_B = total body clearance, Cl_R = renal clearance; D = decreased; I = increased; NC = no change; NR = not reported. *From Refs. 38 and 50.*

results. Consistent with these infectious phenomena, the complete resolution of pulmonary signs and symptoms becomes less and less likely as the disease progresses. *B. cepacia* and *S. maltophilia* generally are resistant to most antibiotics. These bacteria may be susceptible to trimethoprim-sulfamethoxazole or chloramphenicol. *B. cepacia* from cystic fibrosis patients frequently is susceptible to ceftazidime, whereas some strains of *S. maltophilia* may be susceptible to other agents such as doxycycline and piperacillin.

Selection of Dose-Altered Pharmacokinetics. Although altered pharmacokinetics in cystic fibrosis are not limited to antibiotics (Table 30–3), this drug class has been studied most extensively.[50] As is true for theophylline, many cystic fibrosis patients have increased total body clearance for many antibiotics, including the aminoglycosides, some of the β-lactams, and trimethoprim-sulfamethoxazole. Thus higher doses of these agents may be necessary to produce therapeutic concentrations (Table 30–4). Unfortunately, these alterations in pharmacokinetics are neither consistent nor predictable. Why the pharmacokinetics of these antibiotics are different in cystic fibrosis patients is unknown. It appears that for many β-lactam antibiotics, increased total body clearance could be accounted for by increased renal clearance. However, it should be pointed out that renal function, as reflected by glomerular filtration rate and renal blood flow, is not different in cystic fibrosis patients as compared with noncystic fibrosis controls.[51] Moreover, a concomitant increase in renal clearance does not completely explain the increase in total body clearance of aminoglycosides, leading some to speculate about extrarenal pathways for elimination. In any event, increased total body clearance dictates higher doses in many but not all patients. However, a range of dosage requirements should be expected, consistent with a range in the variation of pharmacokinetics in these patients. For example, experience with netilmicin revealed a dosage requirement range of 7–17 mg/kg per day to achieve peak concentrations (one-half hour after the end of a drug infusion) of 8 μg/mL or greater.[52] The mean

TABLE 30–4. Antibiotic Doses in Cystic Fibrosis

Antibiotic	Dose (mg/kg/d)	Regimen	Adult Maximum Dose (g/d)
Parenteral Antibiotics			
Tobramycin,[a] gentamicin,[a] or netilmicin[a]	6–9	q8 h	NA
Amikacin[a]	20–30	q8 h	NA
Azlocillin	400	q4–6 h	24
Aztreonam	200	q6 h	8
Ceftazidime	150	q8 h	6
Colistin	2.5–6.0	q6–8 h	NA
Imipenem	45–100	q6 h	4
Nafcillin	100	q4–6 h	6
Ticarcillin or ticarcillin/clavulanate	400	q4–6 h	18
Piperacillin	400	q4–6 h	18
Oral Antibiotics			
Amoxicillin	20	q8 h	
Amoxicillin/clavulanate	20	q6 h	
Ciprofloxacin[b]	1500 mg/d	q12 h	1.5
Cephalexin	50–100	q6–8 h	6
Dicloxacillin	80–100	q6 h	6
Trimethoprim-sulfamethoxazole	10–15[c]	q12 h	0.64[c]
Inhaled Antibiotics			
Colistin	150 mg/d	q6–12 h	NA
Gentamicin or tobramycin	600–1800 mg/d	q12 h	NA
Polymixin B	250 mg/d	q6–12 h	NA

[a]Starting doses; adjust to desired serum concentrations based on dose/serum concentration relationship.
[b]Adult dose.
[c]Based on trimethoprim.

dosage requirement in this study was approximately 12 mg/kg per day. Peak concentrations of this magnitude are felt to be necessary to adequately treat pneumonia caused by gram-negative bacteria.[53,54] Variations in hepatic metabolic activity or in phenotypic distribution of metabolic polymorphisms may explain some pharmacokinetic differences in cystic fibrosis.[55,56]

Although the pharmacokinetics of antibiotics may correlate with the severity of pulmonary disease,[57,58] it is not possible to predict changes in antibiotic pharmacokinetics in cystic fibrosis patients based on markers of clinical status or disease progression. Attempts to correlate antibiotic pharmacokinetics with Shwachman score (a gross method for quantitation of disease status) have been unsuccessful.[59,60] Attempts to guide aminoglycoside dosing often are based on measured serum concentrations during a course of therapy. However, this method also may meet with mixed success owing to changing pharmacokinetics of this family of antibiotics during an acute pulmonary exacerbation.[61] However, this observation should not deter one from attempts to adjust doses to desirable concentrations based on serum concentration determinations and subsequent pharmacokinetic calculations.

■ *Alternate Routes of Administration.* An additional route of antibiotic administration that is intuitively attractive in patients with cystic fibrosis is by inhalation of aerosolized solution. Such a route of administration should, theoretically, deliver the drug to the actual site of infection and perhaps avoid systemic toxicity. Certainly, many classes of antibiotics including β-lactams, aminoglycosides, and polymyxins have been administered to cystic fibrosis patients in this fashion, often in conjunction with systemic antibiotics. However, until recently, no clear effect or advantage had been demonstrated consistently. Early studies suffered from lack of controls, small sample size, and a failure to ensure that the respiratory equipment used would, in fact, guarantee that the drug is delivered to the small airways. In a subsequent placebo-controlled, multicenter trial, 600 mg tobramycin administered by aerosol three times daily was found to produce a small but statistically significant improvement in FEV_1, forced vital capacity, $FEF_{25-75\%}$, *P. aeruginosa* density in sputum, and peripheral white blood cell count.[62] This being recognized, appropriate clinical circumstances for this form of therapy (type and condition of patient), length of therapy, and frequency of therapy remain to be clarified. One-half of this dose is apparently also effective, and a 300-mg dose is the current norm. If such doses are to be used, preservative-free antibiotic preparations should be used. The efficacy of smaller doses of inhaled aminoglycosides remains unproven.

■ *Bacterial Resistance.* As already noted, emergence of antimicrobial resistance seems to follow the introduction and use of a new antibiotic.[48] *P. aeruginosa* can exhibit many resistance mechanisms, revealed as resistance to quinolones (altered DNA gyrase target site), β-lactams (production of Bush group 1 β-lactamase), aminoglycosides (decreased permeability and modifying enzymes), and carbapenems (decreased permeability). *B. cepacia* is inherently resistant to most antibiotics. Methicillin-resistant staphylococci are increasingly common in institutional settings and will become a more pervasive problem in cystic fibrosis populations. These phenomena require close attention to susceptibility reports in selecting therapy and the avoidance of unnecessary or unnecessarily protracted courses of antibiotic therapy.

■ *Recommendations for Antibiotic Therapy.* Despite these inherent difficulties, a number of recommendations regarding the use of systemic antibiotics in cystic fibrosis can be made. The selection of antibiotics should be based on specific culture and susceptibility results. When instituting empirical therapy in the absence of culture results, the clinician can be guided by the most recent laboratory data or institute therapy based on likely pathogens in the patient's age group. Aminoglycosides should be dosed initially at the upper end of the normal dosage range (e.g., 6–7.5 mg/kg/d for tobramycin), and serum concentrations should be determined so that dosage can be adjusted appropriately to achieve peak concentrations of at least 8 μg/mL. It should be kept in mind that aminoglycoside serum half-lives may lengthen during the course of treatment so that a constant relationship between dose and serum concentration may not exist. Upward adjustments in dosage therefore should be made with some degree of caution and should be followed with further determination of serum concentrations. Once-daily administration of aminoglycosides is gaining popularity, as in other settings. Obviously, such a dosing practice would result in much larger peak concentrations than those mentioned earlier. Comparative efficacy and safety of such dosing regimens in cystic fibrosis patients have not yet been fully elucidated, but this practice is likely to be employed increasingly as cystic fibrosis–specific data are generated.

β-Lactam antibiotics such as extended-spectrum penicillins should be prescribed with aminoglycosides to take advantage of their frequent synergy and prevent the emergence of resistance. These agents should be prescribed in large doses to delay stepwise resistance. Ticarcillin, azlocillin, and piperacillin should be prescribed in a dose of at least 350 mg/kg per day divided into four to six doses. For patients with *P. aeruginosa* and *S. aureus,* the combination of an aminoglycoside and ticarcillin-clavulanate or piperacillin-tazobactam is appropriate. Selection among these agents should be based on local susceptibility patterns and cost considerations. The possible increased incidence of fever and exanthema with the newer pencillins should be kept in mind.[63] Aztreonam would be a safe and effective β-lactam to use in patients experiencing these serum sickness-like reactions to the penicillins.[64] In older patients with *P. aeruginosa* isolates with broad resistance patterns, the clinician should work closely with the microbiology laboratory to identify effective agents or combinations. The potential use of older agents with unique mechanisms of action, such as colistin, should not be overlooked.

Oral antibiotics may be prescribed in symptomatic outpatients with susceptible pathogens in their sputum. Agents with activity against common pathogens such as *S. aureus* and *H. influenzae* are useful in this setting. These typically include such antibiotics as first-generation cephalosporins, trimethoprim-sulfamethoxazole, and amoxicillin–clavulanic acid. The use of such agents on a prophylactic basis is discouraged because the data available at present suggest that a beneficial effect does not outweigh the risk of development of resistance among the common bacterial pathogens of cystic fibrosis.[65] The 4-fluoroquinolone antibiotic ciprofloxacin possesses potent activity against most cystic fibrosis pathogens and has been evaluated in adult patients undergoing pulmonary exacerbations. Although not conclusive because of shortcomings in the studies, available data suggest that this oral agent is as effective as standard intravenous therapy.[66] The availability of a potent oral antipseudomonal agent poses a number of potential uses in the cystic fibrosis population. However, it should be kept in mind that repeated or long-term use likely will lead to resistance and that antibiotics play only a supportive role in the treatment of these patients. Thus oral antibiotic therapy, regardless of efficacy, does not negate the need for other forms of therapy that often are best administered in the hospital setting. It also should be pointed out that although ciprofloxacin appears to be safe in patients less than 18 years of age with little evidence of joint or cartilage toxicity,[67] this agent should be used with caution in the younger population.

Treatment of Other Pulmonary Complications

The drug and/or nondrug treatment of the most serious of pulmonary complications, including pulmonary hypertension, right-sided heart failure, respiratory failure, pneumothorax, and hemoptysis, are beyond the scope of this chapter. In general, the therapeutic approach does not vary substantively from that in other patients.

EVALUATION OF THERAPEUTIC OUTCOMES

GASTROINTESTINAL

The patient's nutritional status should be monitored closely on both short- and long-term bases. Height and weight should be followed with time; anthropometric measurements give more precise information. The adequacy of pancreatic enzyme replacement can be assessed grossly by following stool patterns with the goal of normal number per day and normal consistency. Any evidence of steatorrhea may indicate suboptimal enzyme therapy. A more precise method would involve assessment of fat quantities in the stool. If a patient does not respond to normal doses of enzyme supplement, other factors that can cause similar symptoms (e.g., bloating, abdominal pain, symptomatic steatorrhea) should be considered. These would include lack of adherence with directions for taking the enzymes, outdated enzymes, dietary factors such as excessive fruit juice consumption, high-fat meals, and concomitant gastrointestinal disease (e.g., enteric bacterial or parasitic infection, celiac disease, inflammatory bowel disease). Vitamin status can be assessed through serum monitoring of fat-soluble vitamin concentrations.

PULMONARY

Pulmonary status can be monitored with a combination of clinical observation and examination and a variety of laboratory tests. Over the long run, pulmonary function usually is followed with spirometry, along with assessment of lung volume and oxygenation. Physical examination should focus on signs and symptoms of upper and lower respiratory tract infection. In addition, exercise tolerance, recent character of sputum production, and oxygen requirements are key to long- and short-term assessments. With antibiotic and bronchodilator treatment of acute respiratory exacerbations, a return to preexacerbation clinical status, based on physical examination or pulmonary function testing, becomes a practical end point for antimicrobial treatment. Although the goal of bacterial eradication is desirable, other attainable end points may be more reasonable, as discussed earlier. Bacterial density in sputum, sputum DNA and protein content, and C-reactive protein all have proven value as monitoring parameters but may not be available at many centers. Of the objective parameters, pulmonary function tests correlate best with clinical observations and scoring systems.[68] Response to intravenous antibiotics and aggressive chest physiotherapy, as measured by FEV_1 at the end of 1 week of treatment, has been used to predict total length of therapy necessary. In patients whose FEV had recovered more than 40% at the end of 1 week, a total of 2 weeks of therapy generally was sufficient.[69] Little has been done by way of pharmacodynamic studies in treating cystic fibrosis. Therefore, symptomatic improvement is largely relied on to assess the relative success of antibiotic therapy. Oral antibiotic therapy also should be limited in length with specific end points, such as decreased cough and/or improved pulmonary function, identified as treatment commences.

NEW DIRECTIONS IN THERAPY

Now that the gene and gene product of cystic fibrosis have been identified, gene therapy becomes an obvious potential for treatment.[70] Research to date has centered on introduction of the correct gene into affected tissues. Viral vectors, chiefly adenovirus, have been studied in animal models, and human trials are under way. Liposomes may represent another useful delivery mode to introduce the correct gene.

Other, novel approaches to therapy are currently being investigated and, for the most part, are directed at the inflammatory component of the disease or the basic cellular defect. Protease inhibitors hold potential in this condition for reasons cited earlier. α_1-Antitrypsin administered by aerosol shows promise, as does SLPI and other antiproteases.[71–73] Pentoxifylline, which is known to inhibit tumor necrosis factor-α transcription and its stimulatory effect on polymorphonuclear leukocytes, also shows promise.[74] In an attempt to approach the cellular defect in cystic fibrosis directly, the diuretic amiloride had been shown to possess positive activity in improving respiratory secretion rheology and clearance,[75] presumably by blocking excessive sodium reabsorption, but was found to be no more effective than placebo in a large-scale, controlled trial. At a similar level, the secretagogues adenosine and uridine triphosphate (ATP and UTP) have been shown to increase chloride excretion in epithelial cells of cystic fibrosis patients.[76] The combination of amiloride and UTP (thereby both blocking sodium absorption and stimulating chloride secretion) also may promote clearance of airway secretions.[77] Other experimental therapies interact with the defects in CFTR production or processing. Studies with phenylbutyrate (which increases the amount of functional protein that reaches the cell surface), 8-cyclopentyl-1, 3-dipropylxanthine (CPX), milrinone (a phosphodiesterase inhibitor), and genistein (a tyrosine-kinase inhibitor), each of which activate mutant CFTR, and low concentration gentamicin, which suppresses certain premature stop mutations in CFTR, are all active.

It is hoped that some, if not all, of these approaches will provide viable additions to our pharmacologic armamentarium for this disease. For older, more severely affected patients who may not be able to benefit from such advances, organ transplants (single-lung, double-lung, heart-lung) are more widely available and reasonably successful.[78]

CONCLUSIONS

Pharmacotherapeutic intervention plays an important role in the management of these patients but is complex. The clinician is as yet faced with many unresolved issues in attempting to apply sound therapeutic principles in this population. Although close attention should be paid to pharmacologic treatment, the approach to these patients should be multifaceted and multidisciplinary in character. In addition to the involvement of such pediatric subspecialties as pulmonology, gastroenterology, pharmacology, and infectious diseases, contributions from such areas as nutritional support and social work should be a regular and ongoing part of the management effort.

▶ PRINCIPLES OF PHARMACOTHERAPY

- Cystic fibrosis is a genetic disorder of chloride ion secretion from epithelial cells ultimately causing thickened secretions and affects cells in the lungs, pancreas, intestines, and other exocrine glands/organs.
- Thickened secretions in airways lead to obstruction, infection, and finally, inflammation, leading to most of the morbidity and mortality observed with this disease.
- Pulmonary infections are mainly caused by *P. aeruginosa,* and antibiotic therapy is usually directed at that organism.
- Use of antibiotics and other pharmacologic agents must account for the altered pharmacokinetics often observed in cystic fibrosis patients.
- Maneuvers to aid in airway clearance of thickened sections include respiratory therapy and use of bronchodilators and mucolytic agents.
- Thickened secretions in the pancreas lead to deficiencies in pancreatic digestive enzymes and bicarbonate, which leads to maldigestion, malnutrition, and fat-soluble vitamin deficiency.
- Treatment of the gastrointestinal component of cystic fibrosis includes pancreatic enzyme and vitamin supplementation.
- Complications of cystic fibrosis are mainly secondary to the pulmonary component.
- Experimental therapies are directed at the chloride secretion abnormality and the responsible dysfunctional protein.
- Corrective gene therapy will be the ultimate treatment for this disease.

REFERENCES

1. Steinberg AG, Brown DC. On the incidence of cystic fibrosis of the pancreas. Am J Hum Genet 1960;12:416–424.
2. Wright SE, Morton NE. Genetic studies on cystic fibrosis in Hawaii. Am J Hum Genet 1968;20:157–169.
3. Rommens JM, Iannuzzi MC, Kerem B, et al. Identification of the cystic fibrosis gene: Chromosome walking and jumping. Science 1989;245: 1059–1065.
4. Riordan JR, Rommens JM, Kerem B, et al. Identification of the cystic fibrosis gene: Cloning and characterization of complementary DNA. Science 1989;245:1066–1073.
5. Kerem B, Rommens JM, Buchanan JA, et al. Identification of the cystic fibrosis gene: Genetic analysis. Science 1989;245:1073–1080.
6. Welsh MJ, Smith AE. Molecular mechanisms of CFTR chloride channel dysfunction in cystic fibrosis. Cell 1993;73:1251–1254.
7. Kerem E, Corey M, Kerem B, et al. The relationship between genotype and phenotype in cystic fibrosis: Analysis of the most common mutation (ΔF_{508}). N Engl J Med 1991;323:1517–1522.
8. Mohon RT, Wagener JS, Abman SH, et al. Relationship of genotype to early pulmonary function in infants with cystic fibrosis identified through neonatal screening. J Pediatr 1993;122:550–555.
9. Collins FC. Cystic fibrosis: Molecular biology and therapeutic implications. Science 1992;256:774–779.
10. Feigelson J, Anagnostopoulos C, Poquet M, et al. Liver cirrhosis: Therapeutic implications and long term follow up. Arch Dis Child 1993;68: 653–657.
11. Goldman MJ, Anderson GM, Stolzenberg ED, et al. Human β-defensin-1 is a salt-sensitive antibiotic in lung that is inactivated in cystic fibrosis. Cell 1997;88:553–560.
12. Pier GB, Grout M, Zaida TS, et al. Role of mutant CFTR in hypersusceptibility of cystic fibrosis patients to lung infections. Science 1996;271: 64–67.
13. Wang EEL, Prober CG, Manson B, et al. Association of respiratory viral infections with pulmonary deterioration in patients with cystic fibrosis. N Engl J Med 1984;311:1653–1658.

14. Abman SH, Ogle JW, Butler-Simon N, et al. Role of respiratory syncytial virus in early hospitalizations for respiratory distress of young infants with cystic fibrosis. J Pediatr 1988;113:826–830.
15. Pribble CG, Black PG, Bosso JA, et al. Clinical manifestations of exacerbations of cystic fibrosis associated with nonbacterial infections. J Pediatr 1990;117:200–204.
16. Campbell PW, Parker RA, Roberts BT, et al. Association of poor clinical status and heavy exposure to tobacco smoke in patients with cystic fibrosis who are homozygous for the F_{508} deletion. J Pediatr 1992;120:261–264.
17. May TB, Shinabarger D, Maharaj R, et al. Alginate synthesis by *Pseudomonas aeruginosa:* A key pathogenic factor in chronic pulmonary infections of cystic fibrosis patients. Clin Microbiol Rev 1991;4:191–206.
18. Isles A, Maclusky I, Corey M, et al. *Pseudomonas cepacia* infection in cystic fibrosis: An emerging problem. J Pediatr 1984;104:206–210.
19. Hudson VL, Wielinski CL, Regelmann WE. Prognostic implications of initial oropharyngeal bacterial flora in patients with cystic fibrosis diagnosed before the age of two years. J Pediatr 1993;122:854–860.
20. Triglia JM, Belus JF, Dessi P, et al. Rhinonasal manifestations of cystic fibrosis. Ann Otolaryngol Chir Cervicofac 1993;110:98–102.
21. Lawrence JM, Moore TL, Madson KL, et al. Arthropathies of cystic fibrosis: Case reports and review of the literature. J Rheumatol 1993; 20(Suppl 38):12–15.
22. Rosenstein BJ, Cutting GR. The diagnosis of cystic fibrosis: A consensus statement. J Pediatr 1998;132:589–595.
23. Newborn screening for cystic fibrosis: A paradigm for public health genetics policy development. Proceedings of a 1997 workshop. MMWR Morb Mortal Wkly Rep 1997;46(RR-16):1–24.
24. FitzSimmons SC. The changing epidemiology of cystic fibrosis. J Pediatr 1993;122:1–9.
25. Kerem E, Reisman J, Corey M, et al. Prediction of mortality in patients with cystic fibrosis. N Engl J Med 1992;326:1187–1191.
26. Clinical Practice Guidelines for Cystic Fibrosis Committee. Clinical Practice Guidelines for Cystic Fibrosis. Bethesda, MD, Cystic Fibrosis Foundation, 1997.
27. Riedel BD. Gastrointestinal manifestations of cystic fibrosis. Pediatr Ann 1997;26:235–241.
28. Ramsey BW, Farrell PM, Pencharz P, et al. Nutritional assessment and management in cystic fibrosis. Am J Clin Nutr 1992;55:108–116.
29. FitzSimmons SC, Burkhart GA, Borowitz D, et al. High-dose pancreatic-enzyme supplements and fibrosing colonopathy in children with cystic fibrosis. N Engl J Med 1997;336:1283–1289.
30. Nasr SZ, O'Leary MH, Hillerman C. Correction of vitamin E deficiency with fat-soluble versus water-miscible preparations of vitamin E in patients with cystic fibrosis. J Pediatr 1993;122:810–812.
31. Colombo C, Battezzati PM, Podda M, et al. Ursodeoxycholic acid for liver disease associated with cystic fibrosis: A double-blind multicenter trial. Hepatology 1996;23:1484–1490.
32. Columbo C, Grazia M, Ferrari M, et al. Analysis of risk factors for the development of liver disease associated with cystic fibrosis. J Pediatr 1994;124:393–399.
33. Ramsey BW. Management of pulmonary disease in patients with cystic fibrosis. N Engl J Med 1996;335:179–188.
34. Fuchs HJ, Borwitz DS, Christainsen DH, et al. Effect of aerosolized recombinant human DNase on exacerbations of respiratory symptoms and on pulmonary function in patients with cystic fibrosis. N Engl J Med 1994;331:637–642.
35. Rosenstein BJ, Eigen H. Risks of alternate-day prednisone in patients with cystic fibrosis. Pediatrics 1991;87:245–246.
36. Eigen H, Rosenstein BJ, FitzSimmons S, et al. A multicenter study of alternate-day prednisone therapy in patients with cystic fibrosis. J Pediatr 1995;126:515–523.
37. Konstan MW, Byard PJ, Hoppel CL, et al. Effect of high-dose ibuprofen in patients with cystic fibrosis. N Engl J Med 1995;332:848–854.
38. Spino M. Pharmacokinetics of drugs in cystic fibrosis. Clin Rev Allergy 1991;9:169–210.
39. Gold R, Carpenter S, Heurter H, et al. Randomized trial of ceftazidime versus placebo in the management of acute respiratory exacerbations in patients with cystic fibrosis. J Pediatr 1987;111:907–913.
40. Grimwood K, Semple RA, Rabin HR, et al. Elevated exoenzyme expression by *Pseudomonas aeruginosa* is correlated with exacerbations of lung disease in cystic fibrosis. Pediatr Pulmonol 1993;15:135–139.
41. Beardsmore CS, Thompson JR, Williams A, et al. Pulmonary function in infants with cystic fibrosis: The effect of antibiotic treatment. Arch Dis Child 1994;71:133–137.
42. Jensen T, Pedersen SS, Høiby N, et al. Use of antibiotics in cystic fibrosis: The Danish approach. Antibiot Chemother 1989;42:237–246.
43. Parry MF, Neu HC, Merlino M, et al. Treatment of pulmonary infections in patients with cystic fibrosis: A comparative study of ticarcillin and gentamicin. J Pediatr 1977;90:144–148.
44. Møller NE, Høiby N. Antibiotic treatment of chronic *Pseudomonas aeruginosa* infection in cystic fibrosis patients. Scand J Infect Dis 1981;29(Suppl):87–91.
45. Friis B. Chemotherapy of chronic infections with mucoid *Pseudomonas aeruginosa* in lower airways of patients with cystic fibrosis. Scand J Infect Dis 1979;11:211–217.
46. Krause PJ, Young LS, Cherry JD, et al. The treatment of exacerbations of pulmonary disease in cystic fibrosis: Netilmicin compared with netilmicin and carbenicillin. Curr Ther Res 1979;25:609–617.
47. Aronoff SC, Klinger JD. In vitro activities of aztreonam, piperacillin and ticarcillin combined with amikacin against amikacin-resistant *Pseudomonas aeruginosa* and *P. cepacia* isolates from children with cystic fibrosis. Antimicrob Agents Chemother 1984;25:279–280.
48. Bosso JA, Allen JE, Matsen JM. Changing susceptibility of *Pseudomonas aeruginosa* isolates from cystic fibrosis patients with the clinical use of newer antibiotics. Antimicrob Agents Chemother 1989;33:526–528.
49. Thomassen MJ, Klinger JD, Badger SJ, et al. Cultures of thoracotomy specimens confirm usefulness of sputum cultures in cystic fibrosis. J Pediatr 1984;104:352–356.
50. Lindsay CA, Bosso JA. Optimization of antibiotic therapy in cystic fibrosis patients. Clin Pharmacokinet 1993;24:496–506.
51. Spino M, Chai RP, Isles AF, et al. Assessment of glomerular filtration rate and effective renal plasma flow in cystic fibrosis. J Pediatr 1985;107:64–70.
52. Bosso JA, Townsend PL, Herbst JJ, et al. Pharmacokinetics and dosage requirements of netilmicin in cystic fibrosis patients. Antimicrob Agents Chemother 1985;28:829–831.
53. Moore RD, Smith CR, Lietman PS. Association of aminoglycoside plasma levels with therapeutic outcome in gram-negative pneumonia. Am J Med 1984;77:657–662.
54. Noone P, Parsons MC, Pattison JR, et al. Experience in monitoring gentamicin therapy during treatment of serious gram negative sepsis. Br J Med 1974;1:477–481.
55. Kearns GL. Hepatic drug metabolism in cystic fibrosis: Recent developments and future directions. Ann Pharmacother 1993;27:74–79.
56. Bosso JA, Liu Q, Evans WE, et al. CYP2D6, *N*-acetylation, and xanthine oxidase activity in cystic fibrosis. Pharmacotherapy 1996;16:749–753.
57. MacDonald NE, Anas NG, Peterson RG, et al. Renal clearance of gentamicin in cystic fibrosis. J Pediatr 1983;103:985–990.
58. Nahata MC, Lubion AH, Visconti JA. Cephalexin pharmacokinetics in patients with cystic fibrosis. Dev Pharmacol Ther 1984;7:221–228.
59. Spino M, Chai RP, Isles AF, et al. Cloxacillin absorption and disposition in cystic fibrosis. J Pediatr 1984;105:829–835.
60. Jacobs RF, Trang JM, Kearns GL, et al. Ticarcillin/clavulanic acid pharmacokinetics in children and young adults with cystic fibrosis. J Pediatr 1985;106:1001–1007.
61. Bosso JA, Relling MV, Townsend PL, et al. Intrapatient variations in aminoglycoside disposition in cystic fibrosis. Clin Pharm 1987;6:54–58.
62. Ramsey BW, Dorkin HL, Eisenberg JD, et al. Efficacy of aerosolized tobramycin in patients with cystic fibrosis. N Engl J Med 1993;328:1740–1746.
63. Møller NE, Eriksen KR, Feddersen C, et al. Chemotherapy against *Pseudomonas aeruginosa* in cystic fibrosis: A study of carbenicillin,

azlocillin or piperacillin in combination with tobramycin. Eur J Respir Dis 1982;63:130–139.

64. Jensen T, Koch C, Pedersen SS, et al. Aztreonam for cystic fibrosis patients who are hypersensitive to other β-lactams. Lancet 1987;1:1319–1320.
65. Beardsmore CS, Thompson JR, Williams A, et al. Pulmonary function in infants with cystic fibrosis. Arch Dis Child 1994;71:133–137.
66. Bosso JA. Use of ciprofloxacin in cystic fibrosis patients. Am J Med 1989;87(Suppl 5A):123S–127S.
67. Høiby N, Pedersen SS, Jensen T, et al. Fluoroquinolones in the treatment of cystic fibrosis. Drugs 1993;45(Suppl 3):98–101.
68. Bosso JA, Walker KB. Lack of correlation between objective indicators and clinical-response scores during antimicrobial therapy for acute pulmonary exacerbations of cystic fibrosis. Clin Pharm 1988;7:897–901.
69. Rosenberg SM, Schramm CM. Predictive value of pulmonary function testing during pulmonary exacerbations in cystic fibrosis. Pediatr Pulmonol 1993;16:227–235.
70. Rosenfeld MA, Collins FS. Gene therapy for cystic fibrosis. Chest 1996;109:241–252.
71. McElvaney NG, Hubbard RC, Birrer P, et al. Aerosol α_1-antitrypsin treatment for cystic fibrosis. Lancet 1991;337:392–394.
72. McElvaney NG, Nakamura H, Birrer P, et al. Modulation of airway inflammation in cystic fibrosis: In vivo suppression of interleukin-8 levels on the respiratory epithelial surface by aerosolization of recombinant secretory leukoprotease inhibitor. J Clin Invest 1992;90:296–301.
73. Meyer KC, Kewandeski JR, Zimmerman JJ, et al. Human neutrophil elastase and elastase/alpha 1-antiprotease complex in cystic fibrosis. Am Rev Respir Dis 1991;144:580–585.
74. Aronoff SC, Quinn FJ, Carpenter LS, et al. Effects of pentoxifylline on sputum neutrophil elastase and pulmonary function in patients with cystic fibrosis: Preliminary observations. J Pediatr 1994;125:992–997.
75. Knowles MR, Church NL, Waltner WE, et al. A pilot study of aerosolized amiloride for the treatment of lung disease in cystic fibrosis. N Engl J Med 1990;322:1189–1194.
76. Knowles MR, Clarke LL, Boucher RC. Activation by extracellular nucleotides of chloride secretion in the airway epithelia of patients with cystic fibrosis. N Engl J Med 1991;325:533–538.
77. Bennett WD, Olivier KN, Zeman KL, et al. Effect of uridine 5′-triphosphate plus amiloride on mucociliary clearance in adult cystic fibrosis. Am J Respir Crit Care Med 1996;153:1796–1801.
78. Yankaskas JR, Westerman JH, Thompson JT, et al. Improved results of lung transplantation for patients with cystic fibrosis. J Thorac Cardiovasc Surg 1995;109:224–234.

31
EVALUATION OF THE GASTROINTESTINAL TRACT

Marie A. Chisholm and Mark W. Jackson

The gastrointestinal (GI) tract is comprised of organs and tissues that have diverse forms and functions. It includes the esophagus, stomach, small intestine, large intestine, colon, rectum, biliary tract, gallbladder, liver, and pancreas. Despite the rapid proliferation of technology for the diagnosis of digestive diseases, the patient history and physical examination still hold central roles. When combined with a thorough patient history and physical examination, diagnostic procedures are essential in the evaluation of GI disorders. This chapter describes the most commonly used tools available in clinical practice to evaluate patients with GI diseases.

SYMPTOMS OF GASTROINTESTINAL DYSFUNCTION

There are various symptoms arising from GI dysfunction. Common GI symptoms include heartburn, abdominal pain, dyspepsia, nausea, vomiting, diarrhea, constipation, and gastrointestinal bleeding. Signs and symptoms of malabsorption, hepatitis, and GI infection are also commonly seen. The next sections describe methods that are commonly used to assess patients with GI complaints. For specific details concerning each GI disease state, please consult that particular chapter in this book.

PATIENT HISTORY

A comprehensive patient history is the cornerstone in the evaluation of a patient with digestive complaints. A clear, detailed, chronological account of the patient's problems should be ascertained. This account should include the onset of the problem, the setting in which it developed, and its manifestations. The onset of the problem often provides important information that helps to confirm diagnosis. For example, biliary pain, such as that encountered with symptomatic gallstone disease, typically evolves over minutes and lasts for hours; but pain caused by pancreatitis evolves over hours and lasts for days. The setting is always relevant as it provides clues to the possibilities of origin. For example, is the patient an alcoholic (liver disease, esophageal varices, pancreatitis)? Does the patient have severe atherosclerosis (mesenteric ischemia)? Is the patient immunosuppressed (opportunistic infection)? Also aiding in the differential diagnosis is identification of factors that alleviate or exacerbate the principal symptom. For instance, ingesting a meal often relieves the pain of duodenal ulcer but worsens that of gastric ulcer. Ask questions that address the potential etiologic possibilities, including motility disorders, structural diseases, malignancies, infections, psychosocial factors, dietary factors, and travel-associated diseases.[1,2] Questions concerning past medical and family history detailing illnesses, surgeries, injuries, and habits are extremely valuable (Table 31–1). Because many drugs have been reported to cause GI injury, a patient's medication history is vital (Table 31–2).

PHYSICAL EXAMINATION

Because the organ systems of the body interact and may provide important data needed for diagnosis, it is necessary to perform a thorough physical examination.[3] A global evaluation of the patient should be performed with notable attention to appearances and vital signs because they may suggest clues to the patient's overall condition and stability. Careful examination of the abdomen is also an essential part of the workup. Examination of the abdomen is approached classically by inspection, auscultation, percussion, and palpation. Inspection of the abdomen may reveal scars, hernias, bulges, or peristalsis. Auscultation is mainly focused on analysis of bowel sounds and identification of bruits. Percussion of the abdomen allows for detection of tympani, measurement of visceral organs, and detection of ascites. Palpation may allow the clinician to identify tenderness, rigidity, masses, and hernias. A digital rectal examination is used to detect masses, tenderness, and assess muscle tone. Stool on the examiner's glove obtained during rectal examination is often subjected to hemoccult testing for the indirect detection of occult blood.[1,3]

LABORATORY AND MICROBIOLOGIC TESTS

Laboratory and microbiologic tests may be used to (a) assess organ function, (b) screen for certain GI disorders, and (c) evaluate the effectiveness of therapy.

To achieve an accurate diagnosis and provide the best care, it is important to assess the patient's fluid and electrolyte status, nutritional status, and abdominal organ function. A serum chemistry panel provides clinicians with valuable information. For example, serum creatinine (S_{Cr}) and blood urea nitrogen (BUN) are often used as a measure of hydration status as well as serve as indicators for renal function. Elevations in S_{Cr} and BUN may be indicative of renal dysfunction or dehydration, and bleeding from the GI tract may lead to elevations in BUN. Albumin levels can be used to assess the patient's nutritional and hydration status and provide information concerning hepatic and renal function. Specifically, low albumin may be indicative of malnutrition, hepatic dysfunction, nephrotic syndromes or protein-losing enteropathies such as Crohn's disease and ulcerative colitis. Serum measurements of sodium, chloride, and potassium are

TABLE 31–1. General Questions in a GI History

1. Tell me about the problem that you are experiencing. When did it start?
2. Where is your pain located? Please point to the area where you feel pain. What were you doing when the pain occurred? How rapidly did the pain come on? Is your pain constant or intermittent? What factors exacerbate or alleviate your pain? Does the pain awaken you at night?
3. What medications are you taking to help the pain? How much do you take? Do these medications work?
4. What other medications are you currently taking? Why are you taking them?
5. Have you recently had a change in dietary intake? If so, please describe. Can you draw any correlation between the foods that you eat and your GI complaint?
6. Have you recently had a change in bowel habits? Have you experienced any diarrhea or constipation lately? Do you experience painful bowel movements?
7. Have you experienced any nausea or vomiting lately? If so, please describe conditions centered around this event.
8. Have you experienced any recent change in weight? Was this intentional? How many pounds have you gained or lost and over what time period did this occur? How has your appetite been?
9. Have you passed any blood from your rectum or vomited blood? Have you noticed any dark, tarry stools?
10. Have you had any acid indigestion?
11. Do you have difficulty swallowing?
12. Has anyone in your family experienced similar GI complaints? If so, please describe. Does anyone in your family have a history of GI disorders, including cancer of the GI tract?
13. Describe your past medical history, including illnesses and surgeries.
14. Please describe any past injuries that you have experienced.
15. Have you recently traveled outside of the United States? If so, where? When? How long did you stay? What kind of living conditions did you experience? What foods and drinks did you ingest?

TABLE 31–2. Drugs That May Commonly Cause Gastrointestinal Injury

Gastrointestinal Mucosal Injury	**Liver Damage (Continued)**
Aspirin	Glyburide
Bisphosphonates	Isoniazid
Chemotherapeutic agents	Ketoconazole
Corticosteroids	Methotrexate
Ethacrynic acid	Methyldopa
Ethanol	Monoamine oxidase inhibitors
Gentian violet	Niacin
Isoproterenol	Nifedipine
Nonsteroidal anti-inflammatory agents	Nitrofurantoin
Pancrease supplementation	Phenytoin
Potassium chloride	Propylthiouracil
Reserpine	Pyridium
Warfarin	Rifampin
Jaundice	Salicylates
Acetohexamide	Sulfonamides
Androgens	Tetracycline
Chlorpropamide	Verapamil
Corticosteroids	Warfarin
Erythromycin	Zidovudine
Estrogens	**Pancreatitis**
Ethanol	Azathioprine
Gold salts	Corticosteroids
Nitrofurantoin	Estrogens
Phenothiazines	Ethacrynic acid
Warfarin	Ethanol
Liver Damage	Furosemide
Acetaminophen	Metronidazole
Allopurinol	Opiates
Aminosalicylic acid	Sulindac
Dapsone	Sulfonamides
Erythromycin	Tetracycline
Ethanol	Thiazides

useful to determine electrolyte abnormalities associated with diarrheal illnesses. A complete blood count (CBC) helps to provide information concerning infection, malignancy, bone marrow suppression, anemia, and blood loss.[4]

Specific laboratory blood tests are used as a screening tool for certain GI disorders. For example, measurements of serum aspartate transaminase (AST) and alanine transaminase (ALT) are elevated in most diseases of the liver, and serum alkaline phosphatase and bilirubin are often elevated in hepatobiliary disorders. Because prothrombin time is related to hepatocyte synthesis of vitamin K-dependent clotting factors, it serves as an indirect measure of hepatic function. When evaluating patients with suspected pancreatitis, serum and urine measurements of amylase and lipase are important, because these will be elevated in most patients with acute pancreatitis.

Microbiologic studies are useful in evaluating patients with unexplained diarrhea, abdominal pain, and suspected GI infections. Microbiologic studies of the stool may be used to detect the presence of bacteria and parasites. Pathogens most often responsible for infectious diarrhea and enteritis include bacteria such as *Shigella, Salmonella, Escherichia coli,* and *Yersinia;* viruses such as *cytomegalovirus,* especially in AIDS patients; and parasites such as *Entamoeba histolytica* and *Giardia lambia.*[5]

Because *Helicobacter pylori* is a significant factor associated with peptic ulcer disease and gastritis, identification of this organism is critical in evaluating patients experiencing dyspepsia. Serologic or saliva-based tests are capable of determining the presence of *H. pylori* antibodies in patients. Although serologic *H. pylori* antibody testing can determine whether a patient has been exposed to the organism, it is unable to indicate active infection. The unique capability of *H. pylori* to produce urease enzyme is exploited in certain direct tests of active *H. pylori* infection. At the time of endoscopy, biopsies of the stomach may be used to detect urease activity; for example, the CLO test uses a colored pH indicator that changes when ammonia is generated by *H. pylori.* Carbon[13] and carbon[14] breath tests involve the indirect measurement of urease activity by measuring labeled carbon dioxide in expired air (Fig. 31–1).[6] Tests that detect active *H. pylori* infection may be considered after antibiotic eradication medication use to determine effectiveness of therapy.

DIAGNOSIS

The patient history, physical examination, and routine laboratory tests are extremely useful in establishing a GI diagnosis, but frequently a more specific study is required to confirm or deny a clinical suspicion. The most appropriate diagnostic test depends on the anatomic region involved, the suspected abnormality, patient preferences, patient's overall condition, and clinical manifestation of the patient. The next sections outline the most frequently used diagnostic studies and procedures and their role in evaluating the GI tract.

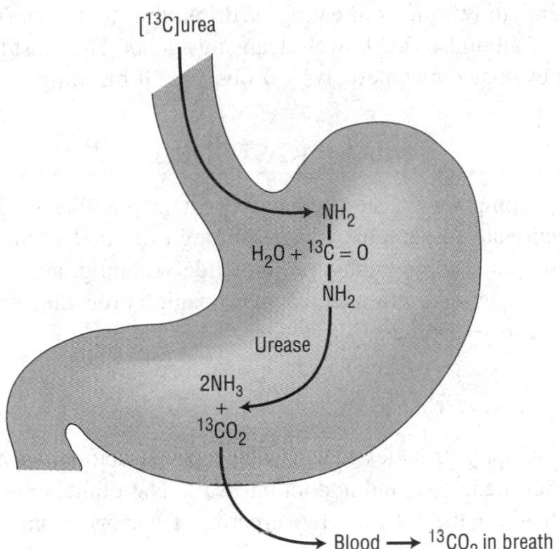

FIGURE 31–1. If urease is present in the stomach during testing with urease ^{13}carbon breath test, urea will be hydrolyzed to form ammonia and labeled carbon dioxide. The labeled carbon dioxide is absorbed into the bloodstream and is detected in expired air.

RADIOLOGY

Radiologic procedures rely on the differential absorption of radiation between adjacent tissues to highlight anatomy and pathology. Radiologic procedures important in evaluating the GI tract include plain radiography, upper GI series, lower GI series, and enteroclysis.[7,8]

PLAIN RADIOGRAPHY OF GI SYSTEM

Radiographic evaluation of the GI tract often starts with plain films of the abdomen, which are straightforward, uncontrasted radiographs.[8] Specific abdominal structures that may be identified include the kidney, ureters, and bladder (KUB); esophagus; stomach; intestine; stones; and vessels. Plain films are often used to evaluate abdominal pain.[9] Clinicians frequently employ plain radiographic fluoroscopy to guide and position other instruments used to evaluate and to treat GI disorders; an example is the manipulation of dilation devices to treat esophageal strictures. Bowel obstruction and perforation are especially well identified by this technique.

CONTRAST AGENTS

Many different types of contrast agents are available. Two types of contrast agents commonly used to enhance visualization of the GI tract are barium sulfate and aqueous iodinated compounds. Barium sulfate is the contrast agent of choice for studying the esophagus, stomach, and intestine except in special clinical situations.[8] Barium sulfate is not generally absorbed, and constipation is the most frequent adverse effect reported with its use. Two widely used iodinated contrast agents for visualizing the GI tract are diatrizoate meglumine and diatrizoate sodium. Unlike barium, these agents are relatively nontoxic if inadvertently introduced into the peritoneal cavity; therefore, the main indications for iodinated agents in GI radiologic films are for suspected bowel perforations. Because iodinated contrast agents are hyperosmolar, they possess the potential to cause severe diarrhea, dehydration, and electrolyte imbalances. Nephrotoxicity associated with iodinated contrast agents may occur and is generally self-limited.[8,10] Allergies and hypersensitivity reactions such as rashes associated with contrast agents are possible and should be monitored and treated accordingly.

UPPER GI SERIES

The upper GI series refers to the radiographic visualization of the esophagus, stomach, and small intestine. Patient preparation for an upper GI usually consists of instructing patients to refrain from eating or drinking 8 to 12 hours prior to testing, thereby allowing the upper GI tract to empty. A contrast agent such as barium sulfate is administered to the patient at the beginning of the study. The observed swallowing of the contrast agent permits visualization and monitoring of esophageal structural and motor functions. This phase of the procedure is most often referred to as a barium swallow. As the contrast medium flows into the stomach and small intestine, several regional radiographic films are taken in order to inspect these areas. This tracking of contrast agents through the small intestine is referred to as the small bowel follow-through. The upper GI series with the small bowel follow-through includes the examination of the esophagus to the distal end of the small intestine and is useful to evaluate and detect obstructions, tumors, ulcers, and abnormal intestinal loops. The upper GI series with small bowel follow-through commonly uncovers gastric cancer, peptic ulcer disease, esophagitis, gastric outlet obstruction, and Crohn's disease (Fig. 31–2).

LOWER GI SERIES

Patients complaining of lower abdominal pain, constipation, or diarrhea are often referred for a lower GI series. Before the procedure the colon is prepared by instructing the patient to refrain from eating or drinking 8 to 12 hours before the procedure and by administering bowel-cleansing agents such as bisacodyl, magnesium citrate, magnesium hydroxide, or polyethylene glycol-electrolyte solution. During a

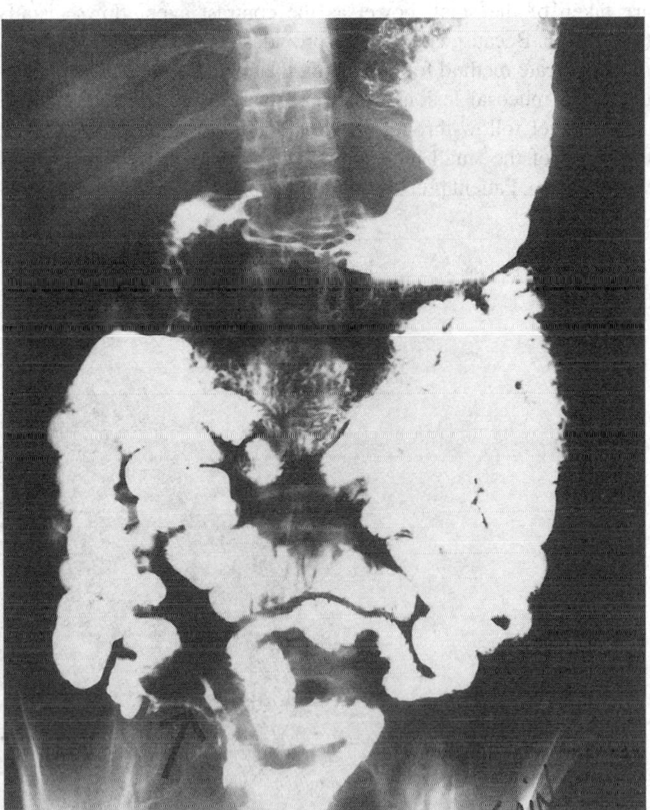

FIGURE 31–2. Upper GI series with small bowel follow-through demonstrating narrowed distal terminal ileum and separation of small bowel loops. These findings are consistent with Crohn's disease.

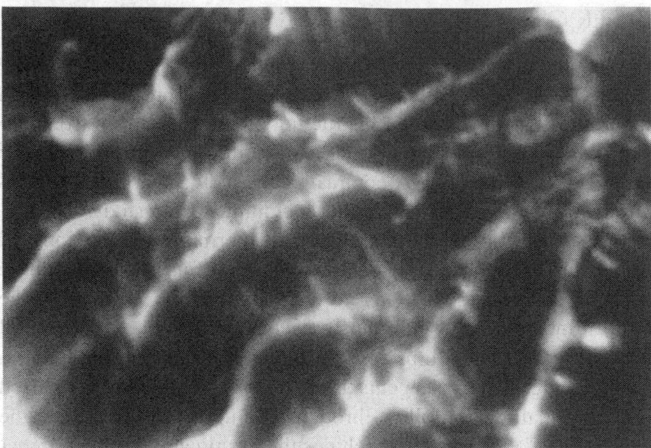

FIGURE 31–3. Normal small bowel enteroclysis. Contrast agents are instilled into the small bowel to highlight tumors, strictures, or other lesions. In this image, one can identify the normal circular folds.

lower GI series, a barium sulfate enema is given to contrast the terminal large intestine and rectum. The lower GI series is useful to detect and evaluate enterocolitis, obstructions, volvulus, and mucosal and structural lesions.[8] The lower GI series is commonly used to diagnose Crohn's disease, ulcerative colitis, colon cancers, and diverticulitis.

SMALL BOWEL ENTEROCLYSIS

Enteroclysis or small bowel enema refers to the technique of direct small bowel introduction of a contrast agent through a tube inserted through the patient's mouth or nose. Intermittent radiographic films are taken of the small bowel as the contrast agent flows distally (Fig. 31–3). Because enteroclysis provides detailed imaging, it is the most accurate method for evaluating the small bowel and for detecting small mucosal lesions that were overlooked on the traditional small bowel follow-through.[11] Methylcellulose is used to enhance the detail of the small intestine in enteroclysis, thereby improving visualization. Patient preparation for this procedure involves instructing patients to refrain from eating or drinking 8 to 12 hours before testing and administering bowel-cleansing agents. The most frequent disorder evaluated by enteroclysis is obscure GI bleeding.

IMAGING STUDIES

By using computer-assisted techniques, it is possible to generate cross-sectional radiographic images through the body. Ultrasonography, computed tomography, radionuclide scanning, and magnetic resonance imaging are frequently used imaging procedures for evaluating digestive disorders.

ULTRASONOGRAPHY

Ultrasonography provides images of deeper structures such as the gallbladder, pancreas, and abdominal wall. The clinician is able to image slices of the GI tract by directing a narrow beam of high-energy sound waves into the body and recording the reflections from the various organs and structures. Because ultrasonography is noninvasive, relatively inexpensive, requires no ionizing radiation, and can be performed with a portable unit, it is a well-accepted and useful technology. It accurately detects gallstones and gallbladder, hepatobiliary, and pancreatic diseases (Fig. 31–4). When combined with Doppler technologies, ultrasonography may image GI vascularity. Ultrasonography is limited by the presence of bowel gas and excessive amounts of body fat.[12,13]

COMPUTED TOMOGRAPHY

Computed tomography (CT) or computed axial tomography (CAT) scans provide detailed images of the GI system in which transverse planes of tissue are swept by a radiographic beam and a computer analysis of the variance in absorption produces a precise reconstructed image of that area.[7,12] Contrast agents may be added in a CT procedure to illuminate specific hollow structures and vascularity of the GI tract. The abdominal CT displays organs from the diaphragm down to the pelvic brim and is especially valuable for detecting GI diseases of the liver, pancreas, spleen, and colon. Patient preparation for CT includes

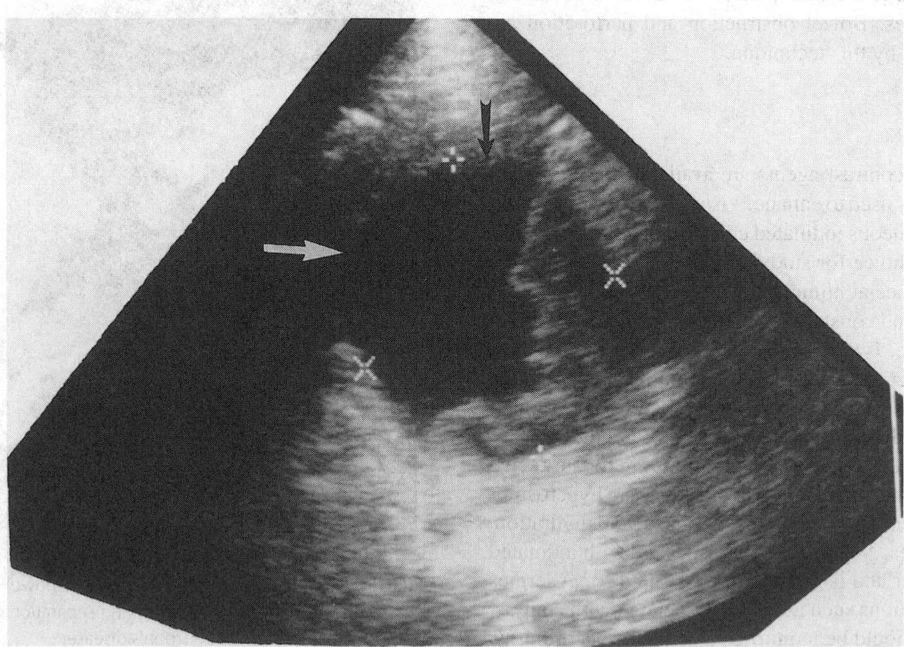

FIGURE 31–4. Abdominal ultrasound demonstrating a chronic pancreatic pseudocyst *(arrows).*

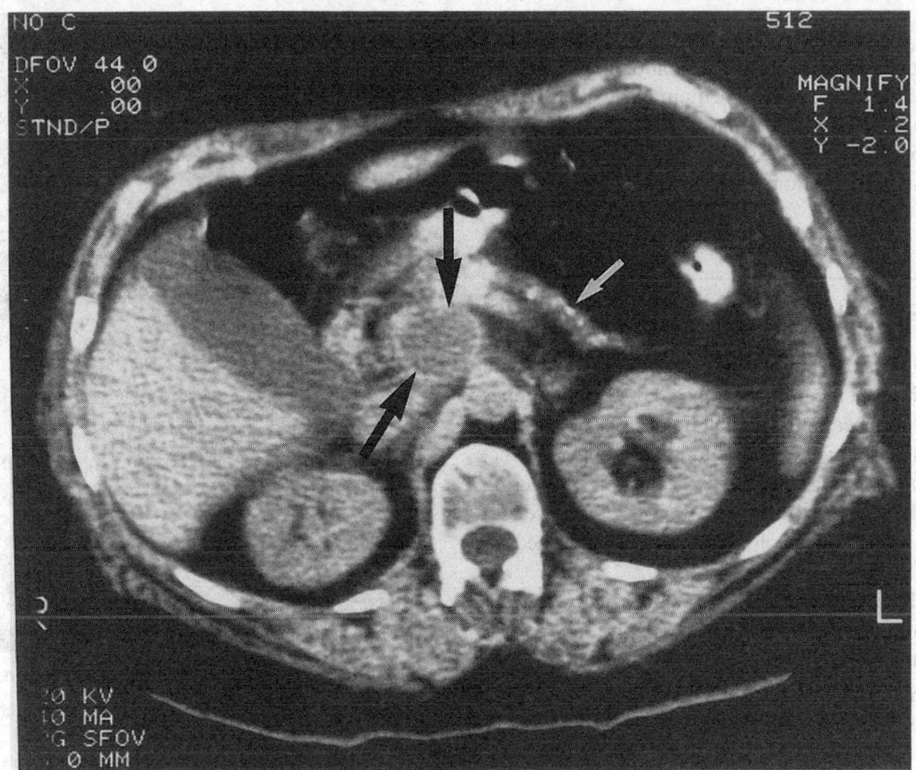

FIGURE 31–5 CT scan of the abdomen showing pancreatitis with calcification *(white arrow)* and pancreatic pseudocyst (*black arrows*).

refraining from eating or drinking for a minimum of 4 hours before the test. The remarkable detail that CT offers in imaging organs and tissues adds to its popularity for evaluation of the GI system. CT is useful in the identification of liver cancer, pancreatitis, pancreatic cancer, intra-abdominal abscesses, and cysts (Fig. 31–5).[12] Unlike ultrasonography, patient body size or the presence of gas does not limit the quality of imaging with CT.

RADIONUCLIDE IMAGING

Radionuclide imaging involves intravenous injections of a radiopharmaceutical imaging agent and the use of a computerized detection camera to gather images. Although the choice of a radiopharmaceutical agent depends on the specific organ or function being studied, the most commonly used agent is technetium (Tc-99m) tagged to a carrier molecule. Radiographic imaging is useful to visualize the liver and spleen (liver-spleen scan), bile ducts, gallbladder (HIDA [hepatoiminodiacetic acid] scan), and gut (bleeding scan).[12] Cysts, abscesses, tumors, and obstructions are detected and displayed as areas of differential uptake of radioactivity (Fig. 31–6).[7] Radionuclide bleeding scans may detect hemorrhages and may assist in localization.

MAGNETIC RESONANCE IMAGING

Magnetic resonance imaging (MRI) places the patient in close proximity to a high-strength magnetic field through which pulses of radiofrequency irradiation are projected, thereby exciting the nuclei of hydrogen, phosphorus, oxygen, and other elements. The radiofrequency signals are manipulated and recorded by computer, and a two-dimensional picture representing a section of the patient is produced.[12] MRI has greater sensitivity to identify liver tumors than ultrasonography, CT, or radionuclide imaging. Although the current use of MRI is not as popular as other imaging techniques because of limited availability, expense, slow scanning time, and problems associated with the use of powerful magnetic fields, its use is predicted to increase in the future.[13]

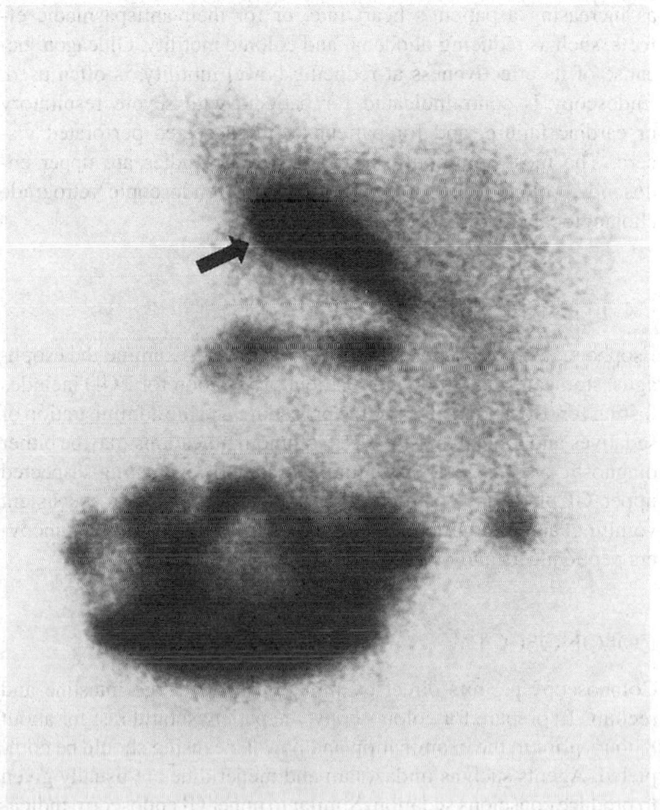

FIGURE 31–6. HIDA scan demonstrating normal gallbladder *(arrow)*.

ARTERIOGRAPHY

Arteriography of the gut defines the configuration of visceral blood vessels after administration of a contrast medium intravenously. Arteriography may be employed for detecting tumors and bleeding lesions and therapeutic applications including embolization of bleeding vessels, fistulas, and inoperable tumors.[12]

ENDOSCOPY

Refinement in optical engineering and fiber optics has made possible the development of the endoscope, which has revolutionized the management of GI disorders. An endoscope is an illuminated optical instrument designed to inspect the interior of the GI tract. Endoscopes enable the practitioner to inspect intraluminal mucosal lesions and to obtain biopsies and washings for cytology studies. The upper GI tract endoscopy (esophagogastroduodenoscopy) is capable of inspecting the esophagus, stomach, and proximal small bowel. The lower GI tract endoscopy of the rectum and colon may be accomplished by colonoscopy or sigmoidoscopy.

Preparation for endoscopic examinations includes instructing patients to refrain from eating or drinking 8 to 12 hours prior to the endoscopic procedures. Bowel cleansing is necessary for colonoscopy and sigmoidoscopy. Topical pharyngeal anesthetics such as viscous lidocaine or benzocaine usually improve patient acceptance of the upper endoscopic tube. Intravenous sedating agents such as meperidine hydrochloride, diazepam, lorazepam, and midazolam hydrochloride are among the most common agents used to induce "conscious sedation" minutes prior to the endoscopy. These sedating agents tend to improve patient acceptance and ease of procedure. With the development of flumazenil, a benzodiazepine antagonist, the popularity of benzodiazepines for mild sedation with GI procedures has increased. In addition, antimuscarinic agents such as atropine sulfate are occasionally used for their cardiovascular effects, such as increasing a patient's heart rate, or for their antispasmodic effects, such as reducing duodenal and colonic motility. Glucagon, because of its effectiveness at reducing bowel motility, is often used. Endoscopy is contraindicated for patients with severe respiratory or cardiac failure, and for patients with suspected perforated viscera. The most commonly used endoscopic studies are upper endoscopy, colonoscopy, sigmoidoscopy, and endoscopic retrograde cholangiopancreatography.

ESOPHAGOGASTRODUODENOSCOPY

Esophagogastroduodenoscopy (EGD) is used to examine the esophagus, stomach, and duodenum. Patient preparation for EGD includes fasting for 6 to 8 hours prior to the procedure and the administration of sedatives and topical anesthetics. Common indications may be either diagnostic or therapeutic in nature, and include evaluating suspected upper GI bleeding, obstructions, upper abdominal pain, persistent vomiting, and radiographic abnormalities.[14] EGD commonly uncovers peptic ulcers and other lesions (Fig. 31–7).

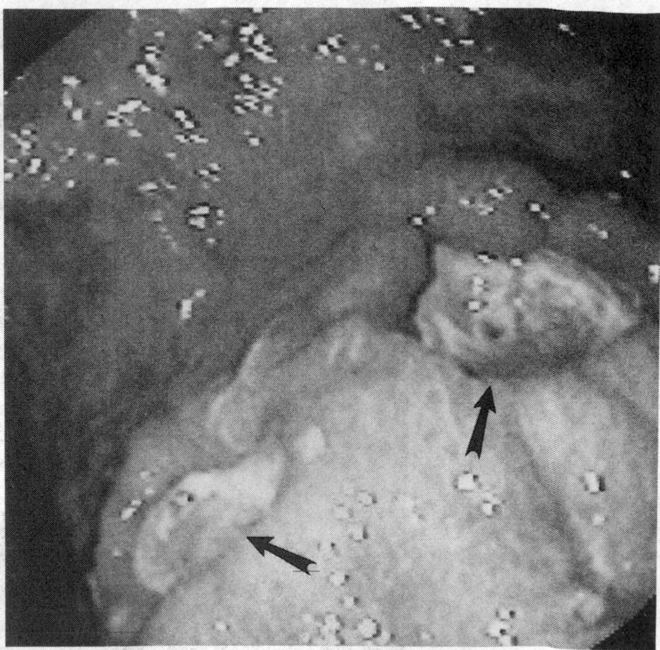

FIGURE 31–7. Deep "punched out" gastric ulcers *(arrows)* as shown by EGD.

COLONOSCOPY

Colonoscopy permits direct examination of the large intestine and rectum. To prepare for colonoscopy, the patient should fast for about 8 hours prior to the examination and bowel cleansing should be completed. Agents such as midazolam and meperidine are usually given to produce conscious sedation. Similar to upper GI endoscopy, indications for lower GI endoscopy can be either diagnostic or therapeutic in nature and include evaluation and detection of abnormalities indicated on radiographic film, GI hemorrhaging, colonic lesions, volvulus, ulcerative colitis, Crohn's disease, diverticulitis, and excision of colonic polyps.[15]

SIGMOIDOSCOPY

Sigmoidoscopy is used to evaluate the sigmoid colon and rectum. Flexible sigmoidoscopy has virtually replaced the rigid sigmoidoscopy because of increased patient comfort and superior examining. The major indication for this examination is to evaluate symptoms related to the colon or rectum and to conduct screening of asymptomatic patients for colon polyps or cancer. Patient preparation involves instructing patients to abstain from eating or drinking 8 to 12 hours prior to the procedure and administering bowel-cleansing agents. Anoscopy is especially useful in evaluating the anus. The major indications for the anoscopic examination include symptoms related to the anus and rectum such as bleeding, protrusions or swelling, pain, and severe itching. Patients undergoing sigmoidoscopy or anoscopy generally do not require sedation.

ENDOSCOPIC RETROGRADE CHOLANGIOPANCREATOGRAPHY

Endoscopic retrograde cholangiopancreatography (ERCP) is an important procedure that is used to evaluate and treat diseases of the biliary tree and pancreas. By injecting contrast agents through a catheter placed in the pancreaticobiliary ducts during ERCP, abnormalities such as obstructions, calculi, and strictures can be examined. Preparation for ERCP consists of conscious sedation and glucagon to relax gut motility. Common reasons for ERCP include detection and evaluation of pancreatic malignancy, pancreatitis, biliary obstruction, bile duct stones, jaundice, and patients whose clinical presentation suggests biliary disease (Fig. 31–8).

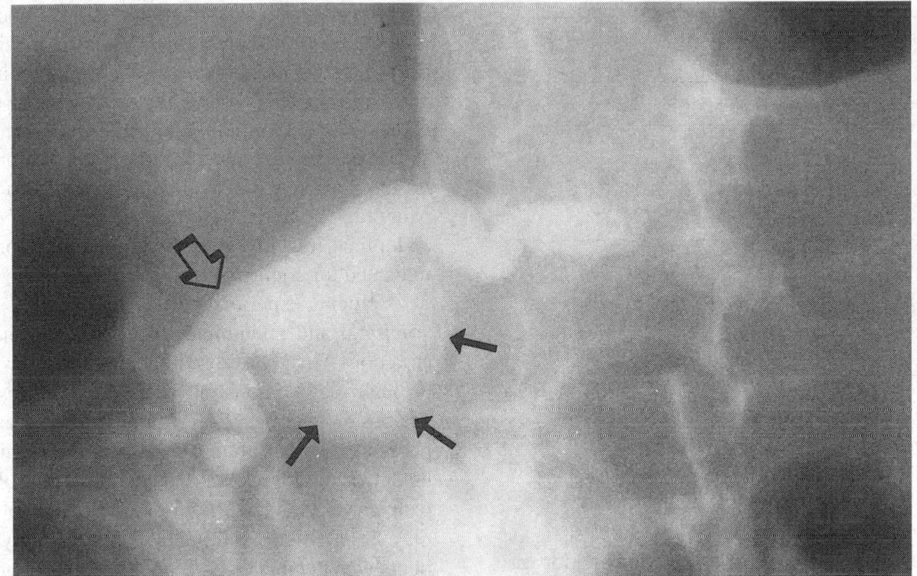

FIGURE 31–8. ERCP demonstrating a dilated, irregular pancreatic duct with areas of stricturing *(large arrow)*. A pancreatic pseudocyst is visible immediately adjacent to the spine *(small arrows)*.

MISCELLANEOUS TESTS

ESOPHAGEAL MANOMETRY

Esophageal manometry is used to evaluate esophageal motor functions. Common indications for this procedure include dysphagia and obscure chest pain. A special catheter equipped with pressure transducers is placed into the esophagus to measure esophageal pressures and peristalsis. Provocative testing with pharmacologic agents such as edrophonium chloride, a cholinergic muscle stimulant, may be used to precipitate esophageal pain during this procedure.[16] Typical reasons for esophageal manometry include evaluating esophageal dysmotility, nonobstructive dysphagia, obscure chest pain, scleroderma, intestinal pseudoobstruction, achalasia, and aiding in positioning instruments such as pH probes.

AMBULATORY pH MONITORING

Gastric fluid pH monitoring in patients who complain of gastroesophageal reflux may be necessary. Indications for pH monitoring include evaluating atypical chest pain and severe or unusual reflux disorders. Ambulatory 24-hour pH monitoring is an elegant way to link esophageal acid exposure, as defined by a probe in the esophagus, with patient's symptoms. The pH probe is placed approximately 5 cm above the distal esophagus. Because intraesophageal pH is normally higher (pH $\geq$ 6) than that of the stomach (pH approximately 1–3), the pH probe will record a decrease in pH if gastroesophageal reflux occurs.

The Bernstein test, another procedure used to measure gastric fluid pH, is less expensive than ambulatory pH monitoring. This procedure requires inserting a nasogastric (NG) tube and administrating alternating dripped solutions of normal saline and 0.1 N hydrochloric acid (HCl) into the esophagus via the NG tube. If patient symptoms are reproduced by the acid perfusion and not the saline, the study is considered abnormal and indicative of acid hypersensitivity.[17]

ENDOSCOPIC ULTRASONOGRAPHY

In recent years, endoscopic ultrasonography has emerged as a useful adjunct in the diagnosis and staging of gastroenterologic disorders. The instrument itself functions very much like a typical upper endoscope but with the added feature of an ultrasound transducer. The examiner is then able to see beneath the mucosa at regional anatomy and pathology. The major advantage of this procedure is its capability to deliver the ultrasound transducer to close proximity of deep tissues for enhanced image resolution. In clinical practice, endoscopic ultrasound is highly useful in detecting and defining gastrointestinal and pancreatic malignancies. It also plays a role in the diagnosis of submucosal lesions and small pancreatic malignancies. Endoscopic ultrasound guidance of fine-needle biopsy is increasingly performed.

LAPAROSCOPY

Laparoscopy uses a tube-like device with an elaborate optical system that permits distinct visualization of the peritoneal cavity. General anesthesia is often given and a surgical incision is made in the abdomen to allow the passage of the laparoscopic instrument. The exterior of the liver, gallbladder, spleen, peritoneum, diaphragm, and pelvic organs may be clearly examined during the laparoscopic examination. Similar to the other endoscopic techniques mentioned, biopsies and therapeutic interventions may occur during the laparoscopy. Reasons for doing laparoscopy include evaluating patients with ascites, abdominal masses, chronic abdominal pain, abnormalities indicated on liver-spleen scan, liver diseases, obstructive jaundice, and hepatic malignancy.

CLINICAL APPLICATIONS OF GI STUDIES

Gastrointestinal evaluations are largely driven by the patient's dominant sign, symptom, or condition. The previous sections of this chapter describe tools used to evaluate the GI tract; the remaining sections outline the application of these tools based on the patient's most

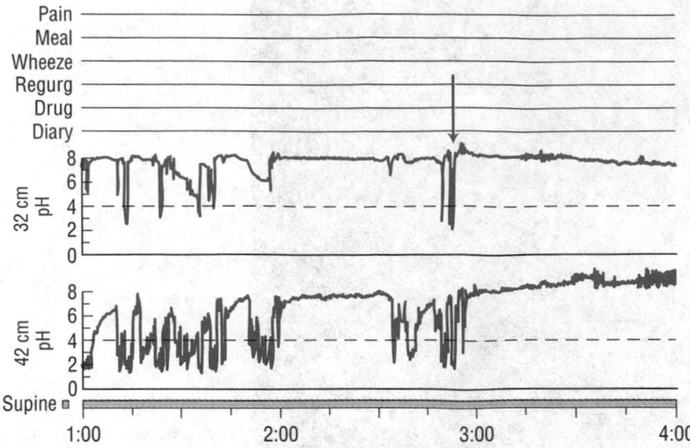

FIGURE 31–9. Ambulatory pH monitoring. The pH recordings from two esophageal probes are plotted over a 3-hour interval. Notice that the patient's symptom of regurgitation correlates with a low pH (<4) event *(arrow)*.

significant mode of presentation. Because of association and for ease of discussion, the modes of GI presentation are grouped as follows: (a) heartburn, dysphagia, and odynophagia; (b) abdominal pain and dyspepsia; (c) nausea and vomiting; (d) diarrhea and constipation; (e) malabsorption; (f) gastrointestinal bleeding; and (g) hepatitis and jaundice.

HEARTBURN, DYSPHAGIA, AND ODYNOPHAGIA

The patient's history is especially useful in evaluating esophageal disease. Cardinal symptoms of the esophagus are heartburn, dysphagia (difficulty in swallowing), and odynophagia (painful swallowing). Heartburn is the most common esophageal complaint and when present is often sufficient to make the diagnosis of gastroesophageal reflux disease (GERD). The ambulatory 24-hour pH study may convincingly link the patient's symptom to an acid event (Fig. 31–9). The role of endoscopy in reflux disease is to evaluate severe or atypical cases and to uncover complications of reflux including esophageal stricture, bleeding, ulcers, and Barrett's esophagus. Dysphagia prompts concern for structural diseases that may be either benign, such as peptic strictures, or malignant, such as esophageal carcinomas. When dysphagia is the dominant symptom, the patient is appropriately referred for a barium swallow. Upper endoscopy offers the capability to inspect the mucosa of the esophagus and to take biopsies.

Esophageal manometry may prove useful in documenting abnormal motility as a basis for dysphagia in those patients who lack evidence for structural disease. Achalasia, also diagnosed with manometry, is an unusual cause of dysphagia because of absent peristalsis in the esophagus. Odynophagia often results from infection and requires biopsy for confirmation.

ABDOMINAL PAIN AND DYSPEPSIA

Abdominal pain is a common reason for patients to seek medical care. A rapid onset of acute pain accompanied by signs of peritonitis, fever, and leukocytosis suggests the possibility of a severe intra-abdominal infection or inflammation. An upright abdominal film may reveal evidence of free peritoneal air under the diaphragm, suggesting a perforated bowel. A serum amylase confirms or denies the possibility of acute pancreatitis. The evaluation may include ultrasonography or CT scans that may be helpful in demonstrating inflammatory or structural diseases such as appendicitis, cholecystitis, diverticulitis, abscesses, or aneurysm.

Patients with long-standing, chronic abdominal pain should undergo a more deliberate evaluation, depending on the location and the temporal patterns of their abdominal pain. For example, nocturnal pain relieved by antacids may suggest peptic ulcer disease. A patient with abdominal pain, early satiety, and weight loss may have gastric cancer, and upper endoscopy and biopsy are particularly useful in diagnosing and evaluating this condition. Persistent attacks of pain radiating to the back may be a result of pancreatic diseases, and abdominal imaging with ultrasonography or CT scans is generally indicated for confirmation.

Patients experiencing abdominal pain associated with nausea, vomiting, and abdominal distention may have a small bowel obstruction. An upper GI radiocontrast study with small bowel follow-through may demonstrate a mechanical obstruction caused by adhesions and hernias. Postprandial bloating and right lower quadrant pain occurs with Crohn's disease of the terminal ileum that also may be detected with a small bowel follow-through. Left lower quadrant pain may reflect diverticulitis; although not always necessary, this may be detected by flexible sigmoidoscopy or barium enema. Patients with anemia or GI blood loss should undergo an evaluation by colonoscopy. Dyspepsia generally refers to a variety of symptoms associated with the ingestion of food and can include such symptoms as belching, burning, epigastric pain, and bloating. Dyspepsia may be the presenting symptom for a variety of disorders including gastric and pancreatic carcinoma, cholelithiasis, intestinal obstruction, and functional disorders. An upper endoscopy can provide visual and histologic information that greatly aids in the differential diagnosis of patients with dyspepsia. An upper GI tract barium series is reasonably accurate in making a diagnosis although it is unable to define mucosal disease. Tests detecting *Helicobacter pylori* should be employed in patients complaining of dyspepsia.

NAUSEA AND VOMITING

As usual, evaluation of nausea and vomiting begins with a careful history. Is the patient pregnant? Is the patient undergoing chemotherapy? Does the patient have a central nervous system disease? Is the patient experiencing an adverse or toxic effect from a drug such as theophylline, digoxin, or an antibiotic? After ruling out the more common causes for persistent nausea and vomiting such as food-borne or viral gastroenteritis, it is advantageous to consider "working up" the patient to detect bowel obstructions. A plain abdominal film may detect bowel obstruction. An upper GI series or an upper endoscopy may show structural lesions or obstructions of the GI tract as well. If an obstruction is not found, serum amylase and lipase should be measured to evaluate the diagnosis of acute pancreatitis. Timing of vomiting relative to meals provides important information. Nausea and vomiting on awakening suggest alcoholic gastritis; vomiting after meals suggests peptic ulcer disease and gastric cancer; vomiting 3 to 8 hours after meals suggests an obstruction in the upper gastrointestinal tract.

DIARRHEA AND CONSTIPATION

Patient history may be useful in identifying diarrhea associated with recent travel, male homosexual activity, antibiotics, or food-borne gastroenteritis. It is helpful to quantify the average number of stools per day, presence of blood and mucus, and stool color. Many patients experience mild abdominal discomfort and diarrhea when taking antibiotics. Other patients may continue to have diarrhea after discontinuing the antibiotics and may continue to experience fever and abdominal tenderness, suggesting antibiotic-associated colitis.

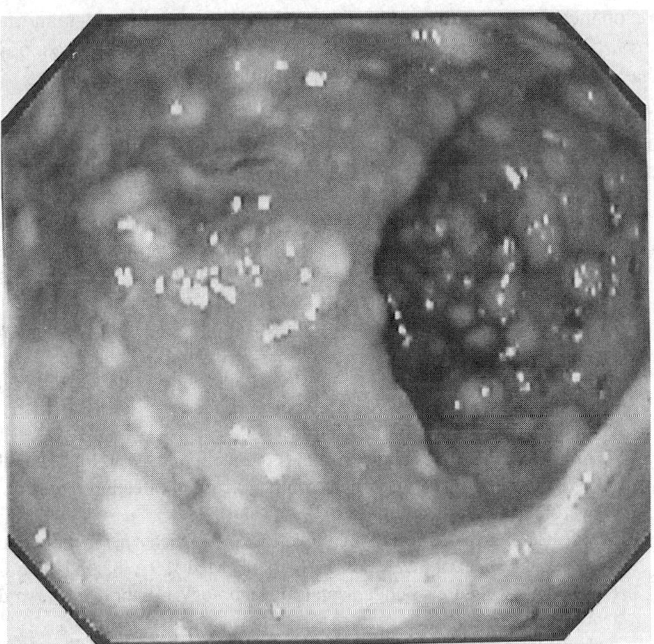

FIGURE 31–10. Sigmoidoscopic photograph revealing the light-raised lesions of antibiotic-associated pseudomembranous colitis.

This diagnosis can be achieved through sigmoidoscopy by observing yellow adherent plaques or "pseudomembranes" (Fig. 31–10). A stool sample may also be examined to detect *Clostridium difficile* toxins. A patient with acute diarrhea who appears feverish and dehydrated, or who has bloody diarrhea, may have an infection and should undergo stool cultures to detect *C. difficile,* ova, and parasites. In addition, evaluation of diarrhea for leukocytes is useful to determine if inflammation is present.

The history and physical examination may provide important clues to direct evaluation of chronic diarrhea. Sigmoidoscopy is reliable for excluding colitis and obstruction caused by cancer or diverticula. A patient with a normal sigmoidoscopy may have the remainder of his or her colon evaluated with an air-contrast barium enema to rule out inflammatory bowel disease or obstruction. A patient with a negative evaluation probably has irritable bowel syndrome ("spastic colon").

Constipation is an imprecise term that implies either infrequent or difficult defecation. It is important for clinicians to obtain a detailed dietary, laxative, and medication history because these may play a role. Appropriate laboratory tests should be performed to exclude metabolic disorders such as hypothyroidism, hypokalemia, hypercalcemia, and hypomagnesemia. If a metabolic disorder cannot be found, an underlying structural abnormality should be sought. Sigmoidoscopy and an air-contrast barium enema are usually the best approaches for evaluation.

MALABSORPTION

Malabsorption is classically manifested by steatorrhea (fat in the stool) and weight loss. Steatorrhea is evaluated by first testing the stool for the presence of fat and, once established, tests are performed to differentiate pancreatic insufficiency from small bowel disease. The d-xylose test is a measure of small bowel absorption that is nearly always abnormal in small bowel malabsorption. A 5-g dose of d-xylose is taken orally by the patient and should normally be absorbed and secreted in the urine. A patient with a normal d-xylose test and steatorrhea probably has pancreatic insufficiency. However, a patient with an abnormal d-xylose test and steatorrhea favors small bowel disease. An upper GI radiocontrast study with small bowel follow-through or small bowel biopsies may prove useful to show the presence of celiac sprue, Whipple disease, lymphoma, or other lesions.

GI BLEEDING

Gastrointestinal bleeding may occur as a life-threatening emergency marked by hematemesis (bloody vomit), hematochezia (bloody stool), or melena (black, tarry stool caused by upper GI bleeding); or, at the other extreme, may be chronic or occult and discovered in the course of evaluating anemia. The goal in evaluating a bleeding patient is to ascertain the site of bleeding (upper versus lower GI tract) and the nature of the bleeding lesion. After the patient is stabilized, endoscopy can be performed to identify bleeding ulcers, erosive gastritis, and esophageal varices. Endoscopy accurately determines the nature of the bleeding lesion in more than 90% of presenting patients, and is often the vehicle for the delivery of therapy (sclerosis injections or cautery). In cases where endoscopy has technically failed to identify or treat the source of the bleeding, or in cases of rapid bleeding, arteriography (angiography) may be advisable. Under these circumstances, arteriography can be used to localize the bleeding site and afford treatment of the bleeding vessel. Barium studies have no role in the management of acute GI bleeding.

HEPATITIS AND JAUNDICE

When the history and physical examination identify active or chronic liver disease, a detailed medication history is critical because numerous agents are known to induce these disorders. When transaminases are 10 or more times normal, viral hepatitis or acute cholangitis is considered, and should prompt further specific diagnostic efforts, including viral markers. Milder elevation of the transaminases is a nonspecific finding and considerations should include alcohol liver disease. In a symptomatic patient with hepatomegaly or clinical signs of liver disease, liver ultrasonography or CT scans may help to exclude cancer. The function of the liver may be measured indirectly by measuring serum albumin and performing coagulation studies.

When hepatocellular disease is suspected, ultrasonography or CT scans of the liver are performed to exclude focal defects such as tumors, abscesses, and vascular lesions prior to performing a percutaneous liver biopsy (Fig. 31–11). Often, a liver biopsy is the best way to resolve questions as to the reason for underlying hepatocellular injury. When alkaline phosphatase is elevated, especially in conjunction with transaminases, one considers cholestatic liver diseases. In suspected biliary disease, an abdominal ultrasound is usually done with special attention to the interhepatic ducts. If the ducts are dilated, one considers an obstructive pancreas, bile duct cancer, bile duct strictures, or common bile duct stones. "Cholestatic" patients without dilated bile ducts may have primary biliary cirrhosis, diagnosed by liver biopsy, or primary sclerosing cholangitis, diagnosed by characteristic bile duct changes on ERCP. Cholestasis may occur with or without jaundice.

Jaundice often, but not always, reflects underlying liver disease. The clinician is commonly faced with the question as to whether the patient's jaundice is a result of an extrahepatic process or an intrahepatic parenchymal liver disease. An extrahepatic lesion is suggested by a disproportionate elevation in alkaline phosphatase and may be confirmed by observing dilated intrahepatic ducts on ultrasonography or CT scan. Often, an ERCP is necessary to visualize the biliary tree and pancreatic ducts so as to identify the precise location and character

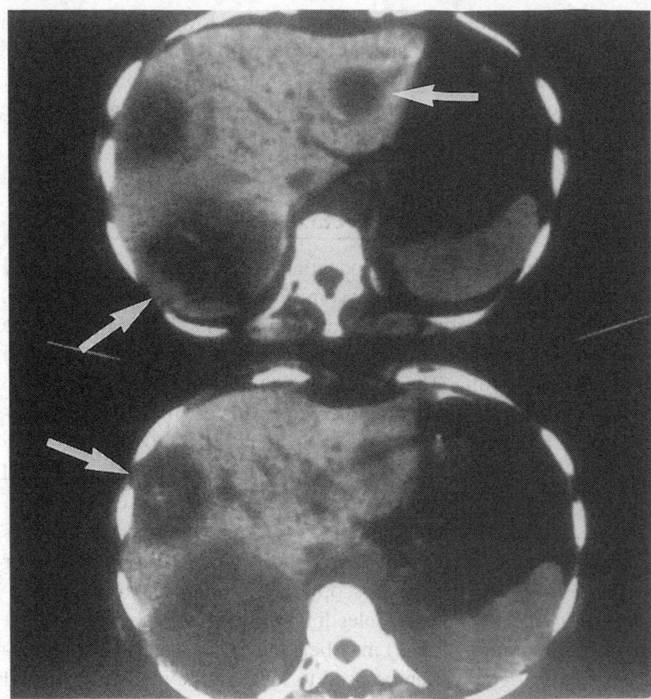

FIGURE 31–11. CT scans of the abdomen showing metastatic cancer of the liver *(arrows).*

of the obstructing lesion. Liver biopsy plays a role in determining the parenchymal role in the cholestatic process.

Hepatomegaly found on physical exam suggests chronic disease. Hepatitis might be the culprit under these circumstances and is easily detected by measurement of serum transaminases. Ultrasonography or CT scans are used to determine if there is focal or diffuse liver disease and obstruction of the biliary tree. A patient with abdominal pain and an enlarged liver may have an abscess, hematoma, or tumor that may be best demonstrated by a CT scan.

CONCLUSIONS

Evaluation of the GI tract begins with a careful history and comprehensive physical examination. It then proceeds in a deliberate and thoughtful manner to establish the correct diagnosis and appropriate management. Laboratory and microbiologic tests, radiography, ultrasonography, computed tomography, radionuclide scanning, magnetic resonance imaging, arteriography, endoscopy, esophageal manometry, pH monitoring, endoscopic ultrasonography, and laparoscopy have definite roles in diagnosing and evaluating GI disorders.

REFERENCES

1. Isselbacher KJ, Podolsky DK. Approach to the patient with gastrointestinal disease. In: Wilson JD, Braunwald E, et al, eds. Harrison's Principles of Internal Medicine. New York, McGraw-Hill, 1991:1213–1216.
2. Janowitz HD. Approach to the patient with gastrointestinal symptoms. In: Sachar DB, Waye JD, et al, eds. Pocket Guide to Gastroenterology. Baltimore, Williams & Wilkins, 1989:1–7.
3. Bates B. A Guide to Physical Examination. Philadelphia, Lippincott, 1994.
4. Jacobs DS, Demott WR, Finley PR, et al. Laboratory Test Handbook. Cleveland, Lexi-Comp, 1994.
5. Guerrant RL. Principles and syndromes of enteric infection. In: Mandell GL, Douglas RG, et al, eds. Principles and Practice of Infectious Diseases. New York, Churchill Livingstone, 1990:837–851.
6. Walsh JH, Peterson WL. The treatment of *Helicobacter pylori* infection in the management of ulcer disease. N Engl J Med 1995;333:984–991.
7. Novelline RA. Squire's Fundamentals of Radiology. Cambridge, Harvard University Press, 1997.
8. Cohen AJ. Radiologic general diagnostic and imaging studies of the small and large bowel. In: Gitnick G, ed. Principles and Practice of Gastroenterology and Hepatology. Stamford, CT, Appleton & Lange, 1994:441–432.
9. Eisenberg RL, Heineken P, Hedgcock MW, et al. Evaluation of plain abdominal radiographs in the diagnosis of abdominal pain. Ann Intern Med 1982;97:257–261.
10. Smith CR, Petty BG. Specific complications of medical management. In: Harvey AM, Johns RT, et al, eds. The Principles and Practice of Medicine. Stamford, CT, Appleton & Lange, 1988:1155–1162.
11. Miller RE, Sellink JL. Enteroclysis: The small bowel enema. How to succeed and how to fail. Gastrointest Radiol 1979;4:269–283.
12. Friedman LS, Needleman L. Hepatobiliary imaging. In: Wilson JD, Braunwald E, et al, eds. Harrison's Principles of Internal Medicine. New York, McGraw-Hill, 1991:1303–1308.
13. Wall SD. Diagnostic imaging procedures in gastro-enterology. In: Bennet JC, Plum F, eds. Cecil Textbook of Medicine. Philadelphia, Saunders, 1996:630–635.
14. Sartor RB. Upper gastrointestinal endoscopy. In: Drossman DA, ed. Manual of Gastroenterologic Procedures. New York, Raven, 1993:131–139.
15. Shinya H, Wolf WI. Colonoscopy. Surg Ann 1976;8:257–295.
16. Benjamin SB, Richter JE, Cordova CM, et al. Prospective manometric evaluation with pharmacologic provocation of patients with suspected esophageal motility dysfunction. Gastroenterology 1983;84:893–901.
17. Sandler RS. Bernstein (acid perfusion) test. In: Drossman DA, ed. Manual of Gastroenterologic Procedures. New York, Raven, 1993:56–60.

32

GASTROESOPHAGEAL REFLUX DISEASE

Dianne B. Williams

Gastroesophageal reflux disease (GERD) is a common medical disorder seen by health care practitioners of all specialties. Although mortality associated with GERD is very low (1 death per 100,000 patients), it has a greater impact on quality of life than do duodenal ulcers, untreated hypertension, mild congestive heart failure, angina, or menopause.[1,2] GERD refers to any symptomatic clinical condition or histologic alteration that results from episodes of gastroesophageal reflux. Gastroesophageal reflux is the retrograde movement of gastric contents from the stomach into the esophagus. When the esophagus is repeatedly exposed to refluxed material for prolonged periods of time, inflammation of the esophagus (reflux esophagitis) occurs, and, in some cases, it can progress to erosion of the esophagus (erosive esophagitis). Gastroesophageal reflux associated with disease processes in organs other than the esophagus, such as the lungs, is referred to as atypical (or extraesophageal) GERD.[3] Severe reflux symptoms associated with a normal endoscopic findings are referred to as endoscopy-negative reflux disease. Many patients suffering from mild GERD do not go on to develop erosive esophagitis and are often managed with lifestyle changes, antacids, and over-the-counter (OTC) histamine (H_2)-receptor antagonists. Those with more severe symptoms (with or without endoscopic findings) predictably follow a course of relapsing disease requiring more intensive treatment with acid-suppressive therapy followed by long-term maintenance therapy.[4] Laparoscopic antireflux surgery offers an alternative to medical management for those patients who fail therapy or for those patients where medical management is undesirable.

EPIDEMIOLOGY

Gastroesophageal reflux disease occurs in both adults and children. The prevalence of GERD is dependent on the geographic region and is highest in Western countries.[1] The prevalence increases in adults older than 40 years of age. Except during pregnancy, there does not appear to be a major difference in incidence between men and women. Heartburn, the hallmark symptom of GERD, is a common complaint during pregnancy, with as many as 25% of women experiencing heartburn on a daily basis.[5] Although gender does not play a major role in the development of GERD, it is an important factor in the development of Barrett's esophagus, a complication of GERD in which the normal squamous epithelium is replaced with columnar epithelium. Barrett's esophagus is most prevalent in white adult males in Western countries.

The true prevalence and incidence of GERD is difficult to assess because (a) many patients do not seek medical treatment, (b) symptoms do not always correlate well with severity of disease, and (c) there is no standardized definition or universal gold standard method for diagnosing the disease.[1]

Approximately 10% of Americans suffer from heartburn daily and more than one-third have intermittent symptoms.[5] Yet many of these patients choose not to seek medical help from a physician and self-treat with OTC medications. Interestingly, as many as 46% of patients with mild disease will heal spontaneously with self-medication, and another 31% will show significant improvement, indicating a relatively benign process in patients with minimal symptoms.[6,7]

Conversely, the presence of symptoms in patients who do seek medical advice does not always correlate well with the presence of esophageal inflammation or erosion, making it extremely difficult to identify which patients will have severe esophageal damage as opposed to those with merely symptoms. Of the 20% to 40% of patients who experience heartburn, approximately 30% to 79% of these patients will have evidence of esophagitis.[8] On the other hand, many patients with esophageal damage may not experience symptoms, or they may present with atypical symptoms.[9]

Finally, the lack of a standardized definition and universal gold standard for diagnosing GERD presents another obstacle in assessing epidemiologic data.

PATHOPHYSIOLOGY

The key factor in the development of GERD is the movement of acid or other noxious substances from the stomach into the esophagus.[10] In many patients with GERD, the problem is not that they produce too much acid, but that the acid produced spends too much time in contact with the esophageal mucosa. A prolonged acid clearance from the esophagus is seen in many patients with gastroesophageal reflux.

In many cases, gastroesophageal reflux is caused by a defective lower esophageal sphincter pressure. Patients may have decreased gastroesophageal sphincter pressures related to (a) spontaneous transient lower esophageal sphincter relaxations, (b) transient increases in intra-abdominal pressure, or (c) atonic lower esophageal sphincter—all of which may lead to the development of gastroesophageal reflux. Problems with other normal mucosal "defense mechanisms" such as anatomic factors, mucosal resistance, and gastric emptying may also contribute to the development of GERD. "Aggressive factors" that may promote esophageal damage upon reflux into the esophagus include gastric acid, pepsin, bile acids, and pancreatic enzymes. Thus, the composition and volume of the refluxate are the most important aggressive factors in determining the consequences of gastroesophageal reflux.

Gastroesophageal reflux may lead to many severe complications, including esophagitis, strictures, and Barrett's esophagus.[10] Strictures are common in the distal esophagus and are generally 1 to 2 cm in length. The use of nonsteroidal anti-inflammatory drugs (NSAIDs) or aspirin has been implicated as an additional risk factor that may contribute to the development or worsening of esophageal strictures.[11] Although GERD may lead to esophageal bleeding, the blood loss is usually chronic and low grade in nature, but can lead to anemia. In some patients, the reparative process leads to the replacement of the squamous epithelial lining of the esophagus by columnar-type epithelium. This condition, known as Barrett's esophagus, is more likely to occur in those patients with a long history (years) of reflux that, in many cases, improves without intervention.[12] It was found in 3.5% of patients undergoing first-time endoscopy for reflux symptoms and is probably higher in patients with more severe or complicated disease.[13] Patients with Barrett's esophagus have a 30% to 80% incidence of esophageal stricture formation. Additionally, the risk of esophageal adenocarcinoma is 30 to 60 times higher in patients with Barrett's esophagus, as compared to the general population.[14] Interestingly, the risk of esophageal adenocarcinoma could be increased, despite the presence or absence of Barrett's esophagus, in patients with long-standing, frequently recurring, reflux symptoms (heartburn and regurgitation).[14]

Rational therapeutic regimens in the treatment of gastroesophageal reflux are designed to maximize normal mucosal defense mechanisms and/or attenuate the aggressive factors.

LOWER ESOPHAGEAL SPHINCTER PRESSURE

The lower esophageal sphincter is a manometrically defined zone of high resting pressure. The sphincter is normally in a tonic state, preventing the reflux of gastric material from the stomach, but relaxes on swallowing to permit the free passage of food into the stomach. Typically, patients with more severe gastroesophageal disease have resting lower esophageal sphincter pressures below 5 mm Hg. Mechanisms by which defective lower esophageal sphincter pressure may cause gastroesophageal reflux are threefold. First, and probably most important, reflux may occur following spontaneous transient lower esophageal sphincter relaxations that are not associated with swallowing.[15] Although the exact mechanism is unknown, esophageal distention, vomiting, belching, and retching have all been shown to cause relaxation of the lower esophageal sphincter. Although not thought to contribute significantly to erosive esophagitis, these transient relaxations, which are normal postprandially, may play an important role in intermittent nonerosive reflux.[4] Transient decreases in sphincter pressure are responsible for approximately 65% of the reflux episodes in patients with GERD. The propensity to develop gastroesophageal reflux secondary to transient decreases in lower esophageal sphincter pressure is probably dependent on numerous factors, including degree of sphincter relaxation, efficacy of esophageal clearance, patient position (more common in recumbent position), gastric volume, and intragastric pressure. Second, reflux may occur following transient increases in intra-abdominal pressure (stress reflux).[10] An increase in intra-abdominal pressure such as that occurring during straining, bending over, coughing, eating, or a Valsalva maneuver may overcome a weak lower esophageal sphincter, and thus may lead to reflux. Third, the lower esophageal sphincter may be atonic, thus permitting free reflux.

Although transient relaxations are more likely to occur when there is substantial lower esophageal sphincter pressure, the latter two mechanisms are more likely to occur when the lower esophageal sphincter pressure is decreased by such factors as fatty foods, gastric distention, smoking, or certain medications.[10] Table 32–1 lists factors and conditions that affect lower esophageal sphincter pressures.[16] Factors that decrease lower esophageal sphincter pressure predispose patients to gastroesophageal reflux. Various foods aggravate esophageal reflux by decreasing lower esophageal sphincter pressure or by precipitating symptomatic reflux by direct mucosal irritation (spicy foods, orange juice, tomato juice, and coffee).[5] Pregnancy, achalasia, and scleroderma are conditions in which reflux is common. There are many postulated reasons for the increased incidence of heartburn during pregnancy including hormonal effects on esophageal muscle, lower esophageal sphincter tone, and physical factors (increased intra-abdominal pressure) resulting from an enlarging uterus.[17]

A decrease in lower esophageal sphincter pressure resulting from any of the previously mentioned causes is not always associated with

TABLE 32–1. Foods and Medications That May Worsen GERD Symptoms

Decrease Lower Esophageal Sphincter Pressure	
Foods	
Carminatives (peppermint, spearmint)	Garlic
Chocolate	Onions
Coffee, cola, tea	
Fatty meal	
Medications	
Anticholinergics	Isoproterenol
Barbiturates	Narcotics (meperidine, morphine)
Benzodiazepines (diazepam)	Nicotine (smoking)
Caffeine	Nitrates
Dihydropyridine calcium channel blockers	Phentolamine
Dopamine	Progesterone
Estrogen	Theophylline
Ethanol	
Direct Irritants to the Esophageal Mucosa	
Foods	
Spicy foods	Tomato juice
Orange juice	Coffee
Medications	
Alendronate	Quinidine
Aspirin	Potassium chloride
Iron	
NSAIDs	

Adapted from Weinberg DS, Kadish SL. The diagnosis and management of gastroesophageal reflux disease. Med Clin North Am 1996;80(2):411–429.

gastroesophageal reflux. Likewise, individuals who experience decreases in sphincter pressures, and subsequently reflux, do not always develop GERD. The other natural defense mechanisms (anatomic factors, esophageal clearance, mucosal resistance, and gastric factors) must be evoked to explain this phenomenon.

ANATOMIC FACTORS

Proposed anatomic factors can be categorized into valvular mechanisms, extrinsic compression, a segment of the esophagus in the abdomen, mucosal choke, and spiral stretch mechanisms. Disruption of the normal anatomic barriers by a hiatal hernia was once thought to be a primary etiology of gastroesophageal reflux and esophagitis. Now it appears that a more important factor related to the presence or absence of symptoms in patients with hiatal hernias is the lower esophageal sphincter pressure. The size of a hiatal hernia is proportional to the frequency of transient lower esophageal sphincter relaxations.[18] Patients with hypotensive lower esophageal sphincter pressures and large hiatal hernias are more likely to experience gastroesophageal reflux following abrupt increases in intra-abdominal pressure as compared to patients with hypotensive lower esophageal sphincter and no hiatal hernia. Although anatomic factors are still considered significant by some, the diagnosis of hiatal hernia is currently considered a separate entity with which gastroesophageal reflux may or may not simultaneously occur.

ESOPHAGEAL CLEARANCE

Approximately 50% of GERD patients with esophagitis have a prolonged acid clearance time from the esophagus.[10] This is not surprising, because the symptoms and/or severity of damage produced by gastroesophageal reflux are partially dependent on the duration of contact between the gastric contents and the esophageal mucosa.[19] This contact time is, in turn, dependent on the rate at which the esophagus clears the noxious material and the frequency of reflux. The esophagus is cleared by primary peristalsis in response to swallowing, secondary peristalsis in response to esophageal distention, and gravitational effects. Swallowing contributes to esophageal clearance by increasing salivary flow. Saliva contains bicarbonate that buffers the residual gastric material on the surface of the esophagus. The production of saliva decreases with increasing age, making it more difficult to maintain a neutral intraesophageal pH. Therefore, esophageal damage due to reflux occurs more often in the elderly and, similarly, in those patients with Sjögren's syndrome.[20]

MUCOSAL RESISTANCE

Within the esophageal mucosa and submucosa there are mucus-secreting glands. The mucus secreted by these glands may contribute to the protection of the esophagus.[21] Bicarbonate moving from the blood to the lumen can neutralize acidic refluxate in the esophagus. When the mucosa is repeatedly exposed to the refluxate in GERD, or if there is a defect in the normal mucosal defenses, hydrogen ions diffuse into the mucosa, leading to the cellular acidification and necrosis that ultimately cause esophagitis.[10] In theory, mucosal resistance may be related not only to esophageal mucus but also to tight epithelial junctions, epithelial cell turnover, nitrogen balance, mucosal blood flow, tissue prostaglandins, and the acid-base status of the tissue.[21]

COMPOSITION OF REFLUXATE

The composition and volume of the refluxate are the most important aggressive factors in determining the consequences of gastroesophageal reflux. In animals, acid has two primary effects when it refluxes into the esophagus. First, if the pH of the refluxate is less than 2, esophagitis may develop secondary to protein denaturation. In addition, pepsin is activated at this pH and may also cause esophagitis. Alkaline esophagitis refers to esophagitis induced by the reflux of bilious and pancreatic fluid. The term "alkaline esophagitis" may be a misnomer in that the refluxate may be either weakly alkaline or acidic in nature. An increase in gastric bile concentrations may be caused by duodenogastric reflux because of a generalized motility disorder or slower clearance of the refluxate.[22] Although bile acids have both a direct irritant effect on the esophageal mucosa and an indirect effect of increasing hydrogen ion permeability of the mucosa, symptoms are more often related to acid reflux than to bile reflux. Esophageal pH monitoring demonstrates that severity of disease is related to degree of esophageal acid exposure and not so much to bile exposure. Specifically, the percentage of time that esophageal pH is below 4 is greater for patients with severe disease as compared to mild disease.[23,24] However, esophageal pH monitoring in conjunction with 24-hour bile monitoring has demonstrated a higher incidence of Barrett's esophagus in patients with both acid and alkaline reflux.[22] More study is needed to substantiate this finding. Nevertheless, the combination of acid, pepsin, and bile is a potent refluxate in producing esophageal damage.

GASTRIC EMPTYING

Delayed gastric emptying contributes to gastroesophageal reflux. An increase in gastric volume may increase both the frequency of reflux and the amount of gastric fluid available to be refluxed. Gastric volume is related to the volume of material ingested, rate of gastric secretion, rate of gastric emptying, and amount and frequency of duodenal reflux into the stomach. Patients with Barrett's esophagus may have a hypersecretory condition that is unresponsive to standard doses of H_2 antagonists. Factors that increase gastric volume and/or decrease gastric emptying, such as smoking and high fatty meals, are often associated with gastroesophageal reflux. This partially explains the prevalence of postprandial gastroesophageal reflux. Fatty foods may increase postprandial gastroesophageal reflux by increasing gastric volume, delaying the gastric emptying rate, and decreasing the lower esophageal sphincter pressure. Patients with gastroesophageal reflux, particularly infants, may have a defect in antral motility. The delay in emptying may promote regurgitation of feedings, which might, in turn, contribute to two common complications of gastroesophageal reflux disease in infants (i.e., failure to thrive and pulmonary aspiration).[25]

The pathophysiology of gastroesophageal reflux is a complex, cyclic process. It is difficult, if not impossible, to determine which occurs first: gastroesophageal reflux leading to a defective peristalsis with delayed clearing, or an incompetent lower esophageal sphincter pressure leading to gastroesophageal reflux. Understanding the factors associated with the development of GERD provides insight into the treatment modalities currently used to manage a patient who suffers from the disease.

CLINICAL PRESENTATION

Patients with GERD may display symptoms described as (a) typical, (b) atypical, or (c) complicated. The hallmark symptom of gastroesophageal reflux and esophagitis is heartburn (i.e., pyrosis), classically described as a substernal sensation of warmth or burning that may radiate to the neck. It is waxing and waning in character, and is often aggravated by activities that worsen gastroesophageal reflux such as supine position, bending over, or eating a meal high in fat. Heartburn is a common complaint of both healthy individuals and of patients with GERD, and is most commonly reported when the gastric pH falls below 4. Other symptoms include water brash (hypersalivation), belching, and regurgitation, which usually occur after eating a large meal (especially a large fatty meal), lying down shortly after eating, or bending over.[26] Regurgitation, the effortless movement of food or liquid from the esophagus into the mouth, is frequently associated with reflux (especially in infants). Typical symptoms generally improve, at least temporarily, with the use of antacids.

Atypical symptoms include nonallergic asthma, chronic cough, hoarseness, pharyngitis, and chest pain that mimics angina.[26] In some cases, these "extraesophageal" symptoms are the only symptoms present, making it more difficult to recognize GERD as the cause, especially when endoscopic studies and x-rays are normal.[12] Further followup is necessary in patients presenting with chest pain to distinguish it from chest pain that is cardiac in nature. Approximately 50% of patients presenting with chest pain who have a normal electrocardiogram (ECG) have GERD.[10] Similarly, 53% of patients with asthma have GERD.[27] Patients presenting with asthma that is poorly responsive to standard medical therapies should be evaluated for GERD as a possible cause for their symptoms.[12] Pulmonary symptoms result from either direct irritation of the vagus nerve when refluxed acid comes in contact with the esophageal mucosa causing bronchospasm (reflex theory) or, less commonly, from aspiration of the refluxate into the lungs causing chemical irritation that manifests as pneumonia or pulmonary fibrosis (reflux theory).[28] Dental erosions have also been reported in patients with gastroesophageal reflux.[29] The severity of the symptoms of gastroesophageal reflux does not usually correlate with the degree of esophagitis, but it does correlate with the duration of reflux.

Patients who are not adequately treated for GERD may go on to develop complications from long-term acid exposure. Continual pain, dysphagia, or odynophagia indicate complicated disease, which usually occurs in patients with more severe esophagitis.[26] Long-term, recurrent reflux symptoms that are not adequately treated may lead to the development of Barrett's esophagus and may be an independent risk factor for the development of esophageal adenocarcinoma.[14] Esophageal strictures may be present in patients presenting with dysphagia. However, these symptoms may occur in other esophageal disorders such as esophageal diverticulum, achalasia, obstruction, esophageal spasm, esophageal infections, scleroderma, and malignancy. Other symptoms suggesting more complicated disease include bleeding, unexplained weight loss, and choking (acid causing cough, shortness of breath or hoarseness).[30] The presence of complicated symptoms should be further investigated to differentiate other diseases as the cause.

DIAGNOSIS

The most useful tool in the diagnosis of gastroesophageal reflux is the clinical history, including both presenting symptomology and associated risk factors. Patients presenting with mild, typical symptoms of reflux (heartburn, regurgitation) do not usually require invasive esophageal evaluation. These patients generally benefit from an initial trial of lifestyle modifications and patient-directed OTC therapies. A clinical diagnosis of GERD can be assumed in patients who respond to appropriate therapy.[30] Further diagnostic testing should be performed in (a) patients who do not respond to empiric (prescription) therapy, (b) patients with warning symptoms suggesting more complicated disease, (c) patients with chronic symptoms who are at risk for Barrett's esophagus, and (d) patients who require continuous, chronic therapy to relieve symptoms.[30]

Patients presenting with atypical symptoms (chest pain, chronic cough, hoarseness, asthma) should first be evaluated to exclude other cardiac or respiratory causes for their symptoms. If cardiac and respiratory systems are normal, esophageal studies are needed to confirm the diagnosis of gastroesophageal reflux.

ENDOSCOPY AND BARIUM RADIOGRAPHY

Patients requiring continuous therapy for long-standing GERD symptoms should undergo endoscopy because of their increased risk of Barrett's esophagus.[30] Endoscopy is the preferred technique for assessing the mucosa for esophagitis and for the presence of complications such as Barrett's esophagus.[30] It enables visualization and biopsy of the esophageal mucosa. Several systems have been used to classify severity of disease; a common grading scale is shown in Table 32–2.[31] Although endoscopy is a highly specific test, it is not extremely sensitive. In mild cases of GERD, the esophageal mucosa may appear relatively normal; however, obtaining mucosal biopsies may increase diagnostic yield. In addition, noninflammatory GERD and major motor disorders may be missed by endoscopy.

Although more cost effective than endoscopy, barium radiography lacks the sensitivity and specificity needed to accurately determine the presence of mucosal injury or to distinguish between Barrett's esophagus and esophagitis.[30] Barrett's esophagus requires histologic confirmation that can only be obtained by endoscopy with biopsy. For these reasons barium radiography has limited use in the routine diagnosis of GERD.[30]

TABLE 32–2. Endoscopic Classification of Esophagitis[31]

Grade 0	Normal esophageal mucosa
Grade 1	Erythema or diffusely red mucosa, edema, causing accentuated folds
Grade 2	Isolated round or linear erosions extending from the gastroesophageal junction upward, and not involving entire circumference
Grade 3	Confluent erosions extending around entire circumference or superficial ulceration without stenosis
Grade 4	Complicated cases; erosions as above plus deep ulcerations, strictures, or columnar epithelium-lined esophagus

PROVOCATIVE AND pH TESTING

Provocative tests such as the acid perfusion (Bernstein) test and gastrointestinal scintiscanning are used to establish a causal relationship between patient symptoms and abnormal acid exposure, especially when esophagitis is not present.[6] In general, provocative tests have limited use in the diagnosis of routine GERD.

Twenty-four-hour ambulatory pH monitoring is most useful in diagnosing gastroesophageal reflux in (a) patients who continue to have symptoms without evidence of esophageal damage, (b) patients who are refractory to standard treatment, and (c) patients who present with atypical symptoms (chest pain or pulmonary symptoms).[30] In patients with atypical symptoms, 24-hour ambulatory pH monitoring may be the only way to objectively prove the symptoms are reflux related. Ambulatory pH monitoring documents the percentage of time the intraesophageal pH is low, determines the frequency and severity of reflux, and is useful in correlating a patient's symptoms with either normal or abnormal esophageal acid exposure.[20,30] Ambulatory pH monitoring may also be useful in patients who are on what is considered adequate therapy but whose symptoms are not improving. However, GERD truly refractory to medical therapy is rare.[30]

Continuous pH monitoring can be performed by passing a small-electrode pH probe intranasally and placing it approximately 5 cm above the lower esophageal sphincter.[20] Patients keep a diary of symptoms and these are correlated with the pH measurement corresponding to the time the symptom was reported. Problems with esophageal pH monitoring arise when different methods are used to perform the test or a patient's baseline differs significantly from the standard baseline. Additionally, pH monitoring is not readily available in many institutions.

ESOPHAGEAL MANOMETRY

Esophageal manometry, to evaluate peristaltic function, should be performed in any patient who is a candidate for antireflux surgery.[30] Esophageal manometry is useful in determining which surgical procedure is best for the patient.

To perform manometry, a multilumen tube is passed into the stomach and the pressures are measured as the tube is pulled back across the lower esophageal sphincter, esophagus, and pharynx.

"OMEPRAZOLE TEST" TO DIAGNOSE GERD

The empiric use of standard dose, or even double-dose, omeprazole as a "therapeutic trial" for diagnosing the presence of GERD may be as beneficial as ambulatory 24-hour pH monitoring in diagnosing GERD. This approach is less expensive, more convenient and more readily available than ambulatory pH monitoring and has shown promise in patients with typical and atypical symptoms of GERD as well.[32–36] It seems especially useful in those patients where other gastrointestinal disorders, such as esophageal erosions, peptic ulcers, and carcinomas, have been ruled out by endoscopy but symptoms are still present. Preliminary results have also been promising in patients with extraesophageal symptoms.[37] Problems with the "omeprazole test" include lack of a standard dosing regimen and duration of the trial.

As compared with endoscopy and ambulatory pH monitoring, the omeprazole test, using 20 mg twice daily, had a sensitivity of approximately 75% and a specificity of approximately 55%.[32]

Traditionally, patients with noncardiac chest pain undergo endoscopy as well as ambulatory pH monitoring to identify noncardiac causes of chest pain. Sensitivity and specificity of omeprazole 60 mg daily for 7 days as the initial diagnostic tool were similar to that obtained with ambulatory pH monitoring.[35] Eighty-four percent of patients were found to be symptom-free at 1 year, as compared with 74% for the strategies that began with an invasive test, and overall costs, as well as use of other diagnostic tests, were significantly lower. Omeprazole 40 mg every morning and 20 mg every evening for 7 days was also relatively sensitive and specific for GERD.[36]

▶ TREATMENT: Gastroesophageal Reflux Disease

DESIRED OUTCOMES

Therapeutic modalities used in the treatment of gastroesophageal reflux are targeted at reversing the various pathophysiologic abnormalities. The goals of treatment are to (a) alleviate or eliminate the patient's symptoms; (b) decrease the frequency or recurrence and duration of gastroesophageal reflux; (c) promote healing of the injured mucosa; and (d) prevent the development of complications. Therapy is directed at augmenting defense mechanisms that prevent reflux and/or decrease the aggressive factors that worsen reflux or mucosal damage (Fig. 32–1). Specifically, therapy is directed at (a) increasing lower esophageal sphincter pressure; (b) enhancing esophageal acid clearance; (c) improving gastric emptying; (d) protecting the esophageal mucosa; (e) decreasing the acidity of the refluxate; and (f) decreasing the gastric volume available to be refluxed.

GENERAL APPROACH TO TREATMENT

The treatment of GERD is categorized into the following modalities: Phase I (lifestyle changes and patient-directed therapy with antacids

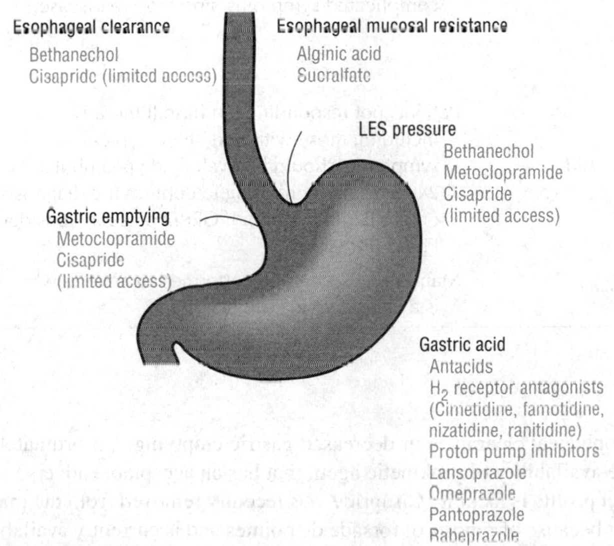

FIGURE 32–1. Therapeutic interventions in the management of gastroesophageal reflux disease. Pharmacologic interventions are targeted at improving defense mechanisms or decreasing aggressive factors. (LES = lower esophageal sphincter).

and/or OTC H_2-receptor antagonists); Phase II (pharmacologic intervention primarily with standard or high-dose antisecretory agents); and Phase III (surgical intervention). The initial therapeutic modality used is in part dependent on the patient's condition (degree of esophagitis, presence of complications). Historically, a step-up approach has been used, starting with noninvasive lifestyle modifications and patient-directed therapy (phase I) and progressing to pharmacologic management (phase II) or surgical intervention (phase III) (Table 32–3).[6,9,10,26] More recent studies show that a step-down approach, starting with a proton pump inhibitor once or twice daily instead of an H_2-receptor antagonist and then stepping down to the lowest acid suppression needed to control symptoms, is also effective. Neither the "step-up" or "step-down" approach has superior efficacy or cost-effectiveness over the other. The clinician should determine the most appropriate approach for an individual patient.[30] Whichever method is used, every attempt should be made to aggressively control symptoms and to prevent relapses early in the course of the patient's disease in order to prevent the long-term complications that are seen with long-standing symptomatic GERD.[38] In patients with moderate to severe GERD, starting with a proton pump inhibitor as initial therapy is advocated because of its superior efficacy over H_2-receptor antagonists.

Dietary and lifestyle modifications and education about factors that may worsen GERD symptoms should be discussed with the patient.[30] Table 32–4 lists many of the lifestyle changes that are included in phase I therapy.[9,39] Although most patients do not respond to lifestyle changes alone, the importance of maintaining these lifestyle changes throughout the course of GERD therapy should be stressed to the patient on a routine basis, no matter what other therapeutic modality is used. Patients with mild symptoms may see improvement with the inexpensive over-the-counter H_2-receptor antagonists, antacids, or alginic acid.

Patients not responding to lifestyle changes and to patient-directed therapy (after 2 weeks) are generally started on a pharmacologic treatment regimen consisting of an acid-suppressing agent. Acid-suppressing therapy with proton pump inhibitors or H_2-receptor antagonists are the mainstay of GERD treatment. Patients presenting with more severe symptoms (with or without esophageal erosions) or with erosive esophagitis should be started on a proton pump inhibitor as initial therapy, because it provides the most rapid symptomatic relief and healing of esophagitis in the highest percent of patients.[30] H_2-receptor antagonists in divided doses are effective in patients with mild GERD.[30] Patients not responding to standard doses of H_2-receptor antagonists may require higher doses and/or more frequent dosing, because improvement correlates with the extent and duration of acid suppression.[12] Standard H_2-receptor antagonist doses may be increased to two to four times the normal dose. If this is necessary, it is more cost effective to switch to a proton pump inhibitor.

TABLE 32–3. Therapeutic Approach to Gastroesophageal Reflux Disease

Patient Presentation	Recommended Treatment Regimen	Comments
Phase I		
Intermittent, mild heartburn	A. Lifestyle changes **PLUS** B. Antacids (Maalox or Mylanta 30 mL as needed or PC & HS, Maalox TC or Mylanta II 15 mL as needed or PC & HS, Gaviscon 2 tabs PC & HS, calcium carbonate 0.5–1 g as needed) **AND/OR** C. Low dose, OTC H_2-receptor antagonists (each taken up to bid) • Cimetidine 200 mg • Famotidine 10 mg • Nizatidine 75 mg • Ranitidine 75 mg	Lifestyle changes should be started initially and continued throughout the course of treatment. If symptoms are unrelieved with lifestyle changes and OTC medications after 2 weeks, begin pharmacologic therapy (Phase II therapy).
Phase II		
Symptomatic relief of GERD	A. Lifestyle modifications **PLUS** B. Standard doses of H_2-receptor antagonists for 6–12 weeks • Cimetidine 400 mg bid • Famotidine 20 mg bid • Nizatidine 150 mg bid • Ranitidine 150 mg bid **OR** B. Proton-pump inhibitors for 4–8 weeks • Esomeprazole 20 mg qd • Lansoprazole 15–30 mg qd • Omeprazole 20 mg qd • Pantoprazole 40 mg qd • Rabeprazole 20 mg qd	For typical symptoms, treat empirically with Phase II therapy. Mild GERD can usually be treated effectively with H_2-receptor antagonists. Patients with moderate to severe symptoms should receive a proton pump inhibitor as initial therapy. If symptoms are relieved, treat recurrences on as-needed basis. If symptoms recur frequently, consider maintenance therapy (MT) with the lowest effective dose. Note: Most patients will require standard doses for MT.
Healing of erosive esophagitis or treatment of patients with moderate to severe symptoms or complications	A. Lifestyle modifications **PLUS** Proton-pump inhibitors for 8–16 weeks (up to bid) • Esomeprazole 20–40 mg qd • Lansoprazole 30 mg qd • Omeprazole 20 mg qd • Rabeprazole 20 mg qd • Pantoprazole 40 mg qd **OR** B. High-dose H_2-receptor antagonist for 8–12 weeks • Cimetidine 400 mg qid or 800 mg bid • Famotidine 40 mg bid • Nizatidine 150 mg qid • Ranitidine 150 mg qid	For atypical symptoms, obtain endoscopy (if possible) to evaluate mucosa. Give a trial of proton-pump inhibitor or H_2-receptor antagonist. If symptoms are relieved, consider MT. Proton pump inhibitor is most effective maintenance therapy in patients with atypical symptoms, complicated symptoms, and erosive disease. Patients not responding to Phase II therapy, including those with persistent atypical symptoms, should be evaluated via ambulatory 24-hour pH monitoring to confirm the diagnosis of GERD (if possible). If GERD present, consider Phase III therapy.
Phase III	Antireflux surgery	Manometry should be performed in anyone who is a candidate for surgery.

Prokinetic agents offer an alternative to standard doses of H_2-receptor antagonists in mild to moderate, nonerosive GERD, but may not be as effective as acid-suppressing agents and can be more expensive. Combining prokinetic agents with acid-suppressing drugs offers only modest improvements in symptoms over standard doses of H_2-receptor antagonists and should not be routinely recommended. These agents improve defects related to esophagogastric motility, such as decreased lower esophageal sphincter pressure, decreased esophageal clearance, or decreased gastric emptying. Unfortunately, the availability of prokinetic agent that has an acceptable adverse effect profile is lacking. Cisapride was recently removed from the market because of reports of torsade de pointes and is currently available only through a limited access program from the manufacturer. For this reason, it is no longer routinely used in managing patients with GERD. The use of other prokinetic agents, such as metoclopramide and bethanechol, is limited by their adverse effect profile.

TABLE 32–4. Nonpharmacologic Treatment of GERD with Lifestyle Modifications

- Elevate the head of the bed (increases esophageal clearance)
  - Use 6–8 inch blocks under the head of the bed
  - Sleep on a foam wedge
- Dietary changes
  - Avoid foods that may decrease lower esophageal sphincter pressure (fats, chocolate, alcohol, peppermint, and spearmint)
  - Avoid foods that have a direct irritant effect on the esophageal mucosa (spicy foods, orange juice, tomato juice, and coffee)
  - Include protein-rich meals in diet (augments lower esophageal sphincter pressure)
  - Eat small meals and avoid eating immediately prior to sleeping (within 3 h if possible) (decreases gastric volume)
  - Weight reduction (reduces symptoms)
- Stop smoking (decreases spontaneous esophageal sphincter relaxation)
- Avoid alcohol (increases amplitude of the lower esophageal sphincter, peristaltic waves, and frequency of contraction)
- Avoid tight-fitting clothes
- Discontinue, if possible, drugs that may promote reflux (calcium channel blockers, beta blockers, nitrates, theophylline)
- Take drugs that have a direct irritant effect on the esophageal mucosa with plenty of liquid if they cannot be avoided (tetracyclines, quinidine, and KCl, iron salts, aspirin, nonsteroidal anti-inflammatory drugs)

Compiled from refs. 9 and 39.

Maintenance therapy is generally necessary to control symptoms and to prevent complications. In patients with more severe symptoms (with or without esophageal erosions), or in patients with other complications, maintenance therapy with a proton pump inhibitor is most effective. Routine use of combination therapy has no role in maintenance therapy of GERD. GERD that is refractory to adequate acid suppression is rare. In these cases, the diagnosis should be confirmed through further diagnostic tests before long-term, high-dose therapy or antireflux surgery is considered.[30]

Antireflux surgery may also be considered a maintenance option in certain patients with established GERD.[30]

NONPHARMACOLOGIC THERAPY

Nonpharmacologic treatment of GERD includes lifestyle modifications, which should be started initially and continued throughout the treatment course for GERD, and surgical intervention.

LIFESTYLE MODIFICATIONS

The most common lifestyle changes that a patient should be educated about include (a) weight loss; (b) smoking cessation; (c) avoidance of alcohol; (d) elevation of the head of the bed; (e) avoidance of foods or medications that exacerbate GERD; and (f) eating smaller meals and avoidance of eating 2 hours prior to sleeping. These and other recommended lifestyle modifications are listed in Table 32–4. Obese patients were 2.8 times more likely to experience GERD symptoms than those patients who were not obese.[40] While there are limited data indicating that reflux occurs more often with obesity, it would seem logical that the increased intra-abdominal pressure and dietary habits of obese patients would predispose them to reflux.[4] Therefore, weight loss is recommended. Smoking can cause aerophagia, which leads to increased belching and regurgitation.[4] However, data are lacking to show that symptoms improve in patients who quit smoking. Nevertheless, patients with GERD should be encouraged to quit smoking. Alcohol, although not thought to play a role in severe disease, decreases lower esophageal sphincter pressure and may exacerbate symptoms such as heartburn.[4] Elevating the head of the bed about 6 to 10 inches with an under mattress foam wedge (not just elevating the head with pillows) decreases nocturnal esophageal acid contact time and should be recommended.[10]

It is important to evaluate patient profiles and to identify potential medications that may exacerbate GERD symptoms. Medications, such as anticholinergics, barbiturates, calcium channel blockers, and theophylline decrease lower esophageal sphincter pressure. Other medications, including aspirin, iron, NSAIDs, quinidine, potassium chloride, and bisphosphonates, act as direct irritants to the esophageal mucosa. Patients taking bisphosphonates (e.g., alendronate) should be instructed to drink 6 to 8 ounces of plain tap water and remain upright for at least 30 minutes following administration. Proper patient education can help prevent dysphagia or esophageal ulceration. Patients should be closely monitored for worsening symptoms when any of these medications are started. If symptoms worsen, alternative therapies may be warranted. The clinician must weigh the risks and benefits of continuing a drug known to worsen GERD and esophagitis. Many foods may also worsen the symptoms of GERD. Fats and chocolates can decrease lower esophageal sphincter pressure, while citrus juice, tomato juice, coffee, and pepper may irritate damaged endothelium.

Many patients are noncompliant with lifestyle modifications, and even those who do comply generally continue to have symptoms requiring acid-suppression therapy. Nonetheless, it is important to regularly stress the value of lifestyle modification.

SURGICAL INTERVENTION

Surgical intervention is a viable alternative for selected patients with well-documented GERD.[30] The goal of antireflux surgery is to reestablish the antireflux barrier, to position the lower esophageal sphincter within the abdomen where it is under positive (intra-abdominal) pressure, and to close any associated hiatal defect.[41] It should be considered in patients (a) who fail to respond to pharmacologic treatment; (b) who opt for surgery despite successful treatment because of lifestyle considerations including age, time, or expense of medications; (c) who have complications of GERD (Barrett's esophagus, strictures, grade 3 or 4 esophagitis); or (d) who have atypical symptoms and reflux documented on 24-hour ambulatory pH monitoring.[41]

Surgical procedures include Nissen, Belsey, Toupet, and Hill operations. The procedure chosen depends on the surgeon's expertise and preference, as well as on anatomic considerations.[41] In general, 90% of patients have symptom resolution following open Nissen fun doplication. Because of the diminished surgical complications with the newer laparoscopic surgical procedures (Nissen fundoplication being one of the most commonly used procedures), the role of surgery in the long-term management of GERD has become more appealing. The major complications with antireflux surgery include gas bloat syndrome (inability to belch or vomit), dysphagia, vagal denervation, splenic trauma, and, very rarely, death.[3] Antireflux surgery has been found to be superior to medical management (with an H_2-receptor antagonist or prokinetic agent). However, similar comparisons with proton pump inhibitors are lacking. A preliminary study of 310 patients who were initially controlled on omeprazole 40 mg daily found antireflux surgery to be slightly superior to omeprazole 20 mg daily at 3 years.[42] Doses of 40 to 60 mg were found to be equally efficacious to antireflux surgery. Long-term effectiveness of antireflux surgery ranges from 5 to 20 years.[30]

PHARMACOLOGIC THERAPY

ANTACIDS AND ANTACID-ALGINIC ACID PRODUCTS

Patients should be educated that antacids are an appropriate component of treating mild GERD, even though documentation of their efficacy in placebo-controlled clinical trials is lacking.[6] Although the literature is somewhat controversial on the superiority of antacids to placebo, physicians and patients clearly consider antacids to be effective for immediate, symptomatic relief, and antacids are often used concurrently with other acid-suppressing therapies. Chewable antacid tablets may be more effective than liquid formulations, possibly as a consequence of prolonged adherence of antacid and saliva to the distal esophagus.[43] Maintaining the intragastric pH above 4 decreases the activation of pepsin from pepsinogen. Also, neutralization of gastric fluid leads to an increased lower esophageal sphincter pressure. Patients who require frequent use of antacids for chronic symptoms should be treated with prescription acid-suppressing therapy because their illness is considered more significant.

An antacid product combined with alginic acid (Gaviscon) is not a potent neutralizing agent and does not enhance lower esophageal sphincter pressure; however, it does form a highly viscous solution that floats on the surface of the gastric contents. This viscous solution serves as a protective barrier for the esophagus against reflux of gastric contents. It also reduces the frequency of the reflux episodes.[44] The combination product (Gaviscon) usually relieves symptoms associated with reflux.[45,46] Efficacy data indicating endoscopic healing are lacking.

Antacid or antacid combination products may cause gastrointestinal adverse effects (diarrhea or constipation depending on the product), alterations in mineral metabolism, and acid-base disturbances. Aluminum-containing antacids may bind to phosphate in the gut and lead to bone demineralization. In addition, antacids interact with a variety of drugs by altering gastric pH, increasing urinary pH, absorbing medications to their surfaces, providing a physical barrier to absorption, or forming insoluble complexes with other medications.[47] Antacids have clinically significant drug interactions with tetracycline, ferrous sulfate, isoniazid, quinidine, sulfonylureas, and quinolone antibiotics. Antacid-drug interactions are influenced by composition, dose, and dosage schedule of the antacid, as well as by the formulation.

Dosage recommendations for antacids in the management of GERD are somewhat difficult to derive from the literature (see Table 32–3 for general dosing guidelines). Doses range from hourly to an as-needed basis. In general, antacids have a short duration of action, which necessitates frequent administration throughout the day to provide continuous neutralization of acid. Typical doses are two tablets or one tablespoonful four times daily—after meals and at bedtime. Taking antacids after meals can increase the duration of action from about 1 hour to about 3 hours; however, nighttime acid suppression cannot be maintained with bedtime doses.

ACID SUPPRESSION WITH H_2-RECEPTOR ANTAGONISTS (CIMETIDINE, FAMOTIDINE, NIZATIDINE, AND RANITIDINE)

Acid-suppressing therapies are the mainstay of treatment of GERD. H_2-receptor antagonists in divided doses are effective in treating patients with mild to moderate GERD.[30] The majority of the trials assessing the efficacy of standard doses of H_2-receptor antagonists indicate that symptomatic improvement is achieved in an average of 60% of patients.[30] However, endoscopic healing rates tend to be lower with an average of 50%.[30] Because H_2-receptor antagonists are equally efficacious, selection of the specific agent to use in the management of GERD should be based on factors such as differences in pharmacokinetics, safety profile, and cost. For symptomatic relief of mild GERD, low-dose, over-the-counter H_2-receptor antagonists may be beneficial. For nonerosive disease, H_2-receptor antagonists are generally given at standard doses twice daily. Patients not responding to standard doses may be hypersecreters of gastric acid, requiring higher doses.[6] For these patients and those with erosive disease, higher doses and/or four times daily dosing (cimetidine 800 mg twice daily, famotidine 40 mg twice daily, nizatidine 150 mg four times daily, or ranitidine 150 mg four times daily) provide better acid control, especially after mealtime acid surges.[4] However, proton pump inhibitors are considered more efficacious and more cost-effective in these patients.

Clinical trials indicate that the efficacy of H_2-receptor antagonists in the management of GERD is extremely variable and is frequently lower than desired.[48–53] Response to the H_2-receptor antagonists appears to be dependent on the (a) severity of disease, (b) duration of therapy, and (c) dosage regimen used. These factors are important to keep in mind when comparing various clinical trials and/or assessing a patient's response to therapy.

Severity of Disease

The severity of esophagitis at baseline has a profound impact on the patient's response to H_2-receptor antagonists. Patients with severe esophagitis (grade 4) who received either ranitidine 150 mg four times daily or famotidine 40 mg twice daily had dramatically lower healing rates (17%) as compared to those with less-severe disease (58%).[54] Following 12 weeks of cimetidine therapy (400 mg four times daily), endoscopic healing was observed in 80% of patients with mild esophagitis (grade 1) and in only 46% of patients with severe disease (grade 3). Clearly, the more severe the esophageal damage, the poorer the response to H_2-receptor antagonists.

Duration of Therapy

Unlike duodenal ulcer disease, in which the duration of therapy is relatively short (e.g., 4–6 weeks), prolonged courses (8 weeks or more) of H_2-receptor antagonists are frequently required in the treatment of GERD. In an open-label trial of famotidine 40 mg daily, endoscopic healing increased as the duration of therapy increased.[52] After 4 weeks of therapy, healing was observed in 50% of patients. The healing rate increased with continued therapy to yield healing rates of 82% and 83% after 12 and 16 weeks of therapy, respectively.

Dosage Regimen Used

H_2-receptor antagonists can be given in low-dose (over-the-counter) regimens, which may give symptomatic relief to patients with mild, typical symptoms of GERD. They can be given in standard doses, usually twice daily, in patients with nonerosive, mild to moderate GERD; or in higher doses (usually given more frequently) for patients not responding to standard doses or for patients with more severe disease.

Low-dose (over-the-counter) H_2-receptor antagonists are effective in treating intermittent heartburn and in preventing meal-provoked heartburn in patients with mild disease (without evidence of esophagitis).[48,53] In one study, 41%, 59%, 70%, 69%, and 62% of heartburn episodes were relieved following as-needed treatment with placebo, famotidine 5 mg, 10 mg, 20 mg, or antacids, respectively.[53]

Standard doses of H_2-receptor antagonists (cimetidine 400 mg four times daily or 800 mg twice daily; ranitidine 150 mg twice daily; famotidine 20 mg twice daily; or nizatidine 150 mg twice daily) are effective in providing symptomatic relief and endoscopic healing in patients with GERD.

Although data identifying the ideal H_2-receptor antagonist dosage regimen to use in the treatment of GERD are lacking, dosage regimens that achieve profound acid suppression may lead to increased healing rates. Higher dosage regimens of H_2-receptor antagonists are potentially more effective than lower doses; this is based on four observations.[50,51] First, gastroesophageal reflux occurs during both daytime and nighttime hours and acid suppression for only part of the day may not be sufficient to prevent the refluxate from injuring the esophageal mucosa, especially postprandially and during the nighttime hours. H_2-receptor antagonists do not easily overcome the stimulus for acid secretion following a meal, and thus postprandial acid secretion may be inadequately suppressed.[24] Dividing the H_2-receptor antagonist dose may provide coverage for both daytime and nighttime acid reflux and may improve symptom control and esophageal healing. However, studies have yielded conflicting results.[24]

Second, high-dose ranitidine (>300 mg daily) provides a greater degree of acid suppression as compared with the standard-dose regimen of 300 mg daily or placebo, and is also associated with higher healing rates.[49,50] Endoscopic healing was shown to be superior following famotidine 40 mg twice daily as compared to famotidine 20 mg twice daily; with healing rates of 58% versus 43% at 6 weeks and 76% versus 67% at 12 weeks, respectively.[51]

Third, a subset of patients with GERD has hypersecretion of gastric acid and may therefore require higher doses of antisecretory agents.[55] Finally, a relationship between the 8-week healing rate of esophagitis and the duration of time that the gastric pH is above 4 has been demonstrated.[24] Based on these findings, one might be able to predict responses to antisecretory regimens based on the regimen's ability to maintain intragastric pH levels above 4.

Although higher doses of H_2-receptor antagonists may provide higher symptomatic and endoscopic healing rates, limited information exists regarding the safety of these regimens and they can be less effective and more costly than once-daily proton pump inhibitors.

In general, the H_2-receptor antagonists are well tolerated. The most common adverse effects are headache, somnolence, fatigue, dizziness, and either constipation or diarrhea. Patients should be monitored for the presence of adverse effects, as well as potential drug interactions, especially when on cimetidine. Cimetidine may inhibit the metabolism of theophylline, warfarin, phenytoin, nifedipine, or propranolol, among others. An alternate H_2-receptor antagonist should be selected if the patient is on any of these medications.

ACID SUPPRESSION WITH PROTON PUMP INHIBITORS (ESOMEPRAZOLE, LANSOPRAZOLE, OMEPRAZOLE PANTOPRAZOLE, AND RABEPRAZOLE)

Proton pump inhibitors are superior to H_2-receptor antagonists in treating patients with moderate to severe GERD. This includes not only those patients with erosive esophagitis or complicated symptoms (Barrett's esophagus, strictures), but also those patients with nonerosive GERD who have moderate to severe symptoms. In these patient populations, relapse is common and long-term maintenance therapy is generally indicated. Comparable doses of proton pump inhibitors are omeprazole 20 mg = esomeprazole 20 mg = lansoprazole 30 mg = rabeprazole 20 mg = pantoprazole 40 mg per day. Symptomatic relief is seen in approximately 83% of patients treated with a proton pump inhibitor while endoscopic healing rate is 78%.[30] All of the proton pump inhibitors are generally well tolerated, while the newer agents, esomeprazole, pantoprazole, and rabeprazole, appear less likely to cause significant drug interactions. In general, all of these agents are safe and effective and the choice of a particular agent will most likely be based on cost.

Proton pump inhibitors block gastric acid secretion by inhibiting gastric H^+/K^+-adenosine triphosphate in gastric parietal cells.[56] This produces a profound, long-lasting antisecretory effect capable of maintaining the gastric pH above 4, even during acid surges seen postprandially.[4,10] While the proton pump inhibitors have the same mechanism of action, there are slight differences in their actual binding to the cysteine residues in the proton pump.

A correlation appears to exist between the percentage of time the gastric pH remains above 4 during the 24-hour period and healing erosive esophagitis. Lansoprazole 15 mg and 30 mg daily, omeprazole 20 mg daily, and ranitidine 150 mg four times daily were compared in suppressing gastric acid secretion in 29 healthy men.[57] After 5 days, the mean 24-hour gastric pH values for lansoprazole 30 mg, 15 mg, omeprazole, and ranitidine were 4.53, 3.97, 4.02, and 3.59, respectively. The percentage of time the pH remained above 4 for the lansoprazole 30 mg, 15 mg, omeprazole, and ranitidine group was 63%, 48%, 51%, and 38%, respectively. This difference was statistically different for the lansoprazole 30-mg group. A similar study also showed that lansoprazole 30 mg maintained a higher 24-hour gastric pH as compared with omeprazole 20 mg.[58]

Rabeprazole appears to have a faster onset of action after the first dose and maintains the gastric pH >4 for a higher percentage of time during a 24-hour period as compared with omeprazole (45% vs 25%). The percentage of time the gastric pH values remained above 4 by day 8 was 60.3% and 50.4%, respectively.[59] Another study showed rabeprazole 20 mg and 40 mg increased mean gastric pH to 4.2 and 4.7, respectively. The percentage of time the esophageal pH was <4 was decreased and fewer reflux episodes were noted with both doses.[60]

During a 5-day study of 38 GERD patients, esomeprazole 20 mg and 40 mg maintained intragastric pH >4 for a significantly longer time as compared to omeprazole 20 mg (18 hours, 13 hours and 11 hours, respectively).[61] The 24-hour median intragastric pH was also significantly higher in both the esomeprazole 20 mg and 40 mg groups as compared with omeprazole 20 mg (4.9, 4.1, and 3.6, respectively).

Proton pump inhibitors are superior to H_2-receptor antagonists in their ability to control symptoms and heal esophagitis in patients with GERD.[62] They are also more cost effective in patients with severe disease. A meta-analysis of 43 double-blind or single-blind trials with various drug classes in patients with erosive esophagitis found that healing was highest with proton pump inhibitors as compared with H_2-receptor antagonists (83.6% vs 51.9%).[62] Symptom relief was achieved in 77% of patients on a proton pump inhibitor as compared with 48% of patients on an H_2-receptor antagonist. Both healing and symptom relief occurred almost twice as fast when a proton pump inhibitor was used. Even with mild esophagitis (grade 1 or 2), omeprazole was still superior to high-dose ranitidine.[63] In a study of 446 patients with grade 1 or 2 esophagitis, omeprazole 20 mg daily was more effective at relieving symptoms than was ranitidine 150 mg four times daily. Sixty-one percent and 74% of patients were symptom-free at 4 weeks and 8 weeks, respectively, in the omeprazole group, as compared with 31% and 50% in the ranitidine group, respectively.

The proton pump inhibitors are efficacious in patients who are refractory to H_2-receptor antagonists.[64,65] The efficacy of omeprazole 20 mg daily versus ranitidine 150 mg twice daily versus ranitidine twice daily with metoclopramide 10 mg four times a day was evaluated for the treatment of poorly responsive, symptomatic GERD that was resistant to H_2-receptor antagonists.[64] Following 8 weeks of treatment, the healing rate was significantly higher for patients receiving omeprazole as compared to those who received ranitidine or ranitidine/metoclopramide (80% vs 40% vs 46%, respectively).

There are a few trials comparing proton pump inhibitors to each other. In general, healing rates at 4 weeks and 8 weeks are similar; lansoprazole and rabeprazole, however, may relieve symptoms faster after the first dose when compared to omeprazole. This is especially true when the higher dose of lansoprazole (30 mg daily) is compared to omeprazole 20 mg.[66] Both daytime and nighttime symptoms, as well as pain severity, were reported to be significantly better with lansoprazole 30 mg, as compared with omeprazole 20 mg or lansoprazole 15 mg, after the first dose. Healing rates at 4 weeks and 8 weeks were similar. Symptom relief was similar when a higher dose of omeprazole (40 mg daily) was compared with lansoprazole 30 mg.[67]

The newest proton pump inhibitor, esomeprazole, is the S-isomer of omeprazole and may offer greater acid suppression and improved healing rates as compared with the other proton pump inhibitors. Esomeprazole was compared with omeprazole in 1960 patients with endoscopy-confirmed reflux esophagitis.[68] The number of patients healed at 8 weeks were 94% (esomeprazole 40 mg), 90% (esomeprazole 20 mg), and 87% (omeprazole 20 mg) ($p < 0.05$). Healing at 4 weeks and improvement in heartburn was also considered superior in the esomeprazole 40 mg group as compared with the omeprazole 20 mg group. More experience with using this agent in clinical practice will clarify its role in the treatment of patients with GERD.

Rabeprazole 20 mg daily was compared with omeprazole 20 mg daily and found to be equally efficacious at 4 and 8 weeks in healing erosive esophagitis. Symptom relief (both frequency and intensity) was similar in both groups.[69]

Similar results were seen when pantoprazole 40 mg was compared with omeprazole 20 mg in 286 patients with mild to moderate reflux esophagitis. Healing rates were 74% and 78%, respectively, after 4 weeks; and 90% and 94%, respectively, after 8 weeks of treatment. Symptom relief was similar for both groups.[70] More published trials are needed with the two newest proton pump inhibitors, pantoprazole and rabeprazole, especially with long-term use.

Omeprazole (40–60 mg daily) and lansoprazole (30–60 mg daily) also appear to be effective in healing esophagitis and esophageal ulcers in patients with gastroesophageal reflux complications.[71,72] When patients with complications of GERD (Barrett's esophagus, strictures, or failed antireflux surgery) who were refractory to high-dose H_2-receptor antagonist therapy received omeprazole 40 mg daily, all patients were healed during 20 weeks of therapy.[71]

Whether proton pump inhibitors can actually reverse Barrett's esophagus remains a topic for debate. The use of high-dose omeprazole (40 mg twice daily) caused partial regression of Barrett's esophagus, but no change was noted in patients receiving ranitidine 150 mg twice daily.[73] Others propose these islands of normal squamous cells that appear in patients with Barrett's esophagus after high-dose proton pump inhibitors may be covering gastric mucosa and may mask the development of cancerous changes in the mucosa.[74] It is unknown whether regression of Barrett's esophagus reduces the risk of adenocarcinoma in someone who already has Barrett's esophagus, but, clearly, aggressive therapy aimed at adequate suppression of acid reflux early in the course of a patient's disease may help to prevent the development of Barrett's esophagus.

The proton pump inhibitors are usually well tolerated; however, potential adverse effects include headache, dizziness, somnolence, diarrhea, constipation, and nausea. The frequency of adverse events appears to be similar to that seen with the H_2-receptor antagonists. Concern and controversy regarding the safety of therapy with a proton pump inhibitor are based on the proton pump inhibitor's ability to produce hypergastrinemia and gastric carcinoid tumors in rats. After nearly a decade of experience with the proton pump inhibitors, gastric carcinoid tumors have not been directly linked to omeprazole use.[6]

Drug interactions with the proton pump inhibitors vary with each agent. All proton pump inhibitors can decrease the absorption of drugs, such as ketoconazole or itraconazole, which require an acidic environment to be absorbed. All proton pump inhibitors are metabolized by the cytochrome P450 system to some extent, specifically by the CYP2C19 and CYP3A4 enzymes. However, no interactions with lansoprazole, pantoprazole, or rabeprazole have been seen with CYP2C19 substrates, such as diazepam, warfarin, or phenytoin.[38] Esomeprazole does not appear to interact with warfarin or phenytoin and an interaction with diazepam is generally not considered clinically relevant. Pantoprazole is also metabolized by a cytosolic sulfotransferase and is therefore less likely to have significant drug interactions, as compared with the other proton pump inhibitors.[75] While generally not causing major concern, omeprazole has the potential to inhibit the metabolism of warfarin, diazepam, and phenytoin; and lansoprazole may decrease theophylline concentrations. Drug interactions with omeprazole are of particular concern in patients who are considered "slow metabolizers," which occurs in approximately 3% of the white population. Unfortunately, it is unclear which patients have the polymorphic gene variation that makes them slow metabolizers.[75] Like omeprazole, the metabolism of esomeprazole may also be altered in patients with this polymorphic gene variation. Rabeprazole increases digoxin trough concentrations by approximately 20%.[75] Patients on potentially interacting drugs should be monitored closely for potential problems.

The proton pump inhibitors degrade in acidic environments and are therefore formulated in a delayed-release capsule or tablet formulation. Lansoprazole and omeprazole contain enteric-coated (pH-sensitive) granules in a capsule form. In patients unable to swallow the capsule, the contents of the capsule can be mixed in applesauce or placed in orange juice. If a patient has a nasogastric tube, the contents should be mixed in 8.4% sodium bicarbonate solution. Patients taking pantoprazole or rabeprazole should be instructed not to crush, chew, or split the delayed-release tablets. Pantoprazole is available in an intravenous formulation, which offers an alternative route of administration for patients unable to take an oral proton pump inhibitor. It should be emphasized that the intravenous product is not more efficacious than oral proton pump inhibitors and will be significantly more expensive. Careful patient selection will be necessary to avoid the tremendous cost anticipated from the use of this product. Patients should be instructed to take their proton pump inhibitor in the morning, 15 to 30 minutes before breakfast to maximize efficacy, because these agents inhibit only actively secreting proton pumps.[4,75] Food may decrease the absorption of lansoprazole. If dosed twice daily, the second dose should be administered approximately 10 to 12 hours after the morning dose and prior to a meal or snack.[38]

PROKINETIC AGENTS

The efficacy of the prokinetic agents cisapride, metoclopramide, and bethanechol has been evaluated in the treatment of GERD. The inferior efficacy and side effect profiles associated with metoclopramide and bethanechol, as compared with cisapride, limit their use in the treatment of GERD. Cisapride, on the other hand, has comparable efficacy to H_2-receptor antagonists in treating patients with mild esophagitis; however, it is less effective than acid suppression in more severe disease.[76] Unfortunately, cisapride is no longer available for routine use because of life-threatening arrhythmias when it is combined with certain medications and other disease states. Prokinetic agents have also been used as adjunctive therapy with an H_2-receptor antagonist. The only scenario in which this combination is appropriate is in a patient with GERD who has a known or suspected motility disorder, or in a patient who has failed high-dose proton pump inhibitor therapy.

Cisapride

The efficacy of cisapride appears similar to that of the H_2-receptor antagonists in patients with mild esophagitis. However, cisapride generally costs more than the H_2-receptor antagonists and offers no real advantage, especially in patients with normal GI motility.[10] Because this agent is no longer available for routine use in GERD, an evaluation of clinical trials is not included. Three treatment protocols are available through the manufacturer, Janssen. One protocol is a pediatric outpatient study, the second protocol is an adult outpatient study, and the third protocol is an inpatient neonatal study. Physicians must register as investigators and patients must be enrolled just as with any other study protocol. More information can be obtained from the company.

Unlike metoclopramide, cisapride is devoid of antidopaminergic effects and, therefore, does not cause extrapyramidal side effects or prolactin secretion.[76] The most commonly reported adverse effects are gastrointestinal in nature and include transient abdominal cramping, borborygmi, diarrhea, and loose stools. Cisapride is contraindicated in patients taking other drugs that inhibit cytochrome P450 3A4, such as fluconazole; ketoconazole; miconazole; itraconazole; clarithromycin; erythromycin; indinavir; ritonavir; or nefazodone, because concurrent use may cause prolongation of the QT interval, leading to ventricular arrhythmias. Cisapride is also contraindicated in patients with a history of prolonged QT intervals; renal failure; history of ventricular arrhythmias; ischemic heart disease; congestive heart failure; uncorrected electrolyte disorders (potassium and magnesium); respiratory failure; and concomitant medications known to prolong the QT interval, including quinidine; procainamide; sotalol; tricyclic antidepressants; maprotiline; sparfloxacin; terodiline; bepridil; certain phenothiazines; and sertindole. These conditions predispose the patient to arrhythmias and increase the risk for QT prolongation, torsade de pointes, cardiac arrest, and even death.

Metoclopramide

Metoclopramide, a dopamine antagonist, increases lower esophageal sphincter pressure in a dose-related manner, and accelerates gastric emptying in gastroesophageal reflux patients.[77] Unlike cisapride, however, metoclopramide does not improve esophageal clearance. Metoclopramide has been shown to provide symptomatic improvement for some patients with gastroesophageal reflux disease; however, substantial data indicating that metoclopramide provides endoscopic healing are lacking.[78]

In addition, metoclopramide's side effect profile and the incidence of tachyphylaxis with continued use limits its usefulness in treating many patients with GERD. Forty-eight percent of patients experienced adverse effects in one study with doses ranging from 10 to 50 mg daily.[79] Seventeen percent of the population withdrew from the study because of adverse effects, such as somnolence, nervousness, fatigue, dizziness, weakness, depression, diarrhea, and rash. The risk of adverse effects is much greater in patients with renal dysfunction because the drug is primarily eliminated by the kidneys. Contraindications include Parkinson's disease, mechanical obstruction, concomitant use of other dopamine antagonists, anticholinergic agents, and pheochromocytoma.

MUCOSAL PROTECTANTS

Sucralfate, a nonabsorbable aluminum salt of sucrose octasulfate, has very limited value in the treatment of GERD. Sucralfate has similar healing rates as H_2-receptor antagonists for patients with mild esophagitis.[80–84] However, sucralfate is less effective than higher doses of H_2-receptor antagonists in patients with refractory esophagitis.[84] Overall, the efficacy of sucralfate varies greatly among the studies. The wide range of response rates may in part be related to patient population, baseline degree of esophagitis, duration of treatment, dose used, or sucralfate formulation used. More studies are needed before sucralfate can be routinely used in the treatment of anything but the mildest cases of GERD.

COMBINATION THERAPY

Combination therapy with an acid-suppressing agent and a prokinetic agent or a mucosal protectant agent would seem logical given the multifactorial nature of the disease, particularly in light of the disappointing results seen with many monotherapy regimens. However, sufficient data to support combination therapy are limited, and this approach should not be routinely recommended unless a patient has esophagitis plus motor dysfunction occurring concurrently or if the patient has failed high-dose proton pump inhibitor therapy. Most studies suggest that combination therapy offers only modest improvements over standard doses of H_2-receptor antagonists alone. Therefore, patients not responding to standard doses of H_2-receptor antagonists should have their dose of H_2-receptor antagonists increased or switched to a proton pump inhibitor instead of adding a prokinetic agent. Monotherapy with a proton pump inhibitor is not only more efficacious in patients not responding to an H_2-receptor antagonist or prokinetic agent alone, but it also improves compliance with once-daily dosing and is ultimately more cost-effective.

MAINTENANCE THERAPY

Although healing and/or symptomatic improvement may be achieved via many different therapeutic modalities, a large percentage of patients with gastroesophageal reflux will relapse following discontinuation of therapy, especially those with more severe disease.[85] Followup studies indicate that 70% to 90% of patients will relapse within 1 year of discontinuation of therapy, regardless of what therapeutic regimen is used.[85] Patients who have symptomatic relapse following discontinuation of therapy or lowering of dose, including patients with complications such as Barrett's esophagus, strictures, or hemorrhage, should be considered for long-term maintenance therapy to prevent complications or worsening of esophageal function.[10] The goal of maintenance therapy is to improve quality of life by controlling the patient's symptoms and preventing complications.[6] These goals cannot generally be achieved by decreasing the dose of the therapeutic modality used for initial healing or switching to a less potent acid-suppressing agent. Most patients will require standard doses to prevent relapses.[71,86,87] Patients should be counseled on the importance of complying with lifestyle changes and long-term maintenance therapy in order to prevent recurrence or worsening of disease.[6]

H_2-receptor antagonists may be effective maintenance therapy for patients with mild disease.[4] Although cisapride was an effective maintenance therapy, it is no longer an option unless it is obtained through the limited access program from the manufacturer. The proton pump inhibitors are the drug of choice for maintenance treatment of moderate to severe esophagitis.[88] Lower doses of a proton pump inhibitor or alternate-day dosing may be effective in some patients with less-severe disease, thereby allowing titration in some cases.[4] Preliminary data with esomeprazole suggest that "on demand" maintenance therapy for patients with endoscopy-negative GERD may be effective.[89,90] However, patients with more severe disease and/or complications should be maintained on omeprazole 20 mg daily, lansoprazole 30 mg daily, rabeprazole 20 mg daily, or esomeprazole 20 mg daily. Long-term, chronic use of higher doses of proton pump inhibitors are not indicated unless the patient has complicated symptoms, has high-grade erosive esophagitis per endoscopy, or has had further diagnostic evaluation to determine level of acid exposure. Many institutions allow the use of normal-dose proton pump inhibitors by all physicians, but limit the use of high-dose proton pump inhibitors to gastroenterologists. Antireflux surgery may also be considered a viable alternative to long-term drug therapy for maintenance of healing in patients who are surgical candidates.

Maintenance Therapy with Proton Pump Inhibitors

In a comparison of maintenance regimens, omeprazole (20 mg daily) alone or in combination with cisapride (10 mg three times daily) was significantly more effective in preventing recurrence than was ranitidine (150 mg three times daily) alone or cisapride (10 mg three times daily) alone.[88] Omeprazole was also effective in patients with complicated forms (grades 4 and 5) of esophagitis.

Omeprazole and lansoprazole in doses of 20 mg and 30 mg daily, respectively, decreased relapse rates significantly.[87,88] At 1 year, relapse rates were 15% and 10%, respectively. Both omeprazole and lansoprazole were superior to H_2-receptor antagonists in maintaining esophageal healing in patients with moderate to severe symptoms.[75,91] Lansoprazole 15 mg daily was compared to lansoprazole 30 mg daily or ranitidine 300 mg twice daily in preventing recurrence of reflux esophagitis.[91] At 12 months, relapse rates were 31%, 20%, and 68% for lansoprazole 15 mg, 30 mg, and ranitidine, respectively. Lansoprazole 15 mg and 30 mg daily were comparable in maintaining remission of reflux esophagitis. A more recent study evaluated patients with mild to moderate GERD (grades 1 to 2 esophagitis).[63] After an acute treatment phase for grade 1 or 2 esophagitis, patients were randomized to receive maintenance therapy with omeprazole 10 mg daily or ranitidine 150 mg twice daily. At 1 year, 68% of patients on omeprazole were in remission, as compared with 39% of patients receiving ranitidine. Even at a lower dose, omeprazole was superior to ranitidine for maintenance therapy.

Preliminary placebo-controlled studies with esomeprazole indicate that maintenance of erosive esophagitis healing occurs in 54% to 94% of patients after 6 months of 10 mg to 40 mg doses of esomperazole.[92,93] Doses of 20 mg to 40 mg were superior to the 10-mg dose. Studies are needed comparing esomeprazole to the other proton pump inhibitors in maintenance therapy for GERD.

Omeprazole 20 mg (given on the weekend) was compared to omeprazole 20 mg daily and ranitidine 150 mg twice daily. The relapse rate at 12 months was 68%, 11%, and 75%, respectively, indicating that weekend regimens are ineffective in preventing recurrence.[86] Alternate-day regimens may be beneficial in patients with mild disease.[94] Long-term studies with the newer agents, especially pantoprazole, are needed but should be effective as maintenance therapy for GERD.

Long-term use of the proton pump inhibitors indicates that they are safe, with no evidence of carcinoid tumors directly linked to their use. Prolonged hypergastrinemia leading to the development of colonic polyps, and potentially, adenocarcinoma was also a concern that has proven unfounded with long-term use of proton pump inhibitors.[95] However, the role of *Helicobacter pylori* status in patients with GERD is a concern. One study showed that patients treated with proton pump inhibitors had a higher incidence of atrophic gastritis that was linked to the development of gastric cancer.[3] In this study, 30% of patients treated with omeprazole over an average of 5 years developed atrophy, whereas none of a cohort group that received antireflux surgery developed atrophy within the same time frame.[96] Most of the patients who developed atrophic gastritis had concomitant *Helicobacter pylori* infection. On the other hand, the presence of *H. pylori* infection may actually have a protective effect against GERD and clearing the infection may be associated with a worsening of GERD symptoms.[97] The FDA recently stated there was insufficient evidence linking proton pump inhibitor use to atrophic gastritis, intestinal metaplasia, or gastric cancer.[98] As a consequence of the controversy surrounding *H. pylori* and GERD, specific guidelines on how to handle these patients are lacking. If found, most clinicians would probably opt to eradicate *H. pylori* infections. Further studies are needed to determine the role of *H. pylori* in patients with GERD.

Maintenance Therapy with H_2-Receptor Antagonists

The studies evaluating the efficacy of the H_2-receptor antagonists in maintaining GERD patients in remission have been disappointing. Currently, ranitidine 150 mg twice daily is the only H_2-receptor antagonist regimen FDA approved for maintenance of healing of erosive esophagitis. The recurrence rates of esophagitis have been shown to be significantly less in patients receiving ranitidine 150 mg twice daily as compared to placebo.[99]

SPECIAL POPULATIONS/CONSIDERATIONS

ATYPICAL GERD SYMPTOMS

Patients presenting with atypical symptoms may require higher doses and longer treatment courses as compared with patients with typical symptoms. These patients are best diagnosed with ambulatory pH testing or an empiric trial with a proton pump inhibitor.[100] In patients presenting with noncardiac chest pain, a short course (1–8 weeks) of omeprazole 20 mg twice daily has been advocated.[100] In patients with asthma, antireflux medications have shown to improve symptoms and even to decrease antiasthma medication use, but had little or no effect on lung function.[101] A trial of 3 months has been advocated using twice-daily proton pump inhibitor therapy for both asthma and laryngeal symptoms thought to be associated with GERD. Doses as high as 60 mg daily have been used.[100] In patients with chronic cough, pH testing is the preferred approach for evaluation of GERD, when available.[102] Maintenance therapy is generally indicated in patients who respond to the therapeutic trial or have endoscopic evidence of reflux. Patients who do not respond to therapy benefit from ambulatory 24-hour monitoring either on or off therapy.[100] Patients not responding to therapy with a positive ambulatory 24-hour monitoring test may need more aggressive therapy. Surgical treatment may be indicated in selected patients not responding to medical management.

ENDOSCOPY-NEGATIVE REFLUX DISEASE

While the integrity of the esophageal mucosa is best evaluated with endoscopy, it does not confirm whether or not the patient's symptoms are related to GERD.[30] In some cases, patients with typical symptoms and increased acid exposure have no evidence of esophageal damage. Many patients with persistent, severe symptoms but normal endoscopy will require therapy similar to those with positive endoscopic findings. This condition is referred to as endoscopy-negative reflux disease.[103] Patients presenting with normal esophageal mucosa on endoscopy may undergo pH testing or a "therapeutic trial" with a proton pump inhibitor to further confirm the diagnosis of GERD. Remember, however, that even when ambulatory pH monitoring or therapeutic trial is used, it does not absolutely rule GERD in or out. In more serious cases, both may be necessary to confirm diagnosis.[30]

The treatment of endoscopy-negative reflux disease has been evaluated in several studies. Patients with normal endoscopy treated with omeprazole had improvement in symptoms, quality of life scores, and antacid use.[104] Treatment with a proton pump inhibitor is more effective than treatment with an H_2-receptor antagonist in these patients, as demonstrated by several clinical trials.[105,106] In a study of 994 patients with heartburn, omeprazole 20 mg once daily was more effective than omeprazole 10 mg once daily, which was more effective than ranitidine 150 mg twice daily at 4 weeks.[105] Symptom relief in patients with normal endoscopy was seen in 61%, 49%, and 40% of patients, respectively. In another study of 221 patients, heartburn was controlled in 66% of patients receiving omeprazole 20 mg once daily, as compared with 31% of those patients receiving cimetidine 400 mg four times daily at 4 weeks.[106] Symptom relief was similar in those with or without esophagitis.

PEDIATRIC PATIENTS WITH GERD

Gastroesophageal reflux occurs in approximately 18% of the infant population. Most have physiologic reflux with no clinical consequence.[107] Complications, although rare, include distal esophagitis, failure to thrive, esophageal peptic strictures, Barrett's esophagus, and pulmonary disease.[108] Chronic vomiting associated with gastroesophageal reflux must be distinguished from other causes such as neurologic, metabolic, eating, and rumination disorders. Developmental immaturity of the lower esophageal sphincter is one suspected cause of gastroesophageal reflux in infants.[108] Like adults, transient lower esophageal sphincter relaxations seem to be the most common cause of gastroesophageal reflux in children. Other causes include impaired luminal clearance of gastric acid, neurologic impairment, and type of infant formula. Uncomplicated gastroesophageal reflux usually resolves without incident by 12 to 18 months and usually responds to supportive therapy, including dietary adjustments, postural management, and reassurance for the parents.[108] Thickened feedings may be useful in milder cases. Smaller, more frequent feedings may also be beneficial. If there is no improvement, medical therapy may be indicated. Combined use of a prokinetic agent and an acid-suppressing agent seems to work the fastest.[108] Unfortunately, there is no longer a readily available prokinetic agent without major problems. H_2-receptor antagonists are commonly used. A dose of ranitidine 2 mg/kg twice daily is effective.[108] The use of proton pump inhibitors is not routinely used in pediatrics. More studies are needed to determine their role in managing gastroesophageal reflux in children.

ELDERLY PATIENTS WITH GERD

Many elderly patients have decreased host defense mechanisms, such as saliva production, which acts as a barrier to the damaging effects of gastric secretions. More aggressive therapy with a proton pump inhibitor may be warranted in patients with symptomatic GERD in those patients older than 60 years of age.[109] These patients have had years of acid reflux that may or may not have been treated adequately. Often, these patients do not seek medical attention because they feel their symptoms are part of the normal aging process. They may present with atypical symptoms such as chest pain, asthma, hoarseness, coughing, wheezing, poor dentition, or jaw pain. Decreased GI motility is a common problem in elderly patients. Unfortunately, there are no good prokinetic agents available to these patients. Cisapride is not available for general use and elderly patients are especially sensitive to the central nervous system (CNS) effects of metoclopramide. They may also be sensitive to the CNS effects of H_2-receptor antagonists. Proton pump inhibitors appear to be the most useful treatment modality because they have superior efficacy and are dosed once daily, which is beneficial in all patients, but is especially beneficial in the elderly.

PHARMACOECONOMIC CONSIDERATIONS

In addition to the traditional clinical end points that demonstrate that a certain therapy is effective, we must also evaluate the cost-effectiveness of the therapy in relation to predicted outcomes and its effects on quality of life.[4] For GERD, one must consider the primary goals of treatment: to relieve symptoms, to prevent recurrence, and to prevent complications. These factors must be evaluated separately, because different costs are associated with achieving each end point. For example, patients with complications associated with GERD, such as strictures, would be more likely to use medical resources as a consequence of revisits and diagnostic tests.[1] Although effects on quality of life may be difficult to evaluate when your goal is preventing recurrence,[4] untreated GERD has a more negative impact on psychological well-being than untreated hypertension, mild heart failure, angina pectoris, or menopause.[2] Improving a patient's quality of life is a measure of treatment success and may help decide which therapy a patient receives.[4]

The proton pump inhibitors are generally more expensive than the H_2-receptor antagonists or prokinetic agents. This is likely to be less of an issue when omeprazole becomes generically available. However, the most expensive therapy is the one that is ineffective.[4] This means that if the H_2-receptor antagonist does not accomplish the treatment goals, then it costs more because the patient must be retreated.

Patient compliance is another factor that will affect the outcome of drug therapy. Drug regimens that are easily managed will improve compliance and, therefore, outcome for the patient. This can especially be a problem in patients who require high-dose therapy with H_2-receptor antagonists. Not only is the patient required to take the drug more often in higher doses, but there is also increased expense associated with such regimens. The patient may be unable to afford the drug. Choosing a drug that is least expensive and provides the greatest benefit related to dosing interval and number of tablets taken is the optimal regimen. Studies comparing various treatment strategies for GERD show that proton pump inhibitors are more cost effective than H_2-receptor antagonists, especially in those patients with moderate to severe disease.[110–112] Decision analysis has been used to evaluate the cost effectiveness of phase I therapy or phase I therapy combined with omeprazole 20 mg daily or ranitidine 150 mg twice daily for patients with persistent symptomatic GERD who failed phase I therapy. A complex model that evaluated the influence of empiric versus definitive therapy, compliance, and efficacy of the three treatment regimens was employed. Although the retail cost of omeprazole was highest among the treatments evaluated, it was the most cost-effective strategy and was associated with the lowest overall cost. Studies also show that proton pump inhibitors improve quality-of-life measures in symptomatic patients with erosive esophagitis.[113] Additional studies are needed evaluating the impact of various treatment regimens on quality-of-life issues, cost, and to compare long-term medical management with antireflux surgery. At least one study showed proton pump inhibitors were equally effective to antireflux surgery and slightly more cost-effective at 5 years. However, the costs were similar after 10 years.[114]

EVALUATION OF THERAPEUTIC OUTCOMES

The long-term benefits of treatment are difficult to assess because of the limited information known about the epidemiology and natural history of GERD. Therefore, successful outcomes are generally measured in terms of three separate end points: (a) relieving symptoms, (b) healing the injured mucosa, and (c) preventing complications.

The short-term goal of therapy is to relieve symptoms, such as heartburn and regurgitation, to the point where they do not impair the patient's quality of life. Patients should be educated regarding lifestyle modifications that should be adhered to throughout the course of therapy including smoking cessation, weight loss, raising the head of the bed, eating smaller meals, and avoiding eating prior to bedtime. Patients should also be instructed to avoid foods that aggravate GERD symptoms, such as fat and chocolate. In addition, the patient's drug profile should be reviewed to identify medications that may contribute to GERD symptoms. These agents should be avoided if possible. Table 32–5 has recommendations for providing pharmaceutical care to patients with GERD.

The health care provider should take an active role in educating the patient about potential adverse effects and drug interactions that may occur with drug therapy. The frequency and severity of symptoms should be monitored and patients should be counseled on symptoms that suggest the presence of complications requiring immediate medical attention, such as dysphagia or odynophagia. Patients with persistent symptoms should be evaluated for the presence of strictures or other complications. Patients should also be monitored for the presence of atypical symptoms such as cough, nonallergic asthma, or chest pain. These symptoms require further diagnostic evaluation. Long-term maintenance treatment is indicated in patients who have strictures because they commonly recur if esophagitis is not treated.[115]

The second goal is to heal the injured mucosa. Again, lifestyle modifications and the importance of complying with the therapeutic regimen chosen to heal the mucosa should be stressed. Patients should be educated about the risk of relapse and the need for long-term maintenance therapy to prevent recurrence or complications.

TABLE 32–5. Recommendations for Providing Pharmaceutical Care to Patients with GERD

1. Assess patient's symptoms to determine whether patient-directed therapy is appropriate or whether the patient should be evaluated by a physician. Determine type of symptoms, frequency, and exacerbating factors. Refer any patient with complicated or atypical symptoms to a physician for further diagnostic workup.
2. Obtain a thorough history of prescription, nonprescription, and natural-drug product use.
3. Counsel patient on lifestyle modifications that will improve symptomatology. These include avoiding foods and medications that worsen GERD, avoiding tight-fitting clothes, eating smaller meals, raising the head of the bed, losing weight, and avoiding tobacco use.
4. Recommend appropriate drug therapy based on patient presentation. Proton pump inhibitors are the drug of choice for patients with moderate to severe symptoms.
5. Develop a plan to assess effectiveness of acid-suppressing therapy after an appropriate amount of time (8–16 weeks). Recommend alternative therapy if necessary.
6. Assess improvement in quality of life measures such as physical, psychological, and social functioning and well-being.
7. Evaluate patient for the presence of adverse drug reactions, drug allergies, and drug interactions.
8. Stress the importance of compliance with therapeutic regimen, including lifestyle modifications. Recommend a therapeutic regimen that is easy for the patient to accomplish.
9. Provide patient education related to disease state, lifestyle modifications, and drug therapy. Patients should be counseled on:
   - What causes GERD and what things to avoid (see #3)
   - When to take their medications
   - What potential adverse effects may occur
   - Which drugs may interact with their therapy
   - What warning signs they should report to their physician (dysphagia, odynophagia, unexplained weight loss, bleeding)

The final, more long-term goal of therapy is to decrease the risk of complications (esophagitis, strictures, and Barrett's esophagus). A small subset of patients may continue to fail treatment, despite therapy with high doses of H_2-receptor antagonists or omeprazole. Maintenance therapy with standard to higher doses of antisecretory agents may be indicated in these acid hypersecretors, because severe esophagitis that is not adequately treated may lead to Barrett's esophagus and its associated risk of adenocarcinoma. Unfortunately, data are lacking that show that effective treatment of esophagitis decreases the risk of developing adenocarcinoma in patients with Barrett's esophagus. Patients should be monitored for the presence of continual pain, dysphagia, or odynophagia.

CONCLUSIONS

Gastroesophageal reflux disease is a common entity that classically presents as heartburn. The pathophysiology of reflux is complex, involving both aggressive factors (acid, pepsin, bile acids, pancreatic enzymes, and prostaglandins) and defense mechanisms (anatomic factors, lower esophageal sphincter pressure, esophageal clearance, and gastric emptying). Therapeutic modalities are designed to minimize the aggressive factors and/or augment defense mechanisms. The pharmacologic critical elements outlined should be considered when evaluating and treating a patient with GERD.

▶ PRINCIPLES OF PHARMACOTHERAPY

- The goals of treatment are to alleviate or eliminate symptoms, decrease the frequency or recurrence and duration of gastroesophageal reflux, promote healing of mucosa, and prevent complications.
- Treatment of GERD often involves a stepwise approach depending on severity of disease and includes Phase I, lifestyle changes and patient-directed therapy; Phase II, pharmacologic treatment; and Phase III, surgical intervention.
- Patients presenting with typical symptoms should be treated with lifestyle modifications and trial of empiric acid-suppression therapy.
- The importance of lifestyle modifications should be stressed throughout a patient's treatment course. Patients who do not respond to empiric therapy or who have more complicated symptoms should undergo diagnostic tests.
- Endoscopy is used to evaluate mucosal damage; 24-hour ambulatory pH or testing or a "therapeutic trial of a proton pump inhibitor" is useful in patients with persistent symptoms or atypical symptoms; and manometry is useful in evaluating motility and before antireflux surgery.
- Acid suppression is the mainstay of GERD treatment. H_2-receptor antagonists in divided doses are used in less severe GERD. Proton pump inhibitors show the greatest relief of symptoms and healing, especially in patients with erosive disease or moderate to severe symptoms.
- Patients who fail H_2-receptor therapy can have their dose and frequency of H_2-receptor antagonist increased or they can be switched to a proton pump inhibitor.
- Many patients will relapse and require long-term maintenance therapy with an H_2-receptor antagonist or a proton pump inhibitor. A proton pump inhibitor is the drug of choice for maintenance of moderate to severe GERD.
- Antireflux surgery offers an alternative for refractory GERD or when pharmacologic management is undesirable.
- Patients should be assessed for relief of symptoms, such as heartburn, and for signs and symptoms of complications that require immediate medical attention, such as dysphagia or bleeding. Patient profiles should also be reviewed for other medications that may aggravate GERD, and these medications should be avoided if possible. Patients should be monitored for adverse drug reactions and potential drug-drug interactions, especially when cimetidine is used. Finally, patients should be assessed for compliance to treatment and maintenance regimens, as well as lifestyle modifications.

REFERENCES

1. Spechler SJ. Epidemiology and natural history of gastro-oesophageal reflux disease. Digestion 1992;51(suppl 1):24–29.
2. Dimenas E. Methodological aspects of evaluation of quality of life in upper gastrointestinal diseases. Scand J Gastroenterol 1993;28:18–21.
3. Kahrilas PJ. Gastroesophageal reflux disease. JAMA 1996;276:983–988.
4. Johnson DA. Medical therapy of GERD: Current state of the art. Hosp Pract (Off Ed) 1996;31:135–148.
5. Nebel OT, Fornes MF, Castell DO. Symptomatic gastroesophageal reflux: Incidence and precipitating factors. Dig Dis 1976;21:953–956.
6. DeVault KR, Castell DO (for the Practice Parameters Committee of the American College of Gastroenterology). Guidelines for the diagnosis and treatment of gastroesophageal reflux disease. Arch Intern Med 1995;155:2165–2173.
7. Ollyo JB, Monnier P, Fontolliet C, Savary M. The natural history, prevalence and incidence of reflux oesophagitis. Gullet 1993;3(suppl):1–10.
8. Richter JE. Severe reflux esophagitis. Gastrointest Endosc Clin N Am 1994;4:677–698.
9. Kitchin LI, Castell DO. Rationale and efficacy of conservative therapy for gastroesophageal reflux disease. Arch Intern Med 1991;151:448–454.
10. Fennerty MB, Castell D, Fendrick AM, et al. The diagnosis and treatment of gastroesophageal reflux disease in a managed care environment. Suggested disease management guidelines. Arch Intern Med 1996;156:477–484.
11. Orenstein SR. Gastroesophageal reflux disease. Semin Gastrointest Dis 1994;5:2–14.
12. Krueger KJ. Changing clinical perspectives toward gastroesophageal reflux. South Med J 1996;89:548–550. Editorial.
13. Cameron AJ, Kamalh PS, Carpenter HA. Prevalence of Barrett's esophagus and intestinal metaplasia at the esophagogastric junction. Gastroenterology 1997;112:A82.
14. Lagergren J, Bergstrom R, Lindgren A, Nyren O. Symptomatic gastroesophageal reflux as a risk factor for esophageal adenocarcinoma. N Engl J Med 1999;340:825–831.
15. Lambert R. Current practices and future perspectives in the management of gastrooesophageal reflux disease. Aliment Pharmacol Ther 1997;11:661–662.
16. Weinberg DS, Kadish SL. The diagnosis and management of gastroesophageal reflux disease. Med Clin North Am 1996;80:411–429.
17. Castell DO. Long-term management of GERD: The pill, the knife or the endoscope? Gastrointest Endosc 1994;40:252–253.
18. Kahrilas P. Hiatal Hernia. Program and abstracts of Digestive Disease Week; 2000 (May); San Diego, California. Session 521.
19. Smith C. Gastroesophageal Reflux Disease. US Pharmacist 1999;24(12):77–86.
20. Bozymski EM. Pathophysiology and diagnosis of gastroesophageal reflux disease. Am J Hosp Pharm 1993;50(suppl 1):S4–S6.
21. Goldstein JL, Schlesinger PK, Mozwecz HL, et al. Esophageal mucosal resistance: A factor in esophagitis. Gastroenterol Clin North Am 1990;19:565–585.
22. Fein M. Duodenogastroesophageal reflux parallels acid and not alkaline exposure in the esophagus and contributes to complications of reflux disease. Am J Gastroenterol 1996;91:1662–1663.
23. Dent J. Roles of gastric acid and pH in the pathogenesis of gastrooesophageal reflux disease. Scand J Gastroenterol 1994;29(suppl 201):55–61.
24. Bell NJV, Burger D, Howden CW, et al. Appropriate acid suppression for the management of gastro-oesophageal reflux disease. Digestion 1992;51(suppl 1):59–67.
25. McCallum RW. Gastric emptying in gastroesophageal reflux and the therapeutic role of prokinetic agents. Gastroenterol Clin North Am 1990;19:551–564.
26. Larsen RR. Gastroesophageal reflux disease. Gaining control over heartburn. Postgrad Med 1997;101:181–187.
27. Kiljander TO, Salomaa ER, Hietanen EK, et al. Gastroesophageal reflux in asthmatics: A double-blind, placebo controlled crossover study with omeprazole. Chest 1999;116(5):1257–1264.
28. Simpson WG. Gastroesophageal reflux disease and asthma. Diagnosis and management. Arch Intern Med 1995;155:798–803.
29. Lazarchik DA, Filler SJ. Dental erosion: Predominant oral lesion in gastroesophageal reflux disease. Am J Gastroenterol 2000;95(suppl 8):S33–S38.
30. DeVault KR, Castell DO and the practice parameters committee of the American College of Gastroenterology. Updated Guidelines for the diagnosis and treatment of gastroesophageal reflux disease. Am J Gastroenterol 1999;94(6):1434–1442.

31. Savary M, Miller G. The esophagus. In: Gassmann SA, ed. Handbook and Atlas of Endoscopy. Solothurn, Switzerland, 1978.
32. Johnnson F, Weywadt L, Sonhaug JN, et al. One-week omeprazole treatment in the diagnosis of gastro-oesophageal reflux disease. Scand J Gastroenterol 1998;33:15–20.
33. Schenk BE, Kuipers EJ, Klinkenberg-Knol EC, et al. Omeprazole as a diagnostic tool in gastroesophageal reflux disease. Am J Gastroenterol 1997;92:1997–2000.
34. Schindlbeck NE, Klauser AG, Voderrholzer WA, Muller-Lissner SA. Empiric therapy for gastroesophageal reflux disease. Arch Intern Med 1995;155(16):1808–1812.
35. Ofman JJ, Gralnek IM, Udani J, et al. The cost-effectiveness of the omeprazole test in patients with noncardiac chest pain. Am J Med 1999;107(3):219–227.
36. Fass R, Fennerty MB, Ofman JJ, et al. The clinical and economic value of a short course of omeprazole in patients with noncardiac chest pain. Gastroenterology 1998;115(1):42–49.
37. Wo JM, Grist WJ, Gussack G, et al. Empiric trial of high-dose omeprazole in patients with posterior laryngitis: A prospective study. Am J Gastroenterol 1997;12(12):2160–2165.
38. Welage LS, Berardi RR. Evaluation of omeprazole, lansoprazole, pantoprazole, and rabeprazole in the treatment of acid-related disorders. J Am Pharm Assoc 2000;40:52–62.
39. Richter JE, Castell DO. Drugs, foods and other substances in the cause and treatment of reflux esophagitis. Med Clin North Am 1981;65: 1223–1234.
40. Locke GR, Talley NJ, Fett SL, et al. Risk factors associated with symptoms of gastroesophageal reflux. Am J Med 1999;106:642–649.
41. Anonymous. Guideline for the surgical treatment of gastroesophageal reflux disease (GERD). Surg Endosc 1998;12(2):186–188.
42. Lundell L, Dalenvack J, Hattlevakk J, et al. Omeprazole or antireflux surgery in the long-term management of gastroesophageal reflux disease: Results of a multicentre, randomized, clinical trial. Gastroenterology 1998;114:A207.
43. Chelikani S, Robinson M, Maton P, et al. Comparison of tablet versus liquid antacids on acidity in the esophagus and stomach. Am J Gastroenterol 1995;90:1570.
44. Washington N, Steele RJ, Jackson SJ, et al. Patterns of food and acid reflux in patients with low-grade oesophagitis—The role of an antireflux agent. Aliment Pharmacol Ther 1998;12(1):53–58.
45. Chevrel B. A comparative crossover study on the treatment of heartburn and epigastric pain: Liquid Gaviscon and a magnesium-aluminum antacid gel. J Med Res 1980;8:300–302.
46. Graham DY, Lanza F, Dorsch ER. Symptomatic reflux esophagitis: A double-blind controlled comparison of antacids and alginate. Curr Ther Res 1977;22:653–658.
47. Welage LS, Berardi RB. Drug interactions with antiulcer agents: Considerations in the treatment of acid-peptic disease. J Pharm Pract 1994;7:177–195.
48. Gottlieb S, Decktor DL, Eckert JM, et al. Efficacy and tolerability of famotidine in preventing heartburn and related symptoms of upper gastrointestinal discomfort. Am J Ther 1995;2:314–319.
49. Johnson NJ, Boyd EJS, Mills JG, et al. Acute treatment of reflux oesophagitis: A multicentre trial to compare 150 mg ranitidine b.d. with 300 mg ranitidine q.d.s. Aliment Pharmacol Ther 1989;3:259–266.
50. Euler AR, Murdock RH, Wilson TH, et al. Ranitidine is effective therapy for erosive esophagitis. Am J Gastroenterol 1993;88:520–524.
51. Wesdorp ICE, Dekker W, Festen HPM. Efficacy of famotidine 20 mg twice a day versus 40 mg twice a day in the treatment of erosive or ulcerative reflux esophagitis. Dig Dis Sci 1993;38:2287–2293.
52. Sekiguchi T, Nishioka T, Kogure M, et al. Once-daily administration of famotidine for reflux esophagitis. Scand J Gastroenterol 1987;22 (suppl 134):51–54.
53. Simon TJ, Berlin RG, Gardner AH, et al. Self-directed treatment of intermittent heartburn: A randomized, multicenter, double-blind, placebo-controlled evaluation of antacid and low doses of an H_2-receptor antagonist (famotidine). Am J Ther 1995;2:304–313.
54. Reynolds JC. Comparative efficacy of famotidine twice daily to ranitidine four times a day in the treatment of erosive esophagitis. Gastroenterology 1995;108(4):A202.
55. Collen MJ, Johnson DA, Sheridan MJ. Basal acid output and gastric acid hypersecretion in gastroesophageal reflux disease. Dig Dis Sci 1994;39:410–417.
56. Horn J. The proton-pump inhibitors: Similarities and differences. Clin Ther 2000;22:266–280.
57. Blum RA, Shi HK, Greski-Rose PA, et al. The comparative effects of lansoprazole, omeprazole and ranitidine in suppressing gastric acid secretion. Clin Ther 1997;19(5):1013–1023.
58. Tolman KG, Sanders SW, Buchi KN, et al. The effects of oral doses of lansoprazole and omeprazole on gastric pH. J Clin Gastroenterol 1997;24:65–70.
59. Williams MP, Sercombe J, Hamilton MI, et al. A placebo-controlled trial to assess the effects of 8 days of dosing with rabeprazole versus omeprazole on 24-h intragastric acidity and plasma gastrin concentrations in young healthy male subjects. Aliment Pharmacol Ther 1998;12:1079–1089.
60. Robinson M, Maton PN, Rodriguez S, et al. Effects of oral rabeprazole on oesophageal and gastric pH in patients with gastro-oesophageal reflux disease. Aliment Pharmacol Ther 1997;11:973–980.
61. Lind T, Kyleback A, Rydberg L, et al. Esomeprazole provides improved acid control vs omeprazole in patients with symptoms of GERD. Aliment Pharmacol Ther 2000;14:861–867.
62. Chiba N, De Cara CJ, Wilkinson JM, Hunt RH. Speed of healing and symptom relief in grade II to IV gastro-oesophageal reflux disease: A meta-analysis. Gastroenterology 1997;112:1798–1810.
63. Festen HP, Schenk E, Tan G, et al. Omeprazole versus high-dose ranitidine in mild gastroesophageal reflux disease: Short- and long-term treatment. The Dutch Reflux Study Group. Am J Gastroenterol 1999;94(4): 931–936.
64. Richter JE, Sabesin SM, Kogut DG, et al. Omeprazole versus ranitidine or ranitidine/metoclopramide in poorly responsive symptomatic gastroesophageal reflux disease. Am J Gastroenterol 1996;91(9):1766–1772.
65. Robinson M, Campbell DR, Sontag S, et al. Treatment of erosive esophagitis resistant to H_2-receptor antagonist therapy. Dig Dis Sci 1995;40:590–597.
66. Castell DO, Richter JE, Robinson MJ, et al. Efficacy and safety of lansoprazole in the treatment of erosive esophagitis. Am J Gastroenterol 1996;91:1749–1757.
67. Mulder CJ, Dekker W, Gerretsen M. Lansoprazole 30 mg versus omeprazole 40 mg in the treatment of reflux oesophagitis grad II, III and IV (a Dutch multicentre trial). Dutch Study Group. Eur J Gastroenterol Hepatol 1996;8:1101–1106.
68. Kahrilas PJ, Falk GW, Johnson DA, et al. Esomeprazole improves healing and symptom resolution as compared with omeprazole in reflux oesophagitis patients: A randomized controlled trial. Aliment Pharmacol Ther 2000;14:1249–1258.
69. Dekkers CP, Beker JA, Thjodleifsson B, et al. Double-blind, placebo-controlled comparison of rabeprazole 20 mg vs omeprazole 20 mg in the treatment of erosive or ulcerative gastro-oesophageal reflux disease. The European Rabeprazole Study Group. Aliment Pharmacol Ther 1999;13:49–57.
70. Mossner J, Holscher AH, Herz R, et al. A double-blind study of pantoprazole and omeprazole in the treatment of reflux oesophagitis: A multicentre trial. Aliment Pharmacol Ther 1995;9:321–326.
71. Klinkenberg-Knol EC, Festen HPM, Jansen JBMJ, et al. Long-term treatment with omeprazole for refractory reflux esophagitis: Efficacy and safety. Ann Intern Med 1994;121:161–167.
72. Sampliner RE. Effect of up to 3 years of high dose lansoprazole on Barrett's esophagus. Am J Gastroenterol 1994;89:1844–1848.
73. Peters FT, Ganesh S, Kuipers EJ, et al. Endoscopic regression of Barrett's oesophagus during omeprazole treatment: A randomised double blind study. Gut 1999;45(4):489–494.
74. Sampliner RE, Camargo E. Normalization of esophageal pH with high-dose proton pump inhibitor therapy does not result in regression of Barrett's esophagus. Am J Gastroenterol 1997;92:582–585.

75. Richardson P, Hawkey CJ, Stack WA. Proton pump inhibitors. Pharmacology and rationale for use in gastrointestinal disorders. Drugs 1998;56(3):307–335.
76. Reynolds JC. Prokinetic agents: A key in the future of gastroenterology. Gastroenterol Clin North Am 1989;18:437–456.
77. Fink SM, Lange RC, McCallum RW. Effect of metoclopramide on normal and delayed gastric emptying in gastroesophageal reflux patients. Dig Dis Sci 1983;28:1057–1061.
78. Ramirez B, Richter JE. Review article: Promotility drugs and the treatment of gastro-oesophageal reflux disease. Aliment Pharmacol Ther 1993; 7:5–20.
79. Taylor DM. Evaluation of the safety of metoclopramide in patients with gastroesophageal reflux disease. Clin Ther 1984;7:28–32.
80. Ross E, Toledo-Pimentel V, Bordas JM, et al. Healing of erosive esophagitis with sucralfate and cimetidine: Influence of pretreatment lower esophageal sphincter pressure and serum pepsinogen I levels. Am J Med 1991;91(suppl 2A):107S–113S.
81. Bremner CG, Marks IN, Segal I, Simjee A. Reflux esophagitis therapy: Sucralfate versus ranitidine in a double-blind multicenter trial. Am J Med 1991;91(suppl 2A):119S–122S.
82. Elsborg L, Jorgensen F. Sucralfate vs. cimetidine in reflux esophagitis: A double-blind clinical study. Scand J Gastroenterol 1991;26:146–150.
83. Jorgensen F, Elsborg L. Sucralfate vs. cimetidine in treatment of reflux esophagitis with special reference to the esophageal motor function. Am J Med 1991;91(suppl 2A):114–117.
84. Pace F, Lazzaroni M, Bianchi-Porro G. Failure of sucralfate in the treatment of refractory esophagitis vs. high dose famotidine: An endoscopic study. Scand J Gastroenterol 1991;26:491–494.
85. Hetzel DJ, Dent J, Reed WD, et al. Healing and relapse of severe peptic esophagitis after treatment with omeprazole. Gastroenterology 1988;95:903–912.
86. Dent J, Yeomans ND, Mackinnon M, et al. Omeprazole v ranitidine for prevention of relapse in reflux oesophagitis: A controlled double blind trial of their efficacy and safety. Gut 1994;35:590–598.
87. Robinson M, Lanza F, Avner D, Haber M. Effective maintenance therapy of reflux esophagitis with low dose lansoprazole: A randomized, double blind placebo-controlled trial. Ann Intern Med 1996;124:859–867.
88. Vigneri S, Termini R, Leandro G, et al. A comparison of five maintenance therapies for reflux esophagitis. N Engl J Med 1995;333:1106–1110.
89. Talley NJ, Lauritsen K, Tunturi-Hihnala H, et al. Esomperazole 20 mg maintains symptom control in endoscopy-negative GERD: A randomized placebo-controlled trial of on-demand therapy for 6 months. Gastroenterology 2000;118(4 Pt 2):A21. Abstract 348.
90. Talley NJ, Venables TL, Green JRB, et al. Esomeprazole 40 mg and 20 mg is efficacious in the long-term management of patients with endoscopy-negative GERD: A placebo-controlled trial of on demand therapy for 6 months. Gastroenterology 2000;118(4 Pt 2):A658. Abstract 3608.
91. Gough AL, Long RG, Cooper BT. Lansoprazole versus ranitidine in the maintenance of reflux oesophagitis. Aliment Pharmacol Ther 1996;10(4):529–539.
92. Vakil NB, Shaker R, Hwang C, et al. Esomeprazole is effective as maintenance therapy in GERD patients with healed erosive esophagitis (EE). Gastroenterology 2000;118(4 Pt 2):A22. Abstract 350.
93. Johnson DA, Benjamin SB, Whipple J, et al. Efficacy and safety of esomeprazole as maintenance therapy in GERD patients with healed erosive esophagitis (EE). Gastroenterology 2000;118(4 Pt 2):A17. Abstract 330.
94. Isal JP, Zeitoun P, Barbier P, et al. Comparison of two dosage regimens of omeprazole—10 mg once daily and 20 mg weekends. Gastroenterology 1990;98:A63. Abstract.
95. Garrett WR. Considerations for long-term use of proton-pump inhibitors. Am J Health Syst Pharm 1998;55:2268–2279.
96. Kuipers EJ, Lundell L, Klinkenberg-Knol EC, et al. Atrophic gastritis and *Helicobacter pylori* infection in patients with reflux esophagitis treated with omeprazole or fundoplication. N Engl J Med 1996;334:1018–1022.
97. O'Connor HJ. *Helicobacter pylori* and gastro-oesophageal reflux disease—Clinical implications and management. Aliment Pharmacol Ther 1999;13:117–127.
98. Anonymous. Proton pump inhibitor relabeling for cancer risk not warranted. FD& C Report 1996;58(Nov 1):T& G 1-2.
99. Euler AR, Murdock RH, Brotherton BJ, et al. Ranitidine 150 mg b.i.d. prevents erosive esophagitis. Gastroenterology 1992;102:A65. Abstract.
100. DeVault KR. Overview of therapy for extraesophageal manifestations of gastroesophageal reflux disease. Am J Gastroenterol 2000;95(8):S39–S44.
101. Field SK, Sutherland LR. Does medical antireflux therapy improve asthma in asthmatics with gastroesophageal reflux? A critical review of the literature. Chest 1998;114;275–283.
102. Irwin RS, Boulet L-P, Cloutier MM, et al. Managing cough as a defense mechanism and a symptom: A consensus panel report of the American College of Chest Physicians. Chest 1998;114(suppl):133S–181S.
103. Van Pinxteren B, Numans ME, Ponis PA, Lau J. Short-term treatment with proton pump inhibitors, H_2-receptor antagonists and prokinetics for gastro-oesophageal reflux disease-like symptoms and endoscopy negative reflux disease. Cochrane Database Syst Rev 2000;(3):1–27.
104. Watson RG, Tham TC, Johnston BT, et al. Double-blind cross-over placebo-controlled study of omeprazole in the treatment of patients with reflux symptoms and physiological levels of acid reflux—The sensitive esophagus. Gut 1997;40:587–590.
105. Venables TL, Newland RD, Patel AC, et al. Omeprazole 10 milligrams once daily, omeprazole 20 milligrams once daily, or ranitidine 150 milligrams twice daily, evaluated as initial therapy for the relief of symptoms of gastro-oesophageal reflux disease in general practice. Scand J Gastroenterol 1997;32(10):965–973.
106. Bate CM, Green JR, Axon AT, et al. Omeprazole is more effective than cimetidine for the relief of all grades of gastro-oesophageal reflux disease-associated heartburn, irrespective of the presence or absence of endoscopic oesophagitis. Aliment Pharmacol Ther 1997;11(4):755–763.
107. Vandenplas Y, Belli D, Benhamou P-H, et al. Current concepts and issues in the management of regurgitation in infants: A reappraisal. Management guidelines from a working party. Acta Paediatr 1996;85:531–534.
108. Faubion WA, Zein NN. Gastroesophageal reflux in infants and children. Mayo Clin Proc 1998;73(2):166–173.
109. Katz PO. Gastroesophageal reflux disease. J Am Geriatr Soc 1998;46:1558–1565.
110. Hillman AL, Bloom BS, Fendrick AM, et al. Cost and quality effects of alternative treatments for persistent gastroesophageal reflux disease. Arch Intern Med 1992;152:1467–1472.
111. Marks RD, Richter JE, Rizzo J, et al. Omeprazole versus H2 receptor antagonists in treating patients with peptic stricture and esophagitis. Gastroenterology 1994;106:907–915.
112. Harris RA, Kuppermann M, Richter JE. Proton pump inhibitors or histamine-2 receptor antagonists for the prevention of erosive reflux esophagitis: A cost-effectiveness analysis. Am J Gastroenterol 1997;92:2179–2189.
113. Revicki D, Wood M, Maton PM, et al. The impact of gastroesophageal reflux disease on health-related quality of life. Am J Med 1998;104:252–258.
114. Heudebert GR, Marks R, Wilcox CM, et al. Choice of long-term strategy for the management of patients with severe esophagitis: A cost-utility analysis. Gastroenterol 1997;112:1078–1086.
115. Dent J. Long-term aims of treatment of reflux disease, and the role of non-drug measures. Digestion 1992;51(suppl 1):30–34.

33

PEPTIC ULCER DISEASE

Rosemary R. Berardi

Acid-related diseases (gastritis, erosions, and peptic ulcer) of the upper gastrointestinal (GI) tract require gastric acid for their formation.[1–4] Peptic ulcer disease (PUD) differs from gastritis and erosions in that ulcers typically extend deeper into the muscularis mucosa.[1] There are three common forms of peptic ulcers: *Helicobacter pylori* (HP)-associated, nonsteroidal anti-inflammatory drug (NSAID)-induced, and stress ulcers (Table 33–1). The term *"stress-related mucosal damage"* (SRMD) is preferred to stress ulcer or stress gastritis, because the mucosal lesions range from superficial gastritis and erosions to deep ulcers.[2] In patients with a suspected ulcer, dyspeptic symptoms are either uninvestigated (dyspepsia) or an ulcer is not confirmed after upper endoscopy (nonulcer dyspepsia).[3]

Peptic ulcers vary in etiology, clinical presentation, and tendency to recur. Acute ulcers (SRMD) develop in critically ill hospitalized patients, whereas chronic ulcers (HP and NSAID-associated) occur primarily in ambulatory patients. Chronic ulcers develop most often in the duodenum and stomach, but occasionally occur in the esophagus, jejunum, ileum, or colon. Peptic ulcers are also associated with Zollinger-Ellison syndrome, radiation, chemotherapy, and vascular insufficiency (Table 33–2).[1,4] This chapter focuses on HP-associated and NSAID-induced ulcers. A brief discussion of SRMD and Zollinger-Ellison syndrome-associated ulcers is included.

The natural course of PUD is characterized by frequent ulcer recurrence. Approximately 50% to 100% of ulcers recur within 1 year of initial ulcer healing with conventional antiulcer regimens.[1] The most important factors that influence ulcer recurrence are HP infection and NSAID use. Other factors include gastric acid hypersecretion, cigarette smoking, a long duration of PUD, ulcer-related complications, and patient noncompliance. The cause of ulcer recurrence is most likely multifactorial.

EPIDEMIOLOGY

Approximately 10% of Americans develop chronic PUD during their lifetime.[1] The incidence varies with ulcer type, age, gender, and geographical location. Race, occupation, genetic predisposition, and societal factors may play a minor role in ulcer pathogenesis, but are attenuated by the importance of HP infection and NSAID use. The overall prevalence of PUD in the United States has shifted from predominance in men to nearly comparable prevalence in men and women. Recent trends suggest a declining rate for younger men and an increasing rate for older women.[1] Factors that have influenced these trends include increased NSAID use in older adults and the declining smoking rates in younger men.

Since 1960, ulcer-related physician visits, hospitalizations, operations, and deaths have declined in the United States by more than 50%, primarily because of decreased rates of PUD among men.[1] The decline in hospitalizations has resulted primarily from a reduction in hospital admissions for uncomplicated duodenal ulcer, with a less dramatic decrease for gastric ulcer.[5] In contrast, hospitalizations of older adults for ulcer related complications (bleeding and perforation) have increased.[1] Mortality from PUD has decreased modestly, but death rates have increased in patients older than 75 years of age, most likely a result of increased consumption of NSAIDs and an aging population. Despite these trends, PUD remains one of the most common gastrointestinal (GI) diseases, resulting in impaired quality of life, work loss, and high-cost medical care.

ETIOLOGY AND RISK FACTORS

Most peptic ulcers occur in the presence of acid and pepsin when HP, NSAIDs, or other factors (Table 33–2) disrupt normal mucosal defense and healing mechanisms (Fig. 33–1).[1,4] Hypersecretion of acid is the primary pathogenic mechanism in hypersecretory states such as Zollinger-Ellison syndrome.[4] Ulcer location appears to be related to a number of etiologic factors. Most duodenal ulcers occur in the first part of the duodenum (duodenal bulb). Benign gastric ulcers can occur anywhere in the stomach, although most are located on the lesser curvature, just distal to the junction of the antral and acid-secreting mucosa.

HELICOBACTER PYLORI

A strong association exists between *Helicobacter pylori* (formerly *Campylobacter pylori*) and PUD (Fig. 33–2).[1,6–8] Most patients with duodenal ulcer or gastric ulcer who are not taking NSAIDs have evidence of HP infection and antral gastritis. Although a causal relationship between HP and chronic superficial gastritis is well established, a similar relationship between HP and PUD has been difficult to confirm because only 15% of individuals infected with HP actually develop clinical manifestations of an ulcer.[1,7] Support for a causal role in PUD is based on the fact that most non-NSAID ulcers are infected with HP, and that HP eradication markedly decreases ulcer recurrence.[1,7] Host-specific cofactors and HP strain variability play an important role in the pathogenesis of PUD.[1,9,10]

Approximately 50% of the world's population is colonized by HP.[1,8] The prevalence of HP is higher in developing countries, where living conditions and hygiene are less than optimal and acquisition occurs during early childhood.[1] In developed countries, there is an age-related increase in the prevalence of HP in adults, but the overall frequency is lower as successive generations have been less likely to acquire the infection as children.[1,9] In the United States, prevalence varies among different ethnic groups of similar socioeconomic status, with infection more common in African and Latin Americans than in whites.[1] One explanation may be that improvement in socioeconomic status for African and Latin Americans has lagged behind that of whites. Infection rates do not appear to differ with gender or smoking status.

HP is potentially transmitted by three different modes.[1,11] First, transmission of the organism in Western countries is thought to be person to person by the fecal-oral route with contaminated water as the source of the infection. The housefly also has the potential to

TABLE 33–1. Comparison of Common Forms of Peptic Ulcer

Characteristic	*Helicobacter pylori*	NSAID	SRMD
Site of damage	Duodenum > stomach	Stomach > duodenum	Stomach > duodenum
Intragastric pH	More dependent	Less dependent	Less dependent
Symptoms	Usually epigastric pain	Often asymptomatic	Asymptomatic
Ulcer depth	Superficial	Deep	Most superficial
GI bleeding	Less severe	More severe	More severe

mechanically transmit HP from human waste to food or children.[11] Members of the same household are likely to become infected when someone in the same household is infected.[1] Second, transmission by the oral-oral route has been postulated because HP has been isolated from the oral cavity. Third, transmission of HP can occur iatrogenically when infected instruments such as endoscopes are used.

Epidemiologic data provide strong evidence that, in some individuals, asymptomatic HP infection is associated with chronic atrophic gastritis, gastric mucosa-associated lymphoid tissue (MALT) lymphoma, and gastric adenocarcinoma (Fig. 33–2).[1,7,12–14] Serologic studies confirm an association between HP and gastric cancer.[1,12] The development of atrophic gastritis and gastric carcinoma is generally a slow process that occurs over 20 years to 40 years. As with PUD, host-specific cofactors and conditions that influence the severity of gastritis are likely to influence the development of chronic atrophic gastritis. A highly specific type of atrophic gastritis (with intestinal metaplasia) is considered to be a precursor of gastric cancer.[7,12] In 1994, the World Health Organization concluded that HP infection is carcinogenic (group I carcinogen) to humans.[7] The relationship between HP and nonulcer dyspepsia remains controversial.[3,15,16]

NONSTEROIDAL ANTI-INFLAMMATORY DRUGS

NSAIDs are one of the most widely prescribed classes of medications in the United States, particularly in individuals 60 years of age and older.[1,17–22] The availability of nonprescription NSAIDs has contributed to their widespread use and associated complications. There is overwhelming evidence linking chronic NSAID (including aspirin) use to a wide variety of GI tract injuries.[1,17–30] Subepithelial gastric hemorrhages occur within 15 minutes to 30 minutes of ingestion, and progress to gastric erosions with continued ingestion.[1,17–22] These lesions heal within a few days with continued NSAID use and do not lead to GI complications. Gastroduodenal ulcers occur in 15% to 30% of regular NSAID users and may develop within a week or with continued treatment (6 months or longer).[17] Gastric ulcers are most common, occur primarily in the antrum, and are of greater concern than erosions because of their potential to bleed or perforate. Duodenal ulcers occur less often and may be produced by a different mechanism. NSAIDs also can cause ulcers in the esophagus or colon and may exacerbate quiescent inflammatory bowel disease.[17,23,24]

TABLE 33–2. Potential Causes of Peptic Ulcer

Helicobacter pylori infection
Nonsteroidal anti-inflammatory drugs
Critical illness (stress-related mucosal damage)
Hypersecretion of gastric acid (e.g., Zollinger-Ellison syndrome)
Viral infections (e.g., cytomegalovirus)
Vascular insufficiency (crack cocaine-associated)
Radiation
Chemotherapy (e.g., hepatic artery infusions)
Rare genetic subtypes
Idiopathic

Hospitalizations, complications, and mortality are dramatically increased in chronic NSAID users.[25–27] Each year, NSAIDs account for at least 16,500 deaths and 103,000 hospitalizations in the United States.[19] Clinically important upper GI events occur in 3% to 4.5% of arthritis patients taking NSAIDs, and 1.5% will have a serious complication (major GI bleed, perforation, obstruction).[17] Ulcer complications occur with prescription and nonprescription NSAIDs, and account for almost all of the NSAID-associated GI mortalities.[25,28] Ulcers have been reported with low doses of aspirin (10–100 mg/d) or nonaspirin NSAIDs, and complications have occurred following a few days of treatment.[1,17–22,25,26,29] Patients with previous PUD, upper GI bleeding, NSAID-related GI complications, or those patients who are taking concurrent corticosteroids, high-dose NSAIDs, or anticoagulants, are at greatest risk for serious GI complications (Table 33–3).[1,17–22,30] Asymptomatic patients taking antacids or H_2-receptor antagonists may be at increased risk for serious GI complications as they appear to mask symptoms related to the complications.[1,31] Cigarette smoking and ethanol ingestion contribute to increased risk but do not appear to be independent factors.[1,19] The high incidence of NSAID-related ulcer complications in individuals older than 60 years of age is associated with age-related changes in gastric mucosal defense.[18] The increased risk of ulcers in older women may be related to increased consumption.[28,31] There is controversy as to whether HP is an independent risk factor for the development of NSAID-induced ulcers, although most of the evidence suggests that HP does not potentiate the risk of ulcer formation in NSAID users.[1,17–21,32,33] However, HP may potentiate the effects of NSAIDs with regard to ulcer bleeding.[17,34]

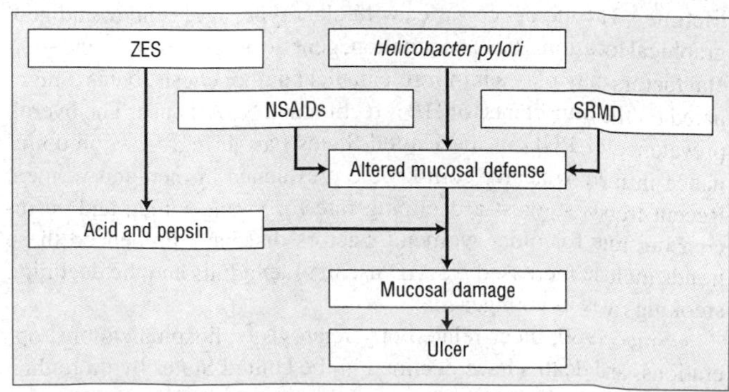

FIGURE 33–1. Pathogenesis of peptic ulcer disease. Acid and pepsin cause ulcers when mucosal defense mechanisms are altered by nonsteroidal anti-inflammatory drugs (NSAIDs), *Helicobacter pylori* (*H. pylori*), or stress-related mucosal damage (SRMD). Hypersecretion of gastric acid causes ulcers in Zollinger-Ellison syndrome (ZES).

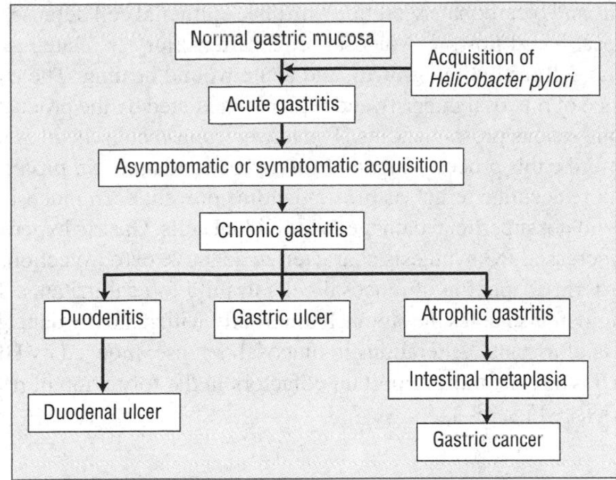

FIGURE 33–2. The natural history of *Helicobacter pylori* infection in the pathogenesis of gastric ulcer and duodenal ulcer and gastric cancer.

CORTICOSTEROIDS

The association between corticosteroids and PUD remains controversial.[1,17–22] Although the use of corticosteroids alone may not increase the risk of ulcer or complications, their concurrent use with NSAIDs does appear to increase the risk of GI events.[1,17,18,20–22] It is possible that corticosteroids either delay or inhibit the healing of ulcers caused by NSAIDs.

UNCOMMON FORMS OF PEPTIC ULCERS

Peptic ulcers may develop in individuals using crack cocaine, in patients with viral infections, and in those patients receiving abdominal radiation or undergoing chemotherapy administered through a hepatic artery pump, such as with 5-fluorouracil (Table 33–2).[1]

CIGARETTE SMOKING

There is strong epidemiologic evidence that links cigarette smoking to PUD, impaired ulcer healing, and ulcer-related GI complications.[1] Cigarette smoking increases ulcer risk and is proportional to the number of cigarettes smoked per day. When antiulcer agents are used to heal or prevent ulcers, smoking impairs ulcer healing and promotes recurrence. The risk of recurrence and impaired healing is modest when fewer than 10 cigarettes are smoked per day. However, smoking does not appear to increase ulcer recurrence after HP eradication.[1] Smoking increases the likelihood of complications and the need for surgery. Death rates are higher among patients who smoke than among nonsmoking patients, although it is not known whether the increase in mortality reflects PUD or the cardiac and pulmonary sequelae of smoking.

The exact mechanism by which cigarette smoking contributes to PUD remains unclear. Possible pathophysiologic mechanisms include delayed gastric emptying of solids and liquids, inhibition of pancreatic bicarbonate secretion, promotion of duodenogastric reflux, and reduction in mucosal prostaglandin (PG) production. Although smoking has been reported to increase gastric acid, it appears to have no consistent effect on acid secretion. It is uncertain whether nicotine or other components of smoke are responsible for these physiologic alterations. It also is possible that cigarette smoking provides a favorable milieu for HP infection.

TABLE 33–3. Risk Factors for Nonsteroidal Anti-Inflammatory Drug (NSAID)-Induced Ulcers and Upper Gastrointestinal Complications

Established risk factors
Age over 60 years
Previous peptic ulcer disease
Previous upper gastrointestinal bleed
Previous NSAID-related gastrointestinal effects
Concomitant corticosteroid therapy
High-dose and multiple NSAID use
Concomitant anticoagulant use or coagulopathy
Chronic major organ impairment (e.g., cardiovascular disease)
Possible risk factors
Cigarette smoking
Alcohol consumption
Poor general health
Asymptomatic patients taking H_2-receptor antagonists or antacids
Helicobacter pylori infection

Compiled from references 1 and 17–22.

GENETIC FACTORS

A number of genetic factors have been proposed to explain familial aggregation of PUD. HP infection, and its association with hypergastrinemia and hyperpepsinogenemia I, offers a more plausible explanation for family clustering than inherited autosomal dominance.[1] Other genetic markers, including blood group O antigen, preceded the recent concept that HP plays a central role in the pathogenesis of PUD. However, certain rare genetic syndromes are associated with peptic ulcers.

PSYCHOLOGICAL STRESS

The importance of psychological factors in the pathogenesis of PUD remains controversial.[1] Clinical observation suggests that ulcer patients are adversely affected by stressful life events. However, results from controlled trials are conflicting and have failed to document a cause-and-effect relationship.[1] Major psychological stress may have an effect on the brain-gut axis resulting in altered acid secretion and GI motility. It is also possible that emotional stress induces behavioral risks such as smoking and the use of NSAIDs or alters the inflammatory response or resistance to HP infection. The role of stress and how it affects PUD is complex and probably multifactorial.

DIETARY FACTORS

The role of diet and nutrition in PUD is uncertain, but may explain regional variations.[1] Coffee, tea, cola beverages, beer, milk, and spices may cause dyspepsia, but do not increase the risk for PUD. In addition, beverage restrictions and bland diets do not alter the frequency of ulcer recurrence. Although caffeine is a gastric acid stimulant, other constituents in decaffeinated coffee or tea, caffeine-free carbonated beverages, beer, and wine are responsible for increasing gastric acid. Ethanol, in high concentrations, is associated with acute gastric mucosal damage and upper GI bleeding; however, there is insufficient evidence to confirm that ethanol causes ulcers.

DISEASES ASSOCIATED WITH PEPTIC ULCERS

Several diseases are associated with peptic ulcers, but many apparent associations are based on inconclusive evidence.[1] The prevalence of PUD among patients with chronic pulmonary disease is increased three- to fivefold, but cigarette smoking may account, in part, for this association. Chronic renal failure with or without hemodialysis or recent transplant is associated with an increased risk for duodenal ulcer. Although the exact mechanism is unknown, viruses related to immunosuppression (Table 33–2) may cause ulcers in renal transplant patients. The increased incidence of PUD in patients with rheumatoid arthritis is most likely related to NSAID and corticosteroid ingestion. The prevalence of PUD is increased in cirrhosis, but a relationship has not been confirmed. Patients with atrophic gastritis, pernicious anemia, Addison's disease, and diabetes appear to have a lower incidence of peptic ulcers.

PATHOPHYSIOLOGY

GASTRIC ACID SECRETION

A minimal level of gastric acid secretion is necessary for the formation of peptic ulcers. Thus, gastric acid serves as a cofactor with HP infection or NSAID use (see Fig. 33–1).[1,36] Basal and nocturnal acid secretion is generally increased in a patient with duodenal ulcer. Factors responsible for acid hypersecretion include increased parietal cell mass, increased basal secretory drive, and increased postprandial secretory drive. Acid hypersecretion may also be a consequence of HP infection.[1,35–37] Patients with Zollinger-Ellison syndrome (described later in the chapter) have basal acid hypersecretion resulting from a gastrin-producing tumor. Unlike patients with duodenal ulcers, patients with gastric ulcers have normal or reduced rates of acid secretion, reflecting a low-normal parietal cell mass. Decreased acid secretion (hypochlorhydria) or an absence of acid secretion (achlorhydria) has been reported in older adults.

Acid secretion is usually expressed as the amount of acid secreted under basal or fasting conditions, as with basal acid output (BAO); after maximal stimulation, as with maximal acid output (MAO); or in response to a meal.[36] Basal, maximal, and meal-stimulated acid secretion varies according to time of day and the individual's psychological state, age, gender, and health status. The lowest acid secretory rates occur between 5 AM and 11 AM, while the highest rates occur between 2 PM and 11 PM. The reason why circadian variations occur is unknown. The BAO is usually higher in men than in women. An increase in the BAO/MAO ratio suggests a basal hypersecretory state such as Zollinger-Ellison syndrome. A review of gastric acid secretion and its regulation can be found elsewhere.[36]

PEPSIN

Pepsin appears to play a critical role in the proteolytic activity involved in ulcer formation.[36] Gastric mucosal cells secrete two types of proteolytic proenzymes. Pepsinogen I (PI) is produced only in the chief and mucous neck cells of the acid-secreting mucosa, whereas pepsinogen II (PII) is found in gastric acid-secreting and antral mucosa. Pepsin is activated by acid pH (optimal pH of 1.8–3.5), inactivated reversibly at pH 4, and irreversibly destroyed at pH 7. Pepsinogen I secretion is directly proportional to the rate of acid secretion. Hypergastrinemia and HP infection increase serum PI concentrations, although HP itself may induce hypergastrinemia.

ALTERED MUCOSAL DEFENSE AND HEALING

Several mechanisms protect the GI mucosa from endogenous and exogenous noxious substances. These defensive mechanisms include mucus and bicarbonate secretion, intrinsic epithelial cell defense, and mucosal blood flow.[1,36] Mucosal repair after injury is related to epithelial cell restitution, growth, and acute wound healing. The maintenance of mucosal integrity and repair is mediated by the production of endogenous prostaglandins. The term *cytoprotection* is often used to describe this process, but *mucosal defense* and *mucosal protection* are more accurate terms, as prostaglandins prevent deep mucosal injury and not superficial damage to individual cells. Gastric hyperemia and increased PG synthesis characterize adaptive cytoprotection, the short-term adaptation of mucosal cells to mild topical irritants. This phenomenon enables the stomach to initially withstand the damaging effects of irritants. Alterations in mucosal defense, induced by HP or NSAIDs, are the most important cofactors in the formation of peptic ulcers (see Fig. 33–1).

ABNORMALITIES IN GASTRIC MOTILITY

Gastric motility determines the rate of delivery of stomach contents to the duodenum, whereas duodenal motility affects the clearance of gastric, biliary, and pancreatic secretions from the duodenum. Accelerated gastric emptying may contribute to a relative increase in the acidity of the proximal duodenum in a subset of duodenal ulcer patients.[1] Abnormal antral-pylorus-duodenal motility patterns permit duodenal contents containing bile salts and pancreatic enzymes to reflux into the stomach. Delayed gastric emptying increases exposure of the stomach to acid, pepsin, and refluxed duodenal contents. It is possible that in a subset of patients, gastric stasis and duodenal reflux may influence the severity of gastric injury induced by HP or NSAIDs.

HELICOBACTER PYLORI

HP is a spiral-shaped, pH-sensitive, gram-negative, microaerophilic bacterium that resides between the mucous layer and surface epithelial cells in the stomach or any location where gastric-type epithelium is found.[37,38] The combination of its spiral shape and flagella permits it to move from the lumen of the stomach, where the pH is low, to the mucous layer, where the local pH is neutral. The acute infection is accompanied by transient hypochlorhydria, which permits the organism to survive in the acidic gastric juice. The exact method by which HP initially induces hypochlorhydria is unclear. One theory is that HP produces large amounts of urease, which hydrolyzes urea in the gastric juice and converts it to ammonia and carbon dioxide.[37,38] The local buffering effect of ammonia protects the organism from the lethal effect of acid. HP also produces acid-inhibitory proteins which allows it to adapt to the low pH environment of the stomach.[37] HP attaches to gastric-type epithelium by adherence pedestals, which prevent the organism from being shed during cell turnover and mucus secretion. Antral organisms colonize gastric metaplastic tissue (which is thought to arise secondary to changes in acid or bicarbonate secretion, products of HP, or host inflammatory responses) in the duodenal bulb leading to duodenitis and duodenal ulcer (see Fig. 33–2).[1]

A number of bacterial and host factors are thought to play a role in the pathogenesis of GI mucosal damage caused by HP infection. HP contributes to gastric mucosal injury by (a) direct mechanisms, (b) alterations in the immune/inflammatory response, and (c) hypergastrinemia leading to increased acid secretion.[35,38–41] In addition, HP enhances the carcinogenic conversion of susceptible gastric epithelial cells.[1,6,7]

Direct mucosal damage is produced by elaborating bacterial enzymes (lipases, proteases, and urease), virulence factors (vacuolating cytotoxin, cytotoxin-associated gene protein, and growth-inhibitory factor), and adherence.[1,39,41] Lipases and proteases degrade gastric mucus, ammonia produced by urease may be toxic to gastric epithelial cells, and bacterial adherence enhances the uptake of toxins into gastric epithelial cells. About 50% of HP strains produce a protein toxin (Vac A) that is responsible for cellular vacuole formation. Strains with cytotoxin-associated gene (cagA) protein are associated with duodenal ulcer, atrophic gastritis, and adenocarcinoma.[1,6,7,39] HP infection alters the inflammatory response and damages epithelial cells directly by cell-mediated immune mechanisms or indirectly by activated neutrophils or macrophages attempting to phagocytose bacteria or bacterial products.[40] HP infection may increase gastric acid secretion in patients with duodenal ulcer, or diminish acid output in patients with gastric cancer.[1,6,7,35,37] Infection of the gastric antrum leads to postprandial hypergastrinemia and hypersecretion of gastric acid. Responsible mechanisms include cytokines, such as tumor necrosis factor (TNF)-α released in HP gastritis; products of HP, such as ammonia; and diminished expression of somatostatin. Why somatostatin is diminished is unclear, but cytokines may be involved.[1,35,41] Corpus (body) gastritis promotes gastric atrophy and decreases acid output.[1,6,7]

NONSTEROIDAL ANTI-INFLAMMATORY DRUGS

NSAIDs cause gastric mucosal damage by two important mechanisms: (a) direct or topical irritation of the gastric epithelium and (b) systemic inhibition of endogenous GI mucosal PG synthesis (Fig. 33–3).[1,18,19,22,42] Although the initial injury is initiated topically by the acidic properties of many of the NSAIDs, systemic inhibition of PGs plays the predominant role in the development of gastric ulcer.[1,18,19,22,42] Cyclooxygenase (COX) is the rate-limiting enzyme in the conversion of arachidonic acid to PGs and is inhibited by NSAIDs (Fig. 33–3). Two similar COX isoforms exist in mammalian cells: cyclooxygenase-1 (COX-1) is found in most body tissue including the stomach, kidney, intestine, and platelets; cyclooxygenase-2 (COX-2) is undetectable in most tissues under normal physiologic conditions, but its expression can be induced during acute inflammation and arthritis (Fig. 33–4).[18,19,22] COX-1 produces protective PGs that regulate physiologic processes such as GI mucosal integrity, vascular homeostasis, and renal function. COX-2 is induced (up regulated) by inflammatory stimuli such as cytokines, and produces PGs involved with inflammation and pain. Adverse effects

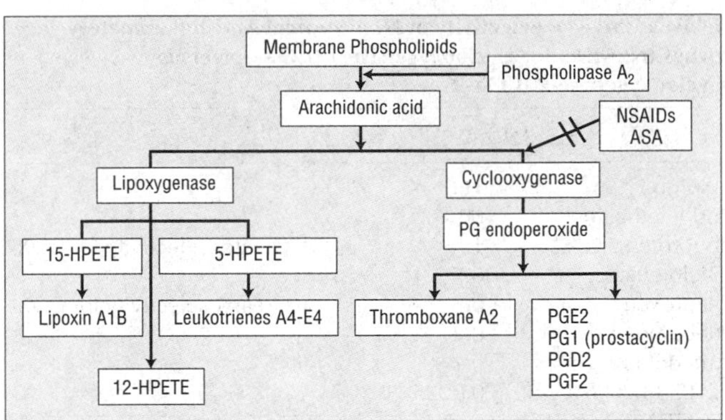

FIGURE 33–3. Metabolism of arachidonic acid after its release from membrane phospholipids. ASA, aspirin; HETE, hydroxyeicosatetraenoic acid; HPETE, hydroperoxyeicosatetraenoic acid; NSAIDs, nonsteroidal anti-inflammatory drugs; PG, prostaglandin; broken arrow indicates inhibitory effects.

(e.g., GI effects, renal toxicity) of NSAIDs are associated with the inhibition of COX-1, whereas anti-inflammatory actions result from NSAID inhibition of COX-2.[18,19,22] NSAIDs inhibit both COX-1 and COX-2 to varying degrees (Table 33–4).[1,18,19,22,43,44]

Other mechanisms may contribute to the development of NSAID-induced mucosal injury. TNF-α may be an important signal for NSAID-induced neutrophil adherence within the gastric microcirculation.[1,18,19,22] Adherence of neutrophils may damage the vascular endothelium and may lead to a reduction in mucosal blood flow, or may liberate oxygen-derived free radicals and proteases. Leukotrienes, products of lipoxygenase metabolism, are inflammatory substances that may contribute to mucosal injury through stimulatory effects on neutrophil adherence (see Fig. 33–3). Topical irritant properties are predominantly associated with acidic NSAIDs (e.g., aspirin) and their ability to decrease the hydrophobicity of the mucous gel layer in the gastric mucosa.[1,18,19,22] Most nonaspirin NSAIDs have topical irritant effects, but aspirin appears to be the most damaging. Although NSAID prodrugs, enteric-coated aspirin tablets or capsules, salicylate derivatives, and parenteral or rectal preparations are associated with less-acute gastric mucosal injury when compared to oral aspirin or NSAID formulations, they can cause peptic ulcers and related GI complications as a result of systemic PG inhibition.

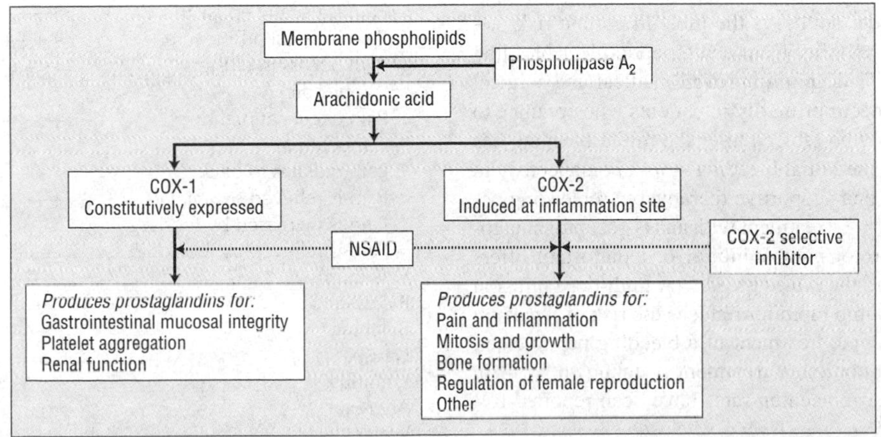

FIGURE 33–4. Synthesis of prostaglandins from arachidonic acid. Currently available nonsteroidal anti-inflammatory drugs (NSAIDs) inhibit cyclooxygenase-1 (COX-1) and cyclooxygenase-2 (COX-2) to varying degrees; broken arrow indicates inhibitory effects.

TABLE 33–4. Selectivity of Nonsteroidal Anti-Inflammatory Drugs (NSAIDs) for Cyclooxygenase-1 (COX-1) Versus Cyclooxygenase-2 (COX-2)

NSAID	COX-2/COX-1[a]	Selectivity
Aspirin	166	
Indomethacin	60	
Ibuprofen	15	↑ Greater selectivity for COX-1
Diclofenac	0.7	
Naproxen	0.6	↓ Greater selectivity for COX-2
Nabumetone	0.2	
Entodolac	0.1	
L745,337[b]	0.0025	

[a]Ratio of mean inhibitory concentration of drug required to inhibit COX-2 by 50% divided by concentration of drug required to inhibit COX-1 by 50%; data obtained from *in vitro* studies.
[b]Selective COX-2 inhibitor.
Adapted from reference 22.

NSAIDs (including aspirin) cause de novo ulcers and can also interfere with the healing of preexisting ulcers by interfering with the process of restitution.[18,22] NSAIDs probably contribute to GI bleeding from current or preexisting ulcers by inhibiting platelet aggregation that results from suppression of thromboxane synthesis.[45] The pathogenesis of small intestinal damage (e.g., duodenal ulcer) and colonic damage is not as well understood as the pathogenesis of NSAID-induced gastropathy.[22,23] Enteric bacteria and enterohepatic recirculation of NSAIDs may play a more important role in the pathogenesis of NSAID-induced injury to the small intestine than does PG inhibition. The mechanisms by which NSAIDs cause or exacerbate preexisting colonic ulcerations and inflammatory bowel disease are attributed to inhibition of colonic PGs, but data are conflicting. A more detailed discussion of the pathogenesis of NSAID-induced small intestinal and colonic injury can be found elsewhere.[22,23]

COMPLICATIONS

Upper GI bleeding, perforation, and obstruction occur with HP and NSAID ulcers and constitute the most serious, life-threatening complications of chronic PUD.[1,34,46–50] Bleeding is caused by the erosion of an ulcer into an artery and is reported to occur in approximately 15% of patients.[1,46] The bleeding may be insidious or may present as melena or hematemesis. Peptic ulcers account for more than one-half of all patients who have an upper GI bleed.[26,46,48] The use of NSAIDs (especially in older adults) is the most important risk factor for GI bleeding. The mortality from acute peptic ulcer bleeding has remained at 6% to 10% despite improved medical and surgical management.[48,50] Deaths occur primarily in patients who continue to bleed, or in those patients who rebleed after the initial bleeding has stopped. In most patients, the initial bleeding stops spontaneously in response to gastric lavage and supportive therapy, but rebleeding occurs in about 15% to 20%.[46,49] Treatment with an H_2-receptor antagonist, sucralfate, antacids, proton pump inhibitor, or somatostatin offers no clear benefit in stopping the *initial* bleed.[46] A high-dose infusion of an intravenous proton pump inhibitor reduces the risk of *recurrent* bleeding following endoscopic treatment of a bleeding peptic ulcer, but the optimal dose and duration of treatment is unknown[46,49,50] In HP-positive patients, lower rebleeding rates have been reported following HP eradication.[46,48]

Ulcer-related perforation into the peritoneal cavity occurs in about 7% of patient with PUD.[1] The incidence of perforation is increasing with the increased use of NSAIDs. Mortality is usually higher for perforated gastric ulcer than duodenal ulcer. The pain of perforation is usually sudden, sharp, and severe, beginning first in the epigastrium, but quickly spreading over the entire abdomen. Most patients experience ulcer symptoms prior to perforation. However, older patients who experience perforation in association with NSAID use may be asymptomatic. Penetration occurs when an ulcer burrows into an adjacent structure (pancreas, biliary tract, liver) rather than opening freely into a cavity.

Gastric outlet obstruction occurs in about 2% of patients with peptic ulcers.[1] Mechanical obstruction is caused by scarring or edema of the duodenal bulb or pyloric channel and can lead to gastric retention. Symptoms usually occur over several months and include early satiety, bloating, anorexia, nausea, vomiting, and weight loss. Perforation, penetration, and gastric outlet obstruction occur most often in patients with long-standing PUD.

Treatment of PUD has improved so dramatically that even the most virulent ulcers can be managed with medication. Intractability to drug therapy is now an infrequent manifestation of PUD and an infrequent indication for surgery.

CLINICAL PRESENTATION

SIGNS AND SYMPTOMS

Abdominal pain is the classic and most frequent dyspeptic symptom of duodenal ulcer and gastric ulcer (Table 33–5 and Fig. 33–5).[1] The pain is often epigastric and described as burning, but may present as vague discomfort, abdominal fullness, or cramping. Many patients with duodenal ulcer describe a typical nocturnal pain that awakens them from sleep (especially between 12 AM and 3 AM).[1] Ulcer-related pain in duodenal ulcer often occurs 1 hour to 3 hours after meals and is usually relieved by food, but this is variable. In gastric ulcer, food may precipitate or accentuate ulcer pain. Antacids usually provide immediate pain relief in most ulcer patients. The abdominal pain usually diminishes or disappears during treatment; however, recurrence of pain after healing often suggests an unhealed or recurrent ulcer.

TABLE 33–5. Signs or Symptoms of Duodenal Ulcer (DU), Gastric Ulcer (GU), and Nonulcer Dyspepsia (NUD)

Sign or Symptom	DU	GU	NUD
Abdominal pain			
Pain is usually epigastric	++++	+++	+++
Pain is frequently severe	++++	+++	++
Pain occurs in clusters (episodic)	+++	+	++
Pain occurs at night (nocturnal)	++++	++	++
Pain radiates to back	++	++	++
Pain is relieved by antacids	++++	++++	+++
Pain is increased by food	++	+	++
Pain is relieved by food	+++	++	++
Heartburn	+++	+	++
Bloating	+++	+++	+++
Belching	+++	+++	+++
Nausea	++	+++	++
Vomiting	++	+++	+
Anorexia	+	++	+
Weight loss	++	++	+

Sign or symptom is: almost always present or occurs almost all of the time (++++); frequently present or occurs most of the time (+++); infrequently present or occurs sometimes (++); rarely present (+). None of the signs or symptoms are always present or always absent in any one patient.

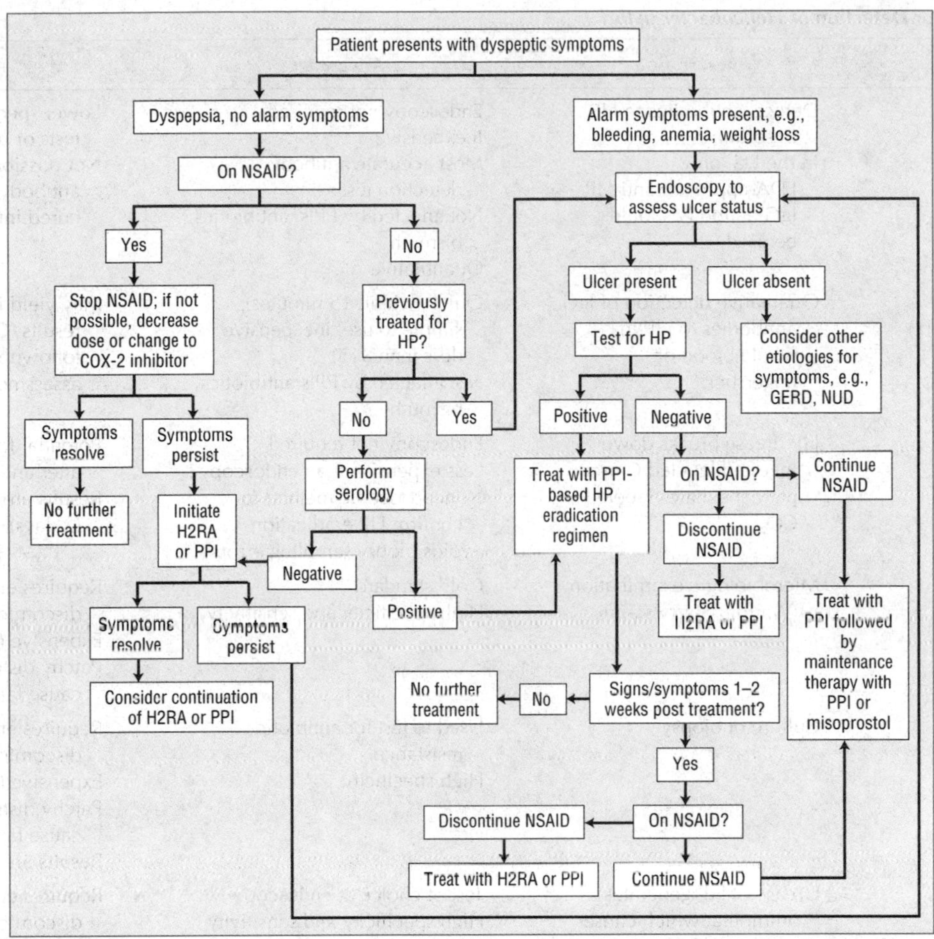

FIGURE 33–5. Algorithm. Guidelines for the evaluation and management of a patient who presents with dyspeptic symptoms. GERD, gastroesophageal reflux disease; H2RA, H2-receptor antagonist; HP, *Helicobacter pylori;* NSAID, nonsteroidal anti-inflammatory drug; NUD, nonulcer dyspepsia; PPI, proton pump inhibitor; COX-2, cyclooxygenase-2.

The severity of ulcer pain varies from patient to patient, and in some patients may be seasonal, occurring more frequently in the spring or fall. Episodes of discomfort usually occur in clusters lasting up to a few weeks followed by a pain-free period or remission lasting from weeks to years. Pain does not always correlate with the presence or absence of acid or an ulcer crater. Asymptomatic patients may have an ulcer at endoscopy, and patients with endoscopically proven healed ulcers may have persistent symptoms. Changes in the character of the pain often suggest the presence of complications. Most patients, particularly older adults, with an NSAID-induced ulcer-related complication do not have prior abdominal symptoms.[19] The reasons for this are unclear, but may result from the analgesic effect of the NSAID or relate to differences in the way older individuals perceive pain.

Patients with PUD also present with other dyspeptic symptoms including heartburn, belching, and bloating (Table 33–5). As many as 50% of patients who take NSAIDs report having "dyspepsia."[19] Dyspepsia may or may not be associated with an ulcer and, in itself, is of little clinical value when trying to identify subsets of patients who are most likely to have an ulcer. Nausea, vomiting, anorexia, and weight loss are more common in patients with gastric ulcers than in patients with duodenal ulcers. Unusual findings may be present when ulcers are associated with hypersecretory states such as Zollinger-Ellison syndrome. Ulcer-like symptoms may occur in the absence of peptic ulceration (nonulcer dyspepsia) and in association with HP gastritis or duodenitis (Table 33–5). It is uncertain whether HP infection plays a role in causing symptoms in patients with nonulcer dyspepsia.[3,16]

DIAGNOSIS

LABORATORY EVALUATION

Routine laboratory tests are not helpful in establishing the diagnosis of uncomplicated PUD.[1] Acid secretory studies and a fasting serum gastrin concentration are only recommended for patients unresponsive to therapy, or for those patients in whom hypersecretory diseases are suspected. The hematocrit, hemoglobin, and stool hemoccult tests are used to detect bleeding.

TESTS FOR *HELICOBACTER PYLORI*

The diagnosis of HP can be made using invasive or noninvasive tests (Table 33–6).[1,51–55] The invasive methods require upper GI endoscopy with a mucosal biopsy taken for histology, culture, or detection of urease activity.[1,51,52,54,55] Recommendations to maximize the diagnostic yield include taking at least three tissue samples from specific areas of the stomach. Histologic identification has a sensitivity and specificity greater than 95% and allows classification of gastritis that may be present. Culture has a specificity of 100% and enables susceptibility testing of antimicrobial agents to detect resistance and permit

TABLE 33–6. Tests for Detection of *Helicobacter pylori*

Test	Description	Advantages	Disadvantages
Antibody detection (laboratory-based)	Detects antibodies to HP in serum; In the US, only FDA-approved anti-HP IgG antibody should be used	Endoscopy not required Inexpensive Most accurate antibody detection test Not affected by PPIs, antibiotics, bismuth Quantitative	Lower specificity than endoscopic tests or urea breath tests Not possible to determine whether antibody is related to active or cured infection
Antibody detection (in office or near patient)	Qualitative detection of IgG antibodies to HP in whole blood or fingerstick	Quick (within 15 minutes), simple to use, inexpensive (less than $15) Not affected by PPIs antibiotics, bismuth	May yield indeterminate or invalid results. Cannot use for early followup testing for quantitative assessment
Urea breath test	HP urease breaks down ingested labeled C-urea; patient exhales labeled CO_2	Endoscopy not required Less expensive than endoscopy Nonendoscopic method to confirm HP eradication Avoids biopsy sampling errors	Potential for false-negative results after antibiotics, bismuth, PPIs Results are not immediate (2 days)
Histology	Microbiologic examination (Warthin-Starry stain)	Gold standard High specificity and sensitivity	Requires endoscopy; patient discomfort Expensive (includes endoscopy) Patchy distribution of HP can cause false-negative results
Culture	Culture of biopsy	Used to test for antibiotic resistance High specificity	Requires endoscopy, patient discomfort Expensive (includes endoscopy) Patchy distribution of HP can cause false-negative results Results are not immediate
Biopsy (rapid) urease	Urease of HP generates ammonia, which causes a color change	Test of choice at endoscopy High specificity and sensitivity Easily performed; rapid results (usually within 24 hours)	Requires endoscopy; patient discomfort Expensive (includes endoscopy) Antibiotics, bismuth, and PPIs can cause false-negative results Patchy distribution of HP can cause false-negative results

PPI = Proton pump inhibitor.
Compiled from references 1 and 51–55.

appropriate treatment. The sensitivity and specificity of the biopsy (rapid) urease test, which detects HP urease enzyme activity, are above 90%. The results of these tests are available within 24 hours, but they do not determine the mucosal status or susceptibility to antibiotics. The CLO test was the first commercially available biopsy urease test. Newer tests, for example, PyloriTek and Hpfast, are now available, but their performance characteristics have not been as extensively defined.[1]

The noninvasive tests (Table 33–6) for HP do not require endoscopy or a mucosal biopsy and include the urea breath test and antibody detection tests.[1,51–55] These tests are simpler and less expensive than endoscopic tests. The urea breath test is based on urease production by HP. The carbon 13 (nonradioactive isotope) and carbon 14 (radioactive isotope) tests require that the patient ingest labeled urea, which is broken down in the stomach to ammonia and labeled bicarbonate. The labeled bicarbonate is absorbed in the blood and excreted in the breath. A mass spectrometer is used to detect carbon 13, whereas carbon 14 is measured using a scintillation counter.

Antibody detection tests (Table 33–6) available in the United States are used to detect circulating immunoglobulin (Ig) G directed against HP. Serologic laboratory-based quantitative tests, such as the enzyme-linked immunosorbent assay (ELISA), have been approved for use by the Food and Drug Administration (FDA) and have a sensitivity and specificity in the range of 90%. Rapid qualitative antibody detection tests (in-office or near patient) use whole blood or fingerstick and are also commercially available. Although a number of these tests have received FDA approval, reports indicate that they are less accurate than the laboratory-based tests and are more likely to yield invalid results because of procedural errors or insufficient blood at fingerstick.[1,51,52,54] Serologic laboratory-based quantitative tests are not usually used to assess HP cure, as antibody titers to HP vary markedly between individuals and take 6 months to 1 year to return to the uninfected range.[1,51,52] However, proportional reductions from pretreatment levels (a 50% decline) may be used to predict treatment success or failure. Other tests, for example, salivary antibody and stool antigen, are under investigation, but are not currently approved for use in the United States.[1,51,53]

Tests for HP (with the exception of antibody detection), may produce false-negative results if antibiotics or bismuth are taken within the previous 4 weeks, or if a proton pump inhibitor is taken within the previous 2 weeks.[1,51,52,54] These agents temporarily suppress HP and cause false-negative results. One report indicates that a false-negative effect is resolved within 5 days after stopping the proton pump inhibitor and that it parallels acid suppression.[52] The urea breath test and antibody detection, as opposed to biopsy-based tests, evaluate the whole stomach without the potential of sampling error.

The selection of a specific HP test depends on patient-specific factors and the clinical situation. Antibody detection tests are the initial screening tests of choice because they are quick, inexpensive, and less invasive than endoscopic biopsy tests. Laboratory-based serology tests are preferred to the rapid qualitative tests because they are more accurate. Although the in-office and near-patient qualitative tests are widely used, it is a matter of opinion as to whether they should be used for the *initial* diagnosis of HP infection.[1] In addition, these tests promote inappropriate or unnecessary HP testing. Patients testing positive often receive HP eradication treatment for a problem that may not be associated with HP, and this promotes the development of antimicrobial resistance.[54]

The urea breath test is used when there is concern regarding a positive antibody test. When endoscopy is indicated, the diagnosis should be established using the biopsy urease test. Patients with gastric ulcers should have extra biopsy samples taken to rule out malignancy. Culturing for antibiotic sensitivity is not practical at this time. Posttreatment assessment, to confirm eradication, is unnecessary in most patients unless they have recurrent symptoms, complicated ulcer, MALT lymphoma, or gastric cancer. The urea breath test is the preferred noninvasive method to verify HP eradication after treatment. To avoid confusing bacterial suppression with eradication, the urea breath test must be delayed at least 4 weeks after the completion of HP eradication treatment. Antibody assays are generally impractical to assess cure because antibody titers remain elevated for at least 6 months after treatment.

IMAGING AND ENDOSCOPY

The diagnosis of PUD depends on visualizing the ulcer crater either by upper GI radiography or by endoscopy.[1] Routine single-barium-contrast techniques can detect 30% of peptic ulcers, whereas it is possible to detect 60% to 80% of ulcers by using optimal double-contrast radiography. Fiber-optic endoscopy detects more than 90% of peptic ulcers and permits direct inspection, biopsy, visualization of superficial erosions, and sites of active bleeding. Because of its lower cost, greater availability, and perhaps greater safety, many physicians believe that radiography should be the initial diagnostic procedure in evaluating patients with suspected uncomplicated PUD. If complications are thought to exist, or if an accurate diagnosis is warranted, endoscopy is the diagnostic procedure of choice. If a gastric ulcer is found on radiography, malignancy should be excluded by direct endoscopic visualization and histology.

CLINICAL COURSE AND PROGNOSIS

The natural history of PUD is characterized by periods of exacerbations and remissions.[1] Ulcer pain is usually recognizable and episodic, but symptoms are variable, especially in older adults and in patients taking NSAIDs. Antiulcer medications, including the H_2-receptor antagonists, proton pump inhibitors, and sucralfate, relieve symptoms, accelerate ulcer healing, and prevent ulcers from recurring, but they do not cure the disease. Both duodenal ulcers and gastric ulcers recur unless the underlying cause (HP or NSAID) is removed. HP eradication alters the natural history of PUD, thereby markedly decreasing ulcer recurrence and complications. NSAIDs increase the risk for ulcers and ulcer-related complications, especially in the older adult. About 20% of all patients with chronic PUD experience upper GI bleeding, perforation, or obstruction. Mortality in patients with gastric ulcer is slightly higher than in duodenal ulcer and the general population. The lifetime risk of gastric adenocarcinoma in HP-infected patients is between 1% and 3%; symptomatic MALT occurs less frequently.[1,14,56]

▶ TREATMENT: Peptic Ulcer Disease

DESIRED OUTCOME

The treatment of chronic PUD varies depending on the etiology of the ulcer (HP or NSAID), whether the ulcer is initial or recurrent, and whether complications have occurred (Fig. 33–5). Overall treatment is aimed at relieving ulcer pain, healing the ulcer, preventing ulcer recurrence, and reducing ulcer-related complications. The goal of therapy in HP-positive patients with an active ulcer, a previously documented ulcer, or a history of an ulcer-related complication, is to eradicate HP and cure the disease with a cost-effective drug regimen.

GENERAL APPROACH TO TREATMENT

Patients with PUD should eliminate or reduce psychological stress, cigarette smoking, and the use of NSAIDs (including aspirin). If possible, alternative agents such as acetaminophen or a nonacetylated salicylate (e.g., salsalate) should be used for analgesia. In patients who cannot discontinue the NSAID, lowering the NSAID dose, using a less-damaging agent (Table 33–4), changing to a COX-2 inhibitor, or coadministering the NSAID with food, an H_2 receptor antagonist, or proton pump inhibitor, may decrease symptoms and mucosal damage.[1,18,43] Although there is no "ulcer diet," the patient should avoid foods and beverages (e.g., spicy foods, caffeine, alcohol) that cause dyspepsia or that exacerbate ulcer symptoms. Antacids may be used in conjunction with other antiulcer medications to relieve occasional ulcer symptoms. Figure 33–5 presents an algorithm for the evaluation and management of a patient with dyspeptic symptoms suggestive of an NSAID or HP-induced ulcer.

Eradication is recommended for all HP-infected PUD patients with (a) an active peptic ulcer, (b) a previously documented ulcer, (c) ulcer-related complications (e.g., upper GI bleeding), or (d) gastric MALT lymphoma.[8,14,54,57] There is no conclusive evidence that HP eradication will reverse the symptoms of dyspepsia or nonulcer dyspepsia.[8,16,54,57,58] Therefore, testing for HP is only recommended if eradication therapy is planned. Treatment of HP is also recommended for HP-positive patients after resection of gastric cancer.[8,57] Asymptomatic patients should not be tested for HP; however, if tested and a positive result is obtained, eradication should be offered after discussing the benefits and risks of therapy.[8,54]

The selection of an HP eradication regimen should be individualized and based on efficacy, tolerability, drug interaction potential,

TABLE 33–7. Comparison of Suggested Drug Regimens Used to Eradicate *Helicobacter pylori*

No	Drug	Dose/Frequency	Duration	Efficacy[a]	Adverse Effects[b]	Compliance[c]
Two-drug regimens						
1.	Clarithromycin	500 mg tid	14 d	Fair-good	Low-medium	Likely
	PPI[d]	qd or bid	14–28 d			
2.	Clarithromycin	500 mg tid	14 d	Fair-good	Low-medium	Likely
	RBC	400 mg bid	14–28 d			
3.	Amoxicillin	1 g bid-tid	14 d	Poor-fair	Low-medium	Likely
	PPI[d]	bid or tid	14–28 d			
Three-drug regimens						
4.	Clarithromycin	500 mg bid	10–14 d	Good-excellent	Low-medium	Likely
	Amoxicillin	1 g bid	10–14 d			
	PPI[d]	bid	10–14 d			
5.	Clarithromycin	500 mg bid	10–14 d	Good-excellent	Medium	Likely
	Metronidazole	500 mg bid	10–14 d			
	PPI[d]	bid	10–14 d			
6.	Amoxicillin	500 mg bid	10–14 d	Good	Medium	Likely
	Metronidazole	500 mg bid	10–14 d			
	PPI[d]	bid	10–14 d			
7.	Clarithromycin	500 mg bid	14 d	Good	Medium	Likely
	Amoxicillin	1 g bid	14 d			
	RBC	400 mg bid	14 d	Good-excellent	Medium	Likely
8.	Clarithromycin	500 mg bid	14 d	Good-excellent	Medium	Likely
	Metronidazole	500 mg bid	14 d			
	RBC	400 mg bid	14 d			
9.	Clarithromycin	500 mg bid	14 d	Good-excellent	Medium	Likely
	Tetracycline	500 mg bid	14 d			
	RBC	400 mg bid	14 d			
Bismuth-based four drug regimens						
10.	BSS	500 mg qid	14 d	Good-excellent	Medium-high	Unlikely
	Metronidazole	250–500 mg qid	14 d			
	Tetracycline	500 mg qid	14 d			
	H2RA or PPI[e]	As directed using conventional ulcer-healing dosages				
11.	BSS	500 mg qid	14 d	Good-excellent	Medium-high	Unlikely
	Metronidazole	250–500 mg qid	14 d			
	Clarithromycin	250–500 mg qid	14 d			
	H2RA or PPI[e]	As directed using conventional ulcer-healing dosages				
12.	BSS	500 mg qid	14 d	Fair-good	Medium-high	Unlikely
	Metronidazole	250–500 mg qid	14 d			
	Amoxicillin	500 mg qid	14 d			
	H2RA or PPI[e]	As directed using conventional ulcer-healing dosages				

PPI, proton pump inhibitor (PPI); H2RA, H2-receptor antagonist; RBC, ranitidine bismuth citrate; BSS, bismuth subsalicylate.
[a]Eradication rate reported in clinical trials = Excellent (>90%); Good (>80%–90%); Fair (>70%–80%); Poor (<70%).
[b]Safety (frequency of clinically important adverse effects) = High; Medium; Low.
[c]Compliance (estimate based on total number of tablets/capsules, frequency of administration, and clinically important adverse effects) = Likely; Unlikely.
[d]Use either omeprazole 20 mg, esomeprazole 20 mg, lansoprazole 30 mg, rabeprazole 20 mg, or pantoprazole 40 mg bid; alternatively, the total PPI daily dosage (e.g., omeprazole 40 mg) may be given qd; only lansoprazole 30 mg is indicated tid (#3).
[e]In the setting of an active ulcer, acid suppression is added to hasten pain relief. When using an H2RA, either cimetidine, ranitidine, famotidine, or nizatidine may be used in ulcer-healing dosages (Table 33–8) for a duration of 4–6 weeks; when using a PPI, either omeprazole, esomeprazole, lansoprazole, rabeprazole, or pantoprazole may be used in ulcer-healing dosages (Table 33–8) for a duration of 2–4 weeks.

antibiotic resistance, cost, and the likelihood of compliance (Table 33–7). Treatment should be initiated with a proton pump inhibitor-based three-drug regimen, as these regimens are most efficacious, better tolerated, simpler, and associated with better compliance. Two-drug regimens are less effective than proton pump inhibitor-based three-drug regimens, and the inclusion of only one antibiotic may lead to antimicrobial resistance. Bismuth-based regimens, although effective, involve a more complicated dosing schedule than the proton pump inhibitor-based three-drug regimens and are associated with a higher incidence of adverse effects. A proton pump inhibitor or H_2-receptor antagonist should be included in the regimen if the patient has an active ulcer, to facilitate the relief of ulcer symptoms. If a second HP treatment course is required, a different antibiotic regimen should be selected. Patients who may not warrant HP eradication include those who are intolerant and those patients who will not comply with the HP drug regimen, as well as those patients with HP-free NSAID ulcers or who have Zollinger-Ellison syndrome. Pharmacists should play an important role in the identification and treatment of patients with HP-associated PUD.[55]

Treatment with a conventional antiulcer drug (H_2-receptor antagonists, proton pump inhibitor, or sucralfate) (Table 33–8), is an alternative to HP eradication, but is discouraged because of the high rate of ulcer recurrence and ulcer-related complications.[1,59] Concomitant therapy (e.g., an H_2-receptor antagonist and sucralfate or an H_2-receptor antagonist and a proton pump inhibitor) adds to drug costs without enhancing efficacy.[1] Low-dose maintenance therapy with an

TABLE 33–8. Oral Drug Regimens Used to Heal Peptic Ulcers or to Maintain Ulcer Healing

Drug	Duodenal or Gastric Ulcer Healing (mg/dose)	Maintenance of Duodenal or Gastric Ulcer Healing (mg/dose)
H2-Receptor Antagonists		
Cimetidine	300 qid, 400 bid, 800 hs	400–800 hs
Famotidine	20 bid, 40 hs	20–40 hs
Nizatidine	150 bid, 300 hs	150–300 hs
Ranitidine	150 bid, 300 hs	150–300 hs
Proton Pump Inhibitors		
Omeprazole	20–40 qd	20–40 qd
Lansoprazole	15–30 qd	15–30 qd
Rabeprazole	20 qd	20 qd
Pantoprazole	40 qd	40 qd
Esomeprazole	20–40 qd	20–40 qd
Mucosal Defense		
Sucralfate (g/dose)	1 qid, 2 bid	1–2 bid or 1 qid

H_2-receptor antagonist or proton pump inhibitor (Table 33–8) should be limited to high risk patients who fail HP eradication, to patients with severe complications, and to those patients with HP-negative ulcers.[1]

NSAID-related dyspepsia should be empirically treated with an H_2-receptor antagonist or with a proton pump inhibitor. If the NSAID is discontinued, most uncomplicated ulcers will heal with standard regimens of an H_2-receptor antagonist, proton pump inhibitor, or sucralfate.[17–19,44,60] If treatment with the NSAID must be continued, or if there is a large ulcer, proton pump inhibitors are the drugs of choice because they accelerate the rate of ulcer healing.[17–19,44,60] At present, patients taking NSAIDs should not be tested to determine HP status. If, however, the patient has an active or prior ulcer, the patient should be tested for HP, and if found positive, treated with an eradication regimen that contains a proton pump inhibitor.[1,19,44] Prophylactic cotherapy with misoprostol or a proton pump inhibitor is indicated for patients who are at increased risk of developing serious ulcer-related complications (Table 33–3).[1,17–19,44,60]

Patients with a complicated ulcer (e.g., upper GI bleeding, obstruction, perforation, or penetration) often require endoscopic or surgical treatment. A definitive diagnosis should be made in these patients as malignancy may be present. Rebleeding post endoscopy may be prevented with an intravenous proton pump inhibitor.[49,50]

NONPHARMACOLOGIC THERAPY

Advances in the medical management of PUD have led to a decline in ulcer-related surgeries.[60] A subset of patients, however, require emergency surgery for bleeding, perforation, or obstruction. Classically, surgical procedures performed for PUD included vagotomy with pyloroplasty or vagotomy with antrectomy. Vagotomy (truncal, selective, or parietal cell) inhibits vagal stimulation of gastric acid. A truncal or selective vagotomy frequently results in postoperative gastric dysfunction and requires a pyloroplasty or antrectomy to facilitate gastric drainage. When an antrectomy is performed, the remaining stomach is anastomosed with the duodenum (Billroth I) or with the jejunum (Billroth II). A vagotomy is unnecessary when an antrectomy is performed for gastric ulcer. The postoperative consequences associated with these procedures include postvagotomy diarrhea, dumping syndrome, anemia, and recurrent ulceration.

PHARMACOLOGIC THERAPY

RECOMMENDATIONS

Patients should eliminate or reduce psychological stress, cigarette smoking, and NSAID use, if possible. Foods and beverages that cause dyspepsia or that exacerbate ulcer symptoms should be avoided. Eradication is recommended for HP-positive patients with an active ulcer, a previously documented ulcer, or a history of ulcer-related complications (e.g., upper GI bleeding) (Table 33–9 and Fig. 33–5). Treatment should be initiated with a 14-day course of a proton pump inhibitor-based three-drug regimen because these regimens have the highest HP eradication rates and the fewest adverse effects. If a second course of eradication therapy is required, the regimen should contain different antibiotics. Maintenance therapy with an H_2-receptor antagonist or proton pump inhibitor is recommended for high-risk patients with ulcer complications, who fail eradication, or who have HP-negative ulcers.

Standard H_2-receptor antagonist, proton pump inhibitor, or sucralfate regimens heal uncomplicated NSAID-induced ulcers if the NSAID is discontinued (Tables 33–8 and 33–9 and Fig. 33–5). A proton pump inhibitor is recommended if the NSAID cannot be discontinued or if the ulcer is large. If HP is present, the ulcer should be healed and the HP eradicated using a proton pump inhibitor-based three-drug regimen. Cotherapy with misoprostol or a proton pump inhibitor is recommended for patients who are at increased risk of developing serious ulcer-related complications.

TREATMENT OF *HELICOBACTER PYLORI*-ASSOCIATED ULCERS

The eradication of HP infection heals ulcers, alters the natural history of HP-positive PUD, and reduces the risk of recurrence to less than 10% in 1 year.[1,59] The term "eradication" is defined as the absence of the organism at least 4 weeks after cessation of antibiotic therapy.[8] Because antibiotics, bismuth preparations, and proton pump inhibitors can suppress the infection, antibiotics and bismuth salts should be stopped 4 weeks prior to HP testing and proton pump inhibitors should be discontinued 1 week prior to testing. An HP-associated ulcer is *cured* when eradication is permanent. The ideal drug regimen is one that achieves an eradication rate of 100% with <1 week of treatment.

TABLE 33–9. Recommendations and Guidelines For Providing Pharmaceutical Care to Patients with *Helicobacter pylori* (HP)-Associated and Nonsteroidal Anti-Inflammatory Drug (NSAID)-Induced Ulcers

***Helicobacter pylori*-Associated Ulcer**

1. Recommend:
   - Testing for HP only in patients with an active ulcer, a past history of documented ulcer, ulcer-related complications (e.g., upper GI bleeding), or gastric MALT lymphoma. Testing for HP infection is *not* indicated in asymptomatic individuals without a history of PUD or in patients on long-term treatment with a PPI for gastroesophageal reflux disease.
   - HP drug regimens with the highest eradication rates and the least potential for adverse effects and noncompliance.
   - Drug treatment regimens that contain two antibiotics in order to increase efficacy and to decrease the possibility of antimicrobial resistance.
   - Discontinuing antibiotics when used for longer than 2 weeks as part of an HP drug-treatment regimen.
   - An H2RA or PPI when a regimen containing bismuth, metronidazole, and tetracycline (or amoxicillin) is used to eradicate HP in a patient with an active ulcer.
   - Posttreatment HP testing only in patients recurrent symptoms, a history of ulcer complications, gastric MALT lymphoma, or gastric cancer.
2. Assure that ampicillin is not substituted for amoxicillin, doxycycline for tetracycline, or azithromycin for clarithromycin. An H2RA should not be substituted for a PPI, and bismuth salts should not be interchanged.
3. Advocate a different antibiotic combination if HP eradication fails and a second treatment is planned.
4. Counsel patients to discontinue or to reduce psychological stress, cigarette smoking, and NSAIDs, and to avoid foods or beverages that cause dyspepsia or that exacerbate ulcer symptoms.
5. Assess likelihood of patient compliance and advocate most effective, but simplest drug regimen.
6. Assess patient allergies to determine if allergic to penicillin (or other antibiotics) so that drug regimens that contain penicillins (or other antibiotics) can be avoided. Avoid regimens that contain tetracycline in children.
7. Discourage patient use of ethanol or ethanol-containing products and counsel about possible disulfiram-like effect when metronidazole is included in the eradication regimen.
8. Assess patient use of oral birth control medications and counsel appropriately when antibiotics are used in the drug regimen.
9. Inform patients of change in stool color when regimens containing bismuth salicylate or ranitidine bismuth citrate are included in an HP eradication regimen.
10. Assess and monitor patient for potential adverse effects, especially those associated with metronidazole, clarithromycin, and amoxicillin.
11. Assess and monitor patients for potential drug interactions, especially those receiving metronidazole, clarithromycin, and cimetidine.
12. Monitor patients for salicylate toxicity, especially in patients receiving cotherapy with other salicylates or anticoagulants, or in patients with renal failure.
13. Assess noncompliance and the possibility of antibiotic resistance to either metronidazole or clarithromycin when a patient fails HP eradication.
14. Provide patient education to patients with PUD who are receiving HP eradication. Information should include:
    - *Cause*—explain that ulcers are associated with bacteria
    - *Treatment*—explain that treatment consists of antibiotics and antiulcer medications
    - *Administration*—instruct the patient on when and how to take medications
    - *Adverse effects*—counsel the patient to report intolerable effects
    - *Complete treatment*—advise the patient to complete treatment even if feeling better
    - *Compliance*—explain the importance of compliance to the drug treatment regimen
    - *Alarm symptoms*—instruct the patient to report bleeding, vomiting, severe abdominal pain
15. Remember that pharmacists can play an important role in the identification and treatment of patients with HP-associated PUD.

NSAID-Induced Ulcer

1. Assess risk factors for NSAID-induced ulcers and ulcer-related complications, and when indicated, recommend appropriate strategies for reducing ulcers/GI complications including cotherapy with a PPI or misoprostol.
2. Recommend either an H2RA or a PPI to heal an NSAID-induced ulcer if the NSAID can be discontinued; larger GU will require a PPI.
3. Recommend a PPI to heal an NSAID-induced ulcer if the NSAID must be continued.
4. Recommend prophylactic cotherapy with either a PPI or misoprostol if the patient is at risk of developing an NSAID-induced ulcer or ulcer-related GI complication.
5. Recommend a three drug PPI-based HP eradication regimen for a HP-positive patient with an active DU or GU taking NSAIDs.
6. Assess likelihood of patient compliance and advocate most effective, but simplest drug regimen for the prevention or treatment of an NSAID-induced ulcer.
7. Monitor patients for signs and symptoms of NSAID-related upper GI bleeding or perforation.
8. Assess and monitor patients for potential drug interactions and adverse effects (especially misoprostol).
9. Provide patient education to patients at risk of NSAID-induced ulcers or GI-related complications as to the following;
   - *Cause*—explain that nonprescription and prescription NSAIDs cause ulcers
   - *Prophylaxis and treatment*—explain that medications are used to both prevent and treat NSAID-induced ulcers/complications.
   - *Administration*—instruct the patient on when and how to take medications
   - *Adverse effects*—counsel the patient to report intolerable effects
   - *Complete treatment*—advise the patient to continue or complete treatment even if feeling better
   - *Compliance*—explain the importance of compliance to the drug treatment regimen
   - *Alarm symptoms*—instruct the patient to report bleeding, vomiting, severe abdominal pain

11. Remember that pharmacists can play an important role in the identification of patients at risk for an NSAID-induced ulcer and in the treatment of NSAID-induced ulcers/complications.

DU, duodenal ulcer; GI, gastrointestinal; GU, gastric ulcer; H2RA, H_2-receptor antagonist; MALT, Mucosa-associated lymphoid tissue; PPI, proton pump inhibitor.

Although the optimal regimen has yet to be identified, acceptable results (efficacy of >80% to 90%) can be obtained by using a number of different drug combinations (Table 33–7).

The selection of an HP eradication regimen should be individualized and take into account efficacy, tolerability, drug-interaction potential, antibiotic resistance, cost, and compliance. The following drugs should not be substituted: ampicillin for amoxicillin, doxycycline for tetracycline, azithromycin for clarithromycin, or an H_2-receptor antagonist for a proton pump inhibitor. Bismuth subsalicylate and ranitidine bismuth citrate should not be interchanged. Amoxicillin should be avoided in penicillin-allergic patients and tetracycline should be avoided in young children. An extensive discussion of the guidelines and recommendations for the evaluation and treatment of HP in adults,[8,54,55,59,65–67] in older adults,[62] and in children[63,64] can be found elsewhere.

Efficacy

Numerous drugs, drug combinations, and dosage regimens have been used to eradicate HP.[8,54–57,59,62–67] The efficacy of the regimens evaluated in clinical trials has been difficult to decipher because of the methods used to analyze the results (intention-to-treat vs per protocol), the methods used to test for HP eradication (endoscopy with biopsy vs urea breath test), the inclusion of patients from different geographic locations (North America versus Europe), and failure to determine pretreatment antimicrobial resistance.[56,65,67]

None of the antiulcer agents (including bismuth salts) have any clinically important effect on HP eradication.[67,68] Clarithromycin is the single most effective antibiotic with an eradication rate of 40% to 70%. Monotherapy with amoxicillin, metronidazole, tetracycline, azithromycin, erythromycin, or the fluoroquinolones is disappointing.[57,67] A discrepancy between high *in vitro* and low *in vivo* efficacy may be related to degradation of the antimicrobial in the acidic environment of the stomach or by insufficient penetration into the gastric mucus.[56,65] Explanations as to why proton pump inhibitors, in particular, enhance the efficacy of antibiotics include possible proton pump inhibitor-induced suppression of HP, better activity or stability of the antibiotic at a higher gastric pH, or enhanced topical antibiotic concentration resulting from decreased gastric secretions.[56,69]

Two-Drug Regimens. The most widely studied two-drug regimen has been a 14-day combination of amoxicillin (1 g twice daily) and omeprazole (20 mg twice daily) (Table 33–7). Early European trials with this regimen suggested that HP eradication rates were >80%; however, when similar clinical trials were conducted in the United States, eradication rates were <60%.[1,65–67] Although it is not known exactly why these rates differ, it may be related to different strains of HP. A 14-day regimen of amoxicillin 1 g three times a day and lansoprazole 30 mg three times a day has an eradication rate of about 70% and was approved by the FDA for patients intolerant or allergic to clarithromycin, or who are known to be resistant to clarithromycin.[1]

Regimens containing clarithromycin (500 mg three times a day) and either a proton pump inhibitor or ranitidine bismuth citrate were the first to be approved by the FDA and are reported to have efficacy rates of 70% to 80% (Table 33–7).[1,59,65–67] Continuation of the proton pump inhibitor or ranitidine bismuth citrate for an additional 14 days is recommended by the FDA but is unnecessary unless the patient has a complicated ulcer or gastroesophageal reflux disease. Despite FDA approval, all two-drug regimens are considered inferior in light of more effective regimens and therefore should not be used as first-line therapy. Because these regimens contain only one antibiotic they are more likely to promote antimicrobial resistance.

Three-Drug Regimens. Proton pump inhibitor-based 14-day regimens with two antibiotics (either clarithromycin and metronidazole or clarithromycin and amoxicillin) are associated with eradication rates of >90% and are reasonably well-tolerated (Table 33–7).[1,54,59,65–67] These three-drug regimens are more effective than regimens that combine amoxicillin and metronidazole (Table 33–7).[1,54,65–67] Although regimens in which the medications are taken twice daily for 10 days versus 14 days appear to have a similar efficacy and have received FDA approval, the 14-day regimen is recommended because the longer duration of treatment favors successful eradication.[1,54,56,65] European trials suggest that a 7-day course of therapy provides eradication rates of >85%, but results of studies conducted in the United States are less convincing.[1,54,65] Thus, a 7-day HP eradication regimen should not be recommended.

European trials suggest that a clarithromycin dose of 250 mg is as effective as 500 mg when given two or three times a day; however, this has not been confirmed in US trials.[64,69] Therefore, the higher clarithromycin dose is recommended for the two- and three-drug regimens. The recommended metronidazole dose is 500 mg when used twice daily and 250 mg when taken four times day, although higher daily dosages have been used (Table 33–7). Ranitidine bismuth citrate may be substituted for the proton pump inhibitor with similar efficacy.[54,66,71]

A number of antibiotics have been evaluated in the three-drug regimens with varying degrees of success.[65] Azithromycin has excellent *in vitro* activity against HP, but *in vivo* studies have yielded disappointing results.[65,72] The drug must be given in high dosages (750 mg) for 14 days, but these regimens require confirmation in larger clinical trials. Until then, azithromycin should not be included as part of the three-drug eradication regimen. Furazolidone (100 mg four times a day) has been used instead of metronidazole and appears to be effective.[65,73] Other antibiotics, including the fluoroquinolones (e.g., ciprofloxacin) have been investigated in a small number of patients.[65] Furazolidone and the fluoroquinolones should not be used as part of a first-line regimen, but may be useful in patients allergic to or intolerant of first-line antibiotics, or in cases of metronidazole or clarithromycin resistance.

Studies that directly compared three-drug regimens that used a proton pump inhibitor with one that included an H_2-receptor antagonist report conflicting results.[69,74] Although regimens containing a higher H_2-receptor antagonist dosage (e.g., famotidine 40 mg twice daily) appear to provide similar eradication rates as those obtained with a standard-dose proton pump inhibitor (e.g., omeprazole 20 mg/d), additional studies are required to confirm these findings. When used as part of a three-drug regimen, an H_2-receptor antagonist should not be substituted for the proton pump inhibitor.

Bismuth-Based Four-Drug Regimens. The original HP eradication regimens in the United States contained a bismuth salt (bismuth subsalicylate) and two antibiotics. The fourth drug, an H_2-receptor antagonist or proton pump inhibitor, is added to the regimen of patients with an active ulcer to hasten symptom relief and to modestly accelerate ulcer healing. HP eradication rates for a 14-day regimen containing bismuth subsalicylate, metronidazole, tetracycline, and an H_2 receptor antagonist (Table 33–7) range from 80% to 85%.[1,54,59,65–67] Substitution of amoxicillin for tetracycline lowers the eradication rate to about 75% and therefore is not recommended.[1,59,65–67] Increasing the duration of treatment to 1 month does not substantially increase eradication. Using a proton pump inhibitor in place of the H_2-receptor antagonist may enhance efficacy and permit a shorter treatment duration. A 7-day course of a regimen containing bismuth subsalicylate, metronidazole tetracycline, and a proton pump inhibitor may provide eradication rates of >90%, but this regimen has not been adequately validated in large in trials in the United States.[1,59,65–67]

Tolerability

Tolerability varies with different regimens.[65] Adverse effects occur in up to 70% of patients receiving bismuth-based four-drug regimens, in 15% to 65% of patients receiving two-drug regimens, and in less than 30% of patients treated with a proton pump inhibitor-based three-drug regimen.[75] Metronidazole-containing regimens increase the frequency of adverse effects (especially when the dose is >1 g/d) and may contribute to a disulfiram-like reaction with ethanol. Common adverse effects include taste disturbances (metronidazole and clarithromycin), nausea, vomiting, abdominal pain, and diarrhea.[65] Antibiotic-associated colitis, a serious complication, occurs infrequently. Vaginal moniliasis occurs in up to 10% of women.[1]

Antimicrobial Resistance

There is increasing concern regarding the emergence of antimicrobial-resistant bacteria. An important determinant of successful HP eradication therapy is the presence of preexisting antimicrobial resistance.[56,76–79] Acquired resistance to metronidazole and clarithromycin is a significant problem. Resistance to tetracycline and amoxicillin has been reported but is uncommon.[1,56] Resistance to bismuth has not been reported. Metronidazole resistance is most common (10% to 60%), but varies depending on prior antibiotic exposure and geographical region.[1,77,79] Secondary (acquired) resistance to failed therapy is higher (80%), especially in women.[1] The clinical importance of metronidazole resistance remains unclear as certain drug combinations render resistance to metronidazole unimportant. Bismuth-based four-drug regimens, which include metronidazole, tetracycline, and a bismuth salt, appear to be effective even against metronidazole-resistant strains.[1,77,79]

Primary resistance to clarithromycin is lower (5% to 10%) than with metronidazole, but it is more likely to affect the clinical outcome.[65,76,79] Secondary resistance occurs in up to two-thirds of treatment failures. When fluoroquinolones were used as single agents to eradicate HP, a high secondary resistance was found. The synergistic effect of more than one antibiotic is likely to render resistance to a single antibiotic less important. However, if antimicrobial sensitivity testing is not available, then patients who have failed HP eradication with metronidazole or clarithromycin should be retreated with alternative regimens that do not include these drugs.

Drug Administration

Patients should be instructed to take all of their medications (except proton pump inhibitors) with meals and at bedtime (if necessary).[65] The proton pump inhibitor should be taken 15 minutes to 30 minutes before meals (see the section "Proton Pump Inhibitors").

Compliance

Compliance with drug treatment has a significant impact on HP eradication and is the single most important factor influencing successful therapy.[65] Compliance decreases with multiple medications, increased frequency of administration, increased length of treatment, and intolerable adverse effects. The patient should be able to comply with at least 80% to 90% of all medication doses over the treatment period.

Immunization

The search for a vaccine against HP is ongoing. A significant problem is the toxicity of currently available mucosal adjuvants (immune-stimulating compounds that produce an immune effect against other substances). New approaches under investigation include the delivery of HP antigens by DNA, live vectors such as attenuated salmonella, and alternate routes of vaccine administration. A detailed discussion of the current status of HP vaccines can be found elsewhere.[80]

CONVENTIONAL TREATMENT OF ACTIVE DUODENAL AND GASTRIC ULCERS

Conventional treatment with an H_2-receptor antagonist, sucralfate, or antacid alleviates ulcer symptoms and heals approximately 70%, 80%, or 90% of duodenal ulcer at 4, 6, or 8 weeks, respectively (Table 33–8).[1] Proton pump inhibitors provide comparable duodenal ulcer healing rates over a shorter treatment period (4 weeks).[1,81,82] A higher daily dose or a longer duration of treatment may be necessary to heal gastric ulcer, because the gastric ulcer is typically larger than the duodenal ulcer. Sucralfate is effective in the treatment of uncomplicated PUD and provides ulcer healing rates at 4 and 8 weeks similar to those obtained with an H_2-receptor antagonist.[1] Antacids, although effective, are not used as single agents to heal ulcers because of their high and frequent doses (100–144 mEq of acid-neutralizing capacity 1 hour and 3 hours after meals and at bedtime) and associated adverse effects.[1] When conventional antiulcer drugs are stopped, most HP-positive patients develop a recurrent ulcer within 1 year.[1]

TREATMENT OF REFRACTORY ULCERS

Ulcers are usually considered refractory to therapy when symptoms, ulcers, or both persist beyond 8 weeks (duodenal ulcer) or 12 weeks (gastric ulcer) despite conventional treatment, or when several courses of HP eradication fail.[1] Poor patient compliance, antimicrobial resistance, cigarette smoking, NSAID use, gastric acid hypersecretion, or tolerance to the antisecretory effects of an H_2-receptor antagonist (see the section "Antiulcer Agents") may contribute to refractory PUD. Because patients with refractory ulcers are infected with HP, upper endoscopy should be performed to confirm a nonhealing ulcer, to exclude malignancy, and to assess HP status. For HP-positive patients, eradication therapy is appropriate (see HP eradication regimens; also see the section "Antimicrobial Resistance"). Higher proton pump inhibitor dosages (e.g., omeprazole 40 mg/d) heal the majority of ulcers proven refractory to standard proton pump inhibitor dosages (e.g., omeprazole 20 mg/d) and standard or high-dose H_2-receptor antagonists.[1,80] Maintenance therapy with the proton pump inhibitor healing dose is often necessary to maintain healing as ulcers usually recur when therapy is discontinued or reduced to lower levels. Changing from one H_2-receptor antagonist or proton pump inhibitor to another is not beneficial. Concurrent therapy with an antisecretory agent and sucralfate or misoprostol may appear rational because of the different mechanisms by which these drugs act, but it is without established benefit. Concurrent treatment with an H_2-receptor antagonist and a proton pump inhibitor offers no proven benefit. Patients with refractory gastric ulcer often require surgery because of the fear of malignancy.

MAINTENANCE OF ULCER HEALING AND PREVENTION OF COMPLICATIONS

Maintenance therapy is aimed at maintaining ulcer healing and at preventing ulcer-related complications (e.g., upper GI bleeding). Because HP eradication offers a cure for HP-associated ulcers and dramatically decreases ulcer recurrence (<10% at 1 year), continuous maintenance therapy has become largely obsolete.[1,81] Maintenance therapy, however, may be indicated for patients who have frequent ulcer recurrences, a history of ulcer-related bleeding, a healed refractory ulcer, failed HP eradication therapy, or who are heavy smokers and require continuous treatment with an NSAID.

Maintenance therapy with lower dosages of all four H_2-receptor antagonists, all five proton pump inhibitors, or sucralfate reduces symptomatic duodenal ulcer recurrence to 20% to 25% at 1 year (Table 33–8).[1,81] Patients with gastric ulcers may require continuation of the full ulcer-healing dose. Maintenance of healing lasts only as long as treatment is continued, as 50% to 90% of ulcers recur after when therapy is withdrawn.[1,81] Continuous long-term maintenance therapy with an H_2-receptor antagonist, proton pump inhibitor, or sucralfate is safe and effective, although sucralfate should be avoided in patients with renal impairment. Ulcer recurrence while on maintenance therapy suggests heavy smoking, noncompliance with the drug regimen, NSAIDs, persistent HP infection, or Zollinger-Ellison syndrome.

TREATMENT OF ACTIVE NSAID-INDUCED ULCERS

NSAIDs should be discontinued if an active ulcer is confirmed. If the NSAID is stopped, most uncomplicated ulcers will heal with standard regimens of an H_2-receptor antagonist, proton pump inhibitor, or sucralfate (Table 33–8).[1,17–19,44,60] Large ulcers require higher proton pump inhibitor dosages or prolonged treatment. If the NSAID must be continued in a patient despite ulceration, consideration should be given to reducing the NSAID dose, or using acetaminophen or nonacetylated salicylates, relatively selective COX-2 inhibitors (e.g., nabumetone, etodolac, meloxicam), or the highly selective COX-2 inhibitors. The proton pump inhibitors are the drugs of choice when the NSAID must be continued, as potent acid suppression is required to accelerate ulcer healing.[17–19,44,60] H_2-receptor antagonists are less effective in the presence of continued NSAIDs; sucralfate does not appear to be effective. If HP is present, treatment should be initiated with an eradication regimen that contains a proton pump inhibitor.[17–19,44,60]

STRATEGIES TO PREVENT NSAID-INDUCED ULCERS

A number of strategies may be used to prevent NSAID-induced ulcers or ulcer-related GI complications. Strategies aimed at reducing the topical irritant effects of NSAIDs—prodrugs, slow-release formulations, enteric-coated products—do not prevent ulcers or clinically important adverse effects such as bleeding or perforation. Medical cotherapy with misoprostol, an H_2-receptor antagonist or a proton pump inhibitor will decrease the chance of ulcer formation and GI complications in high-risk patients (Table 33–3).[1,17–19,44,60,83–89] The development of less injurious NSAIDs, such as the selective COX-2 inhibitors, will decrease the risk of ulcers and complications.[1,17–19,44,60,90–93]

Misoprostol

Misoprostol, 200 μg four times/d, markedly reduces the incidence of NSAID-induced gastric ulcer and duodenal ulcer, but GI adverse effects limit its usefulness.[17–19,44,60,83,84] Lower dosages of 200 μg two or three times/d also prevent ulcer formation, with the 600 μg/d dosage being comparable to 800 μg/d.[1,17–19,44,83] Diarrhea, abdominal cramping, nausea, and flatulence are dose-dependent and can be disabling, necessitating a dosage reduction or discontinuation. A fixed combination of misoprostol 200 μg and diclofenac (50 mg or 75 mg) is available and may enhance compliance, but the flexibility to individualize drug dosage is lost. Although misoprostol reduces NSAID-related ulcer formation, its efficacy in preventing upper GI complications remains controversial. A double-blind clinical trial in rheumatoid arthritis patients receiving misoprostol 200 μg four times/d provides the strongest evidence that serious upper GI complications can be prevented.[44,84] However, the reduction in complications was less than the prevention of endoscopic lesions, indicating that it is not appropriate to extrapolate from ulcer prevention to a reduction in GI complications.

Conventional Antiulcer Agents

Standard H_2-receptor antagonist dosages (e.g., famotidine 40 mg/d) are effective in preventing NSAID-induced duodenal ulcer, but higher dosages (e.g., famotidine 40 mg twice daily) are required to prevent gastric ulcer.[17–19,44,60,85,86] Although the H_2-receptor antagonists are effective in relieving NSAID-related dyspepsia, their use may place the patient at increased risk by masking symptoms of a serious GI complication.[17,31] Standard proton pump inhibitor dosages (e.g., omeprazole 20 mg/d) reduce the incidence of NSAID-induced duodenal ulcer and gastric ulcer.[17–19,44,60,87–89] Omeprazole 20 mg/d is associated with a lower relapse rate than misoprostol 200 μg bid or ranitidine 150 mg bid, and is better tolerated than misoprostol.[87,88] Sucralfate offers no significant benefit in preventing NSAID-induced ulcers and should not should not be used for this purpose.

Selective COX-2 Inhibitors

Two highly selective COX-2 inhibitors, celecoxib and rofecoxib, are currently available in the United States. Double-blind endoscopic trials in arthritic patients indicate that both celecoxib and rofecoxib are associated with fewer ulcers than are nonselective NSAIDs, with rates comparable to placebo over 3 months.[17,19,91–93] Two clinical outcomes trials have reported lower rates of serious upper GI complications indicating that COX-2 inhibitors decrease not only endoscopically visualized ulcers, but GI-related complications.[17,94,95] Patients (e.g., history of GI complications, >65 years old, dyspepsia), may still require a proton pump inhibitor, even after changing to a COX-2 inhibitor. Questions remain regarding the efficacy and long-term safety of the COX-2 inhibitors.[19,93]

Development of Safer NSAIDs that Spare the GI Tract

Nitric oxide-containing NSAIDs (NO-NSAIDs) release exogenous nitric oxide, and in animal studies, appear to protect the mucosa and enhance ulcer healing in the presence of the NSAID.[18,19,22] Studies in humans are needed, however, to confirm these findings. Several other novel strategies that spare GI injury are also under investigation. These include pure R-enantiomers of chiral NSAIDs and NSAIDs preassociated with zwitterionic phospholipids.[18,19,22]

ANTIULCER AGENTS

A comprehensive review of the pharmacology, pharmacokinetics, pharmacodynamics, efficacy, drug interactions, and tolerability of the antiulcer agents can be found elsewhere.[1]

Proton Pump Inhibitors

The proton pump inhibitors (omeprazole, esomeprazole, lansoprazole, rabeprazole, and pantoprazole) dose-dependently inhibit basal and stimulated gastric acid secretion.[1,96–101,103] Under acidic conditions in the parietal cell, the parent compound is protonated and converted to active metabolites, which react covalently with H^+/K^+-ATPase (the proton pump). A sulfhydryl bond is formed that noncompetitively and irreversibly inhibits activity of the enzyme. Full restoration of acid secretion after discontinuing the proton pump inhibitor takes 3 days to 5 days. Because proton pump inhibitors inhibit only those proton pumps that are actively secreting acid, they are most effective when taken 15 minutes to 30 minutes before meals.

The proton pump inhibitors are formulated as gelatin capsules (omeprazole, esomeprazole, and lansoprazole) containing enteric-coated pH-sensitive granules or as an enteric-coated tablets (rabeprazole and pantoprazole), which prevent degradation and premature protonation of the drug in acid. Upon dissolution of the capsule in the stomach, the intact granules pass into the duodenum, where the drug is released and absorbed. The granules may be removed from the capsule and administered in acidic juices (e.g., orange or apple) by mouth, nasogastric tube, or gastrostomy tube; sprinkled on applesauce; or a suspension can be prepared for nasogastric/nasoduodenal use by dissolving the granules in an 8.4% solution of sodium bicarbonate.[102,103]

All five proton pump inhibitors provide similar ulcer-healing rates, maintenance of ulcer-healing rates, and relief of ulcer symptoms when used in recommended dosages (Table 33–8).[1,81,96–101] When higher dosages are indicated, the daily dose should be divided in order to obtain better 24-hour pH control. A dosage reduction is not necessary in renal impairment or older adults, but should be considered in severe hepatic disease.

The short-term (<12 weeks) adverse effects of all five proton pump inhibitors are similar and not unlike those observed with the H_2-receptor antagonists (see the section "H_2-Receptor Antagonists").[1,81,103] Because proton pump inhibitors increase gastric pH, they may alter the bioavailability of orally administered drugs, such as ketoconazole, digoxin, iron, or pH-dependent dosage forms.[81,103,104] Omeprazole selectively inhibits hepatic cytochrome P450 (CYP450) isoenzymes and decreases the elimination of phenytoin, diazepam, and R-warfarin.[1,103,104] Esomeprazole, lansoprazole, rabeprazole, and pantoprazole have a lower potential for CYP-mediated drug interactions. Important hepatic drug interactions with all five proton pump inhibitors are uncommon.

Consequences of Prolonged Hypochlorhydria. All proton pump inhibitors dose-dependently increase serum gastrin concentrations as a function of their potent acid-inhibitory effect (Fig. 33–6).[1,103,105] Fasting gastrin elevations are usually within the normal range and return to baseline within 1 month of discontinuing the drug. A consequence of hypergastrinemia is its trophic effect on enterochromaffin-like (ECL) cells in the gastric epithelium and the development of gastric carcinoid tumors in female rats.[1,103,105] Although proton pump inhibitors may promote gastric mucosal changes in humans that lead to ECL hyperplasia, there is no evidence that these changes result in dysplasia, carcinoid tumors, or gastric adenocarcinoma from 15 years of omeprazole use.[105] Alternatively, long-term proton pump inhibitor therapy in HP-positive patients has been associated with progressive atrophic gastritis of the gastric body.[1,7,105] At this time, there is inadequate evidence to link the long-term use of proton pump inhibitors with gastric cancer in HP-positive patients or to support an association between proton pump inhibitors, colonic polyps, and colorectal cancer.[1] Although bacterial overgrowth occurs in the stomach as a consequence of hypochlorhydria and may lead to carcinogenic *N*-nitroso compounds in animals, it is unlikely to result in significant gastric nitrosation in humans.[103] A decrease in B_{12} was reported in patients receiving long-term (>3 years) omeprazole treatment, but it is not a major concern.

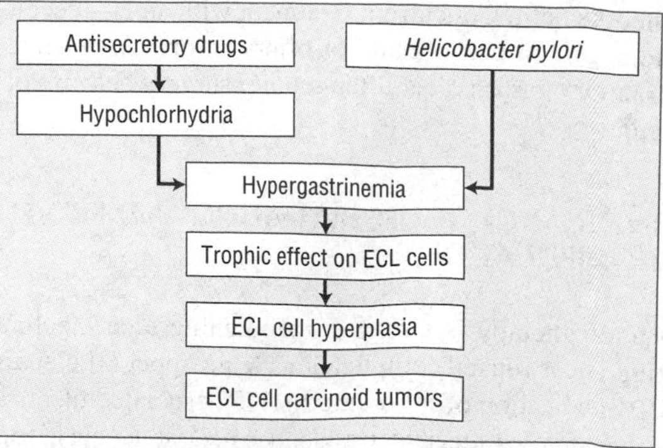

FIGURE 33–6. The gastrin hypothesis suggests that prolonged hypergastrinemia results in hyperplasia of the enterochromaffin-like (ECL) cells of the gastric fundus. The trophic influence of gastrin may be a risk factor for ECL cell carcinoid tumor formation.

H_2-Receptor Antagonists

The H_2-receptor antagonists (cimetidine, famotidine, nizatidine, and ranitidine) competitively and reversibly bind H_2 receptors on the parietal cell, diminishing cytosolic cyclic adenosine monophosphate (cAMP) production and the secretion of histamine-stimulated gastric acid.[1] Ulcer healing is comparable with equipotent multiple daily doses or a single full dose given after dinner or at bedtime, but tolerance to their antisecretory effect may occur (Table 33–8).[1] Twice-daily administration suppresses daytime acid and benefits patients with daytime ulcer pain. Cigarette smokers may require higher doses or a longer duration of treatment. A dosage reduction is recommended in patients with moderate to severe renal failure.

The short- and long-term safety of all four H_2-receptor antagonists is similar.[1] GI disturbances occur most often and usually subside with continued treatment. Central nervous system effects, particularly drowsiness and headache, have been reported with all four H_2-receptor antagonists. Cimetidine is associated with weak antiandrogenic effects that may result in gynecomastia or impotence in men receiving prolonged treatment or high dosages.[1] Thrombocytopenia, the most common hematologic effect, is reversible and occurs with all four H_2-receptor antagonists.[1] The cardiovascular effects and changes in gastric emptying reported with the oral H_2-receptor antagonists are of minimal importance. Cimetidine interferes with the renal tubular secretion of creatinine, but increases in serum creatinine do not represent renal toxicity. Numerous metabolic drug interactions have been reported with cimetidine (e.g., theophylline, phenytoin, warfarin).[1,104] Ranitidine binds less avidly to hepatic CYP450 isoenzymes than does cimetidine, and thus has less potential for drug interactions. Famotidine and nizatidine do not interact with drugs metabolized by hepatic CYPP450 isoenzymes. The H_2-receptor antagonists may alter the bioavailability of orally administered drugs, such as ketoconazole or pH-dependent dosage forms. The effect of cimetidine, ranitidine, nizatidine (but not famotidine) on serum alcohol is unlikely to be clinically important.[1]

Sucralfate

Sucralfate is an aluminum salt of a sulfated disaccharide that, when exposed to gastric acid, forms a viscous adhesive that binds electrostatically to positively charged protein molecules in the ulcer crater, forming a protective barrier that inhibits back-diffusion of hydrogen ions.[1] Attachment to the ulcer crater lasts as long as 6 hours following oral administration. Sucralfate inhibits pepsin, adsorbs bile salts, stimulates endogenous prostaglandins, and may suppress HP.[1] Although aluminum mediates some of these actions, the sucrose moiety plays an important role in ulcer healing. Sucralfate does not have an important effect on acid secretion. The majority of the dose is excreted unchanged in the feces with 3% to 5% excreted in the urine.

Sucralfate should be taken on an empty stomach to prevent binding to dietary protein and phosphate. Deterrents to its use include multiple-doses per day, large tablet size, and the need to separate the drug from meals and potentially interacting medications. Adverse effects are minor and occur <5% of patients. Constipation is most common and develops in about 2% of patients.[1] Nausea, dry mouth, dizziness, and a metallic taste occur infrequently. Seizures may occur in dialysis patients who are also receiving aluminum-containing antacids.[1] Hypophosphatemia may develop with long-term treatment (see the section "Antacids"). Gastric bezoar formation has been reported. The concomitant use of sucralfate with oral fluoroquinolones, phenytoin, digoxin, theophylline, quinidine, amitriptyline, warfarin, ketoconazole, and L-thyroxine may reduce their bioavailability.[1,104] The interaction is minimized by giving the interacting drug at least 2 hours before sucralfate. Alternative antiulcer therapy may be warranted in patients taking oral fluoroquinolones.

Prostaglandins

Misoprostol, a synthetic prostaglandin E_1 (PGE_1) analog, moderately inhibits acid secretion and enhances mucosal defense.[1] Antisecretory effects are dose dependent over the range of 50 μg to 200 μg; cytoprotective effects occur in humans at doses of >200 μg. Because protective effects occur at higher doses, it is difficult to establish the protective effect independent of the antisecretory action. Although not recommended in the United States, a dose of 200 μg four times daily or 400 μg twice daily heals duodenal ulcers and gastric ulcers comparable to standard H_2-receptor antagonist or sucralfate regimens.

Diarrhea, the most troublesome adverse effect, develops in about 30% of patients receiving 800 μg/d, but often subsides over several weeks with continued treatment.[1] Abdominal cramping, nausea, flatulence, and headache typically accompany the diarrhea. Taking the drug with or after meals and at bedtime may minimize the diarrhea. Antacids (other than magnesium) may be taken with misoprostol when needed for abdominal pain. Misoprostol is uterotropic and produces uterine contractions that may endanger pregnancy; therefore, the drug is contraindicated in pregnant women. If misoprostol is prescribed to women in their childbearing years, use of adequate contraceptive measures must be confirmed and a negative serum pregnancy test should be documented within 2 weeks of initiating treatment. Patients should be counseled about the GI effects and the need to avoid magnesium antacids. Young women should be warned about the importance of adequate contraception.

Bismuth Preparations

The most commonly used bismuth salts in the United States are bismuth subsalicylate (Pepto-Bismol) and ranitidine bismuth citrate.[1,68] Bismuth subsalicylate is an insoluble complex that, at a pH below 3.5, reacts with acid to form bismuth oxide and salicylic acid (which is readily absorbed). In the colon, bismuth oxide reacts with hydrogen sulfide to form bismuth sulfide, which blackens the stool. Possible ulcer-healing mechanisms include a local gastroprotective effect, stimulation of endogenous PGs, and suppression of HP. Bismuth salts do not inhibit or neutralize acid.

Bismuth absorption varies with the bismuth salt.[1,68] The bismuth salts (bismuth subsalicylate and ranitidine bismuth citrate) used in the United States are safe and have few adverse effects. Neurologic toxicity has been associated with prolonged bismuth subgallate treatment, but not with bismuth subsalicylate or ranitidine bismuth citrate. Because renal insufficiency may decrease bismuth elimination, bismuth salts should be used with caution in older patients and in renal failure. Bismuth subsalicylate may cause salicylate sensitivity or bleeding disorders, and should be used with caution in patients receiving concurrent salicylate therapy. Patients should be advised that bismuth salts may impart a black color to their stool.

Antacids

Antacids neutralize gastric acid, inactivate pepsin, and bind bile salts. Aluminum-containing antacids also suppress HP and enhance mucosal defense.[1] These latter effects probably contribute to ulcer healing at lower doses. When taken on an empty stomach, the antacid-neutralizing effect lasts for 15 minutes to 30 minutes. When taken 1 hour after a meal, food acts as a buffer for about an hour and prolongs the antacid-neutralizing effect for an additional 2 hours. Magnesium hydroxide has a more prolonged neutralizing effect than either sodium bicarbonate or calcium carbonate. The effects of magnesium oxide and carbonate are similar to magnesium hydroxide. Aluminum hydroxide possesses a low neutralizing capacity; aluminum phosphate has little antacid activity. Magaldrate (hydroxymagnesium aluminate) is transformed to magnesium and aluminum ions in gastric acid. Its effects resemble those of other magnesium/aluminum-containing antacids, but it contains less magnesium per unit of weight. Most antacids have been reformulated to contain only small amounts of sodium.

GI adverse effects are most common and are dose dependent.[1] Magnesium salts cause an osmotic diarrhea, whereas aluminum salts cause constipation. Diarrhea usually predominates with magnesium/aluminum preparations. Antacids are similar in potency, but contain less magnesium, and may cause less diarrhea. Aluminum-containing antacids (except aluminum phosphate) form insoluble salts with dietary phosphorus and interfere with phosphorus absorption.[1] Hypophosphatemia occurs most often in patients with low dietary phosphate intake (e.g., malnutrition, alcoholism). Combined treatment with sucralfate may amplify the hypophosphatemia and the potential for aluminum toxicity (see the section "Sucralfate").

Magnesium-containing antacids should not be used in patients with a creatinine clearance of less than 30 mL/min because magnesium excretion is impaired. Calcium stimulates gastrin, but acid rebound is of questionable clinical importance. Hypercalcemia may occur in patients with normal renal function taking more than 20 g/d of calcium carbonate, and in renal failure patients taking more than 4 g/d. The milk-alkali syndrome (hypercalcemia, alkalosis, renal stones, increased blood urea nitrogen, increased serum creatinine concentration) occurs with high calcium intake in patients with systemic alkalosis produced by either ingestion of absorbable antacids (sodium bicarbonate) or prolonged vomiting. Antacids may alter the absorption and excretion of drugs when administered concomitantly.[1] Important interactions may occur when antacids are administered with tetracycline, warfarin, digoxin, quinidine, isoniazid, ketoconazole, or the fluoroquinolones. Most interactions can be avoided by separating the antacid from the oral drug by 2 hours.

PHARMACOECONOMIC CONSIDERATIONS

HELICOBACTER PYLORI-ASSOCIATED ULCERS

A number of hypothetical cost-effectiveness analyses indicate that for patients with uncomplicated PUD, HP eradication is superior to conventional treatment with an H_2-receptor antagonist.[55,106,107] In addition, prospective reports of "real patients" confirm that HP eradication improves clinical outcomes and decreases the use of health care resources when compared to conventional antisecretory therapy.[108] Thus, it appears that the costs of continued treatment and recurrence far outweigh the cost of HP drug regimens.

NONSTEROIDAL ANTI-INFLAMMATORY-INDUCED ULCERS

Pharmacoeconomic considerations are important in determining the management of GI risks in patients taking NSAIDs, but analysis of the cost-effectiveness of misoprostol has yielded divergent results.[17] A study using data from the MUCOSA trial reported that the cost-effectiveness of misoprostol cotherapy was greatest in patients with the highest risk for NSAID-related GI complications.[109] The cost-effectiveness of using a COX-2 inhibitor only becomes apparent in patients older than 65 years of age who have a history of a clinically important GI event.[17,110] Whether cotherapy with high-dose H_2-receptor antagonist or proton pump inhibitors is cost-effective remains to be determined.

ZOLLINGER-ELLISON SYNDROME

Zollinger-Ellison syndrome is characterized by gastric acid hypersecretion (see Fig. 33–1) and recurrent peptic ulceration that results from a gastrin-producing tumor (gastrinoma).[4,111,112] In the United States, Zollinger-Ellison syndrome accounts for 0.1% of patients with duodenal ulcer. More than 90% of gastrinomas are located in the region of the pancreas, the most common site being the duodenum. Malignant gastrinomas occur in 30% to 50% of patients, with metastases to regional lymph nodes, liver, spleen, and bone.

The most frequent clinical manifestation is severe and recurrent peptic ulceration, typically accompanied by epigastric pain, and often associated with esophagitis, GI bleeding, or perforation. Ulcers occur most often in the duodenum, but may involve the stomach or jejunum. Diarrhea occurs in 30% to 50% of patients and results from high concentrations of acid that overwhelm the duodenum's buffering capacity and damage the mucosa. Intraluminal acid causes steatorrhea by inactivating pancreatic lipase and precipitating bile acids. Vitamin B_{12} malabsorption may result from reduced intrinsic factor activity. Patients may have other symptoms when the parathyroid, pituitary, thyroid, or adrenal glands are involved. The diagnosis is established in patients with a BAO greater than 15 mEq/h (without prior gastric surgery) and when the fasting serum gastrin is higher than 1000 pg/mL.[4,112] Location of the tumor is essential as surgical resection is curative.

Treatment is based on the presence or absence of peptic ulcers, esophagitis, diarrhea, and a gastrinoma, which may be malignant. The proton pump inhibitors are the oral drugs of choice for managing acid hypersecretion, although most experience has been obtained with omeprazole. Treatment should be instituted with omeprazole 60 mg/d (or an equivalent dose of esomeprazole, lansoprazole, rabeprazole, or pantoprazole) and should be adjusted to individual patient response.[4,112] Dividing the daily dose and giving the proton pump inhibitor every 8 hours to 12 hours is most effective in controlling acid output and relieving symptoms. Although doses as high as 360 mg/d of omeprazole have been administered, an average dose of 60–80 mg/d (40–80 mg/d of esomeprazole or rabeprazole; 30–90 mg/d of lansoprazole; or 40–120 mg/d of pantoprazole) reduces basal acid output to target levels. Patients should be evaluated every 6 months to 12 months and the proton pump inhibitor dose adjusted accordingly. A gradual reduction in proton pump inhibitor dose is recommended after the initial dose required for adequate control of gastric acid hypersecretion is achieved.[4] Intravenous pantoprazole is safe and effective for rapid and prolonged acid suppression in patients unable to take oral proton pump inhibitors.[111]

Octreotide directly inhibits gastric acid secretion and the release of gastrin.[4] Although a subcutaneous dose of 100 μg to 250 μg three times/d substantially reduces acid secretion, octreotide is not considered first-line treatment. Patients with metastatic gastrinoma require tumor resection or treatment with chemotherapeutic agents.

STRESS-RELATED MUCOSAL DAMAGE

SRMD (e.g., stress gastritis, stress ulcer) occurs in critically ill patients with risk factors such as multiple trauma or organ system failure, severe burns (>15% of body surface area), increased intracranial pressure, traumatic spinal cord injury or severe medical problems including coagulopathy, and prolonged ventilation (>48 hours).[46,82,113,114] When accompanied by acute upper GI bleeding, SRMD is a cause of significant morbidity and mortality. In contrast to chronic peptic ulcers, these lesions are characteristically asymptomatic, multiple, located in the proximal stomach, unlikely to perforate, and associated with bleeding from superficial mucosal capillaries. The damage is progressive and can result in overt bleeding severe enough to require blood transfusions. The primary pathogenic factor is most likely mucosal ischemia resulting from reduced gastric blood flow (Fig. 33–1).[82,114] Gastric acid appears necessary for the lesions to occur, but acid hypersecretion is not usually present.

Endoscopic evidence of SRMD is present in most critically ill patients within 24 hours of admission to an intensive care unit (ICU), although only 2% to 10% have significant bleeding.[46] Prophylactic therapy to prevent bleeding is most effective if initiated early in the patient's course. However, controversies exist as to the need for prophylaxis, the relative importance of risk factors, the optimal drug regimen, and whether sucralfate is less likely to contribute to nosocomial pneumonia than antacids or H_2-receptor antagonists. Important considerations in the selection of a prophylactic agent include (a) number and severity of risk factors; (b) underlying medical condition of the critically ill patient; (c) comparative efficacy of the drug regimens; (d) adverse effects and potential for drug interactions; (e) overall cost of treatment; and (f) ease of administration.

The need to initiate prophylactic drug therapy in a critically ill patient remains controversial and depends on the number and severity of risk factors and the underlying medical condition of the patient.[113,114] Not all patients admitted to an ICU require prophylactic therapy. Patients with less than two risk factors, in the absence prolonged mechanical ventilation or coagulopathy, do not appear to be at increased risk of bleeding. Patients with at least two risk factors, or individual high-risk factors, for example, coagulopathy, prolonged mechanical ventilation, or multiple organ failure, should receive prophylactic drug therapy. However, prophylaxis may only reduce the incidence of GI hemorrhage by 50%.[113]

Medications used to prevent stress-related mucosal bleeding (SRMB) include antacids (titrated to an intragastric pH > 4), intravenous H_2-receptor antagonists administered intermittently or by continuous infusion, sucralfate (usually given by nasogastric tube), oral proton pump inhibitors (given by nasogastric or nasoduodenal tube) or intravenous proton pump inhibitors.[46,82,113,114] The value of parenteral and enteral nutrition in preventing SRMB remains controversial and requires further investigation.

Numerous clinical trials have documented the efficacy of antacids, intravenous H_2-receptor antagonists (cimetidine, ranitidine, famotidine), and sucralfate in preventing SRMB.[82,113–118] Antacids, although effective, require high doses, frequent administration, and pH monitoring, and are associated with increased adverse effects. H_2-receptor antagonists when given in recommended doses, either intermittently or by continuous infusion, provide similar efficacy. Although maintenance of intragastric pH > 4 is often recommended, especially in high-risk patients, pH control is not the sole factor in determining drug efficacy.

Sucralfate does not requiring pH monitoring or intravenous access, and may decrease the risk of nosocomial pneumonia (when compared to antacids and possibly to H_2-receptor antagonists) in patients requiring ventilation.[113,114,116,117] However, ranitidine, when compared to sucralfate in mechanically ventilated patients, was found to have a lower rate of clinically important GI bleeding with a similar rate of pneumonia.[114,118] When a decision analysis model was used to estimate the cost of cimetidine compared to sucralfate in patients at low risk of bleeding, the cost per bleeding episode averted was 6.5-fold greater with cimetidine than with sucralfate.[119]

A number of small studies suggest that oral proton pump inhibitors may prevent clinically important SRMB, but no large randomized clinical trial has been performed to confirm these findings.[82,113,115] There are no well-controlled clinical trials with intravenous pantoprazole (the only intravenous proton pump inhibitor available in the United States) which evaluates its efficacy in the prophylaxis of SRMB. However, the continuous infusion of this drug should adequately control acid secretion and permit a smooth transition to the oral dosage form. Intravenous pantoprazole can be readily interchanged with the oral dosage form on a mg/mg basis.[120] Although intravenous pantoprazole offers a theoretical advantage in preventing SRMB, recommendations regarding its use await formal trials that will delineate its efficacy, dosage, and safety in critically ill patients.

Improvement in the patient's overall medical condition (discharge from the ICU, extubation, oral intake) suggests that the prophylactic therapy can be discontinued. If a patient develops clinically significant bleeding, endoscopic evaluation of the GI tract is indicated along with aggressive drug treatment. The efficacy of intravenous H_2-receptor antagonists, sucralfate, or a combined regimen of an H_2-receptor antagonist and sucralfate was not superior to placebo in most well-controlled trials. No single study has convincingly demonstrated an overall benefit of an oral or intravenous proton pump inhibitor in the cessation of acute stress-bleeding.[82] However, a continuous infusion of intravenous pantoprazole should be utilized until bleeding stops or surgery is indicated.

EVALUATION OF THERAPEUTIC OUTCOMES

Relief of epigastric pain should be monitored throughout the course of treatment in patients with either HP- or NSAID-induced ulcers. Ulcer pain typically resolves in a few days when NSAIDs are the cause of the symptoms, and within 7 days upon initiation of antiulcer therapy (Fig. 33–5). Most patients with uncomplicated PUD will be symptom-free after treatment with any one of the recommended antiulcer regimens. The persistence, or redevelopment, of symptoms after several weeks of treatment suggests failure of ulcer healing or an alternative diagnosis such as gastroesophageal reflux disease. The majority of patients with uncomplicated HP-positive ulcers do not require confirmation of ulcer healing after HP eradication. When endoscopy is not indicated, the urea breath test is the best test to confirm HP eradication. Assess patient compliance and the possibility of antibiotic resistance in patients who fail therapy.

Ulcer patients, especially older adults or other high-risk patients on NSAIDs, should be closely monitored for signs or symptoms of bleeding, obstruction, penetration, or perforation. Patients who remain symptomatic, have recurrent attacks, or who appear to have ulcer-related complications should be referred for further evaluation. Followup endoscopy to determine whether an ulcer or HP is present can be justified in patients with frequent symptomatic recurrence, refractory disease, complications, or suspected hypersecretory states.

CONCLUSIONS

The discovery of HP has dramatically changed the way in which chronic PUD is treated. However, questions remain regarding methods of transmission, virulence, and pathogenesis. Important issues such as who to test and who to treat require further clarification. In the interim, the search continues for the optimal and most cost-effective drug regimen. Future research will surely provide us with less complicated and safer antimicrobial regimens and perhaps a vaccine. The widespread use of NSAIDs and their associated GI complications is of major concern, especially in older adults. Cotherapy with misoprostol or a proton pump inhibitor reduces NSAID-induced GI events, but the cost-effectiveness of these measures must be compared against the COX-2 inhibitors. Newer drugs that spare the GI tract and decrease NSAID-related morbidity and mortality will soon become available. The pharmacist has the opportunity to play an important role in the successful management of patients with PUD (Table 33–9).

▶ PRINCIPLES OF PHARMACOTHERAPY

- Patients with PUD should reduce psychological stress, cigarette smoking, and NSAID use, and should avoid foods and beverages that exacerbate ulcer symptoms.

- Eradication is recommended for all HP-positive patients with an active ulcer, a documented history of a prior ulcer, or a history of ulcer-related complications. There are no definitive recommendations regarding HP eradication in patients with uninvestigated dyspepsia or nonulcer dyspepsia. Treatment of HP is recommended for HP-positive patients with low-grade MALT lymphoma and after resection of gastric cancer.
- The selection of a HP eradication regimen should be based on efficacy, safety, antibiotic resistance, cost, and the likelihood of compliance. Treatment should be initiated with a proton pump inhibitor-based three-drug regimen. If a second course of HP therapy is required, the regimen should contain different antibiotics.
- Treatment with a conventional antiulcer drug (H_2-receptor antagonist, proton pump inhibitor, or sucralfate) may be an alternative to HP eradication, but is discouraged because of the high rate of ulcer recurrence and ulcer-related complications. Combination therapy adds to drug treatment costs without enhancing efficacy.
- Maintenance therapy with a low-dose H_2-receptor antagonist or proton pump inhibitor is only indicated for high-risk patients who fail HP eradication, patients with severe complications, or those with HP-negative ulcers.
- Prophylactic therapy is indicated for patients at risk of developing NSAID-induced ulcers and related GI complications. H_2-receptor antagonists or proton pump inhibitors relieve dyspeptic symptoms. Standard-dose H_2-receptor antagonists prevent duodenal ulcers, but higher dosages are needed to prevent gastric ulcers. Standard proton pump inhibitor dosages prevent gastric ulcers and duodenal ulcers and are at least as effective as misoprostol cotherapy.
- Patients with PUD, especially those receiving HP eradication or misoprostol cotherapy, require patient education regarding their disease and drug treatment to successfully achieve a positive therapeutic outcome.
- Patients with PUD, who develop recurrent ulcer symptoms or signs or symptoms of GI bleeding or perforation, should be referred for further evaluation. Assess reasons for therapeutic failure, including noncompliance to the drug regimen, antibiotic resistance (HP eradication), heavy smoking, NSAID ingestion, and the need for HP eradication in a patient on conventional antiulcer medications.
- Remember that the determinants of drug treatment costs are often based on the acquisition cost of medications, but this may be erroneous, as the overall cost of the treatment strategy is dependent on its success. Ultimately, the most expensive treatment is the treatment that does not work.

REFERENCES

1. Del Valle J, Cohen H, Laine L, et al. Acid peptic disorders. In: Yamada T, Aplers DH, Laine L, et al, eds. Textbook of Gastroenterology, 3rd ed. Philadelphia, Lippincott Williams & Wilkins, 1999:1370–1444.
2. Yardley JH, Hendrix TR. Gastritis, duodenitis, and associated ulcerative lesions. In: Yamada T, Aplers DH, Laine L, et al, eds. Textbook of Gastroenterology, 3rd ed. Philadelphia, Lippincott Williams & Wilkins, 1999:1463–1499.
3. Talley NJ, Holtmann G. Approach to the patient with dyspepsia and related functional gastrointestinal complaints. In: Yamada T, Aplers DH, Laine L, et al, eds. Textbook of Gastroenterology, 3rd ed. Philadelphia, Lippincott Williams & Wilkins, 1999:660–693.
4. Del Valle J, Scheiman JM. Zollinger-Ellison syndrome. In: Yamada T, Aplers DH, Laine L, et al, eds. Textbook of Gastroenterology, 3rd ed. Philadelphia, Lippincott Williams & Wilkins, 1999:1445–1462.
5. El-Serag HB, Sonnenberg A. Opposing time trends of peptic ulcer and reflux disease. Gut 1998;43:327–333.
6. Williams MP, Pounder RE. *Helicobacter pylori*: from the benign to the malignant. Am J Gastroenterol 1999;94(suppl):S11–S16.
7. Kuipers EJ. Exploring the link between *Helicobacter pylori* and gastric cancer. Aliment Pharmacol Ther 1999;13:(suppl 1):3–11.
8. The Report of the Digestive Health Initiative International Update Conference on *Helicobacter pylori*. Gastroenterology 1997;113(suppl): S4–S8.
9. Go MF. What are the host factors that place an individual at risk for *Helicobacter pylori*-associated disease? Gastroenterology 1997; 113(suppl):S15–S20.
10. Axon AT. Are all Helicobacters equal? Mechanisms of gastroduodenal pathology and their clinical implications. Gut 1999;45(suppl 1):1–4.
11. Megraud F, Broutet N. Have we found the source of *Helicobacter pylori*. Aliment Pharmacol Ther 2000;(suppl 3):7–12. Review.
12. Huang JQ, Hunt RH. *Helicobacter pylori* and gastric cancer—The clinicians' point of view. Aliment Pharmacol Ther 2000;(suppl 3):48–54. Review.
13. Danesh J. *Helicobacter pylori* infection and gastric cancer: Systematic review of the epidemiological studies. Aliment Pharmacol Ther 1999;13:851–856.
14. Bayerdorffer E, Miehlke S, Neubauer A, et al. Gastric MALT-lymphoma and *Helicobacter pylori* infection. Aliment Pharmacol Ther 1997;11:(suppl 1):89–94.
15. Danesh J, Lawrence M, Murphy M, et al. Systematic review of the epidemiological evidence on *Helicobacter pylori* infection and nonulcer or uninvestigated dyspepsia. Arch Intern Med 2000;160:1192–1198.
16. Stanghellini V, Tosetti C, Barbara G, et al. The continuing dilemma of dyspepsia. Aliment Pharmacol Ther 2000;(suppl 3):23–30. Review.
17. Laine L. Approaches to nonsteroidal anti-inflammatory drug use in the high-risk patient. Gastroenterology 2001;120:594–606.
18. Hawkey CJ. Nonsteroidal anti-inflammatory drug gastropathy. Gastroenterology 2000;119:521–535.
19. Wolfe MM, Lichtenstein DR, Singh G. Gastrointestinal toxicity of nonsteroidal antiinflammatory drugs. N Engl J Med 1999;340:1888–1899.
20. Bjorkman DJ. Current status of nonsteroidal anti-inflammatory drug (NSAID) use in the United States: Risk factors and frequency of complications. Am J Med 1999;107(suppl 3A):3S–10S.
21. Raskin JB. Gastrointestinal effects of nonsteroidal anti-inflammatory therapy. Am J Med 1999;106(suppl 5B):3S–12S.
22. Wallace JL. Nonsteroidal anti-inflammatory drugs and gastroenteropathy: The second hundred years. Gastroenterology 1997;112:1000–1016.
23. Wilcox CM, Alexander LN, Cotsonis GA, et al. Nonsteroidal anti-inflammatory drugs are associated with both upper and lower gastrointestinal bleeding. Dig Dis Sci 1997;42:990–997.
24. El-Serag HB, Sonnenberg A. Association of esophagitis and esophageal strictures with diseases treated with nonsteroidal anti-inflammatory drugs. Am J Gastroenterol 1997;92:52–56.
25. Blower AL, Brooks A, Fenn GC, et al. Emergency admissions for upper gastrointestinal disease and their relation to NSAID use. Aliment Pharmacol Ther 1997;11:281–291.
26. Peura DA, Lanza FL, Gostout CJ. The American College of Gastroenterology Bleeding Registry: Preliminary findings. Am J Gastroenterol 1997;92:924–928.
27. Hawkey CJ, Cullen DJ, Greenwood DC, et al. Prescribing of nonsteroidal anti-inflammatory drugs in general practice: Determinants and consequences. Aliment Pharmacol Ther 1997;11:293–298.
28. Tamblyn R, Berkson L, Dauphinee WD. Unnecessary prescribing of NSAIDs and the management of NSAID-related gastropathy in medical practice. Ann Intern Med 1997;127:429–438.
29. Cryer B, Feldman M. Effects of very-low-dose daily, long-term aspirin therapy of gastric, duodenal, and rectal prostaglandin levels and

on mucosal injury in healthy humans. Gastroenterology 1999;117: 17–25.

30. Younossi ZM, Williamson BS, Schatz RA. Effect of combined anticoagulation and low-dose ASA treatment on upper gastrointestinal bleeding. Dig Dis Sci 1997;42:79–82.
31. Singh G. Recent considerations in nonsteroidal anti-inflammatory drug gastropathy. Am J Med 1998;105(1B):31S–38S.
32. Hawkey CJ. *Helicobacter pylori*, NSAIDs and cognitive dissonance. Aliment Pharmacol Ther 1999;13:695–702. Review.
33. Barr M, Buckley M, O'Morain C. Non-steroidal anti-inflammatory drugs and *Helicobacter pylori*. Aliment Pharmacol Ther 2000;(suppl 3): 43–7. Review.
34. Ng TM, Fock KM, Khor JL, et al. Non-steroidal anti-inflammatory drugs, *Helicobacter pylori*, and bleeding gastric ulcer. Aliment Pharmacol Ther 2000;14:203–209.
35. Calam J, Gibbons A, Zoe V, et al. How does *Helicobacter pylori* cause mucosal damage? Its effect on acid and gastrin physiology. Gastroenterology 1997;113(suppl):S43–S49.
36. Del Valle J, Todisco A. Gastric secretion. In: Yamada T, Aplers DH, Laine L, et al, eds. Textbook of Gastroenterology, 3rd ed. Philadelphia, Lippincott Williams & Wilkins, 1999:278–319.
37. Sachs G. Shin M, Munson K, et al. The control of gastric acid and *Helicobacter pylori* eradication. Aliment Pharmacol Ther 2000;14: 1383–401. Review.
38. Peura DA. Ulcerogenesis: Integrating the roles of *Helicobacter pylori* and acid secretion in duodenal ulcer. Am J Gastroenterol 1997;92(suppl):8S–16S.
39. Smoot DT. How does *Helicobacter pylori* cause mucosal damage? Direct mechanisms. Gastroenterology 1997;113(suppl):S31–S34.
40. Ernst PB, Crowe SE, Reyes VE. How does *Helicobacter pylori* cause mucosal damage? The inflammatory response. Gastroenterology 1997;113(suppl):S35–S42.
41. Crabtree JE. Role of cytokines in pathogenesis of *Helicobacter pylori*-induced mucosal damage. Dig Dis Sci 1998;43(suppl):46S–55S.
42. Bjorkman DJ. The effect of aspirin and nonsteroidal anti-inflammatory drugs on prostaglandins. Am J Med 1998;105(suppl 1B):8S–12S.
43. McCarthy DM. Comparative toxicity of nonsteroidal anti-inflammatory drugs. Am J Med 1999;107(suppl 6A):37S–47S.
44. Schoenfeld P, Kimmey MB, Scheiman J, et al. Nonsteroidal anti-inflammatory drug-associated gastrointestinal complications—Guidelines for prevention and treatment. Aliment Pharmacol Ther 1999; 13:1273–85. Review.
45. Schafer AI. Effects of nonsteroidal anti-inflammatory therapy on platelets. Am J Med 1999;106(suppl 5B):25S–36S.
46. Elta GH. Approach to the patient with gross gastrointestinal bleeding. In: Yamada T, Aplers DH, Laine L, et al, eds. Textbook of Gastroenterology, 3rd ed. Philadelphia, Lippincott Williams & Wilkins, 1999:714–743.
47. Hernandez-Diaz S, Rodriguez LA. Association between nonsteroidal anti-inflammatory drugs and upper gastrointestinal tract bleeding/perforation: An overview of epidemiologic studies published in the 1990s. Arch Intern Med 2000;160:2093–2099.
48. Vaira D, Menegatti M, Miglioli M. What is the role of *Helicobacter pylori* in complicated ulcer disease? Gastroenterology 1997;113(suppl): S78–S84.
49. Lau JYW, Sung JJY, Lee KKC, et al. Effect of intravenous omeprazole on recurrent bleeding after endoscopic treatment of bleeding peptic ulcers. N Engl J Med 2000;343:310–316.
50. Bustamante M, Stollman N. The efficacy of proton-pump inhibitors in acute ulcer bleeding: A qualitative review. J Clin Gastroenterol 2000;30:7–13.
51. Vaira D, Holton J, Menegatti M, et al. Invasive and non-invasive tests for *Helicobacter pylori* infection. Aliment Pharmacol Ther 2000; (suppl 3):13–22. Review.
52. Megraud F. How should *Helicobacter pylori* infection be diagnosed? Gastroenterology 1997;113(suppl):S93–S98.
53. Oderda G, Rapa A, Marinello D, et al. Usefulness of *Helicobacter pylori* stool antigen test to monitor response to eradication treatment in children. Aliment Pharmacol Ther 2001;15:203–206.
54. Howden CW, Hunt RH. Guidelines for the management of *Helicobacter pylori* infection. Am J Gastroenterol 1998;93:2330–2338.
55. American Society of Health-System Pharmacists Therapeutic Position Statement on the Identification and Treatment of *Helicobacter pylori*-associated peptic ulcer disease in adults. Am J Health Syst Pharm 2001:58:331–7.
56. Graham DY. Therapy of *Helicobacter pylori*: Current status and issues. Gastroenterology 2000;118(suppl):S2–S8.
57. Lee J, O'Morain C. Who should be treated for *Helicobacter pylori* infection? A review of consensus conferences and guidelines. Gastroenterology 1997;113(suppl):S99–S106.
58. Xia HH, Talley NJ. *Helicobacter pylori* eradication in patients with non-ulcer dyspepsia. Drugs 1999;58:785–792.
59. Peura D. *Helicobacter pylori*: Rational management options. Am J Med 1998;105:424–430.
60. Lanza FL. A guideline for the treatment and prevention of NSAID-induced ulcers. Am J Gastroenterol 1998;93:2037–2046.
61. Seymour NE, Andersen DK. Surgery for peptic ulcer disease and post-gastrectomy syndromes. In: Yamada T, Aplers DH, Laine L, et al, eds. Textbook of Gastroenterology, 3rd ed. Philadelphia, Lippincott Williams & Wilkins, 1999:1530–1548.
62. Anderson J, Gonzalez J. *H. pylori* infection: Review of the guideline for diagnosis and treatment. Geriatrics 2000;55:44–49.
63. Rowland M, Imrie C, Bourke B, et al. How should *Helicobacter pylori*-infected children be managed? Gut 1999;45(suppl 1):36–39.
64. Oderda G. Management of *Helicobacter pylori* infection in children. Gut 1998;43(suppl 1):S10–S13.
65. Chey WD. *Helicobacter pylori*. Curr Treat Option Gastroenterol 1999; 2:171–81.
66. Salcedo JA, Al-Kawas F. Treatment of *Helicobacter pylori* infection. Arch Intern Med 1998;158:842–851.
67. Pounder RE, Williams MP. The treatment of *Helicobacter pylori* infection. Aliment Pharmacol Ther 1997;11(suppl 1):45–41.
68. Lambert JR, Midolo P. The actions of bismuth in the treatment of *Helicobacter pylori* infection. Aliment Pharmacol Ther 1997;11(suppl): 27–33.
69. Peterson WL. The role of antisecretory drugs in the treatment of *Helicobacter pylori* infection. Aliment Pharmacol Ther 1997;11(suppl 1):21–25.
70. Huang J, Hunt RH. The importance of clarithromycin dose in the management of *Helicobacter pylori* infection: A meta-analysis of triple therapies with a proton pump inhibitor, clarithromycin and amoxicillin or metronidazole. Aliment Pharmacol Ther 1999;13:719–729.
71. Van Oijen AH, Verbeek AL, Jansen JD, et al. Treatment of *Helicobacter pylori* infection with ranitidine bismuth citrate or proton pump inhibitor-based triple therapies. Aliment Pharmacol Ther 2000;14:991–999. Review.
72. Chey WE, Fisher L, Barnett J, et al. Low- versus high-dose azithromycin triple therapy for *Helicobacter pylori* infection. Aliment Pharmacol Ther 1998;12:1263–1267.
73. Segura AM, Gutierrez O, Otero W, et al. Furazolidone, amoxicillin, bismuth triple therapy for *Helicobacter pylori* infection. Aliment Pharmacol Ther 1998;11:529–532.
74. Gschwantler M, Dragosics B, Schutze K, et al. Famotidine versus omeprazole in combination with clarithromycin and metronidazole for eradication of *Helicobacter pylori*—A randomized controlled trial. Aliment Pharmacol Ther 1999;1063–1069.
75. Hackelsberger A, Malfertheimer P. A risk-benefit assessment of drugs used in the eradication of *Helicobacter pylori* infection. Drug Saf 1996;15:30–52.
76. Houben MH, Beek DV, Hensen EF, et al. A systematic review of *Helicobacter pylori* eradication therapy—The impact of antimicrobial resistance on eradication rates. Aliment Pharmacol Ther 1999;13:1047–1055.
77. Van Der Wouden EJ, Thijs JC, Van Zwet AA, et al. Nitroimidazole resistance in *Helicobacter pylori*. Aliment Pharmacol Ther 2000;14: 7–14. Review.

78. Megraud F, Doermann HP. Clinical relevance of resistant strains of *Helicobacter pylori*: A review of current data. Gut 1998;43(suppl 1): S61–S65.
79. Graham DY. Antibiotic resistance in *Helicobacter pylori*: Implications for therapy. Gastroenterology 1998;115:1272–1277.
80. Sutton P, Lee A. *Helicobacter pylori* vaccines—The current status. Aliment Pharmacol Ther 2000;14:1107–1118. Review.
81. Welage LS, Berardi RR. Evaluation of omeprazole, lansoprazole, pantoprazole, and rabeprazole in the treatment of acid-related diseases. J Am Pharm Assoc 2000;40:52–62.
82. Wolfe M, Sachs G. Acid suppression: Optimizing therapy for gastroduodenal ulcer healing, gastroesophageal reflux disease, and stress-related erosive syndrome. Gastroenterology 2000;118(suppl):S9–S31.
83. Raskin JB, White RH, Jackson JE, et al. Misoprostol dosage in the prevention of nonsteroidal anti-inflammatory drug-induced gastric and duodenal ulcers: A comparison of three regimens. Ann Intern Med 1995;123:344–350.
84. Silverstein FE. Improving the gastrointestinal safety of NSAIDs: The development of misoprostol—From hypothesis to clinical practice. Dig Dis Sci 1998;43:447–458.
85. Hudson N, Taha AS, Russell RI, et al. Famotidine for healing and maintenance in nonsteroidal anti-inflammatory drug-associated gastroduodenal ulceration. Gastroenterology 1997;112:1817–1822.
86. Taha AS, Hudson N, Hawkey CJ, et al. Famotidine for the prevention of gastric and duodenal ulcers caused by nonsteroidal anti-inflammatory drugs. N Engl J Med 1996;334:1435–1439.
87. Hawkey CJ, Karrasch JA, Szcepanski L, et al. Omeprazole compared with misoprostol for ulcers associated with nonsteroidal anti-inflammatory drugs. N Engl J Med 1998;338:727–734.
88. Yeomans ND, Tulassay Z, Juhasz L, et al. A comparison of omeprazole with ranitidine for ulcers associated with nonsteroidal antiinflammatory drugs. N Engl J Med 1998;338:719–726.
89. Rose P, Huang B, Lukasik N, et al. Evidence that lansoprazole is effective in preventing NSAID-induced ulcers. Gastroenterology 1999;116:G1293. Abstract.
90. Jackson LM, Hawkey CJ. COX-2 selective nonsteroidal anti-inflammatory drugs: Do they really offer any advantages? Drugs 2000;59:1207–1216.
91. Hawkey CJ, Jackson L, Harper SE, et al. The gastrointestinal safety profile of rofecoxib, a highly selective inhibitor of cyclooxygenase-2, in humans. Aliment Pharmacol Ther 2001;15:1–9. Review.
92. Clement D, Goa KL. Celecoxib: A review of its use in osteoarthritis, rheumatoid arthritis, and acute pain. Drugs 2000;59:957–980.
93. Feldman M, McMahon AT. Do cyclooxygenase-2 inhibitors provide benefits similar to those of traditional nonsteroidal anti-inflammatory drugs, with less gastrointestinal toxicity? Ann Intern Med 2000;132: 134–143.
94. Silverstein F, Faich G, Goldstein JL, et al. Gastrointestinal toxicity with celecoxib vs nonsteroidal antiinflammatory drugs for osteoarthritis and rheumatoid arthritis. The CLASS study: A randomized controlled trial. JAMA 2000;284:1247–1255.
95. Bombardier C, Laine L, Reicin A, et al. Comparison of upper intestinal toxicity of rofecoxib and naproxen in patients with rheumatoid arthritis. N Engl J Med 2000;343:1520–1528.
96. Richardson P, Hawkey CJ, Stack WA. Proton pump inhibitors: Pharmacology and rationale for use in gastrointestinal disorders. Drugs 1998;56:307–335.
97. Spencer CM, Faulds D. Esomeprazole. Drugs 2000;60:321–331.
98. Fitton A, Wiseman L. Pantoprazole: A review of its pharmacologic properties and therapeutic use in acid-related disorders. Drugs 1998; 51:460–482.
99. Prakash A, Faulds D. Rabeprazole. Drugs 1998;55:261–267.
100. Langtry HD, Wilde MI. Lansoprazole: An update of its pharmacological properties and clinical efficacy in the management of acid-related disorders. Drugs 1997;54:473–500.
101. Langtry HD, Wilde MI. Omeprazole: A review of its use in *Helicobacter pylori* infection, gastroesophageal reflux disease and peptic ulcer induced by nonsteroidal anti-inflammatory drugs. Drugs 1998;56:447–486.
102. Sharma VK. Comparison of 24-hour intragastric pH using four liquid formulations of lansoprazole and omeprazole. Am J Health Syst Pharm 1999;(suppl 4):518–521.
103. Berardi RR. Proton pump inhibition: An effective, safe approach to GERD management. Postgrad Med 2001; Special Report, October 2001:24–35.
104. Humphries TJ, Minerritt GJ. Drug interactions with agents used to treat acid-related diseases. Aliment Pharmacol Ther 1999;13(suppl 3):18–26.
105. Klingenberg-Knol ED, Nelis F, Dent J, et al. Long-term omeprazole treatment in resistant gastroesophageal reflux disease: Efficacy, safety, and influence on gastric mucosa. Gastroenterology 2000;118:661–669.
106. Taylor JL, Zagari M, Murphy, et al. Pharmacoeconomic comparison of treatments for the eradication of *Helicobacter pylori*. Arch Intern Med 1997;157:87–97.
107. Vakil N, Fennerty MB. Cost effectiveness of treatment regimens for the eradication of *Helicobacter pylori* in duodenal ulcer. Am J Gastroenterol 1996;91:239–245.
108. Sonnenberg A, Schwartz JS, Cutler AF, et al. Cost savings in duodenal ulcer therapy through *Helicobacter pylori* eradication compared with conventional therapies: Results of a randomized, double-blind, multicenter trial. Arch Intern Med 1998;158:852–860.
109. Maetzel A, Ferraz MB, Bombardier C. The cost-effectiveness of misoprostol in preventing serious gastrointestinal events associated with the use of nonsteroidal anti-inflammatory drugs. Arthritis Rheum 1998; 41–16.
110. Watson DJ, Harper S, Ahao P, et al. Treatment with rofecoxib required less gastrointestinal (GI) co-medication and fewer GI procedures than nonspecific cyclooxygenase inhibitors (NSAIDs). Arthritis Rheum 1999;42(suppl):S403. Abstract.
111. Pisegna J. Zollinger-Ellison syndrome. Curr Treat Option Gastroenterol 1999;2:195–203.
112. Hirschowitz BI. Zollinger-Ellison syndrome: Pathogenesis, diagnosis, and management. Am J Gastroenterol 1997;92(suppl 4):44S–50S.
113. Ben-Menachem Tl, Bresalier RS. Prophylaxis for stress-related gastrointestinal hemorrhage. Curr Treat Option Gastroenterol 1999;2:313–319.
114. American Society of Health-System Pharmacists Therapeutic Guidelines on Stress Ulcer Prophylaxis. Am J Health Syst Pharm 1999:56:347–379.
115. Lasky MR, Metzler MH, Phillips JO. A prospective study of omeprazole suspension to prevent clinically significant gastrointestinal bleeding from stress ulcers in mechanically ventilated patients. J Trauma 1998; 44:527–533.
116. Prod'hom G, Leuenberger P, Koerfer J, et al. Nosocomial pneumonia in mechanically ventilated patients receiving antacid, ranitidine, or sucralfate: A randomized controlled trial. Ann Intern Med 1994; 120:653–662.
117. Cook DJ, Reeve BK, Guyatt GH, et al. Stress ulcer prophylaxis in critically ill patients: Resolving discordant meta-analyses. JAMA 1996;275:308–314.
118. Cook D, Guyatt G, Marshall J, et al. Comparison of sucralfate and ranitidine for the prevention of upper gastrointestinal bleeding in patients requiring mechanical ventilation. N Engl J Med 1998;338:791–797.
119. Ben-Menachem T, McCarthy BD, Fogel R, et al. Prophylaxis for stress-related gastrointestinal hemorrhage: A cost-effective analysis. Crit Care Med 1996;24:338–345.
120. Pisegna JR. Switching between intravenous and oral pantoprazole. J Clin Gastroenterol 2001;32:27–32.

34

Inflammatory Bowel Disease

Joseph T. DiPiro and Robert R. Schade

There are two forms of idiopathic inflammatory bowel disease (IBD): (a) ulcerative colitis, a mucosal inflammatory condition confined to the rectum and colon; and (b) Crohn's disease, a transmural inflammation of the gastrointestinal tract that can affect any part, from the mouth to the anus. The etiologies of both conditions are unknown, but they may have some common pathogenetic mechanisms.

EPIDEMIOLOGY

At least 1 million Americans are believed to have IBD, with 15,000 to 30,000 new cases diagnosed annually.[1] Crohn's disease has a reported incidence of 4.3 to 6.8 in the United States, and a prevalence of 20 to 40 per 100,000 people.[2] The rates of IBD are highest in Scandinavia, Great Britain, and North America.[3] The incidence of Crohn's disease varies considerably among studies but has clearly increased dramatically over the last 3 or 4 decades.[3,4] Ulcerative colitis has a reported incidence of 3.7 to 15 and a prevalence of 37 to 212 per 100,000.[4] The incidence of ulcerative colitis has remained relatively constant over many years.[3,4] Although most epidemiologic studies combine ulcerative proctitis with ulcerative colitis, from 17% to 49% of cases are proctitis. The incidence of ulcerative proctitis ranges from 1.1 to 7.1 per 100,000.[4]

Both sexes are affected equally with inflammatory bowel disease,[1,2] although some studies show slightly greater numbers of women with Crohn's disease and males with ulcerative colitis.[5,6] Ulcerative colitis and Crohn's disease have bimodal distributions in age of initial presentation. The peak incidence occurs in the second or third decades of life with a second peak occurring between 50 and 80 years of age.[4] Significantly increased incidence of ulcerative colitis (four to five times normal) has been observed in Ashkenazi Jews, while Blacks and Asians have a relatively low incidence of occurrence.[2]

ETIOLOGY

Although the exact etiology of ulcerative colitis and Crohn's disease is unknown, similar factors are believed responsible for each condition (Table 34–1). The major theories of the cause of IBD involve a combination of infectious or immunologic factors.[7] The inflammatory response with IBD may indicate abnormal regulation of the normal immune response or an autoimmune reaction to self-antigens. The microflora of the gastrointestinal tract may provide an environmental trigger to activate inflammation.[8]

INFECTIOUS FACTORS THEORIES

Microorganisms are likely initiators of the inflammation involved in the pathogenesis of IBD.[9] However, no definitive infectious cause of IBD has been found, even though the presentation is similar to that caused by some invasive microbial pathogens. Suspect agents include the measles virus, protozoans, mycobacteria, and other bacteria. Also, certain strains of bacteria produce toxins (necrotoxins, hemolysins, and enterotoxins) that cause mucosal damage. Bacteria elaborate peptides (e.g., formyl-methionyl-leucyl-phenylalanine [FMLP]) that have chemotactic properties and that cause an influx of inflammatory cells with subsequent release of inflammatory mediators and tissue destruction. Microbes may elaborate super antigens, which are capable of global T-lymphocyte stimulation and subsequent inflammatory response.[9] Through lumenal exposure to potent nonspecific stimulatory bacterial products, the state of activation of the immune system pathways may be up-regulated.[10]

GENETIC FACTORS

Genetic factors are believed to predispose patients to inflammatory bowel diseases, particularly Crohn's disease. In studies of monozygotic twins, there has been a high concordance rate, with both individuals of the pair having an IBD (particularly Crohn's disease). Also, first-degree relatives of patients with IBD had a 13-fold increase in the risk of disease.[11] Other investigators have observed genetic markers that are found more frequently in those with IBD (particularly major histocompatability complex, HLA-DR2 for ulcerative colitis and HLA-A2 for Crohn's disease).[3] A number of genes have been associated with IBDs; however, the nature of the gene products has not been established.

IMMUNOLOGIC MECHANISMS

The immunologic basis of IBD is supported by a number of observations.[8] First is the pathology of the lesions. With Crohn's disease, the bowel wall is infiltrated with lymphocytes, plasma cells, mast cells, macrophages, and neutrophils. Similar infiltration has been observed in the mucosal layer of the colon in patients with ulcerative colitis. Second, many of the systemic manifestations of IBD have an immunologic etiology (e.g., arthritis or uveitis). Finally, IBD is responsive to immunosuppressive drugs (e.g., corticosteroids and azathioprine).

The immune theory of IBD assumes that IBD is caused by an "inappropriate" reaction of the immune system. This may involve an immunodeficiency, such as a defect in cell-mediated immunity or of macrophages or neutrophils. Autoimmunity may be involved. Also, oxidant injury in colon epithelial crypt cells can be demonstrated from inflamed mucosa of patients with inflammatory bowel disease.[12]

Potential immunologic mechanisms include both autoimmune and nonautoimmune phenomena.[9,13] Autoimmunity may be directed against mucosal epithelial cells or against neutrophil cytoplasmic elements. Some patients with IBD have abnormal structural features for colonic epithelial cells even in the absence of active disease. Autoantibodies to these structures have been reported. Also, antineutrophil cytoplasmic antibodies are found in a high percentage of patients with ulcerative colitis (70%) and much less frequently with other forms of colitis (6% with Crohn's disease).[14] Presence of antineutrophil cytoplasmic antibodies in left-sided ulcerative colitis is associated

TABLE 34–1. Proposed Etiologies for Inflammatory Bowel Disease

Infectious Agents
- Viruses (e.g., measles)
- L-Forms of bacteria
- Mycobacteria
- Chlamydia

Genetics
- Metabolic defects
- Connective tissue disorders

Environmental Factors
- Diet
- Smoking (Crohn's disease)

Immune Defects
- Altered host susceptibility
- Immune-mediated mucosal damage

Psychologic Factors
- Stress
- Emotional or physical trauma
- Occupation

with resistance to medical therapy.[15] In contrast, as many as 70% of patients with Crohn's disease have circulating antibody to *Saccharomyces cerevisiae*.[16]

Dysregulation of cytokines is a component of inflammatory bowel disease. Specifically, Th_1 cytokine activity (which enhances cell-mediated immunity and suppresses humoral immunity) is excessive with Crohn's disease, whereas Th_2 cytokine activity (which inhibits cell-mediated immunity and enhances humoral immunity) is excessive with ulcerative colitis.[17] The result is that patients have inappropriate T cell responses to antigens from their own intestinal microflora.[17] Expression of interferon-γ (a Th_1 cytokine) in intestinal mucosa of diseased patients is reported to be increased while interleukin-4 (a Th_2 cytokine) is reduced.[18–20]

TNFα has been identified as a pivotal pro-inflammatory cytokine in Crohn's disease. TNFα can recruit inflammatory cells to inflamed tissues, activate coagulation, and promote the formation of granulomas. Production of TNFα is increased in the mucosa and intestinal lumen with Crohn's disease.[21,22] Eicosanoids such as leukotriene B_4 (LTB4) are increased in rectal dialysates and tissues of IBD patients and are related to disease activity. LTB4 enhances neutrophil adherence to vascular endothelium and acts as a neutrophil chemoattractant. These findings have led to the consideration of leukotriene inhibitor strategies for therapy.

PSYCHOLOGICAL FACTORS

Mental health changes appear to correlate with remissions and exacerbations, especially of ulcerative colitis, but psychological factors overall are not thought to be an etiologic factor. Most rigorous studies conclude that no connection can be made between stress-inducing events and disease symptoms.[23]

DIET AND SMOKING

Changes in diet by people in industrialized countries where Crohn's disease is more common have not been consistently associated with the disease. Studies of increased intake of refined sugars or chemical food additives and reduced fiber intake have provided conflicting results regarding risk for Crohn's disease.

Smoking plays an important but contrasting role in ulcerative colitis and Crohn's disease. Smoking is associated with a lower risk of ulcerative colitis.[24,25] The risk of developing ulcerative colitis in smokers is about 40% of that in nonsmokers.[26] Clinical relapses are associated with smoking cessation, and nicotine transdermal administration has been effective in improving symptoms in patients with ulcerative colitis.[27,28] In contrast, smoking is associated with a twofold increased frequency of Crohn's disease.[3] The mechanisms of these differing effects are not identified.

PATHOPHYSIOLOGY

Ulcerative colitis and Crohn's disease differ in two general respects: anatomic sites and depth of involvement within the bowel wall. There is, however, overlap between the two conditions, with a small fraction of patients showing features of both diseases. Confusion can occur, particularly when the inflammatory process is limited to the colon. Table 34–2 compares pathologic and clinical findings of the two diseases.[29]

ULCERATIVE COLITIS

Ulcerative colitis is confined to the rectum and colon, and affects the mucosa and the submucosa. In some instances, a short segment of terminal ileum may be inflamed; this is referred to as backwash ileitis. Unlike Crohn's disease, the deeper longitudinal muscular layers, serosa, and regional lymph nodes are not usually involved.[5] Because inflammation is usually confined to the mucosa and submucosa, fistulas, perforation, or obstruction are uncommon.

The primary lesion of ulcerative colitis occurs in the crypts of the mucosa (crypts of Lieberkuhn) in the form of a crypt abscess. Here, frank necrosis of the epithelium occurs; it is usually visible only with microscopy but may be seen grossly when coalescence of ulcers occurs. Extension and coalescence ulcers may surround areas of uninvolved mucosa. These islands of mucosa are called pseudopolyps. Other typical ulceration patterns include a "collar-button ulcer," which results from extensive submucosal undermining at the ulcer edge.[5,30] The extensive mucosal damage seen in ulcerative colitis can result in significant diarrhea and bleeding, although a small percentage of patients experience constipation.

Ulcerative colitis can be accompanied by complications that may be local (involving the colon or rectum) or systemic (not directly associated with the colon). With either type the complications may be mild, serious, or even life threatening.

Local complications occur in the majority of ulcerative colitis patients. Relatively minor complications include hemorrhoids, anal fissures, or perirectal abscesses, and are more likely to be present during active colitis. Enteroenteric fistulas are rare.

A major complication is toxic megacolon, a severe condition that occurs in 1% to 3% of patients with active ulcerative colitis or Crohn's disease. With toxic megacolon, ulceration extends below the submucosa, sometimes even reaching the serosa. Vasculitis, swelling of the vascular endothelium, and thrombosis of small arteries occurs; involvement of the muscularis propria causes loss of colonic tone, which leads to dilatation and potential perforation.[5] The patient with toxic megacolon usually has a high fever, tachycardia, distended abdomen, and elevated white blood cell count, and a dilated colon is observed on x-ray. Colonic perforation, however, may occur with or without toxic megacolon and is a greater risk with the first attack. Another infrequent major local complication is massive colonic

TABLE 34–2. Comparison of the Clinical and Pathologic Features of Crohn's Disease and Ulcerative Colitis

Feature	Crohn's Disease	Ulcerative Colitis
Intestinal		
Malaise, fever	Common	Uncommon
Rectal bleeding	Intermittent about 50%	Common
Abdominal tenderness	Common	May be present
Abdominal mass	Very common (especially with ileocolitis)	Not present
Abdominal pain	Very common	Unusual
Abdominal wall and internal fistulas	Very common	Rare
Endoscopic		
Rectal disease	About 20%	Almost 100%
Diffuse, continuous symmetric involvement	Uncommon	Very common
Aphthous or linear ulcers	Common	Rare
Pathologic		
Continuous disease	Rare	Very common
Rectal involvement	Rare	Common
Ileal involvement	Very common	Rare
Strictures	Common	Rare
Fistulas	Very common	Rare
Transmural involvement	Common	Rare
Crypt abscesses	Rare	Very common
Granulomas	Common	Rare
Linear clefts	Common	Rare

hemorrhage. Colonic stricture, sometimes with clinical obstruction, may also complicate ulcerative colitis.

The risk of colonic carcinoma is much greater in patients with ulcerative colitis as compared to the general population. The risk of colon cancer begins to increase 10 years to 15 years after the diagnosis of ulcerative colitis. The absolute risk may be as high as 30% 35 years after diagnosis, and as high as 49% for patients who have a long history of disease and who were less than 15 years of age at the time of diagnosis.[13]

The inflammatory response seen in IBD has also been blamed for the "systemic" complications seen in both Crohn's disease and ulcerative colitis. The systemic extraintestinal complications of ulcerative colitis are summarized in the next section.

HEPATOBILIARY COMPLICATIONS

Approximately 11% of patients with ulcerative colitis are reported to have hepatobiliary complications.[31] However, the reported frequency ranges from 5% to 95% in IBD patients overall.[32] Hepatic complications include fatty liver, pericholangitis, chronic active hepatitis, and cirrhosis. Biliary complications include sclerosing cholangitis, cholangiocarcinoma, and gallstones.

Fatty infiltration of the liver may be a result of malabsorption, protein-losing enteropathy, or concomitant steroid use. The most common hepatic complication is pericholangitis (acute inflammation surrounding the intrahepatic portal venules, bile ducts, and lymphatics), which occurs in up to one-third of ulcerative colitis patients studied. This is associated with progressive fibrosis of intrahepatic and extrahepatic bile ducts in a few percent of ulcerative colitis patients and is referred to as primary sclerosing cholangitis. Cirrhosis may be a sequela of cholangitis or of chronic active hepatitis. Often, the severity of hepatic disease does not correlate with gastrointestinal (GI) disease activity.

Gallstones occur more commonly in patients with Crohn's disease (particularly with terminal ileal disease) and may be related to bile salt malabsorption. Also, cholangiocarcinoma occurs 10 to 20 times more frequently in IBD patients as compared to the general population.[31]

JOINT COMPLICATIONS

Arthritis was found to be present in 4.9% of patients[31] and is typically migratory, involving one or a few, usually large joints. The joints most often affected, in decreasing frequency, are the knees, hips, ankles, wrists, and elbows. Sacroiliitis also occurs commonly. Arthritis associated with ulcerative colitis is generally related to the severity of colonic disease, and resolution without recurrence is seen with proctocolectomy. Also, arthritis in this setting is different from rheumatoid arthritis in that rheumatoid factors are generally not detected. It is nondeforming and nondestructive, even after multiple episodes.

Another potential joint complication is ankylosing spondylitis, which is often unresponsive to treatment. The incidence of ankylosing spondylitis in patients with ulcerative colitis is 30 times that of the general population and occurs most commonly in patients with the HLA-B27 phenotype.

OCULAR COMPLICATIONS

Ocular complications, including iritis, uveitis, episcleritis, and conjunctivitis, occur in up to 10% of patients with IBD. The most commonly reported symptoms with iritis and uveitis include blurred vision, eye pain, and photophobia. Episcleritis is associated with scleral injection, burning, and increased secretions. These complications may parallel the severity of intestinal disease, and recurrence after colectomy with ulcerative colitis is uncommon.

DERMATOLOGIC AND MUCOSAL COMPLICATIONS

Skin and mucosal lesions associated with IBD include erythema nodosum, pyoderma gangrenosum, and aphthous ulceration. Most studies report that 5% to 10% of IBD patients experience dermatologic or mucosal complications.[33]

Raised, red, tender nodules that vary in size from 1 cm to several centimeters are manifestations of erythema nodosum. They are typically found on the tibial surfaces of the legs and arms. These lesions are more commonly observed in Crohn's disease patients and are noted to correlate with disease severity.

Pyoderma gangrenosum occurs more commonly in patients with ulcerative colitis (1% to 5% incidence) and is characterized by discrete skin ulcerations that have a necrotic center and a violaceous color of the surrounding skin.[33] They can be seen on any part of the body but are more commonly found on the lower extremities.

Oral lesions are found in 6% to 20% of patients with Crohn's disease and 8% of patients with ulcerative colitis.[33] The most common lesion is aphthous stomatitis, seen with Crohn's disease. The severity of these lesions tends to parallel GI disease.

CROHN'S DISEASE

Crohn's disease is best characterized as a transmural inflammatory process. The terminal ileum is the most common site of the disorder (14% to 30%), but it may occur in any part of the GI tract from mouth to anus. About two-thirds of patients have some colonic involvement, and 15% to 25% of patients have only colonic disease.[9] Patients often have normal bowel separating segments of diseased bowel; that is, the disease is often discontinuous.

Regardless of the site, bowel wall injury is extensive and the intestinal lumen is often narrowed. The mesentery becomes first thickened and edematous and then fibrotic. Ulcers tend to be deep and elongated and extend along the longitudinal axis of the bowel, at least into the submucosa. The "cobblestone" appearance of the bowel wall results from deep mucosal ulceration intermingled with nodular submucosal thickening.

Complications of Crohn's disease may involve the intestinal tract or organs unrelated to it. Small bowel stricture and subsequent obstruction is a complication that may require surgery. Fistula formation is common and occurs much more frequently than with ulcerative colitis.[9] Fistulae often occur in the areas of worst inflammation, where loops of bowel have become matted together by fibrous adhesions. Fistulae may connect a segment of the GI tract to skin (enterocutaneous fistula), two segments of the GI tract (enteroenteric fistula), or the intestinal tract with the bladder (enterovesicular fistula) or vagina. Crohn's disease fistulae or abscesses associated with them frequently require surgical treatment.

Bleeding with Crohn's disease is usually not as severe as with ulcerative colitis, although patients with Crohn's disease may have hypochromic anemia. Also, as with ulcerative colitis, the risk of carcinoma is increased but not as greatly as with ulcerative colitis.

Systemic complications of Crohn's disease are common, and similar to those found with ulcerative colitis. Arthritis, iritis, skin lesions, and liver disease often accompany Crohn's disease. Renal stones occur in up to 10% of patients with Crohn's disease (less frequently with ulcerative colitis) and are caused by fat malabsorption, which allows for greater oxalate absorption and formation of calcium oxalate stones. Gallstones also occur with greater frequency in patients with ileitis, possibly because of bile acid malabsorption at the terminal ileum.

Nutritional deficiencies are common with Crohn's disease.[34] Reported frequencies of various nutritional parameters are: weight loss, 40% to 80%; growth failure in children, 15% to 88%; iron deficiency anemia, 25% to 50%; vitamin B_{12} deficiency, 20% to 37%; folate deficiency, 13% to 37%; hypoalbuminemia, 25% to 76%; hypokalemia, 33%; and osteomalacia, 36%. There are usually decreased fat stores and lean tissue. Growth failure in children may be associated with hypozincemia.

CLINICAL PRESENTATION

The patterns of clinical presentation of IBD can vary widely. Patients may have a single acute episode that resolves and does not recur, but most patients experience acute exacerbations after periods of remission. With more severe disease, prolonged illness may occur.

ULCERATIVE COLITIS

Although a typical clinical picture of ulcerative colitis can be described, there is a wide range of presentation, from mild abdominal cramping with frequent, small-volume bowel movements to profuse diarrhea. Most patients with ulcerative colitis experience intermittent bouts of illness after varying intervals with no symptoms. Only a small percentage of patients have continuous unremitting symptoms or have a single acute attack with no subsequent symptoms.

Complex disease classifications are generally not used in clinical practice for ulcerative colitis. The arbitrarily determined distinctions of mild, moderate, and severe disease activity are generally used, and these are determined largely by clinical signs and symptoms.[5]

- **Mild**—Less than four stools daily, with or without blood, with no systemic disturbance and a normal erythrocyte sedimentation rate (ESR).
- **Moderate**—More than four stools per day but with minimal systemic disturbance.
- **Severe**—More than six stools per day with blood, with evidence of systemic disturbance as shown by fever, tachycardia, anemia, or ESR of more than 30.

It is also important to determine disease extent; that is, which part of the colon is involved—rectum, descending colon only, or the entire colon.

Two-thirds of patients with ulcerative colitis have mild disease, which almost always starts in the rectum. Occasionally, the mild form may progress to severe disease, which may be called "fulminant" if it occurs acutely. Systemic signs and symptoms of the disease (e.g., arthritis, uveitis, pyoderma gangrenosum) may be present in these patients and, in fact, may be the reason the patient seeks medical attention. Patients with mild disease are believed to be at lower risk of colon cancer. Moderate disease is observed in one-fourth of patients.

With severe disease, the patient is usually found to be in acute distress, has profuse bloody diarrhea, and often has a high fever with leukocytosis and hypoalbuminemia. Often, the patient is dehydrated and, therefore, may be tachycardic and hypotensive. This presentation may have a sudden onset with rapid progression.

The diagnosis of ulcerative colitis is made on clinical suspicion and confirmed by biopsy, stool examinations, sigmoidoscopy or colonoscopy, or barium radiographic contrast studies. The presence of extracolonic manifestations such as arthritis, uveitis, and pyoderma gangrenosum may also aid in establishing the diagnosis.

CROHN'S DISEASE

As with ulcerative colitis, the presentation of Crohn's disease is highly variable. A single episode may not be followed by further episodes, or the patient may experience continuous, unremitting disease. The time between the onset of complaints and the initial diagnosis may be as long as 3 years. The patient typically presents with diarrhea and abdominal pain. Hematochezia occurs in about one-half of the patients with colonic involvement and much less frequently when there is no colonic involvement. Commonly, a patient may first present with a perirectal or perianal lesion. The diagnosis should also be suspected in children with growth retardation, especially with abdominal complaints.

The course of Crohn's disease is characterized by periods of remission and exacerbation. Some patients may be free of symptoms for years, while others experience chronic problems in spite of medical therapy. Nearly all patients have a recurrence of Crohn's disease within 10 years of the initial episode.[12] As with ulcerative colitis, the diagnosis of Crohn's disease involves a thorough evaluation using laboratory, endoscopic, and radiologic testing to detect the extent and characteristic features of the disease. Because of similarities that may exist between ulcerative colitis and Crohn's disease confined to the colon, a definitive diagnosis cannot be made in up to 15% of cases, even with pathologic specimens in hand. Small bowel involvement and strictures detected on radiographs are characteristic of Crohn's disease.

► TREATMENT: Inflammatory Bowel Disease

DESIRED OUTCOME

To treat IBD properly, the clinician must have a clear concept of realistic therapeutic goals for each patient. These goals may relate to resolution of acute inflammatory processes; resolution of attendant complications (e.g., fistulas, abscesses); alleviation of systemic manifestations (e.g., arthritis); maintenance of remission from acute inflammation; or surgical palliation or cure. The approach to the therapeutic regimen differs considerably with varying goals as well as with the two diseases, ulcerative colitis and Crohn's disease.

When determining goals of therapy and selecting therapeutic regimens it is important to understand the natural history of IBD.[35] Some cases of acute ulcerative colitis are self-limited. With mild to moderate acute colitis, without systemic symptoms, 20% of patients may experience spontaneous improvement in their disease within a few weeks; however, a small percentage of patients may go on to experience more serious disease. With severe colitis, improvement without treatment cannot be expected. For instance, the response to medical management of toxic megacolon is variable and emergent colectomy may be required. When remission of ulcerative colitis is achieved, it is likely to last at least 1 year with medical therapy. In the absence of medical therapy, one-half to two-thirds of patients are likely to relapse within 9 months.[35] In some reports, remission rates with placebo have approached those found with active treatment.

A considerable number of patients with active Crohn's disease may achieve at least temporary remission without drug therapy. In two large trials, 26% and 42% of ambulatory patients on placebo achieved remission.[36,37] Once remission is achieved, two-thirds to three-fourths of patients remain in remission up to 2 years without drug therapy.[35] The implication of these data is that up to 40% of patients with active Crohn's disease improve in 3 months to 4 months with observation alone, and that most patients remain in remission for prolonged periods without medical intervention. These observations apply more to mild or moderate disease than to severe disease.

GENERAL APPROACH TO TREATMENT

Treatment of IBD centers on agents used to relieve the inflammatory process. Salicylates, corticosteroids, antimicrobials, and immunosuppressive agents such as azathioprine and mercaptopurine are commonly used to treat active disease and, for some agents, to lengthen the time of disease remission.

In addition to the use of drugs, surgical procedures are sometimes performed when active disease is inadequately controlled or when the required drug dosages pose an unacceptable risk of adverse effects. For most patients with IBD, nutritional considerations are also important, because these patients are often malnourished. Finally, a variety of therapies may be used to address complications or symptoms of IBD. For example, antidiarrheals may be used in some patients, although these are generally to be avoided in severe ulcerative colitis because they may contribute to the development of toxic colonic dilatation. Antimicrobial agents may be used in conjunction with drainage when abscesses are present. Iron may be required, particularly with ulcerative colitis, where blood loss from the colon can be significant.

NONPHARMACOLOGIC THERAPY

NUTRITIONAL SUPPORT

Proper nutritional support is an important aspect of the treatment of patients with IBD, not because specific types of diets are useful in alleviating the inflammatory conditions, but because patients with moderate to severe disease are often malnourished either because the inflammatory process results in significant malabsorption or maldigestion, or because of the catabolic effects of the disease process. Malabsorption may occur in the patient with Crohn's disease with inflammatory involvement of the small bowel, where many nutrients are absorbed, as well as in patients who have undergone multiple small bowel resections with subsequent reduction in absorptive surface ("short gut"). Maldigestion can occur if there is a bile salt deficiency in the gut.

A number of specific diets have been tried in attempts to improve the condition of patients with IBD, but none has gained widespread acceptance. With each individual it is helpful to eliminate specific foods that exacerbate symptoms. This elimination process must be conducted cautiously, as patients have been known to exclude a wide range of nutritious products without adequate justification. Some patients with IBD, although not the majority, have lactase deficiency; therefore, diarrhea may be associated with milk intake. In these patients, avoidance of milk or supplementation with lactase generally improves the patient's symptoms.

Dietary supplementation with fish oil has been proposed to treat IBD. In one placebo-controlled trial, patients with active ulcerative colitis were treated with fish oil supplementation for 4 months and had significant improvements in histologic findings and weight gain.[38] In another trial, 2.7 g/d of fish oil was effective in reducing the rate of relapse in Crohn's disease.[39] Fish oil contains eicosapentaenoic acid, which is metabolized by lipoxygenase and cyclooxygenase (similar to arachidonic acid), and results in lower production of leukotriene B_4 and prostaglandin E_2, which are believed to be important mediators in IBD.

The nutritional needs of the majority of patients can be adequately addressed with enteral supplementation.[40] Patients who have severe disease may require a course of parenteral nutrition to attain a reasonable nutritional status or in preparation for surgery. In one report of patients with severe acute ulcerative colitis, enteral nutrition resulted in a significantly greater increase in serum albumin, fewer adverse effects related to the nutritional regimen, and fewer postoperative infections, as compared to isocaloric, isonitrogenous parenteral nutrition. The regimens were similar with regard to remission rate and the need for colectomy.[41] Consideration should be given to lipid administration for its caloric value as well as in recognition of depleted peripheral fat stores in many IBD patients and the greater potential for fatty acid deficiency.

Parenteral nutrition is an important component of the treatment of severe Crohn's disease or ulcerative colitis. The use of parenteral nutrition allows complete bowel rest in patients with severe ulcerative colitis, which may alter the need for proctocolectomy. Parenteral nutrition has also been valuable in Crohn's disease, because remission may be achieved with parenteral nutrition in about 50% of patients.[42] In some patients, the disease may worsen when parenteral nutrition is stopped. Patients with enterocutaneous fistulas of various etiologies benefit from parenteral nutrition.[42] Parenteral nutrition may also be valuable in children or adolescents with growth retardation associated with Crohn's disease, but surgery is often necessary with severe disease. Finally, when possible, home parenteral nutrition should be used for patients requiring long-term therapy, particularly those with "short gut" as a consequence of surgical resection.

SURGERY

Surgical procedures have an established place in the treatment of IBD. Although surgery (proctocolectomy) is curative for ulcerative colitis, this is not the case for Crohn's disease. Surgical procedures involve resection of segments of intestine that are affected, as well as correction of complications (e.g., fistulas) or drainage of abscesses.

For ulcerative colitis, colectomy may be performed when the patient has disease uncontrolled by maximum medical therapy or when there are complications of the disease such as colonic perforation, toxic dilatation (megacolon), uncontrolled colonic hemorrhage, or colonic strictures. Colectomy may be indicated in patients with long-standing disease (greater than 8 years to 10 years), as a prophylactic measure against the development of cancer, and in patients with premalignant changes (severe dysplasia) on surveillance mucosal biopsies. The most common surgical procedures include proctocolectomy, after which the patient is left with a permanent ileostomy, and abdominal colectomy, with removal of the mucosa of the rectum and anastomosis of an ileal pouch to the anus (ileoanal pull-through). The risk from surgery in these patients is relatively low if the operations are performed on a nonemergent basis.

The indications for surgery with Crohn's disease are not as well established as for ulcerative colitis, and surgery is usually reserved for the complications of the disease. A recognized problem with intestinal resection for Crohn's disease is the high recurrence rate. Surgery may be appropriate in well-selected patients who are documented to continue to have severe or incapacitating disease or obstruction in spite of aggressive medical management. The surgical procedures performed include resections of the major intestinal areas of involvement. In some patients with severe rectal or perineal disease, diversion of the fecal stream is performed with a colostomy. Other indications for surgery include the finding of colon cancer, an inflammatory mass, or intestinal perforations.

PHARMACOLOGIC THERAPY

Drug therapy plays an integral part in the overall treatment of IBD. None of the drugs used for IBD is curative; at best they serve to control the disease process. Therefore, a reasonable goal of drug therapy is resolution of disease symptoms such that the patient can carry on normal daily functions. The major types of drug therapy used in IBD include aminosalicylates; corticosteroids; immunosuppressive agents (azathioprine, mercaptopurine, cyclosporine, and methotrexate); antimicrobials (metronidazole); and agents to inhibit TNFα (anti-TNFα antibodies or soluble TNFα-receptor fusion proteins).

Sulfasalazine, an agent that combines a sulfonamide (sulfapyridine) antibiotic and mesalamine (5-ASA) in the same molecule, has been used for many years to treat IBD but was originally intended to treat arthritis. Sulfasalazine is cleaved by gut bacteria in the colon to sulfapyridine (which is mostly reabsorbed and excreted in the urine) and mesalamine (which mostly remains in the colon and is excreted in stool).[43]

The active component of sulfasalazine is mesalamine.[43] The mechanism of action of mesalamine is not well understood. Cyclooxygenase or lipoxygenase inhibition alone do not account for the agent's effects. Aminosalicylates may inhibit macrophage production of cyclooxygenase, thromboxane synthetase, platelet-activating factor synthetase, and interleukin-1.[44] An alternative theory suggests that mesalamine acts as a superoxide-free radical scavenger.[45]

Because the mechanism of action of sulfasalazine is not related to the sulfapyridine component and since sulfapyridine is believed responsible for many of the adverse reactions to sulfasalazine, mesalamine alone can be used. Mesalamine can be used topically as an enema for the treatment of proctitis or given orally in delayed-release formulations that deliver mesalamine to the small intestine and colon (Table 34–3, Fig. 34–1). Olsalazine is a dimer of two 5-aminosalicylate molecules linked by an azo bond. Mesalamine is released in the colon after colonic bacteria cleave olsalazine. Bisalazide is a mesalamine prodrug that is enzymatically cleaved in the colon to produce mesalamine. The recommended daily doses of the oral mesalamine derivatives are intended to approximate the molar equivalent of mesalamine present in 4 g of sulfasalazine. At present, sulfasalazine is used in preference to oral mesalamine derivatives, mainly because it costs much less. However, it is often not tolerated as well as the mesalamine alternatives. Because the oral mesalamine formulations are coated tablets or granules, they should not be crushed or chewed.

Corticosteroids and adrenocorticotropic hormone (ACTH) have been widely used for the treatment of ulcerative colitis and Crohn's disease. There is a long-standing controversy as to the relative merits of corticosteroids versus ACTH; however, most clinicians

TABLE 34–3. Mesalamine Derivatives for Treatment of Inflammatory Bowel Disease

Product	Trade Name(s)	Formulation	Dose/Day	Site of Action
Sulfasalazine	Azulfidine	Tablet	4–6 g	Colon
Mesalamine	Rowasa, Salofalk, Claversal, Pentasa	Enema	1–4 g	Rectum, terminal, colon
	Asacol	Mesalamine tablet coated with Eudragit-S (delayed-release acrylic resin)	2.4–4.8 g	Distal ileum and colon
	Pentasa	Mesalamine capsules encapsulated in ethylcellulose microgranules	2–4 g	Small bowel and colon
Olsalazine	Dipentum	Dimer of 5-ASA oral capsule	1.5–3 g	Colon
Balsalazide	Colazal	Capsule	6.75 g	Colon

prefer corticosteroids. ACTH may be more effective in patients who have not previously received steroids (steroid-naive patients).[46] Although ACTH is administered parenterally, corticosteroids may be given parenterally, orally, or rectally. The exact mechanism of action of corticosteroids is not known but is believed to involve modulation of the immune system and inhibition of production of cytokines and mediators. It is not clear whether the most important steroid effects are systemic or local (mucosal). Budesonide is gaining attention as a steroid with reduced systemic effects when given by the oral route.

Immunosuppressive agents such as azathioprine and mercaptopurine (a metabolite of azathioprine) or cyclosporine are sometimes used for the treatment of IBD.[47] Azathioprine and mercaptopurine are effective for long-term treatment of Crohn's disease and ulcerative colitis.[48] These agents are generally reserved for patients who are refractory to steroids, and they may be associated with serious adverse effects such as lymphomas, pancreatitis, or nephrotoxicity. The agents are usually used in conjunction with mesalamine derivatives and/or steroids, and must be used for long periods of time (up to 6 months) before benefits may be observed.[49] Remission can be prolonged by azathioprine in steroid-dependent patients with ulcerative colitis.[50] Cyclosporine has also been of short-term benefit in treatment of acute, severe ulcerative colitis when used in a continuous intravenous infusion. Oral doses are ineffective. The agent poses risk of nephrotoxicity and neurotoxicity.

Antimicrobial agents, particularly metronidazole, are frequently used in attempts to control Crohn's disease. Metronidazole is of value in some patients with active Crohn's disease, particularly involving the perineal area or fistulas.[51] The mechanism of metronidazole's effect on Crohn's disease has not been determined but is theorized to relate to interruption of a bacterial role in the inflammatory process. Ciprofloxacin has also been used for treatment of IBD.

Two products inhibit the inflammatory effects of TNFα in the gut. Infliximab is an IgG_1 chimeric monoclonal antibody that binds TNFα, and etanercept is a soluble TNFα-receptor Fc fusion protein that blocks TNFα interaction with cell receptors. Both agents are useful for steroid-dependent or fistulizing disease, but the cost far exceeds other regimens.

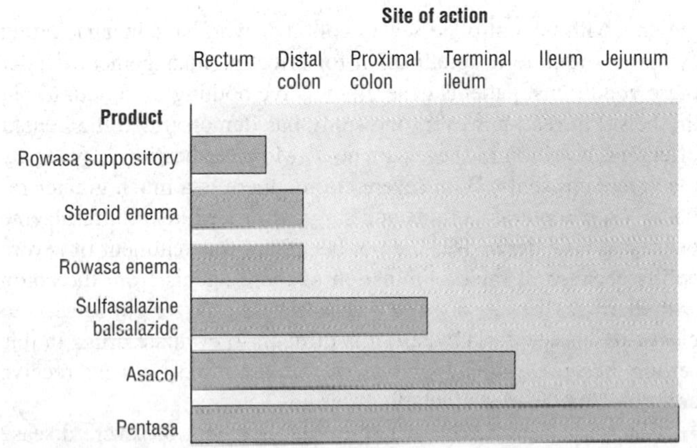

FIGURE 34–1. Site of activity of various agents to treat inflammatory bowel disease.

ULCERATIVE COLITIS

Mild to Moderate Disease

Most patients with active ulcerative colitis have mild to moderate disease and do not require parenteral medications (Fig. 34–2). The first line of drug therapy for these patients is oral sulfasalazine or an oral mesalamine derivative, or, topical mesalamine or steroids for distal disease.[52] When given orally, usually 4 g/d, and up to 8 g/d, of sulfasalazine is required to attain control of active inflammation. There does not appear to be an increased rate of response with increased dosage over 4 g/d, although side effects increase. Even with the use of adequate doses, patient improvement usually takes 2 weeks to 3 weeks, and sometimes longer. The dosage of sulfasalazine that can be given is usually limited by the patient's tolerance of the agent; most adverse effects of sulfasalazine are dose related (GI disturbances, headache, arthralgia).[49] Sulfasalazine therapy should be instituted at 500 mg/d and increased every few days up to 4 g or the maximum tolerated. It should not be used in patients with allergy to sulfa drugs.

Oral mesalamine derivatives (such as those listed in Table 34–3) are reasonable alternatives to sulfasalazine for treatment of ulcerative colitis. Most of these agents are effective for ulcerative colitis, but are no more effective than sulfasalazine.[53] The majority of patients intolerant to sulfasalazine should tolerate one of the other oral mesalamine derivatives. Olsalazine (a dimer of 5-ASA, given orally) is effective for treatment of mild to moderate ulcerative colitis. Of patients taking olsalazine, however, 15% to 25% experience severe diarrhea, often necessitating discontinuation of the drug. This results from a direct osmotic effect of the drug to induce small bowel fluid secretion. For this reason, it is not the drug of first choice. In some patients, combined use of oral sulfasalazine, Pentasa, or olsalazine and rectal steroids or rectal 5-ASA may provide benefits.[54]

Steroids have a place in the treatment of moderate to severe ulcerative colitis. Oral steroids (usually up to 1 mg/kg/d of prednisone equivalent) may be used for patients who do not have an adequate response to sulfasalazine or mesalamine. Prednisone dosages in the

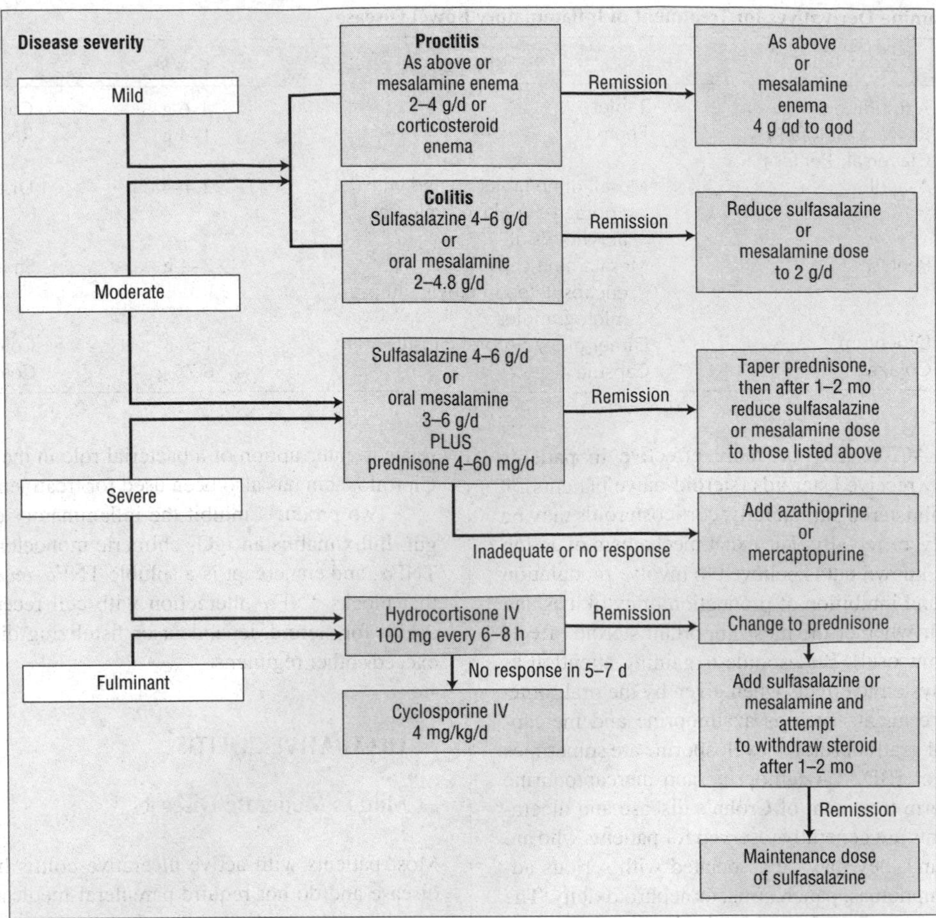

FIGURE 34–2. Treatment approaches for ulcerative colitis.

range of 40–60 mg/d have been superior to regimens of 20 mg/d in inducing remission.[55] Overall, steroids and sulfasalazine appear to be equally efficacious; however, the response to steroids may be evident sooner. The use of oral steroids as initial therapy for mild to moderate ulcerative colitis should be avoided, mainly because of the known risks of steroid use. If steroids are used to attain remission, tapered drug withdrawal should be accomplished to minimize long-term steroid exposure.

Rectally administered steroids or mesalamine can be used as initial therapy for patients with ulcerative proctitis or distal colitis. Rectal agents are also beneficial for treatment of tenesmus. With these agents, local actions are believed to be responsible for drug effects. Rectal steroids are effective in the treatment of active, distal ulcerative colitis. However, rectal mesalamine is more effective than rectal steroids for inducing remission.[56,57]

The choice of rectally administered steroid is a subject of debate as there is varying potential for systemic steroid absorption with different products. Although many steroids have been administered rectally, certain agents such as betamethasone-17-valerate, beclomethasone dipropionate, prednisolone metasulfobenzoate, prednisolone-21-phosphate, and budesonide have been used in attempts to reduce systemic steroid effects. Systemic side effects may be the least severe with beclomethasone dipropionate, because the gut wall and liver rapidly metabolize this agent.[56] Most patients do not experience adrenal suppression from rectal steroids. The use of rectal steroids may often result in reduction of the required oral dose.

Nicotine has been proposed as a treatment for ulcerative colitis (but not as a treatment for Crohn's disease) based on the observation of the onset of a flare of ulcerative colitis after smoking cessation in some individuals. Transdermal nicotine, when used in the highest tolerated dose, improved symptoms of patients with mild to moderate, active ulcerative colitis.[58]

Severe or Intractable Disease

Patients with uncontrolled severe colitis or who have incapacitating symptoms require hospitalization for effective management. Under these conditions, patients generally receive nothing by mouth to put the bowel at rest; however, one study has demonstrated the benefit of enteral nutrition in these patients.[41] Most medication is given by the parenteral route. With severe colitis, there is a much greater reliance on parenteral steroids and surgical procedures. Sulfasalazine or mesalamine derivatives are not beneficial for treatment of severe colitis because of rapid elimination of these agents from the colon with diarrhea, thereby not allowing sufficient time for gut bacteria to cleave the molecules. Overall, it is difficult to evaluate drugs in this setting, because patients with severe disease almost always receive additional medications including steroids.

Steroids have been valuable in the treatment of severe disease because the use of these agents may allow some patients to avoid colectomy. A trial of steroids is warranted in most patients before proceeding to colectomy, unless the condition is grave or rapidly deteriorating. The dose of steroid generally used is 1 mg/kg of prednisone equivalent daily (up to 60 mg/d), although some patients may require much less or much more for satisfactory control. With higher doses, however, steroid side effects may limit drug benefits. The length of the medical trial before consideration of surgery is open to debate. Steroids increase surgical risk, particularly infectious risk, if an operation is required later. After a colectomy is performed, steroids should no longer be required for the disease; however, they must be withdrawn gradually (usually over 3–4 weeks) to avoid hypoadrenal crisis due to adrenal suppression.

A major development in the treatment of severe ulcerative colitis refractory to steroids has been intravenous cyclosporine.[59–61] Continuous intravenous infusion of cyclosporine (4 mg/kg/d) was rapidly effective in steroid-resistant, acute, severe ulcerative colitis and reduced the need for emergent colectomy.[62] Intravenous cyclosporine is recommended for all patients with acute, severe, active ulcerative colitis refractory to steroids.[63]

Maintenance of Remission

After remission from active disease is achieved, the goal of therapy is to maintain remission. The major agents used for maintenance of remission are sulfasalazine and the mesalamine derivatives; steroids do not have a role. The value of sulfasalazine in preventing recurrences has been documented in placebo-controlled trials. One-fourth of patients taking sulfasalazine (2 g/d) had a relapse within 1 year, while three-fourths of patients taking placebo had a relapse.[64]

Olsalazine, Pentasa (a slow-release oral form of mesalamine), and mesalamine enema are also effective for maintaining remission in patients with ulcerative colitis. Pentasa, given 500 mg three times daily, was as effective as sulfasalazine, given 1 g three times daily, in maintaining remission (54% vs 46% in remission at 12 months, respectively).[65] Mesalamine (Asacol), 0.8 or 1.6 g daily, was found effective for prevention of relapses over a 6-month period.[66]

A major question about the use of sulfasalazine for maintenance of remission with ulcerative colitis is the duration of the preventive regimen. Maintenance of remission has been well documented up to 1 year and may last as long as 3 years. The efficacy of sulfasalazine appears to be related to the dose administered, up to a point. Although 4 g/d has a lower recurrence rate than 2 g or 1 g, a 4-g dose will result in intolerable side effects in about one-fourth of patients. Therefore 2 g/d is recommended.

Steroids do not have a role in the maintenance of remission with ulcerative colitis because they are ineffective.[49] Steroids should be gradually withdrawn after remission is induced (over 3–4 weeks). If they are continued, the patient will be exposed to steroid side effects without likelihood of benefits. For patients who require chronic steroid use (>20 mg/d), there is a strong justification for alternative therapies or colectomy. Azathioprine is effective in preventing relapse of ulcerative colitis for periods of up to 2 years.[67] However, 3 months to 6 months may be required before beneficial effects are noted. Oral azathioprine also maintains long-term remission after IV cyclosporine induction.[68]

CROHN'S DISEASE

Management of Crohn's disease often proves more difficult than management of ulcerative colitis, partly because of the greater complexity of presentation with Crohn's disease (Fig. 34–3). The disease may be found to involve any segment of the GI tract, from mouth to anus, and may involve other visceral structures and soft tissues through fistulization. There is a greater reliance on drug therapy with Crohn's disease, because resection of all involved intestine may not be possible and disease recurrence after surgery is common.

Active Crohn's Disease

The goal of treatment for active Crohn's disease is to achieve remission; however, in many patients, reduction of symptoms so that the patient may carry out normal activities, or reduction of the steroid

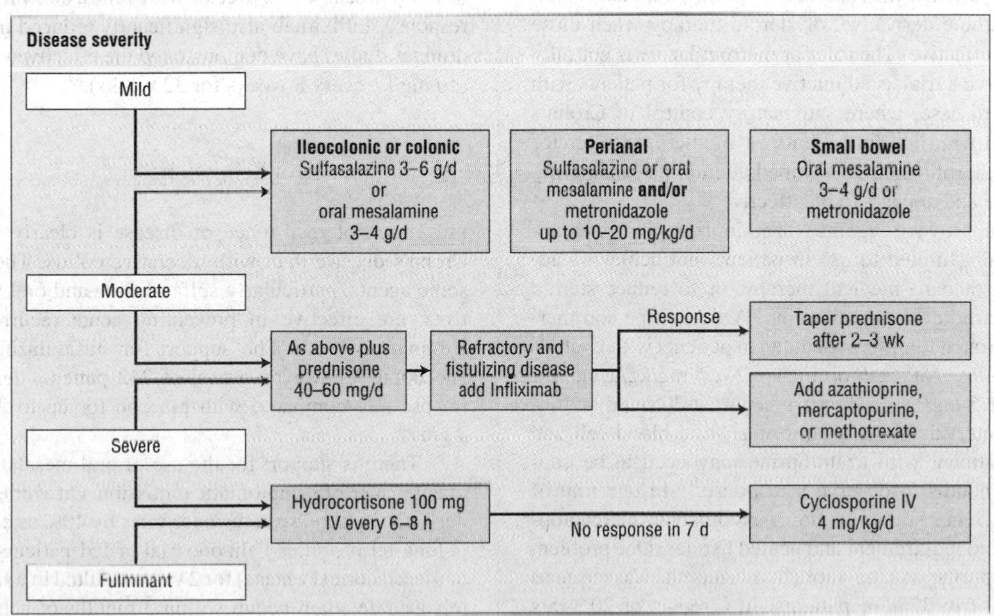

FIGURE 34–3. Treatment approaches for Crohn's disease.

dose required for control, is a significant accomplishment. In the majority of patients, active Crohn's disease is treated with sulfasalazine, mesalamine derivatives, or steroids, although azathioprine, mercaptopurine, methotrexate, or metronidazole are frequently used.

The role of sulfasalazine in the treatment of active Crohn's disease is not as well established as its role in the treatment of ulcerative colitis. Sulfasalazine is more effective when Crohn's disease involves the colon.[36] In these circumstances, sulfasalazine is as effective as prednisone.[36,69] It appears reasonable to initiate a trial of sulfasalazine or oral mesalamine derivative in patients with mild to moderate Crohn's disease, particularly when the colon is involved.

There is limited information also suggesting the benefit of sulfasalazine in ileal Crohn's disease.[70] Other mesalamine derivatives (such as Pentasa or Asacol) that release mesalamine in the small bowel may be more effective than sulfasalazine for ileal involvement. In a trial of 310 patients with active Crohn's disease, Pentasa alone was more effective than placebo in achieving remission in a 16-week trial (43% vs 18%, respectively).[71] This beneficial effect was dose dependent and greatest with a dose of 4 g/d. A course of steroids is appropriate in patients who cannot be controlled with mesalamine. When a patient is maintained on steroids, however, there appears to be no benefit from the addition of sulfasalazine.

Steroids are frequently used for the treatment of active Crohn's disease, particularly with more severe presentations. In the National Cooperative Crohn's Disease Study,[36] prednisone was more effective than placebo in achieving remission (60% remission rate after 17 weeks vs a 30% remission rate for placebo). In this trial, the prednisone doses were 0.25 mg/kg/d for mild disease, 0.5 mg/kg/d for moderate disease, and 0.75 mg/kg/d for severe disease. Prednisone was effective for disease limited to the small bowel. The major limitation of steroids is the risk of adverse effects with long-term use.

Steroids are preferred for treatment of severe Crohn's disease, mainly because these agents can be given parenterally and response to therapy may occur sooner than with other agents. Once remission is achieved, however, it may prove difficult to reduce steroid dosage without a flare of active disease.[44]

Metronidazole (given orally up to 20 mg/kg/d in divided doses) may be useful in some patients with Crohn's disease, particularly in patients with colonic involvement, or in those patients with perineal disease.[51] For most patients, metronidazole would be added to sulfasalazine, a mesalamine derivative, or steroid therapy when those agents alone are not effective. The role for metronidazole is not fully defined. It may deserve a trial as adjunctive therapy for patients with colonic or perineal disease, where satisfactory control of Crohn's disease is not gained with first-line agents, or in attempts to reduce steroid dosage.[38,72] Ciprofloxacin has gained attention as an alternative to metronidazole and appears to be effective.[73]

The immunosuppressive agents (azathioprine and mercaptopurine) are generally limited to use in patients not achieving adequate response to standard medical therapy, or to reduce steroid doses when high steroid doses are required. Azathioprine and mercaptopurine demonstrated long-term benefits in patients with Crohn's disease.[48] The usual doses of azathioprine are 2–2.5 mg/kg/d, and for mercaptopurine, 1–1.5 mg/kg/d. They are begun at 50 mg/d and increased at 2-week intervals while monitoring white blood cell and platelet counts. Treatment with azathioprine may need to be continued for up to 6 months to observe a response.[49] In one trial of patients already receiving sulfasalazine or prednisone, mercaptopurine decreased steroid requirement and healed fistulas. One problem noted with mercaptopurine was that more than 3 months was required to observe a response in 32% of patients. In a report of 20 years of experience with 148 patients, mercaptopurine (50 mg/d, mean 34 months) was judged effective for reduction of steroid dosage or elimination of the need for steroids, healing of fistulas and abscesses, and healing of Crohn's disease of the stomach and duodenum.[74] Some investigators have suggested that azathioprine or mercaptopurine should be started earlier in the course of treatment than has been traditional. Clinical response to mercaptopurine is related to whole-blood concentrations of the metabolite 6-thioguanine, and hepatotoxicity is correlated with another metabolite, 6-methylmercaptopurine.[75] Metabolic inactivation of azathioprine and mercaptopurine occurs by thiopurine S-methyltransferase, which exhibits genetic polymorphism. Enzyme-deficient patients are at greater risk of hepatotoxicity from these agents.[76] Determination of enzyme activity may be necessary to determine which patients require lower doses of these agents.

Cyclosporine has also demonstrated benefit in active Crohn's disease.[59,60] Improvement was noted with cyclosporine in patients who were resistant or intolerant to corticosteroids.[77] In one study, approximately 80% of patients with refractory fistulas responded to intravenous cyclosporine (4 mg/kg/d) within a mean of 7.9 days.[78] The dose of cyclosporine is important in determining efficacy. An oral dose of 5 mg/kg/d was ineffective,[79] whereas 7.9 mg/kg/d was effective.[77] However, toxic effects limit application of the higher dosage. At present, the therapeutic blood or plasma concentration range for cyclosporine has not been established for Crohn's disease, but whole-blood trough concentrations of 200–800 ng/mL (by monoclonal RIA) or 200–400 ng/mL (by high-performance liquid chromatography) have been recommended.[3] When using cyclosporine, however, clinicians should recognize the accompanying long-term risk of renal toxicity as well as the potential for drug interactions.

Methotrexate given as a weekly injection of 25 mg has demonstrated corticosteroid-sparing effects.[80,81] Also, it can induce remission in patients with refractory IBD.[82] It is not clear whether the benefit of methotrexate surpasses the risks (bone marrow suppression, hepatotoxicity, pulmonary toxicity).

Anti-TNFα strategies are gaining interest for treating refractory or fistulizing Crohn's disease. A 5 mg/kg single infusion of infliximab resulted in clinical improvement in 80% of patients with chronic Crohn's disease who were receiving steroids.[83] The benefit lasted 8 weeks to 12 weeks with reinfusion producing a sustained response. Infliximab also significantly reduced fistula drainage. Additional studies have demonstrated the effectiveness of long-term use (10 mg/kg every 8 weeks for 32 weeks).[84]

Maintenance of Remission

Prevention of recurrence of disease is clearly more difficult with Crohn's disease than with ulcerative colitis. There is evidence that some agents, particularly sulfasalazine and oral mesalamine derivatives, are effective in preventing acute recurrences in quiescent Crohn's disease.[85] The support for sulfasalazine has been largely anecdotal;[85] however, a trial of 232 patients demonstrated a lower relapse rate compared with placebo for up to 2 years when given 3 g/d.[86]

There is support for the use of oral mesalamine derivatives for maintenance of symptomatic remission. On average, oral mesalamine derivatives decrease recurrence rates by 40% as compared to placebo in long-term studies.[79] In one trial of 161 patients in remission, 2 g/d of mesalamine (Pentasa) for 2 years resulted in a significantly reduced relapse rate when begun within 3 months of achieving remission.[87] In another trial of mesalamine (Asacol), 125 patients received 2.4 g/d or placebo for 12 months, resulting in a significantly reduced relapse rate with Asacol.[88] Steroids also have no place in the prevention of recurrence of Crohn's disease; these agents do not appear to alter the long-term course of the disease. However, a study of oral budesonide 6 mg/d demonstrated prolongation of time to relapse in ileal and ileocecal disease.[89]

Azathioprine has been studied as an adjunctive agent for the treatment and prevention of Crohn's disease. Although the published data are inconsistent, there is evidence to suggest that azathioprine and mercaptopurine are effective in maintaining remission in Crohn's disease.[49,50] This agent should be reserved for patients who cannot tolerate dosages of steroids required to control their disease and who are not good surgical candidates.

SELECTED COMPLICATIONS

TOXIC MEGACOLON

Toxic megacolon or "toxic colonic dilatation" is a serious complication of IBD that occurs in about 1% or 2% of patients with IBDs, particularly ulcerative colitis. As previously described, the patient with toxic megacolon is usually severely ill with fever, abdominal pain and distention, and decreased bowel sounds; has bloody diarrhea; and is often dehydrated. Immediate and aggressive measures are required to minimize mortality.

The treatment required for toxic megacolon includes general supportive measures to maintain vital functions, consideration for early surgical intervention, and drugs (steroids, cyclosporine, and antimicrobials). Aggressive fluid and electrolyte management is required for dehydration. Fluids and electrolytes may be lost through vomiting, diarrhea, and nasogastric intubation, as well as through fluid accumulation in the bowel. When the patient has lost significant amounts of blood (through the rectum), blood replacement is also necessary. Opiates and anticholinergics should be discontinued because these agents enhance colonic dilatation, thereby increasing the risk of bowel perforation. Broad-spectrum antimicrobials that include coverage for gram-negative bacilli and intestinal anaerobes should be used.

Steroids in high dosages should be administered intravenously to reduce acute inflammation. Doses as high as 2 mg/kg/d of prednisone equivalent have been recommended (generally administered as hydrocortisone).[5] The duration of steroid administration is not certain; however, most clinicians continue the high-dose steroids for up to 2 weeks after improvement is observed and then reduce the dosages (approximately 0.5–1 mg/kg/d) for a few additional weeks. Antimicrobial regimens that are effective against enteric aerobes and anaerobes (e.g., aminoglycoside with clindamycin or metronidazole, imipenem, or extended-spectrum penicillin with β-lactamase inhibitor) should be administered from the time of diagnosis and continued until patient improvement is assured. The duration of the antimicrobial regimen (often 2–3 weeks) should be determined with consideration that there may be significant intra-abdominal contamination with signs and symptoms hidden by steroid effects.

Surgical intervention, mainly an abdominal colectomy with formation of an ileostomy, is an important consideration in patients with toxic megacolon and prevents death in some patients. Early surgical intervention in these patients may result in a reduced mortality rate. In most cases in which colectomy is performed in the face of toxic megacolon, there is a significant risk of operative complications, including postoperative infection.

SYSTEMIC MANIFESTATIONS

The common systemic manifestations of IBD include arthritis; anemia; skin manifestations such as erythema nodosum and pyoderma gangrenosum; uveitis; and liver disease. These problems may be related to the inflammatory process. For some of these manifestations, specific therapies can be instituted, whereas for others, the treatment that is used for the GI inflammatory process also addresses the systemic manifestations.

Anemia occurs when there is significant blood loss from the GI tract. If the patient can consume oral medication, ferrous sulfate should be administered. If the patient is unable to take oral medication and the patient's hematocrit is sufficiently low, blood transfusions may be required. Anemia may also be related to malabsorption of vitamin B_{12} or folic acid, so these may also be required.

There are no consistently recommended therapies for liver disease, skin manifestations, or uveitis associated with IBD. Some reports suggest that these manifestations are worse during exacerbations of the intestinal disease and that measures improving intestinal disease will improve these systemic manifestations. Unfortunately, this association has not been demonstrated consistently. Liver transplantation is being used more frequently for definitive treatment of primary sclerosing cholangitis. For arthritis associated with IBD, aspirin or another nonsteroidal anti-inflammatory drug (NSAID) may be beneficial, as might be steroids.

SPECIAL CONSIDERATIONS

PREGNANCY

Either the occurrence or consideration of pregnancy may cause significant concerns in the patient with IBD. Questions arise as to fertility in patients with IBD, the effect of pregnancy on the disease course, the effect of the disease on the outcome of pregnancy, and the effects of the drugs used in IBD on the fetus.[90]

Patients with IBD do not appear to be less fertile than women in general.[5,91] The rate of normal childbirth is similar to that for healthy populations. Some studies have noted, however, a greater risk of spontaneous abortions in patients with IBD. Also, there is a greater incidence of low-birth-weight infants in mothers with chronic idiopathic ulcerative colitis.[92] Pregnancy does not affect the course of IBD. Patients who are pregnant experience recurrence rates similar to those of nonpregnant females. Also, there is no justification for therapeutic abortion with IBD because termination of the pregnancy has not been observed to improve the disease. There is also unfounded concern that the drugs required to treat IBD may be teratogenic.

Steroids and sulfasalazine should be administered during pregnancy with the same guidelines that would be applied to the nonpregnant patient.[5,92] Steroids given systemically do not appear to be detrimental to the fetus. Sulfasalazine is generally well tolerated; however, there has been suggestion of increased frequency of congenital abnormalities when it is given during pregnancy.[93] Interestingly, sulfasalazine has also been reported to cause decreased sperm counts and reduced fertility in males.[94] This effect is reversible on discontinuation of the drug and it is not reported with mesalamine. Immunosuppressive drugs (azathioprine and mercaptopurine) may be associated with fetal deformities in humans; however, they have been used without detriment in some patients.[91] Metronidazole should not be used in those contemplating pregnancy as it may be teratogenic.

Overall, drug therapy for IBD is not a contraindication for pregnancy, and most pregnancies are well managed in patients with these diseases. The indications for medical and surgical treatment are similar to those in the nonpregnant patient. If a patient has an initial bout of IBD during pregnancy, a standard approach to treatment should be initiated.

Recommendations for use of drugs in nursing mothers vary. Although prednisone and prednisolone can be detected in breast milk, breast-feeding is believed to be safe for the infant when low doses of prednisone are used.[95] Sulfasalazine does not pose a risk of kernicterus, as levels of sulfapyridine in breast milk are low or undetectable. Metronidazole should not be given to nursing mothers because it is excreted into breast milk.[95]

ADVERSE EFFECTS

Drug intolerance often limits the usefulness of agents used to treat IBD. Many patients receiving sulfasalazine, mesalamine, corticosteroids, metronidazole, azathioprine, or mercaptopurine experience some undesired effects. In some cases, these adverse effects can be significant and require discontinuation of the therapy. Knowledge of the common or important adverse reactions will assist in avoiding or minimizing their effects.

Sulfasalazine is often associated with adverse drug effects and these effects may be classified as either dose related or idiosyncratic. Dose-related side effects usually include GI disturbances such as nausea, vomiting, diarrhea, or anorexia, but may also include headache and arthralgia.[44] These adverse reactions tend to occur more commonly on initiation of therapy and decrease in frequency as therapy is continued. Patients may experience these adverse effects at the commonly used dosages. One approach to the management of these reactions is to discontinue the agent for a short period and then reinstitute therapy at a reduced dosage. Some authors suggest that the rate of adverse effects may be related to the concentration of free sulfapyridine in serum, suggesting that the sulfa portion of the molecule is responsible for the adverse effects.[96] Folic acid absorption is impaired by sulfasalazine, which may lead to anemia. Patients receiving sulfasalazine should receive oral folic acid supplementation.

Adverse effects that are not dose related include, most commonly, rash, fever, or hepatotoxicity, as well as relatively uncommon but serious reactions such as bone marrow suppression, thrombocytopenia, pancreatitis, and hepatitis.[44] For most patients with idiosyncratic reactions, sulfasalazine must be discontinued. In some patients who have experienced allergic reactions to sulfasalazine, a desensitization procedure can be instituted. By gradually increasing sulfasalazine dosage over weeks to months, patient tolerance has been improved.[97] Most of the idiosyncratic reactions observed with sulfasalazine are similar to those with the class of sulfonamides in general.

Oral mesalamine derivatives may impose a lower frequency of adverse effects as compared to sulfasalazine. Many patients who are intolerant to sulfasalazine will tolerate oral mesalamine derivatives.[98] Olsalazine, however, may frequently (in as many as 25% of patients) cause watery diarrhea, sometimes requiring drug discontinuation.[99,100]

Adverse reactions to corticosteroids are well recognized and may occur when corticosteroids are used for any indication. There is a greater potential for adverse effects when corticosteroids are used for the treatment of IBD, however, because high doses must often be used for extended periods. In the National Cooperative Crohn's Disease Study, half of patients receiving high-dose steroid therapy experienced side effects, as did one-third of the patients on the lower-dose regimens for maintenance.[101] The well-appreciated adverse effects of corticosteroids include hyperglycemia; hypertension; osteoporosis; acne; fluid retention; electrolyte disturbances; myopathies; muscle wasting; increased appetite; psychosis; and reduced resistance to infection. In addition, corticosteroid use may cause adrenocortical suppression. Specific regimens for withdrawal of corticosteroid therapy have been suggested.[102] To minimize corticosteroid effects, clinicians have used alternate-day steroid therapy; however, some patients do not do well on the days when no steroid is given. For most patients, a single daily corticosteroid dose suffices, and divided daily doses are unnecessary.

Immunosuppressants such as azathioprine and mercaptopurine have a significant potential for adverse reactions. Azathioprine causes bone marrow suppression and has been associated with lymphomas (in renal transplant patients), skin cancer, and pancreatitis (about 3% of patients). Some investigators believe that induction of leukopenia may be necessary for therapeutic effect.[103] Mercaptopurine causes adverse reactions similar to azathioprine; however, there are fewer reports of lymphomas with this agent. Pancreatitis usually occurs within 1 month of initiating therapy with mercaptopurine, and recurs if the patient is rechallenged.[102] In one trial, 10% of patients who received azathioprine or mercaptopurine required discontinuation of treatment because of adverse effects.[104] Allopurinol inhibits the metabolism of mercaptopurine, and a dosage reduction of the latter is required when the two are used in combination.

Most patients receiving metronidazole for Crohn's disease tolerate the agent fairly well; however, mild adverse effects occur frequently. They commonly include paresthesias and reversible peripheral neuropathy, metallic taste, urticaria, and glossitis.[52,105] Other effects include a disulfiram-like reaction if alcohol is ingested in conjunction.

EVALUATION OF THERAPEUTIC OUTCOMES

The success of therapeutic regimens to treat IBD can be measured by patient-reported complaints, signs, and symptoms; by direct physician examination (including endoscopy); by history and physical examination; by selected laboratory tests; and by quality-of-life measures. Evaluation of IBD severity is difficult, because much of the assessment is subjective. To create more objective measures, disease rating scales or indices have been created. The Crohn's Disease Activity Index (CDAI) is a commonly used scale, particularly for evaluation of patients during clinical trials.[106] The scale incorporates eight elements: (a) number of stools in the past 7 days; (b) sum of abdominal pain ratings from the past 7 days; (c) rating of general well-being in the past 7 days; (d) use of antidiarrheals; (e) body weight; (f) hematocrit; (g) finding of abdominal mass; and (h) a sum of symptoms present in the past week. Elements of this index provide a guide for those measures that may be useful in assessing the effectiveness of treatment regimens.

Standardized assessment tools have also been constructed for ulcerative colitis.[27,107] Elements in these scales include (a) stool frequency; (b) presence of blood in the stool; (c) mucosal appearance (from endoscopy); and (d) physician's global assessment based on physical examination, endoscopy, and laboratory data.

Additional studies that are often useful include direct endoscopic examination of affected areas and/or radiocontrast studies. For patients with acute disease, assessment of fluid and electrolyte status is important, because these may be lost during diarrheal episodes. Other laboratory tests, such as serum albumin, transferrin, or other markers of visceral protein status, as well as markers of inflammation (erythrocyte sedimentation rate) may be used.

Assessment of the IBD patient must include consideration of adverse drug effects. Because many of the agents used have a relatively high probability of causing adverse effects, particularly corticosteroids and other immunosuppressive agents, patient assessment should include collection of history and physical and laboratory data that are necessary to prevent or recognize adverse drug effects.

Finally, a patient quality-of-life assessment should be performed regularly.[108] Agents that appear clinically equivalent may differ substantially in resulting quality of life. Inquiry should be made regarding general well being, emotional function, and social function. Social function may include assessment of the ability to perform routine daily functions, maintain occupational activities, sexual function, and recreation.

▶ PRINCIPLES OF PHARMACOTHERAPY

- The exact cause of inflammatory bowel disease is unknown, although there are components that appear to be infectious and other components that suggest immune dysregulation.
- Ulcerative colitis is confined to the rectum and colon, causes continuous lesions, and affects primarily the mucosa and the submucosa. Crohn's disease can involve any part of the GI tract, often causes discontinuous (skip) lesions, and is a transmural process that can result in fistulas, perforations, or strictures.
- Common complications of IBD include rectal fissures, fistulas (Crohn's disease), perirectal abscess (ulcerative colitis), and colon cancer, in addition to hepatobiliary complications, arthritis, uveitis, skin lesions (including erythema nodosum and pyoderma gangrenosum), and aphthous ulcerations of the mouth.
- The severity of ulcerative colitis may be assessed by factors such as stool frequency; presence of blood in stool; fever; pulse; hemoglobin; erythrocyte sedimentation rate; abdominal tenderness; and radiologic or endoscopic findings. The severity of Crohn's disease can be assessed by the Crohn's Disease Activity Index, which includes stool frequency, presence of blood in stool, endoscopic appearance, and physician's global assessment.
- The goals of treatment of IBD are resolution of acute inflammation and complications, alleviation of systemic manifestations, maintenance of remission, and, in some patients, surgical palliation or cure.
- The first line of treatment for mild to moderate ulcerative colitis or Crohn's colitis consists of oral sulfasalazine or mesalamine; mesalamine or steroid enemas may be used for rectosigmoid disease. Delayed-release oral formulations of mesalamine (Pentasa or Asacol) may be used for Crohn's ileitis.
- Corticosteroids are often required for acute ulcerative colitis or Crohn's disease. The duration of steroid use should be minimized and the dose tapered gradually over 3 weeks to 4 weeks.
- Intravenous continuous infusion cyclosporine is effective in treating severe colitis refractory to steroids.
- Sulfasalazine and mesalamine derivatives can prevent recurrence of acute disease in many patients, while steroids are ineffective for this purpose.
- Other drugs that are useful for treatment of Crohn's disease include metronidazole (for perineal disease), azathioprine or mercaptopurine (for inadequate response or to reduce steroid dosage), cyclosporine (for refractory disease), and infliximab for refractory or fistulizing disease.

REFERENCES

1. Kraft SC. Modern clinical aspects of inflammatory bowel disease. Radiol Clin North Am 1987;25:213–224.
2. Whelan G. Epidemiology of inflammatory bowel disease. Med Clin North Am 1990;74:1–12.
3. Andres PG, Friedman LS. Inflammatory bowel disease. Epidemiology and the natural causes of inflammatory bowel disease. Gastroenterol Clinica 1999;28:255–281.
4. Sandler RS. Epidemiology of inflammatory bowel disease. In: Targan SR, Shanahan F, eds. Inflammatory Bowel Disease: From Bench to Bedside. Baltimore, Williams & Wilkins, 1994:5–30.
5. Jewell DP. Ulcerative colitis. In: Feldman M, Scharcchmidt BF, Sleisenger MH, Klein S (eds.) Sleisenger & Fordtran's Gastrointestinal and Liver Disease, 6th ed. Orlando, FL, Saunders, 1998:1735–1761.
6. Russel MG, Stockbtugger RW. Epidemiology of inflammatory bowel disease. Scand J Gastroenterol 1996;31:417–427.
7. Pavli P, Cavanaugh J, Grimm M. Inflammatory bowel disease: Germs or genes? Lancet 1996;347:1198.
8. Kagnoff MF. Immunology and inflammation of the gastointestinal tract. In: Feldman M, Scharcchmidt BF, Sleisenger MH, Klein S, eds. Sleisenger & Fordtran's Gastrointestinal and Liver Disease, 6th ed. Orlando, FL, Saunders, 1998:38–39.
9. Shanahan F. Pathogenesis of ulcerative colitis. Lancet 1993;342:407–411.
10. MacDermott RP. Alterations of the mucosal immune system in inflammatory bowel disease. J Gastroenterol 1996;31:907–916.
11. Peters M, Nevens H, Baert F, et al. Familial aggregation in Crohn's disease: Increased age-adjusted risk and concordance in clinical characteristics. Gastroenterology 1996;111:597.
12. McKenzie SJ, Baker MS, Buffington GD, Doe WF. Evidence of oxidant-induced injury to epithelial cells during inflammatory bowel disease. J Clin Invest 1996;98:136–141.
13. Podolsky DK. Inflammatory bowel disease. Second of two parts. N Engl J Med 1991;325:1008–1015.
14. Yang H, Rotter JI. Genetics of inflammatory bowel disease. In: Targan SR, Shanahan F, eds. Inflammatory Bowel Disease: From Bench to Bedside. Baltimore, Williams & Wilkins, 1994:32–64.
15. Sandborn WJ, Landers CJ, Tremaine WJ, Targan BR. Association of antineutrophil cytoplasmic antibodies with resistance to treatment of left-sided ulcerative colitis: Results of a pilot study. Mayo Clin Proc 1996;71:431–436.
16. Sendid B, Colombel J, Jacquinot P, et al. Specific antibody responses to oligomannosidic epitopes in Crohn's disease. Clin Diagn Lab Immunol 1996;3:219–226.
17. Blumberg RS, Strober W. Prospects for research in inflammatory bowel disease. JAMA 2001;285:643–647.
18. Nielsen OH, Koppen T, Rudiger N, et al. Involvement of interleukin-4 and -10 in inflammatory bowel disease. Dig Dis Sci 1996;41:1786–1793.
19. Parronchi P, Romagnani P, Annunziato F, et al. Type 1 T-helper cell predominance and interleukin-12 expression in the gut of patients with Crohn's disease. Am J Pathol 1997;150:823–832.
20. Niesser M, Volk BA. Altered Th1/Th2 cytokine profiles in the intestinal mucosa of patients with inflammatory bowel disease as assessed by quantitative reversed transcribed polymerase chain reaction (RT-PCR). Clin Exp Immunol 1995;101:428–435.
21. Braegger CP, Nicholls S, Murch SH, et al. Tumour necrosis factor alpha in stool as a marker of intestinal inflammation. Lancet 1992;339:89–91.
22. Van Deventer SJH. Tumor necrosis factor and Crohn's disease. Gut 1997;40:443–448.

23. Talala AH, Drossman DP. Psychosocial factors in inflammatory bowel disease. Gastroenterol Clin North Am 1995;24:699–716.
24. Podolsky DK. Inflammatory bowel disease. First of two parts. N Engl J Med 1991;325:928–937.
25. Boyko ES, Koesell TD, Perera DR, Inui TS. Risk of ulcerative colitis among former and current cigarette smokers. N Engl J Med 1987;316: 707–710.
26. Calkins BM. A meta-analysis of the role of smoking in inflammatory bowel disease. Dig Dis Sci 1989;34:1841–1854.
27. Pullan RD, Rhodes J, Ganesh S, et al. Transdermal nicotine for active ulcerative colitis. N Engl J Med 1994;330:811–815.
28. Sandborn WJ, Tremaine WJ, Offord KP, et al. Transdermal nicotine for mildly to moderately active ulcerative colitis. Ann Intern Med 1997;126: 364–371.
29. Ramming KP. Diseases of the rectum and colon. In: Sabiston DC, ed. Essentials of Surgery. Philadelphia, Saunders, 1987:483.
30. Lichenstein JE. Radiologic-pathologic correlation of inflammatory bowel disease. Radiol Clin North Am 1987;25:3–24.
31. Monsen V, Sorstad J, Hellers G, et al. Extracolonic diagnosis in ulcerative colitis: An epidemiologic study. Am J Gastroenterol 1990;85:711–716.
32. Harmatz A. Hepatobiliary manifestations of inflammatory bowel disease. Med Clin North Am 1994;78:1387–1398.
33. Rankin GB. Extraintestinal and systemic manifestations of inflammatory bowel disease. Med Clin North Am 1990;74:39–50.
34. O'Keefe SJD, Rosser BG. Nutrition and inflammatory bowel disease. In: Targan SR, Shanahan F, eds. Inflammatory Bowel Disease: From Bench to Bedside. Baltimore, Williams & Wilkins, 1994:461–477.
35. Janowicz HD. The "natural history" of inflammatory bowel disease and therapeutic decisions. Am J Gastroenterol 1987;82:498–503.
36. Summers RW, Switz DM, Sessions JT, et al. National Cooperative Crohn's Disease Study: Results of drug treatment. Gastroenterology 1979;77:847–869.
37. Malchow H, Ewe K, Brandes JW, et al. European Cooperative Crohn's Disease Study (ECCDS): Results of drug treatment. Gastroenterology 1984;86:249–266.
38. Stenson WF, Cort D, Rogers J, et al. Dietary supplementation with fish oil in ulcerative colitis. Ann Intern Med 1992;116:609–614.
39. Belluzzi A, Brignola C, Campieri M, et al. Effect of an enteric-coated fish-oil preparation on relapses in Crohn's disease. N Engl J Med 1996;334:1557–1560.
40. Wu S, Craig RM. Intense nutritional support in inflammatory bowel disease. Dig Dis Sci 1995;40:843–852.
41. Gonzalez-Huix F, Fernandez-Banares F, Esteve-Comas M, et al. Enteral versus parenteral nutrition as adjunct therapy in acute ulcerative colitis. Am J Gastroenterol 1993;88:227–232.
42. Lewis JD, Fisher RL. Nutritional support in inflammatory bowel disease. Med Clin North Am 1994;78:1443–1456.
43. Klotz U, Maier K, Fischer C, et al. Therapeutic efficacy of sulfasalazine and its metabolites in patients with ulcerative colitis and Crohn's disease. N Engl J Med 1980;303:1499–1502.
44. Hanauer SB. Inflammatory bowel disease. N Engl J Med 1996;334: 841–848.
45. Ruderman WB. Newer pharmacologic agents for therapy of inflammatory bowel disease. Med Clin North Am 1990;74:133–153.
46. Meyers S, Sachar DB, Goldberg JD, Janowitz HD. Corticotropin versus hydrocortisone in the intravenous treatment of ulcerative colitis. A prospective, randomized, double-blind trial. Gastroenterology 1983;85:351–357.
47. Sandborn WJ. A review of immune modifier therapy for inflammatory bowel disease: Azathioprine, 6-mercaptopurine, cyclosporine. Am J Gastroenterol 1996;91:423–433.
48. Pearson DC, May GR, Fick GH, et al. Azathioprine and 6-mercaptopurine in Crohn's disease: A meta analysis. Ann Intern Med 1995;123:134–142.
49. Hanauer SB, Baert F. Medical therapy of inflammatory bowel disease. Med Clin North Am 1994;78:1413–1426.
50. Hawthorne AB, Logan RFA, Hawkey CJ, et al. Randomized controlled trial of azathioprine withdrawal in ulcerative colitis. BMJ 1992;305: 20–22.
51. Sutherland L, Singleton J, Sessions J, et al. Double-blind, placebo controlled trial of metronidazole in Crohn's disease. Gut 1991;32:1071–1075.
52. Kornbluth A, Sachar DB. Ulcerative colitis practice guidelines in adults. Am J Gastroenterol 1997;92:204–211.
53. Sutherland LR, May GR, Shaffer EA. Sulfasalazine revisited: A meta-analysis of 5-aminosalicylic acid in the treatment of ulcerative colitis. Ann Intern Med 1993;118:540–549.
54. D'Albasio G, Pacini F, Camarri E, et al. Combined therapy with 5-aminosalicylic acid tablets and enemas for maintaining remission in ulcerative colitis: A randomized double-blind study. Am J Gastroenterol 1997;92:1143–1147.
55. Powell-Tuck J, Brown RL, Lennard-Jones JE. A comparison of oral prednisone given as single or multiple daily doses for active proctocolitis. Scand J Gastroenterol 1975;13:833–837.
56. Marshall JK, Irvine EJ. Rectal corticosteroids versus alternative treatments in ulcerative colitis: A meta-analysis. Gut 1997;40:775–781.
57. Lee FI, Jewell DP, Mani V, et al. A randomized trial comparing mesalamine and prednisone foam enemas in patients with acute distal ulcerative colitis. Gut 1996;38:229–233.
58. Sandborn WJ, Tremaine WJ, Offord KP, et al. Transdermal nicotine for mild to moderately active ulcerative colitis. A randomized, double-blind, placebo controlled trial. Ann Intern Med 1997;126:364–371.
59. Sandborn WJ, Tremaine WJ. Cyclosporine treatment of inflammatory bowel disease. Mayo Clin Proc 1992;67:981–990.
60. Present DH, Lichtiger S. Efficacy of cyclosporine in treatment of fistula of Crohn's disease. Dig Dis Sci 1994;39:374–380.
61. Carbonnel F, Boruchowicz A, Duclos B, et al. Intravenous cyclosporine in attacks of ulcerative colitis: Short-term and long-term responses. Dig Dis Sci 1996;41:2471–2476.
62. Lichtiger S, Present DH, Kornbluth A, et al. Cyclosporine in severe ulcerative colitis refractory to steroid therapy. N Engl J Med 1994;330:1841–1845.
63. Present DH. Cyclosporine and other immunosuppressive agents: Current and future role in the treatment of inflammatory bowel disease. Am J Gastroenterol 1993;88:627–630.
64. Misiewicz JJ, Lennard-Jones JE, Connell AM, et al. Controlled trial of sulphasalazine in maintenance therapy for ulcerative colitis. Lancet 1965;1:185–188.
65. Mulder CJ, Tytgat GNJ, Weterman IT, et al. Double-blind comparison of slow-release 5-aminosalicylate and sulfasalazine in remission maintenance in ulcerative colitis. Gastroenterology 1988;95:1449–1453.
66. Mesalamine Study Group. An oral preparation of mesalamine therapy for ulcerative colitis. A randomized, placebo controlled trial. Ann Intern Med 1996;124:204–211.
67. Hawthorne AB, Logan RFA, Hawkey CJ. Randomized controlled trial of azathioprine withdrawal in ulcerative colitis. BMJ 1992;305: 20–22.
68. Fernandez-Banares F, Bertran X, Esteve-Comas M, et al. Azathioprine is useful in maintaining long-term remission induced by intravenous cyclosporine in steroid-refractory severe ulcerative colitis. Am J Gastroenterol 1996;91:2498–2499.
69. Salomon P, Kornbluth A, Aisenberg J, et al. How effective are current therapies for Crohn's disease? A meta-analysis. Am J Gastroenterol 1992;14:211–215.
70. Goldstein F, Farquhar S, Thornton JJ, et al. Favorable effects of sulfasalazine on small-bowel Crohn's disease. A long-term study. Am J Gastroenterol 1987;82:848–853.
71. Singleton JW, Hanauer SB, Gitnick GL, et al. Mesalamine capsules for the treatment of active Crohn's disease: Results of a 16-week trial. Gastroenterology 1993;104:1293–1301.
72. Ewe K, Press AG, Singe CC, et al. Azathioprine combined with prednisolone or monotherapy with prednisolone in active Crohn's disease. Gastroenterology 1993;105:367–372.

73. Colombrel JF, Lemann M, Bouhnik Y, et al. A controlled trial comparing ciprofloxacin with mesalamine for the treatment of active Crohn's disease. Gastroenterology 1997;112:A951.
74. Korelitz BI, Adler DJ, Mendelsohn RA, Sacknoff AL. Long-term experience with 6-mercaptopurine in the treatment of Crohn's disease. Am J Gastroenterol 1993;88:1198–1205.
75. Dubinsky MC, Lamothe S, Yang HY, et al. Pharmacogenomics and metabolite measurement for 6-mercaptopurine therapy in inflammatory bowel disease. Gastroenterology 2000;18:705–713.
76. Yates CR, Krnetski EY, Loennechen T, et al. Molecular diagnosis of thiopurine S-methyltransferase deficiency: Genetic basis for azathioprine and mercaptopurine intolerance. Ann Intern Med 1997;126:608–614.
77. Brynskov J, Freund L, Rasmussen SN, et al. A placebo-controlled, double-blind, randomized trial of cyclosporine therapy in active chronic Crohn's disease. N Engl J Med 1989;321:845–850.
78. Hanauer SB, Smith MB. Rapid closure of Crohn's disease fistulas with continuous intravenous cyclosporin A. Am J Gastroenterol 1993;88: 646–649.
79. Stark ME, Tremaine WJ. Maintenance of symptomatic remission in patients with Crohn's disease. Mayo Clin Proc 1993;68:1183–1190.
80. Feagan BG, Rochon J, Fedorak RN, et al. Methotrexate for the treatment of Crohn's disease. N Engl J Med 1995;332:292–297.
81. Egan LJ, Sandborn WJ. Methotrexate for inflammatory bowel disease: Pharmacology and preliminary results. Mayo Clin Proc 1996;71:69–80.
82. Kozarek RA, Patterson DJ, Gelfand MD, et al. Methotrexate induces clinical and histological remission in patients with inflammatory bowel disease. Ann Intern Med 1989;110:353–356.
83. Targan SR, Hanauer SB, van Deventer SJ, et al. A short-term study of chimeric monoclonal antibody to CA2 to tumor necrosis factor alpha for Crohn's disease. N Engl J Med 1997;337:1029–1035.
84. Rutgeerts P, D'Haens G, Targan S, et al. Efficacy and safety of retreatment with anti-tumor necrosis factor antibody (infliximab) to maintain remission in Crohn's disease. Gastroenterology 1999;117:761–769.
85. Goldstein F. Maintenance treatment for Crohn's disease: Has the time arrived? Am J Gastroenterol 1992;87:551–556.
86. Ewe K, Herfarth C, Malchow H, Jesdinsky HJ. Postoperative recurrence of Crohn's disease in relation to radicality of operation and sulfasalazine prophylaxis: A multicenter trial. Digestion 1989;42:224–232.
87. Gendre JP, Mary JY, Florent C, et al. Oral mesalamine (Pentasa) as maintenance treatment in Crohn's disease: A multicenter placebo-controlled study. Gastroenterology 1993;104:435–439.
88. Prantera C, Pallone F, Brunetti G, et al. Oral 5-aminosalicylic acid (Asacol) in the maintenance treatment of Crohn's disease. Gastroenterology 1992;103:363–368.
89. Lofberg R, Rutgeerts P, Malchow H. Budesonide prolongs time to relapse in ileal and ileocecal Crohn's disease. A placebo controlled, one-year study. Gut 1996;39:82–86.
90. Brostrom O. Prognosis in ulcerative colitis. Med Clin North Am 1990;74:201–218.
91. Hanan IM. Inflammatory bowel disease in the pregnant woman. Compr Ther 1993;19:91–95.
92. Schade RR, Van Thiel DH, Gavaler JS. Chronic idiopathic ulcerative colitis: Pregnancy and fetal outcome. Dig Dis Sci 1984;29:614–619.
93. Willoughby CP, Truelove SC. Ulcerative colitis and pregnancy. Gut 1980;21:469–474.
94. Toovey S, Hudson E, Hendry WF, et al. Sulfasalazine and male infertility: Reversibility and possible mechanism. Gut 1981;22:445–451.
95. Farraye FA. Pregnancy and nursing. In: Peppercorn MA, ed. Therapy of Inflammatory Bowel Disease. New York, Marcel Dekker, 1990.
96. Das KM, Eastwood MA, McManus JPA, et al. Adverse reactions during salicylazosulfapyridine therapy and the relation with drug metabolism and acetylator phenotype. N Engl J Med 1973;289:491–495.
97. Korelitz BI, Present DH, Rubin PH, et al. Desensitization to sulfasalazine after hypersensitivity reactions in patients with inflammatory bowel disease. J Clin Gastroenterol 1984;6:27–31.
98. Linn FV, Peppercorn MA. Drug therapy for inflammatory bowel disease, I. Am J Surg 1992;164:85–89.
99. Feurle GE, Theuer D, Velasco S, et al. Olsalazine versus placebo in the treatment of mild to moderate ulcerative colitis: A randomized double-blind trial. Gut 1989;30:1354–1361.
100. Zinberg J, Molinas S, Das KM. Double-blind placebo-controlled study of olsalazine in the treatment of ulcerative colitis. Am J Gastroenterol 1990;85:562–566.
101. Azad Khan AK, Truelove SC. Circulating levels of sulphasalazine and its metabolites and their relation to the clinical efficacy of the drug in ulcerative colitis. Gut 1980;21:706–710.
102. Haber CJ, Meltzer SJ, Present DH, et al. Nature and course of pancreatitis caused by 6-mercaptopurine in the treatment of inflammatory bowel disease. Gastroenterology 1986;91:982–986.
103. Colonna T, Korelitz BI. The role of leukopenia in the 6-mercaptopurine-induced remission of refractory Crohn's disease. Am J Gastroenterol 1994;89:362–366.
104. O'Brien JJ, Bayless TM, Bayless JA. Use of azathioprine or 6-mercaptopurine in the treatment of Crohn's disease. Gastroenterology 1991;101:39–46.
105. Duffy LF, Daum F, Fisher SE, et al. Peripheral neuropathy in Crohn's disease patients treated with metronidazole. Gastroenterology 1984;88:681–684.
106. Best WR, Becktel JM, Singleton JW, et al. Development of a Crohn's disease activity index. Gastroenterology 1976;70:439–444.
107. Sanborn WJ, Tremaine WJ, Schroeder KW, et al. Cyclosporine enemas for treatment-resistant, mildly to moderately active, left sided ulcerative colitis. Am J Gastroenterol 1993;88:640–645.
108. Irvine EJ, Zhou Q, Thompson AK. The short inflammatory bowel disease questionnaire: A quality of life instrument for community physicians managing inflammatory bowel disease. CERPT investigators. Canadian Crohn's relapse prevention trial. Am J Gastroenterol 1996;91:1571–1578.

35

NAUSEA AND VOMITING

A. Thomas Taylor

Nausea and vomiting are common complaints among many individuals with gastrointestinal (GI) disorders. However, because of the variable etiologies of these problems, management may be quite simple or detailed and complex, essentially innocuous or associated with therapy-induced adverse reactions. This chapter provides an overview of nausea and vomiting, two multifaceted problems.

Nausea is usually defined as the inclination to vomit or as a feeling in the throat or epigastric region alerting an individual that vomiting is imminent. Vomiting is defined as the ejection or expulsion of gastric contents through the mouth and is often a forceful event. Either condition may occur transiently with no other associated signs or symptoms; however, these conditions also may be only part of a more complex clinical presentation.

ETIOLOGY

Nausea and vomiting may be associated with a variety of clinical presentations. In addition to GI diseases, either or both may accompany cardiovascular, infectious, neurologic, or metabolic disease processes. Nausea and vomiting may be a feature of such conditions as pregnancy or may follow operative procedures or administration of certain medications such as those used in cancer chemotherapy. Psychogenic etiologies of these symptoms may be present, especially in young women with an underlying emotional disturbance. Anticipatory etiologies may be involved, such as in patients who have previously received cytotoxic chemotherapy. Specific etiologies associated with nausea and vomiting are presented in Table 35–1.[1]

In addition to identifying conditions associated with nausea and vomiting, it is important to address the specific causative medical problems. For example, nausea and vomiting may occur in as many as 70% of patients with inferior myocardial infarction or diabetic ketoacidosis. As many as 80% to 90% of patients with an Addisonian crisis, acute pancreatitis, or acute appendicitis may present with nausea and vomiting.

The etiology of nausea and vomiting may vary with the age of the patient. For example, vomiting in the newborn during the first day of life suggests upper digestive tract obstruction or an increase in intracranial pressure. Other illnesses associated with vomiting in children include pyloric stenosis, duodenal ulcer, stress ulcer, adrenal insufficiency, septicemia, or diseases of the pancreas, liver, or biliary tree. Also, the hepatocellular failure seen in Reye's syndrome may lead to profound cerebral edema followed by persistent emesis. A common etiology of vomiting in children, however, is viral gastroenteritis caused by rotavirus. Vomiting in infants may be associated with something as simple as overfeeding, rapid feeding, inadequate burping, or lying down too soon after feeding. It should be recognized that these types of vomiting are usually indicative of minor problems and may be altered by changing the approach to feeding.

Drug-induced nausea and vomiting are of particular concern, especially with the increasing number of patients receiving cytotoxic treatment and the number of agents implicated. Included in Table 35–2 are specific cytotoxic agents categorized by their emetogenic potential. Although some agents may have greater emetogenic potential than others, combinations of agents, high doses, clinical settings, psychological conditions, prior treatment experiences, and unusual stimuli to sight, smell, or taste may alter a patient's response to drug treatment. In this setting, nausea and vomiting may be unavoidable and potentially devastating to the patient's desire to continue treatment. Indeed, some patients experience these problems so intensely that chemotherapy is postponed or discontinued. In addition to the emetogenic potential of various cytotoxic regimens, a variety of other common etiologies have been proposed for the development of nausea and vomiting in cancer patients. These are presented in Table 35–3.[2]

PATHOPHYSIOLOGY

The three consecutive phases of emesis include nausea, retching, and vomiting. Nausea, the imminent need to vomit, is associated with gastric stasis and may be considered a separate and singular symptom. Retching is the labored movement of abdominal and thoracic muscles before vomiting. The final phase of emesis is vomiting, the forceful expulsion of gastric contents caused by GI retroperistalsis. The act of vomiting requires the coordinated contractions of the abdominal muscles, pylorus, and antrum, a raised gastric cardia, diminished lower esophageal sphincter pressure, and esophageal dilatation.[3] Vomiting should not be confused with regurgitation, an act in which the gastric or esophageal contents rise to the pharynx because of pressure differences caused by, for example, an incompetent lower esophageal sphincter. Accompanying autonomic symptoms of pallor, tachycardia, and diaphoresis account for many of the distressing feelings associated with emesis.

Vomiting is triggered by afferent impulses to the vomiting center, a nucleus of cells in the medulla. Impulses are received from sensory centers, such as the chemoreceptor trigger zone (CTZ), cerebral cortex, and visceral afferents from the pharynx and GI tract. When excited, afferent impulses are integrated by the vomiting center, resulting in efferent impulses to the salivation center, respiratory center, and the pharyngeal, GI, and abdominal muscles, leading to vomiting.

The CTZ, located in the area postrema of the fourth ventricle of the brain, is a major chemosensory organ for emesis and is usually associated with chemically induced vomiting. Because of its location, bloodborne and cerebrospinal fluid toxins have easy access to the CTZ. Therefore, cytotoxic agents stimulate primarily this area rather than the cerebral cortex and visceral afferents. Similarly, pregnancy-associated vomiting probably occurs through stimulation of the CTZ.

Numerous neurotransmitter receptors are located in the vomiting center, CTZ, and GI tract. Examples of such receptors include cholinergic and histaminic, dopaminergic, opiate, serotonergic, and

TABLE 35–1. Specific Etiologies of Nausea and Vomiting[1]

Gastrointestinal Mechanisms
Mechanical gastric outlet obstruction
- Peptic ulcer disease
- Gastric carcinoma
- Pancreatic disease

Motility disorders
- Gastroparesis
- Drug-induced gastric stasis
- Chronic intestinal pseudo-obstruction
- Postviral gastroenteritis
- Irritable bowel syndrome
- Postgastric surgery
- Idiopathic gastric stasis
- Anorexia nervosa

Intra-abdominal emergencies
- Intestinal obstruction
- Acute pancreatitis
- Acute pyelonephritis
- Acute cholecystitis
- Acute cholangitis
- Acute viral hepatitis

Acute gastroenteritis
- Viral gastroenteritis
- Salmonellosis
- Shigellosis
- Staphylococcal gastroenteritis (enterotoxins)

Cardiovascular Diseases
- Acute myocardial infarction
- Congestive heart failure
- Shock and circulatory collapse

Neurologic Processes
- Midline cerebellar hemorrhage
- Increased intracranial pressure
- Migraine headache
- Vestibular disorders
- Head trauma

Metabolic Disorders
- Diabetes mellitus (diabetic ketoacidosis)
- Addison's disease
- Renal disease (uremia)

Psychogenic Causes
- Self-induced
- Anticipatory

Therapy-induced Causes
- Cytotoxic chemotherapy
- Radiation therapy
- Theophylline preparations (intolerance, toxic)
- Anticonvulsant preparations (toxic)
- Digitalis preparations (toxic)
- Opiates
- Amphotericin
- Antibiotics

Drug Withdrawal
- Opiates
- Benzodiazepines

Miscellaneous Causes
- Pregnancy
- Any swallowed irritant (foods, drugs)
- Noxious odors
- Operative procedures

benzodiazepine receptors. Chemotherapeutic agents, their metabolites, or other emetic compounds theoretically trigger the process of emesis through stimulation of one or more of these receptors. Effective antiemetics are able to antagonize or block the emetogenic receptors.

Anticipatory nausea and vomiting may be elicited either by specific stimuli associated with the administration of noxious, often cytotoxic, agents or by the anxiety associated with these treatments. Many patients demonstrate both types. The most often accepted theory for this pattern of conditioning is that by repeated pairing of

TABLE 35–2. Emetogenic Potential of Cytotoxic Chemotherapy

Most Emetogenic	Moderate	Least Emetogenic
Aldesleukin	Docetaxel	Asparginase
Altretamine	Etoposide	Bleomycin
Carboplatin	Gemcitabine	Busulfan
Carmustine	Mitomycin	Chlorambucil
Cisplatin	Paclitaxel	Cladribine
Cyclophosphamide	Pegaspargase	Cytarabine
Dacarbazine	Procarbazine	Fludarabine
Dactinomycin	Thiotepa	Fluorouracil
Daunorubicin	Topotecan	Hydroxyurea
Doxorubicin		Melphalan
Epirubicin		Mercaptopurine
Idarubicin		Methotrexate
Ifosfamide		Teniposide
Irinotecan		Tamoxifen
Lomustine		Thioguanine
Mechlorethamine		Vinca alkaloids
Mitoxantrone		
Pentostatin		
Streptozocin		

TABLE 35–3. Nonchemotherapy Etiologies of Nausea and Vomiting in Cancer Patients[2]

Fluid and electrolyte abnormalities
- Hypercalcemia
- Volume depletion
- Water intoxication
- Adrenocortical insufficiency

Drug induced
- Opiates
- Antibiotics

Gastrointestinal obstruction
Increased intracranial pressure
Peritonitis
Metastases
- Brain
- Meninges
- Hepatic

Uremia
Infections (septicemia, local)
Radiation therapy

chemotherapy and its aftereffects, previously neutral stimuli such as odors, sounds, and settings acquire the ability to elicit nausea and vomiting.[4,5] These types of stimuli should be expected to be most troublesome in patients receiving agents with the greatest inherent emetogenic potential.

CLINICAL PRESENTATION

Because it is impossible to discuss all clinical settings in which the presence of nausea and vomiting might be a pertinent finding, these processes are presented as they might occur together and also as *simple* or *complex* in presentation. Defined here, the term *simple* applies to those episodes of nausea and/or vomiting that (a) occur occasionally and are self-limiting or relieved by the minimal use of antiemetic methods or medications; (b) account for little patient deterioration such as fluid–electrolyte imbalances, pain, or noncompliance with prescribed therapies; or (c) are not related to the administration of or exposure to noxious agents. Conversely, the term *complex* is used when describing a patient's clinical course as including symptoms that (a) are not adequately or readily relieved by the administration of a single antiemetic method or medication; (b) lead to progressive patient deterioration secondary to fluid-electrolyte imbalances, pain, or noncompliance with prescribed therapies; or (c) are caused by noxious agents or psychogenic events. Psychogenic vomiting is often related to sexual or marital disturbances, health problems of friends or family members, or deeper emotional strains. Pertinent features of this condition may include a positive family history of this condition. Episodes may be induced by meals, are recurrent, are generally not accompanied by nausea, and may be suppressed by the patient. Often these events are not noted to be important by the patient. Unless associated with anorexia nervosa, appetite is usually normal. Many of these conditions subside with reductions in stress.

Most episodes of nausea and vomiting decrease in frequency, duration, and severity as the underlying process resolves. However, during the recovery period, it may be desirable to combat the specific symptoms of nausea and vomiting. Most cases of nausea and vomiting are self-limiting, resolve spontaneously, and only require symptomatic therapy. Antiemetic therapy is indicated in patients with electrolyte disturbances secondary to vomiting, severe anorexia or weight loss, or progression of disease either as a result of refusal of continued therapy or poor nutritional status.

Included in the GI etiologies of nausea and vomiting are a variety of specific disorders associated with mechanical obstruction, motility changes, and infectious diseases of the vital organs within the abdominal cavity. Although each of these conditions may vary in onset, duration, and severity of symptoms, each is, nevertheless, a potential source of nausea and vomiting that may need to be addressed. In this regard, attention to simultaneous signs and symptoms is helpful in making an accurate diagnosis and evaluation of a specific patient. Additional knowledge of a patient's GI history, with particular emphasis on the presence of abdominal pain or discomfort, diarrhea, and blood from the upper or lower GI tract, should always be sought. Knowledge of the patient's tolerance of food is important. Also, the timing of these symptoms in relation to meals as well as the consistency, content, odor, and frequency of the vomitus may be characteristic findings for specific conditions. Further information that may be helpful in understanding a specific clinical presentation includes concomitant findings such as fever or weight loss, a description of precipitating factors, a complete history of recent medication use, and the history or presence of myalgias, behavioral or visual changes, headache, or pain outside the abdomen.

▶ TREATMENT: Nausea and Vomiting

DESIRED OUTCOME

The overall goal of antiemetic therapy is to prevent or to eliminate nausea and vomiting. This should be accomplished without adverse effects or with clinically acceptable adverse effects. Although this goal may be accomplished easily in patients with simple nausea and vomiting, patients with more complex problems require greater assistance. In addition to these clinical goals, appropriate cost issues should be considered, particularly in the management of chemotherapy-induced and postoperative nausea and vomiting.

GENERAL APPROACH TO TREATMENT

The treatment of nausea and vomiting is quite varied depending on the associated medical situation. Even though a number of potentially effective measures are available, most patients receive a medication at some point in their care. For simple nausea and vomiting, patients may choose to do nothing or to select from a variety of over-the-counter (OTC) drugs. As symptoms become worse or are associated with more serious medical problems, patients are more likely to benefit from proven prescription antiemetic drugs. When prescribed according to reliable clinical information, these agents often provide acceptable relief. However, some patients will never be totally free of symptoms. This lack of relief is most disabling to the patient when it is associated with an unresolving medical problem or when the necessary therapy for this condition is the cause, as in the case of patients receiving emetogenic chemotherapy.

NONPHARMACOLOGIC MANAGEMENT

Nonpharmacologic management of nausea and vomiting may include a variety of dietary, physical, or psychological changes consistent with the etiology of symptoms. For patients with simple complaints, perhaps resulting from excessive or disagreeable food or beverage consumption, avoidance or moderation in dietary intake may be preferable. Patients suffering symptoms of systemic illness may improve dramatically as their underlying condition resolves. Finally, patients in whom these symptoms result from labyrinthine changes produced by motion may benefit quickly by assuming a stable physical position.

The variables associated with the development of anticipatory nausea and vomiting include the use of cisplatin, the severity of postchemotherapy vomiting, and the duration of the patient's worst nausea.[6] Although anxiolytic and antiemetic agents offer the most successful treatment for these patients, various relaxation techniques have been reported, including hypnosis, behavior modification, and guided mental imagery.[7–9] However, the efficacy of these nonpharmacologic approaches requires further evaluation. Nevertheless, prevention of these symptoms is extremely important. This may be accomplished through supportive care coupled with potent prophylactic antiemetic regimens prior to chemotherapy treatment.

The management of psychogenic vomiting is greatly dependent on psychological intervention. However, because the underlying problems are so complex and intertwined in personal relationships, psychological therapy may require lengthy, in-depth followup. Pharmacologic therapy offers only minimal benefit in these patients. Surgery, such as gastroenterostomy, is of no value.

PHARMACOLOGIC THERAPY

Although many approaches to the treatment of nausea and vomiting have been suggested, antiemetic drugs (OTC and prescription) are most often recommended. These agents represent a variety of pharmacologic and chemical classes, as well as dosage regimens and routes of administration. With so many treatment possibilities available, factors that enable the clinician to discriminate among various choices must be recognized. These factors include (a) the suspected etiology of the symptoms; (b) the frequency, duration, and severity of the episodes; (c) the ability of the patient to use oral, rectal, injectable, or transdermal topical medications; and (d) the success of previous antiemetic medications. For example, many antiemetics are commercially available as oral agents. Provided a patient can and will adhere to oral dosing, a suitable and effective agent can often be selected; however, for certain other situations, oral medications may be inappropriate because of the patient's inability to retain any appreciable oral ingestions. In these patients, rectal or injectable routes of administration might be preferred. Information concerning commonly available antiemetic preparations is given in Table 35–4.

Some individuals initially experience nausea and vomiting at home or outside formal medical settings. For these symptoms, patients may choose from a lengthy list of OTC products. Although suitable for occasional simple nausea and vomiting, OTC agents are often abandoned by the patient as symptoms continue or become progressively worse. As the patient's condition warrants, prescription medications may be chosen, either as single-agent therapy or in combination. For most conditions, a single antiemetic agent is preferred; however, for those patients who are not responding to such therapy, and for those patients who are receiving highly emetogenic chemotherapy, multiple-agent regimens are usually required. Numerous combinations have been employed through clinical investigation and practice.

The treatment of simple nausea and vomiting usually requires minimal therapy. Products available for self-medication include antacids; histamine$_2$ antagonists such as cimetidine, famotidine, and ranitidine; antihistamine-anticholinergic agents such as cyclizine, dimenhydrinate, diphenhydramine, and meclizine; and phosphorated carbohydrate solutions. Agents requiring physician prescription include some antihistaminic-anticholinergic drugs and phenothiazine agents. The latter agents include benzquinamide, buclizine, parenteral dimenhydrinate and diphenhydramine, hydroxyzine, prochlorperazine, promethazine, and trimethobenzamide. Both OTC and prescription drugs useful in the treatment of simple nausea and vomiting are usually effective in small, infrequently administered doses. Side effects and toxic effects in these settings are also usually minimal.

The management of complex nausea and vomiting may require aggressive drug therapy, often with more than one antiemetic agent. For patients with complex symptoms, effective combinations may include two of the following drugs: benzquinamide, chlorpromazine, dimenhydrinate, droperidol, hydroxyzine, prochlorperazine, promethazine, thiethylperazine, or trimethobenzamide. In combination, each of these drugs is prescribed in small to moderate dosages, achieving symptomatic control through different pharmacologic mechanisms while avoiding the untoward effects caused by high doses. For patients receiving highly emetogenic chemotherapy, antiemetic regimens may include one or more of the following agents: prochlorperazine, metoclopramide, ondansetron, granisetron, dolasetron, dexamethasone, or lorazepam (see "Chemotherapy-Induced Nausea and Vomiting" later in this chapter).

In general, the clinician should evaluate the patient's condition and determine the need for antiemetic treatment of an existing condition or prophylactic therapy to prevent or to lessen anticipated nausea and vomiting episodes, as is seen in patients requiring cytotoxic drugs or operative procedures. After this decision has been made, along with the complete and overall medical evaluation, the antiemetic selection process may proceed. Table 35–4 lists common antiemetic preparations.

ANTACIDS

Patients who are experiencing simple nausea and vomiting may use various antacids. In this setting, single or combination OTC antacid products, especially those containing magnesium hydroxide, aluminum hydroxide, and/or calcium carbonate, may provide sufficient relief, primarily through gastric acid neutralization. Likewise, patients may seek histamine$_2$ antagonists for these symptoms, particularly in the presence of heartburn or brief episodes of gastroesophageal reflux. Patients responding to small, occasional doses of these agents probably do not have significant pathology. However, it is not uncommon for patients with significant GI disease to self-medicate with larger and more frequent doses of antacids with or without a trial of histamine$_2$ antagonist prior to seeking medical care.

Common antacid regimens for the relief of nausea and vomiting include one or more small doses of single- or multiple-agent products. Although antacid therapy may be aggressively applied for the treatment of known ulcer disease, OTC products used by patients are usually taken in response to acute and sporadic episodes of nausea and vomiting. Depending on dose, common products usually supply sufficient ingredients to allow a range of approximately 40–180 mEq of acid-neutralizing capacity.[10–12] Potential adverse effects from antacids are usually related to the presence of magnesium, aluminum, or calcium salts. Specifically, osmotic diarrhea from magnesium and constipation from aluminum or calcium salts may be of concern to patients, particularly those self-medicating with high or frequently administered antacid doses. Generally, however, when used occasionally for acute episodic relief of nausea and vomiting, antacids do not produce serious toxicities.

HISTAMINE$_2$ ANTAGONISTS

Patients may use histamine$_2$ antagonists in low doses to manage simple nausea and vomiting associated with heartburn. Individual dosages of cimetidine 200 mg, famotidine 10 mg, nizatidine 75 mg, or ranitidine 75 mg may be used for brief periods. Except for potential drug interactions with cimetidine, these agents should be expected to cause few side effects when used for episodic relief.

TABLE 35–4. Common Antiemetic Preparations and Adult Dosage Regimens

Drug	Adult Dosage Regimen	Dosage Form/Route	Availability
Antacids			
Antacids (various)	15–30 mL every 2–4 h prn	Liquid	OTC
Histamine H_2 Antagonists			
Cimetidine (Tagament HB)	200 mg bid prn	Tab	OTC
Famotidine (Pepcid AC)	10 mg bid prn	Tab	OTC
Nizatidine (Axid AR)	75 mg bid prn	Tab	OTC
Ranitidine (Zantac 75)	75 mg bid prn	Tab	OTC
Antihistaminic-Anticholinergic Agents			
Benzquinamide (Emete-Con)	25–50 mg every 3–4 h prn	IM, IV	Rx
Buclizine (Bucladin-S)	50 mg twice daily	Tab	Rx
Cyclizine (Marezine)	50 mg every 4–6 h prn	Tab, IM	Rx/OTC
Dimenhydrinate (Dramamine)	50–100 mg every 4–6 h prn	Tab, chew tab, cap, liquid, IM, IV	Rx/OTC
Diphenhydramine (Benadryl)	10–50 mg every 4–6 h prn	Tab, cap, liquid, IM, IV	Rx/OTC
Hydroxyzine (Vistril, Atarax)	25–100 mg every 6 h prn	Tab, cap, liquid, IM	Rx
Meclizine (Bonine, Antivert)	25–50 mg every 24 h prn	Tab, chew tab, cap	Rx/OTC
Promethazine (Phenergan)	12.5–25 mg every 4–6 h prn	Tab, liquid, IM, IV, supp	Rx
Pyrilamine (Nisaval)	25–50 mg 3 to 4 times daily	Tab	Rx/OTC
Scopolamine (Transderm Scop)	0.5 mg every 72 h prn	Transdermal patch	Rx
Trimethobenzamide (Tigan)	200–250 mg 3 to 4 times daily prn	Cap, IM, supp	Rx
Phenothiazines			
Chlorpromazine (Thorazine)	10–25 mg every 4–6 h prn	SR, cap, tab, liquid, IM, IV	Rx
	50–100 mg every 6–8 h prn	Supp	Rx
Fluphenazine (Prolixin)	1.25–2.5 mg every 6–8 h prn	Tab, liquid, IM	Rx
Perphenazine (Trilafon)	8–30 mg/d divided prn	Tab, liquid, IM, IV	Rx
Prochlorperazine (Compazine)	5–10 mg 3 to 4 times daily prn	SR, cap, tab, liquid IM, IV	Rx
	25 mg twice daily prn	Supp	Rx
Promazine (Sparine)	25–50 mg every 4–6 h prn	Tab, IM	Rx
Thiethylperazine (Torecan)	10 mg 3 times daily	Tab, IM, supp	Rx
Cannabinoids			
Dronabinol (Marinol)	5–7.5 mg/m^2 every 2–4 h prn	Cap	Rx (C-II)
Nabilone (Cesamet)	1–2 mg 2 to 3 times daily prn	Cap	Rx (C-II)
Butyrophenones			
Haloperidol (Haldol)	1–5 mg every 12 h prn	Tab, liquid, IM, IV	Rx
Droperidol (Inapsine)	2.5–5 mg every 4–6 h prn	IM, IV	Rx
Corticosteroids			
Dexamethasone (Decadron) for CINV	10 mg prior to chemotherapy, repeat with 4–8 mg every 6 h for total of 4 doses	IV	Rx
Dexamethasone for PONV	10 mg prior to induction of anesthesia	IV	Rx
Methylprednisolone (Solu-Medrol)	125–500 mg every 6 h for total of 4 doses	IV	Rx
Benzodiazepines			
Lorazepam (Ativan)	0.5–4 mg prior to chemotherapy	IV	Rx (C-IV)
Diazepam (Valium)	2–5 mg every 3 h	Tab	Rx (C-IV)
Selective Serotonin Antagonists			
Dolasetron (Anzemet), for CINV	1.8 mg/kg 30 min prior to chemotherapy (undiluted, up to 100 mg over 30 min, or diluted, over 30 min)	IV	Rx
	OR		
	100 mg within 1 h before chemotherapy	Tab	Rx
Dolasetron (Anzemet), for PONV undiluted as single injection	12.5 mg 15 min before the cessation of anesthesia	IV	Rx
	OR		
	100 mg within 2 h before surgery	Tab	Rx
Granisetron (Kytril), for CINV	10 μg/kg prior to chemotherapy (diluted, infuse, over 5 min or undiluted over 30 seconds)	IV	Rx
	OR		
	1 mg up to 1 h prior to chemotherapy and 1 mg 12 h after the first dose, or, 2 mg up to 1 h prior to chemotherapy	Tab	Rx
Granisetron (Kytril) for PONV	20–40 μg/kg 30 min before end of anesthesia	IV	Rx

TABLE 35–4. (continued)

Drug	Adult Dosage Regimen	Dosage Form/Route	Availability
Ondansetron (Zofran), for CINV	32 mg prior to chemotherapy as a single dose (diluted, give over 15 min), or 0.15 mg/kg prior to chemotherapy, repeat at 4 and 8 h	IV	Rx
	OR		
	8 mg 30 min prior to chemotherapy, repeat at 4 and 8 h and every 12 h for 1–2 days after chemotherapy completion	Tab	Rx
Ondansetron (Zofran), for PONV	4 mg prior to induction of anesthesia or postoperatively (undiluted, give over 2–5 min)	IV	Rx
	OR		
	16 mg given 1 h before anesthesia	Tab	Rx
Miscellaneous Agents			
Dextrose, fructose, phosphoric acid (Emetrol)	15–30 mL every 1–3 h prn	Liquid	OTC
Diphenidol (Vontrol)	25–50 mg every 4 h prn	Tab	Rx
Metoclopramide (Reglan), for CINV	1–2 mg/kg every 2 h × 2, then every 3 h × 3	IV	Rx
Metoclopramide (Reglan), for PONV	10–20 mg about 10 min prior to anesthesia	IV	Rx
Metoclopramide (Reglan), for delayed CINV	0.5 mg/kg or 20 mg every 6 h prn, days 2 to 4	Tab	Rx

Rx = prescription; OTC = over the counter; cap = capsule; chew tab = chewable tablet; IM = intramuscular; IV = intravenous; liquid = oral syrup, concentrate, suspension; SR cap = sustained-release capsule; supp = rectal suppository; tab = tablet; CINV = chemotherapy-induced nausea and vomiting; PONV = postoperative nausea and vomiting.

ANTIHISTAMINE-ANTICHOLINERGIC DRUGS

Antiemetic drugs from the antihistaminic-anticholinergic category appear to interrupt various visceral afferent pathways that stimulate nausea and vomiting and may be appropriate in the treatment of simple symptomology. However, when used alone, each provides little efficacy in patients with more complex complaints such as those caused by cytotoxic chemotherapy. Adverse reactions that may be apparent with the use of the antihistaminic-anticholinergic agents primarily include drowsiness, confusion, blurred vision, dry mouth, and urinary retention, and possibly tachycardia, particularly in elderly patients. Also, as doses are increased or are more frequently administered, patients with narrow-angle glaucoma, prostatic hyperplasia, or asthma are at greater risk of complications from the anticholinergic effects of these drugs.

PHENOTHIAZINES

Historically, phenothiazines have been the most widely prescribed antiemetic agents. These agents appear to block dopamine receptors, most likely in the CTZ. Some investigators have found phenothiazines to demonstrate greatest efficacy when compared with placebo and less efficacy when compared with other more potent antiemetics.[13–15] Phenothiazines are marketed in an array of dosage forms, none of which appears to be more efficacious than another; however, there are perhaps some important generalizations concerning their use in overall clinical practice. These agents may be most practical for long-term treatment and are inexpensive in comparison with newer drugs, with the exception of sustained-release products of chlorpromazine or prochlorperazine that may be too costly and of no established clinical advantage. Little distinguishing information is available in the present literature concerning the efficacy of rectal preparations. Rectal administration is most preferred in patients in whom parenteral administration is impractical or in whom oral medications cannot be retained and are therefore ineffective. In many patients, low doses of phenothiazine drugs may not be effective, while larger doses may produce unacceptable risks.[2] Phenothiazines are most useful in patients with simple nausea and vomiting or in those receiving mildly emetogenic doses of chemotherapy. Problems associated with these drugs include troublesome and potentially dangerous side effects, including extrapyramidal reactions, hypersensitivity reactions with possible liver dysfunction, marrow aplasia, and excessive sedation.

BUTYROPHENONES

Two butyrophenone compounds that have antiemetic activity are haloperidol and its congener droperidol. Each agent blocks dopaminergic stimulation of the CTZ. Although each agent is effective in relieving nausea and vomiting, droperidol has been used most often. Depending on its specific indication, the optimal dosage range may vary considerably. For example, preoperative doses of droperidol may range from 2.5 mg to 10 mg, whereas dosage regimens during cytotoxic chemotherapy have been documented as low as 0.5–2.5 mg by intermittent injection to as high as 1.0–1.5 mg/h by intravenous infusion.[16–19] Adverse reactions resulting from the use of the butyrophenone compounds primarily include sedation and the possibility of dystonic reactions. Although dystonia may occur after the initial dose, some patients may experience this problem later in therapy. Injectable diphenhydramine usually rapidly resolves these extrapyramidal reactions.[17]

CORTICOSTEROIDS

Corticosteroids have demonstrated antiemetic efficacy since the initial recognition that patients receiving prednisone as part of their Hodgkin's disease protocol appeared to develop less nausea and vomiting than those patients treated with protocols that excluded this agent. Other corticosteroids showing efficacy include methylprednisolone and dexamethasone. Although the exact mechanism of action for corticosteroids is unknown, the inhibition of prostaglandin synthesis may explain their antiemetic activity.[20] Such an explanation is most appealing in light of the known high emetogenic potential of prostaglandins themselves. However, because of their numerous metabolic effects, a single site of steroid antiemetic activity may be difficult to locate or assess. In addition to the antiemetic benefits of corticosteroids, other desirable effects include increased appetite and an elevation of mood or feelings of well being. Depending on the patient and the drug regimen, these effects may provide the primary benefit of corticosteroid therapy.

Corticosteroids have been used successfully in the management of chemotherapy-induced and postoperative nausea and vomiting with few problems. However, reported adverse effects have included mood changes ranging from anxiety to euphoria, as well as headache, metallic taste, abdominal discomfort, hyperglycemia, and itchy throat.[20] For patients with simple nausea and vomiting, steroids are not indicated and may be associated with unacceptable risks. As with other conditions, steroids should be employed only when the benefit-to-risk ratio is sufficient to warrant a medication with such complex and potentially deleterious effects.

METOCLOPRAMIDE

Metoclopramide, procainamide's congener, provides significant antiemetic effects by blocking the dopaminergic receptors centrally in the CTZ. Peripherally, metoclopramide increases lower esophageal sphincter tone, aids gastric emptying, and accelerates transit through the small bowel, possibly through the release of acetylcholine. Because the adverse reactions of metoclopramide include extrapyramidal effects, IV diphenhydramine 25–50 mg should be prophylactically administered or provided on-call for its anticipated need. Other adverse effects may include restlessness, drowsiness, fatigue, nausea, and diarrhea.[21,22]

SELECTIVE SEROTONIN ANTAGONISTS

Selective serotonin-receptor antagonists have become an increasingly important antiemetic therapy in recent years, particularly in the management of chemotherapy-induced and postoperative nausea and vomiting. Issues involved in the use of ondansetron, granisetron, and dolasetron are reviewed in detail in the sections that follow. Each of these agents may be used in either oral or intravenous dosage forms, depending upon the clinical setting.

OTHER AGENTS

A final group of antiemetic preparations available to patients experiencing nausea and vomiting necessitates some mention. First, the phosphorated carbohydrate solutions (mixtures of fructose, dextrose, and phosphoric acid) are available OTC and may be administered in 15–30-mL doses as often as every 3 hours or as needed. As might be predicted, this mixture is intended only for mild and infrequent symptoms. Because of the inability of these agents to relieve significant symptoms, the solution should not be used in patients with complex problems, especially not in those patients receiving chemotherapy. However, this combination is safe and effective in patients with morning sickness. Adverse reactions to these solutions may include abdominal pain or diarrhea as a consequence of large doses of fructose, or lack of control in diabetic patients because of the dextrose included in the formulations. With the use of small doses, most patients experience little benefit or adversity.

An agent that has received comparatively little attention in the antiemetic literature is diphenidol. Although this agent inhibits the CTZ, as well as conduction in vestibular—cerebellar pathways, and is indicated for the management of nausea and vomiting associated with surgery, malignant neoplasms, antineoplastic chemotherapy, radiation sickness, infectious diseases, and labyrinthine disturbances, it should be used extremely cautiously. Diphenidol should be used only when there is a clear and unquestionable benefit potential. Even though it is an oral agent, this product should be used only in a hospital or under comparable conditions. The primary reason for these required measures with the use of diphenidol is its adverse reaction profile. Auditory and visual hallucinations, disorientation, and confusion have been reported and are the usual warnings against its use. These problems may be even more pronounced in elderly patients, or in those patients with declining renal function, because approximately 90% of diphenidol is excreted in the urine. Last, diphenidol should be avoided during pregnancy or lactation and in children who weigh less than 50 pounds.

Pyridoxine has also been cited as an antiemetic agent; however, its efficacy has not been accepted beyond that of a placebo and it probably has little place in the approach to simple or complex symptoms. Its beneficial mechanism has been suggested to be restoration of depleted pyridoxine body stores.

COMBINATION REGIMENS

The management of nausea and vomiting may require combinations of antiemetic drugs. Most combination protocols are reserved for patients with complex symptoms, especially those patients receiving cytotoxic chemotherapy. Such combinations may include as few as two or as many as five antiemetic agents, each in moderate to high doses. Experienced personnel in a hospital or specialty clinic setting should carefully administer these multiagent regimens. Although oral agents may be used, most regimens are administered intravenously and require continuous patient assessment and feedback for evaluation of efficacy and side effects. Because an increasing number of patients may require such regimens, careful monitoring should be developed and employed to eliminate possibly severe adverse reactions.

The primary goal of combination antiemetic regimens is to select beneficial agents that have different pharmacologic mechanisms as well as toxic effects that are not considered additive or synergistic. These protocols may affect the vomiting center, the CTZ, the cerebral cortex, and/or the peripheral mechanisms that mediate nausea and vomiting.[23] Combinations often include metoclopramide, diphenhydramine, and dexamethasone. Other agents that may be added to the regimen include droperidol, diazepam, thiethylperazine, secobarbital, pentobarbital, chlorpromazine, or prochlorperazine. Dexamethasone may be combined with ondansetron, granisetron, or dolasetron. From this list of possible combinations, it should be apparent that the ideal multiagent antiemetic protocol has not been established. Nevertheless, protocols using injectable metoclopramide or a serotonin antagonist appear to have a high degree of efficacy in preventing nausea and vomiting, even in patients receiving cisplatin.[23–25]

CHEMOTHERAPY-INDUCED NAUSEA AND VOMITING

Information concerning antiemetic drug selection for patients with chemotherapy-induced nausea and vomiting is changing rapidly. Although newer agents may be readily acceptable in clinical practice, older agents may be appropriately prescribed. For example, prior to the use of metoclopramide, phenothiazine antiemetics were frequently chosen in patients with chemotherapy-induced nausea and vomiting. Even with newer therapies, if relief of symptoms is provided and side effects are absent or acceptable, these drugs may be continued. Conversely, failure to achieve adequate antiemetic efficacy during the first course of chemotherapy should prompt the clinician to search for more acceptable agents, possibly combination therapies.[14,15,26] Because of the complexities of chemotherapy-induced nausea and vomiting and the variable patient response, many patients require two or more antiemetic agents, particularly when the cytotoxic regimen includes high-dose cisplatin.

Droperidol, usually given intravenously, has been documented as safe and effective, even in ambulatory cancer patients.[16] Although the optimal antiemetic dose of droperidol for patients receiving chemotherapy may vary, many patients benefit from small doses, particularly when combined with other antiemetic drugs.

A variety of study protocols have been employed in corticosteroid antiemetic clinical trials with variations in drug, dosage regimen, and route of administration. Although studies using steroids in both single- and multiple-agent protocols have demonstrated acceptable efficacy, their exact ranking among antiemetic alternatives is not clear for patients receiving cytotoxic chemotherapy.

Benefits from corticosteroids have been quite variable. Of the corticosteroids studied, the use of dexamethasone has been best defined. During therapy with mildly to moderately emetogenic agents, dexamethasone appeared to be comparable to metoclopramide and superior to prochlorperazine when each was used alone; however, metoclopramide has shown greater efficacy when studied in patients receiving highly emetogenic regimens, especially those regimens that include cisplatin.[27–29] Methylprednisolone has been compared with metoclopramide and thiethylperazine. Benefit appeared to be greater for methylprednisolone than thiethylperazine and comparable to typical metoclopramide doses of less than 2 mg/kg.[30–33] Dosage regimens vary widely among steroid antiemetic protocols. When used alone, dexamethasone has often been administered parenterally as a single dose of 8–20 mg prior to chemotherapy, followed by oral doses of 4–12 mg up to 24 hours after completion of chemotherapy. Methylprednisolone has been administered prior to chemotherapy in a dose of 250 mg. After chemotherapy, up to four subsequent doses have been given. Dexamethasone is effective in patients with delayed nausea and vomiting, particularly when given with metoclopramide and lorazepam.

Metoclopramide is most often prescribed for the prevention and treatment of complex nausea and vomiting in response to chemotherapy administration, particularly cisplatin. For such patients, it has been employed in multiagent combination protocols; however, it has shown efficacy as a single therapy. Alone or in combination, metoclopramide has demonstrated significant efficacy in high doses (1–2 mg/kg IV), with one dose administered approximately 30 minutes prior to chemotherapy. Up to four subsequent doses are given at 2-hour intervals after chemotherapy.

Three selective 5-HT_3 serotonin antagonists—ondansetron, granisetron, and dolasetron—are effective in the management of chemotherapy-induced nausea and vomiting.[35] These agents inhibit emesis by blocking serotonin receptors in the area postrema, as well as those located along vagal afferent nerves in the GI tract.[36] Because these agents do not affect dopamine receptors, they are not associated with akathisia or acute dystonia.[37–39]

Ondansetron is usually administered intravenously 30 minutes prior to chemotherapy at a dose of 0.15 mg/kg over 15 minutes. Similar subsequent doses are given 4 and 8 hours after the first dose. As an alternative, a single 32-mg dose may be used intravenously in adults. Oral doses of 8 mg for adults and 4 mg for children may also be used. Little information is known concerning the dosage in children under the age of 2 years. Although ondansetron is generally well tolerated, reported side effects include diarrhea, headache, fever, constipation, dizziness, and drowsiness.

In adults and children at least 2 years of age, granisetron should be intravenously infused in a dose of 10 μg/kg over 5 minutes, beginning within 30 minutes before the initiation of chemotherapy, only on the day(s) chemotherapy is given. Oral doses of 1 mg may be used in adults. Children under the age of 2 years have not been adequately studied. Reported side effects of granisetron include headache, asthenia, somnolence, diarrhea, and constipation.

Dolasetron, the most recently marketed 5-HT_3 serotonin antagonist, may be administered as a single dose of 1.8 mg/kg, or as a fixed dose of 100 mg intravenously over 30 seconds, or diluted in a compatible solution and infused over a period of 15 minutes. With each method, the dose should be given approximately 30 minutes prior to chemotherapy. For children 2 years to 16 years of age, dolasetron may be given as a single dose of 1.8 mg/kg up to a maximum of 100 mg. However, safety and efficacy for patients younger than 2 years of age have not been established. Side effects most commonly noted in clinical trials include headache, diarrhea, and dizziness.

Although the availability of serotonin antagonists has made a significant impact on the management of patients receiving cytotoxic chemotherapy, these agents have not been effective in adequately controlling delayed emesis in many patients. Furthermore, some patients have experienced a reduction of efficacy with multiple-day chemotherapy or after several cycles of chemotherapy.[40] Because of these problems, most clinicians recommend the addition of dexamethasone or methylprednisolone to the regimen to improve response rates.

The cannabinoids are effective antiemetic agents, even in patients in whom other regimens have failed.[41,42] Dronabinol, Δ-9-tetrahydrocannabinol (THC), is the major psychoactive substance present in marijuana. Cannabinoids are only indicated for nausea and vomiting associated with cancer chemotherapy. Pharmacologic effects on opiate receptors and the cortical and vomiting centers of the brain may explain the beneficial effects of cannabinoids.[41–43] Cannabinoids may be associated with potentially undesirable features and are not equally effective against all stimuli or all doses of the same stimuli. As expected, a number of central nervous system (CNS) effects are common, including mood changes; anxiety; memory loss; fear; confusion; motor incoordination; time distortion; hallucinations; euphoria; relaxation; and hunger. Depending on the severity of these effects, doses should be lowered or discontinued. However, there is a strong correlation between a subjective "high" and antiemetic efficacy. Nabilone has been associated with less euphoric effects than dronabinol. Other potential side effects of the cannabinoids include sedation, blurred vision, hypotension, tachycardia, and paranoid ideation. Tolerance usually develops to most of the side effects, but not to the antiemetic activity.[44,45] Both increased effectiveness and improved tolerance of the cannabinoids may be observed in younger patients. Administration of the cannabinoids should be initiated the night before chemotherapy, because failure to achieve adequate blood concentrations will likely result in vomiting.

Anticipatory nausea and vomiting is a somewhat unique problem sometimes associated with cytotoxic chemotherapy. As many as one in four cancer patients may experience this condition during repeated courses of therapy. According to one study, patients with four or more of the following characteristics may be more likely to develop anticipatory symptoms by their fourth chemotherapy treatment: nausea and/or vomiting experienced after first treatment; nausea after treatment described as "moderate, severe, or intolerable"; vomiting after treatment described as "moderate, severe, or intolerable"; younger than 50 years of age; a susceptibility to motion sickness; feeling warm or hot all over after treatment; sweating following treatment; or feelings of generalized weakness following treatment.[46]

Benzodiazepines represent the best of the therapeutic alternatives in the treatment of anticipatory nausea and vomiting. The most often prescribed agent in this pharmacologic class is lorazepam, administered orally or intravenously for its amnestic effects. Dosage regimens include one dose before and multiple doses after each treatment with cytotoxic chemotherapy. Although some patients appreciate their lack of recall of having received chemotherapy, others find it uncomfortable and unacceptable. The latter patients may refuse lorazepam for subsequent treatments; however, acceptability of this feature of one's care may be highly dependent on the overall severity of symptoms. Similar to other benzodiazepines, lorazepam may display an array of pharmacologic activities including sedation, hypnosis, anxiolysis, and muscle relaxation in doses of 0.5–4.0 mg, with little change in a patient's respiratory or cardiovascular function. Other CNS effects, such as disorientation, hallucinations, incontinence, and amnesia, appear directly related to dose escalation.[47,48]

POSTOPERATIVE NAUSEA AND VOMITING

Nausea and vomiting associated with operative procedures are common problems for some patients. However, not all operative procedures produce these problems to the same degree. Specifically, procedures of the abdomen, eye, ear, nose, and throat are generally associated with higher incidences of nausea and vomiting than other procedures. Women, perhaps related to high gonadotropin levels, appear more susceptible to postoperative problems and experience a threefold higher incidence of nausea and vomiting as compared to men, independent of the type of operation or anesthetic.[49] Children are about twice as susceptible as adults.[49] Other risk factors that may be associated with an increase in postoperative symptoms include patient variables such as obesity, increased age, a history of motion sickness, or prior postoperative emesis. The choice of premedication or general anesthetic agent is also important. For example, inhalational anesthetics such as cyclopropane and nitrous oxide are particularly emetogenic, whereas agents such as isoflurane, enflurane, and halothane cause less, but still significant, postoperative nausea and vomiting. Of the intravenous anesthetics, propofol may be less emetogenic than some agents previously used.[50]

Most patients do not require preoperative prophylactic antiemetic therapy. In 70% to 90% of cases, patients either do not experience these symptoms or may have incomplete resolution when they occur. Simple premedication with atropine may decrease the potential occurrence of these symptoms in some patients. Other anticholinergic agents that may be effective include promethazine, scopolamine, cyclizine, and possibly glycopyrrolate. Although each of these agents has been effective in the prevention of nausea and vomiting in some clinical settings, sedation, dry mouth, and disorientation may limit their usefulness. Few patients will require the administration of additional preoperatively administered therapy.

The use of antiemetic therapy immediately following an operative procedure has been much more aggressively evaluated and applied, either as prophylaxis for potential postoperative symptoms or as acute management of actual nausea and vomiting. A variety of pharmacologic approaches are available and should be prescribed as single or combination therapy in their minimally effective dosage regimens. In doing so, patients will experience fewer adverse effects, some of which may otherwise be very troublesome for the overall recovery of the patient. Among the commonly prescribed antiemetic therapies in the postoperative setting, droperidol has been effective, particularly in patients undergoing obstetric and gynecologic procedures. Limiting effects, however, may include sedation, hypotension, and extrapyramidal signs.

Studies of metoclopramide have provided conflicting results, with some clinical trials documenting control of symptoms and others having concluded little value. Such findings were perhaps a result of metoclopramide's short duration of action, particularly when compared in settings in which patients had received morphine, a known emetogenic analgesic. Metoclopramide in intravenous doses of 10–20 mg administered 10 minutes prior to the induction of anesthesia may be used. Adverse effects of metoclopramide by such regimens include sedation and infrequently extrapyramidal signs. Although possible, extrapyramidal effects appear to be much less likely with the low doses most often prescribed in this setting. Intravenous droperidol in a single dose of 0.625–1.25 mg may be prescribed with or without metoclopramide.

Selective serotonin antagonists are very effective in the prevention of postoperative nausea and vomiting. To date, ondansetron, granisetron, and dolasetron have provided favorable outcomes when compared to placebo, metoclopramide, or droperidol. Ondansetron in oral regimens of 0.15 mg/kg up to a total of 8 mg, or IV regimens of 0.1 mg/kg up to a total of 8 mg, may be effective when given prophylactically prior to surgery. Intravenous granisetron in doses of 20–40 μg/kg given 30 minutes before the end of anesthesia have also been successfully used as postoperative prophylaxis. Similarly, oral doses of dolasetron of 25–100 mg given 1 hour to 2 hours before surgery, or IV doses of 12.5 mg given 15 minutes before the cessation of anesthesia also may be effective. A single IV dexamethasone dose of 8–20 mg may be combined with one of the selective serotonin antagonists to enhance antiemetic efficacy.

Regardless of which drug or regimen is chosen, one of the most often cited reasons for selecting a serotonin antagonist in the postoperative period appears to be the reduction of extrapyramidal effects noted with these agents, particularly as compared to droperidol and metoclopramide. Even so, the true role of serotonin antagonists is controversial. In fact, many clinicians prefer the use of older, more traditional, and less expensive antiemetic therapy. Unlike the more clearly defined etiologies of chemotherapy-induced nausea and vomiting, the unpredictable occurrence and severity of nausea and vomiting for surgical patients depends on the type of surgery, anesthesia, and patient. Therefore, serotonin antagonists are perhaps best reserved for patients who have failed to respond to traditional therapy, or for patients in whom drug allergies or other specific risk factors exist.

Based upon recent evidence, dexamethasone, alone or in combination with other antiemetic drugs, may be used in the management of postoperative nausea and vomiting. When used alone, dexamethasone may have similar efficacy as the selective serotonin antagonists. When used in combination, dexamethasone may enhance the effectiveness of other agents, including the selective serotonin antagonists. Single-dose intravenous administration given immediately before induction of anesthesia seems to be more effective than treatment at the end of anesthesia. However, more studies are needed to more fully determine the appropriate amount and timing of dosage with regard to the type of operative procedure as well as gender and age of the patient.[51,52]

Other antiemetic medications with value in the management of postoperative nausea and vomiting include promethazine, prochlorperazine, scopolamine, diphenhydramine, lorazepam, and ephedrine.

These latter medications may be prescribed in doses similar to those used in other settings and produce similar beneficial and adverse effects. With or without antiemetic therapy, certain nonpharmacologic methods may be effective in reducing the potential for emesis and should be applied universally. These include assisting patients with movement and providing particularly close attention to adequate hydration and pain management.

DISORDERS OF BALANCE

A variety of clinical conditions may be associated with vertigo and dizziness. The etiology of these complaints may include diseases that are infectious; postinfectious; demyelinative; vascular; neoplastic; degenerative; traumatic; toxic; psychogenic; or idiopathic. Therefore, symptoms of imbalance or perceived imbalance by the patient present a particular clinical challenge. Whether associated with a minor or complex disorder, motion sickness may be associated with nausea and vomiting.

Although much progress has been made in the management of other illnesses associated with emesis, motion sickness represents an area in which newer agents have provided little benefit. Studies of serotonin antagonists in motion sickness suggest that the 5-HT_3 receptor is not involved in the neural pathways that bring about motion sickness. In fact, 5-HT_3 serotonin receptor antagonists have provided no beneficial effects in reducing motion sickness when compared to placebo.[53] Interestingly, vertigo has been documented among the adverse reactions of these agents. Therefore, beneficial therapy for patients in this setting can most reliably be found among the antihistaminic-anticholinergic agents. However, their precise mechanisms of action are unknown to date. Neither the antihistaminic nor the anticholinergic potency appears to correlate well with the ability of these agents to prevent or treat the nausea and vomiting associated with motion sickness.

When used for their depressant effects on labyrinth excitability, these agents produce variable efficacy and safety profiles. The most useful antiemetic agent for motion sickness prophylaxis appears to be scopolamine, particularly when used 1 hour to 2 hours prior to symptom-producing exposures.[54] When using the transdermal scopolamine system, the patch should be applied to the hairless area behind one ear at least 4 hours before the antiemetic effect is needed. By delivering a total dose of 1.0 mg of scopolamine, beneficial effects may be recognized for up to 3 days. Oral regimens of antihistaminic-anticholinergic agents given one to several times each day may be effective, especially when the first dose is administered prior to motion.

ANTIEMETIC USE DURING PREGNANCY

More than one-half of pregnant women experience nausea and vomiting to some degree. However, fewer than 1% develop hyperemesis gravidarum, a serious condition marked by severe physical symptoms and/or medical complications. Because drugs may influence embryonic development most during the first 2 months of pregnancy, there has been much interest in the potential maternal and fetal benefits and risks of the antiemetic agents during this early phase.[55–62] Included among the commonly prescribed agents are the phenothiazines (prochlorperazine and promethazine); the antihistaminic-anticholinergic agents (dimenhydrinate, diphenhydramine, meclizine, cyclizine, doxylamine, and scopolamine); metoclopramide; and pyridoxine.

Although many women experience nausea and vomiting during pregnancy, the etiology of hyperemesis gravidarum is not well understood. Numerous mechanisms have been proposed. In addition, the severity of symptoms may vary greatly. In its most severe state, hyperemesis gravidarum may result in volume contraction, starvation, and electrolyte abnormalities; however, as a mild condition, it may be self-limiting and intermittent and may respond favorably to placebo. Other clinical strategies include attention to fluid and electrolyte management, the use of vitamin supplements, reduced intake of dietary fats with increased intake of carbohydrates, and methods aimed at reducing psychosomatic complaints.[59]

Evaluation of teratogenicity of drugs administered during the first trimester of pregnancy is of great importance, particularly in patients with a condition with such variability in its presentation. However, proof of teratogenicity varies among animals and humans. In animals, tests of this nature are performed in the laboratory, may vary with animal strain and breed, and may not be good predictors of human experience. Conversely, the clinical laboratory of patient care is the testing ground for agents used in humans. From this setting, case reports and retrospective epidemiologic reports document the outcome of these human experiences.

Teratogenicity is a major consideration for the use of antiemetic drugs during pregnancy and is the primary factor that dictates this condition's drug of choice. Therefore, both the benefit and side effect profiles for the mother as well as potential fetal risks are important. Of the agents commonly used, those that have demonstrated teratogenicity in animals include diphenhydramine, meclizine, prochlorperazine, and thiethylperazine.[58–64] In humans, however, meclizine has not been shown to have these same effects. Most authors currently do not recommend metoclopramide because its use during pregnancy requires further study. Also, its primary benefit in nonpregnant patients with nausea and vomiting has been in association with cancer, chemotherapy, and high intravenous doses. Although serotonin antagonists have been used during pregnancy and animal studies to date have revealed no harm, these agents are not generally recommended in this setting, particularly as first-line therapy. In addition, these agents may not reduce the severity of nausea, or affect daily weight gain, or affect the number of days required for hospitalization, as compared to other drugs. As a group, the antihistamines, including dimenhydrinate, diphenhydramine, cyclizine, and meclizine, appear to be effective and safe for the treatment of nausea and vomiting during pregnancy. Promethazine may also be considered.[62]

ANTIEMETIC USE IN CHILDREN

Most studies of antiemetic drugs have primarily included adult patients. Appropriate drug and dosage selection as well as the use of combination regimens lead to unique clinical questions in the management of children. For example, children may not require or tolerate the same mg/kg doses of drugs commonly used in adults. This finding is particularly true for metoclopramide. During the 1960s and 1970s, this drug was given as an antiemetic to European children with gastroenteritis. From these populations came numerous reports citing extrapyramidal reactions at cumulative daily doses less than 2.0 mg/kg.[65,66] It is now appreciated that these side effects should be anticipated in children and may occur at intravenous doses as low as 0.5 mg/kg given as repeated doses four times per day. Interestingly, differences in drug disposition, including plasma metoclopramide concentrations, probably do not explain the occurrence of dystonia.[67]

Dosage regimens and anticipated outcome of other antiemetic drugs in children are also unique compared to adults. Phenothiazines appear more likely to produce neuromuscular reactions, particularly dystonias, in children, especially when administered during acute viral illnesses such as chickenpox, measles, and gastroenteritis. Therefore, phenothiazines should be reserved for patients with prolonged vomiting in whom the benefit-to-risk ratio has been examined carefully. Promethazine may be the best agent in this class because its activity is most like that of the antihistamines rather than the phenothiazines.

Antihistaminic-anticholinergic agents may present some difficulty in selection depending on the exact age of the child. For example, the use of benzquinamide, buclizine, cyclizine, and scopolamine is not recommended in children younger than 12 years of age. Dimenhydrinate, however, has been used in children at doses that differ by age for those younger than 2 years, those 2 years to 6 years, and children 6 years to 12 years of age. Interestingly, trimethobenzamide may be used in children orally or rectally but is not recommended for injection. When chosen, it should be prescribed according to weight. Trimethobenzamide is also not recommended by any route for premature or newborn infants. The butyrophenones, haloperidol and droperidol, have been used in children, but not usually in those children younger than 2 years to 3 years of age. In children older than 3 years of age, most patients studied have received droperidol in the preoperative setting as an adjunct to general anesthesia. Fewer children, comparatively, have received droperidol during chemotherapy. Diphenidol, an agent associated with significant adverse effects, is usually not prescribed in children and is not recommended in patients weighing less than 50 pounds. Parenteral lorazepam, although perhaps useful in adults, is not generally recommended for patients younger than 18 years. Likewise, dronabinol is not indicated for children because it has been studied most in patients older than 12 years. Corticosteroids are often included in the anticancer regimens received by children and may be prescribed as antiemetics in this age group, particularly in combination with serotonin antagonists. Finally, serotonin antagonists have been evaluated in children of various ages and have been shown to be both safe and effective, particularly in patients receiving cytotoxic chemotherapy, or in patients in the postoperative period. These agents provide a significant reduction in nausea and vomiting in the absence of extrapyramidal effects.[68–70] However, consistent dosage information is primarily available for children 4 years to 18 years of age. Comparatively little information is available for children 3 years of age and younger.

EVALUATION OF THERAPEUTIC OUTCOMES

In accordance with the information presented concerning age and clinical condition, individualized therapy may be possible through drug selection and dosage adjustment. Monitoring criteria for drug therapy should include the subjective assessment of the patient's severity of nausea as well as objective parameters such as the number of vomiting episodes each day, the volume of vomitus lost, and evaluation of fluid, acid-base balance, and electrolyte status, with particular attention to serum sodium, potassium, and chloride concentrations. In addition, evaluation of renal function may become important, particularly in patients with volume contraction and progressive electrolyte disturbances. Specific parameters include daily urine volume, urine specific gravity, and urine electrolyte concentrations. Physical assessment of patients should include evaluation of mucous membranes and skin turgor, because dryness of these tissues may be indicative of significant volume loss. Table 35–5 lists recommendations for providing pharmaceutical care.

PHARMACOECONOMIC CONSIDERATIONS

As new drugs become accepted into clinical practice, the pharmacoeconomic issues associated with these drugs become increasingly important. Most pharmacoeconomic issues for the antiemetic drugs concern the use of 5-HT_3 antagonists in patients with chemotherapy-induced or postoperative nausea and vomiting. However, regardless of the medical reason associated with these symptoms, the use of expensive medications will always come under scrutiny, particularly because there are numerous potentially effective antiemetic therapies. For example, the routine use of 5-HT_3 antagonists in surgical patients has been questioned because so many procedures produce minimal risk of nausea or vomiting. Depending upon the variables previously reviewed, some patients are at much higher risk of developing these symptoms than are other patients. Clearly, studies are needed that evaluate the pharmacoeconomic issues involved in all common medical situations in which nausea and vomiting pose a clinically significant problem.

There are many important variables to consider when attempting to document the overall costs of using a medication in a particular medical situation. Medication costs alone cannot begin to explain the true pharmacoeconomic outcome associated with the use of antiemetic drugs. For example, the costs associated with an unexpected hospital admission because of vomiting in an outpatient undergoing a surgical procedure quickly offset the savings related to the selection of an inexpensive antiemetic drug. In this and other similar situations, it is economically and clinically important to develop antiemetic protocols based upon appropriate decision analysis and clinical outcomes so that certain patients appropriately receive an expensive drug while other patients appropriately receive a less expensive agent. In developing such protocols, all issues related to nausea and vomiting must be considered. As the number of patients who receive outpatient chemotherapy and surgery increases, the need to prevent subsequent hospitalizations from potentially unsuccessful antiemetic therapy will become increasingly important. However, as the cost of serotonin antagonists declines due to the availability of generic substitutes, greater acceptance of these agents as first-line therapy is more likely.

TABLE 35–5. Recommendations for Providing Pharmaceutical Care To Patients With Nausea and Vomiting

1. Assess patients for specific etiologies associated with nausea and vomiting.
2. Assess cancer patients' drug regimens for the use of emetogenic cytotoxic chemotherapy.
3. Assess cancer patients for potential nonchemotherapeutic etiologies of nausea and vomiting.
4. Assess patient allergies and adverse reactions to previously prescribed medications, including antiemetic drugs. Avoid regimens with previous negative outcomes, if possible.
5. Recommend drug therapy as presented in the chapter text, table, and Principles of Pharmacotherapy for specific patient situations.
6. Provide patient education concerning the etiology of nausea and vomiting as well as the nondrug and drug therapy approaches to overall management.
7. Assess and monitor patients for beneficial and adverse therapeutic outcomes.
8. Adjust recommendations and patient education based upon therapeutic response.

▶ PRINCIPLES OF PHARMACOTHERAPY

- Nausea and vomiting may be a part of the symptom complex for a variety of gastrointestinal, cardiovascular, infectious, neurologic, metabolic, or psychogenic processes.
- Nausea and vomiting may be caused by a variety of medications or other noxious agents, including cytotoxic chemotherapy, analgesics, general anesthetics, antibiotics, theophylline, digitalis, and amphotericin.
- The overall goal of treatment should be to prevent or eliminate nausea and vomiting regardless of etiology.
- Nondrug treatment of nausea and vomiting may include dietary, physical, or psychological management. In each case, the simplest effective therapy should be employed.
- Drug treatment options for the management of nausea and vomiting may be as simple as the use of antacids or as complex as the combination of two or more potent antiemetic drugs.
- Common antiemetic regimens used in patients with cancer should usually include medication prior to chemotherapy, with one or more possible doses after chemotherapy. Common regimens include (a) prochlorperazine with or without lorazepam; (b) ondansetron, granisetron, or dolasetron alone; (c) ondansetron, granisetron, or dolasetron plus dexamethasone or methylprednisolone; and (d) any of the preceding regimens plus dexamethasone or lorazepam as needed.
- Common antiemetic regimens used in patients undergoing surgical procedures might include (a) ondansetron, granisetron, or dolasetron alone; (b) metoclopramide alone; (c) droperidol alone; (d) dexamethasone alone; and (e) ondansetron, granisetron, or dolasetron plus dexamethasone or methylprednisolone.
- The therapeutic end point for antiemetic therapy is an acceptable reduction or absence of nausea and vomiting before and after surgery, chemotherapy, or other symptom-inducing activities.
- Evaluation of adverse reactions from antiemetic therapy includes attention to sedation and extrapyramidal effects.
- The total costs associated with antiemetic therapy should be considered, especially in settings involving the management of complex symptoms or other uses of serotonin antagonists.

REFERENCES

1. Hanson JS, McCallum RW. The diagnosis and management of nausea and vomiting: A review. Am J Gastroenterol 1985;80:210–218.
2. Frytak S, Moertel CG. Management of nausea and vomiting in the cancer patient. JAMA 1981;245:393–396.
3. Feldman M. Nausea and vomiting. In: Sleisenger MH, Fordtran JS, eds. Gastrointestinal Disease. Philadelphia, Saunders, 1983:160–177.
4. Redd WH. Control of nausea and vomiting in chemotherapy patients: Four effective behavioral methods. Postgrad Med 1984;75:105–113.
5. Eyre HJ, Ward JH. Control of cancer chemotherapy-induced nausea and vomiting. Cancer 1984;54:2642–2648.
6. Morrow GR. Prevalence and correlation of anticipatory nausea and vomiting in chemotherapy patients. J Natl Cancer Inst 1982;68:585–588.
7. Lyles JN, Burish TG, Knozely MG, et al. Efficacy of relaxation training and guided imagery in reducing the aversiveness of cancer chemotherapy. J Consult Clin Psychol 1982;50:509–524.
8. Morrow GR, Morrell C. Behavioral treatment for the anticipatory nausea and vomiting induced by cancer chemotherapy. N Engl J Med 1982; 307:1476–1480.
9. Redd WH, Andresen GV, Minagawa RY. Hypnotic control of anticipatory emesis in patients receiving cancer chemotherapy. J Consult Clin Psychol 1982;50:14–19.
10. Dutro MP, Amerson AB. Comparison of liquid antacids. N Engl J Med 1980;302:967.
11. Fordtran JS, Morawski S, Richardson C. *In vitro* and *in vivo* evaluation of antacids. N Engl J Med 1973;288:923–928.
12. Seipler JK, Mahakian K, Trudeau WT. Current concepts in clinical therapeutics: Peptic ulcer disease. Clin Pharm 1986;5:128–142.
13. Edmunds SJ, Prys RC. Pharmacology of drugs used in neuroleptanalgesia. Br J Anaesth 1970;42:207–216.
14. Wampler G. The pharmacology and clinical effectiveness of phenothiazines and related drugs for managing chemotherapy-induced emesis. Drugs 1983;25(suppl):35–51.
15. Lucas VS. Phenothiazines as antiemetics. In: Lazlo J, ed. Antiemetics and Cancer Chemotherapy. Baltimore, Williams & Wilkins, 1983:93–107.
16. Jacobs AJ, Deppe G, Cohen CJ. A comparison of the antiemetic effects of droperidol and prochlorperazine in chemotherapy with *cis*-platinum. Gynecol Oncol 1980;10:55–57.
17. Cersosimo RJ, Bromer R, Hoffer S, et al. The antiemetic activity of droperidol administered by intramuscular injection during cisplatin chemotherapy: A pilot study. Drug Intell Clin Pharm 1985;19:118–121.
18. Paladine W, Price L, Sokol G, et al. Antiemetic trial of droperidol. Proc Am Soc Clin Oncol 1980;21:380.
19. Brown RE, Gregg RE, Hood JC. Droperidol treatment of streptozotocin-induced nausea and vomiting. Drug Intell Clin Pharm 1982;16:775–776.
20. Cersosimo RJ, Karp DD. Adrenal corticosteroids as antiemetics during cancer chemotherapy. Pharmacotherapy 1986;6:118–127.
21. Gralla RJ. Metoclopramide: A review of antiemetic trials. Drugs 1983;25(suppl):63–73.
22. Schyulze-Delriev K. Metoclopramide. Gastroenterology 1979;77:768–779.
23. Strum SB, McDermed JE, Lauer D, et al. Control of acute-onset and delayed-onset chemotherapy-induced nausea and emesis with metoclopramide-based regimens. Intern Med Specialist 1985;6:104–112.
24. Fortner CL, Finley RS, Grove WR. Combination antiemetic therapy in the control of chemotherapy-induced emesis. Drug Intell Clin Pharm 1985;19:21–24.
25. Plezia PM, Alberts DS, Kessler J, et al. Immediate termination of intractable vomiting induced by cisplatin combination chemotherapy using an intensive five-drug antiemetic regimen. Cancer Treat Rep 1984;68:1493–1495.
26. Stoudemire A, Cotanch P, Lazlo J. Recent advances in the pharmacologic and behavioral management of chemotherapy-induced emesis. Arch Intern Med 1984;144:1029–1033.
27. Cognetti F, Pinnaro P, Carlini P, et al. Randomized open crossover trial between metoclopramide and dexamethasone for the prevention of cisplatin-induced nausea and vomiting. Eur J Cancer Clin Oncol 1984;20:183–187.
28. Aapro MS, Plezia PM, Albert DS, et al. Double-blind crossover study of the antiemetic efficacy of high-dose dexamethasone versus high-dose metoclopramide. J Clin Oncol 1984;2:466–471.
29. Markman M, Sheidler V, Ettinger DS, et al. Antiemetic efficacy of dexamethasone. Randomized, double-blind, crossover study with prochlorperazine in patients receiving cancer chemotherapy. N Engl J Med 1984;311:549–552.
30. Kolaric K, Roth A. Methylprednisolone as an antiemetic in patients on *cis*-platinum chemotherapy. Results of a controlled randomized study. Tumori 1983;69:43–46.
31. Giaconne G, Donadio M, Musella R, et al. Comparison of methylprednisolone and metoclopramide in the prophylactic treatment of cisplatin-induced nausea and vomiting. Tumori 1984;70:237–241.
32. Schallier D, Van Belle S, De Greve J, et al. Methylprednisolone as an antiemetic drug. A randomized double-blind study. Cancer Chemother Pharmacol 1985;14:235–237.
33. Ell C, Konig HJ, Brockmann P, et al. Antiemetic efficacy of moderately high-dose metoclopramide in patients receiving varying doses of

cisplatin. Controlled comparison with combination of methylprednisolone and metoclopramide. Oncology 1985;42:354–357.
34. Pope CE II. Acid-reflux disorders. N Engl J Med 1994;331:656–660.
35. Marty M, Pouillart P, Scholl S, et al. Comparison of the 5-hydroxytryptamine$_3$ (serotonin) antagonist ondansetron (GR 38032F) with high-dose metoclopramide in the control of cisplatin-induced emesis. N Engl J Med 1990;322:816–821.
36. Lindley C, Blower P. Oral serotonin type 3-receptor antagonists for prevention of chemotherapy-induced emesis. Am J Health Syst Pharm 2000;57:1685–1697.
37. Bryson JC, Finn AL, Plagge PB, et al. The safety profile of IV ondansetron from clinical trials. Proc ASCL 1990;9:328. Abstract.
38. Smith RN. Safety of ondansetron. Eur J Cancer Clin Oncol 1989;25(suppl):S47–S50.
39. Chaffee BJ, Tankanow RM. Ondansetron—The first of a new class of antiemetic agents. Clin Pharm 1991;10:430–446.
40. Aapro MS. Review of experience with ondansetron and granisetron. Ann Oncol 1993;4(suppl 3):S9–S14.
41. Lazlo J, Lucas VS. Synthetic cannabinoids. In: Lazlo J, ed. Antiemetics and Cancer Chemotherapy. Baltimore, Williams & Wilkins, 1983:116–128.
42. Herman TS, Einhorn LH, Jones SE, et al. Superiority of nabilone over prochlorperazine as an antiemetic in patients receiving cancer chemotherapy. N Engl J Med 1979;300:1295–1297.
43. Tortorice PV, O'Connell MB. Management of chemotherapy-induced nausea and vomiting. Pharmacotherapy 1990;10:129–145.
44. Anderson PO, McGuire GG. Δ-9-Tetrahydrocannabinol as an antiemetic. Am J Hosp Pharm 1981;38:639–646.
45. Neidhart JA, Gagen M. Experimental antiemetic agents (other than cannabinoids and metoclopramide): In: Lazlo J, ed. Antiemetics and Cancer Chemotherapy. Baltimore, Williams & Wilkins, 1983:142–163.
46. Morrow FR, Lindke J, Black PM. Predicting development of anticipatory nausea in cancer patients: Prospective examination of eight clinical characteristics. J Pain Symptom Manage 1991;6:215–223.
47. Lazlo J. Oral lorazepam to improve tolerance of cytotoxic therapy. Lancet 1981;1:1316–1317.
48. Meyer M, Long AM, Natale RB, et al. Phase I, II and III trials of a new antiemetic agent—Lorazepam. Proc Am Soc Clin Oncol 1983;2:88.
49. Mitchelson F. Pharmacological agents affecting emesis: A review. Drugs 1992;43:443–463.
50. Kenny GN. Risk factors for postoperative nausea and vomiting. Anaesthesia 1994;49(suppl):6–10.
51. Wang JJ, Ho ST, Tzeng JI, Tang CS. The effect of timing of dexamethasone administration on its efficacy as a prophylactic antiemetic for postoperative nausea and vomiting. Anesth Analg 2000;91:136–139.
52. Kovac AL. Prevention and treatment of postoperative nausea and vomiting. Drugs 2000;59:213–243.
53. Scott JR, Barnes GR, Wright RJ, Ruddock CJ. The effect on motion sickness and oculomotor function of GR 38032F, a 5-HT$_3$-receptor antagonist with anti-emetic properties. Br J Clin Pharmacol 1989;27:147–157.
54. Wood CD. Antimotion sickness and antiemetic drugs. Drugs 1979;17:471–479.
55. Jarnfelt-Samsioe A, Samsioe G, Velinder GM. Nausea and vomiting in pregnancy—A contribution to its epidemiology. Gynecol Obstet Invest 1983;16:221–229.
56. Tuchmann-Duplessis H. Drugs and xenobiotics as teratogens. Pharmacol Ther 1984;26:273–344.
57. Leathem AM. Safety and efficacy of antiemetics used to treat nausea and vomiting in pregnancy. Clin Pharm 1986;5:660–668.
58. Fairweather DV. Nausea and vomiting during pregnancy. Obstet Gynecol Annu 1978;7:91–105.
59. Kousen M. Treatment of nausea and vomiting in pregnancy. Am Fam Physician 1993;48:1279–1284.
60. Schardein JL. Drugs as Teratogens. Cleveland, OH, CRC Press, 1976;5:130.
61. Koren G, Pastuszak A. Drug therapy : Drugs in pregnancy. N Engl J Med 1998;338:1128–1137.
62. Mazzotta P, Magee LA. A risk-benefit assessment of pharmacological and nonpharmacological treatments for nausea and vomiting of pregnancy. Drugs 2000;59:781–800.
63. Shepard TH. Catalog of Teratogenic Agents, 4th ed. Baltimore, Johns Hopkins University Press, 1983.
64. Nishimura H, Tanimura T. Clinical Aspects of Teratogenicity of Drugs. New York, Elsevier, 1976:212, 241.
65. Low LCK, Goel KM. Metoclopramide poisoning in children. Arch Dis Child 1980;55:310–312.
66. Casteels-Van Daele M, Jaeken J, Van Der Schueren P, et al. Dystonic reactions in children caused by metoclopramide. Arch Dis Child 1970;45:130–133.
67. Bateman DN, Craft AW, Nicholson E, et al. Dystonic reactions and the pharmacokinetics of metoclopramide in children. Br J Clin Pharmacol 1983;15:557–559.
68. Furst SR, Rodarte A, Demars P. Ondansetron reduces postoperative vomiting in children undergoing tonsillectomy. Anesthesiology 1993;79:A1197. Abstract.
69. Lawhorn CD, Brown RE Jr, Schmitz ML, et al. Prevention of postoperative vomiting in pediatric outpatient strabismus surgery. Anesthesiology 1993;79:A1196. Abstract.
70. Stevens RF. The role of ondansetron in paediatric patients: A review of three studies. Eur J Cancer 1991;27(suppl 1):S20–S22.

36

Diarrhea, Constipation, and Irritable Bowel Syndrome

William J. Spruill and William E. Wade

DIARRHEA

In the United States, diarrhea is a troublesome discomfort that is sometimes fatal. Usually, diarrheal episodes begin abruptly and subside within 1 day or 2 days without treatment. This chapter focuses primarily on noninfectious diarrhea, with only minor reference to infectious diarrhea (see Chap. 111). Diarrhea is often a symptom of a systemic disease and not all possible causes of diarrhea are discussed in this chapter.

To understand diarrhea, one must have a reasonable definition of the condition; unfortunately, the literature is extremely variable on this. Simply, diarrhea is an increased frequency and decreased consistency of fecal discharge as compared to an individual's normal bowel pattern. Frequency and consistency are variable within and between individuals. For example, some individuals defecate as often as three times per day, whereas others defecate only two or three times per week. A Western diet usually produces a daily stool weighing between 100 g and 300 g, depending on the amount of nonabsorbable materials (mainly carbohydrates) consumed. Patients with serious diarrhea may have a daily stool weight in excess of 300 g; however, a subset of patients experience frequent small, watery passages. Additionally, vegetable fiber-rich diets, such as those consumed in some Eastern cultures such as Africa, produce stools weighing more than 300 g/d.

Diarrhea may be associated with a specific disease of the intestines or secondary to a disease outside the intestines. For instance, bacillary dysentery directly affects the gut, whereas diabetes mellitus causes neuropathic diarrheal episodes. Furthermore, diarrhea can be considered as acute or chronic disease. Infectious diarrhea is often acute; diabetic diarrhea is chronic. Whether acute or chronic, diarrhea has the same pathophysiologic causes that help identification of specific treatments.

EPIDEMIOLOGY

The epidemiology of diarrhea is different in developed versus developing countries.[1–3] In the United States, diarrheal illnesses are usually not reported to the Centers for Disease Control and Prevention (CDC) unless associated with an outbreak or an unusual organism or condition. For example, AIDS has been identified with protracted diarrheal illness. Diarrhea is a major problem in day care centers and nursing homes, probably because early childhood and senescence plus environmental conditions are risk factors. However, an exact epidemiologic profile in the United States is not available through the CDC or published literature.

In the United States, viral and bacterial organisms account for most episodes of infectious diarrhea. Common causative bacterial organisms include *Shigella, Salmonella, Campylobacter, Staphylococcus,* and *Escherichia coli*. Food-borne bacterial infection is a major concern as the result of several major food poisoning episodes that were traced to poor sanitary conditions in meat-processing plants. Acute viral infections are attributed mostly to Norwalk and rotavirus groups. In developing countries, diarrhea is a leading cause of illness and death in children.[4] Moreover, diarrhea produces an economic burden because of costs related to hospitalization and loss of productivity. It is estimated that 1.3 billion episodes occur annually and that 4 million deaths result from diarrhea in these countries. Factors associated with these findings include poor sanitation, poor nutrition, and age less than 5 years. Worldwide, these children experience an average of three episodes each year (2.7 diarrhea episodes/person/year in Latin America as compared with 1 episode/per person/year in the US and Western Europe).

PATHOPHYSIOLOGY

In the fasting state, 9 L of fluid enters the proximal small intestine each day. Of this fluid, 2 L are ingested through diet; the remainder consists of internal secretions. Because of meal content, duodenal chyme is usually hypertonic. When chyme reaches the ileum, the osmolality adjusts to that of plasma, with most dietary fat, carbohydrate, and protein being absorbed. The volume of ileal chyme decreases to about 1 L/d upon entering the colon. The electrolyte profile of ileal chyme per liter is normally sodium 140 mEq, potassium 8 mEq, chloride 60 mEq, and bicarbonate 70 mEq. In the normal state, the colon absorbs 900 mL of this volume, reducing water loss in the stool to 100 mL daily. Fecal electrolyte content is sodium, 40 mEq/L; chloride, 15 mEq/L; potassium, 90 mEq/L; and bicarbonate, 30 mEq/L.

From the preceding description, one visualizes diarrhea as an imbalance in absorption and secretion of water and electrolytes. In normal volunteers, small intestine water has a maximum rate of absorption. If the small intestine absorption capacity is exceeded, chyme overloads the colon, resulting in diarrhea. In humans, the colon absorptive capacity is about 5 L daily. Colonic fluid transport is critical to water and electrolyte balance.

Absorption from the intestines occurs by three mechanisms: active transport, diffusion, and solvent drag. Active transport means an expenditure of energy is required to move a substrate against a concentration gradient across a membrane. Diffusion, a nonenergy-dependent process, transports substances through a membrane along a concentration gradient. A solvent can "drag" a substrate across a membrane.

Water moves across the gut after the movement of solutes such as sodium and by diffusion.[5] Diffusion obeys the principle of osmosis. For example, when chyme is dilute, water diffuses from the gut into the blood. Also, as ions (e.g., sodium) or nutrients (e.g., glucose) cross a membrane, water quickly "follows" to maintain an isosmotic state. The intestinal mucosa is semipermeable and allows for selective movement of solutes and solvents. For instance, the proximal intestine rapidly makes meal content isosmotic. In the colon, chyme may be hypertonic; bacterial metabolism of carbohydrates partly explains this hypertonic colonic state. Unabsorbed carbohydrates are metabolized into volatile fatty acids and absorbed across the colon. Active transport and diffusion are the mechanisms of sodium transport. Because of the high luminal sodium concentration (142 mEq/L), sodium diffuses from the sodium-rich gut into epithelial cells. Inside the epithelial cell, sodium is actively pumped from a lower concentration (50 mEq/L) to a higher concentration (142 mEq/L) in the blood by sodium-potassium-activated ATPase.

To maintain an isoelectric condition across the epithelial membrane, chloride moves from the lumen into the epithelial cell. The absorption of sodium through the epithelial cells creates an electronegativity in the chyme. To reestablish electric neutrality, positively charged sodium ions pull negatively charged chloride ions into the epithelial cell. In the epithelial cell, chloride channels opened by cyclic adenosine monophosphate (AMP) permit movement of chloride into the intestinal lumen.

Hydrogen ions are transported by an indirect mechanism in the upper small intestine. As sodium is absorbed, hydrogen ions are secreted into the gut. Hydrogen ions then combine with bicarbonate ions to form carbonic acid, which then dissociates into carbon dioxide and water. Carbon dioxide readily diffuses into the blood for expiration through the lung. The water remains in the chyme.

Paracellular pathways are major routes of ion movement. As ions, monosaccharides, and amino acids are actively transported, they create an osmotic pressure, drawing water and electrolytes across the intestinal wall. This pathway accounts for very large amounts of ion transport, especially sodium. Sodium plays an important role in stimulating glucose absorption. Glucose absorption occurs with active transport of sodium from the epithelial cell into the blood. In this process, glucose combines with the transport protein carrying sodium into the blood—a phenomenon referred to as *cotransport*. Another mechanism by which glucose is absorbed is by concentration-dependent diffusion.

Sodium cotransport of amino acids occurs in a similar fashion as described for glucose. Amino acids are transported into most cells against large concentration gradients. When an amino acid combines with extracellular sodium to specific transport protein, both substrates move from the lumen to the blood. Cotransport absorption mechanisms of glucose-sodium and amino acid-sodium are extremely important for treating diarrhea.

Gut motility influences absorption and secretion. Time in which luminal content is in contact with the epithelium is under neural and hormonal control. Neurohormonal substances, such as angiotensin, vasopressin, glucocorticoid, and aldosterone, and neurotransmitters also regulate ion transport.

MECHANISMS

Four general pathophysiologic mechanisms disrupt water and electrolyte balance, leading to diarrhea, and are the basis of diagnosis and therapy. These are (a) a change in active ion transport by either decreased sodium absorption or increased chloride secretion; (b) change in intestinal motility; (c) increase in luminal osmolarity; and (d) increase in tissue hydrostatic pressure. These mechanisms have been related to four broad clinical diarrheal groups: secretory, osmotic, exudative, and altered intestinal transit.

Secretory diarrhea occurs when a stimulating substance either increases secretion or decreases absorption of large amounts of water and electrolytes. Substances that cause excess secretions include vasoactive intestinal peptide (VIP) from a pancreatic tumor, unabsorbed dietary fat in steatorrhea, laxatives, hormones (such as secretin), bacterial toxins, and excessive bile salts. Many of these agents stimulate intracellular cyclic AMP and inhibit Na^+/K^+-ATPase, leading to increased secretion. Also, many of these mediators inhibit ion absorption simultaneously. Clinically, secretory diarrhea is recognized by large stool volumes (>1 L/d) with normal ionic contents and osmolality approximately equal to plasma. Fasting does not alter the stool volume in these patients.

Poorly absorbed substances retain intestinal fluids, resulting in osmotic diarrhea. This process occurs with malabsorption syndromes, lactose intolerance, administration of divalent ions (e.g., magnesium containing antacids), or consumption of poorly soluble carbohydrate (e.g., lactulose). As a poorly soluble solute is transported, the gut adjusts the osmolality to plasma; in so doing, water and electrolytes flux into the lumen. Clinically, osmotic diarrhea is distinguishable from other types as it ceases if the patient resorts to a fasting state.

Inflammatory gut diseases discharge mucus, serum proteins, and blood into the gut. Sometimes bowel movements consist only of mucus, exudate, and blood. Exudative diarrhea probably affects other absorptive, secretory, or motility functions to account for the large stool volume associated with this disorder.

Altered intestinal motility produces diarrhea by three mechanisms: reduction of contact time in the small intestine, premature emptying of the colon, and bacterial overgrowth. Chyme must be exposed to intestinal epithelium for a sufficient time period to enable normal absorption and secretion processes to occur. If this contact time decreases, diarrhea results. Intestinal resection or bypass surgery and drugs (such as metoclopramide) cause this type of diarrhea. On the other hand, an increased time of exposure allows fecal bacteria overgrowth. A characteristic small intestine diarrheal pattern is rapid, small, coupling bursts of waves. These waves are inefficient, do not allow absorption, and rapidly dump chyme into the colon. Once in the colon, chyme exceeds the colonic capabilities to absorb water.

CLINICAL PRESENTATION

Diarrhea is divided into acute and chronic disorders. Usually, acute diarrheal episodes subside with 72 hours of onset. Chronic diarrhea involves frequent attacks over extended time periods. If diarrhea persists or gross blood is present, the patient needs an extensive evaluation.

HISTORY AND PHYSICAL EXAMINATION

Onset and duration differentiate acute and chronic diarrhea. The leading cause of acute diarrhea is viral gastroenteritis. Patients with acute diarrhea complain of an abrupt onset of nausea, vomiting, abdominal pain, headache, fever, chills, and malaise. Bowel movements are frequent and never bloody, and diarrhea lasts 12 hours to 60 hours. Abdominal pain is evaluated for duration, location, and character. Intermittent periumbilical or lower right quadrant pain with cramps and audible bowel sounds is characteristic of small intestinal disease. When pain is present in large intestinal diarrhea, it is a gripping, aching sensation with tenesmus (straining ineffective and painful stooling). Pain localizes to the hypogastric region, right or left lower quadrant, or sacral region. In chronic diarrhea, history of previous bouts, weight loss, anorexia, and chronic weakness are important findings. Certain diarrheal diseases are associated with specific age groups. For example, diarrhea from colon cancer is common with advancing age, whereas diarrhea from viral gastroenteritis is largely a childhood condition. A medication history is extremely important in identifying drug-induced diarrhea (Table 36–1). For example, many agents, including antibiotics and other drugs, cause diarrhea, or, less commonly, pseudomembranous colitis. Self-inflicted laxative abuse for weight loss is popular. Neurotic or psychotic behavior leads to laxative abuse. Drug side effects (e.g., quinidine side effects) often present as diarrhea.

TABLE 36–1. Drugs Causing Diarrhea

Laxatives
Antacids containing magnesium
Antineoplastics
Auranofin (gold salt)
Antibiotics
  Clindamycin
  Tetracyclines
  Sulfonamides
  Any broad-spectrum antibiotic
Antihypertensives
  Reserpine
  Guanethidine
  Methyldopa
  Guanabenz
  Guanadrel
Cholinergics
  Bethanechol
  Neostigmine
Cardiac agents
  Quinidine
  Digitalis
  Digoxin
Nonsteroidal anti-inflammatory drugs
Prostaglandins
Colchicine

Stool characteristics are important in assessing the etiology of diarrhea. A description of the frequency, volume, consistency, and color provides diagnostic clues. For instance, diarrhea starting in the small intestine produces a copious, watery or fatty (greasy), and foul-smelling stool; contains undigested food particles; and is usually free from gross blood. Colonic diarrhea appears as small, pasty, and sometimes bloody or mucoid movements. Rectal tenesmus with flatus accompanies large intestinal diarrhea.

The physical examination of the abdomen in these patients typically demonstrates hyperperistalsis with borborygmi (growling stomach sounds) and generalized or local tenderness. A rectal examination detects masses or possibly fecal impaction, a common cause of diarrhea in the elderly. Checking skin turgor and degree of oral saliva present is useful in assessing the patient's hydration status of the patient. If hypotension, tachycardia, weak radial pulses, or stupor are present, severe dehydration is suggested. Fever usually indicates an infectious cause.

LABORATORY AND ENDOSCOPIC EVALUATION

Spot stool analysis is commonly used for diagnosing unexplained diarrhea, especially in chronic situations.[6] Stool studies include examination for microorganisms, blood, mucus, fat, osmolality, pH, electrolyte and mineral concentration and cultures. Stool test kits are useful for detecting gastrointestinal viruses, particularly rotavirus. Antibody serologic testing shows rising titers over a 3-day to 6-day period, but this test is not practical and nonspecific. Occasionally, total daily stool volume is also determined. Besides stool studies, direct endoscopic visualization and biopsy of the colon may be undertaken to assess for the presence of conditions such as colitis or cancer. Radiographic studies are helpful in neoplastic and inflammatory conditions.

PROGNOSIS

Most acute diarrhea is self-limiting, subsiding within 72 hours. However, infants, young children, the elderly, and debilitated persons are at risk for morbid and mortal events in prolonged or voluminous diarrhea. These groups are at risk for water, electrolyte, and acid-base disturbances, and potentially cardiovascular collapse and death. The prognosis for chronic diarrhea depends on the cause; for example, diarrhea secondary to diabetes mellitus waxes and wanes throughout life.

PREVENTION

Acute viral diarrheal illness often occurs in day care centers and nursing homes. Because person-to-person contact is the mechanism of spreading viral gastroenteritis, isolation techniques must be used to prevent spread between these populations and health care workers. For bacterial, parasite, and protozoal infections, strict food handling, sanitation, water, and other environmental hygiene practices prevent and control their transmission. If diarrhea is secondary to another illness, controlling the primary condition is necessary. Antibiotics and bismuth subsalicylate are advocated for preventing traveler's diarrhea, along with special care with drinking water and fresh vegetables.

▶ TREATMENT: Diarrhea

DESIRED OUTCOME

If prevention is not successful and diarrhea occurs, the therapeutic goals are to (a) manage the diet; (b) prevent excessive water, electrolyte, and acid-base disturbances; (c) provide symptomatic relief; (d) treat curable causes; and (e) manage secondary disorders causing diarrhea (Figs. 36–1 and 36–2). Clinicians must clearly understand that diarrhea, like a cough, may be a body defense mechanism for ridding itself of harmful substances or pathogens. The correct therapeutic response is not necessarily to stop diarrhea at all costs!

NONPHARMACOLOGIC MANAGEMENT

Dietary management is a first priority in the treatment of diarrhea. Most clinicians continue to recommend stopping solid foods for 24 hours and avoiding dairy products. However, fasting is of questionable value because the assumptions based upon this modality have not been extensively studied. In osmotic diarrhea, these maneuvers control the problem. If the mechanism is secretory, the diarrhea persists. When the patient is nauseated or vomiting, a mild, digestible low-residue diet is administered for 24 hours. If vomiting is present and uncontrollable with antiemetics (see Chap. 35), nothing is taken by mouth. As bowel movements decrease, a bland diet is begun. Research shows that feeding should continue in children with acute bacterial diarrhea. Fed children have less morbidity and mortality, whether or not they receive oral rehydration fluids. Studies are not available in the elderly or in other high-risk groups to determine the value of continued feeding in bacterial diarrhea.

WATER AND ELECTROLYTES

Rehydration and maintenance of water and electrolytes are primary treatment goals until the diarrheal episode ends. If the patient is volume depleted, rehydration should be directed to replacing water and

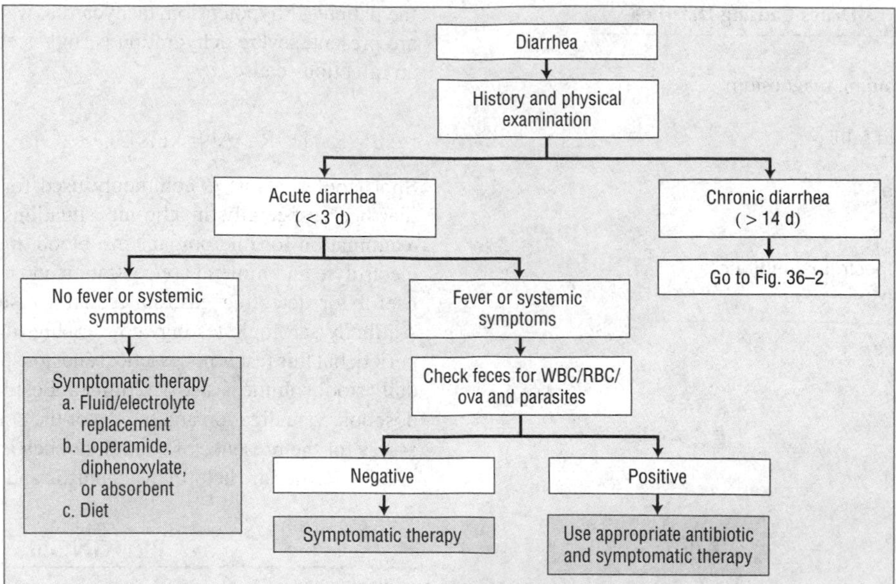

FIGURE 36–1. Recommendations for treating acute diarrhea. Follow these steps: (1) Perform a complete history and physical examination. (2) Is the diarrhea acute or chronic? If chronic diarrhea, go to Fig. 36–2. (3) If acute diarrhea, check for fever and/or systemic signs and symptoms (i.e., toxic patient). If systemic illness (fever, anorexia, volume depletion), check for infectious source. If positive for infectious diarrhea, use appropriate antibiotic/anthelminthic drug, and symptomatic therapy. If negative for infectious cause, use only symptomatic treatment. (4) If no systemic findings, then use symptomatic therapy, based on severity of volume depletion, oral or parenteral fluid/electrolytes, antidiarrheal agents (see Table 36–3), and diet.

electrolytes to normal body composition. Then water and electrolyte deficits are corrected by replacing losses. Many patients will not develop volume depletion and therefore will only require maintenance fluid and electrolyte therapy. Parenteral and enteral routes may be used for supplying water and electrolytes. If vomiting and dehydration are not severe, enteral feeding is the less costly and preferred method. In the United States, many commercial oral rehydration preparations are available (Table 36–2). Because of concerns about hypernatremia, American physicians continue to hospitalize and intravenously correct these deficits in severe dehydration. Oral solutions are strongly recommended.[6,7] In developing countries, the World Health Organization Oral Rehydration Solution (WHO-ORS) saves the lives of millions of children annually (Table 36–2).

During diarrhea, the small intestine retains its ability to actively transport monosaccharides such as glucose. Glucose actively carries sodium with water and other electrolytes. Because the WHO-ORS has a high sodium concentration, US physicians have been reluctant to use it in well-nourished children. This attitude could be changing as controlled comparative studies describe more favorable results with WHO-ORS than with parenteral fluids.[7] Amino acids promote sodium transport and act as an antisecretory agent. Researchers have added glycine to ORS in an attempt to create a "super-ORS." Reports, however, are disappointing, because glycine causes an osmotic diarrhea and diuresis in experimental concentrations. Rice-based oral solution is a hyposmotically active substrate. Rice supplies long-chain molecules and elutes glucose without increasing stool or urine outflows. Pizarro and associates[8] reported effective rehydration of infants with acute diarrhea using a rice-based solution. They also reported decreased stool output and greater absorption and retention of fluid and electrolytes. In summary, oral rehydration solution is a life-saving treatment for millions afflicted in developing countries. Acceptance in the developed countries is less enthusiastic, but preventing hospitalization may win endorsement as a cost-effective alternative, saving millions of dollars.

PHARMACOLOGIC THERAPY

Various drugs have been used to treat diarrheal attacks (Table 36–3). These drugs are grouped into several categories: antimotility, adsorbents, antisecretory compounds, antibiotics, enzymes, and intestinal microflora. Usually, these drugs are not curative but palliative.

OPIATES AND THEIR DERIVATIVES

Opiates and opioid derivatives (a) delay the transit of intraluminal content or (b) increase gut capacity, prolonging contact and absorption. Enkephalins, endogenous opioid substances, regulate fluid movement across the mucosa by stimulating absorptive processes. Most opiates act through peripheral and central mechanisms, except loperamide, which acts peripherally. Loperamide is antisecretory; it inhibits the calcium-binding protein calmodulin, controlling chloride secretion. Loperamide, available as 2-mg capsules or 1 mg/5 mL solution (both are nonprescription products), is suggested for managing acute and chronic diarrhea. The usual adult dose is initially 4 mg orally, followed by 2 mg after each loose stool, up to 16 mg/d. Used correctly, the drug has rare side effects such as dizziness and constipation. If the diarrhea is concurrent with a high fever or bloody stool, the patient should be referred to a physician. Also, diarrhea lasting beyond 48 hours after starting loperamide warrants medical attention.

Loperamide can be also be used in traveler's diarrhea. It is comparable to bismuth subsalicylate for treatment of this disorder.[9] Limitations to the use of opiates include an addiction potential (a real concern with long-term use) and worsening of diarrhea in selected infectious diarrhea.

Paregoric, 2 mg/5 mL morphine, is indicated for managing both acute and chronic diarrhea. However, it is not as widely prescribed today, because of its drug abuse potential. Diphenoxylate is available

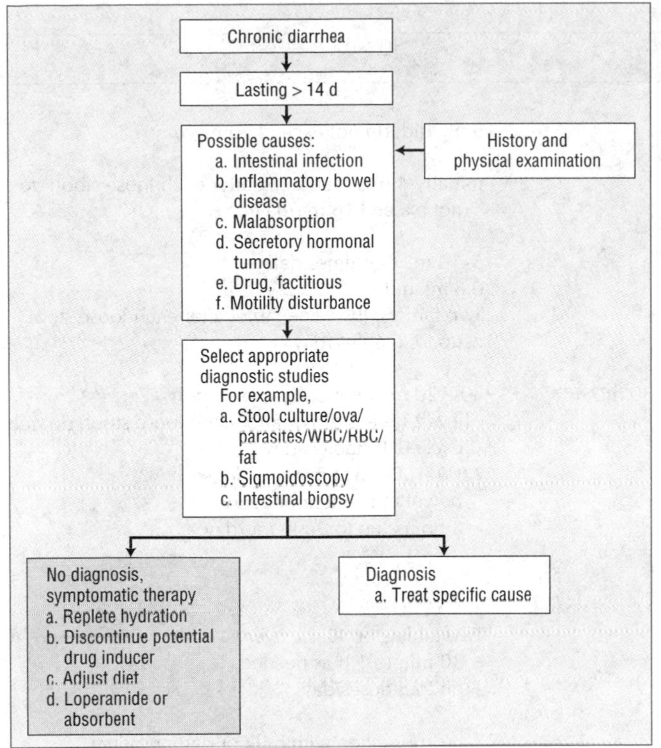

FIGURE 36–2. Recommendations for treating chronic diarrhea. Follow these steps: (1) Perform a careful history and physical examination. (2) The possible causes of chronic diarrhea are many. These can be classified into intestinal infections (bacterial, protozoal); inflammatory disease (Crohn's disease, ulcerative colitis); malabsorption (lactose intolerance); secretory hormonal tumor (intestinal carcinoid tumor, VIPoma); drug (antacid); factitious (laxative abuse); or motility disturbance (diabetes mellitus, irritable bowel syndrome, hyperthyroidism). (3) If the diagnosis is uncertain, selected appropriate diagnostic studies should be ordered. (4) Once diagnosed, treatment is planned for the underlying cause with symptomatic antidiarrheal therapy. (5) If no specific cause can be identified, symptomatic therapy is prescribed.

as 2.5-mg tablets and as a 5-mL solution. A small amount of atropine (0.025 mg) is included to discourage abuse. In adults, when taken as 2.5–5 mg three or four times daily, not to exceed 20 mg total daily dose, diphenoxylate is rarely toxic. Some patients may complain of atropinism (blurred vision, dry mouth, urinary hesitancy). Like loperamide, it should not be used in patients at risk of bacterial enteritis with *Escherichia coli, Shigella,* or *Salmonella*.

A diphenoxylate derivative is difenoxin with atropine and has the same uses, precautions, and side effects. Marketed as 1-mg difenoxin tablet, the adult dosage is 2 mg, then 1 mg after each loose stool, not to exceed 8 mg/d.

ADSORBENTS

Adsorbents are used for symptomatic relief (Table 36–3). These products, many not needing a prescription, are nontoxic, but their effectiveness remains unproven. Adsorbents are nonspecific in their action; they adsorb nutrients, toxins, drugs, and digestive juices. Coadministration with other drugs reduces their bioavailability. The Food and Drug Administration over-the-counter review panel recommends only polycarbophil as an effective adsorbent.

Polycarbophil absorbs 60 times its weight in water and can be used to treat both diarrhea and constipation. Polycarbophil, a nonprescription product, is sold as 500-mg chewable tablets. This hydrophilic, nonabsorbable product is safe and may be taken four times daily, up to 6 g in adults.

ANTISECRETORY AGENTS

Bismuth subsalicylate appears to have antisecretory, anti-inflammatory, and antibacterial effects. As a nonprescription product, it is marketed for indigestion, relieving abdominal cramps, and controlling diarrhea, including traveler's diarrhea. Bismuth subsalicylate dosage strengths are 262-mg chewable tablets, 262 mg/5 mL liquid, and 524 mg/15 mL liquid. The usual adult dose is 2 tablets or 30 mL every 30 minutes to 1 hour up to 8 doses per day.

Bismuth subsalicylate contains multiple components that might be toxic if given excessively to prevent or treat diarrhea. For instance, an active ingredient is salicylate, which may interact with anticoagulants or may cause effects of salicylism (tinnitus, nausea, and vomiting). Bismuth can interfere with tetracycline intestinal absorption and can interfere with some gastrointestinal radiographic studies. Patients may complain of darkening tongue and stools with repeat administration. Salicylate can induce gout attacks in susceptible individuals.

Infectious agents cause many acute diarrheas, which have a strong secretory component. Agents blocking copious fluid flow are

TABLE 36–2. Oral Rehydration Solutions

	WHO-ORS[a]	Pedialyte[b] (Ross)	Rehydralyte[b] (Ross)	Infalyte (Mead Johnson)	Resol[b] (Wyeth)
Osmolality (mOsm/L)	333	249	304	200	269
Carbohydrates[b] (g/L)	20	25	25	30[c]	20
Calories (cal/L)	85	100	100	126	80
Electrolytes (mEq/L)					
Sodium	90	45	75	50	50
Potassium	20	20	20	25	20
Chloride	80	35	65	45	50
Citrate	—	30	30	34	34
Bicarbonate	30	—	—	—	—
Calcium	—	—	—	—	4
Magnesium	—	—	—	—	4
Sulfate	—	—	—	—	—
Phosphate	—	—	—	—	5

[a]World Health Organization Oral Rehydration Solution.
[b]Carbohydrate is glucose.
[c]Rice syrup solids are carbohydrate source.

TABLE 36–3. Selected Antidiarrheal Preparations

	Dose Form	Adult Dose
Antimotility		
Diphenoxylate	2.5 mg/tablet 2.5 mg/5 mL	5 mg qid; do not exceed 20 mg/day
Loperamide	2 mg/capsule 1 mg/5 mL	Initially 4 mg, then 2 mg after each loose stool; do not exceed 16 mg/day
Paregoric	2 mg/5 mL (morphine)	5–10 mL 1–4 times daily
Opium tincture	5 mg/mL (morphine)	0.6 mL qid
Difenoxin	1 mg/tablet	Two tablets, then one tablet after each loose stool; up to 8 tablets/day
Adsorbents		
Kaolin–pectin mixture	5.7 g kaolin + 130.2 mg pectin/30 mL	30–120 mL after each loose stool
Polycarbophil	500 mg/tablet	Chew 2 tablets qid or after each loose stool; do not exceed 12 tablets/day
Attapulgite	750 mg/15 mL 300 mg/7.5 mL 750 mg/tablet 600 mg/tablet 300 mg/tablet	1200–1500 mg after each loose bowel movement or every 2 hours; up to 9000 mg/day
Antisecretory		
Bismuth subsalicylate	1050 mg/30 mL 262 mg/15 mL 524 mg/15 mL 262 mg/tablet	Two tablets or 30 mL every 30 min to 1 h as needed up to 8 doses/day
Enzymes (lactase)	1250 neutral lactase units/4 drops 3300 FCC lactase units per tablet	3–4 drops taken with milk or dairy product 1 or 2 tablets as above
Bacterial replacement (*Lactobacillus acidophilus, Lactobacillus bulgaricus*)		2 tablets or 1 granule packet 3 to 4 times daily; give with milk, juice, or water
Octreotide	0.05 mg/mL 0.1 mg/mL 0.5 mg/mL	Initial: 50 μg subcutaneously 1–2 times per day and titrate dose based on indication up to 600 μg/day in 2–4 divided doses

highly desirable in secretory diarrheas, so bismuth subsalicylate suspension has been studied. When 30 mL of this suspension was given every 30 minutes for eight doses, unformed stools decreased in the first 24 hours in active infection. Bismuth subsalicylate has also been studied to prevent traveler's diarrhea.

Octreotide (Sandostatin), a synthetic octapeptide analog of endogenous somatostatin, is prescribed for the symptomatic treatment of carcinoid tumors and vasoactive intestinal peptide-secreting tumors (VIPomas).[6] Metastatic intestinal carcinoid tumors secrete excessive amounts of vasoactive substances, including histamine, bradykinin, serotonin, and prostaglandins. Primary carcinoid tumors are located throughout the GI tract, with most in the ileum. The predominant clinical signs and symptoms are attributable to excessive 5-hydroxytryptophan and serotonin. The collection of their clinical effects is termed the *carcinoid syndrome*. Paroxysmal vasomotor attacks characterize carcinoid syndrome, most notably sudden red to purple flushing of the face and neck. These attacks are often caused by emotional outbursts or by ingestion of food or alcohol. Some patients have a violent, watery diarrhea with cramping. Initially, diarrhea might be managed with various agents such as codeine, diphenoxylate, cyproheptadine, methysergide, phenoxybenzamine, or methyldopa. Recently, octreotide has become the drug of choice.

Octreotide blocks the release of serotonin and many other active peptides and has been effective in controlling diarrhea and flushing. It is reported to have direct inhibitory effects on intestinal secretion and stimulatory effects on intestinal absorption. Nongastrin-secreting adenomas of the pancreas are tumors associated with profuse watery diarrhea. This condition is termed by various names including Verner-Morrison syndrome; WDHA (watery diarrhea, hypokalemia, achlorhydria) syndrome; pancreatic cholera; watery diarrhea syndrome; and VIPoma. Excessive secretion of VIP from a retroperitoneal or pancreatic tumor causes most of the clinical features. Excessive VIP is isolated in about half of patients along with numerous other peptide hormones (peptide histidine methionine [PHM], serotonin, somatostatin, gastrin, glucagon). Surgical tumor dissection is the treatment of choice. In nonsurgical candidates, however, the profuse watery diarrhea and other symptoms are managed with octreotide.

Octreotide, a parenteral drug, is packaged in vials of 0.05, 0.1, and 0.5 μg/mL. The dosage varies with the indication, disease severity, and variable patient response.[10] For managing diarrhea and flushing associated with carcinoid tumors in adults, the dosage range is 100–600 μg/day in two to four divided doses subcutaneously. In so-called carcinoid crisis, octreotide is given as an IV infusion at 50 μg/h for 8 hours to 24 hours. For controlling secretory diarrhea of VIPomas, the dosage range is 200–300 μg/day in two to four divided doses for 2 weeks. Some patients may need higher doses. Sandostatin LAR, a long-acting octreotide formulation is also available: This product consists of microspheres containing the drug and is administered as 20 μg/day in the gluteus muscle at 4-week intervals for 3 months in both carcinoid tumors and VIPomas. It is recommended that during the first 2 weeks of therapy the short-acting formulation also be administered subcutaneously. Because octreotide inhibits many other gastrointestinal hormones, it has a variety of intestinal side effects. With prolonged use, gallbladder and biliary tract complications, like cholelithiasis, have been reported. About 5% to 10% of patients complain of nausea, diarrhea, and abdominal pain. Local injection pain occurs with about an 8% incidence. With high doses, octreotide may reduce dietary fat absorption, leading to steatorrhea.

Currently two other somatostatin analogs, lanreotide and vapreotide, have been studied.[11] Lanreotide is indicated for patients with carcinoid tumors in a dose of 30 mg intramuscularly (as a depot) every 14 days. If necessary the dose can be increased to 30 mg IM every 7–10 days. Vapreotide is an orphan drug that is indicated for pancreatic and gastrointestinal fistulas.

MISCELLANEOUS PRODUCTS

Lactobacillus preparations replace colonic microflora. A controversial treatment is seeding the gut with this organism. This supposedly restores intestinal functions and suppresses the growth of pathogenic microorganisms. However, a dairy product diet containing 200–400 g of lactose or dextrin is equally effective in recolonization. Again, clinical studies are lacking. The dosage varies depending on the brand and is given with milk, juice, water, or cereal. Intestinal flatus is the primary patient complaint.

Anticholinergic drugs, such as atropine, block vagal tone and prolong gut transit time (Table 36–3). They are available in combination in many nonprescription products and as single entities. Their value in controlling diarrhea is questionable and limited by side effects. To stop diarrhea, clinicians have been falsely taught to dose anticholinergics until they decrease salivary and sweat secretion. Angle-closure glaucoma, selected heart diseases, and obstructive uropathies are relative contraindications to use of anticholinergic agents.

Lactase enzyme products are helpful for patients with lactose intolerance. Lactase is needed for carbohydrate digestion. When a patient lacks this enzyme, eating dairy products causes an osmotic diarrhea. Several products are available for current use each time a dairy product, especially milk or ice cream, is eaten.

EVALUATION OF THERAPEUTIC OUTCOMES

Most patients with acute diarrhea experience mild to moderate distress. In the absence of moderate to severe dehydration, high fever, and blood or mucus in the stool, this illness is usually self-limiting within 3 days to 7 days. Mild to moderate acute diarrhea is usually managed on an outpatient basis with oral rehydration, symptomatic treatment, and diet. Elderly persons with chronic illness and infants may require hospitalization for parenteral rehydration and close monitoring.

In the urgent/emergent situation, restoration of the patient's volume status is the most important outcome. Toxic patients (fever, dehydration, hematochezia, hypotension) require hospitalization, intravenous fluids and electrolyte administration, and empiric antibiotic therapy while awaiting culture and sensitivity results. With timely management, these patients usually recover within a few days.

Therapeutic outcomes are directed toward key symptoms, signs, and laboratory studies. Constitutional symptoms usually improve within 24 hours to 72 hours. Monitoring for changes in the frequency and character of bowel movements on a daily basis in conjunction with vital signs and improvement in appetite are of utmost importance. Also, the clinician needs to monitor body weight, serum osmolality, serum electrolytes, complete blood cell counts, urinalysis, and culture results (if appropriate).

CONTROVERSIES IN DRUG MANAGEMENT

Many experimental drugs have been used to control diarrhea. Phenothiazines, β-blockers, nonsteroidal anti-inflammatory drugs (NSAIDs), calcium channel blockers, and α-adrenergic agonists are only a few agents under investigation in either animals or humans. Nifalatide is an enkephalin analog that delays the onset of castor oil-induced diarrhea and decreases stool frequency. Dizziness and dry mouth are frequent side effects.[12] Enkephalinase inhibitors (e.g., acetorphan or racecadotril) offer another therapeutic choice, by reducing hypersecretion of water and electrolytes into the intestinal lumen. In the search for proabsorption/antisecretory drugs, lidamidine, a prototype α_2-adrenergic agonist, was compared with loperamide and was found to counter diarrhea by either promoting absorption or by preventing secretion. With lidamidine, a clonidine analog, hypotension is a limiting dose-related problem. Prostaglandin inhibitors, aspirin and its analogs, and indomethacin are safe and effective in childhood gastroenteritis; studies in animals support indomethacin in enteropathogen secretory states such as with *Vibrio cholerae*.

Vaccines are a new therapeutic frontier in controlling infectious diarrheas, especially in developing countries.[2,13–16] Cholera vaccine, which is available in the US in the parenteral form of whole-cell inactivated bacteria, yields some protection but is not totally effective and does not prevent transmission. However, live oral vaccine is thought to be protective against *V. cholerae*. This dosage form is currently under investigation. In Europe and Latin America, where oral cholera vaccines are available, studies show this agent to be protective and well tolerated. Oral *Shigella* vaccine, although effective under field conditions, requires five doses and repeat booster doses, thereby limiting its practicality in developing nations. With about 1,500 serotypes for *Salmonella,* a vaccine still is not available. There are three parenteral typhoid vaccine formulations available in the US. In addition, an oral vaccine of *S. typhi* (Tyza) is now available and is administered in 4 doses on days 1, 3, 5, and 7, to be completed at least 1 week before exposure. Rotavirus vaccine is effective in infants and children, and is administered as a three oral dose sequence.

CONSTIPATION

Constipation is a common problem, as evidenced by the tremendous dollar volume spent on laxatives and the prominence they have gained in the advertising media and on the shelves of retail outlets. The patient, often without consultation from a health care professional, initiates most treatments for constipation. One reason why constipation continues to be a frequent problem in the United States is the inadequate diet of many people. Another unfortunate problem is that many people have misconceptions about normal bowel function, and think that daily bowel movements are required for health and well being. Others believe that the lack of a daily bowel movement contributes to the accumulation of toxic substances or is associated with various somatic complaints. These misconceptions lead to the inappropriate use of laxatives by the general public.

Constipation does not have one consistently used definition. When using the term, the lay public or health care professional may be referring to several difficult-to-quantify variables: bowel movement frequency, stool size or consistency, and such symptoms as a feeling of incomplete defecation. Stool frequency is most often used to describe constipation; however, the frequency of bowel movements used to define constipation is not well established.

Normal subjects pass at least three stools per week. Some of the definitions of constipation used in clinical studies include (a) less than three stools per week for women and five stools per week for men despite a high-residue diet, or a period of more than 3 days without a bowel movement; (b) straining at stool greater than 25% of the time and/or two or fewer stools per week; or (c) straining at defecation and less than one stool daily with minimal effort. These varying definitions demonstrate the difficulty in characterizing this problem.

An international committee defined and classified constipation on the basis of stool frequency, consistency, and difficulty of defecation.[17–19] Functional constipation is defined as two or more of the following complaints present for at least 12 months when patients are not taking laxatives: (a) straining at least 25% of the time; (b) lumpy or hard stools at least 25% of the time; (c) feeling of incomplete evacuation at least 25% of the time; or (d) two or less bowel movements in a week. Rectal outlet delay was defined as anal blockage more than 25% of the time and prolonged defecation or manual disimpaction (when necessary).

EPIDEMIOLOGY

As many as 40% of patients older than 65 years of age report symptoms of constipation.[20] The results from 42,375 participants of the National Health Interview Survey on Digestive Disorders demonstrated that there is not an age-related increase in infrequent bowel movements; however, there was an age-related increase in laxative use.[21] The frequency of subjects reporting two or less bowel movements per week was 5.9% for those younger than 40 years of age; 3.8% for subjects 60 to 69 years of age; and 6.3% for subjects older than 80 years of age. In a prospective study of 3,166 people older than 65 years of age in a Florida community,[22] 26% of women and 15.8% of men reported recurrent constipation. Factors found to correlate with self-reported constipation were age, sex (higher frequency in females), total number of drugs taken, abdominal pain, and hemorrhoids.

ETIOLOGY AND PATHOPHYSIOLOGY

Constipation is not a disease but a symptom of an underlying disease or problem. Approaches to treatment of constipation should begin with attempts to determine its cause. Disorders of the GI tract (irritable bowel syndrome or diverticulitis), metabolic disorders (diabetes), or endocrine disorders (hypothyroidism) may be involved. Constipation commonly results from a diet low in fiber or from use of constipating drugs such as opiates. Finally, it is believed that constipation may sometimes be psychogenic in origin.[23] Each of these causes is discussed in the following sections.

Constipation is a frequent problem in the elderly, probably the result of improper diets (low in fiber and liquids), diminished abdominal wall muscular strength, and possibly diminished physical activity. However, the frequency of bowel movements is not decreased with normal aging.[19] In addition, diseases that may cause constipation, such as colon cancers and diverticulitis, are more common with increasing age.

GASTROINTESTINAL DISORDERS

Gastrointestinal disorders are a common cause of constipation. The most frequent GI-related causes of constipation are disorders of the large bowel (irritable bowel syndrome, diverticulitis), but diseases of the upper GI tract (gastroduodenal obstruction from ulceration or cancer) may also be responsible. Irritable bowel syndrome may be associated with constipation, diarrhea, or both. In these patients, objective findings of disease are often absent, but colonic motility is usually abnormal.

Anal and rectal diseases associated with pain on defecation may cause constipation. Hemorrhoids, anal fissures, or ulcerative proctitis may all result in painful elimination and inhibition of the urge to defecate. The result may be a decreased frequency of bowel movements.

Constipation may be an indication of obstruction from tumors that originate in the lumen of the colon or from organs or structures adjacent to the colon. Also, constipation may result from hernias, volvulus of the bowel (torsion or twisting of a loop of intestine), or a variety of diseases (syphilis, tuberculosis, helminthic infections, or lymphogranuloma venereum), all of which may cause stricture of the lumen of the colon.

Neurologic disorders of the GI tract may be a cause of constipation. The most prominent neurologic disorder of the GI tract resulting in constipation is Hirschsprung's disease, also called aganglionosis (congenital absence of neurons to the terminal segments of the bowel).

METABOLIC AND ENDOCRINE DISORDERS

Many metabolic and endocrine disorders affect bowel function. Examples include diabetes mellitus with associated neuropathy, which may affect multiple segments of the GI tract and result in an atonic colon, uremia, and hypokalemia. Hypothyroidism and panhypopituitarism may result in inhibited bowel function. In fact, for some cases of hypothyroidism the presenting symptom is constipation or bowel obstruction. Other disorders such as pheochromocytoma may cause constipation, because catecholamines inhibit GI smooth muscle activity. Hypercalcemia (from any cause) and enteric glucagon excess may also result in inhibited bowel function.

PREGNANCY

Constipation is a frequent problem during pregnancy, possibly resulting from complex factors that include depressed gut motility, increased fluid absorption from the colon, decreased physical activity, and dietary changes. Predisposing dietary factors include inadequate fluid intake, low dietary fiber, and the use of iron salts.

NEUROGENIC CONSTIPATION

In addition to peripheral neurologic disorders that may cause constipation, central nervous system (CNS) disorders also may be responsible. The CNS is an important component in GI regulation, either through reflexes or coordination of other organs. In addition, the CNS modifies GI function in response to conscious effort or emotional stimuli. Many diseases of the CNS can therefore affect GI function. Trauma to the brain (particularly the medulla) or spinal cord may result in inhibited bowel function, as may CNS tumors. Also, cerebrovascular accidents and Parkinson's disease may cause inhibited bowel function.

PSYCHOGENIC CONSTIPATION

The term *psychogenic constipation* has variable acceptance among experts in the field because objective evidence for its existence is slim; however, bowel habits, particularly those developed early in life, may relate to chronic constipation. Ignoring or postponing the urge to defecate may cause blunting of the colonic and rectal

TABLE 36–4. Drugs Causing Constipation

Analgesics
Inhibitors of prostaglandin synthesis
Opiates
Anticholinergics
Antihistamines
Antiparkinsonian agents (e.g., benztropine or trihexaphenidyl)
Phenothiazines
Tricyclic antidepressants
Antacids containing calcium carbonate or aluminum hydroxide
Barium sulfate
Calcium channel blockers
Clonidine
Diuretics (nonpotassium sparing)
Ganglionic blockers
Iron preparations
Muscle blockers (D-tubocurarine, succinylcholine)
Nonsteroidal anti-inflammatory agents
Polystyrene sodium sulfonate

response and may possibly lead to prolonged stool retention. People in certain occupations, such as truck drivers, may be particularly predisposed to this problem. Finally, patients with psychiatric diseases often have constipation. In many instances, improvement in constipation is observed with the onset of psychotherapy.

DRUG-INDUCED CONSTIPATION

Drugs that inhibit the neurologic or muscular function of the GI tract, particularly the colon, may result in constipation (Table 36–4). The majority of cases of drug-induced constipation are caused by opiates, various agents with anticholinergic properties, and antacids containing aluminum or calcium. With most of the agents listed, the inhibitory bowel effects are dose dependent, with larger doses clearly causing constipation more frequently.

Opiates have effects on all segments of the bowel, but effects are most pronounced on the colon. The major mechanism of opiate action has been proposed to be prolongation of intestinal transit time by causing spastic, nonpropulsive contractions. An additional contributory mechanism of action may be an increase in electrolyte absorption.

All opiate derivatives are associated with constipation, but the degree of intestinal inhibitory effects seems to differ between agents. Orally administered opiates appear to have greater inhibitory effects than parenterally administered agents; oral codeine is well known as a potent antimotility agent. Orally administered enkephalins (endogenous opiate-like polypeptides) are recognized to have antimotility properties.

Agents with anticholinergic properties inhibit bowel function by parasympatholytic actions on innervation to many regions of the GI tract, particularly the colon and rectum. Many types of drugs possess anticholinergic action (Table 36–4), and these agents are used commonly in hospitalized and nonhospitalized patients. One study demonstrated that amitriptyline, diphenhydramine, and thioridazine were associated with laxative use in 800 nursing home patients.[15]

In patients older than 65 years of age, the drugs that correlated with constipation were anticholinergics, aspirin, furosemide, nitroglycerin, and amitriptyline.[22] Serum chloride and aspartate aminotransferase, as well as alcohol consumption, were found to be negatively related to constipation. The most important predictors of constipation were age and the total number of medications taken.

CLINICAL PRESENTATION

Constipation may vary from a minor discomfort in an otherwise healthy adult to a symptom of colon cancer or other serious diseases. A basis for evaluation and treatment should be a thorough history including questions about the nature of the "constipation." It is important to ascertain whether the patient perceives the problem as infrequent bowel movements, stools of insufficient size, a feeling of fullness, or difficulty and pain on passing stool. The patient should be asked about the frequency of bowel movements and the chronicity of constipation. Constipation occurring recently in an adult may indicate significant colon pathology such as malignancy; constipation present since early infancy may be indicative of neurologic disorders. The patient also should be carefully questioned about usual diet and laxative regimens. Does the patient have a diet consistently deficient in high-fiber items and containing mainly highly refined foods? What laxatives or cathartics has the patient used to attempt relief of constipation? Finally, the patient should be questioned about other concurrent medications, with interest toward agents that might cause constipation.

For most patients complaining of constipation, a thorough physical examination is not required after it is established that constipation (a) is not a chronic problem, (b) is not accompanied by signs of significant GI disease (e.g., rectal bleeding or anemia), and (c) does not cause severe discomfort. In these circumstances, the patient may be referred directly to the first-line therapies for constipation described in the next section (mainly bulk-forming laxatives and dietary fiber with occasional use of saline or stimulant laxatives). Certain patients, however, require a full examination by a physician to determine the cause of constipation. Patients may then have a series of examinations, proctoscopy, sigmoidoscopy, colonoscopy, or barium enema to determine the presence of colorectal pathology. Also, tests such as thyroid function studies may be performed to determine the presence of metabolic or endocrine disorders.

Chronic constipation can result in a more complex picture. Patients may have long-standing complaints of GI irregularities with a variety of symptoms. The laxative abuser may present with contradictory findings, sometimes diarrhea or weight loss. Laxative abusers may deny laxative use and present with vomiting, abdominal pain, lassitude, thirst, edema, and bone pain (as a consequence of osteomalacia). With prolonged abuse patients may have fluid and electrolyte imbalances (most commonly hypokalemia), protein-losing gastroenteropathy with hypoalbuminemia, and syndromes resembling colitis.

▶ TREATMENT: Constipation

DESIRED OUTCOME

The ultimate goal of treatment for constipation is alteration of lifestyle (particularly diet) to prevent further episodes of constipation. Short term goals include alleviation of acute constipation with relief from symptoms. For patients with chronic constipation, the goals are more long-term and include use of proper diet and decreased reliance on laxatives. Effective treatment of constipation requires the patient to become more knowledgeable about the causes of constipation, proper diet, and appropriate use of laxatives.

GENERAL APPROACH TO TREATMENT

The proper management of constipation requires a number of different modalities; however, the basis for therapy should be dietary modification. The major dietary change should be an increase in the amount of fiber consumed daily. In addition to dietary management, patients should be encouraged to alter other aspects of their life-styles if necessary. Important considerations are to encourage patients to exercise (achieved even by brisk walking after dinner) and to adjust bowel habits so that a regular and adequate time is made to respond to the urge to defecate. Another general measure is to increase fluid intake. This is generally recommended and believed beneficial, although there is little objective evidence of benefit.

If an underlying disease is recognized as the cause of constipation, attempts should be made to correct it. GI malignancies may be removed through a surgical resection. Endocrine and metabolic derangements should be corrected by the appropriate methods. For example, when hypothyroidism is the cause of constipation, cautious institution of thyroid-replacement therapy is the most important treatment measure.

As discussed earlier, many drug substances may cause constipation. After determination of a patient's prescription and nonprescription drug therapy, potential drug causes of constipation should be identified. If the patient is consuming medications well known to cause constipation, consideration should be given to alternative agents. For some medications (e.g., antacids), nonconstipating alternatives exist. If no reasonable alternatives exist to the medication thought to be responsible for constipation, consideration should be given to lowering the dose. If a patient must remain on constipating medications, then more attention must be paid to general measures for prevention of constipation, as discussed next.

NONPHARMACOLOGIC THERAPY

DIETARY MODIFICATION AND BULK-FORMING AGENTS

The most important aspect of the therapy for constipation for the majority of patients is dietary modification to increase the amount of fiber consumed. Fiber, the portion of vegetable matter not digested in the human GI tract, increases stool bulk, retention of stool water, and rate of transit of stool through the intestine. The result of fiber therapy is an increased frequency of defecation. Also, fiber decreases intraluminal pressures in the colon and rectum, which is thought to be beneficial for diverticular disease and for irritable bowel syndrome. The specific physiologic effects of fiber are not well understood. Patients should be advised to include at least 10 g of crude fiber in their daily diets.[19] Fruits, vegetables, and cereals have the highest fiber content. Bran, a byproduct of milling of wheat, is often added to foods to increase fiber content. Raw bran is generally 40% fiber. Medicinal products, often called "bulk-forming agents," such as psyllium hydrophilic colloids (Effersyllium), methylcellulose (Cologel), or polycarbophil (Mitrolan), have properties similar to those of dietary fiber and may be taken as tablets, powders, or granules (Table 36–5).

A trial of dietary modification with high-fiber content should be continued for at least 1 month before effects on bowel function are determined. Most patients begin to notice effects on bowel function 3 days to 5 days after beginning a high-fiber diet, but some patients may require a considerably longer time. Patients should be cautioned that abdominal distention and flatus may be particularly troublesome in the first few weeks of fiber therapy, particularly with high bran consumption. In most patients, these problems resolve with continued use.

TABLE 36–5. Dosage Recommendations for Laxatives and Cathartics

Agent	Recommended Dose
Agents That Cause Softening of Feces in 1–3 d	
Bulk-forming agents	
Methylcellulose	4–6 g/day
Polycarbophil	4–6 g/day
Psyllium	Varies with product
Emollients	
Docusate sodium	50–360 mg/day
Docusate calcium	50–360 mg/day
Docusate potassium	100–300 mg/day
Lactulose	15–30 mL orally
Sorbitol	30–50 g/d orally
Mineral oil	15–30 mL orally
Agents That Result in Soft or Semifluid Stool in 6–12 h	
Bisacodyl (oral)	5–15 mg orally
Phenolphthalein	30–270 mg orally
Cascara sagrada	Dose varies with formulation
Senna	Dose varies with formulation
Magnesium sulfate (low dose)	<10 g orally
Agents That Cause Watery Evacuation in 1–6 h	
Magnesium citrate	18 g 300 mL water
Magnesium hydroxide	2.4–4.8 g orally
Magnesium sulfate (high dose)	10–30 g orally
Sodium phosphates	Varies with salt used
Bisacodyl	10 mg rectally
Polyethylene glycol-electrolyte preparations	4 L

Bulk-forming laxatives have few side effects and minimal systemic effects. The only major caution in the use of bulk-forming laxatives is that obstruction of the esophagus, stomach, small intestine, and colon has been reported when the agents have been consumed without fluid, so these products should not be used without adequate fluids or in patients with intestinal stenosis.

SURGERY

In a small percentage of patients presenting with complaints of constipation, surgical procedures are necessary (with most colonic malignancies and with GI obstruction from a number of causes). In each case, the involved segment of intestine may be resected or revised to allow flow of GI contents through an enterostomy or through the anus. Surgery may be required in some endocrine disorders causing constipation, such as pheochromocytoma, which requires removal of a tumor.

BIOFEEDBACK

The majority of patients with constipation related to pelvic floor dysfunction can benefit from electromyogram-guided biofeedback therapy.[24] The value of biofeedback in children with chronic constipation has not been well demonstrated.[25]

PHARMACOLOGIC THERAPY

DRUG REGIMENS OF CHOICE

Treatment and prevention of constipation should consist of bulk-forming agents in addition to dietary modifications that increase dietary fiber.[23] A variety of products are available that provide adequate bulk. Whichever agent is chosen, it should be used daily and continued indefinitely in most patients, particularly those with chronic constipation. Bulk-forming agents available in combination with diphenylmethane or anthraquinone derivatives should be avoided because the added agents should not be used routinely.

For most nonhospitalized persons with acute constipation, the infrequent use (less than every few weeks) of most laxative products is acceptable; however, before more potent laxative/cathartics are used, relatively simple measures may be tried. For example, acute constipation may be relieved by the use of a tap-water enema or a glycerin suppository; if neither is effective, the use of oral sorbitol, low doses of diphenylmethane or anthraquinone laxatives, or saline laxatives (e.g., milk of magnesia) may provide relief. If laxative treatment is required for longer than 1 week, the person should be advised to consult a physician to determine if there is an underlying cause of constipation that requires treatment with agents other than laxatives.

For some bedridden or geriatric patients, or others with chronic constipation, bulk-forming laxatives remain the first line of treatment, but the use of more potent laxatives may be required relatively frequently. Fiber should be avoided in bedridden patients who are cognitively impaired.[19] When other than bulk-forming laxatives are used, they should be administered in the lowest effective dose and as infrequently as possible to maintain regular bowel function (more than three stools per week). Agents that may be used in these situations include diphenylmethane and anthraquinone derivatives, milk of magnesia, and sorbitol or lactulose. Mineral oil should be avoided, particularly in bedridden patients, because of the risk of aspiration and lipoid pneumonia. Some patients with chronic constipation may present with fecal impactions. Before vigorous oral laxatives can be used, the impaction needs to be removed using mechanical methods, including tap water or saline enemas and digital extraction.

In the hospitalized patient without GI disease, constipation may be related to the use of general anesthesia and/or opiate substances. Most orally or rectally administered laxatives may be used. For prompt initiation of a bowel movement, a tap-water enema or glycerin suppository is recommended, or oral milk of magnesia.

With infants and children, constipation may occur commonly. The approach to the treatment of constipation in young persons should consider neurologic, metabolic, or anatomic abnormalities when constipation is a persistent problem. When not related to an underlying disease, the approach to constipation is similar to that in an adult. Dietary modification should be considered, emphasizing high-fiber food. For acute constipation in most age groups, a tap-water enema or glycerin suppository may be helpful. Occasional use of milk of magnesia or anthraquinone laxatives in low doses is justified for acute constipation.

DRUG CLASSES

The traditional classification system for laxatives and cathartics, by suspected mode of action, is not very useful; the mode of action of many products is not clearly understood. In general, most agents work by promoting some of the mechanisms involved in diarrhea, including active electrolyte secretion, decreased water and electrolyte absorption, increased intraluminal osmolarity, and increased hydrostatic pressure in the gut. Laxatives convert the intestine from primarily an organ that absorbs water and electrolytes to an organ that secretes water and electrolytes. The various classes of laxatives are discussed in this section. The agents are divided into three general classifications: (a) those causing softening of feces in 1 day to 3 days (bulk-forming laxatives, docusates, and lactulose); (b) those that result in soft or semifluid stool in 6 hours to 12 hours (diphenylmethane derivatives and anthraquinone derivatives); and (c) those causing water evacuation in 1 hour to 6 hours (saline cathartics, castor oil, and polyethylene glycol-electrolyte lavage solution).

EMOLLIENT LAXATIVES

Emollient laxatives are surfactant agents, docusate in its various salts, which work by facilitating mixing of aqueous and fatty materials within the intestinal tract. They may increase water and electrolyte secretion in the small and large bowel. These products are generally given orally, although docusate potassium has also been used rectally. These products result in a softening of stools within 1 day to 3 days.

Emollient laxatives are ineffective in treating constipation but are used mainly to prevent constipation. They may be helpful in situations where straining at stool should be avoided, such as after recovery from myocardial infarction, with acute perianal disease, or after rectal surgery. It is unlikely that these agents would be very effective in preventing constipation if major causative factors (e.g., heavy opiate use, uncorrected pathology, inadequate dietary fiber) are not concurrently addressed.

Although docusates are generally safe, a few adverse effects have been noted. They may increase the intestinal absorption of agents administered concurrently and alter toxic potential.

LUBRICANTS

Mineral oil is the only lubricant laxative in routine use. This agent, obtained from petroleum refining, acts by coating stool and allowing easier passage. It inhibits colonic absorption of water, thereby increasing stool weight and decreasing stool transit time. Mineral oil may be given orally or rectally in a dose of 15–45 mL. Generally, the effect on bowel function is noted after 2 days or 3 days of use.

Mineral oil is helpful in situations similar to those suggested for docusates: to maintain a soft stool and to avoid straining for relatively short periods of time (a few days to 2 weeks); however, it possesses a much greater potential for adverse effects and its routine use should be discouraged. Mineral oil may be absorbed systemically and can cause a foreign-body reaction in lymphoid tissue. Also, in debilitated or recumbent patients, mineral oil may be aspirated, causing lipoid pneumonia.[26] For this reason, it should not be used just before bedtime or when a patient is recumbent.

Mineral oil has been reported to decrease the absorption of fat-soluble vitamins (A, D, E, and K) with chronic use by causing retention in the GI tract. Finally, even when given orally, mineral oil may leak from the anal sphincter, causing pruritus and soiling of clothing.

LACTULOSE AND SORBITOL

Lactulose is a disaccharide that is used orally or rectally. It is metabolized by colonic bacteria to low-molecular-weight acids, resulting in an osmotic effect whereby fluid is retained in the colon.[27] The fluid retained in the colon lowers the pH and increases colonic peristalsis. Lactulose is generally not recommended as a first-line agent for the treatment of constipation because it is costly and not necessarily more effective than such agents as sorbitol or milk of magnesia. It may be justified as an alternative for acute constipation, and has been useful particularly in elderly patients. Occasionally, the use of lactulose may result in flatulence, cramps, diarrhea, and electrolyte imbalances.[27] Sorbitol, a monosaccharide, exerts its effect by osmotic action and has been recommended as a primary agent in the treatment of functional constipation in cognitively intact patients.[19] It is as effective as lactulose and much less expensive.

DIPHENYLMETHANE DERIVATIVES

The two commonly used diphenylmethane derivatives are bisacodyl and phenolphthalein. The actions of these agents are believed to be primarily on the colon. Bisacodyl stimulates the mucosal nerve plexus of the colon; the mechanism of action of phenolphthalein is poorly understood (possibly it inhibits active glucose absorption and sodium absorption, resulting in fluid accumulation in the colon by osmotic action). The dose of these agents that is effective in individuals appears to vary greatly. A dose that causes no effects in one patient may result in excessive cramping and fluid evacuation in others. With phenolphthalein, a small portion of the dose undergoes enterohepatic recirculation, which may result in a prolonged laxative action.

These agents are not recommended for regular daily use. Their use is acceptable intermittently (every few weeks) to treat constipation or as a bowel preparation before diagnostic procedures in which cleansing of the colon is necessary. These agents may sometimes cause severe abdominal cramping as well as significant fluid and electrolyte imbalances with chronic use. They should not be used for patients in whom appendicitis is a possibility (perforation of the appendix may result) or during pregnancy or lactation. Finally, the patient taking phenolphthalein-containing laxatives should be cautioned that their urine might turn pink.

ANTHRAQUINONE DERIVATIVES

Anthraquinone derivatives include cascara sagrada, sennosides, and casanthrol. Gut bacteria metabolizes these agents to their active compounds, but the exact mechanisms of action are not understood. Effects are limited to the colon, and stimulation of Auerbach's plexus may be involved. Recommendations for the use of these agents are similar to those for the diphenylmethane derivatives. In most cases, intermittent use is acceptable; daily use should be strongly discouraged.

Most of the concerns with the use of diphenylmethane derivatives (bisacodyl and phenolphthalein) apply to the anthraquinone derivatives. In addition, the anthraquinone derivatives may cause melanosis coli, an accumulation of dark pigment, mainly in the cecum and rectum that is evident after 4 months to 13 months of use. A pathologic effect of melanosis coli has not been demonstrated, and it appears reversible after anthraquinones have been discontinued for 3 months to 6 months.

SALINE CATHARTICS

Saline cathartics are composed of relatively poorly absorbed ions such as magnesium, sulfate, phosphate, and citrate, which produce their effects primarily by osmotic action to retain fluid in the GI tract. Magnesium has been shown to stimulate the secretion of cholecystokinin, a hormone that causes stimulation of bowel motility and fluid secretion. These agents may be given orally or rectally. A bowel movement may result within a few hours after oral doses and in 1 hour or less after rectal administration.

These agents should be used primarily for acute evacuation of the bowel, which may be necessary before diagnostic examinations, after poisonings, and in conjunction with some anthelmintics to eliminate parasites. Such agents as milk of magnesia (an 8% suspension of magnesium hydroxide) may be used occasionally (every few weeks) to treat constipation in otherwise healthy adults. Saline cathartics should not be used on a routine basis to treat constipation. With fecal impactions the enema formulations of these agents may be helpful.

As with most laxatives, these agents may cause fluid and electrolyte depletion. Also, magnesium or sodium accumulation may occur when magnesium-containing cathartics are used in patients with renal dysfunction or when sodium phosphate is used in patients with congestive heart failure.

CASTOR OIL

Castor oil is metabolized in the GI tract to an active compound, ricinoleic acid, which stimulates secretory processes, decreases glucose absorption, and promotes intestinal motility, primarily in the small intestine. Castor oil usually results in a bowel movement within 1 hour to 3 hours of administration. Because the agent has such a strong purgative action, it should not be used for the routine treatment of constipation.

GLYCERIN

Glycerin is usually administered as a 3-g suppository and exerts its effect by osmotic action in the rectum. As with most agents given as suppositories, the onset of action is usually less than 30 minutes. Glycerin is considered a very safe laxative, although it may occasionally cause rectal irritation. Its use is acceptable on an intermittent basis for constipation, particularly in children.

POLYETHYLENE GLYCOL-ELECTROLYTE LAVAGE SOLUTION

Whole-bowel irrigation with polyethylene glycol-electrolyte lavage solution (PEG-ELS) has become popular for colon cleansing before diagnostic procedures or colorectal operations.

Four liters of this solution is administered over 3 hours to obtain complete evacuation of the GI tract. The solution is not recommended for the routine treatment of constipation and its use should be avoided in patients with intestinal obstruction.

OTHER AGENTS

Tap-water enemas may be used to treat simple constipation. The administration of 200 mL of tap water by enema to an adult often results in a bowel movement within 30 minutes. Soapsuds are no longer recommended for use in enemas because their use may result in proctitis or colitis.

PREVENTION

For certain groups of patients, such as those recovering from myocardial infarction or rectal surgery, straining at defecation is to be avoided. For these patients, the basis of preventive therapy should be the use of bulk-forming laxatives. In addition to these products, the use of docusate is popular, although its effectiveness is debated. In pregnant patients, constipation may result because of alterations in anatomy or iron supplementation. As described earlier, bulk-forming laxatives and docusates should be the first line of prevention.

LAXATIVE ABUSE SYNDROME

Misconceptions about normal bowel patterns and the effect of laxatives have contributed to a syndrome of laxative abuse that is relatively common in the United States. The availability of laxatives as chocolates or gums conveys to the public that the use of these agents is without adverse consequences. Abuse of laxatives has occurred traditionally in persons trying to maintain daily bowel function, but more recently has extended to others who use laxatives for the purpose of controlling weight. In either case, the consistent abuse of strong laxatives and cathartics may lead to serious illness.

Laxative abuse for the purpose of maintaining daily bowel function begins with misconceptions about the frequency, quantity, or consistency of stools. With the use of strong purgatives, the colon may be so thoroughly cleansed that a bowel movement may not occur normally until a few days later. This delay reinforces the need for more purgatives and the cycle of laxative dependence is begun. Eventually the patient may require daily laxatives to maintain bowel function.

The laxative abuser may present with contradictory findings of diarrhea and weight loss. In addition, long-term abusers of laxatives tend to have vomiting, abdominal pain, lassitude, weakness, thirst, edema, and bone pain (caused by osteomalacia). With prolonged use of laxatives a number of serious illnesses may arise. These include fluid and electrolyte imbalances (including acid-base imbalances and hypokalemia), protein-losing gastroenteropathy with hypoalbuminemia, and syndromes resembling colitis.

The determination of laxative abuse syndrome can be difficult because many laxative abusers vigorously deny laxative use. Middle-aged women tend to be the most common laxative abusers. The chronic laxative abuse problem should be addressed by a combination of measures, including psychiatric evaluation, dietary modification with reliance on bulk-forming laxatives, and specific guidelines to the patient for the withdrawal of stimulant laxatives.

A variation of laxative abuse is seen in persons who use them as a method of weight loss. It appears from the medical literature and daily news sources that this type of abuse is on the increase. Treatment of patients who abuse laxatives in this way has proven very difficult.

IRRITABLE BOWEL SYNDROME

Irritable Bowel Syndrome (IBS) is one of the most common gastrointestinal disorders encountered in clinical practice. It affects as many as 20% of adults worldwide and is more common in women than men. This latter point is probably a consequence of women being more likely than men to report their symptoms to the medical community. Although a benign disorder, IBS is chronic and recurring in nature. In the United States alone, estimated costs associated with this condition exceeds $8 billion annually.[28,29]

DEFINITION AND MANIFESTATIONS

Irritable bowel syndrome is defined as lower abdominal pain, disturbed defecation (constipation, diarrhea, or an alternating pattern of both) and bloating in the absence of structural or biochemical factors which might explain these symptoms. Abdominal bloating may be accompanied with distension. Abnormal stool frequency is defined as greater than three per day or less than three per week. Stool form may be lumpy and hard, or loose and watery. Abnormal stool passage usually consists of straining, urgency, or feeling of incomplete evacuation. Additionally, patients may experience increased passage of mucus. Nongastrointestinal manifestations include urinary symptoms, fatigue, and dyspareunia. This disorder is thought to be a part of a broader spectrum of symptoms collectively referred to as functional abdominal disorders, and therefore may overlap with conditions such as fibromyalgia, functional dyspepsia and chronic fatigue syndrome. As many as 40% to 60% of patients with IBS have psychological manifestations such as depression and anxiety, or both.[30] The American Gastroenterology Association has stated that (a) GI symptoms are exacerbated by psychological stress; (b) psychological disturbances affect IBS and the behavior of patients with this disorder; and (c) that irritable bowel syndrome can lead to a reduced health-related quality of life.[31]

PATHOPHYSIOLOGY

No single factor can fully explain the pathophysiology of IBS. For many years, it was thought that IBS was the result of motility disorders of the GI tract. However, dysmotility did not explain the symptoms of pain often encountered in patients with this disorder. More recent evidence suggests that visceral hypersensitivity is a major culprit in the pathophysiology of this condition. Balloon distention studies demonstrate that patients with IBS have an increased awareness of gastrointestinal distention and pain at pressures and volumes significantly lower than do control subjects. It appears that this visceral hypersensitivity is a neuroenteric phenomenon that is independent of motility and psychological disturbances. Current theory suggests that visceral hypersensitivity results from alterations in neuroreceptor and afferent spinal neuron function and central nervous system modulation of afferent input in such a way that results in long-term sensitization of pathways involved in the transmission of visceral sensation.[28] Factors known to contribute to these alternations include genetics, motility factors, inflammation, mechanical irritation to local nerves, and psychological factors.

An equally important theory of the pathogenesis of IBS is that normal GI function results from an integration of intestinal sensory, motor, autonomic and central nervous system activity. Gastrointestinal symptoms may relate to dysregulation of these systems. Visceral afferent sensation and intestinal motor function are linked to higher cortical centers that affect GI motility, sensation, and secretion.[28]

DIAGNOSIS

In the past, diagnosis of IBS was based upon identification of the primary complaints of the patient and excluding other medical conditions having a similar clinical presentation. Today, a precise diagnosis is enhanced through the use of symptom-based criteria. This includes either the Manning[28] or Rome II[32] criteria outlined in Table 36–6.

TABLE 36–6. Symptom-Based Criteria

The Manning Criteria[28]

Chronic or recurrent abdominal pain for at least 6 months and two or more of the following:
1. Abdominal pain relieved with defecation
2. Abdominal pain associated with more frequent stools
3. Abdominal pain associated with looser stools
4. Abdominal distention
5. Feeling of incomplete evacuation after defecation
6. Mucus in stools

Rome II diagnostic criteria for IBS[32]

At least 12 weeks, which need not be consecutive, in the preceeding 12 months of abdominal discomfort or pain that has two of three features:
1. Relieved with defecation, and/or
2. Onset associated with a change in frequency of stool; and/or
3. Onset associated with a change in form (appearance) of stool

Additional diagnostic steps that can be taken include sigmoidoscopy or colonoscopy; examination of the stool for occult blood and ova and parasites; complete blood cell count; erythrocyte sedimentation rate; and serum electrolytes. In some cases, radiographic imaging studies, such as computed tomography scans or barium swallows or enemas, may also be necessary if the findings of the above assessment is not typical for IBS.[28]

▶ TREATMENT: Irritable Bowel Syndrome

DESIRED OUTCOME

IBS is usually classified as constipation predominate, diarrhea predominate, or IBS with abdominal pain and bloating. Therapeutic goals in IBS should focus on the patient's chief complaint. Because of the chronicity of the disease, it is imperative that the caregiver develops a therapeutic relationship with the patient. The American Gastroenterology Association recommends patients with IBS undergo psychological treatments such as psychotherapy, relaxation/stress management, cognitive behavior treatment and/or hypnosis.[31]

CONSTIPATION PREDOMINANT DISEASE

In the constipation predominate patient, dietary fiber may be beneficial. Patients should be instructed to begin with 1 tablespoonful with 1 meal daily and gradually increase the dose with 2 meals to 3 meals a day until the desired outcome is achieved. Endpoints that the patient should aim for include bulkier, more easily passed stools. For patients unable to tolerate dietary bran, bulking agents such as psyllium may be substituted.[29] Laxative use is not encouraged in these patients and should only be used in the smallest dose for the least amount of time in cases of severe constipation.

DIARRHEA-PREDOMINANT DISEASE

For patients in whom diarrhea is the primary complaint, avoidance of certain food products may be necessary. Caffeine, alcohol, and artificial sweeteners (sorbitol, fructose, mannitol) are known to irritate the gut and produce a laxative effect. Lactose intolerance should be considered in certain patients; however, the prevalence of this condition may be exaggerated.

Herbal medicines or teas often contain senna, which may produce diarrhea. In patients with disease persistence following dietary modification, loperamide may be used strategically for episodes of urgent diarrhea, or in situations in which the patient wishes to avoid the possibility of an acute onset of symptoms.[29]This drug decreases intestinal transit, enhances water and electrolyte absorption, and strengthens rectal sphincter tone. Some patients may require continuous therapy and careful dosage titration can usually be undertaken to prevent the development of constipation. Cholestyramine may be useful in patients with diarrhea related to idiopathic bile acid malabsorption or following cholecystectomy.[28]

PAIN IN IRRITABLE BOWEL SYNDROME

Select patients with IBS suffer significant pain associated with their disease. Data supporting the use of antispasmodic agents in these patients is conflicting.[29,33,34] In these cases, a trial of low-dose antidepressant therapy is indicated, especially if pain is associated with eating. Both tricyclic compounds and serotonin reuptake inhibitors produce analgesia and may relieve depressive symptoms, if present. Preprandial doses of drugs containing anticholinergic properties may suppress pain (and/or diarrhea) associated with an overactive, postprandial gastrocolonic response. Tricyclic antidepressants should be avoided in patients with pain and constipation.

DRUG CLASSES CURRENTLY UNDER INVESTIGATION FOR THE TREATMENT OF IBS[33]

Numerous agents are currently undergoing investigation for the management of IBS. Selective blockade of the muscarinic M3 receptors as well as β_3-adrenoceptor agonists have been shown to alter gut motility without affecting the cardiovascular system. Other compounds being evaluated include NK_2 receptor antagonists, gut-selective calcium channel blockers, cholecystokinin receptor antagonists, and agents capable of stimulating motilin receptors (motilinomimetics).

▶ PRINCIPLES OF PHARMACOTHERAPY

Diarrhea

- Diarrhea is most often a minor discomfort, not life threatening, and usually self-limited.
- Children, AIDS patients, and the elderly are groups at high risk for severe complications of acute diarrhea. Usually, a diagnosis is based on the history and physical examination, with extensive diagnostic tests reserved for chronic diarrhea.
- Management focuses on preventing excessive water and electrolyte losses, dietary care, relieving symptoms, treating curable causes, and treating secondary disorders.
- The foundation of treatment for diarrhea is fluid and electrolyte replacement, usually by the oral route. A variety of oral rehydration solutions may be used for this purpose.
- Medical referral is indicated when any of these are detected: children younger than 3 years of age; pregnant; frail elderly; moderate to severe (5% to 10% body weight loss) volume depletion; chronic heart, renal, or liver disease; AIDS; moderate

to severe abdominal pain; high fever; bloody or mucoid stool; or chronic diarrhea.

- Patients should be taught the proper use of antidiarrheal medications.

Constipation

- Potential drug causes of constipation should be identified and the regimen altered if possible.
- The foundation of treatment of constipation is dietary fiber or bulk-forming laxatives that provide 10–15 g/d of raw fiber.
- Underlying causes of constipation should be identified when possible and corrective measures taken (e.g., alteration of diet or treatment of diseases such as hypothyroidism).
- Acute constipation may be treated with a tap-water enema or glycerin suppository. If neither is effective, the use of oral sorbitol, low doses of diphenylmethane, or anthraquinone laxatives may provide relief.
- Laxative abuse is a common problem that results from GI complaints or the desire to lose weight. Laxative abusers may deny their condition and may present with constipation or diarrhea.

Irritable Bowel Syndrome

- Therapy for constipation predominant IBS consists primarily of dietary fiber or the use of bulking agents such as psyllium.
- Diarrhea-predominant IBS should be managed by dietary modification and drugs such as loperamide when diet changes alone are insufficient to promote control of symptoms.

REFERENCES

1. DuPont HL. Diarrheal diseases in the developing world. Infect Dis Clin North Am 1995;9:313–324.
2. Feldman R, Banatvala N. The frequency of culturing stools from adults with diarrhea in Great Britain. Epidemiol Infect 1994;113:41–44.
3. Everhart JE, ed. Digestive Disease in the United States: Epidemiology and Impact. NIH Publ 94-1447. Bethesda, MD: National Institutes of Health, 1994.
4. Prado V, O'Ryan ML. Acute gastroenteritis in Latin America. Infect Dis Clin North Am 1994;8:77-106.
5. Kroser JA, Metz DC: Evaluation of the adult patient with diarrhea. Prim Care 1996;23:529–547.
6. The AGA technical review on the evaluation and management of chronic diarrhea Gastroenterology 1999;116:1464–1486.
7. Mahalanabis D. Current status of oral rehydration as a strategy for the control of diarrheal diseases. Indian J Med Res 1996;104:115–124.
8. Pizarro D, Posada G, Sandi L, et al. Rice-based electrolyte solutions for the management of infantile diarrhea. N Engl J Med 1991;324:518–521.
9. Ansdell VE, Ericsson CD. Prevention and empiric treatment of traveler's diarrhea. Med Clin North Am 1999;83:945–973.
10. Harris AG, O'Dorisio TM, Woltering EA, et al. Consensus statement: Octreotide dose titration in secretory diarrhea. Diarrhea Management Conference. Dig Dis Sci 1995;40:1464–1473.
11. Ruszniewski P, Ducreux M, Chayvialle J, et al. Treatment of the carcinoid syndrome with a long acting somatostatin analogue lanreotide: A prospective study of 39 patients. Gut 1996;39:279–283.
12. Viollet C, Prevost G, Maubert E, et al. Molecular pharmacology of somatostatin receptors. Fundam Clin Pharmacol 1995;9:107–113.
13. Thompsom RF, Bass DM, Hoffman SL. Travel vaccine. Infect Dis Clin North Am 1999;13:149–167.
14. Sack DA, Cadoz M. Cholera vaccines. In: Plotkin SA, Mortimer EA Jr, eds. Vaccines, 2nd ed. Philadephia, Saunders, 1994:635–647.
15. Tacket CO, Kotloff KL, Losonsky G, et al. Volunteer studies investigating the safety and efficacy of live oral El Tor Vibrio Cholerae 01 vaccine strain CVD 111. Am J Trop Med Hyg 1997;56:533–547.
16. Rennels MB, Glass RI, Dennehy PH, et al. Safety and efficacy of high-dose rhesus-human reassortant rotavirus vaccines—Report of the national multicenter trial. Pediatrics 1996;97:7–13.
17. Whitehead WE, Chaussade S, Corazziari E. Report of an international workshop on management of constipation. Gastro International 1991; 4:99–113.
18. Koch A, Voldcrholzcr WA, Klauser AG, et al. Symptoms in chronic constipation. Dis Colon Rectum 1997;40:902–906.
19. Romero Y, Evans J, Fleming KC, Phillips SF. Constipation and fecal incontinence in the elderly population. Mayo Clin Proc 1996;71:81–92.
20. Talley NJ, Fleming KC, Evans JM, et al. Constipation in an elderly community. A study of prevalence and potential risk factors. Am J Gastroenterol 1996;91:19–25.
21. Harari D, Gurwith JH, Avorn J, et al. Bowel habit in relation to age and gender. Findings from the National Health Survey and clinical implications. Arch Intern Med 1996;156:315–320.
22. Stewart RB, Moore MT, Marks RG, Hale WE. Correlates of constipation in an ambulatory elderly population. Am J Gastroenterol 1992;87:859–864.
23. Browning SM. Constipation, diarrhea and irritable bowel syndrome. Prim Care 1999;26:113–136.
24. Ko CY, Tong J, Lehman RE, ct al. Biofeedback is effective for fecal incontinence and constipation. Arch Surg 1997;132:829–833.
25. Van der Plas RN, Benninga MA, Buller HA, et al. Biofeedback training in treatment of childhood constipation: A randomised controlled study. Lancet 1996;348:766–767.
26. Gattuso JM, Kamm MA. Adverse effects of drugs used in the management of constipation and diarrhoea. Drug Saf 1994;10:47–65.
27. Clausen MR, Mortensen PB. Lactulose, disaccharides and colonic flora. Clinical consequences. Drugs 1997;53:930–942.
28. Drossman DA. An integrated approach to the irritable bowel syndrome. Aliment Pharmacol Ther 1999;13(suppl. 2):3–14. Review.
29. Thompson WG. Irritable bowel syndrome: A management strategy. Baillieres Best Pract Res Clin Gastroenterol 1999;13:453–460.
30. Farthing MJG. Irritable bowel syndrome: New pharmaceutical approaches to treatment. Baillieres Best Pract Res Clin Gastroenterol 1999;13:461–471.
31. Drossman DA, Whitehead WE, Camilleri M. Irritable bowel syndrome: A technical review for practice guideline development. Gastroenterology 1997;112:2120–2137.
32. Thompson WG, Longstreth GF, Drossman DA, et al. Functional bowel disorders and functional abdominal pain. Gut 1999;45(suppl II):II43–II47.
33. Scarpignato C, Pelosini I. Management of irritable bowel syndrome: Novel approaches to the pharmacology of gut motility. Can J Gastroenterol 1999;13(suppl):50A–65A.
34. Jailwala K, Imperiale TF, Kroenke K. Pharmacologic treatment of the irritable bowel syndrome: A systematic review of randomized, controlled trials. Ann Intern Med 2000;133:136–147.

37

PORTAL HYPERTENSION AND CIRRHOSIS

Edward G. Timm and James J. Stragand

Many chronic inflammatory diseases of the liver result in diffuse hepatocyte necrosis, cellular regeneration and replacement with nodular fibrous tissue. As the number of functioning hepatocytes diminishes and fibrous tissue accumulates a constellation of symptoms and signs develop that is collectively termed *cirrhosis*. The term cirrhosis is derived from the Greek *kirrhos* meaning orange-colored and refers to the yellow-orange hue of the liver seen by the pathologist or surgeon. Histologically, cirrhosis is defined as a diffuse process characterized by fibrosis and a conversion of the normal hepatic architecture into structurally abnormal nodules.[1] Regardless of the mechanism of injury; the end result is the destruction of hepatocytes and their replacement with fibrous tissue. As fibrosis replaces normal hepatic parenchyma, resistance to blood flow results in portal hypertension and the development of varices and ascites.Hepatocyte loss and intrahepatic shunting of blood results in diminished metabolic and synthetic function, which leads to hepatic encephalopathy and coagulopathy.

While cirrhosis has many causes (Table 37–1), in the United States, excessive alcohol intake and chronic viral hepatitis, types B and C, are the most common causes.[1,2] A breakdown of the indications for liver transplantation (Table 37–2) provides an estimate of the clinical frequency for each of the potential causes of cirrhosis, as transplant represents the definitive therapeutic strategy for cirrhosis.[2] This data underestimates alcoholic liver disease, as these patients are often not considered suitable transplant candidates.

This chapter elucidates the pathophysiology of cirrhosis and the resultant effects on the human anatomy and physiology. Treatment strategies for managing the most commonly encountered clinical complications of cirrhosis are discussed.

EPIDEMIOLOGY

Cirrhosis affects 3.6/1,000 adults in the United States and is responsible for 26,000 deaths per year.[3] In 1994, *Morbidity and Mortality Report* ranked cirrhosis as the eleventh leading cause of death.[4] Acute variceal bleeding and spontaneous bacterial peritonitis are among the immediately life-threatening complications of cirrhosis. Associated conditions causing significant morbidity include ascites and hepatic encephalopathy. Approximately 50% of patients with cirrhosis who develop ascites die within 2 years of diagnosis.[5]

ANATOMY AND THE PATHOPHYSIOLOGY OF CIRRHOSIS

Any discussion of cirrhosis must be based on a firm understanding of hepatic anatomy and vascular supply. Conceptually, the liver can be thought of as an elaborate blood filtration system receiving blood from the portal vein and the hepatic artery (Fig. 37–1). Blood enters the liver via the portal triad and drains into the hepatic lobule, the smallest functional unit of this filtration system (Fig. 37–2). The hepatic lobule is hexagonal in shape, at the angles of which are the sites of the portal triads, which contain the smallest branches of the portal vein and hepatic artery, as well as the bile and lymphatic ducts. Within the lobule, individual hepatocytes are arranged in plates, radiating from the periphery to a central vein. The hepatic lobule can be subdivided into functional zones based on relative oxygen supply. The hepatic artery supplies oxygen rich blood to the portal triad.[6,7] Hepatocytes at the periphery therefore receive a higher level of oxygen than the cells near the central vein.

Arterial and venous blood from the portal triad passes through the hepatic lobules to the central veins via the hepatic sinusoids.After passing through the hepatic lobules, blood collects in the central veins, which ultimately coalesce into the hepatic veins, which then enter the inferior vena cava.

In areas of hepatocellular injury, regardless of the nature of the inciting agent, stellate cells become activated, lose their retinoids, and develop features of fibroblasts. They then become a major source of the collagen and other matrix proteins that increase during fibrosis.[9,10] The progressive deposition of fibrous material within the sinusoids disrupts the normal blood flow through the hepatic lobule. Normally the intrahepatic circulation is a low-pressure system with 10 times less resistance to the flow of blood than skeletal muscle.[11,12] As fibrous tissue accumulates, resistance to portal blood flow increases resulting in persistent and progressive elevations in portal blood pressures.

In summary, cirrhosis results in elevation of portal blood pressure because of the increased resistance to blood flow within the hepatic sinusoids. However, with the concept of the portal venous circulation in mind (Fig. 37–1), it can be appreciated how clinically diverse diseases can also result in the development of portal hypertension. Nevertheless, the most common cause of portal hypertension is cirrhosis.[2]

THE PATHOPHYSIOLOGY OF CIRRHOSIS

The anatomic derangements described above result in a number of pathophysiologic abnormalities that are commonly encountered in patients with cirrhosis. These include ascites, portal hypertension and varices, hepatic encephalopathy, and coagulation defects. Additional pathophysiologic abnormalities of chronic liver disease, including hepatorenal syndrome, hepatopulmonary syndrome, and endocrine dysfunction, are discussed under the section dealing with management of complications.

ASCITES

Ascites, the pathologic accumulation of lymph fluid within the peritoneal cavity, is one of the earliest and most common complications of cirrhosis.[13] More than one-half of cirrhotic patients develop ascites within 10 years of the diagnosis of cirrhosis.[14] The pathogenesis of the development of ascites is not completely understood. Several hypotheses regarding the formation of ascites have been proposed, including the older "underfill" and "overflow" concepts.[13,15,16] The most current unifying theory involves the concept of systemic arterial vasodilation which suggests that patients with cirrhosis and portal

TABLE 37–1. Etiology of Cirrhosis[1]

Category	Example
Drugs and toxins	Alcohol, methotrexate, isoniazid, methyldopa, organic hydrocarbons
Infections	Viral hepatitis (types B,C), schistosomiasis
Immune-mediated	Primary biliary cirrhosis, autoimmune hepatitis, primary sclerosing cholangitis
Metabolic	Hemochromatosis, porphyria, α_1-antitrypsin deficiency, Wilson's disease
Biliary obstruction	Cystic fibrosis, atresia, strictures, gallstones
Cardiovascular	Chronic right heart failure, Budd-Chiari syndrome, venoocclusive disease
Cryptogenic	Unknown
Other	Nonalcoholic steatohepatitis, sarcoidosis, gastric bypass

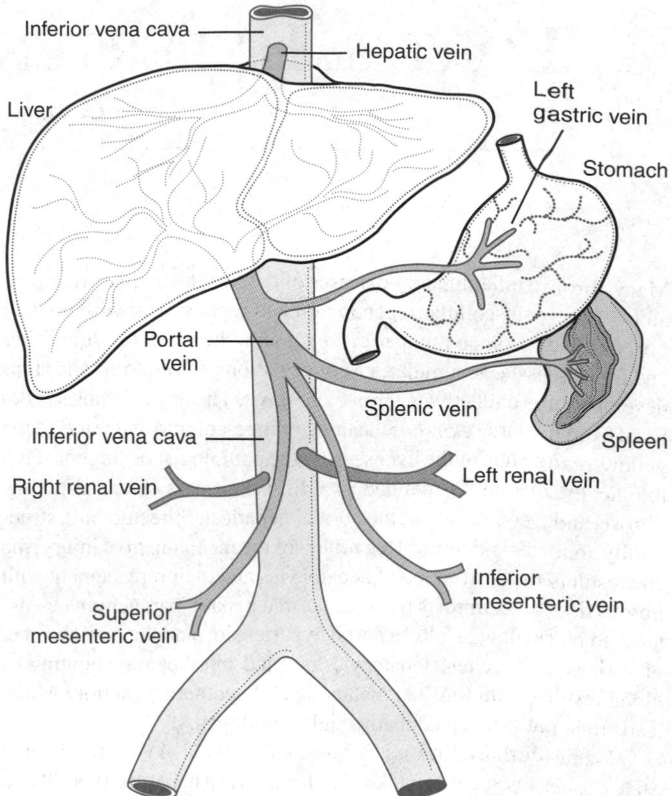

FIGURE 37–1. The portal-venous system.

hypertension have decreased systemic vascular resistance, a reduced mean arterial pressure and an increased cardiac output, which collectively results in a hyperdynamic circulation.[17] Several circulating vasodilators have been proposed including glucagon, vasoactive intestinal peptide, substance P and prostaglandins.[18] Current evidence supports a strong role for nitric oxide as the primary vasodilator in cirrhosis.[19] Increased synthesis of nitric oxide may occur as a result of an increased absorption of bacterial endotoxin from the gut lumen as a consequence of decreased reticuloendothelial activity within the cirrhotic liver.[20] The progressive vasodilation then leads to the activation of the baroreceptors of the kidney and an activation of the renin-angiotensin system with sodium and water retention (Fig. 37–3). The glomerular filtration rate (GFR) is decreased because of vasoconstriction as a result of sympathetic activation and increased activity of angiotensin II, and increased aldosterone synthesis enhances sodium and water retention.[13]

PORTAL HYPERTENSION AND VARICES

Normal portal venous pressure is 5–10 mm Hg.[11] Portal hypertension (PHT) exists when the portal pressure increases to a point where it is 5 mm Hg greater than the pressure in the inferior vena cava. The most important clinical sequelae of PHT is the development of varices or alternative routes of blood flow. Patients with cirrhosis are at risk for varices when portal pressures exceed 12 mm Hg, or greater than vena cava pressure.[11,43] Varices decompress the portal venous system, return blood to the systemic circulation, and can occur at any level of the gastrointestinal (GI) tract. However, the route with the most clinical significance is through the left gastric vein with the development of esophageal varices. Hemorrhage from varices occurs in 25% to 40% of patients with cirrhosis, and each episode of bleeding carries a 30% risk of death.[21,22] Rebleeding can occur in as many as 70% of patients within 1 year.[22] The risk of bleeding from esophageal varices is proportional to the pressure increase within the portal venous system and is related ultimately to the degree of cirrhosis. Increasing portal venous pressure translates into increased variceal pressure and size. As variceal size increases, wall tension also rises, increasing the risk of rupture. According to the Law of Laplace, small increases in a vessels radius results in a large increase in wall tension and increased risk of bleeding.[11] It should be apparent from this understanding that the primary strategy for the treatment of esophageal varices is the reduction of portal hypertension by pharmacologic and surgical approaches.

TABLE 37–2. Indications for Liver Transplant: United Network Organ Sharing Registry 1994

Disease	Frequency (%)
Alcohol	23
Hepatitis C	22.4
Cryptogenic	11
Primary biliary cirrhosis	9.4
Primary sclerosing cholangitis	8.3
Acute hepatic failure	6
Autoimmune hepatitis	5.8
Hepatitis B (chronic)	3.2
Hepatocellular cancer	2.9
Hemochromatosis	1.1
Hepatitis B (acute)	0.9
Budd-Chiari syndrome	0.7
Other	5.3

HEPATIC ENCEPHALOPATHY/PORTAL SYSTEMIC ENCEPHALOPATHY

Hepatic encephalopathy (HE) is a complex neuropsychiatric syndrome with a broad spectrum of clinical signs and symptoms of neurologic impairment that occurs in patients with severe hepatic insufficiency. [23] The term *portal-systemic encephalopathy* (PSE) is often used to describe the encephalopathy that occurs as a consequence of chronic liver disease. The term *portal-systemic* infers a relationship

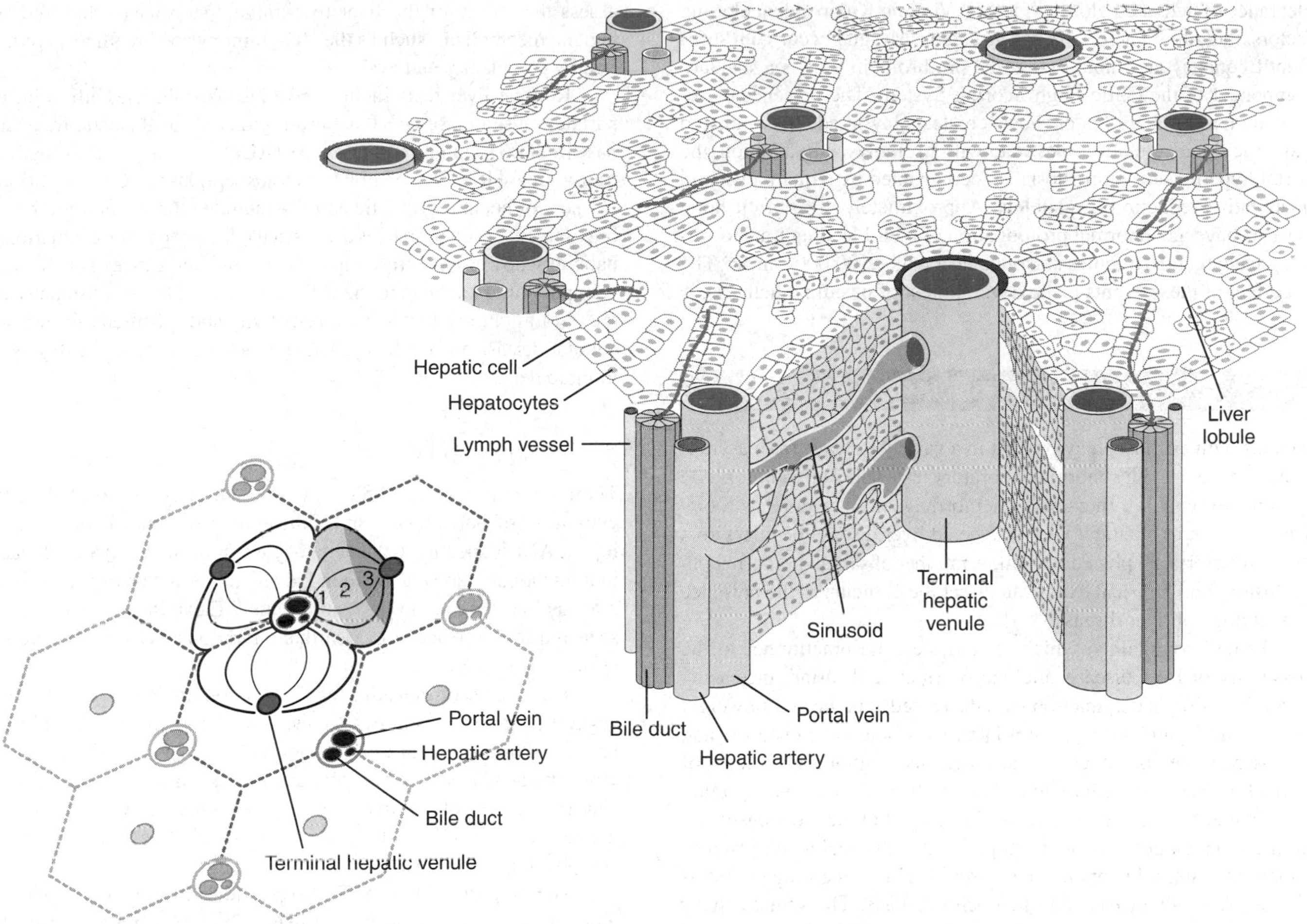

FIGURE 37–2. The hepatic lobule.

between ammonia and other gut metabolites that accumulate in the blood stream as a consequence of shunting through portal-systemic collaterals, and the neurologic abnormalities observed in HE. This is often referred to as the gut:brain connection. For the remainder of this discussion the more common term of hepatic encephalopathy is used.

HE can present in one of three forms: acute, chronic, and subclinical. Acute HE is defined as a distinct event of altered sensorium lasting less than 4 weeks, followed by complete recovery to the baseline mental status. Chronic encephalopathy is defined as cognitive or neuropsychiatric abnormalities that persist for at least 4 weeks. During this time, the severity of the abnormalities fluctuate but no episodes of normal mentation are noted. Subclinical encephalopathy refers to subtle alterations in neuropsychiatric function that are not clinically apparent.[24,25]

A traditional hypothesis suggests that HE is caused by the accumulation of toxic nitrogenous and other toxins that have not been metabolized by the liver. Newer evidence suggests that other mechanisms may be involved, including alterations of the blood-brain barrier; neurotransmitter imbalances; altered cerebral metabolism; impairment of neuronal membrane sodium-potassium ATPase activity; zinc deficiency; and increased endogenous γ-aminobutyric acid/benzodiazepines.[26] That HE occurs as a consequence of elevated arterial ammonia concentrations is the most commonly cited hypothesis, and ammonia levels tend to be elevated in patients with more advanced liver insufficiency. However, ammonia levels are only poorly correlated with the grade of HE.[23] Furthermore, the administration of ammonia failed to induce HE in patients with cirrhosis.[27] Nevertheless, interventions to lower blood ammonia levels are the mainstay of the treatment of HE.

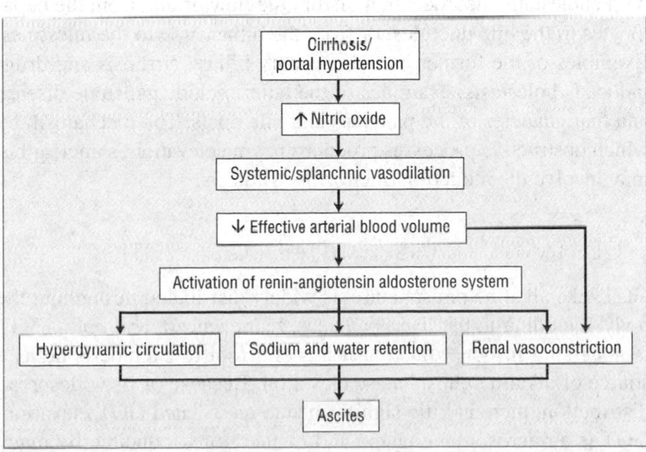

FIGURE 37–3. Pathogenesis of ascites.

COAGULATION DEFECTS

Normal hemostasis is dependent on normal hepatic function. Complex coagulation derangement's can occur in cirrhosis, which are proportional to the degree of hepatic dysfunction. These derangements include the reduction in the synthesis of coagulation factors, and the clearance of activated clotting factors. Vitamin K-dependent clotting factors, including Factor VII, are affected early, and occur with sufficient frequency and rapidity that the prothrombin time is a standard component of the Child-Pugh Scoring System. The presence of activated clotting factors in cirrhosis creates a low-grade disseminated intravascular coagulation-like state with fibrinolysis. In addition, the portal hypertension of cirrhosis is accompanied by a qualitative and quantitative reduction in platelets. Approximately 40% of cirrhotic patients have an abnormal prolongation of their bleeding time to values greater than 10 minutes and platelet counts $<100,000/mm^3$.[28] The net effect of these events is the development of bleeding diathesis.

CLINICAL PRESENTATION

Patients with cirrhosis may present in a variety of ways from asymptomatic patients with abnormal laboratory tests noted on routine blood donation to acute life-threatening hemorrhage in an emergency room. The approach to a patient with suspected liver disease begins with a through history and physical exam. A number of salient points in both the history and physical exam can direct the clinician to the presence and etiology of liver disease.

Patient complaints, which should alert the practitioner to the possibility of liver disease, include pruritus, dark urine, increasing abdominal girth in conjunction with decreased appetite and/or weight loss. Clinical jaundice is often a late manifestation of cirrhosis and its absence does not exclude the diagnosis. A thorough history of alcohol or drug use, with the input of family and friends is important as the patient often underestimates the amount of alcohol consumed. Information about the patient's appetite and physical activity is also important. Family history can also provide clues regarding problems such as Wilson's disease and hemochromatosis. The social history provides information regarding potential occupational exposures to toxic agents such as carbon tetrachloride and other solvents. Symptom duration can provide clues to the etiology of liver disease. A history of acute pain and fever may indicate an obstructive process due to gallstones or an inflammatory condition such as viral or alcoholic hepatitis. The inflammatory conditions cause pain secondary to acute swelling of the hepatic parenchyma with stretching of the Glisson capsule. The patients' past medical and surgical histories need to be explored for prior receipt of blood products. A past history of blood donations is also helpful in pinpointing the duration of problems, as most blood banks would have detected abnormal liver chemistries.

The classic clinical signs of cirrhosis, such as palmar erythema, spider angiomata, and gynecomastia, are neither sensitive nor specific for this disease.[29] Only a combination of physical and laboratory findings provides a reasonable indicator of liver disease. A decreased albumin level was the most common finding in patients with cirrhosis but was nonspecific and occurred in a variety of conditions. An elevated prothrombin time was the single most reliable manifestation of cirrhosis. The combination of thrombocytopenia, encephalopathy, and ascites was found in just over half of cirrhotics, but had the highest predictive value.[29]

LABORATORY ABNORMALITIES

There are no laboratory or radiographic tests of "hepatic function" despite the commonly ordered liver "function" tests. These commonly measured markers are substances produced by the liver and released into the bloodstream during hepatocellular injury and are more correctly termed liver "dysfunction" tests. True liver function tests that assess the ability of the liver to eliminate substances that undergo hepatic metabolism, such as the ^{14}C-aminopyrine breath test are limited by complexity and availability.

Routine liver tests include alkaline phosphatase, bilirubin, aspartate transaminase (AST or serum glutamic-oxaloacetic transaminase [SGOT]), alanine transaminase (ALT or serum glutamic-pyruvic transaminase [SGPT]), γ-glutamyl transpeptidase (GGT). Additional markers of hepatic synthetic activity include albumin and prothrombin time. Liver function tests are often the first step in the evaluation of patients who present with symptoms or signs suggestive of cirrhosis. It is important to understand the cellular source of these substances and the test limitations; that is, their sensitivity and specificity for hepatocellular disease and cirrhosis. The individual liver tests are discussed in more detail.

AMINOTRANSFERASES

The aminotransferases, AST and ALT are enzymes located in the cytoplasm of hepatocytes and will be elevated with hepatocellular injury. ALT is specific to the hepatocyte cytoplasm but AST is located in mitochondria and can be found in any tissue with a high metabolic rate, such as cardiac, kidney, and brain.[30] Elevations of AST can be seen as a consequence of myocardial infarction and ischemic cerebral events.

The degree of elevation of the aminotransferases is helpful in suggesting possible sources for hepatocellular injury. The highest levels (>20-fold increase above normal) are typically seen in acute viral, drug-induced, or ischemic events associated with circulatory catastrophes. Alcoholic liver disease rarely presents with ALT values greater than 500 U/L and higher values should alert the clinician to complicating problems.[30]

The ratio of AST to ALT also provides information in patients with suspected alcoholic liver disease. Seventy percent of patients with alcoholic liver disease had ratios greater than 2 as compared to 4% of patients with viral hepatitis.[31] The low levels of ALT elevation in alcoholic liver disease is thought to be related to pyridoxal 5-phosphate deficiency.[32]

ALKALINE PHOSPHATASE

Alkaline phosphatase is actually a group of isoenzymes widely distributed throughout the body, including the liver, bone, intestine, kidney, and leukocytes.[33,34] Hepatic alkaline phosphatase is located in the sinusoidal and bile canalicular membranes as well as the cytoplasm. The highest level of alkaline phosphatase elevation occurs with cholestatic disorders that disrupt the flow of bile from the hepatocytes to the bile ductules, or from the biliary tree to the intestines. Examples of the former include primary biliary cirrhosis and drug-induced cholestasis; examples of the latter include gallstone disease and malignancies of the pancreas and bile ducts. The mechanism by which obstructive processes produce enzyme elevation is unclear but may involve the induction of enzyme synthesis.[35]

γ-GLUTAMYL TRANSPEPTIDASE (GGT, γGT)

GGT, like alkaline phosphatase, is widely distributed throughout the body, including in the liver, pancreas, kidney, heart, and brain. GGT is not found in bone, making it a useful tool to exclude bone as a source of alkaline phosphatase elevation. Because of its widespread distribution, there is little significance to an isolated GGT elevation. GGT is a microsomal enzyme and is, therefore, inducible by many drugs, such as alcohol, phenytoin, barbiturates, carbamazepine, and warfarin. In liver disease, the levels of GGT correlate well with elevations of the alkaline phosphatase and thus are a sensitive and specific marker for biliary tract disease.[36]

BILIRUBIN

Bilirubin is a breakdown product of hemoglobin derived from senescent red blood cells. Elevations of the serum bilirubin are common in end-stage liver disease, but other causes of hyperbilirubinemia are numerous (Table 37–3).

It is important to understand that not all jaundice is caused by cirrhosis. Understanding the anatomy of the biliary system allows an appreciation of the mechanisms behind the development of jaundice. Bile is actively secreted from the hepatocytes into the bile ducts within the hepatic parenchyma. The ductules coalesce into the intrahepatic bile ducts, and then to the extrahepatic and common bile duct, which passes through the head of the pancreas and enters the proximal small intestine via the ampulla of Vater. The gall bladder, which collects and concentrates bile, connects to the common bile duct via the cystic duct. Obstruction at any level of the biliary tree from the intrahepatic canaliculi to the ampulla of Vater can result in jaundice. Causes of obstruction include malignancies of the pancreas, gallstones within the common bile duct, and drugs that interfere with the passage of bile from the hepatocyte to the canaliculi. Gallstones within the gallbladder do not result in jaundice, as the common bile duct remains open. A combination of reduced hepatic parenchyma and intrahepatic disruption of the smaller bile ducts causes the jaundice of cirrhosis. The net effect is the reduced clearance of bilirubin with the development of clinical jaundice.

When cirrhosis has been established, the degree of bilirubin elevation has prognostic significance and is used as a component of the Child-Pugh scoring system for quantifying the degree of cirrhosis (see below).

Figure 37–4 describes a general algorithm for the interpretation of liver function tests. The algorithm first separates the tests into two categories based on the underlying pathology (pattern of elevations): obstructive (alkaline phosphatase, GGT, and bilirubin) versus hepatocellular (AST and ALT). If a hepatocellular pattern predominates, the magnitude of elevation provides diagnostic assistance. If the degree of elevation is > 20 times normal, the etiology is likely a result

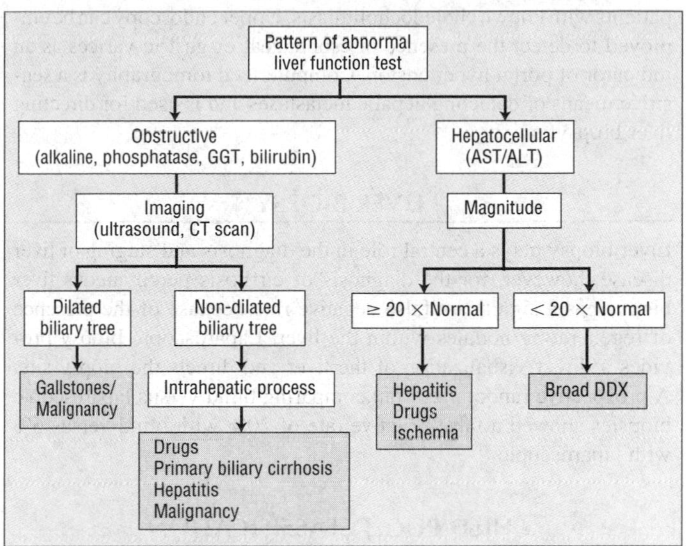

FIGURE 37–4. Interpretation of liver function tests.

of drugs or other toxins, ischemia, or acute viral hepatitis. Elevations < 20 times normal have a broad differential. Unfortunately, most liver enzyme abnormalities will fall into a mixed pattern providing limited diagnostic limited assistance.

ALBUMIN AND COAGULATION FACTORS

These proteins are markers of hepatic synthetic activity and are therefore used to estimate the level of functioning hepatocytes in cirrhosis. They are employed in the Child-Pugh scoring system for liver disease. Albumin levels can be affected by a number of factors including the patient's nutritional status, acute illnesses, which result in redistribution of albumin, and protein losses from renal and intestinal sources.

The liver synthesizes coagulation factors I, II, V, VII, IX, and X.[37] The prothrombin time is prolonged when any of these factors are absent. In acute liver disease the prothrombin time can be used as an outcome measurement in acetaminophen overdose and acute alcoholic hepatitis.[38] In chronic liver disease, the prothrombin time is employed as a marker of decreased synthetic capacity.

THROMBOCYTOPENIA

Thrombocytopenia is a relatively common feature in both acute and chronic liver disease and is proportional to the extent of liver disease.[39] The etiology of thrombocytopenia in liver disease is multifactorial but involves primarily hypersplenism with pooling of platelets, immune-mediated destruction, and the inability of the bone marrow to compensate for the accelerated removal. The bone marrow depression may be related to alcohol, drugs, and nutritional deficiencies associated with the cirrhotic process.[40]

TABLE 37–3. Etiology of Hyperbilirubinemia

Etiology	Diagnosis
Unconjugated	
Excessive production	Hemolysis
Immature enzyme systems	Jaundice of newborn Jaundice of prematurity
Inherited defects	Gilbert's syndrome Crigler-Najjar syndrome
Drug effects	
Conjugated	
Impaired intrahepatic excretion	
Hepatocellular disease	Hepatitis, cirrhosis, drugs
Intrahepatic cholestasis	Drugs, pregnancy
Congenital	Dubin-Johnson syndrome Rotor's syndrome
Obstruction	
Extrahepatic	Calculus, stricture, neoplasm
Intrahepatic	Sclerosing cholangitis, cirrhosis, neoplasm

ENDOSCOPIC AND RADIOGRAPHIC ABNORMALITIES

The use of imaging techniques can provide useful information regarding the presence of liver disease and portal hypertension. The modality chosen is often determined by the clinical presentation. Examples include the use of ultrasound for the detection of gallstones and biliary duct abnormalities in patient's presenting with acute pain and jaundice, or endoscopic retrograde cholangiopancreatography (ERCP) for patients with known choledocholithiasis. Upper endoscopy can be employed to detect the presence of esophageal or gastric varices as an indicator of portal hypertension. Computerized tomography is a sensitive means of detecting hepatic metastases and is used for directing liver biopsy.

LIVER BIOPSY

Liver biopsy plays a central role in the diagnosis and staging of liver disease, however, for the diagnosis of cirrhosis percutaneous liver biopsy has a significant false-negative rate because of the presence of regenerating nodules within the liver. Laparoscopic biopsy provides a direct visualization of the liver and directs the biopsy site. A prospective randomized trail comparing blind versus laparoscopic biopsies showed a false-negative rate of 20% with blind versus 6% with laparoscopic.[41]

CHILD-PUGH CLASSIFICATION

The Child-Pugh classification system has gained widespread acceptance as a means quantifying the myriad effects of the cirrhotic process on the laboratory and clinical manifestations of this disease.[42] The system employs a combination of physical and laboratory findings (Table 37–4). This classification system is important because it is used to assess and define the severity of the cirrhosis and as a predictor for patient survival, surgical outcome, and risk of variceal bleeding.

TABLE 37–4. Criteria and Scoring for the Child-Pugh Grading of Chronic Liver Disease

Score	1	2	3
Bilirubin (mg/dL)	1–2	2–3	>3
Albumin (mg/dL)	>3.5	2.8–3.5	<2.8
Ascites	None	Mild	Moderate
Encephalopathy (grade)	None	1 and 2	3 and 4
Prothrombin time (prolonged seconds)	1–4	4–6	>6

Grade A = <7 points; Grade B = 7–9 points; Grade C = 10–15 points.

MANAGEMENT OF THE COMPLICATIONS OF CIRRHOSIS

The major complications of cirrhosis that require therapeutic intervention include:

- Portal hypertension and variceal bleeding
- Ascites and spontaneous bacterial peritonitis
- Hepatic encephalopathy
- Other systemic complications

▶ TREATMENT: Cirrhosis

GENERAL APPROACHES TO TREATMENT

As is discussed below, the clinical manifestations of cirrhosis are protean and it is difficult to provide overall management guidelines. General approaches to therapy should include:

1. Identify and eliminate where possible the causes of cirrhosis (e.g., alcohol abuse).
2. Assess the risk for variceal bleeding and begin pharmacologic prophylaxis where indicated, reserving endoscopic therapy for high-risk patients or acute bleeding episodes. Variceal obliteration with endoscopic techniques is the recommended treatment of choice in patients with acute bleeding.
3. Evaluate the patient for clinical signs of ascites and manage with pharmacologic therapy (e.g., diuretics and paracentesis). Careful monitoring for spontaneous bacterial peritonitis should be employed in patients with ascites who undergo acute deterioration.
4. Hepatic encephalopathy is a common complication of cirrhosis and requires clinical vigilance and treatment with dietary restriction, elimination of central nervous system (CNS) depressants and therapy to lower ammonia levels.
5. Frequent monitoring for signs of hepatorenal syndrome, pulmonary insufficiency and endocrine dysfunction is necessary.

DESIRED OUTCOMES

Given what has been learned so far regarding the pathophysiology of cirrhosis, it may be intuitive that the desired therapeutic outcomes can be viewed in two categories, *clinical improvement or resolution* of acute complications, such as tamponade of bleeding and resolution of hemodynamic instability for an episode of acute variceal hemorrhage, and *prevention of complications,* such as achieving adequate lowering of portal pressure with medical therapy using β-adrenergic blocker therapy, or supporting abstinence from alcohol. Treatment endpoints and desired therapeutic outcomes are presented for each of the recommended therapies discussed.

PORTAL HYPERTENSION AND VARICEAL BLEEDING

The normal intrahepatic circulation is a low-pressure system with 10 times less resistance to the flow of blood than skeletal muscle. The normal portal venous pressure is 5–10 mm Hg.[11] Portal hypertension exists when portal vein pressure is 5 mm Hg greater than the inferior vena caval pressure, and patients with cirrhosis are at risk for varices when portal pressures exceed 12 mm Hg or greater than vena caval pressure.[11,43] Regardless of the cause of the increased portal pressure, increased collateral blood flow occurs most commonly through four collateral vascular supplies: (a) esophageal submucosal venous plexus; (b) cardiac vein of the stomach; (c) retroperitoneal-umbilical system; and (d) hemorrhoidal system.[43] The collateral flow with the most clinical significance is through the left gastric vein and results in the development of esophageal varices. In a 6-year study of patients with cirrhosis, esophageal varices developed at a rate of 8% per year.[44] In patients with alcoholic cirrhosis, large varices developed in 19% with de novo varices at baseline and in 42% of those with small varices at baseline over a 16-month period of observation.[43]

The propensity of varices to bleed when a threshold pressure is reached is a potentially life-threatening complication. Mortality after the first variceal bleed ranges from 5% to 50% and is dependent upon the severity of the underlying liver disease.[45] Cirrhotic patients who have experienced their first episode of variceal bleeding have a 70% risk of rebleeding.[46] Rebleeding most commonly occurs within the first 2 weeks, but if the patient has not rebled after 6 weeks, the risk of rebleeding drops sharply and approaches that of cirrhotic patients who have never bled.[47]

MANAGEMENT OF PORTAL HYPERTENSION AND VARICEAL BLEEDING

The rationale for therapy is based on the desired reduction of portal venous pressure and the pressure within the varices. Resistance to flow through the liver is a fixed process whereas the vasodilatory effects on splanchnic blood flow are reversible and form the first treatment option. The management of varices involves three strategies: (a) primary prophylaxis (prevention of the first bleeding episode); (b) treatment of acute variceal hemorrhage; and (c) secondary prophylaxis, prevention of rebleeding in patients who have previously bled.[48,49]

Primary Prophylaxis

β-Adrenergic Blockade. The mainstay of primary prophylaxis is the use nonselective β-adrenergic blocking agents such as propranolol or nadolol. These agents block the adrenergic dilatory tone of the mesenteric arterioles resulting in unopposed α-adrenergic-mediated vasoconstriction, and a decrease in portal inflow and portal pressure.[48]

A meta-analysis of nine randomized, controlled trials evaluating the effectiveness of either propranolol or nadolol as primary prophylaxis demonstrated effectiveness in the prevention of bleeding and a trend toward a reduction in mortality.[50–54] A subsequent meta-analysis reported similar findings.[53] The average reduction in the incidence of initial bleeding achieved by nonselective β-adrenergic blockade is approximately 50%.[52] β-Blockade was effective irrespective of the presence of ascites and variceal size, and another study suggested that patients with a higher risk for bleeding, larger varices, or any size varices with a portal pressure >12 mm Hg, are the best candidates for prophylactic β-adrenergic blocker therapy.[52,54] β-Adrenergic blocker therapy should be lifelong, unless it is not tolerated, because bleeding can occur when β-blocker therapy is abruptly discontinued.[55]

Nitrates. Nitrates are known to cause smooth-muscle vasodilation and reduction in portal pressures; however, the role of nitrates in primary prophylaxis is controversial. Isosorbide-5-mononitrate was compared with propranolol for primary prophylaxis in cirrhosis.[56] Equivalent reductions in bleeding were reported, but short-term survival was improved with isosorbide therapy. This report was met with great enthusiasm because it offered an effective alternative for patients who did not tolerate β-adrenergic blockers. Follow up on the patients in the study was continued for up to 7 years with the finding that the early mortality benefit was lost. In fact, the use of isosorbide-5-mononitrate resulted in higher long-term mortality than propranolol in patients >50 years of age.[57] These findings are not entirely surprising because it was appreciated that a potential existed for nitrates to increase portal blood flow and consequently portal pressure by enhancing nitric oxide-mediated vasodilation of the mesenteric vasculature. Considering that vasodilation in liver disease is the hemodynamic expression of liver failure and is a prognostic indicator of morbidity and mortality, this may explain, at least in part, the negative effects on long-term survival.[58] Another therapeutic issue arises because β-adrenergic blockers alone do not adequately lower portal pressure in all patients. A number of trials have shown that the combination of nitrates and β-adrenergic blockers is superior to β-adrenergic blockers alone in lowering portal pressures.[58] β-Adrenergic blocker therapy may suppress the neurohormonal activation associated with the relative hypovolemia induced by the vasodilation from the nitrate therapy and thereby minimize its detrimental effects.[50] With such disparate study findings the role of nitrates in primary prophylaxis is controversial and firm recommendations are difficult. Nevertheless, for patients with an inadequate response to β-adrenergic blockers alone, a long-acting nitrovasodilator should be added to try to achieve adequate lowering of portal pressure. For patients with contraindications or intolerance to β-adrenergic blockers, treatment decisions are uncertain. Groszmann and colleagues suggest that nitrates can probably be used safely in this situation in younger patients who have well-compensated cirrhosis.[50]

Treatment Recommendations: Variceal Bleeding-Primary Prophylaxis

All patients with cirrhosis and portal hypertension should be considered for endoscopic screening, and patients with large varices should receive primary prophylaxis with β-adrenergic blockers. Initiate therapy with oral propranolol 10 mg three times daily or nadolol 20 mg once daily and titrate to a reduction in the resting heart rate of 20% to 25%, an absolute heart rate of 55–60 beats per minute (bpm), or the development of adverse effects. Patients with contraindications or intolerance to β-adrenergic blockers should be considered for trials of alternative prophylactic therapy.[49] Nitrates may be considered for these patients provided they are younger than 50 years of age and have well-compensated cirrhosis. Initiate therapy with isosorbide-5-mononitrate 20 mg orally twice daily and increase to 20 mg three times a day after 1 week if tolerated. Combination therapy with β-blockers and nitrates is recommended for patients with an inadequate lowering of portal pressure in response to β-adrenergic blockers alone. Currently, no evidence supports the use of sclerotherapy, band ligation, surgical shunting, or transjugular intrahepatic portosystemic shunt (TIPS) as primary prophylaxis.[43,49,56] However, one recent study comparing variceal band ligation versus β-blockers as a primary prophylaxis did show a decreased rate of bleeding at 1 year in the banding group.[59]

ACUTE VARICEAL HEMORRHAGE

Variceal hemorrhage typically presents with hematemesis or melena. Important risk factors include active alcohol abuse, use of nonsteroidal anti-inflammatory agents or aspirin, or previous variceal hemorrhage.[49] It is important to note, however, that variceal bleeding secondary to portal hypertension can occur in patients without signs of liver disease; for example, in patients with hepatic splanchnic vein thrombosis. The initial assessment should determine the severity of the bleeding, severity of other organ dysfunction, and the severity of the liver disease. The Child-Pugh scoring system (Table 37–4) is the most reliable means of assessing the severity of chronic liver disease.[49]

MANAGEMENT OF ACUTE VARICEAL HEMORRHAGE

Initial treatment goals include: (a) adequate fluid resuscitation; (b) correction of coagulopathy and thrombocytopenia; (c) control of bleeding; (d) prevention of rebleeding; and (e) preservation of liver function. Prompt stabilization and aggressive fluid resuscitation of patients with active bleeding is followed by endoscopic examination.

General resuscitation measures should be applied in the initial management of variceal hemorrhage following the standard ABC format for airway, breathing, and circulation. Airway management is critical in patients with variceal hemorrhage because of depressed reflexes and/or combative behavior associated with drug and alcohol use. The endoscopic approach to bleeding also requires a quiet and cooperative patient and elective intubation for airway control and adequate sedation is often necessary. Fluid resuscitation involves colloids initially and subsequent blood products after blood bank matching procedures are completed. Packed RBCs, fresh-frozen plasma and platelets may be employed both as volume expanders and corrective therapy for underlying clotting abnormalities. Clinical practice guidelines approved by the American College of Gastroenterology recommend esophagogastroduodenoscopy (EGD) employing endoscopic injection sclerotherapy (EIS) or endoscopic band ligation (EBL) of varices as the primary diagnostic and treatment strategy for upper GI tract hemorrhage secondary to portal hypertension and varices.[60] Vasoactive drug therapy (somatostatin, octreotide, or terlipressin) to stop or slow bleeding is routinely employed early in patient management to allow stabilization of the patient and to permit endoscopy to proceed under more favorable conditions. Antibiotic therapy to prevent sepsis should also be implemented early for patients with signs of infection. Figure 37–5 presents an algorithm for the management of variceal hemorrhage.

DRUG THERAPY

Drug therapy for acute variceal bleeding is based upon the principle that it is possible to reduce portal, and consequently variceal, pressure by reducing portal collateral blood flow via splanchnic vasoconstriction and by decreasing vascular resistance in the intrahepatic circulation via systemic vasodilation.[61] Drugs employed to manage acute variceal bleeding include octreotide or somatostatin, vasopressin, and terlipressin (triglycyl lysine vasopressin).

Somatostatin and Octreotide

Somatostatin is a naturally occurring 14-amino acid peptide and octreotide is a synthetic octapeptide analog that is significantly more potent than native somatostatin. In the gastrointestinal tract somatostatin inhibits glandular secretion, neurotransmission, and smooth-muscle contractility, producing mesenteric vasoconstriction.[62] Octreotide shares four amino acids with somatostatin and these moieties are responsible for its pharmacologic activity. Both somatostatin and octreotide are widely used in the treatment of variceal hemorrhage because of their reported ability to decrease splanchnic blood flow, and to reduce portal and variceal pressures, without significant adverse effects.[46,49] Unlike vasopressin, systemic vasoconstriction and elevations in blood pressure are not seen because the vasoconstriction that occurs with somatostatin and octreotide is selective for the mesenteric circulation. Other reports, however, have failed to demonstrate reductions on gastric mucosal blood flow or intravariceal pressure.[49] Consequently, the precise mechanism of action by which these agents may beneficially impact variceal bleeding still remains unclear.[63] Placebo-controlled clinical trials found somatostatin no more effective than placebo, whereas other studies show a clear benefit with somatostatin.[64–66] A meta-analysis of clinical trials comparing somatostatin and octreotide with vasopressin or terlipressin has demonstrated equivalent efficacy, but the side effect profile of somatostatin and octreotide was superior to vasopressin.[67] This analysis also reported however that somatostatin was more effective in achieving initial and sustained control of bleeding.

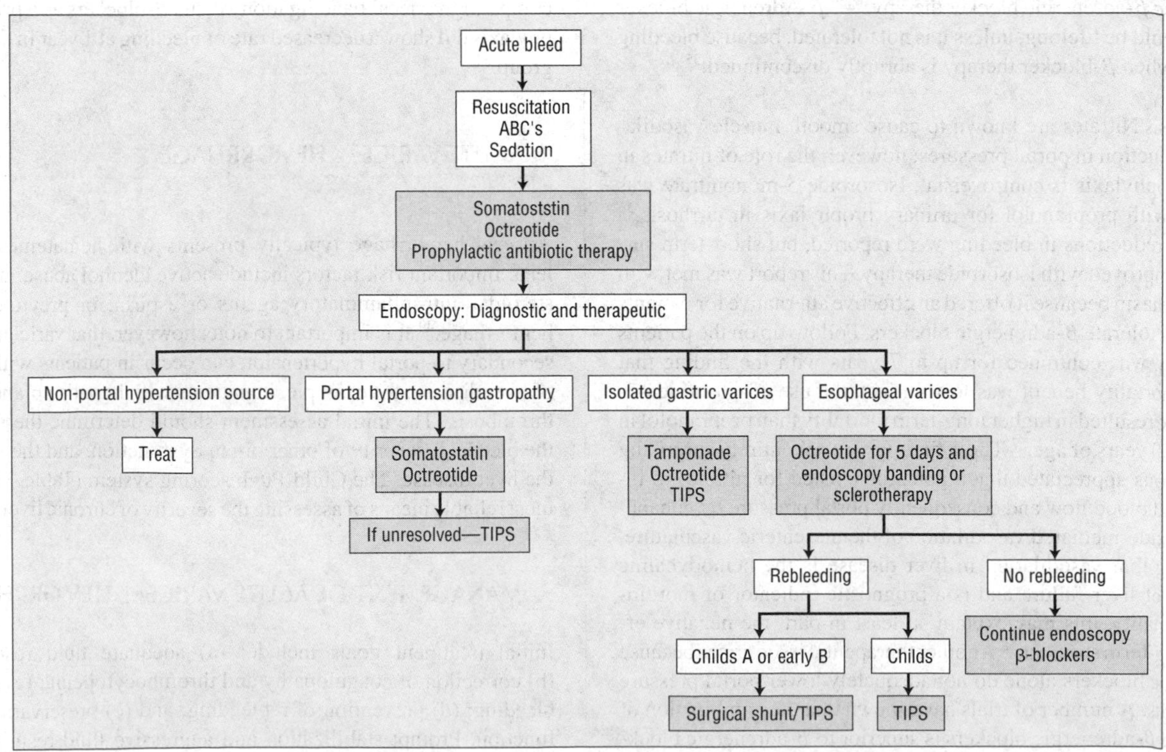

FIGURE 37–5. Management of acute variceal hemorrhage.

Vasopressin (also known as antidiuretic hormone) is a potent, nonselective vasoconstrictor that has been recommended for many years for the management of acute variceal bleeding. Vasopressin reduces portal pressure by causing splanchnic vasoconstriction, which reduces splanchnic blood flow. Unfortunately, the vasoconstrictive effects of vasopressin are nonselective—the vasoconstriction produced is not restricted to the splanchnic vascular bed. Potent systemic vasoconstriction occurs in the coronary and mesenteric circulation as well, resulting in hypertension, severe headaches, coronary ischemia, myocardial infarction and arrhythmias. A meta-analysis of 15 randomized, controlled, clinical trials of vasopressin for variceal hemorrhage demonstrated that vasopressin was significantly more effective than no treatment; however, control of hemorrhage was achieved in only 50% of the bleeding episodes.[46] Adverse effects were reported in 45% of patients, and vasopressin was discontinued in 25% of patients secondary to adverse effects. To minimize adverse effects associated with the peripheral vasoconstriction secondary to vasopressin, and to further lower portal pressure, the combination of vasopressin and intravenous nitroglycerin (NTG) has been evaluated.[68] The combination trended toward improved control of hemorrhage with reduced side effects when compared to vasopressin alone. However, with the recent addition of safer and equally effective treatment alternatives, vasopressin, alone or combined with nitroglycerin, can no longer be recommended as first-line therapy for the management of variceal hemorrhage.[49]

Terlipressin (Glypressin), triglycyl-lysine vasopressin, is a synthetic prodrug of vasopressin with intrinsic vasoconstrictor activity that was developed in an attempt to provide an analogue of vasopressin with lower toxicity. The glycl residues are enzymatically cleaved *in vivo* resulting in the slow conversion into lysine vasopressin. This process results in the availability of lysine vasopressin with a longer half-life permitting bolus dosing every 4 hours.[49] In a number of unblinded clinical trials, terlipressin was associated with a significantly lower rate of adverse effects as compared to vasopressin alone, or as compared to vasopressin combined with nitroglycerin.[49] When compared to octreotide or somatostatin, terlipressin produced a significantly greater reduction in measured variceal pressure. In patients with acute bleeding terlipressin maintained a reduction in variceal pressure, whereas the effects of somatostatin were short-lived.[69] In clinical trials, that have been criticized for small sample size and unclear timing of treatments, terlipressin has demonstrated a beneficial effect on the control of bleeding compared with placebo, and is the only drug that has been shown to reduce mortality.[49] Terlipressin, the preferred drug in Europe for acute variceal bleeding is not currently available in the United States.

Cirrhotic patients with active bleeding are at high risk of infection and sepsis secondary to aspiration, the placement of multiple intravascular access devices, sclerotherapy, translocation, and defects in humoral and cellular immunity.[49] Prophylactic antibiotic therapy to reduce the risk of sepsis during episodes of bleeding is reported to decrease the incidence of rebleeding and to increase short-term survival.[70,71] All patients with variceal hemorrhage should be screened for infection and pan-cultured. Patients should be evaluated at admission and observed throughout therapy for signs and symptoms of spontaneous bacterial peritonitis.[43]

ENDOSCOPIC INTERVENTIONS: SCLEROTHERAPY AND BAND LIGATION

The American College of Gastroenterology published clinical practice guidelines, in 1997, recommending EGD employing EIS or EBL of varices as the primary diagnostic and treatment strategy for upper GI tract hemorrhage secondary to portal hypertension and varices.[72] EIS involves injection of 1–4ml of a sclerosing agent into the lumen of the varices to tamponade blood flow. EBL consists of placement of rubber bands around the varix through a clear plastic channel attached to the end of the endoscope. After the rubber bands are in place, the varix will slough off after 48 hours to 72 hours. Endoscopic approaches can successfully stop bleeding in up to 95% of cases, but rebleeding may occur in 50% of cases. A recent meta-analysis of comparative clinical trials found both techniques equally effective in controlling acute variceal bleeding, but indicated that EBL was superior to EIS in reducing the rebleeding rate, and that EBL was associated with fewer posttreatment complications.[49] Sclerosing agents employed in EIS include ethanolamine, sodium tetradecyl sulfate, polidocanol, and sodium morrhuate. There is no data establishing clinical superiority of any of the sclerosants.[73]

Eight published clinical trials have compared endoscopic sclerotherapy with vasoactive drug therapy for active variceal bleeding. Drug treatment controlled bleeding in 58% to 95% of cases, and sclerotherapy controlled bleeding in 68% to 94% of cases. Rebleeding was slightly less common in patients receiving sclerotherapy and sclerotherapy was associated with a lower mortality rate. Clinical trials of sclerotherapy plus vasoactive drugs versus sclerotherapy alone show a significant advantage for combination therapy, without, however, a beneficial effect on mortality.[49]

INTERVENTIONAL AND SURGICAL TREATMENT APPROACHES

If standard therapy fails to control bleeding (after two failed endoscopic procedures, further attempts are unlikely to be of benefit) a salvage procedure, such as balloon tamponade, TIPS, or surgical shunting, is necessary.

Sengstaken-Blakemore tubes are balloon devices designed to tamponade gastric and esophageal varices from inside the esophagus and can be effective in 70% to 90% of cases of variceal bleeding.[49] However, these devices have a 10% to 30% complication rate and will be ineffective if the bleeding source is nonvariceal, a situation which occurs in 10% to 50% of patients with portal hypertension.[49] Balloon tamponade should be reserved as a temporizing measure until a TIPS procedure or surgical shunt can be performed.[43]

The development of the TIPS provided a major improvement in the management of refractory or severe cases of esophagogastric variceal bleeding and other complications of portal hypertension.[74] The TIPS procedure involves the placement of one or more stents between the hepatic vein and the portal vein (Fig. 37–6). This

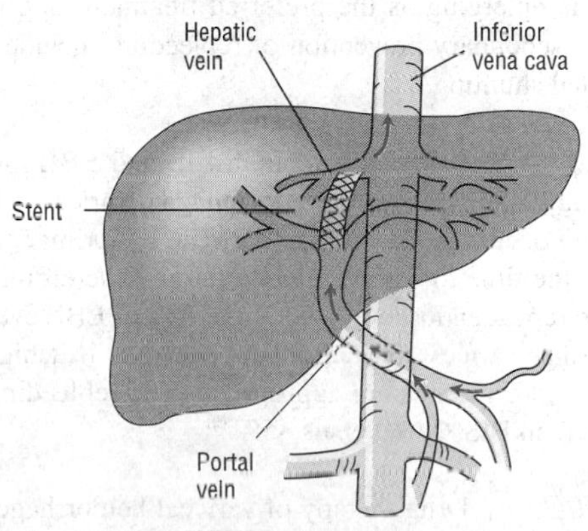

FIGURE 37–6. TIPS.

procedure is widely used because it provides an effective decompressive shunt, without laparotomy, and can be employed regardless of Child-Pugh score. Survival rates with TIPS in patients refractory to endoscopic treatment are comparable to rates achieved with portacaval shunts.[49] Patients undergoing TIPS experience a 30% incidence of encephalopathy, and approximately 50% of shunts dysfunction.[43]

Various surgical shunts have been developed and are effective for the prevention of recurrent variceal hemorrhage in patients refractory to beta-adrenergic blockade and endoscopy. The most commonly employed surgical shunt is the narrow-diameter portacaval shunt. This procedure leaves the portal vein intact in the event that liver transplantation is undertaken in the future.[43]

TREATMENT RECOMMENDATIONS: VARICEAL HEMORRHAGE

Patients require prompt resuscitation with colloids and blood products to correct intravascular losses and to reverse existing coagulopathies. Drug therapy with octreotide or somatostatin should be initiated early to control bleeding and facilitate diagnostic and therapeutic endoscopy. Based upon availability octreotide is preferred. Therapy is initiated with an IV bolus of 50–100 μg and is followed by a continuous infusion of 25 μg/h, up to a maximum rate of 50 μg/h. Monitor patients for hypo- or hyperglycemia, especially patients with diabetes, and assess for cardiac conduction abnormalities. Vasopressin is no longer recommended for control of variceal bleeding. Endoscopy employing EBL or EIS is the primary therapeutic tool in the management of acute variceal bleeding.[46,48,49] Antibiotic prophylaxis is recommended if ascites is present and EIS is planned. Appropriate choices include a third-generation cephalosporin (e.g., ceftazidime or ceftriaxone), a penicillin/β-lactamase inhibitor combination (e.g., piperacillin/tazobactam), or a fluoroquinolone (e.g., ofloxacin). Surgical shunts and TIPS are employed as salvage therapy in patients who have failed repeated endoscopy and vasoactive drug therapy.

Secondary Prophylaxis: Prevention of Rebleeding

Because the risk of rebleeding after initial control of variceal hemorrhage can approach 80%, and rebleeding significantly increases the risk of death, therapy to prevent rebleeding is indicated. It is inappropriate to simply observe patients for evidence of further bleeding. Traditionally, pharmacologic therapy using β-adrenergic blockers was recommended as the initial approach for prevention of rebleeding. A major shift in therapy is underway—endoscopic therapy using EBL or EIS, repeated at regular intervals with the goal of obliteration of varices, is emerging as the preferred treatment option. Alternatives for the secondary prevention of rebleeding include surgical or interventional shunting.

Endoscopy. The objective of both EIS and EBL in prevention of rebleeding is the obliteration of esophageal varices. The majority of rebleeding occurs in the interval between the primary endoscopic session and the time to complete obliteration. Therefore, the patient should have repeat endoscopy with either EIS or EBL every 2 weeks until no further varices are identified. After this is achieved, repeat exams at 3 and 6 months are appropriate. The rebleeding rate after EBL is less than EIS, 27% versus 45%.[68]

Drug Therapy. Drug therapy of variceal hemorrhage is less expensive, offers fewer serious complications, and is usually preferred by patients. In patients without contraindications, β-adrenergic blocking agents should be the initial step in secondary prophylaxis, along with endoscopy.[49,68] A recent meta-analysis of 11 randomized controlled clinical trials demonstrated a significant 21% reduction in rebleeding with β blockers as compared to untreated controls, and a 5.4% improvement in the 2-year overall survival rate.[75] Secondary prophylaxis with β-adrenergic blockade therapy also resulted in a significant 7.4% reduction in death as a consequence of rebleeding. Propranolol was used in 10 trials, nadolol was used in one trial. Patients treated with β-adrenergic blocking agents experienced significantly more adverse events, 22% versus 9%, with 5.7% requiring discontinuation of β-adrenergic blockade therapy. When considering the benefits associated with β-adrenergic blockers, it is important to appreciate that approximately 25% of cirrhotic patients either have contraindications or exhibit intolerance to β-adrenergic blockers, and portal pressures are not adequately lowered in all patients treated with β-adrenergic blockade.[76] Use of a long-acting β blocker is usually recommended to improve compliance, and gradual, individualized, dose escalation may help to minimize side effects. Ideally, portal pressure monitoring can help to assess the response to β-adrenergic blocker therapy and identify nonresponders earlier in the treatment course. This is important because patients with sinusoidal portal hypertension (the type encountered in cirrhosis) do not bleed when the hepatic venous pressure gradient is less than 12 mm Hg. Also, protection against rebleeding has been demonstrated when the hepatic venous pressure gradient is reduced by 20%.[77,78] However, the procedure for measuring portal pressures is invasive, expensive, and not available in most facilities. In addition, the cost-effectiveness of this approach (baseline and post-therapy) has not been compared with simply monitoring heart rate reduction with β blockers.[79] For patients who fail to achieve sufficient reductions in portal pressure with β-blocker therapy alone, combination therapy with nitrates, or spironolactone may more effectively lower portal pressures.[80,81] Combination therapy for secondary prophylaxis, however, has not been evaluated in randomized clinical trials.

Comparisons of β-adrenergic blocker therapy alone with EIS suggest that less variceal rebleeding is seen with EIS, but this benefit is offset by an increase in complications and an increase in sclerosis bleeding.[49,68] A recent study comparing nadolol plus isosorbide mononitrate with EIS suggested that combined drug therapy offered substantial advantages over EIS.[82] Rebleeding was significantly less common with nadolol and isosorbide mononitrate and treatment-associated complications occurred significantly less often as well. However, because EBL is now increasingly preferred over EIS for secondary prophylaxis caused by superior efficacy and safety, data from comparative trials with medical therapy is needed. In one series, the rebleeding rate for EBL was superior to standard medical therapy.[83]

Shunting. TIPS procedures should not have a major role in prevention of rebleeding. When drug therapy and endoscopy fails, alternatives include TIPS placement or shunt surgery. Regular documentation of patency and the requirement of repeat procedures make it an unsuitable long-term solution. In patients with well-compensated hepatic function (Childs-Pugh A or B) surgical shunting is an excellent option.

Treatment Recommendations: Secondary Prophylaxis

The preferred initial approach is currently unsettled and may depend on local experience and expertise.[68] Endoscopy (EIS and EBL) and pharmacologic therapy are both effective in reducing the risk of rebleeding. Either approach alone or the combination of endoscopy with pharmacologic therapy can be considered appropriate initial therapy. Both EIS and EBL provide effective treatment for variceal hemorrhage. As a consequence of decreased complications, bleeding, and possibly mortality, EBL has emerged as the endoscopic treatment of choice.[49,68] Pharmacologic therapy should be initiated with a nonselective β blocker such as propranolol, 20 mg three times a day, or nadolol at a dose of 20–40 mg/once daily and titrated weekly to achieve a goal of a heart rate of 55–60 bpm or a heart rate that is 25% lower than the baseline heart rate. Assessment of portal pressures can identify nonresponders for whom combination therapy with β blockers and nitrates or spironolactone may be attempted to achieve portal pressure gradients <12 mm Hg. Monitor patients for evidence of heart failure, bronchospasm, and glucose intolerance, particularly hypoglycemia in patients with insulin-dependent diabetes. For patients with contraindications to β-adrenergic blockers or in patients who have experienced intolerance or poor compliance, (approximately 25% cannot tolerate β blockers) endoscopy with band ligation is preferred. Patients who fail drug therapy and repeated endoscopic procedures require shunting.

ASCITES AND SPONTANEOUS BACTERIAL PERITONITIS

Patients with cirrhosis fail to maintain normal extracellular fluid volumes secondary to abnormal sodium and fluid retention and an impaired capacity to eliminate water.[13] The development of ascites in patients with cirrhosis is an indication of advanced liver disease and is a poor prognostic sign. Treatment goals for patients with ascites include prevention of serious complications (spontaneous bacterial peritonitis and rupture of an umbilical hernia) and improving the patients sense of well being and quality of life by minimizing respiratory difficulties, loss of appetite, and discomfort from abdominal distention or leg swelling.[84] Treatment of ascites expected to have little affect on survival, however.[85] Patients usually present with ascites, edema, or both, and most commonly complain of discomfort from abdominal or leg swelling, respiratory difficulties, malaise, anorexia, and weight loss. Pleural effusions are common, and in some cases, can be the primary manifestation of the fluid retention. Workup includes a history and physical exam, laboratory tests to assess liver function, abdominal ultrasound to rule out hepatocellular carcinoma, endoscopy to evaluate esophageal and gastric varices, abdominal paracentesis with analysis of ascitic fluid, and a complete evaluation of circulatory and renal function. Treatment of ascites has risks. Depending on the treatment approach and the goals selected, significant adverse reactions can occur including electrolyte disturbances, acid-base abnormalities, hepatic encephalopathy, hypovolemia, and renal insufficiency.

Spontaneous bacterial peritonitis (SBP), infection of preexisting ascitic fluid, in the absence of any evidence of a primary intra-abdominal source of infection, is a common complication in patients with ascites, developing in 10% to 25% of patients followed prospectively for at least 1 year.[85] The incidence of SBP is substantially higher in patients with ascitic fluid protein levels <1g/dL and with serum bilirubin levels above 2.5 mg/dL.[86] Because the antibacterial activity of ascitic fluid is proportional to the level of ascitic fluid protein, patients with low ascitic fluid protein levels are at increased risk of SBP. The pathogenesis of SBP is unknown, but presumably results from hematogenous seeding (cirrhosis permits enteric organisms direct access to the bloodstream via the portosystemic collateral's) of the ascitic fluid which offers a favorable growth medium.[87] Consequently, most episodes of SBP are caused by gram-negative Enterobacteriaceae, with *Escherichia coli* most commonly isolated.

The clinical presentation of SBP can vary from those patients who present with all of the signs and symptoms of peritonitis, including fever, leukocytosis, abdominal pain, hypoactive or absent bowel sounds, and rebound tenderness, to those patients who have no signs or symptoms at all. For this reason, a diagnostic paracentesis with analysis of ascitic fluid should be performed in all patients admitted with ascites or in patients with cirrhosis who suddenly deteriorate.[5,85] SBP is diagnosed when ascitic fluid cell counts show an absolute polymorphonuclear (PMN) leukocyte count of $\geq$250 cells/mm^3, a positive ascitic fluid culture is obtained, or a patient with cirrhotic ascites presents with convincing signs or symptoms of infection.[87]

MANAGEMENT OF ASCITES AND SPONTANEOUS BACTERIAL PERITONITIS

The following treatment guidelines for the management of adult patients with ascites and spontaneous bacterial peritonitis were developed and approved by the Practice Guidelines Committee of the American Association for the Study of Liver Diseases (AASLD).[5]

Ascites

In adult patients with new onset ascites as determined by physical exam or radiographic studies, abdominal paracentesis should be performed and ascitic fluid analysis should include a cell count with differential and a serum-ascites albumin gradient (SAG). If infection is suspected, ascitic fluid cultures should be obtained at the time of the paracentesis. The SAG can accurately determine whether ascites is a result of portal hypertension or another process. If the SAG is >1.1 g/dL, portal hypertension is present with 97% accuracy.[5] If the SAG is <1.1 g/dL, with similar certainty, the patient does not have portal hypertension. This is important because patients without portal hypertension will not respond to salt restriction and diuretics.[88] The treatment of ascites secondary to portal hypertension is relatively straightforward and includes abstinence from alcohol, sodium restriction, and diuretics. This strategy is effective in approximately 90% of patients.[85] Avoiding alcohol provides important benefits. Abstinence from alcohol can result in improvement of the reversible component of alcoholic liver disease and has been shown to actually normalize portal pressures in some patients.[5,89] Even in those patients with cirrhosis from another cause (e.g, autoimmune hepatitis) abstinence from alcohol can reverse alcohol-related effects and result in substantial improvement of the underlying liver disease. Patients with cirrhosis not caused by alcohol abuse have less-reversible liver disease and by the time ascites is present, given the poor prognosis, these patients may be best managed with liver transplantation rather than protracted medical therapy.[5]

Beyond avoidance of alcohol, the primary treatment is salt restriction to 2,000 mg/d and oral diuretic therapy. The traditional approach of fluid restriction and bed rest are no longer recommended.[5] It has been demonstrated that achieving the desired fluid losses in patients with ascites caused by portal hypertension is directly related to sodium balance, not fluid restriction.[90] To monitor these patients, evaluation of urinary sodium excretion, utilizing a 24-hour urine collection, is recommended.[5] Severe hyponatremia, serum sodium <120 mEq/L, does warrant fluid restriction, however, rapid correction of asymptomatic hyponatremia (patients with cirrhosis usually are not symptomatic until their serum sodium concentrations are <110 mEq/L) is not recommended. The conventional recommendations for bed rest in this patient population is not supported by clinical trials and is not considered practical.[5] As the liver disease worsens and urinary sodium excretion progressively falls, diuretic therapy is required to prevent retention of sodium and water.

Diuretic Therapy

The AASLD practice guidelines recommend that diuretic therapy be initiated with single morning doses of spironolactone 100 mg and furosemide 40 mg administered orally with the goal of a 0.5-kg maximum daily weight loss.[5] This combination ratio is used because it usually maintains normokalemia. Previously, spironolactone alone was commonly recommended for initial therapy but clinical trials have demonstrated a 14-day delay in the onset of action as well as the development hyperkalemia when spironolactone is used alone.[91] The dose of each can be increased together maintaining the 100 mg: 40 mg ratio, to a maximum daily dose of 400 mg spironolactone and 160 mg furosemide. Administering spironolactone in single daily doses is justified based on its pharmacokinetics and helps to improve patient compliance.[91] If tense ascites is present, a 4–6 L paracentesis should be performed prior to institution of diuretic therapy and salt restriction.[5] For patients who respond to diuretic therapy, this approach is preferred over the use of serial paracenteses.[92] Laboratory tests for renal function and electrolytes need to be monitored during therapy. Patients who experience encephalopathy, severe hyponatremia (serum sodium <120 mEq/L) despite fluid restriction, or renal insufficiency (serum creatinine >2 mg/dL) should have diuretic therapy discontinued. Alternative approaches for refractory ascites must then be evaluated in these patients.

In patients with refractory ascites, serial paracentesis may be employed as needed. Albumin infusion postparacentesis is controversial but should be employed for volumes exceeding 5 L.[92] Liver transplantation should be considered in patients with refractory ascites. For patients who are not transplant candidates and who fail repeated paracenteses because of loculated ascites, TIPS or peritoneal venous shunts may be considered. Both of these procedures have significant complication rates and are not recommended for the routine treatment of ascites.[5]

Spontaneous Bacterial Peritonitis

Patients with documented or suspected SBP should receive broad-spectrum antibiotic therapy, which must adequately cover the three most commonly encountered pathogens: *Escherichia coli, Klebsiella pneumoniae,* and *Streptococcus pneumoniae.*[5,92] Delaying antibiotic therapy while awaiting evidence of a positive ascitic fluid culture is not recommended and can result in overwhelming infection and death.[5] In some patients, signs and symptoms of infection are present at the bacterascites stage, that is signs and symptoms present before the PMN count in the ascitic fluid is elevated.[93] In these patients, signs and symptoms of infection justify empiric antibiotic therapy, regardless of the PMN count in the ascitic fluid.[93] Cefotaxime 2 g every 8 hours, or a similar third-generation cephalosporin are considered the drugs of choice.[5] Cefotaxime is more effective than aztreonam or the combination of ampicillin and tobramycin.[85] Amoxicillin-clavulanic acid is also effective, but clinical trials comparing it to third-generation cephalosporins have not been reported.[92] Fluoroquinolone antibiotics provide good activity against the usual pathogens encountered in SBP, excellent oral bioavailability, and high penetration into ascitic fluid. Ofloxacin 400 mg every 12 hours administered orally is equivalent to intravenous cefotaxime in terms of resolution of infection as well as survival.[94] For many patients, oral ofloxacin therapy offers a simple, cost-effective alternative to intravenous therapy with third-generation cephalosporins. However, intravenous therapy with an agent such as cefotaxime is preferred for severely ill patients, or for patients with gastrointestinal hemorrhage or ileus, because oral bioavailability may be compromised.[92] Antibiotic therapy should be continued until all signs of infection have resolved and the ascitic fluid PMN count decreases below 250/mm^3.[92] However, routine followup paracentesis to evaluate the ascitic fluid PMN counts is not necessary. A 5-day course of antibiotic therapy was reported to be as efficacious as 10 days of therapy in a randomized trial involving 100 patients with SBP.[92]

Secondary bacterial peritonitis, ascitic fluid infection caused by a treatable intra-abdominal source, can masquerade as SBP and should be considered when multiple or atypical organisms are cultured, a very high ascitic fluid PMN count is seen, or in patients who fail to respond to appropriate antibiotic therapy. Uncomplicated SBP usually responds rapidly to appropriate therapy and the 48-hour PMN count, if obtained, is predictably lower than the initial count.[87] In this setting a followup paracentesis revealing a PMN count that continues to rise despite antibiotic therapy can be helpful in detecting secondary peritonitis.[5]

Antibiotic therapy for the prevention of SBP should be considered in all patients at high risk for this complication, including those who have experienced a prior episode of SBP, or variceal hemorrhage and those with low-protein ascites (<1 g/dL). Norfloxacin 400 mg intravenously once daily, or 400 mg every 12 hours orally or by nasogastric tube; ofloxacin 400 mg intravenously once daily; or the combination of ciprofloxacin and amoxicillin-clavulanic acid markedly reduces the risk of SBP as compared to untreated patients in these high-risk groups.[92] Long-term norfloxacin, 400 mg orally once daily, reduces the risk of recurrent SBP from 70% to 20% at 1 year, primarily by reducing the incidence of SBP caused by gram-negative bacilli from 60% to 3%.[95] However, antibiotic prophylaxis does not prolong survival and it selects out resistant organisms that may subsequently cause SBP.[92,96] Fortunately, episodes of SBP caused by resistant organisms are uncommon.[97–106] Prolonged therapy with ciprofloxacin is a risk factor for fungal infections in patients subsequently undergoing liver transplantation.[92] Intermittent prophylactic strategies, including ciprofloxacin 750 mg orally once a week, trimethoprim-sulfamethoxazole 1 DS tablet five times a week, or inpatient norfloxacin with discontinuation at discharge, are effective and may be less likely to select resistant organisms.[5,92,98]

TREATMENT RECOMMENDATIONS: ASCITES AND SPONTANEOUS BACTERIAL PERITONITIS

Adult patients admitted to the hospital with new-onset ascites should have an abdominal paracentesis performed to establish the serum-ascites albumin gradient, the ascitic fluid PMN count, and to obtain ascitic fluid cultures. Patients who drink alcohol should be strongly discouraged from further alcohol use. Sodium restriction to 2,000 mg/d, together with spironolactone and furosemide, is the mainstay of therapy. Diuretic therapy should be initiated with single morning doses of spironolactone 100 mg and furosemide 40 mg administered orally with the goal of a 0.5-kg maximum daily weight loss. Titrate diuretic therapy using the 100 mg:40 mg ratio, to a maximum daily dose of 400 mg spironolactone and 160 mg furosemide. Fluid restriction, unless the serum sodium is <120 mEq/L, and bed rest are not recommended. Monitor urinary sodium excretion, using a 24-hour urine collection, and monitor serum potassium and renal function frequently. Severe hyponatremia (serum sodium <120 mEq/L) warrants fluid restriction. Avoid rapid correction of asymptomatic hyponatremia in patients with cirrhosis. If tense ascites is present, a 4–6-L paracentesis should be performed prior to institution of diuretic therapy and salt restriction. For patients who respond to diuretic therapy this approach is preferred over the use of serial paracentesis. Discontinue diuretic therapy in patients who experience encephalopathy, severe hyponatremia (serum sodium <120 mEq/L) despite fluid restriction, or renal insufficiency (serum creatinine >2 mg/dL). Serial paracentesis may be considered for patients with refractory ascites with albumin infusion postparacentesis when volumes exceeding 5 L are removed. Liver transplantation should be considered for eligible patients with refractory ascites.[5]

Patients with documented SBP, positive ascitic fluid cultures, or ascitic fluid PMN count ≥250 cells/mm,^{3} regardless of symptoms, should receive broad-spectrum empiric antibiotic therapy with cefotaxime 2 g every 8 hours, or a similar third-generation cephalosporin. Patients with ascitic fluid PMN counts <250 cells/mm^3 but with signs and symptoms of infection (abdominal pain, tenderness, fever, encephalopathy, renal failure, acidosis, or peripheral leukocytosis) should also receive empiric antibiotic treatment with cefotaxime 2 g every 8 hours, or a similar third-generation cephalosporin. Outpatient oral therapy of SBP with fluoroquinolones or amoxicillin/clavulanic acid awaits further clinical trials. Short-term inpatient quinolone therapy should be considered in the prevention of SBP in patients with low-protein ascites (<1 g/dL), variceal hemorrhage, or prior SBP. All patients who have survived an episode of SBP should receive long-term antibiotic prophylaxis.[5]

HEPATIC ENCEPHALOPATHY

The clinical manifestations of HE can range from subtle mental status abnormalities, detectable only with psychomimetic testing, to deep coma.[23] Additionally, different classifications or patterns of HE can also be described. HE is seen in two broad clinical settings, acute fulminant liver failure and chronic liver failure. In patients with chronic liver failure, HE occurs in three patterns, acute, chronic and subclinical.[23,25,99]

HE associated with acute fulminant liver failure has a rapid onset and a short prodrome, patients can progress from drowsiness to delirium, convulsions and finally to coma in as short as 24 hours. The prognosis in these cases is dismal.[23] This pattern of HE usually has no known precipitating factors, and patients who survive the acute insult have an excellent long-term prognosis after a period of acute hepatic support. HE associated with chronic liver failure, as is seen in patients with cirrhosis, has a gradual onset, the severity is often more mild, is commonly associated with known precipitating factors, and has a poor prognosis with the need for long-term treatment of the underlying liver disease.[100] When acute HE develops in a patient with clinically stable cirrhosis it usually is the result of a precipitating cause such as gastrointestinal hemorrhage, infection, electrolyte disorders, dietary excesses, sedative ingestion, or renal insufficiency. Although management strategies are similar for both acute and chronic HE, the urgency of treatment interventions and goals of therapy are different.[23] Patients with subclinical HE often experience only minor motor and attentional deficits and compensate on their own without the need for therapy. Those with more significant deficits that impact activities of daily living can benefit from intervention.[99]

The prevalence of clinically apparent HE is unknown; however, between 50% and 80% of patients with cirrhosis demonstrate neurologic dysfunction by electroencephalography (EEG) or by psychomimetic testing.[101] To determine the severity of HE, a grading system that relates neurologic and neuromuscular signs can be used. (Table 37–5) The pathogenesis of HE is unknown. It is believed to be a multifactorial metabolic/neurophysiologic abnormality.[23]

MANAGEMENT OF HEPATIC ENCEPHALOPATHY

Acute HE usually develops in a clinically stable patient as the result of an acute precipitating event. Table 37–6 lists the most commonly encountered precipitating factors for acute HE and suggests general treatment alternatives. Chronic HE, by definition, occurs and persists in the absence of a precipitating factor. It commonly is encountered in patients who have undergone a TIPS procedure or surgical shunting or in patients with advanced cirrhosis. Patients with acute HE have potentially reversible causes of their encephalopathy, whereas patients

TABLE 37–5. Grading System for Hepatic Encephalopathy

Grade	Level of Consciousness	Personality/ Intellect	Neurologic Abnormalities	EEG Abnormalities
0	Normal	Normal	None	None
Subclinical	Normal	Normal	Psychomimetic only	None
1	Inverted sleep patterns/restless	Forgetful; mild confusion; agitation, irritable	Tremor; apraxia; incoordination; impaired handwriting	Triphasic waves (5 cycles/second)
2	Lethargic, slow responses	Disorientation for time; amnesia; decreased inhibitions; inappropriate behavior	Asterixis, dysarthria; ataxia; hypoactive reflexes	Triphasic waves (5 cycles/second)
3	Somnolent but rousable, confused	Disorientation for place; aggressive	Asterixis; hyperactive reflexes; Babinski's sign; muscle rigidity	Triphasic waves (5 cycles/second)
4	Coma/unrousable	None	Decerebrate	Delta activity (2–3 cycles/second)

TABLE 37–6. Portosystemic Encephalopathy: Precipitating Factors and Therapy

Factor	Therapy Alternatives
Gastrointestinal bleeding	
Variceal	Band ligation/sclerotherapy; octreotide
Nonvariceal	Endoscopic therapy; proton pump inhibitors
Infection/sepsis	Antibiotics; paracentesis
Electrolyte abnormalities	Discontinue diuretics; fluid and electrolyte replacement
Sedative ingestion	Discontinue sedatives/tranquilizers; consider reversal (flumazenil/naloxone)
Dietary excesses	Limit daily protein; lactulose
Constipation	Cathartics; bowel cleansing/enema
Renal insufficiency	Discontinue diuretics; discontinue NSAIDs, nephrotoxic antibiotics; fluid resuscitation

with chronic HE usually do not. Nevertheless, the mediators of the encephalopathy are the same, justifying similar treatment strategies. The major difference is the need for urgent inpatient intervention for management of the precipitating event in acute HE, and the expectation for normal mentation after recovery. Patients with chronic HE typically exhibit a high prevalence of abnormal mentation.[25]

Table 37–7 describes the treatment goals for patients with HE and contrasts the differences between acute and chronic HE. The general approach to the management of HE is to first identify and treat any precipitating factors. For patients with acute HE aggressive management of any precipitating events is essential (see Table 37–6). Treatment of the precipitating often results in prompt resolution of the encephalopathy. Nevertheless, steps to reverse the encephalopathy are undertaken after measures to reverse precipitating events are implemented. The altered sensorium associated with HE itself is associated with increased morbidity and mortality.[25] Although no standards of care have been adopted, it is generally agreed that rapid reversal of HE is recommended.[25] Finally, supportive measures to manage the underlying liver failure need to be implemented. Universal treatment of patients with subclinical HE is not recommended because the consequences of motor and attention deficits are considered minor, and prevention of progression to more severe HE has not been studied.[99] However, treatment of subclinical HE may be undertaken in patients with more significant deficits.

Treatment approaches for HE evolve from the various hypotheses advanced to explain the pathogenesis of HE and include: (a) reducing ammonia blood concentrations by dietary restrictions and drug therapy aimed at inhibiting ammonia production or enhancing its removal; (b) inhibition of the γ-aminobutyric acid-benzodiazepine receptors by flumazenil; and (c) inhibition of false neurotransmitters by optimizing amino acid balance.[23,25,99]

TABLE 37–7. Treatment Goals: Acute and Chronic HE

Acute HE	Chronic HE
Control precipitating factor	Reverse encephalopathy
Reverse encephalopathy	Avoid recurrence
Hospital/inpatient therapy	Home/outpatient therapy
Maintain fluid and hemodynamic support	Manage persistent neuropsychiatric abnormalities
	Manage chronic liver disease
Expect normal mentation after recovery	High prevalence of abnormal mentation after recovery

HYPERAMMONEMIA

Despite criticisms of the ammonia hypothesis, treatment interventions to reduce ammonia blood concentrations have routinely been shown to be beneficial in patients with HE.[25] Decreasing ammonia blood concentrations, by limiting its availability and production, or by enhancing its metabolism, remains a mainstay of therapy for patients with HE.

Decreasing ammonia blood concentrations can be attempted by reducing ammonia production or by decreasing the availability of ammonia in the colon. Limiting dietary protein acutely usually results in a lowering of ammonia concentrations and improvement in HE. In patients with acute HE, protein is withheld or limited to 20 g/d while maintaining the total caloric intake, until the clinical situation improves.[23,25,99] Protein is added back to the diet in 10–20 g/d increments every 3 days to 5 days to a total of 0.8–1 g/kg/d to maintain nitrogen balance.[102] Vegetable-source protein may be preferable to animal-source protein because it contains less aromatic amino acids, which are implicated in generating false neurotransmitters (see below). Also, the higher fiber content of vegetable protein increases colonic transit time and lowers colonic pH secondary to its fermentation by colonic bacteria.[102] In patients with chronic HE, dietary therapy with restricted protein attempts to prevent malnutrition and prevent exacerbation of HE. Protein intolerance is a common problem in patients with chronic liver disease and HE.[25] Vegetable proteins are better tolerated and may result in clinical improvement.[103] The addition of dietary fiber provides clinical improvement in HE and should be included as part of long-term management. As discussed earlier, fiber may act to acidify the colon and to stimulate evacuation of colonic contents.[25] Bowel cleansing using cathartics or lactulose enemas (see below) results in a rapid removal of ammonia substrate from the colon and is effective. Interestingly, tap-water enemas alone are ineffective.[25]

The use of lactulose, a nonabsorbable disaccharide, (and lactitol, not available in the United States) is standard therapy for both acute and chronic HE.[104] Lactulose, when administered orally, passes through the gastrointestinal tract and reaches the colon unchanged. For patients unable to take lactulose orally or via tube administration it may be administered as an enema. In the colon, lactulose lowers colonic pH and exerts a cathartic effect. Fermentation of lactulose by bacteria present in the colon results in the production of organic acids, decreasing colonic pH to approximately 5.[23] Urease-producing bacteria metabolize dietary protein and endogenous protein substrates (epithelial cells) producing ammonia. Acidification of the colon inhibits the viability of these urease-producing bacteria (and may promote the growth of nonurease-producing lactobacilli) decreasing the absorption of ammonia. Acidification also enhances the net movement of ammonia from the blood into the bowel.[23] The cathartic effect of lactulose then eliminates the ammonia as well as protein substrates inhibiting ammonia production.[104] More than 30 clinical trials have demonstrated the efficacy of lactulose in the management of acute HE, and more than 20 studies support its use in chronic HE.[25] Clinical improvement is noted in approximately 86% of patients with acute HE, and in approximately 77% of patients with chronic HE. In acute HE, lactulose is initiated at a dose of 30–60 mL orally every 1 hour to 2 hours (or by retention enema 300 mL lactulose syrup in 700 mL water, held for 30–60 minutes) until catharsis begins. The dose is then decreased to 15–30 mL orally four times daily (enemas every 6 hours to 8 hours) and titrated to produce two to four soft, acidic stools per day.[23,99] In patients with chronic HE, lactulose may be initiated at a dose of 30–60 mL per day with titration to the same endpoint.

Inhibiting the activity of urease-producing bacteria by using neomycin, metronidazole, or vancomycin can decrease production of ammonia.[25,23] Neomycin at doses of 2–8 g daily in divided doses results in clinical improvement in as many as 80% of patients.[103] At these doses, however, bioavailability is 1% to 5% and can result in irreversible ototoxicity and nephrotoxicity.[105] As such, even though efficacy is equivalent to lactulose, it should not be first-line therapy. Metronidazole produces response rates similar to neomycin but side effects, particularly gastrointestinal, limit its use.[23] In patients with an inadequate response to lactulose alone, combination therapy with neomycin and lactulose may provide additive effects and improved clinical response.[23]

Decreasing ammonia production by replacement of urease-producing bacteria in the colon with nonurease producing strains has been attempted with the oral administration of *Lactobacillus acidophilus* and *Enterococcus faecium*.[25] The data supporting this therapy is limited especially for patients with acute HE. However, for patients with less severe HE, *Enterococcus faecium* was as effective as lactulose, treatment effects persisted during drug-free periods, and no adverse effects were reported.[106] Ammonia generated by *Helicobacter pylori* in the stomach has been associated with precipitating or worsening HE in patients with cirrhosis.[107] A recent review recommends routine eradication of *H. pylori* in patients with cirrhosis and a history of HE.[23]

Enhancing ammonia removal by stimulating its detoxification by supporting alternative metabolic pathways can reduce blood-ammonia concentrations. Centrizonal periportal hepatocytes responsible for ammonia metabolism via ureagenesis are impaired in patients with cirrhosis.[108] Clinical trials have shown that L-ornithine L-aspartate (OA) enhances ureagenesis and results in reductions in ammonia concentrations and clinical benefits in patients with grade 1 and grade 2 HE.[25] Clinical response rates similar to lactulose were reported in one trial involving patients with chronic HE.[109] Studies in patients with more severe HE are needed. Zinc deficiency is common in patients with cirrhosis and has been reported to cause overt HE.[110] Zinc is a required cofactor for ammonia metabolism; two of the five metabolic pathways are zinc dependent. Both positive and negative studies evaluating the efficacy of zinc replacement have been published.[23] In a recent controlled trial in cirrhotic patients with mild HE, the administration of zinc sulfate 600 mg/d for 3 months resulted in increased urea formation and lower ammonia levels, along with improvement in psychomimetic test scores.[111] Zinc supplementation is recommended for long-term management in patients with cirrhosis who are zinc deficient.[23,25]

INHIBITION OF γ-AMINOBUTYRIC ACID (GABA)-BENZODIAZEPINE RECEPTORS

The GABA-receptor complex, the primary inhibitory neural network within the central nervous system, is associated with HE.[23,25] This receptor complex is composed of a GABA-binding site, and a benzodiazepine receptor site, which mediate chloride conductance. Based upon evidence of an increase in benzodiazepine receptor ligands in patients with hepatic encephalopathy, flumazenil has been evaluated in uncontrolled studies and has demonstrated significant clinical improvement, with one case report documenting long-term benefit.[112] In these reports, discontinuation of flumazenil resulted in prompt clinical deterioration.[25] Among five prospective, placebo-controlled trials, three reported benefit with flumazenil, whereas two found no difference when compared to placebo. With dosages of 0.2–15 mg IV, response rates were variable, ranging from 17% to 78%; improvements, however, were often transient.[25] Flumazenil, only available in an intravenous dosage form, may be considered for short-term therapy in refractory patients.

FALSE NEUROTRANSMITTERS

A great deal of controversy surrounds the issue of whether or not exogenous protein rich in branched chain aminoacids (BCAAs) is superior to standard protein solutions higher in aromatic amino acids (AAAs).[23,99] Metabolism of AAA's into false neurotransmitters which penetrate the blood-brain barrier (which itself may be perturbed in patients with HE) has been implicated as a cause of HE.[113] A number of clinical trials have evaluated the use of BCAAs in the treatment of HE with conflicting results. Reviews of these trials as well have arrived at different conclusions.[114,115] BCAAs may have a role in the malnourished patient with cirrhosis who is intolerant of protein supplementation, but the current data does not justify routine use of BCAAs for the treatment of HE.[23,99] Impairment of dopaminergic transmission has also been proposed to cause HE, but trials with bromocriptine and levodopa failed to provide any benefit and are not recommended.[23]

TREATMENT RECOMMENDATIONS: HEPATIC ENCEPHALOPATHY

Treatment recommendations depend on the type of HE being managed, acute HE, chronic HE, or subclinical HE. The general approach to the management of HE is to first identify patients with acute HE and then to provide aggressive management of any precipitating events (see Table 37–6). When the precipitating event has been discovered and appropriate therapy initiated, then steps to rapidly reverse the encephalopathy should be implemented. Remember that the altered sensorium associated with HE itself is associated with increased morbidity and mortality.

The mainstay of therapy of HE involves therapy to lower blood ammonia concentrations and includes diet therapy, lactulose, and antibiotics, alone or in combination with lactulose. Other adjunctive therapies include zinc replacement.

In patients with acute HE, protein is withheld or limited to 10–20 g/d while maintaining the total caloric intake, until the clinical situation improves. Titrate protein based on tolerance, increasing intake in increments of 10–20 g/d every 3 days to 5 days to a total of 0.8–1 g/kg/d. In patients with chronic HE, restrict protein to 40 g/d. Vegetable proteins may be better tolerated and may result in clinical improvement. Consider the addition of dietary fiber to animal source protein diets, for patients who find vegetable proteins unpalatable.

The use of lactulose is standard therapy for both acute and chronic HE. In acute HE, lactulose is initiated at a dose of 30–60 mL orally every 1 hour to 2 hours (or by retention enema, 300 mL lactulose syrup in 700 mL water, held for 30–60 minutes) until catharsis begins. The dose is then decreased to 15–30 mL orally four times daily (enemas every 6 hours to 8 hours) and titrated to produce two to four soft, acidic stools per day. In patients with chronic HE, lactulose may be initiated at a dose of 30–60 mL/d with titration to the same endpoint. Monitor electrolytes periodically, follow patients for changes in mental status, and titrate to number of stools as above.

Antibiotic therapy with either metronidazole or neomycin is reserved for patients who have not responded to diet and lactulose therapy where the combination may provide additive effects and improved clinical response. Zinc supplementation at a dose of 600 mg/d is recommended for long-term management in patients with cirrhosis who are zinc deficient.

Other adjunctive therapies that may be considered for patients refractory to standard therapy include eradication of *H. pylori* in patients with cirrhosis and a history of HE, administration of *Lactobacillus acidophilus,* L-ornithine L-aspartate, or flumazenil 0.2 mg up to 15 mg IV. BCAAs may have a role in the malnourished patient with cirrhosis who is intolerant of protein supplementation, but the current data does not justify routine use of BCAAs for the treatment of HE. Universal treatment of patients with subclinical HE is not recommended; however, therapy to improve performance of daily activities, or in patients with more significant deficits, may be considered with close monitoring for adverse effects. Finally, supportive measures to manage the underlying liver failure need to be implemented.

SYSTEMIC COMPLICATIONS

In addition to the more common complications of chronic liver disease discussed above, a number of other complications can occur, including hepatorenal syndrome, hepatopulmonary syndrome, coagulation disorders, and endocrine dysfunction.

Hepatorenal syndrome, functional renal failure in the setting of cirrhosis in the absence of intrinsic renal disease, occurs in patients with cirrhosis as a result of intense vasoconstriction within the renal cortical vasculature. The resultant reduction in blood supply to the kidneys causes avid sodium retention and oliguria. The vasoconstriction that occurs in the kidneys is in stark contrast to the state of systemic vasodilation that is characteristic of chronic liver failure.[116] The pathophysiologic mechanism responsible for these effects is unknown, but is linked to the systemic vasodilation, hypovolemia, and hyperkinetic circulation seen in chronic liver failure.[117] Hepatorenal syndrome is not uncommon and develops in approximately 40% of patients with cirrhosis and ascites within 5 years.[118] Management consists of excluding all other potential nephrotoxins such as nonsteroidal anti-inflammatory agents, and aminoglycosides, and assessment for prerenal azotemia secondary to overaggressive diuretic use.[118] Withholding diuretic therapy and administering a fluid challenge has been recommended for early diagnosis and therapy.[116] Case reports describe successful resolution of hepatorenal syndrome with low-dose dopamine and the combination of dopamine and norepinephrine.[118] Liver transplantation, which if successful results in full recovery of renal function, remains the treatment of choice for refractory hepatorenal syndrome.

Hepatopulmonary syndrome is characterized by alterations in lung mechanics caused by ascites, and by intrapulmonary shunting and gas exchange, and affects 20% to 40% of patients with cirrhosis.[118] These patients present with profound fatigue and dyspnea. In the absence of intrinsic cardiopulmonary disease, cirrhotic patients with these findings should be evaluated for hepatopulmonary syndrome. Physical findings of tense ascites or pleural effusions, not associated with pulmonary parenchymal disease, are suggestive of hepatopulmonary syndrome. A prompt resolution of symptoms after large volume paracentesis is characteristic.[118] Long-term management requires control of ascites (see management of ascites discussed earlier) and supportive therapy with supplemental oxygen, and optimizing of fluid status. The prognosis for these patients is poor. Ultimately, liver transplantation offers the best chance for long-term recovery.

Coagulation disorders are common in patients with chronic liver disease. These disorders increase the risk of bleeding and tend to become more profound as the liver failure becomes more severe. Correction of the coagulopathy is essential for patients actively bleeding (see management of variceal hemorrhage discussed earlier) but present with only minor symptoms such as bruising or nose bleeds in patients not actively bleeding. The pathophysiology of the coagulopathy is complex and involves abnormalities of platelet function, clotting factor deficiencies and fibrinolysis.[119] Acute therapy involves platelet transfusions for thrombocytopenia, and fresh-frozen plasma for prolongation of the prothrombin time because of clotting factor deficiencies. Long-term management of cirrhotic patients with identified coagulopathies is supportive for the management of the underlying cause of cirrhosis; for example, encouraging abstinence from alcohol.

The presence of cirrhosis can produce abnormal regulation and function of multiple endocrine systems.[118] Most common are feminization and hypogonadism, and hypothyroidism. Cirrhosis perturbs the hypothalamic-pituitary-axis (HPA) which is required for normal regulation of sex and thyroid hormones. In men with cirrhosis, testosterone levels are depressed, while estrogen levels are increased. The clinical manifestations of these changes include loss of libido, muscle wasting, and gynecomastia. These clinical findings are not uncommon and have been reported to occur in up to 60% of cirrhotic patients.[118] In women, feminization changes are less well studied. Alcohol use complicates and can worsen sex hormone abnormalities.[118]

Both central and peripheral defects in thyroid secretion are noted in patients with cirrhosis. Again, alcohol plays a major role with direct toxic effects on the thyroid gland. Management includes thyroid hormone replacement for hypothyroidism with usual doses (levothyroxine 50–100 μg/d) and testosterone replacement (testosterone 200 mg three times daily) may be attempted to improve libido, well being, and gynecomastia. Routine hormone replacement has not been shown to impact survival or disease progression.[118]

LIVER TRANSPLANTATION

The complications seen in patients with chronic liver disease are essentially functional as a secondary effect of the circulatory and metabolic changes that accompany liver failure. Consequently, liver transplantation is the only treatment that can offer a cure for complications of end-stage cirrhosis. However, patient selection, evaluation, pre- and postsurgical management is beyond the scope of this review. Refer to Chap. 41.

PHARMACOKINETIC AND PHARMACODYNAMIC CHANGES IN LIVER FAILURE

The liver plays a major role in the absorption, biotransformation, and elimination of many drugs. In addition, patients with cirrhosis may exhibit pharmacodynamic changes with increased sensitivity to the effects of certain drugs.[120] These pharmacodynamic changes are separate and apart from the enhancement of drug effects seen in these patients as a result of the altered serum concentrations of both total and free drug that occur because of the pharmacokinetic changes in these patients. Hepatic drug clearance is primarily dependent upon protein binding, hepatic blood flow, and intrinsic hepatic metabolic activity.[121] The pathophysiologic changes that occur in patients with cirrhosis, including reduced liver blood flow, altered microcirculatory distribution of blood flow within the liver, diminished metabolic and synthetic function, and changes in the endothelial lining of the sinusoids, can have a significant impact on each of these factors. The consequence of these changes is a reduction in intrinsic metabolic activity, a reduction in the delivery of blood to the liver, which decreases clearance and prolongs half-life, and a reduction in the degree of protein binding, which increases in the fraction of unbound drug in the serum. Finally, patients with cirrhosis frequently accumulate large amounts of interstitial fluid resulting in substantial changes in the volume of distribution, which also prolongs drug half-life. These changes occur most commonly in combination in patients with cirrhosis and are dynamic throughout the disease course. The effect that these changes will have depends upon the drug and the type of biotransformation that the drug undergoes.

Drugs with a high extraction ratio (high extraction drugs) are dependent on blood flow for metabolism and the rate of metabolism will be sensitive to changes in blood flow. Drugs with a low extraction ratio (low extraction drugs) are dependent on intrinsic metabolic activity for metabolism and the rate of metabolism will reflect changes in intrinsic clearance.[121] Furthermore, hepatic biotransformation involves two types of metabolic processes: Phase I reactions and Phase II reactions. Phase I reactions involve the cytochrome P450 system and include hydrolysis, oxidation, dealkylation, and reduction reactions. Phase II reactions involve conjugation of the drug with an endogenous molecule such as sulfate or an amino acid rendering it more water soluble, enhancing its elimination. Drugs metabolized by Phase I reactions, especially oxidation, tend to be significantly impaired in patients with cirrhosis, whereas drugs eliminated by conjugation are relatively unaffected.[123]

The variability and complexity of the interaction between the extent and severity of liver disease and individual characteristics of the drug makes it very difficult to predict the degree of pharmacokinetic perturbation in an individual patient. Unfortunately, there are no sensitive and specific clinical or biochemical markers that allow us to quantify the extent of liver insufficiency or the degree of metabolic activity. In addition, renal insufficiency and alterations that commonly accompany cirrhosis further complicate empiric dosing recommendations in these patients.[120] Most of the studies conducted to assess the effects of liver disease on pharmacokinetics have included only patients with Child-Pugh score of A (mild cirrhosis) or B (moderate cirrhosis).[121] Dosing recommendations are most commonly nonspecific with recommendations labeled for patients with mild to moderate liver impairment. Dosing information for patients with more severe liver impairment is not available. As a result, when patients with cirrhosis require therapy with drugs that undergo hepatic metabolism (e.g., benzodiazepines), monitoring response to therapy, anticipating drug accumulation and enhanced effects, is essential. In the case of benzodiazepines, selection of an agent such as lorazepam, an intermediate-acting agent, that is metabolized via conjugation and has no active metabolites is easier to monitor than a drug such as diazepam, a long-acting benzodiazepine, that is oxidized in the liver and has an active metabolite with a long half-life of its own.

A number of recent publications provide an up to date analysis of the pharmacokinetic and pharmacodynamic considerations in patients with liver disease and provide the most recent data on individual drug-dosing recommendations.[121,124,125]

PHARMACOECONOMIC CONSIDERATIONS

Cost-benefit and cost-effectiveness analysis were recently highlighted as a short coming of clinical trials in the field of cirrhosis.[48] However, a number of issues relating to drug therapy of cirrhosis have recently been studied. The cost-effectiveness of long-term antibiotic prophylaxis for the prevention of SBP, especially for high-risk patients as determined by simple laboratory analysis (serum bilirubin ascitic fluid protein levels) was found to provide significant cost savings.[126] In a comparison of propranolol, sclerotherapy, and shunt surgery for prophylaxis against the first variceal bleed, propranolol was the only cost-effective alternative.[127] Because treatment approaches for patients with cirrhosis can range from supportive medical therapy, to repeated endoscopic procedures with serious complications, to liver transplantation, the need for application of economic analysis is obvious. Of critical importance to this question is when in the course of chronic liver disease are the various treatment interventions employed. Should liver transplantation be attempted earlier, avoiding most if not all of the complications discussed in this chapter, and would it prove to be the most cost-effective approach?

EVALUATION OF THERAPEUTIC OUTCOMES

Table 37–8 summarizes the management approach for patients with cirrhosis including monitoring parameters and therapeutic outcomes. Cirrhosis is generally a chronic progressive disease that requires aggressive medical management to prevent or delay common complications. Table 37–8 lists monitoring criteria that need to be carefully followed in order to achieve the maximum benefit from the medical therapies employed and prevent adverse effects. A therapeutic plan including therapeutic endpoints for each medical and diet therapy needs to be developed and discussed with the patient.

► PRINCIPLES OF PHARMACOTHERAPY

- Cirrhosis is a chronic irreversible disease. For patients whose liver disease is secondary to alcohol abuse, attempts to support abstinence are imperative because treating the underlying liver disease through avoidance of alcohol can result in improvement of the reversible component of alcoholic liver disease.
- Liver transplantation is the only approach that is capable of significantly altering the prognosis of cirrhosis, and in patients with advanced disease, this may be preferred over protracted medical therapy in eligible patients.
- The therapy of cirrhosis and portal hypertension primarily involves long-term management of secondary complications that inevitably arise such as variceal bleeding; encephalopathy; ascites; peritonitis; nutritional deficiencies; renal and pulmonary complications; coagulation defects; and endocrine dysfunction.
- All patients with cirrhosis and portal hypertension should be considered for endoscopic screening, and patients with large varices should receive primary prophylaxis with β-adrenergic blockade therapy.
- Octreotide is the preferred vasoactive agent employed in the medical management of variceal bleeding. Vasopressin can no longer be recommended as a first-line agent because of its significant adverse effect profile. Endoscopy employing endoscopic band ligation or endoscopic injection sclerotherapy is the primary therapeutic tool in the management of acute variceal bleeding.
- When nonselective β-adrenergic blocker therapy is used to prevent rebleeding, it is essential that the dose is titrated to achieve a heart rate goal of 60 bpm or a heart rate that is 25% lower than the baseline heart rate.

TABLE 37–8. Management Approach and Outcome Assessments

Complication	Treatment Approach	Monitoring Parameter	Outcome Assessment
Ascites	Diet; diuretics; paracentesis; TIPS	Daily assessment of weight	Prevent or eliminate ascites and its secondary complications
Spontaneous bacterial peritonitis	Antibiotic therapy; prophylaxis if undergoing paracentesis	Evidence of clinical deterioration; e.g., abdominal pain, fever, anorexia, malaise, fatigue	Prevent/treat infection to decrease mortality
Variceal bleeding	Pharmacologic prophylaxis	Child-Pugh score; endoscopy; CBC	Appropriate reduction in heart rate and portal pressure
	Endoscopy; vasoactive drug therapy (octreotide); sclerotherapy; volume resuscitation; pharmacologic prophylaxis	CBC; evidence of overt bleeding	Acute: control acute bleed Chronic: variceal obliteration; reduce portal pressures
Coagulation disorders	Blood products (PPF, platelets); vitamin K	CBC; prothrombin time; platelet count	Normalize PT time; maintain/improve hemostasis
Hepatic encephalopathy	Ammonia reduction (lactulose, cathartics); elimination of drugs causing CNS depression; diet—limit excess protein	Grade of encephalopathy; EEG; psychomimetic testing; mental status changes; concurrent drug therapy	Maintain functional capacity; prevent hospitalization for encephalopathy; decrease ammonia levels; provide adequate nutrition
Hepatorenal syndrome	Eliminate concurrent nephrotoxins (NSAIDs); decrease or discontinue diuretics; volume resuscitation; liver transplantation	Serum and urine electrolytes; concurrent drug therapy	Prevent progressive renal injury by preventing dehydration and avoiding other nephrotoxins Liver transplantation for refractory hepatorenal syndrome
Hepatopulmonary syndrome	Paracentesis; O_2 therapy	Dyspnea; presence of ascites	Acute: relief of dyspnea and hypoxia Chronic: manage ascites as above

NSAIDs = Nonsteroidal anti-inflammatory drugs

- The combination of spironolactone and furosemide is now the recommended initial diuretic therapy for patients with ascites.
- All patients who have survived an episode of spontaneous bacterial peritonitis should receive long-term antibiotic prophylaxis.
- The mainstay of therapy of hepatic encephalopathy involves therapy to lower blood ammonia concentrations and includes diet therapy, lactulose, and antibiotics alone or in combination with lactulose. However, it is important to first identify patients with acute hepatic encephalopathy and to then provide aggressive management of any precipitating events.
- Empiric drug dosing recommendations in patients with cirrhosis are unavailable. When possible, select agents that do not undergo Phase I metabolism and titrate carefully to a desired pharmacodynamic response.

REFERENCES

1. Williams EJ, Iredale JP. Liver cirrhosis. Postgrad Med J 1998;74:193–202.
2. Bell SH, Beringer KC, Detre KM. An update on liver transplant in the US: Recipient characteristics and outcomes. In: Cecka JM, Teraski PL, eds. Clinical Transplants. Los Angeles, UCLA Tissue Type Labs, 1995.
3. Centers for Disease Control. Deaths and hospitalizations from chronic liver disease. JAMA 1993;269:569–572.
4. Current trends mortality patterns—United States, 1992. MMWR Morb Mort Wkly Rep 1994;43:916–917.
5. Runyon BA. AASLD Practice Guidelines: Management of adult patients with ascites caused by cirrhosis. Hepatology 1998;27:264–272.
6. Greenway CV, Stark RD. Hepatic vascular bed. Physiol Rev 1971;51:2–7.
7. Rappaport AM. Anatomic considerations In: Schiff L, ed: Diseases of the Liver. Philadelphia, Lippincott, 1969:1–29.
8. Bissell DM, Maher JJ. Hepatic fibrosis and cirrhosis. In: Zakim DM, Boyer TD, eds. Hepatology: A Textbook of Liver Disease, 3rd ed. Philadelphia, Saunders, 1996:506–525.
9. Friedman SL The cellular basis of hepatic fibrosis: Mechanisms and treatment strategies. N Engl J Med 1993;328:1825–1835.
10. Alcolado R, Arthur MJP, Iredale JP. Pathogenesis of liver fibrosis. Clin Sci 1997;92:103–112.
11. Boyer TD, Henderson JM. Portal hypertension and bleeding esophageal varices. In: Zakim D, Boyer TD, eds. Hepatology: A Textbook of Liver Disease, 3rd ed. Philadelphia, Saunders, 1996:720–763.
12. Grace ND. Prevention of initial variceal hemorrhage. Gastroenterol Clin North Am 1992;21:149–161.
13. Levy M. Pathophysiology of ascites formation. In: Epstein M, ed. The Kidney in Liver Disease, 4th ed. Philadelphia, Hanley and Belfus, 1996:179–204.
14. Gines P, Quintero E, Arroyo V, et al. Compensated cirrhosis: Natural history and prognostic factors. Hepatology 1987;7:122–128.
15. Sherlock S, Shaldon S. The aetiology and management of ascites in patients with hepatic cirrhosis: A review. Gut 1963;4:95.
16. Lieberman FL, Denison FK, Reynolds TB. The relationship of plasma volume, portal hypertension, ascites and renal sodium retention in cirrhosis: The overflow theory of ascites formation. Ann N Y Acad Sci 1970;170:292.
17. Schrier RW, Arroyo V, Bernardi M, et al. Peripheral arterial vasodilation hypothesis: A proposal for the initiation of renal sodium and water retention in cirrhosis. Hepatology 1988;8;1151–1157.
18. Gines P, Fernandez-Esparrach G, Arroyo V, et al. Pathogenesis of ascites in cirrhosis. Semin Liver Dis 1997;17:175–189.
19. Vallance P, Moncada S. Hyperdynamic circulation in cirrhosis: A role for nitric oxide Lancet 1991;337:776–778.
20. Guarner C, Soriano G, Tomas A, et al. Increased serum nitrate and nitrite levels in patients with cirrhosis: Relationship to endotoxemia. Hepatology 1993;18:1139–1143.

21. Bosch J. Prevention of variceal rebleeding: Endoscopes, drugs and more. Hepatology 2000;32:660–662.
22. Gitlin N. Hepatic encephalopathy. In: Zakim D, Boyer TD, eds. Hepatology: A Textbook of Liver Disease, 3rd ed. Philadelphia, Saunders, 1996:605–617.
23. Riordan SM, Williams R. Treatment of hepatic encephalopathy. N Engl J Med 1997;337:473–479.
24. Gitlin N. Subclinical portal systemic encephalopathy. Am J Gastroenterol 1988;82:8–11.
25. Dasarathy S, Mullen KD. Therapy of portosystemic encephalopathy. In: Cohen S, Davis GL, Gianella RA, et al, eds. Therapy of Digestive Disorders: A Companion to Sleisenger and Fordtran's Gastrointestinal and Liver Disease. Philadelphia, Saunders, 2000:385–394.
26. Butterworth RF. The neurobiology of hepatic encephalopathy. Semin Liver Dis 1996;16:235–244.
27. Eichler M, Bessman SP. A double blind study of the effect of ammonium infusion on psychological functioning in cirrhotic patients. J Nerv Ment Dis 1962;134:539–562.
28. Mammen EF. Coagulation defects in liver disease. Med Clin North Am. 1994:78:545–554.
29. Czaja AJ, Wolf AM, Baggenstoss BH. Clinical assessment of cirrhosis in severe chronic active liver disease: Specificity and sensitivity of physical and laboratory findings. Mayo Clinic Proc 1980;55:360–364.
30. Friedman LS, Martin P, Munoz J. Liver function tests and the objective evaluation of the patient with liver disease. In: Zakim D, Boyer TD, eds. Hepatology: A Textbook of Liver Disease, 3rd ed. Philadelphia, Saunders, 1996:764–788.
31. Cohen JA, Kaplan MM. The SGOT:SGPT ratio—An indicator of alcoholic disease. Dig Dis Sci 1979:24:835–838.
32. Lemeng L, Li TK. Vitamin B6 metabolism in chronic alcohol abuse: Pyridoxyl phosphate levels in plasma and the effects of acetaldehyde on pyridoxyl phosphate on synthesis and degradation in human erythrocytes. J Clin Lab Invest 1974;53:693–704.
33. Fishman WH. Perspectives on alkaline phosphatase isoenzymes. Am J Med 1974;56:617–650.
34. Kaplan MM. Alkaline phosphatase. Gastroenterology 1972;62:452–468.
35. Seetharam S, Sussman ML, Komoda T, et al. The mechanism of elevated alkaline phosphatase activity after bile duct ligation in the rat. Hepatology 1986;6:374–380.
36. Chopra S, Griffen PH. Laboratory tests and diagnostic procedures in evaluation of liver disease. Am J Med 1985;79:221–230.
37. Davern TJ, Scharschmidt BF. Biochemical liver tests. In: Feldman M, Scharschmidt BF, Sleisenger MH, eds. Sleisenger and Fordtran's Gastrointestinal and Liver Disease: Pathophysiology/Diagnosis/Treatment, 6th ed. Philadelphia, Saunders, 1998:1112–1122.
38. Clark R, Rake MO, Flute PT, et al. Coagulation abnormalities in acute liver failure. Pathogenetic and therapeutic implications. Scan J Gastroenterol 1973;19(suppl):63–69.
39. de Noronha R, Taylor BA, Wild G, et al. Inter-relationships between platelet count, platelet IgG, serum IgG, immune complexes and the severity of liver disease. Clin Lab Haematol 1991;13:127–135.
40. Aoki, Y, Hirai K, Tanikawa K . Mechanism of thrombocytopenia in liver cirrhosis: Kinetics of indium-111 tropeolin-labeled platelets. Eur J Nucl Med 1993;20:123–129.
41. Pagliaro L, Rinaldi F, Craxi A. Percutaneous blind biopsy vs laparoscopy with guided biopsy in diagnosis of cirrhosis: A prospective randomized trial. Dig Dis Sci 1983;28:39–43.
42. Pugh RNH, Murray-Lyon IM, Dawson JL, et al. Transection of the oesophagus for bleeding oesophagus varices. Br J Surg 1973;60:646–649.
43. Vargas HE, Gerber D, Abu-Elmagd KA. Management of portal hypertension-related bleeding. Surg Clin North Am 1999;79:1–22.
44. Pagliaro L, D'Amico G, Pasta L, et al: Portal hypertension in cirrhosis: Natural history. In: Bosch J, Groszmann RJ, eds. Portal hypertension. Pathophysiology and Treatment. London, Blackwell Scientific, 1994: 72–92.
45. Graffeo M, Buffoli F, Lanzani M, et al. Survival after endoscopic sclerotherapy for oesophageal varices in cirrhotics. Am J Gastroenterology 1994;89:1815–1822.
46. D'Amico G, Pagliaro L, Bosch J. The treatment of portal hypertension: A meta-analytic review. Hepatology 1995;22:332–354.
47. Smith JL, Graham DY. Variceal hemorrhage: A critical evaluation of survival analysis. Gastroenterology 1982;82:968–973.
48. Sharara AJ, Rockey OC. Gastroesophageal variceal hemorrhage. N Engl J Med 2001;345:669–681.
49. Patch D, Burroughs AK. Variceal hemorrhage. In: Cohen S, Davis GL, Gianella RA, et al, eds. Therapy of Digestive Disorders: A Companion to Sleisenger and Fordtran's Gastrointestinal and Liver Disease. Philadelphia, Saunders, 2000:355–372.
50. Lebrec D, Nouel O, Corbic M, et al. Propranolol—A medical treatment for portal hypertension? Lancet 1980;2:180–182.
51. Bosch J, Mastai R, Kravetz D, et al. Effects of propranolol on azygos venous blood flow and hepatic and systemic hemodynamics in cirrhosis. Hepatology 1984;6:1200–1205.
52. Pagliaro L, D'Amico G, Sorensen TA, et al. Prevention of first bleeding in cirrhosis: A meta-analysis of randomized trials of nonsurgical treatment. Ann Int Med 1992;117:59–70.
53. Grace ND Management of portal hypertension. Gastroenterologist 1993; 1:39–58.
54. Poynard T, Cales P, Pasta L, et al. Beta-adrenergic antagonist drugs in the prevention of gastrointestinal bleeding in patients with cirrhosis and esophageal varices. N Engl J Med 1991;324:1532–1538.
55. Grace ND, Conn H, Griszmann R, et al. Propranolol for prevention of first oesophageal variceal hemorrhage: A lifetime commitment? Hepatology 1990;12:407.
56. Angelico M, Carli C, Piatr, C, et al. Isosorbide-5-mononitrate versus propranolol in the prevention of first bleeding in cirrhosis. Gastroenterology 1993;104:1460–1465.
57. Angelico M, Carli C, Piatr C, et al. Effects of isosorbide-5-mononitrate compared with propranolol on first bleeding and long-term survival in cirrhosis. Gastroenterology 1997;113:1632–1639.
58. Groszmann RJ. β-Adrenergic blockers and nitrovasodilators for the treatment of portal hypertension: The good, the bad, and the ugly. Gastroenterology 1997;113:1794–1797.
59. Sarin SK, Lamba GS, Kumar M, et al. Comparison of endoscopic ligation and propranolol for the primary prevention of variceal bleeding. N Engl J Med 1999;340:988–993.
60. Grace ND. Diagnosis and treatment of gastrointestinal bleeding secondary to portal hypertension [practice guidelines] Am J Gastroenterol 1997;92:1082–1091.
61. Groszmann RJ, deFranchis R. Portal hypertension. In: Schiff ER, Sorrell MF, Maddrey WC, eds. Schiff's Diseases of the Liver, 8th ed. Philadelphia, Lippincott-Raven, 1999:387–442.
62. Lamberts S, Van Der Lely A, De Herder W, Hofland L. Octreotide. N Engl J Med 1996;4:246–254.
63. Bosch J, Kravetz D, Rodes J. Effects of somatostatin on hepatic and systemic hemodynamics in patients with cirrhosis of the liver. Comparison with vasopressin. Gastroenterology 1981;80:518–525.
64. Valenzuela JE, Schubert T, Fogel MR, et al. A multicenter, randomized, double-blind trial of somatostatin in the management of acute hemorrhage from esophageal varices. Hepatology 1989;10:958–961.
65. Burroughs AK, McCormick PA, Hughes MD, et al. Randomized, double-blind, placebo-controlled trial of somatostatin for variceal bleeding. Gastroenterology 1990;99:1388–1395.
66. Gotzsche PC, Gjorup I, Bonnen H, et al. Somatostatin vs placebo in bleeding oesophageal varices: Randomized trial and meta-analysis. BMJ 1995;310:1495–1498.
67. Imperiale TF, Teran JC, McCullough AJ. A meta-analysis of somatostatin vs vasopressin in the treatment of acute esophageal variceal hemorrhage. Gastroenterology 1995;109:1289–1294.
68. Bass KM, Somberg KA. Portal hypertension and gastrointestinal bleeding. In: Feldman M, Scharschmidt BF, Sleisenger MH, eds. Sleisenger and Fordtran's Gastrointestinal and Liver Disease: Pathophysiology/ Diagnosis/Treatment, 6th ed. Philadelphia, Saunders, 1998:1284–1309.
69. Monescillo A, Arocena C, Lafuente C, et al. Effects of vasoactive drug therapy on variceal pressure during acute variceal haemorrhage. J Pathol 1995;23:101. Abstract.

70. Goulis J, Armonis A, Patch D, et al. Bacterial infection is independently associated with failure to control bleeding and early rebleeding in cirrhotic patients with gastrointestinal hemorrhage. Hepatology 1998;27:1207–1212.
71. Bernard B, Cadranel J, Valla D. Prognostic significance of bacterial infections in bleeding cirrhotic patients. Gastroenterology 1995;108:1828–1834.
72. Grace ND. Diagnosis and treatment of gastrointestinal bleeding secondary to portal hypertension [practice guidelines]. Am J Gastroenterol 1997;92:1082–1091.
73. Sarin SK, Kumar A. Sclerosants for variceal sclerotherapy: A critical appraisal. Am J Gastroenterol 1990;85:641–649.
74. Richter GM, Noeldge G, Palmaz JC. The transjugular intrahepatic portosystemic stent-shunt (TIPPS): Experience results of a pilot study. Cardiovasc Intervent Radiol 1990;13:200–207.
75. Bernard B, LeBrec D, Mathurin P, et al. Beta-adrenergic antagonists in the prevention of gastrointestinal rebleeding in patients with cirrhosis: A meta-analysis. Hepatology 1997;25:63–70.
76. Garcia-Pagan JC, Feu F, Bosch J. Enhancement of portal pressure reduction by the association of isosorbide-5-mononitrate to propranolol administration in patients with cirrhosis. Hepatology 1990;11:230–238.
77. Feu F, Garcia-Pagan JC, Boscj J. Relation between portal pressure response to pharmacotherapy and risk of recurrent variceal hemorrhage in patients with cirrhosis. Lancet 1995;346:1056–1059.
78. Groszmann R, Bosch J, Grace ND. Hemodynamic events in a prospective randomized trial of propranolol versus placebo in the prevention of a first variceal hemorrhage. Gastroenterology 1990;99:1401–1407.
79. Goulis J, Patch D, Greenslade L, et al. RCT of variceal ligation vs propranolol-isosorbide for variceal rebleeding with target pressure reduction: Methodological problems. Gut 1998;42:F75. Abstract.
80. Garcia-Pagan JC, Feu F, Bosch J Rodes J. Propranolol compared with propranolol with isosorbide-5-mononitrate for portal hypertension in cirrhosis. Ann Intern Med 1991;114:869–873.
81. Nevens F, Lijnene P, VanBilloen H, Fevery J. The effect of long-term treatment with spironolactone on variceal pressure in patients with portal hypertension without ascites. Hepatology 1996;23:1047–1052.
82. Villanueva C, Balanzo J, Novella MT, et al. Nadolol plus isosorbide mononitrate compared with sclerotherapy for the prevention of variceal bleeding. N Engl J Med 1996;334:1624–1629.
83. Chen CY, Chang TT, Lin EY et al. Endoscopic variceal ligation versus conservative treatment for patients with hepatocellular carcinoma and bleeding esophageal varices Gastrointest Endosc 1995;42:535–539.
84. Strauss RM, Boyer TD. Diagnosis and management of cirrhotic ascites. In: Zakim D, Boyer TD, eds. Hepatology: A Textbook of Liver Disease, 3rd ed. Philadelphia, Saunders, 1996:764–788.
85. Gines P, Arroyo V, Rodes J. Therapy of ascites and spontaneous bacterial peritonitis. In: Cohen S, Davis GL, Gianella RA, et al, eds. Therapy of Digestive Disorders: A Companion to Sleisenger and Fordtran's Gastrointestinal and Liver Disease. Philadelphia, Saunders, 2000:373–384.
86. Llach J, Rimola A, Navasa M, et al. Incidence and predictive factors of first episode of spontaneous bacterial peritonitis in cirrhosis with ascites: relevance of ascitic fluid protein concentration. Hepatology 1992;16:724–727.
87. Guarner C, Runyon BA. Spontaneous bacterial peritonitis: Pathogenesis, diagnosis, and treatment. Gastroenterologist 1995;3:311–328.
88. Pockros PJ, Esrason KT, Nguyen C, et al. Mobilization of malignant ascites with diuretics is dependent on ascitic fluid characteristics. Gastroenterology 1992;103:1302–1306.
89. Reynolds TB, Geller HM, Kuzma OT, Redeker AG. Spontaneous decrease in portal pressure with clinical improvement in cirrhosis. N Engl J Med 1960;263:734–739.
90. Eisenmenger WJ, Ahrens EH, Blondheim SH, Kunkel HG. The effect of rigid fluid restriction in patients with cirrhosis of the liver and cirrhosis. J Lab Clin Med 1949;34:1029–1038.
91. Sungalia I, Bartle WR, Walker SE, et al. Spironolactone pharmacokinetics and pharmacodynamics in patients with cirrhotic ascites. Gastroenterology 1992;102;1680–1685.
92. Runyon BA. Ascites and spontaneous bacterial peritonitis. In: Feldman M, Scharschmidt BF, Slisenger MH, eds. Sleisenger and Fordtran's Gastrointestinal and Liver Disease: Pathophysiology/Diagnosis/Treatment, 6th ed. Philadelphia, Saunders, 1998:1310–1333.
93. Runyon BA. Monomicrobial nonneutrocytic bacterascites: A variant of spontaneous bacterial peritonitis. Hepatology 1990;12:710–715.
94. Navasa M, Follo A, Llovet JM, et al. Randomized, comparative study of oral ofloxacin versus intravenous cefotaxime in spontaneous bacterial peritonitis. Gastroenterology 1996;111:1011–1017.
95. Gines P, Rimola A, Planas R, et al. Norfloxacin prevents spontaneous bacterial peritonitis recurrence in cirrhosis: Results of a double-blind, placebo-controlled trial. Hepatology 1990;12:716–724.
96. Dupeyron C, Mangeney N, Sedrati L, et al. Rapid emergence of quinolone resistance in cirrhotic patients treated with norfloxacin to prevent spontaneous bacterial peritonitis. Antimicrob Agents Chemother 1994;38:340–344.
97. Llovet J, Rodriguez-Iglesias P, Moitinho E, et al. Spontaneous bacterial peritonitis in patients with cirrhosis undergoing selective intestinal decontamination. A retrospective study of 229 spontaneous bacterial peritonitis episodes. J Hepatol 1997;26:88–95.
98. Novella M, Sola R, Soriano G, et al. Continuous versus inpatient prophylaxis of the first episode of spontaneous bacterial peritonitis with norfloxacin. Hepatology 1997;25:532–536.
99. Cordoba J, Blei A. Treatment of hepatic encephalopathy. Am J Gastroenterol 1997;92:1429–1439.
100. Mullen KD, Gacad R. Hepatic encephalopathy. Gastroenterology 1996;6:188–202.
101. Gitlin N, Lewis DC, Hinkley L. The diagnosis and prevalence of subclinical hepatic encephalopathy in apparently healthy, ambulant, nonshunted patients with cirrhosis. J Hepatol 1986;3:75–82.
102. Uribe M, Conn HO. Dietary management of portal-systemic encephalopathy. In: Conn HO, Bircher J, eds. Hepatic Encephalopathy: Syndromes and Therapies. Bloomington, IL: Med-Ed Press, 1994:331–349.
103. Bianchi GP, Marchesini G, Fabri A, et al. Vegetable vs animal protein diet in cirrhotic patients with chronic encephalopathy. A randomized crossover comparison. J Intern Med 1993;233:385–392.
104. Clausen MR, Mortensen PB. Lactulose, disaccharides and colonic floras: Clinical consequences. Drugs 1997;53:930–942.
105. Kunin Cm, Chalmers TC, Leevy CM, et al. Absorption of orally administered neomycin and kanamycin with special reference to patients with severe hepatic and renal disease. N Engl J Med 1960;262:380–385.
106. Loguercio C, Abbiati R, Rinaldi M, et al. Long-term effects of *Enterococcus faecium* SF-68 versus lactulose in the treatment of patients with cirrhosis and grade 1–2 hepatic encephalopathy. J Hepatol 1995;23:39–46.
107. Ito S, Miyaji H, Azuma T, et al. Hyperammonemia and *Helicobacter pylori*. Lancet 1995;346:124–125.
108. Stoll B, McNeilly S, Buscher HP, Haussinger D. Functional hepatocyte heterogeneity in glutamate, aspartate and α-ketoglutarate uptake: A histoautoradiographical study. Hepatology 1991;13:247–253.
109. Kircheis G, Nilius R, Held C, et al. Therapeutic efficacy of L-ornithine L-aspartate infusions in patients with cirrhosis and hepatic encephalopathy: Results of a placebo-controlled, double-blind study. Hepatology 1997;25:1351–1360.
110. Van der Rijt CC, Schlam SW, et al. Overt hepatic encephalopathy precipitated by zinc deficiency. Gastroenterology 1991;100:1114–1118.
111. Marchesini G, Fabbri A, Bianchi G, et al. Zinc supplementation and amino acid-nitrogen metabolism in patients with advanced cirrhosis. Hepatology 1996;23:1084–1092.
112. Ferenci P, Grimm G, Meryn S. Successful long-term treatment of portal-systemic encephalopathy by the benzodiazepine antagonist flumazenil. Gastroenterology 1989;96:240–243.
113. Naylor CD, O'Rourke K, Detsky AS, Baker JP. Parenteral nutrition with branched-chain amino acids in hepatic encephalopathy. A meta-analysis. Gastroenterology 1989;97:1033–1042.
114. Charlton MR. Branched chain revisited. Gastroenterology 1996;111:252–255.

115. Nompleggi DJ, Bonkovsky HL. Nutritional supplementation in chronic liver disease: An analytical review. Heatology 1994;19:518–533.
116. Arroyo V, Gines P, Gerbes A. Definition and diagnostic criteria of refractory ascites and hepatorenal syndrome. Hepatology 1996;23;164–176.
117. Badalamenti S, Graziani D, Salerno F, Ponticelli C. Hepatorenal syndrome: New perspectives in pathogenesis and treatment. Arch Intern Med 1993;153:1957–1967.
118. Fitz G. Systemic complications of liver disease. In: Feldman M, Scharsshmidt BF, Sleisinger MH, eds. Sleisinger and Fordtran's Gastrointestinal and Liver Disease: Pathophysiology/Diagnosis/Management, 6th ed. Philadelphia, Saunders, 1999:1284–1309.
119. Mammen EF. Coagulation defects in liver disease. Med Clin North Am 1994:78:545–554.
120. Morgan DJ, McLean AJ. Clinical pharmacokinetic and pharmacodynamic consideration in patients with liver disease. Clin Pharmacokinet 1995;29:370–391.
121. Westphal JF, Brogard JM. Drug administration in chronic liver disease. Drug Saf 1997;1:47–73.
122. Reidenberg MM, Breckenridge A. Drugs and the liver. Clin Pharmacol Ther 1998;64;353–354.
123. Pacifici GM, Viani A, Franchi M, et al. Conjugation pathways in liver disease. Br J Clin Pharmacol 1990;30:427–435.
124. Rodighiero V. Effects of liver disease on pharmacokinetics: An update. Clin Pharmacokinet 1999;37:399–431.
125. Sokol SI, Cheng A, Frishman WH, Kaza CS. Cardiovascular drug therapy in patients with hepatic diseases and patients with congestive heart failure. J Clin Pharmacol 2000;40:11–30.
126. Das A. A cost analysis of long-term antibiotic prophylaxis for spontaneous bacterial peritonitis in cirrhosis. Am J Gastroenterol 1998;93: 895–900.
127. Teran JC, Imperiale TF, Mullen KD, et al. Primary prophylaxis of variceal bleeding in cirrhosis: A cost-effectiveness analysis.

38

Drug-Induced Liver Disease

William R. Kirchain and Mark A. Gill

The number of drugs associated with adverse reactions involving the liver is extensive.[1] The incidence of actual liver injury from most drugs is, fortunately, very low.[2] Chronic liver disease and cirrhosis collectively account for approximately 1% of annual mortality in the United States. Alcohol-induced liver disease accounts for most of these deaths.[3] Still, for an individual patient, drug-induced liver disease is usually a profound, life-changing disease.[4] The liver's function affects almost every other organ system in the body. It is important to know the patterns of drug-related pathology in order to assess adverse reactions when they occur. It is also important to understand how and when to monitor for these reactions.

PATTERNS OF DRUG-INDUCED LIVER DISEASE

IDIOSYNCRATIC REACTIONS

For some drugs, a genetic or acquired abnormality must exist in a particular metabolic pathway for a toxic reaction to take place (Fig. 38–1). In other cases, the reactions are typically associated with a drug concentration and often respond to simply lowering the dose of the drug. Idiosyncratic reactions tend to occur without association to particular blood concentrations or to specifically identified metabolic abnormalities. For example, sulfonylureas, such as glipizide, and antibiotics, such as ciprofloxacin, have caused severe liver disease, resulting in the need for transplantation in a very small group of patients.[5,6] Idiosyncratic reactions are rare and are sometimes described as liver hypersensitivity to a drug.

ALLERGIC HEPATITIS

Allergic reactions in the liver can be caused by many drugs and result in many different kinds of hepatic damage. Trimethoprim-sulfamethoxazole and penicillinase-resistant penicillins, such as dicloxacillin, induce a reaction typical of hepatic hypersensitivity in a few patients. The reaction usually develops within 4 weeks of the start of therapy.[7,8] It is marked by fever, pruritus, rash, eosinophilia, arthritis, and hemolytic anemia. The formation of granulomas within the liver is often seen on biopsy.[9] The reaction reverses with discontinued therapy and reappears on rechallenge. Many other anti-infectives—erythromycin, troleandomycin, trovafloxacin, penicillin, and amoxicillin-clavulanic acid—are associated with this type of reaction.[8,10,11] Allopurinol is also associated with a number of reports of hypersensitivity reactions involving the liver. The onset of symptoms is 1 week to 6 weeks after initiation of therapy. The incidence, like all the allergic liver reactions, is low, estimated at less than 1%. The clinical presentation includes eosinophilia, fever, rash, and arthritis, as previously mentioned. The biopsy may show a pattern of fibrin-ring granulomas similar to those seen in Q fever.[12]

TOXIC HEPATITIS

Toxic reactions are predictable, often dose-related effects in the liver caused by specific agents. Acetaminophen, when taken in overdose, becomes bioactivated to a toxic intermediate, known as *N*-acetyl-*p*-benzoquinoneimine (NAPQI). NAPQI is very reactive, with a high affinity for sulfhydryl groups. The amino acid glutathione provides a ready source of available sulfhydryl groups within the hepatocyte. When the liver's glutathione stores are depleted and there are no longer sulfhydryl groups available to detoxify this metabolite, it begins to react directly with the hepatocyte (Fig. 38–1). Replenishing the liver's sulfhydryl capacity through the administration of N-acetylcysteine early after ingestion of the overdose halts this process.[13] Acetaminophen's toxicity occurs in four stages.[14] During the first hours after ingestion, some patients report mild symptoms of nausea and vomiting, but no elevations of the commonly measured liver enzymes are seen. Not for 40 hours to 50 hours after ingestion do elevations in the liver enzymes begin.[14] *Reye's syndrome* is an aggressive form of toxic hepatitis often associated with aspirin use in children. Valproate toxicity can also present in this pattern. Early in the process of Reye's syndrome, mitochondrial dysfunction leads to the depletion of acyl coenzyme A (CoA) and carnitine. Fatty acids accumulate and gluconeogenesis is impaired, resulting in hypoglycemia. A concurrent disruption of the urea cycle occurs, leading to decrease in the removal of ammonia and a slowing of protein use. A threefold or greater rise in the blood ammonia level and an increase in the prothrombin time are common findings. In advanced stages of Reye's syndrome, many patients develop intracranial hypertension that can be life-threatening and refractory to therapy.[15,16]

CHRONIC ACTIVE TOXIC HEPATITIS

Dantrolene, isoniazid, phenytoin, nitrofurantoin, and trazodone have been reported in association with a type of autoimmune-mediated disease in the liver.[17,18] Patients experience periods of very symptomatic hepatitis followed by periods of convalescence, only to repeat the experience months later. It is a progressive disease with a high mortality rate. It is more common in females than males. Antinuclear antibodies appear in most patients. These drugs appear to form antiorganelle antibodies.[19] The exact identification of a causative agent is sometimes difficult, because diagnosis requires multiple episodes occurring long after exposure to the offending drug.

TOXIC CIRRHOSIS

The scarring effect of hepatitis in the liver leads to the development of cirrhosis. Some drugs tend to cause such a mild case of hepatitis that it may not be detected. Mild hepatitis can be easily mistaken for a more routine generalized viral infection. If the offending drug or agent is not discontinued, this damage will continue to progress. The patient eventually presents not with hepatitis but with cirrhosis. Methotrexate

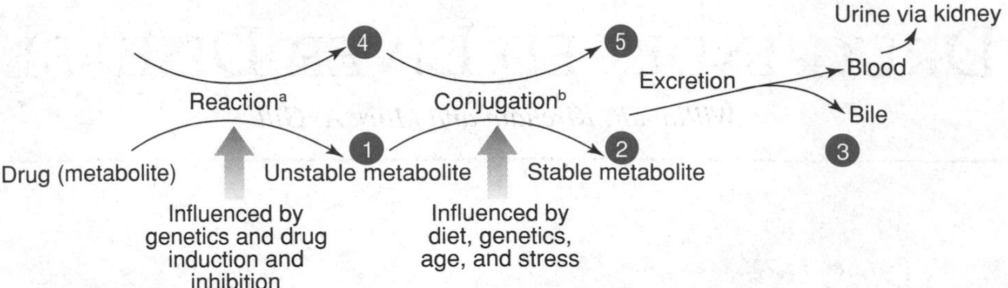

1. Reacts immediately with surrounding cytoplasmic mitochondria, leading to ATP depletion and excessive capase-3 activation
2. Run out of conjugate and allow immediate reactions as in number 1
3. Bile acids accumulate, inducing initiator capase within the hepatocyte
4. Direct stimulation of mitochondrial production of capase-3
5. Indirect stimulation of concurrent metabolic pathways leading to overproduction and ATP or NADPH depletion

[a] Usually oxidative, but can be hydrolytic or reductive, leading to the unstable metabolite
[b] Main conjugates for drugs: glucuronic acid, glycine, glutathione, and water

FIGURE 38–1. The possible mechanisms and pathways through which drugs may induce liver damage.

causes periportal fibrosis in most patients. The lesion results from the action of a bioactivated metabolite produced by cytochrome P450.[20] This process has most commonly been noted in patients treated for psoriasis and arthritis. The extent of damage can be reduced or controlled by increasing the dosage interval to once weekly.[21] Vitamin A, and other forms of β-carotene, is normally stored in liver cells, and causes significant hypertrophy and fibrosis when taken for long periods in high doses. Hepatomegaly is a common finding along with ascites and portal hypertension. In patients with vitamin A toxicity, gingivitis and dry skin are also very common. This is accelerated by ethanol, which competes with retinol for aldehyde dehydrogenase.[22]

LIVER VASCULAR DISORDERS

Focal lesions in hepatic venules, sinusoids, and portal veins occur with various drugs. The most commonly associated drugs are the cytotoxic agents that are used to treat cancer, the pyrrolizidine alkaloids, and the sex hormones. A centralized necrosis often follows and can result in cirrhosis. Azathioprine and herbal teas that contain comfrey (a source of pyrrolizidine alkaloids) have been reported in association with the development of venoocclusive disease. The exact incidence is rare and may be dose related.[23] Peliosis hepatitis is a rare type of hepatic vascular lesion that can be seen as both an acute and a chronic disease. The liver develops large, blood-filled lacunae within the parenchyma. Rupture of the lacunae can lead to severe peritoneal hemorrhage. Peliosis hepatitis is associated with exposure of the liver to androgens, estrogens, tamoxifen, azathioprine, and danazol. Androgens with a 17α-testosterone structure are the most frequently reported agents to cause peliosis hepatitis, usually after at least 6 months of therapy.[24]

MECHANISMS OF DRUG-INDUCED LIVER DISEASE

CENTROLOBULAR NECROSIS

Centrolobular necrosis is often a dose-related, predictable reaction secondary to drugs such as acetaminophen; however, it also can be associated with idiosyncratic reactions, such as those caused by halothane. Also called *direct* or *metabolite-related hepatotoxicity,* centrolobular necrosis is usually the result of the production of a toxic metabolite. The damage spreads outward from the middle of a lobe of the liver.

Patients suffering from centrolobular necrosis tend to present in one of two ways, depending on the extent of necrosis. Mild drug reactions, involving only small amounts of parenchymal tissue, may be detected as asymptomatic elevations in the serum transaminases. If the reaction is diagnosed at this stage, most of these patients will recover with minimal cirrhosis and thus minimal chronic liver impairment. More severe forms of centrolobular necrosis, as documented in cases with bromfenac, trazodone, and piroxicam, are accompanied by nausea, vomiting, upper abdominal pain, and jaundice.[18,25,26]

STEATONECROSIS

Steatonecrosis is a specialized type of acute necrosis resulting from the accumulation of fatty acids in the hepatocyte. Drugs or their metabolites that cause steatonecrosis do so by affecting fatty-acid oxidation within the mitochondria of the hepatocyte. Hepatic vesicles become engorged with fatty acids, eventually disrupting the homeostasis of the hepatocyte. Alcohol is the most common drug that produces steatonecrotic changes in the liver. When alcohol converts into acetaldehyde, the synthesis of fatty acids is increased.[22,27] When the hepatocyte has become completely engorged with microvesicular fat, it often breaks open, spilling into the blood. If enough hepatocytes break open, an inflammatory response begins. If the offending agent is withdrawn before significant numbers of hepatocytes become necrotic, the process is completely reversible without long-term sequelae.

Tetracycline produces steatonecrosis and steatosis.[28] The lesions are characterized by large vesicles of fat found diffused throughout the liver. The development of this reaction is related to the high concentrations achieved when tetracycline is given intravenously and in doses greater than 1.5 g/d. The mortality of tetracycline steatonecrosis is very high (70% to 80%), and those that do survive often develop cirrhosis. Sodium valproate also can produce steatonecrosis through the process of bioactivation. Cytochrome P450 converts valproate to D-4-valproic acid, a potent inducer of microvesicular fat accumulation.[29]

Patients experiencing steatonecrosis may present with abdominal fullness or pain as their only complaint. Patients with more severe steatonecrosis will present with all the symptoms characteristic of alcoholic hepatitis such as nausea, vomiting, steatorrhea, abdominal pain, pruritus, and fatigue.

PHOSPHOLIPIDOSIS

Phospholipidosis is the accumulation of phospholipids instead of fatty acids. The phospholipids usually engorge the lysosomal bodies of the hepatocyte.[30] Amiodarone has been associated with this reaction. Patients treated with amiodarone who develop overt hepatic disease tend to have received higher doses of the drug. These patients also have higher amiodarone to *N*-desethyl-amiodarone ratios, indicating a greater accumulation of the parent compound. Amiodarone and its major metabolite *N*-desethyl-amiodarone remain in the liver of all patients for several months after therapy is stopped. Usually the phospholipidosis develops in patients treated for more than 1 year. The patient can present with either elevated transaminases or hepatomegaly; jaundice is rare.[31,32]

GENERALIZED HEPATOCELLULAR NECROSIS

Generalized hepatocellular necrosis mimics the changes associated with the more common viral hepatitis. The onset of symptoms is usually delayed as much as a week or more after exposure to toxin. Bioactivation is often important for toxic hepatitis to develop, but may not be the immediate cause of damage.[33] Many drugs that are associated with toxic hepatitis produce metabolites that are not inherently toxic to the liver. Instead, they act as haptens, binding to specific cell proteins and inducing an autoimmune reaction.[19] The need for bioactivation by a drug can lead to differences in the incidence of the reaction between males and females. The subspecies of cytochrome P450, *N*-acetyltransferase, and xanthine oxidase vary in abundance and affinities as a function of gender.[34,35]

The long-term administration of isoniazid can lead to hepatic dysfunction in 10% to 20% of those receiving the drug. Yet severe toxic hepatitis develops in only 1% or less of this population.[36] The *N*-acetyltransferase 2 (NAT2) genotype appears to play a role in determining a patient's relative risk. In a recent study, patients with the slow-type NAT2 genotype had a 28-fold greater risk of developing serum aminotransferase elevations than did patients with the fast-type NAT2 genotype.[37] Isoniazid is metabolized by several pathways, acetylation being the major pathway. It is acetylated to acetylisoniazid, which, in turn, is hydrolyzed to acetylhydrazine.[38] The acetylhydrazine and, to a lesser extent, the acetylisoniazid are directly toxic to the cellular proteins in the hepatocyte, but rapid acetylators also detoxify acetylhydrazine very rapidly, converting it to diacetylhydrazine (a nontoxic metabolite).

Ketoconazole produces generalized hepatocellular necrosis or milder forms of hepatic dysfunction in 1% to 2% of patients treated for fungal infections. This reaction has been reported to be fatal in high numbers of HIV-infected patients. The onset is usually early in therapy, although it can be delayed until several months into therapy. In immune-compromised patients where ketoconazole is used for long periods of time, special care should be taken to watch for changes in liver function.[39,40]

CHOLESTATIC JAUNDICE

Cholestatic jaundice, or cholestasis, can be classified by the area of the bile canalicular or ductal system that is impaired. Canalicular cholestasis is very often associated with long-term estrogen therapy. The actual incidence is very low, and is decreasing as the use of high-dose estrogens in oral contraceptives has decreased. Clinically, these patients are often asymptomatic and present with mild to moderate elevations of serum bilirubin.[41] An intravenous form of vitamin E, α-tocopherol acetate, causes cholestatic jaundice, primarily involving the canaliculi, in premature infants. The incidence of this reaction in those receiving this formulation was very high (>10%) and the mortality even higher (>50%).[42] Hepatocellular cholestasis is a much more serious form of cholestatic jaundice that involves both the parenchyma and bile canalicular cells. Floxacillin is associated with this reaction at a rate of 1 per every 15,000 users in Australia and Sweden.[43] Chlorpromazine can precipitate bile salts and decrease total bile flow.[44] The administration of total parenteral nutrition for periods greater than 1 week induces cholestatic changes and nonspecific enzyme elevations in some patients. Patients with low serum albumin concentrations may be at greater risk than patients with normal serum albumin concentrations.[45] This reaction also has been reported to occur rarely with sulfonamides, sulfonylureas, erythromycin estolate and ethylsuccinate, captopril, lisinopril, ticlopidine, and other phenothiazines.[8,46,47]

MIXED HEPATOCELLULAR NECROSIS AND CHOLESTATIC DISEASE

Patients infrequently present with a purely hepatocellular necrosis or cholestatic damage, but rather with a mixed picture of damage. Flutamide causes a mix of lesions that appear at or about the forty-eighth week of treatment.[48,49] Niacin in doses greater than 3 g/d, or in doses greater than 1 g/d of sustained-release formulations, causes the same mixed pattern of damage.[50] These patients often present with only a few signs or symptoms at first but can progress rapidly to fulminant hepatic failure. Additionally, niacin-induced and other drug-induced mixed hepatocellular disease can be misinterpreted as hepatobiliary cancers.[51]

NEOPLASTIC DISEASE

A large body of the current literature on adverse reactions and the liver addresses the development of neoplasms following drug therapy. Both carcinoma- and sarcoma-like lesions have been identified. Fortunately, hepatic tumors associated with drug therapy are usually benign and remit when drug therapy is discontinued. Except in rare instances, these lesions are associated with long-term exposure to the offending agent.[52] Androgens, estrogens, and other hormonal-related agents are the most frequently associated causes of neoplastic disease. The model for drug-induced hepatic cancer is polyvinyl chloride exposure. Used in the production of many types of plastic products, polyvinyl chloride induces angiosarcoma in exposed workers after as few as 3 years of exposure.[53]

ASSESSMENT

The best and most important technique for assessing and monitoring drug-induced liver disease is the patient's history. Questions addressing the patient's drug usage along with a thorough review of systems are essential (Table 38–1). The use of drugs for recreational purposes must not be overlooked. Cocaine has been directly linked to liver disease.[54] Ecstasy, the street name of methylenedioxymethamphetamine (MDMA), has induced fulminant hepatitis, which has led to death in some cases.[55] The more pervasive impact of street drugs on the incidence of hepatic disease is the concomitant injection or

TABLE 38–1. An Approach to Evaluating a Suspected Hepatotoxic Reaction

Step 1	Does the sex or age of the patient increase his or her risk? Does the patient's occupation increase his or her risk? Does the patient's recreational drug use increase his or her risk? Is the patient using any herbal remedies, tonics, or teas that increase risk? Is the patient's diet deficient in vitamins or micronutrients? Is the patient's diet excessive in vitamins or micro-nutrients? Is the patient pregnant? Does the patient have diabetes mellitus?
Step 2	Is there a temporal relationship between the drug and the onset of disease?
Step 3	Is there supporting literature for this type of reaction? Is the clinical evidence consistent with the presentations in the literature? What is the statistical risk for the reaction, and for progression to fulminant failure?
Step 4	Is this a common reaction associated with this drug? Have all more common causes (viruses, alcohol) been ruled out?
Step 5	What happended when the drug was discontinued?
Step 6	Is rechallenge with the drug possible? If so, what happened?
Classifying a Lesion Established as a Case of Hepatotoxicity	
Step 7	What are the biopsy results? What are the CT, MRI, and/or ultrasound results? What is the pattern of enzyme elevation? Is there evidence of recovery or is cirrhosis dominating the clinical outcome?

ingestion of adulterants. Many of these adulterants are either directly toxic or serve to enhance the toxicity of the drug. It is also good to try to determine nondrug hepatic disease risk. Arsenic, for example, is known to induce both acute and chronic hepatic reactions. Arsenic in low concentrations is found in most rot- and insect-resistant lumber.[56] Following Occupational Safety and Health Agency guidelines should decrease the danger of using these products, but will not eliminate it. Even if exposure to an environmental toxin in and of itself does not produce a hepatic reaction, it may predispose a patient to a hepatic reaction when a drug is added. Table 38–2 lists some of the more common hepatic toxins from occupational or environmental exposure that can add to a patient's risk for developing a hepatic lesion.[56] Additionally, a person's use of alternative medicine must be solicited. Many herbal remedies were once wisely abandoned because of their common adverse reactions. Comfrey tea is a common cause of hepatocellular damage.[57] As in the case of the Chinese remedy *jin bu huan,* or as in the case of the more elegantly presented chaparral capsules containing grease wood leaves, the end of therapy with these types of agents is occasionally severe disability or death from fulminant hepatic failure.[58,59] Table 38–3 lists many of the more common herbal remedies that are associated with significant liver disease.[56–59]

The nutritional status of a patient can be as important to the development of a drug-induced liver disease as the hepatotoxin itself.[38,60] Patients who are malnourished because of illness or long-term alcohol abuse make up the most troublesome group.[61] These patients tend to react at lower doses in dose-related reactions and more severely in all types of reactions. A diet heavy in charcoal-grilled meats and vegetables can sometimes induce bioactivation. These patients may be predisposed to or have worse than expected reactions associated with drugs that are metabolized to toxic intermediates.

TABLE 38–2. Environmental Hepatic Toxins[a]

Toxin	Group Associated With Exposure
Arsenic	Chemical, construction, agricultural workers
Carbon tetrachloride	Chemical plant workers, laboratory technicians
Copper	Plumbers, copper foundry workers
Dimethylformamide	Chemical plant workers, laboratory technicians
2,4-Dichlorophenoxyacetic acid	Horticulturalists, gardening enthusiasts
Fluorine	Chemical plant workers, laboratory technicians
Toluene	Chemical and agricultural workers, laboratory technicians
Trichloroethylene	Printers, dye workers, cleaners, laboratory technicians
Vinyl chloride	Plastics plant workers

[a]A partial list of environmental toxins that can cause liver injury. At lower exposure rates, these compounds may also predispose the patient to liver injury from a drug.

All potential drug reactions should be judged as to the timing of the reaction versus drug administration, pharmacokinetic considerations, the literature records of previous reactions, the inclusion of alternative nondrug causes, and close clinical observation when the drug in question is stopped. It is also important to keep in mind that most elevations in liver enzymes will not be associated with a drug. In a study of all patients admitted to a hospital in the United Kingdom with elevated liver transaminase, only 14 of 162 cases involved a drug as the possible cause (2 from alcohol, 9 from acetaminophen overdose, 3 from MDMA).[62] In all cases, titers of serum antibodies to hepatitis A, B, and C should be drawn. Even in cases in which the drug is absolutely targeted as the cause, viral hepatitis may be a complication. Some drugs may even be a facilitator of a viral infection.

Often there is no good clinical test available to determine the exact type of hepatic lesion, short of biopsy. There are still certain patterns of enzyme elevation that have been identified and can be helpful (Table 38–4).[62–64] The specificity of any serum enzyme depends on the distribution of that enzyme in the body. Alkaline phosphatase is found in the bile duct epithelium, bone, and intestinal and kidney cells. 5′-Nucleotidase is more specific for hepatic disease than alkaline phosphatase, because most of the body's store of 5′-nucleotidase

TABLE 38–3. Herbal Remedies Associated with a Relatively High Incidence of Hepatotoxicity

Amanita
Comfrey
Germander
Gordolobo
Grease wood
Margosa oil
Mistletoe
Pennyroyal (squawmint)
Skullcap
Yerba

TABLE 38–4. Relative Patterns of Hepatic Enzyme Elevation Versus Type of Hepatic Lesion

Enzyme	Abreviation(s)	Necrotic	Cholestatic	Chronic
Alkaline phosphatase	Alk phos, AP	↑	↑↑↑	↑
5′-Nucleotidase	5-NC, 5NC	↑	↑↑↑	↑
γ-Glutamyltransferase	GGT, GGTP	↑	↑↑↑	↑↑
Aspartamine transferase	AST, SGOT	↑↑↑	↑	↑↑
Alanine transferase	ALT, SGPT	↑↑↑	↑	↑↑
Lactate dehydrogenase	LDH	↑↑↑	↑	↑

↑ = <100% of normal; ↑↑ = >100% of normal; ↑↑↑ = >200% above normal.

is in the liver. Glutamate dehydrogenase is a good indicator of centrolobular necrosis because it is found primarily in centrolobular mitochondria. Most hepatic cells have extremely high concentrations of transaminases. Aspartate aminotransferase (AST or serum glutamic-oxaloacetic transaminase [SGOT]) and alanine aminotransferase (ALT or serum glutamic-pyruvic transaminase [SGPT]) are commonly measured. Because of their high concentrations and easy liberation from the hepatocyte cytoplasm, AST and ALT are very sensitive indicators of necrotic lesions within the liver.[64,65] After an acute hepatic lesion is established, it may take weeks for these concentrations to return to normal.

Serum bilirubin concentration is a sensitive indicator of most hepatic lesions and has significant prognostic value. High-peak bilirubin concentrations are associated with poor survival. Other important findings that indicate poor survival are a peak prothrombin time greater than 40 seconds, elevated serum creatinine, and low arterial pH. The presence of encephalopathy or prolonged jaundice are not good signs for the survival of the patient and are strong indicators for transplantation.[66]

Bilirubin concentrations and serum enzyme elevations give a static picture of the liver's condition. They do not indicate hepatic function. Clinically available tests to predict hepatic function include measurement of serum proteins (albumin or transferrin). As hepatic function decreases, serum protein concentrations in the body decrease at a rate determined by each protein's own elimination rate. Overhydration and starvation can also decrease serum protein concentrations. Changes in the prothrombin time often occur earlier than the changes in albumin or transferrin. The response of the prothrombin time to the administration of 10 mg of parenteral vitamin K is often used to differentiate between hepatic and extrahepatic disease.

MEASUREMENT OF LIVER FUNCTION

A good compound for a liver function test would theoretically be (a) nontoxic, lacking any pharmacologic effect; (b) either rapidly and completely absorbed orally or easily administered via a peripheral vein; (c) eliminated only by the liver; and (d) easily measured (drug and its metabolite) in blood, saliva, or urine.[67]

Several tests are used in research settings and in liver transplant patients to indicate liver function. Tests, such as sulfobromophthalein, indocyanine green, or sorbitol, measure qualities of hepatic clearance. There are also a few drugs that have been used to test liver function. Sorbitol's advantage over indocyanine green is a much lower incidence of allergic reactions. It is partially cleared by the kidney, and urine levels must also be determined during the test.[68,69] A good estimate of hepatic clearance can be obtained by serial blood levels of a variety of hepatically eliminated drugs if an assay is locally available. Ultrasound pictures and CT scans can be used on a periodic basis to monitor for the development of fibrosis or vascular lesion in the liver and for hepatocellular carcinomas.[70]

If there is a liver biopsy available, the injury should be classified by the histologic findings. In cases in which there is no biopsy, the pattern of liver enzyme elevation can estimate the type of injury. Hepatocellular injuries are marked by elevations in transaminase that are at least two times normal. If the alkaline phosphatase is also elevated, then a hepatocellular lesion is still suspected when the elevation of ALT is notably higher than the elevation of alkaline phosphatase. If the magnitude of elevation is nearly equal between ALT and alkaline phosphatase, then the lesion is likely cholestatic.

A liver injury is acute if it lasts less than 3 months. It is considered chronic after 3 months of consistent symptoms or enzyme elevation. A liver injury is severe if the patient has marked jaundice, if the prothrombin time does not improve by more than 50% after the administration of vitamin K, or if encephalopathy is detectable. If an acute liver injury progresses from normal to severe in a matter of a few days or weeks, it is considered fulminant.[71]

MONITORING

The serum transaminases AST and ALT (SGOT and SGPT) are the most commonly used transaminases in the clinical setting. Concentrations of these enzymes should be obtained about every 4 weeks depending on the reported characteristics of the reaction in question. Methotrexate should be monitored every 4 weeks, because toxicity usually develops over a period of several weeks to months.[72] In addition, some recommend that sulfobromophthalein or indocyanine-green excretion studies be performed on a regular basis and that patients treated for very long periods of time should have a liver biopsy performed every 12 months.[73]

REFERENCES

1. Biour M, Jaillon PJ. Drug-induced hepatic diseases. Pathol Biol (Paris) 1999;47:928–937.
2. Garcia Rodriguez LA, Ruigomez A, Jick H. A review of epidemiologic research on drug-induced acute liver injury using the general practice research data base in the United Kingdom. Pharmacotherapy 1997;17: 721–728.
3. National Center for Health Statistics. Advance report of final mortality statistics 1990. Monthly Vital Statistics Report 1993;41:7.
4. Aithal PG, Day CPJ. The natural history of histologically proved drug-induced liver disease. Gut 1999;44:731–735.
5. Dourakis SP, Tzemanakis E, Sinani C, Kafiri G, Hadziyannis SJJ. Gliclazide-induced acute hepatitis. Eur J Gastroenterol Hepatol. 2000; 12:119–121.
6. Villeneuve JP, Davies C, Cote JJ. Suspected ciprofloxacin-induced hepatotoxicity. Ann Pharmacother 1995;29:257–259.
7. Lindgren A, Olsson R. Liver reactions from trimethoprim. J Intern Med 1994;236:281–284.

8. Olsson R, Wiholm BE, Sand C, Zettergren L, Hultcrantz R, Myrhed M. Liver damage from flucloxacillin, cloxacillin and dicloxacillin. J Hepatol 1992;15:154–161.
9. Pohl LR. Drug-induced allergic hepatitis. Semin Liver Dis 1990;10:305–315.
10. Chen HJ, Bloch KJ, Maclean JA. Acute eosinophilic hepatitis from trovafloxacin. N Engl J Med 2000;342:359–360. Letter.
11. de Haan F, Stricker BH. Liver damage associated with the combination drug amoxicillin-clavulanic acid (Augmentin). Ned Tijdschr Geneeskd 1997;141:1298–1301.
12. Vanderstigel M, Zafrani ES, Deyone JL, et al. Allopurinol hypersensitivity syndrome as a cause of hepatic fibrin granulomas. Gastroenterology 1986;90:188–190.
13. Buckley NA, Whyte IM, O'Connell DL, Dawson AHJ. Oral or intravenous *N*-acetylcysteine: Which is the treatment of choice for acetaminophen (paracetamol) poisoning? J Toxicol Clin Toxicol 1999;37:759–767.
14. Black M. Acetaminophen hepatotoxicity. Gastroenterology 1980;78:382–392.
15. Monto AS. The disappearance of Reye's syndrome—A public health triumph [see comments]. N Engl J Med 1999;340:1423–1424. Editorial; Comment.
16. Belay ED, Bresee JS, Holman RC, Khan AS, Shahriari A, Schonberger LB. Reye's syndrome in the United States from 1981 through 1997. N Engl J Med 1999;340:1377–1382.
17. Lee WM. Drug-induced hepatotoxicity. N Engl J Med 1995;333:1118–1127.
18. Fernandes NF, Martin RR, Schenker S. Trazodone-induced hepatotoxicity: A case report with comments on drug-induced hepatotoxicity. Am J Gastroenterol 2000;95:532–535.
19. Beane PH, Bourdi M. Autoantibodies against cytochrome P450 in drug-induced autoimmune hepatitis. Ann N Y Acad Sci 1993;685:641–645.
20. Hashkes PJ, Balistreri WF, Bove KE, Ballard ET, Passo MHJ. The relationship of hepatotoxic risk factors and liver histology in methotrexate therapy for juvenile rheumatoid arthritis. J Pediatr 1999;134:47–52.
21. Leonard PA, Clegg DO, Carson CC, Cannon GW, Egger MJ, Ward JR. Low-dose pulse methotrexate in rheumatoid arthritis: An 8-year experience with hepatotoxicity. Clin Rheumatol 1987;6:575–582.
22. Leo MA, Lieber CSJ. Alcohol, vitamin A, and beta-carotene: Adverse interactions, including hepatotoxicity and carcinogenicity. Am J Clin Nutr 1999;69:1071–1085.
23. Kumara CR, Ng M, Lin JH, et al. Herbal tea-induced hepatic veno-oclusive disease: Quantification of toxic alkaloid exposure in adults. Gut 1985;26:101–104.
24. Soe KL, Soe M, Gluud CN. Liver pathology associated with anabolic androgenic steroids. Ugeskr Laeger 1994;156:2585–2588.
25. Fontana RJ, McCashland TM, Benner KG, et al. Acute liver failure associated with prolonged use of bromfenac leading to liver transplantation. The Acute Liver Failure Study Group. Liver Transpl Surg 1999;5:480–484.
26. Planas R, DeLeon R, Quer JC, et al. Fatal submassive necrosis of the liver associated with piroxicam. Am J Gastroenterology 1990;85:468–470.
27. Agarwal DP, Goedde HW. Human aldehyde dehydrogenases: Their role in alcoholism. Alcohol 1989;6:517–423.
28. Lee WM. Acute hepatic failure. N Engl J Med 1993;329:1862–1872.
29. Konig SA, Schenk M, Sick C, et al. Fatal liver failure associated with valproate therapy in a patient with Friedreich's disease: Review of valproate hepatotoxicity in adults. Epilepsia 1999;40:1036–1040.
30. Lullman H, Lullman R, Wasserman O. Drug-induced phospholipodosis, II. Tissue distribution of the amphiphilic drug chlorphentermine. CRC Crit Drug Rev Toxicol 1975;4:185–218.
31. Pollak PT, Sharama AD, Charruthers SG. Relation of amiodarone hepatic and pulmonary toxicity to serum drug concentrations and superoxide dimutase activity. Am J Cardiol 1990;65:1185–1191.
32. Chang CC, Petrelli M, Tomashefski JF Jr, McCullough AJJ. Severe intrahepatic cholestasis caused by amiodarone toxicity after withdrawal of the drug: A case report and review of the literature. Arch Pathol Lab Med 1999;123:251–256.
33. Watkins PB. Drug metabolism by cytochrome P450 in the liver and small bowel. Gastroenterol Clin North Am 1992;21:511–526.
34. Hunt CM, Westerkam WR, Stave GM. Effect of age and gender on the activity of human hepatic CYP3A. Biochem Pharmacol 1992;44:275–283.
35. Evans WE, Relling MV. Pharmacogenomics: Translating functional genomics into rational therapeutics. Science 1999;286:487–491.
36. Tsagaropoou-Stinga H, Mataki-Emmanouilidon R, Karida-Kavalioti S, et al. Hepatotoxic reactions in children with severe tuberculosis treated with isoniazid-rifampin. Pediatr Infect Dis 1985;4:270–273.
37. Ohno M, Yamaguchi I, Yamamoto I, et al. Slow N-acetyltransferase 2 genotype affects the incidence of isoniazid and rifampicin-induced hepatotoxicity. Int J Tuberc Lung Dis 2000;4:256–261.
38. Kergueris MF, Bourin M, Larousse C. Pharmacokinetics of isoniazid: Influence of age. Eur J Clin Pharm 1986;30:335–340.
39. Lake-Bakaar G, Scheuer PJ, Sherlock S. Hepatic reactions associated with ketoconazole use in the United Kingdom. Br Med J 1987;294:813–820.
40. Van Puijenbroek EP, Metselaar HJ, Berghuis PH, Zondervan PE, Stricker BHJ. Acute hepatocytic necrosis during ketoconazole therapy for treatment of onychomycosis. National Foundation for Registry and Evaluation of Adverse Effects. Ned Tijdschr Geneeskd 1998;142:2416–2418.
41. Foitl DR, Hyman G, Leftowitch JH. Jaundice and intrahepatic cholestasis following high-dose megestrol acetate for breast cancer. Cancer 1989;63:438–439.
42. Lorch V, Murphy D, Hoersten L, et al. Unusual syndrome among premature infants: Associated with a new intravenous vitamin E product. Pediatrics 1985;75:598–601.
43. Devereaux BM, Crawford DH, Purcell P, Powell LW, Roeser HP. Flucloxacillin-associated cholestatic hepatitis. An Australian and Swedish epidemic? Eur J Clin Pharmacol 1995;49:81–85.
44. Reichel J, Goldberg SB, Ellenberg M, et al. Intrahepatic cholestasis following administration of chlorpropamide. Am J Med 1960;28:654–660.
45. Naji AA, Anderson FH. Relationship between serum albumin and parenteral nutrition-associated cholestasis. J Pediatr Enter Nutr 1984;8:438–444.
46. Crantock L, Prentice R, Powell LJ. Cholestatic jaundice associated with captopril therapy. J Gastroenterol Hepatol 1991;6:528–530.
47. Grimm IS, Litynski JJ. Severe cholestasis associated with ticlopidine. Am J Gastronenterol 1994;89:279–280.
48. Chu CW, Hwang SJ, Luo JC, et al. Flutamide-induced liver injury: A case report. Chung Hua I Hsueh Tsa Chih (Taipei) 1998;61:678–682.
49. Cetin M, Demirci D, Unal A, Altinbas M, Guven M, Unluhizarci KJ. Frequency of flutamide induced hepatotoxicity in patients with prostate carcinoma. Hum Exp Toxicol 1999;18:137–140.
50. Rader JI, Calvert RJ, Hathcock JN. Hepatic toxicity of unmodified and time-release preparations of niacin. Am J Med 1992;92:77–81.
51. Kristensen T, Olcott EWJ. Effects of niacin therapy that simulate neoplasia: Hepatic steatosis with concurrent hepatic dysfunction. J Comput Assist Tomogr 1999;23:314–317.
52. Lee FI, Smith PM, Bennett B, Williams DMJ. Occupationally related angiosarcoma of the liver in the United Kingdom 1972–1994. Gut 1996;39:312–318.
53. Anonymous. Epidemiologic notes and reports: Angiosarcoma of the liver among polyvinyl chloride workers—Kentucky. MMWR Morb Mortal Wkly Rep 1997;46:99–101.
54. Van Thiel DH, Perper JA. Hepatotoxicity associated with cocaine abuse. Recent Dev Alcohol 1992;10:335–341.
55. Jones AL, Simpson KJJ. Mechanisms and management of hepatotoxicity in ecstasy (MDMA) and amphetamine intoxications. Aliment Pharmacol Ther 1999;13:129–33. Review.
56. Wang JS, Groopman JD. Toxic liver disorders. In: Rom WN, ed. Environmental and Occupational Medicine, 3rd ed. Philadelphia, Lippincott-Raven, 1998:831–840.
57. McGuffin M. Self-regulatory initiatives by the herbal industry. 6. Pyrrolizidine alkaloids. Herbal Gram 2000;48:43.
58. Wolf GM, Petrovic LM, Rojter SE, et al. Acute hepatitis associated with the Chinese herbal product jin bu huan. Ann Intern Med 1994;121:729–735.
59. Gordon D, Rosenthal G, Hart J, et al. Chaparral ingestion the broadening spectrum of liver injury caused by herbal medications. JAMA 1995;273:489–490.

60. Wolf R, Strecker M. Endogenous and exogenous factors modifying the activity of human liver cytochrome P-450 enzymes. Exp Toxicol Pathol 1992;44:263–271.
61. Seef LB, Cuccherin BA, Zimmerman HJ, et al. Acetaminophen hepatotoxicity in alcoholics: A therapeutic misadventure. Ann Intern Med 1986;104:399–404.
62. Whitehead MW, Haukes ND, Hainesworth I, Kingham JGC. A prospective study of causes of notably raised aspartate aminotransferase of liver origin. Gut 1999;45:129–133.
63. Zimmerman HJ. Chemical hepatic injury and its detection. In: Plaa G, Hewitt G, eds. Toxicology of the liver: Target organ series. Philadelphia, Raven Press, 1981:1–46.
64. Choppa S, Griffin PH. Laboratory tests and diagnostic procedures in evaluation of liver disease. Am J Med 1985;79:221–230.
65. Yoshida M, Miyajima K, Shiraki K, et al. Hepatotoxicity and consequently increased cell proliferation are associated with flumequine hepatocarcinogenesis in mice. Cancer Lett 1999;141:99–107.
66. O'Grady JG, Alexander GJM, Hayllar KM, Williams R. Early indicators of prognosis in fulminant hepatic failure. Gastroenterology 1989;97:439–445.
67. Barstow L, Smith RE. Liver function assessment by drug metabolism. Pharmacotherapy 1990;10:280–288.
68. Kawasaki S, Sugiyama Y, Iga T, et al. Pharmacokinetic study on the hepatic uptake of indocyanine green in cirrhotic patients. Am J Gastroenterol 1985;80:801–806.
69. Zech J, Lange H, Bosch J, et al. Steady-state extrarenal sorbitol clearance as a measure of hepatic plasma flow. Gastroenterology 1988;95:749–759.
70. Mathieu D, Kobeiter H, Maison P, et al. Oral contraceptive use and focal nodular hyperplasia of the liver. Gastroenterology 2000;118:560–564.
71. Anonymous. Standardization of definitions and criteria of causality assessment of adverse drug reactions, drug-induced liver disorders: Report of an international consensus meeting. Int J Clin Pharmacol Ther Toxicol 1990;28:317–322.
72. Newman M, Auerbach R, Feiner H, et al. The role of liver biopsies in psoriatic patients receiving long-term methotrexate treatment: Improvement in liver abnormalities after cessation of treatment. Arch Dermatol 1989;125:1218–1224.
73. O'Connor GT, Olmstead EM, Sug K, et al. Detection of hepatotoxicity associated with methotrexate therapy for psoriasis. Arch Dermatol 1989;125:1209–1217.

39
PANCREATITIS

Rosemary R. Berardi and Patricia A. Montgomery

Pancreatitis represents either an acute or chronic inflammatory process of the pancreas with variable involvement of regional tissues and remote organs. Acute pancreatitis (AP) is characterized by severe pain in the upper abdomen and increased serum concentrations of pancreatic lipase and amylase. In most instances, patients with mild AP (defined by the absence of organ dysfunction) will have a complete recovery. Severe AP is associated with local complications such as acute fluid collection, pancreatic necrosis, abscess, and pseudocyst. Multiple organ failure—including shock, pulmonary insufficiency, metabolic and cardiac complications, and renal failure—contributes to an unfavorable prognosis. Exocrine and endocrine pancreatic function may remain impaired for variable periods after an acute attack. AP, however, rarely progresses to chronic pancreatitis.[1–5]

Chronic pancreatitis (CP) refers to a syndrome of destructive and inflammatory conditions related to the many sequelae of long-standing pancreatic injury.[6–9] CP is characterized by fibrosis and destruction of exocrine and endocrine tissue. Histologic and functional changes are irreversible, but not invariably progressive. Improvement may occur in a subset of patients when obstruction of the main pancreatic duct is relieved (Fig. 39–1). In the acutely ill, symptomatic exacerbations resemble attacks of AP and may not be distinguishable. Most patients with CP have periods of intractable abdominal pain, maldigestion, and with advancing disease, diabetes mellitus. CP patients with long-standing disease are at an increased risk of developing pancreatic cancer.[6,7] Patients with AP and CP suffer from many of the same complications.

The prevalence of pancreatitis varies widely with geographic area, etiologic factors (e.g., ethanol consumption), and environmental or hereditary factors. The overall prevalence of AP in males and females in the United States is estimated to be less than 1%, whereas the prevalence of CP is about 0.05% in males and 0.01% in females.[1,7] The reported prevalence of overt AP and CP underestimates the true spectrum of these disorders.[7] Alcoholic CP is more common in men and has a peak incidence between 35 and 45 years of age. Black patients are two to three times more likely than white patients to be hospitalized for CP than for alcoholic cirrhosis, but the underlying genetic factor remains elusive.[7]

PHYSIOLOGY OF EXOCRINE PANCREATIC SECRETION

The pancreas possesses both endocrine and exocrine functions. The islets of Langerhans, that contain the cells of the endocrine pancreas, secrete insulin, glucagon, somatostatin, and other polypeptide hormones. The exocrine pancreas is composed of acini that secrete about 1–2 L/d of isotonic fluid that contains water, electrolytes, and pancreatic enzymes necessary for digestion. Bicarbonate is secreted primarily by the centroacinar (ductular) cells, and is the principal ion of physiologic importance. Pancreatic juice is delivered to the duodenum via the pancreatic ducts (Fig. 39–1) where the alkaline secretion (pH about 8.3) neutralizes gastric acid and provides an appropriate pH for maintaining the activity of pancreatic enzymes.[10]

The major pancreatic exocrine enzyme groups are:

Proteolytic: trypsinogen, chymotrypsinogen, procarboxypeptidase, proaminopeptidase
Amylolytic: amylase
Lipolytic: lipase, prophospholipase A_2, carboxylesterase lipase
Nucleolytic: ribonuclease
Other: trypsin inhibitor, colipase

The proteolytic enzymes are secreted as zymogens (inactive enzymes), which are activated in the lumen of the duodenum. Enterokinase, secreted by the duodenal mucosa, converts trypsinogen to trypsin, which then activates all other proteolytic zymogens. Two important mechanisms protect the pancreas from the potential degradative action of its own digestive enzymes. The synthesis of proteolytic enzymes as proenzymes requires extrapancreatic trigger enzymes for activation. In addition, pancreatic juice contains a low concentration of trypsin inhibitor, which inactivates trypsin and partially inhibits chymotrypsin. Proteolytic activity in the intestinal lumen is not inhibited because the concentration is minimal. Lipase, amylase, and nucleases are secreted in their active form by the acinar cells. Colipase facilitates the action of lipase by binding to the bile salt-lipid surface and by lowering the optimum pH of lipase from 8.5 to 6.5, the normal luminal pH in the duodenum.[10]

The regulation of exocrine pancreatic secretion depends on stimulatory and inhibitory factors exerted through hormonal and neuronal mechanisms. Two hormones, secretin (SC) and cholecystokinin (CCK), play an important role in mediating pancreatic secretion and have synergistic effects: SC stimulates ductular cells to increase water and bicarbonate; CCK stimulates acinar cells to secrete a juice that is low in volume and bicarbonate but rich in enzyme content. The release of SC from the intestinal mucosa is pH dependent and occurs when the duodenal pH is approximately 4.5. Below this pH, titratable acid in the duodenum governs pancreatic bicarbonate output. Although the postprandial release of SC is small, nonacid factors, such as products of fat digestion and bile, can also stimulate SC release. The release of CCK from the small intestine depends on the presence of fatty acids and amino acids in the duodenum. Vasoactive intestinal polypeptide (VIP) is structurally similar to SC and exhibits weak secretin-like effects on exocrine pancreatic secretion. Gastrointestinal peptides such as somatostatin inhibit enzyme secretion by modulating cholinergic transmission.[10]

There are three phases of pancreatic exocrine secretion: cephalic, gastric, and intestinal. In the fasted state, basal secretion occurs at a low rate; output fluctuates in cycles with the interdigestive migrating myoelectric complex (IMMC), so that peak secretions occur during phase III of the IMMC.[10] The cephalic phase is stimulated by the sight and smell of food and is mediated by vagal pathways. Gastric distention and the rate of gastric emptying stimulate an increase in enzyme-rich pancreatic fluid. In the intestinal phase, chyme and acid stimulate pancreatic secretion through the release of SC and CCK. A discussion of pancreatic physiology and pancreatic enzymes is found elsewhere.[10]

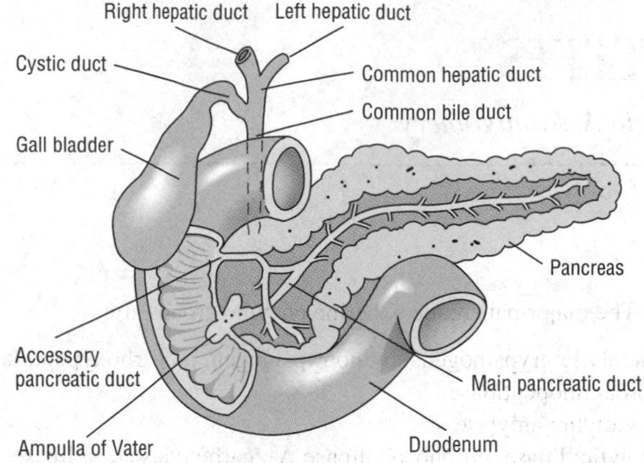

FIGURE 39–1. Anatomic structure of pancreas and biliary tract.

TABLE 39–1. Etiology of Acute Pancreatitis

Structural	Gallstone disease, sphincter of Oddi dysfunction, pancreas divisum, pancreatic tumors
Toxins	Ethanol consumption, scorpion venom, organophosphorus insecticides
Infectious	Bacterial, viral, parasitic
Metabolic	Genetic hypertriglyceridemia, chronic hypercalcemia
Medications	See Table 39–2 for specific drugs
Trauma	Abdominal trauma, postoperative pancreatitis, ERCP*
Vascular	Vasculitis, atherosclerosis, cholesterol emboli, coronary bypass surgery
Other Etiologies	Congenital; idiopathic; hereditary (trypsinogen gene mutations); cystic fibrosis; inflammatory bowel disease; peptic ulcer disease; solid organ transplantation (liver, kidney, heart); refeeding

*ERCP, endoscopic retrograde cholangiopancreatography
(Compiled from references 1–3.)

ACUTE PANCREATITIS

AP varies from mild disease, which is usually self-limiting, to severe disease, in which the severity of the attack correlates with the degree of pancreatic involvement and complications. The morphologic appearance of the pancreas and surrounding tissue ranges from interstitial edema and inflammatory cells (interstitial pancreatitis) to pancreatic and extrapancreatic necrosis (necrotizing pancreatitis), which has a higher risk of infection, organ failure, and mortality.[1–3] The rupture of blood vessels within or around the pancreas may lead to a collection of blood in the retroperitoneal spaces.

ETIOLOGY

The etiologic factors associated with AP are presented in Table 39–1. Gallstone-associated biliary tract disease (30% to 85%) and ethanol use (40%) account for most cases of AP in the United States.[1] The risk of AP after endoscopic retrograde cholangiopancreatography (ERCP) is at least 5%. About 10% to 30% have *idiopathic* pancreatitis, as a cause cannot be determined.[3] Pregnancy is not considered a cause of AP because pregnant women develop pancreatitis as a result of coincident processes, most commonly cholelithiasis. Because of the great functional reserve of the pancreas and the insidious loss of pancreatic function, it is possible that many patients who experience attacks of ethanol-related AP actually have CP.

MEDICATIONS

Many medications have been implicated in AP, but a causal association is difficult to confirm because ethical and practical considerations prevent rechallenge with the suspected agent.[1,3,11–29] Table 39–2 lists medications according to their certainty of causing AP. A "definite" association implies a temporal relationship of drug administration to abdominal pain and hyperamylasemia, or to a positive response to

TABLE 39–2. Medications Associated with Acute Pancreatitis

Definite Association	Probable Association	Possible Association	
5-Aminosalicylic acid	Ampicillin	Acetaminophen	Interleukin-2
Asparaginase	Angiotensin-converting enzyme inhibitors	Amiodarone	Isoniazid
Azathioprine	Bumetamide	Amoxapine	Isotretinoin
Didanosine	Calcium	Carbamazepine	Ketoprofen
Estrogens	Chlorthalidone	Cholestyramine	Ketorolac
Furosemide	Cimetidine	Clarithromycin	Lipid emulsion
Mercaptopurine	Cisplatin	Clonidine	Mefenamic acid
Methyldopa	Clozapine	Cyclosporine	Metolazone
Metronidazole	Corticosteroids	Cyproheptadine	Nitrofurantoin
Pentamidine	Cytarabine	Danazol	Octreotide
Sulfonamides	Ethacrynic acid	Diazoxide	Ondansetron
Sulindac	Ifosfamide	Diphenoxylate	Opiates
Tetracycline	Interferon-α	Ergotamine	Oxyphenbutazone
Thiazides	Meglumine antimoniate	Erythromycin	Paclitaxel
Valproic acid/salts	Procainamide	Famciclovir	Penicillin
	Salicylates	Gold therapy	Piroxicam
	Sodium stibogluconate	Granisetron	Propoxyphene
	Zalcitabine	Hepatitis A vaccination	Ranitidine
		Ibuprofen	Tryptophan
		Indomethacin	Warfarin

(Compiled from Refs. 1, 3, and 11–29.)

rechallenge with the offending agent. Suggestive evidence exists for medications with a "probable" association, whereas evidence is inadequate or contradictory for drugs having a "possible" association. Allergic reactions (e.g., urticaria) usually do not accompany drug-induced AP.

The pathogenesis of drug-induced pancreatitis does not appear to differ from other causes of AP. Exactly how medications induce AP is unknown, but postulated mechanisms include immune-mediated inflammatory response, direct cellular toxicity, pancreatic duct constriction, arteriolar thrombosis, and metabolic effects. It is possible that thiazide diuretics lead to hypotension and pancreatic ischemia. Combination therapy with several medications has also been reported to cause AP.[24,25] Although AP is an infrequent complication of drug therapy, it is prudent to withdraw medication when an association is suspected. Discussion of the specific medications associated with AP can be found elsewhere.[11–29]

PATHOPHYSIOLOGY

The pathophysiology of AP is based on events that initiate the injury and secondary events that establish and perpetuate the injury (Fig. 39–2). The premature activation of pancreatic zymogens within the acinar cells, pancreatic ischemia, or pancreatic duct obstruction initiates AP and leads to a series of secondary events that determine the duration and severity of the injury. Trypsinogen autoactivation and trypsinogen activation by the lysosomal enzyme cathepsin B account for the intracelluar activation of trypsinogen and the zymogen cascade.[1] The release of active pancreatic enzymes directly causes local or distant tissue damage, or may enhance inflammation by activating the alternate complement pathway. Trypsin digests cell membranes and leads to the activation of other enzymes within the pancreas. Lipase damages the fat cells, producing noxious substances that cause further pancreatic and peripancreatic injury. The release of cytokines by the acinar cell or the inflammatory cells directly injures the acinar cell and enhances the inflammatory response. Injured acinar cells liberate chemoattractants that attract neutrophils, macrophages, and other cells to the area of inflammation. Vascular damage and ischemia causes the release of kinins, which makes capillary walls permeable and promotes tissue edema. The release of damaging oxygen-free radicals appears to correlate with the severity of pancreatic injury.[1] Pancreatic infection may result from increased intestinal permeability and translocation of colonic bacteria.

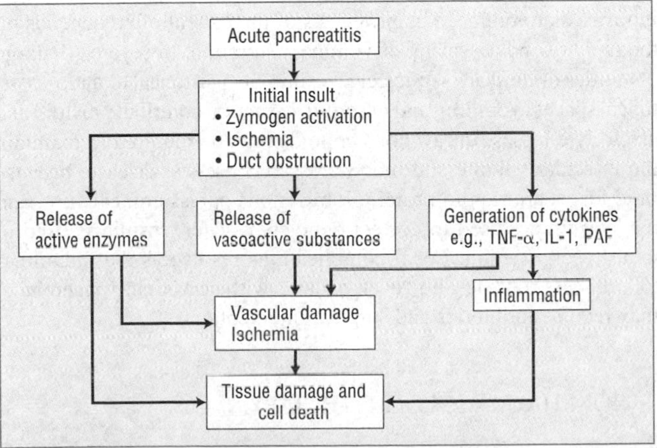

FIGURE 39–2. Pathophysiology of acute pancreatitis—initiating and secondary events. PAF, platelet-activating factor; TNF-α, tumor necrosis factor-α; IL-1, interleukin-1.

COMPLICATIONS

Local complications—including acute fluid collection, pancreatic necrosis, abscess, and pseudocyst (collection of pancreatic juice and tissue debris enclosed by a wall of fibrous or granulation tissue)—develop about 4 weeks after the initial attack. Mortality after a pseudocyst rupture may be as high as 50%.[1] Pancreatic abscess is usually a secondary infection of necrotic tissue or pseudocysts and correlates with the severity of the pancreatitis. Most deaths result from infected necrosis and sepsis.[1,3] Pancreatic ascites occurs when pancreatic secretions spread throughout the peritoneal cavity.

Systemic complications include cardiovascular, renal, pulmonary, metabolic, hemorrhagic, and central nervous system abnormalities.[1] Of the early complications, shock is the main cause of death. Hypotension results from hypovolemia, hypoalbuminemia, the release of kinins, and sepsis. Renal complications are usually caused by hypovolemia. Pulmonary complications develop when fluid accumulates within the pleural space and compresses the lung and the acute respiratory distress syndrome (ARDS) restricts gas exchange. The most common cause of hypoxemia in patients with AP is ARDS. Pleural effusions occur in 4% to 17% of patients with AP and occur more frequently on the left.[1] Gastrointestinal (GI) bleeding occurs secondary to numerous causes including rupture of a pseudocyst. Severe AP is associated with confusion and coma.

CLINICAL PRESENTATION

SIGNS AND SYMPTOMS

The clinical presentation of AP varies depending on the severity of the inflammatory process and whether damage is confined to the pancreas or involves contiguous organs.[1,3] The observation incidence of typical signs and symptoms are:

Abdominal pain: 95%
Radiation of pain to back: 50%
Abdominal distention: 75%
Nausea and vomiting: 80%
Low-grade fever: 75%
Hypotension: 30%
Mental aberrations: 25%
Jaundice: 20%

The initial presentation ranges from moderate abdominal discomfort to excruciating pain, shock, and respiratory distress. Abdominal pain, the major symptom of nearly all patients, is usually epigastric, often radiating to either of the upper quadrants or the back. The onset is usually sudden and the intensity is often described as "knife-like" or "boring." Generally, the pain of AP tends to be steady and usually persists for several days. Repositioning the patient relieves very little of the pain. Nausea and vomiting usually follow the onset of pain. Marked epigastric tenderness, abdominal distention, hypotension, and low-grade fever are observed with widespread pancreatic inflammation and necrosis. In severe disease, bowel sounds are diminished or absent; dyspnea and tachypnea are signs of acute respiratory complications.

DIAGNOSIS

The gold standard for diagnosis of AP is surgical examination of the pancreas or pancreatic histology. In the absence of these procedures, the diagnosis depends on the recognition of an etiologic factor, the clinical signs and symptoms, abnormal laboratory tests, and imaging techniques that predict the severity of the disease. Evaluation of the patient with recurrent acute pancreatitis requires systematic identification and elimination of correctable inciting factors.[30]

LABORATORY TESTS

AP and its complications can be associated with leukocytosis, hyperglycemia, hypoalbuminemia, and mild hyperbilirubinemia. Elevations in serum alkaline phosphatase and liver transaminases are common. Dehydration may lead to hemoconcentration with elevated hemoglobin, hematocrit, blood urea nitrogen (BUN), and serum creatinine concentrations. The total serum calcium is usually normal initially, but hypocalcemia out of proportion to the hypoalbuminemia may develop. Marked hypocalcemia is an indication of severe necrosis and a poor prognostic sign. Some patients with severe AP develop thrombocytopenia and a prolongation in the prothrombin time.

PANCREATIC ENZYMES

A number of laboratory tests are used to detect pancreatic enzymes in the serum and urine. Many of these tests do not provide sufficiently reliable information to be of clinical value. The serum amylase concentration usually rises within 24 hours of the onset of symptoms and returns to normal over the next 3 to 5 days. Persistent elevations suggest extensive pancreatic necrosis and/or related complications; however, serum amylase elevations do not correlate with either the etiology or severity of the disease. In addition, many nonpancreatic diseases may be associated with hyperamylasemia, including salivary, renal, hepatobiliary, metabolic, female reproductive tract, and neoplastic diseases.[1] Pancreatic isoamylase studies assist in determining the origin of elevated serum amylase concentrations, but are not useful for the diagnosis of AP because the diseases that simulate pancreatitis cause pancreatic rather than nonpancreatic amylase concentration to rise.

Serum lipase is specific to the pancreas and concentrations are usually elevated in AP. Serum lipase persists longer than serum amylase elevations and can be detected in the serum after the amylase has returned to normal. The diagnosis of AP is often based on the clinical presentation and an elevated serum amylase or lipase.

IMAGING

A number of radiologic imaging techniques reveal pancreatic abnormalities during the disease course (Table 39–3). None, however, provide a positive diagnosis of AP. The plain film of the abdomen may be useful in ruling out other conditions. Abdominal ultrasonography is indicated in patients with suspected biliary involvement. Computed tomography (CT) is extremely useful in most patients with AP. Contrast-enhanced CT distinguishes interstitial from necrotizing pancreatitis, but does not distinguish between fat necrosis and acute fluid collection. ERCP is used to visualize and remove bile duct stones in patients with gallstone pancreatitis.

CLINICAL COURSE AND PROGNOSIS

The majority of patients with AP recover uneventfully. Mortality rates appear to be influenced by the etiology of the disease and whether the acute attack is an initial or recurrent episode. Mortality is higher during the first attack of AP than during recurrent acute attacks. The severity of an acute attack is predicted using criteria (Ranson's criteria) obtained at the time of admission and during the initial 48 hours of hospitalization (Table 39–4).[1–5] Patients with less than three Ranson criteria have a mortality rate of less than 1%, while those with six or more have a 100% mortality rate.[1,4] The Acute Physiology and Chronic Health Evaluation (APACHE-II) score is more sensitive and specific than Ranson's criteria and can be calculated on admission (Table 39–4).[1,5] Early recognition of severe AP requires aggressive clinical monitoring and therapy. Death during the first few days or weeks often results from systemic complications. When death occurs after this period, it is usually associated with local complications.

► TREATMENT: Acute Pancreatitis

DESIRED OUTCOME

The treatment of AP varies depending on the severity of the attack (Table 39–4, Fig. 39–3). Treatment is aimed at relieving abdominal pain, replacing fluids, minimizing systemic complications, and preventing pancreatic necrosis and infection. In most patients, mild AP is self-limiting and subsides spontaneously within 2 to 7 days of the initiation of supportive care and the reduction of pancreatic secretions. The disease takes a fulminant course in 10% to 15% of patients. Patients with severe AP should be treated aggressively and monitored closely.

GENERAL APPROACH TO TREATMENT

Most patients are initially treated by withholding food or liquids in order to minimize exocrine stimulation of the pancreas. The use of nasogastric aspiration offers no clear advantage in patients with mild AP; however, it is beneficial in patients with profound pain, severe disease, paralytic ileus, and intractable vomiting.[1,3]

Patients with severe AP require aggressive monitoring in an intensive care unit and treatment of cardiovascular, respiratory, renal, and metabolic complications. Fluid resuscitation is essential to correct intravascular volume. The prognosis of the patient often depends on the rapidity and adequacy of volume restoration. In severe AP, large quantities of fluid are sequestered within the peritoneal and retroperitoneal spaces. Vomiting and nasogastric suction contribute to fluid and electrolyte losses. Intravenous colloids may be required to maintain intravascular volume and blood pressure in severe disease, because fluid losses are rich in protein. Intravenous potassium, calcium, and magnesium are used to correct deficiency states. Insulin is used to treat hyperglycemia. Local complications resolve as the inflammatory process subsides; however, patients with necrotizing pancreatitis may require antibiotics and surgical intervention.

NONPHARMACOLOGIC THERAPY

Nutritional deficits develop rapidly in severe AP complicated by tissue necrosis, organ failure, and surgery. Nutritional support should

TABLE 39–3. Practice Guideline Recommendations in Acute Pancreatitis

Practice Parameter	Recommendation
Abdominal Ultrasound	Abdominal ultrasound should be part of the evaluation of the initial episode of acute pancreatitis and should be performed within the initial 24–48 hours of hospitalization. Its use in patients with additional episodes of pancreatitis is to determine whether the cause is gallstones.
Contrast-Enhanced Computed Tomography	Dynamic contrast-enhanced computed tomography (CT) should be performed in patients demonstrated to have severe pancreatitis on the basis of a high APACHE II score and/or evidence of organ failure.
Early Prognostic Signs	The APACHE II score should be generated on the day of admission to help identify patients with severe pancreatitis. After 48 hours, use either the APACHE II score or Ranson's score.
Organ Failure	Monitor closely for the development of organ failure.
Supportive Care	All patients should receive close supportive care including effective pain control, fluid resuscitation, and nutritional support if it is anticipated that oral nutrition will be withheld for >1 week.
Limitation of Systemic Complications	Evidence of significant third space losses require aggressive fluid resuscitation. Patients with severe pancreatitis caused by gallstones should undergo urgent endoscopic retrograde cholangiography. If gallstones are found in the common bile duct, sphincterotomy should be performed and gallstones removed.
Prevention of Pancreatic Infection	In necrotizing pancreatitis associated with organ failure, it is reasonable to initiate treatment with antibiotics with a good spectrum of activity against aerobic and anaerobic bacteria.
Mild Pancreatitis	Fluid resuscitation and careful monitoring are the two most important components of treatment.
Severe Pancreatitis	Dynamic contrast-enhanced CT is recommended after the first 3 days to distinguish interstitial from necrotizing pancreatitis and when pancreatic infection is suspected clinically. (Intravenous contrast should not be used when the creatinine is ≥2 mg/dL; when the creatinine is 1.5–2 mg/dL, intravenous contrast should either not be used or nonionic contrast should be substituted.)
Necrotizing Pancreatitis with Clinical Improvement	If there is symptom improvement in organ failure and general systemic toxicity, medical treatment should be continued, including fluid resuscitation and treatment of systemic complications. Total parenteral nutrition may be required.
Necrotizing Pancreatitis without Clinical Improvement	In the absence of clinical improvement, guided percutaneous aspiration should be performed to distinguish infected necrosis from severe sterile necrosis. Infected necrosis requires surgical débridement. Severe sterile necrosis can usually be treated medically. A subset of patients may require surgical débridement after 4–6 weeks.
Pancreatic Pseudocyst	Asymptomatic pseudocysts require no specific treatment. Symptomatic pseudocysts can be decompressed by surgical, radiologic, or endoscopic methods.

(Adapted from Ref. 5.)

be initiated if it is anticipated that oral nutrition will be withheld for more than 1 week (Table 39–3).[5] Whether to use parenteral or enteral nutrition is controversial.[31–33] Jejunal feedings are at least similar if not superior to parenteral nutrition.[31,32] Animal models of pancreatitis suggest that enteral feeding prevents infection by decreasing translocation of bacteria across the gut wall.[33] Small, controlled clinical trials support the lower rates of infection in patients who received enteral rather than parenteral feedings.[31,32] If enteral feeding is not possible, total parenteral nutrition (TPN) should be implemented before protein and calorie depletion becomes advanced. Intravenous lipids should not be withheld unless the serum triglyceride concentration is greater than 500 mg/dL.[1,5] At present, there is no clear evidence that nutritional support alters outcome in most patients with AP unless malnutrition exists.[32]

Removal of an underlying biliary tract gallstone with ERCP or surgery usually resolves AP and reduces the risk of recurrence.

TABLE 39–4. Recognition of Clinically Severe Acute Pancreatitis

Prognostic Factor	Criterion
APACHE II Score	>8 during initial 24–48 h
On Admission	
Age (years)	>55
White-cell count/mm^3	>16,000
Glucose (mg/dL)	>200
Lactic dehydrogenase (IU/L)	>350
Aspartate aminotransferase (U/L)	>250
Within 48 Hours	
Decrease in hematocrit (% points)	>10
Increase in blood urea nitrogen (mg/dL)	>5
Calcium (mg/dL)	<8
Partial pressure of oxygen (mm Hg)	<60
Base deficit (mmol/L)	>4
Estimated fluid deficit (L)	>6
Organ Failure (Shock)	
Systolic blood pressure (mm Hg)	<90
Pulmonary insufficiency (mm Hg)	≤60
Renal failure, creatinine (mg/dL)	>2
Gastrointestinal bleeding (mL/24 h)	>500
Pancreatitis Necrosis	>30% necrosis by contrast-enhanced computed tomography

(Compiled from Refs. 1–5.)

Surgery may be indicated in AP to treat pseudocyst, pancreatic abscess, and to drain the pancreatic bed if hemorrhagic or necrotic material is present.

PHARMACOLOGIC THERAPY

RECOMMENDATIONS

Whenever possible, discontinue the medications listed in Table 39–2. Patients should receive close supportive care including effective pain control, fluid resuscitation, and nutrition support, if needed (Table 39–3). Antisecretory drugs may be used to prevent stress-related bleeding. Octreotide may be tried in severe AP, but its efficacy remains uncertain (Fig. 39–3). Antibiotics should not be used in the absence of signs of infection except in patients with biliary tract gallstones or in severe AP when pancreatic necrosis or abscess is likely. Patients with life-threatening complications require additional intensive medical therapy or surgery.

RELIEF OF ABDOMINAL PAIN

Analgesics are administered to reduce the severity of abdominal pain. Although the administration of narcotics is associated with mild and transient increases in serum amylase and lipase, these effects are not deleterious to the patient. A traditional approach is to begin with parenteral meperidine (50–100 mg) every 4 hours, because it causes less spasm of the sphincter of Oddi than other narcotic medications.[3,34] Although increased pancreatic duct pressure may correlate with the severity of pain, the difference in the degree of spasm produced by meperidine and equipotent doses of morphine is of questionable clinical importance. The most important factors to consider in selecting an analgesic are efficacy and safety. Morphine should be used in patients who require frequent (e.g., every 2–3 hours) parenteral doses of meperidine, whose pain is unresponsive to large doses (total of >600 mg/d) of meperidine, or whose renal function precludes use of meperidine. Patient-controlled analgesia often achieves adequate pain control. However, it is important to evaluate the need for narcotic medication daily in order to prevent overuse. There is no evidence that antisecretory drugs prevent an exacerbation of abdominal pain.[5]

LIMITATION OF SYSTEMIC COMPLICATIONS AND PREVENTION OF PANCREATIC NECROSIS

Vigorous fluid resuscitation and appropriate pulmonary care are the most important ways to limit systemic complications. It is not clear whether aggressive fluid resuscitation alone is beneficial in preventing

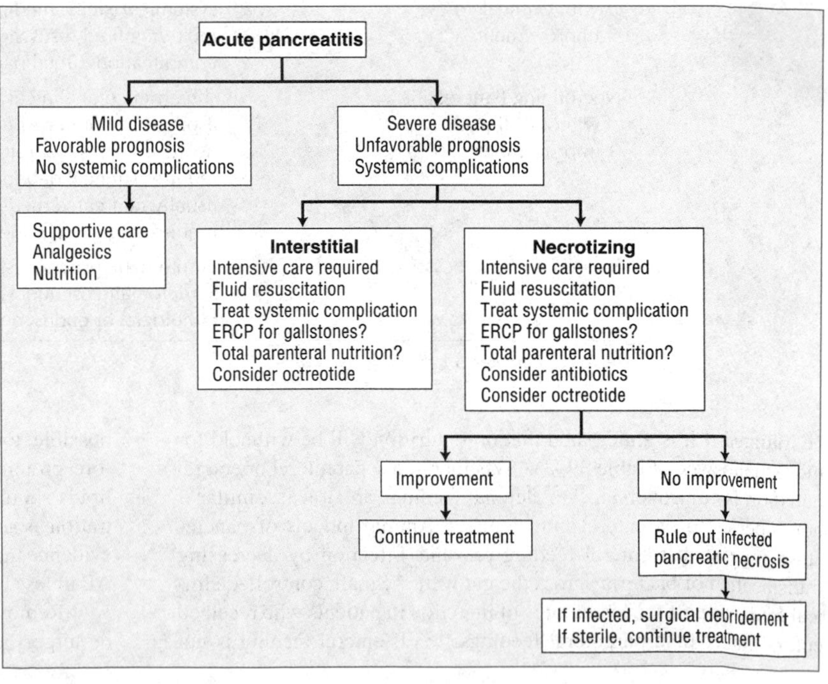

FIGURE 39–3. Guidelines for evaluation and treatment of acute pancreatitis.

pancreatic necrosis. Currently, there is no other available proven method to limit these complications.[5] Potential therapies are aimed at either directly or indirectly reducing pancreatic secretion, inhibiting the action of circulating inflammatory mediators, or increasing pancreatic microcirculation. Procedures such as ERCP, hypothermia, nasogastric suction, pancreatic irradiation, peritoneal lavage, and thoracic duct drainage remain unproven.[1,5]

Antisecretory drugs are no more effective than nasogastric suction or withholding food when used to diminish exocrine secretion. Oral pancreatic enzyme supplementation does not appear to relieve pain, decrease analgesic requirements, or decrease the incidence of complications.[35] Studies fail to confirm the value of protease inhibitors such as aprotinin and gabexate mesilate.[36,37] Drugs such as lexipafant that block circulating inflammatory mediators produced by platelets and white blood cells may have a beneficial effect.[36,38] Low-molecular-weight dextran appears to increase pancreatic microcirculation in experimental animal models, but its efficacy in preventing pancreatic necrosis in humans requires further study.[1,39] Conflicting or inconclusive data exist regarding the efficacy of antioxidants, glucagon, calcitonin, atropine, α-aminocaproic acid, 5-fluorouracil, corticosteroids, and indomethacin.[36]

Somatostatin and Octreotide

The efficacy of somatostatin and its analog octreotide in AP is unclear. Although these agents inhibit pancreatic enzyme secretion, experimental animal models indicate that basal and stimulated pancreatic secretion is reduced in AP.[40,41] Other potential benefits of somatostatin include a possible cytoprotective effect on pancreatic acinus cells and improved intestinal absorption of water and electrolytes. When all patients with pancreatitis are included in clinical trials, octreotide does not appear to be beneficial.[36,40–42] However, in severe AP (patients meeting three or more Ranson's criteria), octreotide 0.1 mg subcutaneously every 8 hours decreased sepsis and length of hospital stay.[43] Reports of this ongoing trial indicate a trend in reduction of mortality. A case-controlled trial in patients with necrotizing pancreatitis also reported a decrease in mortality when octreotide 0.1 mg was given intravenously three times a day.[44] Alternatively, a large, randomized, double-blind trial found that octreotide had no effect on mortality, complications of pancreatitis, or length of stay in patients with moderate to severe AP.[45] High-dose octreotide (0.5 μg/kg/h given by continuous intravenous infusion) provided a more pronounced decrease in serum amylase, greater improvement in pancreatic edema, and earlier return to oral intake than controls.[46] Until there is more definitive data, octreotide use should be limited to patients with severe AP, as it may decrease mortality and possibly the length of hospital stay.

PREVENTION OF INFECTION

The use of prophylactic antibiotics does not offer any therapeutic advantage in patients with mild ethanol-induced AP who do not have necrosis.[2,4,47] Antibiotics may be warranted in patients with biliary or pancreatic duct obstruction, necrotizing pancreatitis, and in patients with likely pancreatic abscess. Early clinical trials found no benefit from use of antibiotics in AP, but studies were flawed as they included patients with all degrees of disease severity and did not have a sufficient number of patients with severe necrotizing AP.[47,48] In addition, the antibiotics employed (including ampicillin) did not penetrate well into pancreatic tissue. The importance of antibiotic penetration into pancreatic tissue has been debated, however, as it is the peripancreatic retroperitoneal necrotic fat and debris, not the pancreas itself, that becomes infected.[36,47] Randomized clinical trials in patients with severe AP have yielded conflicting results.[49–51] Cefuroxime prophylaxis lowered mortality, length of hospital stay, and the overall infection rate, but a decrease in the total number of infections was attributed to fewer urinary tract infections in the antibiotic group.[49] In contrast, prophylaxis with either ceftazidime, amikacin, and metronidazole or imipenem/cilastatin decreased the incidence of sepsis and reduced length of stay, but had no effect on mortality.[50,51] Despite differences among the studies, the results of a meta-analysis demonstrated a reduction in mortality associated with the use of broad spectrum antibiotics in severe AP.[52]

Although somewhat controversial, most experts consider it to be reasonable to use antibiotic prophylaxis for patients with severe AP (Table 39–3, Fig. 39–3).[2,4,5] Because the source of bacterial contamination is most likely the colon, the choice of antibiotic should be broad spectrum, covering the range of enteric aerobic gram-negative bacilli and anaerobic microorganisms.[4,5] The antibiotics selected should be able to penetrate pancreatic tissue and peripancreatic necrotic tissue: for example, with metronidazole, imipenem/cilastatin, mezlocillin, and certain fluoroquinolones; penetration of aminoglycosides is poor.[47,53] In a randomized comparison of perfloxacin and imipenem/cilastin, the fluoroquinolone was associated with a higher rate of infected necrosis.[54] Antibiotics should be started as soon as possible after diagnosis. The duration of treatment remains uncertain, although a 4-week course has been recommended.[47] Selective gut decontamination may be of benefit, but randomized controlled trials are needed to evaluate its efficacy compared to parenteral antibiotics.

CHRONIC PANCREATITIS

CP is an inflammatory condition that usually results in functional and structural damage to the pancreas. In most patients, CP is progressive and loss of pancreatic function is irreversible. Permanent destruction of pancreatic tissue usually leads to exocrine and endocrine insufficiency.[6–9] Cystic fibrosis may be associated with pancreatic exocrine insufficiency in children and is discussed in Chap. 30.

ETIOLOGY

Etiologic risk factors associated with CP are identified in Table 39–5. Prolonged ethanol consumption accounts for 70% of all cases in the United States, 20% are idiopathic, and 10% constitute other less frequent causes.[6–9] Several epidemiologic studies suggest that tobacco smoking is an independent risk factor for CP.[7] Autoimmune pancreatitis may be isolated or occur in association with immune-mediated disorders. Although cholelithiasis may coexist with CP, gallstones rarely lead to chronic disease.

PATHOPHYSIOLOGY

The exact pathogenic mechanism of ethanol-induced CP is uncertain. Inferences can be made from the effects of ethanol on pancreatic tissue and secretion. It appears that ethanol-induced pancreatitis progresses from inflammation to cellular necrosis, and that fibrosis occurs over time. Chronic alcoholism results in a number of changes in pancreatic fluid that creates an environment for the formation of intraductal

TABLE 39–5. Etiologic Risk Factors Associated with Chronic Pancreatitis

Toxic	Ethanol, tobacco, organotin compounds [e.g., di-*n*-butyltin dichloride (DBTC)]
Metabolic	Chronic hypercalcemia associated with hyperparathyroidism, chronic hypertriglyceridemia (controversial), chronic renal failure
Obstructive	Pancreatic divisum, pancreatic duct obstruction (e.g., tumor), sphincter of Oddi (controversial)
Idiopathic	Tropical pancreatitis
Genetic	Autosomal dominant, autosomal recessive/modifier genes (e.g., cystic fibrosis)
Autoimmune	Isolated autoimmune, syndromic autoimmune (e.g., Sjögren's syndrome, inflammatory bowel disease, primary biliary cirrhosis)
Other Etiologies	Postirradiation, postnecrotic pancreatitis, vascular diseases

(Compiled from Refs. 6–9, 55.)

protein plugs that block small ductules.[6] Blockage of the ductules produces progressive structural damage in the ducts and the acinar tissue. Calcium complexes to the protein plugs, first in the small ductules and then in the main pancreatic duct (Fig. 39–1), eventually resulting in injury and destruction of pancreatic tissue. Other theories have been hypothesized, all of which lead to pancreatic destruction and insufficiency.[6]

The pathogenesis of the abdominal pain associated with CP is multifactorial and related, in part, to increased intraductal pressure secondary to continued pancreatic secretion, pancreatic inflammation, and abnormalities involving pancreatic nerves. Malabsorption of protein and fat occurs when the capacity for enzyme secretion is reduced by 90%.[6] Lipase secretion decreases more rapidly than the proteolytic enzymes. Bicarbonate secretion may be decreased leading to a duodenal pH of <4.0.[6] A minority of patients develop complications including pancreatic pseudocyst, abscess, and ascites or common bile duct obstruction leading to cholangitis or secondary biliary cirrhosis. Bleeding is associated with a variety of causes.

CLINICAL PRESENTATION

SIGNS AND SYMPTOMS

The classic features of CP are abdominal pain, malabsorption, weight loss, and diabetes.[6,9] Jaundice occurs in about 10% of patients and results from extrahepatic biliary tract obstruction secondary to fibrosis of the head of the pancreas or stenosis of the common bile duct. Complications, including pancreatic pseudocysts, pleural effusions, and ascites, may be detected on physical examination.

Abdominal pain, either consistent or episodic, is the most prominent clinical feature and is described as dull, epigastric, and radiating to the back. Characteristically, the pain is deep-seated, positional, frequently nocturnal, and unresponsive to medication. The intensity of the pain varies from mild to severe, and does not usually correlate directly with the inflammatory process or other physical findings. Severe attacks last from several days to several weeks and may be aggravated by eating. Most alcoholic patients have chronic pain, while others have intermittent attacks or painless pancreatitis. Nausea, vomiting, and weight loss often accompany the pain. Abstinence from ethanol may provide relief from pain, but does not prevent exocrine dysfunction.[6,9] The course of pain is unpredictable, but frequently lessens as pancreatic insufficiency progresses.[55]

Steatorrhea (excessive loss of fat in the feces) and azotorrhea (excessive loss of protein in the feces) are seen in most patients. Steatorrhea—often associated with diarrhea and bloating—occurs earlier and is most troublesome. About 50% of patients with advanced pancreatic insufficiency present with vitamin B_{12} malabsorption.

Nausea, vomiting, anorexia, and weight loss are often seen in CP patients. Weight loss occurs primarily from avoidance of food because of fear of a painful response to eating. Pancreatic diabetes is usually a late manifestation that is commonly associated with pancreatic calcification. Malabsorption or poorly controlled diabetes may contribute to a reduction in weight. Neuropathy is common and may result from the additive effects of prolonged ethanol ingestion and malnutrition. Ketoacidosis, vascular complications, and nephropathy are uncommon with this form of diabetes.

DIAGNOSIS

Most patients with CP have a history of heavy ethanol use and attacks of recurrent upper abdominal pain. The classic triad of calcification, steatorrhea, and diabetes usually confirms the diagnosis.[6,9] Serum amylase and lipase concentrations usually remain normal unless the pancreatic duct is blocked or a pseudocyst is present. The white blood cell count, fluids, and electrolytes usually remain normal unless fluids and electrolytes are lost as a result of vomiting and diarrhea. Malabsorption of fat can be detected by Sudan staining of the feces or by a 72-hour quantitative measurement of fecal fat.

Surgical biopsy of pancreatic tissue through laparoscopy or laparotomy is the gold standard for confirming the diagnosis of CP.[7] In the absence of histologic samples, imaging techniques are helpful in detecting calcification of the pancreas, other causes of pain (ductal obstruction secondary to stones, strictures, or pseudocysts), and in differentiating CP from pancreatic cancer (see Chap. 31). Ultrasound is the simplest and least expensive of the imaging techniques. The abdominal CT is often used in patients who have a negative or unsatisfactory untrasound examination. ERCP is considered to be the most sensitive and specific test for the diagnosis of CP.[6,56] However, because it is expensive and is associated with complications, it is reserved for patients in whom the diagnosis cannot be established by imaging techniques. Direct tests of pancreatic exocrine function involve the collection of pancreatic fluid after stimulation with exogenous hormones such as secretin or cholecystokinin. These functional tests are not diagnostic of CP, but serve as a sign of CP and a measure or the severity of injury.[6,7] Because these tests are complicated and require intubation and special collection techniques, they are not routinely performed.

CLINICAL COURSE AND PROGNOSIS

Patients with alcoholic CP usually present with an initial acute attack followed by successive attacks that are slower to resolve. Continued ethanol use leads to chronic abdominal pain and progressive exocrine and endocrine insufficiency. In about 50% of patients, the pain diminishes 5 to 10 years after the onset of symptoms.[57] Steatorrhea, calcification, and diabetes usually develop after 10 to 20 years of heavy ethanol ingestion. Most patients present with varying degrees of pain, malnutrition, and glucose intolerance. The mortality rate of CP is approximately 50% within 20 to 25 years of the diagnosis.[9] About 15% to 20% actually die of complications associated with acute attacks. Most deaths occur as a consequence of malnutrition, infection, or ethanol, narcotic, and tobacco use. The clinical course of idiopathic CP is more favorable than alcoholic pancreatitis.[6,7]

▶ TREATMENT: Chronic Pancreatitis

DESIRED OUTCOME

The treatment of uncomplicated CP is aimed primarily at the control of chronic abdominal pain (Fig. 39–4) and the correction of malabsorption with pancreatic enzymes (Fig. 39–5). Diabetes associated with CP may require exogenous insulin.

GENERAL APPROACH TO TREATMENT

The majority of patients with ethanol-related CP require pain control and pancreatic enzyme supplementation.[6,8,9,56–66] Avoidance of alcohol usually decreases pain, but analgesics remain the cornerstone of therapy. Nonnarcotic analgesics such as acetaminophen, nonsteroidal anti-inflammatory drugs (NSAIDs), or tramadol should be tried initially. The dose and frequency of administration should be increased before the patient is switched to a narcotic. Patients unresponsive to nonnarcotic analgesics should be given a trial of pancreatic enzymes prior to using narcotics. Narcotics are required for patients with severe pain. Specific endoscopic or surgical procedures, may be necessary in patients refractory to drug therapy. Patients with malabsorption require pancreatic enzymes to reduce steatorrhea and azotorrhea. Most patients achieve satisfactory results with standard-dosage regimens. In patients who remain symptomatic, dietary fat should be reduced. Consideration may also be given to increasing the pancreatic enzyme dose or switching from an uncoated table to a microencapsulated enteric-coated dosage form. The addition of an antisecretory drug should be reserved for those patients who do not respond to these maneuvers or who have documented low duodenal pH levels.

NONPHARMACOLOGIC THERAPY

Abstinence from ethanol is the most important factor in preventing abdominal pain in the early stages of alcoholic CP, although reports of the effect of abstinence from ethanol have varied.[6,9,57] Small and frequent meals (six meals per day) and a diet restricted in fat (50–75 g/d) are recommended to minimize postprandial pancreatic secretion and resulting pain.[67] Parenteral or enteral nutrition (elemental diets) may be necessary, especially if the patient is chronically debilitated and is unlikely to stimulate pancreatic secretion.[31] When weight loss is refractory to diet and exogenous enzymes, supplementation with medium-chain triglycerides should be considered.

In some patients, pain may be associated with pseudocysts, peptic ulcer, cholelithiasis, biliary or duodenal obstruction, or pancreatic cancer, and if detected, may be amenable to other forms of treatment (Fig. 39–4), including endoscopic procedures such as sphincterotomy, pancreatic duct stenting, and lithotriptic destruction of pancreatic calculi.[6,9,57,59] The most common indication for surgery is abdominal pain refractory to medical therapy. Surgical procedures that alleviate pain include a subtotal pancreatectomy, decompression of the main pancreatic duct, or interruption of the splanchnic nerves.[6,9,57,59] Although the pain may "burn out" as the gland deteriorates, it is unreasonable that a patient wait years for spontaneous relief. A percutaneous injection of a corticosteroid or local anesthetic into the celiac ganglion (celiac nerve block) may be attempted. Unfortunately, pain

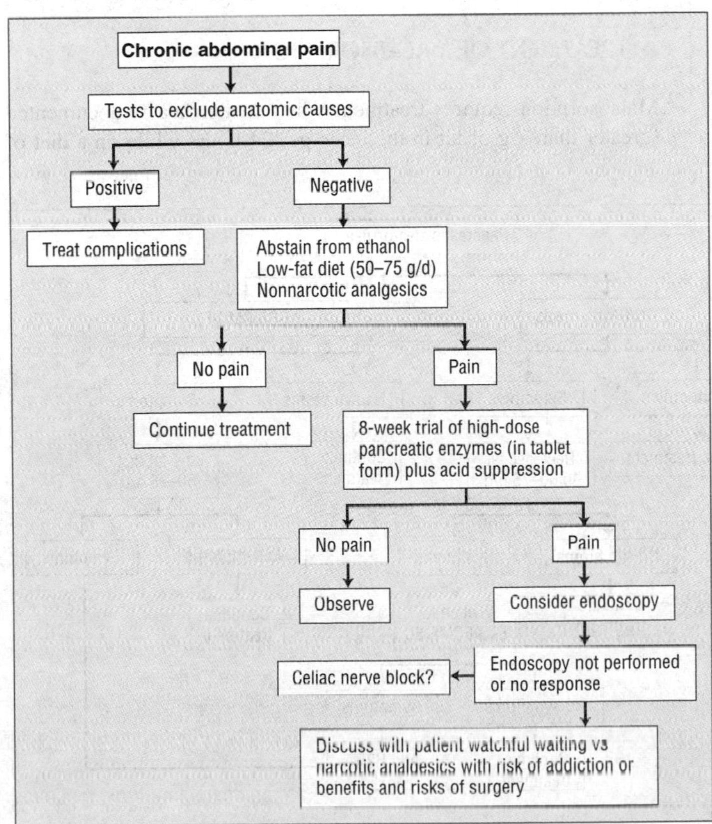

FIGURE 39–4. Guidelines for the treatment of chronic abdominal pain in chronic pancreatitis.

relief obtained by this procedure lasts only a few months, and repeated treatments are not as effective.[57,59]

PHARMACOLOGIC THERAPY

RECOMMENDATIONS

Pain management should begin with nonnarcotic analgesics such as acetaminophen or NSAIDs (Fig. 39–4). If pain persists, the response to exogenous pancreatic enzymes should be evaluated in patients with mild to moderate CP. If these measures fail, the administration of an oral narcotic should be added to the drug regimen. Parenteral narcotics should be reserved for patients with severe pain unresponsive to oral analgesics.

Most patients with malabsorption will require pancreatic enzyme supplementation and a reduction in dietary fat in order to achieve satisfactory nutritional status and become relatively asymptomatic. An initial prandial dose of 30,000 IU of lipase (uncoated tablet, capsule, or powder) is recommended to be given with each meal (Fig. 39–5). Alternatively, the use of microencapsulated enteric-coated dosage forms may be used. The total daily lipase dose should be titrated to reduce steatorrhea. In some patients, a reduction in dietary fat may be necessary. The addition of an antisecretory drug should be reserved for patients resistant to enzyme therapy (Fig. 39–5). If these measures are ineffective, documentation of the diagnosis and exclusion of other diseases should be undertaken.

RELIEF OF CHRONIC ABDOMINAL PAIN

Analgesics

Nonnarcotic analgesics such as acetaminophen or NSAIDs should be given before meals to prevent postprandial exacerbation of pain (Table 39–6).[6,8,56–59] Treatment should be individualized and should begin with the lowest effective dose. The dosage regimen should be maximized before switching to narcotic alternatives. Analgesics should be scheduled around the clock, because they may be more effective and the total amount of medication required over 24 hours may be less. Frequently, severe pain relief necessitates the use of opiate analgesics. Narcotics should not be withheld because of the risk of inducing addiction. Oral agents should be added to the nonnarcotic drug regimen before parenteral narcotics are administered.

Pancreatic Enzymes

The administration of high doses of nonenteric-coated pancreatic enzymes early in the course of the disease may afford pain relief by suppressing pancreatic enzyme secretion through a negative feedback mechanism involving proteases present in the duodenum (Table 39–6). However, results from clinical trials are conflicting especially when nonenteric-coated preparations were compared to enteric-coated enzyme products.[6,8,9,56–62] Possible reasons for failure of enzymes to relieve abdominal pain include insufficient concentrations of trypsin within the pancreatic enzyme preparation, a delayed release of trypsin from pH-dependent dosage forms and gastric acid inactivation or proteolytic destruction of trypsin.[6,8,56–62] Suppression of gastric acid with an antisecretory drug is recommended as it reduces the degradation of proteases in the stomach.[56] Beneficial effects occur in a subset of individuals, primarily those with mild to moderate disease and in patients with a nonethanol etiology.[6,8,57,59]

Other Agents

A number of other agents, including octreotide, allopurinol, and antioxicant therapy (e.g., organic selenium, vitamin E, vitamin C, β-carotene) have been investigated for the purposes of relieving pain in chronic pancreatitis.[6,8,57] There is insufficient evidence to support the use of these agents.

TREATMENT OF MALABSORPTION

Malabsorption requires treatment when steatorrhea is documented (greater than 7 g of fat in the feces per 24 hours while on a diet of

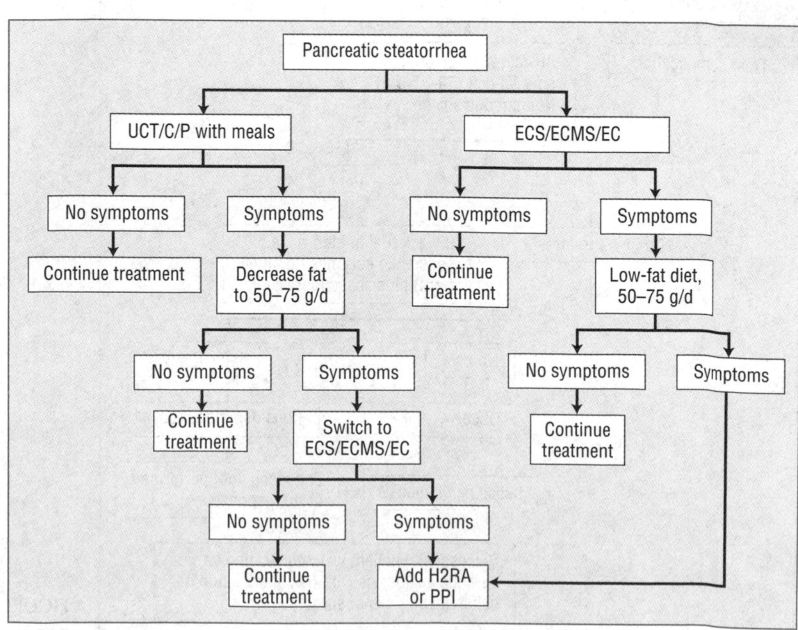

FIGURE 39–5. Guidelines for the treatment of pancreatic steatorrhea in chronic pancreatitis. C, capsule; ECMS, enteric-coated microsphere; ECMT, enteric-coated microtablet; ECS, enteric-coated sphere; H2RA, H2-receptor antagonist; P, powder; PPI, proton pump inhibitor; UCT, uncoated tablet.

TABLE 39–6. Guidelines for the Pharmacologic Treatment of Chronic Pancreatitis

Treatment of Chronic Pain (Oral Drug Regimens)
Nonnarcotic
- Acetaminophen—dosage should be limited to 500 mg four times a day if patient drinks more than two alcoholic beverages per day; increased risk of hepatotoxicty especially in chronic, heavy ethanol use.
- Nonsteroidal anti-inflammatory drugs (NSAIDs)—standard dosage regimens of aspirin, traditional NSAIDs (e.g., ibuprofen), or cyclooxygenase-2 inhibitors (COX-2) NSAIDs; risk of upper gastrointestinal (GI) bleeding in patients with a history of GI bleeding; caution in renal insufficiency.
- Tramadol—50–100 mg every 4–6 hours not to exceed 400 mg/d; has narcotic-like effect; contraindicated in ethanol or hypnotic intoxication; drug interactions; expensive.

Narcotics
- Codeine 30–60 mg every 6 h; hydrocodone 5–10 mg every 4–6 h; oxycodone 5–10 mg every 6 h; fentanyl patch 25–100 μg/h; pentazocine 25–50 mg every 4–6 h; propoxyphene 65 mg every 4–6 h not to exceed 390 mg/d; methadone 2.5–10 mg every 4–6 h; morphine sulfate (extended release) 30–60 mg every 8–12 h; hydromorphone 2–4 mg every 4–6 h.
- Risk of potentiation with ethanol; impaired respiration; constipation; hypotension.
- Dosing is usually based on providing continuous pain relief. consider combining narcotic with acetaminophen or NSAIDs; narcotic dependence is common; narcotic abuse is a concern in alcoholics; tolerance to narcotics may develop.

Pancreatic Enzyme Supplements
- Requires high doses of proteases delivered to the duodenum for relief of pain; nonenteric-coated pancreatic enzymes are recommended; should be taken with each meal and at night if needed; recommend name brands with proven efficacy and safety as generic products have been associated with treatment failure; add antisecretory drug (H_2-receptor antagonist or proton pump inhibitor).
- Viokase, Cotazyme, or Ku-Zyme HP—six to eight with each meal; acid suppression adds to cost.
- May cause nausea, cramping, hyperuricemia; hypersensitivity to pork protein.

Treatment of Maldigestion and Steatorrhea
Nonenteric-Coated Pancreatic Enzymes
- Viokase, Cotazym, or Ku-Zyme HP—six to eight with each meal and at bedtime if needed
- May cause nausea, cramping, hyperuricemia; hypersensitivity to pork protein.
- Addition of antisecretory drug (H_2-receptor antagonist or proton pump inhibitor) may increase efficacy, but will also increase cost.

Enteric-Coated Pancreatic Enzymes
- Enteric-coated spheres, microspheres, and microtablets are available (Table 39–7).
- May cause nausea, cramping, hyperuricemia; hypersensitivity to pork protein.
- Fibrosing colonopathy has occurred in children using preparations that contain the methacrylic acid copolymer coating.
- Usually requires less capsules/tablets per meal; compliance issues.
- Does not usually require additional antisecretory agents; may be less expensive than nonenteric-coated plus antisecretory agent.

Antisecretory Drugs
- May improve enzyme treatment of pain or steatorrhea.
- Proton pump inhibitors may be more effective than H_2-receptor antagonists, but they are also more costly.

(Compiled from Refs. 6, 8, 56–59, and 63.)

100 g/d of fat) and persistent weight loss occurs despite efforts to correct it. The combination of pancreatic enzymes (lipase, amylase, and protease) and a reduction in dietary fat (to less than 25 g/meal) enhances the patient's nutritional status and reduces (but does not totally correct) steatorrhea.

The success of a pancreatic enzyme preparation requires that it contain a high concentration of lipase and proteases, be enteric-coated to avoid destruction by gastric acid, and be the appropriate size to permit efficient delivery of the enzymes to the small intestine.[6,8,62–65,68,69] A critical amount of enzymes must be delivered to the duodenum in sufficient concentrations for digestion to occur. The maximal delivery of pancreatic lipase following a meal is approximately 140,000 IU/h for 4 hours.[6] Malabsorption is minimized if the concentration of enzymes delivered to the duodenum is at least 5% of normal maximal enzyme output. This requires that about 30,000 IU of lipase and 10,000 IU of trypsin be delivered during the 4-hour postprandial period.[6,63]

Most exogenous lipase is rapidly and irreversibly destroyed at an intragastric pH below 4.[6,9,62–65] Enteric-coating is an effective way to protect the acid-labile enzymes, but the enzymes must be emptied from the stomach at the same rate as the ingested food and released in the duodenum. The polymer used to coat the enzyme is pH-dependent and dissolves in the duodenum (pH > 5), where the enzymes are released.[6,63] If a low (<4) intragastric pH prevails, the enteric-coating will remain intact and the enzymes will be released in the upper portion of the small intestine. A low (<4) duodenal pH may prolong dissolution of the enteric coating and release of the enzymes. The size of the enteric-coated enzyme preparation influences the timing of enzyme delivery to the duodenum.[6,63,68,69] Microencapsulated enteric-coated preparations empty from the stomach in synchrony with food and mix with intestinal chyme more thoroughly than large tablets.[6,63] Because the large enteric-coated tablets do not empty with the stomach contents, they are ineffective in treating pancreatic enzyme insufficiency.

Pancreatic Enzyme Supplements

Oral pancreatic enzyme supplements are available as a powder, uncoated or coated tablet, capsule, enteric-coated sphere (ECS) and microsphere (ECMS), or enteric-coated microtablet (ECMT) encased in a cellulose capsule (Table 39–7). Pancreatic enzyme supplements differ in enzyme content and activity, bioavailability, clinical efficacy, patient acceptance, and cost. Compliance is often a problem because of the number of tablets or capsules required per dose, the need to take them with each meal or snack, and the cost of pancreatic enzyme therapy. Consideration should be given to selecting a product that contains higher lipase activity (Table 39–7) so that fewer tablets or capsules are required. Microencapsulated enteric-coated products are not superior to standard doses of conventional nonenteric-coated enzyme preparations such as Viokase.[6,63] Perhaps this is because a lesser quantity of lipase is sometimes administered when an ECS, ECMS, or ECMT is prescribed. The quantity of active lipase delivered to the duodenum appears to be a more important determinant in pancreatic replacement therapy. Generic pancreatic enzyme preparations have been associated with treatment failures when substituted for brand-name products.[70]

Pancreatic enzymes contain nucleic acids and, when given in high therapeutic doses, have been associated with hyperuricosuria, hyperuricemia, and kidney stones.[6,56,58] Impaired folic acid absorption by oral pancreatic enzymes may lead to folic acid deficiency. GI side effects appear to be dose-related, but occur less frequently with the enteric-coated products. Reports of colonic strictures and intestinal obstruction in cystic fibrosis patients taking high-dose pancreatic

TABLE 39–7. Frequently Used Pancreatic Enzyme Preparations

Product	Dosage Form[b]	Enzyme Content (Units)[a]		
		Lipase	*Amylase*	*Protease*
Cotazym	C	8000	30,000	30,000
Cotazym-S	ECS	5000	20,000	20,000
Creon-5	ECMS	5000	16,600	18,750
Creon-10	ECMS	10,000	33,200	37,500
Creon-20	ECMS	20,000	66,400	75,000
Ku-Zyme HP	C	8000	30,000	30,000
Pancrease	ECMS	4500	20,000	25,000
Pancrease MT-4	ECMT	4000	12,000	12,000
Pancrease MT-10	ECMT	10,000	30,000	30,000
Pancrease MT-16	ECMT	16,000	48,000	48,000
Pancrease MT-20	ECMT	20,000	56,000	44,000
Pancrezyme 4X[c]	UCT	12,000	60,000	60,000
Ultrase MT-12	ECMT	12,000	39,000	39,000
Ultrase MT-18	ECMT	18,000	58,500	58,500
Ultrase MT-20	ECMT	20,000	65,000	65,000
Viokase[d]	P	16,800	70,000	70,000
Viokase-8	UCT	8000	30,000	30,000
Viokase-16	UCT	16,000	60,000	60,000

[a]All listed products contain pancrealipase. Pancrealipase contains not less than 24 USP units of lipase activity, not less than 100 USP units of amylase activity, and not less than 100 USP units of protease activity per mg.
[b]C, powder encased in a cellulose capsule; ECMS, enteric-coated microspheres encased in a cellulose capsule; ECMT, enteric-coated microtablets encased in a cellulose capsule; ECS, enteric-coated sphere encased in a cellulose capsule; P, powder; UCT, uncoated tablet.
[c]Vegetable origin (suitable for vegetarians or those with allergies to beef and pork).
[d]Units of 0.7 g of powder.

enzymes (>20,000 IU lipase/capsule) have led to their withdrawal from the market in the United States.[6,56,71] Sensitization and allergic reactions are uncommon but may occur in patients taking the powder.

Adjuncts to Enzyme Therapy

The use of antacids or antisecretory drugs as adjuncts to pancreatic enzyme supplementation does not unequivocally improve their efficacy.[6,63] The use of these agents in conjunction with oral pancreatic enzymes should maintain luminal gastric and duodenal pH above 4 and enhance lipase activity. Increased duodenal pH also prevents bile acid precipitation, increasing fatty acid solubility. In most studies, antacids appear to have little or no added effect in reducing steatorrhea.[6] The beneficial effects of an H_2-receptor antagonist or proton pump inhibitor result from both an increase in pH and a decrease in intragastric volume.[6,72] Divergent results reported may result from differences in the acid secretory status of the patient. Symptomatic patients whose steatorrhea is not corrected by enzyme replacement therapy and a reduction in dietary fat, may benefit from the addition of an H_2-receptor antagonist. A proton pump inhibitor should be considered in patients who fail to benefit from the addition of an H_2-receptor antagonist. The additional cost of antisecretory therapy and the potential for adverse effects and drug interactions should also be considered.

PHARMACOECONOMIC CONSIDERATIONS

The pharmacoeconomic issues associated with the medical treatment of AP and CP have not been extensively examined. Aggressive medical and surgical care decreases mortality in AP, but the overall cost effectiveness of a specific treatment is unknown. The relief of abdominal pain in AP and CP, as well as pancreatic enzyme supplementation in patients with CP, improves quality of life and nutritional status. Although the efficacy of octreotide in AP remains uncertain, its use in severe AP is reasonable and potentially cost effective. Antibiotic prophylaxis of targeted patients may reduce mortality and length of hospital stay, but pharmacoeconomic studies have not confirmed this suspicion. A reduction in the length of stay, however, could offset the cost of antibiotic therapy.

In some cases, medications that cost more may be more cost effective. This is particularly true with pancreatic enzymes and the microencapsulated enteric-coated dosage forms. These latter may cost more, but they offer greater patient acceptance and compliance when compared to uncoated tablets. In addition, when cost is based on the number of tablets or capsules per day, rather than the cost of a single tablet or capsule, the high-potency preparations are usually similar in price. H_2-receptor antagonist or proton pump inhibitor therapy may actually be cost-effective for patients who are not adequately controlled on maximal enzyme therapy.

EVALUATION OF THERAPEUTIC OUTCOMES

ACUTE PANCREATITIS

In patients with mild AP, pain control, fluid and electrolyte status, and nutrition should be assessed periodically depending on the degree of abdominal pain and fluid loss. Patients with severe AP should be transferred to an intensive care unit for close monitoring of vital signs; prothrombin time; fluid and electrolyte status; white blood cell count; blood glucose; lactic dehydrogenase; aspartate aminotransferase; serum albumin; hematocrit; blood urea nitrogen; and serum creatinine. Continuous hemodynamic and arterial blood gas monitoring is essential. Serum lipase, amylase, and bilirubin require less-frequent monitoring. The patient should be monitored for signs of infection, relief of abdominal pain, and adequate nutritional status. Therapeutic outcome depends on the severity of the acute attack, medical management (which is primarily supportive), and prevention or treatment of infection. Despite appropriate supportive therapy, deterioration of respiratory, renal, and cardiovascular function may lead to death.

CHRONIC PANCREATITIS

The severity and frequency of abdominal pain should be assessed periodically in order to determine the efficacy of the patient's pain control regimen. Most patients with abdominal pain can be adequately controlled on acetaminophen or NSAIDs. A trial of pancreatic enzymes plus acid suppression may relieve pain in patients with mild to moderate disease. Patients with severe pain will require narcotics. In these patients, pain should be monitored daily and medications adjusted accordingly. Some patients will require an endoscopic procedure or surgery.

The effectiveness of pancreatic enzyme supplementation to treat malabsorption is measured by improvement in body weight and stool consistency or frequency. The 72-hour stool test for fecal fat may be used when there is concern regarding the adequacy of treatment. Serum uric acid and folic acid concentrations should be monitored yearly in patients prone to hyperuricemia or folic acid deficiency. Blood glucose must be carefully monitored in the diabetic patient. Therapeutic outcome depends in part on the ability of the patient to discontinue alcohol and tobacco and to maintain adequate nutrition. Pain control and pancreatic enzyme supplementation are important therapeutic measures that contribute to the patient's quality of life. A small number of patients die from complications associated with an acute attack.

CONCLUSIONS

Despite modern medical knowledge, much of what we know about the pathophysiologic mechanisms, diagnosis, and treatment of AP and CP is limited. Current research is aimed at ways to reduce the systemic complications of AP and to eliminate the pain and steatorrhea in CP. In the future, answers to the many questions surrounding the mysteries of these diseases will become known. Until then, treatment is largely supportive, and should include the provision of information to the public about the consequences of ethanol-related diseases such as pancreatitis.

▶ PRINCIPLES OF PHARMACOTHERAPY

Acute Pancreatitis

- Discontinue medications that may potentially cause pancreatitis.
- Patients with severe AP require early and aggressive intravenous fluid and electrolyte resuscitation.
- Use parenteral meperidine to control abdominal pain; morphine should be used in patients with renal impairment or those with an inadequate response to high or frequent meperidine doses.
- Octreotide may be used in severe AP, but its efficacy remains uncertain.
- Antibiotics should not be used in the absence of signs of infection except in patients with biliary tract gallstones or in severe AP when pancreatic necrosis or abscess is likely.

Chronic Pancreatitis

- Abstinence from alcohol is an important factor in preventing abdominal pain in the early stages of ethanol-induced CP.
- Initiate pain control with non-narcotic analgesics such as acetaminophen or NSAIDs. The dose and frequency of administration should be increased before the patient is switched to a narcotic. Parenteral narcotics should be reserved for patients with severe pain unresponsive to oral agents. Patients with frequent or constant pain should receive the lowest effective analgesic dose scheduled around the clock.
- A trial of pancreatic enzymes plus acid suppression should be attempted in patients with mild to moderate disease.
- Pancreatic enzyme supplementation and a reduction of dietary fat are used to treat malabsorption and steatorrhea. An initial lipase dose of about 30,000 IU should be given with each meal.
- Symptomatic patients whose steatorrhea is not corrected by pancreatic enzyme supplementation and a reduction in dietary fat may benefit from the addition of an H_2-receptor antagonist or a proton pump inhibitor. An H_2-receptor antagonist should be used before trying a proton pump inhibitor.

REFERENCES

1. Topazian M, Gorelick FS. Acute pancreatitis. In: Yamada T, Aplers DH, Laine L, et al, eds. Textbook of Gastroenterology, 3rd ed. Philadelphia, Lippincott Williams & Wilkins, 1999:2121–2150.
2. Baron TH, Morgan DE. Acute necrotizing pancreatitis. N Engl J Med 1999;340:1412–1417.
3. Grendell JH. Acute pancreatitis. Clin Perspect Gastroenterol 2000;3:327–333.
4. Dervenis C, Johnson CD, Bassi C, et al. Diagnosis, objective assessment of severity, and management of acute pancreatitis. Int J Pancreatol 1999;25:195–220.
5. Banks PA. Practice guidelines in acute pancreatitis. Am J Gastroenterol 1997;92:377–386.
6. Owyang C. Chronic pancreatitis. In: Yamada T, Aplers DH, Laine L, et al, eds. Textbook of Gastroenterology, 3rd ed. Philadelphia, Lippincott Williams & Wilkins, 1999:2151–2177.
7. Etemad B, Whitcomb DC. Chronic pancreatitis: Diagnosis, classification and new genetic developments. Gastroenterology 2001;120:682–707.
8. Toskes PP. Update on diagnosis and management of chronic pancreatitis. Curr Gastroenterol Rep 1999;1:145–153.
9. Steer ML, Waxman I, Freedman S. Chronic pancreatitis. N Engl J Med 1995;332:1482–1490.
10. Owyang C, Williams JA. Pancreatic secretion. In: Yamada T, Aplers DH, Laine L, et al, eds. Textbook of Gastroenterology, 3rd ed. Philadelphia, Lippincott Williams & Wilkins, 1999:355–379.
11. Eland IA, van Puijenbroek EP, Sturkenboom MJCM, et al. Drug-associated acute pancreatitis: Twenty-one years of spontaneous reporting in the Netherlands. Am J Gastroenterol 1999;94:2417–2422.
12. McArthur KE. Review article: Drug-induced pancreatitis. Aliment Pharmacol Ther 1996;10:23–38.
13. Eland IA, Rasch MC, Sturkenboom MJCM, et al. Acute pancreatitis attributed to the use of interferon alpha-2b. Gastroenterology 2000;119:230–233.
14. Gershon T, Olshaker J. Acute pancreatitis following lisinopril rechallenge. Am J Emerg Med 1998;16:523–524.
15. Maringhini A, Termini A, Patti R, et al. Enalapril-associated acute pancreatitis: Recurrence after rechallenge. Am J Gastroenterol 1997;92:166–167.
16. Izraeli S, Adamson PC, Blaney SM, et al. Acute pancreatitis after ifosfamide therapy. Cancer 1994;74:1627–1628.

17. Liviu L, Yair L, Yehuda S. Pancreatitis induced by clarithromycin. Ann Intern Med 1996;125:701. Letter.
18. Goffin E, Horsmans Y, Pirson Y, et al. Acute necrotic-hemorrhagic pancreatitis after famciclovir prescription. Transplantation 1995;59:1218–1219.
19. Hoff PM, Valero V, Holmes FA, et al. Paclitaxel-induced pancreatitis: A case report. J Natl Cancer Inst 1997;89:91–92. Letter.
20. Rodier JM, Pujade-Lauraine E, Batel-Copel L, et al. Granisetron-induced acute pancreatitis. J Cancer Res Clin Oncol 1996;122:132–133. Letter.
21. Balasch J, Martinez-Romain S, Carreras J, et al. Acute pancreatitis associated with danazol treatment for endometriosis. Hum Reprod 1994;9:1163–1165.
22. Domingo P, Ferrer S, Kolle S, et al. Acute pancreatitis associated with sodium stibogluconate treatment in a patient with human immunodeficiency virus. Arch Intern Med 1996;156:1029–1032. Letter.
23. Torrus D, Massa B, Boix V, et al. Meglumine antimonate-induced pancreatitis. Am J Gastroenterol 1996;91:820–821. Letter.
24. Abdul-Ghaffar N, El-Sonbaty MR. Pancreatitis and rhabdomyolysis associated with lovastatin-gemfibrozil therapy. J Clin Gastroenterol 1995;21:340–341.
25. Stricker R, Man K, Bouvier D, et al. Pancreatorenal syndrome associated with combination antiretroviral therapy in HIV infection. Lancet 1997;349:1745–1746.
26. Sammett D, Greben C, Sayeed-Shah U. Acute pancreatitis caused by penicillin. Dig Dis Sci 1998;43:1778–1783.
27. Goyal SB, Goyal R. Ketorolac tromethamine-induced acute pancreatitis. Arch Intern Med 1998;158:411. Letter.
28. Haviv YS, Sharkia M, Galun E, et al. Pancreatitis following hepatitis A vaccination. Eur J Med Res 2000;5:229–230.
29. Eland IA, Alvarez CH, Stricker BHCH, et al. The risk of acute pancreatitis associated with acid-suppressing drugs. Br J Clin Pharmacol 2000;49:473–478.
30. Somogyi L, Martin SP, Venkatesan T, et al. Recurrent acute pancreatitis: An algorithmic approach to identification and elimination of inciting factors. Gastroenterology 2001;120:708–717.
31. Scolapio J, Malhi-Chowla N, Ukleja A. Nutrition supplementation in patients with acute and chronic pancreatitis. Gastroenterol Clin North Am 1999;28:695–707.
32. Lobo DN, Memon MA, Allison SP, et al. Evolution of nutritional support in acute pancreatitis. Br J Surg 2000;87:695–707.
33. Kotani J, Usami M, Nomura H, et al. Enteral nutrition prevents bacterial translocation but does not improve survival during acute pancreatitis. Arch Surg 1999;134:287–292.
34. Isenhower HL, Mueller BA. Selection of narcotic analgesics for pain associated with pancreatitis. Am J Health Syst Pharm 1998;55:480–486.
35. Patankar RV, Chaund R, Johnson CD. Pancreatic enzyme supplementation in acute pancreatitis. HPB Surg 1995;8:159–162.
36. Ulrich CD. Medical management of acute pancreatitis: Strategies, reality, and potential. Curr Gastroenterol Rep 2000;2:115–9.
37. Messori A, Rampazzo R, Scroccaro G, et al. Effectiveness of gabexate mesylate in acute pancreatitis: A meta-analysis. Dig Dis Sci 1995; 40:734–738.
38. Mckay C, Curran FJ, Sharples CE, et al. The use of lexipafant in the treatment of acute pancreatitis. Adv Exp Med Biol 1996;416:365–370.
39. Holtz HG, Schmidt J, Ryschich EW, et al. Isovolemic hemodilution with dextran prevents contrast medium-induced impairment of pancreatic microcirculation in necrotizing pancreatitis of the rat. Am J Surg 1995; 169:161–166.
40. Uhl W, Anghelacopoulos SE, Friess H, et al. The role of octreotide and somatostatin in acute and chronic pancreatitis. Digestion 1999;60 (suppl 2):23–31.
41. Wyncoll DL. The management of severe acute necrotizing pancreatitis: An evidence-based review of the literature. Intensive Care Med 1999;25: 146–156.
42. Jenkins SA, Berein A. The relative effectiveness of somatostatin and octreotide therapy in pancreatic disease. Aliment Pharmacol Ther 1995;9: 349. Review.
43. Paran H, Neufeld D, Mayo A, et al. Preliminary report of a prospective randomized study of octreotide in the treatment of severe acute pancreatitis. J Am Coll Surg 1995;181:121–124.
44. Fiedler F, Jauernig G, Keim V, et al. Octreotide treatment in patients with necrotizing pancreatitis and pulmonary failure. Int Care Med 1996;22:909–915.
45. Uhl W, Buchler MW, Malfertheiner, P et al. A randomized, double blind multicentre trial of octreotide in moderate to severe acute pancreatitis. Gut 1999;45:97–104.
46. Karakoyunlar O, Sivrel E, Tanir N, et al. High-dose octreotide in the management of acute pancreatitis. Hepatogastroenterology 1999;46:1968–1971.
47. Kramer KM, Levy H. Prophylactic antibiotics for severe AP: The beginning of an era. Pharmacotherapy 1999;19:592–602.
48. Ho HS, Frey CF. The role of antibiotic prophylaxis in severe acute pancreatitis. Arch Surg 1997;132:487–493.
49. Sainio V, Kemppainen P, Poulallainen P, et al. Early antibiotic treatment in acute necrotizing pancreatitis. Lancet 1995;346:663–667.
50. Pederzoli P, Bassi C, Vesentini S, et al. A randomized multicenter clinical trial of antibiotic prophylaxis with imipenem. Surg Gynecol Obstet 1993;176:480–483.
51. Delcenserie R, Yzet T, Ducroix JP. Prophylactic antibiotics in treatment of severe acute alcoholic pancreatitis. Pancreas 1996;13:198–201.
52. Golub R, Siddiai F, Pohl D. Role of antibiotics in acute pancreatitis: A meta-analysis. J Gastrointesinal Surg 1994;178:475–503.
53. Bassi C, Pederzoli P, Vesentini S, et al. Behavior of antibiotics during human necrotizing pancreatitis. Antimicrob Agents Chemother 1994;38: 830–836.
54. Bassi C, Falconi M, Talamini G, et al. Controlled clinical trial of pefloxacin versus imipenem in severe acute pancreatitis. Gastroenterology 1998;115:1513–1517.
55. Ammann RW, Muelihaupt B, Zurich Pancreatitis Study Group. The natural history of pain in alcoholic chronic pancreatitis. Gastroenterology 1999;116;1132–1140.
56. Amann ST. Chronic pancreatitis. Curr Treat Option Gastroenterol 1999; 2:401–408.
57. Warshaw A, Banks PA, Fernandez-del C. AGA technical review: Treatment of pain in chronic pancreatitis. Gastroenterology 1998;115:765–776.
58. Whitcomb D, Pfutzer RH, Slivka A. Alcoholic chronic pancreatitis. Curr Treat Option Gastroenterol 1999;2:273–282.
59. Conwell DL, Zuccaro G. Pain management in chronic pancreatitis. Curr Treat Option Gastroenterol 1999;2:295–304.
60. Brown A, Hughes M, Tenner S, et al. Does pancreatic enzyme supplementation reduce pain in patients with chronic pancreatitis: A meta-analysis. Am J Gastroenterol 1997;92:2032–2035.
61. Mossner J. Palliation of pain in chronic pancreatitis: use of enzymes. Surg Clin North Am 1999;79:861–872.
62. Pitchumoni CS. Chronic pancreatitis: Pathogenesis and management of pain. J Clin Gastroenterol 1998;27:101–107.
63. Greenberger NJ. Enzymatic therapy in patients with chronic pancreatitis. Gastroenterol Clin North Am 1999;28:687–693.
64. Apte MN, Keogh GW, Wilson JS. Chronic pancreatitis: Complications and management. J Clin Gastroenterol 1999;29:225–240.
65. Layer P, Keller J. Pancreatic enzymes: Secretion and luminal nutrient digestion in health and disease. J Clin Gastroenterol 1999;28:2–10.
66. Van Hoozen CM, Peeke PG, Taubeneck M, et al. Efficacy of enzyme supplementation after surgery for chronic pancreatitis. Pancreas 1997;14: 174–180.
67. American Gastroenterologic Association Medical Position Statement: Treatment of pain in chronic pancreatitis. Gastroenterology 1998;1155:763–764.
68. Bruno MJ, Borm JJ, Hock FJ, et al. Gastric transit and pharmacodynamics of a two-millimeter enteric-coated pancreatin microsphere preparation in patients with chronic pancreatitis. Dig Dis Sci 1998;43:203–213.

69. Halm U, Loser C, Lohr M, et al. A double-blind randomized, multicentre, crosssover study to prove equivalence of pancreatin minimicrospheres versus microspheres in exocrine pancreatic insufficiency. Aliment Pharmacol Ther 1999;13:951–957.
70. Littlewood JM. Update on intestinal strictures. J R Soc Med 1999;92 (suppl 37):41–49.
71. Hendeles L, Hochhaus G, Kazerounian S. Generic and alternative brand-name pharmaceutical equivalent: Select with caution. Am J Hosp Pharm 1993:323–329.
72. Bruno MJ, Rauws EAJ, Hoek FJ, et al. Comparative effects of adjuvant cimetidine and omeprazole during pancreatic enzyme replacement therapy. Dig Dis Sci 1994;39:988–992.

40
VIRAL HEPATITIS

Marsha A. Raebel and Thomas G. Vondracek

Hepatitis is a major cause of morbidity and mortality in the United States. Viral hepatitis refers to the clinically important hepatotrophic viruses responsible for hepatitis A (HAV), hepatitis B (HBV), delta hepatitis (HDV), hepatitis C (HCV), and hepatitis E (HEV). Hepatitis G virus (HGV) has also been described, however, its role in clinical illness is still not clear.

About 56,000 cases of hepatitis are reported yearly in the United States, but reporting is incomplete, and the actual numbers are much higher.[1] HAV is estimated to cause 130,000 infections yearly, while HBV is considered responsible for 300,000 cases.[1,2] About 150,000 new cases of HCV occur annually, but because of the high rate with which HCV results in chronic infection, almost 4 million Americans (1.8% of the population) are infected with HCV. Between 9% and 14% of all patients infected with HBV develop chronic hepatitis, while chronic disease develops in 80% of patients with HCV. Many of these patients ultimately die of complications of chronic hepatitis such as cirrhosis or hepatocellular carcinoma (HCC).

Outside the United States, viral hepatitis is also a major health problem. Worldwide, 360 million people are infected with HBV.[3] The World Health Organization lists HBV as the ninth leading cause of death in the world.

Viral hepatitis has acute, fulminant, and chronic clinical forms, defined by duration or severity of infection. The clinical, biochemical, immunoserologic, and histologic features of viral hepatitis follow similar patterns regardless of the virus responsible for the patient's illness. Hepatocellular response to injury and the resulting physical signs and symptoms are nonspecific.

ACUTE VIRAL HEPATITIS

Although acute viral hepatitis is usually a self-limiting disease with a low case-fatality rate, it causes significant human suffering and days of work lost. The disease is a systemic viral infection of up to (but not exceeding) 6 months in duration producing inflammatory necrosis of the liver. The natural history of the infection is divided into three stages based on viral serologic markers: incubation, acute hepatitis, and convalescence. Clinical severity of illness varies widely from asymptomatic, anicteric (no jaundice) hepatitis to a systemic illness accompanied by fever, malaise, anorexia, nausea, abdominal discomfort, dark urine and jaundice, to fatal fulminant hepatitis.[2]

Incubation begins shortly after parenteral or oral inoculation with the virus. After the virus reaches the circulation, infective virions accumulate in hepatic sinusoids and are internalized by the hepatocytes. Internalized viral particles replicate within either the cytoplasm or the nucleus with the assistance of the host cellular apparatus. Infective viral particles are shed into blood, bile, and other body secretions during the later phases of the incubation stage. Complete virions and/or viral antigens appear in body fluids and tissues. The duration of the incubation stage differs for each virus (Table 40–1). During the incubation stage, the host is asymptomatic.

The hepatotrophic viruses cause hepatic injury either because of the host immune response or from direct viral damage to hepatocytes. For example, the acute hepatitis stage in HBV begins once the host recognizes the virus and initiates an active immune response against the invading virions. The resulting cellular and humoral immune response is directed against viral antigens found on the host hepatocyte membranes and/or circulating within the vascular compartment.[4]

Acute hepatitis begins with a preicteric phase (before the onset of jaundice), which parallels initiation of the host immune response and occurs before significant liver cell injury. The preicteric phase is frequently associated with nonspecific influenza-like symptoms consisting of anorexia, nausea, fatigue, and malaise.

Most patients with acute viral hepatitis develop only a few mild symptoms and minimal hepatocyte damage. This mild disease is called *acute anicteric hepatitis*. The minimal degree of liver cell damage is reflected by mild elevations of serum bilirubin, γ-globulin, and hepatic transaminase (alanine transaminase [ALT], aspartate transaminase [AST]) values to about twice normal. Subsets of patients experience enough hepatocyte destruction to produce significant liver dysfunction characterized by interruption of bilirubin metabolism and flow. This results in clinical jaundice and *acute icteric hepatitis*. Icteric hepatitis is generally accompanied by fever, right upper-quadrant abdominal pain, nausea, vomiting, dark urine, acholic (light colored) stools, and worsening of systemic symptoms. Clinical symptoms are accompanied by elevations of the serum bilirubin, γ-globulin, and hepatic transaminases from 4 to 10 times above normal. Viral serologic markers and host antibodies are detectable during this stage of the illness.

Most patients with either acute anicteric or icteric hepatitis go through the convalescence stage to complete recovery without developing complications or chronic sequelae. The duration of disease stages and the risk for developing chronic sequelae are different for each virus (Table 40–1).

HEPATITIS A VIRUS

HAV is the primary cause of worldwide hepatitis epidemics throughout history.[5] It remains a significant cause of clinical hepatitis worldwide, although HEV plays a role in many epidemics. Despite the availability of an effective vaccine against HAV, hepatitis A continues to be one of the most frequently reported vaccine-preventable diseases in the United States.[2] In 1997 dollars, the estimated annual direct and indirect costs of HAV in the United States were more than $300 million.[2]

EPIDEMIOLOGY

HAV causes both epidemics and sporadic infections. Both are related to overcrowded conditions and person-to-person spread or ingestion of contaminated food or water. HAV is transmitted by the fecal-to-oral route. The incidence of HAV correlates directly with poor sanitary conditions and hygienic practices.[1] For international travelers, longer

TABLE 40–1. Features of Clinically Important Hepatitis Viruses

	Hepatitis A	Hepatitis B	Hepatitis C	Hepatitis D	Hepatitis E	Hepatitis G
Virus	HAV	HBV	HCV	HDV	HEV	HGBV or HGV*
Family	Picornavirus	Hepadnavirus	Flavivirus	Satellite	Calcivirus	Flavivirus
Size (nm)	27	42	30–60	40	32	?
Genome	ssRNA	dsDNA	ssRNA	ssRNA	ssRNA	ssRNA
Incubation (days)	14–45	40–180	35–84	40–180 coinfection 14–45 superinfection	14–60	? ?
Transmission	Fecal-oral	Parenteral Sexual Perinatal Mucous membrane	Parenteral Sexual Perinatal Mucous membrane	Parenteral Sexual (?) Perinatal	Fecal-oral	Parenteral
Serologic markers						
Antigens	HAVAg**	HBsAg HBcAg HBeAg	HCVAg	HDVAg	Not available ?	Not available ?
Antibodies	Anti-HAV	Anti-HBs Anti-HBc Anti-HBe	Anti-HCV	Anti-HDV	Not available ?	Not available ?
Viral markers	HAV RNA	HBV DNA DNA polymerase	HCV RNA	HDV RNA	Not available	HGBV-C RNA
Clinical illness						
Children	Anicteric	Anicteric 70%	Anicteric 75%	Not known	High % anicteric	Not clear whether associated with clinical illness
Adults	Icteric	Icteric 30%	Most icteric	Icteric 25%	Not known	
Acute mortality (%)	0.3	0.2–1	0.2	2–20	10 (pregnancy)	?
Chronicity (%)	No	2–7 Neonates 90	70–80	2–70	No	
Hepatocellular carcinoma	No	Yes	Yes	Yes	No	?

*Comprised of several RNA viruses: HGBV-A, HGBV-B, HGBV-C.
**Ag = antigen.

lengths of stay in a country with a high rate of hepatitis A also correlates with increased risk. In the United States, groups at increased risk of HAV, in addition to travelers, include men who have sex with men, injecting-drug users, and persons working with nonhuman primates (Table 40–2).[2]

HAV infection in the United States occurs primarily from person-to-person transmission in communitywide outbreaks, in lower socioeconomic groups, and in sporadic common-source outbreaks (outbreaks in which all infected patients contract the infection from a single person or source).[2] Children between 5 and 14 years old are more likely to be involved in communitywide outbreaks, whereas common-source outbreaks primarily involve young adults. Both children and young adults can be infected from common-source outbreaks at day care centers.[1] HAV infection in children is often asymptomatic or unrecognized. Therefore, children serve as an important source for transmitting the infection to others.[2] Rarely, HAV is transmitted by transfusion of contaminated blood products collected while the donor is viremic with HAV.[2] Cases of HAV associated with parenteral drug abuse are increasing.

PATHOPHYSIOLOGY

HAV replication occurs in the liver. Viral antigens are found in the hepatocyte cytoplasm during incubation. They are subsequently shed into bile and feces. The largest concentration of viral particles is found

TABLE 40–2. Groups at Increased Risk of Hepatitis A and Recommended for Preexposure Hepatitis A Vaccination[2]

- Children living in states, counties, or communities where rates of hepatitis A are at least twice the national average (≥20 cases per 100,000 population). For 1987–1997, these states included Arizona, Alaska, Oregon, New Mexico, Utah, Washington, Oklahoma, South Dakota, Idaho, Nevada, and California.
- Children living in states, counties, or communities where rates of hepatitis A are greater than the national average but lower than twice the national average should be considered for routine vaccination (≥10 cases but <20 cases per 100,000 population). For 1987–1997, these states included Missouri, Texas, Colorado, Arkansas, Montana, and Wyoming.
- Persons traveling to or working in countries that have high or intermediate endemicity of infection.*
- Men who have sex with men.
- Illegal-drug users.
- Persons who have occupational risk for infection, e.g., persons who work with HAV-infected primates or HAV in a research laboratory setting.
- Persons who have clotting-factor disorders.
- Persons who have chronic liver disease, e.g., persons with chronic liver disease caused by hepatitis B or C and persons awaiting liver transplants.

*Travelers to Canada, Western Europe, Japan, Australia, or New Zealand are at no greater risk for HAV infection than they are while in the United States. All other travelers should be assessed for hepatitis A risk.

in stool specimens during the 1 to 2 weeks preceding clinical illness or elevation of liver enzymes. Infected persons are at peak infectivity at this time.[2] Viral shedding declines as clinical symptoms appear. Liver injury is immune mediated with cytolytic T cells the most likely effector cells.[4] Death of hepatocytes results in viral elimination and eventual resolution of the clinical illness. Viremia begins soon after infection and continues throughout the time liver enzymes are elevated.[2]

The host antibody response to HAV initially appears as the viral particles begin to disappear from stool. Like most host antibody responses, antibodies of the IgM class appear first and imply recent infection. IgM anti-HAV usually is detectable 5 to 10 days before symptoms appear. The diagnosis of acute HAV infection is confirmed by anti-HAV IgM. After 2 to 6 months, the IgM antibodies are replaced with IgG antibodies, which usually persist throughout life and confer immunity to HAV.[2] Diagnostic tests detect either IgM or total (IgM and IgG) anti-HAV in serum.[2] Patients who receive IG will have low titers of anti-HAV for several weeks after inoculation.[2] Patients who receive hepatitis A vaccine will also have anti-HAV.[2]

CLINICAL PRESENTATION

Asymptomatic or symptomatic infection with HAV occurs after an average incubation period of 28 days, with a range of 15 to 50 days (Table 40–1).[2] Clinical symptoms are age dependent. Children younger than 6 years old are usually asymptomatic or have a mild, influenza-like illness without clinical jaundice.[2] In contrast, more than 70% of infected adults and older children display the characteristic clinical syndrome of acute hepatitis with elevated hepatic transaminase levels and jaundice.[2]

The vast majority of people who become ill with HAV completely recover. HAV infection usually produces a self-limited illness that lasts less than 2 months, although 10% to 15% of patients exhibit a cholestatic illness with predominant elevations of alkaline phosphatase, γ-glutamyl transferase, and total bilirubin that continues or is relapsing for up to 6 months.[2] Rarely, a relapse is associated with cryoglobulinemia, arthritis, and vasculitis. Pruritus is often a major complaint of these patients.[6] No cases of a chronic carrier state or chronic hepatitis have been reported.

Rarely, HAV may cause fulminant hepatitis, resulting in approximately 100 deaths each year in the United States.[2] The case-fatality rate for HAV is 0.3% overall, with higher rates in older age groups and in those in whom acute HAV is superimposed on chronic HCV.[2,7] But, acute HAV causes significant morbidity and human suffering, with an average of 28 days of work lost for each adult who becomes ill.

The clinical diagnosis of acute HAV infection is based on clinical suspicion, characteristic symptoms, and elevated aminotransferases and bilirubin, but confirmation depends on a positive IgM anti-HAV (Table 40–1). HAV infection cannot be differentiated from other types of viral hepatitis by clinical or epidemiological features.[2]

HEPATITIS B VIRUS

EPIDEMIOLOGY

HBV infection is a worldwide public health problem. The prevalence of HBV infection varies in different geographic areas of the world, with carrier rates ranging from 0.1% to 15%. The National Health and Nutrition Examination Surveys III (NHANES III 1988–1994) reported a 4.9% prevalence of HBV infection in the United States. The highest prevalence of disease was in those with a high number of lifetime sexual partners, those of Black race, and those of foreign birth.[8–11]

In highly endemic areas (China, Southeast Asia, the Middle East, and parts of Africa and South America), HBV spread is predominantly by mother-to-infant perinatal transmission and by child-to-child transmission. In highly endemic areas, high rates of chronic viral carriage and virus-associated primary HCC are seen. In parts of the world in which the endemicity of HBV is relatively low (North America, Australia, Western Europe, and temperate South America), the chronic viral carriage rate is correspondingly low, mother-to-infant transmission is relatively uncommon, and HBV transmission occurs either through intimate contact or parenterally. High-risk groups in low endemicity areas include intravenous drug abusers, multitransfused patients, health care providers, male homosexuals, heterosexual partners of HBV-infected people, and heterosexual partners of human immunodeficiency virus (HIV)-infected individuals.[1]

Transmission of HBV in the United States occurs predominantly through contact with infected blood products or body secretions (e.g., saliva, vaginal fluids, and semen). The routine practice of screening blood donors for HBsAg has essentially eliminated HBV as a cause of posttransfusion hepatitis. However, products or concentrates of blood such as clotting factors can remain infective despite prescreening for HBsAg. Excluding cases resulting from clotting factor concentrates, most blood-borne HBV transmissions are a consequence of accidental inoculation by health care workers or the sharing of needles by intravenous drug abusers (percutaneous exposure).[1]

The chief obstacles to eradication of HBV include the carrier state and infections in utero, neither of which is preventable. Individuals who acquire HBV as children (postnatally) have a very high rate of becoming chronic HBsAg carriers.[9] A small percentage of these children develop complications such as cirrhosis or hepatocellular carcinoma within 20 years of being infected.[9] Unfortunately, for infants who acquire HBV in utero, progression to chronic liver disease occurs in about 90%.

PATHOPHYSIOLOGY

The liver injury in HBV infection (like HAV infection) is immune related, and T lymphocytes are important for both the host cellular and humoral responses.[4] Recovery from acute HBV infection depends on both B cell and T cell responses. B cell-dependent antibodies are produced to pre-S and S antigens, and a cytotoxic T lymphocyte (CTL) response is mounted against multiple epitopes in the HBV envelope, nucleocapsid, and polymerase regions.[10] CTL-mediated lysis of infected hepatic cells occurs, resulting in liver injury. Immune clearance of virus is often accompanied by worsening liver disease, known as a flare. An extreme example of this is seen in fulminant hepatitis B when there is often no evidence of HBV replication when the patient presents—the virus has been rapidly and aggressively cleared by the infected individual's immune system. Immune-mediated viral clearance can also occur through noncytolytic pathways via cytokine release.[10]

HBV is not considered a cytopathic virus; in certain circumstances, however, it can cause direct cytotoxic liver injury. Direct cytopathic liver injury can occur when the viral load is very high, as in the rare fibrosing cholestatic hepatitis.[10]

After the HBV enters the vascular compartment, it migrates to the liver, where primary replication occurs. The incubation period of HBV is 1 to 6 months—much longer than HAV.[1] HBV replication occurs in liver cell nuclei, with HBsAg produced in the cell cytoplasm and expressed on the cell surface. These particles are also found circulating

TABLE 40–3. Interpretation of the Laboratory Profile in Hepatitis B Infection[11]

Pattern	Is Patient Infectious?	HBsAg	HBeAg	Anti-HBc Total	Anti-HBs	Anti-HBe
Not infected/early incubation	No	–	–	–	–	–
Early acute HBV infection	Yes	+	–	–	–	–
Acute HBV infection	Yes	+	+	+	–	–
Chronic HBV infection*	Yes	+	+/–	+	–	–
Resolved infection	No	–	–	+	+	+
"Window" period following acute HBV infection	No	–	–	+	–	+

*Patient should be evaluated for complications of chronic infection such as cirrhosis and HCC.

in the plasma of patients with acute HBV, the chronic carrier state, and chronic HBV infection.[1]

In addition to HBsAg from the viral surface region, HBV has antigen markers from the nucleocapsid region (HBcAg and HBeAg) and DNA polymerase from the P region. In acute HBV infection, serologic markers proceed in sequence from the development of HBsAg followed by HBeAg (30 to 60 days prior to onset of clinical symptoms) through to the appearance of anti-HBs in late convalescence (Table 40–3).[11] Antibody to HBsAg (anti-HBs) is initially detected as the concentration of HBsAg in plasma wanes (but is probably present much earlier than detected by standard serologic assays). The presence of anti-HBs without HBsAg indicates protective immunity (Table 40–3).[11] Other antigen markers of HBV infection include pre-S1 and pre-S2 for the envelope, and the functional X protein. These markers are not routinely used clinically.

Anti-HBc, the antibody directed against HBcAg (the inner core viral antigen present in hepatocyte nuclei, not a circulating plasma antigen), is first detected shortly after the onset of acute cellular injury (Table 40–3). Anti-HBc is initially of the IgM class and signifies acute HBV infection. IgG-class anti-HBc antibodies become detectable several months following the acute HBV infection and persist along with HBs antibody for life. Anti-HBc is detectable in essentially all patients who have been exposed to HBV.[11] The presence of plasma anti-HBc IgG antibodies signifies prior infection, but it is not protective (Table 40–3).[4,11]

HBeAg (HBe antigen) is a protein subunit of the viral core detected in plasma immediately prior to or at the onset of hepatocyte injury and correlates with a high degree of infectivity. In contrast, the presence of anti-HBe (HBe antibody) correlates with a very low degree of infectivity and portends complete recovery. Anti-HBe becomes detectable either immediately after the peak of liver injury or in early convalescence, and can persist for years.

CLINICAL PRESENTATION

The clinical course of HBV infection and the associated clinical features cannot be differentiated from other types of viral hepatitis based on symptoms. A wide range of disease expression from asymptomatic infection to fulminant hepatitis occurs. In the typical case of acute HBV infection, the incubation period is followed by a symptomatic prodromal phase consisting of malaise, fatigue, weakness, anorexia, myalgias, and arthralgias. Jaundice develops in about one-third of patients as liver cell destruction increases. Jaundice can persist for several weeks.[1] Extrahepatic manifestations such as neuropathies, glomerulonephritis, pancreatitis, and hematopoietic stem cell suppression (aplastic anemia, thrombocytopenia) are occasionally seen.

Clinical manifestations of acute HBV infection are age dependent. For example, newborns infected with HBV are generally asymptomatic, whereas 25% to 33% of adult patients with acute HBV infection have symptoms; 1% to 2% (of these 25% to 33%) develop fulminant hepatic failure during the acute illness. Of the approximately 65% of adults with subclinical infection, most recover completely.

Acute HBV infection is diagnosed by the presence of anti-HBc IgM (Table 40–3). There are periods during the course of acute HBV infection when specific serologic markers are absent; the lack of such markers complicates diagnosis. These "window" periods can be seen in the early incubation phase when HBsAg and HBeAg are not detectable despite the presence of ongoing viral replication, and early in convalescence when these two antigens are cleared prior to the appearance of anti-HBs antibody. Markers of HBV replication (HBV DNA and DNA polymerase) are sensitive indicators, and are occasionally obtained when a patient is suspected to be in the serologic window period.

HEPATITIS C VIRUS

EPIDEMIOLOGY

HCV is found worldwide and is transmitted primarily through injecting drug use and contaminated blood products. In the United States, HCV is the most common chronic blood-borne infection—40% of chronic liver disease is related to HCV, and an estimated 8,000 to 10,000 HCV-related deaths occur per year.[12,13] Persons at risk for HCV infection in the United States include injecting drug users and health care workers. The Centers for Disease Control and Prevention (CDC) estimates that 1.8% of Americans (3.9 million) have at some time been infected with the hepatitis C virus,[14] with about 2.7 million Americans having chronic infection. The annual incidence of acute HCV infection was stable in the United States throughout the 1980s, at about 230,000 new cases per year.[13] However, the annual incidence rate has declined dramatically since then (to 30,000 to 38,000 new infections per year) as a result of changes in blood-donor selection and screening practices coupled with safer needle-using practices by injecting drug users.[13] Although the number of new cases of acute HCV in injecting drug users has decreased, both the incidence and prevalence of HCV in this group remains high because HCV transmission still occurs in injecting drug users and much HCV transmission has occurred in this group in past decades.[13] Injecting drug use now accounts for about 60% of new HCV cases in the United States.[13] Thirty percent of people with HCV report sexual, hemodialysis, household, occupational, or perinatal exposure.[13] No recognized source of exposure can be determined for the remaining 10% of HCV infections. Other potential methods of transmitting HCV infection include contact with other instruments capable of penetrating the skin or mucous membranes, such as shared contaminated razors, intranasal cocaine use, tattooing, and body piercing. Perinatal transmission rates of HCV are very low (<6%), increase with increasing maternal viral load, and are higher when the mother is coinfected with HIV.[13,15] Sexual transmission rates are much less for HCV than for HBV or HIV (<5%), but transmission is facilitated by concomitant HIV infection.[16,17] The virus is inefficiently spread by sexual contact. In studies of long-term spouses of patients with chronic HCV and no other risk factors, HCV infection prevalence is about 1.5%.[13] Transmission of HCV is higher in those with high-risk sexual practices.[13]

At least 6 major genotypes and over 40 subtypes of HCV have been identified. The genotypes are named by number (1 through 6) and subtypes by letter (1a, 1b, and so forth).[18,19] The different genotypes have considerable genetic and immunogenic variability. The most common HCV genotype in the United States is type 1 (approximately 70% of cases), with subtype 1a being more frequent than type 1b.[19] Genotypes 1a and 1b correlate with more severe liver chronic disease and lower rates of response to IFN therapy.[19]

The virus is constantly undergoing mutation. Consequently, in any one host, the virus actually is a series of quasi-species, each being slightly different from the primary genotype (genetic heterogeneity).

PATHOPHYSIOLOGY

After HCV gains access to the host, the virus enters hepatocytes. The virus then uncoats and releases the genome to begin replication. The viral genome serves as a template for translation of the polyprotein. The processed nonstructural protein forms a complex with the genome and begins synthesis for the negative strand. The negative strand functions as the template for synthesis of the positive strand. The RNA intermediate matures and interacts with the envelope and core proteins to assemble into new virus. Most of the replicative processes are not clearly understood.

In comparison to other viruses, HCV is more likely to cause clinically chronic silent infection in immunocompetent people. HCV accomplishes this despite active humoral and cellular immune responses that are generally targeted against all viral proteins. In acute HCV infection, specific T-cell receptors are activated and HCV-specific helper T cells assist with activation, differentiation, and induction of B cells, as well as stimulating virus-specific cytotoxic T cells.[18] These effects are mediated by various immunoregulatory cytokines. CD8-positive cytotoxic T cells recognize HCV peptides synthesized in infected cells, with resulting lysis of the infected cells.[18] Both the strength and quality of helper T-cell and cytotoxic T-cell responses appear to differ between patients who recover and those who develop chronic HCV infection. HCV elicits only a weak T-cell response in patients who develop chronic infection.[18] Individuals who clear HCV have a stronger type 1 T-helper response which up-regulates cellular immunity. The reasons for this are unclear, but are unrelated to general immune tolerance or immunosuppression.

Virus specific antibodies interfere with viral entry into host cells and opsonize the virus for elimination by macrophages, however they cannot eliminate the virus from infected cells. In addition, the humoral immune response can select HCV variants with sequence changes that allow escape from antibody recognition.[18] Antibodies to one genotype confer no resistance to another genotype. As a consequence of these factors, HCV is able to escape immune surveillance and establish persistent infection more readily. These characteristics of HCV also contribute to poor interferon (IFN) response and make it difficult to develop a vaccine.

HCV can be found in two compartments, the serum and in an intracellular reservoir. Whereas the half-life of HCV in serum is in hours, HCV in the infected cell can have a half-life between 2 and 70 days.[20] HCV production can occur in infected cells at a rate of $>3.7 \times 10^{11}$ virions per day. Therefore, therapy may have to be targeted to eradication of HCV-infected cells or administered for prolonged periods.

CLINICAL PRESENTATION

Acute hepatitis C is clinically indistinguishable from other types of viral hepatitis. The incubation period for HCV ranges from 15 to 150 days (mean, 50 days).[1] The clinical course is generally mild with less than 25% of patients developing jaundice. Major complaints are frequently limited to fatigue and malaise. Similar to other types of viral hepatitis, the hepatic transaminase values in HCV hepatitis vary from mildly to markedly elevated. Unlike the other types, HCV infections characteristically demonstrate a pattern of widely fluctuating enzyme values over the course of the infection. Development of fulminant disease is rare.[17] Infection with HIV results in more severe clinical disease with HCV infection, as does chronic alcohol consumption.[16,17]

An important feature of hepatitis C infection is that 80% to 85% of cases progress to persistent infection and 70% eventually develop chronic hepatitis.[4] The clinical presentation of chronic HCV is discussed in the chronic hepatitis section of this chapter.

Diagnosis of acute HCV depends on clinical symptoms and sequential monitoring of liver transaminase levels until the HCV antibody becomes positive. Seroconversion to anti-HCV appears from 2 to 8 weeks following initial exposure, depending on the assay used.[17] Serologic testing for HCV antibodies by enzyme immunoassay (EIA) is the primary method of initial screening of patients with abnormal liver enzymes.[21] The current immunoassay contains a number of viral antigens and has a sensitivity of 95%.[21] A second test, the recombinant immunoblot assay (RIBA) is used as a supplemental test to confirm EIA results in individuals from low-risk populations because of its high specificity and positive predictive value for HCV.[21] Assays for HCV RNA may be qualitative or quantitative. Qualitative tests are the most sensitive, but should only be used if the detection limit is below 1,000 copies/mL of HCV RNA, otherwise the definition of undetectable HCV RNA varies.

DELTA HEPATITIS VIRUS

EPIDEMIOLOGY

In general, hepatitis delta virus (HDV) infection parallels the transmission patterns and areas of endemicity of HBV. The mortality rate in acute HDV is 2% to 20%. Three forms of HDV infection have been identified and are designated acute HDV-HBV coinfection, acute HDV superinfection, and HDV chronic infection. Coinfection describes simultaneous infection with both HBV and HDV, whereas superinfection occurs when HDV is transmitted after the patient has been exposed to HBV.[1,16] Chronic infection and chronic liver disease occur in approximately 5% of cases of acute HDV-HBV coinfection, but in more than 90% of cases of HDV superinfection.[16]

HDV is primarily transmitted by exposure to infected blood (Table 40–1). Currently, parenteral drug use is the most common risk factor for HDV in the United States;[1] 20% to 50% of HBV infected injecting drug users are also infected with HDV. Sexual transmission of HDV occurs less frequently than with HBV, and perinatal transmission is rare.[16]

ETIOLOGY

HDV is a defective RNA virus that requires the presence of HBV to cause infection. HDV is composed of a single strand of RNA, an internal protein (the delta antigen), and an outer coat of HBsAg. Serologic tests for detection of serum antibodies to the delta antigen (anti-HDV) are useful in diagnosing acute hepatitis and chronic infection.[1,16]

PATHOPHYSIOLOGY

Similar to HBV, replication of the delta virus occurs in the liver. Unlike the typical HBV infection, a biphasic rise in liver transaminase levels can be seen, the first peak attributable to HBV and the second to HDV. The disappearance of HBsAg from serum heralds resolution of both infections and development of specific antibodies to both agents. Lasting immunity to both viruses is provided by the anti-HBs.[16] In HDV superinfection, delta viral replication occurs rapidly because of the persistent HBV infection, providing a ready supply of HBsAg—and a ready source of infectivity.

CLINICAL PRESENTATION

Because of the dependence of HDV on HBV for its infectivity, the natural courses of HDV coinfection and superinfection differ significantly. In coinfection, acute HDV is almost always self-limited, although fulminant hepatitis is reported to occur more frequently with HDV coinfection than with HBV alone. The clinical course may begin with an initial, relatively mild HBV phase followed by a more severe HDV phase.

In HDV superinfection, liver injury and clinical symptoms appear quickly and can be severe, leading to a fulminant course. The majority of these patients develop chronic liver disease, which frequently results in progression to cirrhosis.[16]

Infection with HDV usually worsens the course of the HBV-infected patient. Rapid clinical decompensation in a previously stable HBV carrier should raise the possibility of HDV superinfection. Patients with superinfection in whom both viruses are simultaneously replicating may rapidly develop severe liver disease and progress to liver failure within 2 years.[16]

The diagnosis of HDV infection depends on clinical suspicion, elevated hepatic aminotransferases, and serologic evidence of HBV and HDV infection. In acute superinfection of a chronic HBV carrier, markers for acute HBV are negative. HBsAg, anti-HBc IgG, HDVAg, and anti-HDV IgM are usually present. In acute coinfection, HDVAg, anti-HDV IgM, and anti-HBc IgM are usually present. Anti-HDV IgG follows. HDV RNA may be detected by polymerase chain reaction (PCR) in either serum or in liver tissue.

HEPATITIS E VIRUS

EPIDEMIOLOGY

Hepatitis E virus (HEV) is the second agent responsible for enterically transmitted hepatitis (HAV is the first). HEV is an emerging infectious disease that is the principal cause of enterically transmitted non-A, non-B hepatitis (ET-NANB) in the world. HEV infection occurs commonly in undeveloped countries, but rarely in developed countries.[22] HEV is endemic in Africa, Southeast and Central Asia, Mexico, and Central and South America. Most HEV patients from Western countries are travelers to HEV-endemic areas—and they often have consumed potentially contaminated food and water.[1,22,23] HEV outbreaks often occur during the rainy or monsoon seasons (rain-induced flooding), and are associated with drinking water contaminated with feces.[22] A periodicity of 5 to 10 years has been observed for recurring epidemics.[22]

Neither parenteral nor sexual transmission of HEV has been documented.[22] Vertical transmission from mother to fetus has been reported.[22] HEV acquired during pregnancy has resulted in spontaneous abortion or birth of infants with clinical markers of acute hepatitis.[24]

Most cases of HEV occur in adolescents and young adults.[22] HEV has a low secondary attack rate and relatively low infectivity in comparison to HAV.[22]

PATHOPHYSIOLOGY

Although serologically distinct, HEV infection is virtually indistinguishable from HAV infection. Similar features include enteric transmission; capability to cause epidemics; existence of areas of endemicity relating to poor sanitary conditions; occurrence of primary viral replication in hepatocyte cytoplasm; heavy shedding of viral particles into bile and feces; similarity of incubation period and clinical course; and lack of demonstrated chronic persistent viral infection. The incubation period ranges from 2 to 9 weeks, with a mean of 40 to 45 days.[22,23]

Viremia and fecal shedding occur at onset of clinical illness, peak at the onset of transaminase elevation, and persist for 2 to 4 weeks.[4,24] Peak antibody titers occur at 2 to 4 weeks after infection, with anti-HEV IgM declining within 3 months.[22] Information on the persistence of anti-HEV IgG is conflicting.[22]

CLINICAL PRESENTATION

Infection with HEV is usually self-limited and follows a benign course to complete recovery. Occasionally, HEV is associated with fulminant hepatic failure. Chronic hepatitis does not occur. Pregnant women are the exception to a benign HEV infection course: Women who contract HEV during the third trimester are at risk for developing fulminant hepatitis and/or hepatic failure, with a mortality rate of 10% to 42%.[22,23] As previously mentioned, HEV during pregnancy also increases the risk of complications for the newborn.[22]

During the prodromal phase, HEV-infected patients can have fever and nausea. When the icteric phase occurs, patients have the classic jaundice, dark urine and clay-colored stools, often accompanied by general signs and symptoms (abdominal pain, anorexia, hepatomegaly, malaise and vomiting).[22]

The diagnosis is made on clinical grounds, although serologic tests are available as research tools.[22] Anti-HEV IgG persists for at least 2 years following initial infection and is protective against subsequent infection with HEV.

HEPATITIS G VIRUS (GB VIRUS C, HGV, HGBV, HEPATITIS GBV-C)

HGV is a single-stranded RNA virus of the *Flaviviridae* family (Table 40–1).[25] It is detected in patients with parenteral exposure, for example, in injecting drug users, hemophiliacs, patients on hemodialysis and in those with chronic hepatitis virus infections.[26] HGV can cause persistent infection and viremia, but there is no evidence of hepatitis or hepatocellular injury, and the virus is an unlikely cause of chronic hepatic disease.[26,27] In addition, the presence of HGV does not appear to alter the clinical course of hepatitis A, B, or C.[28] HGV does not appear to cause clinical disease, but can be present in patients with unexplained hepatitis caused by yet unidentified non-A through E viruses.[25]

TT VIRUS (TTV)

TTV, a single-stranded, linear DNA virus, was discovered in 1997. TTV is a transfusion-transmissible virus, but it's association with disease is not clear.[29,30] It is common in patients with chronic HCV.[31]

▶ TREATMENT: Acute Viral Hepatitis

DESIRED OUTCOME

The ultimate goal in treating acute viral hepatitis is to return the individual to the previous state of health, and, in the case of acute HBV, HCV, or HDV infection, to prevent the development of chronic infection. Intermediate goals while the individual is acutely symptomatic and infectious include decreasing morbidity and acute mortality, minimizing the chance the infected person is infecting others, normalizing aminotransferases (cease hepatic inflammation), stopping viral replication in the host, and ultimately eradicating the virus.

GENERAL APPROACH TO THERAPY

Management of acute viral hepatitis is primarily supportive. General measures include a healthy diet, rest, maintaining fluid balance, and avoiding hepatotoxic drugs and alcohol. Special diets are of no benefit. Management includes monitoring for development of chronic liver disease and preventing disease spread. Hospitalization is necessary only for those who have prolonged vomiting, coagulation defects, or fulminant hepatitis.

PHARMACOLOGIC THERAPY

Preliminary trials and case reports of the use of IFN as therapy in acute HBV and HCV infections report promising results.[32] Because not all studies have demonstrated IFN to be useful, further studies are ongoing to define the place of IFN in acute hepatitis treatment, and IFN is not the standard of care for treatment of acute viral hepatitis. If results from these studies demonstrate that a lower rate of chronicity results when treatment is initiated during the acute phase of infection, early identification and treatment could become the primary focus. This would apply to only a few patients, however, because acute HCV infection related to blood transfusion is declining, and most cases of acute community-acquired HCV infection are asymptomatic. Treatments that clearly offer no benefit include corticosteroids and antiemetics.

FULMINANT HEPATITIS (ACUTE LIVER FAILURE)

Liver injury that results in fulminant hepatic necrosis and acute liver failure is relatively rare. When it occurs, death results in days or weeks in nearly 80% of cases.[33] Any potential hepatotoxic agent (e.g., acetaminophen) can be responsible, although viral hepatitis is the most common cause worldwide, especially HBV (1% of patients with acute hepatitis B develop fulminant hepatitis).[11,33,34] Fulminant hepatitis caused by HAV occasionally occurs; acute liver failure caused by HCV is rare.[33]

Patients with fulminant hepatic necrosis typically develop signs and symptoms of viral hepatitis, and then rapidly develop evidence of hepatic failure. The clinical syndrome is usually a 1- to 3-week course of hepatic failure and encephalopathy with coma developing within 8 weeks of the onset of acute hepatitis. Hyperexcitability, insomnia, somnolence, irritability, and impaired mental status are evidence of impending hepatic failure. Ominous signs include rapid decrease in liver size, rapid decline in aminotransferase levels, prolonged international normalized ratio (INR) or prothrombin time, and hypoglycemia. Manifestations of hepatic failure include metabolic encephalopathy, coma, coagulation defects, ascites, and edema. In fulminant liver failure, complications include gastrointestinal (GI) hemorrhage, sepsis, cerebral edema, renal failure, lactic acidosis, and disseminated coagulopathy, with death resulting from bleeding, cerebral edema, hypoglycemia, infection, and/or multisystem organ failure.[33]

Prompt referral for liver transplantation is the therapy of choice for most patients with fulminant hepatic failure.[34] Transplantation should be considered in all cases in which the patient demonstrates progressive clinical deterioration (encephalopathy, hypoglycemia, metabolic acidosis, renal failure, coagulation defects).[34] Patients should be transferred at the first sign of altered mental status, because these patients often worsen very rapidly. One-year survival rates with liver transplantation for fulminant hepatitis are 50% to 80% (as compared to <20% with medical management alone).[34]

There is no specific medical treatment for fulminant hepatic failure. The goal of medical management is to support organ function in the interim until the liver recovers or a donor organ is available.[34] Management therefore focuses on recognition coupled with prevention and aggressive management of complications. Cerebral edema occurs in 75% to 80% of cases that progress to grade IV encephalopathy, and is the leading cause of death in these patients.[34] Management includes intracranial pressure (ICP) monitoring and administration of mannitol (0.3–1 g/kg body weight as a 20% solution administered over 20 minutes) when ICP increases above 20 mm Hg.[34] Pentobarbital lowers ICP, but it also can cause severe hypotension, and its use is limited to cases with elevated ICP unresponsive to mannitol and with good cerebral blood flow.[34] Corticosteroids and hyperventilation are of little value in cerebral edema related to acute liver failure.[34] Fresh-frozen plasma should be administered for bleeding, H_2-blocker therapy should be given to prevent GI bleeding, and aggressive antibiotic therapy should be used for infections. Renal replacement therapy is used for acute renal failure, while fluid replacement (with pulmonary artery wedge pressure and cardiac output monitoring) and vasopressors provide circulatory support.[34] Metabolic abnormalities (e.g., hypoglycemia) should be treated with standard metabolic support. For further information on medical therapy, drug dosing, and adverse effects, the reader is referred to the corresponding topics in appropriate chapters of this textbook. New treatment options being evaluated include artificial liver support systems and hepatocyte transplantation. These options are at an early stage of development and further controlled clinical trials are needed to determine safety and efficacy.[34]

CHRONIC VIRAL HEPATITIS

Chronic viral hepatitis describes continuation of the hepatic necroinflammatory process 6 months or more beyond the onset of the acute illness. The clinical findings, course, and histologic features are similar in all patients with chronic hepatitis regardless of etiology. The current economic impact of chronic viral hepatitis in the United States is huge—estimated anywhere from $1.3 to $15 billion per year. US medical expenditures will almost certainly continue to rise over the next generation.

EPIDEMIOLOGY AND ETIOLOGY

Chronic viral hepatitis is the chief cause of chronic liver disease, cirrhosis, hepatic failure, and HCC throughout the world.[35] It is also the most common reason for liver transplantation.[35] In the United States, chronic liver disease is the tenth leading cause of death among adults each year, with more than half of these deaths being accounted for by HBV and HCV infections. Whereas HCV is most common in the United States, worldwide HBV is most common—more than 300 million people are chronically infected with HBV, 75% of whom are Asian.[10,16] HBV carriers have a relative risk of acquiring HCC that is more than 100-fold that of noncarriers, and 40% of male carriers die of causes related to their liver disease.

In the United States, between one and two million people are chronically infected with HBV resulting in 6,000 deaths annually. The principal reservoir of HBV for infection of others is the chronically infected individual. The primary determinant of chronicity with HBV infection is age when exposed: HBV causes chronic infection in up to 90% of infected neonates, 20% to 50% of infected children younger than 6 years of age, and 6% to 10% of infected adults.[1,16] Chronicity is more likely to occur in patients who had mild, anicteric forms of acute hepatitis.[1] There are six different genotypes of HBV with preliminary data showing that types B and C may be associated with more cirrhosis and HCC.[36]

Over a period of years, about 25% of the adults with chronic HBV infection develop chronic active hepatitis (CAH), a smaller percentage progress to cirrhosis, and a few patients develop HCC. Immunosuppression with HIV results in more severe clinical disease with HBV infection, a higher incidence of both chronic HBV carriers and chronic hepatitis B, and reactivation of HBV in late stages of HIV.

As opposed to HBV, where less than 10% of adult acute disease cases progress to chronic infection, more than 80% of those infected with HCV develop chronic infection. Chronic HCV is often diagnosed decades after the acute illness. Approximately 20% of chronic HCV patients have consistently normal ALT suggesting mild disease, but about the same number have a low-grade, smoldering progression to cirrhosis, with potential for end-stage liver disease and/or HCC. HCV accounts for 60% of HCC in industrialized countries as it develops at a rate of 1% to 4% per year in cirrhotic patients.

In countries where HBV is endemic, hepatitis B vaccination of infants and children has begun to impact the incidence of HCC and death related to HBV. In Taiwan, where a mass vaccination program was launched in 1984, the incidence of HCC in children dropped by 50% from 1981 to 1994.[37]

Close to 4 million Americans, including about a third of HIV-positive individuals, are chronically infected with HCV. The greatest prevalence of anti-HCV is found in the 30- to 49-year-old age group, in which infection is more common in males and in African Americans (6%) versus whites (3%). Genotypes 1a and 1b account for 60% to 80% of the chronic HCV in the United States, and are associated with lower rates of response to treatment.

Among those who develop chronic hepatitis, the extended outcome is uncertain: some have a static form of chronic hepatitis; some progress over a variable period to histologic fibrosis and cirrhosis; some have long-term stable cirrhosis identified only through liver biopsy; some have cirrhosis that progresses to liver failure; and some develop HCC. The uncertainties lie in the relative frequencies and rates of development of these sequelae.[18,38] Major questions exist over whether progression is linear and whether advancement through these manifestations is inevitable. Data available to date suggest that 15% to 20% of those with HCV infection will progress to end-stage liver disease, while the remainder die of other causes.[18]

Because the consequences of chronic HCV may take decades to manifest it is feared that the mortality rate may triple in 10 to 20 years over the current level of 10,000 per year. These fears are somewhat countered by a followup cohort of patients who received blood transfusions 18 years ago in which no difference in overall mortality in HCV patients was observed versus uninfected controls.[39] Also, a recent study showed the 5- and 10-year survival of HCV patients with compensated cirrhosis to be 91% and 79%, respectively. With decompensated cirrhosis the 5-year survival was only 50%.[40]

PATHOPHYSIOLOGY

The host immune response determines the eradication or persistence of HBV infection. In healthy carriers, an absent or poor cell-mediated response results in persistent viral replication, but only minimal liver damage. Healthy carriers have high titers of serum HBsAg and correspondingly high HBsAg concentrations within infected hepatocytes.

In contrast to the vigorous immune response seen in patients who clear HBV after acute infection, patients with chronic HBV infection have a weak HBV-specific cytotoxic lymphocyte (CTL) and CD4-positive T helper cell response that is mounted only against one or a few epitopes.[10] Immune tolerance, manifested by a high rate of progression to chronic infection, little disease activity in the presence of high circulating levels of virus, and low rates of response to IFN therapy is seen in patients with perinatally acquired HBV infection.[10] Patients with chronic HBV infection are deficient in producing, or responding to, IFN, which is needed to stimulate production of HLA class I protein. This lack of HLA class I protein expression on the hepatocyte membrane results in incomplete direction of the lymphocyte to the infected target cell. Persistent HBV infection is more common in immunologically compromised individuals.

Chronic HBV is more likely to occur in individuals with antecedent episodes of mild, anicteric acute hepatitis, suggesting that viral clearance is the ultimate result of hepatic necrosis. This has been demonstrated in patients with acute fulminant hepatitis, for if they survive the acute episode, complete recovery without development of chronic sequelae generally occurs.

There is no known association between the clinical severity of acute HCV hepatitis and subsequent development of chronic HCV. Factors that favor the progression of HCV are virus genotype other than 2 or 3, higher viral load, older age at acquisition, significant ethanol intake, and/or coinfection with HBV or HIV.

In both HBV and HCV, a less-than-complete host immune response may also produce a smoldering inflammatory form of hepatic injury. Although the response is capable of destroying some infected hepatocytes, it is incapable of eliminating the virus entirely. The result is persistent viral replication and continued stimulation of the immune system leading to a decreased number of functioning hepatocytes over time. At this point viral markers can be detected as well as serum transaminases, which represent enzyme leak from hepatocytes undergoing necrosis. Fibrosis resulting from cellular repair mechanisms distorts the basic cellular architecture and hepatic nodules are formed. Widespread hepatic fibrosis with nodule formation is termed cirrhosis, the consequences of which do not differ with regard to etiology and include portal hypertension and ascites. These changes may be detected clinically or on liver biopsy. They occur over time, with cirrhosis and HCC occurring on average 20 or 30 years after HCV infection, respectively.

Primary HCC occurs in a small number of patients with chronic HBV, HCV, or delta hepatitis. The rate of progression to cirrhosis and HCC varies, and depends on factors that include the state of the immune system, geographic and genetic factors, and the serology of the infection.[11] In chronic HCV, HCC is an extension or progression of the disorganized liver architecture in cirrhosis. While HBV may lead to HCC via cirrhosis, some feel that these arise by two separate paths, with integration of HBV into the host genome leading to activation of cellular oncogenes and accounting for HCC.[41]

CLINICAL PRESENTATION

The spectrum of clinical symptoms, course, and histologic features of chronic viral hepatitis is broad. "Healthy" carriers exhibit no symptoms, have normal or near normal liver transaminase values, and minimal nonspecific histologic abnormalities. Unlike acute hepatitis, physical symptoms do not correlate well with the severity of liver injury. Many patients are asymptomatic and are diagnosed only after elevated serum liver transaminases and specific markers of disease are found. An additional group of patients do not present for medical care until they experience a complication of decompensated cirrhosis such as ascites or esophageal variceal bleeding.

Most HBV carriers are HBsAg-positive, HBeAg-negative, and anti-HBe-positive, and do not develop chronic active hepatitis or cirrhosis. They can transmit the disease to others. In contrast to the healthy carriers, chronic HBsAg carriers with markers of ongoing viral replication (HBeAg, and HBV DNA) display persistent hepatic injury. Aminotransferase levels in patients with chronic HBV infection can be minimally elevated or normal. The extent of elevation correlates roughly with the extent of active inflammation. Loss of HBeAg does not indicate cure, but does signify quiescence of disease. When a relatively asymptomatic carrier of HBV experiences an acute exacerbation of hepatitis, several causes must be considered. These include superinfection with another virus, spontaneous reactivation of hepatitis B, or clearance of the HBeAg.

In chronic hepatitis C, there is frequently little clinical evidence that the disease is progressing. The patient is asymptomatic, yet viral RNA remains positive, and if liver biopsy is performed it demonstrates ongoing liver injury and progressive histologic changes. To assess chronic HCV, liver biopsy is the only reliable indicator of disease progression. Serum transaminases are prone to fluctuation and can even normalize, confounding the diagnosis. Unfortunately, the patient can be on an insidious course that progresses to complications after a period of years to decades. It is not uncommon for a patient to present to a physician with cirrhosis or portal hypertension secondary to HCV infection that occurred years to decades prior, yet to have had few or no clinical signs or symptoms during the intervening years. Within 5 years after infection, 30% to 35% of those with chronic HCV develop CAH, 20% to 33% (about 15% of those who have chronic infection) of these patients will progress to cirrhosis.[17] Cirrhosis and hepatic failure usually develop after 10 to 20 years (or longer) of indolent, asymptomatic infection. Whereas subsequent clearance of serum HBsAg may occur at a rate of 1% per year in hepatitis B infection, the spontaneous clearance rate of viral antigen from serum in patients with chronic HCV is extremely low.

In part to address the risk of silent progression of HCV, the National Institutes of Health (NIH) and the American Red Cross have developed a "look back" program for blood banks, hospitals, and other institutions to notify Americans who received blood transfusions prior to June 1992 with intent to identify people who were exposed to tainted blood. The Department of Veterans Affairs has also made the identification and treatment of HCV-infected veterans a priority. In addition to those who received blood products prior to the initiation of routine HCV testing of blood, the following criteria should be used to screen for patients at risk of hepatitis C: hemophilia, hemodialysis, children born to mothers with HCV, organ or tissue donors, and past or present intravenous drug use.

The diagnosis of chronic HCV is made by detecting anti-HCV via EIA. RIBA can be used as a confirmatory test, especially in low-risk populations, to exclude false positives on EIA.

In either chronic HBV or HCV, if the patient is symptomatic, fatigue, malaise, anorexia, and weight loss are common. Many patients have a history of jaundice. On physical examination, hepatomegaly is usually present, but the stigmata of chronic liver disease (spider nevi, splenomegaly, palmar erythema, testicular atrophy, and caput medusa) are generally absent until late in the disease course. Mild but persistent elevations of the serum aminotransferases, bilirubin, and γ-globulin levels can be seen.

Both chronic HBV and chronic HCV are associated with extrahepatic syndromes. Polyarteritis nodosa (inflammation and necrosis of segments of medium-sized or small arteries), other vasculitis-like lesions, and cryoglobulinemic manifestations have been described. In addition, hemolytic uremic syndrome; thrombotic thrombocytopenic purpura; Raynaud's syndrome; Schönlein-Henoch purpura (an eruption of hemorrhaging into the skin that is nonthrombocytopenic; associated with joint pains or swelling and bleeding from the GI tract, as well as other manifestations); infantile papular acrodermatitis (an inflammatory papular eruption of the skin of the extremities of infants); Guillain-Barré syndrome; meningitis; myelitis; and meningoencephalomyelitis have all been reported. Also, other musculoskeletal disorders; erythema multiforme; thrombocytopenia; serum sickness; rash; blood dyscrasias; thyroid abnormalities; arthralgia; glomerulonephritis; and a sicca-like syndrome that resembles Sjögren's syndrome have occurred.[17,42] HBV infection is occasionally associated with renal failure. Treatment of the underlying HBV infection generally improves the extrahepatic disease manifestations.[11]

For patients with chronic viral hepatitis, the presence of ongoing viral replication is the most important factor in evaluating disease progression. However, the prognosis for a patient with chronic viral hepatitis is indicated by the degree of liver damage noted on liver biopsy.

In a patient with a history of blood transfusion, chronically elevated aminotransferase levels, a positive EIA for anti-HCV and CAH on liver biopsy, the diagnosis of chronic HCV is easily made. For patients without risk factors, other potential causes must be ruled out before making the diagnosis of chronic HCV. Serum aminotransferase levels correlate poorly with histologic extent of disease, and liver biopsy provides diagnostic and prognostic information. Most patients with positive anti-HCV will have chronic HCV, even if the aminotransferase levels are normal.

HCC presents as nonspecific right upper quadrant pain in patients with cirrhosis. It is diagnosed via abdominal ultrasound or elevated serum α-fetoprotein levels.

▶ TREATMENT: Chronic Viral Hepatitis

DESIRED OUTCOME

The goal of treatment is to prevent the morbidity and mortality associated with end-stage liver disease by eradicating the HBV or HCV (Table 40–4). Effective treatment of chronic viral hepatitis should also increase the quality of life and prevent infected patients from serving as reservoirs of infection.

Because the complications of chronic hepatitis may take decades to manifest, clinical trials primarily use outcomes of virologic response (clearance of virus), biochemical response (return of transaminases to normal levels), and histologic response (decrease in HAI by at least 2 points), as surrogate markers for decreased risk of cirrhosis, HCC, or death. Long-term outcome studies show that the response to therapy can be maintained for years and that progression of liver disease can be halted. Even regression of fibrosis, once thought to be irreversible, is possible.[43] Sustained virologic or biochemical response is also associated with a reduced risk of HCC.

GENERAL APPROACH TO TREATMENT

Upon the diagnosis of chronic viral hepatitis, the patient should be informed about the disease risks and a program of regular monitoring established. Depending where in the course of infection the disease is diagnosed, monitoring for progression is important for selection of patients for pharmacologic treatment because many more patients die with chronic viral hepatitis than from it. The relative benefits of pharmacologic therapy and their attendant adverse effects and risks need to be discussed as well.

Until recently, monotherapy with IFN was the preferred treatment choice for patients with chronic HBV or HCV. While IFN still is prominent in the treatment of both HBV and HCV, the role of monotherapy has diminished, especially in treatment of HCV.

CHRONIC HBV

Patients considered for treatment are those HBsAg-positive for greater than 6 months with persistent elevations in serum aminotransferases, detectable markers of viral replication (HBeAg, and HBV DNA) in serum, and signs of chronic hepatitis on liver biopsy. Although symptomatic patients are more apt to seek medical attention and to have these irregularities discovered, symptoms alone are not a basis for treatment. To be treated with IFN, patients should not have decompensated liver disease or any specific contraindications to the therapy being considered.

Current strategies to eradicate HBV include the use of antiviral agents that alter viral replication or immunomodulatory agents that modify the host immune response. IFNα-2b was approved by the FDA for use in chronic HBV in 1992. IFN monotherapy now is an option only in selected subgroups of HBV or HCV. Lamivudine (Epivir-HB) was approved for use in chronic HBV in 1998, and has broader indications for use, but questions remain regarding optimal duration of use and management of resistant viruses.

End points of therapy for HBV include disappearance of HBV DNA and elimination of HBeAg (virologic response), resolution of elevated aminotransferases (biochemical response), and improvement of liver histology. HBeAg seroconversion, an even stricter marker of viral response, denotes the loss of both HBeAg and HBV DNA and the appearance of anti-HBe. Loss of HBsAg can occur even years after completion of therapy.

INTERFERONS IN CHRONIC HBV

As compared to a placebo response of 12% to 17%, 33% to 37% of patients respond to IFN therapy by losing HBeAg and HBV DNA. Even though most of these patients will maintain a long-term response, the low overall response rates combined with the adverse effects and need for subcutaneous dosing make IFN a less than ideal agent. Pretreatment predictors of response to IFN include low viral load (HBV DNA <200 copies/mL) and high ALT (>100). For this subset of chronic HBV patients, an IFNα-2a or -2b regimen is a rational option, although these same parameters predict response for lamivudine, an alternative agent.

Resolution of HBV viremia with IFN is associated with a transient exacerbation of the hepatitis, marked by a rise in serum aminotransferase levels during the second or third month of therapy. Although IFN may have direct antiviral effects, this flare is related to IFN immunomodulatory effects resulting in an increased host response (Fig. 40–1). In patients who respond to IFN, HBV DNA levels decrease within days of starting therapy. After 8 to 12 weeks, ALT levels increase, and the patient loses HBV DNA and HBeAg. ALT levels

TABLE 40–4. Goals of Therapy in Patients with Chronic Hepatitis B and Chronic Hepatitis C

Goal	Chronic Hepatitis B	Chronic Hepatitis C
Lose HBV DNA (lose HBV replication)	X	
Lose HBeAg (low infectious potential)	X	
Loss of HBsAg (eradicate HBV)	X	
Lose HCV RNA (lose HCV replication)		X
Lose HCVAg (lose infectious potential)		X
Normalize aminotransferases (cease hepatic inflammation)	X	X
Improve symptoms	X	X
Decrease progression of liver disease	X	X
Reduce cirrhosis	X	X
Reduce hepatocellular carcinoma	X	X
Increase survival	X	X

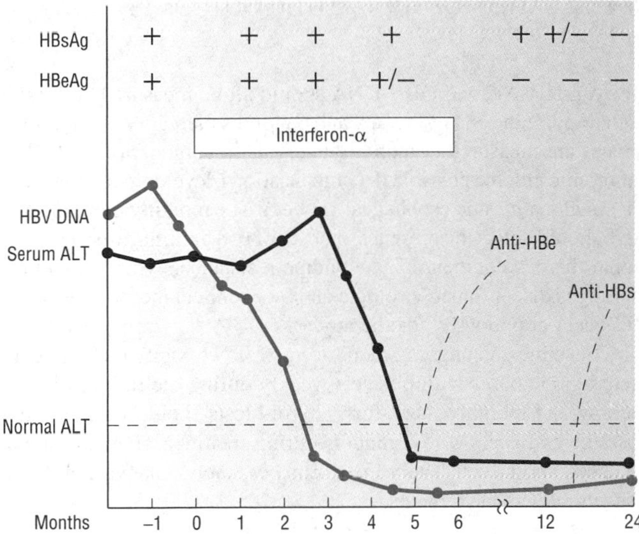

FIGURE 40–1. Typical sustained response to IFN-α in a patient with chronic hepatitis B.

then normalize, and the patient develops anti-HBe.[44] Without the flare, loss of viral replication rarely occurs. Patients infected with precore HBV mutants that prevent HBeAg expression (HBeAg-negative and HBV DNA-positive) are less likely to respond to IFN therapy and have a higher rate of relapse upon discontinuation.[45]

About 10% of the responders to IFN therapy also clear HBsAg in the first year, and although biochemical and histologic responses also occur, they are more frequent in the group responding virologically. Long-term followup of patients treated with IFN has shown that response is sustained in about 90% of patients at least 5 years after therapy and that a distinct survival benefit is present in those who have a virologic response.[46,47]

LAMIVUDINE IN CHRONIC HBV

Lamivudine (Epivir-HB) is a nucleoside analog that competitively inhibits viral reverse transcriptase and terminates proviral DNA chain extension. Because it does not affect host response, it suppresses viral replication but does not directly eliminate the virus from the hepatocytes. Its efficacy is also not associated with, or dependent upon, the flare response seen with IFN. Like IFN though, lamivudine demonstrates higher response rates in patients with elevated transaminases (ALT > 100) and lower viral loads.

Two double-blind randomized controlled trials compared lamivudine 100 mg by mouth daily for 52 weeks versus placebo in previously untreated patients.[48,49] The results are startlingly comparable except that one trial in Asia had a higher biochemical response in both treatment and placebo groups.[48] Both trials demonstrated significant histologic, virologic, and biochemical responses with lamivudine. Lamivudine also prevented histologic worsening or the development of hepatic fibrosis. The results of the Asian trial are especially impressive because it was previously thought that this was a difficult population to treat because of acquisition of disease at an early age.[48] Long-term outcomes are not proven, but the results of these trials are encouraging. Of note, the 32% rate of HBeAg loss in the American trial is similar to the response demonstrated with IFN.

Upon discontinuation of lamivudine HBV DNA tends to rebound, but to levels less than the original baseline. Virologic responses were maintained in about 75% of lamivudine-treated patients 16 weeks posttherapy. Treatment beyond 1 year increases the rate of HBeAg loss and slows the rate and extent of HBV DNA return. Extending duration of therapy would be associated though with a possible increase in adverse effects, increased cost, and increased development of resistance to lamivudine.

Mutations in regions of reverse transcriptase, primarily the YMDD locus, confer resistance against lamivudine. These occur after about 6 months of therapy, are usually accompanied by increases in ALT and HBV DNA, and are more common in patients with elevated baseline viral loads. In the two lamivudine trials, the incidence of these mutations were 14% and 32%, respectively, after 1 year of therapy.[48,49] It is thought that the mutant viruses are relatively less harmful because they are not able to replicate as effectively, but the mutants are replaced by wild-type virus upon treatment discontinuation. Despite the development of resistance, with continued lamivudine therapy the ALT and HBV DNA often remain below baseline levels and some patients may still convert from a HBeAg-positive state.

In the foregoing studies, one reported no association between treatment and transaminase level changes, whereas the other reported posttreatment levels greater than three times baseline in 25% of the treatment group, as compared to 8% in the placebo group. A different cohort of 55 patients had much higher mutation rate (58% after 2 years of lamivudine therapy), with 13 patients (24%) experiencing an ALT spike over 10 times the normal range, and 3 patients (5%) demonstrating hepatic decompensation during the flare.[50,51]

Lamivudine has a much less toxic adverse effect profile than IFN with serious side effects occurring at rates similar to placebo. Most commonly reported are fatigue, nausea and vomiting, headache, cough, and diarrhea. It is administered as a tablet or oral suspension at a dose of 100 mg orally once daily. Lamivudine is well absorbed, and is renally eliminated, requiring dosage adjustment if the creatinine clearance is <50 mL/min. Response to lamivudine is more rapid than with IFN, with HBV DNA levels decreasing by 97% after 2 weeks of therapy, and it has demonstrated success in patient subgroups that typically do not respond to IFN.

Therefore, lamivudine is much more convenient, has fewer adverse effects, and demonstrates at least comparable virologic, histologic, and biochemical activity as compared to IFN. Unsolved with lamivudine is the optimal duration of therapy, especially considering that the correct course upon discovery of resistance is yet unknown. With little comparative data, one is left to choose between a relatively short course of an injectable agent with demonstrated adverse effects but documented long-term outcomes, versus a well-tolerated oral agent with activity across a greater spectrum of patients, but whose long-term effects and optimal duration of therapy are unknown.

COMBINATION THERAPY IN CHRONIC HBV

The newer nucleoside analogs have the potential to change the approach to therapy of chronic HBV from that of a limited course of IFN to long-term suppressive therapy aimed at inhibiting viral replication and ameliorating disease. Combinations of lamivudine with INF have been investigated to treat chronic HBV. A randomized controlled trial of 230 patients failed to show a statistically significant benefit of combination therapy (8 weeks of lamivudine monotherapy followed by 16 weeks of lamivudine plus INF); because of methodological difficulties, however, further study is needed.[52]

Combining therapeutic agents to treat chronic HBV is an area of intense research, but to this point a variety of agents have been combined with IFN with limited success including cyclooxygenase inhibitors, acyclovir, *N*-acetyl cysteine, and levamisole.[53] A meta analysis has also shown the use of prednisone to "prime" the liver prior to IFN therapy to be of little value.[54] Combining famciclovir with lamivudine has shown synergistic inhibitory activity in *in vitro* models and appeared beneficial in a case report.[55] Combinations with lamivudine may be helpful in preventing or slowing the development of resistance.

OTHER THERAPIES IN CHRONIC HBV

Famciclovir, the oral prodrug of penciclovir, decreases HBV DNA levels and is well tolerated, but its HBeAg conversion rate is low and its virologic activity is less rapid and of a lower order of magnitude than lamivudine.[56] It has some benefit in preventing HBV infection after liver or bone marrow transplants at doses of 125–750 mg three times daily for 16 weeks.[52,57] Because HBV may develop resistance to famciclovir, its potential role is limited to combination therapy.

Adefovir is a nucleotide analogue administered as the prodrug adefovir dipivoxil. In addition to achieving loss of HBeAg in 20% to 27% of treated patients, it demonstrated activity versus viral mutants.[58,59]

TREATMENT OF CHRONIC HBV IN SPECIAL POPULATIONS

As opposed to IFN with its significant adverse effect profile, almost all patients are candidates for lamivudine therapy. Patient groups in which lamivudine has shown benefit include various transplant patients, those with decompensated cirrhosis, and patients with precore mutations (HBeAg-negative and HBV DNA-positive). Patients with normal aminotransferase levels should not be treated. Monitoring of this group, with treatment if disease progresses, is more advantageous than treatment, because many will not progress while therapy is associated with cost and risk.

Whereas the use of IFN is discouraged in patients with decompensated cirrhosis, an open trial of 35 such patients with lamivudine demonstrated significant benefit in laboratory and clinical markers in the 23 patients who were maintained on therapy for greater than 6 months. HBV DNA was undetectable in all patients after 6 months and adverse effects were minimal.[60] Lamivudine also shows no decrease in activity in patients who have active replication, but are HBeAg-negative. After a year of treatment, 65% became HBV DNA-negative and had normal transaminases.

Patients coinfected with HIV may not respond as well to IFN, because immunosuppression can block its antiviral actions, but these patients can be considered for therapy if their disease is relatively well controlled.[61] Only a small proportion of cases of HBV infection in the United States are in children. The efficacy of IFN in children seems comparable to that in adults and those with elevated ALT levels at initiation of therapy are more likely to respond. A comparative trial of IFNα-2b 5 MU/m^2 versus 10 MU/m^2 three times weekly for 6 months showed greater HBeAg clearance with the higher dose (53% vs 7%).[62] Children also tend to tolerate IFN therapy better than do adults.

Although some schemes of induction therapy dosing of IFN have been successful in patients who had not responded to previous IFN therapy, it makes sense to try a course of lamivudine first before trying these increased doses.[63]

EVALUATION OF THERAPEUTIC OUTCOMES IN CHRONIC HBV

HBeAg, HBsAg, and HBV DNA should all be measured at the start of therapy, at the end of therapy and 6 months thereafter. Aminotransferases are measured at monthly intervals in conjunction with clinical monitoring for possible decompensation (development of ascites, encephalopathy, and esophageal varices). The monthly monitoring of ALT should detect the presence or absence of a flare, and may also help signal the development of lamivudine resistance. When lamivudine therapy is discontinued virologic and biochemical monitoring should still occur at 6 months posttherapy.

Baseline and ongoing monitoring of IFN toxicity includes complete blood counts with platelets weekly during the first 2 weeks of therapy and monthly thereafter. Thyroid tests should be checked at baseline and every 3 to 6 months during treatment. Patients should be asked about their level of performance, mood changes, ability to concentrate, and symptoms.

CHRONIC DELTA HEPATITIS

In chronic delta hepatitis, high-dose IFNα treatment with 9 MU three times weekly for at least 12 months produces clearance of HDV RNA and normalization of serum aminotransferases in about 50% of patients.[64] Lower doses of IFN are ineffective and relapse can occur more than 1 year after therapy is stopped.[64] Sustained improvement occurs in 15% to 25% of patients.[35] Prolonged, indefinite IFN therapy may be necessary to achieve a sustained response. No predictors of response to IFN have been identified in chronic HDV.

IFN has not been specifically approved for use in chronic HDV and its use should be limited to those patients who have elevated aminotransferases, HBsAg, and anti-HDV in serum, HDVAg in liver; and inflammatory changes on biopsy. A report of five patients with chronic delta hepatitis treated with lamivudine showed that HDV RNA levels dropped in all, but that there was no improvement in HBsAg, ALT levels, or histology.[51,65]

CHRONIC HCV

Patients seropositive for HCV with elevated ALT and inflammation on liver biopsy are candidates for antiviral therapy. A more difficult treatment decision is when patients have elevated ALT, but the histologic changes are mild. In that situation the patient may be closely monitored and treatment withheld. Because relapse frequently occurs shortly after IFN monotherapy is stopped, response to HCV treatment is broken into three general categories:

Response: Reduction of HCV RNA to undetectable levels and normalization of ALT during treatment and 6 months after completion of therapy

Nonresponse: HCV RNA remains detectable or ALT fails to normalize during the course of therapy

Relapse: HCV RNA becomes undetectable and ALT normalizes during treatment, but at least one reemerges in the 6 months after therapy

Occasionally, different time points are used to record results as end-of-therapy responses (ETR) or as sustained response (SR, at least 6 months after therapy).

In 1997, a NIH consensus panel published recommendations on the management of HCV infection.[10,39] Many of the treatment recommendations have been supplanted by comparative data showing the superiority of IFN therapy in conjunction with oral ribavirin as compared to IFN alone. Ribavirin was approved for use in conjunction with IFN for the treatment of chronic HCV in 1998.

INTERFERONS IN CHRONIC HCV

Twelve months of IFN monotherapy was formerly the preferred therapy for chronic HCV. However, with recent data demonstrating the benefit of combination therapy with IFN plus ribavirin, therapy with IFN alone should be reserved for patients with contraindications to ribavirin therapy.

If IFN monotherapy is used, the two most important pretreatment predictors of response are low levels of HCV RNA (less than 2 million copies/mL) and HCV viral genotypes 2 or 3. However, determination of HCV RNA 4 weeks after initiation of therapy predicts outcome even more accurately than the pretreatment variables. Failure to clear HCV RNA by 4 weeks has a 98% negative predictive value for failing to achieve a sustained virologic response.[66] If HCV RNA is negative at that point, then there is a 50% chance of having a sustained virologic response.[66]

In contrast to chronic HBV in which IFN acts as an immunostimulant, in chronic HCV, IFN inhibits HCV replication directly.[6] The pattern of response is also different in HCV. No flare occurs during treatment in those who respond to IFN. In a variety of patient populations attempts to increase the dose of IFN have led to increased end of treatment responses but have done little to increase the sustained response.

IFN decreases the progression of chronic HCV liver disease and the rate of HCC in treated patients.[67,68] It is expected that these beneficial long-term outcomes will be maintained when IFN is used in conjunction with ribavirin.

COMBINATION THERAPY IN CHRONIC HCV

Ribavirin is a synthetic nucleoside analog that shows activity versus both DNA and RNA viruses, but its mechanism of action is unknown. Ribavirin treatment of HCV leads to a transient ALT decrease, but has little effect on HCV RNA levels. Ribavirin is dosed twice daily according to patient weight: 1,000 mg is given if the patient weighs less than 75 kg; 1,200 mg is given if the patient weighs more than 75 kg. It is well absorbed and eliminated renally. Its primary adverse effect is hemolytic anemia that tends to manifest during the first month of therapy and results in hemoglobin levels <10 in about 10% of patients. Contraindications to use are renal failure, anemia, hemoglobinopathies, and severe heart disease. Ribavirin is also a known abortifacient and therefore a pregnancy test is required in women of childbearing age before starting therapy, and strict birth control must be practiced by both men and women during and 6 months after cessation of therapy. The packaged vials of IFNα-2b and oral ribavirin 200-mg tablets in blister packs are purchased as the combination product Rebetron.

Four randomized trials involving more than 2,100 patients have compared the combination of ribavirin plus IFN to IFN monotherapy. Three trials examined initial therapy for chronic HCV; the fourth study included patients who relapsed following a prior course of IFN.[69–72] All studies used doses of IFNα-2b 3 million units three times per week and ribavirin as above. Figure 40–2 summarizes the sustained virologic and biochemical response rates. All trials showed a significant benefit of combination therapy versus IFN monotherapy with at least two-fold increased rates of response in all groups. Across all studies the rate of response was >30% in all combination groups, whereas IFN monotherapy did not reach that mark, and only exceeded 20% twice. The overall benefit was a consequence of an increased end of therapy response and decreased relapse rate in the combination groups. Overall histologic improvement occurred in all treated patients and was more pronounced in the combination treatment. In Fig. 40–2 it appears that increasing the duration of therapy had minor incremental benefit for the combination group.

Both genotype 2 or 3 and low viral load are independent predictors of sustained virologic response.[69,72] The incremental benefit of increasing the duration of combination therapy from 24 to 48 weeks only occurs in the groups with genotype 1 or high viral load. Absence of cirrhosis and a low stage of fibrosis are also independent predictors of sustained virologic response.

Dose reductions are more common with combination therapy. Discontinuation of therapy is more common with combination therapy, but duration of therapy is the biggest factor determining the need

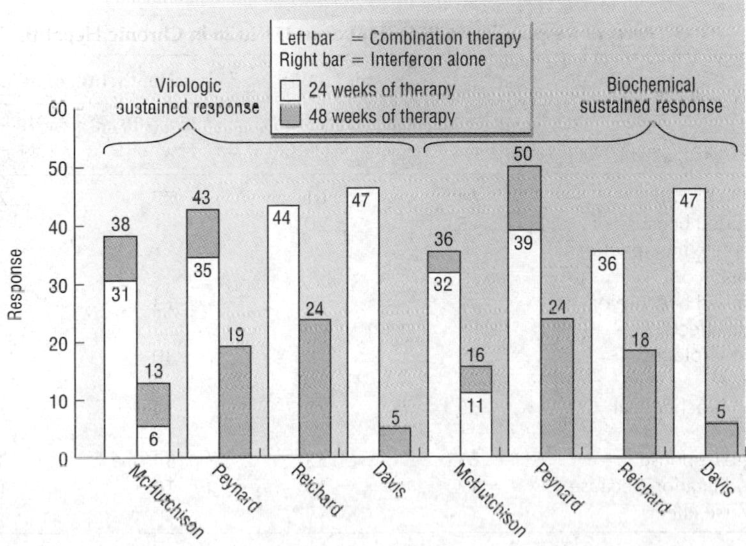

FIGURE 40–2. Combination of ribavirin plus interferon versus interferon alone for chronic hepatitis C.[69–72]

for discontinuation. Combination therapy is associated with increased rash, nausea, dyspnea, pharyngitis, anorexia, and insomnia. Most of the dose reductions with combination therapy are caused by anemia, and the most common reason for drug discontinuations is emotional disturbance.

As a result of this data, 6 months of combination therapy are indicated in patients infected with genotypes 2 or 3, or those with genotype 1 and a low viral load. Patients with genotype 1 and a high viral load would benefit from extending the duration of combination therapy to 12 months.[40] Although one might propose that some subgroups be given a trial of IFN monotherapy first, almost all data indicate that 6 months of combination therapy is more effective than 12 months of IFN. For patients receiving the shorter duration of combination therapy, measuring HCV RNA at 12 weeks is justified to decide whether or not to continue therapy. For the longer course though, 10% of the patients receiving initial combination therapy and demonstrating a sustained virologic response are still HCV RNA-positive at 12 weeks. Therefore, virologic status should be checked at 24 weeks in this group, and therapy stopped if positive.

Although the benefit of combination therapy must be acknowledged, it should also be pointed out that more information is needed. The rate of sustained response is only 35% to 50% and data regarding long-term outcomes are still maturing.[73] Ribavirin therapy is expensive, contributes to adverse effects, and is expected to have poorer compliance and tolerability when used in general practice rather than in clinical trials. Also, more needs to be known in treating patients with cirrhosis, as they made up less than 5% of the population tested.

PEGYLATED (PEG) IFN AND OTHER THERAPIES IN CHRONIC HCV

The conjugation of polyethylene glycol (PEG) to IFN (pegylation) results in a 10- to 100-fold increase in IFN half-life and allows for once weekly SC dosing. PEG-IFN recently received FDA approval for use in chronic HCV. Table 40–5 details the results with Pegasys (Roche), a product of a 40-kDa PEG chain attached to IFNα-2a, versus IFN alone in treatment naive HCV patients and those with cirrhosis.[74,75] The efficacy of the PEG-IFN is comparable to combination therapy with IFN and ribavirin, and the adverse effects are comparable to IFN alone. The impact of pretreatment variables of genotype and viral load are similar in PEG-IFN as with IFN alone. The results of phase III clinical trials of the combination of PEG-IFN plus ribavirin are awaited.

Many other drugs have been tried to treat chronic HCV. Agents that show benefit in conjunction with other therapy include histamine dihydrochloride, thymosin, and amantadine.[20] Histamine dihydrochloride is thought to enhance the efficacy of interleukin (IL)-2 or IFN by suppressing the actions of reactive oxygen metabolites. In a study of 129 HCV patients with poor prognosis, also receiving IFN at standard doses, 72% of the patients demonstrated a response after 12 weeks of therapy.[20] Thymosin, an immunomodulatory peptide, at 1.6 mg subcutaneously twice a week with standard-dose IFN showed biochemical, histologic, and virologic response at the end of therapy greater than IFN alone.[20] Amantadine is an oral antiviral agent that shows conflicting results when given as monotherapy in HCV, but it is relatively well tolerated and therefore could be tried further as part of combination regimens. Triple therapy with ribavirin and IFN shows benefit in pilot studies. Glycyrrhizin has been used as a treatment of chronic hepatitis in Japan for more than 30 years and has produced a decreased incidence of cirrhosis and HCC in comparative trials. Although it is well tolerated, it requires intravenous administration several times per week.

Because lower hepatic iron stores correlate with improved outcome for both chronic HBV and chronic HCV, phlebotomy prior to IFN treatment has been tried in an attempt to improve response rates. Increased hepatic iron facilitates viral replication of HCV, enhances hepatic injury, or decreases the host's immune system ability to clear the virus. Thus far studies have been inconclusive.[20] Treatments that offer no or little long-term benefit include IFNγ, corticosteroids, nonsteroidal anti-inflammatory agents, ursodeoxycholic acid (ursodiol), and acyclovir.

Potential future therapies will likely be aimed at preventing viral replication (e.g., viral enzyme inhibitors, antisense oligonucleotides, and ribozymes), modulating the immune response to HCV (e.g., IL-12 and IL-10) and controlling disease progression in those already infected with HCV.[20] Obviously, development of an effective vaccine is the long-term goal.

TABLE 40–5. Percent Responding to PEG-IFN versus IFNα-2a in Chronic Hepatitis C[74,75]

	Zeuzem, et al. (2000)		Heathcote, et al. (2000)	
	PEG-180 N = 267	IFNα-2a N = 264	PEG-180 N = 88	IFNα-2a N = 264
Completed therapy	84	61	77	73
Discontinued because of incomplete therapeutic response	5	20	1	6
Discontinued because of adverse effects	7	10	13	8
Sustained virologic response	39	19	30	8
Sustained biochemical response	45	25	34	15
Histologic response	63	55	54	31
Dose modification because of adverse effects	19	18	14	14

TREATMENT OF CHRONIC HCV IN SPECIAL POPULATIONS

Many patients with chronic HCV have been treated with IFN and either did not respond to initial therapy or relapsed. Those that have relapsed can receive "high-dose" IFN therapy for 12 months or combination therapy with IFN and ribavirin for 6 months. In either case, therapy should be discontinued if HCV RNA is positive after 3 months of therapy.[40] Pooling data from various trials that measured retreatment of IFN relapsers shows the sustained biochemical response increases from 16% to 29% when the dose of IFN is increased above the standard 3 MU three times a week but the duration of therapy is held at 6 months. If an escalated dose (>3 MU three times weekly) is used for 12 months, the rate increases to 43%.[76] These data also demonstrate that virologic response during the first cycle of IFN is the best predictor of response to retreatment. A recent study also showed impressive results with higher doses of consensus IFN (15 mcg three times weekly for 24 or 48 weeks) to treat relapsed patients.[77] The sustained virologic response was 28% after 24 weeks and 58% after 48 weeks. While these results appear promising, the initial round of treatment was inadequate in about half the patients and could have influenced the "retreatment" results.[78]

When 345 patients who had relapsed received combination therapy versus IFN monotherapy at normal doses, the rates of sustained virologic and sustained biochemical responses favored combination therapy 49% to 5% and 52% to 15% respectively (Fig. 40–2).[70] Other studies show a comparable response rate with escalated dose IFN versus escalated dose IFN plus ribavirin, but clearly demonstrate that patients who relapsed with IFN monotherapy, rather than not responding, have a greater chance to respond to a second round of treatment.[79,80]

The 20% of patients with chronic HCV that demonstrate normal transaminases should not receive treatment. Instead, they should have ALT monitoring at 4- to 6-month intervals. Their sustained response rate is similar to other patients but the relative benefit of therapy can be muted with the relatively benign natural history of progression in this group. Patients with chronic HCV and extrahepatic manifestations of disease such as essential mixed cryoglobulinemia or membranoproliferative glomerulonephritis respond to IFN at rates similar to other groups, and often have improvement in the extrahepatic manifestations.[35] Relapse is frequent after therapy is stopped. Correct diagnosis is important though as IFN can exacerbate autoimmune hepatitis. Long-term maintenance IFN treatment can be considered in this group (if they respond to IFN).

IFN has been used in the treatment of chronic HCV in children at doses of 3–5 MU/m^2 for a 6- to 12-month course in numerous small trials. It appears that children demonstrate a similar response rate, have the same pretreatment predictors of response, and may tolerate therapy better. Until more information is gathered though children are best treated only in clinical trials.

Patients with chronic HCV and cirrhosis present a dilemma as they may have slower and lower response rates than other groups but still derive both histologic and virologic benefit from treatment. One recommendation calls for treating those patients with early cirrhosis who have no signs of portal hypertension as we would any other HCV group, while patients with evidence of portal hypertension should be considered for treatment only in research protocols. A recent meta-analysis suggests that cirrhosis patients respond better to combination ribavirin/IFN therapy.[81]

More than 100 patients with chronic HCV and HIV coinfection have been studied in published trials.[82] It appears that this group responds as most others, but that close monitoring of CD4 and HIV viral load is indicated because ribavirin inhibits phosphorylation of reverse transcriptase inhibitors in vitro. Patient selection is also very important—there are more than 400,000 patients coinfected with HCV and HIV in the United States

EVALUATION OF THERAPEUTIC OUTCOMES

To carry out the plans outlined above requires that viral genotype is performed at baseline and viral load is performed if the patient is a genotype other than 2 or 3. The 1997 NIH recommendations said HCV genotyping should not be considered part of a therapeutic algorithm, but the 1999 European Association for the Study of the Liver (EASL) consensus conference statement recommends genotyping, and states that quantitative HCV RNA testing is helpful with genotype 1.[40] Before treatment all patients should have a liver biopsy, have thyroid function assessed, and women should have a negative pregnancy test.

During treatment, complete blood count (CBC) with platelets should be performed weekly for the first 4 weeks and monthly thereafter. Thyroid tests should be checked every 3 to 6 months during treatment and 6 months after. HCV RNA should be evaluated at 3 or 6 months of combination therapy, depending on the intended duration. Aminotransferase and qualitative HCV RNA should be performed at the end of therapy and 6 and 18 months after the cessation of therapy.[83] Followup biopsy is not indicated.

In patients with established or suspected cirrhosis, screening for HCC with abdominal ultrasound and serum α-fetoprotein is recommended.[40] However, neither the time frame nor cost-effectiveness of such screening has been defined. For patients not started on therapy because of mild histologic disease or normal ALT, liver biopsy should be repeated in 4 to 5 years and ALT at 6-month intervals, respectively.

The side effects of IFN occur frequently enough that the patient should be informed about them before treatment begins (Table 40–6). Many side effects are dose related. The most common and predictable effects are influenza-like and can be counteracted by premedication with a single dose of acetaminophen around the time of injection. Severity decreases with subsequent injections and usually abates in 1 to 2 weeks.[44] Later common adverse effects are fatigue, malaise, and cognitive changes.

Because IFN therapy can exacerbate autoimmune disorders, it is important to exclude autoimmune diagnoses before initiating therapy. Thrombocytopenia and granulocytopenia are more common in patients with cirrhosis and hypersplenism. The psychiatric complications are especially severe in those with severe liver disease, occur in up to 20% of patients, and are the most common dose-limiting side effects. IFN should be discontinued if serious complications occur. The dose of IFN must be reduced in 10% to 40% of patients. Treatment must be discontinued because of adverse effects in 5% to 10% of patients. For many patients, reassurance that the side effects are therapy related, not severe, and will disappear when therapy is stopped is sufficient. It is always important to reassure both patient and family, especially when psychiatric side effects are evident.

Ongoing monitoring of IFN toxicity includes complete blood counts weekly during the first 2 weeks of therapy and monthly thereafter. Patients should be asked about level of performance, mood changes, ability to concentrate, and symptoms. The dose of IFN should be decreased by 50% if any of the following develop: fatigue that interferes with the daily routine, serious mood changes, daily

TABLE 40–6. Side Effects of IFN-α*

Early (in first 2 Weeks of Therapy)	Hematologic	Neuropsychiatric	Autoimmune	Miscellaneous
Fever	Neutropenia	Irritability	Development of autoantibodies	Chronic fatigue
Chills	Thrombocytopenia	Mood lability	Hepatitis	Infections
Myalgias	Anemia	Depression	Thyroid dysfunction	Increased sleep requirement
Fatigue		Tearfulness	Thyroiditis	Anorexia
Malaise		Delirium	Arthropathy	Weight loss
Nausea		Paresthesias	Type I diabetes mellitus	Myalgias
Sleep disturbance		Seizures	Exacerbation of psoriasis or lichen planus	Low-grade fevers
Abdominal pain		Psychosis	Exacerbation of other autoimmune phenomena	Decreased libido
Diarrhea				Alopecia
Headache				Hypertriglyceridemia
Appetite changes				Irritability
				Anxiety
				Depression
				Attention span deficits

*Absolute contraindications to use of IFN include current or past psychosis or severe depression, neutropenia or thrombocytopenia, organ transplant (except liver), symptomatic heart disease, decompensated cirrhosis, and uncontrolled seizures. Relative contraindications to IFN include uncontrolled diabetes and autoimmune disorders.

nausea with occasional vomiting, granulocytopenia (less than 750/mm^3), and/or thrombocytopenia (less than 50,000/mm^3). IFN should be immediately discontinued if fatigue is so severe that it requires bed rest, vomiting occurs more than twice daily, or if profound granulocytopenia (less than 500/mm^3) or thrombocytopenia (less than 30,000/mm^3) occur.[44,45]

Several drugs can potentially interact with IFN. Examples include theophylline (increased theophylline concentration), zidovudine (enhanced hematologic toxicity), vidarabine (vidarabine-induced neurotoxicity), and cytotoxic agents (increased myelosuppression). Careful evaluation for drug interactions with IFN is an integral part of monitoring IFN therapy.

LIVER TRANSPLANTATION

Liver transplantation is an option for patients with end-stage chronic liver disease secondary to viral infection. Unfortunately, recurrent viral hepatitis infection in the transplanted liver is a common problem. All patients with fulminant hepatitis; those with chronic HBV and cirrhosis who do not have markers of viral replication; and patients with HDV infection should be considered transplant candidates.[84] HBV patients who receive liver transplants have 1- and 5-year survival rates of 73% and 44%, respectively.[84] Patients who are positive for HBV DNA and/or HBeAg at the time of liver transplantation should be transplanted only in clinical research trials, as they are at extremely high risk of HBV recurrence and have a more aggressive postoperative course.

Although data are conflicting, in posttransplant patients the best treatment results have been seen with lamivudine 100 mg by mouth once daily given shortly after the appearance of HBsAg.[85] Impressive virologic changes have been seen, although over half the patients have histologic changes consistent with chronic hepatitis. HBIG is often given intravenously postoperatively but does not prevent recurrence in the majority of recipients and it is very expensive.[86] IFN has been used before transplant to decrease HBV DNA and/or to clear HBeAg, and after transplantation to prevent recurrence, but is of marginal benefit and possibly may induce hepatic decompensation.[84]

Current estimates are that 15% to 30% of liver transplants are HCV related.[87] More than 90% of patients develop reinfection of the liver graft,[6] but cumulative survival rates for the HCV-infected patients who receive liver transplantation are similar to HCV-negative transplant recipients.[88] Approximately 45% of patients develop chronic hepatitis C with damage to the graft within 1 to 3 years after transplantation, and within 4 years after transplant, 8% have cirrhosis.[88] Infection with genotype 1b is associated with more severe graft injury.[88] Patients with life-threatening chronic HCV who have a life expectancy of 1 to 2 years without transplant are considered for transplantation.[40]

In treating chronic HCV after liver transplant, IFN monotherapy is associated with an increased risk of rejection, and ribavirin monotherapy is ineffective.[89,90] The combination of the two is becoming first-line therapy although results are inconsistent.[91,92] For a more thorough discussion of liver transplantation the reader is referred to other chapters in this textbook.

Most clinical trial data is with IFNα-2b; it is approved for both HBV and HCV. IFNα-2a differs by only 1 amino acid from IFNα-2b and is also made via recombinant techniques. IFNα-n1 consists of multiple subtypes derived from a human lymphoid cell line. Some of the subtypes are glycosylated. Whether this played a role in a recent trial where it was associated with less HCV relapse than patients treated with IFNα-2b is not known.[93] Consensus IFN was developed by scanning α IFN subtypes and assigning the most common amino acid at each sequence to form this molecule. It has 89% homology with IFNα-2b. Its dosing scheme is different, as 9 μg three times weekly is preferred for HCV treatment.

PATIENT EDUCATION ABOUT CHRONIC HEPATITIS B AND C

After a diagnosis of chronic viral hepatitis is confirmed, patients should be counseled to exercise as tolerated, to avoid alcohol and potentially hepatotoxic drugs (e.g., acetaminophen), and to eat a healthy diet. Patients will feel better if they lead as normal a life as possible, but they should be encouraged to develop a low-stress lifestyle that allows for frequent rest. Vaccination against hepatitis A for patients with chronic HCV or HBV, and against hepatitis B for those with chronic HCV is recommended. We know that hepatitis A virus superinfection in patients with chronic HCV has a substantial risk of fulminant hepatitis A and death.[7] Sexual partners and children of patients with chronic HBV should be vaccinated against hepatitis B. Monitoring for exacerbation of disease should be done periodically (at least once a year), as well as monitoring for spontaneous seroconversion in patients with chronic HBV.

Patients should be told that they could have chronic HBV or HCV for life. Many will feel healthy and have no signs of liver disease, while others will have symptoms, including loss of appetite and nausea. They may or may not have permanent liver disease that can include scarring of the liver, liver cancer, liver failure, and even death. They should be told that they could transmit the disease to others, whether or not they have symptoms. They should tell dentists and other health care professionals that they have HBV or HCV. Patients with chronic HBV or HCV should not donate blood, body organs, semen, or other tissue.[13] Household articles such as toothbrushes, razors, chewing gum, and washcloths should not be shared because of possible contamination with blood.[13] Personal articles such as tissues, menstrual pads, and tampons should be disposed of in a paper bag. Patients should wash their hands well after touching blood or body fluids. Any cuts or open lesions should be covered to prevent the accidental spread of infectious secretions. Safe sex should be recommended for all chronic HBV patients and for those chronic HCV patients with multiple partners. For patients with chronic HCV, it is not necessary to avoid sharing eating utensils.[94] Both pregnancy and breast feeding are acceptable for HCV-infected individuals.[94]

Because certain alternative treatments such as herbs and vitamins can damage the liver, patients with either chronic HBV or chronic HCV should be reminded to ask the pharmacist before using any over-the-counter drug, herbal remedy, or unconventional therapy. These patients should avoid alcohol and not start any medication without first consulting a health care professional. Encourage regular medical followup. Offer self-help groups and additional information sources. Many excellent resources on chronic hepatitis are available (Table 40–7).

For those patients who are being treated with IFN, education about self-administration of subcutaneous injections is necessary. Additionally, the patient and family members or caregiver should be informed about side effects and how to identify serious adverse effects (see above). Methods to decrease the severity of side effects should also be discussed.

Families who are adopting a child from countries where HBV infection is common should have the child tested for HBV as soon as the family arrives home. Even if the child appears healthy, the child can still be infected with HBV and can transmit the infection to others. If the child tests positive, the child should be evaluated for chronic liver disease and possible treatment, and counseled appropriately. All family members should be immunized for hepatitis B before the arrival of the adopted child in the new home.

People with chronic HCV should be told that the disease could attack the liver gradually over a long period of time without them even being aware of it. They should be informed that long-term scarring (cirrhosis), liver cancer, and liver failure are risks, but that we do not know what that means for any given individual.[95] These patients should also be counseled on how to decrease the risk of transmitting the virus to others (similar to patient counseling for patients with chronic hepatitis B). Individuals in long-term, monogamous sexual relationships do not have to change sexual practices. However, because the risk of transmission of HCV is small but real, some may choose to use barrier methods to decrease the transmission risk further. Sexually active people with chronic HCV should discuss the need for counseling and testing with their partners.[13] Pregnancy and breast-feeding need not be avoided in those with HCV infection (although if nipples are cracked/bleeding breast-feeding may need

TABLE 40–7. Viral Hepatitis Information Sources for Health Care Professionals and Patients

Organization Name and Address	Telephone Number	Web Address
American Association for the Study of Liver Diseases (AASLD); 6900 Grove Road; Thorofare, NJ 08086	609-848-1000	http://www.hepar-sjgh.ucsf.edu/
American College of Gastroenterology; 4900 B South 31st Street; Arlington, VA 22206	703-820-7400	http://www.acg.gi.org
American Liver Foundation; 75 Maiden Lane; New York, NY 10038	800-465-4837 or 888-443-7222	http://www.liverfoundation.org
Centers for Disease Control and Prevention (CDC)—Hepatitis Branch; Mailstop G-37, 1600 Clifton Road; Atlanta, GA 30333	888-443-7232	http://www.cdc/gov/hepatitis *or* http://www.cdc.gov/ncidod/diseases/hepatitis/c/index.htm
Digestive Health Initiative; 7910 Woodmont Avenue; Suite 700; Bethesda, MD 20814	800-668-5237	http://www.gastro.org/dhi.html
Hepatitis C Foundation; 1502 Russett Drive; Warminster, PA 18974	215-672-1518	http://www.hepcfoundation.org
Hepatitis Foundation International; 30 Sunrise Terrace; Cedar Grove, JM 07009-1423	800-891-0707	http://www/hepfi.org
Immunization Action Coalition (IAC)/Hepatitis B Coalition; 1573 Selby Avenue; Suite 234; St. Paul, MN 55104	612-647-9009	http://www.immunize.org
National Digestive Diseases Information Clearinghouse (NDDIC); 2 Information Way; Bethesda, MD 20892-3570	301-654-3810	http://www.niddk.nih.gov
National Foundation for Infectious Diseases (NFID); 4733 Bethesda Avenue; Suite 750; Bethesda, MD 20814	301-656-3810	http://www.medscape.com?Affiliates/NFID

to be interrupted temporarily). People can be reassured that HCV is not spread by coughing, sneezing, hugging, sharing eating utensils, or casual contact.[13]

ECONOMIC AND HUMANISTIC OUTCOME CONSIDERATIONS

Because the natural history of chronic hepatitis is not definitively known and because disease progression is not always associated with morbidity or mortality, the relative benefits of treatment are controversial. Considering that cost of care can be expensive and associated with adverse effects, cost effectiveness analysis becomes important. The following are examples of costs of therapies, based on average wholesale prices:[96]

Epivir-HB (lamivudine) 100 mg daily for 1 year = \$1,658
Intron-A (IFNα-2b) 5 MU SC daily × 16 weeks = \$6,784
Intron-A (IFNα-2b) 3 MU SC three times weekly × 6 months = \$2,835
Intron-A (IFNα-2b) 3 MU SC three times weekly × 12 months = \$5,669
Rebetron
Patients weighing <75 kg, 6 months = \$8,640; 12 months = \$17,280
Patients weighing >75 kg, 6 months = \$9,547; 12 months = \$19,094

Despite these costs, analyses demonstrate a benefit in the treatment of hepatitis C not only in previously untreated patients and relapsed patients, but even in those classified as nonresponders. Cost-effectiveness ratios are measured in dollars per year of life gained and are discounted at rates of 3% to 5% per year because future value is less than present value. Cost saving agents, with downstream prevention of cost from morbidity outweighing treatment costs combined with increased life expectancy are desirable, but are infrequently found.

In chronic HCV patients who are previously untreated, IFN monotherapy for 6 to 12 months versus no therapy has been calculated to cost between \$500 and \$6,900 per year of life gained.[97,98] Comparing combination therapy to IFN monotherapy in the same group found \$2,100 to \$2,300 extra dollars were required per year of life gained, depending on duration of therapy and pretreatment variables.[99] In patients who had relapsed with IFN monotherapy, Wong calculated that combination therapy (at three times the cost of IFN monotherapy) would prolong life by 2.8 years and decrease lifetime costs.[100] These projections, based on data presented in Fig. 40–2, also estimate that for combination therapy to *not* be cost-effective would require the virologic SR to be one-sixth of the original estimate. An analysis of combination therapy versus no therapy in previous IFN nonresponders demonstrated that \$8,800 to \$27,800 would have to be spent per quality-adjusted life-year gained.[101] These figures are difficult to reconcile, though, as the costs seem high relative to the benefit in this subgroup—the gain in life expectancy is only from 2 to 4 months.

Each of these analyses is only as good as the underlying assumptions, but the published data are in favor of chronic HCV treatment. In fact, one model showed a favorable effect of empirical IFN monotherapy without recommended pretreatment procedures such as biopsy.[100] Intense scrutiny is required, especially because the natural course of chronic hepatitis C and its impact on morbidity and mortality are still in question. For the time being, patient selection on the basis of predictors of response, coupled with informed patient decision making regarding benefits and risks, is appropriate until better definition is given to the cost effectiveness of treatment of chronic hepatitis C.

It is accepted by most that treatment of chronic HBV in patients with good predictors of response is cost effective, especially among younger individuals.[102–104] Using data from a meta-analysis of 9 trials with 552 chronic HBV patients, it was estimated that IFN treatment would increase life expectancy by 3.1 years and decrease lifetime costs by more than \$2,100.[103] Little data is available with lamivudine, but given that its acquisition cost is one-quarter that of IFN, it would appear to have reasonable cost effectiveness.

Patients with chronic HCV have a significant impairment in quality of life that is unrelated to the severity of disease. Successful treatment of infection increases and recurrence of HCV following liver transplantation decreases quality of life in HCV patients.[105–107] Using a quality of life instrument based on the Medical Outcomes Study short-form health survey (SF-36), patients with chronic HCV score significantly lower than the general population on several of the eight subscales (physical function, physical disability, bodily pain, general health, vitality, social function, emotional disability, and mental health).[108,109] Part of the decrease in quality of life is a result of the disease itself; however, the effect of labeling plays a role as well.[109] This cost must be balanced against the risk, the chance of response, and the expected consequences of untreated chronic hepatitis along with the fact that (especially for chronic HCV) the optimal dose, duration, and combination of therapy are poorly defined.

PREVENTION OF VIRAL HEPATITIS

GOALS OF PREVENTION

The goals of passive and active immunization against viral hepatitis include protecting people from infection, preventing the short-term viremia that can lead to transmission of infection, preventing the morbidity and occasional mortality associated with the disease, avoiding chronic infection, and, ultimately, eliminating transmission.[2,110] The mainstays of hepatitis prevention are risk reduction, education, passive immunization with immune globulins, and active immunization with vaccines. The spread of HAV can be controlled by cautious handling of fomites contaminated with feces coupled with good hand-washing techniques. Universal precautions are used to prevent hepatitis B and C spread within the hospital setting. HBV and HCV spread are reduced, but not eliminated, through screening of blood donors and testing for HBsAg and anti-HCV.

PREVENTION OF HEPATITIS A

General Approach to Prevention of Hepatitis A

Highly effective inactivated vaccines against HAV have been available in the United States since 1995. These vaccines can substantially lower the incidence of HAV infection, and potentially even eradicate the disease.[2]

The most effective means of achieving control of HAV infection is to vaccinate all children by incorporating hepatitis A vaccination into routine childhood immunizations. This is not currently possible because neither a vaccine formulation nor a schedule is available for children younger than 2 years old. Until routine infant vaccination is feasible, the vaccination strategy in the United States includes vaccinating: (a) children in states, counties, and communities with consistently elevated rates of hepatitis A; (b) persons in groups at increased risk for HAV infection, such as international travelers; and (c) persons at risk of adverse outcomes, such as, persons with chronic liver disease.[2]

Even though effective active and passive immunity agents are available for HAV, the importance of avoiding exposure cannot be overemphasized. The most important measures to avoid exposure include good hand-washing techniques and good personal hygiene practices. Travelers can minimize risk by avoiding uncooked shellfish, uncooked fruits and vegetables, and by avoiding drinking water (and other beverages with ice) of unknown purity. If exposure occurs, postexposure prophylaxis is with immune globulin injection.

Immunoglobulin to Prevent Hepatitis A

Immunoglobulin (Ig), formerly immune serum globulin (ISG), provides protection against HAV by passive transfer of concentrated antibodies (immunoglobulins) against the hepatitis A virus (anti-HAV). Ig is effective in modifying the course and preventing the spread of HAV in 85% or more of exposures when used within 2 weeks following the exposure.[2] Ig available in the United States does not contain HBsAg, HIV, or anti-HCV. Pregnancy and lactation are not contraindications to receiving Ig; however, when Ig is administered to pregnant women or infants, thimerosal-free preparations should be used.[2] Both Ig given intramuscularly (IgIM) and Ig for intravenous administration (IgIV) contain anti-HAV, but IgIM is used for prevention of HAV infection.[2]

International travelers are the major group receiving preexposure prophylaxis with Ig. Ig is recommended for susceptible persons traveling to developing countries. The CDC publication, *Health Information for International Travel,* or the CDC Web site (www.cdc.gov) can be consulted for specific recommendations. A single dose of Ig of 0.02 mL/kg IM (in the deltoid or gluteus muscle) is recommended if travel is for less than 3 months. For lengthy stays, 0.06 mL/kg IM should be given every 3 to 5 months.[2] Dosing is the same for adults and children. The concentrations of anti-HAV achieved after administration of Ig (or after active vaccination) are 10 to 100 times lower than those achieved after natural infection and are often below the limits of detection for commercial assays.[2]

The availability of an effective hepatitis A vaccine has reduced the use of Ig in travelers. Ig is less expensive than vaccination, however, and remains an alternative for the traveler who does not need long-term protection. If the interval between the first dose of the hepatitis A vaccine and travel is less than 2 weeks, administration of Ig should be considered to provide passive immunity during the interval before active vaccine-induced immunity develops. In this situation, the lower dose of Ig is used.

The postexposure prophylactic benefit from Ig is greatest early in the incubation period and is of no benefit more than 2 weeks after exposure.[2] In most situations, serologic screening of contacts for anti-HAV is not recommended before Ig administration because screening is costly and delays prophylaxis. A single Ig dose of 0.02 mL/kg IM is used for postexposure prophylaxis. Again, the dose is the same for adults and children. People who have been given one dose of hepatitis A vaccine at least 1 month before exposure do not need Ig.

Ig should be given to previously unvaccinated people who have had (a) close personal contact with a person who has hepatitis A; (b) all staff and attendees of day care centers when hepatitis A is documented; (c) common-source exposures (other food handlers at locations where a food handler has hepatitis A; patrons, if the infected food handler handled food and had diarrhea or poor hygienic practices); (d) classroom contacts of an index case patient; and (e) schools, hospitals, and work settings when close contact occurs with index patients.[2]

Serious adverse events to Ig are rare. Anaphylaxis has been reported in individuals with IgA deficiency who have received repeated doses of Ig.[2] People who need repeat doses while overseas should make sure they receive products that meet US standards for purity.

Ig does not interfere with the immune response to yellow fever vaccine, oral poliovirus vaccine, or inactivated vaccines. Hepatitis A vaccine can be given concomitantly with Ig; however, the antibody titer obtained is lower (but still protective) than when the vaccine is given alone. Ig can interfere with the response to measles, rubella, mumps (MMR), and varicella vaccines.[2] Administration of MMR vaccine should be delayed for at least 3 months after administration of Ig (5 months for varicella vaccine).[2] Conversely, Ig should not be administered within 2 weeks after the administration of MMR (3 weeks for varicella vaccine), unless the benefits of Ig clearly outweigh the benefits of vaccination. If Ig is administered within 2 weeks after administration of MMR (3 weeks for varicella vaccine), the person should be revaccinated—but not sooner than 3 months (5 months for varicella) after Ig.[2]

Vaccines to Prevent Hepatitis A

Inactivated HAV vaccines, Havrix (SmithKline Beecham) and Vaqta (Merck & Co, Inc.) both demonstrate protective efficacy in 94% to 100% of vaccinees within 1 month after primary vaccination.[111,112] When a booster dose is given 6 or more months later, essentially 100% of recipients develop high antibody levels. Both vaccines are indicated for immunization of individuals 2 years of age or older. Groups recommended for preexposure protection against HAV with hepatitis A vaccine are shown in Table 40–2. Hepatitis A vaccine is useful in preventing secondary infection in household contacts of primary cases of HAV infection.[113] No recommendations exist for use of hepatitis A vaccine for postexposure protection, however.

The antigen content of the two vaccines is determined differently, which results in the vaccine units being expressed differently. For Havrix, the vaccine potency is expressed as enzyme-linked immunosorbent assay (ELISA) units, while for Vaqta, the antigen content is expressed as units (U) of HAV antigen.[2]

The two vaccine products have different formulations and the dosing differs according to the person's age. Table 40–8 lists the approved dosing for these vaccines. The primary vaccination is a single dose, with a booster dose 6 to 12 months later for children and adults. Both vaccines are injected intramuscularly into the deltoid muscle. The primary immunization should be given at least 2 weeks (preferably 4 weeks) prior to expected exposure to HAV. The vaccine can be given at the same time as many other vaccines (diphtheria, tetanus, live or inactivated polio, oral and injectable typhoid, cholera, Japanese encephalitis, rabies, yellow fever, and hepatitis B) without interfering with the immune responses. Each vaccine should be given with a different syringe and at a different injection site. Data indicate that if one dose is given with one brand and the other dose given with the other brand, protective antibody levels do not differ;[2] the two brands are interchangeable. Limited data are available on what to do if the patient has a delay in receiving the second vaccine dose. It is

TABLE 40–8. Recommended Dosing of Havrix and Vaqta[2]

Vaccine	Vaccinee's Age (years)	Dose	Volume (mL)	Number of Doses	Schedule (Months)[b]
Havrix	2 to 18	720 ELISA units[a]	0.5	2	0, 6–12
	>18	1440 ELISA units	1	2	0, 6–12
Vaqta	2 to 17	25 Units	0.5	2	0, 6–18
	>17	50 Units	1	2	0, 6

[a]HAVRIX previously was also available as 360 ELISA units per dose. This formulation was administered as a three-dose schedule for persons 2 to 18 years of age. It is no longer available.

[b]0 months represents the timing of the initial dose; subsequent numbers represent months after the initial dose.

known that administering the second (booster) dose up to 35 months after the initial dose results in an adequate response.[2] As with other inactivated vaccines, hepatitis A vaccine can be administered to immunocompromised persons.

Data are limited on long-term persistence of antibody and of immune memory. To date, the vaccines are known to have protective levels of anti-HAV for at least 5 to 8 years.[2,5] Based on kinetic models of antibody decline, it is projected that protective anti-HAV levels should be present for 20 years to life.[2]

The vaccine is safe. Side effects include local reactions at the injection site (soreness, induration, redness, and swelling) and headache.[2] As with all adverse events potentially related to a vaccine, any adverse event temporally related to hepatitis A vaccination should be reported to the Vaccine Adverse Events Reporting System (VAERS, 1-800-822-7967; http://www.fda.gov/cber/vaers/vaers.htm).

Although vaccination of a person who is already immune does not increase the risk of adverse effects, there are certain populations where prevaccination testing should be conducted. Such testing is cost effective in the United States in populations that are expected to have high rates of prior HAV infection. Testing of children is not indicated. The populations for whom prevaccination testing is usually cost-effective include older adolescents and adults (a) who were born or lived for an extended period in geographic areas with a high endemicity of HAV; (b) men who have sex with men; (c) American Indians, Alaskan Natives, Hispanics; (d) injecting drug users; and (e) older adults.[2] Postvaccination testing for serologic response is not indicated because of the high rate of vaccine response.

PREVENTION OF HEPATITIS B

General Approach to Prevention

The two products available for prevention of hepatitis B infection include hepatitis B vaccine (provides long lasting active immunity) and hepatitis B immunoglobulin (HBIg, provides temporary passive immunity).[1] The vaccine is used in preexposure prophylaxis. It is also used in postexposure prophylaxis in combination with HBIg. Vaccination is the most effective method for preventing hepatitis B (Tables 40–9, 40–10, 40–11, and 40–12).

HBIg to Prevent Hepatitis B

HBIg is used only in postexposure prophylaxis. Postexposure prophylaxis for HBV is recommended for perinatal exposure, sexual exposure to HBsAg-positive persons, percutaneous or permucosal exposure to HBsAg-positive blood, and exposure of an infant to a caregiver who has acute hepatitis B.[1] HBIg is given to immunocompromised patients for the same indications and in the same doses as immunocompetent individuals.[115] The recommended dose is 0.06 mL/kg administered intramuscularly. Guidelines for use are listed in Tables 40–9 and 40–10.[1,115,116]

Use of Ig for prophylaxis of HBV infection is only recommended when HBIg is not available. Ig contains anti-HBs in titers of 1:100 to 1:1000, in comparison to the 1:100,000 or greater anti-HBs titer found in HBIg. Ig and HBIg available in the United States do not transmit HBV, HIV, or other viruses.

TABLE 40–9. Recommended Schedule of Immunoprophylaxis to Prevent Perinatal or Sexual Transmission of HBV Infection [1,115,116]

Vaccine Recipient	Immunoprophylaxis	Timing
Infant born to HBsAg-positive mother	Vaccine dose 1	Within 12 hours of birth
	HBIG (0.5 mL, intramuscularly, at a site different from that used for the vaccine)	Within 12 hours of birth
	Vaccine doses 2 and 3	Usual schedule
Infant born to mother not screened for HBsAg	Vaccine dose 1*	Within 12 hours of birth
	HBIG (0.5 mL, intramuscularly, at a site different from that used for the vaccine)	If mother is found to be HBsAg-positive, administer dose to infant as soon as possible, but no later than 1 week after birth
	Vaccine doses 2 and 3*	Usual schedule
Sexual exposure	HBIG (0.06 mL/kg intramuscularly, at a site different from that used for the vaccine)	Single dose within 14 days of sexual contact
	Vaccine dose 1	At time of HBIG treatment
	Vaccine doses 2 and 3	Usual schedule

*The first dose of vaccine is the same as that for the infant of an HBsAg-positive mother. If the mother is found to be HBsAg-positive, that dose is continued. If the mother is found to be HBsAg-negative, the remaining vaccine doses are those appropriate for other infants and children.

TABLE 40–10. Recommendations for Hepatitis B Prophylaxis Following Percutaneous or Permucosal Exposure [1,115,116]

Vaccination Status of Exposed Person	Treatment According to HBsAg Status of Source		
	HBsAg-Positive	HBsAg-Negative	Source Not Tested or Unknown
Unvaccinated	HBIG (one dose of 0.06 mL/kg IM), plus initiate vaccine[a]	Initiate vaccine[a]	Initiate vaccine[a]
Previously vaccinated, known responder	Test exposed person for anti-HBs level If adequate,[b] no treatment If inadequate or titer unknown, 1 vaccine booster dose	No treatment	No treatment
Previously vaccinated, known nonresponder	HBIG (two doses 1 month apart) or HBIG one dose, plus dose of vaccine	No treatment	If known high-risk source, may treat as if source were HBsAg-positive
Previously vaccinated, response unknown	Test exposed person for anti-HBs level If inadequate,[b] HBIG one dose, plus one vaccine booster dose If adequate, no treatment If titer unknown, one vaccine booster dose	No treatment	Test exposed for anti-HBs level If inadequate,[b] vaccine booster dose If adequate, no treatment

[a]Vaccine dosage is given in Table 40–11.
[b]Adequate anti-HBs is ≥10 mIU/mL by radioimmunoassay or enzyme immunoassay.

Vaccines to Prevent Hepatitis B

The comprehensive vaccination strategy in the United States targets interruption of transmission at all age groups through routine infant immunization, continued vaccination of high-risk older adolescents and adults (e.g., HIV-infected individuals), routine screening of pregnant women for HBsAg, and vaccination of all unvaccinated children ages 0 to 18 years of age (Tables 40–11 and 40–12).[116–119] Several states have laws mandating hepatitis B immunization prior to entry into kindergarten or middle school.

In countries where the risk of hepatitis B is relatively low, such as the United States, determining who to vaccinate prior to exposure depends on the risk of infection in that group and the relative cost of pretesting versus the cost of vaccination. Everyone in high-risk, low-prevalence groups (such as health care professionals in training) can be vaccinated without screening.[1] To comply with federal guidelines, employers offer health care workers with potential exposure to blood hepatitis B vaccination at no cost.

In addition to vaccinating health care workers against hepatitis B, other infection control practices are important in preventing transmission of the virus because up to 10% of people do not develop an adequate antibody response to the vaccine. The most important infection control measure is the use of universal precautions. These precautions

TABLE 40–11. Recommended Doses and Schedules of Currently Licensed HB Vaccines

Group	Vaccine		
	Recombivax HB[a] dose, μg (mL)	Engerix-B[a,b] dose, μg (mL)	Comvax[c] dose, μg (ml)
Infants of HBsAg-positive mothers	5 (0.5)	10 (0.5)	Not indicated
All other infants, children, and adolescents ≤19 years of age	5 (0.5)[d]	10 (0.5)	5 (0.5)[e]
Adults age 20 years and older	10 (1)	20 (1)	Not indicated
Dialysis patients and other immunocompromised persons	40 (1)[f]	40 (2)[g,h]	Not indicated

[a]Usual schedules: Infants: Three doses given at birth, at 1 to 2 months, and at 6 to 18 months of age; or, for infants, with other routine immunizations at 1 to 2 months, 4 months, and 6 to 18 months of age. Older children and adults: Three doses given at 0-, 2-, and 6-month or, at 0-, 2-, and 4-month intervals. Higher titers of HBsAb are achieved with the last two doses of vaccine being spaced at least 4 months apart.
[b]Alternative approved schedule: four doses, one given at 0, 1, 2, and 12 month intervals.
[c]Contains 5 μg/0.5 mL hepatitis B surface antigen (HBsAg) and 7.5 μg Hemophilus influenza type B purified capsular polysaccharide fragments conjugated to 125 μg *Neisseria meningitidis* outer membrane protein complex.
[d]An alternate two-dose schedule can be used for adolescents aged 11 to 15 years. If the two-dose schedule is used, the adult dose (1 mL containing 10 μg of HBsAg) is administered with the second dose given 4 to 6 months after the first dose.
[e]Usually given at 2, 4, and 12 to 15 months of age. Comvax is not used when immunizing older children or adolescents.
[f]Special formulation for dialysis patients.
[g]Two 1-mL doses given at different sites.
[h]Four-dose schedule recommended at 0, 1, 2, and 6 month intervals.

TABLE 40–12. Groups Recommended for Preexposure Hepatitis B Vaccination[1,119]

All infants via routine infant vaccination
Unvaccinated 11- to 12-year-old children
Unvaccinated children ages <11 years of age who are Pacific Islanders or who reside in households of first-generation immigrants from countries where HBV is of high or intermediate endemicity
Health care and public safety workers who have occupational exposure to blood
HIV-infected individuals
Injection drug users
Heterosexual individuals who have had more than one sexual partner in the previous 6 months and/or those with a recent episode of a sexually transmitted disease
Sexually active homosexual or bisexual males
Hemodialysis patients
Recipients of certain blood products; i.e., patients with hemophilia and other clotting disorders
Clients and staff of institutions for the developmentally disabled
Household, sexual, and blood exposure contacts of either HBsAg-positive persons or those with acute HBV infection
Household contacts of adoptees from countries where HBV is highly endemic
Populations where HBV is highly endemic (e.g., Alaskan Eskimos)
Inmates of long-term correctional facilities
International travelers to highly endemic HBV regions for > 6 months and who have close contact with the local population; also short-term travelers who have contact with blood, or sexual contact with residents in high- or intermediate-risk areas
Unvaccinated infants under 12 months of age exposed to acute HBV infection through primary care giver

prevent exposure to blood and blood-derived body fluids via use of a variety of barrier precautions, measures to prevent needle sticks, environmental control measures, and good hand-washing techniques. However, if a worker is exposed to material that potentially contains HBV, recommendations for percutaneous exposure to HBV should be followed (Table 40–10).[115,116]

The two recombinant hepatitis B vaccine products available in the United States (Recombivax HB, Merck & Co., Inc.; Engerix-B, SmithKline Beecham) have comparable immune responses and safety profiles.[1] The vaccines contain 5–40 μg HBsAg protein per mL adsorbed onto aluminum.[1] Neither brand of hepatitis B vaccine contains thimerosal.

These vaccines are some of the safest available.[110] Side effects of the vaccine are soreness at the injection site, headache, fatigue, irritability, and fever. The number of patients experiencing adverse reactions decreases with each vaccine dose, and adverse reactions are less common in infants and children than in adults. There is no association between Guillain-Barré syndrome and the recombinant vaccine and the vaccine does not transmit HIV. The hepatitis B vaccine is contraindicated for patients with anaphylaxis to common baker's yeast. Hepatitis B vaccines are inactivated and can be simultaneously administered with other vaccines.[1] Breast-fed infants can be vaccinated with hepatitis B vaccine, as can immunocompromised infants and children.[115,117] The vaccine can be given to pregnant and lactating women.

In the last several years, a small number of claims of serious adverse effects after hepatitis B vaccine administration have occurred. Complaints cover a spectrum of autoimmune and nervous system disorders such as rheumatoid arthritis, optic neuritis, and neurodegenerative disorders similar to multiple sclerosis. Public health officials are confident the vaccine is safe, but because claims of vaccine-induced injury are likely to continue, several epidemiologic studies are underway to evaluate association. Millions of people receive hepatitis B vaccine each year, and some will blame the vaccine for any adverse event that is temporally related to vaccine administration.

HBV vaccine is given as a series of three IM doses into the deltoid (anterolateral thigh in infants) over a period of months. The dose of vaccine to induce the desired antibody response or protective effect varies among the available vaccines (Table 40–11).[116] Specific dosing guidelines for all age groups are listed in Table 40–11.[116,117] All dosing schedules give excellent seroconversion rates, although the postvaccination titer is lower with accelerated dosing and shorter intervals between the second and third dose.[110] The vaccination process does not need to be restarted if doses are missed.[1] If the interval between vaccine doses is greater than recommended, the vaccine series can simply be completed. Partial protection is achieved after the second dose. The purpose of the third vaccine dose is to boost the antibody titers and provide a more durable response.[110] The vaccination series can be started with one vaccine type and completed with another.[117]

Dosing guidelines for infants born to HBsAg-positive mothers and mothers whose HBsAg status is unknown are in Table 40–9.[116,117] Perinatal transmission of HBV occurs in 70% to 90% of infected mothers.[1] Because 20% to 30% of infants infected with HBV die of complications of the infection and a higher percentage experience substantial morbidity, all infants (premature or full term) born to HBsAg-positive women should be vaccinated within 12 hours of birth with HBV vaccine and one dose of HBIg. With this regimen, only 5% to 15% of infants develop the carrier state.[1] Unfortunately, this small percentage of infections occurs in utero and cannot be prevented.

Testing for anti-HBs in a child younger than 1 year of age is not useful because of the persistence of maternal antibody. Pregnant women whose HBsAg status is unknown at delivery should have their blood drawn for testing. If test results cannot be obtained with 12 hours of birth, the infant should be vaccinated. Infants of women determined to be HBsAg-positive should receive HBIg as soon as possible, but always within 7 days of birth. Routine childhood vaccinations can also be given.

For premature infants with birthweights of less than 2000 g born to HBsAg-negative mothers, hepatitis B vaccination should be delayed until just before hospital discharge, until the infant weighs 2000 g or until the infant is 2 months of age.[120] Serologic testing for response is not routinely recommended.

The three-dose vaccination series induces an adequate anti-HBs response in more than 90% of healthy adults and over 95% of infants and children.[1] An adequate response is defined as anti-HBs of 10 mIU/mL or greater, measured 1 to 6 months after completion of the vaccine series.[1] Low (or hypo-) responders (10 to 100 mIU/mL), as well as those with good response (greater than or equal to 100 mIU/mL) have complete protection against clinical infection with the virus. Many factors decrease the immunogenicity of hepatitis B vaccines, including immunocompromised states, smoking, increased age, immunization into the buttock, low dose, renal insufficiency, alcoholism, and increased body mass.[1] A lack of response to the vaccine in immunocompetent adults is genetically determined, and investigational HBV vaccines target the non- and low responders by including other immunogenic domains (pre-S/S components).[121]

Persistence of anti-HBs is directly related to the height of the antibody response.[122] Maintenance of an antibody level above 10 mIU/mL is not essential for protection against infection in immunocompetent individuals. Immunologic memory after primary exposure to the vaccine produces a population of memory B-lymphocytes. With subsequent exposure to HBV, these proliferate, differentiate, and produce anti-HBs within days.[122] Likewise, healthy persons respond to a vaccine booster dose within 3 to 5 days (even if antibody is undetectable prior to the booster dose).[122] For adults and children whose immune status is normal, neither booster doses of vaccine nor serologic testing for immunity are needed. It is not yet known whether the infant hepatitis B immunization series confers lifelong immunity; however, data from long-term studies indicate that most vaccine responders are protected from HBV infection well past adolescence.

Vaccine nonresponders or inadequate responders should be revaccinated with one or two booster vaccine doses, and then given booster doses every year or two thereafter.[1] As many as 50% of nonresponders will develop anti-HBs after two additional doses of vaccine, although the level of antibody achieved is low.[1,110]

Postvaccination testing for immunity is only important for persons at risk for poor antibody response and for those at very high risk for exposure, such as hemodialysis patients, HIV-infected patients, certain public safety personnel, and extremely obese people.[1,110] Other immunosuppressed groups with decreased response to HBV vaccine include alcoholics with clinical liver disease and patients with hematologic malignancies, organ transplants, diabetes, or hemophilia. Hemodialysis patients have decreased seroconversion rates, decreased antibody titers to surface antigens, and a faster rate of loss of antibody after HBV vaccination. Hemodialysis patients require higher vaccine doses or an increased number of doses,[115] and a special high-dose formulation of Recombivax HB (40 μg/mL) is available for them. Protection in this group is maintained only as long as the anti-HBs level remains above 10 mIU/mL. Routine anti-HBs testing (at 12-month intervals) and booster doses to maintain adequate anti-HBs are recommended in hemodialysis patients.[1] Patients with renal disease who will likely need dialysis or transplantation should receive hepatitis B vaccination before dialysis is initiated. For other individuals at risk of poor vaccine response or at high risk of exposure, testing for peak anti-HBs should be conducted 1 to 3 months after completion of the vaccine series. HIV-infected patients are unlikely to respond to revaccination. HIV-infected patients are also prone to have an impaired response to HBV infection and are more likely to become chronic carriers. Testing for antibody response is recommended, with notification of nonresponders of the potential consequences (infection, carrier state, delta virus superinfection).

The vaccine is safe in HBsAg chronic carriers, but ineffective in eliminating HBsAg. Antibody acquired from HBIg or Ig administration or via the placenta will not interfere with development of active immunity; for example, HBIg can be administered concomitantly with the first dose of vaccine.[1]

Postexposure prophylaxis for HBV infection is important for all people not previously vaccinated who are either exposed to blood potentially containing HBsAg or exposed sexually to an HBsAg-positive person. Tables 40–9 and 40–10 have specific recommendations.

PREVENTION OF HEPATITIS C

No vaccine for hepatitis C is available. Vaccine development for HCV is difficult because of the extensive genomic variability of the virus, viral mutants, and the lack of efficacy of serum antibodies. Current recommendations for prevention of HCV include universal precautions for the prevention of blood-borne infections and anti-HCV screening of blood, organ, and tissue donors. Screening of blood donors has virtually eliminated HCV transmission through blood and blood products. Programs that focus on reducing HIV transmission are also likely to decrease transmission of HCV in high-risk groups. No clear policy for counseling women of childbearing age exists.

Benefit associated with identification of HCV infections in health care workers is limited. However, the CDC, in collaboration with the Hospital Infection Control Practices Advisory Committee, recommends that health care institutions consider implementing policies and procedures for followup for HCV infection after percutaneous or permucosal exposures to blood.[123] Followup should include testing the source for anti-HCV; baseline and 6-month followup testing for anti-HCV and AST for the person exposed to an anti-HCV-positive source; confirmation by supplemental anti-HCV testing of all anti-HCV-reactive results; and education of health care workers about blood-borne infections. Postexposure prophylaxis with Ig or IFN is not recommended.

There are no specific recommendations for HCV immune prophylaxis for exposed individuals. Prophylaxis with Ig after needlestick exposure to hepatitis C is not recommended.

PREVENTION OF DELTA HEPATITIS

The delta virus depends on HBV for replication, and thus prevention of HBV infection will prevent HDV.[1] Exposure to HBV and HDV should be treated as an exposure to HBV alone.[1] No products are available to help prevent HDV superinfection in HBsAg carriers.

PREVENTION OF HEPATITIS E

The best prevention method for hepatitis E is avoidance of potentially contaminated food or water and to maintain good sanitary practices.[1] Improvements in drinking water storage, treatment, and distribution, and in sanitation in developing countries, will reduce HEV transmission.[22] There is no evidence that Ig or HBIg will prevent hepatitis E, and it is unlikely that immunoglobulins prepared in the United States would have high concentrations of antibody to hepatitis E, because the disease is rare in the United States. A vaccine would be useful, but it is not clear whether manufacturers are interested in developing a vaccine that would be used primarily in developing countries.

ECONOMIC CONSIDERATIONS IN PREVENTION OF VIRAL HEPATITIS

Vaccination against HAV without prior screening is only cost-saving for groups of young adults who are exposed to a relatively high risk of HAV infection, for example, in communities with high rates of HAV.[2,124] Prior screening for HAV antibodies can only be recommended from a cost-effectiveness point of view at expected levels of natural immunity exceeding 35% (moderately endemic countries or in older travelers).[124] Passive immunization remains the most cost-effective option for occasional short-duration travel to highly endemic areas. Vaccination is cost-effective for individuals who are likely to spend several or prolonged periods in highly endemic countries. On average, vaccination is not going to be cost saving, and the cost per infection prevented can be several thousands of dollars.[124]

Several investigators have examined the cost-effectiveness of the United States hepatitis B vaccination strategies.[125,126] Several studies conclude that universal vaccination of infants, combined with catch-up programs, is cost-effective.[125,126] The cost per life-year-saved compares favorably with programs such as smoking cessation, coronary artery bypass surgery, and pneumococcal vaccination.[125] However, because much of the costs of HBV-related liver disease accrue years into the future, it is important to interpret analyses with caution, and to recognize that not all analyses have found the vaccination to be cost-saving or cost effective.

▶ PRINCIPLES OF PHARMACOTHERAPY

- Viral hepatitis causes significant morbidity and mortality. Despite breakthroughs in diagnosis and management, acute and chronic viral hepatitis infections remain worldwide health problems having tremendous clinical and economic impact.
- Hepatitis A usually does not cause clinical illness in children, but adults with acute HAV can be clinically ill for 1 or more months. It is transmitted by the fecal to oral route. Treatment is symptomatic. Prevention with vaccine or immunoglobulin is encouraged.
- Hepatitis B virus causes acute and chronic disease, with complications that include chronic active hepatitis, cirrhosis, hepatocellular cancer, and death. Some individuals carry the virus and transmit it to others, but are not clinically ill themselves. For patients with chronic hepatitis B, IFNα is the most effective known treatment. A minority of chronic HBV patients are cured with IFNα therapy. Lamivudine is a reasonable alternative therapy.
- Chronic hepatitis C infection is a significant public health problem. The current therapy of choice is a combination of IFNα and ribavirin. Unfortunately, a sustained response is seen in less than half of treated patients.
- Hepatitis E is rarely seen in the United States, except in international travelers. It is similar to HAV in transmission and clinical course.
- More safe and effective therapeutic options and therapeutic combinations are desirable for both chronic HBV and chronic HCV.
- Persons at increased risk for HAV infection or its consequences such as frequent international travelers, should be vaccinated against hepatitis A. Children living in communities with high rates of hepatitis A as well as contacts of case-patients should also receive hepatitis A vaccination.
- All infants should be immunized against hepatitis B. Older children and adults in high-risk groups who have not been previously immunized should also receive the vaccine.
- More widespread use of vaccines provides the best weapon against viral hepatitis. Immunoprophylaxis of viral diseases is one of the most cost-effective medical strategies.
- No effective active or passive immunization measures are available to protect against HCV infection.

REFERENCES

1. Centers for Disease Control and Prevention. Protection against viral hepatitis: Recommendations of the Immunization Practices Advisory Committee (ACIP). MMWR Morb Mortal Wkly Rep 1990; 39:1–26.
2. Centers for Disease Control and Prevention. Prevention of hepatitis A through active or passive immunization: Recommendations of the Advisory Committee on Immunization Practices (ACIP). MMWR Morb Mortal Wkly Rep 1999;48(RR-12):1–37.
3. Margolis HS. Hepatitis B virus infection. Bull World Health Organ 1998:76(suppl 2):152–153.
4. Koziel MJ. Immunology of viral hepatitis. Am J Med 1996;100:98–109.
5. WHO position paper: Hepatitis A vaccines. Wkly Epidemiol Rec 2000; (Feb 4)5:38–44.
6. Kiyasu PK, Caldwell SH. Diagnosis and treatment of the major hepatatrophic viruses. Am J Med Sci 1993;306:248–261.
7. Vento S, Garofano T, Renzini C, et al. Fulminant hepatitis associated with hepatitis A virus superinfection in patients with chronic hepatitis C. N Engl J Med 1998;338:286–290.
8. McQuillan GM, Coleman PJ, Kruszon-Moran D, et al. Prevalence of hepatitis B virus infection in the United States: The National Health and Nutrition Examination Surveys, 1976 through 1994. Am J Public Health 1999;89:14–18.
9. Bortolotti F. Treatment of chronic hepatitis C in children. J Hepatol 1999;31(suppl 1):201–4.
10. Lok ASF. Hepatitis B infection: pathogenesis and management. J Hepatol 2000;32(suppl 1):89–97.
11. Lee WM. Hepatitis B virus infection. N Engl J Med 1997;24:1733–1745.
12. Centers for Disease Control and Prevention. Recommendations for prevention and control of hepatitis C (HCV) infection and HCV-related chronic disease. MMWR Morb Mortal Wkly Rep 1998;47(RR-19): 1–39.
13. Williams I. Epidemiology of hepatitis C in the United States. Am J Med 1999;107(6B):2S–9S.
14. Alter MJ, Kruszon-Moran D, Nainan OV, et al. The prevalence of hepatitis C virus infection in the United States, 1988 through 1994. N Engl J Med. 1999;341:556–562.
15. Zanetti AR, Tanzi E, Newell ML. Mother-to-infant transmission of hepatitis C virus. J Hepatol Suppl 1999;31:96–100.
16. London WT, Evans AA. The epidemiology of hepatitis viruses B, C, and D. Clin Lab Med 1996;16:251–271.
17. Iwarson S, Norkrans G, Wejstal R. Hepatitis C: Natural history of a unique infection. Clin Infect Dis 1995;20:1361–1370.
18. Liang TJ, Rehermann B, Seeff LB, Hoofnagle JH. NIH Conference: Pathogenesis, natural history, treatment, and prevention of hepatitis C. Ann Intern Med 2000;132:296–305.
19. Zein NN, Rakela J, Krawitt EL, et al. Hepatitis C virus genotypes in the United States: Epidemiology, pathogenicity, and response to interferon therapy. Ann Intern Med 1996;125:634–639.
20. Malnick SDH, Beergabel M, Lurie Y. Treatment of chronic hepatitis C virus infection. Ann Pharmacother 2000;34:1156–1164.
21. Fried MW. Diagnostic testing for hepatitis C: Practical considerations. Am J Med 1999;107(6B):31S–35S.
22. Labrique Al, Thomas DL, Stoszek SK, Nelson KE. Hepatitis E: An emerging infectious disease. Epidemiol Rev 1999;21:162–179.
23. Centers for Disease Control and Prevention. Hepatitis E among U.S. travelers, 1989–1992. MMWR Morb Mortal Wkly Rep 1993;42:1–4.
24. Scharschmidt BF. Hepatitis E: A virus in waiting. Lancet 1995;346:519–520.
25. Miyakawa Y, Mayumi M. Hepatitis G virus—A true hepatitis virus or an accidental tourist? N Engl J Med 1997;336:795–796.
26. Slimane SB, Albrecht JK, Fang JWS, et al. Clinical, virological and histological implications of GB virus-C/hepatitis G virus infection in patients with chronic hepatitis C virus infection: A multicentre study based on 671 patients. J Viral Hepat 2000;7:51–55.
27. Meng XW, Komatsu M, Ohshima S, et al. GAB virus C infection: Clinical significance. Can J Gastroenterol 1999;13:814–818.
28. Alter MJ, Gallagher M, Morris TT, et al. Acute non-A-E hepatitis in the United States and the role of hepatitis G virus infection. N Engl J Med 1997;336:741–746.
29. Cossart Y. TTV a common virus, but pathogenic? Lancet 1998;352:164.
30. Kanda Y, Chiba S, Tanaka Y, et al. TT virus in frequently transfused patients. Am J Med 1999;106:116–117.
31. Zein NN, Arslan M, Li H, et al. Clinical significance of TT virus infection in patients with chronic hepatitis C. Am J Gastroenterol 1999;94:3020–3027.
32. Vogel, W. Treatment of acute hepatitis C virus infection. J Hepatol Suppl 1999;31(suppl 1):189–192.
33. Pappas SC. Fulminant viral hepatitis. Gastroenterol Clin North Am 1995;24:161–173.
34. Plevris JN, Schina M, Hayes PC. Review article: The management of acute liver failure. Aliment Pharmacol Ther 1998;12:405–418.

35. Hoofnagle JH, DiBisceglie AM. The treatment of chronic viral hepatitis. N Engl J Med 1997;336:347–356.
36. Kao JH, Chen PJ, Lai MY, Chen DS. Hepatitis B genotypes correlate with clinical outcomes in patients with chronic hepatitis B. Gastroenterology 2000;118:554–559.
37. Chang MH, Chen CJ, Lai MS, et al. Universal hepatitis B vaccination in Taiwan and the incidence of hepatocellular carcinoma in children. N Engl J Med 1997;336:1855–1859.
38. Seeff LB, Miller RN, Rabkin CS, et al. 45-year follow-up of hepatitis C virus infection in healthy young adults. Ann Intern Med 2000;132:105–111.
39. National Institutes of Health consensus development conference panel statement: Management of hepatitis C. Hepatology 1997;26(suppl 1): 2S–10S.
40. EASL international consensus conference on hepatitis C. J Hepatol 1999;30:956–961.
41. Omata M. Treatment of chronic hepatitis B infection. New Engl J Med 1998;339:114–115.
42. McMurray RW. Hepatitis C-associated autoimmune disorders. Rheum Dis Clin North Am 1998;24(2):1–24.
43. Shiratori Y, Imazeki F, Moriyama M, et al. Hepatitis C-associated fibrosis may be reversible. Ann Intern Med 2000;132:517–524.
44. Perillo RP, Mason AL. Therapy for hepatitis B virus infection. Gastroenterol Clin North Am 1994;23:581–601.
45. Perillo RP. Interferon in the management of chronic hepatitis B. Digest Dis Sci 1993;38:577–593.
46. Niederau C, Heinteges T, Lange S, et al. Long-term follow-up of HbeAg-positive patients treated with interferon alpha for chronic hepatitis B. New Engl J Med 1996;334:1422–1427.
47. Krogsgaard K. The long-term effect of treatment with interferon-α2a in chronic hepatitis B. J Viral Hepat 1998;5:389–397.
48. Lai CL, Chien RN, Leung NWY, et al. A one-year trial of lamivudine for chronic hepatitis B. N Engl J Med 1998;339:61–68.
49. Dienstag JL, Schiff ER, Wright TL. Lamivudine as initial treatment for chronic hepatitis B in the United States. N Engl J Med 1999;341:1256–1263.
50. Liaw YF, Chien RW, Yeh CT, et al. Acute exacerbation and hepatitis B clearance after emergence of YMDD motif mutation during lamivudine therapy. Hepatology 1999;30:567–572.
51. Malik AH, Lee WM. Hepatitis B therapy: The plot thickens. Hepatology 1999;30:579–581.
52. Schalm SW, Heathcote J, Cianciara J, et al. Lamivudine and alpha-interferon combination treatment of patients with chronic hepatitis B infection: A randomised trial. Gut 2000;46:562–568.
53. Perillo RP. Antiviral agents in the treatment of chronic viral hepatitis. Prog Liver Dis 1992;10:283–309.
54. Cohard M, Poynard T, Mathurin P, Zarski JP. Prednisone-interferon combination in the treatment of chronic hepatitis B: Direct and indirect meta-analysis. Hepatology 1994;20:1390–1398.
55. Hultgren C, Weiland O, Milich DR, Sallberg M. Cell-mediated immune responses and loss of hepatitis B e-antigen (HBeAg) during successful lamivudine and famciclovir combination therapy for chronic replicating hepatitis B virus infection. Clin Infect Dis 1999;29:1575–1577.
56. Malik AH, Lee WM. Chronic hepatitis B virus infection: treatment strategies for the next millennium. Ann Intern Med 2000;132:723–731.
57. Lau GKK, Liang R, Wu PC, et al. Use of famciclovir to prevent HBV reactivation in HBsAg-positive recipients after allogenic bone marrow transplantation. J Hepatol 1998;28:359–368.
58. Kahn J, Lagakos S, Wulfsohn M, et al. Efficacy and safety of adefovir dipivoxil with antiretroviral therapy; a randomized controlled trial. JAMA 1999;282:2305–2312.
59. Xiong X, Flores C, Yang H, Toole JJ, Gibbs CS. Mutations in hepatitis B DNA polymerase associated with resistance to lamivudine do not confer cross-resistance to adefovir *in vitro*. Hepatology 1998;28:1669–73.
60. Villeneuve JP, Condreay LD, Willems B, et al. Lamivudine treatment for decompensated cirrhosis resulting from chronic hepatitis B. Hepatology 2000,31.207–210.
61. Dieterich DT, Purow JM, Rajapaksa R. Activity of combination therapy with interferon alpha-2b plus ribavirin in chronic hepatitis C patients co-infected with HIV. Semin Liver Dis 1999;19(suppl 1):87–94.
62. Figen G, Nurten K, Hasan O, Aysel Y. Comparison of standard and high dosage recombinant interferon-alpha 2b for treatment of children with chronic hepatitis B infection. Pediatr Infect Dis J 2000;19:52–56.
63. Carreno C, Marcellin P, Hadziyannis S, et al. Retreatment of chronic hepatitis B e antigen-positive patients with recombinant interferon alpha-2a. Hepatology 1999;29:277–282.
64. Farci P, Mandas A, Coiana A, et al. Treatment of chronic hepatitis D with interferon alpha-2a. N Engl J Med 1994;330:88–94.
65. Lau DTY, Doo E, Park Y, et al. Lamivudine for chronic delta hepatitis. Hepatology 1999;30:546–549.
66. Civeira MP, Prieto J. Early predictors of response to treatment in patients with chronic hepatitis C. J Hepatol 1999;31(suppl 1):237–243.
67. International Interferon-α Hepatocellular Carcinoma Study Group. Effect of interferon-α on progression of cirrhosis to hepatocellular carcinoma: A retrospective cohort study. Lancet 1998;351:1535–1539.
68. Yoshida H, Shiratori Y, Moriyama M, et al. Interferon therapy reduces the risk for hepatocellular carcinoma: national surveillance program of cirrhotic and noncirrhotic patients with chronic hepatitis C in Japan. Ann Intern Med 1999;131:174–181.
69. McHutchison JG, Gordon SC, Schiff ER, et al. Interferon alpha-2b alone or in combination with ribavirin as initial treatment for chronic hepatitis C. N Engl J Med 1998;339:1485–1492.
70. Davis GL, Esteban-mur R, Rustigi V, et al. Interferon alpha-2b alone or in combination with ribavirin for the treatment of relapse of chronic hepatitis C. N Engl J Med 1998;39:1493–1499.
71. Reichard O, Norkrans G, Fryden A, et al. Randomised, double-blind, placebo-controlled trial of interferon α-2b with and without ribavirin for chronic hepatitis C. Lancet 1998;351:83–87.
72. Poynard T, Marcellin P, Lee S, et al. Randomised trial of interferon-α2b plus ribavirin for 48 weeks or for 24 weeks versus interferon-α2b plus placebo for 48 weeks for treatment of chronic infection with hepatitis C virus. Lancet 1998;352:1426–1432.
73. Mazzella G, Accogli E, Sottili S, et al. Alpha interferon treatment may prevent hepatocellular carcinoma in HCV-related cirrhosis. J Hepatol 1996;24:141–147.
74. Zeuzem S, Feinman V, Raseanck J, et al. Peginterferon alpha-2a in patients with chronic hepatitis C. N Engl J Med 2000;343:1666–1672.
75. Heathcote EJ, Shiffman ML, Cooksley WG, et al. Peginterferon alpha-2a in patients with chronic hepatitis C and cirrhosis. N Engl J Med 2000;343:1673–1680.
76. Alberti A, Chemello L, Noventa F, Cavalletto L, DeSalvo G. Therapy of re-treatment with alpha interferon. Hepatology 1997;26:137S–142S.
77. Heathcote J, Keef EB, Lee SS. Retreatment of chronic hepatitis C with consensus interferon. Hepatology 1998;27:1136–1143.
78. Buti M, Esteban R. Retreatment of interferon relapse patients with chronic hepatitis C. J Hepatol 1999;31(suppl 1):174–177.
79. Bell H, Hellum K, Harthug S, et al. Treatment with interferon-alpha2a alone or interferon-apha2a plus ribavirin in patients with chronic hepatitis C previously treated with interferon-alpha2a. Scand J Gastroenterol 1999;2:194–198.
80. Bresci G, Parisi G, Bertoni M, Scantena F, Capria A, et al. Interferon plus ribavirin in chronic hepatitis C non-responders to recombinant α-interferon. J Viral Hepat 2000;7:75–78.
81. Schalm SW, Weiland O, Hansen B, et al., and the EUROHEP Study Group for Viral Hepatitis. Interferon/ribavirin for chronic hepatitis C with and without cirrhosis: A meta-analysis of individual patient data. Gastroenterology 1999;117(2):408–413.
82. Pol S, Zylberberg H, Fontaine H, Brechot C. Treatment of chronic hepatitis C in special groups. J Hepatol 1999;31(suppl 1):205–209.
83. Craxi A, Camma C, Giunta M. Definition of response to antiviral therapy in chronic hepatitis C. J Hepatol 1999;31(suppl 1):160–167.
84. Poterucha JJ, Wiesner RH. Liver transplantation and hepatitis B. Ann Intern Med 1997;126:805–807. Editorial.
85. Andreone P, Caraceni P, Grazi GL, et al. Lamivudine treatment for acute hepatitis B after liver transplantation. J Hepatol 1998;29:985–989.

86. Dusheiko GM. New treatments for chronic viral hepatitis B and C. Clin Gastroenterol 1996:10:299–333.
87. Briggs A, Shiell A. Interferon-α in hepatitis C. Pharmacoeconomics 1996;10:205–209.
88. Gane EJ, Portmann BC, Naoumov NV, et al. Long-term outcome of hepatitis C infection after liver transplantation. N Engl J Med 1996;334: 815–820.
89. Feray C, Samuel D, Gigou M, et al. An open trial of IFN alpha recombinant for hepatitis C after liver transplantation. Hepatology 1995;22:1084–1089.
90. Cattral MS, Hemming AW, Wanless IR, et al. Outcome of long-term ribavirin therapy for recurrent hepatitis C after liver transplantation. Transplantation 1999;67:1277–1280.
91. Gotz G, Schon MR, Haefker A, et al. Treatment of recurrent hepatitis C virus infection after liver transplantation with interferon and ribavirin. Transplant Proc 1998;30:2104–2106.
92. Lavezzo B, Rizzetto M. Treatment of recurrent hepatitis C virus infection after liver transplantation. J Hepatol 1999;31(suppl 1):222–226.
93. Farrell GC, Bacon BR, Goldin RD, et al. Lymphoblastoid interferon alpha-n1 improves the long-term response to a 6-month course of treatment in chronic hepatitis C compared with recombinant interferon alpha-2b: Results of an international randomized controlled trial. Hepatology 1998;27:1121–1127.
94. Zarski JP, Leroy V. Counseling patients with hepatitis C. J Hepatol Suppl 1999;31(suppl 1):136–140.
95. Anonymous. The ABCs of hepatitis. Patient notes. Postgrad Med 2000;107:279–280.
96. 2000 Drug Topics Red Book. Montvale, NJ, Medical Economics, 2000:306, 367, 497.
97. Bennett WG, Inoue Y, Beck JR, et al. Estimates of the cost-effectiveness of a single course of interferon-alpha 2b in patients with histologically mild chronic hepatitis C. Ann Intern Med 1997;127:855–865.
98. Kim WR, Poterucha JJ, Hermans JE, et al. Cost-effectiveness of 6 and 12 months of interferon-alpha therapy for chronic hepatitis C. Ann Intern Med 1997;127:866–874.
99. Koff RS. Cost-effectiveness of treatment for chronic hepatitis C. J Hepatol 1999;31(suppl 1):255–258.
100. Wong JB, Bennett WG, Koff RS, Pauker SG. Pretreatment evaluation of chronic hepatitis C. JAMA 1998;280:2088–2093.
101. Kim WR, Poterucha JJ, Dickson ER, Gross JB Jr. Cost effectiveness of ribavirin/interferon treatment among nonresponders to initial interferon for chronic hepatitis C. Hepatology 1998;28:231A.
102. Dusheiko GM, Roberts JA. Treatment of chronic type B and C hepatitis with interferon alpha: An economic appraisal. Hepatology 1995;22:1863–1873.
103. Wong JB, Koff RS, Tine F, Pauker SG. Cost-effectiveness of interferon-alpha 2b treatment of hepatitis B e antigen-positive chronic hepatitis B. Ann Intern Med 1995;122:664–675.
104. Johanson JF. Hepatitis C therapy: is it really worth it? Am J Gastoenterol 1999;94:1412–1413.
105. Foster GR. Hepatitis C virus infection: quality of life and side effects of treatment. J Hepatol 1999;31(suppl 1):250–254.
106. Neary MP, Cort S, Bayliss MS, Ware JE. Sustained virologic response is associated with improved health-related quality of life in relapsed chronic hepatitis C patients. Semin Liver Dis 1999;19(suppl 1): 78–85.
107. Paterson DL, Gayowski T, Wannstedt CF, et al. Quality of life in long-term survivors after liver transplantation: Impact of recurrent viral hepatitis C virus hepatitis. Clin Transplant 2000;14:48–54
108. Carithers RL Jr, Sugano D, Bayliss M. Health assessment for chronic HCV infection. Dig Dis Sci 1996;41:75S–80S.
109. Rodger AJ, Jolley D, Thompson SC, Lanigan A, Crofts N. The impact of diagnosis of hepatitis C virus of quality of life. Hepatology 1999;30:1299–1301.
110. Lemon SM, Thomas DL. Vaccines to prevent viral hepatitis. N Engl J Med 1997;336:196–204.
111. Werzberger A, Mensch B, Kuter B, et al. A controlled trial of a formalin-inactivated hepatitis A vaccine in healthy children. N Engl J Med 1992;327:453–457.
112. Innis BL, Snitbhan R, Kunasol P, et al. Protection against hepatitis A by an inactivated vaccine. JAMA 1994;271:1328–1334.
113. Sagliocca L, Amoroso P, Stroffolini T, et al. Efficacy of hepatitis A vaccine in prevention of secondary hepatitis A infection: A randomised trial. Lancet 1999;353:1136–1139.
114. Thoelen S, Van Damme P, Leentvaar-Kuypers A, et al. The first combined vaccine against hepatitis A and B: An overview. Vaccine 1999;1999:1657–1662.
115. Centers for Disease Control and Prevention. Recommendations of the Advisory Committee on Immunization Practices: Use of vaccines and immune globulins in persons with altered immunocompetence. MMWR Morb Mortal Wkly Rep 1993;42(RR-4):1–18.
116. Centers for Disease Control. Hepatitis B virus: A comprehensive strategy for eliminating transmission in the United States through universal childhood vaccination. MMWR Morb Mortal Wkly Rep 1991;40 (RR-13):1–25.
117. Centers for Disease Control and Prevention. Update: Recommendations to prevent hepatitis B virus transmission—United States. MMWR Morb Mortal Wkly Rep 1995;44:574–575.
118. Centers for Disease Control and Prevention. Update: Recommendations to prevent hepatitis B virus transmission—United States. MMWR Morb Mortal Wkly Rep 1999;48:33–34
119. Centers for Disease Control and Prevention. 1999 USPHS/IDSA guidelines for the prevention of opportunistic infections in persons infected with human immunodeficiency virus. MMWR Morb Mortal Wkly Rep 1999;48(RR10):1–66.
120. Losonsky GV, Wasserman SS, Stephens I, et al. Hepatitis B vaccination in premature infants: A reassessment of current recommendations for delayed immunization. Pediatrics 1999;103(2). http://www.pediatrics.org/cgi/content full/103/2/e14.
121. Bertino JS, Tirrell P, Greenberg RN, et al. A comparative trial of standard or high-dose S subunit recombinant hepatitis B vaccine versus a vaccine containing S subunit, pre-S_1, and pre-S_2 particles for revaccination of healthy adult nonresponders. J Infect Dis 1997;175:678–681.
122. European Consensus Group on Hepatitis B Immunity. Are booster immunisations needed for lifelong hepatitis B immunity? Lancet 2000;355:561–565.
123. Centers for Disease Control and Prevention. Recommendations for follow-up of health-care workers after occupational exposure to hepatitis C virus. MMWR Morb Mortal Wkly Rep 1997;46:603–606.
124. Van Doorslaer E, Tormans G, van Damme P, Beutels P. Cost effectiveness of alternative hepatitis A immunisation strategies. Pharmacoeconomics 1995;8:5–8.
125. Hollinger FB. Comprehensive control (or elimination) of hepatitis B virus transmission in the United States. Gut 1996;38(suppl 2):S24–S30.
126. Margolis HS, Coleman PJ, Brown RE, Mast EE, Sheingold SH, Arevalo JA. Prevention of hepatitis B virus transmission by immunization: An economic analysis of current recommendations. JAMA 1995;274:1201–1208.

41

LIVER TRANSPLANTATION

Jennifer A. Stoffel and Alka Z. Somani

Liver transplantation is a life-saving procedure for patients with severe hepatic disease who have no other medical option. Approximately 115 transplant centers in the United States now perform the operation. Liver transplantation makes up about 20% of all transplant surgeries performed in the United States. The 1-year graft and patient survival rates are 79.6% and 87.5%, respectively, in the United States. In 1998, 4,485 liver transplants were performed, of which 4,413 were cadaveric and 72 were from a living donor. In spite of the number of liver transplantation procedures, about 16,000 patients are still on the waiting list for a liver transplant in the United States. The mean waiting time is 545 days for first-time liver transplant recipients, and 1,317 patients died in 1998 waiting for a liver transplant.[1]

INDICATIONS

The principal indications for transplantation in adults fall into the category of noncholestatic cirrhosis, and account for approximately 60% of liver recipients.[1] This category consists predominately of patients with hepatitis C and alcoholic cirrhosis, but also includes hepatitis B, cryptogenic cirrhosis, and autoimmune hepatitis. In a series of 100 patients, 16 patients had hepatitis C, 14 patients had alcoholic cirrhosis, and 22 patients carried both diagnoses.[2] Other indications for liver transplantation include primary biliary cirrhosis, primary sclerosing cholangitis, acute hepatic failure, primary liver cancer, and inborn errors of metabolism. Pediatric liver transplantation has been performed primarily for biliary atresia and inborn errors of metabolism.

The inborn errors of metabolism that have been treated by liver transplantation are a heterogeneous group of disorders, and correction of the metabolic defect has not always occurred. Liver transplantation has corrected α_1-antitrypsin deficiency; Wilson's disease; tyrosinemia; types I, III, and IV glycogen storage disease; type I hyperoxaluria; and hemophilia A and B. Correction has been incomplete in other disorders such as familial hyperlipidemia. Timing of the transplant is critical for correction of the metabolic disease in order to prevent irreversible damage to the end organ (e.g., central nervous system in ornithine transcarbamylase deficiency) or to prevent hepatocellular carcinoma (e.g., tyrosinemia).

To justify transplantation the patient should have a reasonable life expectancy after transplantation. Age does not appear to be a barrier to liver transplantation, with good 5-year survival rates in patients older than 50 years of age. Unfortunately, hepatitis can reoccur after liver transplantation and can cause hepatic failure in the transplanted liver.[3] Survival following primary orthotopic liver transplantation for hepatitis is favorable, but survival after retransplantation is poor.[4] Table 41–1 summarizes the relative contraindications for liver transplantation and management techniques.

The shortage of donor organs has stimulated work in the area of hepatocyte transplantation[5] and in the development of artificial liver support.[6] Hepatocyte transplantation, where the cells are implanted into the liver or the spleen, may be considered as a temporary bridge to provide liver function in patients with end-stage liver failure until a donor becomes available. Cellular transplantation with hepatocytes is potentially a simpler, less expensive, and less invasive procedure when compared to liver transplantation.

THE PROCEDURE

Liver transplantation is the most technically demanding of the surgical transplant procedures. This difficulty has produced a slow increase in the number of successful centers performing liver transplant procedures. Figure 41–1 shows the anatomic structures critical to liver transplantation.

The first critical step in liver transplantation is the proper procurement of the donor organ. In approximately one-third of human donors, arterial abnormalities in the liver will be encountered that would make the organ useless without special techniques. New preservation solutions have extended the preservation period for livers to as long as 24 hours. This extension in preservation has dramatically affected liver procurement practices and the availability of viable organs.

The recipient operation is roughly conducted in three phases: removal of recipient liver, donor graft revascularization, and biliary reconstruction. The venous hypertension produced by clamping of the inferior vena cava and portal vein during the anhepatic phase can cause edema of the intestinal mucosa, and has been circumvented in adult patients through the use of the venovenous bypass. Graft revascularization involves performing anastomosis of the vena cava above and below the liver (Fig. 41–1, part a) followed by the portal venous anastomosis (Fig. 41–1, part b). Biliary reconstruction can be accomplished in several ways: by end-to-end anastomosis of the donor and recipient common bile ducts over a T-tube stent, by side-to-side choledochostomy after closure of the donor and recipient duct ends, or by anastomosing the graft's common duct to a defunctionalized limb of jejunum (Roux limb, Fig. 41–1, part c). The complete procedure takes many hours, often requires several teams of surgeons, and is frequently accomplished with the replacement of multiple blood volumes for the patient.

One of the most difficult problems in pediatric transplantation is the availability of size-matched allografts. A donor liver allograft has to be within about 20% of the recipient's size. Otherwise the graft can impair breathing or closure of the abdomen if too large and may not be adequate for survival if too small. To overcome this problem, reduced-size liver transplantation has evolved as a technique where the donor liver is surgically reduced in size to meet the needs of the recipient. This technique has been most commonly used in split-liver transplantation in which a donor graft provides livers for two recipients,[7] and in living-related donor operations in which a portion of the left lobe of the healthy liver is taken for the donor graft from the parents.[8] Immunosuppressive therapy is similar to a cadaveric donor graft, but episodes of rejection that are resistant to corticosteroids appear to be less common in the recipient of a living-related donor liver allograft.

TABLE 41–1. Relative Contraindications for Liver Transplantation

Relative Contraindication	Additional Therapy or Management
Primary liver cancer	Chemotherapy
Hepatitis B	Hepatitis B immunoglobulin and lamivudine
Hepatitis C	Interferon α-2b and ribavirin
Multiple abdominal surgeries	New surgical management techniques
HIV	Lowered doses of immunosuppressants

EARLY TRANSPLANT FAILURE

Failure of the newly transplanted liver occurs in 10% to 15% of cases and can result from several different mechanisms. Early graft failure can result from preexisting disease in the donor, and even coagulation defects have been acquired through donor organs. The technical complexity of the operation can produce flaws in revascularization that also lead to graft nonfunction. Surgical complications occur in about 25% of cases and result in a doubling of the hospital expense for the patient.[9] Portal vein thrombosis, hepatic artery thrombosis, and bile duct leaks are all technical problems that have been encountered. Ischemic injury to the donor liver through preservation is difficult to predict, and can produce early graft dysfunction. Perioperative immune events rarely lead to the classic picture of hyperacute rejection in liver transplantation, but graft failure in the first 2 postoperative weeks may still indicate antibody-mediated graft destruction.

CLINICAL PRESENTATION OF THE POSTOPERATIVE LIVER TRANSPLANT PATIENT

The physiologic consequences of liver transplantation are complex, but an oversimplification can be made by combining models of rapidly changing hepatic function, postoperative patients with ileus and biliary tract dysfunction, catabolic patients on high doses of steroids, and immunocompromised patients. The liver transplant patient is represented by all of these models with each intricate component interacting with the other models in an individualized manner. The transition from poor hepatic function to normal liver processes is one that involves changes in both hepatic metabolic and synthetic function. The postoperative patient will have fluid, electrolyte, and nutritional abnormalities that will be combined with biliary tract dysfunction.

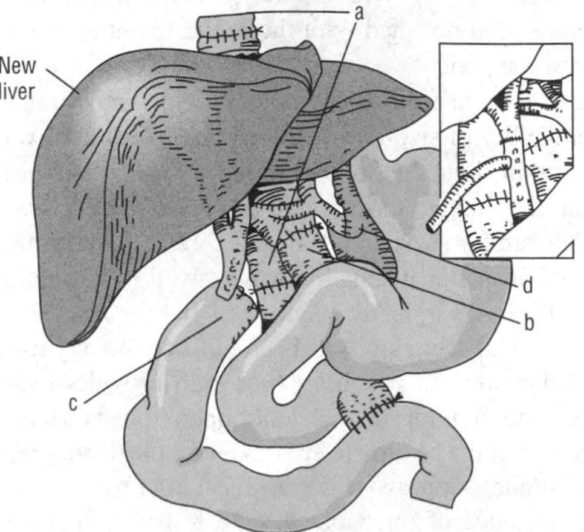

FIGURE 41–1. Orthotopic liver transplantation with (a) suprahepatic and intrahepatic inferior vena cava anastomosis, (b) portal venous anastomosis, (c) choledochojejunostomy, and (d) hepatic arterial anastomosis.

Subsequently there is disruption of bile flow through removal of the gallbladder and, in some cases, temporary placement of a drainage tube (T tube) in the bile duct, which will alter the absorption of fats and fat-soluble drugs. Corticosteroids and the other immunosuppressive drugs have metabolic consequences that affect both endogenous and exogenous substrates. The physiologic changes that the patient is undergoing result in alterations in the biopharmaceutical profile of any agent administered to a liver transplant patient.[10] Changes in drug absorption are quite dramatic in liver transplant patients. After a successful liver transplant operation, the absorption of lipid-soluble compounds is considerably improved. The poor absorption of the lipid-soluble drug cyclosporine A (CSA) improves after successful liver transplantation and reestablishment of bile flow. Vitamin E deficiency and its neurologic complications in liver failure patients are reversed after successful liver transplantation in pediatric patients. In stable adult liver transplant patients, the concentrations of retinol and tocopherol are similar to those seen in normal healthy subjects, indicating recovery of transplanted liver production and excretion of bile salts needed for fat-soluble vitamin absorption.

The protein binding of drugs in liver transplant patients is affected both by the synthetic capacity of the liver and by the pathophysiologic changes associated with the postoperative state. The serum concentration of albumin in liver transplant patients is frequently lower than that observed in normal subjects for months following surgery, resulting in a lower protein-bound fraction for drugs binding to albumin. When compared with patients with chronic liver disease, the binding of agents such as diazepam and salicylic acid is greater in liver transplant patients because of the removal of endogenous binding inhibitors. Studies in liver transplant patients indicate that the concentration of α_1-acid glycoprotein (AAG) increases after surgery and stays at an elevated level for at least 45 days. Correspondingly, the unbound fraction of lidocaine in plasma obtained from stable liver transplant patients is lower than the free fraction values observed in plasma from normal volunteers.

Liver metabolism is altered by a combination of factors related to physiologic changes (preservation injury or decreased effective hepatic blood flow initially), stimulation of hepatic microsomes by some immunosuppressant agents, and inhibition of microsomal drug transformation by other immunosuppressant agents. Metabolism mediated by the cytochrome P450 enzymes is generally depressed during the first month posttransplantation, and then recovers during the next few months. Clear exceptions are the cytochrome P450 isoenzyme CYP2E1, which has enhanced activity in liver transplant patients during the first month, and CYP2D6, which appears to be unaffected by the procedure. The oxidative metabolizing capacity of the liver as determined by antipyrine kinetics is similar in clinically stable liver transplant patients to that observed in normal subjects. First-pass metabolism is also expected to be altered during the transition to normal hepatic function. The conjugative processes of metabolism, as represented by the sulfation and glucuronidation of acetaminophen, normalizes in liver transplant patients, but the renal clearance of the conjugates is altered due to abnormal renal capacity to eliminate the metabolites. Altered biliary function not only affects the absorption of lipophilic compounds, but also affects the elimination of drugs and metabolites. For example, biliary dysfunction in liver transplant patients produces a high concentration of the CSA metabolites in blood.

Renal elimination of drugs in liver transplant patients should not be considered normal in the immediate postoperative period. Earlier studies with liver transplant patients receiving CSA demonstrated that elimination of gentamicin, vancomycin, and the cephalosporin antibiotics is less than would be predicted by serum creatinine. These physiologic alterations in a liver transplant patient must be considered when developing individualized drug regimens.

▶ TREATMENT: Immunosuppressive Measures

DESIRED OUTCOME

1. Prevent acute and chronic rejection of the transplanted organ.
2. Prevent infectious complications of immunosuppression.
3. Prevent adverse drug effects and drug interactions with immunosuppressants.
4. Educate the patient on medications and promote proper medication compliance.

GENERAL APPROACH TO TREATMENT

The goal of immunomodulatory therapy in transplantation is to promote acceptance of donor tissue, while preventing rejection and maintaining the functional status of the immune system with respect to other foreign materials. Immunosuppression with medications following organ transplantation may appear complex because of the varying protocols used by transplant centers throughout the world. Immunosuppressive measures chosen for a liver transplant patient are largely specific for the protocol at an individual transplant center and uses one of several effective drug regimens. Drug combinations provide the most effective therapy by taking advantage of additive or synergistic interaction between agents. The drug protocol should use various agents in combination to produce adequate immunosuppression with minimal adverse drug effects.

NONPHARMACOLOGIC THERAPY

Lymphoid irradiation was one of the earliest nonpharmacologic means of immunosuppression, and is still used in some centers for resistant rejection. Another nonpharmacologic treatment that may influence drug therapy is induction of microchimerism, or the state in which the donor cells are tolerated by the host. To accomplish this, the organ transplant recipient is administered an intravenous infusion of bone marrow from the donor. Adjusting the immunotherapy in the immediate posttransplant period so that the host is not totally suppressed may also facilitate microchimerism. Microchimerism can occur when donor cells migrate from the transplanted organ to establish mutual tolerance with the host's T cells. A small number of donor cells can be identified in the skin biopsies of long-term survivors of liver and kidney transplants.[11] A stable balance of donor cell and recipient cell interaction may be necessary for long-term graft survival. At the present time, nonpharmacologic manipulation must be supplemented with pharmacologic therapy that has been proven to be successful.

Graft versus host disease (GVHD) develops when the graft, which contains immunologically competent cells, recognizes the host as foreign and mounts an immunologic response against the host. This is a rare complication that has been observed in liver and bone marrow transplantation. GVHD clinically presents as fever, rash, and pancytopenia within 4 to 6 weeks of transplantation. The recommended management of GVHD is the aggressive administration of immunosuppressive therapy.[12]

PHARMACOLOGIC THERAPY

DRUG TREATMENTS OF FIRST CHOICE

Commercially available immunosuppressive agents for liver transplantation include:

Immunophilin-binding agents: CSA or tacrolimus (TAC)
Steroids: Methylprednisolone or prednisone (PRED)
Antiproliferative agents: Azathioprine (AZA) or mycophenolate mofetil (MMF)
Anti-T-cell biologic products: Muromonab-CD3 (OKT3) or antilymphocyte (ALG)/antithymocyte globulin (ATG)
Interleukin-2 receptor monoclonal antibody: Daclizumab or basiliximab

TREATMENT PROTOCOLS

Transplant centers use double, triple, or quadruple therapy (Table 41–2). Studies show that the various protocols are equally safe and effective when used by a transplant center that is familiar with medication regimens. Drug combinations should use the lowest effective dose to minimize adverse effects. Deciding which protocol to use may depend on individual patient parameters, including the cause of liver failure, whether the patient has had a previous transplant, sensitization to histocompatability antigens, and side effects caused by the immunosuppressant medications. To avoid the nephrotoxic effects of CSA, initial therapy may include PRED + AZA or MMF and OKT3 or ALG. Cyclosporine therapy is then started 1 to 2 weeks after transplant.

PIVOTAL CLINICAL TRIALS

An open-label randomized multicenter trial comparing CSA and TAC in liver transplantation in the United States found that the actuarial survival rates for patients and grafts were similar between the two groups (1-year graft survival rate was 82% for TAC and 79% for CSA).[13] The patient survival at 1 year was 88% for both groups. The TAC group had significantly lower incidences of acute rejection and corticosteroid-resistant rejection. Nephrotoxicity and neurotoxicity required that more patients be withdrawn from TAC therapy than from CSA therapy. A European trial found similar results in that survival and adverse effects were similar with CSA and TAC in liver transplant patients, but that the incidence of acute, refractory, and chronic rejection was lower in the TAC group.[14] A primary use for TAC in centers that use CSA as their primary immunosuppressant drug is as rescue therapy. Patient survival rates exceeding 80% have been reported in liver transplant patients who were converted from CSA to TAC because of failure of the conventional immunosuppressive therapy, which is considered an outstanding response rate.[15] CSA-associated

TABLE 41–2. Examples of Immunosuppression Protocols

1. CSA or TAC + PRED
2. CSA or TAC + PRED + AZA or MMF or sirolimus
3. CSA or TAC + PRED + AZA or MMF + OKT3 or ALG/ATG
4. Delayed CSA or TAC + PRED + AZA or MMF or sirolimus
5. Delayed CSA or TAC + PRED + AZA or MMF or sirolimus + OKT3 or ALG/ATG

side effects include nephrotoxicity, hypertension, neurologic disorders, and hyperlipidemia, which may lead to posttransplant morbidity. Conversion from CSA to TAC reduces side effects while maintaining stable graft function.[16] Another advantage of TAC is that corticosteroid therapy can frequently be eliminated in the long-term regimen, reducing the adverse effects of prolonged corticosteroid therapy.

ALTERNATIVE TREATMENTS AND OTHER DRUG TREATMENTS

Other pharmacologic agents are often required for the adequate management of a transplant patient. Anti-infective prophylaxis (antibiotic, antifungal, and antiviral) and therapy is used to prevent and treat infections in the immunocompromised patient. The balance between immunosuppression and infection control is critical in the liver transplant patient because of the constant exposure of the graft to intestinal flora. In the presence of rejection, the liver can become an open portal for entry of bacterial organisms from the GI tract. Bacterial or fungal invasion can result in local abscess formation or in general sepsis, both of which represent life-threatening infectious complications of transplantation and immunosuppression. The most frequent cause of death after liver transplantation is severe infection.[17] Table 41–3 shows the routine medications given to a liver transplantation patient upon discharge from the University of Pittsburgh Medical Center in 2000. Antibiotics also need to be given for surgical or dental prophylaxis.

Liver transplant patients have an increased incidence of symptomatic cytomegalovirus (CMV) infection in comparison with renal transplant patients (29% vs 8%, respectively).[18] These infections are most frequently observed from 3 to 8 weeks following transplantation or after an intensive treatment course for rejection. As with other transplants, liver recipients who are seronegative for CMV prior to transplantation are at increased risk for symptomatic CMV infections in comparison with liver recipients who were preoperatively seropositive. Prophylactic regimens may include IV ganciclovir, oral ganciclovir, oral acyclovir, and CMV immunoglobulin. An alternative approach is to follow the patient's leukocyte pp65 antigen concentration and to treat the patient aggressively when the antigen concentration increases.[19] The antigen level can then also be used as a measure of response to therapy in patients undergoing treatment with intravenous ganciclovir. The place of oral ganciclovir in the prophylaxis against CMV disease has not been determined in liver transplant patients.

Patients who are infected with Hepatitis B at the time of liver transplantation are at risk for graft loss secondary to recurrence of the virus. Advances in therapeutic modalities have significantly decreased the recurrence rate. The current standard of care involves combination therapy with hepatitis B immunoglobulin (HBIg) and Lamivudine (Epivir, Glaxo Wellcome). The regimen of HBIg varies among institutions. The regimen at the University of Pittsburgh currently involves 10,000 IU administered as an IV infusion daily for 7 days, and then monthly for 6 months. After 6 months, patients are given an IM injection of 5 mL (1500 IU) every 3 weeks for 18 months. Patients also receive lamivudine 150 mg orally once daily indefinitely.

Other viruses causing significant infections in liver transplant patients include herpes simplex types 1 and 2, adenoviral hepatitis, and Epstein-Barr virus (EBV) diseases ranging from an infectious mononucleosis syndrome to life-threatening lymphoproliferative disease. Lymphomas develop in 1% to 5% of posttransplant patients, which may require decreasing or stopping immunosuppressive therapy. An expanded discussion of the posttransplant lymphoproliferative disease (PTLD) seen in transplant patients and associated with EBV can be found in Chap. 16.

Hypertension (Chap. 12), hyperglycemia (Chap. 74), and hyperlipidemia (Chap. 21) may also be caused or exacerbated by the immunosuppressive medications. Modifying the immunosuppressive therapy may assist in the management of these secondary conditions, but may not result in the desired control. Selection of medications to treat hypertension, hyperglycemia, and hyperlipidemia follow the same guidelines as are used in nontransplant patients. The pharmacotherapist must be aware of the drug interactions in a liver transplant patient and their role in medication selection. Diltiazem increases CSA levels, but diltiazem is considered the drug of choice for hypertension at some transplant centers because it allows the dose of CSA to be reduced.

SPECIAL POPULATIONS: WOMEN AND PREGNANCY

Many women with liver disease have menstrual irregularities and reproductive problems; these problems are corrected by liver transplantation. Healthy infants have been delivered by mothers receiving CSA or receiving TAC, but couples should be counseled about the possible hypertension and graft dysfunction that can accompany pregnancy in a mother with a liver transplant. Medications that are potentially

TABLE 41–3. Routine Medications Orders Upon Discharge for an Adult Liver Transplant Patient (University of Pittsburgh, 2000)

Medication	Usual Dose	Long-term Goal
Immunosuppression		
Tacrolimus	Individualized to level 5–20 ng/mL	Taper dose and level over time if no rejection and stable liver enzymes.
Prednisone	20 mg daily	Taper and discontinue by 6 months if no rejection and stable liver enzymes.
± Mycophenolate mofetil	1 g twice daily	Taper and discontinue after 1 year if no rejection and stable liver enzymes.
± Sirolimus	2–5 mg daily	Minimize tacrolimus-induced nephrotoxicity.
Anti-infective prophylaxis		
Sulfamethoxazole/trimethoprim	SS tab M-W-F	PCP prophylaxis, continue lifelong. Alternative: Pentamidine 300 mg inhaled monthly.
Acyclovir	200 mg twice daily	Herpes virus prophylaxis. Discontinue after 1 month.
Nystatin	5 mL four times daily	For thrush prophylaxis. Taper and discontinue when prednisone decreased to 5 mg.
Gastrointestinal Prophylaxis		
Nizatidine	150 mg twice daily	Change to prn when prednisone reduced to 5 mg daily.

harmful, such as MMF, should be discontinued prior to conception. Pregnancy must be planned and managed as a high-risk situation by both an obstetrician and a surgeon.[20]

DRUG CLASS INFORMATION

Immunophilin-Binding Agents

Tacrolimus inhibits the production of IL-2 in T cells, thereby inhibiting the growth and proliferation of those cells. Tacrolimus binds to the cytoplasmic immunophilin, FK binding protein (FKBP), with subsequent inhibition of the activity of calcineurin. Calcineurin is an enzyme that activates the nuclear factor of activated T cells (NF-AT), which is responsible for cytokine production. Following oral administration, the bioavailability of TAC ranges from 5% to 66%, with a mean of 29% in liver transplant patients. The poor bioavailability of TAC necessitates the use of three to four times higher oral doses than IV doses to obtain similar blood concentrations. Adverse effects that occur with 10% to 20% of patients taking TAC are neurologic, including insomnia, tremors, headaches, photophobia, nightmares, and hypesthesias. Major neurologic side effects occur 8% to 21% of the time, including confusion, seizures, coma, dysarthrias, psychosis, and encephalopathy.

Tacrolimus is metabolized by cytochrome P450 34A, so other medications metabolized by this enzyme can alter TAC concentrations. Macrolide antibiotics, such as erythromycin, and antifungal medications, such as itraconazole and fluconazole, can increase TAC levels, while the anticonvulsants phenytoin and phenobarbital as well as rifampin can lower TAC blood concentration levels. Medications that are nephrotoxic should be used with caution because TAC can also be nephrotoxic. Because TAC decomposes in alkaline media, antacids and medications that increase the pH of the GI tract will decrease TAC absorption, and should be spaced 2 hours apart from TAC administration. Patients should take their TAC doses at a consistent time in relation to meals. Initial intravenous TAC doses range from 0.05 to 0.1 mg/kg/day, and are administered by continuous infusion. Oral doses range from 0.1 to 0.3 mg/kg/day given in two divided doses every 12 hours. Tacrolimus doses are then adjusted according to trough blood levels (5–20 ng/mL), clinical response, and adverse effects. Patients with hepatic dysfunction may require a reduction in dose, but no change is needed with renal dysfunction. Pediatric transplant patients clear the drug more rapidly and require two to four times higher mg/kg doses than adults to maintain equivalent therapeutic concentrations.

Cyclosporine also inhibits T-lymphocyte proliferation by inhibiting the production of interleukin (IL) 2 and other cytokines by T cells. Cyclosporine binds to a cytoplasmic immunophilin called cyclophilin, which blocks the action of calcineurin. Cyclosporine is highly lipophilic and is dependent on bile for intestinal absorption. Following oral administration, the absorption of CSA is incomplete and erratic, especially in liver recipients with T-tube diversion of bile. Cyclosporine is commercially available as either the standard formulation (Sandimmune) or as a microemulsion (Neoral). The two formulations are not bioequivalent and should not be used interchangeably. The microemulsion formulation is less dependent on bile for absorption resulting in higher and more reliable absorption of the drug. In one study of liver recipients with T-tube diversion, the bioavailability of the microemulsion was 6.5 time greater than that of the standard formulation.[21]

Neoral is associated with a lower incidence of rejection compared to Sandimmune.[22] Generic products for both formulations of cyclosporine are now available commercially. For a generic product to be considered bioequivalent, the rate and extent of absorption of the generic formulation should be between 80 % and 125% of the reference product.[23] Additionally, equivalence testing is often done in healthy volunteers. For drugs with a narrow therapeutic index such as cyclosporine, variability in the product supplied may result in serious adverse outcomes. The National Kidney Foundation published a white paper with recommendations regarding the practice of generic substitution for immunosuppressant agents.[24] The authors suggested that the prescribing physician be informed that substitution is to take place so that appropriate monitoring can be completed. Any adverse reactions that occur after a switch should be reported in the patient's medical record and submitted to the FDA.

Adverse reactions to CSA that occur in more than 10% of patients include hypertension, nephrotoxicity, gingival hypertrophy, hirsutism, and tremor. Side effects that occur in less than 10% of patients include seizures, headache, leg cramps, acne, pancreatitis, hepatotoxicity, tachycardia, paresthesias, and sensitivity to temperature extremes. Cyclosporine is also metabolized by cytochrome P450 34A, and shares the same drug interactions as TAC. There are more drug interactions reported with CSA, including with diltiazem and verapamil, but this may be a consequence of greater experience with CSA. The absorption of CSA is enhanced by a meal with a moderate fat content, so the patient should be advised to take CSA with meals. The normal dose range for CSA is 2–5 mg/kg/day as a continuous intravenous infusion, beginning before or after transplantation. Because oral bioavailability averages 30%, initial oral doses are 8–17 mg/kg/day, with long-term dosage reductions to 5 mg/kg/day divided into one or two doses per day. Cyclosporine is excreted in the bile and is nephrotoxic; therefore, dosage adjustments should be made when hepatic dysfunction is present. Similar to TAC, children require higher doses of CSA to maintain therapeutic drug concentrations, which are approximately 100–300 ng/mL.

Sirolimus is a recently approved immunosuppressant agent. Similar to cyclosporine and tacrolimus, sirolimus also binds to immunophilins, specifically, FKBPs. In contrast to tacrolimus, the sirolimus/FKBP complex does not inhibit calcineurin. Instead, the complex binds to the mammalian target of rapamycin (mTOR), which inhibits the signal necessary for IL-2-induced T-cell proliferation.[25] Sirolimus is a lipophilic drug that has poor oral bioavailability, but has extensive tissue distribution. Sirolimus is predominately metabolized by the enzyme cytochrome P450 3A4 (CYP 3A4) and is not renally eliminated to any significant degree. The half life of sirolimus is approximately 60 hours, which allows for once-daily dosing.[26] At present, sirolimus is only approved for use in renal transplant patients receiving immunosuppression with cyclosporine.

Preliminary studies suggest that sirolimus is effective when used in combination with cyclosporine in a steroid-sparing protocol.[27] Additionally, sirolimus used in combination with prednisone and low-dose tacrolimus resulted in a low rate of tacrolimus-related adverse events such as nephrotoxicity and hypertension.[28] The most frequently occurring adverse affects of sirolimus include thrombocytopenia and elevated triglycerides. Hyperlipidemia is reported to occur in 30% to 50% of patients and may require therapy with an 3-hydroxy-3-methylglutaryl coenzyme A (HMG-CoA) reductase inhibitor or fibric acid derivative.[29] Other adverse effects include leukopenia, diarrhea, hypertension, elevated creatinine, and rash. Because sirolimus is metabolized by CYP 3A4, the coadministration with diltiazem and ketoconazole resulted in increased sirolimus concentrations, while rifampin resulted in decreased concentrations. The approved dosing regimen for sirolimus involves a 6-mg loading dose followed by 2 mg once daily. Early clinical trials used daily doses of 4–5 mg.[27,28]

Steroids

Corticosteroids inhibit T-lymphocyte proliferation by blocking gene transcription necessary for the production of several cytokines including IL-1, IL-2, IL-6, gamma interferon, and TNF-alpha.[30] Steroids also inhibit adhesion molecules on endothelial cells necessary for leukocytes to migrate out of the bloodstream. Prednisone is converted to active prednisolone in the body and has multiple effects on the immune system. Prednisone is very well absorbed from the gastrointestinal (GI) tract and has a long biologic half-life, so it can be dosed once daily. The first-line therapy for the treatment of acute graft rejection is high-dose IV methylprednisolone (250–1,000 mg) daily for 3 days or oral prednisone (200 mg). Doses of oral prednisone are then tapered over 5 days to 20 mg/day. Adverse effects of prednisone that occur in more than 10% of patients include increased appetite, insomnia, indigestion (bitter taste), and mood changes. Side effects that occur less commonly, but which are seen with high doses or prolonged therapy, include cataracts, hyperglycemia, hirsutism, bruising, acne, sodium and water retention, hypertension, bone growth suppression, and ulcerative esophagitis. Barbiturates, phenytoin, and rifampin decrease the effectiveness of prednisone, whereas prednisone will decrease the effectiveness of vaccines and toxoids. Prednisone should be taken with food to minimize GI upset. The dose of prednisone varies with the transplant center's protocol but usually is highest immediately following transplant and during treatment for acute rejection. It is becoming frequent practice to taper prednisone with the goal of discontinuation over a period of months. Corticosteroids should never be abruptly discontinued; tapering should be gradual because of suppression of the hypothalamic-pituitary-adrenal axis. Corticosteroids slow the growth rates in children, prompting clinicians to use alternate-day dosing or to withhold steroids until rejection occurs.

Antiproliferative Agents

Azathioprine is an effective antiproliferative agent against both B and T lymphocytes via the inhibition of DNA and RNA synthesis. Azathioprine is metabolized to its active metabolites mercaptopurine, 6-thioinosinic acid, and 6-thioguanine. The immunosuppressive effects of AZA last 12 to 24 hours, making once-daily dosing possible. Azathioprine is used to prevent rejection, but is not used to treat acute graft rejection. Adverse effects that occur in more than 10% of patients include leukopenia, anemia, fever, chills, nausea, and vomiting. Less-common side effects include thrombocytopenia, hepatotoxicity, skin rash, and retinopathy. Because AZA is metabolized by xanthine oxidase, the usual AZA dose should be reduced 67% to 75% in patients also receiving allopurinol. Azathioprine can be taken with food to minimize any gastrointestinal upset. Intravenous doses of AZA are initially 3–5 mg/kg/day, with maintenance IV doses 1–3 mg/ kg/day. The oral AZA maintenance dose may be as low as 0.25–0.5 mg/kg/day. Doses may need downward adjustment when hepatic or renal dysfunction is present or if the white blood cell count (WBC) falls below 3,000–4,000 mm^3.

Mycophenolate mofetil blocks the proliferative responses to T and B lymphocytes by inhibiting antibody formation and the generation of cytotoxic T cells. The adhesion molecules that allow leukocytes to infiltrate tissues are also blocked by MMF. After oral absorption, MMF is hydrolyzed to the active metabolite, mycophenolic acid. Mycophenolic acid is metabolized to a glucuronide conjugate, which is inactive but which may be converted back to the active parent drug in the blood. The drug is 97% bound to albumin in plasma, so that total plasma concentrations will vary in a liver transplant patient as plasma protein concentrations increase with normalizing hepatic synthetic function. Mycophenolate is currently only approved for the prevention of allograft rejection following renal transplantation. Limited data on the effectiveness of MMF in liver transplantation are available, and studies are currently being conducted. Adverse effects with MMF include gastrointestinal disturbances (nausea, vomiting, diarrhea), neutropenia, thrombocytopenia, headache, weakness, dizziness, and insomnia. Antacids decrease the absorption of MMF, and administration of the two agents should be separated by 2 hours. Food delays the absorption of MMF, but it may be necessary to take MMF with food to minimize the GI adverse effects. The dose of MMF for optimizing immunosuppression and minimizing adverse effects is 2 g/d, administered in two divided doses given every 12 hours. Pediatric doses of MMF are approximately 40 mg/kg/d in two doses. Plasma concentration monitoring has been suggested for MMF, but a good correlation with efficacy and adverse effects has not been demonstrated. Mycophenolate appears to be a more specific immunosuppressant for lymphocytes and has less adverse effects than AZA.

Anti-T Cell Antibodies

Muromonab-CD3 is a monoclonal antibody that binds the CD3 receptor on lymphocytes. Circulating T cells become undetectable within minutes of an infusion of OKT3. OKT3 is used as induction therapy following transplantation and treatment of acute cellular rejection. Many transplant centers reserve the use of OKT3 for treating moderate to severe acute rejection that is unresponsive to high-dose corticosteroids. The initial dose of OKT3 may be associated with chills, fever, chest tightness, and wheezing. This first-dose reaction can be minimized by premedication with antipyretics, antihistamines, and corticosteroids. Other adverse effects include fever, headache, neck stiffness, and central nervous system toxicity. The dose of OKT3 is usually 5 mg daily administered IV push for 5 to 14 days, or 2.5 mg in a child who weighs less than 30 kg. A high proportion of patients treated with OKT3 form antibodies to one of the components of OKT3 and may not be able to receive or adequately respond to retreatment.[31]

ALG/ATG globulin is a sterile nonpyrogenic solution of immunoglobulins obtained from either horses (Atgam, Upjohn) or rabbits (Thymoglobulin, SangStat) immunized with human lymphoid cells. ALG/ATG eliminates T cells and decreases the proliferation of newly formed lymphocytes. ALG/ATG is used for induction therapy and for treatment of an acute cellular rejection. Adverse effects include chills and febrile reactions following infusion that can be minimized with premedications (similar to OKT3). Phlebitis and hypotension can be avoided by administering the intravenous infusion over 4 to 6 hours. Thrombocytopenia and increased infectious risks may also occur. The dosing for the two products is significantly different and care must be taken to avoid errors. The dose for Atgam is 10–30 mg/ kg/day for 5 to 14 days for adults. In children, the dose is reduced to 5–25 mg/kg/day. For Thymoglobulin, the dose is 1.5 mg/kg daily for 7 to 14 days for adults. This dose should be reduced for leukopenia or thrombocytopenia.

Interleukin-2 Receptor Monoclonal Antibodies

Daclizumab is a humanized monoclonal antibody comprised of 90% human and 10% murine sequences. The target of this antibody is the CD25 subunit (Tac, p55 α) of the IL-2 receptor. Binding of daclizumab to the IL-2 receptor prevents IL-2-mediated activation and proliferation of T-lymphocytes, a critical step in the development of allograft rejection. Daclizumab is currently approved for the prevention of renal allograft rejection when used in conjunction with cyclosporine and corticosteroid immunosuppression. Clinical experience and research with daclizumab in liver recipients is more limited. Pilot studies have looked at the use of daclizumab as an induction agent used in combination with mycophenolate mofetil and corticosteroid.[32,33] In these studies, calcineurin inhibitor therapy was held for patients with pretransplant renal dysfunction until improvement in clinical parameters was exhibited. The results of these studies suggest that with daclizumab induction, calcineurin inhibitor therapy can be delayed for approximately 7 day and then initiated at low doses. Further studies are needed to determine the place in therapy for daclizumab in liver transplant recipients.

Daclizumab has a half-life of approximately 20 days, which allows for dosing at 2-week intervals. In renal transplantation, the recommended dose is 1 mg/kg, as an intravenous infusion, every 14 days for a total of five doses, with the first dose given on the day of transplant. The dose does not need to be adjusted in renal or hepatic dysfunction. This regimen saturates the IL-2 receptors for approximately 120 days after transplant. The adverse effects noted in patients receiving daclizumab do not appear to be significantly different than those noted with standard immunosuppressive regimens. No significant drug interactions have been reported with daclizumab.

Basiliximab is a chimeric monoclonal antibody that contains approximately 50% human and 50% murine sequences. The target of basiliximab is also the CD25 subunit of the IL-2 receptor, preventing IL-2-mediated T-cell proliferation. Basiliximab is approved for prevention of renal allograft rejection when used in combination with cyclosporine and steroids. Limited data is available on the use of basiliximab in liver transplant patients, further research is necessary to determine the role of basiliximab in this population. The dosing of this drug is more convenient than that for daclizumab. Dosing involves two 20-mg intravenous doses, with the first being given within 2 hours of transplant surgery and the second given on the fourth postoperative day. Because this product contains a greater number of murine sequences than daclizumab, the half-life is only 7 days. Basiliximab appears to have minimal adverse effects at a rate that does not differ significantly from placebo.

PHARMACOECONOMIC CONSIDERATIONS

Liver transplantation is the most expensive of the solid-organ transplant procedures that are routinely performed in a large number of centers. The total average cost for the first year of care after liver transplantation is about $300,000, with average subsequent costs of about $20,000 per year.[34] Actual pharmacy charges make up only approximately 15% of that cost, so that the potential impact of drug therapy on the clinical course, episodes of rejection and infection, and retransplantation is a more important cost determinant than the drug cost alone in the first year following liver transplantation. Long-term maintenance costs are more heavily influenced by the cost of the drugs that are used.

Because liver transplantation is an expensive procedure, the performance of this operation will continue to come under close scrutiny in health care systems with limited resources.[35] Retransplantation of the liver more than doubles the cost of the procedure, and may not be a cost-effective use of scarce donor resources.[36] Managed care approaches to reducing the cost following liver transplantation do affect drug therapy through changes such as the outpatient administration of therapy for treating acute episodes of rejection.[37]

The US FK506 Multicenter Trial reported valuable information on the cost of liver transplantation in the United States, even if the report is not an ideal pharmacoeconomic assessment.[34] The analysis identified a number of areas that significantly affect the cost of the liver transplant procedure, such as the increasing expense associated with steroid and with monoclonal antibody treatment of rejection, and the impact of readmission to the intensive care unit for severe rejection. The study concluded that primary immunosuppression with TAC saved $19,290 in the first year after liver transplantation in comparison with the use of CSA.

The potential for drug therapy to influence the cost of liver transplantation should not be underestimated. Even the use of prostaglandin E_1, which appears to have no impact on mortality or primary nonfunction in liver allografts and may add $5,000 in drug costs, has been claimed to save $50,000 per patient by reducing the morbidity and hospital stay for these patients.[38]

EVALUATION OF THERAPEUTIC OUTCOME

MONITORING OF THE PHARMACEUTICAL CARE PLAN

The pharmacotherapist must attempt to balance drug therapy between adequate immunosuppression to prevent rejection and overimmunosuppression with its concurrent risks. Markers of organ function are important monitoring tools to assess rejection and drug toxicity. Organ tissue biopsies are considered the gold standards in determining the presence, absence, or severity of a rejection episode. Drug concentrations are important general guidelines in preventing rejection and drug toxicity, but patients can exhibit rejection and adverse effects from medications irrespective of drug concentration.

An intensive laboratory assessment program is used to monitor the patient following liver transplantation. Table 41–4 lists the monitoring parameters for following a liver transplant patient. No single test can be interpreted independently; an adequate assessment comes only after considering the clinical, radiologic, and laboratory examinations as a composite representation of the patient's condition. This is particularly true when attempting to assess whether drug therapy, an infection, rejection, or some technical complication of the transplant surgery is causing an adverse event.

The frequency of laboratory and physical monitoring depends on length of time post-transplantation and stability of the patient. When a transplant recipient is in the hospital, laboratory and physical monitoring should be conducted on a daily basis. As an outpatient, monitoring is performed twice weekly for the first few months after transplantation. If the patient remains stable over time, then laboratory monitoring is extended to once weekly, once every other week, and then finally monthly.

GRAFT DYSFUNCTION

The general sequence of events that underlies graft rejection is (a) recognition of the donor's histocompatibility differences by the recipient's immune system; (b) recruitment of activated lymphocytes; (c) initiation of immune effector mechanisms; and (d) destruction of the graft. These processes can take place at varying rates and may involve different mechanisms. Rejection of the transplanted liver can

TABLE 41–4. Monitoring Parameters for a Patient Following Liver Transplantation

Measurement	Application
Serum bilirubin and liver enzymes	Assess functional status of the liver. These tests should improve rapidly unless there is delayed graft function or primary nonfunction. An increase in these values may indicate a technical complication or rejection.
Serum creatinine and BUN (blood urea nitrogen)	Assess renal function. The BUN/creatinine ratio is normally increased in a liver transplant patient. These values should stabilize to the high-normal range in a liver transplant patient; rapid increases may indicate drug toxicity or a change in the hydration status of the patient.
Serum electrolytes	Hypomagnesemia requiring supplementation has been observed. Hyperkalemia requiring fludrocortisone therapy is common. Other abnormalities related to intensive diuretic therapy are also common.
Serum prothrombin time, INR	Assess functional capacity of liver to make coagulation factors. Also important in the event of bleeding episodes due to technical complications.
Blood pressure, weight, vital signs	Prevent hypertensive encephalopathy and the other complications of hypertension. Monitor fluid status and temperature elevations that may accompany infection or graft rejection.
Leukocyte cytomegalovirus (CMV)	Assess CMV status through identification of pp65 marker on cells.
Antigenemia	Allows preemptive antiviral therapy when the level of antigenemia increases.
Physical examination	Assess graft tenderness, neurologic status, and sites of infection on skin incisions or body cavities.
Serum albumin	Assess plasma oncotic pressure and hepatic synthetic function. Albumin supplementation is occasionally prescribed to improve diuretic efficiency until synthesis can restore normal plasma proteins.
Complete blood count	Assess white cell number and differential to monitor for infection. Follow hematocrit to observe for bleeding episodes that may indicate technical complications with the graft.

take place any time following surgery and is classified as either hyperacute, acute cellular, or chronic rejection. Although these processes generally denote a temporal sequence of events, considerable overlap exists in the actual time frame of when each type is observed. The liver appears to be less immunogenic and more likely to promote immunologic tolerance than the other vascularized organs. Hyperacute rejection rarely occurs in patients receiving a liver transplant. The liver's special status for transplantation is not fully understood, but the local release of cytokines may alter the immunologic reaction taking place in the liver.

Hyperacute rejection often occurs within minutes to 2 weeks of the transplant procedure. Early graft dysfunction is treated with supportive care and retransplantation if possible. An immunologic explanation for graft dysfunction becomes more probable as time passes in a patient with an initially functioning liver graft. Initial episodes of acute cellular rejection often occur between 6 days and 6 weeks posttransplantation, but can also occur earlier or later. Other reasons for delayed graft dysfunction include defects in bile duct reconstruction, opportunistic infections, and toxicity from parenteral nutrition, sepsis, or drug-induced hepatotoxicity. The clinical signs of acute cellular rejection are fever, lethargy, graft tenderness, leukocytosis, and a change in the color or quantity of bile. An increased serum bilirubin and increases in hepatic enzymes are the most common biochemical parameters monitored and are sensitive markers of rejection. The liver biopsy is used as definitive evidence of the diagnosis of rejection, but response to antirejection medication has also been used in differentiating rejection from other causes of hepatic dysfunction in a liver transplant patient.

The treatment of acute cellular rejection varies widely from center to center, but generally involves the concepts of (a) optimizing the present immunosuppressive therapy; (b) initially giving high-dose corticosteroids; and (c) the use of OKT3 monoclonal antibody or ALG/ATG for a 7- to 14-day course when steroid resistance is encountered. Figure 41–2 shows a typical flow diagram of the treatment for acute rejections. Increasing the dosage of CSA can be effective in mild cases of rejection, but is infrequently used because of concerns of nephrotoxicity with the drug. The TAC dosage is increased in patients with mild rejection and is effective in some patients. The administration of corticosteroids for rejection can be done as a "pulse" of one to three large doses of methylprednisolone, or can be achieved as a "recycle" of an increased dosage of methylprednisolone, prednisolone, or prednisone for 5 to 10 days. The dosages of other immunosuppressant drugs are often decreased while administering corticosteroids, OKT3, or ALG/ATG therapy. Patients who are deemed steroid resistant are treated with a 7- to 14-day course of OKT3, ALG, or ATG.

Chronic rejection may be a slow and indolent form of cellular rejection. Chronic rejection of the liver is characterized by an obliterative arteriopathy and the loss of bile ducts, which has been referred to as the vanishing bile duct syndrome. These patients experience an asymptomatic rise in the canalicular liver enzymes (alkaline phosphatase and γ-glutamyl transpeptidase) and become jaundiced. These changes can be seen in patients who have not responded adequately to therapy for acute rejection; these changes are considered the result of immunologic and ischemic injury. The changes of chronic rejection are not reversible, and CMV infection has also been implicated in the initiation of the process in transplant patients.

Noncompliance with medications or follow-up care is a preventable cause of graft loss. The reported incidence of noncompliance with medication 3 months after transplantation is about 20%. Patients most likely to become noncompliant are young and in a lower socioeconomic group. In one retrospective study, 91% of patients who were noncompliant with medications or followup care either lost their transplanted organs or died. Noncompliance with medications and the development of chimerism has prompted studies in the weaning of immunosuppression, but withdrawal of medications must be done under the supervision of a transplant physician.[39] The pharmacist can help educate the patient on the importance of medication compliance and help simplify the medication regimen to reduce the incidence of noncompliance in transplant recipients.[40]

CONCLUSIONS

Improved organ preservation techniques have made liver transplantation a more widely available and accepted technique for an expanding list of congenital, autoimmune, and metabolic diseases. New agents

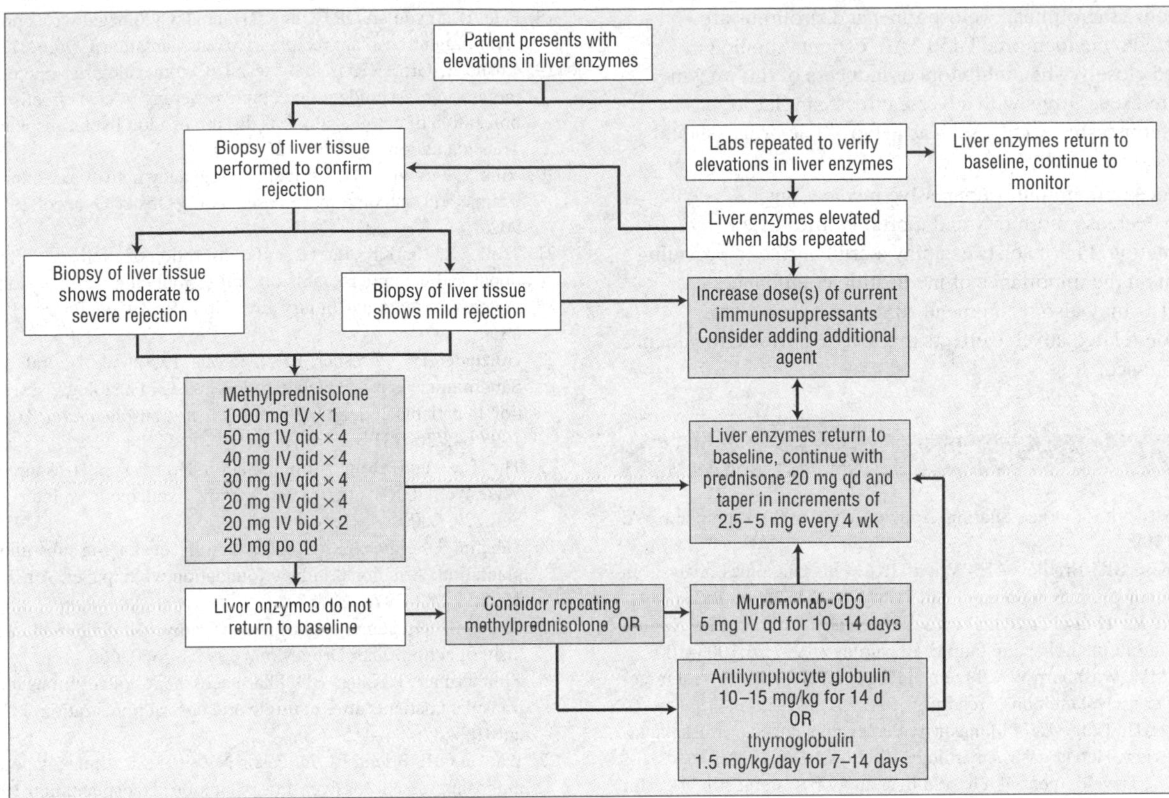

FIGURE 41–2. Flow diagram for the treatment of acute rejection in a liver transplant patient.

such as TAC have improved the immunosuppressive management of liver transplant patients, but the absence of subtle immunologic monitoring techniques means that infection and rejection are persistent clinical problems in these patients. Drug therapy in the liver transplant patient is complicated by rapidly changing hepatic function and the need for intense immunosuppression. The immunosuppressive drug regimen is initially complex and requires intensive monitoring to optimize therapy in the presence of drug interactions and changing drug absorption, distribution, metabolism, and elimination. The pharmacotherapist can make significant contributions to the care of liver transplant patients through the management of complex drug regimens; by managing drug dosing, toxicity, and drug interactions; and by providing patient education and promoting medication compliance.

▶ PRINCIPLES OF PHARMACOTHERAPY

- Liver transplantation is the life-saving procedure in patients with severe hepatic disease and no other medical options. Transplantation may correct metabolic defects initially responsible for liver failure. Recurrence of liver failure due to other etiologies can be minimized with a targeted pharmacologic approach, for example hyperimmunoglobulin plus lamivudine for prevention of recurrent viral hepatitis B.
- A recent liver transplant recipient will experience physiologic changes that may affect the pharmacokinetics of administered medications. The physiologic changes are the result of improved organ function, but typically function is not considered normal. Changes include improved bile salts and serum proteins production, as well as improved liver metabolism.
- The goal of drug therapy for a transplant recipient is to determine a patient-specific regimen that provides an adequate level of immunosuppression to prevent organ rejection and minimizes adverse drug effects and opportunistic infections.
- Immunosuppressive drug protocols include two to four immunosuppressants. The standard immunosuppression regimen is comprised of corticosteroids plus either cyclosporine or tacrolimus. An antiproliferative agent or sirolimus may be added for patients at higher risk of rejection.
- Patients receiving immunosuppression will need prophylactic therapy to prevent infection. Transplant recipients are at risk for infections with *Pneumocystis carinii*, cytomegalovirus, herpes virus, and fungal pathogens.
- Doses of certain immunosuppressants (TAC or CSA) are adjusted according to blood levels, whereas other immunosuppressants (MMF or AZA) are adjusted according to patient response. Doses of the immunosuppressant medications are weaned over time if the patient does not exhibit organ rejection.
- Laboratory tests are essential tools to monitor for the onset of rejection and adverse effects. An elevation in serum bilirubin and liver enzymes may signify the onset of acute rejection. Prothrombin time and serum albumin are also helpful to assess the functional status of the liver. Abnormalities of serum creatinine, blood urea nitrogen (BUN), and electrolytes may indicate nephrotoxic effects of tacrolimus or cyclosporine.
- Organ rejection must be treated aggressively to prevent loss of the transplanted organ. High-dose corticosteroids are typically considered first-line therapy for treatment of rejection. Thymoglobulin or muromonab are used for rejection that is refractory to corticosteroids.
- The pharmacist should be knowledgeable of the management of drug interactions that can occur with the immunosuppressant

medications. Tacrolimus, cyclosporine, and sirolimus are metabolized by cytochrome P450 3A4. Patients should be monitored closely when inhibitors or inducers of this enzyme system are used. Drugs with adverse effects similar to immunosuppressive agents, such as nephrotoxic drugs, should also be used cautiously.

- Compliance with immunosuppressive medications has been shown to decrease morbidity and mortality after liver transplantation. Pharmacists can play a critical role in providing education on the importance of medication compliance. Pharmacists may also recommend strategies to minimize medication related adverse effects that may contribute to patient noncompliance.

REFERENCES

1. United Network for Organ Sharing. Annual Report 1999. Richmond, VA, UNOS, 1999.
2. Geevarghese SK, Bradley AE, Wright JK, et al. Outcomes analysis in 100 liver transplantation patients. Am J Surg 1998;175:448–353.
3. Mohamed R., Hubscher SG, Darius FM, et al. Posttransplant chronic hepatitis in fulminant hepatic failure. Hepatology 1997;25:1003–1007.
4. Johnson MW, Washburn WK, Freeman RB, et al. Hepatitis C viral infection in liver transplantation. Arch Surg 1996;131:284–291.
5. Schmidt HHJ, Tietge UJF, Manns MP. Perspectives of liver transplantation: A review. Hepatogastroenterology 1997;44:1013–1018.
6. Gerlach JC. Development of a hybrid liver support system: A review. Int J Artif Organs 1996;19:645–654.
7. Dunn SP, Haynes JH, Nicolette LA, et al. Split-liver transplantation benefits the recipient of the "leftover liver." Pediatr Surg 1997;32:252–255.
8. Whitington PF, Alonso EM, Piper JB. Pediatric liver transplantation. Semin Liver Dis 1994;14:303–317.
9. Brown RS, Ascher NL, Lake JR, et al. The impact of surgical complications after liver transplantation on resource utilization. Arch Surg 1997;132:1098–1103.
10. Venkataramanan R, Habucky K, Burckart GJ, et al. Clinical pharmacokinetics in organ transplant patients. Clin Pharmacokinet 1989;16:134–161.
11. McDonald JC, Adamashvili I, Zibari GB, et al. Serologic allogenic chimerism. Transplantation 1997:64:865–871.
12. Sanchez-Izquierdo JA, Lumbreras C, Colina F, et al. Severe graft versus host disease following liver transplantation confirmed by PCR-HLA-B sequencing: Report of a case and literature review. Hepatogastroenterology 1996;43:1057–1061.
13. US Multicenter Tacrolimus Liver Study Group. A comparison of tacrolimus (FK-506) and cyclosporine for immunosuppression in liver transplantation. N Engl J Med 1994;331:1110–1115.
14. European Tacrolimus Multicenter Liver Study Group. Randomized trial comparing tacrolimus (FK-506) and cyclosporine in prevention of liver allograft rejection. Lancet 1994;344:423–428.
15. Sher LS, Cosenza CA, Michel J, et al. Efficacy of tacrolimus as rescue therapy for chronic rejection in orthotopic liver transplantation: A report of the US Multicenter Liver Study Group. Transplantation 1997;64:258–263.
16. Pratschke J, Neuhaus R, Tullius SG, et al. Treatment of cyclosporine-related adverse effects by conversion to tacrolimus after liver transplantation. Transplantation 1997;64:938–940.
17. Platz KP, Mueller AR, Rossaint R, et al. Cytokine pattern during rejection and infection after liver transplantation—Improvements in postoperative monitoring? Transplantation 1996;62:1441–1450.
18. Patel R, Snydman DR, Rubin RH, et al. Cytomegalovirus prophylaxis in solid-organ transplant recipients. Transplantation 1996;61:1279–1289.
19. Kusne S, Grossi P, Irish W, et al. Cytomegalovirus pp65 antigenemia monitoring as a guide for preemptive therapy: A cost effective strategy for prevention of cytomegalovirus disease in adult liver transplant recipients. Transplantation 1999;68:1125–1131.
20. Ville Y, Fernandez H, Samuel D. Pregnancy in liver transplant recipients: Course and outcome in 19 cases. Am J Obstet Gynecol 1993;168:896–902.
21. Trull AK, Tan KK, Tan L, et al. Absorption of cyclosporin from conventional and new microemulsion oral formulations in liver transplant recipients with external biliary diversion. Br J Clin Pharm 1995;39:627–631.
22. Graziadei IW, Wiesner RH, Marotta PJ, et al. Neoral compared to Sandimmune is associated with a decrease in histologic severity of rejection in patients undergoing primary liver transplantation. Transplantation 1997;64:726–731.
23. The U.S. and Drug Administration Home Page [resource on World Wide Web]. URL: http://www.fda.gov. Available from Internet. Accessed Sept. 29, 2000.
24. Sabatini S, Ferguson RM, Helderman JH, et al. Drug substitution in transplantation: A national kidney foundation white paper. Am J Kidney Dis 1999;33:389–397.
25. Seghal SN. Rapamune (sirolimus, rapamycin): An overview and mechanism of action. Ther Drug Monit 1995;17:660–665.
26. Zimmerman JJ, Kahan BD. Pharmacokinetics of sirolimus in stable renal transplant patients after multiple oral dose administration. J Clin Pharmacol 1997;37:404–415.
27. Watson CJE, Friend PJ, Jamieson NV, et al. Sirolimus: A potent new immunosuppressant for liver transplantation. Transplantation 1999;67:505–509.
28. McAlister VC, Gao Z, Pelekian K, et al. Sirolimus-tacrolimus combination immunosuppression. Lancet 2000;355:376–377.
29. Vasquez EM. Sirolimus: A new agent for prevention of renal allograft rejection. Am J Health-Syst Pharm 2000;57:437–448.
30. Suthanthiran M, Morris RE, Strom TB. Immunosuppressants: Cellular and molecular mechanisms of action. Am J. Kidney Dis 1996;28:159–172.
31. McIntyre JA, Kincade M, Higgins NG. Detection of IgA anti-OKT3 antibodies in OKT3-treated transplant recipients. Transplantation 1996; 61:1465–1469.
32. Hirose R, Roberts JP, Quan D, et al. Experience with daclizumab in liver transplantation. Transplantation 2000;69:307–310.
33. Eckhoff DE, McGuire B, Sellers M, et al. The safety and efficacy of a two-dose daclizumab (Zenapax)-induction therapy in liver transplant recipients. Transplantation 2000;69:1867–1872.
34. Lake JR, Gorman KJ, Esquivel CP, et al. The impact of immunosuppressive regimens on the cost of liver transplantation-Results from the US FK506 multicenter trial. Transplantation 1995;60:1089–1095.
35. O'Grady JG. Clinical economics review: Liver transplantation. Aliment Pharmacol Ther 1997;11:445–451.
36. Evans RW, Manninen DL, Dong FB, McLynne DA. Is retransplantation cost-effective? Transplant Proc 1993;25:1694–1696.
37. Abouljoud MS, Brown KA, May E, et al. Cost-effective management of acute rejection in liver transplant recipients: A managed care perspective. Transplant Proc 1997;29:1557–1559.
38. Henley KS, Smith D. Prostaglandins in liver transplantation: A $50,000 bonus. Gastroenterology 1997;112:670–671.
39. Mazariegos GV, Reyes J, Marino IR, et al. Weaning of immunosuppression in liver transplant recipients. Transplantation 1997;63:243–249.
40. Schweizer RT, Rovelli M, Palmeri D, et al. Noncompliance in organ transplant recipients. Transplantation 1990;49:374–377.

42

QUANTIFICATION OF RENAL FUNCTION

Thomas J. Comstock

Renal function can be assessed from both a qualitative and a quantitative perspective. Although creatinine clearance is typically considered the clinical standard for assessment of renal function, other tests, such as the urinalysis, radiographic procedures, and biopsy, are also valuable tools in the assessment of renal disease. Quantitative measures, such as clearance, are most useful in establishing the degree of kidney function, or change in function that may occur as a result of disease progression, therapeutic intervention, or toxic insult.[1] Moreover, the design of dosage regimens for drugs eliminated by the kidneys is also dependent on the quantitative measure of kidney function. Determination of the etiology of kidney disease, on the other hand, is dependent on a more qualitative assessment of the kidneys. The urinalysis, for example, may reveal red blood cells or proteinuria, suggestive of glomerular disease. Follow-up studies, such as imaging procedures or kidney biopsy, may then further differentiate the specific cause, thereby pointing to the appropriate therapeutic intervention.

Renal "function" includes the processes of filtration, secretion, and reabsorption, as well as endocrine and metabolic functions. Alterations of all five renal functions, whether declining or improving, have been associated primarily with glomerular filtration rate (GFR). This chapter critically evaluates the various methods that can be used for the quantitative assessment of kidney function (Table 42–1). Where appropriate, discussion regarding the qualitative assessment of the renal function is also presented, including specialized tests such as kidney biopsy.

ENDOCRINE FUNCTION

Secretion of renin by the cells of the juxtaglomerular apparatus, production and metabolism of prostaglandins and kinins, and the production and secretion of erythropoietin by the interstitial cells in response to decreased oxygen tension in the blood are among the kidney's endocrine functions. Because these functions are related to renal mass, decreased endocrine activity is associated with the loss of viable cells. Hematocrit, for example, declines as a function of decreasing GFR, primarily because of a loss of erythropoietin production, leading to the complications associated with anemia, which include fatigue, dyspnea, anorexia, and the development of, or increased, angina.

METABOLIC FUNCTION

The kidneys are capable of a wide variety of metabolic activities, including the activation of vitamin D_3, gluconeogenesis, and metabolism of endogenous compounds such as insulin and steroids, as well as xenobiotics. Impaired renal function results in decreased formation of activated vitamin D_3 and decreased insulin metabolism. It is common for patients with diabetes and chronic renal failure to have reduced requirements for exogenous insulin,[2] and supplemental therapy with activated vitamin D_3 (calcitriol) or other vitamin D analogs (paricalcitol, doxercalciferol) is often necessary in the management of renal osteodystrophy.[3] Numerous enzymes have been identified in the kidneys, primarily the cortex. These include cytochrome P450, *N*-acetyltransferase, glutathione transferase, renal peptidases, and others.[4] The cytochrome P450 system in the kidneys is as active as that in the liver, when corrected for organ mass. Furthermore, the accumulation of uremic toxins is associated with decreased CYP activity for selected isoenzymes. *In vitro* studies demonstrate impaired function of CYP3A4 and 2C9, whereas 1A2, 2C19, and 2D6 are not affected. The clinical importance of these preliminary findings is not fully understood at this time. Reversible metabolism may also be affected by renal disease when normal enzyme function is disrupted. This has been observed with clofibrate[5] and may apply to other compounds eliminated by the same route, such as ketoprofen.[6] See Chap. 50 for more detailed discussion.

EXCRETORY FUNCTION

Although endocrine and metabolic functions are important aspects of the kidney's contribution to maintenance of body homeostasis, it is the excretory function that is often perceived as the "kidney function." Through the combined processes of glomerular filtration, tubular secretion, and tubular reabsorption, the nephron, as the functional unit of the kidney, maintains balance between input and output of water and solutes from the body, and is the key organ responsible for maintenance of homeostasis. This is represented as:

$$\text{Rate of excretion} = \text{Rate of filtration} + \text{Rate of secretion} - \text{Rate of reabsorption}$$

Glomerular filtration occurs through the passive diffusion of water and small-molecular-weight ions and molecules across the glomerular–capillary membrane into Bowman's capsule and the proximal tubule (Fig. 42–1). Because most proteins are too large to be substantially filtered (>60 kDa), or their filtration is impeded by electronegative charges of the glomerulus, compounds presented to the glomerulus in the protein-bound state are not filtered and enter the peritubular circulation. Secretion occurs primarily along the proximal tubule and facilitates elimination of compounds from the plasma into the tubular lumen via active transport. Anionic and cationic transport systems have been characterized and are involved in the transport of many endogenous and exogenous substances. Examples include probenecid, *p*-aminohippurate (PAH), and penicillin as anions, and creatinine, cimetidine, and procainamide as cations.[7] These systems are not mutually exclusive, as probenecid has been observed to compete with

TABLE 42–1. Markers of Renal Function

Renal plasma/blood flow	*p*-Aminohippurate (PAH) ^{131}I-Orthoiodohippurate (^{131}I-OIH) ^{99m}Tc-mercaptoacetyltriglycine (^{99m}Tc-MAG3)
Glomerular filtration rate	Inulin, sinistrin Iothalamate Iohexol ^{99m}Tc-diethylenetriaminepentaacetic acid (^{99m}Tc-DTPA) ^{125}I-Iothalamate Creatinine Cystatin C
Tubular function	*p*-Aminohippurate *N*-1-Methylnicotinamide (NMN) Tetraethyl ammonium (TEA) β_2-Microglobulin Retinol-binding protein (RBP) Protein HC (α_1-microglobulin) *N*-Acetylglucosaminidase (NAG) Alanine aminopeptidase (AAP) Adenosine binding protein (ABP)

the tubular secretion of cimetidine.[8] P-glycoprotein (P-gp), a membrane glycoprotein distributed in tissues including kidney, liver, jejunum, colon, and others, is recognized as an important element in drug elimination by the kidneys.[9] It is located on the apical membrane of the proximal tubule and may play an important role in the elimination of cytotoxic drugs. Blockade of P-gp could result in decreased renal elimination of such compounds, leading to an increased drug exposure. Verapamil, cyclosporine, and the P-gp-specific inhibitor PSC 833 all reduce the activity of this tubular transport mechanism.[10] Further investigations into the exact role of P-gp in drug elimination are presently underway. Reabsorption of water and solutes occurs throughout the nephron, whereas drug reabsorption occurs predominantly along the distal tubule and collecting tubules. Urine flow rate and physicochemical characteristics of the molecule influence these processes. Highly ionized compounds are not reabsorbed unless pH changes within the urine increase the fraction un-ionized, so that reabsorption may be facilitated.

The homeostasis afforded by the kidneys is affected by catecholamines, prostaglandins, renin, antidiuretic hormone, natriuretic hormone, and the number of functioning nephrons. The "intact nephron hypothesis" of Bricker,[11] which was first published more than 30 years ago, proposes that "kidney function" of patients with renal disease is the net result of a reduced number of appropriately functioning nephrons. As the number of nephrons is reduced from the initial complement of 2 million, those unaffected compensate for those damaged by disease or toxic insult. The cornerstone of this hypothesis is that glomerulotubule balance is maintained, such that those nephrons capable of functioning will continue to perform in an appropriate fashion. As GFR declines, tubular reabsorption must decrease to allow for elimination of the solute load. Single nephron GFR (SNGFR) increases in the remaining nephrons, whereas the whole-kidney GFR represents the sum of the SNGFR of the remaining functional nephrons. Based on this, one would presume that a measure of one component of nephron function could be used as an estimate of all renal functions. This, indeed, has been and remains our clinical approach.

Measurement of GFR, however, may not be an appropriate assessment for a drug that undergoes active tubular secretion, or

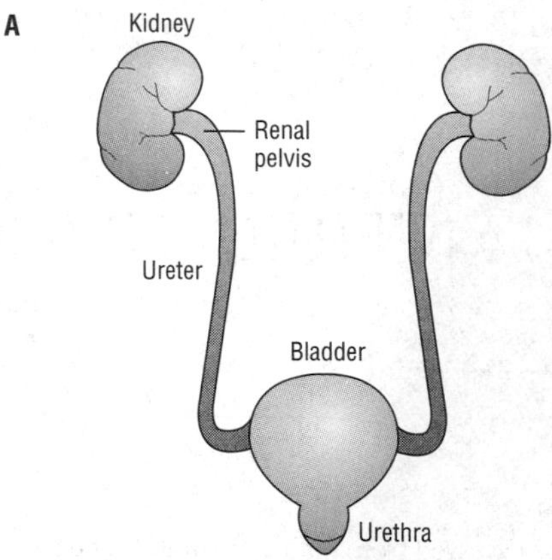

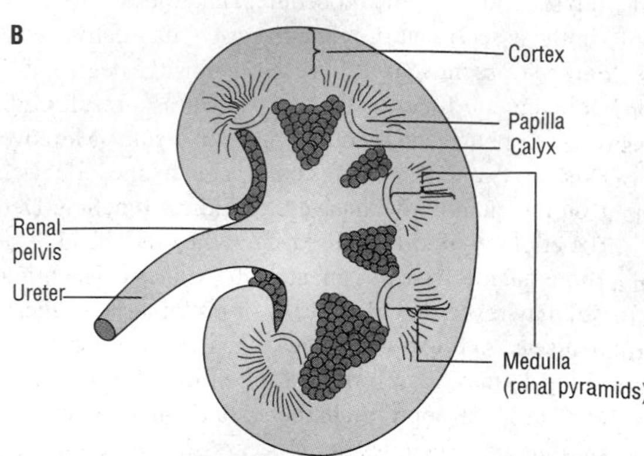

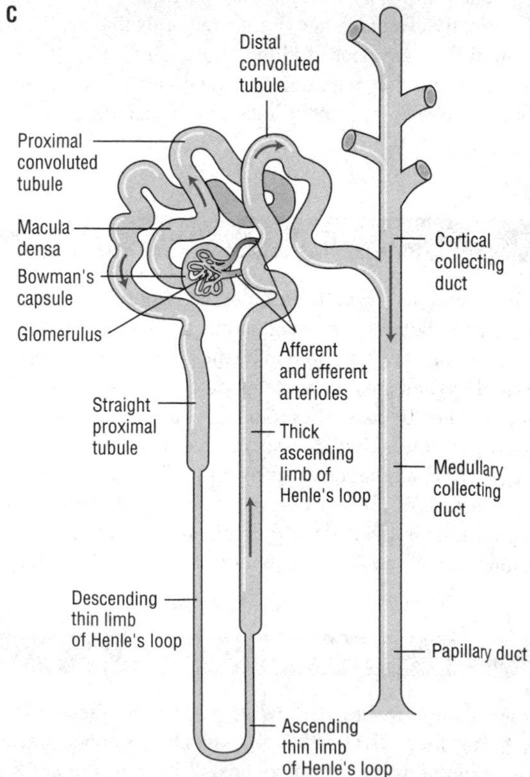

FIGURE 42–1. Structures of the (**A**) urinary system, (**B**) kidney, and (**C**) nephron, the functional unit of the kidney.

for a drug that is extensively reabsorbed. As an example, Hori et al.[12,13] demonstrated that the postfiltration renal handling of ampicillin, which is secreted, and cephalexin, which is secreted and reabsorbed, remained normal in patients with renal failure caused by glomerulonephritis, but was reduced in patients with renal failure associated with tubular dysfunction. They concluded that dosage adjustment based on creatinine clearance would be inappropriate for drugs eliminated by tubular secretion. Maiza and Daley-Yates[14] observed glomerulotubule imbalance in experimentally induced renal failure in rats based on differential effects on inulin (an index of filtration), PAH (an index of anionic secretion), and *N*-1-methylnicotinamide clearance (an index of cationic secretion). Using an experimental nephrotoxic (uranyl nitrate) acute renal failure rat model, Lin and Lin[15] and Gloff and Benet[16] demonstrated differential handling of tetraethylammonium (TEA) bromide and PAH, with greater impairment of tubular secretion than of GFR. Lin and Lin[15] further studied an ischemic acute renal failure model (glycerol) and showed a parallel decline of secretion and GFR for TEA, whereas secretion of PAH decreased at a greater rate than did GFR. These results support the hypothesis that the integrity of different pathways for elimination of compounds may be dependent on the mode of injury as well as the chemical characteristics of the compound. Thus, the kidney should not be considered as a single homogeneously functioning organ, but one with several different, discrete functions. It is thus analogous to the liver in which the multiple metabolic pathways may be impaired to variable degrees dependent on the type of injury or disease. Despite these observations, the clinical impact of the findings has not been fully evaluated.

It is recognized that GFR is dependent on numerous factors, one of which is protein load. Bosch[17] suggested that an appropriate measure of renal function should reflect the "filtration capacity" of the kidney, and not the "resting GFR." Subjects with normal renal function administered an oral or intravenous protein load prior to measurement of GFR have increased their GFR by as much as 50%.[17] As renal function declines, the kidneys compensate by increasing SNGFR. The renal reserve, the maximal degree by which GFR can be increased usually declines, and thus may be a complimentary measure of renal function for these patients.

Quantification of renal function is not only an important diagnostic index, but it also serves as an important parameter for monitoring therapy directed at the etiology of the diminished function itself, thereby allowing for objective measurement of the success or failure of treatment. Measurement of renal function also serves as a useful indicator of the ability of the kidneys to eliminate drugs from the body. Furthermore, alterations of drug distribution and metabolism are associated with the degree of renal function. See Chap. 50 for a discussion of pharmacokinetic changes in renal disease. Although several indices have been used for the quantification of renal function in the research setting, GFR and, more specifically, creatinine clearance are the primary markers of renal function in the clinical arena.[18–20]

SIGNS AND SYMPTOMS OF RENAL DYSFUNCTION

Patients who develop renal disease remain relatively asymptomatic until impairment has progressed to the point that systemic manifestations and/or secondary complications become evident. Diabetes mellitus and hypertension are the two most common causes of end-stage renal disease (ESRD), and as renal function declines, patients may experience development or exacerbation of hypertension, edema, electrolyte abnormalities, anemia, or other complications (see Chaps. 44 and 45). Urine output may increase as the filtration per nephron increases, resulting in a loss of urinary concentrating ability and development of an osmotic diuresis. While a mild metabolic acidosis may be present, patients will typically not demonstrate symptoms, although chronic acidosis will lead to bone demineralization. Hyperkalemia may develop as the GFR drops to 20 mL/min; this may lead to signs of muscle weakness and electrocardiographic (ECG) abnormalities. Additional monitoring of potassium is warranted in those patients also treated with angiotensin-converting enzyme (ACE) inhibitors, as these agents can decrease potassium excretion. The signs and symptoms associated with the progressive loss of renal function are discussed in Chaps. 44 and 45. Decreased erythropoietin production by the kidney leads to decreased red blood cell production, and the accumulation of toxins, as the result of the reduction in GFR, results in a decreased red cell life span. The combination of these events leads to anemia and a multitude of signs and symptoms, including weakness, fatigue, lethargy, impaired mentation, intolerance to cold, and loss of appetite, among others. Occasionally, patients present with mental confusion or severe nausea and vomiting, which is the result of accumulated toxins and is often associated with significantly elevated urea concentrations.

Patients with glomerulonephritis, the third leading cause of ESRD, may present with hematuria, or in some cases, edema. The edema is a result of the nephrotic syndrome, a condition characterized by hypoalbuminemia, loss of more than 3 g of albumin in the urine per day, and edema (see Chap. 49). Hypoalbuminemia contributes to edema formation through a decrease in plasma oncotic pressure. Presence of frothy urine may be suggestive of significant proteinuria. Nonspecific signs that may be associated with renal disease include low-grade fever, rash, arthralgias (vasculitis, interstitial nephritis), auditory impairment (Alport's syndrome or aminoglycoside toxicity), or pulmonary symptoms (Goodpasture's syndrome).

ABNORMALITIES IN PHYSICAL EXAMINATION USED TO DETECT RENAL DYSFUNCTION

Findings on the physical examination are nonspecific for kidney disease, but may be present due to secondary involvement of other organ systems. Fluid overload may be manifest as dependent edema of the lower extremities, congestive heart failure with distended neck veins and presence of an S_3 gallop rhythm, and pulmonary rales. Elevation of blood pressure may also be caused by volume overload, or stimulation of the renin–angiotensin–aldosterone system. Enlarged kidneys may be present with polycystic kidney disease, whereas small kidneys suggest chronic renal failure due to other causes. A palpable suprapubic mass in a patient with a distended bladder is suggestive of urinary tract obstruction.

LABORATORY EVIDENCE FOR RENAL DYSFUNCTION AND ITS INTERPRETATION

The blood urea nitrogen (BUN) and serum creatinine concentrations are the two most common clinical laboratory measurements used for the assessment of kidney function.

BLOOD UREA NITROGEN

Amino acids metabolized to ammonia are subsequently converted in the liver to form urea, the production of which is dependent on protein availability (diet) and hepatic function. Renal handling of urea includes glomerular filtration followed by reabsorption of up to 50%

of the filtered load in the proximal tubule. As urea is able to cross cell membranes by passive diffusion, its reabsorption rate is variable and dependent on the reabsorption of water. The excretion of urea may, therefore, be decreased under conditions of water conservation by the kidneys although the GFR may be reduced only slightly. This condition is evident when a patient exhibits prerenal azotemia, or an increase of the BUN to a greater extent than the serum creatinine. The normal BUN:creatinine ratio is 10 to 15:1, and an elevated ratio is suggestive of a decreased effective circulating volume, which stimulates increased water, and hence, urea reabsorption.[21] Creatinine is not reabsorbed to any significant extent by the kidneys. Despite these limitations, the BUN is often used as a simple screening tool for the detection of renal dysfunction, but particularly in combination with the serum creatinine concentration.

CREATININE

Creatinine is the standard laboratory marker for the detection of kidney disease. The third National Health and Nutrition Examination Survey (NHANES III) revealed a mean serum creatinine of 0.96 mg/dL in women, and 1.16 mg/dL in men in the United States.[22] Values were lower among Mexican-Americans, and higher among non-Hispanic blacks. For all groups, the serum creatinine increased with age. The report also noted that among noninstitutionalized adults, 10.9 million have a serum creatinine greater than 1.5 mg/dL; 3.0 million have a serum creatinine greater than 1.7 mg/dL; and 0.8 million have a serum creatinine greater than 2.0 mg/dL. While the serum creatinine concentration alone is not an optimal measure of kidney function, it is often used as a marker for referral. There is presently no accepted single standard for an "abnormal" serum creatinine, as it is gender, race, and age-dependent.

Creatinine is a product of creatine metabolism from muscle; therefore, its production is directly dependent on muscle mass. At steady state, the "normal" serum creatinine concentration is approximately 0.5–1.5 mg/dL for males and females.[23] Creatinine is eliminated primarily by glomerular filtration, and as GFR declines, the serum creatinine concentration rises (Fig. 42–2).

Several methods are used for the determination of the serum creatinine concentration, most of which are based on the nonspecific Jaffé reaction, a colorimetric method based on the reaction of creatinine with alkaline picrate. This nonspecific method also reacts with noncreatinine chromogens in the serum, which may result in a falsely increased serum creatinine concentration.[23] The noncreatinine chromogens are not present in the urine in sufficient quantities to interfere with the creatinine measurement, which will be several-fold greater than the serum concentration. The impact of this interference is seen with the creatinine clearance (CLcr) calculation:

$$\text{CLcr} = (U_{cr} \times V)/(S_{cr} \times t)$$

where U_{cr} = urine creatinine concentration, V = urine volume, S_{cr} = serum creatinine concentration, and t = duration of the urine collection.

This "normal" interference results in an increase in the serum creatinine concentration of approximately 10% and thereby the creatinine clearance would underestimate the GFR by 10%. In subjects with normal renal function, this tends to counterbalance the effect of the contribution of tubular secretion of creatinine, which increases urine creatinine by nearly 10%. Thus, CLcr may serve as a good measure of GFR in subjects with normal renal function. However, this false increase in serum creatinine becomes less noticeable as the true creatinine concentration rises, due to the increasing contribution of tubular secretion to the renal clearance of creatinine.[24] This becomes important when kidney function is reduced to less than 50% of normal.

Diabetic ketoacidosis may produce increased concentrations of acetoacetate, which serves as a chromophore in the Jaffé reaction, thereby increasing the serum creatinine concentration.[23] Other substances that also react with this procedure in the serum include glucose, protein, pyruvate, fructose, uric acid, and ascorbic acid (Table 42–2).[23] In addition, some cephalosporin antibiotics are associated with a false increase in the serum creatinine concentration, including cephalothin, cefazolin, cephalexin, cefoxitin, cefaclor, and cephradine,[25] whereas other antibiotics, such as the fluoroquinolones (ciprofloxacin, fleroxacin, lomefloxacin, ofloxacin, levofloxacin, sparfloxacin, and temafloxacin), do not produce a false elevation in serum creatinine.[26] The degree of interference is dependent on the serum concentration of the antibiotic, so blood samples for creatinine should be obtained when the antibiotic concentration is lowest (at the end of a dosing interval). These interferences are not observed when the serum creatinine is measured using an enzymatic technique. The antifungal agent 5-flucytosine causes an increase in the serum creatinine when measured using the Ektachem enzymatic system, but does not interact with the Jaffé method.[27] Daly et al.[28] reported a false-negative effect of dobutamine and dopamine on the serum creatinine value when measured using the Ektachem system. The interference is concentration-dependent, and results in a 10% to 100% decrease of the serum creatinine concentration. The authors

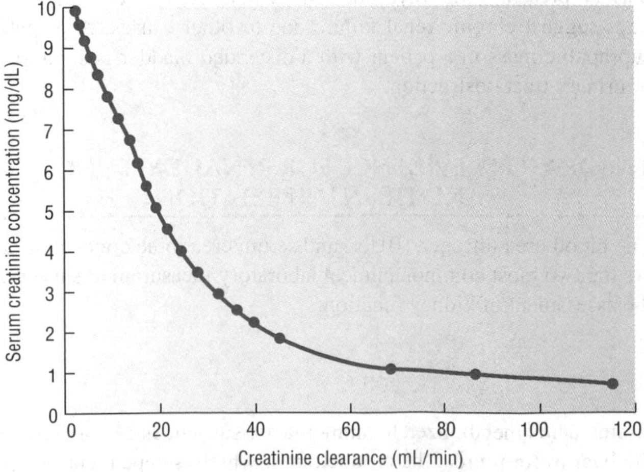

FIGURE 42–2. Relationship between serum creatinine concentration and creatinine clearance.

TABLE 42–2. Factors That May Alter Creatinine Clearance Determinations

Analytical	Physiologic
Acetoacetate	Age, weight, gender
Ascorbic acid	Diet
Cephalosporins (cephalothin, cefazolin, cephalexin, cefoxitin, cefaclor, cephradine)	Diurnal variation
	Drugs (cimetidine, trimethoprim, probenecid)
Dobutamine	Exercise
Dopamine	
5-Flucytosine	
Fructose	
Glucose	
Protein	
Pyruvate	
Uric acid	

hypothesized that both drugs compete with the chromogenic dye for oxidation by hydrogen peroxide in a concentration-dependent manner. The problem is most evident when blood samples are contaminated with residual IV solution containing the interfering drug. These differences emphasize the need to standardize a method within the research or clinic setting, and to be aware of methods employed in the laboratory for the determination of creatinine concentrations.

Other compounds are known to interfere with the serum creatinine concentration, through inhibition of the active tubular secretion of creatinine. Among these are cimetidine and trimethoprim, which compete for creatinine secretion at the cationic transport system.[23] Both trimethoprim and cimetidine demonstrate dose dependency with respect to competition with creatinine for secretion. Ranitidine, an H_2-receptor antagonist similar to cimetidine, was evaluated for its effect on creatinine clearance in 10 healthy subjects. There was no effect following single doses of 300 or 1,200 mg as determined by the ratio of CLcr to CL inulin.[29] Cimetidine, given as a single 400-mg dose in 6 of the same subjects, resulted in a reduction of the CLcr to CL inulin ratio from 1.30 to 1.03, without change in inulin clearance.

The serum creatinine concentration is dependent on the "input" function, or formation rate, and "output" function, or elimination rate. Its formation rate depends on the zero-order production from creatine metabolism, as well as input from other sources, such as dietary intake.[30] Creatine metabolism is directly proportional to muscle mass; therefore, individuals with more muscle mass have a higher serum creatinine concentration at any given degree of kidney function than those with less muscle mass. Exercise is associated with an increase of approximately 10% in the serum creatinine concentration. Cachectic patients, as the result of minimal muscle mass, will have very low serum creatinine concentrations, as do those with spinal cord injuries.[31] Elderly patients and those with poor nutrition may also have low serum creatinine concentrations (<1.0 mg/dL) secondary to decreased muscle mass. Other factors that influence the serum creatinine concentration include the dietary intake of creatine. During the cooking of meat, some creatine is converted to creatinine, which is rapidly absorbed following ingestion. Serum creatinine concentrations may rise as much as 50% within 2 hours of a meat meal and remain elevated for as long as 8 to 24 hours.[30] Ingestion of creatine as an ergogenic dietary supplement is currently popular. There are conflicting reports on the effect of creatine ingestion on the serum creatinine concentration. Poortsmans et al.[32] evaluated a short-term regimen of 20 g creatine per day for 5 days in healthy subjects, and reported no significant change in the serum creatinine, creatinine excretion rate, or creatinine clearance. Robinson et al.,[33] however, reported a 25% to 40% increase in the serum creatinine concentration after ingestion of 20 g creatine per day for either 5 days or 8 weeks. The renal excretion rate of creatinine was not measured. The issue of whether creatine ingestion adversely affects kidney function was studied by Edmonds et al.[34] They noted that creatine supplementation led to an increase in renal disease progression in a rat model for renal cystic disease, suggesting that creatine supplementation may be a risk factor in patients with preexisting renal disease. These conditions present a problem only when a single serum creatinine concentration is used to represent the entire 24-hour collection period, which is usually the case. An alternative is to obtain multiple samples and calculate the area under the serum concentration time curve and divide this by the collection time interval to obtain the average plasma creatinine concentration. This is rarely done in clinical practice, but points out the need to question patients regarding dietary intake for the 24 hours preceding the measurement of CLcr.

Diurnal variation in serum creatinine concentration may also affect the accuracy of the CLcr determination. Although the fluctuation is minimal, the observed peak plasma creatinine concentration generally occurs at approximately 7:00 PM, whereas the nadir is in the morning. To minimize this effect, the CLcr is usually performed over a 24-hour period with the plasma creatinine obtained in the morning, as long as the patient has stable kidney function. Collection of urine remains a limiting factor in the 24-hour CLcr because of incomplete collections, and interconversion between creatinine and creatine that can occur if the urine is not maintained at a pH < 6.

URINALYSIS

Examination of the urine includes assessment of its chemical and physical composition, most of which can be completed with dipstick testing.

pH

The normal urine pH typically ranges from 4.5 to 7.8, and an elevation above this may suggest the presence of urea-splitting bacteria.[23]

Specific Gravity

The measure of urine weight relative to water (1.00) is its specific gravity and is dependent on water intake and urine-concentrating ability. Normal values range from 1.003 to 1.030. Osmolality, which is a measure of the number of solute particles, is a more accurate measure of the kidney's ability to make a concentrated urine. Generally the two values are correlated; however, when large quantities of heavier molecules such as glucose are in the urine, the specific gravity may be elevated relative to the osmolality. These values are used in the assessment of urine concentrating ability and are most informative when interpreted along with the hydration status of the patient and plasma osmolality.[23]

Glucose

Glucose is normally absent in the urine, because the kidney normally completely reabsorbs all the glucose filtered at the glomerulus. In patients with plasma glucose concentrations that exceed the maximum threshold for glucose reabsorption (~180 mg/dL), glucosuria will be present. In the past, patients with diabetes mellitus would use the urine glucose level as a guide to insulin therapy. However, fingerstick methods for direct blood glucose measurements have now replaced the urine tests as a guide to therapy in most clinical settings.[35] Urine glucose testing still remains a valuable tool for the detection of diabetes.

Ketones

Acetoacetate and acetone are excreted in patients with diabetic ketoacidosis. They are also produced under conditions of fasting or starvation.

Nitrite

Nitrite is formed by conversion from nitrate by urinary bacteria. The presence of nitrite may indicate that the patient has a urinary tract infection.

Leukocyte Esterase

Leukocyte esterase is released from lysed granulocytes in the urine; its presence is suggestive of urinary tract infection. If the processing of the urine sample is delayed, a false-positive leukocyte esterase may be reported if the sample is contaminated.

Heme

The heme test indicates the presence of hemoglobin or myoglobin. A positive test without the presence of red blood cells suggests either red cell hemolysis or rhabdomyolysis.[23]

Protein

Protein excretion is normally minimal in healthy individuals (<150 mg/day). Albumin is not significantly filtered because of its size (69 kDa) and anionic character, which results in it being repelled by the negatively charged proteins of the glomerular capillary wall. Albumin excretion is thus usually <30 mg/day in individuals without kidney disease. Smaller proteins, such as β_2-microglobulin, pass through the glomerulus but are reabsorbed in the proximal tubule. Tests for urinary protein include acid precipitation with sulfosalicylic acid, and several dipstick methods. The sulfosalicylic test provides an assessment of total protein in the urine and is performed by the addition of sulfosalicylic acid to urine supernatant in a 1:3 ratio. The resulting turbidity is a semiquantitative approach to estimate the degree of proteinuria. Most dipstick methods that detect protein are not specific for albumin, and, therefore, specific tests were developed for the detection of microalbuminuria, 30–300 mg/day.[36] Measurement of the urine albumin concentration alone is not sufficient, as dilute urine will underestimate excretion, and a concentrated urine overestimate excretion. The 24-hour urine collection and measurement of albumin excretion will avoid these errors, but requires patient compliance for the urine collection. An estimate of daily protein excretion can be made from the ratio of albumin (mg):creatinine (g) in a spot urine from a first-morning collection.[37,38] Because the creatinine production per day is constant in those with stable kidney function, an increased ratio indicates increased albumin excretion. The normal ratio is <30 mg albumin/g creatinine in the urine. Because the ratio is dependent on both the albumin and creatinine concentration, there is an increased variability in the result. Values between 30 and 300 mg/g creatinine are considered to be in the microalbuminuria range.[39] Positive test results should be repeated, particularly in patients without an underlying cause for renal disease, such as diabetes or hypertension. Ruggenenti et al.[40] observed a positive correlation between the degree of proteinuria (using the spot morning protein:creatinine ratio) and rate of progression of renal disease in patients with nondiabetic chronic renal disease.

Formed elements that may be detected in the urine include erythrocytes and leukocytes, casts, and crystals. An important consideration in the assessment of hematuria is whether the cells are of renal origin. More than two cells per high-power field is abnormal, and dysmorphic cells suggest renal parenchymal origin either because of damage as they pass through the glomerulus or during exposure to the varying osmotic environment of the tubular lumen. White blood cells may be present in the urine in association with infection or inflammatory conditions, such as interstitial nephritis. More than one cell per high-power field may be considered abnormal. For both red and white cells, contamination of the sample should also be considered such as during menses, or with inadequate sample collection. Casts are cylindrical forms composed of protein, with or without cells that take the shape of the collecting tubules, where they are formed. Casts without cells are labeled hyaline casts and consist of the Tamm-Horsfall mucoprotein, secreted by the renal tubules. They are nonspecific and may appear in concentrated urine. In the presence of red or white blood cells, casts may be formed that include the cells, indicating that the cells were of renal origin. Solubility of the Tamm-Horsfall protein is increased as urine pH rises; therefore, sample collection for casts should occur with the first morning void when the urine is most acidic. Otherwise, casts may dissolve and elude detection.[21,23]

A variety of crystals may be present in the urine, including uric acid, calcium oxalate, calcium phosphate, calcium magnesium ammonium pyrophosphate, and cystine. Many of these have a unique crystalline form, which permits them to be identified with microscopy.

PROCEDURES USED IN THE ASSESSMENT OF RENAL FUNCTION

The gold standard for the quantitative measure of kidney function is the GFR. Recent observations, however, suggest this measure is not truly reflective of renal functional capacity, because oral protein loading or an amino acid infusion also increases GFR.[17] As a result, inter- and intrasubject variability may limit its use as a longitudinal marker of renal function. Dietary protein intake has been demonstrated to correlate with GFR in healthy subjects. Brändle et al.[41] evaluated renal function in four groups of healthy volunteers, each ingesting a diet controlled for protein over a 4-month period. The GFR was nonlinearly related to the urine nitrogen excretion, with an observed maximum of 181.7 mL/min at a urinary nitrogen excretion rate of 20 g/day, or 125 g/day protein intake. Subjects who are vegetarian will have a low GFR because of reduced dietary protein intake. When challenged with a protein load, these same subjects are able to increase their GFR to the "normal" range.[17] The increased GFR following a protein load is the result of renal vasodilation accompanied by an increased renal plasma flow. The exact mechanism of the renal response to protein is not known, but may be related to extrarenal factors such as glucagon, prostaglandins, and angiotensin II, or intrarenal mechanisms, such as tubular transport and tubuloglomerular feedback.[42,43] Despite the evidence in support of the presence of a renal reserve, standardized evaluation techniques have not been developed; therefore, assessment of the standard GFR measurement technique must consider the dietary protein status of the patient at the time of the study.

MEASUREMENT OF RENAL PLASMA AND BLOOD FLOW

Renal plasma and blood flow are not common clinical measures of renal function but may provide insight into hemodynamic changes related to disease or drug therapy. The kidneys receive approximately 20% of cardiac output and representative values of renal blood flow in men and women of about 1,200 ± 250 and 1,000 ± 180 mL/min/1.73 m^2 have been reported, respectively.[44] Renal plasma flow (RPF) is estimated to be 60% of blood flow if it is assumed that the average hematocrit is 40% and that it can be measured by the use of model compounds that are eliminated from the plasma compartment on a single pass through the kidneys. Because only 20% of the plasma is filtered at the glomerulus, the compound must undergo active tubular secretion and minimal to no reabsorption to be completely eliminated. To accurately reflect RPF, the extraction through the kidney must be nearly 100%. PAH is an organic anion that has been used extensively for the quantitation of renal plasma flow. PAH is approximately 17% bound to plasma proteins and is eliminated extensively by active tubular secretion. Because PAH elimination is active, saturation of the transport processes should be anticipated, and concentrations of PAH in plasma should not exceed 10–20 mg/L.[44] Recently, Dowling et al.[45] used a sequential infusion technique and observed concentration-dependent renal clearance of PAH at concentrations above 100 mg/dL. Furthermore, PAH is also metabolized, possibly within the kidney, to *N*-acetyl-PAH, and it is important for the analytical method to differentiate the parent compound and metabolite.[46] Prescott et al.[47] noted that the renal clearance of PAH alone decreases at low plasma concentrations, while the clearance of the acetyl metabolite increases. Further studies are necessary to evaluate the mechanisms and significance of these findings. The extraction ratio (ER) for PAH is 70% to 90% at plasma concentrations of 10–20 mg/L, hence the term "effective" renal plasma flow (ERPF) has been used when the clearance of PAH is not corrected for the extraction ratio or if it is assumed to be 1.[7] Normal values are about 650 ± 160 mL/min for men and 600 ± 150 mL/min for women.[44] Children will reach normalized adult values by 3 years of age, and ERPF will begin to decline as a function of age after 30 years, reaching about one-half of its peak value by 90 years of age. The method for calculation of ERPF is based on the relationship between organ clearance, extraction ratio (ER), and flow:

$$\text{ERPF} = \text{renal PAH CL} = \text{RPF} \times \text{ER}$$

ERBF can be estimated from ERPF by assuming the extraction ratio is 1 and correcting for the red blood cell volume of the blood (hematocrit, Hct):

$$\text{ERBF} = \text{ERPF}/(1 - \text{Hct})$$

ERPF can also be measured using the radioisotopes ^{131}I-orthoiodohippurate or ^{99m}Tc-mercaptoacetyltriglycine (^{131}I-OIH or ^{99m}Tc-MAG3).[48] One important advantage of this method is its ability to measure ERPF in total or for each kidney independently, as well as its ability to produce renal images. Russell and Dubovsky,[49] using a single-injection technique, compared clearance methods with and without urine collection and showed similar results with each method.

MEASUREMENT OF GLOMERULAR FILTRATION RATE

Normally there are approximately 1 million nephrons per kidney, and each nephron filters independently. The net effect—total GFR—is a representation of the functional renal mass and the factors discussed above. As renal mass declines because of normal physiologic loss of nephrons secondary to the aging process, or because of disease, there is a progressive decline in GFR. Thus, the total GFR represents the functional status of the kidneys.

GFR is expressed as the volume of plasma filtered across the glomerulus per unit time. If the normal RBF were approximately 1.0 L/min, plasma volume was 60% of blood volume, and filtration fraction across the glomerulus was 20%, then the normal GFR is approximately 120 mL/min/1.73 m^2.

Accurate measurement of the GFR requires a compound that has unrestricted diffusion across the glomerulus and into Bowman's capsule without additional clearance by tubular secretion or reduction by reabsorption. Furthermore, renal tubular cells should not metabolize the solute, nor should the solute alter renal function. Given these conditions, the GFR is equivalent to the renal clearance of the solute marker:

$$\text{GFR} = \text{renal CL} = (A_e)/\text{AUC}_{0-t}$$

where renal CL is renal clearance of the marker, A_e is the amount of marker excreted in a specified period of time, t, and AUC_{0-t} is the area under the plasma concentration time curve of the marker.

Under steady-state conditions, the expression simplifies to:

$$\text{GFR} = \text{renal CL} = (A_e)/[(C_{ss}) \times t]$$

where C_{ss} is the steady-state plasma concentration of the marker.

TABLE 42–3. Sensitivity and Clinical Utility of Renal Function Tests

	Accuracy	Clinical Utility	Cost
Inulin clearance	++++	+	$$$$
Radiolabeled markers	+++	+	$$$
Nonisotopic contrast agents	+++	++	$$$
Creatinine clearance	++	+++	$$
Serum creatinine	+	++++	$

+ = least acceptable; ++ = Adequate; +++ = better; ++++ = best.

Several solutes have been used for the measurement of GFR and include both exogenous and endogenous compounds. Those administered as exogenous agents, such as inulin, iothalamate, iohexol, and radioisotopes, require specialized administration techniques and detection methods for the quantitation of function, but generally provide a more accurate measure of GFR. Methods that employ endogenous compounds, such as creatinine, require less-technical expertise, but produce results with greater variability.[25] The marker of choice depends on the purpose and cost of the test; research protocols will generally use a more accurate test than one used in the clinical setting (Table 42–3).

INULIN CLEARANCE

Inulin is a relatively large molecule (5200 daltons) and has the necessary characteristics to serve as a marker for the measurement of GFR. Inulin is a fructose polysaccharide, obtained from plant tubers of the Jerusalem artichoke, dahlia, and chicory plants. It is not bound to plasma proteins, is freely filtered at the glomerulus, is not secreted or reabsorbed, and is not metabolized by the kidney.[25] The volume of distribution of inulin approximates extracellular volume, or 20% of ideal body weight. Because it is eliminated by glomerular filtration, its elimination half-life is dependent on renal function and is approximately 1.3 hours in subjects with normal renal function. For a subject with a GFR of 10 mL/min, the elimination half-life increases to approximately 16 hours. Therefore, a loading dose is essential when using the steady-state continuous infusion approach for measurement of GFR.

The most common technique for determination of GFR with inulin involves intravenous bolus administration followed by a continuous infusion of inulin. The infusion dose must be adjusted in patients with diminished renal function due to the dependence of inulin elimination on GFR. A typical loading dose of 40 mg/kg is administered, followed by a maintenance infusion of 25 mg/min/1.73 m^2 × RF, where RF is the estimated fraction of normal renal function. For such situations, the maintenance infusion is reduced by the fraction of expected GFR based on an estimate of the patient's creatinine clearance. Following a 60-minute equilibration period, sequential measurements of inulin clearance are made over a period of 30 minutes for 3 intervals. Urine is collected, and blood samples bracket each collection period. It is necessary to maintain adequate hydration during the test because GFR is dependent on renal blood flow (RBF) and it assures adequate urine output during the procedure. A relatively constant urine flow will decrease the variability among repeated measurements and should be within the range of 1–10 mL/min. An initial water load of 10–15 mL/kg body weight will usually initiate a diuresis, and additional water equal to the urine output of each interval should be given orally or intravenously to maintain urinary output. It is essential to ensure complete bladder emptying to minimize variability of results. Alternative clearance methods should be employed for patients unable to meet this requirement due to existing conditions (e.g., benign prostatic hypertrophy, neurogenic bladder).

Inulin plasma clearance has been measured following a single-dose intravenous injection with multiple sampling of blood to estimate area under the curve ($AUC_{0-\infty}$). Clearance in this situation was calculated as: CL = Dose/AUC. Continuous infusion of inulin following a bolus injection without urine collection can also provide an assessment of plasma clearance: CL = Infusion rate/C_{ss}. Four or more hours are needed to achieve steady state, and then the results are similar to those obtained using the traditional urine-collection method. Florijn et al.[50] compared the infusion and bolus techniques for both plasma and renal clearance in 14 patients with autosomal-dominant polycystic kidney disease. Variability was lower using plasma clearance and the bolus technique (coefficient of variation of 7.1 ± 3.1% vs 9.7 ± 5.4%), but it overestimated the renal clearance (82.0 ± 30.5 vs 68.3 ± 27.6 mL/min/1.73 m^2). Similar observations were evident for the constant infusion method. The authors provide a regression equation to account for the overestimation; however, measurement of renal clearance precludes the need to introduce additional variability into the assessment of renal function. Orlando et al.[51] evaluated the performance of a single IV bolus injection of inulin in healthy subjects by comparison of plasma and renal clearance. Results were very similar, supporting the single-injection method with standard pharmacokinetic analysis.

Measurement of plasma and urine inulin concentrations can be performed using a colorimetric reaction to detect fructose following acid hydrolysis of inulin, or enzymatically.[52] Glucose cross-reacts with the colorimetric measurement; therefore, it is necessary to correct samples with a "blank" obtained prior to infusion of the inulin. Individuals with elevated plasma glucose concentrations that change during the evaluation will show increased variability in their results.[23] A high-performance liquid chromatographic (HPLC) method using reverse-phase and ultraviolet (UV) detection was recently described. Glucose and drugs commonly administered to patients with renal disease, including corticosteroids, calcitriol, azathioprine, nifedipine, and atenolol, did not interfere with the assay.[53]

Besides kidney function, variability in the inulin clearance can be attributed to body size; the results are less variable if clearance is normalized to body surface area. The normal range will decrease with increasing age, at a rate of approximately 10 mL/min/1.73 m^2 for each decade over 30 years. Gender and differences in renal function, caused by physiologic conditions and/or disease state, may also contribute to the observed variability in the test. Normal inulin clearance is approximately 120 mL/min/1.73 m^2, slightly higher for men and lower for women.

Sinistrin, another polyfructosan, is handled in the same fashion as inulin in humans. It is filtered at the glomerulus and not secreted or reabsorbed to any significant extent. It is a naturally occurring substance derived from the root of the North African vegetable red squill, *Urginea maritime*. Its primary difference from inulin is water solubility. Whereas inulin must be heated prior to administration, sinistrin is soluble at room temperature. Assay methods for sinistrin have been described using enzymatic procedures, as well as HPLC with electrochemical detection.[52,54,55]

IOTHALAMATE CLEARANCE

Alternatives have been sought for inulin as a marker for GFR because of the problems of intermittent availability, high cost, sample preparation, and assay variability. Iothalamate has been commonly used in radiocontrast studies, but is also available in an unlabeled form. This agent is handled in a manner similar to that of inulin. It appears to be freely filtered at the glomerulus and does not undergo substantial tubular secretion or reabsorption.[23] Iothalamate has most commonly been employed in its radiolabeled form, ^{125}I-iothalamate, but recently has been used as a nonisotopic probe. Plasma and urine iothalamate concentrations have been measured using HPLC methods and can be analyzed simultaneously with PAH.[46] Plasma iothalamate clearance has also been evaluated, and was shown to be linearly related to iothalamate renal clearance, but with a positive bias of approximately 10 mL/min. The corrected plasma clearance provided a good estimate of GFR.[56]

IOHEXOL

Iohexol, a nonionic, low osmolar, iodinated contrast agent, has also been used for the determination of GFR. It is eliminated almost entirely by glomerular filtration, and plasma and renal clearance values are similar.[57] Rocco et al.[58] compared iohexol plasma clearance with ^{125}I-iothalamate renal clearance and demonstrated a strong correlation ($r = 0.95$) between the two tests; CL iohexol = 0.90 CL iothalamate + 6.8 mL/min. The plasma iohexol assay was performed using a reverse-phase HPLC method. Lundqvist et al.[59] evaluated a single-sample plasma clearance calculation method using iohexol compared to ^{51}Cr-ethylenediaminetetraacetic acid (EDTA) and demonstrated similar results ($r = 0.918$). These data support iohexol as a suitable alternative marker for the measurement of GFR. Following iohexol administration, a single plasma sample can be used to quantify renal function, provided sufficient time has elapsed since injection in patients with a reduced GFR—more than 24 hours if GFR is less than 20 mL/min.[57] Iohexol has also been assessed for potential renal toxicity in a population of 100 patients, 63 of whom had renal insufficiency. There were no significant changes in renal function as assessed by the serum creatinine concentration and urine protein excretion for up to 1 week after the study.[60]

RADIOLABELED MARKERS

The GFR has also been quantified using radiolabeled markers, such as ^{125}I-iothalamate (614 daltons, radioactive half-life of 60 days), ^{99m}Tc-diethylenetriamine pentaacetic acid (DTPA, 393 daltons, radioactive half-life of 6.03 hours), and ^{51}Cr-EDTA (292 daltons, radioactive half-life of 27 days).[61] These relatively small molecules are minimally bound to plasma proteins and do not undergo tubular secretion or reabsorption to any significant degree. ^{125}I-iothalamate and ^{99m}Tc-DTPA are used in the United States, whereas ^{51}Cr-EDTA is used extensively in Europe. An advantage for the determination of radiolabeled GFR is the ability to determine the individual contribution to overall renal function of each kidney.[62] Various protocols exist for the administration of the marker and subsequent determination of GFR. These protocols center on the issue of plasma clearance versus renal clearance, the latter requiring collection of urine during the evaluation period. The primary concern is whether the marker is cleared solely by filtration in the kidneys, or whether there are other significant routes of elimination. Measurement of radioactivity in plasma samples coupled with standard pharmacokinetic approaches results in plasma clearance, which overestimates GFR if elimination occurs by other routes. The nonrenal clearance of these agents is low (3–8 mL/min), thus plasma clearance should be an acceptable technique except in patients with severe renal insufficiency, GFR < 30 mL/min. Indeed, Morton et al.[63] recently demonstrated that ^{99m}Tc-DTPA plasma clearance and ^{131}I-iothalamate renal clearance were highly correlated in patients with clearance values >20 mL/min: CL DTPA = 0.943 CL iothalamate + 1.12 mL/min ($r = 0.983$). DeSanto et al.[64] observed a better correlation of measured and predicted creatinine clearance to inulin than ^{99m}Tc-DTPA among 15 healthy subjects and 65 patients with renal disease.

CREATININE CLEARANCE

Despite the common use of CLcr to estimate GFR, it is a controversial measurement. Short-duration witnessed CLcr correlates with iothalamate clearance performed using the single-injection technique. In a multicenter study[65] of 136 patients with type I diabetic nephropathy, GFR was assessed using (a) duplicate serum creatinine and 24-hour urine collection, (b) the mean of four iothalamate clearance periods by single-injection technique during water diuresis, and (c) CLcr. CLcr was also estimated for each patient using the Cockcroft-Gault method,[66] corrected for weight and gender. The simultaneous iothalamate and CLcr were 78 ± 35 and 86 ± 35 mL/min, respectively, while the separate 24-hour CLcr was 75 ± 33 mL/min. The Cockcroft-Gault estimate was 79 ± 29 mL/min. Compared to CL iothalamate as the standard, the r^2 values for the simultaneous CLcr, 24-hour CLcr, and Cockcroft-Gault CLcr were 0.81, 0.49, and 0.67, respectively, indicating increased variability with the 24-hour clearance determination. It was not stated whether the 24-hour CLcr measurements were performed as inpatient or ambulatory procedures.[65] In a selected group of 110 patients, measurement of a 4-hour CLcr during water diuresis provided the best estimate of the GFR as determined by the CL iothalamate. Furthermore, the ratio of CLcr to CL iothalamate did not appear to increase as the GFR decreased. These data suggest that a short collection period with a water diuresis may be the best method for estimation of GFR by creatinine clearance.[65]

Creatinine is eliminated by both glomerular filtration and tubular secretion. Tubular secretion augments the filtered creatinine by about 10% in subjects with normal kidney function. If the nonspecific Jaffé reaction is used, which overestimates the serum creatinine concentration by about 10% because of the noncreatinine chromogens, then the creatinine clearance is a very good measure of GFR in patients with normal kidney function. Tubular secretion, however, increases to as much as 100% in patients with renal insufficiency.[24] As renal impairment develops, the remaining nephrons hypertrophy, and the degree of tubular secretion decreases disproportionately (less than) to the decrease in filtration. The result is an overestimation of creatinine clearance as a function of GFR assessed by using inulin clearance. Bauer et al.[24] assessed creatinine clearance as a function of inulin clearance in 123 subjects with various degrees of kidney function. Using a specific assay for the measurement of creatinine, the ratio of CLcr exceeded CL inulin by 14%, which suggested that 14% of the creatinine was eliminated by secretion. The CLcr to CL inulin ratio in subjects with mild impairment was 1.20; for moderate impairment, it was 1.87; and for severe impairment, it was 2.32. Thus, creatinine clearance is a poor indicator of GFR in patients with moderate to severe renal insufficiency.

Creatinine is secreted via the organic cationic pathway, which can be blocked by the coadministration of drugs that compete for the same secretory path, such as cimetidine and trimethoprim. Shemesh et al.[67] studied the effect of an infusion of cimetidine on the tubular secretion of creatinine. The ratio of CLcr to CL inulin was reduced from 1.67 ± 0.10 to 1.16 ± 0.06 within 80 minutes of the start of the cimetidine infusion with no effect on CL inulin. Roubenoff et al.[68] evaluated the potential role of oral cimetidine to improve the accuracy and precision of creatinine clearance as an indicator of GFR. Thirteen patients with lupus nephritis and 24 hour CLcr ranging from 24 to 115.3 mL/min were given 400 mg of cimetidine orally 4 times daily for 2 days before and during a 24-hour CLcr determination. A simultaneous 4-hour ^{99m}Tc-DTPA and CLcr were also determined. Cimetidine reduced the CLcr to CL DTPA ratio from 1.33 with placebo to 1.07 with cimetidine treatment ($P < .05$). No adverse effects were observed from the 2-day cimetidine treatment. Zaltzman et al.[69] administered cimetidine, 800 mg, as a single dose 1 hour prior to a 3-hour timed collection for creatinine and ^{125}I-iothalamate clearances (Table 42–4). The CLcr to CL iothalamate ratio was reduced from 1.53 ± 1.02 to 1.12 ± 0.02, and the authors suggest that this method effectively inhibited the tubular secretion of creatinine. Van Acker et al.[70] demonstrated similar results using multiple doses, although they noted a dose-dependency in the effect of cimetidine; subjects with higher renal cimetidine clearance required larger cimetidine doses for complete blockade of creatinine tubular secretion. A single oral dose of cimetidine, 800 mg, should provide adequate blockade of creatinine secretion to improve the use of the creatinine clearance measurement to estimate GFR. See Table 42–4 for the protocol used by Zaltzman et al.[69]

TABLE 42–4. Protocol for Cimetidine-modified Creatinine Clearance

1. Low-protein breakfast (0.2 g/kg) or fasting for morning test. Obtain height and weight.
2. 800 mg oral cimetidine with 1 L water. Void.
3. Allow 1 hour equilibration.
4. After 1 hour, complete void, ensure at least 3 mL/min (180 mL), replace urine volume with equal volume of water.
5. Begin 3-hour timed urine collection, replacing urine with water in equal volume.
6. Obtain midpoint (1.5 hour) serum creatinine.
7. Calculate timed creatinine clearance, CrCl = (Vol × U_{cr})/(S_{cr} × time). Correct for body surface area.

Derived from Ref. 69.

ESTIMATION OF CREATININE CLEARANCE

Several investigators have developed mathematical relationships between various patient factors as a means to estimate CLcr when urine is unavailable. These factors include age, gender, weight, and serum creatinine concentration. Perhaps the most widely used of these estimators is the one developed by Cockcroft and Gault (CG),[66] which identified age and body mass as factors which significantly improved the estimate of CLcr. Their relationship was based on observations of 249 male patients with stable kidney function whose 24-hour creatinine excretion was greater than 10 mg/kg, except for 23 patients who were included because their 24-hour urine volume was greater than 500 mL. Creatinine clearance ranged from 11 mL/min to normal. Creatinine production (P_{cr}, in mg/kg/day) and excretion significantly decreases with increasing age for males ($P_{cr} = 28 - [0.2 \times \text{Age}]$) and females ($P_{cr} = 0.8 \times P_{cr}$ males). Based on the usual CLcr formula and the relationship of creatinine excretion to age, they derived the following formula to estimate CLcr:

$$\text{CLcr (mL/min)} = [(140 - \text{Age}) \times \text{IBW}]/(S_{cr} \times 72)$$

where age is expressed in years, S_{cr} is the serum creatinine in mg/dL, and IBW is ideal body weight in kg. For females, the result is multiplied by 0.85.

Luke et al.[71] evaluated the ability of the CG method and four other methods to predict CLcr (see Table 42–5), with inulin clearance being considered the standard measure of GFR. Simultaneous inulin and creatinine clearances, and a 24-hour ambulatory CLcr were conducted in 109 patients. The simultaneously determined inulin

TABLE 42–5. Equations for the Estimation of Creatinine Clearance in Adults with Stable Renal Function

Cockroft and Gault[66]	Men: $CLcr = (140-Age)\ IBW/(S_{cr} \times 72)$ Women: $CLcr \times 0.85$
Jelliffe[73]	Men: $CLcr = (100/S_{cr}) - 12$ Women: $CLcr = (80/S_{cr}) - 7$
Jelliffe[74].	Men: $CLcr = 98 - [0.8\ (Age - 20)]/S_{cr}$ Women: $CLcr \times 0.9$
Mawer et al.[72]	Men: IBW $[29.3 - (0.203 \times Age)]$ $[1 - (0.03 \times S_{cr}]/(14.4 \times S_{cr})$ Women: IBW $[25.3 - (0.175 \times Age)]$ $[1 - (0.03 \times S_{cr})]/(14.4 \times S_{cr})$
Hull et al.[75]	Men: $CLcr = [(145 - Age)/S_{cr}] - 3$ Women: $Clcr \times 0.85$
Levey et al. (MDRD)[80]	$GFR = 170 \times (Scr)^{-0.999} \times [Age]^{-0.176} \times [0.762$ if patient is female$] \times [1.180$ if patient is black$] \times [SUN]^{-0.170} \times [Alb]^{0.318}$

CLcr = creatinine clearance in mL/min; IBW = ideal body weight (kg); Scr = serum or plasma creatinine (mg/dL); SUN = serum nitrogen concentration (mg/dL); Alb = serum albumin concentration (gm/dL).

and creatinine clearances correlated best, $r^2 = 0.85$, and the CLcr overestimated CL inulin by approximately 15% due to tubular secretion of creatinine. The correlation coefficient between CL inulin and 24-hour ambulatory CLcr was 0.71. For the five calculated clearances, CG and Mawer et al.[72] correlated the best with inulin clearance. The CG method showed a linear relationship with CL inulin equal to 1.121 of CLcr plus 20.6 mL/min ($r^2 = 0.66$), whereas for Mawer the relationship was CL inulin equal to 1.051 of CLcr plus 18.3 mL/min ($r^2 = 0.66$). The calculated CLcr values from CG and Mawer both appeared to correlate well with the ambulatory and 4-hour CLcr, but the regressions were not reported. Based on their findings, Luke et al.[71] propose continued use of the CG or Mawer method for rapid estimation of CLcr in patients with stable kidney function. The other methods, of Jelliffe[73,74] and of Hull et al.,[75] consistently underestimated the CLcr. As kidney function declined, there was an increase in the fraction of creatinine eliminated by secretion as measured by the CLcr to CL inulin ratio, consistent with earlier reports. This limitation should be taken into consideration when attempting to use CLcr for the estimation of renal function and the individualization of drug dosage regimens. Gault et al.[76] also evaluated the performance of the CG estimator of renal function compared with inulin and ^{99m}Tc-DTPA. Except for conditions of unstable kidney function, it performed similar to the 24-hour creatinine clearance method.

Patients undergoing screening for participation in the African American Study of Kidney Disease (AASK) were evaluated for kidney function based on an estimated CLcr compared with the simultaneous CLcr and ^{125}I-iothalamate, and 24-hour CLcr.[77] The simultaneous CLcr provided the best estimate of GFR. The CG method was the preferred method for estimation of GFR, based on performance and ease of use. This method was noted to underestimate the GFR by 9%, perhaps because of the increased excretion rate of creatinine by black patients.[77,78]

Administration of cimetidine has also resulted in improved performance of CG to predict GFR. Ixkes et al.[79] gave patients three 800-mg doses of cimetidine in 24 hours, and measured creatinine plasma levels from 3 to 7 hours following the final dose. During this 4-hour period, the CL iothalamate was determined as the measure of GFR. The CG calculations were performed with the plasma creatinine measurement 3 hours after the last dose of cimetidine. The ratio of the CG estimated CLcr to CL iothalamateCl ratio decreased from 1.28 ± 0.21 to 0.98 ± 0.11 in the presence of cimetidine.

Although the CG method has stood the test of time, Levey et al.[80] recently devised an improved method based on multiple regression analysis of variables in patients enrolled in the baseline period of the Modification of Diet in Renal Disease Study (MDRD):

$$GFR = 170 \times (P_{cr})^{-0.999} \times [Age]^{-0.176} \times [0.762 \text{ if patient is female}]$$
$$\times [1.180 \text{ if patient is black}] \times [SUN]^{-0.170} \times [Alb]^{0.318}$$

where P_{cr} = plasma creatinine, SUN = serum nitrogen concentration, and Alb = serum albumin concentration. Comparison of prediction equations showed that the new equation ($r^2 = 90.2\%$) provided a more precise estimate of GFR than measured CLcr ($r^2 = 86.6\%$) or the CG ($r^2 = 84.2\%$) equation. Although it is much more cumbersome, it has been recommend as the standard method for the estimation of GFR.

LIVER DISEASE

Renal function in patients with coexisting liver disease and renal impairment was recently reevaluated. Orlando et al.[81] evaluated 10 healthy subjects, 10 patients with mild liver disease, and 10 with severe liver disease, and observed a measured CLcr to CL inulin ratio of 1.05, 1.03, and 1.04 for each group, respectively. When the CLcr of patients with severe liver disease was estimated using the CG equation the resultant ratio (CLcr CG to CL inulin) was 1.23. Lam et al.[82] likewise noted an overprediction by CG of the measured CLcr in patients with severe disease, by 40% to 100%.

Studies of renal function in patients with severe hepatic disease confirm the earlier observations of Hull et al.[75] and Caregaro et al.[83] who reported that measured CLcr overestimated GFR by 50% in hepatic patients with a GFR of 56 ± 19 mL/min/1.73m^2 because of increased tubular secretion of creatinine. DeSanto et al.[84] studied 19 patients with mild liver disease whose inulin and creatinine clearances were 90 ± 4.4 and 122 ± 7 mL/min/1.73 m^2, respectively. The degree of overestimation of GFR by creatinine clearance was inversely correlated with GFR ($r = 0.452$, $P < .04$). Thus, measurement of renal function in patients with hepatic disease should be performed by using a method specific for glomerular filtration, not creatinine clearance.

OTHER SPECIAL POPULATIONS

Davis and Chandler[85] confirmed the accuracy of the CG equation to predict CLcr in trauma patients with stable kidney function, and Thakur and colleagues[31] demonstrated its successful utility in 42 paraplegic subjects. Renal transplant recipients are frequently monitored for renal function, as numerous complications may occur during the life of the allograft. Goerdt et al.[86] assessed the bias and precision with which several nomographic methods predicted GFR (iohexol clearance) in 127 patients with stable kidney function. The CG method performed poorly, overestimating iohexol clearance. This is expected, as iohexol clearance provides a true measure of GFR, whereas the CG CLcr estimate is falsely high because of the tubular secretion of creatinine. Schück et al.[87] compared the CG method with CL sinistrin, a true measure of GFR. The clearance of sinistrin was significantly overestimated by the CG method. These investigators noted significant variability in CG estimates of GFR and concluded that it was an unreliable predictor of GFR. Huang et al.[88] reported the inability of several CLcr equations to predict renal function in hospitalized patients with advanced HIV disease. All methods, including CG, Jelliffe, and Mawer, overestimated the measured 24-hour CLcr. The reasons for the poor predictability of these methods is unclear, although

TABLE 42–6. Equations for the Estimation of Creatinine Clearance in Adults With Unstable Renal Function

		Equations	
Reference	**Units**	***Males***	***Females***
Jelliffe and Jelliffe[90]	mL/min/1.73 m²	$E^{SS} = IBW\,[29.3 - 0.203\,(Age)]$ $E^{SS}_{corr} = E^{SS}\,[1.035 - 0.0337\,(Scr)]$ $E = E^{SS}_{corr} - \frac{[4\,IBW(Scr_2 - Scr_1)]}{\Delta t day}$ $CrCl = \frac{E}{14.4(Scr)}$	$E^{SS} = IBW\,[25.1 - 0.175\,(Age)]$ $E^{SS}_{corr} = E^{SS}[1.035 - 0.0337\,(Scr)]$ $E = E^{SS}_{corr} - \frac{[4\,IBW(Scr_2 - Scr_1)]}{\Delta t day}$ $CrCl = \frac{E}{14.4(Scr)}$
Chiou et al.[91]	mL/min	$V_d = 0.6\,L\,(IBW)$ $CrCl = \frac{2\,IBW\,[28 - 0.2(Age)]}{14.4(Scr_1 + Scr_2)} + \frac{2[V_d\,IBW(Scr_1 - Scr_2)]}{(Scr_1 + Scr_2)\Delta t min} - [CrCl^{NR} \times IBW]$	$V_d = 0.6L\,(IBW)$ $CrCl = \frac{2\,IBW\,[22.4 - 0.16\,(Age)]}{14.4(Scr_1 + Scr_2)} + \frac{2\,[V_d\,IBW(Scr_1 - Scr_2)]}{(Scr_1 + Scr_2)\Delta t min} - [CrCl^{NR} \times IBW]$
Brater[92]	mL/min/70 kg	$CrCl = \frac{[293 - 2.03(Age)] \times [1.035 - 0.01685(Scr_1 + Scr_2)]}{(Scr_1 + Scr_2)\Delta t day} + \frac{49(Scr_1 - Scr_2)}{(Scr_1 + Scr_2)\Delta t day}$	$CrCl = \text{Male value} \times 0.86$

E^{ss} = steady state urinary creatinine excretion, Δt day = time in days between Scr_1 and Scr_2; Δt min = time in minutes between Scr_1 and Scr_2; $CrCl^{NR}$ = nonrenal clearance of creatinine = 0.048 mL/min/kg.

24-hour collection methods result in increased variability, often because of inadequate collection of urine.

Renal function assessment during pregnancy is usually performed using a 24-hour creatinine clearance determination. Quadri and colleagues[89] evaluated the CG method during each trimester in 34 pregnant women and compared these estimates with the measured 24-hour CLcr. Prepregnancy weights were used throughout the study for the CG method, and results correlated well with those for the measured clearance ($r^2 = 0.76$). The maximal CLcr occurred during the second trimester for both methods.

UNSTABLE RENAL FUNCTION

Patients with unstable kidney function present a unique situation because the serum creatinine is changing and the rate of change must be considered in the estimation of CLcr. Table 42–6 lists several equations for estimating renal function under these conditions.[90–92] A change in the serum creatinine concentration of more than 20% over a period of 1 day is suggestive of unstable renal function. Factors previously discussed that may alter the serum creatinine concentration must be evaluated to avoid misinterpretation.

Data regarding which of these methods provide the most accurate estimation of CLcr are lacking. At best, these methods provide an awareness that renal function in patients with acute renal failure is generally markedly lower than one would estimate using steady state methods.

CYSTATIN C

A relatively new marker for renal function has been identified and evaluated in a growing number of populations for its utility as a tool to assess changes in GFR.[93–95] Cystatin C is a nonglycosylated 13.3-kDa basic protein of the cystatin superfamily of inhibitors of cysteine proteases. It is produced by all nucleated cells of the body and is present in stable concentrations, independent of gender, body mass, and acute inflammatory conditions, such as infection. It was initially recommended as a test of kidney function in 1985, on the basis of the fact that serum concentrations were significantly correlated with GFR as well as serum creatinine. Reference ranges of 0.70–1.38 mg/L in children over 1 year of age, and 0.54–1.21 mg/L in adults have been suggested.[95] The recent development of an automated immunoassay technique and validation that it is a more sensitive indicator of reduced renal function than creatinine suggest that cystatin C may have future clinical utility in the assessment of renal function.[94,95] Comparison of ^{125}I-iothalamate with serum creatinine and cystatin C showed that the serum creatinine began to increase when the GFR was 75 mL/min/1.73 m² as compared to 88 mL/min/1.73 m² for cystatin C.[93] Page et al.[96] reported increased concentrations in patients being treated for malignant disease that were independent of CLcr, and pediatric transplant recipients have also been reported to have elevated cystatin C concentrations independent of GFR.[97] These observations suggest that further evaluations of cystatin C in additional populations are necessary before it is accepted as a routine marker for renal function.

RENAL FUNCTION IN CHILDREN

Kidney function in the neonate is difficult to assess because of difficulty in urine and blood collection, the frequent presence of a nonsteady-state serum creatinine, and apparent disparity between development of glomerular and tubular function. Preterm infants demonstrate significantly reduced GFR prior to 34 weeks, which rapidly increases and becomes similar to term infants within the first week of life.[98] Evaluation of GFR in preterm infants on day 3 of life, using an inulin infusion, failed to identify a relationship between patient weight and GFR. Gestational age, which ranged from 23.4 to 36.9 weeks (mean 30.2 weeks), however, correlated with both GFR and reciprocal of serum creatinine. The inulin clearance increased from 0.67 to 0.85 mL/min in those with gestational age <28 weeks versus those of 32 to 37 weeks of age, while S_{cr} decreased from 1.05 to 0.73 mg/dL, respectively. Creatinine was measured using a specific enzymatic method to avoid interference from bilirubin or drugs.[99] Creatinine clearance has also been evaluated in infants less than 1 week of age, and values of 17.8 mL/min/1.73 m² on day 1 increased to 36.4 mL/min/1.73 m² by day 6.[100] In light of these rapid changes in GFR, estimation of GFR is not recommended for infants less than 1 week of age. Kidney function expressed as GFR standardized to body surface area increases with age and stabilizes at approximately 1 year. In older children, GFR is best assessed using standard measurement techniques for GFR. Subcutaneous administration of ^{125}I-iothalamate has been effectively used to measure GFR in children ranging in age from 1 to 20 years.[101]

Estimation of CLcr as described by Schwartz et al.[102] is dependent on the child's age and length:

$$GFR = [\text{length (cm)} \times k]/S_{cr}$$

where k is defined by age group: infant (1 to 52 weeks) = 0.45; child (1 to 13 years) = 0.55; adolescent male = 0.7; and adolescent female = 0.55.

Subsequent studies verified these relationships in children with normal renal function or mild renal impairment. However, variability increases at clearance values <50 mL/min. Al-Harbi and Lireman[103] reported a good correlation of the predicted CLcr with measured 4-hour CLcr and ^{99m}Tc-DTPA ($r = 0.75$) in 48 pediatric renal allograft recipients, aged 3 to 19 years. However, predictive performance measures of bias and precision were not reported. Fong et al.[104] evaluated the method in critically ill children (mean age 5.6 years, range 0.1 to 20.8 years), and concluded that the method significantly overestimated the measured CLcr (bias = 45%). Dose adjustments and other therapeutic decisions based on kidney function warrant appropriate measures of renal status to avoid incorrect decisions. The results of these investigations suggest that further studies will be needed to clarify the value of these predictive methods.

RENAL FUNCTION IN THE ELDERLY

Cross-sectional studies demonstrate decreased GFR as a function of age when GFR is measured as inulin, iothalamate, or creatinine clearance.[66,105] The Baltimore Longitudinal Study on Aging,[106] an evaluation of 254 normal healthy subjects, revealed that creatinine clearance decreases at the rate of approximately 0.75 mL/min/1.73 m^2/y beginning at the fourth decade of life. These subjects were evaluated prospectively for up to 23 years. Interestingly, approximately one-third of the subjects showed no change in renal function from their baseline value, and a small number showed an increased clearance. These changes may be due to normal physiologic changes or to subclinical insults to the kidneys initiating the events leading to chronic progressive loss of renal function. Fliser et al.[107] studied renal functional reserve in healthy young (23 to 32 years) and elderly (61 to 82 years) volunteers using an amino acid infusion technique. Inulin clearance was used as the measure of GFR, which increased 16% in young and 17% in elderly subjects following the infusion. Renal functional reserve thus appears to be maintained in healthy elderly individuals.

Interpretation of the serum creatinine concentration alone is difficult in the elderly patient because of the decreased muscle mass and resultant lower production rate of creatinine. Thus, the serum creatinine often remains within the normal range despite a reduction in the number of functional nephrons. As renal function declines, the kidneys excrete a larger fraction of creatinine. This perpetuates the "normal" serum creatinine. The CG[66] formula can be used to estimate the CLcr of elderly patients. Smythe et al.[108] estimated CLcr in 23 patients >60 years of age using 7 different methods, and compared the results to a measured 24-hour CLcr determination. Estimations were performed with the actual serum creatinine concentration and also with the serum creatinine rounded up to 1.0 mg/dL if the actual value was <1.0 mg/dL. Rounding the serum creatinine to 1.0 mg/dL resulted in a significantly lower (bias = 28.8 mL/min) estimate of GFR, as compared with the actual clearance, than when the unadjusted serum creatinine (bias = 2.3 mL/min) was used. These data strongly suggest that one should not arbitrarily fix the serum creatinine concentration in elderly patients at 1.0 mg/dL. An alternative to the estimation of GFR or a 24-hour clearance determination is a 4-hour clearance performed during water diuresis.[65] This correlated with the inulin clearance as well as an inpatient 24-hour CLcr. However, one must be aware of the potential risk of hyponatremia in the geriatric patient who is unable to tolerate an oral water load, as well as the need for complete bladder emptying to ensure accurate results. O'Connell et al.[109] assessed the accuracy of 2- and 8-hour urine collections compared with 24-hour creatinine clearance determinations in 45 hospitalized patients >65 years old with indwelling urethral catheters. Single, timed urine collections for CLcr showed minimal bias with the 8-hour collection as compared with the 24-hour value, whereas the 2-hour determination was both biased and imprecise. Unfortunately, urinary residual was not determined, the bladder was not rinsed at each collection period, and the mean urine flow was low at 1.23 mL/min; all of these factors may have negatively affected the results of the 2-hour collection.

ASSESSMENT OF PROGRESSION

Chronic progressive kidney disease (see Chap. 44) will eventually lead to ESRD (see Chap. 45), necessitating dialysis or transplantation for survival (see Chaps. 46 and 47). Attempts to slow the rate of progression through dietary modification and blood pressure control, ACE inhibitor or ARB therapy, and improved glucose control in patients with type I diabetes mellitus recently proved successful. These therapeutic interventions can now successfully reduce the rate of renal disease progression and perhaps ultimately decrease the incidence of ESRD. Specific therapies and their effectiveness are discussed in detail in Chap. 44. The efficacy of these and future potential interventions is optimally assessed with regular measurement of accurate and sensitive indices of GFR such as iohexol, iothalamate, or radioisotope clearances.[110] When these are not available, alternative measures, such as reciprocal creatinine ($1/S_{cr}$), should be considered.

A linear decline in the reciprocal of the serum creatinine concentration as a function of time has been used as a simple technique to evaluate the rate of progression of renal disease and to predict the time when dialysis is necessary.[23] Fundamentally, the serum creatinine concentration is a function of input from the breakdown of creatine derived from muscle or dietary sources and its elimination, predominantly through glomerular filtration and tubular secretion. Under steady-state conditions, the formation rate of creatinine equals the elimination rate (R), and CLcr is inversely related to S_{cr} as:

$$S_{cr} = R/CLcr$$

The reciprocal relationship between S_{cr} and CLcr is then expressed as:

$$1/S_{cr} = 1/R \times CLcr$$

Figure 42–3A depicts the reciprocal relationship between S_{cr} and CLcr. As renal function declines, the reciprocal of the serum creatinine concentration decreases as a linear function of the CLcr, and the slope of the relationship is the reciprocal of the elimination rate of creatinine. Under conditions of progressively decreasing kidney function, this relationship assumes that filtration clearance and secretion clearance decrease proportionately, as well as any nonrenal elimination of creatinine. In addition, the rate of input is assumed constant. Based on these assumptions, clinicians can use the reciprocal serum creatinine plotted as a function of time as a prognostic tool, to predict

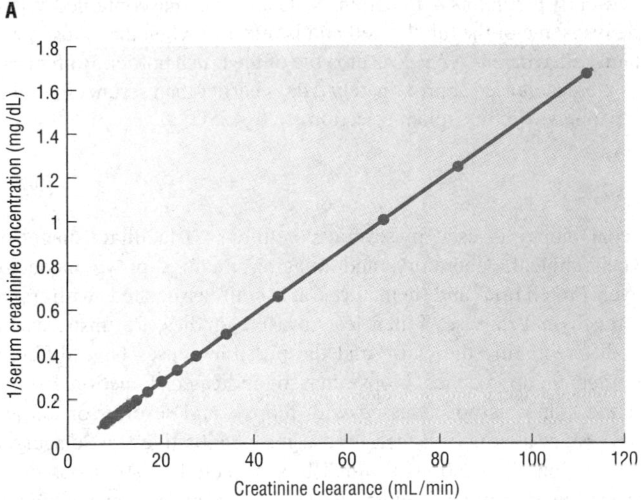

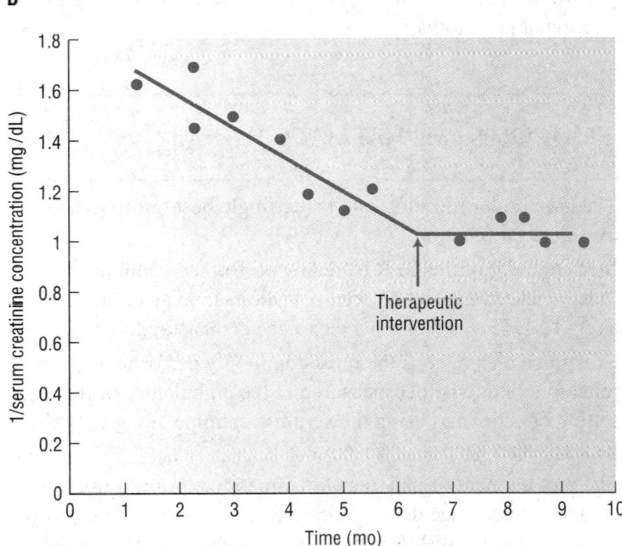

FIGURE 42–3. Linear relationship between 1/serum creatinine concentration and creatinine clearance (A) and 1/serum creatinine concentration as a function of time in a hypothetical patient with progressive renal impairment (B). The arrow indicates a change in the rate of progression, which may be related to a therapeutic intervention.

when dialysis may be needed (when $1/S_{cr} \sim 0.1$) or as a marker for evaluating the success of therapeutic interventions to alter the rate of decline in renal function (Fig. 42–3B). If these assumptions change over time, then the slope of the relationship will also change. Several factors, such as changes in dietary intake of creatinine and decreased muscle mass, which are associated with a reduction in the production of creatinine, may alter the utility of the relationship. Furthermore, if tubular secretion increases in response to nephron hypertrophy or disproportionately to filtration, or if nonrenal routes of elimination of creatinine, such as metabolism by intestinal bacteria, become more important, then changes in the slope of the reciprocal creatinine versus time relationship may be altered. It is most important to be aware of the limitations of serum creatinine measurement and to realize that it is not an adequate test to detect early chronic renal disease or to precisely estimate the disease's rate of progression.

Although not a quantitative measure of renal function, urinary microalbuminuria has been identified as an early marker of renal disease in patients with diabetic nephropathy[111] and numerous other conditions, such as hypertension and obesity.[20,112,113] Patients with microalbuminuria (30–300 mg/d) on at least two or three occasions or overt albuminuria (>300 mg/d) should begin to receive pharmacotherapy. For children, microalbuminuria is considered present if albumin excretion exceeds 0.36 mg/kg/day, and overt albuminuria has been defined as an excretion rate that exceeds 4 mg/kg/day. The urinary albumin to creatinine ratio is also an accurate predictor of 24-hour proteinuria, a marker of renal disease. Guidelines for monitoring indicate that a urine albumin to creatinine ratio of >30 mg/g places the patient at increased risk of developing diabetic nephropathy and is an indication for the initiation of pharmacotherapeutic intervention.[39] Microalbuminuria has also been suggested as a risk factor for renal dysfunction among patients with essential hypertension.[114]

PROCEDURES USED IN THE DIAGNOSIS OF ANATOMIC ABNORMALITIES

RADIOLOGIC STUDIES

Assessment of kidney structure may be accomplished by using several techniques. The standard x-ray of the kidneys, ureters, and bladder (KUB) is useful for a gross estimate of kidney size and the presence of calcifications.[61] Although an easy test to perform, the useful information achieved is minimal, and more detailed evaluations are often necessary. The intravenous urogram (IVU; formerly known as intravenous pyelogram, or IVP) involves the use of a contrast agent to facilitate visualization of the urinary collecting system. It is primarily used in the assessment of structural changes that may be associated with nonglomerular hematuria, pyuria, or flank pain, resulting from recurrent urinary tract infections, obstruction, or stone formation.[61] For patients with insufficient renal filtration, retrograde administration of dye into the ureters may be performed to facilitate visualization of the collecting system. Furthermore, local administration may avoid systemic exposure and associated adverse reactions (see Chap. 48). Contrast agents are also employed during renal angiography for the assessment of renovascular disease. As a test for the diagnosis of renovascular hypertension, the captopril (ACE inhibitor) test is a useful adjunct. Under conditions of unilateral renal artery stenosis, the affected kidney produces large quantities of angiotensin II, which vasoconstricts the efferent arteriole to maintain GFR. The administration of an ACE inhibitor results in reduced uptake of the contrast agent because perfusion of the affected kidney decreases. This occurs as a result of decreased efferent arteriolar vasoconstriction. For patients with bilateral disease, a decrease in uptake is observed in both kidneys.[115]

Ultrasound uses sound waves to generate a two-dimensional image. The echogenicity of the kidney is compared with that of an adjacent organ—liver on the right and spleen on the left—with an increased echogenicity indicating an abnormal finding. Ultrasonography can distinguish the renal pyramids, medulla, and cortex, and abnormalities in structure, such as occurs with obstruction. Renal ultrasound is also used as a guide for site localization during percutaneous kidney biopsy.

Computerized tomography (CT) is a cross-sectional anatomic imaging procedure based on x-ray data. The procedure is frequently performed with contrast to enhance imaging. Spiral, or helical, CT, a more recent technique, provides for three-dimensional reconstruction of tissues. CT is performed as a test for the evaluation of obstructive uropathy, malignancy, and infections of the kidney.

Magnetic resonance imaging (MRI) is based on aligning hydrogen nuclei in the body with the use of a powerful magnet and applying radiofrequency pulses. The signals emitted by the hydrogen nuclei during realignment on repeated pulses allows for generation of the tissue image. Realignment times can also be altered with the use of contrast agents (gadolinium, gadopentetate), leading to increased signal intensity and improved imaging. MRI is useful for the assessment of obstruction, malignancy, and renovascular lesions. The relative advantages and limitations of these procedures are discussed in more detail in several recent reviews.[61,116,117]

SPECIAL PROCEDURES IN THE DIAGNOSIS OF RENAL DYSFUNCTION

MEASUREMENT OF TUBULAR FUNCTION

Although GFR is perhaps the best overall indicator of renal function, it may not be reflective of tubular function, either secretory capacity or cellular function.[118] Tubular secretory function can be assessed by measuring PAH transport as the prototype marker of the organic anion secretory system. *N*-1-Methylnicotinamide (NMN) and TEA are prototype compounds secreted by the cationic transport system and may be used as markers of cationic secretory capacity.[7,119] Edwards et al.[120] demonstrated delayed recovery of NMN clearance among patients with psoriasis treated with low-dose cyclosporine, as compared with the recovery of GFR and renal blood flow. Earlier studies with NMN suggested its use to assess the effects of selected renal diseases on drug handling by the kidneys.[121] Dowling et al.[45] explored the utility of famotidine as a marker for cationic transport, but was unable to demonstrate saturation, perhaps because of other elimination pathways. It should be recognized that these transport systems are not necessarily mutually exclusive. Indeed, probenecid, which is secreted by the anionic pathway, inhibits the secretion of cationic compounds. Quantitative measures of tubular transport capacity are currently limited primarily to the research setting.

Other measures of tubular function are less specific and are regarded primarily as indices of damage within the nephron.[122] Schentag and Plaut[118] demonstrated a delay in the increase of serum creatinine following aminoglycoside toxicity when compared to markers for tubular damage such as the low-molecular-weight protein β_2-microglobulin (11.8 kDa) and urinary enzymes. The rise in β_2-microglobulin is related to an early functional defect in the proximal tubular cell. This is followed by a rise in the excretion of enzymes released as a result of structural damage of the cells, and, finally, by the formation and excretion of cellular casts. Other low-molecular-weight proteins used as markers of tubular function include retinol-binding protein (21 kDa) and protein HC (also known as α_1-microglobulin, 27 kDa).[122] These proteins are normally freely filtered at the glomerulus and then completely reabsorbed by the proximal tubule. Increases in their excretion are thus suggestive of tubular dysfunction but are not diagnostic, as an increased production rate or GFR of less than 30 mL/min may lead to increased excretion. In both cases, the maximal reabsorptive capacity may be exceeded, leading to net excretion of the protein. Retinol-binding protein and protein HC are elevated with tubular damage and may be more appropriate markers than β_2-microglobulin.

Numerous urinary enzymes such as *N*-acetylglucosaminidase (NAG); alanine aminopeptidase (AAP); alkaline phosphatase (AP); γ-glutamyltransferase (GGT); pyruvate kinase; glutathione transferase; lysozyme; and pancreatic ribonuclease have been used as diagnostic markers for renal disease. Jung et al.[123] compared the ability of five enzymes (NAG, AAP, AP, GGT, and lysozyme) to detect early rejection episodes in kidney transplant patients. Only NAG and AAP were early predictors of rejection. NAG is an enzyme contained within the lysosome of the tubular cell and is released when the lysosome is damaged, whereas AAP is an enzyme of the brush border. Both markers were increased approximately 2 days earlier than serum creatinine in patients with transplant rejection.

BIOPSY

Renal biopsy is used in several conditions to facilitate diagnosis when clinical, laboratory, and imaging findings prove inconclusive. Proteinuria and hematuria are both associated with renal parenchymal disease. When less-invasive studies are unsuccessful in differentiating the cause and the possible causes have different therapeutic approaches, biopsy may be indicated. Functional status of the kidney is not assessed with biopsy, and severity of disease and progression is best measured using quantitative tests discussed above. Contraindications to renal biopsy include a solitary kidney, severe hypertension, bleeding disorder, severe anemia, cystic kidney, and hydronephrosis, among others. Complications resulting from biopsy primarily include hematuria, which may last for several days, and perirenal hematoma.[23]

▶ PRINCIPLES OF PHARMACOTHERAPY

- The glomerular filtration rate is the single best test to assess overall renal function.
- Measurement of the GFR is ideally performed using inulin or iothalamate as the test marker, or radioisotope techniques such as ^{99m}Tc-DTPA, when renal clearance is measured.
- Creatinine clearance is the most commonly performed test of renal function, whether measured in the ambulatory or inpatient setting or estimated using the serum creatinine along with the patient's age, gender, and weight.
- The pretreatment of patients with cimetidine prior to the creatinine clearance determination enhances the accuracy of this estimate of true GFR, especially in patients with severe renal dysfunction.
- Caution should be exercised when interpreting the serum creatinine concentration as the sole measure of kidney function. Consideration should be given to patient age, lean body mass, gender, diet, concomitant diseases and drug therapy, circadian rhythm, stability of kidney function, tubular secretion, and analytic method.
- Evaluation of the reciprocal serum creatinine over time is not an acceptable alternative to the measurement of GFR for the assessment of the rate of kidney disease progression. Its use in clinical practice should be limited to those settings where more specific methods are unavailable.
- Non-GFR measures of renal function assessment, including urinalysis, x-ray, CT, MRI, sonography, and biopsy, provide a diagnostic or qualitative assessment of kidney function.

REFERENCES

1. Campens D, Buntinx F. Selecting the best renal function tests. Int J Technol Assess Health Care 1997;13:343–356.
2. Alvestrand A. Carbohydrate and insulin metabolism in renal failure. Kidney Int Suppl 1997;62:S48–S52.

3. Gonzalez EA, Martin KJ. Renal osteodystrophy: Pathogenesis and management. Nephrol Dial Transplant 1995;10(suppl 3):13–21.
4. Elston AC, Bayliss MK, Park GR. Effect of renal failure on drug metabolism by the liver. Br J Anaesth 1993;71:282–290.
5. Meffin PJ, Zilm DM, Veenendaal JR. Reduced clofibric acid clearance in renal dysfunction is due to a futile cycle. J Pharmacol Exp Ther 1983;227:732–738.
6. Verbeeck RK, Wallace SM, Loewen GR. Reduced elimination of ketoprofen in the elderly is not necessarily due to impairment of glucuronidation. Br J Clin Pharmacol 1984;17:783–784.
7. Sica DA, Schoolwerth AC. Renal handling of organic anions and cations: Excretion of uric acid. In: Brenner BM, ed. Brenner and Rector's The Kidney, 6th ed. Philadelphia, W.B. Saunders, 2000:680–700.
8. Hsyu PH, Gisclon LG, Hui AC, Giacomini KM. Interactions of organic anions with the organic cation transporter in renal BBMV. Am J Physiol 1988;254:F56–F61.
9. Bendayan R. Renal drug transport: A review. Pharmacotherapy 1996; 16:971–985.
10. Sikic BI. Pharmacologic approaches to reversing multidrug resistance. Semin Hematol 1997;34:40–47.
11. Bricker NS. On the meaning of the intact nephron hypothesis. Am J Med 1969;46:1–11.
12. Hori R, Okumura K, Kamiya A, et al. Ampicillin and cephalexin in renal insufficiency. Clin Pharmacol Ther 1983;34:792–798.
13. Hori R, Okumura K, Nihira H. A new dosing regimen in renal insufficiency: Application to cephalexin. Clin Pharmacol Ther 1985;38:290–295.
14. Maiza A, Daley-Yates PT. The clearance of drugs in different types of renal disease. Ren Fail 1988;11:67. Abstract.
15. Lin JH, Lin T. Renal handling of drugs in renal failure. I. Differential effects of uranyl nitrate- and glycerol-induced acute renal failure on renal excretion of TEAB and PAH in rats. J Pharmacol Exp Ther 1988;246:896 901.
16. Gloff CA, Benet LZ. Differential effects of the degree of renal damage on *p*-aminohippuric acid and inulin clearances in rats. J Pharmacokinet Biopharm 1989;17:169–177.
17. Bosch JP. Renal reserve. A functional view of glomerular filtration rate. Semin Nephrol 1995;15:381–385.
18. Gaspari F, Perico N, Remuzzi G. Measurement of glomerular filtration rate. Kidney Int Suppl 1997;63:S151–S154.
19. Walser M. Assessing renal function from creatinine measurements in adults with chronic renal failure. Am J Kidney Dis 1998;32:23–31.
20. Rahn KH, Heidenreich S, Bruckner D. How to assess glomerular filtration and damage in humans. J Hypertens 1999;17:309–317.
21. Rose BD, Renneke HG. Renal Pathophysiology—The Essentials. Baltimore, Williams & Wilkins, 1994.
22. Jones CA, McQuillan GM, Kusek JW, et al. Serum creatinine levels in the US population: Third national health and nutrition examination survey. Am J Kidney Dis 1998;32:992–999.
23. Kasiske BL, Keane WF. Laboratory assessment of renal disease: Clearance, urinalysis, and renal biopsy. In: Brenner BM, ed. Brenner and Rector's The Kidney, 6th ed. Philadelphia: W.B. Saunders, 2000:1129–1170.
24. Bauer JH, Brooks CS, Burch RN. Clinical appraisal of creatinine clearance as a measurement of glomerular filtration rate. Am J Kidney Dis 1982;2:337–346.
25. Green AJE, Halloran SP, Mould GP, et al. Interference by newer cephalosporins in current methods for measuring creatinine. Clin Chem 1990,36.2139–2140.
26. Massoomi F, Matthews HG III, Destache CJ. Effect of seven fluoroquinolones on the determination of serum creatinine by the picric acid and enzymatic methods. Ann Pharmacother 1993;27:586–588.
27. Young DS, ed. Effects of Drugs on Clinical Laboratory Tests, 4th ed. Washington, DC, AACC Press, 1995:3.190–3.211.
28. Daly TM, Kempe KC, Scott MG, et al. "Bouncing" creatinine levels. N Engl J Med 1996;334:1749–1750. Letter.
29. Van den Berg, Koopman MG, Arisz L. Ranitidine has no influence on tubular creatinine secretion. Nephron 1996;74:705–708.
30. Mayersohn M, Conrad KA, Achari R. The influence of a cooked meat meal on creatinine plasma concentration and creatinine clearance. Br J Clin Pharmacol 1983;15:227–230.
31. Thakur V, Reisin E, Solomonow M, et al. Accuracy of formula-derived creatinine clearance in paraplegic subjects. Clin Nephrol 1997;47:237–242.
32. Poortsmans JR, Francaux M. Long-term oral creatine supplementation does not impair renal function in healthy athletes. Med Sci Sports Exerc 1999;31:1108–1110.
33. Robinson TM, Sewell DA, Casey A, et al. Dietary creatine supplementation does not affect some haematological indices, or indices of muscle damage and renal function. Br J Sports Med 2000;34:284–288.
34. Edmunds JW, Jayapalan S, DiMarco NM, et al. Creatine supplementation increases renal disease progression in Han:SPRD-cy Rats. Am J Kidney Dis 2001;37:73–78.
35. Goldstein DE, Little RR. Monitoring glycemia in diabetes. Short-term assessment. Endocrinol Metab Clin North Am 1997;26:475–486.
36. Pugia MJ, Lott JA, Clark LW, et al. Comparison of urine dipsticks with quantitative methods for microalbuminuria. Eur J Clin Chem Clin Biochem 1997;35:693–700.
37. Newman DJ, Pugia MJ, Lott JA, et al. Urinary protein and albumin excretion corrected by creatinine and specific gravity. Clin Chim Acta 2000;294:139–155.
38. Parsons M, Newman DJ, Pugia M, et al. Performance of a reagent strip device for quantitation of the urine albumin:creatinine ratio in a point of care setting. Clin Nephrol 1999;51:220–227.
39. Keane WF, Eknoyan G. Proteinuria, albuminuria, risk, assessment, detection, elimination (PARADE): A position paper of the National Kidney Foundation. Am J Kidney Dis 1999;33:1004–1010.
40. Ruggenenti P, Gaspari F, Perna A, Remuzzi G. Cross-sectional longitudinal study of spot morning urine protein:creatinine ratio, 24-hour urine protein excretion rate, glomerular filtration rate, and end stage renal failure in chronic renal disease in patients without diabetes. BMJ 1998;316:504–509.
41. Brändle E, Sieberth HG, Hautman RE. Effect of chronic dietary protein intake on the renal function in healthy subjects. Eur J Clin Nutr 1996;50:734–740.
42. Brenner BM, Lawler EV, Mackenzie HS. The hyperfiltration theory: A paradigm shift in nephrology. Kidney Int 1996;49:1774–1777.
43. Woods LL. Intrarenal mechanisms of renal reserve. Semin Nephrol 1995;15:386–395.
44. Dworkin LD, Sun AM, Brenner BM. The renal circulations. In: Brenner BM, ed. Brenner and Rector's The Kidney, 6th ed. Philadelphia, W.B. Saunders, 2000:277–318.
45. Dowling TC, Frye RF, Fraley DS, Matzke GR. Characterization of tubular functional capacity in humans using para-aminohippurate and famotidine. Kidney Int 2001;59:295–303.
46. Dowling TC, Frye RF, Zemaitis MA. Simultaneous determination of *p*-aminohippuric acid, acetyl-*p*-aminohippuric acid and iothalamate in human plasma and urine by high-performance liquid chromatography. J Chromatogr B Biomed Sci Appl 1998;716(1–2):305–313.
47. Prescott LF, Freestone S, McAuslane JAN. The concentration-dependent disposition of intravenous *p*-aminohippurate in subjects with normal and impaired renal function. Br J Clin Pharmacol 1993;35:20–29.
48. Taylor A, Manatunga A, Morton K, et al. Multicenter trial validation of a camera-based method to measure Tc-99m mercaptoacetyltriglycine, or Tc-99m MAG_3, clearance. Radiology 1997;204:47–54.
49. Russell CD, Dubovsky EV. Comparison of single-injection multisample renal clearance methods with and without urine collection. J Nucl Med 1995;36:603–606.
50. Florijn KW, Barendregt JNM, Lentjes EGWM, et al. Glomerular filtration rate measurement by "single-shot" injection of inulin. Kidney Int 1994;46:252–259.
51. Orlando R, Floreani M, Padrini R, Palatini P. Determination of inulin clearance by bolus intravenous injection in healthy subjects and ascitic patients: Equivalence of systemic and renal clearances as glomerular filtration markers. Br J Clin Pharmacol 1998;46:605 609.

52. Soper CPR, Bending MR, Barron JL. An automated enzymatic inulin assay, capable of full sinistrin hydrolysis. Eur J Clin Chem Clin Biochem 1995;33:497–501.
53. Dall'Amico R, Montini G, Pisanello L, et al. Determination of inulin in plasma and urine by reverse-phase high-performance liquid chromatography. J Chromatogr B Biomed Appl 1995;672:155–159.
54. Buclin T, Pechère-Bertschi A, Séchaud R, et al. Sinistrin clearance for determination of glomerular filtration rate: A reappraisal of various approaches using a new analytical method. J Clin Pharmacol 1997;37:679–692.
55. Ruiz R, Cordova MA, Sierra M, et al. Automated sinistrin measurement. Clin Biochem 1997;30:501–504.
56. Dowling TC, Frye RF, Fraley DS, Matzke GR. Comparison of iothalamate clearance methods for measuring GFR. Pharmacotherapy 1999;19:943–950.
57. Frennby B, Sterner G, Almén T, et al. The use of iohexol clearance to determine GFR in patients with severe chronic renal failure—A comparison between different clearance techniques. Clin Nephrol 1995;43: 35–46.
58. Rocco MV, Buckalew VM Jr, Moore LC, Shihabi ZK. Measurement of glomerular filtration rate using nonradioactive iohexol: Comparison of two one-compartment models. Am J Nephrol 1996;16:138–143.
59. Lundqvist S, Hietala S-O, Groth S, Sjdin J-G. Evaluation of single sample clearance calculations in 903 patients. A comparison of multiple and single sample techniques. Acta Radiol 1997;38:68–72.
60. Lundqvist S, Holmberg G, Jakobsson G, et al. Assessment of possible nephrotoxicity from iohexol in patients with normal and impaired renal function. Acta Radiol 1998;39:362–367.
61. Hricak H, Meux M, Reddy GP. Radiologic assessment of the kidney. In Brenner BM, ed. Brenner and Rector's The Kidney, 6th ed. Philadelphia, W.B. Saunders, 2000:1171–1200.
62. Frennby B, Almén T, Lilja B, et al. Determination of the relative glomerular filtration rate of each kidney in man. Acta Radiol 1995;36:410–417.
63. Morton K, Pisani DE, Whiting JH Jr, et al. Determination of glomerular filtration rate using technitium-99m-DTPA with differing degrees of renal function. J Nucl Med Technol 1997;25:110–114.
64. DeSanto NG, Anastasio P, Cirillo M, et al. Measurement of glomerular filtration rate by the 99m-Tc-DTPA renogram is less precise than measured and predicted creatinine clearance. Nephron 1999;81:136–140.
65. Lemann J, Bidani AK, Bain RP, et al. Use of the serum creatinine to estimate glomerular filtration rate in health and early diabetic nephropathy. Am J Kidney Dis 1990;16:236–243.
66. Cockroft, DW, Gault MH. Prediction of creatinine clearance from serum creatinine. Nephron 1976;16:31–41.
67. Shemesh O, Golbetz H, Kriss JP, et al. Limitations of creatinine as a filtration marker in glomerulopathic patients. Kidney Int 1985;28:830–838.
68. Roubenoff R, Drew H, Moyer M, et al. Oral cimetidine improves the accuracy and precision of creatinine clearance in lupus nephritis. Ann Intern Med 1990;113:501–506.
69. Zaltzman JS, Whiteside C, Cattran D, et al. Accurate measurement of impaired glomerular filtration using single-dose oral cimetidine. Am J Kidney Dis 1996;27:504–511.
70. Van Acker BAC, Koomen GCM, Koopman MG, et al. Creatinine clearance during cimetidine administration for measurement of glomerular filtration rate. Lancet 1992;340:1326–1329.
71. Luke DR, Halstenson CE, Opsahl JA, et al. Validity of creatinine clearance estimates in the assessment of renal function. Clin Pharmacol Ther 1990;48:503–508.
72. Mawer CE, Knowles BR, Lucas SB, et al. Computer-assisted prescribing of kanamycin for patients with renal insufficiency. Lancet 1972;1:12–15.
73. Jelliffe RW. Estimation of creatinine clearance when urine cannot be collected. Lancet 1971;1:975–976.
74. Jelliffe RW. Creatinine clearance: Bedside estimate. Ann Intern Med 1973;79:604–605.
75. Hull JH, Hak LJ, Koch GC, et al. Influence of range of renal function and liver disease on predictability of creatinine clearance. Clin Pharmacol Ther 1981;29:516–521.
76. Gault MH, Longerich LL, Harnett JD, et al. Predicting glomerular function from adjusted serum creatinine. Nephron 1992;62:249–256.
77. Coresh J, Toto RD, Kirk KA, et al. Creatinine clearance as a measure of GFR in screens for the African-American study of kidney disease. Am J Kidney Dis 1998;32:32–42.
78. Goldwasser P, Aboul-Magd A, Maru M. Race and creatinine excretion in chronic renal insufficiency. Am J Kidney Dis 1997;30:16–22.
79. Ixkes MCJ, Koopman MG, van Acker BAC, et al. Cimetidine improves GFR-estimation by the Cockcroft-Gault formula. Clin Nephrol 1997;47:229–236.
80. Levey AS, Bosch JP, Lewis JB, et al. A more accurate method to estimate glomerular filtration rate from serum creatinine: A new prediction equation. Ann Intern Med 1999;130:461–470.
81. Orlando R, Floreani M, Padrini R, Palatini P. Evaluation of measured and calculated creatinine clearances as glomerular filtration markers in different stages of liver cirrhosis. Clin Nephrol 1999;51:341–347.
82. Lam NP, Sperelakis R, Kuk J, et al. Rapid estimation of creatinine clearances in patients with liver dysfunction. Dig Dis Sci 1999;44:1222–1227.
83. Caregaro L, Menon F, Angeli P, et al. Limitations of serum creatinine level and creatinine clearance as filtration markers in cirrhosis. Arch Intern Med 1994;154:201–205.
84. DeSanto NG, Anastasio P, Loguercio C, et al. Creatinine clearance: An inadequate marker of renal filtration in patients with early posthepatitic cirrhosis (Child A) without fluid retention and muscle wasting. Nephron 1995;70:421–424.
85. Davis GA, Chandler MHH. Comparison of creatinine clearance estimation methods in patients with trauma. Am J Health Syst Pharm 1996;53:1028–1032.
86. Goerdt PJ, Heim-Duthoy KL, Macres M, Swan SK. Predictive performance of renal function equations in renal allografts. Br J Clin Pharmacol 1997;44:261–265.
87. Schuck O, Teplan V, Vitko S, et al. Predicting glomerular function from adjusted serum creatinine in renal transplant patients. Int J Clin Pharmacol Ther 1997;35:33–37.
88. Huang E, Hewitt R, Shelton M, Morse GD. Comparison of measured and estimated creatinine clearance in patients with advanced HIV disease. Pharmcotherapy 1996;16:222–229.
89. Quadri KHM, Bernardini J, Greenberg A, et al. Assessment of renal function during pregnancy using a random urine protein to creatinine ratio and Cockcroft-Gault formula. Am J Kidney Dis 1994;24:416–420.
90. Jelliffe RW, Jelliffe SM. A computer program for estimation of creatinine clearance from unstable serum creatinine concentration. Math Biosci 1972;14:17–24.
91. Chiou WL, Hsu FH. A new simple rapid method to monitor renal function based on pharmacokinetic considerations of endogenous creatinine. Res Commun Chem Pathol Pharmacol 1975;10:315–330.
92. Brater DC. Drug Use in Renal Disease. Balgowlah, Australia, ADIS Health Science Press, 1983:22–56.
93. Coll E, Botey A, Alvarez L, et al. Serum cystatin C as a new marker for noninvasive estimation of glomerular filtration rate and as a marker for early renal impairment. Am J Kidney Dis 2000;36:29–34.
94. Price CP, Finney H. Developments in the assessment of glomerular filtration rate. Clin Chim Acta 2000;297:55–66.
95. Randers E, Erlandsen EJ. Serum cystatin C as an endogenous marker of the renal function—A review. Clin Chem Lab Med 1999;37:389–395.
96. Page MK, Bükki B, Luppa P, Neumeier D. Clinical value of cystatin C determination. Clin Chim Acta 2000;297;67–72.
97. Bokenkamp A, Domanetzki M, Zinck R, et al. Cystatin C serum concentrations underestimate glomerular filtration rate in renal transplant recipients. Clin Chem 1999;45:1866–1868.
98. Arant BS Jr. Developmental patterns of renal functional maturation compared in the human neonate. J Pediatr 1978;92:705–712.
99. van den Anker, de Groot R, Broerse HM, et al. Assessment of glomerular filtration rate in preterm infants by serum creatinine: Comparison with inulin clearance. Pediatrics 1995;96:1156–1158.
100. Sertel H, Scopes J. Rates of creatinine clearance in babies less than one week of age. Arch Dis Child 1973;48:717–720.

101. Bajaj G, Alexander SR, Browne R, et al. ^{125}Iodine iothalamate clearance in children. A simple method to measure glomerular filtration. Pediatr Nephrol 1996;10:25–28.
102. Schwartz GJ, Brion LP, Spitzer A. The use of plasma creatinine concentration for estimating glomerular filtration rate in infants, children, and adolescents. Pediatr Clin North Am 1987;34:571–590.
103. Al-Harbi N, Lireman D. Comparison of three different methods of estimating the glomerular filtration rate in children after renal transplantation. Am J Nephrol 1997;17:68–71.
104. Fong J, Johnston S, Valentino T, Notterman D. Length/serum creatinine ratio does not predict measured creatinine clearance in critically ill children. Clin Pharmacol Ther 1995;58:192–197.
105. Lindeman RD. Assessment of renal function in the old. Clin Lab Med 1993;13:269–277.
106. Lindeman RD, Tobin J, Shrock NW. Longitudinal studies on the rate of decline in renal function with age. J Am Geriatr Soc 1985;33:278–281.
107. Fliser D, Ritz E, Franek E. Renal reserve in the elderly. Semin Nephrol 1995;15:463–467.
108. Smythe M, Hoffman J, Kizy K, et al. Estimating creatinine clearance in elderly patients with low serum creatinine concentrations. Am J Hosp Pharm 1994;51:198–204.
109. O'Connell MB, Wong MO, Bannick-Mohrland SD, et al. Accuracy of 2- and 8-hour urine collections for measuring creatinine clearance in the hospitalized elderly. Pharmacotherapy 1993;13:135–142.
110. Agodoa L, Eknoyan G, Ingelfinger J, et al. Assessment of structure and function in progressive renal disease. Kidney Int Suppl 1997;63:S144–S150.
111. Rossing P, Astrup A-S, Smidt UM, et al. Monitoring kidney function in diabetic nephropathy. Diabetologia 1994;37:708–712.
112. Valensi P, Assayag M, Busby M, et al. Microalbuminuria in obese patients with or without hypertension. Int J Obes Relat Metab Disord 1996;20:574–579.
113. Berrut G, Bouhanick B, Fabbri P, et al. Microalbuminuria as a predictor of a drop in glomerular filtration rate in subjects with non-insulin-dependent diabetes mellitus and hypertension. Clin Nephrol 1997;48:92–97.
114. Mimran A, Ribstein J, DuCailar G. Is microalbuminuria a marker of early intrarenal vascular dysfunction in essential hypertension? Hypertension 1994;23:1018–1021.
115. Taylor A, Nally JV. Clinical applications of renal scintigraphy. AJR Am J Roentgenol 1995;164:31–41.
116. Mindell HJ, Fairbank JT. Renal imaging techniques. In: Greenberg A, ed. Primer on Kidney Diseases, 2nd ed. San Diego, Academic Press, 1998:47–53.
117. Lerman LO, Rodriguez-Porcel M, Romero JC. The development of x-ray imaging to study renal function. Kidney Int 1999;55:400–416.
118. Schentag JJ, Plaut ME. Patterns of urinary β_2-microglobulin excretion by patients treated with aminoglycosides. Kidney Int 1980;17:654–661.
119. Nassseri K, Daley-Yates PT. A comparison of N-1-methylnicotinamide clearance with 5 other markers of renal function in models of acute and chronic renal failure. Toxicol Lett 1990;53:243–245.
120. Edwards BD, Maiza A, Daley-Yates PT, et al. Altered clearance of N-1-methylnicotinamide associated with the use of low doses of cyclosporine. Am J Kidney Dis 1994;23:23–30.
121. Maiza A, Daley-Yates PT. Estimation of the renal clearance of drugs using endogenous N-1-methylnicotinamide. Toxicol Lett 1990;53:231–235.
122. Jung K. Urinary enzymes and low-molecular-weight proteins as markers of tubular dysfunction. Kidney Int Suppl 1994;47:S29–S33.
123. Jung K, Diego J, Strobelt V, et al. Diagnostic significance of some urinary enzymes for detecting acute rejection crises in renal transplant recipients: Alanine aminopeptidase, alkaline phosphatase, gamma-glutamyl transferase, N-acetyl-beta-glucosaminidase, and lysozyme. Clin Chem 1986;32:1807–1811.

43
ACUTE RENAL FAILURE

Bruce A. Mueller

Acute renal failure is an abrupt decline in renal function characterized by the inability of the kidney to excrete metabolic waste products (i.e., nitrogenous wastes and water) and maintain acid-base balance. An elevation of the nitrogenous waste products (creatinine and urea nitrogen) is referred to as *azotemia*. *Uremia,* characterized by anorexia, nausea, vomiting and mental status changes, is the clinical syndrome resulting from azotemia. Acute renal failure is not well defined with regards to the presence of uremic symptoms and/or changes in urea nitrogen; thus, most clinical diagnoses are primarily based on an elevation in the serum creatinine concentration. An abrupt (over 24–48 hours) increase of the serum creatinine concentration of more than 50% in a patient with previously normal renal function or an increase of 1.0 mg/dL in a patient with preexisting renal disease (serum creatinine concentration [S_{cr}] >2.0 mg/dL) is a commonly used definition of acute renal failure.[1]

The use of the serum creatinine concentration to define end-stage renal disease (renal failure), although appropriate in chronic renal disease, may by itself be inappropriate to define renal function in a many individuals who develop acute renal failure. Serum creatinine changes may be a poor marker of renal function because a large percentage of patients who develop acute renal failure are critically ill and highly catabolic. Consequently, these patients frequently accumulate non-creatinine waste products (e.g., urea nitrogen and water) out of proportion to the increase in serum creatinine. Therefore, the diagnosis of acute renal failure in critically ill patients should be made whenever the kidneys are unable to maintain acceptable control of body fluid volume, acid-base balance and the levels of nitrogenous waste products (i.e., blood urea nitrogen [BUN]), regardless of whether the serum creatinine concentration has risen significantly. Even though most published studies use a serum creatinine-based definition of acute renal failure, this clinical definition provides a more realistic estimate of patient outcome, anticipation of potential complications, and an increased awareness of the need for early intervention with renal replacement therapy.

EPIDEMIOLOGY

The development of acute renal failure is primarily a phenomenon of hospitalized patients with the diagnosis appearing in their discharge or death summaries, and not in their admitting history. Community-acquired acute renal failure is relatively infrequent, occurring in only 1% of hospital admissions.[2] Prerenal azotemia (as a result of intravascular volume depletion) or postrenal obstruction (as a result of prostatic disease) are common causes of community-acquired acute renal failure.[3] Intrinsic renal damage, although less common than pre- and postrenal causes of community-acquired acute renal failure, is frequently related to infection or medications in patients presenting with acute renal failure.[3] Most patients with community-acquired acute renal failure have a treatable cause of renal failure and their prognosis, although dependent on underlying medical conditions, is generally favorable.[2]

The incidence of hospital-acquired acute renal failure ranges between 2% and 5% of hospitalized patients but it is difficult to quantify because of the lack of agreement on the definition of acute renal failure. The etiologies of acute renal failure in these patients can be separated by the type of patient developing renal failure. For medical/surgical patients on the general hospital ward, the etiology of acute renal failure is frequently prerenal (e.g., intravascular volume depletion or congestive heart failure) and less-often related to renal injury (e.g., medications or radiocontrast agents). Risk factors for the development of acute renal failure on the surgical ward are advanced age (>70 years), diabetes, preexisting renal, pulmonary, or vascular disease.[4,5] For patients in the intensive care unit (ICU), the etiology of acute renal failure is almost always related to multiple insults to the kidney occurring as a consequence of multiple organ failure.[1,6] Risk factors for the development of acute renal failure in the ICU include sepsis, bleeding, volume depletion, chronic liver disease, mechanical ventilation, and surgery.[7] The incidence of acute renal failure acquired in an ICU ranges between 6% and 23%.[8]

The prognosis for patients developing hospital-acquired acute renal failure can best be estimated by dividing the patient population into those who develop acute renal failure who do not require renal replacement therapy, those who develop acute renal failure who do require renal replacement therapy, and those who develop acute renal failure as a result of multiple organ failure (i.e., ICU-acquired acute renal failure). Patients who develop acute renal failure and do not require renal replacement therapy have the most favorable prognosis (Table 43–1). This is because they have recovered renal function, which frequently heralds recovery from the underlying medical condition. Hospitalized patients who develop acute renal failure and require renal replacement therapy, have a less favorable outcome. Multiple investigators have attempted to identify those clinical and demographic factors associated with survival.[1,7,9,10] The mortality rate of patients with acute renal failure who require renal replacement therapy and who have no other major organ system failure ranges from 10% to 25%.[5,11] As the number of failed organ systems increases, so does the mortality rate; for patients with multiple organ failure (≥3 failed organ systems), the mortality rate greatly exceeds 50%.[5,10]

Although there are occasional reports of improvement,[12] the survival rates for hospitalized patients developing acute renal failure have not changed substantially during the last two decades, despite the advances in medicine that have occurred during that period. It is hoped that a better understanding of the pathogenesis of acute renal failure,[13–15] new drug therapies,[16] and improvements in renal replacement technology[17] and techniques[12,18–20] may eventually improve the dismal outcome for these patients.

ETIOLOGY

The classification of acute renal failure into broad categories based on the precipitating factors facilitates the diagnosis and management of patients presenting with this disorder (Table 43–2). Traditionally,

TABLE 43–1. Incidence and Outcomes of ARF Relative to Where ARF Occurs

	Community Acquired	Hospital Acquired	ICU Acquired
Incidence	Low (<1%)	Moderate (2%–5%)	High (6%–23%)
Cause	Single	Single or multiple	Multifactorial
Overall survival rate	70%–95%	30%–50%	10%–30%
Worsened outcome if:	RRT required Poor preadmission health Other failed organ systems	RRT required Poor preadmission health Ischemic ARF cause Other failed organ systems	Intrinsic renal disease Ischemic ARF cause Septic RRT required Poor preadmission health Other failed organ systems
Better outcome if:	Nonoliguric	Nonoliguric Nephrotoxic ARF cause	Prerenal cause Postrenal cause Nonoliguric Nephrotoxic cause

ARF = acute renal failure; RRT = renal replacement therapy.

the causes of acute renal failure have been categorized into prerenal azotemia (resulting from decreased renal perfusion), acute intrinsic renal failure (resulting from structural damage to the kidney), and postrenal obstruction (resulting from the obstruction of urine flow from the kidney out of the body). The addition of the category "functional acute renal failure" aids in the understanding of the pathophysiology of acute renal failure. This category is the result of hemodynamic changes at the level of the glomerulus without decreased perfusion of the kidney or structural damage to it.

PRERENAL AZOTEMIA

Prerenal acute renal failure results from hypoperfusion of the renal parenchyma, with or without systemic arterial hypotension.[21] Renal hypoperfusion with systemic arterial hypotension may be caused by a decline in intravascular volume (e.g., hemorrhage, dehydration) or a decline in effective blood volume (i.e., the blood volume perceived by the arterial baroreceptors). Congestive heart failure and liver failure are two examples of disease states in which there is a decline in effective blood volume without a decrease in intravascular volume. Because the kidney is initially undamaged, the urinalysis will be normal. Eventually, the fractional excretion of sodium will be low, reflecting an increase in the concentrations of the sodium-retentive hormones renin, angiotensin, and aldosterone. Urinary solute will be concentrated as a result of the increased circulating levels of antidiuretic hormone that is released in response to the diminished arterial blood pressure.

Renal hypoperfusion without systemic hypotension most commonly results from bilateral renal artery occlusion, or unilateral occlusion in a patient with a single functioning kidney. In these conditions, the sodium retentive hormones are activated by the decline in renal parenchymal perfusion. However, systemic arterial blood pressure is usually elevated leading to an inhibition of antidiuretic hormone release. Consequently, the urinary indices will reflect enhanced sodium reabsorption (i.e., a low fractional excretion of sodium), but the urinary solute may not be maximally concentrated.

FUNCTIONAL ACUTE RENAL FAILURE

Functional acute renal failure is characterized by a decline in glomerular ultrafiltrate production secondary to a reduced glomerular hydrostatic pressure without damage to the kidney itself. The decline in glomerular hydrostatic pressure is a direct consequence of changes in glomerular afferent (vasoconstriction) and efferent (vasodilation) arteriolar circumference (Fig. 43–1). These clinical conditions most commonly occur in individuals who have reduced effective blood volume (e.g., congestive heart failure, cirrhosis, severe pulmonary disease, hypoalbuminemia) or renovascular disease (e.g., renal artery stenosis) and cannot compensate for changes in afferent or efferent arteriolar tone. Examples of disorders that result in afferent arteriolar vasoconstriction (and an increase in afferent arteriolar resistance) include hypercalcemia and the administration of certain medications (e.g., cyclosporine and nonsteroidal anti-inflammatory drugs [NSAIDs]). A decrease in efferent arteriolar resistance usually results from the administration of an angiotensin- converting enzyme inhibitor (ACEI) or angiotensin II receptor antagonist/blocker (ARB). With correction of the underlying pathologic process or discontinuation of the responsible medication, renal function rapidly returns to baseline. The hepatorenal syndrome is included in this classification scheme because the kidney itself is not damaged and there is intense afferent arteriolar vasoconstriction leading to a decline in glomerular filtration. In all the above conditions, the urinalysis is not different from its baseline state and the urinary indices suggest prerenal azotemia. The urinary solute concentration may be variable depending on circulating levels of antidiuretic hormone.

Functional acute renal failure is very common in individuals with congestive heart failure who receive an ACEI in an attempt to improve left ventricular function. Although the improvement in left ventricular function resulting from the ACEI may take weeks to be clinically significant,[23] the decline in efferent arteriolar resistance resulting from the inhibition of angiotensin II occurs rapidly. Therefore, if the dose of the ACEI is increased too rapidly, there will be a decline in glomerular filtration rate (GFR) with a concomitant rise in the serum creatinine leading to functional acute renal failure. If the increase in the serum creatinine is not too severe (usually <1 mg/dL for those with a baseline S_{cr} less than 3 mg/dL) the medication can be continued. Renal function should gradually improve as renal parenchymal perfusion pressure increases with improvement in left ventricular function.

INTRINSIC RENAL FAILURE

Acute intrinsic renal failure results from damage to the kidney itself. Conceptually, acute intrinsic renal failure can best be discussed on a structural basis; the small blood vessels, glomeruli, renal tubules, and interstitium. Renal failure secondary to small vessel vasculitis (e.g., polyarteritis nodosa, hemolytic uremic syndrome, malignant hypertension) or cholesterol emboli can present with relatively normal urinary sediment because the glomerulus and tubules, at least

TABLE 43–2. Classification of Acute Renal Failure

Category	Classification of Acute Renal Failure	Differential Diagnosis
Prerenal Renal Failure	Systemic Hypoperfusion	Intravascular volume depletion Dehydration Hemorrhage Congestive heart disease Liver disease Nephrotic syndrome Overdiuresis
	Isolated Renal Hypoperfusion	Bilateral renal artery stenosis (unilateral renal artery stenosis in solitary kidney) Emboli Cholesterol Thrombotic
Functional Acute Renal Failure		Medications Cyclosporine ACE inhibitors NSAID Hypercalcemia Hepatorenal syndrome
Acute Intrinsic Renal Failure	Vascular	Vasculitis Polyarteritis nodosa Thrombotic thrombocytopenic purpura (TTP) Hemolytic uremic syndrome Emboli Cholesterol Thrombotic
	Glomerular	Systemic lupus erythematosus Poststreptococcal glomerulonephritis Antiglomerular basement membrane disease
	Acute Tubular Necrosis	Ischemic Hypotension Vasoconstriction Exogenous toxins Contrast dye Heavy metals Drugs (amphotericin B, aminoglycosides, etc) Endogenous toxins Myoglobin Hemoglobin
	Acute Interstitial Nephritis	Drugs Penicillins Ciprofloxacin Sulfonamides Infection Streptococcal
Postrenal Renal failure (Obstruction)	Bladder Outlet Obstruction	Prostatic hypertrophy Improperly placed bladder catheter
	Ureteral (bilateral or unilateral with solitary functioning kidney)	Cervical cancer Retroperitoneal fibrosis
	Renal Pelvis or Tubules	Crystal deposition Oxalate Indinavir Sulfonamides Acyclovir Tumor lysis syndrome

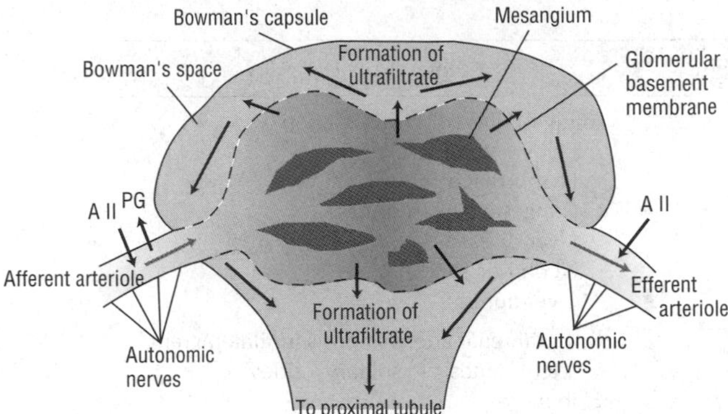

FIGURE 43–1. The formation of glomerular ultrafiltrate is dependent on the surface area of the glomerular capillaries, their permeability, and the net hydrostatic pressure across the capillary wall. As the glomerular capillary surface area increases, secondary to mesangial cell relaxation, the formation of glomerular ultrafiltrate is increased. An increase or decrease in glomerular hydrostatic pressure results in either an increase or decrease in glomerular ultrafiltrate production. Afferent arteriolar vasoconstriction (which is primarily mediated by angiotensin II) or vasodilation (primarily mediated by prostaglandins) can result in a decrease or increase, respectively, in hydrostatic pressure across the capillary. Efferent arteriolar vasoconstriction (primarily mediated by angiotensin II) results in an increase in glomerular hydrostatic pressure. Under conditions in which renal blood flow is diminished, the kidney maintains glomerular ultrafiltration by vasodilating the afferent and vasoconstricting the efferent arterioles. Medications that may interfere with these processes might result in an abrupt decline in glomerular filtration.

initially, are not damaged. When renal failure results from a small vessel vasculitis, the vasculitic process is rarely confined to the kidney. A careful search for diagnostic clues suggesting other organ system involvement usually provides evidence of the diffuse nature of these disease processes.

Acute glomerular inflammation (acute glomerulonephritis) can result from a variety of precipitating causes (e.g., systemic lupus erythematosus, antiglomerular basement membrane disease). In these disorders, the urinalysis usually reveals the presence of heavy proteinuria (>3 g urinary protein per 24-hour collection period) and hemoglobinuria. Microscopic analysis of the urinary sediment frequently shows numerous red blood cells and red blood cell casts, the latter being considered diagnostic for glomerulonephritis. In the early stages of the illness, the fractional excretion of sodium is less than 1 because tubular function is still intact. However, as renal failure becomes more established, the fractional excretion of sodium may increase.

The renal tubules are susceptible to a variety of insults. The tubules contained within the medulla of the kidney are particularly at risk from ischemic injury as this portion of the kidney is very metabolically active and, thereby, has a high oxygen requirement. Severe hypotension or the administration of vasoconstricting drugs preferentially affects the tubules more than any other portion of the kidney. In addition, exogenous toxic substances (e.g., contrast agents, heavy metals, and pharmacologic agents such as aminoglycosides, amphotericin B, foscarnet) and endogenous toxins (e.g., myoglobin, hemoglobin, uric acid) may cause tubular injury. When tubular cells die, they slough off into the tubular lumen forming casts causing increased tubular pressures and reduced glomerular filtration.[14] Regardless of the etiology, tubular injury leads to a loss of urine-concentrating ability, defective distal sodium reabsorption, and a reduction in the GFR. The etiology of acute intrinsic renal failure secondary to tubular injury (referred to as acute tubular necrosis) is usually discernible by reviewing the patient's history and medication list. The urinalysis suggests tubular injury by the presence of coarse "dirty brown" casts. Red blood cells and red blood cell casts are only rarely seen. The urinary indices suggest intrinsic renal dysfunction (i.e., high fractional excretion of sodium, urine osmolality equal to plasma osmolality, and a low urine creatinine to serum creatinine ratio).

Reports of hemolytic uremic syndrome have been on the rise. Hemolytic uremic syndrome is now considered to be one of the most common causes of acute renal failure in children.[24] This syndrome usually is associated with ingestion of foods (especially, undercooked hamburger and other ground meats, unpasteurized goat's milk) contaminated with Shiga toxin-producing strains of *Escherichia coli,* particularly *E. coli* O157:H7. The renal damage associated with this infection is caused by binding of the Shiga toxin to endothelium causing vascular damage and the release of mediators of inflammation. The disease often presents initially with diarrhea; proteinuria may not be seen until later in the course of the disease.[24]

The interstitium of the kidney is also susceptible to injury from a variety of causes. Although acute interstitial nephritis is most commonly caused by medications (see Chap. 48), infections (e.g., streptococcal, leptospirosis, Hantavirus, and HIV infections), and selected autoimmune disorders (systemic lupus erythematosus or mixed connective tissue disease) also may produce a similar syndrome. The presence of white blood cells, white blood cell casts, and coarse granular casts in the urine, suggests interstitial inflammation. The presence of eosinophilia and eosinophiluria also strongly suggest the presence of an interstitial nephritis. Occasionally, low to moderate proteinuria can be seen on urinalysis.

POSTRENAL OBSTRUCTION

Acute renal failure resulting from obstruction may occur at any level within the urinary collecting system from renal tubule to urethra. However, to cause acute renal failure, the obstructing process must involve both kidneys, or one kidney in a patient with a single functioning kidney. Bladder outlet obstruction (e.g., prostatic hypertrophy) is the most common cause of obstructive uropathy. Crystal deposition within the tubules (e.g., secondary to uric acid, oxalate, acyclovir, sulfonamide, indinavir, or methotrexate) and ureteral obstruction (e.g., secondary to shed renal papilla or calculi) are infrequent causes of obstructive acute renal failure. Crystal-induced acute renal failure is often seen in patients who have severe volume contraction or who are receiving large doses of a drug with relatively low solubility. In these cases, patients do not have sufficient urine volume to keep the crystal from precipitating in the urine.[22] The onset of acute anuria, in the absence of a catastrophic event, should suggest acute urinary tract obstruction. However, the development of acute renal failure in a hospitalized patient admitted with normal renal function is rarely secondary to obstruction unless an indwelling urinary catheter has been misplaced. When the obstructing process (e.g., prostatic hypertrophy, cervical cancer) is gradual and incomplete, the patient may present with complaints of a decreased force of the urinary stream and polyuria.

PATHOPHYSIOLOGY

A basic knowledge of renal function facilitates the understanding of how acute renal failure manifests itself clinically. The most logical approach to understanding renal function is to divide the kidney into its four basic component parts: the vasculature; the glomeruli; the tubules; and the interstitium, which surrounds the other three component parts.

RENAL VASCULATURE

Blood flows to each kidney via a main renal artery, which divides in two just prior to entering the renal parenchyma. These two main branches divide into approximately five segmental branches, each of which is the sole provider of blood flow to its respective section. Consequently, arterial occlusion at the level of the segmental branch will result in complete ischemia of that portion of the kidney. In the setting of renal artery occlusion, the creatinine may or may not rise depending on the number of segmental arteries involved. If only a few segmental arteries are occluded, the serum creatinine remains unchanged and the urinalysis is normal. With significant renal infarction, the urinalysis shows hematuria and proteinuria, and the urine indices show an inability to concentrate urinary solutes.

Each segmental renal artery divides into a series of smaller arteries leading to the afferent arterioles of the glomeruli. Lesions at this level of the arterial tree (e.g., cholesterol emboli, vascular lesions, platelet plugs) present as isolated decreased perfusion of multiple glomeruli. The serum creatinine frequently is increased because the lesions are usually diffuse. However, the urinalysis most commonly is normal. The urinary indices often suggest prerenal azotemia (i.e., a low urine sodium concentration and a low fractional excretion of sodium) in the absence of systemic hypotension or a decrease in effective blood volume. The urine volume may or may not be diminished. However, the onset of oliguria secondary to diffuse arterial lesions within the kidney, such as that which occurs with hemolytic uremic syndrome, denotes a poor chance for salvage of renal function.

GLOMERULUS

The glomerulus consists of an enlargement of the proximal end of the renal tubule, which surrounds a vascular tuft connecting the afferent and efferent arterioles (Fig. 43–1). The vascular tuft is encased in the mesangium which consists of mesangial cells and the mesangial matrix. The production of glomerular ultrafiltrate is predominantly dependent on the transcapillary hydrostatic pressure (dictated by the afferent and efferent arteriolar resistance) and the glomerular surface area (primarily governed by the contraction and relaxation of mesangial cells that open and close glomerular capillaries). Afferent arteriolar tone is determined primarily by the local levels of angiotensin II (which induces vasoconstriction) and prostaglandins (which induce vasodilation). Efferent arteriolar tone is predominantly determined by the local concentration of angiotensin II.

Pathophysiologic processes and medications that result in alterations of the afferent and efferent arteriolar tone (i.e., systemic hypotension, hypercalcemia, ACEIs, ARBs, and NSAIDs) reduce glomerular ultrafiltrate production as a result of a decrease in glomerular hydrostatic pressure. Under these conditions, the serum creatinine will rise, the urine sediment will be normal, and the urine indices will suggest prerenal azotemia. However, the urinary solutes may or may not be maximally concentrated depending on the circulating level of antidiuretic hormone. Damage to the glomerular capillary tuft (e.g., acute glomerulonephritis) results in a decline in the glomerular ultrafiltrate production as a result of a decrease in glomerular capillary surface area. Under these conditions the serum creatinine rises. The urinalysis is significant for hematuria and proteinuria because of the increased permeability of the damaged glomerular capillaries. Red cell casts are found often and are considered diagnostic of glomerular capillary injury. The urine indices may suggest prerenal azotemia because the renal tubules are intact. The urinary solutes may or may not be maximally concentrated. Proteinuria exceeding 3 g/d, often referred to as "nephrotic range" proteinuria, may be present and if prolonged results in the nephrotic syndrome.

RENAL TUBULES

Under normal conditions, approximately 180 L/d of glomerular ultrafiltrate are produced, the vast majority of which must be reabsorbed by the renal tubules to maintain homeostasis. Clinically, the renal tubule can be divided into three major sections: the proximal tubule, Henle's loop, and the distal nephron, which includes the distal tubule, the cortical collecting tubule, and the medullary collecting ducts. In the proximal tubule, approximately 60% to 70% of the filtered load of water and solute is isovolemically reabsorbed, as well as the vast majority of filtered amino acids, glucose, and bicarbonate. Isolated injury to the proximal tubule (e.g., as occurs with heavy-metal poisoning or paraproteinemia) results in significant aminoaciduria, glucosuria, and bicarbonaturia. The serum creatinine may rise because of intratubular obstruction, damage to the tubular epithelial cells, or the back leak of glomerular ultrafiltrate across the renal tubule.

In addition to its other functions, Henle's loop is responsible for a significant portion of the total reabsorption of potassium, calcium, and magnesium. It is also responsible for generating/maintaining the osmotic gradient within the kidney necessary for the concentration of urinary solutes. Damage to this portion of the nephron results in wasting of potassium and magnesium by the kidney and an inability of the kidney to concentrate the urine. The medullary portions of Henle's loop are very sensitive to ischemia secondary to hypoperfusion. Consequently, in severe prerenal azotemia with renal hypoperfusion, there may be a loss of urinary concentrating ability despite the continued presence of a low urinary sodium concentration and a low fractional excretion of sodium.

Major functions of the distal nephron include the regeneration of bicarbonate, the excretion of acid (hydrogen ion), the secretion of potassium, and the reabsorption of water. Damage to this portion of the nephron may present as significant acidemia and either hypo- or hyperkalemia, depending on the mechanism of injury. For example, amphotericin B produces small pores in the luminal membrane of distal tubular cells. These pores allow potassium to leak out of the cells into the urine. Consequently, amphotericin B nephrotoxicity is characterized by hypokalemia. Hyperkalemia may occur if the damage to the distal nephron is severe enough to cause oliguria or if the damage disrupts the renin-aldosterone axis. Defects in urine-concentrating ability also are frequent. In addition to the previously mentioned findings, acute tubular necrosis is associated with urinary sediment characterized by the presence of tubular cells, coarse granular casts, and, rarely, red blood cell casts.

INTERSTITIUM

The interstitium of the kidney provides the structural support for the kidney and the environment in which concentrating gradients can be established. In addition, the interstitium of the kidney plays a major role in urinary ammonia handling. To facilitate the regeneration of bicarbonate and the excretion of acid by the distal nephron, the kidney utilizes ammonia as a urinary buffer. When the interstitium of the kidney is damaged (e.g., in acute allergic interstitial nephritis), the concentrating gradient within the kidney may be dissipated and ammonia handling disrupted. Consequently, patients presenting with acute interstitial nephritis frequently are not able to concentrate their urine. They also may have a metabolic acidosis with hyperkalemia, the degree of which is out of proportion to the rise in serum creatinine.

The urinalysis may show mild proteinuria and hematuria. However, the striking finding on microscopic examination of the sediment is the presence of numerous white blood cells and white blood cell casts.

CLINICAL PRESENTATION

Rapid determination of the etiology of acute renal failure is essential. Nearly 90% of patients presenting to the hospital with community acquired acute renal failure have a potentially reversible cause.[2] The most common cause of acute renal failure in hospitalized patients is prerenal azotemia, which may be attenuated with prompt treatment of the renal hypoperfusion. A delayed diagnosis of the acute renal failure etiology may result in a more severe nephrologic injury.

HISTORY

The diagnostic approach to the patient with acute renal failure differs depending on the clinical setting in which the kidneys fail. For patients who present to the outpatient clinic or hospital with an elevated serum creatinine, the first objective is to determine whether the renal failure is acute or chronic. A past medical history of renal disease or of chronic conditions such as poorly controlled hypertension or diabetes mellitus, previous laboratory data documenting the presence of proteinuria or of an elevated serum creatinine, and the finding of bilateral small kidneys on renal ultrasonography, suggests the presence of chronic renal failure. The finding of an elevated parathyroid hormone concentration or evidence of renal osteodystrophy on radiographic bone survey also suggests chronicity.

For patients who do not have the above findings, their renal failure should be considered acute until proven otherwise. In these individuals, a careful review of their recent medications, including over-the-counter medications, complementary and alternative medications, and vitamins, is mandatory (see Chap. 48). The patient's recent history can usually provide an indication of when the renal dysfunction began. Frequently, patients may notice a change in their voiding habits with an increase in urinary frequency or nocturia, both suggesting a urinary concentrating defect. A decrease in the force of the urinary stream may suggest an obstructive process. The presence of cola-colored urine, indicating the presence of blood in the urine, is common in acute glomerulonephritis. If the accompanying proteinuria is severe, the patient may note excessive foaming of the urine in the toilet. The onset of bilateral flank pain may suggest swelling of the kidneys secondary to either acute glomerulonephritis or acute interstitial nephritis. The onset of severe headaches may suggest the development of hypertension as a result of acute renal failure. A recent increase in the patient's weight secondary to salt and water retention also may be helpful in defining the onset of renal failure.

A review of the laboratory data is usually sufficient to define the onset of acute renal failure for patients who develop acute renal failure while hospitalized. However, significant renal injury can occur prior to an increase in the serum creatinine. Consequently, clinicians must pay careful attention to subtle changes in the patient's weight, blood pressure, and urine output if they are to diagnose the onset of acute renal failure. Urine output is one of the easiest parameters to measure and is one of the most useful. In the absence of obstruction, urine output directly correlates with glomerular filtration rate in patients with acute renal failure.[25] Changes in urine output may be helpful in diagnosing the type of renal dysfunction that is present. Acute anuria (<50 mL urine production/24 h) is either secondary to complete urinary obstruction or a catastrophic event (e.g., shock, hemolytic uremic syndrome, acute cortical necrosis). Oliguria (50–400 mL urine production/24 h) suggests prerenal azotemia, functional acute renal failure, or acute intrinsic renal failure. Nonoliguric renal failure (>400 mL urine production/24 h) usually results from acute intrinsic renal failure or incomplete urinary obstruction. As with outpatients who present with acute renal failure, a careful review of the administered medications is also mandatory for individuals who develop acute renal failure while hospitalized.

PHYSICAL EXAMINATION AND URINALYSIS

A physical examination, including assessment of the patient's volume and hemodynamic status, is the next step in evaluating individuals with acute renal failure. Table 43–3 lists common physical findings in patients with acute renal failure. The urinalysis is an extremely important component of the physical examination when the clinician is attempting to classify the cause of renal failure into prerenal azotemia, functional acute renal failure, acute intrinsic renal failure, or obstruction. The finding of a high urinary specific gravity, in the absence of glucosuria or mannitol administration, suggests an intact urinary-concentrating mechanism and that the cause is likely prerenal azotemia or functional acute renal failure. The presence of proteinuria and hematuria indicate glomerular injury. Glucosuria, aminoaciduria, and phosphaturia are associated with acute proximal tubular dysfunction. As noted earlier, the microscopic examination of the urine also is helpful in determining the cause of acute renal failure. Benign urine sediment suggests prerenal azotemia, functional acute renal failure, or urinary obstruction. The presence of red blood cells and red blood cell casts indicates a glomerular injury. The finding of white blood cells and white blood cell casts results from interstitial inflammation (i.e., interstitial nephritis), which can be secondary to an allergic, granulomatous or infectious process.

LABORATORY DATA

A complete blood cell count with differential is essential to rule out infectious processes. Simultaneous measurement of serum and urinary chemistries is often helpful in determining the etiology of acute renal failure (Table 43–4). Calculation of the fractional excretion of sodium (FE_{Na}) from urinary and plasma creatinine and sodium concentrations can yield important information about the patient with acute renal failure:

$$FE_{Na} = (\text{excreted Na/filtered Na}) \cdot 100$$

$$= (U_{vol} \cdot U_{Na})/(GFR \cdot P_{Na}) \cdot 100$$

where

$$GFR = U_{vol} \cdot U_{Cr}/P_{Cr} \cdot \text{time}$$

Thus:

$$FE_{Na} = U_{Na} \cdot P_{Cr} \cdot 100/U_{Cr} \cdot P_{Na}$$

GFR = glomerular filtration rate; P_{Cr} = plasma creatinine; P_{Na} = plasma sodium; time = the time period over which the urine is collected; U_{Cr} = urine creatinine; U_{Na} = urine sodium; U_{vol} = urine volume

The fractional excretion of sodium has clinical utility in differentiating prerenal azotemia and functional acute renal failure from acute intrinsic renal failure. A low urinary sodium concentration and low fractional excretion of sodium (<1%) in a patient with oliguria suggest that there is stimulation of the sodium retentive mechanisms in the kidney and that tubular function is intact. These findings are

TABLE 43–3. Physical Examination Findings in Acute Renal Failure

Physical Examination Finding	Clinical Implication If Present	Possible Diagnoses	Category of Acute Renal Failure	Possible Confounding Factors
Vital signs				
Orthostatic hypotension	Intravascular volume status	Volume depletion	Prerenal azotemia	Antihypertensive therapy Neuropathies (diabetes mellitus)
Skin				
Tenting	Volume status	Volume depletion	Prerenal azotemia	Advanced age
Rash	Allergic reaction	Hypersensitivity reaction	Acute interstitial nephritis	Contact dermatitis
Petechiae	Platelet dysfunction	Thrombotic thrombocytopenic purpura Hemolytic uremic syndrome Sepsis	Acute intrinsic renal failure—vasculitis	Bone marrow suppression Antiplatelet drugs
Splinter hemorrhages Janeway lesions Osler's nodes	Embolic phenomenon	Endocarditis	Acute intrinsic renal failure—acute glomerulonephritis	Small vessel vasculitis
Edema	Volume status	Total body volume overload	Suggests prerenal azotemia unlikely	Right heart failure, deep venous thrombosis
HEENT				
Hollenhorst plaque	Embolic phenomenon	Cholesterol emboli	Acute intrinsic renal failure—vascular	Plaque must be in aorta to affect kidney
Roth spots	Embolic phenomenon	Endocarditis	Acute intrinsic renal failure—acute glomerulonephritis	Other systemic infection
Heart				
S_3 heart sound	Left ventricular function	Congestive heart failure	Prerenal azotemia	Preexisting compensated congestive heart failure
New murmur (particularly diastolic murmurs)	Valvular function	Endocarditis	Acute intrinsic renal failure—acute glomerulonephritis	Preexisting valvular disease Hyperdynamic state
Lung				
Rales	Pulmonary congestion	Pulmonary edema with volume overload or left ventricular dysfunction	Suggests prerenal azotemia unlikely	Compensated CHF
Abdomen				
Renal artery bruit	Arterial integrity	Renal artery stenosis	Prerenal azotemia	Generalized atherosclerosis
Ascites	Elevated venous pressure	Liver failure or right heart failure	Prerenal azotemia Hepatorenal syndrome	Peritoneal membrane disorder (tumor)
Bladder distention	Bladder capacity	Bladder outlet obstruction	Postobstruction renal failure	
GU				
Prostatic enlargement	Prostate size	Prostatic hypertrophy or cancer	Postobstruction renal failure	Nonenlarged prostate dose not exclude obstruction
GYN				
Abnormal bimanual examination	Uterine size Cervical status	Possible bilateral ureteral obstruction or cervical cancer	Postobstruction renal failure	

A variety of physical examination findings may be found in patients with acute renal failure. The first column lists the physical finding, whereas the second column is the clinical implications if these abnormal findings are present. Columns 3 and 4 list the possible diagnoses and category of acute renal failure that is likely to be present. Possible confounding factors that could also explain the physical examination findings are listed in the final column.
CHF = Congestive heart failure.

most characteristic of prerenal azotemia or functional acute renal failure. Similarly, a fractional excretion of sodium exceeding 1% to 2% suggests acute intrinsic renal failure. However, there are a number of causes of acute intrinsic renal failure that are, at least early on, associated with a low fractional excretion of sodium (e.g., contrast nephropathy, myoglobinuria, interstitial nephritis). Diuretic use can limit the diagnostic utility of the fractional excretion of sodium calculation by increasing natriuresis even in hypovolemic patients.

A finding of highly concentrated urine (>500 mOsm/L) suggests stimulation of antidiuretic hormone indicating prerenal azotemia secondary to either hypovolemia or a decrease in effective blood volume. Under these conditions, the urine creatinine to serum creatinine ratio usually exceeds 40. On occasion, some patients may develop an extremely high BUN concentration, while the serum creatinine remains only mildly elevated. In these instances, measurement of the urinary urea nitrogen will enable the clinician to determine whether

TABLE 43–4. Diagnostic Parameters for Differentiating Causes of Acute Renal Failure

Laboratory Test	Prerenal Azotemia	Acute Intrinsic Renal Eailure	Postrenal Obstruction
Urine sediment	Normal	Casts, cellular debris	Cellular debris
Urinary RBC	None	2–4+	Variable
Urinary WBC	None	2–4+	1+
Urine sodium	<20	>40	>40
FE_{Na} (%)	<1	>1–2	Variable
Urine/serum osmolality	>1.5	<1.3	<1.5
Urine/serum creatinine	>40:1	<20:1	<20:1
BUN/S_{cr}	>20	15	15

Common laboratory tests are used to classify the cause of acute renal failure. Functional acute renal failure, which is not included in this table, would have laboratory values similar to those seen in prerenal azotemia. However, the urine osmolality to plasma osmolality ratios may not exceed 1.5 depending on the circulating levels of antidiuretic hormone. The laboratory results listed under acute intrinsic renal failure are those seen in acute tubular necrosis, the most common cause of acute intrinsic renal failure.
RBC = red blood cell; WBC = white blood cell.

the elevated BUN concentration is secondary to the underexcretion of urea nitrogen or to the overproduction of urea nitrogen. A critically ill patient produces approximately 18–19 g of urea nitrogen per day. Excretion of urinary urea nitrogen loads substantially less than that suggests acute renal failure. Excretion of substantially more than that suggests overproduction of urea as the cause for the increased blood urea nitrogen concentration, as might occur with gastrointestinal tract bleeding or excessive protein administration.

DIAGNOSTIC PROCEDURES

Renal ultrasound is rarely helpful in determining the cause of acute renal failure in a hospitalized patient who previously had normal renal function. Insertion of a urinary catheter into the patient's bladder is usually adequate to exclude postrenal obstruction as the cause of acute renal failure. However, for the outpatient who presents with renal failure, the renal ultrasound is instrumental in determining whether the renal failure is acute or chronic and whether or not obstruction is present. A plain film radiograph of the abdomen may be useful in documenting the presence of two kidneys and in checking for renal stones. If the possibility of renal artery obstruction exists, a radioisotope scan or renal angiography may be required. Intravenous pyelography is rarely used in the diagnostic workup of acute renal failure. Cystoscopy with retrograde pyelography may be helpful if the possibility of obstruction exists. This last procedure may be necessary in a patient with the history of a single functioning kidney even if the ultrasound does not demonstrate hydronephrosis. If, despite a careful history, physical examination, and the above diagnostic tests, the etiology of the acute renal failure is unclear, a percutaneous renal biopsy may be indicated. Renal biopsy is not without risk (primarily bleeding) and should only be performed in cases in which the cause of acute renal failure is not evident. In this setting, renal biopsies are useful in determining the cause in greater than 90% of patients.[26]

CLINICAL COURSE AND PROGNOSIS

The clinical course and prognos has been for patients with acute renal failure depends on a number of clinical variables including: (a) the etiology of acute renal failure; (b) the presence of comorbidities; (c) the amount of urine produced by the patient; and (d) whether the patient requires renal replacement therapy.

ETIOLOGY

The etiology of acute renal failure has a major influence on the eventual patient outcome. If the cause of the acute renal failure is determined early and is reversible, the clinical course can be quite short. Hospitalized patients who develop acute renal failure secondary to obstruction (e.g., an improperly placed urinary catheter) rapidly recover renal function following relief of the obstruction. Similarly, if indinavir crystalluria is suspected, prompt discontinuation of the drug and vigorous hydration promptly reverses the nephrotoxicity.[22] Prerenal azotemia, if identified early and treated with aggressive hydration, likewise quickly resolves. Individuals who develop functional acute renal failure recover renal function once the effects of the offending agents resolve. However, the most common cause of acute renal failure in the hospitalized patient is acute tubular necrosis, and its clinical course is quite variable.

The clinical course of acute tubular necrosis has been divided into three distinct phases: an oliguric phase, a diuretic phase, and a recovery phase. The utility of this approach is questionable because recovery from acute tubular necrosis does not begin at a defined time from onset of renal failure. Rather, recovery from acute tubular necrosis occurs 10 to 14 days after the last insult to the kidney. Critically ill patients with acute renal failure often have recurring episodes of hypoxia and hypotension, and are treated with many nephrotoxins that may delay the recovery process. Furthermore, the autoregulation of renal blood flow is deranged in acute renal failure.[14] Renal vasoconstriction results in continued reduced blood flow to the nephron even after the insult to the kidneys is removed and the tubules begin recovering from the acute injury.[27] Actual improvements in GFR are not manifested until tubular cell necrosis is repaired and renal blood flow is normalized.

COMORBIDITY

Patients with acute renal failure who have an increase in their serum creatinine of less than 1–2 mg/dL have an excellent renal prognosis.[2] Their eventual outcome is almost entirely dependent on their associated illnesses and the procedures performed on them (e.g., cardiac catheterization, surgery). Retrospective analyses suggest that these patients have increased mortality rates as compared to those patients that do not have an increase in their creatinine during their hospitalization. However, it is unclear whether this is a cause and effect phenomenon or a selection bias.

The outcome of the patient with acute renal failure is also largely dependent on their comorbid conditions. Liver disease that accompanies acute renal failure is associated with a much higher mortality rate in critically ill patients.[6] Other comorbidities associated with higher mortality rates in patients with acute renal failure include hypoalbuminemia, need for mechanical ventilation, presence of heart failure, and advanced age.[10,26]

Acute renal failure itself has an impact on patient outcome.[28] Patients who receive radiocontrast dye and who develop acute renal failure in the course of their hospitalization, have a mortality rate that is 6.5 times higher than patients who receive dye and do not develop acute renal failure.[9] This higher mortality rate is not wholly explained by differences in comorbidities; consequently, one can conclude that acute renal failure itself contributes to the death of the patient and/or alters the response to other severe illnesses that often result in the death of the patient.

URINE OUTPUT

The presence or absence of oliguria has been suggested to be an independent predictor of eventual patient outcome. Reports of mortality in patients with acute renal failure consistently find that individuals with nonoliguria have significantly higher survival rates than individuals who develop oliguria or anuria.[5] This improved outcome may be partly a result of selection bias, in that patients developing nonoliguric renal failure frequently have more reversible renal insults such as obstruction or prerenal azotemia. Similarly, nonoliguria may be reflective of less kidney damage than what is seen in oliguria. However, the continued ability of the kidney to control volume homeostasis, even in the absence of solute control, may delay the need for renal replacement therapy and its associated risks.

NEED FOR RENAL REPLACEMENT THERAPY

Individuals who require renal replacement therapy for their acute renal failure tend to have a more complicated clinical course and a higher mortality rate.[5] Again, this might be a selection bias, as severe sequelae arising from acute renal failure requiring renal replacement therapy are found in sicker patients. However, the use of renal replacement therapy may delay the recovery of renal function by a variety of mechanisms. Intermittent periods of systemic hypotension associated with hemodialysis may delay the recovery of renal function because this may lead to hypoperfusion of the remaining nephrons and thereby further renal injury.[14] The plastic blood tubing and the composition of the hemodialysis or hemofiltration membrane may activate endogenous inflammatory mediators, which may promote catabolism and enhance organ injury.[17,29] Many of these critically ill patients have coagulation disorders as part of their organ system failure. The anticoagulation required to perform renal replacement increases the risk of bleeding.[9,30] Because of these risks clinicians must carefully consider the benefit to risk ratio of each renal replacement therapy option for each patient.

▶ TREATMENT: Acute Renal Failure

DESIRED GOALS/OUTCOMES

The treatment goals for patients with acute renal failure are driven by the cause of renal failure. In some cases, the primary goals are more supportive in nature. In other cases, very rapid treatment decisions can change the course of the disease. Quantifying or estimating their ever-changing renal function (Chap. 42) is required to facilitate drug dosing and nutritional regimen adjustments, and to assess the patient's response to the therapeutic intervention. The ultimate desired outcomes for patients with acute renal failure are that they survive the insult that damaged their kidneys, experience no further nephrotoxic events, and to regain life-sustaining renal function.

GENERAL APPROACH TO THERAPY

The approach to the patient with acute renal failure is dependent on when, in relation to the course of acute renal failure, the patient is seen. In the case of evolving acute renal failure, efforts must be aimed at preventing further damage to the kidneys. In this scenario, if the offending agent or cause is quickly removed or reversed, the damage to kidney is minimized. In the case of acute tubular necrosis, this "resuscitation" therapy is essential, particularly in the trauma or postsurgery setting, where aggressive ventilation and volume resuscitation can "rescue" hypoxic tubular cells, circumventing acute tubular necrosis. Drug-induced nephrotoxicity often can be reversed if the nephrotoxin is removed. The same is true for acute renal failure that develops secondary to renal artery disease.

The therapeutic priority for those with established acute renal failure is more supportive in nature and designed to prevent further insult to the kidney. This is not always possible because the use of potentially nephrotoxic agents, such as aminoglycosides or dopamine, may be necessary in order for the patient to survive the current situation. If the patient has acute renal failure secondary to other disease states, these conditions must be treated aggressively. Because the prognosis for established acute renal failure in the ICU setting is grim, early diagnosis of cause of acute renal failure is essential.

PREVENTION OF ACUTE RENAL FAILURE—NONPHARMACOLOGIC APPROACHES

Because the presence of acute renal failure significantly increases the mortality of hospitalized patients,[9] efforts should be focused on prevention in patients at high risk. One example of this strategy is to prospectively identify the patient at risk who requires treatment with a known nephrotoxin or who needs to undergo a potentially nephrotoxic procedure. The risk factors for the development of nephrotoxicity after exposure to intravenous contrast medium[31] and to other nephrotoxins, such as aminoglycosides,[32] are well described (see Chap. 48). Common risk factors are preexisting renal or hepatic disease, diabetes mellitus, dehydration, advanced age, and concomitant treatment with other nephrotoxins. Once these patients are identified prospectively, strategies can be implemented to reduce the likelihood of nephrotoxicity. These approaches are detailed in Chap. 48.

NEPHROTOXIN AVOIDANCE

The simplest approach for the prevention of drug-induced acute renal failure is to try to utilize the least-nephrotoxic therapeutic alternatives. Examples of these techniques include initial use of acetaminophen instead of NSAID in at-risk patients with osteoarthritis,[33] and treatment of severe fungal infections with fluconazole[34] or lipid-based amphotericin B in place of the conventional amphotericin B formulation.[35] Many centers substitute low-osmolality contrast media instead of more toxic higher osmolality dyes in selected patients at high risk for nephrotoxicity. However, whether low-osmolality agents are significantly less nephrotoxic than the older high-osmolality agents, particularly in light of their tremendously higher price, has been questioned.[31]

Similarly, it may be possible to use known nephrotoxins in a manner that reduces the risk of kidney damage. When contrast media are to be used in a patient at high risk for nephrotoxicity, the smallest possible effective dose should be used. Similarly, the incidence of nephrotoxicity with once daily aminoglycoside regimens appears to be lower than that seen with traditionally aminoglycoside regimens.[36,37] Consequently, for patients without contraindications for once-daily aminoglycosides (e.g., preexisting renal disease, cystic fibrosis, endocarditis), the preferred regimen is once-daily dosing. New technologies now allow computer systems to identify patients who require dosing adjustments because of their renal function.[38] Systems such as these allow for a proactive approach to pharmacotherapy and may help to prevent the development of acute renal failure in hospitalized patients.[39]

HYDRATION

In the situation in which a nephrotoxic agent must be administered, renal-protective therapies may be used to attenuate the nephrotoxic risk. Given that dehydration is a commonly identified risk factor for the development of acute renal failure, a simple but effective technique is to ensure that the patient is not dehydrated prior to nephrotoxin administration. Volume expansion allows optimal renal perfusion and reduces tubular workload because the kidney doesn't need to vigorously concentrate the urine. This reduction in tubular stress during nephrotoxin exposure may reduce the tubule's susceptibility to damage, but this has not been conclusively demonstrated.[21]

Volume administration prior to nephrotoxin exposure also increases urine output, thereby helping to minimize the kidneys exposure to the toxin. This aspect of volume administration is commonly employed in oncology patients who receive chemotherapy. Tumor lysis syndrome results from the administration of cancer chemotherapeutic agents that destroy large numbers of cells. The intracellular contents of the lysed cells are released into the blood stream, where the kidneys eliminate many of them, including uric acid. If the amount of uric acid present in the urine exceeds the solubility of uric acid, crystals may form in the tubules and result in obstructive nephropathy. Attenuation or prevention of tumor lysis syndrome and uric acid crystal formation can be accomplished with vigorous hydration and urine alkalinization prior to cancer chemotherapy administration. Alkalinization is necessary in this regimen because the solubility of uric acid is pH dependent. The goal of alkalinization in this case is to maintain a urinary pH of greater than 6. The amount of administered sodium bicarbonate in the intravenous solution is adjusted to meet the urinary pH goal. High urinary output is also desirable in order to dilute and eliminate the uric acid from the kidneys. A typical hydration regimen to prevent uric acid crystallization is normal saline 1.5–3 L/m^2/24 h in a patient with normal renal function beginning 24 to 48 hours before the administration of chemotherapy.[40] When therapy will end depends on the chemotherapy regimen and tumor burden, and is guided by monitoring of the patient's serum uric acid concentrations.

Typically, the solution used to hydrate prior to nephrotoxin exposure is normal saline because the goal of this treatment is to expand the intravascular compartment and increase renal perfusion. Solutions such as 5% dextrose are inappropriate for this purpose because they distribute throughout the body. Colloidal solutions stay in the intravascular compartment, but are relatively expensive and not recommended as first-line agents for this purpose.[41] The rate of volume administration for the prevention of nephrotoxin-induced acute renal failure is usually 1–2 mL/kg/h started 3 to 6 hours before the nephrotoxin is administered.[42] Urine output (goal 2 mL/kg/h) is the best indicator as to whether sufficient volume is being given and adequate hydration status has been attained.

SODIUM LOADING

The use of normal saline as the volume expansion agent may yield an added benefit because of its sodium content. A technique frequently employed to mitigate the nephrotoxicity of contrast dye or amphotericin B is to "sodium load" a patient prior to giving the nephrotoxin. Sodium loading may reduce renal damage via the tubuloglomerular feedback mechanism. This regulatory mechanism for GFR is activated when the tubule senses high urine flow or an increased delivery of sodium and results in a decrease in renal blood flow, GFR, and tubular flow.[21,43] These actions may minimize the delivery of a nephrotoxin to the tubule and thus reduce the risk of tubular injury. Hydration regimens administered prior to giving nephrotoxic radiocontrast dyes or amphotericin B typically contain sodium in the form of normal saline.[45] Sodium loading and vigorous hydration are simple interventions and appear to be effective in attenuating the effects of many nephrotoxins (see Table 43–5).

TABLE 43–5. Status of Prophylactic Therapies for the Prevention of Acute Renal Failure Due to Nephrotoxin Exposure

Intervention	Evidence for Prevention of Nephrotoxicity	Situations in Which Intervention Documented to be Effective
Hydration (sodium loading)	Y	Prior to amphotericin or contrast dye administration; tumor lysis syndrome prevention
Mannitol	N	
Loop Diuretics	N	
Dopamine	N	
Calcium Channel Blockers	+/−	Recipient should receive drug prior to transplantation and when kidney is stored in solution containing drug. Not useful for preventing contrast dye nephropathy.
Theophylline	Y	Prior to contrast dye administration
Prostaglandin E_1	Y	Prior to contrast dye administration
Atrial Natriuretic Peptide	N	

Y = some evidence exists for benefit; +/− = evidence equivocal; N = evidence suggests no benefit

PREVENTION OF ACUTE RENAL FAILURE—PHARMACOTHERAPEUTIC ALTERNATIVES

Despite many investigations into the pharmacologic prevention of nephrotoxicity, few studies demonstrate evidence of benefit. Studies with diuretics were a natural follow up to the studies showing the benefits of sodium and volume pretreatment. In theory, the beneficial effects of diuretic therapy should include some of the benefits seen with hydration therapy, as well an increase in renal blood flow via their vasodilating effects. These potential benefits of diuretic therapy, however, may be counteracted when they result in impairment of the tubuloglomerular feedback mechanism. When this feedback loop is blocked, the delivery of nephrotoxins to the kidney may be increased, thereby increasing the risk of the patient developing acute renal failure. Mannitol, an osmotic diuretic theoretically may reduce tubular cell damage by acting as an impermeable solvent, thereby reducing cell swelling. While these theoretical benefits of diuretic therapy appear reasonable, actual documentation of their value in controlled studies is nearly nonexistent.

One of these trials compared the effectiveness of diuretic and/or saline pretreatment in the prevention of nephrotoxicity of contrast dye.[47] This prospective trial was conducted in patients with chronic renal insufficiency who were considered to be at high risk for developing contrast dye nephropathy. These authors compared hydration with 1 mL/kg/h of 0.45% saline to hydration plus either mannitol 25 g or furosemide 80 mg. All subjects received the saline infusion for 12 hours before and after angiography. The mean increase in serum creatinine 48 hours after the dye exposure was significantly higher in the diuretic groups than in the patients who received hydration alone. Similarly, no benefit was observed when furosemide was administered to patients immediately after major surgical procedures that likely would result in reduced renal perfusion.[48] The creatinine clearance in subjects who received continuous infusion furosemide was no different from patients who received placebo.

A double-blind, placebo-controlled comparison of loop diuretics and low-dose dopamine in patients with normal renal function and undergoing cardiac surgery was conducted to determine whether intraoperative drug administration would reduce the incidence of acute renal failure.[49] In this study, subjects were randomized to receive a continuous infusion of furosemide (0.5 μg/kg/min), dopamine (2 μg/kg/min), or normal saline (placebo) as the surgery started. The infusions were maintained for 48 hours or until discharge from the ICU. Subjects in the furosemide group had significantly higher increases in plasma creatinine values and were more likely to develop acute renal failure.[49] No differences in renal function between the dopamine and placebo groups were noted. As a result of this trial and previous work it is evident that diuretics do not have a beneficial effect in preventing the development of acute renal failure. Intravascular volume depletion due to excessive diuresis may in fact increase the risk of acute renal failure in patients about to receive nephrotoxic therapies.

Similarly disappointing results have been reported with other pharmacotherapeutic drug classes.[50] Calcium channel blockers were thought to possibly play a role in preventing the development of acute renal failure because they inhibit the response of the afferent arterioles of the kidney to vasoconstrictive agonists. A subsequent increase in glomerular filtration is noted because the efferent arterioles are relatively resistant to the vasodilating effects of the calcium antagonists. The interventional studies with calcium channel blockers have been equivocal. The most promise has been seen in patients receiving kidney transplants. One of these trials was a nitrendipine study with a 2-year followup period.[51] Patients receiving a kidney transplant and chronic cyclosporine therapy were randomized to receive nitrendipine 5 mg twice daily or placebo. After 24 months, patients treated with nitrendipine had significantly lower serum creatinine values than did the placebo-treated group. This drug benefit persisted even after correcting for possible differences in blood pressure. Acute renal failure prevention studies with calcium channel blockers in other clinical settings have not been nearly as successful.[50]

The adenosine antagonist theophylline has been investigated as a nephroprotective agent prior to the administration of radiocontrast dye. Early studies suggested that theophylline may provide some benefit. In a randomized trial, inulin and creatinine clearances before and after contrast dye administration were unchanged in subjects receiving theophylline (5 mg/kg) prior to the dye infusion while clearances declined significantly in the subjects receiving placebo.[52] However, these same authors performed a follow up trial in 80 vigorously hydrated patients who had preexisting renal dysfunction.[53] Subjects were randomized to receive either 810 mg of theophylline daily or placebo before the infusion of radiocontrast dye. No difference in serum creatinine or creatinine clearance was found between the two groups, although the placebo group did have higher urinary concentrations of N-acetyl-β-glucosaminidase, a marker of tubular damage.[53]

Another study examining the prevention of radiocontrast media-induced nephrotoxicity in patients with preexisting renal dysfunction randomized 60 subjects into 3 different study groups: (a) 0.45% saline infusion 1 mL/kg/h; (b) the saline infusion plus dopamine 2.5 μg/kg/min; and (c) the saline infusion plus intravenous aminophylline administered with a 4 mg/kg loading dose followed by an infusion of 0.4 mg/kg/h.[54] No differences were noted in rates of acute renal failure, need for dialysis, or length of stay.

Prostaglandin E_1 is commercially available and has cytoprotective and vasodilatory effects. Koch et al. administered varying doses of prostaglandin E_1 prior to contrast dye infusion in 130 patients with preexisting renal disease.[55] The mean elevation in serum creatinine caused by contrast dye infusion was significantly higher in the saline-treated subjects as compared with subjects receiving prostaglandin E_1. This is a promising study, particularly because the control arm of the study used hydration with saline, the one therapy that is effective in preventing the development of acute renal failure. However, confirmatory studies are needed before this becomes an accepted preventative measure. Overall, few pharmacologic therapies show much utility in the prevention of acute renal failure. Given the poor prognosis of hospital-acquired acute renal failure, prevention is key. Further studies need to clarify the role of pharmacologic preventative therapy. Until effective preventative drug therapy is found, it appears that adequate hydration with saline is the most appropriate therapy.

ESTABLISHED ACUTE RENAL FAILURE

DESIRED GOALS/OUTCOMES

In patients with established acute renal failure, the goals of therapy are to remove the primary cause of the acute renal failure, to limit further nephrotoxic exposures/events, and to speed up the recovery of renal function. Unfortunately, studies to date show that little can be done with contemporary therapy to hasten renal recovery (Table 43–6). Consequently, therapeutic measures should be supportive in nature. The first goal is to limit future nephrotoxic events until the kidney can recover on its own. Second, efforts must be aimed toward reducing the sequelae that are associated with acute renal failure, mainly volume overload, electrolyte disorders, and elevated BUN

TABLE 43–6. Outcomes of Therapies for the Treatment of Established Acute Renal Failure[54]

Intervention	Improved Renal Function	Improved Azotemia	Improved Mortality
Mannitol	N	+/−	U
Loop diuretics	N	N	N
Dopamine	+/−	+/−	N
Calcium channel blockers	+/−	+/−	N
Atrial natriuretic peptide	+/−	+/−	N
Intensive dialysis	U	N	N
Early dialysis	U	Y	Y
Biocompatible hemodialyzer or hemofilter	U	Y	Y
Insulin-like growth factor I	N	+/−	N

Y = some evidence exists for benefit; +/− = evidence equivocal; N = evidence suggests no benefit; U = unknown

concentration. These therapy goals are accomplished primarily by pharmacologic and renal replacement therapies (Fig. 43–2).

NONPHARMACOLOGIC APPROACHES

VOLUME CONTROL

Probably the most important parameter in acute renal failure is knowledge of the patient's volume status. In the patient with oliguric prerenal azotemia, rapid fluid resuscitation can improve renal perfusion and rescue hypoxic tubules, preventing or ameliorating acute tubular necrosis. However, this same maneuver in a patient with established oliguric acute tubular necrosis would be harmful, resulting in a fluid-overloaded patient. Fluid removal from the volume-overloaded patient needs to be measured in terms of net volume loss rather than in terms of urine output. If the volume given to the patient exceeds urine output, volume overload will worsen despite meeting urine output goals. Sources of excess exogenous fluids that can be minimized in fluid-overloaded patients include reducing the volume of fluid used to administer intravenous medications, reassessing the need for and rate of "keep-open" intravenous solutions, and using concentrated sources

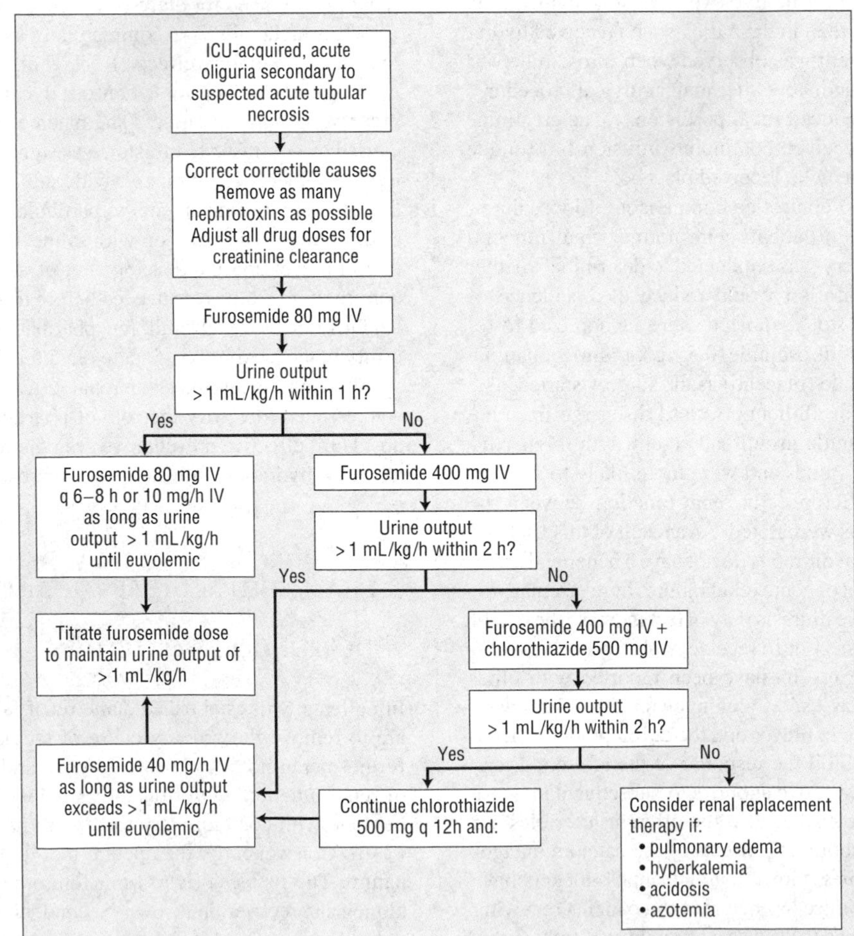

FIGURE 43–2. Treatment algorithm for ICU-acquired oliguric acute renal failure as the result of tubular necrosis.

of enteral and parenteral feedings. Maintenance of euvolemia, tissue perfusion, and electrolyte balance should be the goals of this supportive therapy.

NEPHROTOXIN AVOIDANCE

Exposure to nephrotoxins has been identified as a risk factor for acute renal failure in nearly every epidemiologic study. Avoidance of subsequent nephrotoxic therapies and procedures are essential aspects of the management of patients with established acute renal failure, as well as of the management of those at risk for the development of acute renal failure.[14] Recovery from acute ischemic renal disease usually requires 14 to 21 days from the most recent insult to the kidney, not necessarily the first insult to the kidney. Consequently, repeated exposure to nephrotoxins such as contrast dye, aminoglycosides, NSAIDs, vasoconstrictive agents (e.g., high-dose dopamine, norepinephrine), and others may prolong the duration of acute renal failure. Vasoconstrictors, unfortunately, are often necessary to maintain adequate blood pressure in critically ill patients with acute renal failure. In a prospective report on the outcomes of patients with acute renal failure in Australian ICUs, it was found that 51.7% of patients required epinephrine, 55.1% required norepinephrine, 49.1% required dopamine, and 18.1% required other inotropes.[6] In this report, no difference was noted in the survival rate between patients who did or did not receive these vasoactive substances, but this has been refuted by others who have found that mortality rates were higher in patients requiring catecholamines.[12] This probably is a selection bias, as vasoactive agents are likely to be prescribed for the most critically ill patients.

Judicious use of these agents after carefully considering the risks, benefits, and alternatives is important. Knowledge of the actual nephrotoxic risk of each agent is essential. For example, vancomycin is erroneously considered to be a highly nephrotoxic agent. Much of this nephrotoxic reputation stems from the early formulations of the drug; consequently, clinicians should not avoid its use when it is the most appropriate agent to use for an infection. In other situations, appropriate, less nephrotoxic alternatives can be chosen. Examples include using fluconazole or lipid-based amphotericin B in place of conventional amphotericin B formulations, or using imipenem or third-generation cephalosporins instead of aminoglycosides for susceptible organisms. In many cases, no alternative exists, but all options should be explored before choosing one of these potentially nephrotoxic agents. If they are to be used, careful dosing and close monitoring of serum concentrations, where appropriate, is imperative.

PHARMACOLOGIC ALTERNATIVES

DIURETICS

Nonoliguric acute renal failure is associated with a significantly better prognosis than oliguric acute renal failure.[56] It is unclear whether patients with nonoliguric acute renal failure have less extensive damage to their kidneys or if something is intrinsically therapeutic about having increased urine flow. Nonoliguric patients are often less critically ill than their oliguric counterparts.[56] It is important to remember that the finding of improved survival with nonoliguria does not mean that increasing the urine output to nonoliguria levels with diuretics will improve the oliguric patient's eventual outcome.[57] Nonetheless, diuretics can simplify fluid management in acute renal failure patients by increasing urine output[56,58] and are a mainstay of therapy.[59]

In addition to their diuretic effect, many diuretics have other pharmacologic effects that might be beneficial for the patient with acute renal failure. Tubular obstruction from cellular debris is often associated with vasoconstriction and a reduced GFR that may exacerbate acute renal failure. Because diuretics increase tubule fluid flow, they may prevent tubular obstruction. Loop diuretics increase renal blood flow via their vasodilating effects, a feature that may be beneficial, although clinical studies have not demonstrated this.

Even though diuretics have not been shown to accelerate acute renal failure recovery, most patients with established acute renal failure receive them to augment fluid management. Advantages of increased urine output include easier management of fluid and electrolyte balance, the ability to administer adequate nutrition, reduced risk of developing pulmonary edema, and the reduced need for renal replacement therapy. Fluid overload can be difficult to treat with renal replacement therapy, especially in critically ill patients. Consequently, maximizing urine output is a key objective.

Because maintenance of urine output that results in net fluid loss for the fluid-overloaded patient is a primary therapeutic goal, optimization of diuretic therapy is an important consideration. Typically, either mannitol or loop diuretics are used as first-line agents. The choice between these two therapies is not clear-cut because both have distinct advantages and disadvantages. Both diuretic classes have a long history of safety, and most clinicians are familiar with them. Mannitol, an osmotic diuretic, can only be given parenterally and a typical starting dose is 12.5–25 g of a 20% solution infused intravenously over 3 to 5 minutes. It has almost no nonrenal clearance, so when given to a patient making little urine, it remains in the patient, and in some patients may cause a hyperosmolar state. Additionally, mannitol may cause acute renal failure itself, so its use in acute renal failure must be monitored carefully by measuring urine output and serum electrolytes and osmolality.[60] Because of these limitations, some authors recommend that mannitol be reserved for its nondiuretic uses, such as management of cerebral edema.[61]

The loop diuretics furosemide, bumetanide, torsemide, and ethacrynic acid are frequently used in established acute renal failure. Ethacrynic acid is typically reserved for patients who are allergic to sulfa compounds. Furosemide is the most commonly used loop diuretic because of its low cost, availability in oral and parenteral forms, and good safety and efficacy profiles. Because the oral bioavailability of furosemide is highly variable, initial doses (usually 40–80 mg) are usually given intravenously. Torsemide and bumetanide have better oral bioavailability than furosemide. Torsemide is documented as having an oral bioavailability of 80% to 100% in patients with congestive heart failure, a patient population known to have poor oral furosemide absorption.[62] Torsemide has a longer duration of activity than the other loop diuretics, which allows for less frequent administration but also may make it more difficult to titrate the dose. Loop diuretics should all work equally well in a given patient, provided that they are administered in equipotent parenteral doses so that bioavailability issues are obviated.

Continuous infusion of loop diuretics appears to be more effective than traditional intermittent dosing regimens. Natriuresis is greater when equal doses of loop diuretics are given as a continuous infusion.[63] Furthermore, adverse reactions from loop diuretics (myalgias and hearing loss) occur less frequently in patients receiving continuous infusion as compared to intermittent boluses, ostensibly because lower serum concentrations are attained. However, these adverse effects still may occur with continuous infusion of loop diuretics; thus, patients should be prospectively monitored.[64] The finding that the continuous infusions of loop diuretics have efficacy that is at least as good as intermittent bolus dosing, with less adverse effects, appears to be true for furosemide,[65] bumetanide,[66] and torsemide.[67] When continuous infusion is to be used, an initial loading dose is given (equivalent to furosemide 40–80 mg) prior to the initiation of the continuous infusion at a dose of 10–20 mg/h of furosemide or its equivalent. Patients with low creatinine clearances have much lower rates of diuretic secretion into the tubular fluid; consequently, higher doses are generally used in patients with renal insufficiency.[61]

One drawback of the continuous infusion loop diuretic literature is that few carefully controlled trials in patients with acute renal failure have been conducted. Schuller et al.[65] published the first comparison of continuous infusion and intermittent bolus furosemide in 33 fluid-overloaded patients with chronic renal insufficiency and acute renal failure. The protocol used in this study excluded the use of other diuretics. These investigators found no difference in patient outcome or volume removal rates between the two groups, but the study lacked sufficient statistical power to demonstrate even a 15% difference in fluid loss. Despite the paucity of evidence for diuretic use in this population, many clinicians continue to recommend their use, if for no other reason than increased urine output allows for easier patient management.[56,57,59]

Diuretic Resistance

Diuretic resistance is commonly encountered in acute renal failure patients, especially in those with excessive sodium intake (Table 43–7). Patients with acute tubular necrosis have a reduced number of functioning nephrons on which the diuretic may exert its action. Still other patients may have reduced bioavailability of oral furosemide. Table 43–7 presents possible therapeutic options to counteract each form of diuretic resistance. Combination therapy with loop diuretics plus a diuretic from a different pharmacologic class can be an effective tool in the setting of acute renal failure.[68] Loop diuretics increase the delivery of sodium chloride to the distal convoluted tubule and collecting duct. With time, these areas of the nephron compensate for the activity of the loop diuretic and increase sodium and chloride reabsorption. Diuretics that work at the distal convoluted tubule (thiazides) or the collecting duct (amiloride, triamterene, and spironolactone) may have a synergistic effect when administered with loop diuretics by blocking the compensatory increase in sodium and chloride reabsorption. The combination of loop diuretics and usual doses of thiazide diuretics may be effective in renal disease despite the accumulation of endogenous organic acids in renal disease that block the transport of loop diuretics into the lumen. If oral thiazides cannot be given to the patient, chlorothiazide can be administered parenterally.

Several drug combinations with loop diuretics have been investigated, including the addition of one or more of the following; theophylline, acetazolamide, spironolactone, thiazides, or metolazone.[68] Of these combinations, metolazone is used most frequently with furosemide. Metolazone, unlike other thiazides, produces effective diuresis at a GFR below 20 mL/min. This combination of metolazone and a loop diuretic has been used successfully in the management of fluid overload in patients with congestive heart failure, cirrhosis, and nephrotic syndrome. Additionally, this combination is efficacious in both pediatric patients and adults.[69] The combination of mannitol plus intravenous loop diuretics are used by some practitioners,[56,58] but no convincing evidence of the superiority of this combination regimen to conventional dosing of either diuretic alone exists.

DOPAMINE

The use of dopamine in patients with acute renal failure may be the most controversial therapeutic issue in the intensive care unit. Low-doses (0.5–2 μg/kg/min) of dopamine selectively dilate the renal vasculature and theoretically should result in increased renal blood flow and GFR. At higher doses, the selectivity for the dopamine-1 receptor is lost, as dopamine begins to bind to β- and α-adrenergic receptors, which should result in renal vasoconstriction and a reduction in GFR. Many clinicians attempt to take advantage of this pharmacologic finding by infusing low-dose dopamine in patients with acute renal failure.

Most published studies of low-dose dopamine show that urine output is increased in patients with established acute renal failure.[70]

TABLE 43–7. Common Causes of Diuretic Resistance in Patients With Acute Renal Failure and the Measures Used to Counteract Them

Causes of Diuretic Resistance	Potential Therapeutic Solutions
Excessive sodium intake (sources may be dietary, IV fluids, and drugs)	Remove sodium from nutritional sources and medications
Inadequate diuretic dose or inappropriate regimen	Increase dose, use continuous infusion, or combination therapy
Reduced oral bioavailability (usually furosemide)	Use parenteral therapy; switch to oral torsemide or bumetanide
Nephrotic syndrome	Increase dose, switch diuretics, use combination therapy
Reduced renal blood flow	
Drugs (NSAID, ACE inhibitors, vasodilators)	Discontinue these drugs if possible
Hypotension	Volume and/or vasopressors
Intravascular depletion	Intravascular volume expansion
Increased sodium reabsorption	
Nephron adaptation to chronic diuretic therapy	Combination diuretic therapy, sodium restriction
NSAID use	Discontinue NSAID
Congestive heart failure (CHF)	Treat the CHF, increase diuretic dose, switch to more bioavailable loop diuretic
Cirrhosis	High volume paracentesis
Acute tubular necrosis	Higher dose of diuretic, diuretic combination therapy, add low-dose dopamine

However, dopamine-induced increases in urine formation have not been shown to translate into meaningful improvements in creatinine clearance in acute renal failure patients. Indeed, most investigations of low-dose dopamine in established acute renal failure have found that dopamine is either of no consequence or it is harmful.[73] The placebo arm of the multicenter Auriculin Anaritide Acute Renal Failure Study contained 256 patients who were randomized to the non-Auriculin anaritide arm of the trial.[74] The study's purpose was to evaluate the effect of atrial natriuretic peptide (ANP) on the need for dialysis and mortality in patients with acute tubular necrosis. However in the placebo arm of the trial, the investigators examined the effect that dopamine had on these same factors. At the discretion of the physician, approximately one-third of these 256 subjects received no dopamine, another third received low-dose dopamine (<3 μg/kg/min), and the final third received high-dose dopamine (>3 μg/kg/min). Not surprisingly, sicker patients were more likely to receive dopamine. However, when the authors statistically corrected for selection bias and confounding variables, they reported no significant differences in relative risks of death or need for dialysis between any of the treatment arms. Faced with these findings, these authors called for an end to the routine use of low-dose dopamine in acute renal failure until a prospective, randomized, placebo-controlled trial demonstrated efficacy and safety of the therapy.[74]

The NORASEPT II Study was a multicenter, placebo-controlled trial investigating the activity of a monoclonal antibody to human tumor necrosis factor-α in septic shock.[75] Oliguria was present in 395 of the study subjects. Low-dose dopamine was used in 44% of these subjects, high-dose dopamine was used in 32%, and no dopamine was used in the remaining 24% of study subjects. Similar to the findings of the Auriculin Anaritide Acute Renal Failure Study, no differences were observed in the eventual need for dialysis, incidence of acute renal failure, or 28-day survival.

The results of these studies indicate that the use of dopamine in established acute renal failure has no bearing on patient outcome. However, there may be toxicity associated with even low doses of dopamine, primarily cardiac dysrhythmias and local effects associated with extravasation.[73] Furthermore, low doses of dopamine (2.5 μg/kg/min) have been documented to decrease serum prolactin concentrations by 80% in critically ill oliguric patients.[76] Prolactin is an immunomodulatory hormone involved in the endocrine response to stress. A reduction in prolactin concentrations may suppress cellular immunity and increase the risk of infectious complications in acute renal failure patients. It appears that low-dose dopamine can increase urine output, but it should be used cautiously as it does not improve patient outcome.[70,73]

Ichai et al. recently found that dopamine infusions of 3 μg/kg/min increased fractional excretion of sodium, urine output, and creatinine clearance as compared to a placebo infusion in hemodynamically stable critically ill patients.[71] The increase in diuresis and creatinine clearance was maintained as long as the 48-hour dopamine infusion was maintained; however, the subjects in this study did not have acute renal failure. The mean creatinine clearance of subjects prior to study entry was 67 mL/min. Only one report using low-dose dopamine has shown improvement in patients with stable chronic renal insufficiency and congestive heart failure.[72] In established acute renal failure, low-dose dopamine has been used in conjunction with continuous infusions of loop diuretics and mannitol.[58] This combination may hasten recovery from acute renal failure, but this study lacked a control group using hydration alone. Given that adequate hydration appears to be the best preventative therapy and that the results of this trial are not consistent with most others, combination of diuretics and dopamine as routine therapy for the treatment of established acute renal failure cannot be recommended.

OTHER VASOACTIVE AGENTS

Dobutamine infusions (175 μg/min), unlike low-dose dopamine, are reported to improve creatinine clearance without increasing urine output in critically ill patients with stable creatinine clearances of about 70–80 mL/min.[77] The 18-mL/min increase in creatinine clearance observed in this study was statistically significant as compared to placebo, but probably of little clinical importance in these patients with relatively normal baseline renal function. The mechanism for the improved creatinine clearance appears to be the result of increased cardiac output and renal blood flow because dobutamine does not possess direct effects on the renal vasculature. The effects of dobutamine in patients with oliguric acute renal failure have not been studied.

Fenoldopam is a selective dopamine-1 receptor agonist that causes renal arteriolar vasodilation and natriuresis. Unlike dopamine, however, it does not have α-adrenergic, β-adrenergic, or dopamine-2 activity. In a study of normal volunteers, fenoldopam increased renal blood flow and maintained glomerular filtration rate without adversely affecting systemic blood pressure.[78] Whether these affects will occur in patients with acute renal failure is unknown. Further studies are needed to determine whether fenoldopam has a role in the prevention or treatment of acute renal failure.

EXPERIMENTAL THERAPIES

Our understanding of the pathogenesis of acute renal failure is in its infancy. Most pharmacologic therapies that have been used to either prevent or treat established acute renal failure have been unsuccessful.[16] ANP is one of the latest experimental agents to be studied to pharmacologically improve ischemic acute renal failure patient outcome with somewhat disappointing results.[79] In this trial, overall dialysis-free survival was not different between ANP and placebo-treated patients. Nonoliguric patients actually fared significantly worse if they received ANP instead of placebo. Subgroup analysis of oliguric patients also failed to show a mortality benefit of ANP.[80] Similar studies conducted in Europe also found that the ANP, urodilatin conferred no benefit in patients with acute renal failure treated either with diuretics and low-dose dopamine[81] or with other conventional therapies.[82]

Insulin-like growth factor I appeared to have promise as a preventative therapy for acute renal failure in animals.[83] Increases in GFR are probably mediated through effects on nitric oxide and prostaglandins. These findings prompted a placebo-controlled, multicenter trial using recombinant human insulin-like growth factor I in patients with established acute renal failure.[84] Similar to the findings of other experimental therapies in this population, recombinant human insulin-like growth factor I conferred no advantage to these patients and did not accelerate recovery of renal function. Platelet-activating factor is another inflammation mediator that might be linked to the pathogenesis of acute renal failure.[85] Studies are planned to investigate whether manipulating this mediator might influence the course of acute renal failure.

The development of new renal replacement techniques, and our expanding understanding of the mediators of ischemic acute renal failure will hopefully lead to therapies that can alter its natural course.[14] Therapies directed toward altering the apoptotic pathways that are activated in acute renal failure may result in improved outcomes.[15] Similarly, modifications in the renal replacement therapies used in the these patients may yield a breakthrough.[86]

COMPLICATIONS OF ACUTE RENAL FAILURE

INFECTION

The most common cause of death in patients with acute renal failure is infection.[87] Interestingly, sepsis itself is a very common cause of acute renal failure.[6] Acute renal failure contributes somewhat to the high infection rate by altering leukocyte function and cell-mediated immunity. Other aspects in the care of the patient with acute renal failure can lead to infection. Renal replacement therapy necessitates indwelling vascular or peritoneal access, which can serve as a focus of infection; these sites should be monitored routinely for erythema or purulent drainage. Indwelling urinary catheters also predispose patients with acute renal failure to infection. Therefore, they should be used for no longer than necessary, but in many instances, their use cannot be avoided. Frequent evaluation of urine for signs of infection is warranted.

The comorbidities found in patients with acute renal failure may also play an important role in the development of infection. Concomitant cardiopulmonary failure requiring mechanical ventilation increases the risk of pneumonia. High-dose vasopressor therapy results in reduced blood flow to the gastrointestinal (GI) tract, which may cause ischemia and introduction of gut flora to the bloodstream. The management of a patient with acute renal failure requires (a) prevention of infection where possible; (b) a high index of suspicion in the recognition of infection; and (c) aggressive antibiotic therapy that has been appropriately adjusted for renal disease and renal replacement therapy.

CARDIOVASCULAR

Patients with acute renal failure often have hypertension, intermittent hypotension, heart failure, pericarditis, arrhythmias, and pulmonary edema. The causes of cardiovascular complications in these patients include electrolyte disturbances, impaired acid-base balance, uremia, and volume overload. Volume overload may cause hypertension, which may be best treated with diuretics and renal replacement therapy. Aggressive renal replacement therapy can also alleviate uremic pericarditis and electrolyte and acid-base disorders. Swan-Ganz pressure and clinical monitoring will give an accurate assessment of the patient's volume status, which can be helpful in determining fluid replacement needs.

GASTROINTESTINAL

Critically ill patients with acute renal failure have long been recognized to be at increased risk for GI bleeding. Hypotension, the use of vasoconstrictive agents, and the high catabolic state seen in acute renal failure can contribute to stress ulceration in these patients. The uremic state also may induce bleeding by causing a defect in platelet function. Patients with acute renal failure and additional risk factors for stress-related hemorrhage (e.g., respiratory failure or high-dose corticosteroid use) are at an even higher risk for bleeding. In one series, subjects with acute renal failure were seven times more likely to have a GI bleed than a matched control group.[9] Other common GI complaints in patients with acute renal failure include nausea and vomiting.

NEUROLOGIC

Altered mentation, myoclonus, and lethargy can occur in the setting of acute renal failure. Although these signs/symptoms in the patient with acute renal failure may be caused by extremely elevated BUN, calcium, magnesium, phosphate, and sodium disorders may also cause them. Adverse effects from improperly dosed renally eliminated drugs (such as β-lactam antibiotics, imipenem, histamine-2 blockers) can also manifest as seizures or somnolence. Because acute renal failure often has a sudden onset, electrolyte imbalance and drug accumulation can occur rapidly in these patients. Diligent monitoring of laboratory results, renal replacement schedules, and drug dosing can help to prevent these neurologic sequelae.

RENAL REPLACEMENT THERAPY CONSIDERATIONS IN ACUTE RENAL FAILURE

Renal replacement therapy is not used in all patients presenting with acute renal failure. The usual indications for renal replacement therapy in acute renal failure patients differ somewhat from what they are in patients with end-stage renal disease (ESRD) (Table 43–8; see Chap. 47 for ESRD renal replacement options). Until recently, the patient with acute renal failure who required renal replacement therapy was likely to be treated nearly the same as the patient with ESRD. Most patients with ESRD can be managed with a standard thrice-weekly, 4-hour hemodialysis schedule. In contrast, the patient with acute renal failure who is sick enough to require renal replacement therapy is typically an unstable patient in terms of volume, electrolyte, and BUN control. These patients are not at steady state and are less likely to achieve treatment goals with a standard thrice-weekly dialysis schedule.[88] It is only recently that the nephrology community has begun to earnestly draw a distinction between the renal replacement needs of acute renal failure patients and patients with ESRD.[86]

Mathematical models derived from actual protein catabolic rates measured in patients with acute renal failure have demonstrated that the renal replacement needs for these patients are greater than the needs of their ESRD counterparts.[88] Considerably more renal replacement therapy is required to maintain the prehemodialysis BUN <100 mg/dL in acute renal failure patients than in stable ESRD patients. The higher protein catabolic rate in acute renal failure is the main reason more-intensive therapy is needed. It is not unusual for critically ill patients with acute renal failure to require 4-hour hemodialysis sessions 5 to 7 times per week to maintain the prehemodialysis BUN <100 mg/dL.[88]

Two consequences of this increased need for renal replacement therapy are detailed below. First, relatively new renal replacement techniques, such as continuous hemofiltration and hemodiafiltration, have been developed to meet the needs of hypercatabolic patients and are now commonplace in the ICU. These therapies provide new

TABLE 43–8. The AEIOUs That Describe the Indications for Renal Replacement Therapy

	Indication for Renal Replacement Therapy	Clinical Setting
A	**A**cid-base abnormalities	Metabolic acidosis resulting from the accumulation of organic and inorganic acids
E	**E**lectrolyte imbalance	Hyperkalemia, hypermagnesemia
I	**I**ntoxications	Salicylates, lithium, methanol, ethylene glycol, theophylline, phenobarbital
O	fluid **O**verload	Postoperative fluid gain
U	**U**remia	High catabolism of acute renal failure

challenges in delivering effective pharmacotherapy, particularly in terms of nutritional therapy and in compounding ultrafiltrate replacement solutions. Second, the optimal dosage requirement for the medications prescribed for patients receiving renal replacement therapies that are either relatively new (continuous therapies) or being used in new ways (daily intermittent hemodialysis) are poorly defined. For example, most published dosing recommendations for hemodialysis were derived for patients receiving thrice weekly hemodialysis (see Chap. 50). New dialysis regimens designed to provide adequate azotemic control in acute renal failure[20] likely would require the development of new drug-dosing recommendations.

INTERMITTENT THERAPIES

Renal replacement options for acute renal failure can be divided into two main categories: intermittent and continuous therapies (Table 43–9). Intermittent dialysis remains the most commonly used renal replacement therapy in the United States.[89] Advantages of intermittent therapies are that they are technically simple, the dialysis machines are available at most institutions, and nephrologists and their staff typically have expertise using them.

Intermittent hemodialysis with conventional dialyzers is primarily diffusion based; consequently, it is very efficient in removing solutes of low-molecular-weight (<500 daltons) such as urea, creatinine, most electrolytes, and many drugs. Because diffusional solute removal is so dependent on molecular size and the relative pore size of the dialysis filter, conventional hemodialysis is not very effective in removing solutes of larger molecular weight (e.g., low-molecular-weight proteins and many sepsis mediators) (see Chap. 47). Newer hemodialysis membranes with larger membrane pores have been developed (high-flux membranes) in order to increase the clearance of some of these larger solutes. These new dialysis membranes can partially remove solutes up to approximately 15,000 daltons, but clearances of these large molecules are still considerably lower than small solute clearances. The most clinically relevant aspect of dialysis membrane choice to pharmacists is the marked differences in drug clearance rates with these high-flux membranes. The dialyzer clearance of ceftazidime, cefazolin, tobramycin, and vancomycin is significantly higher when a high-flux dialyzer is used instead of a conventional hemodialyzer.[90–93] For example, acute renal failure patients receiving vancomycin require more frequent dosing if high-flux hemodialyzers are used because about 20% to 30% of the total vancomycin body load is removed with each dialysis treatment.[90]

As blood passes through the hemodialyzer, it comes into contact with chemicals that are found in the dialyzer fibers. Exposure to these substances found in bioincompatible dialyzers—that is, Cuprophan and cellulose—results in complex humoral and cellular host responses that may include anaphylaxis, thromboembolic complications, immunosuppression, and hypercatabolism.[17] These reactions may be deleterious for patients with acute renal failure. High-flux dialyzers composed of synthetic membranes are used commonly in patients with acute renal failure because they tend to be more biocompatible.[91] Although some studies suggest that patients with acute renal failure may have higher survival and renal function recovery rates when biocompatible membranes are used for renal replacement,[92] these findings are controversial.[93,94]

Another drawback of intermittent hemodialysis is that it is not very well tolerated by hemodynamically unstable patients. This problem is compounded in the fluid-overloaded patient who requires extensive volume removal, often 2–3 L or more within the 4-hour dialysis treatment. Most acute renal failure patients are unable to maintain an adequate blood pressure with such rapid fluid removal. It has been hypothesized that these periods of hypotension during the hemodialysis session may actually prolong the duration of acute renal failure because the recovering tubules are now subjected to a hypoxic insult.

TABLE 43–9. Advantages and Disadvantages of Common Renal Replacement Therapies in Acute Renal Failure

	Intermittent Hemodialysis	Intermittent Hemofiltration	Peritoneal Dialysis	Extended Daily Dialysis	Continuous Venovenous Hemofiltration (CVVH)	Continuous Venovenous Hemodiafiltration (CVVHDF)
Solute Control	Usually adequate	Inadequate	Indequate	Adequate	Adequate	Adequate
Volume Control	Variable	Adequate	Adequate	Adequate	Adequate	Adequate
Hemodynamic Stability	Variable	Well tolerated	Well tolerated	Variable	Well tolerated	Well tolerated
Access	Venous	Venous	Peritoneal	Venous	Venous	Venous
Anticoagulation	Short duration	Short duration	None	Long durations	Continuous low dose	Continuous low dose
Technical Complexity	High	High	Low	High	Moderate	High
Workload	Intermittent	Intermittent	Low	Moderate	Moderate	High
Drug-Dosing Ease	Many published recommendations	Difficult	Difficult	Difficult	Many published recommendations	Difficult
Convective Clearance (small & middle molecules)	Mixed	Minimal	Moderate	Moderate	Large	Large
Dialytic Clearance (small molecules)	Large	None	Large	Large	None	Large
Common Complications	Hypotension	Hypotension	Hyperglycemia, atelectasis, peritonitis	Hypotension	Hypotension	↑ Serum lactate, hypotension

Nonetheless, there is a suggestion that earlier[12,95] or more rigorous[96] renal replacement therapy might improve outcome in patients who will eventually require renal replacement therapy.

CONTINUOUS RENAL REPLACEMENT THERAPIES

PERITONEAL DIALYSIS

Peritoneal dialysis is a continuous renal replacement therapy that is usually used for ambulatory patients with chronic renal failure; however, it can also be used in acute renal failure (see Chap. 47). Glucose-containing dialysate solutions are instilled into the patient's peritoneum. The patient's own peritoneal membrane acts as the dialysis membrane. An advantage of peritoneal dialysis in acute renal failure is that it is relatively easy to perform after the dialysis catheter is instilled into patient's peritoneum. The main disadvantage of peritoneal dialysis is that it is not very efficient for volume and solute removal. Its use in acute renal failure is generally limited to children, who tend to have a larger peritoneal membrane surface area relative to their overall body size. This anatomic difference means peritoneal dialysis may be able to provide enough solute removal for children to provide adequate azotemic control. Another common problem with peritoneal dialysis in acute renal failure patients is that it provides a large glucose load to the patient. Patients with acute renal failure who received rapid, frequent (30 to 90-minute dwell times) exchanges of peritoneal dialysate containing 4.25% dextrose, absorbed an average of 1922 kcal/d of glucose from the dialysate, resulting in significant overfeeding.[97]

EXTRACORPOREAL THERAPIES

Several extracorporeal continuous renal replacement therapies have been developed during the last 25 years to address the unique needs of the acute renal failure patient who is hypercatabolic, hypotensive, and volume overloaded. The most commonly used continuous therapies in acute renal failure are continuous hemofiltration and hemodiafiltration. These modalities are more technically difficult and require more nursing time to operate than does intermittent hemodialysis. However, the advantages of continuous therapies are improved fluid and metabolic control, especially in patients unable to tolerate hemodialysis. Continuous therapies generally are better tolerated because the fluid and electrolyte shifts are more gradual.

The continuous therapies have gone by many names over the years, and only recently has consensus been reached on the nomenclature of the therapies.[98] This nomenclature helps differentiate between the many systems in place worldwide. Continuous therapies can take blood from arteries and return them to veins (arteriovenous), allowing the heart to pump blood through the system (Fig. 43–3). Alternatively, blood can be pumped through the hemofilter from a dual-lumen venous catheter (venovenous) (Fig. 43–4). Venovenous systems are preferred if the hardware to run these machines is available, because the cardiovascular systems of critically ill patients often do not provide adequate blood flow through the extracorporeal circuit to allow adequate solute clearance. Systems can be entirely diffusive based (continuous hemodialysis, CVVHD), entirely convective based with no diffusion (continuous hemofiltration, CVVH) or a combination of both (continuous hemodiafiltration, CVVHDF). In the United States, the number of sites using arteriovenous modalities is about the same as the number using venovenous configurations.[89] However, new venovenous machines have entered the market and it is likely that venovenous systems will soon become the most popular.

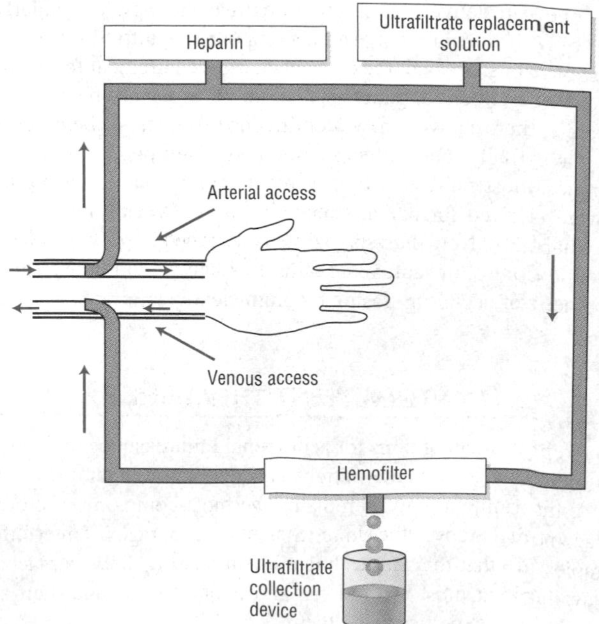

FIGURE 43–3. Schematic of continuous arteriovenous hemofiltration (CAVH). CAVH is the simplest continuous renal replacement therapy, but usually does not provide adequate solute removal for highly catabolic patients with acute renal failure. Blood enters the extracorporeal circuit from the arterial catheter and returns via a separate venous catheter. The hydrostatic force for making ultrafiltrate is provided by the patient's arterial pressure. Blood flow through the circuit and ultrafiltrate production rates are a function of the patient's cardiovascular status. Usually higher heparin doses are required to prevent filter clotting in CAVH versus venovenous systems because of the slower blood flow through the hemofilter in CAVH.

Hemofiltration employs no dialysate, but a high-flux dialyzer or hemofilter with a large pore size is usually used in the system. Solutes dissolved in the plasma water that are small enough to pass through the hemofilter pores are removed as the plasma water they are dissolved in moves across the hemofilter. This plasma water solution is called *ultrafiltrate*, and this type of solute removal is called "*convection.*" Convective solute removal differs from diffusive solute removal in that the solute's molecular weight has little effect on removal. As long as the dissolved solute can fit through the hemofilter pores (<15,000 daltons), it will be removed by convection. Consequently, hemofiltration is more effective than dialytic therapies in the removal of high-molecular-weight substances.[99] Convective removal of higher molecular weight substances may be desirable in patients with diseases such as septic shock because many of the mediators of septic shock have molecular weights of 600 to 30,000 daltons. Consequently, continuous hemofiltration has been proposed as an adjunctive therapy for septic shock.[100]

The continuous nature of these therapies gives them an advantage over intermittent therapies in the treatment of critically ill patients with acute renal failure because solutes and fluid are continually removed as they are produced. Hypotensive, hypervolemic patients that could not tolerate 2–3 L of volume removal over a 4-hour intermittent hemodialysis treatment can usually withstand slow volume removal of 100–200 mL/h for 24 hours (2.4–4.8 L/d).

The convective aspect of continuous hemofiltration or hemodiafiltration allows for optimal volume control. Typically, 1,000 mL/h of ultrafiltrate is formed and discarded and 800–1,000 mL/hr of replacement fluid is infused, depending on the fluid and cardiovascular status of the patient. This intravenous ultrafiltrate replacement

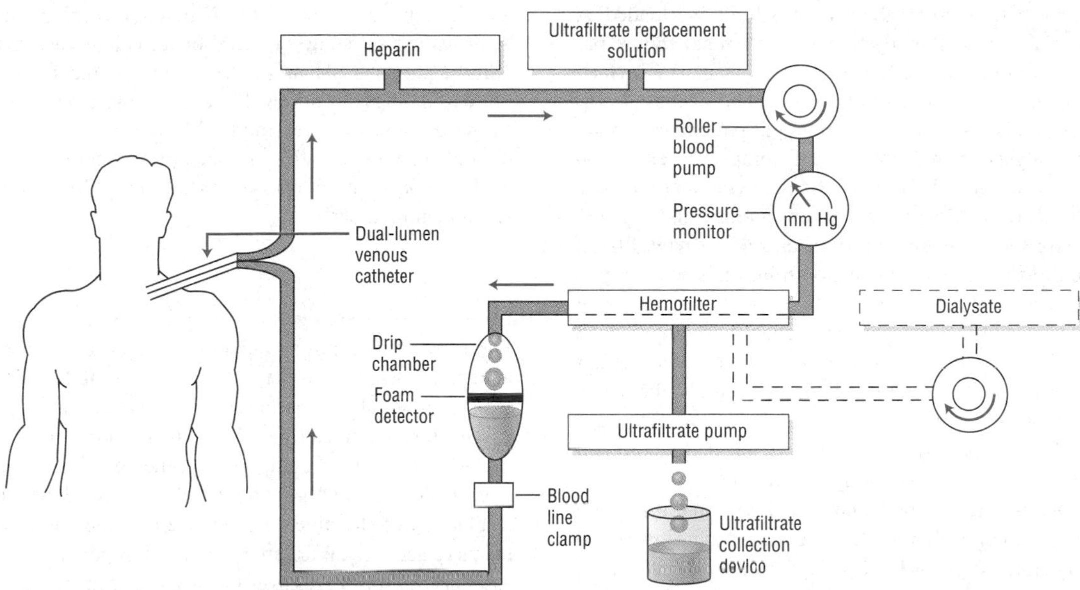

FIGURE 43–4. Schematic of the continuous venovenous renal replacement therapies. The continuous venovenous renal replacement therapies all have the same basic extracorporeal circuit. Blood is pulled into the extracorporeal circuit from a dual-lumen central catheter by a blood pump. Blood is anticoagulated prior to the hemofilter to prevent clotting of the hemofilter. Before the blood returns to the patient through the other lumen of the venous catheter, it travels through a drip chamber and foam detector to prevent accidental air embolization.

In the case of continuous venovenous hemofiltration (CVVH), no dialysate is connected to the right side of the figure, and all fluid and solutes are removed convectively by the pump coming from the hemodiafilter. When continuous venovenous hemodialysis (CVVHD) is used, little or no ultrafiltrate is formed because the pump coming from the hemodiafilter is set at the same rate as the dialysate pump, resulting in mostly diffusive solute removal. Continuous venovenous hemodiafiltration (CVVHDF) occurs when the pump coming from the hemodiafilter is set at a rate much higher than the dialysate pump speed resulting in both diffusive and convective solute removal.

solution contains physiologic concentrations of sodium, potassium, chloride, bicarbonate, and calcium. When the patient is extremely fluid overloaded, less of the volume removed will be replaced in order to achieve the net desired hourly fluid loss for the patient. Some of the ultrafiltrate replacement may be in the form of intravenous medications, blood products, and nutrition. The large hourly fluid removal and subsequent large hourly fluid replacement allows for the administration of drugs, nutrition, and blood products without concern about volume constraints. This luxury is not afforded to patients receiving intermittent hemodialysis or peritoneal dialysis. Consequently, therapies can be administered solely based on patient need instead of on how much volume they will add to the patient. Finally, the drug-dosing considerations for each of these therapies differs greatly from intermittent hemodialysis, and may vary between the different continuous therapies.[98,99,101,102]

At this time, there is no proof of improved patient outcomes between intermittent dialysis and continuous renal replacement therapies. However, subjects that are too hemodynamically unstable to tolerate dialysis may be able to with stand continuous therapies because of their relatively slow but relentless removal of waste products and fluid. Although early comparisons between therapies suggest a higher mortality rate with continuous therapies, this may have been because patients treated with continuous therapies were sicker.[12] In a study that accounted for this difference in disease acuity, survival rates between CVVH and intermittent hemodialysis were not different.[18] Predictors of mortality in this study were severity of illness and not the treatment chosen. Mortality predictors were similar to what has been reported previously—concomitant liver disease, hypotension, older age, infection, and trauma.

NUTRITIONAL THERAPY

Little research has been conducted into what nutritional regimen connotes the best outcome in patients with acute renal failure. Some have questioned whether parenteral nutrition is of any value at all in critically ill patients.[103] While some of this discussion appears in Chap. 139, a few elements bear mention here. For example, the renal replacement therapy chosen for acute renal failure will affect electrolyte, protein, caloric, and vitamin regimens for the patient.[104]

ELECTROLYTES

About the only universally agreed upon aspect of acute renal failure nutritional care is that of electrolyte management. Of the electrolyte abnormalities observed in acute renal failure patients, hyperkalemia is the most common and the most serious. Life-threatening arrhythmias may result from uncontrolled hyperkalemia. The treatment of hyperkalemia is discussed in Chap. 52. Frequent monitoring of potassium serum concentrations is essential. The oliguric acute renal failure patient almost always must be potassium restricted to avoid hyperkalemia. Typically, this means no potassium in parenteral nutrition solutions or a low-potassium diet (<3 g potassium/d) in an enterally fed patient unless serum potassium concentrations (<3.5 mEq/L) warrant supplementation. In patients treated with a continuous renal replacement therapy for extended periods (longer than 1 week), potassium supplementation is commonly required because of the efficient and continuous nature of these therapies.

Sodium restriction (<3 g/d) is also usually indicated in the acute renal failure patient, particularly if the patient is fluid overloaded. A common reason that diuretic therapy fails in acute renal failure patients is excessive sodium intake. For example, 1 L of 0.9% NaCl contains 154 mEq of sodium, or about the equivalent of 3.5 g of dietary sodium. Sodium is also usually restricted in patients receiving intermittent hemodialysis as renal replacement therapy. The exception to this rule is when the critically ill patient is receiving a continuous renal replacement therapy. Most forms of continuous renal replacement therapy are so effective at removing fluid and electrolytes, that an isonatremic (140 mEq/L) parenteral nutrition solution is necessary to keep up with the electrolyte removal by continuous renal replacement therapy. In patients receiving continuous hemodialysis regimens such as CVVHD, the sodium content of the dialysate determines whether sodium needs to be supplemented or restricted. Eventually, the serum sodium concentration will approach that of the dialysate with extended CVVHD. Daily monitoring of serum sodium helps to direct how much sodium to include in the nutritional regimen.

Other electrolytes that must be monitored closely in this population are magnesium and phosphorus. Both are renally eliminated and are not very dialyzable. Typically, their dietary intake is restricted, but in acute renal failure patients with poor nutritional status or in those who receive long durations of continuous renal replacement therapy, they may need to be supplemented. This is particularly true for phosphorus, where acute hypophosphatemia can occur as a result of refeeding syndrome in a critically ill patient who begins to receive nutritional support after a long period of having received none. More frequent is the problem of hyperphosphatemia, especially in the acute renal failure patient with concomitant tissue destruction or catabolism (trauma, rhabdomyolysis, sepsis). Serum phosphorus concentrations may rise, even when no phosphorus is administered to the patient. In these situations, oral phosphate-binding drugs (aluminum hydroxide, calcium carbonate, calcium acetate, or sevelamer HCl) may be used, even in a patient not being enterally fed. As the phosphate binder progresses through the gastrointestinal tract, phosphorus tightly binds to it and is excreted in the stool. Calcium-containing agents are considered first-line therapy, especially in patients being enterally fed. Aluminum-containing antacids are usually reserved for patients with a serum phosphate >7 mg/dL. In these hyperphosphatemic patients, calcium is avoided to reduce the chance of precipitation of calcium and phosphate in the soft tissues. A rule of thumb is to maintain a calcium-phosphate product below 70. The calcium phosphate product is simply calculated by multiplying the serum calcium (mg/dL) by the serum phosphorus (mg/dL). Once the serum phosphorus is reduced to below 7 mg/dL, calcium antacids can be used to maintain normal serum phosphate concentrations.

In contrast to patients with ESRD, calcium balance is usually not a major problem in the patient with acute renal failure. Care must be taken in the hyperphosphatemic patient, as discussed above. However, calcium is an important monitoring parameter in those patients for whom citrate is used for anticoagulation during continuous renal replacement therapy.[105] Citrate is administered in the blood line prefilter, where it binds all free calcium, thereby inhibiting clotting. A calcium replacement solution is administered as soon as the blood leaves the hemofilter so that it has a normal amount of unbound calcium when it reaches the patient. Frequent unbound calcium determinations are necessary to ensure appropriate calcium replacement. Inadequate replacement may result in hypocalcemia and associated tetany, mental status changes, and possible arrhythmias.

The anions—lactate, acetate (which is converted to bicarbonate in the liver), and chloride—are typically given in parenteral nutrition solutions. A 2:1 ratio of chloride:acetate is often used initially; however, this ratio must be adjusted based on the serum electrolytes and the clinical status of the patient. In septic patients with lactic acidosis, extra acetate or bicarbonate is administered to help maintain the patient's pH. In contrast, patients receiving long-term loop diuretic therapy often develop a hypochloremic metabolic alkalosis as the diuretic removes more chloride ion than bicarbonate. Extra chloride supplementation in place of acetate, lactate, or bicarbonate as the anion in the nutritional solution usually corrects the problem when identified early.

PROTEIN

For many years, highly efficient renal replacement therapies were not as readily available in the ICU as they are today. Consequently, the main goal of nutritional therapy in the patient with acute renal failure was to avoid the need for dialysis. To accomplish this, protein restriction was an essential component of the nutrition prescription. Now, a reasonable treatment goal may still be to avoid dialysis, but with the availability of effective renal replacement therapies, we may not need to starve acute renal failure patients. Nitrogenous wastes and volume associated with aggressive nutritional regimens can be removed effectively by continuous renal replacement therapy. Consequently, outcome studies are needed to determine the optimal nutritional regimen in critically ill acute renal failure patients.[106] It may be that aggressive nutrition to meet metabolic needs can be achieved with equally aggressive renal replacement therapies,[107] however studies comparing these regimens to conventional feeding have not been done.

Even with protein restriction, many acute renal failure patients require renal replacement therapy because of the extremely high protein catabolic rate associated with their critical illness. The stressed acute renal failure patient breaks protein down at an accelerated rate and cells do not use amino acids efficiently.[106] The protein catabolic rate in a critically ill patient can easily approach 100 g protein/d.[107] Early studies suggested that adequate protein administration might improve mortality in acute renal failure.[106] The administration of exogenous proteins can improve the net nitrogen balance in the patient, but it is unclear whether a positive nitrogen balance is correlated with positive patient outcome.[107]

Constituents of the administered nutritional regimen may be removed substantially by the renal replacement therapy. This is particularly true in subjects treated with continuous therapies that utilize aggressive ultrafiltration or dialysate flow rates. Measurable amounts of vitamin C, copper, and chromium can be found in the ultrafiltrate of patients treated with CVVH.[108] Extra supplementation of water-soluble vitamins and selected trace elements may be necessary, depending on the duration of continuous renal replacement and the volume of dialysate and ultrafiltrate produced. Similarly, amino acids are removed by any renal replacement therapy, but more are lost with aggressive continuous renal replacement therapy.[109] The amount of amino acids removed is higher when a convective therapy such as CVVH is used, than if dialysis is incorporated into the system.[109] Special notice should be paid to glutamine needs of the patient.[110] Continuous therapies also remove glucose because glucose has a relatively low molecular weight; consequently, plasma glucose should be monitored regularly.[111]

EVALUATION OF THERAPEUTIC OUTCOMES

Key monitoring parameters for patients with acute renal failure differ based on the patient's presentation. Early in the course, the monitoring

TABLE 43–10. Key Monitoring Parameters for Patients With Established Acute Renal Failure

Parameter	Frequency
Fluid ins/outs	Every shift
Patient weight	Daily
Vital signs	Every shift
Blood cultures and sensitivities	Check for results daily; obtain more when clinical signs of infection present
Blood chemistries	
Sodium, potassium, chloride, bicarbonate, calcium, phosphate, magnesium	Daily
BUN/Scr	Daily
Albumin	Once or twice weekly
Complete blood cell count with white cell differential	Daily
Drugs and their dosing regimens	Daily
Nutritional regimen	Daily
Serum concentration data for drugs	After regimen changes and after RRT has been instituted
Times of administered doses	Daily
Doses relative to administration of RRT	Daily
Urinalysis	
Calculate measured creatinine clearance	Every time measured urine collection performed
Calculate fractional excretion of sodium	Every time measured urine collection performed
Plans for renal replacement	Daily
Invasive monitoring parameters	As indicated
Swan–Ganz readings	Every shift

RRT = renal replacement therapy

parameters for the patient with community-acquired acute renal failure differ from those for patients with ICU-acquired acute renal failure. However, once acute renal failure is established, monitoring is similar. Clinicians formulating a care plan for a patient can follow a systematic course of action. The first step is to gather all pertinent data prior to preparing a care plan (Table 43–10). The second step is to estimate the patient's current renal function (see Chap. 42) to determine whether renal replacement therapy is to be instituted or changed if already in place. The addition of renal replacement therapy adds to the number of monitoring parameters that must be followed. For example, the initiation of continuous hemodiafiltration adds the requirements of monitoring glucose, anticoagulation, and ultrafiltrate and dialysate flow rates (Table 43–11). Nutritional regimens must be adjusted to meet the patient's dynamic needs and commonly include adjustment of electrolytes and fluid restriction.

All drug doses must be evaluated in response to the assembled patient database. Diuretic doses may need to be titrated to maintain desired urine output. Most importantly, doses need to be adjusted for changes in renal function and renal replacement therapies. Frequent serum concentration monitoring is necessary because an assumption of a steady-state condition cannot be made in many of these patients, whose renal function changes and, occasionally, whose renal replacement therapy changes. Nonsteady-state creatinine clearance equations and timed urine collections for direct creatinine clearance measurement are often necessary (see Chap. 42). Dosing regimens based on serum concentration results from last week in a patient with oliguria may not apply this week.

TABLE 43–11. Renal Replacement Therapy-Specific Monitoring Parameters

- Hemodialysis
  - Pre- and postdialysis BUN (gives indication of delivered dose of dialysis)
  - Duration of dialysis
  - Type of dialyzer—conventional versus high-flux (especially for vancomycin therapy)
- Continuous renal replacement therapies
  - Inspection of system
    - Clotting of filter
    - Ultrafiltrate/dialysate flow rates
      - Desired rate versus actual rates
      - Nursing notes of overnight ultrafiltrate production and dialysate flow
    - Interruption of therapy for other tests
  - Vascular access (particularly if arterial line used)
    - Signs of bleeding
    - Signs of infection (redness, pus formation)
  - Anticoagulation
    - Partial thromboplastin time (PTT) and platelet count if heparin used for anticoagulation
    - Unbound calcium serum concentration and ECG if citrate used for anticoagulation
    - Signs of bleeding

PHARMACOKINETIC CONSIDERATIONS

Typically, clinicians tend to dose renally eliminated medications in patients with acute renal failure the same as they would dose patients with ESRD. The assumption that patients with acute renal failure or ESRD have the same drug clearance is made because both groups have minimal renal function. Recent evidence suggests that although the renal elimination of drugs is the same between patients with acute renal failure and ESRD, nonrenal elimination may be quite different. The kidney metabolizes many endogenous and exogenous substances in patients with normal renal function.[112,113] The degree of renal metabolism in patients with acute renal failure has not been studied. Nonrenal clearance in patients with acute renal failure is the most difficult clearance parameter to estimate. Although most published dosing guidelines for patients with renal disease do not differentiate between acute or chronic failure, the pharmacokinetics of many agents can differ substantially in these two patient populations. Chronic renal failure is associated with derangements in the hepatic metabolism of many drugs. The mechanism(s) that slow the metabolic pathways responsible for this nonrenal clearance have not been studied extensively, but it appears that retained uremic byproducts are responsible for the reduced enzymatic activity.[112] Only a few investigations have examined whether nonrenal clearance in patients with acute renal failure approximates normal values or values reported in patients with chronic renal failure. For example, the nonrenal clearance of imipenem in adults with acute renal failure lies somewhere between the normal renal function values (130 mL/min) and chronic renal failure values (50 mL/min).[114] In theory, this may occur because uremic byproducts may not have had time to accumulate and affect hepatic function. Further studies are needed to confirm these findings and to evaluate whether this pattern of change is evident with other medications. If nonrenal clearance of some antibiotics in early acute renal failure is greater than anticipated, the resultant serum concentrations would be lower than expected. This could contribute to infection being the primary cause of death in acute renal failure. Clearly, frequent therapeutic drug monitoring is needed in these patients to assess whether nonrenal clearance changes with time with drugs that have substantial nonrenal clearance. Because most of the published dosing guidelines in renal failure were generated from patients with chronic renal failure, future dosing guidelines for drugs with significant nonrenal clearance should specify whether they are for patients with acute or chronic renal failure, particularly if the nonrenal clearance rates differ between patients with acute or chronic renal failure.

PHARMACOECONOMIC CONSIDERATIONS

In 1998, Medicare paid $11 billion to manage patients in the United States with ESRD, but the economic consequences of acute renal failure are poorly defined. Pharmacoeconomic analysis suggests that instituting hemodialysis in the hospital for hospital-acquired acute renal failure costs $128,200 per quality-adjusted life-year saved.[115] These costs range from $61,900 to $274,100, depending on the prognosis of the patient. These figures have been disputed,[116] but highlight the high mortality rate of acute renal failure and the high expense associated with treating these patients.

Economic analysis of the use of specific agents that increase the risk of nephrotoxicity, such as aminoglycosides and intravenous contrast dyes, have been performed, as have the relative costs of various renal replacement therapies to treat acute renal failure. In 1996, it was estimated that the costs of renal replacement therapy in the ICU range from $5,000 to $5,500 per patient per week.[117] The least-expensive therapies are the continuous arteriovenous renal replacement therapies because no pumps and less-skilled nursing personnel are needed. Arteriovenous forms produce less ultrafiltrate production and require less ultrafiltrate replacement solutions and dialysate. The set up costs for buying the machines that run intermittent hemodialysis or continuous venovenous renal replacement are similar; however. the day-to-day costs of continuous therapies are considerably higher.[117] Added costs come from continuous nursing supervision and the ultrafiltrate replacement solutions (usually made by the pharmacy department). When a patient has an ultrafiltrate production rate of 1,000 mL/h, they usually require 20 L of replacement solution that cost about $20/L. With the worldwide trend toward high-volume hemofiltration and new, longer hemodialysis modalities,[20] the societal expense for the management of acute renal failure is likely to increase.

Ancillary costs associated with continuous renal replacement therapy have not been well described but include increased laboratory testing for urea, creatinine, electrolyte, and drug concentrations. Also, pharmacists prepare specialized enteral and parenteral nutritional products to provide adequate caloric and protein intake in minimal volume and with relatively low amounts of undesired electrolytes such as potassium and phosphate. These are added costs of acute renal failure that are indirectly influenced by renal replacement therapy. Because no difference has been definitively demonstrated in patient outcome between intermittent and continuous renal replacement therapies, both will continue to be used to treat patients with acute renal failure. Until quality comparative data are available, the choice of renal replacement will be determined by availability of each of the therapies, caregiver expertise, daily cost, and physician preference.

▶ PRINCIPLES OF PHARMACOTHERAPY

- Prevention of acute renal failure is key because there is little we can do to hasten recovery from established acute renal failure.
- Early resuscitation is essential, especially in the settings of trauma and surgery. If renal perfusion can be quickly reestablished, acute tubular necrosis can be attenuated.
- Find out the cause of the acute renal failure. Therapy is directed by knowing the cause. The optimal therapy for one acute renal failure etiology may complicate another.
- An understanding of the solute (drug)-removal principles of the renal replacement therapy used is essential in order to optimize nutrition and pharmacotherapy.
- Avoid nephrotoxic therapies in at-risk patient populations whenever possible. The duration of acute renal failure may be extended with continued nephrotoxic insults.
- Fluid control is key in acute renal failure. At times you may need to administer fluid (prerenal azotemia) and at other times you may need to restrict fluid (established acute renal failure).
- Strive to eliminate unnecessary fluid administration in oliguric, fluid-overloaded patients. This can be done by maximally concentrating drugs and nutrition and assessing the need for and rate of "keep-open" intravenous solutions.
- Be aggressive early with diuretic dosing. Converting oliguria to nonoliguria may or may not improve outcome, but euvolemic patients are easier to manage than hypervolemic patients. This may require continuous infusions of diuretics or diuretic combination therapy. However, if diuretics do not work in the patient, discontinue their use and consider renal replacement therapy for azotemic and volume control.

REFERENCES

1. Fiaccadori E, Maggiore U, Lombardi M, et al. Predicting patient outcome from acute renal failure comparing three general severity of illness scoring systems. Kidney Int 2000;58:283–292.
2. Kaufman J, Dhakal M, Patel B, Hamburger R. Community-acquired renal failure. Am J Kidney Dis 1991;17:191–198.
3. Obialo CI, Okonofua EC, Tayade AS, Riley LJ. Epidemiology of de novo acute renal failure in hospitalized African Americans: Comparing community-acquired vs hospital-acquired disease. Arch Intern Med 2000;160:1309–1313.
4. Fortescue EB, Bates DW, Chertow GM. Predicting acute renal failure after coronary bypass surgery: Cross-validation of two risk-stratification algorithms. Kidney Int 2000;57:2594–2602.
5. Sural S, Sharma RK, Singhal M, et al. Etiology, prognosis, and outcome of post-operative acute renal failure. Ren Fail 2000;22:87–97.
6. Cole L, Bellomo R, Silvester W, Reeves JH. A prospective, multicenter study of epidemiology, management, and outcome of severe acute renal failure in a "closed" ICU system. Am J Respir Crit Care Med 2000;162:191–196.
7. Briglia A, Paganini EP. Acute renal failure in the intensive care unit. Therapy overview, patient risk stratification, complications of renal replacement, and special circumstances. Clin Chest Med 1999;20:347–366.
8. Elasy TA, Anderson RJ. Changing demography of acute renal failure. Semin Dial 1996;9:438–443.
9. Levy EM, Viscoli CM, Horwitz RI. The effect of acute renal failure on mortality. A cohort analysis. JAMA 1996;275:1489–1494.
10. Lins RL, Elseviers M, Daelemans R, et al. Prognostic value of a new scoring system for hospital mortality in acute renal failure. Clin Nephrol 2000;53:10–17.
11. McMurray SD, Luft FC, Maxwell DR, et al. Prevailing patterns and predictor variables in patients with acute tubular necrosis. Arch Intern Med 1978;138:950–955.
12. Kresse S, Schlee H, Deuber HJ, et al. Influence of renal replacement therapy on outcome of patients with acute renal failure. Kidney Int Suppl 1999;72:S75–S78.
13. Martin PY, Feraille E. Nitric oxide in renal disease. Adv Nephrol Necker Hosp 1999;29:93–113.

14. Kelly KJ, Molitoris BA. Acute renal failure in the new millennium: Time to consider combination therapy. Semin Nephrol 2000;20:4–19.
15. Ueda N, Kaushal GP, Shah SV. Apoptotic mechanisms in acute renal failure. Am J Med 2000;108:403–415.
16. Dishart MK, Kellum JA. An evaluation of pharmacological strategies for the prevention and treatment of acute renal failure. Drugs 2000;59:79–91.
17. Vanholder R, De Vriese A, Lameire N. The role of dialyzer biocompatibility in acute renal failure. Blood Purif 2000;18:1–12.
18. Swartz RD, Messana JM, Orzol S, Port FK. Comparing continuous hemofiltration with hemodialysis in patients with severe acute renal failure. Am J Kidney Dis 1999;34:424–432.
19. Ronco C, Bellomo R, Homel P, et al. Effects of different doses in continuous veno-venous haemofiltration on outcomes of acute renal failure: a prospective randomised trial. Lancet 2000;356:26–30.
20. Kumar VA, Craig M, Depner TA, Yeun JY. Extended daily dialysis: A new approach to renal replacement for acute renal failure in the intensive care unit. Am J Kidney Dis 2000;36:294–300.
21. Blantz RC. Pathophysiology of pre-renal azotemia. Kidney Int 1998;53:512–523.
22. Perazella MA. Crystal-induced acute renal failure. Am J Med 1999;106:459–465.
23. Parmley WW. Pathophysiology and current therapy of congestive heart failure. J Am Coll Cardiol 1989;13:771–785.
24. Trachtman H, Christen E. Pathogenesis, treatment, and therapeutic trials in hemolytic uremic syndrome. Curr Opin Pediatr 1999;11:162–168.
25. Rahman SN, Conger JD. Glomerular and tubular factors in urine flow rates of acute renal failure. Am J Kidney Dis 1994;23:788–793.
26. Haas M, Spargo BH, Wit EJC, Meehan SM. Etiologies and outcome of acute renal insufficiency in older adults: A renal biopsy study of 259 cases. Am J Kidney Dis 2000;35:433–447.
27. Lieberthal W. Biology of acute renal failure: Therapeutic implications. Kidney Int 1997;52:1102–1115.
28. Weisberg LS, Allgren RL, Genter FC, Kurnik BRC. Cause of acute tubular necrosis affects its prognosis. Arch Intern Med 1997;157:1833–1838.
29. Jaber BL, Cendoroglo M, Balakrishnan VS, et al. Impact of dialyzer membrane selection on cellular responses in acute renal failure: A crossover study. Kidney Int 2000;57:2107–2116.
30. Abramson S, Niles JL. Anticoagulation in continuous renal replacement therapy. Curr Opin Nephrol Hyperten 1999;8:701–707.
31. Gerlach AT, Pickworth KK. Contrast medium-induced nephrotoxicity: Pathophysiology and prevention. Pharmacotherapy 2000;20:540–548
32. Swan SK. Aminoglycoside nephrotoxicity. Semin Nephrol 1997;17:27–33.
33. Rehman Q, Lane NE. Getting control of osteoarthritis pain. An update on treatment options. Postgrad Med 1999;106:127–134.
34. Anaissie EJ, Darouiche RO, Abi-Said D, et al. Management of invasive candidal infections: Results of a prospective, randomized, multicenter study of fluconazole versus amphotericin B and review of the literature. Clin Infect Dis 1996;23:964–972.
35. Sorkine P, Nagar H, Weinbroum A, et al. Administration of amphotericin B in lipid emulsion decreases nephrotoxicity: Results of a prospective, randomized, controlled study in critically ill patients. Crit Care Med 1996;24:1311–1315.
36. Murry KR, McKinnon PS, Mitrzyk B, Rybak MJ. Pharmacodynamic characterization of nephrotoxicity associated with once-daily aminoglycoside. Pharmacotherapy 1999;19:1252–1260.
37. Fisman DN, Kaye KM. Once-daily dosing of aminoglycoside antibiotics. Infect Dis Clin North Am 2000;14:475–487.
38. McMullin ST, Reichley RM, Kahn MG, et al. Automated system for identifying potential dosage problems at a large university hospital. Am J Health Syst Pharm 1997;54:545–59.
39. Rind DM, Safran C, Phillips RS, et al. Effect of computer-based alerts on the treatment and outcomes of hospitalized patients. Arch Intern Med 1994;154:1511–1517.
40. Chasty RC, Lin-Yin JA. Acute tumour lysis syndrome. Br J Hosp Med 1993;49:488–492.
41. Bertolissi M. Prevention of acute renal failure in major vascular surgery. Minerva Anestesiol 1999;65:867–877.
42. Hock R, Anderson RJ. Prevention of drug-induced nephrotoxicity in the intensive care unit. J Crit Care 1995;10:33–43.
43. Kribben A, Edelstein CL, Schrier RW. Pathophysiology of acute renal failure. J Nephrol 1999;12(suppl 2):S142–S151.
44. Heidemann HT, Gerkens JF, Spickard WA, et al. Amphotericin B nephrotoxicity in humans decreased by salt repletion. Am J Med 1983;75:476–481.
45. Erley CM. Does hydration prevent radiocontrast-induced acute renal failure? Nephrol Dial Transplant 1999;14:1064–1066.
46. Anderson CM. Sodium chloride treatment of amphotericin B nephrotoxicity standard of care? West J Med 1995;162:313–317.
47. Solomon R, Werner C, Mann D, et al. Effects of saline, mannitol, and furosemide to prevent acute decreases in renal function induced by radiocontrast agents. N Engl J Med 1994;331:1416–1420.
48. Hager B, Betschart M, Krapf R. Effect of postoperative intravenous loop diuretic on renal function after major surgery. Schweiz Med Wochenschr 1996;126:666–673.
49. Lassnigg A, Donner E, Grubhofer G, et al. Lack of renoprotective effects of dopamine and furosemide during cardiac surgery. J Am Soc Nephrol 2000;11:97–104.
50. Conger J. Prophylaxis and treatment of acute renal failure by vasoactive agents: The fact and myths. Kidney Int Suppl 1998;64:S23–S26.
51. Rahn KH, Barenbrock M, Fritschka E, et al. Effect of nitrendipine on renal function in renal-transplant patients treated with cyclosporine: A randomized trial. Lancet 1999;354;1415–1420.
52. Erley CM, Duda SH, Schlepckow S. Adenosine antagonist theophylline prevents the reduction of glomerular filtration rate after contrast media application. Kidney Int 1994;45:1425–1431.
53. Erley CM, Duda SH, Rehfuss D. Prevention of radiocontrast-media-induced nephropathy in patients with pre-existing renal insufficiency by hydration in combination with the adenosine antagonist theophylline. Nephrol Dial Transplant 1999;14:1146–1149.
54. Abizaid AS, Clark CE, Mintz GS, et al. Effects of dopamine and aminophylline on contrast-induced acute renal failure after coronary angioplasty in patients with preexisting renal insufficiency. Am J Cardiol 1999;83:260–263.
55. Koch JA, Plum J, Grabensee B, Modder U. Prostaglandin E1: A new agent for the prevention of renal dysfunction in high-risk patients caused by radiocontrast media. PGE1 Study. Nephrol Dial Transplant 2000;15:43–49.
56. Shilliday IR, Quinn KJ, Allison MEM. Loop diuretics in the management of acute renal failure: A prospective, double-blind, placebo-controlled, randomized study. Nephrol Dial Transplant 1997;12:2592–2596.
57. Kellum JA. Use of diuretics in the acute care setting. Kidney Int Suppl 1998;66:S67–S70.
58. Sirivella S, Gielchinsky I, Parsonnet V. Mannitol, furosemide, and dopamine infusion in postoperative renal failure complicating cardiac surgery. Ann Thorac Surg 2000;69:501–506.
59. Majumdar S, Kjellstrand CM. Why do we use diuretics in acute renal failure? Semin Dial 1996;9:454–459.
60. Better OS, Rubinstein I, Winaver JM, Knochel JP. Mannitol therapy revisited. Kidney Int 1997;52:886–94.
61. Brater DC. Diuretic therapy. N Engl J Med 1998;339:387–395.
62. Vargo DL, Kramer WG, Black PK, et al. Bioavailability, pharmacokinetics, and pharmacodynamics of torsemide and furosemide in patients with congestive heart failure. Clin Pharmacol Ther 1995;57:601–609.
63. Yelton SL, Gaylor MA, Murray KM. The role of continuous infusion loop diuretics. Ann Pharmacother 1995;29:1010–1014.
64. Howard PA, Dunn MI. Severe musculoskeletal symptoms during continuous infusion of bumetanide. Chest 1997;111:359–364.
65. Schuller D, Lynch JP, Fine D. Protocol-guided diuretic management: Comparison of furosemide by continuous infusion and intermittent bolus. Crit Care Med 1997;25:1969–1975.

66. Rudy DW, Voelker JR, Greene PK, et al. Loop diuretics for chronic renal insufficiency: A continuous is more efficacious than bolus therapy. Ann Intern Med 1991;115:360–366.
67. Kramer WG, Smith WB, Ferguson J, et al. Pharmacodynamics of torsemide administered as an intravenous injection and as a continuous infusion to patients with congestive heart failure. J Clin Pharmacol 1996;36:265–270.
68. Ellison DH. Diuretic resistance: Physiology and therapeutics. Semin Nephrol 1999;19:581–597.
69. Segar JL, Chemtob S, Bell EF. Changes in body water compartments with diuretic therapy in infants with chronic lung disease. Early Hum Dev 1997;48:99–107.
70. Harper L, Savage COS. The use of dopamine in acute renal failure. Clin Nephrol 1997;47:347–349.
71. Ichai C, Passeron C, Carles M, et al. Prolonged low-dose dopamine infusion induces a transient improvement in renal function in hemodynamically stable, critically ill patients: A single-blind, prospective, controlled study. Crit Care Med 2000;28:1329–135.
72. Varriale P, Mossavi A. The benefit of low-dose dopamine during vigorous diuresis for congestive heart failure associated with renal insufficiency: Does it protect renal function? Clin Cardiol 1997;20:627–630.
73. Power DA, Duggan J, Brady HR. Renal-dose (low-dose) dopamine for the treatment of sepsis-related and other forms of acute renal failure: Ineffective and probably dangerous. Clin Exp Pharmacol Physiol Suppl 1999;26:S23–S28.
74. Chertow GM, Sayegh MH, Allgren RL, Lazarus JM. Is the administration of dopamine associated with adverse or favorable outcomes in acute renal failure? Am J Med 1996;101:49–53.
75. Marik PE, Iglesias J. Low-dose dopamine does not prevent acute renal failure in patients with septic shock and oliguria. NORASEPT II Study Investigators. Am J Med 1999;107:387–390.
76. Bailey AR, Burchett KR. Effect of low-dose dopamine on serum concentrations of prolactin in critically ill patients. Br J Anaesth 1997;78: 97–99.
77. Duke GJ, Briedis JH, Weaver RA. Renal support in critically ill patients: Low-dose dopamine or low-dose dobutamine? Crit Care Med 1994;22:1919–1925.
78. Mathur VS, Swan SK, Lambrecht LJ, et al. The effects of fenoldopam, a selective dopamine receptor agonist, on systemic and renal hemodynamics in normotensive subjects. Crit Care Med 1999;27:1832–1837.
79. Allgren RL, Marbury TC, Rahman SN, et al. Anaritide in acute tubular necrosis. N Engl J Med 1997;336:828–834.
80. Lewis J, Salem MM, Chertow GM, et al. Atrial natriuretic factor in oliguric acute renal failure. Am J Kidney Dis 2000;36:767–774.
81. Herbert MK, Ginzel S, Muhlschlegel S, Weis KH. Concomitant treatment with urodilatin (ularitide) does not improve renal function in patients with acute renal failure after major abdominal surgery: A randomized controlled trial. Wien Klin Wochenschr 1999;111(4):141–147.
82. Meyer M, Pfarr E, Schirmer G, et al. Therapeutic use of the natriuretic peptide ularitide in acute renal failure. Ren Fail 1999;21:85–100.
83. Hammerman MR. The growth hormone-insulin-like growth factor axis in kidney re-revisited. Nephrol Dial transplant 1999;14:1853–1860.
84. Hirschberg R, Kopple J, Lipsett P, et al. Multicenter clinical trial of recombinant human insulin-like growth factor I in patients with acute renal failure. Kidney Int 1999;55:2423–2432.
85. Lopez-Novoa JM. Potential role of platelet-activating factor in acute renal failure. Kidney Int 1999;55:1672–1682.
86. Kanagasundaram NS, Paganini EP. Critical care dialysis—A Gordian knot. Nephrol Dial Transplant 1999;14:2590–2594.
87. Woodrow G, Turney JH. Cause of death in acute renal failure. Nephrol Dial Transplant 1992;7:230–234.
88. Clark WR, Mueller BA, Kraus MA, Macias WL. Extracorporeal therapy requirements for patients with acute renal failure. J Am Soc Nephrol 1997;8:804–812.
89. Mehta RL, Letteri JM. Current status of renal replacement therapy for acute renal failure. A survey of US nephrologists. The National Kidney Foundation Council on Dialysis. Am J Nephrol 1999;19:377–382.
90. Scott MK, Macias WL, Kraus MA, et al. Intradialytic vancomycin administration: Dialysis membrane effects. Pharmacotherapy 1997;17:256–262.
91. Clark WR, Hamburger RJ, Lysaght MJ. Effect of membrane composition and structure on solute removal and biocompatibility in hemodialysis. Kidney Int 1999;56:2005–2015.
92. Himmelfarb J, Tolkoff Rubin N, Chandran P, et al. A multicenter comparison of dialysis membranes in the treatment of acute renal failure requiring dialysis. J Am Soc Nephrol 1998;9:257–266.
93. Jorres A, Gahl GM, Dobis C, et al. Hemodialysis-membrane biocompatibility and mortality of patients with dialysis-dependent acute renal failure: A prospective randomised multicentre trial. International Multicentre Study Group. Lancet 1999;354:1337–1341.
94. Gastaldello K, Melot C, Kahn RJ, et al. Comparison of cellulose diacetate and polysulfone membranes in the outcome of acute renal failure. A prospective randomized study. Nephrol Dial Transplant 2000;15:224–230.
95. Gettings LG, Reynolds HN, Scalea T. Outcome in post-traumatic acute renal failure when continuous renal replacement therapy is applied early vs. late. Intensive Care Med 1999;25:805–813.
96. Paganini EP, Tapolyai M, Goormastic M, et al. Establishing a dialysis therapy/patient outcome link in intensive care unit acute dialysis for patients with acute renal failure. Am J Kidney Dis 1996;28(suppl 3):S81–S89.
97. Manji N, Shikora S, McMahon M, et al. Peritoneal dialysis for acute renal failure: Overfeeding resulting from dextrose absorbed during dialysis. Crit Care Med 1990;18:29–31.
98. Joy MS, Matzke GR, Armstrong DK, et al. A primer on continuous renal replacement therapy for critically ill patients. Ann Pharmacother 1998;32:362–375.
99. Clark WR, Ronco C. CRRT efficiency and efficacy in relation to solute size. Kidney Int Suppl 1999;72:S3–S7.
100. Sieberth HG, Kierdorf HP. Is cytokine removal by continuous hemofiltration feasible? Kidney Int Suppl 1999;72:S79–S83.
101. Subach RA, Marx MA. Drug dosing in acute renal failure: The role of renal replacement therapy in altering drug pharmacokinetics. Adv Ren Replace Ther 1998;5:141–147.
102. Bohler J, Donauer J, Keller F. Pharmacokinetic principles during continuous renal replacement therapy: Drugs and dosage. Kidney Int Suppl 1999;72:S24–S28.
103. Koretz RL. Does nutritional intervention in protein-energy malnutrition improve morbidity or mortality? J Ren Nutr 1999;9:119–121.
104. Monson P, Mehta RL. Nutritional considerations in continuous renal replacement therapies. Semin Dial 1996;9:152–160.
105. Kutsogiannis DJ, Mayers I, Chin WD, Gibney RT. Regional citrate anticoagulation in continuous venovenous hemodiafiltration. Am J Kidney Dis 2000;35:802–811.
106. Sponsel H, Conger JD. Is parenteral nutrition therapy of value in acute renal failure patients? Am J Kidney Dis 1995;25:96–102.
107. Macias WL, Murphy MH, Alaka KJ, et al. Impact of the nutritional regimen on protein catabolism and nitrogen balance in patients with acute renal failure. JPEN J Parenter Enteral Nutr 1996;20:56–62.
108. Story DA, Ronco C, Bellomo R. Trace element and vitamin concentrations and losses in critically ill patients treated with continuous venovenous hemofiltration. Crit Care Med 1999;27:220–223.
109. Maxvold NJ, Smoyer WE, Custer JR, Bunchman TE. Amino acid loss and nitrogen balance in critically ill children with acute renal failure: A prospective comparison between classic hemofiltration and hemofiltration with dialysis. Crit Care Med 2000;28:1161–1165.
110. Novak I, Sramek V, Pittrova H, et al. Glutamine and other amino acid losses during continuous venovenous hemodiafiltration. Artif Organs 1997;21:359–363.

111. Druml W. Metabolic aspects of continuous renal replacement therapies. Kidney Int Suppl 1999;72:S56–S61.
112. Elston AC, Bayliss MK, Park GR. Effect of renal failure on drug metabolism by the liver. Br J Anaesth 1993;71:282–290.
113. Matzke GR, Frye RF. Drug administration in patients with renal insufficiency. Minimising renal and extrarenal toxicity. Drug Saf 1997;16:205–231.
114. Tegeder I, Bremer F, Oelkers R, et al. Pharmacokinetics of imipenem-cilastatin in critically ill patients undergoing continuous venovenous hemofiltration. Antimicrob Agents Chemother 1997;41:2640–2645.
115. Hamel MB, Phillips RS, Davis RB, et al. Outcomes and cost-effectiveness of initiating dialysis and continuing aggressive care in seriously ill hospitalized adults. SUPPORT Investigators. Study to Understand Prognoses and Preferences for Outcomes and Risks of Treatments. Ann Intern Med 1997;127:195–202.
116. Chertow GM. Dialysis: Cost-effective "SUPPORT" for patients with acute renal failure. Am J Kidney Dis 1998;31:545–549.
117. Moreno L, Heyka RJ, Paganini EP. Continuous renal replacement therapy: Cost considerations and reimbursement. Semin Dial 1996;9:209–214.

44

PATHOPHYSIOLOGY AND THERAPEUTICS OF PROGRESSIVE RENAL DISEASE

Matthew J. Lewis, Wendy L. St. Peter, and Bertram L. Kasiske

The normal human kidneys contain approximately two million functionally integrated glomerulotubular units called nephrons. Under normal conditions these nephrons work in a highly organized fashion to filter, reabsorb, and excrete various solutes and fluid. In addition, the kidney plays an important role in the metabolism of various peptide hormones and in the production of renin, ammonia, erythropoietin (EPO), and 1,25-dihydroxyvitamin D_3.

Renal disease is characterized by disturbances in many of these normal functions. Evidence suggests that even as renal disease develops and adaptations take place, functioning (remnant) nephrons continue to work in a highly organized fashion. Although total kidney glomerular filtration rate (GFR) falls, the GFR of remnant nephrons rises. This adaptation blunts the drop in whole kidney glomerular filtration rate that would occur in the absence of compensatory changes. Unfortunately, this adaptive hyperfiltration process ultimately results in glomerular hypertension, which plays a significant role in glomerular injury. Indeed, in most instances when serum creatinine (S_{Cr}) rises above 2–3 mg/dL or creatinine clearance (Cl_{cr}) falls to approximately 25–40 mL/min, the injury process will progress to end-stage renal failure regardless of the initial etiology of kidney disease.[1]

Solute balance is maintained in chronic renal insufficiency by increases in the fractional excretion of solutes such as sodium, potassium, creatinine, blood urea nitrogen, and phosphorus by remnant nephrons, although the adaptive mechanisms differ in each case. The urinary excretion of any substance is dependent upon the amount of solute filtered at the glomerulus plus the net contribution of tubular secretion and tubular reabsorption.

$$\text{Excretion} = \text{Filtered Load} + \text{Tubular Secretion} - \text{Tubular Reabsorption}$$

$$\text{Filtered Load} = \text{Glomerular Filtration Rate} \times \text{Plasma Concentration}$$

$$\text{Fractional Excretion} = \frac{\text{Amount Excreted}}{\text{Filtered Load}}$$

There are several ways in which remnant nephrons can adapt to maintain solute balance. Plasma concentrations of solutes that undergo minimal tubular secretion or reabsorption, such as creatinine and blood urea nitrogen, rise predictably as renal function declines. This results in an increase in the filtered load presented to each tubule, which allows remnant nephrons to increase excretion proportionally. Serum creatinine rises in proportion to the decline in GFR and can be used clinically to estimate renal function (Chap. 42). Renal tubular reabsorption is the predominant mechanism that regulates excretion for sodium and phosphorus; therefore, in chronic renal insufficiency, tubular reabsorption of these solutes decreases in order to prevent or minimize the increase in plasma concentrations. Potassium balance is maintained via further increases in distal tubular secretion, which is potassium's primary excretory pathway as well as through increased losses through the gastrointestinal tract. Thus, the plasma concentrations of some solutes rise, whereas the plasma concentrations of others remain relatively constant until residual renal function is quite low.

There may be "trade-offs" to many of these adaptations that actually contribute to the uremic state and its complications.[1] An understanding of these renal adaptations is crucial to an understanding of the conservative management of chronic renal insufficiency, because many therapeutic interventions follow logically from the disordered physiology.

Progression of renal disease is a major health care problem throughout the world. A key issue is the early identification of patients with renal insufficiency before they progress to end-stage renal disease (ESRD). The best time to intervene is early in the course of the disease; however, because of a shortage of nephrologists and nurses or pharmacists specializing in nephrology, identification of these patients is a major barrier. Early patient identification and intervention can slow the progression to ESRD, and for many patients, can result in remission of their renal disease.

Pharmacists and other health care providers can play a role in helping to identify the people at risk. Whether in the community, clinic, or hospital setting, health care providers have an opportunity to impact the care and potential outcomes for patients with early renal insufficiency. This chapter provides an overview of the pathophysiology and risk factors for progression of renal disease so that patients can be identified and treated early in the course of their disease to prolong and improve their quality of life.

EPIDEMIOLOGY OF RENAL DISEASE

Many diseases of the kidney, either idiopathic or secondary to systemic illness, can result in ESRD. More than 307,700 Americans were treated for ESRD in 1998.[2] However, ESRD patients represent only a small portion of the estimated 10 million people ($\geq$12 years old) who have kidney disease.[3]

Native Americans and blacks have approximately a three-fold and five-fold greater rate of renal failure, respectively, than do whites. The average life expectancy of a 60-year-old white ESRD patient in the United States is less than 4 years, as compared to 16 to 23 years for a 60-year-old adult without ESRD.[2]

The prevalence of ESRD was projected in 2000 to more than double to an estimated 661,330 patients by 2010 (Fig. 44–1).[2] The largest increase in incidence has been in the Native American and Asian populations. Diabetes, hypertension, and primary glomerulonephritis are the three most common causes of ESRD in the United States. Even though type 1 diabetes accounts for only 5% to 10% of newly diagnosed diabetes in the U.S. population, it accounts for 45.3% of new ESRD patients with a primary diagnosis of diabetes.[4] Patients with type 2 diabetes are generally considered to have a lower risk of renal

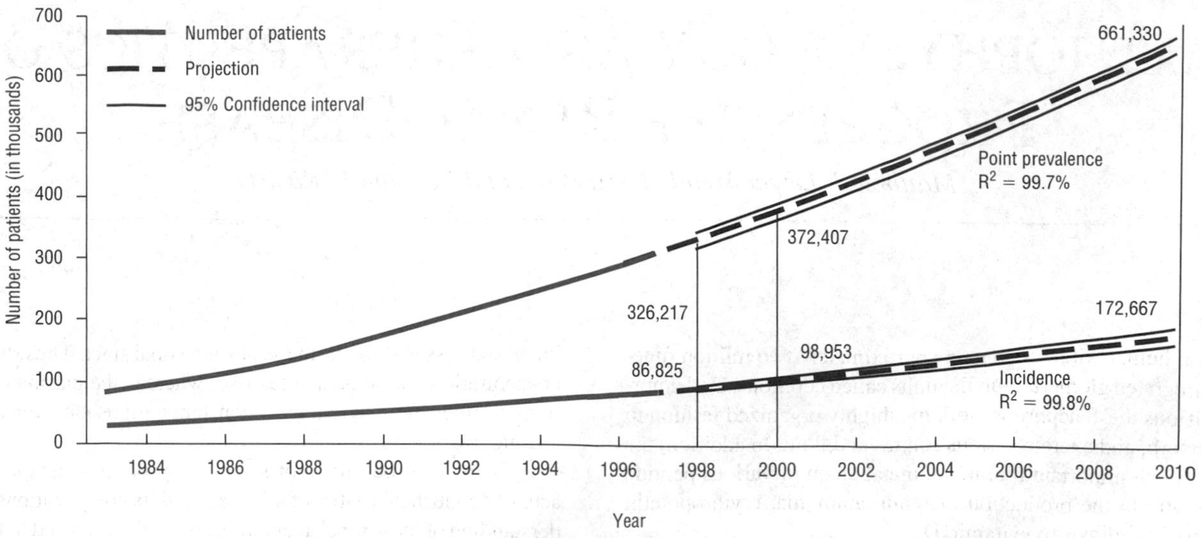

FIGURE 44–1. Number of incidence and point prevalent patients, 1984 to 1998, and projected to 2010. (From Ref. 2.)

complications; however, because they represent more than 85% of the total diabetic population, more patients with type 2 than type 1 diabetes ultimately progress to ESRD.[2,5] Hypertension was the cause of ESRD in 23.5% of newly diagnosed ESRD patients in 1998, and this has increased by about 1% per year during the last decade.[2] Patients who develop ESRD secondary to renal artery stenosis and cholesterol emboli are also categorized under hypertension. Glomerulonephritis and cystic kidney disease account for 12% and 2.7%, respectively, of new ESRD cases. In 1998, the annual Medicare cost to treat an individual with ESRD on dialytic therapy was $53,568.[2] This translated into total medicare expenditures of nearly $11 billion in 1998 for the U.S. ESRD program.[2] The projected medicare costs of this program by the end of the decade (2010) is $28 billion.

The third National Health and Nutrition Examination Survey (NHANES III) assessed serum creatinine levels in the U.S. population.[6] The study evaluated more than 18,000 subjects ≥12 years of age between the years 1988 and 1994. The mean serum creatinine levels for women and men were 0.96 mg/dL and 1.16 mg/dL, respectively.[6] It was estimated that 10.9 million people had a serum creatinine ≥1.5 mg/dL, while 3 million and 800,000 people had values ≥1.7 mg/dL and ≥2.0 mg/dL, respectively.[6] Therefore, it is critical to identify these people with early renal insufficiency to stabilize or to decrease the rise in the incidence in the total number of ESRD patients in the future. The National Kidney Foundation has recognized the importance of early detection and has initiated the Kidney Early Evaluation Program (KEEP). This program was developed to identify, educate, and provide free screening for people at increased risk of developing renal disease.

The U.S. Department of Health and Human Services recognized that renal insufficiency is a major public health issue as evidenced by their inclusion of a focus group on chronic kidney disease in their public health initiative, "Healthy People 2010."[3] One goal for the program includes reducing new cases of chronic kidney disease and its complications. In 1997, there were 289 new cases of ESRD per million population; the goal is to reduce this to 217 new cases per million population by 2010.[3] This goal will only be attained by increasing awareness of both health care providers and the general population of the risk factors for renal disease progression (Table 44–1). In addition, aggressive treatment of glycemic control in diabetics, blood pressure control in hypertensives, screening for microalbuminuria, and use of pharmacotherapeutic agents such as angiotensin-converting enzyme inhibitors (ACEIs) are also indicated.

TABLE 44–1. Risk Factors for Renal Disease Progression

Diabetes
High blood pressure
Environmental exposures
Heavy metals (cadmium, mercury, lead)
Organic compounds (solvents, silica, beryllium)
Proteinuria
Family history of renal disease
Increasing age
African Americans, American Indians, and Alaskan Natives (increased susceptibility with additional risk factors)
Hyperlipidemia
Tobacco use

DISEASE

DEFINITIONS

Currently, there are a variety of definitions / classifications of renal insufficiency within the literature; they are confusing and inconsistent.[7] For practical purposes in this chapter, renal insufficiency is divided into four stages to provide a common framework for the discussion of the clinical course of progressive renal disease. A plot of $1/S_{Cr}$ versus time can be used to evaluate disease progression in individual patients. Unfortunately, the relationship between GFR and $1/S_{Cr}$ is not constant over time; changes in tubular secretion, extrarenal elimination, and rate of generation of creatinine in patients with renal insufficiency can alter the $1/S_{Cr}$ slope without a change in GFR. Therefore, misinterpretation of the rate of decline in renal function can occur if this is the only method used to estimate renal function[8] (see Chap. 42). The accompanying signs and symptoms and laboratory parameters of each stage are described in Fig. 44–2.

- *Mild (Early) renal insufficiency* (CL_{cr} 60–90 mL/min). The GFR, as measured by the CL_{cr}, may decrease by as much as 50% before the plasma concentrations of creatinine (S_{Cr}) or urea nitrogen rise above the normal range. Adaptive increases in solute excretion in remaining nephrons compensate for the decline in functioning kidney mass.
- *Moderate renal insufficiency* (CL_{cr} 30–59 mL/min). A thorough evaluation to determine the etiology of the renal impairment is

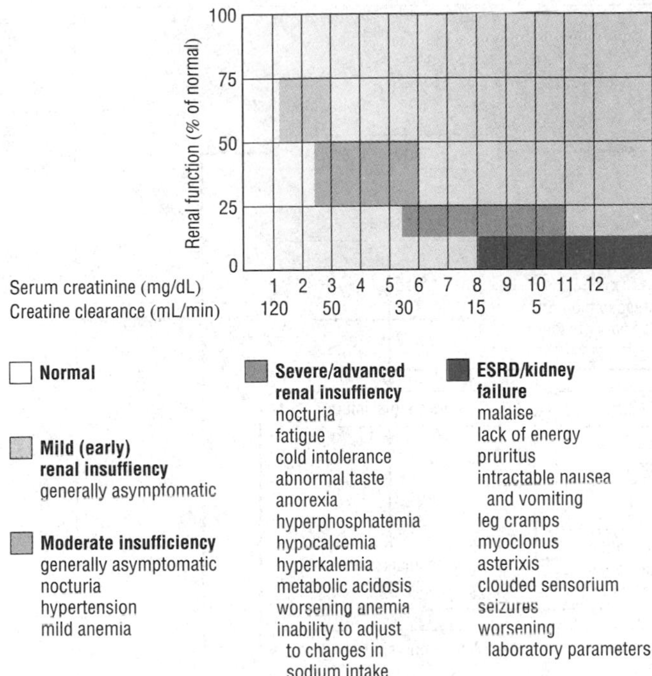

FIGURE 44–2. Staging of chronic kidney disease.

especially critical at this point, because the underlying disease process may reverse or stabilize with appropriate treatment.

- *Severe/advanced renal insufficiency* (CL_{cr} 15–29 mL/min). Patients with this degree of renal dysfunction will progress to ESRD, albeit at individual rates, in 2 to 4 years, unless aggressive pharmacotherapeutic interventions are initiated.
- *ESRD/kidney failure* (CL_{cr} < 15 mL/min). Uremia is a clinical syndrome that develops insidiously as renal function declines. It begins with nonspecific symptoms, which become progressively worse as the creatinine clearance drops below 15 mL/min. It is at this stage that dialysis is indicated to remove the by-products of protein metabolism, such as urea, thought to be largely responsible for this symptom complex (see Chap. 45). The patient requiring chronic dialysis or renal transplantation for relief of uremic symptoms is said to have ESRD.

PATHOPHYSIOLOGY

The mechanisms involved in the pathogenesis of progressive renal insufficiency have not been fully elucidated, but most individuals with creatinine clearance ≤40 mL/min progress to ESRD regardless of the underlying etiology.[9] Multiple risk factors have been identified, including diabetes mellitus or a family history of diabetes; hypertension; degree of proteinuria; hyperlipidemia; obesity; smoking; over 50 years of age; male; and non-white race. Based on experimental animal models, hemodynamic changes at the glomerulus exert a major influence on the rate of progression of renal disease.[10] Increased glomerular capillary plasma flow and glomerular capillary hydraulic pressure lead to glomerular hyperfiltration. Glomerular hyperfiltration and hypertension lead to progressive glomerulosclerosis (scarring within the renal glomeruli) and development of overt proteinuria.[10] In addition, glomerular capillary hypertension contributes directly to the function of remaining intact nephrons. In experimental renal disease, pharmacologic or dietary interventions that decrease glomerular capillary pressure limit the rate and extent of overt proteinuria and glomerulosclerosis.[9] The presence of systemic hypertension is not required for the development of glomerular hyperfiltration and hypertension but, when present, may amplify the pathologic effects of these intrarenal changes.[11] Early hyperfiltration is usually followed by persistent microalbuminuria.[12] Proteinuria is now recognized as an independent risk factor for progression of renal disease.[13] In fact, proteinuria combined with an elevated serum creatinine (>1.4 mg/dL in males and >1.2 mg/dL in females) or increased blood pressure (>140/90 mm Hg) places individuals at a higher risk of renal disease progression.[14] The exact role of proteinuria in promoting renal damage is not clear. One hypothesis involves protein leaking into the tubules, which is then taken up by tubular cells. The tubular cells then produce chemoattractants and cytokines which can react with macrophages and which can ultimately cause interstitial fibrosis and tubular damage.[15] In addition, formation of advanced glycation end-products within the kidney of diabetic patients may also play a role.[16] A reduction of filtration area secondary to glomerular cell injury can lead to hemodynamic changes that increase glomerular capillary pressure and can lead to functional and structural changes in the glomerulus. These pathologic processes lead to glomerulosclerosis, causing an elevation of systemic blood pressure, which may elicit further renal structure damage and consequent worsening of blood pressure control.[11,17,18]

The exact mechanisms involved in the development of ESRD among hypertensive individuals remains controversial. However, two potential mechanisms are a reduction of renal mass secondary to renal tubular ischemia and increased glomerular capillary pressure, which may lead to the development of glomerulosclerosis.[9,19]

Hyperlipidemia is another risk factor associated with progression of renal disease.[20] Experimental studies in rats have demonstrated accelerated glomerulosclerosis when dietary cholesterol supplementation is given in the presence of various renal diseases, whereas pharmacologic therapy or low-fat diets have been shown to limit the progression of renal disease.[9] Lipid abnormalities in patients with normal renal function have not been shown to cause glomerular injury.[21] In patients with diabetes and moderate renal insufficiency, increased low-density lipoprotein (LDL cholesterol) concentrations appear to be predictive of the rate of decline of glomerular function.[22] In nondiabetic patients, elevated total cholesterol, LDL cholesterol, and apolipoprotein B concentrations are associated with a more rapid decline in renal function.[23] Figure 44–3 summarizes the pathophysiology of the progression of renal disease.

CLINICAL PRESENTATION

The signs and symptoms of chronic renal insufficiency are dependent on the patient's degree of residual renal function (Fig. 44–2). The clinical presentation of most patients with early renal insufficiency may be asymptomatic. The primary abnormalities are elevations in serum creatinine and increased urinary protein excretion.

Diabetic nephropathy is characterized by persistent albuminuria/proteinuria (>300 mg/24 h), an increase in blood pressure, and decline in GFR, causing progression of renal disease to ESRD (Fig. 44–4).[14] Clinical studies in diabetic patients demonstrate that persistent microalbuminuria is highly predictive of progression of renal disease and is one of the best early predictors of diabetic nephropathy.[14] Detection of microalbuminuria is also an independent risk factor for heart attack and stroke.[14]

Nondiabetic patients—those with glomerulonephritis, hypertension, polycystic kidney disease, or other causes—may also exhibit proteinuria. Microalbuminuria occurs in 5% to 37% of hypertensive patients, and is a risk factor for an increased overall mortality rate.[25] The Multiple Risk Factor Intervention Trial (MRFIT) found that increased levels of proteinuria in nondiabetics were associated with a high risk of cardiovascular mortality.[24] Increased

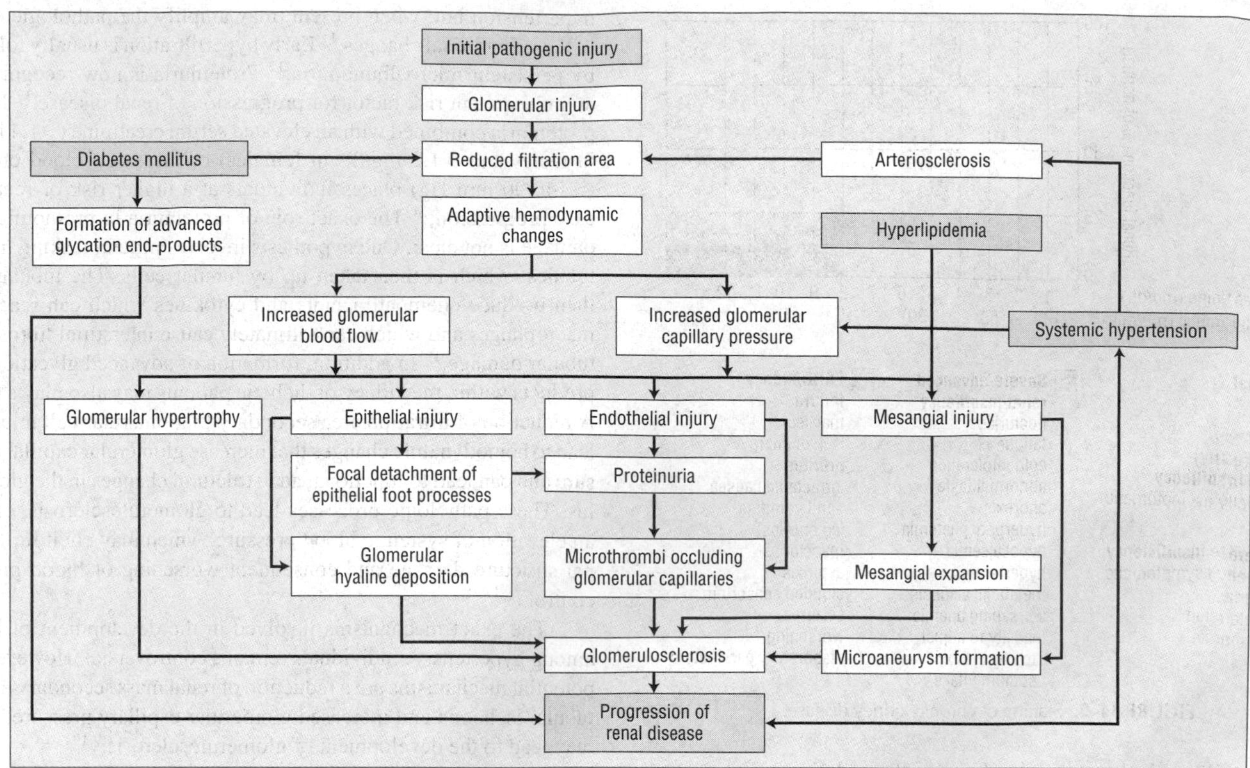

FIGURE 44–3. Proposed mechanisms for progression of renal disease.

urinary albumin excretion (UAE) in hypertensive individuals may be induced by renal hemodynamic changes, glomerular permeability changes, and glomerular structural changes caused by nephrosclerosis (Fig. 44–3). The urinary excretion of protein is generally greater than 2.5 g/day in those with glomerulonephritis. As a consequence, these individuals commonly develop hyperlipidemia and edema. Recent studies confirm that even in nondiabetic patients, proteinuria is an accurate and independent predictor for progression of renal diesease.[26]

DIAGNOSIS

DIABETICS

Type 1 diabetic patients with an elevated UAE are at high risk to develop overt nephropathy within 10 to 14 years.[27] Therefore,

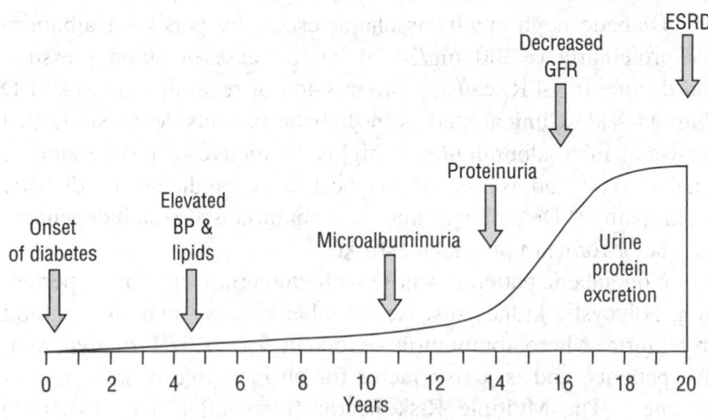

FIGURE 44–4. Clinical course of diabetic nephropathy.

early detection of microalbuminuria facilitates therapeutic intervention that may slow the progression of renal disease and other vascular complications.[14] Diabetic nephropathy is clinically diagnosed if persistent microalbuminuria is present in two of three consecutive urine samples.[14] These samples should be obtained within a 3-month period separated by at least 1 to 2 weeks. If the UAE values are consistently between 30 and 300 mg/24 h, the patient is classified as having persistent microalbuminuria.[14] Another specific and sensitive method of detecting microalbuminuria is a spot albumin:creatinine ratio.[28] If possible, the urine collection should be a first morning void, clean-catch specimen. A ratio of >30 mg urinary albumin/g urine creatinine is considered abnormal (Table 44–2).[14] Accurate assays that can detect UAE between 30 and 300 mg/24 h have been developed.[29] All patients with type 1 diabetes of more than 5 years' duration and all type 2 diabetics should have their urine checked annually for microalbuminuria. Several factors can acutely increase the UAE, including recent heavy exercise; recent ingestion of a high-protein meal; hematuria; sleep apnea; urinary tract infection; fever; uncontrolled hypertension; poor glycemic control; and congestive heart failure. Initial screening or rescreening should be postponed under any of these circumstances.

TABLE 44–2. Testing for Proteinuria/Albuminuria

Test	Normal Range
24-Hour urine albumin collection	<30 mg/24 h
24-Hour urine protein collection	<150 mg/24 h
"Spot" urine albumin:creatinine ratio	<30 mg urine albumin/g urine creatinine
"Spot" urine protein:creatinine ratio	<200 mg urine protein/g urine creatinine

NON-DIABETICS

High risk, non-diabetic patients should be screened on an annual basis for creatinine clearance, serum creatinine, urine protein, blood pressure, cholesterol, and symptoms. These patients include not only those listed in Table 44–1, but also any male with a S_{Cr} >1.5 mg/dL or a female with a S_{Cr} >1.2 mg/dL.[30] Patients with serum creatinine values that meet this criterion should also be evaluated by a nephrologist. As serum creatinine increases the risk for anemia, secondary hyperparathyroidism, metabolic acidosis, and other signs and symptoms also increase (Fig. 44–2). The anemia workup should include monitoring of hemoglobin and hematocrit, red blood cell (RBC) indices, reticulocyte count, and iron studies (serum iron, total iron-binding capacity, % transferrin saturation, and ferritin). To evaluate the extent of secondary hyperparathyroidism, the following labs should be evaluated: calcium, phosphorus, and parathyroid hormone level. Serum bicarbonate concentrations should be monitored occasionally to assess need for bicarbonate replacement therapy (see Chap. 53). The anemia, secondary hyperparathyroidism and metabolic acidosis workup applies to both diabetic and nondiabetic patients with renal insufficiency. Detailed information on treatment of these disorders is found in Chap. 45.

▶ TREATMENT: Progressive Renal Disease

DESIRED OUTCOME

Recent clinical trials have focused on the use of pharmacologic and nonpharmacologic interventions to reverse or delay progressive renal injury before patients develop symptomatic renal insufficiency. It is hoped that prevention and treatment programs that identify patients with early renal disease and focus on major risk factors, such as diabetes and hypertension, will reduce the incidence and prevalence of ESRD. The goals of therapy include stabilizing renal function for those with a GFR above 30 mL/min and the slowing of the rate of progression for those in the range of 15–30 mL/min.

DIABETICS

Nonpharmacologic Therapy

Nutritional Management. Although several small clinical trials have evaluated the role of dietary protein restriction on the rate of chronic renal disease progression, there is still not a clear consensus regarding its efficacy. Pedrini and colleagues evaluated the data from five trials in diabetics (n = 108) via meta-analysis. It was determined that a low-protein diet (range, 0.5–0.85 g/kg/day) reduced the risk of decline in GFR or the increase in urinary albumin excretion rate (relative risk 0.56 [Confidence Interval = 0.4–0.77], $P < 0.001$).[31] It should be noted that the number of patients was very small and a variety of study designs were used; therefore, the results of this analysis only suggest that dietary restriction in diabetic patients may be beneficial. Kasiske and colleagues also performed a meta-analysis of 13 randomized controlled trials (n = 1919) and found that dietary protein restriction was weakly associated with slowing the progression of renal disease.[32] The study population was mainly nondiabetic patients; however, a small subset of diabetic patients (n = 231; note: this meta-analysis does not include patients in the Pedrini study) demonstrated a greater response to the low-protein diet.[32] Overall, it appears that low-protein diet may have some benefit in delaying the progression to ESRD.

The National Kidney Foundation recently published the Kidney Disease Outcomes Quality Initiative (KDOQI) guidelines for nutrition in patients (diabetic and nondiabetic) with chronic renal insufficiency.[33] The recommended protein intake for patients with a GFR <25 mL/min was a diet providing 0.6 g protein/kg/day. This can be increased to 0.75 g protein/kg/day in patients who cannot achieve or maintain an adequate nutritional status with the lower protein diet.[33]

A salt-restricted diet may also slow the progression of renal disease in diabetics and nondiabetics. In certain individuals, a high-salt diet can lead to increased blood pressure, increased glomerular filtration, and a decrease in renal plasma flow.[34] Clinical studies also indicate that an increase in salt intake can limit the antihypertensive and antiproteinuric effects of various antihypertensive agents, including ACEIs and calcium channel blockers.[34]

Pharmacologic Therapy

Intensive Blood Glucose Control. Intensive blood glucose control in patients with type 1 diabetes has been reported to reduce the frequency, decrease the severity, and delay the development or progression of diabetic complications including nephropathy in a number of randomized clinical trials.[35] Although most of these studies included small numbers of subjects (<100) and a short duration of follow-up (<5 years), a meta-analysis of 16 clinical trials demonstrated a statistically significant decreased risk of nephropathy in those on long-term intensive insulin therapy.[35]

The Diabetes Control and Complications Trial (DCCT) was a multicenter (1,441 patients), randomized study designed with sufficient statistical power to compare outcomes associated withintensive versus standard insulin therapy.[36] Intensive insulin therapy was defined as the administration of insulin three or more times daily by injection or by external pump. Intensive insulin therapy reduced the incidence of microalbuminuria and albuminuria as compared to standard therapy in both the primary prevention (no diabetic complications, n = 726) and secondary prevention (preexisting early diabetic complications, n = 715) group.[36] Unfortunately, long-term rigid glycemic control with insulin was associated with a higher incidence of hypoglycemic reactions. There was at least one episode of hypoglycemia in 65% of the patients in the intensive group, as compared to 35% in the standard group.[36] However, decreased diabetic complications in the intensive therapy group outweighed the increased risk of hypoglycemia.[37] A longer follow-up period, however, would have been needed to evaluate the degree by which intensive glucose control would delay the development of diabetic nephropathy.[37] These improved clinical outcomes may not be achievable in clinical practice because many poorly controlled type 1 diabetic patients are reluctant to comply with these recommendations because they fear the risk of hypoglycemia and thus are often lost to follow-up after they are prescribed intensive insulin therapy.[38] The Epidemiology of Diabetes Interventions and Complications (EDIC) study was a 4-year follow-up observational study of DCCT subjects receiving care from primary physicians. The study found that intensive insulin therapy reduced the risk of nephropathy (53% odds ratio reduction in microalbuminuria) for at least 4 years following the DCCT trial.[39]

The United Kingdom Prospective Diabetes Study (UKPDS), a large (n = 3,867) prospective study, assessed the impact of intensive blood glucose and blood pressure control in newly diagnosed patients with type 2 diabetes. The primary end points of the study were microvascular and macrovascular complications including, diabetes-related renal failure and diabetes-related death from renal disease.[40] The therapy in the intensive treatment group included sulfonylureas, metformin, or insulin, while the conventional group was treated with diet therapy alone (see Chap. 74). The hemoglobin A1c in the intensive treatment group was reduced by 11% as compared to the conventional group for the first 10 years following diagnosis.[40] Intensive glucose control, however, did not show a statistically significant decrease in the frequency of microalbuminuria and proteinuria until 9 years after study initiation. The authors concluded that intensive therapy reduced microvascular complications, and that there was also a marked but nonsignificant reduction ($P = 0.052$) in macrovascular complications, specifically myocardial infarction.[40] Diabetes-related mortality, however, was not reduced. It should be noted that the number of renal related events was small and because the subjects were only followed for 15 years from diagnosis, the duration of follow-up may not have been long enough to detect the renal end points.

Antihypertensive Agents. Blood pressure continues to rise or may develop at the onset of diabetic nephropathy and becomes more problematic with the progression of renal insufficiency (Fig. 44–4). Patients diagnosed with both hypertension and diabetes have up to a sixfold higher risk of developing ESRD than do those patients with diabetes mellitus alone.[41] Furthermore, elevated blood pressure is observed more often in type 1 patients with persistent microalbuminuria than in type 1 patients without microalbuminuria. Adequate blood pressure control can reduce the rate of decline in GFR and the degree of albuminuria in hypertensive type 1 or type 2 diabetics.[41] Aggressive β-blocker and diuretic therapy decreased UAE by nearly 50% in a long-term (>6 years) study in type 1 patients with microalbuminuria.[42] ACEIs reduce glomerular capillary pressure and volume, which in animal models of diabetic nephropathy results in preservation of renal function.[43,44] Table 44–3 summarizes the effects of various antihypertensive agents on renal blood flow and GFR.[45,46]

A meta-analysis of 100 controlled and uncontrolled clinical studies assessed the relative effect of several antihypertensive agents on proteinuria and renal function in type 1 and type 2 patients.[47] None of the antihypertensive agents or classes analyzed had a greater effect on blood pressure reduction than any other agent or class. However, only ACEIs decreased proteinuria and preserved GFR independent of the beneficial effects associated with blood pressure reduction.

The results of the multicenter controlled captopril clinical trial indicate that in type 1 patients with nephropathy (n = 409) the progression of renal failure can be reduced.[48] The primary end point of this study was a doubling of the baseline serum creatinine. This pivotal trial proved that captopril can slow the progression of renal disease by providing nearly a 50% reduction in the risk of doubling the serum creatinine.[48] This effect was independent of blood pressure reduction and of greatest benefit in those with the lowest renal function.

A 5-year double-blind trial of enalapril 10 mg every day or placebo in normotensive type 2 patients (n = 103) with microalbuminuria, resulted in stabilization of plasma creatinine concentration and decreased albuminuria in the enalapril group as compared to the placebo group.[49] Another enalapril study in type 2 diabetics reported similar results; a 12.5% absolute risk reduction for the enalapril treatment arm in the development of microalbuminuria over the 6-year followup.[50] Lisinopril has also been reported to decrease proteinuria in normotensive type 1 diabetic patients with microalbuminuria.[51] Recently, the Heart Outcomes Prevention Evaluation (HOPE) study evaluated the effects of ramipril on cardiovascular and renal disease endpoints.[52] This large (n = 9,541), multicentered study included 3,577 subjects with diabetes (98% were type 2 diabetics). The analysis of the patients with diabetes revealed an overall risk reduction of 24% in overt nephropathy in patients treated with ramipril over 4 to 5 years.[52] Compared to the small number of events seen in the UKPDS, the HOPE study had more than 100 events within each group, which increased the power of the analysis. The results of a recent meta-analysis confirm the beneficial effects of ACEI therapy. Progression to proteinuria was reduced by 65% in patients with diabetes and microalbuminuria, and by 40% in patients with overt proteinuria (30% diabetics and 70% nondiabetics) (Fig. 44–5A).[53] The results of this meta-analysis also suggest that ACEIs have a marked impact on the

TABLE 44–3. Effects of Antihypertensive Agents on Renal Blood Flow (RBF) and Glomerular Filtration Rate (GFR)

Antihypertensive Agent	Mechanism of Action	Effects on Renal Hemodynamics
Diuretics	Sodium and volume depletion	Decrease in GFR and RBF
	↑Vasodilatory prostaglandin levels (IV loop diuretics)	Increase in RBF
	Renal vasoconstriction (IV thiazide diuretics)	Decrease in GFR and RBF
β-Adrenergic blockers	↓ Cardiac output	Decrease in GFR and RBF
	↑ Renal vascular resistance (nonselective agents)	Decrease in GFR and RBF
	↓ Renal vascular resistance (β_1-selective agents)	No change in GFR and RBF
Centrally acting antiadrenergic drugs	↓ Renal vascular resistance (methyldopa)	No change in GFR and RBF
	↓ Renal perfusion pressure (clonidine, α_2-adrenergic agonist)	Decrease in GFR and RBF
Peripherally acting antiadrenergic drugs	Direct vasodilation (postsynaptic α_1-adrenoreceptor blocking agents)	No change in GFR and RBF
Direct vasodilator agents	↓ Renal vascular resistance (hydralazine, minoxidil)	Increase in RBF and no effect on GFR
	Arterial vasodilation plus dilatation of venous capacitance vessels (nitroprusside)	Decrease in GFR and RBF (acute effect)
ACE inhibitors/angiotensin-II receptor blockers	Dilation of the efferent arteriole	Decrease in GFR and no change in RBF
Calcium channel blockers	↓ Renal vascular resistance by vasodilation of afferent arterioles (hypertensive patients)	Increase in RBF and no change in GFR

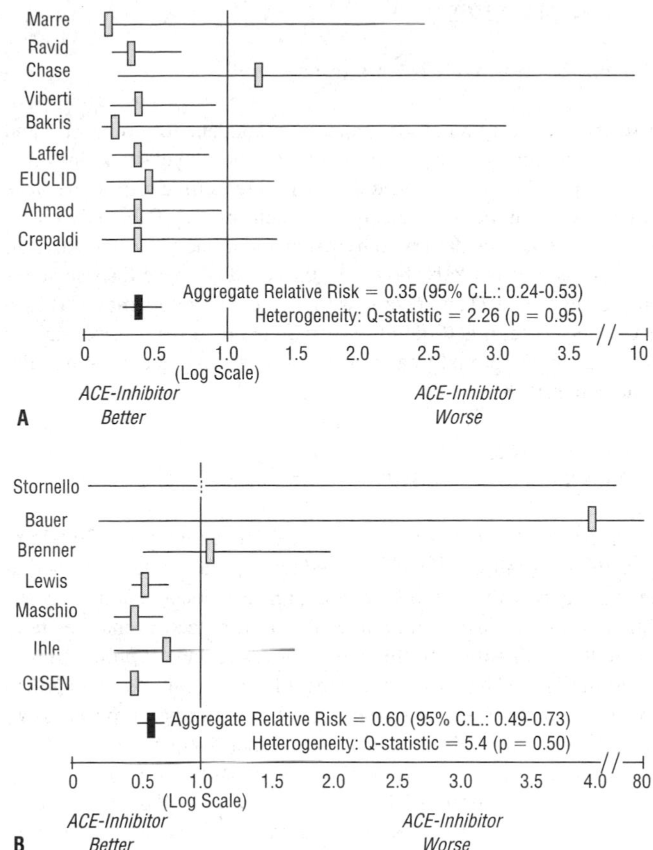

FIGURE 44–5. A. Relative risk for developing microalbuminuria with 95% confidence intervals (CIs) in each study, and the aggregate relative risk with 95% CIs for all studies. (N = 642 with diabetes). **B.** Relative risk for doubling serum creatinine concentration or development of ESRD with 95% CIs in each study, and aggregate relative risk with 95% CIs for all studies. (N = 1,277; 479 with diabetes). (From Ref. 53, used with permission.)

relative risks of doubling of serum creatinine (Fig. 44–5B). These data provide strong support for the use of ACEIs in diabetic patients with or without hypertension.

A variety of ACEIs and doses have been studied, however there is no consensus regarding the optimal ACEI agent or starting dose. The most commonly studied ACEIs in randomized controlled trials are captopril, enalapril, lisinopril, ramipril, and benazepril. It should be noted that ACEIs such as quinapril and moexipril have never been evaluated in any human renal disease progression trials. Although all ACEIs studied have a positive impact on slowing the progression of renal disease, it is not clear that they all yield a similar degree of benefit. Because their pharmacokinetic profiles yield variable plasma and peak/trough ratios, and different tissue concentrations, it is feasible that these characteristics may result in different therapeutic outcomes. Further studies are necessary to answer this question. For normotensive patients with microalbuminuria, one should start with a low ACEI dose and titrate to reduce microalbuminuria by 50% to 80% and yet avoid hypotension. In hypertensive patients, the primary goal is to optimally control the blood pressure and secondarily to minimize urinary protein losses.

The role of angiotensin II receptor blockers (ARBs) in slowing the progression of renal disease is also being investigated. Several experimental models of chronic progressive renal disease have shown similar efficacy to ACEIs. The ARBs candesartan and losartan slow the progression of glomerulopathy in diabetic rats.[54] Recent data on ARB use in humans with progressive renal disease shows favorable results. The Evaluation of Losartan in the Elderly (ELITE) study compared losartan versus captopril in 722 (25% diabetic) patients over 65 years old with heart failure. The study showed that there was no difference in renal dysfunction between groups at both baseline and study completion.[55] The Irbesartan Type II Diabetes Mellitus Nephropathy Trial (IDNT) study included 1,650 patients in 225 clinics worldwide. Patients were assigned to one of three therapies: irbesartan, calcium channel blocker (amlodipine), or placebo.[56] The primary end point of this study was a composite of doubling of baseline serum creatinine, time to ESRD or death. Over a 2.6-year follow-up, the results indicated a 33% reduction in the incidence of the primary end point with irbesartan therapy compared with placebo.[56] Early intervention with irbesartan has also recently been reported to be renoprotective. Parving and colleagues reported that the time to onset of diabetic nephropathy was significantly delayed in type 2 patients who received 300 mg daily for up to 2 years.[57] This beneficial effect was independent of the degree of blood pressure reduction. A similar trend was observed in those who received 150 mg daily, however this did not achieve statistical significance ($P = 0.08$). The Reduction of Endpoints in Non-Insulin Dependent Diabetes Mellitus with the Angiotensin II Antagonist Losartan (RENAAL) study included 1,513 patients from 29 countries.[58] Patients had a history of type 2 diabetes, proteinuria, and renal insufficiency, and were randomized to either losartan (50–100 mg qd) or placebo. The primary end point for this study was also a composite of doubling of the serum creatinine and time to ESRD or death. After 3.4 years of follow-up, the composite end point was reduced by 16% in the losartan group ($P = 0.024$). The relative risk reduction for time to ESRD and doubling of the baseline serum creatinine was reduced with losartan therapy by 28% ($P = 0.002$) and 25% ($P = 0.006$), respectively. However, there was no difference in death between losartan- and placebo-treated subjects.

These findings indicate that the benefit of slowing the progression of renal disease can be seen with the ARBs as well as with the ACEIs. However, until head-to-head trials with these agents are assessed they should not be considered interchangeable.[59]

Bradykinins may play an important role in renal hemodynamics.[60] Because ACEIs prevent the degradation of bradykinins and ARBs lack this effect, more information is necessary before the agents can be considered interchangeable. Combination therapy with ACEIs and ARBs may also be beneficial to further block angiotensin II, yet retain the potential beneficial effects of bradykinin.

Although calcium channel blockers (CCBs) mainly dilate the afferent arteriole and result in no change or an increase in glomerular capillary pressure, some agents in this class decrease glomerular injury without changing renal hemodynamics.[44] The postulated mechanisms for this decrease in renal injury include suppression of glomerular hypertrophy, inhibition of platelet aggregation, and decreased salt accumulation.[44] Two meta-analyses suggest that diabetic patients tended to have either an increase or no reduction in albuminuria if they are treated with dihydropyridine calcium antagonists.[61,62] However, one meta-analysis concluded that nondihydropyridine CCBs may have beneficial effects on proteinuria similar to ACEIs that are independent of blood-pressure reductions.[62] In a prospective study of 52 type 2 diabetics, Bakris et al. reported that the patients treated with nondihydropyridine CCBs (SR verapamil or diltiazem) did as well as those receiving lisinopril, and better than those who received atenolol.[63] The few studies that have evaluated the efficacy of combination therapy with ACEIs and nondihydropyridine CCBs suggest that combination therapy may be more efficacious than either agent alone.[64] Overall, ACEIs and possibly nondihydropyridine CCBs are more effective than other antihypertensive agents at decreasing albuminuria in both type 1 and type 2 diabetics.

The Joint National Committee on Detection, Evaluation, and Treatment of High Blood Pressure (JNC VI) recommends a goal blood pressure of <130/85 mm Hg for patients with renal insufficiency without proteinuria to delay the progression of renal disease.[65] However, some recent large prospective studies, including the Hypertension Optimal Treatment (HOT) trial and the UKPDS, have demonstrated that further reductions in diastolic blood pressure (<80 mm Hg) provides additional benefits.[66,67] These benefits include slowing the progression of renal disease, as well as reduced cardiovascular events. The mean blood pressure in the UKPDS trial tight controlled group (captopril or atenolol) was 144/82 mm Hg versus 154/87 mm Hg in the less-tight group, a statistically significant difference.[67] This difference in blood pressure conferred reductions of 24% in diabetes-related end points, 32% in deaths related to diabetes, 44% in strokes, and 37% in microvascular end points.[67] The study of Lewis and colleagues evaluated the effect of these more rigorous goals on proteinuria and progression of renal disease in type 1 diabetics over 2 years (n = 129).[68] In this study, captopril therapy was titrated to achieve a goal mean arterial pressure (MAP) of ≤92 mm Hg versus 100–107 mm Hg. The authors concluded that more aggressive management of blood pressure to a MAP of ≤92 mm Hg (≤120/80 mm Hg) was optimal to decrease proteinuria.[68] The goal blood pressure for patients with renal insufficiency and >1 g/day of proteinuria remains at 125/75 mm Hg.[65] To achieve these goal blood pressures, three or more different blood pressure medications are likely required.[41] Based on this new information, the National Kidney Foundation Hypertension and Diabetes Executive Committees Working Group has recommended a new target blood pressure, for patients with diabetes and/or renal insufficiency, of <130/80 mm Hg.[41] Figure 44–6 depicts the paradigm they proposed for the management of blood pressure in people with renal insufficiency and diabetes.

NON-DIABETICS

General Approach To Treatment

Patients with early renal insufficiency secondary to glomerular and tubulointerstitial disease, nephrosclerosis, and polycystic kidney disease frequently are grouped together in large clinical trials because of the lower number of subjects with each disease. Patients with renal insufficiency secondary to hypertension alone would also fit into this category. It is likely, however, that each of these disease states progresses to ESRD and responds to therapeutic interventions differently. Therefore, it is difficult to extrapolate data from these trials to define a single optimal treatment pathway for patients with nondiabetic nephropathy.

Nonpharmacologic Therapy

Nutritional Management. Two recent meta-analyses of randomized clinical trials concluded that reducing protein intake in nondiabetic patients with mild to severe renal insufficiency could delay the time to onset of ESRD and reduce the occurrence of renal death by about 40%.[68,69] Although the optimal level of dietary protein intake could not be deduced from the latest of these analyses, the authors concluded that a restricted protein intake should be proposed to all patients. Unfortunately, it is unclear whether adequate nutrition and quality of life can be maintained in patients on low-protein diets.

The Modification of Diet in Renal Disease (MDRD) multicenter study was the largest prospective trial that evaluated the influence of dietary protein and phosphorus restriction on the progression of renal insufficiency in nondiabetic patients.[70] The contribution of blood pressure control was a secondary independent intervention. In this study, 840 patients were enrolled into one of two groups:

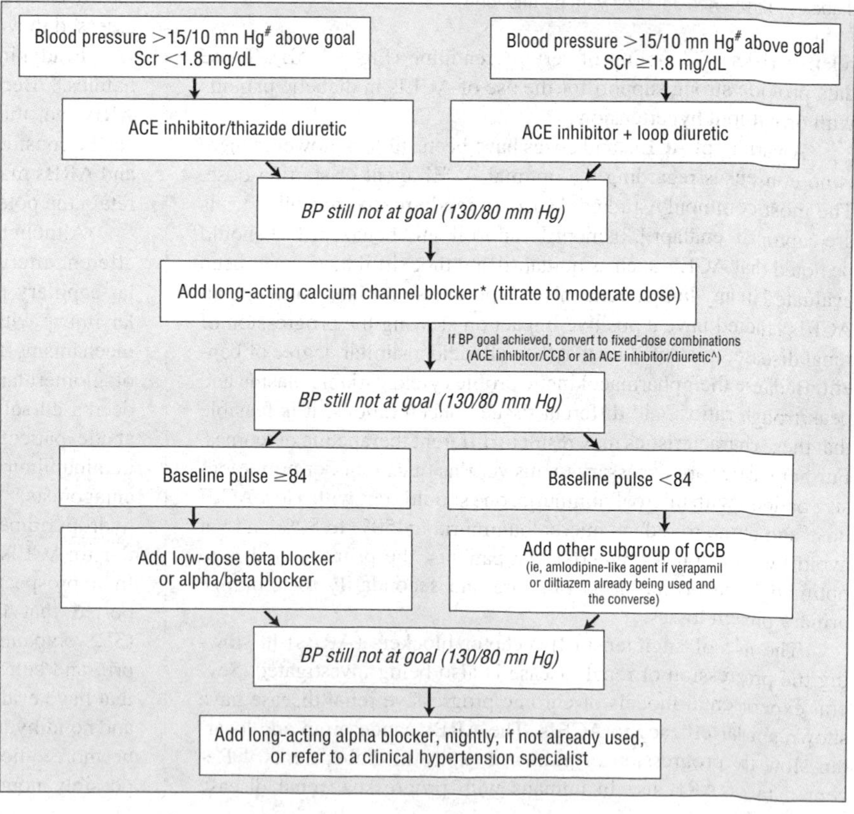

FIGURE 44–6. A suggested paradigm by which blood pressure goals in people with renal insufficiency and/or diabetes can be achieved by the *least-intrusive means possible.* # = Everyone with diabetes and/or renal insufficiency should be instructed on *lifestyle modifications* as per the JNC VI. Everyone, however, should be started on therapy if blood pressure is greater than 130/85 mm Hg. Note that, if blood pressure is <15/10 mm Hg above goal (130/80 mm Hg), then ACEI alone may be used. ^ = ACEI should be the same if two different fixed-dose combinations are used. * = Nondihydropyridine CCBs (verapamil and diltiazem reduce cardiovascular mortality, proteinuria, and diabetic nephropathy progression independent of an ACEI). β-Blockers may be substituted for CCBs if the patient has angina, heart failure, or arrhythmia necessitating their use. (Ref. # 41, used with permission.)

moderate (n = 585) and severe (n = 255) renal dysfunction based on GFR, which was determined by the renal clearance of iothalamate. Subjects in the moderate renal function group (GFR of 25–55 mL/min/1.73 m^2) were randomized into one of four groups: usual or a low-protein diet (1.3 vs 0.58 g/kg/day) with a usual or low MAP goal (107 vs 92 mm Hg). Subjects with severe renal dysfunction (GFR 13–24 mL/min/1.73 m^2) were also randomized to one of four groups: a low-protein diet or very-low-protein diet (0.28 g/kg/day along with a keto acid-amino acid supplement) with a usual or low MAP goal as already described. No significant benefit of protein restriction was demonstrated after 3 years of follow-up in any group. Unfortunately, 24% of the study subjects enrolled had the diagnosis of polycystic kidney disease. This may have confounded the results, because patients with polycystic kidneys tend to progress to renal failure regardless of the intervention.

Secondary analyses of the MDRD study revealed that in those patients with a GFR less than 25 mL/min/1.73 m^2, a protein intake of 0.6 g/kg/day was significantly associated with a decreased rate of progressive renal disease.[71] The rate of progression to ESRD was significantly reduced by 41% for each 0.2 g/kg/day reduction in dietary protein intake. The discrepancy in results can be explained by the different statistical methods used in the two analyses of the data from the MDRD study. The original MDRD study used an intent to treat analysis, which accounted for all patients enrolled regardless of their compliance or follow-up. The secondary analyses only evaluated participants who were compliant with dietary prescription in the high- versus low-protein groups. These analyses demonstrated that if low protein intakes were actually achieved, patients with a GFR less than 25 mL/min/1.73 m^2 would benefit from a protein intake of 0.6 g/kg/day. Recently published nutritional guidelines advocate a protein intake of 0.6 mg/kg/day in patients with a GFR <25 mL/min.[33]

An overall reduction in the rate of GFR decline of 0.53 mL/min/y with the addition of a low-protein diet was recently reported in the meta-analysis of Kasiske et al.[32] The results of protein restriction in nondiabetics indicated a slight overall beneficial effect, however, other more favorable interventions should also be implemented. The use of protein restriction becomes a balancing act between providing too much protein in the diet and therefore risking progression of renal disease versus too little protein and thereby increasing the risk of malnutrition.

Pharmacologic Therapy

Antihypertensive Agents. All hypertensive agents do not preserve renal function to the same degree despite equal blood pressure control. It is important to realize that precipitous falls in blood pressure to normotensive levels may be acutely deleterious to renal function in patients with impaired renal function. This may be especially problematic in the patient treated for hypertensive crisis. Target blood pressure in these patients should be achieved over several weeks so as to allow the kidney to adapt to reduced perfusion pressures.[65] In addition, it is preferable to use antihypertensive agents that maintain renal blood flow and thus do not contribute to declining renal function. An acute but sustained decline in GFR, however, should be expected in patients receiving ACEIs because they reduce intraglomerular pressure, which is the driving force for GFR. S_{Cr} elevations of 25% to 30% within 3 to 7 days after starting therapy should be anticipated and are indicative of the ACEIs pharmacologic effect.[72] If the S_{Cr} rises by more than this the patient may be experiencing hemodynamic-mediated drug-induced acute renal failure, which can be promptly managed by stopping the drug (see Chap. 48).

Several short-term (<1 year) and a few long-term (>2 years) clinical trials have evaluated the effect of three ACEIs (benazepril, enalapril, and ramipril) on renal hemodynamics in nondiabetic patients.[73] Renal function remained stable during short-term ACEI therapy in the majority of these studies and reductions in proteinuria and the rate of progression of renal disease were evident in the others. A large randomized, study compared ramipril plus conventional therapy to placebo plus conventional therapy in 166 nondiabetic patients with nephrotic range proteinuria (>3 g/24 h). Ramipril (1.25–5 mg qd) reduced proteinuria and the rate of GFR decline to a greater extent than what would have been expected from blood pressure reduction alone.[74] Interestingly, the reduction in proteinuria was greatest in those with the highest baseline levels. Unfortunately, the study did not specify which additional antihypertensive agents were administered to study participants. Therefore, if nondihydropyridine CCBs were administered to more patients in one group, the results may have been confounded. A subsequent study by the same group of investigators in patients with a lower degree of proteinuria revealed similar beneficial effects.[75] The relative risk of developing ESRD was 2.3 times higher in the conventional therapy plus placebo group than was the risk for those receiving ramipril. The urinary protein excretion rate was also significantly lower in the treatment group during the 5 years of the study, although the diastolic blood pressures were similar. A recent meta-analysis confirms the results of these two studies and reveals that ACEIs confer a 40% reduction in the risk of developing ESRD or doubling of serum creatinine in patients with overt proteinuria (>330 mg protein/24 h) and renal disease of varying causes (about 50% diabetic patients; see Fig. 44–5B).[53]

With the exception of fosinopril, the clearance of all ACEIs (or their active metabolites) is reduced in renal failure and lower initial doses should be utilized and then later titrated to achieve the optimal therapeutic effect.[76] The antiproteinuric effects of ACEIs have an extended dose-response relationship as compared to the ACEIs antihypertensive action, which tends to plateau sooner. Thus, patients who have reached their goal blood pressure may require further increases in dosage to achieve the maximal reduction in urinary protein excretion. Also, hyperkalemia can complicate ACEI use, especially when patients are concurrently receiving nonsteroidal anti-inflammatory agents.

Studies with ARBs in the progression of nondiabetic renal are limited. Emerging data suggests that these agents may have similar efficacy with ACEIs, particularly in patients with hemodynamically-mediated renal injury.[60] One trial of 188 nondiabetic patients with stable renal insufficiency compared lisinopril (10 mg/day) to valsartan (80 mg/day) over 13 weeks. The data showed that the two agents demonstrated similar efficacy and safety for lowering blood pressure and proteinuria in subjects with a median GFR between 65 and 71 mL/min.[60] A similar study found losartan (50 mg/day) to be as effective as enalapril (20 mg/day) in reducing albuminuria.[77] Combination therapy with ACEIs has been proposed and preliminary data suggest that the combination is safe and results in a greater decrease in proteinuria than that seen with either agent alone.[78]

The calcium channel blocking agents are also effective treatments for hypertension in nondiabetic patients with renal insufficiency and ESRD. However, because all CCBs preferentially dilate pre-glomerular vessels, failure to normalize blood pressure could increase intra-glomerular pressure. There are some experimental data that suggest that nondihydropyridine CCBs may slow the rate of decline of renal function by multiple mechanisms.[61,79] Dosage alterations are unnecessary in renal insufficiency and dosage should be titrated to achieve the desired degree of blood pressure reduction.

Diuretics are commonly used to treat fluid overload and hypertension in patients with renal insufficiency. They may be particularly well suited for treatment of the older patient with compromised renal function who tend to have salt-sensitive blood pressure.[80] Diuretic therapy is clearly indicated in the patient with volume overload, or in patients with fluid retention secondary to other antihypertensive agents. As creatinine clearance falls below 20–30 mL/min, the thiazide diuretics lose their saluretic (increasing the renal excretion of sodium) action but still maintain a modest antihypertensive effect, possibly because of vasodilation.[81] Saluresis in patients with severe renal insufficiency can be maintained through the use of potent loop diuretics such as furosemide, torsemide, or bumetanide. As creatinine clearance declines further, these agents may become ineffective saluretics as well. In such patients, a combination of a loop diuretic plus a thiazide diuretic or metolazone may prove beneficial,[82] although close clinical and laboratory monitoring should be undertaken to prevent profound dehydration and metabolic derangements. Potassium-sparing diuretics, such as spironolactone, triamterene, and amiloride, should be used with extreme caution, if at all, in patients with moderate to severe renal insufficiency (<30 mL/min) because of the risk of hyperkalemia. Triamterene should probably be avoided in renally impaired patients also receiving nonsteroidal anti-inflammatory drugs because of the potential risk of precipitating acute renal failure.[83]

Oral and transdermal clonidine has been used with some success in patients with renal insufficiency.[84] Although the bioavailability of the transdermal system has not been evaluated in this patient population, plasma concentrations are comparable to those achieved with oral dosing.[84] Patients who respond to oral clonidine should maintain blood pressure control when switched to equivalent dosages of the transdermal patch. α_1-Adrenoceptor antagonists (prazosin, terazosin, doxazosin) are also well tolerated and reduce blood pressure in short-term clinical trials in patients with renal insufficiency.[85] There may also be, however, benefit to therapy with α_1-adrenoceptor antagonists in males with benign prostatic hypertrophy. However, there are no data available to determine whether clonidine or α_1-blockers are useful in retarding renal failure progression above and beyond the benefits anticipated to result from blood pressure reduction alone. As a final note, the use of doxazosin in the ALLHAT trial was recently prematurely discontinued because of a higher risk of stroke, congestive heart failure, and angina as compared to patients receiving chlorthalidone.[86] Thus, these agents should be used with extreme caution in patients with renal insufficiency who already have a high risk of cardiovascular death.

Although advocated as first- or second-line therapy in the treatment of essential hypertension, β-blocking agents, with the exception of nadolol and labetalol, may reduce renal blood flow secondary to a reduction in cardiac output in patients with renal insufficiency.[87,88] Even though a deterioration in GFR is unlikely, the availability of multiple other agents relegates these to a lower tier in the therapeutic armamentarium. Hydrophilic β-blockers such as nadolol, acebutolol, and atenolol are mainly eliminated via urinary excretion of unchanged drug, and may require significant dosage adjustment in renally insufficient patients.[89] Minoxidil, when given concurrently with β-adrenoceptor-blocking agents and diuretics (to control tachycardia and fluid retention, respectively), effectively lowers blood pressure in antihypertensive patients with renal insufficiency.[90] However, it is unclear whether minoxidil reduces the rate of decline in renal function.

Large, controlled, randomized prospective studies are needed to determine what degree of blood pressure control is most effective in delaying nondiabetic renal disease, and which antihypertensive agents or combination of agents provide the greatest benefit. Additionally, the issue of control of systemic versus intraglomerular pressure and the potential benefit of specific agents remain to be answered. According to the National High Blood Pressure Education Program, special attention should be paid to hypertensive black patients, those with renal insufficiency, diabetics, and the elderly—groups at the highest risk of progression to ESRD if left untreated. Goal blood pressure defined as 130/85 mm Hg should be sought for all patients, and if tolerated, a lower blood pressure goal of 125/75 may be beneficial for blacks and patients with renal disease and proteinuria above 1 g/24 h.[65,66,91]

Regardless of the treatment regimen, hypertension should be tightly controlled in the patient with underlying renal disease. If proteinuria is present, the use of ACEIs, ARBs, and possibly nondihydropyridine CCBs may be superior to conventional agents in decreasing proteinuria and glomerular hypertension.

HYPERLIPIDEMIA

PATHOPHYSIOLOGY

Hyperlipidemia is associated with progressive renal disease in both animal and human studies.[92] In animal models, use of lipid-lowering agents decreases the extent of glomerular injury when both underlying renal disease and hyperlipidemia are present.[20,22] Therefore, the correction of lipid abnormalities in patients with renal insufficiency may have a beneficial effect on the rate of progression of renal disease. Experimental data indicate that hyperlipidemia may interact with concomitant risk factors such as hypertension, diabetes, and preexisting renal damage to accelerate progression of glomerular injury. The use of a low-fat diet and/or addition of antilipemic agents to the therapeutic regimen may be beneficial in diabetic and nondiabetic patients with renal disease and lipid abnormalities (see Chap. 21). Chronic renal failure with or without nephrotic syndrome is frequently accompanied by abnormalities in lipoprotein metabolism. The prevalence of hyperlipidemia appears to increase as renal function declines.[93] In chronic renal insufficiency without nephrotic syndrome, type IV hyperlipidemia with hypertriglyceridemia (plasma concentrations >200 mg/dL) is seen in approximately 40% to 50% of patients. In addition, 20% to 30% of these patients experience elevations in total cholesterol (TC) >240 mg/dL with 10% to 45% experiencing LDL concentrations >130 mg/dL. Although the concentrations of LDL are not uniformly increased in all patients with renal disease, these patients appear to produce small, dense LDL particles that are more susceptible to oxidation and that are more atherogenic than larger LDL subfractions.[94] Other lipoprotein abnormalities include a reduction in high-density lipoprotein (HDL) concentrations in 25% to 30% of patients, as well as changes in apoprotein (apo) content of lipoprotein molecules (reduction in apo CIII in very-low-density lipoproteins [VLDL]; a decrease in apo A-I in HDL; and elevations in apo B and lipoprotein [a]).[94] Peripheral insulin resistance, carnitine deficiency, and hyperparathyroidism may also contribute to lipid abnormalities.[94] In patients with renal insufficiency and urinary protein excretion greater than 3 g/day, the major lipid abnormalities are elevation of plasma total and LDL cholesterol (prevalence 85% to 90%), with approximately 50% of patients experiencing a low HDL (< 35 mg/dL) cholesterol and 60% of patients showing triglyceride concentrations greater than 200 mg/dL.[93] Figure 44–7 outlines the proposed mechanisms involved

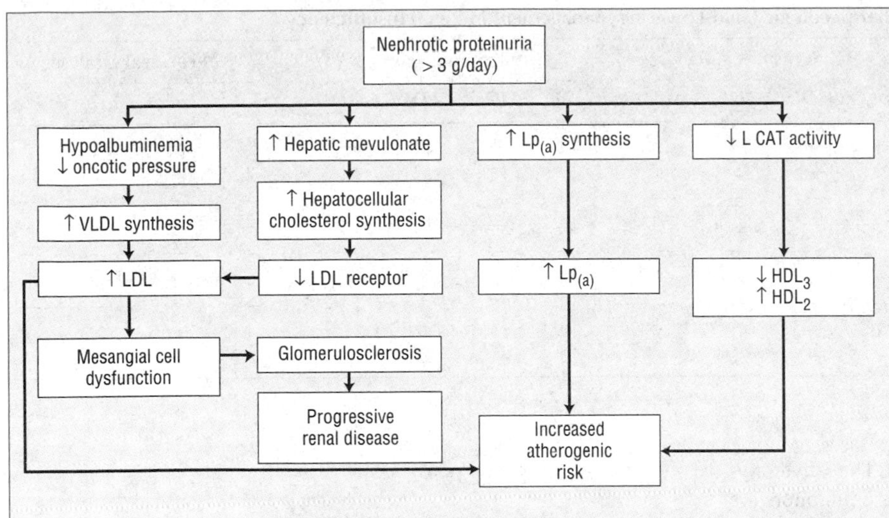

FIGURE 44–7. Potential effects of proteinuria on hyperlipidemia in the nephrotic syndrome. VLDL = very-low-density lipoprotein; LDL = low-density lipoprotein; $LP_{(a)}$ = lipoprotein (a); HDL = high-density lipoprotein; HDL_2 and HDL_3 are subfractions of HDL; LCAT = lecithin cholesterol acyltransferase.

in dyslipidemia of the nephrotic syndrome. Treatment of proteinuria resolves the hyperlipidemia in most patients.

CLINICAL PRESENTATION

Because "myocardial infarction" and "other cardiac causes" are the most commonly reported causes of death in the ESRD population, it would seem prudent to treat patients before their renal disease progresses.[95] Figure 44–2 shows the symptoms associated with decreasing renal function. Unfortunately, many patients are asymptomatic at the time of presentation and the diagnosis is made based on laboratory findings. Whether hypercholesterolemia, hypertriglyceridemia, or other lipoprotein changes contribute to the high incidence of cardiovascular disease or lead to progression of renal disease in these patients is controversial. Clearly, other concomitant risk factors—for example, anemia, diabetes, albuminuria, smoking, hypertension, and left ventricular enlargement—are often present before patients reach ESRD. There are a few epidemiologic studies in chronic kidney disease (CKD) patients with nephrotic syndrome that suggest that the relative risk of coronary death or myocardial infarction is higher in this population as compared with matched controls.[93] Similar analyses have been done in CKD patients without nephrotic syndrome and in patients on dialysis with various lipoprotein abnormalities (low HDL, high triglycerides, high apo B and lipoprotein [a]) correlating with higher risk of cardiovascular disease.[93] Unfortunately, the findings aren't uniform between studies. In addition, hypertriglyceridemia alone has not been shown to be a strong independent risk factor for coronary heart disease in patients with normal renal function following multivariate analysis of several studies.[96] However, hypertriglyceridemia may reduce levels of "protective" HDL, which is now classified as a major risk factor for coronary heart disease.[96] Thus, although hypertriglyceridemia itself may not be atherogenic, it may increase coronary risk through its effects on other lipoproteins.

▶ TREATMENT: Hyperlipidemia

There are no published interventional trials examining whether treatment of the various lipid disorders seen in patients with renal insufficiency reduces the risk of cardiovascular disease. However, there is epidemiologic evidence that lipoprotein abnormalities are associated with higher risk of cardiovascular disease.[93] It is likely that the same lipoprotein abnormalities that confer increased risk of cardiovascular disease in the general population would also be harmful to patients with renal disease. In the absence of specific treatment data for these populations, it seems reasonable to use the most current National Cholesterol Education Program (NCEP) guidelines for classification, treatment decisions and target lipid levels.[96]

In the absence of increased LDL cholesterol levels, high triglyceride or low HDL cholesterol concentrations should be managed with dietary changes (Step 1 NCEP diet) and increased exercise (see Chap. 21). Unfortunately, most patients with moderate to severe chronic renal insufficiency have already been advised to adhere to difficult dietary regimens, which may include protein, phosphorus, sodium, potassium, and fluid restrictions, as well as diabetic exchanges. Thus, although diet therapy is a reasonable first-step approach, it may not be successful in a majority of chronic kidney disease patients because of noncompliance. The use of triglyceride-lowering agents in hypertriglyceridemic CKD patients is controversial because (a) the specific contribution of hypertriglyceridemia to increased coronary artery disease risk in this condition is unknown; (b) a beneficial effect of drugs for reducing coronary artery disease risk in this condition has not been demonstrated; and (c) long-term drug safety has not been proven. Thus, the value of drug therapy remains uncertain at this time.

The best approach to the treatment of hyperlipidemia in patients with nephrotic syndrome is to induce remission of the disease (see Chap. 49) or at least to reduce urine protein excretion by aggressive treatment of concurrent hypertension and/or administration of ACEIs. Reductions of 20% to 25% in total and LDL cholesterol have been reported with strict soy-based vegetarian low-cholesterol and low fat diets,[97] but short-term use of the American Heart Association Step I diet has only minimal effects.[98] Step II diet therapy, as recommended by the NCEP expert panel, may be a reasonable first step in management.[98] However, if LDL cholesterol reduction is suboptimal after 6 months of intensive diet therapy, lipid-lowering drugs should be added.

Five drug classes may prove useful as hypocholesterolemic therapies in patients with renal failure and nephrotic syndrome: the bile acid sequestrants; nicotinic acid; HMG-CoA reductase inhibitors;

TABLE 44–4. Effects of Pharmacologic and Nonpharmacologic Lipid-Lowering Management in Renal Insufficiency

	Nephrotic Syndrome				Renal Insufficiency				Hemodialysis				Peritoneal Dialysis			
	Tot	*HDL*	*LDL*	*Trig*	*Tot*	*HDL*	*LDL*	*Trig*	*Tot*	*HDL*	*LDL*	*Trig*	*Tot*	*HDL*	*LDL*	*Trig*
HMG-CoA	↓↓	↑↑	↓↓	↓↓	↓↓	—	↓↓	↓	↓↓	—	↓↓	↔	↓↓	↑↑	↓↓	↓
Fibrates	↓	—	↑	↓↓	↓↓	—	↓	↓↓	↓↓	↑↑	↓↓	↓↓	↓	—	↓	↓↓
Bile seq	↓	↑	↓	↑↑	—	—	—	—	—	—	—	—	—	—	—	—
Diet	↓↓	—	↓	↑	↑↑	—	↓	↓	↓↓	—	↓↓	↓↓	—	—	—	—
Probocol	↓↓	—	↓	↓	—	—	—	—	—	—	—	—	—	—	—	—
Exercise	—	—	—	—	—	—	—	—	↓↓	—	↑	↓	↓	—	—	↑
Carnitine	—	—	—	—	—	—	—	—	↓↓	↑↑	↓	↓↓	—	—	—	—
Fish oil	↑	—	↑	↓↓	↑↑	—	↑	↓	↓↓	↑↑	↓	↓	↑	—	↑	↓
LMWH	—	—	—	—	—	—	—	—	↓↓	—	↓	↓	—	—	—	—

Double arrows indicate a statistically significant change.

fibric acids (gemfibrozil and clofibrate); and probucol. The 3-hydroxy-3-methylglutaryl coenzyme A (HMG-CoA) reductase inhibitors are the most effective drugs for lowering LDL and total cholesterol in patients with renal disease (with or without nephrotic syndrome) and should generally be regarded as the drugs of first choice.[93] A meta-regression analysis examined usual antihyperlipidemic therapies (with the exception of nicotinic acid) along with carnitine, fish oil, low-molecular-weight heparins, and exercise to determine their effects in nephrotic syndrome, renal insufficiency, hemodialysis, and peritoneal dialysis.[99] Potential limitations always exist with this type of analysis; however, it does help provide a foundation for selecting initial therapy in a specific patient population with specific lipid profiles. Table 44–4 summarizes the results of this study. A more recent prospective study looking at the effects of dyslipidemia on the progression of chronic renal disease found a limited association in 138 patients followed over 13 years.[100] The debate will continue because the most recent meta-analysis (13 prospective controlled trials) concluded that lipid reduction may decrease proteinuria and preserve GFR in patients with renal disease.[101] The rate of GFR decline in the treatment group was 0.156 mL/min/mo lower as compared to the control group.

HMG-CoA reductase inhibitors may have some advantages over other lipid agents. Animal studies have determined that these agents may actually help to delay the progression of renal disease, independent of their lipid effects. The beneficial renal effects include modifying monocyte infiltration, mesangial cell proliferation, and mesangial matrix expansion, in addition to tubulointerstitial inflammation and fibrosis.[102]

ADVERSE EFFECTS

Potential drug interactions and/or side effects can occur with antilipemic therapy in patients with renal insufficiency. The nonselective binding activity of bile acid sequestrants may reduce absorption of corticosteroids, digoxin, thiazide diuretics, warfarin, and other commonly used medications. Myositis and myalgias, along with increased serum creatine phosphokinase (CPK), have been reported in renal failure patients who use clofibrate.[103] Determining the optimal dose of clofibrate in this patient population is difficult, as plasma protein-binding changes markedly affect free concentrations of the active metabolite, clofibric acid, which has a prolonged half-life in renal failure.[104] Gemfibrozil may be a safer alternative, as the half-life is not altered in renal dysfunction.[105] However, some investigators report significant increases in CPK concentrations following usual doses of gemfibrozil in dialysis patients,[106,107] which leads some authors to suggest lower doses of 300 mg bid with close monitoring of CPK levels.[106,108]

Although HMG-CoA reductase inhibitors are remarkably free of adverse effects in otherwise healthy subjects, one should be cognizant of the potential myotoxic effects of these drugs, especially during concomitant cyclosporine, gemfibrozil, and niacin administration, and in the presence of hepatic disease.[109] Large doses of omega-3 polyunsaturated fatty acids (fish oils) lower triglyceride levels in hemodialysis patients,[110,111] but they may interfere with platelet function, predisposing to bleeding. In addition, the high doses necessary to lower triglycerides makes noncompliance more likely.

SMOKING

Considering the well-known adverse effects of smoking on cardiovascular disease, there has been little information published regarding its effects on progression of renal disease. However, interest in this area is increasing. Smokers with type 1 diabetes demonstrate a more rapid progression of nephropathy as compared to nonsmokers with type 1 diabetes.[112] This same study found that "cigarette pack years" was an independent predictive factor for the progression of diabetic nephropathy.[112] Similar studies have shown an approximate twofold increased rate of progression in both type 1 and type 2 diabetics who smoke.[113] The exact physiologic effects of smoking on kidney function have not been fully elucidated; however, recent studies in healthy individuals show that smoking manifests several acute changes, including a drop in GFR and filtration fraction corresponding to an increase in heart rate and blood pressure.[114] This physiologic effect may be a result of nicotine because the same response was reproduced in subjects given nicotine gum. Although some studies show nicotine to have no effect on urinary albumin excretion, other studies link smoking to an increase in albuminuria.[113,114] Regardless of the etiology of the renal disease, it is in the best interest of the patient to stop smoking.

CONSEQUENCES OF CHRONIC RENAL INSUFFICIENCY

ANEMIA

As renal function deteriorates, the kidney produces less EPO. Anemia can ultimately led to left ventricular hypertrophy (LVH) and even heart failure. In fact, nearly three of four patients initiating renal replacement therapy have some degree of heart failure or LVH.[115] The presence of LVH in ESRD patients can increase the risk of mortality almost threefold.[116] Because heart disease is a leading cause of death among ESRD patients, early identification of patients with renal insufficiency will not only help to slow the progression of renal disease but also potentially prevent further cardiovascular injury.[115] Anemia in the patient with chronic renal failure should be evaluated when the hemoglobin is <11 g/dL for premenopausal women and <12 g/dL for postmenopausal women and adult males.[116] Subcutaneous epoetin alfa and oral or parenteral iron therapy should be initiated to maintain a goal hemoglobin of 11–12 g/dL.[116] Appropriate anemia management prevents, and in some cases partially reverses, the LVH found in anemic chronic renal insufficiency and dialysis patients.[117,118] Detailed dosing recommendations and monitoring guidelines are found in Chap. 45.

Recently, an anemia identification and intervention strategy for patients with chronic renal insufficiency was proposed for the Renal Anemia Management Period (RAMP).[119,120] RAMP is defined as "that critical period in the evolution of progressive kidney disease when anemia may be subclinical or asymptomatic, but during which correction of anemia has the potential to alter the complications of chronic renal insufficiency."[119] Although the benefits of such a program have yet to be evaluated the conceptual framework represents a rational approach that addresses current treatment strategies and their economic implications.[120]

HYPERPHOSPHATEMIA/VITAMIN D DEFICIENCY

Serum levels of 1,25-dihydroxy vitamin D begin to decline when CLcr drops below 100 mL/min and are significantly reduced (by about 50%) when CLcr reaches 65 mL/min. Serum phosphorus levels begin to progressively increase when the CLcr drops below 30 mL/min secondary to the kidney's inability to excrete phosphorus. Because serum calcium levels tend to remain in the normal range until the patient approaches ESRD, the product of the serum calcium multiplied by the phosphorus level rises. Elevated calcium-phosphorus products correlate with an increased risk of coronary calcification[121] and systemic vascular and soft tissue calcification. Historic guidelines suggest that this product not exceed 70. However, a recent publication of the relationship of the calcium-phosphorus product with cardiovascular disease has prompted new recommendations for patients with renal failure; a calcium-phosphorus product of <55.[122] The decrease in serum calcium levels, primarily from a lack of active vitamin D production, and the elevation in serum phosphorus levels, are independent stimuli for parathyroid hormone (PTH) release. PTH serum levels are significantly increased in many patients when the CLcr reaches 20–30 mL/min. The development of secondary hyperparathyroidism can have long-term adverse effects on bone. Early detection and management can potentially prevent these cardiovascular and bone complications from developing. The pathophysiology and treatment options for this complex of disorders is described in Chap. 45.

SODIUM AND WATER HOMEOSTASIS

Sodium balance is maintained in most CKD patients until the GFR drops below 30 mL/min. The patient's kidneys compensate for the nonfunctioning nephrons by increasing the FE_{Na} of the remnant nephrons from a normal values of 1% to 3% to values of 10% to 20%. Although water balance is also maintained until the GFR drops below 60 mL/min the ability of the patient to dilute or concentrate urine is impaired. As a result of these adaptations by the kidney, its ability to compensate for abrupt changes in sodium or fluid intake is impaired. Treatment strategies for the management of nocturia, volume overload, and edema, which may develop as a result of CKD, are detailed in Chap. 45.

POTASSIUM HOMEOSTASIS

Potassium balance is maintained in the presence of mild to moderate CKD as the result of the kidney increasing the fractional excretion of this cation. Hyperkalemia is a frequent finding in those CKD patients with GFRs less than 10–15 mL/min. The clinical consequences of hyperkalemia and the management options for this electrolyte abnormality are similar to those for patients with normal renal function (see Chap. 52).

METABOLIC ACIDOSIS

This acid-base abnormality is a frequent finding in CKD patients with GFRs less than 30 mL/min. The pathophysiology, clinical presentation, and therapeutic alternatives for this chronic disorder are discussed in Chap. 53.

PHARMACOECONOMIC CONSIDERATIONS

There have been several evaluations of the pharmacoeconomic impact of screening for microalbuminuria and the subsequent initiation of various pharmacotherapeutic regimens in type 1 diabetic patients. Siegel and colleagues evaluated the cost effectiveness of screening for microalbuminuria.[123] The standard therapy approach they assumed began treatment with hydrochlorothiazide when hypertension was diagnosed. The new program approach assumed three different screening and treatment strategies with ACEIs. Their results suggest that early screening and treatment with ACEIs when persistent microalbuminuria occurs, is likely to be a very cost-effective use of health care dollars, with a cost-effectiveness ratio of $7,900 to $16,500 per year of life saved. This ratio is similar to the cost effectiveness associated with treating hypertension in the general population.

Another group of investigators performed a similar cost-effectiveness analysis of different strategies using the same model.[124] Kiberd et al projected that treating all patients with an ACEI 5 years after diagnosis of diabetes was as cost effective as annual screening for microalbuminuria starting 5 years after diagnosis and the initiation of an ACEI when and if persistent microalbuminuria was detected. The DCCT research group evaluated the cost effectiveness of intensive insulin therapy as compared with conventional diabetes treatment.[125] The analysis demonstrated that implementing intensive insulin therapy would result in an incremental cost per year of life gained of $28,661, which represents a good value to the health care system. Overall, it appears that aggressive insulin therapy, as well as treatment with ACEIs when persistent microalbuminuria is identified, reduces complications, improves quality of life by preserving renal function, and ultimately increases length of life at reasonable costs to society. The results of these simulated analyses remain to be prospectively confirmed.

The UKPDS also performed a cost-effectiveness study that compared tight blood pressure control (ACEI and β-blocker therapy) with less-tight blood pressure control. The main outcomes included use of health care resources and the time free from diabetes related end points. It was concluded that tight blood pressure control in patients with type 2 diabetes and hypertension produced a positive cost-effectiveness ratio with regards to reducing the cost of complications and increasing the interval without complications.[126] A recent study concluded that all middle-aged patients with newly diagnosed type 2 diabetes should be treated with an ACEI rather than be screened for microalbuminuria and then treated.[127] They determined that this treatment method would provide additional benefit with only a modest increase in cost.

EVALUATION OF THERAPEUTIC OUTCOMES

DIABETICS

Based on the available clinical and experimental data, pharmacologic intervention can attenuate hemodynamic adaptations associated with progression of renal disease in diabetic patients. Figure 44–8 summarizes general approaches for the prevention of progression of renal disease in this population.[128] All patients with type 1 diabetes of more than 5 years' duration and all type 2 diabetics should be screened every year for microalbuminuria (annual UAE or urinary albumin-creatinine ratio).[24] Blood glucose should be maintained within or close to normal range either by frequent insulin injections or by use of an insulin pump, while minimizing the risk of hypoglycemia with frequent blood glucose monitoring. If there are no contraindications, ACEI therapy should be initiated in normotensive or hypertensive type 1 diabetic patients with persistent microalbuminuria (30–300 mg/day) or overt albuminuria (>300 mg/day). ACEIs should be titrated every 1 to 3 months to achieve a maximal reduction in UAE. Within 1 week of initiating or increasing a dose of an ACEI, serum creatinine and potassium should be evaluated to detect potential abrupt reductions in GFR or development of hyperkalemia. ACEIs should be prescribed for type 2 patients with or without hypertension who demonstrate persistent microalbuminuria. A nondihydropyridine CCB may be an effective alternative as a single agent or in combination with an ACEI in hypertensive diabetic patients with advanced renal disease and/or proteinuria.

NONDIABETIC PATIENTS

Figure 44–9 summarizes therapeutic interventions for nondiabetic patients with renal insufficiency. Nutritional management should be monitored frequently, regardless of the amount of protein intake prescribed, to avoid complications from malnutrition. Nutrition goals include maintenance of serum albumin above 4 g/dL and transferrin above 200 mg/dL. Based on the results of the MDRD study, a low-protein diet is of questionable benefit in patients with moderate renal function (GFR 25–55 mL/min/1.73 m^2). Therefore, a standard protein diet should be followed unless the patient develops rapid progression of renal failure and/or uremic symptoms.[128] For patients with moderate renal insufficiency as defined by the MDRD study (GFR 13–24 mL/min/1.73 m^2), a low-protein diet of 0.6 g/kg/day may reduce the rate of decline in renal function, time to reach ESRD, and onset of uremic symptoms.[71]

Blood pressure control should target normotensive levels (130/85 mm Hg).[65] If proteinuria above 1 g/day is present, blood pressure should be reduced further (125/75 mm Hg), providing there are

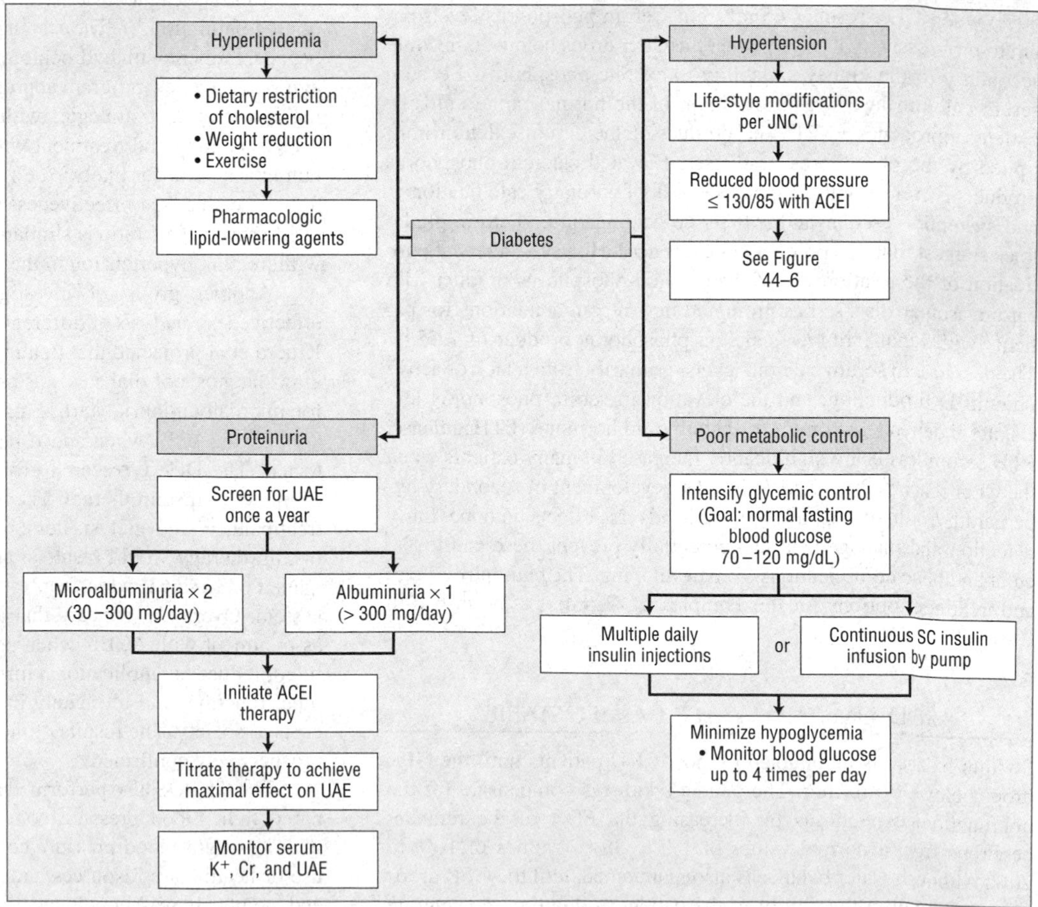

FIGURE 44–8. Therapeutic strategies to prevent progression of renal disease in diabetic individuals. UAE = urinary albumin excretion; CCB = calcium channel blocker; SC = subcutaneous; ACEI = angiotensin-converting enzyme inhibitor; JNC VI = the sixth report of the Joint National Committee on Prevention, Detection, Evaluation, and Treatment of High Blood Pressure.

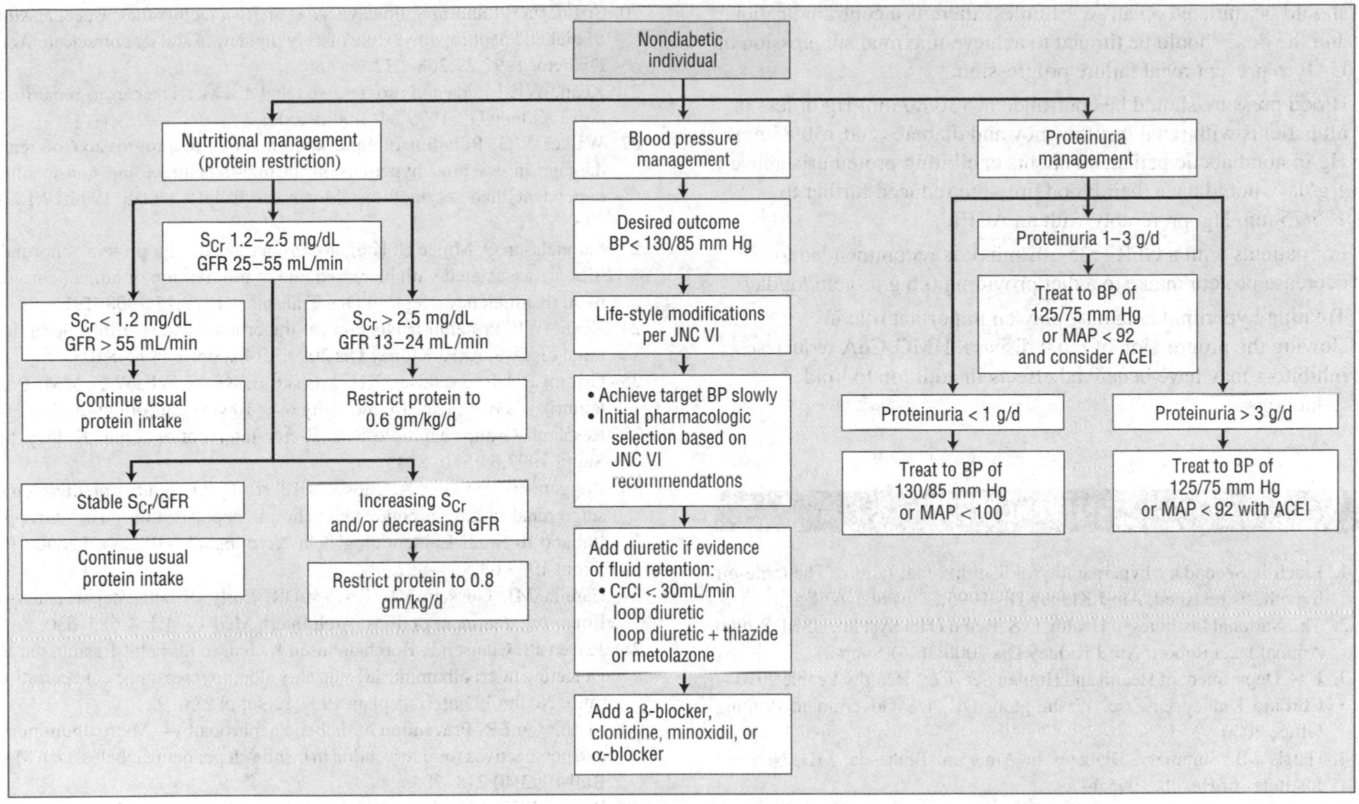

FIGURE 44–9. Therapeutic strategies to prevent progression of renal disease in nondiabetic individuals. ACEI = angiotensin-converting enzyme inhibitor; CCB = calcium channel blocker; BP = blood pressure; S_{Cr} = serum creatinine; GFR = glomerular filtration rate; MAP = mean arterial pressure.

no contraindications. But if the patient has proteinuria above 3 g/day and chronic renal failure, an ACEI, and perhaps a nondihydropyridine CCB, should be considered as first-line therapy.[128]

Nonpharmacologic treatment (weight reduction, alcohol restriction, and increased exercise) should be recommended for all patients with isolated hypertriglyceridemia. Patients with triglyceride concentrations remaining above 1,000 mg/dL after 3 to 6 months of nonpharmacologic treatment should begin gemfibrozil 300 mg bid with dose titration upwards, if necessary (CPK concentrations permitting), to prevent pancreatitis. Nonnephrotic patients with atherogenic concentrations of LDL cholesterol and other risk factors for coronary artery disease should be initiated on HMG-CoA reductase inhibitors. Dosages should be titrated per NCEP panel guidelines for LDL cholesterol concentrations.[96] Nephrotic patients with elevated LDL cholesterol should be placed on a step II diet and/or drug therapy based on NCEP panel guidelines; HMG-CoA reductase inhibitors appear to be a good first choice, with addition of fibric acid derivatives, bile resins, or niacin as appropriate.

If a patient's renal function is deteriorating more rapidly than predicted, a vigorous search for reversible causes is warranted. Potential reasons for acceleration in the rate of decline of renal function in a patient with chronic renal insufficiency include:

- Volume depletion secondary to vomiting, diarrhea, or inappropriate salt restriction or diuretic therapy;
- Uncontrolled hypertension;
- Impaired renal perfusion secondary to hypotension, reduced cardiac output, or renovascular disease;
- Pyelonephritis;
- Urinary tract obstruction (prostatic hypertrophy, papillary necrosis, nephrolithiasis);
- Drug-related effects.

As renal function declines below 25 mL/min and treatable problems have been identified and addressed, the patient should begin to be prepared for the eventuality of renal replacement therapy. Hemodialysis, peritoneal dialysis and renal transplantation options need to be discussed (see Chaps. 46 and 47). Early referral to a nephrologist may allow the proper dialysis access to be placed and dialysis to be initiated before adverse effects of uremia develop. The KDOQI recommends referral for long-term access placement when creatinine clearance is <25 mL/min, or serum creatinine is >4 mg/dL, or if the patient is within 1 year of expected need for dialysis.[116] Early referral may also allow a transplantation to occur without the need for maintenance dialysis.

▶ PRINCIPLES OF PHARMACOTHERAPY

- Type 2 diabetes is a more common cause of ESRD than type 1 diabetes because of an increased prevalence of type 2 diabetes in the general population.
- Diabetic patients should be managed aggressively with intensive insulin therapy to maintain blood glucose within or close to the normal range to prevent progression of renal disease.
- Diabetic patients with or without hypertension who demonstrate persistent microalbuminuria despite intensive insulin therapy

should be initiated on an ACEI unless there is a contraindication, and the dose should be titrated to achieve maximal suppression of UAE to prevent renal failure progression.

- Blood pressure should be controlled at 130/80 mm Hg or less in all patients with renal insufficiency and diabetes and 130/85 mm Hg in nondiabetic patients. Patients exhibiting proteinuria above 1 g/day should have their blood pressure reduced further to 125/75 mm Hg, preferably with an ACEI.
- For patients with a GFR <25 mL/min it is recommended to decrease protein intake to a diet providing 0.6 g protein/kg/day.
- Treating hyperlipidemia may play an important role in slowing the progression of renal disease. HMG-CoA reductase inhibitors may have beneficial effects in addition to lipid reductions.

REFERENCES

1. Llach F. Secondary hyperparathyroidism in renal failure: The trade-off hypothesis revisited. Am J Kidney Dis 1995;25(5):663–679.
2. The National Institutes of Health. U.S. Renal Data System, USRDS 2000 Annual Data Report. Am J Kidney Dis 2000;36(6)(Supp 2).
3. U.S. Department of Health and Human Services. Healthy People 2010—Chronic Kidney Disease. Washington, DC, US Government Printing Office 2000.
4. Harris MI. Summary. Diabetes in America. Bethesda, MD, National Institutes of Health, 1995:1–7.
5. Ritz E, Orth SR. Nephropathy in patients with type 2 diabetes mellitus. N Engl J Med 1999;341(15):1127–1133.
6. Jones CA, McQuillan GM, Kusek JW, et al. Serum creatinine levels in the US population: Third National Health and Nutrition Examination Survey. Am J Kidney Dis 1998;32(6):992–999.
7. Hsu CY, Chertow GM. Chronic renal confusion:Insufficiency, failure, dysfunction, or disease. Am J Kidney Dis 2000;36(2):415–418.
8. Levey AS. Measurement of renal function in chronic renal disease. Kidney Int 1990;38:167–184.
9. Rennke HG, Anderson S, Brenner BM. The progression of renal disease: Structural and functional correlations. In: Tisher CC, Brenner BM, eds. Renal Pathology: With Clinical and Functional Correlations. Philadelphia, J.B. Lippincott, 1994:116–139.
10. Neuringer JR, Brenner BM. Hemodynamic theory of progressive renal disease: A 10-year update in brief review. Am J Kidney Dis 1993;22:98–104.
11. Hostetter TH. Mechanisms of diabetic nephropathy. Am J Kidney Dis 1994;23:188–192.
12. Neuringer JR, Levey AS. Strategies to slow the progression of renal disease. Semin Nephrol 1994;14:261–273.
13. Ruggenenti P, Perna A, Mosconi L, et al. Proteinuria predicts end-stage renal failure in nondiabetic chronic nephropathies. Kidney Int Suppl 1997;63:S54–S57.
14. Keane WF, Eknoyan G. Proteinuria, albuminuria, risk, assessment, detection, elimination (PARADE): A position paper of the National Kidney Foundation. Am J Kidney Dis 1999;33(5):1004–1010.
15. Walls J. Relationship between proteinuria and progressive renal disease. Am J Kidney Dis 2001;37(1 suppl 2):S13–S16.
16. Makino H, Shikata K, Kushiro M, et al. Roles of advanced glycation end-products in the progression of diabetic nephropathy. Nephrol Dial Transplant 1996;11(suppl 5):76–80.
17. Inomata S. Renal hypertrophy as a prognostic index for the progression of diabetic renal disease in non-insulin-dependent diabetes mellitus. J Diabetes Complications 1993;7:28–33.
18. Nath KA. Tubulointerstitial changes as a major determinant in the progression of renal damage. Am J Kidney Dis 1992;20:1–17.
19. Brown TE, Carter BL. Hypertension and end stage renal disease. Ann Pharmacother 1994;28:359–366.
20. Scanferla F, Landini S, Fracasso A, et al. Risk factors for the progression of diabetic nephropathy: Role of hyperlipidemia and its correction. Acta Diabetol 1992;29:268–272.
21. Keane WF. Lipids and progressive renal disease: The cardio-renal link. Am J Kidney Dis 1999;34(2):xliii–xxlvi.
22. Walker WG. Relation of lipid abnormalities to progression of renal damage in essential hypertension, insulin-dependent and non-insulin-dependent diabetes mellitus. Miner Electrolyte Metab 1993;19:137–143.
23. Samuelsson O, Mulec H, Knight-Gibson C, et al. Lipoprotein abnormalities are associated with increased rate of progression of human chronic renal insufficiency. Nephrol Dial Transplant 1997;12:1908–1915.
24. Keane WF. Proteinuria: Its clinical importance and role in progressive renal disease. Am J Kidney Dis 2000;35(4 suppl 1):S97–S105.
25. Grimm RH Jr, Svendsen KH, Kasiske B, Keane WF, Wahi MM. Proteinuria is a risk factor for mortality over 10 years of follow-up. MRFIT Research Group. Multiple Risk Factor Intervention Trial. Kidney Int Suppl 1997;63:S10–S14.
26. Ruggenenti P, Perna A, Mosconi L, et al. Proteinuria predicts end-stage renal failure in nondiabetic chronic nephropathies. The "Gruppo Italiano di Studi Epidemiologici in Nefrologia" (GISEN). Kidney Int Suppl 1997;63:S54–S57.
27. Carella MJ, Gossain VV, Rovner DR. Early diabetic nephropathy—Emerging treatment options. Arch Intern Med 1994;154:625–630.
28. Jensen JS, Clausen P, Borch-Johnsen K, Jensen G, Feldt-Rasmussen B. Detecting microalbuminuria by urinary albumin/creatinine concentration ratio. Nephrol Dial Transplant 1997;12(suppl 2):6–9.
29. Mathiesen ER. Prevention of diabetic nephropathy—Microalbuminuria and perspectives for intervention in insulin-dependent diabetes. Dan Med Bull 1993;40:273–285.
30. Bolton WK, Kliger AS. Chronic renal insufficiency: Current understandings and their implications. Am J Kidney Dis 2000;36(6 suppl 3):S4–S12.
31. Pedrini MT, Levey AS, Lau J, Chalmers TC, Wang PH. The effect of dietary protein restriction on the progression of diabetic and nondiabetic renal diseases: A meta-analysis. Ann Intern Med 1996;124:627–632.
32. Kasiske BL, Lakatua JD, Ma JZ, Louis TA. A meta-analysis of the effects of dietary protein restriction on the rate of decline in renal function. Am J Kidney Dis 1998;31(6):954–961.
33. Clinical practice guidelines for nutrition in chronic renal failure. KDOQI, National Kidney Foundation. Am J Kidney Dis 2000;35(6 suppl 2):S1–S140.
34. Weir MR, Dworkin LD. Antihypertensive drugs, dietary salt, and renal protection: How low should you go and with which therapy? Am J Kidney Dis 1998;32(1):1–22.
35. Wang PH, Lau J, Chalmers TC. Meta-analysis of effects of intensive blood-glucose control on late complications of type I diabetes. Lancet 1993;341:1306–1309.
36. The Diabetes Control and Complication Trial Research Group. Effect of intensive therapy on the development and progression of diabetic nephropathy in the Diabetes Control and Complications Trial. Kidney Int 1995;47:1703–1720.
37. Santiago JV. Perspectives in diabetes—Lessons from the Diabetes Control and Complications Trial. Diabetes 1993;42:1549–1554.
38. Gautier JF, Beressi JP, Leblanc H, Vexiau P, Passa P. Are the implications of the Diabetes Control and Complications Trial (DCCT) feasible in daily clinical practice? Diabetes Metab Rev 1996;22(6):415–419.
39. The Diabetes Control and Complications Trial/Epidemiology of Diabetes Interventions and Complications Research Group. Retinopathy and nephropathy in patients with type 1 diabetes four years after a trial of intensive therapy. N Engl J Med 2000;342(6):381–389.
40. UK Prospective Diabetes Study (UKPDS) Group. Intensive blood-glucose control with sulphonylureas or insulin compared with conventional treatment and risk of complications in patients with type 2 diabetes (UKPDS 33). Lancet 1998;352(9131):837–853.
41. Bakris GL, Williams M, Dworkin L, et al. Preserving renal function in adults with hypertension and diabetes: A consensus approach. Am J Kidney Dis 2000;36(3):646–661.

42. Parving H. Impact of blood pressure and antihypertensive treatment on incipient and overt nephropathy, retinopathy and endothelial permeability in diabetes mellitus. Diabetes Care 1991;14:260–269.
43. Hoelscher D, Bakris G. Antihypertensive therapy and progression of diabetic renal disease. J Cardiovasc Pharmacol 1994;23(suppl 1):S34–S38.
44. Dworkin LD, Benstein JA, Parker M, Tolbert E, Feiner HD. Calcium antagonists and converting enzyme inhibitors reduce renal injury by different mechanisms. Kidney Int 1993;43:808–814.
45. Schlueter WA, Batlle DC. Renal effects of antihypertensive drugs. Drugs 1989;37:900–925.
46. Risler T, Krämer B, Müller GA. The efficacy of diuretics in acute and chronic renal failure: Focus on torsemide. Drugs 1991;41(suppl 3): 69–79.
47. Kasiske BL, Kalil RS, Ma JZ, Liao M, Keane WF. Effect of antihypertensive therapy on the kidney in patients with diabetes: A meta-regression analysis. Ann Intern Med 1993;118:129–138.
48. Lewis EJ, Hunsicker LG, Bain RP, Rohde RD. The effect of angiotensin-converting-enzyme inhibition on diabetic nephropathy. The Collaborative Study Group. N Engl J Med 1993;329:1456–1462.
49. Ahmad J, Siddiqui MA, Ahmad H. Effective postponement of diabetic nephropathy with enalapril in normotensive type 2 diabetic patients with microalbuminuria. Diabetes Care 1997;20(10):1576–1581.
50. Ravid M, Brosh D, Levi Z, Bar-Dayan Y, Ravid D, Rachmani R. Use of enalapril to attenuate decline in renal function in normotensive, normoalbuminuric patients with type 2 diabetes mellitus. A randomized, controlled trial. Ann Intern Med 1998;128(12 Pt 1):982–988.
51. The EUCLID study group. Randomised placebo-controlled trial of lisinopril in normotensive patients with insulin-dependent diabetes and normoalbuminuria or microalbuminuria. Lancet 1997;349:1787–1792.
52. Heart Outcomes Prevention Evaluation Study Investigators. Effects of ramipril on cardiovascular and microvascular outcomes in people with diabetes mellitus: Results of the HOPE study and MICRO-HOPE substudy. Lancet 2000;355(9200):253–259.
53. Kshirsagar AV, Joy MS, Hogan SL, Falk RJ, Colindres RE. Effect of ACE inhibitors in diabetic and nondiabetic chronic renal disease: A systematic overview of randomized placebo-controlled trials. Am J Kidney Dis 2000;35(4):695–707.
54. Mackenzie HS, Ots M, Ziai F, Lee KW, Kato S, Brenner B. Angiotensin receptor antagonists in experimental models of chronic renal failure. Kidney Int Suppl 1997;63:S140–S143.
55. Pitt B, Segal R, Martinez FA, Meurers G, Cowley AJ, Thomas I, et al. Randomised trial of losartan versus captopril in patients over 65 with heart failure (Evaluation of losartan in the elderly study, ELITE). Lancet 1997;349:747–752.
56. Lewis EJ, Hunsicker LG, Clarke WR, et al. Renoprotective effect of the angiotensin-receptor antagonist irbesartan in patients with nephropathy due to type 2 diabetes. N Engl J Med 2001;345:851–860.
57. Parving HH, Lehnert H, Brochner-Mortensen J, et al. The effect of irbesartan on the development of diabetic nephropathy in patients with type 2 diabetes. N Engl J Med 2001;345:870–878.
58. Brenner BM, Cooper ME, Zeeuw DD, et al. Effects of losartan on renal and cardiovascular outcomes in patients with type 2 diabetes and nephropathy. N Engl J Med 2001;345:861–869.
59. Hostetter TH. Prevention of end-stage renal disease due to type 2 diabetes. N Engl J Med 2001;345:910–911.
60. Tarif N, Bakris GL. Angiotensin II receptor blockade and progression of nondiabetic-mediated renal disease. Kidney Int Suppl 1997;63:S67–S70.
61. Maki DD, Ma JZ, Louis TA, Kasiske BL. Long-term effects of antihypertensive agents on proteinuria and renal function. Arch Intern Med 1995;155:1073–1080.
62. Weidmann P, Schneider M, Bohlen L. Therapeutic efficacy of different antihypertensive drugs in human diabetic nephropathy: An updated meta-analysis. Nephrol Dial Transplant 1995;10(suppl 9):39–45.
63. Bakris GL, Copley JB, Vicknair N, Sadler R, Leurgans S. Calcium channel blockers versus other antihypertensive therapies on progression of NIDDM associated nephropathy. Kidney Int 1996;50:1641–1650.
64. Epstein M. Effects of ACE inhibitors and calcium antagonists on progression of chronic renal disease. Blood Press Suppl 1995;2:108–112.
65. The Joint National Committee. The Sixth Report of the Joint National Committee on Prevention, Detection, Evaluation, and Treatment of High Blood Pressure. Arch Intern Med 1997;157(21):2413–2446.
66. Hansson L, Zanchetti A, Carruthers SG, et al. Effects of intensive blood-pressure lowering and low-dose aspirin in patients with hypertension: Principal results of the Hypertension Optimal Treatment (HOT) randomised trial. HOT Study Group. Lancet 1998;351(9118):1755–1762.
67. UK Prospective Diabetes Study Group. Tight blood pressure control and risk of macrovascular and microvascular complications in type 2 diabetes: UKPDS 38. BMJ 1998;317(7160):703–713.
68. Lewis JB, Berl T, Bain RP, Rohde RD, Lewis EJ. Effect of intensive blood pressure control on the course of type 1 diabetic nephropathy. Collaborative Study Group [see comments]. Am J Kidney Dis 1999;34(5):809–817.
69. Fouque D, Laville M, Boissel JP, Chifflet R, Labeeuw M, Zech PY. Controlled low-protein diets in chronic renal insufficiency: Meta analysis. BMJ 1992;304:216–220.
70. Klahr S, Levey AS, Beck GJ, et al. The effects of dietary protein restriction and blood-pressure control on the progression of chronic renal disease. N Engl J Med 1994; 330:877–884.
71. Levey AS, Adler S, Caggiula AW, et al. Effects of dietary protein restriction on the progression of advanced renal disease in the Modification of Diet in Renal Disease study. Am J Kidney Dis 1996;27(5):652–663.
72. Apperloo AJ, de Zeeuw D, de Jong PE. A short-term antihypertensive treatment-induced fall in glomerular filtration rate predicts long-term stability of renal function. Kidney Int 1997;51(3):793–797.
73. Giatras I, Lau J, Levey AS. Effect of angiotensin-converting enzyme inhibitors on the progression of nondiabetic renal disease: A meta-analysis of randomized trials. Ann Intern Med 1997;127(5):337–345
74. The GISEN Group. Randomised placebo-controlled trial of effect of ramipril on decline in glomerular filtration rate and risk of terminal renal failure in proteinuric, nondiabetic nephropathy. Lancet 1997;349:1857–1863.
75. Ruggenenti P, Perna A, Gherardi G, et al. Renoprotective properties of ACE-inhibitors in non-diabetic nephropathies with non-nephrotic proteinuria. Lancet 1999;354:359–364.
76. Sica DA, Gehr TWB. The pharmacokinetics of angiotensin-converting enzyme inhibitors in end-stage renal disease. Semin Dialysis 1994;7:205–213.
77. Nielsen S, Dollerup J, Nielsen B, Jensen HA, Mogensen CE. Losartan reduces albuminuria in patients with essential hypertension. An enalapril controlled 3 months study. Nephrol Dial Transplant 1997; 12(suppl 2): 19–23.
78. Ruilope LM. Is it wise to combine an ACE inhibitor and an angiotensin receptor antagonist? Nephrol Dial Transplant 1999;14:2855–2856.
79. Tarif N, Bakris GL. Preservation of renal function: The spectrum of effects by calcium channel blockers. Nephrol Dial Transplant 1997;12: 2244–2250.
80. Weder AB. The renally compromised older hypertensive. Therapeutic considerations. Geriatrics 1991;46:36–48.
81. Jones B, Nanra RS. Double-blind trial of antihypertensive effect of chlorothiazide in severe renal failure. Lancet 1979;2:1258–1260.
82. Wollam GL, Tarazi RC, Bravo EL, Dustan HP. Diuretic potency of combined hydrochlorothiazide and furosemide therapy in patients with azotemia. Am J Med 1982;72:929–938.
83. Favre L, Glasson P, Vallotton MB. Reversible acute renal failure from combined triamterene and indomethacin: A study in healthy subjects. Ann Intern Med 1982; 96:317–320.
84. Lowenthal DT, Saris SD, Paran E, Cristal N. The use of transdermal clonidine in the hypertensive patient with chronic renal failure. Clin Nephrol 1993;39:37–43.
85. Miura Y, Watanabe M, Yoshinaga K. An evaluation of the efficacy and safety of doxazosin in hypertension associated with renal dysfunction. Am Heart J 1991;121:381–388.
86. ALLHAT Collaborative Research Group. Major cardiovascular events in hypertensive patients randomized to doxazosin vs chlorthalidone: The

antihypertensive and lipid-lowering treatment to prevent heart attack trial (ALLHAT). JAMA 2000;283(15):2013–2014.

87. Innes A, Gemmell HG, Smith FW, Edward N, Catto GRD. The short-term effects of oral labetalol in patients with chronic renal disease and hypertension. J Hum Hypertens 1992;6:211–214.
88. Waal-Manning HJ, Hobson CH. Renal function in patients with essential hypertension receiving nadolol. Br Med J 1980;281:423–424.
89. Wilkinson R. Beta-blockers and renal function. Drugs 1982;23:195–206.
90. Pontremoli R, Robaudo C, Gaiter A, Massarino F, Deferrari G. Long-term minoxidil treatment in refractory hypertension and renal failure. Clin Nephrol 1991;35:39–43.
91. National High Blood Pressure Education Program Working Group. 1995 update of the working group reports on chronic renal failure and renovascular hypertension. Arch Intern Med 1996;156:1938–1947.
92. Mackenzie HS, Brenner BM. Current strategies for retarding progression of renal disease. Am J Kidney Dis 1998;31(1):161–170.
93. Kasiske BL. Hyperlipidemia in patients with chronic renal disease. Am J Kidney Dis 1998;32(5 Suppl 3):S142–S156.
94. Majumdar A, Wheeler DC. Lipid abnormalities in renal disease. J R Soc Med 2000;93(4):178–182.
95. Drüeke TB. Adynamic bone disease, anaemia, resistance to erythropoietin and iron-aluminium interaction. Nephrol Dial Transplant 1993;8(suppl 1):12–16.
96. Expert panel. Executive summary of the third report of the National Cholesterol Education Program (NCEP) expert panel on detection evaluation and treatment of high blood cholesterol in adults (Adult Treatment Panel III). JAMA 2001;285(19):2486–2497.
97. D'Amico G, Gentile MG. Influence of diet on lipid abnormalities in human renal disease. Am J Kidney Dis 1993;22:151–157.
98. Keane WF, St. Peter JV, Kasiske BL. Is the aggressive management of hyperlipidemia in nephrotic syndrome mandatory? Kidney Int Suppl 1992;38:S134–S141.
99. Massy ZA, Ma JZ, Louis TA, Kasiske BL. Lipid-lowering therapy in patients with renal disease. Kidney Int 1995;48:188–198.
100. Massy ZA, Khoa TN, Lacour B, Descamps-Latscha B, Man NK, Jungers P. Dyslipidaemia and the progression of renal disease in chronic renal failure patients. Nephrol Dial Transplant 1999;14(10):2392–2397.
101. Fried L, Orchard T, Kasiske B. Effect of lipid reduction on the progression of renal disease: A meta-analysis. Kidney Int 2001;59:260–269.
102. Oda H, Keane WF. Recent advances in statins and the kidney. Kidney Int Suppl 1999;71:S2–S5.
103. Sherrard DJ, Goldberg AB, Haas LB, Brunzell JD. Chronic clofibrate therapy in maintenance hemodialysis patients. Nephron 1980;25:219–221.
104. Merk W, Graben N, Hartmann H, Nikolaus C, Schlierf G, Schwandt P. Serum levels of free non-protein bound clofibrinic acid after single dosing to patients with impaired renal function of various degrees—A multicenter study. Int J Clin Pharmacol Ther Toxicol 1987;25:59–62.
105. Evans JR, Forland SC, Cutler RE. The effect of renal function on the pharmacokinetics of gemfibrozil. J Clin Pharmacol 1987;27:994–1000.
106. Chan MK. Gemfibrozil improves abnormalities of lipid metabolism in patients on continuous ambulatory peritoneal dialysis: The role of postheparin lipases in the metabolism of high-density lipoprotein subfractions. Metabolism 1989;38:939–945.
107. Pasternack A, Vanttinen T, Solakivi T, Kuusi T, Korte T. Normalization of lipoprotein lipase and hepatic lipase by gemfibrozil results in correction of lipoprotein abnormalities in chronic renal failure. Clin Nephrol 1987;27:163–168.
108. Elisaf MS, Dardamanis MA, Papagalanis ND, Siamopoulos KC. Lipid abnormalities in chronic uremic patients—Response to treatment with gemfibrozil. Scand J Urol Nephrol 1993;27:101–108.
109. Grundy SM. HMG-CoA reductase inhibitors for treatment of hypercholesterolemia. N Engl J Med 1988;319:24–33.
110. Beccari M. Must we treat uremic dyslipidemia? Int J Artif Organs 1993;16:235–244.
111. Azar R, Dequiedt F, Awada J, Dequiedt P, Tacquet A. Effects of fish oil rich in polyunsaturated fatty acids on hyperlipidemia of hemodialysis patients. Kidney Int Suppl 1989;27:S239–S242.
112. Sawicki PT, Didjurgeit U, Muhlhauser I, Bender R, Heinemann L, Berger M. Smoking is associated with progression of diabetic nephropathy. Diabetes Care 1994;17(2):126–131.
113. Ritz E, Benck U, Franek E, Keller C, Seyfarth M, Clorius J. Effects of smoking on renal hemodynamics in healthy volunteers and in patients with glomerular disease. J Am Soc Nephrol 1998;9(10):1798–1804.
114. Halimi JM, Mimran A. Renal effects of smoking: potential mechanisms and perspectives. Nephrol Dial Transplant 2000;15(7):938–940.
115. Pereira BJ. Introduction: New perspectives in chronic renal insufficiency. Am J Kidney Dis 2000;36(6 suppl 3):S1–S3.
116. Eknoyan G, Levin NW, Eschbach JW, et al. National Kidney Foundation—KDOQI 2000 Update. Am J Kidney Dis 2001;37(1):179–194.
117. Hayashi T, Suzuki A, Shoji T, et al. Cardiovascular effects of normalizing the hematocrit level during erythropoietin therapy in predialysis patients with chronic renal failure. Am J Kidney Dis 2000;35:250–256.
118. Wizeman V, Schafer R, Kramer W. Follow-up of cardiac changes induced by anemia compensation in normotensive hemodialysis patients with left-ventricular hypertrophy. Nephron 1993;64:202–206.
119. Besarab A, Levin A. Defining a renal anemia management period. Am J Kidney Dis Suppl 2000;36(6):S13–S23.
120. Kausu A, Obrador GT, Pereira BJG. Anemia management in patients with chronic renal insufficiency. Am J Kidney Dis Suppl 2000;36(6):S39–S51.
121. Goodman WG, Goldin J, Kuizon BD, et al. Coronary-artery calcification in young adults with end-stage renal disease who are undergoing dialysis. N Engl J Med 2000;342(20):1478–1483.
122. Block GA. Prevalence and clinical consequences of elevated Ca-P product in hemodialysis patients. Clin Nephrol 2000;54(4):318–324.
123. Siegel JE, Krolewski AS, Warram JH, Weinstein MC. Cost-effectiveness of screening and early treatment of nephropathy in patients with insulin-dependent diabetes mellitus. J Am Soc Nephrol 1992;3(supp 1):S111–S119.
124. Kiberd BA, Jindal KK. Routine treatment of insulin-dependent diabetic patients with ACE inhibitors to prevent renal failure: An economic evaluation. Am J Kidney Dis 1998;31(1):49–54.
125. The Diabetes Control and Complications Trial Research Group. Lifetime benefits and costs of intensive therapy as practiced in the diabetes control and complications trial. JAMA 1996;276(17):1409–1415.
126. UK Prospective Diabetes Study Group. Cost effectiveness analysis of improved blood pressure control in hypertensive patients with type 2 diabetes: UKPDS 40. BMJ 1998;317(7160):720–726.
127. Golan L, Birkmeyer JD, Welch HG. The cost-effectiveness of treating all patients with type 2 diabetes with angiotensin-converting enzyme inhibitors. Ann Intern Med 1999;131(9):660–667.
128. Jacobson HR, Striker GE. Report on a workshop to develop management recommendations for the prevention of progression in chronic renal disease. Am J Kidney Dis 1995;25(1):103–106.

45

End-Stage Renal Disease

Wendy L. St. Peter, Matthew J. Lewis, and Allan Collins

The spectrum of renal function varies from normal, a creatinine clearance (CLcr) of approximately 120 mL/min, to a point where there is no renal function at all. There are more than 20 terms that have been used to describe the spectrum of reduced glomerular filtration rate in patients with renal disease.[1] Although the terminology is not currently standardized, for the purposes of this chapter, the terms *mild, moderate,* and *severe* chronic kidney disease (CKD) denote CLcr of 60–90, 30–59, and 15–29 mL/min, respectively. In general, the pathology of disease states, which cause renal dysfunction, worsen as renal function declines. Uremia is a clinical syndrome that develops insidiously as renal function declines.[2] It begins with nonspecific symptoms, which become progressively worse as the CLcr drops below 15 mL/min in diabetics and 10 mL/min for other patients. It is at this stage that dialysis is indicated to remove the by-products of protein metabolism, such as urea, that are thought to be largely responsible for this symptom complex, as well as for fluid removal (see Chap. 47). The patient requiring chronic dialysis or renal transplantation for relief of uremic symptoms is said to have end-stage renal disease (ESRD). Chapter 44 focuses on strategies for preventing renal disease from progressing. This chapter focuses on the pathophysiology and pharmacotherapeutic management of ESRD and its complications.

EPIDEMIOLOGY/ETIOLOGY OF END-STAGE RENAL DISEASE

Many primary diseases of the kidney (e.g., glomerulonephritis; see Chap. 49) and systemic diseases (e.g., diabetes mellitus; see Chap. 74) can ultimately result in ESRD. For a thorough discussion of the epidemiology of renal disease see Chap. 44. There were 85,520 incident (new) patients treated for ESRD in 1998, with more than 230,000 patients on dialysis and almost 95,000 patients with a functioning kidney transplant.[3] Although the incidence and prevalence of CKD in the United States is suspected to be even greater than that of ESRD, there is no national registry for CKD as there is for ESRD, thus accurate numbers are unavailable. However, the third National Health and Nutrition Examination Survey (NHANES III) evaluated serum creatinine levels in 18,723 persons aged 12 years and older between 1988 and 1994. Data derived from this survey predicts that over 10.9 and 3.0 million persons in the U.S. noninstitutionalized population have serum creatinine values greater than 1.5 and 1.7 mg/dL, respectively.[4]

The ESRD population in the U.S. has steadily increased during the last decade, as evidenced by the rise in the incident rate (that is those who start dialysis or who received their first transplant in a given year) of 5.2% to 6.7% per year. The incidence is highest in elderly patients, males, and African Americans, as well as in Native Americans. Native Americans and Hispanics have the highest rate of diabetes, whereas Asians are more likely to develop ESRD as the result of glomerulonephritis. The dramatic rise in diabetes in the incident dialysis population during the last decade (from ≈60 to 130 per million population) may be related to obesity, carbohydrate intolerance, and insulin resistance. This increased incidence coupled with improvements in survival of these patients is projected to result in an ESRD population that exceeds 660,000 by 2010. Although the ESRD death rate has declined because of better dialysis therapy, improvement in anemia management, and improved kidney transplant survival, more than 63,000 patients died with ESRD in 1998, with almost half of the dialysis-related deaths attributed to cardiac causes.[3]

Healthy People 2010 is a national health promotion and disease-prevention initiative that has been coordinated by the U.S. Department of Health and Human Services, Office of Disease Prevention and Health Promotion since its inception in 1979. The new Healthy People 2010 goals and objectives were released in January 2000. This update is the first Healthy People initiative to include goals on prevention of chronic kidney disease and attendant problems. One specific objective is to reduce deaths from cardiovascular disease in patients with kidney disease by decreasing risk factors such as smoking, elevated cholesterol, high blood pressure, high calcium-phosphorus product, and improving anemia management in this population. Another goal is to increase the proportion of patients with CKD who receive appropriate counseling on nutrition, ESRD treatment choices, and cardiovascular care at least 12 months before the start of renal replacement therapy.[5] For these national goals to be met, patients with CKD need to be identified, and appropriately diagnosed, and their concomitant diseases addressed.[5]

PATHOPHYSIOLOGY

No single toxin is responsible for all of the abnormalities observed in patients with CKD and ESRD, and the clinical picture likely results from an interplay of multiple factors. Several mechanisms could contribute to the presence of uremic toxins as chronic renal failure progresses. Most likely, the signs and symptoms seen in ESRD patients result from elevations in blood concentrations of various organic compounds (Table 45–1). Accumulation could be the result of increased secretion of biologically active substances such as parathyroid hormone (PTH) and atrial natriuretic peptide, which are overproduced as part of the adaptation to the loss of renal mass; decreased clearance of endogenous substances normally metabolized by the kidney, including PTH, gastrin, growth hormone, glucagon, somatostatin, prolactin, calcitonin, and insulin; and/or decreased clearance of metabolic by-products of protein metabolism.

The ability of uremic toxins to produce clinical manifestations results in large part from their effects at the cellular or metabolic level, which ultimately can affect organ, immune, and other bodily functions.[6] To prove that a substance is a uremic toxin, investigators must show accumulation of the substance, demonstrate toxicity at a cellular or metabolic level upon administration, and show improvement by removal of the toxin by dialysis or other means.[6] Very few of these substances (with the exception of PTH and indoxyl sulfate) have been taken through the process described, so there is still much work to be done in this area.

TABLE 45–1. Potential Uremic Toxins

2,3-Butylene	Indoles
Acetoin	Indoxyl sulfate
Acids	Insulin
Aliphatic amines	Lipochromes
α_2-Glycoprotein	Lysozyme
Amino acids	Mannitol
Aromatic amines	Methylguanidine
β_1-Microglobulin	Middle molecules
β_2-Microglobulin	Myoinositol
Calcitonin	Natriuretic hormone
Chemotaxis inhibiting protein	Other guanidines
Creatinine	Oxalic acid
Cyanate	Parathyroid hormone
Cyclic AMP	P-cresol
Degranulation inhibiting proteins	Phenols
Gastric inhibitory peptide	Potassium
Gastrin	Prolactin
Glucagon	Pyridine derivatives
Glucuronic acid	Renin
Growth hormone	Retinol-binding protein
Granulocyte inhibitory proteins	Ribonuclease
Guanidines	Urea
Hippuric acid	Uric acid
Human pancreatic polypeptide	Water

CLINICAL PRESENTATION

Every major organ system can be affected by ESRD. At the time of referral to a nephrologist patients may present with some but rarely all of the signs and symptoms that are outlined below.

CARDIOVASCULAR SYSTEM

Sodium retention leads to volume expansion, which can result in volume overload and pulmonary edema. Hypertension induced by volume expansion and increased systemic vascular resistance increases myocardial work and results in left ventricular hypertrophy. In addition, hypertension represents a major risk factor for cardiovascular disease, and complications of atherosclerosis are common in these patients. Hyperlipidemia may enhance atherogenesis, while some uremic toxins can decrease myocardial contractility. The high cardiac output state induced by anemia may be poorly tolerated in the face of underlying heart disease. Uremic toxins can induce pericarditis, a potentially fatal complication of CKD.

PULMONARY SYSTEM

The combination of volume overload and uremic toxin-induced increases in capillary permeability can result in noncardiogenic pulmonary edema and pleural serositis.

GASTROINTESTINAL SYSTEM

Anorexia, hiccups, and a metallic taste in the mouth are common in ESRD patients. Nausea, vomiting, diarrhea, or abdominal distention may also occur. Gastric and colonic mucosal ulcerations and telangiectasias with resultant gastrointestinal bleeding are common. Ascites may develop secondary to fluid overload or peritoneal serositis.

NERVOUS SYSTEM

Uremic neuropathy frequently causes sensory and motor dysfunction, particularly affecting leg nerves, resulting in leg cramps and restless leg syndrome. The clinical manifestations of uremic encephalopathy—which include clouded sensorium, coma, seizures, myoclonic jerks, and asterixis—are now rarely seen because of the earlier initiation of dialysis. However, reversal of the sleep-wake cycle is fairly common.

HEMATOLOGIC SYSTEM

A normochromic, normocytic anemia secondary to decreased erythropoietin production and shortened erythrocyte survival is seen in more than 90% of patients. A prolongation in the bleeding time and a bleeding diathesis can result from platelet dysfunction. Gastrointestinal bleeding is common in ESRD, which contributes to anemia. In addition, vitamin and iron deficiency can lead to mixed anemia patterns in this population.

MUSCULOSKELETAL SYSTEM

Renal osteodystrophy (bone disease) is a common manifestation of renal insufficiency that is almost ubiquitously present by the time patients reach ESRD. Calcification of blood vessels or soft tissues may also occur.

ENDOCRINE SYSTEM

A variety of endocrine and metabolic abnormalities are common in ESRD.[7a,b,c,d] Most patients have symptoms of hypothyroidism (low energy, cold intolerance, constipation), but typically the levothyroxine (T_4) concentration is low and the thyroid-stimulating hormone concentration is normal.[7a] Hypothermia is common; body temperatures are approximately 1 °F lower as compared to individuals with normal renal function. Hyperglycemia secondary to peripheral resistance to insulin can occur.[7b] Diabetic patients with CKD may present with more frequent hypoglycemic episodes because the kidney is responsible, in large part, for the degradation of insulin. Insulin doses often must be adjusted downward as renal failure progresses. Primary hypogonadism as well as hypothalamic abnormalities contribute to sexual dysfunction and sterility.[7c,7d]

DERMATOLOGIC SYSTEM

Dry, flaking skin and generalized pruritus are commonly seen in ESRD patients.

IMMUNE SYSTEM

Infectious diseases are common and result in significant morbidity and mortality in patients with ESRD. Although multiple abnormalities in host defenses and an increased susceptibility to infection have been described, the causal link between these observations remains speculative. Absolute lymphopenia and impaired cell-mediated immunity are common in ESRD patients and may be caused by the presence of uremic toxins or protein-calorie malnutrition. Although plasma concentrations of IgG, IgM, and IgA are usually normal, antibody responses appear to be significantly depressed.[8]

▶ TREATMENT: End-Stage Renal Disease

GENERAL APPROACH TO TREATMENT

The therapeutic management of the patient with ESRD hinges on several important principles. First, those treatments known to slow the rate of renal disease progression should be continued and renal function must be monitored closely, even during the first few months to years, while the patient receives dialysis. Second, health care providers need to evaluate each patient for cardiac risk factors and work collaboratively with the patient to reduce or eliminate as many risk factors as possible. This includes aggressive treatment of hypertension, diabetes, and hyperlipidemia, as well as maintaining hematocrit in target range of 33% to 36%. In addition, patients who smoke should be referred to a smoking cessation clinic. Third, patients must receive dietary assessment and instruction to limit protein, potassium, and phosphorus intake, yet maintain adequate caloric intake. Clinical practice guidelines for nutrition therapy in this population were recently published[9] (see Chap. 139). Phosphate-binding medications should be used to control serum phosphorus and calcium concentrations in order to suppress parathyroid hormone secretion and to prevent renal bone disease as well as cardiovascular calcification. Therapy with alkalinizing agents should be administered to patients with systemic acidosis. Finally, each patient's medications should be screened to detect and avoid potential nephrotoxins, as well as to assess appropriateness of the dosage for the patient's level of residual renal function.

NONPHARMACOLOGIC THERAPY

INDICATIONS FOR THE INITIATION OF DIALYTIC THERAPY

Hemodialysis and peritoneal dialysis are the primary renal replacement therapies available for ESRD patients. These nonpharmacologic treatments provide an additional route for the removal of endogenous waste products and water that, coupled with the patient's residual renal function, are life sustaining. The characteristics of these dialysis modalities and the pathophysiology and therapeutic approaches for the management of acute and chronic complications of dialysis are discussed in Chap. 47.

Criteria for the initiation of dialysis in patients with chronic renal insufficiency are largely clinical and include intractable nausea and vomiting; malnutrition; uremic encephalopathy; confusion; asterixis; seizures; myoclonus; uremic pericarditis; development of peripheral neuropathy; development of pruritus; and prophylactic use before major surgery. Currently, early dialysis access placement and initiation of dialysis is being advocated by many nephrologists to prevent symptomatology and to decrease morbidity and mortality.[9–11] After dialysis therapy is initiated, further assessment and intensive dietary instruction using published clinical practice guidelines is necessary, because dietary protein intake can be liberalized.[9] Adequate caloric intake and dietary phosphate restriction remain important goals of dietary management. A no-added-salt diet and fluid restriction to approximately 1,000 mL/d minimizes interdialysis weight gains and hyponatremia. Vitamin D hormone therapy is commonly prescribed to prevent renal osteodystrophy, along with epoetin and iron therapy for treatment of anemia. Aggressive management to reduce cardiac risk factors remains important to prevent future cardiovascular and cerebrovascular mortality.

IMPAIRED WATER AND SODIUM BALANCE

PATHOPHYSIOLOGY

In normal subjects, sodium balance is maintained with sodium intake of 120–150 mEq/d. The fractional excretion of sodium (FE_{Na}) is approximately 1% to 3%. Water balance is also maintained, with a normal range of urinary osmolality of 50–1,200 mOsm/L (see Chap. 51). In patients with chronic renal failure, sodium balance is maintained, but in a volume-expanded state. FE_{Na} increases to as much as 10% to 20%. The exact mechanism whereby FE_{Na} increases is unknown but may be the result of increased concentrations of atrial natriuretic peptide (ANP).[12] The increased secretion of ANP is probably triggered by increased intravascular volume and atrial pressure.

Volume expansion results in hypertension. Increased levels of ANP may interfere with sodium and calcium transport in vascular smooth muscle, resulting in increased resting muscle tone. The resultant increase in peripheral vascular resistance probably contributes to hypertension. Elevated levels of ANP may inhibit sodium and potassium ATPase-dependent pumps in many cells of the body, resulting in altered cellular electrolyte content and membrane potentials.

Water balance is generally maintained but within a limited range. Because the fractional reabsorption of sodium is decreased secondary to ANP, free-water generation by the kidney is impaired. An osmotic diuresis caused by a large solute load per remnant nephron results in obligatory water losses. The ability to dilute or concentrate the urine is impaired and urine becomes isosthenuric (urinary osmolality fixed at that of plasma or approximately 300 mOsm/L).

CLINICAL PRESENTATION

Nocturia is present relatively early in the course of renal insufficiency (CLcr 30–59 mL/min) secondary to the defect in urinary concentrating ability. Total renal sodium excretion decreases despite an increase in sodium excretion by remaining nephrons. Volume overload with pulmonary edema can result, but the most common manifestation of increased intravascular volume is systemic hypertension.[12]

▶ TREATMENT: Volume Overload and Edema

The ability of the kidney to adjust to abrupt changes in sodium intake is greatly diminished in patients with severe CKD and ESRD. Sodium restriction beyond a no-added-salt diet should not be recommended except in the face of hypertension or edema. The kidney maintains the ability to lower urinary sodium content to essentially zero, but this can only be accomplished by very gradual sodium restriction over a period of several days. Hospitalized patients should not routinely be sodium restricted because they have adapted to their outpatient intake. Negative sodium balance and its resultant volume contraction can result in decreased renal perfusion and subsequent further decline in GFR. Saline-containing intravenous solutions should be used cautiously in patients with chronic renal insufficiency because the kidney's ability to excrete a salt load is impaired and such patients are prone to volume overload. Sodium retention and volume expansion contribute to hypertension in many patients with renal insufficiency and ESRD, and diuretic therapy or dialysis may be necessary for control of edema or blood pressure. Alone, thiazide diuretics are ineffective in patients with a CLcr below 30 mL/min. Loop diuretics, particularly when administered by continuous infusion, increase urine volume and renal sodium excretion. A combination of a loop diuretic along with a thiazide diuretic (such as hydrochlorothiazide or metolazone) can result in a more profound excretion of sodium and water.

Fluid restriction is generally unnecessary provided sodium intake is controlled. An intact thirst mechanism maintains total body water and effective plasma osmolality near normal. Because urine volume is relatively fixed at approximately 2 L/d, fluid restriction below this amount should be avoided. Large amounts of free water administered orally or as intravenous fluid may induce hyponatremia and volume overload. When the patient develops ESRD, then dialysis (specifically ultrafiltration) or a renal transplant is necessary to maintain normovolemia.

POTASSIUM HOMEOSTASIS

PATHOPHYSIOLOGY

The kidneys normally excrete 90% to 95% of a daily potassium dietary load, predominately through distal tubular secretion (see Chap. 52). The fractional renal excretion of potassium (FE_K) is approximately 25%. Normally only 5% to 10% of ingested potassium is excreted through the gut. Potassium homeostasis is also maintained by shifting extracellular potassium to intracellular spaces, acutely, following ingestion of a potassium load.[13] In chronic renal insufficiency, potassium balance is maintained by an increase in distal tubular potassium secretion in which aldosterone plays an important role; FE_K can increase to as high as 125%. Thus the serum potassium concentration is usually maintained in the normal range until the patient reaches ESRD (GFR < 10 mL/min). A significant increase in potassium secretion by the colon also contributes to the maintenance of potassium balance, but this adaptation cannot compensate fully for the decrease in renal excretion. An animal study suggests that up-regulated angiotensin II (type AT-1) colonic receptors may be responsible for excretion of potassium in CKD and ESRD.[14]

CLINICAL PRESENTATION

The clinical consequences of hyperkalemia are similar regardless of the patient's renal function. The signs and symptoms of hyperkalemia are discussed in Chap. 52.

▶ TREATMENT: Hyperkalemia

Potassium-sparing diuretics are relatively contraindicated in patients with moderate to severe renal insufficiency because of the high risk of hyperkalemia. β-Blockers, predominantly via β_2-antagonistic effects, interfere with the extrarenal translocation of potassium into cells and may result in a further impairment in potassium handling and life-threatening hyperkalemia. Angiotensin-converting enzyme inhibitor (ACEI) and angiotensin II receptor blocker (ARB) therapy should be monitored closely in patients with moderate to severe renal insufficiency and ESRD because they may provoke hyperkalemia by reducing aldosterone production or by blocking angiotensin II receptors.[14]

The management of hyperkalemia in ESRD can be divided into chronic and acute treatment.[13,15] The goal is to maintain prehemodialysis potassium concentrations of 4.5–5.5 mEq/L. The majority of patients can be managed with a dietary potassium restriction of 50–80 mEq/d and alterations in dialysate potassium concentrations. Constipation in dialysis patients can interfere with colonic potassium excretion; therefore, a good bowel regimen is important. Extrarenal handling of potassium is important in ESRD; therefore, discontinuing ACEI or ARB therapy, or changing to a β_1-selective β-blocker[13] may be necessary in some patients. Pharmacologic treatment is rarely necessary for the ESRD patient on dialysis. Sodium polystyrene sulfonate (with sorbitol), a potassium -sodium exchange resin, can be given orally in doses of 15–30 g between dialysis sessions to increase potassium excretion in the ileum and colon. However, a recent well-designed study questions this practice. In this study, plasma potassium concentrations were either reduced minimally or not at all in hemodialysis patients who were administered single doses of resin with or without the addition of sorbitol or phenolphthalein-docusate.[16] Mineralocorticoids may enhance secretion of potassium into the gut by stimulating aldosterone receptors, although no clinical trials exist to support this. Finally, a short-term study showed that diltiazem 30 mg orally twice daily lessened the rate of increase in plasma potassium between dialysis sessions.[17]

The definitive treatment of severe hyperkalemia in ESRD is hemodialysis. In reality, there is often a delay between diagnosis of hyperkalemia and institution of dialysis, which necessitates the use of other temporizing measures, such as intravenous calcium gluconate, insulin and glucose, nebulized albuterol, and sodium polystyrene sulfonate (see Chap. 52). Unfortunately, shifting potassium into the intracellular fluid compartment with insulin and glucose or with albuterol makes dialysis removal of potassium more difficult.[13] Multiple dialysis sessions may be necessary following potassium redistribution to the extracellular space. Lastly, sodium bicarbonate therapy is no longer advocated in the treatment of ESRD hyperkalemia unless severe metabolic acidosis is also present, because the potassium-lowering effect is unreliable.[18]

METABOLIC ACIDOSIS

PATHOPHYSIOLOGY

People with normal renal function generate enough hydrogen ion to reclaim all filtered bicarbonate and to secrete approximately 1 mEq/kg/d of hydrogen ions, which are generated from the metabolism of dietary proteins (see Chap. 53). As a result they maintain a constant body fluid pH through the buffering of hydrogen ion by proteins, hemoglobin, phosphate, and especially bicarbonate. Renal ammoniagenesis and phosphate excretion buffer the urine and facilitate acid excretion. In severe chronic renal insufficiency, all filtered bicarbonate is reclaimed, but the ability of the kidneys to synthesize ammonia is impaired.[19] This decrease in urinary buffer results in decreased net acid excretion and continuous positive hydrogen ion balance; thus, metabolic acidosis develops. A clinically significant metabolic acidosis is commonly seen when the GFR drops below 20–30 mL/min. The plasma bicarbonate concentration tends to stabilize at 15–20 mEq/L.

CLINICAL PRESENTATION

Metabolic acidosis, through unknown mechanisms, contributes to renal bone disease by altering bone metabolism and vitamin D synthesis.[9,20] The presence of metabolic acidosis may also cause fatigue, decreased exercise tolerance, reduced cardiac contractility, and increased ventricular irritability. Finally, metabolic acidosis appears to stimulate protein catabolism, which can worsen uremia and contribute to a negative nitrogen balance, and lower albumin concentrations, as well as cause growth retardation in children.[9] In addition, lower serum bicarbonate levels in peritoneal dialysis patients are associated with a higher hospitalization rate and longer hospital stays.[9]

▶ TREATMENT: Metabolic Acidosis

The prevention and treatment of severe metabolic acidosis in patients with kidney disease is important for the prevention of the sequelae mentioned above. Metabolic acidosis in both adult and pediatric patients undergoing dialysis can often be managed by using higher concentrations of bicarbonate or acetate in the dialysate (>38 mEq/L bicarbonate is safe and effective). Oral bicarbonate salts (see below) may also be necessary for some patients.[9] The goal of therapy is to maintain a predialysis or stabilized bicarbonate concentration at or above 22 mEq/L.[9]

In patients with moderate to severe renal insufficiency, the use of alkalinizing salts, such as sodium bicarbonate or citrate/citric acid preparations, is useful to replenish depleted body bicarbonate stores. Citrate is metabolized in the liver to bicarbonate, and citric acid is metabolized to CO_2 and water. Sodium bicarbonate tablets are manufactured in 325- and 650-mg strengths (650-mg tablet contains 7.7 mEq sodium and 7.7 mEq bicarbonate). Each mL of Shohl's solution and Bicitra contains 1 mEq sodium and the equivalent of 1 mEq bicarbonate as sodium citrate/citric acid. Polycitra, which contains potassium citrate, should not be used in patients with severe renal insufficiency or ESRD because hyperkalemia may result. Each mL of Polycitra contains 1 mEq of sodium and potassium and 2 mEq of bicarbonate.

The first step in treatment is to calculate a replacement dose of alkali (base) that is needed to restore the serum bicarbonate concentration to normal (24 mEq/L).[20] The amount (mEq) can be approximated by multiplying the volume of distribution of bicarbonate (0.5 L/kg) by the patient's body weight (kg) and by the base deficit (difference between patient's serum bicarbonate value and 24 mEq/L). The calculated amount of bicarbonate replacement therapy should be administered over several days to prevent volume overload from excessive sodium intake.[20] If calcium acetate or calcium carbonate is also being given to the patient, decrease the amount of base administered. After the serum bicarbonate has normalized, reduce bicarbonate therapy to a maintenance regimen designed to neutralize daily acid production (12–20 mEq/d in divided doses).[20] Doses are subsequently titrated to maintain normal plasma bicarbonate concentrations. Patients with renal tubular acidosis (RTA) may require higher doses of alkalinizing agents[21,22] (see Chap. 53). Fluid balance should be monitored carefully because of the sodium content of these agents. Citrate-containing solutions should not be used in combination with aluminum-containing compounds because they can enhance aluminum absorption and increase the risk of aluminum intoxication. Excessive doses of alkalinizing agents may cause metabolic alkalosis, as well as lethargy or cardiac depression secondary to a decrease in ionized serum calcium concentration. Gastrointestinal distress characterized by gastric distention and flatulence is relatively common with high doses of oral sodium bicarbonate.

Laboratory measurement of serum bicarbonate is associated with several technical problems. Blood collection techniques, transportation, and assay methodology can affect the measured concentrations. Blood samples should not have contact with air; process delays should be avoided; and consistent analytical methods should be used with serial measurements to assure accurate measurements.[9]

PHOSPHORUS, CALCIUM, AND VITAMIN D HOMEOSTASIS

RENAL OSTEODYSTROPHY AND SECONDARY HYPERPARATHYROIDISM

Bone disease is a major cause of morbidity and mortality in patients undergoing chronic dialysis treatment. Bone loss can be detected in patients with early stages of renal failure and multiple types of bone lesions have been identified from bone biopsies of patients on dialysis.[23,24] When dialysis therapy was first available in the late 1960s, a high-turnover bone disease called osteitis fibrosa cystica or secondary hyperparathyroidism was the only entity identified. This bone lesion is characterized histologically by areas of peritrabecular fibrosis. Dynamic measurements show a high bone formation rate, which results from high circulating concentrations of PTH. In a random sample of 612 hemodialysis patients, 50% had an intact PTH level more than 3 times the established range.[25] In the 1970s, osteomalacia, characterized by a high volume of osteoid tissue, was first identified in ESRD patients. After several years, aluminum toxicity was implicated as the main cause when histologic stains revealed high levels of aluminum in patients with dialysis-associated osteomalacia. In the 1980s, an adynamic lesion was characterized. Histologically, this lesion shows low amounts of fibrosis or osteoid tissue and low bone formation rates. Initially, adynamic bone disease was also linked to aluminum toxicity as many patients exhibited high amounts of stainable aluminum in bone biopsies. Today, aluminum-containing phosphate binders are not routinely used. However, the incidence of adynamic lesions has increased dramatically over the last 10 years, and may be seen in as many as 50% of dialysis patients.[24] Multiple risk factors for the development of this bone disease have been identified: aluminum toxicity; high concentrations of dialysate calcium along with high doses of calcium-containing phosphate binders; aggressive management with vitamin D therapy; diabetes; and advanced age.[24] Management of PTH, phosphorus, and calcium balance, and minimizing patient exposure to aluminum is important in preventing the development of secondary hyperparathyroidism and slowing or preventing the progression of renal bone disease (renal osteodystrophy).

CARDIOVASCULAR DISEASE

Hyperphosphatemia is present in about 70% of ESRD patients and 40% of ESRD patients have values that exceed 6.5 mg/dL.[26] This increase in serum phosphorus level is associated with an increased risk of cardiovascular mortality, and higher phosphorus levels are associated with increased severity of coronary artery disease.[27] Myocardial calcium content and the degree of vascular calcification in dialysis patients is 4- to 10-fold higher than what has been observed in subjects with normal renal function. The degree of elevation in these two cardiac measures is strongly associated with age and the product of serum calcium multiplied by the serum phosphorus.[28]

ETIOLOGY AND PATHOPHYSIOLOGY

Calcium and phosphorus balance is mediated through a complex interplay of hormones and their effects on bone, gastrointestinal tract, kidney, and parathyroid gland.[29] Phosphate retention inhibits renal activation (1-α-hydroxylation) of vitamin D, which, in turn, reduces gut absorption of calcium. Phosphorus retention directly decreases blood-ionized (free) calcium through a physiochemical interaction, and high serum phosphorus concentrations directly increase PTH synthesis and release through production of prepro-PTH messenger RNA.[30,31] Low blood calcium concentrations provide a major stimulus for PTH secretion. Parathyroid hormone decreases proximal tubular phosphate reabsorption and restores phosphate balance until the GFR falls below 30 mL/min, at which time blood phosphorus concentrations often rise (Fig. 45–1).

The parathyroid glands release PTH in a physiologic attempt to restore normal blood calcium and phosphorus concentrations. However, as functional renal mass declines, serum calcium balance can only be maintained at the expense of increased bone resorption. Decreased production of 1,25-dihydroxyvitamin D_3 (calcitriol) results in impaired intestinal absorption of calcium, provides a stimulus for PTH release, and may contribute to defective bone mineralization.

Secondary hyperparathyroidism, a common manifestation in ESRD patients and those with severe renal insufficiency, can result in osteitis fibrosa cystica if left untreated. Underlying mechanisms are complex but include continued phosphorus retention, which leads to direct stimulation of PTH production, and secretion, as well as subsequent development of hypocalcemia, which stimulates PTH secretion. In addition, declining levels of calcitriol (1,25-dihydroxyvitamin D3) indirectly lead to hypocalcemia and provide further stimulus for PTH secretion (Fig. 45–1). Recently, a new calcium-sensing receptor was discovered on parathyroid cell membranes that may play a role in the pathogenesis of secondary hyperparathyroidism.[29] Parathyroid hyperplasia (nodular or diffuse) is another characteristic feature of secondary hyperparathyroidism. Nodular tissue demonstrates more rapid growth potential and appears to have lower numbers of vitamin D and calcium-sensing receptors, which results in resistance to the effects of calcium and vitamin D therapy.[29] Unfortunately, hyperphosphatemia is hard to control and hypercalcemia may develop in the pharmacologic attempt to achieve suppression of PTH release. High serum phosphorus concentrations and a high calcium-phosphorus product are linked to visceral and vascular calcification and increased mortality in dialysis patients.[29,32,33]

CLINICAL PRESENTATION

Uncontrolled hyperphosphatemia can result in metastatic calcification of joints, vessels, and soft tissue when the calcium phosphorus product is elevated (Table 45–2).[32,33] Clinical bone symptoms are rare in patients with mild to moderate renal insufficiency, although target organs (bone, kidney, and intestine) are affected. Intestinal calcium

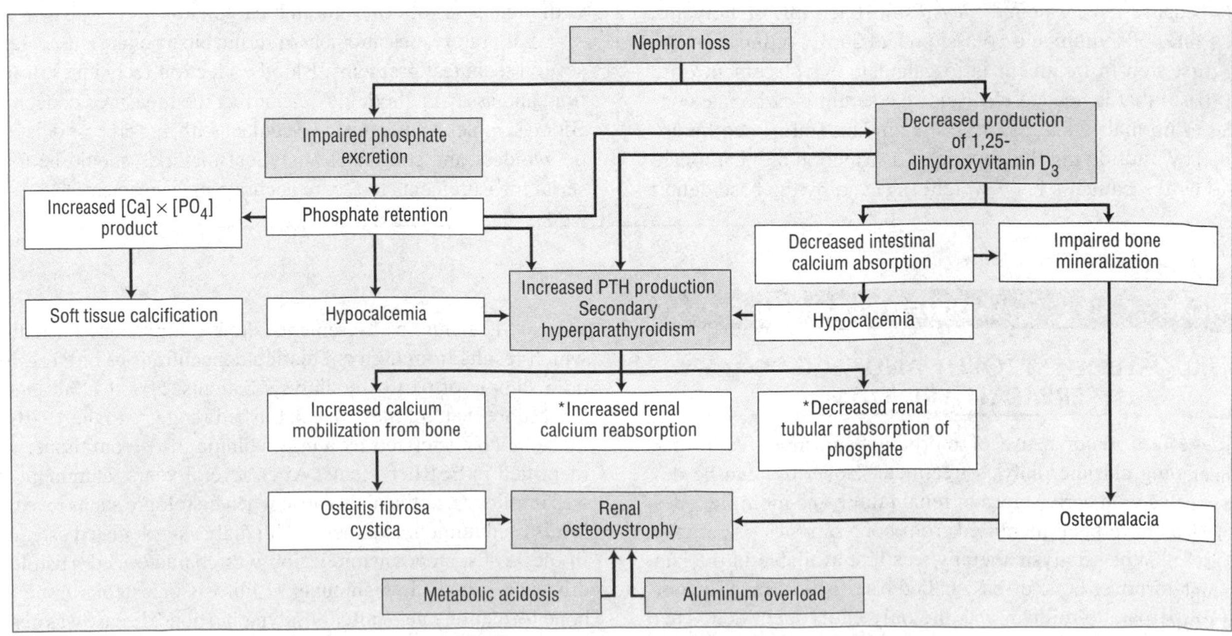

FIGURE 45–1. Pathogenesis of secondary hyperparathyroidism and renal osteodystrophy in patients with chronic renal failure. (*These adaptations are lost as renal failure progresses.)

TABLE 45–2. Laboratory Goals for Prevention and Treatment of Secondary Hyperparathyroidism

	Clcr (mL/min/1.73 m²)		
	>30	*10–30*	*<10 (ESRD)*
Calcium (mg/dL)[a,b,c]	9–11	9–11	9–11
Phosphorus (mg/dL)[c]	2.5–4.0	2.5–4.0	2.5–5.5
Ca × Phos[d]	<55	<55	<55
Intact PTH[e]	Normal range	1–2 × normal range	2–3 × normal range[f]

[a]Corrected calcium for albumin.
[b]Recent review suggests 9.2–9.6 mg/dL in dialysis patients;[30] however, this range has not been evaluated.
[c]Monitor once monthly in most circumstances.
[d]Calcium-phosphorus product; calculated as mg²/dL².
[e]PTH values can be drawn as often as once monthly during dose titration of phosphate binders and vitamin D therapy, or as infrequently as every 3 months after patient is stabilized.
[f]Two to five times normal range for chronic ambulatory peritoneal dialysis patients.

absorption can be decreased even at a GFR of 75 mL/min.[35] Development of secondary hyperparathyroidism and subsequent high circulating concentrations of PTH promotes progression of osteitis fibrosa cystica and may adversely affect lipid metabolism, insulin secretion, and myocardial and skeletal muscle, as well as neurologic and immune functions.[34] Common signs and symptoms of secondary hyperparathyroidism include fatigue and musculoskeletal and gastrointestinal complaints. Bone mineral density and serum calcium and serum 1,25-dihydroxyvitamin D_3 (calcitriol) concentrations decrease progressively, while serum PTH, osteocalcin, bone-specific alkaline phosphatase, and phosphorus concentrations increase as GFR declines.[23] Fifty percent of patients with a GFR less than 50 mL/min have abnormal bone histology.[35] Renal osteodystrophy progresses insidiously for several years before patients become symptomatic. When symptoms such as bone pain and skeletal fractures occur, the disease is not easily amenable to treatment. Bone marrow fibrosis and decreased hematopoiesis are also consequences of severe osteitis fibrosa. Therefore, preventative measures should be initiated in patients with mild to moderate degrees of renal insufficiency.[35]

DIAGNOSIS

Renal osteodystrophy is a generic term; knowledge of the specific underlying bone abnormality is essential to guide therapy. Serum calcium, phosphorus, PTH, alkaline phosphatase, and osteocalcin are serum biochemical markers used in the diagnostic workup and followup of renal osteodystrophy. Immunoradiometric (IRMA) and immunochemiluminescent assays for measurement of serum-intact PTH, the biologically active molecule, are more sensitive in distinguishing between histologic patterns of renal osteodystrophy than older midregion and carboxy-terminal PTH assays.[36,37] However, the Nichols Institute Allegro IRMA (N-IRMA), which is an established assay for intact PTH, measures not only the intact molecule, but also some smaller sections of PTH. A new IRMA manufactured by Scantibodies Laboratory only detects the full-length PTH molecule, which should more accurately reflect the biologically-active PTH molecule.[38] A study of 79 hemodialysis and peritoneal dialysis patients found that intact PTH greater than 450 pg/mL was between 95% and 100% specific for high bone turnover, but that overall, bone turnover could not be predicted in 30% of hemodialysis and 51% of peritoneal dialysis patients with intact PTH values alone.[39] Of note, these results were obtained using the less specific N-IRMA assay. Bone-specific alkaline phosphatase and osteocalcin, a protein synthesized by osteoblasts, are markers for bone formation.[23] Transiliac bone biopsy, although rarely used, is the only technology that clearly differentiates between different etiologies, and thus is the gold standard for evaluation of renal osteodystrophy. Tetracycline administration prior to bone biopsy provides dynamic information about bone turnover.[37] High-resolution x-ray techniques can aid in scoring the severity of bone disease and have been significantly correlated with serum PTH concentrations.[37] Bone-mineral densitometry studies can be used to detect bone loss in patients with CRI and ESRD, and are useful to follow progress after therapeutic intervention.[23,37]

The degree of cardiovascular damage—that is, coronary artery stenosis/calcification—can be quantitated by noninvasive means by using electron beam computed tomography (EBCT; see Chap. 10). Invasive procedures such as coronary angiography can also be used to ascertain the degree of damage if the newer technology is not available.

▶ TREATMENT: Disorders of Phosphorus, Calcium and Vitamin D Homeostasis

DESIRED OUTCOME AND GENERAL APPROACH TO TREATMENT

The overall goal of therapy across the spectrum of renal insufficiency is to prevent secondary hyperparathyroidism and renal osteodystrophy, and to reduce cardiovascular and extravascular calcifications. First, control of serum phosphorus should be achieved, and then serum calcium concentrations and PTH values should be optimized. Currently, there is no consensus on laboratory goals for prevention and treatment. Recent literature suggests that target ranges for serum phosphorus, calcium, calcium-phosphorus product, and PTH should be lowered to prevent an increased risk of cardiovascular morbidity and mortality in this patient population.[32] The National Kidney Foundation, as well as the Renal Physicians Association, has initiatives to develop clinical practice guidelines in this area. In the absence of published guidelines, Table 45–2 can serve as a guide. By the time ESRD develops, most patients require a combination of phosphate-binding medication and vitamin D therapy to prevent the development or progression of secondary hyperparathyroidism, renal osteodystrophy, and cardiovascular and extravascular calcification.

NONPHARMACOLOGIC THERAPY

Dietary phosphorus restriction (6.5–12.0 mg/kg/d) should be initiated in patients with a CLcr of less than 50 mL/min, to prevent early damage and perhaps slow progression of renal disease.[40] This amount of phosphorus restriction is usually achievable with 0.6–0.8 g of protein per kg of body weight. As the number of functioning nephrons decline, dietary restriction alone is usually inadequate to control serum phosphorus, and phosphate-binding agents are instituted. Dietary phosphorus can be liberalized to 900–1,200 mg/d after dialysis is initiated as a single hemodialysis session, or daily peritoneal dialysis treatment can remove up to 700 mg of phosphorus.[40] Examples of foods or beverages that contain high amounts of phosphorus per serving include meats, dairy products, dried beans, nuts, colas, peanut butter, and beer (see Chap. 51).

PHARMACOLOGIC THERAPY

PHOSPHATE-BINDING AGENTS

A variety of calcium-, aluminum-, and magnesium-containing phosphate-binding medications are available along with a nonabsorbable hydrogel phosphate-binding agent, which does not contain calcium, aluminum, or magnesium (Table 45–3). Phosphate-binding agents reduce phosphorus absorption from the gut, thus reducing serum phosphorus concentrations. Prevention of phosphate absorption by phosphate binders may preserve normal synthesis of calcitriol until patients reach ESRD.[41] In addition, lowering phosphate ingestion directly decreases PTH synthesis and secretion.[29] These agents should be administered just before or with meals to maximize their phosphate-binding effect. The dose should be titrated to achieve normal serum phosphorus concentrations in patients with moderate to severe renal insufficiency and concentrations of 2.5–5.5 mg/dL in ESRD patients. There is a linear relationship between the amount of ingested dietary phosphorus and the amount of phosphate-binding agent that is required to achieve goal phosphorus concentrations.[42] Pharmacist counseling is essential with phosphate-binding medications to enhance compliance, as many phosphate binders are marketed as antacids or calcium supplements and many dialysis patients do not know the indicated use.[43] Also, phosphate-binding agents may interfere with the absorption of other oral medications that these patients routinely take.

Aluminum salts were widely used in the 1980's as phosphate-binding agents because of their high binding potency. However, aluminum binders can no longer be recommended as first-line therapy because of the toxicities associated with aluminum accumulation. Aluminum binders should be considered as third-line agents and reserved for acute treatment of severe hyperphosphatemia or used in combination with either calcium-containing binding agents or sevelamer hydrochloride to limit patient exposure to aluminum (Table 45–3).

Oral calcium compounds emerged as first-line agents for controlling both serum phosphorus and calcium concentrations. Calcium carbonate, calcium citrate, and calcium acetate therapies have the potential advantage of partially correcting metabolic acidosis and increasing ionized calcium concentrations, thereby decreasing PTH secretion. Multiple studies have shown that calcium carbonate alone can successfully normalize phosphate concentrations in a high percentage of dialysis patients however, large doses (average 6–14 g/d of calcium carbonate) may be required.[44] Calcium carbonate is marketed in a variety of dosage forms (Table 45–3), and is relatively inexpensive. Unfortunately, many calcium carbonate products fall under the category of food supplements and are not required by law to meet United States Pharmacopeia (USP) disintegration and dissolution requirements. Intact calcium carbonate tablets have been detected in the stool of hemodialysis patients. In general, nationally advertised brands meet United States Pharmacopeia (USP) quality standards for disintegration and dissolution, but it is difficult to determine whether private label or house brands conform to these same standards. In addition, patients with renal failure have been reported to have variability in gastric pH, which may affect disintegration or dissolution. A recent study demonstrated that the disintegration of calcium carbonate products varied tremendously under different pH conditions.[45] Thus, it is prudent to use products with USP labeling. However, if a particular calcium carbonate product appears to be ineffective in a patient, it makes sense to try another product, as USP disintegration tests usually require testing only under one pH condition. Calcium carbonate is more soluble in an acidic medium, and therefore should be administered prior to meals when stomach acidity is highest.[46] In addition, acid-suppressing agents such as ranitidine can reduce the phosphate-binding activity of calcium carbonate by increasing gastric pH.[47]

Single-meal gastrointestinal balance experiments and short-term human trials show that calcium acetate binds approximately twice as much phosphorus as calcium carbonate at comparable doses of elemental calcium.[48,49] Increased binding potency limits gastrointestinal calcium absorption. However, calcium acetate is more soluble, and therefore better absorbed than calcium carbonate in an alkaline pH, which may explain the similar incidence of hypercalcemia when equivalent phosphorus concentrations are achieved.[48,49] Unfortunately, calcium acetate also causes more nausea and diarrhea than does calcium carbonate, which results in poorer medication compliance.[50] A long-term pharmacoeconomic study comparing the cost-effectiveness of calcium acetate versus calcium carbonate on suppression of secondary hyperparathyroidism, bone mass, and metastatic calcification is needed to definitively support calcium carbonate or acetate as the superior phosphate-binding agent.

Although the chloride and citrate salts of calcium may be used as phosphate binders, these agents exhibit several disadvantages compared to the carbonate and acetate salts. The chloride salt is very astringent and unpalatable, and absorbed chloride may contribute to systemic acidosis. The citrate salt binds phosphate poorly *in vitro,* markedly increases intestinal aluminum absorption due to the formation of soluble aluminum citrate complexes, and may contribute to aluminum intoxication.[51] Thus, citrate-containing compounds should not be combined with aluminum-containing compounds. In contrast, calcium acetate does not appear to influence the intestinal absorption of aluminum.[51] In most cases, when calcium binders are used as the primary phosphate binder, a low-calcium dialysate (2.25–2.75 mEq/L) should be used to reduce the potential for hypercalcemia and metastatic calcification.

Although calcium-containing phosphate-binding agents continue to be used as first-line therapy in the management of hyperphosphatemia in patients with renal disease, several recent articles highlight the dangers of giving patients too much calcium in conjunction with high serum phosphate concentrations. An observational cross-sectional analysis of more than 6,000 hemodialysis patients showed that patients with serum calcium-phosphorus product greater than 72 mg^2/dL^2 had a higher risk of death than did patients with a serum calcium-phosphorus product of 42–52 mg^2/dL^2.[26] In addition, investigators evaluated the extent of coronary artery calcification in 39 young patients on dialysis. They found that 14 of 16 patients aged 20 to 30 years had evidence of calcification. Moreover, the mean serum calcium-phosphorus product, phosphorus concentration, and daily intake of calcium were higher in the patients with coronary artery calcification.[33] These data suggest that aggressive use of calcium-containing phosphate binders can place patients at risk for vascular and tissue calcification. Thus, a combination of calcium-containing and noncalcium-containing phosphate binder agents might be used in patients who consistently demonstrate a calcium-phosphorus product greater than 55 mg^2/dL^2.[32]

Magnesium-containing antacids are also fairly effective phosphate binders. Several investigators have shown that magnesium-containing phosphate binders can lessen the amount of calcium-containing binders necessary for optimal phosphorus control,[52] although serum magnesium and potassium concentrations may rise and diarrhea is a problem. Dialysate magnesium concentrations must be reduced to avoid hypermagnesemia when magnesium-binding agents are used.[52] Magnesium carbonate is less-well absorbed and

TABLE 45–3. Phosphate-Binding Agents Used in the Treatment of Hyperphosphatemia of Renal Failure

Agents	Calcium, Aluminum, or Magnesium Content*	Dosage Form	Starting Doses	Comments
Calcium Carbonate (40% calcium)			0.5–1 g (elemental calcium) tid with meals	First-line agent; dissolution characteristics and phosphate-binding effect may vary from product to product. Usual maintenance dosage ranges from 2.4 to 5.6 g (elemental calcium) or 6 to 14 g (calcium carbonate) per day. Available over-the-counter.
Os-Cal 500	500 mg	Tablet, chewable tablet		
Caltrate 600	600 mg	Tablet		
Nephro-Calci	600 mg	Tablet		
CalCarb HD	2400 mg/packet	Powder		To be mixed with food.
Calci-Mix	500 mg	Pull-apart gel capsule		To be mixed with food.
Calci-Chew	500 mg	Tablet		Chewable.
Tums	200, 300, 500 mg	Tablet		Chewable.
Calcium Carbonate	500 mg/5 mL	Suspension		
Many other trade names and generic brands available.				
Calcium Acetate (25% calcium)			0.5–1 g (elemental calcium) tid with meals	First-line agent. Comparable efficacy to calcium carbonate with half the dose of elemental calcium. Prescription product.
Phos-Lo	169 mg	Tablet		
Calcium Citrate (21% calcium)				Citrate enhances absorption of aluminum. Should not be administered concurrently with aluminum binders, antacids, or sulcralfate.
Citracal	200 mg	Tablet		
	500 mg	Effervescent tablet		Contains Aspartame.
Sevelamer Hydrochloride				
Renagel	400 mg	Capsule, tablet	800 mg tid with meals	Second-line agent. Polymer that does not contain calcium, aluminum, or magnesium. Lowers LDL cholesterol. Expensive.
	400, 800 mg			
Aluminum Carbonate			400–500 mg tid with meals	Third-line agent. Do not use concurrently with citrate-containing products.
Basaljel	500 mg	Tablet, capsule		
	400 mg/5 ml	Suspension		
Aluminum Hydroxide			300–600 mg tid with meals	Third-line agent. Do not use concurrently with citrate-containing products.
Amphogel	300, 600 mg	Tablet		
	320 mg/5 mL	Suspension		
AlternaGel	600 mg/5 mL	Suspension		
Magnesium Carbonate				
Mag-Carb	70 mg	Capsule	70 mg tid with meals	Third-line agent. Magnesium concentration in dialysate needs to be reduced to avoid hypermagnesemia.
Magnesium Hydroxide				Serum magnesium concentration should be routinely monitored and kept within the normal range. Diarrhea is a common side effect.
Milk of Magnesia	300,600 mg	Tablet	300–400 mg tid with meals	Third-line agent. Magnesium concentration in dialysate needs to be reduced to avoid hypermagnesemia. Serum magnesium concentration should be routinely monitored and kept within the normal range. Diarrhea is a common side effect.
	400 mg/5 mL	Suspension		
	800 mg/5 mL	Suspension		

*Calcium content expressed as the amount of elemental calcium in each dosage form. The values for aluminum, magnesium, and sevelamer represent total content of the dosage form (e.g., milligrams of aluminum hydroxide).

better tolerated than magnesium hydroxide, and is now commercially available in a capsule formulation (Mag-Carb, R and D Laboratories). Magnesium and potassium serum concentrations must be closely monitored to avoid hypermagnesemia or hyperkalemia.

A nonabsorbable hydrogel phosphate-binding agent, sevelamer hydrochloride, offers a better side effect profile than do magnesium or calcium-containing binders (Table 45–3). This novel agent, which does not contain any aluminum, calcium, or magnesium, effectively lowers phosphorus and PTH concentrations, although large doses are often necessary. In a long-term clinical trial, the mean dosage needed to control serum phosphorus concentration was 6.3 g/d.[53] A comparison of sevelamer with calcium acetate in hemodialysis patients shows a similar decrease in serum phosphorus with a lower incidence of hypercalcemia in the sevelamer group.[54] Interestingly, in one long-term clinical trial, sevelamer also significantly reduced low-density lipoprotein (LDL) cholesterol and elevated high-density lipoprotein (HDL) by a mean of 30% and 18%, respectively.[53] Unfortunately, this new phosphate-binding agent is quite expensive, thus calcium-containing phosphate binders remain first-line therapy.

In summary, patients with renal insufficiency and failure should be initiated on calcium-containing phosphate binders to bind phosphorus and to suppress PTH. If calcium or calcium-phosphorus product rises above target ranges, then sevelamer hydrochloride can be added and the dose of the calcium-containing binders can be reduced. In addition, dialysate calcium can be reduced to lessen exposure to calcium. Magnesium-containing binders are another alternative that can be used in conjunction with calcium-based binders; however, a reduction in dialysate magnesium is necessary to prevent hypermagnesemia. Aluminum-containing binders should be used mainly in the acutely hyperphosphatemic patient; however, if it becomes necessary to use aluminum binders on a chronic basis, then serum aluminum concentrations should be monitored every 3 to 6 months to prevent aluminum toxicity.

Calcium Supplementation

After normophosphatemia is achieved, normocalcemia should be sought by using both dietary and pharmacologic means. Before calcium-containing phosphate binders were routinely used, calcium supplements were often given between meals to optimize total corrected serum calcium concentration at high-normal limits to reduce the stimulus for PTH secretion. Although dietary calcium intake is often subnormal in moderate to severe renal insufficiency patients because of the reduced intake of phosphate-containing dairy products, administration of calcium-containing phosphate binders and the use of vitamin D hormones should ensure a positive calcium balance. Therefore, additional calcium supplementation is no longer necessary in the majority of patients above that which is provided by the phosphate-lowering regimen.

Vitamin D Therapy

Vitamin D therapy should be given to patients who do not achieve normocalcemia or to those with elevated parathyroid hormone and alkaline phosphatase concentrations despite the use of calcium-containing binders alone. It must be emphasized that phosphorus control must be achieved before vitamin D therapy is initiated. There is increasing evidence that hyperphosphatemia causes resistance to the PTH-suppressing effects of vitamin D analogs, as well as directly stimulates PTH release and increases the risk of a high calcium–phosphorus product, which can lead to soft-tissue and vascular calcification.[32,33,55] Many vitamin D analogs are available; however, all but dihydrotachysterol, 1,25-dihydroxyvitamin D_3 (calcitriol), 19-*nor*-1,25 dihydroxy vitamin D_2 (paricalcitol), 1-α-hydroxyvitamin D_2 (doxercalciferol) and 1-α-hydroxyvitamin D_3 (alfacalcidol, not yet available in the United States) require hydroxylation in the kidney to produce the physiologically active hormone. Although biochemical, radiologic, and histologic improvements in renal osteodystrophy have been noted in patients receiving massive doses of vitamins D_2 or D_3, use of these sterols has been rendered obsolete by more physiologically active analogs with shorter half-lives.

Calcitriol has been used for the management of secondary hyperparathyroidism since the 1980s. Calcitriol can suppress PTH secretion by increasing serum calcium concentrations through enhanced gut absorption of calcium as well as by directly decreasing PTH synthesis and secretion by parathyroid cells.[56] Calcitriol can be administered orally as well as by intravenous injection. Controversy exists regarding the most effective route of administration, optimal dose, and dosage interval. Recent reviews nicely summarize the available literature relating to calcitriol for treatment of secondary hyperparathyroidism.[55,56] Calcitriol directly suppresses parathyroid hormone synthesis and secretion, and appears to up-regulate vitamin D receptors, which ultimately may reduce parathyroid hyperplasia.[57] High plasma levels of this sterol, achievable following intermittent (pulse) intravenous dosing two or three times weekly, may more effectively suppress PTH secretion than daily doses of oral calcitriol.[58] In fact, intravenous calcitriol has been safely used in the treatment of patients with hyperparathyroid bone disease in whom hypercalcemia developed during oral calcitriol therapy.[59] Although initial uncontrolled trials suggested that intravenous pulse therapy may be more effective than oral pulse therapy, a review of controlled trials suggests that oral therapy may be just as effective with no greater risks.[60]

The discrepancies between studies that have evaluated parathyroid gland size changes with vitamin D hormone treatment probably can be explained by major differences in study population, such as length of dialytic therapy; dose of calcitriol; use of aluminum versus calcium binders; presence or absence of aluminum bone disease; nodular versus diffuse parathyroid hyperplasia; and dialysate calcium concentration. It also appears that the size of the largest parathyroid gland may be a critical marker for response to calcitriol therapy. It is difficult to suppress PTH in patients with glands greater than 0.5 cm^3 in volume, whereas patients with smaller glands are more easily controlled with calcitriol. Larger glands are more likely to be comprised of nodular tissue, which has lesser density of vitamin D receptors and therefore is less responsive to calcitriol therapy.[61]

Unfortunately, use of calcitriol enhances calcium and phosphorus absorption from the gut, and frequently leads to hypercalcemia and hyperphosphatemia.[60] Conventional daily oral doses of calcitriol (0.25 μg) may be more frequently associated with hypercalcemia and hyperphosphatemia, because calcitriol receptors are located in intestinal mucosa where direct stimulation can occur. Strategies to minimize hypercalcemia while maximizing PTH suppression have included use of oral or intravenous pulse doses of calcitriol and calcitriol administration at bedtime or between meals when gut calcium and phosphorus content is lowest.[56] In addition, the dialysate calcium concentrations can be lowered to 2.25–2.75 mEq/L to limit hypercalcemic episodes.[56] Table 45–4 provides initial dosing guidelines for calcitriol. Intravenous calcitriol can be administered anytime during hemodialysis, as it is highly plasma protein bound and is not removed by the procedure.[62]

TABLE 45–4. Initial Vitamin D Hormone Dosing Guidelines for Prevention and Treatment of Secondary Hyperparathyroidism

Degree of Hyperparathyroidism	Range of Intact PTH (pg/mL)	Calcitriol	Paricalcitol	Doxercalciferol
Mild to moderate	200–600	CKD 0.25 μg PO qd or 0.5 μg PO on alternate days Dialysis: 0.5–1 μg IV or PO biw or tiw	Dialysis: 2 μg IV biw or tiw	CKD or Dialysis: 2.5 μg PO four times weekly or 2 μg IV biw or tiw
Moderate to severe	600–1200	CKD: 0.5 μg PO qd Dialysis: 2–4 μg IV or PO biw or tiw	Dialysis: 4 μg IV biw or tiw	CKD or Dialysis: 7.5 μg PO or 3 μg IV biw or tiw
Severe	>1200	Dialysis: 4–6 μg IV or PO biw or tiw	Dialysis: 8 μg IV biw or tiw	CKD or Dialysis: 10 μg PO or 4 μg IV biw or tiw

biw = two times weekly; tiw = three times weekly.

New vitamin D analogs have been developed that may result in less calcium and phosphorus absorption from the gut, but which retain the positive physiologic actions on bone and parathyroid tissue.[63] The Food and Drug Administration approved 19-*nor*-1-25-dihydroxyvitamin D_2 (paricalcitol) in 1998. Combined data from three identical double-blind, placebo-controlled human trials (n = 78) showed that paricalcitol administered intravenously 3 times a week after hemodialysis significantly reduced PTH over 12 weeks with a mean ending dose of 0.12 μg/kg. The mean serum calcium and phosphorus values did rise slightly during the study in the treatment group. There were 8 episodes of 401 serum calcium measurements that rose >11 mg/dL in the treatment group as compared to 4 of 417 measurements in the placebo group. Elevations of the calcium-phosphorus product >75 occurred in 45 of 395 determinations in the treatment group as compared to 16 of 412 determinations in the placebo group.[64] Interestingly, information about two large comparative trials with calcitriol was submitted in the New Drug Application (NDA) for paricalcitol. The combined results of these studies suggested no major differences in either efficacy or incidence of hypercalcemia between paricalcitol and calcitriol; in fact, one study showed a slightly higher incidence of hypercalcemia in the paricalcitol group.[65] These studies have not been published to date. Oral 1-α-hydroxyvitamin D_2 (doxercalciferol) was tested in a 32-week trial of 99 hemodialysis patients with secondary hyperparathyroidism. Doxercalciferol, in contrast to calcitriol and paricalcitol, is a prohormone that needs to be hydroxylated in the liver to the active 1,25–dihydroxyvitamin D_2 product. This study showed that doxercalciferol effectively reduced PTH. During the double-blind period of the study, 3.26% of serum calcium measurements exceeded 11.2 mg/dL and 7.1% of phosphorus measurements exceeded 8 mg/dL in the doxercalciferol group, as compared to 0.5% and 2.3%, respectively, in the placebo group.

Although the efficacy and safety profile of doxercalciferol looks very promising, a long-term comparative trial with calcitriol will be necessary to conclude that this is a superior agent. Doxercalciferol is now available in both oral and intravenous dosage forms. Table 45–4 lists the initial starting doses of calcitriol, paricalcitol, and doxercalciferol.

The intravenous forms of these vitamin D products are more expensive than their oral versions, and the route of administration does not appear to be important in either efficacy or toxicity. However, the pattern of vitamin D product use in U.S. dialysis units has been strongly influenced by Medicare reimbursement. Currently, intravenous vitamin D products are separately reimbursable expense items for dialysis programs. In fact, dialysis programs often profit from the intravenous administration of vitamin D products given to patients on dialysis. In contrast, oral calcitriol and doxercalciferol are not separately reimbursable and must be purchased by the patient. Thus, even though it appears that oral therapy is as effective as intravenous therapy, and is much less expensive, most dialysis programs continue to administer intravenous vitamin D products, particularly in hemodialysis patients.

Preliminary clinical data are being generated for a new class of compounds, the calcimimetic agents. These compounds mimic the effect of extracellular calcium by stimulating parathyroid cell calcium receptors and may prove useful in the treatment of secondary hyperparathyroidism.[66] Investigations with bisphosphonates, which block osteoclastic bone reabsorption (etidronate also inhibits bone mineralization), show conflicting results; thus, along with calcitonin, their place in therapy is currently confined to the acute treatment of hypercalcemia resulting from hyperparathyroidism (see Chapter 51).

SURGICAL THERAPY

Parathyroidectomy

Parathyroidectomy should be undertaken as the last therapeutic option for patients with secondary hyperparathyroidism. Criteria for surgery include (a) persistent hypercalcemia (serum calcium > 11.5 mg/dL) provided aluminum toxicity has been ruled out; (b) a persistently elevated calcium-phosphorus product and progressive soft-tissue calcification that persists despite vigorous dietary phosphate restriction and phosphate binder use; (c) progressive radiographic lesions of secondary hyperparathyroidism despite aggressive vitamin D therapy, particularly when associated with severe or debilitating symptoms; (d) intractable pruritus recalcitrant to other therapy; and (e) syndrome of calciphylaxis (a rare syndrome characterized by ischemic necrosis of the skin, muscles). Surgical approaches include either subtotal parathyroidectomy or total parathyroidectomy with transplantation of parathyroid tissue to an accessible site, such as the forearm, or ablation therapy with injections of ethanol.[61,67] Postoperative hypocalcemia, hypophosphatemia, and hypomagnesemia may occur because of a marked increase in bone production in relation to bone absorption ("hungry bone syndrome"). The severity of the hypocalcemia depends on the degree of osteitis fibrosa, and preoperative treatment with calcitriol may prevent or minimize the risk. Treatment with supplemental calcium and vitamin D hormones may be necessary for weeks or months. After surgery, continual efforts to prevent hyperphosphatemia and the recurrence of secondary hyperparathyroidism are necessary.

EVALUATION OF THERAPEUTIC OUTCOMES

The therapeutic goals for treatment with dietary phosphate restriction, phosphate-binding agents, and vitamin D therapy are to prevent secondary hyperparathyroidism, vitamin D deficiency, and subsequent renal osteodystrophy without inducing adynamic bone disease from oversuppression of PTH or calcification of vessels and soft tissue. Table 45–2 outlines the specific laboratory treatment goals. Figure 45–2 provides an algorithm approach for the treatment and evaluation of the CKD or ESRD patient on dialysis that uses clinically available noninvasive markers (corrected serum calcium, serum phosphorus, and intact PTH).

ALUMINUM TOXICITY

PATHOPHYSIOLOGY AND CLINICAL PRESENTATION

Although once a major problem, aluminum toxicity occurs less frequently because of use of deionizers and reverse osmosis filters for

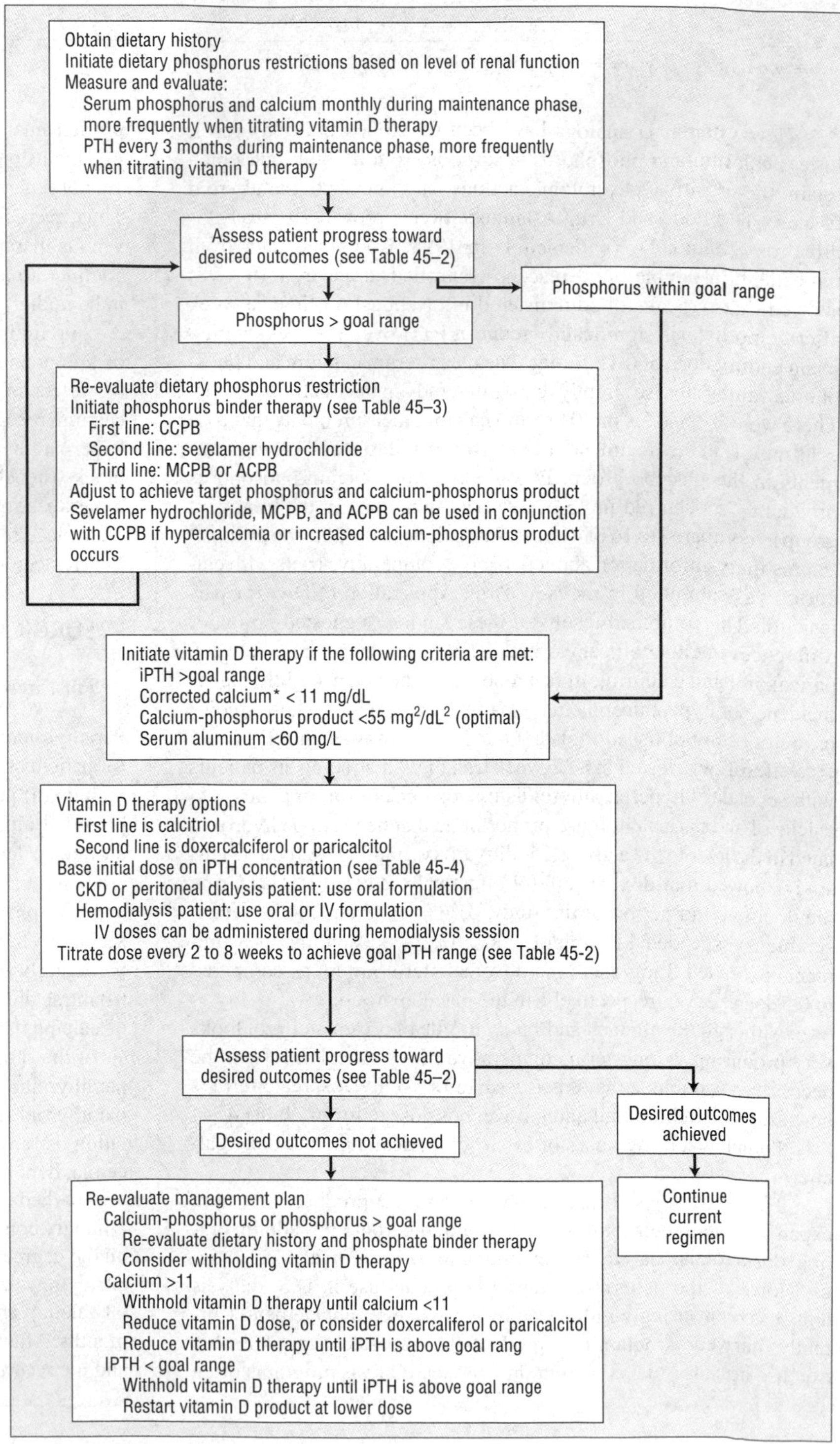

FIGURE 45–2. Approach to prevention and treatment of secondary hyperparathyroidism in patients with renal disease. CCPB = calcium-containing phosphate binder; MCPB = magnesium-containing phosphate binder; *corrected calcium = [(4.0 − pts albumin) × 0.8] + S_{Ca}.

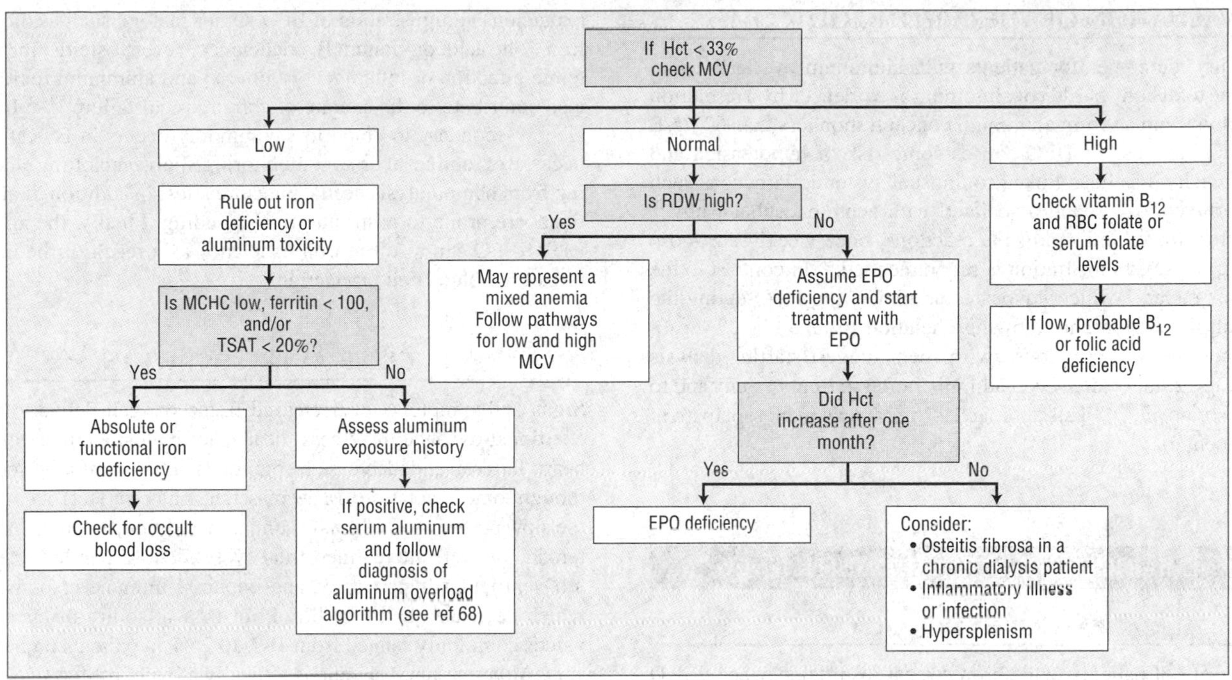

FIGURE 45–3. Diagnostic workup of anemia for CKD or ESRD patient.

dialysate water purification and decreased use of aluminum phosphate binders.[68] Aluminum is renally excreted; thus, accumulation can occur in ESRD patients who are exposed to various sources of aluminum. A recent study showed that the use of aluminum utensils can be a source of aluminum exposure in patients with kidney disease.[69] Aluminum toxicity can contribute to renal osteodystrophy (Fig. 45–1) and can result in decreased hematopoiesis (Fig. 45–3) and encephalopathy. Impaired bone mineralization and altered bone cell proliferation from aluminum excess result in an osteomalacic or adynamic bone histologic pattern.[70] Aluminum and iron compete for the same absorption and cellular uptake pathways. Aluminum may disrupt cellular iron metabolism, causing an iron-deficiency-like pattern and decreased erythropoiesis (microcytic anemia) in the presence of normal iron stores.[70] Interestingly, patients with low serum iron may be predisposed to aluminum toxicity because aluminum binds to transferrin, the major transport protein for iron.[70] Aluminum neurotoxicity can occur insidiously with speech disturbances and can progress to asterixis, myoclonus, visual and auditory hallucinations, seizures, and, ultimately, to death. Rapid manifestations of aluminum toxicity can occur under three circumstances: (a) high concentrations of aluminum in dialysate; (b) concurrent use of aluminum- and citrate-containing products; and (c) acute elevations in plasma and cerebral spinal fluid aluminum concentrations secondary to deferoxamine (DFO) administration.[71,72]

▶ PREVENTION AND TREATMENT: Aluminum Toxicity

Prevention is accomplished (a) by using water purified by deionization or reverse osmosis such that dialysate aluminum concentrations are less than 10 μg/L and (b) by minimizing the use of aluminum-containing phosphate binders or medications and aluminum-containing drinks, foods, and utensils (especially in the presence of citrate). Maintaining adequate iron balance may also lessen the risk for aluminum toxicity.

The gold standard for diagnosis of aluminum-related bone disease is transiliac bone biopsy. Indirect, less-invasive methods such as elevated plasma aluminum, low PTH concentrations, and positive DFO infusion test are also used to identify patients with aluminum overload, but these methods are less specific and sensitive. The DFO infusion test is based on the concept that the amount of aluminum mobilized following a single dose of DFO is representative of the total body burden of aluminum. The change in serum aluminum concentration is the key factor upon which therapeutic decisions are made.[68] Although the DFO infusion test is not entirely reliable in identifying patients with aluminum overload, it continues to be widely used. A negative DFO infusion test plus high PTH concentration may be useful to rule out aluminum toxicity.[73] All patients with symptoms of organ dysfunction from aluminum overload should receive DFO therapy. Hemodialysis alone does not significantly remove aluminum, because it is highly bound to the plasma protein transferrin. However, hemodialysis in combination with DFO therapy can remove substantial amounts of aluminum-DFO complex. High-flux dialysis and hemofiltration (using membranes with high middle molecule clearances) are effective in removing the complex;[74] however, an investigational high-flux dialyzer with immobilized DFO appears to enhance clearance above that of a high-flux dialyzer alone.[75]

EVALUATION OF THERAPEUTIC OUTCOMES

The desired outcomes for patients with aluminum overload are to reduce the total body burden of aluminum as evidenced by a resolution of symptoms and a serum aluminum concentration less than 60 μg/L with DFO. The use of DFO carries some risk of hypotension and ocular toxicity, has been linked to unusual systemic infections such as mucormycosis,[76,77] and associated with acute encephalopathy.[78] In an effort to minimize adverse reactions, once-weekly, low-dose (5 mg/kg) DFO administration is recommended.[68] In contrast to the consensus paper,[68] which advocates administering DFO during the hemodialysis session and allowing chelation to take place over 48 to 72 hours between sessions, two papers suggest starting dialysis within 5 to 12 hours after DFO administration to limit toxicity and to optimize removal.[79,80] This approach is impractical in most outpatient dialysis centers.

ANEMIA OF CHRONIC RENAL INSUFFICIENCY

PATHOPHYSIOLOGY

The majority of patients with chronic renal insufficiency and ESRD exhibit a normochromic, normocytic anemia that progresses as renal function worsens.[81] The primary cause of anemia in patients with chronic renal insufficiency and ESRD is a relative erythropoietin (EPO) deficiency, for which therapy with recombinant human erythropoietin alfa (epoetin alfa) has been available in the United States for more than 10 years. Erythropoietin beta (epoetin beta), another recombinant erythropoietin product with similar pharmacologic effects, is available in other nations.[82] In adults, the kidneys synthesize about 90% of circulating EPO with the remainder synthesized by the liver. EPO is a glycoprotein of approximately 30,000 daltons that is secreted in response to hypoxia.[82] Plasma concentrations of EPO increase exponentially in individuals with normal renal function as hematocrit declines. In contrast, there is no correlation between degree of anemia and EPO concentrations in anemic dialysis patients because they are unable to increase production of EPO in response to hypoxia.[82] Anemia begins to develop when the GFR drops below 50 mL/min and reaches a hematocrit of 30% when GFR is 20–30 mL/min. It is of interest that patients with ESRD secondary to polycystic kidney disease can often maintain a normal hematocrit without exogenous administration of EPO. Other factors, such as blood loss; iron, folic acid, or vitamin B_{12} deficiency; severe osteitis fibrosa; systemic infection or inflammatory illness; and aluminum toxicity may also contribute to the anemia of chronic renal failure.[83,84] Iron deficiency secondary to blood loss commonly occurs in ESRD patients because of routine laboratory monitoring, dialyzer clotting, and bleeding from hemodialysis needle puncture sites. In addition, dialysis patients are prone to gastrointestinal bleeding. Finally, the aggressive use of EPO can result in iron deficiency as a result of the increased rate of red blood cell production.

CLINICAL PRESENTATION

Signs and symptoms of decreased tissue oxygen delivery (fatigue; exertional dyspnea; dizziness; headache; pallor; angina; congestive heart failure; and decreased cognition) are commonly seen even though some adaptation to a decreased hematocrit (Hct) occurs during the slow progression of renal anemia. In addition, anemic patients often demonstrate altered menstrual cycles, loss of penile tumescence, left-ventricular hypertrophy, and impaired immune response, all of which decrease quality of life. Prior to availability of epoetin, Hct values commonly ranged from 18% to 25% in patients on hemodialysis. Although renal anemia is typically a hypoproliferative disorder in which normochromic and normocytic cells are seen on peripheral blood smear, iron deficiency secondary to blood loss or exogenous erythropoietin administration can result in a microcytic, hypochromic pattern. Vitamin B_{12} or folate deficiency can lead to a macrocytic anemia. Because the etiology of anemia in this population is often multifactorial, the workup of an ESRD patient with anemia should be approached in an economical stepwise fashion. An anemia workup should be initiated in CKD patients when the hemoglobin (Hgb) is less than 11 g/dL for premenstrual females and prepubertal patients, or below 12.5 g/dL in adult males and postmenopausal females.[85] The following tests should be completed before the patient begins epoetin: (a) Hct or Hgb; (b) red blood cell (RBC) indices, including mean corpuscular volume (MCV), mean corpuscular hemoglobin concentration (MCHC), and red cell distribution width (RDW); (c) reticulocyte count; (d) iron parameters, including serum iron, total iron-binding capacity (TIBC), ferritin, percent transferrin saturation (TSAT; serum iron divided by TIBC × 100); and (e) a test for occult blood in the stool. Figure 45–3 provides an algorithm to follow once the initial laboratory parameters have been analyzed.

▶ TREATMENT: Anemia of Chronic Renal Insufficiency

The National Kidney Foundation-Dialysis Outcomes Quality Initiative (K/DOQI) was established to improve patient outcomes by formulating recommendations for optimal clinical practices including diagnosis and management of renal anemia.[81] These guidelines were updated in 2001 and are currently known as Kidney Disease Outcomes Quality Initiative (K/DOQI). This was extended to encompass the care of patients with chronic renal insufficiency who were not yet being dialyzed.[85]

DESIRED OUTCOME

The goals of therapy are to prevent or reverse the signs and symptoms of tissue oxygen deprivation and left ventricular hypertrophy (LVH), improve exercise capacity, optimize survival, and ultimately improve the quality of life of patients. Cardiovascular disease is the leading cause of mortality in patients with ESRD[3] and LVH is an independent risk factor for death. In CKD patients, hypertension and hemoglobin concentrations independently predict left ventricular growth.[86] These data suggest that anemia management should begin in the early stages of chronic renal failure. However, data from Health Care Financing Administration (HCFA) Medical Evidence forms show that only 29% of patients who developed ESRD in 1999 received epoetin prior to ESRD diagnosis and the mean hematocrit of these patients was only 30.1%. The mean hematocrit of those patients not receiving epoetin was even more dismal at 28.0%.[87]

Most of the physiologic and quality-of-life studies of epoetin that resulted in resolution of the signs and symptoms of anemia in mainly dialysis patients achieved Hct measurements of 36% or less, and the phase III clinical trials achieved Hct values between 33% and 38%.[81] However, when epoetin alfa was approved in 1989, the target hematocrit range recommended by the FDA (and ultimately incorporated into the package insert) was 30% to 33%. Subsequently, the FDA broadened the range to 30% to 36% in 1994. A study evaluated the effects of a normal Hct (42 ± 3%) as compared with a lower target Hct of 30 ± 3% in more than 1,200 hemodialysis patients with documented heart disease. The study was discontinued when an interim analysis showed that the patients with the higher range experienced a higher death rate than the lower Hct group.[88] Consequently, based on this and many other clinical trials, the DOQI workgroup recommended a target Hct (hemoglobin) range of 33% to 36% (11–12 g/dL).[81,85] Observational studies evaluating the Medicare ESRD database validate this target hematocrit range for ESRD patients by demonstrating that prevalent dialysis patients with hematocrits of 33% to 36% have less risk of hospitalization and death than do patients who fall into lower hematocrit ranges.[89–91] Several studies are in progress that will evaluate the safety of higher Hct levels in ESRD patients. Currently, it is unclear whether the target range of 33% to 36% is adequate for patients with CKD, although the K/DOQI guidelines advocate this range.[85]

GENERAL APPROACH TO TREATMENT

Currently, epoetin is the therapy of choice for long-term correction and maintenance of Hct levels for patients with CKD or ESRD. It is reasonable to begin epoetin therapy in patients with Hct values below 33%; however, current Medicare reimbursement guidelines dictate that Hct levels must fall below 30% before the dialysis center or clinic will be reimbursed. Epoetin therapy results in dose-dependent increases in effective erythropoiesis in both predialysis and dialysis patients. Prior to initiation of epoetin, iron balance should be assessed, as iron deficiency is the most common cause of suboptimal response to epoetin. Because iron, folate, and vitamin B_{12} status should be optimized before or concurrently with the start of EPO, these agents can be considered first-/second-line therapeutic options for renal anemia.

RBC transfusions and androgen therapy are currently third-line treatment options for treatment of renal anemia. RBC transfusions carry many undesirable risks and therefore should only be used in three situations: (a) for acute management of symptomatic anemia; (b) after significant acute blood loss; and (c) prior to surgical procedures that carry a high risk of blood loss. Androgen therapy was also used extensively before epoetin availability, but hemopoietic response was suboptimal in the majority of patients. However, androgen therapy may potentiate the effects of epoetin by increasing the sensitivity of erythroid precursors in some individuals. Although *in vitro* results are encouraging, small human trials testing androgen effects on erythropoiesis yield conflicting results according to two recent reviews.[92,93] A retrospective analysis of 84 patients receiving androgen therapy in Spain showed a correlation between rise in hemoglobin and increased age. The authors concluded that nandrolone decanoate therapy was a less expensive alternative to epoetin and may be particularly suitable in males over 55.[93a] A recent prospective open trial, albeit small (n = 19), convincingly showed that nandrolone decanoate 100 mg IM per week along with epoetin, enhanced Hct response beyond that of epoetin alone, with few side effects.[93b] However, the risks of liver toxicity, malignancy virilization in females, and hypertriglyceridemia outweigh the benefits of androgen therapy in most individuals.[92,93]

PHARMACOLOGIC THERAPY

IRON ASSESSMENT

Iron status is usually assessed by monitoring serum iron, ferritin, TIBC, and TSAT.[94] Plasma ferritin values tend to correlate with body stores of iron located in the liver, bone marrow, and spleen. Unfortunately, ferritin is an acute-phase reactant and serum ferritin values can rise independently of body iron stores in response to inflammation, liver disease, malignancy, or infection. Circulating iron is highly bound to a protein called transferrin. Transferrin-bound iron is readily utilizable by the bone marrow for erythropoiesis. To prevent an absolute (low body stores) or functional (low amount of readily utilizable iron) iron deficiency in renal patients receiving epoetin, it is suggested that ferritin and TSAT values of at least 100 ng/mL and 20%, respectively, be maintained.[85] Another test to evaluate early iron deficiency is an increase in the percentage of hypochromic red blood cells (normally less than 2.5%). This test is not routinely available in the United States, but it is used in Europe. Values greater than 10% are associated with functional iron deficiency. When this methodology is more widely available, it should be incorporated into the workup of anemic patients with CKD.[81,94] Finally, one other marker for predicting functional iron deficiency is reticulocyte hemoglobin content (CHr). In one study, a CHr less than 28 pg at baseline predicted functional iron deficiency and response to iron dextran better than TSAT and ferritin.[95]

Ideally, iron deficiency should be corrected before epoetin therapy is initiated. This can be accomplished rapidly with intravenous iron administration. However, before iron therapy is initiated, several important considerations must be kept in mind: (a) blood losses, therefore iron losses, are higher in hemodialysis patients than in CRI or peritoneal dialysis patients; (b) oral iron is unlikely to be sufficient to maintain adequate iron stores in hemodialysis patients, but may be sufficient in some CKD or peritoneal dialysis patients; (c) epoetin therapy alone will lead to functional and absolute iron deficiency by stimulating erythropoiesis; and (d) maintenance (regular) parenteral doses of iron will likely be required to prevent iron deficiency and promote consistent erythropoiesis in hemodialysis patients.

Oral Iron

Oral iron management should begin with agents that have relatively high bioavailability and low cost. Initially, ferrous salts (sulfate, gluconate, and fumarate) should be prescribed to provide approximately 200 mg of elemental iron per day for adults (2–3 mg/kg for pediatric patients)[85] (see Chap. 99). Patients should be given divided daily doses of iron and instructed to take iron on an empty stomach to maximize absorption. If patients have gastrointestinal complaints (nausea, vomiting, constipation, diarrhea), they can take oral iron with a small snack, try another dosage form such as ferrous sulfate solution, iron-polysaccharide complex, or a sustained-release preparation, or another product such as ferrous fumarate or gluconate. However, the two latter compounds are more expensive and bioavailability is a problem. Administration with meals reduces iron absorption because of the interactions between iron, food, and phosphate binders. Some clinicians suggest giving vitamin C concomitantly with oral iron to enhance absorption. Unfortunately, serum oxalate concentrations rise in dialysis patients who receive more than 250 mg/d of vitamin C;[96] therefore, this maneuver is not recommended.

Intravenous Iron

To achieve the target Hct range, most hemodialysis patients, and many peritoneal and predialysis patients, require intravenous iron. Four IV iron products are currently available in the United States—two composed of iron dextran (INFeD, MW 96,000; and DexFerrum, MW 267,000), ferric gluconate (Ferrlecit, MW 350,000), and iron sucrose (Venofer, MW 43,000). Numerous clinical trials have been conducted with iron dextran preparations, as well as with ferric gluconate and iron sucrose (European data).[97] Parenteral iron improves the responsiveness to epoetin and reduces the amount of epoetin needed to achieve and maintain a target Hct. Initially, many dialysis programs administered IV dextran either as one-time large-dose (500–2,000 mg) infusions or as intermittent courses of therapy (100 mg given during the hemodialysis session for 10 consecutive sessions) to treat iron deficiency. Either of these approaches is reasonable to initially replete patients with an absolute iron deficiency (ferritin < 100 ng/mL).[98] However, many hemodialysis patients become iron deficient before the next treatment is given because of ongoing blood losses. There is mounting support for using smaller maintenance doses of iron dextran (25–100 mg/wk), particularly in hemodialysis patients, to maintain iron balance.[99] The K/DOQI guidelines state: (a) In adult hemodialysis patients with absolute iron deficiency (usually ferritin < 100 ng/mL), administer 100 mg of iron dextran during each dialysis by IV push (over 2 minutes) for 10 sessions (25 mg for pediatric patients weighing less than 10 kg, and 50 mg in those weighing 10–20 kg). (b) To maintain iron balance in adult hemodialysis patients with ferritin values above 100 ng/mL, administer 50 mg each week during dialysis for 10 weeks with measurement of TSAT and ferritin 2 weeks after the 10th dose. Weekly iron doses can then be adjusted (25–100 mg/wk) to maintain goal ferritin and TSAT values as well as optimal erythropoiesis. The weekly dose can be divided and given as one to three doses per week. (c) Predialysis or peritoneal dialysis patients who have an absolute iron deficiency or who cannot maintain iron balance with oral iron alone can be given intermittent total dose infusions of 500–1,000 mg of iron dextran (diluted in 250 mL of normal saline and given over 1 hour).

Iron dextran is not immediately available to the bone marrow for heme synthesis, but must be processed by the reticuloendothelial system (RES) before being released to transferrin or stored within the RES in bone marrow or splenic or hepatic tissue. The incorporation of iron into hemoglobin occurs over weeks, with a plasma disappearance half-time that is dose dependent. Thus, to avoid errors in evaluating iron status, clinicians should wait at least 2 weeks after a loading dose regimen of iron dextran to measure TSAT and perhaps as long as 6 weeks to measure serum ferritin.[99] However, serum iron indices can be evaluated after 1 week if the patient is receiving regular maintenance doses of iron dextran (25–100 mg/wk).[99] Total dose infusions of iron dextran (500–1000 mg administered in one session) are associated with more delayed side effects such as arthralgias, myalgias, and serum-sickness-like symptoms, than are lower doses. However, some investigators report a low incidence of problems with doses equal to or less than 500 mg.[100] Although the need for a test dose is controversial, K/DOQI guidelines recommend that a one-time dose of 25 mg in adults (10–15 mg in pediatric patients) should be administered IV before initiating iron dextran therapy in order to detect the small risk (<0.65%) of anaphylaxis.[85] Two other intravenous iron products (ferric gluconate and iron sucrose) have been used extensively in Europe.[97] Ferric gluconate has undergone clinical trials in the United States and was approved by the FDA in 1999.[101] This product repletes iron stores safely and effectively when given in doses of 62.5–125.0 mg once weekly to three times weekly.[97] European and U.S. clinical data show that allergic reactions with ferric gluconate are rare, and to date, no fatal reactions have been reported, in contrast to iron dextran.[97] In fact, one study showed that patients experiencing allergic reactions to iron dextran could be treated successfully with ferric gluconate.[101] There are some data to suggest that this product has the potential to oversaturate transferrin when given as a rapid infusion; however, this may have more to do with assay methodology rather than actual oversaturation.[97] Current FDA-approved dosage guidelines state that ferric gluconate 125 mg can be administered as an IV infusion over 1 hour or as a single 125-mg dose given over 10 minutes. A recent safety evaluation in more than 1,100 patients of the 10-minute infusion revealed a very low incidence of side effects and only 1 anaphylactoid-like reaction.[102] In contrast to iron dextran, ferric gluconate does not require a test dose. In addition, until further data are available, it should not be administered as a total-dose infusion.

Iron sucrose, which was FDA-approved in 2000, also appears to be a safer alternative than iron dextran.[103] The release characteristics of iron sucrose make it unlikely that oversaturation of transferrin will occur, and it is marketed for administration as 100-mg dose IV push over 5 minutes.[103] The safety profile of this product is excellent as evidenced by the fact that a test done is not required for any patients, including those patients who have demonstrated sensitivity to iron dextran. At this time, iron sucrose is not approved to be given as a total-dose infusion.

Aggressive, long-term use of intravenous iron products can enhance erythropoiesis, but may increase the risk of iron overload and development of such complications as tissue iron accumulation and increased risk of cardiovascular complications, infection, and perhaps even death.[104] The potential long-term risks for parenteral iron therapy are not clearly defined and there are no data that unequivocally confirms that aggressive use of IV iron in CKD or ESRD patients treated with epoetin increases patient morbidity or mortality.[104] However, observational studies have found an association with larger doses of iron dextran (greater than 1,000 mg over a 6-month period in 1 study) and increased mortality in dialysis patients.[105] The K/DOQI workgroup did recognize the potential for these long-term complications; therefore, current guidelines advocate that parenteral iron should be held for at least 3 months in patients who develop a serum ferritin level above 500[106] to 800 ng/mL.[85]

EPOETIN ALFA

Pharmacokinetics and Pharmacodynamics

Understanding the pharmacodynamic profile of epoetin is more important than the pharmacokinetics of this agent. Unlike many drugs where pharmacodynamic action is related to peak or trough concentrations, or half-life can be used to predict the duration of action or time to attainment of steady state, epoetin action must be evaluated on the basis of changes in RBC production rate and the individual's RBC life span.[107] Uremic patients have a shortened RBC life span, which averages 64 days, in contrast to 120 days in normal subjects.[107] Figure 45–4 illustrates the Hct response to the pharmacodynamic effect of epoetin (an increase in Hct). Prior to starting epoetin, the baseline Hct is constant, demonstrating that RBC production is at steady state (the rate at which RBCs are being produced equals the rate at which they are dying). Although the Hct may begin to rise shortly following epoetin initiation as the result of demargination of reticulocytes, it takes approximately 10 days before erythrocyte progenitor cells mature and begin to be continuously released into the circulation at an increased

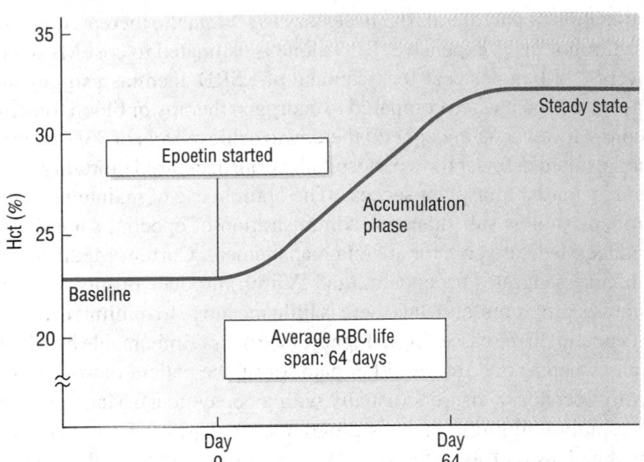

FIGURE 45–4. Pharmacodynamic effect of epoetin or NESP on hematocrit (Hct).

rate. Gradually Hct rises as the RBC production rate exceeds daily RBC death. The Hct continues to increase until the life span of the cells stimulated by epoetin is reached (range, 1–4 months) and a new steady state is achieved. Clinical trials document successful treatment of ESRD anemia with total weekly IV or SC doses of 80–180 U/kg (adults and pediatric patients > 5 years old) or up to 300 U/kg in pediatric patients less than 5 years old.[85]

Epoetin can be administered by either the IV or subcutaneous route. Subcutaneous administration is preferable in chronic ambulatory peritoneal dialysis and CKD patients (these patients usually do not have permanent IV access), and now is being recommended in hemodialysis patients as a way to reduce expenditures for epoetin.[85,108] Although SC administration results in poor bioavailability (approximately 20%), low peak serum concentrations, and a prolonged half-life (approximately 22 hours as compared to 8.3 hours IV),[107] Hct response is at least as good or better than IV administration. This enhanced efficacy is presumed to be caused by a more prolonged physiologic stimulation of erythroid precursors. Although many of these comparative studies suffer from design flaws, the preponderance of data supports the use of SC epoetin, as target Hct may be maintained with lower weekly epoetin doses (15% to 50% lower).[85,108] Once a week, twice a week, and three times a week subcutaneous dosing are all effective. Currently, two formulations of epoetin alfa are available: a single-dose formulation without preservative and a multidose formulation with benzyl alcohol. A clinical trial comparing these two formulations in terms of pain intensity after subcutaneous administration found that the multiple-dose formulation caused less stinging, although several patients did not experience pain with the single-dose preparation.[109]

NOVEL ERYTHROPOIESIS STIMULATING PROTEIN

Novel erythropoiesis-stimulating protein (NESP) was formulated with two additional sialic acid-containing carbohydrates, which required a change of five amino acids from the original epoetin molecule.[110] The increased sialic acid content delays drug clearance; the half-life of NESP when administered IV and SC is thus prolonged to 25.3 hours and 48.8 hours, respectively, when administered to adults.[110a] The half-life of NESP is similar, although the absorption appears to be more rapid in pediatric patients as compared with adult patients with CKD or ESRD.[111] The extended half-life allows for once-a-week or once-every-other-week dosing when given IV or SC in most patients.[111a] NESP was approved by the FDA in September 2001.[111a] This product will be used mainly in CKD or peritoneal dialysis patients due to the convenience of less frequent dosing. Practice guidelines for the use of NESP in these patients and those receiving maintenance HD have recently been proposed by a European working group.[111b] These guidelines and the product labeling propose methods for converting patients from epoetin alfa therapy to NESP.

Resistance to Epoetin

Real or pseudoresistance to epoetin therapy can stem from multiple factors.[81,83,93] Iron deficiency is the most common cause of resistance to epoetin and develops routinely during epoetin therapy.[85] Evaluation and treatment should proceed as previously outlined. Inflammation (localized or systemic infection, active inflammatory disease, surgical trauma) is associated with defective iron utilization known as reticuloendothelial block. Reticuloendothelial block is characterized by a reduction in iron delivery from body stores to the bone marrow, and is generally refractory to iron therapy. Malignancy and autoimmune diseases can cause a resistance to epoetin by decreasing endogenous erythropoietin production, reticuloendothelial block, and reduced bone marrow responsiveness.[81] Cancer cells can invade the bone marrow, and radiation and chemotherapy can damage erythroid progenitor cells. Epoetin therapy can be continued in the infected or postoperative patient, although increased amounts are often required to maintain or slow the rate of decline in Hct.

Hyperparathyroidism is known to cause resistance to epoetin. Erythropoietic response to epoetin therapy in patients with hyperparathyroidism appears to be linked to the severity of bone marrow fibrosis. High concentrations of PTH may also directly inhibit erythropoiesis. Aluminum toxicity, which was discussed earlier, can reduce iron transport. Aluminum also inhibits key enzymes necessary in heme synthesis. Recognition of aluminum toxicity and appropriate chelation therapy with DFO are key steps in improving bone marrow response to epoetin. Unfortunately, DFO also chelates iron, making therapeutic management of anemia more difficult. Hemoglobinopathies are often not responsive or are poorly responsive to epoetin.[85] In patients with sickle cell anemia, epoetin can increase the release of reticulocytes containing mainly hemoglobin S with little or no increase in hemoglobin F (the more stable form). Patients with α-thalassemia may slowly increase their Hct with epoetin following long-term therapy with high doses. Folate and vitamin B_{12} deficiency can also cause epoetin resistance, as both of these are essential for optimal erythropoiesis. Patients on hemodialysis or peritoneal dialysis are routinely prescribed daily vitamins with folate, as this substance is water soluble and dialyzable. Hemodialysis may also be associated with subclinical vitamin C deficiency. Recently, a few small human trials have demonstrated that the administration of IV ascorbic acid can overcome epoetin resistance in some patients who appear to have functional iron deficiency (adequate iron stores but low TSAT).[93] All of these trials have been short-term and there is concern that long-term administration of higher doses of vitamin C may cause accumulation of oxalate. A long-term trial that examines the efficacy and safety of vitamin C is needed before this practice can be widely advocated.

One other factor that may worsen the anemia of chronic renal failure is the use of ACEIs or angiotensin receptor blockers (ARBs). The mechanism has not been elucidated, and several brief reports have been conflicting.[81,112] A recent prospective crossover trial evaluated epoetin doses in 33 patients during 4-month time periods when patients were either receiving an ACEI (usually lisinopril) or an alternative antihypertensive. There was no difference in epoetin doses between time periods. Although the study protocol did not have a specific iron repletion/maintenance protocol in place, ferritin and transferrin saturation values were not different between time periods.[113] Patients currently receiving epoetin and initiating ACEIs or ARBs should have Hct carefully assessed and epoetin dosages increased if necessary to maintain Hct within the target range. Finally, pseudoresistance can occur with occult bleeding or hemolysis. In this case, bone marrow response to epoetin is normal, but blood loss or hemolysis negatively offsets the rate of rise in hematocrit with epoetin. Therefore, a workup of apparent epoetin resistance should always include an evaluation of potential sources of blood loss or hemolysis.

PHARMACOECONOMIC CONSIDERATIONS

Epoetin was a major breakthrough in the therapy of renal anemia, and relegated transfusion therapy to the treatment of acute blood loss and anemia refractory to epoetin. However, this therapy and the increased utilization of parenteral iron necessary to sustain the increased rate of erythropoiesis is expensive. EPO alone is estimated to cost Medicare over $1 billion per year for treatment of ESRD anemia, a significant increase in cost when compared to androgen therapy or blood transfusions. However, using epoetin therapy to achieve Hcts of 33% to 36% has resulted in fewer days of hospitalization, decreased mortality,[89–91] and increased transplant success. The optimal use of maintenance IV iron, as well as subcutaneous administration of epoetin, should also reduce Medicare cost for anemia management. Current Medicare reimbursement rates for epoetin (and IV iron) produce profits for most dialysis programs, and thus there is little incentive to minimize the use of epoetin. In the case of iron therapy, IV iron is reimbursable by Medicare, whereas oral iron is either paid for by the patient out-of-pocket or by secondary insurers (usually with a copayment). Managed care is rapidly infiltrating dialysis programs. Capitation of payments for medications such as epoetin and IV iron therapy will force the dialysis community to change clinical practice to provide for the economic use of both iron and epoetin therapy.

EVALUATION OF THERAPEUTIC OUTCOMES

Figure 45–5 outlines an algorithmic approach to patient evaluation and treatment with epoetin and iron therapy in adults. Effective therapy with epoetin in the treatment of the anemia of CKD decreases hospitalization and morbidity and increases quality of life of dialysis patients.[81,89–91] The mean Hct has been rising in dialysis patients each year since epoetin was introduced and is now stabilizing in the middle of the target range.[114] However, the mean Hct in CKD patients at the diagnosis of ESRD is much less than the target range, and only a minority of these patients receive epoetin.[87] In addition, more than 30% of adult hemodialysis patients had TSAT values less than 20%, and 22% of patients had ferritin concentrations less than 100 ng/mL in 1998.[115] This suggests that epoetin and iron therapy can be further optimized in a sizable percentage of dialysis and CKD patients.

The major side effect of epoetin is a predictable elevation in blood pressure, which occurs in approximately 23% of patients.[81] The exact reason for increased blood pressure is not clear, but may be caused by increased basal and stimulated cytosolic calcium, which increases vascular tone and causes resistance to nitric oxide. In addition, enhanced endothelin production and stimulation of vascular tissue renin-angiotensin system may also contribute.[116] The baseline or final levels of hemoglobin, rate of rise in hemoglobin, or uncontrolled hypertension prior to epoetin use do not appear to be risk factors for development of hypertension.[116] Increases in blood pressure should be treated aggressively and blood pressure should be stable (ideally < 140/90) before epoetin initiation. Epoetin doses should only be reduced or held if aggressive ultrafiltration and antihypertensive management cannot control blood pressure, or if hypertensive encephalopathy occurs. Seizures have occurred in approximately 3% of patients treated with epoetin.[81] Seizure incidence does not appear to be increased over the baseline levels seen in placebo control groups. Because it is controversial whether vascular access thrombosis may be more frequent during epoetin therapy, no increased surveillance is advocated.[85]

UREMIC BLEEDING

PATHOPHYSIOLOGY

Bleeding complications are usually mild, but can result in major hemorrhagic events. The etiology of uremic bleeding is multifactorial. The primary mechanisms underlying the hemostatic problem are platelet biochemical abnormalities and alterations in platelet-vessel wall interactions. Decreased platelet aggregation and adhesiveness have been shown in a number of studies.[117] Additionally, there is a decreased plasma concentration and defective binding of the large multimer of von Willebrand factor (vWF), which results in abnormal platelet-blood vessel wall interactions. Normally platelets flow in a skimming pattern close to the vessel wall, while RBCs occupy the center of the vessel, a situation that is ideal for platelet-vessel wall interaction. Anemia results in dispersion of platelets and RBCs during flow through vessels, which makes it difficult for primary hemostasis to occur.[117] Heparinization during dialysis procedures also increases risk of bleeding. In addition, dialysis patients often receive systemic anticoagulation (warfarin) or antiplatelet therapy (aspirin, Persantine, clopidogrel) for prevention of access clotting or other cardiovascular problems.

CLINICAL PRESENTATION

Uremic patients commonly experience purpura, ecchymoses, epistaxis, and prolonged bleeding from hemodialysis venipuncture sites. Gastrointestinal bleeding occurs less commonly but can be severe and is often related to gastrointestinal telangiectasias. Other severe hemorrhagic complications such as spontaneous retroperitoneal bleeding, hemorrhagic pericarditis, or pleural effusion occur less frequently.[117,118] Subdural hematoma, which may occur in up to 3% of hemodialysis patients, should be suspected when symptoms of headache, vomiting, seizures, somnolence, confusion, or coma occur in conjunction with a hemodialysis treatment.[118] Risk factors for a subdural bleed include head trauma or hypertension. The bleeding time is the clinical test that is most often prolonged in uremia. This test measures the time required for bleeding from a small standardized skin puncture site to cease. Filter paper is used to wipe off the blood from the incision every 30 seconds. This test reflects primary hemostatic function and measures interaction between platelets and the vessel wall following injury. The normal bleeding time averages 4 to 5 minutes (range, 2 to 9 minutes). Unfortunately, this test is not useful in predicting the risk of bleeding in individual patients.[119]

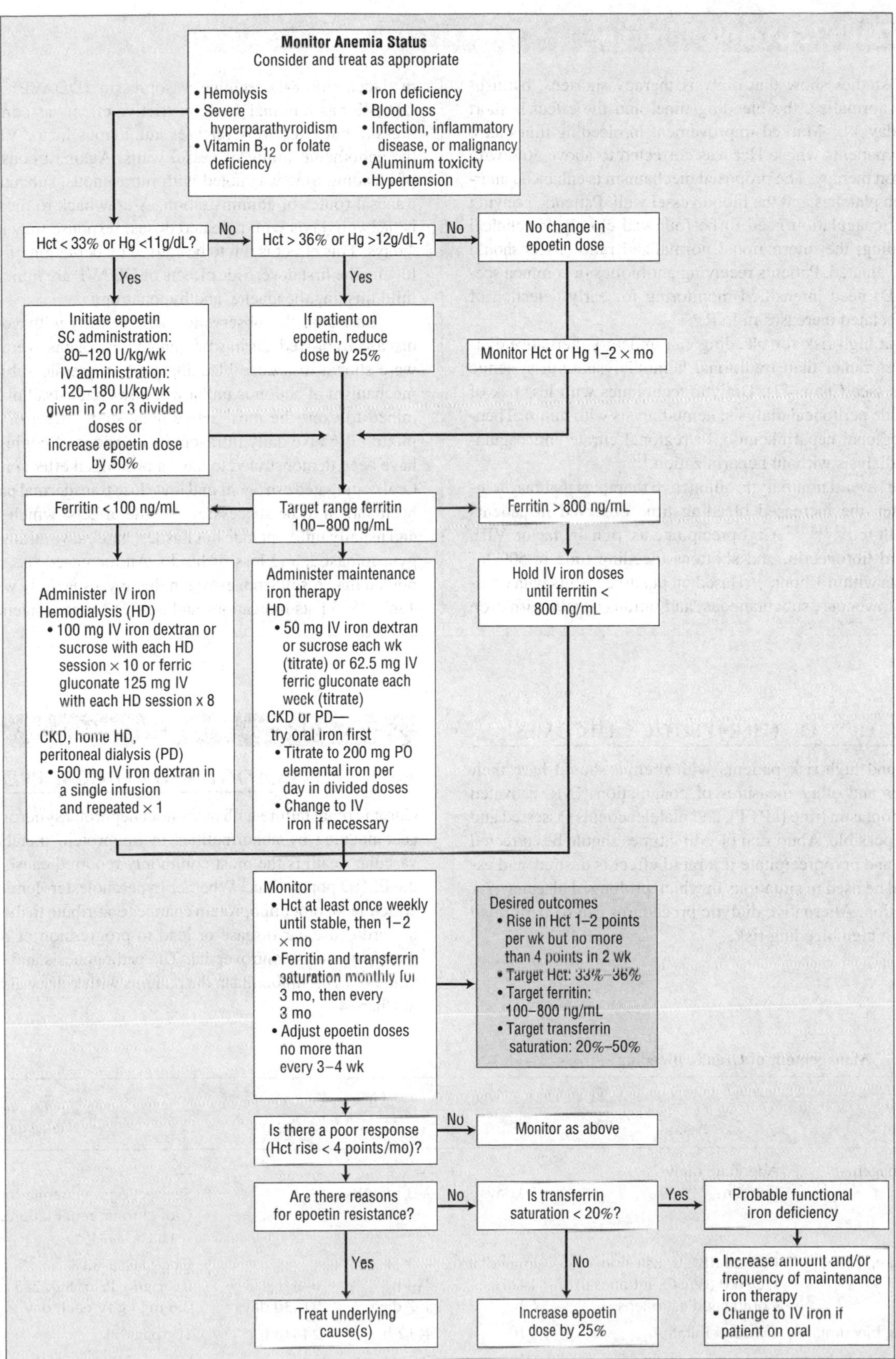

FIGURE 45–5. Approach to epoetin and iron therapy in the treatment of the anemia of chronic renal failure. Where Hg = hemoglobin and Hct = hematocrit.

▶ TREATMENT: Uremic Bleeding

A number of studies show that dialysis therapy shortens, but usually does not normalize, the bleeding time, and the effect is short lived (1 to 2 days).[118] Marked improvement in bleeding times have been found in patients whose Hct was corrected to above 30% with epoetin and iron therapy. The proposed mechanism is enhanced interaction between platelets and the blood vessel wall. Patients receiving Coumadin anticoagulation need to be followed closely for clinical signs of bleeding; the international normalized ratio (INR) should be routinely evaluated. Patients receiving antibiotics (a common scenario in ESRD) need intensified monitoring for early detection of antibiotic-associated increases in INR.

Patients at high risk for bleeding can undergo alternative dialysis procedures rather than traditional hemodialysis with systemic heparinization (see Chap. 47). Dialytic techniques with less risk of bleeding include peritoneal dialysis; hemodialysis with minimal heparinization, regional heparinization, or regional citrate anticoagulation; or hemodialysis without heparinization.[118]

There are several nondialytic adjunctive therapies that may temporarily shorten the increased bleeding time observed in patients with renal failure.[117,118,120] Cryoprecipitate is rich in factor VIII, fibrinogen, and fibronectin, and shortens bleeding time in 50% of uremic patients within 1 hour.[117] Based on positive results with cryoprecipitate, intravenous, subcutaneous, and intranasal administration of 1-deamino-8-D-arginine vasopressin (DDAVP) was evaluated. DDAVP has minimal vasoconstrictive effects as compared to vasopressin, but effectively releases autologous factor VIII (vWF) from the endothelial lining of vessel walls. Again, a consistent lowering of bleeding time was noted with intravenous, subcutaneous, and intranasal routes of administration. A drawback to the use of DDAVP is tachyphylaxis with repeated doses; response may return after 3 to 4 days. This effect is felt to be caused by depletion of vWF stores following the first dose. Side effects of DDAVP are minimal and include mild flushing, headache, and hyponatremia.

Based on the observation that women with von Willebrand's disease improved during pregnancy, estrogens were evaluated and were shown to reduce bleeding time in uremic subjects.[117,121] The mechanism of action is unknown; however, estradiol has been determined to exert the most active hemostatic effect of the conjugated mixture.[122] Five daily intravenous infusions of conjugated estrogens have been demonstrated to have a prolonged effect on bleeding time. Oral conjugated estrogens and low-dose transdermal patches have also been shown to be successful.[117] Side effects, which are uncommon and usually mild, include hot flashes, nausea, vomiting, hypertension, gynecomastia, and loss of libido. An increased risk of thromboembolism may result from estrogen therapy, especially with chronic use. Table 45–5 lists indications and dosage for each agent.

EVALUATION OF THERAPEUTIC OUTCOMES

Preoperative and high-risk patients with uremia should have their bleeding times and other measures of coagulation (INR, activated partial thromboplastin time [aPTT], and platelet counts) assessed and normalized if possible. Abnormal bleeding times should be corrected with DDAVP and cryoprecipitate if a rapid effect is desired, and estrogens should be used in situations in which prolonged bleeding risk is a consideration. Alternative dialytic procedures can be performed in patients with high bleeding risk.

HYPERLIPIDEMIA

PATHOPHYSIOLOGY AND CLINICAL PRESENTATION

Chronic renal failure with or without nephrotic syndrome is frequently accompanied by abnormalities in lipoprotein metabolism. Cardiovascular death is the most commonly reported cause of mortality in the ESRD population.[3] Whether hypercholesterolemia, hypertriglyceridemia, or other lipoprotein changes contribute to the high incidence of cardiovascular disease or lead to progression of renal disease in these patients is controversial. The pathogenesis and clinical presentation of hyperlipidemia in the patients with kidney disease is detailed in Chap. 44.

TABLE 45–5. Management of Uremic Bleeding

Indication	Agent	Effect: *Start*	Effect: *Maximum*	Effect: *End*	Dosage
Long-term management	Adequate dialysis	—	—	—	—
	Epoetin	10 days	2–3 months	—	See section on anemia in discussion of chronic renal failure. Goal: Hct 33%–36%
Acute bleeding episodes	Packed RBC transfusion	Immediate	—	—	Goal: Hct >33%
	DDAVP (IV, SQ, intranasal)	1–2 h	2–4 h	6–8 h	0.3 μg/kg IV or SQ, 2–3 μg/kg intranasal
	Conjugated estrogens	6 h	5–7 days	21–30 days	0.6 mg/kg IV each day × 5 days
Life-threatening bleeding	Cryoprecipitate	1 h	4–12 h	24–36 h	10 "bags" IV
Chronic treatment of telangiectasias	Estrogen/progestin combinations	6 h	5–7 days	—	Various products and dosages used in studies
Management of chronic bleeding tendency	Conjugated estrogens	6 h	5–7 days	—	50 mg orally each day; only studied short-term (<2 wk) 50–100 μg/24 h of transdermal estradiol

▶ TREATMENT: Hyperlipidemia

There are no published interventional trials that document that treatment of the various lipid disorders seen in the ESRD population reduces the risk of cardiovascular disease. However, there is some epidemiologic evidence that demonstrates that lipoprotein abnormalities may be associated with higher risk of cardiovascular disease.[123] It is likely that the same lipoprotein abnormalities that confer increased risk of cardiovascular disease in the general population are also harmful to patients with renal disease. In the absence of specific treatment data for ESRD patients, it seems reasonable to use the most current National Cholesterol Education Program (NCEP) guidelines for classification, treatment decisions, and target lipid levels.[123,124] General guidelines for treatment and evaluation of hyperlipidemia in CKD patients with and without nephrotic syndrome are found in Chap. 44. These guidelines can be applied to patients who are receiving dialysis as well.

Several trials have assessed the effect of L-carnitine supplementation on abnormal lipid metabolism in dialysis patients in, but results have been contradictory. Although L-carnitine supplementation cannot be advocated at this time for hyperlipidemia treatment, carnitine may prove useful for dialysis-related muscle cramps or hypotension, lack of energy, skeletal muscle weakness, cardiomyopathy, or anemia unresponsive to epoetin.[125] Interestingly, reverse flux filtration along with heparin-induced extracorporeal LDL precipitation (HELP) during hemodialysis has been successful in reducing LDL cholesterol in hemodialysis patients with type IIb hyperlipidemia.[126]

ADVERSE EFFECTS

Potential drug interactions and/or side effects with the use of antilipemic therapy in patients with kidney disease are outlined in Chap. 44. Large doses of omega-3 polyunsaturated fatty acids (fish oils) lower triglyceride levels in hemodialysis patients, but they may interfere with platelet function, predisposing to bleeding. In addition, the high doses necessary to lower triglycerides make noncompliance more likely.

HYPERTENSION IN END-STAGE RENAL DISEASE

The pathophysiology and treatment of hypertension is reviewed in detail in Chap. 12. The present discussion focuses on pathophysiology and therapeutic management of hypertension in patients with ESRD.

PATHOPHYSIOLOGY

Hypertension can be a cause or a consequence of renal insufficiency. High blood pressure may also promote renal damage independently of the underlying mechanism of renal disease (Chap. 44). Several morphologic changes, collectively termed *hypertensive nephrosclerosis,* have been noted in kidneys of patients with essential hypertension. Of patients initiating dialysis, approximately 80% to 90% are hypertensive.[127] The pathogenesis is multifactorial but many hypertensive dialysis patients have a volume component to blood pressure elevation (fluid retention promotes high blood pressure).[127] In addition to these factors, increased sympathetic activity, an endogenous digitalis-like substance, elevated levels of endothelin-1, erythropoietin use, hyperparathyroidism, and structural changes in the arteries (e.g., metastatic calcification) may contribute to hypertension in the ESRD patient.[127]

It has been observed that patients with moderate to severe renal insufficiency display an abnormal diurnal rhythm in their blood pressure in that blood pressure does not show a decrease during the nighttime hours.[127] It is unclear what causes this disturbance in the diurnal rhythm, and whether it contributes to the progression of renal insufficiency. High blood pressure can accelerate the rate of decline in renal function as well as cause other end-organ damage. In addition, hypertension is a risk factor for the severe atherosclerosis and cardiovascular disease noted in ESRD.[127] Unfortunately, when 24-hour ambulatory blood pressure monitoring is employed it appears that hypertension is not adequately controlled in a significant number of ESRD patients.[127,128]

▶ TREATMENT: Hypertension in End-Stage Renal Disease

DESIRED OUTCOMES

Cardiovascular disease remains the leading cause of death in patients with ESRD,[3] and it is likely that the high incidence and prevalence of high blood pressure in CKD and ESRD patients contributes to LVH and the high cardiac death rate along with other factors such as anemia, hyperlipidemia, and disorders of calcium and phosphorus metabolism. There are few prospective longitudinal studies of hypertension in dialysis patients, but it appears that hypertension is not well controlled in the dialysis population (particularly in diabetics).[127] Hypertension should be rigorously managed in patients with CKD to prevent progression of renal disease and cardiovascular sequelae. Blood pressure goals and treatment strategies for CKD patients are found in Chap. 44. The goal blood pressure for ESRD patients is controversial. Many clinical trials have used less than 150/90 mm Hg as a treatment goal.[127] The latest National High Blood Pressure Education Working Group recommends a goal blood pressure of 130/85 mm Hg.[129] However, the J-curve phenomena may be an issue in the renal failure population. This may be especially true secondary to the high incidence of ischemic cardiovascular disease in these patients. Therefore, the potential complications of decreasing diastolic blood pressures to below 85 mm Hg may outweigh the benefits in some patients.[130] Thus, different blood pressure goals may need to be set for individual patients based on their clinical status, age, and cardiovascular condition. Blood pressure control should be achieved in a gradual manner to allow for physiologic adaptation.

NON-PHARMACOLOGIC THERAPY

The primary intervention for ESRD patients is to restrict salt (2–3 g/d) and water intake to reduce fluid volume accumulation between dialysis sessions. Massive doses of loop diuretics are generally ineffective in promoting diuresis, and expose the patient to risks of ototoxicity, gastrointestinal upset, muscle cramps, and hyperglycemia. In dialysis patients, achievement of an individual's "dry weight" and control of total-body sodium through the dialytic process results in normalization of blood pressure in 50% to 60% or more of dialysis patients.[131] Interestingly, the Tassin group showed that prolonged hemodialysis (8-hour sessions, 3 times per week) will help to maintain normal blood pressures and will reduce the need for antihypertensive medications in the vast majority of patients.[132] Most importantly, this group has also pointed out that there is a lag phenomenon in blood pressure reduction following achievement of "dry weight." In their group of patients, blood pressure continued to fall over several months while using the dry-weight method of blood pressure control.[133] However, the majority of hemodialysis programs in the United States use shorter dialysis methods (3- to 4-hour sessions, 3 times per week). Patients in whom volume cannot be controlled with standard intermittent hemodialysis may benefit from variable-sodium dialysis or by switching to continuous ambulatory peritoneal dialysis.[127] Antihypertensive medications should be slowly withdrawn except for those medications that are being used to treat underlying cardiovascular disease.

PHARMACOLOGIC THERAPY

Patients in whom salt and water restriction along with aggressive dialysis therapy fail to control high blood pressure may benefit from treatment with medications. Blood pressure control can be achieved by most classes of antihypertensive, and choice should be guided by an individual patient's concomitant disease states. In light of the important role the renin-angiotensin axis plays in the etiology of some cases of dialysis-resistant hypertension, ACEIs can be quite effective. Because the elimination half-lives of the parent compound (captopril, lisinopril) or active metabolite (enalapril, benazepril, ramipril) are prolonged in ESRD patients, lower initial doses may be necessary.[134] Bone marrow depression has been noted in up to 10% of renal failure subjects receiving captopril, especially those with autoimmune diseases.[131] If captopril therapy is initiated in the dialysis patient, close monitoring of white blood cell counts should be undertaken and drug doses kept as low as possible. Other ACEIs, which lack the sulfhydryl group of captopril, may be less likely to cause bone marrow depression and are probably the ACEIs of choice in these patients. ARBs have not been well studied in patients with ESRD. However, they have effectively lowered blood pressure in dialysis patients. As compared to ACEIs, ARBs do not affect bradykinin metabolism, thus, they are not expected to cause anaphylactoid reactions when used in conjunction with polyacrylonitrile (PAN) dialysis membranes.[127] None of the ARBs require dosage adjustment for renal impairment, and none are effectively removed by hemodialysis.[135]

CCBs, particularly the dihydropyridines, which selectively lower systemic vascular resistance, also appear to be effective in the treatment of hypertension in the ESRD patient. In one study, nitrendipine lowered blood pressure effectively in hemodialysis patients with large interdialytic weight gains.[136] This is similar to the observation that a high sodium intake enhances the blood pressure response to calcium channel blockade in essential hypertension. Thus, either ACEI or CCB therapy is an appropriate first-line therapy in the hypertensive ESRD patient in whom achievement of the target postdialysis weight (dry weight) is inadequate to control blood pressure.

A number of other antihypertensive drugs may also be effective in patients with ESRD, including drugs that interfere with renin release such as the β-blockers or the combined α- and β-blockers labetalol or carvedilol. β-Blockers may be particularly useful in hypertensive dialysis patients who have had a myocardial infarction. Agents such as esmolol, timolol, pindolol, metoprolol, or labetalol, which are metabolized and not significantly dialyzable, may be easier to dose titrate than those agents that are both dialyzable and extensively eliminated unchanged by the kidney (acebutolol, atenolol, bisoprolol, nadolol).[131] However, a recent study evaluating the efficacy, safety, and pharmacokinetics of bisoprolol in 6 hemodialysis patients with dialysis-refractory hypertension showed that lowering the daily dose to 2.5 mg/d may prevent dialysis hypotension and bradycardia.[137] Another trial capitalized on the long half-life that atenolol exhibits in patients with ESRD. An investigator administered 25 mg of atenolol to 8 patients following hemodialysis 3 times a week. The antihypertensive effect persisted over 44 hours between dialysis sessions without any increase in intradialytic hypertension.[138]

Sympathetic nervous system active agents, such as prazosin, terazosin, doxazosin, clonidine, guanabenz, and guanfacine, may be required in patients unresponsive to dialytic therapy, plus ACEI, CCB, or β-blocker therapy. Central α_2-agonists such as clonidine appear to be the safest of these agents to use in the dialysis population. Transdermal clonidine, in doses up to 1.2 mg/d (four 0.3-mg patches), has demonstrated success as monotherapy in one short-term study of hypertensive dialysis patients.[139] However, central α_2-agonists can cause bradycardia, as well as dry mouth, which may lead to extra fluid consumption in some patients. Postsynaptic α-blockers (e.g., prazosin) are associated with postural hypotension following hemodialysis.[140] Guanethidine and methyldopa should also be avoided because of potential complications including severe postural hypotension, severe dialysis-related hypotension, and impotence.[131] The addition of vasodilators such as minoxidil or hydralazine may prove useful in patients resistant to combinations of the previously mentioned agents. Hydralazine is often effective as first-line therapy for hypertension and is generally well tolerated. In addition, monotherapy with the drug is well tolerated in diabetic patients because of the underlying autonomic neuropathy that prevents reflex tachycardia. The incidence of drug-induced systemic lupus erythematosus (SLE) does not appear to be increased by the presence of ESRD. Minoxidil therapy may be associated with pericardial effusion and profound reflex tachycardia, which can be suppressed with either the addition of a β-blocker or a central α-adrenoreceptor agonist.

PHARMACOECONOMIC CONSIDERATIONS

Other considerations in selection of antihypertensive therapy in ESRD patients should include compliance and economic factors. In general, most ESRD patients are prescribed an average of 9 to 12 medications. Choosing agents that can be administered once or twice daily may improve patient compliance. In addition, there are now many options within some antihypertensive classes, such as calcium channel blockers, ACEIs, ARBs, and β-blockers. In most cases, no clear therapeutic advantage has been demonstrated with any particular agent within a class. Therefore, selecting the least costly agent that can be administered once or twice daily should have a favorable economic impact over the lifetime of the patient.

EVALUATION OF THERAPEUTIC OUTCOMES

Figure 45–6 is a treatment algorithm for ESRD patients with hypertension that is based on recommendations by the Joint Renal Physicians Association and American Society of Nephrology Clinical Practice Committee.[127] Other guidelines for antihypertensive therapy selection based on other patient characteristics can be found in the JNC-VI report.[141] The mean ambulatory blood pressure goal should be 130/85 mm Hg or less in the majority of dialysis patients, although this may be difficult to achieve because of the significant interdialytic weight gains of many hemodialysis patients. The benefits of achieving this blood pressure goal need to be weighed against the harmful effects of intradialytic hypotension. Blood pressures are always obtained before, during, and after a hemodialysis session. Ambulatory blood pressure monitoring can help to identify dialysis patients with blood pressure profiles that might respond to antihypertensive therapy.[142] Prolonged antihypertensive therapies with a combination of β-blockers, ACEIs, and CCBs result in regression of LVH in hypertensive ESRD patients.[143]

MISCELLANEOUS THERAPEUTIC CONSIDERATIONS

PRURITUS

Despite advances in dialysis treatment, pruritus (itching) remains a vexing problem that occurs in up to 90% of ESRD patients.[144] Pruritus is a manifestation of chronic but not acute renal failure, and usually occurs 6 months or so after dialysis is initiated if it wasn't present prior to starting dialysis.[144,145] The pathogenesis of uremic pruritus is poorly understood, but has been attributed to multiple factors such as inadequate dialysis, skin dryness, secondary hyperparathyroidism, increased vitamin A and histamine plasma concentrations, and increased sensitivity to histamine.[144,145] A small study in hemodialysis and peritoneal dialysis patients showed that patients with pruritus demonstrated higher numbers of degranulated mast cells as compared to patients without pruritus. In addition, higher concentrations of histamine, PTH, and middle-molecular-weight substances, and lower serum iron concentrations were seen in patients with pruritus.[146] ESRD patients with pruritus experience exaggerated itching sensation to exogenous administration of histamine as compared to uremic patients with no pruritus or control patients.[145]

Non-pharmacologic Therapy

Therapy for pruritus is largely empirical. The mainstay of therapy is adequate dialysis treatment. Regular, aggressive dialysis eliminates or improves pruritus in many patients.[144] Poor tolerance to dialysis membranes and sterilants such as ethylene oxide can also cause pruritus in some patients. Thus, using a γ-irradiated membrane or noncomplement-activating membrane such as polymethylmethacrylate may be tried.[144] Other nonpharmacologic therapies include acupuncture and ultraviolet light. Acupuncture has been reported to improve pruritus for months in a small number of patients.[144]

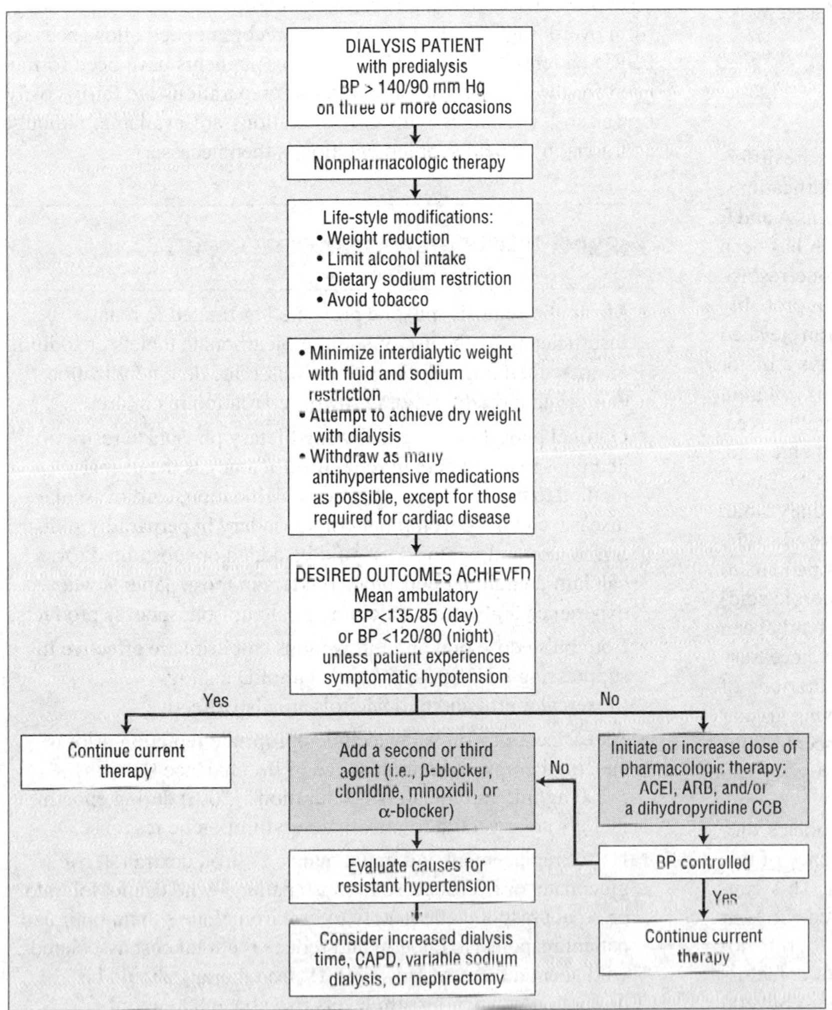

FIGURE 45–6. Treatment algorithm for ESRD patients with hypertension. ACEI = angiotensin-converting enzyme inhibitor; ARB = angiotensin II receptor blocker; CAPD = continuous ambulatory peritoneal dialysis; CCB = calcium channel blocker.

Ultraviolet B therapy benefits a majority of patients in both controlled and uncontrolled studies. The mechanism of response has not been elucidated, but may include reduction in skin content of vitamin A, divalent ions, and/or retinol; reduction in histamine-containing dermal mast cells; detoxification of unknown pathogenic substances; or desensitization of epidermal nerve endings.

Pharmacologic Therapy

Some patients gain relief from topical administration of emollients, although dry skin does not appear to be a predominant factor in pruritus. Numerous drug therapies have been evaluated for the treatment of pruritus. In fact, no single therapy has proven more effective than another therapy in individual patients. Even though elevated plasma histamine concentrations and exaggerated responses to histamine have been noted in uremic patients with pruritus, antihistamine treatment often fails to reduce symptoms. Nonetheless, a 2- to 3-week trial of low-dose regimen may be warranted. Activated charcoal and cholestyramine have also been shown to benefit some patients. However, the binding effects of these two agents on other medications, the extra fluid intake necessary to administer them, and the potential for hyperchloremia with cholestyramine should be weighed against the potential benefits. The beneficial effects of lidocaine, heparin, naloxone, for pruritus treatment have also been described, but more clinical studies are necessary before any of these can be recommended. Recently, ondansetron was evaluated in a placebo-controlled trial in hemodialysis patients because noncontrolled studies had suggested efficacy. Unfortunately, ondansetron did not improve pruritus in this more rigorous evaluation.[147] Robertson and Mueller recently proposed a stepwise process for treating uremic pruritus.[144]

VITAMIN REPLACEMENT

Vitamin requirements for ESRD patients receiving dialysis are different from those of a healthy person because of dietary modifications, renal dysfunction, and dialytic therapy.[96,148,149] Both vitamins A and E have are elevated in ESRD. Hypervitaminosis of vitamin A has been correlated with anemia and hypercalcemia (increased bone resorption) in hemodialysis patients. Vitamin K supplementation is probably unnecessary in most dialysis patients except for those with an elevated INR during or after a course of antibiotics. Vitamin D plays a major role in bone metabolism in ESRD; the dose of 1,25-dihydroxyvitamin D_3 (calcitriol) or other vitamin D analogs needs to be individualized. The water-soluble vitamins (B_1, B_2, B_6, B_{12}, niacin, pantothenic acid, folic acid, biotin, and vitamin C) are low or deficient in the average Western diet. Some of the water-soluble vitamins are dialyzable; others, such as vitamins C and B complex, may be destroyed or the amounts reduced with cooking methods used by dialysis patients to leach out potassium. Vitamins B_6 (pyridoxine) and C (ascorbic acid) as well as folic acid are the three vitamins that have consistently been reported to be deficient in dialysis patients. Vitamin C is necessary for the normal production of oxalic acid. Higher concentrations of oxalate have been reported in hemodialysis patients receiving greater than 250 mg of vitamin C per day. Increased plasma concentrations of oxalate may lead to deposition in soft tissues, muscles, vessels, and organs.

Hyperhomocystinemia is a risk factor for atherosclerotic cardiovascular disease in the normal population, and the prevalence of this disorder is quite high in predialysis and ESRD patients. This condition may be caused by mutations or by deficiencies of enzymes or cofactors that are involved in metabolism of methionine.[150] Serum homocysteine levels can be reduced with supplementation of cofactors involved in its metabolism (folate, vitamin B_{12} and B_6).[150] Several

TABLE 45–6. Recommendated Daily Allowance of Vitamins in ESRD Patients

Vitamin	Recommended Amounts
A	0
E	0
K	0
D	Individualized
B_1	1.5 mg
B_2	1.7 mg
B_6	10 mg
B_{12}	6 μg
Biotin	300 μg
Pantothenic acid	10 mg
Niacinamide	20 mg
Folic acid	>1 mg; 10–15 mg*
C	60 mg

*Administration of doses in this range decreases serum homocysteine levels, a known risk factor for cardiovascular disease.

clinical trials are in progress to evaluate the effects of high doses of these vitamins or other cofactors on homocysteine levels in patients with renal disease. These trials may help to determine whether our current recommendations for folate and vitamin B supplementation in patients with renal disease are adequate.

The goal for vitamin supplementation in this population should be to prevent subclinical and frank deficiency and to avoid pathology from overdosage. Table 45–6 outlines recommended allowances for ESRD patients.[96,149] Special vitamin supplements have been formulated for the dialysis patient, but these preparations are fairly costly. Lower-cost vitamin B with C formulations are available, although additional folic acid supplementation is then necessary.

▶ PRINCIPLES OF PHARMACOTHERAPY

- Metabolic acidosis must be prevented or treated in renal insufficiency by the use of sodium bicarbonate tablets or sodium citrate-containing solutions to prevent bone demineralization, cardiac abnormalities, and growth retardation in children.
- Optimal phosphorus control using dietary phosphate restriction and phosphate binders in renal insufficiency is the primary method to reduce or halt vascular calcification, cardiovascular disease, and the development of secondary hyperparathyroidism. Sevelamer hydrochloride should be added or substituted for calcium-containing phosphate binders in those patients who experience high serum calcium or calcium-phosphorus products.
- Both pulse dose oral and intravenous calcitriol are effective in suppressing PTH release; new vitamin D analogs (doxercalciferol and paricalcitol) are also effective.
- Assessment of iron balance and appropriate repletion prior to epoetin therapy and maintenance of iron balance (ferritin >100 ng/mL and transferrin saturation >20%) during epoetin therapy are essential to maximize erythropoietic response.
- Use of replacement and maintenance IV iron dextran, ferric gluconate, or iron sucrose in those patients who cannot tolerate or do not respond adequately to oral iron alone should optimize patient response to epoetin and reduce the total cost associated with anemia therapy. However, IV iron therapy should be discontinued when ferritin levels rise above 800 ng/mL.

- Blood pressure control should be attained prior to starting epoetin. Antihypertensive agents should be added as necessary to maintain a stable blood pressure.
- Epoetin or NESP should be administered subcutaneously whenever possible. Epoetin doses up to 300 mg/kg/wk can be used in pediatric patients younger than 5 years old. For older children and adult dosage, the initial dosage may range from 80–120 U/kg/wk.
- Following initiation of epoetin or NESP, or after any dose change, steady-state Hct levels will not be attained until one red blood cell life span has occurred (approximately 2 months). Therefore, epoetin or NESP doses should not be adjusted more often than every 3 to 4 weeks.
- The goal Hct for ESRD patients is 33% to 36%. Hct levels should be drawn prior to hemodialysis, or anytime in peritoneal dialysis patients. For consistency, Hct levels should be drawn on the same day each week.
- If the rate of rise in Hct is less than optimal (i.e., less than 4 points in 1 month), or Hct decreases by >3 points during stable epoetin therapy causes for epoetin resistance should be investigated. If no obvious reasons exist, then the dosage can be increased by approximately 25%.
- Hyperlipidemia and hypertension should be aggressively managed in patients with ESRD to reduce cardiovascular morbidity and mortality.

REFERENCES

1. Hsu CY, Chertow GM. Chronic renal confusion: Insufficiency, failure, dysfunction, or disease. Am J Kidney Dis 2000;36(2):415–418.
2. Llach F. Secondary hyperparathyroidism in renal failure: The trade-off hypothesis revisited. Am J Kidney Dis 1995;25(5):663–679.
3. U.S. Renal Data System. USRDS 2000 Annual Data Report. Bethesda, MD, National Institutes of Health, National Institute of Diabetes and Digestive and Kidney Diseases, 2000.
4. Jones CA, McQuillan GM, Kusek JW, et al. Serum creatinine levels in the US population: Third National Health and Nutrition Examination Survey. Am J Kidney Dis 1998;32(6):992–999.
5. Healthy People 2010: Understanding and improving health. Pittsburgh, PA, U.S. Government Printing Office, Superintendent of Documents, 2000:1.
6. Ringoir S. An update on uremic toxins. Kidney Int Suppl 1997;62:S2–S4.

7a. Lim VS. Thyroid function in patients with chronic renal failure. Am J Kidney Dis 2001;38:S80–S84.

7b. Massry SG. Metabolic dysfunction in uremia. Am J Kidney Dis 2001;38:S58–S62.

7c. Bellinghieri G, Santoro D, Lo Forti B, Mallamace A, De Santo RM, Savica, V. Erectile dysfunction in uremic dialysis patients: Diagnostic evaluation in the sildenafil era. Am J Kidney Dis 2001;38:S115–S117.

7d. Savica V, Musolino R, Di Leo R, Santoro D, Vita G, Bellinghieri G. Autonomic dysfunction in uremia. Am J Kidney Dis 2001;38:S118–S121.

8. Cohen G, Haag-Weber M, Hörl WH. Immune dysfunction in uremia. Kidney Int Suppl 1997;62:S79 S82.
9. Anonymous. Clinical practice guidelines for nutrition in chronic renal failure. K/DOQI, National Kidney Foundation. Am J Kidney Dis 2000; 35(6 suppl 2):S1–S140.
10. Anonymous. NKF-DOQI clinical practice guidelines for vascular access. National Kidney Foundation-Dialysis Outcomes Quality Initiative. Am J Kidney Dis 1997;30(4 suppl 3):S150–S191.
11. Hannah R, Levin NW, London R, Osheroff WJ. Renal disease in the managed care setting: Selection and monitoring of outcome criteria. Am J Kidney Dis 1999;33(4 suppl 1):S1–S24.
12. Shemin D, Dworkin LD. Sodium balance in renal failure. Curr Opin Nephrol Hypertens 1997;6:128–32.
13. Allon M, Shanklin N. Effect of albuterol treatment on subsequent dialytic potassium removal. Am J Kidney Dis 1995;26(4):607–613.
14. Hatch M, Freel RW, Vaziri ND. Local upregulation of colonic angiotensin II receptors enhances potassium excretion in chronic renal failure. Am J Physiol 1998;274(2 pt 2):F275–F282.
15. Salem MM, Rosa RM, Batlle DC. Extrarenal potassium tolerance in chronic renal failure: Implications for the treatment of acute hyperkalemia. Am J Kidney Dis 1991;18:421–440.
16. Gruy-Kapral C, Emmett M, Santa AC, Porter JL, Fordtran JS, Fine KD. Effect of single dose resin-cathartic therapy on serum potassium concentration in patients with end-stage renal disease. J Am Soc Nephrol 1998;9(10):1924–1930.
17. Solomon R, Dubey A. Diltiazem enhances potassium disposal in subjects with end-stage renal disease. Am J Kidney Dis 1992;19:420–426.
18. Allon M, Shanklin N. Effects of bicarbonate administration on plasma potassium in dialysis patients: Interactions with insulin and albuterol. Am J Kidney Dis 1996;28(4):508–514.
19. Giovannetti S, Cupisti A, Barsotti G. The metabolic acidosis of chronic renal failure: Pathophysiology and treatment. Contrib Nephrol 1992;100: 48–57.
20. Kraut JA. The role of metabolic acidosis in the pathogenesis of renal osteodystrophy. Adv Ren Replace Ther 1995;2(1):40–51.
21. Sharma AM. Renal tubular dysfunction and acidosis. Nephrol Dial Transplant 1995;10:1544–1545.
22. Zelikovic I. Renal tubular acidosis. Pediatr Ann 1995;24(1):48–54.
23. Rix M, Andreassen H, Eskildsen P, Langdahl B, Olgaard K. Bone mineral density and biochemical markers of bone turnover in patients with predialysis chronic renal failure. Kidney Int 1999;56(3):1084–1093.
24. Kurokawa K, Fukagawa M. Uremic bone disease: Advances over the last 30 years. J Nephrol 1999;12(suppl 2):S63–S67.
25. Salem MM. Hyperparathyroidism in the hemodialysis population: A survey of 612 patients. Am J Kidney Dis 1997;29(6):862–865.
26. Block GA, Hulbert-Shearon TE, Levin NW, Port FK. Association of serum phosphorus and calcium × phosphate product with mortality risk in chronic hemodialysis patients: A national study. Am J Kidney Dis 1998;31(4):607–617.
27. Narang R, Ridout D, Nonis C, Kooner JS. Serum calcium, phosphorus and albumin levels in relation to the angiographic severity of coronary artery disease. Int J Cardiol 1997;27;60(1):73–79.
28. Ribeiro S, Ramos A, Brandao A, et al. Cardiac valve calcification in haemodialysis patients: Role of calcium-phosphate metabolism. Nephrol Dial Transplant 1998;13(8):2037–2040.
29. Slatopolsky E, Brown A, Dusso A. Pathogenesis of secondary hyperparathyroidism. Kidney Int Suppl 1999;73:S14–S19.
30. Almaden Y, Hernandez A, Torregrosa V, et al. High phosphate level directly stimulates parathyroid hormone secretion and synthesis by human parathyroid tissue in vitro. J Am Soc Nephrol 1998;9(10):1845–1852.
31. Slatopolsky E, Dusso A, Brown AJ. The role of phosphorus in the development of secondary hyperparathyroidism and parathyroid cell proliferation in chronic renal failure. Am Med Sci 1999;317(6): 370–376.
32. Block GA, Port FK. Re-evaluation of risks associated with hyperphosphatemia and hyperparathyroidism in dialysis patients: Recommendations for a change in management. Am J Kidney Dis 2000;35(6): 1226–1237.
33. Goodman WG, Goldin J, Kuizon BD, et al. Coronary artery calcification in young adults with end-stage renal disease who are undergoing dialysis. N Engl J Med 2000;342(20):1478–1483.
34. Bro S, Olgaard K. Effects of excess PTH on nonclassical target organs. Am J Kidney Dis 1997;30(5):606–620.
35. Malluche HH, Monier-Faugere M-C. Uremic bone disease: Current knowledge, controversial issues and new horizons. Miner Electrolyte Metab 1991;17:281–296.
36. Kates DM, Sherrard DJ, Andress DL. Evidence that serum phosphate is independently associated with serum PTH in patients with chronic renal failure. Am J Kidney Dis 1997;30(6):809–813.

37. Coen G, Mazzaferro S. Bone metabolism and its assessment in renal failure. Nephron 1994;67:383–401.
38. John MR, Goodman WG, Gao P, Cantor TL, Salusky IB, Juppner H. A novel immunoradiometric assay detects full-length human PTH but not amino-terminally truncated fragments: Implications for PTH measurements in renal failure. J Clin Endocrinol Metab 1999;84(11):4287–4290.
39. Solal M-EC, Sebert J-L, Boudailliez B, et al. Comparison of intact, midregion, and carboxy terminal assays of parathyroid hormone for the diagnosis of bone disease in hemodialyzed patients. J Clin Endocrinol Metab 1991;73:516–524.
40. Brookhyser J, Pahre SN. Dietary and pharmacotherapeutic considerations in the management of renal osteodystrophy. Adv Ren Replace Ther 1995;2(1):5–13.
41. Fournier A, Morinière P, Hamida FB, et al. Use of alkaline calcium salts as phosphate binder in uremic patients. Kidney Int Suppl 1992;38:S50–S61.
42. Slatopolsky E, Weerts C, Norwood K, et al. Long-term effects of calcium carbonate and 2.5 mEq/liter calcium dialysate on mineral metabolism. Kidney Int 1989;36:897–903.
43. Cleary DJ, Matzke GR, Alexander AM, Joy MS. Medication knowledge and compliance among patients receiving long-term dialysis. Am J Health Syst Pharm 1995;52(17):1895–900.
44. Fournier A, Drüeke T, Morinière P, Zingraff J, Boudailliez B, Archard JM. The new treatments of hyperparathyroidism secondary to renal insufficiency. Adv Nephrol Necker Hosp 1992;21:237–306.
45. Stamatakis MK, Alderman JM, Meyer-Stout PJ. Influence of pH on in vitro disintegration of phosphate binders. Am J Kidney Dis 1998;32(5):808–12.
46. Janssen MJA, van der Kuy A, ter Wee PM, van Boven W-PL. Aluminum hydroxide, calcium carbonate and calcium acetate in chronic intermittent hemodialysis patients. Clin Nephrol 1996;45(2):111–119.
47. Tan CC, Harden PN, Rodger RSC, et al. Ranitidine reduces phosphate binding in dialysis patients receiving calcium carbonate. Nephrol Dial Transplant 1996;11:851–853.
48. Schaefer K, Scheer J, Asmus G, Umlauf E, Hagemann J, von Herrath D. The treatment of uraemic hyperphosphataemia with calcium acetate and calcium carbonate: A comparative study. Nephrol Dial Transplant 1991;6:170–175.
49. Morinière P, Djerad M, Boudailliez B, et al. Control of predialytic hyperphosphatemia by oral calcium acetate and calcium carbonate. Nephron 1992;60:6–11.
50. Pflanz S, Henderson IS, McElduff N, Jones MC. Calcium acetate versus calcium carbonate as phosphate-binding agents in chronic haemodialysis. Nephrol Dial Transplant 1994;9:1121–1124.
51. Nolan CR, Califano JR, Butzin CA. Influence of calcium acetate or calcium citrate on intestinal aluminum absorption. Kidney Int 1990;38:937–941.
52. Delmez JA, Kelber J, Norword KY, Giles KS, Slatopolsky E. Magnesium carbonate as a phosphorus binder: A prospective, controlled, crossover study. Kidney Int 1996;49(1):163–167.
53. Chertow GM, Burke SK, Dillon MA, Slatopolsky E. Long-term effects of sevelamer hydrochloride on the calcium × phosphate product and lipid profile of haemodialysis patients. Nephrol Dial Transplant 1999;14(12):2907–2914.
54. Bleyer AJ, Burke SK, Dillon M, et al. A comparison of the calcium-free phosphate binder sevelamer hydrochloride with calcium acetate in the treatment of hyperphosphatemia in hemodialysis patients. Am J Kidney Dis 1999;33(4):694–701.
55. Fernandez E, Llach F. Guidelines for dosing of intravenous calcitriol in dialysis patients with hyperparathyroidism. Nephrol Dial Transplant 1996;11(suppl 3):96–101.
56. Daisley-Kydd RE, Mason NA. Calcitriol in the management of secondary hyperparathyroidism of renal failure. Pharmacotherapy 1996;16(4):619–630.
57. Huraib S, Abu-Aisha H, Abed J, Al Wakeel J, Al Desouki M, Memon N. Long-term effect of intravenous calcitriol on the treatment of severe hyperparathyroidism, parathyroid gland mass and bone mineral density in haemodialysis patients. Am J Nephrol 1997;17:118–123.
58. Slatopolsky E, Delmez J. Pathogenesis of secondary hyperparathyroidism. Miner Electrolyte Metab 1995;21:91–96.
59. Malberti F, Surian M, Cosci P. Effect of chronic intravenous calcitriol on parathyroid function and set point of calcium in dialysis patients with refractory secondary hyperparathyroidism. Nephrol Dial Transplant 1992;7:822–828.
60. Quarles LD, Indridason OS. Calcitriol administration in end-stage renal disease: Intravenous or oral? Pediatr Nephrol 1996;10:331–336.
61. Fukagawa M, Kitaoka M, Kurokawa K. Resistance of the parathyroid glands to vitamin D in renal failure: Implications for medical management. Kidney Int Suppl 1997;62:S60–S64.
62. Levine BS, Song M. Pharmacokinetics and efficacy of pulse oral versus intravenous calcitriol in hemodialysis patients. J Am Soc Nephrol 1996;7:488–496.
63. Slatopolsky E, Dusso A, Brown A. New analogs of vitamin D_3. Kidney Int Suppl 1999;73:S46–S51.
64. Martin KJ, Gonzalez EA, Gellens M, Hamm LL, Abboud H, Lindberg J. 19-nor-1-a-25-dihydroxyvitamin D_2 (paricalcitol) safely and effectively reduces the levels of intact parathyroid hormone in patients on hemodialysis. J Am Soc Nephrol 1998;9:1427–1432.
65. Paricalcitol New Drug Application (NDA No. 20–819). Medical Review, 2000.
66. Goodman WG, Frazao JM, Goodkin DA, Turner SA, Liu W, Coburn JW. A calcimimetic agent lowers plasma parathyroid hormone levels in patients with secondary hyperparathyroidism. Kidney Int 2000;58(1):436–445.
67. Stracke S, Jehle PM, Sturm D, et al. Clinical course after total parathyroidectomy without autotransplantation in patients with end-stage renal failure. Am J Kidney Dis 1999;33(2):304–311.
68. Consensus Conference. Diagnosis and treatment of aluminium overload in end-stage renal failure patients. Nephrol Dial Transplant 1993;8(suppl 1):1–54.
69. Lin J-L, Leu M-L. Aluminum-containing agents may be toxic in predialysis chronic renal insufficiency patients. J Intern Med 1996;240:243–248.
70. Cannata Andía JB. Aluminum toxicity: Its relationship with bone and iron metabolism. Nephrol Dial Transplant 1996;11(suppl 3):69–73.
71. Ellenberg R, King AL, Sica DA, Posner M, Savory J. Cerebrospinal fluid aluminium levels following deferoxamine. Am J Kidney Dis 1990;16:157–159.
72. Alfrey AC. Aluminum toxicity in patients with chronic renal failure. Ther Drug Monit 1993;15:593–597.
73. Mazzaferro S, Coen G, Ballanti P, et al. Deferoxamine test and PTH serum levels are useful not to recognize but to exclude aluminum-related bone disease. Nephron 1992;61:151–157.
74. Day JP, Ackrill P. The chemistry of desferrioxamine chelation for aluminum overload in renal dialysis patients. Ther Drug Monit 1993;15:598–601.
75. Anthone S, Ambrus CM, Kohli R, et al. Treatment of aluminum overload using a cartridge with immobilized desferrioxamine. J Am Soc Nephrol 1995;6:1271–1277.
76. Bentur Y, McGuigan M, Koren G. Deferoxamine (desferrioxamine) new toxicities for an old drug. Drug Saf 1991;6:37–46.
77. Boelaert JR, de Locht M. Side-effects of desferrioxamine in dialysis patients. Nephrol Dial Transplant 1993;8(suppl 1):43–46.
78. McCarthy JT, Milliner DS, Johnson WJ. Clinical experience with desferrioxamine in dialysis patients with aluminum toxicity. Q J Med 1990;74:257–276.
79. Andriani M, Nordio M, Saporitti E. Estimation of statistical moments for desferrioxamine and its iron and aluminum chelates: Contribution to optimisation of therapy in uremic patients. Nephron 1996;72:218–224.
80. Barata JD, D'Haese PC, Pires C, Lamberts LV, Simoes J, De Broe ME. Low-dose (5 mg/kg) desferrioxamine treatment in acutely aluminum-intoxicated haemodialysis patients using two drug administration schedules. Nephrol Dial Transplant 1996;11:125–132.

81. NKF-DOQI Work Group. NKF-DOQI clinical practice guidelines for the treatment of anemia of chronic renal failure. Am J Kidney Dis 1997;30(supp 3)(4):S192–S237.

82. Fisher JW. Erythropoietin: Physiologic and pharmacologic aspects. Proc Soc Exp Biol Med 1997;216(3):358–369.

83. Fishbane S. Hyper-responsiveness to recombinant human erythropoietin in dialysis patients. Dial Transplant 2000;29(9):545, 548, and 581.

84. Gunnell J, Yeun JY, Depner TA, Kaysen GA. Acute-phase response predicts erythropoietin resistance in hemodialysis and peritoneal dialysis patients. Am J Kidney Dis 1999;33(1):63–72.

85. NKF K/DOQI clinical practice guidelines for anemia of chronic kidney disease. Am J Kidney Dis 2001;37(Suppl 1): S182–S238.

86. Levin A, Thompson CR, Ethier J, et al. Left ventricular mass index increase in early renal disease: Impact of decline in hemoglobin. Am J Kidney Dis 1999;34(1):125–134.

87. St. Peter WL, Frazier E, Collins A, et al. Percentage of pre-dialysis and pre-transplant patients receiving erythropoietin and associated hematocrit values. J Am Soc Nephrol 2000;11:167A. Abstract.

88. Besarab A, Bolton WK, Browne JK, et al. The effects of normal as compared with low hematocrit values in patients with cardiac disease who are receiving hemodialysis and epoetin. N Engl J Med 1998;339(9): 584–590.

89. Collins AJ, Ma JZ, Xia A, Ebben J. Trends in anemia treatment with erythropoietin usage and patient outcomes. Am J Kidney Dis 1998;32 (6 suppl 4):S133–S141.

90. Ma JZ, Ebben J, Xia H, Collins AJ. Hematocrit level and associated mortality in hemodialysis patients. J Am Soc Nephrol 1999;10(3): 610–619.

91. Xia H, Ebben J, Ma JZ, Collins AJ. Hematocrit levels and hospitalization risks in hemodialysis patients. J Am Soc Nephrol 1999;10(6): 1309–1316.

92. Johnson CA. Use of androgens in patients with renal failure. Semin Dial 2000;13(1):36–39.

93. Horl WH. Is there a role for adjuvant therapy in patients being treated with epoetin? Nephrol Dial Transplant 1999;14(suppl 2):50–60.

93a. Teruel JL, Aguilera A, Marcen R. et al. Androgen therapy for anaemia of chronic renal failure: Indications in the erythropoietin era. Scand J Urol Nephrol 1996;30:403–408.

93b. Gaughan WJ, Liss KA, Dunn SR, et al. A 6-month study of low-dose recombinant human erythropoietin alone and in combination with androgens for the treatment of anemia in chronic hemodialysis patients. Am J Kidney Dis 1997;30:495–500.

94. Schaefer RM, Bahner U. Iron metabolism in rhEPO-treated hemodialysis patients. Clin Nephrol 2000;53(1 suppl):S65–S68.

95. Mittman N, Sreedhara R, Mushnick R, et al. Reticulocyte hemoglobin content predicts functional iron deficiency in hemodialysis patients receiving rHuEPO. Am J Kidney Dis 1997;30(6):912–922.

96. Makoff R. Vitamin replacement therapy in renal failure patients. Miner Electrolyte Metab 1999;25(4–6):349–51.

97. Bailie GR, Johnson CA, Mason NA. Parenteral iron use in the management of anemia in end-stage renal disease patients. Am J Kidney Dis 2000;35(1):1–12.

98. Auerbach M, Winchester J, Wahab A, et al. A randomized trial of three iron dextran infusion methods for anemia in EPO-treated dialysis patients. Am J Kidney Dis 1998;31(1):81–86.

99. Besarab A, Kaiser JW, Frinak S. A study of parenteral iron regimens in hemodialysis patients. Am J Kidney Dis 1999;34(1):21–28.

100. Rault R, Nespor S, Holley J. Safety and efficacy of 500 mg of iron-dextran as a single IV infusion in patients on chronic dialysis. ASAIO J 1994;23:74. Abstract.

101. Nissenson AR, Lindsay RM, Swan S, Seligman P, Strobos J. Sodium ferric gluconate complex in sucrose is safe and effective in hemodialysis patients: North American Clinical Trial. Am J Kidney Dis 1999;33(3): 471–482.

102. Eschbach JW, Strobos J. Sodium ferric gluconate complex (Ferrlecit): Prospective experience in 1122 hemodialysis patients. J Am Soc Nephrol 2000,11:249A. Abstract.

103. Charytan C, Levin N, Al-Saloum M, Hafeez T, Gagnon S, Van Wyck DB. Efficacy and safety of iron sucrose for iron deficiency in patients with dialysis-associated anemia: North American clinical trial. Am J Kidney Dis 2001;37:300–307.

104. Besarab A, Frinak S, Yee J. An indistinct balance: The safety and efficacy of parenteral iron therapy. J Am Soc Nephrol 1999;10(9):2029–2043.

105. Feldman HI, Santana J, Franklin E, et al. Iron administration and survival in chronic hemodialysis patients. J Am Soc Nephrol 0 AD/9;11:230A. Abstract.

106. Locatelli F, Bommer J, London GM, et al. Cardiovascular disease determinants in chronic renal failure: Clinical approach and treatment. Nephrol Dial Transplant 2001;16:459–468.

107. Uehlinger DE, Gotch FA, Sheiner LB. A pharmacodynamic model of erythropoietin therapy for uremic anemia. Clin Pharmacol Ther 1992;51:76–89.

108. Kaufman JS, Reda DJ, Fye CL, et al. Subcutaneous compared with intravenous epoetin in patients receiving hemodialysis. Department of Veterans Affairs Cooperative Study Group on Erythropoietin in Hemodialysis Patients. N Engl J Med 1998;339(9):578–583.

109. St. Peter WL, Lewis MJ, Macres MG. Pain comparison after subcutaneous administration of single-dose formulation versus multidose formulation of Epogen in hemodialysis patients. Am J Kidney Dis 1998;32(3).470–474.

110. Egrie C, Browne JK. Development and characterization of novel erythropoiesis stimulating protein (NESP). Nephrol Dial Transplant 2001;16(Suppl 3):3–13.

110a. Macdougall IC. An overview of the efficacy and safety of novel erythropoiesis stimulating protein (NESP). Nephrol Dial Transplant 2001;16(Suppl 3):14–21.

111a. www.aranesp.com

111b. The NESP usage guidelines group: Alijama P, Bommer J, Canaud B, Carrera F, Eckardt KU, Hörl WH, Krediet RT, Locatelli F, Macdougall IC, Wikström B. Practice guidelines for the use of NESP in treating renal anaemia. Nephrol Dial Transplant 2001;16(Suppl 3):22–28.

112. Lang SM, Schiffl H. Losartan and anaemia of end-stage renal disease. Lancet 1998;352(9141):1708. Letter.

113. Abu-Alfa AK, Cruz D, Perazella MA, Mahnensmith RL, Simon D, Bia MJ. ACE inhibitors do not induce recombinant human erythropoietin resistance in hemodialysis patients. Am J Kidney Dis 2000;35(6): 1076–1082.

114. St. Peter WL, Roberts T, Ma JZ, et al. Rate of rise in US hematocrit levels and erythropoietin doses may be stabilizing. J Am Soc Nephrol 2000;11:300A. Abstract.

115. Health Care Financing Administration. 1999 Annual Report, End Stage Renal Disease Clinical Performance Measures Project. Baltimore, MD, Health Care Financing Administration, Office of Clinical Standards and Quality, 1999:1.

116. Vaziri ND. Mechanism of erythropoietin-induced hypertension. Am J Kidney Dis 1999;33(5):821–828.

117. Weigert AL, Schafer AI. Uremic bleeding: Pathogenesis and therapy. Am J Med Sci 1998;316(2):94–104.

118. Lohr JW, Schwab SJ. Minimizing hemorrhagic complications in dialysis patients. J Am Soc Nephrol 1991;2:961–975.

119. George JN, Shattil SJ. The clinical importance of acquired abnormalities of platelet function. N Engl J Med 1991;324:27–39.

120. Eberst ME, Berkowitz LR. Hemostasis in renal disease: Pathophysiology and management. Am J Med 1994;96:168–179.

121. McCarthy ML, Stoukides CA. Estrogen therapy of uremic bleeding. Ann Pharmacother 1994;28:60–62.

122. Sloand JA. Long-term therapy for uremic bleeding. Int J Artif Organs 1996;19(8):439–440.

123. Kasiske BL. Hyperlipidemia in patients with chronic renal disease. Am J Kidney Dis 1998;32(5 suppl 3):S142–S156.

124. Expert panel. Executive summary of the third report of the National Cholesterol Education Program (NCEP) expert panel on detection evaluation and treatment of high blood cholesterol in adults (Adult Treatment Panel III). JAMA 2001;285(19):2486–2497.

125. AAKP Carnitine Renal Dialysis Consensus Group. Role of L-carnitine in treating renal dialysis patients. Dial Transplant 1994;23:177–181.
126. Bosch T, Samtleben W, Thiery J, et al. Reverse flux filtration: A new mode of therapy improving the efficacy of heparin-induced extracorporeal LDL precipitation in hyperlipidemic hemodialysis patients. Int J Artif Organs 1993;16:75–85.
127. Mailloux LU, Haley WE. Hypertension in the ESRD patient: Pathophysiology, therapy, outcomes, and future directions. Am J Kidney Dis 1998;32(5):705–719.
128. Grekas D, Bamichas G, Bacharaki D, Goutzaridis N, Kasimatis E, Tourkantonis A. Hypertension in chronic hemodialysis patients: Current view on pathophysiology and treatment. Clin Nephrol 2000;53(3):164–168.
129. National High Blood Pressure Education Program Working Group. 1995 update of the working group reports on chronic renal failure and renovascular hypertension. Arch Intern Med 1996;156:1938–1947.
130. Rosansky SJ. Treatment of hypertension in renal failure patients: When do we overtreat? When do we undertreat? Blood Purif 1996;14:315–320.
131. Campese VM, Chervu I. Hypertension in dialysis subjects. In: Henrich WL, eds. Principles and Practice of Dialysis. Baltimore, MD, Williams and Wilkins, 1994:148–169.
132. Charra B, Calemard E, Ruffet M, et al. Survival as an index of adequacy of dialysis. Kidney Int 1992;41:1286–1291.
133. Charra B, Bergstrom J, Scribner BH. Blood pressure control in dialysis patients: Importance of the lag phenomenon. Am J Kidney Dis 1998;32(5):720–724.
134. Sica DA, Gehr TWB. The pharmacokinetics of angiotensin-converting enzyme inhibitors in end-stage renal disease. Semin Dialysis 1994;7:205–213.
135. Song JC, White CM. Pharmacologic, pharmacokinetic, and therapeutic differences among angiotensin II receptor antagonists. Pharmacotherapy 2000;20(2):130–139.
136. London GM, Marchais SJ, Guerin AP, et al. Salt and water retention and calcium blockade in uremia. Circulation 1990;82:105–113.
137. Kanegae K, Hiroshige K, Suda T, et al. Pharmacokinetics of bisoprolol and its effect on dialysis refractory hypertension. Int J Artif Organs 1999;22(12):798–804.
138. Agarwal R. Supervised atenolol therapy in the management of hemodialysis hypertension. Kidney Int 1999;55(4):1528–1535.
139. Rosansky SJ, Johnson KL, McConnell J. Use of transdermal clonidine in chronic hemodialysis patients. Clin Nephrol 1993;39:32–36.
140. Harter HR, Delmez JA. Effects of prazosin in the control of blood pressure in hypertensive dialysis patients. J Cardiovasc Pharmacol 1979;1(suppl):S43–S55.
141. The Joint National Committee. The Sixth Report of the Joint National Committee on Prevention, Detection, Evaluation, and Treatment of High Blood Pressure. Arch Intern Med 1997;157(21);2413–2446.
142. Townsend RR, Ford V. Ambulatory blood pressure monitoring: Coming of age in nephrology. J Am Soc Nephrol 1996;7:2279–2287.
143. Cannella G, Paoletti E, Delfino R, Peloso G, Molinari S, Traverso GB. Regression of left ventricular hypertrophy in hypertensive dialyzed uremic patients on long-term antihypertensive therapy. Kidney Int 1993;44:881–886.
144. Robertson KE, Mueller BA. Uremic pruritus. Am J Health Syst Pharm 1998;53:2159–2170.
145. Stahle-Bäckdahl M. Pruritus in hemodialysis patients. Skin Pharmacol 1992;5:14–20.
146. Dimkovic N, Djukanovic L, Radmilovic A, Bojic P, Juloski T. Uremic pruritus and skin mast cells. Nephron 1992;61:5–9.
147. Ashmore SD, Jones CH, Newstead CG, Daly MJ, Chrystyn H. Ondansetron therapy for uremic pruritus in hemodialysis patients. Am J Kidney Dis 2000;35(5):827–831.
148. Makoff R. Water-soluble vitamin status in patients with renal disease treated with hemodialysis or peritoneal dialysis. J Renal Nutrition 1991;1:56–73.
149. Makoff R, Dwyer J, Rocco M. Folic acid, pyridoxine, cobalamin and homocysteine and their relationship to cardiovascular disease in ESRD. J Ren Nutr 1996;6:2–11.
150. Tremblay R, Bonnardeaux A, Geadah D, et al. Hyperhomocystinemia in hemodialysis patients: Effects of 12-month supplementation with hydrosoluble vitamins. Kidney Int 2000;58(2):851–858.

46

RENAL TRANSPLANTATION

Heather J. Johnson and Karen L. Heim-Duthoy

Each year the number of patients diagnosed with end-stage renal disease (ESRD) increases by more than 70,000, totaling 300,000 patients in 1998. The primary therapeutic options for these individuals are hemodialysis, peritoneal dialysis, and/or renal transplantation. The most commonly reported causes of renal failure include diabetes mellitus, hypertension, chronic glomerulonephritis of various etiologies, and polycystic kidney disease.[1] Renal transplantation is the preferred long term therapeutic option for most patients with ESRD because it provides patients with the greatest potential improvement in overall quality of life. Dialysis catheter-related infections, continuous ambulatory peritoneal dialysis (CAPD) associated peritonitis, and scheduled dialysis treatments are avoided, and dietary restrictions are fewer. While the analysis of quality of life is complex, patients generally report improved quality of life following transplantation as compared to patients on maintenance dialysis.[3] However, transplantation is a treatment, rather than a cure, for ESRD. Patients and clinicians are to be reminded that there are several adverse consequences/complications that have been associated with transplantation.

Patient and graft survival rates following renal transplantation have improved significantly over the past 30 years as a result of advances in pharmacotherapy, surgical techniques, organ preservation, and the postoperative management of patients. Although success rates vary among transplant centers, 1-year graft survival rates are about 94% for living-related (LRT), and 89% for cadaveric renal transplantation (CRT). Five-year graft survival rates are about 77% and 63% for LRT and CRT, respectively.

Because of continuous improvements in clinical outcomes, cost effectiveness, and quality of life, renal transplantation is the treatment option that provides patients with renal failure the best chance of survival and return to a normal or near-normal life-style.[4] Patients with medical conditions, such as unstable cardiac disease or recently diagnosed malignancy, for whom the risk of surgery or chronic immunosuppression would be greater than the risks associated with chronic dialysis, are excluded from renal transplantation. The most frequent reason for patient exclusion is unstable cardiac disease or recently diagnosed malignancy. Some transplant centers also exclude patients who are human immunodeficiency virus (HIV) antibody positive and patients with a history of drug abuse or noncompliance with medical regimens.

EPIDEMIOLOGY

In spite of efforts to increase public awareness about organ donation, the waiting list continues to grow and reached almost 50,000 by the end of 1999.[2] In 1996, median waiting time for white recipients exceeded 680 days and was nearly double for nonwhite recipients. In 1999, 12,483 kidney transplants were performed in the United States, a third of which were from living donors. Efforts to expand the donor pool include relaxing the absolute age limitations for organ donation, transplantation of two pediatric kidneys into adult recipients, and the use of living-unrelated donors. Despite these efforts to expand the donor pool, more than 2,300 patients died in the United States waiting for a kidney transplant in 1998.

This chapter discusses the pharmacotherapy required for the management of patients following renal transplantation, including immunosuppressive, anti-infective, and other treatments.

PHYSIOLOGIC CONSEQUENCES OF RENAL TRANSPLANTATION

The glomerular filtration rate (GFR) of a successfully transplanted kidney may be near normal almost immediately after transplantation. In some patients, however, the concentration of standard biochemical indicators of renal function, such as serum creatinine and blood urea nitrogen (BUN), may remain elevated for several days. Standard formulae used to predict drug dosing rely on stable serum creatinine and may be inaccurate immediately following transplantation.

Although the allograft is able to remove uremic toxins from the body, it may take several weeks for other physiologic complications of chronic renal failure, such as anemia, calcium and phosphate imbalance, and altered lipid profiles, to resolve. The renal production of erythropoietin and 1-hydroxylation of vitamin D may return toward normal early in the postoperative period. Because the onset of physiologic effects may be delayed, continuation of pretransplant calcitriol, calcium supplementation, and/or phosphate binders may be warranted in some patients.

PATHOPHYSIOLOGY

FACTORS AFFECTING THE SUCCESS OF RENAL TRANSPLANTATION

The success of renal transplantation can be measured in terms of length of graft and patient survival, the half-life of transplanted kidneys, or quality of life. The factors that influence the success of renal transplantation include HLA- and DR-antigen matching between donor and recipient, donor age and serum creatinine, donor cardiac instability, and prolonged cold ischemia time. The estimated half-lives for kidneys are 26.9 years for HLA-identical grafts and 12.2 and 10.8 years, respectively, for grafts from a sibling or parent who are 1-haplotype matches. The estimated half-life for HLA-matched grafts was 17.3 years and 7.8 years for mismatched kidneys.[5] Recipient factors associated with diminished success of transplantation include age < 15 or > 50 years, retransplantation, black race, and the presence of preformed anti-HLA antibodies. Size mismatching between donor and recipient has also been implicated. Multiparous women are also at increased risk for immunologic graft loss. These factors contribute to the major determinants of graft survival: rejection and delayed graft function (Table 46–1).

TABLE 46–1. Impact of Delayed Graft Function (DGF) and Acute Rejection (AR) on Length of Stay and Renal Allograft Survival

	I −DGF/−AR	II +DGF	III +AR	IV +DGF/+AR
Median length of stay (days)[1]	10	17	15	21
1-year graft survival (%)[2]	88	74	72	56
5-year graft survival (%)[3]	66	53	48	35

[1] ANOVA $P = 0.05$.
[2] I vs II, $P < 0.001$; I vs III, $P < 0.001$; IV vs I, II, and III, $P < 0.01$.
[3] I vs II and III, $P < 0.001$; IV vs II and III, $P < 0.001$.
Data from Ref. 6.

DELAYED GRAFT FUNCTION

Primary nonfunction of a renal allograft or delayed graft function (DGF) may result in postoperative anuria. The primary cause is acute tubular necrosis (ATN). The incidence of ATN increases when kidneys are harvested from donors following cardiac arrest, from donors who are hypotensive or on vasopressors, or from older donors. Prolonged periods of warm and cold ischemia, greater than 40 minutes and 48 hours, respectively, increase the risk of ATN. The management of patients with ATN may be difficult because serum creatinine, the major parameter used to monitor for acute rejection, remains elevated. Cyclosporine (CSA) and tacrolimus (TAC) may be implicated in the prolongation of ATN, but a clear cause-and-effect relationship has not been established.

Delayed graft function is defined by the need for dialysis in the postoperative period or the failure of the serum creatinine to fall below 4 mg/dL or by 30% of the pretransplant value. The incidence of DGF in primary cadaveric renal transplantation ranges from 8% to 50% and results in a slower return of the kidney's excretory, metabolic, and synthetic functions. Delayed graft function is associated with prolonged hospital stays, higher costs, difficulty in the management of immunosuppressive therapy, slower patient rehabilitation, and poor graft survival. Urinary complications such as ureteral obstruction, thrombosis, or leak, or vascular complications, including arterial or venous stenosis or thrombosis, may also result in early graft dysfunction.

Persistently elevated serum creatinine and BUN levels confound the perioperative management of renal transplant recipients. Among the differential diagnoses are acute rejection, ATN, and/or CSA or TAC toxicity. These processes are not mutually exclusive. Definitive diagnosis is made by renal biopsy. In the presence of elevated serum creatinine, clinicians may reduce the dose of CSA or TAC to minimize the potential for drug nephrotoxicity and hasten the recovery from ATN. This practice may result in subtherapeutic immunosuppressant concentrations and hasten the occurrence of acute rejection. Delayed graft function is a factor predisposing patients to acute rejection. Induction therapy using the strategy of delayed CSA or TAC administration may be useful in this setting.

GRAFT REJECTION

Allograft rejection depends on the activation of alloreactive T cells and antigen-presenting cells such as B lymphocytes, macrophages, and dendritic cells. Acute allograft rejection is primarily caused by the infiltration of T cells into the allograft, which triggers inflammatory and cytotoxic effects on the graft. Complex interactions between the allograft and cellular cytokines, cell-to-cell interactions, $CD4^+$ and $CD8^+$ T cells, and B cells ultimately lead to chronic rejection and graft loss if adequate immunosuppression is not maintained.[7]

The sequence of events that underlies graft rejection is (a) recognition of the donor's histocompatibility differences by the recipient's immune system; (b) recruitment of activated lymphocytes; (c) initiation of immune effector mechanisms; and (d) destruction of the graft. Rejection of the transplanted tissue can take place at anytime following surgery and is clinically classified as hyperacute rejection, acute cellular rejection, or chronic rejection.

HYPERACUTE REJECTION

Hyperacute rejection may occur when preformed donor-specific antibodies are present in the recipient at the time of the transplant and may be evident within minutes of the transplant procedure. Hyperacute rejection can be induced by immunoglobulin G (IgG) antibodies that bind to antigens on the vascular endothelium, such as class I major histocompatibility complex (MHC), ABO, and vascular endothelial cell antigens. Tissue damage can be mediated through antibody-dependent, cell-mediated cytotoxicity, or through the activation of the complement cascade. The ischemic damage to the microvasculature rapidly produces tissue necrosis.

Hyperacute rejection has become uncommon because transplant donors are matched for ABO blood groups and cross-match testing is done to determine the presence of donor-specific lymphocytotoxic antibodies. A positive cross-match presents a serious risk factor for graft failure even if hyperacute rejection does not occur. A negative lymphocytotoxicity cross-match does not entirely rule out the possibility of hyperacute rejection because non-MHC antigens on the vascular endothelium can serve as targets of donor-specific antibodies.

ACUTE CELLULAR REJECTION

Although the earliest episodes have been observed within days postoperatively, acute cellular rejection may occur at anytime after transplantation. Cellular rejection is mediated by alloreactive T lymphocytes that appear in the circulation and infiltrate the allograft through the vascular endothelium. After the graft is infiltrated by lymphocytes, the cytotoxic cells can specifically kill allograft targets, whereas the local release of lymphokines will attract and stimulate macrophages to produce tissue damage through a delayed hypersensitivity-like mechanism.

Acute rejection is usually evidenced by a prompt rise in serum creatinine. A specific histologic diagnosis can be obtained via biopsy of the allograft and is often used to guide therapy for rejection. A biopsy specimen with a diffuse infiltrate of lymphocytes is consistent with acute cellular rejection. After the diagnosis of rejection has been confirmed, the potential risks and benefits of specific antirejection therapies must be evaluated. Hypertension often worsens during an episode of rejection. Patients may experience edema and weight gain as a result of sodium and fluid retention. Symptomatic azotemia may also develop in severe cases. In addition, patients may experience graft tenderness, fever, and malaise. Appropriate adjustments in pharmacotherapy are warranted in the face of diminished renal function.

CHRONIC REJECTION

The prevention and treatment of chronic rejection is perhaps the most important problem to be addressed in transplantation. Although advances have been made in the management of acute rejection, the half-life of kidney transplantation has remained largely unchanged.

Chronic rejection is the most common cause of graft loss in the late post-transplant period (>1 year). Although acute rejection is a strong predictor of chronic rejection, it is unclear why reduction in the incidence of acute rejection associated with the widespread adoption of CSA and TAC has not had an impact on the incidence of chronic rejection. The current tendency to decrease doses of CSA and TAC in the face of "good" graft function without dynamic measurement of immunologic factors may lead to subclinical rejection. Although chronic rejection may simply be a slow and indolent form of cellular rejection, the involvement of the humoral immune system and antibodies against the vascular endothelium appears to play a role. The pathogenesis of chronic rejection is difficult to dissect because of prolonged exposure to multiple drugs, and because of the presence of other abnormalities that may predispose the patient to similar pathologic changes in organ function.

Chronic rejection can occur early (within 3 to 6 months) or late (>1 year) in the post-transplant course. Hypertension, proteinuria, and a progressive decline in renal function present as a classic triad in chronic rejection. Manifestations of chronic rejection are generally dependent on the degree of renal insufficiency and hypoalbuminemia. Classic symptoms of uremia occur as end-stage renal disease develops. These processes are very difficult to treat because their presentation is slow and indolent and the changes in renal function are usually not reversible.

▶ TREATMENT: Renal Transplantation

IMMUNOSUPPRESSIVE THERAPY

GOALS OF IMMUNOSUPPRESSION

Transplant immunosuppression must be balanced in terms of graft and patient survival (the prevention of rejection versus the risk of adverse effects associated with therapy including life-threatening infection or malignancy). A multidrug approach is rational from the immunomechanistic viewpoint because the agents may have overlapping and potentially synergistic mechanisms. Furthermore, multidrug immunosuppression may allow the use of lower doses of individual agents associated with different side effect profiles to minimize the severity of expected adverse effects.

The goals of immunosuppression vary depending on the time interval since transplantation. Immediately following surgery, the primary goal of therapy is to prevent hyperacute and acute rejection. The high doses of immunosuppressants required to achieve this goal may result in serious complications (e.g., infection, thrombocytopenia, and drug-induced diabetes) if maintained long-term. Rapid tapering may minimize these effects.

Acute graft rejection affects 30% to 40% of patients during the first 1 to 3 months following transplantation. Therefore, the doses of immunosuppressants are usually kept high to prevent rejection during this high-risk period. The doses of immunosuppressants are generally reduced if the patient develops serious adverse effects such as opportunistic infections, nephrotoxicity, or hepatotoxicity. The goal of maintenance immunosuppression is to prevent acute and chronic rejection while minimizing drug-related toxicity. In the long-term management of the transplant patient, the doses of immunosuppressants are gradually reduced (over 6 to 12 months) in an effort to minimize adverse effects. Many institutions may completely withdraw specific immunosuppressives in select patients to reduce long-term toxicity as well as cost. It is important to recognize that while the goals of transplant immunosuppression are universal, protocols for immunosuppressive therapy vary widely among institutions. Table 46–2 details immunosuppressive options for induction, maintenance, and the management of acute rejection.

INDUCTION THERAPY

Induction therapy involves the utilization of a high level of immunosuppression at the time of transplantation with or without the immediate introduction of CSA or TAC. Historically, induction consisted of the use of polyclonal or monoclonal antibodies, azathioprine (AZA), and high-dose corticosteroids at the time of transplantation. CSA administration was delayed until the establishment of graft function. This type of induction strategy is based on the following rationale: (a) the newly transplanted kidney is susceptible to nephrotoxic injury from CSA or TAC; (b) CSA and TAC dosage adjustment to maintain target concentrations is difficult in the perioperative period; and (c) immunologic benefit from initial, more intensive immunosuppression is added with the use of a polyclonal or monoclonal antibody preparation.[8,9] The prophylactic use of antibody preparations (ATG or OKT3) during induction therapy is controversial. OKT3 induction with AZA, steroids, and delayed CSA has been compared to conventional therapy (AZA, steroids, and CSA). OKT3 use is associated with significantly fewer rejection episodes (51% vs 66%) and a longer time to initial rejection (46 days vs 8 days).[10] Furthermore, the prophylactic use of OKT3 has resulted in improved graft survival at 5 years post-transplant (73% with OKT3 vs 64% with conventional therapy).[11] Induction strategies that include antibody therapy are preferred by about 50% of transplant centers. Figure 46-1 illustrates one strategic approach to the use of induction therapy with either ATG or OKT3. Sequential induction strategies with IL-2 receptor antagonists are not clearly defined. Currently available agents are summarized below.

MONOCLONAL ANTIBODIES

Muromonab (OKT3)

OKT3 is a murine monoclonal antibody to the CD3 receptor on mature human T cells. Minutes following the administration of OKT3, $CD3^+$ cells are rapidly removed from the circulation. OKT3 should be given as a rapid IV bolus. Although its rapid intravenous administration is an advantage over ATG infusions, OKT3 administration is associated with significant first-dose adverse reactions. The cytokine-release syndrome related to OKT3, including fever, chills, rigors, pruritus, and alterations in blood pressure, may occur with the first several doses. Methylprednisolone, acetaminophen, diphenhydramine, indomethacin, and pentoxifylline may be used as premedications. Pulmonary edema is associated with OKT3 use in transplant patients who are significantly fluid overloaded; therefore, patients may need to be dialyzed prior to administration. Aseptic meningitis is another potential complication of OKT3 therapy. If encephalitic symptoms develop, OKT3 should be discontinued and appropriate care initiated. Finally, some believed that the potential for development of host antibodies after induction administration might preclude its use as an effective rejection therapy. However, it has been demonstrated that OKT3 can be safely and successfully used as rejection therapy in patients who have undergone previous OKT3 induction.[10,12] Specifically, these studies

TABLE 46–2. Summary of Immunosuppression Options for Induction, Maintenance, and Rejection Therapy

Agent	Induction	Maintenance	Rejection
Monoclonal antibodies			
Basiliximab	20 mg IV day 0, 4	—	—
Daclizumab	1 mg/kg IV q14d × 5	—	—
Muromonab (OKT3)	2.5–5 mg/d IV × 7–14 days		5–10 mg/d IV qd × 7–10 days *Check human antimurine antibodies before second course*
Polyclonal antibodies			
Antithymocyte globulin (equine–ATGAM)	10–30 mg/kg/d IV × 7–14 days	—	15–30 mg/kg IV qd × 7–14 days
Antithymocyte globulin (rabbit-thymoglobulin)	Unapproved; 50 mg up to 2.5 mg/kg/d	—	1.5 mg/kg IV qd × 7–14 days
Corticosteroids			
Prednisone	Perioperative taper: 50 mg qid × 4 doses; 40 mg qid × 4 doses; 30 mg qid × 4 doses; 20 mg qid × 4 doses; 10 mg qid × 4 doses; then 20 mg/d	20–60 mg/d tapering by 2.5–5 mg q 2–4 wk *or* 0.5–0.75 mg/kg/d tapering to 0.15 mg/kg/d @ 6 months	5-day oral "cycle": 100 mg, 80 mg, 60 mg, 40 mg, 20 mg; taper slowly from 20 mg
Methylprednisolone	1000 mg × 1 then Prednisone *or* 1,000 mg × 1; 500 mg × 1; 250 mg × 1; then prednisone *or* 1,000 mg × 1; 50 mg qid × 4 doses; 40 mg qid × 4; 30 mg qid × 4; 20 mg qid × 4; 30 mg bid × 2; 20 mg × 1; then prednisone	—	IV: 500 mg/d × 3 *or* 1,000 mg × 2; 500 mg × 2; 250 mg × 2; then prednisone
Antiproliferative agents			
Azathioprine	3–5 mg/kg po/IV qd	1–3 mg/kg IV/po qd	—
Mycophenolate Mofetil	1–1.5 g po bid	1–1.5 g po bid	Conversion from AZA; doses up to 3.5 g/d
Calcineurin inhibitors			
Cyclosporine	5–6 mg/kg/d IV until GI function resumes *or* 6–20 mg/kg/d po divided bid	5–15 mg/kg/d po divided bid *Initial Neoral doses are usually lower than Sandimmune; adjust doses based on target concentrations.*	
Tacrolimus	0.05–0.1 mg/kg/d IV until GI function resumes	0.1–0.3 mg/kg/d divided bid	Conversion from CSA in refractory rejection
Rapamycin derivatives			
Sirolimus	Loading dose: 6 mg po within 24–48 hours posttransplant	2 mg po qd	

confirm that the presence of low anti-OKT3 antibody titers (≤1:100) does not preclude successful retreatment with OKT3 for rejection.

Induction with the conventional OKT3 dose (5 mg/d for 7 to 14 days) effectively prevents rejection in renal transplant recipients.[10] However, there are also data demonstrating the utility of low-dose (2.5-mg) OKT3 induction therapy.[13,14] Darby et al. administered conventional or reduced doses of OKT3, based on CD3 counts, to renal allograft recipients with plasma reactive antibodies (PRA) >50%.[22] The total OKT3 doses for the conventional and low-dose groups were 64.4 and 38.3 mg, respectively. There were no differences in acute rejection, serum creatinine, and graft and patient survival (1 year) between the conventional and low-dose OKT3 groups.[13] Although adverse events were not directly assessed, they appear to occur less frequently with reduced OKT3 doses.[14] A sequential induction protocol using OKT3 is more cost effective than conventional therapy in renal transplantation.[15] Furthermore, low-dose administration of OKT3 in this setting may additionally enhance cost effectiveness. The exact role of OKT3 in induction therapy needs to be further defined (i.e., high- vs low-risk patients and conventional vs reduced dosing).

IL-2 Receptor Antagonists

Basiliximab and daclizumab exert their immunosuppressive effects by binding to and blocking the α subunit of the IL-2 receptor on the surface of activated T-lymphocytes. They, thereby, inhibit IL-2-mediated activation of lymphocytes, a necessary step for the clonal expansion of T cells. Clinical trials in renal transplant patients using daclizumab or basiliximab versus placebo in combination with CSA-based immunosuppression demonstrated significant reductions

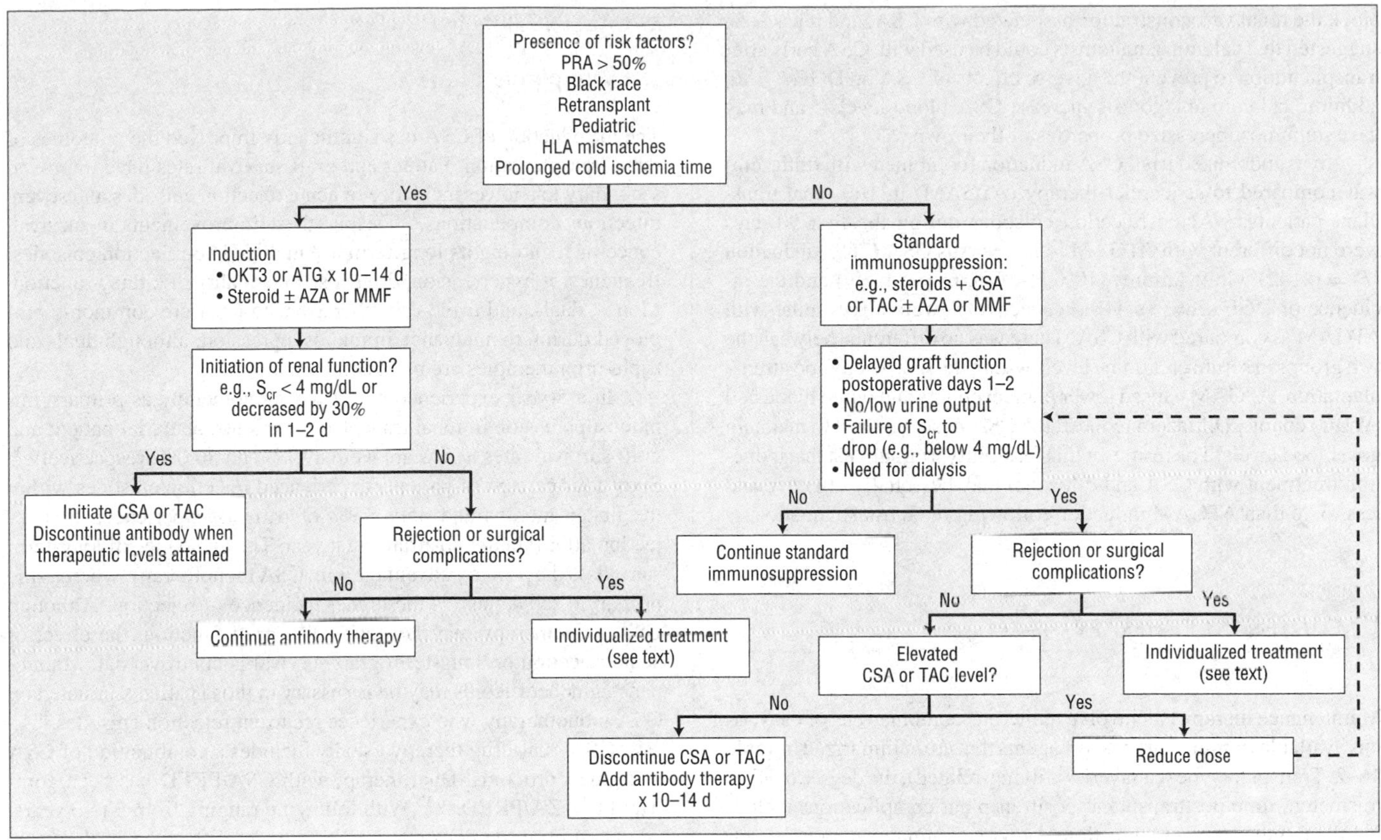

FIGURE 46–1. Decision tree for antibody induction therapy with ATG or OKT3.

in the incidence of biopsy-proven rejection in the first 6 months posttransplantation: daclizumab, 22% versus 35%; basiliximab, 30% versus 44%.[16,17] Trials evaluating the IL-2 receptor antagonists in CSA- or TAC-sparing regimens are ongoing.

Basiliximab (Simulect, Novartis), a chimeric (murine/human) antibody, is given as 2 intravenous infusions for induction therapy: 20 mg over 20 to 30 minutes just prior to transplantation, followed by 20 mg on the fourth postoperative day. Daclizumab (Zenapax, Hoffman-LaRoche) is a humanized antibody given in 5 intravenous doses of 1 mg/kg every 14 days starting from the time of transplantation. Both agents can be administered via a peripheral or central venous catheter.

The side effects reported in the clinical trials of the agents were comparable to those reported in the placebo arms. Importantly, this greater degree of immunosuppression did not seem to confer an increased risk of infection. Although experience is limited, no drug interactions with the IL-2 receptor antagonists have been reported. Few patients have developed anti-idiotype antibodies to basiliximab and daclizumab, but readministration of these agents has not been studied and the risks of anaphylaxis are unknown. Even though these agents have not been associated with the infusion-related adverse effects that are common with other antibody preparations, there are an increasing number of reports of anaphylactic reactions following administration of the second dose of basiliximab.

POLYCLONAL ANTIBODIES

Two polyclonal antithymocyte globulin preparations are in commercial use in the United States: ATGAM (equine) and Thymoglobulin (rabbit). These agents produce complement-mediated lysis of lymphocytes, facilitate lymphocyte removal by the reticuloendothelial system, and alter T-cell function. These agents are associated with dose-limiting thrombocytopenia and leukopenia, and with an increased risk of viral infections and malignancy. ATGAM doses range from 10–30 mg/kg/d for 7 to 14 days for the induction of immunosuppression or the treatment of rejection. Doses must be filtered and administered over 4 to 6 hours via a central venous access.[10] Thymoglobulin is currently approved only for the treatment of rejection. Like ATGAM, Thymoglobulin must be administered slowly (over 4 to 6 hours) through an inline filter. For the treatment of rejection, Thymoglobulin, 1.5 mg/kg/d for 7 to 14 days has been compared to ATGAM 15 mg/kg/d for 7 to 14 days.[18] In this study, Thymoglobulin had a higher rejection reversal rate (88% vs 76%, $P = 0.027$) and was also associated with greater T-cell depletion. Although the authors concluded that Thymoglobulin is superior to ATGAM, these differences might not have been significant if higher doses of ATGAM had been used. Thymoglobulin has also been used as part of sequential induction strategies. Intermittent administration of Thymoglobulin based on $CD3^+$ T-lymphocyte count has been evaluated as a strategy to minimize the adverse effects and costs of Thymoglobulin. Djamali et al. evaluated intermittent (50 mg/d × 3 days followed by Thymoglobulin for $CD3^+$ T-lymphocytes $>10/mm^3$), versus daily administration (50 mg/d) as part of a quadruple immunosuppression induction regimen also containing CSA, AZA, and prednisone (PRED). They demonstrated no differences in graft function, acute rejections, or ATG-related side effects between intermittent and daily therapies. There was a difference, however, of $760/patient in treatment costs.[19]

OTHER INDUCTION STRATEGIES

Use of CSA as an induction agent is controversial. Decreased renal blood flow secondary to CSA constriction of the renal vasculature may exacerbate delayed graft function and negate some of the beneficial effects of starting CSA early after transplantation. Calcium antagonists block the renal vasoconstriction associated with CSA, and it has been suggested that calcium antagonists could be used with CSA early after transplantation to prevent the adverse effects of CSA on DGF.[20–23] In addition, calcium antagonists increase CSA blood levels[24] and may have immunosuppressive properties of their own.[24–26]

In a randomized trial, CSA induction (combined with diltiazem) was compared to sequential therapy (ATGAM) in 100 renal transplant patients.[27] Acute rejection episodes during the first 90 days were not different with ATGAM (42%) versus CSA (28%) induction ($P = 0.142$). Graft failures (10% vs 16%, respectively) and the incidence of DGF (28% vs 34%, respectively) were also similar with ATGAM as compared with CSA. There was no difference between the two groups in serum creatinine levels within the first 90 days posttransplantation. ATGAM caused lower platelet counts and white blood cell (WBC) counts. Diltiazem reduced the CSA dose required to maintain goal blood levels. The results of this feasibility trial suggest that induction treatment with CSA and diltiazem may be equally effective and less toxic than ATGAM induction following renal transplantation.[27]

MAINTENANCE THERAPY

Maintenance therapy can involve numerous combinations of the various available immunosuppressive agents that are summarized in Table 46–2. Transplant type (cadaveric vs living-related), the degree of HLA mismatch, time posttransplant, posttransplant complications including the number of acute rejections, previous immunosuppressive adverse reactions, compliance, and financial considerations are among the patient-specific factors considered in individualizing maintenance immunosuppression. CSA or TAC is generally a central component in most maintenance regimens. Renal transplant patients may receive mono-, dual-, or triple-drug therapy during the maintenance phase. In the early posttransplant period ($\leq$ 6 months), most cadaveric renal transplant recipients are maintained on triple-drug therapy (CSA or TAC, AZA or MMF, and prednisone). In contrast, recipients of living-related grafts may receive only dual-drug therapy, such as AZA or mycophenolate mofetil (MMF) and prednisone. As patients progress through the posttransplant course, the risk of acute rejection decreases; therefore, maintenance immunosuppression is tapered, and, in some cases, certain agents may be discontinued.

GLUCOCORTICOIDS

An intravenous glucocorticoid, commonly high-dose methylprednisolone, is given during the perioperative period. The dose of methylprednisolone is rapidly tapered and discontinued as oral PRED is initiated. Prednisone doses are tapered progressively over time to a baseline dose of 10–15 mg/d by the sixth month posttransplant. At 1-year posttransplant, maintenance doses may be less than 10 mg/d in some patients. In patients receiving TAC, PRED may be tapered even lower and eventually discontinued. As doses are tapered, it is preferable to administer steroids every other day and between 7 and 8 AM to mimic the body's diurnal release of cortisol. Although conversion to alternate-day regimens or complete withdrawal of PRED in patients with stable posttransplant courses has been used with success in some transplant centers, steroids are often continued for the entire life of the functional graft. Long-term steroid use and its associated deleterious effects are well-recognized and particularly troublesome in transplant patients. Table 46–3 summarizes the specific adverse effects of glucocorticoids that are commonly encountered in transplant patients.

CALCINEURIN INHIBITORS

Cyclosporine

The introduction of CSA has significantly improved the outcomes of renal transplantation. Patient and graft survival rates have improved secondary to a lower incidence of acute rejection episodes and severe infectious complications.[28] Despite these improvements in survival, concerns regarding its long-term use include late-rejection episodes, frequency of hypertension, drug cost, and quality of kidney function. Mono-, dual-, and triple-drug therapy with CSA are commonly employed during maintenance immunosuppression, although dual- and triple-drug therapies are most common.

In a 5-year experience with CSA monotherapy as primary immunosuppression in renal transplant recipients, actuarial patient and graft survival rates at 5 years were 89.7% and 80.0%, respectively.[29] Sixty-four percent of patients experienced rejection episodes within the first 6 months and only 3.9% of patients experienced first rejection after the first posttransplant year. The avoidance of long-term steroids is the primary advantage with CSA monotherapy, whereas the primary disadvantage is the higher incidence of rejection. Although CSA monotherapy may not jeopardize graft function, the effect of acute rejection on long-term graft survival is controversial. Maintenance glucocorticoids may be necessary in those patients initiated on CSA monotherapy who experience recurrent rejection episodes.[30]

CSA dual-drug therapy usually includes a combination of CSA and glucocorticoids. Dual therapy with CSA/PRED has been compared to AZA/PRED.[31,32] With follow-up ranging from 3 to 6 years, Ghoneim et al. demonstrated no significant difference in the overall frequency of acute rejection episodes or graft survival between the two living-related transplant groups; however, the number of patients experiencing two or more rejection episodes was greater in the AZA/PRED group.[31] In contrast, Amend et al. observed significant differences in graft survival between CSA/PRED- and AZA/PRED-treated CRT patients. Graft survival for all study periods during the 5-year follow-up was greater for both diabetics (20% to 22%) and nondiabetics (35% to 40%) in the CSA/PRED group.[32] The different outcomes of these two studies could be attributed to the difference in study subjects and the source of the kidney, cadaveric versus living-related, because survival rates are improved following living-related transplants.

CSA triple-drug therapy consists of CSA, glucocorticoids, and AZA. Eventual tapering and/or elimination of glucocorticoids or CSA is attempted in some patients. CSA dual-drug therapy (CSA/PRED and CSA/AZA) has been compared to CSA triple-drug therapy (CSA/AZA/PRED) in CRT patients. Although the CSA/AZA group had more frequent early rejection, no significant differences in 1-year patient or graft survival, morbidity, and mortality were identified.[33] The long-term (4-year follow-up) effects of CSA dual-drug versus CSA triple-drug immunosupp-ression therapy have been evaluated. Both studies reported no differences in graft and patient survival. However, Isoniemi et al. demonstrated other parameters of follow-up including graft function and chronic allograft damage index from renal biopsy to be significantly better in the triple-drug therapy group, whereas Lindholm et al. reported no difference in renal function determined by serum creatinine between groups.[34,35]

The impact of CSA on long-term ($\geq$5 years) renal allograft function has been analyzed. Although patient survival did not differ between treatment groups, Monaco et al. demonstrated a significantly greater 5-year graft survival in CSA-treated patients (triple-drug therapy).[36] Another retrospective study demonstrated no difference in 5-year actual survival in patients who had received either AZA or steroids or CSA mono-, dual-, or triple-drug therapy (88% vs 90%, respectively).[37] The 5-year actual graft survival rate

TABLE 46–3. Adverse Effects of Immunosuppressive Agents

Adverse Effects	AZA	MMF	Steroids	CSA	TAC	SRL	IL2RA	ATG	OKT3	Management
Acne			+	+						Dose reduction; increased hygiene; topical agents (e.g., retinoic acid)
Adrenal suppression			+							Taper doses slowly; administer every other day; patient identification card
Anaphylaxis							+	+		
Cataracts/glaucoma			+							Annual eye examinations
Electrolyte abnormalities				+ (↑K) (↓Mg)	++ (↑K), (↓Mg)	+ (↓K)				Monitor serum electrolytes
Gastrointestinal abnormalities	++ Nausea, vomiting	++ Diarrhea, nausea, abdominal pain	+ GI bleeding	+	++ Diarrhea, nausea, vomiting, anorexia			+	++	AZA: administer after meals; MMF: decrease or divide dose, administer with food; TAC/PRED: administer with food; ulcer prophylaxis
Gingival hyperplasia				++						Patient education; dental hygiene; consider TAC
Glucose alterations			++	+	++					Monitor glucose; adjust doses of hypoglycemics or immunosuppressants
Headache				+	++			+	+	Check drug concentration; adjust dose
Hepatotoxicity	+			+	++					Monitor liver enzymes; adjust dose and discontinue as needed
Hirsutism				++						Patient education; consider TAC
Hyperlipidemia			++	++	+	++				Dietary counseling; pharmacotherapy as needed
Hypertension			++	++	++				+	Monitor blood pressure; sodium restriction and antihypertensive medications as needed
Leukocytosis			++		++					Monitor WBCs
Leukopenia	++	++		+		++		++	+	Monitor WBCs; dose-dependent and reversible with AZA/MMF
Nephrotoxicity				++	++	+				Monitor serum creatinine/BUN; adjust dose and discontinue as needed
Osteoporosis/aseptic necrosis			+/++							Annual bone examinations; weight-bearing exercise
Personality changes			++							Patient and family education
Pruritus					++					Treatment as appropriate (see Chap. 45)
Respiratory abnormalities					++				+	TAC: pleural effusion, dyspnea OKT3: pulmonary edema
Seizures				+	+			+	+	
Thrombocytopenia	++	+			+	++		++	+	Monitor platelets
Tremor				++	++				+	Adjust dose as needed
Weight gain			++							Patient education; exercise

++ = >10% incidence; + = <10% incidence.

was not different between the AZA and CSA. In fact, 5-year graft survival after the development of chronic graft dysfunction was 34% in AZA patients and 53% in CSA patients. Similarly, Slaton et al. compared 1- and 5-year patient and graft survival in cadaveric renal transplant recipients treated with either AZA or CSA as the primary immunosuppressive agent.[38] Although patient survival rates did not differ between groups, the 5-year graft survival rate was greater in the CSA than AZA group (61% vs 29%); the mean serum creatinine concentration at 5 years was significantly greater in the CSA group (CSA 1.79 vs AZA 1.30 mg/dL, $P < 0.05$). In contrast, the results of a meta-analysis evaluating chronic immunosuppression in renal transplant patients refute these reports.[39] One- and 5-year graft and patient survival, rejection rate per patient, and infection rate were analyzed; no statistical differences between CSA triple-drug therapy over dual-drug therapy (CSA/PRED) were detected.

Burke et al. reported the results of a multicenter, long-term efficacy and safety of CSA evaluation in renal transplant patients. Graft survival was 78% after a median follow-up of 36 months. In the 1,663 patients evaluated, there were 279 grafts lost. The leading cause of graft loss was acute rejection (68 patients) and chronic graft dysfunction (125 patients).[40] The optimal immunosuppressive regimen is not always clear-cut; further study in terms of longer follow-up may help determine which maintenance regimen(s) are preferred.

Formulations. CSA, a highly lipophilic cyclic polypeptide, was initially released as Sandimmune. Use of the original formulation was associated with clinically significant interpatient and intrapatient variability in pharmacokinetic parameters secondary to unpredictable bioavailability. Subsequently, CSA was reformulated using a microemulsion delivery system to improve its bioavailability. This formulation, Neoral, is self-emulsifying and spontaneously forms a microemulsion with aqueous fluids in the GI tract. With Neoral, the rate and extent of CSA absorption is significantly greater and intraindividual variability in pharmacokinetic parameters is reduced.

In recent years, generic formulations of CSA have been developed. Based on the improved bioavailability and reduced pharmacokinetic variability of Neoral, generic formulations were tested for pharmacokinetic and therapeutic equivalence to the reference formulation of Neoral. The first generic CSA product to be FDA approved was SangCya [Cyclosporine Oral Solution, USP (MODIFIED) 100 mg/mL].[41] Initially, this formulation was shown to be bioequivalent to Neoral oral solution.[42] However, this product was recalled by the FDA in July 2000.[43] The recall was prompted by new clinical evidence demonstrating a reduction in bioavailability, relative to Neoral oral solution, when SangCya was coadministered with apple juice (labeling suggested that SangCya could be taken with apple or orange juice). The FDA allowed the product to remain in pharmacies and hospitals so that patients could smoothly transition from SangCya to another CSA formulation. In 2000, two generic formulations of cyclosporine capsules [USP (MODIFIED)] were approved by the FDA.[44,45] These formulations are copromoted by Eon Labs/Mylan and SangStat/Abbott Laboratories (Gengraf). Both formulations have received AB ratings from the FDA, indicating that the products are therapeutically equivalent to, or interchangeable with, the reference drug. If conversion from Neoral is desired, patients should be converted on a 1 mg:1 mg basis. After the conversion is made, follow-up is required to assess for changes in trough concentrations and adverse effects.

CSA is an important part of immunosuppression in transplant patients. The cost of CSA, as well as the cost of other immunosuppressive drugs, is substantial, considering that these patients will require long-term immunosuppression (Table 46–4).[46] Substantial cost savings may be achieved with the use of FDA-approved generic CSA formulations.

Dosing. Initiation of oral CSA therapy generally begins with a dose of 8–18 mg/kg/d divided into 2 daily doses. Higher CSA doses are more commonly used in dual-drug therapy regimens, whereas lower doses are part of triple-drug therapy regimens. Doses are adjusted on the basis of whole-blood concentrations of the drug and the clinical response of the patient. The desired blood concentration range is dependent on assay methodology and individual risk factors

TABLE 46–4. Cost Comparison of Immunosuppressive Agents (2001 AWP)

Medication	Initial Dose[a]	Daily Cost	Maintenance	Daily Cost
Polyclonal antibodies				
ATGAM (ATG)	20 mg/kg/d × 7–10 days	$1,470.00	—	
Thymoglobulin	1.5–2.5 mg/kg/d × 14 days	$1,391.25		
Monoclonal antibodies				
OKT3	5 mg/kg/d × 7–10 days	$780.00	—	
Simulect (basiliximab)	20 mg × 2 doses	$1,419.75	—	
Zenapax (daclizumab)	1 mg/kg × 5 doses	$250.92	—	
Corticosteroids				
Solu-Medrol	500 mg	$9.50		
Deltasone (PRED)	20 mg/d	$0.20	7.5 mg/d	$0.04
Prednisone (generic)	20 mg/d	$0.20	7.5 mg/d	$0.04
Calcineurin inhibitors				
Neoral (Novartis, CSA)	7 mg/kg/d	$30.50	3.5 mg/kg/d	$15.24
Sandimmune (Novartis, CSA)	7 mg/kg/d	$34.65	3.5 mg/kg/d	$17.32
Gengraf (Abbott, CSA)	7 mg/kg/d	$27.50	3.5 mg/kg/d	$13.75
Cyclosporin capsules, USP-modified (Eon, CSA)	7 mg/kg/d	$27.50	3.5 mg/kg/d	$13.75
Prograf (Fugisawa, TAC)	0.2 mg/kg/d	$42.04	0.1 mg/kg/d	$21.02
Antiproliferative agents				
Imuran (AZA)	2 mg/kg/d	$4.80	1 mg/kg/d	$2.40
Azathioprine (generic)	2 mg/kg/d	$3.93	1 mg/kg/d	$1.96
CellCept (MMF)	2 g/d	$20.24	2 g/d	$20.24
Rapamune (SRL)	2 mg/d	$13.70	2 mg/d	$13.70

[a]Starting doses for a 70-kg patient.

for rejection such as time posttransplant. As the risk for acute rejection decreases with time, oral CSA doses are reduced and may be as low as 3 mg/kg/d or less during maintenance therapy. If oral administration is not possible, CSA may be administered intravenously at one-third the oral dosage.

Therapeutic Drug Monitoring. The absorption, distribution, and metabolism of CSA are highly variable; many factors contribute to this intrapatient and interpatient variability.[47,48] As these factors change in the posttransplant course, CSA pharmacokinetic parameters change.[49] Therefore, CSA blood concentrations are routinely measured in an attempt to optimize therapy.[50] Radioimmunoassay (RIA) and fluorescence polarization immunoassay are the most commonly used methods; however, high-performance liquid chromatography (HPLC) is recognized as the reference procedure.[51] It is important to determine which assay methodology the laboratory is using because target ranges vary between specific (which quantitates parent CSA) and nonspecific (which quantitates parent plus metabolite concentration) assays. The therapeutic range for whole blood RIA is 375–400 ng/mL versus 100–200 ng/mL for HPLC. In serum or plasma, the therapeutic range for RIA is 175–250 ng/mL; for HPLC, it is 75–150 ng/mL. Moreover, it is extremely important to interpret CSA concentrations in the context of relevant clinical and laboratory data, along with the appropriate reference ranges.

The most common and practical method of CSA monitoring is the measurement of trough blood concentrations.[50] CSA trough concentrations are measured frequently (daily or three times per week) following the initiation of the drug and during the stabilization period after transplantation. An alternative to the assessment of CSA trough concentrations is the characterization of the individual's CSA pharmacokinetic profiles.[52] Theoretically, a pharmacokinetic profile consisting of serial samples collected throughout a CSA dosage interval is more reflective of overall CSA exposure than are individual trough concentrations. Sequential CSA profiles provide a more comprehensive pharmacokinetic characterization, and area under the curve (AUC) has been suggested to correlate with graft outcome.[53] However, because of the intrapatient variability in the pharmacokinetics of CSA, the usefulness of a single pharmacokinetic profile to predict long-term dosing strategies is controversial. Unlike the ease of obtaining CSA trough concentrations, measurement of CSA pharmacokinetic profiles is a more complicated procedure. The cost of additional blood samples and practicality of using these profiles for therapeutic monitoring at individual institutions must be considered. In patients receiving Neoral, the use of limited sampling strategies has resulted in an excellent correlation with drug exposure.[54] The relationship between trough and total exposure to CSA appears to be stronger with Neoral than with Sandimmune. This relationship may be particularly useful to minimize the potential for increased toxicity secondary to greater drug exposure.

CSA concentrations may be markedly increased as the result of drug interactions. Diltiazem and ketoconazole, for example, inhibit the hepatic elimination of CSA via inhibition of cytochrome P450 3A4 and have been used to achieve desired concentrations of CSA with lower CSA doses. A complete discussion of CSA drug interactions is found elsewhere;[55] see Chap. 18, Table 18–6.

Adverse Effects. Table 46–3 summarizes CSA adverse effects and management in the renal transplant patient. The clinician is frequently required to differentiate between allograft rejection and CSA nephrotoxicity, which is generally a diagnosis of exclusion. Typically, nephrotoxicity is defined as an increase in serum creatinine of 25% over several days that reverses following a CSA dose reduction. Because the clinical features of acute allograft rejection and CSA nephrotoxicity may overlap considerably, a renal biopsy continues to be the diagnostic gold standard (Table 46–5). Differentiating between CSA nephrotoxicity and chronic rejection is also difficult because the clinical signs and symptoms may be similar. Because biopsy findings are similar in patients with CSA nephrotoxicity and with chronic rejection, this is a much more difficult differential diagnosis.

CSA discontinuation in renal transplant patients may be considered in some cases of chronic nephrotoxicity or uncontrolled hypertension. In these patients, immunosuppression is generally maintained with PRED and AZA, or by the addition of TAC. Improved renal function may result from such a change in therapy, but it may take several weeks for the beneficial effects to be fully realized. However, CSA discontinuation may precipitate an episode of acute graft rejection and should be completed in conjunction with careful monitoring. The financial impact of additional monitoring during the conversion period and the potential adverse effects of TAC including hyperkalemia and neurologic effects must also be considered.

Tacrolimus

TAC, formerly FK506, was initially approved by the FDA in 1994 for patients undergoing orthotopic liver transplantation. Most of the early experience with TAC in renal transplantation was as rescue therapy for refractory rejection. The FDA approved TAC as primary therapy for renal transplantation in 1997. Jordan et al. converted 169 patients with biopsy-confirmed, steroid-resistant rejection from CSA-based immunosuppression to TAC in an attempt to salvage failing allografts. This practice resulted in a success rate of 74% with a mean follow-up of 30 months.[56] Others reported graft survival rates ranging from 60% to 98% with follow-up ranging from 4 to 9 months.[57]

TABLE 46–5. Differential Diagnosis of Acute Rejection versus CSA or TAC Nephrotoxicity

	Acute Rejection	CSA or TAC Nephrotoxicity
History	Often <4 weeks postop	Often >6 weeks postop
Clinical presentation	Fever Hypertension Weight gain Graft swelling/tenderness Decreased daily urine volume	Afebrile Hypertension Graft nontender Good urine output
Laboratory	Rapid rise in serum Cr ($\geq$ 0.3 mg/dL/d) Normal CSA or TAC concentration	Gradual rise in serum Cr (> 0.15 mg/dL/d) Elevated CSA or TAC concentration
Biopsy	Interstitial lymphocytic infiltrates	Interstitial fibrosis, tubular atrophy, glomerular thrombosis, arterial inflammation

The early experience using TAC in renal transplantation was derived from an unblinded randomized trial comparing TAC with CSA in patients undergoing retransplantation or who had failed conventional immunosuppressive regimens. One-year actuarial patient survival for individuals receiving TAC ($n = 240$) was 90% versus 94% for patients receiving CSA ($n = 196$), whereas the 1-year graft survival for both groups was similar—74% for TAC versus 77% for CSA. Although not statistically significant, 44% ($n = 105$) of TAC-treated patients were able to have steroids withdrawn as compared to no patients treated with CSA; and fewer patients treated with TAC required antihypertensive therapy as compared to CSA-treated patients (57% vs 75%). Finally, the mean serum cholesterol in TAC-treated patients was significantly lower (187 mg/dL) than in the CSA patients (236 mg/dL) ($P < 0.0001$).[58]

A phase III multicenter trial in the United States compared CSA ($n = 207$) to TAC ($n = 205$) in regimens consisting of antilymphocytic therapy and AZA/PRED. Although no differences were reported at 1 year in patient (95.6% vs 96.6%) or graft (91.2% vs 87.9%) survival, significantly fewer TAC-treated patients experienced biopsy-proven acute rejection (30.7% vs 46.4%, $P = 0.001$). Follow-up at 3 years showed similar rates of patient and graft survival, but there were fewer graft failures in the TAC group. In a similar European trial, TAC ($n = 303$) was compared to CSA ($n = 145$) in combination with AZA and in combination with low-dose corticosteroids. At 1 year, TAC was associated with a reduction in acute rejection (25%) as compared to CSA (45.7%). As in the U.S. trial, there were no differences in patient or graft survival.[57]

Limited data are available with TAC in comparison to Neoral alone or in combination with MMF. One-year follow-up evaluating AZA/TAC, MMF/TAC, and CSA/MMF in CRT showed similar graft survival and rates of rejection, but a trend toward a lower rate of steroid-resistant rejection in the MMF/TAC arm.[59] Whether the decreased incidence of acute rejection noted with TAC will translate into a long-term benefit remains to be determined. In an analysis of UNOS data, however, Gjertson et al. compared allograft half-lives between 544 TAC- and 35,147 CSA-treated patients. They reported a half-life of 13.8 years in TAC-treated patients as compared to 8.8 years with CSA.[60]

Dosing and Monitoring. In a 6-week trial designed to define the optimal trough blood concentrations of TAC, 120 patients were randomized to CSA-based immunosuppression or 1 of 3 TAC groups based on target trough concentrations: low (5–14 ng/mL), medium (15–25 ng/mL), or high (26–40 ng/mL). All patients also received AZA and PRED. Primary outcomes were biopsy-proven acute rejection or toxicity of any type. There were no differences in rejection between the three TAC groups, but patients receiving TAC had a lower incidence of rejection as compared to patients receiving CSA (14% vs 32%, $P = 0.048$). Neurologic and gastrointestinal side effects occurred more frequently at higher concentrations of TAC.[57] One-year follow-up of these same patients showed a similar incidence of rejection between TAC- and CSA-treated patients: 32% versus 33%. Although nephrotoxicity occurred with a similar frequency, the incidence of neurologic and gastrointestinal side effects remained higher in TAC-treated patients.[61] A recent review of the role of TAC in renal transplantation suggests an oral starting dose of 0.2–0.3 mg/kg/d and target 12-hour whole-blood trough concentrations of 15–20 ng/mL (0 to 1 month posttransplant), 10–15 ng/mL (1 to 3 months posttransplant), and 5–12 ng/mL (>3 months posttransplant). Like CSA, TAC pharmacokinetics exhibit wide variation: oral bioavailability ranging from 5% to 67% (mean 29%), and half-life from 4 to 41 hours.[62] Tacrolimus is metabolized by the cytochrome P450 3A enzyme system. As such, there is a great potential for drug interactions with other substrates as well as inhibitors and inducers of this system. Tacrolimus is subject to pH-mediated degradation by sodium bicarbonate and magnesium oxide, whereas aluminum hydroxide gel adsorbs TAC. Tacrolimus administration should, therefore, be separated from these compounds by at least 2 hours.

Adverse Effects. The adverse effects associated with TAC in renal transplantation patients include neurologic toxicity, nephrotoxicity, and electrolyte disturbances such as hyperkalemia and hypomagnesemia.[58] Neurotoxicity including coma, tremor, headaches, paresthesias, and insomnia is more common in patients treated with >0.3 mg/kg/d of TAC or TAC blood concentrations > 25 ng/mL. Nephrotoxicity associated with TAC varies from 18% to 42% in liver transplant recipients, but the incidence is not well defined in renal transplant recipients. In a series of 128 patients undergoing renal biopsy for the investigation of renal dysfunction, Katari et al. reported that TAC nephrotoxicity, defined primarily by the absence of rejection and a fall in serum creatinine following dose reduction, accounted for graft dysfunction in 17% of patients.[63] Tacrolimus nephrotoxicity was accompanied by hyperglycemia, hyperkalemia, and tremors in several patients. Posttransplant lymphoproliferative disorder is also associated with TAC. As observed with CSA, most adverse effects related to TAC improve with dosage reduction or discontinuation.

In comparison to CSA, TAC is associated with increased occurrence of neurologic complications including tremor, paresthesias, and anxiety. Tacrolimus is also associated with less hypercholesterolemia.[57,64] Hirsutism, acne, and gingival hyperplasia are infrequently associated with TAC therapy. The incidence of posttransplant diabetes is approximately 20%, but is often reversible when doses of TAC and/or steroids are reduced.[57,51]

ANTIPROLIFERATIVE AGENTS

Azathioprine

Azathioprine, a prodrug for 6-mercaptopurine, is commonly used following renal transplantation. The immunosuppressive activity of AZA is correlated with its reduction in WBCs. Initial doses of 3–5 mg/kg/d are given with subsequent individualization (0.5–3 mg/kg/d) to maintain a stable serum creatinine and a WBC count of $3.5–5 \times 10^3$ cells/mm^3. Dose-limiting adverse effects of AZA are often hematologic in origin (Table 46–3). Leukopenia, anemia, and thrombocytopenia are common adverse effects and can be managed by dose reduction or discontinuation of AZA. Hepatotoxicity and pancreatitis are less common adverse effects of AZA; they are generally reversible on dose reduction or discontinuation.[9,28,30,34]

Mycophenolate Mofetil

MMF is the morpholinoethyl ester of the immunosuppressant mycophenolic acid (MPA). Following oral administration, MMF is rapidly and completely converted to MPA. MPA exerts its immunosuppressive effect through noncompetitive binding to inosine monophosphate dehydrogenase, ultimately leading to a reduction in guanosine nucleotide synthesis. This eventually results in diminished DNA polymerase activity and a reduction in lymphocyte proliferation via both the de novo and salvage pathways.[65]

MMF has been studied for the prevention of acute rejection in approximately 1,500 patients in three randomized controlled trials

TABLE 46–6. Summary of Pivotal Mycophenolate Mofetil Rejection Prophylaxis Trials

	U.S. Trial			Tricontinental Trial			European Trial		
	MMF 2 g	*MMF 3 g*	*AZA*	*MMF 2 g*	*MMF 3 g*	*AZA*	*MMF 2 g*	*MMF 3 g*	*Placebo*
n	167	166	166	173	164	166	165	160	166
6-month									
Biopsy-proven rejection (%)[a]	19.8	17.5	38.0	19.7	15.9	35.5	17.0	13.8	46.4
Graft survival (%)	98.2	93.3	91.4	96.0	98.2	97.0	95.7	93.7	91.0
Patient survival (%)	96.4	94.5	97	99.4	98.2	98.8	97.6	97.5	98.8
Opportunistic infections (%)	44.8	45.7	47.5				38.2	34.4	27.7
Invasive CMV (%)	9.1	10.8	6.1				3.0	6.9	2.4
Malignancy (%)	3.6	0	1.2						
Lymphoma (%)	0.6	1.2	0						
Diarrhea (%)	31.5	37.3	23.8				12.7	15.6	12.7
Leukopenia (%)							10.9	13.8	4.2
12-month									
Graft survival (%)	95.8	91.0	90.2	91.2	92.0	88.8			
Patient survival (%)	94.5	94.0	95.7	96.5	95.7	95.7			
Opportunistic infections (%)				46.0	46.0	44.0			
Invasive CMV (%)				7.0	11.0	6.0			
Malignancy skin/nonskin (%)				9.0/2.0	5.0/4.0	5.0/3.0			
Lymphoma (%)	0.6	0.6	0	1.2	1.2	0.6			
Diarrhea (%)				28.0	31.0	17.0			
Leukopenia (%)				19.0	35.0	30.0			
Costs per patient ($)	27,807		29,158	29,294		28,857			
3-year									
Graft survival (%)	87.3	84.3	83.5	81.9	84.8	80.2			
Patient survival (%)	89.7	88.0	88.4	93.0	91.5	87.7			
Invasive CMV (%)	2.3	1.7	0						
Malignancy (%)				2.9	6.1	3.7			
Lymphoma (%)	0.6	1.8	0.6	1.2	1.8	0.6			
Diarrhea (%)	16.8	26.4	16.9						
Anemia (%)	16.0	20.7	12.1						

[a]MMF 2 g vs. AZA, $P = 0.0036$; MMF 3 g vs. AZA, $P = 0.0006$; MMF 2 g vs. AZA/placebo, $P = 0.004$; MMF 3 g vs. AZA/placebo, $P = 0.043$.

summarized in Table 46–6. These trials compared MMF (plus CSA and steroids) to regimens that included either placebo or AZA. In the European Trial, significantly fewer patients had biopsy-proven rejection or treatment failure during the first 6 months after transplantation with MMF 2 g/d (30.3%) or MMF 3 g/d (38.8%), than with placebo (56%).[66] Similar results were reported in the U.S. Trial and the Tricontinental Trial.[67,68] Among the three trials there were no differences in patient or graft survival at 1 year.[69] Pooled analysis of these trials showed a reduction in the number of patients at 1 year with biopsy-proven rejection or treatment failure in the MMF 2 g/d (36.8%) and MMF 3 g/d group (39.6%), in comparison with patients who received AZA or placebo (53.8%).[70] Based on these results, many transplant centers added MMF to or replaced AZA in existing immunosuppression protocols. However, 3-year follow-up of the U.S. Trial failed to demonstrate a significant difference in the combined end point of graft and patient survival: MMF 2 g/d (81.2%); MMF 3 g/d (78.3%); AZA (75%).[71] Analysis of 3-year graft survival in the Tricontinental Trial produced similar results: MMF 2 g/d (81.9%); MMF 3 g/d (84.8%); AZA (80.2%).[68]

Dosing and Monitoring. Unlike other immunosuppressive agents, there is no compelling indication that MMF should be dosed in adult patients on a mg/kg basis given the weak correlation between MPA AUC and body weight.[65] In contrast to CSA and TAC, plasma appears to be the most appropriate medium for measuring MPA. Therapeutic drug monitoring and pharmacodynamic monitoring are not routinely done; however, MPA AUC seems to correlate with outcome.[65]

MMF is currently available in both oral and intravenous formulations. Although IV administration of equal doses closely mimics oral administration, the two cannot be considered bioequivalent.[73] MPA AUC is unchanged in patients with renal impairment. MPAG, the inactive glucuronide metabolite, is renally eliminated and accumulates in patients with renal dysfunction. Doses should be limited to 2 g/d in patients with CLcr <25 mL/min because this group may be more prone to adverse effects associated with MMF.[74] MMF doses up to 3.5 g/d have been used for the treatment of acute rejection, but should be titrated based on efficacy and toxicity. MPA is not significantly removed by hemodialysis. Given its high degree of protein binding (97.5%), MPA is unlikely to be affected significantly by peritoneal dialysis. Pharmacokinetic studies in renal transplant recipients showed an increase in AUC and C_{max} in patients who are at least 3 months posttransplant when compared to those patients who are less than 40 days posttransplant. The clinical significance of this finding remains to be determined. Dose reduction in the first year posttransplant based on the pharmacokinetic and pharmacodynamic properties of MMF has not been evaluated.[75]

Numerous drug interactions have been documented with MMF. Food delays the absorption and decreases MPA C_{max} by 25% but has no effect on MPA AUC. Prescribing information indicates that MMF should be taken on an empty stomach, but MMF is often given with food in clinical practice to minimize gastrointestinal (GI) effects.

Administration with aluminum- and magnesium-containing antacids, however, significantly decreases both C_{max} (37%) and AUC (15%), and should be avoided.[65] It has been suggested that administration of iron may produce similar results, but this has not been tested.

Acyclovir, commonly used in renal transplant recipients for the treatment and prevention of viral infections, competes with MPAG for renal tubular secretion. AUCs of both entities are increased with concomitant acyclovir and MMF administration. Patients with severe renal insufficiency may be at increased risk of seizures and delirium because of the accumulation of acyclovir, although no cases have been reported with concomitant MMF administration.[65] Single-dose intravenous ganciclovir in combination with MMF produced no change in the disposition of ganciclovir, MPA, or MPAG.[76] Although no pharmacokinetic interaction was demonstrated, there is potential for additive pharmacodynamic effects such as bone marrow suppression.

CSA appears to have no effect on MPA pharmacokinetics, whereas concomitant administration of TAC and MMF may result in increased MPA trough levels and AUC. MPA AUC increased by greater than 50%, whereas the MPA 12-hour trough doubled in TAC-treated patients. Although studies evaluating the efficacy of different doses of MMF in combination with TAC have not been conducted, clinicians should note that patients receiving MMF and TAC may be at greater risk for MMF-associated side effects such as bone marrow suppression and GI effects. These patients may require lower doses of MMF than CSA-treated patients to achieve a similar pharmacodynamic effect. MMF does not affect the pharmacokinetics of either CSA or TAC.[62]

Adverse Effects. Unlike CSA and TAC, MMF is not associated with nephrotoxicity, neurotoxicity, or hypertension. GI side effects such as nausea, vomiting, diarrhea, and abdominal pain, however, occur more frequently in MMF-treated patients as compared to those receiving AZA or placebo.[66,67] In addition, GI symptoms occur with similar frequency during intravenous and oral therapy. Clinically, however, dose reduction, dividing the total daily dose into three, administration with food, and upward titration from lower doses during initial therapy may alleviate some of these GI symptoms. MMF also has hematologic effects resulting in leukopenia and anemia. Tissue-invasive cytomegalovirus (CMV) was also more common in MMF-treated patients.[66–68] Malignancy and posttransplant lymphoproliferative disease (PTLD) are of significant concern with greater amounts of immunosuppression. At the 3-year follow-up of the U.S. Trial, there was a greater prevalence of lymphoma in the MMF 3 g/d group (1.8%) as compared with the MMF 2 g/d and AZA groups (each 0.6%).[71] Similar analysis of the European data showed a 1.8% prevalence of PTLD in the MMF 3 g/d group as compared with 1.2% and 0.6% in the MMF 2 g/d and AZA groups, respectively. Other malignancies also occurred in more patients receiving MMF 3 g/d than in the MMF 2 g/d and AZA-treated patients, 6.1% versus 2.9% and 3.7%, respectively.[72] Given the small numbers, these findings did not reach statistical significance. Longer follow-up of patients receiving MMF is required to characterize the lifelong risk of malignancy. Because peripheral intravenous MMF administration is associated with local edema and inflammation, central venous administration may be the preferred route.

Cost. The average wholesale price of MMF 2 g/d is $5,475 for yearly maintenance therapy, as compared to $1,277 for AZA 150 mg/d. Sullivan et al. evaluated the pharmacoeconomic impact of MMF therapy in the first year posttransplant using data from the U.S. Trial. This analysis showed a difference of approximately $1,300 (4.6%) per patient per year in favor of MMF 2 g/d versus AZA.[77] In a similar analysis of the data from the Tricontinental Trial, Keown et al. reported lower costs associated with the treatment of rejection, dialysis, and graft failure in patients receiving MMF, but mean first-year costs were higher on average in the MMF patients, $29,294 versus $28,857 for AZA-treated patients. Routine use of MMF 2 g/d would be associated with a cost of $14,268 per graft year gained.[78] Given the lack of difference in patient and graft survival at 1 and 3 years discussed previously, the cost-effectiveness demonstrated by Sullivan and Keown may not persist beyond the first year. The high annual cost of MMF therapy may not translate into a pharmacoeconomic advantage given the small differences in graft loss demonstrated after the first year. The most appropriate length of therapy with this new and costly agent remains to be determined. Currently, trials are underway to evaluate the effect of MMF withdrawal on acute rejection in renal transplant patients. Preliminary animal studies suggested that MPA may prevent or slow the progression of chronic rejection.[79,80] Although attempts to demonstrate the potential of MMF to change the course of ongoing chronic rejection in a clinical setting (as measured by a change in the slope of $1/S_{cr}$ vs time) and the 3-year follow-up of clinical trials did not produce promising results, a recent evaluation of the U.S. Scientific Renal Transplant Registry showed a superior 4-year survival of MMF-treated recipients ($n > 8{,}000$) versus AZA. This improvement in survival was independent of reduction in acute rejection.[81,82]

RAPAMYCIN DERIVIATIVES

Sirolimus

Sirolimus (SRL), also known as rapamycin, is a macrolide immunosuppressant that inhibits T-cell activation via suppression of IL-2- and IL-4-driven proliferation. This mechanism of action is distinct from CSA or TAC. Like TAC, SRL binds to FK binding protein (FKBP). This complex then binds to the mammalian target of rapamycin (mTOR) to inhibit IL-2-mediated signal transduction. Whereas CSA and TAC inhibit cytokine production, SRL appears to inhibit the response to these cytokines.[83]

Sirolimus has been evaluated in CSA-based regimens. The primary endpoint for these trials was the combined incidence of biopsy-proven rejection, graft loss or patient death at 6 months. Kahan et al. compared SRL/CSA/PRED to AZA/CSA/PRED. Although patient survival was similar in all groups, the incidence of biopsy-proven rejection was significantly lower in SRL-treated patients.[84]

Dosing and Formulation. The recommended dosing schedule is an oral loading dose of 6 mg as soon as possible after transplantation, followed by 2-mg/d maintenance doses. Higher doses may be warranted in African Americans. In patients with hepatic failure, the dose should be reduced by one-third.

Sirolimus is currently available as Rapamune in a 1 mg/mL solution. The oral solution must be protected from light and refrigerated. When stored properly, the solution is stable for 12 months. Once opened, the solution should be used within 30 days. If left at room temperature, the solution is stable for 24 hours. A capsule formulation is in development.[83]

Therapeutic Drug Monitoring. Sirolimus appears to be subject to the same pharmacokinetic variability that has been observed with CSA and TAC. Sirolimus is poorly absorbed from the GI tract with an oral bioavailability of about 15%. Peak concentrations are reached in approximately 1.4 ± 1.2 hours. In early studies, trough concentrations correlated with AUC. Thus, sirolimus trough concentrations may be useful for guiding therapy. The volume of distribution of sirolimus ranges from 5.6–16.7 L/kg. Partitioning between blood and plasma is extensive and widely variable, but does not appear to be concentration or temperature dependent. In the plasma, SRL is highly bound to proteins including albumin, α_1-acid glycoprotein, and lipoproteins.[83]

Like CSA and TAC, SRL is extensively metabolized by the cytochrome P450 3A4 isoenzyme. Only 2% of SRL is renally eliminated unchanged. The half-life of SRL ranges from 57 to 63 hours in renal transplant patients. Clearance appears to be slightly slower among males, but no dosage adjustment is recommended based on gender. Clearance among black recipients is significantly higher than among non-black recipients, but no differences were observed in mean trough concentrations.

Sirolimus AUC and trough concentrations are significantly increased by concomitant CSA administration. Patients should take SRL 4 hours following CSA to minimize this interaction. No data are available for TAC. Drug interaction studies with diltiazem and ketoconazole demonstrate significant increases in SRL exposure. The pharmacokinetic parameters of diltiazem and ketoconazole were not evaluated. It is recommended that ketoconazole be avoided if possible. Rifampin increases the clearance of SRL. Alternative agents should be used. Studies with acyclovir, digoxin, glyburide, nifedipine, norgestrel, ethynyl estradiol, prednisolone, and trimethoprim/sulfamethoxazole (TMP/SMX) showed no significant effects of coadministration. Although corticosteroids, ganciclovir, gemfibrozil, and HMG-CoA reductase inhibitors have been used concomitantly with SRL without an observed increase in side effects, caution is warranted.[83]

Limited data suggest that trough blood concentrations of 10–15 ng/mL are associated with favorable outcomes. At present, however, the routine therapeutic drug monitoring of SRL levels is not indicated for all patients. Children, African Americans, or patients with hepatic impairment, who may exhibit altered pharmacokinetics, may benefit from SRL trough blood monitoring to minimize toxicity and optimize efficacy. Patients receiving other medications metabolized by P450 3A4 or *p*-glycoprotein substrates may also benefit from therapeutic drug monitoring. Whole blood is the preferred medium for assessing SRL concentrations. Trough samples should be collected in EDTA tubes and protected from light. Currently, HPLC and HPLC-mass spectroscopy are the assays of choice. An immunoassay is in development.[83]

To overcome the pharmacokinetic limitations of sirolimus, SDZ-RAD, a rapamycin derivative, was developed. This compound exhibits comparable in vitro immunosuppressive activity to sirolimus. The pharmacokinetics of SDZ-RAD evaluated in Neoral-treated patients demonstrate linearity from 2.5–25 mg oral doses, with an elimination half-life of 24 to 35 hours. No changes in steady-state CSA kinetics were demonstrated in this study. Thrombocytopenia occurred at doses of 15–25 mg. Currently, studies are underway to evaluate its efficacy in renal transplant recipients.[79,85]

Adverse Effects.

Leukopenia, thrombocytopenia, and hypercholesterolemia are the primary dose-limiting toxicities of SRL. Initial studies indicated no nephrotoxicity, but data from the Phase III clinical trials show an increase in serum creatinine and decrease in glomerular filtration rate in some patients receiving SRL. Herpes simplex virus infections appear to occur with greater frequency in SRL-treated patients, particularly at doses of 5 mg/d. There does not appear to be an increase in the risk of CMV, fungal, or bacterial infections, or in the risk of PTLD.

ACUTE REJECTION THERAPY

The management of transplant rejection should be individualized. A specific histologic diagnosis should be made because treatment is often individualized based on histology. Prophylactic agents such as ganciclovir, nystatin, TMP/SMX, H_2-receptor antagonists, and/or antacids may be used to minimize adverse effects associated with intensive immunosuppression.[86]

Acute cellular rejection is the only type of rejection that responds well to therapy. High-dose steroids continue to be first-line therapy. Specific protocols vary between transplant centers; the general practice is to increase the steroid dose for 3 to 7 days, tapering down to the maintenance level or prerejection dose, whichever is higher. One option is to give 250–1,000 mg IV methylprednisolone for 3 days. Another approach is to use an "oral cycle" of steroids consisting of 200 mg oral PRED, decreasing the dose by 40 mg each day until a maintenance dose of 20 mg/d is achieved. Although no corticosteroid regimen has been shown to be superior to another, oral steroid cycles are less costly and easier to administer than intravenous therapy.

The use of MMF for the treatment of rejection has been recently evaluated.[87] MMF was assessed as rescue therapy versus intravenous corticosteroids in 150 renal transplant recipients with biopsy-proven rejection refractory to antilymphocyte therapy. Patients were randomized to methylprednisolone 5 mg/kg for 5 days or MMF 1.5 g bid, which could be increased to 3.5 g/d as needed for efficacy. The primary efficacy variable, graft loss, and patient death at 6 months was 26% in the steroid-treated patients versus 14% in the MMF group ($P = 0.081$). Secondary analysis at 1 year showed a difference in graft loss or death: 31.5% (steroids) versus 18% (MMF, $P = 0.042$). The number of patients reporting adverse events, primarily gastrointestinal (70.1% vs 33.8%) and hematologic (50.6% vs 25.5%), was significantly higher in the MMF group.[87] In patients receiving immunosuppression consisting of CSA, AZA, and PRED, Pirsch et al. evaluated conversion to MMF 1.5 g bid versus AZA 1 to 2 mg/kg/d in combination with intravenous corticosteroids for the treatment of first biopsy-proven acute rejection within 6 months posttransplant. Primary end points were first use of antibody therapy during 6 months and patient/graft survival at 1 year. MMF decreased the use of ATG/ALG/OKT3 (16.8% vs 41.7%, $P < 0.0001$) and was associated with a nonsignificant improvement in patient and graft survival (92% vs 85.2%). More patients in the MMF group, however, withdrew secondary to adverse events (17.7% vs 10.2%).[88] MMF, with or without corticosteroids, should be considered for the treatment of acute rejection in MMF-naive patients.

OKT3 therapy may also be used as a first-line treatment of acute cellular rejection. The reversal rate for acute rejection in patients treated with OKT3 is more than 80%, compared to a reversal rate of 65% to 75% achieved with high-dose steroids.[89] In addition, it has been suggested that long-term graft survival may be higher when OKT3 is used as primary treatment for first episodes of rejection.[90] Two factors that must be considered with OKT3 use are the added potential for infectious and/or central nervous system (CNS) toxicity and increased cost when compared to high-dose steroids. As a result of these factors and the good to excellant responsiveness of acute cellular rejections to steroid treatment, OKT3 is usually reserved as a second-line agent.[91] Although corticosteroids are generally considered the first-line therapy for acute rejection, recent data indicate that African Americans do not respond as well to glucocorticoids as non-African Americans. Other therapies, such as OKT3, may thus be preferable for this patient population.[92]

STRATEGIES TO MINIMIZE IMMUNOSUPPRESSIVE COMPLICATIONS

STEROID WITHDRAWAL

Because of the many detrimental effects associated with chronic steroid therapy, dose minimization has been the goal of therapy. The availability of CSA, TAC, and MMF has permitted complete withdrawal of corticosteroids in some patients. Factors to consider when evaluating studies of these alternative strategies in transplant patients include patient selection criteria, timing and rapidity of withdrawal, and duration of follow-up.

There is evidence that the continuation of steroids is beneficial in transplant patients receiving CSA-based immunosuppression. With a follow-up period of 1 year, Matl et al. demonstrated no difference in rejection in patients receiving triple-drug therapy (CSA, AZA, and steroids) versus those patients withdrawn from steroids and receiving CSA and AZA.[93] A randomized, controlled trial of steroid withdrawal between 1 and 6 years posttransplant in 100 patients receiving CSA, AZA, and steroids was conducted.[94] Eighty-six percent (42 of 49 patients) randomized to steroid withdrawal were successfully withdrawn. However, steroid withdrawal was followed by a 25% increase in serum creatinine at 1 year in 53% of patients (18% in control group; $P < 0.001$).

Long-term outcome may differ from short-term results following steroid withdrawal. Sanfey et al. describe their experience of steroid withdrawal in patients initially receiving CSA, AZA, and steroids.[95] They report successful steroid withdrawal in 67% (29 of 43 patients) with a follow-up of 38.3 ± 11.0 months (mean ± SD). Furthermore, they report a graft loss of 7% (3 of 43 patients). Similarly at long-term follow-up (mean of 4 years), Dunn et al. report 42% (5 of 12 patients) experiencing at least 1 episode of biopsy-proven rejection following the withdrawal of steroids from CSA-based immunosuppression.[96] Of the five patients who experienced rejection, one recovered, three lost their graft, and one developed chronic rejection. Patient and graft survival were 92% and 58%, respectively.

Steroid withdrawal in patients receiving dual-drug therapy has also been evaluated. Patients receiving CSA and steroids were withdrawn from steroids and randomized to continue with CSA alone or with the addition of AZA.[97] Although the CSA/AZA regimen was more effective than CSA alone in reducing the incidence of acute rejection, graft loss from chronic rejection did not differ at 5 years following steroid withdrawal. Hollander et al. reported an increase in rejection rate 26% versus 2% in those CSA/steroid patients who were withdrawn from steroids at 1 year posttransplant and had a 14-month follow-up.[98] Patients who were successfully withdrawn from steroids, reported beneficial effects on hypertension, hypercholesterolemia, hyperglycemia, and appearance.

A meta-analysis of steroid withdrawal in CSA-based immunosuppression was completed.[99] Seven randomized controlled trials, including three steroid withdrawal and four steroid avoidance, were used in the analysis. The collective incidence of acute rejection was 48% and 30% for the steroid-free (n = 681) and steroid maintenance (n = 592) groups, respectively ($P = 0.012$). These results are similar to the recently published meta-analysis of Kasiske et al.[100] In the assessment of prednisone withdrawal trials, the proportion of patients with acute rejection was greater and the relative risk of graft failure was increased following steroid withdrawal.

Steroid withdrawal in patients receiving TAC-based therapy has also been studied. Shapiro et al. evaluated 379 patients who were randomized to receive either double (TAC and steroids) or triple (TAC, AZA, and steroids)-drug therapy.[101] Patients were categorized into two groups: those withdrawn from steroids and those who continued on steroids. Two hundred eighty-nine (76%) patients were withdrawn from prednisone. In the steroid withdrawal group, serum creatinine at 2 years was 1.7 ± 0.7 mg/dL. Three-year actuarial patient and graft survival rates for the steroid withdrawal versus steroid continuation group were 98% and 94% versus and 80% and 50%, respectively. Although these results were unexpected, steroid withdrawal was not randomized but only a theoretical goal. These outcomes may have been the result of a group that did well versus a group that had ongoing complications following transplantation. However, steroid withdrawal with TAC-based immunosuppression was possible in the majority of patients and it appears to be relatively safe within the first 3 years post-transplantation in a selected patient population.

In an uncontrolled trial, 26 renal allograft recipients receiving MMF, CSA, and prednisone underwent steroid withdrawal.[102] Mean steroid withdrawal time was 17 months posttransplant and steroid free follow-up time was 10 months. No rejection episodes occurred following steroid withdrawal. Similarly, Kupin et al. reported relatively low acute rejection rates following steroid withdrawal, with a 2-year follow-up, in kidney transplant patients receiving MMF/CSA (5%) versus an historical control group on AZA/Neoral (14%) or AZA/Sandimmune (22%; $P < 0.05$).[103]

A large European multicenter study investigated the safety of reducing steroid doses in renal transplant patients receiving CSA and MMF.[104] At 1-year posttransplant, the patient and graft survival rates were 98% and 94% for the withdrawal group and 97% and 93% in the control group. The withdrawal group experienced a reduction in cardiovascular risk factors and an enhancement in bone density. In a multicenter, prospective, randomized, double-blind trial, steroid withdrawal at 3 months posttransplant was evaluated in 266 patients receiving CSA, MMF, and prednisone.[105] The cumulative incidence of rejection or treatment failure within 1 year posttransplant for the maintenance and withdrawal groups was 9.8% and 30.8%, respectively. The study was discontinued early as a result of the difference in incidence of acute rejection. There was no difference between groups in patient and graft survival. Long-term follow-up will help to determine the ultimate consequences of acute rejection. However, withdrawal patients had lower cholesterol levels and less need for antihypertensives. Long-term follow-up assessing steroid withdrawal from MMF immunosuppression is needed.

Special concerns exist regarding the long-term use of corticosteroids in children, including abnormal growth rates. Some transplant centers withhold prednisone therapy in children until a first-rejection episode occurs. Alternate-day steroids may improve growth rates in patients who require corticosteroids to maintain allograft function. Steroid withdrawal may reduce blood pressure and lipids while improving growth in children. The use of steroid withdrawal in pediatric transplant patients receiving TAC-based immunosuppression was recently reported.[106] Data from this study indicate that steroid withdrawal in children is associated with reasonable patient and graft survival for the first 5 years posttransplant.

Although steroid withdrawal is still considered controversial, steroid withdrawal protocols are routinely utilized. However, it must be initiated and completed with caution to avoid graft rejection and loss. When considering steroid withdrawal protocols, the posttransplant course should be reviewed. Transplant patients who have had a favorable course without rejection and/or who have significant steroid-related adverse effects may benefit from steroid withdrawal. Specifically, patients with stable graft function and serum creatinine of less than 2 mg/dL and no history of previous rejection or signs of interstitial fibrosis or vascular sclerosis, patients with high risk for cardiovascular disease, and children may be optimal candidates for steroid withdrawal or avoidance. Potential contraindications for these alternative strategies may include patients at high risk for rejection and patients with posttransplant oligoanuria where high-dose CSA may result in vasoconstriction and exacerbation of delayed graft function. With steroid withdrawal, doses should be tapered slowly in a stepwise fashion. Frequent monitoring of creatinine and CSA concentrations should be implemented.[107]

CSA WITHDRAWAL

Concerns about chronic CSA nephrotoxicity and the high cost of prolonged therapy have led to examination of several strategies for electively withdrawing CSA. Unfortunately, there are major differences in the designs, results, and conclusions of these studies. A meta-analysis of elective CSA withdrawal in renal transplant patients, revealed that the rate of acute rejection was higher in patients undergoing CSA withdrawal than in those patients who continued to receive CSA.[108] Although there was no evidence that the higher incidence of acute rejection following CSA withdrawal led to increased graft loss or patient mortality, it is possible that the duration of follow-up was too brief to have allowed the detection of these outcomes. The second meta-analysis of Kasiske et al. corroborates these data; acute rejection is increased and there appears to be no decrease in graft survival following CSA withdrawal.[100] This finding was in direct contrast to the results of steroid withdrawal.

Elective CSA withdrawal at 1 year posttransplantation was evaluated in renal transplant recipients receiving CSA, AZA, and prednisone.[109] CSA was withdrawn in 192 patients who had been rejection free for 12 months. Thirty-four patients elected to continue CSA. Initially, CSA was tapered over a 6-week period. However, this taper schedule was discontinued when 8 of the first 27 (29.6%) patients developed acute rejection within 6 months. Subsequently, CSA was tapered over a 12-week period, preceded by an increase in AZA and prednisone dosage. With the slow CSA taper, the incidence of acute rejection within 6 months was 9.1% among 165 patients ($P < 0.01$ versus 6-week taper). Actuarial 5-year graft survival for patients continuing CSA, undergoing 6-week CSA taper, and undergoing 12-week CSA taper was 81.7%, 88.9%, and 81.5%, respectively. Lastly, the relative risk of acute rejection within 6 months of CSA withdrawal was approximately two times greater for each donor-recipient HLA mismatch ($P < 0.001$).

CSA withdrawal was also reported to be successful from a retrospective study conducted by Smith et al.[110] Patients received CSA, AZA, and prednisone. The median time of CSA discontinuation was 22 months posttransplantation. Acute rejection within 6 months of CSA discontinuation was evident in 12 of 97 patients (12.4%). Six-year graft survival in the withdrawal group was 84%. Other studies have also yielded positive results following CSA withdrawal.[111,112]

Keitel et al. published a long-term evaluation of elective CSA withdrawal in 64 renal transplant recipients receiving CSA, AZA, and prednisone.[113] Time of withdrawal ranged from 3 to 24 months following transplant. Follow-up was at 5 years posttransplantation. The incidence of chronic rejection was significantly increased in patients who experienced acute rejection following CSA withdrawal (83.3% versus 36.5%; $P = 0.004$).

Immunosuppressive protocols vary widely and often are individualized based on the number and severity of acute rejections. Similarly, long-term immunosuppression should be individualized. The strategy of CSA withdrawal remains controversial. For those patients who can be successfully discontinued from CSA, there are substantial advantages in terms of economics and absence of long-term adverse effects. However, potential long-term negative consequences may result from the increased incidence of acute rejection episodes following CSA withdrawal. Data indicate that a large percentage of patients do not require continued CSA immunosuppression. The challenge is to identify which patients would benefit from CSA withdrawal. Genetics, tissue matching, socioeconomic factors, and posttransplant course may influence the risk/benefit ratio of CSA withdrawal. Furthermore, when considering withdrawal for economic reasons, the cost of additional monitoring and the treatment of potential rejection episodes must be included in the analysis.

CONVERSION

Replacement of CSA/prednisone by AZA/prednisone or discontinuation of prednisone resulting in CSA monotherapy may also be used as alternative strategies. Hilbrands et al. employed this strategy at 3 months posttransplantation in a randomized, prospective study.[114] Although both immunosuppressive regimens were associated with relatively high acute rejection rates, AZA/prednisone and CSA monotherapy regimens were comparably effective immunosuppressive regimens as measured by patient and graft survival. Furthermore, an improvement in GFR within 1 week following conversion from CSA to AZA has been reported.[115] Two other prospective, randomized conversion trials converting a CSA/prednisone regimen to AZA/prednisone demonstrated no difference in patient or graft survival at 5 to 10 years.[116,117] Furthermore, positive effects on blood pressure as well as renal allograft function were demonstrated.

Conversion of CSA/prednisone to MMF/prednisone has been evaluated in 17 stable renal transplant recipients.[118] Two patients' participation in the study was stopped during the transition of low-dose CSA to MMF (one because of diarrhea and one because of steroid responsive rejection). Following complete conversion to MMF/prednisone, the remaining 15 patients experienced no acute rejections. The conversion was associated with an improvement in blood pressure, kidney function, uric acid, and lipid profiles at 1-year follow-up. After 1 year, two additional patients discontinued MMF (one because of Kaposi's sarcoma and one because of recurrent infections). Long-term follow-up to assess graft and patient survival is needed.

COMPLICATIONS

Infectious complications following transplantation are generally classified according to the causative organism, site of the infection, and time of appearance following surgery. Bacterial infections occur most frequently within the first month posttransplantation and generally affect the urinary tract, respiratory tract, wound, or vascular access sites. Viral infections are most commonly caused by herpes simplex (early posttransplant), herpes zoster (late posttransplant), or CMV. Other infections caused by nocardia, fungi, or protozoa occur rarely in renal transplant recipients.[119] Chapter 120 discusses the treatment of infection in the immunocompromised host. Special considerations of therapy in renal transplant patients for CMV, herpes, and *Pneumocystis carinii* infections are described in the following sections.

Noninfectious complications following transplantation include exacerbation of preexisting conditions such as diabetes and hypertension. However, some of these problems are posttransplant complications. The treatment of anemia, diabetes, gastrointestinal disease, hyperlipidemia, hypertension, malignancy, and osteoporosis are discussed elsewhere in this text. Some of the special considerations for renal transplant recipients, however, are detailed in Table 46–7.

CYTOMEGALOVIRUS INFECTIONS

In individuals with a normal immune system, CMV rarely produces symptoms. However, in patients with a suppressed immune system, CMV is usually symptomatic and can be quite serious. Cytomegalovirus is the most important viral pathogen affecting transplant patients; 50% to 60% of patients have been infected with the virus. CMV is responsible for 30% of febrile episodes, 35% of leukopenia, 20% of graft failure, and 25% of mortality in kidney transplantation.[120,121] Following transplantation, patients may develop symptomatic primary or secondary CMV infections. A previously CMV-seronegative patient who receives an organ or blood product from a CMV-seropositive donor is considered to have a primary CMV infection. A secondary infection is characterized by reactivation of the latent virus or reinfection in a previously seropositive patient. Patients with primary infections are generally more symptomatic than patients with secondary infections.

Typically, patients with CMV infection present between 4 and 10 weeks following transplantation with general malaise, gastritis, fever, elevated liver function studies, leukopenia, thrombocytopenia, and atypical lymphocytes on a WBC differential. Deterioration in renal function may also be observed. CMV retinitis is a rare manifestation in transplant patients, whereas CMV gastritis is a common complication. The leading cause of death associated with CMV infection is pneumonia.

The incidence and severity of symptomatic CMV infections in transplant recipients are related to the intensity of immunosuppression required to prevent graft rejection. Patients treated on multiple occasions with high-dose steroids or patients receiving OKT3 or ATGAM are at high risk for developing symptomatic CMV disease.[120] Poor HLA matching, cadaveric allografts, and CMV-positive donor serology are associated with more severe CMV disease.[122,123]

Because many transplant patients have primary CMV infections or reinfections, it would be ideal to limit the transplantation of CMV-positive organs, but given the high prevalence of CMV in most donor pools, this is not possible. Therefore, multiple strategies have been proposed for the prevention of CMV, including both prophylactic (to prevent disease) and preemptive (to prevent disease when it is likely to occur based on the detection of CMV infection without the presence of symptoms) interventions. Because of the conflicting results reported by various trials, there is controversy as to which agent(s), if any, should be used in renal transplant recipients.

PROPHYLAXIS OF CYTOMEGALOVIRUS INFECTIONS

High-dose acyclovir has been reported to reduce the incidence and severity of CMV disease in renal allograft recipients.[124] This widely quoted study was a prospective, double-blind, 12-week evaluation of 104 kidney transplant patients. Patients were randomized to receive either placebo or high-dose oral acyclovir (800 mg qid with dose adjustment based on renal function) for 12 weeks posttransplantation. There was a significant reduction in CMV isolation from blood (11% vs 41%) and disease requiring ganciclovir therapy (4% vs 13%) in patients receiving acyclovir. The greatest benefit was demonstrated in seronegative recipients of seropositive donor kidneys; however, there were only 13 patients in this subgroup.[124] Birkeland et al. demonstrated the efficacy of high-dose acyclovir prophylaxis in all patients, regardless of serology before transplant; in addition, these patients received preemptive ganciclovir during treatment with monoclonal antibodies.[125] In another case-controlled study of cadaveric kidney transplant patients who received high-dose acyclovir for 3 months, only seropositive patients had a significantly lower incidence of CMV disease.[126]

Other studies of prophylactic acyclovir, however, failed to produce similar results.[127] The failure of acyclovir in these reports is consistent with *in vitro* data suggesting that CMV is unlikely to be inhibited by levels of acyclovir that are achievable *in vivo*. Some investigators suggest that acyclovir prophylaxis is less effective in patients who receive antilymphocyte antibodies.[128] Discrepancies between studies may result from institutional differences in prevalence of CMV, immunosuppressive regimens, and definitions of CMV disease or infection.

Acyclovir therapy, if used, should be given for the first 12 weeks following transplantation because the risk for developing CMV is greatest during this period. Because acyclovir is primarily excreted unchanged via the kidney, the dose of acyclovir should be individualized based on renal function (see Chap. 50). Oral acyclovir is usually well tolerated; headache and nausea are the most commonly reported adverse effects. With high-dose therapy, adverse effects are more common and include nausea, severe headaches, and neurologic toxicity, such as tremor, delirium, and paresthesias, which improve with dose reduction. High-dose oral acyclovir costs range from $300 to $1,200 per 12-week course.[123] This additional cost may not produce enough benefit to warrant routine prophylaxis in all renal transplant patients.

Valacyclovir is an oral prodrug formulation of acyclovir with increased bioavailability that results in higher systemic concentrations of acyclovir. Administration of valacyclovir 500 mg 4 times daily provides an AUC equal to that of 10 mg/kg of intravenous acyclovir.[129] Trials are currently underway to examine the efficacy and safety of valacyclovir as CMV prophylaxis in renal transplant recipients.

Immunoglobulins, including polyclonal (IVIG) and CMV hyperimmune (CMVIG) immunoglobulin, have demonstrated variable efficacy for preventing CMV. Polyclonal immunoglobulin preparations are not standardized with regard to CMV-antibody content. As a result, high doses of polyclonal immunoglobulin preparations are generally required to deliver an effective amount of CMV antibodies. The administration of large fluid volumes may be difficult in renal transplant patients, who may be fluid overloaded.

One pediatric study demonstrated the benefit of polyclonal immunoglobulin (Gammagard) as prophylaxis in CMV-negative recipients of CMV-positive allografts. Symptomatic disease developed in 17% of IVIG-treated patients versus 71% of control patients. Although results were statistically significant, the study population was small and the control group received more treatments with monoclonal antibodies (46% vs 71%, NS).[130] Conti et al. demonstrated that conventional immunoglobulin was superior to placebo and equivalent to low-dose intravenous ganciclovir for the prophylaxis of CMV disease in CMV-negative renal transplant recipients of CMV-positive organs. However, the cost of IVIG was significantly greater than that of ganciclovir ($4,000/patient vs $350/patient).[131] The high cost and availability of other agents makes the use of polyclonal IVIG as a prophylactic agent for CMV uncommon.

TABLE 46–7. Special Pharmacotherapy Considerations in Renal Transplant Recipients

Problem	Pharmacotherapy	Special Considerations
Infection		
Perioperative prophylaxis	1st Generation cephalosporin × 24 to 48 h Bowel decontamination	Donor culture results Penicillin allergy: use vancomycin
Pneumocystis carinii Pneuomonia prophylaxis	TMP/SMX 400/80 qd; Pentamidine 300 mg inhaled q mo *or* Dapsone 50–100 mg po qd	avoid sulfa allergy
Fungal—Prophylaxis or treatment	Nystatin, clotrimazole, fluconazole, itraconazole, ketoconazle, amphotericin B	Inhibit P450 3A4, monitor CSA and TAC levels, decrease doses Consider liposomal products; decrease or stop CSA or TAC to minimize nephrotoxicity
Delayed graft function		Remember to adjust doses of renally eliminated drugs; e.g., acyclovir, ganciclovir, TMP/SMX
Prolonged uremia		
Hyperphosphatemia	Phosphorous binders; restrict dietary intake	
Hypocalcemia	Calcium supplementation; calcitriol	
Metabolic acidosis	Sodium bicarbonate; Shol's solution	
Hyperkalemia	See Chap. 52	May be exacerbated by CSA, TAC, or ACEIs, acidosis; fludricortisone acetate 0.1 mg po qd to bid for refractory hyperkalemia
Anemia	Continue erythropoietin until excretory function resumes Iron supplementation	In patients with graft function, HCT should return to normal by 3–4 months posttransplant; if patient has good function and anemia persists, evaluate for folate, vitamin B_{12} deficiency
Hyperglycemia		
Diabetes pretransplant	Insulin	Insulin requirements will increase with improving renal function
	Oral hypoglycemics	Glucocorticoids, TAC, CSA also increase hypoglycemic requirements Avoid Metformin
Post-transplant diabetes	Insulin Oral hypoglycemics	Risk factors: obesity, family history, African American race, cadaveric kidney, TAC > CSA May resolve/improve as immunosuppressive doses decrease
GI ulcer prophylaxis	H_2-Receptor antagonists Sucralfate Proton pump inhibitors Consider CMV gastritis	Renally eliminated If DGF: caution aluminum content No DGF: may cause hypophosphatemia
Hyperlipidemia	Diet HMG-CoA reductase inhibitors ("statins")	If on CSA, consider switch to TAC; discontinue or hold SRL CSA/TAC may increase "statin" levels; start at lowest dose Monitor for muscle cramps, and increased CPK levels Monitor LFTs
	Gemfibrozil	Adjust for renal impairment Caution with concomitant "statin"
Hypertension	Calcium channel blockers	Diltiazem, verapamil inhibit CSA/TAC metabolism Dihydropyridines may potentiate CSA-gingival hyperplasia
	ACE inhibitors; angiotensin II receptor blockers	May exacerbate hyperkalemia Monitor K^+, S_{cr} to assess for renal allograft vascular disease; may be useful in posttransplant erythrocytosis (HCT >55%)
Osteoporosis	Oral calcium supplementation (1,000–1,500 mg/d)	If daily intake <1,000 mg elemental calcium
	Oral vitamin D	Documented deficiency
	Calcifediol (1,000 IU/d)	If kidney functioning
	Calcitriol (0.5 μg/d)	If kidney not functioning
	Hormone replacement therapy	Postmenopausal women without contraindications
	Calcitonin or oral bisphosphonates	Documented loss in bone mineral density >3% Data lacking for bisphosphonates in patients with renal insufficiency
Malignancy		
Prevention	Minimize immunosuppressant doses; avoid sun exposure (sun block, hats, clothing); routine self-examinations (skin, lymph nodes); yearly gynecologic/prostate exams	AZA particulary associated with skin cancers CSA/TAC may be associated with lymphoproliferative disorders (lymphomas)
Treatment	Discontinue or minimize immunosuppressants Surgical, radiologic, or antineoplastic therapy	Do not abruptly withdraw corticosteroids

The safety and efficacy of preventive CMVIG was evaluated in a prospective, controlled, randomized, multicenter trial in seronegative renal transplant patients receiving seropositive grafts.[132] Patients received 550 mg/kg over a 16-week period and were followed for up to 1 year. Patients who received CMVIG had significantly fewer confirmed CMV syndromes (21% vs 60%), less marked leukopenia (4% vs 37%), and fewer fungal and protozoal infections (0 vs 20%) as compared to controls. Furthermore, the incidence of serious CMV disease was reduced in the CMVIG group. Adverse effects associated with CMVIG are rare but include flushing; anxiety; nausea; a metallic taste; headache; shortness of breath; palpitations; backache; and muscle cramps. Currently, CMVIG is approved in the United States for attenuation of primary CMV disease in high-risk patients (donor positive/recipient negative).[133] The calculated cost for a 7-dose regimen of Cytogam for a 70-kg patient is $11,825 (2001 AWP).

Combination strategies using CMVIG and antiviral agents for CMV prevention are used in some institutions.[134] Contrasting results have been obtained. Carrieri et al. retrospectively compared patients who received acyclovir plus CMVIG to acyclovir alone and demonstrated a reduction in the incidence of CMV disease from 47% to 23% with the combination in high-risk patients.[135] Further evaluations need to be performed to assess the absolute benefit of combination regimens.

Ganciclovir triphosphate, the active metabolite of ganciclovir, is a potent inhibitor of the replication of human herpes viruses, including CMV. Ganciclovir has been used prophylactically and preemptively in renal transplant patients. Rondeau et al. evaluated intravenous ganciclovir 5 mg/kg initiated on day 14 posttransplantation in seronegative patients receiving seropositive grafts. Although there was no difference in incidence of CMV infection or disease between ganciclovir and control patients, ganciclovir use was associated with a delayed onset and decreased severity of CMV.[136] When used in renal transplant patients receiving monoclonal antibodies, the concurrent use of ganciclovir significantly reduced the incidence and severity of symptomatic disease.[137,138] Some studies suggest that the administration of ganciclovir to patients who are CMV antigen-positive reduces the incidence of symptomatic disease;[139] other studies, however, don't support this conclusion.[140]

Ganciclovir is currently available in both an intravenous and oral dosage form. Oral ganciclovir has a low mean bioavailability of 8.4%.[141] Food increases the bioavailability of oral ganciclovir. Table 46–8 lists dosage guidelines for oral ganciclovir. Following oral administration, peak plasma concentrations occur in 2 to 4 hours. Oral ganciclovir administration results in plasma concentrations within the IC_{50} range for most susceptible strains of CMV, whereas those observed with intravenous administration are usually above the IC_{50}. Ganciclovir is extensively renally eliminated as unchanged drug. Therefore dosage adjustment is required in patients with renal impairment (see Chap. 50). Side effects of ganciclovir include neutropenia (50%) and thrombocytopenia (20%). Because neutropenia is frequently observed as a consequence of CMV, it is often difficult to ascertain the precise cause. In general, the adverse hematologic effects of ganciclovir are reversible within 3 to 7 days following discontinuation of therapy. Less common toxicities associated with ganciclovir therapy include CNS toxicity (headache, tremor, confusion, seizures, and hallucinations). Fever, rash, and alterations in liver function have also been reported, but these side effects are uncommon and a definite cause-and-effect relationship has not been established. Future studies that evaluate monotherapy as well as combination strategies are needed to determine the optimal dose and duration for preventative therapy.

Foscarnet prophylaxis is not advocated in renal transplant patients because of the potential additive nephrotoxicity that may occur when it is concurrently administered with agents such as CSA, TAC, and amphotericin B. Future options for the prevention of CMV disease include the use of CMV vaccines. The Towne strain of human CMV reduced the incidence of severe CMV disease in seronegative patients.[142] Such vaccines, when perfected, may prove to be less costly and more effective than current prophylactic strategies.

TABLE 46–8. Oral Ganciclovir Dosage Guidelines

Normal renal function	
Creatinine clearance ≥ 70 mL/min	3,000 mg/d (1,000 mg po tid)
Impaired renal function	
Creatinine clearance	
50–69 mL/min	1,500 mg/d (500 mg po tid)
25–49 mL/min	1,000 mg/d (500 mg po bid)
10–24 mL/min	500 mg po qd
< 10 mL/min	500 mg po 3 times/wk following dialysis

TREATMENT OF CYTOMEGALOVIRUS INFECTIONS

Until the development of ganciclovir, withholding immunosuppression was the mainstay of therapy for active CMV disease. Currently, intravenous ganciclovir is the therapy of choice for the treatment of CMV infections in renal transplant patients. Jordan et al. reported their experience treating 36 renal transplant patients with tissue invasive CMV disease.[143] Patients received ganciclovir (2.5 mg/kg every 12 hours) until they were asymptomatic and afebrile for 5 days. CMV disease was classified as mild in 75%, moderate in 17%, and severe in 8% of the patients. The average length of treatment was 12.2 days. Viral blood cultures were negative 7.5 days after treatment in all evaluable cases, and 9 of 11 urine cultures were negative in 8 days. All patients were asymptomatic after the initial course of treatment. The 1-year patient and graft survival rates were 100% and 56%, respectively. Ganciclovir was well tolerated with side effects limited to transient leukopenia, thrombocytopenia, and rash.

Foscarnet is generally reserved for the treatment of CMV infections that are unresponsive to therapy with ganciclovir. Andersson et al. used foscarnet as a continuous IV infusion (0.15 mg/kg/min) in eight renal transplant recipients. Seven of the patients were CMV virus culture negative 1 week after starting the foscarnet. Side effects included an increase in serum creatinine (5 of 8 patients), hypocalcemia (4 of 8 patients), and confusion (1 of 8 patients). All side effects were reversible after dosage reduction or discontinuation of the drug.[144] A rise in serum creatinine may be secondary to foscarnet or other clinical factors. For the present, foscarnet may be used cautiously in patients unresponsive or intolerant to therapy with ganciclovir.

HERPES VIRUS INFECTIONS

Herpes simplex virus (HSV) infections in renal transplant patients are most commonly the result of reactivation of a previous infection. Symptomatic HSV infection usually presents as labial or oral lesions in the first 1 to 3 months posttransplantation, but patients may also present with reactivation of varicella zoster as "shingles." Prophylactic therapy with low-dose oral acyclovir delays the development of HSV infections in patients following renal transplantation.[145] Intravenous acyclovir is indicated for those patients who develop disseminated HSV infections.

PNEUMOCYSTIS CARINII PNEUMONIA

The incidence of *Pneumocystis carinii* pneumonia (PCP) within the first year posttransplantation is reported to be 3% to 5%.[146] Low-dose TMP/SMX (400/80 mg daily) is effective in the prevention of *Pneumocystis* infections in renal transplant patients. Furthermore, after 3 months of therapy, it is frequently possible to reduce therapy from once daily to three times per week.[147]

Aerosolized pentamidine (300 mg every month) may be used alternatively in patients with allergies or intolerable adverse effects to sulfonamides.[148] Although it is generally well tolerated and has a relatively low incidence of nephrotoxicity and myelotoxicity, the prophylactic use of aerosolized pentamidine is expensive. In addition, its aerosolized administration is associated with difficulty in sputum and bronchoalveolar lavage collection, making the diagnosis of breakthrough PCP more difficult to establish, and cough secondary to the irritating effects, which increases the risk of spreading transmissible agents.[149] The use of inhaled albuterol prior to aerosolized pentamidine may minimize cough and bronchospasm.[148] Dapsone may also be used as an alternative for PCP prophylaxis. Its use has been evaluated in patients with HIV and appears to be promising.[150]

The duration of *Pneumocystis* prophylaxis is unclear. The risk of infection caused by *P. carinii* is likely to decrease as immunosuppression is reduced; therefore, prophylaxis is generally discontinued within 6 to 12 months following transplantation. The reinstitution of prophylaxis in patients requiring treatment for acute rejection may be appropriate. The therapy of choice for the treatment of PCP continues to be TMP/SMX.

CARDIOVASCULAR DISEASE

Cardiovascular disease is a leading cause of morbidity and mortality in renal transplant patients.[151] Hypertension, hyperlipidemia, and diabetes contribute significantly to cardiovascular disease and are common complications in transplant recipients. Impaired graft function, corticosteroids, CSA, and TAC may cause posttransplant hypertension. It seems appropriate to use recommendations from the Joint National Commission (JNC-VI) and the National Kidney Foundation Task Force on Cardiovascular Disease.[152,153] The goal of antihypertensive therapy is dependent on the patient's degree of residual renal function and proteinuria (see Chaps. 12 and 44). Most classes of antihypertensive medications effectively reduce blood pressure in renal transplant patients. Special precautions, however, are required in this population.

Calcium channel blockers are considered first-line agents in this population. In addition to their ability to control blood pressure, calcium channel blockers may ameliorate the nephrotoxic effects of CSA, improve renal hemodynamics, decrease the incidence of delayed graft function, and provide some immunosuppression. Calcium channel blockers, however, may also contribute to gingival hyperplasia that is often associated with CSA-based immunosuppression. Diltiazem, verapamil, nicardipine, and amlodipine inhibit CSA metabolism via the CYP 450 3A4 system (see Chap. 18).[154] This interaction may lead to CSA-induced nephrotoxicity and neurotoxicity if left unchecked. However, with proper monitoring and CSA dosage adjustments, agents such as diltiazem and verapamil, can be used to decrease the daily dose of CSA.

Angiotensin-converting enzyme inhibitors (ACEIs) and angiotensin II receptor blockers (ARBs) are effective for reducing blood pressure in many renal transplant recipients. ACEIs and ARBs have a special niche in the management of posttransplant erythrocytosis. However, the combination of efferent arteriolar vasodilation caused by the ACEI or ARB and afferent vasoconstriction caused by CSA or TAC may result in a decrease in glomerular filtration when these agents are used together. Hyperkalemia caused by CSA and TAC is frequently aggravated by concomitant therapy with an ACEI. When ACEIs or ARBs are used in patients posttransplantation, close monitoring of serum creatinine and potassium is required.

Hyperlipidemia may be exacerbated by CSA, corticosteroids, diuretics, and β-adrenergic blockers.[155] Furthermore there is indirect evidence suggesting that posttransplant hyperlipidemia may influence the progression of chronic renal allograft rejection.[156] It is controversial whether the management of hyperlipidemia in renal transplant recipients should be more aggressive than current guidelines for the general population, which are discussed in Chap. 21. Aggressive lipid lowering may not only arrest the progress or prevent the complications of atherosclerosis, but may also promote renal graft survival in this specific population. With the use of lipid-lowering agents, potential interactions with immunosuppressive regimens must be considered.

Dietary intervention, although safe, may be relatively ineffective for the treatment of hyperlipidemia in the transplant population. Along with dietary modification, dose reduction or withdrawal of CSA and/or steroids may assist in minimizing hyperlipidemia. For most patients, the combination of dietary intervention and an HMG-CoA reductase inhibitor should be considered the treatment of choice. HMG-CoA reductase inhibitors are highly effective in the treatment of hyperlipidemia, specifically increased low-density lipoprotein (LDL), in renal transplant patients. These agents should be used with caution because of several reports of rhabdomyolysis resulting in renal failure when lovastatin was combined with CSA. Safety measures, including the use of low HMG-CoA reductase inhibitor doses and avoiding inappropriately high CSA or TAC concentrations, should be taken. The concurrent use of medications known to increase the risk of myopathy (such as gemfibrozil) should be avoided.

Patients should be informed of the signs and symptoms of rhabdomyolysis. Baseline and follow-up creatine phosphokinase (CPK) measurements (every 6 months) have been used to identify patients who develop subclinical rhabdomyolysis when cholesterol-lowering therapy is used. In addition, because of the potential for hepatotoxicity from HMG-CoA reductase inhibitors, close monitoring of liver function is indicated.[155]

Bile acid binding resins may be used to lower cholesterol in renal transplant patients, but adequate doses are difficult to achieve without the development of GI adverse effects. Because the absorption of CSA is dependent on the presence of bile in the GI tract, patients should be instructed to separate dosing of bile acid binding resins and CSA by at least 2 hours. For those transplant patients who have hypertriglyceridemia refractory to dietary intervention, fish oil and fibric acid derivatives are well-tolerated, effective alternatives. Gemfibrozil is most effective in lowering serum triglyceride concentrations, but the dose must be reduced in patients with decreased renal function.[155]

Corticosteroids, CSA, and TAC can impair glucose control in previously diabetic patients as well as cause new-onset posttransplant diabetes mellitus (PTDM) in 4% to 20% of patients. Corticosteroids seem to induce insulin resistance and impair peripheral glucose uptake, whereas CSA and TAC appear to inhibit insulin production.[157] Tacrolimus seems to be more diabetogenic than CSA (20% vs 7%).[62] Patients with PTDM should be referred for nutritional counseling and advised on the merits of weight loss (if appropriate). There are, however, some special considerations in renal transplant patients. Up to 40% of patients with PTDM will require insulin therapy.[157] In diabetic patients who can be managed with an oral hypoglycemic agent, glipizide, which is extensively metabolized by the liver, may be preferred over renally eliminated agents such as glyburide. Metformin should be avoided because of the risk of accumulation and lactic acidosis in those with moderate renal impairment. Regardless of therapy, frequent blood glucose monitoring is imperative in the early postoperative phase, both to improve glucose control and to identify those with PTDM. Early posttransplant, variable renal function secondary to DGF or rejection is common. Changes in renal function affect the elimination of many hypoglycemic agents, including insulin, and may result in hyper- or hypoglycemia. Patients and clinicians should also be aware that dose changes of immunosuppressant drugs also affect glycemic control. Tapering of immunosuppressive medications may result in reduced insulin requirements, whereas steroid pulses for the treatment of rejection may result in increased insulin requirements.

MALIGNANCY

Advances in immunosuppression have decreased the incidence of acute rejection and increased patient survival, thus increasing the patient's lifetime exposure to immunosuppression. While the precise mechanism is unclear, posttransplant malignancy seems to be related to the level of immunosuppression, as evidenced by a difference in the rates of malignancy associated with quadruple versus triple versus dual immunosuppressant regimens.[158] Although the introduction of CSA was associated with an increased prevalence of lymphoma in transplant patients versus AZA-based regimens, it is unclear whether this is a direct affect of CSA or is merely related to the level of immunosuppression achieved. Posttransplant malignancies are often divided into three classes: de novo malignancy, recurrent disease, and directly transmitted from donor to recipient. The overall incidence of cancer in renal transplant recipients is 6%, ranging from 4% to 18%. Malignancy increases with the length of follow-up and may affect as many as 72% of patients surviving greater than 20 years. Although the risk of lung, breast, colon, and prostate cancer does not appear to be increased over the general population, Kaposi's sarcoma, squamous cell carcinoma, non-Hodgkin's lymphoma, skin cancer, and cancers of the vulva and perineum do occur more commonly in transplant recipients. In patients with a history of cancer prior to transplantation, recurrence is dependent on both the length of time since cancer treatment and the type of cancer. Most cancers recur in patients who were treated less than 2 years prior to transplantation. Malignancies that recur most frequently are renal carcinoma, malignant melanoma, sarcomas, and nonmelanoma skin cancers. The risk of transmitting a cancer from donor to recipient has decreased secondary to exclusion of donors with a history of malignancy. In the event that a donor malignancy comes to light, postrenal transplant, transplant nephrectomy, and return to dialysis is the most prudent course.[159]

CONCLUSION

Renal transplantation remains the therapy of choice for most patients with ESRD. The development of new immunosuppressive agents and improved immunologic monitoring methods have reduced complications and prolonged graft survival. The importance of pharmacotherapy in the successful management of renal transplant patients has created an opportunity for pharmacists to enhance patient outcomes. Pharmacists are involved in the management of renal transplant patients along the continuum of care. Pharmacists provide patient medication counseling for pretransplant patients in the dialysis unit or pretransplant renal clinic. In the perioperative period, pharmacists assist in the early postoperative management of fluids, electrolytes, infection, hypertension, diabetes, immunosuppression, and general drug dosing in these patients with continuously changing renal function. Long-term, pharmacists manage many of the complications experienced by these patients, including anemia, diabetes, GI disease, hypertension, hyperlipidemia, infection, and osteoporosis. Pharmacists provide patients and family with medication education and compliance monitoring and are frequently an invaluable source of information regarding payment and reimbursement for medication. Although there may be a direct link between these activities and improved patient outcomes, documentation is limited and remains a fertile area for future research.

ACKNOWLEDGMENTS

The authors wish to thank Tracy Anderson, PharmD, and Janice Lovick for their assistance in the preparation of this chapter.

▶ PRINCIPLES OF PHARMACOTHERAPY

- Acute rejection and delayed graft function are the major determinants of graft survival.
- Chronic rejection, the most common cause of late graft loss, is unresponsive to currently available immunosuppressive agents.
- Patient and graft survival rates for renal transplantation have improved significantly so that it is difficult to show differences between treatment regimens. The high cost of new therapies relative to expected improvements needs to be continually evaluated.
- Given the number of immunosuppressive agents currently and soon to be available, immunosuppressive combinations can be tailored based on individual response, adverse effects, cost, and patient acceptance.
- Infection (e.g., CMV, PCP) prophylaxis should be tailored to patient and donor characteristics in addition to the degree of immunosuppression.
- Nephrotoxic agents and those with significant effect on cytochrome P450 3A4 should be used with caution. In addition, they require enhanced monitoring (e.g., S_{cr}, CSA, or TAC levels). In addition to immunologic complications posttransplant, renal transplant recipients are at increased risk for hypertension, hyperlipidemia, and impaired glucose metabolism, all of which are associated with coronary artery disease.
- As the length of patient survival increases, malignancy becomes a significant cause of morbidity and mortality.

REFERENCES

1. U.S. Renal Data System. USRDS 2000 Annual Data Report. Bethesda, MD, National Institutes of Health, National Institute of Diabetes and Digestive and Kidney Diseases, 2000.
2. United Network for Organ Sharing, 1999.
3. Pablo R, Ortega F, Baltar JM, et al. Health-related quality of life (HRQOL) of kidney transplanted patients: Variables that influence it. Clin Transplant 2000;14:199–207.
4. Wolfe RA, Ashby VB, Milford EL, et al. Comparison of mortality in all patients on dialysis, patients on dialysis awaiting transplantation, and recipients of a first cadaveric transplant. N Engl J Med 1999;341:1725–1730.

5. Hariharan S, Johnson CP, Bresnahan BA, Taranto SE, McIntosh MJ, Stablein D. Improved graft survival after renal transplantation in the United States, 1988 to 1996. N Engl J Med 2000;342:605–612.
6. Ojo A, Wolfe RA, Held PJ, Port FK, Schmouder RL. Delayed graft function: Risk factors and implications for renal allograft survival. Transplantation 1997;63:968–974.
7. Suthanthiran M, Strom TB. Renal transplantation. N Engl J Med 1994;331:365–376.
8. Opelz G. Efficacy of rejection prophylaxis with OKT3 in renal transplantation. Collaborative Transplant Study. Transplantation 1995;60:1220–1224.
9. Indudhara R, Khauli RB, Menon M, Stoff JS. Simultaneous quadruple immunosuppression with cyclosporine induction therapy in high-risk renal transplant recipients. J Urol 1994;152:307–311.
10. Burk ML, Matuszewski KA. Muromonab-CD3 and antithymocyte globulin in renal transplantation. Ann Pharmacother 1997;31:1370–1377.
11. Norman DJ, Kahana L, Stuart FP Jr, et al. A randomized clinical trial of induction therapy with OKT3 in kidney transplantation. Transplantation 1993;55:44–50.
12. Shield CF III. Consequences of anti-OKT3 antibody development: OKT3 reuse and long-term graft survival. Transplant Proc 1993;25(suppl 1): 81–82.
13. Darby CR, Moore RH, Shrestha B, et al. Reduced dose OKT3 prophylaxis in sensitised kidney recipients. Transpl Int 1996;9:565–569.
14. Parlevliet KJ, ten Berge RJ, Raasveld MH, et al. Low-dose OKT3 induction therapy following renal transplantation: A controlled study. Nephrol Dial Transplant 1994;9:698–703.
15. Shield CF III, Jacobs RJ, Wyant S, Das A. A cost-effective analysis of OKT3 induction therapy in cadaveric kidney transplantation. Am J Kidney Dis 1996;27:855–864.
16. Vincenti F, Kirkman R, Light S, et al. Interleukin-2-receptor blockade with daclizumab to prevent acute rejection in renal transplantation. N Engl J Med 1998;338:161–165.
17. Nashan B, Moore R, Amlot P, et al. Randomised trial of basiliximab versus placebo for control of acute cellular rejection in renal allograft recipients. Lancet 1997;350:1193–1198.
18. Gaber AO Results of the double-blind, randomized, multicenter phase III clinical trial of Thymoglobulin versus Atgam in the treatment of acute rejections episodes after renal transplantation. Transplantation 1998; 66:29–37.
19. Djamali A, Turc-Baron C, Portales P, et al. Low dose antithymocyte globulins in renal transplantation: Daily versus intermittent administration based on T-cell monitoring. Transplantation 2000;69:799–805.
20. Chagnac A, Zevin D, Ori Y, et al. The effect of high-dose nifedipine on renal hemodynamics of cyclosporine-treated renal allograft recipients. Transplantation 1992;53:766–769.
21. Sorenson SS, Skovbon H, Eiskjr H, Thomsen K, Pedersen EB. Effect of felodipine on renal haemodynamics and tubular sodium handling in cyclosporin-treated renal transplant recipients. Nephrol Dial Transplant 1992;7:69–78.
22. Suthanthiran M, Haschemeyer RH, Riggio RR, et al. Excellent out come with a calcium channel blocker—Supplemented immunosuppressive regimen in cadaveric renal transplantation. Transplantation 1993;55:1008–1013.
23. Khauli RB, Wilson JM, Baker SP, et al. Triple therapy in cadaveric renal transplantation: Role of induction cyclosporine and targeted levels to avoid rejection. J Urol 1995;153:1805–1810.
24. Brockmoller J, Neumayer HH, Wagner K, et al. Pharmacokinetic interaction between cyclosporin and diltiazem. Eur J Clin Pharmacol 1990;38:237–242.
25. Weir MR, Peppler R, Gomolka D, Handwerger BS. Additive inhibition of afferent and efferent immunological responses of human peripheral blood mononuclear cells by verapamil and cyclosporine. Transplantation 1991;51:851–857.
26. Dumont L, Chen H, Daloze P, Xu D, Garceau D. Immunosuppressive properties of the benzothiazepine calcium antagonists diltiazem and clentiazem, with and without cyclosporine, in heterotic rat heart transplantation. Transplantation 1993;56:181–184.
27. Kasiske BL, Johnson HJ, Goerdt PJ, et al. A randomized trial comparing cyclosporine induction with sequential therapy in renal transplant recipients. Am J Kidney Dis 1997;30:639–645.
28. Najarian JS, Fryd DS, Strand M, et al. A single institution, randomized, prospective trial of cyclosporine versus azathioprine-antilymphocyte globulin for immunosuppression in renal allograft recipients. Ann Surg 1985;201:142–157.
29. Andreu J, Campistol JM, Oppenheimer F, et al. Cyclosporine monotherapy as primary immunosuppression in renal transplantation—Five-year experience. Transplant Proc 1994;26:337–340.
30. Tarantino A, Aroldi A, Stucchi L, et al. A randomized prospective trial comparing cyclosporine monotherapy with triple-drug therapy in renal transplantation. Transplantation 1991;52:53–57.
31. Ghoneim MA, Sobh MA, Shokeir AA, et al. Prospective randomized study of azathioprine versus cyclosporin in live-donor kidney transplantation. Am J Nephrol 1993;13:437–441.
32. Amend W, Soskin T, Vincenti F, et al. Long-term experience in primary cadaver renal transplants using cyclosporine. Clin Transplant 1990;4:341–346.
33. Hardie IR, Tiller DJ, Mahony JF, et al. Optimal combination of immunosuppressive agents for renal transplantation: First report of a multicentre, randomized trial comparing cyclosporine+prednisolone with cylcosporine+azathioprine and with triple therapy in cadaver renal transplantation. Transplant Proc 1993;25:583–584.
34. Lindholm A, Albrechtsen D, Tufveson G, et al. A randomized trial of cyclosporine and prednisone versus cyclosporine, azathioprine, and prednisolone in primary cadaveric renal transplantation. Transplantation 1992;54:624–631.
35. Isoniemi H, Ahonen J, Tikkanen MJ, et al. Long-term consequences of different immunosuppressive regimens for renal allografts. Transplantation 1993;55:494–499.
36. Monaco AP, Sahyoun AI, Madras PN, et al. Cyclosporine in multidrug therapy in living-related kidney transplantation. Clin Transplant 1990;4:347–356.
37. Montagnino G, Colturi C, Tarantino A, et al. The impact of azathioprine and cyclosporine on long-term function in kidney transplantation. Transplantation 1991;51:772–776.
38. Slaton JW, Kropp KA, Jhunjhunwala JS, Selman SH. Cyclosporine versus azathioprine: A 5-year follow-up of 200 consecutive cadaver renal transplant recipients. J Urol 1994;151:582–585.
39. Helderman JH, Van Buren DH, Amend WJC Jr, Pirsch JD. Chronic immunosupression of the renal transplant patient. J Am Soc Nephrol 1994;4(suppl 1):S2–S9.
40. Burke JF, Pirsch JD, Ramos EL, et al. Long-term efficacy and safety of cyclosporine in renal- transplant recipients. N Engl J Med 1994;331:358–363.
41. SangCya. FDA approval. RL Williams letter to SangStat Medical Corporation, October 31, 1998. http://www.fda.gov/cder/foi/appletter/1998/64195ltr.pdf.
42. First MR, Alloway R, Schroeder TJ: Development of Sang-35: A cyclosporine formulation bioequivalent to Neoral. Clin Transplant 1998;12:518–524.
43. SangCya. FDA recall. Drugs in the News, News Along the Pike, 2000;6(7):11. http://www.fda.gov/cder/pike/july2000htm.
44. New generic cyclosporine formulations FDA approval. G Buehler letter to Abbott Laboratories dated May 12, 2000. http://www.fda.gov/cder/foi/appletter/200/65003ltr.pdf.
45. J Woodcock letter to Eon Labs Manufacturing, Inc. dated Jan 13, 2000. http://www.fda.gov/cder/foi/appletter/2000/65017ltr.pdf.
46. Drug Topics Redbook. Montvale, NJ, Medical Economics Data, 2001.
47. Lindholm A, Welsh M, Alton C, Kahan BD. Demographic factors influencing cyclosporine pharmacokinetic parameters in patients with uremia: Racial differences in bioavailability. Clin Pharmacol Ther 1992;52:359–371.
48. Ohlman S, Lindholm A, Hagglund H, Sawe J, Kahan BD. On the intraindividual variability and chronobiology of cyclosporine pharmacokinetics in renal transplantation. Eur J Clin Pharmacol 1993;44:265–269.

49. Awni WM, Kasiske BL, Heim-Duthoy KL, Rao KV. Long-term cyclosporine pharmacokinetic changes in renal transplant recipients: Effects of binding and metabolism. Clin Pharmacol Ther 1989;45: 41–48.
50. Kahan BD, Shaw LM, Holt D, Grevel J, Johnston A. Consensus document: Hawk's Cay meeting on therapeutic drug monitoring of cyclosporine. Clin Chem 1990;36:1510–1516.
51. Dumont RJ, Ensom MH. Methods for clinical monitoring on cyclosporin in transplant patients. Clin Pharmacokinet 2000;38:427–447.
52. Grevel J, Kahan BD. Abbreviated kinetic profiles in area-under-the-curve monitoring of cyclosporine therapy. Clin Chem 1991;37:1905–1908.
53. Lindholm A, Kahan BD. Influence of cyclosporine pharmacokinetics, trough concentrations, and AUC monitoring on outcome after kidney transplantation. Clin Pharmacol Ther 1993;54:205–218.
54. Serafinowicz A, Gaciong Z, Majchrzak J, et al. Abbreviated kinetic profiles to estimate exposure to CyA in renal allograft recipients treated with Sandimmun-Neoral. Transplant Proc 1997;29:277–279.
55. Campana C, Regazzi MB, Buggia I, Molinaro M. Clinically significant drug interactions with cyclosporin: An update. Clin Pharmacokinet 1996;30:141–179.
56. Jordan ML, Naraghi R, Shapiro R, et al. Tacrolimus rescue therapy for renal allograft rejection—Five-year experience. Transplantation 1997; 63:223–228.
57. Laskow DA, Neylan JFIII, Shapiro RS, et al. The role of tacrolimus in adult kidney transplantation: A review. Clin Transplant 1998;12:489–503.
58. Shapiro R, Jordan M, Scantlebury VP. Renal transplantation at the University of Pittsburgh: Impact of FK 506. In: Terasaki PI, Cecka JM, eds. Clinical Transplants. Los Angeles, UCLA Tissue Typing Laboratory, 1995:229–236.
59. Johnson C, Ahsan N, Gonwa T, et al. Randomized trial of tacrolimus (Prograf) in combination with azathioprine or mycophenolate mofetil versus cyclosporine (Neoral) with mycophenolate mofetil after cadaveric kidney transplantation. Transplantation 2000;69:834–841.
60. Gjertson DW, Cecka JM, Terasaki PI. The relative effects of FK506 and cyclosporine on short- and long-term kidney graft survival. Transplantation 1995;60:1384–1388.
61. Vincenti F, Laskow DA, Neylan JF, Mendez R, Matas AJ. One-year follow-up of an open-label trial of FK506 for primary kidney transplantation. Transplantation 1996;61:1576–1581.
62. Plosker GL, Foster RH. Tacrolimus: A further update of is pharmacology and therapeutic use in the management of organ transplantation. Drugs 2000;59:323–389.
63. Katari SR, Magnone M, Shapiro R, et al. Clinical features of acute reversible tacrolimus (FK506) nephrotoxicity in kidney transplant recipients. Clin Transplant 1997;11:237–242.
64. Hohage H, Arlt M, Brückner D, et al. Effects of cyclosporin A and FK 506 on lipid metabolism and fibrinogen in kidney transplant recipients. Clin Transplant 1997;11:225–230.
65. Bullingham RES, Nicholls AJ, Kamm BR. Clinical pharmacokinetics of mycophenolate mofetil. Clin Pharmacokinet 1998;34:429–455.
66. European Mycophenolate Mofetil Cooperative Study Group. Placebo-controlled study of mycophenolate mofetil combined with cyclosporin and corticosteroids for prevention of acute rejection. Lancet 1995;345:1321–1325.
67. The Tricontinental Mycophenolate Mofetil Renal Transplantation Study Group. A blinded, randomized clinical trial of mycophenolate mofetil for the prevention of acute rejection in cadaveric renal transplantation. Transplantation 1996;61:1029–1037.
68. Sollinger HW. Mycophenolate mofetil for the prevention of acute rejection in primary cadaveric renal allograft recipients. Transplantation 1995;60:225–232.
69. Gonwa TA. Mycophenolate mofetil for maintenance therapy in kidney transplantation. Clin Transplant 1996;10:128–130.
70. Halloran P, Mathew T, Tomlanovich S, et al. Mycophenolate mofetil in renal allograft recipients: A pooled efficacy analysis of three randomized, double-blind, clinical studies in prevention of rejection. Transplantation 1997;63:39–47.
71. Tomlanovich S, Cho S, Hodge E, et al. Mycophenolate mofetil in cadaveric renal transplantation: 3-year data. Am Soc Transpl Physicians 1997;361. Abstract.
72. The International Mycophenolate Mofetil Study Group. A long-term randomized multicenter study of mycophenolate mofetil (MMF) in cadaveric renal transplantation: Results at 3 years. Am Soc Transpl Physicians 1997;362. Abstract.
73. Pescovitz MD, Conti D, Dunn J, et al. Intravenous mycophenolate mofetil: Safety, tolerability, and pharmacokinetics. Clin Transplant 2000; 14:179–188.
74. Johnson HJ, Swan SK, Heim-Duthoy KL, et al. The pharmacokinetics of a single dose of mycophenolate mofetil in patients with various degrees of renal function. Clin Pharmacol Ther 1998;63:512–518.
75. Simmons WD, Rayhill SC, Sollinger HW. Preliminary risk-benefit assessment of mycophenolate mofetil in transplant rejection. Drug Saf 1997;17:75–92.
76. Wolfe EJ, Mathur V, Tomlanovich S, et al. Pharmacokinetics of mycophenolate mofetil and intravenous ganciclovir alone and in combination in renal transplant recipients. Pharmacotherapy 1997;17:591–598.
77. Sullivan SD, Garrison LP Jr, Best JH, Members of the U.S. Renal Transplant Mycophenolate Mofetil Study Group. The cost effectiveness of mycophenolate mofetil in the first year after primary cadaveric transplant. J Am Soc Nephrol 1997;8:1592–1598.
78. Keown PA, Sullivan SD, Best JH, Garrison LP, Krueger H. Economic evaluation of mycophenolate mofetil (MMF) for prevention of acute graft rejection after cadaveric renal transplantation in Canada. Am Soc Transpl Physicians 1997;620. Abstract.
79. Morris RE, Wang J, Blum JR, et al. Immunosuppressive effects of the morpholinoethyl ester of mycophenolic acid (RS-61443) in rat and nonhuman primate recipients of heart allografts. Transplant Proc 1991;23(suppl 2):19–25.
80. Steele DM, Hullett DA, Bechstein WO, et al. Effects of immunosuppressive therapy on the rat aortic allograft model. Transplant Proc 1993;25 (pt 1):754–755.
81. Smith MT, Newby BS, Rao RN, et al. Response to MMF in patients with chronic renal allograft rejection. American Society of Transplant Physicians, Annual Meeting, Chicago, May 10–14, 1997. Abstract.
82. Ojo AO, Meier-Kriesche HU, Hanson JA, et al. Mycophenolate mofetil reduces late renal allograft loss independent of acute rejection. Transplantation 2000;69:2405–2409.
83. Vasquez EM. Sirolimus: A new agent for prevention of renal allograft rejection. Am J Health Syst Pharm 2000;57:437–451.
84. Kahan BD. Efficacy of sirolimus compared with azathioprine for reduction of acute renal allograft rejection: A randomised multicentre study. Lancet 2000;356:194–202.
85. Neumayer H-H, Paradis K, Korn A, et al. Entry-into-human study with the novel immunosuppressant SDZ RAD in stable renal transplant recipients. Br J Clin Pharmacol 1999;48:694–703.
86. Suthanthiran M, Strom TB. Mechanisms and management of acute renal allograft rejection. Surg Clin North Am 1998;78:77–94.
87. The Mycophenolate Mofetil Renal Refractory Rejection Study Group. Mycophenolate mofetil for the treatment of refractory, acute, cellular renal transplant rejection. Transplantation 1996;61:722–729.
88. Mele TS, Halloran PF. The use of mycophenolate mofetil in transplant recipients. Immunopharmacology 2000;47:215–245.
89. Ortho Multicenter Transplant Study Group. A randomized clinical trial of OKT3 monoclonal antibody for acute rejection of cadaveric renal transplants. N Engl J Med 1985;313:337–342.
90. Tesi RJ, Elkhammas EA, Henry ML, Ferguson RM. OKT3 for primary therapy of the first rejection episode in kidney transplants. Transplantation 1993;55:1023–1029.
91. Oh C-S, Stratta RJ, Fox BC, et al. Increased infections associated with the use of OKT3 for treatment of steroid-resistant rejection in renal transplantation. Transplantation 1988;45:68–73.
92. Vasquez EM, Benedetti E, Pollak R. Ethnic differences in clinical response to corticosteroid treatment of acute allograft rejection. Transplant 2001;71:229–233.

93. Matl I, Lacha J, Lodererova A, Simova M, Teplan V, Lanska V, Vitko S: Withdrawal of steroids from triple-drug therapy in kidney transplant patients. Nephrol Dial Transplant 2000;15:1041–1045.
94. Ratcliffe PJ, Dudley CR, Higgins RM, Firth JD, Smith B, Morris PJ: Randomised controlled trial of steroid withdrawal in renal transplant recipients receiving triple immunosuppression. Lancet 1996;348:643–648.
95. Sanfey H, Haussman G, Isaacs I, Ishitani M, Lobo P, McCullough C, Pruett T: Steroid withdrawal in kidney transplant recipients: Is it a safe option? Clin Transplant 1997;11:500–504.
96. Dunn T, Asolati M, Holman D, et al. Long-term outcome of kidney transplantation after steroid withdrawal. Transplant Proc 1998;30:1788–1789.
97. Sandrini S, Maiorca R, Scolari F, et al. A prospective randomized trial on azathioprine addition to cyclosporine versus cyclosporine monotherapy at steroid withdrawal, 6 months after renal transplantation. Transplantation 2000;69:1861–1867.
98. Hollander AA, Hene RJ, Hermans J, van Es LA, van der Woude FJ. Late prednisone withdrawal in cyclosporine-treated kidney transplant patients: A randomized study. J Am Soc Nephrol 1997;8:294–301.
99. Hricik DE, O'Toole MA, Schulak JA, Herson J. Steroid-free immunosuppression in cyclosporine-treated renal transplant recipients: A meta-analysis. J Am Soc Nephrol 1993;4:1300–1305.
100. Kasiske BL, Chakkera HA, Louis TA, Ma JZ. A meta-analysis of immunosuppression withdrawal trials in renal transplantation. J Am Soc Nephrol 2000;11:1910–1917.
101. Shapiro R, Jordan ML, Scantlebury VP, et al. Outcome after steroid withdrawal in renal transplant patients receiving tacrolimus-based immunosuppression. Transplant Proc 1998;30:1375–1377.
102. Grinyo JM, Gil-Vernet S, Seron D, et al. Steroid withdrawal in mycophenolate mofetil-treated renal allograft recipients. Transplantation 1997;63:1688–1690.
103. Kupin W, Venkat KK, Goggins M, et al. Improved outcome of steroid withdrawal in mycophenolate mofetil-treated primary cadaveric renal transplant recipients. Transplant Proc 1999;31:1131–1132.
104. Lebranchu Y, Aubert P, Bayle F, et al. Could steroids be withdrawn in renal transplant patients sequentially treated with ATG, cyclosporine, and CellCept? One-year results of a double-blind, randomized, multicenter study comparing normal dose versus low-dose and withdrawal of steroids. French Study Group. Transplant Proc 2000;32:396–397.
105. Ahsan N, Hricik D, Matas A, et al. Prednisone withdrawal in kidney transplant recipients on cyclosporine and mycophenolate mofetil—A prospective randomized study. Steroid Withdrawal Study Group. Transplantation 1999;68:1865–1874.
106. Chakrabarti P, Wong HY, Scantlebury VP, et al. Outcome after steroid withdrawal in pediatric renal transplant patients receiving tacrolimus-based immunosuppression. Transplantation 2000;70:760–764.
107. Tarantino A, Montagnino G, Ponticelli C. Corticosteroids in kidney transplant recipients. Safety issues and timing of discontinuation. Drug Saf 1995;13:145–156.
108. Kasiske BL, Heim-Duthoy K, Ma JZ. Elective cyclosporine withdrawal after renal transplantation. A meta-analysis. JAMA 1993;269:395–400.
109. Heim-Duthoy KL, Chitwood KK, Tortorice KL, Massy ZA, Kasiske BL. Elective cyclosporine withdrawal 1 year after renal transplantation. Am J Kidney Dis 1994;24:846–853.
110. Smith SR, Minda SA, Samsa GP, et al. Late withdrawal of cyclosporine in stable renal transplant recipients. Am J Kidney Dis 1995;26:487–494.
111. Chew-Wong A, Alberu J, Abasta-Jimenez M, Alvarez-Sandoval E, Gabilondo-Navarro F, Correa-Rotter R. Withdrawal versus continuous cyclosporine therapy in kidney transplant recipients of one-haplotype-matched donors. Transplant Proc 19999;31:1106–1109.
112. Saadi MG, Francis MR, Selim OE. Five-year follow-up of early post-renal transplantation cyclosporin withdrawal: Do we benefit from a state of tolerance? Transplant Proc 1997;29:2593–2595.
113. Keitel E, Michelon T, Dominguez V, et al. Long-term evaluation of two protocols of elective cyclosporine withdrawal in renal transplant recipients. Transplant Proc 1999;31:3013–3015.
114. Hilbrands LB, Hoitsma AJ, Koene KA. Randomized, prospective trial of cyclosporine monotherapy versus azathioprine-prednisone from three months after renal transplantation. Transplantation 1996;61:1038–1046.
115. Hilbrands LB, Hoitsma AG, Wetzels JF, Koene RA. Detailed study of changes in renal function after conversion from cyclosporine to azathioprine. Clin Nephrol 1996;45:230–235.
116. MacPhee IA, Bradley JA, Briggs JD, et al. Long-term outcome of a prospective randomized trial of conversion from cyclosporine to azathioprine treatment one year after renal transplantation. Transplantation 1998;66:1186–1192.
117. Hollander AA, van Saase JL, Kootte AM, et al. Beneficial effects of conversion from cyclosporin to azathioprine after kidney transplantation. Lancet 1995;345:610–614.
118. Schrama YC, Joles JA, van Tol A, Boer P, Koomans HA, Hene RJ. Conversion to mycophenolate mofetil in conjunction with stepwise withdrawal of cyclosporine in stable renal transplant recipients. Transplantation 2000;69:376–383.
119. Fishman JA, Rubin RH. Infection in organ-transplant recipients. N Engl J Med 1998;338:1741–1751.
120. Hebart H, Kanz L, Jahn G, Einsel H. Management of cytomegalovirus infection after solid-organ or stem-cell transplantation. Drugs 1998;55: 59–72.
121. Uber L, Cofer J, Baliga P, Rajagopalan PR. Effectiveness of combination prophylaxis with cytomegalovirus hyperimmune globulin and acyclovir in the high-risk kidney transplant recipient. Transplant Proc 1995;27:42–43.
122. Patel R, Snydman DR, Rubin RH, et al. Cytomegalovirus prophylaxis in solid organ transplant recipients. Transplantation 1996;61:1279–1289.
123. Dickinson BI, Gora-Harper ML, McCraney SA, Gosland M. Studies evaluating high-dose acyclovir, intravenous immune globulin, and cytomegalovirus hyperimmunoglobulin for prophylaxis against cytomegalovirus in kidney transplant recipients. Ann Pharmacother 1996;30:1452–1464.
124. Balfour HH Jr, Chace BA, Stapleton JT, Simmons RL, Fryd DS. A randomized, placebo-controlled trial of oral acyclovir for the prevention of cytomegalovirus disease in recipients of renal allografts. N Engl J Med 1989;320:1381–1387.
125. Birkeland S, Gahrn-Hansen B, Andersen H, el al. Cytomegalovirus prophylaxis in antibody-treated renal transplanted patients. Transplant Proc 1995;27:3473–3476.
126. Legendre C, Ducloux D, Ferroni A, et al. Acyclovir in preventing cytomegalovirus infection in kidney transplant recipients: A case-controlled study. Transplant Proc 1993;25:1431–1433.
127. Kletzmayr J, Kotzmann H, Popow-Kraupp T, Kovarik J, Klauser R. Impact of high-dose oral acyclovir prophylaxis on cytomegalovirus (CMV) disease in CMV high-risk renal transplant recipients. J Am Soc Nephrol 1996;7:325–330.
128. Rubin RH, Tolkoff-Rubin NE. Antimicrobial strategies in the care of organ transplant recipients. Antimicrob Agents Chemother 1993;37:619–624.
129. Product Information. Valtrex (valacyclovir hydrochloride) caplets. Glaxo SmithKline 1997.
130. Flynn JT, Kaiser BA, Long SS, et al. Intravenous immunoglobulin prophylaxis of cytomegalovirus infection in pediatric renal transplant recipients. Am J Nephrol 1997;17:146–152.
131. Conti DJ, Freed BM, Gruber SA, Lempert N. Prophylaxis of primary cytomegalovirus disease in renal transplant recipients. Arch Surg 1994;129:443–447.
132. Snydman DR, Werner BG, Heinze-Lacey B, et al. Use of cytomegalovirus immune globulin to prevent cytomegalovirus disease in renal transplant recipients. N Engl J Med 1987;317:1049–1054.
133. Product Information. CytoGam (cytomegalovirus immune globulin intravenous—human). Med Immune 1996.
134. Tsevat J, Snydman DR, Pauker SG, et al. Which renal transplant patients should receive cytomegalovirus immune globulin? A cost-effective analysis. Transplantation 1991;52:259–265.

135. Carrieri G, Jordan ML, Shapiro R, et al. Acyclovir/cytomegalovirus immune globulin combination therapy for CMV prophylaxis in high-risk renal allograft recipients. Transplant Proc 1995;27:961–963.
136. Rondeau E, Bourgeon B, Peraldi MN, et al. Effect of prophylactic ganciclovir on cytomegalovirus infection in renal transplant recipients. Nephrol Dial Transplant 1993;8:858–862.
137. Gomez E, de Ona M, Aguado S, et al. Cytomegalovirus preemptive therapy with ganciclovir in renal transplant patients treated with OKT3. Nephron 1996;74:367–372.
138. Hibberd PL, Tolkoff-Rubin NE, Conti D, et al. Preemptive ganciclovir therapy to prevent cytomegalovirus disease in cytomegalovirus antibody-positive renal transplant recipients—A randomized controlled trial. Ann Intern Med 1995;123:18–26.
139. Gotti E, Suter F, Baruzzo S, et al. Early ganciclovir therapy effectively controls viremia and avoids the need for cytomegalovirus (CMV) prophylaxis in renal transplant patients with cytomegalovirus antigenemia. Clin Transplant 1996;10:550–555.
140. Brennan DC, Garlock KA, Lippmann BA, et al. Control of cytomegalovirus-associated morbidity in renal transplant patients using intensive monitoring and either preemptive or deferred therapy. J Am Soc Nephrol 1997;8:118–125.
141. Noble S, Faulds D. Ganciclovir. An update of its use in the prevention of cytomegalovirus infection and disease in transplant recipients. Drugs 1998;56:115–146.
142. Plotkin SA, Higgins RM, Kurtz JB, et al. Multicenter trial of Towne strain attenuated virus vaccine in seronegative renal transplant recipients. Transplantation 1994;58:1176–1178.
143. Jordan ML, Hrebinko RL Jr, Dummer JS, et al. Therapeutic use of ganciclovir for invasive cytomegalovirus infection in cadaveric renal allograft recipients. J Urol 1992;148:1388–1392.
144. Andersson J, Akesson-Johansson A, Brattstrom C. Evaluation by immune scanning electron microscopy of foscarnet treatment of cytomegalovirus infection in patients with renal transplants. Scand J Infect Dis 1989;21:605–610.
145. Seale L, Jones CJ, Kathpalia S, et al. Prevention of herpesvirus infections in renal allograft recipients by low-dose oral acyclovir. JAMA 1985;254:3435–3438.
146. Higgins RM, Bloom SL, Hopkin JM, Morris PJ. The risks and benefits of low-dose cotrimoxazole prophylaxis for *Pneumocystis* pneumonia in renal transplantation. Transplantation 1989;47:558–560.
147. Hughes WT, Rivera GK, Schell MJ, Thornton D, Lott L. Successful intermittent chemoprophylaxis for *Pneumocystis carinii* pneumonitis. N Engl J Med 1987;316:1627–1632.
148. Saukkonen K, Garland R, Koziel H. Aerosolized pentamidine as alternative primary prophylaxis against *Pneumocystis carinii* pneumonia in adult hepatic and renal transplant recipients. Chest 1996;109:1250–1255.
149. Levine SJ, Masur H, Gill VJ, et al. Effect of aerosolized pentamidine prophylaxis on the diagnosis of *Pneumocystis carinii* pneumonia by induced sputum examination in patients infected with the human immunodeficiency virus. Am Rev Respir Dis 1991;144:760–764.
150. Kemper CA, Tucker RM, Lang OS, et al. Low-dose dapsone prophylaxis of *Pneumocystis carinii* pneumonia in AIDS and AIDS-related complex. AIDS 1990;4:1145–1148.
151. Kasiske BL. Cardiovascular disease after renal transplantation. Semin Nephrol 2000;20:176–187.
152. Mailloux LU, Levey AS. Hypertension in patients with chronic renal disease. Am J Kidney Dis 1998;32:S120–S141.
153. The sixth report of the Joint National Committee on prevention, detection, evaluation, and treatment of high blood pressure. Arch Intern Med 1997;157:2413–2446.
154. Pesavento TE, Jones PA, Julian BA, Curtis JJ. Amlodipine increases cyclosporine levels in hypertensive renal transplant patients: Results of a prospective study. J Am Soc Nephrol 1996; 7:831–835.
155. Massy ZA, Kasiske BL. Post-transplant hyperlipidemia: Mechanisms and management. J Am Soc Nephrol 1996; 7:971–977.
156. Massy ZA, Guijarro C, Wiederkehr MR, Ma JZ, Kasiske BL. Chronic renal allograft rejection: Immunologic and nonimmunologic risk factors. Kidney Int 1996;49:518–524.
157. Jindal RM, Sidner RA, Milgrom ML. Post-transplant diabetes mellitus: The role of immunosuppression. Drug Saf 1997;16:242–257.
158. Opelz G, Schwarz V, Wujciak T, et al. Analysis of non-Hodgkin's lymphomas in organ transplant recipients. Transplant Rev 1995;9:231–240.
159. Penn I. The problem of cancer in organ transplant recipients: An overview. Transplant Sci 1994;4:23–32.

47

HEMODIALYSIS AND PERITONEAL DIALYSIS

Gary R. Matzke and George R. Bailie

Hemodialysis (HD) and peritoneal dialysis (PD) are the major treatment options for patients with end-stage renal disease (ESRD). During the 1980s, the use of PD showed a steep increase; however, from 1988 to 1996, the percent increase per year for PD and HD patients was nearly the same.[1] The proportion of patients started on PD has declined each year since 1996. Thus, at the end of 1999 about 210,000 patients in the United States received maintenance hemodialysis. Just over 22,000 patients received some form of peritoneal dialysis. The percent of dialysis patients who receive peritoneal dialysis varies enormously among countries, from 5% to 10% in Japan and Germany, to over 30% in New Zealand, Australia, and Canada.[2] There are several reasons for these differences, including the difference in costs between PD and HD, availability of equipment and trained personnel, political pressures, and physician and patient preferences.[3]

In the United States, it is projected that the number of dialysis patients will exceed 600,000 by the year 2010, assuming that the growth rate of about 7% to 9% per year observed during the 1990s continues.[4] The number of kidney transplants performed each year has remained relatively static over the last 5 to 10 years at about 8,000 to 10,000, while the number of patients with ESRD awaiting transplants has increased sharply from 10,000 in 1986 to more than 39,000 in 1998.[4] The limited availability of transplantation as a treatment option for patients with ESRD has thus compounded the demand for chronic renal replacement therapy.

Although there are several major mechanical and technical differences between HD and PD, comparative mortality studies have shown inconsistent results.[5–10] Bloembergen et al.[5,6] found that there was a 19% increase in the relative risk of death of U.S. peritoneal dialysis patients as compared to those receiving hemodialysis, and that peritoneal dialysis patients had more deaths as a result of infections, acute myocardial infarctions, other cardiac causes, and cerebrovascular diseases. The results of two Canadian studies highlight the extent of the current controversy. Fenton et al.[7] retrospectively compared mortality rates of HD and continuous ambulatory (CAPD) or continuous cycling peritoneal dialysis (CCPD) patients who started therapy between 1990 and 1994. They reported that the mortality rate in CAPD/CCPD patients was significantly lower than that observed in HD patients; the mortality rate ratio (MRR) was 0.73 (PD/HD). This protective effect was most evident in the first 2 years of therapy, as demonstrated by the finding of similar 5-year survival probabilities of approximately 35%. Foley and colleagues[8] prospectively followed a cohort of PD and HD patients who initiated dialysis therapy between 1984 and 1991. They reported that there was no difference in mortality rate among PD patients during the first 2 years (17.8% of PD patients versus 16.5% of HD patients died during the first 2 years). However, after 2 years the mortality rate in the PD group was significantly greater than in the HD patients (MRR = 1.57). These "differences" in outcome may be related to a multiplicity of factors, such as the dose of dialysis, physician bias in selection of the initial mode of therapy, patient compliance, and unmeasured comorbidities, such as hyperlipidemia or degree of diabetic control.[9] Cardiovascular events account for 25% to 40% of deaths in HD and PD patients, whereas peritonitis is the second most common cause of mortality among peritoneal dialysis patients. Of patients leaving PD, the major reasons are death or transfer to hemodialysis because of inadequacy or frequent episodes of peritonitis.[8,10] Thus, the selection of the optimal therapy for a given patient must be individualized.

Irrespective of the mode of chronic renal replacement therapy, the life expectancy of U.S. dialysis patients is markedly lower than that of healthy subjects of the same age and gender. Although, age- and sex-matched ESRD patients have about 20% to 25% of the expected remaining lifetime of the general population,[11] their first year mortality rate has fallen 38.5% in the last decade from a rate of 29.9% in 1988.[12] The data from the Canada-USA PD study group indicate that the 2-year survival probability was 79.7% for Canadian patients and 63.2% for U.S. patients.[13] The relative risk of death was, thus, almost twofold higher for U.S. patients. Possible reasons for these observations include increased age, the number of comorbid conditions including cardiovascular diseases and diabetes, modality selection bias, and malnutrition among U.S. patients. The higher acceptance rate for dialysis in the United States may also be a factor, as well as the dose of the dialytic therapy.[14]

Morbidity can be grossly assessed by the number of hospitalizations per patient-year, the number of days hospitalized, or the incidence of certain complications such as cardiovascular events.[15] Early comparative studies demonstrated more hospitalized days with PD (21.9 vs. 17.3 per year), but the policy at that time was for inpatient treatment of peritonitis. Because many PD infections are now treated on an outpatient basis, the number of hospital days is dramatically lower than for HD patients in some centers.[16] Hospitalizations are more frequent for whites than for blacks, and the frequency and duration increase with age in both groups. Vascular access problems and cardiovascular complications are now the most common reasons for hospital admission. Cardiovascular morbidity (especially arrhythmias and hypotensive episodes) is significantly reduced with PD, and cardiac performance appears to be improved, as evidenced by decreases in intraventricular septum and left ventricular mass index and the lower incidence of pericarditis.[8]

In recognition of the high morbidity and mortality of dialysis patients, the Health Care Financing Administration (HCFA), in 1993, developed a series of health-care quality improvement programs to evaluate various aspects of dialysis care. Now called the Clinical Performance Measures Project, it examines markers of the quality of care (anemia management, serum albumin, vascular access (for hemodialysis), and adequacy of dialysis). The most recent annual report studied a sample population of about 8,838 HD and 1,650 PD patients. Although improvements in the indicators have been reported, there is still much opportunity for further improvement.[17] For example, in 1998, only 52% of PD patients had hematocrit values in the target range (hemoglobin of 11–12 g/dL). More than 40% of PD patients had an inadequate nutritional status, defined as a serum albumin of less than 3.5 g/dL (bromcresol green [BCG] method of assay), or 35%, if defined as less than 3.2 g/dL (bromcresol purple [BCP] method).

The pharmacotherapy regimens of ESRD patients are extremely complicated because of the multiplicity of concomitant diseases, as well as the dialysis-associated complications that develop. Although the average hemodialysis and peritoneal dialysis patient is prescribed eight scheduled and three or more as-needed medications,[18,19] the efficacy of these agents may be limited by inappropriate duplications[20] and poor compliance because of a lack of understanding by the patient of why, when, and how they should take their medication.[18,21] The number of drug-related problems in the dialysis population is large,[22] and is exacerbated when dialysis outpatients undergo hospitalization.[23] In the 1990s, several models of pharmaceutical care were implemented to enhance the outcome of ESRD patients in the institutional and ambulatory environment.[24,25] The success of these programs remains to be determined.

This chapter is a primer on the principles and practice of dialysis. The multiple types of catheters and other accesses for HD and PD are described. The variants of HD and PD are detailed in light of the fact that dialysis by either route is not a generic procedure. The "optimal" dose of dialysis for each patient population is reviewed, and methodologies to quantitate what dose of dialysis an individual patient receives are described. Finally, the complications of both dialytic therapies are presented, along with pertinent nonpharmacologic and pharmacologic therapeutic alternatives.

INDICATIONS FOR DIALYSIS

Dialysis should be initiated electively rather than urgently in patients with chronic renal disease (see Chap. 45). Because of the progressive nature of the disease, the need for dialysis should begin to be planned for once the patient's creatinine clearance (CLcr) drops below 25 mL/min. Although some patients may be symptom free with this degree of renal function, many patients reduce their dietary protein intake and this reduction may result in malnutrition.[26] Beginning the preparation process at this point, if possible, should allow adequate time for proper education of the patient and family and for the creation of a suitable vascular or peritoneal access.

The primary criterion for initiation is the patient's clinical status: the presence of persistent anorexia, nausea, and vomiting, especially if accompanied by weight loss, declining serum albumin levels, uncontrolled hypertension or congestive heart failure, and neurologic deficits or pruritus (see Chap. 45). Patients are generally not started on dialysis until their serum creatinine or blood urea nitrogen (BUN) level reaches a critical value. However, if they have one or more of the signs or symptoms listed above, the National Kidney Foundation's Dialysis Outcomes Qualitative Initiative (NKF-K/DOQI) guidelines suggest that nondiabetic patients should be started when their CLcr is 9–14 mL/min/1.73 m^2. Diabetics may need to be started earlier.[26] Table 47–1 lists the advantages and disadvantages of hemodialysis while those for peritoneal dialysis are delineated in Table 47–2. These factors along with the patients' concomitant diseases, preferences, and support environments are the principle determinants of the dialysis mode they will receive. Finally, the initiation of dialysis in the ambulatory setting before the onset of severe complications such as pericarditis, encephalopathy, or pulmonary edema will also result in significant cost savings as compared with the initiation of dialysis in an acute care environment.

TABLE 47–1. Advantages and Disadvantages of Hemodialysis

Advantages

1. Higher solute clearance allows intermittent treatment.
2. Parameters of adequacy of dialysis are better defined and therefore underdialysis can be detected early.
3. Technique failure rate is low.
4. Even though intermittent heparinization is required, hemostasis parameters are better corrected with hemodialysis than peritoneal dialysis.
5. In-center hemodialysis enables closer monitoring of the patient.

Disadvantages

1. Requires multiple visits each week to the hemodialysis center, which translates into loss of control by the patient.
2. Disequilibrium, dialysis hypotension, and muscle cramps are common. May require months before the patient adjusts to hemodialysis.
3. Infections in hemodialysis patients may be related to the choice of membranes, the complement-activating membranes being more deleterious.
4. Vascular access is frequently associated with infection and thrombosis.
5. Decline of residual renal function is more rapid compared to peritoneal dialysis.

TABLE 47–2. Advantages and Disadvantages of Peritoneal Dialysis

Advantages

1. More hemodynamic stability (blood pressure) due to slow ultrafiltration rate.
2. Increased clearance of larger solutes, which may explain good clinical status in spite of lower urea clearance.
3. Better preservation of residual renal function.
4. Convenient intraperitoneal route of administration of drugs such as antibiotics and insulin.
5. Suitable for elderly and very young patients who may not tolerate HD well.
6. Freedom from the "machine" gives the patient a sense of independence (for continuous ambulatory peritoneal dialysis).
7. Less blood loss and iron deficiency, resulting in easier management of anemia or reduced requirements for erythropoietin and parenteral iron.
8. No systemic heparinization requirement.
9. Subcutaneous versus intravenous erythropoietin or darbepoetin is usual, which may reduce overall doses and be more physiologic.

Disadvantages

1. Protein and amino acid losses through peritoneum and reduced appetite owing to continuous glucose load and sense of abdominal fullness predispose to malnutrition.
2. Risk of peritonitis.
3. Catheter malfunction, exit site, and tunnel infection.
4. Inadequate ultrafiltration and solute dialysis in patients with a large body size, unless large volumes and frequent exchanges are employed.
5. Patient burnout and high rate of technique failure.
6. Risk of obesity with excessive glucose absorption.
7. Mechanical problems such as hernias, dialysate leaks, hemorrhoids, or back pain may occur.
8. Extensive abdominal surgery may preclude peritoneal dialysis.
9. No convenient access for intravenous iron administration.

HEMODIALYSIS

PRINCIPLES OF HEMODIALYSIS

Fundamentally, hemodialysis consists of the perfusion of heparinized blood and physiologic salt solution on opposite sides of a semipermeable membrane. Nitrogenous waste products such as urea and creatinine and other uremic toxins move from the blood into the dialysate by passive diffusion along concentration gradients and or convection. The rate of diffusion depends on the difference between the concentrations of solute in blood and dialysate, solute characteristics, the dialyzer composition, and blood and dialysate flow rates. The second process that occurs during dialysis is convection or ultrafiltration; this is the primary means for removal of excess body water. Convection (expressed as mL of plasma water removed per hour per mm Hg of pressure within the dialyzer) can be maximized by increasing the hydrostatic pressure gradient across the dialysis membrane, or by changing to a dialyzer that is more permeable to water transport. Those solutes that are dissolved in plasma water will be removed along with water if the pores in the dialyzer are large enough to allow them to pass. These two processes can be controlled independently, and thus a patient's hemodialysis prescription can be individualized to attain the desired degree of solute (urea) removal and fluid balance.

VASCULAR ACCESS

Permanent access to the bloodstream for hemodialysis may be accomplished by several techniques[27] (Fig. 47–1). The native arteriovenous fistula (AV fistula) has the longest survival of all blood-access devices and is associated with the lowest rate of complications. However, this access requires about 2 months or more for the venous limb of the access to "mature," that is, to dilate as the result of the increased pressure, before it can be used. This type of access is now used less frequently than in the past, especially in diabetic patients, because of peripheral vascular disease and indiscriminate use of the peripheral veins.

Synthetic arteriovenous vascular grafts are now the chronic access initially used for most patients. Although these grafts can be made from multiple materials, polytetrafluoroethylene (PTFE) is the agent of choice and is now used as the initial access in more than 60% of patients.[28] PTFE grafts require only 2 to 3 weeks to endothelialize before they can be routinely used. The primary disadvantages of this type of access are the shorter survival and the fact that they have higher rates of infection and thrombosis than do native AV fistulas.

Double-lumen or twin single-lumen catheters with Dacron cuffs are now commonly used for long-term, temporary or permanent vascular access. These catheters are excellent choices for small children, diabetic patients with severe vascular disease, the morbidly obese, and those patients who have no remaining sites for arteriovenous access. The addition of Dacron cuffs was designed to stabilize the catheter placement, to reduce the incidence of infection, and to prolong the time period of use from several weeks to 6 months or more.

The choice of vascular access type is dependent not only on the adequacy of the patient's vasculature but also on how soon the patient will require hemodialysis.[29] Acute dialysis access can be achieved by the insertion of a dual-lumen or two single-lumen catheters into the internal jugular, subclavian, or femoral vein. Once placed, these devices can be used immediately and for up to several months as the bridge between temporary and permanent access for patients with ESRD. The primary complications associated with all vascular accesses are infection, thrombosis, and stenosis.[27,29] Optimal approaches for the treatment of these complications have been proposed and Table 47–3 outlines the specific recommendations of the NKF-K/DOQI working group for the treatment of infection.

HEMODIALYSIS PROCEDURES

Hemodialysis consists of an external vascular circuit through which the patient's blood is transferred in sterile polyethylene tubing to the dialysis filter (dialyzer) via a mechanical pump (Fig. 47–2). The patient's blood then passes through the dialyzer on one side of the

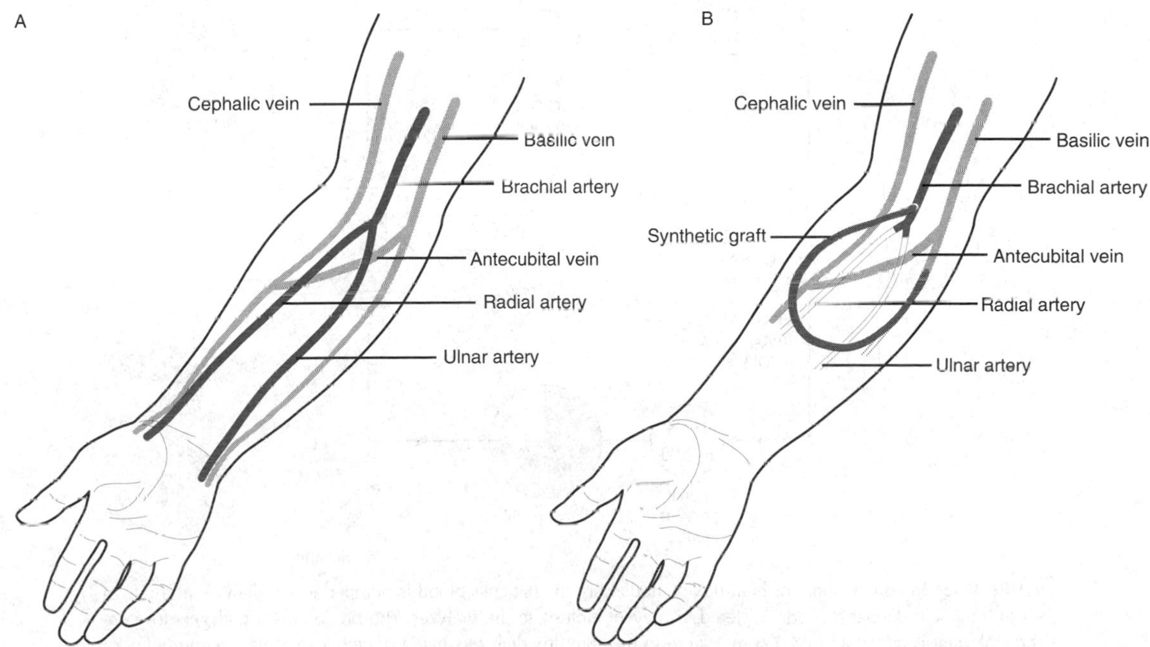

FIGURE 47–1. The predominant types of vascular access for chronic dialysis patients are (**A**) the arteriovenous fistula and (**B**) the synthetic arteriovenous forearm graft. The first primary arteriovenous fistula is usually created by the surgical anastomosis of the cephalic vein with the radial artery. The flow of blood from the higher pressure arterial system results in hypertrophy of the vein. The most common AV graft is between the brachial artery and the basilic or cephalic vein.

TABLE 47–3. Guidelines for the Treatment of Hemodialysis Access Infections

I. Primary Arteriovenous Fistula
  A. Treat as subacute bacterial endocarditis for 6 weeks.
  B. Initial antibiotic choice should always cover gram-positive organisms, e.g., vancomycin 20 mg/kg IV with serum concentration monitoring or cefazolin 20 mg/kg IV 3 times per week.
  C. Gram-negative coverage is indicated for patients with diabetes, HIV infection, prosthetic valves, or those receiving immunosuppressive agents, gentamicin 2 mg/kg IV with serum concentration monitoring.

II. Synthetic Arteriovenous Grafts
  A. Local infection—empiric antibiotic coverage for grampositive, gram-negative, and *Enterococcus*, e.g., gentamicin plus vancomycin then individualized after culture results available. Continue for 2 to 4 weeks.
  B. Extensive infection—antibiotics as above plus total resection.
  C. If access is less than 1 month old, antibiotics as above plus remove the graft.

III. Tunneled Cuffed Catheters (Internal Jugular, Subclavians)
  A. Infection localized to catheter exit site.
    1. No drainage—topical antibiotics, e.g., mupirocin ointment.
    2. Drainage present—gram-positive antibiotic coverage, e.g., cefazolin 20 mg/kg IV 3 times per week.
  B. Bacteremia with or without systemic signs or symptoms.
    1. Gram-positive antibiotic coverage as in III A2.
    2. If symptomatic at 36 hours, remove the catheter.
    3. If stable and asymptomatic, change catheter and provide culture-specific antibiotic coverage for a minimum of 3 weeks.

semipermeable membrane and is returned to the patient. The dialysate solution, which consists of purified water and electrolytes, is pumped through the dialyzer countercurrent to the flow of blood on the other side of the semipermeable membrane. The dialysate circuit, unlike the vascular circuit, is not sterile and is a potential source of infection for the patient, particularly if the membrane were to rupture.

In conventional or standard hemodialysis, low-permeability (low- to medium-flux) membranes (Table 47–4) are used and diffusion is the primary mechanism by which uremic waste products such as urea are removed from the patient. Blood flows through the dialyzer at a rate of 200–350 mL/min, and the dialysate flow rate is generally fixed at 500 mL/min. Under this set of clinical conditions, the clearance of urea by the dialyzer rarely exceeds 200 mL/min, and the duration of therapy required to deliver the desired amount of dialysis is usually 4 to 5 hours per session.

High-flux dialysis (HFD) gained increased acceptance during the 1990s. The higher efficiency of HFD resulted in a shortening of the duration of dialysis therapy from approximately 4 to 5 hours 3 times per week to 2 to 3 hours 3 times per week.[30,31] The features of HFD are procedure times usually less than 3 hours, blood flow rates greater than 400 mL/min, dialysate flow rates greater than 500 mL/min, urea clearances that are usually in excess of 250 mL/min, and the use of strict controls on the rate of fluid removal. The clearance of low-molecular-weight solutes such as urea is increased dramatically in HFD as the result of the increased blood and dialysate flow rates, and the contribution of convective transfer of the solute dissolved in the ultrafiltrate. Middle- and high-molecular-weight solutes including many drugs are cleared at a higher rate because of the larger pore size (>70 angstroms) and the higher ultrafiltration coefficient (K_{uf}); (generally in the range of 20–60 mL/h/mm Hg) of this type of dialyzer membrane, which facilitates their transport (see Chap. 50).[32–35]

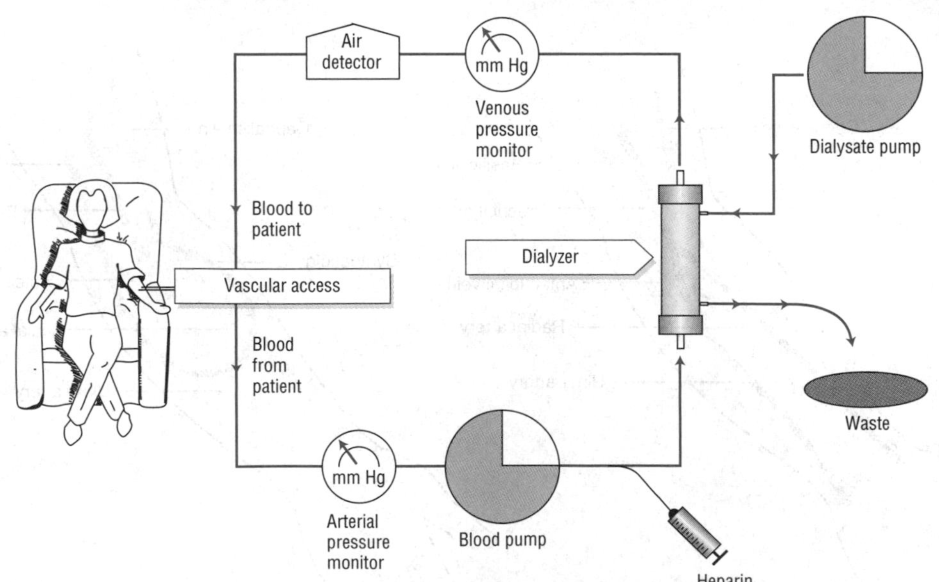

FIGURE 47–2. In conventional or high-flux hemodialysis, the patient's blood is pumped to the dialyzer at a rate of 300–600 mL/min. Heparin is administered to prevent clotting in the dialyzer. The predominant dialyzers for conventional dialysis are small (0.8–1.5 m^2), low- to medium-flux dialyzers made of cellulose acetate, cuprophan, or hemophan. High-flux hemodialysis systems incorporate a synthetic dialyzer made of polysulfone, polyacrylonitrile, polymethylmethacrylate, or a high-flux cellulosic-based filter; for example, cellulose triacetate of variable size (0.65–2.1 m^2). The dialysate, which is usually bicarbonate buffered, is pumped at a rate of 500–1,000 mL/min through the dialyzer countercurrent to the flow of blood. The rate of fluid removal from the patient is controlled by adjusting the pressure in the dialysate compartment.

TABLE 47–4. Characteristics of Selected Dialyzers Frequently Used in the United States

Manufacturer	Membrane	Type	Surface Area (m^2)	Priming Volume (mL)	K_{uf}	Biocompatibility	Urea CL at Q_B of 300 mL/min	Vitamin B_{12} CL at Q_B of 200 mL/min
Low Flux								
Baxter CA 110	CA	HF	1.1	70	4.8	+	212	50
Terumo NT120L	CL	HF	1.2	88	6.0	−	239	63
Fresenius F6	PS	HF	1.2	83	5.5	++	234	56
Toray B 3 1.0A	PMMA	HF	1.0	61	7.0	++	212	70
Medium Flux								
Gambro LA 700	CL	PP	1.3	93	11.2	−	246	74
Baxter DICEA 210G	DA	HF	2.1	125	15.5	+	268	105
Terumo T220	CL	HF	2.2	148	8.0	−	268	87
High Flux								
Fresenius F80A	PS	HF	1.8	110	65	++	259	110
Baxter CT190G	CTA	HF	1.9	115	36	++	273	143
Toray BK2.1U	PMMA	HF	2.1	135	19	++	263	125

CL = cellulose; CA = cellulose acetate; CDA = cellulose diacetate; PS = polysulfone; CTA = cellulose triacetate; PMMA = polymethylmethacrylate; HF = hollow fiber; PP = parallel plate; ND = no data; − = bioincompatible; + = somewhat biocompatible; ++ = biocompatible.

Typically, these dialyzers, which are composed of polysulfone (PS), polymethylmethacrylate (PMMA), polyamide (PA), cellulose triacetate (CTA), and polyacrylonitrile (PAN), have higher middle-molecule clearances than are attainable with standard hemodialysis.[36] There are currently more than 100 dialyzers available in the United States. The dialyzers differ in the composition of the membrane and ultrafiltration coefficient as described above, as well as in structural design (hollow fiber vs flat parallel plate), membrane surface area, sterilization method, and degree of biocompatibility (see Table 47–4). If the dialysis filter membrane does not induce an adverse reaction, such as activation of the complement system (C3a and C5a) when it comes in contact with the patient's blood, it is considered to be biocompatible. In the acute setting, the incidence of hypotension, fever, bronchoconstriction, and thrombocytopenia are lower in patients dialyzed with biocompatible filters. The most biocompatible dialyzers use a synthetic membrane of PS, PAN, or PMMA, and may have a low, medium, or high ultrafiltration coefficient. In addition, these dialyzers also have minimal chronic effects on the immune system, cytokine release (interleukin-1 and -6 and tumor necrosis factor), and production of β_2-microglobulin and, thus, are associated with a reduced risk of morbidity and mortality.[37] Furthermore, the nutritional status of patients receiving HD with biocompatible filters may be improved[38] and residual renal function preserved, relative to patients receiving dialysis with bioincompatible filters.[39,40]

Although little attention has focused on patient selection criteria for HFD versus standard hemodialysis, the best candidates for HFD are those with a vascular access that can deliver at least 400 mL/min, and absence of severe cerebrovascular or cardiovascular disease. In addition to patient factors, the economics of the individual dialysis unit enter into the selection process.

THE HEMODIALYSIS PRESCRIPTION

The goal is to prescribe and deliver the "optimal" dose of dialysis for each individual patient, that is, the amount of therapy above which there is no cost-effective increment in the patient's quality-adjusted life expectancy.[41] The two key goals of the prescription are to achieve the desired dry weight (an index of optimal fluid status) and adequate removal of endogenous waste products such as urea, elevations of which are associated with many of the complications of ESRD. Unfortunately, many nephrologists still prescribe dialysis by specifying a dialyzer manufacturer, size of the dialyzer, blood and dialysate flow rate, and the amount of weight to be removed within a certain time period with no a priori expectation as to the amount (dose) of dialysis being delivered.

During the past 5 to 7 years, multiple studies, mostly retrospective analyses, have reported that U.S. patient survival is improved when the dose of dialysis is increased.[14,42–44] The critical role of the dialysis dose is evident from the data of Hakim et al.[45] In this prospective trial, as the dose of dialysis was increased by 62% over a 3-year period, the annual mortality rate declined from 22.8% in 1988 to 9.1% in 1991 and the number of hospital days per patient per year decreased from 15.2 to 10.3. Although the optimal dose remains to be determined, the dose of dialysis has steadily increased by 3.5% to 5% per year during the late 1990s.[44]

The desired dose of dialysis can be expressed as a urea-reduction ratio (URR), which is calculated as the predialysis BUN minus the postdialysis BUN multiplied by 100, divided by the predialysis BUN,[28] or the *Kt/V*, which is the ratio of the dialyzer clearance of urea (K) in L/h multiplied by the duration of dialysis (t) in hours, divided by the urea distribution volume of the patient (V) in liters.[47] *Kt/V* is a unitless parameter that quantitates the fraction of the patient's total body water that is cleared of urea during a dialysis session. Patient mortality decreases as the *Kt/V* increases.[14,48] Mortality risk from all causes is reduced by 8% for every 0.1 increase in *Kt/V*,[48] and no significant differences are evident among the major causes of death, that is, coronary artery disease, other cardiac causes, cerebrovascular disease, or infections.[43] This translates into a 24% decrease in mortality if the *Kt/V* was increased from 1.0 to 1.3 or, in other words, 18 rather than 24 deaths per 100 patient years. Thus, many nephrologists now recommend a target *Kt/V* of at least 1.2 for nondiabetic patients receiving standard dialysis and 1.4 to 1.5 or greater for diabetics and/or patients receiving HFD therapy.[26,31]

After the desired *Kt/V* is selected for a patient, the duration of each treatment (t), which is dependent on the patient's urea volume of distribution (V) and the dialyzer clearance of urea (K), can be calculated. The time on dialysis can also be impacted by the need for fluid removal owing to interdialytic weight gain and the patient's residual renal function.[46,49]

CLINICAL ASSESSMENT OF THE DELIVERED DIALYSIS DOSE

The URR is an easy and frequently used measure of the delivered dialysis dose.[26] It, however, does not account for the contribution of convective removal of urea, and errors in delivered dose are difficult to detect in the target range of URR of ≥65% owing to the curvilinear relationship between the URR and *Kt/V*.[50] Thus, while URR is a practical tool for epidemiologic outcome studies, its relative inaccuracy and incomplete characterization of key prescription variables limit its usefulness as a guide to individualize hemodialysis therapy.[26,42]

Urea kinetic modeling of measured BUN levels is the optimal means to determine the delivered dose of dialysis.[26,47,51] Although simplified single-compartment models have been used and may still be applicable for patients receiving standard dialysis, with the introduction of HFD, the limitations of these simplified approaches are quite evident.[47] When the urea clearance of the dialyzer exceeds 180 mL/min and blood sampling is rigorous, one can clearly see that urea kinetics are best characterized by a two-compartment model with a central compartment volume that increases during the time between dialysis treatments.[50,52] As the result of this kinetic behavior, a marked rebound in urea concentrations is seen after dialysis, as has been described for many drugs (see Chap. 50).

The easiest way to assess the dose of dialysis actually delivered to the patient is to determine the ratio of serum BUN_{post} to BUN_{pre} (R) and from it, the *Kt/V*:[47]

$$Kt/V = \ln(R - 0.008t) + [(4 - 3.5R)(UF/Wt_{\text{post}})]$$

where, t is the duration of dialysis in hours, and UF is the predialysis minus the postdialysis weight.

This equation provides the best estimate of kinetically modeled *Kt/V* because it considers the effect of the efficiency of the treatment as a function of the treatment time, and the convective removal of urea in the ultrafiltrate (UF/Wt). Alternatively, urea kinetic modeling can be used to calculate the *Kt/V* using a two-compartment model.[47]

Because of the two-compartment behavior of urea, the timing of the post-treatment BUN sample is critical.[47,52] If the sample is obtained immediately after the end of the treatment, equilibration between the two compartments is incomplete and the sample will overestimate the magnitude of the treatment administered. The only "true" sample is the one obtained after the two compartments reach equilibrium. In the majority of cases, an almost complete equilibration between compartments is reached within 15 to 30 minutes after the end of the treatment. At this time, the sample is representative of the concentration of BUN in the body water. It is possible to calculate *Kt/V* using a sample immediately after the treatment if appropriate corrections are made to transform that sample into an equilibrated value (eKt/V).[53] This correction considers the urea clearance of the dialyzer used during the treatment, since the magnitude of the rebound is proportional to the efficiency of the treatment. These are among the multiple situations that may contribute to variances between the prescribed and delivered dose of dialysis.

The deficiency in delivered hemodialysis therapy may also be related to patient compliance with dialysis prescription.[54,56] Sherman et al.[54] reported that 50% of the patients they reviewed had either missed or ended their treatment early in the 3-month study period. Because compliance with the dialysis prescription is important for patient survival, different behavioral compliance styles need to be devised and evaluated.[55] Finally, reuse of the dialyzer[25,56–58] may affect the delivery of an adequate dose of dialysis. More than 80% of dialysis facilities reuse dialyzers. Because the effective volume of the dialyzer may decrease because of the clotting of the individual fibers, NKF-K/DOQI guidelines recommend that they be discarded if the volume loss exceeds 20%.[26] Compliance with this guidance does not assure the adequate delivery of HD,[57,58] and thus there is a need to routinely (every 1 to 3 months) measure the dose of dialysis patients receive. Optimal anticoagulation via heparin modeling appears to improve the urea clearance of polysulfone dialyzers and increase the delivered *Kt/V* despite extensive reuse of the filters.[59] Thus, dialyzer urea clearance may be preserved and patient care improved if anticoagulation is rigorously monitored.

INTRADIALYTIC COMPLICATIONS

Patients with ESRD develop several sequelae as the result of the reduction in functioning nephron mass. The pathophysiology and management of complications such as anemia, acid-base and electrolyte disorders, aluminum overload, uremic bleeding, and hyperparathyroidism are discussed in Chap. 45. In addition to these disorders, the primary pathology responsible for the patient's development of ESRD, such as hypertension, diabetes mellitus, or hyperlipidemia, may progress and contribute significantly to the patient's morbidity and risk of death.[60]

Intradialytic complications such as hypotension; acute hemorrhage caused by dialyzer rupture; hemolysis; cardiac arrhythmia; muscle cramps; nausea and vomiting; air embolism; chest or back pain; and pruritus are relatively frequently reported in hemodialysis patients. Despite the use of higher blood flow rates and dialyzers with increased K_{uf}, the incidence of most of these complications is lower in patients receiving HFD as compared to standard hemodialysis.[31,61] The replacement of acetate with bicarbonate as the dialysate buffer has been a major reason for the decrease in hypotension and nausea and vomiting. The use of volumetric ultrafiltration controllers during HFD, as well as individualized dialysate sodium levels, has likely also contributed to the lower incidence of these symptoms.[31] The incidence of pruritus and headache appear to be similar among the types of hemodialysis. Table 47–5 delineates the incidence and etiology or predisposing factors for the five most commonly observed intradialytic complications.

TABLE 47–5. Common Complications During Hemodialysis

	Incidence (%)	Etiology/Predisposing Factors
Cramps	2–50	Hypotension Idiopathic Dehydration Sodium level in dialysate too low
Headache	5	For most, mechanism unknown Acute caffeine withdrawal owing to dialytic removal Vasodilatation secondary to acetate dialysate solution
Hypotension	15–50	Excessive ultrafiltration Target weight too low Vasodilation secondary to acetate dialysate solution Autonomic neuropathy Patient unable to compensatorily increase cardiac output
Itching	50–90	Uremic toxins Elevated calcium-phosphorus product Dry skin Allergy to heparin, plasticizers in dialysis tubing, sterilant, or any other medication
Nausea and vomiting	5–15	Hypotension May be an early sign of disequilibrium syndrome

▶ TREATMENT: Complications

HYPOTENSION

The incidence of symptomatic hypotension during or immediately following dialysis ranges from 15% to 50%. The etiology of these episodic events is multifactorial (see Table 47–5) and includes ingestion of antihypertensive medications or food in the hours prior to or during dialysis, as well as severe hypocalcemia and high dialysate magnesium concentrations. Acute management of hypotension includes placing the patient in the Trendelenburg position, decreasing the ultrafiltration rate, and/or administering normal or hypertonic saline.[62,63]

Numerous nonpharmacologic and pharmacotherapeutic interventions have been used to prevent/reduce the incidence of symptomatic dialysis hypotension (Table 47–6). Randomized, blinded prospective trials are rare and thus comparisons between therapeutic alternatives are difficult to quantify. Nonpharmacologic therapies should be the first line of therapy among patients who are unresponsive to these measures, and hematocrit should be optimized to 33% to 36%. If they remain symptomatic, oral mitodrine, an α_1-adrenergic agonist prodrug with vasoconstrictive properties and minimal direct cardiac or central nervous system effects should be considered.[64] Two recent trials indicate that this agent, when administered in doses ranging from 2.5 to 25 mg prior to dialysis, significantly increased the minimal systolic (from 93–96.6 to 107–114 mm Hg) and diastolic (from 52–53.2 to 58–59 mm Hg) blood pressures during dialysis.[65,66] Furthermore, the dialysis symptoms of cramps, fatigue, dizziness, and weakness were subjectively reduced.[66] Although further studies with long-term follow-up are necessary to characterize this drug's efficacy and safety profile in dialysis patients, it appears to be the most rational and useful prophylactic pharmacologic therapy for hypotension.

The preventive use of two other pharmacologic alternatives is associated with significant reductions in the incidence of intradialytic hypotension. The intravenous administration of carnitine (20 mg/kg at the end of each dialysis) was reported by Ahmad et al.[67] to have reduced the number of hypotensive episodes from 17 to 7 ($P < 0.02$) in a pool of 38 patients. In contrast, the placebo group ($n = 44$) demonstrated no significant change in the number of episodes (9 baseline vs 11 treatment). The high cost and need for intravenous administration, however, relegate this agent to a third- to fourth-line alternative.

TABLE 47–6. Management of Hypotension

Acute treatment	Trendelenburg position placement
	Decrease ultrafiltration rate
	100–200 mL bolus of normal saline
	10–20 mL of hypertonic saline (23.4%) over 3–5 min
	12.5 g mannitol
Prevention	
Nonpharmacologic	Accurately set "dry weight"
	Use steady constant UFR
	Keep dialysate sodium > serum sodium
	Use bicarbonate dialysate
	Avoid food before or during HD
Pharmacologic	Caffeine 250 mg po 2 h into dialysis session
	Carnitine 20 mg/kg IV during dialysis
	Ensure hematocrit is >33%
	Midodrine 5–10 mg 30 min before HD

Caffeine administration has also been reported to decrease the incidence of dialysis-associated hypotension. Shinzato et al.[68] observed a significantly lower frequency of sudden-onset (1.7 ± 1.5 times/4 weeks in the caffeine group versus 4.4 ± 1.5 times/4 weeks in the placebo group) but no effect on gradual-onset hypotension. The proposed mechanism for these differential responses is speculative, and the separation of hypotension into two types of clinical presentations makes it difficult to compare the results of this trial to other studies. Caffeine has a minimal likelihood of adverse events and can be easily administered, and thus it is a reasonable alternative to midodrine.

MUSCLE CRAMPS

Skeletal muscle cramps complicate 25% to 50% of hemodialysis treatments.[63] Although the pathogenesis of cramps is multifactorial, plasma volume contraction caused by excessive ultrafiltration is frequently the initiating event. This perspective is supported by the fact that the incidence increases as the fractional reduction in body weight increases and the fact that acute onset of cramps during hemodialysis may be relieved by an intravenous infusion of saline, hypertonic saline, or mannitol.[63] Idiopathic nocturnal cramping has frequently been reported in hemodialysis patients. Although there are no comparative data regarding the efficacy of nonpharmacologic and pharmacologic therapy, the former should be the first line of treatment because the adverse consequences are minimal (Table 47–7).

Vitamin E and quinine are the most frequently used pharmacotherapeutic interventions. Roca et al.[69] reported that both vitamin E and quinine significantly reduce the incidence of cramps (from 10.4 and 10.9 per month to 3.3 and 3.6 per month, respectively ($P < 0.0005$). Quinine is usually well tolerated, but occasionally it may cause temporary sight and hearing disturbances, thrombocytopenia, or gastrointestinal distress. Furthermore, it tends to increase plasma digoxin levels and may enhance the effect of warfarin. This constellation of adverse events prompted the withdrawal of over-the-counter (OTC) and prescription quinine products from the U.S. market.[70] Hydroquinine was recently reported to be "safe" short-term therapy for the prevention of ordinary muscle cramps[71] and, where available, may be a reasonable therapeutic option. Prazosin also appears to significantly reduce the incidence of cramps during hemodialysis.[72] Unfortunately, its use was associated with a significant increase in the incidence of hypotension that required therapeutic intervention

TABLE 47–7. Management of Cramps

Acute treatment	100–200 mL bolus of normal saline
	10–20 mL of hypertonic saline (23.4%) over 3–5 min
Prevention	50 ml of hypertonic glucose (50%)
Nonpharmacologic	Accurately set "dry weight"
	Keep dialysate sodium > serum sodium
	Riding stationary bike before bedtime
	Stretching exercises
Pharmacologic	Diphenhydramine 12.5–50 mg qhs
	Hydroquinine 300 mg po qd
	Oxazepam 5–10 mg po 2 hrs before HD
	Prazosin 0.25 mg po at start of HD
	Quinine 200–300 mg po qhs or as tonic water
	Vitamin E 400 IU qhs

during and after dialysis. Thus, vitamin E appears to be the safest choice among these therapeutic options.

PRURITUS

Pruritus is one of the most common, frustrating, and potentially disabling symptoms of renal insufficiency.[63,73] Although it may be evident prior to the initiation of dialysis, it is more common in dialyzed patients (15% to 49% of predialysis patients versus 50% to 90% of dialysis patients). Episodic presentation after 6 or more months of dialysis is classic, with localization predominantly to the back. The severity may worsen during dialysis, and for up to 25% of patients, the itching persists after dialysis. The pathogenesis of this symptom complex is multifactorial and is associated with dry skin; hyperphosphatemia and increased calcium phosphate deposition in the skin; inadequate dialysis; anemia; neuropathy; and hypervitaminosis A.[73] Although histamine is classically considered to be one of the mediators of the itching sensation, the poor clinical responses that patients with generalized pruritus have with antihistamine therapy suggests that it may not be the only or even the predominant mediator. In fact, recent data suggest that the perception of this symptom may be mediated via activation of opioid receptors.[74]

There are many therapeutic alternatives for the management of this condition however most have limited clinical utility (Table 47–8). The optimization of the delivered dose of dialysis is a logical and often useful intervention.[73] The use of biocompatible dialyzers may further enhance this therapeutic option. Compliance with the patient's prescribed dietary restrictions on phosphate intake and optimization of phosphate binder therapy (see Chap. 45) may also result in marked improvement. Ultraviolet B light treatment elicits a beneficial response in many patients and is a logical option for those who are not receiving photosensitizing drug therapy.[73]

Pharmacologic alternatives range from the topical application of emollients or capsaicin to the oral administration of antihistamines, cholestyramine, or activated charcoal. Although no comparative trials have been rigorously conducted, each of these has demonstrated beneficial responses relative to placebo. Dry skin is a frequent finding in hemodialysis and peritoneal dialysis patients, and the regular application of hydrating/occlusive emollients (e.g., Aquaphor, aqueous cream BP) reduces the severity of pruritus.[75] Antihistamine therapy may also be beneficial, and the choice of agent from among the myriad of options will likely depend on the patient's past history of responsiveness and sensitivity to the central nervous system (CNS) depressant effects associated with classic agents.[76] Nonsedating antihistamines, such as loratadine or fexofenadine, may be used for those patients with extreme sensitivity to the sedative effects of the classic agents. The therapeutic options listed in order of preference (see Table 47–8) should be evaluated for a period of 4 to 6 weeks prior to switching to another option or initiating combination therapy.

TABLE 47–8. Therapeutic Alternatives for the Management of Pruritus in Dialysis Patients

Nonpharmacologic Therapy

1. Assure the delivery of adequate dialysis (*Kt/V* of 1.4).
2. Use biocompatible dialyzers.
3. Encourage compliance with dietary phosphate restrictions.
4. Ultraviolet B light therapy.
5. Acupuncture.

Pharmacologic Therapy

1. Maintain hematocrit of >33%
2. Topical emollient therapy—twice a day application at a minimum.
3. Initiate a 4–6-wk trial of an oral H_1 antihistamine: hydroxyzine 25–50 mg po q8–12h, cyproheptadine 2–4 mg po q8–12h. If the patient has a history of drowsiness with these agents, a nonsedating agent, e.g., loratadine or fexofenadine, can be tried.
4. If no response, start cholestyramine 5 g po bid with doses scheduled to minimize drug-absorption interactions.
5. Activated charcoal 1.0–1.5 g po qid for 6–8 wk.
6. Combination therapy of two or more of the agents listed above.

DIALYZER REACTIONS

Dialyzer reactions encompass a broad range of clinical symptoms that include anaphylactic (type A) and nonspecific (type B) events.[63,77] In the past, these two types of reactions were considered to be part of the "first-use" syndrome because they presented much more frequently when new, as opposed to reprocessed, dialyzers were used. Although reprocessing may reduce the incidence of type B events, it has little to no benefit for patients who have experienced a type A reaction.[78] The symptom complex associated with type A reactions is similar to a drug-induced anaphylactic reaction and may be a result of hypersensitivity to ethylene oxide (a common dialyzer sterilant), heparin, or formaldehyde and glutaraldehyde (common reuse sterilants). This type of reaction has also been associated with activation of the bradykinin system by some dialyzer membranes (especially the AN69), particularly in patients receiving angiotensin-converting enzyme (ACE) inhibitors, because these agents block bradykinin inactivation.[63,79] The dialysis procedure should be stopped immediately for those patients who experience this type of reaction. The blood in the dialyzer should not be returned to them, and resuscitative therapy with epinephrine, antihistamines, and steroids is likely to be required.

Type B reactions are more common than type A reactions, but are less severe (3–5/100 treatments vs 5/100,000 treatments). Chest and back pain are the most frequently reported symptoms and they may be noted within minutes of the start of dialysis or delayed (up to 1 to 2 hours). Complement activation and subsequent anaphylatoxin formation are associated to some degree with all dialysis membranes. Synthetic high-flux membranes have the least potential to produce this syndrome, followed by modified cellulose membranes (such as Hemophan and cellulose triacetate), whereas Cuprophan and cellulose acetate membranes have the greatest potential to produce this syndrome. Although no specific treatment is warranted and the patient can continue with dialysis treatment, the patient should be switched to a more biocompatible dialyzer and/or put on a reprocessing program because this may minimize the occurrence of this reaction in the future.[63]

OTHER DIALYSIS/ESRD-ASSOCIATED COMPLICATIONS

Complications associated with hemodialysis therapy that began after and/or that persist during the inter-dialytic period include hypertension,[80,81] hyperlipidemia,[82] immune system dysfunction,[83] disequilibrium syndrome,[84] and amyloidosis.[85,86] ESRD patients demonstrate several abnormalities of immune function, some of which are aggravated by the mode of dialysis therapy they receive. For example, granulocyte phagocytic ability, natural killer cell functions, and lymphocyte interleukin-2 receptor density were impaired to a greater extent when dialysis was performed using bioincompatible filters relative to certain biocompatible synthetic filters.[83] Furthermore, Hornberger and colleagues[87] reported a significant reduction (almost 50%) in mortality and infection-related hospital admissions for patients treated with high-flux biocompatible membranes as compared to patients treated with standard hemodialysis.

Because the dialysate-delivery circuit of hemodialysis machines is not sterile, inadequate water treatment at the municipal and/or dialysis center, poor dialysis machine design, or lack of quality control may result in acute infectious and toxic adverse effects among this population of patients.[88,89] The acuity and severity of problems like these, which are unique to hemodialysis patients, is evidenced by the fact that 81% of patients (101 of 124) who underwent hemodialysis at a Brazilian dialysis center during February 1996 had acute liver injury, and 50 died of acute liver failure secondary to exposure to the hepatotoxins (microcystins produced by algae) that were detected in the municipal water supply and the dialysate at the dialysis center.

Hypertension is present in about 70% of ESRD patients at the start of hemodialysis and is a major contributor to their high rate of cardiovascular mortality.[90] Although excessive sodium and fluids are significant contributors to the development and maintenance of hypertension, the pathogenesis is clearly multifactorial. In addition to an optimized dialysis prescription designed to achieve the patient's "dry weight," the vast majority of new patients (75% to 83%) require antihypertensive therapy[19,20,90] (see Chaps. 12 and 45 for therapeutic alternatives). Calcium channel blockers are the most frequently used antihypertensive class; more than 50% of new patients received one of these agents in 1996 to 1997.[20] ACE inhibitors were prescribed for 24%, whereas β-blockers and central α_2-receptor antagonists were used by 17% and 14% of patients, respectively. Despite the extensive use of these agents alone or in combination, more than 70% of patients still have inadequately controlled blood pressure.[80,91] Compliance, rather than a lack of efficacious alternatives, may be the major factor limiting the attainment of the desired therapeutic goals.[21]

Hyperlipidemia is a common finding in dialysis patients. Elevated triglycerides have been noted in 30% to 70% of hemodialysis patients, whereas hypercholesterolemia is more likely to be seen in peritoneal dialysis patients. Although glucose absorption and protein losses via the peritoneum may explain the derangements of lipid metabolism in peritoneal patients, no such initiating event has been identified that would explain the findings in hemodialysis patients.[82,92] Therapeutic options for dialysis patients are similar to non-ESRD patients and include nonpharmacologic, such dietary, as well as pharmacologic approaches (see Chaps. 21 and 44).

Disequilibrium syndrome is characterized by a set of systemic and neurologic symptoms, as well as EEG changes that may occur during but generally soon (hours) after the end of dialysis.[63,84] It has been reported in the acute and chronic setting and may be caused by an acute increase in brain water content. In mild cases, one may observe only nonspecific symptoms such as nausea, vomiting, headache, or restlessness. Severe disequilibrium is characterized by the development of seizures, obtundation, or coma. Prevention is the key to the management of this syndrome. The incidence of the syndrome can be minimized by the adjustment of dialysate sodium (at least 140 mEq/L) and glucose (at least 200 mg/dL) levels and a reduction in ultrafiltration rate and the target URR.

Dialysis-related amyloidosis is commonly seen in ESRD patients who have received dialysis for more than 8 to 10 years secondary to the accumulation of β_2-microglobulin.[93] The first and most prominent clinical manifestation of this syndrome is carpal tunnel syndrome. Approximately 20% to 25% of dialysis patients develop it after 5 years and the incidence increases to around 80% after 10 years.[86] Other clinical manifestations include shoulder, knee, ankle, elbow, and hip pain and stiffness with soft-tissue swelling. Radiologic lesions are usually evident before the onset of pain.

Serum β_2-microglobulin levels are significantly elevated in the presence of renal insufficiency; however, serum levels do not continuously rise, a finding that is compatible with its deposition in tissues.[85] Although the role of the dialyzer membrane is controversial, Cuprophan and cellulose acetate membranes stimulate β_2-microglobulin production, and because of their small pores, the clearance of this compound is negligible. In contrast, high-flux biocompatible membranes produce little to no stimulus of β_2-microglobulin production. Furthermore, owing to their high porosity and the absorption of β_2-microglobulin to some of the membranes, postdialysis levels may be 50% lower than those prior to dialysis. Despite these beneficial effects, no progressive decrease in predialysis levels has been reported. This may be the result of the short-term nature of some of the evaluations and the massive tissue stores that would need to be removed before one could see progressive declines. The prevalence of carpal tunnel syndrome was recently reported to be on the decline.[86,94] The confirmatory results at two centers (one in Germany and one in Japan) are encouraging and suggest that the use of high-flux dialyzers and/or highly purified dialysate water may reduce the risk of morbidity and mortality associated with β_2-microglobulin amyloidosis. At present, there is no adequate definitive treatment for this syndrome. Symptomatic treatment with nonsteroidal anti-inflammatory agents, systemic corticosteroids, therapeutic ultrasound, and physical therapy may be of benefit for some patients.[93]

PERITONEAL DIALYSIS

The first patients treated with CAPD were described in 1975, and the number receiving this form of dialysis increased slowly until the early 1980s. Mechanical and clinical improvements to the delivery system, such as improved catheters and dialysate bags, led to a rapid increase in the use of CAPD as a viable alternative to hemodialysis for the treatment of ESRD up until 1996. Some patients—such as those with more hemodynamic instability (angina, hyper- or hypotension) or significant residual renal function and perhaps patients who desire to maintain a significant degree of self-care may be better suited to CAPD or one of the other peritoneal dialysis variants rather than to HD. Table 47–2 shows the advantages and disadvantages of peritoneal dialysis.

PRINCIPLES OF PERITONEAL DIALYSIS

The three basic components of dialysis—namely, a blood-filled compartment separated from a dialysate-filled compartment by a semipermeable membrane—are also used for peritoneal dialysis. In peritoneal dialysis, the dialysate-filled compartment is the peritoneal cavity, into which dialysate is instilled via a permanent peritoneal catheter that traverses the abdominal wall. The contiguous peritoneal membrane surrounds the peritoneal cavity. The cavity, which normally contains about 100 mL of lipid-rich lubricating fluid, can expand to a capacity of several liters. The peritoneal membrane that lines the cavity functions as the semipermeable membrane, across which diffusion and ultrafiltration occur. The membrane is classically described as a monocellular layer of mesothelial cells. However, in reality, the dialyzing membrane is also comprised of the basement membrane and underlying connective and interstitial tissue. The peritoneal membrane has a total area that approximates body surface area (about 1–2 m^2). Blood vessels supplying and draining the abdominal viscera, musculature, and mesentery constitute the blood-filled compartment.

Solutes and water to be removed from blood during PD are not in intimate contact with the dialysis membrane as they are in hemodialysis and must therefore travel a considerable distance to the dialysate-filled compartment. Unlike hemodialysis, there is no easy method to regulate blood flow to the surface of the peritoneal membrane, nor is there a countercurrent flow of blood and dialysate to increase diffusion and convection via changes in hydrostatic pressure. For these reasons, PD is a much less efficient process per unit time as compared with hemodialysis and must therefore be a virtually continuous procedure to achieve acceptable goals for solute and water removal (such as in CAPD).

During most peritoneal dialysis modalities, the solute profile is markedly different from what is observed in hemodialysis patients. In intermittent hemodialysis, there is a "sawtooth" pattern of solute concentration over time. Because CAPD is essentially continuous, conditions similar to a steady state occur, and solute profiles are more level over time. CAPD, therefore, may represent a more physiologic process that is similar to endogenous renal function. Furthermore, the massive swings in body water content and high peak concentrations of uremic toxins in hemodialysis patients are less than optimal. CAPD may therefore be more beneficial for patients with cardiovascular instability.

The peritoneal membrane has different transport characteristics than conventional (Cuprophan), high-efficiency (cellulose acetate), or high-flux (cellulose triacetate, polysulfone, and the like) hemodialysis membranes (Table 47–9). The peritoneal membrane permits the passage of larger-molecular-weight solutes than the older, low-flux conventional type of hemodialysis membranes. However, this difference is less marked for newer, high-flux membranes. These differences not only aid our understanding of the relative efficiency of each system in the removal of endogenous solutes but also helps us to predict the dialyzability of exogenously administered drugs.

PERITONEAL ACCESS

Access to the peritoneal cavity is via the placement of an indwelling catheter. Many types are available, and a typical example is shown in Figure 47–3. Most catheters are manufactured from a silastic material, which is soft, flexible, and biocompatible. A typical adult catheter is about 40–45 cm long, 20–22 cm of which are inside the peritoneal cavity. Placement of the catheter is such that the distal end lies low in a pelvic gutter. The center section of the catheter has one or two cuffs, made of a porous material. This section is tunneled inside the anterior abdominal wall so that the cuffs provide mechanical support and stability to the catheter, a mechanical barrier to skin organisms, and prevent their migration along the catheter into the peritoneal cavity. The cuffs are placed at different sites surrounding the abdominal rectus muscle. The remainder of the central section of the catheter is tunneled subcutaneously before exiting the abdominal surface, usually a few centimeters below and to one side of the umbilicus.

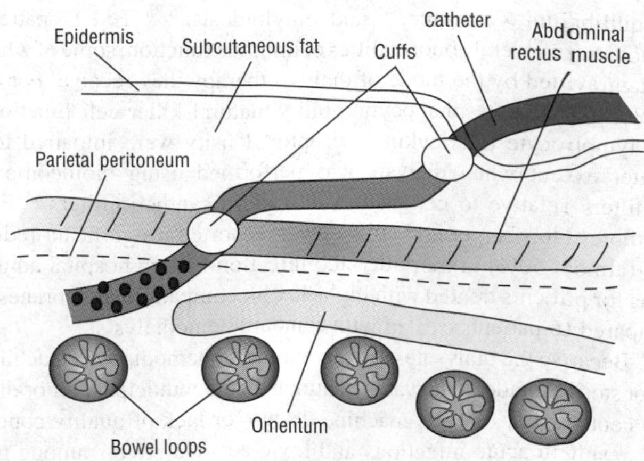

FIGURE 47–3. Diagram of the placement of a peritoneal dialysis catheter through the abdominal wall in the peritoneal cavity.

The placement of the exit site of the catheter is one of the factors related to the development or prevention of exit-site infections and peritonitis. Many new catheters and surgical techniques for catheter placement have recently been developed. The driving forces for this development are to enhance patient comfort and to reduce infectious risk. The external section of most peritoneal catheters ends with a Luer-lock, which can be connected to a variety of administration sets.[95] These catheters can be used immediately if necessary, provided small initial volumes are instilled; however, a maturation period of 2 to 6 weeks is preferred.

PERITONEAL DIALYSIS PROCEDURES

There are several types of peritoneal dialysis, of which CAPD remains the most common. Others include a variety of automated systems (collectively termed automated peritoneal dialysis [APD]), including continuous cycling PD (CCPD), nocturnal tidal PD (NTPD), and nightly intermittent PD (NIPD) (Fig. 47–4).[96] In recent years,

TABLE 47–9. Comparison of Weekly Clearances of Solutes by Peritoneal and Hemodialysis Membranes

Solute	MW	Peritoneum[a] (L/wk)	Cuprophan[b] (L/wk)	Cellulose Triacetate[b] (L/wk)
Urea	60	64	119	139
Creatinine	113	57	96	126
Vitamin B_{12}	1355	37	27	86
Inulin	5200	17	14	51
β_2-Microglobulin	11,800	8	0	38

[a]Based on four 2-L exchanges daily.
[b]Based on three 3-h dialyses per week.

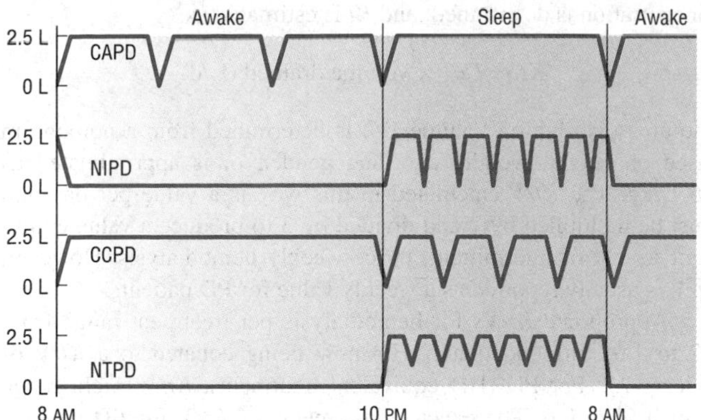

FIGURE 47–4. Comparison of peritoneal dialysis modalities. Continuous ambulatory peritoneal dialysis (CAPD). Patients perform three 2.5-L peritoneal dialysate exchanges during waking hours (8 AM to 10 PM), with each dialysate dwell lasting approximately 4 hours. Before bedtime, they perform an exchange and instill 2.5 L of dialysate overnight (10 PM to 8 AM). The following morning, the patient performs an exchange and the process begins again.

Nocturnal intermittent peritoneal dialysis (NIPD). Patients are free from performing dialysate exchanges during their waking hours (8 AM to 10 PM). Prior to bedtime, they attach their catheter to a cycling machine and receive six to eight 2.5-L exchanges of dialysate while they sleep. Each dialysate dwell time is approximately 2 hours long. The following morning, the patients unhook their catheters from the cycler and go about normal activities with an empty peritoneum.

Continuous cyclic peritoneal dialysis (CCPD). Patients instill 2.5 L of dialysate into their peritoneal cavity upon waking and allow it to dwell for the remainder of their waking hours (8 AM to 10 PM). Prior to bedtime, they drain the daytime dwell and attach their catheter to a cycling machine and receive three to five dialysate exchanges while they sleep. Each dialysate dwell time is approximately 2 hours long. The following morning, a 2.5-L dwell is instilled in the peritoneal cavity and the patient carries it during waking hours (8 AM to 10 PM).

Nocturnal tidal peritoneal dialysis (NTPD). Patients are free from performing dialysate exchanges during their waking hours (8 AM to 10 PM). Prior to bedtime, they attach their catheter to a cycling machine and instill a constant volume of 1,200–1,500 mL of dialysate into their peritoneal cavity. Over and above this constant volume, six to eight exchanges of 1,250 mL (total 2.5 L of dialysate) are carried out approximately every hour. The following morning, the patients unhook their catheters from the cycler and go about normal activities with an empty peritoneum. *(Adapted from Ref. 96, with permission.)*

there has been a substantial increase in the number of PD patients being treated with the APD systems, and they may soon be used to treat more patients than CAPD. The prototypic form of APD is usually a hybrid between CAPD and CCPD, in which some of the daily exchanges (usually the overnight exchange) are completed using an automated device. All variants of PD require the placement of a dialysis solution in the peritoneal cavity, allowing it to remain in situ for some period of time (called the *dwell time*), removing the spent dialysate, and then repeating the process. All forms use the same dialysate, which is commercially available in volumes of 1–3 L in a flexible polyvinyl chloride plastic bag. The constituents of commercial PD solutions include sodium 132 mEq/L (132 mmol/L), chloride 102 mEq/L (102 mmol/L), lactate 35 mEq/L, and magnesium 1.5 mEq/L (0.75 mmol/L). Solutions have traditionally contained calcium 3.5 mEq/L (1.75 mmol/L), although there is a current trend to use low calcium-containing solutions of 2.5 mEq/L (1.25 mmol/L) to reduce the risk of hypercalcemia, aluminum bone disease, or metastatic calcification. The osmotic load is provided by dextrose, in concentrations ranging from 1.5% to 4.25%, which provides osmolarities of 350–480 mOsmol, as compared to that of serum, which is 280 mOsmol. Other osmotic agents have been used, including mannitol, glycerol, glucose polymers such as icodextrin, and amino acids, but are not widespread because of expense or difficulty in manufacture.[98,99] It should be recognized that dextrose is not the ideal osmotic agent for peritoneal dialysate because these solutions are not biocompatible with peritoneal mesothelial cells or with peritoneal leukocytes.[100] The cytotoxic effects on these cells are mediated by the osmolar load and the low pH of the solutions, as well as the peritoneal sclerosis thought to result from the leaching of a plasticizer from the dialysate container.

In a basic CAPD system, dialysate is permitted to flow into the peritoneal cavity under gravity. The dialysate is preheated to body temperature and inflow occurs over a period of about 15 minutes. A typical dwell period for daytime exchanges in CAPD is 4 to 6 hours, using one of the lower-dextrose-concentration dialysate solutions. At the end of the prescribed dwell period, the empty dialysate bag is placed in a dependent position, the administration set is unclamped, and the dialysate is permitted to flow out of the peritoneal cavity via the catheter and administration set into the original container. The bag containing the spent fluid is detached and discarded. A new bag of dialysate is attached, and the process is repeated. The process of outflow, aseptic manipulation of the administration set and catheter, and inflow requires a total time of about 30 minutes. Thus, dialysis actually occurs for about 3.5 hours out of a prescribed 4-hour period. Typically a patient instills a 2–3-L exchange of dialysate three times during the day and then a single exchange using a higher-dextrose-concentration dialysate for an overnight, 8 to 12 hour dwell.

The prescribed dose of dialysis may be altered by changing the number of exchanges per day, by altering the volume of each exchange, or by altering the strength of dextrose in the dialysate for some or all exchanges. Increasing any one of these variables increases the effective osmotic gradient across the peritoneum, leading to increased ultrafiltration and diffusion (solute removal). If the dwell time is extended, an equilibrium will be reached, after which time there will be no further water or solute removal. Indeed after a critical period, reverse water movement may occur.

Alternative PD systems have been designed for patients who are unable or unwilling to perform the necessary aseptic manipulations, and for those who require more dialysis.[96] APD provides an automated cycler that performs the exchanges. The device is set up in the evening, and the patient attaches the peritoneal catheter to it at bedtime. The machine performs several short-dwell exchanges (usually 1 to 2 hours) during the night and this permits a long cycle-free daytime dwell of up to 12 to 14 hours. Thus, APD provides an exchange profile in reverse of that of CAPD. Typical APD regimens involve total 24-hour exchanges of about 12 L, which include one or more daytime dwells.[97] This type of regimen is sometimes referred to as APD with a "wet" day. The APD variant, NIPD, has a similar theme, except that the peritoneal cavity tends to be dialysate free during the day. This type of regimen is frequently referred to as APD with a "dry" day. A number of variants exist and depend largely on equipment availability, patient and prescriber preference, and whether the patient retains any residual renal function, which influences the quantity of dialysis prescribed (see Fig. 47–4).

A paramount factor that influences the rate of peritonitis in PD patients is the type of administration set and its method of connection to the peritoneal catheter. Early systems used a simple plastic spike to connect these sections. However, the rate of peritonitis was excessive, resulting from touch contamination of the catheter. During the past decade, significant steps have been made to minimize this risk.[95]

Newer systems have Y tubing on the bag side of the system. One of these newer systems, the double-bag system, permits both a flush-before-fill procedure and disconnection during the dwell. Although the number of steps is reduced, the risks of biofilm formation and peritonitis remain high.[101] Such systems sacrifice cost for the benefit of decreased infection risk.

ADEQUACY OF PERITONEAL DIALYSIS

Peritoneal dialysis patients may have numerous metabolic and nutritional abnormalities, such as sustained uremia (BUN levels sufficiently elevated to produce symptoms); accumulation of "middle molecule" toxins; amino acid and albumin loss into the dialysate; glucose absorption from the dialysate; loss of muscle mass and increased adipose tissue; and poor appetite. Although the nutritional status of CAPD patients may improve for up to 1 year following the initiation of CAPD, long-term deterioration in nutritional status, as measured by serum albumin, plasma amino acid concentrations, and anthropometric parameters, is seen in more than 40% of patients.[102,103] Poor nutritional status correlates with poor clinical outcome.[103]

Many PD patients may be malnourished when they start PD, especially if they had been receiving a low-protein diet as a means of slowing the progression of renal failure (see Chap. 44), together with the general loss of appetite that accompanies ESRD.[102] In addition, some renal diseases (such as glomerulonephritis) are treated using corticosteroids, which may increase net protein catabolism. The recommended daily protein intake for CAPD patients is $\geq$1.2 g/kg body weight, which exceeds that for normal individuals (0.75–1.0 g/kg/d), because there may be a substantial loss of albumin (5–15 g/d) in the dialysate. The BUN concentration is the net result of both a patient's nutritional status (in terms of dietary protein intake and protein catabolic rate) and the quantity of dialysis the patient has received. For these reasons, the assessment of the adequacy of dialysis requires more than a simple examination of the BUN profile.

What constitutes "adequate" versus "optimal" dialysis is controversial. The NKF-K/DOQI[26] recommends the use of two criteria to assess the dose of dialysis delivered: Kt/V_{urea} per week, and total weekly creatinine clearance (L/wk) normalized to 1.73 m^2. As in hemodialysis, Kt/V is a unitless value that correlates the patient's peritoneal membrane urea clearance (K) with the duration of dialysis (t) and the volume of distribution (V) of urea.

Several major studies[104,105] used multivariate analysis to assess the association between adequacy of peritoneal dialysis and survival. The largest of these, the Canada-USA cooperative study (CANUSA),[105] studied 680 PD patients in 14 centers who began dialysis between 1990 and 1992. Decreases of 0.1 in weekly Kt/V_{urea} or 5 L/1.73 m^2/wk in CLcr were associated with 5% to 7% increases in the risk for death. No plateau was observed. Thus, the greater the urea and creatinine clearances, the greater is the rate of patient survival. For this reason, optimal doses of dialysis are impossible to define; rather, the more dialysis delivered, the better. The lower threshold of dialysis dose that constitutes an acceptable risk for patient outcome has been termed "adequate dialysis," and the values for the primary adequacy indices are discussed below.

Kt/V

Calculation of Kt/V for PD requires that the total volume of drained effluent per day be determined (this value is the volume instilled plus volume of water ultrafiltered). A dialysate to plasma (D/P) urea concentration is determined, and Kt is estimated as:

$$Kt = D/P \times \text{volume drained (L/d)}$$

The urea distribution volume (V) is determined from a nomogram based on height, weight, age, and gender, or is approximated as 0.6 L/kg. The Kt/V calculated in this way is a value per day and must be multiplied by 7 and divided by 3 to produce a value equivalent to that of intermittent, thrice-weekly hemodialysis. However, Kt/V is usually reported as a weekly value for PD patients.

Appropriate Kt/Vs for hemodialysis per treatment range from 1.2 to 1.6, with "adequate" HD now being equated to a Kt/V of at least 1.2. For PD (HD equivalent treatment), Kt/V might range from 0.54 to 0.6. The exact requirements of Kt/V for PD patients remain unknown because of the lack of definitive published data. However, the recent NKF-DOQI clinical practice guidelines recommend that, in CAPD patients, Kt/V values should exceed 2.0, or 0.67 in terms of HD equivalents.[26] For APD with a dry day and wet day, the Kt/V values should exceed 2.2 and 2.1, respectively. This difference may be because of the differences in efficiency of hemodialysis and different variants of PD in clearing small- and middle-sized molecules.

One problem associated with the determination of Kt/V for PD patients is the impracticality of 24-hour collections of dialysis effluent. Abbreviated collection periods have been used, and calculations based on the first morning exchange after an overnight dwell correlated well ($r = 0.92$) with a 24-hour collection.[106] It is important to note that residual renal function may provide a significant component of the total Kt/V. Patients may commence PD with a residual creatinine clearance of about 9–12 mL/min, which might equate to a Kt/V_{renal} of 0.2–0.4. Over a period of 1 to 2 years, residual renal function tends to progressively deteriorate to zero. Because Kt/V_{total} is the sum of Kt/V_{PD} and Kt/V_{renal}, the Kt/V_{total} will progressively diminish unless Kt/V_{PD} is increased (by increasing the prescribed dose of PD) to compensate for the reduced Kt/V_{renal}. Thus, unless Kt/V_{PD} is increased, Kt/V_{total} may diminish from 2.0 to 1.7 over this period of time.

CREATININE CLEARANCE

Weekly measured CLcr, normalized to 1.73 m^2, is also used to assess adequacy of PD,[107,108] because it correlates well ($r = 0.71$) with Kt/V. For CAPD patients, the total CLcr should be at least 60 L/wk/1.73 m^2, which is approximately equivalent to a weekly Kt/V_{urea} of 1.96.[26] For APD with a dry day or wet day, the corresponding values are 66 and 63 L/wk/1.73 m^2, respectively. Such values are the sum of both peritoneal and residual renal clearance and are influenced by body muscle mass.

Patients may start PD with a significant residual CLcr, which will diminish over the following several years. This loss of residual renal function is the major cause of decreased total clearance in PD patients over time. Unfortunately, the standard regimen of four 2-L exchanges per day in CAPD may provide inadequate clearances in some patients, especially heavier patients.[106] A reevaluation of data from the CANUSA study[105] examined the influence of body surface area and residual renal function. It was suggested that clearances might be maximized by adopting larger fill volumes (2.5–3 L), more frequent exchanges (5–6/d), and the use of wet days in APD patients. A wet day is a regimen that includes a prolonged dwell during the daytime, between the frequent, automated nighttime exchanges. Also, based on peritoneal membrane characteristics, patients with low-transport membranes should be considered for hemodialysis.

PERITONEAL EQUILIBRATION TEST

The peritoneal equilibration test (PET) is a diagnostic test designed to determine an individual PD patient's peritoneal membrane clearance and ultrafiltration characteristics. It quantitates the ease with which solutes and water can transfer across the membrane. Because the peritoneal membrane permits movement of solutes in both directions, the PET simultaneously determines the passage of creatinine from blood to dialysate, glucose from dialysate to blood, and free water transfer in both directions across the peritoneal membrane. The objective of the PET is to determine which variant of PD is appropriate for an individual patient and to predict the daily dialysis requirement. Solute transport is defined as high, high average, low average, or low, and ultrafiltration rates as poor, adequate, good, or excellent. To perform a PET, a patient receives a standardized exchange, and simultaneous blood and dialysate samples are obtained at intervals throughout the exchange. Dialysate-to-plasma ratios of creatinine and glucose are plotted, and the rate and magnitude of the change over 4 hours predicts the permeability of the membrane. A highly permeable membrane allows easy passage of both creatinine and glucose. Because the glucose concentration in the dialysate is the primary force that results in ultrafiltration, it follows that patients who have a high solute transport rate (in other words, a high dialysis clearance of creatinine) also have a poor ultrafiltration rate, because there is also a high transfer of glucose to blood. The prognostic interpretation of PET results is depicted in Table 47–10.

CHANGING THE PD PRESCRIPTION

Recent NKF-DOQI clinical practice guidelines suggest that the adequacy of PD be assessed by using measured *Kt/V* and CLcr three times in the first 6 months of dialysis, that is, at months 1, 4, and 6.[26] The reasoning behind this frequency is to accurately establish a baseline creatinine and urea excretion rate. Thereafter, the *Kt/V* and CLcr should be measured every 4 months, at months 10, 14, and so on. The rationale for this is that it is imperative to detect subtle decreases in residual renal function and noncompliance and to make the necessary alterations to the prescribed PD dose to compensate for them. In addition, every 4 months is a compromise between frequent enough to be clinically helpful, yet not so frequent as to be overly intrusive. It is recommended that the first PET be conducted within the first month of treatment.

COMPLICATIONS

Mechanical, medical, and infectious problems complicate peritoneal dialysis therapy.[95] Mechanical complications include kinking of the catheter and inflow and outflow obstruction; excessive catheter motion at the exit site leading to induration and possible infection and aggravation of tissues; pain from impingement of the catheter tip on the viscera; or inflow pain resulting from a jet effect of too rapid dialysate inflow.

TABLE 47–10. Prognostic Value of Peritoneal Equilibration Test Results

Solute Transport	Ultrafiltration Rate	Solute Clearance	Appropriate Dialysis Modality
High	Low	Adequate	APD, CAPD
High Average	Adequate	Adequate	APD, CAPD
Low Average	Good	Adequate ±	APD or CAPD with high daily volumes
Low	Excellent	Inadequate	Hemodialysis

TABLE 47–11. Medical Complications of Peritoneal Dialysis

Cause	Complication	Treatment
Glucose load	Exacerbation of diabetes mellitus	IP insulin
Fluid overload	Exacerbation of CHF Edema Pulmonary congestion	Increase ultrafiltration
Electrolyte abnormalities	Hyper- and hypocalcemia	Alter dialysate content
PD additives	Chemical peritonitis	Discontinue PD additives
Malnutrition	Albumin loss Loss of amino acids Muscle wasting Increased adipose tissue	Dietary changes, parenteral nutrition, discontinue PD
Unknown	Fibrin formation in dialysate	IP heparin

CHF = chronic heart failure; IP = intraperitoneal; PD = peritoneal dialysis.

Table 47–11 lists the numerous medical complications of PD. An average PD patient absorbs up to 60% of the dextrose in each exchange. This continuous supply of calories leads to increased adipose tissue deposition, decreased appetite, malnutrition, and altered requirements for insulin in diabetic patients. Infectious complications of PD are a major cause of morbidity and mortality and are the leading cause of technique failure and transfer from PD to hemodialysis.[109,110] The two predominant infectious complications are peritonitis and catheter-related infections, which include both exit-site and tunnel infections. Some 40% to 60% of patients develop their first episode of peritonitis within 1 year of starting CAPD, although the incidence is significantly lower in APD patients.[111] Peritonitis is a major cause of catheter loss in PD patients. In one series, peritonitis was responsible for the loss of 17% of all catheters in PD patients younger than 50 years of age, and for 25% of all catheters in patients older than 60 years of age.[112] Together, catheter-related infections plus peritonitis are the most common cause of catheter loss in this population, being responsible for 61% and 60% of catheters lost in the <50 and >60 years old age groups, respectively.

A statistically significant correlation between infectious complications and death rates has been reported.[113] Of patients who had more than 1 peritonitis episode per year, 0.5–1 episode per year, or less than 0.5 episode per year, 50% died after 3, 4, and 5 years of therapy, respectively. It is important to note that these relationships are not necessarily cause and effect, because many of these patients succumb to cardiovascular events.

PERITONITIS

The incidence of peritonitis is influenced by connector technology, by the composition of patient populations, and by the use of APD versus CAPD. Elderly and diabetic individuals have a higher incidence of peritonitis.[110,112] The mean incidence of peritonitis for most dialysis centers in the United States is about one episode every 12 to 24 patient-months, although it may vary from as frequent as one episode every 5 to 6 patient-months, to as infrequent as one episode every 60 to 72 patient-months.

The typical signs and symptoms of peritonitis are abdominal tenderness (76%), cloudy effluent (98%), abdominal pain (78%), fever

(38%), nausea and vomiting (25%), and chills (18%). Peritonitis has several imprecise definitions, but most recent guidelines suggest that an elevated dialysate white blood cell count >100/mm^3, of which at least 50% are polymorphonuclear neutrophils, is necessary to confirm the diagnosis of peritonitis.[114] A patient who presents with abdominal pain and a cloudy effluent is usually given a provisional diagnosis of peritonitis. Inherent in this definition is a number of false-positive and false-negative diagnoses, because 5% of patients with culture-proven peritonitis will have clear dialysate,[114] and some patients, such as menstruating females, may have cloudy PD effluent without clinical infection. Sterile culture peritonitis remains problematic; it is defined as an episode in which there is clinical suspicion of peritonitis, but for which the culture of the dialysate reveals no organism. There are several postulates for the high incidence (up to 20% of episodes) of culture-negative peritonitis. Many peritonitis-producing organisms are slime producers[101] and may adhere to the peritoneal membrane or to the catheter surface and be protected from exogenous antibiotics. Sufficient numbers of these bacteria may proliferate to cause peritoneal membrane inflammation and clinical peritonitis, but an inadequate number may seed into the peritoneal cavity to be recovered by conventional microbiologic techniques. In addition, planktonic bacteria may be rapidly phagocytosed by peritoneal white blood cells (WBCs), thereby rendering them unavailable for culture.

Most of the organisms producing peritonitis adhere to the peritoneal membrane, with a relatively smaller number appearing as free-floating planktonic bacteria in dialysate. There may be as few as 10^4 planktonic organisms per milliliter of effluent. Removal of a small volume of dialysate from the bag may thus result in too few organisms to culture. Contemporary methods have increased the recovery rate of organisms and decreased the culture-negative rate.[114] These methods all use some type of concentrating technique. Centrifugation is commonly employed, by which a large volume of dialysate (100 mL) is centrifuged and the resultant pellet may be cultured on plates or in broth. Filtration of a large volume through a 0.44-μm filter can be used for clear effluent, which contains few WBCs or fibrin that would otherwise clog the filter. The filter can subsequently be divided and cultured as above. Other methods that have been used for very cloudy effluent include attempts to lyse WBCs to release bacteria trapped within them using water, surfactants, and ultrasound. Blood-culturing methods also decrease the sterile culture rate.

TABLE 47–12. Organisms Causing Peritonitis

Organisms	% Episodes
Gram positive	40–50
Staphylococcus epidermidis	30–45
Staphylococcus aureus	10–20
Streptococci	10–15
Enterococci	3–5
Diphtheroids	<5
Gram negative	25–35
Escherichia coli	5–12
Pseudomonas aeruginosa	5–8
Enterobacter	2–3
Acinetobacter	2–3
Klebsiella	2–3
Proteus	2–3
Mixed gram positive and negative	10–15
	5–10
Fungi	5–20
Sterile culture, presumed bacterial	5

The majority of infections (40% to 50%) are caused by gram-positive bacteria in CAPD, of which *Staphylococcus epidermidis* is the predominant organism (Table 47–12).[115] There is no single predominant gram-negative organism. Together, gram-positive and gram-negative organisms account for 65% to 90% of all episodes of peritonitis and constitute the spectrum against which initial empiric therapy is directed. In APD, there is a relative increase in the percentage of infections caused by polymicrobial and fungal organisms.

▶ TREATMENT: Peritonitis

The International Society of Peritoneal Dialysis Ad Hoc Advisory Committee on Peritonitis Management evaluates the diagnostic and therapeutic data every few years.[114] Their most recent report includes a series of tables that provide guidelines for diagnosis and pharmacotherapy of peritoneal dialysis-associated infections. The guidelines have changed significantly from previous versions and are now reflective of recently available information pertaining to the increasing prevalence of vancomycin-resistant enterococci, the effect of residual renal function on the pharmacokinetics of antibiotics, and evidence of the adverse effects of aminoglycosides on residual renal function.

Initial empiric therapy for peritonitis, regardless of whether a Gram stain was performed or organisms identified, should include agents effective against both gram-positive and gram-negative organisms (Fig. 47–5). Intraperitoneal (IP) administration is favored over the intravenous route, and combinations of a first-generation and a third-generation cephalosporin are recommended. Dosing recommendations were generated for intermittent (one large dose into one exchange per day) and continuous therapy (antibiotic addition to each exchange), and sub-categorized on the basis of the patients residual renal function.

The choice between these regimens requires careful consideration for several reasons. The dialysate and serum concentrations achieved after intermittent and continuous therapies are very different. The pharmacokinetics of intermittent intraperitoneal ceftazidime and cefazolin have been well described since the previous update in 1996.[116,117] Single daily doses of 15 mg/kg of cefazolin and ceftazidime in CAPD are effective in achieving serum concentrations greater than the minimum inhibitory concentration for sensitive organisms over 48 hours. In CAPD, it is usual to add the single daily dose into the exchange with the longest dwell, to ensure maximal bioavailability. APD dosing strategies are different, because of the increased clearances of solutes in such systems. In APD, it is suggested that a single daily dose of 20 mg/kg is required to maintain adequate serum cefazolin concentrations over 24 hours, if the single dose is added to a daytime, ambulatory exchange.[118] In addition, recent studies have identified dosing recommendations for several other antibiotics in APD, including tobramycin (1.5 mg/kg LD then 0.5 mg/kg qd IP),[118] piperacillin (4 g IV bid),[119] and vancomycin (35 mg/kg LD then 15 mg/kg qd IP).[120]

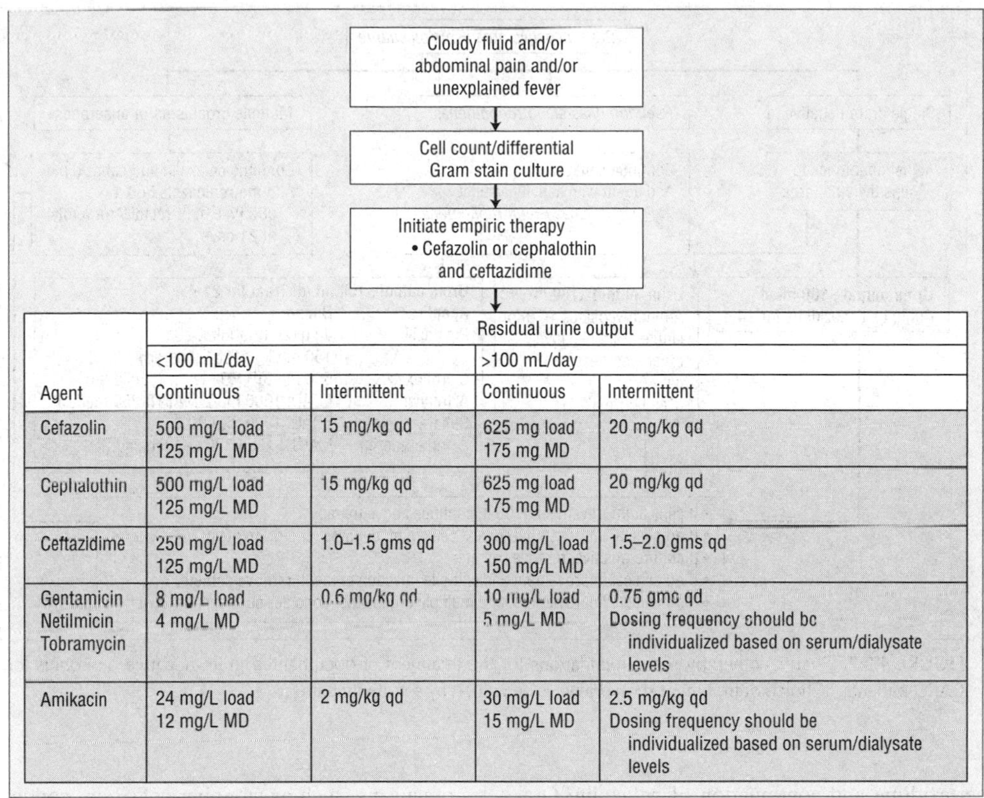

Agent	Residual urine output			
	<100 mL/day		>100 mL/day	
	Continuous	Intermittent	Continuous	Intermittent
Cefazolin	500 mg/L load 125 mg/L MD	15 mg/kg qd	625 mg load 175 mg MD	20 mg/kg qd
Cephalothin	500 mg/L load 125 mg/L MD	15 mg/kg qd	625 mg load 175 mg MD	20 mg/kg qd
Ceftazidime	250 mg/L load 125 mg/L MD	1.0–1.5 gms qd	300 mg/L load 150 mg/L MD	1.5–2.0 gms qd
Gentamicin Netilmicin Tobramycin	8 mg/L load 4 mg/L MD	0.6 mg/kg qd	10 mg/L load 5 mg/L MD	0.75 gms qd Dosing frequency should be individualized based on serum/dialysate levels
Amikacin	24 mg/L load 12 mg/L MD	2 mg/kg qd	30 mg/L load 15 mg/L MD	2.5 mg/kg qd Dosing frequency should be individualized based on serum/dialysate levels

FIGURE 47–5 Empiric pharmacotherapy selection for CAPD patients with suspected peritonitis. MD = maintenance dose.

The Ad Hoc Advisory Committee's recommendations for treatment of a dialysate culture- positive gram-positive infection are detailed in Fig. 47–6. The presence of Enterococcus would indicate the replacement of the cephalosporin with IP ampicillin, with the possible addition of an aminoglycoside, depending on sensitivities. In addition, if the Enterococcus is ampicillin-resistant, recommendations are supplied for starting vancomycin or clindamycin. The presence of *Staphylococcus aureus* (methicillin sensitive) would warrant the

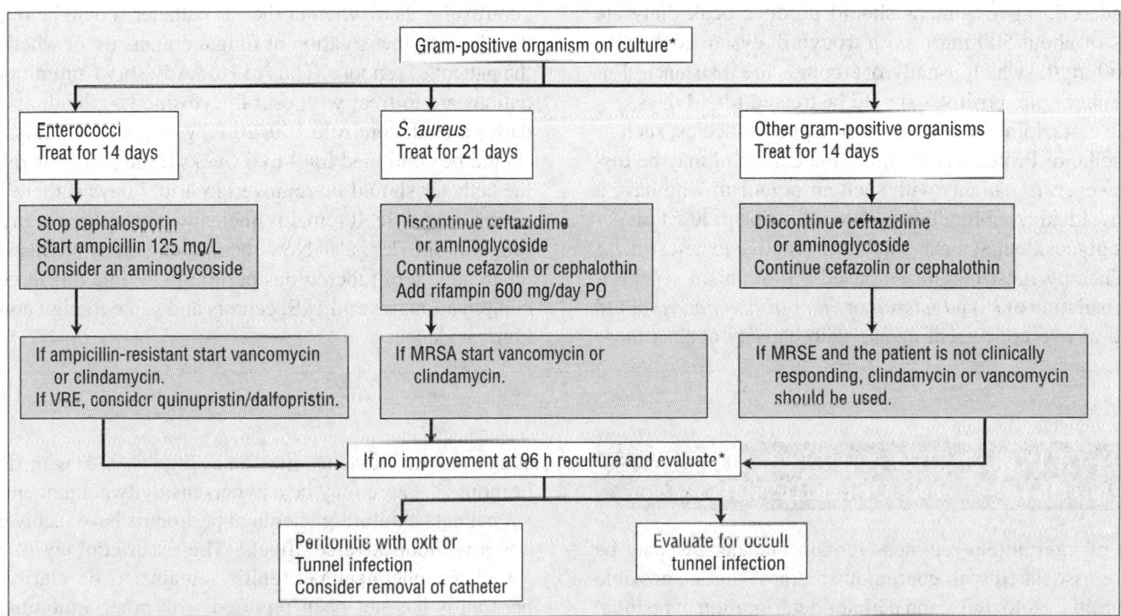

FIGURE 47–6. Pharmacotherapy recommendations for the treatment of documented gram-positive peritonitis in CAPD patients.
*Choice of therapy should always be guided by sensitivity patterns

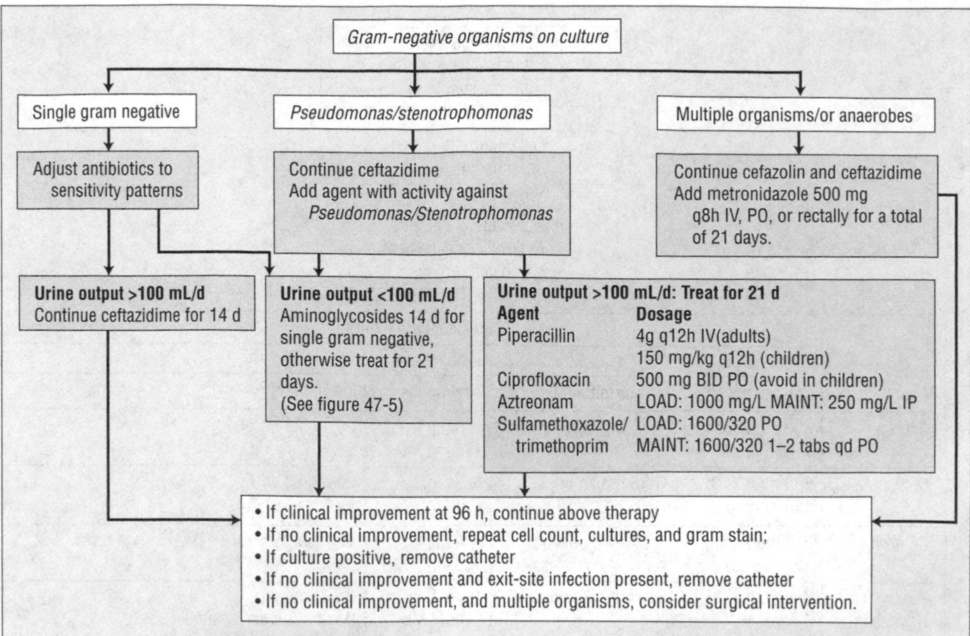

FIGURE 47–7. Pharmacotherapy recommendations for the treatment of documented gram-negative peritonitis for CAPD patients. *Choice of treatment should always be guided by sensitivity patterns.

discontinuation of ceftazidime and continuation of cefazolin. Oral rifampin might be added if there was an inadequate clinical response, defined as continued cloudy dialysate, abdominal pain, and elevated dialysate white blood cells. If the organism is methicillin-resistant *S. aureus*, then the entire regimen should be changed to one of oral rifampin and IP vancomycin or clindamycin. *S. aureus* infections should be treated for 21 days. The presence of any other gram-positive species can usually be treated by the continuation of IP cefazolin alone. *S. epidermidis* is often reported as resistant to cephalosporins. The resistance is often relative, with minimum inhibitory concentrations (MICs) in the 16–32 mg/L range. However, the recommended dosage regimens should produce peak dialysate concentrations of about 500 mg/L with trough dialysate concentrations of 50–100 mg/L, which usually overcomes the resistance. Enterococci and other gram positives should be treated for 14 days.

If a single ceftazidime-sensitive gram-negative species, such as *E. coli*, Klebsiella, or Proteus, is cultured, the cefazolin may be discontinued. However, in patients with such an organism who have a low degree of residual renal function (<100 mL urine production per day), an aminoglycoside may be a suitable alternative to ceftazidime (Fig. 47–7). Therapy must be chosen based on organism sensitivities. However, isolation of *Pseudomonas* or *Stenotrophomonas* should dictate the use of two concurrent agents with activity against these organisms, such as stopping cefazolin, continuing ceftazidime, and adding an aminoglycoside (if <100 mL urine/d) or oral ciprofloxacin (if >100 mL urine/d). Isolation of multiple gram-negative organisms would warrant the continuation of both cephalosporins and the addition of metronidazole.

Fungal peritonitis is associated with a poor prognosis and high morbidity and mortality. One problem with prospective assessment of antifungal regimens is the infrequency with which these infections occur. This makes it difficult to design and implement comparative studies. Most literature about antifungal treatment is therefore retrospective or limited to reports of local experience.[121,122] There is controversy as to whether the PD catheter should be removed immediately upon the isolation of fungal organisms, or whether to observe the patient's response. The Ad Hoc Advisory Committee recommendations are to treat with oral flucytosine (2-g loading dose then 1 g daily) plus fluconazole 100–200 mg orally or IP daily.[114] Treatment should be continued for 4 to 6 weeks if the patient is responding, but the catheter should be removed in 4 to 7 days if there is inadequate clinical response. It remains unclear whether there is any benefit from fungal prophylaxis.[123] New recommendations are also provided for the treatment of tuberculous peritonitis. While this infection is a rare complication, several U.S. centers and some foreign countries have a high incidence.

TOXICITY OF INTRAPERITONEAL DRUG-THERAPY FOR THE TREATMENT OF PERITONITIS

The toxicities of intermittent regimens remain unclear, but may be similar to those associated with continuous therapy, that is, possible chemical peritonitis, ototoxicity, and perhaps deterioration of residual renal function. A series of early reports of chemical peritonitis with vancomycin suggested that the problem may be brand-specific or associated with large doses (1–2 g). One recent prospective study suggested the incidence may be as high as 23% with IP doses of 1 g or more.[124] There may be a hypersensitivity component to the effect, yet patients exhibiting chemical peritonitis have received subsequent doses without adverse effects. The exact etiology of vancomycin-associated chemical peritonitis remains to be clarified. Chemical peritonitis has not been reported with other antibiotics. Increasing evidence suggests that either intravenous or intraperitoneal aminoglycosides increase the rapidity of decline in patients' residual renal function, leading to a recommendation that patients that have significant residual renal function should not receive aminoglycosides if other antibiotic choices are available.[124]

CATHETER-RELATED INFECTIONS

The incidence of exit-site infections is about 0.8–1.2 episodes per patient-year.[125] The incidence is lower in older (<60 years of age) patients.[112] Causative organisms are different from those associated with peritonitis; the most common is S. *aureus* (about 40% to 50% of episodes), followed by *S. epidermidis, Pseudomonas aeruginosa,* and other enteric gram-negative bacilli (about 15% to 20% each).[115] The diagnostic characteristics of these infections are also vague but generally include the presence of purulent drainage and erythema. The risk of exit-site infections is increased several-fold in patients who are nasal carriers of *S. aureus.*[126] The use of topical antibiotics and disinfectants to treat catheter-related infections is controversial,[127,128] and there are few adequately controlled studies to determine the effectiveness of systemic antibiotics. Current recommendations suggest that gram-positive organisms should be treated with an oral penicillinase-resistant penicillin or first-generation cephalosporin for 2 to 3 weeks. Rifampin may be added if necessary, in slowly resolving or particularly severe appearing *S. aureus* infections (Fig. 47–8). Vancomycin should be avoided in routine or empiric treatment of gram-positive infections. Gram-negative organisms should be treated with oral quinolones. The effectiveness of this approach may be diminished owing to the chelation drug interactions with divalent and trivalent metal ions, which are commonly taken by dialysis patients.

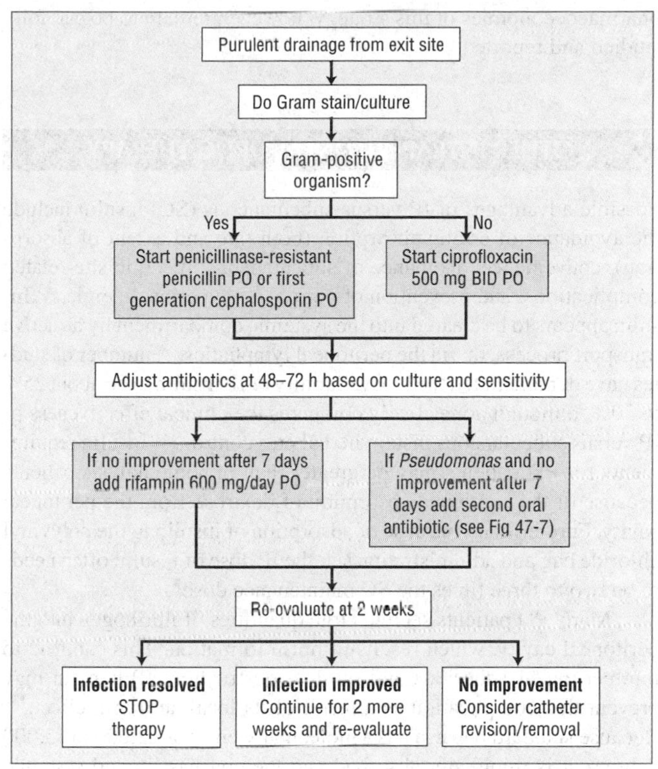

FIGURE 47–8. Management strategy of exit-site infections for peritoneal dialysis patients.

▶ TREATMENT: Prophylaxis of Peritonitis and Catheter-Related Infections

Attempts to prevent peritonitis and catheter-related infections have included refinement of connector system technology and the use of prophylactic antibiotic regimens and vaccines. Several studies have examined the impact of antibacterial agents as prophylaxis against both peritonitis and tunnel-related infections. Intermittent rifampin, 300 mg orally twice a day for 5 days, repeated every 3 months appears to decrease in the onset and number of catheter-related infections, but not peritonitis. The efficacy of other antibiotic prophylaxis for peritonitis and catheter-related infections is limited. Long-term, extended duration prophylaxis with penicillins or cephalosporins has not been shown to be effective.

Nasal carriage of S. *aureus* is associated with an increased risk of catheter-related infections and peritonitis. In addition, diabetic patients and those on immunosuppressive therapy are at increased risk for *S. aureus* catheter infections. Prophylaxis with intranasal mupirocin (bid for 5 days every month), mupirocin (daily) at the exit site, or oral rifampin can effectively reduce *S. aureus* exit-site infections.[129] Because of the minimal toxicity of mupirocin and the risk of rifampin resistance, mupirocin regimens are preferred.

PHARMACOKINETICS OF INTRAPERITONEAL DRUG THERAPY

The pharmacokinetics of intraperitoneal drug therapy have become more clearly defined in recent years.[130] Drugs may be added to dialysate to produce a local effect with limited systemic absorption. Alternatively, high systemic bioavailability may be desired for a systemic effect, or to ensure there is an adequate systemic reservoir, which would produce appropriate dialysate concentrations in subsequent drug-free exchanges (as with intermittent IP antibiotics). The primary pharmacokinetic factor that influences the bidirectional transfer of drugs is the magnitude of the ratio of systemic volume of distribution compared to the dialysate volume. The greater the ratio of the systemic volume to dialysate volume, the more readily will a drug molecule pass into the systemic circulation from the dialysate under the influence of a large concentration gradient. Conversely, drugs will more readily pass from the blood into the dialysate if the ratio of the systemic volume to the dialysate volume is small. Thus, drug regimens can be manipulated depending on whether one desires adequate clearance from dialysate into blood, or into dialysate from blood. Attempts have also been made to correlate peritoneal drug clearances with peritoneal membrane solute transport characteristics.[131]

Over the past decade, sound pharmacokinetic information has become available for a number of drugs in CAPD patients, and, to a lesser extent, for APD. Significant systemic bioavailability has been reported for some agents. In addition to their local effects for the management of peritonitis, as a result of their excellent systemic bioavailability, IP antibiotics can be used to treat systemic infections.[132] Potential benefits of the IP versus IV route for the management of systemic infections include use of an already existing access for administration, ability to treat infections on an outpatient basis, avoidance of costs for intravenous lines, possible avoidance of intravenous drug-related toxicities (such as thrombophlebitis and possibly red-neck syndrome), and improved patient acceptance. The pharmacoeconomics of this strategy, however, remain to be carefully studied and reported.

OTHER INTRAPERITONEAL DRUG THERAPY

Possible advantages of IP versus subcutaneous (SC) insulin include the avoidance of erratic absorption (both rate and extent of absorption), convenience, avoidance of subcutaneous injection site-related complications, and prevention of peripheral hyperinsulinemia.[133] Insulin appears to be cleared into the systemic compartment by an active transport process, or via the peritoneal lymphatics. A number of studies have demonstrated the bioavailability of IP insulin to be about 25% to 30%, although none clearly compares the clinical effectiveness of IP versus subcutaneous insulin in diabetes control.[133] Insulin requirements for PD patients may be greater than in hemodialysis patients because of the continued absorption of dextrose from the peritoneal cavity. Furthermore, because of adsorption of insulin to the polyvinyl chloride bag and administration set, the IP dose of insulin often needs to be two to three times the SC maintenance dose.

Many PD patients secrete large quantities of fibrinogen into the peritoneal cavity, which results in fibrin formation. This can lead to intraperitoneal adhesions and outflow obstruction. IP heparin may prevent this complication as a result of its local antifibrin effect.[134] Because standard heparin has a molecular weight of 12,000 to 15,000 daltons, it is minimally absorbed and thereby has limited systemic effects. The absorption of IP erythropoietin has also been studied. Its bioavailability is low, but may be increased when added into a dry peritoneum.[135]

STABILITY OF INTRAPERITONEAL ADDITIVES

There have been relatively few stability studies of drug additives to peritoneal dialysate, and the majority of those completed have been for antibiotics.[136] It appears that most antibiotic additives are stable (usually defined as retaining at least 90% of initial activity) for about 1 week if refrigerated or 1 to 2 days at room temperature. It is important to note that some studies may not be stability indicating, that is, they may assay total concentration of an agent, some of which may be from parent-drug degradation products and which may not therefore maintain the same degree of pharmacologic activity. Thus, appropriate studies would be those that also determine the concentrations of known degradation products. Clinicians must recall that chemical stability does not imply microbiological sterility.

NUTRITION AND PERITONEAL DIALYSIS

For many years it has been clear that CAPD patients were protein malnourished, on the basis of biochemical, anthropometric, and subjective measurements.[102] It has been estimated that 20% to 70% of PD patients may be malnourished.[137] Malnutrition has a significant impact on patient outcome,[102] and low serum albumin concentrations may be the strongest single predictor of decreased survival.[103] The mortality in those CAPD patients who have a serum albumin of less than 3.5 g/dL is increased by 3.5-fold. There is also a strong interrelationship between nutritional status and adequacy of dialysis. As *Kt/V* increases, serum albumin increases and mortality and morbidity decrease. Recently, a distinction was made between malnutrition without concomitant inflammation (Type 1) and malnutrition with an inflammatory process (Type 2).[138]

Intraperitoneal nutrition (IPN) has been attempted in an effort to address the nutritional needs of PD patients.[139] IPN usually contains both amino acids and glucose and is differentiated from practices of IP administration of amino acids only (IPAA). Both are normally 1% to 1.1% solutions. Thus, assuming a 75% absorption, 2 L of 1% IPAA would provide about 15 g of amino acid to the patient (about 0.2 g/kg body weight). Unfortunately, the majority of studies are of relatively short duration (1 to 2 months), although several have examined the influence of IPN and IPAA therapy for up to 6 months.[140] The results appear equivocal, some demonstrating improvements in certain nutritional parameters, and others not. There does not appear to be a consensus that these therapies positively influence patient survival or longevity. Potential adverse effects include acidosis, exacerbation of uremia, and loss of appetite. These issues, together with the significant costs of IP amino acid-based solutions, warrant further careful, long-term study before this approach is used clinically.

PATIENT OUTCOMES

During the past two decades, the renal community has focused much of its attention on technologically advancing the dialysis procedure, devising methods to quantitate the dose of dialysis delivered, and assessing the impact of the therapy on the morbidity and mortality of patients. During this time frame, the demographics of the U.S. dialysis population changed dramatically. The median age of ESRD patients increased from 55 to 61 years since 1980, and currently the United States has the oldest dialysis population of any industrialized nation.[141] These older patients have a larger number of coexistent medical conditions, many of which independently are associated with marked morbidity and mortality and, thereby, significantly contribute to the higher mortality seen in U.S. ESRD patients. The nutritional status of the patients at the time of dialysis initiation has also been shown to be a strong predictor of mortality.[137]

The optimal success of medical care has traditionally been defined as "curing" the disease. Recently, the paradigm has shifted in many settings to the prevention of a disease. In light of the persistent increase in the incidence of ESRD, these should remain avenues of avid research for the foreseeable future. For the patient with ESRD, however, the ultimate outcome may not be attainable, that is, decreasing annual mortality must surely have a finite limit based on the patient's concomitant disease states and life-style. Thus, a focus on quality of life [142,143] and rehabilitation[144,145] may be a valuable and viable goal toward which the nephrology community should redirect its research resources.

Some efforts in these fields have been initiated recently, but much remains to be done. The NKF-K/DOQI suggests a series of clinical outcome goals for PD patients. Although some of these are definitive statements, such as the hematocrit or serum albumin goals, others remain rather vague. For example, it is suggested that patient quality of life and pediatric growth and development be measured, but no specific goals are cited. This is because of the lack of published literature that might indicate an appropriate goal. Under these circumstances, pharmacists along with others on the health-care team need to become involved with the development, validation, and use of quality of life assessments, so that they can quantitate the contributions of their innovative interventions.

REFERENCES

1. U.S. Renal Data System 2001 Annual Data Report. Bethesda, MD, The National Institutes of Diabetes and Digestive and Kidney Diseases, 2001:70.
2. U.S. Renal Data System 1998 Annual Data Report. Bethesda, MD, The National Institutes of Diabetes and Digestive and Kidney Diseases, 1998:161.
3. Ismail N, Hakin RM, Oreopoulos DG, Patrikarea A. Renal replacement therapies in the elderly: Part 1. Hemodialysis and chronic peritoneal dialysis. In-depth review. Am J Kidney Dis 1993;22:759–782.
4. U.S. Renal Data System 2000 Annual Data Report. Bethesda, MD, The National Institutes of Diabetes and Digestive and Kidney Diseases, 2000:71.
5. Bloembergen WE, Port FK, Mauger EA, Wolfe RA. A comparison of mortality between patients treated with hemodialysis and peritoneal dialysis. J Am Soc Nephrol 1995;6:177–183.
6. Bloembergen WE, Port FK, Mauger EA, Wolfe RA. A comparison of cause of death between patients treated with hemodialysis and peritoneal dialysis. J Am Soc Nephrol 1995;6:184–191.
7. Fenton SSA, Schaubel DE, Desmeules M, et al. Hemodialysis versus peritoneal dialysis: A comparison of adjustment mortality rates. Am J Kidney Dis 1997;30:334–342.
8. Foley RN, Parfrey PS, Harnett JD, et al. Mode of dialysis therapy and mortality in end-stage renal disease. J Am Soc Nephrol 1998;9:267–276.
9. Wu MS, Yu CC, Yang CW, et al. Poor pre-dialysis glycaemic control is a predictor of mortality in type II diabetic patients on maintenance haemodialysis. Nephrol Dial Transplant 1997;12:2105–2110.
10. de Fijter CWH, Oe LP, Nauta JJP, et al. Clinical efficacy and morbidity associated with continuous cyclic compared with continuous ambulatory peritoneal dialysis. Ann Intern Med 1994;120:264–271.
11. U.S. Renal Data System 1993 Annual Data Report. Bethesda, MD, The National Institutes of Diabetes and Digestive and Kidney Diseases, 1993:13.
12. U.S. Renal Data System 2000 Annual Data Report. Bethesda, MD, The National Institutes of Diabetes and Digestive and Kidney Diseases, 2000:129.
13. Churchill DN, Thorpe KE, Vonesh EF, Keshaviah PR, for the Canada-USA (CANUSA) Peritoneal Dialysis Study Group. Lower probability of patient survival with continuous peritoneal dialysis in the United States compared with Canada. J Am Soc Nephrol 1997;8:965–971.
14. Held PJ, Port FK, Wolfe RA, et al. The dose of hemodialysis and patient mortality. Kidney Int 1996;50:550–556.
15. Habach G, Bloembergen WE, Mauger EA, et al. Hospitalization among United States dialysis patients: Hemodialysis versus peritoneal dialysis. J Am Soc Nephrol 1995;5:1940–1948.
16. McMurray SD, Miller J. Impact of capitation on freestanding dialysis facilities: Can you survive? Am J Kidney Dis 1997;30:542–548.
17. Health Care Financing Administration. 1999 Annual Report, End Stage Renal Disease Clinical Performance Measures Project. Baltimore, MD, Department of Health and Human Services, Health Care Financing Administration, Office of Clinical Standards and Quality, 1999.
18. Cleary DJ, Matzke GR, Alexander ACM, Joy MS. Medication knowledge and prescription-drug-taking behavior of patients receiving chronic dialysis. Am J Health Syst Pharm 1995;52:1895–1900.
19. U.S. Renal Data System 1998 Annual Data Report. Bethesda, MD, The National Institutes of Diabetes and Digestive and Kidney Diseases, 1998:51–62.
20. Kaplan B, Mason NA, Shimp LA, Ascion FJ. Chronic hemodialysis patients. Part I: Characterization and drug-related problems. Ann Pharmacother 1994;28:316–319.
21. Curtin RB, Svarstad BL, Andress D, Keller T, Sacksteder P. Differences in older versus younger hemodialysis patients' noncompliance with oral medications. Geriatr Nephrol Urol 1997;7:35–44.
22. Grabe DW, Low CL, Bailie GR, Eisele G. Evaluation of drug-related problems in an outpatient hemodialysis unit and the impact of a clinical pharmacist. Clin Nephrol 1997;47:117–121.
23. Possidente CJ, Bailie GR, Hood VL. Disruptions in drug therapy in long-term dialysis patients who require hospitalization. Am J Health Syst Pharm 1999;56:1961–1964.
24. Tang I, Vrahnos D, Hatoum H, Lau A. Effectiveness of clinical pharmacists interventions in a hemodialysis unit. Clin Ther 1993;15:459–464.
25. Pahre S. Nephrology pharmacy practice in the outpatient dialysis setting. Adv Ren Replace Ther 1997;4:179–181.
26. NKF-K/DOQI Clinical Practice Guidelines for Dialysis Adequacy. Update 2000. Am J Kidney Dis 2001;37(suppl 1):S65–S136.
27. Besarab A, Raja RM. Vascular access for hemodialysis. In: Daugirdas JT, Blake PG, Ing TS, eds. Handbook of Dialysis, 3rd ed. Philadephia, Lippincott Williams & Wilkins, 2001:67–101.
28. U.S. Renal Data System 1997 Annual Data Report. Bethesda, MD, The National Institutes of Diabetes and Digestive and Kidney Diseases, 1997:55.
29. NKF-K/DOQI. Clincial Practice Guidelines for Vascular Access: Update 2000. Am J Kidney Dis 2001;37(suppl 1):S137–S181.
30. Acchiardo SR. High-flux hemodialysis. In: Bosch JP, ed. Contemporary Issues in Nephrology: Hemodialysis High-Efficiency Treatments, Vol. 27. New York, Churchill Livingstone, 1993:105–117.
31. Collins AJ. High-flux, high-efficiency procedures. In: Henrich WE, ed. Principles and Practice of Dialysis. Baltimore, Williams & Wilkins, 1994:22–37.
32. Matzke GR, Palevsky PM, Frye RF. In vitro model for tobramycin disposition during hemodialysis with conventional and high flux biocompatible membranes. J Am Soc Nephrol 2000;11:286A.
33. Woffindin C, Hoenich NA. Hemodialyzer performance: A review of the trends over the past two decades. Artif Organs 1995;19:1113–1119.
34. Amin NB, Padhi ID, Touchette MA, et al. Characterization of gentamicin pharmacokinetics in patients hemodialyzed with high-flux polysulfone membranes. Am J Kidney Dis 1999;34:222–227.
35. Agarwal R, Cronin RE. Heterogeneity in gentamicin clearance between high-efficiency hemodialyzers. Am J Kidney Dis 1994;23:47–51.
36. Daugirdas JT, van Stone JC, Boag JT. Hemodialysis apparatus. In: Daugirdas JT, Blake PG, Ing TS, eds. Handbook of Dialysis, 3rd ed. Philadephia, Lippincott Williams & Wilkins, 2001:46–66.
37. van Ypersele de Strihou C. Are biocompatible membranes superior for hemodialysis therapy? Kidney Int 1997;52:S101–S104.
38. Ikizler TA. Biocompatibility and nutrition in hemodialysis. Semin Dial 1998;11:7–9.
39. Hartman J, Fricke H, Schiffl H. Biocompatible membranes preserve residual renal function in patients undergoing regular hemodialysis. Am J Kidney Dis 1997;30:366–373.
40. McCarthy JT, Jenson BM, Squillace DP, Williams AW. Improved preservation of residual renal function in chronic hemodialysis patients using polysulfone dialyzers. Am J Kidney Dis 1997;29:576–583.
41. Hornberger JC. The hemodialysis prescription and cost effectiveness. J Am Soc Nephrol 1993;4:1021–1027.
42. Helgerson SD, McClelland WM, Frederick PR, et al. Improvement in adequacy of delivered dialysis for adults in-center hemodialysis patients in the United States, 1993 to 1995. Am J Kidney Dis 1997;29:851–861.
43. Bloembergen WE, Stannard DC, Port FK, et al. Relationship of dose of hemodialysis and cause-specific mortality. Kindey Int 1996;50:557–565.
44. U.S. Renal Data System 2000 Annual Data Report: Atlas of End-Stage Renal Disease in the United States. Bethesda, MD, National Institutes of Health, National Institute of Diabetes and Digestive and Kidney Diseases, 2000:78.
45. Hakim RM, Breyer J, Ismail N, et al. Effects of dose of dialysis on morbidity and mortality. Am J Kidney Dis 1994;23:661–669.
46. Daugirdas JT, Kjellstrand CM. Chronic hemodialysis prescription: A urea kinetic approach. In: Daugirdas JT, Blake PG, Ing TS, eds. Handbook of Dialysis, 3rd ed. Philadelphia, Lippincott Williams & Wilkins, 2001:121–147.

47. Daugirdas JT, van Stone JC. Physiologic principles and urea kinetic modeling. In: Daugirdas JT, Blake PG, Ing TS, eds. Handbook of Dialysis, 3rd ed. Philadelphia, Lippincott Williams & Wilkins, 2001:15–45.
48. Held PJ, Carroll CE, Liska DW, et al. Hemodialysis therapy in the United States: What is the dose and does it matter? Am J Kidney Dis 1994;24:974–980.
49. Abuelo JG. Large interdialytic weight gains: Causes, consequences, and corrective measures. Semin Dial 1998;11:25–32.
50. Depner TA. Approach to hemodialysis urea modeling. In: Henrich WL, ed. Principles of Practice of Dialysis. Baltimore, Williams & Wilkins, 1994:47–62.
51. Daugirdas JT, Depner TA. A nomogram approach to hemodialysis urea modeling. Am J Kidney Dis 1994;23:33–40.
52. Pearson P, Lew S, Abramson F, Bosch J. Measurement of kinetic parameters for urea in end-stage renal disease patients using a two-compartment model. J Am Soc Nephrol 1994;4:1869–1873.
53. Daugirdas JT. Estimation of the equilibrated *Kt/V* using the unequilibrated postdialysis BUN. Semin Dial 1995;8:283–284.
54. Sherman RA, Cody RP, Matera JJ, et al. Deficiencies in delivered hemodialysis therapy due to missed and shortened treatments. Am J Kidney Dis 1994;24:921–923.
55. Kimmel PL, Peterson RA, Weihs KL, et al. Behavioral compliance with dialysis prescription in hemodialysis patients. J Am Soc Nephrol 1995;5:1826–1834.
56. U.S. Renal Data System 2000 Annual Data Report. Atlas of End-Stage Renal Disease in the United States. Bethesda, MD, National Institutes of Health, National Institutes of Diabetes and Digestive and Kidney Diseases, 2000:78.
57. Cheung AK, Agodoa LY, Daugirdas JT, et al. Effects of hemodialysis reuse on clearance of urea and β_2-microglobulin. J Am Soc Nephrol 1999;10:117–127.
58. Scott MK, Mueller BA, Sowinski KM. The effects of peracetic acid-hydrogen peroxide reprocessing on dialyzer solute and water permeability. Pharmacotherapy 1999;19:1042–1049.
59. Ouseph R, Brier ME, Ward RA et al. Improved dialyzer reuse after use of a population pharmacodynamic model to determine heparin doses. Am J Kidney Dis 2000;35:89–94.
60. Consensus Development Conference Panel. Morbidity and mortality on renal dialysis: NIH Consensus Conference Statement. Ann Intern Med 1994;121:62–70.
61. Bregman H, Daugirdas JT, Ing TS. Complications during hemodialysis. In: Daugirdas JT, Ing TS, eds. Handbook of Dialysis, 2nd ed. Boston, Little, Brown, 1994:149–168.
62. Pastan S, Bailey J. Dialysis therapy. N Eng J Med 1998;338:1428–1437.
63. Bregman H, Daugirdas JT, Ing TS. Complications during hemodialysis. In: Daugirdas JT, Blake PG, Ing TS, eds. Handbook of Dialysis, 3rd ed. Philadelphia, Lippincott Williams & Wilkins, 2001:148–168.
64. Blowey DL, Balfe JW, Gupta I, Gajaria MM, Koren G. Midodrine efficacy and pharmacokinetics in a patient with recurrent intradialytic hypotension. Am J Kidney Dis 1996;28:132–136.
65. Flynn JJ, Mitchell MC, Caruso FS, McElligott MA. Midodrine treatment for patients with hemodialysis hypotension. Clin Nephrol 1996;45: 261–267.
66. Cruz DN, Mahnensmith RL, Perazella MA. Intradialytic hypotension: Is midodrine beneficial in symptomatic hemodialysis patients? Am J Kidney Dis 1997;30:772–779.
67. Ahmad SA, Robertson HT, Golper TA, et al. Multicenter trial of L-carnitine in maintenance hemodialysis patients. II. Clinical and biochemical effects. Kidney Int 1990;38:912–918.
68. Shinzato T, Miwa M, Shigeru N, et al. Role of adenosine in dialysis-induced hypotension. J Am Soc Nephrol 1994;4:1987–1994.
69. Roca AO, Jarjoura D, Blend D, et al. Dialysis leg cramps. Efficacy of quinine versus vitamin E. ASAIO J 1992;38:M481–M485.
70. Federal Register, April 19, 1995.
71. Jansen PH, Veenhuiezen KC, Wesseling AI, et al. Randomised controlled trial of hydroquinine in muscle cramps. Lancet 1997;349:528–532.
72. Sidhom OA, Odeh YK, Krumlovsky FA, et al. Low-dose prazosin in patient with muscle cramps during hemodialysis. Clin Pharmacol Ther 1994;56:445–451.
73. Robertson KE, Mueller BA. Uremic pruritus. Am J Health Syst Pharm 1996;53:2159–2170.
74. Peer G, Kivity S, Agami O, et al. Randomised crossover trial of naltrexone in uraemic pruritus. Lancet 1996;348:1552–1554.
75. Morton CA, Lafferty M, Hau C, et al. Pruritus and skin hydration during dialysis. Nephrol Dial Transplant 1996;11:2031–2036.
76. Estelle F, Simons R. H_1-receptor antagonists: Comparative tolerability and safety. Drug Saf 1994;10:350–380.
77. Salem M, Ivanovich PT, Ing TS, et al. Adverse effects of dialyzers manifesting during the dialysis session. Nephrol Dial Transplant 1994;9 (suppl 2):127–137.
78. Kaufman AM, Godmere RO, Levin NW. Dialyzer reuse. In: Daugirdas JT, Blake PG, Ing TS, eds. Handbook of Dialysis, 3rd ed. Philadelphia, Lippincott Williams & Wilkins, 2001:169–181.
79. Pegues DA, Beck-Sague CM, Woollen SW, et al. Anaphylactoid reactions associated with reuse of hollow-fiber hemodialyzers and ACE inhibitors. Kidney Int 1992;42:1232–1237.
80. Cannella G, Paoletti E, Ravera G, et al. Inadequate diagnosis and therapy of arterial hypertension as causes of left ventricular hypertrophy in uremic dialysis patients. Kidney Int 2000;58:260–268.
81. Schomig M, Eisenhardt A, Ritz E. Controversy on optimal blood pressure on haemodialysis: Normotensive blood pressure values are essential for survival. Nephrol Dial Transplant 2001;16:469–474.
82. Wheeler DC. Should hyperlipidemia in dialysis patients be treated? Nephrol Dial Transplant 1997;12:19–21.
83. Deschamps-Latscha B, Herbelin A. Long-term dialysis and cellular immunity: A critical survey. Kidney Int 1993;43(suppl 41):S135– S142.
84. Arieff AI. Dialysis disequilibrium syndrome: Current concepts on pathogenesis and prevention. Kidney Int 1994;45:629–635.
85. Hakim RM, Wingard RL, Husni L, Parker RA, Parker TF. The effect of membrane biocompatibility on plasma β_2-microglobulin levels in chronic hemodialysis patients. J Am Soc Nephrol 1996;7:472–478.
86. Schwalbe S, Holzhauer M, Schaeffer J, et al. β_2-Microglobulin associated amyloidosis: A vanishing complication of long-term hemodialysis? Kidney Int 1997;52:1077–1083.
87. Hornberger JC, Chernew M, Peterson J, Garber AM. A multivariate analysis of mortality and hospital admissions with high-flux dialysis. J Am Soc Nephrol 1992;3:1227–1237.
88. Outbreaks of gram-negative bacterial blood stream infections traced to probable contamination of hemodialysis machines—Canada 1995; United States, 1997; and Israel, 1997. MMWR Morb Mortal Wkly Rep 1998;47:55–59.
89. Jochimsen EM, Carmichael WW, An J, et al. Liver failure and death after exposure to microcystins at a hemodialysis center in Brazil. N Engl J Med 1998;338:873–878.
90. Zoccali C, Dunea G. Hypertension. In: Daugirdas JT, Blake PG, Ing TS, eds. Handbook of Dialysis, 3rd ed. Philadelphia, Lippincott Williams & Wilkins, 2001:466–476.
91. Salem M. Hypertension in the hemodialysis population: A survey of 649 patients. Am J Kidney Dis 1995;26:461–468.
92. Kasiske BL. Hyperlipidemia in patients with chronic renal disease. Am J Kidney Dis 1998;32(5 Suppl 3):S142–S156.
93. Kay J, Hano JE. Musculoskeletal and rheumatic diseases. In: Daugirdas JT, Blake PG, Ing TS, eds. Handbook of Dialysis, 3rd ed. Philadelphia, Lippincott Williams & Wilkins, 2001:637–651.
94. Koda Y, Nishi SI, Miyazaki S, et al. Switch from conventional to high-flux membrane reduces the risk of carpal tunnel syndrome and mortality of hemodialysis patients. Kidney Int 1997;52:1096–1101.
95. Buoncristiani U. Continuous ambulatory peritoneal dialysis connection systems. Perit Dial Int 1993;13(suppl 2):5139–5145.
96. Brophy DF, Mueller BA. Automated peritoneal dialysis: New implications for pharmacists. Ann Pharmacother 1997;31:756–764.
97. Frankenfield DL, Prowant BF, Flanigan MJ, et al. Trends in clinical indicators of care for adult peritoneal dialysis patients in the United States from 1995 to 1997. Kidney Int 1999;55:1998–2010.

98. La Greca, Feriani M, Ronco C, et al. Proceedings of the 6th International Course on PD. Perit Dial Int 1997;17(suppl 2):S47–S83.
99. Peers E, Gokal R. Icodextrin: Overview of clinical experience. Perit Dial Int 1997;17:22–26.
100. Holmes CJ. Biocompatibility of peritoneal dialysis solutions. Perit Dial Int 1993;13:88–94. Editorial.
101. Dasgupta MX, Ward K, Noble PA, et al. Development of bacterial biofilms on silastic catheter materials in peritoneal dialysis fluid. Am J Kidney Dis 1994;23:709–716.
102. Ikizler TA, Wingard RL, Hakim RM. Future approaches to the treatment of malnutrition. Malnutrition in peritoneal dialysis patients: Etiologic factors and treatment options. Perit Dial Int 1995:15(suppl):S63–S66.
103. Dombros NV, Digenis GE, Oreopoulos DG. Is malnutrition a problem for the patient on peritoneal dialysis? Nutritional markers as predictors of survival in patients on CAPD. Perit Dial Int 1995:15(suppl):S10–S19.
104. Maiorca R, Brunori G, Zubani R, et al. Predictive value of dialysis adequacy and nutritional indices for mortality and morbidity in CAPD and hemodialysis patients. A longitudinal study. Nephrol Dial Transplant 1995;10:2295–2305.
105. Churchill DN, Taylor DW, Keshaviah PR, et al. Adequacy of dialysis and nutrition in continuous peritoneal dialysis: Association with clinical outcomes. J Am Soc Nephrol 1996;7:198–207.
106. Dumler F, Schmidt R, Cruz C. Abbreviated method for urea kinetic modeling in continuous ambulatory peritoneal dialysis patients. Perit Dial Int 1993;13(suppl 2):S50–S52.
107. Keshaviah R. Adequacy of CAPD: A quantitative approach. Kidney Int 1992;42(suppl 38):S160–S164.
108. Tzamoloukas AR, Murata GH, Sena R. Assessing the adequacy of peritoneal dialysis. Perit Dial Int 1993;13:236–237.
109. de Fijter CWH, Oe LP, Nauta JJP, et al. Clinical efficacy and morbidity associated with continuous cyclic compared with continuous ambulatory peritoneal dialysis. Ann Intern Med 1994:120:264–271.
110. Port FK. Risk of peritonitis and technique failure by CAPD connection technique. A national study. Kidney Int 1992:42:967–974.
111. Rodriguez-Carmona A, Fonatn MP, Falcon TG, Rivera CF, Valdes F. A comparative analysis of the incidence of peritoneal and exit site infection in CAPD and automated peritoneal dialysis. Perit Dial Int 1999;19: 253–258.
112. Holley JL, Bernardini J, Perlmutter JA, Piraino B. A comparison of infection rates among older and younger patients on continuous peritoneal dialysis. Perit Dial Int 1994;14:66–69.
113. Maiorca R, Giovanni CC, Giulio B, et al. Morbidity and mortality of CAPD and hemodialysis. Kidney Int 1993;43(suppl 40):S4–S15.
114. Keane WF, Bailie GR, Boeschoten E, et al. Adult peritoneal dialysis-related peritonitis treatment recommendations: 2000 update. Perit Dial Int 2000;20:396–411.
115. Vas SI. The diagnosis of peritonitis in patients on continuous ambulatory peritoneal dialysis. Semin Dial 1995;8:232–237.
116. Manley HJ, Bailie GR, Asher RD, Eisele G, Frye RF. Pharmacokinetics of intermittent intraperitoneal cefazolin in continuous ambulatory peritoneal dialysis patients. Perit Dial Int 1999;19:65–70.
117. Grabe DW, Bailie GR, Eisele G, Frye RF. Pharmacokinetics of intermittent intraperitoneal ceftazidime. Am J Kidney Dis 1999;33:111–117.
118. Manley HJ, Bailie GR, Frye RF, Hess LD, McGoldrick MD. Pharmacokinetics of intermittent intravenous cefazolin and tobramycin in patients treated with automated peritoneal dialysis. J Am Soc Nephrol 2000;11:1310–1316.
119. Manley HJ, Bailie GR, Frye RF, McGoldrick MD. Intermittent intravenous piperacillin pharmacokinetics in automated peritoneal dialysis patients. Perit Dial Int 2000;20:686–693.
120. Manley HJ, Bailie GR, Frye RF, McGoldrick MD. Intravenous vancomycin pharmacokinetics in automated peritoneal dialysis patients. Perit Dial Int 2001;21:378–385.
121. Goldie SJ, Kiernan-Troidle L, Torres C, et al. Fungal peritonitis in a large chronic peritoneal dialysis population: A report of 55 episodes. Am J Kidney Dis 1996;28:86–91.
122. The Turkish Multicenter Peritoneal Dialysis Study Group. The rate, risk factors, and outcome of fungal peritonitis in CAPD patients: Experience in Turkey. Perit Dial Int 2000;20:338–341.
123. Williams PF, Moncrief N, Marriott J. No benefit in using nystatin prophylaxis in peritoneal dialysis patients. Perit Dial Int 2000;20:352–353.
124. Shemin D, Maaz D, St. Pierre D, Kahn SI, Chazan JA. Effect of aminoglycoside use on residual renal function in peritoneal dialysis patients. Am J Kidney Dis 1999;34:14–20.
125. Flanagan MJ, Hochstetler LA, Langholdt D, Lim VS. CAPD catheter infections: Diagnosis and management. Perit Dial Int 1995;15:248–254.
126. Piraino B, Perlmutter JA, Holley JL, Bernardini J. *Staphylococcus aureus* peritonitis is associated with *Staphylococcus aureus* nasal carriage in peritoneal dialysis patients. Perit Dial Int 1993;13(suppl 2):5332–5334.
127. Piraino B, Bernardini J, Lutes R, et al. Randomized trial of mupirocin at exit-site vs oral rifampin to prevent *S. aureus* catheter infections. Perit Dial Int 1994;14(suppl 1):527. Abstract.
128. Waite NM, Webster N, Laurel M, et al. The efficacy of exit-site povidone-iodine ointment in the prevention of early peritoneal dialysis-related infections. Am J Kidney Dis 1997;29:763–768.
129. Piraino B, Lu VL. Nasal mupirocin: Its role in dialysis patients. Semin Dial 1997;10:145–147.
130. Taylor CA, Abdel-Rahman E, Zimmerman SW, Johnson CA. Clinical pharmacokinetics during continuous ambulatory peritoneal dialysis. Clin Pharmacokinet 1996;31:293–308.
131. Elwell RJ, Bailie GR, Manley HJ. Correlation of intraperitoneal antibiotic pharmacokinetics and peritoneal membrane transport characteristics. Perit Dial Int 2000;20:694–698.
132. Gorman T, Eisele G, Bailie GR. Intraperitoneal antibiotics effectively treat non-dialysis-related infections. Perit Dial Int 1995;15:283–284.
133. Chan E, Montgomery PA. Administration of insulin via continuous ambulatory peritoneal dialysis. Pharmacotherapy 1993;13:455–460.
134. Tabata T, Shimada H, Emoto M, et al. Inhibitory effect of heparin and/or antithrombin III on intraperitoneal fibrin formation in continuous ambulatory peritoneal dialysis. Nephron 1990;56:391–395.
135. Taylor CA, Kosorok MR, Zimmerman SW, Johnson CA. Pharmacokinetics of intraperitoneal epoetin alfa in patients on peritoneal dialysis using an 8-hour "dry dwell" dosing technique. Am J Kidney Dis 1999;34: 657–662.
136. Bailie GR, Kane MP. Stability of drug additives to peritoneal dialysate: A review. Perit Dial Int 1995;15:328–335.
137. Kopple JD. Effect of nutrition on morbidity and mortality in maintenance dialysis patients. Am J Kidney Dis 1994;24:1002–1009.
138. Stenvinkel P, Lindholm B, Heimburger O. New strategies for management of malnutrition in peritoneal dialysis patients. Perit Dial Int 2000; 20:271–275.
139. Jones MR. Intraperitoneal amino acids: A therapy whose time has come? Perit Dial Int 1995:15(suppl):S67–S74
140. Maurer O, Saxenhofer H, Jaeger P, et al. Six-month overnight administration of intraperitoneal amino acids does not improve lean mass. Clin Nephrol 1996;45:303–309.
141. Kurtin P, Nissenson AR. Variation in end-stage renal disease patient outcomes: What do we know, what should we know, and how do we find it out? J Am Soc Nephrol 1993;3:1738–1747.
142. Hays RD, Kallicli JD, Mapes DL, et al. Development of the kidney disease quality of life (KDQOL) instrument. Qual Life Res 1994;3:329–338.
143. Chapman MM, Meyer KB. Assessing health status in a dialysis clinic. Am J Health Syst Pharm 1995:52(suppl 3):531–532.
144. Proceedings from Renal Rehabilitation and Health Care Reform: Strategies for a changing era. Am J Kidney Dis 1994:24(suppl 1):S1–S32.
145. Holley JL, Nespor S. An analysis of factors affecting employment of chronic dialysis patients. Am J Kidney Dis 1994;23:681–685.

48

DRUG-INDUCED RENAL DISEASE

Thomas D. Nolin, Paul A. Abraham, and Gary R. Matzke

Drug-induced renal disease or nephrotoxicity (DIN) is a relatively common complication of several diagnostic and therapeutic agents. It is seen in both inpatient and outpatient settings with variable presentations depending on the drug and clinical setting. Manifestations of DIN include acid-base abnormalities, electrolyte imbalances, urine sediment abnormalities, proteinuria, pyuria, and/or hematuria. For example, hypokalemia and hypomagnesemia may be seen with both aminoglycoside antibiotic and diuretic therapy.[1] Diuretics may also induce metabolic alkalosis. However, the most common manifestation of DIN is a decline in the glomerular filtration rate, which results in a rise in the serum creatinine (S_{cr}) and blood urea nitrogen (BUN). Thus, initial diagnosis of DIN typically involves detection of elevated S_{cr} and BUN, for which there is a temporal relationship between the toxicity and use of a potentially nephrotoxic drug. Numerous quantitative definitions of DIN and/or acute renal failure have been published.[2] Thus, it is difficult to ascertain the "true" incidence of DIN for any drug. As a result, broad ranges of incidence have been reported in various studies of the same agent. DIN is often reversible on discontinuation of the offending agent, but may also lead to chronic and/or end-stage renal failure (see Chaps. 44 and 45). Many different mechanisms are involved in the pathogenesis of DIN. The development of drugs with novel mechanisms of action provides the potential for the presentation and identification of new unique nephropathies. This chapter reviews the epidemiology, pathophysiology, risk factors, and basic principles of prevention of drug-induced nephrotoxicity. Detailed discussions of these issues plus management strategies are presented for widely used agents that have been associated with moderate to high likelihood of DIN.

EPIDEMIOLOGY

Drug-induced nephrotoxicity occurs in all settings in which drugs are ingested or administered. It is a significant source of morbidity and mortality in the acute care hospital setting. DIN accounts for nearly 7% of all drug toxicity and up to 29% of all cases of acute renal failure in hospitals.[3,4] Overall, in-hospital drug use may contribute to 35% of all cases of acute tubular necrosis (ATN), most cases of allergic interstitial nephritis (AIN), as well as to nephropathy caused by alterations in renal hemodynamics and postrenal obstruction.[5] Aminoglycoside antibiotics, radiocontrast media, nonsteroidal anti-inflammatory drugs (NSAIDs), angiotensin-converting enzyme inhibitors (ACEIs), and diuretics are frequently implicated.[2,4]

The incidence and characteristics of outpatient- or community-acquired DIN are less-well understood because mild toxicity is often unrecognized. However, the pharmacoepidemiology of these effects has become more important as care increasingly shifts to the outpatient setting. Although as many as 3% to 6% of hospital admissions have been attributed to adverse drug effects during outpatient therapy,[6] 20% of hospital admissions for acute renal failure have been attributed specifically to community-acquired DIN.[2] NSAID nephrotoxicity is common and well defined. Prescribed and over-the-counter (OTC) NSAID therapy has been associated with a fourfold-increased risk of hospitalization for acute renal failure during the first month of therapy. The predominant risk factors include males > 65 years old, high drug dose, cardiovascular disease, recent hospitalization for nonrenal disease, and concomitant use of other potentially nephrotoxic drugs.[7] ACEIs are also associated with transient acute renal failure, and long-term therapy with the immunosuppressants cyclosporine and tacrolimus,[8] and abuse of combination analgesics,[9] have resulted in interstitial nephritis. Several recent reports indicate that unregulated OTC health foods and nutritional supplements can also cause renal failure, including chromium picolinate,[10] L-lysine,[11] creatine,[12] and Chinese herbal products containing aristolochic acid.[13]

ASSESSMENT OF RENAL TOXICITY

Because the most common manifestation of DIN is a decline in the glomerular filtration rate leading to a rise in the S_{cr} and BUN, the onset of toxicity in hospitalized acutely ill patients is most often recognized by routine laboratory monitoring of the two chemistries. Decreased urine output may also be an early sign of toxicity, particularly with radiographic contrast media, NSAIDs, and ACE inhibitors. In the outpatient setting, nephrotoxicity is often recognized by symptoms such as malaise, anorexia, and vomiting, or volume overload (shortness of breath or edema), which develop as the result of severe renal insufficiency. Serum creatinine or BUN concentrations and urine collection for creatinine clearance may subsequently be measured to quantify the degree of loss of glomerular filtration. A change in S_{cr} of at least 0.5 mg/dL for subjects with a S_{cr} < 2.0 mg/dL and an increase of 30% for those with $S_{cr} \geq 2.0$ mg/dL in a temporal fashion to the initiation of drug therapy is a common threshold for the identification of DIN. Marked intrasubject between-day variability of S_{cr} values has been noted (±20% for values within the normal range) (see Chap. 42). Furthermore, S_{cr} may be altered as the result of dietary changes and initiation of drug therapy, which may interfere with the assay procedure.

Nephrotoxicity may be evidenced by alterations in renal tubular function without loss of glomerular filtration. Indicators of proximal tubular injury include metabolic acidosis with bicarbonaturia; glycosuria in the absence of hyperglycemia; and reductions in serum phosphate, uric acid, potassium and magnesium due to increased urinary losses. Indicators of distal tubular injury include polyuria from failure to maximally concentrate urine, metabolic acidosis from impaired urinary acidification, and hyperkalemia from impaired potassium excretion. Urinary excretion of enzymes and low-molecular weight proteins, including *N*-acetyl-βD-glucosaminidase and β_2-microglobulin, respectively, are also indices of early tubular injury. However, these indicators are rarely measured in clinical practice. Rather, they are a sensitive means to assess toxicity, particularly in clinical research investigations.

PATHOPHYSIOLOGICAL MECHANISMS OF NEPHROTOXIC SUSCEPTIBILITY

The kidneys are more sensitive than many other organs to drug toxicity. Immune-mediated, drug-induced nephrotoxicities include glomerulonephritis and allergic interstitial nephritis, either with or without nephrotic syndrome. The kidney is highly susceptible to this type of injury because its large vascular surface area yields extensive exposure to circulating immune mediators and intrinsic immune function of glomerular mesangial cells and renal cytokine activation. Nonimmunologic mechanisms of DIN relate to several specialized characteristics of normal renal physiology, including regulation of blood flow, intrarenal drug metabolism, tubular transport processes, and urine concentration and acidification abilities (Fig. 48–1).

AUTOREGULATION OF RENAL BLOOD FLOW

The kidneys constitute only 0.4% of body weight, but receive 20% to 25% of resting cardiac output. This enhances the kidney's exposure to circulating drugs. Within each nephron, blood flow and pressure are regulated by glomerular afferent and efferent arterioles to maintain capillary hydrostatic pressure and glomerular filtration (Fig. 48–2A). This specialized blood flow is precisely regulated by interrelations between renal prostaglandins, atrial natriuretic factor, the sympathetic nervous system, the renin-angiotensin system, and the macula densa response to distal tubular solute delivery. In this unique vascular setting, β-blockers[14] and NSAIDs may reduce total renal blood flow, radiographic contrast media may shunt intrarenal blood flow away from superficial nephrons,[15] osmotic diuresis secondary to mannitol therapy may reduce glomerular blood flow caused by tubuloglomerular feedback,[16] and ACEIs dilate glomerular efferent arterioles and result in a decrease in glomerular filtration pressure. Finally, dietary salt restriction can activate neurohumoral renal hemodynamic control systems that increase renal susceptibility to these drug nephrotoxicities.[17]

INTRARENAL DRUG METABOLISM

Multiple renal enzymes contribute to drug metabolism. These include cytochrome P450 and mixed function oxidases in proximal tubular epithelial cells, which have activity similar to their counterparts in the liver. In contrast, prostaglandin endoperoxide synthetase activity is more localized to the renal papilla and medulla. The kidney may thus transform a drug to a nephrotoxic metabolite. As an example, acetaminophen can be oxidized to reactive species that contribute to acute tubular necrosis following acute overdose and to analgesic nephropathy with chronic consumption.[18]

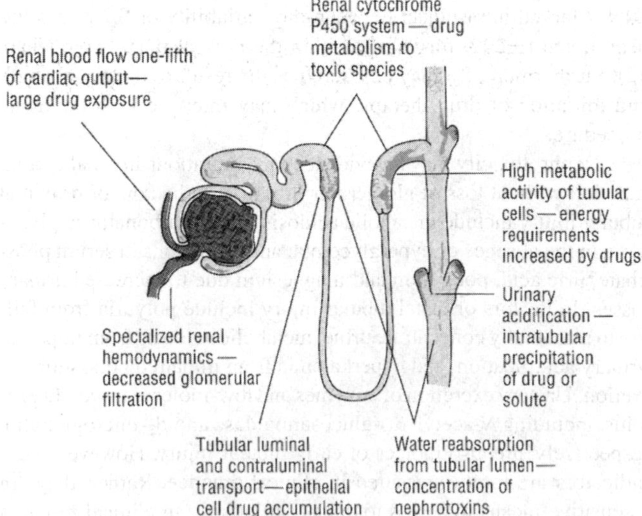

FIGURE 48–1. Mechanisms of renal susceptibility to drug toxicity. See text for discussion.

TUBULAR TRANSPORT PROCESSES

Tubular transport systems within the kidney, including the organic cation transporter 1 (OCT1), organic anion transporter 1 (OAT1), and P-glycoprotein (P-gp), play a vital role in the elimination of drugs and their metabolites from the body.[19–21] Proximal tubule cells are the primary site of active carrier-mediated transport of organic ions from blood to urine.[21] The concentration of drugs in the proximal tubule can thus be several-fold higher than systemic concentrations, resulting in local cytotoxicity, which may eventually manifest as clinical nephrotoxicity. OAT1 is implicated in the cellular uptake, accumulation, and nephrotoxicity of the acyclic nucleotide antivirals adefovir and cidofovir,[22] and some cephalosporin antibiotics.[23] Administration of OAT1 inhibitors such as probenecid markedly reduce cytotoxicity induced by these agents. Conversely, P-gp has been called the molecular "vacuum cleaner" because of the varied substrates it is known to pump out of cells, including anticancer agents, calcium-channel blockers, steroids, digoxin, cyclosporine and tacrolimus.[19,24] Unlike OCT1 and OAT1, overexpression of P-gp in the renal tubular cells prevents nephrotoxicity induced by cyclosporine, and inhibition of the protein leads to toxicity.[19] Elevated intracellular drug concentrations may cause cytotoxicity as the result of impairment of mitochondrial function and decreased adenosine triphosphate (ATP) synthesis, increased oxidative stress, depletion of reduced glutathione and other antioxidants, inhibition of phospholipid metabolism, or disruption of protein synthesis. Aminoglycosides, cyclosporine, and cisplatin appear to mediate nephrotoxicity by increasing the formation of superoxide ion and hydrogen peroxide, which in the presence of iron subsequently generates its hydroxyl radical, a reactive oxygen species that contributes to cellular oxidative stress and nephrotoxicity.[25]

CONCENTRATION OF SOLUTE IN THE TUBULAR LUMEN

Ninety-nine percent of the water filtered by the glomerulus is reabsorbed. Normally, 50% to 85% of water reabsorption occurs in the proximal tubule, while the remainder occurs in the descending loop of Henle and collecting duct. Systemic volume depletion increases the percent of water reabsorption in the proximal tubule. As water reabsorption increases, the concentration of drugs increase within the tubular lumen. Thus, the luminal surfaces of cells, particularly in the proximal tubule, can be exposed to higher concentrations of potential toxins and for a longer time than most other tissues in the body. This enhances binding of drugs to tubular epithelial cells and promotes active and passive transport into cells. The enhancement of aminoglycoside nephrotoxicity by systemic volume depletion is an example.[26]

HIGH ENERGY REQUIREMENTS

Renal tubular epithelial cells have high energy requirements because of active tubular transport and metabolic processes. These high energy needs are precariously supplied to medullary tubular epithelial cells, which function in a state of chronic hypoxia because of their

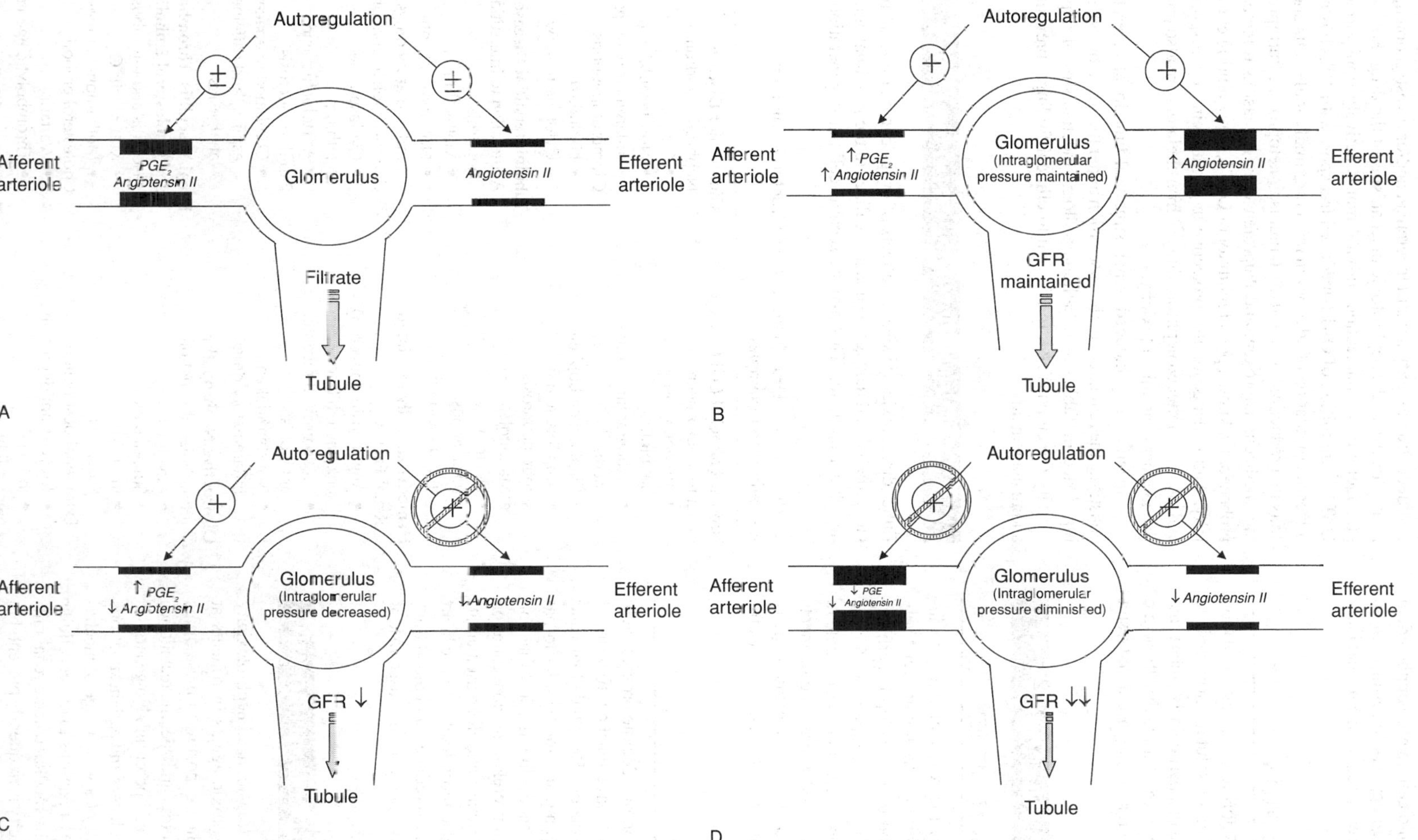

FIGURE 126–2. **A.** Normal glomerular autoregulation serves to maintain intraglomerular capillary hydrostatic pressure, glomerular filtration rate (GFR), and, ultimately, urine output. This is accomplished by modulation of afferent and efferent arterioles. Afferent and efferent arteriolar vasoconstriction are primarily mediated by angiotensin II whereas afferent vasodilation is primarily mediated by prostaglandins. **B.** The kidney maintains GFR by dilating the afferent arteriole and constricting the efferent arteriole, specifically in response to a decrease in renal blood flow. During states of reduced blood flow the juxtaglomerular apparatus increases renin secretion. Plasma renin converts angiotensinogen to angiotensin I, and, ultimately, to angiotensin II (AII) by angiotensin-converting enzyme. AII constricts the afferent and efferent arterioles resulting in a net increase in intraglomerular pressure. Additionally, renal prostaglandins, prostaglandin E_2 (PGE_2) in particular, are released and induce a net dilation of the afferent arteriole, thereby improving blood flow into the glomerulus. Together these processes maintain glomerular filtration rate and urine output. **C.** ACE inhibitor nephropathy often occurs in the setting of reduced blood flow. When ACE inhibitor therapy (e.g., enalapril, ramipril) is initiated, the synthesis of angiotensin II is decreased, thereby preferentially dilating the efferent arteriole. This reduces outflow resistance from the glomerulus and decreases hydrostatic pressure in the glomerular capillaries, which alters Starling's forces across the glomerular capillaries to decrease intraglomerular pressure and GFR. **D.** NSAIDs inhibit vasodilatory prostaglandins at the afferent arteriole, resulting in net constriction of the arteriole and a subsequent decrease in intraglomerular pressure and GFR. Combined use of NSAIDs and ACEIs commonly induces hemodynamically mediated renal failure because of a dramatic decrease in intraglomerular pressure.

perfusion with venous blood returning from the deep medulla. As a consequence these medullary tubular epithelial cells are especially sensitive to drugs that increase energy demands or decrease oxygen delivery, which can result in ischemic cell death. Amphotericin B-induced medullary tubular cell damage appears to result from an imbalance between increased cellular energy requirements and inadequate oxygen delivery.[27]

URINE ACIDIFICATION

Urine pH decreases to approximately 4.5 during maximal stimulation of renal tubular hydrogen ion secretion. Certain solutes can precipitate and obstruct the tubular lumen at this acid pH, particularly when urine is concentrated. For example, in the presence of a maximally acidic urine, intratubular precipitation of methotrexate may occur and result in acute renal failure.[28]

SUSCEPTIBLE PATIENT POPULATIONS

CHRONIC RENAL INSUFFICIENCY

Chronic renal insufficiency develops as the result of injury to involved glomerular and tubular units while others remain relatively intact. The remaining functional nephron units develop hyperfiltering glomeruli and hyperfunctioning tubules to compensate for the damaged nephrons. These residual nephrons are more susceptible to nephrotoxic injury because of their increased energy requirements and exposure to elevated concentrations of drugs. The nephrotoxicity of radiographic contrast media in patients with chronic renal insufficiency is such an example.[29]

ELDERLY

Renal blood flow and glomerular filtration rate decline progressively with age, particularly in males once they have reached 40 years of age.[30] Progressive sclerosis of glomeruli occurs. Residual glomerular and tubular units increase function in compensation, similar to patients with chronic renal insufficiency. This decline in renal function is not accompanied by a rise in the serum creatinine concentration due to the age-related decline in muscle mass and decreased creatinine generation. Older individuals are also more likely to have heart failure and hepatic insufficiency, which also reduce renal blood flow. Together, these processes predispose the elderly to increased risk of nephrotoxicity.[31]

PRINCIPLES FOR PREVENTION OF DRUG NEPHROPATHY

The primary principle for prevention of drug-induced nephrotoxicity is to avoid the use of potentially nephrotoxic agents in patients at increased risk for toxicity. However, when exposure to these drugs cannot be avoided, recognition of risk factors and specific techniques may be used to reduce the drugs nephrotoxic potential. No generalizable risk factors are applicable to all drug classes and patient situations because drug toxicity develops as a result of a wide range of mechanisms, from idiosyncratic hypersensitivity reactions to direct cellular toxicity. An exception is hemodynamically mediated acute renal failure due to NSAIDs and ACEIs. Their toxicity is frequently preventable by recognizing pre-existing renal insufficiency and decreased effective renal blood flow caused by volume depletion, heart failure, or liver disease. Elderly patients with hypertension or heart failure may be especially sensitive to the combined use of ACEIs and NSAIDs.

Certain approaches to reduce drug toxicity are prudent and generally effective; for example, careful and adequate hydration to establish high renal tubular urine flow rates. However, other strategies to reduce drug toxicity are still theoretical and/or investigational, and relate directly to the nephrotoxic mechanisms of the drug. For example, adefovir is a nucleotide antiviral that is actively transported by OAT1.[22] Inhibition of OAT1-mediated transport with NSAIDs minimizes accumulation of adefovir in renal proximal tubule cells and results in a reduction in toxicity.[32] Diflunisal, ketoprofen, flurbiprofen, indomethacin, naproxen, and ibuprofen were at least as effective as probenecid, a known potent inhibitor of OAT1, at preventing cytotoxicity. Antioxidants are also protective in gentamicin-, cyclosporine-, and cisplatin-induced nephrotoxicity.[25] Iron chelators are also protective against gentamicin toxicity.

Specific drug-induced renal structural-functional alterations constitute the remainder of this discussion under the seven broad headings listed in Table 48–1. Pathophysiologic mechanisms of nephrotoxicity are emphasized, in addition to clinical findings, prevention, and management.

TUBULAR EPITHELIAL CELL DAMAGE

Either direct toxic or ischemic effects of drugs can cause renal tubular epithelial cell damage. Damage localizes in the proximal and distal tubular epithelia. This may be seen as cellular degeneration and

TABLE 48–1. Drug-Induced Renal Structural-Functional Alterations and Examples

Tubular Epithelial Cell Damage
- Acute tubular necrosis
  - Aminoglycoside antibiotics
  - Radiographic contrast media
  - Cisplatin/carboplatin
  - Amphotericin B
- Osmotic nephrosis
  - Mannitol
  - Dextran
  - Intravenous immunoglobulin

Hemodynamically-Mediated Renal Failure
- Angiotensin-converting enzyme Inhibitors
- Angiotensin II receptor antagonists
- Nonsteroidal anti-inflammatory drugs

Obstructive Nephropathy
- Intratubular obstruction
  - Acyclovir
  - Sulfadiazine
  - Indinavir
  - Foscarnet
- Extra renal obstruction
  - Tricyclic antidepressants
  - Indinavir
- Nephrolithiasis
  - Triamterene
  - Indinavir

Glomerular Disease
- Nephrotic syndrome
  - Gold
  - Nonsteroidal anti-inflammatory drugs
- Glomerulonephritis
  - Hydralazine
  - Cytokine therapy

Tubulointerstitial Disease
- Acute allergic interstitial nephritis
  - Methicillin
  - Nonsteroidal anti-inflammatory drugs
- Chronic interstitial nephritis
  - Cyclosporine
  - Lithium
  - Aristolochic acid
- Papillary necrosis
  - Combined phenacetin, aspirin, and caffeine analgesics

Renal Vasculitis, Thrombosis, and Cholesterol Emboli
- Vasculitis and thrombosis
  - Mitomycin C
  - Methamphetamines
- Cholesterol emboli
  - Warfarin
  - Thrombolytic agents

Pseudo Renal Failure
- Corticosteroids
- Trimethoprim
- Cimetidine

sloughing from proximal and distal tubular basement membranes in ATN, or swelling and vacuolization of proximal tubular cells in osmotic nephrosis. ATN is the most common presentation of DIN in the inpatient setting. The primary agents implicated are radiocontrast media, aminoglycosides, cisplatin, amphotericin B, foscarnet, and osmotically active agents such as immunoglobulins, dextrans, and mannitol.[1,33]

ACUTE TUBULAR NECROSIS

AMINOGLYCOSIDE NEPHROTOXICITY

Incidence

Nephrotoxicity has been reported in 1.7% to 58% of patients receiving aminoglycoside therapy. The large variance is in part because of the use of different definitions of toxicity and variability between agents in the class, as well as the risk factors in the study population.[34]

Clinical Presentation

A gradual rise in the serum creatinine concentration and decrease in creatinine clearance after 6 to 10 days of therapy are the initial clinical manifestations of toxicity. Increased renal tubular proteinuria (β_2-microglobulin) and brush-border enzymuria precede the creatinine rise by several days, but are not usually detected clinically.[26] Patients typically present with nonoliguria, maintaining urine volumes greater than 500 mL/d. Renal magnesium and potassium wasting can occur. Renal failure is usually mild if aminoglycoside therapy is stopped, but may be severe and require dialysis therapy. Aminoglycoside-associated nephropathy must be evaluated carefully because not all renal failure during a course of therapy is caused by the aminoglycoside. Dehydration, sepsis, ischemia, and other nephrotoxic drugs frequently contribute.

Pathogenesis

The pathogenesis of reduced glomerular filtration rate in patients receiving aminoglycosides is predominantly the result of proximal tubular epithelial cell damage leading to obstruction of the tubular lumen and backleak of the glomerular filtrate across the damaged tubular epithelium.[35] The toxicity of various aminoglycosides is related to cationic charge, which facilitates binding of filtered aminoglycosides to renal tubular epithelial cell luminal membranes. For instance, neomycin has six cationic amino groups and is the most nephrotoxic aminoglycoside, whereas streptomycin, with three groups, is least toxic. Gentamicin and tobramycin, with five amino groups, have similar and intermediate toxicity, whereas amikacin and netilmicin, with four and three amino groups, respectively, may be less toxic. Binding to tubular epithelial cells is followed by intracellular transport and concentration in lysosomes. Subsequent binding to acidic phospholipids (phosphatidylinositol) causes their aggregation and inhibits phospholipase activity.[26,35] This presents histopathologically as myeloid bodies within lysosomes of renal tubular epithelial cells. The membrane function of mitochondria and other cell organelles is also affected.[26] Cellular dysfunction and death may result from release of lysosomal enzymes into the cytosol, generation of reactive oxygen species, altered cellular metabolism, and alterations in cell membrane fluidity leading to reduced activity of membrane-bound enzymes, including Na^+/K^+-ATPase, dipeptidyl peptidase IV, and neutral aminopeptidase.[26] Although binding of aminoglycosides to tubular epithelial cells is facilitated by the number of cationic groups present, inherent risks of toxicity are also a factor

TABLE 48–2. Potential Risk Factors for Aminoglycoside Nephrotoxicity

Related to aminoglycoside dosing:
- Large total cumulative dose
- Prolonged therapy
- Trough concentration exceeding 2 mg/L
- Recent previous aminoglycoside therapy

Related to synergistic nephrotoxicity. Aminoglycosides in combination with:
- Cyclosporine
- Amphotericin B
- Vancomycin
- Diuretics

Related to predisposing conditions in the patient:
- Preexisting renal insufficiency
- Increased age
- Poor nutrition
- Shock
- Gram-negative bacteremia
- Liver disease
- Hypoalbuminemia
- Obstructive jaundice
- Dehydration
- Potassium or magnesium deficiencies

Risk Factors

Multiple risk factors for aminoglycoside nephrotoxicity have been identified. These relate to aminoglycoside dosing, synergistic toxicity in combination with other drugs, and predisposing conditions in the patient (Table 48–2). These risk factors have been consistently identified in all investigations and the reader is referred to the in-depth reviews on this issue.[26,35] Although combined vancomycin and aminoglycoside therapy has been reported by some to be highly nephrotoxic, a meta-analysis suggests only a 1% to 7% increased risk of toxicity with combination therapy compared to aminoglycoside therapy alone.[36]

Prevention

The prevention of aminoglycoside-induced nephrotoxicity has received considerable attention in recent years. Alternative antibiotics should be used whenever possible and changes from empiric therapy made as soon as microbial sensitivities are known. Commonly used alternatives include fluoroquinolones (e.g., ciprofloxacin, levofloxacin) and third-generation cephalosporins (e.g., ceftazidime, cefepime). When aminoglycosides are necessary, the specific drug used does not appear to significantly affect the risk of nephrotoxicity, and therapy should be selected to optimize antimicrobial efficacy. Furthermore, it is imperative to avoid volume depletion, to limit the total aminoglycoside dose administered, and to avoid concomitant therapy with other nephrotoxic drugs.

Prospective, individualized pharmacokinetic monitoring has been used for more than 25 years. Although many have reported a decrease in the incidence of aminoglycoside-induced nephrotoxicity the studies were often small and statistically underpowered. Recently, Streetman et al. estimated that pharmacokinetic monitoring decreased costs associated with aminoglycoside nephrotoxicity by more than $900 per patient.[38] High intermittent dosing of aminoglycosides, often called "once-daily" dosing, used in combination with other antibiotics, has been intensively investigated as a practical cost-effective method to maintain antimicrobial efficacy while potentially reducing nephrotoxicity, vestibular and ototoxicity.[26,37,39,40] Historically, high 1 hour postdose concentrations such as those obtained during once-daily dosing were thought to contribute to the renal and auditory toxicity. Recent data suggests otherwise, and in fact, even calls into question the utility of monitoring peak concentrations.[37,39] Nephrotoxicity may be reduced because proximal tubular aminoglycoside uptake appears to be limited during the transient, high-peak serum concentrations caused by saturation of binding sites. The achievement of low aminoglycoside concentrations for a greater proportion of the dosing interval facilitates excretion of the aminoglycoside. A recent meta-analysis suggests greater clinical efficacy and reduced nephrotoxicity with once-daily dosing, as compared to standard dosing.[37] Seriously ill, immunocompromised, renal-insufficient, and elderly patients, however, are not ideal candidates for this approach.[37] Indeed, nephrotoxicity was more common in elderly patients who received once daily versus conventional gentamicin or tobramycin.[41] Another method of preventing aminoglycoside nephrotoxicity may include the administration of agents that decrease aminoglycoside binding to lysosomal phospholipids in the kidney.[35] The administration of polyaspartic acid, an investigational polyanionic peptide, has been shown to decrease the interaction of aminoglycosides with anionic phospholipids and thereby cell injury.[26]

Management

Serum creatinine concentrations should be measured frequently (every 2 to 4 days) during therapy. Aminoglycoside use should be discontinued or the dosage regimen revised if the S_{cr} increases by >0.5 mg/dL during a course of therapy. Other nephrotoxic drugs should be discontinued if possible, and the patient should be maintained adequately hydrated and hemodynamically stable. Dialysis may be necessary, but renal failure due solely to aminoglycoside toxicity is usually reversible.

RADIOGRAPHIC CONTRAST MEDIA NEPHROTOXICITY

Incidence

Nephrotoxicity induced by radiographic contrast media is the third-leading cause of hospital-acquired acute renal failure.[42] The incidence rises from <1% in patients with low risk to 20% to 30% in patients with preexistent renal insufficiency.[29,43] The risk of contrast nephropathy increases as the number of risk factors increases, and diabetic patients with renal insufficiency have the greatest risk.[29,43,44] Mortality from radiocontrast nephrotoxicity is reported to be 29%.[45] A decrease in renal function following contrast administration may also be caused by concomitant medical illness and dehydration, often a result of fluid restriction and cathartics used for study preparation. The presence of a "prerenal" state of acute renal failure may be the primary cause or a contributing risk factor to the observed decrease in renal function.[43,44]

Clinical Presentation

Toxicity ranges from transient tubular enzymuria to irreversible oliguric (urine volume < 500 mL/d) renal failure requiring dialysis therapy.[29,43] Severe toxicity is most frequent in diabetic patients with preexistent severe renal insufficiency. The typical course is an initial transient osmotic diuresis followed by tubular proteinuria and enzymuria. The serum creatinine rises and peaks between 2 and 5 days after exposure with recovery after 4 to 10 days. Oliguria is present in about 50% of cases. Urinalysis typically reveals only hyaline and granular casts, but may also be completely bland.[44] Importantly, the urine sodium concentration and fractional excretion of sodium are frequently low.[29,43] Although toxicity has generally been considered to be mild and reversible, a retrospective cohort analysis revealed a 34% mortality rate in 174 patients with contrast media-associated acute renal failure (rise in serum creatinine of ≥25% from baseline and ≥2.0 mg/dL) as compared to 7% mortality in a cohort without acute renal failure.[46] Death was attributable to sepsis, respiratory failure, delirium, and bleeding that intensified after the onset of acute renal failure.

Pathogenesis

Contrast nephropathy appears to be caused by direct tubular toxicity and by renal ischemia.[15,29,43] Direct tubular toxicity is suggested by renal tubular enzymuria and biopsy findings of proximal tubular epithelial cell vacuolization and acute tubular necrosis. In addition to the direct toxic effects of contrast media, the nonselective proteinuria induced by contrast media may indirectly damage tubular epithelial cells. In contrast to these findings, the low urine sodium concentration and low fractional excretion of sodium frequently observed suggest preserved renal tubular function and participation of renal ischemia more than tubular toxicity. Renal ischemia may result from systemic hypotension associated with contrast injection, as well as renal vasoconstriction mediated by imbalance of humoral agents including prostaglandins, adenosine, atrial natriuretic peptide, nitric oxide, and endothelin.[29,43,44] Renal ischemia may also result from dehydration as a result of osmotic diuresis accompanying use of hyperosmolar agents (900–1,780 mOsm/kg) and increased blood viscosity caused by red blood cell crenation and aggregation.

Risk Factors

Pre-existent renal insufficiency, particularly diabetic nephropathy with renal insufficiency, is the major risk factor. Conditions associated with decreased renal blood flow, including congestive heart failure and dehydration, also confer risk. The presence of multiple myeloma has been considered a relative contraindication for contrast use, but the risk appears to be associated with concomitant dehydration, renal insufficiency, or hypercalcemia, rather than with the diagnosis itself. Both larger doses of contrast and use of older hyperosmolar contrast agents promote risk in susceptible patients.[29]

Prevention

The importance of strategies aimed at preventing radiocontrast-induced nephrotoxicity cannot be overemphasized. All patients scheduled to receive radiocontrast media should be assessed for risk factors, and the risk:benefit ratio should be considered.[47] Nephrotoxicity can be predicted in the majority of patients at risk, which justifies the use of procedures with even minimal benefit.[48] High-risk patients should be identified, primarily by medical history and indication for the contrast study, but also by prestudy serum creatinine concentrations.[29] Nephrotoxicity is best prevented in high-risk patients by using alternative imaging procedures (e.g., ultrasound, magnetic resonance imaging, and nuclear medicine scans). However, if contrast media must be used, the smallest adequate dose should be administered. Dose reduction proportional to the level of renal insufficiency may be protective, but may limit the adequacy of imaging.[47]

The utility of lower osmolar nonionic (iohexol and iopamidol) and ionic (ioxaglate) contrast agents to prevent nephrotoxicity remains unclear. Standard contrast media are not reabsorbed in the kidney and cause osmotic diuresis, which contributes to the renal toxicity observed with these agents. The second generation of contrast agents have half the osmolality of standard agents, and have been associated with a decreased incidence of contrast nephropathy, especially when used in patients with pre-existing renal insufficiency.[44] The largest prospective trial of 1,196 patients revealed that a 0.5-mg/dL or greater rise in S_{cr} occurred 55% less often in patients with preexisting renal insufficiency and 30% less often in patients with diabetic nephropathy who received iohexol (a second-generation agent) as compared to diatrizoate.[49] However, use of low-osmolar agents does not eliminate nephrotoxicity, and the preventative measures outlined below should be utilized with these agents. Because these agents are considerably more expensive than standard higher osmolar ionic agents, their true cost-benefits remain controversial. A cost-effective strategy may be to use low-osmolar contrast agents in patients with preexisting renal insufficiency, particularly those with diabetic nephropathy, and standard agents in patients with normal renal function. Additionally, the low-osmolar agents cause less histamine release and may be advantageous for hemodynamically unstable patients or those with a history of hypersensitivity to contrast media. Dialysis to remove contrast media after administration does not appear to prevent toxicity.[50]

Dehydration should be corrected before contrast administration, other nephrotoxic drugs discontinued if possible, and subsequent contrast studies appropriately timed to avoid cumulative toxicity. Saline hydration before and after contrast administration may reduce the incidence of toxicity in high-risk patients.[44] In addition to the obvious correction of dehydration, saline administration may lessen the impact of contrast induced osmotic diuresis. Additional beneficial effects of saline prehydration may include dilution of contrast media, prevention of renal vasoconstriction leading to ischemia, and avoidance of tubular obstruction. Use of mannitol and furosemide to prevent toxicity remains controversial. Investigators recently treated high-risk patients undergoing cardiac catheterization with either saline alone or a combination of furosemide, low-dose dopamine, and mannitol. No difference in renal function indices was observed between the groups.[48] Dopamine appears to offer some protection against contrast nephropathy in select patients,[51] but it should not be used in diabetic patients.[44] A recent study of the efficacy of atrial natriuretic peptide for the prevention of contrast nephropathy showed no benefit as compared to control.[42] The administration of theophylline,[44,47] fenoldopam[52a,52b] and prostaglandin E_1[53] prior to exposure may also be protective.

Management

Currently, there is no specific therapy available for managing established contrast nephropathy[44] (See Chap. 43). Care is supportive with dialysis as needed in selected patients. Careful attention must be given to preventing infection and bleeding and providing respiratory support in view of the high association of these complications with death.[46]

CISPLATIN AND CARBOPLATIN NEPHROTOXICITY

Incidence

Platin-containing compounds are important chemotherapeutic agents that frequently cause renal tubular damage.[28,54] The incidence of cisplatin nephrotoxicity was 50% to 100% in the 1980s. Subsequently, the incidence of toxicity decreased to 6% to 13%, primarily by limiting the total drug dose and reducing the rate of administration. However, when used in combination with other nephrotoxins, high-dose cisplatin appears to contribute to acute renal failure (ARF), which occurs in >50% of patients who receive a bone marrow transplant for advanced breast cancer.[55] Carboplatin, a second-generation platinum analog, is associated with a lower incidence of nephrotoxicity than cisplatin.[28]

Clinical Presentation

Nephrotoxicity manifests early during therapy as transient proximal tubular cell brush border and lysosomal enzymuria.[28] Peak serum creatinine concentrations occur approximately 10 to 12 days after initiation of therapy, with recovery by 21 days. However, renal damage can be cumulative with subsequent cycles of therapy and the serum creatinine concentration may continue to rise. Irreversible chronic renal insufficiency may result. Renal magnesium wasting is common and can be accompanied by hypocalcemia and hypokalemia.[28] Hypomagnesemia may be severe, causing seizures, neuromuscular irritability, or personality changes, and may persist long after chemotherapy has ended. Hypomagnesemia results primarily from urinary losses caused by renal tubular damage, as well as by the magnesuric effects of saline hydration and diuretic therapy to prevent toxicity. Anorexia and diarrhea also contribute to hypomagnesemia, because of decreased intake and increased loss of magnesium, respectively.

Pathogenesis

Proximal tubular damage appears acutely after administration of platin-containing compounds, as the result of impairment of cell energy production, possibly by binding to proximal tubular cellular proteins and sulfhydryl groups with disruption of cell enzyme activity and uncoupling of oxidative phosphorylation.[28,56] The initial proximal tubular damage is followed by a progressive loss of glomerular filtration and impaired distal tubular function.[54] Renal biopsies generally show sparing of glomeruli with necrosis of both proximal and distal tubules and collecting ducts.[28,56]

Risk Factors

Risk factors include increased age, dehydration, renal irradiation, concurrent use of aminoglycoside antibiotics, and alcohol abuse.[54,56]

Prevention

Toxicity is best prevented by dose reduction and decreased frequency of administration, which usually requires using the platin compounds in combination with other chemotherapeutic agents. Vigorous saline hydration is important and should be used in all patients; doses range from 1 to 4 L within 24 hours of cisplatin treatment, to as high as 3 L/m^2 within 24 hours for high-dose carboplatin.[54] Although protective roles, per se, for furosemide or mannitol diuresis are less clear,[29] their use is often necessary to maintain volume homeostasis. Amifostine, an organic thiophosphate that is converted to an active metabolite, chelates cisplatin in normal cells and reduces the nephrotoxicity, neurotoxicity, ototoxicity, and myelosuppression associated with cisplatin and carboplatin therapy.[57] The renoprotective effect of amifostine administration was recently demonstrated in patients receiving cisplatin/ifosfamide based chemotherapy.[58] Thirty-one patients with solid tumors were randomized to receive chemotherapy with and without amifostine 1,000 mg. Amifostine fully preserved GFR after administration of two cycles of chemotherapy as compared to a 30% reduction in GFR in the control group. In addition, less-severe hypomagnesemia and decreased tubular damage were observed in the amifostine group. Pretreatment with amifostine should be considered in patients at risk for renal dysfunction.[54] Promising investigational techniques include the use of hypertonic saline to reduce tubular cisplatin uptake; reduced renal exposure by use of localized intraperitoneal administration in conjunction with systemic administration of sodium thiosulfate for those with peritoneal tumors; and use of *N*-acetylcysteine, a sulfhydryl donor, and disulfiram metabolite diethyldithiocarbamate.[28,54,56] Recently, the protective effect of melatonin,[59] and the ability of cisplatin-incorporated polymeric micelles to maintain antitumor activity while reducing nephrotoxicity were demonstrated.[60]

Management

Acute renal failure because of cisplatin therapy is usually partially reversible with time and supportive care, including dialysis. Serum magnesium concentrations should be monitored frequently and hypomagnesemia corrected. Hypocalcemia and hypokalemia may be difficult to reverse until hypomagnesemia is corrected. Progressive chronic renal failure caused by cumulative toxicity may not be reversible, and in some cases, requires chronic dialysis support.

AMPHOTERICIN B NEPHROTOXICITY

Incidence

Amphotericin B remains the antifungal drug of choice for most systemic infections, but dose-dependent nephrotoxicity occurs to varying degrees in many patients.[61] Toxicity is seen initially with cumulative doses as low as 300–400 mg and reaches an incidence of 80% when cumulative doses approach 4 g.[62] Several liposomal amphotericin B formulations are now available. Although numerous studies demonstrate lower rates of nephrotoxicity with liposomal formulations as compared to conventional amphotericin B, it is difficult to compare rates of toxicity between products and studies because of varying study populations enrolled, different doses administered, and inconsistent definitions of nephrotoxicity and methods of assessment.[63]

Clinical Presentation

Toxicity is often initially manifest by abnormalities of renal tubular function including potassium, sodium, and magnesium wasting; impaired urine-concentrating ability; and distal renal tubular acidosis caused by a leak of hydrogen ions back out of the tubular lumen.[61] Substantial potassium and magnesium replacement may be necessary. Renal blood flow and glomerular filtration rate decreases are common, and result in a rise in serum creatinine and blood urea nitrogen concentrations.[61]

Pathogenesis

Renal pathologic findings include focal vacuolization of small arterial and arteriolar smooth-muscle cells, as well as proximal and distal tubular epithelial cell damage. The mechanisms of renal dysfunction include direct tubular epithelial cell toxicity with increased tubular permeability and necrosis, as well as arterial vasoconstriction and ischemic injury.[64] Tubular membrane permeability to solutes such as sodium and potassium increases when amphotericin binds to membranes and acts as an ionophore. Renal vasoconstriction occurs by unclear mechanisms, possibly including direct effects of amphotericin B on cellular calcium fluxes and activation of vasoconstrictor prostaglandins. Overall, the combined effects of increased cell energy and oxygen requirements due to greater cell membrane permeability and reduced cellular oxygen delivery because of renal vasoconstriction results in renal medullary tubular epithelial cell necrosis and renal failure.[27,61]

Risk Factors

Risk factors include baseline renal insufficiency, higher average daily doses, diuretic use, volume depletion, and concomitant administration of other nephrotoxins (cyclosporine, in particular).[61,62] Rapid infusions of amphotericin B have the potential to increase toxicity. A recent comparison of 24-hour continuous infusions with conventional 4-hour infusions revealed a significant reduction of toxicity, attributed to decreased "pretubular" effects (e.g., effects on renal blood flow and glomerular filtration rate).[65]

Prevention

Nephrotoxicity is best minimized by limiting the cumulative dose and avoiding concomitant administration of other nephrotoxins. Additionally, providing hydration with a high sodium diet and 1 L intravenous 0.9% sodium chloride daily appears to reduce toxicity.[61,66] Mannitol infusion to induce an osmotic diuresis has not been protective.[61] Pretreatment with a calcium channel blocker may prove useful.[67] Administration of low-dose dopamine to bone marrow transplant and leukemia patients showed no reduction of nephrotoxicity compared to controls.[68] Several liposomal amphotericin B formulations are now available and have been reported to reduce nephrotoxicity by enhancing drug delivery to sites of infection and away from mammalian cell membranes.[69] Overall, however, the safety and efficacy of liposomal formulations remains to be unequivocally established and their judicious use is warranted.[70]

Management

Amphotericin nephrotoxicity is best treated by discontinuation of therapy and substitution of alternative antifungal therapy, if possible. Renal tubular dysfunction and glomerular filtration will improve gradually to some degree in most patients, but damage may be irreversible.

PENTAMIDINE NEPHROTOXICITY

Pentamidine therapy for *Pneumocystis carinii* infections is also limited by nephrotoxicity. Prospective studies show azotemia in 60% to 90% of treated patients.[71] Hyperkalemia, metabolic acidosis, hypomagnesemia, and hypocalcemia may also occur. Toxicity is more frequent in patients with AIDS than in patients without this immune deficiency, and may be accentuated by concomitant amphotericin B therapy. The mechanism of toxicity is unknown, but tubular degeneration has been seen histopathologically. The primary alternative therapy for *P. carinii,* trimethoprim-sulfamethoxazole, may also cause renal dysfunction because of allergic interstitial nephritis and inhibition of tubular secretion of creatinine, but the incidence is lower than with pentamidine.[71]

FOSCARNET NEPHROTOXICITY

Foscarnet, an antiviral pyrophosphate analog used in AIDS and other immunosuppressed patients to treat cytomegalovirus (CMV) retinitis and life-threatening CMV infections, is a well known nephrotoxic agent.[71,72] As many as 66% of patients treated with foscarnet develop renal insufficiency.[72] The mechanism appears to be complexation of foscarnet with ionized calcium and precipitation of calcium-foscarnet salt crystals in renal glomeruli causing a crystalline glomerulonephritis. Foscarnet crystals may also precipitate in the renal tubules causing tubular necrosis. Foscarnet nephrotoxicity can be minimized by administering the appropriate dose after vigorously prehydrating the patient. Intravenous hydration provides better nephroprotection than oral hydration.[73] In addition, cidofovir, a potent nucleotide analog administered intravenously for CMV infection in AIDS patients, is associated with renal proximal tubular cell injury and renal failure.[74] Probenecid blocks renal tubular epithelial cell uptake of cidofovir, and when combined with saline hydration, can reduce the incidence of nephrotoxicity.[74]

OSMOTIC NEPHROSIS

Several drugs, including mannitol, low-molecular-weight dextran, and radiographic contrast media, or drug vehicles, including sucrose and propylene glycol, are associated with vacuolization, swelling, and ultimately necrosis of proximal tubular epithelial cells with a decline in renal function.[75] The decline in renal function may be a result of the hypertonic and osmotically active nature of these agents. However, they have not been shown to be actually contained within cellular vacuoles. Intravenous immunoglobulin solutions contain hyperosmolar sucrose and may cause osmotic nephrosis and acute renal failure, which is rapidly reversible on discontinuing therapy.[76] Toxicity may be prevented by diluting the solution and reducing the rate of infusion. Hydroxyethylstarch (HES), used as a plasma volume expander, is implicated in the development of osmotic nephrosis.[77] Recently, 129 patients with severe sepsis or septic shock were randomly assigned to receive either 6% HES or 3% fluid-modified gelatin. The frequencies of ARF (42% vs 23%) and oliguria (56% vs 37%) were significantly greater in the HES group, and regression analysis revealed HES to be an independent risk factor for ARF.[77]

Mannitol may rarely cause oligoanuric renal failure with proximal tubular cell vacuolization on biopsy. Mechanisms include pinocytosis of mannitol into cells, causing swelling and tubular lumen obstruction.[17] Mannitol can also cause direct renal vasoconstriction or induce an osmotic diuresis with increased solute delivery to the macula densa and subsequent tubuloglomerular feedback leading to vasoconstriction of the glomerular afferent arteriole and decreased renal blood flow. Risk factors for mannitol DIN include excessive doses, preexistent renal insufficiency, and concomitant diuretic or cyclosporine therapy.[16,78] Nephrotoxicity may be prevented by limiting the dose and avoiding dehydration and concomitant diuretic therapy. The serum mannitol concentration should be maintained <1,000 mg/dL (as evidenced by an osmolal gap <55 mOsm/kg water). Maintenance of an osmolal gap of 20 mOsm/kg water or greater is usually adequate.[16,78] Patients usually recover normal renal function when elevated mannitol concentrations decrease following drug withdrawal or hemodialysis. Mannitol-induced osmotic diuresis and volume depletion could increase the nephrotoxicity of other drugs, particularly NSAIDs, ACE inhibitors, and cyclosporine.

HEMODYNAMICALLY MEDIATED RENAL FAILURE

Hemodynamically mediated renal insufficiency results from a decrease in intraglomerular pressure. Mechanisms commonly include a decrease in renal blood flow, vasoconstriction of glomerular afferent arterioles, and vasodilation of glomerular efferent arterioles.

ANGIOTENSIN II-CONVERTING ENZYME INHIBITORS AND ANGIOTENSIN II RECEPTOR BLOCKERS

INCIDENCE

The incidence of ACEI- or angiotensin II receptor blocker (ARB)-induced nephrotoxicity has not been established. However, this appears to be one of the most common causes of drug-induced nephrotoxicity in hospitalized as well as ambulatory patients. Patients with severe atherosclerotic renal artery stenosis, patients hospitalized with congestive heart failure or renal insufficiency with serum creatinine >1.6 mg/dL, and patients with primary renal disease, including diabetic nephropathy, and serum creatinine >3.0 mg/dL are most likely to experience a significant decline in renal function with these agents.

CLINICAL PRESENTATION

Therapy with ACEIs and ARBs can acutely reduce glomerular filtration rate, manifesting as a rise in serum creatinine.[79,80] Importantly, a distinction must be made between a potentially detrimental reduction in GFR and a normal, predictable rise in serum creatinine. Dose-related changes in serum creatinine should be anticipated in most patients with ACEIs based upon their pathophysiologic effects.[81,82] An increase in serum creatinine of up to 30% within 2 to 5 days of initiating therapy is an indication that the drug has begun to exert its desired pharmacologic effect.[81] The increase in creatinine usually stabilizes within 2 to 3 weeks and is usually reversible upon stopping the drug. Furthermore, an association exists between acute increases in serum creatinine of ≤30% from baseline which stabilize within the first 2 months of initiating therapy and preservation of renal function.[81]

A decline in renal function has been reported in the presence and absence of renal artery stenosis. The rise is often minimal in renovascular disease if only one renal artery is stenotic, but is more apparent in patients with a single kidney with renovascular disease, congestive heart failure, volume depletion, or bilateral renal small vessel disease.[80] Up to one-third of patients with bilateral renal artery stenosis demonstrate a rise in serum creatinine >30% after starting ACEI therapy.[83]

PATHOGENESIS

The pathogenesis of ACEI or ARB nephropathy is a decrease in glomerular capillary hydrostatic pressure sufficient to reduce glomerular ultrafiltration.[1] This often occurs in settings in which glomerular afferent arteriolar blood flow is reduced and the efferent arteriole is vasoconstricted to maintain sufficient glomerular capillary hydrostatic pressure for ultrafiltration (Fig. 48–2B). ACEI or ARB therapy reduces angiotensin II synthesis or activity, respectively, thereby dilating the efferent arteriole and reducing glomerular capillary hydrostatic pressure (Fig. 48–2C). This decreases glomerular ultrafiltration and GFR.

RISK FACTORS

Patients at greatest risk are those dependent on angiotensin II to maintain blood pressure and renal efferent arteriolar constriction. These include patients with hemodynamically significant renal artery stenosis, particularly bilateral stenosis, and those with decreased effective arterial renal blood flow, particularly those with congestive heart failure, volume depletion from excess diuresis or gastrointestinal fluid loss, hepatic cirrhosis with ascites, and the nephrotic syndrome.[1,83]

PREVENTION

A common strategy for at-risk patients who are hospitalized is to initiate therapy with very low doses of a short-acting ACEI, then gradually up titrate the dose and convert to a longer-acting agent after therapy is tolerated. Outpatients may be started on low doses of long-acting ACEIs with gradual dose titration. Renal function and serum potassium concentrations must be monitored carefully, daily for hospitalized patients and every 2 to 3 days for outpatients. Monitoring may need to be more frequent during outpatient initiation of ACEI or ARB therapy for patients with preexisting renal insufficiency, congestive heart failure, or suspected renovascular disease. Concurrent hypotensive agents and diuretics should be used cautiously and dehydration avoided.[83]

MANAGEMENT

Acute decreases in renal function and hyperkalemia usually resolve over several days after ACEI or ARB therapy is discontinued. Occasional patients will require management of severe hyperkalemia, usually with sodium polystyrene sulfate (see Chap. 52). ACEI or ARB therapy may frequently be reinitiated, particularly for patients with congestive heart failure, after intravascular volume depletion has been corrected or the diuretic dose reduced. The development of mild renal insufficiency (serum creatinine concentration of 2–3 mg/dL) may be an acceptable trade-off for hemodynamic improvement in certain patients with severe congestive heart failure or renovascular disease not amenable to invasive management. Congestive heart failure patients with greater renal insufficiency may be best treated by substitution of hydralazine and nitrates for afterload reduction.

NONSTEROIDAL ANTI-INFLAMMATORY DRUGS

INCIDENCE

NSAIDs have an overall favorable safety profile, resulting in OTC availability in the United States of ibuprofen, naproxen, and ketoprofen for short-term therapy. While potential adverse renal effects from OTC NSAIDs are a concern,[84] activity of vasodilatory prostaglandins is not necessary to maintain renal function in healthy individuals. NSAIDs are unlikely to impair renal function in the absence of renal ischemia or excess renal vasoconstrictor activity. Nevertheless, people receiving NSAID therapy have a fourfold higher risk for hospitalization.[7]

CLINICAL PRESENTATION

Renal failure can occur within days of initiating therapy, particularly with a short-acting NSAID such as ibuprofen.[85] Urine volume and sodium concentration are usually low. The urine sediment is usually unchanged from baseline, but may show granular casts. Parenteral NSAID therapy with ketorolac is associated with a transient decline in renal function, even after a single dose.[86] However, in a retrospective cohort analysis, parenteral ketorolac therapy was not identified as a risk for acute renal failure in hospitalized patients.[87] Topically administered NSAIDs can also cause nephropathy.[88]

PATHOGENESIS

NSAIDs inhibit cyclooxygenase (COX)-catalyzed prostaglandin production and impair renal function by decreasing synthesis of vasodilatory prostaglandins from arachidonic acid.[89] Renal prostaglandins are synthesized in the renal cortex and medulla by vascular endothelial and glomerular mesangial cells. Their effects are primarily local and result in renal vasodilation (particularly prostacyclin and PGE_2). They have limited activity in states of normal renal blood flow, but in states of decreased renal blood flow, their synthesis is increased and they protect against renal ischemia and hypoxia by antagonizing renal vasoconstriction caused by angiotensin II, norepinephrine, endothelin, and vasopressin. Administration of NSAIDs in the setting of renal ischemia and compensatory increased prostaglandin activity may thus alter the balance of activity between renal vasoconstrictors and vasodilators. This leaves the activity of renal vasoconstrictors unopposed and promotes renal ischemia with loss of glomerular filtration. This hemodynamically mediated acute renal failure is the most common adverse renal effect of NSAIDs.

RISK FACTORS

Persons at greatest risk for NSAID hemodynamic nephropathy generally have preexisting renal insufficiency, medical problems associated with high plasma renin activity (hepatic disease with ascites, decompensated congestive heart failure, or intravascular volume depletion), or systemic lupus erythematosus. Additional risk factors include atherosclerotic cardiovascular disease and diuretic therapy. The elderly are also at higher risk because of interaction of prevalent medical problems, multiple drug therapies, and reduced renal function. Advanced age, however, has not been shown to be an independent risk factor for toxicity in limited trials in otherwise healthy elderly subjects.[89,90] Combined NSAID and ACEI or ARB therapy is also a concern and should be avoided (see Fig. 48–2D).

PREVENTION

NSAID-induced acute renal failure can be prevented by recognizing high-risk patients and by using analgesics with less prostaglandin inhibition, such as acetaminophen, nonacetylated salicylates, aspirin, and possibly nabumetone. Nonnarcotic analgesics (e.g., propoxyphene, tramadol) may also be useful, but do not provide anti-inflammatory activity.[89] When NSAID therapy is essential for high-risk patients, management of predisposing medical problems should be optimized and renal function monitored. Sulindac may be useful in high-risk patients because it is a potent NSAID that may have lesser effects on renal prostaglandin synthesis and function. The mechanism of renal prostaglandin sparing is unclear, but may involve intrarenal metabolism of the active drug, sulindac sulfide, by cytochrome P450-dependent mixed-function oxidases to an inactive metabolite, sulindac sulfoxide. However, this favorable effect of sulindac has not been consistently observed, especially at higher therapeutic doses, in patients with hepatic disease, or during prolonged therapy. The oral prostaglandin E analog, misoprostol, may be useful to prevent NSAID nephropathy.[91]

Whereas traditional, nonselective NSAIDs inhibit COX 1 and COX 2, the selective NSAIDs meloxicam, celecoxib, and rofecoxib preferentially inhibit COX-2.[92] COX-2 inhibitors were anticipated to have less renal toxicity in high-risk patients. However, recent data indicates they effect renal function similar to nonselective NSAIDs and thus caution is warranted with their use, particularly in high risk patients.[92–94]

MANAGEMENT

Acute renal failure caused by NSAIDs is treated by discontinuation of therapy and supportive care. Renal failure may be severe, but recovery is usually rapid and dialysis is rarely necessary. Occasionally the hemodynamic insult is sufficiently severe to cause frank tubular necrosis, which can prolong recovery. The differential diagnosis of NSAID hemodynamically mediated acute renal failure must include NSAID-induced acute interstitial nephritis, with or without the nephrotic syndrome, because steroid therapy may benefit this type of renal injury.

SULFINPYRAZONE

Sulfinpyrazone, a uricosuric congener of phenylbutazone, also causes hemodynamically mediated acute renal failure.[95] Sulfinpyrazone inhibition of renal prostaglandin synthesis or reduction of renal kallikrein-kinin activity may imbalance renal hemodynamics, causing renal ischemia. Renal insufficiency may be transient despite continued sulfinpyrazone administration or prolonged and oliguric with a low urinary sodium concentration.

CYCLOSPORINE AND TACROLIMUS

Cyclosporine and tacrolimus have dramatically enhanced organ transplantation.[96] Nephrotoxicity is a major dose-limiting adverse effect of both drugs. Early, acute, hemodynamically mediated renal insufficiency and delayed chronic interstitial nephritis have both been observed (see "Chronic Interstitial Nephritis," later in this chapter).[96]

INCIDENCE

Historically, reversible acute renal insufficiency occurred frequently in transplant recipients during the first 6 months of cyclosporine therapy. The combined effects of lower-dose therapy and use of pharmacokinetic monitoring have reduced the incidence of acute renal dysfunction. Nevertheless, most patients with apparently stable renal function will experience increased renal blood flow and glomerular filtration rates following withdrawal of therapy.[97] Irreversible chronic interstitial nephritis with end-stage renal disease developed in 10% of heart transplant recipients following initial high-dose therapy.[97] Chronic nephropathy has been observed in as many as 67% of bone marrow transplant recipients receiving cyclosporine for 8 years.[96]

CLINICAL PRESENTATION

Acute renal toxicity may occur within days of initiating therapy. Serum creatinine concentration rises and creatinine clearance decreases. Hypertension, hyperkalemia, sodium avidity, and hypomagnesemia may occur. No urine sediment abnormalities are seen. Urinary enzyme excretions increase, but are not reliable indicators of toxicity. Renal biopsy reveals thickening of arterioles, mild focal glomerular sclerosis, proximal tubular epithelial cell vacuolization and atrophy, and interstitial fibrosis. Biopsy is useful to distinguish acute cyclosporine nephrotoxicity from renal allograft rejection, the latter being evidenced by cellular infiltration.[96]

Chronic toxicity becomes apparent after 6 to 12 months of therapy as a slowly rising serum creatinine concentration and decreased creatinine clearance. However, the rise in serum creatinine concentration and decreased creatinine clearance may be delayed and not reflect the severity of histopathologic changes. Urinalysis reveals few red and white blood cells with low-range proteinuria. Renal biopsy shows progressive renal arteriolar hyalinosis, glomerular sclerosis, and a striped pattern of interstitial fibrosis. Biopsy cannot easily distinguish chronic cyclosporine toxicity from chronic rejection.[97,98]

PATHOGENESIS

A dose-related hemodynamic mechanism is likely during the initial months of therapy because renal function improves rapidly following dose reduction. Reversible vasoconstriction and injury to glomerular afferent arterioles occurs, possibly because of increased activity of vasoconstrictors, including thromboxane A2, endothelin, and the sympathetic nervous system, or diminished activity of vasodilators, nitric oxide, or prostacyclin.[97,99] Vasoconstriction caused by increased renin-angiotensin system activity may also contribute.[100] In contrast, renal arteriolar hyalinization and chronic renal ischemia, as well as increased extracellular matrix synthesis, appear to contribute to cyclosporine induced chronic renal failure.[97,98]

RISK FACTORS

Risk factors include increased age and higher initial cyclosporine dose, as well as renal graft rejection; hypotension; infection; and concomitant therapy with nephrotoxic drugs such as aminoglycosides, amphotericin B, acyclovir, NSAIDs, and radiocontrast agents; as well as drugs that inhibit cyclosporine hepatic metabolism.[96] The high incidence of acute renal insufficiency with potential progression to chronic nephropathy has decreased with current lower dose therapy, but concern remains for a slow, dose-dependent decline in glomerular filtration.[97]

PREVENTION

Because acute DIN appears to be dose related, pharmacokinetic and pharmacodynamic monitoring is an important means of preventing toxicity. However, the persistent presence of therapeutic or low cyclosporine concentrations cannot preclude nephrotoxicity. Calcium channel blockers may antagonize the vasoconstrictor effect of cyclosporine by dilating glomerular afferent arterioles and preventing acute decreases in renal blood flow and glomerular filtration.[96] In addition, decreased doses of cyclosporine or tacrolimus, primarily when used in combination with other nonnephrotoxic immunosuppressants, may minimize the risk of toxicity, but this may increase the risk of chronic rejection.[96]

MANAGEMENT

Acute renal insufficiency usually improves with dose reduction, and treatment of contributing illness or the discontinuation of interacting drugs. Chronic renal failure is usually irreversible, but progressive toxicity may be limited by discontinuation of cyclosporine therapy or dose reduction with the continuation of other immunosuppressants (e.g., prednisone, azathioprine).

TRIAMTERENE

Triamterene, a potassium-sparing diuretic, is associated with transient decreases in creatinine clearance and abnormal urinary sediment in normal subjects and hypertensive patients.[101] In combination with hydrochlorothiazide, triamterene has caused reversible acute renal failure in elderly patients. In combination with indomethacin, triamterene has induced acute renal failure in normal subjects and patients at risk for NSAID nephropathy. A hemodynamic mechanism is most likely as suggested by the apparent increased risk for nephrotoxicity during combined triamterene and indomethacin therapy. Presumably, triamterene causes renal vasoconstriction that is counterbalanced by increased renal synthesis of vasodilatory prostaglandins. Concomitant NSAID therapy may induce renal ischemia by preventing the compensatory increase in renal prostaglandin synthesis. The implications of these observations are unclear because triamterene and NSAIDs are frequently used together without apparent nephrotoxicity.

PROPRANOLOL

Propranolol, a nonselective β-adrenergic receptor blocker, reduces renal blood flow 10% to 20% in hypertensive patients.[14] The glomerular filtration rate is less consistently reduced.[14] In contrast, nadolol, another nonselective β-blocker, increases renal blood flow, whereas other β-blockers do not appear to alter renal hemodynamics.[102] The mechanism of the propranolol-induced decrease in renal blood flow is unknown. Because renal function does not decrease with other

β-blockers, the effect is unlikely to result from blockade of β-receptors or decreased cardiac output. Other postulated mechanisms include renal vasoconstriction because of unopposed β-adrenergic activity or inhibition of renal vasodilator activity, possibly mediated by the kallikrein-kinin system.[14] The clinical significance of these effects is unknown. However, it may be prudent to avoid propranolol therapy in patients with renal insufficiency.

OKT3

OKT3 therapy for the prevention and treatment of acute renal and cardiac allograft rejection is often accompanied by a rise in the serum creatinine concentration that returns toward baseline after 3 to 5 days.[99] Renal biopsy findings of mild interstitial edema or no abnormalities suggest the mechanism is increased vascular permeability due to a renal capillary leak. This renal dysfunction is believed to be part of a cytokine syndrome associated with OKT3 therapy. OKT3 causes lymphocyte activation and release of cytokines, particularly tumor necrosis factor, γ-interferon, and interleukins-2 and -6, which may induce secretion of group II secretory phospholipase A_2 as a mediator of nephrotoxicity.[103] Renal function often improves spontaneously despite continued OKT3 therapy.

OBSTRUCTIVE NEPHROPATHY

Obstructive nephropathy is the result of mechanical obstruction to urine flow following glomerular filtration. This may be caused by intratubular obstruction from crystal precipitation within the tubules of the kidney or extrarenal obstruction of the ureters or bladder.[104] Pain, hematuria, and infection may precede a significant rise in serum creatinine.

RENAL TUBULAR OBSTRUCTION

Drug-induced acute renal tubular obstruction can be caused by intratubular precipitation of tissue degradation products, as well as by drugs or their metabolites. Acute uric acid nephropathy following cancer chemotherapy, is the most common cause of renal failure due to obstruction by tissue degradation products. Acute oliguric or anuric renal failure develops rapidly. The diagnosis is supported by a urine uric acid to creatinine ratio greater than one. Pretreatment hydration, urinary alkalinization to pH 7.0, and allopurinol can prevent uric acid precipitation.

Drug-induced rhabdomyolysis leads to intratubular precipitation of myoglobin, and if severe, it leads to acute renal failure.[105] The most common cause of drug-induced rhabdomyolysis is direct myotoxicity from 3-hydroxy-3-methylglutaryl coenzyme A (HMG-CoA) reductase inhibitors, including lovastatin and simvastatin.[105–107] The risk of rhabdomyolysis is increased when this class of drugs is administered concurrently with gemfibrozil, niacin, or inhibitors of the CYP3A4 metabolic pathway (e.g., cyclosporine, erythromycin, itraconazole). Rhabdomyolysis may also result from pressure necrosis during stupor or coma following ingestion of central nervous system (CNS) depressants (e.g., alcohol, narcotics), or extreme neuromuscular agitation and associated metabolic demands with abuse of CNS stimulants (e.g., amphetamines, cocaine, ecstasy, phencyclidine).

Intratubular precipitation of drugs (e.g., sulfonamides) or their metabolites can also cause acute renal failure.[104] Sulfadiazine when used at high doses for toxoplasmosis in AIDS patients,[108] acetazolamide[109] and methotrexate and its less soluble metabolite, 7-hydroxymethotrexate,[28] also precipitate in acid urine and can cause oligoanuric renal failure. Intravenous and high-dose oral acyclovir therapy for acute herpes zoster is also associated with intratubular precipitation in dehydrated oliguric patients.[104] This can be diagnosed by the presence of birefringent needle-shaped crystals within urine leukocytes using polarized light microscopy. Massive administration of ascorbic acid can also result in obstruction of renal tubules with calcium oxalate crystals. Oxalate, a poorly soluble ascorbic acid metabolite, can also precipitate and worsen renal function when ascorbic acid is administered to patients with acute renal failure or the congenital nephrotic syndrome. Low-molecular-weight dextran therapy for volume expansion and rheologic effects has also caused renal failure, possibly by intratubular precipitation of filtered dextran. Triamterene may also precipitate in renal tubules and cause renal failure.[104] Foscarnet complexation with ionized calcium may result in precipitation of calcium-foscarnet salt crystals in renal glomeruli causing primarily a crystalline glomerulonephritis. The salt crystals may then secondarily precipitate in the renal tubules causing tubular necrosis.[72]

Renal failure as a result of intratubular precipitation of most tissue-degradation products or drugs and their metabolites can be largely prevented, and possibly treated, by administering the appropriate dose after vigorously prehydrating the patient, maintaining a high urine volume and urinary alkalinization.

EXTRARENAL URINARY TRACT OBSTRUCTION

Drug therapy may also cause renal insufficiency because of lower urinary tract obstruction. Calculi or retroperitoneal fibrosis can cause ureteral obstruction. Bladder dysfunction with urinary outflow obstruction can result, particularly in males with prostatic hypertrophy, from anticholinergic drugs, including tricyclic antidepressants and disopyramide. Bladder outlet and ureteral obstruction may result from bladder fibrosis following hemorrhagic cystitis with cyclophosphamide or ifosfamide therapy. Mesna cotherapy can prevent cystitis and this complication.

NEPHROLITHIASIS

Nephrolithiasis (formation of kidney stones) does not present as classic nephrotoxicity because GFR is usually not decreased. Drug-induced nephrolithiasis represents abnormal crystal precipitation in the renal collecting system potentially causing pain, hematuria, infection, or, occasionally, urinary tract obstruction with renal insufficiency.

Renal stone formation, possibly also accompanied by intratubular precipitation of crystalline material, is a rare complication of drug therapy. Until the AIDS era, triamterene had been the drug most frequently associated with renal stone formation, with an incidence approximating 1 in 1,500 users of triamterene-hydrochlorothiazide.[101] However, it is unclear whether triamterene or its metabolites actually cause stone formation, or whether they are passively absorbed onto the organic matrix of preexisting calculi. Sulfadiazine, a poorly soluble sulfonamide used to treat *Toxoplasma gondii* infection in AIDS patients, causes symptomatic acetylsulfadiazine crystalluria with stone formation and flank or back pain, hematuria, or renal insufficiency in 1.9% to 7.5% of AIDS patients.[110] A high urine volume and urinary alkalinization to pH > 7.15 may be protective. Similarly, the protease inhibitor indinavir is associated with crystalluria, dysuria, urinary frequency, back and flank pain, and nephrolithiasis in approximately 10% of AIDS patients.[111] Acute renal failure due to intratubular precipitation of crystalline indinavir and collecting system obstruction from nephrolithiasis have occurred.[112] Because indinavir is more water soluble at acid pH, urine acidification could be protective, but is not practical. Maintaining a high urine volume may be most protective. Allopurinol may rarely cause xanthine, hypoxanthine, and oxypurinol stones during therapy for conditions having excess uric acid production.[113] Allopurinol inhibits xanthine oxidase and increases the urinary excretion of poorly soluble xanthine, hypoxanthine, and oxypurinol. Massive ingestion of magnesium trisilicate-aluminum hydroxide for gastric symptoms is associated with magnesium ammonium phosphate (struvite) stone formation, possibly because of hypermagnesuria and increased urinary pH.[114] Laxative abuse may lead to the unusual formation of ammonium urate stones, possibly because of increased urinary pH and ammonium concentration.[115] Recently, nephrolithiasis was reported to be a complication of the ingestion of various products containing ephedrine, norephedrine, and pseudoephedrine.[116]

GLOMERULAR DISEASE

Proteinuria with or without a decline in the glomerular filtration rate is a hallmark sign of glomerular injury (see Chap. 49). Several different glomerular lesions may occur, mostly by immune mechanisms rather than direct toxicity. Although drug-induced glomerular disease is uncommon, a variety of agents have been implicated.

Minimal change glomerular injury with nephrotic range proteinuria (i.e., >3.5 g/d) caused by drugs is frequently accompanied by interstitial nephritis and is most common during NSAID therapy.[117] Ampicillin, rifampin, phenytoin, and lithium have also been implicated. The pathogenesis is unknown, but nephrotic-range proteinuria caused by NSAID therapy is frequently associated with a T-lymphocytic interstitial infiltrate, suggesting disordered cell-mediated immunity. These cells may release lymphokines that increase glomerular capillary permeability to proteins. Proteinuria usually resolves rapidly after discontinuation of the offending drug. Prednisone therapy, in doses ranging from 0.5–1 mg/kg body weight for 2 to 4 weeks, may help resolve the lesion.[118]

Focal segmental glomerulosclerosis is characterized by patchy areas of glomerular sclerosis with interstitial inflammation and fibrosis (see Chap. 49). Chronic heroin abuse is the most common drug cause of this lesion.[117] The pathogenesis is unknown but may include direct toxicity by heroin or adulterants and injury from bacterial or viral infections accompanying intravenous drug use. End-stage renal failure develops in most cases. No specific therapy is available, although discontinuation of heroin use may prevent progression. Focal segmental glomerulosclerosis is the predominant renal lesion in AIDS patients and may result from human immunodeficiency virus infection or heroin abuse. Glomerulosclerosis caused by HIV infection may be distinguished from heroin nephropathy by tubuloreticular structures in endothelial cells on electron microscopy and a more rapid course and poorer prognosis. Focal segmental sclerosis has also been attributed to therapy with lithium and α-interferon.[119]

Membranous nephropathy, the most common drug-induced glomerular lesion, is characterized by immune complex deposition along glomerular capillary loops. Parenteral gold is the most common cause, with an incidence of 1% to 10% in patients treated for rheumatoid arthritis.[120] Oral gold therapy has a lesser incidence. The pathogenesis may involve damage to proximal tubule epithelium with antigen release, antibody formation, and glomerular immune complex deposition. Gold has been identified in proximal tubular cells, but not in the glomerular deposits. Genetic factors appear to be important because patients with human leukocyte antigens (HLAs) DR3 or B8 have increased susceptibility. Renal function is preserved and proteinuria resolves 6 to 39 months after discontinuing gold therapy.[120] Similarly, mercury found in diuretics, topical skin preparations, and industrial vapors as well as D-penicillamine cause membranous nephropathy.[117] NSAIDs also cause membranous nephrotic syndrome, accounting for 10% of membranous nephropathy in adults.[121] The prognosis appears favorable with resolution after discontinuing NSAID use.

Membranoproliferative glomerulonephritis is a rare consequence of drug therapy associated with hydralazine-induced systemic lupus erythematosus.[117] Rapidly progressive or crescentic glomerulonephritis may result from propylthiouracil-induced systemic lupus erythematosus, penicillamine, and combined interleukin-2 and interferon-α use.[117] Proliferative glomerulonephritis may result from chlorpropamide use. Crescentic IgA glomerulonephritis may follow recombinant interleukin-2 therapy. Glomerular amyloidosis occurs with heroin abuse, particularly by subcutaneous injection, causing immune stimulation from chronic skin inflammation.

TUBULOINTERSTITIAL DISEASE

These diseases involve the renal tubules and their surrounding interstitial tissue. The presentation may be "acute" and reversible, with interstitial inflammatory cell infiltrates, rapid loss of renal function, and systemic symptoms, or "chronic" and irreversible, with interstitial fibrosis, slow loss of renal function, and no systemic symptoms. Papillary necrosis, a variant of chronic interstitial nephritis, originates deep in the renal medulla involving the papillae.

ACUTE ALLERGIC INTERSTITIAL NEPHRITIS

INCIDENCE

AIN is common and the underlying cause for 3% to 15% of all cases of acute renal failure.[122,123] Multiple drugs have been implicated (Table 48–3).

CLINICAL PRESENTATION

Penicillins

Methicillin-induced allergic interstitial nephritis is the prototype for most presentations of AIN.[122] Clinical signs present 17 days (range, 2 to 44 days) after initiation of therapy and include (with their approximate incidence) fever (75%); maculopapular rash (25%); eosinophilia (80%); pyuria and hematuria (90%); low-level proteinuria (90%); and oliguria (18%). Systemic hypersensitivity findings of fever, rash, eosinophilia, and eosinophiluria suggest the diagnosis, but this constellation of findings is not consistently reliable because one or more are frequently absent. Eosinophiluria, an important marker of drug-induced AIN, is frequently absent,[122] possibly because of the fragility of eosinophils in urine and inadequate laboratory methodology. Anemia, leukocytosis, and elevated IgE levels may occur. Tubular dysfunction may be manifested by acidosis, hyperkalemia, salt wasting, and concentrating defects.

NSAIDs

Fenoprofen-allergic interstitial nephritis, the prototype for NSAID-induced AIN, has a different clinical presentation than that seen with most other drugs.[118] Patients are older (reflecting NSAID use for degenerative joint disease) and the onset is delayed, a mean of

TABLE 48–3. Drugs Associated with Allergic Interstitial Nephritis

Antibiotics	Nonsteroidal Anti-Inflammatory Drugs
Acyclovir	Indomethacin
Aminoglycosides	Naproxen
Amphotericin B	Ibuprofen
Aztreonam	Diflunisal
Cephalosporins	Piroxicam
Ciprofloxacin	Ketoprofen
Erythromycin	Diclofenac
Ethambutol	**Miscellaneous**
Indinavir	Acetaminophen
Penicillins	Allopurinol
Rifampin	Interferon-α
Sulfonamides	Aspirin
Tetracyclines	Azathioprine
Trimethoprim-sulfamethoxazole	Captopril
Vancomycin	Cimetidine
Diuretics	Clofibrate
Acetazolamide	Cyclosporine
Amiloride	Glyburide
Chlorthalidone	Gold
Furosemide	Methyldopa
Triamterene	*P*-Aminosalicylic acid
Thiazides	Phenylpropanolamine
Neuropsychiatric	Propylthiouracil
Carbamazepine	Radiographic contrast media
Lithium	Ranitidine
Phenobarbital	Sulfinpyrazone
Phenytoin	Warfarin sodium
Valproic acid	

5.4 months from initiation of therapy. Systemic signs of an allergic reaction (rash, fever, and eosinophilia) are infrequent, occurring in only 19% of cases. Concomitant nephrotic syndrome (proteinuria greater than 3.5 g/d) caused by minimal-change glomerulopathy is characteristic.

Prompt diagnosis of allergic interstitial nephritis is important because discontinuation of the offending drug may prevent irreversible renal damage. Renal biopsy is the most specific method for diagnosis, but is usually not possible in acutely ill patients. Gallium-67 renal imaging is a sensitive diagnostic technique, but is nonspecific and of limited usefulness because acute pyelonephritis, nil-lesion nephrotic syndrome, and cholesterol embolization also give positive scans.[122]

PATHOGENESIS

The pathology of allergic interstitial nephritis is a diffuse or focal interstitial infiltrate of lymphocytes, plasma cells, eosinophils, and occasional neutrophils.[122] Granulomas and tubular epithelial cell necrosis, are relatively common with drug-induced AIN. The pathogenesis is an allergic hypersensitivity response.[122,123] Occasionally, a humoral antibody-mediated mechanism is implicated by the presence of circulating antibody to a drug hapten-tubular basement membrane complex, low serum-complement levels, and deposition of IgG and complement in the tubular basement membrane. More commonly, a cell-mediated immune mechanism is suggested by the absence of these findings and the presence of a predominantly T-lymphocyte infiltrate with an increased helper to suppressor cell ratio. In particular, NSAID interstitial nephritis involves T lymphocytes, possibly in response to altered prostaglandin synthesis.

RISK FACTORS

No specific risk factors have been identified because these are idiosyncratic hypersensitivity reactions. Individuals with other drug allergies may have increased risk and warrant close monitoring.

PREVENTION

Because of the idiosyncratic nature of these reactions, no specific prevention is known. Patients must be monitored carefully to recognize the signs and symptoms and discontinue therapy promptly.

MANAGEMENT

No prospective treatment trials have been reported. However, prednisone therapy in a dose of 0.5–1 mg/kg body weight for 1 to 4 weeks has been used and may improve the rate and extent of renal recovery.[122]

CHRONIC INTERSTITIAL NEPHRITIS

Lithium, cyclosporine, and few other drugs can cause chronic interstitial nephritis, which is usually a progressive and irreversible lesion. Streptozotocin and other antineoplastic nitrosoureas also cause dose-dependent chronic interstitial disease.[28] In addition, mesalazine, 5-aminosalicylic acid, and ifosfamide may cause chronic interstitial nephritis, which can reverse when drug use is discontinued promptly.[28]

LITHIUM

Incidence

Several renal tubular lesions are associated with lithium therapy. The most common lesion is an impaired ability to concentrate urine (nephrogenic diabetes insipidus), which is seen in as many as 87% of patients.[124] Acute tubular necrosis, and chronic tubulointerstitial nephritis, are less frequently noted and incomplete distal renal tubular acidosis is rarely reported. The most important question for lithium use is whether long-term lithium therapy, with lithium concentrations maintained in the therapeutic range, causes chronic tubulointerstitial nephritis with renal insufficiency. Although mild nonprogressive renal insufficiency has been reported in 10% or more of patients during long-term therapy, the role for lithium has not been established because occurrences have been infrequent and studies suggesting nephrotoxicity were frequently uncontrolled.[125] Chronic toxicity is also questioned because renal function has not declined during short- and long-term lithium therapy in studies when lithium concentrations have been maintained in the therapeutic range.[126]

Clinical Presentation

Patients with nephrogenic diabetes insipidus often have polydipsia and polyuria (see Chap. 51). They adapt well to their urinary-concentrating defect and these concerns are usually minimal. Acute tubular necrosis is frequent in the setting of acute lithium toxicity. The patient is generally asymptomatic. Urinalysis may show moderate proteinuria, a few red and white blood cells, and granular casts. Renal function usually returns to baseline values after lithium concentrations are reduced to the therapeutic range. Chronic renal insufficiency may develop insidiously and be recognized by rising BUN or creatinine concentrations or the onset of hypertension. The urinalysis may show mild proteinuria, and a few red and white blood cells.

Pathogenesis

Impaired ability to concentrate urine is the result of a dose-related decrease in collecting duct response to antidiuretic hormone. This results from impaired formation of cellular cAMP in response to antidiuretic hormone. Lithium-induced acute renal failure occurs predominantly during episodes of acute lithium intoxication.[125] The pathogenesis includes dehydration secondary to nephrogenic diabetes insipidus as well as direct proximal and distal tubular cell toxicity. Chronic tubulointerstitial nephritis attributed to lithium is evidenced by biopsy findings of interstitial fibrosis, focal tubular atrophy, and glomerular sclerosis.[125] The pathogenesis may involve cumulative damage from lithium-induced acute tubular necrosis. Alternatively, cumulative direct lithium toxicity may occur because duration of therapy correlates with the decline in the glomerular filtration rate. Finally, some patients may have increased susceptibility to lithium toxicity. Although the reason for this is unknown, this could explain the difficulty in characterizing the nephrotoxic effects of chronic lithium therapy.

Risk Factors

The major risk factor for acute renal failure is an elevated lithium concentration, particularly in association with dehydration. Concomitant therapy with neuroleptic agents[125] and ACE inhibitors[127] may contribute. Chronic nephrotoxicity may result from cumulative damage caused by repeated episodes of acute renal injury.

Prevention

Prevention of acute and chronic toxicity includes maintaining lithium concentrations as low as therapeutically possible, avoiding dehydration, and monitoring renal function. It is unknown whether progression to severe renal failure can be prevented by stopping lithium use when mild renal insufficiency is first recognized. This poses a dilemma because lithium is highly effective for affective disorders and the risks and potential benefits of discontinuing such a beneficial drug need to be carefully considered. However, if lithium therapy is continued, renal function must be monitored and therapy discontinued if it continues to decline.

Management

Symptomatic polyuria and polydipsia can be reversed by discontinuation of lithium therapy or ameliorated with amiloride or NSAIDs during continued lithium therapy[128] (see Chap. 51). Acute renal failure is usually reversible with supportive care, including dialysis to reduce toxic blood-lithium concentrations. Progressive chronic interstitial nephritis is treated by discontinuation of lithium therapy, adequate hydration, and avoidance of other nephrotoxic agents.

CYCLOSPORINE

Cyclosporine causes both acute hemodynamically mediated renal failure and chronic interstitial nephritis after 6 to 12 months of therapy. This can result in irreversible renal insufficiency and biopsy findings of arteriolar hyalinosis, glomerular sclerosis, and a striped pattern of interstitial fibrosis.[96–98] Chronic cyclosporine toxicity has become the more important of these two entities because reduced cyclosporine dosages and monitoring of drug concentrations has decreased acute toxicity. Chronic interstitial nephritis is a major concern for therapy because as many as 10% of cardiac transplant patients developed end-stage renal failure with prolonged high-dose therapy.[97] The pathogenesis appears to involve sustained renal arteriolar endothelial cell injury causing chronic renal ischemia.[98] Cyclosporine may also induce synthesis and accumulation of interstitial matrix, apparently caused by increased activity of cytokines, peptide growth factors, or thromboxane.[97] Nephrotoxicity has been dose-dependent in some, but not all analyses,[98] and occurs even following low-dose therapy. The risk of chronic interstitial renal disease appears to be reduced in those receiving low-dose therapy.

ARISTOLOCHIC ACID (CHINESE HERB NEPHROPATHY)

Incidence

In early 1993, nine cases of women with rapidly progressive kidney failure leading to end-stage renal disease were reported in Brussels, Belgium.[129] Eight of nine patients had strikingly similar pathologic findings of interstitial fibrosis with tubular atrophy on renal biopsy. All patients had presented for dialysis treatment between 1991 and 1992. Further investigation revealed that all the women were patients of the same weight loss clinic and had received a "slimming" treatment containing Chinese herbs. Subsequent analysis of the herb-based treatment demonstrated significant amounts of *Aristolochia fangchi* (Guang fang ji), known to contain aristolochic acid (AA), the major alkaloid of the botanical species *Aristolochia*.[130] The term *Chinese herb nephropathy* (CHN) was established and associated with AA exposure after confirmatory renal biopsies were obtained from additional Belgian renal failure patients with prior exposure to the same Chinese herb-based treatment.[130] By 1998, more than 100 cases of CHN had been identified in Belgian women who had used products containing Chinese herbs in an effort to lose weight.[131] Numerous additional cases of nephropathy and ESRD associated with the use of *Aristolochia* species have been reported from around the globe.[132]

Clinical Presentation

Patients with CHN typically present with mild to moderate hypertension, mild proteinuria, glycosuria, and subacute renal failure evidenced by elevated serum creatinine concentrations.[133,134] Anemia and shrunken kidneys are also common on initial presentation. The overwhelming majority of cases reported have been in women. The main pathologic lesions observed in the kidneys of CHN patients are interstitial fibrosis with atrophy and destruction of tubules throughout the renal cortex.[134] In general, the glomeruli are not affected. However, collapse of the capillaries, wrinkling of the basement membrane, and thickening of Bowman's capsule and afferent arteriolar walls are evident. These findings suggest that the primary lesion is located in the vessel walls, which leads to renal ischemia, tubular necrosis, interstitial nephritis, and, ultimately, to the extensive interstitial fibrosis that is observed. Atypical urothelial cells are also apparent. Perhaps the most remarkable feature of CHN is the rate at which it progresses. In most instances nephropathy progresses to ESRD requiring dialysis or transplantation within 6 to 24 months of exposure to AA.[133] Several cases of malignancy have also been reported in CHN patients.[135–137] An alarming 40% to 46% prevalence of urothelial transitional cell carcinoma has been observed in nephroureterectomy specimens obtained from Belgian CHN patients who underwent renal transplantation.[135,137]

Pathogenesis

Although the precise mechanism of aristolochic acid-induced nephropathy and urothelial carcinoma is yet to be characterized, recent data indicates direct DNA damage may be the cause. The major components of AA, are metabolized to mutagenic compounds called aristolactam I and aristolactam II, respectively, which form DNA adducts in humans.[137–139] Direct cellular toxicity is an unlikely mechanism because the onset is delayed and progression of renal failure continues after AA exposure.[133]

Risk Factors

Possible risk factors for the development of AA-induced toxicity remain only speculative. More than 1,700 patients were exposed to AA in the Belgian weight-loss clinic, yet only 100 patients with nephropathy were identified.[135] Furthermore, why is this type of nephropathy not prevalent in China and other Eastern cultures, where use of *Aristolochia* species is commonplace? Possible explanations include differences in dose and duration of use, because batch-to-batch variability in the composition of herbs in the "slimming" regimen was evident.[135] The concurrent use of other medications may also contribute. Many individuals receiving the herbal regimen were also prescribed the appetite stimulants dexfenfluramine and/or phentermine. It is possible the sympathomimetic agents induced renal ischemia, which then potentiated the AA toxicity. Lastly, interindividual differences in drug metabolism cannot be ruled out, because the AA metabolites have been implicated in the development of toxicity.

Prevention

The primary means of preventing CHN appears to be limiting exposure to compounds containing aristolochic acids. Several countries, including the United Kingdom, Canada, Australia, and Germany have banned the use of *Aristolochia*-containing herbs.[140]

PAPILLARY NECROSIS

Papillary necrosis is a form of chronic interstitial nephritis characterized by necrosis of the renal papillae, which are the regions of the kidney where the collecting ducts enter the renal pelvis. Analgesic use is the most common cause of papillary necrosis, accounting for 36% of all cases.[141]

ANALGESIC NEPHROPATHY

Incidence

"Classic" analgesic nephropathy, characterized by chronic tubulointerstitial nephritis with papillary necrosis,[142] was initially reported in 1953 and was subsequently recognized as a worldwide public health concern. The incidence of analgesic nephropathy among dialysis patients in the United States, Europe, and Australia has been reported to be 0.8%, 3%, and 9%, respectively.[143] Chronic excessive consumption of combination analgesics, particularly those containing phenacetin, was believed to be the major cause and led to the removal of phenacetin and phenacetin mixtures from most world markets. It was subsequently thought, however, that abuse of contemporary analgesics, aspirin, acetaminophen, and NSAIDs, alone or in combinations, also result in analgesic nephropathy regardless of phenacetin content.[142,143] This controversial issue is still being scrutinized, and a recent review of the subject suggests that there is insufficient evidence to associate nonphenacetin-combined analgesics with nephropathy.[144]

Clinical Presentation

Analgesic nephropathy evolves insidiously over years. It is difficult to recognize and may be underdiagnosed as a cause of end-stage renal failure. The most sensitive and specific diagnostic criteria include (a) a history of chronic daily "habitual" analgesic ingestion (classically this equated to a cumulative phenacetin ingestion of 3 kg or more); (b) intravenous pyelography, renal ultrasound, or renal computerized tomography imaging, which reveals decreased renal mass and bumpy renal contours; and (c) papillary calcifications.[145] Frequently, however, imaging only demonstrates "chronic pyelonephritis," small kidneys with thin renal cortices and blunted calyces. Analgesics are taken most commonly for chronic headaches.[146] Women are affected more than men. Upper gastrointestinal irritation from analgesics with blood loss leading to anemia has been characteristic. Hypertension and atherosclerotic cardiovascular disease are common. Early renal manifestations include impaired maximal urinary concentration, sterile pyuria, microscopic hematuria, and low levels of proteinuria. Urinary tract infection is common. Creatinine clearance declines slowly. Renal biopsy reveals nonspecific chronic interstitial inflammation and scarring. The incidence of lower urinary tract transitional cell carcinoma is increased with heavy phenacetin use.

Pathogenesis

Mechanisms of analgesic nephropathy remain unclear and difficult to study. This is partly a result of a lack of diagnostic markers of evolving renal damage *in vivo*. In addition, animal models of analgesic nephropathy are difficult to establish. The increased risk with analgesic mixtures containing phenacetin or acetaminophen and salicylates or NSAIDs is based on the following observations.[146,147] The renal lesion begins in the papillary tip as a result of accumulated toxic metabolites, decreased blood flow, and impaired cellular energy production. The metabolism of phenacetin to acetaminophen, which is then oxidized to toxic free radicals that are concentrated in the papilla, appears to be the initiating factor that causes toxicity by mechanisms analogous to acetaminophen hepatotoxicity. Toxicity is prevented by availability of reduced glutathione. However, salicylates deplete renal glutathione and thereby facilitate phenacetin and acetaminophen toxicity. In addition, renal medullary and papillary ischemia may contribute due to decreased synthesis of vasodilatory renal prostaglandins by salicylates and NSAIDs. Evidence for nephrotoxicity from chronic ingestion of single analgesics, acetaminophen or NSAIDs alone, challenge these concepts.[148,149]

Risk Factors

The epidemiology of analgesic use and analgesic nephropathy continues to evolve.[144,150] The classic concept persists that risk for end-stage renal disease increases with cumulative consumption of combination analgesics, phenacetin, or acetaminophen and aspirin or NSAIDs.[143] Caffeine contained in combination analgesics may increase risk, but its role is not clear.[147] Chronic use of therapeutic doses of NSAIDs alone, but not aspirin or salicylates alone, can cause analgesic nephropathy with end-stage renal failure.[148] Case-control studies associate high-dose acetaminophen use alone with an increased risk for end-stage renal disease. However, this association remains inconclusive because of study design flaws and because acetaminophen is the preferentially prescribed analgesic for patients with chronic kidney disease.[144]

Prevention

Prevention has depended primarily on public health efforts to restrict the sale of phenacetin and combination analgesics. This has effectively reduced analgesic nephropathy in Australia and Europe. However, risk continues with continued availability of OTC combination analgesics containing aspirin, acetaminophen, and caffeine in the United States and throughout the world.

Individuals requiring chronic analgesic therapy may reduce risk by limiting the total dose, avoiding combined use of two or more analgesics, and maintaining good hydration to prevent renal ischemia and decrease the papillary concentration of toxic substances. Acetaminophen remains the preferred nonopiate analgesic for renal-insufficient patients.

Management

Treatment of established nephrotoxicity requires cessation of analgesic consumption. This can prevent progression and may improve renal function. Persistent surreptitious analgesic abuse should be considered if renal function continues to decline. Patients should also be monitored for associated transitional cell carcinoma of the renal pelvis, calyces, ureters, and bladder, which may present years after analgesic nephropathy is diagnosed.

RENAL VASCULITIS, THROMBOSIS AND CHOLESTEROL EMBOLI

Systemic polyarteritis nodosa, a vasculitis with involvement of small- and medium-sized renal arteries, has been described following methamphetamine abuse.[151] Patients may have hematuria, proteinuria, renal insufficiency, and hypertension. Renal and visceral vascular aneurysms can be demonstrated by angiography. The pathogenesis may be a toxic reaction to methamphetamine or the result of associated hepatitis B infection. Penicillin and sulfonamide therapies are also considered as causes of polyarteritis nodosa, although these associations are less clear.[151]

Oral contraceptive agents, cyclosporine, mitomycin C, cisplatin, and quinine can cause a thrombotic microangiopathy (hemolytic-uremic syndrome, thrombotic thrombocytopenic purpura) manifested by endothelial proliferation and thrombus formation in the renal and central nervous system vasculature.[152–154] The association with mitomycin C is notable because the pathogenesis appears to be a direct toxic effect with a predictable incidence: 1.6% in patients receiving less than 50 mg/m^2 and 27.8% in patients receiving more than 70 mg/m^2.[153] Nephrotoxicity has occurred following chemotherapy with mitomycin C alone or with 5-fluorouracil, cisplatin, bleomycin, a Vinca alkaloid, and tamoxifen.[154] Microangiopathic hemolytic anemia and thrombocytopenia are usually present. Systemic endothelial damage with multisystem organ failure has occurred.[154] Renal failure can be severe and irreversible, although corticosteroids, antiplatelet agents, vincristine sulfate, plasma exchange, plasmapheresis, and high-dose intravenous IgG have each induced clinical improvement.

Anticoagulants and thrombolytics, particularly warfarin, can systemically embolize cholesterol particles from aortic atherosclerotic plaques to small arteries and arterioles, including renal arterioles. These agents remove or prevent thrombus formation over ulcerative plaques, causing emboli.[155] Cholesterol emboli induce an inflammatory obliterative vascular response, causing renal ischemia. Purple discoloration of the toes and mottled skin over the legs are important clinical clues.

PSEUDO-RENAL FAILURE

Pseudo-renal failure occurs when either the BUN or creatinine concentration rises, suggesting a decrease in renal function, despite maintenance of the glomerular filtration rate. The BUN concentration commonly increases without an increase in creatinine concentration during corticosteroid or tetracycline therapy. These drugs cause protein catabolism, and thereby increase ureagenesis and the BUN concentration as the result of tissue breakdown. The glomerular filtration rate is unchanged and is accurately reflected by the creatinine clearance and creatinine concentration.

Similarly, the serum creatinine concentration may rise while the BUN concentration remains unchanged by either of two mechanisms. First, drugs, including trimethoprim, cimetidine, or pyrimethamine, competitively inhibit secretion of creatinine into the proximal tubular lumen.[156,157] This effect is minimal during therapy in patients with normal renal function in whom the serum creatinine concentration usually remains in the normal range because tubular secretion of creatinine contributes only 5% to 10% to creatinine excretion.[156] In contrast, in renal-insufficient patients, the rise in serum creatinine is greater because tubular secretion of creatinine contributes a proportionately greater amount to urinary creatinine excretion.[156] Ranitidine and famotidine do not inhibit tubular secretion of creatinine at therapeutic doses.[157] Competitive inhibition of creatinine secretion has been considered useful in the evaluation of renal function because creatinine clearance usually overestimates true glomerular filtration rate in the presence of renal insufficiency. Administration of cimetidine during urine collection decreases creatinine secretion and provides a creatinine clearance value that more closely approximates true glomerular filtration, particularly in patients with renal disease (see Chap. 42).[156,157] Second, several drugs, particularly cefoxitin and other cephalosporin antibiotics, can increase the serum creatinine concentration by direct interference with the enzymatic measurement of creatinine by the Jaffé method.[156] The incidence of this effect is unknown, but it is uncommon; it is most prevalent among patients with decreased renal function. These drugs do not appear to interfere with determination of creatinine clearance.

COSTS OF DRUG-INDUCED NEPHROTOXICITY

The pharmacoeconomics of drug-induced nephrotoxicity are not well defined. An analysis of aminoglycoside therapy in the acute care environment for 1984 to 1985 revealed that the mean additional cost for each episode of toxicity (in 1984 dollars) was $2,501. The management of aminoglycoside nephrotoxicity was estimated to cost $4,500 per patient in 1998.[34] Individualized pharmacokinetic monitoring for those with reduced renal function[34] and alternative dosage strategies[37] have been reported to reduce the incidence and thereby the economic impact of aminoglycoside nephrotoxicity. Outpatient care costs of NSAID toxicity have also been evaluated. Costs for hospital care for NSAID-induced acute hemodynamically mediated renal failure and interstitial nephritis combined are estimated at $990 million per year.[159] The risk of ESRD stemming from immunosuppressant-induced nephrotoxicity contributes substantially to the cost of heart transplantation.[96] The estimated cost per transplant patient is $6,700 within 5 years, increasing to $14,200 within 8 years post-transplantation. Finally, patients who develop ESRD require dialysis, which typically costs more than $50,000 per year.

▶ PRINCIPLES OF PHARMACOTHERAPY

- Know the potential nephrotoxicity of diagnostic and therapeutic pharmacologic agents.
- Compare the potential risks and expected benefits for each course of treatment.
- Consider alternative diagnostic and therapeutic approaches.
- Use the lowest dose and shortest course of therapy that is efficacious.
- Monitor appropriately for potential toxicity.
- Modify therapy if toxicity occurs.

REFERENCES

1. Choudhury D, Ahmed Z. Drug-induced nephrotoxicity. Med Clin North Am 1997;81:705–717.
2. Elasy TA, Anderson. RJ. Changing demography of acute renal failure. Semin Dial 1996;9:438–443.
3. Leape LL, Brennan TA, Laird N, et al. The nature of adverse events in hospitalized patients. Results of the Harvard medical practice study II. N Engl J Med 1991;324:377–384.
4. Davidman M, Olson P, Kohen J, et al. Iatrogenic renal disease. Arch Intern Med 1991;151:1809–1812.
5. Thadhani R, Pascual M, Bonventre JV. Acute renal failure. N Engl J Med 1996;334:1448–1460.
6. Strom BL, Tugwell P. Pharmacoepidemiology: Current status, prospects, and problems. Ann Intern Med 1990;113:179–181.
7. Gutthan SP, Rodriguez LAG, Raiford DS, Oliart AD, Romeu JR. Nonsteroidal anti-inflammatory drugs and risk of hospitalization for acute renal failure. Arch Intern Med 1996;156:2433–2439.
8. Josephson MA, Chiu MY, Woodle ES, et al. Drug-induced acute interstitial nephritis in renal allografts: Histopathologic features and clinical course in six patients. Am J Kidney Dis 1999;34:540–548.
9. Elseviers MM, de Broe ME. Analgesic Nephropathy: Is it caused by multi-analgesic abuse or single substance use? Drug Saf 1999;20:15–24.
10. Wasser WG, Feldman NS. Chronic renal failure after ingestion of over-the-counter chromium picolinate. Ann Intern Med 1997;126:410.
11. Lo JC, Chertow GM, Rennke H, Seifter JL. Fanconi's syndrome and tubulointerstitial nephritis in association with l-lysine ingestion. Am J Kidney Dis 1996;28:614–617.
12. Pritchard NR, Kalra PA. Renal dysfunction accompanying oral creatine supplements. Lancet 1998;351:1252–1253.
13. Vanherweghem JL, Tielemans C, Simon J, Depierreux M. Chinese herbs nephropathy and renal pelvic carcinoma. Nephrol Dial Transplant 1995;10:270–273.
14. Epstein M, Oster JR. Beta blockers and renal function: A reappraisal. J Clin Hypertens 1985;1:85–99.
15. Porter GA. Effects of contrast agents on renal function. Invest Radiol 1993;28(suppl 5):S1–S5.
16. Dorman HR, Sondheimer JH, Cadnapaphornchai P. Mannitol-induced acute renal failure. Medicine (Baltimore) 1990;69:153–159.
17. Bennett WM. Drug interactions and consequences of sodium restriction. Am J Clin Nutr 1997;65(suppl):678S–681S.
18. Duggin GG. Combination analgesic-induced kidney disease: The Australian experience. Am J Kidney Dis 1996;28:S39–S47.
19. Del Moral RG, Olmo A, Aguilar M, O'Valle F. P glycoprotein: A new mechanism to control drug-induced nephrotoxicity. Exp Nephrol 1998;6:89–97.
20. Zhang L, Brett CM, Giacomini KM. Role of organic cation transporters in drug absorption and elimination. Annu Rev Pharmacol Toxicol 1998;38:431–460.
21. Van Aubel R, Masereeuw R, Russel F. Molecular pharmacology of renal organic anion transporters. Am J Physiol Renal Physiol 2000;279:F216–F232.
22. Ho ES, Lin DC, Mendel DB, Cihlar T. Cytotoxicity of antiviral nucleotides adefovir and cidofovir is induced by the expression of human renal organic anion transporter 1. J Am Soc Nephrol 2000;11:383–393.
23. Takeda M, Tojo A, Sekine T, et al. Role of organic anion transporter 1 (OAT1) in cephaloridine (CER)-induced nephrotoxicity. Kidney Int 1999;56:2128–2136.
24. Yu DK. The contribution of P-glycoprotein to pharmacokinetic drug-drug interactions. J Clin Pharmacol 1999;39:1203–1211.
25. Baliga R, Ueda N, Walker PD, Shah SV. Oxidant mechanisms in toxic acute renal failure. Drug Metab Rev 1999;31:971–997.
26. Swan SK. Aminoglycoside nephrotoxicity. Semin Nephrol 1997;17: 27–33.
27. Brezis M, Rosen S. Hypoxia of the renal medulla—Its implications for disease. N Engl J Med 1995;332:647–655.
28. Berns JS, Ford PA. Renal toxicities of antineoplastic drugs and bone marrow transplantation. Semin Nephrol 1997;17:54–66.
29. Rudnick MR, Berns JS, Cohen RM, Goldfarb S. Contrast media-associated nephrotoxicity. Semin Nephrol 1997;17:15–26.
30. Ali H. Renal disease in the elderly. Postgrad Med 1996;100:44–57.
31. Bennett WM. Drug-related renal dysfunction in the elderly. Geriatr Nephrol Urol 1999;9:21–25.
32. Mulato AS, Ho ES, Cihlar T. Nonsteroidal anti-inflammatory drugs efficiently reduce the transport and cytotoxicity of adefovir mediated by the human renal organic anion transporter 1. J Pharmacol Exp Ther 2000;295:10–15.
33. Nolan CR, Anderson RJ. Hospital-acquired acute renal failure. J Am Soc Nephrol 1998;9:710–718.
34. Slaughter RL, Cappelletty DM. Economic impact of aminoglycoside toxicity and its prevention through therapeutic drug monitoring. Pharmacoeconomics 1998;14:385–394.
35. Mingeot-Leclercq M, Tulkens PM. Aminoglycosides: Nephrotoxicity. Antimicrob Agents Chemother 1999;43:1003–1012.
36. Goetz MB, Sayers J. Nephrotoxicity of vancomycin and aminoglycoside therapy separately and in combination. J Antimicrob Chemother 1993;32:325–334.
37. Freeman CD, Nicolau DP, Belliveau PP, Nightingale CH. Once-daily dosing of aminoglycosides: Review and recommendations for clinical practice. J Am Antimicrob Chemother 1997;39:677–686.
38. Streetmen DS Nafziger AN, Destache CJ, Bertino AS Jr. Individualized pharmacokinetic monitoring results in less aminoglycoside-associated nephrotoxicity and fewer associated costs. Pharmacotherapy 2001;21:443–451.
39. McCormick JP. An emotional-based medicine approach to monitoring once-daily aminoglycosides. Pharmacotherapy 2000;20:1524–1527.
40. Prins JM, Weverling GJ, Be Blok K, et al. Validation and nephrotoxicity of a simplified once-daily aminoglycoside dosing schedule and guidelines for monitoring therapy. Antimicrob Agents Chemother 1996;40:2494–2499.
41. Koo J, Tight R, Rajkumar V, Hawa Z. Comparison of once-daily versus pharmacokinetic dosing of aminoglycosides in elderly patients. Am J Med 1996;101:177–183.
42. Kurnik BRC, Allgren RL, Genter FC, et al. Prospective study of atrial natriuretic peptide for the prevention of radiocontrast-induced nephropathy. Am J Kidney Dis 1998;31:674–680.
43. Solomon R. Contrast-medium-induced acute renal failure. Kidney Int 1998;53:230–242.
44. Murphy SW, Barrett BJ, Parfrey PS. Contrast nephropathy. J Am Soc Nephrol 2000;11:177–182.
45. Nash K, Hafeez A, Abrinko P, Hou S. Hospital-acquired renal insufficiency 1996. J Am Soc Nephrol 1996;7:1376.
46. Levy EM, Viscoli CM, Horwitz RI. The effect of acute renal failure on mortality. A cohort analysis. JAMA 1996;275:1489–1494.
47. Gerlach AT, Pickworth KK. Contrast medium-induced nephrotoxicity: Pathophysiology and prevention. Pharmacotherapy 2000;20:540–548.
48. Stevens MA, McCullough PA, Tobin KJ, et al. A prospective randomized trial of prevention measures in patients at high risk for contrast nephropathy: Result of the P.R.I.N.C.E. study. Prevention of Radiocontrast Induced Nephropathy Clinical Evaluation. J Am Coll Cardiol 1999;33:403–411.
49. Rudnick MR, Goldfarb S, Wexler L, et al. Nephrotoxicity of ionic and nonionic contrast media in 1196 patients: A randomized trial. Kidney Int 1995;47:254–261.
50. Lehnert T, Keller E, Gondolf K, et al. Effect of haemodialysis after contrast medium administration in patients with renal insufficiency. Nephrol Dial Transplant 1998;13:358–362.
51. Hans SS, Hans BA, Dhillon R, et al. Effect of dopamine on renal function after arteriography in patients with pre-existing renal insufficiency. Am Surg 1998;64:432–436.
52. Tepel M, Van Der Giet M, Schwarzfeld C, et al. Prevention of radiographic-contrast-agent-induced reductions in renal function by acetylcysteine. N Engl J Med 2000;343:180–184.

52a. Chu VL, Cheng JWM. Fenoldopam in the prevention of contrast media-induced acute renal failure. Ann Pharmacother 2001;35:1278–1282.

52b. Murphy MB, Murray C, Shorteri GD. Fenoldopam-a selective peripheral domamine-receptor agonist for the treatment of severe hypertension. N Engl J Med, Vol 345, No. 21.

53. Koch JA, Plum J, Grabensee B, Modder U. Prostaglandin E1: A new agent for the prevention of renal dysfunction in high risk patients caused by radiocontrast media? PGE1 Study Group. Nephrol Dial Transplant 2000;15:43–49.

54. Kintzel PE. Anticancer drug-induced kidney disorders: Incidence, prevention, and management. Drug Saf 2001;24:19–38.

55. Merouani A, Shpall EJ, Jones RB, Archer PG, Schrier RW. Renal function in high dose chemotherapy and autologous hematopoietic cell support treatment for breast cancer. Kidney Int 1996;50:1026–1031.

56. Anand AJ, Bashey B. Newer insights into cisplatin nephrotoxicity. Ann Pharmacother 1993;27:1519–1525.

57. Foster-Nora JA, Siders R. Amifostine for protection from antineoplastic drug toxicity. Am J Health Syst Pharm 1997;54:787–800.

58. Hartmann JT, Knop S, Fels LM, et al. The use of reduced doses of amifostine to ameliorate nephrotoxicity of cisplatin/ifosfamide-based chemotherapy in patients with solid tumors. Anticancer Drugs 2000; 11:1–6.

59. Sener G, Satiroglu H, Kabasakal L, et al. The protective effect of melatonin on cisplatin nephrotoxicity. Fundam Clin Pharmacol 2000;14:553 560.

60. Mizumura Y, Matsumura Y, Hamaguchi T, et al. Cisplatin-incorporated polymeric micelles eliminate nephrotoxicity, while maintaining antitumor activity. Jpn J Cancer Res 2001;92:328–336.

61. Sawaya BP, Briggs JP, Schnermann J. Amphotericin B nephrotoxicity: The adverse consequences of altered membrane properties. J Am Soc Nephrol 1995;6:154–164.

62. Fisher MA, Talbot GH, Maislin G, et al. Risk factors for amphotericin B-associated nephrotoxicity. Am J Med 1989;87:547–552.

63. Wingard JR, White MH, Anaissie E, et al. A Randomized, double-blind comparative trial evaluating the safety of liposomal amphotericin B versus amphotericin B lipid complex in the empirical treatment of febrile neutropenia. Clin Infect Dis 2000;31:1155–1163.

64. Fanos V, Cataldi L. Amphotericin B- induced nephrotoxicity: A review. J Chemother 2000;12:463–470.

65. Eriksson U, Siefert B, Schaffner A. Comparison of effects of amphotericin B deoxycholate infused over 4 or 24 hours: Randomised controlled trial. BMJ 2001;322:1–6.

66. Anderson CM. Sodium chloride treatment of amphotericin B nephrotoxicity. Standard of care? West J Med 1995;162:313–317.

67. Brouhard BH, Baetz-Greenwalt B. Calcium-channel blocking agents as therapy for amphotericin B nephrotoxicity. Cleve Clin J Med 1992;59:263–264.

68. Camp MJ, Wingard JR, Gilmore CE, et al. Efficacy of low-dose dopamine in preventing amphotericin B nephrotoxicity in bone marrow transplant patients and leukemia patients. Antimicrob Agents Chemother 1998;42:103–106.

69. Leenders ACAP, de Marie S. The use of lipid formulations of amphotericin B for systemic fungal infections. Leukemia 1996;10:1570–1575.

70. Harrell CC, Hanf-Kristufek L. Comparison of nephrotoxicity of amphotericin B products. Clin Infect Dis 2001;32:990–991.

71. Peter BS, Carlin E, Weston RJ, et al. Adverse effects of drugs used in the management of opportunistic infections associated with HIV infection. Drug Saf 1994;10:439–454.

72. Maurice-Estepa, L, Daudon M, Katlama C, et al. Identification of crystals in kidneys of AIDS patients treated with foscarnet. Am J Kidney Dis 1998;32:392–400.

73. Cheung TW, Jayaweera DT, Pearce D, et al. Safety of oral versus intravenous hydration during induction therapy with intravenous foscarnet in AIDS patients with cytomegalovirus infections. Int J STD AIDS 2000;11:640–647.

74. Cundy KC. Clinical pharmacokinetics of the antiviral nucleotide analogues cidofovir and adefovir. Clin Pharmacokinet 1999;36:127 143.

75. Yorgin PD, Theodorou AA, Al-Uzri A, et al. Propylene glycol-induced proximal renal tubular cell injury. Am J Kidney Dis 1997;30:134–139.

76. Haskin JA, Warner DJ, Blank DU. Acute renal failure after large doses of intravenous immune globulin. Ann Pharmacother 1999;33:800–803.

77. Schortgen F, Lacherade J, Bruneel F, et al. Effects of hydroxyethylstarch and gelatin on renal function in severe sepsis: A multicenter randomised study. Lancet 2001;357:911–916.

78. Visweswaran P, Massin EK, Dubose TD Jr. Mannitol-induced acute renal failure. J Am Soc Nephrol 1997;8:1028–1033.

79. Saine DR, Ahrens ER. Renal impairment associated with losartan. Ann Intern Med 1996;124:775.

80. Textor SC. Renal failure related to angiotensin-converting enzyme inhibitors. Semin Nephrol 1997;17:67–76.

81. Bakris GL, Weir MR. Angiotensin-converting enzyme inhibitor-associated elevations in serum creatinine: Is this a cause for concern? Arch Intern Med 2000;160:685–693.

82. Reardon LC, Macpherson DS. Hyperkalemia in outpatients using angiotensin-converting enzyme inhibitors. How much should we worry? Arch Intern Med 1998;158:26–32.

83. Wynckel A, Ebikili B, Melin J, et al. Long term follow-up of acute renal failure caused by angiotensin converting enzyme inhibitors. Am J Hypertens 1998;11:1080–1086.

84. Whelton A. Renal effects of over-the-counter analgesics. J Clin Pharmacol 1995;35:454–463.

85. Whelton A, Stout RL, Spilman PS, Klassen DK. Renal effects of ibuprofen, piroxicam, and sulindac in patients with asymptomatic renal failure: A prospective, randomized, crossover comparison. Ann Intern Med 1990;112:568–576.

86. Schoch PH, Ranno A, North DS. Acute renal failure in an elderly woman following intramuscular ketorolac administration. Ann Pharmacother 1992;26:1233–1236.

87. Feldman HI, Kinman JL, Berlin JA, et al. Parenteral ketorolac: The risk for acute renal failure. Ann Intern Med 1997;126:193–199.

88. O'Callaghan CA, Andrews PA, Ogg CS. Renal disease and use of topical non-steroidal anti-inflammatory drugs. BMJ 1994;308:110–111.

89. Whelton A. Nephrotoxicity of nonsteroidal anti-inflammatory drugs: Physiologic foundations and clinical implications. Am J Med 1999; 106:13S–24S.

90. Solomon DH, Gurwitz JH. Toxicity of nonsteroidal anti-inflammatory drugs in the elderly: Is advanced age a risk factor? Am J Med 1997; 102:208–215.

91. Nesher G, Sonnenblick M, Dwolatzky T. Protective effect of misoprostol on indomethacin-induced renal dysfunction in elderly patients. J Rheumatol 1995;22:713–716.

92. Brater DC. Effects of nonsteroidal anti-inflammatory drugs on renal function: Focus on cyclooxygenase-2-selective inhibition. Am J Med 1999;107:65S–71S.

93. Swan SK, Rudy DW, Lasseter KC, et al. Effect of cyclooxygenase-2 inhibition on renal function in elderly persons receiving a low-salt diet: A randomized, controlled trial. Ann Intern Med 2000,133:1–139.

94. Perazella MA, Eras J. Are selective COX-2 inhibitors nephrotoxic? Am J Kidney Dis 2000;35:937–940.

95. Walls M, Goral S, Stone W. Acute renal failure due to sulfinpyrazone. Am J Med Sci 1998;315:319–321.

96. de Mattos AM, Oyaei AJ, Bennett WM. Nephrotoxicity of immunosuppressive drugs: Long-term consequences and challenges for the future. Am J Kidney Dis 2000;35:333–346.

97 Bennett WM, DeMattos A, Meyer MM, et al. Chronic cyclosporine nephropathy: The Achilles' heel of immunosuppressive therapy. Kidney Int 1996;50:1089–1100.

98. Falkenhain ME, Cosio FG, Sedmak DD. Progressive histologic injury in kidneys from heart and liver transplant recipients receiving cyclosporine. Transplantation 1996;62:364–370.

99. Olyaei AJ, de Mattos AM, Bennett WM. Immunosuppressant-induced nephropathy: Pathophysiology, incidence and management. Drug Saf 1999;21:471–488.

100. Lee DBN. Cyclosporine and the renin-angiotensin axis. Kidney Int 1997;52:248–260.

101. Sica DA, Gehr TWB. Triamterene and the kidney. Nephron 1989;51: 454–461.
102. Danesh BJZ, Brunton J, Sumner DJ. Comparison between short-term renal hemodynamic effects of propranolol and nadolol in essential hypertension: A crossover study. Clin Sci 1984;67:243–248.
103. Wever PC, Roest RW, Wolbink-Kamp AM, et al. OKT3-induced nephrotoxicity is associated with release of group II secretory phospholipase A2. Eur J Clin Invest 1996;26:873–878.
104. Perazella MA. Crystal-induced acute renal failure. Am J Med 1999;106:459–465.
105. Vanholder R, Sever MS, Erek E, Lameire N. Rhabdomyolysis. J Am Soc Nephrol 2000;11:1553–1561.
106. Al Shohaib S. Simvastatin-induced rhabdomyolysis in patient with chronic renal failure. Am J Nephrol 2000;20:212–213.
107. Grunden JW, Fisher KA. Lovastatin-induced rhabdomyolysis possibly associated with clarithromycin and azithromycin. Ann Pharmacother 1997;31:859–863.
108. Hein R, Brunkhorst R, Thon WF, et al. Symptomatic sulfadiazine crystalluria in AIDS patients: A report of two cases. Clin Nephrol 1993;39: 254–256.
109. Rossert J, Rondeau E, Jondeau G, et al. Tamm-Horsfall protein accumulation in glomeruli during acetazolamide-induced acute renal failure. Am J Nephrol 1989;9:56–57.
110. Becker K, Jablonowski H, Haussinger D. Sulfadiazine-associated nephrotoxicity in patients with the acquired immunodeficiency syndrome. Medicine (Baltimore) 1996;75:185–194.
111. Kopp JB, Miller KD, Mican JAM, et al. Crystalluria and urinary tract abnormalities associated with indinavir. Ann Intern Med 1997;127:119–125.
112. Berns JS, Cohen RM, Silverman M, Turner J. Acute renal failure due to indinavir crystalluria and nephrolithiasis: Report of two cases. Am J Kidney Dis 1997;30:558–560.
113. Kranen S, Keough D, Gordon RB, Emerson BT. Xanthine-containing calculi during allopurinol therapy. J Urol 1985;133:658–659.
114. Millette CH, Snodgrass GL. Acute renal failure associated with chronic antacid ingestion. Am J Hosp Pharm 1981;38:1352–1355.
115. Dick WH, Lingeman JE, Preminger GM, et al. Laxative abuse as a cause for ammonium urate renal calculi. J Urol 1990;143:244–247.
116. Powell T, Hsu FF, Turk J, Hruska K. Ma-huang strikes again: Ephedrine nephrolithiasis. Am J Kidney Dis 1998;32:153–159.
117. Adler SG, Cohen AH, Glassock RJ. Secondary glomerular diseases In: Brenner BM, ed. Brenner and Rectors' The Kidney, 5th ed. Philadelphia, WB Saunders, 1996:1563–1566.
118. Abraham PA, Keane WF. Glomerular and interstitial disease induced by nonsteroidal anti-inflammatory drugs. Am J Nephrol 1984;4:1–6.
119. Coroneos E, Petrusevska G, Varghese F, Truong LD. Focal segmental glomerulosclerosis with acute renal failure associated with alpha-interferon therapy. Am J Kidney Dis 1996;28:888–892.
120. Hall CL. Gold nephropathy. Nephron 1988;50:265–272.
121. Radford MG Jr, Holley KE, Grande JP, et al. Reversible membranous nephropathy associated with the use of nonsteroidal anti-inflammatory drugs. JAMA 1996;276:466–469.
122. Toto RD. Review: Acute tubulointerstitial nephritis. Am J Med Sci 1990;299:392–410.
123. Michel DM, Kelly CI. Acute intestinal nephritis. J Am Soc Nephrol 1998;9:506–515.
124. Markowitz GS, Radhakrishnan J, Kambham N, et al. Lithium nephrotoxicity: A progressive combined glomerular and tubulointerstitial nephropathy. J Am Soc Nephrol 2000;11:1439–1448.
125. Walker RG. Lithium nephrotoxicity. Kidney Int 1993;44(suppl 42):S93–S98.
126. Kallner G, Petterson U. Renal, thyroid and parathyroid function during lithium treatment: Laboratory tests in 207 people treated for 1–30 years. Acta Psychiatr Scand 1995;91:48–51.
127. Lehmann K, Ritz E. Angiotensin-converting enzyme inhibitors may cause renal dysfunction in patients on long-term lithium treatment. Am J Kidney Dis 1995;25:82–87.
128. Lam SS, Kjellstrand C. Emergency treatment of lithium-induced diabetes insipidus with nonsteroidal anti-inflammatory drugs. Ren Fail 1997;19:183–188.
129. Vanherweghem JL, Depierreux M, Tielemans C, et al. Rapidly progressive interstitial renal fibrosis in young women: Association with slimming regimen including Chinese herbs. Lancet 1993;341:387–391.
130. Cosyns JP, Jadoul M, Squifflet JP, et al. Chinese herbs nephropathy: A clue to Balkan endemic nephropathy? Kidney Int 1994;45:1680–1688.
131. Vanherweghem JL. Misuse of herbal remedies: The case of an outbreak of terminal renal failure in Belgium. J Altern Complement Med 1998;4: 9–16.
132. Vanherweghem JL. Nephropathy and herbal medicine. Am J Kidney Dis 2000;35:330–332.
133. Reginster F, Jadoul M, van Ypersele DS. Chinese herbs nephropathy presentation, natural history and fate after transplantation. Nephrol Dial Transplant 1997;12:81–86.
134. Depierreux M, Van Damme B, Vanden Houte K, Vanherweghem JL. Pathologic aspects of a newly described nephropathy related to the prolonged use of Chinese herbs. Am J Kidney Dis 1994;24:172–180.
135. Cosyns JP, Jadoul M, Squifflet JP, et al. Urothelial lesions in Chinese-herb nephropathy. Am J Kidney Dis 1999;33:1011–1017.
136. Yang CS, Lin CH, Chang SH, Hsu HC. Rapidly progressive fibrosing interstitial nephritis associated with Chinese herbal drugs. Am J Kidney Dis 2000;35:313–318.
137. Nortier JL, Martinez MC, Schmeiser HH, et al. Urothelial carcinoma associated with the use of a Chinese herb (*Aristolochia fangchi*). N Engl J Med 2000;342:1686–1692.
138. Bieler CA, Stiborova M, Wiessler M, et al. 32P-post-labelling analysis of DNA adducts formed by aristolochic acid in tissues from patients with Chinese herbs nephropathy. Carcinogenesis 1997;18:1063–1067.
139. Krumme B, Endmeir R, Vanhaelen M, Walb D. Reversible Fanconi syndrome after ingestion of a Chinese herbal "remedy" containing aristolochic acid. Nephrol Dial Transplant 2001;16:400–402.
140. Kessler DA. Cancer and herbs. N Engl J Med 2000;342:1742–1743.
141. Griffin MD, Larson TS, Bergstralh EJ. Renal papillary necrosis—A sixteen-year clinical experience. J Am Soc Nephrol 1995;6:248–256.
142. Henrich WL, Agodoa LE, Barrett B, et al. Analgesics and the kidney: Summary and recommendations to the scientific advisory board of the National Kidney Foundation from an ad hoc committee of the National Kidney Foundation. Am J Kidney Dis 1996;27:162–165.
143. Elseviers MM, de Broe ME. Analgesic nephropathy: Is it caused by multi-analgesic abuse or single substance use? Drug Saf 1999;20:15–24.
144. Feinstein AR, Heinemann LAJ, Curhan GC, et al. Relationship between nonphenacetin-combined analgesics and nephropathy: A review. Kidney Int 2000;58:2259–2264.
145. Elseviers MM, De Broe ME. Combination analgesic involvement in the pathogenesis of analgesic nephropathy: The European perspective. Am J Kidney Dis 1996;28:S48–S55.
146. Duggin GG. Combination analgesic-induced kidney disease: The Australian experience. Am J Kidney Dis 1996;28:539–547.
147. DeBroe ME, Elseviers MM. Analgesic nephropathy. N Engl J Med 1998;338:446–452.
148. Bennett WM, Henrich WL, Stoff JS. The renal effects of nonsteroidal anti-inflammatory drugs: Summary and recommendations. Am J Kidney Dis 1996;28:S56–S62.
149. Buckalew VM. Habitual use of acetaminophen as a risk factor for chronic renal failure: A comparison with phenacetin. Am J Kidney Dis 1996;28:S7–S13.
150. Michielsen P, de Schepper P. Trends of analgesic nephropathy in two high-endemic regions with different legislation. J Am Soc Nephrol 2001;12:550–556.
151. Porter GA, Bennett WM. Nephrotoxin-induced acute renal failure. In: Brenner BM, Stein JH, eds. Contemporary Issues in Nephrology, Vol 6. New York, Churchill Livingstone, 1980:123–162.

152. Lakkis FG, Campbell OC, Badr KF. Microvascular diseases of the kidney. In: Brenner BM, ed. Brenner and Rectors' The Kidney, 5th ed. Philadelphia, WB Saunders, 1996:1712–1730.
153. Valavaara R, Nordman E. Renal complications of mitomycin C therapy with special reference to the total dose. Cancer 1985;55: 47–50.
154. Groff JA, Kozak M, Boehmer JP, et al. Endotheliopathy: A continuum of hemolytic uremic syndrome due to mitomycin therapy. Am J Kidney Dis 1997;29:280–284.
155. Lye WC, Cheah JS, Sinniah R. Renal cholesterol embolic disease. Case report and review of the literature. Am J Nephrol 1993;13:489–493.
156. Lafayette RA, Perrone RD, Levey AS. Laboratory evaluation of renal function. In: Schrier RW, Gottschalk CW, eds. Diseases of the Kidney, 6th ed. Boston, Little, Brown, 1997:307–354.
157. Andreev E, Koopman M, Arisz L. A rise in plasma creatinine that is not a sign of renal failure: Which drugs can be responsible. J Intern Med 1999;246:247–252.
158. Eisenberg JM, Koffer H, Glick HA, et al. What is the cost of nephrotoxicity associated with aminoglycosides? Ann Intern Med 1987;107:900–909.
159. McGoldrick MD, Bailie GR. Nonnarcotic analgesics: Prevalence and estimated economic impact of toxicities. Ann Pharmacother 1997;31:221–227.

49
GLOMERULONEPHRITIS

Alan H. Lau

Clinical and pathologic findings associated with primary glomerular injury were first reported in the 19th century. The natural history of many glomerular diseases was not described until the 1950s, when percutaneous diagnostic kidney biopsy became available. The development of immunofluorescence microscopy and advances in immunopathology in the 1960s and 1970s further expanded our understanding of the antibody-related immune mechanisms that are responsible for the different types of glomerular injury.[1] Recent advances in cell and molecular biology afford us a plethora of new information concerning the disease processes.[2] However, the precise pathogenetic mechanisms for many glomerular diseases remain unknown and the available therapeutic regimens are still far from optimal. In 1998, glomerulonephritis was the third most common cause of end-stage renal disease (ESRD), accounting for 9.1% of all the cases, or about 7,500 patients each year.[3]

This chapter provides an overview of the pathophysiologic mechanisms of glomerular injury and the clinical presentations of glomerulonephritis. The specific characteristics of and the treatment approach for each of the more common forms of glomerulonephritis are also discussed. Although diabetes mellitus and amyloidosis are important secondary causes of glomerular diseases, the scope of this chapter is limited to the primary causes of glomerulonephritis.

PATHOPHYSIOLOGY

NORMAL ANATOMY AND FUNCTION

The glomerulus, which is enclosed within the Bowman's capsule, consists of two important components: the filtration barrier and the mesangium (Fig. 49–1). Blood flow in the glomerular capillary bed is supplied by the afferent arteriole, while the efferent arterioles channel the flow leaving the glomerular tuft. The capillary wall, which serves as a filtration barrier, consists of three well-defined layers: fenestrated endothelium, glomerular basement membrane (GBM), and epithelial cells. The epithelial cells, also known as podocytes, have specialized foot processes embedded in the outer layer of the GBM. It is across this barrier that fluid flows and ultimately forms ultrafiltrate. Under normal conditions, the GBM appears to function as a compact hydrated gel of matrix proteins with a pore-like structure. The mesangium provides support for the glomerular capillaries and also modulates blood flow through the capillaries. It consists of mesangial cells embedded in an extracellular matrix.

The unique capillary bed of the glomerulus allows small nonprotein plasma constituents up to the size of inulin, which has a molecular weight of 5,200 daltons, to pass freely while excluding macromolecules equal to or larger than albumin, which has a molecular weight of 69,000 daltons (Fig. 49–2). Both the size and charge of the molecules affect the ease of passage through the glomerular membrane.[4] For molecules with similar effective molecular radii, those that are anionic tend to experience more difficulties in passing through than molecules that are cationic.[4]

Fixed, negatively charged sites are found within the glomeruli in all three layers of the capillary wall: the endothelium, the epithelium, and the GBM. Biochemical and cytochemical studies show that the epithelial cell coat is composed of a negatively charged glycoprotein (podocalyxin), made up largely of sialic acid. The GBM contains an abundance of negatively charged sulfated glycosaminoglycans that can affect the passage of ionic molecules through the capillary wall. The movement of negatively charged molecules is restricted more than that of neutral or positively charged molecules.[4] Different glomerular diseases affect this size- and charge-selective barrier to different extent, and glomerulopathies therefore present with varied clinical features and solute-excretion patterns.

Aside from being a barrier for solute excretion, some of the glomerular cells, such as the epithelial cells, have phagocytic function that can remove macromolecules trapped within the filtration barrier. They are also capable of synthesizing the GBM. In contrast, the mesangial cells regulate glomerular hemodynamics by responding to angiotensin II and producing prostaglandins. They also synthesize and respond to various cytokines and thus play a key role in immune-mediated glomerular diseases. There are also resident phagocytes in the mesangium. They remove macromolecules trapped in the basement membrane and move them into the urinary space. These phagocytes are involved in the development of both immune and nonimmune glomerular injury.[5]

ETIOLOGY

The etiology of most human glomerulonephritides is unknown. However, humoral and cellular immunologic mechanisms are implicated in the pathogenesis. Abnormalities in coagulation and metabolism, as well as hereditary and vascular diseases, also contribute to glomerular damage. The histopathologic manifestations vary substantially among the different types of glomerulonephritis. An overview of the primary pathogenetic mechanisms is presented in this section, and specific abnormalities for each of the primary types of glomerulonephritis are presented in subsequent sections.

PATHOGENESIS OF GLOMERULAR INJURY AND PATHOLOGIC MANIFESTATIONS

The glomerular lesion may be diffuse (involving all glomeruli), focal (involving some but not all glomeruli), or segmental, also known as local (involving part of the individual glomeruli). The pathologic manifestations may also be described as proliferative (overgrowth of epithelium, endothelium, or mesangium), membranous (thickening of GBM), and/or sclerotic.

The glomerular capillary wall is particularly susceptible to immune-mediated injury. Antigen and antibody tend to localize in the glomerulus probably because of its high blood flow and capillary hydrostatic pressure. Parenchymal damage can be induced as a result of humoral- and cell-mediated immune reactions (Table 49–1).

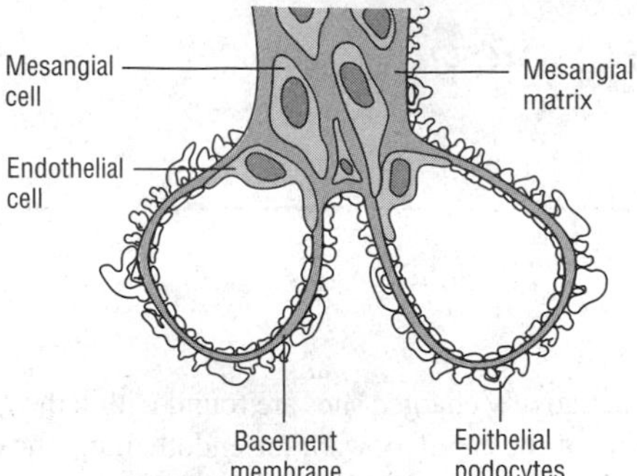

FIGURE 49–1. Microanatomy of glomerulus.

TABLE 49–1. Immunologic Mechanisms of Glomerular Injury

Circulating immune complexes
In situ antigen–antibody interaction
Intrinsic glomerular antigen; e.g., GBM antigens
Exogenous planted antigens
Cell-mediated mechanism

Antibodies and sensitized T lymphocytes are the primary mediators of glomerular injury.[6–8]

Production of antibodies to endogenous or exogenous antigens that are recognized as foreign by the host is the first step in humoral immunologic damage to the glomerulus. Endogenous antigens may be intrinsic glomerular antigens, such as Heymann's antigen on the epithelial cell or Goodpasture's antigen on the GBM, or previously sequestered antigens, such as DNA or thyroglobulin. Exogenous antigens are most often viral, bacterial, parasitic, or fungal in origin (Table 49–2). Antineutrophil cytoplasmic autoantibodies (ANCAs), autoantibodies that react to the cytoplasmic components of neutrophils and monocytes, have been found in patients with idiopathic crescentic glomerulonephritis and also in the accompanying vasculitis.[9]

Classically, it was considered that complexes of antigens and antibodies were formed in the circulation and then passively entrapped in the glomerular capillary or mesangium. However, experimental data shows that antibodies may combine with endogenous glomerular antigens or exogenous antigens entrapped in the glomerulus to form complexes locally, or *in situ.*[7] Regardless of the mechanism of formation, these antigen–antibody complexes are often localized along the capillary loop or the mesangium (Fig. 49–1) and can be detected by immunofluorescence microscopy. The type and extent of glomerular damage is dependent on the location of the immune complex formation and the rate at which it is removed. Impaired removal facilitates the growth of the complex and thus increases the likelihood of glomerular damage.

Subsequent to antigen-antibody formation, a series of biologic events is triggered that ultimately leads to glomerular injury. Both inflammatory and noninflammatory lesions can be induced by antibody deposition. Noninflammatory lesions can be a result of noncomplement-fixing antibody binding to the glomerular epithelial cell (mechanism 1), or activation of the complement system to form the C5b-9 membrane attack complex (mechanism 2).[7,8] Both mechanisms can damage the glomerular epithelial cell and result in capillary wall injury and proteinuria (Fig. 49–3). Inflammatory lesions are induced by glomerular infiltration of circulating inflammatory cells such as neutrophils, monocytes/macrophages, and platelets (mechanism 3), or proliferation of resident glomerular mesangial cells (mechanism 4), resulting in GBM damage[7] (Fig. 49–3). The migration of neutrophils and monocytes to the glomerular tufts is promoted by chemoattractants such as complement fragments (C3a, C5a), platelet-activating factor, interleukin-8, and monocyte chemotactic protein-1.[10] Various cytokines, chemokines, and growth factors are then released to participate in the inflammatory process.[6]

T cells sensitized to glomerular antigen, macrophages, and resident mesangial cells are important participants in cell-mediated injury. Sensitized T cells can cause glomerular hypercellularity in the absence of antibody deposition.[6–8,10] Cytotoxic T cells may bind with the target cells and destroy them. Alternatively, a delayed-type

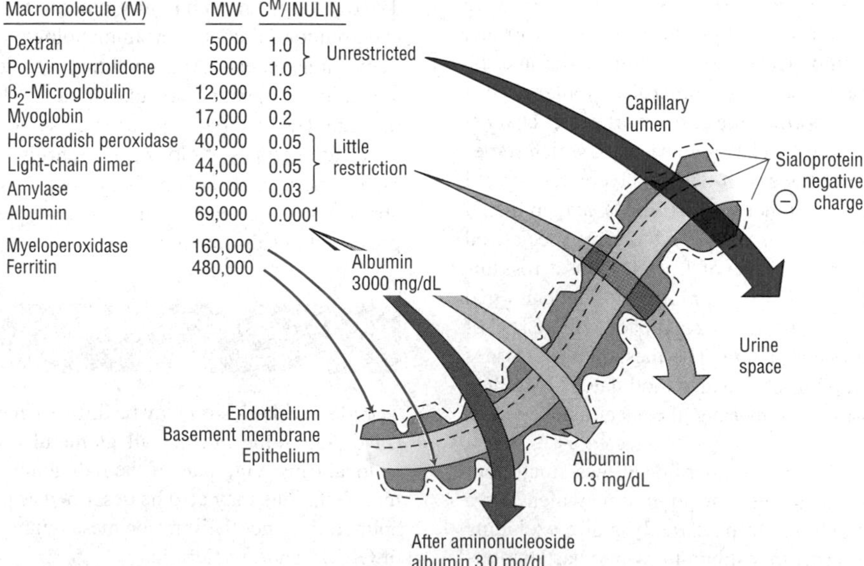

FIGURE 49–2. Movement of various macromolecules across the glomerular capillary. The fractional clearance of each macromolecule as compared to inulin (C^M/INULIN) decreases as molecular weight (MW) increases. The disproportionately greater restriction of albumin movement indicates inportance of factors other than size, such as negative charge of albumin. *(From Hutt MP, Kelleher SP. Proteinuria and the nephrotic syndrome. In: Schrier RW, ed. Renal and Electrolyte Disorders, 3rd ed. Boston, Little, Brown, 1986, with permission.)*

TABLE 49–2. Antigens Possibly Involved in Immune-Mediated Glomerular Injury

Source of Antigen	Clinical Example
Endogenous Antigens	
Released sequestered cellular antigens	DNA, thyroglobulin
Endogenous antigens modified by exogenous source	IgG modified by streptococcal neuraminidase
Tumor antigens	CEA in bronchial and other solid tumors
Intrinsic glomerular antigens	Goodpasture's syndrome
Neutrophil granule constituents	ANCA-associated glomerulonephritis
Exogenous	
Viral	Hepatitis B
Bacterial	Streptococcal organisms
Parasitic	Malaria
Fungal	Candida

CEA = carcinoembryonic antigen; ANCA = antineutrophil cytoplasmic antibody.

hypersensitivity reaction may be initiated by activated T cells, through the release of lymphokines, to attract, activate, and transform monocytes into macrophages.[7] These humoral and cellular mediators, in conjunction with a host of toxic molecular entities, including reactive oxygen species, proteinases, eicosanoids, and procoagulants, which are secreted by neutrophils, macrophages, platelets, and resident glomerular cells, can alter the permeability, blood flow, and function of the glomeruli. Vascular constriction and occlusion follow and result in the eventual destruction of the glomeruli.

Acute forms of glomerular injury may frequently lead to chronic and persistent renal dysfunction, even though the original immune factors that induce glomerular injury have resolved. Progression to end-stage renal failure may be inevitable. Experimental and clinical investigations suggest that a variety of factors may participate in the progression of renal injury.[11] These factors include systemic and glomerular hypertension;[12] high dietary protein intake; proteinuria;[13–15] glomerular hypertrophy; hyperlipidemia;[16] activation of the coagulation system;[12] abnormalities of calcium and phosphorus balance;[12] and tubulointerstitial injury.[14] Tubulointerstitial injury is an important factor in the progression of glomerular disease (Fig. 49–4). Much interest has been focused on the role of proteinuria in causing glomerular and tubulointerstitial damage. The degree of proteinuria not only is an index of the severity of glomerular diseases, but also provides a measure of the rate of progression of renal injury. Heavy proteinuria is an indicator of poor prognosis in various glomerular diseases.[15] Although there is no direct evidence to substantiate that proteinuria per se results in progression of renal impairment,[13,14] there are many possible mechanisms through which proteinuria directly or indirectly causes renal damage. Proximal tubular uptake and metabolism of albumin may lead to unregulated intracellular release of potentially toxic fatty acids, which may provoke secretion of a lipid macrophage chemotactic factor, resulting in interstitial inflammation.[15] Tubular hypermetabolism may lead to increased reactive oxygen species production and renal ammoniagenesis, resulting in complement activation and consequent tubular injury.[14] Proteinuria is also accompanied by an increased flux of macromolecules across the mesangium. The mesangial overload may then lead to structural damage. The passage of serum components, such as complement, across the GBM may have a pathophysiologic effect on the glomerular epithelial cells and alter the integrity of the glomerular filtration barrier.[13] The damaging effects of macromolecules other than albumin, such as immunoglobulins, lipoproteins, transferrin, and complement, remain to be characterized.[14]

CLINICAL PRESENTATION

Patients with glomerular disease may present with a nephritic or a nephrotic syndrome (Table 49–3). Nephritic syndrome reflects glomerular inflammation and frequently results in hematuria. White cells and cellular and granular casts are commonly found in the urine. In contrast, nephrotic syndrome reflects noninflammatory injury to the glomerular structures, and results in few cells or cellular casts in the urine. Initially, there may be limited or no reduction in renal excretory function.

Hematuria occurs when red blood cells leak through the openings of the GBM. The presence of red cell casts is highly indicative

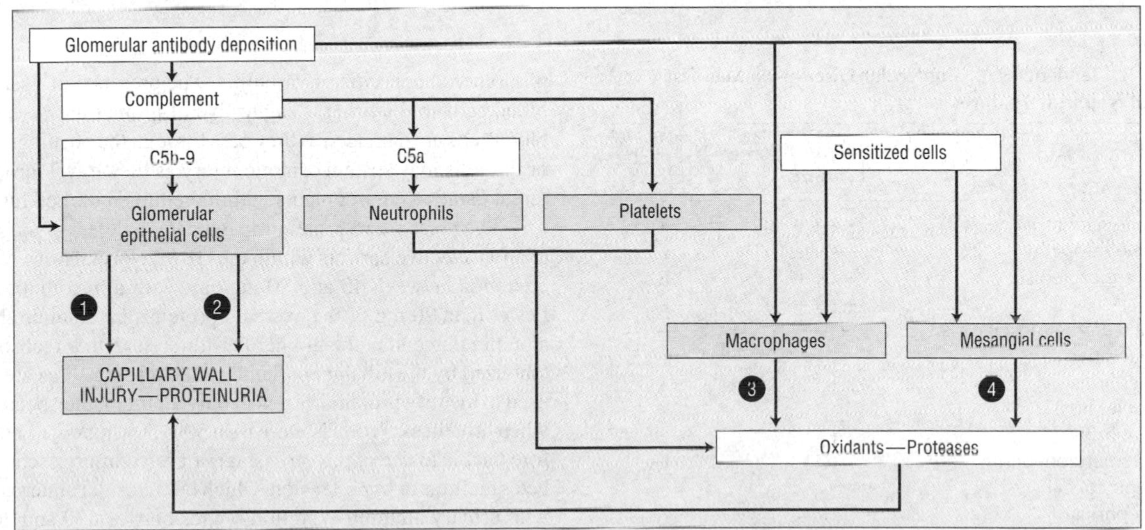

FIGURE 49–3. The major pathways of immune-mediated glomerular injury. Mechanisms 1 and 2 primarily act on the glomerular epithelial cell and result in noninflammatory lesions. Mechanisms 3 and 4 involve participation of effector cells and result in glomerular inflammation and structural damage. *(Adapted from Ref. 7.)*

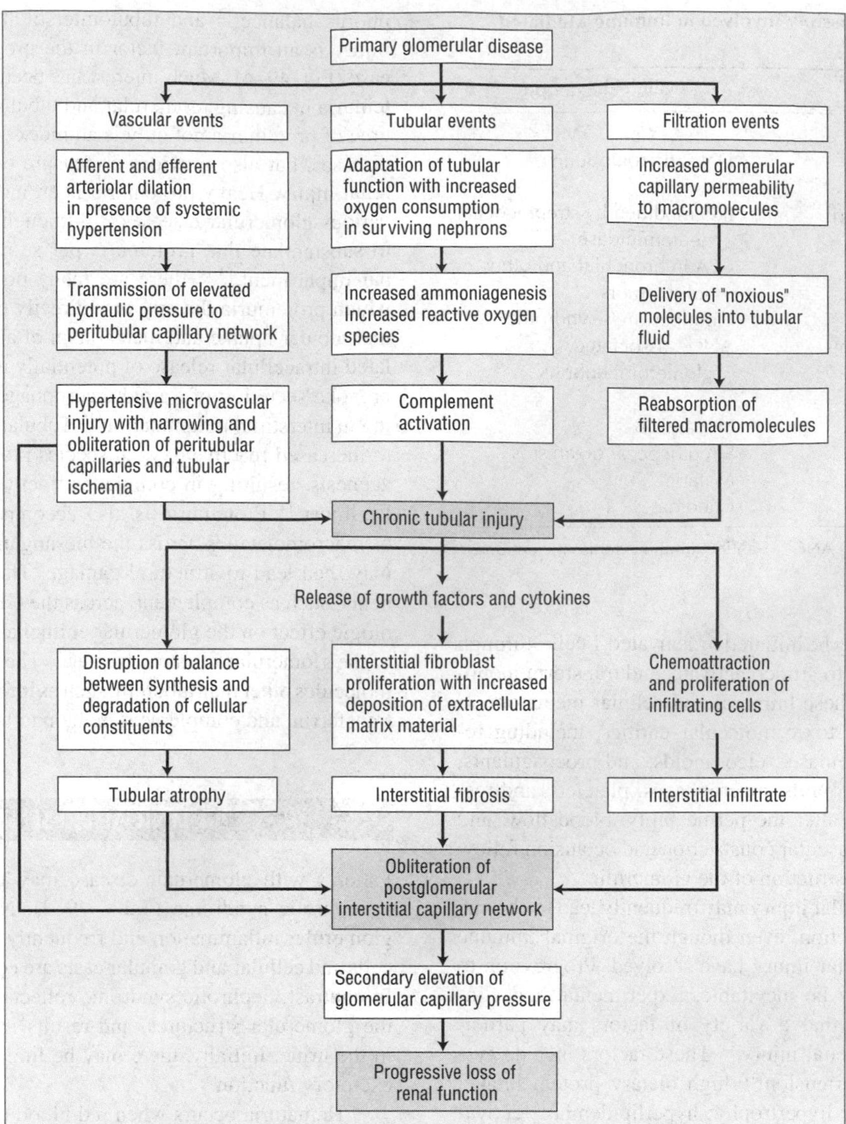

FIGURE 49–4. Proposed sequence of events leading from primary glomerular disease to progressive loss of renal function through tubulointerstitial injury. *(Modified from Ref. 14, with permission.)*

TABLE 49–3. Tendencies of Glomerular Diseases to Manifest Nephrotic and Nephritic Features

	Nephrotic Features	Nephritic Features
Minimal-change nephropathy	++++	−
Membranous nephropathy	++++	+
Diabetic glomerulosclerosis	++++	+
Amyloidosis	++++	+
Focal segmental glomerulosclerosis	+++	++
Mesangioproliferative glomerulonephritis	++	++
Membranoproliferative glomerulonephritis	++	+++
Proliferative glomerulonephritis	++	+++
Acute poststreptococcal glomerulonephritis	+	++++
Crescentic glomerulonephritis[a]	+	++++

[a]Can be immune complex–mediated, antiglomerular basement membrane antibody–mediated, or associated with antineutrophil cytoplasmic autoantibodies.

of glomerulonephritis or vasculitis. The presence of dysmorphic red blood cells in the urine is suggestive of glomerular disease. The red blood cells are damaged as they pass through the openings in the GBM or the cells may sustain osmotic injury as they travel through the different osmotic environments within the lumen of the kidney tubules.

The presence of proteinuria indicates a defect of the size- and/or charge-selective barriers within the GBM. Normal urinary protein excretion is between 40 and 80 mg/day, with a maximum of 150 mg. Fewer than 20 mg of the excreted proteins are albumin. Most of the albumin that enters the glomerular filtrate is either reabsorbed or catabolized by the tubular epithelium. The dipsticks that are commonly used to identify proteinuria detect only albumin; they become positive when protein excretion is more than 300–500 mg/day. They are therefore unable to detect the early stages of renal injury secondary to diabetes mellitus or hypertension, which often result in microalbuminuria with urinary albumin excretion ranges between 30 and 300 mg/day. Micral (Boehringer Mannheim Diagnostics), a simple immunoassay on a dipstick, permits specific and semiquantitative determination of urinary albumin concentrations at five levels: 0, 10, 20, 50, and

100 mg/L. It shows no cross-reactivity with other human proteins that may possibly be present in urine. The test may be used reliably for a urine specimen that has been stored for up to 7 days at 4°C (39.2°F) and even in the presence of bacterial contamination. Another qualitative test, Microbumintest (Ames), registers a positive reading when the urine albumin concentration is greater than 40 mg/L.[17]

Hypertension is a common feature in patients with glomerular diseases. Expansion of plasma volume as a result of renal salt retention is frequently the cause of hypertension, especially during acute disease. In contrast, increased activity of vasoconstrictors, such as angiotensin II, is often the cause in patients with chronic glomerular diseases.[18] Scarring of the glomerulus resulting in regional ischemia is thought to be responsible for the hypertension. Activation of the sympathetic nervous system and the release of vasoconstrictor substances may also contribute.

NEPHRITIC SYNDROME

Glomerular bleeding resulting in hematuria is a typical finding in nephritic syndrome. Dysmorphic red cells, especially acanthocytes, are a sensitive and specific marker of glomerular bleeding. The presence of pus and cellular and granular casts in the urine is common. The extent of proteinuria is variable, typically about 1–3 g/day, but it may be in the nephrotic range (>3 g/day). Patients with severe nephritic glomerular injury have renal function impairment because of the reduced glomerular surface area available for filtration. The latter is a result of constriction of the capillary lumen by proliferating mesangial cells or inflammatory cells. As renal function declines, hypertension and edema may develop or preexisting conditions may worsen.

NEPHROTIC SYNDROME

Nephrotic syndrome is characterized by proteinuria greater than 3.5 g/day/1.73 m^2, hypoproteinemia, edema, and hyperlipidemia. A hypercoagulable state may also be present in some patients. The syndrome may be the result of primary diseases of the glomerulus or associated with systemic diseases such as diabetes mellitus, lupus, amyloidosis, and preeclampsia. Hypoproteinemia, especially hypoalbuminemia, results from increased urinary loss of albumin and an increased rate of catabolism of filtered albumin by proximal tubular cells. The compensatory increase in hepatic synthesis of albumin is insufficient to replenish the protein loss, probably because of malnutrition.

Edema formation in patients with nephrotic syndrome was traditionally thought to be driven by the reduced plasma oncotic pressure secondary to hypoalbuminemia. If the oncotic pressure is low, the movement of fluid from the vascular space to the interstitial compartment results in a reduction of the plasma volume, which can trigger compensatory renal sodium and water retention through the activation of renin-angiotensin-aldosterone axis, vasopressin and the sympathetic nervous system (the "underfill" mechanism). However, experimental data suggest that the plasma volume is actually normal or elevated.[19] This may be because hypoalbuminemia does not cause edema until the serum albumin concentration is less than 2 g/dL. In addition, the transcapillary oncotic pressure gradient is not as high as previously thought because increased lymphatic flow reduces the interstitial oncotic pressure by removing protein and fluid from the interstitium thereby reducing the transcapillary oncotic pressure gradient.[20] Thus, fluid retention is likely mediated by a primary increase in sodium reabsorption at the distal nephron, which is probably caused by tubular resistance to the action of atrial natriuretic peptide (the "overflow" mechanism).[21] At present, the sensitivity of methods for plasma volume measurements in distinguishing underfill from overfill mechanisms is still questionable. It is likely that both mechanisms may contribute to nephrotic edema in different patients.[21]

Although albuminuria below the nephrotic range appears to have a minor influence on serum cholesterol in patients with primary glomerular disease, daily urinary albumin excretion of greater than 3 g is associated with a significant increase in serum cholesterol concentrations.[22] Hyperlipidemia in nephrotic syndrome is characterized by elevated serum total cholesterol and triglyceride concentrations, with increased very-low-density lipoprotein (VLDL) and low- density lipoprotein (LDL) cholesterol concentrations. Although high-density lipoprotein (HDL) cholesterol concentrations are normally distributed, there is a maldistribution of HDL subtypes, with a reduction in HDL_2 and an increase in HDL_3.[23,24] Furthermore, lipoprotein (a) levels may also be increased. Oval fat bodies and fatty casts are also found in the urine. The mechanisms for nephrotic hyperlipidemia are not well defined. A reduction in plasma oncotic pressure as a result of hypoalbuminemia may stimulate hepatic synthesis of lipids and lipoproteins. The increased VLDL production and increased liver cholesterol synthesis along with a decrease in LDL receptor activity can then lead to an increase in LDL cholesterol concentrations. In addition, reduced serum albumin or the loss of a liporegulatory substance may result in reduced VLDL clearance[23,24] Nephrotic patients with hyperlipidemia, especially those with concomitant hypertension, are presumed to have an increased risk for atherosclerotic vascular disease. Hyperlipidemia also promotes the progression of glomerular injury, as evidenced by glomerulosclerosis, mesangial expansion, and hyalinosis.[16,23]

Many patients with nephrotic syndrome have a hypercoagulable state caused by defects of several control proteins in the coagulation cascade. The concentration of the coagulation inhibitor antithrombin III is reduced because of increased loss in the urine.[25] A reduced amount of the coagulation inhibitors protein C and S, along with increased concentrations of factors V and VIII, increased fibrinogen concentrations, and abnormal platelet function, may also contribute to the hypercoagulable state.[25] The net result of these alterations in coagulation is an increased risk for arterial and venous thrombosis, especially in the deep veins and renal veins. As many as 25% of patients with membranous nephropathy may have renal vein thrombosis.

DIAGNOSIS

Patients with suspected glomerular disease should first be evaluated for a potential systemic cause. An extensive medical history should be obtained to identify symptoms of diabetes mellitus, amyloidosis, systemic lupus erythematosus (SLE), and other familial conditions associated with renal disease. Reduced appetite, fatigue, weight gain, and edema are all suggestive of nephrotic syndrome. Thorough medication, environmental, and occupation histories should be obtained to identify possible exposure to drugs, toxins, or chemicals that are known to be nephrotoxic. A carefully conducted physical examination may reveal signs and symptoms associated with systemic diseases, such as hypertension, rash, arthritis, retinopathy, neuropathy, lymphadenopathy, and hepatomegaly, as well as evidence of malignancy.

Examination of urine for active sediments, such as red blood cells, white blood cells, and casts, can differentiate the nephrotic and nephritic nature of the disease. The patient may present with normal urinalysis, isolated hematuria, or proteinuria, or significant abnormalities, such as nephrotic–range proteinuria, hematuria, pyuria, lipiduria, and the presence of different casts. Nephrotic sediment is

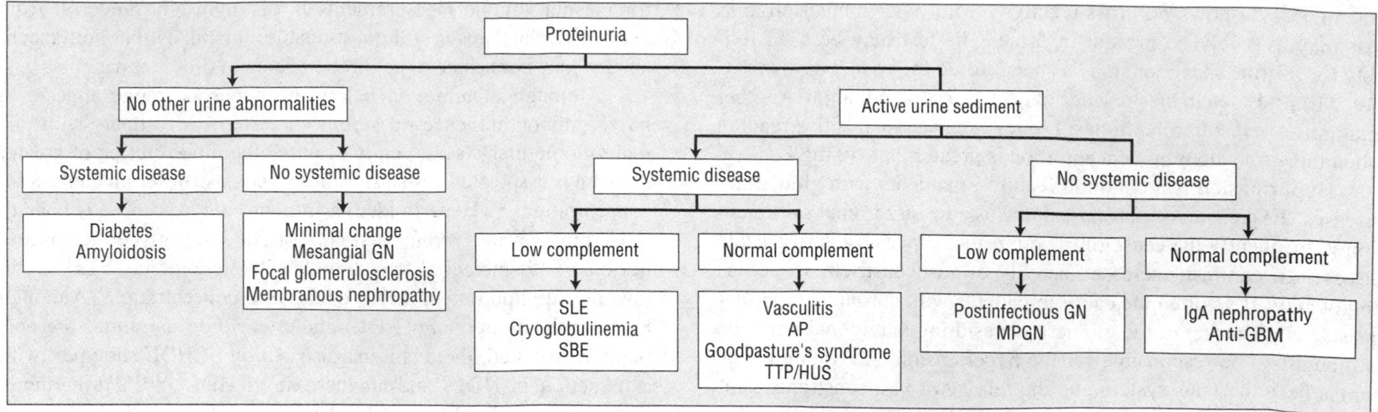

FIGURE 49–5. Clinical presentations of glomerulonephritis. AP = anaphylactoid purpura; GBM = glomerular basement membrane; GN = glomerulonephritis; HUS = hemolytic-uremic syndrome; MPGN = membranoproliferative glomerulonephritis; SBE = subacute bacterial endocarditis; SLE = systemic lupus erythematosus; TTP = thrombotic thrombocytopenic purpura.

characterized by heavy proteinuria (usually more than 3 g/d) and lipiduria. The patient's total urinary protein excretion can be quantified by a 24-hour urine collection or estimated by measuring the total protein:creatinine ratio in a random daytime urine specimen. This ratio correlates closely with the total urinary protein excretion. A ratio of 250 mg/dL:100 mg/dL represents 2.5 g of protein excreted a day per 1.73 m^2 of body surface area.[26] In contrast, nephritic sediment includes hematuria, pyuria, cellular and granular casts, and variable degrees of proteinuria. When glomerular diseases progress to advanced renal insufficiency and result in a significant reduction in the glomerular filtration rate (GFR), urinalysis may show less proteinuria and hematuria. In patients with chronic glomerular disease, broad waxy casts may be present in the urinary sediment.

GFR in patients with glomerular disease may be variable. In the early stages of the disease, the GFR may remain normal. Initial injury to the glomerulus primarily lowers the permeability coefficient (K_f) of the GBM, by reducing the surface area available for filtration and/or the unit permeability of the membrane. The reduced permeability is compensated by an elevation in the glomerular capillary hydrostatic pressure through afferent arteriolar dilation and efferent arteriolar constriction. Extensive glomerular damage may therefore be present before a substantial reduction of total GFR is evident.

Patients who present with glomerulonephritis may be categorized according to the presence or absence of evidence for systemic disease (Fig. 49–5). Determination of the serum complement concentration is frequently helpful in defining the specific type of glomerular disease (Table 49–4). Measurement of antinuclear and anti-DNA antibodies, antistreptolysin antibodies, circulating anti-GBM antibodies, and cryoglobulins is useful in identifying the etiology.

TABLE 49–4. Categorization of Renal Diseases Based on Serum Complement Levels

Low Serum Complement Level	Normal Serum Complement Level
Systemic Diseases	**Systemic Diseases**
Systemic lupus erythematosus	Vasculitis group
Infection-related glomerulonephritis	Polyarteritis nodosa
	Hypersensitivity vasculitis
Subacute bacterial endocarditis	Wegener's granulomatosis
"Shunt" nephritis	Henoch–Schönlein purpura
Cryoglobulinemia	Goodpasture's syndrome
Primary Renal Diseases	**Primary Renal Diseases**
Acute poststreptococcal glomerulonephritis	IgA nephropathy
	Idiopathic rapidly progressive glomerulonephritis
Membranoproliferative glomerulonephritis	Idiopathic nephrotic syndrome

The patient's age is often helpful in pinpointing the specific type of glomerular disease. Many of the conditions are more prevalent in certain age groups, although they may occur at any age. Benign hematuria, for example, is primarily a disease of children. Lupus and idiopathic membranoproliferative glomerulonephritis (MPGN) are seen primarily in 15- to 40-year-old patients, and primary amyloidosis affects adults over the age of 40. Figure 49–6 indicates the distribution of the different causes of nephrotic-range proteinuria relative to the age of patients undergoing renal biopsy.

Although the cause of proteinuria and glomerular disease may be established from clinical and laboratory evaluation, more often uncertainty persists. Specific treatment of the glomerular disease depends on the underlying pathology. Percutaneous renal biopsy is, therefore,

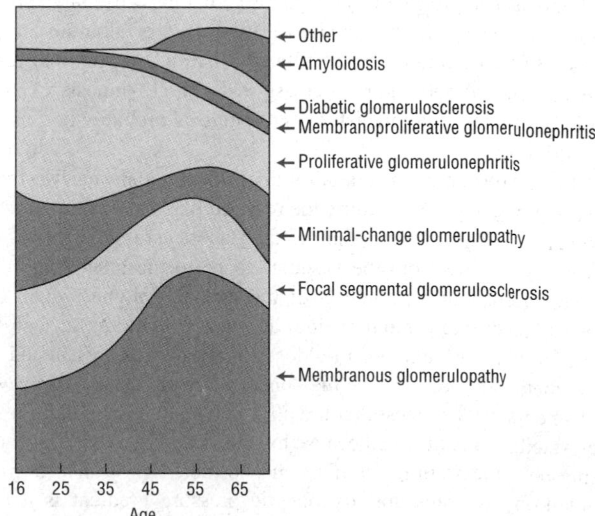

FIGURE 49–6. Frequency of various causes for nephrotic-range proteninuria (>3 g/day) relative to age in patients undergoing renal biopsy evaluation at the University of North Carolina Nephropathology Laboratory. The full vertical height of the bar represents 100% of the patients. The patients with proliferative glomerulonephritis generally presented with nephritic features in addition to the proteinuria and included patients with lupus nephritis, IgA nephropathy, and postinfectious glomerulonephritis. *(From Ref. 53, with permission.)*

often needed to provide a definitive diagnosis. One notable exception is minimal-change disease (lipoid nephrosis), which is the most common etiology for nephrotic syndrome in children between 1 and 6 years of age. An empiric trial of corticosteroids is indicated for these patients without the need for histologic diagnosis. Biopsy is indicated only for those who fail to respond to a therapeutic course of corticosteroids.

The decision to perform a biopsy should be based on an evaluation of the potential risks of the procedure against the anticipated benefits of knowing the underlying pathology as the basis for rational therapy. The most common complication of biopsy is bleeding, which may present as hematuria or perinephric hematoma. About 10% of the patients have gross hematuria, which usually resolves in several days. However, blood transfusion may be needed in up to 1.0% of patients and nephrectomy or therapeutic embolic infarction may be necessary in 0.1% of the patients because of severe bleeding. Mortality from renal biopsy is probably less than 0.1%. Biopsy is contraindicated in patients with a solitary kidney, polycystic kidney disease, uncontrolled hypertension, coagulation defects, or poor cooperation. Morphologic diagnosis can usually be made if tissue is examined with light, immunofluorescence, and electron microscopic techniques.

▶ TREATMENT: Glomerulonephritis

GENERAL APPROACH TO TREATMENT

The management of patients with glomerulonephritis involves specific pharmacologic therapy for the glomerular disease, and supportive measures to prevent and/or treat the pathophysiologic sequelae, namely, hypertension, edema, and progression of renal disease. In patients with nephrotic syndrome, supportive therapy should also address the management of extrarenal complications of heavy proteinuria, namely, hypoalbuminemia, hyperlipidemia, and thromboembolism.

Immunosuppressive agents, alone or in combination, may be used to alter the different immune processes that are responsible for the glomerulonephritides. Corticosteroids, in addition to their immunosuppressive effect, also possess anti-inflammatory activities. They reduce the production and/or release of many substances that mediate the inflammatory process, such as prostaglandins, leukotrienes, platelet-activating factors, tumor necrosis factors (TNFs), and interleukin-1 (IL-1). Movement of leukocytes and macrophages to the site of inflammation is also inhibited. The immunosuppressive effects of corticosteroids are mediated through the inhibition of the release of IL-1 and TNF by activated macrophages, and IL-2 by activated T cells. In addition, the actions of migration-inhibitory factor and γ-interferon are inhibited. Processing of antigens is thus affected by the presence of corticosteroids. Cytotoxic agents, such as cyclophosphamide, chlorambucil, or azathioprine, may be used occasionally to treat glomerular diseases. Cyclosporine is also used to treat certain glomerulonephritis. It can reduce lymphokine production by activated T lymphocytes and it can decrease proteinuria by improving the permselectivity of the GBM.

Because many immune factors are implicated in the pathogenesis of glomerulonephritis, plasmapheresis may be used to remove these mediators. Platelets are activated in glomerular disease and platelet factors can cause arteriolar smooth-muscle cell proliferation and alter vascular permeability. Antiplatelet agents are therefore used in some patients. Nonsteroidal anti-inflammatory agents (NSAIDs) are often used to reduce proteinuria because of their antiplatelet effect and their ability to alter capillary wall permeability. They may also affect arachidonic acid metabolism; however, the specific mechanisms of these beneficial effects remain to be established.

SUPPORTIVE THERAPY

In patients with nephrotic syndrome, dietary measures involve restriction of sodium intake to 50–100 mEq/day,[20,27] protein intake of 0.8–1.0 g/day,[27,28] and a low-lipid diet of less than 200 mg cholesterol. Total fat should account for less than 30% of daily total calories.[27] Sodium restriction is important not only in the control of edema, but also in the control of hypertension and proteinuria. Similarly, protein restriction not only helps to reduce proteinuria, but also has a potential role in retarding the progression of renal disease. Patients should also stop smoking because a dose-dependent increase in risk for developing ESRD was observed in men with primary inflammatory (IgA glomerulonephritis) or non-inflammatory (polycystic kidney disease) renal diseases.[29]

EDEMA

Management of nephrotic edema involves salt restriction, bedrest, and use of support stockings and diuretics. However, severe salt restriction is difficult to achieve in patients who are sodium-avid and prolonged bedrest could predispose nephrotic patients to thromboembolism. Hence, use of a loop diuretic, such as furosemide, is frequently required. Although the delivery of diuretic to the kidney tubules is normal, the presence of large amounts of protein in the urine promotes drug binding and thereby reduces the availability of the diuretic to the luminal receptor sites. In addition, reduced sodium delivery to the distal tubule secondary to decreased glomerular perfusion may also alter diuretic effectiveness. Large doses of the loop diuretic, such as 160–480 mg of furosemide, may be needed for patients with moderate edema (see Chap. 51). In some patients, a thiazide diuretic or metolazone, may be added to enhance natriuresis.[27,30] Alternatively, continuous intravenous infusion of a loop diuretic, such as furosemide 160–480 mg/day, may be employed and is more effective than intermittent bolus injections in inducing urinary sodium excretion.[31] In patients with morbid edema, albumin infusion may be used to expand plasma volume and to increase diuretic delivery to the renal tubules, thus enhancing diuretic effect. However, it may precipitate congestive heart failure and may also reduce therapeutic response to steroid in minimal change nephropathy. In patients with significant edema, the goal of treatment should be a daily loss of 1–2 lb of fluid until a reasonable weight has been obtained.

HYPERTENSION

Optimal control of hypertension in patients with glomerular disease is important in reducing both the progression of renal disease and the risk for cardiovascular disease[28,32] (see Chaps. 12 and 44). The target blood pressure is suggested to be 130/80–85 mm Hg. In patients with chronic renal insufficiency (GFR of 15–55 mL/min) and proteinuria greater than 1 g/day, the mean arterial pressure should be reduced further to no more than 92 mm Hg, which is equivalent to 125/75 mm Hg or less.[32,33] For patients with chronic renal insufficiency and proteinuria of 0.25–1.0 g/day, the mean arterial pressure should be less than 98 mm Hg, which is equivalent to 130/80 mm Hg.[33] However, aggressive blood pressure reduction may increase the risk for stroke and myocardial infarction in susceptible patients.

Thiazide or loop diuretics with salt restriction are often used for initial blood pressure control. Angiotensin-converting enzyme (ACE) inhibitors or angiotensin II receptor blockers (ARBs) may be added if blood pressure control is not adequate. The ACE inhibitors and the ARBs reduce renal protein excretion, have renoprotective effects, and are well tolerated and effective.[33,34] Alternatively, nondihydropyridine calcium channel blockers (e.g., diltiazem) may have proteinuria-reduction properties and could be used as an additional agent. The dihydropyridine calcium channel blockers (e.g., nifedipine, amlodipine, nisoldipine) can also be used to lower blood pressure but without the benefit of urinary protein reduction.[35]

PROTEINURIA

Dietary protein restriction reduces proteinuria and may retard renal function deterioration. The intent to treat analysis of the Modification of Diet in Renal Disease (MDRD) study in patients with moderate renal insufficiency (GFR of 25–55 mL/min/1.73 m^2), did not show that a low-protein diet was able to slow renal disease progression. However, the secondary analysis revealed that protein intake of 0.66 g/kg/day reduced the rate of GFR deterioration in patients with severe renal insufficiency, GFR of 13–24 mL/min/1.73 m^2.[36] In view of the lack of definitive proof about the benefit of protein restriction on disease progression, a standard protein diet—greater than 0.8 g/kg/day—is recommended for patients with moderate renal insufficiency. However, the patients should be made aware of the potential benefits of reducing protein intake to 0.6 g/kg/day. Decreasing dietary protein will also reduce the intake of phosphorus and potassium. In many instances, the potential benefits of protein restriction have to be balanced against the need for protein intake to overcome nutritional deficiencies. For nondialyzed patients who have GFRs of less than 25 mL/min/1.73 m^2, dietary protein intake should be reduced to 0.6 g/kg/day because it can retard the rate of renal function loss and also the time to reach end-stage renal disease.[28,33]

Because heavy proteinuria is the underlying cause for hypoalbuminemia and other complications of nephrotic syndrome, various strategies—including protein restriction to 0.8–1.0 g/kg/day, plus an additional gram of protein for each gram of protein lost in the urine,[28] ACE inhibitors,[37,38] and NSAIDs[39]—are used to reduce proteinuria (see Chap. 44). Although blood pressure reduction decreases proteinuria, the reduction of proteinuria by ACE inhibitors exceeds what can be expected by their antihypertensive effect.[35,37] An additive antiproteinuric effect has been shown by combining a low-protein diet with ACE inhibition,[38] as well as combined therapy with ACE inhibitors and NSAIDs.[40] Serum albumin concentrations were also improved during treatment.[37,38] ACE inhibition may also allow the use of a high-protein diet without risks of decreased albumin synthesis.[41] Although a reduction in proteinuria is usually apparent within the first few weeks of therapy, the maximal effect is attained after 8 to 12 weeks.[42] The initial antiproteinuric effect of ACE inhibitors is associated with a fall in filtration fraction, suggesting a reduction in intraglomerular pressure. However, an improvement of GBM permselectivity may be responsible for the long-term effect of ACE inhibitors.[42]

NSAIDs probably reduce proteinuria through an alteration of intrarenal hemodynamics, a decrease in GFR, and also restoration of the barrier size-selectivity of the GBM.[27,42] Indomethacin and meclofenamate are the two NSAIDs that have been evaluated the most. Their antiproteinuric effect occurs within 1 to 2 weeks of the initiation of therapy.[27,43] NSAID therapy is indicated for patients with severe steroid-resistant nephrotic syndrome who have greater than 50% residual renal function.[43] The agents should be avoided in those with poor renal function because of their potential detrimental effect on kidney function and also the increased susceptibility of these patients to nephrotoxicity.[27,43] Long-term treatment is indicated for those who have greater than 40% reduction in urinary protein excretion and/or those whose serum albumin concentrations are doubled during therapy.[43] In conjunction with dietary sodium restriction, the antiproteinuric efficacy of protein restriction, ACE inhibition, and NSAIDs is enhanced.[42]

HYPERLIPIDEMIA

Abnormal lipoprotein profile increases the risk of atherosclerosis and coronary heart disease in patients with nephrotic syndrome.[44] It is therefore prudent to treat patients with persistent nephrotic syndrome and sustained dyslipidemia, especially those with high VLDL and LDL cholesterol levels in the presence of a normal or low HDL cholesterol level. Therapy is especially needed for those with concurrent atherosclerotic cardiovascular disease, or with additional risk factors for atherosclerosis, such as smoking and hypertension.[23] Whether correction of lipoprotein abnormalities will slow the progression of renal disease as demonstrated in animal studies requires clinical confirmation.[23,33]

A low-fat diet is usually not sufficient to correct hyperlipoproteinemia.[16,27,45] Lipid-lowering agents are usually required. Probucol, bile acid resins, fibric acid derivatives, and hydroxymethylglutaryl coenzyme A (HMG-CoA) reductase inhibitors have been evaluated in patients with nephrotic syndrome.[23] HMG-CoA reductase inhibitors, also known as the statins such as lovastatin, pravastatin, simvastatin, and fluvastatin, are considered the treatment of choice.[16,23,27] These agents inhibit the rate-limiting step in cholesterol biosynthesis, namely, the conversion of HMG-CoA to mevalonate. In short-term studies, they reduce total plasma cholesterol concentration by 22% to 36%, LDL cholesterol by 27% to 45%, and total plasma triglyceride concentration by 19% to 40%.[23] The increase in HDL cholesterol and/or decrease in atherogenic lipoprotein (a) is variable.[42,46,47] Meta-analysis showed that use of HMG-CoA reductase inhibitors resulted in the greatest and most consistent decrease in LDL cholesterol levels.[45] Recent experimental data reveal that the statins may modulate intracellular signaling systems that involve in cell proliferation, inflammation and fibrogenic responses. These findings suggest that the statins may also have beneficial effects on the progression of renal disease.[48]

When ACE inhibitors are used to reduce proteinuria, it is common to see an accompanying decrease in total plasma cholesterol and the lipoprotein (a) level.[36,49] Combined use of an ACE inhibitor with an HMG-CoA reductase inhibitor may therefore be more effective in controlling nephrotic hyperlipidemia. In all the patients, consistent use of a prudent diet, modest exercise, cessation of smoking, and adequate blood pressure control should be the cornerstone of hyperlipidemia management. They may offer as much or more benefit than the lowering of cholesterol levels by pharmacologic means.

ANTICOAGULATION

Intravascular thrombosis is a serious and common complication of nephrotic syndrome, particularly in membranous nephropathy. Patients are at risk for developing renal vein thrombosis, pulmonary emboli, or other thromboembolic events. Although it is generally agreed that patients who have documented thromboembolic episodes should be anticoagulated with warfarin until remission of nephrotic syndrome, the use of prophylactic anticoagulation is controversial. A decision analysis study suggested that prophylactic anticoagulation is beneficial in patients with membranous nephropathy.[50] However, prospective controlled studies should be conducted to confirm these findings. Anticoagulation should also be considered in patients with increased risks for thrombosis, such as prolonged bedrest, surgery, episodes of dehydration, or use of high-dose intravenous steroids.[27] As an example, low-dose, subcutaneous heparin may be given prophylactically for a limited duration in patients with severe nephrotic syndrome who are placed on bedrest. For patients with a history of thromboembolic episode, warfarin should be given, after an initial course of standard or low-molecular-weight heparin, for as long as heavy proteinuria and hypoalbuminemia are present. The role of low-molecular-weight heparin in preventing thromboembolism is uncertain, but preliminary results are encouraging.[51]

DISEASE PROGRESSION AND TREATMENT CONSIDERATIONS

The course and prognosis of the different glomerular diseases are extremely variable and depend on the underlying etiology. In glomerular diseases with a secondary cause, such as poststreptococcal glomerulonephritis, after the initiating factor is removed, the prognosis of the renal disease is often good. In contrast, the rates of renal function deterioration among the primary glomerulonephritides vary according to the form of glomerulonephritis. Most patients with minimal-change disease, IgA nephropathy, and membranous nephropathy have a fairly good prognosis. However, those with focal segmental glomerulosclerosis who are resistant to therapy, as well as those with rapidly progressive glomerulonephritis who are untreated, are likely to experience rapid loss of renal function. In some instances, half of the renal function may be lost within a 3-month period. Certain glomerulonephritides, such as minimal-change nephropathy, are very responsive to treatment. In contrast, for some other types of glomerulonephritis, such as membranous proliferative glomerulonephritis, consistently effective therapy is yet to be found.

Because of the variable courses exhibited by the different glomerulonephritides, specific treatment approaches have been developed for each disease. The natural history of the glomerulonephritis has to be well delineated before a promising regimen can be evaluated, from both therapeutic and economic perspectives. Otherwise, patients will be exposed to unnecessary treatment-related toxicities if they have a type of glomerulonephritis that is likely to undergo spontaneous remission. Many of the drugs that are used to treat glomerular diseases are potentially toxic. The many adverse effects associated with steroids are well known, and cytotoxic agents have potentially serious toxicities. Long-term use of cyclosporine may compromise renal function and nullify the renoprotection derived from treatment. The potential therapeutic benefits of treatment regimens should always be weighed against the risks to which the patients are being exposed. It is therefore imperative to identify patients who are most likely to benefit from treatment, especially those who have other risk factors that may contribute to the deterioration of their renal function. In those instances in which satisfactory regimens are not available to treat the primary disease, appropriate supportive measures should be employed. Optimization of systemic and glomerular pressure, reducing proteinuria, and possibly controlling hyperlipidemia may all improve the long-term outcome as well as the quality of life of these patients.

TREATMENT MONITORING

Patients should be monitored closely for therapeutic response as well as the development of treatment-related toxicities. While the rate of renal function deterioration is an important indicator of the long-term success of treatment, resolution of nephrotic and nephritic signs and symptoms associated with the glomerulopathies are important short-term therapeutic targets.

Serum creatinine concentration as well as creatinine clearance ought to be evaluated prior to and during treatment; 24-hour urine outflow should be collected to determine the extent of proteinuria. Alternatively, the daily urine protein excretion may be estimated by the urinary total protein:creatinine concentration ratio. After establishing the correlation between the 24-hour urinary protein excretion with the protein:creatinine ratio, single random urine specimens may be used in place of a 24-hour urine collection. Blood pressure should be monitored periodically to assess the need for and also the adequacy of antihypertensive therapy. The pressures should also be evaluated in conjunction with clinical signs and symptoms of edema and fluid overload to gauge the need for volume control as well as diuretic use. For patients with nephrotic syndrome, serum lipid concentrations should be monitored. If the patient has hematuria, urinalysis and complete blood count ought to be obtained. The clinician should also be aware of the patient's appetite and energy level because these are indicators of the patient's overall state of well-being. At times, renal biopsy is needed to assess response to treatment and disease progression, to determine future treatment strategy, and to confirm the initial diagnosis.

Patients receiving cytotoxic drug treatment ought to be evaluated for drug-related toxicities every week during the initial treatment period. After 1 month of treatment, the frequency of monitoring may be reduced. When the patient is on long-term steroid treatment, monthly visits are often required for assessment of both efficacy and toxicities. If a favorable response is obtained after a course of treatment, the patient may be evaluated every 3 to 4 months. The patient's renal function, proteinuria, urinalysis, blood pressure, lipid profile, and the overall state of health should be assessed during these regular follow-up visits.

OUTCOME AND ECONOMIC EVALUATION

Prospective, randomized, controlled comparative trials need to be conducted in a sizable patient population before the efficacy and economic implications of a new regimen can be established. This type of large-scale study is potentially feasible for the more common forms of glomerulonephritis such as minimal-change disease, IgA nephropathy, and membranous nephropathy. In contrast, prospective, controlled trials are difficult to conduct for the relatively uncommon glomerulonephritides such as membranous proliferative glomerulonephritis. After defining the natural history and the optimal drug regimen for each glomerulonephritis, in conjunction with the incidence of drug-induced complications, the economic implication of the individual treatment approach can be assessed. However, the optimal approaches for treating most types of glomerulonephritis have not been identified and the economic implications of the individual treatment regimens are yet to be established.

PATHOPHYSIOLOGY AND PHARMACOTHERAPY OF INDIVIDUAL GLOMERULOPATHIES

MINIMAL-CHANGE NEPHROPATHY

Minimal-change nephropathy (also termed minimal-change disease) is commonly found in children between 3 months and 6 years of age. It is one of the most common chronic diseases in childhood. In children between 1 and 4 years of age, minimal-change disease accounts for more than 90% of all cases of nephrotic syndrome. The percentage drops gradually to less than 50% after age 10 years, and only accounts for 10% to 15% of all cases of idiopathic nephrotic syndrome in adults. Secondary causes of minimal-change nephropathy caused by NSAIDs, lymphoproliferative disorders, and the like, are rare. They are responsible for up to 13% of all cases of minimal-change nephropathy in adults.

PATHOPHYSIOLOGY

Minimal-change disease is also known as "*nil*" disease primarily because of the absence of definitive pathologic changes observed under light and immunofluorescence microscopy. The characteristic lesion in patients with minimal-change disease, as visualized under electron microscopy, is the spreading and fusion of the foot processes of epithelial cells over an unchanged GBM. *Lipoid nephrosis* is another term that has been used to describe this type of glomerular disease because lipids, as well as renal tubular cells, are found in the urine. The pathogenesis of minimal-change disease is still unknown. Altered cell-mediated immunologic response, specifically T-cell dysfunction, is suspected to be responsible. The activated lymphocytes are thought to secrete lymphokines that reduce the production of anions in the GBM. The permeability of the GBM to plasma albumin is therefore increased through a reduction of electrostatic repulsion. The loss of anionic charges also results in fusion of the foot processes of the epithelial cells. Other conditions that involve T-cell abnormalities, such as Hodgkin's disease, T-cell lymphoma, and nephritis induced by NSAIDs, are also associated with minimal-change disease.

CLINICAL PRESENTATION

Most patients present initially with edema, frequently acute in onset, following a nonspecific upper respiratory tract infection, allergic reaction, or vaccinations, which might have activated the T lymphocytes. Nephrotic syndrome with massive proteinuria (substantially more than 40 mg/m^2/h for children and 3 g/day for adults), edema, hypoalbuminemia, and hyperlipidemia is common. The patient's weight may be increased dramatically because of sodium and fluid retention. Nephrotic features, such as gross hematuria, are uncommon. However, microscopic hematuria may be seen in up to 20% to 25% of patients. Hypertension and decreased renal function are uncommon in children but are more common in older adults.[52] In some patients, volume depletion may result in mild to moderate azotemia.

▶ TREATMENT: Minimal-Change Nephropathy

PHARMACOLOGIC THERAPY

STEROIDS

Minimal-change disease is the most responsive to initial treatment with corticosteroids. In children, steroid therapy is expected to reduce proteinuria in about 90% of the patients. The 10-year renal survival is greater than 95%.[53] Because of the excellent response to initial therapy with steroids and the prevalence of this glomerular disease in children, reduction of proteinuria secondary to steroid treatment is considered diagnostic for minimal-change disease without the need for biopsy. In the International Study of Kidney Disease in Children (ISKDC), remission was induced, as evidenced by diuresis, loss of edema, and resolution of proteinuria, within 8 weeks of therapy in more than 93% of the 363 children.[54] Prednisone was administered at a dose of 60 mg/m^2/day, with a maximum of 80–100 mg daily, in divided doses during the first 4 weeks. The dose was then reduced to 40 mg/m^2/day, or a maximum of 60 mg daily, in divided doses for 3 consecutive days every 7 days for another 4 weeks. An alternate-day dosage regimen can be used instead in the second 4 weeks, after which the prednisone dosage is tapered over several months (Fig. 49–7).[53,55] Single daily doses of prednisone, instead of multiple daily doses, may result in faster and more sustained response with less-frequent and less-severe side effects.[53] Proteinuria will disappear in 50% of patients after 1 week and in 90% of patients after 4 weeks of treatment. Studies conducted to evaluate the effectiveness of longer and shorter courses of steroid therapy for initial treatment, as well as recurrences,[55] showed that longer therapy (6 weeks of daily prednisone followed by 6 weeks of alternate-day treatment) results in lower incidence of relapse (36%) than both standard-course (4 weeks; 61%) and short-course (3 weeks; 81%) therapy. However, the cumulative doses of steroid received for the initial treatment and subsequent relapses during the entire follow-up period were not different between the long and standard courses. As a result, many centers now use the long course therapy during the initial episode and short-course treatment for relapses.[56]

For adults, the dose of prednisone is 1 mg/kg/day during the initial 4 weeks with a reduction to 0.75 mg/kg/day every other day for the next 4 weeks. Proteinuria will disappear in 50% to 60% of patients after 8 weeks of treatment, and complete remission will be attained in 80% of patients after 28 weeks of therapy.[52] In some patients, 16 weeks of therapy may be needed before remission is induced.[52,54] Use of lower doses of steroids may increase relapse rate and alternate-day high dose steroid therapy may reduce the rate of total remission.

Relapse

As many as 75% to 85% of the patients who respond to initial steroid therapy (steroid sensitive) will experience a relapse of proteinuria, mostly within 6 to 12 months after disease onset. However, some patients may not have the first relapse until 24 to 30 months later.[57] The risk of relapse is affected by the duration of initial steroid therapy.[27,55] Children who were asymptomatic with proteinuria diagnosed on a urinary screening program tend to have less frequent relapses and a more favorable clinical course.[58] In those who relapse, 50% to 65% may have steroid-responsive relapse episodes over the subsequent

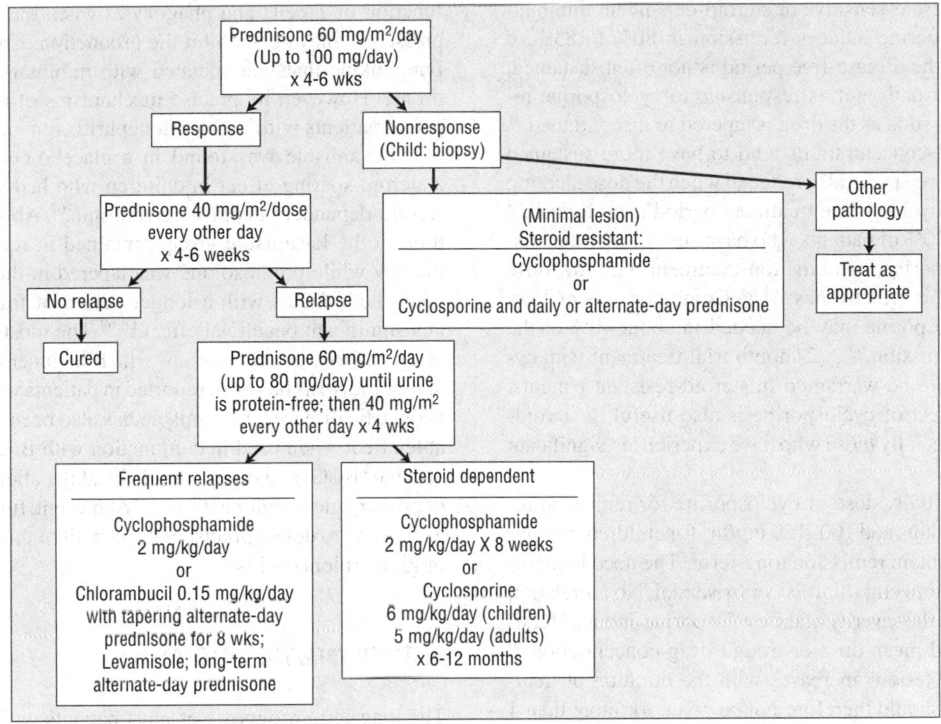

FIGURE 49–7. Treatment algorithm for minimal-change nephropathy. *(Modified from Ref. 55.)*

3- to 5-year period.[57] The dose and duration of steroid treatment for the relapse do not influence the subsequent rate of relapse.[27,55] The current regimen for relapse consists of 60 mg/m^2/day, up to 80 mg/day of prednisone until the urine is free of protein for 3 days. Four weeks of alternate day prednisone at 40 mg/m^2/dose will then be used.[55] Giving the initial daily doses of prednisone for 4 weeks instead of until the urine is clear of protein may induce a more prolonged remission, however, the cumulative dose of prednisone will be doubled. Because most patients will relapse soon, it is preferred to treat until the urine is free of protein for 3 days and then proceed with the tapering regimen as described earlier.[55]

Frequent Relapse

About 10% to 20% of children experience 3 or 4 relapses that are responsive to steroid. However, half of these patients will relapse frequently and become steroid dependent, requiring continuous low-dose alternate-day prednisone to maintain an extended relapse-free period.[55] A small number of patients eventually develop resistance to steroids and a biopsy done at that time often reveals another pathology such as focal segmental glomerular sclerosis. It is controversial whether minimal-change disease progresses into focal segmental glomerular sclerosis or whether the glomerulosclerosis that was present at the time of initial diagnosis was inadvertently diagnosed as minimal-change nephropathy because of tissue-sampling error during the renal biopsy.

For patients who are steroid resistant, as well as for those patients who require large doses of steroids to sustain remission (steroid dependent), alternative therapy should be considered. Furthermore, in pediatric patients, the growth inhibition associated with long-term steroid use often necessitates the use of alternative agents. Cyclophosphamide at 2.0 mg/kg/day for 12 weeks given alone or with prednisone (50–75 mg/m^2) is very effective in inducing remission and restoring steroid responsiveness in patients who were previously steroid dependent and then became steroid resistant. Alternatively, chlorambucil at 0.1–0.2 mg/kg/day may be used. This agent, however, is associated with more adverse effects than cyclophosphamide. Azathioprine has also been used; however, treatment for 6 to 12 months is often needed before any favorable response is apparent.[59] Because of the risk for adverse reactions, use of these cytotoxic agents should be reserved for patients who are clearly steroid resistant, or who are steroid dependent (two consecutive relapses during therapy or relapse within 14 days after dosage reduction or termination of steroid treatment) with significant adverse effects; or for those patients who have two or more relapses within 6 months after the first episode, or who had three or more relapses within 12 months.[27]

The immunosuppressive effect of cytotoxic agents, with or without the concurrent use of steroids, can result in serious infections, which are the primary cause of death in patients with minimal-change nephropathy.[60] Other toxicities associated with cyclophosphamide include gonadal fibrosis, which results in sterility, hemorrhagic cystitis, alopecia, and a potential to develop malignancy in those on long-term treatment. Patients on chronic steroid therapy often develop growth retardation, osteoporosis, obesity, and cataracts.[55]

CYCLOSPORINE

Cyclosporine has been used in adult and pediatric patients. The drug decreases lymphokine production by activated T lymphocytes and thereby reduces proteinuria by reversing the lymphokine-induced alterations in the anionic charge and permeability of the GBM to albumin. Cyclosporine can also reduce proteinuria by improving the permselectivity of the GBM.

In patients with steroid-sensitive or steroid-dependent minimal-change disease, cyclosporine induces remission in 80% to 85% of the patients. However, the disease-free period is not often sustained, and relapse, which is usually not as responsive to cyclosporine retreatment, may occur as soon as the drug is tapered or discontinued.[61] Patients with high IL-2 concentrations tend to have more sustained remission.[62] The rate of relapse is also reduced when the dose tapering is gradual or when the cyclosporine treatment period is prolonged.[63] Although only 10% to 20% of patients who have steroid-resistant disease respond to cyclosporine, combination treatment with low-dose steroid may increase the effectiveness.[61,64] Combined use of low-dose steroid with cyclosporine may be needed in about 40% of the patients to maintain remission.[65] A 2-month trial treatment with cyclosporine may therefore be warranted in steroid-resistant patients. The steroid-sparing effect of cyclosporine is also useful in steroid-dependent patients, especially those who have experienced significant adverse effects.

The usual starting daily dose of cyclosporine for remission induction is 5 mg/kg for adults and 100–150 mg/m^2 for children. Similar dosages are used to maintain remission long-term. The need to monitor cyclosporine blood concentrations is controversial. No correlation has been found between the severity of the cyclosporine-induced tubulointerstitial lesions and mean dose or trough drug concentration.[60] The incidence of these lesions increases with the duration of treatment and cyclosporine should therefore not be given for more than 4 months in the absence of any beneficial effect.[61] However, a recent retrospective study reported that use of cyclosporine for up to 7.5 years resulted in pathologic changes in kidney biopsy specimens in only a small number of patients but without deterioration in renal function.[66] Other nonrenal adverse effects associated with cyclosporine treatment are hypertrichosis, gingival hyperplasia, gastrointestinal symptoms, and hypertension.

Currently, cyclosporine is indicated for patients (a) who relapse frequently or are steroid dependent, after failing to respond to a course of cyclophosphamide; (b) for whom cyclophosphamide is contraindicated or when gonadal toxicity is a concern; (c) who are steroid dependent when a "steroid holiday" is needed for catch-up growth and puberty; or (d) who have steroid-resistant disease.[55]

LEVAMISOLE

Levamisole, an immunostimulant, has been evaluated for the treatment of patients with steroid-dependent nephrotic syndrome. The agent can promote the maturation of young T cells and restore the function of T cells and phagocytes when the immune system is depressed. It may also inhibit the production of an immunosuppressive lymphokine that is associated with minimal-change nephrotic syndrome. However, its precise mechanisms of action in immunocompetent patients with glomerulonephritis remain to be identified.

Levamisole was found in a placebo-controlled study to have a steroid-sparing effect in children who had steroid-responsive and steroid-dependent nephrotic syndrome.[67] About half of the 31 children in the levamisole group remained in remission 16 weeks into therapy while prednisolone was tapered in the initial 8 weeks. Two controlled studies with a longer period of follow-up did not reveal any significant beneficial effect.[68,69] The most serious adverse effect of levamisole is neutropenia, which is generally reversible. Rarely, agranulocytosis has been reported in patients with connective tissue or neoplastic diseases. Levamisole has also been shown to have a favorable effect when used in conjunction with Bacillus Calmette-Guérin vaccine (BCG) and dipyridamole in adult patients with different types of primary glomerulonephritis.[70] At present, further controlled studies are needed to define precisely the benefit of this agent in the treatment of glomerulonephritis.

THERAPEUTIC OUTCOMES

The long-term prognosis of most patients with minimal-change disease is good. The majority of pediatric patients will not experience any relapse of the disease 10 years after the initial onset, and most will be free of the proteinuria after puberty.[57] In adults, an 85% to 90% survival rate is seen 10 years after the disease onset.[57] Although this condition may spontaneously remit in up to 70% of untreated adults,[71] life-threatening complications may be associated with untreated nephrotic syndrome. Development of renal failure is uncommon in both adult and pediatric patients. Significant deterioration of renal function is observed only in those patients who are steroid resistant or steroid dependent. Because of the overall favorable outcome of the disease and the relatively uncommon progression into chronic renal failure, aggressive use of cytotoxic agents is not indicated even in most patients with frequent relapses. Toxicities associated with aggressive therapy do not justify the need to induce remission in those patients who fail to respond to steroids and the nonaggressive use of cytotoxic agents. Symptomatic therapy with diuretics to control edema, in conjunction with a low-salt diet and albumin infusion as needed for acute development of anasarca, is often a more rewarding therapeutic approach. NSAIDs and ACE inhibitors may also be used to reduce the proteinuria.

FOCAL SEGMENTAL GLOMERULOSCLEROSIS

Focal segmental glomerulosclerosis (FSGS) is a histologic lesion that can be idiopathic (primary) or secondary to a variety of causes. Conditions such as sickle cell disease, cyanotic congenital heart disease, and morbid obesity can induce hemodynamic stress on an initially normal nephron population and result in FSGS.[72] Severe glomerular injury can also be seen in patients with nephropathy associated with heroin abuse and human immunodeficiency virus (HIV) infection.[72,73] The primary and secondary sclerotic lesions may be morphologically similar, but they represent diseases with different courses and responses to therapy.

PATHOPHYSIOLOGY

Sclerotic lesions are characteristically found in some of the glomeruli (focal) and usually involve only a portion of the glomeruli (segmental).[74] Similar to the minimal-change disease, fusion of foot processes is commonly seen in those glomeruli that are not sclerotic. It is thought that both minimal-change disease and FSGS share similar pathogenetic mechanisms, with FSGS resulting in severe injury to the glomerular epithelial cells. During the early stage of FSGS, only a small number of glomeruli may have the segmental sclerotic lesion and the disease may be confined to the juxtamedullary region. If an inadequate number of glomeruli are sampled during renal biopsy, the diagnosis of FSGS may be missed, or the patient may be thought to have minimal-change disease. Resistance to steroid therapy may thus be one of the first clues that the patient indeed has FSGS rather than minimal-change disease. Alternatively, a patient may have the steroid-sensitive minimal-change disease initially, which subsequently progresses to steroid-resistant FSGS. In those patients who have cellular lesions, such as collapse of glomerular capillaries, or hypertrophy and hyperplasia of surrounding glomeruli epithelial cells, the risk for developing renal failure is increased.[75]

CLINICAL PRESENTATION

FSGS accounts for less than 15% of the cases of idiopathic nephrotic syndrome in children and about 15% to 20% in adults. Almost all the patients present with proteinuria, and many of them have all the features of nephrotic syndrome.[76] The proteinuria is nonselective, containing albumin and other higher-molecular-weight proteins, and is usually less severe when compared to patients who have minimal-change disease. Hypertension, microscopic hematuria, and renal dysfunction may be seen in up to half of the patients. The reduced renal function becomes more prevalent as the disease progresses.

The presenting clinical features in nephrotic adults with minimal-change nephropathy can be indistinguishable from that of FSGS, renal biopsy is therefore critical in the treatment of adults with nephrotic syndrome. FSGS is 2 to 4 times more common in black patients than in white patients. They tend to present with proteinuria more frequently in the nephrotic range and are more likely to experience a rapid decline in renal function.

▶ TREATMENT: Focal Segmental Glomerulosclerosis

PHARMACOLOGIC THERAPY

STEROIDS

Because the pathophysiology of primary FSGS is unknown, it is impossible to direct pharmacologic treatment against any specific pathologic processes. Furthermore, the treatment of FSGS remains controversial because of the lack of data from randomized, prospective, controlled trials. A course of prednisone (1–2 mg/kg/day) with tapering after 3 to 4 months of treatment may be used for nephrotic patients.[74] Urinary protein excretion and serum albumin concentration should be monitored to assess efficacy. The average time to induce complete remission is 3 to 4 months, and 5- to 9 months may be needed in some patients.[76] A longer duration of treatment (6 months or more) has resulted in complete remission in more than 40% of patients; older studies reported a response rate of less than 20% using regimens of a shorter duration.[76–78] In general, treatment should be given for 6 months before the patient is considered steroid resistant.[63,79] For patients who are not nephrotic, the relative favorable prognosis does not support the use of steroid or other immuno suppressive agents. However, close followup and good blood pressure control with ACE inhibitors are necessary to minimize disease progression.[74]

CYTOTOXIC AGENTS

Cytotoxic agents such as cyclophosphamide, chlorambucil, and azathioprine historically have been ineffective in the treatment of FSGS. However, Ponticelli recently reported that treatment with the immunosuppressive agents chlorambucil and cyclophosphamide, for more than 1 year was successful in inducing remission in those patients receiving their first treatment, as well as in those patients who did not respond initially.[78] In another study, combining prednisone therapy with cyclophosphamide and/or azathioprine over an extended period of time resulted in complete or partial remission in 60% of 59 adult patients.[77] Using an aggressive regimen incorporating pulse methylprednisolone infusions with long-term immunosuppression using oral alternate-day prednisone and an alkylating agent, a remission rate of 65% was observed in children who had steroid-resistant FSGS.[56,72]

CYCLOSPORINE

Short-term cyclosporine may reduce proteinuria in some patients who have FSGS resistant to corticosteroid and cytotoxic agents.[76,79] However, relapse of proteinuria is frequent, especially if treatment is withdrawn abruptly.[81] The relapse may occur within 2 months of tapering or drug discontinuation.[76] A prolonged period of treatment with slow tapering may result in longer periods of remission.[63] Long-term cyclosporine therapy was evaluated in 21 black and Hispanic children (who tend to have more rapid renal function deterioration than do white children) who had steroid-resistant FSGS.[82] The cyclosporine dosage was titrated to the serum cholesterol concentration with higher doses given to patients with severe hypercholesterolemia.[82,83] This aggressive regimen (4–20 mg/kg/day for 3 to 97 months) reduced proteinuria from 6.2–2.0 g/day and the percentage of patients who developed ESRD (78% in historical controls to 24% in treated patients).[82] Although histologic evidence of cyclosporine nephrotoxicity was not seen in this study, the drug was found by others to be more nephrotoxic in steroid-resistant than in steroid-responsive disease.[56] In a recent randomized, controlled study, combined treatment of cyclosporine with low-dose prednisone for 26 weeks was found to induce partial or complete remission of proteinuria in 70% of steroid-resistant patients. Renal function was also better preserved than treatment with steroid alone. However, the relapse rate was still high upon treatment discontinuation.[84]

SYMPTOMATIC THERAPY

Because of the lack of a consistently effective regimen for primary FSGS, many patients with mild disease are treated conservatively for symptomatic control. ACE inhibitors have been found to be effective in reducing proteinuria and in stabilizing renal function in patients with primary or secondary FSGS.[42,72] The dilation of efferent arterioles by these agents reduces intraglomerular pressure, which may diminish the potential effect of glomerular hypertension on the development of FSGS.[42] The driving force for proteinuria may also be reduced without necessarily correcting the primary defect in glomerular wall permselectivity.[72] The NSAID meclofenamate is effective in reducing proteinuria in patients with steroid-resistant FSGS.[43] These favorable results have, however, not been confirmed in studies using a larger number of patients. Thus, their role in the overall scheme of therapy remains to be defined. For patients with more severe disease, corticosteroids with or without immunosuppressive agents should be considered. Treatment should not be continued for more than 3 to 4 months unless the patient experiences a remission. In this case, therapy may be continued for 12 to 24 months to maintain the therapeutic response.[77]

THERAPEUTIC OUTCOME

Patients with primary FSGS are at risk for developing ESRD. For the 30% to 50% of adults and children who had attained complete remission, ESRD develops in about 10% or less of these patients at 10 years.[76,85] For those patients who are resistant to therapy, the rate of renal function deterioration to ESRD may be rapid, within 1 year, or slow, over as long as 10 to 20 years. About 50% of them develop ESRD in 10 years.[85] Those patients with severe proteinuria (>10–15 g/day), high serum creatinine concentration at diagnosis, initial steroid resistance, or interstitial fibrosis on renal biopsy are likely to have a more rapid decline in renal function.[74] A kidney transplantation is often indicated for those patients who develop ESRD; however, FSGS has recurred in 20% to 50% of the renal allografts soon after transplantation. Children and those with severe disease or rapid progression to ESRD prior to transplantation are more likely to experience a recurrence. The proteinuria may reappear within hours after transplantation and graft failure may occur in one-third to one-half of the patients. The median time to recurrence was reported to be 14 days in one study.[86] Although cyclosporine is ineffective in preventing the recurrence of nephrotic syndrome after transplantation, a high dose of the agent (up to 35 mg/kg/day) induces a remission of the recurrent disease.[87] ACE inhibitors and plasmapheresis are also used to prolong graft survival. The effectiveness of these therapies and the rapid recurrence of the disease in the transplanted kidney substantiate the possibility that a circulating humoral mediator is responsible for the nephropathy.[88]

MEMBRANOUS NEPHROPATHY

Membranous nephropathy is the most common disorder responsible for idiopathic nephrotic syndrome in adults, accounting for about 20% to 25% of cases.[89] The hallmark histologic features of membranous nephropathy are glomerular capillary wall thickening with subepithelial deposits under light and electron microscopy. Most cases are idiopathic, but about 25% of adults and 80% of children have secondary causes.[89,90] In the United States, the most common etiologies are autoimmune diseases (e.g., lupus), infection (e.g., hepatitis B), syphilis, neoplasm (e.g., carcinoma of the lung, breast, gastrointestinal tract, or kidney),[91] and medications (e.g., organic gold, penicillamine, mercury, or captopril). Malaria and schistosomiasis are common causes in other parts of the world. De novo membranous nephropathy can also occur in the allografts of renal transplant patients.[92] Because the response to therapy as well as the prognosis for idiopathic and secondary membranous nephropathy are different, it is important to identify any potential underlying causes for the nephropathy prior to treatment. Although this glomerular disease can occur at any age, the peak incidence is between 30 and 50 years and is especially likely in patients over 50 years old who present with nephrotic syndrome.[89]

PATHOPHYSIOLOGY

Examination of kidney tissue under light microscopy reveals normal mesangium and normocellularity. The glomerular capillary wall may be thickened in well-developed lesions. Trichome stain shows subepithelial deposits, and silver stain reveals spike-like projections between deposits. These projections gradually fuse to engulf the deposits such that, in the advanced stage, the capillary wall is markedly thickened and intramembranous deposits are found. Progressive changes in capillary lumen patency parallel those in the GBM, resulting in glomerulosclerosis with capillary collapse and tubular atrophy in end-stage membranous nephropathy. Immunofluorescence microscopy shows strong capillary wall staining of IgG and C3 on the epithelial side of the basement membrane. Secondary membranous nephropathy exhibits similar lesions except for the additional presence of mesangial expansion and hypercellularity with fewer deposits. In patients with membranous nephropathy induced by lupus, subendothelial and extraglomerular deposition can also be seen.

Antibody-mediated immune injury appears to be the main pathogenetic mechanism. Animal models of membranous nephropathy, particularly Heymann nephritis in rats, provide evidence that it is an autoimmune disease with immune complex deposition in the subepithelium of the GBM.[93] The immune complex can be formed *in situ* or deposited from circulating immune complexes. In Heymann nephritis, the intrinsic antigen is megalin (formerly gp330), a glycoprotein produced by the visceral epithelial cells. The antimegalin antibodies traverse the glomerular basement membrane to form immune complexes in the coated pits of the glomerular epithelial cells. These antimegalin immune complexes then become anchored to the glomerular basement membrane and detached from the podocyte cell membrane. These processes repeat themselves, resulting in accumulation of more immune complexes in the GBM until they become morphologically apparent.[93] Although the antigen responsible for primary human membranous nephropathy is not known, the mechanism for disease progression is thought to be similar.

CLINICAL PRESENTATION

Most patients with membranous nephropathy present with heavy proteinuria exceeding 3.5 g/day. The signs and symptoms are usually insidious in onset and may consist of anorexia, malaise, edema, anasarca, or ascites, and pericardial and pleural effusions may also be present. As a result of a hypercoagulable state, pulmonary embolism may develop, but rarely results in death.[94] The incidence of renal vein thrombosis varies from 5% to 62%,[25,90,94] and membranous nephropathy should be suspected when there is a sudden onset of hematuria; loin pain; pulmonary embolus; fluctuating or worsening proteinuria or glomerular filtration rate; renal tubular acidosis; or an increase in leg edema. Hypertension is found in about 30% of patients and is more common in the presence of renal insufficiency or until the disease is advanced.

In addition to heavy proteinuria, urinalysis often reveals lipiduria and oval fat bodies. Microhematuria is seen in fewer than 25% of patients, and gross hematuria and red cell casts are rare. In idiopathic membranous nephropathy, the serum complement concentrations are normal. Low levels of complement should alert one to search for secondary causes, such as lupus, hepatitis B infection, or an alternative diagnosis. Similarly, antinuclear antibodies, anti-DNA antibodies, rheumatoid factor, hepatitis B serologies, and serum cryoglobulins are generally negative in idiopathic membranous nephropathy. Occult malignancy has been found in as many as 10% of elderly patients with membranous nephropathy.[91]

The natural course of idiopathic membranous nephropathy is variable. About 25% of patients experience spontaneous remission of the disease over a mean of 5.5 years.[90] Less than 10% of the nonnephrotic patients and about one-third to one-half of the nephrotic patients will progress to end-stage renal failure over 10 to 15 years.[89] Some other patients have various degrees of renal insufficiency and persistent proteinuria. Heavy proteinuria (>10 g/day); male gender; elevated serum creatinine concentration at the time of presentation; poorly controlled hypertension; old age at onset of disease; non-Asian race; certain HLA antigens; and tubulointerstitial fibrosis on initial renal biopsy are associated with progressive renal disease.[89,90] Overall, patients with idiopathic membranous nephropathy have a relatively benign course. The mean 10-year survival is about 70%. Those who present with persistent nonnephrotic proteinuria seldom develop renal insufficiency and have a normal life expectancy. Fewer than 10% of patients develop a remitting and relapsing course.[90] The prognosis for secondary membranous nephropathy depends on the underlying cause. Remission occurs when the infection resolves or when the causative medication is withdrawn.

▶ TREATMENT: Membranous Nephropathy

The treatment of idiopathic membranous nephropathy is controversial and ranges from supportive therapy to immunosuppression with steroids alone, or in combination with alkylating agents. Conservative management of membranous nephropathy includes the control of edema with salt restriction and diuretics[20] and reduction of proteinuria with protein restriction and ACE inhibitors (Fig. 49–8).[95] Management of hypertension and hyperlipidemia is required for most patients, whereas prophylactic anticoagulation, despite having benefits shown to outweigh the risks, is usually given only for patients with renal vein thrombosis or documented pulmonary embolus.[50,90]

PHARMACOLOGIC THERAPY

STEROIDS

Remission of proteinuria, whether spontaneously or treatment related, may confer a good prognosis. Corticosteroids alone were ineffective in increasing the remission rate of proteinuria in all controlled trials and in preventing progression in all but one study.[90] The result of a meta-analysis also supported the lack of efficacy of steroids alone.

CYTOTOXIC AGENTS

Cytotoxic agents, when used in conjunction with corticosteroid, are effective in inducing the remission rate of nephrotic syndrome and reducing the frequency of ESRD at 10 years.[90,97] Ponticelli devised such a regimen by combining intravenous methylprednisolone (1 g) for 3 days followed by oral methylprednisolone (0.4 mg/kg) for the subsequent 27 days of months 1, 3, and 5. Oral chlorambucil (0.2 mg/kg) is to be given daily in months 2, 4, and 6.[97] He has also substituted cyclophosphamide (2.5 mg/kg/day) for chlorambucil, which resulted in similar rates of proteinuria remission and relapse, but with fewer serious side effects in those who received cyclophosphamide.[96]

A meta-analysis was conducted to evaluate the data from prospective trials using steroids and cytotoxic agents. The cytotoxic agents, but not steroids, were found to be effective in reducing

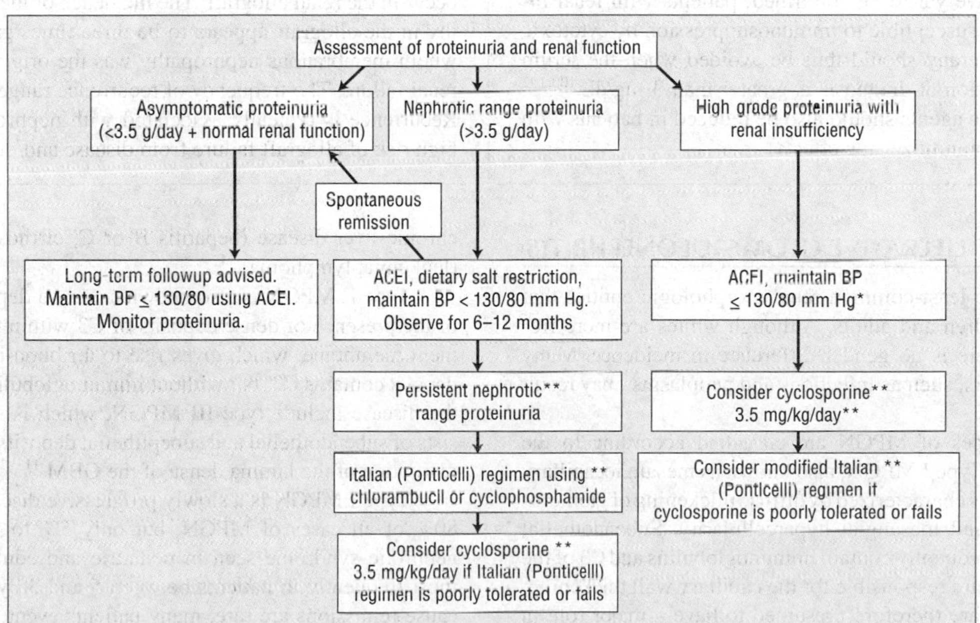

FIGURE 49–8. Treatment algorithm for idiopathic membranous nephropathy. Patients may change from one category to another during the course of follow-up.* = Supported by evidence from controlled trials; ACEI = angiotensin-converting enzyme inhibiting drug; ** = introduction of risk reduction strategies for both secondary effects of disease and adverse effects of immunotherapy. *(Modified from Ref. 90.)*

nephrotic-range proteinuria as well as increasing the likelihood of complete or partial remission.[98]

THERAPEUTIC OUTCOME

Because spontaneous remission is common and only about 25% of patients with new-onset idiopathic membranous nephropathy ultimately develop ESRD in 20 to 30 years, it is prudent not to aggressively treat all patients at the onset of the disease.[99–101] Patients who have a low likelihood for renal disease progression can be managed with observation and symptomatic therapy. Normalizing the blood pressure and reducing proteinuria with ACE inhibitors is reasonable because both hypertension and proteinuria are independent risk factors for the progression of renal failure.[90] Patients with low risk for renal disease progression include children 2 to 16 years of age, adult males with proteinuria less than 2 g/day, or adult females with proteinuria less than 5 g/day and normal renal function.[99,102] In contrast, patients who have a high risk of developing renal failure, including those with proteinuria greater than 10 g/day with or without impaired renal function, and patients with symptomatic nephrotic syndrome with a plasma albumin of less than 2 g/dL, should be aggressively treated to induce remission.[91,99,101] An alkylating agent such as chlorambucil or cyclophosphamide, combined with steroids[101,102] or the high-dose steroid regimen used in the study by Ponticelli,[97] can be given to induce remission after considering the benefits and risks of treatment.[27,102]

In patients with deteriorating renal function, steroids alone do not have a proven role in delaying the progression of renal disease. When a slightly modified version of the regimen by Ponticelli (methylprednisolone plus chlorambucil) was used in patients with renal insufficiency, improvement in renal function was reported in some small, uncontrolled studies.[90,104] However, more than half of the patients experienced significant myelosuppression secondary to chlorambucil. When cyclophosphamide was used with steroid, beneficial effects were observed in a small case series, but not in a randomized, controlled trial.[90,103] Although the therapeutic effects of cytotoxic agents for these patients have yet to be confirmed, patients with renal insufficiency are more susceptible to immunosuppression by cytotoxic agents. Cytotoxic therapy should thus be avoided when the serum creatinine concentration at diagnosis is greater than 3 mg/dL.[100,102] The dose of cytotoxic agents should also be reduced in patients with renal impairment to minimize side effects.

For patients with severe nephrotic syndrome who did not respond to cytotoxic therapy, cyclosporine treatment should be considered.[89] The drug may offer some benefits to these patients; however, the risk for cyclosporine nephrotoxicity is of concern, especially during long- term therapy. A 12-month course of cyclosporine (mean dose of 3.8 mg/kg/day) was found to reduce proteinuria as well as the rate of renal deterioration.[106] In a recent study of 41 patients who received cyclosporine, many with concurrent steroid and ACE inhibitor, the median treatment time to complete remission was 225 days among the 34% of patients who attained complete remission.[107] At present, the beneficial effects of cyclosporine are not well substantiated and the optimal duration of treatment is also not known. For many patients, hypertension may be exacerbated during therapy and the serum creatinine concentration may be elevated because of the nephrotoxic effect. When the renal function declines, the dose of cyclosporine should be reduced. In addition, proteinuria may recur when the cyclosporine treatment is stopped.

Because aggressive treatment is not warranted for patients with mild disease and the risk of immunosuppression by cytotoxic agents, is high there has been attempt to identify, early in the developed using data from 184 patients in Toronto.[108] The probability of progression to renal insufficiency was calculated from the level of proteinuria, creatinine clearance at the beginning of observation as well as the slope of renal function decline over a 6-month period. Although the model was validated retrospectively using patient data from Italy and Finland, the applicability of this model in clinical practice remains to be confirmed prospectively.

The treatment of secondary membranous nephropathy is directed at removing the underlying cause. For instance, membranous nephropathy secondary to syphilis can be treated with penicillin. α-Interferon is beneficial in the management of hepatitis B-induced membranous nephropathy.[109] Corticosteroids are of no benefit in this setting, and have been shown to induce transient viral replication to result in increased serum concentrations of hepatitis B virus antigen and hepatitis B virus DNA.[110]

Both de novo[92] and recurrent membranous nephropathy may occur in the renal allograft. The incidence of membranous nephropathy in the allograft appears to be three times greater in patients for whom membranous nephropathy was the original primary cause of renal failure. The frequency of recurrence ranges from 2% to 7%.[111] Recurrence is typically associated with nephrotic syndrome and a high risk of allograft failure from disease and/or rejection.

MEMBRANOPROLIFERATIVE GLOMERULONEPHRITIS

MPGN is one of the least-common renal morphologic entities that occurs in older children and adults. Although whites are more frequently affected, there is no gender difference in incidence. Many diseases and disorders, such as infections and neoplasms, may result in secondary MPGN.

The several types of MPGN are classified according to the pathologic features. Type I MPGN, also known as mesangiocapillary glomerulonephritis, is characterized by diffuse thickening of glomerular capillary walls and mesangial hypercellularity. Subendothelial dense deposits that frequently contain immunoglobulins and C3 of the complement system are responsible for the capillary wall thickening. Immune complexes are therefore presumed to have a major role in the pathogenesis of type I MPGN, which is the most common type of primary, idiopathic MPGN. Type I MPGN may also be secondary to systemic immune-complex-mediated disease (lupus), chronic infection (infected ventriculoatrial shunt, endocarditis, malaria), chronic liver disease (hepatitis B or C, cirrhosis), and malignancy (leukemia, lymphoma).[112]

Type II MPGN is also known as dense-deposit disease because of the presence of dense deposits of C3 within the glomerular basement membrane, which gives rise to a ribbon-like appearance. The deposit contains C3, but without immunoglobulins. Other variants of the disease include type III MPGN, which is seen rarely and consists of subendothelial and subepithelial deposits with lamination and disruption of the lamina densa of the GBM.[113]

Type I MPGN is a slowly progressive disease that accounts for 80% of all cases of MPGN, but only 5% to 15% of all cases of nephrotic syndrome seen in pediatric and adult patients. It occurs most frequently in patients between 5 and 30 years of age, and because remissions are rare, many patients eventually develop ESRD. The renal survival is 60% to 65% at 10 years, and the presence of nephrotic syndrome, interstitial disease, and hypertension are poor prognostic indicators.[114] Type II MPGN is a more aggressive disease that constitutes about 15% of all patients with MPGN. Only 20% of patients remain stable for more than a few years and the median time before the development of ESRD is 7 years. There is an impression that the incidence of idiopathic MPGN has declined recently worldwide.

Nephrotic syndrome is the most common presenting condition and some patients may also have a nephritic component (hematuria), hypertension, and renal insufficiency. Hypocomplementemia is commonly seen.

▶ TREATMENT: Membranoproliferative Glomerulonephritis

The efficacy of corticosteroids, cyclophosphamide, antiplatelet drugs, and anticoagulants has been evaluated in patients with MPGN. In children, prednisone 40 mg/m^2 given on alternate days, is effective, when compared with placebo, in reducing the decline in GFR.[115] This observation was confirmed by other uncontrolled studies.[114] Prednisone should therefore be given for 6 to 12 months to children with MPGN, proteinuria (more than 3 g/day), and/or impaired renal function.[114] Other recent studies suggest that this regimen may also be beneficial in children with mild proteinuria.

While the effect of steroid has not been proven in adults, antiplatelet drugs, such as dipyridamole and aspirin, as well as warfarin, were found in randomized, controlled trials to reduce proteinuria, but had no effect on GFR.[114] However, an increased incidence of bleeding was observed in the treatment groups.[116] Adults patients with idiopathic MPGN, heavy proteinuria, and/or impaired renal function should be given dipyridamole or aspirin. Unfortunately, no controlled study comparing the effect of steroid with antiplatelet agents is yet available.

Cyclophosphamide and azathioprine were found to have no beneficial effect Cyclosporine was evaluated in a limited number of patients with MPGN. Some beneficial effect was suggested; however, the trials were not controlled or randomized.[117] In addition, the risks for developing adverse effects were high. Figure 49–9 presents an algorithm for treatment and followup.

It is difficult to conduct large-scale controlled trials for MPGN because of the low incidence of the disease. Based on the available studies, many of the drugs evaluated do not have any consistent, beneficial effect on renal function and proteinuria. Renal transplantation is an alternative; however, recurrence rate is close to 100% for type II MPGN and is about 20% to 30% for type I MPGN. Nonetheless, fewer than 10% of the transplanted patients have graft failure as a result of recurrence.

IMMUNOGLOBULIN A NEPHROPATHY

Immunoglobulin A nephropathy, also known as Berger's disease, was first described by Berger and Hinglais in France in 1968. It is now recognized to be the most common primary glomerulonephritis in the world and accounts for 10% of patients with ESRD in many countries. The prevalence among patients with glomerulonephritis or patients who had kidney biopsy varies around the world from as high as 50% in Japan and East Asia to 10% to 30% in Europe. In the United States, the overall prevalence is about 10% to 15%, but is as high as 35% among Native Americans living in New Mexico.[118] These differences in prevalence may reflect the more conservative diagnostic approach in the U.S. patients with isolated hematuria or mild proteinuria are generally not referred for kidney biopsy in the United States.

IgA nephropathy has a male predominance, two to six times more common than females, and is more frequently seen in younger adults. It is uncommon in blacks both in the United States and in Africa.[118] IgA nephropathy was once thought to be a benign disease presenting with asymptomatic hematuria; however, it is now recognized that IgA nephropathy can present with any clinical syndrome associated with glomerular disease, and some of the patients will develop ESRD over variable periods of time.

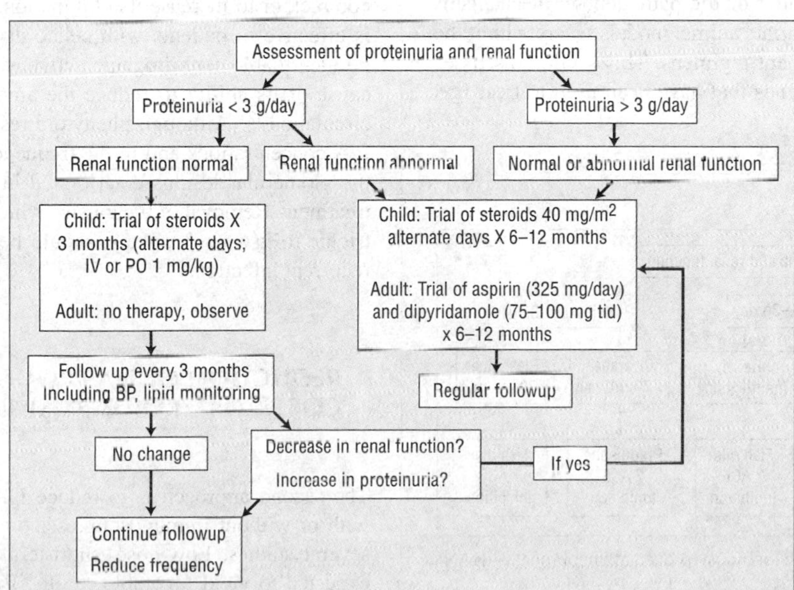

FIGURE 49–9. Treatment algorithm for membranoproliferative proliferative glomerulonephritis (MPGN). *(Modified from Ref. 114.)*

PATHOPHYSIOLOGY

Henoch-Schönlein purpura (HSP) is a systemic disease that is believed to be closely linked to IgA nephropathy because they share similar immunohistologic features. HSP may be the systemic form of the disease process causing IgA nephropathy in which only the joints, skin, and gastrointestinal tract are involved rather than the kidneys. Mesangial deposition of IgA immune complex is also seen in patients with celiac disease and dermatitis herpetiformis, possibly due to an increased exposure to antigens. Patients with chronic liver disease may have IgA nephropathy because of reduced clearance of IgA immune complexes. Secondary IgA nephropathy may be present in patients with different connective tissue diseases, carcinomas, and HIV infection.

The diagnosis of IgA nephropathy can be established by immunofluorescence examination of the kidney biopsy. The hallmark feature is the dominance or codominance of IgA deposition in the mesangium. IgG and/or IgM as well as C3 may also be present. The IgA immune complex, composed of IgA antibody bound with an *environmental* antigen, such as virus, bacteria, or food substances, is presumed to be deposited from the systemic circulation. Alternately, the complex may be formed in situ, with the IgA antibody bound with an *endogenous* antigen in the mesangium. Another theory postulates that abnormal IgA, produced in excess by B cells during upper respiratory infection, self-aggregates or causes production of autoantibodies and immune complexes, which deposit in the mesangium. In the mesangium, IgA can bind with receptors on the mesangial cells to induce proliferation and cytokine production. In addition, it can activate complement through the alternate pathway to induce glomerular damage.[119]

Conditions that stimulate the release of IgA are believed to cause IgA deposition in the mesangium. In fact, infections of the upper respiratory tract or intestinal mucosa are known to correlate with the onset or exacerbation of IgA nephropathy. IgA production is likely to be increased through antigenic stimulation of IgA-producing mucosal lymphoid tissue by microorganisms as well as ingested or inhaled substances.

CLINICAL PRESENTATION

IgA nephropathy commonly presents in the second and third decades of life, but it can occur at any age. Many of the patients have gross hematuria concurrent with an infection, most commonly pharyngitis or tonsillitis and less often pneumonia, gastroenteritis, or urinary tract infection.[118] In contrast to the 10- to 14-day delay after the pharyngitis in poststreptococcal glomerulonephritis, the hematuria of IgA nephropathy occurs 1 to 2 days after the onset of infection symptoms. The hematuria lasts from 24 hours to a few days, and it may recur with a febrile illness months or years later. Frequently, there is persistent microscopic hematuria between episodes of gross hematuria. Proteinuria is common and sometimes it can be in the nephrotic range. In contrast, hypertension and edema that are frequent in poststreptococcal glomerulonephritis are infrequent in IgA nephropathy. Renal dysfunction is uncommon at the initial presentation; however, about 10% to 20% of the patients develop ESRD within 10 years, and 30% develop it after 20 years.[120] Hypertension, severe proteinuria, renal function impairment, old age, and the severity of histologic lesions are all predictive factors for poor long-term outcome.[119,120] The alternative, but less common, clinical presentations are asymptomatic, microscopic hematuria with variable degrees of proteinuria or nephrotic syndrome.

▶ TREATMENT: Immunoglobulin A Nephropathy

Spontaneous remission is seen in only 10% to 25% of children and 5% to 7.5% of adults. Unfortunately, no therapy is known to be consistently effective for the treatment of IgA nephropathy. Because of the slow progression of the disease to ESRD, it is very difficult to conduct trials to evaluate the long-term effectiveness of specific treatments. The lack of understanding of the pathogenetic mechanisms and the unavailability of appropriate animal models severely limit the development of rational treatment regimens. This section discusses the several therapeutic approaches that have been used to treat IgA nephropathy (Fig. 49–10).

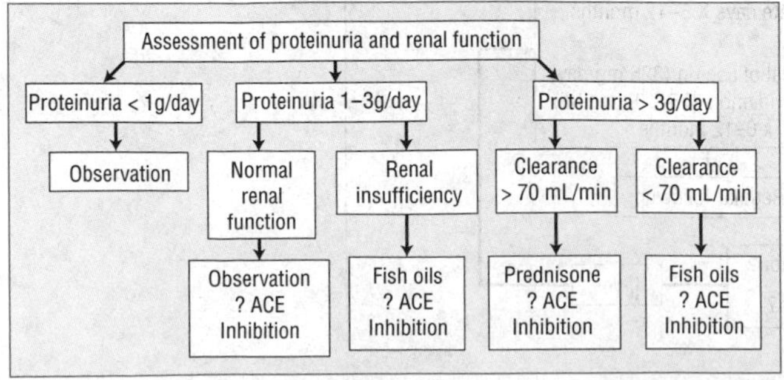

FIGURE 49–10. Treatment algorithm for biopsy-proven IgA nephropathy (IgAN). *(Modified from Ref. 120.)*

REDUCTION OF IgA IMMUNE COMPLEX: LOW GLUTEN DIET, PHENYTOIN

The first approach is to prevent the formation of the IgA immune complex or to increase its elimination. Restriction of dietary gluten is effective in patients with celiac disease but not in patients with no identifiable nephritogenic antigens. Phenytoin was evaluated because of its ability to reduce the amount of polymeric IgA in the circulation.[121] Although phenytoin resulted in a reduction in serum IgA concentrations and in the frequency of macroscopic hematuria, the glomerular lesions deteriorated in some of the patients despite treatment. Removal of the tonsils, which produce IgA_1 and may contribute to IgA nephropathy, should be considered for patients with recurrent infections.[122]

REDUCTION OF IgA PRODUCTION: CORTICOSTEROIDS, IMMUNOSUPPRESSANTS

The second approach is to reduce IgA production. Corticosteroids with or without immunosuppressive agents have been evaluated in several studies. Low-dose, short-term (<3 months) therapy is not expected to yield favorable results. Patients with progressive renal failure will not generally benefit from steroid therapy. In contrast, early treatment of proteinuric patients using an intensive and prolonged regimen (IV methylprednisolone and oral prednisolone combination for 6 months) may have a modest effect on proteinuria reduction, but its effect on renal function preservation is not as clear.[120,123] A meta-analysis of randomized trials reveals that heavy proteinuria (greater than 3 g/day) may be reduced by steroids and/or cytotoxic drugs in 66.7% of the patients.[124] The combination of cyclophosphamide, dipyridamole, and warfarin was shown to reduce proteinuria; however, renal function continued to decline on long-term followup.[120] A recent study showed that the azathioprine, prednisolone, heparin, and warfarin combination was better than heparin and warfarin alone in preserving renal function and reducing proteinuria at 2 years.[125] However, long-term follow-up data are not yet available.

REDUCTION OF GLOMERULAR INFLAMMATION: FISH OIL

The third approach is to reduce glomerular inflammation induced by IgA deposits. Anti-inflammatory agents, antiplatelet drugs, and anticoagulants have been tried without success to decrease the production or action of mediators responsible for IgA immune complex-induced glomerular damage. However, the *n*-3 fatty acids in fish oil, which limit the production or action of cytokines and eicosanoids, delay the progression of renal failure and reduce proteinuria slightly in patients with marked proteinuria and serum creatinine concentrations less than 3 mg/dL prior to study enrollment.[126] A meta-analysis of five controlled studies indicated that a minor, but not statistically significant, beneficial effect on renal function may be observed.[127] Donadio recently reported that fish oil was effective in reducing renal function deterioration over a 2-year period in patients with severe disease.[129] However, reduction in proteinuria, a key cause for renal injury, was only modest. Some of the fish oil preparations are rich in cholesterol, it is therefore appropriate to monitor the low-density lipoprotein cholesterol levels in patients receiving fish oil therapy.

ACE INHIBITION

ACE inhibitors can reduce proteinuria in patients with IgA nephropathy through their effect on the filtration barrier in the glomerular membrane.[129] In addition, they have been shown to be superior to other antihypertensive agents, including β-adrenergic antagonists, in reducing the progression of renal failure as well as proteinuria in both normotensive and hypertensive patients with IgA nephropathy.[129,130] Interestingly, the reduction in proteinuria is seen only in patients with a deletion polymorphism in the ACE gene, the DD genotype.[132] The angiotensin receptor antagonist irbesartan was also shown to have a similar effect on proteinuria reduction with no change on the GFR.[132] Combined use of ACE inhibitors and angiotensin receptor antagonist may have an additive effect on proteinuria reduction.[133] However, their total effect on renal function preservation is not known.[134] Because hypertension is a negative prognostic indicator of IgA nephropathy and many of these patients already had left ventricular diastolic malfunction, despite being normotensive, early antihypertensive intervention with ACE inhibitors should be instituted.[119,133]

OTHER THERAPEUTIC APPROACHES

Patients with IgA nephropathy have abnormal production of IgA and several different immunoglobulins. High-dose immunoglobulins, initially administered intravenously, followed by the intramuscular route, for over 9 months arrested the decline of renal function and reduced hematuria and proteinuria in all of the 11 patients evaluated.[134] The efficacy of this regimen must be confirmed in a larger number of patients before it is used as primary therapy.

Urokinase, danazol, dapsone, sodium cromoglycate, and plasma exchange have also been evaluated but none is consistently effective and had not been shown to affect renal function.[120] Cyclosporine treatment for 12 weeks was evaluated in nine patients. Proteinuria was reduced and plasma albumin concentrations increased. However, the creatinine clearance decreased during treatment and did not return to baseline after termination of cyclosporine therapy.[136] Cyclosporine is not, therefore, indicated for patients with IgA nephropathy.

Recently, the HMG-CoA reductase inhibitor fluvastatin was reported to reduce urinary protein excretion in moderately proteinuric (0.6–1.6 g/day) in patients who had IgA nephropathy with normal renal function.[137] Creatinine clearance remained stable during the 6-month study. Longer-term evaluation in a larger patient population will be needed to confirm the effect of this class of agents.

THERAPEUTIC OUTCOME

Normotensive patients with normal renal function, isolated microhematuria and proteinuria less than 1 g/day should be observed closely without specific treatment.[119] Because corticosteroids reduce proteinuria, a course of alternate-day prednisone (1 mg/kg/day) with subsequent tapering is indicated for patients with proteinuria greater than 3 g/d who have good renal function (>70 mL/min).[120] The more aggressive IV/PO steroid regimen described above may also be considered, even though its efficacy has not been definitively established. For patients with a slow progressive decline in creatinine clearance (<70 mL/min), fish oil should be given. Some clinicians may also consider using azathioprine, mycophenolate mofetil, or dipyridamole/warfarin therapy, although the efficacy of these agents has not been established. If the patient experiences rapid GFR decline of more than 2 mL/min/mo, immunoglobulin therapy may be considered despite the fact that only limited data are available. Other therapies that may be considered for these patients include pulse steroids, cyclophosphamide/steroid combination, mycophenolate mofetil, and plasmapheresis.[119,120,136]

If the patient is hypertensive, ACE inhibitors, instead of other antihypertensive agents, ought to be used to control the blood pressure as well as the proteinuria. The target blood pressure should be <125/80 mm Hg. Some clinicians recommend using ACE inhibitors or angiotensin-receptor blockers for all patients with >1 g/day proteinuria.[134] In patients with recurrent macroscopic hematuria in conjunction with tonsillitis, tonsillectomy should be considered.[120,122] In all of the patients, smoking should be avoided because of the dose-dependent increase in risk for developing ESRD.[29]

For those patients who develop end stage renal failure secondary to IgA nephropathy, transplantation is an effective alternative, especially for young adults. However, disease recurrence and subsequent graft loss are now recognized to be a clinically significant concern. Recurrence of IgA mesangial deposits in the renal allograft may occur in up to 50% of patients in 5 years and be universally present at 10 years or more post-transplant; but the recurrence of clinical disease is only about 10% to 15%.[118,119] The frequencies of graft survival for living related donor and cadaveric donor are not different. There is also no correlation between the aggressiveness of the primary disease and the rate of recurrence.[118] Immunosuppression using corticosteroids, azathioprine, and/or cyclosporine is not expected to prevent the recurrent nephropathy.

LUPUS NEPHRITIS

Glomerulonephritis is one of the most serious complications of SLE and accounts for much of the morbidity and mortality of patients afflicted with the disease.[138] The renal manifestations of lupus nephritis are variable and encompass a wide spectrum of histopathologic lesions.[138,139] The underlying histopathology is associated with different prognosis and response to therapy, which cannot be predicted solely based on clinical manifestations. A renal biopsy is therefore required to assess the severity of the disease and to predict the short-term and long-term outcomes associated with therapy. Drugs, such as hydralazine and procainamide, are known to precipitate a lupus syndrome; however, they are unlikely to cause disease that affects the kidney.

PATHOPHYSIOLOGY

Lupus nephritis is the prototype of all immune complex–mediated glomerulonephritis. It is characterized by the pleomorphic histologic presentations. Immune complex deposits, whether formed in the circulation or *in situ*, can be found in the mesangial, subendothelial, and subepithelial regions of the glomerulus, as well as the peritubular interstitium and vasculature outside the glomerulus.[139] Based on light, immunofluorescence, and electron microscopy findings, lupus nephritis can be categorized into six World Health Organization (WHO) classes: I—normal; II—mesangial; III—focal proliferative; IV—diffuse proliferative; V—membranous; and VI—advanced sclerosing.[140,141] In an attempt to enhance the predictive values of the histologic findings, semiquantitative assessment of active lesions and sclerotic changes are used to determine activity index and chronicity index, respectively.[139] Although the usefulness of these indices is still controversial, class IV patients are generally found to have the worst overall prognosis with 5-year renal survival of 60% to 80%, or 90% with recent aggressive treatment.[140]

The hallmark feature in the pathogenesis of SLE is the dysregulated production of antibodies against multiple antigens in the body.[138] Circulating immune complexes can be deposited in the glomerulus or formed *in situ*. The size and location of the immune complexes in the glomerulus correlate with the nature and severity of renal injury.[139] Deposition of small numbers of stable immune complexes of intermediate size in the mesangium tends to produce less-severe inflammation in the glomerulus. The sequestration of the immune complexes in the mesangium prevents them from activating inflammatory mediators. Hence, the lesion is noninflammatory in nature. In contrast, large numbers of intermediate-sized or large immune complexes can overload the mesangial clearing system. The eventual accumulation of these complexes in the subendothelial region allows them access to plasma inflammatory mediators, resulting in infiltration of inflammatory cells and release of necrotizing enzymes. Because subepithelial deposits are denied access to circulating inflammatory mediators, there is disproportionately more disturbance of glomerular capillary permeability than inflammatory response. Heavy proteinuria is, therefore, the primary clinical picture in lupus-induced membranous nephropathy.[139]

CLINICAL PRESENTATION

Females have a higher risk for developing lupus, especially in the adult years. The onset of nephritis is usually seen within the first 4 years of diagnosis of SLE but may also be the first manifestation of the disease. The clinical presentation ranges from minimal hematuria and proteinuria to severe, rapidly progressive diffuse glomerulonephritis. Proteinuria is very common and nephrotic syndrome is seen in most patients with membranous lesions. Microscopic hematuria is almost always present while macroscopic hematuria is rare.[140] Active urinary sediments (red cell casts, dysmorphic red cells, hematuria) are suggestive of the diffuse proliferative lesion; however, they do not reliably reflect the underlying glomerular lesion.[138] Hypertension is present in 25% to 45% of patients, and is associated with a worse prognosis.[143] Other conditions found to be associated with poor prognosis include elevated serum creatinine concentration, heavy proteinuria, anemia (hematocrit <26%), black race, and disease onset during childhood, or in those >60 years of age. Most patients have hypocomplementemia and increased antibody titers for anti-double-stranded DNA, particularly those with focal or diffuse proliferative lesions.[89] Serum creatinine concentration at the time of diagnosis is most predictive of short-term outcome.[139]

▶ TREATMENT: Lupus Nephritis

The treatment of lupus nephritis has evolved over the past several decades. The choice of therapy depends on the underlying lesion, and the activity, as well as the chronicity indices. Acute life-threatening diseases involving multiple organs require induction treatment that can suppress the disease promptly. In contrast, long-term management of chronic, indolent diseases requires therapy with more acceptable side-effect profiles. Corticosteroids are the cornerstone of therapy. However, for severe lupus nephritis, primarily the diffuse proliferative type, alkylating agents may be needed to reduce or prevent the progression to ESRD.

Patients with normal renal function and less than 2 g of proteinuria usually do not require therapy, except for the management of extrarenal lupus manifestations. The prognosis of these patients is generally good and renal biopsy can be delayed. However, close followup of renal function and urinalysis is required.

ACUTE INDUCTION TREATMENT

Patients with more than 2 g of proteinuria, deteriorating renal function, and/or active urinary sediments require a renal biopsy to define the underlying lesion and determine the activity and chronicity of disease. Those with classes II, III, and V lesions can be treated with oral steroids for 12 to 16 weeks with subsequent tapering to 'low doses' to maintain remission. The concurrent use of an immunosuppressive agent was found in meta-analysis to be more effective in reducing the incidence of ESRD than steroid alone.[144] Patients with class IV lesions, and those with class III lesions associated with subendothelial deposits and signs of severe disease activity, should be treated with 'pulse' intravenous methylprednisolone followed by low-dose oral steroid. Cyclophosphamide is used concurrently because it is a powerful B cell inhibitor and can suppress the resynthesis of autoantibodies to normal levels.[140] Combined use of intravenous cyclophosphamide and methylprednisolone is more effective than either agent alone in inducing remission.[145] However, the risk for adverse events, such as infection, amenorrhea, and cervical dysplasia, is increased with the cytotoxic regimens.[149]

Investigators at the National Institutes of Health (NIH) have used Fludarabine, which targets lymphoid cells, with cyclophosphamide.[151] Favorable results have been obtained thus far with respect to proteinuria reduction. Also being investigated is the use of immunoablative high-dose cyclophosphamide with reinfusion of autologous stem cells. Alternately, granulocyte-stimulating factor may be used without stem-cell rescue.[151]

CHRONIC MAINTENANCE TREATMENT

Oral steroid is most frequently used for maintenance treatment (prednisolone 5–15 mg/day or equivalent).[140] Alternate-day regimens, although not evaluated, are often used in children to minimize growth retardation. Monthly 'pulse' steroid has also been used, but its toxicity and efficacy have not been evaluated. The concurrent use of a cytotoxic agent was shown by meta-analysis to be more beneficial.[144] Cyclophosphamide, because of its bladder and gonadal toxicity, should not be given for more than 12 weeks.[140] Instead, it has been given as monthly and then bimonthly intravenous injection for up to 2 or more years. However, toxicity is still a concern and azathioprine is therefore more commonly used long-term. Cyclosporine has been evaluated in a few studies with varied results.[153] There are recent data to suggest that it may reduce proteinuria and lupus activity, stabilize renal function, and improve kidney morphology. A randomized trial is currently underway at NIH to evaluate its effectiveness.

Mycophenolate mofetil has been used in place of azathioprine and in small studies, has yielded good results.[146,151] However, its efficacy needs to be confirmed in larger controlled trials. Other therapeutic measures that have been used for lupus nephritis include plasmapheresis, intravenous γ-globulin, fish oil, total lymphoid irradiation, and intravenous thromboxane antagonists.[152] None of these modalities was effective in controlled trials. Promising investigational agents that may be used in the future include LJP-394, composed of four double-stranded oligodeoxynucleotides, which can render specific B-lymphocytes unresponsive to immunogen. It can reduce anti-DNA antibody production in SLE-prone animals. A recent Phase II/III clinical trial showed that LJP-394 increased time to renal flares, reduced number of renal flares, time to institution of high-dose corticosteroids and/or cyclophosphamide, and decreased anti-ds-DNA levels.[147,152] A definitive trial is in progress. Anti-C5A is a monoclonal antibody that is being evaluated for membranous nephropathy and is potentially beneficial for lupus nephritis. Anti-CD40 ligand, which exerts immunosuppression by blocking communication between B and T cells, is being evaluated in patients.[148] Also being investigated is bindarit, which blocks the production of monocyte chemoattractant protein MCP-1. As a result, the inflammation in the glomeruli is reduced.[149]

In patients who do not respond to cyclophosphamide and steroid therapy, cyclosporine has produced favorable results in some.[152] However, the number of patients studied was small and the follow-up period was short. Treatment with plasmapheresis in addition to a standard regimen consisting of a short course of oral cyclophosphamide and oral prednisone did not improve the clinical outcome of patients with severe lupus nephritis when compared to standard regimen alone.[153]

The survival of patients with lupus nephritis has improved during the last two to three decades, and now ranges from 74% to 80% at 10 years.[143] This improvement cannot be explained solely by the use of cytotoxic agents. The lower steroid dosage and better management of complications such as hypertension, infections, hyperlipidemia, and other metabolic complications of the disease also likely have contributed to the more favorable long-term outcome. Lupus patients with ESRD on dialysis fare as well as those with non–lupus-related renal disease. In those patients who received a renal transplant, the allograft outcome of patients with lupus nephritis is favorable.[154] Recurrence of lupus in the renal allograft can occur, but is usually of minor clinical importance.

RAPIDLY PROGRESSIVE GLOMERULONEPHRITIS

Rapidly progressive glomerulonephritis (RPGN) describes a clinicopathologic syndrome of rapid loss of renal function—usually a greater than 50% decrement of the glomerular filtration rate within 3 months. The predominant histologic finding of RPGN is extensive crescent formation, usually in more than 50% of the glomeruli. Hence, it is also known as crescentic glomerulonephritis. RPGN accounts for 2% to 7% of all renal biopsy findings, and is responsible for up to 5% of patients with ESRD. Although a rare disease, RPGN usually leads to renal demise within weeks or months if left untreated.

RPGN is not a single-disease entity. A variety of glomerulonephritides with or without systemic diseases may present as RPGN, including anti-GBM glomerulonephritis; Goodpasture's syndrome; lupus nephritis; poststreptococcal glomerulonephritis; membranoproliferative glomerulonephritis; IgA nephropathy; polyarteritis nodosa; Wegener's granulomatosis; and idiopathic crescentic glomerulonephritis.[155] RPGN may also be found superimposed on an underlying primary glomerulopathy such as membranous nephropathy.

Besides the hallmark feature of extensive crescents, severe endocapillary proliferation and segmental necrosis can also be seen on light microscopy. Based on immunofluorescence microscopic findings, three types of primary RPGN can be identified. Type I RPGN is characterized by the linear localization of immunoglobulins, mainly IgG, along the GBM, signifying anti-GBM antibody–induced injury. Type II is defined by the coarse granular deposition of immunoglobulins and complement within the capillary walls and mesangium, denoting immune–complex–mediated injury. Type III is characterized by scanty or lack of immune complex deposits; therefore, it is also known as pauci-immune RPGN. Circulating ANCAs are often detected in type III RPGN. This immunohistologic classification of RPGN reflects the immunopathogenesis of the different types of crescentic glomerulonephritis.

PATHOPHYSIOLOGY

Although the causal relationships are not firmly established, several etiologic factors are implicated for RPGN, including toxins, drugs, viral and bacterial infections, neoplasm, autoimmune mechanisms, and various immunogenetic factors.[155]

Irrespective of the etiology and type of RPGN, the disruption in the glomerular capillary wall seems to be the common lesion in crescentic glomerulonephritis.[155] Various mechanisms have been proposed to account for the severe damage to the capillary wall. Both humoral and cellular pathways of inflammation are involved. Activation of the terminal C5b-9 (membrane-attacking complex) of the complement system produces severe capillary wall injury. Both neutrophils and macrophages release proteinases and reactive oxygen species and may thereby produce severe glomerular injury. Platelets and the coagulation system are activated and result in capillary thrombosis.[156] Fibrinogen and procoagulants that are released from ruptured capillaries may come into contact with thrombogenic tissue debris and lead to fibrinoid changes.[156] In anti-GBM glomerulonephritis, the direct attack of the anti-GBM antibody on the noncollagenous region of the type IV collagen molecule of the GBM is responsible for the capillary wall injury.[155] ANCAs may also play an important role in mediating the vascular injury in patients with ANCA-associated disease.[9] The interaction of ANCAs with neutrophils and monocytes, which have been primed by concurrent infections or inflammatory processes, can lead to activation of these leukocytes and release of toxic oxygen species and lytic enzymes, resulting in vascular injury.[9,157]

The disruption of the capillary wall allows movement of macrophages and other plasma constituents into Bowman's space and stimulates the formation of crescents, which are composed mainly of parietal epithelial cells, as well as macrophages and fibroblasts. Crescent formation indicates the severity of the glomerular capillary disease but not its pathogenesis. The age of crescents can serve as a marker for disease duration and the likelihood of successful therapeutic intervention.[155]

CLINICAL PRESENTATION

Among the crescentic glomerulonephritides, the pauci-immune RPGN is the most frequent, accounting for more than 50% of cases, whereas the anti-GBM antibody–mediated RPGN is the least frequent, occurring in roughly 10% to 20% of patients. Sixty percent to 70% of patients with type I RPGN may have concurrent pulmonary hemorrhage and Goodpasture's syndrome, which is caused by antibodies directed against the pulmonary alveolar basement membrane.[156] Most patients with immune complex-mediated RPGN have collagen vascular disease, systemic infections, or a severe form of primary glomerular disease. Approximately 70% of patients with type III RPGN also present with evidence of systemic vasculitis, such as Wegener's granulomatosis and polyarteritis nodosa. They often have insidious onset with initial symptoms such as fatigue, fever, night sweats, and arthralgias.[157] Other patients have only renal manifestations, and they are said to have idiopathic crescentic glomerulonephritis or renal vasculitis.[155,156]

The clinical presentation is dominated by progressive renal insufficiency with complaints of tea-colored urine, malaise, anorexia, low-grade fever, and migratory polyarthropathy. Mild hypertension is usually present. Uremic signs and symptoms may develop as renal function worsens. Type I RPGN is more commonly found in the third and sixth decades of life, while patients with ANCA-mediated disease tend to be older, with peak incidence occurring between 50 and 60 years of age. The age-related incidence varies among the immune complex–mediated RPGN; for example, poststreptococcal glomerulonephritis and Henoch–Schönlein purpura nephritis are more common in young children, whereas membranoproliferative glomerulonephritis is more frequently seen in older children.[156] Urinalysis commonly shows nephritic sediments with hematuria, erythrocyte casts, and proteinuria. However, overt nephrotic syndrome is rare.

Serologic analysis is very useful in distinguishing the different types of RPGN. The detection of serum anti-GBM antibodies with the appropriate clinical presentation confirms the diagnosis of anti-GBM glomerulonephritis. More than 80% of patients with pauci-immune or idiopathic crescentic glomerulonephritis have circulating ANCAs.[9,156] ANCAs are autoantibodies specific for the cytoplasmic constituents of neutrophil granules and monocyte lysosomes. Patients with ANCA-associated disease limited to renal involvement often have P-ANCA (perinuclear staining), whereas patients with Wegener's granulomatoses tend to have C-ANCA (cytoplasmic staining).[9,156] Both the anti-GBM antibody and the ANCAs are absent in patients with type II RPGN. Measurements of circulating immune complexes are not useful for making a specific diagnosis, but detection of specific serum antibodies known to mediate immune complex–associated nephritis is helpful: anti-DNA antibody as a marker for lupus nephritis and elevated anti-streptolysin-O titers for poststreptococcal glomerulonephritis. The serum complement levels are normal in RPGN, although they can be low in the immune complex–mediated category.

▶ TREATMENT: Rapidly Progressive Glomerulonephritis

Early aggressive therapy has improved the renal prognosis of patients with crescentic glomerulonephritis. The rapid deterioration of renal function and the paucity of large patients make randomized controlled studies very difficult to conduct. Based on the available data, immunosuppressive therapy alone appears to be ineffective for type I RPGN while types II and III RPGN respond well to high-dose steroid therapy.[155,159] Irrespective of the type of RPGN, poor response to therapy and an ominous renal survival are expected if the patient presents with oliguria, has a serum creatinine concentration greater than 6 or 7 mg/dL, is dialysis dependent, or has a renal biopsy showing advanced chronic parenchymal disease.[156]

ANTI-GBM GLOMERULONEPHRITIS (TYPE I)

Research data on the treatment of anti-GBM glomerulonephritis are limited. Pulse intravenous administration of corticosteroids has been used successfully to alleviate pulmonary hemorrhage, but the results are not as convincing for glomerulonephritis.[155,159] When used, the immunosuppression should be maintained for 8 weeks to prevent antibody rebound.[155] Plasmapheresis, in combination with steroids and cytotoxic agents, was found to be more beneficial than immunosuppression alone.[136,159] Plasmapheresis may confer its benefits by removing the circulating pathogenetic anti-GBM antibody and is therefore used for 2 weeks or until the antibody disappears.[159,160] The treatment was found to be useful in treating pulmonary hemorrhage; however, the long-term benefits on renal function are unknown. Because of the rapid decline in renal function, diagnosis should be established early so that therapy can proceed without delay. When the serum creatinine concentration is 6 mg/dL or above, or the patient is oliguric or requires dialysis, the response to therapy is usually poor and the patient should be treated conservatively.[155,159] Poor response should also be expected when crescents are found in more than 85% of the glomeruli.

IMMUNE COMPLEX-MEDIATED GLOMERULONEPHRITIS (TYPE II)

The treatment of this type of RPGN varies with the underlying glomerulonephritis. Patients with postinfectious RPGN generally have a favorable prognosis even without treatment. Complete spontaneous recovery occurs in 50% of cases, whereas chronic renal failure develops in 32%.[155] Pulse doses of methylprednisolone, followed by oral prednisone and then tapering, have been shown to be beneficial in type II RPGN, with a response rate of 85% in patients with acute disease and 70% in those with more chronic disease.[159] Plasmapheresis does not appear to provide any additional benefit.[159]

ANTINEUTROPHIL CYTOPLASMIC AUTOANTIBODY (ANCA)-ASSOCIATED GLOMERULONEPHRITIS (TYPE III)

Type III RPGN has been treated successfully with pulse doses of intravenous methylprednisolone, followed by oral prednisone for 1 month and then tapering over the next 6 to 12 months.[155,159] The recognition that pauci-immune necrotizing crescentic glomerulonephritis is part of the spectrum of necrotizing vasculitides, especially with the detection of ANCAs in these patients, have led to the use of cyclophosphamide with steroids.[9,159] Cyclophosphamide should be given for 6- to 12 months either orally (2 mg/kg/day) adjusted to maintain leukocyte count between 3,000 and –5,000/mL, or intravenously starting at 0.5 g/m^2/mo and increased monthly by 0.25 g to a maximum of 1 g/m^2/mo.[159,161] The dose should be adjusted to maintain a nadir in the leukocyte count of 3,000–5,000/mL 2 weeks after treatment. Vigilant monitoring of the white cell count is necessary to prevent severe leukopenia. The combined use of cyclophosphamide and steroid resulted in higher remission rate and less risk for relapse than steroid alone. This regimen is indicated even for patients with advanced disease, dialysis dependence as well as for relapse. During treatment, the serum ANCA levels can be monitored to determine the efficacy of therapy. However, the precise role of ANCA monitoring is not clear.

At present, plasmapheresis is not expected to have any additional benefits for patients with mild to moderate disease who are receiving immunosuppressive therapy.[160] However, there are limited data to suggest that, when used as an adjunct to immunosuppressive therapy, plasmapheresis may be beneficial for patients with severe disease.[136,159] In those patients presenting with pulmonary hemorrhage, early and aggressive use of plasmapheresis has reduced substantially the nearly 50% mortality rate.[161]

Several other agents have been used to prevent recurrence of ANCA-associated diseases.[161] Mycophenolate mofetil has been used anecdotally with favorable results. Methotrexate has also been used; however, it should not be given when the creatinine clearance is less than 50 mL/min. Trimethoprim–sulfamethoxazole was found to reduce ACNA-associated vasculitis, especially in the upper respiratory tract.

RENAL TRANSPLANTATION

Anti-GBM nephritis may recur in up to 55% of patients who received a renal transplant. However, only 25% of these patients showed clinical disease activity, with rare allograft failure. Because the frequency of recurrence and its severity are related to the presence of circulating anti-GBM antibody, it is recommended that transplantation should not be performed until the anti-GBM antibody is undetectable for at least 6 to 12 months.[111] The recurrence rate of ANCA-associated nephritis is 17%, based on the pooled analysis of 127 patients.[162] The average time to relapse from transplantation is 31 months. The chronic use of immunosuppressants to prevent rejection might have lowered the relapse rate.

POSTSTREPTOCOCCAL GLOMERULONEPHRITIS

Poststreptococcal glomerulonephritis (PSGN) and glomerulonephritis caused by other infectious agents, such as bacteria, viruses, and parasites, were once common. Improved sanitation, personal hygiene, medical care, and public health measures helped to decrease the incidence of group A streptococcal infection both in the United States and other developed countries, resulting in a decline of PSGN. However, PSGN is still common in developing countries. In contrast, glomerulonephritis secondary to other infectious agents, such as hepatitis C and HIV viruses, is seen with increasing frequency in developed countries.

It was more than 200 years ago when hematuria and proteinuria were found to be associated with epidemics of scarlet fever. Certain strains of group A streptococci were identified in the 1950s to be responsible for the glomerular disease. PSGN is now the most common form of glomerulonephritis in children, but is less common than the other types of glomerulonephritis in adults. It normally follows pharyngeal or skin infection caused by the nephritogenic strains of group A streptococci; however, other strains of streptococci, such as group C and G, have also been reported to cause PSGN. Streptococcal pharyngitis is more common in winter and early spring, whereas skin infection is frequently found in the summer. The risk for developing acute glomerulonephritis secondary to the nephritogenic strains of bacteria is about 10% to 15% in infected patients. However, three to four times more patients may experience a subclinical form of the disease.

PATHOPHYSIOLOGY

Despite decades of research, the characteristics of the antigens responsible for the production of the nephritogenic immune complexes remain unclear. It has been postulated that the streptococcal antigens may induce changes in the glomerular components so that they become immunogenic or that autologous IgG may be altered to become antigenic. Alternately, the streptococcal antigens may induce antibodies that react with glomerular antigens. *In situ* immune complexes are then formed and result in a complement-mediated inflammatory response. The kinin and coagulation cascades are activated and chemotactic factors are released to recruit neutrophils and monocytes, resulting in acute glomerular lesions.

Examination of the acute PSGN kidneys reveals hypercellular glomerulus with proliferation of mesangial and endothelial cells. Infiltration of neutrophils, monocytes, and eosinophils is apparent within the capillary lumen and also in the mesangial areas. Crescent formation may be seen in patients with severe disease, and if found in more than 30% of the glomeruli, RPGN may be present concurrently.[163] The prognosis is generally poor for these patients and complete recovery is unlikely. When the tissue is examined under electron microscope, "humps," which are multiple large, discrete, electron-dense, dome-shaped deposits, can be found beneath the epithelial foot processes. Immunofluorescence examination reveals diffuse granular deposits of IgG and C3 along the glomerular basement membrane and also in the mesangium.

CLINICAL PRESENTATION

PSGN is seen mostly in children aged between 5 and 15 years, with a peak incidence between ages 6 and 7 years. It is uncommon in children younger than 2 years of age and in adults older than 50 years of age. Males are twice as likely to be affected as females. The nephritis is preceded by a latent period following a streptococcal infection. The latent period is commonly 7 to 14 days for pharyngitis and 14 to 28 days for skin infection. In patients with preexisting nephritis such as IgA nephropathy and membranoproliferative glomerulonephritis, the streptococcal infection may exacerbate the nephritis and result in hematuria.

Following the latent period, an acute nephritic syndrome develops with hematuria and edema being the most common characteristics. Gross hematuria is seen in 70% of patients, and microscopic hematuria can be found in all patients. Edema, which is often worse in the morning, is found commonly in the periorbital area and around the eyelids. Hypertension is usually mild to moderate and results from sodium and water retention; at times, it may be severe enough to cause hypertensive encephalopathy. Many patients have signs and symptoms associated with volume overload, which include dyspnea, orthopnea, and cough. In some instances, progression to overt congestive heart failure may be seen. Severe hypertension may also result in neurologic abnormalities.

Urinalysis of patients with PSGN reveals hematuria, dysmorphic red blood cells, and red cell casts. Proteinuria is common, but often not in the nephrotic range. Renal function is frequently mildly impaired, and serum creatinine concentration is often normal. However, blood urea concentration may be disproportionately high.

Throat or skin culture may be positive for group A streptococci, despite the latent period following the initial infection. However, antibiotic therapy may render the culture result negative. Serologic measurements of antibodies to different streptococcal antigens can confirm recent exposure to the infection. Titers that can be measured include the antistreptolysin (ASO), antistreptokinase, antihyaluronidase (AHase), antideoxyribonuclease B (ADNase B), and antinicotyladenine dinucleotidase (NADase).[164] In most patients with streptococcal pharyngitis, the ASO titers begin to rise about 10 to 14 days later, peak at 3 to 4 weeks, and persist for several months before decreasing. The rise in ASO titers can be reduced by antibiotic treatment and may not be seen in patients with streptococcal skin infection where the streptolysin may be bound to skin lipids. ADNase B and AHase titers should be used instead because they are specific and are positive in the majority of patients. The streptozyme test is a combined assay for ASO, ADNase B, NADase, and AHase. It has a high rate of false-positive and false-negative results, and the antibody levels do not correlate with nephritogenicity or disease severity. Recently, antizymogentiters were found to be the best marker to diagnose streptococoal associated nephritis.[165] Increased availability of this test may facilitate early and accurate diagnosis of nephritis.

Serum complements may also be measured in patients with PSGN. Hemolytic complement activity (CH_{50}) and C3 levels are reduced in more than 90% of the patients for 4 to 6 weeks. If the C3 level is depressed for more than 6 to 8 weeks, MPGN, lupus nephritis, or glomerulonephritis related to endocarditis or occult visceral abscess should be suspected.

Renal biopsy is not normally indicated for PSGN unless the patient has severe renal dysfunction, severe proteinuria, significant hypertension, and/or prolonged oliguria, which are not typical for PSGN. If the hematuria is prolonged or proteinuria or depressed C3 level persists, renal biopsy is needed to detect other types of glomerulonephritis such as lupus, RPGN, or MPGN.

► TREATMENT: Poststreptococcal Glomerulonephritis

The treatment of PSGN is mainly supportive and symptomatic. Early antibiotic therapy does not prevent subsequent PSGN, but it may reduce the severity of the disease.[166] It can, however, prevent the spread of the streptococcal infection to other family members. Antibiotic prophylaxis is not recommended because infected patients will develop long-lasting, often lifelong immunity against the strain of streptococci. Exposure to another nephritogenic strain of streptococci is possible, but unlikely.

Supportive measures, as discussed earlier in this chapter, should be used to control fluid volume and blood pressure. Because the hypertension is of the low-renin type, ACE inhibitors and β-blockers are not expected to be useful. If the patient has crescentic disease, use of pulse steroids and/or immunosuppressive agents can be considered;[155] however, the efficacy and safety of these agents have not been established for this condition.

The acute manifestations of PSGN are normally self-limited, and more than 95% of the patients have renal function restored within 3 to 6 weeks. Diuresis usually begins 7 to 10 days after onset of the acute episode, whereas hypertension and azotemia resolve in 1 to 2 weeks. Gross hematuria lasts for 1 to 2 weeks and proteinuria usually resolves within 6 months in more than 90% of children. However, microscopic hematuria may persist for up to 2 years. Children, in general, have more rapid recovery than adults. Prognosis is often better when PSGN occurs during an epidemic than in those found sporadically. Most of the children will recover fully and be free from chronic complications of PSGN if they have no preexisting renal disorder, heavy proteinuria, or crescentic glomerular lesions or did not require hospitalization during the acute episode.[167] In contrast, adult patients have a less favorable long-term outcome. As many as 50% of the patients had persistent proteinuria, hypertension, and renal insufficiency.[168,169] Some of the patients may develop end-stage renal failure.

CONCLUSIONS

A better understanding of the pathogenetic mechanisms leading to glomerular injury has improved the treatment of glomerulonephritis. However, the glomerulonephritides are a heterogeneous group of immune disorders with different clinical courses, prognoses, and responses to current immunologic and nonimmunologic therapies. The clinician should understand the natural history and prognosis of each subgroup of glomerulonephritis, the efficacy of different immunomodulating regimens in inducing disease remission and preserving renal function, and the characteristics of at-risk patients who warrant aggressive therapy. Judicious use of immunosuppressive agents with careful monitoring of their adverse effects cannot be overemphasized. In addition, treatment of the disease complications and control of factors that lead to progression of renal disease are important in reducing the morbidity and mortality of patients with glomerulonephritis.

REFERENCES

1. Couser WG. Research opportunities and future directions in glomerular disease. Semin Nephrol 1993;13:457–471.
2. Miller DE, Noble NA, Yu X, Border WA. Molecular and cellular biological techniques in the study of glomerular diseases. Semin Nephrol 1992;12:506–515.
3. U.S. Renal Data System 2000 Annual Data Report. Bethesda, MD, National Institutes of Health and National Institute of Diabetes and Digestive and Kidney Diseases, 2000.
4. Bohrer MP, Baylis C, Humes HD, et al. Permselectivity of the glomerular capillary wall: Facilitated filtration of circulating polycations. J Clin Invest 1978;61:72–78.
5. Schreiner GF. The mesangial phagocyte and its regulation of contractile cell biology. J Am Soc Nephrol 1992;2:S74–S82.
6. Schena FP, Gesualdo L, Grandaliano G, Montinaro V. Progression of renal damage in human glomerulonephritides: Is there sleight of hand in winning the game? Kidney Int 1997;52:1439–1457.
7. Couser WG. Mediation of immune glomerular injury. J Am Soc Nephrol 1990;1:13–29.
8. Makker SP. Mediators of immune glomerular injury. Am J Nephrol 1993; 13:324–336.
9. Jennette JC, Falk RJ. Antineutrophil cytoplasmic autoantibodies and associated diseases: A review. Am J Kidney Dis 1990;15:517–529
10. Remuzzi G, Zoja C, Perico N. Proinflammatory mediators of glomerular injury and mechanisms of activation of autoreactive T cells. Kidney Int Suppl 1994;44:S8–S16.
11. Klahr S, Schreiner G, Ichikawa I. The progression of renal disease. N Engl J Med 1988;318:1657–1666.
12. Ritz E, Orth S, Wennich T, et al. Systemic hypertension versus intraglomerular hypertension in progression. Kidney Int 1994;45:438–442.
13. Williams JD, Coles GA. Proteinuria: A direct cause of renal injury morbidity? Kidney Int 1994;45:443–450.
14. Ong ACM, Fine LG. Loss of glomerular function and tubulointerstitial fibrosis: Cause or effect? Kidney Int 1994;45:345–351.
15. Thomas ME, Schreiner F. Contribution of proteinuria to progressive renal injury: Consequences of tubular uptake of fatty acid bearing albumin. Am J Nephrol 1993;13:385–398.
16. Keane WF. Lipids and the kidney. Kidney Int 1994;46:910–920.
17. Kasiske BL, Keene WF. Laboratory assessment of renal disease: Clearance, urinalysis and renal biopsy. In: Brenner BM, ed. The Kidney, 5th ed. Philadelphia, WB Saunders, 1996:1137–1174.
18. Rodríguez-Iturbe B, Colic D, Parra G, Gutkowska J. Atrial natriuretic factor in the acute nephritic and nephrotic syndromes. Kidney Int 1990;38: 512–517.
19. Geers AB, Koomans HA, Roos JC, Dorhout Mees EJ. Preservation of blood volume during edema removal in nephrotic subjects. Kidney Int 1985;28:652–657.
20. Humphreys MH. Mechanisms and management of nephrotic edema. Kidney Int 1994;45:266–281.
21. Schrier RW, Fassett RG. A critique of the overfill hypothesis of sodium and water retention in the nephrotic syndrome. Kidney Int 1998;53: 1111–1117.
22. Warwick GL, Fox JG, Boulton-Jones JM. The relationship between urinary albumin excretion rate and serum cholesterol in primary glomerular disease. Clin Nephrol 1994;41:135–137.
23. Wheeler DC, Bernard DB. Lipid abnormalities in the nephrotic syndrome: Causes, consequences, and treatment. Am J Kidney Dis 1994;23:331–346.
24. Kaysen GA, De Sain-van der Verlden M. New insights into lipid metabolism in the nephrotic syndrome. Kidney Int Suppl 1999;71: S18–21.
25. Llach F. Hypercoagulability, renal vein thrombosis, and other thrombotic complications of the nephrotic syndrome. Kidney Int 1985;28:429–439.
26. Ginsberg JM, Chang BS, Matarese RA, et al. Use of single voided urine samples to estimate quantitative proteinuria. N Engl J Med 1983;309: 1543–1546.
27. Ponticelli C, Passerini P. Treatment of the nephrotic syndrome associated with primary glomerulonephritis. Kidney Int 1994;46:595–604.
28. Klahr S, Levey A, Beck G, et al. The effects of dietary protein restriction and blood pressure control on the progression of chronic renal disease. N Engl J Med 1994;330:877–884.
29. Orth SR, Stockmann A, Conradt C, et al. Smoking as a risk factor for end-stage renal failure in men with primary renal disease. Kidney Int 1998;54: 926–31.
30. Fliser D, Schroter M, Neubeck M. Coadministration of thiazides increases the efficacy of loop diuretics even in patients with advanced renal failure. Kidney Int 1994;46:482–488.
31. Rudy DW, Voelker JR, Greene PK, et al. Loop diuretics for chronic renal insufficiency: A continuous infusion is more efficacious than bolus therapy. Ann Intern Med 1991;115:360–366.
32. Ruggenenti P, Perna A, Gherardi G, et al. Chronic proteinuric nephropathies: Outcomes and response to treatment in a prospective cohort of 352 patients with different patterns of renal injury. Am J Kidney Dis 2000;35:1155–1165.
33. Burgess E. Conservative treatment to slow deterioration of renal function: Evidence-based recommendations. Kidney Int Suppl 1999;70:S17–25.
34. Hostetter, TH. Prevention of end-stage renal disease due to type 2 diabetes. N Engl J Med 2001;345:910–11.
35. Gansevoot R, Slinter W, Hemmelder M, et al. Antiproteinuric effect of blood pressure lowering agents: A meta analysis of comparative trials. Nephrol Dial Transplant 1995;10:1963–1974.
36. Levey AS, Adler S, Caggiula AW, et al. Effects of dietary protein restriction on the progression of advanced renal disease in the Modification of Diet in Renal Disease Study. Am J Kidney Dis 1996;27:652–663.
37. Praga M, Hernandez E, Montoyo C, et al. Long-term beneficial effects of angiotensin-converting enzyme inhibition in patients with nephrotic proteinuria. Am J Kidney Dis 1992;20:240–248.
38. Gansevoort RT, de Zeeuw D, de Jong PE. Additive antiproteinuric effect of ACE inhibition and a low-protein diet in human renal disease. Nephrol Dial Transplant 1995;10:497–504.
39. Vriesendorp R, Donker AJM, de Zeeuw D, et al. Effects of nonsteroidal anti-inflammatory drugs on proteinuria. Am J Med 1986;81(suppl 2B): 84–94.
40. Heeg JA, de Jong PE, de Zeeuw D. Additive antiproteinuric effect of angiotensin-converting enzyme inhibition and non-steroidal anti-inflammatory drug therapy: A clue to the mechanism of action. Clin Sci 1991;81:367–372.
41. Don BR, Kaysen GA, Hutchinson FN, et al. The effect of angiotensin-converting enzyme inhibition and dietary protein restriction in the treatment of proteinuria. Am J Kidney Dis 1991;27:10–7.
42. ter Wee PM, Donker AJM. Pharmacologic manipulation of glomerular function. Kidney Int 1994;45:417–424.

43. Velosa JA, Torres VE. Benefits and risks of nonsteroidal antiinflammatory drugs in steroid-resistant nephrotic syndrome. Am J Kidney Dis 1986;8:345–350.
44. Ordonez JD, Hiatt RA, Killebrew EJ, Fireman BH. The increased risk of coronary heart disease associated with nephrotic syndrome. Kidney Int Suppl 1993;44:638–642.
45. Massy ZA, Ma JZ, Louis TA, Kasiske BL. Lipid-lowering therapy in patients with renal disease. Kidney Int 1995;48:188–198.
46. Coleman JE, Watson AR. Hyperlipidemia, diet and simvastatin therapy in steroid-resistant nephrotic syndrome of childhood. Pediatr Nephrol 1996;10:171–174.
47. Thomas ME, Harris KPG, Ramaswamy C, et al. Simvastatin therapy for hypercholesterolemic patients with nephrotic syndrome or significant proteinuria. Kidney Int 1993;44:1124–1129.
48. Oda H, Keane WF. Recent advances in statins and the kidney. Kidney Int Suppl 1999;71:S2–S5.
49. Keilani T, Schlueter WA, Levin ML, et al. Improvement of lipid abnormalities associated with proteinuria using fosinopril, an angiotensin-converting enzyme inhibitor. Ann Intern Med 1993;118:246–254.
50. Sarasin FP, Schifferli JA. Prophylactic oral anticoagulation in nephrotic patients with idiopathic membranous nephropathy. Kidney Int 1994;45: 578–585.
51. Rostoker G, Durand-Zaleski I, Petit-Phar M, et al. Prevention of thrombotic complications of the nephrotic syndrome by the low-molecular-weight heparin enoxaparin. Nephron 1995;69:20–28.
52. Nolasco F, Cameron JS, Heywood EF, et al. Adult-onset minimal-change nephrotic syndrome: A long-term follow-up. Kidney Int 1986;29: 1215–1223.
53. Jennette JC, Mandal AK. The nephrotic syndrome. In: Mandal AK, Jennette JC, eds. Diagnosis and Management of Renal Disease and Hypertension, 2nd ed. Durham, NC, Carolina Academic Press, 1994:235–272.
54. A report of the International Study of Kidney Disease in Children: The primary nephrotic syndrome in children. Identification of patients with minimal change nephrotic syndrome for initial response to prednisone. J Pediatr 1981;98:561–564.
55. Bargman JM. Management of minimal lesion glomerulonephritis: Evidence-based recommendations. Kidney Int Suppl 1999;70:S3–S16.
56. Tune BM, Mendoza SA. Treatment of the idiopathic nephrotic syndrome: Regimens and outcomes in children and adults. J Am Soc Nephrol 1997;8:824–832.
57. Siegel NJ. Minimal change nephropathy. In: Greenberg A, Cheung AK, Coffman TM et al., eds. Primer on Kidney Diseases, 2nd ed. San Diego, Academic Press, 1998:149–152.
58. Hiraoka M, Takeda N, Tsukahara H, et al. Favorable course of steroid-responsive nephrotic children with mild initial attack. Kidney Int 1995;47:1392–1393.
59. Cade R, Mars D, Privette M, et al. Effect of long-term azathioprine administration in adults with minimal-change glomerulonephritis and nephrotic syndrome resistant to corticosteroids. Arch Intern Med 1986;146:737–741.
60. A report of the International Study of Kidney Disease in Children: Minimal change nephrotic syndrome in children: Deaths during the first 5 to 15 years' observation. Pediatrics 1984;73:497–501.
61. Niaudel P, Habib R. Cyclosporine in the treatment of idiopathic nephrosis. J Am Soc Nephrol 1994;5:1049–1056.
62. Tejani A, Suthanthiran M, Pomrantz A. A randomized controlled trial of low-dose prednisone and ciclosporin versus high-dose prednisone in nephrotic syndrome of children. Nephron 1991;59:96–99.
63. Meyrier A, Noel H, Auriche P, Gallard P, and the Collaborative Group of the Societe de Nephrologie. Long-term renal tolerance of cyclosporin A treatment in adult idiopathic nephrotic syndrome. Kidney Int 1994;45: 1446–1456.
64. Meyrier A, Condamin M-C, Broneer D, and the Collaborative Group of the French Society of Nephrology. Treatment of adult idiopathic nephrotic syndrome with cyclosporin A: Minimal-change disease and focal-segmental glomerulosclerosis. Clin Nephrol 1991;35(suppl 1): S37–S42.
65. Hulton SA, Neuhans TJ, Dillon MJ, Barratt TM. Long-term cyclosporin A treatment of minimal-change nephrotic syndrome of childhood. Pediatr Nephrol 1994;8:401–403.
66. Hino S, Takemura T, Okada M, et al. Follow-up study of children with nephrotic syndrome treated with a long-term moderate dose of cyclosporine. Am J Kidney Dis 1998;31:932–9.
67. British Association for Paediatric Nephrology. Levamisole for corticosteroid-dependent nephrotic syndrome in childhood. Lancet 1991; 337:1555–1557.
68. Weiss R. Randomized, double-blind, placebo controlled trial of levamisole for children with frequently relapsing/steroid dependent nephrotic syndrome. J Am Soc Nephrol 1993;4:289.
69. Dayal U, Dayal A, Shastry JCM, Raghupathy P. Use of levamisole in maintaining remission in steroid-sensitive nephrotic syndrome in children. Nephron 1994;66:408–412.
70. Xu J, Qian T, Jiang J, et al. Clinical studies in the use of BCG and levamisole in the treatment of glomerulonephritis. Nephrol Dial Transplant 1991;6:548–553.
71. Black DA, Rose G, Brewer DB. Controlled trial of prednisone in adult patients with the nephrotic syndrome. Br Med J 1970;3:421–426.
72. D'Agati V. The many masks of focal segmental glomerulosclerosis. Kidney Int 1994;46:1223–1241.
73. Rennke HG, Klein PS. Pathogenesis and significance of nonprimary focal and segmental glomerulosclerosis. Am J Kidney Dis 1989;13:443–456.
74. Korbet SM. Primary focal segmental glomerulosclerosis. J Am Soc Nephrol 1998;9:1333–1340.
75. Schwartz MM, Evans J, Bain R, Korbet SM. Focal segmental glomerulosclerosis: Prognostic implications of the cellular lesion. J Am Soc Nephrol 1999;10:1900–1907.
76. Korbet SM, Schwartz MM, Lewis EJ. Primary focal segmental glomerulosclerosis: Clinical course and response to therapy. Am J Kidney Dis 1994;23:773–783.
77. Banfi G, Moriggi M, Sabadini E, et al. The impact of prolonged immunosuppression on the outcome of idiopathic focal-segmental glomerulosclerosis with nephrotic syndrome in adults. A collaborative retrospective study. Clin Nephrol 1991;36:53–59.
78. Ponticelli C, Villa M, Banfi G, et al. Can prolonged treatment improve the prognosis in adults with focal segmental glomerulosclerosis? Am J Kidney Dis 1999;34:618–25.
79. Burgess E. Management of focal segmental glomerulosclerosis: Evidence-based recommendations. Kidney Int Suppl 1999;70:S26–32.
80. Tune BM, Lieberman E, Mendoza SA. Steroid-resistant nephrotic focal segmental glomerulosclerosis: A treatable disease. Pediatr Nephrol 1996; 10:772–778.
81. Ponticelli C, Rizzoni G, Edefonti A, et al. A randomized trial of cyclosporine in steroid-resistant idiopathic nephrotic syndrome. Kidney Int 1993;43:1377–1384.
82. Ingulli E, Singh A, Baqi N, et al. Aggressive, long-term cyclosporine therapy for steroid-resistant focal segmental glomerulosclerosis. J Am Soc Nephrol 1995;5:1820–1825.
83. Ingulli E, Tejani A. Severe hypercholesterolemia inhibits cyclosporin A efficacy in a dose-dependent manner in children with nephrotic syndrome. J Am Soc Nephrol 1992;3:254–259.
84. Cattran DC, Appel GB, Hebert LA, et al. A randomized trial of cyclosporine in patients with steroid-resistant focal segmental glomerulosclerosis. Kidney Int 1999;56:2220–2226.
85. Cattran DC, Rao P. Long-term outcome in children and adults with classic focal segmental glomerulosclerosis. Am J Kidney Dis 1998;32:72–79.
86. Tejani A, Stablein DH. Recurrence of focal segmental glomerulosclerosis posttransplantation: A special report of the North American Pediatric Renal Transplant Cooperative Study. J Am Soc Nephrol 1992;2:S258–S263.
87. Mowry J, Marik J, Cohen A, et al. Treatment of recurrent focal segmental glomerulosclerosis with high-dose cyclosporine A and plasmapheresis. Transplant Proc 1993;25:1345–1346.
88. Artero M, Biava C, Amend W, et al. Recurrent focal glomerulosclerosis: Natural history and response to therapy. Am J Med 1992;92:375–383.

89. Wasserstein AG. Membranous glomerulonephritis. J Am Soc Nephrol 1997;8:664–674.
90. Geddes CC, Cattran DC. The treatment of idiopathic membranous nephropathy. Semin Nephrol 2000;20:299–308.
91. Burstein DM, Korbert SM, Schwartz MM. Membranous glomerulonephritis and malignancy. Am J Kidney Dis 1993;22:5–10.
92. Heidet L, Gagnadoux ME, Beziau A, et al. Recurrence of de novo membranous glomerulonephritis on renal grafts. Clin Nephrol 1994;41:314–318.
93. Kerjaschi D. Molecular pathogenesis of membranous nephropathy. Kidney Int 1992;41:1090–1105.
94. Bernard DB. Extrarenal complications of the nephrotic syndrome. Kidney Int 1988;33:1184–1202.
95. Rostoker G, Maadi AB, Remy P, et al. Low-dose angiotensin-converting-enzyme inhibitor captopril to reduce proteinuria in adult idiopathic membranous nephropathy: A prospective study of long-term treatment. Nephrol Dial Transplant 1995;10:25–29.
96. Ponticelli C, Altieri P, Scolari F, et al. A randomized study comparing methylprednisolone plus chlorambucil versus methylprednisolone plus cyclophosphamide in idiopathic membranous nephropathy. J Am Soc Nephrol 1998;9:444–450.
97. Ponticelli C, Zucchelli P, Passerini P, et al. A 10–year follow-up of a randomized study with methylprednisolone and chlorambucil in membranous nephropathy. Kidney Int 1995;48:1600–1604.
98. Imperiale TF, Goldfarb S, Berns JS. Are cytotoxic agents beneficial in idiopathic membranous nephropathy? A meta-analysis of the controlled trials. J Am Soc Nephrol 1995;5:1553–1558.
99. Glassock RJ. Therapy of idiopathic nephrotic syndrome in adults. A conservative or aggressive approach? Am J Nephrol 1993;13:422–428.
100. Cameron JS. Membranous nephropathy is still a treatment dilemma. N Engl J Med 1992;327:638–639.
101. Hebert LA. Therapy of membranous nephropathy: What to do after (meta) analyses. J Am Soc Nephrol 1995;5:1543–1545.
102. Piccoli A, Pillon L, Passerini P, et al. Therapy for idiopathic membranous nephropathy: Tailoring the choice by decision analysis. Kidney Int 1994; 45:1193–1202.
103. Branten AJ, Reichert LJ, Koene RA, et al. Oral cyclophosphamide versus chlorambucil in the treatment of patients with membranous nephropathy and renal insufficiency. QJM 1998;91:359–66.
104. Warwick GL, Geddes CG, Boulton-Jones JM. Prednisolone and chlorambucil therapy for idiopathic membranous nephropathy with progressive renal failure. QJM 1994;87:223–229.
105. Falk RJ, Hogan SL, Muller KE, et al. Treatment of progressive membranous glomerulopathy. A randomized trial comparing cyclophosphamide and corticosteroids with corticosteroids alone. The Glomerular Disease Collaborative Network. Ann Intern Med 1992;116:438–445.
106. Cattran DC, Greenwood C, Ritchie S, et al. A controlled trial of cyclosporine in patients with progressive membranous nephropathy. Kidney Int 1995;47:1130–1135.
107. Fritsche L, Budde K, Farber L, et al. Treatment of membranous glomerulopathy with cyclosporin A. How much patience is required? Nephrol Dial Transplant 1999;14:1036–1038.
108. Cattran DC, Pei Y, Greenwood CM, et al. Validation of a predictive model of idiopathic membranous nephropathy: Its clinical and research implications. Kidney Int 1997;51:901–907.
109. Lin CY. Treatment of hepatitis B virus-associated membranous nephropathy with recombinant alpha-interferon. Kidney Int 1995;47: 225–230.
110. Lai KN, Tam JS, Lin HJ, et al. The therapeutic dilemma of the usage of corticosteroid in patients with membranous nephropathy and persistent hepatitis B virus surface antigenaemia. Nephron 1990;54:12–17.
111. Ramos EL, Tisher CC. Recurrent diseases in the kidney transplant. Am J Kidney Dis 1994;24:142–154.
112. Rennke HG. Secondary membranoproliferative glomerulonephritis. Kidney Int 1995;47:643–656.
113. D'Amico G, Ferrario F. Mesangiocapillary glomerulonephritis. J Am Soc Nephrol 1992;2:S159–S166.
114. Levin A. Management of membranoproliferative glomerulonephritis: Evidence-based recommendations. Kidney Int Suppl 1999;70:S41–46.
115. Tarshish P, Bernstein J, Tobin JN, et al. Treatment of mesangiocapillary glomerulonephritis with alternate-day prednisone—A report of the International Study of Kidney Disease in Children. Pediatr Nephrol 1992; 6:123–130.
116. Zimmerman SW, Moorthy AV, Dreher WH, et al. Prospective trial of warfarin and dipyridamole in patients with membranoproliferative glomerulonephritis. Am J Med 1983;75:920–927.
117. Cattran DC. Current status of cyclosporin A in the treatment of membranous, IgA and membranoproliferative glomerulonephritis. Clin Nephrol 1991;35(suppl 1):S43–S47.
118. Donadio JV, Grande JP. Immunoglobulin A nephropathy: A clinical perspective. J Am Soc Nephrol 1997;8:1324–1332.
119. Floege J, Feehally J. IgA nephropathy: recent developments. J Am Soc Nephrol 2000;11:2395–2403.
120. Nolin L, Courteau M. Management of IgA nephropathy: Evidence-based recommendations. Kidney Int Suppl 1999;70:S56–S62.
121. Egido J, Rivera F, Sancho J, Barat A, Hernando L. Phenytoin in IgA nephropathy: A long-term controlled trial. Nephron 1984;38:30–39.
122. Béné MC, Hurault de Ligny B, Kessler M, et al. Tonsils in IgA nephropathy. Contrib Nephrol 1993;104:153–161.
123. Pozzi C, Bolasco PG, Fogazzi GB, et al. Corticosteroids in IgA nephropathy: A randomized controlled trial. Lancet 1999;353:883–887.
124. Schena FR, Montenegro M, Scivittaro V. Meta-analysis of randomized controlled trials in patients with IgA nephropathy (Berger's disease). Nephrol Dial Transplant 1990;5(suppl 1):47–52.
125. Yoshikawa N, Ito H. Combined therapy with prednisolone, azathioprine, heparin-warfarin, and dipyridamole for paediatric patients with severe IgA nephropathy: Is it relevant for adult patients? Nephrol Dial Transplant 1999;14:1097–1099.
126. Donadio JV, Bergstralh EJ, Offord KP, et al. A controlled trial of fish oil in IgA nephropathy. N Engl J Med 1994;331:1194–1199.
127. Dillon JJ. Fish oil therapy for IgA nephropathy: Efficacy and interstudy variability. J Am Soc Nephrol 1997;8:1739–1744.
128. Strihou CY. Fish oil for IgA nephropathy. N Engl J Med 1994;331: 1227–1229.
129. Donadio JV, Larson TS, Bergstralh EJ, et al. A randomized trial of high-doe compared with low-dose omega-3 fatty acids in severe IgA nephropathy. J Am Soc Nephrol 2001;12:791–799.
130. Cattran DC, Greenwood C, Ritchie S. Long-term benefits of angiotensin-converting enzyme inhibitor therapy in patients with severe immunoglobulin A nephropathy: A comparison to patients receiving treatment with other antihypertensive agents and to patients receiving no therapy. Am J Kidney Dis 1994;23:247–254.
131. Hunley T, Julian B, Phillips J. Angiotensin converting enzyme gene polymorphisms: Potential silencer motif and impact on progression in IgA nephropathy. Kidney Int 1996;49:571–577.
132. Perico N, Remuzzi A, Sangalli F, et al. The antiproteinuric effect of angiotensin antagonism inhuman IgA nephropathy is potentiated by indomethacin. J Am Soc Nephrol 1998,9:2308–2317.
133. Russo D, Pisani A, Balletta MM, et al. Additive antiproteinuric effect of converting enzyme inhibitor and losartan in normotensive patients with IgA nephropathy. Am J Kidney Dis 1999;33:851–856.
134. Dillon JJ. Treating IgA nephropathy. J Am Soc Nephrol 2001;12: 846–847.
135. Rostoker G, Desvaux-Belghiti D, Pilatte Y, et al. High-dose immunoglobulin therapy for severe IgA nephropathy and Henoch-Schönlein purpura. Ann Intern Med 1994;120:476–484.
136. Sanz-Guajardo D. Plasmapheresis in the treatment of glomerulonephritis: indications and complications. Am J Kidney Dis 2000;36:liv–lvi.
137. Buemi M, Allegra A, Corica F, et al. Effect of fluvastatin on proteinuria in patients with immunoglobulin A nephropathy. Clin Pharmacol Ther 2000;67:427–431.
138. Mills JA. Systemic lupus erythematosus. N Engl J Med 1994;330: 1871–1879.
139. Kashgarian M. Lupus nephritis: Lessons from the path lab. Kidney Int 1994;45:928–938.

140. Cameron JS. Lupus nephritis. J Am Soc Nephrol 1999;10:413–424.
141. Berden JHM. Lupus nephritis. Kidney Int 1997;52:538–558.
142. Schwartz MM, Lan SP, Bernstein J, et al. Role of pathology indices in the management of severe lupus glomerulonephritis. Kidney Int 1992;42: 743–748.
143. Gruppo Italiano per lo Studio della Neffrite Lupica (GISNEL). Lupus nephritis: Prognostic factors and probability of maintaining life-supporting renal function 10 years after the diagnosis. Am J Kidney Dis 1992;19:473–479.
144. Bansal VK, Beto JA. Treatment of lupus nephritis: A meta-analysis of clinical trials. Am J Kidney Dis 1997;29:193–199.
145. Gourley MF, Austin HA, Scott D, et al. Methylprednisolone and cyclophosphamide, alone or in combination, in patients with lupus nephritis. A randomized, controlled trial. Ann Intern Med 1996;125:549–557.
146. Dooley MA, Cosio FG, Nachman PH. Mycophenolate mofetil therapy in lupus nephritis: Clinical observations. J Am Soc Nephrol 1999;10: 833–839.
147. Wallace DJ. Clinical and pharmacological experience with LJP-394. Expert Opin Investig Drugs 2001;10:111–117.
148. Kalled SL, Cutler AH, Datta SK, Thomas DW. Anti-CD40 ligand antibody treatment of SNF1 mice with established nephritis: Preservation of kidney function. J Immunol 1998;160:2158–65.
149. Zoja C, Corna D, Benedetti G, et al. Bindarit retards renal disease and prolongs survival in murine lupus autoimmune disease. Kidney Int 1998; 53:726–734.
150. Boumpas DT, Austin HA, Vaughan EM, et al. Risk for sustained amenorrhea in patients with systemic lupus erythematosus receiving intermittent pulse cyclophosphamide therapy. Ann Intern Med 1993;119:366–369.
151. Austin HA, Balow JE. Treatment of lupus nephritis. Semin Nephrol 2000; 20:265–276.
152. Balow JE, Boumpas DT, Austin HA. New prospects for treatment of lupus nephritis. Semin Nephrol 2000;20:32–39.
153. Clark WF, Jevnikar AM. Renal transplantation for end-stage renal disease caused by systemic lupus erythematosus nephritis. Semin Nephrol 1999; 19:77–85.
154. Clark WF, Jevnikar AM. Renal transplantation for end-stage renal disease caused by systemic lupus erythematosus nephritis. Semin Nephrol 1999; 19:77–85.
155. Couser WG. Rapidly progressive glomerulonephritis: Classification, pathogenetic mechanisms, and therapy. Am J Kidney Dis 1988;11: 449–464.
156. Jennette JC, Falk RJ. Diagnosis and management of glomerulonephritis and vasculitis presenting as acute renal failure. Med Clin North Am 1990; 74:893–908.
157. Kallenberg CGM, Brouwer E, Weening JJ, et al. Anti-neutrophil cytoplasmic antibodies: Current diagnostic and pathophysiological potential. Kidney Int 1994;46:1–15.
158. Jindal KK. Management of idiopathic crescentic and diffuse proliferative glomerulonephritis: Evidence-based recommendations. Kidney Int Suppl 1999;70:S33–40.
159. Bolton WK. Treatment of glomerular disease: ANCA-negative RPGN. Semin Nephrol 2000;20:244–255.
160. Madore F, Lazarus MJ, Brady HR. Therapeutic plasma exchange in renal disease. J Am Soc Nephrol 1996;7:367–385.
161. Falk RJ, Nachman PH, Hogna SL, et al. ANCA glomerulonephritis and vasculitis: A Chapel Hill perspective. Semin Nephrol 2000;20:233–243.
162. Nachman PH, Segelmark M, Westman K, et al. Recurrent ANCA-associated small-vessel vasculitis after transplantation: A pooled analysis. Kidney Int 1999;56:1544–1550.
163. Couser WG, Johnson RJ. Postinfective glomerulonephritis. In: Neilson EG, Couser WG, eds. Immunologic Renal Diseases. Philadelphia, Lippincott-Raven, 1997:915–944.
164. Rodriguez-Iturbe B, Parra G. Glomerulonephritis associated with infection: Poststreptococcal glomerulonephritis. In Massry SG, Glassock RJ, ed. Massry & Glassock's Textbook of Nephrology, 4th ed. Philadelphia, Lippincott Williams & Wilkins, 2001;667–671.
165. Parra G, Rodriguez-Iturbe B, Batsford S, et al. Antibody to streptococcal zymogen in the serum of patients with acute glomerulonephritis: a multicentric study. Kidney Int 1998;54:509–517.
166. Weinstein L, Le Frock J. Does antimicrobial therapy of streptococcal pharyngitis or pyoderma alter the risk of glomerulonephritis? J Infect Dis 1971;124:229–231.
167. Moudgil A, Bagga A, Fredrich R, et al. Poststreptococcal and other infection-related glomerulonephritides. In: Greenberg A, ed. Primer on Kidney Diseases, 2nd ed. San Diego, Academic Press, 1998:193–199.
168. Baldwin DS. Post-streptococcal glomerulonephritis: A progressive disease? Am J Med 1977;62:1–11.
169. Pinto SW, Sesso R, Vasconcelos E, et al. Follow-up of patients with epidemic poststreptococcal glomerulonephritis. Am J Kidney Dis 2001; 38:249–255.

50

Drug Therapy Individualization for Patients with Renal Insufficiency

Reginald F. Frye and Gary R. Matzke

Patients with renal insufficiency are commonly encountered in clinical practice. Reductions in renal function can be associated with disease states, drug effects (e.g., drug-induced nephrotoxicity), or the result of the known age-related maturation or diminution of renal function. In children, renal function does not mature to adult values until approximately 1 year of age. In older adults, age-related declines in renal function combined with the increased use of medications make this patient group particularly susceptible to adverse effects secondary to inappropriate pharmacotherapy.[1] The presence of compromised renal function in any patient age group, ranging from pediatric to geriatric, requires that the clinician understand the aspects of drug disposition that are altered in the presence of renal insufficiency and the appropriate methods to individualize drug therapy.[2,3]

Renal insufficiency is accompanied by progressive alterations in several other organ systems and results in the development of anemia, hyperparathyroidism, bleeding abnormalities, hyperlipidemia, hypertension, and changes in gastrointestinal (GI) tract integrity (see Chaps. 44 and 45). There are now many reports that document changes in the disposition of some drugs in patients with renal insufficiency as the result of changes in bioavailability,[4] protein binding,[5,6] distribution volume,[7] and metabolic activity.[8]

Drug therapy individualization for patients with renal insufficiency may require only a simple dose adjustment based on the fractional reduction in creatinine clearance.[9] However, the use of medications that are extensively metabolized or for which dramatic changes in protein binding and/or distribution volume have been noted may require a more complex adjustment.[7,9] Furthermore, because of the physiologic and biochemical changes associated with progressive renal insufficiency, patients may respond to a given dose or serum concentration of a drug differently than patients with normal renal function.[10]

Knowledge of basic pharmacokinetic principles combined with the drug disposition properties of a particular compound and the degree and type of pathophysiologic alterations associated with renal insufficiency makes it possible for the pharmacotherapist to design an individualized therapeutic regimen. This chapter describes the influence of renal insufficiency on drug absorption, distribution, metabolism, and elimination, and provides a practical approach for drug dosage individualization for patients with reduced renal function as well as those receiving continuous renal replacement therapy, continuous ambulatory peritoneal dialysis, or hemodialysis.

EFFECT ON DRUG ABSORPTION

There is little quantitative information regarding the influence of impaired renal function on drug absorption and bioavailability. Drug bioavailability in this patient population may be altered by several factors, including changes in GI transit time and gastric pH; edema of the GI tract; vomiting and diarrhea (frequent complications of severe renal insufficiency); and antacid administration. The assessment of bioavailability in this patient population is further complicated, because most patients with severe renal insufficiency receive multiple medications, many of which cannot be discontinued during the course of a bioavailability study.

Some of the drug absorption "bioavailability" studies in patients with renal failure have not provided an assessment of absolute bioavailability (i.e., they have not included intravenous administration of the drug). Rather, they have documented alterations in the peak concentration (C_{max}), time at which the peak concentration was attained (t_{max}), or in the fractional amount of drug recovered in the urine in a finite time period. Unfortunately, this limited information has been extrapolated to suggest that drug absorption is slowed and/or that the extent of absorption is reduced.[5]

The absolute bioavailability of only a few drug compounds is affected. An increase in bioavailability as the result of a decrease in metabolism during the drug's first pass through the GI tract and liver has been noted for a few agents.[5,7] The increased bioavailability of four β-blockers (tolamolol, bufuralol, oxprenolol, and propranolol), dextropropoxyphene, and dihydrocodeine are because of this mechanism. Although the bioavailability of these compounds is increased, clinical consequences (development of excessive or unexpected adverse effects) have been demonstrated only with dextropropoxyphene and dihydrocodeine. The lack of association between the pharmacokinetic profile and clinical consequences of the β-blockers may be a result of an alteration in the responsiveness of patients with renal disease to these agents, as has been reported with propranolol in the elderly.[11]

EFFECT ON DRUG DISTRIBUTION

The volume of distribution of many drugs may be significantly increased or decreased in patients with renal insufficiency (Table 50–1).[7,12,13] Alterations in distribution volume may result from increased or decreased protein binding; altered tissue binding; or pathophysiologic alterations in body composition, for example, the fractional contribution of total body water to total body weight; or they may be an artifact of the volume term used in the comparison.

Generally, the plasma protein binding of acidic drugs (e.g., warfarin, phenytoin) is decreased in uremia[6,14] (Table 50–2), whereas the binding of basic drugs (quinidine, lidocaine) is usually normal or slightly decreased or increased[6,15,16] (Table 50–3). The decrease in binding of acidic drugs in uremic plasma has been attributed to qualitative changes in the binding sites, accumulation of endogenous inhibitors of binding, and decreased concentrations of albumin. The first two of these mechanisms appear to account for most of the observed changes in binding. In addition, the high concentrations of metabolites of some compounds that accumulate in patients with renal insufficiency may interfere with the protein binding of the parent compound.

TABLE 50–1. Effect of ESRD on the Volume of Distribution of Selected Drugs*

	Normal	ESRD	Change from Normal (%)
Increased			
Amikacin	0.20	0.29	45
Azlocillin	0.21	0.28	33
Bretylium	3.58	4.48	25
Cefazolin	0.13	0.17	31
Cefonicid	0.11	0.14	27
Cefoxitin	0.16	0.26	63
Cefuroxime	0.20	0.26	30
Clofibrate	0.14	0.24	71
Cloxacillin	0.14	0.26	86
Dicloxacillin	0.08	0.18	125
Erythromycin	0.57	1.09	91
Furosemide	0.11	0.18	64
Gentamicin	0.20	0.32	60
Isoniazid	0.6	0.8	33
Minoxidil	2.6	4.9	88
Nalmefene	7.9	14.7	86
Naproxen	0.12	0.17	42
Phenytoin	0.64	1.4	119
Trimethoprim	1.36	1.83	35
Vancomycin	0.64	0.85	33
Decreased			
Chloramphenicol	0.87	0.60	−31
Digoxin	7.3	4.0	−45
Ethambutol	3.7	1.6	−57
Methicillin	0.45	0.30	−33
Pindolol	150 L	80 L	−47
Pipemidic acid	2.0	0.84	−58

*All data are in liters per kilogram unless otherwise stated.

TABLE 50–2. Change in Percent Unbound of Acidic Drugs in Patients with Normal Renal Function and End-Stage Renal Disease (ESRD)

	Normal	ESRD	Change from Normal (%)
Abecarnil	4	15	275
Azlocillin	62.5	75	20
Cefazolin	16	29	81
Cefoxitin	27	59	119
Ceftriaxone	10	20	100
Clofibrate	3	9	200
Cloxacillin	5	20	300
Diazoxide	6	16	167
Dicloxacillin	3	9	200
Diflunisal	12	44	267
Doxycycline	12	28	133
Furosemide	4	6	50
Methotrexate	57.2	63.8	12
Metolazone	5	10	100
Moxalactam	48	64	33
Naproxen	0.2	0.8	300
Pentobarbital	34	41	21
Phenylbutazone	5.5	16	191
Phenytoin	10	21.5	115
Piretanide	6	12	100
Salicylate	8	20	150
Sulfamethoxazole	34	58	71
Valproic acid	8	23	188
Warfarin	1	2	100
Zomepirac	1.3	3.8	192

TABLE 50–3. Change in Percent Unbound of Basic Drugs in Patients with Normal Renal Function and End-Stage Renal Disease (ESRD)

	Normal	ESRD	Change from Normal (%)
Decreased			
Bepridil	0.3	0.1	−67
Clonidine	55.6	47.6	−14
Disopyramide	32	28	−13
Propafenone	3.4	2.4	−29
Increased			
Amphotericin B	3.5	4.1	17
Chloramphenicol	45	64	42
Clonazepam	13.9	16	15
Clorazepate	2	5	150
Diazepam	2	8	300
Fluoxetine	5.5	6.5	18
Ketoconazole	1	1.5	50
Morphine	65	71	9
Prazosin	6	10.1	68
Triamterene	19	43	126

Although the fraction of unbound drug increases in patients with renal insufficiency, a new equilibrium is established as a result of increased drug elimination/distribution such that the free concentrations remain comparable. However, total concentrations are reduced because of an increase in drug clearance. Thus, the net effect of changes in protein binding is an alteration in the relationship between total drug concentrations and effect. This can be illustrated with the anticonvulsant phenytoin. The protein binding of this acidic drug, which binds to albumin, is significantly reduced as a result of endogenous substances that accumulate in renal failure and compete for binding, as well as by conformational changes in albumin in patients with end-stage renal disease.[17] This change in protein binding alters the relationship between total phenytoin concentration and effect or toxicity. The resulting increase in unbound fraction, from the normal of 0.1 to 0.2 or more, results in increased hepatic clearance and decreased total concentrations. Thus, in patients with renal insufficiency, the therapeutic range (normal, 10–20 μg/mL) shifts downward as the degree of renal impairment increases. Although the unbound concentration therapeutic range is unchanged in the presence of renal failure, unbound concentrations are often not measured. However, unbound concentration measurements provide the best means for individualizing phenytoin therapy in patients with renal insufficiency. Methods have been presented to equate an observed total concentration in patients with end-stage renal disease receiving hemodialysis treatment to what would be expected in patients with normal renal function.

Predicting the degree of protein binding in individuals improves the ability to interpret total drug concentrations. Liponi et al.[17] suggested a method by which the total phenytoin concentration (C_m^{total}) in patients with creatinine clearance values of 10–24 mL/min or less than 10 mL/min can be equated to the concentration that would be observed if plasma protein concentrations and phenytoin-binding characteristics were normal. A patient's "equated" total phenytoin concentration (C_e^{total}) would thus equal:

$$C_e^{total} = \left(\frac{1}{[1] + [(nK_a)(p)]}\right)\left(C_m^{total}\right)(10)$$

where nK_a is the binding parameter based on the patient's renal function (10–24 mL/min = 1.5, and <10 mL/min = 1.0), and p is the measured serum albumin concentration. This methodology allows one to approximate the equivalent "total" phenytoin concentration in a patient with reduced renal function and can be used to predict dosage requirements via a standard nonlinear approach (see Chap. 4).

The principal binding protein for several basic drug compounds is α_1-acid glycoprotein (AAG), an acute-phase reactant whose plasma concentration is increased in a wide variety of patients, including renal transplant patients and hemodialysis patients.[7] The fraction of those drugs principally bound to AAG may be significantly increased in uremic patients.[6] Thus, patients with renal insufficiency may experience increased or decreased protein binding depending on the principal binding protein for the drug in question.

Altered tissue binding may also affect the apparent volume of distribution of a drug. The distribution volume of digoxin has been reported to be reduced by 30% to 50% from normal values in patients with renal disease.[18] It has been postulated that this reduction in the distribution volume is secondary to a decrease in tissue binding as a result of competitive inhibition by endogenous or exogenous substances. This factor must therefore be considered when designing individualized dosage regimens. Multiple methods have been proposed to estimate the degree of reduction in digoxin's distribution volume.[18] The volume of distribution of digoxin can be estimated as follows:

$$V_{\mathrm{D(liters)}} = [226] + \left[\frac{(298)(\mathrm{CLcr})}{29.1 + \mathrm{CLcr}}\right]$$

For a patient weighing 60 kg with a creatinine clearance (CLcr) of approximately 15 mL/min, the volume of distribution for digoxin would be:

$$V_{\mathrm{D(liters)}} = [226] + \left[\frac{(298)(15)}{29.1 + 15}\right] = 327\ \mathrm{L\ or\ 5.5\ L/kg\ TBW}$$

This represents a 30% reduction from the volume of distribution that would have been anticipated in a patient with normal renal function. Acidosis or the presence of digoxin-like immunoreactive substances that bind to and inhibit membrane ATPase may also contribute to this phenomenon.[19] In this situation, the absolute amount of digoxin bound to the receptor is reduced and the resultant serum digoxin concentration from any dose would be greater.

Knowledge of protein and tissue binding changes in patients with renal insufficiency is critically important in the interpretation of serum drug concentrations. Numerous investigations show that the unbound concentration of several drugs in plasma correlates more closely with the concentration of drug at the receptor site and, therefore, with the pharmacologic effect, than does the total concentration of drug in plasma.[20] Because an alteration in plasma protein or tissue binding of a drug will likely alter the total drug concentration, the usual expected relationship between total drug concentration and pharmacologic response will be perturbed, but the relationship to unbound drug should be unaffected.

Thus, in patients with renal insufficiency, particularly those with end stage renal disease (ESRD), a "normal" total drug concentration may be associated with either serious adverse reactions secondary to elevated unbound drug concentrations or subtherapeutic responses because of an altered plasma to tissue drug concentration ratio. The monitoring of unbound drug concentrations in this patient population is therefore suggested for those drugs that have a narrow therapeutic range, are highly protein bound (free fraction of $<20\%$), and for which marked variability in the free fraction has been reported, for example, phenytoin and disopyramide.

Finally, the method used to calculate the volume of distribution may be influenced by renal disease. The three most commonly used volume of distribution terms are volume of the central compartment (V_c), volume of the terminal phase (V_β, V_{area}), and volume of distribution at steady state (V_{ss}). The central compartment volume is calculated as the intravenous bolus dose divided by the initial plasma concentration. V_c for many drugs approximates extracellular fluid volume and thus may be increased or decreased by shifts in this physiologic volume. Renal insufficiency, especially oliguric acute renal failure, is often accompanied by fluid overload and a resultant increased V_c due to reduced renal elimination of water and sodium. V_{area} or V_β is calculated as the total body clearance divided by the terminal elimination rate constant (k or β). This volume term represents the proportionality constant between plasma concentrations in the terminal elimination phase and the amount of drug remaining in the body. V_β is affected by both distribution characteristics, as well as by the elimination rate constant. The third volume term, the steady-state volume of distribution (V_{ss}), is calculated as (AUMC × Dose)/AUC^2, where AUMC is the area under the first moment of the concentration-time curve and AUC is the area under the concentration-time curve (see Chap. 4). V_β and V_{ss} will often be similar in magnitude, with V_β being slightly larger. In situations in which V_β is much larger than V_{ss}, V_β may reflect the elimination rate more than the distribution volume. Because V_{ss} has the advantage of being independent of drug elimination, it may be the most appropriate volume term to use when one desires to compare drug distribution volumes between patients with renal insufficiency and those with normal renal function.[21]

EFFECT ON METABOLISM

Although the role of the kidneys as an excretory organ for drugs and chemicals and their polar metabolites is well described, the fact that the kidney is very metabolically active in the biotransformation of a variety of drugs is not well appreciated.[7,8] The renal cytochrome P450 (CYP) system catalyzes the metabolism of a variety of chemicals and drugs with an activity that may equal that of the liver on an activity per gram of tissue basis. Whole-kidney homogenate CYP activity has varied from 14% to 18% of that observed in the liver. Glucuronide, glutathione, and sulfate conjugation activity has also been documented in kidney homogenates. Prescott and associates[22] demonstrated that *p*-aminohippurate (PAH), a compound frequently used to estimate effective renal plasma flow, is converted to *N*-acetyl-PAH by the human kidney and liver. This metabolism accounts for up to 25% of the total elimination of PAH. These studies clearly suggest that the kidney possesses considerable drug-metabolizing capability. However, the contribution to the total metabolic activity is generally low, because total kidney weight is far less than liver weight.

Investigations of the effect of chronic renal failure on hepatic enzyme activity in animals have demonstrated reductions in some, but not all pathways of drug metabolism.[8] The mechanism by which chronic renal failure may affect hepatic drug metabolism is not clearly known. However, it has been shown in rat models of chronic renal failure that protein expression of several CYP enzymes, including CYP3A1 and CYP3A2 (corresponding to human CYP3A4), is reduced in the liver by as much as 75%. The mechanism of this decrease in protein content is reduced mRNA expression, indicating transcriptionally mediated down-regulation.[23] The *in vivo* relevance of these effects was demonstrated in rats with chronic renal failure using enzyme-selective breath tests; the results showed that chronic renal failure has differential effects on enzyme activity with CYP2C11 and CYP3A2 being significantly reduced (by 35%), while CYP1A2 activity was not different from control animals.[24] Collectively, these data indicate that chronic renal impairment has

TABLE 50–4. Effect of ESRD on Nonrenal Clearance

Decreased			
Acyclovir	Aztreonam	Bufuralol	Captopril
Cefmenoxime	Cefmetazole	Cefonicid	Cefotaxime
Cefotiam	Cefsulodin	Ceftizoxime	Cilastatin
Cimetidine	Ciprofloxacin	Cortisol	Encainide
Erythromycin	Erythromycin	Imipenem	Isoniazid
Methylprednisol	Metoclopramide	Moxalactam	Nicardipine
Nimodipine	Nitrendipine	Procainamide	Quinapril
Verapamil	Zidovudine		
Unchanged			
Acetaminophen	Chloramphenicol	Clonidine	Codeine
Diflunisal	Indomethacin	Insulin*	Isradipine
Lidocaine	Morphine	Metoprolol	Nisoldipine
Nortriptyline	Pentobarbital	Propafenone	Quinidine
Theophylline	Tocainide	Tolbutamide	
Increased			
Bumetanide	Cefpiramide	Fosinopril	Nifedipine
Phenytoin	Sulfadimidine		

*May be unchanged or decreased.

a detrimental effect on drug metabolism in the kidney, as well as on drug metabolism within the liver. Clinical data to support this premise include observations of reduced nonrenal clearance for several drugs in patients with renal insufficiency.[10] The observed reductions in nonrenal clearance are generally proportional to the reductions in glomerular filtration rate (GFR). The effect(s) of renal failure on nonrenal drug clearance may also depend on whether the renal failure is acute or chronic. Effects observed in acute renal failure do not appear to be as great as those observed in chronic renal failure, potentially due to less accumulation of or exposure to metabolic inhibitors.[10]

Drug metabolism may be increased, decreased, or unaffected by renal failure depending on the drug and the species (animals versus man) investigated[22,25,26] (Table 50–4). These studies should be interpreted cautiously because concurrent drug intake, age, smoking habit, and alcohol intake often were not controlled. Furthermore, the possibility of pharmacogenetic variation must be considered. Prediction of the effect of renal impairment on the metabolism of a particular drug is thus difficult; for example, nifedipine, nitrendipine, and nisoldipine are all apparently metabolized *in vivo* by CYP3A4, yet the metabolism of nifedipine is increased,[27] the metabolism of nitrendipine is decreased,[28] and the metabolism of nisoldipine is unaffected by renal failure.[29] The effect of renal insufficiency on other CYP enzymes has not been fully evaluated, but preliminary data suggest a differential effect on the individual isozymes with the activity of some enzymes (CYP2C19) being reduced, while others (CYP2D6) are not affected.[30] This differential effect on individual enzymes may help to explain some of the conflicting reports of whether drug metabolism is altered in the presence of renal disease. If the metabolism of a drug is known to be increased or decreased in patients with renal failure, then the dose will need to be adjusted appropriately to achieve the desired effect. If the effect of renal failure on metabolism is unknown, then the agent should be used with extreme caution.

Patients with severe renal insufficiency receiving chronic treatment with some agents may experience accumulation of metabolite(s) as well as parent compound. Metabolites of several drugs have been reported to have significant pharmacologic and/or toxicologic activity. However the pharmacokinetics and pharmacology of metabolites are not often fully elucidated in humans. In a sense, the patient with severe renal impairment is being exposed to a "new pharmacologic entity" if the serum concentrations of the metabolite exceed those reported in patients with normal renal function.

The metabolite may have pharmacologic activity similar to that of the parent drug and thus contribute significantly to clinical response; for example, oxypurinol and desacetyl cefotaxime.[46] Alternatively, the metabolite may have qualitatively dissimilar pharmacologic action; for example, normeperidine has a central nervous system (CNS)-stimulatory activity that reportedly produces seizures, whereas meperidine has CNS-depressant actions.[31] Because of the multiplicity of potential interactions of compounds that are primarily metabolized, the practical consequences of metabolite accumulation are difficult to predict and are most often identified in those patients at risk by trial and error (Table 50–5).

EFFECT ON RENAL EXCRETION

Net renal excretion (CL_R) of a drug is the composite of glomerular filtration, tubular secretion, and reabsorption ($CL_R = (GFR \times f_u) + CL_{secretion} - CL_{reabsorption}$), where f_u is the fraction of the drug unbound to plasma proteins. Drug elimination by filtration occurs by a diffusion process, but tubular secretion and reabsorption are bidirectional processes that involve carrier-mediated renal transport systems. The two primary renal transport systems—termed the anionic and cationic pathways—are responsible for the transport of a number of organic acids and basic drugs, respectively. Other important renal transport systems include the nucleoside and *p*-glycoprotein transporters, which are involved in the renal tubular transport of dideoxynucleosides (e.g., zidovudine, dideoxyinosine) and digoxin, respectively.[32] A reduction in glomerular filtration rate results in a decrease in renal drug clearance. For drugs that are extensively renally secreted ($CL_R > 300$ mL/min), the loss of filtration clearance (up to 120 mL/min) will have less of an impact than for those primarily dependent on GFR. Alterations in one or more of the three renal processes (filtration, secretion, reabsorption) secondary to reductions in functional nephron mass may have a dramatic effect on the pharmacokinetics of a drug.

Although it was once thought that the mechanisms of renal elimination declined in a parallel manner in the presence of renal disease, it is now known that this may not be a valid assumption. Kamiya et al.[33] and Hori et al.[34] demonstrated that the type of renal disease may explain in part the differences in pharmacokinetic parameters observed among patients with similar reductions in glomerular filtration rate. The disposition of antibiotic agents extensively secreted by the proximal renal tubules (e.g., ampicillin, cephalexin) was altered to a greater degree in patients with tubulointerstitial disease as compared to those with primary glomerular disease. Quantitative investigations of renal handling of new drugs will be required to elucidate the relative contribution of tubular and glomerular function to renal drug clearance. The availability of these data should provide a more rational approach to dosage regimen design for those agents that undergo extensive tubular secretion or reabsorption.

In the absence of data delineating the contribution of tubular function to renal elimination, the clinical measurement or estimation of creatinine clearance remains the guiding factor for drug-dosage regimen design.[7,9] The importance of an alteration in renal function on drug elimination thus depends on two factors: the fraction of drug normally eliminated by the kidney unchanged and the degree of renal insufficiency.

TABLE 50–5. Pharmacologic Activity of Selected Drug Metabolites

Parent Drug	Metabolite	Pharmacologic Activity of Metabolites
Acetaminophen	*N*-Acetyl-*p*-benzoquinoneimine	Responsible for hepatotoxicity
Allopurinol	Oxypurinol	Metabolite primarily responsible for suppression of xanthine oxidase
Azathioprine	Mercaptopurine	All of the immunosuppressive activity resides in the metabolite
Cefotaxime	Desacetyl cefotaxime	Similar antimicrobial spectrum, but one-fourth to one-tenth as potent
Chlorpropamide	2-Hydroxychlorpropamide	Similar *in vitro* insulin-releasing activity
Clofibrate	Chlorophenoxyisobutyric acid	Primarily responsible for hypolipidemic effect and direct muscle toxicity
Codeine	Morphine-6-glucuronide	Possibly more active than parent compound; may contribute to prolonged narcotic effect in renal failure patients
Imipramine	Desmethylimipramine	Similar antidepressant activity
Ketoprofen	Ketoprofen glucuronide	Accumualtion of acyl glucuronide may worsen toxic effects (gastrointestinal disturbances and impairment of renal function)
Meperidine	Normeperidine	Less analgesic activity than parent, but more CNS-stimulatory effects
Morphine	Morphine-6-glucuronide	Possibly more active than parent compound; may contribute to prolonged narcotic effect in renal failure patients
Mycophenolic acid	Mycophenolic acid glucuronide	Lacks pharmacologic activity but may be associated with dose-limiting (gastrointestinal) side effects
Procainamide	*N*-Acetyl procainamide	Distinct antiarrhythmic activity, the mechanism of which is different from that of the parent compound
Sulfonamides	Acetylated metabolites	Devoid of antibacterial activity, but elevated concentrations are associated with toxicity
Theophylline	1,3-Dimethyl uric acid	Cardiotoxicity has been demonstrated
Zidovudine	Zidovudine triphosphate	Primarily responsible for antiretroviral activity

Quantitation of the patient's renal function can be accomplished by measurement of creatinine clearance or estimation based on the stable serum creatinine (see Chap. 42). Because of the time delay involved and problems in obtaining complete urine collections, measured creatinine clearance values are infrequently used for initial drug-dosage regimen design. Therefore, the calculation of initial drug dosage regimens relies on the estimation of creatinine clearance (CLcr) in adults and children from such routinely available clinical data as age, gender, height, weight, and serum creatinine. These relationships are most accurate for individuals of average muscle mass for their age, weight, and height. The creatinine clearance of emaciated and obese adult patients is difficult to predict, and incorrect estimates have been obtained with most methods.

Several methods are also available for estimating creatinine clearance in adults with acute renal insufficiency using age, height, weight, serum creatinine, and time data (see Chap. 42). These methods have not been as rigorously validated as the equations for patients with stable renal function. However, they are one of the few methods we have to approximate renal function in this complex patient situation.

DRUG-DOSAGE REGIMEN DESIGNS

PATIENTS WITH RENAL INSUFFICIENCY

Most dosage adjustment guidelines have proposed the use of a fixed dose or interval for patients with broad ranges of renal function.[13,35–37] For example, moderate renal insufficiency may encompass a creatinine clearance range of 30–50 mL/min, severe renal insufficiency is often defined as a creatinine clearance of 10–29 mL/min and end-stage renal disease is defined by a creatinine clearance <10 mL/min. These categories encompass up to a 10-fold range in renal function and, thus, the drug regimen may not be optimal for all patients whose renal function lies within the range.

The design of the optimal dosage regimen for patients with renal insufficiency requires an individualized assessment and is dependent on the availability of an accurate characterization of the relationship between the pharmacokinetic parameters of the drug and renal function and an accurate assessment of the patient's renal function (creatinine clearance). Secondary references such as the *AHFS Drug Information*,[35] and textbooks[38] are excellent sources of information about a drug's pharmacokinetic characteristics in subjects with normal renal function. However, they often do not provide the explicit relationships of the kinetic parameters of interest (total body clearance, elimination rate constant, and distribution volume) with a continuous index of renal function, such as creatinine clearance. To find this information, you may need to identify the original research study that assessed the drug's disposition or a comprehensive review article on the class of drugs of interest. Ideally, one should be able to identify a relationship between total body clearance (CL), elimination rate constant (k), or distribution volume (V_D) with CLcr (see Table 50–6). This information, along with the patient's CLcr, will enable prediction of the patient's kinetic parameters and then formulation of a therapeutic regimen to attain the desired therapeutic outcome.

If specific literature recommendations and/or the relationship of kinetic parameters to CLcr are not available, then one can estimate the kinetic parameters of the patient with the method of Rowland and Tozer,[9] provided you know the fraction of the drug that is eliminated renally unchanged (f_e) in subjects with normal renal function. These approaches assume that the change in CL and k are proportional to CLcr, that renal disease does not alter the drug's metabolism, that the metabolites if formed are inactive and nontoxic, that the drug obeys first-order (linear) kinetic principles, and that it is adequately described by a one-compartment model. If these assumptions are true then the kinetic parameter/dosage adjustment factor (Q) can be calculated as:

$$Q = 1 - [f_e(1 - KF)]$$

TABLE 50–6. Relationship Between Renal Function and Pharmacokinetic Parameters of Selected Drugs

Drug	Total Body Clearance (mL/min)
Acyclovir	CL = 3.37 (CLcr) + 0.41
Amikacin	CL = 0.60 (CLcr) + 9.6
Cefmetazole	CL = 1.18 (CLcr) − 0.29
Ceftazidime	CL = 1.15 (CLcr) + 10.6
Ciprofloxacin	CL = 2.83 (CLcr) + 363
Digoxin	CL = 0.88 (CLcr) + 23
Gentamicin	CL = 0.98 (CLcr)
Netilmicin	CL = 0.65 (CLcr) + 3.72
Ofloxacin	CL = 1.04 (CLcr) + 38.7
Piperacillin	CL = 1.36 (CLcr) + 1.50
Procainamide	CL = 3.00 (CLcr) + 0.23 (ABW)
Teicoplanin	CL = 7.09 (CLcr) − 16.2
Tobramycin	CL = 0.80 (CLcr)
Vancomycin	CL = 0.69 (CLcr) + 3.7

(Compiled from Refs. 12, 37, and 38.)

where KF is the ratio of the patient's CLcr to the assumed normal value of 120 mL/min. Thus, for a drug that is 85% eliminated renally unchanged in a patient who has a CLcr of 10 mL/min, the Q factor would be:

$$\begin{aligned} Q &= 1 - [0.85(1 - (10/120))] \\ &= 1 - [0.85(0.92)] \\ &= 1 - 0.78 \\ &= 0.22 \end{aligned}$$

The estimated total body clearance for this patient would then be calculated as $CL_{PT} = CL_{norm} \times Q$, where CL_{norm} is the mean value in patients with normal renal function as reported in the literature.

After the kinetic parameters for the patient are estimated, the best method for dosage regimen adjustment should be selected. Specifically, one must determine whether the desired goal is the maintenance of a similar peak, trough, or average steady-state drug concentration. If there is a significant relationship between peak concentration and clinical response[39] (e.g., aminoglycosides) or toxicity[37] (e.g., quinidine, phenobarbital, and phenytoin), then attainment of the specific target values is critical. If, however, no specific target values for peak or trough concentrations have been reported (e.g., antihypertensive agents, benzodiazepines, and cephalosporins), then a regimen goal of attaining the same average steady-state concentration may be appropriate.

Although several methods have been proposed to attain the desired average steady-state concentration profile, the principal choices are to decrease the dose or prolong the dosing interval. If the size of the dose is reduced while the dosing interval remains unchanged, the desired average steady-state concentration will be similar; however, the peak will be lower and the trough higher (Fig. 50–1). Alternatively, if the dosing interval is increased and the dose size remains unchanged, the peak and trough concentrations in the patient with reduced renal function will be similar to those in the patient with normal renal function. This dosage adjustment method is often preferred because it is likely to yield significant cost savings as a result of a reduction in nursing and pharmacy time, as well as a reduction in the supplies associated with frequent drug administration. Finally, the dose and dosing interval may both need to be changed to attain a desired peak or trough serum concentration time profile.

Regardless of the approach chosen to adjust the dosage regimen, the first step in the process, as previously mentioned, is to estimate

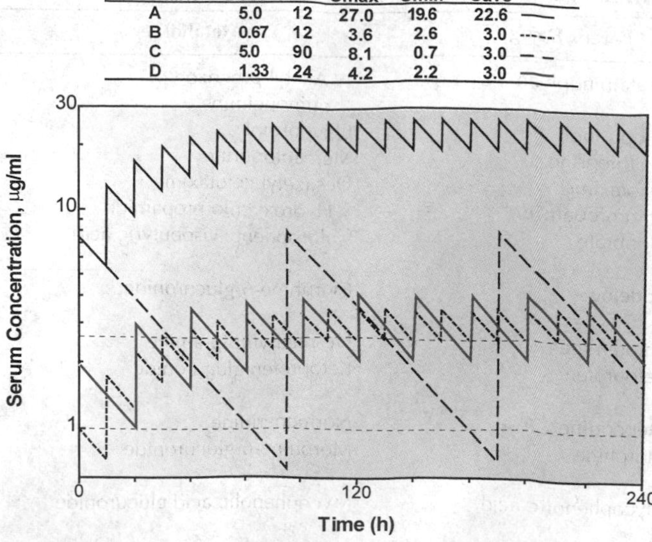

FIGURE 50–1. Without a change in dosage regimen this patient would achieve excessive steady-state serum concentrations (Scenario A). Although the average steady-state concentrations (C_{ave}) are identical, the concentration-time profile will be markedly different if one changes the dose and maintains the dosing interval (τ) constant (Scenario B), versus changing the dosing interval (τ) and maintaining the dose constant (Scenario C) or changing both (Scenario D).

the drug disposition parameters in the patient with renal insufficiency. The ratio (Q) of the estimated elimination rate constant or total body clearance of the patient relative to subjects with normal renal function (CLcr > 120 mL/min) may then be calculated. This parameter may be used to determine the dose or dosing interval alterations necessary for the patient.

For example, the following relationship between total clearance (CL) and creatinine clearance has been reported for ganciclovir:[40]

$$CL(mL/min/1.8\,m^2) = 1.25(CLcr) + 8.57$$

Thus, CL for a subject with normal renal function (CL_{norm}) would be calculated as:

$$\begin{aligned} CL_{norm} &= [1.25(120)] + 8.57 \\ CL_{mean} &= 158.6\ mL/min/1.8\,m^2 \end{aligned}$$

Clearance (CL_{fail}) for a patient with a creatinine clearance of 10 mL/min would be:

$$\begin{aligned} CL_{fail} &= [1.25(10)] + 8.57 \\ CL_{fail} &= 21.1\ mL/min/1.8\,m^2 \end{aligned}$$

Ganciclovir is commonly used in solid organ transplant patients as prophylaxis against or treatment for cytomegalovirus infection.[41] The IC_{50} of ganciclovir against most clinical isolates of cytomegalovirus is between 0.5 and 1.0 μg/mL (approximately 2.0–4.0 μmol/L). Therefore, trough concentrations should exceed these values, but caution is warranted because neutropenia is associated with the attainment of ganciclovir trough concentrations exceeding 2.6 μg/mL (10 μmol/L).[42] If a patient with reduced renal function received the typical ganciclovir dose for a patient with normal renal function, the predicted trough concentrations would approach 20 μmol/L. Therefore, a dosage modification in this patient is necessary to avoid potential toxicity. The dosing regimen can be modified using the ratio of the predicted clearance values. Therefore, the quotient or Q, for this patient is calculated as:

$$Q = CL_{fail}/CL_{norm}$$
$$Q = 21.1/158.6$$
$$Q = 0.133$$

where CL_{norm} is the clearance in a patient with normal renal function and CL_{fail} is the clearance of the patient with impaired renal function.

The maintenance dose (D_f) for the patient or the adjusted dosing interval (τ_f) may then be calculated from the following relationships, where D_n is the normal dose and τ_n is the normal dosing interval:

$$D_f = D_n \times Q$$
$$\tau_f = \tau_n/Q$$

For this patient situation, the normal dose and dosing interval of ganciclovir would be 5 mg/kg and 12 hours, respectively. If we wanted to maintain the dosing interval at 12 hours, then D_f would be calculated as:

$$D_f = (5\text{ mg/kg}) \times (0.133) = 0.67\text{ mg/kg}$$

This regimen would result in decreased peak and trough concentrations compared to a patient with this degree of renal insufficiency who received a normal dosage regimen (Fig. 50–1).

If we want to maintain D_n and extend the dosing interval, τ_f would be calculated as:

$$\tau_f = \tau_n/Q = 12/0.133 = 90\text{ hours}$$

This regimen would yield similar peak and trough concentrations in the renally impaired patient as in the normal renal function patient, but there is a risk of missed doses with such an unorthodox interval (Fig. 50–1, scenario C). In addition, the prolonged period below the C_{ss} average concentration may be less than optimal.

Finally, a practical dosing interval may be selected and then a dose based on that interval can be calculated (Fig. 50–1, scenario D). If a dosage interval τ_f of 24 hours were selected, because in many institutions there is an increased risk of missed doses with longer dosing intervals, then the D_f would be calculated as follows:

$$\begin{aligned} D_f &= [D_n \times Q \times \tau_f]/\tau_n \\ &= [(5\text{ mg/kg}) \times (0.133) \times (24)]/12 \\ &= 1.33\text{ mg/kg} \end{aligned}$$

This method would likely be most appropriate in this case; prolonged subtherapeutic concentrations are avoided and troughs are reduced from the first method. The selection of which dosage adjustment method to use to calculate an optimal regimen depends on the drug characteristics and the patient care situation. This dosage adjustment method assumes that the protein binding and volume of distribution of the drug are not significantly altered by renal insufficiency. Thus, this approach cannot be used with accuracy for those drugs with demonstrated differences in these pharmacokinetic parameters.

If the volume of distribution (V_D) of a drug is significantly altered in patients with renal insufficiency or in whom one desires to attain a specific maximum or minimum concentration, the estimation of a dosage regimen becomes more complex. If the relationship between V_D and creatinine clearance has been characterized, then V_D may be estimated. If one assumes that a one-compartment linear model can describe the drug, the predicted V_D may then be used with the predicted elimination rate constant (k) of the drug to yield an adjusted dosing interval and intravenous or oral dose.

For orally administered drugs, the τ_f can be calculated as:

$$\tau_f = [(-1/k_f)(\ln[C_{min}/C_{max}])] + t_{peak}$$

and the dose can be approximated as:

$$\text{Dose}_{po} = \left[\text{SFC}_p^t V_D(k_a - k)\right]/\left[k_a\left(e^{-kt}/1 - e^{-k\tau}\right)\left(e^{-kat}/1 - e^{-ka\tau}\right)\right]$$

where, S equals the salt fraction, F equals bioavailability, C_p^t equals the desired plasma concentration at time t, and k_a is the absorption rate constant. This approach allows for the individualization of a dosage regimen for attainment of specific peak and trough serum concentrations. If the drug is absorbed extremely rapidly, one can approximate the τ_f as: $\tau_f = (-1/k_f)(\ln[C_{min}/C_{max}])$ and the dose as Dose $= V_D \times (C_{max} - C_{min})$.

Digoxin is a frequently used oral medication for which the V_D is decreased in patients with renal insufficiency and for which one usually desires to closely control the plasma concentration time profile. The V_D and CL_{fail} of digoxin can be estimated for a 70-kg patient with a CLcr of 12 mL/min as follows previously described.[18]

$$\begin{aligned} V_D &= 226 + [(298(\text{CLcr}))/(29.1 + \text{CLcr})] \\ &= 226 + [(298(12))/(29.1 + 12)] \\ &= 226 + 87.0 \\ &= 313\text{ L} \end{aligned}$$

$$\begin{aligned} CL_{fail} &= (0.88 \times \text{CLcr}) + 23\text{ mL/min} \\ &= 10.6 + 23 \\ &= 33.6\text{ mL/min} \end{aligned}$$

$$\begin{aligned} k_f &= CL_{fail}/V_D \\ &= (33.6\text{ mL/min} \times 1440\text{ min/d})/313\text{ L} \\ &= 48.3\text{ L/d}/313\text{ L} \\ &= 0.154\text{ day}^{-1} \end{aligned}$$

The t_{peak} is generally at 2 hours and the k_a from the literature is about 0.76 per hour or 18 per day.[38] Thus, one now has all the information needed to calculate the τ_f and dose for this patient:

$$\begin{aligned} \tau_f &= [(-1/k_f)(\ln[C_{min}/C_{max}]) + t_{peak} \\ &= [(-1/0.154)(\ln[0.8/1.4]) + 2\text{ hours} \\ &= [(-6.49)(-0.56)] + 2\text{ hours} \\ &= 3.6\text{ days} + 2\text{ hours} \\ &\approx 4\text{ days} \end{aligned}$$

$$\begin{aligned} \text{Dose}_{po} = {} & [(1.4)(313)(18 - 0.154)]/[18(e^{-0.154(0.083)}/1 - e^{-0.154(4)}) \\ & - (e^{-18(0.083)}/1 - e^{-18(4)})] \end{aligned}$$

$$\text{Dose} = 0.226\text{ mg or one 0.25 mg oral capsule every 4 days}$$

Alternately, the predicted volume of distribution and elimination rate constant or the total body clearance may be used to calculate a dose regimen that will maintain the desired average steady-state concentration of the drug (C_{ss}).

$$\text{Dose (mg/h)} = C_{ss}\,[(k_f \times V_D)\text{ or }(CL_f)]$$

Depending on how much variance about the average steady state one desires, the dosing interval may range from hourly to as infrequently as every 48 hours or longer. For example, if the calculated dose were 10 mg/h, the desired average steady-state concentration would be maintained with a dosing interval of 60 mg every 6 hours or 480 mg every 48 hours.

PATIENTS RECEIVING CONTINUOUS RENAL REPLACEMENT THERAPY

Continuous renal replacement therapy (CRRT) is used for the management of fluid overload and the removal of uremic toxins in patients with acute renal failure and other conditions.[43] The several forms of CRRT are extensively described in Chap. 43. Which of these therapies will be optimal for a given patient is dependent on several factors, including bleeding risk, degree of hypercatabolism, acid-base balance, and experience of the health-care provider.

Drug therapy individualization for the patient receiving CRRT is complicated by the fact that patients with acute renal failure may have a higher residual nonrenal clearance of some drugs than patients with chronic renal insufficiency who have a similar CLcr.[44–46] For example, the nonrenal clearance of imipenem in patients with acute renal failure (95 mL/min) is between the values observed in chronic renal failure patients (50 mL/min) and those with normal renal function (130 mL/min).[45] This may occur because of less exposure to or accumulation of uremic by-products that may alter hepatic function. A nonrenal clearance value in a patient with acute renal failure that is higher than anticipated based on chronic renal failure data would result in lower than expected, possibly subtherapeutic, serum concentrations.

In addition to patient-specific differences, there are marked differences between intermittent hemodialysis and the three primary types of CRRT (continuous arteriovenous or venovenous hemofiltration [CAVH/CVVH]), continuous arteriovenous or venovenous hemodialysis (CAVHD/CVVHD), and continuous arteriovenous or venovenous hemodiafiltration (CAVHDF/CVVHDF)] with regard to drug removal.

During CAVH/CVVH drug removal primarily occurs via convection/ultrafiltration (the passive transport of drug molecules at the concentration at which they exist in plasma water into the ultrafiltrate). The clearance of a drug by either of these methods is thus a function of the membrane permeability for the drug, which is called the sieving coefficient (SC) and the rate of ultrafiltrate formation (UFR). The SC can be calculated as:

$$SC = (2C_{UF})/[(C_a/1 - \theta) + (C_v/1 - \theta)]$$

where C_a and C_v are the concentration of the drug in the plasma going into and returning from the filter, respectively, C_{UF} is the concentration in the ultrafiltrate and θ is 0.0107 times the total protein concentration in plasma. The SC is often approximated by the fraction unbound (f_u) because this information may be more readily available. Thus, the clearance by these two modes of CRRT can be calculated as:

$$CL_{CVVH} = UFR \times SC$$

or

$$CL_{CVVH} = UFR \times f_u$$

Clearance of a drug by CAVHDF/CVVHDF (CL_{CAVHDF}/CL_{CVVHDF}) is generally greater than by CAVH/CVVH because in addition to the convection/ultrafiltration process, drug is removed by diffusion from the plasma water into the dialysate. The CL_{CVVHDF} can be mathematically approximated providing the blood flow rate is greater than 100 mL/min and dialysate flow rate (DFR) is between 8 and 33 mL/min as:

$$CL_{CVVHDF} = (UFR \times f_{ub}) + CL_{diffusion}$$

In the clinical setting, it is not possible to separate these two components of CL_{CVVHDF}. In essence the CL_{CVVHDF} is calculated as the product of the combined ultrafiltrate and dialysate volume (V_{df}) and the concentration of the drug in this fluid (C_{df}) divided by the plasma concentration (C_p^{mid}) at the midpoint of the V_{df} collection period.

There are differences in the rate of drug removal not only between the three primary modes of CRRT but also within each mode.[43] This is a result of differences in the filter membrane composition as the result of variable degrees of drug binding to the membrane and the permeability characteristics of the membrane.[47–50] The primary factors that influence drug clearance during CRRT are thus ultrafiltration rate, blood flow rate, and dialysate flow rate. For example, clearance in CAVH/CVVH is directly proportional to the ultrafiltration rate, whereas clearance in CAVHDF/CVVHDF, which depends on both the ultrafiltration rate and the dialysate flow rate, increases as either flow rate increases. Changes in blood flow rate generally have only a minor effect on drug clearance by any mode of CRRT. These effects are shown for ceftazidime clearance in Fig. 50–2, with different ultrafiltration flow rates (5 and 45 mL/min) and increasing dialysate flow rates (8.3–33.3 mL/min).[48]

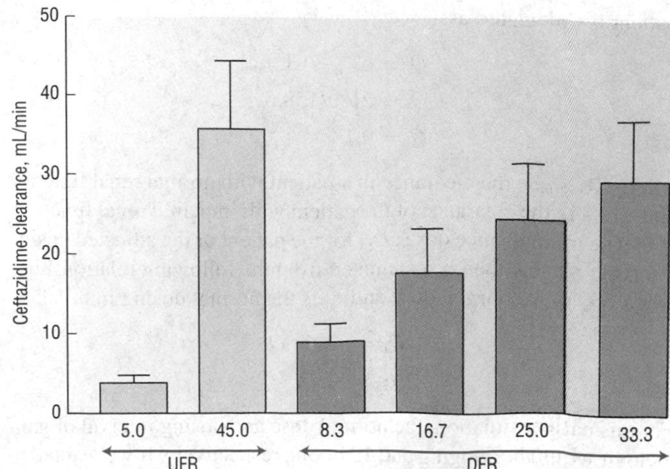

FIGURE 50–2. The effect of increasing ultrafiltration rate (UFR; ml/min) and dialysate flow rate (DFR; ml/min) on the clearance of ceftazidime.

An algorithmic approach for drug dosage adjustment in patients undergoing CRRT has been proposed.[43] Individualization of therapy for a patient receiving CRRT therapy is dependent on the patient's residual renal function and the clearance of the drug by the mode of CRRT they are receiving. The patient's residual drug clearance can be predicted as described in the previous section of this chapter. The CRRT clearance can also be ascertained from published literature reports.[43,51,52] The SCs of frequently used drugs are summarized in Table 50–7, and the clearance of selected drugs by CAVH/CVVH or CAVHD/CVVHD is listed in Table 50–8. These data can be used to design initial dosage regimens for patients receiving CRRT.

For example, WT is a 48-year-old, 60-kg male in acute renal failure with a serum creatinine that has increased from 2.3 mg/dL to 7.2 mg/dL over 3 days. The residual creatinine clearance value in this patient, calculated using the Jelliffe and Jelliffe equation for changing serum creatinines (see Chap. 42), is 4.8 mL/min. The consulting nephrologist recommends that CVVHDF be initiated using a Fresenius F-40 filter at blood and dialysate flow rates of 100 and 33.3 mL/min, respectively. The patient is to receive ceftazidime while on CVVHDF. The patient's residual ceftazidime clearance can be estimated using the regression equation in Table 50–6 relating CLcr and clearance:

$$CL_{RES}\ (mL/min) = [1.15 \times (CLcr)] + 10.6$$

$$CL_{RES} = [1.15 \times (4.8)] + 10.6 = 16.1\ mL/min$$

The total clearance while on CVVHDF would be the sum of the patient's residual clearance and the ceftazidime clearance associated with CVVHDF (Table 50–8) as follows:

$$CL_T = CL_{RES} + CL_{CVVHDF}$$

$$CL_T = 16.1\ mL/min + 15.2\ mL/min = 31.3\ mL/min$$

TABLE 50–7. Predicted and Measured Sieving Coefficients of Selected Drugs

Drug	Predicted	Measured
Amikacin	0.95	0.88
Amphotericin	0.01	0.32–0.4
Ampicillin	0.8	0.6–0.69
Cefoperazone	0.10	0.27–0.69
Cefotaxime	0.62	0.55–1.1
Cefoxitin	0.30	0.32
Ceftazidime	0.90	0.38–0.78
Ceftriaxone	0.10	0.71–0.82
Clindamycin	0.25	0.49–0.98
Digoxin	0.75	0.96
Erythromycin	0.25	0.37
5-Flurocytosine	0.96	0.98
Gentamicin	0.95	0.81–0.95
Imipenem	0.80	0.78
Metronidazole	0.80	0.80
Mezlocillin	0.68	0.68
Nafcillin	0.20	0.47
N-Acetyl procainamide	0.80	0.92
Netilmicin	—	0.85
Oxacillin	0.05	0.02
Phenobarbital	0.60	0.86
Phenytoin	0.10	0.45
Procainamide	0.80	0.86
Theophylline	0.47	0.85
Tobramycin	0.95	0.78–0.86
Vancomycin	0.90	0.5–0.8

(Adapted from Ref. 43.)

This patient clearance value can be used to adjust the ceftazidime dose as described earlier. The ceftazidime clearance in a patient with normal renal function would be calculated as:

$$CL_{norm}\ (\text{mL/min}) = [1.15 \times (CLcr)] + 10.6$$

$$CL_{norm} = [1.15 \times (120)] + 10.6 = 148.6\ \text{mL/min}$$

The dosage adjustment factor would then be:

$$Q = CL_T/CL_{norm}$$

$$Q = 31.3/148.6 = 0.21$$

For this patient situation, the normal regimen of ceftazidime would be 1,000 mg (D_n) every 8 hours (τ_n). If one wanted to maintain D_n and extend the dosing interval, then τ_f would be calculated as:

$$\tau_f = \tau_n/Q$$

$$\tau_f = 8\ \text{hours}/0.21$$

$$\tau_f = 38\ \text{hours or a more practical 36 hours}$$

Therefore, this patient should receive 1,000 mg every 36 hours. If the additional clearance associated with CVVHDF (15.2 mL/min) was not considered, the dosing interval would have been considerably longer at approximately 72 hours.

PATIENTS RECEIVING CHRONIC AMBULATORY PERITONEAL DIALYSIS

Although the majority of patients with ESRD receive treatment with hemodialysis, approximately 15% of dialysis patients receive one of the multiple variants of continuous peritoneal dialysis (CPD). Peritoneal dialysis, like other dialysis modalities, has the potential to affect drug disposition; however, drug therapy individualization is often less complicated in these patients owing to the continuous nature of the procedure (see Chap. 47).

Many of the factors that are important in determining drug dialyzability for other treatment modalities pertain to peritoneal dialysis as well.[53] Peritoneal dialysis involves the instillation of 1–3 L of dialysis solution into the peritoneal cavity. Waste products and other substances, including drugs, move from the blood and surrounding tissues into the dialysis solution by means of diffusion and ultrafiltration. Factors that influence drug dialyzability in peritoneal dialysis include drug-specific characteristics such as molecular weight, solubility, degree of ionization, protein binding, and volume of distribution. The intrinsic properties of the peritoneal membrane that affect drug removal include blood flow, pore size, and peritoneal membrane surface area, which is approximately equal to the body surface area. There is an inverse relationship between peritoneal drug clearance and molecular weight, protein binding, and volume of distribution. Also, drug compounds that are ionized at physiologic pH will diffuse across the membrane more slowly than un-ionized compounds. In general, hemodialysis is more effective in removing drug substances than peritoneal dialysis such that if a drug is not removed by hemodialysis, it

TABLE 50–8. Clearance of Selected Drugs by CAVH/CVVH and/or CAVHD/CVVHD

	CAVH/CVVH		CAVHD/CVVHD		
				DFR 1 L/hr	DFR 2 L/hr
Drug	*SC*	*Clearance*	*SC*	*Clearance*	
Amikacin	0.93 ± 0.16	10.1			
Amrinone	0.80–1.4	2.4–14.4			
Cefuroxime		11.0 ± 5.2	0.90 ± 0.30	14.0 ± 2.2	16.2 ± 3.4
Ceftazidime			0.86 ± 0.07	13.1 ± 1.3	15.2 ± 1.3
Cilastatin	0.77	4.0 ± 2.3	0.68 ± 0.08	10.0 ± 3.0	18.0 ± 4.0
Ciprofloxacin				16.3	19.9
Digoxin				6.4–10.0	11
Gentamicin		3.5 ± 1.9		5.2 ± 1.8	
Imipenem	0.80	13.3	1.05 ± 0.19	16.0 ± 7.0	
Phenytoin	0.37 ± 0.08	1.0		6.5	
Theophylline				14.8	
Tobramycin		3.5 ± 1.9		11.1–29	14.9
Vancomycin	0.80	6.7–13.3	0.66 ± 0.08	12.1 ± 5.7	16.6 ± 5.7

Clearance is in ml/min. SC = sieving coefficient; DFR = dialysate flow rate; NR = not reported.
(From Ref. 43.)

TABLE 50–9. Comparison for Selected Drugs of Residual Drug Clearance in ESRD (CL_{ESRD}) to Clearance By Continuous Ambulatory Peritoneal Dialsysis (CL_{CAPD}), Intermittent Peritoneal Dialysis (CL_{IPD}), and Hemodialysis (CL_{HD})*

Drug	CL_{ESRD}	CL_{CAPD}	CL_{IPD}	CL_{HD}
Aztreonam	1.44	0.13	0.13	2.6
Cefazolin	0.30	0.06		2.1
Cefotaxime	7.13 ± 0.74	0.40 ± 0.08		1.6
Ceftazidime	0.74 ± 0.20	0.10 ± 0.02	0.50	2.3
Gentamicin	0.24	0.17	0.75	2.1
Mezlocillin	6.0		0.44	1.7
Pipericillin	3.90 ± 0.77	0.22		4.4
Ticarcillin	0.96		0.43	2.0
Vancomycin	5.0	0.85 ± 0.22		0.8

*All data (mean ± SD) are in liters per hour.
(*From Refs. 7, 20, and 53.*)

is not likely to be removed by peritoneal dialysis. As shown in Table 50–9, the contribution of peritoneal dialysis to total body clearance is often low and, for most drugs, markedly less than the contribution of hemodialysis. Detailed reviews of the disposition of other drugs in CAPD patients are reported elsewhere.[7,53] Anti-infective agents are the most commonly studied drugs due to their primary role in the treatment of peritonitis.[54] Most other drugs can generally be dosed according to the residual renal function of the patient because additional clearance by peritoneal dialysis is so small.

CHRONIC HEMODIALYSIS PATIENTS

The number of patients with ESRD who receive chronic hemodialysis has steadily increased since the early 1970s and currently over 200,000 patients receive this life-sustaining therapy.[55] Although many new hemodialyzers have been introduced in the past 20 years and the efficiency of the hemodialysis procedure has been increased, the effect of hemodialysis on drug disposition is rarely reevaluated after initially reported. Thus, most of the literature probably represents an underestimation of the impact of hemodialysis on drug disposition.

The impact of hemodialysis on a patient's drug therapy is dependent on several factors, including the characteristics of each drug, the dialysis conditions, and the clinical situation for which dialysis is performed. Drug-related factors that affect dialyzability include the molecular weight, protein binding, and distribution volume of each drug.[7] The impact of distribution volume (V_D) on drug removal by dialysis is evident in the following example, where drug A has a 10-L V_D, but drug B has a V_D of 80 L. Neither drugs is bound to plasma proteins. They are exclusively eliminated unchanged by the kidney and both drugs have a molecular weight of 300 and a dialyzer clearance of 40 mL/min (2.4 L/h). The half-life in an anuric patient during dialysis [$t_{1/2} = (V_D \times 0.693)/\text{CL}$] will be markedly different for these two drugs (2.9 hours vs 23 hours) and thus approximately 50% of drug A but only 10% of drug B will be removed during 3 hours of dialysis as a direct result of the larger distribution volume. Prior to the mid-1980s these were the primary factors that needed to be known to assess the degree of dialyzability of a given drug because the vast majority of dialysis filters were composed of cellulose, cellulose acetate, or regenerated cellulose (cuprophane). These "conventional" filter materials were generally impermeable to drugs with a molecular weight over 1,000 and the clearance by hemodialysis tended to decline dramatically (by up to 60%) as molecular weight increased from 100 to 500.[56] Drugs that are small but highly protein bound are also not well dialyzed because both of the principal binding proteins, AAG and albumin, have a very high molecular weight. Finally, those drugs

TABLE 50–10. Drug Disposition During Dialysis Depends on Dialyzer Characteristics

Drug	Hemodialysis Clearance (mL/min)		Reference(s)
	Conventional	*High-Flux*	
Ceftazidime	55–60	155	59
Cefuroxime	NR	103	12
Foscarnet	183	253	64
Gentamicin	58	116	62
Netilmicin	46	87–109	12
Tobramycin	31–73	117–151	60
Ranitidine	43	67	63
Vancomycin	9–21	40–150	12, 58, 61

that are widely distributed throughout the body are poorly removed by hemodialysis.

The dialysis prescription for the patient can also dramatically affect the degree of drug removal. The primary factors that can vary between patients are the type of hemodialysis they are prescribed, which is primarily reflected in the composition of the dialysis membrane, the filter surface area, blood and dialysate flow rates, and whether or not the dialysis unit reuses the dialysis filter. Dialysis membranes are composed of cellulose-based, semisynthetic or synthetic materials (e.g., polysulfone, polymethylmethacrylate, or acrylonitrile). The synthetic filter materials are now available for low-, medium-, and high-flux modes of dialysis (see Chap. 47), with the principal difference between modes being in the filter pore size, which can range from 25 to greater than 60 angstrom and the degree of water transport (ultrafiltration coefficient). The dialysis membranes used in high-flux hemodialysis (HFD) have the greatest pore sizes and more closely mimic the filtration characteristics of the human kidney than the filters used to deliver conventional hemodialysis. This allows the passage of most solutes, including drugs, that have a molecular weight of 20,000 or less.[56] Thus, high-molecular-weight drugs such as vancomycin are likely to be removed by this mode of dialysis, although they are not by conventional dialysis. An increase in removal has also been reported with several other drugs that have lower molecular weights (Table 50–10).[57–64] Figure 50–3 shows the plasma concentration time profile of gentamicin in patients receiving dialysis using either a low-flux [cellulose acetate (CA170)] or a high-flux [polysulfone (F80)] dialyzer. The net result is that the patient receiving high-flux dialysis will require larger postdialysis doses relative to the patient receiving low-flux dialysis to maintain similar concentrations. The final component of the dialysis prescription that may affect drug clearance by dialysis is whether or not the patient has authorized the unit to reuse his or her dialyzer. Currently, more than 75% of all dialysis units in the United States use this procedure to reduce the cost of chronic hemodialysis.[55] The effect of dialysis filter reuse on the clearance of endogenous molecules such as urea, creatinine, and β_2-microglobulin has been evaluated for many dialyzers.[65] A decrease in urea and creatinine clearances and an increase in β_2-microglobulin clearance was observed with some but not all dialyzers. Only one center has evaluated the effect of reuse on drug clearance (cefazolin, ceftazidime, tobramycin, and vancomycin) following the first, and tenth use of cellulose acetate, cellulose triacetate, and polysulfone dialyzers.[66] No change was noted with the cellulose acetate dialyzer. Ceftazidime and vancomycin clearance decreased by up to 13% with the polysulfone filter. In contrast, significant decreases in clearance were observed with the cellulose triacetate dialyzer (24% to 43%) for all four drugs.

The impact of hemodialysis on drug therapy should thus not be viewed as a generic procedure such that a certain percentage of drug in the body is removed with each dialysis session; neither should

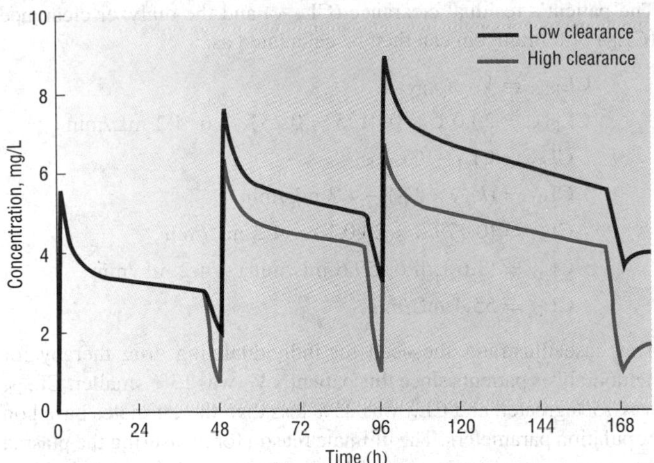

FIGURE 50–3. Clearance of gentamicin by low- and high-clearance dialyzers in patients given the same gentamicin dose. Concentrations in the patient receiving dialysis with a low-clearance dialyzer will continue to accumulate, whereas concentrations in the patient receiving dialysis with the high-clearance dialyzer will be maintained at the same peak, and predialysis concentrations will be observed after the third dose.

simple "yes-no" answers on the dialyzability of drug compounds be considered sufficient information for therapeutic decisions. Reference materials that indicate "yes-no" status regarding the dialyzability of drug compounds provide no quantification of the impact of hemodialysis and are thus of little value to the clinician who needs to design a rational dosing regimen for a patient. Compounds considered non-dialyzable with low-flux dialyzers may in fact be significantly removed by high-flux hemodialyzers. Characteristics of the dialysis prescription such as membrane composition and surface area, and blood and dialysis flow rates, are thus critical data for the design of drug dosing regimens for chronic hemodialysis patients.

The effect of hemodialysis on drug disposition can be estimated in several ways.[7] The determination of drug concentrations at the start and end of dialysis, with the subsequent calculation of the half-life during dialysis ($t_{1/2,\mathrm{onHD}}$), has frequently been used as an index of drug removal by dialysis. Unfortunately, the $t_{1/2,\mathrm{onHD}}$ may not be interpretable because declining plasma drug concentrations during dialysis represent elimination by the body as well as by dialysis. Furthermore, if significant rebound in drug concentrations after dialysis has been reported, the removal of drug by the dialysis procedure may be artificially high depending on when, after dialysis, the concentration is determined (Table 50–11).[67–71]

An alternative and more accurate means of assessing the effect of hemodialysis is to calculate the dialyzer clearance of the drug.[7] The dialyzer clearance (CL_D) can be calculated by several approaches. The CL_D^b from blood can be calculated as $CL_D = Q_b[(A_b - V_b)/A_b]$, where Q_b is blood flow through the dialyzer, A_b is the concentration of drug in blood going into the dialyzer, and V_b is the blood concentration of drug leaving the dialyzer. This equation is valid only if the drug concentrations are measured in whole blood and if the drug rapidly and completely distributes into red blood cells. Because drug concentrations are generally determined in plasma, the previous equation is usually modified to $CL_D^p = Q_p[(A_p - V_p)/A_p]$ where p represents plasma and Q_p is plasma flow, which equals Q_b (1 − hematocrit). This clearance calculation accurately reflects dialysis drug clearance only if the drug does not penetrate red blood cells or bind to formed blood elements.

Because of potential problems in accurately determining Q_b or Q_p, the dialysate recovery method is widely used. In addition, venous plasma concentrations may be concentrated, because plasma water is generally removed from the blood at a faster rate than drug when ultrafiltration is performed simultaneously with diffusion during dialysis.

The recovery clearance approach, the benchmark for the determination of dialyzer clearance, can be calculated as:[7]

$$CL_D^r = R/AUC_{0-t}$$

where R is the total amount of drug recovered unchanged in the dialysate and AUC_{0-t} is the area under the predialyzer plasma concentration-time curve during hemodialysis. To determine the AUC_{0-t}, at least two, and preferably three to four, plasma concentrations should be obtained during dialysis.

The hemodialysis clearance values reported in the literature may vary significantly depending on which of the previous methods was used to calculate CL_D. The principal reason for this is that for most medications we do not know the degree and rapidity with which the drug crosses the red blood cell (RBC) membrane. Because the CL_D^r method incorporates no assumption of the degree of RBC permeability, it can be reliably used as the benchmark value. Comparisons of CL_D^p and CL_D^b values to the CL_D^r benchmark thus provide valuable insight to a drug's dialyzability.

The following principles may be applied to drug-dosage regimen design by using a value of CL_D that is reported in the literature.[7,12,13,37] Because clearance terms are additive, the total clearance during dialysis can be calculated as the sum of the patient's residual clearance during the interdialytic period (CL_{RES}) and dialyzer clearance (CL_D):

$$CL_T = CL_{RES} + CL_D$$

The half-life during the period between dialysis treatments and during dialysis can then be calculated from the following relationships using an estimate of the drug's distribution volume (V_D), which can be obtained from review articles:[7,12,13,37]

$$t_{1/2,\,\mathrm{offHD}} = 0.693\,[V_D/CL_{RES}]$$
$$t_{1/2,\,\mathrm{onHD}} = 0.693\,[V_D/(CL_{RES} + CL_D)]$$

Once the key pharmacokinetic parameters have been estimated/calculated, they may be used to simulate the plasma concentration-time profile of the drug for the individual patient and ascertain how much drug to administer and when. This approach to drug therapy individualization can be accomplished in a stepwise fashion assuming first-order elimination of the drug and a one-compartment model. For example, a 34-year-old male with ESRD was admitted to a hospital from the outpatient hemodialysis unit, where he experienced shaking and chills and had a temperature of 40°C (104°F). He weighed 70 kg and was 69 inches tall, had a residual creatinine clearance of 3 mL/min, and received conventional dialysis for 4 hours three times a week on a CA210 cellulose acetate dialyzer. He received 140 mg of tobramycin at the end of his hemodialysis treatment.

The first step is to estimate this patient's pharmacokinetic parameters of tobramycin on the basis of published population data. The volume of distribution in this patient is 23.1 L (0.33 L/kg × 70 kg) and

TABLE 50–11. Rebound in Drug Concentrations after the End of Hemodialysis

	t_{max}	% Rebound
Cefmetazole	0.9	17.9
Ceftibuten	0.58	45.9
Gentamicin	1.3	23.3
Netilmicin	1.9	38.3
Tobramycin	1.7	18.3
Vancomycin	6.4	52.4

his residual total body clearance (CL_{RES}) estimated from the relationship between CL and creatinine clearance [$CL_{RES} = CLcr \times 0.98$] as 3 mL/min or 0.144 L/hr. The elimination rate constant can be approximated as:

$$\begin{aligned} K &= CL_{RES} \div V_D \\ &= 0.144 \text{ L/hr} \div 23.1 \text{ L} \\ &= 0.0062 \end{aligned}$$

The hemodialysis clearance of tobramycin is dependent on the dialyzer, and a value of 73 mL/min has recently been reported by Matzke et al.[60] for the CA210 dialyzer.

One now can predict what the plasma concentrations of tobramycin will be over the next 24 to 48 hours. The concentration at the end of the 30-minute infusion (C_{max}) would be:

$$C_{max} = \frac{(\text{Dose}/t')1 - e^{-kt'}}{CL_{RES}}$$

$$C_{max} = \frac{(140 \text{ mg}/0.5 \text{ hr})1 - e^{-(CL_{RES}/V_D)t'}}{0.144 \text{ L/hr}}$$

$$C_{max} = \frac{(280 \text{ mg/hr})\,1 - e^{-(0.0062)0.5}}{0.144 \text{ L/hr}}$$

$$C_{max} = (1944 \text{ mg/L})\,(0.003) = 5.8 \text{ mg/L}$$

The plasma concentration prior to the next dialysis session (C_{bD}), which is 44 hours away, and the concentration after dialysis (C_{aD}) can be calculated as:

$$\begin{aligned} C_{bD} &= C_{max} \times e^{-(CL_{RES}/V_D)\times t} \\ &= 5.8 \times e^{-0.0062\times 44} \\ &= 4.4 \text{ mg/L} \\ C_{aD} &= C_{bD} \times e^{-((CL_{RES}+CL_D)/V_D)\times t} \\ &= 4.5 \times e^{-((0.144+4.38)/23.1)\times 4} \\ &= 4.5 \times e^{-0.195\times 4} \\ &= 2.1 \text{ mg/L} \end{aligned}$$

On the basis of these data, no further therapy will likely be required until after the next dialysis treatment. During this interdialytic interval, however, several blood samples should be collected to characterize this patient's residual tobramycin clearance, distribution volume, and the clearance of tobramycin during dialysis. Blood samples were therefore collected at the following times after the first dose:

Day 1	7 PM (2 hours after dose)	6.5 mg/L
Day 2	8 AM (39 hours after dose)	4.1 mg/L
Day 3	12 noon (after HD)	2.0 mg/L

The C_{max} can be calculated by back-extrapolation to the end of the infusion. The elimination rate during the interdialytic period (k_{ID}) and during dialysis (k_{DD}), and the V_D can be calculated as:

$$k_{ID} = (\ln C_1/C_2)/\Delta t$$

$$k_{ID} = (\ln 6.5/4.1)/37 = 0.0125/\text{h}$$

$$k_{DD} = (\ln C_2/C_3)/\Delta t$$

$$k_{DD} = (\ln 4.1/2.0)/4 = 0.179/\text{h}$$

$$V_D = \frac{\text{Dose}/t'}{k_{ID}} \frac{1 - e^{-k_{ID}\,t'}}{(C_{max} - C_{min}e^{-k_{ID}\,t'})}$$

$$V_D = \frac{140/0.5}{0.0125} \frac{1 - e^{-(0.0125)0.5}}{(6.7 - 0.0\ e^{-(0.0125)0.5})}$$

$$V_D = \frac{134.4}{6.7} = 20 \text{ L}$$

The patient's residual clearance (CL_{RES}) and the dialyzer clearance (CL_D) of tobramycin can then be calculated as:

$$\begin{aligned} CL_{RES} &= V_D \times k_{ID} \\ CL_{RES} &= 20.0 \text{ L} \times 0.0125 = 0.25 \text{ L/h or } 4.2 \text{ mL/min} \\ CL_D &= CL_T - CL_{RES} \\ CL_D &= (k_{DD} \times V_D) - 4.2 \text{ mL/min} \\ CL_D &= (0.179/\text{h} \times 20.0 \text{ L}) - 4.2 \text{ mL/min} \\ CL_D &= (3.6 \text{ L/h or } 59.6 \text{ mL/min}) - 4.2 \text{ mL/min} \\ CL_D &= 55.4 \text{ mL/min} \end{aligned}$$

This case illustrates the need for individualizing drug therapy for hemodialysis patients since this patient's V_D was 13% smaller, CL_{RES} was 75% greater, and CL_D was 25% less than the estimates based on population parameters. The ultimate reason for measuring the plasma concentrations of aminoglycosides and several other agents is to individualize the patient's dosage regimen. Thus, there remains one important step in our evaluation: the calculation of the dose this patient should receive next. The two factors that enter into this decision are the desired peak and trough concentrations and the degree of rebound in drug concentrations, after the end of dialysis. Because tobramycin concentrations have been noted to increase by about 20% within 1.5 to 2 hours after the end of hemodialysis (Table 50–11), the trough concentration of this patient can be considered to be 2.4 mg/L (2.0 mg/L × 1.2). Although this value is higher than one might like to maintain in an individual with normal renal function, a prolonged period of almost 24 hours would be required just to have the concentration drop below 2.0 mg/L. It is frequently necessary in critically ill individuals to redose the patient even though the postdialysis trough values are between 2 and 3 mg/L. Assuming the desired peak concentration was 7.0 mg/L, the postdialysis dose this patient would need can then be calculated as follows because the elimination half-life is extremely prolonged relative to the infusion time and thus minimal drug is eliminated during the infusion period:

$$\begin{aligned} \text{Dose} &= V_D \times (C_{max} - C_{min}) \\ &= 20.0 \text{ L} \times (7.0 - 2.4) = 92 \text{ mg} \end{aligned}$$

Combination antibiotic therapy with aminoglycosides and extended-spectrum penicillins are frequently prescribed for ESRD patients to provide wider antibacterial coverage against gram-negative bacilli through a synergistic effect. The combined use may result in *in vitro* chemical inactivation of the aminoglycoside, leading to a loss in antibiotic activity. The rate of inactivation is related to the incubation period, temperature, presence of solutes, and β-lactam concentration.

The extent of aminoglycoside inactivation *in vivo* may not be clinically significant in human subjects with normal or slightly impaired renal function due to the short contact time. However, in patients with severe renal insufficiency, subtherapeutic aminoglycoside concentrations and a decreased aminoglycoside elimination half-life have been reported. Patients will require appropriate dosage modification to maintain the desired serum concentrations. Inactivation of gentamicin and tobramycin by ticarcillin[72,73] and pipercillin[74,75] has been reported in patients receiving chronic dialysis therapy. The disposition of netilmicin and isepamicin, however, is unaffected by piperacillin administration.[74,75] No significant changes in V_D were noted for any of the aminoglycosides, and thus the inactivation clearances of netilmicin and isepamicin were significantly less than those of tobramycin and gentamicin. From these data tobramycin appears to be affected to the greatest degree followed by gentamicin, netilmicin, and isepamicin in descending order.

Thus, the elimination of aminoglycosides in ESRD patients also receiving antipseudomonal penicillins will be increased; therefore, frequent serum concentration monitoring should be performed. To minimize any *in vitro* inactivation of aminoglycosides that would complicate assessment of the *in vivo* effects, serum samples should be assayed as soon as possible after collection. If this is not possible, serum samples should be frozen (preferably at −70°C, or −94°F) until they can be assayed.

CONCLUSIONS

Subtherapeutic or supratherapeutic responses to drugs in patients with renal insufficiency are often misinterpreted and not recognized as such. The adverse outcomes associated with inappropriate drug use and dosing have not been quantified but do warrant future investigations. Sound pharmacokinetic principles as illustrated in this chapter, used in concert with reliable population pharmacokinetic estimates, should ultimately yield the optimal approach to drug dosage regimen design for patients with renal insufficiency. Individualization of therapy should be undertaken whenever clinical therapeutic monitoring tools are available.

REFERENCES

1. Vestal RE. Aging and pharmacology. Cancer 1997;80:1302–1310.
2. Hammerlein A, Derendorf H, Lowenthal DT. Pharmacokinetic and pharmacodynamic changes in the elderly. Clinical implications. Clin Pharmacokinet 1998;35:49–64.
3. Milsap RL, Jusko WJ. Pharmacokinetics in the infant. Environ Health Perspect 1994;102(suppl 11):107–110.
4. Sagraves R. Pediatric dosing information for health-care providers. J Pediatr Health Care 1995;9:272–277.
5. Ritschel WA, Denson DD. Influence of disease on bioavailability. In: Ritschel WA, ed. Pharmacokinetics: Regulatory, Industrial, Academic Perspectives. New York, Marcel Dekker, 1995.
6. Grandison MK, Boudinot FD. Age-related changes in protein binding of drugs: implications for therapy. Clin Pharmacokinet 2000;38:271–290.
7. Matzke GR, Millikin SP. Influence of renal disease and dialysis on pharmacokinetics. In: Evans WE, Schentag JJ, Jusko WJ, eds. Applied Pharmacokinetics: Principles of Therapeutic Drug Monitoring, 3rd ed. Spokane, WA, Applied Therapeutics, 1992:8-1 to 8-49.
8. Elston AC, Bayliss MK, Park GR. Effect of renal failure on drug metabolism by the liver. Br J Anaesth 1993;71:282–290.
9. Rowland M, Tozer TN. Clinical Pharmacokinetics: Concepts and Applications, 3rd ed. Philadelphia, Lea & Febiger, 1995.
10. Matzke GR, Frye RF. Drug administration in patients with renal insufficiency: Minimizing renal and extrarenal toxicity. Drug Saf 1997;16:205–231.
11. Vestal RE, Wood AJ, Shand DG. Reduced β-receptor sensitivity in the elderly. Clin Pharmacol Ther 1979;26:181–186.
12. St Peter WL, Redickill KA, Halstenson CE. Clinical pharmacokinetics of antibiotics in patients with impaired renal function. Clin Pharmacokinet 1992;22:169–210.
13. St Peter WL, Halstenson CE. Pharmacologic approach in patients with renal failure. In: Chernow B, ed. The Pharmacologic Approach to the Critically Ill Patient. Baltimore, Williams & Wilkins, 1994:41–79.
14. Vanholder R, Van Landsehoot N, De Smet R, et al. Drug protein binding in chronic renal failure: Evaluation of nine drugs. Kidney Int 1988;33:996–1004.
15. Chan GL, Axelson JE, Price JD, et al. In vitro protein binding of propafenone in normal and uraemic human sera. Eur J Clin Pharmacol 1989;36:495–499.
16. Pritchard JF, Matzke GR, Opsahl JA, et al. Effects of hemodialysis on plasma protein binding of bepridil. J Clin Pharmacol 1995;35:137–141.
17. Liponi DF, Winter ME, Tozer TN. Renal function and therapeutic concentrations of phenytoin. Neurology 1984;34:395–397.
18. Job ML. Digoxin. In: Murphy JE, ed. Clinical Pharmacokinetics Pocket Reference, 2nd ed. Bethesda, MD, American Society of Hospital Pharmacists, 2001;143–162.
19. Malini PL, Strocchi E, Feliciangeli G, Buscaroli A, Bonomini V. Digitalis receptors and digoxin sensitivity in renal failure. Clin Exp Pharmacol Physiol 1985;12:115–120.
20. Lam YW, Barnerji S, Hatfield C, Talbert RL. Principles of drug administration in renal insufficiency. Clin Pharmacokinet 1997;32:30–57.
21. Koup J. Disease states and drug pharmacokinetics. J Clin Pharmacol 1989;29:674–679.
22. Prescott LF, Freestone S, McAuslane JA. The concentration-dependent disposition of intravenous p-aminohippurate in subjects with normal and impaired renal function. Br J Clin Pharmacol 1993;35:20–29.
23. Leblond F, Guevin C, Demers C, et al. Downregulation of hepatic cytochrome P450 in chronic renal failure. J Am Soc Nephrol 2001;12:326–332.
24. Leblond FA, Giroux L, Villeneuve JP, Pichette V. Decreased in vivo metabolism of drugs in chronic renal failure. Drug Metab Dispos 2000; 28:1317–1320.
25. Touchette MA, Slaughter RL. The effect of renal failure on hepatic drug clearance. DICP 1991;25:1214–1224.
26. Kim YG, Shin JG, Shin SG, et al. Decreased acetylation of isoniazid in chronic renal failure. Clin Pharmacol Ther 1993;54:612–620.
27. Van Bortel L, Bohm R, Mooij J, et al. Total and free steady-state plasma levels and pharmacokinetics of nifedipine in patients with terminal renal failure. Eur J Clin Pharmacol 1989;37:185–189.
28. Aronoff GR. Pharmacokinetics of nitrendipine in patients with renal failure: Comparison to normal subjects. J Cardiovasc Pharmacol 1984; 6:S974–S976.
29. Van Harten J, Burggraaf J, van Brummelen P, et al. Influence of renal function on the pharmacokinetics and cardiovascular effects of nisoldipine after single and multiple dosing. Clin Pharmacokinet 1989;16:55–64.
30. Frye RF, Matzke GR, Alexander ACM, et al. Effect of renal insufficiency on CYP activity. Clin Pharmcol Ther 1996;59:155.
31. Wolfert AI, Sica DA. Narcotic usage in renal failure. Int J Artif Organs 1988;11:411–415.
32. Bendayan R. Renal drug transport—A review. Pharmacotherapy 1996; 16:971–985.
33. Kamiya A, Okumura K, Hori R. Quantitative investigation of renal handling of drugs in dogs with renal insufficiency. Pharm Sci 1984;74:892–896.
34. Hori R, Okumura K, Kamiya A, et al. Ampicillin and cephalexin in renal insufficiency. Clin Pharmacol Ther 1983;34:792–798.
35. McEvoy GK, Litvak K, Welsh OH, et al. American Hospital Formulary Service, Drug Information. Bethesda, MD, American Society of Hospital Pharmacists, 2001.
36. Aronoff GR, Berns JS, Brier ME, et al. Drug Prescribing in Renal Failure: Dosing Guidelines for Adults, 4th ed. Philadelphia, American College of Physicians, 1998.
37. Murphy JE. Clinical pharmacokinetics pocket reference, 2nd ed. Bethesda, MD, American Society of Hospital Pharmacists, 2001.
38. Benet LZ, Williams RL. Design and optimization of dosage regimens: Pharmacokinetic data. In: Goodman GA, Rall TW, Nies AS, Taylor P, eds. The Pharmacological Basis of Therapeutics, 8th ed. Elmsford, NY, Pergamon Press, 1990:1650–1735.
39. Craig WA. Pharmacokinetic/pharmacodynamic parameters: Rationale for antibacterial dosing of mice and men. Clin Infect Dis 1998;26:1–12.
40. Sommadossi JP, Bevan R, Ling T, et al. Clinical pharmacokinetics of ganciclovir in patients with normal and impaired renal function. Rev Infect Dis 1988;10:S507–S514.
41. Pescovitz MD, Pruett TL, Gonwa T, et al. Oral ganciclovir dosing in transplant recipients and dialysis patients based on renal function. Transplantation 1998;27:1104–1107.

42. Balfour HH. Management of cytomegalovirus disease with antiviral drugs. Rev Infect Dis 1990;12:S849–S860.
43. Joy MS, Matzke GR, Armstrong DK, Marx MA, Zarowitz BJ. A primer on continuous renal replacement therapy for critically ill patients. Ann Pharmacother 1998;32:362–375.
44. Macias WL, Mueller BA, Scarim SK. Vancomycin pharmacokinetics in acute renal failure: Preservation of non-renal clearance. Clin Pharmacol Ther 1991;50:688–694.
45. Mueller BA, Scarim SK, Macias WL. Comparison of imipenem pharmacokinetics in patients with acute or chronic renal failure treated with continuous hemofiltration. Am J Kidney Dis 1993;21:172–179.
46. Heinemeyer G, Link J, Weber W, et al. Clearance of ceftriaxone in critical care patients with acute renal failure. Intensive Care Med 1990;16:448–453.
47. Kronfol NO, Lau AH, Barakat MM. Aminoglycoside binding to polyacrylonitrile hemofilter membranes during continuous hemofiltration. ASAIO Trans 1987;33:300–303.
48. Matzke GR, Frye RF, Joy MS, Palevsky PM. Determinants of ceftazidime clearance by continuous venovenous hemofiltration and continuous venovenous hemodialysis. Antimicrob Agents Chemother 2000;44:1639–1644.
49. Joy MS, Matzke GR, Frye RF, Palevsky PM. Determinants of vancomycin clearance by continuous venovenous hemofiltration and continuous venovenous hemodialysis. Am J Kidney Dis 1998;31:1019–1027.
50. Lau AH, Kronfol NO. Determinants of drug removal by continuous hemofiltration. Int J Artif Organs 1994;17:373–378.
51. Reetze-Bonorden P, Bohler J, Keller E. Drug dosage in patients during continuous renal replacement therapy. Clin Pharmacokinet 1993;24:362–379.
52. Bressolle F, Kinowski JM, de la Coussaye JE, et al. Clinical pharmacokinetics during continuous hemofiltration. Clin Pharmacokinet 1994;26:457–471.
53. Taylor CA, Abdel-Rahman E, Zimmerman SW, Johnson CA. Clinical pharmacokinetics during continuous ambulatory peritoneal dialysis. Clin Pharmacokinet 1996;31:293–308.
54. Keane WF, Baile GR, Boeschoten E, et al. Adult peritoneal dialysis-related peritonitis treatment recommendations: 2000 update. Perit Dial Int 2000;20:396–411.
55. U.S. Renal Data Systems. USRDS 2000 Annual Data Report. Bethesda, MD, The National Institutes of Health, Institute of Diabetes and Digestive and Kidney Diseases, 2000.
56. Konstantin P. Newer membranes: Cuprophan versus polysulfone versus polyacrylonitrile. In: Bosch JP, ed. Contemporary Issues in Nephrology. Hemodialysis: High Efficiency Treatments, vol 27. New York, Churchill Livingstone, 1993:63–78.
57. Golper TA, Vincent HH, Gleason JR, Vos MC. Drug removal during high efficiency and high-flux hemodialysis. In: Bosch JP, ed. Contemporary Issues in Nephrology. Hemodialysis: High Efficiency Treatments, vol 27. New York, Churchill Livingstone, 1993:175–209.
58. Pollard TA, Lampasona V, Mullins RE, et al. Vancomycin redistribution: Dosing recommendations following high flux hemodialysis. Kidney Int 1994;45:232–237.
59. Matzke GR, Palevsky P.M., Frye, RF. In-vitro model for ceftazidime disposition during hemodialysis with conventional and high-flux biocompatible membranes. Annual Meeting of the American Association of Pharmaceutical Scientists. Indianapolis, IN, November 1, 2000.
60. Matzke GR, Palevsky PM, Frye RF. In-vitro model for tobramycin disposition during hemodialysis with conventional and high flux biocompatible membranes. J Am Soc Nephrol 2000;11:286A.
61. Matzke GR, Frye RF, Nolin TD, et al. Vancomycin removal by low- and high-flux hemodialysis with polymethylmethacrylate dialyzers. J Am Soc Nephrol 1999;10:193A.
62. Amin NB, Padhi ID, Touchette MA, et al. Characterization of gentamicin pharmacokinetics in patients hemodialyzed with high-flux polysulfone membranes. Am J Kidney Dis 1999;34:222–227.
63. Tsuruoka S, Sugimoto KI, Hayasaka T, et al. Ranitidine clearance during hemodialysis with high-flux membrane: Comparison of polysulfone and cellulose acetate hemodialyzers. Eur J Clin Pharmacol 2000;56:581–583.
64. Aweek FT, Jacobson MA, Martin-Munley S, et al. Effect of renal disease and hemodialysis on foscarnet pharmacokinetics and dosing recommendations. J Acquir Immune Defic Syndr 1999;20:350–357.
65. Cheung AK, Agodoa LY, Daugirdas JT, et al. Effects of hemodialyzer reuse on clearances of urea and β_2-microglobulin. J Am Soc Nephrol 1999;10:117–127.
66. Palevsky PM, Frye RF, Matzke GR. Effect of dialyzer reprocessing on the clearance of low and intermediate molecular weight solutes. J Am Soc Nephrol 2001;12:273A.
67. Barbhaiya RH, Knupp CA, Forgue ST, et al. Pharmacokinetics of cefepime in subjects with renal insufficiency. Clin Pharmacol Ther 1990;48:268–276.
68. Halstenson CE, Guay DR, Opsahl JA, et al. Disposition of cefmetazole in healthy volunteers and patients with impaired renal function. Antimicrob Agents Chemother 1990;34:519–523.
69. Matzke GR, O'Connell ME, Collins AJ, Keshaviah PR. Disposition of vancomycin during hemofiltration. Clin Pharmacol Ther 1986;40:425–430.
70. Kelloway JS, Awni WM, Lin CC, et al. Pharmacokinetics of ceftibuten-*cis* and its *trans* metabolite in healthy volunteers and in patients with chronic renal insufficiency. Antimicrob Agents Chemother 1991;35:2267–2274.
71. Halstenson CE, Berkseth RO, Mann HJ, Matzke GR. Aminoglycoside redistribution phenomenon after hemodialysis: Netilmicin and tobramycin. Int J Clin Pharmacol Ther Toxicol 1987;25:50–55.
72. Russo ME, Atkin-Thor E. Gentamicin and ticarcillin in subjects with end-stage renal disease. Clin Nephrol 1981;15:175–180.
73. Matzke GR, Luckham DR, Collins AJ, Halstenson CE. Effect of ticarcillin on gentamicin and tobramycin pharmacokinetics in a patient with end-stage renal disease. Pharmacotherapy 1984;4:158–160.
74. Halstenson CE, Wong MO, Herman CS, et al. Effect of concomitant administration of piperacillin on the dispositions of isepamicin and gentamicin in patients with end-stage renal disease. Antimicrob Agents Chemother 1992;36:1832–1836.
75. Halstenson CE, Hirata CA, Heim-Duthoy KL, Abraham PA, Matzke GR. Effect of concomitant administration of piperacillin on the dispositions of netilmicin and tobramycin in patients with end–stage renal disease. Antimicrob Agents Chemother 1990;34:128–133.

51

DISORDERS OF SODIUM, WATER, CALCIUM, AND PHOSPHORUS HOMEOSTASIS

Melanie S. Joy and Gerald A. Hladik

Homeostasis of fluid and electrolytes is necessary for the body's normal physiologic functions. Disorders of sodium, water, calcium, and phosphorus are common complications of multiple acute and chronic diseases. These disorders are frequently associated with the acute care setting; however, they are clearly present in a less-severe state in the ambulatory care environment. The consequences of electrolyte disorders can range from asymptomatic to life-threatening requiring hospitalization. The maintenance of fluid and electrolyte homeostasis requires adequate functioning of feedback mechanisms, hormones, and multiple organ systems. It is necessary to understand the pathophysiology of these disorders in order to classify and develop appropriate treat plans.

From a pharmaceutical care perspective, disorders of electrolytes can result from drug therapy. In addition, with some drug therapies, toxicity can be enhanced when underlying electrolyte disorders are present. Drug-induced disorders respond well to discontinuation of the offending agent(s); however, additional therapies are sometimes required to correct the disorder. This chapter reviews the etiology, classification, clinical presentation, and therapy for disorders of sodium, water, calcium, and phosphorus.

SODIUM AND WATER HOMEOSTASIS

Two-thirds of total body water is distributed intracellularly while one-third is contained in the extracellular space.[1] Sodium and its accompanying anions, chloride and bicarbonate, comprise more than 90% of the total osmolality of the extracellular fluid (ECF), while intracellular osmolality is primarily dependent on the concentration of potassium and its accompanying anions (mostly organic and inorganic phosphates). The differential concentrations of sodium and potassium in the intra- and extracellular fluid is maintained by the Na^+-K^+-ATPase pump.[2] Most cell membranes are freely permeable to water, and thus the osmolality of intra- and extracellular body fluids is the same. Symptoms in patients with hypo- and hypernatremia are primarily related to alterations in cell volume.[3] It is therefore essential to understand the factors that cause changes in cell volume.

Solutes that cannot freely cross cell membranes, such as sodium, are referred to as "effective osmoles." The concentration of effective osmoles in the ECF determines the tonicity of the ECF, which directly effects the distribution of water between the extra- and intracellular compartments.[4] Addition of an isotonic solution to the ECF will result in no change in intracellular volume because there will be no change in the effective osmolality of the ECF. Addition of a hypertonic solution to the ECF, however, will result in a decrease in cell volume, whereas addition of a hypotonic solution to the ECF will result in an increase in cell volume. Table 51–1 summarizes the composition of commonly used intravenous solutions and their respective distribution into extracellular and intracellular compartments following infusion.

Hypo- and hypernatremia are syndromes of altered tonicity and cell volume caused by changes in water balance. Thus, an understanding of factors that effect tonicity and water balance is essential in order to understand the pathogenesis and evaluation of these syndromes. The serum sodium concentration is tightly regulated, and usually varies by no more than 2% to 3%. The kidney regulates water excretion through a feedback mechanism with the hypothalamus, such that the serum osmolality remains relatively constant (275–290 mOsm/kg) despite day-to-day variations in water intake. The serum osmolality is comprised primarily of sodium and the accompanying anions chloride and bicarbonate, and may be estimated by:

$$\text{Sosm} = (2 \times S_{Na}) + (B_{glucose}/18) + (BUN/2.8)$$

where Sosm = serum osmolality in mOsm/kg; S_{Na} = serum sodium concentration in mEq/L; $B_{glucose}$ = glucose concentration in mg/dL; and BUN = blood urea nitrogen concentration in mg/dL.[5]

Antidiuretic hormone (ADH) is released from the posterior pituitary when the plasma osmolality rises by 1% to 2% or more.[6] ADH binds to the vasopressin-2 (V2) receptors on the basolateral surface of renal tubular epithelial cells, and through a series of second messenger reactions, a water channel (aquaporin-2) is inserted into the apical tubular lumen surface of the cell.[7] Water may then pass through the cell into the peritubular capillary space, and is then reabsorbed into the systemic circulation. A rise in serum osmolality sensed in the hypothalamus results not only in ADH release, but also in stimulation of thirst. The combination of an increase in water intake and a decrease in water excretion results in a decrease in the serum osmolality and inhibition of ADH secretion once the plasma osmolality is restored to normal.

Nonosmotic release of ADH occurs when the effective arterial blood volume (EABV) decreases by approximately 5% to 10%.[8] The EABV is the vascular component of the ECF that is responsible for organ perfusion.[9] A change in the EABV promotes an afferent response from baroreceptors in the chest and neck and activation of the renin-angiotensin system, leading to synthesis of angiotensin II. Angiotensin II then stimulates both nonosmotic release of ADH and thirst. The volume stimulus overrides osmotic inhibition of ADH release, and conservation of water fosters restoration of blood pressure and EABV at the expense of hypo-osmolality.

The proper assessment of a patient with an abnormal serum sodium concentration requires recognition that the serum sodium level may bear no relationship to the ECF volume and sodium content. Hypernatremia and hyponatremia may be associated with conditions of high, low, or normal ECF sodium and volume. Abnormalities in the serum sodium concentration are thus a result of an alteration in the normal ratio between the total sodium and water content in the ECF.

TABLE 51–1. Composition of Intravenous Replacement Solutions

Solution	Dextrose (gm/dL)	[Na^+] (mEq/L)	[C^-] (mEq/L)	Tonicity	Distribution %ECF	%ICF	Free Water/L
5% Dextrose in Water (D_5W)	5	0	0	Hypotonic	40	60	1,000 mL
0.45% saline (½ normal saline)	0	77	77	Hypotonic	73	37	500 mL
0.9% saline (normal saline)	0	154	154	Isotonic	100	0	0 mL
3% saline (hypertonic saline)	0	513	513	Hypertonic	100*	0	−2,331 mL

*This solution will result in osmotic removal of water from the intracellular space.

HYPONATREMIA

EPIDEMIOLOGY/ETIOLOGY

Hyponatremia (serum sodium <135 mEq/L) is the most common electrolyte abnormality in hospitalized patients, with a reported incidence of about 2.5%.[10] Brain injury results from either the acute effects of hypo-osmolality or from too rapid correction of hypo-osmolality in patients with symptomatic hyponatremia, and is associated with a 20% incidence of significant morbidity and a mortality rate as high as 25%.[11] Hyponatremia is predominantly the result of an excess of extracellular water relative to sodium because of impaired water excretion. The kidney normally has the capacity to excrete large volumes of dilute urine after ingestion of a water load. Nonosmotic release of ADH, however, can lead to retention of water and to a drop in serum sodium concentration, despite a fall in both serum and intracellular osmolality. The causes of nonosmotic release of ADH include hypovolemia, decreased EABV as seen in patients with CHF, nephrosis, and cirrhosis, and the syndrome of inappropriate ADH (SIADH) release. The pathophysiology, clinical features, and management of hyponatremia are detailed below.

PATHOPHYSIOLOGY

Hyponatremia in patients with normal serum osmolality may be caused by hyperlipidemia or hyperproteinemia. If serum sodium concentration is measured by flame photometry, the volume of serum is overestimated because the elevated lipids or proteins account for a greater proportion of the total volume of the sample (Fig. 51–1).[12] Because the sodium is distributed in only the water component of serum, the measured serum sodium concentration is falsely decreased.

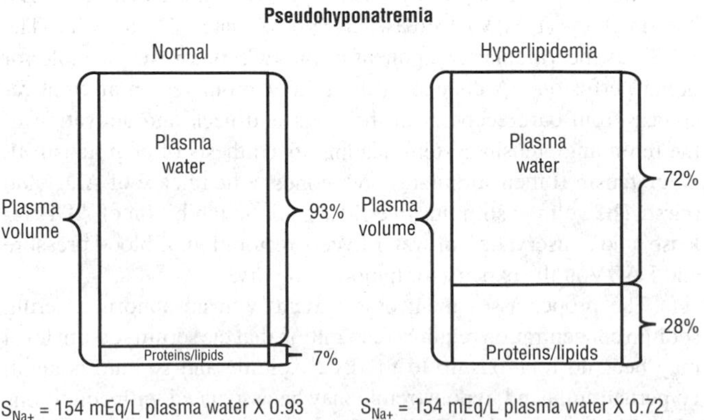

FIGURE 51–1. Elevated lipids or proteins result in a larger discrepancy between the volume of the sample and plasma water, leading to a falsely low measurement of the serum sodium concentration when using the method of flame photometry.

The measurement of serum osmolality, however, is not significantly affected leading to a discrepancy between the calculated and measured serum osmolality. Because the serum sodium level is falsely decreased, this condition has been termed *pseudohyponatremia*. This laboratory artifact is uncommon today and has been overcome with the use of ion-specific electrodes to measure the serum sodium concentration.[13]

Hyponatremia in the presence of an elevated serum osmolality suggests the presence of excess effective osmoles in the ECF. This is most frequently encountered in patients with hyperglycemia, but is also seen in patients who have received irrigation with glycine during surgery, or in patients who have been treated with osmotic diuretics such as mannitol.[14,15] The presence of glucose, glycine, or mannitol leads to diffusion of water from the cells into the extracellular compartment resulting in hyponatremia. For every 100 mg/dL rise in the serum glucose concentration, the serum sodium level decreases by 1.7 mEq/L[16] and the serum osmolality rises by 2 mOsm/kg.[17] Unmeasured osmoles should be suspected in patients with hypertonic hyponatremia when the difference between the measured and calculated osmolality, the "osmolal gap," exceeds 15 mOsm/kg.[18]

In patients with a low plasma osmolality (hypotonicity), the most important step in the diagnostic evaluation of hyponatremia is the clinical assessment of the extracellular fluid volume.[19] Categorization of patients with hypotonic hyponatremia into one of three groups (decreased, increased, or clinically normal ECF volume) is crucial in order to identify the pathophysiologic mechanisms responsible for the hyponatremia and thereby propose an appropriate treatment regimen (Fig. 51–2).

HYPOVOLEMIC HYPOTONIC HYPONATREMIA

Most patients with ECF volume contraction lose fluids that are hypotonic relative to plasma and thus may be transiently hypernatremic. This includes patients with fluid losses caused by diarrhea, excessive sweating, and diuretics. This "transient" hypernatremic hyperosmolality results in osmotic release of ADH and stimulation of thirst. If sodium and water losses continue, more ADH is released as a result of hypovolemia. Patients who then drink water or who are given hypotonic fluids intravenously retain water and develop hyponatremia. Urine osmolality is generally greater than 450 mOsm/kg, reflecting the presence of ADH and formation of a concentrated urine.[19] The urine sodium concentration is <20 mEq/L when sodium losses are extrarenal, as in patients with diarrhea, and >20 mEq/L in patients with renal sodium losses, as occurs in the setting of diuretic use or adrenal insufficiency.[20]

Diuretic-induced hyponatremia occurs more frequently in patients treated with thiazide diuretics than in those patients who are receiving loop diuretics.[21] In addition to causing extracellular volume depletion and nonosmotic stimulation of ADH, thiazides interfere with urinary dilution and water excretion by blocking tubular sodium

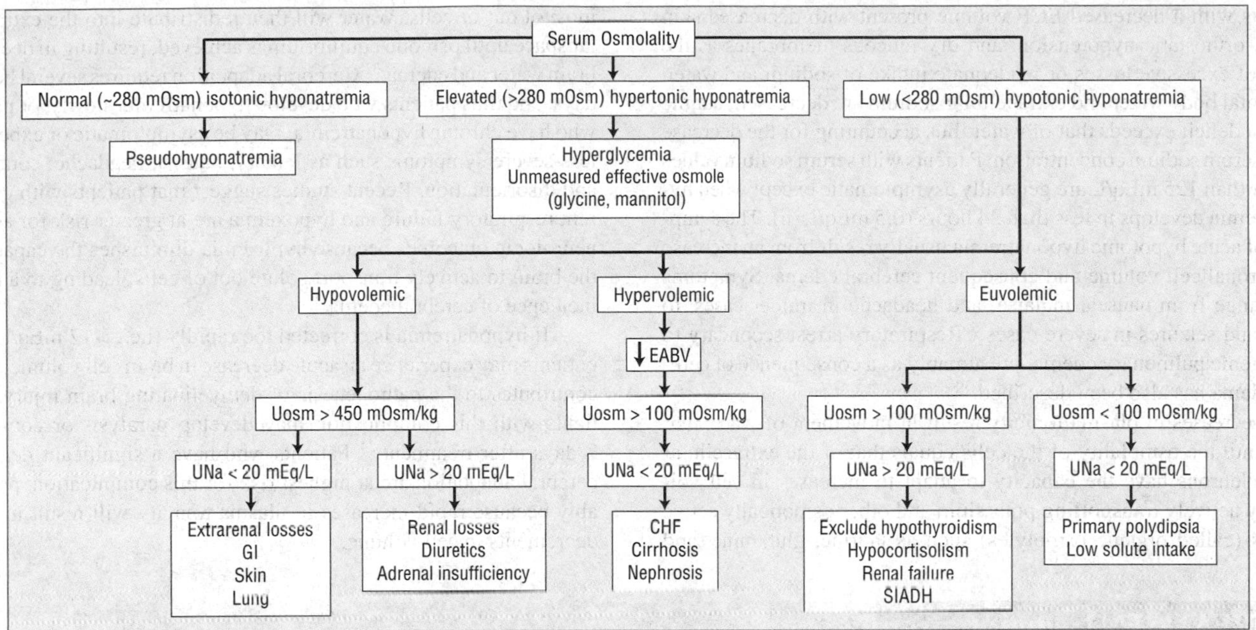

FIGURE 51–2. Diagnostic algorithm for the evaluation of hyponatremia. CHF = congestive heart failure; UNa = urine sodium concentration; Uosm = urine osmolality; SIADH = syndrome of inappropriate antidiuretic hormone secretion.

and potassium reabsorption in the distal tubule. Water is then retained in excess of sodium by virtue of nonosmotic release of ADH and excretion of urine with a concentration of sodium and potassium that exceeds that of the plasma.

Hyponatremia occurs less commonly with loop diuretics for several reasons. First, most loop diuretics have a shorter half-life than that of thiazides, and patients can therefore replete the urinary sodium and water losses prior to taking the next dose, thereby minimizing the degree of nonosmotic ADH stimulation. Loop diuretics also interfere with both urinary dilution and concentration. The latter is disrupted through inhibition of solute transport into the medulla, which interferes with creation of the medullary osmotic gradient. Thus, relatively less water is retained in the presence of ADH.

EUVOLEMIC HYPOTONIC HYPONATREMIA

Euvolemic hyponatremia is associated with a normal or slightly decreased ECF sodium content and increased total body water and ECF volume. The increase in ECF volume is usually not sufficient to cause peripheral or pulmonary edema, and thus patients appear clinically euvolemic. Euvolemic hyponatremia is most commonly caused by SIADH secretion. In this syndrome, water intake exceeds capacity of the kidneys to excrete water either because of enhanced renal sensitivity to ADH or because of an increased release of ADH via nonosmotic and/or nonphysiologic processes.[22] The urine osmolality in SIADH is generally greater than 100 mOsm/kg, and the urine sodium concentration is greater than 20 mEq/L as a result of the ECF volume expansion. The most common causes of SIADH include tumors such as oat cell cancer of the lung, central nervous system (CNS) disorders (e.g., head trauma, stroke, meningitis, and pituitary surgery), as well as pulmonary disease. Drugs such as chlorpropamide, carbamazepine, cyclophosphamide, and nonsteroidal anti-inflammatory drugs (NSAIDs) induce SIADH by enhancing the sensitivity of the kidney to ADH.[23–26] Selective serotonin reuptake inhibitors and methylenedeoxymethamphetamine, a drug of abuse commonly known as Ecstasy, also induce nonosmotic release of ADH.[27,28] Patients with renal insufficiency, adrenal insufficiency, and hypothyroidism may also present with euvolemic hyponatremia, and the evaluation of patients with suspected SIADH should always include exclusion of these disorders.

The differential diagnosis of euvolemic hypotonic hyponatremia also includes primary or psychogenic polydipsia. Patients with this disorder drink more water (usually >20 L/day) than the kidneys can excrete as solute-free water. Unlike SIADH, however, ADH is suppressed resulting in a urine osmolality that is less than 100 mOsm/kg. The urine sodium is typically low (<15 mEq/L) as a result of urinary dilution.[29] Hyponatremia may develop with more modest water intake in patients on a very low solute diet, such as a sodium-free vegetarian diet.

HYPERVOLEMIC HYPOTONIC HYPONATREMIA

Hyponatremia associated with an increase in ECF volume occurs in conditions in which renal sodium and water excretion are impaired. Patients with cirrhosis, congestive heart failure, and nephrotic syndrome have an expanded ECF volume and edema, but a decreased EABV. The decreased EABV results in renal sodium retention and, eventually, ECF volume expansion and edema. At the same time, there is nonosmotic release of ADH and retention of water in excess of sodium thus perpetuating the hyponatremia.

CLINICAL PRESENTATION

Most patients with hyponatremia are asymptomatic, and the laboratory finding is often uncovered in the routine evaluation of patients presenting with symptoms attributable to another medical condition such as volume depletion or congestive heart failure.[5] Hyponatremic patients with a decreased ECF volume present with decreased skin turgor, orthostatic hypotension, and dry mucous membranes as the result of excessive losses or inadequate intake of sodium and water. Both total body water and extracellular sodium are decreased, but the sodium deficit exceeds that of water thus accounting for the decrease in the serum sodium concentration. Patients with serum sodium values greater than 125 mEq/L are generally asymptomatic except when hyponatremia develops in less than 24 hours (0.5 mEq/L/h). The symptoms of acute hypotonic hyponatremia usually result from an increase in neuronal cell volume and consequent cerebral edema. Symptoms may range from nausea, malaise, and headache in milder cases, to coma and seizures in severe cases.[5] Respiratory arrest secondary to neurogenic pulmonary edema, presumably as a consequence of cerebral edema has also been described.[30]

Decreases in plasma tonicity result in movement of water into cells until the osmolality of the cells equals that of the extracellular fluid. Neurons have the capacity to adapt to increases in cell volume by actively transporting potassium and other osmotically active solutes (called organic osmolytes) such as taurine, glutamine, and inositol out of cells. Water will then redistribute into the extracellular space until osmotic equilibrium is achieved, resulting in decreased brain water and edema.[31] Cerebral adaptation requires several hours to days, and thus patients who develop hyponatremia slowly, or patients who have chronic hyponatremia, may be asymptomatic or experience less-severe symptoms such as lethary, nausea, headache, confusion, and disorientation. Recent studies suggest that patients with concurrent respiratory failure and hypoxemia are at greater risk for adverse neurologic outcomes because hypoxemia diminishes the capacity of the brain to actively transport solute out of cells, leading to a higher incidence of cerebral edema.[32]

If hyponatremia is corrected too rapidly (i.e., >12 mEq/L/day), patients may experience an acute decrease in brain cell volume, which contributes to the pathogenesis of demyelinating brain injury.[33] Patients with this complication may develop paralysis or coma 5 to 7 days after treatment.[34] Patients who have a significant degree of cerebral adaptation are at highest risk for this complication, presumably because rapid increases in plasma tonicity will result in larger decrements in cell volume.

▶ TREATMENT: Hyponatremia

DESIRED OUTCOME

The goal of treating patients with hypovolemic hypotonic hyponatremia is to correct the ECF volume deficit, which will then lead to correction of the hyponatremia and restoration of organ perfusion. The treatment goals for hypervolemic and euvolemic hypotonic patients depend on the underlying cause of the hyponatremia and whether the patient is symptomatic. Patients who develop hyponatremia rapidly have the highest risk for cerebral edema, and thus require more aggressive therapy to correct the hypotonicity. The goal for these patients is to increase the tonicity at a rate appropriate to restore and maintain cell volume as close to normal as possible. Asymptomatic patients do not require rapid correction of the serum sodium, and the treatment is dictated by the underlying etiology. In all cases the goal is to avoid a rise in the serum sodium concentration greater than 12 mEq/L in 24 hours.

ACUTE SYMPTOMATIC HYPOTONIC HYPONATREMIA

The patient with symptoms attributable to hypotonicity regardless of fluid status should initially be treated with either a 0.9% or a 3% concentrated solution of sodium chloride until symptoms resolve, which generally requires that the serum sodium be increased to approximately 120 mEq/L. The serum sodium concentration should be titrated upward at a rate of 1.5–2 mEq/L/h for the first several hours in patients with severe symptoms (seizures, coma). However, the total correction still should not exceed 12 mEq within the first 24 hours.

The relative concentrations of urine sodium and potassium (osmotically effective urine cations) must be compared with that of the infusate in planning a treatment regimen for patients with hypotonic hyponatremia. For the serum sodium to rise after infusion of a solution of sodium chloride, the concentration of sodium in the infusate must exceed the sum of the sodium and potassium concentration in the urine in order to effect net free water excretion. Patients with SIADH often have urinary concentrations of osmotically effective urine cations that exceed the sodium concentration of 0.9% saline (154 mEq/L), and thus patients should be preferentially treated with 3% saline (513 mEq/L). Use of isotonic saline, in this case, carries the potential hazard of actually worsening hyponatremia.[35] The relatively high concentration of urinary sodium in patients with SIADH stems from the fact that the ECF is expanded, thus minimizing reabsorption of sodium along the nephron. When the urine osmolality exceeds 300 mOsm/kg, it is generally advisable to add an intravenous loop diuretic not only to increase the excretion of solute free water, but also to prevent volume overload, which may result from infusion of hypertonic saline. Intravenous furosemide, initially at a dose of 40 mg every 6 hours, is generally sufficient to prevent volume overload and to decrease the concentration of osmotically active urine cations to less than 150 mEq/L.

Patients with hypovolemic hypotonic hyponatremia, on the other hand, should be treated with normal saline because the concentration of osmotically effective urine cations is invariably less than that of isotonic saline. In contrast to patients with SIADH, sodium is avidly reabsorbed throughout the nephron when the effective circulating blood volume is decreased. The urine osmolality, then, is primarily comprised of urea and the concentration of urine sodium is often less than 20 mEq/L.

Hypervolemic patients are particularly problematic to manage acutely because the sodium and volume required to minimize the risk of cerebral edema or seizures may worsen their already compensated hepatic, cardiac, or renal function. It is generally agreed that these patients should be treated with hypertonic saline and prompt initiation of fluid restriction. Loop diuretic therapy will also likely be required to facilitate urinary excretion of free water.

CALCULATION OF RATE OF ADMINISTRATION OF HYPERTONIC SALINE

Several methods have been developed to determine the correct volume of 3% saline to administer, but it is important to keep in mind that these formulas do not account for ongoing solute and water excretion, and only provide a rough estimate of the correct dose. The change in plasma sodium resulting from the infusion of 3% saline can be estimated as:[5]

$$\text{Change in } S_{Na} \text{ with 1 liter of infusate} = [IV_{Na} - S^1_{Na}] \div (BW + 1 \text{ liter})$$

where S^1_{Na} = patient serum sodium concentration; IV_{Na} = sodium concentration of infusate; IV_{vol} = volume of 3% saline infused; and BW = total body water (in liters), which may be estimated as a fraction of total body weight (kilograms) as follows:[36]

0.6 × Body weight for children and men < 70 years old
0.5 × Body weight for men ≥ 70 years old and females < 70 years old
0.45 × Body weight for women ≥ 70 years old

The serum sodium of a 50-kg 80-year-old female with SIADH presenting with confusion and a serum sodium level of 108 mEq/L, for example, should be corrected to approximately 120 mEq/L over the first 24 hours of hospitalization. The change in serum sodium of 12 mEq/L may be calculated as follows:

$$\begin{aligned}\text{Change in } S^1_{Na} &= (513\,\text{mEq/L} - 108\,\text{mEq/L}) \\ &\quad \div [(0.45\,\text{kg} \times 50\,\text{kg}) + 1.0\,\text{L}] \\ &= [405\,\text{mEq/L}] \div 23.5\,\text{L} \\ \text{Change in } S^1_{Na} &= 17\,\text{mEq/L}\end{aligned}$$

Because 1 L of 3% saline results in a 17 mEq/L rise in the serum sodium, one can extrapolate that each 100 mL would increase the serum sodium by 1.7 mEq/L. Thus, the total dose required to achieve a change of 12 mEq/L in 24 hours will be approximately 705 mL. In the presence of symptoms, the serum sodium should be raised by approximately 1.5 mEq/L/h over the first 2 to 4 hours (for a total of 6 mEq/L) or until the symptoms have resolved. Thus, an initial infusion rate of 88 mL/h [1.5 mEq/L/h ÷ 1.7 mEq/L/100 mL] for the first 2 to 4 hours, followed by an infusion rate of approximately 17.5–22 mL/h for the next 20 to 22 hours respectively would be a reasonable initial treatment plan.

EVALUATION OF THERAPEUTIC OUTCOMES

Patients with symptomatic hypotonic hyponatremia should be admitted to the intensive care unit or to a highly monitored setting for close monitoring of neurologic and volume status. Serial physical examinations of the heart, lungs, and neurologic status should be performed several times over the initial 12 hours of hospitalization. The serum sodium concentration should be measured every 2 to 4 hours, and the urine osmolality, sodium, and potassium should be measured every 4 to 6 hours over the first day of therapy. The rate of administration of the infusate should then be adjusted to avoid exceeding a rise in the serum sodium greater than 12 mEq/L/day.

HYPOVOLEMIC HYPOTONIC HYPONATREMIA

Because this condition is rarely associated with symptoms the desired outcomes can generally be achieved with restoration of the blood pressure to the normal range, absence of postural changes in blood pressure, or increases in the central venous pressure or pulmonary capillary wedge pressure to greater than 10 cm H_2O as assessed by central venous or pulmonary artery catheter. A 0.9% solution of sodium chloride, which has a tonicity that approximates that of the ECF, should be infused to correct the volume deficit, because all of the infused solution will remain in the ECF.

ECF volume deficit (ECFVd), is dependent on the patient's weight, age, and the degree of volume depletion, and is difficult to precisely estimate. An ECFVd loss that is equal to a 10% to 15% decrease in body weight is associated with the development of postural hypotension. An ECFVd loss as low as 5%, however, can result in hyponatremia caused by nonosmotic ADH release as a result of stimulation of baroreceptors located in the chest and neck. The ECFVd of patients can be estimated as illustrated in this case: a 42-year-old male weighs 70 kg on initial examination and presents with postural hypotension and has a serum sodium of 125 mEq/L:[37]

$$\begin{aligned}\text{ECFVd} &= \text{ECFV}_{norm} - \text{ECFV}_{current} \\ \text{ECFVd} &= [\text{TBW}_{norm} \times 0.6\,\text{L/kg} \times 0.33] \\ &\quad - [\text{TBW}_{current} \times 0.6\,\text{L/kg} \times 0.33]\end{aligned}$$

Where TBW_{norm} is 15% greater than $\text{TBW}_{current}$:

$$\begin{aligned}\text{ECFVd} &= [80.5\,\text{kg} \times 0.6\,\text{L/kg} \times 0.33] \\ &\quad - [70\,\text{kg} \times 0.6\,\text{L/kg} \times 0.33] \\ \text{ECFVd} &= 15.9\,\text{L} - 13.9\,\text{L} \\ \text{ECFVd} &= 2\,\text{L}\end{aligned}$$

A 0.9% solution of sodium choride is considered to be isotonic and thus is optimal to correct the volume deficit because it will remain in the ECF space (see Table 51–1).

The expected rise in the serum sodium concentration following infusion of 2 L 0.9% saline (154 mEq/L) may be estimated as:

$$\text{Change in } S_{Na} \text{ with 1 liter of infusate} = \left[IV_{Na} - S^1_{Na}\right] \div (BW + 1 \text{ liter})$$

$$\begin{aligned}\text{Change in } S_{Na} \text{ with 1 liter of infusate} &= [154\,\text{mEq/L} - 125\,\text{mEq/L}] \\ &\quad \div \{(0.6 \times 70\,\text{kg}) + 1.0\,\text{L}\} \\ &= [29\,\text{mEq/L}] \div 43\,\text{L} = 0.67\,\text{mEq/L}\end{aligned}$$

Therefore, the change in S_{Na} with infusion of 2 liters of 0.9% saline would be:

$$2 \times 0.67\,\text{mEq/L} = 1.34\,\text{mEq/L}$$

Thus, the final serum sodium concentration is 125 mEq/L + 1.34 mEq/L = 126 mEq/L.

Because the over-riding initial treatment goal is to restore vital organ perfusion, it is generally necessary to infuse 0.9% saline at 200–400 mL/h until hemodynamic stability is restored. The infusion rate can then be decreased to 100–150 mL/h such that the serum sodium level rises no more than 12 mEq/L over the initial 24 hours. Infusion of 0.9% saline at rates greater than 250 mL/h, however, should be used cautiously in patients with a history of left ventricular dysfunction or renal insufficiency. Once the ECF volume is restored, ADH secretion will cease, and a rapid water diuresis may ensue, which may potentially result in a rise in the serum sodium at a rate greater than 12 mEq/L/d. If this occurs, the infusate should be changed to 0.45% saline at a rate that approximates urine output (approximately 1.5–2 mL/kg/h is a reasonable initial rate), in order to decrease the rate of rise in the serum sodium concentration.[5]

EVALUATING THERAPEUTIC OUTCOMES

Patients presenting with evidence of volume depletion should be reexamined frequently during the initial few hours of the resuscitation phase until hemodynamic stability is restored. Intravenous 0.9% saline should be administered judiciously in patients with a history of congestive heart failure or renal insufficiency, with frequent assessments of the cardiopulmonary examination so the infusion rate may be appropriately decreased when pulmonary congestion is detected.

The serum sodium concentration should be measured every 2 to 4 hours to allow timely adjustment of the rate and composition of intravenous fluids in order to avoid a rise in the serum sodium to greater than 12 mEq/L/d.

ASYMPTOMATIC EUVOLEMIC HYPOTONIC HYPONATREMIA

The treatment of SIADH always involves water restriction and correction of the underlying cause. Drugs that could be contributing should be identified and discontinued when possible. The goal is to induce negative water balance by restricting water intake to approximately 1,000–1,200 mL/day, such that water losses from insensible sources (skin and lung) and from obligate urine and fecal losses exceed intake. Daily insensible water losses, via skin and lungs are approximately 700 mL/day, while approximately 100–200 mL and 1,500 mL/day is lost in stool and in urine output respectively. Because approximately 850 mL of water per day is ingested in food, and an additional 350 mL are generated from oxidative processes, the water intake reduction should result in a negative water balance of several hundred milliliters per day.[38] Other goals include maintenance of the serum sodium level above 125 mEq/L to prevent symptoms of hypotonicity, and avoidance of iatrogenic hypo- or hypervolemia.

Patients with chronic SIADH who are unable to restrict water sufficiently to maintain the serum sodium greater than 120–125 mEq/L may be treated by increasing solute intake with either urea or sodium chloride and/or loop diuretics.[39] Sodium chloride or urea tablets increase the obligatory daily solute excretion, which augments the capacity for renal water excretion. The goal is to increase the daily solute intake and excretion to approximately 900 mOsm per day. Because an average diet contains approximately 600 mOsm, 9 g of sodium chloride would be required to increase the osmolar excretion to 900 mOsm/d (each 1 g sodium chloride tablet contains 17 mmol of sodium and 17 mmol of chloride). Because extracellular volume expansion is an expected adverse effect, a loop diuretic should be administered concurrently to avoid pulmonary congestion and peripheral edema. Loop diuretics also enhance water excretion by limiting the formation of the medullary concentration gradient.[40]

Other treatment options include demeclocycline therapy and investigational ADH receptor antagonists. Demeclocycline (initially 900–1,200 mg/day, then decreased to 600–900 mg/day total daily dose given in 3 to 4 divided doses), interferes with tubular ADH activity, and is yet another option for patients with chronic SIADH.[41] Because of its delayed onset of action (3 to 6 days), this agent has no role in the acute management of severe hyponatremia. It should not, however, be used in patients with liver disease and cirrhosis, who are at high risk for demeclocycline-induced renal tubular toxicity and acute renal failure. Several V2 receptor antagonists of ADH are currently under investigation, and show promise for the treatment of chronic hypo-osmolal syndromes such as chronic SIADH.[42]

EVALUATION OF THERAPEUTIC OUTCOMES

The serum sodium level should be measured every 24 to 48 hours after the water restriction is initiated until it stabilizes at a concentration of greater than 125 mEq/L. A continued decline in the serum sodium level would indicate either noncompliance with the prescribed restriction or the need for a more stringent restriction. Once the serum sodium level has stabilized above 125 mEq/L, patients should then be seen every 2 to 4 weeks to assess neurologic status and to obtain serum and urine for sodium, potassium, and osmolality. Again attention should be given to volume status (i.e., blood pressure, skin turgor, heart and lung exam), particularly in patients who are being treated with sodium chloride tablets and loop diuretics.

ASYMPTOMATIC HYPERVOLEMIC HYPOTONIC HYPONATREMIA

The goals of treatment of asymptomatic hyponatremic patients with an expanded ECF volume include minimizing rapid changes in cell volume and effecting negative water balance until the serum sodium is greater than 125 mEq/L. This entails correction of the underlying cause when possible, as well as restriction of water intake to a volume less than 1,000–1,200 mL/day. Dietary intake of sodium chloride should be restricted to 1,000–2,000 mg/day, depending on the degree of ECF volume expansion and edema.

Patients with hypervolemic hypotonic hyponatremia caused by congestive heart failure should be treated with measures that can potentially improve cardiac contractility and improve the EABV, thereby limiting the nonosmotic release of ADH. Therapeutic options include digitalis, or afterload reduction with angiotensin-converting enzyme inhibitors (ACEIs) or angiotensin II receptor blockers. Of these, only ACEIs have been shown in clinical trials to be of benefit in partially correcting hyponatremia in patients with congestive heart failure.[43] No specific ACE inhibitor offers any particular advantage for this indication, and the dose should be titrated to keep the systolic blood pressure in the 110 to 130 mm Hg range. Dose-limiting adverse effects include hyperkalemia (serum potassium > 5.5 mEq/L), as well as a decline in renal function. The benefits and risks of continuing ACE inhibition must be weighed carefully in each case, but in general, an acute increase in the serum creatinine greater than 30% would require either a decrease in dose or discontinuation of the ACE inhibitor.

Other potentially treatable causes of asymptomatic hyponatremia associated with an expanded ECF volume include nephrotic syndrome and cirrhosis. ACEIs may be used to decrease proteinuria in patients with nephrotic syndrome, leading to partial correction of hypoalbuminemia and to a decrease in nonosmotic release of ADH. Patients with advanced cirrhosis may benefit from placement of a transjugular intrahepatic portosytemic shunt, which can increase the EABV and thus reduce the nonosmotic release of ADH. This procedure can potentially exacerbate or precipitate hepatic encephalopathy, and should be avoided in patients with a history of encephalopathy.

EVALUATION OF TREATMENT OUTCOMES

Patients should initially be evaluated on a daily basis with a thorough physical exam to assess for lung congestion, ascites and peripheral edema. The serum sodium concentration should be measured daily until it stabilizes above 125 mEq/L following initiation of water restriction. Patients should then be assessed 1 week following discharge, and then every 2 to 4 weeks to assess compliance with the water restriction and to reassess volume status.

HYPERNATREMIA

EPIDEMIOLOGY/ETIOLOGY

Hypernatremia (serum sodium > 145 mEq/L) is always associated with hypertonicity and results from a deficit of water relative to ECF sodium content. Hyperosmolar states are a potent stimulus for thirst, and therefore hypernatremia is most commonly observed in patients with an impaired thirst response or in those without access to water. Infants, comatose patients, as well as the elderly or disabled patients with an impaired sensorium or functional status are therefore at highest risk for this disorder.[44] Hypernatremia occurs in approximately 0.3% to 1.0% of hospitalized patients.[45] Outcome generally depends upon the rapidity with which the hypernatremia developed. Mortality from acute hypernatremia in children, which develops in less than 72 hours, ranges from 10% to 70%. In contrast, chronic hypernatremia in children, defined as that which develops over 3 or more days, has a mortality rate of 10%.[46] An acute increase in serum sodium in adults to greater than 160 mEq/L is associated with a 75% mortality rate. Adults in whom the hypernatremia developed chronically also have a high mortality in the 60% range.[47] Hypernatremia in adults is often associated with a serious underlying illness, which may contribute to the high mortality rates.

PATHOPHYSIOLOGY

Hypernatremia may result from either loss of water or hypotonic fluids, or, less commonly, from administration of hypertonic fluids or ingestion of sodium (Fig. 51–3). Water loss commonly occurs as a result of insensible losses (evaporative losses of water through the skin and lungs) in patients deprived of water. Hospitalized patients, especially those who are febrile or receiving mechanical ventilation, are often treated with intravenous fluids containing insufficient free water to replace insensible losses. Hypernatremia may be observed in patients with hypotonic gastrointestinal losses (diarrhea or vomiting) or in patients who have been exposed to high temperatures who suffer large water losses from both sweat and insensible losses.

Patients with diabetes insipidus (DI), or those undergoing an osmotic diuresis, may also have large urinary losses of water. DI is classified as either central (characterized by deficient secretion of ADH) or nephrogenic (characterized by resistance to ADH activity). Table 51–2 summarizes the causes of DI. Patients with central DI often present with sudden onset of polyuria, whereas patients with nephrogenic DI develop polyuria more gradually.

Administration of hypertonic saline can result in hypernatremia and an expanded ECF volume. This is typically iatrogenic, and may follow administration of sodium bicarbonate, use of hypertonic saline enemas, or intrauterine injection of hypertonic saline. Rarely, patients with hyperaldosteronism spontaneously present with an expanded ECF and mild hypernatremia.[48]

TABLE 51–2. Causes of Diabetes Insipidus

Central DI	Nephrogenic DI
Idiopathic	Lithium toxicity
Familial	Hypercalcemia
Neurosurgery	Hypokalemia
Head trauma	Cidofavir
CNS malignancy	Foscarnet
Hypoxic encephalopathy	Inherited Aquaporin-2 defect
Sheehan's syndrome	Inherited ADH-V2 receptor defect
	Demeclocycline

CLINICAL PRESENTATION

The symptoms of hypernatremia are primarily caused by a decrease in neuronal cell volume, and may include weakness, restlessness, confusion, and coma. Hypernatremia results in movement of water from the intracellular space to the extracellular fluid. Neurons can adapt to hypertonicity in the ECF by generating intracellular organic osmolytes within 24 hours of onset. This increase in intracellular fluid (ICF) tonicity then draws water into the neurons, thus limiting the decrease in cell volume. Patients with chronic hypernatremia are less likely to present with symptoms caused by this cerebral adaptation.

Hypernatremia is often associated with serious underlying illness, and thus symptoms may also be because of coexisting disorders. Patients with a history of severe diarrhea or vomiting may present with ECF volume depletion. Elderly patients deprived of water after sustaining a stroke or hip fracture often present with mental status changes and signs of ECF volume depletion. Clinically detectable extracellular fluid volume depletion, however, may not be evident until the serum sodium concentration exceeds 160 mEq/L, because these patients primarily have water loss, two-thirds of which is derived from the intracellular space. The urine is concentrated with an osmolality greater than 450 mOsm/kg as a result of both osmotic and nonosmotic release of ADH. The first step in evaluating patients with hypernatremia is the clinical assessment of the ECF volume, urine volume, and urine osmolality (Fig. 51–4).

Patients with a contracted ECF volume and a low urine output include those who have sustained insensible water losses that exceed intake, as well as those with extrarenal losses of hypotonic fluids. On

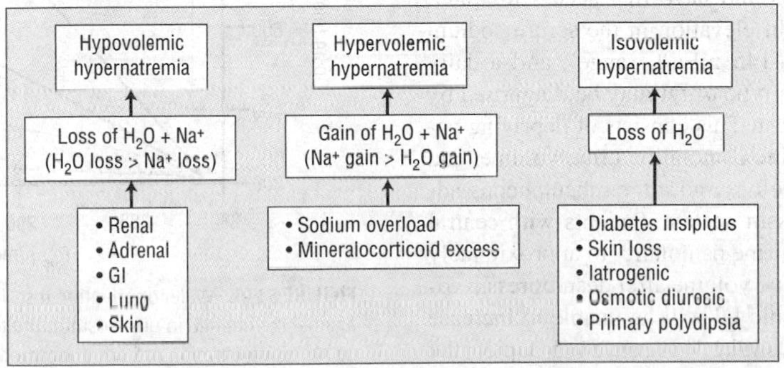

FIGURE 51–3. Common etiologies of hypernatremia.

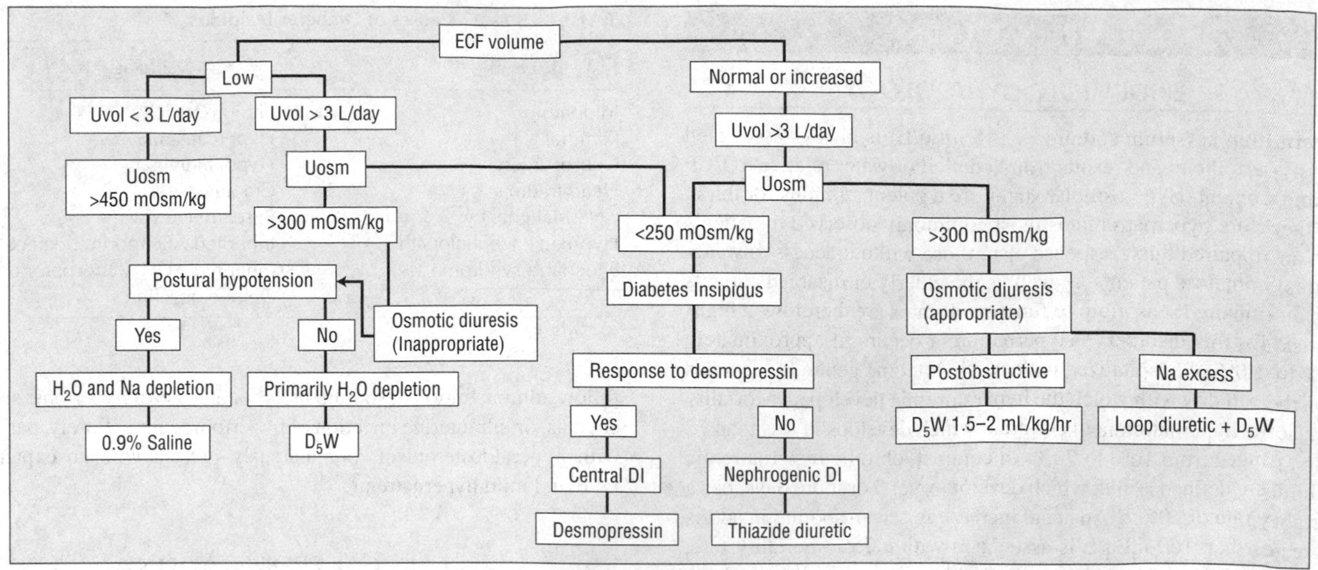

FIGURE 51–4. Diagnostic and treatment algorithm for hypernatremia. ECF = extracellular fluid; Uvol = daily urine volume; Uosm = urine osmolality; H_2O = water; Na = sodium; D_5W = 5% dextrose in water. See text for guidelines regarding calculations of infusion rates for intravenous solutions.

physical exam, one should search for postural hypotension, diminished skin turgor, and delayed capillary refill. The daily urine output is typically less than 1 L.

OSMOTIC DIURESIS

Patients undergoing an osmotic diuresis generally have urine volumes greater than 3 L/day. Excessive urinary excretion of glucose, sodium, urea, or an exogenously administered solute such as mannitol, are identified either by history or by direct measurement of serum and urinary concentrations of the suspected solute. Patients with postobstructive diuresis, such as those with bladder outlet obstruction due to prostatic hypertrophy, are usually volume expanded as a result of retained excess solute due to a decline in the glomerular filtration rate (GFR).[49] The osmotic diuresis that follows alleviation of the obstruction is appropriate in that it promotes excretion of the excess retained solute. Patients with severe hyperglycemia, on the other hand, present with signs of volume depletion, and the diuresis is, therefore, inappropriate, further exacerbating the degree of ECF volume contraction.

Diabetes Insipidus

Patients with diabetes insipidus tend to maintain a normal ECF volume as long as they are conscious and have free access to water. Patients typically have only a slight elevation in the serum sodium concentration (usually in the 141–145 mEq/L range), and a daily urine volume greater than 3 L. The type of DI may be diagnosed by performing the water deprivation test. This consists of depriving patients of water for 8–12 hours. Urine osmolality, urine volume, and body weight, are then measured before and after subcutaneous administration of 5 μg of desmopressin acetate. Patients with central DI will show a prompt increase in urine osmolality to approximately 600 mOsm/kg and a decrease in urine volume after desmopressin administration. Those with nephrogenic DI will be unable to increase the urine osmolality above 300 mOsm/kg.[49] Figure 51–5 depicts the changes in plasma and urine osmolality observed in the water deprivation test. Direct measurement of vasopressin levels after infusion of 5% saline at a rate of 0.05 mL/kg/min for no more than 2 hours improves the accuracy of diagnosis, but carries a high risk of ECF volume overload.[50] Furthermore, measurement of serum vasopressin levels, is complicated by the fact that the molecule is unstable, and inappropriate specimen handling and processing often results in falsely low values.

Sodium Overload

Patients who have ingested large amounts of sodium [>4 tablespoons (1,400 mEq Na^+) of sodium chloride] or who have received greater than 5 L of hypertonic fluids are volume expanded, although this may not always be clinically evident as edema. This results in an osmotic diuresis, polyuria, and a urine osmolality greater than 300 mOsm/kg. The excess sodium will be excreted in the urine in patients with normal renal function.

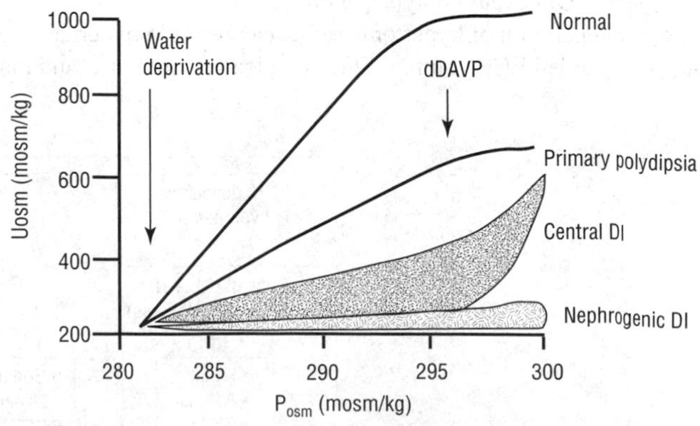

FIGURE 51–5. Water deprivation test. The change in plasma osmolality is plotted against the change in urine osmolality following water deprivation and subcutaneous administration of 5 μg of desmopressin acetate. U_{osm} = urine osmolality; P_{osm} = plasma osmolality; DI = diabetes insipidus. *(Adapted from Ref. 51).*

► TREATMENT: Hypernatremia

DESIRED OUTCOME

The goals in treating patients with hypernatremia include correction of the serum sodium concentration at a rate that restores and maintains cell volume as close to normal as possible, as well as normalizing the ECF volume in states of ECF volume depletion and expansion. Adequate treatment should result in the resolution of symptoms associated with hypovolemia. Careful titration of fluids and medications should minimize the adverse effects from too rapid correction. Modulation of dietary sodium intake and sodium replacement may be necessary to prevent recurrence of hypernatremia.

PHARMACOLOGIC THERAPY

Hypovolemic Hypernatremia

Hypovolemic hypernatremia (postural hypotension, tachycardia, decreased skin turgor), should initially be treated with 0.9% saline until hemodynamic stability is restored. An initial infusion rate of 200–300 mL/h will likely be appropriate for many patients. Once intravascular volume is restored, 0.45% saline or D_5W can then be infused to correct the water deficit, the volume of which may be estimated as:

$$\text{Water Deficit} = \text{Present TBW} \times \left[\left(S^{p}_{Na}/140 - 1\right)\right]^{37}$$

where TBW = total body water; S^{p}_{Na} = patient serum sodium concentration (mEq/L); and 140 = normal or goal S_{Na} (mEq/L).

The rate of correction depends on the rapidity with which the hypernatremia developed. Hypernatremia that has developed over a few hours may be corrected at a rate of approximately 1 mEq/L/h, whereas a rate of 0.5 mEq/L/h should be used when it has developed more slowly.[48]

Treatment of hyperglycemia-induced osmotic diuresis consists of correcting the hyperglycemia with insulin, as well as administering 0.9% saline until signs of ECF volume depletion resolve. Once hemodynamic stability is restored, the water deficit should be corrected in a manner analogous to that described for patients with hypovolemic hypernatremia above. The corrected serum sodium level should be calculated by adding 1.7 mEq/L for every 100 mg/dL rise in the serum glucose concentration before estimating the water deficit.[5]

Hypernatremia in patients undergoing a postobstructive diuresis should be treated with infusion of hypotonic fluids such as 0.45% saline at maintenance rates of approximately 1.5 mL/kg/h. It is important to avoid the temptation to administer fluids to replace urine output on a 1 mL:1 mL volume basis, because this tends to perpetuate the diuresis.

The serum sodium concentration and fluid status should be monitored every 2 to 3 hours over the first 24 hours of admission in patients with symptomatic hypernatremia to permit appropriate adjustment in the rate of infusion of hypotonic fluids. After symptoms resolve and the serum sodium is less than 148 mEq/L, serum sodium determinations every 6 to 12 hours and fluid status assessment every 8 to 24 hours are generally sufficient to follow the course of therapy.

Central DI

Patients with central DI are usually treated with intranasal desmopressin, beginning at a dose of 10 μg once daily. A dose of 10 μg twice daily is typically required in adults. Because of variable absorption of oral desmopressin, DI is best treated with the intranasal formulation 1-deamino-8-D-arginine vasopressin (DDAVP). Each insufflation of intranasal DDAVP delivers 10 μg of desmopressin acetate at a concentration of 100 μg/mL.[51] Drugs with antidiuretic properties have been successful in the management of central and nephrogenic DI (Table 51–3). They may be used as an alternative to DDAVP or adjunctively.

The desmopressin dose should be adjusted to achieve adequate urinary concentration during sleep to prevent nocturia, to result in a daily urine volume of approximately 1.5–2 L and to maintain the serum sodium concentration in the 137–142 mEq/L range. The serum sodium concentration should be measured every 3 to 4 days during the initial dose titration period, and then every 2 to 4 months.

Nephrogenic DI

Initially the underlying cause of the nephrogenic DI should be addressed. Hypercalcemia and hypokalemia should be corrected and medications that may contribute to the pathogenesis should be discontinued. One key goal in treating nephrogenic DI is to induce mild ECFVd (1–1.5 L) with a thiazide diuretic and dietary sodium restriction (85 mEq Na^+ or 2,000 mg sodium chloride per day), which often can decrease urine volume by as much as 50% (Table 51–3). This will increase proximal water reabsorption and therefore decrease the volume of filtrate delivered to the distal nephron, thus resulting in decreased urine volume. NSAIDs such as indomethacin at a dose of 50 mg tid may be used as adjunctive therapy by potentiating the activity of ADH.[52] Patients with lithium-induced nephrogenic DI may derive particular benefit from amiloride at a dose of 5–10 mg daily, which directly inhibits uptake of lithium from the tubular lumen into principle cells in the cortical collecting duct.[53]

TABLE 51–3. Drugs Used to Manage Central and Nephrogenic DI

Drug	Indication	Dose
Desmopressin acetate (DDAVP)	Central and nephrogenic DI	5–20 μg intranasally q 12–24 h
Chlorpropamide	Central DI	125–250 mg po daily
Carbamazepine	Central DI	100–300 mg po bid
Clofibrate	Central DI	500 mg po qid
Hydrochlorothiazide	Central and nephrogenic DI	25 mg po q 12–24 h
Amiloride	Lithium-related nephrogenic DI	5–10 mg po daily
Indomethacin	Central and nephrogenic DI	50 mg po q 8–12 h

EVALUATION OF TREATMENT OUTCOMES

Physical examination with attention to volume status and measurement of serum and urine sodium concentration and osmolality should be assessed every 2 to 3 months. A 24-hour urine collection to measure urine volume and sodium excretion will help guide therapy with diuretics and determine compliance with sodium restriction.

SODIUM OVERLOAD

Treatment of sodium overload consists of administration of loop diuretics to facilitate excretion of the excess sodium, as well as intravenous D_5W. The latter should be infused at a rate that will decrease the serum sodium at approximately 0.5 mEq/L/h, or 1 mEq/L/h in cases in which the hypernatremia developed rapidly over several hours.[48] The volume of infusate may be estimated as described previously. Furosemide should be administered at a dose of 20–40 mg intravenously every 6 hours.

The serum sodium should initially be measured every 2 to 4 hours, and the diuretic continued until signs of ECF volume overload (pulmonary congestion, edema) resolve. The serum sodium concentration can be determined every 6 to 12 hours once the serum sodium level is less than 148 mEq/L and symptoms of hypertonicity resolve.

EDEMA

The kidney responds to changes in the EABV, rather than directly sensing/measuring the sodium content of the ECF. A decline in the EABV results in decreased sodium and water excretion.[9] Under these conditions, the kidneys retain all of the water and sodium ingested until the EABV is restored to normal. An increase in dietary sodium is accompanied by an increase in water intake caused by the initial increase in serum osmolality and stimulation of thirst. The resultant increase in ECF volume augments renal perfusion, effecting a transient increase in GFR which leads to enhanced sodium filtration and excretion.[54] These homeostatic mechanisms are crucial in maintaining sodium balance, as retention of just a few milliequivalents of sodium per day can eventually lead to an expanded ECF volume and edema formation.

PATHOPHYSIOLOGY

Edema is clinically detectable in adults when the interstitial volume increases by approximately 2.5–3 L, which correlates with a 4–4.5-L increase in ECF volume, and a 500–600 mEq increase in ECF sodium.[55] Edema develops when excess sodium is retained either as a primary defect in renal sodium excretion, or as a response to a decrease in the EABV despite an already expanded or normal ECF volume. An increase in the capillary hydrostatic pressure because of an expansion in the ECF volume, or an increase in central venous pressure may lead to edema formation. Edema may also occur when there is an alteration in Starling forces within the capillary.[56] The Starling equation denotes the relationship between factors affecting the movement of fluid between the capillary and interstitium and is discussed in detail in Chap. 24.

An acute decompensation in myocardial contractility leads to an elevation in pulmonary venous pressure that is transmitted back to the pulmonary capillaries resulting in pulmonary edema. On a chronic basis, renal sodium and water retention due to diminished EABV leads to a rise in the ECF volume and edema formation in both peripheral and pulmonary interstitial tissues.

Edema formation in patients with nephrotic syndrome is primarily related to renal sodium and water retention. A decrease in capillary oncotic pressure does not appear to play a major role until the serum albumin concentration falls to less than 2 g/dL. This is explained by the fact that both capillary and interstitial oncotic pressure decrease proportionately above a serum albumin concentration of 2 g/dL, and thus the transcapillary oncotic gradient is not significantly altered.[57]

Patients with cirrhosis initially develop ascites as a result of an increase in the pressure in the portal circulation proximal to the diseased liver. Sequestration of fluid in the abdominal cavity (ascites) and peripheral vasodilation as a consequence of increased levels of circulating cytokines, result in a decrease in the effective circulating volume, activation of the sympathetic nervous system and secondary hyperaldosteronism. Therefore, renal sodium retention leads to worsened ascites and edema.

CLINICAL PRESENTATION

Edema is usually first detected in the feet or pretibial area of ambulatory patients and in the presacral area of bed-bound individuals. Edema is described as pitting when a depression created by exerting pressure over a bony prominence such as the tibia for several seconds does not rapidly refill. The severity of the edema may be quantified based on the depth of the pit as outlined below: 1+ = 2 mm, 2+ = 4 mm, 3+ = 6 mm, and 4+ = 8 mm.

The extent of the edema should also be quantified according to the area of involvement. Pretibial edema, for example, should be quantified according to how far it extends up the lower leg (e.g., one-third up the lower leg). Pulmonary edema, defined as an increase in lung interstitial and alveolar water, is manifest as end inspiratory rales, initially localized to the dependent portions of the lungs.

▶ TREATMENT: Edema

GENERAL APPROACH TO TREATMENT

The goals of diuretic therapy are to minimize tissue edema and thus improve organ function, as well as to relieve symptoms of edema such as dyspnea in patients with congestive heart failure (CHF) or abdominal distention in patients with ascites. It is important to emphasize that the presence of edema does not always dictate the need for instituting pharmacologic (diuretic) therapy. Only pulmonary edema requires immediate pharmacologic treatment because it is life-threatening. Other forms of edema may be treated gradually, with a comprehensive approach that includes not only

TABLE 51–4. Maximal Effective Dose and Dosing Interval for Edema Management with Loop Diuretics

Diuretic	Dosing Interval	Normal	Cirrhosis	CHF	Nephrotic Syndrome	GFR 10–50 mL/min	GFR <10 mL/min
Furosemide							
IV	6–8 h	10–40 mg	40 mg	40–80 mg	120 mg	80 mg	200 mg
Oral	6–8 h	20–80 mg	80 mg	80–160 mg	240 mg	160 mg	320–400 mg
Bumetanide							
IV/Oral	6–8 h	1 mg	1 mg	2–3 mg	3 mg	2–3 mg	8–10 mg
Torsemide							
IV/Oral	24 h	15–20 mg	10–20 mg	20–50 mg	50 mg	20–50 mg	50–100 mg

(Adapted from Ref. 59.)

diuretics, but also sodium restriction and treatment of the underlying disease state. Sodium chloride intake should generally be restricted to 1,000–2,000 mg/day. A slow, more judicious approach in non–life threatening situations will help to minimize complications of diuretic therapy and excessive fluid removal. These may include impaired vital organ perfusion, azotemia, and impaired cardiac output due to a fall in the left ventricular end diastolic filling pressure.

PHARMACOLOGIC THERAPY

Diuretics are the primary pharmacologic therapy for the management of edema. Patients with expanded ECF volume and edema often require treatment with diuretics when treatment of the underlying disease and daily sodium restriction are insufficient to relieve the edema. Diuretics can be categorized according to the site in the nephron where sodium reabsorption is inhibited. Loop diuretics inhibit the Na^+-K^+-$2Cl^-$ carrier in the loop of Henle. Thiazide diuretics inhibit the Na^+-Cl^- carrier in the distal tubule. Finally, potassium-sparing diuretics inhibit the sodium channel in the cortical collecting duct either directly (triamterene, amiloride), or by interfering with aldosterone activity (spironolactone). The efficacy of a diuretic depends on the presence of several factors including the amount of filtered solute normally reabsorbed at the site of action, the amount of solute reabsorbed distal to the site of action, and adequate delivery of drug to the site of action in the nephron.

Loop diuretics are the most potent diuretics, as evidenced by the fact that they increase peak fractional excretion of sodium (FeNa) to 20% to 25%. Thiazide- and potassium-sparing diuretics are less potent and increase peak FeNa to 3% to 5% and 1% to 2%, respectively.[58] Although a large portion of the filtered sodium is reabsorbed in the proximal nephron, the efficacy of proximal acting diuretics such as acetazolamide are limited by reabsorption of the excess fluid and sodium in the loop of Henle.

The effectiveness of thiazide and loop diuretics is dependent on the concentration of the drug in the tubular lumen. Diuretics are delivered to the tubular lumen of the kidney by active transport by the proximal tubular cells. Osmotic diuretics, on the other hand, are freely filtered into the tubular lumen in the proximal tubule, whereas spironolactone gains access to mineralocorticoid receptors in the cortical collecting duct through diffusion from the systemic circulation.

A threshold concentration of loop or thiazide diuretic must be delivered to the active site (e.g., loop of Henle, distal tubule) in order to achieve a natriuresis.[59] Once this concentration is achieved, further increases in diuretic dose will not elicit an increase in diuretic response. Thus, a ceiling dose of diuretic is recognized. Administration of 40 mg of intravenous furosemide to a normal subject will result in excretion of 200–250 mEq of sodium in 3–4 L over a 3 to 4 hour period.[59] Table 51–4 summarizes the maximal effective doses and dosing intervals for loop diuretics in patients with cirrhosis, CHF, and nephrotic syndrome with normal and decreased glomerular filtration rates. Patients with renal insufficiency require larger doses of diuretics to achieve adequate concentration of the drug to the active site. The natriuretic response is decreased in patients with renal insufficiency because the filtered load of sodium falls proportionately as GFR declines. This may be partially overcome by dosing diuretics more frequently, as well as by using continuous infusions in critically ill hospitalized patients.[60] The latter will maintain more consistent levels of the diuretic above the threshold concentration. Patients that are diuretic resistant should be treated with both a loop and a thiazide-type diuretic.

Patients with CHF and a normal GFR have impaired oral absorption of furosemide. An adequate diuresis is most readily sustained by increasing the frequency of diuretic administration (Fig. 51–6). Patients with nephrotic syndrome commonly develop diuretic resistance. Increased uptake of sodium in the distal tubule, impaired delivery of diuretics to the site of action, as well as decreased intrinsic diuretic activity have been demonstrated. Animal studies have demonstrated binding of furosemide to albumin in the tubular lumen, which decreases the availability of the drug to the active site.[61] Human studies, however, have demonstrated that when albumin binding is inhibited by concurrent administration of sulfasoxazole, diuretic resistance persists, suggesting a decrease in intrinsic tubular sensitivity to loop diuretics.[62] This impaired natriuretic response may be overcome by using higher diuretic doses to increase the delivery of free drug to the secretory site in the nephron (Fig. 51–7).[60]

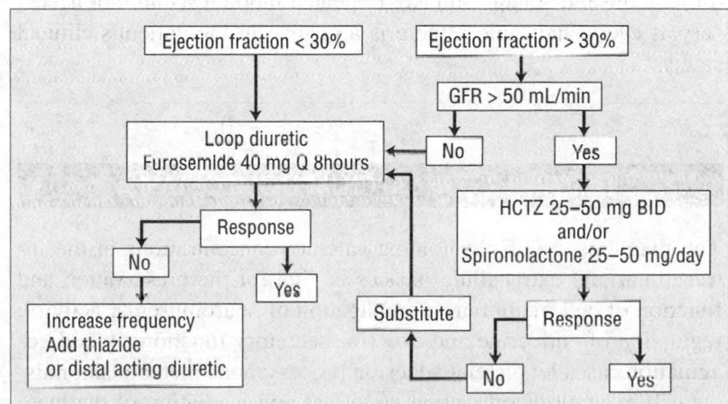

FIGURE 51–6. Therapeutic algorithm for diuretic use in patients with congestive heart failure. GFR = glomerular filtration rate; HCTZ = hydrochlorothiazide.

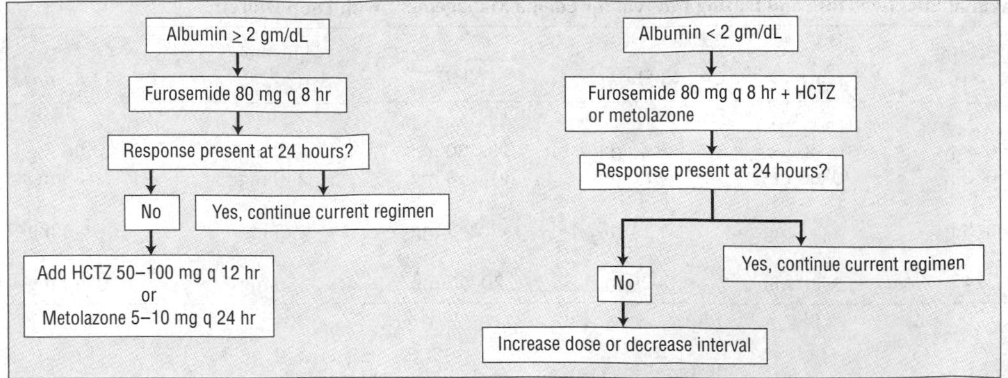

FIGURE 51–7. Therapeutic algorithm for diuretic therapy in patients with nephrotic syndrome. HCTZ = hydrochlorothiazide.

Combinations of loop diuretics with distally acting diuretics are generally necessary to promote a natriuresis that exceeds tubular sodium reabsorption.

Secondary hyperaldosteronism plays a major role in the pathogenesis of edema in patients with cirrhosis. These patients, therefore, should initially be treated with spironolactone in the absence of impaired GFR and hyperkalemia (Fig. 51–8). Thiazides may then be added for patients with a creatinine clearance > 50 mL/min. For those patients who remain diuretic resistant, a loop diuretic may replace the thiazide. Patients with impaired GFR (Clcr ≤ 30 mL/min) generally will require a loop diuretic, with addition of a thiazide in those who do not achieve adequate diuresis.[60] Care should be taken to avoid hypokalemia, which may precipitate hepatic encephalopathy by increasing ammoniagenesis.[63]

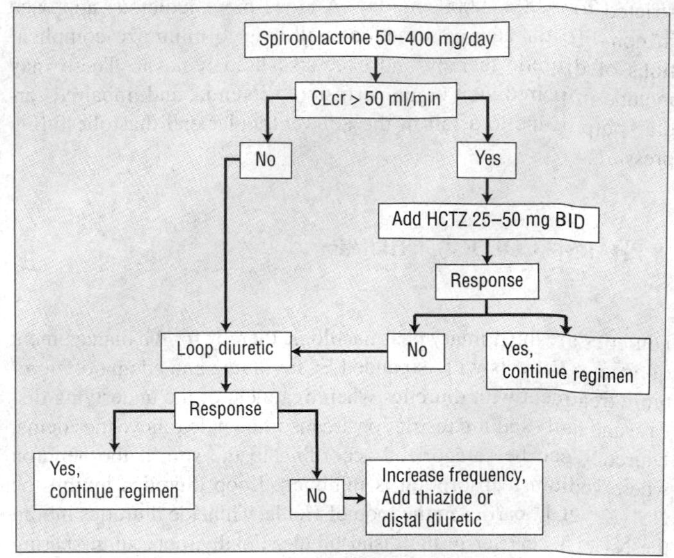

FIGURE 51–8. Therapeutic algorithm for diuretic use in patients with cirrhosis. Clcr = creatinine clearance; HCTZ = hydrochlorothiazide.

EVALUATION OF THERAPEUTIC OUTCOMES

Patients should be monitored by serial physical examinations, including measurement of blood pressure and pulse in both supine or seated positions and after standing for 2 to 3 minutes. ECF volume may be estimated based on the height of the jugular venous pressure, extent of edema, auscultation of the heart and lungs, and skin turgor. Followup monitoring (10 to 14 days after initiation of therapy) should include determinations of serum sodium, potassium, chloride, bicarbonate, magnesium, calcium, blood urea nitrogen, serum creatinine, and uric acid. A new steady state will have developed over that time period and further fluctuations in ECF volume and electrolyte balance should not occur in the absence of a change in clinical status, diuretic dose, or dietary intake. Repeated blood tests are not necessary at every visit unless there is a change in the patient's clinical status.

Complications of loop and thiazide diuretic therapy include hypokalemia, excess depletion of ECF volume, hyponatremia, hypokalemia, hypomagnesemia, metabolic alkalosis, and hyperuricemia. Thiazides can also cause hypercalcemia, particularly in patients with mild subclinical hyperparathyroidism. Chronic therapy with potassium sparing diuretics, including triamterene, amiloride, and spironolactone may cause a mild metabolic acidosis and can precipitate hyperkalemia. Patients with renal insufficiency or those receiving NSAIDs, ACEIs, or angiotensin II receptor blockers are at highest risk for this complication. In addition, spironolactone may cause reversible gynecomastia in patients receiving therapy for more than several weeks.

DISORDERS OF CALCIUM HOMEOSTASIS

The maintenance of physiologic calcium concentrations in the intracellular and extracellular spaces is vital for the preservation and function of cell membranes; propagation of neuromuscular activity; regulation of endocrine and exocrine secretory functions; blood coagulation cascade; platelet adhesion process; bone metabolism; muscle cell excitation/contraction coupling; and mediation of the electrophysiologic slow-channel response in cardiac and smooth-muscle tissue.

The disorders of calcium homeostasis are related to the calcium content of the extracellular fluid, which contains less than 0.5% of the total body stores of calcium. Skeletal bone contains more than 99% of total body stores of calcium.[64] ECF calcium is moderately bound to plasma proteins (46%), primarily albumin.[65] Unbound or ionized calcium is the physiologically active form and is the fraction that is homeostatically regulated.[66] Extracellular calcium, however, is most commonly measured as the total serum calcium level, which includes both bound and unbound calcium.[65] The normal total calcium serum concentration range is 8.5–10.5 mg/dL.[66]

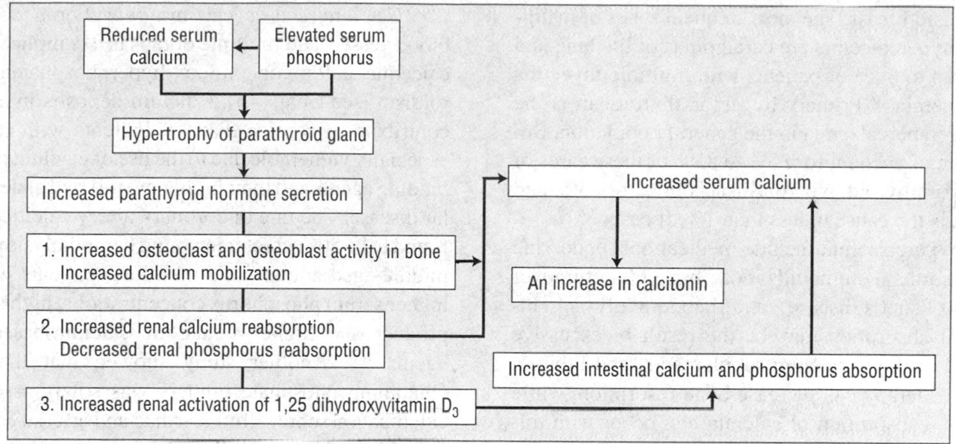

FIGURE 51–9. Homeostatic mechanisms to maintain serum calcium concentrations.

The concentration of ionized calcium is closely regulated by the interactions of parathyroid hormone (PTH), phosphorus, vitamin D, and calcitonin (Fig. 51–9). Parathyroid hormone increases serum calcium concentrations by stimulating calcium release from bone, reducing renal excretion, and enhancing absorption in the gastrointestinal tract secondary to increased renal production of 1,25-dihydroxyvitamin D_3. Vitamin D directly increases serum calcium, as well as phosphorus concentrations, by increasing gastrointestinal absorption. Indirectly, it can also lead to calcium release from bone and reduced renal excretion. Calcitonin inhibits osteoclastic bone resorption. Its plasma concentrations are increased when ionized calcium concentrations are high as the body attempts to return the calcium level to the normal range. Disruption of these homeostatic mechanisms results in the clinical manifestations of hypercalcemia or hypocalcemia.

Any factor that alters the concentration of albumin or its binding of calcium may be expected to change the fraction of total serum calcium in the ionized form. The most significant cause of changes in calcium binding to albumin is a change in extracellular fluid pH. In the presence of metabolic alkalosis the fraction of calcium bound to albumin is increased, thus reducing the plasma concentration of ionized calcium. This may result in symptomatic hypocalcemia; that is, paresthesias, muscle cramping and spasms, memory loss, and seizures.[61] Conversely, metabolic acidosis decreases calcium binding to albumin and results in increased ionized calcium. Hypoalbuminemic states are probably the most common cause of "laboratory" hypocalcemia. When the albumin level is decreased, ionized calcium concentration may be normal even though total concentration is reduced. Each 1 g/dL drop in the serum albumin concentration below 4 g/dL, will result in a decrease of total serum calcium concentration by 0.8 mg/dL.[64,65]

HYPERCALCEMIA

Hypercalcemia (total serum calcium >10.5 mg/dL) may be induced by a multitude of causes (Table 51–5). The most common causes of hypercalcemia are cancer and primary hyperparathyroidism. The incidence of primary hyperparathyroidism is approximately 270 new cases per million persons per year.[67] Hypercalcemia of cancer occurs in approximately 20% to 40% of cancer patients at some time during the course of their disease.[68] Cancer-associated hypercalcemia is predominantly encountered in hospitalized patients, while primary hyperparathyroidism accounts for the vast majority of cases in the outpatient setting.[69,70]

PATHOPHYSIOLOGY

Hypercalcemia is the result of one of three primary mechanisms: increased bone resorption, increased gastrointestinal absorption, or decreased elimination by the kidneys (Fig. 51–9). Many tumors secrete parathyroid hormone-related protein (PTHrP) which binds to the parathyroid hormone receptors in bone and renal tissues, leading to increased bone resorption and renal tubular reabsorption.[71] Tumors may also secrete substances, such as vitamin D, transforming growth factor, interleukins, prostaglandins, interferon, tumor necrosis factor, and granulocyte-macrophage colony stimulating factor, which are associated with the development of hypercalcemia.[68] Hypercalcemia of malignancy is a common complication of squamous cell carcinomas of the lung, head, and neck, hematologic malignancies such as multiple myeloma and T-cell lymphomas, and carcinomas of

TABLE 51–5. Etiologies of Hypercalcemia

Neoplasms	**Medications**
Bone metastasis	Thiazides
Breast	Lithium
Multiple myeloma	Vitamin D
Lymphoma	Vitamin A
Leukemia	Calcium
Humoral induced	Aluminum/magnesium antacids
Ovary	Theophylline
Kidney	Tamoxifene
Pheochromocytoma	Gancyclovir
Multiple endocrine neoplasia	**Granulomatous Disease**
Lung	Sarcoidosis
Head and neck	Tuberculosis
Esophagus	Cryptococcus
Cervix	Berylliosis
Lymphoproliferative disease	Histoplasmosis
	Coccidiodomycosis
Hyperparathyroidism	Leprosy
Primary	**Endocrine Disease**
Tertiary	Adrenal insufficiency
Miscellaneous	Hyperthyroidism
Immobilization	Acromegaly
Paget's disease	
Familial hypocalciuric hypercalcemia	
Adolescence	
Rhabdomyolysis	

ovary, kidney, bladder, and breast. The most frequent types of malignancy associated with hypercalcemia are carcinomas of the lung and breast.[65] Furthermore up to 40% of patients with multiple myeloma may develop hypercalcemia.[70] Primary hyperparathyroidism is the most common cause of hypercalcemia in the general population. Benign parathyroid adenomas account for 80% to 85% of these cases of hyperparathyroidism, parathyroid hyperplasia accounts for 15%, and parathyroid carcinoma is the cause in less than 1% of cases.[68,69]

Other causes of hypercalcemia include medications, endocrine and granulomatous disorders, immobilization, high bone-turnover states (adolescence and Paget's disease), and rhabdomyolysis.[72] Increased gastrointestinal absorption may be the result of excessive ingestion of vitamin D analogs, calcium supplements, and lithium. Lithium and vitamin A therapy can increase bone resorption, while increased renal tubular reabsorption of calcium can occur with thiazide and lithium therapy. Aluminum antacids prevent calcium deposition, thereby increasing serum concentrations.[73] Addison's disease, acromegaly, and thyrotoxicosis are endocrine disorders that may lead to hypercalcemia due to increased renal tubular reabsorption and increased bone resorption. Finally the granulomatous disorders (sarcoidosis, tuberculosis, histoplasmosis, leprosy) are associated with hypercalcemia caused by an increase in gastrointestinal absorption.[73]

CLINICAL PRESENTATION

Patients with mild to moderate hypercalcemia, that is, serum calcium concentrations of less than 13 mg/dL, may often be asymptomatic. This is usually the case in drug-induced hypercalcemia and the vast majority of patients with primary hyperparathyroidism.[74] The signs and symptoms of hypercalcemia that are usually present if the total serum calcium concentration is >13 mg/dL may differ depending on the acuity of onset.[65] Hypercalcemia of malignancy usually develops quickly and is accompanied by a classic symptom complex of anorexia, nausea and vomiting, constipation, polyuria, polydipsia, and nocturia.[74] Polyuria and nocturia secondary to a urinary-concentrating defect constitute some of the most frequent renal effects of hypercalcemia.[74] Hypercalcemic crisis, is characterized by an acute elevation of serum calcium to a value >15 mg/dL, acute renal insufficiency, and obtundation (inability to arouse).[74] If untreated, hypercalcemic crisis may progress to oliguric renal failure, coma, and life-threatening ventricular arrhythmias, which may lead to death.[74] Complications associated with chronic hypercalcemia (hyperparathyroidism) include metastatic calcification, nephrolithiasis, and chronic renal insufficiency.[74]

Calcium and/or calcium-phosphorus complex deposition in blood vessels and multiple organs is a complication of chronic hypercalcemia and/or concomitant hyperphosphatemia and hyperparathyroidism (see Chap. 45). Calcium deposits in atherosclerotic lesions contribute to cardiac disease. Patients with renal insufficiency are especially vulnerable due to the use of calcium products as phosphate-binding agents and their higher overall risk of developing cardiovascular disease. The rate of coronary artery calcification progression was found to be 50% greater in young hemodialysis patients versus normal middle-aged adults.[75] Furthermore, patients with calcifications had higher serum phosphorus concentrations, higher calcium-phosphorus product and higher intake of calcium-based, phosphate-binding agents.[75,76] Another study showed that the intake of calcium-containing phosphate binders was solely associated with vascular calcification score.[77] Intracardiac and arterial calcifications have been found in patients with Paget's disease who have normal renal function. These calcifications were found to be five times more common than in the general population. Although usually asymptomatic, these lesions can result in heart block and valvular disease.[78]

The electrocardiographic changes associated with hypercalcemia include shortening of the QT interval and coving of the ST-T wave.[74] Very high serum calcium concentrations may cause T-wave widening, indicating a repolarization defect that may be associated with spontaneous ventricular tachyarrhythmias.[74] Hypertension and arrhythmias have occurred in the setting of hypercalcemia. Sensitivity to the pharmacologic and toxic actions of digitalis may be enhanced in the setting of hypercalcemia.[68]

Nephrolithiasis (kidney stones) and nephrocalcinosis (calcium deposits in the kidney) are the primary renal complications arising from long-standing hypercalcemia, as the result of primary hyperparathyroidism. It is estimated that hyperparathyroidism accounts for 2% to 8% of all patients with calcium stones.[79] Sarcoidosis is the other hypercalcemic condition frequently associated with calcium stones.[79] Other causes of nephrolithiasis with calcium-containing stones include hypocitraturia, renal tubular acidosis, hyperoxaluria, and hyperuricosuria.[80,81] Stone formers who have primary hyperparathyroidism are more likely to be female, over age 50 years, and have a family history of multiple endocrine disorders.[79] High dietary sodium intake can also raise urinary calcium concentrations, thus predisposing patients to calcium stones. The proposed mechanism is a reduction in calcium reabsorption in the kidney. Although chronic renal failure can be the ultimate result of persistent stones, it is the primary cause of renal disease in <2% of the end-stage renal disease population.[82] A patient's first renal symptom is a loss of medullary concentrating ability.[79]

▶ TREATMENT: Hypercalcemia

DESIRED OUTCOME

The indications for the treatment of acute hypercalcemia are dependent on the degree of hypercalcemia, acuity of its development, and presence or absence of symptoms (Fig. 51–10). The objectives of treatment are reversal of signs and symptoms, restoration of normocalcemia, treatment of the underlying cause of hypercalcemia, and prevention of long-term consequences. Chronic hypercalcemia is usually caused by an underlying medical condition or prescribed therapies. The treatment of malignancies may help mitigate acute hypercalcemic episodes. The goals of treatment of hyperparathyroidism are to reduce serum calcium concentrations as well as to reduce long-term complications such as vascular complications, chronic renal insufficiency, and kidney stones. Medications including thiazides, lithium, antacids and vitamins A and D need to be recognized as potential reversible causes of hypercalcemia.

NONPHARMACOLOGIC THERAPY

Hypercalcemic crisis and acute symptomatic severe hypercalcemia should be considered medical emergencies and treated immediately. These patients may require immediate acting interventions to promptly reduce the serum calcium concentration. Hemodialysis

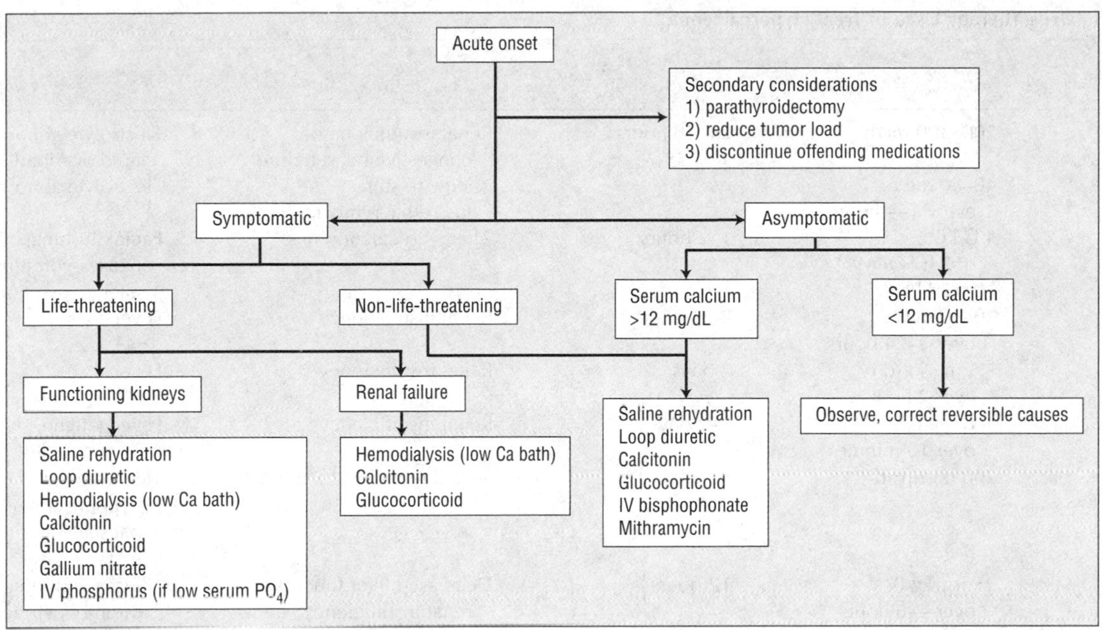

FIGURE 51–10. Pharmacotherapeutic options for the acutely hypercalcemic patient. Ca = calcium; PO_4 = phosphorus.

against a zero or low calcium dialysate solution is considered the treatment of choice, especially in patients with impaired renal function or life-threatening hypercalcemia.[72] However, because there may be considerable delays in initiating dialysis due to the need for evaluation by a nephrologist and placement of a vascular access device, pharmacologic therapy consisting of volume expansion and calciuresis (when not contraindicated by renal dysfunction) and/or calcitonin is usually initiated in the interim. Effective treatment of moderate to severe hypercalcemia in the absence of life-threatening symptoms begins with attention to the underlying disorder and correction of associated fluid and electrolyte abnormalities. Patients with primary hyperparathyroidism may ultimately need surgery, particularly if they have had calcium nephrolithiasis. Patients with malignancy often require reduction of tumor load to control the exogenous supply of cytokines and hormones that cause the hypercalcemia. In contrast, patients with drug-induced hypercalcemia generally respond to discontinuation of the offending agent.

PHARMACOLOGIC THERAPY

Table 51–6 reviews the treatment options for hypercalcemia. For those patients with normal to moderately impaired renal function, the cornerstone of initial treatment of hypercalcemia is volume expansion to increase urinary calcium excretion. Patients with severe renal insufficiency usually do not tolerate volume expansion; they may be initiated on therapy with calcitonin. Patients with symptomatic hypercalcemia are often dehydrated secondary to vomiting and polyuria; thus, rehydration with saline-containing fluids is necessary to interrupt the stimulus for sodium and calcium reabsorption in the renal tubule.[83] Rehydration can be accomplished by the infusion of normal saline at rates of 200–300 mL/h, depending on concomitant conditions (primarily cardiovascular and renal) and extent of hypercalcemia. Adequacy of hydration is assessed by measuring fluid intake and output or by central venous pressure monitoring.[70,72] Loop diuretics such as furosemide (40–80 mg IV every 1 to 4 hours) or ethacrynic acid (for patients with sulfa allergies) may also be instituted to increase urinary calcium excretion and to minimize the development of volume overload from the administration of saline[70](see Table 51–6). Loop diuretics, such as furosemide, block calcium (and sodium) reabsorption in the thick ascending limb of the loop of Henle and augment the calciuric effect of saline alone. The importance of rehydration prior to loop diuretic use is reiterated because dehydration may lead to increased serum calcium because of enhanced proximal tubule calcium reabsorption.[65] Potassium chloride should be added to the saline solution after rehydration is accomplished to maintain normokalemia in the presence of diuretic therapy. Serum magnesium levels should also be monitored, and magnesium replacement instituted if magnesium levels begin to trend downward. Rehydration with saline and administration of furosemide can result in a decrease of 2–3 mg/dL in total serum calcium within 24 to 48 hours.[70]

In those patients in whom saline hydration therapy may be contraindicated (e.g., CHF, moderate to severe renal dysfunction), short-term therapy with calcitonin is effective in reducing serum calcium levels within hours. Calcitonin decreases serum calcium concentrations primarily by inhibiting bone resorption. It may also reduce renal tubular reabsorption of calcium, thus promoting calciuresis. Calcitonin may be administered subcutaneously or intramuscularly (for larger volumes) in a starting dose of 4 U/kg every 12 hours, or intravenously at a rate of 10–12 U/h. The side effects from intravenously administered calcitonin (facial flushing, nausea, and vomiting) limit patient acceptability. Allergic reactions, although rare, do occur, therefore, a test dose (intradermal injection of 0.1 mL of a 10-U/mL solution) is recommended prior to starting therapy. If marked erythema and/or wheal formation does not occur within 15 minutes after administration, therapy can begin. Calcitonin has a rapid onset of action (within 1 to 2 hours); however, the degree and extent of serum calcium level reduction are often unpredictable.[65] Calcitonin therapy is frequently associated with tachyphylaxis caused by antibody formation to foreign proteins or molecules resembling the calcitonin polypeptide.[84] The addition of corticosteroid therapy or conversion to human calcitonin increase effectiveness.[65] Subcutaneous administration of salmon calcitonin in doses of 50–100 IU daily or three times weekly have been prescribed in patients with Paget's disease. The intranasal formulation of calcitonin has been used in the treatment of

TABLE 51–6. Drug Therapy Used to Treat Hypercalcemia

Drug	Starting Dosage	Time Frame to Initial Response	Contraindications	Adverse Effects
0.9% saline ± electrolytes	200–300 mL/h	24–48 hours	Renal insufficiency; congestive heart failure	Electrolyte abnormalities; fluid overload
Loop diuretics	40–80 mg IV every 1–4 hours	n/a	Allergy to sulfas (use ethacrynic acid)	Electrolyte abnormalities
Calcitonin	4 U/kg q12 h SQ/IM 10–12 U/h IV	1–2 hours	Allergy to calcitonin	Facial flushing nausea/vomiting allergic reaction
Pamidronate	30–90 mg IV over 2–24 hours	2 days	Renal insufficiency	Fever
Etidronate	7.5 mg/kg/d IV over 2 hours	2 days	Renal insufficiency	Fever
Zoledronate	4–8 mg IV over 15 minutes	1–2 days	Renal insufficiency	Fever, fatigue, skeletal pain
Gallium nitrate	200 mg/m²/d	?	Severe renal insufficiency	Nephrotoxicity; hypophosphatemia; nausea/vomiting/diarrhea; metallic taste
Mithramycin	25 μg/kg IV over 4–6 hours	12 hours	Decreased liver function; renal insufficiency; thrombocytopenia	Nausea/vomiting; stomatitis; thrombocytopenia; nephrotoxicity; hepatotoxicity;
Glucocorticoids	40–60 mg oral prednisone equivalents	?	Serious infections; hypersensitivity	Diabetes; osteoporosis; infection

Paget's disease, in doses of 200–400 IU daily; unfortunately, this has resulted in only mild decreases in serum calcium. The lack of significant efficacy of the synthetic intranasal formulation is a result of the lower potency and shorter duration of action as compared to salmon calcitonin.

Bisphosphonates block bone resorption very efficiently, render the hydroxyapatite crystal of bone mineral resistant to hydrolysis by phosphatases, and also inhibit osteoclast precursors from attaching to the mineralized matrix thus blocking their transformation into mature functioning osteoclasts.[70,74,85] Pamidronate is very effective in controlling hypercalcemia associated with malignancy and slightly more effective than etidronate.[68] The usual dose of pamidronate is 30–90 mg as an IV infusion given over 2 to 24 hours. Pamidronate also has the advantage of single-day therapy and is currently the bisphosphonate of choice.[70] Etidronate, when administered in doses of 7.5 mg/kg/day by slow intravenous infusion over at least 2 hours for 3 days, is effective in the therapy of hypercalcemia of malignancy.[70] Zoledronate is the newest bisphosphonate that has shown efficacy for the treatment of hypercalcemia of malignancy. It is considered to be the most potent drug in its class and has been found to induce higher rates of response than pamidronate (complete responses of 88.4% to 86.7% for zoledronate versus 69.7% for pamidronate).[86,87] Intravenous doses of 4 mg to 8 mg given over five minutes have resulted in normalization of serum calcium concentrations.[87] Intravenous infusions of 0.02 or 0.04 mg/kg diluted in 5% dextrose (given over 20 to 50 minutes) have also been effective.[88]

The onset of serum calcium concentration decline is slower with bisphosphonate therapy (concentrations begin to decline in 2 days and reach a nadir in 7 days); thus, calcitonin therapy may be necessary if rapid serum level reduction is required.[70,89] Duration of normocalcemia varies, but usually does not exceed 2 weeks, depending on the severity and treatment response of the underlying malignancy.[65] The duration of response has been suggested to be longer with zoledronate (4–5 weeks).[88] Fever is a common side effect of intravenous bisphosphonate therapy. Data on the use of these agents for maintenance intravenous therapy are limited; however, pamidronate has demonstrated more promise than etidronate. Although oral bisphosphonates are useful for the treatment of bone turnover in Paget's disease, there is insufficient data to suggest their use for the initial treatment of hypercalcemia. The use of oral bisphosphonates for maintenance therapy in patients predisposed to hypercalcemia (malignancy) has been successful in some cases.[90] The safety of continuous bisphosphonate therapy in patients with moderate to severe renal insufficiency is currently unknown.

Gallium nitrate is indicated for the treatment of symptomatic hypercalcemia of malignancy not responsive to hydration therapy. However, because of its adverse effect profile, it is generally reserved for those who fail to respond to less-toxic agents. Gallium nitrate inhibits bone resorption, and may be superior to calcitonin in inducing normocalcemia. It may provide a longer duration of normocalcemia as compared to etidronate. The initial dose is usually a continuous IV infusion of 200 mg/m²/day for 5 consecutive days. Because gallium nitrate is nephrotoxic, use caution if it is coadministered with other nephrotoxic drugs. Other common adverse effects include hypophosphatemia, nausea, vomiting, diarrhea, hypocalcemia, and metallic taste.

Mithramycin (plicamycin) is a potent cytotoxic antibiotic that inhibits osteoclast-mediated bone resorption and thereby reduces hypercalcemia. Mithramycin may be administered at a dose of 25 μg/kg via intravenous infusion over 4 to 6 hours in saline or 5% dextrose solutions. This therapy may be repeated daily for 3 to 4 days or on alternating days for 3–8 doses.[70,91] Serum calcium levels begin to fall within 12 hours of a mithramycin dose with the peak effect generally occurring within 48 to 96 hours.[65,70] Single doses are usually well tolerated.[91] Adverse effects of mithramycin include nausea, vomiting, stomatitis, thrombocytopenia, inhibition of platelet function, renal, and hepatotoxicity.[65] Because these adverse effects are more commonly associated with multiple doses, mithramycin is usually limited to short-term therapy in patients who have not responded to alternative therapies. Monitoring parameters include complete blood count, liver function, and renal function. Mithramycin should be avoided in patients with thrombocytopenia, and liver and renal insufficiency.[70]

Glucocorticoids are usually effective in the treatment of hypercalcemia resulting from multiple myeloma, leukemia, lymphoma, sarcoidosis, and hypervitaminoses A and D.[65,85,91] The mechanisms of glucocorticoid-induced reductions in serum calcium include reduced gastrointestinal absorption, defective vitamin D metabolism causing hypercalciuria, increased bone resorption, decreased osteoblast proliferation, and reduction in sex hormone (estrogen and testosterone) concentrations.[92] Daily doses of 40–60 mg of prednisone or the equivalent is effective.[65] The disadvantages of glucocorticoid therapy are its relatively slow onset of action and the potential for diabetes mellitus, osteoporosis, and increased susceptibility to infection.[67,84]

Finally, intravenous phosphate may rapidly reduce ionized calcium concentrations through the formation of insoluble calcium-phosphate salts. However, intravenous phosphate is extremely hazardous because extraskeletal precipitation of calcium-phosphate may result in metastatic calcification, hypotension, acute renal failure, or death.[65,75] Therefore, intravenous phosphates should be reserved for the extraordinary patient with severe hypercalcemia and concomitant hypophosphatemia.[65] Oral phosphorus is not used chronically for the treatment of hypercalcemia because calcium-phosphate crystals may precipitate in the kidneys or other major organs when the calcium-phosphorus product is >50–60 mg^2/dL^2.[93] Serum calcium, phosphorus, and creatinine should be monitored closely. Oral phosphorus treatment is only indicated when there is concomitant hypophosphatemia (<2 mg/dL).

Other miscellaneous treatments for hypercalcemia are available, but clinical experience is limited. Inhibitors of prostaglandin synthesis, such as indomethacin, are rarely effective and thus not currently recommended. Asymptomatic patients with mild hypercalcemia may be carefully observed, especially if treatment for the underlying condition (malignancy) is initiated. The calcimimetic agents (currently investigational) may prove to be an alternative treatment for hypercalcemia.[94] These agents mimic the role of calcium, bind to calcium receptors on the parathyroid gland (and possibly osteoblastic precursors) and result in reduced parathyroid hormone and serum calcium concentrations.[94]

HYPOCALCEMIA

The incidence of hypocalcemia (total serum calcium less than 8.5 mg/dL) in intensive care unit (ICU) patients ranges from 70% to 90% based on total, to 15% to 50% based on ionized calcium concentrations.[66] Hypocalcemia is more commonly seen in hospitalized patients than in outpatients.

PATHOPHYSIOLOGY

Hypocalcemia is the result of alterations in the effect of parathyroid hormone and vitamin D on the bone, gut, and kidney (Fig. 51–8). The primary causes of hypocalcemia are postoperative hypoparathyroidism and vitamin D deficiency. Other causes include magnesium deficiency, thyroid surgery, medications, and hypoalbuminemia.[95] Parathyroid hormone concentrations are elevated in conditions of hypocalcemia, with the exception of hypoparathyroidism and hypomagnesemia[96] (Fig. 51–11).

A symptomatic rapid fall in serum calcium concentrations (often to values <7.0 mg/dL) is common in patients who have had a parathyroidectomy or thyroidectomy. Hypocalcemia in these postsurgical patients is generally transient in nature.[97] The "hungry bone syndrome" is a condition of profound hypocalcemia whereby the bone avidly incorporates calcium and phosphorus from the blood

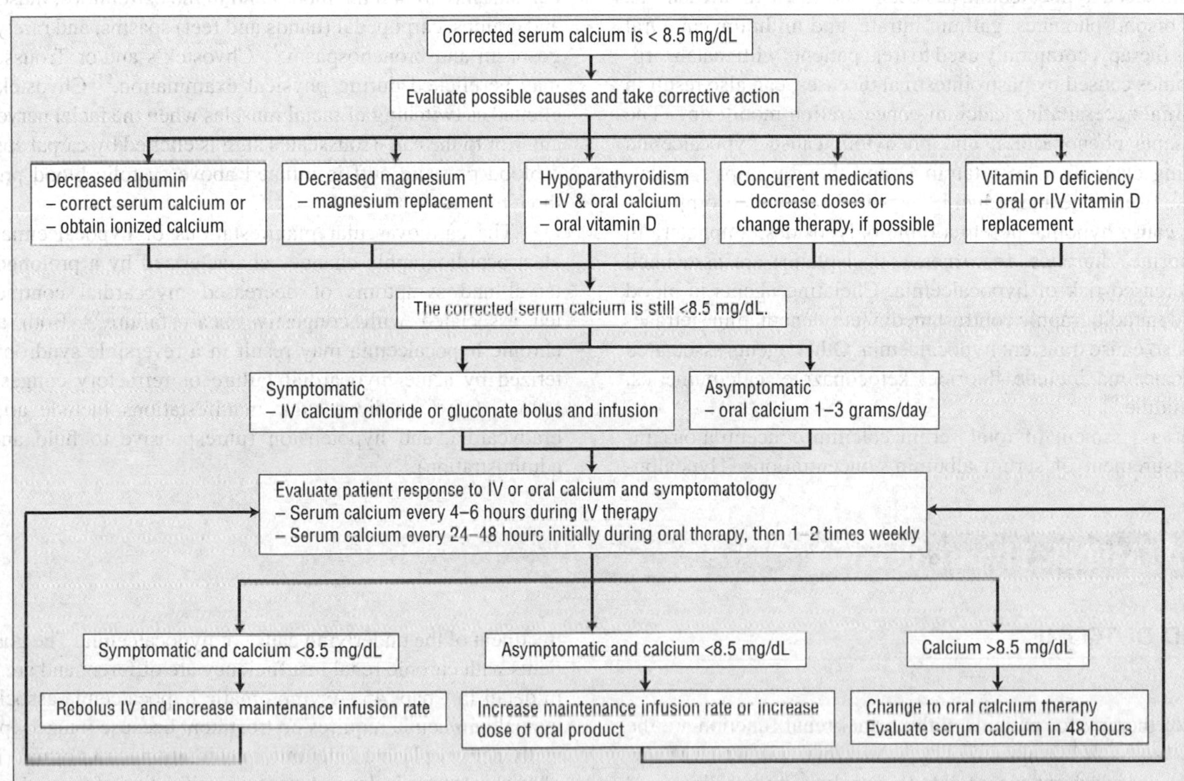

FIGURE 51–11. Hypocalcemia treatment algorithm.

in an attempt to recalcify bone. This is common after correction (usually surgery) of prolonged states of hyperparathyroidism and/or hyperthyroidism. Serum calcium concentrations should be monitored every 6 hours during the 24 to 48 hours following such surgeries and pharmacologic doses of calcium may be necessary to prevent or minimize the drop in serum calcium (see the treatment discussion).

Vitamin D and its metabolites play an important role in the maintenance of extracellular calcium concentrations and in normal skeletal structure and mineralization. Vitamin D is necessary for the optimal absorption of calcium and phosphorus. On a worldwide basis, the most common cause of hypocalcemia is nutritional vitamin D deficiency. In malnourished populations, manifestations include rickets and osteomalacia. Nutritional vitamin D deficiency is uncommon in Western societies because of the fortification of milk with ergocalciferol.[97] The most common cause of vitamin D deficiency in Western societies is gastrointestinal (GI) disease.[74] Gastric surgery, chronic pancreatitis, small-bowel disease, intestinal resection, and bypass surgery are associated with decreased concentrations of vitamin D and metabolites.[74] Vitamin D replacement therapy may need to be administered by the intravenous route if poor oral bioavailability is noted. Decreased production of 1,25-dihydroxyvitamin D_3 may occur as a result of a hereditary defect resulting in vitamin D-dependent rickets. It also can occur secondary to chronic renal insufficiency where insufficient production of the 1-α-hydroxylase enzyme is available for the production of the most active metabolite, 1,25-dihydroxyvitamin D_3.[98] Treatment of hypocalcemia associated with chronic renal failure is reviewed in Chap. 45.

Hypomagnesemia of any cause may be associated with severe symptomatic hypocalcemia that is unresponsive to calcium replacement therapy (see Chap. 52). Reduced serum magnesium concentrations can impair PTH secretion and induce resistance of target organs to the actions of PTH.[95] Normalization of serum calcium concentrations in these patients is thus dependent on appropriate replacement of magnesium.

Drug-induced hypocalcemia has been reported with furosemide, calcitonin, bisphosphonates, gallium nitrate, and mithramycin. Oral phosphorus therapy, commonly used to treat patients with malabsorption syndromes caused by gastrointestinal diseases, can also result in hypocalcemia, necessitating calcium-concentration monitoring. The anticonvulsants phenobarbital and phenytoin cause hypocalcemia by increasing catabolism of vitamin D and thereby impairing calcium release from bone and reducing intestinal calcium absorption.[95] Drugs that cause hypomagnesemia (aminoglycosides, amphotericin B, cyclosporine, diuretics, foscarnet, and cisplatin) are associated with an increased risk of hypocalcemia. Chelating agents in blood (citrate) and in radiographic contrast media (ethylenediamine tetraacetate) can also cause transient hypocalcemia. Other agents associated with hypocalcemia include fluoride, ketoconazole, calcimimetics, and pentamidine.[95]

Proper assessment of total serum calcium concentrations includes measurement of serum albumin concentrations. Hypoalbuminemia, which may be associated with many chronic disease states, is probably the most common cause of "laboratory hypocalcemia." Patients remain asymptomatic because the ionized fraction of serum calcium remains normal (reference range 4.4–5.4 mg/dL). A corrected total serum calcium concentration can be calculated based on the measured total serum calcium and the difference between a patient's measured albumin concentration and the normative value of 4 g/dL by the following equation:

$$\text{Corrected } S_{ca}(\text{mg/dL}) = \text{measured } S_{ca}(\text{mg/dL}) + (0.8 \times 4.0 \text{ g/dL} - \text{measured albumin (g/dL)})$$

CLINICAL PRESENTATION

The clinical manifestations of hypocalcemia are quite variable. The acuteness of the development of hypocalcemia plays a large role in whether or not symptoms will occur.[97] The more acute the drop in ionized calcium concentration, the more likely the patient will develop symptoms. Thus, acid-base balance plays a significant role in the likelihood of the development of hypocalcemic symptoms, with alkalosis predisposing to symptom development. Concomitant hypomagnesemia, hypokalemia, hyponatremia, and additive side effects from prescribed medications also increase the likelihood of symptomatic presentation.

Hypocalcemia may manifest as neuromuscular, CNS, dermatologic, and cardiac sequelae.[74] Acute hypocalcemia is more likely to manifest as neuromuscular (paresthesias, muscle cramps, tetany, and laryngeal spasm) and cardiovascular symptoms, whereas chronic hypocalcemia often presents as CNS (depression, anxiety, memory loss, confusion, hallucinations, and tonic-clonic seizures) and dermatologic symptoms (hair loss, grooved and brittle nails, and eczema).[95] The hallmark sign of acute hypocalcemia is tetany caused by enhanced peripheral neuromuscular irritability.[74] Tetany manifests as paresthesias around the mouth and in the extremities, muscle spasms and cramps, carpopedal (hands and feet) spasms, and rarely as laryngospasm and bronchospasm.[74] Chvostek's and/or Trousseau's sign may be elicited during physical examination.[95] Chvostek's sign is elicited as twitching of facial muscles when the facial nerve is tapped anterior to the ear. Trousseau's sign is elicited by carpal spasm when a blood pressure cuff is inflated above systolic blood pressure for three minutes.

The cardiovascular manifestations of hypocalcemia result in electrocardiographic changes characterized by a prolonged QT interval and symptoms of decreased myocardial contractility often associated with congestive heart failure.[95] Both acute and chronic hypocalcemia may result in a reversible syndrome characterized by acute myocardial failure or refractory congestive heart failure. Other cardiovascular manifestations include arrhythmias, bradycardia, and hypotension (unresponsive to fluid and pressor administration).[95]

▶ TREATMENT: Hypocalcemia

DESIRED OUTCOME

The goals of therapy for patients with normal renal function are the resolution of signs and symptoms of hypocalcemia, restoration of normocalcemia, management of associated electrolyte abnormalities, and treatment of the underlying cause of hypocalcemia. The goals for patients with chronic renal insufficiency are different and are discussed in detail in Chap. 45. Asymptomatic hypocalcemia associated with hypoalbuminemia requires no treatment because ionized (physiologically active) plasma calcium concentrations are normal. Treatment of hypocalcemia is dependent on identification of the pathogenesis of the underlying disorder, acuteness of onset, and presence and severity of symptoms. Acute, symptomatic hypocalcemia requires parenteral administration of soluble calcium salts (Fig. 51–11).

PHARMACOLOGIC THERAPY

The initial therapeutic intervention for patients with acute symptomatic hypocalcemia is to administer 100–300 mg of elemental calcium intravenously over 5 to 10 minutes.[99] This may be provided by the administration of 1 g of calcium chloride (27% elemental calcium) or 2–3 g of calcium gluconate (9% elemental calcium). Calcium gluconate is generally preferred over calcium chloride for peripheral venous administration because calcium gluconate is less irritating to veins. Disadvantages to the use of calcium gluconate are the lower percentage of elemental calcium per volume and the less predictable, slightly smaller increase in plasma ionic calcium compared with calcium chloride. Calcium should not be infused at a rate greater than 60 mg of elemental calcium per minute because severe cardiac dysfunction may result.[99] Intravenous calcium administration should be used with caution in patients receiving digitalis glycosides, because of the possibility of cardiac arrhythmias.[66] Calcium should not be added to bicarbonate- or phosphate-containing solutions because of the possibility of precipitation. The bolus dose of calcium is only effective for 1 to 2 hours and should be followed by a continuous infusion of elemental calcium at a rate of 0.5–2.0 mg/kg/h.[66] The calcium concentrations should be monitored every 4 to 6 hours during the intravenous infusions. The ionized calcium concentration usually normalizes within 4 hours, and the maintenance infusion rate of elemental calcium can then be decreased to 0.3–0.5 mg/kg/h.[65] The maintenance infusion can be adjusted to maintain the desired concentration of calcium.

Once acute hypocalcemia is corrected by parenteral administration, further treatment modalities should be individualized according to the cause of hypocalcemia. If hypomagnesemia is present, magnesium supplementation is indicated (see Chap. 52). Asymptomatic and chronic hypocalcemia associated with hypoparathyroidism and vitamin D-deficient states may be managed by oral calcium and vitamin D supplementation (see Tables 45–3 and 45–4). Therapy is begun with 1–3 g/d of elemental calcium.[64] Average maintenance doses range from 2 g to 8 g of elemental calcium per day in divided doses. If serum calcium does not normalize, a vitamin D preparation may need to be added.

Treatment of hypocalcemia associated with vitamin D-deficient states should be individualized. In patients with malabsorption, vitamin D requirements vary markedly, and large doses may be required. In contrast, vitamin D deficiency associated with anticonvulsant medication may be corrected with smaller doses of vitamin D. Oral doses of 1,25-dihydroxyvitamin D_3 usually range from 0.5 μg to 3 μg daily. The usual initial oral dose of ergocalciferol is 50,000 IU daily.[99] Vitamin D doses are usually adjusted approximately every 4 weeks. The treatment of vitamin D deficiency associated with chronic renal failure generally requires the administration of 1,25-dihydroxyvitamin D_3 or another synthetic analog, such as paricalcitol or doxercalciferol. Situations in which 25-hydroxylase activity is reduced (e.g., hepatic disease) may also require treatment with calcitriol (1,25-dihydroxyvitamin D). The newer vitamin D analogs (paricalcitol and doxercalciferol) were developed to preferentially suppress PTH secretion with less effect on serum calcium concentration. Their efficacy in treating hypocalcemia may thus be less apparent. In selected cases, calcium supplementation may be required if vitamin D replacement alone is ineffective in returning calcium concentrations to normal.

Adverse effects of oral calcium and vitamin D supplementation include hypercalcemia and hypercalciuria, especially in the hypoparathyroid patient, where the renal calcium-sparing effect of parathyroid hormone is absent. Hypercalciuria may increase the risk of calcium stone formation and nephrolithiasis in susceptible patients. One maneuver to help prevent calcium stones is to maintain the calcium at a low normal concentration. Monitoring 24-hour urine collections for total calcium concentrations (goal < 300 mg/24 h) may also minimize the occurrence of hypercalciuria. The addition of thiazide diuretics for patients at risk for stone formation may result in a reduction of both urinary calcium excretion and vitamin D requirements.[99]

DISORDERS OF PHOSPHORUS HOMEOSTASIS

Phosphorus is an essential element in phospholipid cell membranes, nucleic acids, and phosphoproteins required for mitochondrial function.[100] Phosphorus regulates the intermediary metabolism of carbohydrates, fats, and proteins. Phosphorus also regulates enzymatic reactions including glycolysis, ammoniagenesis, and the 1-hydroxylation of 25-hydroxyvitamin D_3.[100] In addition, phosphorus is required for the generation of 2,3-diphosphoglycerate (2,3-DPG) in red blood cells, which is required for normal oxygen-hemoglobin dissociation and delivery of oxygen to the tissues.[101] Phosphorus is the source of the high-energy bonds of adenosine triphosphate (ATP), thus fueling a wide variety of physiologic processes, including muscle contractility, electrolyte transport, neurologic function, and other important biochemical reactions.[100] Considering its diverse biologic importance, it is not difficult to appreciate the clinical implications of disorders of phosphorus homeostasis.

Phosphorus is present in living organisms mainly as inorganic phosphate and organic phosphate esters. Phosphorus is the major intracellular anion. The majority of intracellular phosphorus exists as organic esters, mainly 2,3-DPG, adenosine and guanosine triphosphate, and fructose 1,6-diphosphate.[100] Only a small fraction of intracellular phosphorus exists as inorganic phosphate; however, this fraction is critical because it is the source from which ATP is resynthesized.[100] The majority of inorganic phosphate is located in the extracellular space. Normal serum phosphorus concentration in the adult is 2.5–4.5 mg/dL. Extracellular inorganic phosphate is the prime determinant of intracellular phosphate; thus, small increments in the organic phosphate pool can profoundly alter both the extracellular and intracellular phosphate pools. Metabolic disturbances (acidosis and alkalosis, ketoacidosis), hydrogen ion shifts, and hormones (PTH, calcitonin, cortisol, vitamin D) all can cause shifts in phosphorus concentrations. Because of these phenomena, the serum phosphorus level does not accurately reflect total body stores.[101]

The typical western diet provides a daily intake of 800–1,600 mg of phosphorus. Approximately 60% to 80% of this is absorbed in the gastrointestinal tract by passive and active transport (vitamin D mediated). PTH, 1,25-dihydroxyvitamin D_3, and low-phosphate diets mediate increased absorption. Decreased absorption occurs under conditions of increased dietary intake of phosphorus and magnesium, glucocorticoid therapy, and hypothyroidism. Excretion by the kidney is the single most important regulator of steady-state serum phosphorus concentrations. Renal excretion of phosphorus is regulated by glomerular filtration and proximal tubular reabsorption by passive transport coupled to sodium (sodium-phosphate cotransport). Under normal conditions, 85% to 90% of filtered phosphate is reabsorbed, the majority in the early proximal tubule. Renal tubular reabsorption of phosphorus is inhibited by parathyroid hormone and 1,25-dihydroxyvitamin D_3.[100] Conversely, phosphorus reabsorption in the renal tubule is increased by growth hormone.[100] Internal phosphorus balance (transcellular phosphate distribution) is also of importance in the maintenance of normal serum phosphorus. The serum phosphorus level may vary by as much as 2 mg/dL throughout the day, as the result of acute changes in transcellular distribution of phosphate influenced primarily by carbohydrate intake, insulin secretion, and diurnal variation.[101]

HYPERPHOSPHATEMIA

Serum phosphorus concentration is so closely regulated by the kidneys that it is unusual for hyperphosphatemia (serum phosphorus concentration greater than 4.5 mg/dL) to develop in patients with normal renal function. The most frequent causes of hyperphosphatemia are decreases in urinary phosphorus excretion, and increases in phosphate entrance into the extracellular fluid via either exogenous administration or endogenous intracellular phosphate release.

PATHOPHYSIOLOGY

The most common cause of hyperphosphatemia is a decrease in urinary phosphorus excretion secondary to decreased glomerular filtration rate.[102] Retention of phosphorus decreases vitamin D synthesis and induces hypocalcemia, which leads to an increase in PTH. This physiologic response inhibits further tubular reabsorption of phosphorus to correct hyperphosphatemia and normalize serum calcium concentrations. Patients with excessive exogenous phosphorus administration or endogenous intracellular phosphorus release in the setting of acute renal failure may develop profound hyperphosphatemia.[100] Severe hyperphosphatemia is commonly encountered in patients with renal disease, especially those with glomerular filtration rates less than 15 mL/min/1.73 m^2 (see Chap. 45).

Hypoparathyroidism results in increased renal tubular reabsorption of phosphorus and may result in hyperphosphatemia. Hyperphosphatemia associated with hypoparathyroidism is usually less severe than that associated with severe renal failure or excessive exogenous or endogenous introduction of phosphorus into the ECF space. Hypoparathyroidism is the most important cause of increased tubular phosphorus reabsorption. Acromegaly and thyrotoxicosis may also cause hyperphosphatemia by reducing urinary phosphorus excretion.

Iatrogenic causes of hyperphosphatemia have been widely reported, and awareness of the phosphorus content of intravenous, oral, and rectally administered phosphorus-containing products can aid in its prevention. It is often recognized that large doses of phosphorus administered intravenously to treat hypercalcemia can result in severe life-threatening hyperphosphatemia. Although less-well recognized, oral and rectal administration of phosphate-containing solutions can also result in severe and life-threatening hyperphosphatemia, especially in patients with moderate and severe renal insufficiency.[102] The risk of mortality (because of sudden hypocalcemia with tetany and hyperphosphatemia) is dependent on the amount of phosphorus absorbed from the administered product; a 25% mortality rate has been observed with serum phosphorus concentrations greater than or equal to 33 mg/dL.[102]

Any disorder that results in necrosis of skeletal muscle cells, that is, rhabdomyolysis, can result in the release of large amounts of intracellular phosphorus into the systemic circulation. This condition is frequently associated with acute renal failure and thus severe hyperphosphatemia may develop due to increased endogenous phosphorus release coupled with decreased renal phosphorus excretion. Bowel infarction, malignant hyperthermia, and severe hemolysis are also conditions that may increase endogenous release of phosphorus.

Hyperphosphatemia is not uncommonly observed in patients undergoing treatment for acute leukemia and lymphomas.[103] Chemotherapeutic treatment of acute lymphoblastic leukemia may result in the release of large amounts of phosphorus into the systemic circulation secondary to lysis of lymphoblasts. Initiation of chemotherapy for Burkitt's lymphoma results in a rapid lysis of malignant cells, resulting in hyperphosphatemia, hyperuricemia, hyperkalemia, and hypocalcemia. This syndrome is commonly referred to as tumor lysis syndrome.[103]

Acid-base disorders such as lactic acidosis and diabetic ketoacidosis can release endogenous intracellular phosphorus and cause hyperphosphatemia. In one study, hyperphosphatemia was present in 94.7% of patients with diabetic ketoacidosis prior to the initiation of treatment.[104] After the institution of treatment, serum phosphorus levels decrease and patients may ultimately develop hypophosphatemia.

Medications are another cause of hyperphosphatemia. Excessive intravenous or oral administration of phosphorus is an obvious potential cause of elevated serum phosphate concentrations. Phosphate-containing enemas increase concentrations, especially in those with renal insufficiency. Intravenous or oral vitamin D therapy can increase absorption of phosphorus in the gastrointestinal tract by up to 50%. Bisphosphonate therapy is associated with increased serum phosphate concentrations. Acute phosphorus poisoning as a result of ingestion of laundry detergents is a rare and often unrecognized cause of elevated phosphate concentrations.

CLINICAL PRESENTATION

Some of the signs and symptoms of hyperphosphatemia are a result of the low solubility of the calcium-phosphate complexation product. It has been estimated that calcium-phosphate crystals are likely to form *in vivo* when the product of the serum calcium and phosphate concentrations exceeds 50–60 mg^2/dL^2.[93] Recent evidence suggests that the calcium-phosphorus product should be maintained at less than 55 mg^2/dL^2 to reduce cardiovascular morbidity and mortality secondary to arterial calcification.[75,93] Furthermore, serum phosphorus concentrations greater than 6.5 mg/dL, but not serum calcium concentrations, are associated with increased morbidity and mortality.[93]

The major effects of hyperphosphatemia are related to the development of hypocalcemia (caused by phosphate inhibition of renal 1α-hydroxylase) and its related consequences, as well as vascular and organ damage resulting from the deposition of calcium-phosphate crystals. Extravascular calcification can result in band keratopathy, "red eye," pruritus periarticular calcification especially in renal failure patients (see Chaps. 44 and 45). In addition, soft-tissue calcifications in the conjunctiva, skin, heart, cornea, lung, gastric mucosa, and kidney have been observed primarily in chronic renal failure patients.[100] Hyperphosphatemia associated with chronic renal disease may result in renal osteodystrophy because of overproduction of parathyroid hormone. This condition is discussed in detail in Chap. 45.

▶ TREATMENT: Hyperphosphatemia

DESIRED OUTCOME

The treatment of hyperphosphatemia should be directed at the correction of reversible factors, treatment of the disease states associated with its development, the management of associated signs and symptoms, management of associated electrolyte abnormalities, and the return of serum phosphate concentrations to the normal range.

PHARMACOLOGIC THERAPY

Severe symptomatic hyperphosphatemia manifesting as hypocalcemia and tetany should be treated by the intravenous administration of calcium salts (see the discussion of hypocalcemia). Although this may seem counterintuitive in a patient with a phosphorus of 16 mg/dL and a calcium of 7 mg/dL (the calcium-phosphorus product is 112 mg^2/dL^2), correction of severe hypocalcemia is of primary importance because of the critical nature of this disorder. In general, the most effective way to treat asymptomatic chronic hyperphosphatemia is to decrease phosphate absorption in the lumen of the GI tract by the use of phosphate-binding agents.[100] Antacids containing divalent and trivalent cations (calcium, magnesium, and aluminum) or sevelamer are the agents most frequently used in the prevention and treatment of hyperphosphatemia (see Table 45–3). Long-term treatment with aluminum hydroxide and aluminum carbonate should be discouraged because of the association with anemia, CNS disorders, and bone disease. Short-term therapy with these agents is effective and safe. The most frequent adverse effect from phosphate-binding agents (especially calcium) is constipation. Calcium salts are the preferred phosphate-binding agents except when there is concomitant hypercalcemia. Therapy with the new polymer agent (sevelamer) may avoid the detrimental effects associated with aluminum, magnesium, or calcium therapy.

HYPOPHOSPHATEMIA

Mild to moderate hypophosphatemia is defined as a serum phosphorus concentration of 1.0–2.0 mg/dL, whereas severe hypophosphatemia is defined as a serum phosphorus concentration of less than 1.0 mg/dL.[105] Hypophosphatemia is found in approximately 1% to 3% of hospital admissions.[101] The incidence in hospitalized critically ill patients is 18% to 28%.[105] Unlike its severe form, mild or moderate hypophosphatemia seldom causes recognizable signs and symptoms.[103]

PATHOPHYSIOLOGY

Hypophosphatemia may be the result of decreased gastrointestinal absorption, increased urinary excretion, or extracellular to intracellular redistribution[100] (Table 51–7). Although mild to moderate hypophosphatemia is common and can occur in inpatients and outpatients, severe hypophosphatemia is predominantly encountered in the acute care setting and can be associated with life-threatening symptoms.

Phosphate-binding substances such as sucralfate, calcium carbonate, and aluminum/magnesium-containing antacids have the potential to bind large amounts of phosphorus in the gut, thereby preventing absorption. If phosphate-binding agents are ingested on a chronic basis in conjunction with a dietary phosphorus deficiency, hypophosphatemia may result.[103] Patients who are receiving long-term phosphate-binding agents, those with peptic ulcer disease or chronic renal insufficiency, and those who may be predisposed to moderate hypophosphatemia (alcoholics) are at highest risk for the development of severe hypophosphatemia. Hyperparathyroidism may cause hypophosphatemia as a result of decreased gastrointestinal absorption of dietary phosphorus. Table 51–7 lists other conditions causing decreased gastrointestinal absorption.

Increased renal losses of phosphorus can occur in hyperparathyroid (primary and secondary) patients with normal renal function and those with vitamin D deficiency. Elevated parathyroid hormone levels lead to an increase in serum calcium concentrations and decreased serum phosphorus concentrations. Serum phosphorus is

TABLE 51–7. Conditions Causing Hypophosphatemia

Decreased Gastrointestinal Absorption
- Phosphate-binding drugs
  - Sucralfate
  - Calcium carbonate
  - Aluminum/magnesium antacids
  - Sevelamer
- Decreased dietary phosphorus intake
- Glucocorticoids
- Vitamin D deficiency/resistance
- Hypoparathyroidism
- Chronic diarrhea
- Steatorrhea

Increased Urinary Excretion
- Hyperparathyroidism (primary and secondary)
- Recovery from burns
- Rickets
- Malignant neoplasms
- Fanconi's syndrome
- Acute volume expansion
- Metabolic acidosis
- Renal transplantation
- Vitamin D deficiency and/or resistance
- Diuretics
  - Acetazolamide
  - Osmotic agents
- Glucocorticoids
- Sodium bicarbonate

Internal Redistribution
- Refeeding syndrome
- Parenteral nutrition
- Parathyroidectomy (hungry bone syndrome)
- Alcoholism
- Respiratory alkalosis
- Diabetic ketoacidosis (correction)
- Dextrose solutions
- Insulin
- Catecholamines
- Anabolic steroids
- Glucagon
- Calcitonin
- Erythropoietin

decreased as the result of a reduction in renal tubular reabsorption.[106] Recovery from extensive third-degree burns is associated with a marked diuretic phase associated with an impressive renal loss of phosphate.[103] This recovery may also be associated with the development of an anabolic state as stress levels decrease and nutritional therapies take effect. Because phosphorus is rapidly incorporated into the new cells this may contribute to the severity of the hypophosphatemia. Drugs that cause increased renal elimination of phosphorus include diuretics (acetazolamide and osmotic diuretics), glucocorticoids, and sodium bicarbonate.

Rapid refeeding of malnourished patients with high-carbohydrate, high-calorie nutritional diets with inadequate amounts of supplemental phosphorus may result in severe symptomatic hypophosphatemia. This phenomenon is especially prevalent in patients with other underlying risk factors for the development of hypophosphatemia, such as alcoholism.[106] The etiology of severe hypophosphatemia associated with hyperalimentation and nutritional recovery may be separated into two phases: acute, rapid hypophosphatemia secondary to intracellular shifts of phosphorus resulting from glucose-induced insulin secretion; and the gradual decrease in serum phosphorus concentration over 5 to 10 days secondary to tissue repair in the presence of phosphorus deprivation.[107] The development of severe hypophosphatemia secondary to hyperalimentation can be prevented by the administration of 12–15 mmol of phosphorus per liter of hyperalimentation solution or 15 mmol per 1,000 calories of dextrose.[108] Transcellular shifts in phosphorus also occur after parathyroidectomy, causing severe hypocalcemia and hypophosphatemia because of hungry bone syndrome (deposition of phosphorus and calcium in the bone).

Severe and prolonged respiratory alkalosis (a result of hyperventilation, pain, anxiety, and sepsis) can cause hypophosphatemia.[101] Respiratory alkalosis is thought to contribute significantly to the hypophosphatemia observed during alcohol withdrawal.[101] Although patients with diabetic ketoacidosis may present with hyperphosphatemia, the institution of therapy to correct it may cause serum phosphorus concentrations to decrease rapidly as phosphorus shifts back into the intracellular compartment. In addition, the acidosis associated with the diabetic ketoacidotic state can cause a decomposition of organic compounds inside the cell and a release of inorganic phosphorus into the plasma and subsequently into the urine.[107] The combination of intracellular phosphorus breakdown and the shift of phosphorus into cells on initiation of treatment may lead to severe hypophosphatemia. Drugs associated with transcellular shifts in phosphorus include dextrose solutions, glucagon, insulin, catecholamines, calcitonin, erythropoietin, and anabolic steroids.

Chronic ethanol abusers are prone to a variety of serum electrolyte disorders including hypocalcemia, hypomagnesemia, hypokalemia, and hypophosphatemia. The etiology of hypophosphatemia in the alcoholic patient is multifactorial. Malnutrition, poor dietary intake, diarrhea, vomiting, and the use of phosphate-binding antacids may all contribute to the hypophosphatemia of alcoholism.[107] In addition, serum phosphorus concentrations may decrease after hospitalization in the alcoholic patient with the institution of dextrose-containing intravenous fluids, as a result of an intracellular shift of phosphorus.[108,109] Hyperventilation associated with the alcohol withdrawal syndrome may also contribute to the development of hypophosphatemia.[103] Alcoholic patients are particularly susceptible to the complications of hypophosphatemia such as rhabdomyolysis, which is often seen during withdrawal or refeeding.[103,109] Thus, serum phosphorus concentrations should be routinely monitored in alcoholic patients.

TABLE 51–8. Manifestations of Severe Hypophosphatemia

Neurologic	**Hematologic**
Irritability	Decreased 2,3-DPG
Apprehension	Hemolysis
Weakness	WBC dysfunction
Numbness	Platelet dysfunction
Paresthesias	**Bone**
Dysarthria	Osteopenia
Confusion	Osteomalacia
Obtundation	Bone pain
Seizures	**Pulmonary**
Coma	Acute respiratory failure
Apathy	Slow weaning from ventilator
Delirium	Respiratory muscle fatigue
Hallucinations	**Renal**
Paranoia	Acute tubular necrosis
Peripheral neuropathy	(rhabdomyolysis)
Muscular	**Cardiac**
Myalgia	Congestive cardiomyopathy
Weakness	Decreased contractility
Rhabdomyolysis	Arrhythmias
Dysphagia	
Ileus	

CLINICAL PRESENTATION

The clinical manifestations of severe hypophosphatemia are diverse and may affect many organ systems (Table 51–8). It is likely that two primary biochemical abnormalities are responsible for most of the clinical manifestations of severe hypophosphatemia.[100] First, intracellular energy stores may be decreased secondary to depletion of intracellular ATP, which is dependent on inorganic intracellular phosphate. This can result in disruptions in cellular function. Second, reduced red blood cell (RBC) 2,3-DPG concentrations are associated with a shift to the left of the oxyhemoglobin saturation curve. This shift is associated with a decrease in the release of oxygen to peripheral tissues (increased oxygen affinity for hemoglobin) and may result in tissue hypoxia.[100] These metabolic disorders can be seen in a wide variety of organ systems.

Neurologic (CNS) manifestations of severe hypophosphatemia result in a metabolic encephalopathy syndrome.[107] This progressive syndrome of irritability, apprehension, weakness, numbness, paresthesias, dysarthria, confusion, obtundation, seizures, and coma has been described in patients with severe hypophosphatemia.[103,106] Neuropsychiatric disturbances include apathy, delirium, hallucinations, and paranoia. Peripheral neuropathy and symptoms resembling Guillain-Barré syndrome have also been reported.[106]

Severe hypophosphatemia may result in significant dysfunction of skeletal muscle ranging from myalgia, bone pain, and weakness, with chronic hypophosphatemia, to potentially fatal rhabdomyolysis, with severe, acute hypophosphatemia.[106] Laboratory evaluations can help to distinguish between chronic and acute on chronic hypophosphatemia. Elevated alkaline phosphatase, normal creatine phosphokinase, and normal to low phosphorus and calcium are present in cases of chronic hypophosphatemia. In contrast, hyperkalemia, hyperuricemia, elevated blood urea nitrogen and creatinine, hypercalcemia, and myoglobinuria are present in cases in which rhabdomyolysis complicates the acute or chronic hypophosphatemia.[106] Hypophosphatemia can result in acute respiratory failure secondary to respiratory muscle weakness and diaphragmatic contractile dysfunction. Thus, frequent assessment of serum phosphorus concentration is indicated in patients at risk for respiratory failure. Likewise, adequate treatment of hypophosphatemia in respiratory failure may aid in successful weaning from the ventilator.[101] Dysphagia and ileus have also been attributed to hypophosphatemia.[101]

Cardiac muscle function has been reported to be impaired in the setting of hypophosphatemia and has resulted in congestive cardiomyopathy.[110] This has been reported in alcoholics, and postoperative and intensive care patients. A depletion in cardiac ATP stores has been hypothesized as the cause of this syndrome.[106] Arrhythmias have also been reported in patients with hypophosphatemia. Because hypophosphatemia is a potentially reversible cause of heart failure, it should be considered in patients who experience an acute deterioration in ventricular function.

Hematologic manifestations of hypophosphatemia include decreased levels of 2,3-diphosphoglycerate, decreased red blood cell ATP, and membrane rigidity.[100] When red blood cell ATP decreases to below 15% of normal, cells become spherocytic and rigid, and are trapped and destroyed in the spleen.[107] Therefore, hemolysis may be a manifestation of severe hypophosphatemia. Reduction in ATP content of white blood cells (WBC) may result in mobility, chemotaxis, phagocytosis, and bactericidal dysfunction.[103] These changes may contribute to an increased risk of infection in hypophosphatemic patients. Animal studies also demonstrate platelet abnormalities in the setting of hypophosphatemia.[106] The implications of hypophosphatemia on human platelet function, however, have not been determined.

Finally, prolonged hypophosphatemia may result in osteopenia and osteomalacia because of enhanced osteoclastic resorption of bone. Glucose intolerance from hypophosphatemia caused by tissue insensitivity to insulin has also been described.

▶ TREATMENT: Hypophosphatemia

DESIRED OUTCOME

The goals of therapy are the reversal of signs and symptoms of hypophosphatemia, normalization of serum phosphorus concentrations, and management of underlying conditions. Awareness of the clinical situations in which hypophosphatemia may be anticipated (alcoholism, diabetic ketoacidosis, parenteral nutrition) is of vital importance in preventing iatrogenic hypophosphatemia. The routine addition of phosphorus in concentrations of 12–15 mmol/L to intravenous hyperalimentation solutions is of utmost importance for the prevention of severe hypophosphatemia in hospitalized patients.

PHARMACOLOGIC THERAPY

Severe (<1 mg/dL) or symptomatic hypophosphatemia should be treated with parenteral phosphorus replacement. Oral phosphorus supplementation is usually reserved for patients who are asymptomatic or who exhibit mild to moderate hypophosphatemia. Estimation of total body phosphorus deficit is difficult because phosphorus is an intracellular electrolyte. Dosage and infusion recommendations, as well as response to parenteral phosphorus replacement, are highly variable.[105] The infusion of 15 mmol of phosphorus in 250 mL 5% dextrose or 0.9% sodium chloride over 3 hours is a safe and effective treatment for severe hypophosphatemia.[105] Mean increases in serum phosphate of 0.5–0.8 mg/dL have been reported. Doses of 15–30 mmol of phosphorus can be given over 1 to 3 hours in patients without hypercalcemia (serum calcium > 10.5 mg/dL).[105] Other authors recommend a wider dosage range of 0.08–0.64 mmol/kg body weight (5–45 mmol in a 70-kg patient) given over 4–12 hours.[111,112] Intravenous phosphate therapy produces the desired increase in serum phosphorus at 24 hours in 20% to 80% of patients. Response is dependent on the degree of phosphate depletion and replacement dose administered.[100] Furthermore, the initial success is often followed in 48 to 72 hours by recurrent hypophosphatemia, necessitating close monitoring of serum phosphorus and repeated administration of phosphorus products as warranted.

Parenteral phosphorus supplementation (Table 51–9) is associated with risks of hyperphosphatemia, metastatic soft tissue deposition of calcium-phosphate product, hypomagnesemia, hypocalcemia, and hyperkalemia or hypernatremia (caused by intravenous phosphorus salt). Inappropriate administration of large doses of parenteral phosphorus over relatively short time periods has resulted in symptomatic hypocalcemia and soft-tissue calcification.[100] The rate of infusion and choice of initial dosage should, therefore, be based on severity of hypophosphatemia, presence of symptoms, and coexistent medical conditions. Patients should be closely monitored with frequent (every 6 hours) serum phosphorus determinations for 48 to 72 hours after starting intravenous therapy. It may be necessary to continue administration of intravenous phosphorus for several days in some patients, while other patients may be able to tolerate an oral maintenance regimen. Monitoring should also include assessment of serum potassium, calcium, and magnesium concentrations. Hypomagnesemia secondary to intracellular shifts occurs frequently (27% to 80%) in severely hypophosphatemic patients.[105] Therapy with parenteral phosphorus should be undertaken with great

TABLE 51–9. Phosphorus Replacement Therapy

Product (Salt)	Phosphate Content
Oral Therapy	
Neutra-Phos (7 mEq/L each of Na and K)	250 mg/packet
Neutra-Phos K (14.25 mEq/mL K)	250 mg/capsule
K-Phos Neutral (13 mEq/tablet Na and 1.1 mEq/tablet K)	250 mg/tablet
Uro-KP Neutral (10.9 mEq/tablet Na and 1.27 mEq/tablet K)	250 mg/tablet
Intravenous Therapy	
Sodium PO_4 (4.0 mEq/mL Na)	3.0 mmol/mL
Potassium PO_4 (4.4 mEq/mL K)	3.0 mmol/mL

caution and at reduced dosage for patients with hypercalcemia or renal dysfunction.[103,109]

Mild to moderate or asymptomatic hypophosphatemia can be treated by the administration of oral phosphorus salts in doses of 1.5–2.0 g (50–60 mmol) daily in divided doses (Table 51–9). Phosphorus concentrations should be monitored daily, with the goal of correcting the reduced phosphorus concentration in approximately 7 to 10 days. The primary dose-limiting adverse effect associated with oral phosphorus replacement is the development of osmotic diarrhea. Patients with mild to moderate hypophosphatemia and moderate to severe renal insufficiency should receive reduced daily oral doses (i.e., 1 g or approximately 30 mmol of phosphorus) with careful monitoring of serum phosphorus concentration, because they are predisposed to phosphorus retention. In addition to phosphorus supplementation for hypophosphatemia, dipyridamole may decrease renal phosphate leaking and increase serum phosphorus. Doses of 75 mg four times daily have resulted in increases in serum 1,25-dihydroxyvitamin D_3 and decreases in serum calcium and urolithiasis events.[113]

CONCLUSIONS

The pharmacist can play an integral part in the management of underlying fluid and electrolyte abnormalities and thus improve the patient's outcome. Most importantly, the pharmacist is responsible for reviewing the patient's medication history and determining whether any of the patient's current drug therapy may have contributed to the existing abnormalities. The pharmacist should also assume responsibility for drug therapy recommendations to reduce the risk of developing new electrolyte problems and to optimize the outcome of the current management plan.

Pharmacists in ambulatory settings may identify existing or potential drug-related fluid and electrolyte abnormalities and then suggest dosage adjustments or new drug therapies when appropriate. It is hoped that this proactive interventional approach will facilitate the management of mild disorders in the community and reduce the need for hospitalization. It is critical that the pharmacist be aware of the signs and symptoms of fluid and electrolyte problems that patients may have. Pharmacists should attempt to ascertain the presence of mild symptoms in those patients at high risk [e.g., the elderly and those with significant organ disease (renal, cardiac, and hepatic impairment)].

▶ PRINCIPLES OF PHARMACOTHERAPY

- Patients with symptomatic hyponatremia are at high risk of neurologic complications, and the serum sodium concentration in these patients should be raised 1.5–2 mEq/L/h for the first 3 to 4 hours, but no more than 12 mEq/L/d to avoid cerebral demyelination.
- Patients with hypotonic hyponatremia caused by volume depletion should initially receive normal saline followed by 0.45% saline once signs of ECF volume depletion abate in order to avoid overly rapid correction of the serum sodium concentration.
- Hypoxemic respiratory insufficiency impairs the cerebral compensatory mechanisms for adapting to hypo-osmolality, and also identifies patients at high risk for poor neurologic outcomes.
- In patients with SIADH and symptomatic hypotonic hyponatremia, the most efficient means of correcting the hyponatremia involves use of 3% saline in conjunction with a loop diuretic. Use of normal saline in this setting can potentially worsen the hyponatremia, particularly if the urine sodium plus urine potassium concentration exceeds 154 mmol/L.
- The various formulas for calculating the 3% saline dose are only estimates, and patients should be monitored with frequent blood chemistries (generally every 2 to 4 hours over the first 12 hours).
- Treatment of asymptomatic hyponatremia should be dictated by the underlying etiology. Patients with chronic SIADH may be successfully managed with increased solute intake, often in conjunction with a loop diuretic.
- The serum sodium concentration should be corrected at a rate of approximately 0.5 mEq/L/h in patients with hypernatremia. The serum sodium concentration in patients who develop hypernatremia over the course of several hours (such as following hypertonic saline infusion) should be corrected at approximately 1 mEq/L/h.
- Patients with central DI should be treated with intranasal desmopressin acetate, with a goal of restoring water balance such that the urine volume decreases to less than 2 L/d and the serum sodium concentration is maintained in the 137–142 mEq/L range.
- Patients with nephrogenic DI should be treated by correcting the underlying cause when possible, and through use of sodium chloride restriction in conjunction with a thiazide diuretic to decrease the ECF volume by approximately 1–1.5 kg.
- The fluid and electrolyte complications of diuretic therapy occur within the first 2 weeks of diuretic therapy, and repeated monitoring of serum chemistries is generally not necessary in the absence of a change in clinical status, diuretic dose, or dietary intake.
- Patients with renal insufficiency require larger doses of diuretics to achieve adequate delivery of the drug to the active site. The natriuretic response is decreased in patients with renal failure due to the decrease in the filtered load of sodium. This may be overcome by dosing diuretics more frequently, as well as by using continuous infusions in critically ill, hospitalized patients. Patients that remain diuretic resistant should be treated with both a loop and a thiazide-type diuretic.
- Patients with congestive heart failure and a normal GFR have impaired absorption of diuretics. An adequate diuresis is most readily sustained by increasing the frequency of diuretic administration.
- Patients with nephrotic syndrome commonly develop diuretic resistance. Increased distal tubular sodium avidity, as well as impaired delivery of diuretics to the site of action have been demonstrated. The impaired natriuretic response may be overcome by using higher doses to increase the delivery of free drug to the secretory site in the proximal nephron. Combinations of a loop diuretic with a distal diuretic are generally necessary to promote a natriuresis that exceeds tubular sodium reabsorption.
- Patients with cirrhosis should initially be treated with spironolactone in the absence of impaired GFR and hyperkalemia. Thiazides may then be added for patients with a creatinine clearance >50 mL/ min. For those patients who remain diuretic resistant, a loop diuretic may replace the thiazide.

- Hypercalcemia and hypocalcemia effect several important organ systems, necessitating the prompt identification of these disorders and initiation of corrective therapy.
- The correction of hypercalcemia includes multiple treatment modalities including hydration, diuretics, bisphosphonates, and steroids.
- Hypophosphatemia can result from decreased gastrointestinal absorption, increased urinary excretion, and intracellular redistribution.
- The treatment for hypophosphatemia consists of intravenous phosphate salts in doses of 0.08–0.64 mmol/kg for acute therapy and oral doses of 50–60 mmol/d for maintenance therapy.

REFERENCES

1. Berl T, Robertson GL. Pathophysiology of water metabolism. In: Brenner BM, ed. The Kidney, 6th ed. Philadelphia, WB Saunders, 2000:866–924.
2. Andreoli TE. Water: Normal balance, hyponatremia, and hypernatremia. Ren Fail 2000;2:711–735.
3. McManus ML, Churchwell KB, Strange K. Regulation of cell volume in health and disease. N Engl J Med 1995;333:1260–1266.
4. Gennari FJ. Serum osmolality: Uses and limitations. N Engl J Med 1984;310:102–105.
5. Androgué HJ, Madias NE. Hyponatremia. N Engl J Med 2000;342:1581–1589.
6. Baylis PH. Osmoregulation and control of vasopressin secretion in healthy adults. Am J Physiol 1987;253(5 pt 2):R671–R678.
7. Deen PM, Verdijk MA, Knoers NV, et al. Requirement of human renal water channel aquaphorin-2 for vasopressin dependent concentration of urine. Science 1994;264(5155):92–95.
8. Bourque CW, Oliet SH, Richard D. Osmoreceptors, osmoreception, and osmoregulation. Front Neuroendocrinol 1994;15:231–274.
9. Skorecki KL, Brenner BM. Body fluid homeostasis. A contemporary overview. Am J Med 1981;70:77–88.
10. Anderson RJ. Hospital-associated hyponatremia. Kidney Int 1986; 29: 1237–1247.
11. Sterns RH. Severe symptomatic hyponatremia: Treatment and outcome: A study of 64 cases. Ann Intern Med 1987; 07:656–664.
12. Oster JR, Singer I. Hyponatremia, hyposmolality, and hypotonicity: Tables and fables. Arch Intern Med 1999;159:333 336.
13. Maas AHJ, Siggard-Andersen O, Weisberg HF, Zijlstra WG. Ion-selective electrodes for sodium and potassium: A new problem of what is measured and what should be reported. Clin Chem 1985;31:482–485.
14. Star RA. Hyperosmolar states. Am J Med Sci 1990;300:402–412.
15. Agarwal R, Emmett M. The post-transurethral resection of prostate syndrome: Therapeutic proposals. Am J Kid Dis 1994;24:108–111.
16. Arieff AI. Management of hyponatremia. Br Med J 1993;307:305–308.
17. Aabakken L, Johansen KS, Rydningen EB, Bredesen JE, Ovrebo S, Jacobsen D. Osmolal and anion gaps in patients admitted to an emergency medical department. Hum Exp Toxicol 1994;13:131–134.
18. Arieff AI, DeFronzo RA. Disorders of sodium metabolism—hyponatremia. In: Arieff AI, DeFronza eds. Fluid, Electrolyte, and Acid-Base Disorders, 2nd ed. New York, Churchill Livingstone, 1995:255–303.
19. Sterns RH, Narins RG. Hypernatremia and hyponatremia: Pathophysiology, diagnosis, and therapy. In: Androgué HJ, ed. Contemporary Management in Critical Care. Vol. 1, No. 2. Acid-Base and Electrolyte Disorders. New York, Churchill Livingstone, 1991:161–191.
20. Kamel KS, Ethier JH, Richardson RM, Bear RA, Halperin ML. Urine electrolytes and osmolality: When and how to use them. Am J Nephrol 1990;10:89–102.
21. Friedman E, Shadel M, Hakim HM, Farfel Z. Thiazide-induced hyponatremia. Reproducibility by single-dose challenge and an analysis of pathogenesis. Ann Intern Med 1989;110(1):24–30.
22. Smith DM, McKenna K, Thompson CJ. Hyponatraemia. Clin Endocrinol 2000;52:667–678.
23. Hensen J, Haenelt M, Gross P. Water retention after oral chlorpropamide is associated with an increase in renal papillary arginine vasopressin receptors. Eur J Endocrinol 1995;132(4):459–464.
24. Kamiyama T, Iseki K, Kawazoe N, Takishita S, Fukiyama K. Carbamazepine-induced hyponatremia in a patient with partial central diabetes insipidus. Nephron 1993;64(1):142–145.
25. Bressler RB, Huston DP. Water intoxication following moderate dose intravenous cyclophosphamide. Arch Intern Med 1985; 145:548.
26. Rault RM. Case report: hyponatremia associated with nonsteroidal anti-inflammatory drugs. Am J Med Sci 1993; 305:318–320.
27. Liv BA, Mittman N, Knowles SR, Shear NH. Hyponatremia and the syndrome of inappropriate secretion of antidiuretic hormone associated with the use of selective serotonin reuptake inhibitors: A review of spontaneous reports. Can Med Assoc J 1996;155(5):519–527.
28. Holden R, Jackson MA. Near-fatal hyponatremic coma due to vasopressin over-secretion after "ecstasy" (3,4-MDMA). Lancet 1996;347 (9007):1052.
29. Hairprasad MK, Eisinger RP, Nadler IM, Padmanabhan CS, Nidus BD. Hyponatremia in psychogenic polydipsia. Arch Intern Med 1980; 140(12):1639–1642.
30. Ayus JC, Arieff AI. Pulmonary complications of hyponatremic encephalopathy—Non-cardiogenic pulmonary edema and hypercapnic respiratory failure. Chest 1995;107(2):517–521.
31. Verbalis JG, Gullans SR. Hyponatremia causes large sustained reductions in brain content of multiple organic osmolytes in rats. Brain Res 1991;567:274–282.
32. Ayus JC, Arrief AI. Chronic hyponatremic encephalopathy in post-menopausal women—Association of therapies with morbidity and mortality. JAMA 1999;281(24):2299–2304.
33. Sterns RH. Severe symptomatic hyponatremia: Treatment and outcome: A study of 64 cases. Ann Intern Med 1987;107:656–664.
34. Sterns RH, Riggs JE, Schochet SS Jr. Osmotic demyelination syndrome following correction of hyponatremia. N Engl J Med 1986;314:1535–1542.
35. Gross P, Reimann D, Neidel J, et al. The treatment of severe hyponatremia. Kidney Int Suppl 1998;64:S6–S11.
36. Fanestil DD, Moore FD. Compartmentation of body water. In: Narins RG, ed. Maxwell and Kleeman's Fluid and Electrolyte Metabolism, 5th ed. New York, McGraw-Hill, 1994:1–20.
37. Mange K, Matsuura D, Cizman B, et al. Language guiding therapy: The case of dehydration versus volume depletion. Ann Intern Med 1997;127:848–853.
38. Inadomi DW, Kopple JD. Fluid and electrolyte complications in total parenteral nutrition. In: Narins RG, ed. Maxwell and Kleeman's Fluid and Electrolyte Metabolism, 5th ed. New York, McGraw-Hill, 1994:1446–1447.
39. Lauriat SM. Berl T. The hyponatremic patient: Practical focus on therapy. J Am Soc Nephrol 1997;8(10):1599–607.
40. Decaux G, Waterlot Y, Genette F, Mockel J. Treatment of the syndrome of inappropriate secretion of antidiuretic hormone with furosemide. N Engl J Med 1981;304(6):329–330.
41. Verbalis JG. Hyponatremia and hyposmolar disorders. In: Greenberg A, ed. Primer on Kidney Diseases, 2nd ed. San Diego, CA. Academic Press, 1998:57–63.
42. Saito T, Ishikawa S, Abe K, et al. Acute aquaresis by the nonpeptide arginine vasopressin (AVP) antagonist OPC-31260 improves hyponatremia in patients with syndrome of inappropriate secretion of antidiuretic hormone (SIADH). J Clin Endocrinol Metab 1997;82:1054–1057.
43. Elisaf M, Theodorou J, Pappas C, Siamopoulos K. Successful treatment of hyponatremia with angiotensin-converting enzyme inhibitors in patients with congestive heart failure. Cardiology 1995;86:477–480.
44. Oh MS, Carroll HJ. Regulation of intracellular and extracellular volume. In: Arieff AI, DeFronzo RA, eds. Fluid, Electrolyte, and Acid-Base Balance Disorders, 2nd ed. New York, Churchill Livingstone, 1995:1–28.

45. Fried LF, Palevsky PM. Hyponatremia and hypernatremia. Med Clin North Am 1997; 81:585–609.
46. Moritz ML, Ayus JC. The changing pattern of hypernatremia in hospitalized children. Pediatrics 1999;104:435–439.
47. Oh MS, Carroll HJ. Disorders of sodium metabolism: Hypernatremia and hyponatremia. Crit Care Med 1992;20:94–103.
48. Androgué HJ, Madias NE. Hypernatremia. N Engl J Med 2000;342: 1493–1499.
49. Rose BD, Post TW. Hyperosmolar states—Hypernatremia. In: Rose BD, Post TW, eds. Clinical Physiology of Acid-Base and Electrolyte Disorders, 5th ed. New York, McGraw-Hill, 2001:746–793.
50. Zerbe RL, Robertson GL. A comparison of plasma vasopressin measurements with a standard indirect test in the differential diagnosis of polyuria. N Engl J Med 1981:304:1539–1546.
51. Physicians Desk Reference, 55th ed. Montvale, NJ, 2001:702–704.
52. Monnens L, Jonkman A, Thomas C. Response to indomethacin and hydrochlorothiazide in nephrogenic diabetes insipidus. Clin Sci 1984;66:709–715.
53. Battle DC, Von Riotte AB, Gaviria M, Grupp M. Amelioration of polyuria by amiloride in patients receiving long-term lithium therapy. N Engl J Med 1985;312:408–414.
54. Bonventre JV, Leaf A. Sodium homeostasis: Steady states without a setpoint. Kidney Int 1982;21(6):880–883.
55. Rose BD. Clinical Physiology of Acid-Base and Electrolyte Disorders, 5th ed. New York, McGraw-Hill, 2001:478.
56. Taylor AE. Capillary fluid filtration: Starling forces and lymph flow. Circ Res 1981;49(3):557–575.
57. Schrier RW. Pathogenesis of sodium and water retention in high-output and low-output cardiac failure, nephrotic syndrome, cirrhosis, and pregnancy. N Engl J Med 1988;319(17):1127–1134.
58. Rose BD. Diuretics. Kidney Int 1991;39:336–352.
59. Brater DC. Diuretic therapy. N Engl J Med 1998;339:387–395.
60. Rudy DW, Voelker JR, Greene PK, Esparza FA, Brater DC. Loop diuretics for chronic renal insufficiency: A continuous infusion is more efficacious than bolus therapy. Ann Intern Med 1991;115:360–366.
61. Kirchner, KA, Voelker, JR, Brater, DC. Intratubular albumin blunts the response to furosemide—A mechanism for diuretic resistance in the nephrotic syndrome. J Pharmacol Exp Ther 1990;252(3):1097–1101.
62. Agarwal R, Gorski JC, Sundblad K, Brater DC. Urinary protein binding does not effect response to furosemide in patients with nephrotic syndrome. J Am Soc Nephrol 2000;11:1100–1105.
63. Weiner ID. Wingo CS. Hypokalemia—Consequences, causes, and correction. J Am Soc Nephrol 1997;8(7):1179–1188.
64. Reber PM, Heath H III. Hypocalcemic emergencies. Med Clin North Am 1995;79:93–106.
65. Nussbaum SR. Pathophysiology and management of severe hypercalcemia. Endocrinol Metab Clin North Am 1993;22:343–362.
66. Zaloga GP. Hypocalcemia in critically ill patients. Crit Care Med 1992;20:251–262.
67. Potts JT. Hyperparathyroidism and other hypercalcemic disorders. Adv Intern Med 1996;41:165–212.
68. Zojer N, Keck AV, Pecherstorfer M. Comparative tolerability of drug therapies for hypercalcaemia of malignancy. Drug Saf 1999;21(5):389–406.
69. Rude RK. Hyperparathyroidism. Otolaryngol Clin North Am 1996; 29:663–679.
70. Chisholm MA, Mulloy AL, Taylor AT. Acute management of cancer-related hypercalcemia. Ann Pharmacother 1996;30:507–513.
71. Strewler GJ. The physiology of parathyroid hormone-related protein. N Engl J Med 2000;342(3):177–185.
72. Deftos LJ. Hypercalcemia, mechanisms, differential diagnosis, and remedies. Postgrad Med 1996;100:119–126.
73. Schmidt-Gayk H, Haerdt H. Differential diagnosis of hypercalcemia: Laboratory assessment. Recent results in cancer research 1994;137:122–137.
74. Agus ZS, Wasserstein A, Goldfarb S. Disorders of calcium and magnesium homeostasis. Am J Med 1982;72:473–488.
75. Goodman WG, Goldin J, Kuizon BD, et al. Coronary-artery calcification in young adults with end-stage renal disease who are undergoing dialysis. N Engl J Med 2000;342:1478–1483.
76. Goldsmith DJ, Covic A, Sambrook PA, Ackrill P. Vascular calcification in long-term haemodialysis patients in a single unit: A retrospective analysis. Nephron 1997;77:37–43.
77. Guerin AP, London GM, Marchais SJ, Metivier F. Arterial stiffening and vascular calcifications in end-stage renal disease. Nephrol Dial Transplant 2000;15:1014–21.
78. Singer FR, Krane SM. Paget's disease of bone. In: Avioli LV, Krane SM, eds. Metabolic Bone Disease and Clinically Related Disorders, 3rd ed. New York, Academic Press, 1998:545–605.
79. Rodman JS, Mahler RJ. Kidney stones as a manifestation of hypercalcemic disorders. Hyperparathyroidism and sarcoidosis. Urol Clin North Am 2000;27(2):275–285.
80. Dretler SP. The physiologic approach to the medical management of stone disease. Urol Clin North Am 1998;25(4):613–623.
81. Parks JH, Coe FL. Pathogenesis and treatment of calcium stones. Semin Nephrol 1996;16(5):398–411.
82. U.S. Renal Data System. 1999 Annual Data Report. Bethesda, MD, The National Institutes of Health, National Institute of Diabetes and Digestive and Kidney Diseases, 1999.
83. Mundy GR, Guise TA. Hypercalcemia of malignancy. Am J Med 1997;103:134–145.
84. Singer FR, Ginger K. Resistance to calcitonin. In: Singer F, Wallach S, eds. Paget's Disease of Bone. Clinical Assessment, Present and Future Therapy. New York, Elsevier, 1991:75–85.
85. Barri YM, Knochel JP. Hypercalcemia and electrolyte disturbances in malignancy. Hematol Oncol Clin North Am 1996;10:775–790.
86. Body JJ. Clinical research update: zoledronate. Cancer 1997;80(8): 1699–1701.
87. Major P, Lortholary A, Hon J, et al. Zoledronic acid is superior to pamidronate in the treatment of hypercalcemia of malignancy: a pooled analysis of two randomized, controlled clinical trials. J Clin Oncol 2001;19(2):558–567.
88. Body JJ, Lortholary A, Romieu G, et al. A dose-finding study of zoledronate in hypercalcemic cancer patients. J Bone Miner Res 1999; 14(9):1557–1561.
89. Watters J, Gerrard G, Dodwell D. The management of malignant hypercalcemia. Drugs 1996;52:837–848.
90. Rastad J, Benson L, Johansson H, et al. Clodronate treatment in patients with malignancy-associated hypercalcemia. Acta Med Scand 1987;221:489–494.
91. Edelson GW, Kleerekoper M. Hypercalcemic crisis. Med Clin North Am 1995;79:79–92.
92. Manolagas SC, Weinstein RS. New developments in the pathogenesis and treatment of steroid-induced osteoporosis. J Bone Min Res 1999;14(7):1061–1066.
93. Block GA, Port FK. Re-evaluation of risks associated with hyperphosphatemia and hyperparathyroidism in dialysis patients: Recommendations for a change in management. Am J Kidney Dis 2000;35(6):1226–1237.
94. Collins MT, Skarulis MC, Bilezikian JP, et al. Treatment of hypercalcemia secondary to parathyroid carcinoma with a novel calcimimetic agent. J Clin Endocrinol Metab 1998;83(4):1083–1088.
95. Guise TA, Mundy GR. Evaluation of hypocalcemia in children and adults. J Clin Endocrinol Metab 1995;80(5):1473–1478.
96. Singer FR. Medical management of nonparathyroid hypercalcemia and hypocalcemia. Otolaryngol Clin North Am 1996;29(4):701–710.
97. Juan D. Hypocalcemia: Differential diagnosis and mechanisms. Arch Intern Med 1979;139:1166–1171.
98. Fouser L, Disorders of calcium, phosphorus and magnesium. Pediatr Ann 1995;24:38–46.
99. Tohme JF, Bilezikian JP. Hypocalcemic emergencies. Endocrinol Metab Clin North Am 1993;22:363–375.
100. Hruska K, Gupta A. Disorders of phosphate homeostasis. In: Avioli LV, Krane SM, eds. Metabolic Bone Disease and Clinically Related Disorders, 3rd ed. New York, Academic Press, 1998:207–236.

101. Weisinger JR, Bellorin-Font E. Magnesium and phosphorus. Lancet 1998;352:391–396.
102. Fine A, Patterson J. Severe hyperphosphatemia following phosphate administration for bowel preparation in patients with renal failure: Two cases and a review of the literature. Am J Kidney Dis 1997;29(1):103–105.
103. Bourke E, Yanagawa N. Assessment of hyperphosphatemia and hypophosphatemia. Clin Lab Med 1993;13:183–207.
104. Kelsler R, McDonald RD, Cadnapaphornchai P. Dynamic changes in serum phosphorus levels in diabetic ketoacidosis. Am J Med 1985;79:571–576.
105. Perreault MM, Ostrop NJ, Tierney MG. Efficacy and safety of intravenous phosphate replacement in critically ill patients. Ann Pharmacother 1997;31:683–688.
106. Subramanian R, Khardori R. Severe hypophosphatemia. Pathophysiologic implications, clinical presentation, and treatment. Medicine (Baltimore) 2000;79:1–78.
107. Knochel JP. The pathophysiology and clinical characteristics of severe hypophosphatemia. Arch Intern Med 1977;137:203–220.
108. Silvis SE, DiBartolomeo AG, Aaker HM. Hypophosphatemia and neurological changes secondary to oral caloric intake. Am J Gastroenterol 1980;73:215–222.
109. Hoggson SF, Hurley DL. Acquired hypophosphatemia. Endocrinol Metab Clin North Am 1993;22:397–409.
110. Michiels JP, Dive A, Donckier J, Installe E. Reversible myocardial dysfunction in a patient with alcoholic ketoacidosis. Am J Emerg Med 1998; 16:371–373.
111. Lentz RD, Brown DM, Kjellstrand CM. Treatment of severe hypophosphatemia. Ann Intern Med 1978;89:941–944.
112. Clark CL, Sacks GS, Dickerson RN, Kudsk KA, Brown RO. Treatment of hypophosphatemia in patients receiving specialized nutrition support using a graduated dosing scheme: Results from a prospective clinical trial. Crit Care Med 1995;23:1504–1511.
113. Prie D, Blanchet FB, Essig M, Jourdain JP, Friedlander G. Dipyridamole decreases renal phosphate leak and augments serum phosphorus in patients with low renal phosphate threshold. J Am Soc Nephrol 1998;9:1264–1269.

52

DISORDERS OF POTASSIUM AND MAGNESIUM HOMEOSTASIS

Donald F. Brophy and Todd W.B. Gehr

Potassium and magnesium are electrolytes that are responsible for numerous metabolic activities. Disorders of these electrolytes are frequently seen in both the acute care and community ambulatory care settings. Clinicians should have a firm understanding of the etiology, pathophysiology, symptoms, pharmacotherapy, and monitoring of these disorders. This chapter describes the homeostatic mechanisms that are responsible for the maintenance of normal potassium and magnesium serum concentrations. The clinical disorders responsible for the development of hyperkalemia or hypermagnesemia and hypokalemia or hypermagnesemia are also reviewed.

POTASSIUM

Potassium is the most abundant cation in the body, with estimated total body stores of 3,000–4,000 mEq.[1] Ninety-eight percent of this amount is contained within the intracellular compartment, and the remaining 2% is distributed within the extracellular compartment. The Na^+/K^+ ATPase pump located in each cell membrane is responsible for the compartmentalization of potassium. This pump is an active transport system that mobilizes sodium out of the cell, and potassium into the cell at a ratio of 3:2. Consequently, the pump maintains a higher concentration of potassium inside the cell.

The normal serum concentration range for potassium is 3.5–5.0 mEq/L, whereas, the intracellular potassium concentration is usually about 140 mEq/L.[2] Approximately 70% of the intracellular potassium is located in skeletal muscle; the remaining 30% is located in the liver and red blood cells. Extracellular potassium is distributed throughout the serum and interstitial space. Potassium is dynamic in that it is constantly moving between the intracellular and extracellular compartments according to the body's needs.[3] Therefore, the serum potassium concentration alone does not accurately reflect the total body potassium content.

Potassium has many physiologic functions within cells, including protein and glycogen synthesis, cellular metabolism and growth. It is also a determinant of the electrical action potential across the cell membrane.[1] The ratio of the intracellular to extracellular potassium concentration is the major determinant of the resting membrane potential across the cell membrane. Thus, the resting membrane potential is greatly affected by variations in extracellular potassium concentration. Serum potassium concentrations outside the normal range can have disastrous effects on neuromuscular activity, in particular, cardiac conduction. Hypo- and hyperkalemia are both associated with potentially fatal cardiac arrhythmias, along with other neuromuscular disturbances.

CONTROL OF POTASSIUM HOMEOSTASIS

Potassium homeostasis and the maintenance of serum potassium within the normal range are regulated by dietary intake, gastrointestinal and urinary excretion, hormones, acid-base balance, and body fluid tonicity.[4]

The recommended daily allowance for dietary potassium intake is approximately 50 mEq/d.[2] Potassium is found in abundance in fruits and vegetables, and meats. The typical American ingests approximately 50–150 mEq of potassium daily.[4] Nearly all of this is absorbed, with only 10–20 mEq, or 20%, eliminated in feces. The amount eliminated in the feces increases, however, in patients with diarrhea, and perhaps in those with underlying chronic renal insufficiency.[5]

The kidney is the primary route of potassium elimination. Potassium is freely filtered with almost all of it being reabsorbed passively in the proximal tubule and the thick ascending limb of the loop of Henle.[6] Urinary potassium excretion, therefore, is primarily determined by potassium secretion from the luminal cells of the distal tubule and collecting duct. The normal amount of potassium excreted in the urine is generally 40–90 mEq/L,[2] but it can vary based on dietary intake, serum potassium concentration and aldosterone activity.

Hormones such as insulin, catecholamines, and aldosterone dramatically affect potassium homeostasis. Insulin may be the most important hormonal mediator of potassium balance because it stimulates the cellular Na^+/K^+ ATPase pump to increase cellular potassium uptake in the liver, muscle and adipose tissue.[4] Evidence suggests that a complex negative feedback loop exists where insulin secretion tightly regulates potassium concentrations.[1] Indeed, serum potassium increases of only a few tenths of a milliequivalent stimulate pancreatic insulin secretion into the portal circulation in an attempt to prevent hyperkalemia from occurring.[1] If hyperkalemia occurs, glucagon is released from the liver to protect against insulin-induced hypoglycemia. Conversely, hypokalemia inhibits insulin secretion, which explains why some patients receiving diuretics develop hyperglycemia.[7]

Circulating catecholamines such as epinephrine also result in an intracellular movement of potassium by two mechanisms.[8] They stimulate the β-receptor, which directly activates the Na^+/K^+ ATPase pump. Secondly, they stimulate glycogenolysis, which raises blood glucose levels, thereby increasing insulin secretion. This dual mechanism is often used therapeutically in patients with hyperkalemia to normalize serum potassium concentrations.

Aldosterone is a mineralocorticoid that is secreted from the adrenal glands in response to high serum potassium concentrations. Aldosterone promotes potassium excretion through the kidneys. Aldosterone works at the distal tubule and collecting duct to promote the reabsorption of sodium and water, in exchange for potassium. The net result is potassium secretion into the urine. Aldosterone may also have extrarenal activity by stimulating cellular Na^+/K^+ ATPase pump activity.[8]

Changes in acid-base status significantly affect the serum potassium concentration. For example, in an acidotic state, the body compensates for excessive hydrogen ions by moving them from the serum into the cell, in exchange for intracellular potassium, to maintain electroneutrality. The efflux of potassium into the serum can result in hyperkalemia. A commonly quoted approximation of the pH effect is that for every 0.1 unit decrease in pH, there is a corresponding increase in serum potassium of 0.6–0.8 mEq/L (with a wide range of 0.2–1.7).[6] This is often referred to as false hyperkalemia because there isn't a true excess of total body potassium. Only metabolic inorganic acids, such as hydrochloric acid, result in an increase in serum potassium. Metabolic acidoses caused by organic acids, such as lactic acidosis and ketoacidosis, do not result in hyperkalemia, because both cation and anion enter the cell, thus maintaining electroneutrality.[1] Respiratory acidosis does not significantly affect the serum potassium concentration.[8]

Metabolic alkalosis, conversely, results in hypokalemia as a result of a net loss of hydrogen ion in the serum. In response, the body releases intracellular hydrogen ion into the serum to increase the acidity of the blood in exchange for extracellular potassium ions. This creates a relative deficiency of serum potassium. Serum potassium falls approximately 0.6 mEq/L for each 0.1 unit rise in blood pH. Similarly, this is frequently termed false hypokalemia because there isn't a true deficiency in total body potassium.

Finally, hyperosmolality results in enhanced movement of potassium from the cell into the extracellular fluid. This occurs most likely because of the associated cell shrinkage and water loss, which increases the intracellular to extracellular potassium gradient.[4] This is seen most commonly in conditions such as diabetic ketoacidosis. Conversely, hypo-osmolality does not seem to affect potassium distribution.

HYPOKALEMIA

Hypokalemia is one of the most commonly encountered electrolyte abnormalities in clinical practice.[9] Hypokalemia can be described as mild (serum potassium 3.0–3.5 mEq/L), moderate (serum potassium 2.5–3.0 mEq/L), or severe (less than 2.5 mEq/L). When hypokalemia is detected, a diagnostic workup that evaluates the patient's comorbid disease states and concomitant medications should be initiated.

PATHOPHYSIOLOGY

Hypokalemia results when there is a total body potassium deficit, or when serum potassium is shifted into the intracellular compartment. Total body deficits occur in the setting of poor dietary intake of potassium, or when there are excessive renal and gastrointestinal losses of potassium from the body.

Maintaining a consistent dietary intake of potassium is important because the body has no effective method for storing potassium. Approximately 5% of the total body potassium content is turned over daily,[2] underscoring the importance of eating a well-balanced diet. Elderly patients with chronic diseases, and patients undergoing surgery are at increased risk for developing hypokalemia because of insufficient intake or losses resulting from surgery.

Many drugs may cause hypokalemia by a variety of mechanisms. These mechanisms include intracellular potassium shifting and increased renal or stool losses (Table 52–1). Nonpotassium-sparing diuretic administration is the most common cause of drug-induced hypokalemia.[9] Loop and thiazide diuretics inhibit renal sodium reabsorption, which results in increased sodium delivery to the distal tubule. Consequently, hypokalemia develops because the distal tubule selectively reabsorbs sodium, and excretes potassium down its concentration gradient. Secondly, because diuretics result in volume contraction, aldosterone is secreted which further promotes the renal excretion of potassium. If concomitant potassium supplements are not provided to patients receiving loop and thiazide diuretics, hypokalemia is inevitable.

The second most common etiology of hypokalemia is loss of potassium rich gastrointestinal (GI) fluid through diarrhea and vomiting. The typical potassium loss in feces is approximately 10 mEq per day.[9] In diarrheal states, this amount increases proportionally with the volume of stool output. Vomiting also accounts for substantial potassium losses, which have been estimated to be as high as 30–50 mEq/L.[2] Metabolic alkalosis can also occur in cases of severe diarrhea and vomiting due to loss of HCO_3-rich fluids. As discussed above, this causes an intracellular shifting of potassium, which lowers the serum concentration of potassium even further. Prolonged diarrhea

TABLE 52–1. Drug-Induced Hypokalemia by Mechanism

Hypokalmeia Caused by Transcellular Shift	Hypokalemia Caused by Enhanced Renal Excretion	Hypokalemia Caused by Enhanced Fecal Elimination
β_2-Receptor agonists	**Diuretics**	**Sodium polystyrene sulfonate**
Epinephrine	Acetazolamide	**Phenolphthalein**
Albuterol	Thiazides	**Sorbitol**
Terbutaline	Indapamide	
Pirbuterol	Metolazone	
Salmeterol	Furosemide	
Isoproterenol	Torsemide	
Ephedrine	Bumetanide	
Pseudoephedrine	Ethacrynic Acid	
Tocolytic agents	**High-dose penicillins**	
Ritodrine	Nafcillin	
Nylidrin	Ampicillin	
Theophylline	Penicillin	
Caffeine Insulin overdose	**Mineralocorticoids**	
	Miscellaneous	
	Aminoglycosides	
	Amphotericin B	
	Cisplatin	

Adapted from Ref. 9.

and vomiting can significantly affect children and elderly patients because their kidneys are unable to effectively maintain an adequate fluid status.

Hypomagnesemia can also contribute to the development of hypokalemia because it reduces the intracellular potassium concentration, and promotes renal potassium wasting.[10] The intracellular potassium concentration falls because hypomagnesemia impairs the function of the Na^+/K^+ ATPase pump. The mechanism of the accelerated renal loss of potassium is unknown.[10] It is unclear whether hypomagnesemia directly causes hypokalemia because the two are often found together as a result of drugs (diuretic administration) or disease states (diarrhea). When concomitant hypokalemia and hypomagnesemia occur, the magnesium deficiency must be corrected first, otherwise full repletion of the potassium deficit is difficult.[10]

CLINICAL PRESENTATION

The signs and symptoms of hypokalemia are usually nonspecific and highly variable between patients. The severity of symptoms appears to be related to the degree of hypokalemia and its rapidity of onset.[9] Fortunately, most normal, healthy patients with mild hypokalemia are asymptomatic. Patients with underlying cardiac conditions, however, are at increased risk of developing life-threatening cardiac arrhythmias, even in cases of mild hypokalemia.[9,11]

Potassium is necessary for the normal transmission and conduction of nerve impulses throughout neuromuscular tissue, such as cardiac and skeletal muscle. Hypokalemia results in hyperpolarization of the resting membrane potential, which impairs muscular contraction. Most signs and symptoms, therefore, involve impaired cardiovascular and/or muscular activity.

The two primary cardiovascular signs and symptoms of hypokalemia are hypertension and cardiac arrhythmias.[11] Data from several epidemiologic and clinical trials implicate hypokalemia in the pathogenesis and maintenance of essential hypertension.[12–19] Although the exact mechanism of this is unknown, it appears that potassium depletion leads to sodium and water retention, and to intravascular volume expansion. African Americans seem to be most sensitive to the hypertensive effects of hypokalemia.[19] A recent meta-analysis suggests that the reduction of systolic blood pressure after potassium supplementation was nearly three times greater in African Americans as compared to whites.[18] The relationship between potassium and hypertension was noted by the most recent Joint National Committee on the Prevention, Detection, Evaluation, and Treatment of High Blood Pressure,[17] which recommended increased potassium intake as a means for the prevention and treatment of hypertension.

Arrhythmias are the second major cardiac complication of hypokalemia. The elderly, and patients with underlying ischemic heart disease,[11] or congestive heart failure,[20] appear to have the highest risk of developing hypokalemia-related arrhythmias. Indeed, sudden cardiac death from ventricular fibrillation has been reported in patients receiving hydrochlorothiazide for the treatment of hypertension.[21] The electrocardiographic (ECG) effects of hypokalemia are characterized by ST segment depression or flattening, T-wave inversion, and U-wave elevation. Consequently, a widening of the QRS complex and PR-interval may also occur. Hypokalemia-associated arrhythmias include bradycardia, heart block, atrial flutter, paroxysmal atrial tachycardia, and ventricular fibrillation. It is well known that hypokalemia predisposes patients to digitalis induced cardiac arrhythmias.[9]

Muscle weakness, cramping, easy fatigability, and myalgias characterize the neuromuscular effects of hypokalemia. These effects are the result of hyperpolarization of skeletal muscle cells, which impairs their ability to depolarize and contract, and decreased blood flow to skeletal muscles.[11]

▶ TREATMENT: Hypokalemia

DESIRED OUTCOME

The goals of hypokalemia management are to prevent and to treat serious life-threatening complications, to normalize the serum potassium concentration, to identify and correct the underlying cause of hypokalemia, and to prevent overcorrection of the potassium concentration.

GENERAL APPROACH TO THERAPY

The general approach to therapy depends on the degree and rapidity of hypokalemia, and the presence of symptoms. Serum potassium concentrations between 4.0 and 3.5 mEq/L are a sign of early potassium depletion. No pharmacologic therapy is recommended at this point; however, these patients should be encouraged to increase their dietary intake of potassium-rich foods. When the serum potassium concentration is between 3.5 and 3.0 mEq/L, it is still debatable whether pharmacologic therapy should be initiated for all patients. Oral potassium supplementation should be initiated in patients with underlying cardiac conditions that predispose them to cardiac arrhythmias. This includes patients receiving concomitant digoxin therapy.[21] Patients with serum potassium concentrations below 3.0 mEq/L should always be treated to achieve values >4 mEq/L. In asymptomatic patients, oral therapy is the preferred route of administration. Intravenous potassium may be necessary in symptomatic patients with severe depletion, or in patients who are intolerant to oral supplementation. In patients with concomitant hypomagnesemia, the magnesium deficit should be corrected before potassium supplementation, to prevent refractory hypokalemia.[20]

NONPHARMACOLOGIC THERAPY

Various nonpharmacologic therapies exist to prevent and treat hypokalemia. Probably the best and most abundant source of potassium comes from dietary sources, in particular, fresh fruits and vegetables, fruit juices, and meats.[20] Table 52–2 lists foods that are excellent sources of potassium. Salt substitutes are another effective, inexpensive source of potassium. Increased dietary intake of potassium should not be used long-term because it may add unwanted calories to the patient. Moreover, dietary potassium is almost entirely coupled with phosphate, rather than chloride, so it isn't as effective in correcting potassium loss associated with hypochloremic conditions such as vomiting, nasogastric suctioning, and diuretic therapy.[20]

TABLE 52–2. Foods That Are High in Potassium

Highest Content (>1,000 mg/100 g)
- Dried figs
- Molasses

Very High Content (>500 mg/100 g)
- Dried fruits (dates, prunes)
- Nuts
- Avocados
- Bran cereals
- Lima beans

High Content (>250 mg/100 g)
- Vegetables
  - Spinach
  - Tomatoes
  - Broccoli
  - Squash
  - Beets
  - Cauliflower
  - Carrots
  - Potatoes
- Fruits
  - Bananas
  - Cantaloupe
  - Kiwi
  - Oranges
  - Mangos
- Meats
  - Ground beef
  - Steak
  - Pork
  - Lamb
  - Veal

From Refs. 9 and 20, with permission.

PHARMACOLOGIC THERAPY

Guidelines for potassium supplementation were recently published by the National Council on Potassium in Clinical Practice.[20] These guidelines provide a comprehensive framework for potassium prophylaxis and replacement in many distinct patient populations. When deciding on appropriate pharmacotherapy to replete potassium, five factors must be considered: (a) the patient's normal baseline potassium concentration; (b) underlying medical conditions that may affect potassium balance; (c) concomitant medications that may affect potassium balance; (d) the patient's dietary and salt intake; and (e) the patient's ability to comply with the therapeutic regimen.[20] Table 52–3 summarizes the committee's general guidelines.

A general rule for potassium replacement is that for every 1 mEq/L fall of potassium from 3.5 mEq/L, there is a corresponding total body potassium deficit of 100–150 mEq. In patients receiving loop or thiazide diuretics, 40–100 mEq of potassium is generally needed to correct mild deficits. Doses up to 120 mEq may be required in more severe deficiencies. The total daily dose should be divided into three to four doses to prevent GI side effects. Patients receiving diuretics may become chronically hypokalemic and may benefit from combination potassium-sparing diuretic therapy.

Whenever possible, potassium supplementation should be administered by mouth. Three salts are available for oral potassium supplementation: chloride, phosphate, and bicarbonate. Potassium phosphate should be used when patients are both hypokalemic and hypophosphatemic; potassium bicarbonate is most commonly used when potassium depletion occurs in the setting of metabolic acidosis. Potassium chloride, however, is the primary salt form used because it is the most effective treatment for the common causes of potassium depletion (e.g., diuretic-induced hypokalemia). Potassium chloride can be administered in either tablet or liquid formulations (Table 52–4). The liquid forms are generally less expensive; however, patient compliance may be low because of their strong, unpleasant taste.[20] Two

TABLE 52–3. General Consensus Guidelines for Potassium Replacement

Guideline	Comment
Potassium replacement therapy should accompany dietary consumption of potassium-rich foods.	Potassium-rich foods often cannot completely replace potassium associated with chloride losses (vomiting, diuretics, nasogastric suction) because it is almost entirely coupled to phosphate. Furthermore, increasing dietary intake of these foods may lead to unwanted weight gain.
Potassium replacement is recommended in patients who are sodium sensitive, and in hypertensive patients.	A high-sodium diet often results in excessive urinary potassium excretion.
Potassium replacement is recommended in patients who are subject to vomiting, diarrhea, or diuretic/laxative abuse.	These conditions promote excessive renal and GI potassium loss.
Potassium supplementation is best administered orally in divided doses over several days to achieve full repletion.	
Laboratory measurement of serum potassium is convenient, but not always accurate.	Clinicians should be aware of the factors that result in transcellular potassium shifts. Monitoring 24-hour urinary potassium excretion may be necessary in high-risk patients.
Patient adherence to potassium replacement may be increased with compliance-enhancing regimens.	Microencapsulated products have no bitter smell or aftertaste and have much better GI tolerance. Regimens should be made as simple as possible to follow.
A potassium dosage of 20 mEq/day is usually sufficient to prevent hypokalemia from occurring. Doses of 40–100 mEq are usually sufficient to treat hypokalemia.	

Adapted from Ref. 20.

TABLE 52–4. Differentiation of Available Potassium Supplements

Supplement	Comment
Controlled-release microencapsulated tablet	Disintegrates better in GI tract. Fewer GI erosions as compared to wax-matrix tablets.
Encapsulated controlled-release microencapsulated particles	Fewer erosions as compared to wax-matrix tablets.
Potassium chloride elixir	Inexpensive, poor taste, poor compliance, immediate effect.
Potassium chloride effervescent tablets for solution	More expensive than elixir, convenient.
Wax-matrix extended-release tablets	Easier to swallow. More GI erosions as compared to other therapies.

sustained-release preparations are currently available in the United States: a wax-matrix formulation, and a microencapsulated formulation. The microencapsulated tablet disintegrates better in the stomach as compared to the wax-matrix preparation, and is associated with less GI erosion.[9,20] Regardless of preparation used, potassium is generally well absorbed.

Intravenous potassium use should be limited to (a) severe cases of hypokalemia (serum concentration < 2.5 mEq/L); (b) patients exhibiting signs and symptoms of hypokalemia such as ECG changes or muscle spasms; or (c) patients unable to tolerate oral therapy. Intravenous supplementation is more dangerous than oral therapy because it is more likely to result in hyperkalemia and thrombophlebitis and pain at the site of infusion are common adverse events.

The vehicle in which intravenous potassium is administered is important. Whenever possible, potassium should be mixed in saline containing solutions (e.g., 0.9% NaCl, 0.45% NaCl), and not dextrose-containing solutions. Dextrose-containing solutions stimulate insulin secretion, which causes further intracellular shifting of potassium. Indeed, there are reports of enhanced hypokalemia in patients being repleted with potassium in dextrose infusions.[23] Generally, 10–20 mEq of potassium is diluted in 100 mL 0.9% NaCl for intravenous administration. These concentrations are generally safe when administered through a peripheral vein over 1 hour. When infusion rates exceed 10 mEq/h, ECG monitoring should be performed to detect cardiac signs of hyperkalemia. The serum potassium concentration should be evaluated following the infusion of each 30–40 mEq, to direct further potassium replacement requirements. Multiple doses of potassium can be repeated as needed until the serum potassium concentration normalizes.

In cases of severe potassium depletion, patients may require as much as 300–400 mEq/d. In this instance, it is common practice to dilute 40–60 mEq in 1,000 mL 0.45% NaCl and infuse at a rate not exceeding 40 mEq/h. If possible, this should be performed in an intensive care unit under continuous ECG monitoring. Because of the high potassium concentration, and the risk for burning pain and peripheral venous sclerosis, the infusion should be through a central intravenous line into a large vein (e.g., superior vena cava). Frequent serum potassium monitoring should be performed to avoid the development of hyperkalemia.

ALTERNATIVE THERAPIES

Potassium-sparing diuretics are an alternative to exogenous potassium supplementation, especially when patients are concomitantly receiving drugs that are known to deplete potassium (e.g., diuretics, amphotericin B). Spironolactone inhibits the effect of aldosterone in the distal convoluted tubule, thereby decreasing potassium elimination in the urine. Spironolactone is especially effective as a potassium-sparing agent in patients with primary or secondary hyperaldosteronism. Amiloride and triamterene act by an aldosterone-independent mechanism, however the complete mechanism of their potassium sparing is unknown.

Spironolactone is available as 25-mg, 50-mg, and 100-mg tablets. The usual starting dose is 25–50 mg daily, and can be titrated to a maximum dose of 400 mg/d. The potassium-retaining effects generally take about 48 hours to occur. Important side effects include hyperkalemia, gynecomastia, breast tenderness, and impotence in men.[22]

Triamterene is available as 50-mg and 100-mg capsules. The usual starting dose is 50 mg twice daily, which can be titrated to 100 mg twice daily. Triamterene 50 mg is available as a combination product with hydrochlorothiazide 25 mg and is commonly used for the treatment of stage I to II hypertension. Common side effects include hyperkalemia, sodium depletion, and metabolic acidosis.[22]

Amiloride is available as a 5-mg tablet. The usual starting dose is 5 mg daily, however, 10 mg can be given in those with severe hypokalemia. This is also available as a combination product with hydrochlorothiazide 50 mg. The most common side effects are hyperkalemia and metabolic acidosis.[22]

Generally, concomitant use of potassium supplementation with potassium-sparing diuretics is not necessary. However, conditions that result in excessive urinary potassium wasting, such as congestive heart failure, cirrhosis, or the nephrotic syndrome may require dual therapy.[22] There is a significant risk of hyperkalemia during combination therapy, especially in patients with underlying renal insufficiency or diabetes mellitus.

PHARMACOECONOMIC CONSIDERATIONS

To date, there have been no pharmacoeconomic evaluations of the different pharmacotherapeutic alternatives to manage hypokalemia. The most economical source of potassium is from the diet. Thus, patients receiving diuretic therapy should be instructed to increase their dietary intake of potassium-rich foods. By doing so, they may avert the need for exogenous potassium therapy. Additionally, oral potassium supplementation is much less expensive than intravenous supplementation by virtue of its ease of administration and lack of need for EKG monitoring. The pharmacoeconomic difference between the oral products is dependent on several variables, including patient tolerance and compliance.

EVALUATION OF THERAPEUTIC OUTCOMES

Serum potassium concentrations should be monitored regularly while the patient is receiving potassium supplementation. For patients receiving long-term prophylactic potassium supplementation during diuretic therapy, the serum potassium and magnesium concentrations, as well as renal function should be monitored during each clinic visit. In hospitalized patients receiving therapy for mild hypokalemia, the potassium concentration should be monitored daily. This usually isn't a problem because of the frequent laboratory monitoring performed in hospitalized patients. Generally, the potassium concentration begins to rise within 72 hours. If it doesn't rise appreciably within 96 hours, the clinician should suspect concomitant magnesium depletion.[22] If present, correcting the magnesium deficit generally results in normalization of potassium. In patients receiving IV potassium supplementation, close ECG monitoring is required for infusions above 10 mEq/h, in addition to patient complaints of burning pain or thrombophlebitis at the site of infusion.

HYPERKALEMIA

Hyperkalemia is defined as a serum potassium concentration greater than 5.5 mEq/L. It can be further classified according to its severity: mild hyperkalemia (serum potassium 5.5–6 mEq/L); moderate hyperkalemia (6.1–6.9 mEq/L); and severe hyperkalemia (greater than 7 mEq/L).[22] Hyperkalemia is much less common than hypokalemia. In fact, if all patients with acute and chronic renal failure were excluded, the true prevalence of hyperkalemia would be insignificant.[22]

PATHOPHYSIOLOGY

Hyperkalemia develops when potassium intake exceeds excretion (i.e., elevated total body stores), or when the transcellular distribution of potassium is disturbed (i.e., normal total body stores). Generally, there are four primary causes of true hyperkalemia: (a) increased potassium intake; (b) decreased potassium excretion; (c) tubular unresponsiveness to aldosterone; and (d) redistribution of potassium into the extracellular space. The four major causes of true hyperkalemia are discussed below.

Hyperkalemia Associated with Increased Potassium Intake

Hyperkalemia in this setting is almost always associated with renal insufficiency. Predialysis and dialysis patients that are noncompliant with dietary potassium restrictions often present with life-threatening hyperkalemia. Many of these patients don't realize that fresh fruits and vegetables contain large amounts of potassium. Anecdotally in many dialysis centers, the incidence of hyperkalemia peaks during the summer months when fresh garden produce is available. Another common dietary source of hyperkalemia is potassium chloride salt substitutes. Many dialysis patients are instructed to use salt substitutes to avoid excessive sodium intake in an attempt to control volume overload. These patients unwittingly become hyperkalemic because these products contain approximately 10–15 mEq potassium per gram, or 200 mEq per tablespoon. Educating renal insufficiency patients on dietary modifications is of paramount importance to prevent them from becoming hyperkalemic.

Hyperkalemia Associated with Decreased Renal Potassium Excretion

The kidneys excrete 80% of the daily potassium intake. Therefore when the kidney is unable to excrete potassium appropriately, as in acute and chronic renal failure, potassium retention results in hyperkalemia. Moreover, many drugs can inhibit the kidney's ability to excrete potassium by inhibiting aldosterone.

Severe hyperkalemia is more common in acute renal failure (ARF) than in chronic renal failure because ARF patients are often hypercatabolic and can have underlying disorders, such as rhabdomyolysis or tumor lysis syndrome, which result in release of potassium from injured or lysed cells.[25] Severe hyperkalemia is rare in stable chronic renal failure, perhaps because of enhanced GI potassium excretion.[22]

Renal excretion of potassium is also inhibited by various endocrinology disorders, including adrenal insufficiency, Addison's disease and selective hypoaldosteronism. All of these disorders involve a decreased production of aldosterone, which results in the retention of potassium. In addition, several drugs have profound effects on the kidney's ability to secrete potassium. Four drug classes in particular have specific effects at the kidney, and include angiotensin-converting enzyme inhibitors (ACEIs), angiotensin receptor blockers (ARBs), potassium-sparing diuretics, and prostaglandin inhibitors such as nonsteroidal anti-inflammatory drugs (NSAIDs). Other miscellaneous drugs that cause hyperkalemia are trimethoprim-sulfamethoxazole, heparin, and pentamidine.

Tubular Unresponsiveness to Aldosterone

Certain medical conditions, such as sickle cell anemia, systemic lupus erythematosus, and amyloidosis can produce a defect in tubular potassium secretion, possibly as the result of an alteration in the aldosterone-binding site. The exact mechanism of the tubular unresponsiveness is unknown.

Redistribution of Potassium into the Extracellular Space

The efflux of potassium into the ECF is to be expected in the presence of metabolic acidosis, secondary to diabetes mellitus, chronic renal failure, or lactic acidosis. β-Blockers can also result in a transcellular potassium shift.

The serum potassium concentration may also be falsely elevated in some conditions, and not reflect the actual *in vivo* potassium concentration. This is termed *pseudohyperkalemia*. Pseudohyperkalemia occurs most commonly in the setting of extravascular hemolysis of red blood cells.[24] When a blood specimen is not processed promptly, and cellular destruction occurs, intracellular potassium is released into the serum. Pseudohyperkalemia can also occur in conditions of thrombocytosis or leukocytosis. If severe hyperkalemia is found in a patient who is asymptomatic with an otherwise normal laboratory report, the hyperkalemia is most likely pseudohyperkalemia,[22] and a repeat blood sample should be evaluated. Elevated potassium concentrations are normally associated with other laboratory abnormalities, such as low CO_2 (acidosis) or elevated BUN and creatinine concentrations (indicating renal insufficiency).

CLINICAL PRESENTATION

The clinical signs and symptoms of hyperkalemia are related to the effects of excessive potassium on neuromuscular, cardiac, and smooth muscle. Cardiac arrhythmias are the most life-threatening symptom of hyperkalemia. Elevated potassium concentrations decrease the resting membrane potential of myocardial cells, thereby slowing their action potential. The cardiac rhythm disturbances associated with hyperkalemia pose the greatest danger to the patient, because they may lead to ventricular fibrillation or cardiac standstill (asystole). The earliest ECG changes are peaked T-waves and shortening of the QT interval, reflecting an increased rate of repolarization with occasional ST-segment depression.[25] These changes are typically seen when serum potassium concentrations are 5.5–6 mEq/L. With serum concentrations between 6 and 7 mEq/L, the PR-interval and QRS duration are prolonged (Fig. 52–1). When the serum concentration exceeds 7–8 mEq/L, ECG manifestations of delayed depolarization occur, resulting in slowed cardiac conduction,

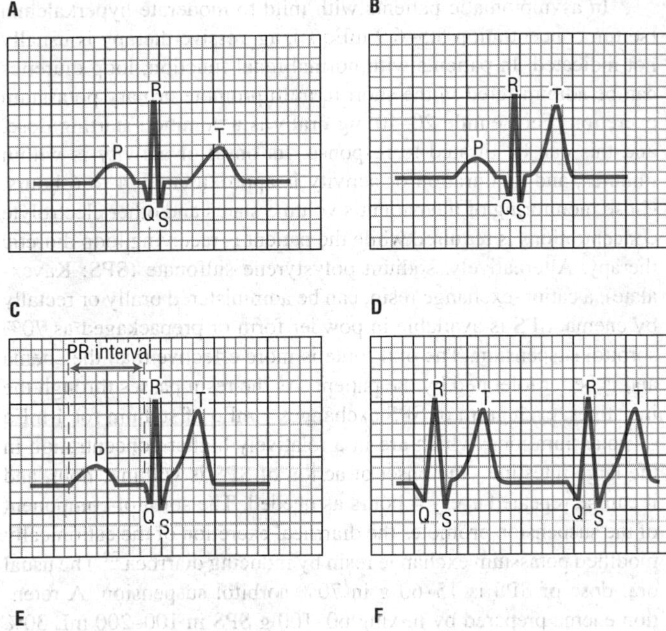

FIGURE 52–1. The earliest ECG manifestation of hyperkalemia is an increase in the rate of ventricular repolarization, which results in a "peaking" of the T wave at serum potassium concentrations of ≈5.5 to 6.0 mEq/L (**B**), relative to the normal ECG presentation (**A**). Further increases in the serum potassium concentration above 6 mEq/L result in conduction delays through the His–Purkinje system, the atrial myocardium, and the ventricular myocardium. The ECG manifestations of these conduction delays and the sequence in which they occur are a widening of the PR interval (**C**), delay through the His–Purkinje system, a loss of the P wave (**D**), delay through the atrial myocardium, and a widening of the QRS complex (**E**), delay through the ventricular myocardium. Finally, there is a merging of the QRS complex with the T wave (**F**), which results in a sine-wave appearance to the tracing.

widening of the QRS complex and decreased amplitude, widening, and eventual loss of the P-wave.[25] When serum concentrations exceed 9–10 mEq/L, the QRS complex merges with the T-wave, resulting in a sine-wave pattern, which may deteriorate to ventricular fibrillation or asystole at concentrations from 10–12 mEq/L.[22] Note that the serum concentrations at which the characteristic electrocardiographic changes occur are variable, because hypocalcemia, acidosis, hyponatremia, and the rapidity of elevation of serum potassium all may enhance the cardiotoxicity of hyperkalemia. Acute hyperkalemia is generally more dangerous than chronic hyperkalemia, because the protective mechanisms for rapid intracellular movement of potassium may be overwhelmed. Rapid increases in potassium concentration predominately affect conduction and heart rate rather than the T-wave or ST segment.[22]

▶ TREATMENT: Hyperkalemia

DESIRED OUTCOME

The goals of therapy for the treatment of hyperkalemia are to antagonize adverse cardiac effects, reverse any symptoms that may be present, and to return the serum and total body stores of potassium to normal. Severe hyperkalemia (>7 mEq/L) or moderate hyperkalemia (6.1–6.9 mEq/L), when associated with clinical symptoms or electrocardiographic changes, requires immediate treatment. Initial treatment of hyperkalemia is focused on antagonism of the membrane actions of hyperkalemia (calcium). Secondarily, one should attempt to decrease extracellular potassium concentration by promoting its intracellular movement (glucose, insulin, β_2-receptor agonists, sodium bicarbonate). Finally, removal of potassium from the body by hemodialysis and/or cation-exchange resins may need to be implemented.[26] The underlying cause of hyperkalemia should be identified and reversed, and exogenous potassium must be withheld.

GENERAL APPROACH TO TREATMENT

Figure 52–2 describes the general treatment approach to hyperkalemia. In patients who are symptomatic, calcium should be administered to prevent or treat any cardiac manifestations of hyperkalemia. When the patient is hemodynamically stabilized, the serum potassium concentration should be rapidly decreased within minutes by administering drugs that result in an intracellular shift. If the patient is asymptomatic, rapid correction is not necessary. The clinician can administer an ion exchange resin, e.g. sodium polystyrene sulfonate that results in removal of potassium from the body over several hours

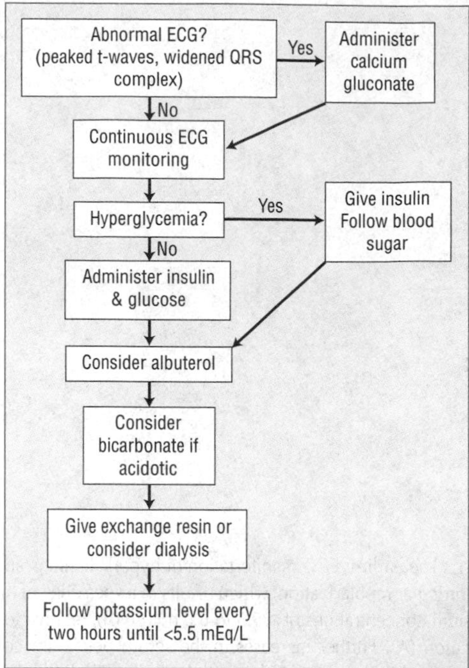

FIGURE 52–2. Treatment algorithm for hyperkalemia. The first step is to evaluate the patient's ECG. If peaked T-waves or widened QRS complexes are present, administer 1 ampule IV calcium gluconate 10% and repeat every 30 to 60 minutes until ECG normalizes. If the ECG is normal, continue to monitor for cardiac complications. Next, decide on the best therapeutic approach based on the underlying patient symptoms; for example, underlying diabetes or acid-base status, and immediacy for correction. For nonacidotic conditions, IV insulin and glucose is preferred for nondiabetic patients with normal blood glucose. If the patient is diabetic with elevated blood glucose, only IV insulin is required. If the patient is unresponsive to this therapy after 30 to 60 minutes, albuterol via nebulizer is considered adjunctive second-line therapy. Sodium bicarbonate should only be administered when the hyperkalemia is secondary to metabolic acidosis. Potassium exchange resins or dialysis should be used last line for acute situations. If the patient has end-stage renal disease, dialysis may be the preferred first-line therapy. In nonacute situations where rapid onset is not required, potassium exchange resins are considered a first-line therapy. The patient should be monitored every 2 hours until the serum potassium concentration falls below 5.5 mEq/L.

NONPHARMACOLOGIC THERAPY

ESRD patients who present with severe hyperkalemia, or with cardiac manifestations of hyperkalemia should undergo immediate hemodialysis. Dialysis is the most rapid means of lowering potassium, compared to bicarbonate, epinephrine or insulin/glucose therapy.[26] Other forms of dialysis can be performed (e.g., peritoneal dialysis or continuous renal replacement therapy), although they appear to be less effective in acute therapy.[26]

PHARMACOLOGICAL THERAPY

Various drug therapies exist for lowering the serum potassium concentration. The optimal regimen for a given patient is dependent on the rapidity and degree of lowering that is necessary. Table 52–5 provides an overview of the available therapies, and their respective onset and the degree of change one can expect.

In asymptomatic patients with mild to moderate hyperkalemia (serum concentration 5.5–6.9 mEq/L), aggressive therapy is usually not indicated. In patients with normal renal function, loop diuretics can be administered in the short term to promote urinary potassium excretion. Furosemide 20–40 mg orally is a common starting dose, and this can be titrated to response. Its onset of activity is within minutes, and its duration of activity is approximately 4 to 6 hours. Close monitoring of the patient's volume status and other electrolyte concentrations is required while the patient is receiving loop diuretic therapy. Alternatively, sodium polystyrene sulfonate (SPS; Kayexalate), a cation-exchange resin, can be administered orally or rectally by enema. SPS is available in powder form or prepackaged as 70% sorbitol suspension. The oral route is more effective than the enema and is better tolerated by the patient. As the resin passes through the intestines, each gram of SPS exchanges 1 mEq of sodium for 1 mEq of potassium ions, which are in a relatively higher concentration in the large intestine. The onset of action of SPS is within 1 hour, and it can be repeated every 4 hours as needed. The sorbitol component of the suspension promotes the diarrheal excretion of the cationically modified potassium exchange resin by inducing diarrhea.[22] The usual oral dose of SPS is 15–60 g in 70% sorbitol suspension. A retention enema prepared by mixing 60–100 g SPS in 100–200 mL 30% sorbitol or 10% dextrose warmed to body temperature will usually remove 0.5 mEq of potassium per gram of SPS.[22] The enema may be retained in the rectum for several hours as tolerated by the patient.

In symptomatic patients, or in those with severe hyperkalemia (serum potassium > 7 mEq/L), emergency care is indicated. Initial therapy in this setting is the administration of intravenous calcium to protect the heart from life-threatening arrhythmias.[24–26] Calcium antagonizes the cardiac membrane effect of hyperkalemia and reverses EKG changes within minutes. Its duration of action is 30–60 minutes, and it can be repeated as needed based on EKG findings. Intravenous calcium can be given as either the chloride or gluconate salt; each are available as a 10% solution by weight. Calcium chloride provides approximately three times more calcium than equal volumes of the gluconate salt, however, it can cause tissue necrosis if extravasation occurs. For this reason, calcium gluconate is more commonly administered with the standard dose being one 10-mL ampule IV bolus over 5 to 10 minutes.

Rapid correction of hyperkalemia, may necessitate the administration of drugs that result in an intracellular shift of potassium, such as insulin and dextrose, sodium bicarbonate, and the β_2-receptor agonist albuterol. The treatment of choice depends upon the underlying medical disorders accompanying hyperkalemia. For example, in patients with concomitant metabolic acidosis, a sodium bicarbonate bolus or infusion is the preferred therapy. Sodium bicarbonate helps to correct the metabolic acidosis by raising the extracellular pH, in addition to causing a rapid intracellular potassium shift. It should be noted that sodium bicarbonate is much less effective when hyperkalemia is not related to metabolic acidosis.[25] Sodium bicarbonate is also less effective in patients with ESRD, in whom a decrease in serum potassium can take as long as 4 hours.[27] It can also lead to sodium overload and eventual volume overload in this population. Insulin and dextrose therapy is an effective method of reducing potassium. Insulin increases the activity of the Na^+/K^+ ATPase pump, thereby intracellularly shifting potassium. Glucose should be given with insulin unless the serum glucose is greater than 250 mg/dL because hypoglycemia can develop with unopposed insulin therapy. Albuterol is a β_2-adrenergic agonist that has a dual mechanism for lowering serum potassium. First, it stimulates the Na^+/K^+ ATPase pump to promote intracellular potassium uptake. Second, it stimulates pancreas β receptors to increase insulin secretion. Albuterol can be administered

TABLE 52–5. Therapeutic Alternatives for the Management of Hyperkalemia

Treatment Options for Hyperkalemia						
Medication	*Dose*	*Route of Administration*	*Onset/Duration of Action*	*Acuity*	*Mechanism of Action*	*Expected Result*
Calcium	1g (1 ampule)	IV over 5–10 min	1–2 min/10–30 min	Acute	Raises cardiac threshold potential	Reverses ECG effects
Furosemide	20–40 mg	IV	5–15 min/4–6 hours	Acute	Inhibits renal Na^+ reabsorption	Increased urinary K^+ loss
Regular insulin	5–10 U	IV or SC	30 min/2–6 hours	Acute	Stimulates intracellular K^+ uptake	Intracellular K^+ redistribution
Dextrose 10%	1,000 mL (100 g)	IV over 1–2 hours	30 min/2–6 hours	Acute	Stimulates insulin release	Intracellular K^+ redistribution
Dextrose 50%	50 mL (25 g)	IV over 5 min	30 min/2–6 hours	Acute	Stimulates insulin release	Intracellular K^+ redistribution
Sodium bicarbonate	50–100 mEq	IV over 2–5 min	30 min/2–6 hours	Acute	Raises serum pH	Intracellular K^+ redistribution
Albuterol	10–20 mg	Nebulized over 10 min	30 min/1–2 hours	Acute	Stimulates intracellular K^+ uptake	Intracellular K^+ redistribution
Hemodialysis	4 hours	N/A	Immediate/variable	Acute	Removal from plasma	Increased K^+ elimination
Sodium polystyrene sulfonate	15–60 g	Oral or rectal	1 hour/variable	Non-acute	Resin exchanges Na^+ for K^+	Increased K^+ elimination

by IV or via nebulizer; however, IV administration is not FDA approved in the United States. The problems with nebulized albuterol therapy are frequent underdosing and, subsequently, poor response in as many as 33% of patients.[27] Moreover, cardiac side effects such as tachycardia may be undesirable in patients who already have abnormal ECGs. In summary, albuterol should be reserved as adjunctive therapy in patients already receiving insulin and dextrose therapy, due to its synergistic activity on the Na^+/K^+ Atpase pump.

DISORDERS OF MAGNESIUM HOMEOSTASIS

Magnesium plays a central role in cellular function and is an important cofactor for a variety of enzymes and receptors, especially those systems dependent on ATP.[28,29] Mitochondrial function, protein synthesis, cell membrane function and parathyroid hormone (PTH) secretion are just a few important functions affected by magnesium. It is the fourth most abundant extracellular cation and second most abundant intracellular cation. Disorders of magnesium homeostasis are commonly encountered clinical problems and most frequently are manifested as alterations in cardiovascular and neuromuscular function. Life-threatening conditions such as paralysis and cardiac arrhythmias may occur, making the proper recognition and treatment of these problems of paramount importance.

Magnesium is distributed in three major compartments: extracellular, 1.3%; intracellular, 13%; and bone, 67%.[30] Because of its predominant intracellular distribution, measurement of magnesium in the extracellular compartment may not accurately reflect the total body magnesium content. The majority of magnesium in the ECF is in the ionized form; only 20% to 30% is protein bound. The normal range for serum magnesium is 1.4–1.7 mEq/L, which equates to 1.7–2.1 mg/dL or 0.7–0.85 mmol/L.

The maintenance of magnesium homeostasis depends on the balance between intake and output. Thirty percent to 40% of ingested magnesium is absorbed in the small bowel. A small amount is secreted in intestinal secretions and reabsorbed in the sigmoid colon. The kidneys play a major role in maintaining magnesium balance. Renal magnesium handling is unique in that only 15% to 25% of the filtered magnesium is reabsorbed in the proximal tubule; the majority of reabsorption occurs in the loop of Henle.[30] This explains why loop diuretics often cause profound urinary magnesium wasting. Unlike most other important electrolytes, magnesium has no hormonal regulation of the distribution of magnesium between bone and circulating or intracellular magnesium pools. Because of this, both hypomagnesemia and hypermagnesemia commonly occur.

HYPOMAGNESEMIA

The prevalence of hypomagnesemia in outpatients and hospitalized patients is approximately 6 to 12%.[32] In patients with concomitant hypokalemia, the incidence rises to nearly 42%.[32] The incidence in critically ill patients may be as high as 65% principally because of the concomitant use of diuretics and aminoglycosides.[33] Although serum magnesium concentrations are not a reliable index of total body magnesium content, they remain the primary diagnostic tool to evaluate body stores.

PATHOPHYSIOLOGY

Hypomagnesemia is usually associated with disorders of the intestinal tract or kidney. Drugs or conditions that interfere with intestinal absorption, or increase renal excretion of magnesium can result in hypomagnesemia (Table 52–6). Decreased intestinal absorption as a

TABLE 52–6. Causes of Hypomagnesemia

Gastrointestinal	**Renal (continued)**
Reduced intake	Pyelonephritis
Protein-calorie malnutrition	Nephrotic syndrome
Total parenteral nutrition without magnesium	Drug-induced renal losses
Prolonged parenteral fluid administration without magnesium	Aminoglycosides
Alcoholism	Amphotericin B
Reduced absorption	Cyclosporine
Primary hypomagnesemia	Diuretics
Malabsorption syndromes (e.g., tropical sprue, celiac disease, radiation enteritis, intestinal lymphectasia)	Digitalis
	Cisplatin
Short-bowel syndrome (e.g., small-bowel resection, ileal bypass)	Alcohol
Pancreatic insufficiency	Hormone-induced renal losses
Increased loss	Hyperparathyroidism
Excessive vomiting	Hyperthyroidism
Prolonged nasogastric suction	Aldosteronism
Excessive laxative use	Hypoparathyroidism
Intestinal and biliary fistulas	"Hungry bone syndrome" after parathyroidectomy
Prolonged diarrhea (ulcerative colitis, Crohn's disease, cancer of the colon)	**Internal Redistribution**
	Diabetic ketoacidosis
Renal	Glucose, amino acid, insulin administration
Primary tubular disorders	Massive blood transfusion (citrate)
Primary renal magnesium wasting	Pancreatitis with lipidemia (magnesium soap)
Bartter's syndrome	**Other**
Renal tubular acidosis	Excessive sweating and lactation
Diuretic phase of acute tubular necrosis	Hypercalcemia and hypercalciuria
Postobstructive diuresis	Phosphate depletion
Postrenal transplant diuresis	Chronic alcoholism
Glomerulonephritis	ECF volume expansion

result of small bowel diseases is the most common cause of hypomagnesemia worldwide.[34] These disorders include regional enteritis; radiation enteritis; ulcerative colitis; acute and chronic diarrhea; pancreatic insufficiency and other malabsorptive syndromes; small-bowel bypass surgery; and chronic laxative abuse.[34]

Hypomagnesemia is commonly associated with alcoholism, and occurs in as many as 30% of hospitalized patients.[35] The etiology is often multifactorial including reduced intake, pancreatic insufficiency, chronic vomiting and diarrhea and urinary magnesium wasting. In addition, patients who are hospitalized for acute alcohol withdrawal often receive IV glucose administration and may experience even greater reductions in the serum magnesium concentration.[36] Because hypomagnesemia may contribute to the development of delirium tremens associated with alcohol withdrawal, frequent monitoring and aggressive magnesium replacement is indicated for these patients, especially those with tachyarrhythmias, hypocalcemia or hypokalemia.

Primary renal magnesium wasting may be due to a defect in renal tubular magnesium reabsorption, or inhibition of sodium reabsorption in those segments in which magnesium transport follows passively. The former condition is associated with hypercalciuria, nephrolithiasis, and progressive renal disease.[34] The latter is associated with Gitelman's and Bartter's syndromes.[34] Much more common than these is renal magnesium wasting secondary to diuretics. Hypomagnesemia occurs with both thiazide and loop diuretics, and may be present in as many as 37% of diuretic users.[37] Other commonly used drugs which may cause renal magnesium wasting include aminoglycosides, amphotericin B, cyclosporine, tacrolimus, cisplatin, pentamidine, and foscarnet.[37]

CLINICAL PRESENTATION

Because hypomagnesemia is often associated with a variety of other electrolyte abnormalities such as hypokalemia and hypocalcemia, it is difficult to ascribe specific clinical manifestations solely to magnesium deficiency. The dominant organ systems involved in hypomagnesemia include the neuromuscular and cardiovascular systems.[34] The typical symptoms of hypomagnesemia include tetany, positive Chvostek's and Trousseau's signs, and generalized convulsions.[34] Chvostek's sign is a facial twitch produced by tapping on the cheek over the branches of the facial nerve. Trousseau's sign is a hand spasm produced by placing a blood pressure cuff over the forearm and inflating the pressure above the systolic pressure for 3 minutes. Tremor and neuromuscular irritability are the most common signs and symptoms; tetany is less common.

Magnesium deficiency has been implicated in cardiac arrhythmias, hypertension, and sudden death. ECG changes include widening of the QRS complex and peaked T-waves with mild hypomagnesemia, and prolonged PR-interval, progressive widening of the QRS complex and flattening of T-waves with more severe magnesium deficiency.[34] Hypomagnesemia may predispose patients to digoxin-induced arrhythmias by increasing digoxin uptake in the myocardium, and potentiating the effect of digoxin on the myocardium. Digoxin-induced arrhythmias associated with magnesium deficiency are refractory to the usual antiarrhythmic agents but responsive to magnesium administration.[37,38]

The most important and potentially life-threatening cardiovascular effect of hypomagnesemia is the induction of ventricular arrhythmias. Patients who have concomitant myocardial ischemia or those who have undergone cardiopulmonary bypass procedures appear to be at highest risk for arrhythmias.[34] Magnesium may also play an important etiologic role in torsades de pointes, an atypical form of ventricular arrhythmias treatable with magnesium infusion.

A number of clinically significant electrolyte disturbances commonly occur with hypomagnesemia. Hypokalemia occurs in 40% to 60% of patients with hypomagnesemia,[10] in part because conditions that cause hypomagnesemia, such as diuretic use and diarrhea, are also associated with hypokalemia. Hypomagnesemia also causes renal potassium wasting, probably as a result of it reducing Na^+/K^+

ATPase activity, thus promoting potassium secretion in the loop of Henle. Hypokalemia observed in the setting of hypomagnesemia is thus generally refractory to potassium supplementation and requires correction of the magnesium deficit.[10]

Hypocalcemia is one of the most prominent symptoms of hypomagnesemia.[34] Hypocalcemia is usually detected first because it is more commonly measured in clinical practice. The etiology of hypocalcemia is not entirely clear, but probably is caused by decreased secretion of PTH, low 1,25-$(OH)_2$ vitamin D concentrations, and skeletal resistance to PTH.[34] As with hypokalemia, hypocalcemia accompanied by hypomagnesemia is most effectively treated with magnesium administration.

▶ TREATMENT: Hypomagnesemia

DESIRED OUTCOME

The treatment goals in the management of hypomagnesemia are: (a) resolution of the corresponding signs and symptoms; (b) restoration of normal magnesium concentrations; (c) correction of concomitant electrolyte abnormalities; and (d) identifying and correcting the underlying cause of magnesium depletion.

PHARMACOLOGIC THERAPY

Magnesium supplementation can be given by either the oral, intramuscular (IM), or IV route. Table 52–7 outlines one approach to the hypomagnesemic patient. The severity of the magnesium depletion and the presence of severe signs and symptoms should dictate the route of administration. Because IM administration is painful, it should be reserved for those patients with severe hypomagnesemia and limited venous access. IV bolus administration is associated with flushing, sweating, and a sensation of warmth; thus, bolus administration should be avoided if possible. Even if severe magnesium depletion is present, approximately 50% of the administered dose is excreted in the urine. Consequently, magnesium replacement should be performed over 3 to 5 days, and continued supplementation should be provided for patients unable to eat and for those patients with continued magnesium wasting.

Asymptomatic patients, or those patients with serum concentrations greater than 1 mEq/L (1.2 mg/dL), can be treated with oral supplements, such as antacids or laxatives. Diarrhea is the most common dose-limiting side effect of oral therapy, however, and can greatly reduce patient compliance.

If cases of severe magnesium depletion (serum levels less than 1 mEq/L), or if signs and symptoms are present regardless of the serum level, IV magnesium should be administered. A 50% solution of $MgSO_4$ is available for injection in 2-mL or 10-mL ampules (4 mEq/mL). The 50% solution should be diluted to 20% before injection to prevent venous sclerosis and pain. Therapy should be continued until the signs and symptoms have resolved completely. In patients with renal insufficiency, the dose should be reduced by 50%, and serum concentrations should be monitored every 6 to 12 hours for the first 24 hours and then daily until stable.

HYPERMAGNESEMIA

Hypermagnesemia (serum magnesium > 2 mEq/L) is a rare occurrence. It is generally seen in the setting of advanced renal failure when magnesium intake exceeds the excretory capacity of the kidneys. The prevalence of hypermagnesemia in hospitalized patients has been estimated to range from approximately 6% to 9%.[39,40] Elderly patients are prone to hypermagnesemia because of their reduced GFR and because of their consumption of magnesium-containing antacids and vitamins.[31]

PATHOPHYSIOLOGY

Because absolute magnesium excretion falls as GFR declines, serum magnesium concentrations rise in patients with moderate to severe renal insufficiency. Indeed, magnesium concentrations steadily rise as the GFR falls below 30 mL/min.[41] As long as the patient maintains a normal diet, the serum magnesium concentration typically stabilizes at approximately 2.5 mEq/L. If patients with renal insufficiency are taking concomitant magnesium-containing antacids, the serum level can approach 6 mEq/L, a value associated with signs and symptoms

TABLE 52–7. Guidelines for Treatment of Magnesium Deficiency in Adults

1. Serum Magnesium < 1 mEq/L (1.2 mg/dL) with Life-threatening Symptoms (seizure, arrhythmia)

Day 1

2 g $MgSO_4$ (1 g $MgSO_4$ = 8.1 mEq Mg^{2+}) mixed with 6 mL 0.9% NaCl in 10-mL syringe and administer IV push over 1 min

Follow with 0.5 mEq Mg^{2+}/kg lean body weight IV infusion over 5–6 h, then 0.5 mEq Mg^{2+}/kg lean body weight IV infusion over 17–18 h

Days 2–5

0.5 mEq Mg^{2+}/kg lean body weight per day divided in maintenance IV fluids

2. Serum Magnesium < 1 mEq/L (1.2 mg/dL) without Life-threatening Symptoms

Day 1

Total of 1 mEq Mg^{2+}/kg lean body weight per day as continuous IV infusion, or divided and given IM every 4 h for five doses

Days 2–5

Total of 0.5 mEq Mg^{2+}/kg lean body weight IV infusion per day as continuous IV infusion or divided and given IM every 6–8 h

3. Serum Magnesium > 1 mEq/L (1.2 mg/dL) and < 1.5 mEq/L (1.8 mg/dL) without Symptoms

As in no. 2, above, or

Milk of Magnesia 5 mL four times daily as tolerated, or

Magnesium-containing antacid 15 mL three times daily as tolerated, or

Magnesium oxide tablets 300 mg four times daily, increase to two tablets four times daily as tolerated

TABLE 52–8. Causes of Hypermagnesemia

Decreased Renal Excretion
Acute renal failure
Chronic renal failure with exogenous intake
Excessive Intake
Treatment of toxemia of pregnancy
Ureteral irrigants (hemiacidrin)
Cathartics
Other
Lithium therapy
Hypothyroidism
Milk–alkali syndrome
Addison's disease
Viral hepatitis
Acute diabetic ketoacidosis

of toxicity.[31] Critically ill patients with multiorgan system failure receiving enteral or parenteral nutrition are also prone to develop hypermagnesemia. Finally, the parenteral treatment of eclampsia with magnesium sulfate can lead to hypermagnesemia. Table 52–8 lists other causes of hypermagnesemia.

CLINICAL PRESENTATION

The signs and symptoms of hypermagnesemia reflect magnesium's action on the neuromuscular and cardiovascular systems (Fig. 52–3). Although there is wide interpatient variability between magnesium concentration and symptoms, they are rare when the serum concentration is less than 4 mEq/L. Deep-tendon reflexes are usually lost when the magnesium concentration exceeds 6 mEq/L. Central nervous system depression, manifested as drowsiness, lethargy, and somnolence occur at levels of 7–9 mEq/L; respiratory muscle paralysis, and severe cardiac rhythm abnormalities are usually not seen until the magnesium concentration approaches 12 mEq/L.[28,41,42] Complete heart block and death usually occur when concentrations exceed 15 mEq/L.[31]

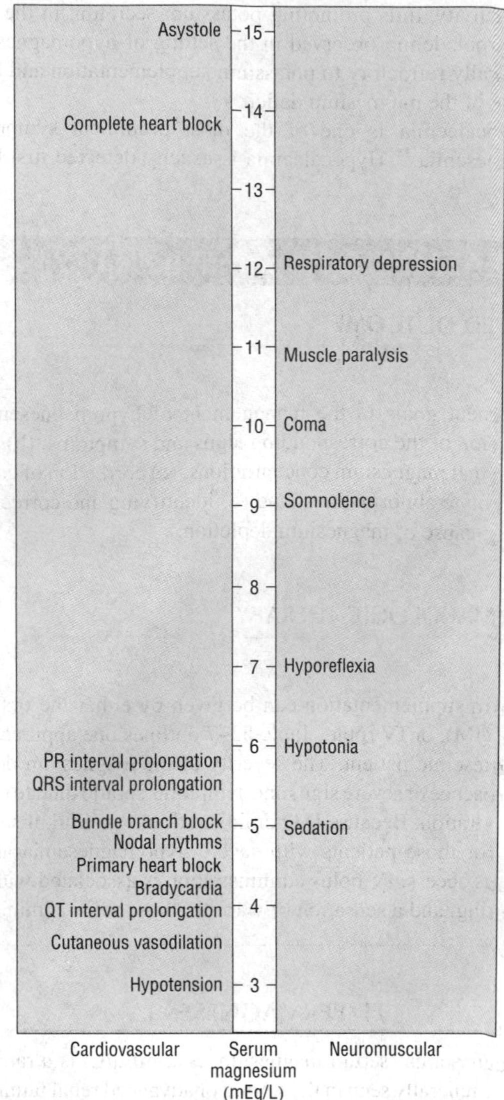

FIGURE 52–3. Clinical findings associated with hypermagnesemia.

▶ TREATMENT: Hypermagnesemia

DESIRED OUTCOME

The goals of therapy are to (a) reverse the neuromuscular and cardiovascular manifestations of hypermagnesemia; (b) decrease the magnesium concentration towards normal values; and (c) diagnose and reverse the underlying cause of hypermagnesemia.

PHARMACOLOGIC THERAPY

The treatment of hypermagnesemia depends on the presence of signs and symptoms, and degree of serum concentration elevation. Intravenous calcium in doses of 100–200 mg of elemental calcium directly antagonizes the neuromuscular and cardiovascular effects of hypermagnesemia. The clinical effect of calcium is immediate but the effect is transient; hence, repeated intravenous doses of 100–200 mg elemental calcium can be administered hourly until the hypermagnesemic symptoms abate and the magnesium concentration is normalized. Supportive care with cardiac pacing, vasopressors and mechanical ventilation may be necessary in life-threatening situations. In patients with adequate renal function, forced diuresis with saline and loop diuretics can promote magnesium elimination. An initial loop diuretic bolus of furosemide 40 mg intravenously can be used for immediate effects. Subsequent dosing can be determined based on the patient's clinical response. Patients with chronic renal insufficiency may require long-term loop diuretic therapy to maintain adequate fluid and electrolyte balance. In patients with ESRD, hemodialysis with a magnesium free dialysate should be emergently undertaken.

REFERENCES

1. Peterson LN, Levi M. Disorders of potassium metabolism. In: Schrier RW, ed. Renal and Electrolyte Disorders, 5th ed. Philadelphia, Lippincott-Raven, 1997:192–240.
2. Lee CAB, Barrett CA, Ignatavicius DD. Fluids and Electrolytes: A Practical Approach, 4th ed. Philadelphia, FA Davis, 1996:57–71.
3. Cogan MG. Fluid and Electrolytes. Physiology and Pathophysiology. Norwalk, CT: Appleton & Lange, 1991:125–163.
4. Sharma K, Cox M. Potassium homeostasis. In: Szerlip HM, Goldfarb S, eds. Workshops in Fluid and Electrolyte Disorders. New York, Churchill Livingstone, 1993:71–96.
5. Agarwal R, Afzalpurkar R, Fordtran JS. Pathophysiology of potassium absorption and secretion by the human intestine. Gastroenterology 1994; 107:548–571.
6. Rose BD, Rennke HG. Renal Pathophysiology—The Essentials. Baltimore, MD: Williams & Wilkins, 1994:169–190.
7. Krishna GG. Hypokalemic states: Current clinical issues. Semin Nephrol 1990;10:515–524.
8. Kamel KS, Halperin ML, Faber MD, et al. Disorders of potassium balance. In: Brenner BM, ed. The Kidney, 5th ed. Philadelphia, WB Saunders, 1996:999–1037.
9. Gennari FJ. Hypokalemia. N Eng J Med 1998;339:451–458.
10. Ryan MP. Interrelationships of magnesium and potassium homeostasis. Miner Electrolyte Metab 1993;19:290–295.
11. Weiner ID, Wingo CS. Hypokalemia—Consequences, causes, and correction. J Am Soc Nephrol 1997;8:1179–1188.
12. Krishna GG, Kapoor SC. Potassium depletion exacerbates essential hypertension. Ann Intern Med 1991;115:77–83.
13. Barri YM, Wingo CS. The effects of potassium depletion and supplementation on blood pressure: A clinical review. Am J Med Sci 1997;314: 37–40.
14. Geleijnse JM, Witteman JCM, den Breeijen JH, et al. Dietary electrolyte intake and blood pressure in older subjects: The Rotterdam Study. J Hypertens 1996;14:737–741.
15. INTERSALT Cooperative Research Group. INTERSALT: An international study of electrolyte excretion and blood pressure. Results for 24-hour urinary sodium and potassium excretion. BMJ 1988;297:319–328.
16. Ascherio A, Hennekens C, Willett WC, et al. Prospective study of nutritional factors, blood pressure, and hypertension among US women. Hypertension 1996;27:1065–1072.
17. The Sixth Report of the Joint National Committee on Prevention, Detection, Evaluation, and Treatment of High Blood Pressure. Arch Intern Med 1997;157:2413–2446.
18. Whelton PK, He J, Cutler JA, et al. Effects of oral potassium on blood pressure: Meta-analysis of randomized controlled clinical trials. JAMA 1997;277:1624–1632.
19. Langford HG. Dietary potassium and hypertension: Epidemiologic data. Ann Intern Med 1983;98:770–772.
20. Cohn JN, Kowey PR, Whelton PK, Prisant LM. New guidelines for potassium replacement in clinical practice: A contemporary review by the National Council on Potassium in Clinical Practice. Arch Intern Med 2000;160:2429–2436.
21. Siscovick DS, Raghunathan TE, Psaty BM, et al. Diuretic therapy for hypertension and the risk of primary cardiac arrest. N Eng J Med 1994;330:1852–1857.
22. Mandal AK. Hypokalemia and hyperkalemia. Med Clin North Am 1997;81:611–639.
23. Agarwal A, Wingo CS. Treatment of hypokalemia. N Eng J Med 1999;340:154–155. Letter.
24. Weiner ID, Wingo CS. Hyperkalemia: A potential silent killer. J Am Soc Nephrol 1998;9:1535–1543.
25. Chmielewski CM. Hyperkalemic emergencies:Mechanisms, manifestations and management. Crit Care Nurs Clin North Am 1998;10:449–458.
26. Greenberg A. Hyperkalemia: Treatment options. Semin Nephrol 1998; 18:46–57.
27. Wong SL, Maltz HC. Albuterol for the treatment of hyperkalemia. Ann Pharmacother 1999;33:103–106.
28. Toto KH, Yucha CB. Magnesium homeostasis, imbalances, and therapeutic uses. Crit Care Nurs Clin North Am 1994;6:767–783.
29. Wicks TC. AANA Journal course. Update for nurse anesthetists—Magnesium homeostasis and deficiency. AANA J 1999;67:171–179.
30. Quamme GA. Renal magnesium handling: New insights in understanding old problems. Kidney Int 1997;52:1180–1195.
31. Hruska KA, Slatopolsky E. Disorders of phosphorus, calcium and magnesium metabolism. In: Schrier RW, Gottschalk CW, eds. Diseases of the Kidney, Vol. 3, 6th ed. Boston, MA, Little, Brown and Company, 1997:2477–2526.
32. Wong ET, Rude RK, Singer FR, Shaw ST Jr. A high prevalence of hypomagnesemia in hospitalized patients. Am J Clin Pathol 1983;79:348–352.
33. Ryzen E. Magnesium homeostasis in critically ill patients. Magnesium 1989;8:201–212.
34. Kelepouris E, Agus ZS. Hypomagnesemia: Renal magnesium handling. Semin Nephrol 1998;18:58–73.
35. Elisaf M, Merkouropolous M, Tsianos EV, et al. Pathogenetic mechanisms of hypomagnesemia in alcoholic patients. J Trace Elem Med Biol 1995;9:210–214.
36. Kobrin SM, Goldfarb S. Magnesium deficiency. Semin Nephrol 1990; 10:525–535.
37. Tso EL, Barish RA. Magnesium: Clinical considerations. J Emerg Med 1992;10:735–745.
38. Whang R, Hampton EM, Whang DD. Magnesium homeostasis and clinical disorders of magnesium deficiency. Ann Pharmacother 1994;28:220–226.
39. Whang R, Ryder KW. Frequency of hypomagnesemia and hypermagnesemia requested vs. routine. JAMA 1990:263;3063–3064.
40. Wong ET, Rude RK, Singer FR, et al. A high prevalence of hypomagnesemia and hypermagnesemia in hospitalized patients. Am J Clin Pathol 1983;79:348–352.
41. Van Hook JW. Endocrine crises. Hypermagnesemia. Crit Care Clin 1991; 7:215–223.
42. Clark BA, Brown RS. Unsuspected morbid hypermagnesemia in elderly patients. Am J Nephrol 1992;12:336–343.

53

ACID-BASE DISORDERS

Paul M. Palevsky and Gary R. Matzke

Acid-base disorders are common, and often serious, disturbances that may result in significant morbidity and mortality. This chapter reviews the mechanisms responsible for the maintenance of acid-base balance and the laboratory analyses that aid clinicians in their assessment of acid-base disorders. The pathophysiology of the four primary acid-base disturbances is presented, the therapeutic options are critiqued, and guidelines for assessment of the achievement of the desired therapeutic outcomes are presented. Because many drugs affect acid-base homeostasis and many acid-base abnormalities are potentially preventable, pharmacists may have a significant impact on patient outcomes. The pharmacist's responsibility includes anticipation of drug-related problems, avoidance or minimization of clinical consequences, and the design of appropriate treatment regimens. To provide this level of pharmaceutic care, one must understand the physiology of respiratory and metabolic acid-base regulation.

ACID-BASE CHEMISTRY

An acid is a substance that can donate protons (hydrogen ions, H^+):

$$HCl \rightarrow H^+ + Cl^-$$

A base is a substance that can accept protons (hydrogen ions):

$$NH_3 + H^+ \rightarrow NH_4^+ \text{(base)}$$

Table 53–1 lists the acid-base pairs commonly encountered in clinical practice.

The acidity of body fluids is quantified in terms of the hydrogen ion concentration. By convention, the degree of acidity is expressed as pH, or the negative logarithm (base 10) of the hydrogen ion concentration. Thus, hydrogen ion concentration and pH are inversely related. Normally, the pH of blood is maintained at 7.40 ($[H^+]$ of 4×10^{-8} M) with a range of 7.35–7.45. A pH of less than 6.7 ($[H^+]$ of 2×10^{-7} M), representing a fivefold increase in hydrogen ion concentration, or greater than 7.7 ($[H^+]$ of 2×10^{-8} M), representing a 50% decrease in hydrogen ion concentration, are considered incompatible with life.

The hydrogen ion concentration in blood may not be indicative of that in other body compartments. For example, the pH within cells, within the cerebrospinal fluid, or on the surface of bone may all be altered without causing an alteration in blood pH.[1] Recognizing this caveat, the acid-base status of the body is usually analyzed based on measurement of blood pH. Alterations in blood pH serve as the basis for the diagnosis of acid-base disorders.

Because the dissociation of acid-base pairs is an equilibrium reaction, the relationship between hydrogen ion concentration or pH and the relative concentrations the acid and base can be described mathematically in terms of the dissociation constant for the acid-base buffer pair. When expressed as a logarithmic relationship, where p*K* is the negative logarithm of the dissociation constant, *K*, this is known as the Henderson-Hasselbalch equation:

$$pH = pK + \log([\text{base}]/[\text{acid}])$$

BUFFERS

The ability of a weak acid and its corresponding anion (base) to resist change in the pH of a solution upon the addition of a strong acid or base is referred to as buffering. An acid-base pair is most efficient in functioning as a buffer at a pH close to its pK. The principal extracellular buffer is the carbonic acid/bicarbonate (H_2CO_3/HCO_3^-) system. Other physiologic buffers include plasma proteins, hemoglobin, and phosphates. Because the isohydric principle requires that all buffer systems remain in chemical equilibrium, the complex buffering of biologic fluids can be analyzed based on a single buffer pair.

The carbonic acid/bicarbonate buffer system plays a unique role in acid-base homeostasis. In addition to being the most abundant extracellular buffer, the components of this buffer pair are under dynamic regulation by the body. In the presence of carbonic anhydrase, carbonic acid, $[H_2CO_3]$ is in equilibrium with CO_2 gas. Changes in ventilation, which alter the partial pressure of CO_2 (P_{CO_2}) in the blood, regulates the carbonic acid level in the blood. The bicarbonate concentration is independently regulated by the kidney. because the p*K* for the carbonic acid/bicarbonate system is 6.1, the relationship between pH, carbonic acid, and bicarbonate concentrations can be described by the Henderson-Hasselbalch equation. The concentration of carbonic acid is directly proportional to the amount of CO_2 dissolved in blood, which is equal to the product of P_{CO_2} and its solubility in physiologic fluids, ($P_{CO_2} \times 0.03$). This term can therefore be substituted into the above equation in place of $[H_2CO_3]$.

$$pH = 6.1 + \log([HCO_3^-]/[H_2CO_3])$$
$$pH = 6.1 + \log([HCO_3^-]/(P_{CO_2} \times 0.03))$$

Thus, hydrogen ion concentration and pH are determined not by the absolute amounts of bicarbonate and P_{CO_2}, but by their ratio.[1] Under normal physiologic conditions, the kidneys maintain the serum bicarbonate at about 24 mEq/L, while the lungs maintain the P_{CO_2} at approximately 40 mm Hg. The normal physiologic pH is, thus, 7.40:

$$pH = 6.1 + \log[24/(0.03 \times 40)]$$
$$pH = 6.1 + 1.3 = 7.4$$

If, in response to an acid load, the serum bicarbonate concentration were to fall to 12 mEq/L, the predicted pH would be:

$$[HCO_3^-] = 12\,\text{mEq/L}$$
$$P_{CO_2} = 40\,\text{mm Hg}$$
$$pH = 6.1 + \log[12/(0.03 \times 40)]$$
$$pH = 6.1 + 1.0 = 7.1$$

However, the normal respiratory response to an acid load is hyperventilation. As a result, if the P_{CO_2} fell to approximately 26 mm Hg, the change in pH would be less:

$$[HCO_3^-] = 12\,\text{mEq/L}$$
$$P_{CO_2} = 26\,\text{mm Hg}$$
$$pH = 6.1 + \log[12/(0.03 \times 26)]$$
$$pH = 6.1 + 1.19 = 7.29$$

TABLE 53–1. Acid-Base Pairs

Carbonic acid/bicarbonate	H_2CO_3/HCO_3^-
Monobasic/dibasic phosphate	H_2PO_4/HPO_4^-
Ammonium/ammonia	NH_4^+/NH_3
Lactic acid/lactate	$H_6C_3O_2/H_5C_3O_2^-$

Thus, the physiologic regulation of both P_{CO_2} and $[HCO_3^-]$ permit the carbonic acid/bicarbonate system to provide more effective buffering of the extracellular fluids than could be achieved on the basis of chemical buffering alone.

REGULATION OF ACID-BASE HOMEOSTASIS

Cellular metabolism results in the production of large quantities of hydrogen that need to be excreted in order to maintain acid-base balance. In addition, small amounts of acid and alkali are also presented to the body through the diet. The bulk of acid production is in the form of CO_2, produced from the metabolism of carbohydrates, proteins, and lipids. When respiratory function is normal, the amount of CO_2 produced metabolically is equal to the amount lost by respiration, and the blood CO_2 concentration remains constant. The average adult produces approximately 15,000 mmol of CO_2 each day from the catabolism of carbohydrate, protein, and fat.[2]

Digestion of dietary substances and tissue metabolism also results in the production of nonvolatile acids. These acids are derived primarily from the sulfur-containing amino acids cysteine and methionine, as well as from ingested sulfur. In addition, phosphates are generated from the metabolism of proteins and phospholipids. Neutral substances such as glucose may also be incompletely metabolized to intermediates, such as lactic and pyruvic acid, and fatty acids may be incompletely metabolized to acetoacetic acid and β-hydroxy-butyric acid. These dietary and metabolic fixed-acids are excreted, primarily by the kidney, to maintain acid-base homeostasis. On average, daily fixed-acid excretion is approximately 0.8 mEq/kg/d or 50–100 mEq.[3]

Three mechanisms collectively maintain acid-base balance: extracellular buffering, ventilatory regulation of carbon dioxide elimination, and renal regulation of hydrogen ion and bicarbonate excretion. Extracellular buffering is the body's first and fastest defense against a sudden increase in hydrogen ion concentration. Hyperventilation will then result in a decrease in P_{CO_2}, returning blood pH toward normal. Finally, the kidney will excrete the excess hydrogen ion, and return acid-base balance to normal.

EXTRACELLULAR BUFFERING

The body's buffering system can be divided into three components: bicarbonate/carbonic acid, proteins, and phosphates. The bicarbonate buffer is the most important of the body's buffers, because (a) there is more bicarbonate present in the extracellular fluid (ECF) than any other buffer component; (b) the supply of carbon dioxide is unlimited; and (c) the acidity of ECF can be regulated by controlling either the bicarbonate concentration or the P_{CO_2}.

Carbonic acid represents the respiratory component of the buffer pair because its concentration is directly proportional to the P_{CO_2}, which is determined by ventilation. Bicarbonate represents the metabolic component because the kidney may alter its concentration by reabsorption, generating new bicarbonate, or altering elimination.[4] The bicarbonate buffer system easily adapts to changes in acid-base status by alterations in ventilatory elimination of acid (P_{CO_2}) and/or renal elimination of base (HCO_3^-).

The phosphate buffer system consists of serum inorganic phosphate (3.5–5.0 mg/dL), intracellular organic phosphate, and calcium phosphate in bone. Extracellular phosphate is present only in low concentrations so that its usefulness as a buffer is limited; however, as an intracellular buffer, phosphate is more useful. Calcium phosphate in bone is relatively inaccessible as a buffer, but prolonged metabolic acidosis will result in the release of phosphate from bone.

Intracellular and extracellular proteins also act as buffering systems. The charged side chains of amino acids provide the buffering action. Because the concentration of protein is much greater intracellularly than extracellularly, protein is much more important as an intracellular buffer.

RESPIRATORY REGULATION

The second mechanism for maintenance of acid-base homeostasis is control of ventilation. Both the rate and depth of ventilation can be varied to allow for excretion of CO_2 generated by diet and tissue metabolism. Medullary chemoreceptors in the brain stem sense changes in P_{CO_2} and in pH and modulate the control of breathing. Increasing minute ventilation, by increasing either or both respiratory rate or tidal volume will increase CO_2 excretion and decrease the blood P_{CO_2}. Conversely, decreasing minute ventilation decreases CO_2 excretion and increases blood P_{CO_2}. This system rapidly adjusts, within minutes, to changes in acid-base balance[2].

RENAL REGULATION

The kidney plays a central role in the regulation of acid-base homeostasis through the excretion or reabsorption of filtered HCO_3^-, the excretion of metabolic fixed-acids and generation of new HCO_3^- to replace that which was lost through the titration of acid or as the result of losses in gastrointestinal fluids.

Because bicarbonate is a small ion, it is freely filtered at the glomerulus. The bicarbonate load delivered to the nephron is approximately 4,500 mEq/d. To maintain acid-base balance, this entire filtered load must be reabsorbed. Bicarbonate reabsorption occurs primarily in the proximal tubule (Fig. 53–1). In the tubular lumen, filtered bicarbonate combines with hydrogen ion secreted by the apical Na^+,H^+-exchanger to form carbonic acid. The carbonic acid is rapidly broken down to CO_2 and water by carbonic anhydrase located on the luminal surface of the brush border membrane. The CO_2 then diffuses into the proximal tubular cell, where it reforms carbonic acid in the presence of intracellular carbonic anhydrase. The carbonic acid dissociates to form hydrogen ion, that can again be secreted into the tubular lumen, and bicarbonate that exits the cell across the basolateral membrane and enters the peritubular capillary.

Excretion of metabolic fixed-acids and generation of new HCO_3^- is achieved through renal ammoniagenesis and distal tubular hydrogen ion secretion. Ammoniagenesis plays a critical role in acid-base homeostasis with ammonium ($NH4^+$) excretion comprising approximately 50% of renal net acid excretion. Ammonium is generated from the deamination of glutamine in the proximal tubule. For each ammonium ion excreted in the urine, one bicarbonate ion is regenerated and returned to the circulation.[5]

Distal tubular hydrogen ion secretion accounts for the remaining 50% of net acid excretion (Fig. 53–2). In the distal tubular cell, CO_2 combines with water in the presence of intracellular carbonic anhydrase to form carbonic acid, which dissociates to H^+ and HCO_3^-. The H^+ is actively transported into the tubular lumen by a H^+-ATPase. The bicarbonate exits the cell across the basolateral membrane and enters the circulation.[5]

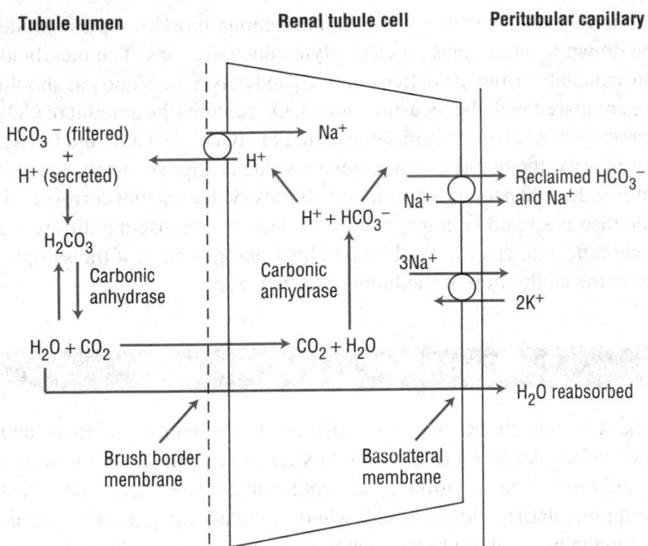

FIGURE 53–1. Proximal tubular bicarbonate reabsorption. In the tubular lumen, filtered bicarbonate combines with hydrogen ion secreted by an apical Na^+,H^+-exchanger to form carbonic acid. The carbonic acid is rapidly broken down to CO_2 and water by carbonic anhydrase located on the luminal surface of the brush border membrane. The CO_2 then diffuses into the proximal tubular cell, where it reforms carbonic acid in the presence of intracellular carbonic anhydrase. The carbonic acid dissociates to form hydrogen ion, that can again be secreted into the tubular lumen, and bicarbonate that exits the cell across the basolateral membrane and enters the peritubular capillary.

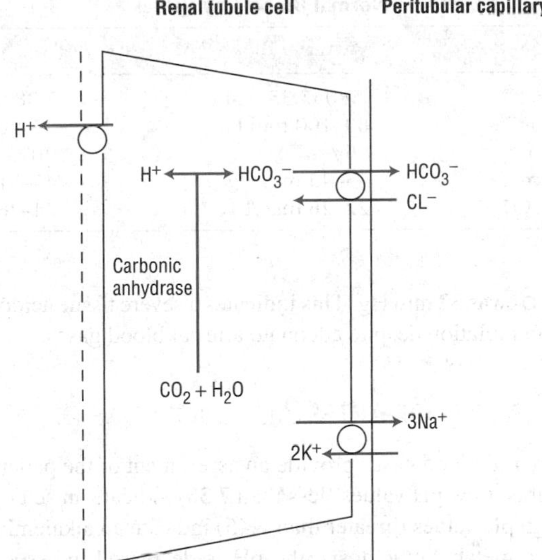

FIGURE 53–2. Collecting duct acid excretion. Hydrogen ion and bicarbonate are generated intracellularly from CO_2 and water, in the presence of intracellular carbonic anhydrase. The hydrogen ion is actively secreted into the tubular lumen by H^+- ATPases located in the apical (luminal) membrane. Bicarbonate exits the cell across the basolateral membrane and enters the peritubular capillary.

ACID-BASE DISTURBANCES

Alterations in blood pH are designated by the suffix "emia": acidemia is an arterial blood pH < 7.35 and alkalemia is an arterial blood pH > 7.45. The pathophysiologic processes that result in alterations in blood pH are designated by the suffix "osis". These disturbances are classified as either metabolic or respiratory in origin. In metabolic acid-base disorders, the primary disturbance is in the plasma bicarbonate concentration. Metabolic acidosis is characterized by a decrease in the plasma bicarbonate concentration while in metabolic alkalosis the plasma bicarbonate concentration is increased. Respiratory acid-base disorders are caused by alterations in alveolar ventilation that produce corresponding changes in the arterial carbon dioxide tension ($Paco_2$). In respiratory acidosis, the $Paco_2$ is elevated; in respiratory alkalosis it is decreased. Each disturbance has a compensatory (secondary) response which corrects the $[HCO_3^-]/Paco_2$ ratio toward normal and mitigates the change in pH (Table 53–2). Although the time-course of the compensatory responses to metabolic disturbances is rapid, the metabolic compensation for respiratory disturbances is slow. As a result, respiratory disturbances are characterized as acute (minutes to hours in duration), indicating that there has not been sufficient time for metabolic compensation, or chronic (days), indicating sufficient time for metabolic compensation has occurred.

CLINICAL ASSESSMENT OF ACID-BASE STATUS

Arterial blood gases, along with serum electrolytes, physical findings, medical and medication history, and the clinical condition of the patient, are the primary tools to determine the cause of an acid-base disorder and to design a course of therapy.

ARTERIAL BLOOD GASES

Blood gases are measured to determine the patient's oxygenation and acid-base status. Under normal circumstances, there is no clinically significant difference in pH between arterial and mixed venous blood. Arterial samples are designated with the letter "*a*" (Pao_2 and $Paco_2$), while mixed venous samples are labeled with the letter "*v*" or not labeled (Pvo_2 and $Pvco_2$). The normal values for arterial and venous blood gases are shown in Table 53–3. Arterial blood provides the added information of how well the lungs are oxygenating the blood (an accurate measurement of Po_2). Arterial blood rather than venous blood should be used whenever possible because venous blood obtained from an extremity may provide misleading information. If metabolism in the extremity is altered by hypoperfusion, exercise, infection, or some other cause, the differences between arterial and venous blood can be dramatic. Weil and associates[6] reported average mixed venous pH of 7.15 and Pco_2 of 74 mm Hg during cardiopulmonary resuscitation, even though the arterial pH was 7.41 and arterial

TABLE 53–2. Interpretation of Simple Acid-Base Disorders

Acid-Base Disorder	pH	Primary Disturbances	Compensation
Acidosis			
Respiratory	Decrease	Increase $Paco_2$	Increase HCO_3^-
Metabolic	Decrease	Decrease HCO_3^-	Decrease $Paco_2$
Alkalosis			
Respiratory	Increase	Decrease $Paco_2$	Decrease HCO_3^-
Metabolic	Increase	Increase HCO_3^-	Increase $Paco_2$

TABLE 53–3. Normal Blood Gas Values

	Arterial Blood	Mixed Venous Blood
pH	7.40 (7.35–7.45)	7.38 (7.33–7.43)
Po_2	80–100 mm Hg	35–40 mm Hg
Sao_2	95%	70%–75%
Pco_2	35–45 mm Hg	45–51 mm Hg
HCO_3^-	22–26 mEq/L	24–28 mEq/L

Pco_2 was 32 mm Hg. This indicates a severe tissue acidosis from CO_2 accumulation despite adequate arterial blood gases.

ANALYSIS OF ARTERIAL BLOOD GAS DATA

Arterial blood gases provide an assessment of the patient's acid-base status. Low pH values (less than 7.35) indicate an acidemia, whereas high pH values (greater than 7.45) indicate an alkalemia (Fig. 53–3). In a metabolic acidosis, the pH is decreased in association with a decreased serum bicarbonate concentration and a compensatory fall in $Paco_2$. In a respiratory acidosis, the pH is decreased; the $Paco_2$, however, is elevated. The serum bicarbonate concentration is variable, depending upon whether it is an acute disturbance (minimal increase in serum bicarbonate) or a chronic respiratory acidosis (substantial increase in serum bicarbonate). In a metabolic alkalosis, the pH is elevated in association with an increased bicarbonate concentration and a compensatory rise in $Paco_2$. In respiratory alkalosis, the pH is also elevated; the $Paco_2$, however, is decreased. As with respiratory acidosis, the metabolic compensation is variable, with a minimal decrease in serum bicarbonate in acute respiratory alkalosis and a larger decrease in $[HCO_3^-]$ in chronic respiratory alkalosis.

Table 53–4 lists the degree of expected compensatory response for each primary disturbance. If the observed compensatory response is substantially different than that predicted by these empiric relationships, a mixed acid-base disturbance (i.e., more than one primary disorder) may be present. Nomograms, such as the one shown in Fig. 53–4, may also be used to differentiate between the various acid-base disorders.[4,7] In this nomogram, each pathologic acid-base disorder, together with the appropriate range of *in vivo* physiologic compensation, is represented as a shaded band. Blood gas values—serum bicarbonate, pH, and carbon dioxide tension—falling within a band usually represent a single disturbance; however, a mixed disturbance may occasionally present in this way. Acid-base values falling outside any band almost certainly represent a mixed acid-base disturbance.[7]

When arterial blood gases differ significantly from those expected on the basis of the patient's clinical condition and previous laboratory determinations, additional venous blood samples should be drawn to assess plasma electrolyte concentrations. The bicarbonate calculated from the patient's $Paco_2$ and pH on the blood gas should be compared with the measured total CO_2 content (the amount of CO_2 gas extractable from plasma, consisting of HCO_3^-, H_2CO_3, and Pco_2). Ordinarily, the blood gas bicarbonate value is approximately 1.0–2.0 mEq/L less than total CO_2 content.[8] If these values do not correspond, the results should be interpreted with caution because the difference may reflect an error in the blood collection or storage of the sample, or in the calibration of the blood-gas analyzer.

METABOLIC ACID-BASE DISORDERS

The two metabolic acid-base disorders, metabolic acidosis and metabolic alkalosis, are generated by a primary change in the serum bicarbonate concentration. In metabolic acidosis, bicarbonate is lost or a nonvolatile acid is gained, whereas metabolic alkalosis is characterized by a gain in bicarbonate or a loss of nonvolatile acid.

METABOLIC ACIDOSIS

PATHOPHYSIOLOGY

Metabolic acidosis is characterized by a decrease in pH as the result of a primary decrease in serum bicarbonate concentration. This can result from the buffering (consumption of HCO_3^-) of an exogenous acid, an organic acid accumulating because of a metabolic disturbance (e.g., lactic acid, ketoacids) or the progressive accumulation of endogenous acids secondary to impaired renal function (e.g., phosphates, sulfates).[9] The serum HCO_3^- can also be decreased as the result of a loss of bicarbonate-rich body fluids (e.g., diarrhea, biliary drainage, pancreatic fistula) or occur secondary to the rapid administration of nonalkali-containing intravenous fluids (dilutional acidosis).

The serum anion gap (AG), as defined below, may be used to help differentiate between etiologies of metabolic acidosis. To maintain electroneutrality, the total concentration of cations in the serum must equal the total concentration of anions. The cation concentration is equal to the sodium concentration plus that of "unmeasured" cations (UCs), predominantly magnesium, calcium, and potassium. The anion concentration is equal to the concentrations of chloride, bicarbonate, and "unmeasured" anions (UAs), including proteins, sulfates, phosphates, and organic anions. Therefore,

$$[Na^+] + [UCs] = ([Cl^-] + [HCO_3^-]) + [UAs]$$

$$\text{Anion gap} = [Na^+] - ([Cl^-] + [HCO3^-]) = [UAs] - [UCs]$$

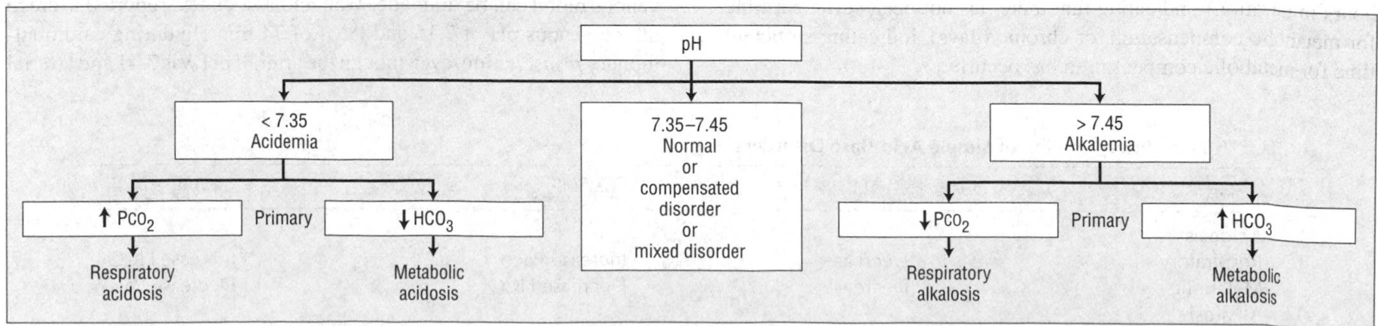

FIGURE 53–3. Analysis of arterial blood gases.

TABLE 53–4. Guidelines for Initial Interpretation of Acid-Base Disorders

Metabolic acidosis	Pa_{CO_2} (in mm Hg) should fall by 1.0–1.5 times the fall in plasma [HCO_3^-] (in mEq/L)
Metabolic alkalosis	Pa_{CO_2} (in mm Hg) should increase by 0.25–1.0 times the rise in plasma [HCO_3^-] (in mEq/L)
Acute respiratory acidosis	The plasma [HCO_3^-] should rise by 0.1 times the increase in Pa_{CO_2} ± 3
Acute respiratory alkalosis	The plasma [HCO_3^-] should fall by 0.1–0.3 times the decrease in Pa_{CO_2} but usually not to less than 18 mEq/L
Chronic respiratory acidosis	The plasma [HCO_3^-] should rise by 0.4 times the increase in Pa_{CO_2} ± 4
Chronic respiratory alkalosis	The plasma [HCO_3^-] should fall by 0.2–0.5 times the decrease in Pa_{CO_2} but usually not to less than 14 mEq/L

From Ref. 4, with permission.

The normal serum AG is approximately 9 mEq/L, with a range of 3–11 mEq/L. This value is lower than the value of 12 mEq/L cited in the literature in the past because of changes in the instrumentation for measurement of serum electrolytes during the past decade.[10] Increases in the anion gap to values in excess of 17–20 mEq/L are indicative of the accumulation of unmeasured anions in ECF.

These unmeasured anions are generated as the result of the consumption of HCO_3^- by endogenous organic acids such as lactic acid, acetoacetic acid, or β-hydroxybutyric acid or from the ingestion of toxins such as methanol or ethylene glycol. The degree of elevation in the serum AG is dependent on the clearance of the anion, as well as the multiple factors that influence HCO_3^- concentrations. Thus, the serum AG is a relative rather than an absolute indication of the cause of metabolic acidosis. The anion gap may also be elevated in the metabolic acidosis due to renal failure from the accumulation of various organic anions, phosphates and sulfates.

In hyperchloremic metabolic acidosis, bicarbonate losses from the ECF are replaced by chloride and the anion gap remains normal. This decrease in bicarbonate results from losses from the gastrointestinal tract, dilution of bicarbonate in the ECF space by the addition of sodium chloride solutions, or the addition of chloride-containing acids to the ECF. Common causes of metabolic acidosis with an increased anion gap or a normal anion gap are listed in Table 53–5.

HYPERCHLOREMIC METABOLIC ACIDOSIS

Hyperchloremic metabolic acidosis may result from increased gastrointestinal bicarbonate loss, renal bicarbonate wasting, impaired renal acid excretion or exogenous acid gain. Gastrointestinal disorders such as diarrhea, biliary drainage, and pancreatic fistula may result in the loss of large volumes of bicarbonate-containing fluids, with diarrhea being the most common cause for hyperchloremic metabolic acidosis. Severe diarrhea can lead to a daily loss of 5–10 L of fluid containing 100–140 mEq/L of sodium, 20–40 mEq/L of potassium, 80–100 mEq/L of chloride, and 30–50 mEq/L of bicarbonate.[4] Patients who have undergone ureteral diversion into the sigmoid colon or isolated ileal loop may also develop a hyperchloremic metabolic acidosis. In these patients, chloride is reabsorbed and the bicarbonate secreted by the gastrointestinal epithelial cells while urine is retained in the colon or bowel loop, results in a net loss of bicarbonate. Hyperchloremic metabolic acidosis caused by renal bicarbonate wasting is the defining disturbance in proximal renal tubular acidosis and is a complication of therapy with carbonic anhydrase inhibitors. During the treatment of diabetic ketoacidosis, renal losses of β-hydroxybutyrate and acetoacetate, which would otherwise be metabolized to yield bicarbonate, may contribute to the development of hyperchloremic metabolic acidosis. Impaired renal acid excretion as a result of distal tubular dysfunction characterizes the distal renal tubular acidoses. Impaired renal acid excretion is also characteristic of moderate to severe renal insufficiency. Initially, the metabolic acidosis of renal insufficiency is hyperchloremic progressing to an anion-gap acidosis as the renal insufficiency worsens and sulfates, phosphates, and other anions accumulate. Hyperchloremic metabolic acidosis may also result from the exogenous administration of acid as hydrochloric acid or ammonium chloride or the unbuffered administration of acid salts of amino acids in hyperalimentation fluids.

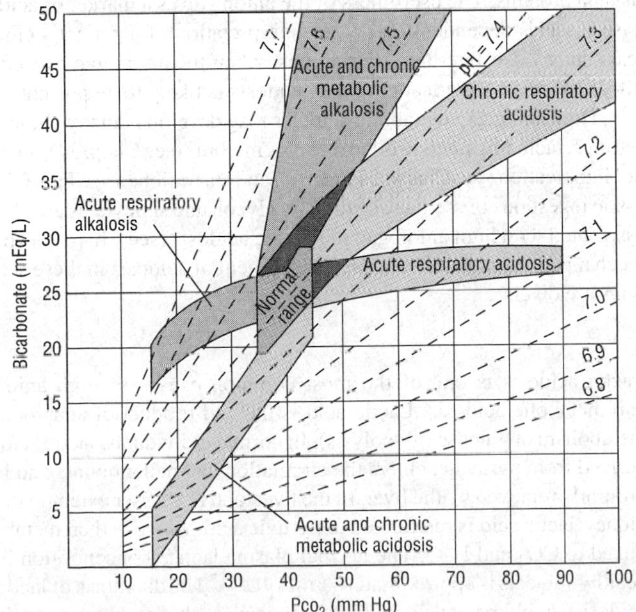

FIGURE 53–4. Acid-base nomogram. (Reprinted from Ref. 2, with permission.)

RENAL TUBULAR ACIDOSIS

Renal tubular acidosis (RTA) refers to a group of disorders characterized by impaired tubular renal acid handling despite normal or near-normal glomerular filtration rates. These patients often present with hyperchloremic metabolic acidosis. These disorders may involve the proximal tubule, with a resultant failure to reabsorb filtered bicarbonate, or affect acid excretion in the distal tubule.

TABLE 53–5. Common Causes of Metabolic Acidosis

Increased Anion Gap	Normal Anion Gap/ Hyperchloremic States
Alcoholic ketoacidosis	Acid ingestion (hydrochloric acid or ammonium chloride)
Diabetic ketoacidosis	Carbonic anhydrase inhibitors
Lactic acidosis	Cholestyramine
Renal failure (acute or chronic)	Diarrhea
Methanol ingestion	Dilutional acidosis
Ethylene glycol ingestion	Gastrointestinal disorders
Salicylate overdose	Pancreatic fistula
Starvation	Potassium-sparing diuretic
	Renal tubular acidosis
	Ureterosigmoidostomy, ileostomy

The distal RTAs are the most common and are all characterized by impaired net acid excretion (NAE). The distal RTAs are subdivided into those that are associated with hypokalemia (Type I) and those associated with hyperkalemia (Type IV). Patients with classic distal (Type I) RTA have impaired H^+ ion secretion, and are unable to excrete the daily acid load necessary to maintain acid-base balance.[4] These patients are unable to maximally acidify their urine (i.e., attain urine pH of <5.5) even in the face of an acid challenge. Type I RTA may be the result of a primary tubular defect or develop secondary to a wide variety of disorders including hypercalcemia, multiple myeloma, lupus erythematosus, Sjögren's syndrome, sickle-cell disease, and renal transplant rejection, or following the administration of amphotericin B or ingestion of toluene. The primary form of this disorder usually occurs in children and can result in severe acidosis, growth retardation, nephrocalcinosis, and kidney stones.[11] In adults, clinical complications include osteomalacia, nephrocalcinosis, and recurrent kidney stones. The hypokalemia associated with classic distal (Type I) RTA results from secondary hypoaldosteronism associated with volume depletion. The renal potassium wasting decreases considerably when bicarbonate therapy is begun.

The hyperkalemic distal (Type IV) RTAs are a heterogeneous group of disorders characterized by hypoaldosteronism or generalized distal tubule defects. The most common form of Type IV RTA is hyporeninemic hypoaldosteronism. This syndrome is most commonly associated with mild renal insufficiency caused by diabetic nephropathy, but may also be seen in a variety of other disorders including chronic interstitial nephritis, sickle-cell disease, HIV nephropathy, and obstructive uropathy. The clinical presentation of this syndrome is often exacerbated by pharmacologic therapy with agents that can interfere with the renin-angiotensin-aldosterone axis such as β-adrenergic blockers, angiotensin-converting enzyme inhibitors, angiotensin receptor blockers, and nonsteroidal anti-inflammatory drugs. Heparin may induce the syndrome by inhibiting adrenal aldosterone biosynthesis. Patients with this form of RTA are able to maximally acidify their urine (urine pH < 5.5).[4] The primary defect in acid excretion is impaired ammoniagenesis caused by mild renal insufficiency. Hyperaldosteronism predisposes to the development of hyperkalemia, which results in further impairment of ammoniagenesis. Treatment to control the hyperkalemia is usually sufficient to reverse the metabolic acidosis, and mineralocorticoid replacement is frequently unnecessary.

Hyperkalemic distal (Type IV) RTA resulting from generalized distal tubule defects is less common than hyporeninemic-hypoaldosteronism, but is more common than classic distal (Type I) RTA. Patients with this defect have impaired tubular potassium secretion in addition to impaired urinary acidification (urine pH > 5.5 despite acidemia or acid loading). Urinary obstruction is the most frequent cause of this disorder which may also be associated with sickle-cell nephropathy, lupus erythematosus, HIV nephropathy, analgesic abuse nephropathy, amyloidosis, renal transplant rejection, and chronic cyclosporine nephrotoxicity.

Proximal (Type II) RTA is characterized by defects in proximal tubular reabsorption of bicarbonate. Normally, more than 85% of filtered bicarbonate is reabsorbed in the proximal tubule. Defects in proximal tubular bicarbonate reabsorption result in increased delivery of bicarbonate to the distal nephron, which has a limited capacity for bicarbonate reabsorption. As a result, at a normal serum bicarbonate concentration, the filtered bicarbonate load is incompletely reabsorbed, and is lost in the urine. As the serum bicarbonate concentration falls, the filtered load of bicarbonate is proportionately decreased. A new equilibrium is established where the kidney is able to reabsorb the filtered bicarbonate load, albeit at a reduced serum bicarbonate concentration. Thus, patients with proximal RTA present with a chronic, nonprogressive hyperchloremic metabolic acidosis. These patients are able to acidify their urine in response to an acid load, but develop bicarbonaturia at a reduced serum bicarbonate concentration following bicarbonate loading. The impaired bicarbonate reabsorption results in salt wasting and secondary hyperaldosteronism. Hypokalemia, which may be severe, develops as a result of the hyperaldosteronism and bicarbonaturia.[4,11] Unlike patients with classic distal (Type I) RTA, the hyperkalemia in proximal RTA is exacerbated by alkali replacement. Proximal RTA may develop as an isolated defect or it may be associated with generalized proximal tubular dysfunction (Fanconi's syndrome), with impaired proximal tubular glucose, phosphate, and amino acid reabsorption. Proximal RTA usually presents as an acquired disorder, secondary to a variety of diseases (amyloidosis, multiple myeloma, or nephrotic syndrome) or exposure to toxins (lead, cadmium, mercury, or outdated tetracyclines). Pharmacologic therapy with carbonic anhydrase inhibitors produces an iatrogenic form of proximal RTA.

ELEVATED ANION GAP METABOLIC ACIDOSIS

Metabolic acidosis with an increased anion gap commonly results from increased endogenous organic acid production. In lactic acidosis, lactic acid accumulates as a byproduct of anaerobic metabolism. Accumulation of the ketoacids β-hydroxybutyric acid and acetoacetic acid defines the ketoacidosis of uncontrolled diabetes mellitus, alcohol intoxication and starvation (see Table 53–5). In advanced renal failure, accumulation of phosphate, sulfate and organic anions is responsible for the increased anion gap, which is usually less than 24 mEq/L.[12] The severe metabolic acidosis seen in myoglobinuric acute renal failure caused by rhabdomyolysis may be caused by the metabolism of large amounts of sulfur-containing amino acids released from myoglobin.[14]

The presence of mild elevations in the anion gap cannot be automatically attributed to the presence of a high anion gap metabolic acidosis. Elevations in the anion gap have been observed in as many as 47% of hospitalized patients.[14] A variety of factors may contribute to this nonspecific elevation in the anion gap, including the presence of alkalemia, which increases the anionic charge of albumin and other plasma proteins. The usefulness of the anion gap as a marker of acid-base status is dependent on proper interpretation of a patient's clinical status.[15] Despite these limitations, when the anion gap exceeds 20–25 mEq/L a significant organic acidosis is likely to be present.[16]

High anion gap metabolic acidosis may develop in many clinical settings, including uncontrolled diabetes mellitus (see Chap. 74), alcohol intoxication (see Chaps. 37 and 67), and starvation (see Chap. 64). Toxic ingestions of methanol, ethylene glycol, and salicylates are also associated with high anion gap metabolic acidosis (see Chap. 9). The mechanisms responsible for the development of acidosis in these settings are diverse.

Lactic Acidosis

Lactic acidosis is one of the most common causes of high anion gap metabolic acidosis. Lactic acid is the end product of anaerobic metabolism of glucose (glycolysis). In normal individuals, lactic acid, derived from pyruvate, enters the circulation in small amounts and is promptly removed by the liver. In the liver, and to a lesser extent in the kidney, lactic acid is reoxidized to pyruvic acid, which is then metabolized to CO_2 and H_2O. The normal plasma lactate concentration in healthy subjects is approximately 1 mEq/L.[9,17] The diagnosis of lactic acidosis should be considered in all patients with metabolic acidosis associated with an increased anion gap. Lactic acidosis is considered

TABLE 53–6. Causes of Lactic Acidosis

Primary decrease in tissue oxygenation
Shock
Severe anemia
Congestive heart failure
Asphyxia
Carbon monoxide poisoning
Deranged oxidative metabolism
Diabetes mellitus
Liver failure
Malignancy
Seizures
Medications (iron, isoniazid, metformin, salicylates)
Methanol, ethanol, ethylene glycol
Disorders associated with inborn errors of metabolism

to be present when lactate concentrations exceed 4–5 mEq/L in an acidemic patient.

Classically, lactic acidosis has been differentiated into disorders associated with tissue hypoxia (type A lactic acidosis) and disorders associated with deranged oxidative metabolism (type B lactic acidosis), although the distinction between them is blurred (Table 53–6). The etiologies of lactic acidosis can also be categorized on the basis of changes in lactate production and/or utilization.[4,18] Metabolic disturbances can result in increased tissue pyruvate production or impaired utilization, with proportional increases in lactate concentrations. Increased lactate production is more commonly associated with alterations in tissue redox state, resulting in preferential conversion of pyruvate to lactate. During anaerobic metabolism, nicotinamide adenine dinucleotide (NADH) accumulates, driving the conversion of pyruvate to lactate and increasing the lactate to pyruvate ratio. States of enhanced metabolic activity (e.g., grand mal seizures, strenuous exercise, hyperthermia), decreased tissue oxygen delivery (e.g., severe anemia, hypoxia, circulatory shock, carbon monoxide poisoning) or impaired oxygen utilization (e.g., cyanide toxicity) all are associated with lactic acidosis. Impaired hepatic clearance of lactate, as seen in hypoperfusion states, liver failure, and alcohol intoxication may also result in lactic acidosis.

Cardiovascular and septic shock, with resultant tissue hypoperfusion are the most common causes of lactic acidosis. Poor tissue perfusion and hypoxia influence enzymatic pyruvate and lactate metabolism to stimulate anaerobic glycolysis and to decrease lactate utilization. This leads to hyperlactatemia and lactic acidosis. Although the mortality rate of this type of lactic acidosis may be as high as 80% and correlates with the degree of hyperlactatemia, the acidemia and blood lactate levels are more likely markers of severity of illness than mediators of morbidity and mortality.

Lactic acidosis associated with liver disease, drugs (e.g., metformin), toxins, and congenital enzyme deficiency may be due to deranged oxidative metabolism or impaired lactate clearance.[4] The exact role of diabetes mellitus in the induction of lactic acidosis is not clear. It may involve a decrease in pyruvate dehydrogenase activity, the enzyme responsible for pyruvate metabolism. Lactic acidosis in neoplastic disease is uncommon and reported mostly in patients with myeloproliferative disorders. Leukocytes and neoplastic cells in general have high rates of glycolysis. In the case of a large tumor or tightly packed bone marrow, oxygenation can be decreased, favoring the accumulation of lactate. Lactic acidosis has been reported in patients with massive liver tumors, and it has been postulated that the liver uptake of lactate is decreased in these patients. Lactic acidosis associated with seizures is usually transient and occurs because of excessive muscle activity.[9]

CLINICAL PRESENTATION

Chronic metabolic acidosis is usually not associated with severe acidemia and is relatively asymptomatic. The major manifestations are on the bones, where chronic acidemia causes bone demineralization with the development of rickets in children and osteomalacia and osteopenia in adults. In infants and children, chronic metabolic acidosis is associated with growth failure and short stature and may be associated with nonspecific symptoms including anorexia, nausea, weight loss, and muscle weakness.

Severe metabolic acidosis is usually associated with acute processes. The manifestations of severe acidemia (pH < 7.15–7.20) involve the cardiovascular, respiratory, and central nervous systems (Table 53–7). Hyperventilation is often the first sign of metabolic acidosis. At a pH of 7.2, pulmonary ventilation increases about fourfold and an eightfold increase has been noted at a pH of 7.0.[19] Respiratory compensation may occur as Kussmaul's respirations—the deep, rapid respirations seen commonly in patients with diabetic ketoacidosis. In extremely severe acidosis (pH < 6.8), central nervous system (CNS) function is disrupted to such a degree that the respiratory center is depressed.

CNS depression correlates more closely with spinal fluid pH than with blood pH. For this reason, neurologic symptoms tend to occur more frequently and to a greater degree in patients with respiratory acidosis, because the CO_2 accumulated in the respiratory form readily crosses the blood-brain barrier to cause acidosis in the CNS.[1] Because of the slow penetration of administered bicarbonate into the CNS, the CNS pH fails to normalize as rapidly as blood pH. Therefore, patients continue to hyperventilate because of sustained CNS acidity and severe respiratory alkalosis may occur. Sustained lowering of Pa_{CO_2} within 12 to 36 hours is to be anticipated during the correction of any metabolic acidosis.[1]

Systemic acidosis can cause peripheral arteriolar dilatation characterized by flushing, a rapid heart rate, and wide pulse pressure. Initially, cardiac output may be increased, but as acidosis becomes more

TABLE 53–7. Major Adverse Consequences of Severe Acidemia

Cardiovascular
Impairment of cardiac contractility
Arteriolar dilatation, venoconstriction
Increased pulmonary vascular resistance
Reductions in cardiac output, arterial blood pressure, and hepatic and renal blood flow
Sensitization to reentrant arrhythmias and reduction in threshold of ventricular fibrillation
Attenuation of cardiovascular responsiveness to catecholamines
Respiratory
Hyperventilation
Decreased strength of respiratory muscles and promotion of muscle fatigue
Dyspnea
Metabolic
Increased metabolic demands
Insulin resistance
Inhibition of anaerobic glycolysis
Reduction in ATP synthesis
Hyperkalemia
Increased protein degradation
Cerebral
Inhibition of metabolism and cell-volume regulation
Obtundation and coma

Adapted from Ref. 17.

severe, myocardial contractility becomes impaired and cardiac output falls. Experimental work in animals has demonstrated that cardiac contractility decreases as pH declines to values of 7.0 or less by infusion of lactic acid.[20] In contrast, the effects of vagal stimulation were enhanced at pH levels lower than 7.1, probably as a consequence of inhibition of acetylcholinesterase. This increases the danger of vagally mediated bradycardia and heart block during acidosis.

Gastrointestinal symptoms of metabolic acidosis include loss of appetite, nausea, and vomiting. Severe acidosis (pH < 7.1) interferes with carbohydrate metabolism and insulin utilization, and results in hyperglycemia. Metabolic acidosis alters potassium homeostasis and contributes to the development of hyperkalemia. The magnitude of the effect on serum potassium depends on the type of acidosis: Acidosis caused by mineral acids (e.g., hydrochloric acid) are associated with a greater change in potassium levels than acidosis caused by organic acids (e.g., lactic acidosis), in which the increase in potassium attributable to the acidosis per se is minimal.

COMPENSATION

The patient's primary means to compensate for metabolic acidosis is to increase carbon dioxide excretion by increasing respiratory rate. This results in a decrease in Pa_{CO_2}. This ventilatory compensation results from stimulation of the respiratory center by changes in cerebral bicarbonate concentration and pH.[1] Respiratory compensation begins rapidly (within 15 to 30 minutes) but does not reach a steady state for 12 to 24 hours after the onset of metabolic acidosis. For every 1 mEq/L decrease in bicarbonate concentration below the average of 24, the Pa_{CO_2} decreases by about 1.0–1.5 mm Hg from the normal value of 40 (see Table 53–4).

The anticipated Pa_{CO_2}, associated with a given bicarbonate concentration, for patients with uncomplicated metabolic acidosis can be more precisely calculated as:[21]

$$Pa_{CO_2} = (1.5 \times [HCO_3^-]) + 8 \pm (2 \times SEM)$$

where 1.0 is the standard error of the mean (SEM) of the relationship of HCO_3^- to Pa_{CO_2}. For example, 95% of patients with a plasma bicarbonate of 16 mEq/L should have an arterial P_{CO_2} of 30–34 mm Hg. An observed arterial P_{CO_2} within this range is consistent with physiologic respiratory compensation for a metabolic acidosis and suggests that there is no respiratory disturbance. In contrast, if the P_{CO_2} is less than 30 mm Hg, a superimposed respiratory alkalosis could be diagnosed, whereas if the P_{CO_2} is greater than 34 mm Hg, a superimposed respiratory acidosis is present.

▶ TREATMENT: Metabolic Acidosis

CHRONIC METABOLIC ACIDOSIS

Asymptomatic patients with mild to moderate degrees of acidemia (plasma bicarbonate of 12–20 mEq/L; pH of 7.2–7.4) do not require emergent therapy. They can usually be managed with gradual correction of the acidemia, over a period of days to weeks, using oral sodium bicarbonate or other alkali preparations (Table 53–8). A systemic approach to the management of metabolic acidosis in patients with renal failure is described in Chap. 45.

In all forms of chronic metabolic acidosis, primary therapy should be directed at treating the underlying disease state.

TABLE 53–8. Therapeutic Alternatives for Oral Alkali Replacement

Generic Name	Trade Name(s)	mEq Alkali	Dosage Form (s)	Comment
Shohl's solution Sodium citrate/citric acid	Bicitra (Willen)	1 mEq Na/mL; equivalent to 1 mEq bicarbonate	Solution (500 mg Na citrate, 334 mg citric acid/5 mL)	Citrate preparations increase absorption of aluminum
Sodium bicarbonate	Various (e.g., Rugby)	3.9 mEq bicarbonate/tablet (325 mg) 7.8 mEq bicarbonate/tablet (650 mg)	325 mg tablet 650 mg tablet	Bicarbonate preparations may cause bloating owing to CO_2 production
	Baking soda (various)	60 mEq bicarbonate/tsp (5 g/tsp)	Powder	
Potassium citrate	Urocit-K (Mission)	5 mEq citrate/tablet	5 mEq tablet	See above
Potassium bicarbonate/potassium citrate	K-Lyte (Bristol) K-Lyte DS (Bristol)	25 mEq bicarbonate/tablet 50 mEq bicarbonate/tablet (DS)	25 mEq tablet (effervescent) 50 mEq tablet (effervescent)	See above
Potassium citrate/citric acid	Polycitra-K (Willen)	2 mEq K/mL;equivalent to 2 mEq bicarbonate 30 mEq bicarbonate/UD packet	Solution (1100 mg K citrate, 334 mg citric acid/5 mL) Crystals for reconstitution (3300 mg K citrate, 1002 mg citric acid/UD packet)	See above
Sodium citrate/potassium citrate/citric acid	Polycitra (Willen) Polycitra-LC (Willen)	1 mEq K, 1 mEq Na/mL; equivalent to 2 mEq bicarbonate	Syrup (Polycitra) Solution (Polycitra-LC) (Both contain 550 mg K citrate, 500 mg Na citrate, 334 mg citric acid/5 mL)	See above

Gastrointestinal pathology should be treated to reduce ongoing bicarbonate losses, and factors that exacerbate RTA should be treated. If acidemia persists, alkali therapy should be instituted, with the goal of normalization of blood pH. The loading dose of alkali to initially correct the acidemia can be calculated as follows:[22]

$$\text{Loading dose (mEq)} = (V_DHCO_3^- \times \text{body weight [BW]})\ (\text{desired }[HCO_3^-] - \text{current }[HCO_3^-])$$

For a 60-kg patient with a serum bicarbonate of 15 mEq/L,

$$\begin{aligned}\text{Loading dose (mEq)} &= (0.5\text{ L/kg} \times 60\text{ kg}) \times (24\text{ mEq/L} \\ &\quad -15\text{ mEq/L}) \\ &= 30\text{ L} \times 9\text{ mEq/L} \\ &= 270\text{ mEq}\end{aligned}$$

The calculated loading dose of alkali should be administered over several days to avoid volume overload from the accompanying sodium load. For this scenario, a regimen of 60–70 mEq tid for 3 to 5 days should result in an increase in HCO_3 levels toward normal. In addition to the calculated loading dose, supplemental alkali must also be provided to replace ongoing losses, which can be approximated to be 2 mEq/kg/d (the mean of the range) or 40 mEq tid. In patients with associated volume depletion, bicarbonate replacement can be provided simultaneous with volume resuscitation by substituting bicarbonate for chloride in intravenous crystalloid solutions.

In patients with chronic metabolic acidosis because of gastrointestinal bicarbonate losses, maintenance therapy should provide sufficient alkali to replace ongoing bicarbonate losses. The magnitude of this replacement is variable and substantial (>10 mEq/kg/d). In addition, associated losses of other electrolytes, such as potassium and magnesium, may be required.

Proximal (type II) RTA is a bicarbonate-wasting disorder that requires the administration of large maintenance doses of alkali (10–15 mEq/kg/d). As alkali replacement raises the serum bicarbonate concentration toward normal, the proximal tubule's capacity to reabsorb bicarbonate is overwhelmed and renal bicarbonate wasting increases. Potassium supplementation is always necessary, as the bicarbonaturia resulting from alkali therapy increases the renal potassium wasting. In children, aggressive therapy of proximal RTA is necessary to avoid growth retardation and osteopenia. Because this is generally a mild, nonprogressive acidosis in adults, the benefit of alkali therapy is frequently outweighed by the risks of increased potassium wasting.

In patients with classic distal (type I) RTA, maintenance therapy usually requires only enough alkali to buffer the amount of acid generated from dietary intake and metabolism. This usually approximates 1–3 mEq/kg/d. After initial potassium deficits are replaced, ongoing potassium supplementation may not be required, as renal potassium losses decrease following initiation of appropriate alkali therapy. The use of potassium alkali salts may, however, be desirable in patients with associated nephrolithiasis, because sodium salts may increase urinary calcium excretion.

The metabolic acidosis associated with hyperkalemic distal (type IV) RTA with hyporeninemic-hypoaldosteronemia, often seen in patients with diabetes mellitus, may be corrected by the treatment of hyperkalemia alone (see Chap. 52). The use of supplemental alkali (1–2 mEq/kg/d) to increase sodium intake and stimulate distal tubular potassium secretion may be beneficial. A minority of patients requires the administration of pharmacologic amounts of fludrocortisone.[1] Type IV RTA resulting from a generalized distal tubular often responds to low doses of alkali (1.5–2.0 mEq/kg/d).[23] Corrections of the acidosis along with modest dietary potassium restriction (to 1 mEq/kg/d) will often result in the maintenance of serum potassium levels of 5 mEq/L or less.

ACUTE SEVERE METABOLIC ACIDOSIS

The management of patients with life-threatening acute metabolic acidosis (plasma bicarbonate of ≤ 8 mEq/L and pH < 7.20) is dependent on the underlying cause and the patient's cardiovascular status. Effective treatment of the underlying cause of some organic acidoses (e.g., ketoacidosis) can result in the regeneration of bicarbonate within hours, thus mitigating the need for alkali therapy. Patients with hyperchloremic acidosis (e.g., diarrhea induced) are unable to regenerate bicarbonate, and the generation of new bicarbonate by the kidneys may require several days before one can observe a meaningful change in their status.[17] Thus, intravenous alkali therapy is often required for these patients. The role of alkali therapy in patients with severe lactic acidosis is controversial. Although conventional wisdom recommends the use of alkali replacement in patients with severe acidemia caused by the deleterious effects of acidemia on circulatory function,[9,17,18] studies have not demonstrated improved outcome with alkali replacement.[26–29]

There are several therapeutic alternatives available for the acute correction of severe metabolic acidosis. Sodium acetate, sodium citrate, and sodium lactate are unreliable sources of alkali because their alkalinizing effect is dependent on their oxidative conversion to bicarbonate. This process is often impaired in critically ill patients, especially those with liver disease or circulatory failure. Although sodium bicarbonate is the most widely used intravenous alkalitic agent,[17] several studies suggest that it is frequently ineffective and may actually be deleterious, especially in patients with lactic acidosis.[26–29] Two of the three remaining alternatives (Carbicarb and dichloroacetate) are investigational and not routinely available in most clinical practice settings. Tromethamine, or THAM, is a carbon dioxide-consuming, commercially available solution that buffers respiratory as well as metabolic acids.

SODIUM BICARBONATE

Although it has been recommended that sodium bicarbonate be administered to raise the arterial pH to about 7.15–7.20, there are no controlled clinical trials demonstrating that sodium bicarbonate administration is significantly better than general supportive care in reducing morbidity and mortality in these patients.[4,17,26–29] In theory, sodium bicarbonate administration provides fluid and electrolyte replacement and increases arterial pH, thereby improving cardiac function, perfusion and oxygenation of peripheral tissues, and intracellular pH, and should therefore decrease lactate production and increase clearance. However, sodium bicarbonate administration can actually have an adverse effect on intracellular pH. When bicarbonate is given by IV infusion, the carbon dioxide generated diffuses more readily than bicarbonate across cell membranes and into cerebrospinal fluid. Therefore, the intracellular pH can actually be decreased by administration of bicarbonate.[4]

Excessive sodium bicarbonate administration may result in (a) a shift of the oxyhemoglobin saturation curve to the left and, thereby, impaired oxygen release from hemoglobin to tissues; (b) sodium and water overload, with subsequent pulmonary congestion and hypernatremia; (c) paradoxical acidosis as a result of the production of CO_2 that freely diffuses into myocardial and cerebral cells;[31] and (d) decreased ionized calcium with resultant decreased myocardial contractility. If there is an endogenous source of bicarbonate, such as can occur in the case of ketoacidosis or lactic acidosis, a bicarbonate "overshoot" may develop because the ketoacids (acetoacetic acid and β-hydroxybutyric acid) or lactic acid are converted in the liver to bicarbonate once the underlying cause of acidosis is corrected.[17,32] Alkalosis may also result if too much is given too fast.[17]

If intravenous sodium bicarbonate is to be used, one must be mindful that the goals are to increase, not normalize, pH (to approximately 7.20) and plasma bicarbonate (to 8–10 mEq/L). There is no calculative method that will assure attainment of these goals with a given dose of sodium bicarbonate because of the multiplicity of competing processes that can affect acid-base status (vomiting, potential increases in endogenous acid production, renal failure) and the marked variability in the volume of distribution of bicarbonate (50% of BW in patients with mild acidosis to approximately 100% in those with severe acidosis).[22] Adrogue and Madias[17] recently recommended that the dose of sodium bicarbonate be calculated using a distribution volume of 50% of BW for all patients to avoid overtreatment. The total dose calculated as described previously in the RTA section should be administered as an infusion over one-half to several hours. Followup monitoring of arterial blood gases beginning no sooner than 30 minutes after the end of the infusion should be used to guide further therapeutic decisions.

Bicarbonate therapy is generally not necessary in the routine patient with cardiac arrest, even if the initial arrest was unmonitored. The standards and guidelines from the National Conference on Cardiopulmonary and Emergency Cardiac Care state that sodium bicarbonate is most useful in cardiac life support when combined with ventilation in an attempt to maintain near-normal arterial pH during an arrest.[33] During a cardiac arrest, sodium bicarbonate (initial dose 1 mEq/kg) may be administered by rapid, direct intravenous injection. It should be used only after more proven interventions such as defibrillation, cardiac compression, support of ventilation including intubation, and drug therapies such as epinephrine and antiarrhythmic agents have been employed. Subsequent doses of sodium bicarbonate should be based on measurements of arterial blood pH and $PaCO_2$.

TROMETHAMINE

THAM, available as a 0.3 N solution, is a highly alkaline, sodium-free organic amine that acts as a proton acceptor to prevent or correct acidosis.[34] Tromethamine combines with hydrogen ions from carbonic acid to form bicarbonate and a cationic buffer. THAM also acts as an osmotic diuretic to increase urine flow, urine pH, and the excretion of fixed acids, CO2, and electrolytes. At pH 7.4, 30% of THAM is not ionized and therefore is capable of reaching equilibrium with total body water. This portion may penetrate into cells and may neutralize acidic anions of the intracellular fluid. Intracellular pH increases have been noted within 1 hour after the infusion of THAM. There is, however, no clinical or physiologic evidence that this action is beneficial, or that THAM is more efficacious than sodium bicarbonate.[17,25]

When THAM is used, it must be administered slowly, with careful monitoring to avoid alkalosis. The usual empiric dosage range for tromethamine is 1–5 mmol/kg administered intravenously over 1 hour, but doses up to 1.25 mmol/kg may be given over 5 to 15 minutes in acute situations. The dose of THAM can be individualized using the following equation:[34]

$$\text{Dose of 0.3 N THAM (in mL)} = 1.1 \times \text{BW (in kg)} \times \left(\text{normal } \left[\text{HCO}_3^-\right] - \text{current } \left[\text{HCO}_3^-\right]\right)$$

The need for additional THAM is determined by serial measurements of the serum bicarbonate concentration and calculation of the base deficit: normal $[HCO_3^-]$ − current $[HCO_3^-]$. Large doses may cause respiratory depression as a result of an increase in blood pH and a decrease in $PaCO_2$ concentration.[25] Tromethamine solution is highly alkaline and may cause severe inflammation, vascular spasm, or tissue damage (necrosis, sloughing, pain, chemical phlebitis, thrombosis) if infiltration occurs. Hyperkalemia, hypoglycemia, hypocalcemia, and impaired coagulation have also been reported.[25,35] This agent should only be used with extreme caution in patients with severe liver or kidney failure.

CARBICARB

Carbicarb is an equimolar mixture of sodium carbonate (Na_2CO_3) and sodium bicarbonate ($NaHCO_3$).[36,37] It is no longer commercially available in Canada, and its use in the United States is still investigational. The carbonate ion is a stronger base than is bicarbonate and, thus, preferentially buffers hydrogen ions. The result of this reaction is the formation of bicarbonate rather than CO_2. Thus, Carbicarb limits, but does not eliminate, the generation of CO_2. Unlike bicarbonate, which can produce a paradoxical intracellular acidosis and thereby impair cardiac function, Carbicarb appears to correct intracellular acidosis if present.[38,39] In a prospective, double-blind, randomized, multicenter trial, Leung and colleagues[36] compared Carbicarb to sodium bicarbonate in surgical patients with mild intraoperative metabolic acidosis. Carbicarb proved as effective as sodium bicarbonate in correcting mild metabolic acidosis. Furthermore, cardiac output increased with Carbicarb as compared to sodium bicarbonate. Carbicarb also appears to be beneficial in the management of lactic acidosis.[38]

Although the optimal dosage of Carbicarb has not been determined, it can be approximated as:[36]

$$\text{Dose (in mEq of Na)} = 0.2 \text{ L/kg} \times \text{BW (in kg)} \times \text{(base deficit)}$$

The risk of hypervolemia and hypertonicity after Carbicarb administration is similar to that of bicarbonate. The small number of trials reporting the clinical utility of this agent and its continued investigational status in most of the world limits its use/availability for the foreseeable future.

DICHLOROACETATE

Dichloroacetate (DCA), another investigational agent, significantly lowers serum lactate levels and increases blood pH in patients with lactic acidosis.[40,41] DCA facilitates aerobic lactate metabolism by stimulating the activity of lactate dehydrogenase, reverses hyperlactatemia, and decreases morbidity in acquired and congenital forms of lactic acidosis. In a randomized, multicenter, placebo-controlled trial, Stacpoole et al.[40] studied the effects of DCA (50–100 mg/kg) in 252 patients with lactic acidosis. Serum lactate was significantly lowered and blood pH increased, but there was no improvement in patient outcome as compared to conventional management. A subsequent study in patients undergoing liver transplantation demonstrated that DCA attenuated lactate acid accumulation and reduced the need for bicarbonate therapy in this high-risk patient population.[30] The drug also improves cardiac output and left ventricular mechanical efficiency under conditions of myocardial ischemia or failure, probably by facilitating myocardial glucose utilization and inhibiting gluconeogenesis. DCA administration has also been reported to reverse the abnormal glucose metabolism, branch chain amino acid utilization, and muscle catabolism in septic patients.[42] DCA can cause a reversible peripheral neuropathy that may be ameliorated or prevented with thiamine supplementation. Mild drowsiness has been reported in approximately half of the adult recipients, but no other drug-related adverse effects have been reported.[40] The future role of DCA in the management of metabolic acidosis, particularly lactic acidosis, remains to be clarified. For the present, its use is limited by its investigational status.

METABOLIC ALKALOSIS

PATHOPHYSIOLOGY

Metabolic alkalosis is a simple acid-base disorder that presents as alkalemia (increased arterial pH) with an increase in plasma bicarbonate. It is an extremely common entity that is observed in 33% to 51% of hospitalized patients with acid-base disturbances.[43,44] Under normal circumstances, the kidney is readily able to excrete an alkali load. Thus, evaluation of patients with metabolic alkalosis must consider two separate issues: (a) the initial process that generates the metabolic alkalosis; and (b) alterations in renal function that maintain the alkalemic state.

Generation

The generation of metabolic alkalosis can result from excessive losses of H^+ via the gastrointestinal tract or kidneys or from the gain of exogenous, bicarbonate-rich fluids. The most common initiating event is the loss of chloride-rich, bicarbonate-poor fluid from the body as seen with diuretic use, nasogastric suctioning, or vomiting. Gastric secretory volume is usually less than 50 mL/h in the basal state but may increase fivefold with stimulation. The gastric juice is rich in chloride and H^+. In the gastric parietal cells, hydrogen ion and bicarbonate are generated from CO_2 and water.[46] The hydrogen ion is secreted into gastric fluid and the bicarbonate is retained in the ECF. Normally, an amount of bicarbonate equal to the bicarbonate generated in the stomach is eliminated in the alkaline pancreatic and small-bowel secretions, maintaining hydrogen ion balance. With vomiting and nasogastric suctioning, hydrogen ion is lost externally and metabolic alkalosis results. Chloride diarrhea, as seen with secretory villous adenomas and other secretory diarrheas may also result in gastrointestinal loss of chloride-rich, bicarbonate-poor fluid and the generation of metabolic alkalosis.

Diuretic therapy, with agents acting on the thick ascending limb of the loop of Henle (e.g., furosemide, bumetanide, and torsemide) and distal convoluted tubule (thiazides), is also a common mechanism for generation of metabolic alkalosis. These agents promote the excretion of sodium and potassium almost exclusively in association with chloride without a proportionate increase in bicarbonate excretion. Collecting duct hydrogen ion secretion is stimulated directly by the increased luminal flow rate and sodium delivery, and indirectly by intravascular volume contraction, which results in secondary hyperaldosteronism. Renal ammoniagenesis may also be stimulated by concomitant hypokalemia, further augmenting net acid excretion.

Increased renal acid excretion may also be the result of excess mineralocorticoid activity. Elevated mineralocorticoid levels directly stimulate collecting duct hydrogen ion secretion and indirectly increase ammoniagenesis by causing hypokalemia.[19] Increased mineralocorticoid activity may result from Cushing's syndrome, primary hyperaldosteronism, or hyperaldosteronism secondary to increased renin activity (e.g., malignant hypertension). In Bartter's and Gitelman's syndromes, defects in sodium transport in the loop of Henle (Bartter's) or distal convoluted tubule (Gitelman's) lead to hypokalemia, secondary hyperaldosteronism, and metabolic alkalosis,[53–55] In Liddle's syndrome, enhanced sodium reabsorption by the cortical collecting duct epithelial sodium channel results in a syndrome of pseudohyperaldosteronism.[45] The enzyme 11-β-hydroxysteroid dehydrogenase (11βOHSD) converts cortisol to cortisone, which is unable to bind to the mineralocorticoid receptor. Inhibition of 11βOHSD by glycyrrhizic acid, a major component of black licorice, or by carbenoxalone, permits activation of the mineralocorticoid receptor in the kidney by physiologic concentrations of glucocorticoids.[47]

Administration of high doses of doses of penicillins (e.g., ticarcillin) may produce metabolic alkalosis because they act as nonreabsorbable anions. High concentrations of poorly reabsorbable anions in the distal renal tubule increase luminal flow rate and luminal electronegativity, which enhance the secretion of potassium and hydrogen ion and result in hypokalemia and metabolic alkalosis.

Metabolic alkalosis may also be generated by the gain of exogenous alkali. This may be seen as a result of bicarbonate administration or from the infusion of organic anions that are metabolized to bicarbonate, such as acetate, lactate, and citrate. The milk-alkali syndrome was a previously common cause of metabolic alkalosis, in which patients with peptic ulcer disease developed metabolic alkalosis, nephrolithiasis, and nephrocalcinosis from the ingestion of large quantities of milk products and oral alkali. This syndrome has become increasingly uncommon with the advent of effective therapy for dyspeptic syndromes.

Maintenance

No matter which condition initiated the metabolic alkalosis, abnormalities in renal function underlie its maintenance. Normally, the kidneys are capable of excreting all of the excess bicarbonate presented to them, even during periods of increased bicarbonate loads.[4] As the serum bicarbonate concentration increases, the filtered bicarbonate load exceeds the maximal rate for bicarbonate reabsorption, and the excess bicarbonate is excreted in the urine. Under normal circumstances, the excess bicarbonate is rapidly excreted and metabolic alkalosis does not occur, or is corrected in a matter of hours.[46]

Several mechanisms may impair renal bicarbonate excretion, and contribute to the maintenance phase of metabolic alkalosis.[45] In general, these mechanisms can be divided into volume mediated processes (sodium chloride responsive) and volume-independent processes (sodium chloride resistant) that are predominately associated with excess mineralocorticoid activity and hypokalemia. The patient's response to volume replacement may be predicted by the urine chloride concentration, and permits the differential diagnosis of metabolic alkalosis as shown in Table 53–9.

Intravascular volume depletion maintains metabolic alkalosis through a number of mechanisms. Decreases in glomerular filtration

TABLE 53–9. Courses of Metabolic Alkalosis Differentiated on the Basis of Their Responsiveness to Sodium Chloride

Sodium chloride responsive (urinary chloride concentration < 10 mEq/L)
Gastrointestinal disorders
Vomiting
Gastric drainage
Villous adenoma of the colon
Chloride diarrhea
Diuretic therapy
Correction of chronic hypercapnia
Cystic fibrosis
Excessive bicarbonate therapy of an organic acidosis
Mild/moderate potassium deficiency
Sodium chloride resistant (urinary chloride concentration > 20 mEq/L)
Excess mineralocorticoid activity
Hyperaldosteronism
Cushing's syndrome
Bartter's syndrome
Gitelman's syndrome
Excessive black licorice intake
Profound potassium depletion
Magnesium deficiency
Liddle's syndrome
Unclassified
Alkali administration
Milk–alkali syndrome
Massive blood or plasmanate transfusion
Nonparathyroid hypercalcemia
Carbohydrate refeeding after starvation
Large doses of penicillin

rate reduce the filtered load of bicarbonate at any given serum concentration, thereby decreasing the kidney's ability to excrete a bicarbonate load. While this may play a role in patients with chronic renal insufficiency, it is also an important factor in patients in whom intravascular volume contraction accompanies metabolic alkalosis. Decreased effective arterial blood volume also enhances proximal and distal tubular sodium reabsorption. Sodium reabsorption must be coupled with reabsorption of an anion, such as chloride or bicarbonate, or exchange with a cation, such as potassium or hydrogen, in order to maintain charge neutrality. In the proximal tubule, increased sodium reabsorption stimulates bicarbonate reabsorption. In the distal nephron, enhanced sodium reabsorption, particularly in the setting of hypokalemia, stimulates hydrogen ion secretion.

Mineralocorticoid excess also plays a significant role in the maintenance of metabolic alkalosis. In patients with volume-responsive metabolic alkalosis, intravascular volume depletion stimulates aldosterone secretion. As discussed earlier, excess mineralocorticoid activity may also underlie the generation of metabolic alkalosis. In either situation, the increased mineralocorticoid effect stimulates collecting duct H^+-secretion. Metabolic alkalosis may also be maintained by persistent hypokalemia, Hypokalemia has a multitude of effects on renal acid-base homeostasis, enhancing proximal tubular bicarbonate reabsorption, stimulating ammoniagenesis and increasing distal tubular H^+ secretion[46].

CLINICAL PRESENTATION

There are no unique signs or symptoms associated with mild to moderate metabolic alkalosis, but patients may complain of symptoms related to the underlying cause of the disorder (e.g., muscle weakness with hypokalemia or postural dizziness with volume depletion). They may have a history of vomiting, gastric drainage, or diuretic use, all of which contribute to the development of metabolic alkalosis. Severe alkalemia (blood pH > 7.60) has been associated with cardiac arrhythmias, particularly in patients with heart disease, and hyperventilation with hypoxemia.[48] Neuromuscular irritability may be present, with signs of tetany or hyperactive reflexes, possibly caused by the decreased ionized calcium concentration that occurs secondary to the increase in pH. This decrease in ionized calcium may be caused by a conformational change in the albumin molecules, to which the calcium is bound, resulting in increased binding, or by decreased competition from hydrogen ions for binding sites on the albumin molecule. Mental confusion, muscle cramping, and paresthesia may also occur.

COMPENSATION

The respiratory response to metabolic alkalosis is hypoventilation, which results in an increased $Paco_2$. Using the Henderson Hasselbalchh equation, one can see that an increase in the $Paco_2$ will return the $[HCO_3^-]/Paco_2$ ratio, and therefore the pH, toward normal. Respiratory compensation is initiated when the central and peripheral chemoreceptors sense an increase in pH and occurs within hours. The $Paco_2$ increases 6–7 mm Hg for each 10 mEq/L increase in bicarbonate, up to a $Paco_2$ of about 50–60 mm Hg (see Table 53–4) before hypoxia sensors react to prevent further hypoventilation. If the $Paco_2$ is normal or less than normal, one should consider the presence of a superimposed respiratory alkalosis, which may be secondary to fever, gram-negative sepsis, or pain.

▶ TREATMENT: Metabolic Alkalosis

Treatment of metabolic alkalosis should be aimed at correcting the factor(s) responsible for the maintenance of the alkalosis. If the factors responsible for its generation are unresolved, interventional efforts should also focus on reducing or correcting them. For example, vomiting should be treated with antiemetics, gastric losses of H^+ during nasogastric suction may be modulated by giving H_2-histamine blockers such as ranitidine, or proton-pump inhibitors such as omeprazole, and reducing or discontinuing diuretic therapy.[45,48,51,52] Metabolic alkalosis will persist until the renal mechanism responsible for maintaining the disorder is corrected, despite the fact that the original cause of the elevated plasma bicarbonate may have resolved. For example, hypovolemia should be treated with sodium chloride (i.e., diuretic abuse, nasogastric suction) to allow excretion of bicarbonate by the kidney. However, patients with severely compromised cardiovascular function may not be able to tolerate this therapeutic approach. In situations such as this and/or the presence of life-threatening alkalosis, some have advocated reduction in pH by control of ventilation.[4] Although controlled hypoventilation, sometimes using inspired CO_2, with supplemental oxygen to prevent hypoxia, may be lifesaving,[4] this approach is not universally accepted.[45,48] Therapy for metabolic alkalosis can be conceptualized on the basis of the sodium chloride responsiveness of the disorders as shown in Fig. 53–5.

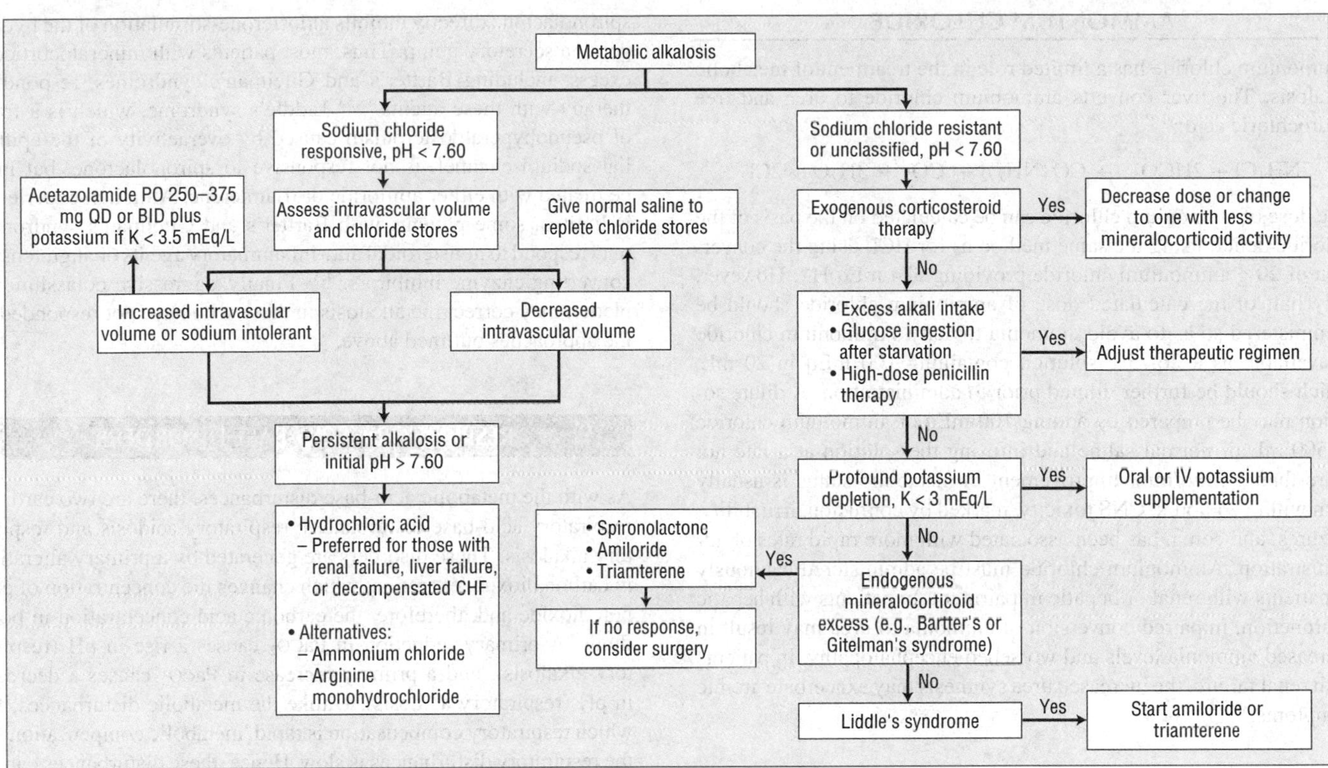

FIGURE 53–5. Treatment algorithm for patients with primary metabolic alkalosis.

SODIUM CHLORIDE-RESPONSIVE DISORDERS

Sodium chloride-responsive disorders usually result from volume depletion and chloride loss, which may accompany severe vomiting, prolonged nasogastric suction and diuretic therapy. Initially, therapy is directed at expanding intravascular volume and replenishing chloride stores. Sodium and potassium chloride containing solutions should be administered to patients who can tolerate the volume load.[45,48] Patients with metabolic alkalosis who are volume overloaded or intolerant to volume administration because of congestive heart failure, may benefit from the carbonic anhydrase inhibitor acetazolamide. This agent inhibits the action of carbonic anhydrase, thereby inhibiting renal bicarbonate reabsorption. Unfortunately, it also increases the renal losses of potassium and phosphate. Administration of acetazolamide (250–375 mg once or twice daily) may promote a sufficient bicarbonate diuresis and return the pH toward normal. However, because the clinical effectiveness of the drug declines as the HCO_3^- concentration falls, only rarely will this approach fully correct the alkalosis.[45]

Acidifying agents, including hydrochloric acid, ammonium chloride, and arginine monohydrochloride may be used to treat severe (pH > 7.6) symptomatic metabolic alkalosis. In general, this management is reserved for patients who are unresponsive to conventional fluid and electrolyte management or who are unable to tolerate the requisite volume load because of decompensated CHF or advanced renal failure.[45,48] Alternatively, hemodialysis using a low-bicarbonate dialysate may be used for the rapid correction of metabolic acidosis.

HYDROCHLORIC ACID

Hydrochloric acid is usually infused intravenously via a large central vein as a 0.1–0.25 N HCl solution in either 5% dextrose or normal saline, although sterile water has also been used. Extemporaneously prepared solutions can be made by adding 100–250 mEq of HCl through a 0.22-mm filter into a glass container of saline or dextrose. Hydrochloric acid may also be added to parenteral nutrient solutions and administered via a central line without serious degradation of proteins.[50] The rate of infusion should be 100–125 mL/h (10–25 mEq/h), with frequent monitoring of arterial blood gases. To prevent overcorrection, the infusion should be stopped when the arterial pH falls to 7.50.[46]

The dose of hydrochloric acid may be based on an estimate of the total body chloride deficit:[34]

$$\text{Dose HCl (mEq)} = [0.2\ \text{L/kg} \times \text{BW (kg)}] \times [103 - \text{observed serum chloride}]$$

where the estimated chloride space is 0.2 times the body weight and the average serum chloride is 103 mEq/L. Alternatively, the dose may be calculated based on the estimated base deficit:[48]

$$\text{Dose HCl (mEq)} = [0.5\ \text{L/kg} \times \text{BW (kg)}] \times (\text{desired } [HCO_3^-] - \text{observed } [HCO_3^-])$$

At present, there are no comparative data that address the relative accuracy of these two formulas for determining the dose of acid. The dose of hydrochloric acid is usually infused intravenously over 12 to 24 hours. Improvement is usually seen within 24 hours of initiating therapy. Arterial blood gases and serum electrolytes should be drawn every 4 to 12 hours to evaluate and adjust therapy. If the Pa_{CO_2} is markedly elevated because of respiratory compensation, the estimated dose of hydrochloric acid should be infused over at least 24 hours.[49] Otherwise, a severe transient respiratory acidosis may occur because of the slower reduction of the elevated bicarbonate concentration in the cerebrospinal fluid than in the extracellular fluid.

AMMONIUM CHLORIDE

Ammonium chloride has a limited role in the treatment of metabolic alkalosis. The liver converts ammonium chloride to urea and free hydrochloric acid:[34]

$$2NH_4Cl + 2HCO_3^- \rightarrow CO(NH_2)_2 + CO_2 + 3H_2O + 2Cl^-$$

The dose of ammonium chloride can be calculated on the basis of the chloride deficit using the same method as for HCl, using the conversion of 20 g ammonium chloride providing 374 mEq H^+. However, only half of the calculated dose of ammonium chloride should be administered so as to avoid ammonia toxicity. Ammonium chloride is available as a 26.75% solution containing 100 mEq in 20 mL, which should be further diluted prior to administration. A dilute solution may be prepared by adding 100 mEq of ammonium chloride to 500 mL of normal saline and infusing the solution at a rate not more than 1 mEq/min. Improvement in metabolic status is usually seen within 24 hours. CNS toxicity, marked by confusion, irritability, seizures, and coma, has been associated with more rapid rates of administration. Ammonium chloride must be administered cautiously to patients with renal or hepatic impairment. In patients with hepatic dysfunction, impaired conversion of ammonia to urea may result in increased ammonia levels and worsened encephalopathy. In patients with renal failure, the increased urea synthesis may exacerbate uremic symptoms.[34]

ARGININE MONOHYDROCHLORIDE

Arginine monohydrochloride at a dose of 10 g/h given intravenously has been used to treat metabolic alkalosis, although it was never FDA-approved for this purpose.[34] Although it has been stated that it was taken off the market because of the risk of severe hyperkalemia,[45] it is still commercially available. Like ammonium chloride, arginine must undergo metabolism by the liver to produce hydrogen ions, with a conversion of 100 g to 475 mEq. Unlike ammonium chloride, arginine combines with ammonia in the body to synthesize urea; thus, it may be used in patients with relative hepatic insufficiency. Patients with renal insufficiency should not receive arginine monohydrochloride because it may significantly elevate BUN and is associated with severe hyperkalemia.[34,35] The increase in potassium is caused by arginine-induced shifts of potassium from the intracellular to the extracellular space.

SODIUM CHLORIDE-RESISTANT DISORDERS

Sodium chloride-resistant disorders are commonly associated with hypermineralocorticoidism and are characterized by a high urinary chloride concentration. Life-threatening alkalemia is a very rare occurrence with these disorders. Management of these disorders usually consists of treatment of the underlying cause of mineralocorticoid excess. In patients in whom the mineralocorticoid excess cannot be corrected, chronic pharmacologic therapy may be required. Patients who are taking corticosteroids may require a dosage reduction or may need to be switched to a corticosteroid with less mineralocorticoid activity. Patients with an endogenous source of excess mineralocorticoid activity may require surgery or the administration of spironolactone, amiloride, or triamterene.[45,48]

Spironolactone is a competitive antagonist of the mineralocorticoid receptor. Amiloride and triamterene are potassium-sparing diuretics that inhibit the epithelial sodium channel in the distal convoluted tubule and collecting duct. All three agents inhibit aldosterone-stimulated sodium reabsorption in the collecting duct. In addition, spironolactone directly inhibits aldosterone-stimulation of the hydrogen ion secretory pump. Thus, most patients with mineralocorticoid excess, including Bartter's and Gitelman's syndromes, respond to therapy with these agents.[45,53] Liddle's syndrome, which is a form of pseudohyperaldosteronism caused by overactivity of the epithelial sodium channel, is not responsive to spironolactone, but may be treated with either amiloride or triamterene. Although experience is limited, some patients with Bartter's and Gitelman's syndromes may respond to nonsteroidal anti-inflammatory agents or angiotensin-converting enzyme inhibitors.[54,55] Finally, aggressive potassium repletion may correct the alkalosis in those who have not responded to the approaches outlined above.

RESPIRATORY ACID-BASE DISORDERS

As with the metabolic acid-base disturbances, there are two cardinal respiratory acid-base disturbances: respiratory acidosis and respiratory alkalosis. These disorders are generated by a primary alteration in carbon dioxide excretion, which changes the concentration of carbon dioxide and, therefore, the carbonic acid concentration in body fluids. A primary reduction in $Pa{CO_2}$ causes a rise in pH (respiratory alkalosis), and a primary increase in $Pa{CO_2}$ causes a decrease in pH (respiratory acidosis). Unlike the metabolic disturbances, for which respiratory compensation is rapid, metabolic compensation for the respiratory disturbances is slow. Hence, these disturbances can be further divided into acute disorders, with duration of minutes to hours that is too short for metabolic compensation to have occurred, and chronic disorders, that have been present long enough for metabolic compensation to be complete.

RESPIRATORY ALKALOSIS

Respiratory alkalosis is characterized by a primary decrease in $Pa{CO_2}$ that leads to an elevation in pH. The $Pa{CO_2}$ falls when the excretion of CO_2 by the lungs exceeds the metabolic production of CO_2. It is the most frequently encountered acid-base disorder, occurring physiologically in normal pregnancy and in persons living at high altitudes. Respiratory alkalosis also occurs frequently among hospitalized patients (Table 53–10).

PATHOPHYSIOLOGY

A decrease in $Pa{CO_2}$ occurs when ventilatory excretion exceeds metabolic production. Because endogenous production of CO_2 is relatively constant, negative CO_2 balance is primarily caused by an increase in ventilatory excretion of CO_2 (hyperventilation). The metabolic production of CO_2, however, may be increased during periods of stress or with excess carbohydrate administration (e.g., parenteral nutrition). Hyperventilation may develop from an increase in neurochemical stimulation via either central or peripheral mechanisms or be the result of voluntary or mechanical (iatrogenic) hyperventilation.

A decrease in $Pa{CO_2}$ may occur in patients with cardiogenic, hypovolemic, or septic shock because oxygen delivery to the carotid and aortic chemoreceptors is reduced. This relative deficit in $Pa{O_2}$ stimulates an increase in ventilation. The hyperventilation in sepsis is also mediated via a central mechanism. Hyperventilation-induced respiratory alkalosis with an elevation in cardiac index and hypotension without peripheral vasoconstriction may therefore be an early sign of sepsis.

TABLE 53–10. Causes of Respiratory Alkalosis

Central stimulation of respiration
Anxiety
Pain
Fever
Brain tumors, vascular accidents
Head trauma
Pregnancy
Progesterone
Catecholamines, theophylline, nicotine
Salicylates
Peripheral stimulation of respiration
Pulmonary emboli
Congestive heart failure
Altitude
Asthma
Pulmonary shunts
Hypotension
Pneumonia
"Stiff lungs" without hypoxemia
Multiple mechanisms
Hepatic cirrhosis
Gram-negative sepsis
Mechanical or voluntary hyperventilation

CLINICAL PRESENTATION

Respiratory alkalosis may cause adverse neuromuscular, cardiovascular, and gastrointestinal effects. During periods of decreased $PaCO_2$, there is a decrease in cerebral blood flow, which may be responsible for symptoms of light-headedness, confusion, decreased intellectual functioning, syncope, and seizures. Nausea and vomiting may occur, probably as a result of cerebral hypoxia. In severe respiratory alkalosis, cardiac arrhythmias may occur, owing to sensitization of the myocardium to the arrhythmogenic effects of circulating catecholamines.[2] Acute respiratory alkalosis has no effect on blood pressure or cardiac output in awake individuals. Anesthetized patients, however, may experience a decrease in both cardiac output and blood pressure, possibly owing to the lack of a tachycardic response.[56]

The concentration of serum electrolytes may also be altered secondary to the development of respiratory alkalosis. The serum chloride concentration is usually slightly increased, and serum potassium concentration may be slightly decreased. Clinically significant hypokalemia can be a consequence of extreme respiratory alkalosis, although the effect is usually very small or negligible.[2,56] Serum phosphorus concentration may decrease by as much as 1.5–2.0 mg/dL because of the shift of inorganic phosphate into cells. Reductions in the blood ionized calcium concentration may be partially responsible for symptoms such as muscle cramps and tetany. Approximately 50% of calcium is bound to albumin, and an increase in pH results in an increase in binding secondary to increased dissociation in carboxyl groups on the albumin molecule.[56]

COMPENSATION

The initial response of the body to acute respiratory alkalosis is chemical buffering. Hydrogen ions are released from the body's buffers—intracellular proteins, phosphates, and hemoglobin—and titrates down the serum bicarbonate concentration. This process occurs within minutes. Acutely, the bicarbonate concentration is decreased by a maximum of no more than 3.0 mEq/L for each 10 mm Hg decrease in $PaCO_2$[19] (see Table 53–4). When only the physicochemical buffering has occurred, the disturbance is referred to as acute respiratory alkalosis.

Metabolic compensation occurs when respiratory alkalosis persists for more than 6 to 12 hours. In response to the alkalemia, proximal tubular bicarbonate reabsorption is inhibited and the serum bicarbonate concentration falls. Renal compensation is usually complete within 1 to 2 days. The renal bicarbonaturia, as well as decreased NH_4^+ and titratable acid excretion, are direct effects of the reduced $PaCO_2$ and pH on renal reabsorption of chloride and bicarbonate.[2] The acuity of the respiratory alkalosis can be assessed on the basis of the degree of renal compensation (see Table 53–4). In fully compensated respiratory alkalosis, the bicarbonate concentration falls by 4 mEq/L below 24 for each 10 mm Hg drop in $PaCO_2$. For example, a sustained decrease in $PaCO_2$ of 20 mm Hg will lower serum bicarbonate from 24 to 14 mEq/L with a resultant pH of 7.46. Bicarbonate concentrations differing from those anticipated using the preceding guidelines suggest a mixed acid-base disorder (refer to Fig. 53–4).

▶ TREATMENT: Respiratory Alkalosis

Because most patients with respiratory alkalosis, especially chronic cases, have few or no symptoms and pH alterations are usually mild (pH not exceeding 7.50), treatment is often not required.[48] The first consideration in the treatment of acute respiratory alkalosis with pH > 7.50 is the identification and correction of the underlying cause. Relief of pain, correction of hypovolemia with intravenous fluids, treatment of fever or infection, treatment of salicylate overdose, and other direct measures may prove effective. A rebreathing device, such as a paper bag, may be useful in controlling hyperventilation in patients with the anxiety/hyperventilation syndrome. Oxygen therapy should be initiated in patients with severe hypoxemia. Patients with life-threatening alkalosis (pH > 7.60) and complications such as arrhythmia or seizures may require mechanical ventilation with sedation and/or paralysis to control hyperventilation. Simple respiratory alkalosis rarely requires such aggressive therapy, but it may be necessary for patients with mixed respiratory and metabolic alkalosis.

Respiratory alkalosis in patients receiving mechanical ventilation is usually iatrogenic. It may often be corrected by decreasing the minute ventilation (i.e., the number of mechanical breaths per minute times the volume delivered), although other measures can also be employed. The use of a capnograph and spirometer in the breathing circuit enables a more precise adjustment of the ventilator settings. Another method of treating respiratory alkalosis is to increase the amount of dead space in the ventilator circuit by placing a known length of tubing between the artificial airway and the "Y" piece of the ventilator. This results in "rebreathing" of expired gas and, therefore, an increase in the inspired carbon dioxide concentration, which should increase the carbon dioxide tension of the patient, correcting the respiratory alkalosis. In patients breathing more rapidly than the ventilator settings, sedation with or without paralysis may be beneficial.

TABLE 53–11. Causes of Acute Respiratory Acidosis

Perfusion abnormalities
Massive pulmonary embolism
Cardiac arrest
Airway and pulmonary abnormalities
Severe pulmonary edema
Severe pneumonia
Smoke inhalation
Pneumothorax
Severe bronchospasm
Adult respiratory distress syndrome
Airway obstruction: foreign body, laryngeal edema
Aspiration of vomitus
Neuromuscular abnormalities
Trauma, stroke
Narcotic or sedative overdose
Brainstem or cervical cord injury
Guillain-Barré syndrome
Myasthenia gravis
Status epilepticus
Mechanical ventilator
Ventilator malfunction
Inadequate frequency or tidal volume settings
Large dead space
Total parenteral nutrition (increased CO_2 production)

RESPIRATORY ACIDOSIS

PATHOPHYSIOLOGY

Respiratory acidosis, a primary retention of carbon dioxide that lowers the pH, results from a failure of the lungs to excrete carbon dioxide normally. This may be the result of neuromuscular diseases that inhibit central control of ventilation or neuromuscular function, intrinsic airway or parenchymal pulmonary disease, or interruption in pulmonary perfusion (Table 53–11). Acute respiratory acidosis with hypoxemia, hypercarbia, and acidosis is life-threatening. Those disorders that produce an increase in $Paco_2$ and hypoxemia to a degree compatible with life (e.g., chronic obstructive pulmonary disease), with or without oxygen therapy, may result in chronic respiratory acidosis (Table 53–12). These patients can function normally without noticeable neurologic defects with $Paco_2$ concentrations in the range of 90–100 mm Hg (normal, 40 mm Hg), provided adequate oxygenation is maintained.[56]

CLINICAL PRESENTATION

Respiratory acidosis may produce neuromuscular symptoms, including altered mental status, abnormal behavior, seizures, stupor, and coma. Hypercapnia may mimic stroke or CNS tumors by producing headache, papilledema, focal paresis, and abnormal reflexes. Carbon dioxide acts as a vasodilator in the brain, thus causing an increase in cerebral blood flow.[2] This increase in cerebral blood flow is thought to be partially responsible for the CNS symptoms. The CNS response to hypercapnia is extremely variable between patients and is also

TABLE 53–12. Causes of Chronic Respiratory Acidosis

Neuromuscular abnormalities
Brainstem infarct
Obesity–hypoventilation (Pickwickian) syndrome
Tumors
Poliomyelitis
Multiple sclerosis
Diaphragmatic paralysis
Pulmonary abnormalities
Chronic obstructive pulmonary disease
Kyphoscoliosis
Interstitial pulmonary disease
Overzealous parenteral feeding

influenced by the acuity of presentation. Chronic hypercapnia blunts the usual respiratory stimulus resulting from increased $Paco_2$. In patients with severe chronic respiratory acidosis, hypoxemia rather than hypercapnia provides the primary ventilatory stimulus.[56]

The degree to which cardiac contractility and heart rate are altered depends on the severity of the acidosis and the rapidity with which it develops. Modest acute hypercapnia ($Paco_2$ of 50–55 mm Hg) stimulates a stress-like response, with elevated catecholamines and corticosteroid hormone levels, and can result in increased cardiac output and pulmonary artery pressure.[57] As the severity increases, cardiac output declines and vascular resistance decreases. Refractory hypotension may be present in some patients.[2]

In respiratory acidosis, the serum potassium concentration increases modestly secondary to cellular shifts. The increases are less than those seen with inorganic metabolic acidosis and are difficult to predict for individual patients.[56]

COMPENSATION

The body responds to acute respiratory acidosis with chemical buffering. The increase in $Paco_2$ results in increased carbonic acid levels. The carbonic acid dissociates, releasing hydrogen ions, which are buffered by nonbicarbonate buffers (i.e., proteins, phosphate, Hemoglobin) and bicarbonate. Thus, on the basis of physicochemical factors, increases in $Paco_2$ raise the serum bicarbonate concentration. In general, in acute respiratory acidosis, the bicarbonate concentration increases by 1 mEq/L above 24 for each 10 mm Hg increase in $Paco_2$ above 40 (see Table 53–4).

Metabolic compensation occurs when respiratory acidosis is prolonged beyond 12 to 24 hours. In response to hypercapnia and acidemia, proximal tubular bicarbonate reabsorption, ammoniagenesis, and distal tubular hydrogen secretion are enhanced, resulting in an increase in serum bicarbonate concentration and raising the pH toward normal. Renal compensation for chronic hypercapnia generally results in the plasma bicarbonate concentration increasing by 4 mEq/L above 24 for each 10 mm Hg increase in $Paco_2$ above 40 (see Table 53–4). The new steady state in acid-base values is generally achieved within 5 days of the onset of hypercapnia in dogs; the time interval necessary for compensation in humans has not been established.

▶ TREATMENT: Respiratory Acidosis

The treatment of respiratory acidosis is dependent on the chronicity of the patient's condition. Respiratory decompensation in patients with chronic elevations in $Paco_2$ are frequently seen in those with acute infections and those recently started on narcotic analgesics or oxygen therapy.[48] Aggressive treatment of these conditions can offer considerable benefit and should be initiated. Furthermore, tranquilizers and sedatives should be avoided and supplemental oxygen, if used, should be minimized. Acute respiratory acidosis and acute respiratory acidosis superimposed on chronic respiratory acidosis are discussed in detail below.

ACUTE RESPIRATORY ACIDOSIS

When carbon dioxide excretion is severely impaired ($Pa{CO_2} > 80$ mm Hg) and/or life- threatening hypoxia is present ($Pa{O_2} < 40$ mm Hg), the immediate therapeutic goal is to provide adequate oxygenation. Under these circumstances, hypoxia, not acidemia, is the principle threat to life. A patent airway needs to be established, which may necessitate intubation. Excessive secretions must be cleared from the airway and oxygen administered to restore adequate oxygenation. Mechanical ventilation is likely to be required.

The underlying cause of the acidosis should be treated aggressively (e.g., bronchodilators for treatment of severe bronchospasm; discontinuing or reversing the effects of respiratory depressant drugs such as narcotics and benzodiazepines). Bicarbonate administration is rarely necessary in the treatment of respiratory acidosis. Furthermore, rapid correction of acidosis with bicarbonate may eliminate the patient's respiratory drive or precipitate a metabolic alkalosis. Cautious use of alkali (bicarbonate or THAM) can restore the responsiveness of bronchial muscles to β-adrenergic agonists and thus may be beneficial for those patients with severe bronchospasm.[58] Arterial blood gases should be monitored closely to ensure that the respiratory acidosis is resolving without creating a metabolic alkalosis as the result of compensatory elevation in HCO_3^- and decrease in $Pa{CO_2}$. Arterial blood gases should be obtained every 2 to 4 hours during the acute phase and less frequently (every 12 to 24 hours) as the acidosis improves.

ACUTE RESPIRATORY ACIDOSIS IN A COMPENSATED CHRONIC RESPIRATORY ACIDOTIC PATIENT

Patients with a history of chronic respiratory acidosis (e.g., those with chronic obstructive pulmonary disease) may experience an acute worsening of their respiratory acidosis. This may result in severe life-threatening hypoxemia. As with acute respiratory acidosis, the goals of therapy are maintenance of a patent airway and adequate oxygenation. Individuals with chronic respiratory acidosis are routinely able to tolerate a low $Pa{O_2}$ and an elevated $Pa{CO_2}$ because of compensation (increased number of red blood cells, hemoglobin content, and 2,3-diphosphoglycerate). The drive to breathe in these patients is dependent on hypoxemia rather than hypercarbia. Administration of oxygen to a patient with chronic respiratory acidosis can eliminate this drive to breathe and result in the syndrome of carbon dioxide narcosis. In this case, if the $Pa{O_2}$ is ≥ 50 mm Hg, no oxygen treatment is necessary. If the $Pa{O_2}$ is <50 mm Hg, oxygen therapy should be initiated carefully using a controlled flow of oxygen.[2]

Arterial blood gases should be checked periodically to ensure adequate oxygenation. If the $Pa{CO_2}$ increases during oxygen therapy, it may be a sign of impending carbon dioxide narcosis and oxygen therapy may need to be discontinued. The underlying cause of the acute exacerbation should be aggressively managed. Pulmonary infections should be treated with the appropriate antibiotics and bronchodilators administered as necessary. Excess secretions should be cleared from the airway to allow proper gas exchange. This may involve increasing oral fluid intake to decrease the viscosity of secretions, deep breathing, and postural drainage, suction, or bronchoscopy.

MIXED ACID-BASE DISORDERS

When two or more primary acid-base disturbances occur simultaneously, a mixed acid-base disorder results. A mixed disturbance can be suspected from the clinical setting and medical history, and can be diagnosed with this information together with arterial blood gas and electrolyte data.[2,17,48]

DIAGNOSIS

The diagnosis of a mixed disorder depends on an understanding of the appropriate quantitative response of the compensatory mechanisms for each of the simple acid-base disturbances. To diagnose mixed disorders, one must know how each of the four simple disorders alters pH, $Pa{CO_2}$, and $[HCO_3^-]$ (see Table 53–4). If a given set of blood gases does not fall within the range of expected responses for a simple acid-base disturbance (see Fig. 53–4), a mixed disorder should be suspected. In addition to laboratory information, a clinical evaluation of the patient is crucial. A thorough history and physical examination will often lead to the diagnosis, even before the laboratory data are available. Examples of common mixed disturbances follow.

MIXED RESPIRATORY ACIDOSIS AND METABOLIC ACIDOSIS

In mixed respiratory and metabolic acidosis, there is a failure of compensation. The respiratory disorder prevents the compensatory decrease in $Pa{CO_2}$ expected in the defense against metabolic acidosis. The metabolic disorder prevents the buffering and renal mechanisms from raising the bicarbonate concentration as expected in the defense against respiratory acidosis. In the absence of compensatory mechanisms, the pH decreases markedly.

Mixed respiratory and metabolic acidosis may develop in patients with cardiorespiratory arrest, in those with chronic lung disease who are in shock, and in metabolic acidosis patients who develop respiratory failure. This mixed disorder should be treated by responding to both the respiratory and metabolic acidosis. Improved oxygen delivery must be initiated to improve hypercarbia and hypoxia. Mechanical ventilation may be needed to reduce $Pa{CO_2}$. During the initial stage of therapy, appropriate amounts of alkali should be given to reverse the metabolic acidosis (see "Treatment: Metabolic Acidosis," earlier in this chapter).

MIXED RESPIRATORY ALKALOSIS AND METABOLIC ALKALOSIS

The combination of respiratory and metabolic alkalosis is the most common mixed acid-base disorder. This mixed disorder occurs frequently in critically ill surgical patients with respiratory alkalosis caused by mechanical ventilation, hypoxia, sepsis, hypotension, neurologic damage, pain, or drugs, and with metabolic alkalosis caused by vomiting or nasogastric suctioning and massive blood transfusions. It may also occur in patients with hepatic cirrhosis who hyperventilate, receive diuretics, or vomit, as well as in patients with chronic respiratory acidosis and an elevated plasma bicarbonate concentration who are placed on mechanical ventilation and undergo a rapid fall in $Pa{CO_2}$.

The decrease in bicarbonate concentration that usually compensates for respiratory alkalosis is prevented by the complicating metabolic alkalosis. Likewise, the increase in $PaCO_2$ expected to compensate for metabolic alkalosis is prevented by primary respiratory alkalosis. The failure of compensation that occurs with mixed respiratory and metabolic alkalosis may result in a severe alkalemia.

Correction of the metabolic component by administration of sodium chloride and potassium chloride solutions should be undertaken, and readjustment of the ventilator or treatment of an underlying disorder causing hyperventilation may correct or ameliorate the respiratory component of this mixed disorder.

MIXED METABOLIC ACIDOSIS AND RESPIRATORY ALKALOSIS

This mixed disorder is often seen in patients with advanced liver disease, salicylate intoxication, and pulmonary-renal syndromes. The respiratory alkalosis decreases the $PaCO_2$ beyond the appropriate range of the respiratory compensation for metabolic acidosis. The plasma bicarbonate concentration also falls below the level expected in compensation for a simple respiratory alkalosis. In a sense, the defense of pH for either disorder alone is enhanced; thus, the pH may be normal or close to normal, with a low $PaCO_2$ and a low $[HCO_3^-]$. Treatment of this disorder should be directed at the underlying cause. Because of the enhanced compensation, the pH is usually closer to normal than in either of the two simple disorders.

MIXED METABOLIC ALKALOSIS AND RESPIRATORY ACIDOSIS

This mixed disorder often occurs in patients with chronic obstructive pulmonary disease (COPD) and chronic respiratory acidosis who are treated with salt restriction, diuretics, and, possibly, glucocorticoids. When diuretics are initiated, the plasma bicarbonate may increase because of increased renal bicarbonate generation and reabsorption, providing mechanisms for both generating and maintaining metabolic alkalosis. The elevated pH diminishes respiratory drive and may therefore worsen the respiratory acidosis.

Although the pH may not deviate significantly from normal, treatment may need to be initiated to maintain PaO_2 and $PaCO_2$ at acceptable levels. Because it is often difficult to correctly identify this mixed disorder, it is helpful to observe the patient's response to discontinuation of diuretics and administration of sodium and potassium chloride.[2] If the patient has a simple metabolic alkalosis, the $PaCO_2$ will normalize, but it will only minimally affect the $PaCO_2$ if it is a mixed disorder. Treatment should be aimed at decreasing the plasma bicarbonate with sodium and potassium chloride therapy, thereby allowing the renal excretion of retained bicarbonate from the diuretic-induced metabolic alkalosis. This therapy should be used cautiously to avoid exacerbating any underlying congestive heart failure.

EVALUATION OF THERAPEUTIC OUTCOMES

Because acid-base disorders are such a common and widespread problem, pharmacists may play a key role in identifying, preventing, and properly treating acid-base abnormalities. Acid-base disorders do not occur only in the intensive care unit setting. Patients in ambulatory and extended care settings have many chronic conditions and drug therapies that commonly affect acid-base balance. Thus, pharmacists in all practice settings should use their knowledge to identify patients at high risk for developing drug-related problems and to undertake appropriate prevention and treatment measures to improve the quality of life of the patients they care for.

► PRINCIPLES OF PHARMACOTHERAPY

- Primary therapy of most acid-base disorders must include treatment or elimination of the underlying cause, not just correction of the pH and electrolyte disturbances.
- Loss of gastric acid from vomiting or nasogastric suctioning is often responsible for the development of a metabolic alkalosis, characterized by hypochloremia and hyperbicarbonatemia.
- Diarrhea and laxative abuse are common causes of metabolic acidosis, owing to the loss of bicarbonate in the stool.
- Aggressive diuretic therapy may produce a metabolic alkalosis, and the accompanying hypokalemia may be serious.
- Overly aggressive sodium bicarbonate therapy for the treatment of metabolic acidosis can frequently result in "overshoot" alkalosis, paradoxical transient CNS acidosis, hypernatremia, and hyperosmolality.
- The presence of a large anion gap metabolic acidosis may be the result of lactic acidosis, diabetic ketoacidosis, or substance intoxication (methanol, ethylene glycol, aspirin).
- In most cases of acute respiratory acidosis, such as following cardiopulmonary arrest, sodium bicarbonate therapy is not indicated and may be detrimental. Blood gas analysis should guide therapy.
- Significant drug-induced acid-base disorders are usually the result of an overdose; however, some medications can affect acid-base balance when ingested in therapeutic amounts; for example, progesterone derivatives; respiratory stimulants; barbiturates; benzodiazepines; opiates; β-blockers; lithium; metformin;, carbonic anhydrase inhibitors; diuretics;, and nitroprusside.

REFERENCES

1. Narins RG. Acid-base disorders: Definitions and introductory concepts. In: Narins RG, ed. Maxwell & Kleeman's Clinical Disorders of Fluid and Electrolyte Metabolism, 5th ed. New York, McGraw-Hill, 1994:765–768.
2. Kaehny WD. Pathogenesis and management of respiratory and mixed acid-base disorders. In: Schrier RW, ed. Renal and Electrolyte Disorders, 5th ed. Philadelphia, Lippincott-Raven, 1997:172–191.
3. Laski ME. Normal regulation of acid-base balance. Med Clin North Am 1983;67:771–780.
4. Shapiro JI, Kaehny WD. Pathogenesis and management of metabolic acidosis and alkalosis. In: Schrier RW, ed. Renal and Electrolyte Disorders, 5th ed. Philadelphia, Lippincott-Raven, 1997:130–169.
5. Halperin ML, Jungas RL, Cheema-Dhadli S, Brosnan JT. Disposal of the daily acid load: An integrated function of the liver, lungs and kidneys. Trends Biochem Sci 1987;12:197–199.
6. Weil MH, Rackow EC, Trenio R, et al. Difference in acid-base state between venous and arterial blood during cardiopulmonary resuscitation. N Engl J Med 1986;315:153–155.
7. Arbus GS. An in-vivo acid-base nomogram for clinical use. Can Med Assoc J 1973;109:291–293.
8. Broughton JO. Understanding Blood Gases. Madison, WI, Ohmeda, 1980.
9. Narins RG, Krishna GG, Yee J, et al. The metabolic acidoses. In: Narins RG, ed. Maxwell & Kleeman's Clinical Disorders of Fluid and Electrolyte Metabolism, 5th ed. New York, McGraw-Hill, 1994:769–826.
10. Winter SD, Pearson JR, Gabow PA, Schultz AL, Lepoff RB. The fall of the serum anion gap. Arch Intern Med 1990;150:311–313.
11. Halperin ML, Carlisle EJ, Donnelly S, et al. Renal tubular acidosis. In: Narins RG, ed. Maxwell & Kleeman's Clinical Disorders of Fluid and Electrolyte Metabolism, 5th ed. New York, McGraw-Hill, 1994:875–910.

12. Oster JR, Perez GO, Materson BJ. Use of the anion gap in clinical medicine. South Med J 1988;81:229–237.
13. McCarron DA, Elliot WC, Rose JS, et al. Severe mixed metabolic acidosis secondary to rhabdomyolysis. Am J Med 1979;67:905–908.
14. Lolekha PH, Lolekha S. Value of the anion gap in clinical diagnosis and laboratory evaluation. Clin Chem 1983;29:279–283.
15. Salem MM, Mujais SK. Gaps in the anion gap. Arch Intern Med 1992;152:1625–1629.
16. Gabow PA, Kaehny WD, Fennessey PV, et al. Diagnostic importance of an increased serum anion gap. N Engl J Med 1980;303:854–858.
17. Adrogue HJ, Madias NE. Management of life-threatening acid-base disorders. N Engl J Med 1998;338:26–34.
18. Kraut JA, Madias NE. Lactic acidosis. In: Adrogue HJ, ed. Contemporary Management in Critical Care, Vol 1. Baltimore, Williams & Wilkins, 1995:449–457.
19. Narins RG, Emmett M. Simple and mixed acid-base disorders: A practical approach. Medicine (Baltimore) 1980;59:161–187.
20. Teplinsky K, O'Toole M, Olman M, et al. Effect of lactic acidosis on canine hemodynamics and left ventricular function. Am J Physiol 1990;258:H1193–H1199.
21. Albert MS, Dell RB, Winters RW. Quantitative displacement of acid-base equilibrium in metabolic acidosis. Ann Intern Med 1964;66:312–322.
22. Kraut JA. The role of metabolic acidosis in the pathogenesis of renal osteodystrophy. Adv Ren Replace Ther 1995;2:40–51.
23. Morris RC, Ives HE. Inherited disorders of the renal tubule. In: Brenner BM, ed. Brenner and Rector's The Kidney, Vol II, 5th ed. Philadelphia, WB Saunders, 1996:1764–1827.
24. Kamel KS, Briceno LF, Sanchez MI, et al. A new classification for renal defects in net acid excretion. Am J Kidney Dis 1997;29:136–146.
25. Moon PF, Gabor L, Gleed RD, Erb HN. Acid-base, metabolic, and hemodynamic effects of sodium bicarbonate or tromethamine administration in anesthetized dogs with experimentally induced metabolic acidosis. Am J Vet Res 1997;58:771–776.
26. Sing RF, Branas CA, Sing RF. Bicarbonate therapy in the treatment of lactic acidosis: Medicine or toxin? J Am Ostepath Assoc 1995;95:52–57.
27. Cooper DJ, Walley KR, Wiggs BR, Russell JA. Bicarbonate does not improve hemodynamics in critically ill patients who have lactic acidosis: A prospective controlled clinical study. Ann Intern Med 1990;112:492–498.
28. Mizock BA. Lactic acidosis in critical illness. Crit Care Med 1992;20:80–93.
29. Forsythe SM, Schmidt GA. Sodium bicarbonate for the treatment of lactic acidosis. Chest 2000;117:260–267.
30. Shangraw RE, Winter R, Hromco J, Robinson ST, Gallaher EJ. Amelioration of lactic acidosis with dichloroacetate during liver transplantation in humans. Anesthesiology 1994;81:1127–1138.
31. Adrogue HJ, Rashad MN, Gorin AB, Yacoub J, Madias NE. Assessing acid-base status in circulatory failure: Differences between arterial and central venous blood. N Engl J Med 1989;320:1312–1316.
32. Faber MD, Kupin WL, Heiling CW, Narins RG. Common fluid-electrolyte and acid-base problems in the intensive care unit: Selected issues. Semin Nephrol 1994;14:8–22.
33. Emergency Cardiac Care Committee and Subcomittees, American Heart Association. Guidelines for cardiopulmonary resuscitation and emergency cardiac care. JAMA 1992;268:2171–2302.
34. Drug Information. American Hospital Formulary Service. 1998.
35. Marmarou A, Holdaway R, Ward JD, et al. Traumatic brain tissue acidosis: Experimental and clinical studies. Acta Neurochir 1993;57:160–164.
36. Leung JM, Landow L, Franks M, et al. Safety and efficacy of intravenous Carbicarb in patients undergoing surgery: Comparison with sodium bicarbonate in the treatment of mild metabolic acidosis. Crit Care Med 1994;22:1540–1549.
37. Shapiro JI. Functional and metabolic responses of the isolated heart during acidosis: Effects of sodium bicarbonate and Carbicarb. Am J Physiol 1990;258:H1835–H1839.
38. Shapiro JI. Pathogenesis of cardiac dysfunction during metabolic acidosis: Therapeutic implications. Kidney Int 1997;51:47–51.
39. Bersin RM, Arieff AI. Improved hemodynamic function during hypoxia with Carbicarb, a new agent for the management of acidosis. Circulation 1988;77:227–233.
40. Stacpoole PW, Wright EC, Baumgartner TG, et al. A controlled clinical trial of dichloroacetate for treatment of lactic acidosis. N Engl J Med 1992;327:1564–1569.
41. Stacpoole PW. The pharmacology of dichloroacetate. Metabolism 1989;38:1124–1144.
42. Vary TC, Siegel JH, Zechnich A, et al. Pharmacologic reversal of abnormal glucose regulation, BCAA utilization, and muscle catabolism in sepsis by dichloroacetate. J Trauma 1988;28:1301–1311.
43. Hodgkin JE, Soeprono FF, Chan DM. Incidence of metabolic alkalosis in hospitalized patients. Crit Care Med 1980;8:725–728.
44. Wilson RF, Gibson D, Percinel AK, et al. Severe alkalosis in critically ill patients. Arch Surg 1972;105:197–203.
45. Palmer BF, Alpern RJ. Metabolic alkalosis. J Am Soc Nephrol 1997;8:1462–1469.
46. Sabatini S, Kurtzman NA. Metabolic alkalosis. In: Narins RG, ed. Maxwell & Kleeman's Clinical Disorders of Fluid and Electrolyte Metabolism, 5th ed. New York, McGraw-Hill, 1994:933–956.
47. Farese RV Jr, Biglieri EG, Shackleton CH, et al. Licorice-induced hypermineralocorticoidism. N Engl J Med 1991;325:1223–1227.
48. Adrogue HJ, Madias NE. Management of life-threatening acid-base disorders II. N Engl J Med 1998;338:107–111.
49. Brimioulle S, Berre J, Dufaye P, et al. Hydrochloric acid infusion for treatment of metabolic alkalosis associated with respiratory acidosis. Crit Care Med 1989;17:232–236.
50. Mirtallo JM, Rogers KR, Johnson JA, et al. Stability of amino acids and the availability of acid in total parenteral nutrition solutions containing hydrochloric acid. Am J Hosp Pharm 1981;38:1729–1731.
51. Rowlands BJ, Tindall SF, Elliot DJ. The use of dilute hydrochloric acid and cimetidine to reverse severe metabolic alkalosis. Postgrad Med J 1978;54:118–123.
52. Barton CH, Vaziri ND, Ness RL, et al. Cimetidine in the management of metabolic alkalosis induced by nasogastric drainage. Arch Surg 1979;1:70–74.
53. Colussi G, Rombola G, De Ferrari ME, Macaluso M, Minetti L. Correction of hypokalemia with antialdosterone therapy in Gitelman's syndrome. Am J Nephrol 1994;14:127–135.
54. Hene RJ, Koomans HA, Dorhout Mees EJ, et al. Correction of hypokalemia in Bartter's syndrome by enalapril. Am J Kidney Dis 1987;9:200–205.
55. Vinci JM, Gill JR Jr, Bowden RE, et al. The kallikrein-kinin system in Bartter's syndrome and its response to prostaglandin synthetase inhibition. J Clin Invest 1987;61:1671–1682.
56. Gennari FJ. Respiratory acidosis and alkalosis. In: Narins RG, ed. Maxwell & Kleeman's Clinical Disorders of Fluid and Electrolyte Metabolism, 5th ed. New York, McGraw-Hill, 1994:957–990.
57. Giebisch G, Berger L, Pitts RF. The extrarenal responses to acute acid-base disturbances of respiratory origin. J Clin Invest 1955;34:231–245.
58. Respiratory pump failure: Primary hypercapnia (respiratory acidosis). In: Adrogue HJ, Tobin MJ, eds. Respiratory Failure. Cambridge, MA, Blackwell Science, 1997:125–134.

54

EVALUATION OF NEUROLOGIC ILLNESS

Susan C. Fagan and Fenwick T. Nichols

In the past decade, many novel pharmacologic agents for previously untreatable neurologic diseases have been introduced, along with better treatments for other neurologic illnesses. It is therefore essential that the pharmacist understands the tools used to diagnose and manage neurologic disease.[1,2]

The assessment of the neurologic patient follows an orderly progression that may differ from assessment in other specialties. The diagnostic steps of the clinical method are as follows[3]:

1. *Initial assessment.* Identification of clinical data by history and neurologic examination.
2. *Localization.* Interpretation of signs and symptoms in terms of anatomy, physiology, and pathophysiology to localize the anatomic site of the disease process.
3. *Synthesis.* Consideration of lesion location, course of the illness, relevant past history and family history, other medical illnesses, and the results of laboratory investigations to arrive at a cause of illness (etiologic diagnosis)

SIGNS AND SYMPTOMS FROM HISTORY AND PHYSICAL EXAMINATION

As in all of medicine, obtaining an accurate and complete history is of utmost importance in the evaluation of neurologic diseases. In many instances, the diagnosis can be made on the basis of the history, and the neurologic examination can be tailored to optimally evaluate the patient and confirm the diagnosis. The clinician is dependent on the patient or family for the details of the illness. Care must be taken to avoid "leading" the patient. Obtaining an accurate history may be difficult because a number of neurologic diseases may affect patients' speech and memory.

The physical examination is important in revealing evidence of systemic disease that may have secondarily affected the nervous system (e.g., a seizure in a patient with elevated temperature and stiff neck may suggest meningitis). The neurologic examination is only one component of a complete general physical examination.

THE NEUROLOGIC EXAMINATION

The neurologic examination consists of six main components: higher cortical function (mental status), cranial nerves, motor function, reflexes, sensory function, and gait. Table 54–1 describes the common approaches to assessing each of the six domains and includes examples of the diseases in which abnormal findings are common. Table 54–2 describes the cranial nerve examination in more detail. The reader is encouraged to consult a patient assessment resource to better understand the intricacies of the neurologic examination.

LABORATORY TESTS AND PROCEDURES FOR DIAGNOSIS

In addition to the neurologic examination, certain imaging techniques and procedures may be essential in the diagnosis of neurologic disorders. Some of the more commonly used procedures are described next.[2]

Lumbar puncture (LP) is used to obtain cerebrospinal fluid (CSF). It is used most often as an evaluation of central nervous system infections such as meningitis and encephalitis, but it is also useful in subarachnoid hemorrhage, multiple sclerosis, and dementia. Opening pressure, cell count and differential, glucose, total protein, and culture and sensitivity are obtained routinely. A space-occupying lesion in the brain with mass effect is a relative contraindication to LP because herniation could result. Prior to performing an LP, the patient should be checked for papilledema, which may indicate increased intracranial pressure. The opening CSF pressure usually is less than 180 mm H_2O. Normal CSF is clear and colorless and should not contain any red blood cells (RBCs) or polymorphonuclear cells. The presence of up to five mononuclear cells is considered normal. Total protein in the CSF usually is 45 mg/dL or less. Protein may increase with infection, breakdown of the blood-brain barrier (tumors, stroke, and trauma), and diabetes.

Electroencephalography (EEG) records the electrical activity of the brain. The record is interpreted by observing the basic rhythms and waveforms, the symmetry of the recording, and abnormal electrical discharges. It also may be used to assess the response to photic stimulation or hyperventilation. It is used primarily in the diagnosis of seizures and may be helpful in the evaluation of patients with altered mental status. EEG also may be used to measure evoked potentials (EPs). The EPs are the EEG response to repetitive stimuli (visual, auditory, or tactile) and provide information about the presence of abnormalities and disturbances (but not the cause) in the specific pathways tested.

Electromyography (EMG) and nerve conduction velocities (NCVs) are used to assess the function of the peripheral nerves, neuromuscular junction, and muscles. NCVs are measured by stimulating the nerve and recording the speed of conduction of the impulse. NCVs can be used to detect the presence of localized peripheral nerve injuries (carpal tunnel, etc.) or diffuse symmetrical neuropathies (which may be inherited or acquired). EMG assesses muscle dysfunction due to primary muscle disease or secondary to nerve injury. This test is used to diagnose peripheral neuropathies (inherited and acquired), Guillain-Barré syndrome, myasthenia gravis, amyotrophic lateral sclerosis, radiculopathies, and muscle diseases.

The cerebral circulatory system can be imaged or evaluated in a number of different ways, depending on the type and location of the abnormality suspected. Imaging techniques can be used to identify local arterial stenosis, aneurysms, or arteriovenous malformations.

TABLE 54–1. The Neurological Examination

Domain	Tests Performed	Diseases
Mental status	While obtaining the history: general mental and emotional status, speech, memory, alertness, abstract reasoning, ability to follow commands (motor integration), ability to communicate	Dementias, stroke, metabolic encephalopathies
Cranial nerves	Visual acuity, visual fields, eye movements, jaw strength, corneal reflex, facial symmetry, auditory acuity, gag reflex, shoulder and neck strength	Myasthenia gravis, Parkinson's disease, stroke, amyotrophic lateral sclerosis (ALS)
Motor Function	Motor strength with and without resistance, coordination (rapid alternating movements, finger-to-nose), tremors, atrophy, fasiculations	Stroke, myasthenia gravis, Parkinson's disease, ALS
Reflexes	Biceps, triceps, tendon reflexes, plantar response (Babinski sign is an upgoing toe and is abnormal), superficial cutaneous reflexes (abdominal)	Stroke, spinal cord lesions, endocrine diseases (e.g., diabetes, hypothyroidism), peripheral neuropathy
Sensory function	Asymmetry to pin-prick, vibration,temperature	Stroke, peripheral neuropathy, migraine aura, diabetes, spinal cord lesions
Gait	Walking, standing (Romberg test = eyes closed will accentuate disequilibrium)	Stroke, Parkinson's disease, spinal cord lesions

Atherosclerosis of the extracranial arteries, a frequent cause of stroke, can be evaluated using ultrasound (referred to as duplex sonography, carotid Doppler, color-flow Doppler), magnetic resonance angiography (MRA), spiral computed tomography angiography (CTA), or intraarterial angiography. The intracranial arterial circulation can be evaluated using transcranial Doppler (TCD), MRA, CTA, or intraarterial angiography. Each technique has its own advantages and disadvantages. Intraarterial angiography provides the best imaging of the smaller arteries of the cerebral circulation but is more invasive than the other measures.

Computed tomography (CT) uses x-rays to produce images of "slices" of the brain that are 1.5 to 10 mm in thickness. CT revolutionized the practice of neurology by allowing a direct image of the brain. CT is currently available in most communities and is used to evaluate patients with intracranial disease. CT scans are used to identify

TABLE 54–2. Cranial Nerve Function and Examples of Testing

I. Olfactory nerve. Smell: Identify odors (coffee, cinnamon, lemon; test each nostril separately).
II. Optic nerve. Visual acuity: Eye card; Visual fields: Peripheral vision and blind spot; Funduscopic exam; Pupil size and reaction; Color vision (rarely done).
III. Oculomotor. (Cranial nerves III, IV, and VI have similar functions and are tested as a unit.) Eye movements: Patient is asked to watch a light as it moved up, down, and on both sides, while eye movements are observed.
IV. Trochlear. See III.
V. Trigeminal nerve. Motor: Tests power of jaw opening and sideways deviation against the resistance of a hand placed against the jaw. Sensory: Test corneal reflex by touching cornea (also nasal mucosa) with a wisp of cotton.
VI. Abducens. See III.
VII. Facial nerve. Observe asymmetry of face at rest or on speaking, baring teeth, raising eyebrows, or wrinkling forehead. Reflex eye closure to a threatening movement. Glabellar tap: Repetitive tapping over bridge of nose—initial blinking should cease after the first few taps.
VIII. Auditory nerve. Vestibular division: Observe for nystagmus, positional testing. Auditory division: Test acuity with light sound; watch, whisper, rubbing of fingers close to ear.
IX. Glossopharyngeal nerve. Test for gag reflex by touching back of throat with tongue depressor; test swallowing and coughing and note any drooling or pooling of saliva. Test symmetry of palate movement on vocalizing "ah."
X. Vagus nerve. Test gag reflex as in IX.
XI. Spinal accessory nerve. Trapezius and sternomastoid muscles: Test power of shrugging shoulders and turning the head to one side against resistance.
XII. Hypoglossal nerve. Motor function of tongue. Look for wasting and abnormal movements.

TABLE 54–3. General Principles Guiding the Evaluation of Neurologic Illness

1. Patients must cooperate with the examiner; therefore, patient reliability and effort must be considered in the interpretation of the findings.
2. The neurologic examination of a patient is often adapted to focus on the patient's specific problem. For example, a patient with Bell's palsy (facial involvement) will have a thorough cranial nerve examination but a less extensive evaluation of hand strength.
3. The importance of symmetry cannot be overemphasized. Rather than comparing a patient's neurologic function to a "normal" standard, asymmetry of strength, sensation, and coordination are often of great importance in detecting neurologic deficits.
4. Although the neurologic examination is important in diagnosing and quantifying neurologic deficits in patients, functional assessment (what the patient can do compared to baseline state—activities of daily living) is also important in making decisions about therapy. For this purpose, functional assessment scales are used with increasing frequency but are usually disease specific, in that they incorporate functions that are most commonly affected by the disease. Often, knowledge of the disease-specific functional scale is necessary to interpret clinical trials of new treatments for neurologic diseases (e.g., Barthel Index for acute ischemic stroke, Expanded Disability Status Scale (EDSS) in multiple sclerosis).

tumors, hemorrhages, infarctions, hydrocephalus, and atrophy. Intravenous contrast agents (a contrast-enhanced scan) can be administered to enhance the image of blood vessels and areas of blood-brain barrier damage that may be caused by abscesses, tumors or stroke.

Magnetic resonance imaging (MRI) uses the magnetic properties of the hydrogen atom nucleus and proton to produce computer-processed scans that provide improved anatomic accuracy when compared with CT scans. MRI offers the advantages of differentiating between white and gray matter, delineating lesions close to bone (brain stem and cerebellum), and no radiation risk; however, it is not as readily available as CT and is more expensive. MRI has a proven advantage over CT in detecting plaques in multiple sclerosis and is also useful in the diagnosis of tumors and very early ischemic stroke (diffusion-weighted imaging, or DWI). Imaging of the spinal cord can be accomplished either by MRI (MRI myelography) or CT (CT myelography).

Other imaging techniques such as positron-emission tomography (PET) and single-photon-emission computed tomography (SPECT) are considered tests of brain function. These tests are being studied extensively in epilepsy as well as in cerebrovascular disorders, cerebral tumors, movement disorders, and dementia. PET scans use a positron-emitting isotope to display chemical activity and the rates of biologic processes within the brain. This method can assess regional metabolic changes in the brain. The expense, technical complexity (a cyclotron is needed), and limited availability of this technique limit its clinical utility.

SPECT scans measure radiotracer uptake by tissues and provide cross-sectional images of the brain. This technique has been used extensively to assess cerebral blood flow. Although the resolution of SPECT is not as good as PET, the availability has led to wide clinical use in disorders such as stroke, dementia, and epilepsy.

General principles guiding the evaluation of neurologic illness are summarized in Table 54–3.

REFERENCES

1. Adams RD, Victor M, Ropper AH. Principles of Neurology, 6th ed. New York, McGraw-Hill, 1997:3–11.
2. Adams RD, Victor M, Ropper AH. Principles of Neurology, 6th ed. New York, McGraw-Hill, 1997:12–40.
3. Adams RD, Victor M, Ropper AH. Principles of Neurology, 6th ed. Companion Handbook. New York, McGraw-Hill, 1998:3–9.

55

MULTIPLE SCLEROSIS

Jacquelyn L. Bainbridge, John R. Corboy, and Barry E. Gidal

Multiple sclerosis (MS) is an inflammatory disease of the central nervous system (CNS) that affects between 250,000 and 350,000 persons in the United States.[1] It is one of the major causes of neurologic disability in young and middle-aged adults. The term *multiple sclerosis* refers to two characteristics of the disease: the numerous affected areas of the brain and spinal cord producing multiple neurologic symptoms that accrue over time and the characteristic plaques or sclerosed areas that are the hallmark of the disease.

Although MS was first described almost 130 years ago, the cause remains a mystery, and a cure is still unavailable. Nevertheless, many advances have been made in treating and managing the complications of the disease and improving the quality of life of those individuals affected by MS.

EPIDEMIOLOGY

MS is usually diagnosed in patients between the ages of 20 and 45 years (although cases in children have been reported), with the peak incidence occurring in the fourth decade.[2] Onset can occur as early as age 10 and as late as the eighth decade.[3] Women are afflicted more than men by a ratio of approximately 2:1.[3] Men usually develop the first signs of MS at a later age than women and are also more likely to develop the chronic progressive form of the disease.[3,4] The most important factors in the determination of individuals at risk for developing the disease are geography, age, environmental influences, and genetics.[2,5,6]

Based on rates of prevalence of MS, the world can be divided into three geographic zones.[7] In general, the greater the distance from the equator, the higher is the prevalence of the disease.[2,7,8] Within the United States, the prevalence of MS is higher in those states above the thirty-seventh parallel. Ethnic differences in prevalence are also observed within the described geographic areas, with MS occurring more frequently in whites of Scandinavian ancestry than in other ethnic groups.[8,9] Asian-Americans, African-Americans, American Hispanics living in California, Australian aborigines, Polynesian Maoris, Lapps, and Hungarian gypsies are among the ethnic groups that have a very low reported incidence of MS, sometimes despite being located in what are considered high-risk areas.[8,9] MS is considered a rare disease in Africa.

It is thought that a crucial environmental agent that may predispose one to developing MS is contracted by susceptible individuals between the ages of 10 and 15 years[4,10] who have usually lived in a high-risk area for at least 2 years.[4] Interestingly, an individual who migrates from a low- to a high-risk area prior to the age of 15 years has the same chance of developing MS as those who live in a high-risk area all their lives.[11] If the move is made in the opposite direction, from a high- to a low-risk area, the individual retains the high risk if the move is made after the age of 15 years but acquires the lower risk if the move is made prior to this age.[10,11]

The familial recurrence rate of MS is approximately 10%, with siblings being the most commonly reported relationship.[9] Concordance data show a higher prevalence of MS between monozygotic than between dizygotic twins.

Genetic studies also have determined an association between MS and the major histocompatibility complex (MHC) and, in particular, with the human leukocyte antigen (HLA) region on the sixth chromosome that is associated with the genetic control of immune mechanisms.[9,12,13] This association between HLA haplotype and MS susceptibility may vary between ethnic groups. In whites, the strongest association appears to be with the MHC class II allele DR2 haplotype. The relative risk of developing MS is approximately four times as great in $DR2^+$ versus $DR2^-$ individuals.[13] This association is not specific enough to be used for diagnostic purposes, given a 30% to 50% false-negative rate and that the $DR2^+$ haplotype is found in at least 20% of the healthy white population. Although the significance of the association between MS and the HLA region remains unclear, the fact that certain HLA antigens are neither necessary nor sufficient to lead to the development of MS suggests that inheritance is most likely polygenic in nature and that there may only be a genetic susceptibility to developing this disease following an as-yet-unknown etiologic challenge.

ETIOLOGY

AUTOIMMUNE THEORY

In the autoimmune theory (Fig. 55–1), MS results from an autoimmune attack against self-myelin or self-oligodendrocyte antigens. The actual mediator of myelin destruction has not been established, but this activity has been attributed to the action of macrophages, killer T cells, lymphokines, antibodies, or a combination of these elements.[14] T-helper cells ($CD4^+$) appear to be key initiators of myelin destruction in MS. These autoreactive $CD4^+$ cells are activated in the periphery, perhaps following a viral infection, and recognize myelin basic protein (MBP), proteolipid protein, myelin oligodendrocyte glycoprotein, and myelin-associated glycoprotein in the blood of patients with MS. These antigens are presented by HLA class II molecules on both macrophages and astrocytes. This cellular recognition initiates an inflammatory cascade where $CD4^+$ cells are activated and proliferate. During this process, various cytokines are secreted, and B cells and macrophages are activated. Activated T cells are then able to cross the blood-brain barrier (BBB). Once across the BBB, these cells can interact with specific MHC class II molecules on antigen-presenting cells and thereby induce an autoimmune response that eventually will lead to the destruction of myelin.[14] Impaired T-suppressor cell function also may play a role in the immunologic process.[15] A reduction in T-suppressor cells, or supressor activity, has been reported during active MS and in patients with progressive disease; however, a relative increase in the T-helper/suppressor ratio is not found consistently and does not always correlate with disease activity.[16,17]

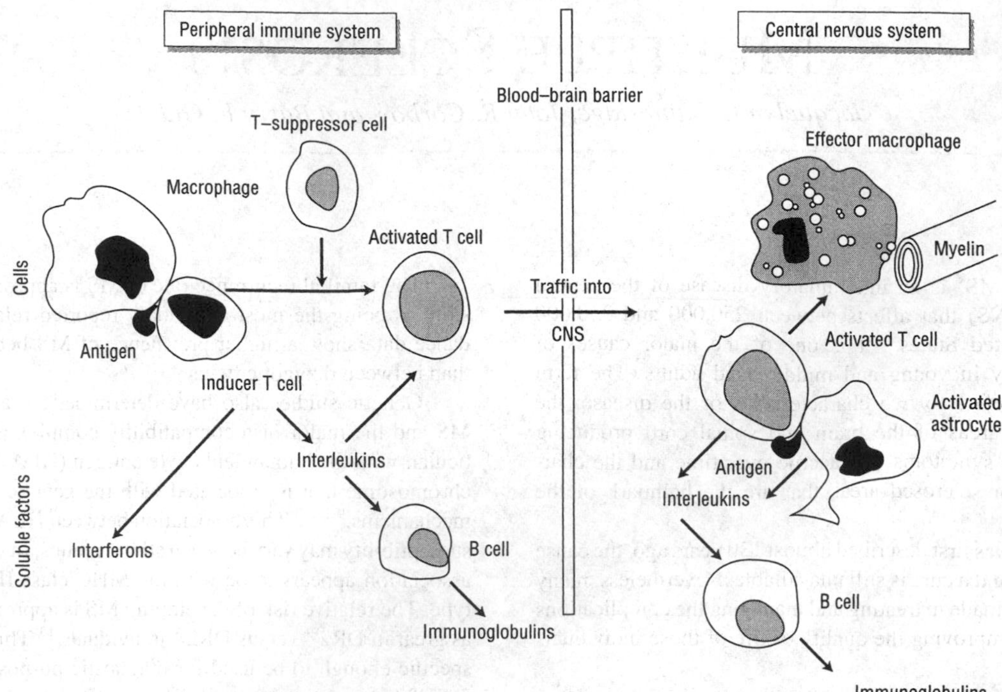

FIGURE 55–1. Autoimmune theory of the pathogenesis of MS. The immune response is initiated in the peripheral immune compartment when antigen is processed and presented to an inducer cell by a macrophage or antigen-presenting cell. The inducer cell becomes activated and releases a number of soluble factors including interleukins and interferons, which act on both B cells and T cells to augment the immune response. T-suppressor cells act to dampen the immune response. Activated T cells traffic into the central nervous system, where they again release factors, presumably after having antigen presented to them. In this regard, astrocytes are capable of presenting antigens to T cells. Other cellular elements also enter the CNS (macrophages, B cells), where the potential for a local immune response occurs. B cells are known to produce immunoglobulin locally within the CNS, and macrophages function within the CNS to phagocytose myelin, in addition to their antigen-presenting properties.
(Reprinted with permission from Ann Neurol, vol 23, p 214, 1988.)

ROLE OF CYTOKINES

Cytokines are molecules whose physiologic functions are numerous and include modulating inflammatory and anti-inflammatory responses in the immune system. Cytokines such as tumor necrosis factor alpha (TNF-α), interleukin-2 (IL-2), and interferon-gamma (INF-γ) have been alleged as contributors to the pathogenesis of MS. TNF-α may contribute to demyelinization by up-regulation of MHC class I expression, direct injury of oligodendrocytes, and/or promotion of BBB breakdown.[18] INF-γ is produced predominantly by CD4$^+$ cells and is involved in antiviral responses. Because of this, INF-γ was at one time evaluated as a potential MS disease-modifying agent. Clinical trials, however, clearly demonstrated that treatment with this compound resulted in an unexpected increase in disease exacerbation.[19] INF-γ up-regulates MHC class II expression on macrophages, microglia, and astrocytes, leading to an inflammatory response. INF-γ also upregulates adhesion molecules, which are crucial in the early stages of inflammation by facilitating the migration of T cells across the endothelial cells of the BBB.[20]

In contrast, the role of modulating, or down-regulating, cytokines has been described recently. In patients with stable or mild disease, increased numbers of cells are found that express mRNA for transforming growth factor beta (TGF-β) and IL-10 as compared with patients with severe disease.[21,22]

QUESTIONABLE MICROBIAL ETIOLOGY

Although no clear association with any microbial agent has been identified, there are several ways in which a virus or bacteria could play a role in the pathogenesis of MS. These might include either a direct attack on myelin and/or the oligodendrocyte or stimulation of an autoimmune response leading to demyelination.[14,23] Evidence to support a viral etiology includes increased immunoglobulin G (IgG) synthesis in the CNS, increased antibody titers to certain viruses, and epidemiologic studies indicating a childhood exposure factor and suggesting that "viral" infections may precipitate exacerbations. In addition, viruses have been shown to cause diseases with prolonged incubation periods, myelin destruction, and a relapsing/remitting course in humans and in experimental animal models.[2,24]

The most compelling evidence against a microbial etiology is the fact that no single infectious agent has been identified as the cause of MS. Many possibilities have been implicated, including mycoplasma, spirochetes, rabies virus, herpes simplex, canine distemper virus, coronavirus, human T-cell leukemia virus (HTLV)-1, MS-associated retrovirus, measles, and most recently, human herpes virus-6 (HHV-6)[25] and *Chlamydia pneumoniae.*[26] However, studies have been unable to establish a causal relationship.[24]

PATHOPHYSIOLOGY

The basic physiologic derangement in MS is the stripping of the myelin sheath surrounding neurons in the CNS. Demyelination, coupled with an inflammatory response, leads to the formation of the characteristic MS lesions or plaques that are found primarily in the brain, spinal cord, and optic nerves. Initially, neuronal axons, although stripped bare of their myelin sheath, are usually well preserved.[23] Recent studies, however, have shown that damage to axons can be significant, even early in the course of the illness.[27] Axonal damage may be seen as a hypointense lesion, or T1 hole, on magnetic resonance imaging (MRI) scans, and these seem to correlate well with disability.[28]

Demyelination and axonal transection cause disruption in the transmission of nerve impulses, which leads to neurologic symptoms reflecting the area of the brain or spinal cord that is affected. Demyelinated nerve fibers have prolonged refractory periods that will impair conduction of electrical impulse volleys. Maximal electrical impulse frequency may be reduced substantially before impulse conduction is interrupted entirely. A single plaque may extend across several nerve pathways, producing symptoms involving several nervous system functions. Smaller plaques may cause isolated disturbances; however, typically several plaques develop at the same time, causing multiple but unrelated problems such as disturbed vision and decreased sensation.

The pathology of MS lesions is different in early stages of the disease, during chronic MS, and during acute exacerbations.[29] Active and inactive lesions can be found side by side in the brain. Both types of lesions display some degree of perivascular inflammation, but inflammation is much more pronounced and usually associated with BBB damage in active lesions.[29]

Decreased numbers of oligodendrocytes (myelin-producing cells) are observed within the MS plaques, causing speculation as to whether myelin or the oligodendrocyte is the target of an immunologic attack.[16,23,30] Oligodendrocyte destruction appears to occur in a nonspecific manner in early or acute MS, whereas selective destruction of myelin and oligodendrocytes occurs in chronic stages of MS.[29] Although the etiology and pathogenesis of MS remain unclear, it appears that the immune system is crucial in this disease. Many investigators consider MS to be an autoimmune or immunopathologic disorder, whereby an immune response is directed toward myelin antigens. Although the triggering event for this autoimmune response remains a mystery, an initial viral process is suspected.[14,31]

CLINICAL PRESENTATION

The clinical presentation of MS is extremely variable among patients and may vary over time in a given patient. The signs and symptoms of MS usually are divided into three categories (Table 55–1). Primary symptoms are a direct consequence of conduction disturbances produced by demyelination and axonal damage and reflect the area of the brain or spinal cord that is damaged. Secondary symptoms are complications resulting from primary symptoms. For example, urinary retention, a primary symptom, may lead to frequent urinary tract infections, considered a secondary symptom. Tertiary symptoms relate to the effect of the disease on the patient's everyday life.[32] The most widely used clinical rating scale in MS is the Expanded Disability Status Scale (EDSS), in which a numerical value ranging from 0 (no disability) to 10 (death from MS) is assigned based on the evaluation of several neurologic functions.[33] The limitations to this scale are

TABLE 55–1. Common Symptomatology of Multiple Sclerosis

Primary Symptoms	Secondary Symptoms	Tertiary Symptoms
Visual complaints	Recurrent urinary tract infections	Financial problems
Gait problems	Urinary calculi	Personal/social problems
Paresthesias	Decubiti	Vocational problems
Pain	Muscle contractures	Emotional problems
Spasticity	Respiratory infections	
Weakness	Poor nutrition	
Ataxia		
Speech difficulty		
Psychological changes		
Cognitive changes		
Fatigue		
Bowel/bladder dysfunction		
Sexual dysfunction		
Tremor		

the relative insensitivity to clinical changes that do not involve impairment of gait and ambulation, such as changes in cognition, fatigue, and affect. This scale is not linear, and therefore, functional changes from 1.0 to 2.0 are not the same as changes from 6.0 to 7.0. This scale is also subject to interevaluator inconsistency. Increasingly, MRI is being used as an index of both disease activity and progression.[34,35] Specifically, the appearance of new lesions or changes in lesion number, size, and volume (burden of disease) are being used as outcome measures. It is important to note, however, that the correlation between MRI lesion load and clinical disability is modest at best.[36]

The unpredictable nature of MS makes it impossible to anticipate when an exacerbation will occur. However, certain factors have been reported to aggravate symptoms or even lead to an acute attack (new episode of demyelination). These implicated factors include infections, hyperventilation, heat (including fever), sleep deprivation, stress, malnutrition, anemia, concurrent organ dysfunction, exertion, and childbirth.[2–4,37] Interestingly, many patients experience a significant reduction in acute relapses during the third trimester of pregnancy, followed by a relative increase postpartum.[37] Physical trauma probably does not play a major role in the onset or exacerbation of MS.[38]

CLINICAL COURSE AND PROGNOSIS

The clinical course of MS is variable but seems to follow a general pattern of exacerbations and remissions (Fig. 55–2). MS can be classified into four clinical categories.[39] About 85% of patients have attacks—new symptoms lasting at least 24 hours and separated from other symptoms by at least 30 days—followed by remissions (complete or incomplete) at the outset of the illness. This is typically called *relapsing-remitting MS* (RRMS). In RRMS patients, attacks frequency tend to decrease over time, independent of the development of worsening disabilities.[39] Neurologic recovery following an acute exacerbation is usually quite good early in the disease course, but following repeated relapses, recovery tends to be less complete. Given these features, interpretation and evaluation of potential therapeutic interventions must be done quite cautiously, and control groups are essential in the design of clinical studies.

A benign course—characterized by an abrupt onset, few exacerbations, and no permanent disability—is seen in at most 20% of RRMS patients, but the majority eventually enter a progressive phase

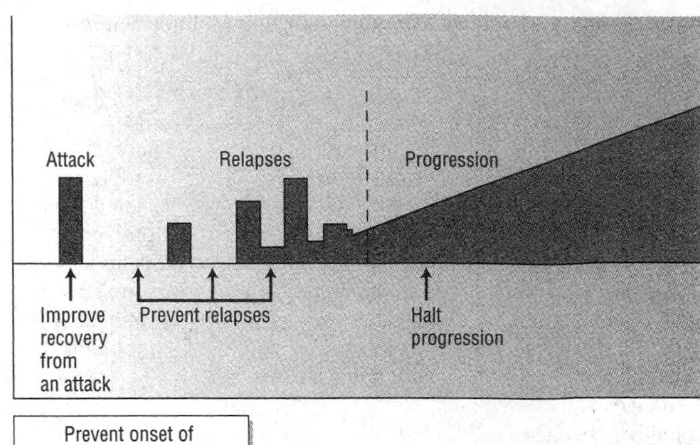

FIGURE 55–2. Clinical course and treatment of multiple sclerosis. The horizontal axis represents time, and the vertical axis represents level of disability. The vertical dotted line represents the onset of the progressive disease phase. The progressive phase may evolve after a number of relapses or, in a subcategory of patients, may be the clinical course of the disease from the onset.
(Reprinted with permission from Ann Neurol, vol 23, p 212, 1988.)

in which acute attacks and remissions are difficult to identify. This is commonly referred to as *secondary progressive MS* (SPMS). Disability tends to accumulate more significantly during this phase of the illness. In distinction, about 15% of patients have *primary progressive MS* (PPMS) from the outset, characterized by the slow onset of symptoms, without attacks, and disability that continually worsens over time. In general, PPMS patients tend to have a worse prognosis than those who initially present with RRMS. Finally, a small percentage of patients might have a mixture of both progression and relapses, referred to as *progressive-relapsing MS* (PRMS).[39]

MS itself usually does not directly diminish life expectancy, but the development of complications such as pneumonia or septicemia (secondary to decubitus ulcers or urinary tract infections) may lead to a shorter than expected life span. Most of this decrease in life span is seen in patients with progressive disease. Suicide rates as high as seven times that expected in the general population have been reported.[39] Clinical and demographic factors that have been used to predict prognosis of MS are listed in Table 55–2.[39–41] Most likely reflecting improvements in overall care, World Health Organization (WHO) statistics suggest that mortality from MS has decreased up to 25% during the past 30 years.[42]

DIAGNOSIS

MS symptoms frequently can be attributed to other neurologic diseases, just as many syndromes can mimic MS. In the past, the unpredictable nature of MS and the lack of laboratory tests and imaging techniques specific for the disease led to difficulties in making this diagnosis, especially in the early stages of the disease. The diagnosis remains primarily a clinical one that requires the demonstration of "lesions separated in space and time," referring to the occurrence of at least two episodes of neurologic disturbance reflecting distinct sites of damage in the CNS that cannot be explained by another mechanism.[43] Advances in MRI scanning have begun to stretch the diagnostic criteria and ultimately may allow us to make a diagnosis of definite MS based on a single, typical attack in association with two or more typical lesions seen on brain MRI scans (see below).

LABORATORY STUDIES

To date, there are no tests specific for MS. Tests that are used frequently include MRI, cerebrospinal fluid (CSF) evaluation, and evoked potentials. Evidence provided by these studies, used in conjunction with the clinical history, aids in establishing the diagnosis of MS.

IMAGING STUDIES

MRI, especially with gadolinium enhancement, is much more sensitive than computed tomographic (CT) scans in the detection of MS lesions and is currently considered the preferred imaging method.[40,44] It is extremely helpful not only for diagnosis but also for prognosis. Patients with a single, typical attack of demyelination (e.g., optic neuritis) and three or more T2-weighted lesions on the brain MRI scan have a greater than 80% likelihood of developing a second attack (clinically definite MS) over 10 years.[45] In contrast, similar individuals with normal brain MRI scans have about an 11% to 15% likelihood of having a second attack over 10 years. Total volume of T2-weighted lesions (burden of disease) at onset also appears to correlate with development of disability.[45] Lesions that enhance with gadolinium indicate new lesions and disruption of the BBB. Lesions are observed on MRI in up to 95% of patients with clinically definite MS. More important, they are observed in 65% to 85% of patients with suspected MS.[40] New, experimental MRI measures, such as brain atrophy, magnetization transfer, and magnetic resonance spectroscopy, may add to our understanding of the relationship of imaging abnormalities and progression of disease.

CEREBROSPINAL FLUID EVALUATION

In MS patients, CNS synthesis of IgG is increased, whereas serum IgG levels are normal. Electrophoretic studies of the CSF show that the IgG separates into a small number of discrete bands called *oligoclonal bands*.[40] Although oligoclonal banding of IgG is present in 90% to 95% of patients with clinically definite, established MS, it is significant only if banding is not found in the serum.[40,46] It is important to remember that CSF IgG elevations are not specific for MS and may be seen in a variety of other diseases. Early on (e.g., after initial symptoms), CSF may be positive in only 30% to 50%. Increasingly, with advances in MRI scanning, CSF analysis is reserved only for atypical cases. Myelin basic protein is detected in the CSF of 90% of patients

TABLE 55–2. Prognostic Indicators In Multiple Sclerosis

Indicator	Favorable Prognosis	Unfavorable Prognosis
Age at onset	<40 years	>40 years
Gender	Female	Male
Initial symptoms	Optic neuritis or sensory symptoms	Motor or cerebellar symptoms
Attack frequency in early disease	Low	High
Course of disease	Relapsing/remitting	Progressive

shortly after an acute attack. Additional CSF abnormalities may include increased CSF protein concentrations in approximately 25% of patients and a mild CSF leukocytosis.[40] The presence of greater than 50×10^6 mononuclear cells in the CSF usually indicates a diagnosis other than MS.[46]

EVOKED POTENTIALS

Evoked potentials may be helpful in establishing areas of demylination that are clinically silent. Slowed conduction of visual, brain stem, and somatosensory potentials can be identified, although the sensitivity and specificity of these tests seem to be somewhat less than that seen with MRI evlauation.

MIMICS OF MS

A number of disorders can mimic MS. Thus most patients are screened with blood tests for rheumatologic, collegan-vascular, and infectious diseases.

▶ TREATMENT: Multiple Sclerosis

To date, no therapy has been shown to cure MS, and only recently has any therapy shown the ability to slow the progression of the disease. Symptomatic management of the disease is of utmost importance to maintain the patient's quality of life. A number of different treatment modalities have been studied, but many trials had a flawed design.[47] The lack of specific indicators for disease activity and the unpredictable course of the disease make assessment of various therapies difficult. There are no universally accepted treatment protocols, and treatments vary among clinicians and treatment centers. Perhaps more important, treatment decisions frequently are based on the wishes and goals of individual patients. One potential algorithm for the treatment of RRMS is shown in Figure 55–3.

DESIRED OUTCOME

Therapy of MS may be attempted at different stages during the course of the disease, as shown in Figure 55–2. The basic goals of therapy are to decrease the severity, intensity, and duration of exacerbations; enhance recovery from exacerbations; prevent relapses and the onset of progressive disease; halt or even reverse progressive disease; and provide symptomatic relief from the complications of MS.

DISEASE-MODIFYING MODALITIES

TREATMENT OF ACUTE EXACERBATIONS

Various immunosuppressive agents have been evaluated for disease-modifying activity in MS.[48–50] Treatment of an acute exacerbation varies depending on the severity of the attack. Mild exacerbations that do not produce functional decline may not require any treatment.[48] When functional ability is affected, treatment is usually started with corticosteroids. Treatment varies between clinicans. In milder cases, some clinicans use oral prednisone in a variety of dosing regimens.[48] Results from a large trial of optic neuritis suggest, and the American Academy of Neurology recommends, however, that if treatment with steroids is warranted, it is best to use intravenous methylprednisolone.[51–53] Optic neuritis is characterized on MRI by lesions in the optic nerve. Patients with optic neuritis generally complain of variable degrees of visual loss, blurring vision, or hazy vision. The onset of symptoms typically is quite sudden and progressive. A majority of optic neuritis patients eventually will be diagnosed with MS. Because effects of corticosteroids may be transient and tend to diminish with repeated use, some clinicians stress that steroid therapy should not be used for symptom fluctuations without any functional consequence.

The mechanism of action for corticosteroids in MS is unknown, but it is speculated that steroids improve recovery by decreasing edema in the area of demyelination.[48] In addition, steroids have been shown to reduce BBB abnormalities observed by CT scan, reduce CSF IgG synthesis, and decrease concentrations of MBP during acute exacerbations. Unfortunately, the relationship between these parameters and disease activity has not been established.

High-dose methylprednisolone has been shown to shorten the duration of acute exacerbations,[54–56] although it has not been shown to affect the progression of disease.[18,48,57] Comparative trials of adrenocorticoid hormone (ACTH) and high-dose intravenous steroids suggest that steroids produce a quicker and more predictable improvement in acute exacerbations. Although the reasons for this are not entirely clear, differences between agents may be due to the variable adrenal secretion of endogenous glucocorticoids following ACTH stimulation.[58] The use of ACTH, therefore, has been largely supplanted by methylprednisolone.

Methylprednisolone doses may range from 500 to 1000 mg/d, given intraveneously. The duration of therapy is variable and may range from 3 to 10 days depending on clinical response. If improvement occurs, it is usually seen in the first 3 to 5 days; therefore, parenteral therapy may be continued for up to 5 days, followed by an oral steroid taper. Oral steroid regimens typically begin with 60 to 80 mg of prednisone for 3 to 7 days, and then the dosage is tapered over 7 days or longer depending on the patient's symptoms.[58] Depending on the duration of steroid use, some practitioners may not use a steroid taper.

A very small number of patients have very severe attacks, manifested by hemiplegia, paraplegia, or quadriplegia. If these patients fail to improve with aggressive steroid therapy, a recent study suggests that treatment with plasma exchange may be beneficial for about 40% of patients.[59,60]

PREVENTION OF RELAPSES AND PROGRESSION (ABC THERAPY—AVONEX, BETASERON, COPAXONE)

Interferon-β-1b and Interferon-β-1a

Interferon-β-1b (Betaseron) was the first agent shown to have an effect on the course of the illness.[61] Interferon-β-1b is a nonglycosylated synthetic analog of recombinant interferon-β produced in *Escherichia coli.* Although the exact mechanism of action is unknown, its effect in MS may be due to its immunomodulating properties, including the ability to augment suppressor cell function and reduce interferon-β secretion by activated lymphocytes, its macrophage-activating effect, and its ability to down regulate the expression of interferon-β-induced class II MHC gene products on antigen-presenting glial cells.[47,62–64]

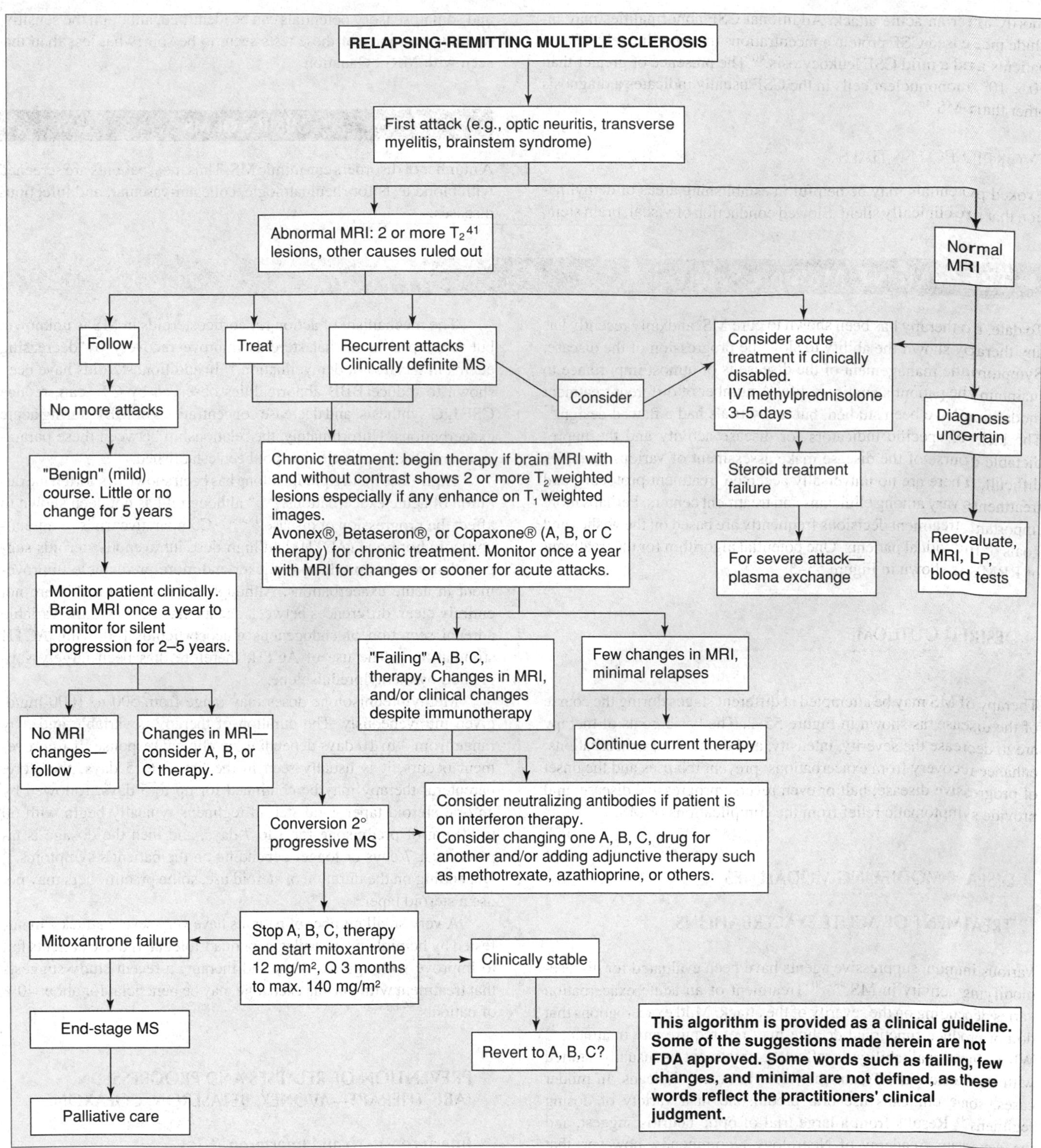

FIGURE 55–3. Algorithm for management of relapsing-remitting multiple sclerosis.

Interferon-β-1b also suppresses T-cell proliferation and may decrease BBB permeability.[64] The clinical relevance of the interferons' viral inhibiting effects is unclear.

Interferon-β-1b is administered every other day subcutaneously at a dose of 8 million IU. Clinical trials have demonstrated that at these doses, interferon-β-1b can reduce annual relapse rate significantly as compared with placebo. In addition, comparison of serial MRI data showed that at 3 years, placebo-treated patients tended to have an increase in total lesion area of about 20%, whereas interferon-treated patients had no significant increases. With respect to clinical disability, however, no significant differences were noted between the interferon- and placebo-treated groups.[65]

Baseline complete blood counts, platelet determinations, and liver function tests should be documented before starting therapy with interferon-β-1b. The most common adverse effects include injection-site redness and swelling and possibly necrosis, as well as flulike symptoms (fever, chills, myalgias). These symptoms can be mild or severe and are seen in the majority of patients. The flulike side effects typically occur for up to 24 hours after injection and are seen for 1 to 2 months after starting the shots. Injection-site reactions may occur at anytime and be lessened by using appropriate injection technique, including site rotation (thighs and buttocks) and hydrocortisone cream. Ice applied before and/or after the injection also may decrease the pain and the redness, as may the use of an autoinjector. Nonsteroidal anti-inflammatory agents (NSAIDs) or acetaminophen taken before and at regular intervals for 24 hours after administration may alleviate the flulike symptoms. Initiation of one-quarter or one-half the standard dose and then increasing to full dosage over 1 to 2 months also may be beneficial in reducing flulike side effects.[66] Some authors suggest that because of the transient immune activation that may occur following the introduction of interferon-β, a short burst of oral prednisone may alleviate some adverse effects.[66] Less commonly reported side effects include shortness of breath, tachycardia, and depression. Clinicians must monitor patients carefully for signs of depression and treat accordingly. Although depression is a common finding in MS patients, recent studies tend to support the notion that interferon-β-1b treatment may be provocative. Patients who develop depressive symptoms should be monitored closely because there may be a risk for suicide. The other side effects are usually transient. Most patients will not feel better when taking this drug, and many will experience side effects; thus compliance may become a major issue. Patients should be reminded that some of the side effects are transient, and they should be counseled to minimize problems associated with local reactions.

Interferon-β-1a (Avonex) is a natural-sequence glycosolated product derived from recombinant Chinese hamster ovary cells. When given 30 μg intramuscularly once weekly for 2 years, patients receiving interferon-β-1a demonstrated statistically significant reductions in annual relapse rate (by approximately one-third) as well as disease progression, which was defined as a progression of 1.0 point on the EDSS. Disease progression also was assessed by MRI studies, where it was found that patients receiving active drug had significantly fewer new enhancing lesions as compared with placebo-treated patients.[67] More recent studies reveal significant effects on slowing brain atrophy[68] and the progression of cognitive decline[69] in patients treated with Avonex. Taken together, these observations show that interferon-β-1a possesses significant disease-modifying activity. Although the adverse effect profile of interferon-β-1a resembles that of interferon-β-1b, interferon-β-1a may hold several advantages, including markedly fewer local injection-site reactions and once-weekly administration versus subcutaneous injection every other day. Treatment-emergent depression was no more common with interferon-β-1a than with placebo.

Finally, safety data of interferon-β in pregnancy and lactation are lacking. Abortifacient activity in primates has been noted, however. Until adequate safety data are available, women should be counseled as to appropriate contraception while using these products.

Glatiramer Acetate (Copaxone)

Glatiramer acetate (Copaxone, formerly known as copolymer-1) is a synthetic polypeptide consisting of L-alanine, L-glutamic acid, L-lysine, and L-tyrosine. Although the precise mechanism of action of this compound is unknown, glatiramer acetate appears to mimic the antigenic properties of MBP.[70] This agent also may act by directly binding to MHC class II receptors and inhibiting binding of MBP peptides to T-cell receptor complexes.[70] Recently, glatiramer acetate has demonstrated that it induces Th2 (anti-inflammatory) lymphocytes in experimental allergic encephalomyelitis (EAEs).[70,71] This is thought to contribute to "bystander" suppression at the site of the MS lesion and thereby reduce inflammation, demylination, and axonal damage.[71] Glatiramer acetate also may suppress T-cell activation. Glatiramir acetate is given as a daily 20-μg subcutaneous dose. Glatiramer acetate appears to have a relatively mild adverse-effect profile, with mild pain and pruritus at the injection site being the most frequent patient complaints. Approximately 10% of patients will experience a transient reaction consisting of chest tightness, flushing, and dyspnea beginning several minutes after injection and lasting usually no longer than 20 minutes. If patients have no history or evidence of coronary artery disease, they may be assured that these reactions are almost always self-limiting and appear benign. Several adverse effects that have been associated with the interferons, including flulike symptoms and depression, do not appear to be provoked by glatiramer acetate. Multicenter trials with glatiramer acetate have demonstrated statistically significant reductions in mean annual relapse rate ($\sim$25%) that is comparable with the interferons. An extension trial, completed after the original, pivotal 2-year study, suggests that glatiramer acetate slows the progression of disability in patients with RRMS.[72] Unfortunately, no clinical trials have compared the interferons with glatiramer acetate. In order to determine which agent is truly superior, head-to-head clinical trials comparing these three agents need to be completed.

Remaining Questions for ABC Therapy

Despite encouraging results from well-conducted clinical trials, several relevant questions remain. A concern with both interferon products is the development of neutralizing antibodies. In clinical trials, 38% of patients receiving interferon-β-1b developed antibodies.[73] In these patients, the exacerbation rate was similar to that in placebo-treated patients. With interferon-β-1a, neutralizing antibodies were found in 22% of treated patients. Because assays for these antibodies differ, it is difficult to judge the relative significance of these data. The long-term clinical significance of these findings is still unclear. Whether these antibodies are cross-reactive between products is unknown. The clinical relevance of neutralizing antibodies must be evaluated prospectively. Neutralizing antibodies have not been seen with glatiramer acetate.

Intriguingly, in vitro data suggest potential synergism between glatiramer acetate and interferon-β. Given the cost of these therapies, as well as the potential for additive adverse effects, this therapeutic combination cannot be recommended until clinical evidence demonstrating benefit is available. This combination is currently under discussion by many investigators.

All three of the ABC drugs are FDA-approved only for relapsing forms of the disease. It is unclear whether the beneficial effects seen with the ABC products in RRMS will be evident in patients with SPMS or PPMS. Clinical trials of Betaseron and Rebif (interferon-β-1a marketed in Europe and Canada and given subcutaneously three times per week) in SPMS have had mixed results. There is a suggestion that patients with SPMS and ongoing attacks or enhancing MRI lesions may benefit, whereas those without such findings will not benefit. An Avonex trial in patients with SPMS is still underway, with patients receiving twice the usual dose or placebo. Trials of Avonex and Copaxone are being conducted in patients with PPMS. Alternative delivery routes, including nasal and oral, are being studied. The optimal dosage and duration of therapy with the interferon agents are unclear, and the lack of comparative trials clouds the question of which agent is superior. Finally, determination of "treatment failure" and what to do in the event of progression of disease while on ABC therapy remains a difficult question.

The most important question in the use of the ABC drugs is when to begin therapy. The Medical Advisory Board of the National Multiple Sclerosis Society has adopted recommendations regarding the use of the current MS disease-modifying agents, and these are summarized in Table 55–3.[74] Clearly, these drugs are only partial therapies that slow the course of the illness but do not suppress it. They also require injections and have side effects and costs that limit their use. There is now, however, overwhelming evidence that the natural history of MS is that the vast majority of patients will have progressive disease over time. Pathologic data clearly show that even in acute lesions there is significant axonal damage that is essentially irreversible. MRI data show that 80% to 90% of all new, enhancing lesions are asymptomatic, suggesting that a "quiet" clinical course does not necessarily mean there is not ongoing disease activity. Thus the view that a significant number of patients have "benign" MS is probably not accurate.

Furthermore, it is now known that very early therapy is effective. In patients with a single clinical episode consistent with demyelination and two or more lesions on brain MRI (i.e., at high risk for developing clinically definite MS), treatment with Avonex produced a 44% reduction compared with placebo in the likelihood of patients going on to have a second clinical attack over a 2-year period of study. Several MRI measures also were significantly better in treated patients.[41] Thus not only is very early therapy warranted, but it is also effective. The "watch and wait" attitude so prevalent after the original introduction of Betaseron in 1993 does not appear defensible at this point in time. Indeed, the National MS Society recommends patients with relapsing disease be placed on ABC therapy immediately after the diagnosis of relapsing disease.[74]

Other Therapies

Short-term, intensive, pulse doses of corticosteroids, similar to those used in acute exacerbations, initially may decrease disability, but prolonged steroid therapy has no established effects on the progression of disease.[57] If progression continues, an immunosuppressive agent may be tried.[49,50]

Mitoxantrone (Novantrone), a member of the anthracenediene family, has now been approved by the FDA for reducing neurologic disability and/or the frequency of clinical relapses in patients with SPMS (chronic), PRMS, or worsening RRMS.[75] Mitoxantrone is the only approved agent for SPMS.[76–78] Mitoxantrone is administered as a short (5- to 15-minute) intravenous infusion dosed at 12 mg/m^2 every 3 months. An evaluation of left ventricular ejection fraction is recommended prior to administration of the initial dose and if signs or symptoms of congestive heart failure develop. The left ventricular ejection fraction also should be evaluated in patients who have received a cumulative dose of 100 mg/m^2 or more. The lifetime cumulative dose of mitoxantrone is 140 mg/m^2.[75] Other potential side effects noted with this agent are nausea, alopecia, menstrual disorder, amenorrhea, upper respiratory tract infection, urinary tract infection, and leukopenia.[75] Please see the package insert for a complete listing of side effects documented with mitoxantrone. What role mitoxantrone will play in the treatment of MS remains unclear because potential cardiac toxicity appears to limit its long-term use. Currently, there are no proven therapies for the treatment of PPMS.[79]

Cyclophosphamide has been studied alone and in combination with other treatment modalities in attempts to slow progression of MS.[80] Maintenance therapy with intermittent (monthly) pulse doses of cyclophosphamide may slow the progression of disease in younger patients with secondary progressive disease, but further study is required to confirm benefit in these patients. Prolonged therapy with cyclophosphamide usually is intolerable, but it appears that some form of maintenance is necessary.[80] Although cyclophosphamide appears beneficial, toxicities may limit its use to patients with an unusually severe disease course.[49] Due to the toxicity profile of this agent, its use has fallen out of favor.

Conflicting results have been seen when azathioprine is used alone or in combination with other therapies. Reductions in the exacerbation rate and slowing of disease progression are only modest.[50] It is usually given in doses of 2 to 3 mg/kg until the white blood cell count drops to less than 4000/mm.[3] It is then followed with corticosteroid therapy.[48,50] Although not without serious side effects, azathioprine may be less toxic than cyclophosphamide and may be tolerated for a longer period of time. Methotrexate (MTX) given as 7.5 mg orally each week also has shown modest benefit in slowing disease progression.[48]

TABLE 55–3. Disease Management Consensus Statement (Abridged)

- Initiation of therapy is advised as soon as possible following a definite diagnosis of MS and determination of a relapsing course.
- Patients' access to medication should not be limited by the frequency of relapses, age, or level of disability.
- Treatment is not to be stopped during evaluation for continuing treatment.
- Therapy is to be continued indefinitely, unless there is clear lack of benefit, intolerable side effects, new data that reveal other reasons for cessation, or better therapy becomes available.
- All three agents should be included in formularies and covered by third-party payers so that physicians and patients may determine the most appropriate agent on an individual basis.
- Movement from one immunomodulating drug to another should be permitted.
- Most concurrent medical conditions do not contraindicate use of any of these therapies.

Modified from Ref. 74.

TABLE 55–4. Treatment of Selected Primary MS Symptoms

Spasticity	Bladder Symptoms	Sensory Symptoms	Fatigue
Baclofen	Propantheline	Carbamazepine	Amantadine
Dantrolene	Oxybutinin	Phenytoin	Pemoline
Diazepam	Dicyclomine	Amitriptyline or other TCAs	Antidepressants
Tizandine	DDAVP		Modafanil
Tiagabine	Self-catheterization	Gabapentin	Methylphenidate
Gabapentin	Imipramine or amitriptyline	Lamotrigine	Dextroamphetamine
	Prazosin		
	Botulinum toxin type A		

Cyclosporine appears to produce only a modest delay in the progression of disability in chronic progressive MS. A significant number of patients may develop severe side effects, in particular nephrotoxicity and hypertension,[81] which may limit the usefulness of this agent.

Other experimental modalities include total lymphoid irradiation (TLI), interferon-α, monoclonal antibodies, cladribine, and intravenous immune globulin (IVIG).[48] IVIG may stimulate remyelinization of neurons in established MS lesions. Further studies are required to confirm the observation of reduced exacerbations and improved neurologic function.

SYMPTOMATIC MANAGEMENT

Many of the symptoms of MS do not require pharmacologic management or do not respond to it. This section covers those primary symptoms in which pharmacologic management may be of benefit (Table 55–4). See the preceding section on the treatment of acute exacerbation for a discussion on optic neuritis.

GAIT DIFFICULTIES AND SPASTICITY

Problems with gait may be due to spasticity, weakness, ataxia, defective proprioception, or a combination of these factors. Spasticity is amenable to pharmacologic intervention, whereas physical therapy may be required in treating gait disturbances due to any of the other factors. Spasticity is commonly encountered and tends to affect the legs more markedly than the arms. Spasticity may result in falls; however, in the later stages of the disease, the increased muscle tone of a spastic limb often lends strength to patients with underlying weakness. Therefore, when using muscle relaxants, one must be careful not to decrease the tone to an extent where ambulation is actually hindered.[32,82] Baclofen (Lioresal), a γ-aminobutyric acid (GABA) analog, is the preferred agent and is usually started in dosages of 10 mg tid and titrated upward to achieve the desired response. Most patients will achieve a satisfactory response with dosages between 40 and 80 mg/d; however, dosages higher than the recommended daily maximum of 80 mg are required by some patients.[32,82] Continuous intrathecal administration of baclofen may be an option for those patients unable to tolerate or those who do not respond to oral therapy. Baclofen should not be discontinued abruptly to avoid the possibility of seizures.[82] Small doses of diazepam (e.g., 0.5 to 1 mg) are often added to baclofen in patients in whom optimal response has not been achieved. A newer agent, tizanidine (Zanaflex), is a short-acting, centrally acting α-adrenergic agonist that can reduce spasticity by increasing presynaptic inhibition of motor neurons. Tizanidine appears to have efficacy comparable with that of baclofen.[83] Dosage of this medication must be titrated slowly over 2 to 4 weeks, starting with 4 mg at bedtime and adjusting based on clinical response. Effective tolerated dosages have ranged from 2 to 36 mg/d. Sedation, dizziness, and dry mouth are the most commonly reported adverse effects of this agent. Hypotension also can occur, as well as a rare but severe hepatotoxicity. Increased aminotransferase activity was noted in 5% of patients during clinical trials. In patients who are unable to tolerate baclofen or tizanidine, diazepam (Valium), clonazepam (Klonopin), or dantrium sodium (Dantrolene) may be considered as alternatives, but they generally are less effective than either baclofen or tizanidine. Mild spasticity also may respond to moderately high doses of gabapentin (Neurontin). Tiagabine (Gabitril) may be useful in some patients with spasticity, but side effects may prohibit its use.

TREMOR

Cerebellar symptoms such as tremor can be troubling and difficult to control. Medications that may be helpful include propranolol, primidone, and isoniazid.

BOWEL AND BLADDER SYMPTOMS

Patients commonly complain of incontinence, urgency, frequency, and nocturia, which are indications of a hyperreflexic bladder (i.e., inability to store urine). A number of anticholinergic agents including oxybutynin chloride (Ditropan, 10 to 20 mg/d), tolterodine (Detrol, 2 to 4 mg/d), propantheline bromide (Probanthine, 45 to 90 mg/d) and dicyclomine hydrochloride (Bentyl, 30 to 80 mg/d) are used to treat this problem if symptoms are mild.[84] Ditropan is now also available in an extended-release formulation (5 and 10 mg). In addition, tricyclic antidepressants, such as imipramine (Tofranil) and amitriptyline (Elavil), also have been used for their anticholinergic properties. With all anticholinergic agents, great care must be used to avoid the problem of constipation, which is worsened by the patient's natural instinct to limit fluid intake (due to increasing the urge to urinate). As an alternative, the synthetic antidiuretic hormone preparation desmopressin (DDAVP) has been reported to be effective in the treatment of urgency and incontinence.[84] Use of DDAVP is probably best limited to bedtime so as to improve sleep because there may be significant problems with hyponatremia and possible seizures if overused. Patients with significant sphincter activity may benefit from the oral use of α-adrenergic blockers such as prazosin (Minipress) or intramuscular use of botulinum toxin type A (Botox).

Intermittent self-catheterization with or without a concomitant anticholinergic agent is recommended in patients with large postvoid urine residual volumes (>100 mL) or when the urinary problem is hyporeflexic in nature (failure to empty).[65] Patients with large postvoid residual volumes are at risk for developing urinary tract infections and often are prescribed urinary acidifiers such as vitamin C or antiseptics such as methenamine mandelate to prevent infections. For more severe symptoms, urologic referral and urodymanic testing should be considered prior to treatment.

Constipation due to either inactivity or medication side effects is the most common bowel complaint. Increases in dietary fiber and hydration may alleviate this problem, but in some instances laxatives or enemas may be necessary.[32]

MAJOR DEPRESSION

Major depression is common in patients with MS, and the risk of suicide may be increased markedly as compared with healthy subjects.[85,86] Patients should be monitored closely for the development of major depressive symptomatology and treated accordingly (see Chap. 69). Interferon products should be used cautiously in patients with significant depression.

SENSORY SYMPTOMS

Numbness and paresthesias are frequent sensory complaints but usually do not require treatment. Some MS patients may develop acute or chronic pain syndromes,[87] such as trigeminal neuralgia and painful dysasthesias, for which treatment is necessary. Carbamazepine (Tegretol) is the preferred agent for the treatment of trigeminal neuralgia and is used in the same doses that are used for the treatment of seizure disorders. Painful dysasthesias are burning sensations that commonly occur in the extremities. These pains often respond to treatment with tricyclic antidepressants, carbamazepine, gabapentin (Neurontin), or other anticonvulsant medications such as lamotrigine (Lamictal).

SEXUAL DYSFUNCTION

Sexual dysfunction in both men and women is also common in MS, and counseling should be offered to both partners. Sildenafil citrate (Viagra) is very effective for men with MS who have erectile dysfunction. Viagra is currently being studied in the female population with MS and sexual dysfunction.

FATIGUE

Fatigue, one of the most common complaints in MS patients, can be severely disabling. Although typically present in the late to middle afternoon, it may increase with heat exposure, exertion, or intercurrent infection. The cause of fatigue is unclear. Spasticity, weakness, and depression also may contribute to MS-related fatigue. Amantadine hydrocholoride (100 mg bid) often is used and may offer significant relief.[82] Pemoline (Cylert) also has been used in doses starting at 18.75 to 37.5 mg/d,[82] but its use is limited by an FDA advisory suggesting very frequent monitoring of liver function tests due to potential toxicity. Methylphenidate (Ritalin) and dextroamphetamine (Dexedrine) also are commonly used for fatigue in MS. Modafanil (Provigil), a recently approved medication for the treatment of narcolepsy, at 100 mg bid, now has been shown to also be helpful for MS-related fatigue. Antidepressants may be helpful, but only if the patient exhibits symptoms of depression. Otherwise, the sedating effects may worsen fatigue.

The aminopyridines, 4-aminopyridine and 3,4-diaminopyridine,[88] are potassium channel blockers that are currently under investigation in the symptomatic treatment of MS. These agents appear to improve conduction in demyelinated axons and may improve strength and decrease heat sensitivity.[48]

Each symptom should be assessed individually, and therapy with available agents should be tried and modified when needed. In addition to counseling patients regarding the adverse effects associated with medications, pharmacists also should actively encourage patients to comply with their prescribed regimens.

PHARMACOECONOMIC CONSIDERATIONS

As with many therapeutic decisions, economic cost both to the individual and society must be considered. Currently, the annual cost of the new potentially disease-modifying therapies is considerable. The cost to the pharmacist of glatiramer and both currently available interferons is between $10,000 and $11,000 per patient per year. Given this expense, it must be remembered that these therapies are not curative and that individual patients may experience variable results. Future investigations evaluating these therapeutic modalities clearly will need to address both economic and humanistic outcomes.

EVALUATION OF THERAPEUTIC OUTCOMES

Response to treatment of acute exacerbations of MS are seen commonly within days. With respect to disease-modifying treatments, it is important for the clinician to recognize that over the short term (days to weeks), little or no apparent benefit may be noted by either patient or clinician. Evaluation of therapeutic outcomes, such as decreased MS exacerbations and hospitalizations or perhaps slowed disease progression and disability (as measured using scales such as EDSS), must be conducted over a period of months to years. Patients should be provided with realistic goals and expectations of these treatment options and encouraged to participate in the evaluation of therapeutic response. Initially, it may be important to reevaluate patients at relatively short time intervals to monitor for adverse effects.

CONCLUSIONS

MS is an inflammatory disease of the CNS that appears to strike young, genetically susceptible individuals living in high-risk geographic areas. Although the exact etiology of MS is unknown, it is likely that MS is an autoimmune disease triggered by a viral infection. There is no cure for MS, but quality of life can be improved through symptomatic management. Because of the relapsing-remitting nature of

MS, it is often difficult to assess whether improvement is due to treatment or due to the course of the disease. The paucity of conclusive evidence for many of the described treatments and the lack of specific guidelines make treatment choices difficult.

▶ PRINCIPLES OF PHARMACOTHERAPY

- The etiology of MS is unknown, and currently there is no cure.
- MS appears to be an immunologic disorder, which is characterized by CNS demyelination and axonal damage.
- Diagnosis of MS is made primarily on the basis of clinical examination and MRI findings.
- Acute exacerbations or relapses usually are treated with high-dose glucocorticoids, such as methylprednisolone.
- In most patients suffering from an acute exacerbation, a clinical response to steroid treatment can be expected within 3 to 5 days.
- Treatment with interferon-β or glatiramer acetate (ABC therapy) can reduce annual relapse rate, slow progression of disability, slow cognitive decline, and slow changes seen on the brain MRI scans.
- Treatment with immunomodulating ABC therapy should begin promptly after the diagnosis of relapsing MS is made, probably after just a single attack if the MRI is suggestive of high risk of further attacks. Therapy after ABC "treatment failure" and in patients with SPMS and PPMS is not clear.
- The only treatment approved for SPMS is mitozantrone.
- Patients suffering from MS frequently will have symptoms such as spasticity, bladder dysfunction, fatigue, pain, and depression that may require treatment. Patients must be counseled that therapies such as interferon-β and glatiramer acetate will not relieve these symptoms.
- Depression is common in MS and may pose the risk of suicide.

ACKNOWLEDGMENT

We would like to acknowledge Ruth C. Taggart, MSN, ANP-C, for her contribution to this chapter.

REFERENCES

1. Anderson DW, Ellenberg JH, Leventhal CM, et al. Revised estimate of the prevalence of multiple sclerosis in the United States. Ann Neurol 1992;31:333–336.
2. Wynn DR, Rodriguez M, O'Fallon WM, et al. Update on the epidemiology of multiple sclerosis. Mayo Clin Proc 1989;64:808–817.
3. Sadovnick AD, Ebers GC. Epidemiology of multiple sclerosis: A critical overview. Can J Neurol Sci 1993;20:17–29.
4. Lechtenberg R. Multiple Sclerosis Fact Book. Philadelphia, Davis, 1988.
5. Ebers GC, Bulman D. The geography of MS reflects genetic susceptibility. Neurology 1986;36(Suppl 1):108.
6. Compston A. Risk factors for multiple sclerosis: Race or place? (Editorial). J Neurol Neurosurg Psychiatry 1990;53:821–823.
7. Kurtzke JF. Epidemiologic contributions to multiple sclerosis: An overview. Neurology (NY) 1980;30(Suppl 2):61–79.
8. Ebers GC. Genetics and multiple sclerosis: An overview. Ann Neurol 1994;36:S12–S14.
9. Compston A. The epidemiology of multiple sclerosis: Principles, achievements, and recommendations. Ann Neurol 1994;36:S211–S217.
10. Wolfson C, Wolfson EB, Zielinski JM. On the estimation of the distribution of the latent period of multiple sclerosis. Neuroepidemiology 1989;8:239–248.
11. Detels R, Visscher BR, Haile RW, et al. Multiple sclerosis and age at migration. Am J Epidemiol 1978;108:386–393.
12. Hillert J. Human leukocyte antigen studies in multiple sclerosis. Ann Neurol 1994;36:S15–S17.
13. Genetics and immunology. In: Kesselring J, ed. Multiple Sclerosis. Cambridge, UK, Cambridge, University Press, 1997:30–48.
14. Lucchinetti CF, Rodriguez M. The controversy surrounding the pathogenesis of the multiple sclerosis lesion. Mayo Clin Proc 1997;72:665–678.
15. De Keyser J. Autoimmunity in multiple sclerosis. Neurology 1988;38:371–374.
16. McDonald WI. The mystery of the origin of multiple sclerosis. J Neurol Neurosurg Psychiatry 1989;49:113–323.
17. Poser CM. Pathogenesis of multiple sclerosis: A critical reappraisal. Acta Neuropathol 1986;71:1–10.
18. Sharief MK, Thompson EJ. In vivo relationship of tumor necrosis factor alpha to blood-brain barrier damage in patients with active multiple sclerosis. J Neuroimmunol 1992;38:27–33.
19. Panitch HS, Hirsch RL, Schindler J, Johnson KP. Treatment of multiple sclerosis with gamma interferon: Exacerbation associated with activation of the immune system. Neurology 1987;37:1097–1102.
20. Hartung HP, Archelos JJ, Zievasek J, et al. Circulating adhesion molecules and inflammatory mediators in demyelination: A review. Neurology 1995;45(Suppl 6):22–32.
21. Link J, Soderstrom M, Olsson T. Increased TGFβ, IL-4 and INFα in multiple sclerosis. Ann Neurol 1994;36:379–386.
22. Rieckman P, Albrecht M, Kitze B, et al. Cytokine mRNA levels in mononuclear blood cells from patients with multiple sclerosis. Neurology 1994;44:1523–1526.
23. Sobel RA. The pathology of multiple sclerosis. Neurol Clin 1995;13:1–16.
24. Johnson RT. The virology of demyelinating diseases. Ann Neurol 1994;36:S54–S60.
25. Berti R, Soldan SS, Akhyani N, et al. Extended observations on the association of HHV-6 and multiple sclerosis. J Neurovirol 2000; 6(Suppl 2):S85–S87.
26. Sriram S, Stratton CW, Yao S, et al. *Chlamydia pneumoniae* infection of the central nervous system in multiple sclerosis. Ann Neurol 1999; 46(1):6–14.
27. Trapp BD, Peterson J, Ransohoff RM, et al. Axonal transection in the lesions of multiple sclerosis. N Engl J Med. 1998;338:278–285.
28. Truyen L, van Wuesberghe JHTM, Barkof F, et al. Accumulation of hypointense lesions ("blackholes") on T1 spin echo MRI correlates with disease progression in multiple sclerosis. Neurology 1996;47:1469–1476.
29. Lassman H, Suchanek G, Ozawa K. Histopathology and the blood–cerebrospinal fluid barrier in multiple sclerosis. Ann Neurol 1994;36:S42–S46.
30. Rodriguez M. Multiple sclerosis: Basic concepts and hypothesis. Mayo Clin Proc 1989;64:570–576.
31. Weiner HL, Hafler DA. Immunotherapy of multiple sclerosis. Ann Neurol 1988;23:211–222.
32. Schapiro RT. Symptom management in multiple sclerosis. Ann Neurol 1994;36:S123–S129.
33. Kurtzke JF. Rating neurologic impairment in multiple sclerosis: An expanded disability status scale (EDSS). Neurology 1983;33:1444–1452.
34. Noseworthy JH. Clinical scoring methods for multiple sclerosis. Ann Neurol 1994;36:S80–S85.
35. Miller DH. Magnetic resonance imaging in monitoring the treatment of multiple sclerosis. Ann Neurol 1994;36:S91–S94.
36. Filippi M, Paty DW, Kappos L, et al. Correlations between changes in disability and T2 weighted brain activity in multiple sclerosis: A follow-up study. Neurology 1995;45:255–260.
37. Abramsky O. Pregnancy and multiple sclerosis. Ann Neurol 1994;36:S38–S41.
38. Kurland LT. Trauma and multiple sclerosis. Ann Neurol 1994;36:S33–S37.

39. Weinshenker BG. Natural history of multiple sclerosis. Ann Neurol 1994;36:S6–S11.
40. Swanson JW. Multiple sclerosis: Update in diagnosis and review of prognostic factors. Mayo Clin Proc 1989;64:577–586.
41. Jacobs LD, Beck RW, Simon JH, et al. Intramuscular interferon beta-1a therapy initiated during a first demyelinating event in multiple sclerosis. N Engl J Med 2000;343:898–904.
42. Williams ES, Jones DR, McKeran RO. Mortality rates from multiple sclerosis: Geographical and temporal variations revisited. J Neurol Neurosurg Psychiatry 1991;54:104–109.
43. McDonald WI, Silberberg DH. The diagnosis of multiple sclerosis. In: McDonald WI, Silberberg DH, eds. Multiple Sclerosis. Boston, Butterworth, 1986:1.
44. McFarland H, Frank JA, Albert PS, et al. Using gadolinium-enhanced magnetic resonance imaging lesions to monitor disease activity in multiple sclerosis. Ann Neurol 1992;32:758–766.
45. O'Riordan JI, Thompson AJ, Kingsley DP, et al. The prognostic value of brain MRI in clinically isolated syndromes of the CNS: A 10-year follow-up. Brain 1998;121(Pt 3):495–503.
46. Olsson T. Cerebrospinal fluid. Ann Neurol 1994;36:S100–S102.
47. Myers LW, Ellison GW. The peculiar difficulties of therapeutic trials for multiple sclerosis. Neurol Clin 1990;8:119–141.
48. Hunter SF, Weinshenker BG, Carter JL, Noseworthy JH. Rational clinical immunotherapy for multiple sclerosis. Mayo Clin Proc 1997;72:765–780.
49. Becker C, Gidal BE, Flemming JO. Immunotherapy in multiple sclerosis, part 2. Am J Health Syst Pharm 1995;52:2105–2120.
50. Becker C, Gidal BE, Flemming JO. Immunotherapy in multiple sclerosis, part 1. Am J Health Syst Pharm 1995;52:1985–2000.
51. Kaufman DI, Trobe JD, Eggenberger ER, Whitaker JN. Practice parameter: The role of corticosteroids in the management of acute monosymptomatic optic neuritis. Report of the quality standards subcommittee of the American Academy of Neurology. Neurology 2000;54:2039–2044.
52. Beck RW, Cleary PA, Trobe JD, et al. The effect of corticosteroids for acute optic neuritis on the subsequent development of multiple sclerosis. N Engl J Med. 1993;329:1764–1769.
53. Beck RW, Cleary PA, et al. Optic Neuritis Treatment Trial: One-year follow-up results. Arch Ophthalmol 1993;111:773–775.
54. Rose AS, Kuzma JW, Kurtzke JF, et al. Cooperative study in the evaluation of therapy in multiple sclerosis: ACTH versus placebo, final report. Neurology 1970;20(Suppl):1–19.
55. Durelli L, Cocito A, Riccio C, et al. High-dose intravenous methylprednisolone in the treatment of multiple sclerosis: Clinical immunologic correlations. Neurology 1986;36:238–243.
56. Milligan NM, Newcombe R, Compston DAS. A double-blind controlled trial of high-dose methylprednisolone in patients with multiple sclerosis: 1. Clinical effects. J Neurol Neurosurg Psychiatry 1987;50:511–516.
57. Goodin DS. The use of immunosuppressive agents in the treatment of multiple sclerosis: A critical review. Neurology 1991;41:980–985.
58. Kappos L. Therapy. In: Kesselring J, ed. Multiple Sclerosis. Cambridge, UK, Cambridge University Press, 1997:148–167.
59. Weinshenker BG, O'Brian PC, Petterson TM, et al. A randomized trial of plasma exchange in acute central nervous system inflammatory demyelinating disease. Ann Neurol 1999;46(6):878–886.
60. Weinshenker BG. Therapeutic plasma exchange for acute inflammatory demyelinating syndromes of the central nervous system. J Clin Apheresis 1999;14(3):144–148.
61. The IFNB Multiple Sclerosis Study Group. Interferon beta-1b is effective in relapsing-remitting multiple sclerosis: 1. Clinical results of a multicenter, randomized, double-blind, placebo-controlled trial. Neurology 1993;43:655–661.
62. The IFNB Multiple Sclerosis Study Group. Interferon beta-1b is effective in relapsing-remitting multiple sclerosis: 2. MRI analysis results of a multicenter, randomized, double-blind, placebo-controlled trial. Neurology 1993;43:662–667.
63. Goodkin DE. Interferon β-1b. Lancet 1994;344:1057–1060.
64. Arnason BG, Reder AT. Interferons and multiple sclerosis. Clin Neuropharmacol 1994;17:495–547.
65. The INFB Multiple Sclerosis Study Group and the University of British Columbia MS/MRI Analysis Group. Interferon β-1b in the treatment of multiple sclerosis. Neurology 1995;45:1277–1285.
66. Guttman-Weinstock B, Rudick RA. Prescribing recommendations for interferon-beta in multiple sclerosis. CNS Drugs 1997;8:102–112.
67. Jacobs LD, Cookfair DL, Rudick RA, et al. Intramuscular interferon beta-1a for disease progression in relapsing multiple sclerosis. Ann Neurol 1996;39:285–294.
68. Simon JH, Jacobs L, Campion M, et al. A longitudinal study of brain atrophy in relapsing MS. Neurology 1999;58:139–145.
69. Fischer JS, Priore RL, Jacobs LD, et al. Neuropsychological effects of interferon β-la in relapsing multiple sclerosis. Ann Neurol 2000;48:885–892.
70. Aharoni R, Teitelbaum D, Sela M, et al. Copolymer 1 induces T cells of the T helper type 2 that cross-react with myelin basic protein and suppress experimental autoimmune encephalomyelitis. Proc Natl Acad Sci USA 1997;94:10821–10826.
71. Johnson KP. Therapy of relapsing forms. In: Burks JS, Johnson KP, eds. Multiple Scelerosis: Diagnosis, Medical Management, and Rehabilitation. New York, Demos Medical Publishing, 2000:167–175.
72. Johnson KP, Brooks BR, Cohen JA, et al. Extended use of glatiramir acetate (Copaxone) is well tolerated and maintains its clinical effect on multiple sclerosis relapse rate and degree of disability. Neurology 1998;50:701–708.
73. The INFB Multiple Sclerosis Study Group and the University of British Columbia MS/MRI Analysis Group. Neutralizing antibodies during treatment of multiple sclerosis with interferon beta 1b: Experience during the first three years. Neurology 1996;47:889–894.
74. van den Noort S, Eidelman B, Rammohan K, et al., for the National Multiple Sclerosis Society (NMSS). Disease Management Consensus Statement: Clinical Bulletin. National MS Society, New York, 1998:1–8.
75. Immunex Corporation. Novantrone (mitoxantrone concentrate for injection) package insert. Seattle, WA, October, 2000.
76. Hartung HP, Gonsett R. Mitoxantrone in progressive multiple sclerosis (MS): A placebo-controlled, randomized, observer-blind European phase III multicenter study. Clinical results. Multiple Sclerosis 1998;4:325.
77. Edan G, Miller D, Clanet M, et al. Therapeutic effect of mitoxantrone combined with methylprednisolone in multiple sclerosis: A randomised multicentre study of active disease using MRI and clinical criteria. J Neurol Neurosurg Psychiatry 1997;62:112–118.
78. Hartung H, Gonsett R, and the MIMS Study Group. Mitoxantrone in progressive multiple sclerosis (MS): Clinical results and three-year follow-up of the MIMS trial (Abstract 56). Multiple Sclerosis 1999;5(Suppl 1):S15.
79. Noseworthy JH, Lucchinetti C, Rodriguez M, Weinshenker BG. Multiple sclerosis. N Engl J Med 2000;343:938–952.
80. Goodkin DE, Plencner S, Palmer-Saxerud J, et al. Cyclophosphamide in chronic progressive multiple sclerosis: Maintenance versus nonmaintenance therapy. Arch Neurol 1987;44:823–827.
81. The Multiple Sclerosis Study Group. Efficacy and toxicity of cyclosporine in chronic progressive multiple sclerosis: A randomized, double-blinded, placebo-controlled clinical trial. Ann Neurol 1990;27:591–605.
82. Mitchell G. Update on multiple sclerosis therapy. Med Clin North Am 1993;77:231–249.
83. Wagstaff AJ, Bryson HM. Tizanidine. Drugs 1997;53:435–452.
84. Kinn AC, Larsson PO. Desmopressin: A new principle for symptomatic treatment of urgency and incontinence in patients with multiple sclerosis. Scand J Urol Nephrol 1990;24:109–112.
85. Schubert DS, Foliart RH. Increased depression in multiple sclerosis patients: A metaanalysis. Psychosomatics 1993;34:124–130.
86. Stenager EN, Stenager E, Koch Henriksen N, et al. Suicide and multiple sclerosis: An epidemiological investigation. J Neurol Neurosurg Psychiatry 1992;55:542–545.
87. Moulin DE. Pain in multiple sclerosis. Neurol Clin 1989;7:321–331.
88. Beaver CT Jr. The current status of studies of aminopyridine in patients with multiple sclerosis. Ann Neurol 1994;36:S118–S121.

56

EPILEPSY

Barry E. Gidal, William R. Garnett, PharmD, and Nina Graves, PharmD

Epilepsy has been recognized for at least 2400 years. It is derived from the Greek *epilepsia,* meaning "to come upon, to be grabbed hold of or thrown down, to attack, to seize hold of." Hughlings Jackson, in 1861, first developed the theory that seizures were caused by an excessive discharge of the gray matter of the brain.

Today, epilepsy is viewed as a symptom of disturbed electrical activity in the brain caused by a wide variety of disorders. *Epilepsy* is a general name given to the wide range of symptoms that reflect the many functions of the brain in a pathologically disturbed manner. It is a collection of many different types of seizures that vary widely in severity, appearance, cause, consequence, and management. Epilepsy implies a periodic recurrence of seizures with or without convulsions.[1] Seizures that are prolonged or repetitive can be life-threatening. The effect epilepsy has on patients' lives can be extremely frustrating. Indeed, studies have shown that patients with epilepsy who do not experience complete seizure control have lower self-reported quality-of-life scores than patients who are seizure-free.

In the early 1980s, the primary drugs used for epilepsy were phenobarbital, phenytoin, carbamazepine, and valproic acid. During the 1990s, eight newer drugs were approved for use in epilepsy: felbamate, gabapentin, lamotrigine, topiramate, tiagabine, zonisamide, levetiracetam, and oxcabazepine. The newer agent vigabatrin, which is widely available outside the United States, failed to be approved by the Food and Drug Administration (FDA) due largely to concerns over neurophthamalogic toxicities including visual field deficits.[2] The availability of new drugs for epilepsy offers new opportunities to improve treatment and makes it essential that clinicians review all their patients to ensure that they are achieving the best outcomes possible.

EPIDEMIOLOGY

Each year, 120 per 100,000 people in the United States come to medical attention because of a newly recognized seizure. At least 8% of the general population will have at least one seizure in a lifetime. However, it is possible to have a seizure and not have epilepsy.[3] Recurrence of a first unprovoked seizure within 5 years ranges between 23% and 80%. Children with an idiopathic first seizure and a normal electroencephalogram (EEG) have a particularly favorable prognosis.[4] Some seizures may occur as single events resulting from withdrawal of central nervous system (CNS) depressants (e.g., alcohol, barbiturates, and other drugs) or during acute illnesses (e.g., meningitis or encephalitis) or toxic conditions (e.g., uremia or eclampsia). Some patients will have seizures only associated with fever. These febrile seizures do not constitute epilepsy.

Epilepsy is a chronic disorder characterized by recurrent seizures.[1] The age-adjusted incidence of epilepsy is 44 per 100,000 person-years. Each year, about 125,000 new epilepsy cases occur; of these, 30% are in people under the age of 18 at the time of diagnosis. There is a bimodal distribution in the occurrence of the first seizure, with one peak occurring in newborn and young children and the second peak occurring in patients older than age 65.[5] The relatively high frequency of epilepsy in the elderly is now being recognized. At least 10% of patients in long-term care facilities are taking at least one antiepileptic drug (AED).[6] At this time, it is unknown if these AEDs are used for seizures or other conditions.[1] The seizure type and the cause of the seizure change with age.[5]

ETIOLOGY

Seizures occur because small numbers of neurons discharge abnormally. Anything that disrupts the normal homeostasis of the neuron and disturbs its stability may trigger abnormal activity and seizures. A genetic predisposition to seizures has been suggested. Patients with mental retardation and cerebral palsy are at increased risk for seizures. The more profound the degree of mental retardation as measured by intelligence quotient (IQ), the greater the incidence of epilepsy. However, mental retardation is not synonymous with epilepsy. In the elderly, 67% of seizures are partial in onset. The causes of seizures in the elderly may be multifactorial and include cerebrovascular disease (both ischemic and hemorrhagic stroke), neurodegenerative disorders, tumor, head trauma, metabolic disorders, and CNS infections.[5] In some cases, if an etiology can be found, it can be corrected, and the patient will not require chronic AEDs; however, most patients who present with seizures do not have an identifiable cause and thus have idiopathic epilepsy.[5] The incidence of idiopathic epilepsy is higher in children.[7]

Many factors have been shown to precipitate seizures in susceptible individuals.[1] Hyperventilation may precipitate absence seizures. Sleep, sleep deprivation, sensory stimuli, and emotional stress may initiate seizures. Hormonal changes occurring around the time of menses, puberty, or pregnancy have been associated with the onset of or an increased frequency of seizures. A history for theophylline, alcohol, phenothiazine, antidepressant (especially maprotiline), and street drug use should be obtained from patients presenting with seizures. Also, AEDs in toxic concentrations may cause seizures in certain patients. Perinatal factors and subsequent events have been identified as risk factors for the later development of epilepsy. Children who are small for gestational age or with neonatal seizures are at increased risk for developing epilepsy. The most clearly established risk factors for epilepsy in all age groups are head trauma, especially in cases where the dura mater has been breached and where there is evidence of loss of conciousness, CNS infections, and stroke. Immunizations have not been associated with an increased risk of epilepsy.[5] However, pertussis immunization has been associated with an increase in febrile seizures.

PATHOPHYSIOLOGY

Seizure activity is characterized by paroxysmal discharges occurring synchronously in a large population of cortical neurons. This is characterized on the EEG as a sharp wave or "spike." The basic physiology of a seizure episode is traceable to an unstable cell membrane or its surrounding supportive cells. The seizure originates from the gray matter of any cortical or perhaps subcortical area. Initially, a small number of neurons fire abnormally. Normal membrane conductances and inhibitory synaptic currents break down, and excess excitability spreads, either locally to produce a focal seizure or more widely to produce a generalized seizure.[8] This onset propagates by physiologic pathways to involve adjacent or remote areas. The clinical manifestations depend on the site of the focus, the degree of irritability of the surrounding area of the brain, and the intensity of the impulse. An abnormality of potassium conductance, a defect in the voltage-sensitive ion channels, or a deficiency in the membrane ATPases linked to ion transport may result in neuronal membrane instability and a seizure. Selected neurotransmitters (e.g., glutamate, aspartate, acetylcholine, norepinephrine, histamine, corticotropin-releasing factor, purines, peptides, cytokines, and steroid hormones) enhance the excitability and propagation of neuronal activity, whereas γ-aminobutyric acid (GABA) and dopamine inhibit neuronal activity and propagation. A relative deficiency of inhibitory neurotransmitters such as GABA or an increase in excitatory neurotransmitters such as glutamate would promote abnormal neuronal activity. Normal neuronal activity also depends on an adequate supply of glucose, oxygen, sodium, potassium, chloride, calcium, and amino acids. Systemic pH is also a factor in precipitating seizures. The different kinds of epilepsies probably arise from different neurophysiologic abnormalities.

Control of abnormal neuronal activity with AEDs is accomplished by elevating the threshold of neurons to electrical or chemical stimuli or by limiting the propagation of the seizure discharge from its origin. Raising the threshold most likely involves stabilization of neuronal membranes, whereas limiting the propagation involves depression of synaptic transmission and reduction of nerve conduction.[8]

During a seizure, there is a large increase in the demand for blood flow to the brain to carry off CO_2 and to bring substrates for neuronal metabolic activity. The brain has a limited capacity to increase blood flow, and during a seizure, the brain may use more energy than it can manufacture. The more prolonged the seizure, the more likely the brain is to suffer ischemia that may result in neuronal destruction and brain damage. The developing brain is especially vulnerable to damage. Although individual seizures as such do not cause a significant decrease in intelligence, it has been suggested that patients suffering a large number of generalized tonic-clonic (GTC) seizures (e.g., >100 GTC seizures) or who have multiple episodes of status epilepticus may be at risk for eventual cognitive declines. Seizures beget seizures. There appears to be a positive correlation between the early initiation of appropriate AED therapy and the ability to control seizure activity. The failure to control seizures seems to lead to an increase in seizure activity and also to the occurrence of other seizure types. Therefore, appropriate therapy should be initiated early after the diagnosis of epilepsy.

CLINICAL PRESENTATION

The International League Against Epilepsy (ILAE) has proposed two major schemes for classification of seizures and epilepsies: the International Classification of Epileptic Seizures[9] and the International Classification of the Epilepsies and Epilepsy Syndromes.[10]

The International Classification of Epileptic Seizures (Table 56–1) combines the clinical description with certain electrophysiologic findings in order to classify epileptic seizures. Seizures are divided into two main pathophysiologic groups—partial seizures and generalized seizures—by EEG recordings and clinical symptomatology.

TABLE 56–1. International Classification of Epileptic Seizures

I. Partial seizures (seizures begin locally)
   A. Simple (without impairment of consciousness)
      1. With motor symptoms
      2. With special sensory or somatosensory symptoms
      3. With psychic symptoms
   B. Complex (with impairment of consciousness)
      1. Simple partial onset followed by impairment of consciousness—with or without automatisms
      2. Impaired consciousness at onset—with or without automatisms
   C. Secondarily generalized (partial onset evolving to generalized tonic-clonic seizures)
II. Generalized seizures (bilaterally symmetrical and without local onset)
   A. Absence
   B. Myoclonic
   C. Clonic
   D. Tonic
   E. Tonic-clonic
   F. Atonic
   G. Infantile spasms
III. Unclassified seizures
IV. Status epilepticus

Compiled from Ref. 9.

Partial (focal) seizures begin in one hemisphere of the brain and—unless they become secondarily generalized—result in an asymmetric clinical manifestation. Partial seizures manifest as alterations in motor functions, sensory or somatosensory symptoms, or automatisms. Partial seizures with no loss of consciousness are classified as *simple partial.* The symptoms (aura) often experienced prior to a GTC seizure may be a simple partial seizure that secondarily generalizes. Partial seizures with an alteration of consciousness are described as *complex partial.* With complex partial seizures, the patient may have automatisms, periods of memory loss, or aberrations of behavior.[1] Some patients with complex partial epilepsy have been mistakenly diagnosed as having psychotic episodes. Complex partial seizures may progress to a generalized seizure.[1] Partial epilepsy may begin in infancy and may be difficult to recognize in an elderly population. Patients with complex partial seizures are typically amnestic to these events.

Generalized seizures have clinical manifestations that indicate involvement of both hemispheres. Motor manifestations are bilateral, and there is a loss of consciousness. Generalized seizures may be further subdivided by EEG and clinical manifestations.[1] A partial seizure that becomes generalized is referred to as a *secondarily generalized seizure.*

Generalized absence seizures are manifested by a sudden onset, interruption of ongoing activities, a blank stare, and possibly a brief upward rotation of the eyes. They generally occur in young children through adolescence. The EEG during the seizure has a characteristic 2- to 4-cycle/s spike and slow-wave complex.[1] It is important to differentiate absence seizures from complex partial seizures.

Generalized tonic-clonic seizures, formerly known as *grand mal,* are what many people think of as epilepsy. Although they may be preceded by premonitory symptoms (auras), the majority of patients lose consciousness without warning. The seizure results in a sudden sharp tonic contraction of muscles followed by a period of rigidity and clonic movements. The patient may fall and be injured. During the seizure, the patient may cry or moan, lose sphincter control, bite the tongue, or develop cyanosis. After the seizure, the patient may be unconscious for a variable period of time and frequently goes into a deep sleep. Tonic and clonic seizures may occur separately.[1] Brief shocklike muscular contractions of the face, trunk, and extremities are known as *myoclonic jerks.* They may be isolated events or rapidly repetitive.[1] A sudden loss of muscle tone is known as an *atonic seizure.* This may be described as a head drop, the dropping of a limb, or a slumping to the ground.[1] These patients often wear protective headware to prevent trauma.

The International Classification of Epilepsies and Epilepsy Syndromes[10] adds components such as age of onset, intellectual development, findings on neurologic examination, and results of neuroimaging studies to more fully define epilepsy syndromes. Syndromes can include one or many different seizure types (e.g., Lennox-Gastaut syndrome). The syndromic approach includes seizure type(s) and possible etiologic classifications (idiopathic, symptomatic, cryptogenic, or unknown). *Idiopathic* describes syndromes that are presumably genetic but also those in which no underlying etiology is documented or suspected. A family history of seizures is commonly present, and neurologic function is essentially normal except for the occurrence of seizures. *Symptomatic* cases involve evidence of brain damage or a known underlying cause. A *cryptogenic* syndrome is assumed to be symptomatic of an underlying condition that cannot be documented. *Unknown* or *undetermined* is used when no cause can be identified. This syndromic classification is more important for prognostic determinations than as a classification based simply on seizure type. The syndrome classification scheme requires more information and, in return, provides a more powerful tool for comprehensive clinical management. A patient's epilepsy is classified based on seizure type (generalized versus partial) and syndromic type (idiopathic, symptomatic, cryptogenic).

▶ TREATMENT: Epilepsy

DESIRED OUTCOME

The ultimate goal of treatment for epilepsy is no seizures and no side effects with an optimal quality of life. The best quality of life is associated with a seizure-free state.[11] Often, however, a balance between efficacy and side effects must be reached, because with the older AEDs used as monotherapy, fewer than 50% of patients become seizure-free.

Because therapy is extended for many years (often a lifetime), chronic side effects must be considered.[12] If the patient is overly sedated or develops other significant side effects, some seizure control may have to be sacrificed to improve functioning.[13] The patient should be involved in deciding what balance between frequency of seizures and the occurrence of side effects is most appropriate. The newer AEDs offer alternatives for balancing seizure frequency and drug side effects.

Providing optimal quality of life goes beyond balancing seizures and side effects. It involves assessing all the concerns of a patient with epilepsy. For example, patients with epilepsy are concerned about driving, their future, forming relationships, safety, social isolation, social stigma, and so on.[14] Despite public awareness programs, there are still many misconceptions about epilepsy. These misconceptions often liken epilepsy to mental retardation, possession by demons, or punishment by God. Patients may be encouraged to contact or join the Epilepsy Foundation of America (1-800-EFA-1000) or other support groups that encourage patients with epilepsy to lead normal lives. Knowledge about epilepsy has been correlated with an improved quality of life. It is also important to recognize that patients with epilepsy may have other neuropsychiatric comorbidities such as depression, anxiety, and sleep disturbances.[15] Clinicians should be aware of these potential problems and consider therapy where appropriate.

GENERAL APPROACH TO TREATMENT

The general approach to treatment involves identification of goals, assessment, development of a care plan, and a follow-up evaluation. During the assessment phase, it is critical to establish an accurate diagnosis of the seizure type and classification.[16] This diagnostic step will help determine the appropriate initial AEDs. Patient-specific treatment goals must be identified, and these may change over time. In patients with new-onset epilepsy, the goal should be "no seizures, no side effects," and an optimal quality of life. Patients with chronic epilepsy ideally have this same goal, but it may not be possible to achieve it immediately, and thus the goal at a specific point in time must be established (e.g., decrease the number of seizures or alleviate toxicity). Identification of specific goals will help in the development of the short- and long-term treatment plans. Patient characteristics such as age, medical condition, ability to comply with a prescribed regimen, and insurance coverage also should be explored because these may influence AED choices or help explain lack of response or unexpected side effects. Once the assessment is complete, the advantages and disadvantages of appropriate AEDs are compared. For patients with new-onset seizures, the choice is whether to use drug therapy and, if so, which one. For a patient with long-standing epilepsy, adequacy of the current medication regimen must be evaluated. An AED should not be considered ineffective unless the patient has experienced some concentration-dependent side effects with continued seizures. If a decision is made to start AED therapy, monotherapy is preferred, and about 70% of all patients with epilepsy can be maintained on one drug.[7] However, many of these patients are not seizure-free. The percentage of patients who are seizure-free on one drug varies by seizure type. The prognosis for 12-month seizure freedom is best for those who have only GTC seizures (48% to 55%), worst for those who have only complex partial seizures (23% to 26%), and intermediate for those with mixed seizure types (25% to 32%).[17] Drugs may be combined in an attempt to help the patient become seizure-free. Combining AEDs with different mechanisms of action may be advantageous, although this approach is as yet unproven. Approximately 65% of patients can be expected to be maintained on one AED and be considered well controlled, although not necessarily seizure-free. Of the 35% with unsatisfactory control, 10% will be well controlled with a two-drug treatment. Of the remaining 25%, 20% of these will continue to have unsatisfactory control despite multiple-drug treatment. Fifteen percent of these will become surgical candidates.[18] For some patients, an implantable device such as the vagal nerve stimulator (see below) may be an additional nondrug option.

Once the care plan is established, a prescription is generated for a specific AED. Usually this includes a dose titration schedule. At this point, patient education and assurance of patient understanding of the plan are essential. Detailed directions regarding titration, what to do in the event of a treatment-emergent side effect, and what to do if a seizure occurs must be provided to patients. Documentation of the assessment, care plan, and educational process is essential. Providing the patient with a seizure and side-effect diary will assist in the follow-up and evaluation phase. At the follow-up stage of treatment (which can be done in the hospital, clinic, pharmacy, or by phone), the treatment goals must be reviewed. If the goal has been achieved, new goals should be identified. For example, if the GTC seizures are now controlled, the goal may be to control partial seizures. If a patient fails to respond to the first AEDs, trials with other AEDs should be attempted. Completion of the evaluation often requires a reassessment of the patient and development of a new care plan. The assessment at this point should evaluate compliance, efficacy, and safety of the initial treatment.

Noncompliance may be the single most common reason for treatment failure. It is estimated that up to 60% of patients with epilepsy are noncompliant.[19] The rate of noncompliance is increased by the complexity of the drug regimen and by doses taken three and four times a day.[19] Noncompliance is not influenced by age, sex, psychomotor development, seizure type, or seizure frequency.[20]

WHEN TO START AEDs

Drug treatment may not be indicated in patients whose seizures have minimal impact on their lives or those who have had only a single seizure. If a patient presents after a single isolated seizure, one of three treatment decisions can be made: treat, possibly treat, or do not treat. These decisions are based on the probability of the patient having a second seizure (Table 56–2). For patients with no risk factors, the probability of a second seizure is less than 10% in the first year and approximately 24% by the end of 2 years. If risk factors are present, this recurrence rate can increase dramatically and can be as high as 80% after 5 years.[1] Are these rates high enough to warrant AED therapy? That decision often depends on the patient's lifestyle. Patients who have had two or more seizures generally should be started on AEDs. One study examined whether treatment affected the recurrence rate after a single unprovoked GTC seizure. The treated group had a 25% risk of seizure recurrence at 24 months compared with 51% for the untreated group.[23]

TABLE 56–2. Recurrence Risk for Patients Experiencing One Unprovoked Seizure

Type of Patient	1st-Yr Risk (%)	5th-Yr Risk (%)
Adults with single unproved seizure		34
No CNS insult	10	29
Influence of family history		
Sibling with seizure	29	46
No sibling with seizures	7	27
EEG patterns		
GSW on EEG	15	58
Normal EEG	9	26
Occurrence of previous seizure	10	39
Due to an illness or childhood febrile seizure		
Remote symptomatic with Todd's paresis	26 41	48 75
Status epilepticus at onset	37	56
Prior acute seizure	60	80
Idiopathic	10	29

CNS = central nervous system; EEG = electroencephalogram; GSW = generalized spikes and waves.

Compiled from Ref. 150.

WHEN TO STOP AEDs

The AEDs initially used to control seizures may not need to be given for a lifetime. Polypharmacy may be reduced, and some patients can discontinue AEDs altogether. In reducing polypharmacy, the drug considered less appropriate for the seizure type (or the agent deemed most responsible for adverse effects) should be discontinued first. In some cases, decreasing the number of AEDs a patient is receiving can decrease side effects and increase cognitive abilities.[24] This improvement in cognition may be small, especially if the patient is on a drug that primarily affects psychomotor speed with less effect on higher-order cognitive functioning.

Factors favoring successful withdrawal of AEDs include a seizure-free period of 2 to 4 years, complete seizure control within 1 year of onset, an onset of seizures after age 2 but before age 35 years, and a normal neurologic examination and EEG. Factors associated with a poor prognosis in discontinuing AEDs, despite a seizure-free interval, include a history of a high frequency of seizures, repeated episodes of status epilepticus, a combination of seizure types, and development of abnormal mental functioning. Children who have irregular generalized spike and wave activity in EEG recordings prior to discontinuation of treatment may have a higher relapse rate (67%) compared with children without epileptiform activity (33%) or children with other types of epileptiform activity (33%) in their last EEG recordings before discontinuation.[25] A 2-year seizure-free period is suggested for absence and rolandic epilepsy, whereas a 4-year seizure-free period is suggested for simple partial, complex partial, and absence associated with tonic-clonic convulsions. Withdrawal is generally not suggested for patients with juvenile myoclonic epilepsy or absence with clonic-tonic-clonic seizures.The American Academy of Neurology has issued guidelines for discontinuing AEDs in seizure-free patients[26] (Table 56–3). When the factors likely to be associated with successful withdrawal are present, the relapse rate is expected to be less than 32% for children and 39% for adults.[26] A recent study examined patients who had had a seizure recurrence after randomization to either AED withdrawal or continued AED therapy.[27] The authors suggested that the population that develops epilepsy and then enters a period of remission for 2 or more years may be divided into two groups: (1) patients whose epilepsy has ceased and (2) patients with long interictal intervals but epilepsy that is still active. Patients are divided about evenly between the two groups.

If the decision is made to attempt AED withdrawal, this should be done gradually. This may be particularly true for patients with profound developmental disabilities. Some patients will have a recurrence of seizures as the AEDs are withdrawn. Sudden withdrawal is associated with the precipitation of status epilepticus. Withdrawal seizures are of particular concern for agents such as benzodiazepines and barbiturates. Seizure relapse has been reported to be more common if the AEDs are withdrawn over 1 to 3 months than over 6 months.

TABLE 56–3. American Academy of Neurology Guideline for Discontinuing AEDs in Seizure-Free Patients

After assessing the risks and benefits to both patient and society from a recurrent seizure, the discontinuance of antiepileptic drugs may be considered by the physician and informed patient or parent/guardian if the patient meets the following profile:

- Seizure-free 2 to 5 years on AEDs (mean, 3.5 years)
- Single type of partial seizure (simple partial, complex partial, or secondary generalized tonic-clonic seizure) or single type of primary generalized tonic-clonic seizures
- Normal neurologic examination/normal IQ
- EEG normalized with treatment

The risk of seizure relapse has been estimated at 10% to 70%. A meta-analysis determined that the relapse rate was 25% after 1 year and 29% after 2 years.[28] Withdrawal doubles the risk of seizure recurrence for the first 1 to 2 years but does not modify the long-term prognosis of a person's epilepsy. If seizures recur after AED withdrawal, AEDs should be restarted. Ninety percent of patients will regain at least another 2-year remission.[27] In addition to seizure relapse, the withdrawal of AEDs has been associated with the emergence of anxiety and depression.[29]

The patient should agree to the plan to reduce or withdraw AED therapy. Some patients may be reluctant to stop medications because of fear of a seizure or the potential interference with activities of daily living such as driving. There may be a significant psychosocial benefit to the patient from AED withdrawal.[30] Withdrawal may need to be scheduled at the convenience of the patient (e.g., during a summer vacation). A follow-up of 5 years is suggested for any patient withdrawn from AED therapy.

NONPHARMACOLOGIC THERAPY

Nonpharmacologic therapy for epilepsy includes diet, surgery, and implantation of a vagal nerve stimulator.[31] Vagus nerve stimulation (VNS) is an implanted medical device approved for use in epilepsy. The NeuroCybernetic Prosthesis (NCP) system was approved by the FDA in 1997 and is "indicated for use as an adjunctive therapy in reducing the frequency of seizures in adults and adolescents over 12 years of age with partial-onset seizures, which are refractory to antiepileptic medications." The device consists of an implantable, programmable pulse generator connected to a helical lead. The generator is implanted in a subcutaneous infraclavicular pocket and is powered by a lithium battery. The lead is attached to the left vagus nerve and delivers a biphasic current through the skin to the nerve that can be programmed to different parameters by the physician. In addition, the patient can use a magnet placed over the generator to activate the generator during a seizure or aura.

The mechanisms of antiseizure actions of VNS are unknown, but recent studies have indicated that VNS acutely causes widespread, bilateral cortical and subcortical alterations in blood flow, suggesting that it affects synaptic activity in humans.[32]

The VNS device is relatively safe. The most common side effect associated with stimulation is hoarseness during stimulation (up to 72% in one study). Other commonly occurring adverse events include voice alteration (50%), increased cough (41%), pharyngitis (28%), dyspnea (18%), dyspepsia (12%), and nausea (19%). Serious adverse effects reported included infection, nerve paralysis, hyesthesia, facial paresis, left vocal chord paralysis, left facial paralysis, left recurrent laryngeal nerve injury, urinary retention, and low-grade fever.

In a large multicenter, add-on, double-blind, randomized, active-control study of VNS therapy for partial-onset seizures, all patients were implanted with the device. Patients were randomized to receive "low" stimulation (pseudoplacebo) versus "high" stimulation (active) ($n = 95$ "high" stimulation; $n = 103$ "low" stimulation). The mean decrease in total seizure frequency from baseline was 15.2% in the "low" group versus 27.9% in the "high" group ($P = .04$).[33]

Over all the VNS studies, the percentage of patients who achieved a 50% or greater reduction in their seizure frequency ("responders") ranged from 23% to 50%.

Surgery is the most widespread and most useful nonpharmacologic therapy.[34] The use of surgery for intractable epilepsy that significantly interferes with patients' lives and functioning is increasing in both adult and pediatric patients. The success rate is reported to be between 80% and 90% in properly selected patients.[34] A focus in the temporal lobe has the best chance for a positive outcome, but extratemporal foci may be excised successfully in more than 75% of the patients. The procedure is not without risk. Learning and memory are most susceptible to impairment postoperatively, and general intellectual abilities are also affected in a small number of patients. It may be particularly useful in children with intractable epilepsy. Patients may still need to receive AED therapy for a period of time following successful epilepsy surgery in order to prevent seizure recurrence.[35]

The ketogenic diet was devised in the 1920s. It is high in fat and low in carbohydrates and protein and thus leads to acidosis and ketosis. Protein and calorie intake are set at levels that will meet requirements for growth. Most of the calories are provided in the form of heavy cream and butter. No sugar is allowed. Vitamins and minerals are supplemented.[36] Medium-chain triglycerides may be substituted for the dietary fats. Fluids are also controlled. It requires strict control and parent compliance. Although some centers find this useful for refractory patients, others have found that it is poorly tolerated by patients. Long-term effects are unknown.

PHARMACOLOGIC THERAPY

DRUG TREATMENTS OF FIRST CHOICE

The drug treatments of first choice depend on the type of epilepsy (Table 56–1) as well as on the interface between drug-specific adverse effects and patient preferences. Few guidelines or treatment protocols have been published. Figure 56–1 is a suggested algorithm for a general approach to the treatment of epilepsy.

Because the majority of adults have localization-related (partial-onset) seizures, the most widely used AEDs traditionally have been carbamazepine, phenobarbital, phenytoin, and valproic acid. For complex partial seizures, these AEDs have similar efficacy.[37] However, carbamazepine and phenytoin may be preferred, based on two pivotal trials conducted through the Veterans Administration (VA) Epilepsy Cooperative Study Group. In the first of these trials, patients with new-onset partial or generalized epilepsy were randomized to receive either carbamazepine, phenobarbital, phenytoin, or primidone.[38] Doses were titrated upward until seizures were controlled or unacceptable toxicity occurred. At the end of 3 years, patients who received either carbamazepine or phenytoin were equally likely and patients on phenobarbital or primidone were least likely to have remained on their originally assigned treatment. Thus carbamazepine and phenytoin were considered the drugs of first choice in patients with new-onset partial or generalized seizures. A follow-up study, using almost identical methods, compared carbamazepine and valproic acid.[39] Carbamazepine- and valproic acid–treated groups had equal retention rates for tonic-clonic seizures. Carbamazepine was superior to valproic acid for partial seizures. Valproic acid caused slightly more adverse effects.

These VA cooperative studies directly compared widely used AEDs available at the time the studies were designed, and they are among the very few comparative studies. In clinical trials of newer AEDs, the comparison is between active drug and placebo in patients who continue to have seizures despite current treatment with standard AEDs. Thus it is difficult to directly compare the efficacy of the newer with that of the older AEDs. Recently, European trials have been conducted that compare the older AEDs such as carbamazepine and

TABLE 56–4. Drugs of Choice for Specific Seizure Disorders

Seizure Type	First-Line Drugs	Alternative Drugs
Partial seizures	Carbamazepine Phenytoin Lamotrigine Valproic acid Oxcarbazepine	Gabapentin Topiramate Levetiracetam Zonisamide Tiagabine Primidone, phenobarbital Felbamate
Generalized seizures		
Absence	Valproic acid, ethosuximide	Lamotrigine
Myoclonic	Valproic acid, clonazepam	Lamotrigine, topiramate, felbamate
Tonic-clonic	Phenytoin, carbamazepine, valproic acid	Lamotrigine, topiramate, phenobarbital, primidone, oxcarbazepine

phenytoin with newer entities including lamotrigine and gabapentin. A meta-analysis has been published recently that attempts to indirectly compare some of the newer AEDs.[40] Because of wide and overlapping confidence intervals for both efficacy and tolerability outcome measures, however, no statistically significant differences between agents could be found. Generally speaking, the newer AEDs appear to have comparable efficacy with the older agents and perhaps are better tolerated. What has become obvious is that individuals may

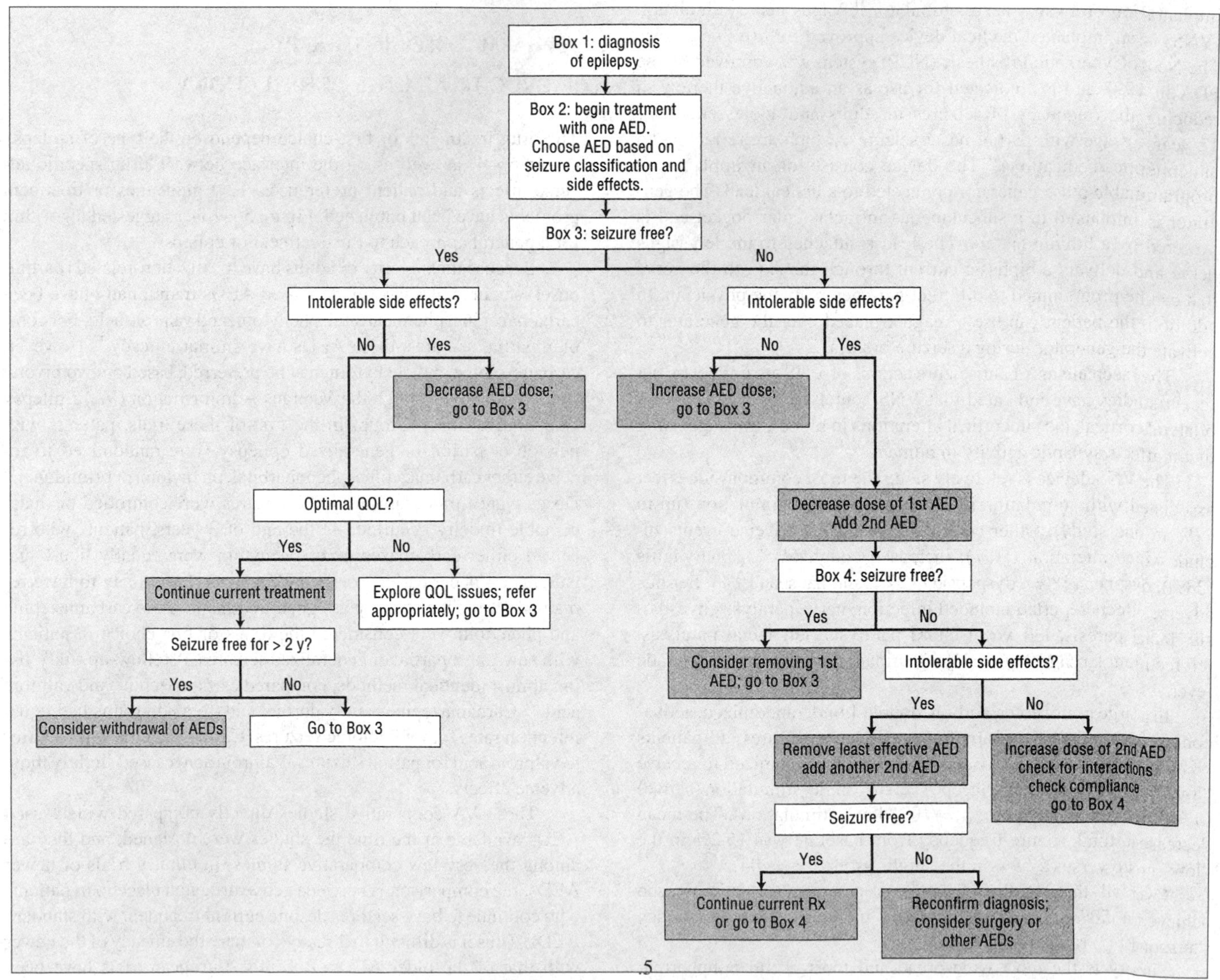

FIGURE 56–1. Algorithm for treatment of epilepsy.

respond differently to each AED, and that an understanding of each of these newer agents is needed to optimize therapy for individual patients.

ALTERNATIVE DRUG TREATMENTS

Some benzodiazepines (e.g., diazepam, lorazepam, and midazolam) are used in the acute treatment of status epilepticus. On a chronic basis, other benzodiazepines such as clonazepam can be useful, especially in the treatment of seizure types that occur primarily in children, although tolerance may develop. Recently, a rectal formulation of diazepam gel has been approved for acute repetitive seizures.

Acetazolamide has possible efficacy in a variety of seizure disorders, including GTC, absence, and complex partial seizures. Due to rapid emergence of tolerance, intermittent use has been more effective, and it may be particularly useful in treating the increase in seizure frequency present during menses (catamenial epilepsy).[41] Adrenocorticotropic hormone (ACTH) is often used for infantile spasms.

SPECIAL CONSIDERATIONS IN THE FEMALE PATIENT

Many hormones influence brain electrical excitability, and the steroid hormones estrogen and progesterone may interact in complex ways to alter neuronal excitability and protein synthesis. Estrogen has a seizure-activating effect, whereas progesterone exerts a seizure-protective effect. Estrogen has an inhibitory effect on GABA receptors, potentiates excitatory glutaminergic activity, and may promote the development of kindling. Progesterone has the opposite effects and appears to potentiate GABA receptor activity and reduce neuronal discharge rates. AEDs, especially hepatic metabolizing enzyme inducers, also affect hormones by increasing the metabolism of steroid hormones and inducing the production of sex hormone–binding globulin. This may lead to decreases in the unbound fraction of the hormone. Enzyme-inducing AEDs, including topiramate, may cause treatment failures in females taking oral contraceptives; thus treatment with a moderate or high hormonal dose oral contraceptive ($\geq$50 μg) is necessary.[42] A supplemental form of birth control in addition to oral contraceptives is advised if breakthrough bleeding occurs. Valproic acid, benzodiazepines, and most of the newer AEDs are not enzyme inducers and have not been associated with this effect.[43] In some women, vulnerability to seizures is highest just before and during the menstrual flow (catamenial seizures) and at the time of ovulation. The risk of catamenial epilepsy is estimated at 12.5% but may occur in as many as 50% of women with epilepsy.[44] This pattern of seizure exacerbation may be related to progesterone withdrawal and changes in the estrogen-to-progesterone ratio. Conventional AEDs should be tried first in these women. As noted previously, intermittent acetazolamide also has been used, but with variable and limited success. Hormonal therapy with progestational agents, particularly cyclic natural progesterone therapy, also may be effective.[45] Reproductive endocrine disorders are common in women with epilepsy and include menstrual irregularity, infertility, sexual dysfunction, and possibly an increased risk of polycystic ovary syndrome. Potential mechanisms for these disturbances include disruptuion of the hypothalamic-pituitary-adrenal (HPA) axis via seizure discharges in limbic structures and/or AEDs. AEDs, particularly the enzyme-inducing agents (e.g., carbamazepine, phenytoin, phenobarbital), also may affect HPA axis function by altering the metabolism of the neuroactive sex hormones, including testosterone. Although a definitive causal relationship has not yet been established, an apparent increased incidence of polycystic ovary syndrome has been suggested for women with epilepsy who are receiving valproic acid.[46]

Pregnancy raises several concerns, including the possibility of increased maternal seizures, pregnancy complications, and adverse fetal outcome. About 25% to 30% of women have increased seizures during pregnancy, whereas seizures decrease in a similar number. Increased seizure activity may result from either a direct effect on seizure threshold or a reduction in AED concentration. An increase in clearance has been reported for phenytoin, carbamazepine, phenobarbital, ethosuximide, and clorazepate. Protein binding also may be altered. The altered disposition of AEDs may begin as early as the first 10 weeks of pregnancy and may take up to 4 weeks postpartum to return to normal.

There is a higher incidence of adverse pregnancy outcomes in women with epilepsy. Although the risk of congenital malformations is 4% to 6% (twice as high as in nonepileptic women), more than 90% of pregnancies in epileptic mothers have satisfactory outcomes. Barbiturates and phenytoin are associated with congenital heart malformations, orofacial clefts, and other malformations. Valproic acid and carbamazepine are predominantly associated with spina bifida (neural tube defect) and hypospadias. The risk of neural tube defect with valproic acid and carbamazepine has been estimated to be 1% to 2% and 0.5% to 1%, respectively, and appears to be related to drug exposure during gestational days 0 to 28. Other adverse pregnancy outcomes associated with maternal seizures, but not necessarily caused by AEDs, are growth, psychomotor, and mental retardation. Women with epilepsy are also more likely to have miscarriages, and 10% to 20% of infants are born with low birth weight.[47] Guidelines have been developed for counseling and managing the pregnant woman with epilepsy.[48] The North America pregnancy registry (1-888-233-2334) has been established for reporting any pregnancy in women taking AEDs. Many of these teratogenic effects can be prevented by adequate folate intake; therefore, prenatal vitamins with folic acid (~0.4 to 1 mg/day) should be given to any woman of childbearing potential who is taking AEDs. Higher AED doses and concentrations, polytherapy, and a family history of birth defects appear to increase the teratogenic risk. Therefore, deciding on the most effective single-drug treatment prior to conception is vitally important. New AEDs are reported to be less teratogenic, and animal reproductive toxicology studies appear to be favorable. At present, clinical data are quite limited, and more experience is needed before the true risk (or lack thereof) can be determined. AEDs also can lead to neonatal hemorrhagic disorder. Vitamin K (10 mg orally, given daily during the last month of pregnancy) should be given to the mother in order to prevent this coagulopathy.[42] Although AEDs pass into the breast milk, the concentrations are very low, and the infant receives a subtherapeutic dose. In general, the knowledge of the degree of protein binding of a given AED can allow for prediction of breast milk accumulation, with drugs with less protein binding partitioning more. Treatment with AEDs is not necessarily a reason to discourage breast feeding.[49] It is advisable that women taking any AED (particularly barbiturates or benzodiazepines) closely observe their infants for signs of excess sedation, irritability, or poor feeding.

Little is known regarding the effect of menopause on epilepsy. The perimenopausal period may be associated with worsening of seizures, possibly due to fluctuations in sex hormones. At menopause, seizures actually may improve, particularly in women who previously presented with a catamenial pattern. The effect of hormone-replacement therapy on seizure control is still unclear, but clinicians should monitor for seizure exacerbation in women receiving supplemental estrogen.

DRUG CLASS INFORMATION

Pharmacology and Mechanism of Action

The mechanism of action of most AEDs can be categorized as either affecting ion channels, augmenting inhibitory neurotransmission, or modulating excitatory neurotransmission.[50] The ion channels affected include the sodium and calcium channels. Increases in inhibitory neurotransmission affect CNS concentrations of GABA, whereas efforts to decrease excitatory neurotransmission are focused primarily on glutatmate and aspartate. AEDs that are effective against GTC and partial seizures probably reduce sustained repetitive firing of action potentials by delaying recovery of sodium channels from activation. Drugs that reduce corticothalamic T-type calcium currents are effective against generalized absence seizures.[50]

Pharmacokinetics

Awareness of pharmacokinetic properties can aid in the optimization of AED therapy (Table 56–5). Ideally, an AED used chronically should have a relatively prolonged absorption profile to avoid large peak-trough differences. Volumes of distribution of most AEDs are similar, with the exception of valproic acid. Protein binding less than 90% generally is not clinically important. Several commonly used AEDs are bound more than 90%; thus determination of unbound concentrations may be helpful in some clinical situations. The unbound or "free" concentration is the active drug capable of penetrating the blood-brain barrier and interacting at the receptor site. In patients who are not responding or having side effects at "therapeutic" concentrations of total drug, an unbound concentration may explain the unusual response. For populations known to have conditions that alter plasma protein binding (chronic renal failure, liver disease, hypoalbuminemia, burns, pregnancy, malnutrition, neonates, elderly, and displacing drugs), unbound rather than total drug concentrations should be measured for highly protein-bound drugs.[51] Unbound concentration monitoring is especially useful for phenytoin.

Many AEDs are metabolized extensively through various enzyme systems. The most common is the cytochrome P450 system, although through different subtypes. Several AEDs have active metabolites. Several of the newer AEDs have significant renal elimination.

Neonates may metabolize drugs more slowly but eliminate unchanged drug more rapidly. Infants and children may metabolize drug rapidly.[1] The volume of distribution changes as children grow. The ability to metabolize drugs decreases with age, and lower doses of AEDs are required in the elderly.[1] Although pharmacokinetic

TABLE 56–5. Antiepileptic Drug Pharmacokinetic Data

AED	$T_{1/2}$(h)[a]	Time to Steady State (d)	Unchanged (%)	V_D (L/kg)	Clinically Important Metabolite	Protein Binding (%)
Carbamazepine	12 M; 5–14 Co	21–28 for completion of auto-induction	<1	1–2	10,11-epoxide	40–90
Ethosuximide	A 60 C 30	6–12	10–20	0.67	No	0
Felbamate	16–22	5–7	50	0.73–0.82	No	~25
Gabapentin[b]	5–40[d]	1–2	100	0.65–1.04	No	0
Lamotrigine	25.4 M	3–15	0	1.28	No	40–50
Levetiracetam	7–10	2		0.7	No	<10%
Oxcarbazepine	3–13	2		0.7	10-Hydroxy carbazepine	40%
Phenobarbital	A 46–136 C 37–73	14–21	20–40	0.6	No	50
Phenytoin	A 10–34 C 5–14	7–28	<5	0.6–8.0	No	90
Primidone	A 3.3–19 C 4.5–11	1–4	40	0.43–1.1	PB[c] PEMA[c]	80
Tiagabine	5–13		Negligible		No	95
Topiramate	18–21	4–5	50–70	0.55–0.8 (male) 0.23–0.4 (female)	No	15
Valproic acid	A 8–20 C 7–14	1–3	<5	0.1–0.5	May contribute to toxicity	90–95 binding saturates
Zonisamide	24–60	5–15		0.8–1.6	No	40–60%

[a]A = adult; C = child; M = monotherapy; Co = combination therapy.
[b]The bioavailability of gabapentin is dose dependent.
[c]PB = phenobarbital; PEMA = phenylethylmalonamide.
[d]Half-life depends on renal function.

differences can be anticipated, pharmacodynamic changes have not been studied as extensively in the elderly. However, the elderly may have increased sensitivity to CNS drugs such as benzodiazepines.[52] A change in the pharmacodynamics would mean that the therapeutic range for younger patients would be invalid in the elderly. Because of pharmacokinetic and potential pharmacodynamic changes in the elderly, patient response rather than blood levels is the most important clinical outcome for patients of all ages.

Disease states may alter the pharmacokinetics of AEDs. Liver disease may decrease drug metabolism and protein binding. Patients with chronic renal failure may have decreased elimination of unchanged drug as well as altered protein binding.

Role of Serum Drug Concentration Monitoring

Although most older AEDs have published therapeutic ranges, the serum concentration should be viewed as a tool with which to optimize therapy for an individual patient, not, however, as a therapeutic end point in and of itself.[54] The serum concentration is a target that should be correlated with clinical outcome.[20] The desired response is the cessation of seizures without side effects. Seizure control may occur before the "minimum" of the published range is achieved, and side effects may appear before the "maximum" of the range is achieved. Some patients may need and tolerate concentrations beyond the "maximum." The therapeutic range for AEDs may be different for different seizure types. Serum concentrations may need to be higher to control complex partial seizures than to control tonic-clonic seizures.[53] Clinicians should define a therapeutic range for an individual patient, above which there are side effects and below which the patient experiences seizures. The pharmacodynamic response to AEDs may change as the patient ages, in that elderly patients may be more sensitive to various neurocognitive adverse effects of these drugs.

Efficacy

Classification of seizure types and epilepsy syndromes has improved the ability of clinicians to select drugs of choice for specific seizures (see Table 56–4). Primarly generalized seizures such as absence seizures may respond pharmacologically differently from other seizure types. Phenytoin, phenobarbital, and carbamazepine, although effective in GTC and partial seizures, are ineffective in treating absence seizures and in some cases may precipitate an increase in seizure activity. Absence seizures are best treated with ethosuximide, valproic acid, or perhaps lamotrigine. Gabapentin and tiagabine do not appear to be effective in this setting. If the patient has a combination of absence and other generalized or partial seizures, valproic acid is the preferred first choice because it is the only AED effective against absence and other seizure types. If valproic acid is ineffective in treating a mixed seizure disorder that includes absence, ethosuximide should be used in combination with another AED.[12] The traditional treatment of tonic-clonic seizures is phenytoin or phenobarbital, but the use of carbamazepine and valproic acid is increasing because these AEDs have a lower incidence of side effects and equal efficacy. Valproic acid is the drug of first choice for atonic seizures and for juvenile myoclonic epilepsy.[12] Lamotrigine and perhaps top iramate may be alternative agents for these seizure types. The newer agent zonisamide also may prove to be a valuable agent in primary generalized seizure types.

Carbamazepine traditionally has been recognized as the AED of first choice for partial seizures. Alternatives to carbamazepine are phenytoin, valproic acid, gabapentin, lamotrigine, tiagabine, topiramate, levatiracetam, oxcarbazepine, and zonisamide.The newer antiepileptic drugs were first approved as adjunctive therapy for patients with refractory partial seizures. Monotherapy trials with several of these newer agents including lamotrigine, gabapentin, topiramate, and oxcarbazepine have been completed. To date, only lamotrigine and oxcarbazepine have received FDA approval for use in monotherapy in patients with partial seizures. Phenobarbital and primidone are also useful in partial seizures, but adverse effects limit their utility. Felbamate, which has monotherapy approval, is effective but has been associated with some significant side effects.

Adverse Effects

Adverse drug reactions (ADRs) of AEDs can be divided into acute and chronic (Table 56–6). Acute effects can be dose-related (concentration-related) or idiosyncratic. Concentration-dependent effects are common and troublesome but not usually life threatening. Neurotoxic ADRs are encountered commonly and can include sedation, dizziness, blurred or double vision, difficulty with concentration, and ataxia. In many cases these effects can be alleviated by decreasing drug dose. Most idiosyncratic reactions due to an allergic reaction are mild, but they can be more serious if the hypersensitivity involves one or more organ systems. Other idiosyncratic side effects including hepatitis and blood dyscrasias are rare but can be serious.

Acute organ failure, if it is going to occur, generally occurs within the first 6 months of AED therapy. Unfortunately, laboratory screening of blood and urine typically is not helpful in predicting or detecting the early stage of severe reactions and generally is not recommended in asymptomatic patients. Laboratory assessment may be reasonable if the patient reports an unexplained illness (e.g., lethargy, vomiting, fever, or rash).[55]

Chronic side effects can occur despite serum concentrations within the therapeutic range, and multiple organ systems can be affected.[7] The incidence of chronic side effects is greatest with phenytoin (33%), phenobarbital (23%), carbamazepine (15%), and valproic acid (12%). The type and incidence of possible chronic side effects with the newer AEDs are mostly unknown at this time. The incidence of any side effects is lowest in patients on monotherapy and increases with each polytherapy.

The comparative effects of AEDs on cognition have been difficult to evaluate because of differences in study design, seizure types, control of drug concentrations, and neuropsychological tests used. In general, there are not large differences between the older drugs,[56] although the barbiturates phenobarbital and primidone appear to cause more cognitive impairment than other commonly used AEDs. Phenytoin, particularly when serum concentrations are above the commonly accepted therapeutic range, may have a greater effect on motor function and speed. Among the older AEDs, valproic acid may cause less impairment of cognition. Improvement in cognition has been reported in patients switched from phenytoin or phenobarbital to these agents. However, these effects are subtle and may not be pronounced if patients are in the same relative area of the therapeutic range.[57] Patients reduced from polytherapy to monotherapy also demonstrate improvement in cognition.[58] Some of the newer agents are believed to cause fewer neurobehavioral or cognitive effects. Among the newer AEDs, gabapentin and lamotrigine have been shown in several studies to cause fewer cognitive impairments as compared with older agents such as carbamazepine.[59] Conversely, topiramate may cause substantial cognitive impairment, particularly when used at high doses

TABLE 56–6. Antiepileptic Drug Side Effects

	Acute Side Effects		
AED	*Concentration Dependent*	*Idiosyncratic*	Chronic Side Effects
Carbamazepine	Diplopia Dizziness Drowsiness Nausea Unsteadiness Lethargy	Blood dyscrasias Rash	Hyponatremia
Ethosuximide	Ataxia Drowsiness GI distress Unsteadiness Hiccoughs	Blood dyscrasias Rash	Behavior changes Headache
Felbamate	Anorexia Nausea Vomiting Insomnia Headache	Aplastic anemia Acute hepatic failure	Not established
Gabapentin	Dizziness Fatigue Somnolence Ataxia		Weight gain
Lamotrigine	Diplopia Dizziness Unsteadiness Headache	Rash	Not established
Levetiracetam	Sedation Behavioral Disturbance (?)	Not established	Not established
Oxcarbazepine	Sedation Dizziness Ataxia Nausea	Rash	Hyponatremia
Phenobarbital	Ataxia Hyperactivity Headache Unsteadiness Sedation Nausea	Blood dyscrasias Rash	Behavior changes Connective tissue disorders Intellectual blunting Metabolic bone disease Mood change Sedation
Phenytoin	Ataxia Nystagmus Behavior changes Dizziness Headache Incoordination Sedation Lethargy Cognitive impairment Fatigue Visual blurring	Blood dyscrasias Rash Immunologic reaction	Behavior changes Cerebellar syndrome Connective tissue changes Skin thickening Folate deficiency Gingival hyperplasia Hirsutism Coarsening of facial features Acne Cognitive impairment Metabolic bone disease Sedation
Primidone	Behavior changes Headache Nausea Sedation Unsteadiness	Blood dyscrasias Rash	Behavior change Connective tissue disorders Cognitive impairment Sedation

TABLE 56–6. (Continued)

AED	Acute Side Effects: *Concentration Dependent*	Acute Side Effects: *Idiosyncratic*	Chronic Side Effects
Tiagabine	Dizziness Fatigue Difficulties concentrating Nervousness Tremor Blurred vision Depression Weakness	Not established	Not established
Topiramate	Difficulties concentrating Psychomotor slowing Speech or language problems Somnolence, fatigue Dizziness Headache	Not established	Kidney stones
Valproic acid	GI upset Sedation Unsteadiness Tremor Thrombocytopenia	Acute hepatic failure Acute pancreatitis	Polycystic ovary-like syndrome(?) Alopecia Weight gain Hyperammonemia
Zonisamide	Sedation Dizziness Cognitive impairment Nausea	Rash Oligohydrosis	Kidney stones

or during rapid dose escalation. Finally, in some cases, AED treatment itself has been suggested to cause worsening of seizures. This may result from either improper selection of an AED for a specific seizure type or syndrome or may represent a paradoxical toxic effect of the drug.[60]

Drug-Drug and Drug-Food Interactions

The AEDs frequently interact with each other via complex mechanisms. Interactions can occur in any of the pharmacokinetic processes: absorption, distribution, or elimination. Caution should be used when AEDs are added to or withdrawn from a drug regimen (Fig. 56–2). Some specific interactions are listed in Tables 56–7 and 56–8. Knowledge of which cytochrome P450 (CYP) subtype is involved can help predict interactions.

Phenobarbital, phenytoin, primidone, and carbamazepine are potent inducers of CYP, epoxide hydrolase, and uridine diphosphate glucuronosyltransferase (UGT) enzyme systems. Valproic acid can inhibit several CYP isozymes as well as UGT. In addition, valproic acid can displace some drugs from plasma albumin. Felbamate, topiramate, and oxcarbazepine can act as inducers with some isoforms and inhibitors of others. Ethosuximide, gabapentin, lamotrigine, tiagabine, levitiracetam, and zonisamide have little clinically significant effect on hepatic drug metabolism. Other than levitiracetam and gabapentin, which are mainly eliminated unchanged by the renal route, all other AEDs are metabolized wholly or in part by hepatic enzymes, and their disposition may be altered by metabolic changes. Some interactions are clinically unremarkable and some need only careful clinical monitoring, but others require prompt dosage adjustment.

Dosing and Administration

Almost all AEDs are associated with depressed CNS function (e.g., drowsiness, lethargy, tiredness) early in the course of treatment, but some tolerance usually develops in 7 to 10 days. Therefore, except in life-threatening situations (e.g., status epilepticus), AEDs should be started in low doses and increased gradually until seizure control is achieved or intolerable side effects occur. A general rule is to initiate therapy with one-fourth to one-third of the anticipated maintenance dose and increase the dose to maintenance over 3 to 4 weeks.[20] This allows the clinician to treat the patient and find the therapeutic range for that patient and not just dose to published values.

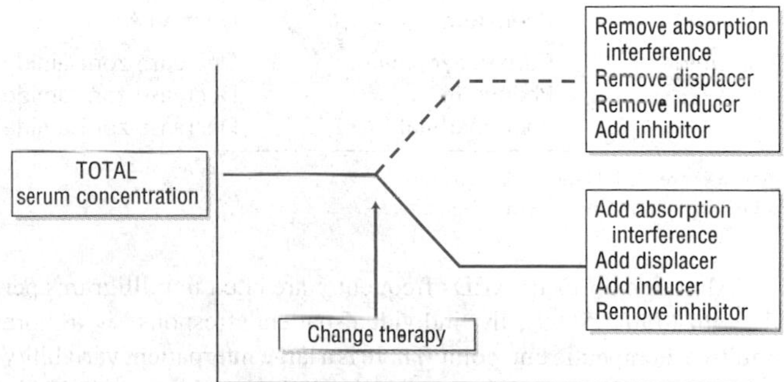

FIGURE 56–2. Effect of drug interactions. If a medication is added to or withdrawn from a patient's AED regimen, serum concentrations of the AED may change. Total serum concentrations will decrease *(bottom line)* if a compound is added that interferes with absorption, displaces from protein binding sites, or induces metabolism. If an inhibitor is removed from the regimen, concentrations will also decrease. Total concentrations will increase *(upper, dashed line)* if a compound is removed that interferes with absorption, displaces from protein binding sites, or induces metabolism, or if an enzyme inhibitor is added.

TABLE 56–7. Interactions Between Antiepileptic Drugs

AED	Added Drug	Effect[a]
Carbamazepine (CBZ)	Felbamate	Incr. 10,11 epoxide
	Felbamate	Decr. CBZ
	Phenobarbital	Decr. CBZ
	Phenytoin	Decr. CBZ
Felbamate (FBM)	Carbamazepine	Decr. FBM
	Phenytoin	Decr. FBM
	Valproic acid	Incr. FBM
Gabapentin	No known interactions	
Lamotrigine (LTG)	Carbamazepine	Decr. LTG
	Phenobarbital	Decr. LTG
	Phenytoin	Decr. LTG
	Primidone	Decr. LTG
	Valproic acid	Incr. LTG
Levetiracetam	No known interactions	
Oxcarbazepine	Carbamazepine	Decrease MHD[b]
	Phenytoin	Decrease MHD[b]
	Phenobarbital	Decrease MHD[b]
Phenobarbital (PB)	Felbamate	Incr. PB
	Phenytoin	Incr. or decr. PB
	Valproic acid	Incr. PB
Phenytoin (PHT)	Carbamazepine	Decr. PHT
	Felbamate	Incr. PHT
	Methsuximide	Incr. PHT
	Phenobarbital	Incr. or decr. PHT
	Valproic acid	Decr. Total PHT
	Vigabatrin	Decr. PHT
Primidone (PRM)	Carbamazepine	Decr. PRM Incr. PB
	Phenytoin	Decr. PRM Incr. PB
	Valproic acid	Incr. PRM Incr. PB
Tiagabine (TGB)	Carbamazepine	Decr. TGB
	Phenytoin	Decr. TGB
Topiramate (TPM)	Carbamazepine	Decr. TPM
	Phenytoin	Decr. TPM
	Valproic acid	Decr. TPM
Valproic acid (VPA)	Carbamazepine	Decr. VPA
	Lamotrigine	Decr. VPA
	Phenobarbital	Decr. VPA
	Primidone	Decr. VPA
	Phenytoin	Decr. VPA
Zonisamide	Carbamazepine	Decrease zonisamide
	Phenytoin	Decrease zonisamide
	Phenobarbital	Decrease zonisamide

[a]Incr. = increased; Decr. = decreased.
[b]MHD = 10-monohydroxymetabolite.

Although doses of AEDs frequently are cited in milligrams per kilogram (Table 56–9), the individual patient's response is a more definitive therapeutic end point. There is a large interpatient variability in pharmacokinetic parameters, which results in a large variation in the milligram per kilogram dose required to achieve adequate blood concentrations and response.[20] Therefore, the concentration of the drug in the serum or plasma may be a guideline in assessing drug dosing. In compliant patients with low plasma concentrations who are receiving a usual milligram per kilogram dose, the dosage may need to be increased if there are no side effects and seizures are continuing.

SPECIFIC DRUG INFORMATION

Carbamazepine

Pharmacology and Mechanism of Action. Animal studies indicate that carbamazepine depresses transmission in the nucleus ventralis anterior of the thalamus. This area has been associated with the generalization and spread of seizure discharge. The exact mechanism by which carbamazepine suppresses seizure spread is obscure, although it is believed to act primarily through inhibition of voltage-gated sodium channels. There is some depression of posttetanic potentiation (PTP) by carbamazepine, but it is of a lesser magnitude than occurs with phenytoin. It affects ionic conductance only at concentrations far above those normally produced in humans. It may inhibit an increase in cyclic AMP. Other biochemical effects are unknown.[50]

Pharmacokinetics. The absorption of carbamazepine from immediate-release tablets is slow and erratic because of its low water solubility. Because absorption is dissolution-rate-dependent, dose-dependent absorption may occur, resulting in less bioavailability at higher doses. The variable absorption results in times to peak of 2 to 24 hours (average 6 hours). There is also a large variability in the peak-to-trough concentrations of up to 40%. There is no first-pass metabolism. Food may enhance the bioavailability of carbamazepine. The suspension dosage form is absorbed faster than the tablets.[20] Controlled-release (Tegretol XR) and sustained-release (Carbatrol) preparations are also available. These are bioequivalent in twice-daily dosing to dosing four times daily with immediate-release carbamazepine.

Carbamazepine is a neutral and highly lipophilic drug that results in high body tissue binding. Carbamazepine binds to α_1-acid glycoprotein and to albumin. The usefulness of free carbamazepine concentrations remains to be defined.

Most (98% to 99%) of an administered dose of carbamazepine is metabolized by the liver, primarily by CYP 3A4.[61] Although 33 metabolites have been identified, the major metabolite is carbamazepine-10,11-epoxide.[62] This metabolite has anticonvulsant activity in animals and humans. The formation of the 10,11-epoxide is influenced by other enzyme-inducing or enzyme-inhibiting drugs. The 10,11-epoxide concentration may change with no change in parent carbamazepine concentration.[63]

Carbamazepine has the unique ability to induce its own metabolism (autoinduction).[64] The half-life after a single dose is much longer than the half-life after chronic therapy. The presence of enzyme-inducing drugs reduces the half-life even more. The enzyme-induction effect begins within 3 to 5 days after the initiation of therapy and takes 21 to 28 days to complete. Therefore, it is possible to achieve initial concentrations that are within the therapeutic range but have concentrations fall despite continued therapy with good compliance. Some patients who respond well to initial therapy may be labeled refractory or noncompliant if the autoinduction phenomenon is not considered. The autoinduction rapidly reverses if therapy with carbamazepine is temporarily discontinued.[64] This would be very important in epilepsy-monitoring units where all drugs are stopped in an attempt to precipitate seizures in patients being evaluated for seizure surgery.

Efficacy. Carbamazepine's relative lack of side effects compared with phenytoin and phenobarbital has resulted in an increased use for a variety of seizure disorders. It also may be useful in selected psychiatric disorders and in trigeminal neuralgia. Carbamazepine is considered an AED of first choice for partial seizures, especially complex partial seizures. It is also useful for generalized tonic-clonic seizures.

TABLE 56–8. Interactions With Other Medications

AED	Altered By	Result	Alters	Result
Carbamazepine	Cimetidine	Incr. CBZ	Oral contraceptives (OC)	Decr. efficacy of OC
	Erythromycin	Incr. CBZ	Doxycycline	Decr. doxycycline
	Fluoxetine	Incr. CBZ	Theophylline	Decr. theophylline
	Isoniazid	Incr. CBZ	Warfarin	Decr. warfarin
	Propoxyphene	Incr. CBZ		
Oxcarbazepine			OC	Decr. efficacy of OC
Phenobarbital	Acetazolamide	Incr. PB	OC	Decr. efficacy of OC
Phenytoin	Antacids	Decr. absorption of PHT	Oral contraceptives	Decr. efficacy of oral contraceptives
	Cimetidine	Incr. PHT	Bishydroxycoumarin	Decr. anticoagulation
	Chloramphenicol	Incr. PHT	Folic acid	Decr. folic acid
	Disulfiram	Incr. PHT	Quinidine	Decr. quinidine
	Ethanol (acute)	Incr. PHT	Vitamin D	Decr. vitamin D
	Fluconazole	Incr. PHT		
	Isoniazid	Incr. PHT		
	Propoxyphene	Incr. PHT		
	Warfarin	Incr. PHT		
	Ethanol (chronic)	Decr. PHT		
Primidone	Isoniazid	Decr. metabolism of primidone	Chlorpromazine	Decr. chlorpromazine
	Nicotinamide	Decr. metabolism of primidone	Corticosteroids	Decr. corticosteroids
			Quinidine	Decr. quinidine
			Tricyclics	Decr. tricyclics
			Furosemide	Decr. renal sensitivity to furosemide
Topiramate			OC	Decr. efficacy of OC
Valproic acid	Cimetidine	Incr. VPA		
	Salicylates	Incr. free VPA		

Incr. = increased; decr. = decreased.

Adverse Effects. Side effects (see Table 56–6) of carbamazepine may fluctuate daily, paralleling the rise and decline of serum concentrations. The side-effect profile also may follow a circadian rhythm. Neurosensory side effects (e.g., diplopia, blurred vision, nystagmus, ataxia, unsteadiness, dizziness, and headache) are the most common, occurring in 35% to 50% of patients. These side effects are more common during initiation of therapy and may dissipate with continued treatment. Patients have variable threshold concentrations for the occurrence of CNS side effects. If the carbamazepine serum concentration is kept below the individual threshold, the CNS side effects can be minimized. Dosage manipulation, including the use of the controlled- or sustained-release preparations, should be tried before the patient is considered to be intolerant of carbamazepine. An analog of carbamazepine, oxcarbazepine, may lead to fewer ADRs.

Carbamazepine may induce a hyponatremic hypoosmolar condition that is similar to the syndrome of inappropriate antidiuretic hormone secretion.[65] The incidence may increase with age. Periodic determinations of serum sodium are recommended, especially in the elderly.

The concern over carbamazepine-induced bone marrow suppression has been reinforced by a "black box" warning in the package insert requiring frequent complete blood count (CBC) monitoring. However, only a few cases of aplastic anemia, the most serious complication, have been reported since 1964. In many cases, there were confounding factors that precluded a definite cause-and-effect relationship. Thrombocytopenia and anemia have an incidence of less than 5% and usually respond to a cessation of drug therapy. Leukopenia is the most common hematologic side effect. An incidence as high as 10% has been reported. Leukopenia is usually transient even when the drug is continued and may be due to a redistribution of white blood cells (WBCs) rather than a decrease in their production. In about 2% of patients, the leukopenia is persistent, but even patients with WBC counts of $3000/mm^3$ or less do not seem to have an increased incidence of infection. A clinical guide is to continue carbamazepine therapy unless the WBC count drops to less than $2500/mm^3$ and the absolute neutrophil count drops to less than $1000/mm^3$.

Rashes are the most frequent hypersensitivity response. An incidence of 9.9% has been reported.[66] These are usually mild but may progress to a Stevens-Johnson syndrome. Other rare side effects reported with carbamazepine include hepatitis, osteomalacia, cardiac conduction defects, and lupuslike reactions. Carbamazepine appears to have modest effects on cognitive functioning.

Drug-Drug and Drug-Food Interactions. Because of concentration-dependent efficacy and side effects, drug interactions with carbamazepine are often clinically very significant. Valproic acid increases 10,11-epoxide metabolite concentrations without affecting the concentration of carbamazepine via inhibition of epoxide hydrolase. The interaction of erythromycin or clarithromycin with carbamazepine (CYP 3A4 inhibition) is particularly significant. Carbamazepine may interact with other drugs by inducing their metabolism; for example, carbamazepine increases the metabolism of valproic acid, theophylline, warfarin, and ethosuximide (see Tables 56–7 and 56–8). The absorption of carbamazepine suspension is slower and diminished when it is given during nasogastric (NG) feeding. This may result from adherence to the NG tube. It is recommended that carbamazepine suspension be mixed with an equal volume of diluent before being administered through NG feeding tubes.[67]

TABLE 56-9. AED Dosing and Target Serum Concentration Ranges

	Trade Name	Manufacturer	Year Introduced	Usual Initial Dose	Usual Maximum Daily Dose	Target Serum Concentration Range
Barbiturates						
Mephobarbital	Mebaral	Sanofi Winthrop	1935	50–100 mg/day	400–600 mg	Not defined
Phenobarbital	Various	Generic	1912	1–3 mg/kg/day (10–20 mg/kg LD)	180–300 mg	10–40 μg/mL
Primidone	Mysoline	Wyeth-Ayerst	1954	100–125 mg/day	750–2000 mg	5–10 μg/mL
Benzodiazepines						
Clonazepam	Klonopin	Roche	1975	1.5 mg/day	20 mg	20–80 ng/mL
Clorazepate	Tranxene	Abbott	1981	7.5–22.5 mg/day	90 mg	Not defined
Diazepam	Valium	Roche/generic	1968	PO: 4–40 mg IV: 5–10 mg	PO: 4–40 mg IV: 5–30 mg	100–1000 ng/mL
Lorazepam	Ativan	Wyeth-Ayerst generic		PO: 2–6 mg IV: 0.05 mg/kg IM: 0.05 mg/kg	PO: 10 mg IV: 0.044 mg/kg	10–30 ng/mL
Hydantoins						
Ethotoin	Peganone	Abbott	1957	<1000 mg/day	2000–4000 mg with food	15–50 μL
Mephenytoin	Mesantoin	Sandoz	1947	50–100 mg/day	200–800 mg	25–40 μg/mL
Phenytoin	Dilantin	Pfizer	1938	PO: 3–5 mg/kg (200–400 mg) (15–20 mg/kg LD)	PO: 500–600 mg	Total: 10–20 μg/mL Unbound: 0.5–3 μg/mL
Succinimides						
Ethosuximide	Zarontin	Pfizer	1960	500 mg/day	500–2000 mg	40–80 μg/mL
Methsuximide	Celontin	Pfizer	1957	300 mg/day	300–1200 mg	*N*-desmethyl metabolite 10–40 μg/mL
Other						
Carbamazepine	Tegretol	Novartis, generic	1974	400 mg/day	400–2400 mg	4–14 μg/mL
Felbamate	Felbatol	Carter Wallace	1993	1200 mg/day	3600 mg	40–100 μg/mL[a]
Gabapentin	Neurontin	Pfizer	1993	900 mg/day	4800 mg	4–16 μg/mL[a]
Lamotrigine	Lamictal	Glaxo SmithKline	1994	25 mg qod if on VPA; 25–50 mg/day if not on VPA	100–150 mg if no VPA; 300–500 mg if not on VPA	4–20 μg/mL[a]
Levetiracetam	Keppra	UCB-Pharma	2000	500–1000 mg/day	3000–4000 mg	Not defined
Oxcarbazepine	Trileptal	Novartis	2000	300–600 mg/day	2400–3000 mg	12–30 μg/mL[a] (MHD)
Tiagabine	Gabitril	Abbott	1997	4–8 mg/day	80 mg	Not defined
Topiramate	Topamax	Ortho McNeil	1997	25–50 mg/day	200–1000 mg	Not defined
Valproic acid	Depakene Depakote Depacon	Abbott	1978	15 mg/kg (500–1000 mg)	60 mg/kg (3000 5000 mg)	50–150 μg/mL[a]
Zonisamide	Zonegran	Elan	2000	100–200 mg/day	600 mg	10–40 μg/mL[a]

[a]Based on data from clinical trials–no established therapeutic ranges.

Dosing and Administration. The variable contributions of the 10,11-epoxide metabolite and free carbamazepine concentrations have restricted a precise definition of the therapeutic range. Loading doses of carbamazepine typically are not used. There are significant CNS-depressant effects and gastrointestinal complaints (e.g., nausea and vomiting) associated with large initial doses.

During dosage titration, it should be remembered that carbamazepine clearance increases with time. Doses may be started at one-fourth to one-third of the anticipated maintenance dose and increased every 2 to 3 weeks.Because of the auto- and heteroinduction of carbamazepine metabolism, it is necessary to administer the drug two to four times per day. Although some patients, especially those on monotherapy, can be maintained on twice-a-day therapy, others may require more frequent dosage administration. Children are likely to need more frequent administration. Annoying CNS and gastrointestinal side effects may be minimized by giving larger doses at bedtime. A controlled-released dosage form (Tegretol XR) given twice a day has comparable pharmacokinetics to immediate-release carbamazepine given four times a day.[68] The sustained-release Carbatrol capsules can be opened and used as a sprinkle on food. Carbamazepine tablets should not be stored in places where they would be exposed to high heat and high humidity.

Advantages. This drug has been approved as an AED since 1974 and has been well studied. There are oral solid and liquid dosage forms available. The oral solid dosage form is available as an immediate-release tablet, a sustained-release capsule, and a controlled-release tablet. The sustained- and controlled-release dosage forms allow for twice-a-day dosing to reduce the peak-to-trough fluctuations. Compared with other first-generation AEDS, carbamazepine causes minimal cognitive impairment.

Disadvantages. Carbamazepine has an active metabolite that can contribute to efficacy and toxicity. Other drugs can alter the concentration of this metabolite without changing the concentration of the parent carbamazepine. Carbamazepine induces its own metabolism, which requires careful dosage titration. Carbamazepine induces the metabolism of other medications, and other drugs may interact with it and/or the active metabolite. There is no parenteral formulation. CNS side effects including sedation are associated with the immediate-release formulations. These side effects may be less with the sustained-release or controlled-release formulations, but this has not been prospectively evaluated. In utero exposure to carbamazepine has been associated with a 1% risk of spina bifida. The generic formulations available have been associated with breakthrough seizures when brands have been switched.

Place in Therapy. Carbamazepine is considered a first-line therapy for patients with newly diagnosed partial seizures and for patients with primary generalized convulsive seizures who are not in an emergent situation.

Ethosuximide

Pharmacology and Mechanism of Action. The exact mechanism of action of ethosuximide remains elusive. Ethosuximide inhibits NADPH-linked aldehyde reductase necessary for the formation of γ-hydroxybutyrate, which has been associated with the induction of absence seizures. It also may inhibit the sodium-potassium ATPase system. Ethosuximide is not believed to have a direct membrane effect or to affect brain metabolism.[69]

Pharmacokinetics and Efficacy. Metabolism occurs in the liver by hydroxylation, and the metabolites are believed to be inactive. There is some evidence of a nonlinear metabolic process at higher concentrations. Ethosuximide has a chiral center, and there may be some stereochemical aspects to its metabolism.[69]

The only indication for the use of ethosuximide is the treatment of absence seizures, for which it is the treatment of choice. It may be used in combination with valproic acid for difficult-to-control absence patients.[69]

Adverse Effects, Drug-Drug Interactions, and Drug-Food Interactions. Ethosuximide is a relatively benign anticonvulsant. The most frequently reported side effects are nausea and vomiting (up to 40%), and these symptoms may be minimized by administration of smaller doses and more frequent dosing. Other common side effects include drowsiness, fatigue, lethargy, dizziness, hiccoughs, and headaches. Rarely, idiosyncratic reactions such as rashes, lupus, and blood dyscrasias have been reported.[69]

Because ethosuximide is not protein-bound, displacement interactions cannot occur. The metabolism of ethosuximide may be induced by carbamazepine. A complex interaction between valproic acid and ethosuximide has been reported. Valproic acid may inhibit the metabolism of ethosuximide, but only if the metabolism of ethosuximide is near saturation.[20]

Dosing and Administration. The therapeutic range of ethosuximide was defined in a relatively small number of patients. Many unresponsive patients became responders when their drug concentrations were raised to equal those of the responsive patients. A loading dose of ethosuximide is not required. Titration over 1 to 2 weeks to maintenance doses of 20 mg/kg per day usually results in concentrations of approximately 50 μg/mL. Data suggest that patients can be managed successfully on once-a-day therapy; however, gastrointestinal distress appears to be dose-related, and the total daily dose is usually divided into two equal doses.[69]

Advantages. This drug is very effective in the treatment of absence seizures. It is generally well tolerated and has few pharmacokinetic interactions.

Disadvantages. Ethosuximide has a very narrow spectrum of activity.

Place in Therapy. Ethosuximide is still a first-line treatment for absence seizures.

Felbamate

Pharmacology and Mechanism of Action. Felbamate is a structural analog of meprobamate, but its use does not result in the tolerance or dependence associated with meprobamate. Felbamate appears to act as an antagonist of the glycine receptor site on the *N*-methyl-D-aspartate (NMDA) receptor. This action inhibits the initiation and propagation of seizures. It also may inhibit NMDA-glycine-stimulated increases in intracellular Ca^{2+}.[70]

Pharmacokinetics. Felbamate is rapidly and well absorbed. The absorption is unaffected by food or antacids. About 40% to 50% of a dose of felbamate is metabolized by hydroxylation and conjugation pathways in the liver, with the rest being excreted unchanged in the urine. In patients taking enzyme-inducing drugs, the elimination half-life is shorter. Felbamate displays linear pharmacokinetics, and the concentrations are dose-proportional.

Efficacy. Felbamate has been approved for use in patients 14 years of age and older as monotherapy and as adjunctive therapy in patients with partial seizures with and without secondary generalization and for children 2 years of age and older as adjunctive therapy for the Lennox Gastaut syndrome.[71] Because of the association of aplastic anemia and acute liver failure with felbamate postmarketing, felbamate is now only recommended for patients refractory to other AEDs.

Adverse Effects. The most frequently reported side effects with felbamate prior to marketing were anorexia, weight loss, insomnia, nausea, and headache. Less common side effects included diarrhea, rash, diplopia, ataxia, rhinitis, and taste disturbances. The side effects of felbamate are more common with polytherapy than with monotherapy.[71] After about 1 year of general use and 100,000 patient-care exposures, the use of felbamate was found to be associated with aplastic anemia and acute liver failure. The onset was between 68 and 354 days of therapy. The approximate rate of occurrence of aplastic anemia is 1 in 3000 and of hepatitis is 1 in 10,000.[1] Initially, no relationship with dose and no predictors of who is more likely to develop these life-threatening reactions were apparent. Data are now emerging suggesting an increased risk for aplastic anemia in patients with a history of cytopenia, AED allergy or significant toxicity, viral infection, and/or immunologic problems.

Drug-Drug and Drug-Food Interactions. Significant drug interactions have been reported with felbamate. Felbamate inhibits the clearance and increases the concentration of phenytoin, valproic acid, and phenobarbital.[72] The concentration of carbamazepine decreases in patients on concurrent therapy with felbamate secondary to enzyme induction, and the concentration of the 10,11-epoxide metabolite increases.[73] It is recommended that the dose of phenytoin, carbamazepine, and valproic acid be decreased by about 30% when felbamate is added.[71] These interactions are dose-proportional, and there is a further change in clearance with each dosage increase of felbamate. Felbamate does not appear to interact with either gabapentin or lamotrigine. Phenytoin and carbamazepine are enzyme inducers and have been shown to increase the clearance of felbamate.

Dosing and Administration. A therapeutic range for felbamate has not been established. The drug is dosed to clinical response. If felbamate is used as monotherapy, the dose is initiated at 1200 mg/day (15 mg/kg in children) and then is increased by 600 mg every 2 weeks up to a maximum dose of 3600 mg (45 mg/kg in children).

Advantages. Felbamate has a unique mechanism of action. It is approved for treating atonic seizures in patients with the Lennox-Gastaut syndrome and is effective in treating patients with partial seizures.

Disadvantages. The use of felbamate is limited by the association with aplastic anemia and hepatotoxicity as well as multiple drug interactions.

Place in Therapy. This agent should be reserved for patients not responding to other AEDs.

Gabapentin

Pharmacology and Mechanism of Action. Structurally, gabapentin incorporates the inhibitory neurotransmitter GABA into a cyclohexane ring.[74] Gabapentin was designed to be a GABA agonist, but its exact mechanism of action is still unclear. It has been demonstrated that gabapentin does not react at either GABA receptor, alter GABA uptake, or interfere with GABA transaminase. Gabapentin appears to bind to an amino acid carrier protein and act at a unique receptor. Gabapentin also may modulate specific voltage-sensitive Ca^{2+} channels.[50] It elevates human brain GABA levels, possibly via alterations in GABA synthesis or reversal of the neuronal GABA transporter, resulting in nonvesicular release of GABA.[75]

Pharmacokinetics. Gabapentin is a substrate of the L-amino acid carrier protein in the gut (system L) as well as in the CNS.[76] This amino acid carrier protein transports the drug across the gut membrane by an active process. The binding of gabapentin to this system is saturable, and gabapentin therefore displays dose-dependent bioavailability that appears to vary considerably between individuals.[77] The percent of dose excreted unchanged in the urine is 47%, 34%, 33%, and 27% for daily doses of 1200, 2400, 3600, and 4800 mg.[78] At single doses greater than 1200 mg three times per day, there appears to be a plateauing of the concentration achieved.[79] Food, including protein-rich meals, does not appear to interfere with gabapentin oral absorption.[80]

Because gabapentin is eliminated exclusively by renal elimination, dosage adjustments will be necessary in patients with significantly impaired renal function. In anuric patients maintained on hemodialysis, the mean elimination half-life on nondialysis days is 132 hours. Approximately 35% of gabapentin is recovered in dialysate. Gabapentin half-life during dialysis is approximately 4 hours.[81]

Efficacy. Gabapentin is approved as adjunctive therapy for partial seizures with or without secondary generalization in adults with epilepsy.[82] Recent clinical trials conducted in less refractory or medically intractable patients with partial seizures have confirmed that the adjunctive use of this agent is both efficacious and well tolerated.[83] Although placebo-controlled trials of gabapentin monotherapy in refractory patients have been inconclusive, monotherapy trials comparing gabapentin with carbamazepine in new-onset epilepsy have suggested effectiveness. Gabapentin does not appear to be as efficacious in the treatment of primarly generalized seizure types.

Gabapentin has been used as adjunctive therapy in children with refractory partial seizures[84] and with benign epilepsy with centrotemporal spikes (BECTS).[85] One case study reported an increase in absence and myoclonic seizures when gabapentin was used in a patient with Lennox-Gastaut syndrome.[86]

Gabapentin also has been used for treatment of neuropathic pain[87,88] and various psychiatric disorders including bipolar affective disorder and anxiety.[89]

Adverse Effects, Drug-Drug Interactions, and Drug-Food Interactions. Fatigue, somnolence, dizziness, and ataxia are the most frequently reported side effects. Rash is uncommon with this agent. Other side effects reported include nystagmus, tremor, and diplopia. Aggressive behavior has been reported in children.[90] The CNS effects of gabapentin are generally less than those of traditional AEDs.[77] Some clinicians have noted that patients may gain weight while on gabapentin.

Gabapentin does not induce or inhibit liver enzymes. Therefore, drug interactions are not likely to occur with gabapentin.[77] There is a 10% reduction in the clearance of gabapentin in patients taking cimetidine and a 20% reduction in the bioavailability if aluminum antacids are taken simultaneously with gabapentin.

Dosing and Administration. The manufacturer recommends a gabapentin dose of 300 mg at bedtime on the first day, increasing to 900 mg/day over 3 days. Faster titration rates (e.g., starting at 300 to 900 mg tid) have been well tolerated.[91] The manufacturer recommends maintenance doses of 1800 to 2400 mg/day, but higher doses (5000 to 10,000 mg/day) have been used safely. Most clinicians are using doses of 2400 to 4800 mg/day for epilepsy. It is unclear if higher doses of gabapentin should be given more frequently than three times per day because of saturable absorption, however.[92] Gabapentin does not appear to be absorbed rectally. Patients with end-stage renal disease maintained on hemodialysis should receive an initial 300- to 400-mg dose with 200 to 300 mg gabapentin given after every 4 hours of hemodialysis.[81]

Advantages. Gabapentin has multiple mechanisms of action and is mechanistically different from the first-generation AEDs. Gabapentin is not metabolized and is excreted unchanged by the kidney. It has the additional advantages of a broad therapeutic index, minimal CNS adverse effects, and no drug interactions. Gabapentin doses can be escalated rapidly.

Disadvantages. Gabapentin is absorbed by an active process that saturates at higher doses. This may require more frequent daily dosing for patients who need doses greater than 3600 mg/day. Doses exceeding the 3600 mg/d maximum listed in the package insert may be required in some patients to achieve seizure remission. There is no parenteral formulation.

Place in Therapy. Gabapentin is an adjunctive agent for patients with partial seizures who have failed initial treatment. Although monotherapy trials have not proven effective in previously diagnosed refractory patients, there may be a role for this drug in patients with less severe seizure disorders, such as new-onset epilepsy. Gabapentin has been shown to be useful in the treatment of chronic pain and other nonepileptic conditions.

Lamotrigine

Pharmacology, Mechanism of Action, and Pharmacokinetics. A primary mechanism of action for lamotrigine appears to be blockade of neuronal sodium channels that is both voltage- and use-dependent. In addition to sodium channels, lamotrigine produces dose-dependent inhibition of high-voltage activation Ca^{2+} currents, possibly through inhibition of presynaptic N-type Ca^{2+} channels. Release of excitatory amino acid neurotransmitters such as glutamate and aspartate is blocked by lamotrigine during sustained repetitive firing. Animal models also suggest that lamotrigine inhibits ischemia-induced release of excitatory neurotransmitters, suggesting a neuroprotective action.[93]

Lamotrigine is completely and rapidly absorbed, with a bioavailability of 98%.[94] Food does not significantly affect drug absorption. Lamotrigine is also absorbed following rectal administration, although mean area under the curve (AUC) is approximately 50% of corresponding oral administration values. Lamotrigine is approximately 55% bound to plasma proteins, and binding is unaffected by phenytoin, phenobarbital, carbamazepine, or valproate. Lamotrigine is extensively hepatically metabolized by uridine diphosphate glucuronosyltranferase. This glucuronide metabolite is pharmacologically inactive. Renal elimination of unchanged drug accounts for a minor fraction of administered dose (<10%). When given as monotherapy in adults, lamotrigine elimination half-life is approximately 24 to 29 hours. Oral clearance averages 0.35 to 0.59 ml/min/kg. Lamotrigine clearance is higher in children and lower in the elderly as compared with young adults. There are only modest differences in the pharmacokinetics of lamotrigine in the elderly versus younger subjects.[95] In a group of elderly volunteers, aged 65 to 76 years, lamotrigine clearance was 37% lower when compared with a group of young adults. Hepatic disease, depending on severity, can influence lamotrigine pharmacokinetics. Approximately 17% of a lamotrigine dose may be removed by hemodialysis, with half-life being reduced to about 13 hours. A well-defined concentration-effect serum range has not been established for this agent. The half-life is prolonged in patients with renal failure. For patients on dialysis, the half-life is much more prolonged between dialyses (57.4 hours) but shorter during dialysis (13 hours).[94]

Efficacy. Lamotrigine is approved as adjunctive therapy and monotherapy in adult patients with partial epilepsy refractory to other agents.[94,96] Lamotrigine is also approved for use in controlling seizures associated with the Lennox-Gastuat sysndrome. In several controlled trials, lamotrigine also has demonstrated effectivness against generalized seizures such as absence seizures.[97] Lamotrigine may lead to improvements in the patient's mood. Comparisons between lamotrigine and older agents including carbamazepine and phenytoin as initial monotherapy have been conducted in Europe, and the results would suggest comparable effectiveness and perhaps better tolerability, particularly in elderly patients.[98]

Adverse Effects. The most frequently reported side effects of lamotrigine include diplopia, drowsiness, ataxia, and headache. Adverse effects are more common when lamotrigine is given in combination with other AEDs (e.g., diplopia when given concomitant carbamazepine or tremor with valproic acid) as compared with monotherapy and thus may be pharmacodynamic in nature. It may cause rash, which usually appears in the first 3 to 4 weeks of therapy. The rash is typically generalized, erythematous, and morbilliform and generally is mild to moderate in severity. However, the Stevens-Johnson reaction also has been reported. Some of these rashes, especially a rash that develops early, may necessitate the withdrawal of lamotrigine.[99] Risk factors for the emergence of more serious rashes appear to be concomitant use of valproic acid and situations where high initial doses or too rapid dosage escalation is used. The incidence also may be higher in children than in adults.

Drug-Drug and Drug-Food Interactions. Lamotrigine does not inhibit or induce liver enzymes. The potential for this agent causing pharmacokinetic interactions is low, and accordingly, lamotrigine has been shown not to interfere with the metabolism of the other AEDs or oral contraceptives.[100] The addition of lamotrigine was associated with a small (25%) decrease in steady state valproate acid plasma concentrations.

The metabolism of lamotrigine does display substantial interpatient variability in plasma clearance, however, and may be altered by concurrent therapy with other drugs. Lamotrigine elimination half-life is reduced by approximately 50% in the presence of inducing drugs, such as carbamazepine, phenobarbital, primidone, and phenytoin. Lamotrigine clearance also may be increased by oxcarbazepine. Valproic acid inhibits the clearance of lamotrigine. Inhibition of lamotrigine metabolism by valproic acid is substantial and appears to occur even at very low serum concentrations. Clinically, this implies that in order to achieve any given plasma concentration, larger maintenance doses of lamotrigine (as compared with monotherapy) may be required in the presence of an inducer, whereas lower doses may be necessary when given with valproic acid. Felbamate does not appear to interfere with lamotrigine matabolism. A pharmacodynamic interaction may occur with carbamazepine, leading to an increase in CNS side effects.

Dosing and Administration. A definitive therapeutic range for lamotrigine has not been established. Measurement of serum concentrations may be useful in assessing the impact of pharmacokinetic interactions, however. In patients who are taking enzyme-inducing drugs, lamotrigine can be started more rapidly than in patients receiving valproic acid. The maintenance doses are also different (see Table 56–9). These different doses are critical due to the relationship between rash, concomitant valproic acid, and the dose escalation rate. Removal of inducers from a lamotrigine regimen may necessitate decreases in lamotrigine doses, whereas removal of valproic acid may necessitate an increase in the lamotrigine dose.

Advantages. Lamotrigine is potentially a broad-spectrum AED having efficacy in partial seizures as well as several types of generalized seizures. A pediatric dosage form is available. It does not induce or inhibit the metabolism of other AEDs. Lamotrigine has linear pharmacokinetics and is not highly protein-bound. It appears to be generally well tolerated, and may have mood stabilizing effects .

Disadvantages. Lamotrigine is associated with skin rash in patients who start at a high dose, have rapid dose escalation, and/or are taking concurrent valproic acid, which significantly prolongs its half-life. Therefore, the initial doses must be low (lower if the patient is on valproic acid) and escalated slowly in order to maximize patient safety. There is no parenteral dosage form.

Place in Therapy. Lamotrigine is useful as both adjunctive treatment in patients with partial seizures and monotherapy. Lamotrigine may have comparable effectiveness as more traditional AEDs such as carbamazepine and phenytoin in these patients when used as monotherapy. In addition, lamotrigine may be useful alternative therapy in patients with primary generalized seizure types such as absence seizures.

Levetiracetam

Pharmacology, Mechanism of Action, and Pharmacokinetics. Levetiracetam, an *S*-enantiomer pyrolidone derivative, is chemically unrelated to other available AEDs. While the precise mechanism of action of levetiracetam has yet to be delineated, it is known that this drug is not active in the classical models of maximal electroshock and pentylenetetrazol seizures in mice. It is also not active against seizures induced by classical chemoconvulsants and does not interact with benzodiazepine or GABA receptors. Levetiracetam does appear to be effective in genetic and kindled animal models of epilepsy. This agent therefore may have a unique mechanism of action.[101] There is some evidence that levetiracetam may have *antiepileptogenic* effects, meaning that this compound may be able to prevent the development of epilepsy in certain circumstances. Clinical confirmation of these animal experiments are still needed, however.

Levetiracetam is rapidly and completely absorbed following oral administration and displays negligible protein binding (<10%). Renal elimination of unchanged parent drug accounts for the majority of drug clearance (66%), with the remainder being metabolized in blood via enzymatic hydrolysis of an acetamide group to inactive metabolites.[102] This metabolic pathway does not involve either the CYP or UGT isozyme systems. The plasma half-life of this drug is approximately 7 hours. Because this drug is renally eliminated, clinicians should anticipate age-related reductions in clearance in the elderly patient. Conversely, levetiracetam clearance in children appears to be approximately 40% higher than in adults. Currently, there are no data regarding concentration-effect relationships, so the role of therapeutic drug level monitoring is unknown.

Efficacy. Levetiracetam has demonstrated efficacy in the adjunctive treatment of partial seizures in adults with refractory epilepsy.[103] Currently, there are insufficient data to evaluate the utility of this agent in primary generalized seizures or as monotherapy.

Adverse Effects. Adverse effects appear to be modest, with sedation, fatigue, and coordination difficulties being the most common CNS effects. Using a slower rate of dose escalation may be helpful in minimizing this effect. Formal studies evaluating the cognitive effects of this medication have not yet been conducted. An increase in infections as well as a slight yet statistically significant decline in red and white blood cell counts also was noted during clinical trials. The clinical significance of this is not known.

Drug-Drug and Drug-Food Interactions. Levetiracetam is not an inhibitor or inducer of either CYP, UGT, or epoxide hydrolase enzyme systems, and in vitro data would predict a low potential for causing pharmacokinetic interactions.[104] It does not appear to interact with other AEDs,[105] warfarin, or digoxin. Levetiracetam may be given without regard to meals.

Dosing and Administration. The manufacturer's recommendation is to initiate dosing at 500 mg orally twice daily, titrating at 1000 mg/day increments every 2 weeks to a maximum recommended dose of 3000 mg/day (1500 mg bid). In order to minimize CNS effects, clinicians might consider initiating the drug at one-half this rate.

Advantages. Levetiracetam has a novel, although unknown, mechanism of action. It has linear pharmacokinetics and is not metabolized by the CYP system. No significant drug interactions, including oral contraceptives, have been reported. Initial doses may be effective. The drug appears to be well tolerated.

Disadvantages. There have been limited patient exposures to levetiracetam. The dose needs to be adjusted for patients with decreased renal functioning, and slower dose escalation may be needed to avoid CNS adverse effects. There is no parenteral formulation.

Place in Therapy. Currently, levetiracetam is indicated for patients with partial seizures who have failed initial therapy.

Oxcarbazepine

Pharmacology and Mechanism of Action. Oxcarbazepine is structurally related to carbamazepine. However, it is rapidly converted to a monohydrate derivative (MHD) that is the active component.[106] Therefore, oxcarbazepine can be considered a prodrug. The mechanism of action of oxcarbazepine is similar to that of carbamazepine and perhaps lamotrigine. Oxcarbazepine (as the MHD) blocks voltage-sensitive sodium channels, modulates the voltage-activated calcium currents, and increases potassium conductance. It has no significant interactions with brain neurotransmitters or modulation of receptor sites.

Pharmacokinetics. Oxcarbazepine is completely absorbed and is extensively metabolized by noninducible cytosolic ketoreductases to its pharmacologically active 10-monohydroxy metabolite (MHD).[107] The concentration of MHD peaks in 4 to 6 hours after a dose of oxcarbazepine. MHD is inactivated by glucuronide conjugation and is also eliminated by the kidneys. The plasma half-life of MHD is 9.3 ± 1.8 hours. The half-life of MHD does not change with repeated dosing, and there is no autoinduction. The half-life of MHD is shorter in patients taking enzyme-inducing drugs. The relationship between dose and concentration is linear. Oxcarbazepine is 67% protein-bound, and MHD is 35% to 40% protein-bound. Both oxcarbazepine and MHD cross the blood-brain barrier and the placenta. The pharmacokinetics of MHD are similar in children, adolescents, and adults. Children 2 to 6 years of age need larger doses to achieve the same concentration, suggesting a more rapid clearance. The C_{max} and bioavailability of MHD in elderly volunteers were higher than in younger volunteers, and the elimination rate was slower, possibly reflecting decreased renal elimination. Patients with significant renal impairment may require a dosage reduction. The target concentration that has been suggested for MHD is 20 to 200 μmol/L.

Efficacy. Oxcarbazepine has been compared with phenytoin, valproic acid, carbamazepine, and placebo.[108] In these monotherapy, double-blind comparative trials in newly diagnosed patients, oxcarbazepine is as effective as phenytoin, valproic acid, and carbamazepine. However, it was better tolerated with fewer side effects. All placebo-controlled trials were positive in favor of oxcarbazepine. Oxcarbazepine is indicated for use as monotherapy or adjunctive therapy in the treatment of partial seizures in adults and as adjunctive therapy in the treatment of partial seizures in children aged 4 to 16 years with epilepsy.

Adverse Effects. Oxcarbazepine has been in clinical use since 1990 and was marketed in over 50 countries before it was approved for use in the United States.[109] In the U.S. clinical trials, the most frequently reported adverse events were dizziness, nausea, headache, diarrhea, vomiting, upper respiratory tract infections, constipation, dyspepsia, ataxia, and nervousness. In comparative trials, oxcarbazepine generally caused fewer side effects than phenytoin, valproic acid, or carbamazepine. Dizziness may be more common in elderly patients. Hyponatremia, defined as a plasma sodium level of less than 125 mmol/L, has been reported in up to 25% of patients taking oxcarbazepine. Similar to carbamazepine, hyponatremia appears to occur more often in elderly patients. While the incidence of hyponatremia is higher than what is seen with carbamazepine, data from clinical trials suggest that many patients have been asymptomatic and about 80% have been taking sodium-depleting medications. Nevertheless, clinicians should consider monitoring serum sodium levels following initiation of oxcarbazepine, as well as instructing patients on the symptoms of hyponatremia. About 25% to 30% of patients who develop a rash with carbamazepine will experience a similar reaction with oxcarbazepine.

Drug-Drug and Drug-Food Interactions. Oxcarbazepine decreases the bioavailability of ethinyl estradiol and levonorgestrel.[110] Concurrent use of oxcarbazepine with oral contraceptives containing ethinyl estradiol and levonorgestrel may render these agents less effective. Women taking oral contraceptives should be counseled about failure. The metabolism of oxcarbazepine is slightly altered by verapamil. There are no interactions between cimetidine, erythromycin, or warfarin and oxcarbazepine. The administration of oxcarbazepine in doses greater than 1200 mg with phenytoin has resulted in a 40% increase in the concentration of phenytoin, consistent with inhibition of CYP 2C19. Oxcarbazepine treatment also may cause declines in lamotrigine serum concentrations, suggesting induction of UGT isozymes.[111]

Enzyme-inducing drugs increase the clearance of the active MHD and decrease MHD concentrations. The replacement of carbamazepine with oxcarbazepine may result in a drug interaction because an enzyme-inducing drug is being removed. The administration of oxcarbazepine with food causes a 16% increase in the AUC and a 23% increase in the C_{max} of MHD.

Dosing and Administration. In adults, the starting dose of oxcarbazepine as monotherapy is 300 mg twice a day. The dose is titrated upward at a rate of 600 mg/day per week to a maximum dose of 2400 mg/day. Some patients may require a slower titration rate. For children aged 4 to 16 years, the starting dose is 8 to 10 mg/kg given twice a day, not to exceed 600 mg/day. The dose is titrated to the target dose over 2 weeks. The recommended daily dose according to weight is 20 to 29 kg, 900 mg/day; 29.1 to 39 kg, 1200 mg/day; and more than 39 kg, 1800 mg/day. In patients being converted from carbamazepine, the typical maintenance doses of oxcarbazepine are 1.5 times the carbamazepine dose.

Advantages. This is a prodrug that is rapidly converted to the active MHD, which has a mechanism action similar to carbamazepine. There is no autoinduction associated with oxcarbazepine. The efficacy of oxcarbazepine has been shown to be comparable with that of carbamazepine, phenytoin, and valproic acid. This drug was approved in 50 other countries before it was approved in the United States, so broad international experience has been gained.

Disadvantages. Oxcarbazepine is more expensive than comparable doses of carbamazepine. About 30% of patients who have had a skin rash with carbamazepine have a cross-reaction with oxcarbazepine. There are more reports of hyponatremia with oxcarbazepine. Replacing carbamazepine with oxcarbazepine may result in interactions with the removal of carbamazepine. Enzyme-inducing drugs may increase the clearance of MHD. This drug is not likely to be effective in seizure types in which carbamazepine is ineffective.

Place in Therapy. Oxcarbazepine is a potential first-line drug for patients with partial seizures and primary generalized convulsive seizures. However, it is more expensive than carbamazepine, to which it is closely related.

Phenobarbital and Primidone

Phenobarbital and primidone may be considered together because primidone is metabolized to phenobarbital. Primidone is an active AED and has a second metabolite that may be active—phenylethylmalonamide (PEMA). In general, because of costs and dosing frequency, phenobarbital should be tried before primidone. In some refractory patients, primidone will be effective where phenobarbital has failed because of additional AED activity.

Mechanism of Action and Pharmacokinetics. Phenobarbital and primidone elevate seizure threshold by decreasing postsynaptic excitation, possibly by stimulating postsynaptic GABA-ergic inhibitory responses.[50] Phenobarbital is rapidly and completely absorbed regardless of whether it is given orally, intramuscularly, or rectally.[20] It has a biphasic distribution. Initially, phenobarbital penetrates highly perfused organs including the brain. It penetrates the brain at a rate comparable with that of phenytoin, and peak concentrations are achieved 3 to 20 minutes after an intravenous dose. Phenobarbital distributes evenly to all body tissues including fat. Decreasing systemic pH drives phenobarbital into body tissues. Phenobarbital is about 50% bound to plasma proteins, but the free fraction was reported to be 93% in a burn patient with uremia.[20]

Drugs affecting liver enzymes may alter phenobarbital metabolism, but phenobarbital clearance is not affected by liver blood flow. Despite the fact that phenobarbital is a potent enzyme inducer, there is no evidence in humans that it is an autoinducer. The elimination of phenobarbital is linear. Because tubular reabsorption of phenobarbital is pH-dependent, the amount excreted renally can be increased by giving diuretics and urinary alkalinizers.

Primidone is metabolized to phenobarbital and PEMA. The primidone-to-phenobarbital ratio is highly variable. A significant portion of primidone is excreted unchanged. The half-life of primidone may become shorter after chronic therapy because the phenobarbital metabolite may induce the metabolism of primidone.

Efficacy. Phenobarbital is the drug of choice for neonatal seizures. It is also useful in generalized seizures (except absence) and may be useful in patients with partial seizures. Primidone shares the same indications but is less useful in partial seizures.[112] Neither drug is a drug of first choice because of their adverse effects. The widespread use of phenobarbital in the prophylaxis of febrile seizures has been questioned.[113] Although efficacy of these agents is comparable with that of other traditional AEDs, the significant adverse cognitive effects of these drugs limit their utility.

Adverse Effects, Drug-Drug Interactions, and Drug-Food Interactions. As noted previously, CNS side effects are the primary factors limiting the use of phenobarbital. Tolerance usually develops to initial complaints of fatigue, drowsiness, sedation, and depression. In children, paradoxically, the primary side effect is hyperactivity. Phenobarbital impairs higher cortical function and depresses cognitive performance.[113] In susceptible patients, phenobarbital may precipitate porphyria. Other adverse effects include rashes (including serious rashes such as Stevens-Johnson syndrome), osteomalacia, and hypotension (see Table 56–6).

The side effects of primidone and phenobarbital are similar and may be difficult to separate. The initial side effects of sedation, nystagmus, and ataxia may be minimized by starting at a low dose and gradually increasing the dose.

Phenobarbital is a potent enzyme inducer and may increase the elimination of any drug metabolized by both CYP- and UGT-mediated metabolism. Valproic acid, phenytoin, felbamate, cimetidine, and chloramphenicol inhibit phenobarbital metabolism, necessitating a decrease in dose. Ethanol increases the metabolism of phenobarbital. The drug interactions of primidone are similar to those of phenobarbital.

Dosing and Administration. At therapeutic primidone concentrations, most patients have a phenobarbital concentration that is in the therapeutic range. It is rare that a patient on primidone needs supplemental doses of phenobarbital. PEMA concentrations are not monitored routinely.

In nonacute situations, phenobarbital should be started in low doses and titrated upward. The dose-concentration relationship is linear. Because the half-life of phenobarbital is long, doses can be given once daily. Bedtime dosing sometimes minimizes the consequences of CNS depression. Because of its long half-life, phenobarbital takes 3 to 4 weeks to reach steady state. Therefore, rapid dosage adjustments should be avoided in a nonacute situation. Primidone is not administered as a loading dose. An initial dose of 50 to 125 mg may be increased every 2 to 4 days until the desired concentration is reached. Because of the short half-lives of primidone and PEMA, the drug should be given in divided doses.

Advantages. Phenobarbital has linear and predictable pharmacokinetics. If the dose is doubled, the resulting serum concentrations double. It also has the advantage of having multiple dosage forms (e.g., oral solid, oral liquid, intramuscular, and intravenous) so that the route of administration can be varied according to patient need, including emergent conditions. It is the most inexpensive AED.

Disadvantages. Phenobarbital is associated with significant side effects. These include delayed intellectual development, hyperactivity in children, and cognitive impairment in adults. The mental slowing is of particular concern in older patients, who may fall while taking phenobarbital. Also, phenobarbital is an enzyme inducer and interacts with many other drugs metabolized by the CYP system. Phenobarbital has a very long half-life and takes a long time to achieve steady state. Dosage adjustments should not be made more often than every 2 to 3 weeks.

Place in Therapy. Phenobarbital is reserved for patients who have failed other AEDs. It may be useful in refractory status epilepticus.

Phenytoin

Pharmacology and Mechanism of Action. Phenytoin blocks PTP by influencing synaptic transmission. Proposed mechanisms include altering ion fluxes associated with depolarization, repolarization, and membrane stability; altering calcium uptake in presynaptic terminals; influencing calcium-dependent synaptic protein phosphorylation and transmitter release; altering the sodium-potassium ATP-dependent ionic membrane pump; and preventing cyclic nucleotide buildup and cerebellar stimulation.[50]

Pharmacokinetics. Absorption of phenytoin is primarily from the duodenum, and it may be saturable. Absorption is almost complete, with dissolution being the rate-limiting step. Absorption may be prolonged, and secondary peaks may be seen. Enterohepatic cycling of phenytoin occurs, but there is no first-pass metabolism.[114]

The absorption of orally administered phenytoin is affected by the particle size of the formulation. Therefore, some brands may be absorbed faster than others, and the brand that a patient receives should not be changed without careful monitoring.[20] The intramuscular administration of phenytoin is problematic and best avoided. Fosphenytoin can be administered safely intravenously and intramuscularly.

Phenytoin enters the brain quickly, where it is redistributed to other body tissues, including saliva and breast milk. It crosses the placenta to reach an equilibrium between mother and fetus. Phenytoin is bound to serum and tissue proteins. Obesity may increase the volume of distribution.

For most patients, phenytoin binding to albumin is predictable and proportional throughout the therapeutic range. Equations have been developed to normalize the phenytoin concentration in patients with hypoalbuminemia or renal failure. A good correlation has been shown between the free phenytoin concentration and the ratio of total phenytoin to albumin in patients with normal albumin or hyperalbuminemia. The ratio was not predictive for patients with hypoalbuminemia. A recent recalculation[115] of this equation was more reliable in elderly nursing home and trauma patients:

$$C_{\text{calc}} = C_{\text{obs}}/0.25ALB + 0.1$$

where C_{calc} is the calculated serum concentration, C_{obs} is the observed concentration, and ALB is albumin concentration.

Phenytoin is metabolized in the liver primarily by parahydroxylation to 5-(p-hydroxyphenyl)-5-phenylhydantoin (HPPH). The major isoform responsible for phenytoin's metabolism is CYP 2C9, but CYP 2C19 is also involved.[61] HPPH is conjugated and excreted in the urine as a glucuronide. About 80% of an oral dose of phenytoin appears in the urine as HPPH. Abnormally low percentages of HPPH in the urine would indicate a problem with absorption. Phenytoin is a low-extraction drug, and its metabolism is not greatly influenced by changes in liver blood flow; however, because the major route of metabolism is hydroxylation, the clearance may be influenced by drugs that stimulate or inhibit liver microsomal enzymes.[114]

Phenytoin displays Michaelis-Menten elimination (the metabolism changes from first-order to zero-order) because the enzyme system is saturable. When the enzyme system is saturated, any change in dosage produces significantly disproportional changes in serum concentrations. The process may be described by the equation

$$D = V_{max} \times C_p / K_m + C_p$$

where D is the dose (in mg/d), V_{max} is the maximum rate of metabolism, K_m is the serum concentration at which the rate of metabolism is half-maximal, and C_p is the serum concentration.

Because V_{max} and K_m are both highly and independently variable, the metabolism of phenytoin may saturate at any concentration, and this may occur at doses used clinically. V_{max} has been shown to decline with age, and K_m may be affected by concurrent drug therapy. It is very difficult to predict the resulting outcome of a dosage increase of phenytoin. Also, serum concentrations do not decline by a constant percentage on discontinuation. Therefore, any dosage change should be followed by careful patient monitoring and serum concentration determinations.[114]

Because of the saturable metabolism, the clinically useful concept of half-life may be inappropriate for phenytoin. Half-life assumes concentration-independent elimination. A more relevant term for phenytoin is the time required to eliminate 50% ($t_{50\%}$) of the serum concentration. The average $t_{50\%}$ for phenytoin is 22 hours, but it may range from 7 to 42 hours. Because of saturation, the $t_{50\%}$ increases with increasing serum concentrations, and the time to reach steady state may be prolonged.[114]

Less than 5% of a dose of phenytoin is excreted unchanged. Renal impairment does not affect the excretion of HPPH. Although an inhibitory effect of HPPH on phenytoin metabolism has been suggested, it has not been documented in humans. Neither hemodialysis nor peritoneal dialysis affects the clearance of phenytoin. Clinically insignificant amounts of phenytoin are removed by plasmapheresis.[20]

Efficacy and Adverse Effects. Phenytoin may be used for any generalized seizure type except absence seizures because it may worsen absence seizures. Partial seizures also may be treated with phenytoin.

When phenytoin is initiated, the CNS depressant effects may result in lethargy, fatigue, incoordination, blurred vision, higher cortical dysfunction, and drowsiness (see Table 56–6). These effects are usually transient and may be minimized by slow dosage titration.

When serum concentrations exceed 20 μg/mL, a significant number of patients exhibit nystagmus at a 45-degree lateral gaze. Ataxia frequently occurs at concentrations greater than 30 μg/mL. At concentrations greater than 40 μg/mL, mental status changes including coma occur. At very high concentrations, phenytoin can exacerbate seizures or precipitate generalized status epilepticus.[55,116]

It is difficult to determine whether the chronic side effects of phenytoin are concentration- or duration-dependent. One of the more common chronic side effects is gingival hyperplasia, which occurs in up to 50% of patients. Good oral hygeine should be promoted to possibly minimize the gingival hyperplasia. Suppression of cognitive abilities is also a concern. Other chronic effects include hirsutism, acne, coarsening of facial features, vitamin D deficiency, osteomalacia, folic acid deficiency, carbohydrate intolerance, immunologic disturbances, hypothyroidism, and peripheral neuropathy. Phenytoin is associated with rare hypersensitivity or idiosyncratic reactions resulting in rashes, Stevens-Johnson syndrome, pseudolymphoma, bone marrow suppression, lupuslike reactions, and hepatitis.[55,116]

Drug-Drug and Drug-Food Interactions. Phenytoin is prone to many drug interactions (see Tables 56–7 and 56–8), and these have been reviewed extensively. The effects of phenytoin may be enhanced or reduced by drugs that affect its pharmacokinetic parameters. Drug interactions affecting absorption, metabolism, or excretion are potentially more significant because total and free concentrations are affected. The rate of absorption of phenytoin may be decreased if it is given simultaneously with food. The bioavailability of phenytoin suspension may be decreased in patients receiving continuous enteral nutrient tube feedings. A single-dose study of simultaneous administration of enteral feeding found no difference in phenytoin bioavailability, indicating that the mechanism was something other than physical contact.[20] Phenytoin is highly protein-bound and may be displaced by other highly protein-bound drugs, resulting in an increase in free phenytoin. The initial increase in free phenytoin is followed by an increase in clearance, a fall in total phenytoin concentrations, and the reestablishment of normal free phenytoin concentrations. Usually no dosage adjustment is necessary. Problems arise when clinicians react to the lower total phenytoin concentration without considering the free concentration. If protein-binding interactions are suspected, free rather than total phenytoin concentrations are a better therapeutic guideline. The metabolism of phenytoin can be inhibited (as by cimetidine) as well as increased (by phenobarbital). Phenytoin may alter the pharmacokinetics of other drugs.

A complex interaction of phenytoin with folic acid also has been described, making vitamin ingestion an important part of the drug history. Phenytoin reportedly decreases folic acid absorption, but folic acid enhances the clearance of phenytoin.[117] Replacement of folic acid can reduce phenytoin concentrations and result in loss of efficacy.

Dosing and Administration. Three dosage forms are used for oral administration of phenytoin (Table 56–10). The salt content should be considered in dosage form changes. If given in equal amounts of

TABLE 56–10. Phenytoin Dosage Forms

Dosage Form	Salt or Acid	Extended or Prompt	Amount of Acid Available
Dilantin capsules	Phenytoin sodium	Extended	
100 mg			92 mg
30 mg			27 mg
Dilantin suspension 125 mg/5 mL	Phenytoin acid	Prompt	125 mg/5 mL
Dilantin Infatabs 50 mg	Phenytoin acid	Prompt	46 mg
Phenytoin injectable 50 mg/mL	Phenytoin sodium	Prompt	46 mg/ml
Fosphenytoin 50 mg PE/ml			50 mg PHT equivalents/mL
Phenytoin capsules (generic)	Phenytoin sodium	Prompt	92 mg

PHT = phenytoin.

phenytoin acid, the tablets, capsules, and suspension have the same bioavailability. Changes between dosage forms may lead to changes in phenytoin concentration. Phenytoin capsules are designated as immediate-release and extended-release forms. Only the extended-release capsules should be used in once-a-day dosing. Particle size rather than formulation may determine the rate of absorption. Phenytoin suspension settles, but resuspension can be accomplished without overzealous agitation.

If oral administration is not feasible, intravenous administration of phenytoin is preferred over intramuscular administration. Fosphenytoin is a prodrug for phenytoin and is available as a parenteral dosage form (see Chap. 57). It is very water-soluble and is rapidly converted to phenytoin systemically. Fosphenytoin can be given rapidly intravenously and intramuscularly with reliable absorption and minimal pain.

Dosing of phenytoin should start at about 5 mg/kg per day for adults. Subsequent dosage adjustments should be done cautiously due to its nonlinearity in elimination. One author has suggested that if the patient's concentration is less than 7 μg/mL, the dose should be increased by 100 mg/day. If the concentration is between 7 and 12 μg/mL, the dose can be increased by 50 mg/day. If the concentration is greater than 12 μg/mL, dose increases of 30 mg/day or less should be made. These increases will result in less than 10% of patients achieving a phenytoin serum concentration greater than 25 μg/mL.[118]

Advantages. Phenytoin has been used for over 60 years, and its risk-to-benefit ratio is well developed. It is available as an oral solid, an oral liquid, and a parenteral (phenytoin and fosphenytoin) dosage form, allowing flexibility in dosing and use in emergent conditions.

Disadvantages. Phenytoin displays Michaeles-Menten pharmacokinetics, and the metabolism saturates at doses given clinically. This makes phenytoin a difficult drug to dose. Also, phenytoin is an inducer of CYP, is metabolized by CYP, and is highly protein-bound.

Therefore, there are many drug interactions with phenytoin. Phenytoin is also associated with multiple side effects, including cognitive slowing at higher concentrations, gingival hyperplasia, cosmetic alterations, and teratogenicity, among others.

Place in Therapy. Phenytoin is a first-line AED for primary generalized convulsive and partial seizures. Its use in therapy may be reevaluated as more experience is gained with newer AEDs.

Tiagabine

Pharmacology and Mechanism of Action. Tiagabine hydrochloride is a novel AED that is a potent and specific inhibitor of GABA uptake into glial and other neuronal elements. Thus tiagabine enhances the action of GABA by decreasing its removal from the synaptic space.[119]

Pharmacokinetics. Tiagabine is quickly and nearly completely absorbed after oral administration. There is a linear relationship between daily doses and serum concentrations. Tiagabine is oxidized in the liver by CYP 3A4 enzymes. Enzyme inducers increase its clearance. Children eliminate tiagabine slightly faster than adults. Subjects with hepatic impairment have higher and more prolonged plasma concentrations of total and unbound drug. Renal dysfunction does not change its pharmacokinetics.[119]

Efficacy. Tiagabine is approved for adjunctive use in patients with partial seizures. Five add-on, placebo-controlled trials and six noncomparative, open-label, long-term multicenter trials have been or are being conducted in Australia, Europe, and the United States. The results of these trials involving 2261 patients indicate that tiagabine is efficacious as add-on therapy in patients with refractory partial seizures. Efficacy of tiagabine is sustained with long-term treatment. These studies included a wide age range of patients, including adolescents and the elderly.[120] There is only limited experience with tiagabine monotherapy, and it currently does not have FDA approval for this indication.

Adverse Effects. Discontinuation resulting from adverse events in clinical trials was infrequent, occurring in 15% of patients receiving tiagabine compared with 5% receiving placebo. The most frequently reported adverse event was dizziness. Adverse events that were significantly more common with tiagabine than with placebo were dizziness, asthenia, nervousness, tremor, diarrhea, and depression. Rash is uncommon with tiagabine. Adverse events usually were mild to moderate in severity and transient, and most were associated with dose titration. CNS side effects may be diminished by taking tiagabine with food, thus slowing the absorption rate. Serious adverse events were uncommon, and no idiosyncratic events, including visual field defects, were reported.[121]

Drug-Drug and Drug-Food Interactions. Enzyme inducers, such as carbamazepine and phenytoin, increase tiagabine clearance and decrease the half-life. Food decreases the rate, but not the extent, of absorption. Tiagabine is displaced from protein by naproxen, salicylates, and valproate. However, tiagabine does not displace phenytoin, valproic acid, amitryptyline, tolbutamide, and warfarin. The AUC of valproic acid is reduced 10% to 12% when tiagabine is added. There is approximately a 5% increase in tiagabine AUC when cimetidine is added.[119]

Dosing and Administration. A clear dose response has been demonstrated, and the minimal effective dose level is 30 mg/day. The initial dose is 4 mg/day, and this can be titrated up to 56 mg/day in intervals of 4 to 8 mg/wk. The dosage range typically employed is 32 to 56 mg daily,[119] and this can be explained in part by the presence of concomitant enzyme-inducing AEDs. Slow dosage titration is essential to decrease adverse CNS effects.

Advantages. Tiagabine has a specific, known mechanism of action. It is the first drug marketed in the United States that acts only on GABA reuptake. This drug has linear pharmacokinetics and does not cause pharmacokinetic interactions.

Disadvantages. Initially high and rapid dosage escalation is associated with increased CNS side effects. Therefore, the drug must be started at a low dose and gradually titrated to patient response. Lower doses may be needed in patients with liver disease. Tiagabine is metabolized by CYP 3A4, and other drugs may alter its clearance. There is no parenteral formulation.

Place in Therapy. Tiagabine is a second-line therapy for patients with partial seizures who have failed initial therapy. This drug does not appear to have a role in primary generalized seizure types.

Topiramate

Mechanism of Action and Pharmacokinetics. Topiramate is a sulfamate-substituted monosaccharide that has multiple modes of action involving voltage-dependent sodium channels, GABA receptors, and antagonism of AMPA subtype glutamate receptors.

Mean values for maximal plasma concentration (C_{max}) and AUC increased linearly with dose; however, a greater than proportional increase in both parameters was observed, probably due to saturable binding of the drug to erythrocytes.[122] Topiramate does not display significant protein binding. Approximately 50% of the dose is excreted renally in patients on no other drugs, but metabolism is increased approximately 50% when topiramate is given with enzyme-inducing AEDs. Renal tubular reabsorption may be prominently involved in the renal handling of topiramate.[123–125]

Efficacy. Topiramate is approved as adjunctive therapy in adults with partial seizures. Its efficacy as adjunctive treatment in refractory partial epilepsy in both adults and children appears good.[126] In adult patients, over 40% of patients have a 50% or greater reduction in seizure frequency when topiramate is added to their regimen, with up to 7% becoming seizure-free. Topiramate also may be used in seizures associated with Lennox-Gastaut syndrome and may be useful in other primary generalized seizures.[127] Currently, although clinical experience and limited controlled data suggest the effectiveness of topiramate as monotherapy for partial seizures, it does not have FDA approval for this indication.

Adverse Effects, Drug-Drug Interactions, and Drug-Food Interactions. The main adverse events of topiramate are ataxia, impaired concentration, memory difficulties, attentional deficits, confusion, dizziness, fatigue, paresthesia, somnolence, and "thinking abnormally," which rarely has included psychosis. Word-finding difficulties are a somewhat unique and specific problem with topiramate and may occur in a significant number of patients. Most of these occurred during rapid titration and higher doses.[128] There may be an increased incidence of cognitive dysfunction in patients receiving concomitant therapy with topiramate and valproic acid. During long-term treatment, weight loss can occur and may be dose-dependent. Nephrolithiasis has occurred in 1.5% of patients receiving topiramate, which is two to four times the incidence in the general population. Patients should be encouraged to maintain adequate fluid intake to reduce this problem.

Food slightly reduces the rate but not the extent of absorption.[123] Topiramate does not change plasma levels of carbamazepine, carbamazepine-epoxide, or lamotrigine. Oral clearance of digoxin is slightly increased when topiramate is added. Phenytoin serum concentrations may increase in some patients,[124] an effect consistent with in vitro studies showing an inhibitory effect of topiramate on the CYP 2C19 isoform. Topiramate can modestly increase the oral clearance of valproic acid and increase the formation of the 4-ene-valproic acid. The clinical significance of this interaction is unclear.[129] Adjustments in topiramate dose may be needed when potent enzyme inducers, such as phenytoin or carbamazepine, are added or discontinued from a topiramate regimen.

Dosing and Administration. Topiramate should be titrated slowly in order to avoid adverse events. Starting doses are 25 to 50 mg/day, increasing by 25 to 50 mg/day every week or every other week. The minimally effective dose of topiramate is approximately 200 mg/day.[130] For patients on other AEDs, doses greater than 600 mg/day do not appear to lead to improved efficacy and may lead to increased side effects. However, higher doses may prove beneficial to individual patients who tolerate them. Monotherapy doses of 1000 mg/day have been used successfully.

Advantages. Topiramate has multiple mechanisms of action and may be a broad-spectrum AED. It is eliminated mainly by the kidney but is partly metabolized by the liver. It has linear pharmacokinetics and few drug interactions.

Disadvantages. With rapid dosage escalation, topiramate is associated with depressed cognitive functioning, including word-finding skills. Therefore, low initial doses should be used, and the dose must be titrated slowly. Renal stones and weight loss also have been associated with topiramate. The dose should be altered in patients with renal failure. There is no parenteral formulation.

Place in Therapy. Topiramate is an adjunctive AED for patients with partial seizures who have failed initial therapy. Its role as a primary AED and in other seizure types is being evaluated.

Valproic Acid/Divalproex Sodium

Mechanism of Action. Initially it was believed that valproic acid increased GABA by inhibiting its degradation or by activating its synthesis. Although this may explain some of valproic acid effects, the time course for the increase in GABA compared with anticonvulsant effects of valproic acid indicates that effects on synthesis and degradation of GABA do not fully explain how valproic acid prevents seizures. It has been proposed that valproic acid may potentiate postsynaptic GABA responses, may have a direct membrane-stabilizing effect, and may affect potassium channels.[131]

Pharmacokinetics. Valproic acid appears to be completely absorbed from available oral dosage forms when administered on an empty stomach.[131] The rate of absorption differs between preparations. Peak concentrations occur in 0.5 to 1 hour with the syrup, 1 to 3 hours with the capsule, and 2 to 6 hours with the enteric-coated tablet.[131] There is a diurnal decrease in absorption of the enteric-coated preparation following an evening dose. Food delays but does not decrease the amount of valproic acid absorbed.[20]

Valproic acid distributes widely throughout the body. The binding sites for valproic acid are saturable, and the free fraction may increase as the total concentration increases. The saturable binding may indicate that the free concentration is a better monitoring parameter than the total valproic acid concentration, especially at higher concentrations or in patients with hypoalbuminemia.[20,21] The protein binding of valproic acid is decreased in patients with head trauma.

Valproic acid is metabolized primarily by the liver. There is no first-pass metabolism, and the clearance is independent of hepatic blood flow. As with other highly protein-bound drugs, an increase in free drug results in an increase in clearance. Thus the clearance of valproic acid changes at higher concentrations.[20]

The primary route of valproic acid metabolism is β-oxidation, although up to 40% of a dose may be excreted as the glucuronide. At least 10 metabolites of valproic acid have been identified. Some of these may have weak anticonvulsant activity, and at least 1 metabolite may be responsible for the hepatotoxicity reported with valproic acid. One of the lesser oxidative metabolites, 4-en-valproic acid, causes significant hepatotoxicity in rats. The formation of this metabolite is increased when valproic acid is given with enzyme-inducing drugs.[131]

Efficacy and Adverse Effects. Valproic acid is the drug of first choice for most generalized seizures including absence and myoclonic seizures[131] and is approved for both adjunctive and monotherapy treatment of partial seizures.[132] Although not currently approved, the parenteral administration of valproic acid may be useful in the treatment of status epilepticus.[133] It also may be useful in neonatal seizures.[131]

The most common side effects are usually mild.[131] The most frequently reported side effects are gastrointestinal complaints (up to 20%), including nausea, vomiting, anorexia, and weight gain. Pancreatitis is very rare. The gastrointestinal complaints may be minimized but not totally alleviated with the enteric-coated formulation or by giving the drug with food. Other frequently reported side effects (drowsiness, ataxia, postural tremor) may respond to a modification of dose (see Table 56–6). Alopecia and hair changes are temporary. Weight gain can be significant for many patients and may involve stimulation of appetite and/or inhibition of fatty acid β-oxidation, leading to reduced metabolic rate.[134] Valproic acid causes minimal cognitive impairment.[131] As discussed previously, it also has been suggested that valproic acid may be associated with polycystic ovary syndrome.

The most serious side effect reported with valproic acid is hepatotoxicity. Hyperammonemia is common (50%) but does not necessarily imply liver damage; however, at least 67 fatalities have been attributed to valproic acid hepatotoxicity. Most deaths have occurred in patients who were less than 2 years of age, mentally retarded, and receiving multiple AED therapy. The hepatotoxicity occurs early in the course of therapy.[135] Patients who complain of nausea, vomiting, lethargy, anorexia, and edema in the first 6 to 12 months of therapy should have liver function tests drawn. Multiple AED therapy may alter the normal metabolism, leading to increased formation of the potentially liver-toxic 4-en-valproic acid. Valproic acid has been shown to alter carnitine metabolism,[136] and it has been postulated that a deficiency of carnitine alters fatty acid oxidation that could lead to both liver toxicity and hyperammonemia. However, valproic acid hepatotoxicity has occurred in a patient taking supplemental carnitine, and a prospective study demonstrated no effect on well-being when carnitine was added. While carnitine may partially ameliorate hyperammonemia,[137] it is expensive, and there are only limited data to support routine supplemental use in patients taking valproic acid.[136]

Thrombocytopenia, as well as alterations in platelet aggregation, occurs in the patients receiving valproic acid and is related to serum concentration.[138] Other hematologic toxicities have been reported, including leukopenia with transient neutropenia, transient erythroblastopenia, and bone marrow changes.

Drug-Drug and Drug-Food Interactions. Drugs that induce liver enzymes may alter valproic acid kinetics by increasing metabolism; for example, phenytoin, phenobarbital, primidone, and carbamazepine all increase valproic acid clearance. Topiramate may modestly reduce valproic acid serum concentrations. Because it is highly protein-bound, other highly protein-bound drugs may displace valproic acid. Free fatty acids and aspirin may alter valproic acid binding. Felbamate may impair valproic acid clearance, via inhibition of β-oxidation.

Valproic acid is an enzyme inhibitor and can inhibit specific CYP isozymes, epoxide hydrolase, and UGT isozymes. The addition of valproic acid to phenobarbital results in a 30% to 50% decrease in the clearance of phenobarbital and toxicity if the dose of phenobarbital is not reduced.[131] Valproic acid may increase concentrations of 10, 11-carbamazepine epoxide without affecting concentrations of the parent drug, via inhibition of epoxide hydrolase. Valproic acid is also a potent inhibitor of lamotrigine, via inhibition of UGT enzymes, and can result in a doubling of half-life. It does not appear to cause clinically significant pharmacokinetic interactions with any of the other newer AEDs.

Dosing and Administration. The minimal effective concentration of valproic acid is 50 μg/mL; however, there is disagreement on the upper end of the therapeutic range.[131] Although 100 to 120 μg/mL is widely quoted as the upper end of the therapeutic range, experience indicates that a significant number of patients have improved seizure control when the concentration is increased. Although some reports have linked tremor, drowsiness, stupor, and decreases in fibrinogen to concentrations greater than 80 to 100 μg/mL, there are very few clearly defined concentration-dependent side effects of valproic acid. In refractory or partially responding patients, the concentration of valproic acid may be titrated upward cautiously, provided the patient is monitored closely. As the concentration is increased, protein binding may become saturated, and concentration monitoring of free drug may be helpful.[20]

Although some patients may have a half-life sufficiently long to permit once-a-day dosing with enteric-coated divalproex, more frequent dosing is the norm. Based on half-life data, twice-daily dosing is feasible with any valproic acid dosage form; however, children and other patients taking enzyme inducers may require dosing three to four times daily. The serum concentration-dose relationship is curvilinear (i.e., the concentration-dose ratio decreases with increasing dose), probably because of increasing free concentrations and a resulting increase in clearance.

Valproic acid is available as a soft gelatin capsule, an enteric-coated tablet, a syrup, a "sprinkle," and a parenteral formulation (intravenous) solution for replacement of oral therapy or in situations where rapid loading is deemed necessary.[22] This parenteral formulation must not be given intramuscularly due to tissue necrosis. The sprinkle formulation is designed to be opened and mixed with food. The sprinkle formulation has a slower rate of absorption, which results in less fluctuations in the peak-to-trough ratio. Its absorption is unaffected by food.[20] The soft gelatin capsule is available in several generic forms. The syrup is absorbed more rapidly than either solid. The enteric-coated tablet is not a sustained-release dosage form; it consists of sodium divalproex, which must be metabolized in the gut to valproic acid, and is enteric coated to reduce the incidence of gastrointestinal distress. The enteric coating does cause delayed absorption, although once the enteric coating dissolves, sodium divalproex has absorption, metabolism, and elimination rates similar to those for other dosage forms. Absorption of the enteric-coated preparation is decreased following an evening dose. Recently, a sustained-release formulation of valproic acid has been marketed (Depakote ER), but clinicians may need to monitor serum drug concentrations if converting patients from divalproex (Depakote) to this product because of possible differences in bioavailability.

Advantages. Valproic acid is available as an oral solid, liquid, and sprinkle formulation and as an intravenous dosage form. The intravenous formulation may be useful in patients with refractory status epilepticus. A sustained-release formulation has been approved for once-a-day dosing in patients with migraine headaches. Valproic acid has a wide therapeutic index, is effective in a variety of seizure types, and is a broad-spectrum AED.

Disadvantages. Some patients report significant weight gain with valproic acid, and this may limit compliance. It is also associated with other side effects such as alopecia, tremors, pancreatitis, polycystic ovary disease, and thrombocytopenia. The gastrointestinal side effects may be minimized by using the enteric-coated formulation. Valproic acid is an enzyme inhibitor and interacts with other drugs.

Place in Therapy. Valproic acid is first-line therapy for generalized seizures such as myoclonic, atonic, and absence seizures. It is also useful in partial seizures and in primary generalized convulsive seizures.

Zonisamide

Pharmacology and Mechanism of Action. Zonisamide is a synthetic 1,2-benzisoxazole derivative classified as a sulfonamide and is chemically different for other AEDs. It has shown anticonvulsant activity in several experimental animal models, suggesting that zonisamide is a broad-spectrum AED. It is believed to exert its antiepileptic effect by reducing repetitive neuronal firing via blockade of voltage-sensitive sodium channels and by reducing voltage-dependent T-type Ca^{2+} channels.[139] Zonisamide also facilitates dopaminergic and serotonergic neurotransmission, weakly inhibits carbonic anhydrase, and blocks K^+ evoked glutamate release.[140] It is also postulated that zonisamide may protect the neurons from free-radical damage.

Pharmacokinetics. Zonisamide is completely absorbed, reaching the maximum peak concentration in 2 to 6 hours. It is only about 40% protein-bound and has a very long half-life (e.g., 63 to 69 hours in uninduced subjects).[141] With once-a-day dosing there is about 28% variability in the steady-state concentration, but with twice-a-day dosing there is only about 14% variation. Zonisamide is metabolized by both CYP 3A4 (50%) and *N*-acetylation (20%).[142] Eight inactive metabolites have been identified. Studies in patients with liver impairment have not been reported. About 30% is excreted unchanged. Marked renal impairment (C_{Cr} <20 mL/min) was associated with an increase in the AUC of zonisamide of 35%. Zonisamide is found in most tissues, but the concentration in red blood cells, liver, kidney, and adrenal gland is twice as high as in plasma. Zonisamide crosses the placenta. The concentration in breast milk is similar to that in the plasma. Although not firmly established, a target concentration range of 10 to 40 μg/mL has been suggested.

Efficacy. Zonisamide has been approved in Japan and North Korea for over 11 years, and there are over 250,000 patient exposures in these countries. Recently, there have been three pivotal clinical trials in the United States and Europe involving 1336 total patients with partial seizures with or without secondary generalization. These studies revealed that 28% to 42% of the patients had 50% or greater reduction in seizure frequency, 27% of the patients had a 75% or greater reduction in seizure frequency, and 8% of the patients were seizure-free. There does not appear to be any tolerance to the long-term antiepileptic effect. In Japan, zonisamide has been shown to be effective in patients with tonic-clonic, tonic, absence, myoclonic, and atonic seizures.

Adverse Effects. The most common adverse effects occurring during the clinical trails of zonisamide mainly involved the CNS (e.g., somnolence, dizziness, anorexia, headache, nausea, agitation, and irritability).[143] The side effects were more common with a more rapid dose escalation. Because zonisamide is a sulfonamide, hypersensitivity reactions (0.02%) may occur, and a history of allergy to sulfonamide compounds should be a contraindication to zonisamide use. A 2.6% incidence of symptomatic kidney stones has been reported in U.S. trials. Because of reports of modest, reversible declines in renal function in some patients, monitoring of renal function status may be advisable for certain patients. Oligohydrosis has been reported.

Drug-Drug and Drug-Food Interactions. Zonisamide does not inhibit or induce the CYP system. CYP inducers and CYP 3A4 inhibitors can affect the concentration of zonisamide.[144] Treatment with enzyme inducers can reduce zonisamide half-life to 27 to 36 hours. The administration of zonisamide with food delays the time to peak concentration but does not decrease the extent of absorption.

Dosing and Administration. In adults, the initial recommended dose of zonisamide is 100 mg/day. Doses should be titrated by 100 mg every 2 weeks to patient response. The dosage range in adults is 100 to 600 mg/day. In children in Japan, zonisamide is initiated at a dose of 2 to 4 mg/kg per day and titrated to 4 to 8 mg/kg per day up to a maximum of 12 mg/kg per day. Concentrations may increase or decrease if a coadministered inducer or inhibitor is withdrawn, thus necessitating a dosage adjustment.

Advantages. Zonisamide has multiple mechanisms of action and may be a broad-spectrum AED. There is broad international experience with this drug. Zonisamide has a very long half-life and is suitable for once- or twice-a-day dosing.

Disadvantages. The dose of zonisamide should be slowly titrated to patient response. This drug is a sulfonamide derivative and should not be used in patients with a sulfa allergy. Renal stones and weight loss also have been associated with zonisamide.

Place in Therapy. Zonisamide is currently approved for patients with partial seizures who have failed initial therapy. Its use as a primary AED is being evaluated currently. Zonisamide is potentially effective in a variety of partial and primary generalized seizure types.

PHARMACOECONOMIC CONSIDERATIONS

The direct costs of epilepsy include the cost of the drug, treatment for adverse events, emergency room visits, drug levels, laboratory tests, physician visits, rehabilitation, and transportation. Indirect costs include the costs associated with time lost from work, the inability to get a job, decreased productivity, and mortality.

It has been difficult to assess the entire cost of epilepsy to society. Pashko and coworkers[145] used a cohort of Pennsylvania Medicaid patients to estimate that the total direct cost of epilepsy is in excess of $10 billion annually, with the majority of the per-patient cost incurred for inpatient hospitalization (uncontrolled seizures or treatment-related toxicity). Another study suggested that the direct costs of epilepsy made up about 37% of the total costs, with indirect costs accounting for about 63% of the total costs.[146] This study also indicated that the costs were much less for a patient who is well controlled than for a patient who is poorly controlled. Drug costs in the Pashko study accounted for about 10% of the total costs of epilepsy. In another study, the cost-effectiveness of some of the newer drugs (e.g., lamotrigine, vigabatrin, and gabapentin) was estimated for the first year of drug therapy. There was little difference in initial costs, but gabapentin, with fewer side effects, resulted in cost savings.[147] The methodology used in this study has been criticized. There have been no pharmacoeconomic studies comparing the older, less expensive AEDs with the newer, more expensive drugs.

Providing the best quality of life possible is a treatment goal for patients with epilepsy. This concept entails more than a balance between side effects and the number of seizures. Quality of life takes into account all the concerns of patients with epilepsy, including their social and economic concerns. This can best be assessed by the patient. Seizure freedom leads to the best quality of life.[11] In one study, driving was listed as the most important concern by 28% of patients, followed by employment (21%), independence (9%), safety (6%), AED side effects (5%), seizure unpredictability (5%), and seizure avoidance (5%).[148] Assessment of quality of life as a therapeutic outcome ultimately may be more meaningful than measuring blood levels of the AEDs.

It is clear that the cheapest drugs in epilepsy (e.g., phenobarbital) are not the best because of the number of side effects. Further, drug therapy that would control seizures, decrease side effects, improve the quality of life, and reduce the use of other health care resources would be cost effective. Because epilepsy treatment continues to be very patient-specific, the drug or combination of drugs that controls seizures with the least number of side effects will be the drug(s) of choice for a given patient, no matter how expensive the drug acquisition cost.

Because many patients with epilepsy require minimal variation in blood concentrations to prevent seizures and avoid side effects, generic prescribing for epilepsy remains controversial. One study suggested that the money saved by generic prescribing is outweighed by negative health gain for the person with epilepsy, increased work in general practice, and increased social costs.[149]

EVALUATION OF THERAPEUTIC OUTCOMES

An individual therapeutic serum concentration range should be established for a given patient. This range should be the upper and lower limits of plasma concentrations that result in minimal side effects and optimal seizure control. This therapeutic plasma concentration range should be used to identify the appropriate patient-specific dose. Patients should be chronically monitored for seizure control, social adjustment, drug interactions, compliance, dosage adjustments, and toxicity. Patient response is more important than the serum drug concentration.

Outcomes can be assessed by prospective clinical monitoring, drug utilization review, and quality-of-life assessments. Clinical monitoring involves identifying the number and type of seizures. Patients should be given a seizure diary, and the severity as well as the frequency of seizures should be monitored. There should be a decrease in the number or severity of seizures. Patients should be questioned to determine if they are seizure-free. If not, they may be candidates for combination therapy. Other clinical monitoring parameters include side effects, dosing, compliance, and drug interactions. Drug utilization reviews can be done for a given drug, or a disease utilization review could be done for all patients with epilepsy. In a utilization review, criteria for acceptable practice are developed, and a given population is measured to determine if these standards are met. Finally, there is a disease-specific quality-of-life rating scale for epilepsy, and the quality of life of epilepsy patients can be screened or assessed in depth. Uncontrolled seizures can be socially devastating, resulting in impaired progress in school or loss of employment. If the seizures are repetitive and prolonged, there is the possibility of brain injury or death.

CONCLUSIONS

The treatment of epilepsy begins with a careful identification of the seizure type and selection of the most appropriate AED. Therapy should be initiated slowly, except in life-threatening situations, to avoid acute toxicity. Although most patients can be managed successfully on monotherapy, some patients' seizures remain uncontrolled despite use of multiple AEDs. The newer AEDs offer more opportunity for complete seizure control. There is a continuing need for new AEDs and additional research in this area.

► PRINCIPLES OF PHARMACOTHERAPY

- Accurate diagnosis and classification of seizure/syndrome type are critical to selection of appropriate pharmacotherapy (see Table 56–4).
- Patient-specific treatment goal(s) should be identified. Often a balance between efficacy and side effects must be reached. Treatment goals may change over time.
- Patient characteristics such as age, medical condition, ability to comply with prescribed regimen, and insurance coverage also may influence choice of AED(s).
- Pharmacotherapy of epilepsy is highly individualized and requires titration of dose to optimize AED therapy (maximal seizure control with minimal or no side effects). About 70% of patients can be maintained on one AED.
- If the therapeutic goal is not achieved, a second drug may be added or a switch to an alternative single AED can be made (see Fig. 56–1).
- When pharmacotherapy is initiated, assurance of patient understanding of the plan is essential to successful treatment. Patient education must be continuously addressed and patient compliance continuously reinforced.
- After assessing risks and benefits, discontinuance of AEDs may be considered if specific criteria are met (see Table 56–3).

REFERENCES

1. Leppik IE. Contemporary Diagnosis and Management of the Patient with Epilepsy, 2d ed. Newtown, PA, Handbooks in Health Care, 1996.
2. Gidal BE, Privitera M, Sheth R, Gilman J. Vigabatrin: A novel therapy for seizure disorders. Ann Pharmacother 1999;33:1277–1286.
3. Hauser W. The prevalence and incidence of convulsive disorders in children. Epilepsia 1994;35(Suppl 2):S1–S6.
4. Shinnar S, Berg A, Moshe S, et al. Risk of seizure recurrence following a first unprovoked seizure in childhood. Pediatrics 1990;85:1076–1085.
5. Hauser W. Seizure disorders: The changes with age. Epilepsia 1992;33 (Suppl 4):S6–S14.
6. Cloyd JC, Lackner TE, Leppik IE. Antiepileptics in the elderly. Arch Fam Med 1994;3:589–598.

7. Chadwick D. Epilepsy. J Neurol Neurosurg Psychiatry 1994;57:264 277.
8. Dichter MA. Emerging insights into mechanisms of epilepsy: Implications for new antiepileptic drug development. Epilepsia 1994;35:S51–S57.
9. Commission on Classification and Terminology of the International League Against Epilepsy. Proposal for revised clinical and electroencephalographic classification of epileptic seizures. Epilepsia 1981;22: 489–501.
10. Commission on Classification and Terminology of the International League Against Epilepsy. Proposal for revised classification of epilepsies and epileptic syndromes. Epilepsia 1989;30:389–399.
11. Vickrey BG, Hays RD, Rausch R, et al. Quality of life of epilepsy surgery patients as compared with outpatients with hypertension, diabetes, heart disease, and/or depressive symptoms. Epilepsia 1994;35:597–607.
12. Chadwick D. Standard approach to antiepileptic drug treatment in the United Kingdom. Epilepsia 1994;35:S3–S510.
13. Meador KJ. Cognitive side effects of antiepileptic drugs. Can J Neurol Sci 1994;21:S12 S16.
14. Gilliam F, Kuzniecky R, Faught E, et al. Patient-validated content of epi- lepsy specific quality of life measurement. Epilepsia 1997;38:233–236.
15. Wiegartz P, Seidenberg M, Woodard A, et al. Co-morbid psychiatric disorder in chronic epilepsy: Recognition and etiology of depression. Neurology 1999;53(Suppl 2):S3–S8.
16. Brodie MJ, French JA. Management of epilepsy in adolescents and adults. Lancet 2000;356:323–328.
17. Mattson RH, Cramer JA, Collins JF. Prognosis for total control of complex partial and secondarily generalized tonic clonic seizures. Department of Veterans Affairs Epilepsy Cooperative Studies No. 118 and No. 264. Neurology 1996;47:68 76.
18. Mattson R. Current challenges in the treatment of epilepsy. Neurology 1994;44(Suppl 5):S4–S9.
19. Garnett WR. Antiepileptic drug treatment: Outcomes and adherence. Pharmacotherapy 2000;20:191S–199S.
20. Garnett WR. Antiepileptics. In: Schumacher GE, ed. Therapeutic Drug Monitoring. Norwalk, CT, Appleton & Lange, 1995;345–395.
21. Gidal BE, Collins DM, Beinlich B. Valproic acid neurotoxicity in a hypoalbuminemic patient. Ann Pharmacother 1993;27:32–34.
22. Limdi NA, Faught E. The safety of rapid valproic acid infusion. Epilepsia 2000;41:1342–1345.
23. First Seizure Trial Group. Randomized clinical trial on the efficacy of antiepileptic drugs in reducing the risk of relapse after a first unprovoked tonic-clonic seizure. Neurology 1993;43:478–483.
24. Duncan JS, Shorvon SD, Trimble MR. Effects of removal of phenytoin, carbamazepine, and valproate on cognitive function. Epilepsia 1990;31:584–591.
25. Andersson T, Braathen G, Persson A, Theorell K. A comparison between one and three years of treatment in uncomplicated childhood epilepsy. A prospective study: 2. The EEG as predictor of outcome after withdrawal of treatment. Epilepsia 1997;38:225–232.
26. Quality Standards Subcommittee of AAN. Practice parameter: A guideline for discontinuing antiepileptic drugs in seizure-free patients—Summary statement. Neurology 1996;47:600–602.
27. Chadwick D, Taylor J, Johnson T. Outcomes after seizure recurrence in people with well-controlled epilepsy and the factors that influence it. The MRC Antiepileptic Drug Withdrawal Group. Epilepsia 1996;37:1043–1050.
28. Berg AT, Shinnar S. Relapse following discontinuation of antiepileptic drugs: A meta-analysis. Neurology 1994;44:601–608.
29. Ketter TA, Malow BA, Flamini R, et al. Anticonvulsant withdrawal: Emergency psychopathology. Neurology 1994;44:55–61.
30. Jacoby A, Johnson A, Chadwick D. Psychosocial outcomes of antiepileptic drug discontinuations. Epilepsia 1992;33:1123–1131.
31. Salinsky MC, Uthman BM, Ristanovic RK, et al. Vagus nerve stimulation for the treatment of medically intractable seizures. Results of a 1-year open-extension trial. Arch Neurol 1996;53:1176–1180.
32. Henry TR, Bakay Ra, Votaw JR, et al. Brain blood flow alterations induced by therapeutic vagus nerve stimulation in partial epilepsy: I. Acute effects at high and low levels of stimulation. Epilepsia 1998;30:983–990.
33. Handforth A, DeGiorgio CM, Schachter SC, et al. Vagus nerve stimulation therapy for partial-onset seizures: A randomized active-control trial. Neurology 1998;51:48–55.
34. Engel J. Surgery for seizures. N Engl J Med 1996;334:647–652.
35. Schiller Y, Casino GD, So EL, Marsh R. Discontinuation of antiepileptic drugs after successful epilepsy surgery. Neurology 2000;54:346–349.
36. Nordli DRJ, De Vivo DC. The ketogenic diet revisited: Back to the future. Epilepsia 1997;38:743–749.
37. Heller AJ, Chesterman P, Elwes RD, et al. Phenobarbitone, phenytoin, carbamazepine, or sodium valproate for newly diagnosed adult epilepsy: A randomised comparative monotherapy trial. J Neurol Neurosurg Psychiatry 1995;58:44–50.
38. Mattson RH, Cramer JA, Collins JF, et al. Comparison of carbamazepine, phenobarbital, phenytoin, and primidone in partial and secondarily generalized tonic-clonic seizures. N Engl J Med 1985;313:145–151.
39. Mattson RH, Cramer JA, Collins JF, et al. A comparison of valproate with carbamazepine for the treatment of complex partial seizures and secondarily generalized tonic-clonic seizures in adults. N Engl J Med 1992;327:765–771.
40. Marson AG, Kadir ZA, Chadwick DW. New antiepileptic drugs: A systematic review of their efficacy and tolerability [See comments]. Br Med J 1996;313:1169–1174.
41. Resor SR, Resor LD, Woodbury DM, Kemp JW. Sulfonamides and derivatives: Acetazolamide. In: Mattson RH, Meldrum BS, Levy RH, eds. Antiepileptic Drugs, 4th ed. New York, Raven, 1995;969–985.
42. Morrell MJ. The new antiepileptic drugs and women: Efficacy, reproductive health, pregnancy, and fetal outcome. Epilepsia 1996;37:S34–S44.
43. Wilbur K, Ensom MH. Pharmacokinetic drug interactions between oral contraceptives and second-generation anticonvulsants. Clin Pharmacokinet 2000;38:355–365.
44. Duncan S, Read CL, Brodie MJ. How common is catamenial epilepsy? Epilepsia 1993;34:827–831.
45. Herzog AG. Progesterone therapy in women with epilepsy: A 3 year follow-up. Neurology 1999;52:1917–1918.
46. Isojarvi JT, Rattya J, Myllyla VV, et al. Valproate, lamotrigine, and insulin-mediated risks in women with epilepsy. Ann Neurol 1998;43: 446–451.
47. Liporace JD. Womens issues in epilepsy. Postgrad Med 1997;102:123–138.
48. Practice parameter. Management issues for women with epilepsy: Summary statement. Neurology 1998;51:944–948.
49. Brodie MJ. Management of epilepsy during pregnancy and lactation. Lancet 1990;336:426–427.
50. Rho JM, Sankar R. The pharmacological basis of antiepileptic drug action. Epilepsia 1999;40:1471–1483.
51. Commission on Antiepileptic Drugs, International League Against Epilepsy. Guidelines for therapeutic monitoring on antiepileptic drugs. Epilepsia 1993;34:585–587.
52. Albrecht S, Ihmsen H, Hering W, et al. The effect of age on the pharmacokinetics and pharmacodymanics of midazolam. Clin Pharmacol Ther 1999;65:630–639.
53. Schmidt D, Einicke I, Haenel F. The influence of seizure type on the efficacy of plasma concentrations of phenytoin, phenobarbital and carbamazepine. Arch Neurol 1986;43:263–265.
54. Snodgrass SR, Parks BR. Anticonvulsant blood levels: Historical review with a pediatric focus. J Child Neurol 2000;15:734–746.
55. Camfield P, Camfield C. Acute and chronic toxicity of antiepileptic medications: A selective review. Can J Neurol Sci 1994;21:S7–S11.
56. Vermeulen J, Aldenkamp AP. Cognitive side effects of chronic antiepileptic drug treatment: A review of 25 years of research. Epilepsy Res 1995;22:65–95.
57. Meador KJ, Loring DW, Huh K, et al. Comparative cognitive effects of anticonvulsants. Neurology 1990;40:391–394.

58. Ludgate J, Keating J, O'Dwyer R, et al. An improvement in cognitive function following polypharmacy reduction in a group of epileptic patients. Acta Neurol Scand 1985;71:448–452.
59. Meador KJ, Loring DW, Ray PG, et al. Differential cognitive effects of carbamazepine and gabapentin. Epilepsia 1999;40:1279–1285
60. Elger CE, Bauer J, Scherrmann J, Widman G. Aggrevation of focal epileptic seizures by antiepileptic drugs. Epilepsia 1998;39(Suppl 3): S15–S18.
61. Levy RH. Cytochrome P450 isozymes and antiepileptic drug interactions. Epilepsia 1995;36:S8–S13.
62. Tomson T, Almkvist O, Nilsson BY. Carbamazepine-10,11-epoxide in epilepsy: A pilot study. Arch Neurol 1990;47:888–892.
63. Robbins DK, Wedlund PJ, Buhn R, et al. Inhibition of epoxide hydrolase by valproic acid in epileptic patients receiving carbamazepine. Br J Clin Pharmacol 1990;29:759–762.
64. Schaffler L, Bourgeois BRD, Luders HO. Rapid reversibility of autoinduction of carbamazepine metabolism after temporary discontinuation. Epilepsia 1994;35:195–198.
65. VanAmelsvoort TH, Bakshi R, Devaus CB, Schwabe S. Hyponatremia associated with carbamazepine and oxcarbazepine therapy: A review. Epilepsia 1994;35:181–188.
66. Konishi T, Naganuma Y, Hongo K, et al. Carbamazepine-induced skin rash in children with epilepsy. Eur J Pediatr 1993;152:605–608.
67. Clark-Schmidt AL, Garnett WR, Lowe DR, et al. Loss of carbamazepine suspension through nasogastric feeding tubes. Am J Hosp Pharm 1990;47:332–372.
68. Thakker KM, Mangat S, Garnett WR, et al. Comparative bioavailability and steady state fluctuations of Tegretol commercial and carbamazepine OROS tablets in adult and pediatric epileptic patients. Biopharm Drug Dispos 1992;24:839–841.
69. Wolff D. Ethosuximide. In: Wyllie E, ed. The Treatment of Epilepsy: Principles and Practice, 2d ed. Baltimore, Williams & Wilkins, 1996;856–864.
70. Taylor LA, McQuade RD, Tice MA. Felbamate, a novel antiepileptic drug, reverses *N*-methyl-D-aspartate/glycine-stimulated increases in intracellular Ca^{2+} concentration. Eur J Pharmacol 1995;289:229–233.
71. Graves N. Felbamate. Ann Pharmacother 1993;27:1073–1081.
72. Graves MN, Holmes GB, Fuerst RH, et al. Effect of felbamate on phenytoin and carbamazepine serum concentrations. Epilepsia 1989;30: 225–229.
73. Wagner ML, Remmel RP, Graves NM, Leppik IE. Effect of felbamate on carbamazepine and its major metabolites. Clinl Pharmacol Ther 1993; 53:536–543.
74. McLean MJ. Gabapentin. Epilepsia 1995;36:S73–86.
75. Taylor CP, Gee NS, Su TZ, et al. A summary of mechanistic hypothesis of gabapentin pharmacology. Epilepsy Res 1998;29:233–249.
76. Luer MS, Hamani C, Dujovny M, et al. Saturable transport of gabapentin at the bloodbrain barrier. Neurol Res 1999;21:559–562.
77. Gidal BE, Radulovic LL, Kruger S, et al. Inter- and intra-subject variability in gabapentin (GBP) absorption and absolute bioavailability. Epilepsy Res 2000;40:123–127.
78. Bockbrader HN, Breslin EM, Underwood BA, et al. Multiple-dose, dose-proportionality study of Neurontin (gabapentin) in healthy volunteers. Epilepsia 1996;37:159.
79. McLean MJ. Clinical pharmacokinetics of gabapentin. Neurology 1994; 44:S17–S22.
80. Gidal BE, Maly MM, Kowalski J, et al. Gabapentin absorption: Effect of mixing with foods of varying macronutrient content. Ann Pharmacother 1998;32:405–408.
81. Wong MO, Eldon MA, Keane WF, et al. Disposition of gabapentin in anuric subjects on hemodialysis. J Clin Pharmacol 1995;35:622–626.
82. Leiderman DB. Gabapentin as add-on therapy for refractory partial epilepsy: Results of five placebo-controlled trials. Epilepsia 1994;35: S74–S76.
83. Morrell MJ. Dosing to efficacy with Neurontin: The STEPS trial. Epilepsia 1999;40(Suppl 6):S23–S26; McLean MJ, Morrell MJ, Willmore LJ, et al. Safety and tolerability of gabapentin as adjunctive therapy in a large, multicenter study. Epilepsia 1999;40:965–972.
84. Khurana DS, Riviello J, Helmers S, et al. Efficacy of gabapentin therapy in children with refractory partial seizures. J Pediatr 1996;128:829–833.
85. Trudeau VL, Kilgore MB, Poulter CJ, et al. A multicenter, open-label extension study of gabapentin (Neurontin) monotherapy in pediatric patients with benign epilepsy with centrotemporal spikes (BECTS). Epilepsia 1996;37:111.
86. Vossler DG. Exacerbation of seizures in Lennox-Gastaut syndrome by gabapentin. Neurology 1996;46:852–853.
87. Backonja M, Beydoun A, Edwards KR, et al. Gabapentin for the symptomatic treatment of painful neuropathy in patients with diabetes mellitus. JAMA 1998;280:1831–1836.
88. Rowbotham M, Harden N, Stacey B, et al. Gabapentin for the treatment of postherpetic neuralgia. A randomized controlled trial. JAMA 1998;280:1837–1842.
89. Letterman L, Markowitz JS. Gabapentin: A review of published experience in the treatment of bipolar disorder and other psychiatric conditions. Pharmacotherapy 1999;19:565–572.
90. Lee DO, Steingard RJ, Cesena M, et al. Behavioral side effects of gabapentin in children. Epilepsia 1996;37:87–90.
91. Fisher RS, Sachdeo FC, Pellock J, et al. Dose intitiation of gabapentin (CI-945) add-on therapy: A multicenter, randomized, double-blind, comparative study. Epilepsia 1996;37:158.
92. Gidal BE, DeCerce J, Bockbrader HR, et al. Gabapentin bioavailability: Effect of dose and frequency of administration in adult patients with epilepsy. Epilepsy Res 1998;31:91–99.
93. Coulter DA, Antiepileptic drug cellular mechanism of action: Where does lamotrigine fit in? J Child Neurol 1997;12:S2–S9.
94. Messenheimer JA. Lamotrigine. Epilepsia 1995;36:S87–S94.
95. Posner J, Holdich CP. Comparison of lamotrigine pharmacokinetics in young and elderly healthy volunteers. J Pharm Med 1991;1:121–128.
96. Gilliam F, Vazquez B, Sackellares JC, et al. An active-control trial of lamotrigine monotherapy for partial seizures. Neurology 1998;51:1018–1025.
97. Frank LM, Enlow T, Holmes GL, et al. Lamictal (lamotrigine) monotherapy for typical absence seizures in children. Epilepsia 1999;40:973–979.
98. Brodie MJ, Overstall PW, Giorgi L, The UK Lamotrigine Elderly Study Group. Multicenter, double blind randomized comparison between lamotrigine and carbamazepine in elderly patients with newly diagnosed epilepsy. Epilepsy Res 1999;37:81–87.
99. Messenheimer JA, Rash in adult and pediatric patients treated with lamotrigine. Can J Neurol Sci 1998;25:S14–S18.
100. Holdrich T, Whiteman P, Orme M, et al. Effect of lamotrigine on pharmacology of the combined oral contraceptive pill [Abstract]. Epilepsia 1992;32(Suppl 1):96.
101. Klitgaard H, Matagne A, Gobert J, Wulfert E. Evidence for a unique profile of levetiracetam in rodent models of seizures and epilepsy. Eur J Pharmacol 1998;353:191–206.
102. Cloyd J, Remmel R. Antiepileptic drug pharmacokinetics and interactions: Impact on the treatment of epilepsy. Pharmacotherapy 2000;20:139S–151S.
103. Shorvon SD, Lowenthal A, Bielen E, Loiseau P. Multicenter double blind, randomized placebo-controlled trial of levetiracetam as add-on therapy in patients with refractory partial seizures. Epilepsia 2000;41:1179–1186.
104. Nicolas JM, Collart P, Gerin B, et al. In vitro evaluation of potential drug interactions with LEV, a new antiepileptic agent. Drug Metab Dispos 1999;27:250–254.
105. Perucca E, Gidal BE, Ledent E, Baltes E. Levetiracetam does not interact with other antiepileptic drugs. Epilepsia 2000;41(Suppl 7):254–255.
106. Mclean MJ, Schmutz M, Wamil AW, et al. Oxcarbazepine: mechanisms of action. Epilepsia 1994;35(Suppl 3):S5–S9.
107. Lloyd P, Flesch G, Dieterle W. Clinical pharmacology and pharmacokinetics of oxcarbazepine. Epilepsia 1994;35:10–13.
108. Reinikainen KJ, Keranen T, Halonen T, et al. Comparison of oxcarbazepine and carbamazepine: A double blind study. Epilepsy Res 1987; 1:284–289.

109. Schachter SC. Oxcarbazepine: current status and clinical applications. Exp Opin Invest Drugs 1999;8:1103–1112.
110. Klosterkov, Jensen P, Saano V, et al. Oxcarbazepine: Pharmacokinetic interaction and their clinical relevance. Epilepsia 1993;35:S14–S19.
111. May TW, Ramback B, Jurgens U. Influence of oxcarbazepine and methsuximide on lamotrigine concentrations in epileptic patients with and without valproic acid comedication: Results of a retrospective study. Ther Drug Monit 1999;21:175–181.
112. Painter MJ. Benzodiazepines and the barbiturates in the treatment of childhood epilepsy. In: Dodson WE, Pellock JM, eds. Pediatric Epilepsy: Diagnosis and Treatment. New York, Demos, 1993:281–289.
113. Farwell JR, Lee YJ, Hirtz DG, et al. Phenobarbital for febrile seizures effects on intelligence and on seizure recurrence. N Engl J Med 1990; 322:364–369.
114. Tozer TN, Winter ME. Phenytoin. In: Evans WE, Schentag JJ, Jusko WJ, eds. Applied Pharmacokinetics, 3d ed. Spokane, WA, Applied Therapeutics, 1992:25-1–25-44.
115. Anderson GD, Pak C, Doane KW, et al. Revised Winter-Tozer equation for normalized phenytoin concentrations in trauma and elderly patients with hypoalbuminemia. Ann Pharmacother 1997;31:279–284.
116. Bourgeois BFD. Pharmacologic intervention and treatment of childhood seizure disorders: Relative efficacy and safety of antiepileptic drugs. Epilepsia 1994,35.S18–S23.
117. Berg MJ, Fincham RW, Ebert BE, et al. Decrease of serum folates in healthy male volunteers taking phenytoin. Epilepsia 1988;29:67–73.
118. Privitera MD. Clinical rules for phenytoin dosing [See comments]. Ann Pharmacother 1993;27:1169–1173.
119. Schachter SC. Tiagabine: Current status and potential clinical applications. Exp Opin Invest Drugs 1996;5:1377–1387.
120. Ben-Menachem E. International experience with tiagabine add-on therapy. Epilepsia 1995;36:S14–S21.
121. Leppik IE. Tiagabine: The safety landscape. Epilepsia 1995;36:S10–S13.
122. Gidal BE, Lensmeyer GL. Therapeutic drug monitoring of topiramate: Evaluation of the saturable distribution between erythrocytes and plasma in whole blood using an optimized HPLC method. Ther Drug Monit 1999; 21:567–576.
123. Doose DR, Walker SA, Gisclon LG, Nayak RK. Single-dose pharmacokinetics and effect of food on the bioavailability of topiramate, a novel antiepileptic drug. J Clin Pharmacol 1996;36:884–891.
124. Gisclon LG, Curtin CR, Kramer LD. The steady-state pharmacokinetics of phenytoin (Dilantin) and topiramate (Topamax) in epileptic patients on monotherapy and during combination therapy [Abstract]. Epilepsia 1994:35(Suppl 8):54.
125. Langtry HD, Gillis JC, Davis R. Topiramate: A review of its pharmacodynamic and pharmacokinetic properties and clinical efficacy in the management of epilepsy. Drugs 1997;54:752–773.
126. Elterman RD, Glauser TA, Wylie E, et al. A double-blind, randomized trial of topiramate as adjunctive therapy for partial-onset seizures in children. Neurology 1999;52:1338–1344.
127. Biton V, Montouris GD, Ritter F et al. A randomized, placebo controlled study of topiramate in primary generalized tonic clonic seizures. Neurology 1999;52:1330–1337.
128. Shorvon SD. Safety of topiramate: adverse events and relationship to dosing. Epilepsia 1996;37(Suppl 2):S18–S22.
129. Rosenfeld WE, Liao S, Kramer LD, et al. Comparison of the steady-state pharmacokinetics of topiramate and valproate in patients with epilepsy during monotherapy and concomitant therapy. Epilepsia 1997;38:324–333.
130. Faught E, Wilder BJ, Ramsay RE, et al. Topiramate placebo-controlled dose-ranging trial in refractory partial epilepsy using 200-, 400-, and 600-mg daily dosages. Neurology 1996;46:1684–1690.
131. Davis R, Peters DH, McTavish D. Valproic acid: A reappraisal of its pharmacological properties and clinical efficacy in epilepsy. Drugs 1994; 47:332–372.
132. Beydoun A, Sackellares JC, Shu V. Safety and efficacy of divalproex sodium monotherapy in partial epilepsy: A double-blind, concentration-response design clinical trial. Depakote Monotherapy for Partial Seizures Study Group. Neurology 1997;48:182–188.
133. Giroud M, Gras D, Escousse A, Venaud G. Use of valproic acid injection in status epilepticus. Drug Invest 1993;5:154–159.
134. Gidal BE, Anderson GD, Spencer NW, et al. Valproate associated weight gain in patients with epilepsy: Potential relationship to energy expenditure and metabolism. J Epilepsy 1996;9:234–241.
135. Dreifuss FE, Santilli N. Valproic acid hepatic fatalities: A retrospective review. Neurology 1987;37:379–385.
136. Kelley RI. The role of carnitine supplementation in valproic acid therapy. Pediatrics 1994;93:891–892.
137. Gidal BE, Inglese CM, Meyer JM, et al. Diet and valproate mediated transient hyperammonemia: Effect of L-carnitine supplementation in children with epilepsy. Pediatr Neurol 1997;16:301–305.
138. Gidal BE, Spencer NW, Collins DM, et al. Valproate mediated disturbances of hemostasis: Relationship to concentration and dose. Neurology 1994;44:1418–1422.
139. Suzuki S, Kawakami K, Nishimura S, et al. Zonisamide blocks T-type calcium channel in cultured neurons of rat cerebral cortex. Epilepsy Res 1992;12:21–27.
140. Okada M, Kaneko S, Hirano T, et al. Effects of zonisamide on dopaminergic system. Epilepsy Res 1995;22:193–205.
141. Kochak GM, Page JG, Buchanan RA, et al. Steady-state pharmacokinetics of zonisamide, an antiepileptic agent for the treatment of refractory complex partial seizures. J Clin Pharmacol 1998;38:166–171.
142. Nakasa H, Komiya M, Ohmori S, et al. Characterization of human liver microsomal cytochrome P450 involved in the reductive metabolism of zonisamide. Mol Pharmacol 1993;44:216–221.
143. Harden CL. Therapeutic safety monitoring: What to look for and when to look for it. Epilepsia 2000;41(Suppl 8):S37–S44.
144. Perucca E, Bialer M. The clinical pharmacokinetics of the newer antiepileptic drugs: Focus on topiramate, zonisamide and tiagabine. Clin Pharmacokinet 1996;1:29–46.
145. Pashko S, McCord A, Sena MM. The cost of epilepsy and seizures in a cohort of Pennsylvania Medicaid patients. Med Interface 1993;November:79–84.
146. Begley CE, Annegers JF, Lairson DR, et al. Cost of epilepsy in the United States: A model based on incidence and prognosis. Epilepsia 1994;35:1230–1243.
147. Hughes D, Cockerell OC. A cost minimization study comparing vigabatrin, lamotrigine, and gabapentin for the treatment of intractable partial epilepsy. Seizure 1996;5:89–95.
148. Gilliam F, Kuzniecky R, Faught E, et al. Patient-validated content of epilepsy-specific quality-of-life measurement. Epilepsia 1997;38:233–236.
149. Crawford P, Hall WW, Chappell B, et al. Generic prescribing for epilepsy: Is it safe? Seizure 1996;5:1–5.
150. Hauser WA, Rich SS, Annegers JF, Anderson VE. Seizure recurrence after a first unprovoked seizure: An extended follow-up. Neurology 1990;40:1163–1170.

57

STATUS EPILEPTICUS

Stephanie J. Phelps, Collin A. Hovinga, and Bradley A. Boucher

Status epilepticus (SE) is a common neurologic emergency that may be associated with brain damage and death. Convulsive SE accounts for between 1% and 8% of all hospital admissions[1] and between 3% and 5% of admissions to neurologic intensive care units.[2] Although there is no consensus on the definition of SE, for practical purposes, SE may be defined as recurrent seizures without an intervening period of consciousness before the next seizure or any seizure lasting longer than 30 minutes whether or not consciousness is impaired.[3–6] SE can present in several forms (Table 57–1) and is classified according to the revised International Classification of Epileptic Seizures.[3] The syndrome most commonly associated with the term *status epilepticus* is tonic-clonic or generalized *convulsive* SE (GCSE). This type of SE is characterized by repeated primary or secondary generalized seizures that are associated with a persistent postictal state. *Nonconvulsive* SE (NCSE) is characterized by a fluctuating or continuous "twilight" state that produces altered consciousness (i.e., absence SE or complex partial SE) or by repeated simple partial seizures. Simple partial seizures are manifested as focal motor convulsions, focal sensory symptoms, or focal impairment of function not associated with altered consciousness.[7]

EPIDEMIOLOGY

Because most studies do not consider the seizure duration or type, etiology, or patient's age, the incidence of SE is difficult to determine. Previous studies using older definitions for SE (seizure lasting longer than 60 minutes) have suggested that between 50,000[1] and 160,000[4] individuals in the United States have an episode of SE yearly. However, a recent community-based study estimated that the incidence of SE in the United States may be as high as 250,000[8] cases per year. It is estimated that the global incidence of convulsive SE ranges between 1.2 and 5 million cases per year.[9] The most common and severe form of SE (GCSE) accounts for approximately 75% of cases, and NCSE accounts for 25%.[10] DeLorenzo and associates reported that more than 70% of adults and 50% of children with GCSE initially presented with partial seizures that became secondarily generalized.[10] The annual incidence of absence SE and complex partial SE is 1 and 35 cases per million, respectively.[11] It is likely that the incidence of NCSE is actually higher than this figure because of underdiagnosis.[7]

SE may be the initial presentation of epilepsy in 12% to 60% of all patients[12,13] and may be the initial presentation of epilepsy in as high as 48% to 75% of children[14] and 70% of elderly individuals.[1,10] In children, 21% and 64% of cases are reported by the first and fifth years of age, respectively.[15,16] The incidence of GCSE is higher in nonwhites than in whites across all ages.[10]

Although most reports note that the incidence of SE in previously diagnosed epileptics ranges between 0.5%[1] and 6.6%,[17] a recent study noted that the incidence might be as high as 42%.[10] Others have reported that within 5 years of the diagnosis of epilepsy, 20% of patients will have an episode of SE.[5]

ETIOLOGY

Although there has been no change in the pattern of etiologies during the past two decades,[18] precipitating events for SE vary from study to study and generally reflect various populations and referral patterns. Common etiologies and mortality rates for pediatric and adult populations are shown in Table 57–2.[8,10]

Precipitating events for GCSE are divided into two groups. Type I etiologies are not associated with any new structural lesions and include epileptic patients with SE.[19] A variety of prescription, over-the-counter, and recreational medications also must be considered in any patient with new-onset SE. Type II etiologies are associated with structural lesions and have a poor prognosis. These include brain tumor, anoxic encephalopathy, meningitis, stroke, and hemorrhage.

There are major differences in pediatric and adult etiologies. In patients less than 1 year old, the major causes of seizures are acute encephalopathy or metabolic disease (amino acid disturbances).[20] During the neonatal period, it is imperative to consider drug withdrawal-induced seizures (addicted mothers). Although infrequent, a pyridoxine deficiency may exist, and the electroencephalogram (EEG) should normalize within several hours following treatment with an intravenous dose of pyridoxine (100 mg). In young children, the cause is frequently idiopathic but may be associated with fever or a viral illness.[20] Generally, fever-induced SE is not associated with sequelae unless accompanied by an underlying neurologic abnormality.[21] In a study of 44 normal children with fever-induced GCSE, there was no increase in the risk of subsequent febrile or afebrile seizures within 12 months following the episode. However, there was a risk of recurrent seizures in patients with a prior neurologic abnormality.[22]

In adults, the most frequent precipitating factors are cerebrovascular disease, withdrawal of antiepileptic drugs (AEDs), and low anticonvulsant serum concentrations. Interestingly, infection is not a major cause of SE in adults; however, there have been increasing reports of SE associated with the human immunodeficiency virus (HIV).[6] In elderly patients who have their first seizures after age 60, cerebrovascular disease is the leading cause of SE. The initiating events of NCSE have not been well characterized.[7] Absence SE has been associated with carbamazepine therapy[23] and benzodiazepine withdrawal.[24]

PATHOGENESIS

Human studies investigating the mechanisms of SE are difficult; hence scientists have relied largely on experimental animal models. Although the exact mechanisms responsible for GCSE are unknown, it appears that there is an activated cascade of changes in excitatory amino acid neurotransmission, gamma-aminobutyric acid (GABA) inhibition, and *N*-methyl-D-aspartate (NMDA) receptor-mediated channel events[25–29] (Fig. 57–1). It is unlikely that a single mechanism is responsible for SE but that multiple interrelated events occur simultaneously at the cellular, brain, and systemic levels.

TABLE 57–1. International Classification of Status Epilepticus

Convulsive		Nonconvulsive	
International	*Traditional Terminology*	*International*	*Traditional Terminology*
Primary generalized SE • Tonic-clonic[a,b] • Tonic[a,c] • Clonic[c] • Myoclonic[b] • Erratic[d]	Grand mal, epilepticus convulsivus	Absence[c]	Petit mal, spike-and-wave stupor, spike-and-slow-wave or 3/s spike-and-wave, epileptic fugue, epilepsia minora continua, epileptic twilight, minor SE
Secondary generalized SE[a,b] • Tonic • Partial seizures with secondary generalization		Partial SE[a,b]	Focal motor, focal sensory, epilepsia partialis continuans, adversive SE
		Simple partial Somatomotor Dysphasic Other types	Elementary
		Complex partial	Temporal lobe, psychomotor, epileptic fugue state, prolonged epileptic stupor, prolonged epileptic confusional state, continuous epileptic twilight state

[a]Most common in older children.
[b]Most common in adolescents and adults.
[c]Most common in infants and young children.
[d]Most common in neonates.

Neurotransmitters released from the presynaptic terminal may cause either an excitatory or inhibitory effect on neuronal discharge. An increase in excitatory (e.g., glutamate and acetylcholine) or a decrease in inhibitory (e.g., GABA) neurotransmitters can cause sustained seizures with subsequent neuronal death.[30]

The ionic events that occur during SE are associated with opening of ion channels coupled with excitatory amino acid receptors. During GCSE, glutamate activation of the NMDA receptor causes processes that normally suppress the NMDA receptor-coupled channels to be overcome, resulting in opening of the gated calcium channels. This causes cell depolarization and calcium entry, which further depolarizes the cell. Sustained depolarization may not only sustain GCSE but also may eventually cause neuronal death. However, because NMDA receptor antagonists are no more effective than traditional anticonvulsants, it is unlikely that glutamate is the sole mechanism for GCSE.[31] Likewise, certain NMDA receptor antagonists may decrease rather than increase the seizure threshold. A second theory suggests that the excitatory amino acid-induced depolarization causes a passive flux of anion, cations, and water into the neuron, producing an osmotic cell lysis. If adenosine triphosphate production also decreases, the sodium pump fails, membrane ion exchange increases, and neurons swell further.

Other non-NMDA receptors (e.g., α-amino-3 hydroxy-5 methyl-4 isoxazolepropionate [AMPA], kainate) are activated by quisqualate and kainic acid, producing fast excitatory postsynaptic potentials. Neuronal damage in the hippocampus, similar to that noted after GCSE, has been reported following kainic acid-induced SE. This supports the theory that neuron destruction is independent of the systemic metabolic factors discussed in the next section. Antagonists of non-NMDA glutamate transmission can stop or prevent seizures, suggesting that glutamate agonism is an important etiologic event during GCSE.

The mechanisms that normally terminate seizures are poorly understood. The leading candidate, GABA, binds to postsynaptic receptors to regulate the opening and closing of the GABA channel. GABA binds to two distinct receptor subtypes. $GABA_A$ receptors are postsynaptic receptors that control chloride channels to produce hyperpolarization of the postsynaptic cell membrane. These receptors have binding sites for GABA as well as for select anticonvulsants (e.g., phenobarbital, benzodiazepines) and enhance $GABA_A$ currents. $GABA_B$ receptors are located pre- and postsynaptically and couple with calcium and potassium to inhibit the presynaptic membrane release of excitatory amino acids.

TABLE 57–2. Etiology and Mortality for Pediatric and Adult Cases of Status Epilepticus

Etiology	Pediatric ($n = 200$) % SE cases (% mortality)	Adult ($n = 512$) % SE cases (% mortality)
Type I (no structural lesion)		
Infection	55 (5)	6 (35)
CNS infection	11 (0)	2 (20)
Metabolic	20 (5)	12 (36)
Low AED levels	16 (0)	24 (7)
Alcohol	0 (0)	13 (8)
Idiopathic	6 (0)	13 (18)
Type II (structural lesion)		
Anoxia/hypoxia	27 (13)	14 (65)
CNS tumor	3 (50)	5 (22)
CVA	5 (0)	26 (27)
Drug overdose	5 (0)	3 (23)
Hemorrhage	5 (11)	4 (35)
Trauma	13 (0)	3 (23)
Remote causes[a]	33 (5)	7 (13)

Percentages do not add up to 100% because some patients had multiple etiologies. (AED = antiepileptic drug; CVA = cerebrovascular accident)
[a]More than half of remote causes were congential malformations and CVA in pediatric and adult patients, respectively.
Data modified from Refs. 8 and 10.

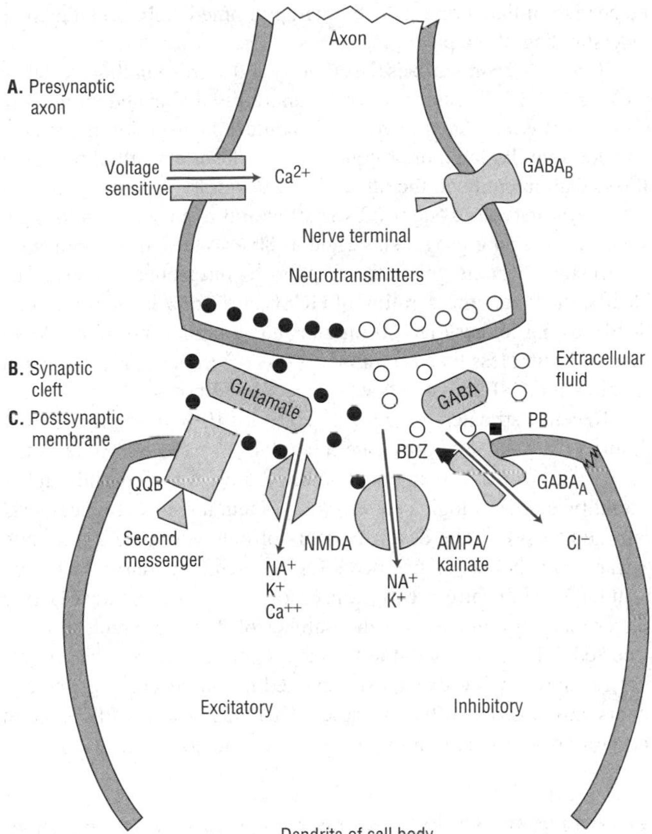

FIGURE 57–1. Neurotransmitters, receptors, and ion channels at nerve synapses. (A) Presynaptic axon. When axon action potential arrives at presynaptic nerve terminal, voltage-sensitive calcium (CA^{2+}) channels activate and cause release of neurotransmitter into the synaptic cleft. Presynaptic nerve terminals may be excitatory (glutamate) or inhibitory (GABA). $GABA_B$ receptors, activated by presynaptic axo-axonic synapses, decrease Ca^{2+} channel influx through a second-messanger pathway and can inhibit presynaptic neurotransmitter release into the synaptic cleft. (B) Synaptic cleft. Neurotransmitters (glutamate, GABA) move across the synaptic cleft. (C) Postsynaptic membrane of nerve dendrite or cell body. Excitatory neurotransmitters depolarize the postsynaptic membrane. Glutamate receptors are more often on the neuron dendrite than on the neuron cell body. There are four subtypes of receptors: (1) α-amino-3 hydroxy-5 methyl-4 isoxazolepropionate (AMPA), (2) kainate subtypes that are Na^+ and K^+ channels, (3) NMDA subtypes permeable to NA^+, K^+, and Ca^{++} and also voltage dependent, and (4) a quisqualate B (QQB) subtype that activates a second-messenger pathway. Inhibitory neurotransmitters: $GABA_A$ receptors are more often on the neuron cell body than on the dendrite and cause Cl^- influx that stabilizes the postsynaptic membrane. The $GABA_A$ receptors have additional binding sites for benzodiazepines (BDZ) and barbiturates (PB) that enhance binding of GABA to the receptor. Glycine, not shown, is an inhibitory neurotransmitter active only in the spinal cord at the postsynaptic membrane.

During SE, the GABA system does not function to inhibit seizures. GABA levels increase during the early phases of GCSE and continue to be elevated during late SE. This may represent increased synthesis or diminished breakdown. Immediately prior to the onset of chemically induced seizures, there is a progressive loss of $GABA_A$ receptor sensitivity to GABA. A diminution of GABAergic inhibition in the hippocampus has been reported in animals after a single, brief seizure.[27] Additionally, many $GABA_A$ antagonists can precipitate SE, and $GABA_A$ agonists (e.g., benzodiazepines) can abort SE. Likewise, abrupt withdrawal of a GABA agonist can induce SE. There is growing evidence that $GABA_A$ receptors are modified during SE and that the modification contributes to persistent seizures. Although the role of $GABA_B$ receptor agonists in SE is unknown, inhibition of the presynaptic receptors may inhibit GABA release, causing SE. Although GABA is important, it is unlikely that loss of GABA inhibition is the sole mechanism for SE.

PATHOPHYSIOLOGY

As GCSE progresses, there are systemic alterations, progression of motor phenomena, and specific EEG findings.[32] Two distinct and predictable phases have been identified.[2,20,26,32–36] Phase I occurs during the first 30 minutes of seizure activity, and phase II begins 60 minutes later. Although the presence of systemic complications affects the prognosis of SE, one must remember that SE may destroy neurons independent of these systemic events.[37] In fact, the systemic effects of experimentally induced seizures in animals can be blocked, but the damage to the neocortex, cerebellum, and hippocampus persists.

During phase I, each seizure produces marked increases in plasma epinephrine, norepinephrine, and steroid concentrations that may cause hypertension, tachycardia, and cardiac arrhythmias.[35] Within minutes, arterial systolic pressures may rise to values above 200 mm Hg, and heart rate may increase by 83 beats per minute. Although blood pressure returns to normal within 60 minutes, mean arterial pressure (MAP) does not fall below 60 mm Hg; hence cerebral perfusion pressure (CPP) is not compromised. In animals, cerebral blood flow (CBF) is also increased by 200% to 600%, thereby protecting neurons.

Seizure-induced increases in sympathetic and parasympathetic stimulation of the heart, in the presence of a hypoxic myocardium, may result in ventricular arrhythmias. Arrhythmias are seen frequently early in GCSE and may prove fatal.[35] Autonomic neuron stimulation also can cause a release of insulin and glucagon. Concurrently, circulating catecholamines cause an elevation of hepatic cyclic adenosine monophosphate (cAMP), producing glycogenolysis. Although the patient may be hyperglycemic initially, serum glucose begins to fall.

Seizure-induced muscular contractions and hypoxia cause lactic acid release that can cause a severe acidosis that may be accompanied by hypotension and shock. Muscle contractions can be so severe that rhabdomyolysis with secondary hyperkalemia and acute tubular necrosis may occur. Excessive heat is generated by increased muscle activity, and a correlation has been shown between increased body temperature and severity of brain injury.[38]

The airway may be obstructed, and the patient may become cyanotic or hypoxic at any time. Additionally, an increase in salivation and tracheal and pulmonary secretions may result in aspiration pneumonia. Although transient pleocytosis (white blood cells up to 20,000/mm^3) may occur, it should not be attributed to SE until infectious causes have been eliminated.

Between seizures, the EEG slows, and blood pressure normalizes. Although metabolic demands are increased, the brain is able to adequately compensate for these increased demands. If seizure activity exceeds 60 minutes (phase II), the EEG ictal discharge and clonic motor activity become continuous, and the patient begins to decompensate. Despite elevated levels of catecholamines, blood pressure is no longer increased, and the patient may become hypotensive. During the late phase, autoregulation of CBF becomes dependent on MAP and begins to fail. There continues to be an excessive consumption of oxygen and glucose; however, compensatory mechanisms are no longer able to keep up with demands.[37]

During phase II, serum glucose may be normal or decreased. Profound hypoglycemia, secondary to hyperinsulinemia, can occur in patients with hepatic dysfunction or in those with reduced glycogen stores (e.g., elderly, neonates). Hyperthermia and respiratory deterioration with hypoxia and ventilatory failure may develop. There also may be metabolic and biochemical complications, including respiratory and metabolic acidosis, hyperkalemia, hyponatremia, and azotemia. There is increased sweating and salivation. Marked elevations in plasma prolactin, glucagon, growth hormone, and adrenocorticotropic hormone also have been identified.[33]

OUTCOMES OF GCSE

MORBIDITY

Two theories exist regarding GCSE-associated morbidity. Both theories recognize that GCSE is harmful to the brain, but the first theory contends that morbidity occurs from the underlying etiology that caused GCSE.[1] The second theory contends that GCSE itself is responsible for morbidity.[32,39] Although histopathologic changes in animal neurons are evident following 30 minutes of GCSE, it is hard to establish a relationship between long-term outcome and SE because it is difficult to weigh the effects of seizure type, duration, etiology, concurrent physiologic events, and therapy or lack thereof.

Reports suggest that GCSE may decrease cognitive function in adults and that simple or complex partial SE lasting for days may cause prolonged memory deficits and neuronal death.[6,40,41] Some practitioners believe that there is an association between GCSE and deterioration in intellectual function,[32] but others have disputed the significance of the association.[39] Animal studies have shown that both single and refractory seizures inhibit brain growth and protein synthesis, causing permanent reduction in brain cell number.[36] Likewise, animal studies have noted that seizures inhibit cell multiplication and reduce the accumulation of myelin and synaptic markers. Importantly, these effects have been observed in the absence of neuronal necrosis. Although extrapolation of these results to humans is difficult, studies have noted that following GCSE, patients may experience a decrease in performance on intelligence quotient and subtle neuropsychometric tests.[39] Development of an epileptic focus (epilepsy) is more likely in patients who have experienced GCSE.[1,32,39] Additionally, these patients are less likely to experience remission of their epilepsy.[1,32,39]

Age,[14] seizure duration,[4] and severe preexisting brain disease[42] are related to SE-induced morbidity. In a study of 239 children with a 60-minute duration of GCSE, 67% of survivors had sequelae of epilepsy, mental retardation, or neurologic deficits.[14] Conversely, another study reported neurologic deficits in only 9.1% of patients with GCSE for a 30-minute or greater duration.[16] Both studies found that the younger the child, the greater was the chance of sequelae.[14,16] The mean duration of GCSE in patients who did not have neurologic sequelae was 1.5 hours compared with 10 hours in patients with neurologic sequelae.[4] Both human and animal studies support the premise that seizures exceeding 60 minutes can cause neuronal damage. Finally, morbidity also may be higher in patients with preexisting epilepsy.[16]

MORTALITY

The mortality from GCSE depends on the etiology, time from onset of SE to initiation of treatment, seizure duration, and patient age.[8] Using mortality data from the Richmond study, one would project the U.S. mortality rate to be between 22,000 and 42,000 individuals per year.[10] The decreasing mortality rate for SE probably reflects a change in the definition of GCSE (60 to 30 minutes), recognition of the need to initiate presequenced therapy immediately, and a greater understanding of the pathogenesis.

Table 57–2 summarizes the etiology and corresponding mortality rates for GCSE.[8,10] Interestingly, the mortality associated with many etiologies was significantly greater in adults than in children. Patients may die from SE, but more frequently they die as a result of the acute illness that precipitated the attack.[5] For example, patients with serious central nervous system (CNS) structural changes (hemorrhage, stroke) have a poor prognosis, whereas 80% to 90% of patients with no structural lesions generally respond to intravenous phenytoin.[5] Clearly, the longer the duration of GCSE, the worse is the prognosis. GCSE lasting longer than 60 minutes has a higher mortality (32%) than SE lasting less than 60 minutes (2.5%).[8] In one study, the mean duration of GCSE in patients who died was 13 hours.[4]

Recent estimates suggest a 2.5% to 10% mortality rate in children,[10,43] a 14% to 30% rate in adults,[6,10] and a 38% rate in the elderly.[10] Seizures in the neonatal period are associated with higher mortality and neurologic sequelae (e.g., mental retardation, cerebral palsy, epilepsy).[44] The best predictors of outcome were a 5 minute Apgar score below 7, the need for resuscitation during the first 5 minutes after birth, early onset of seizures, seizures lasting longer than 30 minutes, and the number of days on which seizures occurred.[44] DeLorenzo and associates reported that race had an effect on mortality but that gender exerted no influence.[8] Conversely, others have noted no effect of race.[45] There also was no difference in mortality between community hospitals and major medical centers.[8]

CLINICAL PRESENTATION AND DIAGNOSIS

Most generalized tonic-clonic seizures are self-limiting and stop within 5 to 7 minutes. Diagnosis includes observation, physical examination, laboratory assessment, EEG, and neurologic imaging. A careful history of the nature and duration of the seizure should be obtained.[46]

Physical examination should assess language, motor, sensory, and reflex abnormalities. A diagnosis of GCSE should not be made until a trained clinician has observed at least one generalized tonic-clonic seizure in a patient with a history of repeated seizures and impaired consciousness. For NCSE, the diagnosis should not be made until 30 minutes of continuous seizure activity has been observed.[47] For patients without a previous history of NCSE, an EEG is required for diagnosis.

Clinical features of NCSE may vary. Approximately 20% of patients may present mildly obtunded. Marked clouding occurs in two-thirds of patients, and marked lethargy and somnolence with pronounced eyes-open unresponsiveness and waxy rigidity occur in 15% of patients.[11] Language disturbance (e.g., mutism, paucity of speech) and inappropriate behavior (e.g., agitation, aggressiveness, hallucinations, emotional liability) can occur.[11] Motor features may include minor eyelid, face, and limb twitching.[11] It also should be remembered that patients with NCSE and patients with GCSE who are comatose or who have been given neuromuscular blockers may not have clinical SE but may continue to have electrical SE.[48]

Laboratory tests are important in the diagnosis of various etiologies. Hypoglycemia, hyponatremia (<120 meq/L), hypernatremia, hypomagnesemia, hypocalcemia, and renal failure all can cause seizures. Although hypomagnesemia in alcoholics is often cited as an etiology, its importance is probably overstated. A urine drug screen should be obtained in all patients to rule out the possibility of illicit drug use, drug overdose, or drug withdrawal. It is also necessary to determine serum AED concentration(s) in a patient on chronic anticonvulsants because loading doses may or may not require adjustment. Likewise, high concentrations of AEDs can induce seizures, and low or nondetectable levels may reflect noncompliance or rapid withdrawal of anticonvulsants. Assessment of parameters (e.g., albumin, renal function, hepatic function) affecting anticonvulsant dosing also may be useful.

A second phase of diagnostic tests is conducted after the seizures have stopped. It is important to determine if the patient is febrile or has a systemic or CNS infection. Many physiologic consequences of SE (e.g., leukocytosis, pleocytosis, and hyperthermia) produce symptoms that may be confused with other conditions such as infections. If a CNS infection is suspected, empirical antibiotics should be started, and a spinal tap should be obtained once the patient is stable.

An EEG is a valuable diagnostic tool, but treatment should not be delayed while awaiting results. Patients who do not awaken after clinical control of their seizures should have an EEG performed to rule out NCSE or recurrent subclinical seizures. NCSE patients frequently have abnormalities that begin in one area of the cortex and produce waxing and waning rhythmic activity in one or several brain regions. A trial of benzodiazepines, with concurrent EEG assessment, may be necessary to make a diagnosis of NCSE. Most patients with GCSE have organized discharges that start over the entire cortex simultaneously. Postictal slowing or depressed amplitude may help determine a focal cause of seizures.

In order to rule out vascular, neoplastic, or infectious etiologies, computed tomography (CT) or magnetic resonance imaging (MRI) should be performed in any patient with new-onset seizures. Although MRI is preferred, the use of ancillary technologies (e.g., infusion pumps) may preclude this test. The CT scan is generally adequate and can be done in emergency situations.

If the patient is refractory to treatment, one must consider pseudoseizures. Clinical features of pseudoseizures include resistance to passive eye opening, persistence of a positive conjunctival reflex, downgoing plantar reflexes, and the occurrence of repeated, apparently generalized seizures without cyanosis.[49]

▶ TREATMENT: Status Epilepticus

Although a diagnosis of SE technically cannot be made until seizure activity has persisted for greater than 30 minutes, therapy should not be withheld waiting for this period to pass. Any tonic-clonic seizure that does not stop automatically within 10 minutes should be treated during the diagnostic workup. Anytime doubt exists regarding the diagnosis, the patient should be treated as if he or she had SE.[5] Additionally, any person experiencing more than three major seizures within 24 hours may be at risk to progress to SE and should be treated aggressively.[40] An algorithm of the choice of anticonvulsants, timing, and dosing for the treatment of GCSE in hospitalized patients is given in Figure 57–2. Occasionally, patients with a history of frequent prolonged seizures may receive acute treatment at home. For example, rectal diazepam and intramuscular midazolam are administered easily and are effective rapidly.[50,51] However, repeated doses can lead to serious cardiorespiratory complications and generally are discouraged in the home environment.

DESIRED OUTCOME

It is imperative that a clear, presequenced management plan be initiated rapidly. There are four immediate goals in the management of SE. The first is patient stabilization and includes adequate oxygenation, preservation of cardiorespiratory function, and management of systemic complications. The second goal is correct diagnosis of the subtype of SE and identification of precipitating factors. Correct diagnosis prevents a delay in initiation of effective therapy and avoids the administration of large doses of unnecessary medications. The third and primary goal is to stop clinical and electrical seizure activity as soon as possible. The fourth and final goal is to prevent seizure recurrence.

NONPHARMACOLOGIC THERAPY

Concurrent with initiation of AEDs, vital signs should be assessed, and an adequate airway with ventilation should be established and maintained. The patient should be positioned to protect the airway from aspiration, and oxygen should be administered. If the patient is experiencing poor air exchange, he or she should be intubated and ventilated mechanically and managed using arterial blood gas determinations. A short-acting neuromuscular blocker may be required to facilitate intubation; however, it may mask the clinical symptoms of SE but not the electrical activity. EEG monitoring may be necessary in patients on neuromuscular blockers. Because hyperpyrexia can occur following prolonged SE, temperature should be monitored frequently. If fever occurs, a source of infection should be sought and antipyretics given. Antipyretics usually are not effective in SE-induced hyperthermia, and a cooling blanket may be required.[6]

Several anticonvulsants can cause tissue damage on extravasation; therefore, a secure intravenous line should be placed, and an infusion of normal saline should be started. Because all patients have some degree of cerebral edema, overhydration should be avoided.[43] Because cerebral perfusion depends on blood pressure, it is imperative that normal to high-normal blood pressure be maintained. Benzodiazepines, phenytoin, fosphenytoin, and phenobarbital can cause hypotension[5]; however, it generally can be controlled by slowing the rate of infusion or by administering dopamine.

Although hypoglycemia is a rare cause of SE, all patients should receive glucose. Wernicke's encephalopathy can develop in alcoholics; hence thiamine (100 mg) should be given prior to glucose in adults.[43] Initially, adults should receive 50 mL of a 50% solution, and children should be given 1 mL/kg of a 25% solution.[43] Serum glucose should be determined to assess the need for further glucose supplementation.

Most patients who have been seizing for prolonged periods will develop metabolic and/or respiratory acidosis. For this reason, an arterial blood gas should be obtained to determine pH, PaO_2, $PaCO_2$, and HCO_3. Metabolic acidosis resolves quickly following termination of SE; however, if the pH is below 7.2 secondary to a metabolic acidosis, sodium bicarbonate should be given. Persistent metabolic acidosis can be treated with 0.5–1 meq/kg[52] or 50 meq of sodium bicarbonate to pediatric or adult patients, respectively. If the patient has respiratory acidosis, assisted ventilation should correct the imbalance.

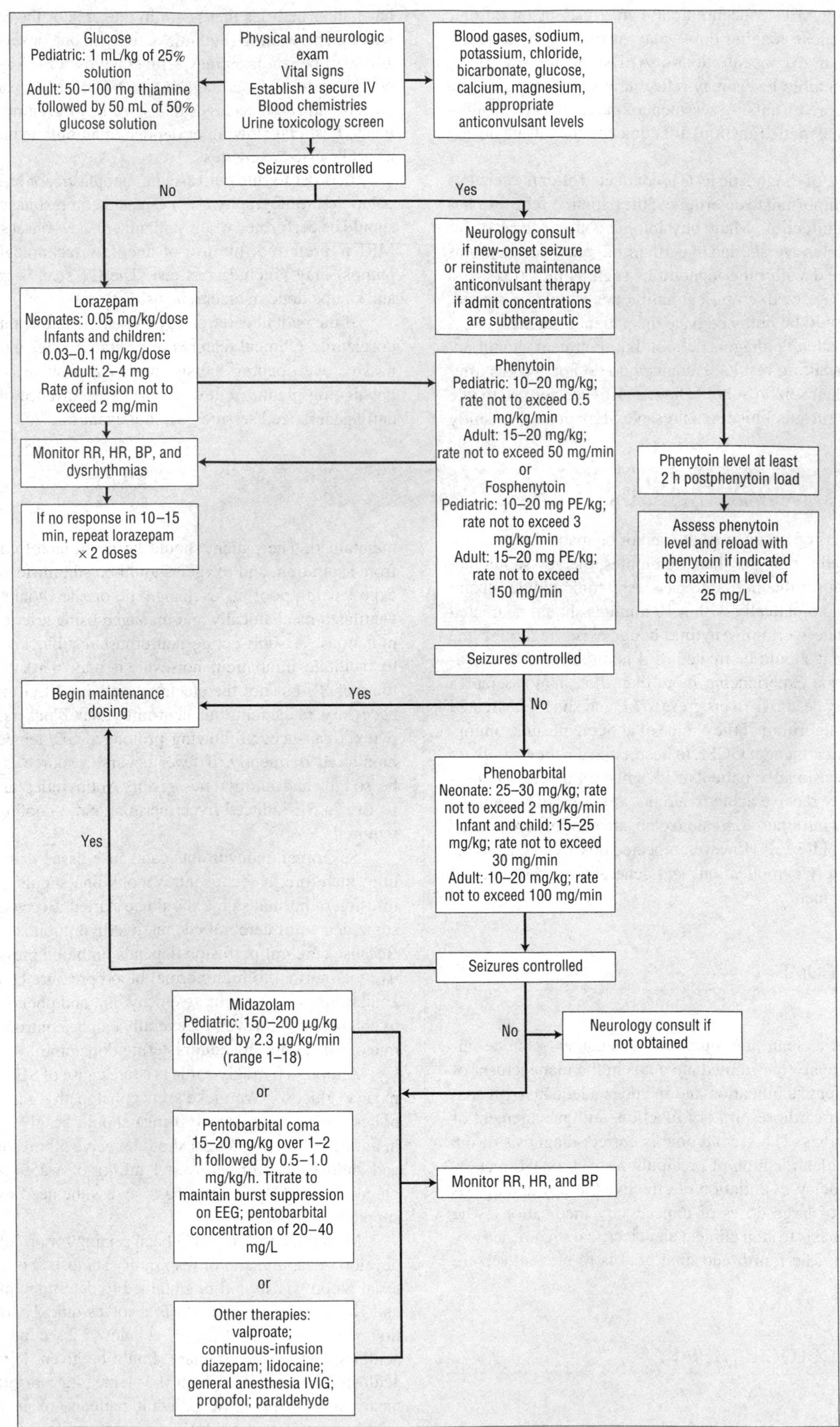

FIGURE 57–2. Algorithm for the management of GCSE.

PHARMACOLOGIC THERAPY

The three most commonly used classes of anticonvulsants for the treatment of GCSE are the benzodiazepines, phenytoin/fosphenytoin, and barbiturates. It should be noted that only five prospective, randomized studies have compared therapies for GCSE.[53–57] The first two studies were a blinded comparison of lorazepam versus diazepam in adults[53] and children.[55] The third study was a randomized comparison of phenobarbital with phenytoin plus diazepam.[56] The fourth study compared lorazepam with phenytoin.[54] The fifth study was a multicenter, prospective, randomized, double-blind comparison of phenytoin and diazepam, phenytoin alone, lorazepam, or phenobarbital.[57] Therefore, Figure 57–2 is a compilation of the results of limited studies,[53–57] a report of an advisory committee,[43] and clinical observations of the authors.

GENERAL CONVULSIVE STATUS EPILEPTICUS

Benodiazepines

The benzodiazepines are very effective in the initial treatment of SE and should be administered as soon as possible to patients who are actively seizing. If seizures have stopped, a benzodiazepine is not indicated, and a longer-acting anticonvulsant should be given.[43] Generally, one or two doses of an intravenous benzodiazepine will stop seizures within minutes.[55,58] Treiman reported lasting control of SE with benzodiazepines in 79% of 1455 patients from 47 clinical trials.[59] Diazepam, lorazepam, and midazolam are the only benzodiazepines available in the United States in a parenteral dosage form. Because these are equally effective in GCSE,[53,59,60] the preferred benzodiazepine is determined by differences in the pharmacokinetic and pharmacoeconomic profiles of the available agents.

Diazepam is an extremely lipophilic drug with a large volume of distribution (1–2 L/kg).[43] Following a single intravenous dose, 58% of adults had cessation of seizures by a median time of 2 minutes (range, immediate to 10 minutes),[53] and 65% of children had cessation of seizures by a mean time of 26 seconds (range, 20–51 seconds).[55] Although its initial distribution phase into the brain is extremely quick (10 seconds), it redistributes rapidly into body fat.[5] This causes its half-life in the brain to be less than 1 hour and results in an extremely short duration of effect (0.25–0.5 hours).[43] This rapid fall in concentration may result in seizure recurrence if diazepam is the sole anticonvulsant. For this reason, a longer-acting anticonvulsant (e.g., phenytoin, phenobarbital) should be given immediately after diazepam. The recommended initial diazepam doses in neonates, infants, and children, and adults are 0.15–0.75, 0.1–0.5, and 0.15–0.25 mg/kg, respectively.[43,61] If the patient does not respond within 5 minutes, the dose should be repeated.[43] The maximum total dosage is 5 mg in children under age 5 years,[62] 10 mg in children 5 years or older,[62] and 40 mg in adults.[7] Although plasma concentrations of 0.2–0.8 mg/L have been associated with seizure control,[5] assays are not readily available; hence therapeutic drug monitoring is impractical.

Although lorazepam is not approved by the Food and Drug Administration (FDA) for SE, it is currently the benzodiazepine of choice.[43,58] In fact, Treiman and associates reported that lorazepam was as effective in overt SE as diazepam plus phenytoin.[57] Lorazepam is less lipid soluble and takes slightly longer to reach peak levels in the brain than diazepam. Following a single intravenous dose, 78% of adults had cessation of seizures by a median time of 3 minutes (range, immediate to 15 minutes)[53] and 70% of children by a mean time of 29 seconds (range, 25–60 seconds).[55] Redistribution is minimal, leading to a longer duration of action (>12–24 hours). Lorazepam also has a higher-affinity binding to the benzodiazepine receptor than diazepam.[43] For these reasons, significantly fewer patients treated with lorazepam require additional anticonvulsants for seizure termination.[55] Data suggest that a single dose produces serum concentrations above 200 ng/mL and provides seizure protection for 24 hours.[5] The dose of lorazepam is 0.05-0.5 mg/kg in pediatric patients and 0.1 mg/kg in adults.[43] If the seizure continues after 5 minutes, a second dose may be given.[43] If there is still no response after 5 minutes, a third (final) dose may be given. The maximum total dosage of lorazepam is 4 mg in pediatric patients and 8 mg in adults.[43] It should be remembered that patients chronically on benzodiazepines (such as Klonopin) may have developed tolerance; hence they may require very large doses before response.

Diazepam and lorazepam cause vein irritation and should be diluted with an equal volume of compatible diluent before administration. The diluent for both diazepam and lorazepam contains propylene glycol, which may cause dysrhythmia and hypotension if administered too rapidly.[43] Therefore, the administration of diazepam and lorazepam should not exceed 5 and 2 mg/min, respectively.[63] If an intravenous line cannot be established, lorazepam and diazepam can be given rectally.[64] Intramuscular administration of the these agents may result in delayed or inadequate peak concentrations. This is especially true for diazepam, which has a slow and erratic absorption following intramuscular injection into the gluteal area.[5] For rectal administration, a Foley catheter is inserted rectally, the bulb is inflated, and the catheter is pulled back slightly. Diazepam (0.2 0.7 mg/kg) is mixed in an equal volume of saline, injected through the Foley catheter, and flushed with 5–10 mL of saline. Peak concentrations occur in 6 to 10 minutes in children and 10 to 20 minutes in adults.[5] A rectal diazepam gel (Diastat) has been approved by the FDA for the treatment of recurrent seizures in patients 2 years of age or older. Although it is expensive, it should be considered in those with frequent seizures or in those who reside far from a medical center. Because diazepam gel is provided in standard strengths (i.e., 5, 10, 15, and 20 mg), the desired dose is rounded up to the nearest commercially available strength. Using this method, patients will receive 90% to 180% of the dose calculated on a weight and age basis. For geriatric or debilitated patients, the dose of the rectal gel should be adjusted downward to reduce the likelihood of ataxia and oversedation. Clinical studies have shown this to be safe.

Midazolam is a water-soluble benzodiazepine that diffuses rapidly into the CNS. However, it has an extremely short half-life (0.8 hour), which requires it to be given by continuous infusion when giving it chronically. Its cost limits its use as a first-line benzodiazepine in hospitalized patients. However, recently there has been increased interest in using midazolam in acute situations in which intravenous access cannot be obtained readily. Various routes of administration (e.g., buccal, intranasal, and intramuscular) have been used successfully to rapidly (<10 min) terminate seizures. Typically, intranasal midazolam is given in doses ranging from 0.1-0.2 mg/kg.[65] The dose can be repeated one time if necessary. Resulting peak concentrations occur within 1 to 3 minutes and exceed those required for sedation in adults (40–70 ng/mL). Unfortunately, heavy breathing and increased nasal discharge may limit or delay absorption in a seizing patient. Buccal midazolam and rectal diazepam have shown equal efficacy in the termination of prolonged seizures in children.[66] Clinical cessation of seizures was achieved in 75% and 59% of cases for midazolam and diazepam, respectively. Median response time between the medications also was similar (midazolam, 6 minutes; diazepam, 8 minutes). Buccal administration is performed easily by drawing up the desired volume of midazolam injection or syrup, parting the patient's lips, and squirting it into the mouth. If the patient's jaws are clenched, there should be no attempt to separate them. The volume of fluid is small enough (e.g., 2–5 mL) to be placed in the cavity between the cheek and gum without significant concern for aspiration. Because of its increased solubility, intramuscular midazolam has a more reliable absorption (mean bioavailabilty approximately 90%) than either diazepam or lorazepam.[67] Doses of 0.15–0.3 mg/kg have stopped seizures successfully in 1 to 10 minutes. In fact, some practitioners have recommended intramuscular midazolam as first-line treatment in the out-of-hospital setting by emergency medical technicians.[51] Midazolam has been well tolerated with all the aforementioned routes with minimal changes in blood pressure or respiration.

All benzodiazepines can impair consciousness and interfere with neurologic assessment.[43] A brief period of cardiorespiratory depression (30-60 s) may occur in 12.5% of patients and can necessitate assisted ventilation or require intubation.[53] This is especially true if benzodiazepines are used concomitantly with barbiturates.[59] Hypotension secondary to a reduction in vasomotor tone may occur following high doses of benzodiazepines.

Phenytoin

According to some practitioners, the hydantoins are the long-acting anticonvulsants of choice for GCSE.[68] Intravenous phenytoin is effective in terminating GCSE (40% to 91%),[43] has a relatively long half-life (20–36 hours),[69] and lacks significant CNS depression[43]; however, it cannot be delivered rapidly enough to be considered a first-line single agent. Treiman and colleagues reported that phenytoin alone was inferior to lorazepam, phenobarbital, or diazepam plus phenytoin at stopping overt SE within 20 minutes of infusion.[57] It takes longer to control seizures than the benzodiazepines because it is less lipid soluble and enters the brain more slowly.[69] The distribution half-life of phenytoin is 2 to 5 minutes, and complete distribution occurs within 20 to 60 minutes.[69] Phenytoin is also associated with administration-related cardiovascular toxicity and is ineffective in some forms of NCSE.[34]

Although a number of loading doses have been recommended, doses less than 18 mg/kg usually do not achieve and maintain serum concentrations in the therapeutic range for 24 hours.[34] Provided the patient has not been on phenytoin prior to admission, standard loading doses for adults are 15–20 mg/kg and for pediatric patients 20 mg/kg.[43] Reduced doses of 15 mg/kg are recommended for elderly patients.[43] The average volume of distribution of phenytoin in the adult and pediatric patient is 0.75–0.6 L/kg, respectively.[34] This means that an 18 mg/kg loading dose in an adult will result in serum concentration immediately after the end of the infusion of approximately 24 mg/L. Very obese patients will require larger loading doses than nonobese patients. In obese patients, loading doses should be calculated on adjusted body weight:[70]

$$\text{Weight (kg)} = \text{ideal body weight (IBW)} + 1.33\,(\text{weight} - \text{IBW})/\text{IBW}$$

If the patient has been on phenytoin prior to admission and the admission phenytoin concentration is known, the following equation can be used to calculate a loading dose (LD):

$$\text{LD}_{\text{ADULT}} = (\text{concentration}_{\text{desired}} - \text{concentration}_{\text{admission}}) \times 0.75\,\text{L/kg} \times \text{weight (kg)}$$

As mentioned earlier, phenytoin fully equilibrates in to the brain within 20 to 60 minutes.[71] This delayed effect is the reason for waiting 60 minutes for response before administering a second partial LD. If seizures continue after the initial LD, some practitioners have recommended an additional LD of 5 mg/kg[40]; however, additional phenytoin may result in toxic serum concentrations and exacerbation of seizures. Additionally, there is no evidence that doses above 20 mg/kg will be of benefit in patients uncontrolled with the initial LD.[5] In order to maintain serum concentrations within the therapeutic range, maintenance dosing should be started within 12 to 24 hours of the LD. For a review of the distribution and elimination pharmacokinetics of phenytoin, see Chapter 56.

The complications associated with intravenous phenytoin are related primarily to the rate of administration and product pH. The vehicle (propylene glycol) may cause hypotension, especially in older patients with preexisting heart disease and in critically ill patients with marginal blood pressure.[43] Injectable phenytoin must be diluted to 5 mg/mL or less in normal saline. If it is mixed in a glucose-containing solution, microcrystals will precipitate. The maximum rate of infusion is 50 mg/min in adults[69] and 1 mg/kg per minute in children under 50 kg.[43] The rate of infusion should not exceed 25 mg/min in elderly patients or those with a history of atherosclerotic cardiovascular disease.[72] Vital signs and an electrocardiogram should be obtained during administration and the rate slowed if hypotension develops, the QT interval widens, or arrhythmias develop.[43] In all patients, the rate should be reduced once seizures have stopped.[43] Phenytoin causes less respiratory depression and sedation than the benzodiazepines or phenobarbital.

Because phenytoin has a pH of approximately 13, its intravenous infusion is associated with discomfort. Catheter infiltration during an infusion can cause tissue necrosis. Intramuscular administration is not recommended because it produces extreme pain and may cause tissue necrosis. Crystallized phenytoin also has been found at the injection site for more than 24 hours.[5] Additionally, absorption following intramuscular administration is delayed and erratic. Oral loading has been used in patients not actively seizing; however, 4 to 12 hours may be required before adequate blood concentrations are obtained.[68]

Fosphenytoin

Fosphenytoin is a water-soluble phosphate ester of phenytoin that has no known pharmacologic activity prior to its conversion to phenytoin.[73] It is rapidly and completely converted to phenytoin after intravenous and intramuscular dosing.[73] Reported fosphenytoin conversion half-lives following intravenous administration have ranged from 8 to 15 minutes.[74–76] This inherent delay in conversion to phenytoin was initially a major concern in the use of fosphenytoin for SE. However, protein binding for fosphenytoin is exceedingly high (unbound fraction 0.01–0.05) and is nonlinear.[77] Hence, fosphenytoin displaces phenytoin from albumin, transiently increasing the unbound phenytoin concentration. This increase in the unbound concentration (the pharmacologically active form of phenytoin) offsets the delay in phenytoin formation from the prodrug, making it bioequivalent to phenytoin at 50 mg/min.[76] Following conversion of fosphenytoin to phenytoin, the fraction unbound and concentrations of unbound phenytoin return to baseline.

Limited studies of fosphenytoin in SE are available. Allen and colleagues reported an open-label study where 54 patients with GCSE received a single intravenous fosphenytoin LD of 18 mg phenytoin equivalents (PE) per kilogram.[78] Mean rate of administration was 121 mg PE per minute (range, 36–218 mg PE/min). Benzodiazepine pretreatment was allowed as a standard of care for GCSE. Seizures were aborted in 93% of patients. In another study, 17 adult patients with acute seizures received intravenous doses of fosphenytoin, whereas 6 patients received intravenous phenytoin.[76] Adverse events required adjustment of the infusion rate in 4 of 6 phenytoin-treated patients compared with 2 of 17 fosphenytoin-treated patients. Pain or phlebitis at the injection site occurred in 5 patients receiving phenytoin compared with no patients receiving fosphenytoin. Complaints of transient, generalized itching and warmth occurred in 9 of 17 fosphenytoin-treated patients. These findings are consistent with other clinical studies that generally have demonstrated that fosphenytoin is safe and significantly better tolerated than phenytoin when administered intravenously.[79,80]

The most frequently observed adverse events reported with parenteral fosphenytoin use are nystagmus, dizziness, and ataxia. These adverse events likely represent effects of the parent drug following conversion. Two side effects that occur more frequently with fosphenytoin than phenytoin are paresthesia and pruritus. These sensations typically have a distribution to the face and groin areas and are associated with dose and infusion rate. Symptoms subside with lowering of the infusion rate. Dissipation of symptoms usually occurs within minutes to 1 hour postinfusion. These adverse events do not appear to be allergic reactions (no skin manifestations or vasodilatation) and alone do not warrant cessation of therapy.

In order to minimize dosing errors, all doses and dosing rates are determined using PE, thereby obviating the need for interconversion of doses between phenytoin sodium and fosphenytoin. Pediatric and adult patients with GCSE should receive fosphenytoin LDs of 15–20 mg PE per kilogram. In adults, the rate of adminis- tration should be 100–150 mg PE per minute. Pediatric patients should receive fosphenytoin at a rate between 1 and 3 mg PE per kilogram per minute. Recently, fosphenytoin has been shown to be safe when administered in neonates.[81] Loading doses (14.5–24.3 mg PE/kg) have produced average 8-hour phenytoin concentrations of 21.6 mg/L (range 10.5–34.5 mg/L). No electrocardiographic or blood pressure changes were noted; however, rates (0.6 PE/kg/min) were slower than recommended for pediatric patients. SE ceased in 50% of neonates, and an additional 37% had lowering of seizure rate. In some infants and neonates receiving fosphenytoin, phenytoin concentrations have been difficult to maintain despite above-average dosing (>10 mg PE/kg/day).[82] The mechanism for this phenomenon is unknown. This stresses the need to individualize doses carefully in this population.

Patients being treated for GCSE should not be loaded with intramuscular fosphenytoin except when intravenous access is impossible because of delays in achieving maximum phenytoin concentrations. Fosphenytoin should be diluted prior to intravenous administration in 5% dextrose or normal saline to a concentration of 1.5–25 mg PE per milliliter. Continuous electrocardiographic, blood pressure, and respiratory status monitoring is required for all LDs of fosphenytoin. Fosphenytoin serum concentrations are not available commercially and are of no value in therapeutic drug monitoring. Serum phenytoin concentrations are the end point for therapeutic drug monitoring, and the desired concentration range in patients receiving fosphenytoin is the same as that for phenytoin (10–20 mg/L). Because fosphenytoin cross-reacts with several immunoassays for phenytoin to cause falsely elevated phenytoin concentrations, serum phenytoin concentrations should not be obtained for at least 2 hours or more following fosphenytoin dosing.[83]

Phenobarbital

There are three different opinions regarding the use of phenobarbital in GCSE. The most widely held contention is that because barbiturates cause CNS and respiratory depression, phenobarbital should be the third-line agent when benzodiazepines plus phenytoin have failed.[5] The second group contends that the barbiturates are as safe and effective as other anticonvulsants and argues that phenobarbital should be the initial drug of choice.[56] This belief is especially evident in pediatric institutions with large emergency departments. Clearly, the barbiturates continue to be the anticonvulsant of choice for neonatal seizures.[84] The third emerging opinion is that continuous-infusion midazolam should be the third-line anticonvulsant before the barbiturates.[9]

Two studies have compared the efficacy of phenobarbital to other anticonvulsants. Shaner and colleagues compared phenobarbital alone with diazepam plus phenytoin in adult patients with GCSE.[56] Phenobarbital acted more rapidly and was as safe and effective as the combination of diazepam plus phenytoin.[56] Likewise, Treiman and colleagues reported that phenobarbital was as effective as lorazepam alone or diazepam plus phenytoin in overt SE and was not associated with serious adverse effects.[57]

Although no one is technically right or wrong, for the present time the Working Group on Status Epilepticus has recommended that phenobarbital be given after benzodiazepines and phenytoin have failed.[43] Currently, most practitioners agree that phenobarbital is the long-acting anticonvulsant of choice in patients with a hypersensitivity to the hydantoins or in those with cardiac conduction abnormalities.

Although phenobarbital penetrates into the brain slowly,[69] the highest brain concentrations occur 5 to 15 minutes after an intravenous infusion.[85] On average, seizures are controlled within 5.5 minutes after initiating the LD.[56] Phenobarbital exhibits first-order linear pharmacokinetics, and there is no maximum dose beyond which further doses are likely to be ineffective.

Patients should be given a 20–25 mg/kg load of phenobarbital.[43,85] Higher LDs (30 mg/kg) have been used in neonates without adverse effects.[84] Because the volume of distribution of the barbiturates is 1 L/kg, each milligram per killogram administered as an LD will increase the serum phenobarbital concentration by 1 mg/L.[40] Therefore, a 20 mg/kg LD should produce a serum phenobarbital concentration of approximately 20 mg/L. If the initial LD does not stop the seizures within 20 to 30 minutes, an additional 10–20 mg/kg dose may be given. If the seizures continue, a third 10 mg/kg load may be given.[86] In patients with refractory GCSE, some practitioners have advocated continued escalation of phenobarbital dosing without reference to a predetermined maximum concentration.[86] Once GCSE is controlled, the maintenance dose should be started within 12 to 24 hours.

Although injectable phenobarbital, like injectable phenytoin, contains propylene glycol, it can be given more rapidly than phenytoin. The rate of administration should not exceed 100 mg/min in adults[43] and 2 mg/kg per minute[40] or 30 mg/min in pediatric patients.[69] Although phenobarbital can be given intramuscularly, its rate of absorption is too slow to be effective in GCSE.[5]

Phenobarbital may cause depression of consciousness and respiration. The risk of apnea and hypopnea may be more profound in patients treated initially with benzodiazepines.[43] Medical personnel should be ready to provide respiratory support whenever the two agents are used together. If significant hypotension develops, the infusion should be slowed or stopped.[43]

REFRACTORY GCSE

Approximately 10% to 15% of patients with overt GCSE will fail therapy with a benzodiazepine, phenytoin, and phenobarbital.[18] Likewise, about 30% of patients with subtle manifestations of GCSE remain in SE after administration of these anticonvulsants.[9] When adequate doses of a benzodiazepine, phenytoin, and phenobarbital have failed, the condition is termed *refractory*.[9] When a patient develops refractory GCSE, a neurologist with expertise in epilepsy should be consulted, and an intense search should be performed for an acute or progressive cause.[43]

It should be remembered that the longer GCSE lasts, the harder it is treat[5,43] and that failure to aggressively treat early in the course of SE increases the likelihood of nonresponse.[43] The optimal therapeutic approach for patients with refractory GCSE has not been determined. Approaches used include the benzodiazepines, barbiturate coma, valproate, paraldehyde, propofol, lidocaine, and inhaled anesthetics. Regardless of therapy, the goal is to stop electrical epileptiform activity.

Benzodiazepines

Although refractory GCSE has been treated with a variety of agents, some practitioners have advocated not only that midazolam should be the first-line agent in refractory GCSE but that it also should be the third-line agent in patients unresponsive to lorazepam plus phenytoin.[9] A large number of midazolam loading (0.02–0.38 mg/kg) and maintenance doses (range, 1–18 μg/kg/min) have been given to pediatric patients.[82,88,89] It has been suggested that children receive an initial 0.15 mg/kg LD followed by a 1 μg/kg per minute continuous infusion that is increased every 15 minutes until seizures are controlled.[89] Once SE is terminated, dosages can be decreased by 1 μg/kg per minute every 2 hours. This dosing method has proven effective, with response rates of 95% within 65 minutes. Currently, studies have shown significant differences in the time to termination of seizures (0.8–65 min). This probably reflects the heterogeneity in the doses given and the differences in the patient populations studied. Four adult patients were given a midazolam LD (0.2 mg/kg) and a continuous infusion of 0.75–11 μg/kg per minute for 8 hours to 10 days.[90] Clinical examination and scalp EEG documented termination of seizures in all patients within minutes. Because tachyphylaxis can develop, frequent increases in the infusion rate may be necessary, and dosing should be guided by EEG response.[9] Hypotension and poikilothermia can occur and may require supportive therapies.[9] Once seizures are controlled, the midazolam infusion should be discontinued gradually. Bleck recommends that successful discontinuation is enhanced by keeping the patient's phenytoin serum concentration near 20 mg/L and phenobarbital concentration above 40 mg/L.[9] Generally, continuous infusions of midazolam have been well tolerated with few cases of hypotension and respiratory depression. Because of midazolam's short half-life, patients may return to consciousness more rapidly (approximately 4 hours) than those receiving higher doses of more sedating anticonvulsants (e.g., phenytoin, phenobarbital).[88]

Labar and colleagues treated nine episodes of refractory GCSE with high-dose intravenous lorazepam.[91] Doses ranged from 0.3–9 mg/h with as little as 2 mg/6 h to as much as 9 mg/h. Seizures were terminated in all patients, and lorazepam was discontinued slowly over 24 to 48 hours. Another controlled report also noted that continuous-infusion diazepam can control GCSE successfully in patients unresponsive to phenytoin or phenobarbital.[92]

Barbiturate Coma

If there is an inadequate response to high doses of midazolam after 1 hour, anesthetizing the patient to suppress the cerebral ictal discharge is recommended.[9,43] Although it is likely that the patient is already being mechanically ventilated, intubation and respiratory support may be required during barbiturate coma. Likewise, continuous monitoring of vital signs is essential because hypotension is a concern.

Barbiturate coma usually is achieved with either phenobarbital or pentobarbital. Crawford and colleagues reported the use of very high-dose phenobarbital in refractory GCSE.[86] Phenobarbital (10 mg/kg) was given every 30 minutes regardless of serum concentration until seizures stopped or hypotension occurred. Although very high-dose phenobarbital stops refractory GCSE successfully, the long half-life of phenobarbital (90–120 hours) produces coma for several days after the anticonvulsant is discontinued. Therefore, a short-acting barbiturate such as pentobarbital ($t_{1/2}$ of 11–23 hours), which allows more rapid reversal of coma, generally is preferred.

Although several sources note that the initial LD of pentobarbital is 5 mg/kg,[43] this dose is inadequate because it will not produce the concentrations (30–40 mg/L) necessary to induce an isoelectric EEG. Pentobarbital should be initiated with an LD of at least 15–20 mg/kg over 40 to 60 minutes.[5] Should hypotension occur during the LD, the rate of administration should be slowed or dopamine should be administered. The LD should be followed immediately by an infusion of 0.5–3 mg/kg per hour.[43] The maintenance infusion should be increased gradually until there is evidence of burst suppression on EEG (i.e., flat EEG) or adverse effects occur. Although the duration of barbiturate coma in most studies has been 2 to 3 days, pentobarbital coma has been used safely for 53 days in an 18-year-old patient.[93] In order to avoid complications (e.g., pneumonia, pulmonary edema), the pentobarbital should be discontinued as soon as possible. Twelve hours after a burst suppression pattern is obtained, the rate of pentobarbital infusion should be titrated downward every 2 to 4 hours to enable the clinician to determine if the patient's GCSE is in remission.

Valproate

Limited human data exist regarding the use of valproate in refractory GCSE. Holle and associates reviewed the literature regarding the use of valproate in SE.[94] Animal data suggest that even high-dose valproate is not effective because of its delayed access to the site of action.[94] This has not proven to be true in human studies. Most of the experience with valproate in GCSE has been with the rectal route of administration. Studies have reported that 200 mg every 6 hours or 600–4000 mg/day (average dose, 600 mg qid) as a rectal suppository terminated or reduced clinical SE.[94] Snead and Miles described a series of seven pediatric patients who had not responded to benzodiazepines, phenytoin, and phenobarbital.[95] Patients received an LD of 10–15 mg/kg given as a 1:1 dilution of tap water and valproate syrup enema. Five patients became seizure-free within 3 to 12 hours. The Working Group on Status Epilepticus recommends an LD of 20 mg/kg.[43]

Although an intravenous dosage form of valproate has been approved recently by the FDA, it is not labeled for SE. Giroud and colleagues evaluated the use of intravenous valproate in 23 adults with SE.[96] Patients received an LD of 12 mg/kg followed by a continuous infusion of 0.5 mg/kg per hour; however, serum concentrations were lower than projected, and subsequent patients received an LD of 15 mg/kg followed by a continuous infusion of 1 mg/kg per hour.

Seizures ceased in 11 of the 12 patients within 20 minutes, and partial SE ceased in less than 20 minutes in 8 of 11 patients. Mean valproate concentration before tapering was 67.4 mg/L. Another study used a similar dosing regimen (15 mg/kg LD, continuous infusion 1 mg/kg/h) and observed comparable response rate (80% of patients in less than 30 minutes).[97] Price and colleagues evaluated valproate's effectiveness in two groups of adults ($n = 24$) with diazepam-resistant GCSE.[98] In one group, a 400-mg LD was given over 5 minutes, followed by a continuous infusion starting at 100 mg/h and increased based on clinical response. The second group received a 15 mg/kg LD administered at 1000 mg/h, followed by a continuous infusion started at 400 mg/h that was titrated downward when seizures ceased. Although valproate was effective (14 of 15 patients) in the first group, responses were delayed up to 4 hours. Valproate was similarly effective in the second group (7 of 9 patients), but they experienced more rapid (<1 hour) termination of seizures. Currently, only one study accounted for the effects of enzyme-inducing anticonvulsants when dosing valproate.[99] In pediatric patients, it is recommended that all patients receive a 20 mg/kg LD administered at 2 mg/kg per minute to achieve a total valproate concentration of 75 mg/L. The continuous infusion rate is determined by the presence of concurrent anticonvulsant (no inducers present, 1 mg/kg/h), one or more inducers (phenytoin, phenobarbital, 2 mg/kg/h), and inducers and pentobarbital coma (4 mg/kg/h). Although the manufacturer currently recommends intravenous valproate be given at no faster than 20 mg/min, much faster rates (2–6 mg/kg/min) are being used to administer LDs in practice.[99,100] In general, intravenous valproate has been well tolerated, with no cases of respiratory depression. One case of hypotension was noted in a pediatric patient given valproate 30 mg/kg (0.5 mg/kg/min).[101] Although this is a rare phenomenon, monitoring patients at risk for hemodynamic instability is warranted.

Propofol

Propofol is an extremely lipid soluble and has a large volume of distribution. It has a very rapid onset of action and an extremely short half-life (2–4 min), which promotes rapid awakening on drug discontinuation. Although there are reports of its effectiveness in both GCSE and NCSE, it is not licensed by the FDA for these indications, and it has not been compared with other anticonvulsants. Patients have been given a 100-mg LD, followed by continuous infusions ranging from 5–11.33 mg/kg per hour.[102,103] Infusion for up to 18 days has been reported.[102] Propofol does not have to be diluted. It may cause respiratory and cerebral depression, bradycardia, and metabolic acidosis. Seizures also have been reported.[104] Additionally, normal adult doses may provide over 1000 calories per day as lipid, and the cost to the patient may exceed $1000 per day.

Lidocaine

Although lidocaine has been used in refractory GCSE,[105] its use is not recommended unless other agents have failed. It is administered intravenously and has a rapid onset of action (20–30 s). The recommended initial dose is 50–100 mg (1–3 mg/kg) over 2 minutes.[5,105] Because of the short half-life, a lidocaine infusion is initiated at a rate of 1.5–3.5 mg/kg per hour in adults or 6 mg/kg per hour in infants.[5,105] Although the therapeutic serum concentration range for the antiarrhythmic effects of lidocaine is 2-6 mg/L,[106] the therapeutic range for SE has not been established. Serum lidocaine concentrations should be monitored to avoid drug accumulation and toxicity. CNS toxicity (e.g., fasiculations, visual disturbances, tinnitus) may occur at concentrations between 6 and 8 mg/L; seizures and obtundation may develop when concentrations exceed 8 mg/L.[106]

Paraldehyde

Historically, rectal or intravenous paraldehyde has been used for refractory GCSE.[5,85] Although effective, it is extremely difficult to administer and is associated with serious adverse effects (e.g., hypotension, tachycardia, pulmonary edema, and polyethylene emboli). Intravenous paraldehyde is no longer manufactured in the United States. The only available formulation currently licensed is an enteral product that is difficult to obtain in a timely manner. A dose of 0.3–0.5 mL/kg can be given every 20 minutes rectally via a rubber catheter.[43] For rectal administration, it should be diluted 1:1 in vegetable oil. Additional references should be consulted before using this product.[5,107,108]

Other Agents

One report noted excellent clinical and EEG results following rectal chloral hydrate administration (30 mg/kg) in five adult patients who were refractory to intravenous diazepam, phenytoin, phenobarbital, and valproate.[109]

Halothane, isoflurane, ketamine, and other inhaled anesthetics produce EEG suppression.[5,110] However, these gases are difficult to deliver outside the operating room and require the presence of an anesthesiologist. They have no proven advantages over traditional anticonvulsants (e.g., barbiturate coma or continuous-infusion benzodiazepines) and can raise intracranial pressure.[5] If used, dosing is titrated to obtain EEG burst suppression. Although there are no controlled trials, some practitioners have postulated that magnesium has anticonvulsant properties and may be neuroprotective by interacting with the NMDA receptor.[111] Additionally, magnesium deficiency lowers the seizure threshold.

NONCONVULSIVE SE

Absence SE

Although absence SE is the most frequent type of nonconvulsive SE, only 3% of all patients with absence seizures develop SE.[7] The clinical manifestations of this disorder include an altered state of consciousness and/or behavior (e.g., lethargy, decreased mental function). In one series of 38 patients, the duration of absence SE ranged from 30 minutes to 2 days.[7] The longest reported episode of absence SE is 60 days.[41] The most important diagnostic and management tool in patients with suspected absence SE is an EEG because absence SE will have a classic three per second spike-and-slow-wave pattern.[7]

Although the likelihood of morbidity secondary to absence SE is not known, it is not considered life-threatening. Long-acting anticonvulsants (e.g., ethosuximide and clonazepam) are effective, but they are not available in a parenteral dosage form; hence absence SE has been treated traditionally with intravenous diazepam/lorazepam or rectal valproate. Studies have shown that intravenous valproate is rapidly effective in nonconvulsive SE.[99,112] Higher doses may be required to maintain valproate concentrations in patients on medications known to induce valproate's metabolism and in children. Intravenous acetazolamide (250–500 mg) has been used to terminate absence SE; however, it is less effective than the benzodiazepines.[7] Intravenous phenytoin/fosphenytoin or phenobarbital may be tried in patients who do not respond to the other therapies.[7] Currently, general anesthesia or barbiturate coma are not appropriate.[7]

Atypical Absence and Myoclonic SE

Minor motor seizures are difficult to treat. Valproate remains the drug of choice for atypical absence. Refractory patients should be tried on a combination of valproate plus ethosuximide or clonazepam.[7] Generalized myoclonic SE is rare but may occur during absence or atypical SE. Again, valproate is the drug of first choice.[7]

Complex Partial SE

Complex partial SE occurs when a patient experiences clinical and electrical activity that is focal in onset and associated with altered consciousness. Although it is often difficult to differentiate complex partial SE from absence SE, there are some important differences. Unlike absence SE, which is associated with a single prolonged event, complex partial SE is a continuous series of repeated seizures. Additionally, patients with complex partial SE experience phases of total unresponsiveness with stereotypical automatisms, whereas individuals with absence SE do not. Complex partial SE should be treated aggressively because clinical and experimental data suggest that memory and behavioral alterations may be associated with this type of SE.[7] Management of complex partial SE is similar to that described for GCSE. Although the combination of intravenous lorazepam or diazepam plus phenytoin is effective, phenytoin alone may be more beneficial because it does not cause sedation.[7] Should the patient continue to experience complex partial SE, administration of phenobarbital is warranted.[7] It is essential that EEG monitoring be performed to evaluate response.

PHARMACOECONOMIC CONSIDERATIONS

Although no prospective pharmacoeconomic studies have been performed in the area of SE, a number of economic issues may have an impact on formulary considerations. Clearly, there are intra- and interclass differences in medication costs and in ancillary tests or technologies associated with select therapies. For example, if one assumes five treatment options[57] and hypothetically initiates anticonvulsant therapy in a patient weighing 70 kg, the following differences in average wholesale prices are noted:

- Lorazepam alone (8 mg): $36.46
- Diazepam (20 mg) plus generic phenytoin (1 g): $15.01
- Phenobarbital (20 mg/kg) alone: $28.22
- Generic phenytoin (1 g) alone: $13.33
- Diazepam (20 mg) plus fosphenytoin (1 g): $181.68
- Valproate (15 mg/kg load, 1 mg/kg/h): $53.78

Although many practitioners have heralded the arrival of fosphenytoin as an important therapeutic advancement, it has created a fiscal and ethical dilemma for many institutions. Fosphenytoin is associated with less infusion pain, intravenous-site complications, and hemodynamic adverse effects than phenytoin; however, the cost of this agent ($180 versus $13.33 per gram) has caused many practitioners and administrators to struggle with the practical and ethical importance of the increased safety profile relative to the cost of the product to an institution. When evaluating the difference in cost of these two agents, it is important to remember that phenytoin requires the placement of two intravenous catheters because of its incompatibility with many solutions and medications that are given concurrently. Additionally, some institutions are giving fosphenytoin intramuscularly in the emergency room and avoiding the placement of a catheter and use of an infusion device. Likewise, many institutions do not consider the expense associated with a tissue infiltration of phenytoin. Should an infiltration of phenytoin cause tissue necrosis that necessitates plastic surgery or amputation, the expense of a single million-dollar lawsuit likely will offset the difference between phenytoin and fosphenytoin cost to several institutions.

If one advocates midazolam as third-line therapy over phenobarbital (20 mg/kg) and administers an LD of midazolam (0.15 mg/kg) followed by only a 1-hour continuous infusion (2.3 μg/kg per minute), midazolam will cost $608.26 more than phenobarbital. Conversely, one might argue that should a patient experience phenobarbital-induced respiratory depression and require mechanical ventilation, phenobarbital ultimately would be more expensive. Finally, a 24-hour infusion of propofol to the same patient will cost in excess of $1000.

EVALUATION OF THERAPEUTIC OUTCOMES

Initial success is defined as termination of all clinical and electrical activity, but ultimate success is measured by the patient's quality of life. The morbidity and mortality associated with SE is affected by the underlying etiology; however, these can be minimized by the rapid implementation of a rational therapeutic plan. An EEG is an extremely important tool that not only may allow the practitioner to determine when abnormal electrical activity has been aborted but also may assist in determining which AED was effective. Because many of the AEDs affect the cardiorespiratory system, it is imperative that vital signs (e.g., heart rate, respiratory rate, and blood pressure) be monitored during drug infusion. It also may be necessary to monitor the electrocardiogram in some patients. Finally, it is imperative that the infusion site be assessed for any evidence of infiltration before and during administration of phenytoin.

CONCLUSIONS

Our understanding of the cellular basis, physiology, and neuropathology of SE continues to evolve. Over the past decade, research into an activated cascade of pathophysiologic changes in neurotransmission, GABAergic inhibition, and NMDA receptor channel-mediated events has enhanced our understanding of SE significantly. Although anticonvulsants will continue to be the mainstay of therapy in terminating SE, specific agents including antagonists of excitatory amino acid neurotransmitters (e.g., glutamate and calcium channel blockers) and agonists of inhibitory neurotransmitters (GABA) may help to block neuronal damage. Likewise, additional trials investigating the role of newer anticonvulsants in SE are warranted.

▶ PRINCIPLES OF PHARMACOTHERAPY

- SE is a neurologic emergency that may be associated with brain damage and death.
- For practical purposes, SE is defined as recurrent seizures without an intervening period of consciousness before the next seizure begins or any seizure lasting longer than 30 minutes whether or not consciousness is impaired.
- Although a diagnosis of SE does not officially occur until seizure activity has persisted for greater than 30 minutes, anticonvulsant therapy should not be withheld waiting for this period to pass. Any tonic-clonic seizure that does not stop automatically within 10 minutes should be treated.
- Although the pathophysiology of SE is unknown, experimental models have shown that there is a loss of GABA-mediated inhibitory synaptic transmission and that glutamatergic excitatory synaptic transmission sustains SE.
- The first goal of treatment is patient stabilization and includes adequate oxygenation, preservation of cardiorespiratory function, and management of systemic complications.
- The primary goal of therapy is to stop all clinical and electrical seizure activity as soon as possible.
- Lorazepam is the benzodiazepine of choice in SE because of its rapid onset and long duration of action.
- Currently, the hydantoins (phenytoin and fosphenytoin) are the long-acting anticonvulsants of choice. One of these should be given concurrently with benzodiazepines.
- The maximum rate of infusion for phenytoin is 50 mg/min in adults and 1 mg/kg per minute in pediatric patients. The maximum rate of infusion should not exceed 25 mg/min in elderly patients or those with a history of atherosclerotic cardiovascular disease. The maximum rate of infusion for fosphenytoin in adults and pediatric patients is 150 and 3 mg phenytoin equivalents per minute, respectively.
- Phenobarbital may cause hypotension or respiratory depression and arrest, especially if given in conjunction with the benzodiazepines.

REFERENCES

1. Hauser WA. Status epilepticus: Epidemiologic considerations. Neurology 1990;40:S9–S13.
2. Shorvon S. Tonic clonic status epilepticus. J Neurol Neurosurg Psychiatry 1993;56:125–134.
3. Commission on Classification of Terminology, International League Against Epilepsy. Proposal for revised clinical and electroencephalographic classification of epileptic seizures. Epilepsia 1981;22:489–501.
4. Delgado-Escueta AV, Wasterlain CG, Trieman DM, Porter RJ. Management of status epilepticus. N Engl J Med 1982;306:1337–1340.
5. Ramsey RE. Treatment of status epilepticus. Epilepsia 1993;34:S71–S81.
6. Treiman DM. Generalized convulsive status epilepticus in the adult. Epilepsia 1993;34:S2–S11.
7. Cascino GD. Nonconvulsive status epilepticus in adults and children. Epilepsia 1993;34:S21–S28.
8. DeLorenzo RJ, Towne AR, Pellock JM, Ko D. Status epilepticus in children, adults, and the elderly. Epilepsia 1992;33:S15–S25.
9. Bleck TP. Advances in the management of refractory status epilepticus. Crit Care Med 1993;21:955–957.
10. DeLorenzo RJ, Pellock JM, Towne AR, Boggs J. Epidemology of status epilepticus. J Clin Neurophysiol 1995;12:316–325.
11. Kaplan PW. Nonconvulsive status epilepticus. Semin Neurol 1996;16:33–40.
12. Rowan AJ, Scott DF. Major status epilepticus: A series of 42 patients. Acta Neurol Scand 1970;46:573–584.
13. Gross-Tsur V, Shinnar S. Convulsive status epilepticus in children. Epilepsia 1993;34:S12–S20.
14. Aicardi J, Chevrie JJ. Convulsive status epilepticus in infants and children: A study of 239 cases. Epilepsia 1970;11:187–197.
15. Granner MA, Lee SI. Nonconvulsive SE: EEG analysis in a large series. Epilepsia 1994;34:42–47.
16. Maytal J, Shinnar S, Moshe SL, Alvarez LA. Low morbidity and mortality of status epilepticus in children. Pediatrics 1989;83:323–331.
17. Pellock JM. Status epilepticus. In: Dodson WE, Pellock JM, eds. Pediatric Epilepsy: Diagnosis and Therapy. New York, Demos, 1993:197–206.
18. Lowenstein DH, Alldredge BK. Status epilepticus at an urban public hospital in the 1980s. Neurology 1993;43:483–488.
19. Barry E, Hauser WA. Status epilepticus and antiepileptic levels. Neurology 1994;44:47–50.
20. Brown JK, Hussian IHMI. Status epilepticus: 1. Pathogenesis. Dev Med Child Neurol 1991;33:3–17.
21. Verity CM, Ross EM, Golding J. Outcome of childhood status epilepticus and lengthy febrile convulsions: Findings of national cohort study. Br Med J 1993;307:225–228.
22. Maytal J, Shinnar S. Febrile status epilepticus. Pediatrics 1990;86:611–616.
23. Callahan DJ, Noetzel MJ. Prolonged absence status epilepticus associated with carbamazepine therapy, increased intracranial pressure, and transient MRI abnormalities. Neurology 1992;42:2198–2201.
24. Thomas P, Lebrun C, Chatel M. De novo absence status epilepticus as a benzodiazepine withdrawal syndrome. Epilepsia 1993;34:355–358.
25. Ditcher MA, Ayala GF. Cellular mechanism of epilepsy: A status report. Science 1987;237:157–164.
26. Fountain NB, Lothman EW. Pathophysiology of status epilepticus. J Clin Neurophysiol 1995;12:326–342.
27. Kapur J, Stringer JL, Lothman EW. Evidence that repetitive seizures in the hippocampus causes a lasting reduction in GABAergic inhibition. J Neurophysiol 1989;61:417–426.
28. Meldrum BS. Anatomy, physiology, and pathology of epilepsy. Lancet 1990;336:231–234.
29. Johnston MV. Neurotransmitters and epilepsy. In: Wyllie E, ed. The Treatment of Epilepsy: Principles and Practice. Philadelphia, Lea & Febiger, 1993:111–125.
30. Lipton SA, Rosenberg PA. Excitatory amino acids as a final common pathway for neurologic disorders. N Engl J Med 1994;330:613–622.
31. Bertram EH, Lothman EW. NMDA receptor antagonists and limbic status epilepticus: A comparison with standard anticonvulsants. Epilepsy Res 1990;5:177–184.
32. Lothman E. The biochemical basis and pathophysiology of status epilepticus. Neurology 1990;40:13–23.
33. Kapur J, MacDonald RL. Status epilepticus: A proposed pathophysiology. In: Shorvon S, Dreifuss F, Fish S, Thomas D, eds. The Treatment of Epilepsy. Cambridge, MA, Blackwell Science, 1996:258–268.
34. Leppik IE. Status epilepticus: The next decade. Neurology 1990;40:4–9.
35. Walton NY. Systemic effects of generalized convulsive status epilepticus. Epilepsia 1993;34:S54–S58.
36. Wasterlain CG, Fujikawa DG, Penix L, Sankar R. Pathophysiological mechanisms of brain damage from status epilepticus. Epilepsia 1993;34:S37–S53.
37. Meldrum BS, Nilsson B. Cerebral blood flow and metabolic rate early and late in prolonged epileptic seizures induced in rats by bicuculline. Brain 1976;99:523–542.

38. Liu Z, Gatt A, Mikati M, Holmes GL. Effect of temperature on kainic acid-induced seizures. Brain Res 1993;63:51–58.
39. Dodill CD, Wilensky AJ. Intellectual impairment as an outcome of status epilepticus. Neurology 1990;40:23–27.
40. Leppik IE. Status epilepticus. In: Wyllie E, ed. The Treatment of Epilepsy: Principles and Practice. Philadelphia, Lea & Febiger, 1993: 678–685.
41. Jagoda A. Nonconvulsive seizures. Emerg Med Clin North Am 1994; 12:963–971.
42. Oxbury JM, Whitty CWM. Causes and consequences of status epilepticus in adults: A study of 86 cases. Brain 1971;94:733–744.
43. Working Group on Status Epilepticus. Treatment of convulsive status epilepticus: Recommendations of the Epilepsy Foundation of America's Working Group on Status Epilepticus. JAMA 1993;270:854–859.
44. Gal P. Anticonvulsant therapy after neonatal seizures: How long should it continue? A case for early discontinuation of anticonvulsants. Pharmacotherapy 1985;5:268–273.
45. Towne AR, Pellock JM, Ko D, DeLorenzo RJ. Determinations of mortality in status epilepticus. Epilepsia 1994;35:27–34.
46. DeLorenzo RJ. Status epilepticus: Concepts in diagnosis and treatment. Semin Neurol 1990;10:396–405.
47. Treiman DM. General principles of treatment: Responsive and intractable status epilepticus in adults. In: Delgado-Escueta AV, Wasterlain CG, Treiman DM, Porter RJ, eds. Status Epilepticus. New York, Raven Press, 1983:377–384.
48. Munn RI, Farrell K. Failure to recognize status epilepticus in a paralyzed patient. Can J Neurosci 1993;20:234–236.
49. Howell SJL, Owen L, Chadwick DW. Pseudostatus epilepticus. Q J Med 1989;71:507–519.
50. Camfield CS, Camfield PR, Smith E, et al. Home use of rectal diazepam to prevent status epilepticus in children with convulsive disorders. J Child Neurol 1989;4:125–126.
51. LeDuc TJ, Goellner WE, Sanadi NE. Out-of-hospital midazolam for status epilepticus. Ann Emerg Med 1996;28:3.
52. Standards and guidelines for cardiopulmonary resuscitation (CPR) and emergency cardiac care (ECC): 6. Pediatric advanced life support. JAMA 1992;268:2262–2275.
53. Leppik IE, Derivan AT, Homan RW, et al. Double-blind study of lorazepam and diazepam in status epilepticus. JAMA 1983;249:1452–1454.
54. Treiman DM, De Giorgio CM, Ben-Menachem E, et al. Lorazepam versus phenytoin in the treatment of generalized convulsive status epilepticus: Report of an ongoing study. Neurology 1985;35:284.
55. Appleton R, Sweeney A, Choonara I, et al. Lorazepam versus diazepam in the acute treatment of epileptic seizures and status epilepticus. Dev Med Child Neurol 1995;37:682–688.
56. Shaner DM, McCurdy SA, Herring MO, Gabor AJ. Treatment of status epilepticus: A prospective comparison of diazepam and phenytoin versus phenobarbital and optional phenytoin. Neurology 1988;38: 202–207.
57. Treiman DM, Meyers PD, Walton NY, et al. A comparison of four treatments for generalized convulsive status epilepticus: Veterans Affairs Status Epilepticus Cooperative Study Group. N Engl J Med 1998;339:792–798.
58. Treiman DM. The role of benzodiazepines in the management of status epilepticus. Neurology 1990;40:32–42.
59. Treiman DM. Pharmacokinetics and clinical use of benzodiazepines in the management of status epilepticus. Epilepsia 1989;30:S4–S10.
60. Giang DW, McBride MC. Lorazepam versus diazepam for the treatment of status epilepticus. Pediatr Neurol 1988;4:358–361.
61. Siberry GK, Iannone R, ed. The Harriet Lane Handbook, 15th ed. St. Louis, Mosby, 2000.
62. Diazepam. In: Physicians' Desk Reference, 51st ed. Oradell, NJ, Medical Economics, 1997:2334–2337.
63. Cascino GD. Generalized convulsive status epilepticus. Mayo Clin Proc 1996;71:787–792.
64. Albano A, Reisdorff EJ, Wiegenstein JG. Rectal diazepam in pediatric status epilepticus. Am J Emerg Med 1989;70:168–172.
65. Kendall JL, Reynolds M, Goldberg R. Intranasal midazolam in patients with status epilepticus. Ann Emerg Med 1997;29:415–417.
66. Scott RC, Besag F, Neville B. Buccal midazolam and rectal diazepam for treatment of prolonged seizures in childhood and adolescence: A randomised trial. Lancet 1999;353:623–626.
67. Towne AR, DeLorenzo RJ. Use of intramuscular midazolam for status epilepticus. J Emerg Med 1999;17:323–328.
68. Cloyd JC, Gumnit RJ, McLain W. Status epilepticus: The role of intravenous phenytoin. JAMA 1980;244:1479–1481.
69. Browne TR. The pharmacokinetics of agents used to treat status epilepticus. Neurology 1990;40:28–32.
70. Abernethy DR, Greenblatt DJ. Phenytoin disposition in obesity: Determination of loading dose. Arch Neurol 1985;42:468–471.
71. Wilder BJ, Ramsey E, Willmore J, et al. Efficacy of intravenous phenytoin in the treatment of status epilepticus: Kinetics of central nervous system penetration. Ann Neurol 1977;1:511–518.
72. Donovan PJ. Phenytoin administration by constant intravenous infusion: Selective rates of administration. Ann Emerg Med 1991;20: 139–142.
73. Boucher BA. Fosphenytoin: A novel phenytoin prodrug. Pharmacotherapy 1996;16:777–791.
74. Boucher BA, Bombassaro AM, Rasmussen SN, et al. Phenytoin prodrug 3-phosphoryloxymethyl phenytoin (ACC-9653): Pharmacokinetics following intravenous and intramuscular administration. J Pharm Sci 1989;78:929–932.
75. Eldon MA, Loewen GR, Voightman RE, et al. Pharmacokinetics and tolerance of fosphenytoin and phenytoin administered intravenously to healthy subjects. Can J Neurol Sci 1993;20:S180.
76. Andrews CO, Turnbull MD, Paloucek FP, et al. Safety and pharmacokinetics of fosphenytoin following intravenous loading dose administration. Pharmacotherapy 1994;14:367.
77. Hussey EK, Dukes GE, Messenheimer JA, et al. Protein binding of phenytoin and a phenytoin prodrug. Pharm Res 1988;5:S214.
78. Allen FH, Runge JW, Legarda S, et al. Safety, tolerance, and pharmacokinetics of intravenous fosphenytoin (Cerebyx) in status epilepticus. Epilepsia 1995;36:S90.
79. Jamerson BD, Dukes GE, Brouwer KLR, et al. Venous irritation related to intravenous administration of phenytoin versus fosphenytoin. Pharmacotherapy 1994;14:47–52.
80. Ramsay RE, Philbrook B, Fischer JH, et al. Safety and pharmacokinetics of fosphenytoin (Cerebyx) compared with Dilantin following rapid intravenous administration. Neurology 1996;46:A245.
81. Gustafson MC, Ritter FJ. Fosphenytoin for status epilepticus in the neonate. Epilepsia 1999;40:S124.
82. Takeoka M, Krishnamoorthy KS, Soman TB, Caviness VS Jr. Fosphenytoin in infants. J Child Neurol 1998;13:537–540.
83. Kugler AR, Olson SC, Webb CL, et al. Cross-reactivity of fosphenytoin (Cerebyx) in two human phenytoin immunoassays. Pharm Res 1994;11:S102.
84. Donn SM, Grasela TH, Goldstein GW. Safety of a higher loading dose of phenobarbital in the term newborn. Pediatrics 1985;75:1061–1064.
85. Ramsey RE. Pharmacokinetics and clinical use of parenteral phenytoin, phenobarbital, and paraldehyde. Epilepsia 1989;30:S1–S3.
86. Crawford TO, Mitchell WG, Fishman LS, Snodgrass SR. Very-high-dose phenobarbital for refractory status epilepticus in children. Neurology 1988;38:1035–1040.
87. Rivera R, Segnini M, Baltodano A, Perez V. Midazolam in the treatment of status epilepticus in children. Crit Care Med 1993;21:991–994.
88. Holmes GL, Riviello JJ. Midazolam and pentobarbital for refractory status epilepticus. Pediatr Neurol 1999;20:259–264.
89. Koul RL, Aithala GR, Chacko A, et al. Continuous midazolam infusion as treatment of status epilepticus. Arch Dis Child 1997;76:445–448.
90. Parent JM, Lowenstein DH. Treatment of refractory generalized status epilepticus with continuous infusion of midazolam. Neurology 1994; 44:1837–1840.
91. Labar DR, Ali A, Root J. High-dose intravenous lorazepam for the treatment of refractory status epilepticus. Neurology 1994;44:1400–1403.

92. Bell HE, Bertino JS Jr. Constant diazepam infusion in the treatment of continuous seizure activity. Drug Intell Clin Pharm 1984;18: 965–970.
93. Mirski MA, Williams MA, Hanlet DF. Prolonged pentobarbital and phenobarbital coma for refractory generalized status epilepticus. Crit Care Med 1995;23:400–404.
94. Holle LM, Gidal BE, Collins DM. Valproate in status epilepticus. Ann Pharmacother 1995;29:1042–1043.
95. Sneed OC, Miles MV. Treatment of status epilepticus in children with rectal sodium valporate. J Pediatr 1985;106:323–325.
96. Giroud M, Gras D, Escousse A, et al. Use of injectable valproic acid in status epilepticus. Drug Invest 1993;5:154–159.
97. Czapinski P, Terczynski A. Intravenous valproic acid administration in status epilepticus. Neurol Nerochir Pol 1998;32:11–22.
98. Price DJ. Intravenous valproate: experience in neurosurgery. Fourth Int Symp Sodium Valproate in Epilepsy. Roy Soc Med Int Congr Sympt Ser 1989;152:197–203.
99. Hovinga CA, Chicella MF, Rose DF, et al. Use of intravenous valproate in three pediatric patients with nonconvulsive or convulsive status epilepticus. Ann Pharmacother 1999;33:579–584.
100. Venkataraman V, Wheless JW. Safety of rapid intravenous infusion of valproate loading doses in epilepsy patients. Epilepsy Res 1999;35:147–153.
101. White JR, Santos CS. Intravenous valproate associated with significant hypotension in the treatment of status epilepticus. J Child Neurol 1999;14:822–823.
102. Wood PR, Browne GPR, Pugh S. Propofol infusion for the treatment of status epilepticus. Lancet 1988;1:480–481.
103. Pitt-Miller PL, Elcock BJ, Maharaj M. The management of status epilepticus with a continuous propofol infusion. Anesth Analg 1994;78:1193–1194.
104. Makela JP, Iivanainen M, Pieninkeroinen, et al. Seizures associated with propofol anesthesia. Epilepsia 1993;34:832–835.
105. Aggarwal P, Wali JP. Lidocaine in refractory status epilepticus: A forgotten drug in the emergency department. Am J Emerg Med 1993;2:243–244.
106. Pieper JA, Johnson KE. Lidocaine. In: Evans WE, Schentag JJ, Jusko WJ, eds. Applied Pharmacokinetics, 3d ed. Spokane, WA, Applied Therapeutics, 1992:21-1–21-37.
107. Curless RG, Holzman BM, Ramsay RE. Paradehyde therapy in childhood status epilepticus. Arch Neurol 1983;40:477–480.
108. Giacoia GP, Gessner PK, Zaleska MM, Boutwell WC. Pharmacokinetics of paraldehyde disposition in the neonate. J Pediatr 1984;104:291–296.
109. Lampl Y, Eshel Y, Gilad R, Sarova-Ponchas I. Chloral hydrate in intractable status epilepticus. Ann Emerg Med 1990;19:674–676.
110. Meeke RI, Soifer BE, Gelb AW. Isoflurane for the refractory management of status epilepticus. Drug Intell Clin Pharm 1989;23:579–581.
111. Dimple HL. Drugs in status epilepticus. Anaesthesia 1995;50:824–825.
112. Chez MG, Hammer MS, Loeffel M, et al. Clinical experience of three pediatric patients and one adult case of spike and wave status epilepticus treated with injectable valproic acid. J Child Neurol 1999;14:239–242.

58

ACUTE MANAGEMENT OF THE HEAD INJURY PATIENT

Bradley A. Boucher and Stephanie J. Phelps

An increasing level of interest in neurotrauma has been spurred largely by a greater understanding of the pathophysiology of severe head injury and a belief that outcome can be improved through use of evidence-based management guidelines and administration of neuroprotective agents. This chapter will summarize current understanding of central nervous system (CNS) trauma and highlight guidelines and systematic reviews of the literature pertaining to management of the severe head injury patient.

EPIDEMIOLOGY

It is estimated that nearly 2 million persons annually sustain a nonfatal head injury in the United States resulting in 373,000 hospital admissions and 75,000 deaths based on the 1985–1987 National Health Information Survey.[1] While the frequency of head injury remains high, the mortality rate following traumatic brain injury has decreased from nearly 25 per 100,000 to below 20 per 100,000 population per year since 1979.[2] Motor vehicle accidents account for about 50% of all adult cases, whereas falls, assaults, gunshot wounds, sports and recreational accidents, and other miscellaneous causes account for the remaining cases.[3] Most head trauma occurs in early adulthood in persons who are free of medical problems; peak age for acute neurotrauma is 15 to 24 years.[3]

PATHOPHYSIOLOGY

PRIMARY HEAD INJURY

The neurologic sequelae of head trauma can occur instantaneously as a consequence of the primary injury or can result from secondary injuries that follow within minutes, hours, or days.[4] Primary injury involves the external transfer of kinetic energy to various structural components of the head [e.g., nerve cells, nerve synapses, supporting cells of the brain (glial cells), and cerebral blood vessels]. The biomechanical forces responsible for primary head injury can be broadly classified as concussive/compressive (e.g., blunt-object blow, penetrating-missile injuries) and acceleration/deceleration (e.g., instantaneous head movements following motor vehicle accidents). Primary injuries are further categorized as focal or diffuse. The latter usually are associated with shearing forces, which affect axons within the brain.[5]

SECONDARY BRAIN INJURY

A complex sequence of pathophysiologic events precipitated by primary head injury may seriously disrupt the normal CNS balance between oxygen supply and demand.[4] The end result of this imbalance is cerebral ischemia, the key pathophysiologic event triggering secondary injury. Figure 58–1 is a simplified schematic of the processes that constitute secondary brain injury and their various interrelationships. Readers are referred to a recent review and the cited reference chapters in the textbook, *Neurotrauma,* for a more detailed discussion of these complex events.[6] The brain is particularly susceptible to ischemia because of its normally high resting energy requirement and its limited capacity to store oxygen, glucose, and high-energy phosphate compounds [e.g., adenosine triphosphate (ATP)].[4] Study of ischemia following head injury has documented that it is typically an early event that occurs less than 6 hours after the insult.[7] Patients studied after this 6-hour window frequently have hyperemia (i.e., "luxury perfusion"). This latter phenomenon is the result of an uncoupling of oxygen delivery (CDO_2) and consumption ($CMRO_2$) in the brain, a process that is closely autoregulated under normal circumstances.[4] Factors that can diminish cerebral oxygen supply following head injury include cerebral edema, expanding mass lesions (e.g., epidural, subdural, and intracerebral hematomas), cerebral vasospasm, and loss of vasoregulatory control.[4] Hypoxia can further exacerbate local decreases in cerebral oxygen supply following acute respiratory failure and systemic hypotension. Metabolic demand also can increase following neurotrauma secondary to seizures, agitation, and temperature elevation.

Brain tissue affected by focal ischemia has a dense core surrounded by a marginally viable region referred to as the *ischemic penumbra*.[6] Cells in this area are electrically silent and unable to perform normal neurologic functions. If adequate cerebral blood flow (CBF) is restored, the affected tissue may recover; however, sustained ischemia can result in further loss of cellular integrity and eventual cell death. The loss of ionic homeostasis is postulated to be a key event in fostering secondary brain injury within the ischemic penumbra. Cellular influx of sodium, chloride, and water with a corresponding efflux of potassium and magnesium begins with Na^+, K^+-ATPase pump dysfunction.[4] An influx of calcium into the presynaptic terminal ends of damaged neurons is mediated by N type voltage sensitive calcium channels. This, in turn, stimulates excessive release of the excitatory amines glutamate and aspartate from the affected neurons.[6,8] Influx of calcium and additional sodium is stimulated by activation of the *N*-methyl-D-aspartate (NMDA) receptor.

Calcium influx and its intracellular accumulation initiate a number of events that amplify and perpetuate secondary neuronal injury. High intracellular concentrations of calcium result in mitochondrial dysfunction, which further inhibits cellular respiration, a process already affected by ischemic and/or hypoxic insults.[9] A second major deleterious effect of calcium is to stimulate activation of proteases and phosphatases, including calpains and phospholipase A_2.[6,9] The effect of phospholipase A_2 stimulation includes formation of several arachidonic acid metabolites derived from membrane lipids: thromboxane A_2, prostaglandins, and leukotrienes.[9] The subsequent effects of these metabolites include platelet aggregation, vasodilation, vasoconstriction, and lipid peroxidation. A by-product of lipid peroxidation is

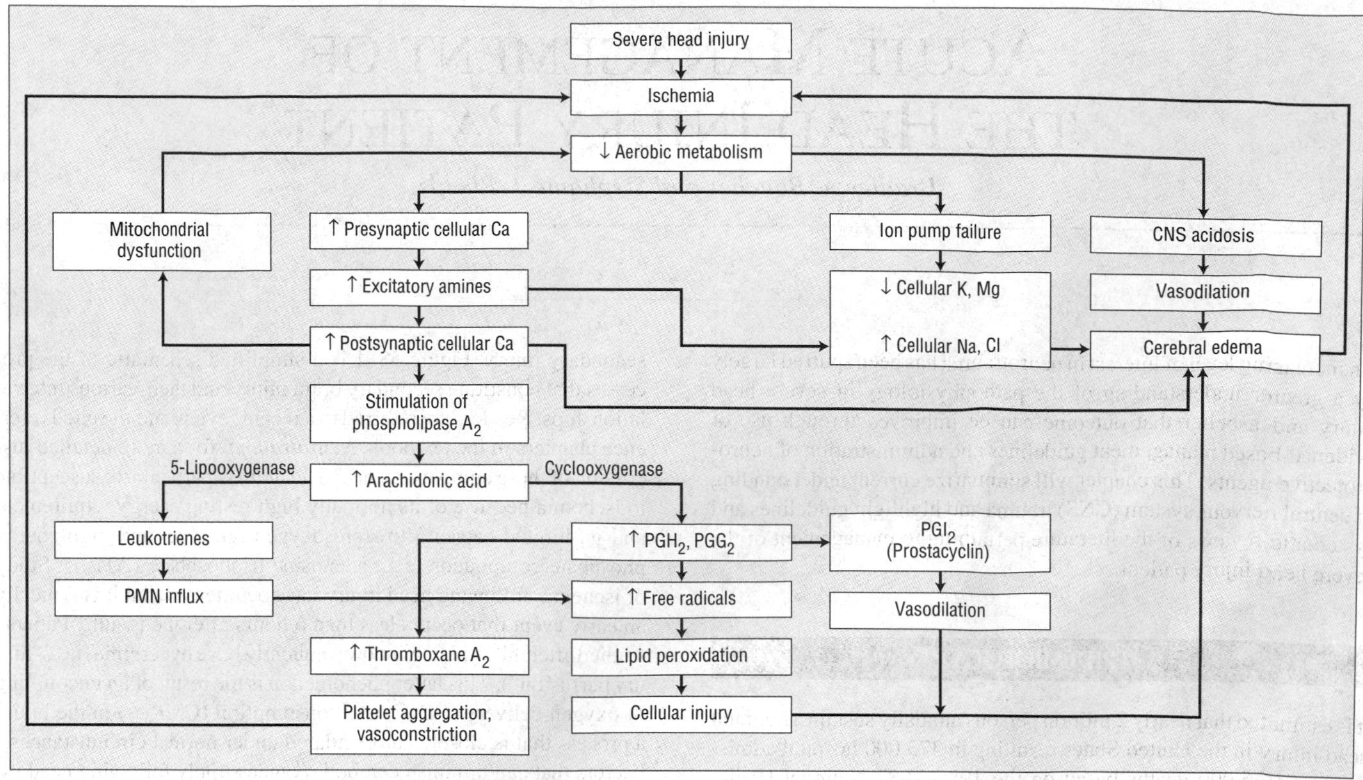

FIGURE 58–1. Schematic illustration of the cascade of biochemical events proposed to occur following severe neurotrauma (secondary brain injury).

the formation of oxygen free-radical species.[10] Lipid peroxidation is an especially damaging event because the formation of oxygen free radicals can propagate itself, resulting in further cellular membrane damage unless quenched by endogenous antioxidants (e.g., vitamin E, ascorbic acid, superoxide dismutase).[6,10] Finally, calcium influx also can stimulate nucleases that break down DNA, resulting in programmed cell death (i.e., apoptosis).[9] Cell-mediated injury involving inflammatory mediators (e.g., cytokines, platelet-activating factor, etc.), nitric oxide, and cell adhesion molecules is yet another possible mechanism involved in secondary neuronal injury.[11] Among the cell lines implicated are polymorphonuclear neutrophils, platelets, endothelial cells, and macrophages.

Additionally, vasogenic cerebral edema can develop as a consequence of cerebral capillary endothelial damage.[4] With cytotoxic and vasogenic edema comes expansion of the intracellular and extracellular fluid spaces, respectively. Elevated intracranial pressure (ICP) is the most detrimental consequence of cerebral edema formation and occurs as the brain tissue volume increases within the nondistensible skull. A significant increase in ICP may further compromise CBF and extend cytotoxic edema. Hence an increase in ICP can be self-perpetuating unless this cycle is reversed.

CLINICAL PRESENTATION

An initial neurologic examination is essential for assessing the extent of brain injury and establishing a baseline for future comparison. The level of consciousness on admission ranges from awake and alert to completely unresponsive. The Glasgow Coma Scale (GCS) is the most widely used system to grade the arousal and functional capacity of the cerebral cortex.[12] The GCS defines the level of consciousness according to eye opening, motor response, and verbal response (Table 58–1). A GCS of 15 corresponds to a normal neurologic examination. A GCS of 3–8, 9–12, and 13–14 is consistent with severe, moderate, and minor head injury, respectively.[13] The possibility of ethanol or drug intoxication, hypotension, hypoxia, postictal state, or hypothermia altering the neurologic examination always should be considered. Because narcotic and muscle relaxants affect the neurologic

TABLE 58–1. Glasgow Coma Scale

	Response	Score
Eyes	Open spontaneously	4
	To verbal command	3
	To pain	2
	No response	1
Best motor response		
To verbal command	Obeys	6
To painful stimulus (pressure to nailbeds)	Localizes pain	5
	Flexion, withdrawal	4
	Flexion, abnormal (decorticate rigidity)	3
	Extension (decerebrate rigidity)	2
	No response	1
Best verbal response (Arouse patient with painful stimulus if necessary)	Oriented and converses	5
	Disoriented and converses	4
	Inappropriate words	3
	Incomprehensible sounds	2
	No response	1
	TOTAL	3–15

examination, they should not be administered until the initial examination is complete. Significant posttraumatic amnesia (e.g., > 1 hour), increasing dizziness, a moderate to severe headache, limb weakness or paresthesia, cerebral spinal fluid (CSF) otorrhea or rhinorrhea, and seizures indicate more severe injury.[14] A rapid deterioration in mental status strongly suggests the presence of an expanding lesion within the skull. Computed tomography (CT) of the head is an important diagnostic tool for detecting the presence of mass lesions. Simple, rapidly attainable clinical variables that are predictive of survival include patient age, GCS, Injury Severity Score, pupil reactivity, and presence or absence of a hematoma found on CT of the head.[15]

In addition to a profoundly abnormal neurologic examination, patients with severe head injury also may have significant alterations or instability in their vital signs, including abnormal breathing patterns (e.g., apnea, Cheyne-Stokes respiration, tachypnea), hypotension, or bradycardia. Hypotension and/or hypoxia, although observed in the majority of patients, usually occurs as a result of blood loss, spinal cord injury (e.g., neurogenic shock), impaired cardiac function, or compromised ventilation.[14] After stabilization of vital signs, a thorough physical examination should be performed in order to identify injuries that may contribute to secondary brain injury. For example, airway obstruction and aspiration may compromise pulmonary gas exchange, chest trauma may affect both pulmonary and cardiac function (e.g., rib fractures, tension pneumothorax, cardiac tamponade), and substantial blood loss from intraabdominal or vascular injuries may decrease the blood's oxygen-carrying capacity. Initial and follow-up laboratory tests should include determination of serum electrolytes and blood glucose, a complete blood count (CBC), an arterial blood gases (ABG) determination, a blood ethanol level (EtOH), and a urine drug screen.[14]

▶ TREATMENT: Head Injury

In July 1995, the Brain Trauma Foundation (BTF) published an extensive document entitled, *Guidelines for the Management of Severe Head Injury,* as a joint initiative with the Guidelines Committee of the American Association of Neurological Surgeons (AANS) and the Joint Section on Neurotrauma and Critical Care of the AANS and the Congress of Neurologic Surgeons.[16] This landmark publication established for the first time a comprehensive series of evidence-based standards, guidelines, and options for the care of the severe head injury patient and resulted in a significant change in management of these patients by neurosurgeons.[17] In 2000, these guidelines were revised and expanded to include early indicators of prognosis.[18] Additionally, a series of systematic reviews emanating from The Cochrane Library have been published.[19–25] These reviews have rigorously evaluated the literature for essentially all the major conventional head injury treatment strategies. The recommendations emanating from the BTF and these reviews will be highlighted throughout the remaining portion of this chapter. Until further clinical studies become available, recommendations from these three sources should serve as the foundation on which all clinical decisions in managing severe head injury are based.

DESIRED OUTCOMES

The overall goal in head injury management is not only reduction in morbidity and mortality but also optimization of long-term functional outcome for these patients. This requires careful attention to the following short-term therapeutic goals: (1) establishment of an adequate airway and maintenance of breathing and circulation during the initial period of evaluation, (2) maintenance of balance between CDO_2 and $CMRO_2$, (3) prevention or attenuation of secondary neuronal injury, and (4) prevention and/or treatment of associated medical complications.

INITIAL RESUSCITATION

The first priority in the unconscious patient is the establishment of an airway, which ensures adequate oxygenation and prevents aspiration. Thereafter, restoring and maintaining systemic blood pressure to a mean arterial pressure (MAP) of 90 mm Hg or greater is of utmost importance. Correcting and preventing early hypotension (systolic blood pressure <90 mm Hg) and hypoxia ($PaO_2 < 60$ mm Hg) is essential because these two factors are among the most powerful predictors of outcome.[5] Isotonic saline [0.9% normal saline (NS)] remains the most commonly used and least expensive resuscitation fluid. While there has been some interest in using hypertonic saline in the resuscitation of head injury patients, clinical studies have yielded equivocal results relative to superiority over isotonic solutions.[26–28] Vasopressors and inotropic agents may be needed to maintain an adequate MAP if hypotension persists after adequate restoration of intravascular volume. Figure 58–2 is an algorithm summarizing treatment priorities in the initial management of acute head injury.

POSTRESUSCITATIVE CARE

Following successful resuscitation, priorities shift toward diagnostic evaluation of intracranial and extracranial injuries and emergent surgical intervention as needed. Approximately 40% of patients with severe head injury have an intracranial mass. Evacuation of intracranial hematomas (i.e., epidural, subdural, and intracerebral hematomas), elevation of depressed skull fractures, and debridement of penetrating wound tracts are essential to control ICP and improve outcome. Continuous ICP monitor placement (e.g., ventricular catheter, parenchymal fiberoptic catheter, or subarachnoid, subdural, and epidural monitors) is indicated in patients with a GCS of ≤ 8 with an abnormal admission CT scan or in high-risk severe head injury patients with a normal CT scan (i.e., age > 40 years, motor posturing, systolic blood pressure < 90 mm Hg).[18] Ventricular catheters have a therapeutic advantage over the other alternatives. Specifically, CSF can be drained using this device as a means to lower ICP. Continuous ICP monitoring is the most important means to objectively evaluate the success of therapies used to decrease ICP. Normal ICP ranges from 0 to 10 mm Hg; once ICP exceeds 20 to 25 mm Hg, therapy should be initiated to decrease ICP below this range.[18] Jugular venous saturation monitoring is strongly advocated by some practitioners for detection of cerebral hypoxia, although it is not currently addressed within the BTF guidelines.[29,30] Hence its use remains limited at present.

The principal monitoring parameter for severe head injury patients within the intensive care environment is the cerebral perfusion pressure (CPP), which is the difference between MAP and ICP

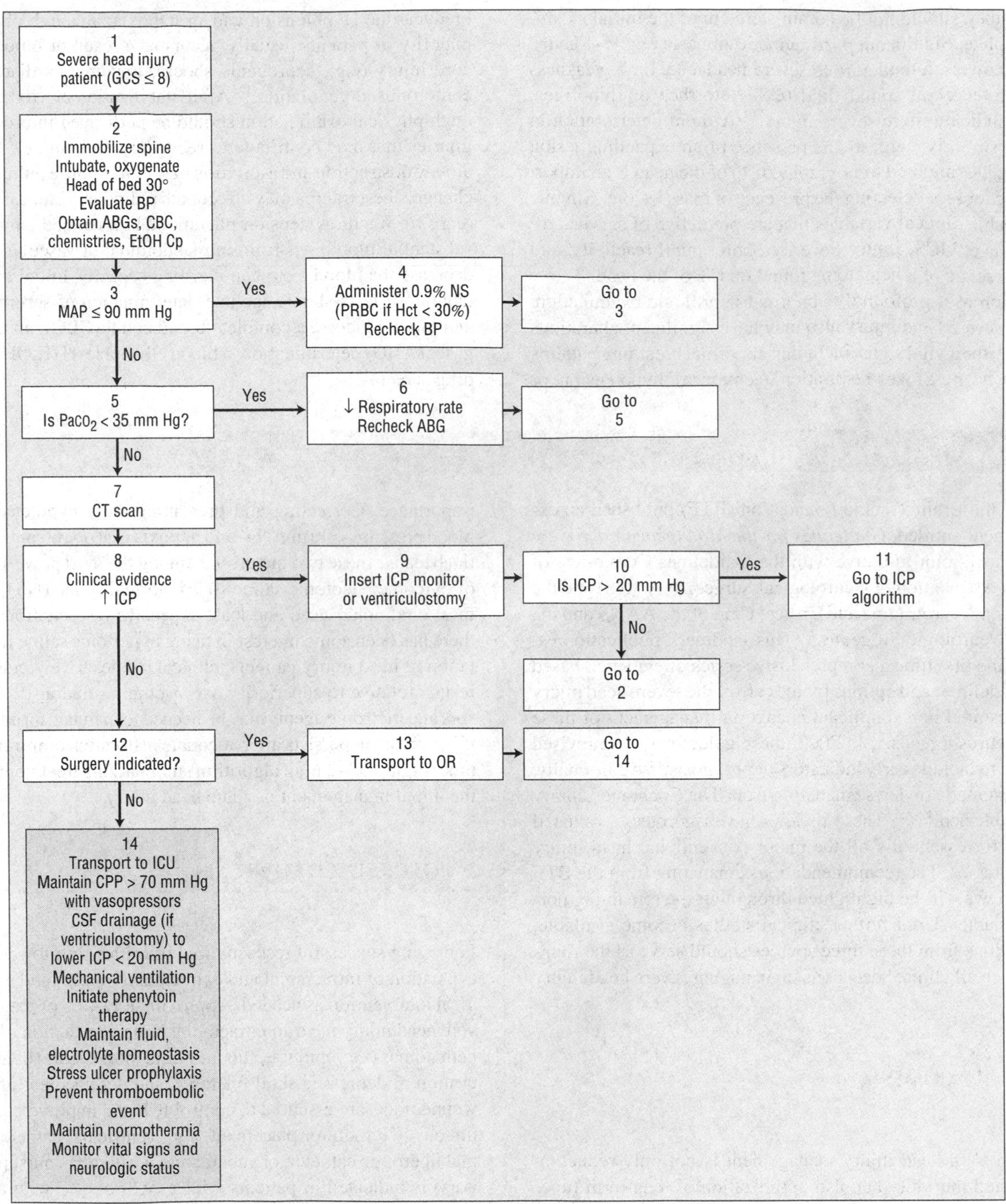

FIGURE 58–2. Algorithm for the acute management of the head injury patient. *(Adapted from Boucher BA. Neurotrauma: Pharmacotherapy Self Assessment Program, 3d ed., Module 2: Critical Care, pp 215–238, 1995. By permission of the American College of Clinical Pharmacy.)*

(i.e, CPP = MAP − ICP). The CPP is essentially the pressure gradient driving CBF. Therefore, maintenance of an acceptable CPP is critical in reducing cerebral ischemia and secondary injury. The BTF guidelines recommend that CPP be maintained at greater than 70 mm Hg based on a number of studies that have demonstrated decreased morbidity and mortality in patients when CPP was actively sustained above 70 to 80 mmHg.[18,31] A recent study, however, refutes this benchmark, suggesting that a CPP of more than 60 mm Hg may be adequate.[32] Regardless of the goal value, CPP can be sustained by increasing MAP or by lowering elevated ICP.

The MAP can be increased through normalization of the intravascular volume combined with pharmacologically inducing systemic hypertension as needed. The goal of volume expansion should be euvolemia and avoidance of a hypoosmolar state. If the hematocrit is below 30%, transfusion of packed red blood cells (PRBCs) is indicated. Volume status should be targeted to a central venous pressure of 5 to 10 mm Hg or a pulmonary artery wedge pressure between 10 and 14 mm Hg.[13] After achievement of euvolemia, the patient's head should be elevated at 30 degrees to promote venous drainage and decrease ICP. If restoration of the intravascular volume is inadequate in elevating MAP to an acceptable level, hypertension should be induced using vasopressors or inotropic support. While concern has been raised as to the potential for induced hypertension to increase ICP, studies have shown that this does not occur in most patients and that ICP actually may fall.[33] The drugs employed most commonly to induce hypertension are the sympathomimetic amines, dopamine, norepinephrine, and phenylephrine. While none of these agents has shown superiority, norepinephrine is a reasonable selection at a starting dose of 0.02 μg/kg per minute.[13] Patients should be monitored for renal dysfunction, lactic acidosis, and signs of peripheral ischemia when these agents are used, especially at high doses.

TREATMENT OF INTRACRANIAL HYPERTENSION

GENERAL PHARMACOLOGIC STRATEGIES

Pain, agitation, excessive muscle movement, and resisting mechanical ventilation can cause transient increases in ICP.[34] As such, use of analgesics, sedatives, and paralytics has an important primary role in the management of intracranial hypertension (Fig. 58–3). Nonetheless, there have been no studies of the effect of sedation on outcome in patients with severe head injury.[18] Morphine sulfate is the most commonly used analgesic and sedative in this setting.[34,35] Alternative sedatives include short-acting opiates (e.g., remifentanil),[36] propofol,[37] etomidate, intermittent low-dose pentobarbital, and short-acting benzodiazepines (e.g., midazolam), especially if there is a reasonable suspicion of alcohol withdrawal as the underlying etiology of the agitation.[34,35] The potential for these agents to decrease MAP and CPP must be monitored closely. The use of any sedative agent also must be weighed against their potential to obscure the neurologic examination of the patient. Cautious reversal of the effect of benzodiazepines with flumazenil can be used to allow examination of the patient.[35] Interference with the neurologic examination also is associated with paralytic agents. Prophylactic neuromuscular blockade (i.e., unrelated to ICP control) is not recommended based on evidence indicating increased complications and length of stay following paralytic use.[38] Hyperthermia also should be avoided because patients with elevated temperatures may have a poorer outcome than normothermic patients.[39] Hence maintenance of a core temperature of less than 37.5°C using acetaminophen and cooling blankets is indicated for patients following severe neurotrauma.[13]

HYPERVENTILATION

The practice of aggressive hyperventilation ($PaCO_2$ of 25–30 mm Hg) to decrease ICP is no longer recommended.[18] Hyperventilation acutely decreases systemic and cerebral $PaCO_2$. The resulting hypocapnia, in turn, induces cerebral vasoconstriction, thereby decreasing CBF and cerebral blood volume (CBV).[40] For decades it was a widely held belief that a reduction in CBV and any accompanying decrease in ICP were beneficial. Nonetheless, two systematic reviews of the literature concluded that data are inadequate to ascertain potential benefit or harm from hyperventilation.[24,41] Other studies have determined that severe head injury patients with normocapnia versus those receiving aggressive hyperventilation have an improved outcome at 3 and 6 months.[18] Hence the BTF guidelines recommend that $PaCO_2$ be maintained near 35 mm Hg, especially during the first 24 hours.[18] Thereafter, a $PaCO_2$ in the range of 30 to 35 mm Hg may be used if ICP control is inadequate.[13]

HYPOTHERMIA

While hypothermia has been used for nearly 50 years as a cerebral protective maneuver in head injury patients, recent interest has been fueled by the results of several preliminary studies in the early 1990s demonstrating trends in improvement in mortality and morbidity rates in severe head injury patients randomized to receive mild to moderate hypothermia (34–35°C).[41] However, in the most extensive follow-up investigation to date, hypothermia did not improve outcome significantly in a group of severe head injury patients at 12 months despite improvement at 3 and 6 months.[43] Another investigation was unable to discern any difference in clinical outcomes between normothermia and mild hypothermia in severe head injury patient groups whose ICPs were maintained below 20 mm Hg using conventional therapies despite beneficial effects in select patient subsets with elevated ICP.[44,45] These negative results were confirmed in a recently published randomized multicenter study of 392 acute head injury patients.[46] No significant difference in functional status 6 months after the injury was observed in those patients with hypothermia (body temperature of 33°C) compared with normothermic patients in this trial.[46] In actuality, hypothermic patients had more hospital days with complications than normothermic patients.[46] Prior to this pivotal trial, a systematic review of the literature did discern potential benefits of hypothermia on attenuating severe disability or death based on data combined from several small trials.[25] The mechanism underlying any protective effect of hypothermia is likely multifactorial, although a reduction is $CMRO_2$ is offered most frequently as the basis of any therapeutic benefits. Potential side effects of hypothermia include coagulation disturbances, sepsis, cardiac arrhythmias, hypokalemia, acid-base imbalances, pancreatitis, decreased creatinine clearance, and shivering.[43,47] Considering these latter risks and data from the most recent investigation, hypothermia should be considered an investigational treatment that is reserved for patients with elevated ICP refractory to all other forms of therapy.

DIURETICS

Although a variety of osmotic diuretics (e.g., urea, glycerol) can be used to decrease ICP, mannitol is unquestionably the most widely employed.[35,48] Despite the common practice of administering mannitol to patients with suspected or actual increase in ICP following head injury, no clinical trials comparing its effects against placebo have been performed.[23,41] The mechanisms responsible for mannitol's beneficial effects likely relate to (1) an immediate plasma-expanding effect that reduces blood viscosity and increases CBF and (2) establishing an osmotic concentration gradient across an intact blood-brain barrier; as water diffuses from the brain into the intravascular compartment, ICP decreases.[18,35] If the blood-brain barrier is disrupted as a result of injury or "opened" with prolonged use of the osmotic agent, rebound elevations of ICP may occur as mannitol accumulates in the brain tissue, resulting in an increase in intracellular brain volume.[35]

Effective doses of mannitol range from 0.25–1 g/kg intravenously every 4 hours.[18,35] Increased ICP is reduced within minutes following mannitol administration, and the duration of action ranges from 90 minutes to 6 hours depending on the dose and the clinical conditions present.[18] In order to maximize benefit and minimize adverse events, it generally is recommend that mannitol should not be administered as a continuous infusion in this setting.[18] However, no clinical trials have compared different mannitol dosages or types

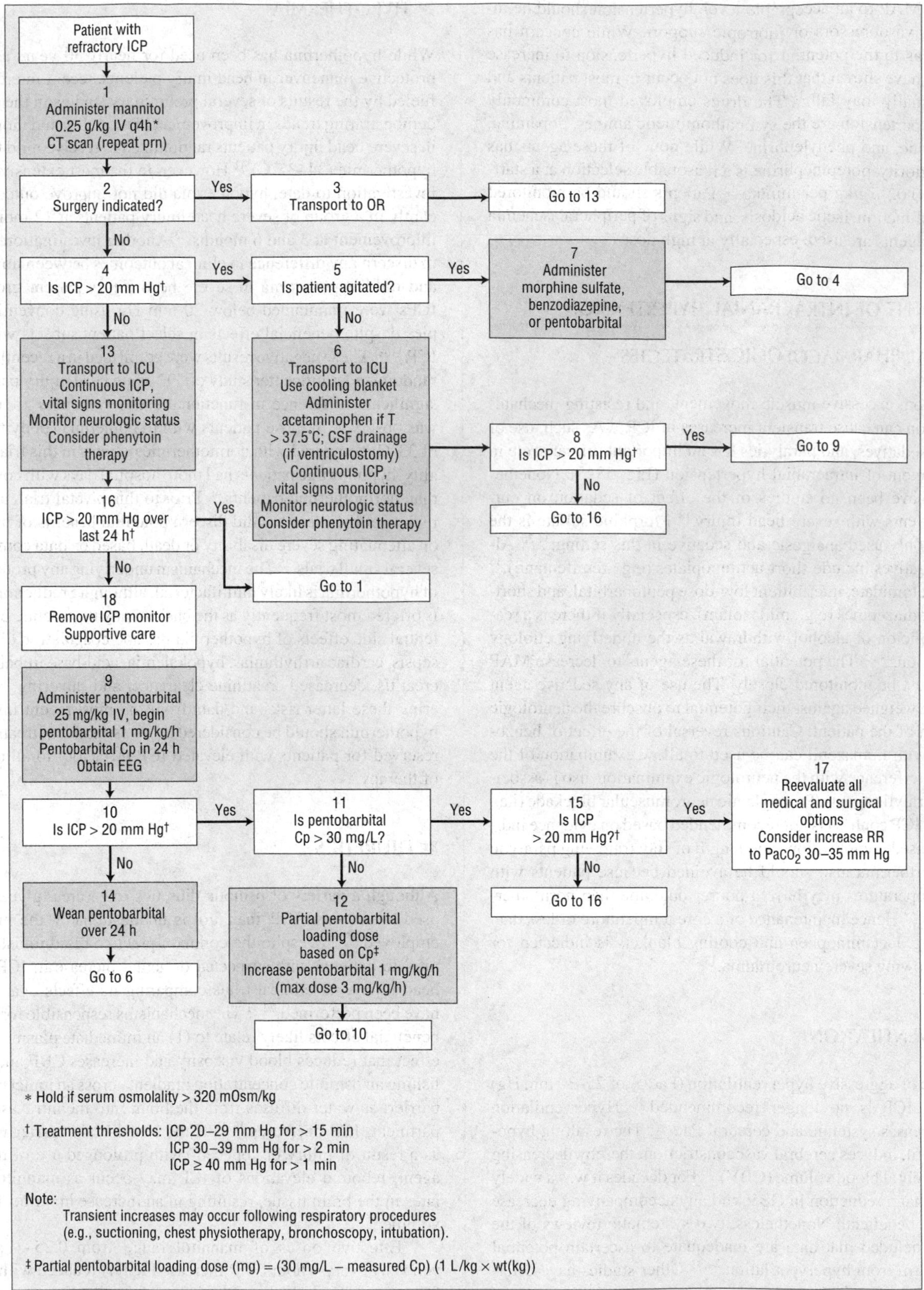

FIGURE 58–3. Algorithm for the management of ICP. *(Adapted from Boucher BA. Neurotrauma: Pharmacotherapy Self Assessment Program, 3d ed., Module 2: Critical Care, pp. 215–238, 1995. By permission of the American College of Clinical Pharmacy.)*

of administration.[23] Monitoring and maintaining serum osmolality at less than 320 mosm/kg is important relative to minimizing adverse events.[35] Intravenous furosemide (0.5–1 mg/kg) may be used in conjunction with mannitol in refractory cases.

Several adverse effects are associated with mannitol. In addition to hypotension resulting from its diuretic effect, a reversible acute renal dysfunction may occur in patients with previously normal renal function after long-term, high-dose administration, especially if serum osmolality exceeds 320 mosm/kg.[18,35] Acute exacerbation of underlying congestive heart failure and pulmonary edema also may occur following rapid intravascular volume expansion. Furosemide is recommended as an alternative diuretic for lowering ICP in these latter patient groups.

CORTICOSTEROIDS

Although corticosteroids are effective in preventing or reducing cerebral edema in patients with structural brain damage (e.g., tumors), the majority of studies in patients with severe head injury have not demonstrated that they lower ICP or improve outcome.[18] In addition, use of corticosteroids following head injury has been associated with increased complications, including gastrointestinal bleeding, glucose intolerance, electrolyte abnormalities, and infection.[13] Based on six major randomized trials, the BTF guidelines strongly recommend that corticosteroids not be used.[18] Recent systematic reviews nonetheless have concluded that neither moderate benefits nor moderate harmful effects of corticosteroids in head injury patients can be excluded after review of all clinical trial data collected to date.[19,49] Thus the controversy over corticosteroid use in severe head injury patients continues. Estimates from one of the systematic reviews indicated that a randomized clinical trial of over 20,000 participants would be needed to resolve this issue definitively.[49] An ambitious international investigation known as the Corticosteroid Randomization after Significant Head Injury (CRASH) study has been initiated in an attempt to finally resolve the debate concerning the merits of corticosteroid therapy in patients with severe head injury.[50] In this study, patients are randomized to receive a 48-hour continuous infusion of methylprednisolone or placebo.

BARBITURATES

High-dose barbiturate therapy (i.e., barbiturate coma) has been used for decades in the management of increased ICP despite a lack of evidence documenting beneficial effects on patient morbidity and mortality.[21] Nonetheless, based largely on beneficial outcomes observed in a randomized clinical trial published in 1988, the BTF guidelines recommend that high-dose barbiturate therapy be considered in hemodynamically stable severe head injury patients refractory to maximal medical and surgical ICP lowering therapy.[18,51] Prophylactic use of barbiturates is not advocated in light of insufficient evidence supporting this practice and the potential for adverse events (e.g., hypotension).[18,21] Several mechanisms responsible for the cerebral protective effects of barbiturates have been proposed. These include (1) lowering the regional $CMRO_2$ with a coupled reduction in CBF to these areas, (2) inhibition of lipid peroxidation, and (3) altering cerebral vascular tone.[35]

Prior to inducing a barbiturate coma, the severe head injury patient must be mechanically ventilated with continuous monitoring of arterial blood pressure, electrocardiogram (ECG), and ICP. Pentobarbital is the most commonly used barbiturate for this indication, although thiopental also has been used over the years. Pentobarbital should be administered as an intravenous loading infusion totaling 25 mg/kg (i.e., 10 mg/kg over 30 minutes, then 5 mg/kg/h for 3 hours), followed by an initial maintenance infusion of 1 mg/kg per hour.[18] The maintenance infusion can be titrated upward if needed to a maximum of 2–3 mg/kg per hour.[35] If the systolic blood pressure falls during the loading or maintenance infusions, the rate should be slowed temporarily and blood pressure support initiated. The goal of a barbiturate coma is to maintain ICP and CPP at the previously discussed target thresholds in addition to achieving a pentobarbital steady-state concentration between 30 and 40 mg/L and electroencephalogram burst suppression.[18] Initiation of barbiturate therapy withdrawal can occur when ICP has been controlled satisfactorily for 24–48 hours.[18] Barbiturates should be tapered over 24–72 hours to prevent ICP spikes.

Side effects associated with high-dose barbiturate therapy involve primarily the cardiovascular system. Hypotension, caused by peripheral vasodilation, may occur and necessitate decreasing the barbiturate dose or the administration of fluids and vasopressors to maintain blood pressure. A recent systematic review of the literature revealed that for every four patients receiving barbiturate therapy, one will develop hypotension.[21] Gastrointestinal (GI) effects of barbiturates include decreased GI muscular tone and decreased amplitude of contraction. On emergence from coma, there may be a period of GI hypermotility. Care should be taken to avoid extravasation of pentobarbital and thiopental solutions because severe tissue damage may occur. Barbiturates should be administered by continuous infusion through a central line dedicated to this purpose. The potential for barbiturates to induce the hepatic drug metabolism of concurrent medications also should be considered.

TREATMENT AND PROPHYLAXIS OF POSTTRAUMATIC SEIZURES

Seizures greatly increase $CMRO_2$. Therefore, it is generally agreed that patients who have experienced 1 or more seizures following a moderate to severe head injury should receive anticonvulsant therapy to avoid further increases in $CMRO_2$. Initial therapy in these persons should consist of incremental intravenous doses of diazepam (5–40 mg adults, 0.1–0.5 mg/kg infants and children) or lorazepam (2–8 mg adults, 0.03–0.1 mg/kg infants and children) to terminate any seizure activity, followed by intravenous phenytoin to prevent seizure recurrence. The merits of preventive anticonvulsant therapy in patients who have not had a seizure postinjury historically has been more controversial. Risk factors for early posttraumatic seizures (< 7 days postinjury) include a GCS of less than 10, cortical contusion, depressed skull fracture, subdural hematoma, epidural hematoma, intracerebral hematoma, penetrating head wound, or a seizure within the first 24 hours of injury.[18] In a landmark randomized, placebo-controlled study, the incidence of early posttraumatic seizures in patients receiving placebo was 14.2% compared with 3.6% in patients receiving phenytoin ($P < .05$) without a significant increase in drug-related side effects.[52,53] A recent systematic review of the literature corroborated these findings, estimating a pooled relative risk for early seizure prevention of 0.34 (95% confidence interval, 0.21–0.54) in those patients receiving anticonvulsants.[22] Thus it is recommended that phenytoin (or alternatively, carbamazepine) be used to prevent seizures in head injury patients at high risk within the first 7 days.[18] Valproate therapy is not recommended based on a trend for higher mortality in a study comparing valproate-treated patients with those receiving phenytoin short-term therapy.[54] The benefits of prophylactic anticonvulsants beyond 7 days has not been demonstrated, and thus their use for this indication is not recommended.[18,22,52] Unfortunately, despite reducing the incidence of early seizures following head injury, no beneficial effects have been documented for anticonvulsants on patient mortality or long-term disability.[22]

SUPPORTIVE CARE

While maintaining an adequate CPP and normalizing ICP are the highest priorities in preventing secondary injury following severe neurotrauma, attention also must be given to preventing and/or treating systemic and extracranial complications. This includes careful ongoing fluid and electrolyte management.[55] Common electrolyte disturbances in head injury patients that should be monitored and treated aggressively include hyponatremia, hypomagnesemia, hypokalemia, and hypophosphatemia.[35,56] Aggressive nutritional support of the head injury patient is another important therapeutic consideration.[57] Infectious complications commonly encountered in severe head injury patients include nosocomial pneumonia, sepsis, urinary tract infections, meningitis, and brain abscesses.[58,59] Treatment of these potentially devastating infections should be aggressive, with careful attention to antibiotic blood-brain barrier penetration for intracranial infections. Adjunctive administration of granulocyte colony-stimulating factor also has received limited attention relative to preventing nosocomial infections in these patients.[60,61] Other important therapeutic interventions include correction of any documented coagulopathy,[62] acute gastritis prophylaxis, prevention of thromboembolic events,[62] and fever control.[63]

INVESTIGATIONAL THERAPY

The steady decrease in morbidity and mortality following severe neurotrauma over the last 30 years can be attributed largely to expeditious and aggressive management of those events resulting in secondary injury (i.e., ischemia, hypoxia, increased ICP) using conventional treatment strategies. Numerous neuroprotective agents targeting specific pathophysiologic processes that are theorized to occur following severe head injury have been investigated over the last decade in an attempt to further enhance the prospects for a meaningful recovery. A review of these investigations is outlined below. Unfortunately, none of these agents to date has been able to demonstrate a significant reduction in morbidity or mortality following severe head injury in phase III clinical trials, with the exception of nimodipine in a subset of patients. Numerous explanations have been offered as to the variance between benefits observed in animal models of head injury using a variety of neuroprotective drugs and their lack of effectiveness in patients. These include mechanistic differences in secondary head injury between animal models and patients,[64,65] patient heterogenicity relative to intracranial and extracranial pathology,[64,65] inadequate sample size,[66] poor drug penetration into the brain,[67,68] insensitive outcome measures,[67,68] patient enrollment imbalances,[67,68] and unrealistic improvement expectations.[65,68] Other issues that require careful attention in future clinical trials to maximize the utility of these agents are the dose, timing, and sequencing of drug administration; duration of therapy relative to the traumatic event; and possibly combination therapy.[64,65] Despite the investigational study failures to date, the search is likely to continue for neuroprotective agents that eventually may improve the long-term outcome in severe head injury patients by avoiding some of the pitfalls in study design present in previous negative investigations.

MODULATION OF CALCIUM INFLUX

Calcium Antagonists

The calcium antagonists are obvious candidates for potentially attenuating the deleterious effects of calcium influx in acute neurotrauma patients. Nimodipine, a dihydropyridine, has been studied most extensively among the calcium antagonists that block the postsynaptic L-type calcium channel. Unfortunately, two major trials of nimodipine in head injury patients did not demonstrate a statistically significant improvement in outcome compared with placebo.[69] A significant benefit was observed in the subgroup of patients with posttraumatic subarachnoid hemorrhage (tSAH) receiving nimodipine that was corroborated in a follow-up investigation.[70] The nimodipine dosage used in the latter investigation was 2 mg/h intravenously for 7–10 days, followed by 360 mg daily administered orally until day 21 of treatment.[70] A recent sytematic review of the literature concluded that nimodipine may be beneficial in tSAH patients, although there is insufficient evidence to support use of calcium antagonists in unselected head injury patients.[20] Systemic hypotension is a relative limitation with the use of other L-type calcium channel antagonists for this indication.

Another target for calcium modulation is the presynaptic N-type voltage-sensitive calcium channels. Omega conotoxin (SNX-111, ziconotide) is one such antagonist that has been evaluated in head injury patients. Unfortunately, a major phase III trial of omega conotoxin was halted prematurely after an interim analysis deemed the likelihood for a favorable outcome to be very small compared with placebo.[64] Profound systemic hypotension requiring vasopressor support was a major concern with the use of this agent.

Glutamate Antagonists

A significant amount of experimental evidence has been accumulated confirming the efficacy of NMDA receptor antagonists in attenuating secondary injury events following model head injury. Based on these results, both competitive and noncompetitive NMDA receptor antagonists have been developed as neuroprotective agents. D-CPP-ene and CGS 19755 (Selfotel) are investigational NMDA antagonists competing with glutamate at the receptor site (i.e., competitive antagonists). Results of two phase III Selfotel clinical trials involving 693 patients did not demonstrate increased efficacy compared with placebo and possible increased mortality and serious brain-related adverse events in the treatment groups during interim analysis of the data.[71] As such, the trials were stopped prematurely.[71] Noncompetitive NMDA antagonists or receptor channel blockers bind to the open NMDA receptor, thereby blocking the ionic current.[6] Compounds within this group include ketamine, phencyclidine, dextromethorphan, dextrorphan, and the investigational agents dizocilpine (MK-801), dexanabinol, and aptiganel (Cerestat).[6] A phase III trial of aptiganel also was discontinued prematurely based on limited benefit (1.1%) in favor of the treatment over placebo in the first 340 patients studied.[68] Another NMDA receptor antagonist that selectively blocks the NR2B regulatory site on the postsynaptic receptor that has undergone clinical investigation is CP-101,606.[72] A phase III study involving 600 severe head injury patients randomized to receive either CP-101,606 or placebo was completed recently. Results of this investigation are expected in the near future.

ANTIOXIDANTS/FREE-RADICAL SCAVENGERS

The potential role of oxygen free radicals in the pathophysiology of head injury has stimulated interest in the use of antioxidants to interrupt the self-perpetuating cycle of membrane destruction in these patients. Tirilazad (Freedox), a 21-aminosteroid, is one such antioxidant that has undergone phase III testing in head injury, stroke, and tSAH patients. An attractive feature of this steroid analog is that although it is a potent inhibitor of lipid peroxidation, it is essentially devoid of glucocorticoid activity. Unfortunately, two major trials of tirilazad in head injury patients were unable to demonstrate efficacy compared with placebo.[68,73] An enzymatic free-radical scavenger that has undergone clinical trials in severe head injury patients is superoxide dismutase conjugated to a polyethylene glycol polymer (PEG-SOD; pegorgotein, Dismutec). While results of the preliminary phase II trial were promising, no statistically significant improvement in outcome or mortality was observed in the larger phase III trial in severe head injury patients receiving two doses of pegorgotein compared with placebo.[74,75]

OTHER TREATMENT STRATEGIES

Formation of inflammatory mediators including the metabolites of arachidonic acid have been implicated in the latter stages of secondary injury following neurotrauma. As such, both cyclooxygenase inhibitors (e.g., nonsteroidal anti-inflammatory drugs)[76] and mixed cyclooxygenase-lipooxygenase inhibitors (e.g., BW7544C) have been studied in experimental neurotrauma models with limited success. Furthermore, the immunosuppressant cyclosporin A has received some attention relative to attenuation of cortical damage in animal models of traumatic brain injury.[77] Inhibitors of inflammatory mediators are also under consideration as neuroprotective agents. These include antagonists to bradykinin,[78] platelet-activating factor, cytokines, and leukotriene LT_4. Lastly, various growth factors and cofactors such as insulin-like growth factor-1[79] and GM_1 ganglioside may have a future role in the management of head injury by promoting nerve cell regeneration and differentiation.[5,80]

EVALUATION OF THERAPEUTIC OUTCOMES

Achievement of the aforementioned short-term goals and eventually returning severe head injury patients to their preinjury neurologic status are the benchmarks on which all therapies are measured. One of the most commonly used assessment tools for this purpose in head injury patients is known as the Glasgow Outcome Scale (GOS).[81,82] This straightforward scale categorizes patient outcome as (1) death, (2) persistent vegetative state, (3) severe disability (conscious but disabled), (4) moderate disability (disabled but independent), and (5) good recovery. The Disability Rating Scale (DRS) is another measurement instrument used extensively in head injury studies that incorporates the GOS in addition to grading activities of daily living (e.g., feeding, toileting, grooming), cognitive functioning, and employability in assessing long-term outcome for these patients.[83] These objective outcome measures, typically measured at 3 and 6 months postinjury, are useful not only to scientists and clinicians but also to payers in evaluating the relative merits of costly available rehabilitation programs for these patients.[84] Estimates of medical spending on injury exceeded $65 billion (1993 dollars) in the United States based on data from 1987.[85] Use of a clinical pathway also may be beneficial relative to reducing resource utilization from an institutional perspective.[86] Unfortunately, no difference in the incidence of complications or functional outcomes was observed in a controlled investigation using such a clinical pathway for severe traumatic brain injury patients.[86]

CONCLUSIONS

Publication of the *Guidelines for the Management of Severe Head Injury* published by the BTF in 1995 and its revision in 2000 were landmark events in establishing evidence-based standards, guidelines, and options for conventional management of the severe head injury patient. Attenuation of secondary neuronal injury through adherence to the recommendations contained in these reports offers the greatest likelihood for a meaningful recovery in these patients at present. Combining an ever-increasing understanding of the pathophysiologic processes occurring following a severe head injury with advances in neuroprotective pharmacology offers the greatest promise for further reduction of morbidity and mortality. Unfortunately, despite numerous attempts, no investigational therapy has been associated with a significant improvement in functional outcome following severe head injury to date.

▶ PRINCIPLES OF PHARMACOTHERAPY

- Cerebral ischemia is the key pathophysiologic event triggering secondary neuronal injury following severe head injury.
- Intracellular accumulation of calcium is postulated to be a central pathophysiologic process in amplifying and perpetuating secondary neuronal injury via inhibition of cellular respiration and enzyme activation.
- *Guidelines for the Management of Severe Head Injury* published by the BTF serves as the foundation on which clinical decisions in managing neurotrauma patients are based.
- Correcting and preventing early hypotension (systolic blood pressure < 90 mm Hg) and hypoxia (PaO_2 < 60 mm Hg) are paramount goals during the initial resuscitative and intensive care of severe head injury patients.
- The principal monitoring parameter for severe head injury patients within the intensive care environment is the CPP (CPP = MAP - ICP); CPP should be maintained higher than 70 mm Hg through the use of fluids, vasopressors, and/or ICP normalization therapy.
- Nonspecific pharmacologic treatment in the management of intracranial hypertension should include analgesics, sedatives, anxiolytics, antipyretics, and paralytics under selected circumstances.

- Specific pharmacologic treatment in the management of intracranial hypertension includes mannitol, furosemide, and high-dose pentobarbital.
- Neither corticosteroids nor aggressive hyperventilation (i.e., $PaCO_2 < 35$ mm Hg) should be used in the management of intracranial hypertension.
- Use of phenytoin for the prophylaxis of posttraumatic seizures should be discontinued after 7 days if no seizures are observed.
- Numerous investigational strategies (e.g., calcium antagonists, glutamate antagonists, antioxidants, and free-radical scavengers) targeted at interrupting the pathophysiologic cascade of events occurring following severe head injury are being studied.

REFERENCES

1. Collins JG. Types of injuries by selected characteristics. Vital Health Stat 1990;10:1–68.
2. Sosin DM, Sniezek JE, Waxweiler RJ. Trends in death associated with traumatic brain injury, 1979 through 1992: Success and failure. JAMA 1995;273:1778–1780.
3. Kraus JF, McArthur DL, Silverman TA, Jayaraman M. Epidemiology of brain injury. In: Narayan RK, Wilberger JE Jr, Povlishock JT, eds. Neurotrauma. New York, McGraw-Hill, 1996:13–30.
4. Veremakis C, Lindner DH. Central nervous system injury: Essential physiologic and therapeutic concerns. In: Civetta JM, Taylor RW, Kirby RR, eds. Critical Care. Philadelphia, Lippincott-Raven, 1997:273–289.
5. Teasdale GM, Graham DI. Craniocerebral trauma: protection and retrieval of the neuronal population after injury. Neurosurgery 1998;43:723–737.
6. Luer MS, Rhoney DH, Hughes M, Hatton J. New pharmacologic strategies for acute neuronal injury. Pharmacotherapy 1996;16:830–848.
7. Bouma GJ, Muizelaar JP, Choi SC, et al. Cerebral circulation and metabolism after severe traumatic brain injury: the elusive role of ischemia. J Neurosurg 1991;75:685–693.
8. Smith DH, McIntosh TJ. Traumatic brain injury and excitatory amino acids. In: Narayan RK, Wilberger JE Jr, Povlishock JT, eds. Neurotrauma. New York, McGraw-Hill, 1996:1445–1458.
9. Young W. Death by calcium: A way of life. In: Narayan RK, Wilberger JE Jr, Povlishock JT, eds. Neurotrauma. New York, McGraw-Hill, 1996:1421–1431.
10. Hall ED. Free radicals and lipid peroxidation. In: Narayan RK, Wilberger JE Jr, Povlishock JT, eds. Neurotrauma. New York, McGraw-Hill, 1996:1405–1419.
11. Hsu CY, Hu ZY, Doster SK. Cell-mediated injury. In: Narayan RK, Wilberger JE Jr, Povlishock JT, eds. Neurotrauma. New York, McGraw-Hill, 1996:1433–1444.
12. Jennett B, Teasdale G. Aspects of coma after severe head injury. Lancet 1977;1:878–881.
13. Kelly DF, Doberstein C, Becker DP. General principles of head injury management. In: Narayan RK, Wilberger JE Jr, Povlishock JT, eds. Neurotrauma. New York, McGraw-Hill, 1996:71–101.
14. Valadka AB, Narayan RK. Emergency room management of the head-injured patient. In: Narayan RK, Wilberger JE Jr, Povlishock JT, eds. Neurotrauma. New York, McGraw-Hill, 1996:119–135.
15. Signorini DF, Andrews PJ, Jones PA, et al. Predicting survival using simple clinical variables: A case study in traumatic brain injury. J Neurol Neurosurg Psychiatry 1999;66:20–25.
16. Bullock R, Chesnut RM, Clifton GL, et al. Guidelines for the management of severe head injury. Brain Trauma Foundation, American Association of Neurological Surgeons, Joint Section on Neurotrauma and Critical Care. J Neurotrauma 1996;13:641–734.
17. Marion DW, Spiegel TP. Changes in the management of severe traumatic brain injury: 1991–1997. Crit Care Med 2000;28:16–18.
18. Brain Trauma Foundation. The American Association of Neurological Surgeons. The Joint Section on Neurotrauma and Critical Care. Management and prognosis of severe traumatic brain injury. J Neurotrauma 2000;17:449–627.
19. Alderson P, Roberts I. Corticosteroids for acute traumatic brain injury. Cochrane Database Syst Rev 2000;2.
20. Langham J, Goldfrad C, Teasdale G, et al. Calcium channel blockers for acute traumatic brain injury. Cochrane Database Syst Rev 2000;2.
21. Roberts I. Barbiturates for acute traumatic brain injury. Cochrane Database Syst Rev 2000;2.
22. Schierhout G, Roberts I. Antiepileptic drugs for preventing seizures following acute traumatic brain injury. Cochrane Database Syst Rev 2000;2.
23. Schierhout G, Roberts I. Mannitol for acute traumatic brain injury. Cochrane Database Syst Rev 2000;2.
24. Schierhout G, Roberts I. Hyperventilation therapy for acute traumatic brain injury. Cochrane Database Syst Rev 2000;2.
25. Signorini DF, Alderson P. Therapeutic hypothermia for head injury. Cochrane Database Syst Rev 2000;2.
26. Freshman SP, Battistella FD, Matteucci M, Wisner DH. Hypertonic saline (7.5%) versus mannitol: a comparison for treatment of acute head injuries. J Trauma 1993;35:344–348.
27. Qureshi AI, Suarez JI, Castro A, Bhardwaj A. Use of hypertonic saline/acetate infusion in treatment of cerebral edema in patients with head trauma: experience at a single center. J Trauma 1999;47:659–665.
28. Shackford SR, Bourguignon PR, Wald SL, et al. Hypertonic saline resuscitation of patients with head injury: A prospective, randomized clinical trial. J Trauma 1998;44:50–58.
29. Cruz J. The first decade of continuous monitoring of jugular bulb oxyhemoglobin saturation: Management strategies and clinical outcome. Crit Care Med 1998;26:344–351.
30. Woodman T, Robertson CS. Jugular venous oxygen saturation monitoring. In: Narayan RK, Wilberger JE Jr, Povlishock JT, eds. Neurotrauma. New York, McGraw-Hill, 1996:519–537.
31. Lang EW, Chesnut RM. Intracranial pressure and cerebral perfusion pressure in severe head injury. New Horiz 1995;3:400–409.
32. Juul N, Morris GF, Marshall SB, Marshall LF. Intracranial hypertension and cerebral perfusion pressure: Influence on neurological deterioration and outcome in severe head injury. The Executive Committee of the International Selfotel Trial. J Neurosurg 2000;92:1–6.
33. Bouma GJ, Muizelaar JP, Bandoh K, Marmarou A. Blood pressure and intracranial pressure-volume dynamics in severe head injury: Relationship with cerebral blood flow. J Neurosurg 1992;77:15–19.
34. Duhaime AC. Conventional drug therapies for head injury. In: Narayan RK, Wilberger JE Jr, Povlishock JT, eds. Neurotrauma. New York, McGraw-Hill, 1996:365–374.
35. Chesnut RM. Treating raised intracranial pressure in head injury. In: Narayan RK, Wilberger JE Jr, Povlishock JT, eds. Neurotrauma. New York, McGraw-Hill, 1996:445–469.
36. Tipps LB, Coplin WM, Murry KR, Rhoney DH. Safety and feasibility of continuous infusion of remifentanil in the neurosurgical intensive care unit. Neurosurgery 2000;46:596–601.
37. Kelly DF, Goodale DB, Williams J, et al. Propofol in the treatment of moderate and severe head injury: A randomized, prospective, double-blinded pilot trial. J Neurosurg 1999;90:1042–1052.
38. Hsiang JK, Chesnut RM, Crisp CB, et al. Early, routine paralysis for intracranial pressure control in severe head injury: Is it necessary? Crit Care Med 1994;22:1471–1476.
39. Gopinath SP, Robertson CS, Contant CF, et al. Jugular venous desaturation and outcome after head injury. J Neurol Neurosurg Psychiatry 1994;57:717–723.
40. Diringer MN, Yundt K, Videen TO, et al. No reduction in cerebral metabolism as a result of early moderate hyperventilation following severe traumatic brain injury. J Neurosurg 2000;92:7–13.
41. Roberts I, Schierhout G, Alderson P. Absence of evidence for the effectiveness of five interventions routinely used in the intensive care management of severe head injury: A systematic review. J Neurol Neurosurg Psychiatry 1998;65:729–733.
42. Clifton GL, Hayes RL. Hypothermia for the treatment of head injury. In: Narayan RK, Wilberger JE Jr, Povlishock JT, eds. Neurotrauma. New York, McGraw-Hill, 1996:401–412.

43. Marion DW, Penrod LE, Kelsey SF, et al. Treatment of traumatic brain injury with moderate hypothermia. N Engl J Med 1997;336:540–546.
44. Shiozaki T, Kato A, Taneda M, et al. Little benefit from mild hypothermia therapy for severely head injured patients with low intracranial pressure. J Neurosurg 1999;91:185–191.
45. Shiozaki T, Sugimoto H, Taneda M, et al. Selection of severely head injured patients for mild hypothermia therapy. J Neurosurg 1998;89: 206–211.
46. Clifton GL, Miller ER, Choi SC, et al. Lack of effect of induction of hypothermia after acute brain injury. N Engl J Med 2001;344:556–563.
47. Metz C, Holzschuh M, Bein T, et al. Moderate hypothermia in patients with severe head injury: Cerebral and extracerebral effects. J Neurosurg 1996;85:533–541.
48. Ghajar J, Hariri RJ, Narayan RK, et al. Survey of critical care management of comatose, head-injured patients in the United States. Crit Care Med 1995;23:560–567.
49. Alderson P, Roberts I. Corticosteroids in acute traumatic brain injury: Systematic review of randomised controlled trials. Br Med J 1997;314: 1855–1859.
50. Roberts I. Design of CRASH trial: Trial is best way to elucidate effectiveness of corticosteroids in acute severe head injury. Br Med J 1999;319:1069.
51. Eisenberg HM, Frankowski RF, Contant CF, et al. High-dose barbiturate control of elevated intracranial pressure in patients with severe head injury. J Neurosurg 1988;69:15–23.
52. Temkin NR, Dikmen SS, Wilensky AJ, et al. A randomized, double-blind study of phenytoin for the prevention of posttraumatic seizures. N Engl J Med 1990;323:497–502.
53. Haltiner AM, Newell DW, Temkin NR, et al. Side effects and mortality associated with use of phenytoin for early posttraumatic seizure prophylaxis. J Neurosurg 1999;91:588–592.
54. Temkin NR, Dikmen SS, Anderson GD, et al. Valproate therapy for prevention of posttraumatic seizures: A randomized trial. J Neurosurg 1999;91:593–600.
55. Andrews BT. Fluid and electrolyte management in the head-injured patient. In: Narayan RK, Wilberger JE Jr, Povlishock JT, eds. Neurotrauma. New York, McGraw-Hill, 1996:331–344.
56. Polderman KH, Bloemers FW, Peerdeman SM, Girbes AR. Hypomagnesemia and hypophosphatemia at admission in patients with severe head injury. Crit Care Med 2000;28:2022–2025.
57. Young B, Ott L. Nutritional and metabolic management of the head-injured patient. In: Narayan RK, Wilberger JE Jr, Povlishock JT, eds. Neurotrauma. New York, McGraw-Hill, 1996, pp 345–363.
58. Girou E, Stephan F, Novara A, et al. Risk factors and outcome of nosocomial infections: Results of a matched case-control study of ICU patients. Am J Respir Crit Care Med 1998;157:1151–1158.
59. Greenberg SB, Atmar RL. Infectious complications after head injury. In: Narayan RK, Wilberger JE Jr, Povlishock JT, eds. Neurotrauma. New York, McGraw-Hill, 1996:703–722.
60. Heard SO, Fink MP, Gamelli RL, et al. Effect of prophylactic administration of recombinant human granulocyte colony-stimulating factor (filgrastim) on the frequency of nosocomial infections in patients with acute traumatic brain injury or cerebral hemorrhage. The Filgrastim Study Group. Crit Care Med 1998;26:748–754.
61. Ishikawa K, Tanaka H, Takaoka M, et al. Granulocyte colony-stimulating factor ameliorates life-threatening infections after combined therapy with barbiturates and mild hypothermia in patients with severe head injuries. J Trauma 1999;46:999–1007.
62. Lazio BE, Simard JM. Anticoagulation in neurosurgical patients. Neurosurgery 1999;45:838–847.
63. Bruder N, Raynal M, Pellissier D, et al. Influence of body temperature, with or without sedation, on energy expenditure in severe head-injured patients. Crit Care Med 1998;26:568–572.
64. Bullock MR, Lyeth BG, Muizelaar JP. Current status of neuroprotection trials for traumatic brain injury: Lessons from animal models and clinical studies. Neurosurgery 1999;45:207–217.
65. Teasdale GM, Maas A, Iannotti F, et al. Challenges in translating the efficacy of neuroprotective agents in experimental models into knowledge of clinical benefits in head injured patients. Acta Neurochir Suppl 1999;73:111–116.
66. Dickinson K, Bunn F, Wentz R, et al. Size and quality of randomised controlled trials in head injury: Review of published studies. Br Med J 2000;320:1308–1311.
67. Doppenberg EM, Choi SC, Bullock R. Clinical trials in traumatic brain injury: What can we learn from previous studies? Ann NY Acad Sci 1997;825:305–322.
68. Maas AI, Steyerberg EW, Murray GD, et al. Why have recent trials of neuroprotective agents in head injury failed to show convincing efficacy? A pragmatic analysis and theoretical considerations. Neurosurgery 1999;44:1286–1298.
69. Murray GD, Teasdale GM, Schmitz H. Nimodipine in traumatic subarachnoid haemorrhage: A reanalysis of the HIT I and HIT II trials. Acta Neurochir 1996;138:1163–1167.
70. Harders A, Kakarieka A, Braakman R. Traumatic subarachnoid hemorrhage and its treatment with nimodipine. German tSAH Study Group. J Neurosurg 1996;85:82–89.
71. Morris GF, Bullock R, Marshall SB, et al. Failure of the competitive *N*-methyl-D-aspartate antagonist Selfotel (CGS 19755) in the treatment of severe head injury: Results of two phase III clinical trials. The Selfotel Investigators. J Neurosurg 1999;91:737–743.
72. Merchant RE, Bullock MR, Carmack CA, et al. A double-blind, placebo controlled study of the safety, tolerability and pharmacokinetics of CP-101,606 in patients with a mild or moderate traumatic brain injury. Ann NY Acad Sci 1999;890:42–50.
73. Marshall LF, Maas AI, Marshall SB, et al. A multicenter trial on the efficacy of using tirilazad mesylate in cases of head injury. J Neurosurg 1998;89:519–525.
74. Muizelaar JP, Marmarou A, Young HF, et al. Improving the outcome of severe head injury with the oxygen radical scavenger polyethylene glycol-conjugated superoxide dismutase: A phase II trial. J Neurosurg 1993;78:375–382.
75. Young B, Runge JW, Waxman KS, et al. Effects of pegorgotein on neurologic outcome of patients with severe head injury: A multicenter, randomized controlled trial. JAMA 1996;276:538–543.
76. Slavik RS, Rhoney DH. Indomethacin: A review of its cerebral blood flow effects and potential use for controlling intracranial pressure in traumatic brain injury patients. Neurol Res 1999;21:491–499.
77. Scheff SW, Sullivan PG. Cyclosporin A significantly ameliorates cortical damage following experimental traumatic brain injury in rodents. J Neurotrauma 1999;16:783–792.
78. Marmarou A, Nichols J, Burgess J, et al. Effects of the bradykinin antagonist Bradycor (deltibant, CP-1027) in severe traumatic brain injury: Results of a multicenter, randomized, placebo-controlled trial. American Brain Injury Consortium Study Group. J Neurotrauma 1999;16:431–444.
79. Hatton J, Rapp RP, Kudsk KA, et al. Intravenous insulin-like growth factor-I (IGF-I) in moderate-to-severe head injury: A phase II safety and efficacy trial. J Neurosurg 1997;86:779–786.
80. Faden AI. Pharmacologic treatment approaches for brain and spinal cord trauma. In: Narayan RK, Wilberger JE Jr, Povlishock JT, eds. Neurotrauma. New York, McGraw-Hill, 1996:1479–1490.
81. Jennett B, Bond M. Assessment of outcome after severe brain damage. Lancet 1975;1:480–484.
82. Choi SC, Marmarou A, Bullock R, et al. Primary end points in phase III clinical trials of severe head trauma: DRS versus GOS. The American Brain Injury Consortium Study Group. J Neurotrauma 1998;15:771–776.
83. Rappaport M, Hall KM, Hopkins K, et al. Disability rating scale for severe head trauma: Coma to community. Arch Phys Med Rehabil 1982;63: 118–123.
84. Hannay HJ, Sherer M. Assessment of outcome from head injury. In: Narayan RK, Wilberger JE Jr, Povlishock JT, eds. Neurotrauma. New York, McGraw-Hill, 1996:723–747.
85. Miller TR, Lestina DC. Patterns in U.S. medical expenditures and utilization for injury, 1987. Am J Public Health 1996;86:89–93.
86. Spain DA, McIlvoy LH, Fix SE, et al. Effect of a clinical pathway for severe traumatic brain injury on resource utilization. J Trauma 1998;45:101–104; discussion 104–105.

59

PARKINSON'S DISEASE

Merlin V. Nelson, Richard C. Berchou and Peter A. LeWitt

While its clinical manifestations previously had escaped attention, *paralysis agitans* had an unmistakable presence following the 1817 publication by an obscure British physician, James Parkinson.[1] Parkinson provided vivid descriptions of such features as an "involuntary tremulous motion" and the tendency to "pass from a walking to a running pace." Later observers added a variety of signs and symptoms, among them rigidity and instability of balance, to define idiopathic Parkinson's disease (IPD) as we know it today.

EPIDEMIOLOGY

The annual incidence of IPD increases with age from about 20 per 100,000 in the fifth decade of life to about 90 per 100,000 in the seventh decade of life, with the usual age of onset at about age 60.[2] Extensive research into the epidemiology of IPD suggests that environmental factors such as rural living, drinking well water, and heavy metal and hydrocarbon exposure may contribute to the cause.[3,4] Interestingly, cigarette smoking and caffeine consumption are associated with a slight protection against the illness.[5,6]

The onset of IPD in later life implies that cumulative exposures to putative toxins, factors associated with central nervous system aging, or other as yet uncharacterized cell death mechanisms may be responsible for the onset and progression of the disease. While IPD is sporadic in most instances, genetic factors also may have a role in its etiology, particularly if the disease begins before age 50.[7] Mutations in *α-synuclein* (a presynaptic protein) and *parkin* genes have been identified in autosomal-dominant and autosomal-recessive kindreds, respectively, with early-onset familial Parkinson's disease, but phenotypes and pathologic findings are different from those in IPD.[8,9]

ETIOLOGY

The pathogenesis of IPD is not known. Neurotoxins highly selective to substantia nigra pars compacta (SNc) dopaminergic neurons are instructive because animal models of parkinsonism can be created with 6-hydroxydopamine and with 1-methyl-4-phenyl-1,2,3,6-tetrahydropyridine (MPTP). The latter compound is converted by monoamine oxidase (MAO) type B to the toxic 1-methyl-4-phenylpyridinium (MPP^+) ion. Oxidase inhibition by selegiline eliminates the toxicity of MPTP. MPP^+ is toxic to neurons by interfering with mitochondrial metabolism. Another controversial mechanism of toxicity that has received consideration for the pathogenesis of IPD is cellular damage from oxyradicals.[10,11] Dopamine metabolism generates free radicals from autooxidation and from MAO metabolism (Fig. 59–1). Several antioxidative mechanisms are present within and outside neurons to limit any damage that might be produced by free-radical attack, but it is possible that such protection might be overwhelmed or impaired in IPD.

PATHOPHYSIOLOGY

Dopaminergic projections from the SNc to the striatum (putamen and caudate) synapse on two populations of efferent neurons[12] (Fig. 59–2). The direct pathway involves activation of striatal D_1 dopamine receptors that stimulate inhibitory gamma-aminobutyric acid (GABA)/substance P efferents to the globus pallidus interna (GPi) and substantia nigra pars reticulata (SNr). The indirect pathway involves activation of striatal D_2 dopamine receptors that inhibit inhibitory GABA/enkephalin efferents to the globus pallidus externa (GPe). The GPe projects inhibitory GABA neurons to the subthalamic nucleus (STN). Here, excitatory glutaminergic neurons project to the GPi. GPi output is inhibitory on the ventroanterior and ventrolateral thalamic projections to the frontal cortex. Thus loss of nigrostriatal dopamine neurons in IPD results in reduction of cortical activation (see Fig. 59–2). Virtually all the motor deficits of IPD are attributable to the marked loss in dopaminergic neurons projecting to the putamen.

In reality, the pathways and interactions involved are even more complex than those described but are beyond the scope of this text.[13] The synaptic organization of the basal ganglia involves a variety of neurotransmitters, including acetylcholine, dopamine, GABA, glutamate, substance P, and serotonin. These are all possible targets for interventions in IPD. Drugs enhancing dopaminergic neurotransmission and inhibiting acetylcholine effects have been successful in IPD therapeutics; the role for drug modulation of other neurotransmitters active in the basal ganglia has not been explored completely.

The model of dopaminergic depletion or blockade in producing parkinsonian features provided much of the impetus for development of therapies to augment stimulation of striatal dopamine receptors. Stimulation of D_1 dopamine receptors activates adenylate cyclase. D_2 dopamine receptors are coupled to a guanosine triphosphate (GTP)-binding protein that opens potassium channels to hyperpolarize neurons, thereby reducing the excitability of striatal cells.[14] In IPD, activation of the D_2 receptor appears to be of primary importance for mediating both clinical improvements and some adverse effects (such as hallucinations). Dyskinesias are more likely to occur with L-dopa therapy (D_1 and D_2 agonism) than with dopamine agonist therapy (primarily D_2 agonism), suggesting D_1 receptor involvement in producing dyskinesia.

Pathologic findings reveal a markedly decreased number of nigrostriatal dopamine neurons and a positive correlation between the degree of nigrostriatal dopamine loss and the severity of clinical features. The threshold for onset of parkinsonism appears to be the loss of 80% or more of these neurons.[15] [^{18}F]Fluorodopa positron-emission studies clearly demonstrate decreased uptake and use of fluorodopa in IPD.[16] A compensatory increase in striatal dopamine receptors in response to decreased dopamine release has not been supported by positron-emission studies that have shown no difference in dopamine receptor density between sides in hemiparkinsonian subjects.[17] Progressive supranuclear palsy (PSP) and other "Parkinson-plus" disorders are not responsive to dopamine replacement or dopamine agonist

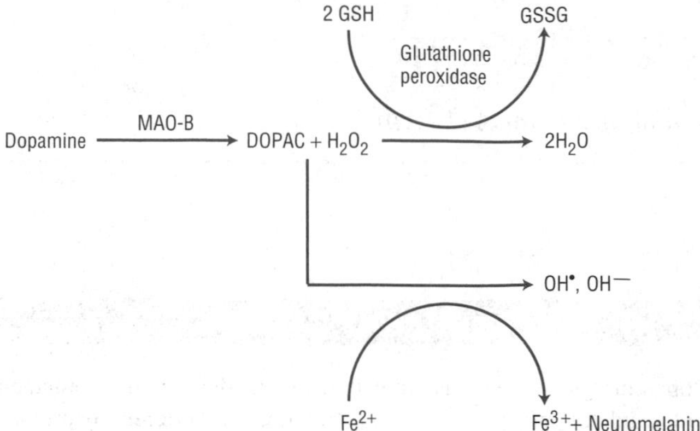

FIGURE 59–1. Dopamine metabolism results in hydrogen peroxide (H_2O_2) formation. If the glutathione system is deficient or excess hydrogen peroxide is present, hydrogen peroxide accepts an electron from ferrous iron (Fe^{2+}) forming ferric iron (Fe^{3+}) and the hydroxyl free radical (OH*). The hydroxyl free radical can cause lipid peroxidation, thereby damaging neuronal cell membranes. MAO-B = monoamine oxidase B; DOPAC =3,4-dihydroxyphenylacetic acid; H_2O = water; GSH = glutathione; GSSG = glutathione disulfide; OH^- = the hydroxide ion.

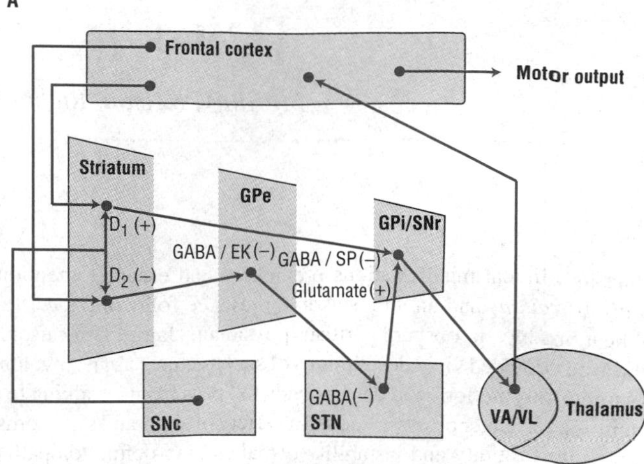

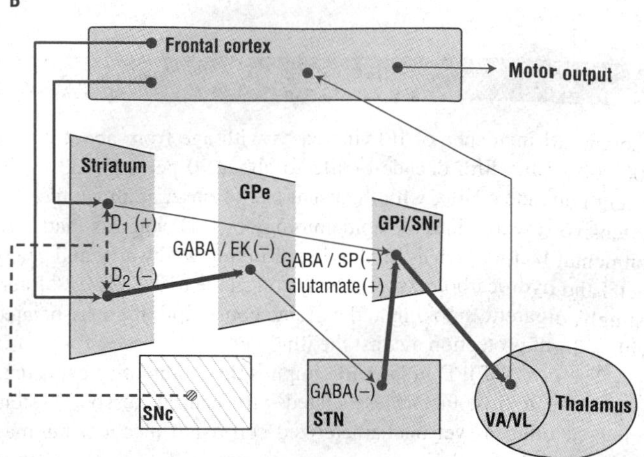

FIGURE 59–2. *A.* The normal balance of the basal ganglia-thalamocortical circuit. GPe = globus pallidus externa; GPi = globus pallidus interna; SNr = substantia nigra pars reticulata; SNc = substantia nigra pars compacta; VA = ventroanterior and VL = ventrolateral nuclei of the thalamus; STN = subthalamic nucleus. *B.* With nigrostriatal degeneration (dashed line), there is loss of inhibition of the GPi by the direct pathway and activation of the GPi via the indirect pathway resulting in decreased activation of the cortex. See text for full details.

therapies, presumably on the basis of decreased dopamine receptors due to damage to postsynaptic elements and other neuropathologic changes beyond those found in IPD.

Dopamine metabolism is shown in Figure 59–3, and the range of therapeutic interventions for IPD are summarized in Table 59–1. Tyrosine, the metabolic precursor of dopamine, is converted by tyrosine hydroxylase (TH) to L-dihydroxyphenylalanine (L-dopa) in a highly regulated synthetic process. L-Dopa is decarboxylated to dopamine by the enzyme L-amino acid decarboxylase (L-AAD). L-AAD is present outside the central nervous system and in some nonaminergic neurons, whereas TH is found exclusively in aminergic neurons. Peripheral L-AAD can be blocked by administering antagonists such as carbidopa or benserazide that do not pass the blood-brain barrier. Use of these drugs with L-dopa increases the central nervous system penetration of exogenously administered L-dopa and decreases adverse effects from the peripheral metabolism to dopamine. Dopamine is stored in synaptic vesicles until stimulated to be released into the synapse by calcium-dependent mechanisms. Dopamine activity is terminated primarily by reuptake into the presynaptic neuron by means of a specific dopamine transporter. In the presynaptic neurons, sequestration into the storage granules or the actions of catabolic pathways involving MAO or catechol-*O*-methyltransferase (COMT) lead to inactivation of dopamine.

Since dopamine tonically inhibits acetylcholine neurons in the striatum, the degeneration of nigrostriatal dopamine neurons results in a relative increase of striatal cholinergic interneuron activity. This increased cholinergic activity contributes especially to the tremor of IPD, as evidenced by symptomatic improvement with the use of anticholinergics and worsening with cholinergic agents.

IPD has a characteristic neuropathologic picture that permits differentiation from similar clinical syndromes. In the SNc, loss of neurons and the Lewy body (a neuronal inclusion body composed of amyloid neurofilaments) are always found. Lewy bodies appear in degenerating neurons in association with adjacent gliosis. The loss of pars compacta neurons is the basis for loss of dopamine projections to the striatum. Lewy bodies can be found in other neurologic disorders and in normal aging. The occurrence of Lewy bodies in patients without parkinsonism indicates that the disease can exist as a pathologic entity with less involvement than necessary for causing clinical signs and symptoms (incidental Parkinson's disease). Even patients whose clinical features strongly suggest IPD may lack its characteristic pathology.

CLINICAL PRESENTATION

While the disorder is unmistakable in its advanced form, distinguishing mild IPD from changes seen with normal aging can be challenging. Diagnostic criteria specify that at least two of the following be present: limb muscle rigidity, resting tremor (at 3–6 Hz and abolished by movement), bradykinesia, or postural instability.[18] For the diagnosis of IPD, other conditions must be excluded (Table 59–2). Medication-induced parkinsonism can mimic the idiopathic disorder, so it is important to establish if such medications have been used (e.g., antipsychotics, antiemetics, or metoclopramide). Several neurodegenerative conditions resemble the clinical picture of IPD, including PSP, striatonigral degeneration, olivopontocerebellar degeneration, and rarely, Huntington's or Wilson's disease. In order to distinguish IPD from secondary parkinsonism, other diagnostic

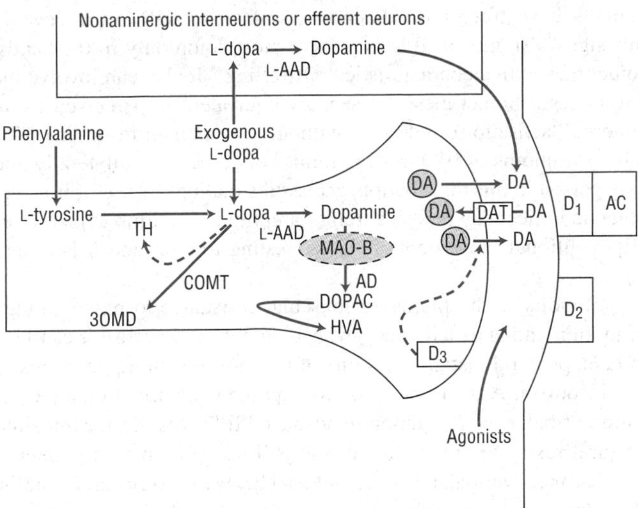

FIGURE 59–3. Dopamine metabolism in presynaptic dopamine neuron (see text for full details). 3OMD = 3-*O*-methyldopa; AC = adenylate cyclase; AD = aldehyde dehydrogenase; COMT = catechol-*O*-methyl transferase; D1–D3 = dopamine receptors; DA = dopamine; DAT = dopamine transporter; DOPAC = 3,4-dihydroxyphenylacetic acid; HVA = homovanillic acid; L-AAD = L-aromatic amine decarboxylase; MAO-B = monoamine oxidase B; TH = tyrosine hydroxylase.

criteria include lack of other neurologic impairments and responsiveness to L-dopa.

IPD develops insidiously and progresses slowly in most patients, although progression sometimes arrests. Initial complaints may include sensory symptoms, but as the disease progresses, the patient exhibits one or more classic clinical features: resting tremor, rigidity, bradykinesia, or change in posture. Characteristic problems, even in mildly affected patients, include small handwriting (micrographia), decreased facial animation (hypomimia) and blink rate, diminished arm swing while walking, shuffling gait, soft or indistinct speech (hypophonia), and decreased dexterity in everyday activities. Symptoms can progress to severe functional impairment, where patients require nursing home placement and are confined to bed or wheelchair.

Other clinical characteristics of IPD are listed in Table 59–3. Bradykinesia refers to slowness of movement. Movement in IPD is often slow throughout an intended action, but initiation of movement may display a hesitation out of proportion to slowness affecting completion of the movement. A progressive slowing and decline in dexterity with repetition may impair tasks such as finger tapping. Intermittent immobility (*freezing*) is another common characteristic. Freezing is especially likely to occur in situations such as when walking in a crowd or when walking through a narrow doorway. Patients also may experience a slow shuffling gait with difficulty halting their steps while walking, or *festination*.

The pathophysiology of bradykinesia appears to be an impairment in the execution of learned or semireflex sequential motor plans. This has been attributed to a disconnection between basal ganglia structures and the supplementary motor cortex. Many inputs influence the functioning of this system. For example, bradykinesia can on occasion be reversed by sudden changes in emotional state. This type of response, termed *kinesia paradoxica,* suggests that the intrinsic program for movement is intact in IPD.

Tremor occurring at rest is highly typical of IPD and often is the sole presenting complaint; however, only two-thirds of parkinsonian

TABLE 59–1. Mechanisms for Potential IPD Treatments

Increase Endogenous Dopamine
L-Dopa
- Inhibit peripheral metabolism by dopa decarboxylase
  - Carbidopa
  - Benserazide
- Sustained-release products
- Infusions
  - Intravenous
  - Duodenal/jejunal
- Inhibit catechol-*O*-methyl-transferase
  - Entacapone (peripheral only)
  - Tolcapone (peripheral and central)
- Inhibit central and peripheral metabolism by monoamine oxidase B
  - Selegiline (deprenyl)

Dopamine Agonists
D_2-specific
- Bromocriptine
- Lisuride
- Cabergoline

D_2- and D_3-specific
- Pramipexole
- Ropinirole

D_1- and D_2-nonspecific
- Pergolide
- Apomorphine
  - Intravenous
  - Subcutaneous infusions
  - Intranasal
  - Sublingual

Partial agonists
- Terguride

Anticholinergic
Benztropine
Trihexyphenidyl

TABLE 59–2. Differential Diagnosis of Parkinsonism

Idiopathic parkinsonism (Parkinson's disease, Lewy body parkinsonism)
Secondary parkinsonism
- Drug-induced
  - Antipsychotics (phenothiazines, butyrophenones, risperidone, others)
  - Antiemetics (metoclopramide, prochlorperazine)
  - Other drugs (reserpine, alpha-methyldopa)
- Toxic
  - Carbon monoxide poisoning
  - Hydrogen sulfide
  - Manganese
  - Methanol
  - MPTP (1-methyl-4-phenyl-1-2-5-6-tetrahydropyridine)
  - Petrochemicals
- Neoplasms or strokes in the regions of the nigrostriatal pathways
- Traumatic lesions interrupting substantia nigra projections
- Normal pressure hydrocephalus

Parkinsonism with other neuronal system degenerations
- Wilson's disease (copper deposition in the brain)
- Progressive supranuclear palsy
- Pallidonigral degeneration
- Corticobasalganglionic degeneration
- Alzheimer's disease
- Multiple system atrophy
  - Striatonigral degeneration
  - Shy-Drager syndrome
  - Olivopontocerebellar atrophy

TABLE 59–3. Clinical Features

Primary
Bradykinesia
Postural instability
Resting tremor (may have postural and action components)
Rigidity
Motor Symptoms
Decreased dexterity
Dysarthria
Dysphagia
Festinating gait
Flexed posture
"Freezing" at initiation of movement
Hypomimia
Hypophonia
Micrographia
Slow turning
Autonomic Symptoms
Bladder and anal sphincter disturbances
Constipation
Diaphoresis
Orthostatic blood pressure changes
Paroxysmal flushing
Sexual disturbances
Mental Status Changes
Confusional state
Dementia
Psychosis (paranoia, hallucinosis)
Sleep disturbance
Other
Fatiguability
Oily skin
Pedal edema
Seborrhea
Weight loss

patients have tremor on diagnosis, and some will never develop this sign.[19] Tremor in IPD is present most commonly in the hands, sometimes with a characteristic "pill-rolling." It also can involve the jaw or legs. Sometimes, the sensory equivalent is perceived as an "internal" sensation of vibration without outward manifestations. Like other symptoms of IPD, resting tremor often begins unilaterally and may persist in this distribution. Stressful situations or use of limbs in other activities may increase tremor amplitude in a limb at rest. Usually, volitional movement abolishes resting tremor, and it is absent during sleep.

Rigidity is the increased muscular resistance to passive range of motion and is usually "cog-wheel" in nature. Because it can lead to falls, postural instability is one of the most disabling problems of parkinsonism. A disturbance of appropriate responses to the perturbation of balance is common in advanced IPD. Testing for impaired postural responses by means of the pull test (in which a patient is unable to recover balance after sudden backward displacement at the shoulders) can help to identify the risk for falling. Many patients with impaired postural responses also have tendencies for propulsive gait (festination) and a forward flexed posture of their axial structures along with partial flexion of the extremities.

IPD is predominantly a disorder of motor capabilities; however, neuropsychological abnormalities can be detected even in patients with early or mild forms of the disorder with full cognitive abilities. Although intellectual deterioration is not inevitable in IPD, some patients deteriorate in a manner indistinguishable from Alzheimer's disease and other dementing conditions. It is difficult to estimate the number of patients at risk because medications and concomitant illnesses can confound analysis of the degree of cognitive decline due specifically to IPD. IPD patients are also at increased risk for depression. While the disabilities of IPD may provoke some instances of depression, the biochemical changes in the brain due to IPD also may predispose for endogenous depression.

▶ TREATMENT: Parkinson's Disease

SURGICAL THERAPY

The most promising surgical technique at this time is deep brain stimulation (DBS) of the GPi and STN, which decreases outflow from these areas (as shown in Fig. 59–2*B*) and thus reduces input to the thalamus.[20] Thalamic DBS and thalamotomy (focal destructive lesion of the thalamus) can reduce disabling tremor. Pallidotomy (a focal destructive lesion of the GPi) and GPi DBS can help with severe dyskinesias and on/off fluctuations but is not as helpful for bradykinesia. STN DBS may provide the most improvement in bradykinesia but is still investigational. Destructive lesions are immediate and permanent, whereas DBS requires lifelong maintenance. Transplantation of autologous adrenal medulla tissue has been abandoned, and fetal tissue transplants are still investigational.

PHARMACOLOGIC THERAPY

Treatment algorithms for early and advanced IPD are shown in Figures 59–4 and 59–5; however, more complete algorithms covering virtually every aspect of IPD management have been published.[21] The optimal management of IPD is best determined by individualized considerations of a patient's disability. The only established pharmacologic therapy for IPD is medication that can transiently reverse signs and symptoms. Vitamin E (2000 IU/day) and other agents aimed at neuroprotection have not proven useful in preventing progression of the disease. In patients with mild features of IPD, use of symptomatic medications often is not needed if disabilities have not evolved. Many patients with nothing more than mild slowness and resting tremor often can be managed effectively with only anticholinergics or amantadine.

The most efficacious treatment for IPD is replacement of the natural neurotransmitter dopamine by the use of its immediate precursor, L-dopa. Although L-dopa is more effective than other medications currently available, there has been concern with possible long-term risks. Some clinicians minimize use of L-dopa for this reason. As indicated in the treatment algorithm shown in Figure 59–4, anticholinergic drugs or amantadine can be used for treating resting tremor as an alternative to L-dopa. Long-acting propranolol (160 mg/day), an effective agent in essential tremor, also has shown benefit in parkinsonian tremor; however, primidone (250 mg/day) and clonazepam (4 mg/day) have not.[22] While not highly effective against bradykinesia, gait disturbance, or other features of advanced parkinsonism, these medications can be useful for relieving mild disabilities experienced by patients in the first few years after the onset of parkinsonism. The decision to incorporate L-dopa or dopamine

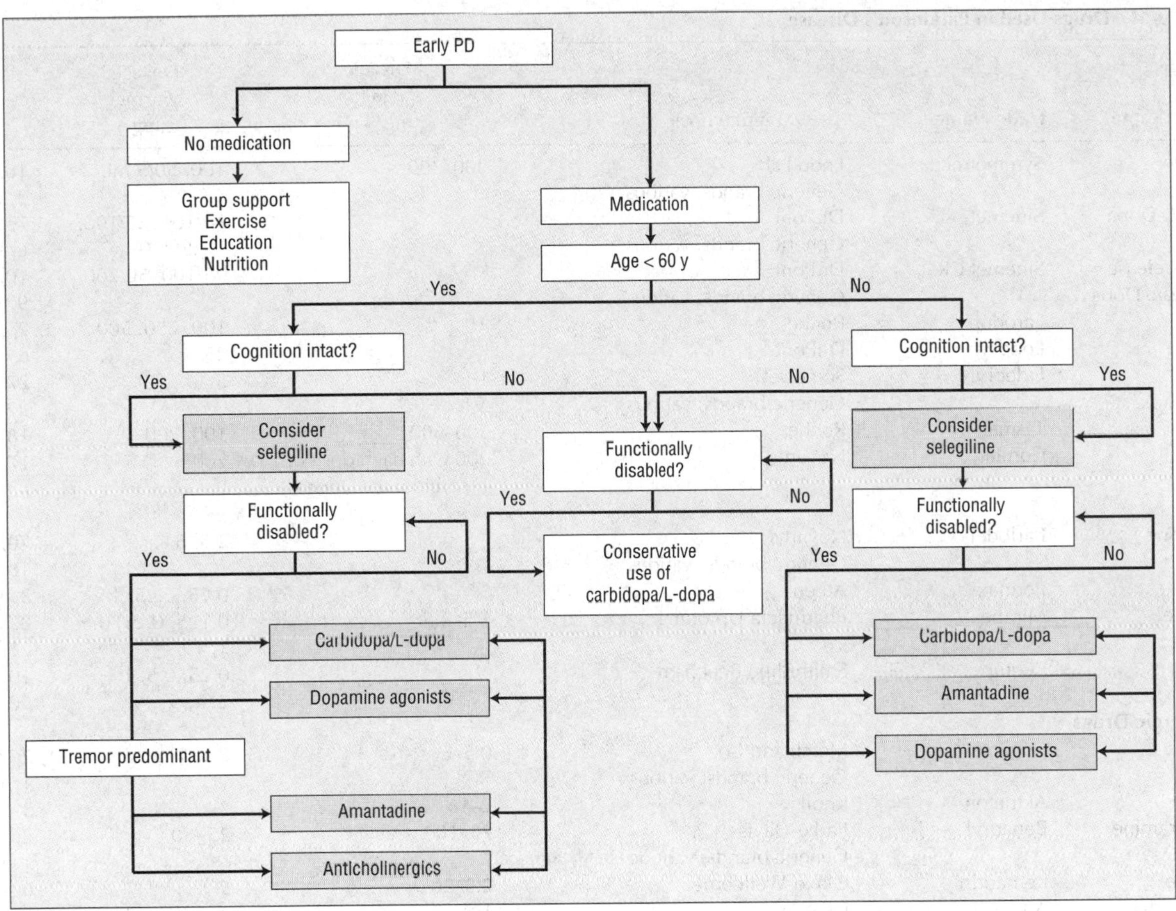

FIGURE 59–4. General algorithm for treating early IPD.

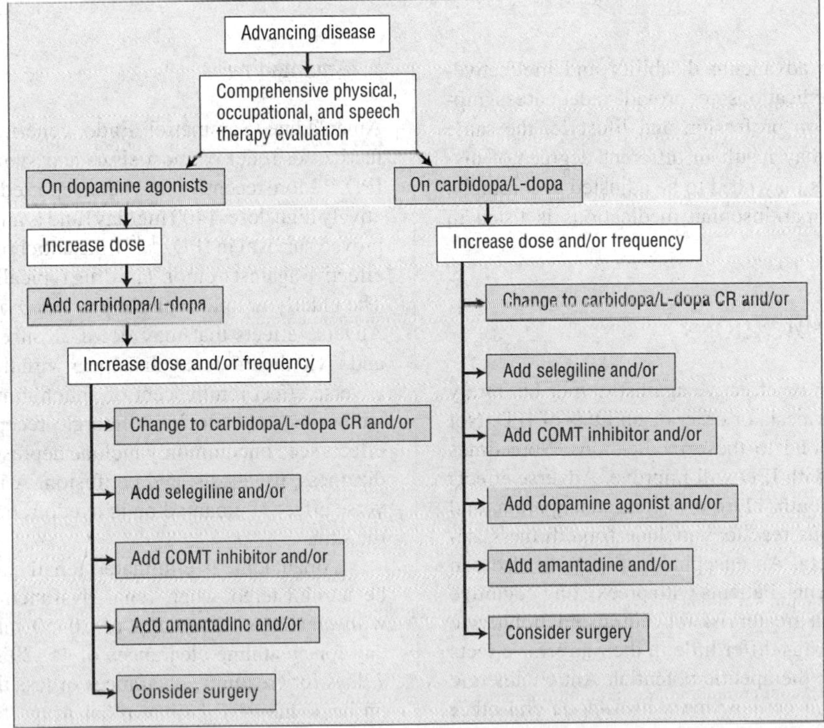

FIGURE 59–5. Algorithm for treating advanced IPD.

TABLE 59–4. Drugs Used in Parkinson's Disease

Generic Name	Trade Name	Manufacturer	Dosage Range (mg/day)	Dosage Forms (mg)	Cost Index[a]
Amantadine	Symmetrel	Endo Labs	200–300	100, 50/5 mL	10, 10
		Generic brands, various			3, 6
Carbidopa/L-Dopa	Sinemet	DuPont	[b]	10/100, 25/100, 25/250	7, 8, 10
		Generic brands, various			6, 6, 8
Controlled-release carbidopa/L-Dopa	Sinemet CR	DuPont	[b]	25/100, 50/200	10, 19,
		Generic brands, various			9, 17
L-Dopa	Larodopa	Roche	[b]	100, 250, 500	2, 3, 6
Carbidopa	Lodosyn	DuPont	[b]	25	6
Selegiline	Eldepryl	Somerset	10	5	27
		Generic brands, various			22
Tolcapone	Tasmar	Roche	300–600	100, 200	18, 20
Entacapone	Comtan	Novartis	200 with each dose of carbidopa/L-Dopa	200	17
Agonists					
Bromocriptine	Parlodel	Novartis	[b]	2.5, 5	20, 31
		Generic brands, various			18, 27
Pergolide	Permax	Athena	[b]	0.05, 0.25, 1	3, 13, 40
Pramipexole	Mirapex	Pharmacia Upjohn	1.5–4.5	0.125, 0.25, 0.5	8, 11, 21
				1, 1.5	21, 21
Ropinirole	Requip	SmithKline Beecham	[b]	0.25, 0.5, 1	10, 10, 10
				2, 4, 5	10, 20, 20
Anticholinergic Drugs					
Benztropine	Cogentin	Merck and Co.	0.5–6	0.5, 1, 2	2, 2, 3
		Generic brands, various			1, 1, 1
Biperiden	Akineton	Knoll	2–16	2	3
Diphenhydramine	Benadryl	Parke-Davis	25–100	25, 50	2, 3
		Generic brands, various			1, 1
Procyclidine	Kemadrin	Glaxo-Wellcome	2.5–20	5	6
Trihexyphenidyl	Artane	Lederle	1–15	2, 5, 2/5 mL	2, 4, 4
		Generic brands, various			1, 3

[a]Cost index calculated from June 2000 average wholesale price per 100. Approximate cost per 100 (or per pint for solutions) equivalent to index × $10.00
[b]Dosage must be individualized.

agonist therapy comes from advancing disability and ineffectiveness of these alternative medications to provide adequate symptomatic control. Depending on profession and lifestyle, the same basic parkinsonian features may result in different degrees of disability, and drug therapy goals may need to be adjusted accordingly. A summary of available antiparkinsonian medications is listed in Table 59–4.

ANTICHOLINERGIC MEDICATIONS

The anticholinergic drugs can be effective against tremor but rarely show much benefit for bradykinesia or other disabilities of IPD. Not all patients with tremor respond to these medications. Sometimes dystonic features associated with IPD will improve. Adverse effects of these drugs include dry mouth, blurred vision, constipation, and urinary retention. More serious reactions include forgetfulness, sedation, depression, and anxiety. An encephalopathic state also can evolve gradually in some patients. Patients with preexisting cognitive deficits and advanced age are at greater risk for central anticholinergic effects. The anticholinergic drugs differ little in their adverse effects and have essentially the same therapeutic potential. Anticholinergic drugs can be used alone or in conjunction with L-dopa and other antiparkinsonian agents.

Amantadine

Amantadine (Symmetrel, Endo, generic brands, various) is often effective for relief of most signs and symptoms in patients with mild IPD.[23] More recently it has been reported to decrease dyskinesia at relatively high doses (400 mg/day) and is an independent predictor of improved survival in IPD.[24,25] Like anticholinergics, it can be especially effective against tremor. The drug typically is used at 200–300 mg/day. The elderly are particularly prone to confusion at the higher doses. Adverse effects that may occur at onset of the drug (e.g., sedation and vivid dreams) may disappear with time. Dry mouth is a common adverse effect reminiscent of anticholinergic drugs, although amantadine does not block cholinergic receptors. Other adverse central effects seen uncommonly include depression, hallucinations, anxiety, dizziness, psychosis, and confusion. A frequent (and reversible) adverse effect of amantadine is livedo reticularis, a diffuse mottling of the skin.

Amantadine is eliminated renally, and a decreased dose should be administered when renal dysfunction is present (100 mg/day with creatinine clearances of 30–50 mL/min, 100 mg every other day for creatinine clearances of 15–29 mL/min, and 200 mg every 7 days for creatinine clearances of less than 15 mL/min and patients on hemodialysis). Unlike other drugs for IPD, the precise mechanism of action of amantadine is unknown, but it may involve either dopaminergic or nondopaminergic mechanisms such as inhibition of *N*-Methyl-D-aspartate receptors.[26]

L-Dopa and Carbidopa/L-Dopa

L-Dopa (Larodopa, Roche) was first studied for parkinsonism in the 1960s, and recognition of its unequivocal benefit was reported in 1967.[27] It is still the most effective drug in the management of IPD. L-Dopa is the immediate precursor of dopamine. It crosses the blood-brain barrier, whereas dopamine does not. In the striatum and elsewhere, L-dopa is converted by L-AAD to dopamine. Peripherally formed dopamine is responsible for adverse effects such as nausea, vomiting, cardiac arrhythmias, and postural hypotension. By combining L-dopa with the peripherally acting L-amino acid decarboxylase inhibitors carbidopa (Sinemet, DuPont, generic brands, various) or benserazide (Madopar, not available in the United States), peripheral conversion of L-dopa to dopamine is blocked. As a result, increased amounts of L-dopa are transported into the brain, and peripheral adverse effects of dopamine are reduced.[28]

Today, L-dopa is used almost exclusively as a combination product with decarboxylase inhibitors. Starting L-dopa doses of 200–300 mg/day often are adequate for relief of disability. Some patients require larger amounts on a daily basis; however, the usual maximal dose of L-dopa needed by patients even with severe parkinsonism is 800 mg/day. Slow buildup of dose (e.g., increments of 100 mg L-dopa per week) can help to assess the lowest effective dose and minimizes the risk for adverse effects, such as postural hypotension, nausea, vomiting, sedation, and vivid dreams.

Generally about 75 mg carbidopa is required to prevent peripheral adverse effects, but some patients may benefit from as much as 150 mg/day. Carbidopa/L-dopa is most widely used in a 25-mg/100-mg tablet form, although 25-mg/250-mg and 10-mg/100-mg forms are also available. Controlled-release preparations of carbidopa/L-dopa are available in 50-mg/200-mg and 25-mg/100-mg forms. If peripheral adverse effects are prominent, 25-mg carbidopa (Lodosyn, DuPont) tablets are available.

Motor Complications. Between 5% and 10% of IPD patients will develop involuntary movements or short-duration responses with each year of L-dopa treatment.[29] Movement complications associated with long-term treatment with carbidopa/L-dopa and their suggested treatments are listed in Table 59–5 and have been reviewed recently.[30] Debate exists whether these complications are related to treatment or are intrinsic to disease progression. Initiating therapy with the controlled-release form of carbidopa/L-dopa did not reduce motor complications compared with standard-release carbidopa/L-dopa in a 5-year trial.[31]

Wearing Off. End-of-dose deterioration (the "wearing off" effect) has been related to increasing loss of neuronal storage capability for dopamine. Initially, exogenous L-dopa is taken up by the remaining presynaptic neurons, converted to dopamine, and stored in synaptic vesicles. With progressive loss of presynaptic neurons, storage capacity declines, and patients become more dependent on the rate of L-dopa delivery to the brain for the generation of dopamine. Hence the peripheral pharmacokinetics of L-dopa increasingly become the determinants of dopamine synthesis.

TABLE 59–5. Motor Fluctuations and Possible Interventions in IPD

Effect	Possible Treatments
End of dose deterioration ("wearing off")	Increase frequency of doses; controlled-release carbidopa/L-dopa; consider agonists, selegiline, COMT inhibitors, or amantadine; duodenal or intravenous L-dopa infusions; carbidopa/L-dopa oral solution; subcutaneous apomorphine infusions; transdermal dopamine agonists
Delayed onset of response	Give on empty stomach before meals; crush or chew and take with a full glass of water; reduce dietary protein intake; antacids; morning standard-release carbidopa/L dopa if on sustained release carbidopa/L-dopa; infusions of L-dopa; dopamine agonists
Drug-resistant "off" periods	Increase carbidopa/L-dopa dose and/or frequency; give on empty stomach before meals; crush or chew and take with a full glass of water; infusions of L-dopa or dopamine agonists; apomorphine intranasal spray
Random oscillations ("on/off")	Dopamine agonists; controlled-release carbidopa/L-dopa, selegiline; COMT inhibitors; infusions of L-dopa or dopamine agonists; consider drug holiday
Start hesitation ("freezing")	Increase carbidopa/L-dopa dose; dopamine agonists; gait modifications (tapping, rhythmic commands, stepping over objects, rocking)
Peak-dose dyskinesia (I-D-I response[a])	Smaller more frequent doses of carbidopa/L-dopa; controlled-release carbidopa/L-dopa; dopamine agonist; consider amantadine, propranolol, fluoxetine, buspirone, clozapine, surgical treatment
Diphasic dyskinesias (D I D response[b])	Reduce anticholinergic medication
Dystonia	Baclofen; nighttime carbidopa/L-dopa; morning standard-release carbidopa/L-dopa if on sustained-release carbidopa/L-dopa; dopamine agonists; anticholinergics; selective denervation with botulinum toxin
Myoclonus	Decrease nighttime L-dopa doses; clonazepam
Akathisia	Benzodiazepines; propranolol

[a]I-D-I is the improvement-dyskinesia/dystonia improvement pattern of response.
[b]D I D is the dyskinesia-improvement-dyskinesia pattern of response.

With advancement of IPD, a single carbidopa/L-dopa dose may produce benefits for as little as 1.5 to 2 hours. As a result, carbidopa/L-dopa needs to be given more frequently in order to prevent the "wearing off" of its benefits. Alternatively, a controlled-release product is available (Sinemet CR, DuPont) that can extend the duration of L-dopa effect. A more gradual "wearing off" of L-dopa effect and the need for fewer daily doses are associated with this product.[32] Some patients will require an increase in L-dopa intake when switched to the sustained-release form because of its decreased bioavailability. Patients maintained on the sustained-release product also may require a conventional carbidopa/L-dopa dose in the morning for its more rapid absorption and response.[33]

Dopamine agonists also can be added to a carbidopa/L-dopa regimen in an attempt to treat "wearing off." In addition, either intravenous or duodenal L-dopa infusions will produce constant serum L-dopa concentrations (and presumably striatal dopamine concentrations) and thus reduce response fluctuations.[34,35] Although some patients have been maintained on duodenal and intravenous infusions for long periods of time, these invasive methods of administration require careful planning and generally are not used outside the research setting. Sipping small amounts of carbidopa/L-dopa solution is an easier way to noninvasively titrate drug intake to optimal effect.[36] A solution that is stable for 24 hours can be prepared by adding 10 tablets of carbidopa/L-dopa and 2 g crystalline ascorbic acid to 1 liter of tap water. Finally, MAO-B inhibitors such as selegiline and the COMT inhibitors tolcapone (Tasmar, Roche) and entacapone (Comtan, Novartis) extend the action of L-dopa.

Drug-Resistant Off Periods. Drug-resistant "off" periods or delayed response to carbidopa/L-dopa can be due to delayed stomach emptying or decreased absorption in the upper gastrointestinal tract. Chewing a tablet or crushing it and then drinking a full glass of water may decrease disintegration time and facilitate gastric emptying.

Rapid Fluctuations. Rapid fluctuations from "on" to "off" motor states (*yo-yoing*) can develop in patients receiving L-dopa chronically. Rapid transitions from normal or dyskinetic "on" motor activity to bradykinetic or "off" states may just be an extension of "wearing off." Nonmotor symptoms also may fluctuate.[37] Concentration versus effect data reveal nonlinear (sigmoid E_{max} model) relationships such that small changes in serum L-dopa concentrations may lead to large effect responses, even if the sustained-release product is used.[38] Differences in the pharmacodynamic parameters EC_{50} (concentration at half-maximal effect), K_{eo} (elimination rate constant from the effect compartment), and N (the sigmoidicity constant) have been found between stable and fluctuating IPD patients with no change in pharmacokinetic parameters.[39] These same pharmacodynamic parameters have been found to change significantly in individual patients followed longitudinally over 4 years.[40] With progression of IPD, motor skill performance decreases so that there will be larger differences between baseline capabilities and maximum therapeutic effect; hence there will be an even steeper slope at the EC_{50} and more clinically noticeable dose-by-dose effects. These circumstances contribute to rapid fluctuations in motor responses. Simulations of the number of times a patient could alternately tap two levers 25 cm apart using mean pharmacodynamic and kinetic values for stable and fluctuating patients are shown in Figure 59–6 to illustrate further the dramatic differences between these groups. These pharmacodynamic mechanisms have been reviewed in detail by Nutt and Holford.[41]

Infusions of L-dopa or regimens of drugs with long-acting dopaminergic effects tend to alleviate these fluctuations. Dopaminergic agonists also can be added to L-dopa to treat on/off fluctuations. Other strategies include MAO inhibitors and inhibitors of COMT that decrease the clearance of L-dopa. A drug-free period (drug holiday) has been investigated in an attempt to modify postsynaptic dopamine receptors and thus decrease on/off fluctuations. Because of the discomforts and risks, as well as the limited gains for most patients, drug holidays have not been useful as a therapeutic intervention.

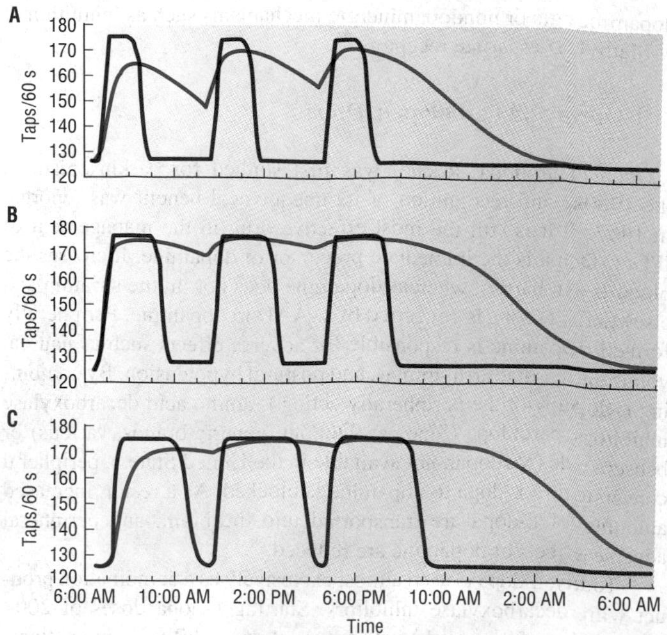

FIGURE 59–6. Effect of change in carbidopa/L-dopa dosage form on tapping effect in stable (*blue line*) and fluctuating (*black line*) patients using pharmacodynamic parameters obtained from Ref. 39. *A.* Carbidopa/L-dopa 25 mg/100 mg (K_{el} of 1.242 h^{-1}, K_a of 3.384 h^{-1}, and V/f of 35.4 L) administered at typical administration times of 7 A.M., 12 noon, and 5 P.M. *B.* Carbidopa/L-dopa 50 mg/200 mg (same pharmacokinetic parameters as in *A*) administered at the same times. *C.* Carbidopa/L-dopa 50 mg/200 mg with a longer half-life of absorption of 1.4 h (K_a = 0.5) simulating the controlled-release form.

Dyskinesias. Another complication of L-dopa therapy is dyskinesias (choreiform abnormal involuntary movements involving usually the neck, trunk, and upper extremities). These involuntary movements usually are associated with peak antiparkinsonian benefit (peak-effect dyskinesia or improvement-dyskinesia/dystonia-improvement), although they also can develop during the rise and fall of L-dopa effects (the dyskinesia-improvement-dyskinesia or diphasic pattern of response). In the case of peak-effect dyskinesias or dystonias, smaller, more frequent doses of L-dopa, use of the sustained-release preparations, or addition of dopamine agonists sometimes can be beneficial. The optimal treatment for the dyskinesia-improvement-dyskinesia pattern is unknown and actually can worsen with strategies useful for extending L-dopa effect.

Simplistically, dyskinesias can be thought of as too much movement secondary to extension of the pharmacologic effect or too much striatal dopamine receptor stimulation. However, the phenomenology is far more complex, as demonstrated by the occasional patient simultaneously demonstrating parkinsonian features and dyskinesias. An interaction between different classes of dopamine receptors may be involved. A partial dopamine agonist, terguride, has been found to suppress dyskinesias without worsening parkinsonian symptoms, suggesting that some pharmacologic approaches may differentiate the effects of dopaminergic stimulation on different aspects of motor system activation.[42]

Dystonias, Myoclonus, Akathisia. Dystonias (sustained muscle contractions or abnormal postures) are especially common in the distal lower extremities. Clenching of the toes or involuntary turning of the foot can precede the development of IPD. Dystonias often occur in the early morning hours or on awakening and improve with the first L-dopa dose of the day. Remedies for this problem include bedtime administration of sustained-release L-dopa, dopaminergic agonists, baclofen, or selective denervation with botulinum toxin. Another problem that can occur during sleep is myoclonus. Lowering nighttime L-dopa doses or use of clonazepam can be beneficial. Akathisia (the sensation of inner restlessness resulting in the need to make movements) can be treated with benzodiazepines or propranolol.

Psychosis. L-Dopa and dopaminergic agonists not only act on the nigrostriatal system but also facilitate mesolimbic dopaminergic projections. This may result in psychiatric symptoms, including delirium, agitation, paranoia, delusions, or hallucinations. These effects occur even more frequently in older patients and in those with underlying confusion or dementia.[43] Management guidelines have been published.[44,45] These are summarized in Table 59–6. The atypical antipsychotic clozapine at low doses can be quite effective for psychotic symptoms while also improving tremor and other motor symptoms; however, weekly monitoring for leukopenia is required.[46] Quetiapine initiated at a dose of 12.5 mg/day and titrated upward by 12.5 mg per week is also safe and effective.[47] Other antipsychotics, including olanzapine and risperidone, also can improve psychotic symptoms but worsen parkinsonian features.[48]

When to Start Treatment. The decision to start L-dopa early (as soon as the diagnosis of IPD is made) or late (only when symptoms compromise social, occupational, or psychological well-being) has generated controversy.[49,50] Proponents for delaying treatment point to evidence suggesting that long-term L-dopa therapy is associated with increased risk of response fluctuations, increased risk of dementia, and loss of L-dopa efficacy.[51] L-Dopa therapy hypothetically could increase oxidative stress in dopaminergic neurons and thus increase dopaminergic neuronal loss; however, there is no firm evidence that this mechanism actually causes IPD.

The counterargument is that response fluctuations are secondary to disease progression, not L-dopa.[52] A multicenter study found that withholding L-dopa therapy for more than 3 years after diagnosis resulted in a doubling of the excess mortality rate compared with early treatment.[53]

A 40-week randomized, double-blind, placebo-controlled clinical trial comparing earlier versus later L-dopa (ELLDOPA) is now underway to address this issue.[54] At this time, the general consensus is that the proper time to initiate L-dopa therapy is at least when the disease interferes with the patient's occupation or activities of daily living or when the patient wishes to begin therapy after considering all risks and benefits.

Pharmacokinetics and Pharmacodynamics. L-Dopa pharmacokinetic properties help explain some of the clinical effects seen. There is marked intra- and intersubject variability in the time to peak plasma concentrations after oral L-dopa. Often there may be more than one peak plasma concentration after a single dose, which is attributed to erratic gastric emptying. Meals delay gastric emptying, whereas antacids (which decrease gastric acidity) promote gastric emptying.[55] L-Dopa is absorbed primarily in the proximal duodenum by a saturable large neutral amino acid (LNAA) transport system. Competition for this site by dietary or supplemental LNAAs can reduce L-dopa plasma concentrations. The gut wall also contains a saturable decarboxylase, which limits bioavailability of L-dopa unless it is combined with a peripheral decarboxylase inhibitor such as carbidopa.

L-Dopa is not bound to plasma proteins. It crosses the blood-brain barrier by stereospecific saturable facilitated diffusion and competes with LNAA for transport into the brain. High-dose infusions of phenylalanine and leucine decrease clinical response to L-dopa without altering L-dopa plasma concentrations.[56] This has led to special diets being recommended for these patients, although reduction in protein intake generally is not needed to maintain good L-dopa effect.[57] A metabolite of L-dopa, 3-*O*-methyldopa (3OMD), also competes for transport, but it is not clear how this affects L-dopa clinical response. Drug holidays may allow the body to clear this longer half-life metabolite, thus restoring L-dopa responsiveness.

L-Dopa elimination is primarily by decarboxylation to dopamine. Additional pathways are by 3-*O*-methylation and transamination. With adequate decarboxylase inhibition, increased amounts of L-dopa are metabolized by the other pathways. The elimination half-life of L-dopa is about 1 hour, and this is extended to about 1½ hours with the addition of carbidopa. 3OMD has a half-life of about 15 hours and accumulates with chronic dosing. There are no peripheral pharmacokinetic differences between patients with stable responses, response fluctuations, and on/off fluctuations.

L-Dopa should not be administered with MAO-A inhibitors because of a risk for hypertensive crisis or with traditional

TABLE 59–6. Stepwise Approach to Drug-Induced Psychosis in Parkinson's Disease

1. Simplify the antiparkinsonian regimen as much as possible by discontinuing the medications with the highest risk-benefit ratio first.
   a. Discontinue anticholinergics, including other nonparkinsonian medications with anticholinergic activity such as antidepressants, e.g., amitriptyline.
   b. Discontinue selegiline.
   c. Taper and discontinue dopamine agonists.
   d. Taper and discontinue amantadine, being aware that amantadine withdrawal delirium has been reported.[94]
   e. Discontinue COMT inhibitors.
2. Consider atypical antipsychotic medication if psychosis persists.
   a. Quetiapine 12.5 mg at bedtime and gradually increased upward by 12.5 mg per week until psychosis controlled, *or*
   b. Clozapine 6.25 mg at bedtime and gradually increased upward by 6.25 mg per week until psychosis controlled with weekly monitoring for leukopenia.

antipsychotic agents because of possible antagonism of L-dopa effect.

Selegiline

Selegiline (Eldepryl, Somerset), an irreversible MAO-B inhibitor, also known as deprenyl, is marketed for extending L-dopa effects. By blocking dopamine breakdown, it modestly extends the duration of action from each dose of L-dopa. Patients with "wearing off" of L-dopa actions experience up to 1 hour of increased action from each L-dopa dose. Selegiline also increases the peak effects of L-dopa and can worsen preexisting dyskinesias or psychiatric symptoms such as delusions and hallucinations. Often use of selegiline permits reduction of L-dopa intake to as little as one-half its previous optimal dose.

Selegiline has been used widely at a dose of 10 mg/day, although its irreversible inhibition of MAO-B can be achieved at lower doses.[58] In addition, renewal of the enzyme proceeds at a slow rate, so the effect of the drug lingers for weeks. Selegiline is lipophilic and penetrates the blood-brain barrier rapidly. The metabolic pathway of selegiline leads to end products of L-methamphetamine and L-amphetamine.[59] Adverse effects of selegiline are minimal and include insomnia and jitteriness. The hypertensive "cheese effect," which occurs from ingesting tyramine with the use of MAO-A inhibitors, does not occur with selegiline.[60] Rarely, concomitant selective serotonin reuptake inhibitors can cause the serotonin syndrome (i.e., hypertension, diaphoresis, and shivering).[61] A similar reaction has been reported with meperidine.[62]

Selegiline has been investigated for neuroprotective properties. It inhibits the oxidative deamination of dopamine, which generates hydrogen peroxide and ultimately oxyradicals capable of damaging nigrostriatal neurons (see Fig. 59–1). Since MAO-B inhibition diverts dopamine catabolism to an alternate route not generating peroxide, selegiline therapy was proposed as a means for sparing these neurons from oxidative stress. Studies evaluating its neuroprotective properties have shown that it can delay the need for L-dopa by about 9 months and has symptomatic effects, but there is no firm evidence that it can slow neurodegeneration.[63] A report of increased mortality when selegiline is combined with L-dopa as compared with L-dopa alone is of concern,[64] but the study has methodologic flaws[65] and has not been confirmed in other studies.[66]

COMT Inhibitors

COMT inhibitors tolcapone (Tasmar, Roche) and entacapone (Comtan, Novartis) have no effect on IPD by themselves. They are used in conjunction with carbidopa/L-dopa to prevent the peripheral conversion of levodopa to 3OMD and thus prolong the action of carbidopa/L-dopa. These agents significantly decrease "off" time and decrease L-dopa requirements by increasing the L-dopa area under the curve (AUC) by about 50% without increasing C_{max} or T_{max}.[67] This may offer a theoretical advantage over controlled-release carbidopa/L-dopa by not delaying the time to maximal effect. Concomitant use of nonselective MAO inhibitors should be avoided to avoid inhibition of the majority of the pathways for normal catecholamine metabolism. It remains to be seen whether the use of these adjunctive agents will be more beneficial and cost-effective than maximizing therapy with carbidopa/L-dopa alone.

Tolcapone has effects on both peripheral and central COMT, but it is unclear what role central COMT inhibition has. Its use is limited by a few cases of fatal hepatotoxicity such that strict monitoring is required, as outlined in the package insert. Tolcapone should be discontinued if there is any elevation in liver function tests above the upper limit of normal or if any sign or symptoms develop suggesting hepatic failure (e.g., persistent nausea, fatigue, lethargy, anorexia, jaundice, dark urine, pruritus, or right upper quadrant abdominal tenderness). An informed consent is included in the package insert to ensure that patients are informed of the risk of adverse effects. The starting and recommended dose is 100 mg three times per day as an adjunct to carbidopa/L-dopa. Delayed onset of diarrhea at 6 to 8 weeks also can occur in up to 5% of patients. Since an alternative similar but safer medication is available, any role for tolcapone is unclear.

Entacapone has a shorter half-life than tolcapone, and 200 mg needs to be given with each dose of carbidopa/L-dopa up to 8 times per day. In two large clinical trials, entacapone increased "on" time by about 1 hour and decreased "off" time by about 1 hour while the average daily dose of levodopa was decreased by about 12%.[68,69] Dopaminergic adverse effects may occur and are managed easily by carbidopa/L-dopa dosage reduction. Brownish orange urinary discoloration may occur, as with tolcapone, but there is no evidence of hepatotoxicity from entacapone.

Dopamine Agonists

The dopamine agonists pergolide (Permax, Athena), bromocriptine (Parlodel, Novartis), and the nonergots pramipexole (Mirapex, Pharmacia Upjohn) and ropinirole (Requip, SmithKline Beecham) are beneficial as adjuncts to L-dopa therapy in patients with deteriorating response to L-dopa, in patients who are experiencing fluctuations in response to L-dopa, and in patients with limited clinical response to L-dopa secondary to inability to tolerate higher doses. The dopamine agonists decrease the frequency of "off" periods and provide an L-dopa-sparing effect. Crossover studies suggest that pergolide with L-dopa is similar or possibly more efficacious with fewer adverse effects than bromocriptine with L-dopa.[70] Pergolide may improve functional status in patients with deteriorating response to bromocriptine,[71] whereas bromocriptine does not appear to improve function in patients with a deteriorating response to pergolide.[72]

Bromocriptine monotherapy in previously untreated IPD patients is limited by a high incidence of adverse effects and treatment failures necessitating either lowering the dose or the addition of L-dopa.[73,74] Pergolide, pramipexole, and ropinirole seem to be more effective as monotherapy alternatives to L-dopa, but only pramipexole and ropinirole are approved for monotherapy.[75] Investigations of the combination of L-dopa with dopamine agonists or a dopamine agonist alone as initial therapy revealed a decreased risk for the development of response fluctuations.[76–79] This has generated controversy as to whether initial treatment of IPD should be with dopamine agonist monotherapy.[80,81] Younger patients are more likely to develop motor fluctuations because they have a longer life expectancy, and therefore, dopamine agonists may be preferred. Older patients are more likely to suffer from psychosis from the dopamine agonists and have a shorter life expectancy, and thus carbidopa/L-dopa may be the best starting medication, particularly if there is any dementia present. There is no rationale at this time to choose one dopamine agonist over another based on receptor specificity; however, choice of agonist depends on cost issues and physician experience.

A recommended initial dose of bromocriptine is 1.25 mg once or twice daily. The dose of bromocriptine should be escalated slowly by 1.25 to 2.5 mg/day every week and maintained at the minimum amount necessary to accomplish the desired therapeutic effect. Average daily dosages of less than 30 mg may be effective for several years in many patients; however, some patients may require dosages up to 120 mg/day.

A recommended initial dose of pergolide (which is about 13 times more potent than bromocriptine) is 0.05 mg/day for 2 days, gradually increasing the dose by approximately 0.1–0.15 mg/day every 3 days over a 12-day period. Should more drug be needed, the dose may then be increased by 0.25 mg every 3 days until symptoms are eliminated or adverse effects occur. The mean therapeutic dose in most clinical trials was approximately 3 mg/day.

Pramipexole is initiated at a dose of 0.125 mg three times a day and increased every 5 to 7 days as tolerated. In a fixed-dose study, daily doses of 3, 4.5, and 6 mg were not more effective than 1.5 mg/day, and the higher doses were associated with a higher frequency of adverse effects.[82] If switching from bromocriptine or pergolide to pramipexole, a 10:1 and 1:1 direct dosage substitution is recommended, respectively.[83] Ropinirole is initiated at 0.25 mg three times a day and increased by 0.25 mg three times a day on a weekly basis.

The limiting factor in dopamine agonist therapy is adverse effects. These occur in 30% to 50% of patients and are more frequent at higher doses and with rapid escalation of dose. Nausea is the most frequently reported gastrointestinal effect, occurring in greater than 50% of patients taking the drug; vomiting occurs rarely. Cardiovascular effects occur infrequently, with the exception of postural hypotension, which is common. Central nervous system effects are most commonly dose limiting and occur in as many as one-third of patients taking dopamine agonists. These include confusion, hallucinations, and sedation. Guidelines addressing sleep episodes in IPD and with agonists have been published.[84] The addition of a dopamine agonist to L-dopa therapy can increase the frequency and severity of dyskinesias during periods of good functional status but can allow reduction in carbidopa/L-dopa dose. Seventeen of 300 (6%) patients receiving pramipexole had peripheral edema that seemed to be dose-related, nonresponsive to diuretics, and resolved with stopping the medication.[85] The ergot dopamine agonists are associated rarely with pleuropulmonary fibrosis.[86]

Bromocriptine is fairly rapidly absorbed, exhibits high first-pass metabolism, is highly protein bound, and has multiple metabolites excreted primarily through the bile.[87] The elimination half-life is about 3 hours. A slow release bromocriptine product has been investigated but is not available clinically.[88] A significant increase in bromocriptine plasma concentrations has been documented with erythromycin.[89] Pergolide has approximately the same duration of action as bromocriptine. Pramipexole is primarily renally excreted with an 8- to 12-hour half-life. The initial dosage must be adjusted in renal insufficiency (0.125 mg twice daily for creatinine clearances of 35–59 mL/min, 0.125 mg once daily for creatinine clearances of 15–34 mL/min). Ropinirole has a 6-hour half-life and is metabolized by cytochrome P450 1A2.[90] Potent inhibitors (fluroquinolones) and inducers (smoking) of this enzyme likely will lead to alterations in ropinirole clearance.

Apomorphine and lisuride are dopamine agonists being investigated but not available in the United States. Cabergoline is a selective D_2 ergot agonist with a long half-life (70 hours) that is as effective as bromocriptine but dosed up to 4 mg once a day.[91] It is available in the United States only as a 0.5-mg tablet (Dostinex, Pharmacia Upjohn) for the treatment of hyperprolactinemia. Transdermal delivery forms of potent dopamine agonists are being investigated. Apomorphine and lisuride have both been administered as subcutaneous infusions, and a number of formulations including sublingual and intranasal apomorphine are being investigated. Specific D_1 receptor agonists do not appear to have much antiparkinsonian effect. Domperidone is a peripheral dopamine receptor blocker (not available in the United States) that can be used to block some of the adverse effects of the dopamine agonists.[92]

PHARMACOECONOMIC CONSIDERATIONS

Few pharmacoeconomic assessments have been reported in IPD treatment. Treatment with anticholinergic medications, amantadine, and carbidopa/L-dopa is inexpensive. For cost-effectiveness, the lowest dose giving adequate results should be used and optimization of the carbidopa/L-dopa regimen attempted before adding more costly medications. In early IPD, a long duration response can be seen such that a carbidopa/L-dopa dose every 3 days may be all that is required.[93] Initial therapy with the more expensive sustained-release product (Sinemet CR) in the absence of response fluctuations is not indicated. As symptoms progress, the addition or continued use of dopamine agonists, selegiline, or COMT inhibitors can add considerable expense, sometimes with minimal or no benefit.

EVALUATION OF THERAPEUTIC OUTCOMES

A list of monitoring parameters is given in Table 59–7. It is important to educate patients and caregivers that IPD is a neurodegenerative disease that will progress with time. They can participate in treatment by recording medication administration times as well as duration of "on" and "off" times that can be reviewed on each office visit. If a bothersome symptom such as dystonia occurs only infrequently, it can be videotaped by the family to be reviewed with the physician.

The history always should include a detailed medication history because patients often may improvise and adjust their own medication schedule. It is important to determine the times of the day that may be most difficult for them to function. Assessment of general level of functioning including activities of daily living will help determine when L-dopa or dopamine agonists should be added. A history of falls should be investigated further as to the circumstances surrounding the falls to determine whether falls are secondary to IPD or some other etiology. The patient should be questioned about common adverse effects of the antiparkinsonian medications including nausea, hypotension, and psychiatric difficulties. The patient also should be observed for dyskinesias and, if present, educated about them. Recommendations should always be made in view of the patient's perception of the severity of symptoms.

CONCLUSIONS

Although the cause of Parkinson's disease remains unknown, the identification of a neurotoxin and a mechanism to protect against the neurotoxin have advanced the knowledge of this disease. Pharmacologic therapy through manipulation of the dopaminergic system can improve a patient's functional status significantly and prolong meaningful life. Despite problems associated with L-dopa, it remains the standard of therapy for patients with Parkinson's disease. The goal of management remains maintaining acceptable functional control with the minimum amount of antiparkinsonian drug necessary.

TABLE 59–7. Monitoring Parkinson's Disease Therapy

1. Determine medications, medication administration times, relationship to meals, and the time of the last dose. Educate the patient that carbidopa/L-dopa is absorbed best on an empty stomach.
2. Assess patient's general impression of function, and address any specific concerns the patient may have.
3. Inquire specifically about dose-by-dose effects of medication, wearing off of medication, inadequate response to a single dose of medication, "freezing," abnormal involuntary movements, cramps or spasms, hallucinations (particularly visual hallucinations), and nausea, vomiting, or light-headedness. Offer suggestions to help alleviate these.
4. Inquire about the preceding symptoms from the caregivers, and address any concerns they may have with specific attention to psychotic features and dyskinesias that may not be apparent to the patient.
5. Observe the patient and determine if dyskinetic movements are present and if the patient is aware of them. If present, educate the patient about dyskinesias and recommend appropriate interventions.
6. Ensure that the patient and/or caregivers understand the recommended medication regimen.

▶ PRINCIPLES OF PHARMACOTHERAPY

- Carbidopa/L-dopa is the standard of therapy in IPD.
- Dosages of carbidopa/L-dopa and dopamine agonists must be individualized.
- Most carbidopa/L-dopa-treated patients will eventually develop response fluctuations.
- Response fluctuations may be partially explained by pharmacokinetic and pharmacodynamic properties of L-dopa.
- Medication administration times and dose-by-dose therapeutic and adverse effects must be determined in assessing therapeutic outcomes in order to optimize treatment.
- Selegiline, COMT inhibitors and controlled release carbidopa/L-dopa decrease response fluctuations through pharmacokinetic mechanisms.
- Anticholinergics should be used with caution in the elderly or those with preexisting cognitive difficulties.
- Amantadine is useful for relieving mild features of IPD even in the elderly.
- The optimal time to start carbidopa/L-dopa is controversial, but in general treatment should be started when the disease interferes with the patient's occupation or activities of daily living.
- Dopamine agonists are L-dopa-sparing and decrease response fluctuations but are more likely to cause neuropsychiatric symptoms.

REFERENCES

1. Tyler KL. A history of Parkinson's disease. In: Koller WC, ed. Handbook of Parkinson's Disease, 2d ed. New York, Marcel Dekker, 1992:1–34.
2. Bower JH, Maraganore DM, McDonnell SK, Rocca WA. Incidence and distribution of parkinsonism in Olmsted County, Minnesota, 1976–1990. Neurology 1999;52:1214–1220.
3. Pezzoli G, Canesi M, Antonini A, et al. Hydrocarbon exposure and Parkinson's disease. Neurology 2000;55:667–673.
4. Gorell JM, Johnson CC, Rybicki BA, et al. The risk of Parkinson's disease with exposure to pesticide, farming, well water and rural living. Neurology 1998;50:1346–1350.
5. Morens DM, Grandinetti A, Reed D, et al. Cigarette smoking and protection from Parkinson's disease: False association or etiologic clue. Neurology 1995;45:1041–1051.
6. Ross GW, Abbott RD, Petrovitch H, et al. Association of coffee and caffeine intake with the risk of Parkinson disease. JAMA 2000;283:2674–2679.
7. Tanner CM, Ottman R, Goldman SM. Parkinson disease in twins: An etiologic study. JAMA 1999;281:341–346.
8. Polymeropoulos MH, Lavedan C, Leroy E, et al. Mutation in the α-synuclein gene identified in families with Parkinson's disease. Science 1997;276:2045–2047.
9. Lucking CB, Durr A, Bonifati V, et al. Association between early-onset Parkinson's disease and mutations in the *parkin* gene. New Engl J Med 2000;342:1560–1567.
10. Calne DB. The free radical hypothesis in idiopathic parkinsonism: Evidence against it. Ann Neurol 1992;32:799–803.
11. Fahn S, Cohen G. The oxidant stress hypothesis in Parkinson's disease: Evidence supporting it. Ann Neurol 1992;32:804–812.
12. Meara RJ. Review: The pathophysiology of the motor signs in Parkinson's disease. Age Ageing 1994;23:342–346.
13. Smith Y, Bevan MD, Shink E, Bolam JP. Microcircuitry of the direct and indirect pathways of the basal ganglia. Neuroscience 1998;86:353–387.
14. Mercuri NB, Calabresi P, Bernardi G. Physiology and pharmacology of dopamine D_2 receptors: Their implications in dopamine-substitute therapy for Parkinson's disease. Neurology 1989;39:1106–1108.
15. Bernheimer H, Birkmayer W, Hornykiewicz O, et al. Brain dopamine and the syndrome of Parkinson's and Huntington: Clinical, morphological, and neurochemical correlations. J Neurol Sci 1973;20:415–455.
16. Calne DB, Snow BJ. PET imaging in parkinsonism. Adv Neurol 1993;60:484–487.
17. Rutgers AWF, Lakke JPWF, Paans AMJ, et al. Tracing of dopamine receptors in hemiparkinsonism with positron emission tomography. J Neurol Sci 1987;80:237–248.
18. Gelb DJ, Oliver E, Gilman S. Diagnostic criteria for Parkinson disease. Arch Neurol 1999;56:33–39.
19. Martin WE, Loewenson RB, Resch JA, Baker AB. Parkinson's disease: Clinical analysis of 100 patients. Neurology 1973;23:783–790.
20. Hallett M, Litvan I, Task Force on Surgery for Parkinson's Disease. Evaluation of surgery for Parkinson's disease: A report of the therapeutics and technology assessment subcommittee of the American Academy of Neurology. Neurology 1999;53:1910–1921.
21. Olanow CW, Koller WC. An algorithm (decision tree) for the management of Parkinson's disease: Treatment guidelines. Neurology 1998;50(Suppl 3):S1–S57.
22. Koller WC, Herbster G. Adjuvant therapy of parkinsonian tremor. Arch Neurol 1987;44:921–923.
23. Fahn S, Isgreen W. Long-term evaluation of amantadine and levodopa combination in parkinsonism by double-blind crossover analysis. Neurology 1975;25:695–700.
24. Metman LV, Del Dotto P, LePoole K, et al. Amantadine for levodopa-induced dyskinesias: A 1-year follow-up study. Arch Neurol 1999;56:1383–1386.
25. Uitti RJ, Rajput AH, Ahlskog JE, et al. Amantadine treatment is an independent predictor of improved survival in Parkinson's disease. Neurology 1996;46:1551–1556.

26. Jackisch R, Link T, Neufang B, Koch R. Studies on the mechanism of the antiparkinsonian drugs memantine and amantadine: No evidence for direct dopaminomimetic or antimuscarinic properties. Arch Int Pharmacodyn Ther 1992;320:21–42.
27. Cotzias CG, Van Woert MH, Schiffer LM. Aromatic amino acids and modification of parkinsonism. New Engl J Med 1967;276:374–379.
28. Papavasilou PS, Cotzias GC, Duby SE, et al. Levodopa in parkinsonism: Potentiation of central effects with a peripheral inhibitor. New Engl J Med 1972;285:8–14.
29. Poewe WH, Wenning GK. The natural history of Parkinson's disease. Neurology 1996;47(Suppl 3):S146–S152.
30. Ahlskog JE. Medical treatment of later stage motor problems of Parkinson disease. Mayo Clin Proc 1999;74:1239–1254.
31. Koller WC, Hutton JT, Tolosa E, et al. Immediate-release and controlled release carbidopa/levodopa in PD: A five year randomized multicenter study. Neurology 1999;53:1012–1019.
32. LeWitt PA, Nelson MV, Berchou RC, et al. Controlled-release carbidopa/levodopa (Sinemet 50/200 CR4): Clinical and pharmacokinetic studies. Neurology 1989;39(Suppl 2):45–53.
33. Stocchi F, Quinn NP, Barbato L, et al. Comparison between a fast and a slow release preparation of levodopa and a combination of the two: A clinical and pharmacokinetic study. Clin Neuropharmacol 1994;17: 38–44.
34. Quinn N, Parkes JD, Marsden CD. Control of on/off phenomenon by continuous intravenous infusion of levodopa. Neurology 1984;34:1131–1136.
35. Kurth MC, Tetrud JW, Tanner CM, et al. Double-blind, placebo-controlled crossover study of duodenal infusion of levodopa/carbidopa in Parkinson's disease patients with "on-off" fluctuations. Neurology 1993;43:1698–1703.
36. Kurth MC, Tetrud JW, Irwin I, et al. Oral levodopa/carbidopa solution versus tablets in Parkinson's patients with severe fluctuations: a pilot study. Neurology 1993;43:1036 1039.
37. Hillen ME, Sage JI. Nonmotor fluctuations in patients with Parkinson's disease. Neurology 1996;47:1180–1183.
38. Nelson MV, Berchou RC, LeWitt PA, et al. Pharmacodynamic modeling of concentration-effect relationships after controlled release carbidopa/levodopa (Sinemet CR4) in Parkinson's disease. Neurology 1990;40:70–74.
39. Contin M, Riva R, Martinelli P, et al. Pharmacodynamic modeling of oral levodopa: Clinical application in Parkinson's disease. Neurology 1993;43:367–371.
40. Contin M, Riva R, Martinelli P, et al. Longitudinal monitoring of the levodopa concentration effect relationship in Parkinson's disease. Neurology 1994;44:1287–1292.
41. Nutt JG, Holford NHG. The response to levodopa in Parkinson's disease: Imposing pharmacological law and order. Ann Neurol 1996;39:561–573.
42. Rascol O. Medical treatment of levodopa-induced dyskinesias. Ann Neurol 2000;47(Suppl 1):S179–S188.
43. Aarsland D, Larsen JP, Cummings JL, Laake K, et al. Prevalence and clinical correlates of psychotic symptoms in Parkinson disease: A community based study. Arch Neurol 1999;56:595–601.
44. Juncos JL. Management of psychotic aspects of Parkinson's disease. J Clin Psychiatry 1999;60(Suppl 8):42–53.
45. Friedman JH, Factor SA. Atypical antipsychotics in the treatment of drug induced psychosis in Parkinson's disease. Mov Disord 2000;15:201–11.
46. The Parkinson Study Group. Low dose clozapine for the treatment of drug-induced psychosis in Parkinson's disease. New Engl J Med 1999;340:757–763.
47. Hernandez HH, Friedman JH, Jacques C, Rosenfeld M. Quetiapine for the treatment of drug-induced psychosis in Parkinson's disease. Mov Disord 1999;14:484–487.
48. Wolters EC, Jansen ENH, Tuynman-Qua HG, Bergmans PLM. Onlanzapine in the treatment of dopaminomimetic psychosis in patients with Parkinson's disease. Neurology 1996;47:1085–1087.
49. Fahn S, Bressman SB. Should levodopa therapy for parkinsonism be started early or late? Evidence against early treatment. Can J Neurol Sci 1984;11:200–206.
50. Muenter MD. Should levodopa therapy be started early or late? Can J Neurol Sci 1984;11:195–199.
51. Rajput AH, Stern W, Laverty WH. Chronic low-dose levodopa therapy in Parkinson's disease: An argument for delaying levodopa therapy. Neurology 1984;34:991–996.
52. Agid Y. Levodopa: Is toxicity a myth? Neurology 1998;50:858–863.
53. Diamond SG, Markham CH, Hoehn MM, et al. Multicenter study of Parkinson mortality with early versus later dopa treatment. Ann Neurol 1987;22:8–12.
54. Fahn S. Parkinson disease, the effect of levodopa, and the ELLDOPA trial. Arch Neurol 1999;56:529–535.
55. Rivera-Calimlim L, Dujovne CA, Morgan JP, et al. L-Dopa treatment failure: Explanation and correction. Br Med J 1970;4:93–94.
56. Nutt JG, Woodward WR, Hammerstad JP, et al. The "on-off" phenomenon in Parkinson's disease: Relation to levodopa absorption and transport. New Engl J Med 1984;310:483–488.
57. Berry EM, Growdon JH, Wurtman JJ, et al. A balanced carbohydrate:protein diet in the management of Parkinson's disease. Neurology 1991;41:1295–1297.
58. Mahmood I. Is 10 milligrams selegiline essential as an adjunct therapy for the symptomatic treatment of Parkinson's disease? Ther Drug Monit 1998;20:717–721.
59. Heinonen EH, Myllyla V, Sotaniemi K, et al. Pharmacokinetics and metabolism of selegiline. Acta Neurol Scand 1989;80(Suppl 126):93–99.
60. Elsworth JD, Glover V, Reynolds GP, et al. Deprenyl administration in man: A selective MAO-B inhibitor without "cheese-effect." Psychopharmacology 1987;57:33–38.
61. Richard IH, Kurlan R, Tanner C, et al. Serotonin syndrome and the combined use of deprenyl and an antidepressant in Parkinson's disease. Neurology 1997;48:1070–1077.
62. Zornberg GL, Bodkin JA, Cohen BM. Severe adverse interaction between pethidine and selegiline. Lancet 1991;337:246.
63. Shoulson I, Parkinson Study Group. DATATOP: A decade of neuroprotective inquiry. Ann Neurol 1998;44(Suppl 1):S160–S166.
64. Lees AJ on behalf of the Parkinson's Disease Research Group of the United Kingdom. Comparison of therapeutic effects and mortality data of levodopa and levodopa combined with selegiline in patients with early mild Parkinson's disease. Br Med J 1995;311:1602–1606.
65. Ahlskog JE. Treatment of early Parkinson's disease: Are complicated strategies justified? Mayo Clinic Proc 1996;71:659–670.
66. Parkinson Study Group. Mortality in DATATOP: A multicenter trial in early Parkinson's disease. Ann Neurol 1998;43:318–325.
67. Ruottine HM, Rinne UK. COMT inhibition in the treatment of Parkinson's disease. J Neurol 1998;245(Suppl 3):25–34.
68. Rinne UK, Larsen JP, Siden A, Worm-Peterson J. Entacapone enhances the response to levodopa in parkinsonian patients with motor fluctuations. NOMECOMT Study Group. Neurology 1998;51:1309–1314.
69. The Parkinson Study Group. Entacapone improves motor fluctuations in levodopa-treated Parkinson's disease patients. Ann Neurol 1997;42:747–755.
70. Pezzoli G, Martinoni E, Pacchetti C, et al. A crossover, controlled study comparing pergolide with bromocriptine as an adjunct to levodopa for the treatment of Parkinson's disease. Neurology 1995;45(Suppl 3):S22–S27.
71. Lieberman A, Neophytides A, Liebowitz M, et al. Comparative efficacy of pergolide and bromocriptine in patients with advanced Parkinson's disease. Adv Neurol 1983;37:95–108.
72. Olanow CW. Pergolide, Parlodel crossover study. Neurology 1988; 38:314–316.
73. Tashiro K, Goto I, Kanazawa I, et al. Eight-year follow-up study of bromocriptine monotherapy for Parkinson's disease. Eur Neurol 1996;36(Suppl 1):32–37.
74. Hely MA, Morris JGL, Reid WGJ, et al. The Sidney multicentre study of Parkinson's disease: A randomised, prospective five year study comparing low dose bromocriptine with low dose levodopa-carbidopa. J Neurol Neurosurg Psychiatry 1994;57:903–910.
75. Factor SA. Dopamine agonists. Med Clin North Am 1999;83:415–443.
76. Przuntek H, Welzel D, Gerlach M, et al. Early institution of bromocriptine in Parkinson's disease inhibits the emergence of levodopa associated

motor side effects: Long term results of the PRADO study. J Neurol Transm 1996;103:699–715.
77. Montastruc JL, Rascol O, Senard JM, Rascol A. A randomised controlled study comparing bromocriptine to which levodopa was later added, with levodopa alone in previously untreated patients with Parkinson's disease: A five year follow up. J Neurol Neurosurg Psychiatry 1994;57:1034–1038.
78. Rascol O, Brooks DJ, Korczyn AD, et al. A five-year study of the incidence of dyskinesia in patients with early Parkinson's disease who were treated with ropinirole or levodopa. New Engl J Med 2000;342:1491.
79. Parkinson Study Group. A randomized controlled trial comparing pramipexole with levodopa in early Parkinson's disease: Design and methods of the CALM-PD study. Clin Neuropharmacol 2000;23:34–43.
80. Weiner WJ. The intial treatment of Parkinson's disease should begin with levodopa. Mov Disord 1999;14:716–724.
81. Montastruc JL, Rascol O, Senard JM. Treatment of Parkinson's disease should begin with a dopamine agonist. Mov Disord 1999;14:725–730.
82. Parkinson Study Group. Safety and efficacy of pramipexole in early Parkinson disease: A randomized dose-ranging study. JAMA 1997;278:125–130.
83. Goetz CG, Blasucci L, Stebbins GT. Switching dopamine agonists in advanced Parkinson's disease: Is rapid titration preferable to slow? Neurology 1999;52:1227–1229.
84. Olanow CW, Schapira AHV, Roth T. Waking up to sleep episodes in Parkinson's disease. Mov Disord 2000;15:212–215.
85. Tan E, Ondo W. Clinical characteristics of pramipexole-induced peripheral edema. Arch Neurol 2000;57:729–732.
86. Ling LH, Ahlskog JE, Munger TM, et al. Constrictive pericarditis and pleuropulmonary disease linked to ergot dopamine agonist therapy (cabergoline) for Parkinson's disease. Mayo Clin Proc 1999;74:371–375.
87. Cedarbaum JM. Clinical pharmacokinetics of anti-parkinsonian drugs. Clin Pharmacokinet 1987;13:141–178.
88. Mannen T, Mizuno Y, Iwata M, et al. A multicenter, double-blind study on slow release bromocriptine in the treatment of Parkinson's disease. Neurology 1991;41:1598–1602.
89. Nelson MV, Berchou RC, Kareti D, LeWitt PA. Pharmacokinetic evaluation of erythromycin and caffeine administered with bromocriptine. Clin Pharmacol Ther 1990;47:694–697.
90. Bloomer JC, Clarke SE, Chenery RJ. In vitro identification of the P450 enzymes responsible for the metabolism of ropinirole. Drug Metab Dist 1997;25:840–844.
91. Inzelberg R, Nisipeanu P, Rabey JM, et al. Double-blind comparison of cabergoline and bromocriptine in Parkinson's disease patients with motor fluctuations. Neurology 1996;47:785–788.
92. Barone JA. Domperidone: a peripherally acting dopamine2-receptor antagonist. Ann Pharmacother 1999;33:429–440.
93. Quattrone A, Zappia M. Oral pulse levodopa therapy in mild Parkinson's disease. Neurology 1993;43:1161–1166.
94. Factor SA, Molho ES, Brown DL. Acute delirium after withdrawal of amantadine in Parkinson's disease. Neurology 1998;50:1456–1458.

60
PAIN MANAGEMENT

Terry J. Baumann

Although the world is full of suffering, it is also full of the overcoming of it.

Helen Keller[1]

Humans have always known and sought relief from pain. The act of relieving pain is probably as old as the medical profession itself. Today, pain's impact on society is still great, and indeed, pain complaints remain a primary reason patients seek medical advice.[2]

Regrettably, many health care providers do not receive adequate training in this area, and new information is not widely disseminated and/or understood. Clearly, pain management is enhanced when a multidisciplinary approach is applied. Thus, understanding the pathophysiology of pain therapy and maintaining a working knowledge of individual pain regimens are important to clinicians and are key factors in reversing the problem of inadequate pain control.

DEFINITION

An acceptable definition of pain remains an enigma. Once thought to be a punishment from the gods, the word is derived from the Latin *peone* and the Greek *poine,* meaning "penalty" or "punishment."[3] Aristotle considered pain a feeling and classified it as a passion of the soul, where the heart was the source or processing center of pain.[3] This Aristotelian concept predominated for the next 2000 years, although Descartes, Galen, and Vesalius postulated that pain was a sensation in which the brain played an important role. In the nineteenth century, Mueller, Van Frey, and Goldscheider hypothesized the concepts of neuroreceptors, nociceptors, and sensory input.[3] These theories developed into the current definition of pain: "an unpleasant sensory and emotional experience associated with actual or potential tissue damage or described in terms of such damage."[4] Pain is often so subjective, however, that many clinicians define pain as whatever the patient says it is. The best care is achieved when (1) the patient comes first and (2) when in doubt remember number 1.[5]

EPIDEMIOLOGY

Fifty million Americans are partially or totally disabled because of pain.[2] The annual cost of pain to American society can be estimated in the billions of dollars.[6] These numbers are expected to rise as more and more Americans work beyond 60 years of age and survive into their eighties.[6]

Unfortunately, pain often remains undertreated and continues to be a problem in hospitals, long-term care facilities, and the community. Seriously ill hospitalized patients have reported a 50% incidence of pain; 15% had extremely or moderately severe pain occurring at least 50% of the time, and 15% were dissatisfied with overall pain control.[7] In a follow-up report 4 years later, the author states that pain control persists as a major problem in hospitalized patients, and some of these patients are still in pain many months after hospitalization and experience pain even on their deathbeds.[8] In addition, problems with inadequate use of analgesics have been reported in cancer patients residing in nursing homes[9]; in the Michigan pain study, 70% of chronic pain patients claimed to have pain despite treatment, with 22% believing treatment worsened pain.[6]

PATHOPHYSIOLOGY

The pathophysiology of pain involves a complex array of neural networks in the brain that are acted on by afferent stimuli to produce the experience we know as pain. These peripheral and central mechanisms are dynamic and are modulated by changes that occur secondary to tissue damage. In acute pain, this modulation is short-lived, but in some situations, the changes may persist and chronic pain develops.[10] Classification by inferred pathology in terms of nociceptive and neuropathic pathways gives one a better understanding of both acute and chronic pain.[11] Nociceptive pain best outlines the pathophysiology of acute pain, whereas neuropathic pathophysiology is why some chronic pain develops.

NOCICEPTIVE PAIN

Nociceptive pain typically is classified as either somatic (arising from skin, bone, joint, muscle, or connective tissue) or visceral (arising from internal organs such as the large intestine or pancreas). While somatic pain most often presents as throbbing and well localized, visceral pain can manifest as pain feeling as if it is coming from other structures (referred) or as a well-localized phenomenon.[11] We can think of nociception in terms of stimulation, transmission, perception, and modulation[11] (Table 60–1).

STIMULATION

The first step leading to the sensation of pain is stimulation of free nerve endings known as *nociceptors*. These receptors are found in both somatic and visceral structures, distinguish between noxious and innocuous stimuli, and are activated and sensitized by mechanical, thermal, and chemical impulses.[11] The underlying mechanism of these noxious stimuli (which and in of themselves may sensitize/stimulate the receptor) may be the release of bradykinins, K^+, prostaglandins, histamine, leukotrienes, serotonin, and substance P (among others) that sensitize and/or activate the nociceptors.[12,13] Receptor activation leads to action potentials that are transmitted along afferent nerve fibers to the spinal cord[11] (Fig. 60–1).

TRANSMISSION

Nociceptive transmission takes place in A-delta and C afferent nerve fibers.[11] Stimulation of large-diameter, sparsely myelinated A delta fibers evokes sharp, well-localized pain, whereas stimulation of unmyelinated, small-diameter C fibers produces dull, aching, and poorly localized pain.[11] These afferent, nociceptive pain fibers synapse in

TABLE 60–1. Nociception: Basic Process of Pain Transmission

1. *Stimulation.* Noxious stimulus sensitizes and/or stimulates nociceptors and causes the release of neural chemicals that also sensitize and/or stimulate nociceptors. This activation leads to the production of an action potential.
2. *Transmission.* The action potential continues from the site of noxious stimulus to the dorsal horn of the spinal cord and then ascends to higher centers. Transmission takes place in at least five pathways:
   a. Spinothalamic tract
   b. Spinoreticular tract
   c. Spinomesencephalic tract
   d. Dorsal column postsynaptic spinomedullary pathway
   e. Propriospinal multisynaptic ascending systems
3. *Perception.* Conscious experience of pain.
4. *Modulation.* Inhibition of nociceptive impulses. Neurons from the brain stem descend to the spinal cord and release substances such as endogenous opioids, serotonin, and norepinephrine that inhibit transmission of nociceptive impulses.

Compiled from Refs. 11, 12, and 13.

various layers (laminae) of the spinal cord's dorsal horn,[13] releasing a variety of neurotransmitters, including glutamate, substance P, and calcitonin gene-related peptide.[14] The complex array of events that influence pain can be partially explained by the conversations between neuroreceptors and neurotransmitters that take place in this synapse. For example, by stimulating large sensory myelinated fibers (e.g., A-beta) that mutually connect in the dorsal horn with pain fibers, both noxious and nonnoxious stimuli can have an inhibitory effect on pain transmission[15] (see Fig. 60–1). Functionally, the importance of the interplay between these different fibers and various neurotransmitters and neuroreceptors is evident in the analgesic response produced by topical irritants or transcutaneous electrical nerve stimulation. These pain-initiated processes reach the brain through a complex array of at least five ascending spinal cord pathways, which include the spinothalamic tract[16] (see Table 60–1). Information other than pain is also carried along these pathways. Thus pain is influenced by many factors supplemental to nociception and precludes simple schematic representation. It is postulated that the thalamus acts as a relay station as these pathways ascend and pass the impulses to central structures where pain can be processed further.[11]

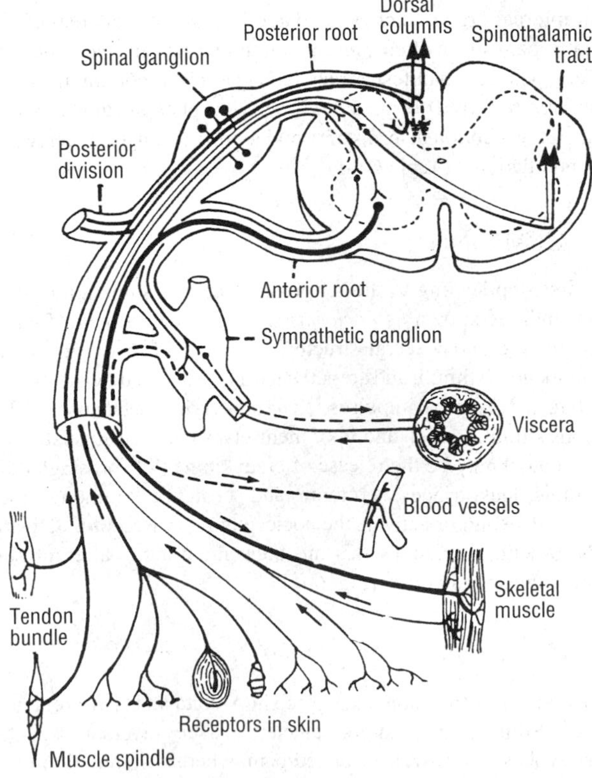

FIGURE 60–1. Schematic representation of dorsal horn nociceptive modulation. *(Adapted from Ref. 13.)*

PAIN PERCEPTION

At this point in transmission, pain is thought to become a conscious experience that takes place in higher cortical structures. The brain may only accommodate a limited number of pain signals; thus cognitive and behavioral functions can modify pain. Relaxation, distraction, meditation, and guided mental imagery may decrease pain by limiting the number of processed pain signals.[11]

MODULATION

The body modulates pain through a number of complex processes. One, known as the *endogenous opiate system,* consists of neurotransmitters (e.g., enkephalins, dynorphins, and β-endorphins) and receptors (e.g., mu, delta, kappa) that are found throughout the central nervous system (CNS).[16] Like exogenous opioids, endogenous opioids bind to opioid receptor sites and inhibit the transmission of pain impulses.[11] Other receptor types also can influence this system. Activation of *N*-methyl-D-aspartate (NMDA) receptors, found in the dorsal horn, can decrease the mu receptors' responsiveness to opiates.[16]

The CNS also contains a highly organized descending system for control of pain transmission. This system can inhibit synaptic pain transmission at the dorsal horn and originates in the brain.[11] Important neurotransmitters here include endogenous opioids, serotonin, norepinephrine, γ-aminobutyric acid (GABA), and neurotensin.[11]

NEUROPATHIC PAIN

Neuropathic pain is distinctly different from nociceptive pain. It is pain sustained by abnormal processing of sensory input by the peripheral or central nervous system. A large number of neuropathic pain syndromes exist (Fig. 60–2), and they are often difficult to treat.[11]

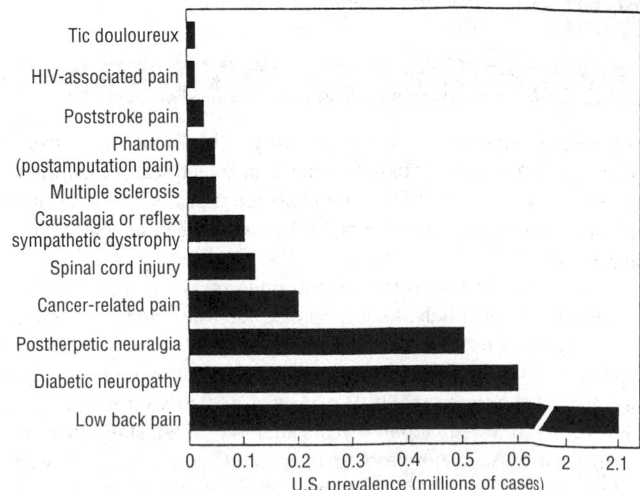

FIGURE 60–2. Estimated prevalence of neuropathic pain. *(Adapted from Ref. 14.)*

In addition, the pain reported often is not evident by examining physical findings.[11]

The mechanism responsible may be the nervous system's endogenous dynamic nature. Nerve damage or persistent stimulation may cause pain circuits to rewire themselves both anatomically and biochemically.[14] This produces spontaneous nerve stimulation, autonomic neuronal pain stimulation, and a progressive increase in discharge of dorsal horn neurons.[11,14]

Clinically, patients present with spontaneous pain transmission (often described as burning, tingling, shock-like, or shooting), exaggerated painful response to normally noxious stimuli (hyperalgesia), or painful response to normally nonnoxious stimuli (allodynia).[11,17] This change over time may help explain why this type pain often manifests long after the actual nerve-related injury.

CLINICAL PRESENTATION

Clinical presentation of pain is best addressed by proper pain assessment. A patient-oriented approach is essential, and evaluation methods should not differ from those used in other medical conditions.[3] Therefore, a comprehensive history and physical examination are imperative to thoroughly evaluate underlying diseases and possible contributing factors.[3] A baseline characterization of pain can be obtained by assessing PQRST characteristics[18] (Table 60–2). Attention also must be given to mental factors that alter the pain threshold. Anxiety, depression, fatigue, anger, and fear in particular are noted to lower this threshold, whereas rest, mood elevation, sympathy, diversion, and understanding raise the pain threshold.[18]

Clinicians must evaluate all components of the pain experience, e.g., behavioral (part of our reaction to pain is learned),[19] cognitive (thinking processes alter pain experiences),[20] social (pain expression differs in accordance with social environments),[21] and cultural (cultural background may influence pain tolerance).[21] In addition, separating pain with neuropathic pathophysiology (see Fig. 60–2) from

TABLE 60–2. PQRST Characteristics of Pain

P	Palliative factors	What makes the pain better?
	Provocative factors	What makes the pain worse?
Q	Quality	Describe the pain.
R	Radiation	Where is the pain?
S	Severity	How does this pain compare with other pain you have experienced?
T	Temporal factors	Does the intensity of the pain change with time?

Modified from Ref. 18.

that caused by a known nociceptive pathophysiology (e.g., posttrauma pain) allows for improved treatment regimens. Nociceptive pain is often acute, localized, well described, and relieved with conventional analgesic therapy (e.g., opioids, acetaminophen, nonsteroidal anti-inflammatory drugs), whereas neuropathic pain is often chronic, not well recognized, and not easily treated with conventional analgesics. Proper patient assessment also must include an evaluation of pain management. Pain intensity, pain relief, and medication side effects must be assessed and reassessed on a regular basis. The timing and regularity of this assessment will depend on the type of pain and the medications administered. Postoperative pain and acute exacerbation of cancer pain may need to be assessed every hour, whereas chronic nonmalignant pain may need only daily assessment. Quality of life also must be assessed on a regular basis in all patients.

The clinician must remember, however, that "pain is always subjective. Objective observations of grimacing, limping, and tachycardia may be useful in assessing the patient, but these signs are often absent in patients with chronic pain known to be caused by structural lesions. There is no neurophysiological or chemical test that can measure pain. The clinician does well in the absence of strong contrary evidence to accept the patient's report of pain"[22]

▶ TREATMENT: Acute and Chronic Pain

Acute pain may be a useful physiologic process warning individuals of disease states and potentially harmful situations. Unfortunately, severe, unremitting, undertreated, acute pain, when it outlives its biologic usefulness, can produce many deleterious effects (e.g., psychological problems). When acute pain is not treated effectively, the stress and concurrent reflex reactions often cause hypoxia, hypercapnia, hypertension, excessive cardiac activity, and emotional difficulties.

Under normal conditions, acute pain subsides quickly as the healing process decreases the pain-producing stimuli; however, in some instances, pain persists for months to years, leading to a chronic pain state with features quite different from those of acute pain (Table 60–3). Chronic pain can be divided into four subtypes: pain that persists beyond the normal healing time for an acute injury, pain related to a chronic disease, pain without identifiable organic cause, and pain that involves both the chronic and acute pain associated with cancer.[23] Patients in chronic pain often develop severe psychological problems caused by fear and memory of past pain. In addition, chronic pain patients may develop dependence on and tolerance to analgesics, have trouble sleeping, and more readily react to environmental changes that can intensify the pain response. Distinguishing between chronic and acute pain states is very important because of differing management techniques.[22]

ACUTE PAIN MANAGEMENT

The obvious way to relieve pain is to eliminate the underlying cause. This is often not possible, however, and symptomatic relief is usually indicated. Therapeutic interventions include pharmacologic treatment, stimulation therapies, and psychological therapies.

NONPHARMACOLOGIC THERAPY

Stimulation Therapy

Transcutaneous electrical nerve stimulation (TENS) has shown moderate success in managing surgical, traumatic, and oral-facial pain.[15] Although opioid-like side effects are certainly prevented, this technique has not gained wide acceptance in acute pain.

Psychological Intervention

Even though the cognitive, behavioral, and social aspects of pain are well established, psychological techniques for the treatment of acute

TABLE 60–3. Characteristics of Acute and Chronic Pain

Characteristic	Acute Pain	Chronic Pain
Relief of pain	Highly desirable	Highly desirable
Dependence and tolerance to medication	Unusual	Common
Psychological component	Usually not present	Often a major problem
Organic cause	Common	Often not present
Environmental contributions and family involvement	Small	Significant
Insomnia	Unusual	Common component
Treatment goal	Cure	Functionality

Modified from Ref. 3, p. 256.

pain are not employed widely. Simple interventions (e.g., introductory information about sensations to expect after certain procedures) reduce patient distress and greatly reduce postprocedure suffering.[24] Other successful psychological techniques include relaxation training, imagery, and hypnosis.[24]

PHARMACOLOGIC TREATMENT

Nonopioid Agents

Analgesia should be initiated with the most effective analgesic agent having the fewest side effects. Acetaminophen, acetylsalicylic acid (aspirin), and nonsteroidal anti-inflammatory drugs (NSAIDs), often are preferred over opiates in the treatment of acute mild to moderate pain (Tables 60–4 and 60–5). These drugs (with the exception of acetaminophen) affect the prostaglandins produced by the arachidonic acid cascade in response to noxious stimuli,[25] thereby decreasing the number of pain impulses received by the CNS. Therapeutic outcomes are also less than desired in those who do not expect "mild" analgesics to relieve pain. Studies comparing the efficacy of these agents have been inconsistent. Therefore, the choice of a particular agent often depends on availability, cost, pharmacokinetics, pharmacologic characteristics (see Tables 60–4 and 60–5), and the side-effect profile (Table 60–6). It should be noted that all NSAIDs have some analgesic effects, but only those which are approved by the Food and Drug Administration (FDA) for the treatment of pain are compared in the tables (agents approved exclusively for the treatment of osteoarthritis and/or rheumatoid arthritis are not included in this table). There appears to be a great deal of interpatient variability in the therapeutic response to the NSAIDs. After an adequate drug trial of any of these agents, it is considered rational therapy to switch to another member of this drug group for an additional trial period.

Opioid Agents

Most clinicians consider the use of opioids to be the next logical step in the management of acute pain. The classification of these agents, their equianalgesic doses, and dosing guidelines are outlined in Tables 60–7 and 60–8.

The pharmacologic activity of opioids depends on their affinity for opiate receptors.[26] Therapeutic activities and side effects range from those exhibited by the pure opiate agonists (e.g., morphine) to those seen with the pure opiate antagonists (e.g., naloxone). Partial agonists and antagonists (e.g., pentazocine) compete with agonists for opiate receptor sites and, depending on the inherent agonist and antagonist properties, exhibit mixed agonist-antagonist activity. Mixed agonist-antagonist agents with analgesic activity appear to exhibit selectivity for analgesic receptor sites.[26] This may result in analgesia with fewer undesirable side effects.

TABLE 60–4. Pharmacokinetic and Pharmacodynamic Profiles of FDA-Approved Nonopioid Analgesics (does not include agents approved only for osteoarthritis or rheumatoid arthritis)

Agent	Time to Peak Concentration (h)	Elimination Half-Life (h)	Analgesic Onset (h)	Analgesic Duration (h)
Aspirin	0.25–2	0.25–0.33	0.5	3–6
Choline salicylate	1.5–2	—[a]	—[a]	4
Magnesium salicylate	1.5–2	—[a]	—[a]	4
Sodium salicylate	0.67	—[a]	—[a]	4
Diflunisal	2–3	8–12	1	8–12
Acetaminophen	0.5–2	1.25–3	0.5–1	3–6
Meclofenamate	0.5–2	0.8–5.3	—[a]	4–6
Mefenamic acid	2–4	2–4	—[a]	6
Etodoloc	1	7	0.5–1	6–8
Diclofenac potassium	1	—[a]	0.5	6–8
Ibuprofen	1–2	1–2.5	0.5	4–6
Fenoprofen	1–2	2–3	0.25–0.5	4–6
Ketoprofen	0.5–2	2–4	1	4–8
Naproxen	2–4	12–17	1	Up to 12
Naproxen sodium	1–2	12–13	0.5–1	Up to 12
Ketorolac (parenteral)	0.5–1	4–6	0.17	6
Ketorolac (oral)	0.5–1	4–6	0.5–1	4–6
Rofecoxib	2–3	17	0.5–1	Up to 24
Celecoxib	3	11	1	12–24

[a]Data not available to author.
Compiled from Refs. 33, 34, 52, 53, 54, 55, 56, 57, 58, and 61.

TABLE 60–5. FDA Approved Nonopioid Analgesics in Adults (does not include agents approved only for osteoarthritis or rheumatoid arthritis)

Class and Generic Name	Usual Dosage Range (mg)	Maximal Dose (mg/day)
Salicylates		
Acetylsalicylic acid[a] (aspirin)	325–650 every 4 h	4000
Choline[a]	870 every 3–4 h	5220
Magnesium[a]	300–600 every 4 h	3500
Sodium[a]	325–650 every 4 h	5400
Diflunisal	500–1000 initial	
	250–500 every 8–12 h	1500
para-Aminophenol		
Acetaminophen[a]	325–1000 every 4–6 h	4000
Fenamates		
Meclofenamate	50 every 4–6 h	400
Mefenamic acid	Initial 500	
	250 every 6 h (maximum of 7 days)	1000[b]
Pyranocarboxylic Acid		
Etodoloc	200–400 every 6–8 h	1200
Acetic Acid		
Diclofenac potassium	In some patients, initial 100	150[c]
	50 three times a day	
Propionic Acids		
Ibuprofen[a]	200–400 every 4–6 h	3200
		1200[d]
Fenoprofen	200 every 4–6 h	3200
Ketoprofen[a]	25–50 every 6–8 h	300
	12.5–25 every 4–6 h[d]	75[d]
Naproxen	500 initial	
	500 every 12 h or 250 every 6–8 h	1000[b]
Naproxen sodium[a]	In some patients, 440 initial[d]	
	220 every 8–12 h[d]	660[d]
Naproxen delayed-release[e]	375–500 every 12 h	1000
Naproxen controlled-release[e]	750–1000 every 24 h	1500
Pyrrolizine Carboxylic Acid		
Ketorolac (parenteral)	30–60 (single dose only)	30–60
	15–30 every 6 h (maximum of 5 days)	120
Ketorolac (oral) (indicated for continuation with parenteral only)	In some patients, initial oral dose 20 10 every 4–6 h (maximum of 5 days, which includes parenteral doses)	40
Cyclooxygenase 2 Inhibitors		
Rofecoxib	50 mg every 24 h[f] (maximum 5 days)[f]	50[f]
Celecoxib	Initial 400 followed by another 200 on first day[f]	400[f]
	200 twice daily[f]	

[a]Available both as an over-the-counter preparation and as a prescription drug.
[b]Up to 1250 mg on the first day.
[c]Up to 200 mg on the first day.
[d]Over-the-counter.
[e]Not for the initial treatment of acute pain.
[f]For acute pain.
Compiled from Refs. 33, 34, 58, and 61.

The effects of the opioid analgesics are relatively selective, and at normal therapeutic concentrations, these agents do not decrease sensitivity to touch, sight, or hearing[27]; however, as the dosage increases, so do the undesirable side effects (Table 60–9). Patients in severe pain may receive very high doses of opioids with no unwanted side effects, but as the pain subsides, they will not tolerate even very low doses.[27] Frequently, when opioids are administered, pain is not eliminated, but its unpleasantness is decreased.[77] Patients report that although their pain is still present, it no longer bothers them.

Opioids share related pharmacologic attributes and exert a profound effect on the CNS and gastrointestinal tract.[27] Mood changes, sedation, respiratory depression, nausea, vomiting, decreased gastrointestinal motility, dependence, and tolerance are evident in varying degrees with all agents. Consideration of efficacy and side-effect profile assists in the selection of the most appropriate agent.

The route of administration depends on individual patient needs. Peak analgesic effect usually occurs 1.5 to 2 hours after oral administration, and this delay must be a consideration when immediate relief is needed.[22] The opioids differ greatly in equianalgesic dose (see Table 60–7). Table 60–7 should be used only as a guide because the nature of pain makes it necessary to individualize pain regimens. True opioid allergies are rare, but Table 60–7 also can be used when treating a patient who is hypersensitive to opiates. Although caution is always advised, a decrease in potential cross-sensitivity exists when staying in one class. The classes are morphine-like agonists, meperidine-like agonists, and methadone-like agonists. When considering

TABLE 60–6. Relative Side Effects of FDA-Approved Nonopioid Analgesics (does not include agents approved only for osteoarthritis or rheumatoid arthritis)

Agent	GI Irritation	CNS Effects	Hepatic Toxicity	Renal Toxicity
Aspirin	++++++	+	++	++
Choline salicylate	+++	—[a]	—[a]	—[a]
Magnesium salicylate	+++	—[a]	—[a]	—[a]
Sodium salicylate	+++	—[a]	—[a]	—[a]
Diflunisal	++	+	+	+
Acetaminophen	+	+	++	+
Meclofenamate	++	+	+	++
Mefenamic acid	++	+	+	++
Etodolac	++	+	+	++
Diclofenac potassium	++	+	+	++
Ibuprofen	++	+	+	++
Fenoprofen	++	++	+	++
Ketoprofen	++	+	+	++
Ketorolac[b]	++	+	+	+
Naproxen	++	+	+	++
Rofecoxib[b]	+	+	+	+
Celecoxib	+	+	+	++

[a]No data available to author.
[b]Five-day use only.
Compiled from Refs. 33 and 34.

cross-sensitivity, the mixed agonist-antagonist class acts much like the morphine-like agonists.[28]

In the initial stages of acute pain, analgesics should be given around the clock. This should commence after administering a typical starting dose and titrating up or down depending on the patient's degree of pain and demonstrated side effects (e.g., sedation).[22] As-needed schedules often produce wide swings in analgesic plasma concentrations that create wide swings in pain and sedation. This may initiate a vicious cycle where increasing amounts of pain medications are needed for relief. As the painful state subsides and the need for medication decreases, however, as-needed schedules can be used. Continuous intravenous and subcutaneous methods of opioid infusion are effective in some postoperative pain,[22] but the probability of unwanted side effects is high. An alternative method that has gained prominence is patient-controlled analgesia (PCA). With this technique, patients can self-administer preset amounts of intravenous opioids via a syringe pump electronically interfaced with a timing device. Using this procedure, patients balance pain control with sedation.

Administration of opiates directly into the CNS (i.e., epidural and intrathecal/subarachnoid routes) has shown considerable promise in the control of acute pain[29] (Table 60–10) and is becoming prominent in both large and small institutions throughout the United States. Because of reports of marked sedation, respiratory depression, pruritus, nausea, vomiting, urinary retention, and hypotension,[30] these methods of analgesia require careful monitoring and are best employed by experienced practitioners. Respiratory depression is of concern and can occur within the first half hour or manifest as late as 12 hours after a single dose of epidural morphine.[30] Naloxone is used to antagonize this effect, but continual infusion may be required.[30] Analgesia as well as side effects are evident at lower doses when the opioids are administered intrathecally instead of epidurally. Intrathecally, single morphine doses of 0.1–0.3 mg are common, whereas epidurally, doses of 1–6 mg are the norm.[29] These intrathecal and epidural opioids often are administered on a continuous-infusion and/or patient-contolled basis, and when given simultaneously with intrathecal or epidural local anesthetics such as bupivacaine, they have been proven safe and effective.[31] All agents administered directly into the CNS should be preservative-free.

Morphine and Congeners. Despite the availability of several newer agents, morphine remains the prototype opiate analgesic. As new opioid and nonopioid compounds are developed, their efficacy and side-effect profiles are compared with morphine as the standard. Many clinicians consider morphine the first-line agent when treating moderate to severe pain. Morphine can be given parenterally, orally, or rectally.

Morphine's CNS effects are numerous. Through direct stimulation of the chemoreceptor trigger zone, morphine causes nausea and vomiting.[27] Opioid-induced nausea is observed most frequently after the initial dose and often subsides with subsequent doses.[32] Although euphoria and dysphoria have been reported, morphine's unpleasant effects are more prominent when administered to those not experiencing pain.[27] As doses of morphine are increased, the respiratory center becomes less responsive to carbon dioxide, resulting in progressive respiratory depression. This effect is less pronounced in those being treated for severe pain. Respiratory depression often manifests as a decrease in respiratory rate (although minute volume and tidal volume are also affected) and is further compounded because the cough reflex is also depressed. Morphine-induced respiratory depression can be reversed by pure opioid antagonists.[27] In patients with underlying pulmonary dysfunction, caution must be employed when using morphine or any related opioid. Although these patients may be functioning normally, they are already using compensatory breathing mechanisms and are at risk for further respiratory compromise.[27] Precaution is also urged when using opiate analgesics with alcohol or other CNS depressants. This combination amplifies CNS depression and is potentially harmful and possibly lethal.

Therapeutic doses of morphine have minimal effects on blood pressure, cardiac rate, or cardiac rhythm when patients are supine; however, morphine does produce venous and arteriolar vessel dilatation, and orthostatic hypotension may result. Hypovolemic patients are more susceptible to morphine-induced cardiovascular changes (e.g., decreases in blood pressure).[27] Because morphine prompts a

TABLE 60–7. Opioid Analgesics

Class and Generic Name	Route	Equianalgesic Dose (mg)
Morphine-Like Agonists		
Morphine	IM	10
	PO	30
Hydromorphone	IM	1.5
	PO	7.5
Oxymorphone	IM	1.0
	R	5[a]
Levorphanol	IM (acute)	2.0
	PO (acute)	4.0
	IM (chronic)	1.0
	PO (chronic)	1.0
Codeine	IM	15–30[b]
	PO	15–30[b]
Hydrocodone	PO	5–10[b]
Oxycodone	PO	20 30[c]
Meperidine-Like Agonists		
Meperidine	IM	75
	PO	300[c]
Fentanyl	IM	0.1–0.2
	Transdermal	25 μg/h[d]
	Transmucosal for breakthrough pain only	
Methadone-Like Agonists		
Methadone	IM (acute)	10
	PO (acute)	10–20
	IM (chronic)	2–4
	PO (chronic)	2–4
Propoxyphene	PO	65[b]
Agonist-Antagonist Derivatives		
Pentazocine	IM, SQ	30–60
	PO	50[b]
Butorphanol	IM	2
	Intranasal	1[b] (one spray)
Nalbuphine	IM	10
Buprenorphine	IM	0.4
Dezocine	IM	10
Antagonists		
Naloxone	IV	0.4–1.2[e]
Central Analgesic		
Tramadol	PO	50–100[b]

[a]Reference 58 considers 5 mg rectal morphine = 5 mg rectal oxymorphone.
[b]Starting dose only (equianalgesia not shown).
[c]Starting doses lower (oxycodone, 5–15 mg; meperidine, 50 mg).
[d]Equivalent IM morphine dose = 8–22 mg day.
[e]Starting doses to be used in cases of opioid overdose.
Compiled from Refs. 27, 34, and 58.

decrease in myocardial oxygen demand in ischemic cardiac patients, it is often considered the drug of choice when using opioids to treat pain associated with myocardial infarction.

Morphine decreases the propulsive contractions of the gastrointestinal tract, and biliary and pancreatic secretions are reduced.[27] The end result, especially when morphine is administered over extended time periods, is constipation. Morphine-induced spasms of the sphincter of Oddi have been observed.[27] However, the clinical significance of such an occurrence should be assessed on an individual basis. Although morphine's effect on the urinary bladder varies, urinary retention can become a problem; tolerance develops to this effect over time.[27] Morphine-induced histamine release often manifests as pruritus, and although not seen often, it may exacerbate bronchospasm in patients with a history of asthma.[27] Therapeutic doses of morphine do not directly affect cerebral circulation, but drug-induced respiratory depression can increase intracranial pressure. Thus caution is advised in head trauma patients who are not ventilated because morphine may exaggerate this pressure[27] while clouding the neurologic examination results.

Hydromorphone is more potent, has better oral absorption characteristics, and is more soluble than morphine, but its overall pharmacologic profile parallels that of morphine. Oxymorphone can be administered rectally and by injection. Although it is more potent than morphine, it offers no real pharmacologic advantages. Although levorphanol has an extended half-life, its overall therapeutic effects are similar to those of morphine.

Codeine is an analgesic that is effective in the treatment of mild to moderate pain. It is often combined with other analgesic products and enjoys a popularity that makes it the standard for other oral narcotics. Unfortunately, codeine has the same propensity to produce tolerance, dependence, and constipation as morphine. Hydrocodone, a derivative of codeine, also is seen most often in combination products and has pharmacologic properties similar to those of morphine. Oxycodone has a similar potency to morphine and is an excellent oral analgesic for moderate to severe pain. This is especially true when the product is used in combination with nonopioids; however, its predilection for causing tolerance and dependence, along with its basic opioid characteristics, likens it to morphine. It should be noted that sustained-release oxycodone is also available.

Meperidine and Congeners (Phenylpiperidines). The prototype phenylpiperidine, meperidine, has a pharmacologic profile comparable with that of morphine; however, it is not as potent and has a shorter analgesic duration. This necessitates larger doses that often must be administered more frequently for satisfactory pain relief. Although meperidine is effective orally, larger doses must be administered to achieve the same effect as obtained with the parenteral form (see Table 60–7). With high doses or in patients with renal failure, the metabolite normeperidine accumulates, causing CNS excitability, manifested as tremor, muscle twitching, and possibly seizures.[33] The combination of monoamine oxidase inhibitors and meperidine should not be used because this mixture can produce severe respiratory depression or excitation, delirium, hyperpyrexia, and convulsions.[27] In most clinical settings, meperidine offers no real advantage over morphine and is largely being displaced by other opioids.

Fentanyl is a synthetic opioid structurally related to meperidine and is used often in anesthesiology as an adjunct to general anesthesia.[33] This agent is more potent and shorter acting than meperidine (see Tables 60–7 and 60–11). Transdermal fentanyl is also available for the treatment of chronic pain in patients requiring opioid analgesics. One patch can provide analgesic support for 72 hours, but it takes 12 to 24 hours to obtain optimal analgesic effect after a patch is applied. In addition, it may take 6 days after increasing a dose before new steady-state levels are achieved. Thus the patch should not be used in patients with acute pain.[34] A fentanyl lozenge on a stick is available for the treatment of breakthrough cancer pain.[34]

Methadone and Congeners. Methadone has gained considerable popularity because of its oral efficacy, extended duration of action, and ability to suppress withdrawal symptoms in heroin addicts. With repeated doses, the analgesic duration of action is prolonged,[34] but

TABLE 60–8. Dosing Guidelines

Agent	Doses (Titrate Up or Down Based on Patient Response)	Notes
NSAIDs/acetaminophen/aspirin	Dose to maximum before switching to another agent (see Table 60–5)	Used in mild to moderate pain May use in conjunction with narcotic agents to decrease doses of each Regular alcohol use and high doses of acetaminophen may result in liver toxicity Care must be exercised to avoid overdose when combination products containing these agents are used
Morphine	PO 5–30 mg q 3–4 h[a] IM 5–10 mg q 3–4 h[a] IV 1–2.5 mg q 5 min prn[a] SR 15–30 mg q 12 h (may need to be q 8 h in some patients) Rectal 10–20 mg q 4 h[a]	Drug of choice in severe pain Use immediate-release product with SR product to control "breakthrough" pain in cancer patients Every 24 hour product available
Hydromorphone	PO 2–4 mg q 3–6 h[a] IM 1–4 mg q 4–6 h[a] IV 0.1–0.5 mg q 5 min prn[a] Rectal 3 mg q 6–8 h[a]	Use in severe pain More potent than morphine; otherwise, no advantages
Oxymorphone	IM 1–1.5 mg q 4–6 h[a] IV 0.5 mg initially Rectal 5 mg q 4–6 h[a]	Use in severe pain No advantages over morphine
Levorphanol	PO 2–3 mg q 6–8 h[a] IM 1–2 mg q 6–8 h	Use in severe pain Extended half-life useful in cancer patients In chronic pain, wait 3 days between dosage adjustments
Codeine	PO 15–60 mg q 3–6 h[a] IM 15–60 mg q 3–6 h[a] IV 15–60 mg q 3–6 h[a] (max. 360 mg q day)	Use in moderate pain Weak analgesic; use with NSAIDs or aspirin or acetaminophen
Hydrocodone	PO 5–10 mg q 3–6 h[a]	Use in moderate/severe pain Most effective when used with NSAIDs or aspirin or acetaminophen
Oxycodone	PO 5–15 mg q 3–6 h[a] Controlled release, 10–20 mg q 12 h	Use in moderate/severe pain Most effective when used with NSAIDs or aspirin or acetaminophen Use immediate-release product with controlled-release product to control "breakthrough" pain in cancer patients
Meperidine	PO 50–150 mg q 3–4 h[a] IM 50–150 mg q 3–4 h[a] IV 5–10 mg q 5 min prn[a]	Use in severe pain Oral not recommended Do not use in renal failure May precipitate tremors, myoclonus, and seizures Monoamine oxidase inhibitors can induce hyperpyrexia and/or seizures
Fentanyl	IM 0.05–0.1 mg q 1–2 h[a] Transdermal 25 μg/h q 72 h Transmucosal 200 μg may repeat ×1 30 minutes after first dose is given then titrate	Used in severe pain Do not use in acute pain Transmucosal for "breakthrough" cancer pain
Methadone	PO 2.5–10 mg q 3–4 h (acute) IM 2.5–10 mg q 3–4 h (acute) PO 5–20 mg q 6–8 (chronic)	Effective in severe chronic pain Sedation can be major problem Some chronic pain patients can be dosed every 12 hours
Propoxyphene	PO 100 mg q 4 h[a] (napsylate) PO 65 mg q 4 h[a] (HCl) (max. q day 600 mg of napsylate, 390 mg HCl)	Use in moderate pain Weak analgesic; most effective when used with NSAIDs or aspirin or acetaminophen Will cause carbamazepine levels to increase 100 mg of napsylate salt = to 65 mg of HCl salt
Pentazocine	PO 50–100 mg q 3–4 h[b] (max. 600 mg q day) IM 30 mg q 3–4 h[b] (max 360 mg q day)	Third-line agent for moderate to severe pain May precipitate withdrawal in opiate dependent patients

TABLE 60–8. (continued)

Agent	Doses (Titrate Up or Down Based on Patient Response)	Notes
Butorphanol	IM 1–4 mg q 3–4 h[b] IV 0.5–2 mg q 3–4 h[b] Intranasal 1 mg (1 spray) q 3–4 h[b] If inadequate relief after initial spray, may repeat in other nostril ×1 in 60–90 minutes Max 2 sprays (one per nostril) q 3–4 h[b]	Second-line agent for moderate to severe pain May precipitate withdrawal in opiate dependent patients
Nalbuphine	IM/IV 10 mg q 3–6 h[b] (max 20 mg dose, 160 mg q day)	Second-line agent for moderate to severe pain May precipitate withdrawal in opiate dependent patients
Buprenorphine	IM 0.3 mg q 6 h[b] Slow IV 0.3 mg q 6 h[b] May repeat ×1, 30–60 min after initial dose	Second-line agent for moderate to severe pain May precipitate withdrawal in opiate dependent patients
Dezocine	IM 5–20 mg q 3–6 h[b] IV 2.5–10 mg q 2–4 h[b]	Second-line agent for moderate to severe pain May precipitate withdrawal in opiate dependent patients
Naloxone	IV 0.4–1.2 mg	When reversing opiate side effects in patients needing analgesia, dilute and titrate (0.1–0.2 mg q 2–3 min) so as not to reverse analgesia
Tramadol	PO 50–100 mg q 4–6 h[a]	Maximum dose is 400 mg/24 h Decrease dose in renal impairment and in the elderly

[a]May start with an around-the-clock regimen and switch to prn if/when the painful signal subsides or is episodic.
[b]May reach a ceiling analgesic effect.
Compiled from Refs. 24, 26, 33, 34, and 58.

excessive sedation also may result. Although methadone is effective in acute pain,[34] it is usually used to treat chronic pain. The pharmacologic profile resembles that of morphine. However, a property unique to methadone when compared with other opioids may be its ability to antagonize NMDA receptors.[35] This property may prove useful in the treatment of neuropathic pain.

Propoxyphene is one-half as potent as codeine and is more effective than placebo when 65–100 mg is ingested.[36] It is usually used in combination with acetaminophen in the treatment of moderate pain. The toxicity profile of propoxyphene is similar to that of codeine.

TABLE 60–9. Major Adverse Effects of the Opioid Analgesics

Effect	Manifestation
Mood changes	Dysphoria, euphoria
Somnolence	Lethargy, drowsiness, apathy, inability to concentrate
Stimulation of chemoreceptor trigger zone	Nausea, vomiting
Respiratory depression	Decreased respiratory rate
Decreased gastrointestinal motility	Constipation
Increase in sphincter tone	Biliary spasm, urinary retention (varies among agents)
Histamine release	Urticaria, pruritus, rarely exacerbation of asthma (varies among agents)
Tolerance	Larger doses for same effect
Dependence	Withdrawal symptoms upon abrupt discontinuation

Compiled from Refs. 3, 26, and 27.

Opioid Agonist-Antagonists Derivatives

Analgesic agents that stimulate the analgesic portion of opioid receptors while blocking or having no effect on the toxicity portion would be considered ideal. The agonist-antagonist derivatives were developed with this in mind. The analgesic class produces analgesia and has a ceiling effect on respiratory depression.[26] These agents also have a lower abuse potential than morphine, but psychotomimetic responses (e.g., hallucinations and dysphoria, as seen with pentazocine), a ceiling analgesic effect, and a propensity to initiate withdrawal in opioid-dependent populations[26] have diminished their widespread clinical use.

Opioid Antagonists

The pure opioid antagonist naloxone binds competitively to opioid receptors but does not produce an analgesic response. Therefore, it is used most often to reverse the toxic effects of agonist- and agonist-antagonist-derived opioids.

Central Analgesic

Tramadol has two basic modes of action: mu opiate receptor binding and weak inhibition of norepinephrine and serotonin reuptake. It is indicated for the relief of moderate to moderately severe pain.[37]

Although associated with less respiratory depression than morphine at recommended doses, tramadol has a side-effect profile similar to that of the previously mentioned opioid analgesics. Tramadol alone may enhance the risk of seizures. In addition, concomitant use with serotonin reuptake inhibitors, opioids, tricyclic antidepressants,

TABLE 60–10. Intraspinal Opioids

Agent	Dose (mg) (Single)	Onset of Pain Relief (min)	Duration of Pain Relief (h)	Continual Infusion Dose (mg/h)
Epidural Route				
Morphine	1–6	30	6–24	0.1–1
Hydromorphone	1–2	15	6–16	0.1–0.2
Fentanyl	0.025–0.1	5	1–4	0.025–0.1
Subarachnoid Route				
Morphine	0.1–0.3	15	8–24 +	—
Fentanyl	0.005–0.025	5	3–6	—

Modified from Ref. 29.

monoamine oxidase inhibitors, neuroleptics, or other drugs that can reduce the seizure threshold, and use in patients with seizure disorders may increase the risk of seizures.[37]

Tramadol may have a place in treating patients with chronic pain, especially that of neuropathic origin.[38] However, this agent has little advantage over the previously mentioned opioid analgesics when treating patients for acute pain.

Combination Therapy

The combination of opioid and nonopioid oral analgesics often results in analgesia superior to that produced by either agent alone.[24] Attacking pain on two fronts, prostaglandins and opiate receptors, enhances pain relief and facilitates the use of lower doses of each agent. This frequently produces a more favorable side-effect profile and is the reason there are so many aspirin- and/or acetaminophen-opioid analgesic combination products marketed. The addition of an injectable NSAID (ketorolac) makes this combination possible also in patients who cannot take oral medications. The clinician should not be limited by the availability of commercially established fixed-ratio combinations. For example, the administration of NSAIDs in combination with scheduled opioid regimens is often very effective in the treatment of pain resulting from bone metastases in advanced cancer.[39]

Agents shown to potentiate the analgesic efficacy of parenteral opioids include hydroxyzine and dextroamphetamine.[39] Promethazine and chlorpromazine, once thought to possess this potentiating property, apparently offer no inherent analgesic or potentiating characteristics when combined with narcotics, although unwanted sedation may be increased.[24] Methotrimeprazine, a phenothiazine derivative, does induce analgesia but also produces sedation, orthostatic hypotension, and dizziness.[34]

REGIONAL ANALGESIA

Regional analgesia with properly administered local anesthetics can provide relief of both acute and chronic pain[31] (Table 60–12). These agents can be positioned by injection (i.e., in joints, in the epidural or

TABLE 60–11. Opioid Analgesic Pharmacokinetics[a]

Agent	Time to Peak (h)	Half-Life (h)	Analgesic Onset (min)	Analgesic Duration (h)
Morphine	0.5–1	2	10–20	3–5
Hydromorphone	0.5–1	2–3	10–20	3–5
Oxymorphone	0.5–1	2–3	10–20	4–6
Levorphanol	0.5–1	12–16	10–20	5–8
Hydrocodone (PO)	1	4	30–60	4–6
Codeine	0.5–1	3	10–20	4–6
Oxycodone (PO)	0.5–1	2–3	30–60	4–6
Meperidine	0.5–1	3–4	10–20	2–5
Fentanyl	10–20	3–4	7–15	1–2
Methadone	0.5–1	15–30	10–20	4–5 (acute) >8 (chronic)
Propoxyphene (PO)	2.0–2.5	6–12	30–60	4–6
Pentazocine	0.5–1	4–5	15–20	3–6
Butorphanol	0.5–1	2.5–3.5	10–20	4–6
Nalbuphine	0.5–1	2–5	<15	4–6
Buprenorphine	0.5–1	5	10–20	4–8
Dezocine	0.17–1.5 (IM)	0.6–5 (IV)	15–30 (IV)	2–4 (IV)
Naloxone[c] (IV/IM)	—[b]	1–1.5	1–2 (IV) 2–5 (IM)	0.5–2 (IV) IM may last longer
Tramadol (PO)	2–3	6–7	<60	4–6

[a]Based on intramuscular data unless otherwise indicated.
[b]No data available to author.
[c]Narcotic antagonist.
Compiled from Refs. 27, 32, 33, and 34.

TABLE 60–12. Local Anesthetics[a]

Agent	Onset (min)	Duration (h)
Esters		
Procaine	2–5	0.25–1
Chloroprocaine	6–12	0.50
Tetracaine	≤15	2–3
Amides		
Mepivacaine	3–5	0.75–1.5
Bupivacaine	5	2–4
Lidocaine	<2	0.5–1
Prilocaine	<2	≥1
Etidocaine	3–5	5–10
Ropivacaine[b]	11–26	1.7–3.2
Levobupivacaine[b]	2–18	6–12

[a]Unless otherwise indicated, values are for infiltrative anesthesia.
[b]Epidural administration in cesarean section.
Compiled from Refs. 34, 59, and 60.

intrathecal space, along nerve roots, in a nerve plexus) or topically. Regional anesthetics relieve pain by blocking nociceptive transmission and interrupting sympathetic reflexes.[31] Their lipid solubility, pK_a, percentage of un-ionized drug, drug concentration, vasodilator behavior, and amount of vasoconstrictor (commonly epinephrine) used concomitantly determine the mechanism of action.[31] High plasma concentrations can cause signs of CNS excitation and depression, including dizziness, tinnitus, drowsiness, disorientation, muscle twitching, seizures, and respiratory arrest.[33] Cardiovascular effects include myocardial depression, hypotension, decreased cardiac output, heart block, bradycardia, ventricular arrhythmia, and cardiac arrest.[34] Disadvantages of such methods include the need for skillful technical application, the need for frequent administration, and highly specialized follow-up procedures.

CHRONIC PAIN MANAGEMENT

CANCER PAIN

Managing the pain of malignant diseases encompasses both acute and chronic management techniques. Thus pharmacologic treatment and psychological therapies are best combined with surgical methods, anesthetic procedures, and supportive care measures in a multidisciplinary approach to pain relief.[40] The goal is to provide patients with enough pain amelioration to tolerate diagnostic and therapeutic manipulation and permit them to function at a level that will allow freedom of movement and choice.[40] Unfortunately, a number of patients with cancer may die without significant relief of pain.[9,40] Assessment techniques described in Table 60–2 apply to these patients. Special attention must be given to continual reassessment of the painful state, and individualization of therapy is always required.[39]

Nonpharmacologic Treatment

Psychological and Supportive Care. Previously mentioned psychological techniques (e.g., relaxation training, controlled mental imagery) are very helpful in relieving pain experienced in malignant disease[39] and prove especially useful in conjunction with pharmacologic therapy.

Supportive care, in and outside the hospital, using programs such as hospice is one of the cancer patient's greatest allies not only in coping with pain but also in accepting the disease. The positive effect this has on the patient cannot be overstated.

Pharmacologic Treatment

Pharmacologic management is the mainstay of therapy, and a typical progression of analgesic use is outlined in Figure 60–3. The objective is to prevent the patient from experiencing constant fluctuation between severe pain and pain relief. This is best accomplished by around-the-clock administration schedules that inhibit serum analgesic concentrations from falling below the point at which a patient experiences the suffering of pain. As-needed (prn) schedules are to be employed in conjunction with around-the-clock regimens and are used only when patients experience breakthrough pain. Again, nonopioid agents are used as first-line agents, with NSAIDs being especially effective in treating bone pain.[39] Bone pain also can be treated with radiopharmaceuticals. Both strontium-89 and samarium SM 153 lexidronam have been shown to provide pain relief.[34] The choice of opiate remains controversial but should be based on patient acceptance, analgesic effectiveness, and pharmacokinetic, pharmacodynamic, and side-effect profiles. Many clinicians have found morphine both safe and effective when administered by the oral (sustained-release, liquid, and fast-release), subcutaneous, rectal, continual intravenous infusion, patient-controlled intravenous, epidural, or intrathecal route.[39] Epidural clonidine is also effective with epidurally administered opioid analgesics for the treatment of refractory pain.[34] The fentanyl patch may provide a more convenient dosing alternative in patients on stable regimens. Although heroin has shown analgesic and side-effect characteristics equal to those of morphine, it has no proven superiority.[41] Meperidine is not recommended for long-term use because of its relatively short duration of action and the CNS hyperirritability of normeperidine, one of its metabolites.[39] Anticonvulsant drugs and tricyclic antidepressants have been shown to be effective in pain of neuropathic origin.[42] Antihistamines, amphetamines, and steroids are used as adjuvant pain medications[39]; however, they have enjoyed only limited success as pain relievers.

Anesthetic and neurosurgical approaches have proven successful in alleviating pain but require special expertise and usually are reserved for patients who are refractory to conventional analgesics. They most commonly involve either sectioning or stimulation of the spinal cord, brain, or peripheral nerves. These techniques block pain pathways and subsequently alleviate pain.[39]

NONMALIGNANT CHRONIC PAIN

The numerous etiologies that produce nonmalignant chronic pain make treatment complex, and its management assumes multidisciplinary aspects. As pain becomes gradually more chronic, it loses many of the autonomic characteristics evident in the acute stage, and additional symptoms such as depression, sleep disturbances, anxiety, irritability, work problems, and family instability tend to dominate.[3] Patients should not be told that the pain they are feeling is "psychosomatic" or in their head. In most cases, etiology is not as important as symptomatic relief. Objectives in evaluation include establishing an accurate diagnosis, identifying iatrogenic factors, obtaining a comprehensive psychiatric and psychosocial assessment, paying special attention to family and social problems, and obtaining a description of factors that alleviate or exacerbate pain.[3]

Pharmacologic approaches to patient care do not differ from those described previously; however, neuropathic pain may require

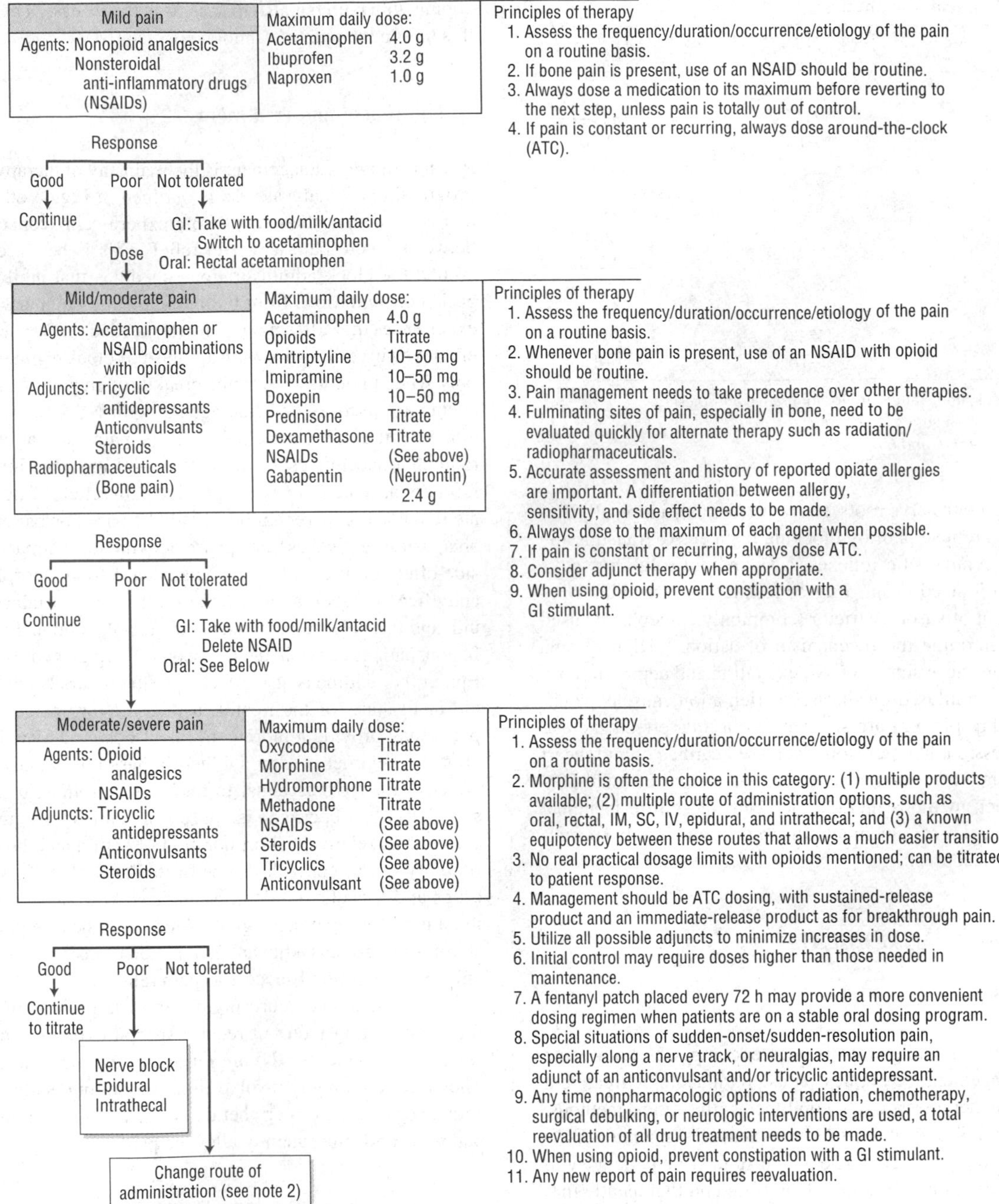

FIGURE 60–3. Algorithm for pain management in oncology patients. *(Adapted from the Kaiser Permanente Algorithm for Pain Management in Patients with Advanced Malignant Disease, and Ref. 39.)*

medications not normally thought of as analgesics. Topically applied capsaicin (which deplete nerves of substance P), tricyclic antidepressants (which block the reuptake of serotonin and norepinephrine, thus enhancing pain inhibition), anticonvulsants (e.g., gabapentin, which may decrease neuronal excitability), and NMDA receptor antagonists (e.g., dextromethorphan, which may enhance opioid effectiveness and decrease neuronal excitability) all have been proven effective in neuropathic pain.[42–45] In addition, it is important to remember that chronic pain patients often have received many pharmacologic regimens. Adding another traditional analgesic (e.g., opioids) to their therapy may promote dependence and not improve pain control.[3] Other nonpharmacologic therapies (e.g., spinal cord stimulation) or psychological techniques may prove more successful. Nevertheless, many times a trial of opioids is warranted, but such a trial should not be done without a complete assessment of the pain complaint.[46] In all cases, an integrated, systematic approach often provided by pain clinics, with a strong emphasis on patient-clinician relationships, is essential. The goal is to improve or maintain the patient's level of functioning, decrease the rate of physical deterioration, decrease pain perception, improve the patient's sense of well-being, improve family and social relationships, and decrease dependency on drug therapy.[3] Patients and clinicians must realize that maximum effective treatment may take months or even years.

PHARMACOECONOMIC CONSIDERATIONS

One cannot overemphasize the "suffering" component of pain. Most of us know how devastating pain can be to our daily lives. Swift relief from acute and cancer pain and well-planned treatment regimens in chronic nonmalignant pain will allow patients to concentrate on recovery and regaining control of their lives. Although few well-designed pharmacoeconomic studies have been performed,[47,48] most pain clinicians believe that this approach leads to decreased time in the hospital, decreased time away from work, and overall increased quality of life.

EVALUATION OF THERAPEUTIC OUTCOMES

The key to treating pain effectively is to consistently monitor effectiveness (pain relief) versus side effects (e.g., sedation) and titrate treatment accordingly (see Table 60–8). In acute pain this often needs to be done several times a day (in the early stages, hourly), whereas in chronic pain this may take place daily or even weekly. The frequency of evaluation also depends on the drug, the administration route, and other therapies being used. When patients cannot be asked about their pain (e.g., coma), monitoring agitation and heart rate is appropriate. Given the subjective nature of pain, the most successful therapies will involve not only frequent patient assessment but also a large degree of patient control (as with PCA).

All opioids can cause constipation. The best management of constipation is prevention. Patients should be counseled on the proper intake of fluids and fiber. A laxative may be added if needed. As noted earlier, CNS depressants (e.g., alcohol, benzodiazepines) amplify CNS depression when used with narcotic analgesics and should be monitored closely and discouraged when possible.

CONCLUSIONS

Pharmacologic agents to treat pain are not always used appropriately. Inadequate dose titration, fear of analgesic side effects, varying analgesic requirements, inadequate application of currently available therapies, and failure to appreciate the complications of untreated pain contribute to ineffective and inappropriate pain management. Adherence to the basic principles of pharmacotherapy will promote rational pain-control decisions. Analgesic agents should be given an adequate trial and often require individual dosage titration. Even in acute pain, administering analgesics as needed (prn) may promote anxiety and contribute to future drug dependence. These drugs should be administered on a regular dosing schedule and not on an as-needed schedule. However, as-needed regimens can be used in breakthrough pain (pain despite regular dosing of analgesics) or when acute pain displays great variability or has subsided greatly. Capsaicins, tricyclic antidepressants, and/or anticonvulsants should be considered for neuropathic pain. Side effects of all medications being used should be well understood and excessive sedation avoided. Finally, placebo therapy never should be used to diagnose psychogenic pain, and the route of administration always should be geared to the analgesic needs of the patient.

It must be remembered that pain is whatever the patient says it is. In acute pain and cancer pain, when patients say they are hurting, aggressive drug therapy should be considered. In chronic pain, aggressive assessment, special diligence in the diagnosis and treatment of neuropathic pain, and understanding may be more appropriate. If acute pain does not subside within the anticipated duration of the insult (often 1 to 2 weeks), further investigation of the cause is warranted. Cancer pain and chronic pain may need treatment for years.

Clinicians must keep in mind that the risk of dependency is real but often overstated and can promote inappropriate pain management. In addition, the elderly and the young are at a higher risk for undertreatment because of misunderstandings regarding the pathophysiology of their pain. Although care must be taken in these populations to ensure proper individualized treatment plans following accepted guidelines,[49,50] the general principles of pharmacotherapy as outlined in this chapter are the guiding tenets of management.

Poor training of health care practitioners in pain assessment and management, improper patient education, and inadequate communication among health care professionals have been suggested as reasons for inadequate pain relief.[51] The better use of an integrated approach, employing the expertise of many disciplines, as well as individualized pharmacologic and nonpharmacologic strategies, may well be the most overlooked principle of pharmacotherapy.[51] Indeed, it is the responsibility of the pharmacist and all health care professionals who deal with pain to communicate therapies and ensure proper management in an effort to relieve treatable suffering and pain.

▶ PRINCIPLES OF PHARMACOTHERAPY[3]

- Always ask the patient if he or she has pain and assess the characteristics of pain (see Table 60–2).
- Identify the source of pain.
- Select the most effective analgesic with the fewest side effects.
- Properly titrate the dose for each individual and administer for an adequate duration.
- Always consider around-the-clock regimens for acute and chronic pain.
- Use as-needed regimens for breakthrough pain or when acute pain displays great variability and/or has subsided greatly.
- Assess for side effects of analgesics, particularly the constipation seen with the opioids.
- Avoid excessive sedation by titrating the opioids carefully.
- Adjust the route of administration to the needs of the patient; whenever possible, use oral medication.
- When converting from one agent to another, use equianalgesic doses and then titrate.
- Do not use placebo therapy to diagnose psychogenic pain.
- Consider the use of capsaicins, tricyclic antidepressants, and anticonvulsants when treating neuropathic pain.
- Use a multidisciplinary approach and nonpharmacologic strategies whenever possible.

REFERENCES

1. *www.river.org/dHawk/keller-quotes.html*. Selected quotes from Helen Keller. David Hawkins Quote Page, 1998.
2. Joint Commission on Accreditation of Healthcare Organizations (JCAHO). Pain Assessment and Management an Organizational Approach. Oakbrook Terrace, IL, JCAHO, 2000:1.

3. Stimmel B. Pain, Analgesia and Addiction: The Pharmacology of Pain. New York, Raven Press, 1983.
4. Turk DC, Okifuji A. Pain terms and taxonomies of pain. In: Loeser JD, Butler SH, Chapman CR, et al., eds. Bonica's Management of Pain. Philadelphia, Lippincott Williams & Wilkins, 2000:17–25.
5. Partners Against Pain News, Vol. 4, No. 3. Norwalk, CT, Purdue Pharma L.P., 2000:1.
6. Gallagher RM. Primary care and pain medicine: A community solution to the public health problem of chronic pain. Med Clin North Am 1999;83(3):555–583.
7. Desbiens NA, Wu AW, Broste SK, et al. Pain and satisfaction with pain control in seriously ill hospitalized adults: Findings from the SUPPORT research investigations. Crit Care Med 1996;24(12):1953–1961.
8. Desbiens NA, Wu AW. Pain and suffering in seriously ill hospitalized patients. J Am Geriatr Soc 2000;48:S183–S186.
9. Bernabei R, Gambassi G, Lapane K, et al. Management of pain in elderly patients with cancer. JAMA 1998;279:1877–1882.
10. Loeser JD, Melzack R. Pain: An overview. Lancet 1999;353:1607–1609.
11. Pasero C, Paice JA, McCaffery M. Basic mechanisms underlying the causes and effects of pain. In: McCaffery M, Pasero C, eds. Pain. St. Louis, Mosby, 1999:15–34.
12. Johnson BW. Pain mechanisms: Anatomy, physiology, and neurochemistry. In: Raj PP, Abrams BM, Hahn MB, et al., eds. Practical Management of Pain. St. Louis, Mosby, 2000:117–143.
13. Byers MR, Bonica JJ. Peripheral pain mechanisms and nociceptor plasticity. In: Loeser JD, Butler SH, Chapman CR, et al., eds. Bonica's Management of Pain. Philadelphia, Lippincott Williams & Wilkins, 2000: 26–72.
14. Bennett GJ. Neuropathic pain: New insights, new interventions. Hosp Pract 1998;October:95–114.
15. Chabal C. Trancutaneous electrical nerve stimulation. In: Loeser JD, Butler SH, Chapman CR, et al., eds. Bonica's Management of Pain. Philadelphia, Lippincott Williams & Wilkins, 2000:1842–1847.
16. Terman GW, Bonica JJ. Spinal mechanisms and their modulation. In: Loeser JD, Butler SH, Chapman CR, et al., eds. Bonica's Management of Pain. Philadelphia, Lippincott Williams & Wilkins, 2000:73–152.
17. Elliott, KJ. Taxonomy and mechanisms of neuropathic pain. Semin Neurol 1994;(14)3:195–205.
18. Twycross RG. Pain and analgesics. Curr Med Res Opin 1978;5:497–505.
19. Fordyce WE. Learning processes in pain. In: Sternbach RA, ed. The Psychology of Pain. New York, Raven Press, 1978:49–72.
20. Chapman CR. New directions in the understanding and management of pain. Soc Sci Med 1984;19:1261–77.
21. Craig KD. Social modelling influences on pain. In: Sternbach RA, ed. The Psychology of Pain. New York, Raven Press, 1978:73–109.
22. American Pain Society. Principles of analgesic use in the treatment of acute pain and chronic cancer pain. Clin Pharm 1990;9:601–611.
23. Chapman CR, Bonica JJ. Chronic pain: Current Concepts. Kalamazoo, MI, Scope Publications, 1985:4.
24. Clinical Practice Guideline. Acute pain management: Operative or medical procedures and trauma. U.S. Department of Health and Human Services, Public Health Service, Agency for Health Care Policy and Research, (now called Agency for Healthcare Research and Quality), 1992.
25. Cashman J, McAnulty G. Nonsteroidal anti-inflammatory drugs in perisurgical pain management. Drugs 1995;49(1):51–70.
26. Miyoshi HR, Leckband SG. Systemic opioids and analgesics. In: Loeser JD, Butler SH, Chapman CR, et al., eds. Bonica's Management of Pain. Philadelphia, Lippincott Williams & Wilkins, 2000:1682–1709.
27. Reisine T, Pasternak G. Opioid analgesics and antagonists. In: Hardman JG, Limbird LE, Molinoff PB, et al., eds. The Pharmacological Basis of Therapeutics. New York, McGraw-Hill, 1995:521–555.
28. Baumann TJ. Analgesic selection when the patient is allergic to codeine. Clin Pharm 1991;10:658.
29. Ready BL. Regional analgesics with intraspinal opioids. In: Loeser JD, Butler SH, Chapman CR, et al., eds. Bonica's Management of Pain. Philadelphia, Lippincott Williams & Wilkins, 2000:1953–1966.
30. Littrell RA. Epidural analgesia. Am J Hosp Pharm 1991;48:2460–2474.
31. Buckley PF. Regional anesthesia with local anesthetics. In: Loeser JD, Butler SH, Chapman CR, et al., eds. Bonica's Management of Pain. Philadelphia, Lippincott Williams & Wilkins, 2000:1893–1952.
32. Pasero C, Portenoy RK, McCaffery M. Opioid analgesics. In: McCaffery M, Pasero C, eds. Pain. St. Louis, Mosby, 1999:161–299.
33. Anonymous. American Hospital Formulary Service. In: McVoy GK, ed. Drug Information. Bethesda, MD, American Society of Hospital Pharmacists, 1987, 1991, 1994, 1997, 1999, 2001.
34. Anonymous. Facts and Comparisons. Philadelphia, Lippincott, 1986, 1991, 1994, 1997, 2000.
35. Sang CN. NMDA-receptor antagonists in neuropathic pain: Experimental methods to clinical trials. J Pain Symptom Manag 2000;19(1 Suppl):S21–S25.
36. Beaver WT. Mild analgesics: A review of their clinical pharmacology, part II. Am J Med Sci 1966;251:576–599.
37. Package insert. Tramadol, Ortho-McNeil, December 1999.
38. Sindrup SH, Andersen G, Madsen C, et al. Tramadol relieves pain and allodynia in polyneuropathy: A randomized, double-blind, controlled trial. Pain 1999;83(1):85–90.
39. Clinical Practice Guideline No. 9. Management of Cancer Pain. Washington, U.S. Department of Health, Public Health Service, Agency for Health Care Policy and Research, (now called Agency for Healthcare Research and Quality), 1994.
40. Foley KM. The treatment of cancer pain. New Engl J Med 1985;313: 84–95.
41. Health and Public Policy Committee, American College of Physicians. Drug therapy for severe chronic pain in terminal illness. Ann Intern Med 1983;99:870–873.
42. Sindrup SH, Jensen TS. Efficacy of pharmacologic treatments of neurophatic pain: An update and effect related to mechanism of drug action. Pain 1999;83(3):389–400.
43. Nelson KA, Park KM, Robinovitz E, et al. High dose dextromethorphan versus placebo in painful diabetic neuropathy. Neurology 1997;48 (5):1212–1218.
44. Semenchuk, M. Adjuvant analgesics for management of neuropathic pain. In: Beizer JL, ed. Clinical Pharmacy Newswatch, Vol. 6. Parke-Davis, 1999:1.
45. Katz NP. MorpiDex (ms:dm) double-blind, multiple-dose studies in chronic pain patients. J Pain Symptom Manag 2000;1(19):S37–S41.
46. The use of opioids for the treatment of chronic pain: A consensus statement from the American Academy of Pain Medicine and American Pain Society. Approved 1996, American Pain Society Web Site: *www.ampainsoc.org*.
47. Tugwell P. Economic evaluation of the management of pain in osteoarthritis. Drugs 1996;52(Suppl 3):48–58.
48. Portenoy RK. Issues in the economic analysis of therapies for cancer pain. Oncol Huntint 1995;9(Suppl 11):71–78.
49. Clinical Practice Guideline, American Geriatrics Society Panel on Chronic Pain in Older Persons. The management of chronic pain in older persons. J Am Geriatr Soc 1998;46:635–651.
50. Clinical Practice Guideline. Acute pain management in infants, children and adolescents: Operative and medical procedures. Washington, U.S. Department of Health and Human Services, Public Health Service, Agency for Health Care Policy and Research (now called Agency for Healthcare Research and Quality), 1992.
51. News: Panel cites need for improved pain management. Clin Pharm 1986;5:777–778.
52. Amadio P. Peripherally acting analgesics. Am J Med 1984;77:17–26.
53. Hopkinson JH, Smith MT, Bare WW, et al. Acetaminophen (500 mg) versus acetaminophen (325 mg) for relief of pain in episiotomy patients. Curr Ther Res 1974;16:194–200.
54. Levy G. Comparative pharmacokinetics of aspirin and acetaminophen. Arch Intern Med 1981;141:279–281.
55. Gaston GW, Mallow RD, Frank JE. Comparison of etodolac, aspirin, and placebo for pain after oral surgery. Pharmacotherapy 1986;6:199–205.

56. Package insert. Diclofenac potassium, Geigy Pharmaceuticals, Ardsley, NJ, Feb. 1996.
57. Package insert. Rofecoxib, Merck & Co., Whitehouse Station, NJ, 2000.
58. Principles of Analgesic Use in Treatment of Acute Pain and Cancer Pain. 4th ed. American Pain Society, Glenview, IL, 1999.
59. Package insert. Ropivicaine, Astra, Westborough, MA, January 1999.
60. Package insert. Levobupivacaine, Pudue Pharma L.P., Norwalk, CT, December 1999.
61. Package insert. Celeeoxib, Pharmacia/Pfizer, New York, NY, October, 2001.

61
HEADACHE DISORDERS

Brian E. Beckett and Katherine C. Herndon

Headache is one of the most common complaints encountered by health care practitioners, accounting for 18 million outpatient visits annually.[1] As one of the top 10 presenting complaints in ambulatory medical care, headache may be symptomatic of a distinct pathologic process or may occur without an underlying cause. In 1988, the International Headache Society (IHS) published a classification system for headache disorders, cranial neuralgias, and facial pain to facilitate their diagnosis in clinical practice and research (Table 61–1).[2] The IHS classification provides more precise definitions and standardized nomenclature for both the primary (migraine, tension-type, and cluster headache) and secondary (symptomatic of organic disease) headache disorders. This chapter focuses on the management of migraine and cluster headaches.

Migraine, the most common of the chronic primary headache disorders, is a recurring headache of moderate to severe intensity that is associated with gastrointestinal, neurologic, and autonomic symptoms. The most common migraine variants are migraine without aura (formerly called common migraine) and migraine with aura (formerly called classical migraine) in which a complex of focal neurologic symptoms precedes or accompanies the attack. According to the American Migraine Study, approximately 24 million Americans suffer from migraines, and more than one-half of all migraineurs report significant disability with their headaches.[3] Despite the prevalence of migraine and its associated disability, studies indicate that the majority of migraine sufferers have not been diagnosed by a physician and take over-the-counter medications, rather than prescription drugs, for headache relief.[3,4] An improved understanding of the diagnosis and pathophysiologic mechanisms of migraine has lead to the development of migraine-specific medications capable of providing rapid relief from moderate to severe attacks. However, a thorough evaluation of the headache history is essential to establish an accurate diagnosis of migraine and identify patients who may benefit from these newer therapeutic options.

MIGRAINE HEADACHE

EPIDEMIOLOGY

Results of the American Migraine Study indicate that 18% of women and 6% of men in the United States experience one or more migraine headaches per year.[3] The prevalence of migraine varies considerably by age and gender. Before the age of 12 years, migraine is more common in boys than in girls, but prevalence increases more rapidly in girls after puberty.[4] After age 12, women are two to three times more likely than men to suffer from migraine. Gender differences in migraine prevalence have been linked to menstruation, however these differences persist beyond menopause. Prevalence is highest in both men and women between the ages of 35 and 45 years.[3] The usual age of onset is 10 to 29 years of age, but onset of migraine in early childhood is not uncommon.[5] Migraine headaches are more common in lower socioeconomic groups, perhaps the result of stress, poor diet, misuse of over-the-counter medications, or reduced access to health care. In the American Migraine Study, 86% of women and 82% of men with migraine reported some headache-related disability, and approximately one-third were severely disabled or needed bed rest during an attack.[3,6] The economic burden of migraine is substantial; however, the direct medical costs associated with migraine treatment are far exceeded by the indirect costs that result from work-related disability.[7,8] In the United States, Hu and colleagues estimated the annual costs of migraine-related missed workdays and reduced productivity at $13 billion.[8] A number of neurologic and psychiatric disorders, including epilepsy, major depression, and anxiety disorder, show increased comorbidity with migraine.[4,9] Whether this relationship is causal or representative of a common pathophysiologic mechanism is unknown.

PATHOPHYSIOLOGY

The etiologic and pathophysiologic mechanisms of migraine are not completely understood. According to the vascular hypothesis proposed by Harold Wolff in 1938, the migraine aura is caused by intracerebral arterial vasoconstriction that is followed by reactive extracranial vasodilation and associated headache.[4] Although studies of regional blood flow in the brain do not support the vascular hypothesis, the aura phase of migraine is associated with a reduction in cerebral blood flow that begins in the occipital region and moves across the cerebral cortex at a rate of 2–3 mm/min.[10] However, most clinicians now believe that the positive and negative symptoms of the migraine aura are caused by neuronal dysfunction, not ischemia. The neurologic changes of the aura parallel those that occur during spreading depression, a neuronal event characterized by a wave of depressed electrical activity that advances across the brain cortex at a rate that is consistent with the spread of aura symptoms.[10] To date, spreading depression has been demonstrated only in animal models.

Migraine pain is believed to result from activity within the trigeminovascular system, a network of visceral afferent fibers that arise from the trigeminal ganglia and project peripherally to innervate the pain-sensitive intracranial extracerebral blood vessels, dura mater, and large venous sinuses (Fig. 61–1).[11] These fibers also project centrally, terminating in the trigeminal nucleus caudalis in the brainstem and upper cervical spinal cord, and thus provide a pathway for nociceptive transmission from meningeal blood vessels into higher centers of the central nervous system. Activation of trigeminal sensory nerves triggers the release of vasoactive neuropeptides, including calcitonin gene-related peptide (CGRP), neurokinin A, and substance P, from perivascular axons. The released neuropeptides interact with dural blood vessels to promote vasodilation and dural plasma extravasation, resulting in perivascular inflammation.[11] Orthodromic conduction along trigeminovascular fibers transmits pain impulses to the trigeminal nucleus caudalis where the information is relayed further to higher cortical pain centers. Continued afferent input may result in sensitization of these central sensory neurons, producing a hyperalgesic state that prolongs and intensifies headache pain as the attack progresses.[12]

TABLE 61–1. International Headache Society Classification System: Focus on Migraine Headache

1. Migraine
   - 1.1 Migraine without aura
   - 1.2 Migraine with aura
     - 1.2.1 Migraine with typical aura (aura lasting less than 1 hour)
     - 1.2.2 Migraine with prolonged aura (aura lasting more than 1 hour and less than 1 week)
     - 1.2.3 Familial hemiplegic migraine
     - 1.2.4 Basilar migraine
     - 1.2.5 Migraine aura without headache
     - 1.2.6 Migraine with acute onset aura (aura develops fully in less than 5 minutes)
   - 1.3 Ophthalmoplegic migraine (associated with paresis of one or more ocular cranial nerves)
   - 1.4 Retinal migraine (attacks of monocular scotoma or blindness for less than 1 hour and associated with headache)
   - 1.5 Childhood periodic syndromes that may be precursors to or associated with migraine
     - 1.5.1 Benign paroxysmal vertigo of childhood (brief attacks of vertigo in otherwise healthy children)
     - 1.5.2 Alternating hemiplegia of childhood (attacks of hemiplegia involving each side alternately)
   - 1.6 Complications of migraine
     - 1.6.1 Status migrainosus (headache lasting more than 72 hours despite treatment)
     - 1.6.2 Migrainous infarction (aura symptoms not fully reversible within 7 days and/or associated ischemic infarction)
   - 1.7 Migrainous disorder not fulfilling above criteria
2. Tension-type headache
3. Cluster headache and chronic paroxysmal hemicrania
4. Miscellaneous headaches unassociated with structural lesion
5. Headache associated with head trauma
6. Headache associated with vascular disorders
7. Headache associated with nonvascular intracranial disorder
8. Headache associated with substances or their withdrawal
9. Headache associated with noncephalic infection
10. Headache associated with metabolic disorder
11. Headache or facial pain associated with disorder of cranium, neck, eyes, ears, nose, sinuses, teeth, mouth, or other facial or cranial structures
12. Cranial neuralgias, nerve trunk pain, and deafferentation pain
13. Headache not classifiable

Adapted from Ref. 2.

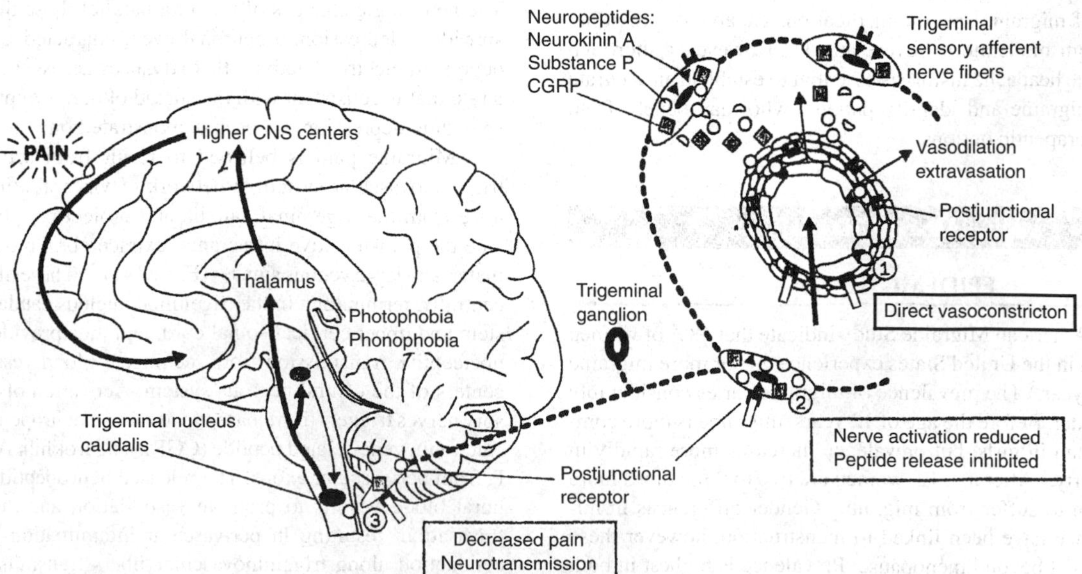

FIGURE 61–1. The pathophysiology of migraine headache. Vasodilation of intracranial extracerebral blood vessels (possibly the result of an imbalance in the brainstem) results in the activation of the perivascular trigeminal nerves which release vasoactive neuropeptides to promote neurogenic inflammation. Central pain transmission may activate other brainstem nuclei, resulting in associated symptoms (nausea, vomiting, photophobia, phonophobia). The antimigraine effects of the 5-HT$_{1B/ID}$ receptor agonists are highlighted at areas 1, 2, and 3. *(Adapted with permission from Ferrari MD. Migraine. Lancet 1998;351:1043–1051 © by The Lancet Ltd.)*

Despite recent advances in the understanding of the pathophysiology of headache pain, there is still a considerable lack of knowledge regarding the mechanisms that are involved in the initiation of a migraine attack. Neuronal dysfunction is now accepted as the primary basis of migraine pathophysiology. Activity within the trigeminovascular system may be regulated in part by noradrenergic and, most importantly, serotonergic neurons within the brainstem. A recent neuroimaging study revealed selective activation of specific brainstem nuclei (the locus ceruleus and dorsal raphe nucleus) during spontaneous migraine attacks.[13] Brainstem activation persisted following an injection of sumatriptan despite reversal of cortical activation and relief of headache pain and associated symptoms. Thus, the pathogenesis of migraine may be related to an imbalance in the activity of serotonin-containing neurons and/or noradrenergic pathways in brainstem nuclei that modulate cerebral vascular tone and nociception.[11] This imbalance may result in vasodilation of intracranial extracerebral blood vessels and consequent activation of the trigeminovascular system. Future research may further delineate the role of the brainstem as the "migraine generator."

Genetic factors appear to play an important role in an individual's susceptibility to migraine attacks. Studies in monozygotic twins suggest that up to 50% of the contribution to the common migraine variants is genetically based with a substantial influence from environmental factors.[14] While it may be possible for any individual to experience a migraine attack, it is the recurrence of attacks in the migraineur that is abnormal. Attack occurrence and frequency are governed by the sensitivity of the central nervous system to migraine-specific triggers. Migraineurs appear to have a lowered threshold of response to specific triggers as a result of genetic factors that govern the balance of excitation and inhibition at various levels in the central nervous system.[10] Thus, trigger factors can be viewed as modulators of the genetic set point that predisposes to migraine headache. The hyperresponsiveness of the migrainous brain may be the result of an inherited abnormality in P/Q-type calcium channels that regulate cortical excitability through the release of serotonin and other neurotransmitters.[4] Low levels of magnesium or dopamine, increased levels of excitatory amino acids, and alterations in levels of endogenous opioids may also affect the migraine threshold.[10]

Serotonin (5-hydroxytryptamine or 5-HT) has long been implicated as an important mediator of migraine headache. Specific populations of the seven subfamilies of 5-HT receptors (5-HT_1 to 5-HT_7) appear to be involved in the pathophysiology and treatment of migraine headache.[15] Specific acute antimigraine drugs such as the ergot alkaloids and triptan derivatives are agonists of vascular and neuronal 5-HT_1 receptor subtypes, resulting in vasoconstriction of meningeal blood vessels and inhibition of vasoactive neuropeptide release and pain signal transmission.[11] Drugs used for migraine prophylaxis appear to stabilize serotonergic neurotransmission and raise the migraine threshold by antagonizing or down-regulating 5-HT_2 receptors, or by modulating serotonergic neuronal discharge.[15]

CLINICAL PRESENTATION

The migraine attack has been divided into several phases which merit description. The premonitory symptoms of the *prodrome* are experienced by approximately 60% of migraineurs in the hours or days before the onset of headache.[16] Prodromal symptoms vary widely among migraineurs, but are usually consistent within an individual. Neurologic symptoms (phonophobia, photophobia, hyperosmia, difficulty concentrating) are most common, but psychologic (anxiety, depression, euphoria, irritability, drowsiness, hyperactivity, restlessness), autonomic (polyuria, diarrhea, constipation), and constitutional symptoms (stiff neck, yawning, thirst, food cravings, anorexia) are also reported.[4,16]

The migraine *aura,* a complex of positive and negative focal neurologic symptoms that precedes or accompanies an attack, is experienced by approximately 20% of migraineurs.[16] The aura typically evolves over 5 to 20 minutes and lasts less than 60 minutes. Headache usually occurs within 60 minutes of the end of the aura. Occasionally, aura symptoms begin at the onset of headache or during the attack. The aura is most often visual and frequently affects half of the visual field.[4,16] Visual auras vary in their complexity, and can include both positive (scintillations, photopsia, teichopsia or fortification spectrum) and negative (scotoma, hemianopsia) features. Sensory and motor aura symptoms, such as paresthesias or numbness involving the arms and face, dysphasia or aphasia, weakness, and hemiparesis, are also reported.

The average migraineur experiences between one and four attacks per month.[17] Migraine *headache* may occur at any time of the day or night, but most often occurs in the early morning hours upon awakening. Pain is usually gradual in onset, peaking in intensity over a period of minutes to hours and lasting between 4 and 72 hours in adults. The intensity of head pain is typically reported as moderate to severe with a rating of 5 or greater on a 0 to 10 pain scale.[18] Pain may occur anywhere in the face or head, but most often involves the frontotemporal region. The headache is typically unilateral and throbbing or pulsating in nature; however, pain may be bilateral at onset or become generalized during the course of an attack.[10] Gastrointestinal symptoms almost invariably accompany a migraine headache. During an attack, as many as 90% of migraineurs experience nausea, and emesis occurs in approximately one-third of patients.[17] Other systemic symptoms associated with the headache phase include anorexia, food cravings, constipation, diarrhea, abdominal cramps, nasal stuffiness, blurred vision, diaphoresis, facial pallor, and localized facial, scalp, or periorbital edema. Sensory hyperacuity, manifested as photophobia, phonophobia, or osmophobia, is frequently reported. As headache pain is usually aggravated by physical activity, most migraineurs seek a dark, quiet room for rest and relief. Impaired concentration, depression, irritability, fatigue, or anxiety will often accompany the headache. Once headache pain wanes, patients may experience a *postdromal* phase characterized by exhaustion, malaise, irritability, and recurrence of pain with sudden head movement.[18] The reader is referred to the IHS classification and recent reviews for descriptions of the classical migraine variants and other migraine subtypes (Table 61–1).[2,4,10]

Although headache may be a manifestation of a serious or life-threatening condition, patients presenting with even the most severe and chronic symptoms rarely suffer from underlying organic disease.[19] A comprehensive headache history is the most important element in establishing the clinical diagnosis of migraine.[10] Secondary headache can be identified or excluded based on the headache history, as well as the results of general medical and neurologic examinations. Diagnostic and laboratory testing may also be warranted in the setting of suspicious headache features or an abnormal examination. The routine use of neuroimaging (computed tomography or magnetic resonance imaging) is generally not indicated in patients with migraine and a normal neurologic examination, but it should be considered in patients with an unexplained abnormal neurologic examination or an atypical headache history.[20,21] Because migraine headaches usually begin by the second or third decade of life, headaches beginning after age 50 suggest an organic etiology such as a mass lesion, cerebrovascular disease, or temporal arteritis. Table 61–2 summarizes the headache evaluation, including the essential elements of the headache history. Table 61–3 lists the IHS diagnostic criteria for migraine with and without aura.[2]

TABLE 61–2. Evaluation of the Headache Patient

Obtain a thorough headache history
- Age at onset
- Attack frequency and timing
- Duration of attacks
- Precipitating or aggravating factors
- Ameliorating factors
- Description of the aura (if present)
- Quality, intensity, location, and radiation of headache pain
- Associated signs and symptoms
- Treatment history
- Family and social history
- Impact of headaches

Perform general medical and neurologic physical examination
- Vital signs (fever, hypertension)
- Fundoscopy (papilledema, hemorrhage, exudates)
- Palpation and auscultation of the head and neck (masses, sinus tenderness, hardened or tender temporal arteries, trigger points, temporomandibular joint tenderness, bruits, nuchal rigidity, cervical spine tenderness)
- Neurologic exam (identify abnormalities or deficits in mental status, cranial nerves, deep-tendon reflexes, motor strength, coordination, gait, cerebellar function)

Identify diagnostic alarms in the headache evaluation
- Acute onset of the "first" or "worst" headache ever (thunderclap headache)
- Accelerating pattern of headache following subacute onset
- Onset of headache after age 50
- Headache associated with systemic illness (fever, nausea, vomiting, stiff neck, rash)
- Headache with focal neurologic symptoms or papilledema
- New-onset headache in a patient with cancer or HIV

If headache alarms are present, diagnostic testing may be indicated*
- Laboratory studies to identify metabolic or electrolyte abnormalities, infection, medication overuse, drug effects, temporal arteritis (headache onset after age 50)
- Neuroimaging for suspected mass lesion, stroke, hemorrhage, or abscess
- Lumbar puncture for suspected infection or increased intracranial pressure

*The diagnostic workup should be based on the headache history and physical examination in order to identify or exclude secondary headache.
Compiled from Refs. 4, 10, and 19.

TABLE 61–3. IHS Diagnostic Criteria for Migraine

Migraine without Aura

A. At least five attacks fulfilling B through D below
B. Headache attacks lasting 4 to 72 hours (untreated or unsuccessfully treated)
C. Headache has at least two of the following characteristics:
   1. Unilateral location
   2. Pulsating quality
   3. Moderate or severe intensity (inhibits or prohibits daily activities)
   4. Aggravation by walking stairs or similar routine physical activity
D. During headache, at least one of the following:
   1. Nausea and/or vomiting
   2. Photophobia and phonophobia
E. At least one of the following:
   1. History, physical, and neurologic examinations do not suggest an organic disorder
   2. History and/or physical and/or neurologic examinations do suggest such disorder, but it is ruled out by appropriate investigations
   3. An organic disorder is present, but migraine attacks do not occur for the first time in close temporal relation to the disorder

Migraine with Aura

A. At least two attacks fulfilling B through C below
B. At least three of the following four characteristics:
   1. One or more fully reversible aura symptoms indicating focal cerebral cortical and/or brainstem dysfunction
   2. At least one aura symptom develops gradually over more than 4 minutes, or two or more symptoms occur in succession
   3. No aura symptom lasts more than 60 minutes (if >60 minutes, then diagnosis is migraine with prolonged aura). If more than one aura symptom is present, accepted duration is proportionally increased
   4. Headache follows aura with a free interval of less than 60 minutes. (It may also begin before or simultaneously with the aura)
C. At least one of the following:
   1. History, physical, and neurologic examinations do not suggest an organic disorder
   2. History and/or physical and/or neurologic examinations do suggest such disorder, but it is ruled out by appropriate investigations
   3. An organic disorder is present, but migraine attacks do not occur for the first time in close temporal relation to the disorder

Adapted from Ref. 2.

▶ TREATMENT: Migraines

DESIRED OUTCOME

Clinicians who care for migraineurs must appreciate the impact of this painful and debilitating disorder on the life of the patient, the patient's family, and the patient's employer. Treatment strategies must address both immediate and long-term goals. Acute migraine therapies should provide consistent, rapid relief, and enable the patient to resume his or her normal activities at home, school, or work. Recurrence of symptoms and treatment-related adverse effects should be minimal. Ideally, patients should be able to effectively manage their own headaches without a visit to a physician's office or emergency room. In addition, migraineurs should take an active role in the creation of a long-term formal management plan. An individualized approach to treatment can result in a reduction in attack frequency and severity, thus minimizing headache-related disability and emotional distress, and improving the patient's quality of life.

GENERAL APPROACH TO TREATMENT

Nonpharmacologic and pharmacologic interventions are available for the management of migraine headache, however drug therapy remains the mainstay of treatment for most patients. Pharmacotherapeutic management of migraine may be acute (symptomatic or abortive) or preventive (prophylactic). When choosing acute or preventive therapies, the clinician should consider the patient's response to specific medications and their tolerability, as well as coexisting illnesses that may limit treatment choices. Abortive therapies can be migraine-specific (ergots and triptans) or nonspecific (analgesics, antiemetics, nonsteroidal anti-inflammatory drugs, corticosteroids), and are most effective at relieving pain and associated symptoms when administered at the onset of migraine (Table 61–4).[6,22] A stratified care approach, in which the selection of initial treatment is based on headache-related disability and symptom severity, is the preferred treatment strategy for the migraineur.[21,23] Because attack severity

TABLE 61–4. Acute Migraine Therapies[a]

Medication	Dosage	Comments
Analgesics		
Acetaminophen	1000 mg at onset; repeat q4–6 h as needed	Maximum daily dose is 4 g
Acetaminophen 250 mg/aspirin 250 mg/caffeine 65 mg	2 tablets at onset and q6 h	Available over-the-counter as Excedrin Migraine
Aspirin or acetaminophen with butalbital, caffeine[b]	1–2 tablets q4–6 h	Limit dose to 4 tablets/day and usage to 2days/wk
Isometheptene 65 mg/dichloralphenazone 100 mg/acetaminophen 325 mg (Midrin)	2 capsules at onset; repeat 1 capsule every hour as needed	Maximum of 6 capsules/day and 20 capsules/mo
Nonsteroidal Anti-inflammatory Drugs		
Aspirin	500–1000 mg q4–6 h	Maximum daily dose is 4g
Ibuprofen	200–800 mg q6 h	Avoid doses >2.4 g/day
Naproxen sodium	550–825 mg at onset; may repeat 220 mg in 3–4 hours	Avoid doses >1.375 g/day
Diclofenac potassium	50–100 mg at onset; may repeat 50 mg in 8 hours	Avoid doses >150 mg/day
Ergotamine tartrate[b]		
Oral tablet (1 mg) with caffeine 100 mg	2 mg at onset, then 1–2 mg q30 min as needed	Maximum dose is 6 mg/day or 10 mg/wk; consider pretreatment with an antiemetic
Sublingual tablet (2 mg)		
Rectal suppository (2 mg) with caffeine 100 mg	Insert ½ to 1 suppository at onset; repeat after 1 hour as needed	Maximum dose is 4 mg/day or 10 mg/wk; consider pretreatment with an antiemetic
Dihydroergotamine		
Injection 1 mg/mL	0.25–1 mg at onset IM or SQ; repeat every hour as needed	Maximum dose is 3 mg/day or 20 mg/wk
Nasal spray	One spray (0.5 mg) in each nostril at onset; repeat sequence 15 minutes later (total dose is 2 mg or 4 sprays)	Maximum dose is 3 mg/day; prime sprayer 4 times before using; do not tilt head back or inhale through nose while spraying; discard open ampules after 8 hours
Serotonin Agonists (Triptans)		
Sumatriptan		
Injection	6 mg SQ at onset; may repeat after 1 hour if needed	Maximum daily dose is 12 mg
Oral tablets	25, 50, or 100 mg at onset; may repeat after 2 hours if needed	Optimal dose is 50–100 mg Maximum daily dose is 200 mg
Nasal spray	5, 10, or 20 mg at onset; may repeat after 2 hours if needed	Optimal dose is 20 mg; maximum daily dose is 40 mg; single-dose device delivering 5 or 20 mg; administer one spray in one nostril
Zolmitriptan	2.5 or 5 mg tablet at onset; may repeat after 2 hours if needed	Optimal dose is 2.5 mg; maximum daily dose is 10 mg
Naratriptan	1 mg or 2.5 mg tablet at onset; may repeat after 4 hours if needed	Optimal dose is 2.5 mg; maximum daily dose is 5 mg
Rizatriptan	5 or 10 mg at onset as regular or orally disintegrating tablet; may repeat after 2 hours if needed	Optimal dose is 10 mg; maximum daily dose is 30 mg; onset of effect is similar with standard and orally disintegrating tablets; use 5 mg dose (15 mg/day max) in patients receiving propranolol
Almotriptan	6.25 or 12.5 mg at onset; may repeat after 2 hours if needed	Optimal dose is 12.5 mg; maximum daily dose is 25 mg
Miscellaneous		
Butorphanol nasal spray	1 spray in 1 nostril (1 mg) at onset; repeat in 1 hour if needed	Limit to 4 sprays/day; consider use only when nonopioid therapies are ineffective or not tolerated
Metoclopramide	10 mg IV at onset	Useful for acute relief in the office or emergency department setting
Prochlorperazine	10 mg IV or IM at onset	Useful for acute relief in the office or emergency department setting

[a]Limit use of symptomatic medications to 2 days/wk when possible to avoid medication misuse headache
[b]Commonly implicated in rebound headache. Adhere to dosing guidelines and limit usage to 2 days/wk
Compiled from Refs. 6, 22, 24, 25, 28, 64, and 76.

varies in individuals, patients may be advised to use nonspecific agents for mild to moderate headache, while reserving migraine-specific medications for more severe attacks. The absorption and efficacy of orally administered drugs may be compromised by the gastric stasis or nausea and vomiting that often accompany migraine.[9,16] Pretreatment with antiemetic agents or the use of nonoral treatment (suppositories, nasal spray, injections) may be advisable when nausea and vomiting are severe. Administration of the prokinetic agent metoclopramide enhances the absorption of oral medications, in addition to its antiemetic effects.[9,16]

The frequent or excessive use of acute migraine medications can result in a pattern of increasing headache frequency and drug consumption known as *medication-overuse headache* (or rebound headache).[21,24,25] The syndrome appears to evolve as a self-sustaining, headache-medication cycle in which headache returns as the medication effect wears off, leading to the consumption of more drug for relief. The headache history often reflects the gradual onset of an atypical daily or near daily headache with superimposed episodic migraine attacks. Medication overuse is one of the most common causes of chronic daily headache.[4] Agents most commonly implicated in this syndrome include simple and combination analgesics, opiates, ergotamine tartrate, and triptans.[21,24–27] Discontinuation of the offending agent leads to a gradual decrease in headache frequency and severity, and a return of the original headache characteristics. While detoxification can usually be accomplished on an outpatient basis, hospitalization may be necessary for the control of refractory rebound headache and other withdrawal symptoms (nausea, vomiting, asthenia, restlessness, and agitation). Regulation of nociceptive systems and renewed responsiveness to therapy may not occur for 3 to 12 weeks following medication withdrawal.[4,25] Most experts recommend limiting use of acute migraine therapies to *2 days per week* in order to avoid the development of medication misuse headache.[21,24,28]

Prophylactic migraine therapies are administered on a daily basis to reduce the frequency, severity, and duration of attacks, and increase responsiveness to symptomatic migraine therapies (Table 61–5).[22,24] Preventive therapy should be considered in the setting of recurring migraines that produce significant disability; frequent attacks requiring symptomatic medication more than twice per week; symptomatic therapies that are ineffective, contraindicated, or produce serious side effects; and uncommon migraine variants that cause profound disruption and/or risk of neurologic injury (e.g., hemiplegic migraine, basilar migraine, migraine with prolonged aura).[21,28,29] Preventive therapy may also be administered intermittently when headaches recur in a predictable pattern (e.g., menstrual migraine). The efficacy of the various agents used for migraine prophylaxis appears to be similar, however the quality of published data is limited for many commonly used drugs.[29] Thus, the selection of an agent is typically based on its side effect profile and comorbid conditions of the patient.[21] Individual response to a particular agent cannot be predicted, and it may be necessary to try multiple therapies before successful prophylaxis is achieved.[29] A therapeutic trial of 2 to 3 months is necessary to judge the efficacy of each medication, however, some reduction in attack frequency may be evident by the first month of therapy.[21,29] Drug therapy should be initiated with low doses and advanced slowly until a therapeutic effect is achieved or side effects become intolerable. Drug doses for migraine prophylaxis are often lower than those that are necessary for other indications.[4] Because patient adherence to prescribed regimens is frequently poor, once-daily dosing is preferred when possible.[30] Overuse of acute headache medications will interfere with the therapeutic effects of preventive treatment.[28] Prophylactic treatment is usually continued for at least 3 to 6 months after the frequency and severity of headaches has diminished, and then gradually tapered and discontinued. Many migraineurs experience fewer and less severe attacks for lengthy periods following discontinuation of prophylactic medications or taper to a lower dose.[4] Successful prophylaxis is generally viewed as a reduction in headache symptoms by at least 50%.[22,24] However, this level of benefit will be achieved in only approximately one-half of the patients prescribed these therapies.[9,29]

TABLE 61–5. Prophylactic Migraine Therapies

Medication	Dose
β-Adrenergic Antagonists	
Atenolol	25–100 mg/day
Metoprolol[a]	50–300 mg/day in divided doses
Nadolol	80–240 mg/day
Propranolol[ab]	80–240 mg/day in divided doses
Timolol[b]	20–60 mg/day in divided doses
Antidepressants	
Amitriptyline	25–150 mg at bedtime
Doxepin	10–200 mg at bedtime
Imipramine	10–200 mg at bedtime
Nortriptyline	10–150 mg at bedtime
Protriptyline	5–30 mg at bedtime
Fluoxetine	10–80 mg/day
Phenelzine[c]	15–60 mg/day in divided doses
Valproic Acid/Divalproex Sodium[b]	500–1500 mg/day in divided doses
Verapamil[a]	240–360 mg/day in divided doses
Methysergide[bc]	2–8 mg/day in divided doses with food
Nonsteroidal Anti-Inflammatory Drugs[c]	
Aspirin	1300 mg/day in divided doses
Ketoprofen[a]	150 mg/day in divided doses
Naproxen sodium[a]	550–1100 mg/day in divided doses
Vitamin B_2	400 mg/day

[a]Sustained-release formulation available
[b]FDA approved for prevention of migraine
[c]Daily or prolonged use limited by potential toxicity
Compiled from Refs. 6, 21, 24, 28, 29, 96, 97, and 109.

NONPHARMACOLOGIC THERAPY

Nonpharmacologic therapy of acute migraine headache is limited, but may include application of ice to the head and periods of rest or sleep, usually in a dark, quiet environment.[16] Preventive management of migraine should begin with the identification and avoidance of factors that consistently provoke migraine attacks in susceptible individuals (Table 61–6).[16] Changes in estrogen levels associated with menarche, menstruation, pregnancy, menopause, oral contraceptive use, and hormone replacement therapy can trigger, intensify, or alleviate migraine.[31–34] Attacks are linked exclusively to menstruation in approximately 14% of women (i.e., true menstrual migraine).[6,31] A headache diary that records the frequency, severity, and duration of attacks may facilitate the identification of migraine triggers. Patients may also benefit from adherence to a wellness program that includes regular sleep, exercise, and eating habits, smoking cessation, and limited caffeine intake.[16] Behavioral interventions, such as relaxation therapy, biofeedback (often used in combination with relaxation therapy), and cognitive therapy, are preventive treatment options for patients who prefer nondrug therapy or when symptomatic therapies are poorly tolerated, contraindicated, or ineffective.[21,35–37]

ACUTE MIGRAINE TREATMENT

ANALGESICS AND NONSTEROIDAL ANTI-INFLAMMATORY DRUGS (NSAIDS)

Simple analgesics and NSAIDs are effective medications for the management of mild to moderate migraine attacks (Table 61–4).[6,21] Efficacy of acetaminophen was demonstrated in a randomized, placebo-controlled study in which approximately 60% of patients had migraine headache of moderate intensity.[38] Of the NSAIDs, aspirin, ibuprofen,

TABLE 61–6. Precipitating Factors Associated with Migraine

Psychological Factors
Anxiety
Depression
Stress
Environmental Factors
Bright or flickering lights
High altitude
Glare
Loud noise
Strong odors
Tobacco smoke
Weather changes
Dietary Factors
Alcohol
Aspartame
Caffeine
Chocolate
Citrus fruit
Monosodium glutamate
Sodium nitrite (preserved meats and fish, food coloring)
Tyramine (aged cheeses, sour cream, wine, beer, liver, bananas, avocado, chocolate, yogurt, pods of broad beans)
Medications
Cocaine
H_2-receptor antagonists
Hormone replacement therapy
Indomethacin
Mestranol
Nicotine
Nifedipine
Nitrates
Oral contraceptives
Reserpine
Theophylline
Hormonal Factors
Menopause
Menstruation
Pregnancy
Lifestyle
Excessive or insufficient sleep
Fatigue
Fasting or dieting
Skipped meals
Smoking
Strenuous exercise
Stress

Compiled from Refs. 16, 20, and 24.

naproxen sodium, naproxen, diclofenac-potassium, and flurbiprofen have demonstrated efficacy in at least one placebo-controlled study; however, the relative efficacy of the different NSAIDs has not been established.[39–45] Comparisons with other pharmacotherapeutic classes are limited. Naproxen sodium was comparable to oral ergotamine in a double-blind study by Treves and colleagues.[46] Diclofenac-potassium provided similar acute headache relief to oral sumatriptan in a placebo-controlled study.[43] Aspirin plus metoclopramide was equivalent to oral sumatriptan in the first of three headache attacks treated over a 3-month period; sumatriptan was superior, however, for the second and third attacks.[47]

NSAIDs appear to prevent neurogenically-mediated inflammation in the trigeminovascular system through the inhibition of prostaglandin synthesis.[43] Long-acting, slow-release NSAIDs (e.g., oxaprozin, piroxicam, nabumetone) are less useful for acute headache management than faster-acting first-line agents.[48] NSAIDs are not commonly associated with rebound headaches, and they have been used successfully during the withdrawal period in rebound headache.[45] Combination therapy with metoclopramide can speed the absorption of analgesics and NSAIDs and alleviate migraine-related nausea and vomiting.[25] Suppository analgesic preparations and intramuscular ketorolac are also options when nausea and vomiting are severe.[6] Effervescent formulations may offer the advantage of enhanced absorption.[25] Acute NSAID therapy is associated with gastrointestinal (dyspepsia, nausea, vomiting, diarrhea) and central nervous system side effects (somnolence, dizziness). NSAIDs should be used cautiously in patients with previous ulcer disease, renal disease, or hypersensitivity to aspirin.[45]

The over-the-counter combination of acetaminophen, aspirin, and caffeine was approved for the treatment of migraine in the United States because of its proven efficacy in relieving migraine pain and associated symptoms.[49] Aspirin and acetaminophen are also available in prescription combination products containing a short-acting barbiturate (butalbital) or narcotic (codeine, propoxyphene). Midrin, a combination of acetaminophen, isometheptene mucate (a sympathomimetic amine), and dichloralphenazone (a chloral hydrate derivative), has demonstrated modest benefits in placebo controlled studies and is generally viewed as an alternative for patients with mild to moderate migraine attacks.[21,50] Although frequent consumption of aspirin or acetaminophen alone can result in medication overuse headache, combination analgesics appear to pose a greater risk.[24,28] Analgesics containing butalbital and narcotics also carry the risk of habituation and dependence, in addition to their sedative side effects.

OPIATE ANALGESICS

Narcotic analgesic drugs (e.g., meperidine, butorphanol, oxycodone, hydromorphone) provide effective relief of intractable migraine, but they should generally be reserved for patients with severe infrequent headache in whom conventional therapies are contraindicated or as "rescue medication" after patients have failed to respond to conventional therapies. Frequent use of narcotic analgesics may lead to the development of addiction and rebound headache. The intranasal formulation of butorphanol, a synthetically derived opioid agonist-antagonist, may provide an alternative to frequent office or emergency department visits for injectable migraine therapies. Onset of analgesia occurs within 15 minutes of administration. Pain relief with transnasal butorphanol was statistically superior to placebo and comparable to intramuscular methadone in randomized, placebo-controlled trials.[51] Adverse effects with butorphanol are common and include dizziness, nausea and/or vomiting, drowsiness, and taste perversion. Butorphanol is a controlled substance that carries the potential for dependence and addiction. Thus, it should be prescribed with care, and long-term therapy should be closely supervised.[22]

ANTIEMETICS

Adjunctive antiemetic therapy is useful for combating the nausea and vomiting that accompany migraine headaches and the medications used to treat acute attacks (e.g., ergotamine tartrate). A single dose of an antiemetic, such as metoclopramide, chlorpromazine, or prochlorperazine, administered 15 to 30 minutes before ingestion of oral abortive migraine medications is often sufficient. Suppository preparations are available when nausea and vomiting are particularly prominent. In addition to their antiemetic effects, dopamine antagonist drugs have also been used successfully as monotherapy for the treatment of intractable headache. Prochlorperazine administered by the intravenous and intramuscular routes and intravenous metoclopramide provided more effective pain relief than placebo.[52,53] Chlorpromazine has also provided relief of migraine headache comparable to intravenous metoclopramide and dihydroergotamine (DHE) when administered parenterally.[54] The precise mechanism of action for these agents is unknown. The dopamine antagonists offer an alternative to the narcotic analgesics for the treatment of refractory migraine. Drowsiness and dizziness were occasionally reported with the use of dopamine antagonists in migraineurs. Extrapyramidal side effects were infrequently reported in migraine trials.

MISCELLANEOUS NONSPECIFIC MEDICATIONS

Corticosteroids may be an effective acute migraine treatment when other therapies have failed or are contraindicated, however controlled clinical trials are lacking.[55,56] Short courses of orally or parenterally administered agents such as prednisone, dexamethasone, and hydrocortisone appear to be useful in the management of refractory headache that has persisted for several days.

Studies suggest a role for intranasal lidocaine 4% in the treatment of acute migraine headache.[57,58] Intranasal lidocaine provides effective pain relief within 5 minutes of administration, but headache recurs in approximately 20% to 40% of patients, usually within 1 hour. Adverse effects are generally limited to local irritation of the nose or eye, unpleasant taste, and numbness of the throat.

Preliminary investigations of intramuscular droperidol, nitrous oxide, and intravenous propofol have yielded favorable results in the treatment of acute migraine headache.[59–61] Future studies may establish a more defined role for these agents in migraine management.

ERGOT ALKALOIDS AND DERIVATIVES

Ergotamine tartrate and DHE are useful for the treatment of moderate to severe migraine attacks.[21] These drugs are nonselective 5-HT_1 receptor agonists that constrict intracranial blood vessels and inhibit the development of neurogenic inflammation in the trigeminovascular system.[62] Central inhibition of the trigeminovascular pathway is also reported.[63] They also display activity at α-adrenergic, β-adrenergic, and dopaminergic receptors. Venous and arterial constriction occur with therapeutic doses, but ergotamine tartrate exerts more potent arterial effects than DHE.[62,64]

Ergotamine tartrate is available for oral, sublingual, and rectal administration (Table 61–4). Oral and rectal preparations contain caffeine to enhance absorption and potentiate analgesia.[64] Ergotamine has poor bioavailability as a consequence of extensive first-pass metabolism. Rectal administration is preferred because it produces blood levels that are 20- to 30-fold higher than identical oral doses.[6,64] Dosage requirements should be strictly titrated to establish an effective, but subnauseating, dose for future attacks. Some clinicians recommend ergotamine titration (i.e., one-fourth of a suppository administered at hourly intervals) on a headache-free day to determine the subnauseating dose. Once patients establish the ergotamine dose that alleviates an evolving migraine, therapy for subsequent attacks should be initiated with that single effective dose. It is most effective when administered early in the migraine attack.[25] Evidence supporting the efficacy of ergotamine tartrate is lacking, despite its use in migraineurs since 1925. Many published studies are difficult to interpret because of the use of various, nonvalidated outcome measures and methodologic flaws in early investigations.[63] However, ergotamine appeared to be comparable to combination analgesics and NSAIDs in single-dose studies, and its use is supported by extensive clinical experience.[46,64,65]

DHE is available for intranasal and parenteral administration by the intramuscular, subcutaneous, and intravenous routes (Table 61–4).[64] Parenteral DHE was previously viewed as outpatient or emergency department treatment for moderate to severe migraine, but patients can be trained to self-administer DHE intramuscularly or subcutaneously.[6,24,66] Subcutaneous DHE was less effective than subcutaneous sumatriptan at 2 hours (relief in 73.1% and 85.3% of patients, respectively), but the therapies were equivalent at 3 and 4 hours.[67] Headache recurrence was significantly lower with subcutaneous DHE (17.7% versus 45% in sumatriptan-treated patients). Patients with intractable headache have been managed safely and effectively with inpatient administration of repetitive intravenous DHE for 3 to 7 days.[64] The bioavailability of DHE is approximately 30% following intranasal administration, and maximum plasma concentration is achieved in 30 to 60 minutes.[68] The efficacy of DHE nasal spray has been consistently demonstrated in multiple placebo-controlled studies.[69,70] In a double-blind, placebo-controlled trial conducted by The Dihydroergotamine Working Group, 61% and 70% of patients receiving 2 mg of intranasal DHE experienced headache relief at 2 and 4 hours, respectively (23% and 28% with placebo).[69] Statistically superior pain relief may not be achieved until 4 hours postdose.[69,70] Subcutaneous and intranasal sumatriptan provided superior relief of headache pain and nausea when compared to intranasal DHE at 2 hours.[71,72] Rates of headache recurrence were lower with DHE than with sumatriptan in these studies.[71,72] DHE is packaged in amber glass ampules to maintain product stability. It is dispensed with an assembly kit that facilitates ampule breakage and sprayer assembly.

Nausea and vomiting (resulting from stimulation of the chemoreceptor trigger zone) are among the most common adverse effects of the ergotamine derivatives; however, ergotamine is 12 times more emetic than DHE.[62] Pretreatment with an antiemetic agent should be considered with ergotamine and intravenous DHE therapy. Other common side effects include abdominal pain, weakness, fatigue, paresthesias, muscle pain, diarrhea, and chest tightness. Occasionally, symptoms of severe peripheral ischemia (ergotism) including cold, numb, painful extremities; continuous paresthesias; diminished peripheral pulses; and claudication may result from the vasoconstrictor effects of the ergot alkaloids. Gangrenous extremities, myocardial infarction, hepatic necrosis, and bowel and brain ischemia have been rarely reported.[64] DHE is rarely associated with such side effects.[64,73] Triptans and ergot derivatives should not be used within 24 hours of each other, and prophylactic therapy with methysergide is not recommended.[63,64] Recently, reports of severe vasospasm during concomitant therapy with ergotamine and protease inhibitors have appeared in the literature.[74,75] These cases are attributed to the inhibitory effects of the protease inhibitors on the CYP3A4 isoenzyme, and a consequent rise in ergotamine blood levels. Ergotamine derivatives are contraindicated in patients with renal or hepatic failure; coronary, cerebral, or peripheral vascular disease; uncontrolled hypertension; sepsis; and women who are pregnant or nursing.[64] DHE does not appear to cause rebound headache, however dosage restrictions for ergotamine tartrate should be strictly observed to prevent this complication.[64]

SEROTONIN RECEPTOR AGONISTS (TRIPTANS)

Introduction of the serotonin receptor agonists or "triptans" represented a significant advance in migraine pharmacotherapy. The first member of this class, sumatriptan, and the second-generation agents, zolmitriptan, naratriptan, rizatriptan, and almotriptan are selective agonists of the 5-HT_{1B} and 5-HT_{1D} receptors. Relief of migraine headache is the result of three key actions: vasoconstriction of pain-producing intracranial blood vessels through stimulation of vascular 5-HT_{1B} receptors, inhibition of vasoactive neuropeptide release from trigeminal perivascular nerves through stimulation of presynaptic 5-HT_{1D} receptors, and interruption of pain signal transmission within the brainstem trigeminal nuclei through stimulation of 5-HT_{1D} receptors (centrally acting agents).[9,11] Individual affinities for 5-HT_{1B} and 5-HT_{1D} receptors vary somewhat but are comparable.[11,76] These agents also display varying affinity for 5-HT_{1A}, 5-HT_{1E}, and 5-HT_{1F} receptors. The triptans are appropriate first-line therapy for patients with moderate to severe migraine, or rescue therapy when nonspecific medications are ineffective.[6,21]

Sumatriptan, the most extensively studied antimigraine therapy, is available for subcutaneous, oral, and intranasal administration.[9] Subcutaneous sumatriptan is consistently superior to placebo in alleviating migraine headache and associated symptoms with relief reported in 71% of patients at 1 hour (43% pain free) and 79% at 2 hours (60% pain free) in meta-analysis of placebo-controlled studies.[9,76] The subcutaneous injection is packaged as an autoinjector device for self-administration by patients.[77] The efficacy of the 50-mg and 100-mg doses of oral sumatriptan is comparable in meta-analysis, with 59% of patients reporting relief at 2 hours with either dose.[9,76,78] In addition to enhanced efficacy, subcutaneous sumatriptan has a more rapid onset of action (10 minutes) when compared to the oral formulation (30 minutes).[6,76] Intranasal sumatriptan provides a faster onset of effect (15 minutes) than the oral formulation, and produces similar rates of response (relief in 61% of patients at 2 hours) in placebo-controlled studies.[76] Approximately 30% to 40% of patients who respond to sumatriptan experience headache recurrence within 24 hours.[76] This has been attributed to the drug's short half-life, but recurrence is a problem with most acute migraine therapies.[9,76] A second dose given at the time of recurrence is usually effective. Routine administration of a second dose by the oral or subcutaneous routes does not improve initial efficacy or prevent subsequent recurrence.[79] Administration of sumatriptan during the aura has no effect on aura duration or subsequent headache development.[80]

The second-generation triptans—zolmitriptan, naratriptan, and rizatriptan—appear to offer an improved pharmacokinetic and pharmacodynamic profile as compared to sumatriptan.[9,76,81] These agents have higher oral bioavailability and longer half-lives than oral sumatriptan, which could theoretically improve within-patient treatment consistency and reduce headache recurrence (Table 61–7).[9] Naratriptan has the longest half-life of the triptans, but the slowest onset of action. Penetration of the blood-brain barrier, as a result of increased lipophilicity, allows for a central site of action within the trigeminal nuclei and may hasten the onset of therapeutic effect of the second-generation agents.[9,11] Sumatriptan does not cross the intact blood-brain barrier in experimental systems. However, evidence suggests that the blood-brain barrier may be disrupted during a migraine attack, allowing central access for sumatriptan, as well.[11] Results of placebo-controlled studies with each of the second-generation agents reveal somewhat comparable 2-hour response rates; however, comparative clinical trials are necessary to determine their relative efficacy. Two-hour headache response ranged from 62% to 67% in placebo-controlled studies of zolmitriptan, with recurrence rates of approximately 30%.[82,83] Rizatriptan provided relief in 62% to 77% of patients at 2 hours in placebo-controlled studies.[84,85] Headache recurred in 41% to 47% of patients. The relatively slower onset of naratriptan results in somewhat lower response rates at 2 hours (49%), but 4-hour response rates approach 60% to 68%, and recurrence rates ranged from 17% to 33%.[81,86–88]

Studies comparing the second-generation agents with sumatriptan have also been published. Rizatriptan (5 mg and 10 mg) provided similar headache relief to oral sumatriptan (50 mg and 100 mg) with similar recurrence rates, but time to headache relief, pain-free response rates at 2 hours, and relief of selected associated symptoms was superior with rizatriptan.[89–91] In a comparative trial, zolmitriptan 5 mg was at least as effective as sumatriptan 25 mg or 50 mg, and was superior to sumatriptan on selected headache response outcome measures.[92] Sumatriptan 100 mg was superior to naratriptan 2.5 mg when 4-hour headache response was assessed in a comparative study (80% vs 63%; $p < .05$).[88] Recurrence rates were lower with naratriptan than with sumatriptan (17% versus 44%, respectively; p value not reported), but 24-hour overall efficacy (headache relief at 24 hours without worsening, rescue medication, or recurrence) was similar. In a trial comparing optimal doses of rizatriptan and naratriptan, rizatriptan provided superior headache response rates at 2 hours and shorter time to onset of relief of headache and associated symptoms.[93] Four-hour response rates were not reported in this study. Clinical response to the triptans can vary considerably among individual patients, and lack of response to one agent does not preclude effective therapy with another member of the class.[94,95]

Side effects to the triptans are common, but usually mild to moderate in nature and of short duration. Adverse effects are consistent among the class, and include paresthesias, fatigue, dizziness, flushing, warm sensations, and somnolence. Local side effects are reported with the subcutaneous (minor injection site reactions) and intranasal (taste perversion, nasal discomfort) routes. Doses that provide the best ratio of efficacy and safety are considered optimal (Table 61–4). The tolerability profile of naratriptan was similar to placebo and superior to

TABLE 61–7. Pharmacokinetics of the 5-$HT_{1B/1D}$ Agonists in Patients with Migraine

Drug	Bioavailability	T_{max}	Half-life	Elimination
Sumatriptan			2 h	MAO-A; inactive metabolites
SC injection	97%	12 min		
Oral tablets	14%	2.5 h		
Nasal spray	17%	1.5–2.5 h		
Zolmitriptan	40%	2 h	3 h	CYP1A2, MAO-A; 1 active metabolite
Naratriptan	70%	3–4 h	6 h	50% excreted unchanged by kidneys; CYP-450; inactive metabolites
Rizatriptan	45%	1–1.5 h[a] 1.6–2.5 h[b]	2–3 h	MAO-A; 1 active metabolite
Almotriptan	70%	1–3 h	3–4 h	40% excreted unchanged by kidneys; CYP3A4, CYP2D6, MAO-A; inactive metabolites

MAO, monoamine oxidase
[a]Regular tablets
[b]Orally disintegrating tablets
Compiled from Refs. 76 and 81.

rizatriptan in published clinical studies.[86–88,93] Up to 15% of patients receiving a triptan consistently report "chest symptoms," including tightness, pressure, heaviness, or pain in the chest, neck, or throat.[6,9] The mechanism of these symptoms is unknown, but a cardiac source of pain seems unlikely in most patients.[9] However, all triptans are partial agonists of human coronary arteries in vitro, resulting in a small, but significant, vasoconstrictor response.[9,81] Adverse cardiac events are rare because 5-HT_{2A} receptors mediate most of the effects of serotonin on coronary vessels.[6] Isolated cases of myocardial infarction and coronary vasospasm with ischemia have been reported, but myocardial ischemia is unlikely in patients with normal coronary vasculature.[81] The triptans are contraindicated in patients with a history of ischemic heart disease (angina pectoris, Prinzmetal's angina, previous myocardial infarction), uncontrolled hypertension, and cerebrovascular disease. Patients at risk for unrecognized coronary artery disease (e.g., postmenopausal women, men over 40 years of age, and patients with multiple risk factors) should receive a cardiovascular assessment prior to triptan use. Their initial dose should be administered under medical supervision. Triptans are also contraindicated in patients with hemiplegic and basilar migraine. The triptans should not be given within 24 hours of the ergotamine derivatives. Administration of sumatriptan, rizatriptan, and zolmitriptan within 2 weeks of therapy with monoamine oxidase inhibitors is not recommended. Concomitant therapy with the selective serotonin reuptake inhibitors (SSRIs) should be carefully monitored because of isolated reports of serotonin syndrome in sumatriptan-treated patients. Frequent use of the triptans has been associated with the development of medication misuse headache.[26,27]

PROPHYLACTIC THERAPY

β-ADRENERGIC ANTAGONISTS

β-Adrenergic antagonists are the most widely used drugs for migraine prophylaxis, and are generally regarded as the treatment of choice for this indication.[6,28,96] Propranolol, nadolol, timolol, atenolol, and metoprolol have proven efficacy in controlled clinical trials, reducing the frequency of attacks by 50% in up to 60% of patients.[6,97] Because the relative efficacy of the individual agents has not been established, selection of a β-blocker may be based on β selectivity, convenience of the formulation, and tolerability. Atenolol and nadolol have long half-lives, permitting once-daily dosing which may improve adherence to therapy.[30] β-Blockers with intrinsic sympathomimetic activity are ineffective for migraine prophylaxis.[97] Although their precise mechanism of antimigraine action is unknown, they may raise the migraine threshold by modulating serotonergic neurotransmission in cortical or subcortical pathways. β-Blockers are particularly useful in patients with comorbid anxiety, hypertension, or angina. Side effects can include fatigue, sleep disturbances, vivid dreams, memory disturbance, depression, gastrointestinal intolerance, impotence, bradycardia and hypotension. Use of nonlipophilic β-blockers may lessen central nervous system side effects.[97] β-Blockers should be used with caution in patients with congestive heart failure, peripheral vascular disease, atrioventricular conduction disturbances, asthma, depression, and diabetes. Bronchoconstrictive and hyperglycemic effects may be minimized with β_1-selective agents.

ANTIDEPRESSANTS

Because the efficacy of amitriptyline has been demonstrated in placebo-controlled studies, it appears to be the antidepressant of choice for migraine prophylaxis. Amitriptyline reduces the frequency, severity, and duration of migraine attacks.[98] Other tricyclic antidepressants (TCAs) that have been used successfully for migraine prophylaxis include doxepin, nortriptyline, protriptyline, and imipramine.[21,97] The beneficial effects of TCAs in migraine are independent of their antidepressant activity, and may be related to antagonism of 5-HT_2 receptors on cerebral vessels or suppression of serotonergic neuronal activity in the brainstem.[28] TCAs are generally well-tolerated at the lower doses typically required for migraine prophylaxis. Anticholinergic side effects are common, and limit use of these agents in patients with benign prostatic hyperplasia and glaucoma. Evening doses are preferred because of associated sedation. Increased appetite and weight gain may occur. Orthostatic hypotension, and cardiac toxicity (slowed AV conduction) are also occasionally reported. The more favorable side effect profile of nortriptyline and protriptyline could prove advantageous in patients who are particularly intolerant of the anticholinergic and sedative side effects of amitriptyline.

SSRIs have not been extensively studied for the preventive treatment of migraine headaches, but clinicians have used them nonetheless.[6,96,97] Fluoxetine was efficacious in an early placebo-controlled study, but a subsequent evaluation did not confirm benefit in migraineurs.[99,100] Prospective data evaluating the other SSRIs (sertraline, paroxetine, fluvoxamine, citalopram) are lacking.[21] The SSRIs are considered to be less effective than TCAs for migraine prophylaxis, but have gained favor with some clinicians as a result of their more favorable adverse effect profile.[4] These agents should not be considered as first- or second-line medications for the management of migraine; however, they may be of some use when depression is a significant contributor to headache.[28,97]

Monoamine oxidase inhibitors(MAOs), such as phenelzine, have been used in the management of refractory headache, but their complex adverse effect profile limits use to experienced prescribers.[6,96] Strict adherence to a tyramine-free diet (Table 61–5) is necessary to avoid potentially life-threatening hypertensive crisis.

ANTICONVULSANTS

Valproic acid and divalproex sodium (a 1:1 molar combination of valproate sodium and valproic acid) can reduce the frequency of headaches by at least 50% in up to 65% of migraineurs.[101–103] Efficacy of valproic acid, a facilitator of γ-aminobutyric acid (GABA) neurotransmission, may be partly a result of the inhibition of serotonergic neurons of the dorsal raphe nuclei.[18] Nausea and vomiting, the most common early side effects, are self-limited and appear to be less common with divalproex sodium and gradual titration of doses (e.g., begin with 250 mg of divalproex sodium at bedtime and titrate slowly). Tremor, weight gain, and hair loss are also common complaints. Hepatotoxicity is the most serious, although rare, side effect of valproate therapy. Silberstein has published clinical guidelines for the use of valproate in migraineurs.[104] Clinical monitoring for symptoms suggestive of hepatotoxicity (e.g., nausea, vomiting, anorexia, lethargy, abdominal pain, bruising, bleeding, rash, and jaundice) is preferable to routine laboratory screening in patients whose risk of developing valproate hepatotoxicity is negligible (e.g., patients older than 10 years of age who are receiving monotherapy and have no underlying metabolic or neurologic disorder).[104] However, baseline laboratory studies (complete blood count with differential, serum chemistries, liver function tests) and patient evaluation every 1 to 2 months during the first 6 to 9 months of therapy is recommended. Although valproate levels may be useful for assessing compliance and toxicity, rigid adherence to the anticonvulsant therapeutic range of valproate (50–100 μg/mL) is unlikely to benefit the migraine patient.[104]

Divalproex sodium is particularly useful in patients with comorbid seizures or manic-depressive disorder. Studies suggest a possible role for other anticonvulsants, including gabapentin and topiramate; however, further clinical studies are needed to confirm their utility in migraine prophylaxis.[4,21]

METHYSERGIDE

Methysergide is one of the oldest and most effective agents for migraine prophylaxis.[6] This semisynthetic ergot alkaloid is a potent 5-HT_2 receptor antagonist that appears to stabilize serotonergic neurotransmission in the trigeminovascular system to block the development of neurogenic inflammation.[105] Although methysergide is an effective preventive medication in 60% or more of migraineurs, it is reserved for patients with refractory headaches, as rare (1 in 2500 patients), but potentially serious, retroperitoneal, endocardial, and pulmonary fibrotic complications have occurred during long-term, mostly uninterrupted, use.[97,105] Consequently, a medication-free interval of 4 weeks is recommended following each 6-month treatment period.[105] Dosage should be tapered over a 1-week period to prevent rebound headaches. Monitoring for fibrotic complications should include periodic auscultation of the heart, as well as yearly chest roentgenography, echocardiography, and abdominal imaging (e.g., ultrasound, CT, or MRI).[105] Patients should report clinical symptoms of flank pain, dysuria, chest pain, or shortness of breath. Methysergide is best tolerated when taken with meals. In addition to gastrointestinal intolerance, insomnia, vivid dreams, hallucinations, claudication, and muscle cramps are also reported with its use. It is contraindicated in patients with uncontrolled hypertension, coronary or peripheral vascular disease, hepatic or renal dysfunction, peptic ulcer disease, and in pregnant women. Peripheral vasospasm and severe claudication have been reported, occasionally in patients without a prior history of vascular disease. In addition to clinical monitoring for possible vasospastic effects (progressive claudication and cold, numb, painful extremities), monthly checks of peripheral pulses have been recommended by some clinicians.[96]

CALCIUM CHANNEL BLOCKERS

Among the calcium channel blockers, verapamil is considered the agent of choice for the prevention of migraines; however, it provided only modest benefit in decreasing the frequency of attacks in two placebo-controlled studies.[106,107] Verapamil has little effect on the severity of migraine attacks. The therapeutic effect of verapamil, which is thought to be a result of the inhibition of 5-HT release, may not be noted for up to 8 weeks after the initiation of therapy.[97] It is generally considered a second- or third-line prophylactic agent when other drugs with established clinical benefit are ineffective or contraindicated.[6] Side effects of verapamil may include constipation, hypotension, bradycardia, atrioventricular block, and exacerbation of congestive heart failure.

NONSTEROIDAL ANTI-INFLAMMATORY DRUGS (NSAIDS)

NSAIDs are modestly effective for reducing the frequency, severity, and duration of migraine attacks, however, potential gastrointestinal and renal toxicity limit the daily or prolonged use of these agents.[55] Consequently, NSAIDs have been used intermittently to prevent headaches that recur in a predictable pattern, such as menstrual migraine. Administration of NSAIDs in the perimenstrual period may be beneficial in women with true menstrual migraine.[108] NSAIDs should be initiated 1 to 2 days prior to the time of headache vulnerability and continued over a period of 5 to 7 days. Prostaglandin production may be enhanced in women with menstrual migraine, and the preventive mechanism of NSAIDs is thought to involve inhibition of prostaglandin synthesis.[4,31] If long-term NSAID therapy is initiated, monitoring of renal function and occult blood loss is necessary.

MISCELLANEOUS PROPHYLACTIC AGENTS

A recent double-blind, placebo-controlled study demonstrated the efficacy of vitamin B_2 (400 mg) in migraine prophylaxis. Vitamin B_2 was associated with 50% or greater improvement in attack frequency in 59% of patients.[109] Additional interventions for the prophylactic management of menstrual migraine may include perimenstrual ergotamine tartrate and hormonal adjustment with estrogen replacement, bromocriptine, tamoxifen, or danazol. The reader is referred to recent reviews for further discussion of these treatment modalities.[4,108] Studies with the herbal medication feverfew have yielded conflicting results in migraineurs, but beneficial effects were demonstrated in a controlled clinical trial.[110] Other medications have been suggested as effective alternatives for migraine prophylaxis, including clonidine, guanfacine, cyproheptadine, magnesium, and carbamazepine.[21] Although the clinical utility of these agents has not been adequately studied, they may prove useful for patients who are intolerant of standard prophylactic therapies.

PHARMACOECONOMIC CONSIDERATIONS

Although migraine is widely recognized as a disease that exacts an enormous toll on the sufferer, the direct and indirect costs associated with migraine headache impose a substantial burden on society as well. The direct costs associated with migraine diagnosis and treatment are substantial. The volume of health care services used by migraineurs is two to five times that of nonmigraineurs, with 90% of patients reporting visits to a medical clinic and up to 50% reporting visits to an emergency department.[111,112] However, the indirect costs of the illness related to work absenteeism, decreased productivity, and impairment greatly exceed the direct cost of medical care.[7,8] The estimated indirect cost of migraine-related disability, the most important determinant of the economic impact of migraine, is approximately $13 billion each year.[8]

According to the American Migraine Study, only 41% of women and 29% of men with clear symptoms of migraine were diagnosed by a physician.[113] Although 95% of severe migraine sufferers take some medication for their headaches, only 40.1% of women and 28.2% of men with moderate to severe headache-related disability take prescription medication.[113] Because many migraineurs who receive inadequate care experience substantial levels of pain and disability, improvement in migraine diagnosis, care, and treatment could potentially result in lower direct and indirect costs of the disease.

Education of headache patients regarding required behavior changes and effective use of acute and prophylactic pharmacotherapy might be time-consuming, but it is extremely cost-effective. Oversights may lead to decreased efficacy of medications resulting in repeat dosing and polypharmacy, decreased compliance, increased emergency department use, increased doctor shopping, and, perhaps, increased use of expensive diagnostic procedures and inpatient services.[97] Recent studies demonstrate that effective migraine treatment with sumatriptan can reduce productivity loss during a migraine attack.[114] Health care resource use and time lost from workplace productivity and nonworkplace activity were also significantly reduced 3 to 6 months after the initiation of sumatriptan therapy in a managed care population.[115] Health-related quality of life also improved in these patients. These studies demonstrate that the clinical benefits of effective migraine therapy may ultimately translate into reduced indirect migraine-related costs. Further studies should be conducted to demonstrate the value of effective migraine pharmacotherapies in reducing the overall costs of managing the migraineur.

SUMMARY

Acute and preventive pharmacotherapy for migraine should be individualized based on the individual patient response, tolerability of the available agents, and the presence of comorbid conditions. Migraine management should be individualized on the basis of the patient's clinical presentation and medical history. Analgesics and NSAIDs may be considered the drugs of choice for infrequent mild to moderate attacks. The triptans or DHE can be used as secondary agents if initial therapies prove ineffective, or as first-line therapy in moderate to severe migraine headache. Abortive therapy should be instituted early in the course of the attack to optimize efficacy and minimize migraine-related pain and disability. Preventive therapy should be considered in the setting of recurring migraines that produce significant disability, frequent attacks requiring symptomatic medication more than twice per week, symptomatic therapies that are ineffective, contraindicated, or produce serious side effects, and uncommon migraine variants that cause profound disruption and/or risk of neurologic injury. Efficacy of a prescribed prophylactic regimen should be reassessed periodically. Prolonged headache-free intervals could allow for gradual dosage reduction and discontinuation of therapy.

CLUSTER HEADACHE

EPIDEMIOLOGY

Cluster headache, the most severe of the primary headache disorders, is characterized by attacks of severe, unilateral head pain which occur in series lasting for weeks or months (i.e., cluster periods) separated by remission periods usually lasting months or years.[4,116] Cluster headaches may be episodic or chronic (Table 61–8).[2] It is relatively uncommon among the primary headache disorders, with an estimated prevalence of approximately 0.4% for men and 0.08% for women.[116] Unlike migraine, men are four to seven times more likely than women to suffer from cluster headache.[4] Onset can occur at any age, but is most common in the late twenties. Recent evidence suggests that a genetic predisposition for cluster headache may exist in certain families.[4]

PATHOPHYSIOLOGY

The etiologic and pathophysiologic mechanisms of cluster headache are not completely understood. Similar to migraine headache, the head pain of cluster attacks is thought to involve activation of trigeminovascular neurons with resultant release of vasoactive neuropeptides and the development of sterile, neurogenic inflammation.[116] The characteristic location of head pain appears to implicate the cavernous sinus as the site of the inflammatory process.[10] Triggers of cluster headache attacks may cause periodic discharges of the trigeminovascular system that result in headache pain; however, the mechanisms that activate the trigeminovascular system are not yet understood. The periodicity and regularity of attacks may implicate hypothalamic dysfunction and resulting alterations in circadian rhythms in the pathogenesis of cluster headache.[4,116] Hypothalamus-induced changes in cortisol, prolactin, testosterone, growth hormone, β-endorphin, and melatonin have been demonstrated during periods of cluster headache attack.[116] Neuroimaging studies performed during acute cluster headache attacks have demonstrated activation of the ipsilateral hypothalamic gray.[10] This region may be the fundamental "driver" of the cluster attack. Because serotonergic systems modulate activity in

TABLE 61–8. Diagnostic Criteria for Episodic and Chronic Cluster Headache

A. At least five attacks fulfilling B through D below.
   Episodic cluster headache: Cluster periods last (untreated) 7 days to 1 year, separated by remissions of at least 14 days
   Chronic cluster headache: Attacks occur for more than 1 year without remission or with remission lasting less than 14 days
B. Severe unilateral orbital, supraorbital and/or temporal pain lasting 15 to 180 minutes untreated
C. Headache is associated with at least one of the following signs which have to be present on the painful side:
   1. Conjunctival injection
   2. Lacrimation
   3. Nasal congestion
   4. Rhinorrhea
   5. Forehead and facial sweating
   6. Miosis
   7. Ptosis
   8. Eyelid edema
D. Frequency of attacks: from one every other day to eight per day
E. At least one of the following:
   1. History, physical, and neurologic examinations do not suggest an organic disorder
   2. History and/or physical and/or neurologic examinations do suggest such disorder, but it is ruled out by appropriate investigations
   3. An organic disorder is present, but cluster headache does not occur for the first time in close temporal relation to the disorder

Adapted from Ref. 2.

both the hypothalamus and trigeminovascular neurons, 5-HT may play a significant role in cluster headache pathophysiology. The association of cluster headache with high-altitude hypoxia, rapid-eye movement sleep, and vasodilator therapy, as well as the efficacy of oxygen inhalation therapy in aborting cluster attacks, suggest that hypoxemia may also play a role in the pathogenesis of cluster headache.[116]

CLINICAL PRESENTATION

Attacks occur in cluster periods lasting 2 weeks to 3 months in most patients, followed by long, pain-free intervals.[4,116] Periods of remission average 2 years in length, but have been reported from 2 months to 20 years in duration. Approximately 10% of patients have chronic symptoms with no remission periods. Cluster headache attacks occur at night in more than 50% of patients and appear to be more common in the spring and fall.[116] Attacks occur suddenly with pain peaking quickly after onset and generally lasting 15 to 180 minutes.[2] Auras are not present with cluster headaches. The pain is excruciating and penetrating, but usually nonthrobbing, and is most often unilateral in orbital, supraorbital, or temporal locations.[4,116] The headache is associated with autonomic features consistent with sympathetic system paresis and parasympathetic overdrive. These features are present on the pain side and include conjunctival injection, lacrimation, and nasal stuffiness or rhinorrhea. Ipsilateral scalp and facial tenderness, ptosis, miosis, and periorbital swelling are also described. During the cluster period, attacks occur from once every other day to eight times per day.[4] Whereas migraine patients retreat to a quiet dark room, cluster headache patients generally move about during an attack and may rub or beat their heads against objects in an attempt to alleviate the pain.[116] Male patients often have a history of heavy tobacco and/or alcohol use.[116] Table 61–8 lists the IHS diagnostic criteria for cluster headaches.[2]

▶ TREATMENT: Cluster Headaches

As in migraine, therapy for cluster headaches involves both abortive and prophylactic therapy. Abortive therapy is directed at managing the acute attack. Prophylactic therapy is intended to shorten the duration of episodic cluster attacks, in addition to reducing the frequency and severity of attacks in both episodic and chronic cluster headache. Prophylactic therapies are started early in the cluster period and administered daily until the patient is headache-free for at least 2 weeks. The medication is then tapered, but may be restarted with the next cluster period. Patients with chronic cluster headache may require prophylactic medications indefinitely.

ABORTIVE THERAPY

OXYGEN

The standard acute treatment of cluster headache is inhalation of 100% oxygen by facial mask at a rate of 7–10 L/min for 10 to 15 minutes.[4,116,117] Oxygen inhalation relieves pain almost immediately and is effective in approximately 70% of adult patients.[117] Repeat administration may be necessary because of recurrence, as oxygen appears to merely delay, rather than abort, the attack in some patients.[116] No side effects have been reported. The beneficial effect of oxygen is thought to be a result of cerebral vasoconstriction, but this has not been confirmed.[116,118]

ERGOTAMINE DERIVATIVES

Intravenous or intramuscular DHE provides effective relief for acute attacks of cluster headache.[4,116] Onset of effect usually occurs within 10 minutes following intravenous administration.[116] Intramuscular administration is effective within 30 minutes and patients may be trained to self-administer the IM injection.[116] Repeated IV administration of DHE for 3 to 7 days can break the cycle of frequent cluster headache attacks with minimal side effects.[64,116] Ergotamine tartrate has also provided effective relief of cluster headache attacks when administered sublingually or rectally, however the pharmacokinetics of these preparations frequently limit their clinical utility.[4,116] Dosing guidelines are similar to those for migraine headache therapy.

SUMATRIPTAN

Subcutaneous sumatriptan is a safe and effective acute treatment for cluster headaches.[119,120] Headache relief is reported within 15 minutes of administration in approximately 75% of patients.[119] Adverse events reported in cluster headache patients are similar to those seen in migraineurs. Sumatriptan has been used in the management of cluster headaches for up to 1 year without evidence of tachyphylaxis or increased toxicity.[120] Orally administered sumatriptan has limited use in cluster attacks because of its relatively long onset of action; oral zolmitriptan, however, was efficacious in patients with episodic cluster headache with 60% of patients experiencing relief (mild or no pain) at 30 minutes.[121]

PROPHYLACTIC THERAPY

VERAPAMIL

Verapamil, the preferred calcium channel blocker for the prevention of cluster headaches, is effective in approximately 70% of patients.[4,117] The beneficial effects of verapamil often appear after 1 week of therapy. Effective doses usually range from 240 mg/day to 360 mg/day for episodic attacks, but higher doses may be necessary to control chronic cluster headache.

LITHIUM

Lithium carbonate is effective against episodic and chronic cluster headache attacks, with beneficial effects often appearing during the first week of therapy. A positive response is seen in up to 78% of patients with chronic cluster headache, and in up to 63% of patients with episodic cluster headache.[4] The usual dose of lithium for cluster headache is 600–900 mg/day administered in divided doses. Tachyphylaxis to lithium has occasionally been reported during prolonged therapy.[4,116] Optimal plasma lithium levels for prevention of cluster headache have not been established, but efficacy has been reported at relatively low serum concentrations (0.3–0.8 mEq/L).[4,116]

Initial side effects are mild and include tremor, lethargy, nausea, diarrhea, and abdominal discomfort. Lithium treatment has been associated with headache symptoms described as episodes of moderately severe, throbbing occipital pain lasting 6 to 12 hours, but these headaches are easily distinguishable from the cluster headache and disappear when lithium is withdrawn. Lithium should be administered with caution to patients with significant renal or cardiovascular disease, dehydration, pregnancy, or concomitant diuretic use. For a complete review of lithium use, refer to Chap. 70.

ERGOTAMINE

Ergotamine can be an efficacious agent for prophylactic as well as abortive therapy of cluster headaches.[4,118] A 2-mg bedtime dose is often beneficial for the prevention of nocturnal headache attacks. Daily use of 1–2 mg of ergotamine alone or in combination with verapamil or lithium may provide effective headache prophylaxis in patients refractory to other agents with little risk of ergotism or rebound headache.[4,116]

METHYSERGIDE

In patients unresponsive to other therapies, methysergide 4–8 mg/day in divided doses is usually effective in shortening the course of cluster headaches.[116,118] Response to treatment usually occurs within 1 week of initiation of the drug. Response rates in patients with episodic cluster headache approach 70%, but chronic cluster headache patients receive less benefit.[116] Precautions regarding methysergide use were described earlier in this chapter.

CORTICOSTEROIDS

Corticosteroids are useful for chronic cluster headaches refractory to verapamil, lithium, ergotamine, and methysergide, or combinations of these agents.[4,116] Therapy is initiated with 40–60 mg/day of prednisone and tapered over approximately 3 weeks. Relief appears within 1 to 2 days of initiating therapy. To avoid steroid-induced complications, long-term use is not recommended. Headaches may recur when therapy is tapered or discontinued.

MISCELLANEOUS AGENTS

Other therapies that have been used in the acute management of cluster headache include intranasal lidocaine, intranasal capsaicin, and intramuscular leuprolide.[116,122] Preliminary evidence may also support the use of divalproex sodium, gabapentin, baclofen, topiramate, and phototherapy treatments, but well-designed, controlled studies are lacking.[4,116,123,124] Neurosurgical intervention may be necessary for patients with chronic cluster headache that is resistant to all medical therapies.[4,116]

EVALUATION OF THERAPEUTIC OUTCOMES

Because of the prevalence of migraine and cluster headaches, pharmacists need to be actively involved in patient care issues. Patients should be monitored for frequency, intensity, and duration of headaches, as well as any change in the headache pattern. To this end, migraineurs should be encouraged to keep a headache diary to document the frequency, severity, and duration of migraine attacks, as well as response to medication and potential trigger factors. Careful monitoring is essential to initiate the most appropriate pharmacotherapy, document therapeutic successes and failures, identify medication contraindications, and prevent or minimize adverse events. Patients taking abortive therapy should be monitored for frequency of use of prescription and over-the-counter medications in order to identify potential medication misuse headache. Patient counseling is necessary to allow for proper medication use (e.g., self-injection with sumatriptan), to encourage early use of medications in the headache cycle, and to enhance patient compliance. Strict adherence to dosing guidelines should be stressed to minimize potential toxicity. Patterns of abortive medication use can be documented to establish the need for prophylactic therapy. Prophylactic therapies should also be monitored closely for adverse reactions, abortive therapy needs, adequate dosing, and compliance. Consultation with other health care practitioners should be encouraged when changes in headache patterns or medication use occur.

CONCLUSIONS

Although migraine and cluster headaches appear to occur as a result of neuronal dysfunction, the precise etiology and nature of the dysfunction are unknown. Serotonergic neurotransmission and the trigeminovascular system appear to play important roles. A careful patient workup, including patient history, physical examination, and appropriate laboratory tests, should identify most headache patients with major disease. A variety of strategies can be helpful for managing both migraines and cluster headaches (Figs. 61–2 and 61–3).

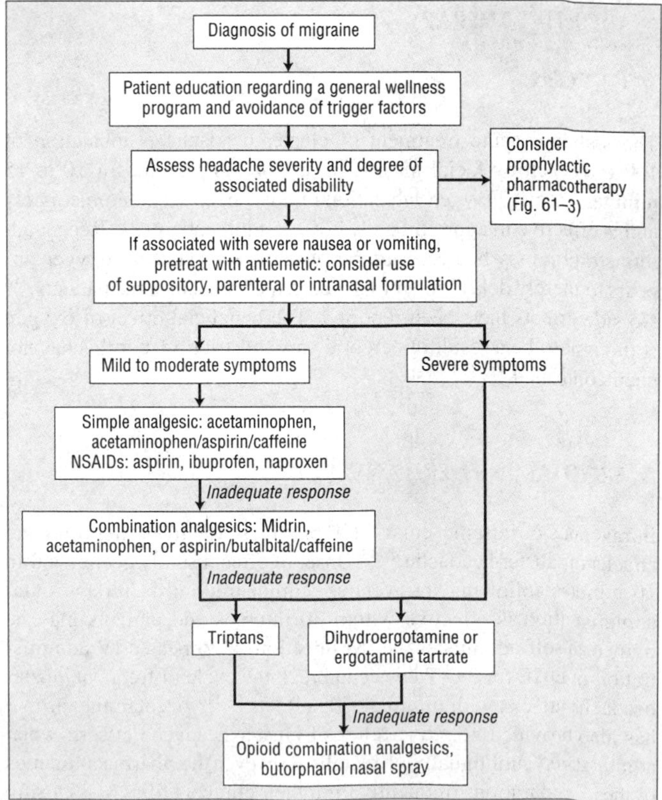

FIGURE 61–2. Treatment algorithm for migraine headaches.

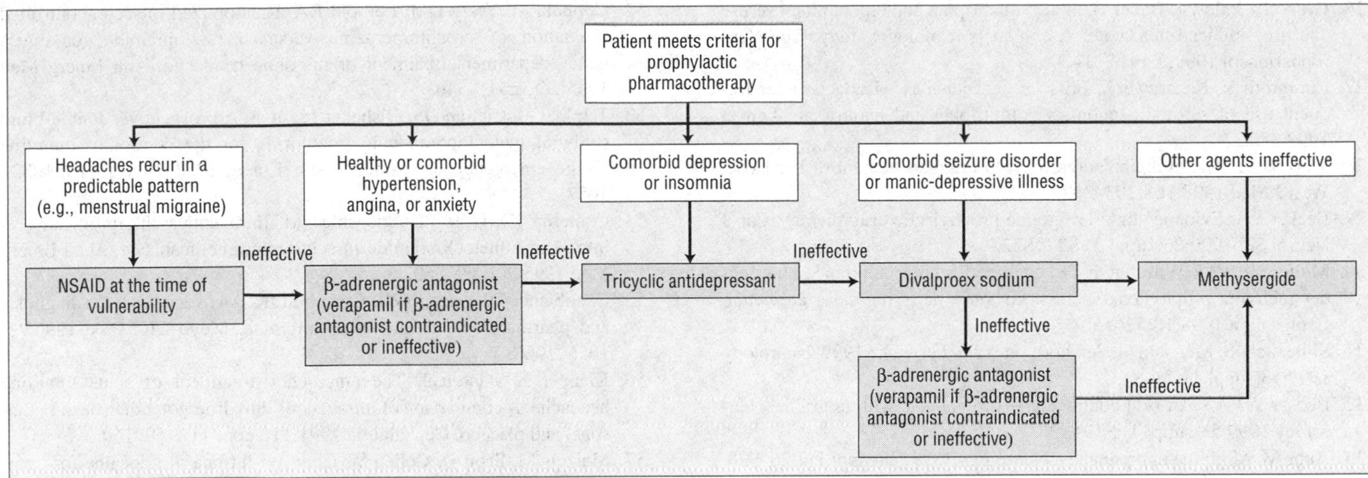

FIGURE 61–3. Treatment algorithm for prophylactic management of migraine headaches.

Management of primary headache disorders is directed at suppressing an acute attack and preventing recurrences. Continuing research into the problem of headache disorders will better define pathophysiologic mechanisms and aid the search for less toxic and more efficacious pharmacologic agents.

▶ PRINCIPLES OF PHARMACOTHERAPY OF MIGRAINE

- A general wellness program and avoidance of migraine triggers should be included in the management plan.
- Abortive therapy should be given early in the migraine attack.
- After an effective abortive agent and dose have been identified, subsequent treatments should begin with that same regimen.
- Strict adherence to maximum daily and weekly doses of antimigraine medications is essential.
- Preventive therapy should be considered in the setting of recurring migraines that produce significant disability; frequent attacks requiring symptomatic medication more than twice per week; symptomatic therapies that are ineffective, contraindicated, or produce serious side effects; and uncommon migraine variants that cause profound disruption and/or risk of neurologic injury.
- The selection of an agent for migraine prophylaxis should be based on individual patient response, tolerability, convenience of the drug formulation, and comorbid conditions of the patient.
- Each prophylactic medication should be given an adequate therapeutic trial to judge its efficacy, usually 2 to 3 months.

REFERENCES

1. Dubose CD, Cutlip AC, Cutlip WD. Migraines and other headaches: An approach to diagnosis and classification. Am Fam Physician 1995;51:1498–1504.
2. Headache Classification Committee of the International Headache Society. Classification and diagnostic criteria for headache disorders, cranial neuralgias, and facial pain. Cephalalgia 1988;8(suppl 7):1–96.
3. Stewart WF, Lipton RB, Celentano DD, Reed ML. Prevalence of migraine headache in the United States: Relation to age, income, race, and other sociodemographic factors. JAMA 1992;267:64–69.
4. Silberstein SD, Lipton RB, Goadsby PJ. Headache in Clinical Practice. Oxford, UK, Isis Medical Media, 1998:11–58, 61–90, 115–124.
5. Dahlof CGH. Current concepts of migraine and its treatment. Neurologia 1999;14:67–77.
6. Silberstein SD, Goadsby PJ, Lipton RB. Management of migraine: An algorithmic approach. Neurology 2000;55(suppl 2):S46–S52.
7. Stewart WF, Lipton RB, Simon D. Work-related disability: Results from the American migraine study. Cephalalgia 1996;16:231–8.
8. Hu XH, Markson LE, Lipton RB, et al. Burden of migraine in the United States. Arch Intern Med 1999;159:813–818.
9. Ferrari MD. Migraine. Lancet 1998;351:1043–1051.
10. Lance JW, Goadsby PJ. Mechanism and Management of Headache, 6th ed. Oxford, UK, Butterworth Heinemann, 1998:9–16, 25–157, 176–205, 291–298.
11. Hargreaves RJ, Shepheard SL. Pathophysiology of migraine—New insights. Can J Neurol Sci 1999;26(suppl 3):S12–S19.
12. Edvinsson L. On migraine pathophysiology. In: Edvinsson L, ed. Migraine and Headache Pathophysiology. London, Martin Dunitz, 1999: 3–15.
13. Weiller C, May A, Limmroth V, et al. Brain stem activation in spontaneous human migraine attacks. Nat Med 1995;1:658–660.
14. Gardner K. The genetic basis of migraine: How much do we know? Can J Neurol Sci 1999;26(suppl 3):S37–S43.
15. Hamel E. The biology of serotonin receptors: Focus on migraine pathophysiology and treatment. Can J Neurol Sci 1999;26(suppl 3):S2–S6.
16. Saper JR. Diagnosis and symptomatic treatment of migraine. Headache 1997;37(suppl 1):S1–S14.
17. Dahlof CGH, Solomon GD. The burden of migraine to the individual sufferer: A review. Eur J Neurol 1998;5:525–533.
18. Silberstein SD, Lipton RB. Overview of diagnosis and treatment of migraine. Neurology 1994;44(suppl 7):S6–S16.
19. Dalessio DJ. Diagnosing the severe headache. Neurology 1994.44 (suppl 3):S6–S12.
20. Firshberg BM. The utility of neuroimaging in the evaluation of headache in patients with normal neurologic examinations. Neurology 1994;44: 1191–97.
21. Silberstein SD. Practice parameter: evidence-based guidelines for migraine headache (an evidence-based review). Neurology 2000;55: 754–763.
22. Weitzel KW, Thomas ML, Small RE, Goode JV. Migraine: A comprehensive review of new treatment options. Pharmacotherapy 1999;19(8): 957–973.
23. Lipton RB, Stewart, WF, Stone AM, et al. Stratified care vs step care strategies for migraine: The disability in strategies of care study. JAMA 2000;284:2599–2605.
24. Bartleson JD. Treatment of migraine headaches. Mayo Clin Proc 1999;74:702–708.
25. Moore KL, Noble SL. Drug treatment of migraine: Acute therapy and drug rebound headache. Am Fam Physician 1997;56(8):2039–2048.

26. Evers S, Gralow I, Bauer B, et al. Sumatriptan and ergotamine overuse and drug-induced headache: A clinicoepidemiologic study. Clin Neuropharmacol 1999;22(4):201–206.
27. Limmroth V, Kazarawa Z, Fritsche G, Diener H. Headache after frequent use of serotonin agonists zolmitriptan and naratriptan. Lancet 1999:353:378.
28. Maizels M. The clinician's approach to the management of headache. West J Med 1998;168:203–212.
29. Becker WJ. Evidence based migraine prophylactic drug therapy. Can J Neurol Sci 1999;26(suppl 3):S27–S32.
30. Mulleners WM, Whitmarsh TE, Steiner TJ. Noncompliance may render migraine prophylaxis useless, but once-daily regimens are better. Cephalalgia 1998;18:52–56.
31. Silberstein S, Merriam G. Sex hormones and headache 1999. Neurology 1999;53(suppl 1):S3–S13.
32. Becker WJ. Use of oral contraceptives in patients with migraine. Neurology 1999;53(suppl 1):S19–S25.
33. Aube M. Migraine in pregnancy. Neurology 1999;53(suppl 1):S26–S28.
34. Fettes I. Migraine in menopause. Neurology 1999;53(suppl 1):S29–S33.
35. McGrath PJ. Clinical psychology issues in migraine headaches. Can J Neurol Sci 1999;26(suppl 3):S33–S36.
36. Andrasik F. Behavioral management of migraine. Biomed Pharmacother 1996;50:52–57.
37. Reid GJ, McGrath PJ. Psychological treatments for migraine. Biomed Pharmacother 1996;50:58–63.
38. Lipton RB, Baggish JS, Stewart WF, et al. Efficacy and safety of acetaminophen in the treatment of migraine: Results of a randomized, double-blind, placebo-controlled, population-based study. Arch Intern Med 2000;160:3486–3492.
39. Boureau F, Joubert JM, Lasserre V, et al. Double-blind comparison of an acetaminophen 400 mg-codeine 25 mg combination versus aspirin 1,000 mg and placebo in acute migraine attack. Cephalalgia 1994;14(2):157–161.
40. Kloster R, Nestvold K, Vilming ST. A double-blind study of ibuprofen versus placebo in the treatment of acute migraine attacks. Cephalalgia 1992;12(3):169–171.
41. Johnson ES, Ratcliffe DM, Wilkinson M. Naproxen sodium in the treatment of migraine. Cephalalgia 1985;5(1):5–10.
42. Andersson PG, Hinge HH, Johansen O, et al. Double-blind study of naproxen vs placebo in the treatment of acute migraine attacks. Cephalalgia 1989;9(1):29–32.
43. Diclofenac-K/Sumatriptan Migraine Study Group. Acute treatment of migraine attacks: efficacy and safety of a nonsteroidal anti-inflammatory drug, diclofenac-potassium, in comparison to oral sumatriptan and placebo. Cephalalgia 1999;19:232–240.
44. Awidi AS. Efficacy of flurbiprofen in the treatment of acute migraine attacks: A double-blind cross-over study. Curr Ther Res 1982;32(3):492–497.
45. Pfaffenrath V, Scherzer S. Analgesics and NSAIDs in the treatment of the acute migraine attack. Cephalalgia 1995;suppl 15:14–20.
46. Treves TA, Streiffler M, Korczyn AD. Naproxen sodium versus ergotamine tartrate in the treatment of acute migraine attacks. Headache 1992;32:280–282.
47. Oral Sumatriptan and Aspirin-plus-Metoclopramide Comparative Study Group. A study to compare oral sumatriptan with oral aspirin plus oral metoclopramide in the acute treatment of migraine. Eur Neurol 1992;32(3):177–184.
48. Von Seggern RL, Adelman JU. Cost considerations in headache treatment Part 2: Acute migraine treatment. Headache 1996;38:493–502.
49. Lipton RB, Stewart WF, Ryan RE, et al. Efficacy and safety of acetaminophen, aspirin, and caffeine in alleviating migraine headache pain: Three double-blind, randomized, placebo-controlled trials. Arch Neurol 1998;55:210–217.
50. Diamond S. Treatment of migraine with isometheptene, acetaminophen, and dichloralphenazone combination: A double-blind, crossover trial. Headache 1976;15(4):282–287.
51. Hoffert MJ, Couch JR, Diamond S, et al. Transnasal butorphanol in the treatment of acute migraine. Headache 1995;35(2):65–69.
52. Coppola M, Yealy DM, Leibold RA. Randomized, placebo-controlled evaluation of prochlorperazine versus metoclopramide for emergency department treatment of migraine headache. Ann Emerg Med 1995;26(5):541–546.
53. Tek DS, McClellan DS, Olshaker JS, et al. A prospective, double-blind study of metoclopramide hydrochloride for the control of migraine in the emergency department. Ann Emerg Med 1990;19(10):1083–1087.
54. Cameron JD, Lane PL, Speechley M. Intravenous chlorpromazine vs intravenous metoclopramide in acute migraine headache. Acad Emerg Med 1995;2(7):597–602.
55. Capobianco DJ, Chesire WP, Campbell JK. An overview of the diagnosis and pharmacologic treatment of migraine. Mayo Clin Proc 1996;71:1055–1066.
56. Klapper J, Stanton J. The emergency treatment of acute migraine headache: A comparison of intravenous dihydroergotamine, dexamethasone, and placebo. Cephalalgia 1991;11(suppl 11):159–160.
57. Maizels M, Scott B, Cohen W, Chen W. Intranasal lidocaine for treatment of migraine: A randomized, double-blind, controlled trial. JAMA 1996;276:319–321.
58. Maizels M, Geiger AM. Intranasal lidocaine for migraine: A randomized trial and open-label follow-up. Headache 1999;39:543–551.
59. Richman PB, Reischel U, Ostrow A, et al. Droperidol for acute migraine headache. Am J Emerg Med 1999;17(4):398–400.
60. Krusz JC, Scott V, Belanger J. Intravenous propofol: Unique effectiveness in treating intractable migraine. Headache 2000;40:224–230.
61. Triner WR, Bartfield JM, Birdwell M, Robak N. Nitrous oxide for the treatment of acute migraine headache. Am J Emerg Med 1999;17(3):278–281.
62. Silberstein SD. The pharmacology of ergotamine and dihydroergotamine. Headache 1997;37(suppl 1):15–25.
63. Tfelt-Hansen P, Saxena PR, Dahlof C, et al. Ergotamine in the acute treatment of migraine: A review and European consensus. Brain 2000;123:9–18.
64. Silberstein SD, Young WB. Safety and efficacy of ergotamine tartrate and dihydroergotamine in the treatment of migraine and status migrainous. Neurology 1995;45:577–584.
65. Hakkarainen H, Quiding H, Stockman O. Mild analgesics as an alternative to ergotamine in migraine. A comparative trial with acetylsalicylic acid, ergotamine tartrate, and a dextropropoxyphene compound. J Clin Pharmacol 1980;20(10):590–595.
66. Weisz MA, El-Raheb M, Blumenthal HJ. Home administration of intramuscular DHE for the treatment of acute migraine headache. Headache 1994;34:371–373.
67. Winner P, Ricalde O, Le Force B, et al. A double-blind study of subcutaneous dihydroergotamine vs subcutaneous sumatriptan in the treatment of acute migraine. Arch Neurol 1996;53:180–184.
68. Logemann CD, Rankin LM. Newer intranasal migraine medications. Am Fam Physician 2000;61:180–186.
69. Gallagher RM and the Dihydroergotamine Working Group. Acute treatment of migraine with dihydroergotamine nasal spray. Arch Neurol 1996;53:1285–1291.
70. Dihydroergotamine Nasal Spray Multicenter Investigators. Efficacy, safety, and tolerability of dihydroergotamine nasal spray as monotherapy in the treatment of acute migraine. Headache 1995;35(4):177–184.
71. Touchon J, Bertin L, Pilgrim AJ, et al. A comparison of subcutaneous sumatriptan and dihydroergotamine nasal spray in the acute treatment of migraine. Neurology 1996;47:361–365.
72. Boureau F, Kappos L, Schoenen J, et al. A clinical comparison of sumatriptan nasal spray and dihydroergotamine nasal spray in the acute treatment of migraine. Int J Clin Pract 2000;54(5):281–286.
73. Lipton R. Ergotamine tartrate and dihydroergotamine mesylate: Safety profiles. Headache 1997;37(suppl 1):S33–S41.
74. Rosenthal E, Sala F, Chichmanian RM, et al. Ergotism related to the concurrent administration of ergotamine tartrate and indinavir. JAMA 1999;281(11):987.
75. Liaudet L, Buclin T, Jaccard C, Eckert P. Severe ergotism associated with interaction between ritonavir and ergotamine. BMJ 1999;318:771.

76. Tfelt-Hansen P, DeVries P, Saxena PR. Triptans in migraine: A comparative review of pharmacology, pharmacokinetics, and efficacy. Drugs 2000;60(6):1259–1287.
77. The Sumatriptan Auto-Injector Study Group. Self-treatment of acute migraine with subcutaneous sumatriptan using an auto-injector device. Eur Neurol 1991;31:323–331.
78. Pfaffenrath V, Cunin G, Sjonell J, et al. Efficacy and safety of sumatriptan tablets (25 mg, 50 mg, 100 mg) in the acute treatment of migraine: Defining the optimum doses of oral sumatriptan. Headache 1998;38: 184–190.
79. Ferrari MD, James MH, Bates D, et al. Oral sumatriptan: Effect of a second dose, and incidence and treatment of headache recurrences. Cephalalgia 1994;14:330–338.
80. Bates D, Ashford E, Dawson R, et al. Subcutaneous sumatriptan during the migraine aura. Neurology 1994;44:1587–1592.
81. Deleu D, Hanssens Y. Current and emerging second-generation triptans in acute migraine therapy: A comparative review. J Clin Pharmacol 2000;40:687–700.
82. Rapoport AM, Ramadan NM, Adelman JU, et al. Optimizing the dose of zolmitriptan for the acute treatment of migraine: A multicenter, double-blind, placebo-controlled, dose range-finding study. Neurology 1997;49(5):1210–1218.
83. Solomon GD, Cady MD, Klapper JA, et al. Clinical efficacy and tolerability of 2.5 mg zolmitriptan for the acute treatment of migraine. Neurology 1997;49:1219–1225.
84. Kramer MS, Matzura BS, Polis A, et al. A placebo-controlled crossover study of rizatriptan in the treatment of multiple migraine attacks. Neurology 1998;51:773–781.
85. Teall J, Tuchman M, Cutler N, et al. Rizatriptan for the acute treatment of migraine and migraine recurrence. A placebo-controlled, outpatient study. Headache 1998;38(4):281–287.
86. Mathew NT, Asgharnejad M, Peykamian M, Laurenza A. Naratriptan is effective and well tolerated in the acute treatment of migraine. Neurology 1997;49(6):1485–1490.
87. Klassen A, Elkind A, Asgharnejad M, et al. Naratriptan is effective and well tolerated in the acute treatment of migraine: Results of a double-blind, placebo-controlled, parallel-group study. Headache 1997;37:640–645.
88. Havanka H, Dahlof C, Pop PH, et al. Efficacy of naratriptan tablets in the acute treatment of migraine: A dose-ranging study. Clin Ther 2000;22:970–980.
89. Goldstein J, Ryan R, Jiang K, et al. Crossover comparison of rizatriptan 5 mg and 10 mg versus sumatriptan 25 mg and 50 mg in migraine. Headache 1998;38:737–747.
90. Visser WH, Terwindt GM, Reines SA, et al. Rizatriptan vs sumatriptan in the acute treatment of migraine: A placebo-controlled, dose-ranging study. Arch Neurol 1996;53:1132–1137.
91. Tfelt-Hansen, P, Teall J, Rodriguez F, et al. Oral rizatriptan versus oral sumatriptan: A direct comparative study in the acute treatment of migraine. Headache 1998;38:748–755.
92. Gallagher Rm, Dennish G, Egilius LH, et al. A comparative trial of zolmitriptan and sumatriptan for the acute oral treatment of migraine. Headache 2000;40:119–128.
93. Bomhof M, Paz J, Legg N, et al. Comparison of rizatriptan 10 mg vs. naratriptan 2.5 mg in migraine. Eur Neurol 1999;42:173–179.
94. Mathew N, Kailasam J, Gentry P, Chernyshev O. Treatment of nonresponders to oral sumatriptan with zolmitriptan and rizatriptan: A comparative open trial. Headache 2000;40:464–465.
95. Stark S, Spierings E, McNeal S, et al. Naratriptan efficacy in migraineurs who respond poorly to oral sumatriptan. Headache 2000;40:513–520.
96. Noble SL, Moore KL. Drug treatment of migraine: Preventive therapy. Am Fam Physician 1997;56(9):2279–2286.
97. Adelman JU, Von Seggern RL. Cost considerations in headache treatment Part 1: prophylactic migraine treatment. Headache 1995;35:479–487.
98. Ziegler DK, Hurwitz A, Hassanein RS, et al. Migraine prophylaxis: A comparison of propranolol and amitriptyline. Arch Neurol 1987;44(5):486–489.
99. Adly C, Strumanis, Chesson A. Fluoxetine prophylaxis of migraine. Headache 1992;32(2):101–104.
100. Saper JR, Silberstein SD, Lake AE, Winters ME. Double-blind trial of fluoxetine: Chronic daily headache and migraine. Headache 1994;34(9): 497–502.
101. Jensen R, Brinck T, Olesen J. Sodium valproate has a prophylactic effect in migraine without aura: A triple-blind, placebo-controlled crossover study. Neurology. 1994;44:647–651.
102. Mathew NT, Saper JR, Silberstein SD. Migraine prophylaxis with divalproex. Arch Neurol 1995;52:281–286.
103. Silberstein SD, Collins SD. Safety of divalproex sodium in migraine prophylaxis: An open-label, long-term study. Headache 1999;39:633–643.
104. Silberstein SD. Divalproex sodium in headache: Literature review and clinical guidelines. Headache 1996;36:547–555.
105. Silberstein SD. Methysergide. Cephalalgia 1998;18:421–435.
106. Markley HG, Cheronis JC, Piepho RW. Verapamil in prophylactic therapy of migraine. Neurology 1984;34(7):973–976.
107. Solomon GD, Steel JG, Spaccavento LJ. Verapamil prophylaxis of migraine: A double-blind, placebo-controlled study. JAMA 1983; 250(18):2500–2502.
108. Boyle C. Management of menstrual migraine. Neurology 1999;53 (suppl 1):S14–S18.
109. Schoenen J, Jacquy J, Lenaerts M. Effectiveness of high-dose riboflavin in migraine prophylaxis: A randomized controlled trial. Neurology 1998;50(2):466–470.
110. Murphy JJ, Heptinstall S, Mitchell JR. Randomised double-blind placebo-controlled trial of feverfew in migraine prevention. Lancet 1988;2(8604):189–192.
111. Stang PE, Osterhaus JT, Celentano DD. Migraine: Patterns of healthcare use. Neurology 1994;44(suppl 4):S47–S55.
112. Kozma CM, Mauch RP, Reeder CE, Lawrence BJ. A literature review comparing the economic, clinical, and humanistic attributes of dihydroergotamine and sumatriptan. Clin Therapeutics 1994;16:1037–1049.
113. Lipton RB, Stewart WF. Migraine in the United States: A review of epidemiology and health care use. Neurology 1993;43(suppl 3):6–12.
114. Cady RC, Ryan R, Jhingram P, et al. Sumatriptan injection reduces productivity loss during a migraine attack: Results of a double-blind, placebo-controlled trial. Arch Intern Med 1998;158:1013–1018.
115. Lofland JH, Johnson NE, Batenhorst AS, Nash DB. Changes in resource use and outcomes for patients with migraine treated with sumatriptan: A managed care perspective. Arch Intern Med 1999;159:857–863.
116. Mendizabal JE, Umana E, Zweifler RM. Cluster headache: Horton's cephalalgia revisited. South Med J 1998;91(7):606–617.
117. Kudrow L. Response of cluster headache attacks to oxygen inhalation. Headache 1981;21:1–4.
118. Ekbom K. Treatment of cluster headache: Clinical trials, design and results. Cephalalgia 1995;(suppl 15)8:33–36.
119. The Sumatriptan Cluster Headache Study Group. Treatment of acute cluster headache with sumatriptan. N Engl J Med 1991;325:322–326.
120. Gobel H, Lindner V, Heinz A, et al. Acute therapy for cluster headache with sumatriptan: Findings of a one-year long-term study. Neurology 1998;51:430–435.
121. Bahra A, Gawel MJ, Hardebo JE, et al. Oral zolmitriptan is effective in the acute treatment of cluster headache. Neurology 2000;54:291–296.
122. Marks DR, Rapoport A, Padla D, et al. A double-blind placebo-controlled trial of intranasal capsaicin for cluster headache. Cephalalgia 1993;13:114–116.
123. Hanit-Hering R, Gadoth N. Baclofen in cluster headache. Headache 2000;40:48–51.
124. Wheeler SD, Carrazana EJ. Topiramate-treated cluster headache. Neurology 1999;53:234–236.

62
EVALUATION OF PSYCHIATRIC ILLNESS

Patricia A. Marken and Mark E. Schneiderhan

Certain patient assessment skills are common across specialties; however, psychiatry uses additional procedures that are less objective than traditional laboratory tests and physical examination techniques. Mental health clinicians need training in psychiatric assessment in order to participate meaningfully on the treatment team and to provide quality patient care. Additionally, patients with mental illness are treated routinely in the general medical settings; thus good psychiatric assessment skills can no longer be limited to psychiatric pharmacy specialists. This chapter provides an overview of appropriate assessment techniques used by clinicians when working with psychiatric patients to develop pharmaceutical care plans.

OVERVIEW OF THE *DIAGNOSTIC AND STATISTICAL MANUAL OF MENTAL DISORDERS*

The *Diagnostic and Statistical Manual of Mental Disorders,* first edition (DSM-I) provides a common language for mental health practitioners to describe psychiatric disorders.[1] Common language is essential because there is considerable overlap of symptoms between many diagnoses. DSM-I was introduced in 1952 and was the first manual on mental disorders to contain a description of diagnostic categories. The most recent edition, DSM-IV-TR (Text Revision), was released in 2000. The DSM-IV-TR uses essentially the same diagnostic criteria sets as DSM-IV.[1] Its purpose it to correct factual errors in DSM-IV and update the text sections (e.g., associated features, prevalence, differential diagnosis) with more contemporary empirical evidence. The major overhaul of diagnostic criteria and introduction of new diagnoses will occur with the DSM-V, which probably will not be available until 2006.[1,2]

The DSM-IV-TR is widely accepted as the most important diagnostic reference for mental illness. It contains many components that provide a comprehensive understanding of the illness and assist clinicians in making an accurate diagnosis. For example, the multiaxial patient evaluation ensures that most factors that could contribute to, or modify, the condition are considered during a patient assessment. The Axis I diagnosis lists the principal psychiatric disorder or disorders or provisional diagnoses present. On Axis II, developmental and personality disorders are listed. On Axis III, existing physical disorders or conditions are listed. On Axis IV, the severity of psychosocial stressors that may have contributed to a new or recurrent mental disorder or exacerbation of an existing condition are described. Stressors are rated on a scale of 1 (none) to 6 (catastrophic) and can be acute (lasting less than 6 months) or enduring (lasting longer than 6 months). Examples of stressors include difficulties with interpersonal relationships, parenting, occupation, living circumstances, finances, the legal system, and health. The Axis V diagnosis describes the global assessment of functioning (GAF), rated on a scale from 1 (persistent danger to self or others) to 90 (minimal or absent symptoms). A GAF rating should be made for the current level of functioning and the highest level of functioning in the past months to a year prior to the current evaluation. By documenting the baseline level of functioning, the GAF helps in establishing ultimate therapeutic goals.

DSM-IV-TR provides information on all mental disorders recognized by the American Psychiatric Association and includes age of onset, clinical course, complications, predisposing factors, prevalence, and differential diagnoses. The specific diagnostic criteria for each mental illness and the number of symptoms required to establish a diagnosis are also listed. The DSM-IV-TR also includes decision trees for differential diagnosis and a glossary of technical terms. *The Clinical Interview Using the DSM-IV* is a companion book that provides extensive information on interviewing techniques to allow the clinician to establish the presence of a DSM-IV diagnosis.[2]

Additional information besides the DSM-IV-TR diagnosis is required before a comprehensive treatment plan is developed. The *American Psychiatric Association Practice Guidelines for Psychiatric Evaluation of Adults* offers a more comprehensive approach to patient assessment and will yield the information needed for appropriate treatment planning. It includes a full discussion of the domains of a thorough clinical evaluation including history of present illness, past psychiatric history, general medical history, social and occupational history, physical and mental status examinations, and diagnostic tests. It further describes issues of privacy, evaluations in the elderly, and techniques in working in multidisciplinary teams.[3]

MENTAL STATUS EXAMINATION

The mental status examination (MSE) in psychiatry can be conceptualized as the counterpart to the physical examination in medicine. However, conducting a MSE does not obviate the need for a physical examination in a psychiatric patient. The MSE creates a description of current patient behavior, thoughts, perceptions, and functioning and provides an objective evaluation used for diagnosis, assessment of the course of the illness, and response to treatment. The interview should be completed in a quiet, private, and comfortable area where the patient and the interviewer feel at ease. The interviewer should introduce himself or herself and explain the procedure in order to facilitate establishment of a trusting relationship. Generally, open-ended questions should come first, followed by questions focused on more specific or personal data. Open-ended questions ask the patient to provide descriptions and other information in his or her own words. Even though more specific questions may then be necessary to fill in the gaps, beginning in this manner minimizes the risk of "leading" the patient. Patients may respond to specific questions and "yes" or "no" questions with answers they think the interviewer wants to hear.

The interviewer must be nonjudgmental in order to develop trust and rapport with the patient and to ensure completeness and accuracy of the information. An MSE has several components.[2,3]

APPEARANCE AND ATTITUDE TOWARD EXAMINER

The appearance of the patient throughout the interview should be noted, including age, dress, grooming and hygiene, use of cosmetics, and facial expressions. A description of appearance also should include unusual physical characteristics and the general state of physical health. The interviewer should note whether the patient is cooperative, mute, hostile, paranoid, or withdrawn.

ACTIVITY

Changes in motor activity include overactivity, underactivity, and catatonia. Overactivity includes an increase in purposeful movements or agitation, where the movements appear purposeless to the observer. Examples of overactivity include pacing; hand wringing; picking at clothing, skin, or hair; inability to sit still during the interview; and excessive hand gestures. Underactive patients move less than expected. Patients with rigid posture, an absence of movement, and failure to communicate may be catatonic.

SPEECH AND LANGUAGE

The quantity, content, and speed of speech and whether the patient makes eye contact should be noted. Speech should be assessed as to whether it proceeds logically in a goal-directed manner or the content is vague and poorly organized. Abnormal speech characteristics include *blocking,* whereby the person suddenly stops speaking without any obvious reason. *Thought blocking* usually occurs when a hallucination or delusion intrudes into the person's thinking or when upsetting issues are discussed. *Circumstantial speech* lacks a clear direction because of excess unnecessary information, but the circumstantial patient eventually will make his or her point. In *tangential speech,* however, the ultimate point is never made. *Perseveration* is repetition of speech despite the patient trying to produce a new answer. *Flight of ideas* is overproductive, rapid speech during which the patient jumps rapidly from one idea to the next. *Mutism* is when the patient does not respond even though he or she is aware of the discussion.

MOOD AND AFFECT

Affect describes the prevailing emotional tone, whereas mood describes more sustained feelings. To properly evaluate a patient's mood and affect, their appearance and the content of speech must be considered. Change in facial expression and the presence of tears, flushing, sweating, or tremors should be noted. Affect can be described further by its range, appropriateness, intensity, and stability. For example, in schizophrenia or depression, the affect may be flat, whereby no change in expression occurs throughout the interview. In contrast, during a manic episode, the affect is very intense and often labile. The range of emotional expression is reduced but not absent with blunted affect. An example of inappropriate affect is when a patient laughs when he or she is depressed or cries when stating that he or she is happy. A rapidly shifting affect from one extreme to the other is described as labile.

THOUGHT AND PERCEPTUAL DISTURBANCES

A variety of thought disturbances can occur in mental illness. *Delusions* are fixed, false beliefs that are not based in reality or consistent with the patient's religion or culture. Delusions can be paranoid, somatic, or grandiose in nature, and patients may be delusional in that they believe they are controlled by an outside force. Delusions are often unshakable, and one should not attempt to talk a patient out of a delusion. *Obsessions* are unwanted thoughts or ideas that intrude into a person's thinking. *Compulsions* are actions often performed in response to the obsessions or to control anxiety associated with the obsession. *Thought broadcasting* is the belief that one's thoughts are audible to others. *Hallucinations* are false sensory impressions or perceptions that occur in the absence of an external stimulus. Hallucinations may be auditory, visual, olfactory, or gustatory and may be continuous or intermittent. In contrast, *illusions* are visual perceptions that are misinterpreted but have a real sensory stimulus. For example, a patient who perceives a chair sitting in a dark corner to be a threatening figure is experiencing an illusion.

NEUROPSYCHIATRIC EVALUATIONS

A neuropsychiatric evaluation assesses sensorium, attention, concentration, memory, and higher cognitive functions such as orientation, abstraction, and calculation. Prior to initiation of the neuropsychiatric evaluation, it should be documented whether the patient has been prescribed medications with sedative properties because the outcome of the examination could be altered if central nervous system depressants have been taken.

Sensorium, or level of consciousness, refers to the alertness of the patient and, if he or she is not fully alert, the amount of stimulation needed to awaken the patient. Attention and concentration can be assessed using serial 7s or 3s, whereby the patient subtracts backward from 100 in increments of 7 or 3, respectively. Another concentration test is to have a patient spell a five-letter word backward. Language skills are assessed initially by having a patient read something aloud and silently. General intelligence can be assessed loosely by asking factual information about current news items, recent presidents, or popular television shows or sporting events. Memory is the ability to recall past experiences and is classified as immediate, recent (past events leading to the patient's current situation), and remote (historical facts). Orientation to time, place, person, and situation assesses immediate and recent memory. Asking a patient to recall three objects 5 minutes after they are learned is another test for recent memory. Remote memory is assessed by asking the patient to recall old facts of their life, such as where they were born or where they went to school. Remote memory usually stays intact the longest in patients with intellectual decline. Abstraction is the ability to interpret information such as a proverb ("People in glass houses shouldn't throw stones") or identify similarities or differences between words (apple and orange). Abstraction ability is influenced by education and linguistic fluency; thus inability to abstract is not always a sign of a thought disorder.

INSIGHT AND JUDGMENT

Insight refers to patients' awareness that they have a mental illness and the consequences of that illness on their life. Patients typically have a lack of insight when they are psychotic. Patients with poor insight are often noncompliant with prescribed medications. Judgment is the ability to make decisions appropriate to the situation and may be impaired in a variety of mental illnesses.

An MSE is usually completed on admission to a hospital or intake into a psychiatric facility. The MSE should be used to identify initial target symptoms that are monitored during the course of drug therapy. Table 62–1 provides examples of questions that can be used to gather some information in the MSE. Note that these are additional

TABLE 62–1. Examples of Interview Questions for Assessing Mental Illnesses

Mania
1. Do your thoughts go faster than you can say them?
2. Have you noticed a change in the amount of sleep that you require?
3. Have you spent a lot of money lately? What did you spend it on?
4. Do you have a lot of extra energy?
(To assess hallucinations and delusions, see Schizophrenia section in this table.)

Depression
1. Do you cry without any reason?
2. Do you still enjoy the same hobbies/activities that you once did?
3. Has your weight changed recently?
4. Have you had changes in your energy level recently?
5. Do you have any guilty feelings?
6. Do you find it difficult to remember phone numbers, names of friends, appointments, and so forth?
(To assess sleep and suicidal potential, see Sleep and Suicide Potential sections in this table.)

Schizophrenia

Delusions
1. Do you feel that people plot against you?
2. Do you ever feel that you are watched or spied on?
3. Do you have any special abilities?
4. Does anyone ever try to mess with you or bother you?
5. Do others read your thoughts?

Hallucinations
1. Does the TV or radio ever tell you things?
2. Do you hear voices that other people don't hear?
3. What do they say? How many voices?
4. How often do they bother you?
5. Do the voices ever tell you to hurt yourself or someone else?
6. Have you ever heard your name called when there is no one there?
7. Have you ever seen anything strange that you can't explain?
8. Do you ever see things that bother you and no one else?
9. Do you want to act on what the voices say?

Thought Broadcasting/Insertion
1. If I stood by you could I hear your thoughts?
2. Does your head ever act like a radio?
3. Do you feel that others can put thoughts in your head?

Insight
1. What reasons did your family give you for coming here?
2. What brought you here?
3. Do you consider yourself in need of help?
4. What does your medication do for you?

Sleep
1. Tell me about your sleep.
2. How many hours do you sleep each night at present?
3. How many hours do you usually sleep at night?
4. Do you sleep all through the night?
5. Is there a reason for your waking up?
6. Do you have trouble falling asleep?
7. How do you feel when you wake up?

Suicide Potential
1. Do you feel your life is worth living?
2. Do you ever think of hurting yourself?
3. Do you see things improving in the future?
4. Do you think you will try to hurt yourself now?
5. How would you do it?
6. Do you have the means to hurt yourself?

questions that can be asked for probing and clarification after as much information as possible has been gathered using open-ended (nonleading) questions.

SYSTEMATIC MEASUREMENT OF COGNITIVE FUNCTION

Neuropsychiatric rating scales provide specific information such as the rate of change and severity of cognitive decline or improvement. They are useful in situations where repeated measurements of a patient's mental status are needed because they allow the clinician to determine response to an intervention (e.g., medication) in a more systematic manner. In addition, some cognitive function measures are useful screens for Alzheimer's and other dementias, cerebral infarction, and encephalitis or encephalopathies. A number of cognitive rating scales are available, with the most common being the Mini-Mental State Exam (MMSE). The MMSE globally assesses many cognitive domains including orientation, visuospatial organization, memory, and reasoning to determine an overall score of cognitive function. The MMSE takes 5 to 10 minutes to administer and is used routinely in a clinical setting.[4] Other examples of cognitive rating scales include the Information-Memory-Concentration Test (IMC), the Dementia Rating Scale (DRS), and the Clock Drawing and Alzheimer's Disease Assessment Scale.[4,5] Some scales are useful for identifying deficits in specific cognitive domains such as orientation, speech and language, visuospatial, visuoperceptual and visuomotor skills, memory, arithmetic calculations, and reasoning. (Table 62–2).

Most of the rating scales involve a structured interview that requires clinician training to ensure accurate administration. Noise and distraction can affect the patient's performance ability; therefore, the interview should be conducted in a quiet area with adequate lighting. The interviewer should speak slowly and clearly to the patient when providing instructions or asking questions.

Both the patient's and the family's histories of mental illness provide important information when formulating a diagnosis. Information should be descriptive and include the current and previous psychiatric diagnoses, presentation of each illness, time frame between episodes, level of functioning between episodes, length of each episode, total duration of illness, and treatment given during each episode. Baseline functioning or the highest level of functioning achieved in the past few years is important information because it provides a target or goal for treatment. Information on the history of the current episode and reasons for coming to the clinician also should be gathered. A family history should include a medication history of the immediate relatives because a family member's response to a given medication may predict an individual patient's response to that same medication.

A social history should include educational and occupational background, religion, marital status, substance use patterns including smoking, and current living situation. By understanding a patient's living environment and social situation, strategies to prevent noncompliance and to reduce stress and increase social support can be developed.

MEDICATION HISTORY

A thorough medication history is one of the most important contributions a pharmacist can make to treatment planning. The history should include medication for both psychiatric and medical conditions. The medication history should note not only which medications have been

TABLE 62–2. Selected Neuropsychiatric Measures

Rating Scale	Type	Scoring	Comments
Mini-Mental State Exam	Structured interview	Maximum score is 30. 23 or less is indicative of cognitive impairment. Level of consciousness also listed	5–10 minutes to administer Global assessment of orientation, attention, recall and language, memory
Dementia Rating Scale	Structured interview	Total scores range form 0 to 144 (perfect score)	30–40 minutes to administer. Global measure of dementia using 5 subscales: attention, initiation and perseveration, construction, conceptualization, memory
Neurobehavioral Cognitive Status Examination (NCSE, COGNISTAT)	Structured interview	Eight separately scored cognitive domains (11 subsets). The 8 domains are scored and plotted on a graph provided.	5–10 minutes in non-impaired and up to 30 minutes in impaired patients. Distinguishes confusional states from dementias by using separate domain scores such as: language, memory, calculations, etc. Requires some practice, however easy to administer
Clock Drawing	Instructional	Qualitative assessment (template matching) Quantitative scoring Points awarded for correctness of design	Assessment at bedside which involves either copying a clock, putting hands on a clock and/or showing a specific time. Cognitive domains: comprehension, conceptualization, visuospatial skills
Alzheimer's Disease Assessment Scale (ADAS)	Structured interview	21 items total: 11 items in the cognitive (COG) subset. 10 items in the non-cognitive behavioral subset. Each subsets may be scored separately from the total ADAS score	Takes 45 minutes to administer the ADAS and 35 minutes for the ADAS-COG. The ADAS-COG refers to the cognitive assessment subset commonly used to measure cognitive function in clinical drug trials. Requires training for administration and scoring

Adapted from Refs. 4 and 5.

taken but also how they were tolerated and how well the patient responded to them. Because most psychiatric medications have a delay in the onset of effect and many mental illnesses are chronic, it is important to determine whether an adequate trial (adequate duration and adequate dose) was provided before the patient was considered nonresponsive. If a patient has a history of noncompliance, specific causes such as cost, complicated dosing schedules, lack of insight, and adverse effects should be investigated.

MEDICAL ASSESSMENT IN PSYCHIATRY

A careful medical assessment of patients who present with psychiatric symptoms is important for many reasons.[3,6,7] Both medical illnesses and medications can cause psychiatric symptoms, making an accurate diagnosis very difficult. Patients with psychiatric illnesses, especially depressive and anxiety disorders, may describe only physical complaints. Many patients with chronic psychiatric illnesses receive poor medical care and need a medical referral. Finally, psychotropic medications can cause or exacerbate medical conditions, such as diabetes mellitus or cardiac arrhythmia's, necessitating an understanding of patients' other risk factors for these conditions before medication is selected.

Medical illnesses may be misdiagnosed or undiagnosed in patients with psychiatric conditions for many reasons, including patient appearance or behavior prohibiting a thorough evaluation, inaccurate information from the patient, and incomplete data to make an appropriate diagnosis and treatment recommendation.[8]

An important clue that a physical illness may be causing or contributing to psychiatric symptoms is rapidity of onset of psychiatric symptoms. Most chronic mental illnesses have a prodromal period, whereas medically based psychiatric symptoms often have a more rapid onset of symptoms. Patients over age 40 at first presentation are more likely to have a medical cause for their psychiatric symptoms because major psychiatric illnesses such as schizophrenia and bipolar affective disorder usually first present at an earlier age. A family history of physical illnesses with a psychiatric component, such as Huntington's chorea and systemic lupus erythematosus, provides an additional clue. Patients with fluctuating levels of consciousness, disorientation, memory impairment, or visual, tactile, or olfactory hallucinations, substance abuse, and serious medical conditions are more likely to have a medical basis for their illness.

There is no consensus about specific diagnostic tests needed in the evaluation of a patient with mental illness.[3] Pharmacists will want diagnostic tests to help evaluate the relative safety of specific medications (e.g., renal status when selecting a mood stabilizer or electrocardiogram when selecting an antidepressant) or when baseline information is needed to identify future adverse effects from medications (e.g., lithium-induced hypothyroidism, clozapine-induced diabetes mellitus). General laboratory screening is useful for ruling out medical causes of psychiatric illnesses, but extensive testing is usually unnecessary and not cost-effective. Laboratory tests should be individualized to the age, medical history, and physical health of the patient. A complete physical examination, along with a detailed medical and medication history, vital signs, weight and body mass index, and routine blood chemistry, is recommended by many clinicians.[3,6,8] Urine drug screens and blood alcohol tests play an important role in identifying the contribution of substances of abuse to the presenting symptoms. If available, recent laboratory tests can be used to evaluate medical status, provided that no change in physical status has occurred since they were taken. A blood chemistry panel and a complete blood count are usually needed to assess contraindications and complications to drug therapy. A fasting glucose determination is preferred over a random measure when a patient takes medications known to cause significant weight gain and/or induced diabetes mellitus.[9] Serum concentration monitoring of selected medications is also helpful in increasing probability of response and minimizing the likelihood of adverse effects.

In patients for whom a medical cause for the psychiatric symptoms is suspected, more extensive medical testing is indicated. Almost any test can be considered, with the decision based on the proposed cause of the symptoms. Additional testing can include an electroencephalogram (EEG) to evaluate for the presence of seizure activity or other neurologic conditions, computed tomography (CT) or magnetic resonance imaging (MRI) to detect structural abnormalities, sedimentation (SED) rate and antinuclear antibodies (ANA) for autoimmune disorders, an HIV test, thyroid function tests, or B_{12} and folate concentrations for anemias.[10]

The identification of biologic markers as diagnostic tools and predictors or indicators of drug response is of great interest but currently of little clinical utility. The most promising was the dexamethasone suppression test (DST), which was proposed to be a marker for endogenous melancholic depression. Its lack of sensitivity and specificity has limited its utility as a routine screening tool during a workup for depression.[10,11]

PSYCHOLOGICAL TESTING

Although pharmacists are not involved directly in psychological testing, they can use the results to evaluate the role of medication in relationship to the diagnosis. Psychological testing alone cannot establish a firm diagnosis but can be a useful diagnostic tool when coupled with clinical judgment. Types of psychological testing include personality tests, intelligence tests, and neuropsychological tests.[12] Table 62–3 describes common psychological tests.

TABLE 62–3. Common Psychological Tests

Wechsler Intelligence Scales (WAIS-R for adults; WISC-R for children)
Measures abstract thinking, learning from experience, problem solving, adjustment to new situations
Score less than 70 denotes mental retardation
Bender Visual Motor Gestalt Test
Screening test for brain damage, learning problems, emotional difficulties, nonverbal intelligence
Person is asked to reproduce nine geometric designs
Interpretation of Projective Drawings
Patient draws a person, house-tree-person, family
Used to assess unconscious feeling, conflicts, and strengths
Rorschach
Patient interprets 10 inkblots and explains what they mean
Assesses personality structure
Minnesota Multiphasic Personality Inventory (MMPI-2)
Measures personality traits from 567 true/false questions
Can be affected by intelligence, education, socioeconomic status

PSYCHIATRIC RATING SCALES

Psychiatric rating scales have multiple uses including research, patient care, and education.[13] The purpose of a rating scale is to provide objective data to answer a clinical or research question. A single psychiatric rating scale score provides only a limited picture or snapshot of a complex clinical situation. However, repeated ratings can objectively describe longitudinal change over a defined treatment period. For example, the Hamilton Anxiety Rating Scale (HAM-A) can be used to assess baseline symptoms of anxiety and the change produced by an intervention or time.[14] The HAM-A can detect features of somatic and psychic anxiety (e.g., anxious mood, tension, fears, insomnia, somatic, and cardiovascular symptoms).

Global rating scales, such as the Clinical Global Impression (CGI) scale, assess the overall severity of illness based on a rater's clinical experience.[15] The rating scale will not determine the reason for the symptoms; for example, a patient's anxiety may be secondary to paranoia or a primary anxiety disorder. Second, a patient may have a 15% drop in a rating scale score from one week to the next but remain severely ill. Sensitivity, specificity, reliability, and validity are important considerations when selecting a rating scale. The sensitivity of a test refers to its ability to detect a symptom or illness, given that the symptom or illness is present. Specificity refers to a test's ability to determine that a symptom or illness is absent given that the person does not have the illness.

Rating scales are also available to measure adverse side effects. Global and specific assessments of adverse effects are a federal requirement in clinical drug trials. Also in clinical practice, medical professionals should report significant adverse medication reactions to the U.S. Food and Drug Administration (FDA) using MEDWatch.[16] Often, important adverse effects are realized only after a medication product has been prescribed to a large population in the postmarketing period. Specific adverse side-effect measures may be used for specific categories of medications. For example, patients treated with antipsychotic agents may be susceptible to extrapyramidal side effects (EPSs). Tardive dyskinesia is a potentially irreversable movement disorder (please refer to the Chap. 68) that requires close monitoring approximately every 3 to 6 months during treatment with antipsychotic agents.[17] Table 62–4 provides a summary of the most common rating scales used to assess and quantify the presence and severity of adverse effects.

Reliability is the extent to which the score on the scale reflects the hypothetical "true" score and how much interference occurs from outside influences.[18] Reliability is reported by the correlation coefficient, which represents a chance correlation (zero) or perfect correlation (one). Rating scales with correlation coefficients of less than 0.7 are usually considered unreliable for clinical studies. Interrater reliability—agreement in rating scores among clinicians—is important to achieve when multiple people rate the same patient or population. Interrater reliability is established by having all raters independently rate individual patients at the same time to determine the correlation of their scores. Other types of reliability include test-retest reliability (assesses the stability of the scale in producing the same results with repeated use) and internal consistency (degree to which

TABLE 62–4. Adverse Effects Measures[16,17]

Rating Scale	Type	Scoring	Comments
Systematic Assessment for Treatment Emergent Events—General Inquiry (SAFTEE-GI)	Structured interview and global assessment	Summary scores of a number of events, average severity and impairment	5–10 minutes to complete. Baseline and weekly evaluations. Easy to administer. The specific reported information may be more useful than an overall summary score
MEDWatch	Global assessment	No scoring involved	Minutes to complete. The one-page form requires a narrative description of the problem or adverse reaction.
Abnormal Involuntary Movement Scale (AIMS)	Tardive dyskinesia assessment	12-item 5-point severity scale. Items 1–4 orofacial movement; 5–7 extremity and truncal movement; 8–10 global severity; 11 and 12 problems with teeth or dentures (yes or no)	5–10 minutes to complete. Commonly used in most clinical settings for dyskinesia assessment. Requires training and clinical experience to make diagnosis. Diagnostic criteria: at least 3-months of antipsychotic treatment, Mild severity score (2) in two discrete areas or moderate severity (3) in one area (i.e., orofacial)
Dyskinesia Identification System: Condensed User Scale (DISCUS)	Tardive dyskinesia assessment	15-item 5-point severity scale. Items 1, 2 face; 3 eyes; 4, 5 oral; 6–9 lingual; 10, 11 head/neck/trunk; 12, 13 upper limb; 14, 15 lower limb	10–15 minutes to complete. More descriptive criteria for scoring severity than the AIMS. Scoring based on three dimensions: frequency, detectability and intensity. A flowchart is provided in the user's manual to assign an item score
Rating Scale for Extrapyramidal Side Effects (Simpson-Angus EPS Scale)	Drug-induced Parkinson's and dystonia assessments	10-item 5-point anchored severity scale. Mean score is obtained by adding all scores and dividing by 10. A mean score of 0.3 is the upper limit for no EPS	10 minutes to complete. Item domains include: gait, arm dropping, shoulder shaking, elbow rigidity, wrist rigidity, leg pendulousness, head dropping, glabella tap, tremor, and salivation. Requires training and practice to administer
Barnes Akathisia Rating Scale (BARS)	Drug-induced akathisia	4 items including three 4-point anchored severity scored items and a 5-point global rating score item. Total score of 12 possible	10 minutes to complete. Items 1–3 (objective akathisia, subjective awareness of restlessness, and subjective distress related to restlessness). Diagnostic criteria: requires both objective and subjective ratings of at least 1 in either two subjective items. Psuedoakathisia is suggested with a positive objective rating but no subjective score is noted

Adapted from Refs. 16 and 17.

items in the scale measure different aspects of the same condition without overlap).

Validity, in contrast, is the ability of a scale to measure what it was designed to measure. Content validity measures the extent to which the scale assesses appropriate aspects of the illness. Concurrent validity is a measure of the correlation of the rating scale with an external measure such as diagnosis or clinical change. Construct validity is the extent to which the test appears to measure symptom traits in contrast to measuring a more limited, specific symptom.

Psychiatric rating scales should not be confused with psychological tests such as neuropsychological and intellectual assessments and are best used as only one part of a comprehensive diagnostic plan. Tables 62–5, 62–6, and 62–7 describe commonly used patient-rated and clinician-rated scales for a variety of disease states.[19–24] In clinical research, a combination of clinician- and self-rated rating scales and diagnostic tests provides the most accurate measurement of drug efficacy and treatment outcome.

CONCLUSIONS

Patient assessment is the backbone from which a pharmaceutical care plan evolves. Problem identification and therapeutic monitoring cannot occur unless a thorough assessment is completed first. The initial assessment is also the basis for evaluating response to therapy throughout the course of treatment. Psychiatric assessment requires sensitivity and good listening skills on the part of the clinician because it is based primarily on a subjective interview and not objective tests. With careful data collection, pharmacists can make substantial contributions to care that improve patient outcomes.

TABLE 62–5. Schizophrenia Rating Scales

Rating Scale	Type	Scoring	Comments
Brief Psychiatric Rating Scale (BPRS)	Clinician rated	18 items, 7-point severity scale. Total ≥38 indicates moderate severity	The anchored BPRS provides descriptions of each severity rating to increase the interrater reliability The BPRS has four clusters of symptoms: thinking disturbance, anxious depression, withdrawal-retardation, and hostility-suspiciousness
Scale for Assessment of Negative Symptoms (SANS)	Clinician rated	30 items, 6-point severity scale: 0 = normal 5 = severe	Measures degree of affect, alogia, avolition, anhedonia, and attention
Schedule for Affective Disorders and Schizophrenia—Change version (SADS-C)	Clinician rated	29 items, 6-point scale and Global Assessment Scale. Subsets of items can be combinded to score specific affective symptoms	Structured interview to measure change in symptoms and assess anxiety, depression, manic features, and delusions or disorganization
Positive and Negative Syndrome Scale (PANSS)	Clinician rated	30 items, 7-point severity scale	Based on the 18-item Brief Psychiatric Rating Scale
Nurses Observations Scale for Inpatient Evaluation (NOSIE)	Observational	30 items, 4-point severity scale: 0 = never 1 = sometimes 2 = often 3 = usually 4 = always	Patients behavior is rated daily
Clinical Global Impression Scale (CGI)	Observational	Severity of illness, 7-point rating scale Global improvement, 7-point rating scale Efficacy index: 1–4 = marked improvement 5–8 = moderate improvement 9–12 = minimal improvement 13–16 = unchanged/worse	Observational rating scale to compare severity of illness compared to other similar patients and measures improvement from baseline. The efficacy index measures therapeutic effect and side effects to determine the score.

TABLE 62–6. Depression Rating Scales

Rating Scale	Type	Scoring	Comments
Hamiltion Psychiatric Rating Scale for Depression (HAM-D)	Clinician rated	17-item scale: ≤6 = normal mood 17–25 = mild depression >25 = severe depression	Used to screen patients for drug studies and to determine severity of symptoms and treatment outcome The standard to compare other depression rating scales
Montgomery-Asberg Depression Rating Scale (MADRS)	Clinician rated	10 items, 7-point scale. For each item: 0 = no symptoms 6 = severe symptoms	Differentiates between all the intermediate grades of depression Decreases bias in patients with other medical illness and increased somatization
Beck Depressive Inventory (BDI)	Patient rated	21-item scale: 0–9 = normal 10–15 = mild depression 16–19 = mild to moderate 20–29 = moderate to severe 30–63 = severe depression	The standard for self-rating scales and an objective measure of change in symptoms as a result of treatment
Zung Self-rating Depression Scale (SDS)	Patient rated	20 items, 4-point severity scale: <50 = normal 50–59 = minimal to mild 60–69 = moderate to marked ≥70 = severe depression	Severity rated by frequency of occurrence of symptoms. May not be as sensitive in measuring changes in severity of symptoms
Raskin's Mood Scales and Modified Mood Scales for Depression (RMS)	Patient rated	53-item scale	Measures the presence or absence of symptoms. Sensitive in measuring changes resulting from treatment

TABLE 62–7. Anxiety Rating Scales

Rating Scale	Type	Scoring	Comments
Hamilton Anxiety Scale (HAM-A, HAM-AS, or HAMRS)	Clinician rated	14 items, 5-point scale. Scores of ≥18–20 = moderate anxiety	Consists of subscales to measure somatic and psychic anxiety
Self-rating Anxiety Scale (SAS) (Zung)	Patient rated	20-item scale, 4-point intensity ratings	Correlates with the clinician-rated Anxiety Status Inventory (ASI); however, there is little information on the validity of either test
State-Trait Anxiety Inventory (STAI)	Patient rated	20-item state anxiety (A-state) and 20-item trait anxiety (A-trait) 4-point intensity ratings Total scores range from 20 to 80	A-trait scale reflects the patients general or baseline anxiety. A-state scale reflects the patients most current anxiety and measures changes in anxiety. The A-state score is sensitive to stress-induced testing
Sheehan Panic and Anticipatory Anxiety Scale (SPAAS)	Patient and clinician rated	3-part scale	Measures panic attacks, anticipatory anxiety, and limited symptom attacks. Patient and clinician rated
Yale-Brown Obsessive Compulsive Scale (YBOCS)	Clinician rated	Semistructured interview	Consists of several clusters of obsessions and compulsions. Used to assess change in treatment studies

REFERENCES

1. American Psychiatric Association. Diagnostic and Statistical Manual of Mental Disorders, 4th ed Text Revision (DSM-IV-TR). Washington, American Psychiatric Press, 2000.
2. Othemer E, Othmer SC. The Clinical Interview Using DSM-IV, Vol. 1: Fundamentals. Washington, American Psychiatric Press, 1994.
3. Fogel BS, Shellow R. Practice guideline for psychiatric evaluaiton of adults. In: McIntyre, JS, Charles SC, Zarin DA, eds. American Psychiatric Association Practice Guidelines for the Treatment of Psychaitric Disorders. Compendium 2000. Washington, American Psychiatric Association, 2000;5–26.
4. Schneider LS, Tariot Pierre N, Olin JT. Brief assessments of cognitive function. In: Manual of Rating Scales for the Assessment of Geriatric Mental Illnesses, Vol. 5. Wilmington, DE, Astra-Zeneca, 2000;19–21.
5. Salmon DP. Neuropsychiatric measures for cognitive disorders. In: Rush AJ, Pincus HA, First MB, et al., eds. Handbook of Psychiatric Measures, Vol. 21. Washington, American Psychiatric Association, 2000;417–455.
6. Strauss GD. The psychiatric interview, history and mental status examination. In: Kaplan HI, Sadock BJ, eds. Comprehensive Textbook of Psychiatry, Vol.1, 6th ed. Baltimore, Williams & Wilkins, 1995;521–531.
7. Rosse RB, Deutsch LH, Deutsch SI. Medical assessment and laboratory testing and psychiatry. In: Kaplan HI, Sadock BJ, eds. Comprehensive Textbook of Psychiatry, Vol. 1, 6th ed. Baltimore, Williams & Wilkins, 1995;601–619.
8. Sternberg DE. Testing for physical illness in psychiatric patients. J Clin Psychiatry 1986;47(Suppl 1):3–9.
9. Henderson DC, Caliero E, Gray C, et al. Clozapine, diabetes mellitus, weight gain and lipid abnormalities: A five-year naturalistic study. Am J Psychiatry 2000;157:975–81.
10. Morihisa JM, Rossr RB, Cross, CD, et al. Laboratory and other diagnostic tests in psychistry. In: Hales RE, Yudofsky SC, eds. Essentails of Clinical Psychiatry, 3d ed. Washington, American Psychiatric Press, 1999;119–146.
11. Carroll BJ. The informed use of the dexamethasone suppression test. J Clin Psychiatry 1986;47:10–12.
12. Bulter RW, Satz P. Personality assessment of adults and children. In: Kaplan HI, Sadock BJ, eds. Comprehensive Textbook of Psychiatry, Vol. 1, 6th ed. Baltimore, Williams & Wilkins, 1995;544–562.
13. Marder SR. Psychiatric rating scales. In: Kaplan HI, Sadock BJ, eds. Comprehensive Textbook of Psychiatry, Vol. 1, 6th ed. Baltimore, Williams & Wilkins, 1995;619–637.
14. Hamilton M. The assessment of anxiety states by rating. Br J Med Psychol 1959;32:50–55.
15. Guy W. ECDEU Assessment Manual for Psychopharmacology, rev. ed. DHWE Publication (ADM) 76-338. Washington, U.S. Government Printing Office, 1976;158–169.
16. Schooler NR, Chengappa KNR. Adverse effect measures. In: Rush AJ, Pincus HA, First MB, et al., eds. Handbook of Psychiatric Measures, Vol. 11. Washington, Americal Psychiatric Association, 2000;151–168.
17. Sprague RL, Kalachnik JE. Reliability, validity, and a total score cutoff for the dyskinesia identification system: Condensed user scale (DISCUS) with mentally ill and mentally retarded populations. Psychopharm Bull 1991;27:51–58.
18. Thompson C. Introduction. In: Thompson C, ed. The Instruments of Psychiatric Research. New York, Wiley, 1989;1–16.
19. Fankhauser MP, German ML. Understanding the use of behavioral rating scales in studies evaluating the efficacy of antianxiety and antidepressant drugs. Am J Hosp Pharm 1987;44:2087–2100.
20. Andreasen NC. The scale for assessment of negative symptoms (SANS): Conceptual and theoretical foundations. Br J Psychiatry 1989;155(Suppl 7):49–58.
21. Kay SR, Opler LA, Lindenmayer JP. The positive and negative syndrome scale (PANSS): Rationale and standardization. Br J Psychiatry 1989;155(Suppl 7):59–65.
22. Montgomery SA, Asberg M. A new depression scale designed to be sensitive to change. Br J Psychiatry 1979;134:382–389.
23. Sheehan DV. The Anxiety Disease. New York, Bantam, 1983:114–115.
24. Goodman WK, Price LH, Rasmussen SA, et al. The Yale-Brown Obsessive Compulsive Scale (Y-BOCS): II. Validity. Arch Gen Psychiatry 1989;46:1006–1011.

63

CHILDHOOD DISORDERS

Julie A. Dopheide and Karen A. Theesen

Treating children with psychotropic drugs requires a very different approach than treating adults. A child's neurologic, physiologic, and psychosocial status is undergoing constant changes throughout the developmental period. Age-related pharmacodynamic and pharmacokinetic differences can alter drug disposition and response. Well-defined diagnostic criteria guide drug selection[1]; however, frequent comorbid disorders present treatment challenges. In addition, children may not be able to verbalize symptom response or adverse effects of a medication. All factors considered, children generally are given psychotropic drugs to control a group of symptoms or behaviors in order to facilitate the child's learning and development.

The psychiatric assessment of a child requires obtaining information from the child, parents, caregivers, and teachers. The overall diagnostic impression is formed from psychiatric, social, neuropsychological, and educational evaluations. Before the initiation of psychotropic drugs, the child, family, and caregivers need to be familiar with the risks and benefits of both drug and nondrug therapies. In addition, an explanation of drug monitoring techniques and possible adverse effects, including those of drug withdrawal, should be presented. The risks associated with untreated illness and the possibly related issues of low self-esteem and impaired academic and social functioning also should be discussed.[2]

The past decade has brought greater acceptance of pharmacotherapeutic treatments for behavioral disorders in children. Psychotropic prescribing has increased significantly in all age groups. For example, from 1991 to 1995, the number of antidepressants prescribed to toddlers doubled, stimulant rates tripled, and clonidine prescriptions increased 28-fold.[3] Despite increased prescribing, suboptimal treatment of children with attention deficit-hyperactivity disorder (ADHD) and other psychiatric disorders is documented across several studies.[4,5] Clearly, a multimodal treatment approach (e.g., family therapy, behavioral therapy) that includes appropriate prescribing is associated with the best outcome.[2,6,7]

ATTENTION DEFICIT-HYPERACTIVITY DISORDER

CLINICAL PRESENTATION AND EPIDEMIOLOGY

The three essential features of ADHD are signs of developmentally inappropriate inattention, impulsivity, and hyperactivity. Inattention typically involves failing to finish tasks, not seeming to listen, being easily distracted, having difficulty concentrating on schoolwork, and having difficulty sticking to a play activity. Impulsivity often is manifested as acting before thinking, shifting excessively from one activity to another, difficulty in organizing work, needing much supervision, frequently calling out in class, and difficulty awaiting a turn in games or group situations. Hyperactivity generally includes excessive running about or climbing on things, difficulty sitting still or staying seated, and excessive movement during sleep. Symptom presence and severity vary with the situation. It is unusual for a child to display signs of the disorder in all settings or even in the same setting at all times.[1] The onset of ADHD is typically by the age of 3 years and must occur by age 7, although the disorder may not require professional attention until the child enters school. The National Institutes of Health (NIH) estimate the prevalence in school- age children to be 3% to 5%; however, community sample estimates average 2.9% for girls and 9.2% for boys.[6] Girls display more inattention and less hyperactive and impulsive symptomatology.[6,8] Symptoms may persist across the life cycle for both sexes, but hyperactivity usually does not present beyond middle childhood.[6,8]

It is critical to clarify the diagnosis of ADHD in individuals with these symptoms. Inattention and distractibility can be symptoms of an anxiety disorder, depression, or bipolar disorder.[2,6,8] In other cases, these anxiety or mood disorders can coexist with ADHD, just as learning deficiencies and conduct or oppositional disorders are common comorbid conditions.[2,8,9] The presence of multiple comorbid conditions, particularly conduct or oppositional disorder, may increase the likelihood of ADHD chronicity.[6,8] Overdiagnosis of ADHD and overprescribing of stimulants are considered problems in some communities, pointing to the need for careful documentation that functionally impairing symptoms are indeed attributed to ADHD.[10–12]

ETIOLOGY AND PATHOPHYSIOLOGY

ADHD is a clinical diagnosis with multiple heterogeneous causes.[2,6,8] Both genetic and nongenetic factors are involved. The child of a parent with ADHD has up to a 50% chance of developing ADHD; monozygotic twins have up to a 92% concordance rate for ADHD.[8,13,14] In addition, children with fetal alcohol syndrome, lead poisoning, and meningitis have a higher incidence of ADHD symptomatology.[2,6,8] Although not a primary cause, a positive association exists between adverse factors in the family (e.g., severe marital discord, low social class, large family size, paternal criminality, maternal mental disorder, foster care) and ADHD.[15] Dietary causes are unlikely.[2,6,8]

Although brain studies show no definitive pathophysiologic markers of ADHD, the prefrontal cortex and the basal ganglia are consistently reported as abnormal, typically smaller.[13,16] In addition, adults and some youths with ADHD display overexpression of the dopamine transporter gene (*DAT*) and altered dopamine$_4$ (D_4) receptor polymorphisms; implications of these findings are being studied.[17,18]

A prevailing pathophysiologic explanation for ADHD symptoms involves deficits in prefrontal cortex-mediated executive brain function also known as *response inhibition*. Children with ADHD are unable to "edit" their behavior, resist distractions, and develop an awareness of space and time.[13,18] In addition, a dysregulation of arousal in frontosubcortical pathways has been proposed. Children with ADHD display insufficient alertness during dull and repetitive tasks alternating with overarousal during exciting activities.[19] Effective treatments modulate dopamine (DA) and norepinephrine (NE) to improve executive functioning and regulate arousal for improved performance. The clinical response associated with stimulants is not paradoxical and is not diagnostic for ADHD because asymptomatic children also experience increased attention, decreased motor activity, and improvement on learning tasks when given stimulants.[2,8,20]

▶ TREATMENT: Attention Deficit-Hyperactivity Disorder

PHARMACOLOGIC THERAPY

Pharmacotherapy should be considered whenever a thorough diagnostic assessment indicates symptoms of ADHD and/or a comorbid condition that causes significant functional impairment. Several studies demonstrate superiority of stimulants compared with behavioral interventions in alleviating core symptoms of ADHD.[2,7,8] Stimulants have not been shown to improve social and academic functioning reliably; therefore, multimodal treatment, individualized to the specific needs of the child and family, is crucial for overall positive therapeutic outcome.[2] Multimodal treatment includes parent training, family therapy, classroom interventions, and contingency management (e.g., rewards for good behavior).[2,7,8] Figure 63–1 provides an algorithm for drug selection in the treatment of ADHD.

Stimulants (e.g., methylphenidate, mixed amphetamine salts, dextroamphetamine, pemoline) are the most effective drug treatment options, with efficacy ranging from 70% to 96% when a trial of each drug is given using wide dosage ranges.[2,6,8] Adderal, a combination of dextroamphetamine and D,L-amphetamine salts, is a longer-acting alternative to methylphenidate.[21] Caffeine has been found to be inferior in efficacy to dextroamphetamine, methylphenidate, and pemoline.[22] Pemoline is not considered to be a first-line therapy because of the risk of hepatic toxicities.

Despite knowledge of the effects of stimulants on neurotransmitter activity, how these drugs affect the primary symptoms of ADHD is unclear. The central nervous system (CNS) stimulants, in varying degrees, inhibit the reuptake of DA and NE, enhance release of DA and NE from the presynaptic neuron, or inhibit the enzyme monoamine oxidase (MAO). Because stimulants work through slightly different mechanisms, lack of response to one stimulant does not preclude response to another.[23]

Dosing of the stimulants should be titrated for maximum individual efficacy and minimum side effects. Although initiation and dosage titration procedures vary, the following scheme is based on published recommendations of experienced clinicians.[7,24] The initial dose is 2.5 mg dextroamphetamine or mixed amphetamine salts or 5.0 mg methylphenidate. Drug response is maximal during the absorption phase, is evident in 15 to 30 minutes, and lasts 2 to 6 hours. Future dosing increments should be 2.5 and 5 mg, respectively. The dosing schedule can be determined by observing when the loss of positive drug effect occurs during the 2 to 6 hours after an oral dose. Most patients require a two- or three-times-daily dosing schedule due to the short half-lives of these drugs (2 to 4 hours for methylphenidate and approximately 6 hours for dextroamphetamine). Controlled studies show substantial symptom reduction from the late afternoon dose with no untoward effects on sleep.[25,26] Single daily doses of Adderal may be as effective as multiple daily doses of methylphenidate in some children.[21,27]

Sustained-release products are reported to be either equally or less effective than short-acting products. The convenience of once-daily dosing must be weighed against the potential for difficulty falling asleep with sustained-release products.[23,28] Doses range from 0.3–1 mg/kg/day for methylphenidate. Maximum daily doses are 40 mg dextroamphetamine/mixed amphetamine salts (Adderal) and 60 mg methylphenidate.[8,21,22] A new extended-release preparation of

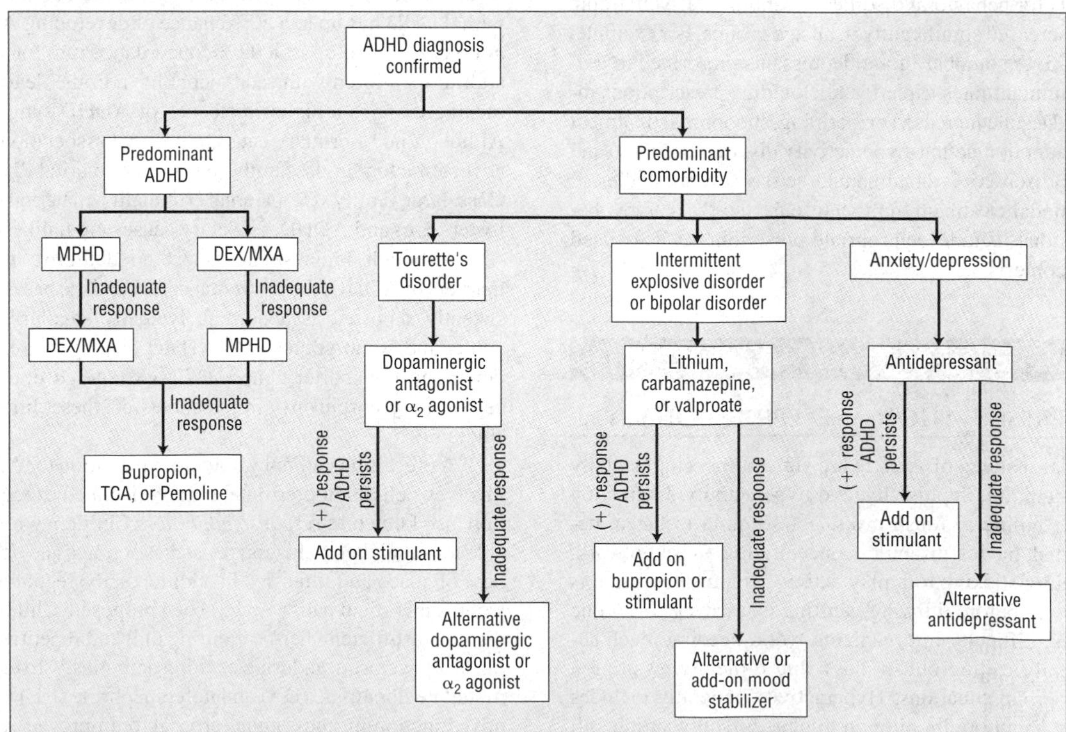

FIGURE 63–1. Algorithm for management of ADHD. Treat predominant disorder first, reassess, and consider alternative or "add on" medications for optimal symptom control. MPHD = methylphenidate; DEX = dextroamphetamine; MXA = mixed amphetamine salts; TCA = tricyclic antidepressant. *(Adapted from Refs. 2, 8, 22, 24, 27, and 51.)*

methylphenidate with the osmotic controlled-release delivery system (OROS technology, Concerta) is available in 18- and 36-mg tablets with recommendations for once-daily dosing up to a maximum of 54 mg/day.[29] Adults with ADHD also are responsive to methylphenidate using doses up to 1 mg/kg/day.[22,24]

The recommended starting dose of pemoline is 37.5 mg, with dosing increments ranging from 18.75–37.5 mg/day. Optimal benefit usually is achieved with 56.25–75 mg/day, and the maximum dose is 112.5 mg/day. Onset of therapeutic effect is 2 hours postdose.[24] A potential advantage of pemoline is a longer duration of action, allowing once-daily dosing. Pemoline displays wide interindividual variability in metabolism. The plasma half-life varies from 2 to 12 hours acutely and extends to 14 to 34 hours with chronic dosing. Pemoline may accumulate for weeks to months with chronic dosing.[30]

Imipramine and desipramine are the most systematically studied antidepressants (TCAs) in the treatment of ADHD, although nortriptyline is also effective.[8,24] The onset of TCA clinical response occurs within the first 2 weeks, and full response is achieved by week 3. The initial dose of TCA is 10 mg twice daily or 25 mg in the morning. Therapeutic doses of TCA are 1–5 mg/kg/day administered in divided doses.[8,24] Variability in dosage requirements may be due to the 10-fold interpatient variability in resulting drug plasma concentration achieved at a given dose. If tolerance seems to develop after months of therapy, a dosage adjustment may be necessary to compensate for age-related changes in distribution and metabolism.

TCAs and bupropion are second-line alternatives to the stimulants for treatment of ADHD. The potential benefits of TCAs in comparison with stimulants include a longer duration of action, less sleep disturbance, and reduced risk of abuse. Their negative aspects include decreased efficacy, more adverse effects, and the risk of death in overdose.[8,22,24] TCAs are also effective for adults with ADHD.[22,31]

Bupropion, a monocyclic antidepressant, is a DA and NE reuptake inhibitor with no significant direct effect on serotonin or MAO. Its active metabolites augment noradrenergic and dopaminergic function. Investigations with bupropion at doses of 3–6 mg/kg/day titrated over a 2-week period have demonstrated efficacy greater than placebo in a controlled trial[32] and efficacy comparable with methylphenidate ($n = 15$ children) in another controlled trial.[24,33] Advantages of bupropion include less toxicity compared with TCAs and less appetite suppression compared with stimulants. Bupropion also may be effective in adults at antidepressant doses.[22] The monoamine oxidase inhibitor (MAOI) tranylcypromine is effective but used infrequently due to the potential for dangerous drug and dietary interactions.[22] Serotonergic-specific reuptake inhibitors (SSRIs) are not effective for ADHD.[8,24]

Clonidine and guanfacine are less effective alternatives to stimulant monotherapy, but they are prescribed more frequently as adjuncts to control aggression or to improve sleep.[8,24,34] Clonidine and guanfacine, central α_2-adrenergic agonists, inhibit noradrenergic activity by decreasing the release of NE from the presynaptic neuron. Both reduce the firing rate within the locus ceruleus and decrease excessive arousal. Clonidine may be initiated at 0.05 mg at bedtime with slow upward titration to an average dose of between 0.15 and 0.3 mg/day.[22] Guanfacine may be initiated at 0.5 mg qhs with slow upward titration to a dose within 1–4 mg/day. Guanfacine has a longer elimination half-life (18 hours) compared with clonidine (2.5 hours).[35]

Lithium and anticonvulsants are used increasingly to control aggression and explosive behavior in patients with a diagnosis of ADHD. These patients actually may have childhood-onset bipolar disorder or combined ADHD-intermittent explosive disorder.[9,24] Lithium, valproate, and carbamazepine are effective for explosive behavior, aggression, and impulsivity, but they are not appropriate treatments for a child with the inattentive subtype of ADHD. Dosing starts in low divided doses with titration over 1 to 2 weeks to therapeutic response.[8,24,36]

Conventional antipsychotics improve symptoms of hyperactivity and impulsivity, but negative effects on learning and cognitive functioning as well as extrapyramidal side effects (e.g., dystonia and tardive dyskinesia) limit their usefulness.[22,24] The atypical antipsychotic risperidone has been used to control severe aggression in refractory cases of ADHD, but more studies are needed to clarify its place in therapy.[24]

Stimulants are considered first-line therapy in most cases of ADHD; however, comorbid conditions have an impact on the drug-selection process, calling for a careful, systematic approach. If multiple drugs are started simultaneously, it is impossible to determine the impact of each drug. The predominance of symptoms guides the drug-selection process (see Fig. 63–1). For example, if a child presents as severely anxious/depressed with associated attentional problems, then an antidepressant should be initiated first with monitoring to determine if attentional symptoms improve.[37] When a child presents with severe ADHD and associated anxiety/depression, a stimulant should be initiated to treat the more severe ADHD. If ADHD symptoms improve significantly but anxiety/depression persists, then an antidepressant can be added. Careful monitoring is needed to detect drug interactions leading to higher stimulant plasma levels and increased adverse effects.[24] Recent studies show that stimulants do not routinely make anxiety disorders worse, but they may not improve symptoms either.[8,24] In children with epilepsy, methylphenidate is effective; however, the child must be stabilized and seizure-free on an anticonvulsant prior to initiation of the stimulant.[38] Patients with seizure disorders should not receive bupropion.

PHARMACOECONOMIC CONSIDERATIONS

No cost-benefit studies on the treatment of ADHD have been published. Methylphenidate and dextroamphetamine appear to provide the most effective and economic therapy due to relatively low drug cost and monitoring requirements. The cost of Adderal is approximately twice that of dextroamphetamine, and Concerta is twice the cost of Adderal. Pemoline's acquisition cost is greater than that of Adderal and less than that of Concerta, but laboratory monitoring further increases overall costs. Imipramine, desipramine, clonidine, and mood stabilizers are relatively inexpensive, but ongoing electrocardiographic and blood-level monitoring and adverse events (if they occur) increase costs significantly.

EVALUATION OF THERAPEUTIC OUTCOMES

Careful documentation of baseline symptoms and complaints over a 1-month predrug period is essential to the evaluation of therapeutic and adverse outcomes. Baseline symptoms can be measured using videotapes, clinician rating scales, or both. In addition, height, weight, and eating and sleeping patterns should be recorded. After the initiation and titration of any drug treatment, it is necessary that parents, teachers, and clinicians assess the overall functioning of the child using objective rating scales to determine if significant therapeutic benefit justifies continuing medication.[23,24] Therapeutic effects of the stimulants include decreased motor activity and impulsivity and increased attention span. Improved cognitive performance may result from an overall improvement in attention and concentration and may not be a direct effect on cognition.[13,20] This suggests that stimulants are indicated for target behaviors and not for primary learning disorders.

The benefits of drug therapy must outweigh the adverse effects. Anorexia, insomnia, stomach aches, and headaches are frequent but usually mild with stimulant use in children. Anorexia and stomach aches can be minimized by giving the stimulant with or after meals. Insomnia, specifically a delay in onset of sleep, can be minimized by adjusting the dosing schedule and/or the child's bedtime.[23] Occasionally, insomnia persists, and dosage reduction is necessary. Methylphenidate typically is better tolerated with less adverse CNS reactions, including insomnia, when compared with dextroamphetamine.[39] The relative tolerability of mixed amphetamine salts requires study. Clonidine has been described as an effective treatment for insomnia, but cardiovascular adverse effects may limit acceptability.[24,34,40] Stimulant-induced headache, abdominal pain, and new onset or exacerbation of tics may require dosage reduction or drug discontinuation. Rare effects include hallucinations (visual or tactile) or delusions, which require dosage reduction or discontinuation. Heart rate and blood pressure may increase with stimulants, but the magnitude is rarely of clinical importance.[8,22]

Pemoline is not a first-line agent due to the risk of hepatic failure. Over 20 cases have been reported to the Food and Drug Administration (FDA), with severity of outcomes ranging from full recovery to liver transplantation or death.[24,41–43] Although not predictive of the onset of liver disease, routine liver function tests are recommended every 3 to 6 months or as clinical symptoms (i.e., fatigue, nausea, vomiting, anorexia) warrant during pemoline therapy. Hepatotoxicity is less likely in children older than age 10 on pemoline only.[24]

Growth delay is a possibility with stimulant use, but studies in children indicate that effects are temporary, with normalization in height and weight occurring through midadolescence.[2,8] Proposed mechanisms include alterations in growth hormone secretion and suppression of appetite leading to reduced calorie intake. Heights and weights should be assessed every 3 months for all patients receiving stimulants. Some evidence exists attributing maturational delays to ADHD itself.[44]

A more controversial aspect of stimulant use concerns drug holidays and duration of treatment. Drug holidays are important because they provide time to reassess treatment. All children should be given a drug-free trial every year. Consideration must be given to the risks of negative effects on learning, socialization, and self-image while off of stimulant in determining the frequency and duration of drug holidays. Drug dosage often varies from year to year, largely due to age-related pharmacokinetic changes. As a child develops, hepatic metabolism slows and volume of distribution increases.

The impact of ADHD and its treatment on the development of substance abuse has been investigated in epidemiologic studies. A diagnosis of ADHD confers a greater risk of adolescent and adult substance abuse.[45] The risk is greater if conduct disorder, antisocial personality, or bipolar disorder coexists.[8,46] There is no evidence linking therapy with CNS stimulants for ADHD with substance abuse disorders, and effective treatment may facilitate functioning and participation in substance abuse recovery.[45,47] Nevertheless, practitioners need to pay attention to the presence of an active substance abuse disorder in weighing the risk versus benefit of treatment with stimulants. Alternative therapies may be more appropriate.

TCAs are effective for control of impulsivity and hyperactivity, but they are not as effective as stimulants in increasing attention.[22,23] Parents should provide doses of TCAs throughout the week and not just during school days. TCA withdrawal effects are common in children and include nausea, vomiting, and diarrhea.

Common adverse effects of TCAs in children are similar to those seen in adults and include sedation and anticholinergic and cardiovascular effects. Toxic effects include the potential for various arrhythmias and first-degree heart block.[8,24] The effects of TCAs on the electrocardiogram should be monitored carefully. Of more concern are reports of sudden death in seven children taking desipramine. Children and adolescents given TCAs should have pretreatment and follow-up electrocardiograms to assess the effects of TCA therapy on cardiac rate and rhythm.[23,24] Possible CNS effects include dizziness, aggressiveness, excitement, nightmares, insomnia, forgetfulness, and irritability. Signs of CNS toxicity are confusion, impaired concentration, hallucinations, and delusions.

Bupropion's adverse effects include nausea, which may resolve over time or with slower dosage titration, and rash, which may require discontinuation of therapy if severe. Bupropion is associated with exacerbation of tics and therefore should be used with caution in individuals with tics or a family history of tics.[48]

The most common side effect of clonidine is dose-dependent sedation that usually subsides after 2 to 3 weeks of therapy.[22,24] Of concern are reports of bradycardia, rebound hypertension, heart block, and sudden death.[24,40] Four children have died on the combination of methylphenidate and clonidine; however, complicating factors make it impossible to link the drug combination directly with the cause of death.[24] Concurrent clonidine and stimulant administration, as well as missed doses of clonidine, adds to the risk of adverse cardiovascular events. When clonidine therapy is warranted due to past positive response or treatment resistance, careful clinical monitoring for fatigue, dizziness, and autonomic changes (e.g., blood pressure, pulse) is recommended.[24] The American Heart Association has stated that electrocardiographic monitoring is not required for clonidine treatment in children, although many clinicians continue to assess for electrocardiogram changes. Similar adverse-effect monitoring is necessary with guanfacine, although its α_{2a} selectivity may result in less sedation and hypotension than clonidine.[49] When discontinuing treatment, clonidine and guanfacine should be withdrawn slowly (0.05 mg clonidine/0.5 mg guanfacine every 3 days) to prevent rebound hypertension or behavioral dyscontrol.[40]

CONCLUSIONS

At this time, the best drug therapy for ADHD is either methylphenidate, mixed amphetamine salts, or dextroamphetamine. Bupropion and TCAs are good options for those unresponsive to or unable to tolerate stimulants. Clonidine and guanfacine are third-line options that require careful cardiovascular monitoring. Mood stabilizers (e.g., lithium, divalproex, and carbamazepine) are adjuncts for control of aggression or comorbid bipolar disorder). Other agents require further investigation before their status in the treatment of ADHD can be fully determined.

TOURETTE'S DISORDER

EPIDEMIOLOGY AND CLINICAL PRESENTATION

Once considered rare, Tourette's disorder is present in approximately 1% of boys and 0.4% of girls.[50,51] The essential features of this CNS disorder are multiple motor tics and one or more vocalizations. A tic is a sudden, rapid, recurrent, nonrhythmic, stereotyped motor movement or vocalization. Motor tics include eye blinking, facial twitching, lip licking, shoulder shrugging, moving hair out of eyes, and coughing. Vocal tics include throat clearing, hissing, barking, snorting, echolalia, and coprolalia.[1] Tics may be suppressed voluntarily for minutes to hours. The clinical presentation may vary from being just noticeable to debilitating, and the type of tic expressed may change over time.[51,52]

Presence of both motor and vocal tics is necessary for more than 1 year before the diagnosis of Tourette's disorder is made. The median age of onset of motor tics is 7 years, with most patients having the onset of symptoms before age 14. Transient tic disorder is diagnosed if motor or vocal tics occur for less than 1 year. If either motor or vocal tics are present for longer than 1 year, chronic motor or vocal tic disorder is diagnosed.[1]

Tics are most prominent during childhood, with some plateau and attenuation of symptoms during adolescence. The early twenties frequently bring stabilization of symptoms, although exacerbations occur during adulthood with characteristic waxing and waning or fluctuating symptom severity.[51]

Over 90% of children with Tourette's disorder have coexisting conditions such as ADHD (75%), mood disorders (60%), obsessive-compulsive disorder (40%), other anxiety disorders, or a combination of comorbidities.[53] Tourette's disorder itself does not cause diminished intellectual functioning; however, the severity of tics and associated illnesses can result in significant functional impairment sometimes requiring hospitalization.[51,53]

ETIOLOGY AND PATHOPHYSIOLOGY

Tourette's disorder is transmitted in a complex polygenic pattern, whereas symptoms and severity of the disorder vary from one generation to another.[51,54] The neurochemical pathophysiology involves an imbalance in the interaction of dopaminergic, serotonergic, and noradrenergic systems in multiple brain regions. The imbalance may cause a lack of regulation of the brain's inhibitory mechanisms, resulting in tics and associated behavior disorders. This multisystem etiology best explains the success of a variety of treatment options.[51,55]

▶ TREATMENT: Tourette's Disorder

PHARMACOLOGIC THERAPY

Whenever symptoms are severe enough to impair the child's ability to function, drug therapy should be initiated. Haloperidol and pimozide (D_2 receptor antagonists) are approved by the FDA and highly effective with a relatively rapid onset. Clonidine is significantly less effective but has no risk of extrapyramidal side effects. Psychotherapy and behavioral treatment are useful adjuncts.

Therapy with haloperidol or pimozide should be initiated at very low doses of 0.25–0.5 mg/day given at bedtime and then increased gradually. Gradual titration over 2 to 3 weeks helps minimize extrapyramidal and sedative effects while permitting careful assessment of response. Symptoms may regress within 48 to 72 hours after an effective dose is reached. Doses less than 5 mg/day are effective in controlling tics for most patients, but occasionally doses approaching 10 mg/d are required.[51,56] Pimozide is considered comparable or possibly superior to haloperidol in efficacy when equivalent doses are used.[56]

Risperidone, a 5-HT_2/D_2 receptor antagonist, was effective in 58% of children and adults in an open trial at an average dose of 2.7 mg/day titrated from a starting dose of 0.5 mg once or twice daily.[57] Ziprasidone, another 5-HT_2/D_2 antagonist, showed significant efficacy versus placebo in a controlled study at an average dose of 30 mg/day titrated from a starting dose of 5 mg/day. One case report describes partial control of tics with olanzapine.[55] Clozapine, a 5-HT_2 antagonist with minimal D_1-blocking and no significant D_2-blocking effects, was found to be ineffective with worsening of symptoms in some Tourette's patients.[51,55]

Clonidine is prescribed widely for the treatment of Tourette's disorder, but its efficacy is not well established.[51,55] In some patients, the response is limited to attentional and behavioral problems with no changes in the frequency of tics. A clonidine trial should be initiated carefully, usually 0.025–0.05 mg given in the morning with gradual titration every 4 to 7 days to the usual therapeutic trial dose of 0.15–0.25 mg/day (maximum 0.5 mg/day).[51,55] Doses usually are divided during maintenance therapy for more continuous symptom control and to minimize adverse effects. The onset of therapeutic effects is slow, ranging from 2 weeks to a few months. Although the clonidine patch is not well studied, Comings and associates recommend it over oral dosage forms. The starting dose is one-fourth of a 0.1-mg transdermal patch applied every 4 to 7 days and gradually increased over weeks to months as needed.[58]

COMORBIDITY AND ALTERNATIVES

Pharmacotherapy of Tourette's disorder is challenging due to multiple coexisting disorders typically requiring medication combinations. Often the behavioral problems precede and are more disturbing than the involuntary movements, making them a treatment priority.

TOURETTE'S AND ADHD

Pharmacotherapy with stimulants increases dopaminergic and noradrenergic activity, which has the potential to aggravate or precipitate tics. One study examined the comparative effects of methylphenidate and dextroamphetamine on tics in children and found the majority experienced improvement in ADHD symptoms with acceptable effects on tics.[59] Methylphenidate was better tolerated than dextroamphetamine. This study confirms previous reports of methylphenidate efficacy and superior tolerability compared with other stimulants in treating attentional disorders in patients with comorbid Tourette's and ADHD.[60] Patients and caregivers should be aware of the risks of using stimulants in children with Tourette's disorder. Careful monitoring is essential, and worsening of tics is reversible once the stimulant is discontinued.[22,51]

Reports of TCA therapy for comorbid ADHD and tics show significant improvement in attention without worsening of tics.[22] TCAs may be preferred to clonidine. A controlled trial in children aged 7 to 13 years with Tourette's disorder and ADHD found that desipramine 100 mg/day was superior to clonidine 0.2 mg/day in improving attention. Neither desipramine nor clonidine demonstrated efficacy for tics or caused worsening of tics.[61]

Clonidine is a less effective alternative to stimulants in the treatment of children with Tourette's disorder and ADHD (see ADHD section for dosing). Guanfacine, a central α_{2a}-selective noradrenergic receptor agonist, was administered to 10 children with ADHD and Tourette's disorder over a 4- to 20-week open trial at a dose of 1.5 mg/day. Significant decreases in motor and phonic tics as well as improvements in attention were noted, with side effects reported as transient sedation and headache.[49] Due to its similarity to clonidine, guanfacine's cardiovascular effects warrant careful clinical monitoring.[8,22,24]

Nicotine administration by gum or patch may potentiate the effects of dopamine-blocking agents in relieving tics, according to small open trials and case reports.[62] ADHD symptoms may improve as well.[63] The adverse effects of nicotine on overall health may limit usefulness, and further investigations are needed.

TOURETTE'S AND ANXIETY/MOOD DISORDERS

Therapeutic trials (6–8 weeks) of fluoxetine, fluvoxamine, sertraline, paroxetine, or clomipramine should be tried when obsessive-compulsive, anxiety, or depressive symptoms cause functional impairment in patients with Tourette's disorder.[51,53,64] Careful monitoring for behavioral activation, disinhibition, and motor restlessness is essential during therapy because these symptoms occur in 20% to 40% of children and may require drug discontinuation.[64]

PHARMACOECONOMIC CONSIDERATIONS

No pharmacoeconomic studies have been published on Tourette's disorder. Haloperidol provides the most economic therapy due to high efficacy and low drug cost. Pimozide is more expensive than generic haloperidol. Although generic clonidine is inexpensive, delayed onset of effect and significantly lower efficacy substantially increase total costs of treatment. The clonidine patch (Catapres TTS) is approximately ten times the cost of generic clonidine tablets on a weekly basis. 5-HT_2/D_2 antagonists such as risperidone are expensive alternatives due to high medication costs.

EVALUATION OF THERAPEUTIC OUTCOMES

Once a drug is selected, Comings' general principles for pharmacologic management of patients with Tourette's disorder are useful.[52]

1. Tourette's disorder patients are very sensitive to medication. Low doses should be started, with gradual (weekly) increases as tolerated.
2. A plateau effect is normal. At first, tics may remit at a very low dose. However, as the body adjusts to this state, tics may return slowly, requiring upward adjustments after 2 to 4 weeks.
3. The treatment goal is not necessarily total elimination of all tics.
4. If tics disappear for a number of weeks, the dose can be decreased.
5. Medication should not be stopped abruptly. Withdrawal effects can be intolerable.[52]

Medication does not impair neuropsychological performance according to one controlled study; however, assessment of individual risk versus benefit is necessary.[65] The use of regular videotaped assessments in conjunction with a standardized rating scale (Yale Global Tic Severity Scale) is helpful in objectively evaluating symptoms and side effects.[55] Adult patients with Tourette's disorder still may be responsive to drug treatments that were effective during childhood, although the dose and schedule may require adjustment.[51]

Typical antipsychotic side effects have been reported with haloperidol doses of 2 mg/day or greater. In one review of 24 patients treated with haloperidol for Tourette's disorder, 66.7% discontinued treatment due to intolerable side effects (e.g., dysphoria, akathisia, nervousness, sedation, dystonia, and cognitive dulling or feeling drugged).[62] Lowering the dose may alleviate side effects. An antiparkinsonian agent such as benztropine (at a starting dose of 0.5 mg orally twice daily) generally will reverse extrapyramidal side effects. Whether a patient with Tourette's disorder is developing a new symptom or is developing tardive dyskinesia can be difficult to determine. Dosage titration of the medication and careful monitoring will assist in this clinical decision-making process.

Pimozide is less likely to cause extrapyramidal side effects than haloperidol. Anticholinergic side effects may occur in addition to drowsiness and, occasionally, anxiety. Electrocardiographic changes, including T- and U-wave abnormalities and prolongation of the QT (corrected) interval, are found rarely in recommended therapeutic doses for Tourette's disorder; however, patients given pimozide should receive baseline and follow-up electrocardiograms.[51,52,56]

Adverse effects reported during clinical studies with risperidone include light-headedness, sedation, akathisia or agitation, weakness, insomnia, depressed mood, aggressive behavior, weight gain, and extrapyramidal effects including tardive dyskinesia.[57,67] Eighteen cases of risperidone-associated liver abnormalites have been reported to the FDA in children aged 8 to 18 years; therefore, liver function monitoring every 3 months or when clinical signs and symptoms warrant (e.g., weakness, fatigue, nausea, jaundice) is recommended.[68]

For clonidine and guanfacine, the most common adverse effect is sedation. Fortunately, tolerance usually develops to this effect over days to weeks. The most potentially serious side effects are cardiovascular (see the ADHD section earlier in the chapter).[40] Other clonidine side effects include dry mouth, headache, mood changes, and even a temporary worsening of tics in 10% of patients. The clonidine patch also may cause skin irritation, which can be minimized by changing the location of the patch every few days or pretreating the skin with beclomethasone dipropionate aerosolized spray.[58]

Drugs that inhibit cytochrome P450 isoenzyme 3A4 (e.g., macrolide antibiotics, some antidepressants) should not be combined with pimozide due to the risk of excessive pimozide blood levels and lethal QT (corrected) prolongation.[70] Antidepressants that inhibit cytochrome P450 isoenzymes can increase levels of dopamine-blocking drugs, leading to intolerable extrapyramidal side effects in some patients.

CONCLUSIONS

Pimozide and haloperidol have the advantage of greatest efficacy and rapid onset in the treatment of Tourette's disorder. Risperidone and ziprasidone show promise; however, comparison studies with haloperidol and pimozide are needed to determine their relative safety and efficacy. Clonidine and guanfacine have the advantage of no extrapyramidal side effects, but they are significantly less effective and require ongoing cardiovascular monitoring. Drug treatment must be highly individualized, considering comorbid disorders, side-effect sensitivity, and drug interactions.

ENURESIS

ETIOLOGY, PATHOPHYSIOLOGY, AND CLINICAL PRESENTATION

The essential feature of enuresis is repeated involuntary or intentional voiding of urine by day or night that is not caused by any physical disorder. Rare physical causes of enuresis (e.g., diabetes mellitus, diabetes insipidus, seizure disorders, or urinary tract infections) should be ruled out. Diagnostic criteria for enuresis include the repeated voiding of urine that is characterized by either a frequency of at least twice per week for at least 3 months or the presence of clinically significant distress or impairment in social, academic, or other important areas of functioning. The child must be at least 5 years of age.[1] Enuresis may be primary or secondary. Primary enuresis, the most common type, is diagnosed if the child has never established urinary continence. Secondary enuresis follows an established period (3–6 months) of urinary continence.

At age 5, prevalence is 15% to 20%; at age 10, it is 5%; for adolescents, it is 2% to 3%, and 0.5% to 1% of adults wet the bed at least once a month. The ratio of males to females with enuresis is 3:2.[71,72] Factors that predispose a child to either type of enuresis include a positive family history, reduced functional bladder capacity,[73] delayed or lax toilet training, constipation,[74] psychological factors, and developmental delay.[75] Some children with nocturnal enuresis lack the normal circadian variation in urine excretion rate, urine osmolality, and antidiuretic hormone (ADH) secretion. Nocturnal enuresis is not associated with a particular sleep stage, although children with enuresis are more difficult to arouse.[71,75,76]

▶ TREATMENT: Enuresis

The first step in treating the child with enuresis is to educate the family about the high frequency of the problem, dispel any misconceptions, provide emotional support, and strongly discourage punishment. For younger children who have not been toilet trained properly, the conditioning technique of dry bed training should be tried first. This technique encourages extra fluids during the day and restricts fluids close to bedtime. Children are encouraged to use the toilet before bedtime. If this method is unsuccessful, then a bed-wetting alarm can be used. Teaching continence skills and various behavioral and conditioning methods remain the primary treatments for enuresis, and drug treatment remains a secondary approach.[71,77,78] Combined treatment with an enuresis alarm and desmopressin can be particularly successful for severe enuresis.[79]

PHARMACOLOGIC THERAPY

Desmopressin acetate, a synthetic analog of the natural human ADH arginine vasopressin is available currently in a nasal spray and oral tablet for the treatment of nocturnal enuresis. Desmopressin raises overnight urinary osmotic concentration by increasing water reabsorption and reducing the volume of urine entering the bladder.[76,80] For children 6 years of age and older, the initial recommended nasal dose is 20 μg at bedtime, increasing to 40 μg at bedtime after 3 days if there is no response. Some patients may respond to as little as 10 μg. One-half of each dose is administered in each nostril. About 10% of the dose of desmopressin is absorbed from the nasal mucosa, and plasma concentrations reach a maximum about 45 minutes after administration. Less than 1% of oral desmopressin is absorbed, with effective dosages ranging from 200–400 μg/day.[80–83] The 400-μg dose provides greater efficacy with comparable tolerability.[77,80] Biologic half-life is 4 to 6 hours, and the duration of action varies from 6 to 24 hours.[80]

The exact mechanism of action of TCAs in treating enuresis is unknown; proposed mechanisms include an anticholinergic effect, an α-adrenergic agonist effect, and an increase in ADH.[76] Imipramine is the most studied TCA, although desipramine, amitriptyline, and nortriptyline are also effective. For children 6 years of age and older, the initial dose of imipramine should be 25 mg at bedtime, with weekly increases of 25 mg if necessary. A nightly dose greater than 75 mg is rarely necessary, although doses up to 150 mg have been required in teenagers.[84,85]

PHARMACOECONOMIC CONSIDERATIONS

No pharmacoeconomic studies on enuresis are available. The use of a bed-wetting alarm provides the highest overall cure rate, and drugs are a secondary approach. However, insurance companies commonly reimburse drug therapy, whereas they do not for alarms. The most inexpensive drug therapy is low-dose TCAs. Higher doses require more extensive monitoring of plasma levels and electrocardiograms, which increases overall cost. Therapy with desmopressin is substantially more expensive than with TCAs.

EVALUATION OF THERAPEUTIC OUTCOMES

Before treatment begins, an accurate baseline of bed-wetting frequency must be established. It usually takes 3 to 4 months of using a bed-wetting alarm, but more than 70% of the children are cured using this method.[82] Drug treatment is necessary when nondrug methods fail. Unfortunately, therapeutic efficacy does not extend beyond drug administration.[77,81,84,87–89] If drug treatment is required for more than several weeks, attempts to discontinue the drug every 3 to 6 months are advisable to assess for spontaneous remission. Slow tapering of the medication may decrease the frequency of relapse.[90]

Desmopressin is effective in reducing the number of wet nights in 70% of children. In a short-term (2 week) controlled study, 24.5% of adolescents/adults became completely dry,[87] whereas in a naturalistic 6-week trial, 22% of children became completely dry.[91] Predictors of best response to desmopressin include older age (>9 years), fewer initial wet nights, and larger bladder capacity.[86,92] Patients with colds or allergies that affect the nasal mucosa may have a less than optimal response to desmopressin nasal spray. Infrequent adverse effects of the spray include nasal irritation, epistaxis, rhinitis, and nasal congestion, whereas tablet or spray may cause transient headache, chills, dizziness, nausea, and abdominal pain. Rare effects of water intoxication, hyponatremia, and subsequent tonic-clonic seizures have been reported,[93] particularly in children with concurrent physical disorders, intentional overdoses, or excessive fluid intake. When desmopressin is administered, evening fluid should be limited to 8 ounces to prevent hyponatremia or water intoxication.[81,94,95]

TCA efficacy often is immediate and usually is evident within 7 days. Drug plasma concentrations of imipramine plus desipramine correlate with clinical response, and although individual variation exists, a higher percentage of patients responds to higher plasma levels (>116 ng/mL). In addition, true nonresponders exist at therapeutic doses and plasma levels.[84] Imipramine significantly increases the number of dry nights for 70% to 80% of children with enuresis.[84] An initially effective dose often becomes ineffective in 2 to 6 weeks, but increasing the dose usually reestablishes control. One week is needed to evaluate the efficacy of a new dose. Refer to the ADHD section and the TCAs for monitoring parameters and adverse effects.

CONCLUSIONS

Overall, both desmopressin and TCAs are effective in the treatment of nocturnal enuresis so long as the drug is maintained. Drug selection is based on adverse-effect profiles, ease of administration, and cost. Imipramine has a higher incidence of adverse effects than desmopressin, and the risk of accidental overdose is of concern, especially in very disorganized families. In contrast, desmopressin is markedly more expensive than imipramine.

▶ PRINCIPLES OF PHARMACOTHERAPY

- Careful documentation of baseline symptoms and complaints over a 1-month predrug period is essential to the evaluation of therapeutics and adverse outcomes in ADHD.
- Stimulants are the most effective treatment for ADHD.
- Symptoms of inattention and impulse control can continue in adolescence and adulthood and may require continued treatment.
- Disorders comorbid with ADHD have an impact on drug selection. For a child with ADHD and major depression or an anxiety disorder, an antidepressant may be needed adjunctively. Bupropion should be avoided in patients with seizure disorder.
- Tourette's disorder presents with both motor and vocal tics, which are present during childhood, plateau during adolescence, and may remit during adulthood with a characteristic fluctuating course.
- The decision to medicate for Tourette's disorder is based on the degree of concern perceived by the patient, symptom severity, and comorbid disorders.
- Individuals with Tourette's disorder are particularly sensitive to medication side effects, so medication dosing must be individualized carefully, and close monitoring is essential.
- Nondrug approaches to enuresis management, such as dry-bed training using moisture-sensitive alarms, are preferred because of higher cure rates and avoidance of drug side effects.
- Desmopressin is effective orally and intranasally for enuresis, but it is expensive and works better in older than younger children.
- Imipramine is effective in enuresis at wide dosage ranges. It has rapid onset, but side effects may be problematic for some patients.

REFERENCES

1. American Psychiatric Association. Diagnostic and Statistical Manual of Mental Disorders, 4th ed. (DSM-IV). Washington, American Psychiatric Press, 1994:37–121.
2. NIH Consensus Development Conference Statement on the Diagnosis and treatment of ADHD. J Am Acad Child Adolesc Psychiatry 2000; 39(2):182–193.
3. Zito JM, Safer DJ, dosReis S, et al. Trends in the prescribing of psychotropic medications to preschoolers. JAMA 2000;283:1025–1030.
4. Jensen PS, Kettle L, Roper MS, et al. Psychoactive medication prescribing practices for U.S. children: Gaps between research and clinical practice. J Am Acad Child Adolesc Psychiatry 1999;38(5):557–565.
5. Hoagwood K, Kelleher KJ, Feil M, et al. Treatment services for children with ADHD: A national perspective. J Am Acad Child Adolesc Psychiatry 2000;39(2):198–206.
6. American Academy of Pediatrics. Clinical practice guideline: Diagnosis and evaluation of the child with attention-deficit/hyperactivity disorder. Pediatrics 2000;105(5):1158–1170.
7. MTA Cooperative Group. A 14-month randomized clinical trial of strategies for attention-deficit/hyperactivity disorder. Arch Gen Psychiatry 1999;56:1073–1086.
8. Goldman LS, Genel M, Bezman RJ, et al. Diagnosis and treatment of attention-deficit/hyperactivity disorder in children and adolescents. JAMA 1998;279(14):1100–1107.
9. Sachs GS, Baldassano CF, Truman CJ et al. Comorbidity of attention deficit hyperactivity disorder with early and late onset bipolar disorder. Am J Psychiatry 2000;157:466–468.
10. LeFever GB, Dawson KV, Morrow AL. The extent of drug therapy for attention deficit-hyperactivity disorder among children in public schools. Am J Public Health. 1999;89(9):1359–1364.
11. Angold A, Alaattin E, Egger HL, et al. Stimulant treatment for children: a community perspective. J Am Acad Child Adolesc Psychiatry 2000;39(8):975–984.
12. Mota VL, Schachar RJ. Reformulating attention-deficit/hyperactivity disorder according to signal detection theory. J Am Acad Child Adolesc Psychiatry 2000;39(9):1144–1151.
13. Barkley, RA. Attention-deficit hyperactivity disorder. Sci Am 1998;279: 66–71.
14. Stage MW, Lombroso PJ, Pauls DL, et al. The genetics of childhood psychiatric disorders: A decade of progress. J Am Acad Child Adolesc Psychiatry 2000;39(8):946–962.
15. Biederman J. Family-environment risk factors for attention-deficit hyperactivity disorder. Arch Gen Psychiatry 1995;52:464–470.

16. Hendren RL, De Backer I, Pandina GJ. Review of neuroimaging studies of child and adolescent psychiatric disorders from the past 10 years. J Am Acad Child Adolesc Psychiatry 2000;39(7):815–828.
17. Dougherty, DD, Bonab AA, Spencer TJ, et al. Dopamine transporter density in patients with attention deficit-hyperactivity disorder. Lancet 1999;354:2132–2133.
18. Arnsten AFT. Genetics of childhood disorders: XVIII. ADHD: 2. Norepinephrine has a critical modulatory influence on prefrontal cortical function. J Am Acad Child Adolesc Psychiatry 2000;39(9):1201–1203.
19. Biederman J, Spencer T. Attention-deficit/hyperactivity disorder (ADHD) as a noradrenergic disorder. Biol Psychiatry 1999;46(9):1234–1242.
20. Pliszka SR, McCracken JT, Maas JW. Catecholamines in attention-deficit hyperactivity disorder: Current perspectives. J Am Acad Child Adolesc Psychiatry 1996;35:264–272.
21. Pliszka SR, Browne RG, Olvera RL, et al. A double-blind, placebo-controlled study of Adderall and methylphenidate in the treatment of ADHD. J Am Acad Child Adolesc Psychiatry 2000;39(5):619–626.
22. Spencer T, Biederman J, Wilens T. Pharmacotherapy of attention deficit hyperactivity disorder across the life cycle. J Am Acad Child Adolesc Psychiatry 1996;35:409–432.
23. Theesen K. The Handbook of Psychiatric Drug Therapy for Children and Adolescents. Binghamton, NY, Haworth, 1995:1–39.
24. Pliszka SR, Greenhill LL, Crismon ML, et al. The Texas medication algorithm project: Report of the Texas consensus conference panel on medication treatment of childhood attention-deficit/hyperactivity disorder, parts 1 and 2. J Am Acad Child Adolesc Psychiatry 2000;39(7):908–927.
25. Greenhill LL, Abikoff HB, Arnord E, et al. Medication treatment strategies in the MTA study: Relevance to clinicians and researchers. J Am Acad Child Adolesc Psychiatry 1996;35:1304–1313.
26. Kent JD, Blader JC, Koplewicz HS, et al. Effects of late-afternoon methylphenidate administration on behavior and sleep in attention-deficit hyperactivity disorder. Pediatrics 1995;96:320–325.
27. Manos MJ, Short EJ, Findling RL. Differential effectiveness of methylphenidate and Adderall in school-age youths with attention-deficit/hyperactivity disorder. J Am Acad Child Adolesc Psychiatry 1999;38(7):813–819.
28. Pelham WE, Greenslade KE, Vodde-Hamilton M, et al. Relative efficacy of long-acting stimulants on children with ADHD: A comparison of standard methylphenidate, sustained-release methylphenidate, sustained-release dextroamphetamine, and pemoline. Pediatrics 1990;86:226–237.
29. Modi NB, Lindemulder B, Gupta SK. Single- and multiple-dose pharmacokinetics of an oral once-a-day osmotic controlled-release OROS (methylphenidate HCL) formulation. J Clin Pharmacol 2000;40(4):379–88.
30. Sallee F, Stiller R, Perel J, Bates T. Oral pemoline kinetics in hyperactive children. Clin Pharmacol Ther 1985;37:606–609.
31. Wilens TE, Biederman J, Prince J, et al. Six-week, double-blind, placebo-controlled study of desipramine for adult attention deficit hyperactivity disorder. Am J Psychiatry 1996;153:1147–1153.
32. Conners CK, Casat CD, Gualtieri CT, et al. Bupropion hydrochloride in attention deficit disorder with hyperactivity. J Am Acad Child Adolesc Psychiatry 1996;34:1314–1321.
33. Barrickman LL, Perry PJ, Allen AJ, et al. Bupropion versus methylphenidate in the treatment of attention-deficit hyperactivity disorder. J Am Acad Child Adolesc Psychiatry 1995;34:649–657.
34. Prince JB, Wilens TE, Biederman J, et al. Clonidine for sleep disturbances associated with attention-deficit hyperactivity disorder. A systematic chart review of 62 cases. J Am Acad Child Adolesc Psychiatry 1996;35:599–605.
35. Hunt RD, Arnsten AFT, Asbell MD. An open trial of guanfacine in the treatment of attention-deficit hyperactivity disorder. J Am Acad Child Adolesc Psychiatry 1995;34:50–54.
36. Silva R, Munoz D, Alpert M. Carbamazepine use in children and adolescents with features of attention-deficit hyperactivity disorder: A meta-analysis. J Am Acad Child Adolesc Psychiatry 1996;35:352–358.
37. Hughes CW, Emslie GJ, Crismon ML, et al. The Texas children's medication algorithm project: Report of the Texas consensus conference panel on medication treatment of childhood major depressive disorder. J Am Acad Child Adolesc Psychiatry 1999;38(11):1442–1454.
38. Gross-Tsur V, Manor O, van der Meere J, et al. Epilepsy and attention deficit hyperactivity disorder: Is methylphenidate safe and effective? J Pediatr 1997;130:40–44.
39. Efron D, Jarman F, Barker M, Grad D. Side effects of methylphenidate and dexamphetamine in children with ADHD: A double-blind, crossover trial. Pediatrics 1997;100(4):662–666.
40. Cantwell DP, Swanson J, Connor DF. Case study: Adverse response to clonidine. J Am Acad Child Adolesc Psychiatry 1997;36:539–544.
41. Berkovitch M, Pope E, Phillips J, et al. Pemoline-associated fulminant liver failure: Testing the evidence for causation. Clin Pharmacol Ther 1995;57:696–698.
42. Marotta PJ, Roberts E. Pemoline hepatotoxicity in children. J Pediatr 1998;132:894–897.
43. Rosh JR, Dellert SF, Narkewicz M, et al. Four cases of severe hepatotoxicity associated with pemoline: Possible autoimmune pathogenesis. Pediatrics 1998;101:921–923.
44. Kramer JR, Loney J, Ponto LB, et al. Predictors of adult height and weight in boys treated with methylphenidate for childhood behavior problems. J Am Acad Child Adolesc Psychiatry 2000;39(4):517–524.
45. Biederman J, Wilens T, Mick E, et al. Pharmacotherapy of ADHD reduces risk for substance use disorder. Pediatrics 1999;104(2):293–294.
46. Disney ER, Elkins IJ, McGue M, Iacono WG. Effects of ADHD, conduct disorder, and gender on substance use and abuse in adolescence. Am J Psychiatry 1999;156(10):1515–1521.
47. Horner BR, Scheibe KE. Prevalence and implications of attention-deficit hyperactivity disorder among adolescents in treatment for substance abuse. J Am Acad Child Adolesc Psychiatry 1997;36:30–36.
48. Spencer T, Biederman J, Steingard R, Wilens T. Bupropion exacerbates tics in children with attention-deficit hyperactivity disorder and Tourette's syndrome. J Am Acad Child Adolesc Psychiatry 1993;32:211–214.
49. Chappell PB, Riddle MA, Scahill L, et al. Guanfacine treatment of comorbid attention-deficit hyperactivity disorder and Tourette's syndrome: Preliminary clinical experience. J Am Acad Child Adolesc Psychiatry 1995;34:1140–1146.
50. Kadesjo B, Gillberg C. Tourette's disorder: Epidemiology and comorbidity in primary school children. J Am Acad Child Adolesc Psychiatry 2000;39(5):548–555.
51. Peterson BS. Considerations of natural history and pathophysiology in the psychopharmacology of Tourette's syndrome. J Clin Psychiatry 1996;57:24–34.
52. Comings DE. Tourette Syndrome and Human Behavior. Duarte, CA, Hope Press, 1990:1–792.
53. Coffey BJ, Biederman J, Geller D, et al. Distinguishing illness severity from tic severity in children and adolescents with Tourette's disorder. J Am Acad Child Adolesc Psychiatry 2000;39(5):556–551.
54. Comings DE. Tourette's syndrome genetics. Child Psychiatry Hum Dev 1997;27:139–150.
55. Sallee FR, Kurlan R, Goetz CG, et al. Ziprasidone treatment of children and adolescents with Tourette's syndrome: A pilot study. J Am Acad Child Adolesc Psychiatry 2000;39(3):292–299.
56. Sallee FR, Nesbitt L, Jackson C, et al. Relative efficacy of haloperidol and pimozide in children and adolescents with Tourette's disorder. Am J Psychiatry 1997;154:1057–1062.
57. Bruun RD, Budman CL. Risperidone as a treatment for Tourette's syndrome. J Clin Psychiatry 1996;57:29–31.
58. Comings DE, Comings BG, Tacket T, Li SZ. The clonidine patch and behavior problems (Letter). J Am Acad Child Adolesc Psychiatry 1990;29:667–668.
59. Castellanos FX, Giedd JN, Elia J, et al. Controlled stimulant treatment of ADHD and comorbid Tourette's syndrome: Effects of stimulant and dose. J Am Acad Child Adolesc Psychiatry 1997;36:589–596.
60. Gadow KD, Sverd J, Sprafkin J. Efficacy of methylphenidate for attention-deficit hyperactivity disorder in children with tic disorder. Arch Gen Psychiatry 1995;52:444–455.
61. Singer HS, Brown J, Quaskey S, et al. The treatment of attention deficit hyperactivity disorder in Tourette's syndrome: A double-blind, placebo-

controlled study with clonidine and desipramine. Pediatrics 1995;95: 74–81.
62. Silver AA, Shytle D, Philipp MK. Case study: Long-term potentiation of neuroleptics with transdermal nicotine in Tourette's syndrome. J Am Acad Child Adolesc Psychiatry 1996;35:1631–1636.
63. Conners CK, Levin ED, Sparrow E, et al. Nicotine and attention in adult attention deficit hyperactivity disorder (ADHD). Psychopharmacol Bull 1996;32:67–73.
64. Leonard HL, March J, Rickler KC, et al. Pharmacology of the selective serotonin reuptake inhibitors in children and adolescents. J Am Acad Child Adolesc Psychiatry 1997;36:725–736.
65. Bornstein RA, Yang V. Neuropsychological performance in medicated and unmedicated patients with Tourette's disorder. Am J Psychiatry 1991;148:468–471.
66. Silva RR, Munoz DM, Daniel W, et al. Causes of haloperidol discontinuation in patients with Tourette's disorder: Management and alternatives. J Clin Psychiatry 1996;57:129–135.
67. Feeney DJ, Klykylo W. Risperidone and tardive dyskinesia (Letter). J Am Acad of Child Adolesc Psychiatry 1996;35:1421–1422.
68. Kumra S, Herion D, Jacobsen LK, et al. Case study: Risperidone-induced hepatotoxicity in pediatric patients. J Am Acad Child Adolesc Psychiatry 1997;36:701–705.
69. Kumra S, Grothe D. Risperidone hepatotoxicity (Letter). J Am Acad Child Adolesc Psychiatry 1998;37(3):247.
70. DeVane CL, Nemeroff CB. Psychotropic drug interactions 2000. TEN 2000;2(1):55–75.
71. Norgaard, JP, Djurhuus H, Watanabe H, et al. Experience and current status of research into the pathophysiology of nocturnal enuresis. Br J Urol 1997;79:825–835.
72. Hjalmas K. Nocturnal enuresis: Basic facts and new horizons. Eur Urol 1998;33:53–57.
73. Robson WL. Enuresis treatment in the U.S. Scand J Urol Nephrol 1999;S202:56.
74. Issenman, RM, Filmer RB, Gorski PA. A review of bowel and bladder control development in children: How gastrointestinal and urologic conditions relate to problems in toilet training. Pediatrics 1999;103:1346–1352.
75. Skoog SJ. Primary nocturnal enuresis: An analysis of factors related to its etiology (Editorial). J Urol 1998;159:1338–1339.
76. Gimpel GA, Warzak WJ, Kuhn BR, Walburn JN. Clinical perspectives in primary nocturnal enuresis. Clin Pediatr 1998;37:23–30.
77. Moffatt MEK. Nocturnal enuresis: A review of the efficacy of treatments and practical advice for clinicians. Dev Behav Pediatr 1997;18:49–56.
78. Lackgren G, Hjalmas K, van Gool J, et al. Nocturnal enuresis: a suggestion for a European treatment strategy. Acta Paediatr 1999;88:679–690.
79. Bradbury MG, Meadow SR. Combined treatment with enuresis alarm and desmopressin for nocturnal enuresis. Acta Paediatr 1995;84:1014–1018.
80. Janknegt RA, Zweers HM, Delaere KP, et al. Oral desmopressin as a new treatment modality for primary nocturnal enuresis in adolescents and adults: A double-blind, randomized, multicenter study. Dutch Enuresis Study Group. J Urol 1997;157:513–517.
81. Moffatt ME, Harlos S, Kirshen AJ, Burd L. Desmopressin acetate and nocturnal enuresis: How much do we know? Pediatrics 1993;92:420–425.
82. Rushton HG. Nocturnal enuresis: Epidemiology, evaluation and currently available treatment options. J Pediatr 1998;114:691–696.
83. Stenberg A, Laackgren GL. Desmopressin tablet treatment in nocturnal enuresis. Scand J Urol Nephrol 1995;173:95–99.
84. Fritz GK, Rockney RM, Yeung AS. Plasma levels and efficacy of imipramine treatment for enuresis. J Am Acad Child Adolesc Psychiatry 1994;33:60–64.
85. Daly JM, Wilens T. The use of tricyclic antidepressants in children and adolescents. Pediatr Clin North Am 1998;45:1123–1135.
86. Rushton HG, Belman AB, Skoog S, et al. Predictors of response to desmopressin in children and adolescents with monosymptomatic nocturnal enuresis. Scand J Urol Nephrol 1995;173:109–111.
87. Monda JM, Husmann DA. Primary nocturnal enuresis: A comparison among observation, imipramine, desmopressin acetate and bedwetting alarm systems. J Urol 1995;154:745–748.
88. Dobson P. Enuresis treatment in the U.K. Scand J Urol Nephrol 1999;S202:61–65.
89. Kahan E, Morel D, Amir J, Zelcer C. A controlled trial of desmopressin and behavioral therapy for nocturnal enuresis. Medicine 1998;77:384–388.
90. Riccabona M, Oswald J, Glauninger P. Long-term use and tapered dose reduction of intranasal desmopressin in the treatment of enuretic children. Br J Urol 1998;81(Suppl 3):S24–S25.
91. Hjalmas K, Hanson E, Hellstrom AL, et al. Long-term treatment with desmopressin in children with primary monosymptomatic nocturnal enuresis: An open multicentre study. Swedish Enuresis Trial (SWEET) Group. Br J Urol 1998;82:704–709.
92. Eller DA, Austin PF, Tanguay S, Homsy YL. Daytime functional bladder capacity as a predictor of response to desmopressin in monosymptomatic nocturnal enuresis. Eur Urol 1998;S33:25–29.
93. Donoghue MB, Latimer E, Pillsbury HL, Hertzog JH. Hyponatremic seizure in a child using desmopressin for nocturnal enuresis. Arch Pediatr Adolesc Med 1998;152:290–292.
94. Robson WL, Norgaard JP, Leung AK. Hyponatremia in patients with nocturnal enuresis treated with DDAVP. Eur J Pediatr 1996;155:959–962.
95. Owens RG, Karram MM. Comparative tolerability of drug therapies used to treat incontinence and enuresis. Drug Saf 1998;19:123–139.

64
EATING DISORDERS

Patricia A. Marken and Roger W. Sommi

The initial descriptions of anorexia nervosa (AN) were published over a century ago[1,2]; however, bulimia nervosa (BN) was described as a distinct disorder in 1979.[3] Extensive research has improved our understanding of these severely disabling and potentially fatal disorders. Eating disorders encompass several biologic, psychological, and developmental etiologies. Pharmacologic management remains only a piece of a comprehensive plan that emphasizes cognitive-behavioral therapy and psychotherapy.

EPIDEMIOLOGY

ANOREXIA NERVOSA (AN)

AN occurs predominantly in females (90%) and usually presents in late adolescence. The median age of onset is 17, with new cases rarely occurring after age 40. The reported prevalence of AN in the United States ranges from 1 in 100 to 1 in 800 for females between the ages of 12 and 18 years.[4] The prevalence of AN may have increased recently, as noted by one epidemiologic study that reported a sixfold increase in the number of documented cases of AN for the period of 1970 to 1976 compared with the period of 1960 to 1969.[5]

BULIMIA NERVOSA (BN)

BN also occurs predominantly in females (90%) and usually presents in adolescence or early adult life.[4] BN has been studied primarily in college students, and therefore, knowledge of its prevalence may be limited by the lack of data from other populations. Between 1% and 3% of adolescent and young adult females meet diagnostic criteria for BN, with the prevalence being about one-tenth that in males.[4]

EATING DISORDER NOT OTHERWISE SPECIFIED/BINGE EATING DISORDER

The American Psychiatric Association's *Diagnostic and Statistical Manual of Mental Disorders,* fourth edition, test revision (DSM-IV-TR), includes the diagnosis of eating disorder not otherwise specified (NOS).[4] Individuals with eating disorder NOS manifest symptoms characteristic of eating disorders, but they do not meet the diagnostic criteria for a specific eating disorder. Up to 50% of patients admitted to tertiary care settings have this diagnosis.[6] In addition, research diagnostic criteria have been established for further consideration of a binge eating disorder (BED). The diagnostic criteria for BED describe binge eating without the purging behavior requisite for the bulimia diagnosis. The epidemiology of these disorders is unknown but is likely to be reflective of eating disorders in general.[6]

ETIOLOGY AND PATHOPHYSIOLOGY

The potential etiologic or exacerbating factors for eating disorders represent an array of physiologic, biochemical, developmental, psychological, and psychiatric phenomena. It is difficult to delineate the biologic basis for eating disorders because it is unclear whether the observed biologic changes are causing the aberrant eating behavior or are a result of the eventual starvation.

Abnormalities of the hypothalamic-pituitary-gonadal (HPG), hypothalamic-pituitary-adrenal (HPA), and hypothalamic-pituitary-thyroid (HPT) axes have been described as potential causes of AN. An extensive review of the psychoendocrinology of AN is provided by the Work Group on Eating Disorders.[6] Although many endocrine abnormalities occur in other forms of starvation, a primary difference with AN is that the dysfunction may not correct despite weight normalization. The finding of amenorrhea in the majority of females with AN supports the role of the HPG axis and in particular the function of the gonadotropins luteinizing hormone (LH), follicle-stimulating hormone (FSH), and gonadotropin-releasing hormone (GnRH).[7] It should be noted that up to 25% of females had amenorrhea before the onset of AN, and the return of menses lags behind weight normalization.

The role of the neurotransmitter serotonin in eating disorders has been investigated extensively because it plays an important role in feeding. The primary location of serotonin-mediated eating activity is the medial hypothalamus. Serotonin activity in the paraventricular and ventromedial nuclei controls energy balance, whereas activity in the suprachiasmatic nucleus controls the circadian pattern of feeding. Stimulation of serotonin receptors in these areas decreases carbohydrate intake, enhances satiety, and terminates feeding. In contrast, stimulation of presynaptic serotonin autoreceptors initiates feeding, presumably by inhibiting the release of serotonin. In anorexia, plasma tryptophan (a serotonin precursor), urinary concentration of the major serotonin metabolite 5-hydroxyindoleacetic acid (5-HIAA), platelet serotonin binding, and basal cerebrospinal fluid (CSF) 5-HIAA concentrations are reportedly decreased. These abnormalities all correct with weight normalization.[8]

The role of other neurotransmitters also should be considered. In the presence of decreased food intake, norepinephrine is released in the paraventricular nucleus, which inhibits satiety, while at the same time release of norepinephrine is inhibited at the lateral hypothalamus, which increases the sensation of hunger. Dopamine is associated with self-administration and self-stimulatory behaviors in other disorders and similarly may be related etiologically to the eating binges observed in BN. Taste and food cues also are regulated by neurotransmitters within the hypothalamus. Hypothalamic dysfunction may account for the food preferences present in BN and the food dislikes exhibited by persons with AN.

A great deal of emphasis is placed on psychological and developmental issues in the pathogenesis of eating disorders, especially regarding the role of the family. Issues surrounding family separations, losses, and dysfunction may trigger abnormal eating behavior.[6,9] Whether family-related issues are truly etiologic for eating disorders remains controversial. It is interesting, however, to note that the prognosis is better in persons with a relatively healthy family environment.[10] Eating disorder patients also commonly have a history of physical and sexual abuse. Finally, athletes are at special risk for eating disorders, especially female gymnasts, figure skaters, distance runners, and swimmers and male wrestlers and body builders.[11] Attention should be given to these variables when diagnostic and treatment decisions are considered.

Eating disorders are very complex and probably will not be explained by any simple physiologic, biochemical, developmental, psychological, or psychiatric model. Instead, a multifaceted view of potential etiologies will best serve the clinician in making decisions about treatment alternatives.

DIAGNOSTIC CRITERIA AND CLINICAL PRESENTATION

Figure 64–1 lists the common clinical signs and symptoms for AN and BN. AN and BN occur together in about 30% to 64% of patients with eating disorders and may not be distinct diagnostic entities but rather occur along a continuum of symptoms.[12–15] Many patients initially present with either AN or BN and alternate from one eating disorder to the other. The clinician should pay particular attention to these fluctuations and alter therapy accordingly because patients with AN and BN need different treatment interventions.

Medical consequences of an eating disorder are vast and are related primarily to self-induced starvation and purging. Patients commonly present with vague complaints of lethargy and pain. Metabolic and electrolyte disturbances along with dehydration are common and occur because of poor dietary intake, self-induced vomiting, or chronic laxative and diuretic abuse. Severe electrolyte disturbances can cause cardiac disturbances and even sudden death. Abnormalities of the hypothalamic-pituitary axes are likely the result of starvation. These abnormalities include effects on estradiol, the gonadotropins (e.g., LH, FSH, and GnRH), thyroid function, adrenal function, and growth hormone.[7] Osteoporosis and infertility are potential long-term complications of endocrine changes. Vomiting can cause dental problems, including decalcification, erosion of the enamel and dentin layers, and staining of the surfaces of the teeth.[4] Chronic starvation can cause brain atrophy visible on computed tomographic (CT) scan as an increase in ventricular-to-brain ratio. Decreases in white matter and CSF volumes return to normal after a healthy weight is achieved, but gray matter loss may continue to persist. The loss of gray matter can be demonstrated during neuropsychological testing.[6,17,17] A thorough physical and laboratory evaluation, as described in Table 64–1, is needed to determine the severity of medical complications.[18,19] The

TABLE 64–1. Physical and Laboratory Assessment of Eating Disorders

Evaluation	Target Symptoms
Pulse	Sinus bradycardia
Blood pressure	Hypotension, orthostasis
Respiratory rate	Rapid if heart failure occurs during refeeding
Temperature	Hypothermia, cold intolerance
ECG	ST depression, flat T waves, U waves, increased QT, AV block
GI	Hypoactive bowel sounds, gastritis, abdominal distention, bloating, diarrhea, constipation
Skin	Dry, scaling, lanugo, hair loss, callus on fingers and hands (Russel's sign), bruising
Menses	Amenorrhea
CBC	Leukopenia, anemias, thrombocytopenia
Electrolytes	Hypokalemia, hypomagnesemia, hypo/hyper-phosphatemia
pH	Metabolic alkalosis (acidosis if laxative abuse)
Amylase	Elevated, pancreatitis rare
Liver	Hypoalbuminemia, gamma-glutamyl transpeptidase if alcohol abuse
Thyroid	Decreased T_3 and T_4 but not true disease
Cortisol	Elevated with lack of dexamethasone suppression test
Bone density	Osteoporosis
CT	Ventricular enlargement
Dental	Loss of tooth enamel

Modified from Ref. 26.

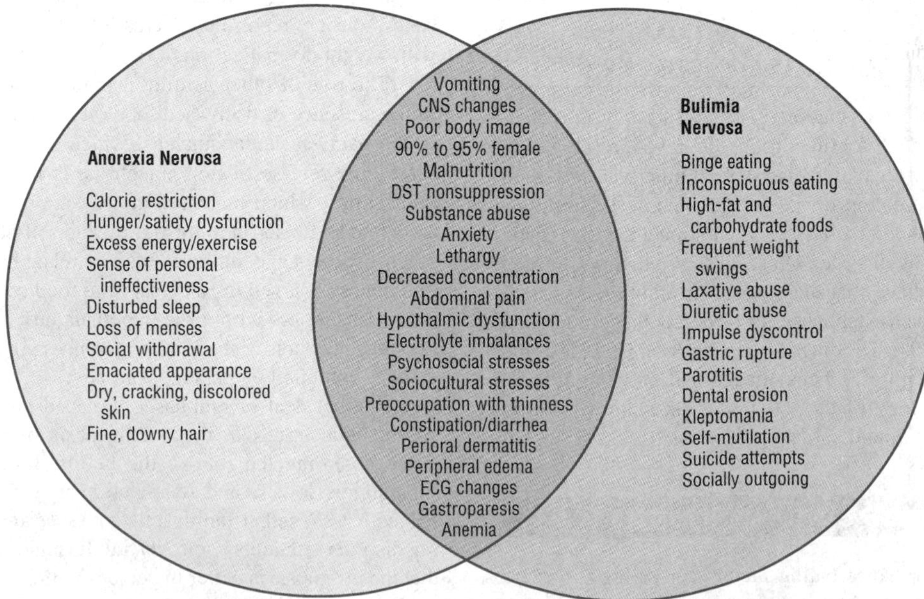

FIGURE 64–1. Signs and symptoms of anorexia nervosa and bulimia nervosa.

presence of a particular medical complication depends on whether the patient engages in starvation or purging (vomiting, laxative abuse) and the frequency and severity of the behavior.

Depression, schizophrenia, obsessive-compulsive disorder, and conversion disorders should be included in the differential diagnosis of AN and BN because eating abnormalities can be a component of these illnesses. The salient difference between these psychiatric disorders and eating disorders is the overriding drive for thinness, a disturbed body image, increased energy level directed toward losing weight, and binge-eating episodes that are relatively specific for the eating disorders. Additionally, many patients will experience relief of the psychiatric symptoms on refeeding and not require psychotropics.[6]

ANOREXIA NERVOSA

The core features of AN include refusal to maintain a minimal normal body weight (e.g., > 85% normal body weight or body mass index >17.5 kg/m^2), intense fear and obsession about weight gain or being "fat," a distorted body image, and amenorrhea. Patients typically lack an appreciation for the degree of weight loss experienced or are preoccupied with the idea that a part of their body is too large, the key feature of a distorted body image. The DSM-IV-TR further classifies AN into restricting type or binge-eating/purging type. The AN patient has difficulty in sensing when he or she is full (satiety) and commonly complains of feeling bloated soon after he or she starts eating. Patients also feel as though they are not in control of various aspects of their life and, in particular, of caloric intake. When patients with AN are underweight, they often present with features of major depression, but these symptoms are more likely the consequence of starvation than a true case of a mood disorder. Specific DSM-IV-TR criteria for AN and its subtypes can be found in Table 64–2.

Cormorbidity is also an issue because up to 75% of treated patients have a primary mood disorder.[19] A link between AN and anxiety disorders, especially social phobia (fear of eating in public) and obsessive-compulsive disorder (OCD), has been noted. For example, the lifetime prevalence of OCD in patients with AN is reported to be as high as 25%, much higher than the lifetime prevalence of 2.5% in the general population.[19,20] Substance abuse appears to be less of a problem than with BN. Personality disorders are also more common among people with AN, especially the avoidant and obsessive-compulsive types, than in the general population.[21]

The course of AN most commonly consists of a single episode with subsequent return to normal weight. These patients may still experience issues with disturbed body image, disordered eating, and other psychiatric problems.[6] Some patients may experience an unremitting course leading to death or episodic periods of anorexic behavior.[4] A recent study found that 50% of AN patients had a "good" outcome, 30% had a "medium" outcome, and 20% a "poor" outcome.[22] A poorer prognosis is associated with a longer duration of illness, having a lower initial weight, having a premorbid history of poor family relationships, and the presence of BN or additional symptoms such as vomiting and laxative abuse.[6,23] Varying numbers exist on the mortality of AN, but it is clear that it is among the highest of all psychiatric disorders. Long-term follow-up shows that between 10% and 18% of AN patients eventually died, primarily from cardiac arrest or suicide.[4,23,24]

TABLE 64–2. DSM-IV Diagnostic Criteria for Anorexia Nervosa and Bulimia Nervosa

Anorexia Nervosa

1. Refusal to maintain body weight over a minimal normal weight for age and height; or failure to make expected weight gain during period of growth, leading to a body weight 15% lower than expected normal weight for age and height.
2. Intense fear of gaining weight or becoming fat, even though underweight.
3. Disturbance in the way one's body weight, size, or shape is experienced, undue influence of body weight or shape on self-evaluation, or denial of the seriousness of the current low body weight.
4. In postmenarchal females, amenorrhea (absence of at least three consecutive menstrual cycles when otherwise expected to occur [primary or secondary amenorrhea]).

Subtypes are based on findings during the current episode with regard to binge-eating or purging behavior (self-induced vomiting or the misuse of laxatives, diuretics, or enemas):

Restricting type: The person has not regularly engaged in binge-eating or purging behavior.

Binge-eating/purging type: The person has regularly engaged in binge-eating or purging behavior.

Bulimia Nervosa

1. Recurrent episodes of binge eating characterized by both of the following:
   A. Eating, in a discrete period of time, an amount of food that is definitely larger than most people would consume during a similar period of time and under similar circumstances.
   B. A feeling of lack of control over eating behavior during the episode.
2. Recurrent compensatory behavior to prevent weight gain such as self-induced vomiting; misuse of laxatives, diuretics, enemas, or other medications; strict dieting or fasting; or vigorous exercise.
3. Binge-eating episodes and compensatory behaviors occur on average at least twice weekly for 3 months.
4. Self-evaluation is unduly influenced by body shape and weight.
5. Symptoms do not occur exclusively during episodes of AN.

Subtypes are based on findings during the current episode with regard to binge-eating or purging behavior (self-induced vomiting or the misuse of laxatives, diuretics, or enemas).

Purging type: The person has regularly engaged in self-induced vomiting or the misuse of laxatives, diuretics, or enemas

Nonpurging type: The person has used other inappropriate compensatory behaviors, such as fasting or excessive exercise, but has not engaged in self-induced vomiting or the misuse of laxatives, diuretics, or enemas.

Modified and reprinted from the Diagnostic and Statistical Manual of Mental Disorders, 4th ed-Text Revision. Copyright 2000 American Psychiatric Association.

BULIMIA NERVOSA

The core feature of BN is binge eating—an excessive intake of calorie-laden food over a short period of time. Persons with BN, as with AN, are overly sensitive about their weight and have a distorted body image. Most have normal weight, although some may be slightly underweight or overweight for body size and age. DSM-IV-TR further differentiates an episode of BN into purging type or nonpurging type, depending on the patient's recent use of purging methods to offset the effects of binge eating. The DSM-IV-TR diagnostic criteria for BN and its subtypes are listed in Table 64–2.

Patients typically binge one or more times daily and vomit at least once daily. Patients may consume 5000 to 20,000 calories during a single binge, although caloric intake can be smaller. Patients tend to consume foods that are easy to ingest, do not require much chewing or preparation, and are high in carbohydrates or fat (e.g., ice cream, bread, candy, or doughnuts). Binge eating typically is secretive, and episodes are often precipitated by a stressful event. Patients experience a loss of control over their eating behavior and are often remorseful perafter a binge. Although binges typically last less than 2 hours, they have been reported to last for more than 8 hours. To compensate for the excessive caloric intake, many patients fast for prolonged periods, exercise compulsively, purge, or abuse laxatives, resulting in frequent weight fluctuations.

Psychiatric comorbidity includes depression (up to 80%), impulse-control problems, and substance abuse. Approximately 30% to 37% of bulimic patients have a personal history of substance abuse.[25] Kleptomania (another impulse-control disorder) is reported more commonly in patients with BN than in the general public.[26] Personality disorders, especially borderline and avoidant types, are more common in these patients that in the general population.[21]

The prognosis of BN has not been well studied. On average, a 70% reduction in binge eating and purging episodes has been reported following any treatment intervention. Patients with milder presenting symptoms who are treated on an outpatient basis tend to do better. A 6-year follow-up of patients who received intensive treatment found that 60% were "good," 29% had "intermediate" response, 10% were doing "poorly," and 1% had died.[27]

▶ TREATMENT: Eating Disorders

DESIRED OUTCOME

Various treatment modalities are used to improve the quality of life for patients with AN and BN. Although the approach to individual patients may differ, the basic goals of treatment are to reduce distorted body image, restore and maintain healthy body weight, reestablish normal eating patterns, improve associated psychological and physical problems, resolve contributory family problems, and prevent relapse.

GENERAL APPROACH TO TREATMENT

The initial step in treatment is engaging the patient and important parties into a collaborative treatment plan. Denial is a common problem, and without active patient participation, treatment will not be a success. An individualized treatment plan is based on the specific core and associated features of the eating disorder and will provide for a team approach to care. Clinicians who provide care to patients with eating disorders include psychiatrists, nutrition specialists, psychologists, specially trained counselors, nurses, and pharmacists. Hospitalization should be based on the criteria outlined in Table 64–3,[6] because most patients can be managed in an outpatient setting. Medications are never indicated as a sole treatment for eating disorders.[11]

ANOREXIA NERVOSA

NONPHARMACOLOGIC THERAPY

Nondrug treatments are the cornerstone of AN treatment. Nondrug treatments include behavioral management, cognitive-behavioral therapy (CBT), interpersonal psychotherapy, nutritional counseling, and group and family therapy.[28] CBT helps the patient overcome distorted thinking, self-worth being measured by body image, feelings of being fat despite evidence to the contrary, and denial of the seriousness of the condition. Interpersonal psychotherapy focuses on interpersonal relationships, whereas behavioral therapy provides positive reinforcements for weight gain.[19] CBT has emerged as the preferred strategy in most eating disorder programs. Treatment based on an addiction model (twelve-step program) is not well studied and should be avoided unless it also manages the medical and other psychiatric features of AN as part of the program.[6] Initially, treatment is directed toward restoring a healthy weight and treating food phobias. After the patient is medically stable, therapy addresses interpersonal problems, and finally, skill development for relapse prevention is targeted.[29] Appropriate oral refeeding is also pivotal to the successful outcome in these patients. A controlled weight gain of 2 to 3 pounds a week for inpatients is recommended. Patients will need a slow upward titration of their caloric intake to amounts as high as 70 to 100 kcal/kg per day in order to minimize both medical and psychological consequences that can occur with a more rapid refeeding.[6]

PHARMACOLOGIC THERAPY

ANTIDEPRESSANTS

The goals of antidepressant therapy in AN is to improve depression, anxiety, and obsessional thought patterns and promote weight gain,

TABLE 64–3. Criteria for Hospitalization of Patients With Eating Disorders

1. Significant weight loss (25% less than normal weight or greater), particularly if weight loss has been recent and rapid, severe starvation symptoms are present or the patient has been ill for more than 2 years
2. Medical complications and metabolic abnormalities from bingeing, purging, and starvation (e.g., HR < 40 bpm, BP < 90/60 mm Hg, glucose < 60 mg %, K < 3 mEq/L, T° < 97° F
3. Suicidal ideation
4. Nonresponsiveness to outpatient treatment (after 3 to 4 months) and poor motivation to recover
5. Demoralization, nonfunctional family
6. Continuous supervision required to prevent purging (vomiting, laxative abuse)

Modified from Ref. 6 and 11.

although benefit has not been demonstrated in all areas.[30] A double-blind comparison of 100 mg clomipramine at bedtime and placebo in 16 subjects found that the clomipramine-treated subjects had significantly more hunger and energy than the placebo subjects. Rate of weight gain was slower in clomipramine-treated subjects, perhaps due to increased activity.[31] Subjects maintained a more stable weight than the placebo patients after discontinuation of the study. Open trials with 20 to 60 mg/day fluoxetine found a reduction in obsessions and depression, maintenance of the target body weight, and restoration of normal eating behavior; however, controlled and long-term trials are needed before fluoxetine can be recommended routinely.[32,33] A controlled trial found that fluoxetine added no benefit to nutrition and psychosocial measures in hospitalized malnourished patients.[34]

Since symptom response is generally limited, the overall role of antidepressants in managing AN remains secondary to nondrug treatments.[6] Antidepressants should be initiated only if depression, obsessions, or compulsions persist after the target weight has been achieved, since many symptoms will resolve as weight improves.[6] This may be particularly important because of a report describing additional weight loss in acutely ill, severely underweight patients (mean body mass index of 15.6 kg/m^2) taking citalopram for symptoms of AN.[34] Selective serotonin reuptake inhibitors (SSRIs) are usually used as first-line antidepressants because they are better tolerated and have greater cardiovascular safety than tricyclic antidepressants (TCAs), especially in low-weight patients.[30] Patients with AN are sensitive to anticholinergic and cardiovascular effects, and if TCAs are used, low starting doses and a slow titration toward an effective dose are needed. The risk of cardiotoxicity in a malnourished population must not be underestimated, especially in chronic purgers, who may have hypokalemia. A baseline electrocardiogram (ECG) must be obtained before beginning an antidepressant. Cyproheptadine, an agent evaluated in the 1980s and early 1990s, is no longer recommended as an option in the current practice guidelines.[6]

ANTIPSYCHOTICS

Typical antipsychotics were the first medications used to treat AN, based on reports of weight gain and reduced eating-related anxiety, agitation, and obsessions.[35] Clinical experience has found little specific improvement from using the typical antipsychotics in AN patient and that risks outweigh the benefits. Interest in using the atypical agents with SSRIs in patients with severe obsessions and compulsions has been reported anecdotally but never studied in a systematic manner.

MISCELLANEOUS AGENTS

Metoclopramide (Reglan) may be helpful in increasing the gastric emptying rate and reducing bloating and abdominal pain common in AN.[36,37] Short-acting benzodiazepines, given before meals, are useful when severe anxiety limits eating.[6] Estrogen replacement (conjugated estrogens 0.3 to 1.25 mg/d) has been used, but refeeding and restoring menses are a better approach to minimizing bone density loss.[38,39] Total parenteral nutrition (TPN) is sometimes needed during the initial management of severely malnourished patients or when oral refeeding fails; however, the decision to administer TPN must be made carefully because of the potentially devastating psychological effect on patients who do not wish to gain weight.

BULIMIA NERVOSA

NONPHARMACOLOGIC THERAPY

Nondrug strategies are similar to those used with AN and play an equally important role in treatment success. Cox and Merkel evaluated 32 studies of individual and group therapy techniques used to manage BN.[40] Most studies had methodologic shortcomings such as failure to use a control group, overreliance on self-reporting as an outcome, and small sample sizes. However, about 40% of patients were totally abstinent from binge eating and purging at follow-up. No intervention was found to be clearly superior to any other. A trial not included in the Cox and Merkel analysis found that interpersonal psychotherapy and CBT were equally effective and superior to behavioral therapy alone.[41] More recently, CBT was found to be superior to interpersonal psychotherapy for improving BN symptoms.[42]

Nutritional counseling, planned meals, and family therapy are also important components of treatment. The role of twelve-step programs for both AN and BN is controversial because their efficacy has not been systematically evaluated, and there is great variability in the treatment from site to site. Concern exists because patients may not have the medical or behavioral complications of the illness addressed by this model of care. Experts recommend that twelve-step programs never be the sole initial treatment modality for patients with eating disorders.[6]

PHARMACOLOGIC THERAPY

ANTIDEPRESSANTS

Antidepressants have been extensively evaluated in BN, although benefit is not universal, and design problems are present in several trials. It is also important to note that the literature evaluating the role of antidepressants in BN has not grown much since the early to middle 1990s. Antidepressants are reported to reduce binge eating, vomiting, anxiety, obsessions, impulsivity, and depression and improve eating habits, although their impact on body dissatisfaction remains unclear. Response varies across trials, but reduction of binge/purge behavior has been as high as 75% with antidepressant therapy.[6] Placebo-treated patients tended to have a response of about half that seen in antidepressant-treated patients. Reduction in vomiting episodes tends to mirror reductions in binge episodes. The prevalence of major depression is 15% or less in most studies, suggesting an antibulimic effect independent of an antidepressant effect.[30]

Imipramine, desipramine, and phenelzine demonstrated superiority over placebo in double-blind trials for treating specific symptoms of BN.[43–49] Doses for BN are the same as those used to treat depression, although slow titration is needed to allow time to develop tolerance to adverse effects. Serum concentration monitoring of TCAs is recommended to ensure that absorption is not compromised by purging. The same plasma concentration ranges used in depression are used for patients with BN. Phenelzine should be used only if the patient will reliably follow the dietary and medication restrictions. Trazodone, up to 400 mg/day, also has been beneficial and generally well tolerated.[50] Bupropion is not used in patients with BN because of an unacceptably high risk of seizures.

Fluoxetine is the only antidepressant with Food and Drug Administration (FDA) approval for treatment of BN. The Fluoxetine Bulimia Nervosa Collaborative Study Group conducted the largest trial evaluating an antidepressant in BN. It should be noted that there was no active control group. Fluoxetine (60 mg/day) was found to be superior to both placebo and fluoxetine (20 mg/day) for reducing vomiting, bingeing, depression, carbohydrate craving, and pathologic eating habits. The drug was well tolerated, and weight changes were minimal, even at 60 mg/day.[51] In a 16-week study, 60 mg fluoxetine per day had a similar benefit. The subjects receiving active drug had significantly more of the common fluoxetine adverse effects (e.g., insomnia, nausea, anxiety, decreased libido) than the placebo subjects. Placebo subjects had more depression, myalgia, and emotional lability as adverse effects. About 11% of fluoxetine subjects dropped out due to adverse effects versus about 6% of placebo subjects.[52] Fluvoxamine, mean dose 182 mg/day, also has demonstrated efficacy in a placebo-controlled trial.[53]

Tolerability is the basis for selecting an antidepressant in BN because of heightened sensitivity to adverse effects and lack of a clear difference in efficacy between the classes. For these reasons, SSRIs are usually first-line agents. A careful baseline physical examination and laboratory workup are essential because underlying electrocardiographic changes (U waves, prolonged Q-T interval, flattened T waves) secondary to hypokalemia or bradycardia and arterioventricular block from starvation may be present. All antidepressants can cause seizures; thus a careful risk-benefit assessment is warranted if the patient has predisposing factors such as a personal or family history of seizures, cerebrovascular disease, or alcohol or sedative-hypnotic withdrawal.[54]

Antidepressants also have been evaluated in BED. A significant reduction in binge episodes has been found, although the response to placebo also was high, suggesting the need for further evaluation before antidepressants become a standard of care.[55,56]

MOOD STABILIZERS

The pharmacotherapy of BN is based on two pathophysiologic models: a relationship to seizure disorders and a relationship to affective disorders. Anticonvulsants were the first medications specifically targeted to treat BN. Green and Rau noted that 38 of 59 patients with binge eating had abnormal electroencephalograms. They subsequently administered phenytoin (Dilantin) to 47 BN patients in an open trial and achieved a 57% improvement in bulimic symptoms.[57] Wermuth and colleagues conducted a double-blind, placebo-controlled trial in 20 subjects and found no significant difference between the placebo and phenytoin-treated groups.[58] Kaplan and colleagues, in a placebo-controlled, double-blind trial of 6 BN patients treated with carbamazepine (Tegretol), found a dramatic response in one patient in both bulimic and affective symptoms.[59] Valproic acid (Depakene) produced a dramatic response in a patient with concurrent bulimia and bipolar affective disorder in a single case report. Subsequent bulimic episodes occurred only after the serum concentration decreased to apparent subtherapeutic values.[60] Anticonvulsants are reserved for the subgroup of BN patients with a comorbid bipolar affective disorder. Doses used and serum concentrations sought are similar to those used for patients with seizure disorders. Lithium is reserved for patients with comorbid bipolar affective disorder. It must be used cautiously because the risk of toxicity increases as a result of purging and laxative abuse. Serum concentrations should be maintained between 0.6 and 0.8 mEq/L.[61] The adverse effect of weight gain often makes mood stabilizers unacceptable to patients in the long term.

MISCELLANEOUS AGENTS

TPN is occasionally needed in metabolically disturbed patients, although the decision to use it must be weighed against the psychological risks of forced refeeding. Low-dose benzodiazepines, such as 0.25 mg alprazolam three times a day administered before meals, may help reduce anxiety associated with refeeding, although long-term use is not warranted for most patients because of the risk of abuse.

COMBINATION THERAPY

A comparison of imipramine and psychotherapy found that the three groups receiving active treatment (imipramine alone, imipramine plus psychotherapy, or placebo plus psychotherapy) showed a better response than did those receiving placebo alone and that combination treatment was superior to imipramine alone. Imipramine reduced depression and anxiety but did not improve eating behavior.[62] Angras and associates compared the effectiveness of desipramine (mean dose 168 mg/d; mean serum concentration 130.8 μg/mL), CBT, and their combination for 16 or 24 weeks in outpatients with BN. The combination of desipramine and CBT for 24 weeks was found to be superIor to any other treatment or duration for reducing bingeing, purging, dietary preoccupation, and hunger.[63] Walsh and colleagues compared the following treatments: CBT and desipramine (mean dose 143 mg/day), CBT and placebo, supportive psychotherapy and desipramine (mean dose 220 mg/day), supportive psychotherapy and placebo, and desipramine alone (mean dose 198 mg/day). Fluoxetine (mean dose 55 mg/day) was substituted in the case of inadequate response or poor tolerance to desipramine. Patients receiving CBT and medication had the best response. CBT was the superior psychotherapy intervention, and medication added a modest benefit to nondrug measures. Patients receiving supportive psychotherapy and medication had no better response than those receiving medication alone. A significant difference existed in desipramine doses between the CBT and supportive psychotherapy groups, whereas no difference was found in fluoxetine dose across groups. Finally, two-thirds of patients had to be switched to fluoxetine.[64] In summary, the combination of pharmacologic and nonpharmacologic measures appears to produce the best outcome for patients with BN. Overall, the combination of antidepressants and CBT seems to provide better coverage for both disordered eating (bingeing, purging, eating attitudes), mood, and anxiety symptoms than either treatment alone.

EVALUATION OF THERAPEUTIC OUTCOMES

ANOREXIA NERVOSA

The overall goals of treatment for a patient with AN are to restore healthy weight and eating habits; prevent and resolve physical complications; correct behavioral problems, dysfunctional thoughts, and psychological problems; improve family relationships; and prevent relapse.[6] A diary that records exercise frequency, menses, food intake, patterns of eating, and associated feelings while eating is helpful to monitor progress. Weekly weigh-ins on the same scale, preferably at a clinician's office, help monitor progress early in treatment and reduce the focus on weight and anxiety from variability found among different scales.[29] A healthy weight gain of no more than 2 to 3 pounds per week toward a goal of 90% of normal weight or a body mass index greater than 18.5 kg/m^2 is a critical sign of treatment success. A patient's use of coping skills and contingencies also should be assessed. Antidepressants are likely to assist in alleviation of persistent depression, anxiety, and obsessions. Their benefit for restoration and maintenance of a target weight is unclear, and this should not be the primary reason for the use of antidepressants. Improvement in mood should occur within approximately 8 weeks. Patients receiving TCAs should be evaluated for anticholinergic effects, especially dry mouth and constipation, hypotension, and sedation. Patients receiving fluoxetine should be monitored for agitation, drug-induced anorexia, nausea, weight loss, and insomnia. Follow-up laboratory tests and electrocardiograms are not part of routine monitoring unless signs and symptoms persist necessitating their collection or the patient continues to lose weight despite treatment. The decision to use long-term medication must be based on specific and sustained improvement in the target symptoms mentioned balanced against tolerance of adverse effects.

BULIMIA NERVOSA

Treatment can produce a reduction in target behaviors such as bingeing and purging, but total absence of these behaviors is a less common outcome. The actual definition of recovery varies, since once-a-month binge/purge episodes are considered by some to be recovery, whereas others consider a patient recovered only when complete absence of these behaviors occurs.[23] Of concern is that ongoing symptoms may predispose patients to relapse.[65] Any individual treatment plan using medication should carefully describe frequency and severity of medication-responsive target symptoms and routinely assess changes from baseline in mood, anxiety, eating behaviors, and laxative abuse.[6] Figure 64–2 describes a proposed treatment algorithm for BN, but it should be noted that no consensus for treatment has been endorsed.[30,65] The time to onset of effect is unclear, but a 4- to 6-week trial at a therapeutic dose should be tried to fully determine response. Bewteen 20% and 40% of subjects are estimated to have a poor or inadequate response to antidepressants, and there are few data on predictors of response or whether switching to another class in an unresponsive patient is effective.[66] Optimal duration of treatment after response is also poorly defined. Most clinicians will treat for 6 months to 1 year and then reevalaute the need for ongoing treatment. If the symptoms return within a few months after the antidepressant is discontinued, then the treatment may need to be reinitiated. The impact of antidepressants on the long-term prognosis of BN is also ill defined. Careful evaluation for binge/purge behavior is necessary to ensure that treatment failure is not secondary to vomiting. Evaluation of previously described adverse effects also should be part of the treatment plan. Supportive counseling that encourages compliance may be needed early in treatment while the patient becomes tolerant to adverse effects.

The eating disorder patient presents a challenge to clinicians in ambulatory care. Impulsivity associated with BN may increase the risk for suicide. Prescriptions of the more toxic medications should be limited to small supplies. In addition, the pharmacist should be alert to identify persons who make large or frequent purchases of laxatives or ipecac syrup. If such activity is noted, possible laxative abuse and bulimic behaviors should be considered. Finally, a single case of fluoxetine abuse was reported in a patient with AN, indicating the need for attention to the frequency of refills.[67]

There are no formal evaluations looking at the economic impact of eating disorders on an individual patient level, on global health care costs, or on indirect costs such as unemployment, premature death, or disability payments. Certainly, the chronic nature, the medical and psychological disability found in severe cases, and the lack of improvement in up to a third of patients suggest a significant cost impact. A pharmacist can contribute to the appropriate use of resources by ensuring that medications are used in situations where there is evidence demonstrating their benefit and that they are never used as the sole treatment modality. For example, antidepressants are started after normal weight is restored in AN patients and not to treat depressive symptoms in significantly malnourished patients.

CONCLUSIONS

Our understanding of the pathophysiology and symptomatology of eating disorders has improved significantly over the past several years. Although various models are used to explain the etiology of eating

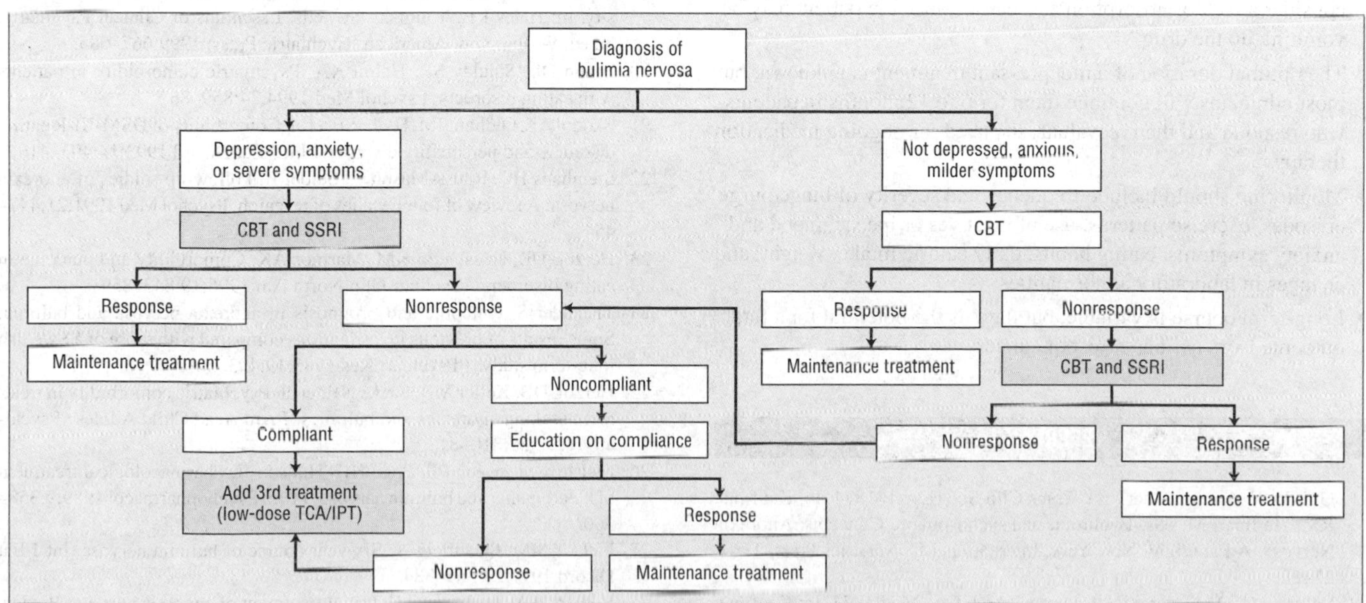

FIGURE 64–2. Proposed treatment algorithm for bulimia nervosa.

disorders, it is unlikely that any single model will sufficiently explain these complex disorders. Medication serves an adjunctive role to a variety of psychosocial therapies in AN, whereas it plays a more central role in the treatment of BN. By gaining a greater understanding of the underlying physiologic changes and the psychosocial complications associated with eating disorders, treatment plans can be specifically designed for an individual patient with the goal of improving the quality of life.

▶ PRINCIPLES OF PHARMACOTHERAPY

- The cause of eating disorders is complex; thus ongoing multidisciplinary treatment is needed to ensure a positive outcome.
- Careful medical and psychiatric assessments are needed at baseline to determine severity of illness and comorbid conditions.
- Outpatient treatment is appropriate for the majority of patients.
- The cornerstone of treatment is nonpharmacologic measures such as CBT, nutritional counseling, and interpersonal psychotherapy.
- In patients with AN, one goal is to achieve and maintain a body weight within 85% of the normal weight for age and height. If the patient is malnourished, oral refeeding with the daily caloric intake slowly titrated upward to 2000 to 3000 kcal/day is preferred. Parenteral refeeding is a treatment of last resort.
- Antidepressants in AN are reserved for patients with mood, anxiety, and obsessional symptoms that persist after weight has improved.
- Antidepressants can improve both mood and specific target symptoms in BN, but they remain adjunctive to nonpharmacologic treatments.
- SSRIs are considered first-line agents when drugs are indicated because of improved tolerability and safety, but they do not have superior efficacy compared with other antidepressant classes. The dose of fluoxetine in BN is higher (60 mg/day) than the dose usually used in depression.
- An adequate drug therapy trial is 4 to 6 weeks. If treatment fails, consider a lack of absorption as a cause, since the patient may be vomiting up the drug.
- The optimal duration of antidepressant treatment is unknown, but most clinicians will continue them for 6 to 12 months in patients who respond and then reevaluate the need for ongoing medication therapy.
- Monitoring should include frequency and severity of binge/purge episodes, exercise patterns, use of laxatives or ipecac, mood and anxiety symptoms, eating habits, daily caloric intake, weight, and changes in laboratory abnormalities.
- Long-term course is variable, but there is the potential for a fatal outcome from cardiac arrest or suicide.

REFERENCES

1. Gull WW. Anorexia nervosa. Trans Clin Soc (Lond) 1874. In: Kaufman RM, Heifman M, eds. Evolution of Psychosomatic Concepts. Anorexia Nervosa: A Paradigm. New York, International Universities Press, 1964: 22–28.
2. Lesegue C. De l'anorexic hysterique. Arch Gen Med 1873. In: Kaufman RM, Heifman M, eds. Evolution of Psychosomatic Concepts. Anorexia Nervosa: A Paradigm. New York, International Universities Press, 1964: 385.
3. Russel G. Bulimia nervosa: An ominous variant of anorexia nervosa. Psychol Med 1979;9:429–448.
4. American Psychiatric Association. Diagnostic and Statistical Manual of Mental Disorders, 4th ed Test Revision (DSM-IV-TR). Washington, American Psychiatric Press, 2000:583–596.
5. Jones DJ, Fox MM, Babigian HM, Hutton HE. Epidemiology of anorexia nervosa in Monroe County, New York, NY: 1960–1976. Psychosom Med 1980;42:551–558.
6. Work Group on Eating Disorders. American Psychiatric Association Practice Guidelines. Practice guidelines for eating disorders. Am J Psychiatry 2000;157(Suppl):1–39.
7. Weiner H. Psychoendocrinology of anorexia nervosa. Psychiatr Clin North Am 1989;12:187–206.
8. Liebowitz SF. The role of serotonin in eating disorders. Drugs 1990;39(Suppl 3):33–48.
9. Garfinkel PE. Eating disorders. In: Kaplan HI, Sadock BJ, eds. Comprehensive Textbook of Psychiatry, 6th ed. Baltimore, Williams & Wilkins, 1995:1361–1372.
10. Rosenvinge JH, Mouland SO. Outcome and prognosis of anorexia nervosa. Br J Psychiatry 1990;156:92–97.
11. Powers PS. Initial assessment and early treatment options for anorexia nervosa and bulimia nervosa. Psychiatr Clin North Am 1996;19:639–655.
12. Casper RC, Hedeker D, McClough JF. Personality dimensions in eating disorders and their relevance for subtyping. J Am Acad Child Adolesc Psychiatry 1992;31:830–840.
13. Eckert ED, Halmi KA, Marchi P, et al. Ten-year follow-up of anorexia nervosa: Clinical course and outcome. Psychol Med 1995;25:143–156.
14. Garner DM, Olmsted MP, Garfinkel PE. Does anorexia nervosa occur on a continuum? Subgroup of weight-preoccupied women and their relationship to anorexia nervosa. Int J Eating Disord 1983;2:11–20.
15. Garner DM, Garfinkel PE, O'Shaughnessy M. Validity of the distinction between bulimia with and without anorexia nervosa. Am J Psychiatry 1985;142:581–587.
16. Kingston K, Szmukler G, Andrews D, et al. Neuropsychological and structural brain changes in anorexia nervosa before and after refeeding. Psychol Med 1996;26:15–28.
17. Lambe EK, Katzman DK, Mikulis DJ, et al. Cerebral gray matter volume deficits after weight recovery from anorexia nervosa. Arch Gen Psychaitry 1997;54:537–542.
18. Carney CP, Anderson AE. Eating disorders: Guide to medical evaluation and complications. Psychiatr Clin North Am 1996;19:657–679.
19. Halmi KA. Eating disorders: Anorexia nervosa, bulimia nervosa, and obesity. In: Hales RE, Yudofsky SC, eds. Essentials of Clinical Psychiatry, 3d ed. Washington, American Psychiatric Press, 1999:667–685.
20. Braun DL, Sunday SR, Halmi KA. Psychiatric comorbidity in patients with eating disorders. Psychol Med 1994;24:859–867.
21. Skodol AE, Oldham JM, Hyler SE, et al. Comorbidity of DSM-III-R eating disorders and personality disorders. Int J Eat Disord 1993;14:403–416.
22. Steinhaus HC, Rauss-Mason C, Seidel R. Follow-up studies of anorexia nervosa: A review of four decades of research. Psychol Med 1991;21:447–454.
23. Herzog DB, Nussbaum KM, Marmor AK. Comorbidity and outcome in eating disorders. Psychiatr Clin North Am 1996;19:843–859.
24. Theander S. Outcome and prognosis in anorexia nervosa and bulimia: Some results of previous investigations compared with those of a Swedish long-term study. J Psychiatr Res 1985;19:493–508.
25. Herzog DB, Keller MB, Sacks NR, et al. Psychiatric comorbidity in treatment seeking anorexics and bulimics. J Am Acad Child Adolesc Psychiatry 1992;31:810–818.
26. McElroy SL, Keck PE, Pope HG, Hudson JI. Pharmacological treatment of kleptomania and bulimia nervosa. J Clin Psychopharmacol 1989;9:358–360.
27. Fichter MM, Quadfleig N. Six year course of bulimia nervosa. Int J Eat Disord 1997;22:361–384.
28. Bowers WA, Anderson AE. Initial treatment of anorexia nervosa: Review and recommendations. Harvard Rev Psychiatry 1994;2:193–203.

29. Kleifield EI, Wagner S, Halmi KA. Cognitive-behavioral treatment of anorexia nervosa. Psychiatr Clin North Am 1996;19:715–737.
30. Jimerson DC, Wolfe BE, Brotman AW, Metzger ED. Medication in the treatment of eating disorders. Psychiatr Clin North Am 1996;19:739–754.
31. Lacey JH, Crisp AH. Hunger, food intake and weight: The impact of clomipramine on refeeding an anorexia nervosa population. Postgrad Med J 1980;56:79–85.
32. Gwirtsman HE, Guze BH, Yager J, Gainsley B. Fluoxetine treatment of anorexia nervosa: An open clinical trial. J Clin Psychiatry 1990;51:378–382.
33. Kaye WH, Weltzin TE, Hsu G, Bulik CM. An open trial of fluoxetine in patients with anorexia nervosa. J Clin Psychiatry 1991;52:464–471.
34. Berg C, Eriksson M, Lindberg G, Sodersten P. Selective serotonin reuptake inhibitors in anorexia. Lancet 1996;348:1459–1450.
35. Dally PJ, Sargant W. A new treatment for anorexia nervosa. Br Med J 1960;1:1770–1773.
36. Saleh JW, Lebwohl SF. Metoclopramide-induced gastric emptying in patients with anorexia nervosa. Am J Gastroenterol 1980;74:127–132.
37. Stacher G, Abatzi-Wentzel TA, Wiesnagrotzki S, et al. Gastric emptying, body weight, and symptoms in primary anorexia nervosa: Long-term effects of cisapride. Br J Psychiatry 1993;162:398–402.
38. Bachrach LK, Guido D, Katzman DK, et al. Decreased bone density in adolescent girls with anorexia nervosa. Pediatrics 190;86:40–447.
39. Treasure JL, Russell GF, Fogelman I, Murphy B. Reversible bone loss in anorexia nervosa. Br Med J (Clin Res Ed) 1987;295:474–475.
40. Cox GL, Merkel WT. A qualitative review of psychosocial treatments for bulimia. J Nerv Ment Dis 1989;177:77–83.
41. Fairburn CG, Jones R, Peveler RC, et al. Psychotherapy and bulimia nervosa: Longer-term effects of interpersonal therapy, behavior therapy and cognitive behavioral therapy. Arch Gen Psychiatry 1993;50:419–428.
42. Angras WS, Walsh BT, Fairburn CG, et al. A multicenter comparison of cognitive-behavioral therapy and interpersonal psychotherapy for bulimia nervosa. Arch Gen Psychiatry 2000;57:459–466.
43. Pope HG, Hudson JI, Jonas JM, Yurgelun-Todd D. Bulimia treated with imipramine: A placebo-controlled, double-blind study. Am J Psychiatry 1983;140:554–558.
44. Pope HG, Hudson JI, Jonas JM, Yurgelun-Todd D. Antidepressant treatment of bulimia: A two-year follow-up study. J Clin Psychopharmacol 1985;5:320–327.
45. Mitchell JE, Pyle RL, Eckert ED, Hatsakami D, et al. Response to alternative antidepressants in imipramine nonresponders. J Clin Psychopharmacol 1989;9:291–293.
46. Barlow J, Blouin J, Blouin A, Perez E. Treatment of bulimia with desipramine: A double-blind crossover study. Can J Psychiatry 1988;33:129–133.
47. Hughes PL, Wells LA, Cunningham CJ, Ilstrup DM. Treating bulimia with desipramine: A double-blind, placebo controlled trial. Arch Gen Psychiatry 1986;43:182–186.
48. McCann UD, Angras WS. Successful treatment of nonpurging bulimia nervosa with desipramine: A double-blind, placebo-controlled study. Am J Psychiatry 1990;147:1509–1513.
49. Walsh BT, Gladis M, Roose SP, et al. Phenelzine vs placebo in 50 patients with bulimia. Arch Gen Psychiatry 1988;45:471–475.
50. Pope HG, Keck PE, McElroy SL, Hudson JI. A placebo-controlled study of trazodone in bulimia nervosa. J Clin Psychopharmacol 1989;9:254–259.
51. Fluoxetine Bulimia Nervosa Collaborative Study Group. Fluoxetine in the treatment of bulimia nervosa: A multicenter, placebo-controlled, double-blind trial. Arch Gen Psychiatry 1992;49:139–147.
52. Goldstein DJ, Wilson MG, Thompson VL, et al. Long-term fluoxetine treatment of bulimia nervosa. Br J Psychiatry 1995;166:660–666.
53. Fitcher MM, Kruger R, Rief W, et al. Fluvoxamine in prevention of relapse in bulimia nervosa: Effects on eating-specific psychopathology. J Clin Psychopharmacol 1996;16:9–18.
54. Betts TA, Kabra PL, Cooper R, Jeavons DM. Epileptic fits as a probable side effect of amitriptyline. Lancet 1968;1:390–392.
55. McElroy SL, Casuto, LS, Nelson EB, et al. Placebo-controlled trial of sertraline in the treatment of binge eating disorder. Am J Psychiatry 2000;157:1004–1006.
56. Hudson J, McElroy SL, Raymond NC, et al. Fluvoxamine in the treatment of binge eating disorder: A multicenter, placebo-controlled, double-blind trial. Am J Psychiatry 1998;155:1756–1762.
57. Green RS, Rau JH. Treatment of compulsive eating disorders with anticonvulsant medication. Am J Psychiatry 1974;131:428–432.
58. Wermuth BM, Davis KL, Hollister LE, Stunkard AJ. Phenytoin treatment of binge eating syndrome. Am J Psychiatry 1977;136:1249–1253.
59. Kaplan AS, Garfinkel PE, Darby PL, Garner DM. Carbamazepine in the treatment of bulimia. Am J Psychiatry 1983;140:1225–1226.
60. Herridge PL, Pope HG. Treatment of bulimia and rapid cycling bipolar disorder with sodium valproate: A case report. J Clin Psychopharmacol 1985;5:229–230.
61. Hsu LKG, Clement L, Santhouse R. Treatment of bulimia with lithium: A preliminary study. Psychopharmacol Bull 1987;2:45–48.
62. Mitchell JE, Pyle RL, Eckert ED, et al. A comparison study of antidepressants, structured interview and group psychotherapy in the treatment of bulimia nervosa. Arch Gen Psychiatry 1990;47:149–157.
63. Angras WS, Rossiter EM, Arnow B, et al. Pharmacological and cognitive-behavioral treatment for bulimia nervosa: A controlled comparison. Am J Psychiatry 1992;149:82–87.
64. Walsh BT, Wilson GT, Loeb KL, et al. Medication and psychotherapy in the treatment of bulimia nervosa. Am J Psychiatry 1997;154:523–531.
65. Crow SJ, Mitchell JE. Integrating cognitive therapy and medications in bulimia nervosa. Psychiatr Clin North Am 1996;19:755–760.
66. Solyom L, Solyom C, Ledwidge B. The fluoxetine treatment of low-weight chronic bulimia nervosa. J Clin Psychopharmacol 1990;10:421–425.
67. Wilcox JA. Abuse of fluoxetine by a patient with anorexia nervosa. Am J Psychiatry 1987;144:1100.

65

ALZHEIMER'S DISEASE

Jennifer L. Defilippi, M. Lynn Crismon, and William R. Clark

I now begin the journey that will lead me into the sunset of my life.

Ronald Reagan

Alzheimer's disease (AD), first characterized by Alois Alzheimer in 1907, is a gradually progressive dementia affecting both cognition and behavior. The exact pathophysiologic mechanisms underlying AD are not entirely known, and no cure exists.[1] Although drugs may reduce Alzheimer's symptoms for a time, the disease is eventually fatal. This disease profoundly affects the family as well as the patient. A person with AD eventually loses his or her very identity, not just memories, but all associated cognitive, analytical, and physical functioning.[1] Persons with AD experience something akin to traveling through a time warp, dropped into a foreign universe in which they no longer know how to function. They gradually lose sense of time, date, or year, and become unable to operate simple appliances. Simple day-to-day activities such as paying bills, mailing letters, and grocery shopping become beyond their capabilities. Language skills are lost, beginning with the ability to remember less commonly used words and names, and progressing over time to total loss of speech. Calculation of simple figures becomes impossible, such as how much change to expect when paying for a $4 item with a $5 bill. Behavioral problems emerge, and the personality slowly erodes. Men and women with AD slowly become strangers in their own environments, increasingly unable to recognize their homes, neighborhoods, friends, or family members. Personality, memory, and functional ability fade away until the person becomes essentially like a small child, robbed of the ability to dress, feed, bathe, or even use the bathroom without help. The need for supervision and assistance increases until the late stages of the disease, when Alzheimer's sufferers become totally dependent on a family member, spouse, or other caregiver for all of their basic needs. These are all experiences of the more than 4 million people in the United States who have AD.[1]

In the *Diagnostic and Statistical Manual for Mental Disorders,* 4th edition, Text Revised (DSM-IV-TR),[2] AD is classified under the heading of Delirium, Dementia, and Amnestic and Other Disorders. Dementias are neuropsychiatric disorders defined by widespread symptoms of memory loss and deficits in cognition and reasoning. Dementia is a nonspecific term describing a significant decline in cognitive function, regardless of cause. Dementias, synonymous with the popular lay term "senility," result from underlying disease, and are not part of normal aging. Delirium differs from dementia in that it develops over a short period of time (hours to days), and involves an acute change in the level of consciousness in addition to a decline in cognition. Because the severity, prognosis, and treatment of dementia depends almost entirely on the underlying cause, an accurate diagnosis is essential.

EPIDEMIOLOGY

AD is the most common cause of dementia, accounting for over 60% of all cases of late-life cognitive dysfunction[1] and Table 65–1 lists etiology-based subclasses of dementia. This chapter focuses exclusively on dementia of the Alzheimer's type. However, the reader is encouraged to use the nonspecific treatment portions of this chapter to assist in management of noncognitive behavioral problems associated with other forms of dementia.

AD is generally thought of as a disease of old age, because most cases present in persons older than age 65, but in about 5% of cases onset can be as early as age 40, resulting in the arbitrary age classifications of early onset (ages 40 to 64 years) and late-onset ($\geq$ age 65 years) disease.[3] Studies using standardized diagnostic criteria, gathered by actual patient evaluation, and not limited to institutionalized populations are thought to provide the best estimates of prevalence. One such study found an overall disease prevalence of 10.3% in a large community sample of persons older than age 65 years.[4] Both the prevalence and the incidence of AD increase exponentially with age, affecting approximately 3% (incidence, $\approx$1%) of individuals aged 65 to 74 years, and rising dramatically to 47% (incidence, $\approx$8.4%) of persons aged 85 years and older.[4–7] AD affects two times as many women as men, and although genetic inheritance is the primary mode of transmission, several environmental factors may contribute. Factors determining age of onset and rate of progression remain largely undefined. AD is the fourth leading cause of death in US elderly persons.[8] This is somewhat of a misrepresentation, as AD does not cause death directly, but indirectly by predisposing patients to sepsis, pneumonia, choking and aspiration, nutritional deficiencies, and trauma.[8] Severe cognitive impairment and cachexia worsen the prognosis.[9] Approximately 100,000 individuals with AD die every year. As most individuals with Alzheimer's do not seek medical attention early in the illness, it is difficult to estimate survival time after onset. Survival following AD onset is estimated to be 3 to 20 years. However, in a recent Canadian study among a largely elderly cohort, the adjusted median life expectancy after physician diagnosis was 3.3 years.[10]

The economic and social costs of AD are staggering. It is the third most expensive illness in the United States after heart disease and cancer. However, much of the cost of caring for these patients is left to their families. The total national cost of Alzheimer's disease is estimated at approximately $100 billion annually.[11] To put these numbers in perspective, in 1991, the estimated medical cost of acquired immunodeficiency syndrome (AIDS) was $4.2 billion. The Medicaid costs alone for institutionalized AD patients was estimated at $5.7 billion.[12]

The average life expectancy in 1900 was 47 years. Few people lived long enough to experience the onset of AD. Life expectancy is now 75 years; 4 million people are afflicted with AD, and 250,000 more cases are diagnosed annually.[12,13] By the year 2050, one of five people will be over age 65 years, and the number of Alzheimer's patients is projected at 14 million (Fig. 65–1). AD has become a major public health concern, yet in comparison to other major illnesses such as AIDS, heart disease, and cancer, it has received relatively little attention. The potential financial burden of this disease on the health care system could reach crisis proportions unless more effective avenues are developed to provide care for these individuals, to prevent the disease from occurring, or to slow its progress.

TABLE 65–1. Classification of Dementia

- Dementia of the Alzheimer's type
- Vascular dementia (formerly multi-infarct dementia)
- Dementia as a consequence of HIV disease
- Dementia as a consequence of head trauma
- Dementia as a consequence of Lewy body disease
- Dementia as a consequence of normal-pressure hydrocephalus
- Dementia as a consequence of idiopathic Parkinson's disease
- Dementia as a consequence of cortico-basal ganglionic degeneration (CBGD)
- Dementia as a consequence of progressive supranuclear palsy (PSP)
- Dementia as a consequence of Huntington's disease
- Dementia as a consequence of Pick's disease
- Dementia as a consequence of Creutzfeldt-Jakob disease
- Dementia as a consequence of other general medical disorders (indicate disorder, e.g., B_{12} deficiency, hypothyroidism)
- Substance-induced persisting dementia (persistent dementia resulting from exposure to toxins, drugs of abuse or medications)
- Dementia as a consequence of multiple etiologies
- Dementia not otherwise specified (reserved for dementia that cannot be attributed to any other subtype)

Adapted from Refs. 2, 3, and 38.

ETIOLOGY

The exact etiology of AD is unknown. Genetic, environmental, and infectious etiologies have been explored as potential causes of AD.

GENETICS

Genetic factors have been investigated in both early onset and late-occurring Alzheimer's disease. Almost all early onset cases of AD can be attributed to alterations on chromosome 1, 14, or 21. Approximately 5% of the cases of AD are early onset.[14] The majority and most aggressive early onset cases are attributed to mutations of an Alzheimer's gene located on chromosome 14, which produces a protein called presenilin 1.[15] Similar in structure to presenilin 1 is a protein produced by a gene on chromosome 1 called presenilin 2. Presenilin 2 is responsible for early onset AD in a family of Germans living in Russia's Volga Valley.[14] Both presenilin 1 and presenilin 2 encode for membrane proteins that may be involved in amyloid precursor protein (APP) processing. It has been suggested, but not proven, either that presenilins actually are γ-secretase or that presenilins affect γ-secretase activity.[15] As a group, presenilins account for approximately 50% of all early onset AD cases.

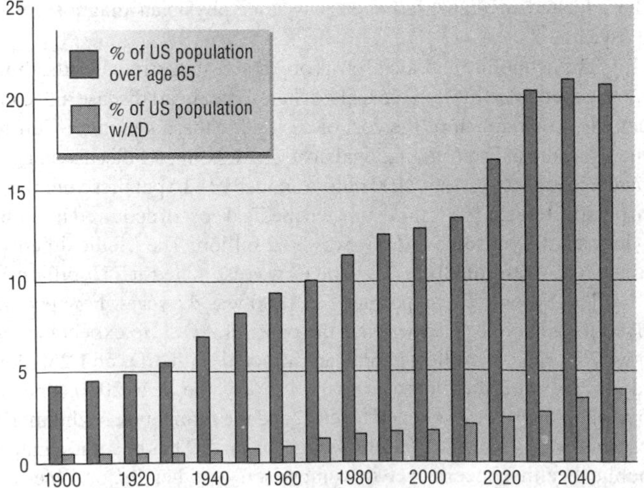

FIGURE 65–1. Our aging population: Increasing percentage of total US population over age 65 years and estimated percent with AD from the year 1900 projected to the year 2050. Estimates based on data from references 4 and 12.

APP is encoded on chromosome 21. Only a small number of early onset, familial AD cases have been associated with mutations in the APP gene, resulting in overproduction of β-amyloid protein (βAP).[14,15]

Genetic susceptibility to late-onset AD is thought to be primarily influenced by the apolipoprotein E (apo E) genotype. The gene responsible for the production of apo E is located on chromosome 19 in a region previously associated with late-onset AD. Three major subtypes or alleles of apo E occur, and are termed apo E2, apo E3, and apo E4.[14,15] Humans inherit one copy of the apo E gene from each parent. Apo E3 is the most common type, occurring in 40% to 90% of the population, with apo E2 and apo E4 occurring less frequently.[15] However, rather than being causative, the apo E4 allele is a risk factor for development of AD.

Inheritance of the apo E4 isoform increases risk for late-onset AD; however, the degree of risk depends on such factors as number of apo E4 copies, age, ethnicity, and gender.[15,16] Overall, about 40% of patients with late onset AD have at least one copy of apo E4. Individuals homozygous for apo E4 are at increased risk, and as many as 90% of persons inheriting two copies of apo E4 will develop AD by age 80 years. Moreover, onset of symptoms occurs at a relatively younger age as compared to patients having no or only one copy of apo E4 in their genotype.[15,16] In whites, inheriting a single copy of apo E4 increases AD risk, whereas inheriting the apo E2 allele protects against AD.[15,17] However, this may not be true in African Americans. Differences also exist with regard to gender; inheriting one copy of apo E4 increases risk in females more than in males.

Although inheritance of the apo E4 allele increases the risk of AD, it is not diagnostic or even essential for disease presence. AD occurs in persons with no copies of apo E4, and the apo E4 genotype is also more common in other dementias involving abnormal tau protein such as Pick's disease and progressive supranuclear palsy.[18] Not all persons with two alleles of apo E4 develop AD. If a person homozygous for apo E4 does not develop AD by age 80 years, it is unlikely to occur.

Lastly, a mutation in the tau gene on chromosome 17 is associated with an abnormality in tau protein and development of the rare frontotemporal dementia.[15]

ENVIRONMENTAL FACTORS

A number of environmental factors have been associated with increased risk of AD, including stroke, alcohol abuse, small head circumference, repeated or severe head trauma, and lower levels of education.[45] In particular, traumatic head injury in combination with the apo E4 genotype has been associated with an increased risk of AD.[19]

PATHOPHYSIOLOGY

STRUCTURAL CHANGES

AD is defined by both neuropathologic and clinical criteria. Neuropathologically, AD destroys neurons in the cortex and limbic structures of the brain, particularly the basal forebrain, amygdala, hippocampus, and cerebral cortex. These areas are responsible for higher learning, memory, reasoning, behavior, and emotional control. Anatomically, four major alterations in brain structure are seen: cortical atrophy; degeneration of cholinergic and other neurons; presence of neurofibrillary tangles (NFTs); and the accumulation of neuritic plaques.[1,15,18] Neurofibrillary tangles and neuritic plaques are considered the signature lesions of AD; without them, AD does not occur. But plaques and tangles may also be present in other diseases and even in normal aging. To understand the causes of AD, researchers must discern the circumstances in which these lesions lead to the clinical picture of AD.[19]

NFTs are comprised of paired helical filaments that aggregate in dense bundles, appearing microscopically like tiny flames filling the neuronal cell body. Paired helical filaments are formed from tau protein. Tau protein provides structural support to microtubules, the cell's transportation and skeletal support system.[15,19] When tau filaments undergo abnormal phosphorylation at a specific site, they cannot bind effectively to microtubules, and the microtubules collapse. Without an intact system of microtubules, the cell cannot function properly and eventually dies.[19] Overactivity of kinases such as microtubule affinity-regulating kinase (MARK), or underactivity of phosphatases could theoretically produce or prevent breakdown of abnormally phosphorylated tau protein.[15,19] NFTs are found in other dementing illnesses besides AD, and may represent a common method by which various inciting factors culminate in cell death.[15]

Neuritic plaques (also termed amyloid or senile plaques) are extracellular lesions found in the brain and cerebral vasculature (amyloid angiopathy). Plaques are comprised of βAP, and an entwined mass of broken neurites (axon and dendrite projections of neurons).[1,15,19] Many of these broken neurites contain neuropil filaments made up of the abnormally phosphorylated tau protein found in NFTs.[15,19] Two types of glial cells, astrocytes and microglia, are also found in plaques.[1,15,19] Among other functions, glial cells secrete inflammatory mediators and serve as scavenger cells, which may be important in considering inflammatory processes in of AD. While the number of NFTs are strongly correlated with the severity of dementia, the number of neuritic plaques are not.[15] Clinical development of AD may correlate inversely with the number of normal neurons and synapses remaining despite plaque presence,[15,18,19] thus introducing the concept of neurologic reserve.

Forming the center of the neuritic plaque are aggregates of a 39- to 43-amino acid protein segment called βAP.[15] The amyloidoses are a set of diseases marked by amyloid protein deposition in various target organs. The βAP accumulating in the brain and cerebral blood vessels in AD is different from other disease producing amyloid proteins.[15]

β-Amyloid protein is cleaved from the APP, a transmembrane protein.[1,15,19] Proteases cleave APP in several different ways (Fig. 65–2). In the normal secretory pathway APP is cleaved through the βAP region, first using an enzyme called α secretase, and then by an enzyme termed γ secretase. The resulting product, p3, is soluble and harmless.[15] In the potentially pathologic pathway, the endosomal pathway cleaves on both sides of βAP, first with β-secretase and

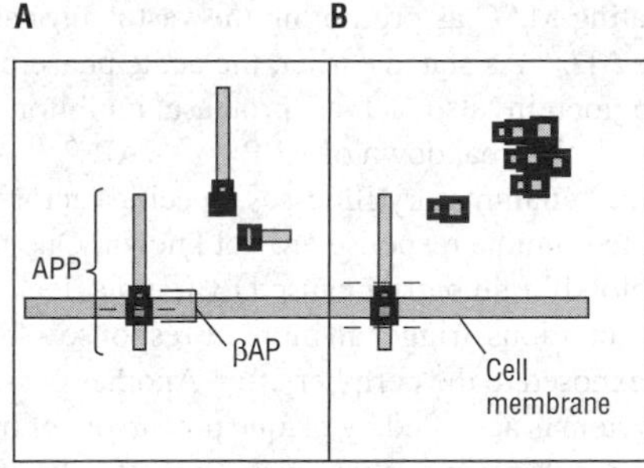

FIGURE 65–2. Representation of two physiologic cleavage sites of APP. APP is pictured as a transmembrane protein, with the βAP subunit anchored within the membrane. In section **A,** α secretase and then γ secretase cut APP through the βAP region. In section **B,** β secretase and then γ secretase cut βAP on either side of the βAP subunit. βAP is then released intact into the extracellular fluid, where it can aggregate, forming insoluble preamyloid plaques. *Adapted from Ref. 15 and 19.*

then with γ-secretase, resulting in the formation of βAP (Cpp-bAPP) to be released into the extracellular space.[15,19] Most of these βAP strings contain 40 amino acids, but it was recently determined that a version of βAP containing 42 amino acids damages nerve cells. Although it is not exactly known how βAP causes neuronal damage, it does cause dysregulation in calcium and damage to mitochondria.[15] In turn, this may trigger inflammatory mediators. Taken as a whole, these data suggest βAP deposition occurs early in the disease process, rather than being simply an end-product of neuronal death, and likely initiates the process of plaque formation and nerve cell destruction.

INFLAMMATORY MEDIATORS

Inflammatory mediators and other immune system constituents are present near areas of plaque formation, suggesting that the immune system plays an active role in the pathogenesis of AD. Although perhaps not the disease-initiating event, an immune response generated against some brain insult could facilitate neuronal destruction. Evidence supporting significant involvement of the immune system includes the increased presence of acute phase proteins, such as α_1-antichromotrypsin (ACT) and α_2-macroglobulin, both in the serum and within amyloid plaques of patients with AD.[20] Glial cells (microglial cells and astrocytes), cytokines (e.g., interleukin-1 and interleukin-6), and components of the classic complement cascade are also markedly increased in plaque-infested areas.[20] These inflammatory mediators increase βAP toxicity and aggregation. Chronic production of cytotoxic agents and free radicals by activated microglia can result in accelerated neurodegeneration.

Epidemiologic studies suggest that patients who take nonsteroidal anti-inflammatory drugs (NSAIDs) have a lower risk of developing AD. However, present data are insufficient to determine how long, at what dose, or at what point prior to the development of AD symptoms a person must take NSAIDs to achieve the greatest therapeutic benefit. At this point, it is too early to recommend that all patients with AD take NSAIDs, and more details must be known before NSAIDs can be recommended to prevent AD.

Microglial cells located around and within amyloid plaques are thought to release inflammatory mediators, which locally destroy neuronal tissue. Glial cells also function as phagocytes, similar to macrophages and monocytes in the periphery. Another component of the complement cascade, the membrane attack complex (MAC), is found associated with broken neurites and areas containing

NFTs, implicating MAC as promoting the vast neuronal destruction characterizing AD.[20] As stated earlier, the acute phase proteins ACT and α_2-macroglobulin also act as protease inhibitors, and could influence proteolytic breakdown of APP into βAP.[15,20] As is the case in many chronic inflammatory illnesses, specific factors responsible for initiating the immune response are not known. One theory is that breaks in the blood-brain barrier caused by trauma, leaky endothelial cells, or other conditions, trigger an immune response to brain proteins previously unexposed to the periphery.[20,21] Another possibility is that the immune system is activated by plaque precursors or byproducts of damaged cells, resulting in further destruction of adjacent neurons.[21]

THE CHOLINERGIC SYSTEM

Multiple neuronal pathways are destroyed in AD. Damage occurs in any nerve cell population located in or traveling through plaque-laden areas.[15] Widespread cell destruction results in a variety of neurotransmitter deficits. Most profoundly damaged are the cholinergic pathways, particularly a large system of neurons located at the base of the forebrain in the nucleus basalis of Mynert, a brain area believed to be involved in thought integration.[1,15] Axons of these cholinergic neurons project to the frontal cortex and hippocampus, areas strongly associated with memory and cognition.

The discovery of vast cholinergic cell loss led to the development of a cholinergic hypothesis. The cholinergic hypothesis targeted cholinergic cell loss as the source of memory and cognitive impairment in AD. Therefore, it was presumed that increasing cholinergic function would improve symptoms of memory loss, much the same way that dopamine replacement improves tremor and rigidity in Parkinson's disease. This approach is flawed for two reasons. First, cholinergic cell loss appears to be a secondary consequence of Alzheimer's pathology, not the disease-producing event; second, cholinergic neurons are only one of many neuronal pathways destroyed in AD. Simple addition of acetylcholine cannot compensate for the loss of neurons, receptors, and other neurotransmitters consumed during the course of the illness. Enhancing cholinergic activity no more cures AD than dopamine replacement cures Parkinson's disease.[22] The principle is the same, however: to minimize or improve dementia symptoms through augmentation of cholinergic transmission at remaining synapses.

An additional theoretical rationale for the use of cholinesterase inhibitors in AD is the fact that acetylcholinesterase, perhaps butylcholinesterase, is thought to play a role in plaque development.[19]

OTHER NEUROTRANSMITTER ABNORMALITIES

Although the cholinergic system has received a lion's share of attention in AD pharmaceutical research, deficits exist in other neuronal pathways as well. Serotonergic neurons of the raphe nuclei and noradrenergic cells of the locus ceruleus are also lost, while monoamine oxidase type B (MAO-B) activity is increased. MAO-B is found predominately in the brain and in platelets, and is responsible for metabolizing dopamine. The presence of increased MAO-B concentrations may seem counterintuitive considering the vast neuronal loss in AD, unless one considers that MAO-B is also contained in glial cells whose populations are increased. Increased platelet and brain MAO-B concentrations are also seen in Parkinson's disease, but not multi-infarct dementia.[15,23] Other abnormalities appear in glutamate pathways of the cortex and limbic structures, where a loss of neurons leads to a focus on excitotoxicity models as possible contributing factors to AD pathology.

Glutamate is a major excitatory neurotransmitter in the cortex and hippocampus. Many neuronal pathways essential to learning and memory use glutamate as a neurotransmitter, including the pyramidal neurons (a layer of neurons with long axons carrying information out of the cortex), hippocampus, and entorhinal cortex. Glutamate and other excitatory amino acid neurotransmitters have been implicated as potential neurotoxins in AD.[24,25] If glutamate is allowed to remain in the synapse for extended periods of time, it can act as a toxin, destroying nerve cells. Toxic effects are thought to be mediated through increased intracellular calcium and accumulation of free radicals.[1,24,25] The presence of βAP renders cells more susceptible to glutamate-mediated excitotoxicity *in vitro*. Dysregulated glutamate activity is thought to be one of the primary mediators of neuronal injury after stroke or acute brain injury. Although intimately involved in cell injury, the role of excitatory amino acids in AD is as yet unclear.

ESTROGEN

Estrogen is thought to be involved in promoting neuronal growth, and in preventing oxidative damage, which would benefit cells exposed to β-amyloid.[26] Estrogen receptors are present in the brain, and are distributed in a pattern consistent with areas destroyed in AD.[27,28] In the hippocampus, cerebral cortex, and basal forebrain, estrogen receptors colocalize with receptors for nerve growth factor on cholinergic nerve terminals.[28,29] The presence of estrogen increases the number of nerve growth factor receptors. The ability of estrogen to interact with nerve growth factor may explain estrogen's ability to promote synaptic growth, stimulating axons and dendrites to sprout new terminals. Estrogen supplementation also prevents decrements in choline uptake and choline acetyltransferase (ChAT) concentrations, occurring in rats following ovariectomy. This suggests estrogen is important in maintaining normal cholinergic neurotransmission.[28] Estrogen may also increase *N*-methyl-D-aspartate (NMDA) receptor numbers in brain areas involved in recording new memory. In addition to promoting growth, estrogen prevents cell damage. Estrogen acts as an antioxidant.[26] In culture, estrogen protects hippocampal neurons exposed to glutamate and β-amyloid from cytotoxic and free radical damage. Progesterone[26] was also effective in preventing cell damage, but less effective than estrogen in specifically preventing damage following exposure to βAP. Estrogen may prevent formation of neuritic plaques by facilitating preferential degradation of APP by α-secretase into soluble products, as opposed to β-secretase, which is potentially amyloidogenic.[27]

In addition to the *in vitro* experiments summarized above, conflicting data exist regarding the risk of AD in women who take estrogen replacement therapy (ERT).[30] While several epidemiologic studies have shown a lower risk of AD in women who take ERT, other well-controlled cohort studies have not.[31] The potential role of estrogen in the etiology or prevention of AD remains to be elucidated.

A single common mechanism for producing AD does not exist. Regardless of the source, however, the features remain the same: degeneration of neurons in higher brain areas; accumulation of NFTs and neuritic plaques; profound destruction of cholinergic pathways; and an insidious dementia, slowly progressive until death.

CLINICAL PRESENTATION

The onset of AD is almost imperceptible, without abrupt changes in cognition or function. Deficits occur progressively over time and are global, affecting multiple areas of cognition.[1,32,33] For treatment

TABLE 65–2. Fundamental Symptom Categories in Alzheimer's Disease

Cognitive Deficits[a]	Noncognitive Psychiatric Symptoms and Disruptive Behavior[b]
• Memory Loss *Poor recall; agnosia; losing items* • Dysphasia *Anomia; circumlocution; aphasia* • Dyspraxia • Disorientation *Impaired perception of time; direction; cannot recognize acquaintances, family, or self* • Impaired calculation • Impaired judgment and problem solving skills	• Depression • Psychotic Symptoms *Hallucinations; delusions; suspiciousness* • Nonpsychotic Disruptive Behaviors *Physical and verbal aggression; motor hyperactivity; uncooperativeness; wandering; repetitive mannerisms/activities; combativeness*

[a] Cognitive deficits: symptoms occurring in all patients as disease progresses
[b]Noncognitive symptoms: symptoms that are variably present, consisting mainly of psychiatric and behavioral problems
Compiled from Ref. 34.

and assessment purposes, it is helpful to divide Alzheimer's symptoms into two basic categories: cognitive symptoms and noncognitive (behavioral) symptoms (Table 65–2).[33] Cognitive symptoms are present throughout the illness, whereas behavioral symptoms are less predictable.[33]

Loss of memory is typically the presenting patient complaint, and is frequently brought to the clinician's attention by a family member. Memory is a nonspecific term representing many diverse areas of cognitive function (e.g., recall, recognition, calculation, and orientation). Crucial to understanding the plight of persons with AD is to understand that "loss of memory" means the inability to extract and use all previously learned information, activity, and experience. Patients' initial complaints of "memory loss" typically refer to disorientation for time or an inability to recall recent events. In early AD, the ability to lay down new memory (learn) and to recall recent events is impaired, whereas recall for remote events (childhood/adolescent years) is spared until later in the disease process. Common early problems include forgetting appointments, misplacing items such as keys, getting lost traveling to familiar locations, and difficulties handling money or balancing a checkbook. Patients may notice an increasing need for lists, problems recalling the date or day of the week, and difficulty performing routine tasks at home or work. Anomia is a problem, with difficulty recalling names of familiar objects or people. Speech becomes difficult as details and content words are lost, and patients resort to confabulation or circumlocution (nonspecific, evasive speech) to compensate for their deficits. Problems with speech, recall of events, and comprehension result in decreased socialization and withdrawal from casual conversation.

Persons with AD often conceal their memory problem well at first, and may deny or "forget" that they have a memory problem. Common symptoms of moderate dementia include the inability to use objects (apraxia); loss of the ability to draw complex figures or to conceptualize their orientation in space (constructional apraxia); inability to identify common objects (agnosia); inability to work or do routine household chores; forgetting to eat or to change clothes; disorientation to place; and difficulty initiating activities. Patients also become unable to determine the appropriate time of day for accomplishing activities and are generally unable to plan or independently follow a daily schedule. As dementia progresses, patients may become lost in their own homes, unable to recognize family or spouses, and unable to speak (aphasia). Judgment and reasoning are extremely impaired, and without supervision, patients may burn themselves on appliances, leave water running, wander outside and become lost, or engage in other dangerous activities. Wandering, combativeness, and incontinence are common reasons for placement in a long-term care facility. In the final stages of the disease, patients lose the ability to eat, walk, or communicate. Choking, aspiration, or infection generally results in death within 3 to 20 years of disease onset.

Noncognitive symptoms, such as mood disturbances, changes in personality, disruptive behavior, and psychosis, are present at one time or another in most patients and can pose significant management problems for caregivers. Patients frequently experience "sundowning," or worsening of symptoms at night because of decreased sensory input and fewer orienting stimuli. Early in the course of the illness, the patient may become depressed, frustrated, or irritable. Anxiety, hostility, misinterpretations, and delusions are common in the moderate stage of AD. Disruptive behavior and psychosis are most often seen in the moderate to severe stages of AD, with severity fluctuating over time.

Common disruptive behaviors include wandering, agitation, aggression, resistance to care, and purposeless activity. Suspiciousness, nonsystematized paranoid delusions, and misinterpretation of actual phenomena (illusions) are the most common psychotic symptoms in demented patients. Delusions in AD more often appear to be an attempt to explain things that have been forgotten. Other delusions may stem from an inability to recognize friends and family members, combined with preferential loss of recent memories. As a consequence of these phenomena, the patient may become agitated, physically or verbally aggressive, or attempt to leave the residence in search of missing persons or to "go home."[34]

Persons with AD become extraordinarily dependent on those around them. Family and direct caregivers may experience considerable psychological distress through role changes, time commitments, cost, and the hassles of day-to-day care. It is extremely difficult for caregivers to cope with the transformation of someone from an able-bodied companion or parent to a dependent stranger. Any attempts at therapeutic management must take into account the effect of treatment on the caregiver, both with respect to cost and ease of use versus expected therapeutic gain.

DIAGNOSIS

Minor memory loss, sometimes called age-associated memory impairment, is a common complaint associated with normal aging and is not a cause for concern. However, if memory loss affects social or occupational functioning, or is noticed by friends and coworkers, patients should be encouraged to visit a neurologist for a formal evaluation. At present, the only way to definitively diagnose AD is through direct examination of brain tissue at autopsy or biopsy. Great interest exists in screening patients for early recognition of AD. To date, there is no tool available for screening, and the best approach to successful treatment is with early recognition.[35] Because no definitive diagnostic laboratory, clinical, or imaging tests are available, AD remains a diagnosis of exclusion, although there is growing consensus that it should be a diagnosis of inclusion. To design criteria that would minimize inaccurate diagnoses, a workgroup was established, in 1984, by the National Institute of Neurological and Communicative Disorders and Stroke (NINCDS) and the Alzheimer's Disease and Related Disorders Association (ADRDA). Use of the workgroup's explicit criteria has reduced the percentage of erroneously diagnosed AD cases to

TABLE 65–3. NINCDS-ADRDA Criteria and Diagnostic Workup for Probable Alzheimer's Disease

I. History of progressive cognitive decline of insidious onset
- In-depth interview of patient and caregivers

II. Deficits in at least two or more areas of functioning

III. No disturbance of consciousness
- Confirmation with use of dementia rating scale (e.g., Mini-Mental Status Exam [MMSE*] or Blessed Dementia Scale)

IV. Age between 40 and 90 years (usually >65 years)

V. No other explainable cause of symptoms
- Normal laboratory tests including hematology, full chemistries, B_{12} and folate, thyroid function tests, VDRL (to rule out venereal disease or syphilis)
- Normal electrocardiogram and electroencephalogram
- Normal physical exam, including thorough neurological exam
- Neuroimaging: CT or MRI scanning: No focal lesions signifying other possible causes of dementia are present. Abnormalities which are common, but not diagnostic for AD include general cerebral wasting, widening of sulci, widening of the ventricles, and lesions of white matter surrounding the ventricle deep in the brain

*The Folstein Mini-Mental Status Exam[40] is a commonly used scale that measures orientation, recall, short-term memory, concentration, constructional praxis, and language. The MMSE is scored from 0 to 30, with a score of 10 to ~28 typical of very early to moderate Alzheimer's disease.
Adapted from Ref. 36.

less than 10%, and the NINCDS-ADRDA criteria (Table 65–3) are the standard.[36] Patient's fulfilling these criteria are given a diagnosis of probable AD. The Agency for Health Care Research and Quality has also published guidelines for the recognition and assessment of AD that are useful tools in the primary care setting.[37]

Evaluation of a patient with suspected Alzheimer's disease should include a history and physical exam with appropriate laboratory tests, neurologic and psychiatric exams, standardized rating assessments, functional evaluation, a caregiver interview, and possibly neuroimaging scans. The history should be obtained from the patient and reliable caregivers, and should confirm a slowly progressive, but not precipitous, deterioration in cognition. Information regarding prescription drug use, history of alcohol or other substance use, family medical history, and history of trauma, depression, or head injury should be obtained. It is important to rule out medication use as contributing to dementia symptoms, especially medications with anticholinergic or other central nervous system side effects.

Routine laboratory tests and physical, psychiatric, and neurologic exams should rule out other disorders including other neurologic causes of dementia, pseudodementia related to a mood disorder, long-standing substance abuse, and medical conditions such as hypothyroidism and vitamin B_{12} deficiency. Imaging tools help rule out multi-infarct dementia or tumors, and although atrophy ventricular dilatation or other nonspecific abnormalities are often seen on computed tomography (CT) scans or magnetic resonance imaging (MRI), these alone are insufficient to confer an AD diagnosis. Positron emission tomography (PET) and single-photon emission computed tomography (SPECT) have been suggested as potential diagnostic tools for AD, but at present they remain research probes.[38,39]

An established dementia screening scale, such as the Folstein Mini-Mental Status Exam (MMSE),[40] can aid in confirming a history of deficits in two or more areas of cognition and establish a baseline to evaluate change in severity.[36,40] The average expected decline in MMSE score in an untreated patient is two to four points per year.[41] Thorough neuropsychological testing is generally unnecessary, but it may be helpful if a diagnosis of dementia is in doubt.[38,39] Following diagnosis, AD is staged using a scale such as the Global Deterioration Scale (GDS) (Table 65–4).[42] This seven-point system is widely used, has been validated as correlating to psychometric measures and changes in CT or PET scans, and is useful to monitor the

TABLE 65–4. Stages of Cognitive Decline: The Global Deterioration Scale (GDS)

Stage		Description
Stage 1	Normal	No subjective or objective change in intellectual functioning.
Stage 2	Forgetfulness	Complaints of losing things or forgetting names of acquaintances. Does not interfere with job or social functioning. Generally a component of normal aging.
Stage 3	Early confusion	Cognitive decline causes interference with work and social functioning. Anomia, difficulty remembering right word in conversation, and recall difficulties are present and noticed by family members. Memory loss may cause anxiety for patient.
Stage 4	Late confusion (early AD)	Patient can no longer manage finances or homemaking activities. Difficulty remembering recent events. Begins to withdraw from difficult tasks and to give up hobbies. May deny memory problems.
Stage 5	Early dementia (moderate AD)	Patient can no longer survive without assistance. Frequently disoriented with regard to time (date, year, season). Difficulty selecting clothing. Recall for recent events is severely impaired; may forget some details of past life (e.g., school attended or occupation). Functioning may fluctuate from day to day. Patient generally denies problems. May become suspicious or tearful. Loses ability to drive safely.
Stage 6	Middle dementia (moderately severe AD)	Patients need assistance with activities of daily living (e.g., bathing, dressing, and toileting). Patients experience difficulty interpreting their surroundings; may forget names of family and caregivers; forget most details of past life; have difficulty counting backward from 10. Agitation, paranoia, and delusions are common.
Stage 7	Late dementia	Patient loses ability to speak (may only grunt or scream), walk, and feed self. Incontinent of urine and feces. Consciousness reduced to stupor or coma.

Adapted from Ref. 42.

global changes in the patient with AD. Functional assessment can be obtained from the patient and caregiver using the Functional Activities Questionnaire (FAQ).[43]

Genetic markers for Alzheimer's disease would be useful in identifying patients at risk for Alzheimer's disease. Although apo E4 is a risk factor for development of Alzheimer's disease, not all individuals with apo E4 develop AD, including some who are homozygous for the allele. Also, some patients with postmortem confirmed AD do not possess the apo E4 allele. Recently published epidemiologic studies and meta-analyses show that although the presence of the apo E4 allele increases the odds of having AD, genotyping of patients does not significantly improve diagnostic accuracy over clinical diagnosis based on established criteria.[44–47] Most epidemiologic studies have been conducted on largely white populations. Some evidence suggests that differences in ethnicity affect the association between the apo E4 allele and the risk of developing AD.[47,48] Because the data are inconclusive, apo E4 typing as a screening tool is not recommended. Better population-based estimates of risk are needed in order to provide appropriate genetic counseling.[14,39] Concern also exists regarding potential discrimination by insurance companies and employers toward individuals who possess one or more copies of apo E4.

As the course of Alzheimer's progresses, a sudden worsening in cognition may occur. While it is common to attribute this to a worsening in symptoms, diagnostic evaluation of delirium should be considered because the symptomatology is similar. Delirium is under-recognized and under-diagnosed. Estimates of the incidence of delirium range as high as 56% in hospitalized elderly patients with only 10% to 30% having symptoms upon admission.[49] Delirium can coexist or be superimposed upon dementia and can often confound the clinical picture of a confused elderly patient. As defined in the *DSM-IV-TR*, delirium is a disturbance of consciousness accompanied by a change in cognition that cannot be attributed to preexisting or evolving dementia.[2] Cognitive disturbance in the form of memory impairment, disorientation, and speech disturbances (e.g., anomia), as well as disorganized thinking, inability to focus or maintain attention, disturbed psychomotor activity, and abnormal sleep-wake cycle, are generally present in delirium as well as dementia. Hallucinations and illusions can also be present. Bizarre psychomotor behaviors can occur including both hyper- and hypoactivity.[49–51] The salient features that help to distinguish delirium from dementia are a reduced clarity of awareness of the environment, an abrupt onset, fluctuating course over time, and evidence of a direct physiologic cause.[2]

Delirium is usually reversible once the precipitating factor is addressed, but symptoms may persist for days or even weeks before complete resolution. Unfortunately, some patients experience permanent impairment, which may be a harbinger of new onset or worsening dementia.[49–51] A multitude of factors have been reported to cause delirium including metabolic disturbances (electrolyte imbalances or glucose fluctuations), infections, and recent addition or withdrawal of medication or alcohol.[2,49,51] Medications with anticholinergic properties are generally implicated in delirium and include well-known classes such as antiparkinson agents, many antipsychotic agents, tricyclic antidepressants, and sedating antihistamines. Additive effects from medications with low anticholinergic properties such as digoxin, furosemide, cimetidine, ranitidine, corticosteroids, and theophylline may also be a concern.[52] Antihypertensives, narcotics, sedative-hypnotics, and antibiotics have also been associated with cases of delirium.[50,51]

▶ TREATMENT: Alzheimer's Disease

DESIRED OUTCOMES

None of the current treatments for AD are curative or are known to directly reverse or halt the pathophysiologic processes of the disorder. Therefore, the primary goal of treatment in AD is to maintain patient function as long as possible. Secondary goals are aimed toward treating the psychiatric and behavioral sequelae that occur as a result of the disease.

GENERAL APPROACH TO TREATMENT

Treatment of AD must include both nonpharmacologic and pharmacologic approaches because this illness has a profound effect on the patient and the family. It is emphasized that nonmedication interventions are the current primary interventions for management of AD, and medications should be used in the context of multimodal interventions. Upon initial diagnosis, the patient and caregiver should be educated on the course of illness, available treatments, legal decisions, and quality of life issues. Communication between the patient and family members is essential in order to minimize stress on everyone. Current pharmacotherapeutic interventions for AD are for the most part symptomatic attempts to either improve or maintain cognition. However, there is some evidence that some interventions (e.g., cholinesterase inhibitors, vitamin E) may prolong the time to critical functional end points. Secondary pharmacotherapeutic interventions are aimed at treating depression, psychosis, and agitation in the Alzheimer's patient. No medications are available to change the course of illness or cure AD at this time.

NONPHARMACOLOGIC THERAPY

Nonpharmacologic treatment is a key component in treating AD. Once a patient has been given a diagnosis of AD, treatment should begin with education of the patient, and especially the family or other caregivers, regarding the disease, prognosis, and changes in lifestyle that are necessary as the disease progresses. Table 65–5 lists basic principles of care for the Alzheimer's patient. While encouraging as much

TABLE 65–5. Basic Principles of Care for the Alzheimer's Patient

- Keep requests and demands of the patient simple, and avoid complex tasks that might lead to frustration
- Avoid confrontation, and defer requests that lead to frustration
- Remain calm, firm, and supportive if the patient becomes upset
- Maintain a consistent environment and avoid unnecessary changes
- Provide frequent reminders, explanations, and orientation cues
- Recognize declines in capacity and adjust expectations for patient performance
- Bring sudden declines in function and the emergence of new symptoms to professional attention

Adapted from Ref. 38.

function and self-reliance as possible, the life for the Alzheimer's patients must become progressively more simple and structured in order to compensate for the deficits in cognition and to ensure safety. Education and guidance need to be provided regarding the patient's independence in conducting activities of daily living, including use of power tools, household repairs, cooking, and especially driving. Latches may need to be installed on doors and cabinets to prevent wandering or rummaging through household items. The patient will need frequent reminders in the beginning, and assistance later, with personal hygiene and other personal activities of daily living. A night-light and a bedside commode may help prevent confusion and wandering when the patient awakens in the middle of the night for toileting.

Caregiver communication is essential at all stages of AD. For example, overly technical or detailed directions may confuse and upset patients. Family members may not realize at first the degree of impairment of the Alzheimer's patient's memory and ability to reason. Simple instructions or a demonstration of the desired activity improves patient understanding. Caregivers with good intentions may try to push patients to continue doing familiar tasks in the hope that this will preserve existing function as long as possible. As the patient becomes increasingly unable to accomplish a task because of disease progression, the patient may easily become frustrated and upset. A simple change to a less demanding lifestyle may decrease agitated behaviors substantially. The patient, for example, may accuse a family member of stealing an item that has been misplaced. The family member becomes upset at this accusation and attempts to rationalize or argue with the patient. This frequently causes agitated behavior to escalate. Although difficult, the caregiver may find that by ignoring accusations or changing the subject, the patient will calm down.

The caregiver must be prepared to face the changes in life that will occur, and acceptance of this does not come easily. Denial on the part of the patient and rationalization on the part of the family are common. The clinician should encourage the family to address legal and financial matters and designate a durable power of attorney for execution of financial and medical decisions once the patient is incompetent. The caregiver will need to address issues such as respite services to provide time for rest, relaxation, and conduct of personal business. Eventually, the caregiver will need to face critical questions with respect to institutionalization. The two primary reasons for institutionalization are behavioral disturbances and incontinence, problems secondary to Alzheimer's that most caregivers find difficult to manage in the home. This is probably the most difficult decision for the caregiver, and clinician support and referral to social services is important in assisting the caregiver. The family should be referred to local resources, such as the Alzheimer's Association, that can provide detailed information regarding support services. Table 65–6 lists some referral sources and references for caregivers.

TABLE 65–6. Resources for Caregivers of Persons With Alzheimer's Disease

The following organizations provide educational literature, information on diagnosis, treatment, social support, and ongoing research in Alzheimer's disease:

- Administration on Aging
  Department of Health and Human Services
  330 Independence Avenue, SW
  Washington, DC 20201
  202-619-7501
  FAX: 202-260-1012
  Internet address: http://www.aoa.dhhs.gov
- Alzheimer's Disease Education and Referral Center (ADEAR)
  PO Box 8250
  Silver Springs, MD 20907-8250
  1-800-438-4380
  e-mail: adear@alzheimers.org
- Alzheimer's Disease and Related Disorders Association (ADRDA or The Alzheimer's Association)
  919 North Michigan Avenue, Suite 100
  Chicago, IL 60611-1676
  1-800-272-3900 (24-hour line)
  Internet address: http://www.alz.org
- Alzheimer's Disease Society of Canada
  491 Lawrence Ave. West, #501
  Toronto, Ontario, Canada M5M1C7
- American Association of Retired Persons (AARP)
  Washington, DC
  1-800-424-3410
- Corporation for National Service
  Office of Public Liaison
  1201 New York Avenue, NW
  Washington, DC 20525
  202-1606-5000
- Elder Care Locator
  1-800-667-1116

Further Reading:

- Failure-Free Activities for the Alzheimer's Patient. San Francisco, CA: Cottage Books, 1987.
- Reminiscence: Uncovering a Lifetime of Memories. San Francisco, CA: Elder Press, 1991.
- Living in the Labyrinth. A Personal Journey Through the Maze of Alzheimer's. San Francisco, CA: Elder Press, 1993.
- The 36-Hour Day. Baltimore, MD: Johns Hopkins University Press, 1981.

PHARMACOLOGIC THERAPY

PHARMACOTHERAPY OF COGNITIVE SYMPTOMS

Currently, the cholinesterase inhibitors are the only class of medication indicated for treatment of AD and are used as first-line agents. None of the agents in this class have been compared in head-to-head clinical trials; therefore, no conclusions on the effectiveness of one agent versus another can be made. The latest treatment guidelines were published prior to the approval of rivastigmine and galantamine; however, both guidelines recommend the use of cholinesterase inhibitors in patients with mild-moderate stages of dementia.[53,54] Additionally, the American Psychiatric Association guidelines recommend consideration for concomitant treatment with vitamin E. Based on the approval of the newest cholinesterase inhibitors, additional treatment guidelines are necessary. With the exception of tacrine, any of the cholinesterase inhibitors are appropriate as initial treatment. Donepezil is preferred by some clinicians because more data are available on long-term use, and it can be given once daily. If the decline in MMSE score is greater than two to four points after treatment for 1 year with the initial cholinesterase inhibitor, it is reasonable to change to a different cholinesterase inhibitor. Otherwise, treatment should be continued with the initial medication. Cholinesterase inhibitors should be used throughout the course of illness because of the cognitive benefits, possible treatment of behavioral symptoms, and economic factors. Additionally, vitamin E should be used adjunctively with the cholinesterase inhibitors throughout treatment. Figure 65–3 shows pharmacotherapeutic treatment algorithms for AD. These recommendations are made based upon available efficacy, safety, and tolerability data.

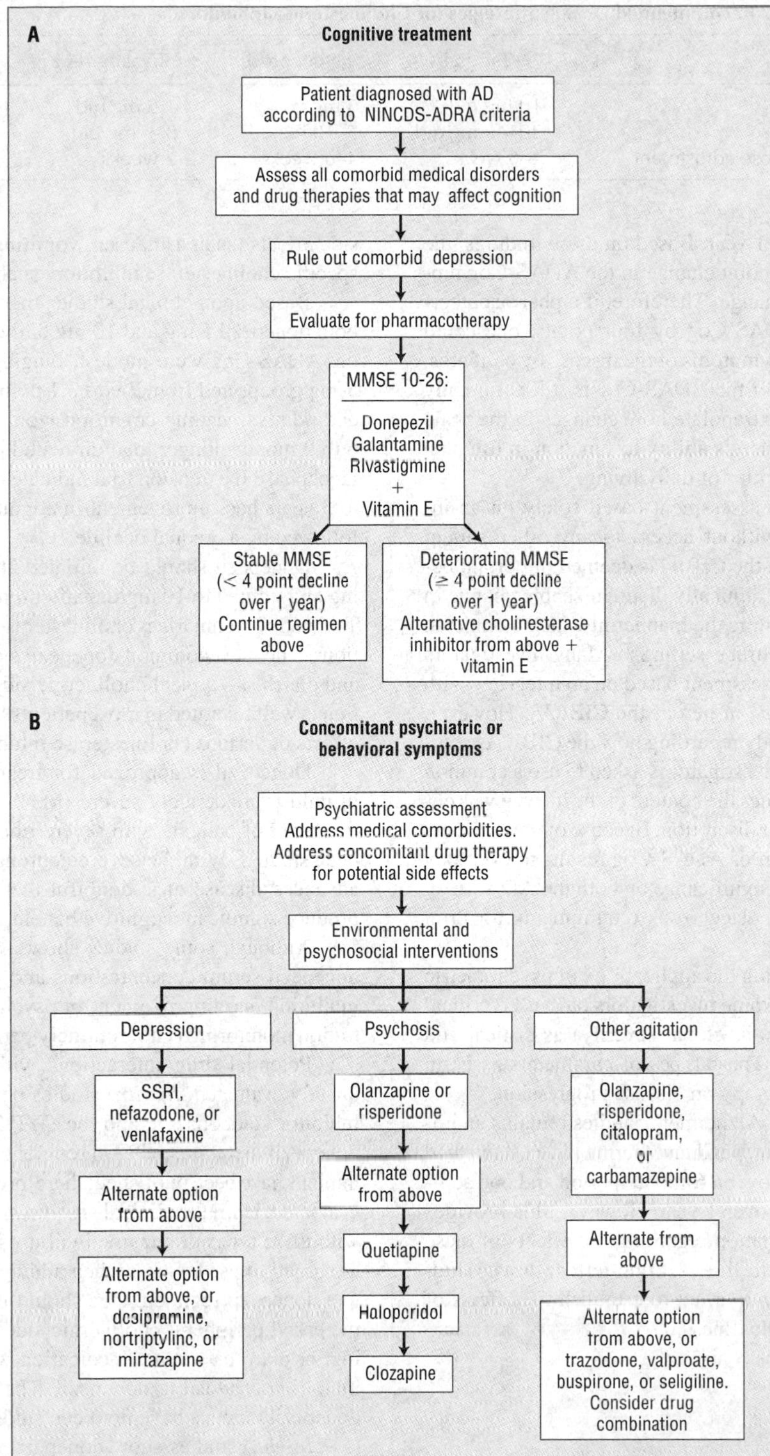

FIGURE 65–3. Proposed treatment algorithms for Alzheimer's disease: **A,** Cognitive treatment and **B,** concomitant psychiatric or behavioral symptoms.

Research Methodology for Pharmacotherapeutic Studies of Cognition-Enhancing Agents

The Food and Drug Administration (FDA) developed minimum, uniform criteria for conducting efficacy studies in Alzheimer's patients. At a minimum, studies in support of a New Drug Application (NDA) for treatment of AD must be double-blind, placebo controlled, randomized, and of parallel group design. Efficacy must be indicated by statistically significant differences between groups on both the Alzheimer's Disease Assessment Scale Cognitive Portion (ADAS-Cog) and the Clinical Interview-Based Impression of Change (CIBIC).[55] The ADAS-Cog is a structured psychometric assessment measuring patient performance on multiple, discrete areas of cognitive function. A decrease in ADAS score indicates improved cognition. In natural disease progression studies, scores on the ADAS-Cog have been shown to worsen (increase) by an average of four points over

TABLE 65–7. Recommended Dosing Strategies for Cholinesterase Inhibitors

	Tacrine	Donepezil	Rivastigmine	Galantamine
Starting dose	10 mg qid	5 mg qd	1.5 mg bid	4 mg bid
Maintenance dose	20–40 mg qid	5–10 mg qd	3–6 mg bid	8–16 mg bid
Time between dose adjustment	4–6 weeks	4–6 weeks	2 weeks	4 weeks

6 months and seven points over 1 year. Based on these findings, the general consensus is that a four-point change in the ADAS-Cog represents a clinically significant change. Therefore, if a pharmacotherapeutic agent decreases the ADAS-Cog by four points, one could think of this as having reversed symptoms of the disease by 6 months. However, the clinical relevancy of the ADAS-Cog is still commonly questioned, as it is difficult to extrapolate how changes in the scale reflect potential changes in a patient's ability to function in life on a daily basis and to complete activities of daily living.

The CIBIC is a clinician's assessment based solely on an interview with the patient, and without access to any other patient information.[56] Efficacy based on the CIBIC is deemed important because it is thought to represent a clinically distinguishable change in cognition and to more closely mimic the manner in which a clinician might evaluate a patient in the office setting.[57] Many investigators use the CIBIC-Plus, a clinical assessment based on an interview with both the patient and the caregiver, in lieu of the CIBIC.[57] However, guidelines vary from study to study regarding how the CIBIC is actually conducted. Sometimes the investigator is asked to use a common structured interview and other times the content of the interview is entirely up to individual investigator discretion. Because of the concerns noted regarding the extrapolation of ADAS-Cog results to everyday life, the FDA requires statistical significance on both the ADAS-Cog and the CIBIC (compared with placebo) as requirements for drug approval.

Because of concerns regarding the applicability of psychometric tests to routine clinical practice, some investigators have used critical outcomes (e.g., institutionalization, global severity) as critical end points in Alzheimer's studies.[58] These types of parameters assist in examining the effects of drug therapy on disease progression.

The appropriate duration of Alzheimer's studies remains an important question. Studies with donepezil and tacrine have established efficacy as compared to placebo over a 6-month period and one additional donepezil trial conducted over 1 year. However, this provides the clinician with limited information regarding the effects of these medications over the duration of the illness. Long-term followup studies of medication treatment are important to establish the effects of these agents over the course of the illness.

Cholinesterase Inhibitors

Just as levodopa was developed as replacement therapy for dopaminergic deficiency in Parkinson's disease, in the early 1980s, researchers began to examine means in which to enhance cholinergic activity in patients with AD. Tacrine was the first such drug to be examined in a systematic fashion. However, tacrine is fraught with significant side effects, including hepatotoxicity, that severely limit the ability of patients to adhere to treatment. For all practical purposes, the use of tacrine has been replaced by the advent of safer, more tolerable cholinesterase inhibitors.

Donepezil[59] is a piperidine, cholinesterase inhibitor with specificity for inhibition of acetylcholinesterase as compared to butyrylcholinesterase. This specificity is claimed to result in fewer peripheral side effects (such as nausea, vomiting, and diarrhea) than with nonspecific cholinesterase inhibitors such as tacrine.[60]

Based upon clinical studies that led to donepezil approval,[61–64] both donepezil 5 mg and 10 mg daily are efficacious. Effect sizes on the ADAS-Cog were modest, ranging from 1.5 to 2.5 points in the 5-mg groups and from 2.9 to 3.1 points in the 10-mg groups at study end points, meaning cognition would be improved or stabilized for 6 to 9 months longer than untreated patients. Results from an open-label phase II extension trial indicate that patients on donepezil for up to 5 years had improvement in cognition for the first 6 to 9 months, followed by a gradual decline.[65]

Donepezil should be initiated at a 5-mg/day dose in the morning and titrated to 10 mg/day after 4 to 6 weeks if it is well tolerated. Table 65–7 summarizes cholinesterase inhibitor dosing recommendations. The most common donepezil side effects are nausea, vomiting, and diarrhea—typical cholinergic side effects; however, the medication is well tolerated in most patients.[60] Table 65–8 compares the side effects of various cholinesterase inhibitors.

Donepezil is approved for treatment of cognitive impairment in mild to moderately severe (MMSE 10 to 26) AD. Its efficacy in treatment of patients with severe impairment (MMSE <10) has not been studied. With the severe neuronal degeneration associated with advanced disease, it is doubtful that a cholinesterase inhibitor will produce significant cognitive benefit in such patients.

Although some studies show a high correlation between both donepezil serum concentrations and percent of acetylcholinesterase inhibition and improvement in psychometric scores, serum concentration monitoring is not routinely performed in clinical practice.[61–63]

Potential drug interactions with donepezil have been inadequately evaluated. *In vitro* studies demonstrate that the CYP 3A3/4 inhibitor ketoconazole and the CYP 2D6 inhibitor quinidine inhibit donepezil metabolism.[66] No reports of these potential interactions in humans have been published; therefore, clinical significance cannot be evaluated. Until the clinical significance of potential drug interactions with these types of enzyme inhibitors is better elucidated, clinicians are urged to use caution when adding CYP 2D6 or 3A3/4 inhibitors to a donepezil regimen. One should monitor the patient for possible increased peripheral cholinergic side effects such as nausea, vomiting, or diarrhea when a medication with potent CYP 2D6 or 3A3/4 inhibition is added to donepezil. The effects of enzyme inducers on donepezil kinetics have not been studied.

In vitro studies show donepezil to have a low affinity for CYP 2D6 and 3A4, thus making clinically significant drug interactions through these isoenzymes unlikely.[66] In humans, donepezil is reported by the manufacturer to have no effect on the kinetics of theophylline, warfarin, digoxin, or cimetidine.

Butyrylcholinesterase is thought to play an important role in acetylcholine degradation following the depletion of acetylcholinesterase. Additionally, acetylcholinesterase is found in two forms: globular G4 and G1. The highest concentrations of globular G1 can be found in the hippocampus and cortex, two regions known to be affected in Alzheimer's disease. Interestingly, although the globular G4 form is significantly depleted in postmortem studies, globular G1 remains abundant. By blocking this particular form of the

TABLE 65–8. Comparative Common Adverse Effects of the Cholinesterase Inhibitors from Clinical Trials Data

Adverse event	Tacrine (n = 634)	Donepezil (n = 747)	Rivastigmine (n = 1189)	Galantamine (n = 1040)
Elevated Liver function tests	29%	NR	NR	NR
Nausea or vomiting	28%	NR	NR	NR
Nausea	NR	11%	47%	24%
Vomiting	NR	5%	31%	13%
Diarrhea	16%	10%	19%	9%
Headache	11%	10%	17%	8%
Dizziness	12%	8%	21%	9%
Muscle cramps	9%	6%	NR	NR
Insomnia	6%	9%	9%	5%
Fatigue	4%	5%	9%	5%
Anorexia	9%	4%	17%	9%
Depression	4%	3%	6%	7%
Abnormal dreams	NR	3%	NR	NR
Weight decrease	3%	3%	3%	7%
Somnolence	4%	2%	5%	4%
Abdominal pain	8%	NR	13%	5%
Tremor	2%	NR	4%	3%
Agitation	7%	NR	NR	NR
Rhinitis	8%	NR	NR	NR

NR, not reported
Compiled from Package insert data Refs. 59, and 106–108.

acetylcholinesterase enzyme, higher concentrations of acetylcholine may be obtained.[67]

Rivastigmine recently became available as the third cholinesterase inhibitor. Rivastigmine has central activity at acetylcholinesterase and butyrylcholinesterase, but low activity at these sites in the periphery. At least theoretically, this should result in a lower incidence of peripheral side effects.[60] Rivastigmine activity at the acetylcholinesterase globular G1 site is higher than at G4, and may be theoretically advantageous because it may prevent degradation of acetylcholine via this enzyme over the course of the disease as compared to other cholinesterase inhibitors without this activity. It is difficult to say what this means clinically, and long-term head-to-head trials with other cholinesterase inhibitors are needed.

Clinical studies leading to the approval of rivastigmine indicate that doses of 6–12 mg/day are efficacious.[68–70] It should be noted that with an intent-to-treat analysis in the European rivastigmine study,[70] statistical significance was not achieved on the ADAS-Cog. Statistical significance was obtained only in the high-doses group with a last observation carried forward (LOCF) analysis, with an effect size of 2.07 points on the ADAS-Cog. Dropout rates because of adverse effects or worsening of symptoms may have contributed to the lack of efficacy in the intent-to treat analysis; whereas, the LOCF analysis is more representative of patients who were able to tolerate treatment and complete most or all evaluation points. In the second study,[68] the change in ADAS-Cog score was statistically significant in the intent-to-treat high-dose rivastigmine group with an effect size of 3.78 points. This means cognition would be improved or stabilized for about 6–12 months longer than untreated patients. Activities of daily living were measured using the Progressive Deterioration Scale and showed a significantly higher score (i.e., improved) for patients in the 6–12-mg group.[70] Rivastigmine has not been evaluated in patients with severe dementia or for treatment of behavioral symptoms.

Rivastigmine should be initiated at a dose of 1.5 mg bid and titrated upward at a minimum of 2 week intervals to a maximum daily dose of 12 mg. Tolerability and absorption are improved when rivastigmine is given with food. The potential for drug interactions is low because of low protein binding, and it is not metabolized through the cytochrome P450 enzyme system.[67,71] Cholinergic side effects are the most common adverse effects with rivastigmine, but it was well tolerated in clinical studies.[68–70] Table 65–8 compares the side effects of the cholinesterase inhibitors.

Galantamine is the fourth approved cholinesterase inhibitor, and it also has activity as a nicotinic receptor agonist. Galantamine has been studied in two randomized placebo-controlled trials.[72,73] The first study[73] was a 6-month, double-blind trial with an additional 6-month open-label extension. Patients were initiated at 8 mg/day followed by weekly titration of 8 mg/day to a maintenance dose of 24 mg/day or 32 mg/day. Both dosage groups were significantly improved at the end of 6 months on the ADAS-Cog and CIBIC-plus. The effect sizes as measured by using the ADAS-Cog for the 24 mg/day and 32 mg/day groups were 3.9 and 3.4 points, respectively. Therefore, one could expect improvement or stabilization occurring for about 9 months longer in patients receiving galantamine, than in patients who did not receive treatment. At the end of the extension phase, no difference was seen from baseline scores in the galantamine 24 mg/day group. Patients who were switched from galantamine 32 mg/day to 24 mg/day actually had a significant worsening in symptoms. This suggests that if a patient's cognition is not deteriorating and the patient is tolerating a given dose of galantamine, that dosage should be maintained throughout treatment to avoid an accelerated decline in cognitive function. Activities of daily living were assessed using the Disability Assessment for Dementia scale and improvements at 6-months were seen with both dosages.

The second study enrolled 978 patients to receive either placebo or galantamine 8, 16, or 24 mg/day for 5 months. ADAS-Cog and CIBIC-plus scores in the 16- and 24-mg/day groups were statistically different from those in the placebo group and in the 8-mg/day group. The Neuropsychiatric Inventory (NPI) was used to evaluate the effect on behavioral and psychotic symptoms. Both the 16- and 24-mg/day groups were significantly different than the placebo and 8-mg/day groups; but there was actually no improvement over baseline score. An activities of daily living assessment was conducted using the AD

Cooperative Study Activities of Daily Living Inventory. Galantamine 16- and 24-mg/day groups showed less deterioration in activities of daily living. Galantamine was initiated at 8 mg/day with dosage titration of 8 mg/day occurring at 4-week intervals. Dropout rates because of adverse drug reactions (ADRs) were much higher in the first study than in the second study. Slower titration resulted in better patient tolerance and fewer reported ADRs; therefore, adjustment at 4-week intervals is recommended in clinical practice.

Antioxidants

Based upon pathophysiologic theories involving free radicals, significant interest has evolved regarding the use of antioxidants in the treatment of AD. One study compared the use of vitamin E 1,000 IU bid, selegiline 5 mg bid, the combination, and placebo in the treatment of moderately impaired AD patients.[74] Instead of using cognition on psychometric assessments as their primary outcomes, time to critical end points (i.e., death, institutionalization, loss of ability to perform activities of daily living, or severe dementia) was used as a measure of efficacy. Both vitamin E and selegiline were superior to placebo, and the combination was actually slightly inferior to either treatment alone. The net result of treatment was a delay of 7 months in reaching one of the specified critical end points. However, the study has been criticized because the placebo and active treatment groups had significantly different baseline MMSE scores, and because efficacy could be demonstrated only when the baseline scores were used as a covariate. Although not statistically significant, vitamin E showed slight superiority to either selegiline alone or the combination. Based upon these findings, vitamin E's favorable side effect profile, and low cost, it is considered the preferred treatment, and it can be continued indefinitely. Although potential benefits of vitamin E combined with a cholinesterase inhibitor have not been evaluated, there are no known complications from their combined use.

Selegiline's use in AD has been evaluated in other studies. In a 15-month double-blind study in mildly demented patients, the only demonstrated effect with selegiline 10-mg daily was a mild decrease in Brief Psychiatric Rating Scale scores. The clinical significance of this effect was questioned by the investigators.[75] Other studies with selegiline alone have shown mixed results. Some studies show improvement in cognition, while others show improvement in behavior or mood.[75,76] Patients who are more severely demented, particularly those with behavioral symptoms, may be more likely to receive benefit than patients with milder disease presentation. Further research is necessary to elucidate its role in treating AD.

Estrogen

Interest in estrogen use has increased over the last decade. Most, but not all epidemiologic studies show a lower incidence of AD in women who took ERT postmenopausally. Results from these epidemiologic trials, prompted researchers to look at the use of estrogen as a treatment for cognitive decline.

Recently, two randomized, double-blind, placebo-controlled trials evaluated estrogen as a treatment for cognitive decline.[77] In the first study, 42 women with mild to moderate Alzheimer's disease were enrolled to receive either 1.25 mg of conjugated estrogens or placebo. Improvement on the ADAS-Cog was the primary outcome measure, but behavioral and functional outcomes were also assessed. No difference was seen between treatment groups at 4 or 16 weeks in any of the outcome assessments.

Similarly, in the second trial, 120 women with mild to moderate Alzheimer's disease were enrolled to receive 0.625 mg/day or 1.25 mg/day of conjugated estrogens, or placebo.[78] The primary outcome measure in this study was improvement on the Clinical Global Impression of Change scale with other cognitive, behavioral, and functional outcomes as secondary measures. Again, no difference was seen in the primary or secondary outcomes between the two groups at 2, 6, 12, or 15 months with the exception of the Clinical Dementia Rating Scale, which actually showed a worsening in score in the combined analysis of both estrogen groups.

These two studies do not support a role for estrogen in treating symptoms of AD. Ongoing clinical trials are being conducted to determine the potential role of estrogen as a preventative treatment for AD. The risk-benefit ratio of estrogen replacement to prevent AD should be weighed prior to initiating treatment. Because data for prevention are inconclusive at this time, estrogen should only be used in those patients who have another medical reason for ERT.

Anti-Inflammatory Agents

A number of epidemiologic studies show either a lower incidence of AD or higher MMSE scores in AD if NSAIDs were taken on a regular basis.[79] In a 15-year longitudinal analysis, use of NSAIDs was associated with a lower incidence of AD.[80] Patients with reported use of NSAIDs for more than 2 years had a relative risk of AD of 0.4 as compared to a relative risk of 0.65 for those taking NSAIDs for less than 2 years.

Indomethacin was studied in a small, double-blind AD treatment trial with positive results.[81] Although patients treated with indomethacin 100–150 mg/day did not appear to show cognitive decline during the 6-month trial, about one-third dropped out because of gastrointestinal (GI) side effects. The outcome measures in this study were poorly defined, and it is difficult to know whether these changes were clinically significant.

Prednisone was evaluated in a double-blind, placebo-controlled trial in 138 patients with probable Alzheimer's disease randomized to receive either prednisone 20 mg/day, tapered to 10 mg/day after 4 weeks, or placebo for 1 year.[82] No significant difference between groups existed in the primary outcome measure, change in ADAS-Cog score. Behavioral symptoms measured by the Brief Psychiatric Rating Scale actually worsened significantly in the prednisone group. Even at low doses, adverse events commonly associated with glucocorticoids occurred in some patients. Higher doses may have produced a significant effect on cognition; however, it is unlikely that they would be tolerated in this population; and data from other patient populations suggest that prednisone may be associated with cognitive impairment.[83,84] Thus, prednisone is not recommended for treating AD. Similarly, a randomized trial of diclofenac/misoprostol was not effective for treatment of AD.[85]

NSAIDs have a significant incidence of adverse effects, particularly gastritis and the possibility of GI bleeds. Because of the absence of multicenter, controlled trials to support efficacy and the side effect potential, NSAIDs are not recommended for general use in the treatment or prevention of AD at the present time. Clinical trials with COX-2 inhibitors in AD are currently underway.

Ginkgo Biloba

Egb 761, an extract of ginkgo biloba, is claimed to improve memory. Although it is thought to be an antioxidant and to affect inflammation and neuromodulation, the mechanisms of the multiple compounds in Egb 761 have not been elucidated. A recent meta-analysis determined that only 4 of 57 ginkgo biloba studies that were identified met minimal scientific standards for clinical trials.[86] The effect size at 12 weeks for a total of 212 patients treated with ginkgo and 212 with placebo was 0.41 (confidence interval [CI] 0.22–0.61). Although this is comparable to the effect size seen in a 24-week donepezil study,[62] the clinical relevance is minimal. Standardized doses of gingko ranged from 120 to 240 mg/day. No significant adverse events were reported; however, two case reports have been associated with hemorrhaging. Obvious limitations exist with the meta-analysis, including pooling of data from heterogeneous populations, differences in methodology, and potential reviewer bias in study selection. However, it reveals the paucity of well-designed studies in this area while suggesting that gingko may have some therapeutic effect and should be evaluated in future clinical studies.

Even if the herbal extract is effective, significant problems exist with its use. The content of herbal products is poorly standardized, and significant variation in supposed active ingredient content for some herbals exists from lot to lot and among manufacturers. Until these products are better standardized and their manufacturing and stability better assured, it is recommended that they be used with caution. Furthermore, little is known about potential adverse reactions, drug interactions, or long-term toxicity with their use.

PHARMACOTHERAPY OF NONCOGNITIVE SYMPTOMS

The majority of patients with AD manifest noncognitive symptoms at some point in the illness.[33,34] These symptoms can be roughly divided into three categories: psychotic symptoms, inappropriate or disruptive behavior, and depression. Effective management of these problems is important because behavioral symptoms are distressing to both the patient and the caregiver, necessitate increased caregiver supervision and patience, and are a leading reason for nursing home placement. In fact, presence of neuropsychiatric symptoms increases caregiver burden more than loss of cognition or self-care.

Strategies for treatment of psychotic or behavioral symptoms should include both environmental and pharmacologic interventions (e.g. antipsychotics, antidepressants, mood stabilizers, and anxiolytics). The potential harm to the patient or caregiver should be used as a guide for selecting the appropriate intervention. For example, hallucinations or delusions that are of a nonstressful, nonthreatening nature can generally be ignored or redirected by family members. Nonaggressive behaviors can generally be managed with environmental interventions, such as distracting the patient from the behavior, creating a structured environment, providing reassurance to calm the patient, and attending support groups for the caregiver. Patients with aggressive behaviors should be approached similarly; however, pharmacologic treatment is often an additional necessity.

Despite the widespread nature of noncognitive symptoms in AD, until recently, little research has been conducted in these patients. Data from clinical trials of antidepressants and antipsychotics are now emerging, although more research is needed. Because of limited clinical data, side effect profiles have been used as a guide in selecting the appropriate treatment. Psychotropic medications with anticholinergic effects should be avoided because they may actually worsen cognition. Other side effects in the elderly include sedation, medication-induced postural instability, and extrapyramidal side effects, which can decrease the clinical utility of traditional psychotropic agents.

General guidelines governing therapy can be summarized as follows: Use reduced doses, monitor closely, titrate dosage slowly, and document carefully. Caregivers often have erroneous expectations regarding the effects of psychotropic medications, and the anticipated benefits and risks of therapy should be clearly explained. Disruptive behaviors and delusions wax and wane with disease progression. Attempts to slowly taper and discontinue antipsychotic medication should be undertaken in minimally symptomatic patients at least every 3 months, because many patients who initially respond to these medications show no change in symptoms and occasionally improve on medication withdrawal.[87] Table 65–9 outlines suggested doses of medications.

Antipsychotics

Antipsychotic medications have traditionally been used to treat disruptive behaviors and psychosis in AD patients. Symptoms responding to antipsychotics include assaultiveness, extreme agitation and hyperexcitability, hallucinations, delusions, suspiciousness, hostility, and uncooperativeness.[88,89] Symptoms not responding include withdrawal, apathy, cognitive deficits, wandering, and incontinence.[71]

Until the advent of the atypical antipsychotics, conventional agents were widely used, although available placebo-controlled studies suggested that they were moderately effective at best.[88–90] More recently, risperidone has been used both in clinical trials and practice in patients with psychotic symptoms or behavioral disturbances associated with dementia.[38] In a double-blind, placebo controlled trial, 45% of patients receiving risperidone 1 mg/d and 50% of patients receiving 2 mg/day had a 50% reduction in total (BEHAVE-AD) scores.[91] It should be noted that although risperidone demonstrated statistically significant efficacy in this study, there was a high placebo response rate (33%). Side effects, particularly extrapyramidal effects and somnolence, increased with increased dose, and they were most prominent with risperidone 2 mg daily. Balancing efficacy with adverse effects, it is recommended to begin with 0.25 mg daily and to titrate in 0.25–0.5-mg increments to 1 mg daily. If response is inadequate, further titrating to a maximum of 2 mg daily may be necessary if the patient is tolerating the medication.

Olanzapine has been studied in a 6-week double-blind, placebo-controlled trial with fixed doses of 5, 10, and 15 mg/day of olanzapine.[92] Reduction in total NPI score was statistically significant in the 5-mg/day and 10-mg/day groups; however, 15 mg/day did not separate from placebo. When assessing response rates as defined by a 50% reduction in total score from baseline, 66% of patients in the 5-mg/day group, 57% in the 10-mg/day group, and 36% in the placebo group achieved this end point. Because the pharmacologic profile of olanzapine includes cholinergic blockade, some concern has been raised as to the utility of this agent in the AD population. Peripheral anticholinergic side effects were statistically significant in the 15-mg/day group, but no differences were seen in central effects. It is important to note that MMSE scores were unchanged after 6 weeks in all treatment groups; however, these results cannot be extrapolated over the long-term.

No placebo-controlled trials are currently available evaluating quetiapine in psychosis of dementia. However, open-label studies suggest good tolerability. For patients who respond inadequately or who have unacceptable side effects with risperidone or olanzapine, quetiapine is a reasonable alternative.

Patients with AD are more sensitive to antipsychotic side effects than other patient groups. Increased sensitivity to antipsychotic side effects in the elderly appears to be the result of altered pharmacodynamics rather than altered pharmacokinetics.[93,94] Particularly problematic side effects are extrapyramidal side effects, postural instability caused by α-adrenergic blockade, and anticholinergic effects,

TABLE 65–9. Medications Used in Treating Noncognitive Symptoms of Dementia

Drugs	Suggested Dosage in Dementia (mg/day)	Indications
Antipsychotics		Psychosis: hallucinations, delusions, suspiciousness
Clozapine	12.5–100 mg	Disruptive behaviors: agitation, aggression
Haloperidol	0.5–4 mg	
Olanzapine	2.5–10 mg	
Quetiapine	12.5–200 mg	
Risperidone	0.25–2 mg	
Antidepressants		Depression: poor appetite, insomnia, hopelessness, anhedonia, withdrawal, suicidal thoughts, agitation
Citalopram	10–20 mg	
Desipramine	50–150 mg[ab]	
Fluoxetine	5–20 mg	
Nortriptyline	25–150 mg[ab]	
Paroxetine	10–40 mg	
Sertraline	50–200 mg	
Trazodone	75–400 mg[a]	
Anticonvulsants		Agitation or aggression
Carbamazepine	100–1,000 mg[ab]	
Valproic Acid	1,000–2,500 mg[ab]	
Others		
Buspirone	10–45 mg	Disruptive behaviors
Oxazepam	10–60 mg[a]	Disruptive behaviors
Selegiline	10 mg	Disruptive behaviors, agitation, anxiety, depression

[a]Administer in divided doses

[b]Dosage adjustment should be guided by drug serum concentrations.

Adapted from Refs. 38, 75, 76, 87, 93, and 95.

including increased confusion, urinary retention, constipation, and dry mouth.[93,94] For a more detailed description of antipsychotic side effects, see Chap. 68. Overall, fewer side effects are seen with the newer atypical antipsychotics, making them a preferred choice for treatment of psychosis or aggression in the AD patient.[95] Effective doses of antipsychotic medications are much lower than those typically used to treat schizophrenia (see Table 65–8). The rule of thumb is to "start low and go slow."

Depression

Prevalence estimates of depression in AD differ widely, ranging from less than 10% to 80%. Actual prevalence rates of major depression in AD are probably 5% to 15% in community-based patients and 15% to 20% among institutionalized patients.[87] The inconsistency in these figures is largely attributed to symptom overlap, diagnostic differences, and the patient population sampled. Early in the course of AD, depression presents much the same as in other elderly persons; while later in the disease course diagnosis can be difficult. Apathy, decreased initiative and socialization, decreased concentration, psychomotor retardation, agitation, and changes in appetite and sleep patterns are all symptoms intrinsic to both dementia and depression.[87,93] In determining whether or not a patient with these symptoms is also depressed, it is particularly important to assess the patient's affect and ability to experience pleasure. Affective signs of depression might include crying spells, staying in bed, decreased food intake, asking to be killed, moaning, or sorrowful facial expression. An interview with the patient's caregiver can be helpful in obtaining a more accurate record of symptoms. Depression may be more common in the early stages of AD as the patient attempts to adjust to limitations associated with cognitive loss.

The bulk of literature examining antidepressant use in AD is made up of case reports and uncontrolled studies. Most of these report a favorable response to antidepressants.[93,94] The only available placebo-controlled study, an 8-week trial of imipramine versus placebo, showed significant response in both treatment groups but no advantage of imipramine over placebo.[95] One other controlled trial compared fluoxetine 10 mg/d and amitriptyline 25 mg/day and found that both were equally effective; however, the fluoxetine group tolerated the medication much better and had significantly lower dropout rates.[96] The available literature also suggests that antidepressant response, as measured by reductions in Hamilton Depression Rating (HAM-D) scores, is not as dramatic as in depressed nondemented patients. Because depressive target symptoms are difficult to distinguish from dementia, it is unclear whether this modest decrease in HAM-D scores is a result of poor drug response or of difficulty in assessing symptoms in this population.[93,95] Some clinicians have noted that a longer duration of treatment (e.g., up to 12 weeks) is required before elderly patients experience an antidepressant effect.

It is desirable to document symptoms of depression for several weeks prior to initiating antidepressant therapy in a patient with AD. A significant nonspecific treatment response occurs in this population, and it is possible that simply visiting with a clinician or increasing the patient's activity level may be sufficient to improve symptoms. Should this approach fail, a trial of an antidepressant may be initiated. Pharmacotherapy should be initiated with an antidepressant possessing a favorable side effect profile. Acceptable first line antidepressants in this population include selective serotonin reuptake inhibitors (SSRIs) such as citalopram, fluoxetine, paroxetine, or sertraline; serotonin/norepinephrine reuptake inhibitors such as venlafaxine; or the triazolopyridine, nefazodone.[94] Trazodone, the more sedating of the triazolopyridines, reportedly decreases insomnia, agitation, and dysphoria in AD patients. Although lacking anticholinergic effects, trazodone tends to cause orthostasis and excess sedation at antidepressant doses. Because of their low propensity to cause anticholinergic effects, orthostatic hypotension, and sedation, the SSRIs are often considered the preferred antidepressants in this population. SSRIs can usually be dosed once daily. These medications are not risk free, however. Gastrointestinal adverse effects, confusion, agitation, dizziness, and insomnia have been reported in patients with AD taking fluoxetine, especially at higher doses (>20 mg of fluoxetine daily).[97] Paroxetine reportedly causes more anticholinergic effects than other SSRIs. For a more complete discussion of treatment of depression, refer to Chap. 69.

Miscellaneous Therapies

Because antipsychotic therapy has shown only modest efficacy and poses a substantial risk of undesirable side effects, medications traditionally used to treat disruptive behaviors and aggression in other psychiatric and neurologic disorders have been suggested as potential alternatives. These alternatives include benzodiazepines, buspirone, carbamazepine, selegiline, valproate, and SSRIs. Table 65–9 lists doses of selected medications.

In addition to antipsychotics, placebo-controlled studies of two different medications have been reported. A controlled study comparing citalopram and fluphenazine for psychosis and behavioral disturbances of dementia found citalopram 10–20 mg/day at least equally efficacious as fluphenazine in improving scores on the Neurobehavioral Rating Scale (E-BEHAVE-AD), and both were statistically superior to placebo.[94] One controlled trial with carbamazepine (mean dose = 300 mg/d; mean Cp = 5.3 μg/mL) showed a significant reduction in Brief Psychiatric Rating Scale scores as compared to placebo. Carbamazepine was well tolerated in AD patients.[98]

Benzodiazepines, particularly oxazepam, have been used to treat anxiety, agitation, and aggression, but they generally show inferior efficacy when compared to antipsychotics. Because benzodiazepines impair cognition, can result in disinhibition, and may increase the risk of falls in AD patients, their routine use is not advised.[38,93] Conversely, the 5-HT_{1A} partial agonist buspirone has shown benefit in treating agitation and aggression in a limited number of patients with minimal adverse effects.[99,100] Selegiline decreases anxiety, depression, and agitation in open-label and controlled studies.[75,101,102] Although a longer-term, double-blind study using selegiline in mildly demented patients showed no benefit, the more typical patient with AD (greater disease severity) may be more likely to respond.[76] Should antipsychotics fail to manage noncognitive behaviors, available evidence suggests that a trial of citalopram or carbamazepine may be appropriate second-line alternatives. Only minimal evidence exists to support the use of valproate in this population. Lithium has shown no benefit and frequent toxicity.[38,93] Clearly, more rigorous placebo-controlled studies are needed to determine the relative efficacy and place in therapy for these medication alternatives.

Interest has grown regarding the potential use of cholinesterase inhibitors for treatment of psychiatric symptoms in AD. Studies assessing noncognitive symptoms in clinical trials with tacrine, donepezil, and galantamine suggest that these agents have positive effects on psychiatric and behavioral symptoms.[103] Unfortunately, these have been posthoc analyses or small open-label trials, making it difficult to draw conclusions. The most compelling data come from the metrifonate clinical trials, in which the NPI was used in a prospective, placebo-controlled trial to determine differences in psychiatric symptoms between the treatment groups.[103] Significant differences were seen in hallucination and apathy scores. Additional research is needed in this area before specific treatment recommendations can be made with confidence.

PHARMACOECONOMIC CONSIDERATIONS

The cost of caring for an individual with AD is significant, not only from the perspective of dollars expended but also from the viewpoint of uncompensated hours spent in caring for the patient and the effects of the illness on quality of life of both the patient and caregiver. Considering both formal and informal costs, Rice and colleagues estimated that the annual costs for caring for an Alzheimer's patient were $47,000, regardless of whether the person was living at home or in a nursing home. Formal costs are those expenses associated with payment to a care provider, whereas informal costs are costs associated with noncompensated time spent by family caregivers in providing for the patient. Clearly, the economic burden for the home-living AD patient is the time spent in caring for the patient, whereas in the nursing home, it is money spent for others to provide care.

Few attempts have been made to evaluate the pharmacoeconomics of available medications in Alzheimer's disease. This situation arises because clinical trials of AD agents are usually a maximum of 3 to 6 months in duration, whereas treatment of the patient may last for years. Attempts have been made to use modeling and simulation studies to predict the pharmacoeconomic implications of treatment. Lubeck and coworkers modeled data from the 30-week tacrine trial to predict costs over the course of the illness.[104] They estimated average annual cost savings with tacrine treatment to be $2,243 for patients taking 80–160 mg daily and $4,052 for patients taking 160 mg/day. These formal costs were primarily saved by a projected delay in the time to nursing home placement. A major flaw in this study is an assumption in their model that the patient decline over the course of the illness would be the same as projected from the 30-week study. Ernst and associates modeled potential cost savings of cholinesterase inhibitor treatment, and found potential cost savings for most mild or severely ill patients to be small. However, for home-dwelling patients with a baseline MMSE score of 7, potential cost savings from treatment were significant, with prevention of a two-point decline saving $3,700 annually.[105] The extent to which these types of studies predict economic outcomes in real practice is unclear.

As multiple treatments for AD have been introduced into clinical practice, these types of modeling studies need to be verified by retrospective database analyses and prospective pharmacoeconomic studies. If AD treatments delay cognitive decline and time to nursing home placement, then they not only have potential economic benefit, but significant effects on the quality of life of patients and caregivers. Not only should total formal costs associated with the disease be evaluated in such studies, but studies evaluating informal, uncompensated costs for the caregiver and quality of life for both the patient and caregiver need to be performed.

EVALUATION OF THERAPEUTIC OUTCOMES

An evaluation of therapeutic outcomes in the patient with AD begins with a thorough assessment at baseline and a clear definition of therapeutic goals. Cognitive status, physical status, functional performance, mood, thought processes, and behavior all need to be evaluated before initiation of drug therapy. The clinician should interview both the patient and the caregiver to assess response to drug therapy. Because caregivers often have difficulty giving honest and frank information about their loved one's condition in his or her presence, it is often necessary to interview family caregivers separately. In evaluating response to cognitive agents, the clinician should ask questions about the patient's ability to perform daily functional tasks and about mood and behavior, as well as questions about memory and orientation. Objective assessments, such as the MMSE for cognition and the Functional Activities Questionnaire for activities of daily living, should be used to quantify changes in symptoms and function.[37]

Because target symptoms of psychiatric disorders may respond differently in demented patients, a detailed list of symptoms to be treated should be documented in the pharmacotherapy plan to aid in monitoring. These could include, for example, "striking at spouse because patient believes spouse is an impostor," "verbal threats and refusal to allow clothes to be changed," and so on, as opposed to documenting vague symptoms such as "aggression" or "delusions." To make an accurate assessment of depression, multiple symptoms—including sleep, appetite, and activity and interest levels—need to be assessed in addition to the patient's stated mood.

The patient should be observed carefully for potential side effects of drug therapy. Depending on the therapeutic agent being employed, patients should be assessed for potential side effects such as diarrhea, GI distress, dizziness, sedation, extrapyramidal side effects, or worsening of behavior. The specific side effects to be monitored and the method and frequency of monitoring should be documented. Periodic assessments for drug effectiveness, side effects, compliance, need for dosage adjustment, or change in treatment should occur at least monthly. However, patients need to be treated for an adequate duration to see a therapeutic effect from a given intervention. Because the effects of cognition-enhancing medications are not great, a treatment period of several months to a year may be necessary before it can be determined whether therapy is beneficial. Cognitive effects of the drug are often noticed only as a plateauing during treatment or as deterioration following drug discontinuation. In general, cognitive agents should be continued if the patient is demonstrating no change in clinical status. However, if there is doubt, the medication can be slowly tapered and discontinued, and the patient monitored off the drug for 4 to 6 weeks to determine the need for continued therapy.

▶ PRINCIPLES OF PHARMACOTHERAPY

- A thorough patient evaluation to determine the cause of dementia and to rule out other disorders should occur before considering drug therapy.
- The etiology of AD is as yet unknown, and pharmacotherapy neither cures nor arrests the pathophysiology.
- Nondrug therapy and social support for the patient and family are the primary treatment interventions for AD.
- Thorough family and caregiver education should occur regarding the disease prognosis and limitations of treatments. Appropriate referral to social and legal support services should be made.
- Pharmacotherapy is primarily oriented toward treating symptoms and decreasing the rate of cognitive decline.
- A thorough baseline assessment, using rating scales, should be performed before initiating drug therapy for cognitive or behavioral symptoms.
- Slow medication dosage titration with careful monitoring should occur to minimize the incidence of severe adverse drug reactions.
- A thorough behavioral assessment and plan with careful examination of environmental factors should be conducted before initiating drug therapy for behavioral symptoms.
- Pharmacotherapy for behavioral symptoms should be self-limited, and medication tapering and discontinuation attempted in patients with stable symptoms.

REFERENCES

1. Crismon ML, Eggert AE. Alzheimer's disease. In: Pharmacist Care: Mental Health. Institute for Pharmacist Care Outcomes, 2000:ALZ1–ALZ29.
2. Diagnostic and Statistical Manual for Mental Disorders, 4th ed, Text Revised. Washington, DC, American Psychiatric Association, 2000.
3. Rocca WA, Amaducci LA, Schoenberg BS. Epidemiology of clinically diagnosed Alzheimer's disease. Ann Neurol 1986;19:415–424.
4. Evans DA, Funkenstein HH, Albert MS, et al. Prevalence of Alzheimer's disease in a community population of older persons: Higher than previously reported. JAMA 1989;262:2551–2552.
5. Rice DP, Fox PJ, Max W, et al. Datawatch: The economic burden of Alzheimer's disease care. Health Affairs 1993;12:164–176.
6. Evans DA. Estimated prevalence of Alzheimer's disease in the United States. Milbank Q 1990;68:267–289.
7. Hebert LE, Scherr PA, Beckett LA, et al. Age-specific incidence of Alzheimer's disease in a community population. JAMA 1995;273:1354–1359.
8. Chandra V, Bharucha NE, Schoenberg BS. Conditions associated with Alzheimer's disease at death: Case-control study. Neurology 1986;36:209–211.
9. Evans DA, Smith LA, Scherr PA, et al. Risk of death from Alzheimer's disease in a community population of older persons. Am J Epidemiol 1991;134:403–412.
10. Wolfson C, Wolfson DB, Asgharian M, et al. A reevaluation of the duration of survival after the onset of dementia. N Engl J Med 2001;344:1111–1116.
11. Johnson N, Davis T, Bosanquet N. The epidemic of Alzheimer's disease: How can we manage the costs? Pharmacoeconomics 2000:18:215–223.
12. Ernst RL, Hay JW. The US economic and social costs of Alzheimer's disease revisited. Am J Pub Health 1994;84:1261–1264.
13. US Bureau of the Census. Current Population Reports, Special Studies P23–190,65+ in the United States. Washington DC, US Government Printing Office, 1996.
14. Blacker D. New insights into genetic aspects of Alzheimer's disease. Postgrad Med 2000;108:119–122, 125, 126, 129.
15. St George-Hyslop PH. Piecing together Alzheimer's. Sci Am 2000;283 (6):76–83.
16. Tang MX, Maestre G, Tsai WY, et al. Effect of age, ethnicity, and head injury on the association between Apo E genotypes and Alzheimer's disease. Ann N Y Acad Sci 1996;802:7–15.
17. Corder EH, Saunders AM, Risch NJ, et al. Protective effect of apolipoprotein E type 2 allele for late-onset Alzheimer's disease. Nat Genet 1994; 7:180–184.
18. Mirra SS. Alzheimer's disease and other dementias: Neuropathological considerations. In: Heston LL, ed. Progress in Alzheimer's Disease and Similar Conditions. Washington, DC, American Psychiatric Press, 1997:21–34.
19. Mortimer JA. Is Alzheimer's disease a lifelong illness? Risk factors for pathological and clinical disease. In: Heston LL, ed. Progress in Alzheimer's Disease and Similar Conditions. Washington, DC, American Psychiatric Press, 1997:9–20.
20. McGeer EG, Mcgeer PL. Innate immunity in Alzheimer's disease: A model for local inflammatory reactions. Mol Interventions 2001;1:22–29.
21. Blass JP. Pathophysiology of the Alzheimer's syndrome. Neurology 1993;43(suppl 4):S25–S38.

22. Schneider LS. Clinical Pharmacology of aminoacridines in Alzheimer's disease. Neurology 1993;43(suppl 4):S64–S79.
23. Piccini GL, Finali G, Piccirilli M. Neuropsychological effects of L-deprenyl in Alzheimer's type dementia. Clin Neuropharmacol 1990:13:147–163.
24. Francis PT, Sims NR, Procter AW, Bowen DM. Cortical pyramidal neuron loss may cause glutamatergic hypoactivity and cognitive impairment in Alzheimer's disease: Investigative and therapeutic perspectives. J Neurochem 1993;60:1589–1604.
25. Pomara N, Singh R, Deptula D, et al. Glutamate and other CSF amino acids in Alzheimer's disease. Am J Psychiatry 1992;149:251–254.
26. Goodman Y, Bruce AJ, Cheng B, et al. Estrogens attenuate and corticosterone exacerbates excitotoxicity, oxidative injury, and amyloid B-peptide toxicity in hippocampal neurons. J Neurochem 1996;66:1836–1844.
27. Jaffe AB, Toran-Allerand CD, Greengard P, Gandy SE. Estrogen regulates metabolism of Alzheimer amyloid B precursor protein. J Biol Chem 1994;269:13065–13068.
28. Simpkins JW, Singh M, Bishop J. The potential role for estrogen replacement therapy in the treatment of the cognitive decline and neurodegeneration associated with Alzheimer's disease. Neurobiol Aging 1994;15:S195–S197.
29. Wickelgren I. Estrogen stakes claim to cognition. Science 1997;276:675–678.
30. Tang MX, Jacobs D, Stern Y, et al. Effect of estrogen during menopause on risk and age at onset of Alzheimer's disease. Lancet 1996;348:429–432.
31. Seshadri S, Zornberg GL, Derby LE, et al. Postmenopausal estrogen replacement therapy and the risk of Alzheimer disease. Arch Neurol 2001;58:435–440.
32. McKhann G, Drachman D, Folstein M, et al. Clinical diagnosis of Alzheimer's disease. Neurology 1984;34:939–944.
33. Mohs RC. Neuropsychological assessment of patients with Alzheimer's disease. In: Bloom FE, Kupfer DJ, eds. Psychopharmacology: The Fourth Generation of Progress. New York, Raven, 1995:1377–1388.
34. Raskind MA. Geriatric psychopharmacology: Management of late-life depression and the noncognitive behavioral disturbances of Alzheimer's disease. Psychiatry Clin North Am 1993;16:815–827.
35. Doraiswamy PM. Early recognition of Alzheimer's disease: What is consensual? What is controversial? What is practical? J Clin Psychiatry 1998;59(suppl 13):6–18.
36. McKhann G, Drachman D, Folstein M, et al. Clinical diagnosis of Alzheimer's disease: Report of the NINCDS-ADRDA work group under the auspices of the department of health and human services task force on Alzheimer's disease. Neurology 1984;34:939–944.
37. Costa PT Jr., Williams TF, Somerfield M, et al. Recognition and Initial Assessment of Alzheimer's Disease and Related Dementias. Clinical Practice Guideline No. 19. Rockville, MD, US Department of Health and Human Services, Public Health Service, Agency for Health Care Policy and Research, 1996. AHCPR no. 97–0702.
38. Rabins P, Blacker D, Bland W, and the Workgroup on Alzheimer's Disease and Related Dementias. Practice guideline for the treatment of patients with Alzheimer's disease and other dementias of late life. Am J Psychiatry 1997;154(suppl 5):1–39.
39. Geldmacher DS, Whitehouse PJ. Differential diagnosis of Alzheimer's disease. Neurology 1997;48(suppl 6):S2–S9.
40. Folstein MF, Folstein SE, McHugh PR. Mini mental state: A practical method for grading the cognitive state of patients for the clinician. J Psychiatr Res 1975;12:189–198.
41. Doraiswamy PM. Current cholinergic therapy for symptoms of Alzheimer's disease. Prim Psychiatry 1996;3:56–68.
42. Reisberg B, Ferris SH, DeLeon MJ, Crook T. The global deterioration scale for assessment of primary degenerative dementia. Am J Psychiatry 1982;139:1136–1139.
43. Pfeffer RI, Kurosaki TT, Harrah CH, et al. Measurement of functional activities of older adults in the community. J Gerontol 1982;37:323–329.
44. Jonker C, Schmand B, Lindeboom, et al. Association between apolipoprotein E4 and the rate of cognitive decline in community-dwelling elderly individuals with and without dementia. Arch Neurol 1998;55:1065–1069.
45. Tsuang D, Larson E, Bowen J, et al. The utility of apolipoprotein E genotyping in the diagnosis of Alzheimer's disease in a community-based case series. Arch Neurol 1999;56:1489–1495.
46. Mayeux R, Saunders A, Shea S, et al. Utility of the apolipoprotein E genotype in diagnosis of Alzheimer's disease. N Engl J Med 1998;338:506–511.
47. Farrer LA, Cupples LA, Haines JL, et al. Effects of age, sex and ethnicity on the association between apolipoprotein E genotype and Alzheimer's disease: A meta-analysis. JAMA 1997;278:1349–1356.
48. Ganguli M, Chandra V, Kamboh MI, et al. Apolipoprotein E polymorphism and Alzheimer disease. Arch Neurol 2000;57:824–830.
49. Jacobson, SA. Delirium in the elderly. Psychiatr Clin North Am 1997;20(1):91–110.
50. Caine ED. Delirium, dementia, amnestic and other cognitive disorders. In: Saddock BJ, Saddock VA, eds. Comprehensive Textbook of Psychiatry, 7th ed. Philadelphia, Williams & Wilkins, 2000:320–321.
51. Inouye SK. The dilemma of delirium: Clinical and research controversies regarding diagnosis and evaluation of delirium in hospitalized elderly medical patients Am J Med 1994;97:278–288.
52. Tune LE, Carr S, Hoag E, Cooper T. Anticholinergic effect of drugs commonly prescribed for the elderly: Potential means for assessing risk of delirium. Am J Psychiatry 1992;149:1393–1394.
53. Rabins P. Practice guideline for the treatment of patients with Alzheimer's disease and other dementias of late life. Am J Psychiatr 1997;154(suppl 5):1–39.
54. Small GW, Rabins PV, Barry PP, et al. Diagnosis and treatment of Alzheimer disease and related disorders: Consensus statement of the American Association for Geriatric Psychiatry, the Alzheimer's Association, and the American Geriatrics Society. JAMA 1997;278:1363–1371.
55. Cognex expanded access proposed by FDA as part of "program of further study"; Warner-Lambert will support NDA studies with other data by April 1. FDC Rep, March 25, 1991, 4–9.
56. Knopman DS, Knapp MJ, Gracon SI, Davis CS. The clinical interview-based impression (CIBI): A clinician's global change rating scale in Alzheimer's disease. Neurology 1994;44:2315–2321.
57. Crismon ML. Tacrine: First drug approved for Alzheimer's disease. Ann Pharmacother 1994;28:744–751.
58. Sano M, Ernesto C, Thomas RG, et al. A controlled trial of selegiline, alpha-tocopherol, or both as treatment for Alzheimer's disease. N Engl J Med 1997;336:1216–1222.
59. Eisai. Aricept (donepezil hydrochloride) package insert. Teaneck, NJ, September 1998.
60. Nordberg A, Svensson A. Cholinesterase inhibitors in the treatment of Alzheimer's disease: A comparison of tolerability and pharmacology. Drug Saf 1998;19(6):465–480.
61. Rogers SL, Friedhoff LT, donepezil study group. The efficacy and safety of donepezil in patients with Alzheimer's disease: Results of a US multicentre, randomized, double-blind, placebo-controlled trial. Dementia 1996;7:293–303.
62. Rogers SL, Doody RS, Mohs RC, et al. Donepezil improves cognition and global function in Alzheimer disease. Arch Intern Med 1998;158:1021–1031.
63. Rogers SL, Farlow MR, Doody RS, et al. A 24-week, double-blind, placebo-controlled trial of donepezil in patients with Alzheimer's disease. Neurology 1998;50:136–145.
64. Burns A, Rossor M, Hecker J, et al. The effects of donepezil in Alzheimer's disease—Results from a multinational trial. Dement Geriatr Cogn Disord 1999;10:237–244.
65. Rogers SL, Doody RS, Pratt RD, Ieni JR. Long-term efficacy and safety of donepezil in the treatment of Alzheimer's disease: Final analysis of a US multicentre open-label study. Eur Neuropsychopharmacol 2000;10:195–203.
66. Crismon ML. Pharmacokinetics and drug interactions of cholinesterase inhibitors used in Alzheimer's disease. Pharmacotherapy 1998;18(2 Pt 2):47S–54S.

67. Jann MW. Rivastigmine, a new-generation cholinesterase inhibitor for the treatment of Alzheimer's disease. Pharmacotherapy 2000;20:1–12.
68. Corey-Bloom, Anand R, Veach J. A randomized trial evaluating the efficacy and safety of ENA 713 (rivastigmine tartrate), a new acetylcholinesterase inhibitor, in patients with mild to moderately severe Alzheimer's disease. Int J Geriatr Psychopharmacol 1998;1:55–65.
69. Agid Y, Dubois B. Efficacy and tolerability of rivastigmine in patients with dementia of the Alzheimer type. Curr Ther Res 1998;59:837–845.
70. Rosler M, Anand R, Cicin-Sain A, et al. Efficacy and safety of rivastigmine in patients with Alzheimer's disease: International randomized controlled trial. BMJ 1999;318:633–640.
71. Spencer CM, Noble S. Rivastigmine: A review of its use in Alzheimer's disease. Drugs Aging 1998;13:391–441.
72. Tariot PN, Erb R, Podgorski CA, et al. Efficacy and tolerability of carbamazepine for agitation and aggression in dementia. Am J Psychiatry 1998;155:54–61.
73. Raskind MA, Peskind ER, Wessel T, et al. Galantamine in AD: A 6-month randomized, placebo-controlled trial with a 6-month extension. Neurology 2000;54:2261–2268.
74. Sano M, Ernesto C, Thomas RG, et al. A controlled trial of selegiline, alpha-tocopherol, or both as treatment for Alzheimer's disease. N Engl J Med 1997;336:1216–1222.
75. Burke WJ, Roccaforte WH, Wengel SP, et al. L-Deprenyl in the treatment of mild dementia of the Alzheimer type: Results of a 15-month trial. J Am Geriatr Soc 1993;41:1219–1225.
76. Schneider LS, Tariot PN. Emerging drugs for Alzheimer's disease: Mechanisms of action and prospects for cognitive enhancing medications. Med Clin North Am 1994;78:911–934.
77. Henderson VW, Paganini-Hill A, Miller BL, et al. Estrogen for Alzheimer's disease in women: Randomized, double-blind, placebo-controlled trial. Neurology 2000;54:295–301.
78. Mulnard RA, Cotman CW, Kawas C, et al. Estrogen replacement therapy for treatment of mild to moderate Alzheimer disease: A randomized controlled trial. JAMA 2000;283:1007–1015.
79. McGeer PL, Shculzer M, McGeer EG. Arthritis and anti-inflammatory gents as possible protective factors for Alzheimer's disease: A review of 17 epidemiologic studies. Neurology 1996;47:425–432.
80. Stewart WF, Kawas C, Corrada M. Risk of Alzheimer's disease and duration of NSAID use. Neurology 1997;48:626–632.
81. Rogers J, Kirby LC, Hempelman SR, et al. Clinical trial of indomethacin in Alzheimer's disease. Neurology 1993;43:1609–1611.
82. Aisen PS, Davis KL, Berg JD, et al. A randomized controlled trial of prednisone in Alzheimer's disease. Neurology 2000;54:588–593.
83. Schmidt LA, Fox NA, Goldberg MC. Effects of acute prednisone administration on memory, attention and emotion in healthy human adults. Psychoneuroendocrinology 1999;24:461–483.
84. Keenan PA, Jacobson MW, Soleymani RM, et al. The effect on memory of chronic prednisone treatment in patients with systemic disease. Neurology 1996;47:1396–1402.
85. Scharf S, Mander A, Ugoni A, et al. A double-blind, placebo-controlled trial of diclofenac/misoprostol in Alzheimer's disease. Neurology 1999;53:197–201.
86. Oken BS, Storzbach DM, Kaye JA. The efficacy of ginkgo biloba on cognitive function in Alzheimer disease. Arch Neurol 1998;55:1409–1415.
87. Borson S, Raskind MA. Clinical features and pharmacologic treatment of behavioral symptoms of Alzheimer's disease. Neurology 1997;48:S17–S24.
88. Schneider LS, Pollock VE, Lyness SA. A meta-analysis of controlled trials of neuroleptic treatment in dementia. J Am Geriatr Soc 1990;38:553–563.
89. Tune LE, Carr S, Hoag E, Cooper T. Anticholinergic effect of drugs commonly prescribed for the elderly: Potential means for assessing risk of delirium. Am J Psychiatry 1992;149:1393–1394.
90. Lanctot KL, Best TS, Mittman N, et al. Efficacy and safety of neuroleptics in behavioral disorders associated with dementia. J Clin Psychiatry 1998;59:550–561.
91. Katz IR, Jeste DV, Mintzer JE, et al. Comparison of risperidone and placebo for psychosis and behavioral disturbances associated with dementia: A randomized, double-blind trial. J Clin Psychiatry 1999;60:107–115.
92. Street JS, Clark WS, Gannon KS, et al. Olanzapine treatment of psychotic and behavioral symptoms in patients with Alzheimer disease in nursing care facilities. Arch Gen Psychiatry 2000;57:968–976.
93. Raskind MA, Peskind ER, Wessel T, et al. Galantamine in AD: A 6-month randomized, placebo-controlled trial with a 6-month extension. Neurology 2000;54:2261–2268.
94. Pollock BG. A placebo-controlled trial of citalopram and fluphenazine in behavioral problems of dementia. Abstracts of the 2000 Annual Meeting of the American Psychiatric Association, May 2000.
95. Defilippi JL, Crismon ML. The use of antipsychotic agents in patients with dementia. Pharmacotherapy 2000;20:23–33.
96. Taragano FE, Lyketsos CG, Mangone CA, et al. A double-blind, randomized, fixed-dose trial of fluoxetine vs. amitriptyline in the treatment of major depression complicating Alzheimer's disease. Psychosomatics 1997;38:246–252.
97. Geldmacher DS, Waldman AJ, Doty L, Heilman KM. Fluoxetine in dementia of the Alzheimer's type: Prominent adverse effects and failure to improve cognition. J Clin Psychiatry 1994;55:161.
98. Schneider LS, Pollock Lyness SA. A meta-analysis of controlled trials of VE, neuroleptic treatment in dementia. J Am Geriatr Soc 1990;38:553–563.
99. Sakuye KM, Camp CJ, Ford PA. Effects of buspirone on agitation associated with dementia. Am J Geriatr Psychiatry 1993;1:82–84.
100. Hermann N, Eryavec G. Buspirone in the management of agitation and aggression associated with dementia. Am J Geriatr Psychiatry 1993;1:249–253.
101. Tariot PN, Cohen RM, Sunderland T, et al. L-Deprenyl in Alzheimer's disease. Arch Gen Psychiatry 1987;44:427–433.
102. Schneider LS, Pollock VE, Zemansky MF, et al. A pilot study of low-dose L-deprenyl in Alzheimer's disease. J Geriatr Psychiatry Neurol 1991;4:143–148.
103. Cummings JL. Cholinesterase inhibitors: A new class of psychotropic compounds. Am J Psychiatry 2000;157:4–15.
104. Lubeck DP, Mazonson PD, Bowe T. Potential effect of tacrine on expenditures for Alzheimer's disease. Med Interface 1994;7:130–138.
105. Ernst RL, Hay JW, Fenn C, et al. Cognitive function and the costs of Alzheimer disease: An exploratory study. Arch Neurology 1997;54:687–693.
106. Janssen Pharmaceutica. Reminyl (galantamine hydrobromide) package insert. Titusville, NJ, February 2001.
107. Novartis Pharmaceuticals. Exelon (rivastigmine tartrate) package insert. East Hanover, NJ, January 2001.
108. Parke Davis Division of Warner-Lambert. Cognex (tacrine hydrochloride tablets) package insert. Morris Plains, NJ, May 1998.

66

SUBSTANCE-RELATED DISORDERS: OVERVIEW AND DEPRESSANTS, STIMULANTS, AND HALLUCINOGENS

Paul L. Doering

Abuse of alcohol, tobacco, and other drugs (ATOD) is the nation's number one health problem, according to a Robert Wood Johnson (RWJ) health care report prepared by the Institute for Health Policy, Brandeis University.[1] The economic cost of substance abuse to the U.S. economy each year is staggering, and it is estimated at over $414 billion.[1] A heavy smoker will stay 25% longer when hospitalized than a nonsmoker, and a problem drinker will stay four times as long as a nondrinker.[1] According to RWJ, "Without a reduction in ATOD abuse, health care costs cannot be curtailed effectively." Each year, there are more deaths and disabilities from ATOD abuse than from any other preventable cause.[1] Of the more than 2 million deaths each year in the United States, approximately one in four is attributable to alcohol, illicit drug, or tobacco use: 100,000 people die as a result of alcohol, 16,000 from illicit drug use and related AIDS deaths, and 430,700 from tobacco-related illness.

RWJ also reports a direct link to crime and arrests, with one-half to two-thirds of homicides and serious crimes involving alcohol. Nearly one-half of men arrested for homicide and assault actually test positive for an illegal drug.[1] ATOD abuse contributes to family problems, with one in four Americans reporting that alcohol has been a cause of trouble in the family and alcohol abuse playing a part in one of three failed marriages.[1]

This and the next chapter focus on the problems associated with the abuse of chemical substances and the things clinicians can do to help deal with these problems.

TERMINOLOGY

The lack of a common vocabulary in substance abuse treatment and prevention leads to several problems. There is a large array of terms in common use, many without precise meaning. A number of professional disciplines are involved in research, treatment, and education regarding alcohol and other drug-related problems, and each discipline tends to use its own terminology. This lack of universal agreement on language hampers effective communication among professionals and leads to difficulties in formulating public policy and administering third-party reimbursement programs.

To remedy this situation, the American Medical Association's Council on Scientific Affairs, Panels on Alcoholism and Drug Abuse recommended establishment of a task force to develop standard definitions. Representatives from 23 professional organizations used a four-stage Delphi survey of substance abuse experts to help achieve greater clarity and uniformity in terminology associated with alcohol and other drug-related problems. Their efforts resulted in a list of 50 most important substance abuse terms and their definitions.[2] The following are a few of the terms agreed on by the panel:

- *Abstinence.* Cessation of use of a psychoactive substance previously abused or on which the user has developed drug dependence.
- *Abuse potential.* The property of a substance that, by its physiologic or psychological effects, or both, increases the likelihood of an individual's abusing or becoming dependent on the substance.
- *(Drug) addiction.* A chronic disorder characterized by the compulsive use of a substance resulting in physical, psychological, or social harm to the user and continued use despite that harm.
- *Alcohol abuse.* Use of ethyl alcohol in a quantity and with a frequency that cause the individual significant physiologic, psychological, or sociologic distress or impairment.
- *Alcohol dependence.* Chronic loss of control over the consumption of alcoholic beverages despite obvious psychological or physical harm to the person. Increasing amounts are required over time, and abrupt discontinuance may precipitate a withdrawal syndrome. Following abstinence, relapse is frequent.
- *Alcoholism.* A chronic, progressive, and potentially fatal biogenetic and psychosocial disease characterized by tolerance and physical dependence and manifested by a loss of control, as well as diverse personality changes and social consequences.
- *(Drug) dependence.* A generic term that relates to physical or psychological dependence, or both. It is characteristic for each pharmacologic class of psychoactive drugs. Impaired control over drug-taking behavior is implied.
- *Drug abuse.* Any use of drugs that causes physical, psychological, economic, legal, or social harm to the individual user or to others affected by the drug user's behavior.
- *Drug misuse.* Any use of a drug that varies from a socially or medically accepted use.
- *Physical dependence.* A physiologic state of adaptation to a drug or alcohol, usually characterized by the development of tolerance to drug effects and the emergence of a withdrawal syndrome during prolonged abstinence.
- *Psychological dependence.* The emotional state of craving a drug either for its positive effect or to avoid negative effects associated with its absence.
- *Substance abuse.* The use of a psychoactive substance in a manner detrimental to the individual or society but not meeting criteria for substance or drug dependence.

- *Tolerance.* Physiologic adaptation to the effect of drugs so as to diminish effects with constant dosages or to maintain the intensity and duration of effects through increased dosage.
- *Withdrawal syndrome.* The onset of a predictable constellation of signs and symptoms involving alerted activity of the central nervous system after the abrupt discontinuation of or rapid decrease in dosage of a drug.

EPIDEMIOLOGY

NATIONAL HOUSEHOLD SURVEY ON DRUG ABUSE

The National Household Survey on Drug Abuse[3] is the primary source of statistical information on the use of illegal drugs by the U.S. population. Conducted by the federal government since 1971, the survey collects data from a representative sample of the population at their place of residence. Since October 1992, the survey has been supported and directed by the Substance Abuse and Mental Health Services Administration (SAMHSA).

At the time of this writing, the most recent data available from the Household Survey are from 1999. These data show that an estimated 14.8 million Americans were current illicit drug users (i.e., they had used an illicit drug in the month prior to interview). This represents 6.7% of the population 12 years old and older. Marijuana is the most commonly used illicit drug, used by 75% of current illicit drug users. About 43% of current illicit drug users in 1999 (an estimated 6.4 million Americans) were current users of illicit drugs other than marijuana and hashish.[3]

The overall use of illicit drugs among Americans of all ages remained unchanged in 1999, but the decline in illicit drug use among young people ages 12 to 17 that began in 1997 has continued through 1999. Among teens, there has been a consistent, downward trend from 11.4% in 1997 to 9.9% in 1998 to 9.0% in 1999—a statistically significant decline. The number of illicit drug users was at its highest level in 1979 (25.4 million, 14.1%), declined until 1992 (12.0 million, 5.8%), and remained at approximately the same level through 1999.[3]

The highest rate of illicit drug use was found among persons aged 18 to 20 years, with rates of current use between 20% and 21%. As in prior years, men continued to have a higher rate of current illicit drug use than women (8.7% versus 4.9%) in 1999. Among adults aged 18 and older in 1999, college graduates had the lowest rate of current use (4.8%). The rate was 7.1% among adults who had not completed high school. This is despite the fact that adults who had completed 4 years of college were more likely to have tried illicit drugs in their lifetime than adults who had not completed high school (45.6% versus 30.0%).

THE MONITORING THE FUTURE STUDY

Every year the Institute for Social Research of the University of Michigan conducts its Monitoring the Future Study (MTFS), supported under a series of research grants from the National Institute on Drug Abuse.[4] The project has many purposes. Among them is to study changes in the beliefs, attitudes, and behavior of young people in the United States. This study focuses on youth because of their significant involvement in today's social changes and, most important, because youth in a very literal sense will constitute our future society.[4]

In 1999, approximately 45,000 eighth, tenth, and twelfth grade students in 433 public and private secondary schools were surveyed. After one or two years of decline, overall illicit drug use among teens remained steady in 1999 in all three grades. Marijuana is the most widely used illicit drug. The annual prevalence rates in grades 8, 10, and 12, respectively, are 17%, 32%, and 38%, and current daily prevalence rates (defined as the proportion using it on 20 or more occasions in the prior 30 days) are 1.4%, 3.8%, and 6.0%. Other interesting trends have emerged for the following drugs:

Ecstasy. Use of this so-called club drug showed a sharp rise in 1999 among older teens. About 1 in 20 tenth and twelfth grade students indicated using ecstasy at some time during the prior 12 months (4.4% and 5.6%, respectively).

Anabolic steroids. Use of steroids among younger male teens increased in 1999. Roughly 1 in every 40 boys in the eighth (2.5%) and tenth (2.8%) grades indicated some steroid use during the prior year, a statistically significant increase over 1998.

Inhalants. Inhalant use continued a gradual decline, one that has been ongoing for the past 4 years. Inhalants, the only class of drug that tends to be more popular among younger teens than older ones, include a wide variety of common household products that youngsters inhale or "huff" in order to get high, such as glues, solvents, butane, gasoline, and aerosols. The annual prevalence rates for eighth, tenth, and twelfth graders in 1999 were 10%, 7%, and 6%, respectively.

Crack cocaine. Use of crack cocaine declined in 1999 among eighth graders for the first time in some years and leveled off among tenth graders. Annual prevalence for crack stands at 1.8%, 2.4%, and 2.7% at grades 8, 10, and 12.

Crystal methamphetamine. Use of this stimulant drug exhibited a significant decline in 1999 among twelfth graders (the only grade level at which use is asked). The annual prevalence of methamphetamine use in twelfth grade fell from 3.0% in 1998 to 1.9% in 1999.

TRENDS IN SUBSTANCE ABUSE EMERGENCIES: THE DAWN PROGRAM

Since the early 1970s, the Drug Abuse Warning Network (DAWN),[5] an ongoing national survey of hospital emergency departments (ED) has collected information on patients seeking hospital ED treatment related to their use of an illegal drug or the nonmedical use of a legal drug. The survey provides data that describe the impact of drug use on hospital ED in the United States. More important, it serves as an early warning system to the ever-changing patterns of use of illegal drugs. These data allow health care professionals to be better prepared to react to medical emergencies arising from illegal drug use and to target prevention and education programs to specific drug-using groups or populations.

DAWN defines a *drug-related episode* as an ED visit that was induced by or related to the use of an illegal drug(s) or the nonmedical use of a legal drug for patients aged 6 years and older. A *drug mention* refers to a substance that was mentioned during a drug-related ED episode. Because up to four drugs can be reported for each drug-related episode, there are more mentions than episodes cited in DAWN's reports.

In 1999, there were an estimated 554,932 drug-related ED episodes and 1,015,206 ED drug mentions in the United States. Cocaine-related episodes constituted 30% of all ED drug-related episodes in 1999, more than any other illicit substance measured by DAWN. This figure was relatively unchanged from 1998.

Heroin/morphine-related episodes were relatively stable from 1998 (77,645 mentions) to 1999 (84,409). Heroin/morphine was mentioned in 15% of ED episodes.

ECONOMIC IMPACT OF SUBSTANCE ABUSE

Substance abuse and addiction have an enormous impact on the economy. In a 1996 study, the Center on Addiction and Substance Abuse (CASA) at Columbia University found that 21 cents of every tax dollar paid to the City of New York was attributable to substance abuse and addiction.[6] Additionally, in 1994, substance abuse and addiction cost New York City more than $20 billion. Of that $20 billion, less than 4% ($735 million) went toward the actual treatment of substance abuse and addiction, and only 0.4% ($80 million) was spent on ways to prevent it. The other $19.2 billion paid for the consequences of the problem.[6]

Another CASA study showed that the total impact of substance abuse on federal entitlement programs (e.g., Medicare, Medicaid, Veterans Administration, federal employee and other health programs, SSDI, AFDC, food stamps, SSI, and unemployment compensation) could be estimated conservatively to be $77.6 billion. Of this amount, $66.4 billion represents costs directly attributed to substance abuse.[7] The public assistance expenditure for recipients whose substance abuse or addiction must be addressed before they become self-sufficient amounts to $11.2 billion. Although 92% of substance abuse–related health entitlement costs is spent to treat the consequences of tobacco, alcohol, and drug abuse, only 8% is spent to treat alcohol, drug, or tobacco dependence.[7]

CASA also has examined the cost of substance abuse and addiction to our Medicaid[8] and Medicare[9] programs. Nearly 1 of every 5 dollars ($7.4 billion out of $41 billion) spent by Medicaid in 1994 on inpatient services and more than 1 of every 4 dollars ($20 billion out of $87 billion) spent by Medicare during the same period on inpatient hospital care were attributable to ATOD abuse and addiction. One of every five Medicaid hospital days is attributable to substance abuse. More than 70 conditions that require hospitalization in the Medicaid population are attributable in whole or in part to ATOD abuse.[8,9]

The majority of the substance abuse–related diseases in the Medicaid population are linked to tobacco and illicit drugs, many related to birth complications resulting from cocaine use. More than 60 Medicare ailments are attributable to ATOD abuse. The majority of the substance abuse–related diseases in the Medicare population are associated with tobacco, which accounts for 80% of these diseases. If substance abuse and addiction do not decrease, it will cost the Medicare program alone more than $1 trillion over the next 20 years.[9]

Substance abuse is a major complicating factor in our correctional system today. A study published in 1998 found that 80% of the total population in federal prisons were substance-related offenders; that is, they committed a drug offense and/or were substance users whose use of alcohol or drugs was somehow related to their crime. In state prisons, 81% were substance-related offenders. Nearly ten times as many inmates were serving time for drug offenses in 1993 as in 1980. Involvement in criminal activity varied directly with the prevalence, frequency, and seriousness of drug use. Persons testing positive for drugs at the time of arrest have a higher probability of being rearrested. Addicted offenders who receive little or no treatment for their substance abuse problem appear to show an accelerating pattern of criminal activity over time.[10]

ACUTE VERSUS CHRONIC PROBLEMS

Misuse of chemical substances causes problems of two types: those which occur acutely and those which arise after continued use of a drug. Acute problems are usually predictable, given the pharmacology of the drug. Acute drug intoxications usually occur at doses in excess of that normally taken. Chronic abuse of chemical substances can cause a wide array of physical, psychological, and psychiatric ailments. The substance-induced disorders to be discussed here mainly include intoxication and withdrawal. Psychiatric problems associated with substance abuse, including dementia, psychosis, mood disorders, and anxiety, are discussed elsewhere. Physical illnesses associated with chronic use of chemicals (e.g., alcoholic liver disease) are likewise covered in other chapters.

The essential feature of substance dependence is the continued use of the substance despite adverse substance-related problems. The criteria for substance dependence are the same for each of the drugs or drug classes, varying only to fit the unique pharmacologic properties of each drug. Patients who take prescribed drugs for appropriate medical indications and in correct dose may still show tolerance, physical dependence, and withdrawal symptoms if the drug is stopped abruptly rather than being tapered. Tolerance and physical dependence are inevitable consequences of chronic treatment with opioids and certain other drugs, but tolerance and physical dependence, by themselves, do not imply "addiction." To meet criteria for the diagnosis of substance dependence, at least three of the following must be present at any time in a 12-month period:

1. Tolerance.
2. Withdrawal, indicated by the appearance of the characteristic withdrawal syndrome or the use of the same or related drug to relieve or avoid withdrawal symptoms.
3. Substance taken in larger amounts or over a longer period of time than was intended.
4. Persistent desire or unsuccessful efforts to cut down or control substance use.
5. Time spent in activities necessary to obtain the substance, use the substance, or recover from its effects.
6. Social, occupational, or recreational activities given up or reduced because of substance use.
7. Substance use continued despite knowledge of having a persistent or recurrent physical or psychological problem caused or exacerbated by the substance.

The characteristic feature of substance abuse is a maladaptive pattern of substance use indicated by repeated adverse consequences related to the repeated use of the substance. Examples include failure to fulfill important obligations at work, school, or home; repeated use in situations in which it is physically dangerous, such as driving under the influence; legal problems; and social or interpersonal problems such as arguments and fights.

Intoxication refers to the development of a substance-specific syndrome after recent ingestion and presence in the body of a substance, and it is associated with maladaptive behavior during the waking state caused by the effect of the substance on the central nervous system (CNS). Examples include belligerence, mood lability, impaired judgment, and impaired social or occupational functioning. Evidence for recent intake of the substance can be obtained from the history, physical examination, or laboratory examination. The most common changes involve disturbances in perception, wakefulness, attention, thinking, judgment, motor behavior, and interpersonal behavior.

In addition to the previous definition, *withdrawal* can be further described as the development of a substance-specific syndrome after cessation of or reduction in intake of a substance that was used regularly by the individual to induce a state of intoxication. Withdrawal causes significant distress to the individual and is associated with impairment in social, occupational, or other areas of functioning. Withdrawal is usually associated with substance dependence. Withdrawal generally is also associated with a craving to readminister the drug to relieve the symptoms.

As with most illnesses, the course and prognosis of the disorders of substance use and dependence are variable. Untreated physical withdrawal from the CNS depressants is potentially life-threatening, but withdrawal almost always can be managed successfully with proper medical care. Getting patients who are drug dependent to stop using drugs is very difficult, and many patients return to drug use even after treatment. As many as 75% of treated substance-dependent patients relapse at least once. Many patients, however, are able to obtain recovery with treatment and continued care in programs such as Alcoholics Anonymous (AA) or Narcotics Anonymous (NA). Substance dependence or addiction can be viewed as a chronic illness that can be controlled successfully with treatment but cannot be cured and is associated with a high relapse rate. Without treatment, the course can progress to life-threatening severity, resulting from the effects of the drug, drug contaminants, or medical complications of use.

CNS DEPRESSANTS

BENZODIAZEPINES AND OTHER SEDATIVE–HYPNOTICS

In clinical practice, the benzodiazepines largely have replaced the short-acting barbiturates and other nonbarbiturate sedative-hypnotics. Benzodiazepines with faster onset (e.g., diazepam) tend to be preferred by the recreational drug user because they are reinforcing. A few years ago, flunitrazepam burst on the scene as a "party drug" and a "date-rape drug."[11] It will be discussed in a separate section later. Because all benzodiazepines have abuse and dependence liability, patients cannot be switched from one benzodiazepine to another in hopes of decreasing a pattern of drug abuse or dependence behavior. Zolpidem, a nonbenzodiazepine, nonbarbiturate sedative, has been suggested to have little liability for physical dependence, but tolerance and withdrawal have been reported in association with its use as well.[12]

Benzodiazepines generally do not cause significant respiratory depression, as do the barbiturate-like drugs.[13] Signs and symptoms of withdrawal are similar in many respects to those of alcohol withdrawal, but the time courses may be quite different. While withdrawal from shorter-acting agents (e.g., lorazepam and alprazolam) has an onset within 12 to 24 hours of the last dose, others (e.g., diazepam, chlordiazepoxide, clorazepate, phenobarbital, and amobarbital) have elimination half-lives or active metabolites with elimination half-lives of 24 to over 100 hours. As a result, the onset of withdrawal symptoms may be delayed for several days after discontinuation of the drug.[14] Dependence on sedative-hypnotics and benzodiazepines is summarized in Table 66–1.

Long-term use of even therapeutic doses of benzodiazepines may cause physical dependence and withdrawal symptoms after abrupt discontinuation.[14] The likelihood and severity of withdrawal are a function of both dose and duration of exposure. Gradual tapering of dosage is also associated with less withdrawal and rebound anxiety than abrupt discontinuation. Patients who have taken benzodiazepines for the treatment of anxiety often experience a rebound increase in anxiety after discontinuation of the antianxiety drug. The heightened autonomic activity of severe anxiety can be mistaken easily for drug withdrawal. A combination of withdrawal and increased anxiety also may occur, and each may intensify the other. Occurrence of hallucinations or seizures would indicate severe physical withdrawal. For additional information on benzodiazepine withdrawal, refer to Chapter 71.

FLUNITRAZEPAM

Flunitrazepam emerged in the mid-1990s as an illegal drug in the United States that was predominantly abused recreationally and

TABLE 66–1. Dependence on Sedative–Hypnotics[a]

Generic Name	Common Trade Names (Manufacturer)	Oral Sedating Dose (mg)	Physical Dependence Dose and Time Needed to Produce Dependence	Time Before Onset of Withdrawal (h)	Peak Withdrawal Symptoms (d)
Benzodiazepines					
Diazepam	Valium (Roche)	5–10	40–100 mg × 42–120 d	12–24	5–8
Chlordiazepoxide	Librium, Libritabs (Roche)	10–25	75–600 mg × 42–120 d	12–24	5–8
Clorazepate	Tranxene (Abbott)	7.5–15	45–180 mg × 42–120 d (est.)	12–24	5–8
Alprazolam	Xanax (Upjohn)	0.25–8	8–16 mg × 42 d (est.)	8–24	2–3
Flunitrazepam	Rohypnol (Roche)	1–2	8–10 mg × 42 d (est.)	24–36	2–3
Barbiturates					
Secobarbital	Seconal, Seco-8 (Lilly)	100	800–2200 mg × 35–37 d	6–12	2–3
Pentobarbital	Nembutal (Abbott)	100	Same	6–12	2–3
Equal parts of secobarbital and amobarbital	Tuinal (Lilly)	100	Same	6–12	2–3
Amobarbital	Amytal (Lilly)	65–100	Same	8–12	2–5
Nonbarbiturate Sedative–Hypnotics					
Ethchlorvynol	Placidyl (Abbott)	200	1–1.5 g × 30 d	6–12	2–3
Chloral hydrate	Noctec (various)	250	Exact dose unknown; 12 g/d chronically has led to delirium upon sudden withdrawal	6–12	2–3
Meprobamate	Equanil, Miltown, Meprotabs (various)	400	1.6–3.2 g × 270 d	8–12	3–8

Withdrawal symptoms are tremor, tachycardia, diaphoresis, nausea, vomiting, blood pressure delirium, seizures, and hallucinations.

associated with sexual assaults. Medically, this benzodiazepine is used in the short-term treatment of insomnia and as a preanesthetic medication. It has physiologic effects similar to those of diazepam. A comprehensive review of this drug has been published and will serve as a basis for the discussion below.[11]

Marketed under the trade name Rohypnol, flunitrazepam is manufactured worldwide, including Europe and Latin America, in 1- and 2-mg tablets by Hoffman-LaRoche. However, the drug is neither manufactured nor approved for medical use in the United States.

Flunitrazepam is ingested orally, frequently in conjunction with alcohol or other drugs, including heroin. The drug's effects begin within 30 minutes, peak within 2 hours, and may persist for up to 8 hours or more depending on the dosage.[11] Adverse effects associated with the use of flunitrazepam include decreased blood pressure, memory impairment, drowsiness, visual disturbances, dizziness, confusion, gastrointestinal disturbances, and urinary retention.

Flunitrazepam use causes dependence in humans. Once dependence has developed, abstinence induces withdrawal symptoms, including headache, muscle pain, extreme anxiety, tension, restlessness, confusion, and irritability. Numbness, tingling of the extremities, loss of identity, hallucinations, delirium, convulsions, shock, and cardiovascular collapse also may occur. Withdrawal seizures can occur 1 week or more after cessation of use. As with other benzodiazepines, treatment for flunitrazepam dependence includes a gradual tapering of the drug.[11]

Flunitrazepam is often combined with alcohol, marijuana, or cocaine to produce a rapid and very dramatic "high." Even when used by itself, the drug can cause users to appear extremely intoxicated, with slurred speech, poor coordination, swaying, and bloodshot eyes, with no odor of alcohol. The drug has been added to punch and other drinks at fraternity parties and college social gatherings, where it is reportedly given to female party participants in hopes of lowering inhibitions and facilitating potential sexual conquest. Police departments in several parts of the country say that after ingestion of flunitrazepam, several young women have reported waking up in strange surroundings with no clothes on or actually having been sexually assaulted while under the influence of the drug.[15] For this reason, flunitrazepam has come to be called the "date rape drug."

Flunitrazepam and other benzodiazepines are often detected in biologic samples from driving under the influence (DUI) offenders. Data collected over a 3½-year period in Miami-Dade County, Florida, showed that flunitrazepam was present in up to 10% of DUI cases in 1995 and 1996 and had fast become the most frequently encountered benzodiazepine. However, a dramatic drop in case numbers followed the legal reclassification of the drug as a schedule I substance in Florida in February 1997. A recent rise in clonazepam cases coincides with the decrease in flunitrazepam confirmation and may indicate a new trend in abuse of the benzodiazepines.[16]

γ-HYDROXY BUTYRATE

γ-Hydroxybutyric acid (GHB) is a chemical compound structurally similar to the inhibitory brain neurotransmitter γ-amino butyric acid (GABA). Powdered forms of GHB were marketed in health food stores as a "nutritional supplement" before being removed from the retail market by the Food and Drug Administration (FDA) in 1991. At that time it was used primarily by body builders for its purported ability to increase growth hormone, but it proved to cause serious illness and death when taken in excess doses or in combination with alcohol or other drugs. With the exception of investigational research, it is not approved for any use in the United States. Primary groups using GHB include party and nightclub attendees. Like flunitrazepam, GHB is also characterized as a "date rape drug."[15] From August 1995 to September 1996, poison control centers in New York and Texas received reports of 69 acute poisonings and one death attributed to ingestion of GHB.[17]

Although some of the neurophysiologic actions of GHB could involve alterations in dopaminergic transmission in the basal ganglia, both its physiologic and pharmacologic actions probably are mediated through specific brain receptors for GHB. In addition, GHB might mediate some of its effects through interaction with the $GABA_B$ receptor.[18] Manifestations of acute GHB toxicity include coma, seizures, respiratory depression, and vomiting. Other documented effects of GHB include amnesia and hypotonia (associated with doses of 10 mg/kg of body weight), abnormal sequence of rapid eye movement (REM) and non-REM sleep (doses of 20 to 30 mg/kg), and anesthesia (doses of approximately 50 mg/kg). Doses greater than 50 mg/kg can decrease cardiac output and produce severe respiratory depression, seizurelike activity, and coma[19]; coma and respiratory depression may be potentiated by concomitant use of alcohol.[20] There is no antidote for GHB overdose, and treatment is restricted to nonspecific supportive care. Figure 66-1 shows a protocol recommended for treating suspected GHB overdoses.

In the United States, GHB has been produced clandestinely in widely varying degrees of purity. Today, GHB is sold mostly as a liquid under such names as "grievous bodily harm," "Georgia home boy," "liquid ecstasy," "liquid X," "liquid E," "GHB," "soap," "scoop," "easy lay," "salty water," "G-riffick," and "organic quaalude."

In Dallas, GHB use has been associated with events at which several persons have been found comatose. Some persons who have sustained adverse effects of GHB have reported being given the drug surreptitiously (e.g., having it slipped into their drink), whereas others have admitted to intentional use. In March 2000, GHB was placed into schedule I of the Controlled Substances Act. Until recently, the major source of GHB sold on the streets was manufacture from inexpensive kits obtained over the Internet. It is mixed largely by nonchemists from recipes that can be flawed or incomplete, and finished products are often of questionable purity and, more important, unknown potency. Improper preparation of GHB can result in a mixture of GHB and sodium hydroxide that can be severely toxic because of the combined effects of the GHB and the direct caustic effects of sodium hydroxide. Since there is no way to tell the strength of homemade GHB, what might be a safe dose today (e.g., "one capful") could produce a toxic dose tomorrow if a different batch is used. Fortunately, crackdowns in 1997 by the FDA, the Department of Justice, and other enforcement groups has led to a decreased availability of ready-made kits on the Internet. Despite the FDA's action, GHB remains available to consumers.

The decreased Internet availability of kits to make GHB has been accompanied by an increased availability of chemical precursors to GHB as well as GHB analogs. Also available in gyms and health food stores, these substances include γ-butyrolactone (GBL) and 1,4-butanediol. GBL is converted in the body to GHB. Labels of marketed products may use unfamiliar synonyms to disguise the actual content. GBL is also known by the chemical names 2(3H)-furanone dihydro, butyrolactone, γ-butyrolactone, 4-butyrolactone, dihydro-2(3H) furanone; 4-butanolide, 2(3H)-furanone, dihydro, tetrahydro-2-furanone, and butyrolactone-γ. Marketed as "nutritional" or "dietary" supplements, these products claim to fight stress and depression, relieve anxiety, induce deep sleep, stimulate growth hormone, aid in muscle building, enhance athletic performance, combat aging, and enhance sexual performance. They are available under an ever-increasing list of proprietary names, including Renewtrient, Blue Nitro, and Revivarant.[19]

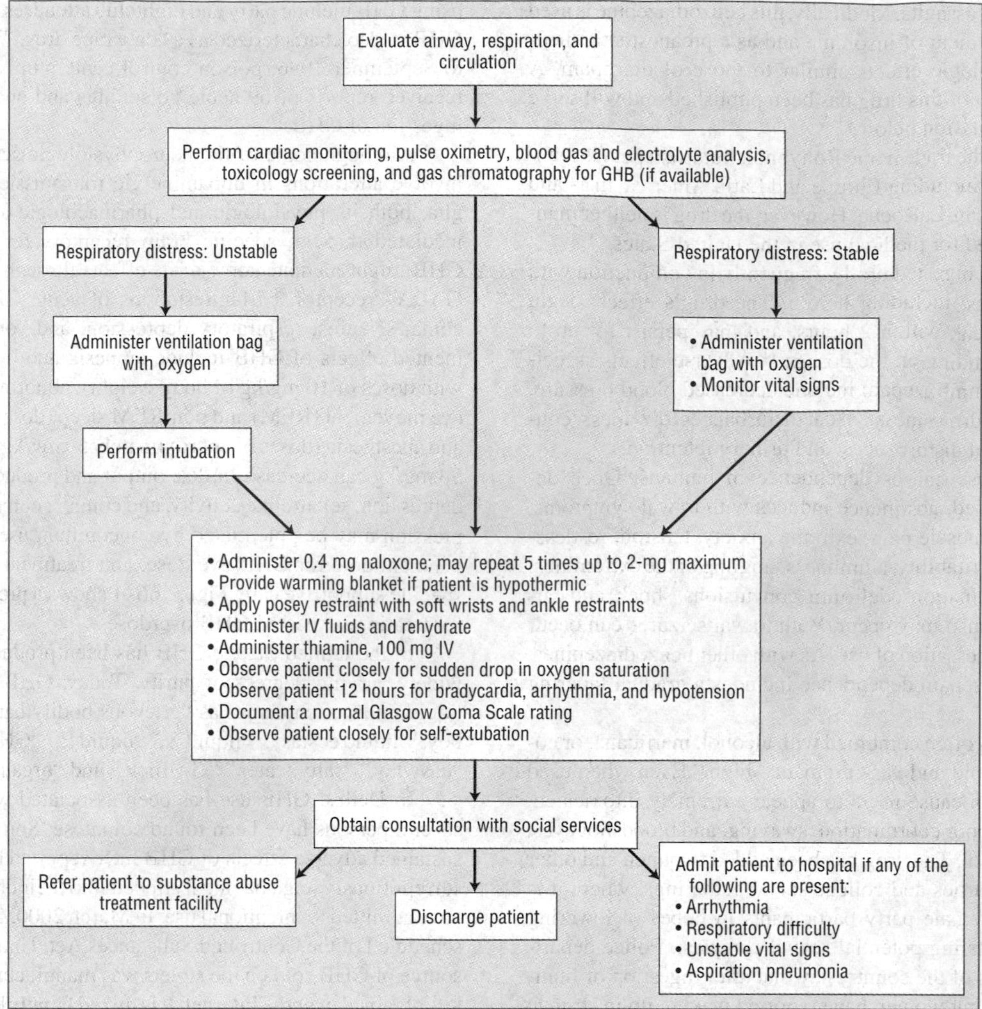

FIGURE 66–1. Protocol for treatment of suspected GHB overdose.

Most clinically significant effects of GHB, even when mixed with other drugs, fade within hours. Respiratory suppression, leading to hypoxia and death, is the most serious of these effects. As stated earlier, treatment is complicated by the fact that precise dosing information is usually not available because GHB purchased on the street may vary in potency. In general, treatment is symptomatic and supportive.

Withdrawal resulting in severe agitation, mental status changes, elevated blood pressure, and tachycardia has been reported hours after stopping chronic use of GHB. In one case, the patient admitted to substantial GHB abuse on a daily basis for 2.5 years. Previous attempts at cessation reportedly resulted in diaphoresis, tremors, and agitation. The patient required 507 mg lorazepam and 120 mg diazepam over 90 hours to control agitation.[21] Given the increasing use of GHB, more cases of severe GHB withdrawal should be anticipated.

OPIATES

Incidence and prevalence of opiate use are widely variable depending on the drug. Heroin gained widespread notoriety during the 1960s and 1970s and remains the single most commonly used illicit opiate. In 1999, an estimated 200,000 Americans were current heroin users. Among past year users of heroin, 35% were dependent on heroin.[3] In Florida, the Medical Examiner's Commission reported that heroin-related deaths skyrocketed from 28 in 1993 to 206 in 1998, an increase of more than 600%. Collectively, use of opiates other than heroin is far more common. Approximately 6% of adults have tried an opiate or opiatelike analgesic for nonmedical use, with around 1% having used an opiate analgesic within 1 month.[3] Hydromorphone has become widely used among the opiate-using population, with single 4-mg tablets selling for as much as $70.[22] Hydromorphone has a pharmaceutical profile very similar to heroin, with the advantage of purity. Drug combinations involving opiates are quite popular. Opiates are commonly combined with stimulant drugs, especially cocaine, a combination known as a "speedball." Opiate users frequently also drink alcohol, especially when their use of opiate drugs declines because of lack of availability or sometimes following treatment.

Many of the complications of opiate use, especially intravenous use, are related not only to the drug itself but also to varying purity, contaminants, and techniques of administration such as dirty equipment and use of shared needles. Overdoses, anaphylactic reactions to impurities, nephrotic syndrome, septicemia, endocarditis, and acquired immune deficiency syndrome (AIDS) are examples.

Signs and symptoms of opioid intoxication and withdrawal are summarized in Table 66–2.[23] Onset of the acute phase of withdrawal varies with the drug consumed but ranges from a few hours after stopping heroin to 3 to 5 days after stopping methadone. The duration of withdrawal ranges from 3 to 14 days. Opioid withdrawal is

TABLE 66–2. Signs and Symptoms of Opioid Intoxication and Withdrawal

Intoxication	Withdrawal
Euphoria	Lacrimation
Dysphoria	Rhinorrhea
Apathy	Mydriasis
Motor retardation	Piloerection
Sedation	Diaphoresis
Slurred speech	Diarrhea
Attention impairment	Yawning
Miosis	Fever
	Insomnia
	Muscle aching

significantly different from withdrawal from alcohol or other sedative-hypnotics. The biggest difference is that opioid withdrawal is not fatal unless there is a concurrent medical problem of major concern. This has significant treatment implications. Although patients in opioid withdrawal may be in great discomfort and incapacitated, they are not delirious. The presence of delirium should raise the question of concurrent withdrawal from another drug, such as alcohol, or another cause of delirium possibly secondary to drug use.

Some researchers have noted that snorting and smoking heroin may be growing in popularity as alternatives to injecting the drug.[3] Regardless of how users take the drug, an increase in the purity of heroin could be one reason for the increase in hospital ED visits. During the last decade, the purity of street heroin ranged from 1% to 10%; more recently, the purity of heroin, especially that from South America, has skyrocketed to rates as high as 98%, with the national purity average at 41%.[24]

Another form of heroin known as "black tar" is available in the western United States. Black tar heroin, which is produced only in Mexico, may be sticky like roofing tar or hard like coal, and its color may vary from dark brown to black. The color and consistency of black tar heroin result from the crude processing methods used to illicitly manufacture heroin in Mexico. Black tar heroin is often sold on the street in its tarlike state at purities ranging from 20% to 80%. It is most frequently dissolved, diluted, and injected.[24]

CNS STIMULANTS

COCAINE

Cocaine is perhaps the most behaviorally reinforcing of all drugs of abuse. Clinicians estimate that approximately 10% of people who begin to use the drug "recreationally" will go on to serious, heavy use. Once having tried cocaine, an individual cannot predict or control the extent to which he or she will continue to use the drug.

The most characteristic systemic effect of cocaine is stimulation of the CNS.[25] In the CNS, cocaine appears to mediate its effects primarily by blocking reuptake of catecholamine neurotransmitters such as norepinephrine and dopamine. The most common clinical manifestations of cocaine stimulation of the CNS are intense euphoria, decreased fatigue, and increased alertness.

In 1999, an estimated 1.5 million Americans were current cocaine users. This represents 0.7% of the population aged 12 and older. The estimated number of current crack cocaine users (see below) was 413,000 in 1999.[3]

Cocaine is absorbed rapidly from virtually all sites of application. For many years, cocaine has been administered as the hydrochloride salt form, usually by inhalation, but also by injection. In the last 15 to 18 years as the purity of cocaine hydrochloride obtained on the street declined, many users converted the cocaine hydrochloride to cocaine base, also known as "crack" or "rock." Crack cocaine receives its name from the crackling sound that occurs when the rocks are melted into vapors and smoked. Smoking the drug leads to almost instant absorption and intense euphoria. Peak plasma concentrations of greater than 900 ng/mL have been achieved following inhalation of cocaine base vapors compared with concentrations of only 150 to 200 ng/mL achieved after inhalation of similar amounts of pure cocaine hydrochloride powder.[25]

The high from snorting may last 15 to 30 minutes, whereas that from smoking may last 5 to 10 minutes. Increased use can reduce the period of stimulation. Some users of cocaine report feelings of restlessness, irritability, and anxiety. An appreciable tolerance to the high may be developed, and many addicts report that they seek but fail to achieve as much pleasure as they did from their first exposure. Scientific evidence suggests that the powerful neuropsychological reinforcing property of cocaine is responsible for an individual's continued use despite harmful physical and social consequences. In rare instances, sudden death can occur on the first use of cocaine or unexpectedly thereafter. However, there is no way to determine who is prone to sudden death.

High doses of cocaine and/or prolonged use can trigger paranoia. Smoking crack cocaine can produce a particularly aggressive paranoid behavior in users. When addicted individuals stop using cocaine, they often become depressed. This may lead to further cocaine use to alleviate depression. Prolonged cocaine snorting can result in ulceration of the mucous membranes of the nose and can damage the nasal septum enough to cause it to collapse. Cocaine-related deaths are often a result of cardiac arrest or seizures followed by respiratory arrest.

Recent research has helped clarify certain patterns of cocaine use such as combining cocaine and alcohol. Such drug use would seem counterintuitive because cocaine is a CNS stimulant and alcohol a CNS depressant. In the presence of alcohol, cocaine is metabolized to cocaethylene, a longer-acting but potent psychoactive compound as compared with the parent drug.[26] The risk of death from cocaethylene is greater than from cocaine.[27] The cocaine-alcohol combination is one of the most commonly identified among individuals who come to hospital EDs with acute substance abuse problems.

Cocaine is metabolized and eliminated rapidly. The elimination half-life of cocaine is approximately 1 hour, and the duration of effect is very short.[25] The short duration of effect provides a powerful incentive for repeated use of the drug. Many users experience intense drug use cycling, sometimes lasting days, characterized by rapidly repeating doses of cocaine until their supply is exhausted. Laboratory monkeys, given a choice between food and cocaine around the clock for 8 days, consistently choose cocaine.[28]

Complications of cocaine use frequently involve cardiovascular events.[29] At higher doses, it increases heart rate because of an overall systemic increase in sympathetic tone. At toxic doses, cocaine causes cardiac failure due to a direct effect on myocardial contractility. Cocaine is also pyrogenic, and hyperthermia is observed frequently in cocaine poisoning. Death is usually related to arrhythmias, shock, or convulsions.

Cocaine is a psychotomimetic drug, sometimes even at systemically nontoxic doses. A kindling phenomenon has been described with cocaine in which neuronal function becomes altered with each dose of the drug. This causes a type of reverse tolerance with increased receptor sensitivity to cocaine, and psychosis may be caused by doses that formerly did not cause psychosis. The toxic psychosis is characterized by auditory, visual, and frequently tactile hallucinations, paranoid thinking, and looseness of associations. The psychosis is qualitatively very similar to a paranoid schizophrenic psychosis.[30]

Recently, research has been conducted to better understand the mechanisms by which cocaine produces its pleasurable effects as they are occurring. Volkow and colleagues[31] have found a significant relationship between the intensity and duration of the "high" induced by cocaine and the degree to which the drug blocks one of the major mechanisms to control the amount of dopamine in the brain. There is a clear relationship between the degree to which cocaine blocks the dopamine transporter and the cocaine abuser's experience of euphoric feelings.

Previously, animal studies[32] have suggested that cocaine works in large part by occupying or blocking dopamine transporter (DAT) sites, thereby preventing reuptake of dopamine by the brain cells that release it. It is this abnormally long presence of dopamine at the synapse that is believed to cause the high and other effects associated with cocaine use.

To study the relationship between the subjective effects of cocaine and its activity in the brain of humans, Volkow[31] gave injections of cocaine to 17 volunteers who were current cocaine users. Using positron emission tomographic (PET) scans, they produced images of the volunteers' brains showing the concentrations of cocaine occupying DAT sites. They found that doses of cocaine commonly abused by humans blocked about 60% to 77% of the cocaine users' DAT sites. The researchers were able to document a significant relationship between the intensity and duration of the high induced by the cocaine and the concentration of the drug at DAT sites seen in the PET scans. In order for the subjects to perceive cocaine's effects, at least 47% of the DAT sites had to be blocked by cocaine. With a better understanding of the mechanism by which the "high" from cocaine is produced, perhaps specific drugs can be developed that block these subjective effects of the drug, allowing easier detoxification and drug avoidance.

Signs and symptoms of cocaine intoxication are summarized in Table 66–3. Although there is some controversy as to whether cocaine is associated with physical withdrawal on abrupt discontinuation, most clinicians feel that there is a characteristic syndrome of withdrawal effects, although they are not life-threatening.[33] Cocaine withdrawal consists primarily of fatigue, sleep disturbance, nightmares, and depression; it begins within hours of discontinuing the drug and lasts up to several days.

AMPHETAMINES AND OTHER STIMULANTS

During World War II, methamphetamine was used by soldiers as an aid to fight fatigue and enhance performance. In Japan, intravenous methamphetamine abuse reached epidemic proportions immediately after World War II, when supplies stored for military use became available to the public.

TABLE 66–3. Signs and Symptoms of Cocaine Intoxication and Withdrawal

Intoxication	Withdrawal
Motor agitation	Fatigue
Elation/euphoria	Sleep disturbance
Grandiosity	Nightmares
Loquacity	Depression
Hypervigilance	Increased appetite
Tachycardia	
Mydriasis	
Elevated or lowered blood pressure	
Sweating or chills	
Nausea and vomiting	

In the United States in the 1950s, legally manufactured tablets of methamphetamine were used nonmedically by college students, truck drivers, and athletes, who usually did not become severely addicted. This pattern changed drastically in the 1960s with the increased availability of injectable methamphetamine.

According to the Drug Enforcement Administration (DEA),[22] methamphetamine has been the most prevalent clandestinely produced controlled substance in the United States since 1979. Initially, the clandestine manufacture of methamphetamine was based primarily in the West and Southwest. Today, methamphetamine can be found in cities across the United States. There were an estimated 378,000 new methamphetamine users in 1998, up from 149,000 in 1990.[3]

Street methamphetamine is referred to by many names, such as "speed," "meth," and "crank." Methamphetamine hydrochloride, clear chunky crystals resembling ice, which can be inhaled by smoking, is referred to as "ice," "crystal," and "glass." Methamphetamine is manufactured clandestinely using the ephedrine or pseudoephedrine reduction method. In this process, ephedrine or pseudoephedrine is extracted from over-the-counter (OTC) cold and allergy tablets. Using recipes learned from friends or taken off the Internet, the ephedrine or pseudoephedrine is converted into high-quality methamphetamine in makeshift, illegal labs by untrained individuals. Pharmacists should be wary of persons wishing to purchase large quantities of products containing OTC sympathomimetic products.

The physiologic and psychological effects of amphetamines and other stimulants are qualitatively similar to those of cocaine—they diminish fatigue, increase alertness, and suppress appetite. Pharmacologically, amphetamines increase the activity of catecholamine neurotransmitters (e.g., norepinephrine and dopamine) by blocking reuptake, increasing release of neurotransmitters, and inhibiting the degradative enzyme monoamine oxidase.[34] The longer duration of effect of methamphetamine has led to a shift away from cocaine and toward the longer-acting drug.

Methamphetamine is taken orally or intranasally, by intravenous injection, and by smoking. Immediately after inhalation or intravenous injection, the methamphetamine user experiences an intense sensation, called a "rush" or "flash," that lasts only a few minutes and is described as extremely pleasurable.

Because methamphetamine elevates mood, people who experiment with it tend to use it with increasing frequency and in increasing doses, although this was not their original intent. The CNS actions that result from taking even small amounts of methamphetamine include increased wakefulness, increased physical activity, decreased appetite, increased respiration, hyperthermia, and euphoria. Other CNS effects include irritability, insomnia, confusion, tremors, convulsions, anxiety, paranoia, and aggressiveness. Hyperthermia and convulsions can result in death.

Cardiovascular side effects, which include chest pain and hypertension, also can result in cardiovascular collapse and death. In addition, methamphetamine causes increased heart rate and blood pressure and can cause irreversible damage to blood vessels in the brain, producing strokes. Other effects of methamphetamine include respiratory problems, irregular heartbeat, and extreme anorexia.

DESIGNER DRUGS

A *designer drug* is a chemical compound that is similar in structure and effect to another drug of abuse but differs slightly chemically.

Originally, designer drugs were produced in clandestine laboratories to mimic the psychoactive effects of controlled drugs yet be different enough so as not to be illegal. Although this legal loophole has been closed, the number of potential synthetic analogs that can be made and distributed is very large. The most commonly known types of analog drugs available through the illicit drug market include analogs of fentanyl and meperidine, phencyclidine (PCP), amphetamine, and methamphetamine. The street names of designer drugs vary according to time, place, and manufacturer, and they change frequently.

FENTANYL ANALOGS

Fentanyl was introduced in 1968 as a synthetic narcotic to be used as an analgesic in surgical procedures because of its minimal effect on the heart. In the early 1980s, however, crude clandestine laboratories began manufacturing fentanyl derivatives that were pharmacologically similar to heroin and morphine.[35] These fentanyl analogs create addiction similar to that of the opiate narcotics and present a significant drug abuse problem, including an increased potential for overdose. The most commonly known fentanyl analog is α-methylfentanyl, which is known on the streets as "China white." Other fentanyl analogs on the street include 3-methylfentanyl (TMF), known on the street as "synthetic heroin," "tango and cash," and "goodfella."

As with other narcotic analgesics, respiratory depression is the most significant acute toxic effect of the fentanyl derivatives. Fentanyl analogs are 80 to 1000 times more potent than morphine, depending on how they are made, and are 200 times more potent than heroin. They are intended to duplicate the euphoric effects of heroin. Fentanyl analogs have a very rapid onset (1 to 4 minutes) and a short duration of action (approximately 30 to 90 minutes), which varies according to the drug.[35] Because of the potency and quick onset, even a very small dose of a fentanyl analog can lead to sudden death.

α-Methylfentanyl, which appeared in Orange County, California, in 1979, was the first synthetically produced fentanyl that resulted in overdose deaths. Between 1980 and 1985, China white and several other fentanyl analogs were responsible for 100 unintentional overdose deaths in California.[35]

In 1988, TMF was identified in 16 unintentional overdose deaths in Allegheny County, Pennsylvania. Multiple-drug use was common in most of these cases. Because TMF is a powerful opiate, it is possible that it compounded the respiratory suppressant effects of the other drugs ingested, thereby causing death. In 1991, the fentanyl analog tango and cash was implicated in at least 28 deaths, primarily in New York and other Northeast areas. In 1992, China white was found to be the cause of death in 21 overdoses during 2 months in Philadelphia. To date, fentanyl analogs are responsible for the drug overdose deaths of more than 150 people in the United States.[35]

The most common route of administration is by injection. Authorities report that a victim can die so suddenly from respiratory paralysis that the needle may still be in the dead user's arm. Recent data indicate that smoking and sniffing are two means of ingestion that are becoming more popular—perhaps because of the attempt on the part of users to avoid the transmission of HIV and AIDS.[22]

MEPERIDINE ANALOGS

Over the past decade, the illicit use of meperidine has increased during periods when heroin was scarce. Two meperidine analogs that have appeared on the streets include 1-methyl 4-phenyl-4-propionoxypiperidine (MPPP) and 1 [2 phenylethyl]-4-acetyloxy-piperdine (PEPAP).[35]

An impurity formed during the clandestine manufacture of MPPP, called 1-methyl-4-phenyl-1,2,3,6,-tetrahydropyridine (MPTP), has been shown to be a potent neurotoxin and has caused irreversible brain damage in several individuals. The damage is manifested in a syndrome resembling a very severe parkinsonism, which results in increased muscle tone, difficulty in moving and speaking, drooling, and cogwheel rigidity of the upper extremities. Tremor in such patients characteristically involves the proximal muscles and is more pronounced than the typical involuntary resting tremor occurring in idiopathic parkinsonism.[35]

METHAMPHETAMINE ANALOGS

Several dozen analogs of amphetamine and methamphetamine are hallucinogenic. The methamphetamine analogs currently of concern include 3,4-methylenedioxy-amphetamine (MDA) and especially 3,4-methylenedioxy-methamphetamine (MDMA).[40] Use of this latter drug has skyrocketed in recent years. The drug is particularly popular among young people at all-night dance parties sometimes referred to as "raves," and the drug is classified among the "club drugs." Data from the most recent MTFS show the use of MDMA, known most commonly on the street as "ecstasy," rose among older teens (tenth and twelfth graders). Some 4.4% of the 1999 tenth graders reported some use of ecstasy during the prior 12 months (up from 3.3% in 1998) and 5.6% of the twelfth graders (up from 3.6% in 1998).[3]

In the first 7 months of 2000, nearly 8 million dosage units of MDMA were seized by the U.S. Customs Service and the DEA, dwarfing the 750,000 doses seized in 1998 and exceeding the 3.5 million confiscated in 1999. In July 2000, federal agents in Los Angeles seized $40 million worth of the drug, the largest such confiscation in U.S. history and an ominous sign of the increasing popularity and profitability of this drug. The record-setting shipment seized contained about 2.1 million tablets.

MDMA is structurally similar to methamphetamine and mescaline and stimulates the CNS, producing a mild hallucinogenic effect. Known most commonly on the street as ecstasy, it is also called "Adam," "X," "X-TC," "Stacy," "beans," "essence," "lover's speed," "Eve," or "e." Users under the influence of MDMA are said to be "rolling." Those taking both MDMA and lysergic acid diethylamide (LSD) are referred to as "trolling," a combination of the slang terms "tripping" and "rolling." MDMA is usually taken by mouth in tablet, capsule, or powder form, but it also may be smoked, snorted, or injected. Ecstasy sells for $20 to $40 per tablet and is estimated to cost about 20 cents each to make.

MDMA was first synthesized in 1912 by a German company, but it went largely unnoticed for 40 years until research resumed on the compound. Despite the renewed interest in this compound, the drug still has no therapeutic use, although various claims have been made by a small number of mental health practitioners for the usefulness of MDMA in enhancing psychotherapy. Illicit use of the drug did not become popular until the late 1980s and early 1990s. MDMA is classified as a schedule I controlled substance.

The effects of MDMA usually last approximately 4 to 6 hours. Users of the drug say that it produces profoundly positive feelings, empathy for others, elimination of anxiety, and extreme relaxation. MDMA is also said to suppress the need to eat, drink, or sleep, enabling users to endure 2- to 3-day parties. Consequently, MDMA use sometimes results in severe dehydration or exhaustion. MDMA generally reduces inhibitions and creates a sense of euphoria, but it also can evoke anxiety and paranoia. Heavier doses generate depression, irrationality, and psychosis. Users claim they experience feelings of closeness with others and a desire to touch them.

MDMA can result in a variety of acute psychiatric disturbances, including panic, anxiety, depression, and paranoid thinking.[36] Physical symptoms include muscle tension, nausea, blurred vision, faintness, chills, and sweating. MDMA also increases the heart rate and blood pressure. Other effects include hyperthermia, dehydration, vomiting, tremors, loss of control over body movements, insomnia, convulsions, rapid eye movements, and teeth and jaw clenching.

MDMA is perceived to be a harmless drug by many of its users, based in part on the fact that the risk of death is low compared with other drugs like heroin and cocaine. However, mounting evidence points to a neurotoxic effects of MDMA involving a complex and incompletely understood mechanism. MDMA has been shown clearly to destroy serotonin-producing neurons in animals.[37] Doses of MDMA that produce neurotoxicity are only two or three times more than the minimum dose needed to produce a psychotropic response. This suggests that individuals who are self-administering the drug may be getting a neurotoxic dose.[38]

The first direct evidence that chronic use of MDMA causes brain damage in humans was published in 1998.[39] Using PET imaging techniques, researchers studied 14 previous users of MDMA who were currently abstaining from use and 15 controls who had never used MDMA. The PET scanning technique used selectively labels the serotonin transporter. The study analyzed whether there were differences in serotonin transporter binding between abstinent MDMA users and participants in the control group. MDMA users showed decreased global and regional brain serotonin transporter binding compared with controls. Decreases in serotonin transporter binding positively correlated with the extent of previous MDMA use. This research shows direct evidence of a decrease in a structural component of brain serotonin neurons in human MDMA users.

In a related study,[40] researchers found that heavy MDMA users have memory problems that persist for at least 2 weeks after they have stopped using the drug. The authors compared 24 abstinent MDMA users and 24 control subjects on several standardized tests of memory, after matching subjects for age, gender, educational level, and vocabulary score (a surrogate of verbal intelligence). The authors also explored correlations between changes in memory function and decrements in cerebrospinal fluid (CSF) 5-hydroxyindoleacetic acid (5-HIAA), which serves as a marker of central serotonin neural function. These researchers were able to show that greater use of MDMA (total milligrams per month) was associated with greater impairment in immediate verbal memory and delayed visual memory. Furthermore, lower vocabulary scores were associated with stronger dose-related effects, with men having greater dose-related deficits than women. Lastly, lower concentrations of CSF 5-HIAA were associated with poorer memory performance. The authors concluded that abstinent MDMA users have impairment in verbal and visual memory and that the extent of memory impairment correlates with the degree of MDMA exposure and the reduction in brain serotonin, as indexed by CSF 5-HIAA.

McCann and coworkers[41] conducted a study to determine the effects of MDMA use on cognitive performance. Twenty-two MDMA users who had not used MDMA for at least 3 weeks and 23 control subjects were tested repeatedly with a computerized cognitive performance assessment battery while participating in a 5-day controlled inpatient study. CSF measures of monoamine metabolites also were collected as an index of brain monoaminergic function. MDMA users and controls were found to perform similarly on several cognitive tasks. However, MDMA subjects had significant performance deficits on a sustained-attention task requiring arithmetic calculations, a task requiring complex attention and incidental learning, a task requiring short-term memory, and a task of semantic recognition and verbal reasoning. MDMA users also had significant selective decreases in CSF 5-HIAA. The authors believe that their data provide further evidence that MDMA is neurotoxic to brain serotonin neurons in humans, and the behavioral data suggest that brain serotonin injury is associated with subtle but significant cognitive deficits.

Manufacturers of illicit drugs sometimes substitute other, potentially more dangerous substances for the one the buyer is expecting. Other suppliers produce products adulterated with chemical byproducts of the incomplete synthesis of active ingredients. One such chemical, *para*-methoxyamphetaime (PMA), is a drastically more potent hyperthermic agent than MDMA.[42] Deaths from the drug likely will rise as a result of these poor-quality tablets.

PHENCYCLIDINE AND KETAMINE

PCP, commonly referred to as "angel dust" and "crystal," was popular in the 1970s, but as its adverse effects became better known, use declined. PCP is most often a substitute for or contaminant of other drugs, and its most common pattern of use may now be unintentional. The actual extent of its use is unclear. It is often misrepresented as LSD or Δ^9-tetrahydrocannabinol (THC). With the exception of the pharmaceutical dosage form of dronabinol, THC is virtually unavailable on the street because it is highly unstable when isolated from the marijuana plant. When used intentionally, PCP is commonly smoked with marijuana and referred to as a "crystal joint," but it also may be taken orally or intravenously.

PCP has widely varied actions including CNS stimulation, depression, and hallucinogenic properties. Pharmacologically, it is known to block reuptake of serotonin, dopamine, and norepinephrine, but neurotransmitter antagonists do not effectively block its effects. In low doses, PCP causes sedation, ataxia, nystagmus, slurred speech, and paresthesias. At higher doses, users experience an increase in heart rate, blood pressure, temperature, diaphoresis, and muscle rigidity. At acutely toxic doses, coma and seizures may occur.[43]

Behavioral effects of PCP range from sleep to catatonic detachment to paranoid psychosis to violent hostility. Users are sometimes amnestic for events that occur under the influence of the drug. Psychoses sometimes last for weeks. Users with a previous history of schizophrenia are especially susceptible to the psychotomimetic effects of the drug. The only truly characteristic behavioral effect of PCP use is its high unpredictability. The signs and symptoms of PCP intoxication are summarized in Table 66–4.

Ketamine, a compound chemically related to PCP, is used primarily as a veterinary anesthetic but has gained popularity recently as a recreational drug.[44] Once used extensively in human medicine, it has fallen out of favor because of "emergence delirium," characterized by hallucinations, delirium, vivid dreams, and other psychiatric effects. This untoward effect as a medicinal agent is precisely the effect that recreational users are seeking. Previously, ketamine was not a controlled substance in the United States and hence it was often the target

TABLE 66–4. Signs and Symptoms of Phencyclidine Intoxication

Nystagmus	Euphoria
Increased blood pressure	Motor agitation
Tachycardia	Anxiety and emotional lability
Paresthesias	Hostility
Ataxia	Delusions
Slurred speech	Hallucinations
Muscle rigidity	

of drug-diversion schemes or thefts from physicians' or veterinarians' offices. Effective August 12, 1999, ketamine was placed in schedule III of the Controlled Substances Act.[45] As a result of this rule, the regulatory controls and criminal sanctions of schedule III will be applicable to the manufacture, distribution, dispensing, importation, and exportation of ketamine and products containing ketamine.

Known as "special K," "jet," "green," and other names on the street, ketamine usually is injected but can be evaporated to solid crystals, powdered, and smoked, snorted, or swallowed. Marijuana cigarettes are sometimes soaked in the ketamine solution, allowed to dry, and then smoked. Ketamine has become popular as a "rave" club drug. Side effects include significant transient increases in blood pressure and heart rate, respiratory depression, airway obstruction, apnea, muscular hypertonus, psychomotor and psychotomimetic effects, and acute dystonic reactions. Following overdose, seizures, polyneuropathy, increased intracranial pressure, respiratory arrest, and cardiac arrest may occur.[44]

The effects of a ketamine "high" usually last an hour, but they can last for 4 to 6 hours, and 24 to 48 hours are generally required before the user will feel completely "normal" again. Effects of chronic use of ketamine may take from several months to 2 years to disappear completely. Low doses (25 to 100 mg) produce psychedelic effects quickly. Large doses can produce vomiting and convulsions and may lead to hypoxia of the brain and muscles; 1 g can cause death. Flashbacks may even occur 1 year after use. Long-term effects include tolerance and possible physical and/or psychological dependence.

HALLUCINOGENS

The drugs commonly classified as hallucinogens are LSD, psilocybin, dimethyltryptamine (DMT), mescaline, and other related compounds. LSD is one of the most potent mood-changing chemicals. It is manufactured from lysergic acid, which is found in ergot, a fungus that grows on rye and other grains.

Pharmacologically, LSD and related drugs stimulate both presynaptic (5-HT_{1A}, 5-HT_{1B}) and postsynaptic (5-HT_2) serotonin recognition sites in the brain, which functionally may cause either agonist or antagonist effects on serotonin activity.[46] Precisely how the hallucinogens exert their effects remains unclear. LSD, often referred to as "acid," is an extraordinarily potent compound, producing observable CNS effects at doses as low as 25 μg.[46]

LSD is sold on the street in tablets, capsules, and occasionally, liquid form. It is odorless, colorless, and tasteless and usually is taken by mouth. Often LSD is added to absorbent paper, such as blotter paper, and divided into small, decorated squares, with each square representing one dose.

The DEA[22] reports that the strength of LSD samples obtained currently from illicit sources ranges from 20 to 80 μg LSD per dose. This is considerably less than the levels reported during the 1960s and early 1970s, when the dosage ranged from 100 to 200 μg or higher per unit.

The effects of LSD are unpredictable. They depend on the amount taken; the user's personality, mood, and expectations; and the surroundings in which the drug is used. Usually, the user feels the first effects of the drug 30 to 90 minutes after taking it. The physical effects include dilated pupils, higher body temperature, increased heart rate and blood pressure, sweating, loss of appetite, sleeplessness, dry mouth, and tremors.

Sensations and feelings change much more dramatically than the physical signs. The user may feel several different emotions at once or swing rapidly from one emotion to another. If taken in a large enough dose, the drug produces delusions and visual hallucinations. The user's sense of time and self changes. Sensations may seem to "cross over," giving the user the feeling of hearing colors and seeing sounds. These changes can be frightening and can cause panic.

TABLE 66–5. Signs and Symptoms of Hallucinogen Intoxication

Psychologic	Physical
Perceptual intensification	Mydriasis
Depersonalization	Tachycardia
Derealization	Diaphoresis
Illusions	Palpitations
Hallucinations	Blurred vision
Synesthesias	Tremor
	Incoordination
	Dizziness
	Weakness
	Drowsiness
	Paresthesias

Many LSD users experience flashbacks, recurrence of certain aspects of a person's experience, without the user having taken the drug again. A flashback occurs suddenly, often without warning, and may occur within a few days or more than a year after LSD use. Flashbacks usually occur in people who use hallucinogens chronically or have an underlying personality problem; however, otherwise healthy people who use LSD occasionally also may have flashbacks.

Most users of LSD voluntarily decrease or stop its use over time. LSD is not considered an addictive drug because it does not produce compulsive drug-seeking behavior. However, in common with many of the addictive drugs, LSD produces tolerance, so some users who take the drug repeatedly must take progressively higher doses to achieve the state of intoxication that they had achieved previously.

Signs and symptoms of hallucinogen intoxication are summarized in Table 66–5. Psychological symptoms of intoxication include a subjective intensification of perceptions, depersonalization, illusions, hallucinations, and synesthesias, the overflow of one sensory modality to another (colors are heard, sounds are seen). Among the hallucinogenic drugs, LSD is the most potent and long acting; it is hundreds of times more potent than both psilocybin and mescaline. DMT is inactive when ingested orally but can be smoked, inhaled, or injected. There is cross-tolerance among LSD, psilocybin, and mescaline. There is not an observable physical withdrawal syndrome after abrupt discontinuation of hallucinogenic drugs.[47]

Complications from hallucinogen use are primarily psychological. Users sometimes experience prolonged episodes of panic—the so-called bad trip. The flashbacks noted are common, occurring in approximately 15% of users and occurring episodically up to several years after the last exposure to the drug. Flashbacks may occur spontaneously but are also triggered by other drugs, including marijuana, and by anxiety-provoking stimuli. Physical effects of hallucinogen use are relatively nontoxic. Contrary to a widely held notion in the 1960s and early 1970s, there is no reliable evidence that hallucinogen use causes chromosome damage or genetic defects.[46]

MARIJUANA

Marijuana, referred to as "reefer," "pot," "grass," or "weed," remains the most commonly used illicit drug. It is used by 75% of current illicit drug users, or 11.1 million Americans. Approximately 57% of current illicit drug users consumed only marijuana, 18% used marijuana and another illicit drug, and the remaining 25% used an illicit

TABLE 66–6. Signs and Symptoms of Marijuana Intoxication

Tachycardia	Euphoria
Conjunctival congestion	Sensory intensification
Increased appetite	Apathy
Dry mouth	Hallucinations

drug but not marijuana in the past month.[3] *Cannabis sativa,* the marijuana plant, has been produced with increasingly sophisticated growing techniques to produce a plant of greater potency.[22] The principal psychoactive component of marijuana is THC. Hashish, the dried resin of the top of the plant, is much more potent than the plant itself.

Marijuana has been used widely and is believed by many to be a relatively harmless, nonaddictive intoxicant. Chronic low doses of marijuana usually are not associated with significant physical withdrawal on abrupt discontinuation, but many chronic users exhibit compulsive drug-seeking and drug-use behaviors characteristic of addiction or dependence. Acutely, marijuana has many of the effects of alcohol—sedation, a decrease in reactivity and ability to perform complex tasks, and disinhibition. Marijuana also causes hallucinations with high enough doses. Chronic use is associated with all the risks of tobacco smoking, although marijuana smokers are commonly also tobacco smokers, and thus differentiation of effects is often difficult. Endocrine effects including amenorrhea, decreased testosterone production, and inhibition of spermatogenesis have been demonstrated. Marijuana is associated with an amotivational syndrome characterized by a behavioral pattern of apathy, dullness, impaired judgment, decreased concentration and memory, loss of interest in personal hygiene, and a general reduction of goal-directed behavior.[48]

The signs and symptoms of marijuana intoxication are summarized in Table 66–6. Cardiovascular effects and reddened conjunctivae are the most prominent physical effects with acute use (tachycardia, increased blood pressure with large orthostatic changes). Although the duration of effect of marijuana may be only several hours, THC is detectable on toxicologic screening for up to 4 to 5 weeks, especially in chronic users.

It has been observed that some people experience a more "pleasurable" effect from marijuana than others, and researchers believe that this is heavily influenced by heredity.[49] A recent study[50] demonstrated that identical male twins were more likely than nonidentical male twins to report similar responses to marijuana use, indicating a genetic basis for their sensations.

Environmental factors such as the availability of marijuana, expectations about how the drug would affect them, the influence of friends and social contacts, and other factors that would be different even for identical twins also were found to have an important effect; however, it also was discovered that the twins' shared or family environment before age 18 had no detectable influence on their response to marijuana.

Taking the environmental and genetic influences together, these results suggest that although exposure to marijuana by factors such as social contacts is important, there are individual differences, perhaps in the brain's reward system, associated with genetic factors that influence whether one will continue using marijuana.

These physiologic differences coupled with the observation that individuals who find pleasure in using marijuana are more likely to use it repeatedly lead to the conclusion that heredity plays a significant role in determining susceptibility to continuing marijuana use.

Researchers have found that the daily use of one to three marijuana joints appears to produce approximately the same lung damage and potential cancer risk as smoking five times as many cigarettes.[51] The study results suggest that the way smokers inhale marijuana, in addition to its chemical composition, increases the adverse physical effects. The study findings refute the argument that marijuana is safer than tobacco because users smoke only a few joints a day.

A series of in-depth case studies[52] found that adults who smoked marijuana daily believed it helped them function better, improving self-awareness and relationships with others. However, researchers found that users were more willing to tolerate problems, suggesting that the drug served as a buffer for those who would rather avoid confronting problems than make changes that might increase their satisfaction with life. The study indicated that these subjects used marijuana to avoid dealing with their difficulties, and the avoidance inevitably made their problems worse.

In 1988, it was discovered that the membranes of certain nerve cells contain protein receptors that bind THC. Subsequent research has shown that two major cannabinoid receptor subtypes exist and that subtype 1 (CB1) is expressed primarily in the brain, whereas subtype 2 (CB2) is expressed primarily in the periphery. Once securely bound to its receptors, THC triggers a series of cellular reactions that ultimately lead to the high that users experience when they smoke a marijuana cigarette.[53] It was reasoned that an endogenous THC-like compound must exist and bind to these receptors. In 1992, researchers identified a naturally occurring chemical in the body that binds to these same receptors. Named anandamide, this and related compounds behave chemically like THC and are referred to by some as *endocannabinoids.*[54] Studies will continue with anandamide and its analogs to understand how it interacts with THC receptors to affect memory, movement, hunger, pain, and other functions that are altered by marijuana use.[55]

The issue of whether or not marijuana use is a "gateway" to the use of other drugs has been hotly debated for many years. Research shows that long-term use of marijuana produces changes in the brain that are similar to those seen after long-term use of other major drugs of abuse such as cocaine, heroin, and alcohol. Moreover, these changes may increase a user's vulnerability to addiction to other abusable drugs by "priming" the brain to be more easily changed by drugs in the future.[56] A substantial number of chronic, high-dose marijuana users become addicted, and previous research with animals has shown that stopping heavy marijuana use suddenly can cause distinct withdrawal symptoms in these individuals.

The purpose of the above-referenced study was to discover whether corticotropin-releasing factor (CRF), the neurochemical that increases during emotional times and periods of stress, plays a role in dependence on marijuana. Earlier studies have suggested that CRF plays a role in the neurobiologic and behavioral effects of withdrawal from addiction to cocaine, alcohol, and opiates and possibly a role in drug dependence in general.[56]

Rats were injected with HU-210, a potent substance that mimics the effects of marijuana. An analysis of the rats' brains showed that one injection of HU-210 reduced the release of CRF in the amygdala, that part of the brain which controls emotions.[56]

After 14 days of HU-210 treatment, the researchers induced drug withdrawal by injecting rats with the antagonist SR 141716A, a substance that blocks many effects of marijuana. The HU-210-treated rats showed many withdrawal symptoms after marijuana antagonist injection. Moreover, these rats showed an increased release of CRF at the same time they demonstrated dramatic behavioral withdrawal symptoms. Importantly, the specific brain areas that were activated during cannabinoid withdrawal are quite active during withdrawal from other drugs of abuse and play a key role in stress responses in general.[56]

Researchers believe that the findings from this and other studies suggest that addiction to one drug may make a person more vulnerable to abuse of and addiction to other drugs. Cannabinoid abuse, by activating CRF mechanisms, may lead to a subtle disruption of brain processes that are then "primed" for further and easier disruption by other drugs of abuse.[56]

Clearly, there is much more work to be done before the precise health and psychological effects of marijuana use are well understood. In fact, many of these health issues remain the subject of much debate. Undoubtedly, opinions on its risks are polarized along the lines of proponents' views on what its legal status should be. This polarization of opinion has prevented the development of any consensus on what health information the medical profession should give to patients who are users or potential users of marijuana. There is conflicting evidence about many of the effects of marijuana use. Readers are referred to an excellent article that attempts to summarize in a dispassionate way the evidence on the most probable adverse health and psychological consequences of acute and chronic use of marijuana.[57]

INHALANTS

Inhalants are CNS depressants, and symptoms of intoxication are similar to those of alcohol. Intoxication is often accompanied by headache and nausea, and users may experience hallucinations and delusions. The most serious physical risk of acute use is sudden death, usually from cardiac arrhythmias. Some users die from suffocation by plastic bags that contain the solvent. With chronic use, the drugs are toxic to virtually all organ systems. Psychological impairment; impaired pulmonary, renal, and hepatic function; neuropathies; encephalopathy; and brain damage have all been observed.[58]

Inhalation of organic solvents including gasoline, glue, aerosols, amyl nitrite, and nitrous oxide has remained fairly constant over the past few years. Approximately 7.8% of persons over age 12 have tried inhalant drugs.[3] The rate of first use of inhalants among youths aged 12 to 17 rose significantly from 1990 to 1998 from 11.6 to 28.1 per 1000 potential new users.[3]

MECHANISMS OF TOLERANCE, DEPENDENCE, AND WITHDRAWAL

Drug dependence depends on the reinforcing properties of the drug being used (the drug satisfies a need that demands repetition). Drug dependence most likely evolves in a phasic manner. The euphoriant or other pleasant properties of a drug act initially as reinforcers of drug-seeking behavior; but as tolerance develops, the pleasant effects of the drug are reduced, and higher doses are required to produce the same desirable feelings. Also, the user becomes aware of the need to avoid the pain and discomfort associated with the abstinence syndrome, or drug withdrawal. Many drug-dependent individuals state that their principal motivation for drug use turns relatively quickly from seeking of pleasurable effects to avoidance of unpleasant effects.

Mechanisms of physical dependence involve homeostasis. Drugs disturb biochemical and physiologic systems, which adapt to reduce those effects. Such compensatory adaptation leads to the development of tolerance. Therefore, when the drug is withdrawn, the compensatory changes dominate, and the user experiences withdrawal symptoms. The clinical manifestations of withdrawal syndromes generally are opposite to those effects produced by the drugs. In many cases, the disturbance in homeostatic mechanisms may be long lasting. Withdrawal may consist of an acute, relatively short phase lasting several days, followed by a more subacute, protracted withdrawal syndrome. Protracted withdrawal has been reported most consistently for alcohol and opiates. Opiate dependence, for example, is associated with a "conditioned abstinence syndrome" lasting up to several months or longer after cessation of intake and may be precipitated by environmental stimuli previously associated with drug use.[59] Opiate-dependent individuals have reported the onset of physical withdrawal symptoms after merely coming into contact with their previous environment (e.g., the user's neighborhood, the sight of heroin, or the observation of other individuals using drugs). Conditioned abstinence may be described as a heightened sensitivity to stimuli, abnormal autonomic responses, dysphoria, and intense craving for the effects of the drug.

There are two types of physiologic tolerance to drugs.[59] The first, *pharmacokinetic tolerance,* also called *metabolic* or *dispositional tolerance,* results from changes in the pharmacokinetics of drugs. Usually, this type of tolerance is related to increased metabolism. Examples of drugs associated with dispositional tolerance are barbiturates and alcohol. The second type of tolerance is *pharmacodynamic tolerance,* also known as a *cellular* or *functional tolerance.* Pharmacodynamic tolerance results from adaptive changes at the site of action of drugs, such as changes in receptor system binding sensitivity. Examples of drugs that exhibit pharmacodynamic tolerance are alcohol and the opiates.

TOLERANCE TO CNS DEPRESSANTS

The principal mechanism of barbiturate tolerance appears to be pharmacokinetic.[59] All barbiturates are potent inducers of liver enzymes and induce their own metabolism. Tolerance to benzodiazepines appears to be primarily pharmacodynamic.[59] The precise cellular mechanism of tolerance to benzodiazepines is not clear but may be a decrease in the number or sensitivity of benzodiazepine receptors.

Tolerance to opiates appears to be pharmacodynamic.[59] The primary center in the brain for both opiate and noradrenergic-mediated neurons appears to be the locus ceruleus in the midbrain. Neurons from the locus ceruleus project throughout the cerebral cortex. Although there are multiple subtypes of opiate receptors, the opiate receptor appears to be primarily a presynaptic receptor and has an inhibitory effect on the noradrenergic nerve terminal (i.e., stimulation of the presynaptic opiate receptor inhibits neuronal release of norepinephrine). The endogenous ligand for the opiate receptor is enkephalin. Another presynaptic receptor that serves as an inhibitory receptor for noradrenergic activity is the α_2-adrenergic receptor. The presynaptic α_2-receptor is a norepinephrine autoreceptor.

Chronic use of exogenous opiates, such as heroin, hydromorphone, and methadone, causes a decrease in production of the endogenous substance enkephalin, just as administration of exogenous corticosteroids causes a decrease in endogenous production of cortisol. Greater than normal activity at the receptor is associated with a compensatory decrease in the binding sensitivity of the opiate receptor system, also known as *downregulation.* Because the opiate receptor is inhibitory to noradrenergic activity, a downregulation effect would diminish the effect of opiates; thus larger doses would be required to achieve the same degree of inhibition of noradrenergic activity. Abrupt discontinuation of exogenous opiates produces a downregulated inhibitory opiate receptor system in the presence of diminished levels of endogenous ligand enkephalin. Therefore, opiate withdrawal can be conceptualized as a syndrome of noradrenergic hyperactivity.[60]

TOLERANCE TO CNS STIMULANTS

Tolerance to the stimulants, including cocaine, is pharmacodynamic in nature,[59] but the precise cellular mechanism is unclear. Tolerance to different pharmacologic effects of stimulants develops at different rates. Tolerance to appetite suppression, for example, develops within days to weeks, whereas tolerance to the euphoric effects and increased alertness develops more slowly. A type of reverse pharmacodynamic tolerance, *kindling,* has been observed with both cocaine and amphetamines. The neuropharmacology of cocaine and amphetamine withdrawal is not well understood; however, such withdrawal effects as depression, fatigue, and increased sleep and appetite are the opposite of the usual effects of the drug, as is the case with most drugs. Chronic cocaine use may cause a catecholamine depletion in the brain.

Tolerance develops to PCP and the LSD-type hallucinogens, although the mechanisms are not clearly understood. PCP may be associated with a dispositional tolerance. Tolerance to marijuana appears to be more pharmacodynamic than dispositional, although marijuana is known to induce microsomal liver enzymes.[61] The mechanism of tolerance to inhalants is not understood.

► TREATMENT: Substance-Related Disorders

ACUTE DRUG INTOXICATIONS

Treatment of drug intoxication, summarized in Table 66–7, is primarily supportive, and vital functions are maintained while waiting for the drug to be eliminated. When absolutely necessary, physical restraint may be required temporarily while a diagnostic evaluation is initiated to rule out other causes for the behavior (e.g., metabolic or fluid and electrolyte disturbances). Whenever possible, drug therapy should be avoided because psychotropic drug therapy has the potential for worsening a toxic reaction to another psychoactive agent; however, when patients are agitated, combative, assaultive, hallucinatory, or delusional, drug therapy may be required. Drug therapy also may be indicated in the treatment of an acute, potentially fatal drug overdose. Toxicology screens are useful in the evaluation and treatment process, but knowledge of the metabolism of the suspected drug and its excretion patterns is important for proper interpretation of test results. When toxicology screens are desired, blood or urine should be collected immediately on the patient's arrival.

For alcohol and barbiturate intoxication, supportive treatment is the rule. For benzodiazepine intoxication, the benzodiazepine antagonist flumazenil (Mazicon, Roche) can be used to reverse toxic effects. It is not indicated in all cases of suspected drug overdosage, however, and is specifically contraindicated in cases in which cyclic antidepressant involvement is known or suspected because of the risk of seizures. In addition, it should be used with caution in patients when benzodiazepine physical dependence is suspected because of the risks of induction of benzodiazepine withdrawal.[62] In the case of opiate intoxication, if the patient is unconscious and respiration is depressed, the opiate antagonist naloxone (Narcan, DuPont) can be used to revive the patient. The usual dosage for naloxone in acute opiate toxicity is 0.4 to 2.0 mg intravenously, given approximately every 3 minutes as necessary.[63] Although naloxone is effective in reversing opiate overdose, it also may precipitate physical withdrawal in physically dependent patients. Patients who fail to respond to a total dosage of 10 mg naloxone probably have a cause of acute intoxication other than an opiate.

Intoxication with stimulants, including cocaine, is treated pharmacologically only if the patient is overtly psychotic and agitated. Injectable benzodiazepines, usually lorazepam (Ativan, Wyeth-Ayerst) 2 to 4 mg intramuscularly every 30 minutes to 6 hours as necessary, can be used for agitation. As a backup to lorazepam, antipsychotic drugs can be used on a short-term basis, primarily in patients with psychotic symptoms, and usually at relatively low doses, such as haloperidol (Haldol, McNeil) 2 to 5 mg intramuscularly every 30 minutes to 6 hours as necessary, followed by 5 to 15 mg orally per day in single or divided doses if the patient is still psychotic after initial treatment.[33] Cardiovascular complications are treated symptomatically with antiarrhythmic agents or other interventions as necessary. Seizures generally are treated supportively. Intravenous lorazepam or diazepam can be used if seizures progress to status epilepticus.

Hallucinogen intoxication is treated in a manner similar to stimulant intoxication. Drug therapy often can be avoided because patients may respond to careful reassurance, or so-called talk-down therapy. When necessary, short-term antianxiety and/or antipsychotic drug therapy can be used, as described previously. The same approach applies to marijuana and inhalant intoxication.

PCP intoxication is more unpredictable and more difficult to treat than other psychosis-producing drugs. Most clinicians suggest that sensory input be minimized to the extent possible; thus talk-down therapy is not recommended and may in fact make the patient worse. If PCP intoxication is suspected, patients should be left alone in a quiet, dimly lit room. If behavior is uncontrollable, antianxiety and/or antipsychotic drug therapy may be necessary.

TABLE 66–7. Treatment of Substance Intoxication

Drug Class	Pharmacologic Therapy	Nonpharmacologic Therapy
Benzodiazepines	Flumazenil 0.2 mg/min IV initially, repeat up to 3 mg maximum	Support vital functions
Alcohol, barbiturates, and sedative–hypnotics (nonbenzodiazepines)	None	Support vital functions
Opiates	Naloxone 0.4–2.0 mg IV every 3 min	Support vital functions
Cocaine and other CNS stimulants	Lorazepam 2–4 mg IM q 30 min to 6 h prn agitation Haloperidol 2–5 mg (or other antipsychotic agent) every 30 min to 6 h prn psychotic behavior	Monitor cardiac function
Hallucinogens, marijuana, and inhalants	Lorazepam and/or haloperidol as above	Reassurance; "talk-down therapy"; support vital functions
Phencyclidine	Lorazepam and/or haloperidol as above	Minimize sensory input

TABLE 66–8. Treatment of Withdrawal From Some Common Drugs of Abuse

Drug or Drug Class	Pharmacologic Therapy
Benzodiazepines	
Short to intermediate acting	Chlordiazepoxide 50 mg tid-qid or lorazepam 2 mg tid-qid; taper over 5–7 d
Long acting	Chlordiazepoxide 50 mg tid-qid or lorazepam 2 mg tid-qid; taper over additional 5–7 d
Barbiturates	Pentobarbital tolerance test; initial detoxification at upper limit of tolerance test; decrease dosage by 100 mg every 2–3 d
Opiates	Methadone 20–80 mg PO daily; taper by 5–10 mg daily or clonidine 2 μg/kg tid × 7 d; taper over additional 3 d
Mixed-substance withdrawal	
Drugs are cross-tolerant	Detoxify according to treatment for longer-acting drug used
Drugs are not cross-tolerant	Detoxify from one drug while maintaining second drug (cross-tolerant drugs), then detoxify from second drug
CNS stimulants	Supportive treatment only; pharmacotherapy often not used; bromocriptine 2.5 mg tid or higher may be used for severe craving associated with cocaine withdrawal

WITHDRAWAL

Treatment of drug withdrawal is the primary indication for drug therapy in substance-related disorders. Goals of drug therapy include prevention of progression of withdrawal to life-threatening severity, enabling the patient to be sufficiently comfortable and functional in order to participate in a behavioral treatment program, and supportive drug therapy. The clinician should remember that withdrawal is usually part of a substance dependence disorder. Patients with drug dependence generally cope with almost any stress through the use of a drug. In drug therapy for withdrawal, it is important to avoid reinforcing the patient's drug-seeking and drug-use behavior to the extent possible. Drug withdrawal in the best of circumstances is uncomfortable. Patients must be educated to deal with the stress of withdrawal without seeking drugs. The use of drugs as needed for anxiety or insomnia should be avoided. Treatment of drug withdrawal is summarized in Table 66–8.

CNS DEPRESSANT WITHDRAWAL

Benzodiazepines

Treatment of benzodiazepine withdrawal is very similar to the treatment of alcohol withdrawal, and the same drugs and dosages may be used.[14] The major difference in management is the length of treatment. The onset of withdrawal symptoms in patients physically dependent on the long-acting benzodiazepines may be delayed up to 7 days after discontinuation of the drug.[64] A common approach in detoxification of such patients is to initiate treatment at usual dosages (chlordiazepoxide 50 mg three times a day; lorazepam 2 mg three times a day) and to maintain the initial dosage for 5 days, with gradual tapering over an additional 5 days. Detoxification in patients physically dependent on shorter-acting benzodiazepines is similar to treatment of alcohol withdrawal. Among the benzodiazepines, alprazolam has been suggested to be more difficult to taper and discontinue than the other benzodiazepines.[68] Whether the difficulty is related to a different patient population commonly treated with alprazolam (e.g., panic disorder) or to intrinsic differences between alprazolam and other benzodiazepines is not clear. A longer, more gradual taper of the benzodiazepine used for detoxification may be needed. With all benzodiazepines, protracted minor abstinence symptoms—such as anxiety, insomnia, irritability, sensitivity to light and sound, and muscle spasms—may remain for several weeks in patients with a history of long exposure, even after the acute phase of benzodiazepine withdrawal is complete.

Barbiturates and Other Sedative-Hypnotic Drugs

While once used extensively, barbiturates and other nonbenzodiazepine sedating medications have been replaced largely by safer and more effective medications. Abuse problems with barbiturates resemble those seen with benzodiazepines in many ways. Withdrawal from barbiturates should be handled similarly to interventions for the abuse of alcohol and benzodiazepines.[59]

Opiates

Opiate withdrawal is not life-threatening unless there is a concurrent life-threatening medical condition. Although most patients complain of symptoms of withdrawal, such as cramping or insomnia, these symptoms are tolerable, and initiation of drug therapy may be avoided in many cases. Because opiate withdrawal is not life-threatening, observable signs of withdrawal, such as mydriasis, pilomotor erection, diaphoresis, or diarrhea, should be noted before initiation of drug therapy.

The conventional drug therapy for opiate withdrawal has been methadone, a synthetic opiate. Usual starting dosages have been 20 to 40 mg/d orally. The dosage of methadone can be tapered in decrements of 5 to 10 mg/d until discontinued. Most patients in withdrawal continue to complain of mild symptoms after detoxification is completed. Some patients who are unable to discontinue methadone completely or habitually return to drug use when methadone is discontinued are placed in methadone-maintenance treatment programs and receive methadone chronically.[65]

L-Methadyl acetate hydrochloride (LAAM, Orlaam, Biometric Research Institute) was approved by the FDA in 1993 as a potential alternative to methadone maintenance. LAAM forms two long-acting metabolites, which allow three-times-a-week dosing.[66]

Heroin-dependent individuals reduced their use of heroin by nearly 90% after 16 weeks of LAAM treatment.[67] In a clinical trial comparing different LAAM doses in the treatment of opiate addiction, researchers found that heroin use was reduced for individuals taking a regimen of low, medium, or high doses of LAAM, with effectiveness increasing substantially at the highest dose. This suggests that treatment programs need to get patients to the most effective dosage levels as quickly as possible.[67]

An increasingly accepted method of opiate detoxification is the use of clonidine. Clonidine can attenuate the noradrenergic hyperactivity of opiate withdrawal without interfering significantly with activity at the opiate receptors. Production of enkephalin and the return of receptors to normal levels of sensitivity can occur as rapidly as possible. Advantages of detoxification with clonidine include a somewhat more rapid detoxification and an absence of the euphoria sometimes observed with methadone.[68]

For rapid detoxification in the management of opiate withdrawal in opiate-dependent individuals, various dosage regimens of oral clonidine have been used. Dosages must be individualized carefully according to the patient's response and tolerance, and patients must be monitored and supervised closely. Clonidine is often given in an initial dosage of 6 μg/kg per day in three divided doses. Dosage can be increased if necessary to as high as 17 μg/kg per day. The patient is maintained on the same dosage for 7 days, which is then tapered and discontinued over the next 3 days. A common clonidine side effect is orthostatic hypotension, and the patient's blood pressure should be monitored in the supine and standing positions at least daily. If blood pressure drops to an unacceptably low level (e.g., lying systolic blood pressure less than 90 mm Hg), the dose should be held. If blood pressure has risen in time for the next dose, clonidine can be resumed. Clonidine for treatment of opiate withdrawal also has been administered transdermally, but this method has not been well studied.[68]

Less well established opiate detoxification strategies include the combination of clonidine and naltrexone. Naltrexone, an opiate antagonist, is used to rapidly induce withdrawal that is then attenuated with clonidine. The potential advantage of this method is the shortening of detoxification to as little as 2 days.[66] A similar detoxification regimen using buprenorphine, a partial opiate agonist, and naltrexone has been tried.[66] Buprenorphine has been used as an alternative to methadone maintenance as well.[69]

A rapid detoxification (RD) technique has been developed that is designed to shorten detoxification by precipitating withdrawal through the administration of opioid antagonists such as naloxone hydrochloride or naltrexone.[70] This approach is thought to have the advantage of getting patients though detoxification rapidly to minimize the risk of relapse and initiating treatment more quickly with naltrexone maintenance combined with suitable psychosocial interventions. Ultrarapid opioid detoxification (URD) represents a variant of this technique in which patients undergo opioid antagonist–precipitated withdrawal while under general anesthesia or heavy sedation. Although it is difficult to estimate the extent of their clinical use, these techniques are becoming increasingly available in response to rising demand for opioid-dependence treatment services. In the United States there has been a rapid proliferation of programs offering URD, with some programs charging up to $7500 per treatment.[70]

A recent meta-analysis was performed to assess the evidence for the efficacy of both RD and URD to determine their role among the available treatment options for opioid dependence. Analysis was performed on 12 studies of RD and 9 studies of URD. The authors concluded that more research is needed using more rigorous research methods, longer-term outcomes, and comparisons with other methods of treatment for opioid dependence before these techniques can gain widespread acceptance.[70]

WITHDRAWAL FROM OTHER SUBSTANCES

Withdrawal from other drugs, including cocaine and other stimulants, is primarily supportive. Pharmacotherapy recently has assumed a greater role in treating cocaine withdrawal and dependence, however. Bromocriptine (Parlodel, Sandoz), a dopamine antagonist at low dosages and an agonist at high dosages, is usually used in the treatment of parkinsonism and hyperprolactinemia and has been used to treat cocaine withdrawal symptoms and to reduce the craving for cocaine. Use of bromocriptine is based on the hypothesis that chronic use of cocaine causes dopamine depletion; therefore, higher dosages should be used (i.e., 2.5 mg three times daily or higher). Despite initially promising pilot studies, recent evidence does not support the efficacy of bromocriptine to reduce cocaine use or craving.[71]

SUBSTANCE DEPENDENCE

The treatment of drug dependence is primarily behavioral. The patient generally is taught that complete abstinence is the only realistic alternative to a life of uncontrollable drug use and despair that ultimately will end in death and that there is no intermediate, controllable level of drinking or use of another drug. However, complete and permanent abstinence as the sole route to recovery is controversial. There may be an extremely few individuals who can return to controllable levels of drinking alcohol, but it is impossible to predict who these individuals are; thus most treatment programs continue to advocate complete abstinence. The prospect of life without alcohol or other drugs is incomprehensible to many patients. Entry into treatment often is facilitated by some type of leverage that the drug-dependent person associates with negative consequences, such as potential loss of job, divorce, legal problems, or deteriorating physical health. Early treatment is directed at penetrating the denial of a problem that is always present. The patient must be educated as to the disease of addiction, the effects of drugs, and the permanence of the condition.

In recent years, there has been a trend toward outpatient treatment for drug dependence, due in part to cost-containment efforts. Inpatient treatment programs can cost as much as $20,000 for a 4-week stay. When withdrawal symptoms are mild to moderate and there are no other medical indications for hospitalization, outpatient treatment may be an attractive alternative to inpatient treatment. One critical criterion for outpatient treatment is the patient's compliance with complete abstinence from the dependence-producing drug during the treatment experience.

Families must be involved in treatment. The course of the patient's illness often has a devastating effect on other family members. Severely depleted self-esteem, denial of the family member's addiction, feelings of responsibility for the family member's drug use, and other behaviors that parallel the addiction process are often present. Treatment must be a lifelong process. Aftercare, or what is now being called *continued care,* should include regular and frequent treatment in some form. Most drug-dependence treatment programs embrace a treatment approach based on the twelve steps to recovery. Alcoholics Anonymous (AA) is one of the most successful of all self-help groups. Associated groups include Alanon (a group for family members of alcoholics), Narcotics Anonymous (self-help groups based on the AA concept for users of other drugs), Overeaters Anonymous (a group for individuals with eating disorders), Gamblers Anonymous, and several other similar programs. Among chemically dependent health care professionals, treatment that incorporates both AA and peer-led self-help groups may be most effective.[72]

COEXISTENT DRUG DEPENDENCE AND PSYCHIATRIC DISORDERS: THE DUAL-DIAGNOSIS PATIENT

Although the majority of chemical dependence is primary (no evidence of a preexisting major psychiatric problem prior to the first life problem related to addiction), a significant percentage coexists with another psychiatric disorder. One way to conceptualize this is that there are two broad categories of persons who receive diagnoses of two or more conditions that occur together. In one type, chemical dependence might be secondary to a complication of a psychiatric disorder. In these individuals, the onset of the psychiatric disorder significantly predated the regular abuse of substances.

A second type has two concurrent primary diagnoses, chemical dependence and a psychiatric disorder. Recognition of this type of patient has been increasing in recent years. The prevalence of this comorbidity varies remarkably depending on the perspectives of the assessment team, the clinical situation in which the evaluation takes place, the severity of the disorders, and the patient's perspective. As a result, the data on the prevalence of comorbid conditions are quite variable and by no means are definitive.[73]

Results of one large study[74] suggest that more than half of people who abuse drugs other than alcohol have at least one comorbid mental illness, with cocaine abusers demonstrating an additional psychiatric illness in 76% of cases. In another study,[75] approximately 25% of those with an anxiety disorder were diagnosed as having a substance abuse disorder. Prevalence rates for psychiatric disorders for those in substance abuse treatment generally were double the rates for those who were not in treatment.

When dual problems of a psychiatric disorder and substance use disorder coexist, they are interactive and may be interdependent. This may be particularly true when personality disorder and substance abuse or dependence coexist.[73] Of the personality disorders, antisocial personality disorder (APD) has been subject to the most extensive validity and reliability testing in patients with substance abuse.[73] Even so, there continues to be controversy about the reliability and stability in the APD diagnosis, particularly when substance abuse is involved.

Treatment of the patient with coexisting substance use and psychiatric disorders involves initial treatment of the substance use disorder, especially when the patient is in physical withdrawal. If symptoms of psychiatric disorder continue after the patient has been drug-free for a minimum of 2 weeks, then treatment of the psychiatric disorder must be considered. Psychotropic drug therapy appropriate to the diagnosis may be indicated. Improved relations between psychiatrists and chemical-dependence treatment professionals have led to cooperative efforts to treat all aspects of the patient's illness.

DRUG ABUSE INFORMATION AND THE INTERNET

With the recent growth of the Internet, information about drug abuse is available with a click of the mouse. Many Web sites have been developed to provide factual, reliable information covering a wide array of topics related to abuse of chemical substances. Unfortunately, there are numerous sites where incomplete, misleading, blatantly incorrect, or even dangerous information can be found. Browsing just a few newsgroups, Web sites, or listserves shows that much of the information is unreliable. It may be useful for the clinician working in the substance abuse area to periodically check the "pro-drug" Web sites to see what is being discussed. In this manner, the practitioner can remain up to date on the latest drug fads and can better respond to questions from clients. Appendix 66–1 contains Web addresses useful in providing drug abuse prevention and treatment information to professionals and laypersons alike.

CONCLUSIONS

Substance use disorders remain one of the great public health issues of contemporary society. Dependence on drugs is a powerful emotional and political issue. Because we live in a chemically oriented society, everyone is affected in some way by drug abuse and drug dependence. Health care professionals must be particularly vigilant for problems associated with drug use not only for our patients but also for ourselves.

▶ PRINCIPLES OF PHARMACOTHERAPY

- Problems related to abuse of chemical substances can occur acutely (e.g., respiratory arrest from using heroin) or after some length of time (e.g., dependence, withdrawal from continued use of an opiate). The treatment approach is distinctly different depending on the type of problem.
- Pharmacotherapy of substance-related disorders is most often adjunctive to other modes of therapy such as counseling and intense psychotherapy.
- Withdrawal from certain classes of drugs (e.g., benzodiazepines, barbiturates) can be life-threatening, and steps must be taken to ensure that withdrawal is gradual and that it takes place in closely supervised settings.
- While there is much research focusing on drugs to treat the underlying addictive processes, to date the successes have been few. Whereas methadone and L-methadyl acetate hydrochloride (LAAM) are used for narcotic maintenance, clonidine is used to treat withdrawal symptoms, and naltrexone is used to prolong abstinence, the logical approach at present should center on prevention. Because of their knowledge of pharmacology and the actions of drugs on the body, pharmacists can play a key role in education of young people on the dangers of recreational drug use.

REFERENCES

1. Schneider Institute for Health Policy, Brandeis University. Substance Abuse: The Nation's Number One Health Problem. Key Indicators for Policy—Update. Princeton, Robert Wood Johnson Foundation, 2001
2. Rinaldi RC, Steindler EM, Wilford BB, Goodwin D. Clarification and standardization of substance abuse terminology. JAMA 1988;259:555–557.
3. National Household Survey on Drug Abuse. Rockville, MD, U.S. Department of Health and Human Services, Substance Abuse and Mental Health Services Administration, 1999.
4. Monitoring the Future Study: National High School Senior Drug Abuse Survey, Rockville, MD, U.S. Department of Health and Human Services, National Institute on Drug Abuse, 1999.
5. Substance Abuse and Mental Health Services Administration, Office of Applied Studies, Drug Abuse Warning Network. DAWN Series D-15, DHHS Publication No. (SMA) 00-3462, August 2000.
6. National Center on Addiction and Substance Abuse at Columbia University. Substance Abuse and Urban America: Its Impact on an American City. New York, February 1996.
7. National Center on Addiction and Substance Abuse at Columbia University. Substance Abuse and Federal Entitlement Programs. New York, February 1995.

8. National Center on Addiction and Substance Abuse at Columbia University. The Cost of Substance Abuse to America's Health Care System: Medicaid. New York, July 1993.
9. National Center on Addiction and Substance Abuse at Columbia University. The Cost of Substance Abuse to America's Health Care System: Medicare. New York, May 1994.
10. National Center on Addiction and Substance Abuse at Columbia University. Behind Bars: Substance Abuse and America's Prison Population. New York, January 1998.
11. Woods JH, Winger G. Abuse liability of flunitrazepam. J Clin Psychopharmacol 1997;17(Suppl 2):1S–57S.
12. Bottlender R, Schutz C, Moller HJ, Soyka M. Zolpidem dependence in a patient with former polysubstance abuse. Pharmacopsychiatry 1997; 30:108.
13. Hobbs WR, Rall TW, Verdoorn TA. Hypnotics and sedatives: Ethanol. In: Hardman JG, Limbird LE, eds. Goodman and Gilman's The Pharmacological Basis of Therapeutics, 9th ed. New York, McGraw-Hill, 1996:361–396.
14. Smith DE, Wesson DR. Benzodiazepines and other sedative-hypnotics. In: Galanter M, Kleber HD, eds. Textbook of Substance Abuse Treatment. Washington, American Psychiatric Press, 1994:179.
15. Schwartz RH, Milteer R, LeBeau MA. Drug-facilitated sexual assault ("date rape"). South Med J 2000;93:558–561.
16. Raymon LP, Steele BW, Walls HC. Benzodiazepines in Miami-Dade County, Florida, driving under the influence (DUI) cases (1995–1998) with emphasis on Rohypnol: GC-MS confirmation, patterns of use, psychomotor impairment, and results of Florida legislation. J Anal Toxicol 1999;23:490–499.
17. CDC. Gamma-hydroxy butyrate use—New York and Texas, 1995–1996. MMWR 1997;46:281–283.
18. Tunnicliff G. Sites of action of gamma-hydroxybutyrate (GHB)—A neuroactive drug with abuse potential. J Toxicol Clin Toxicol 1997;35: 581–590.
19. CDC. Adverse events associated with ingestion of gamma-butyrolactone—Minnesota, New Mexico, and Texas, 1998–1999. MMWR 1999; 48:137–40.
20. Kam PC, Yoong FF. Gamma-hydroxybutyric acid: An emerging recreational drug. Anaesthesia 1998;53:1195–1198.
21. Craig K, Gomez HF, McManus JL, Bania TC. Severe gamma-hydroxybutyrate withdrawal: A case report and literature review. J Emerg Med 2000;18:65–70.
22. Drug Enforcement Administration, Department of Justice. Drugs of Abuse. Washington, U.S. Government Printing Office, 1996.
23. American Psychiatric Association. Diagnostic and Statistical Manual of Mental Disorders, 4th ed (DSM-IV). Washington, American Psychiatric Press, 1994.
24. U.S. Department of Justice, Drug Enforcement Administration. The Supply of Illicit Drugs to the United States. National Narcotics Intelligence, Consumers Committee, August 1996.
25. Gold MS, Miller NS. Cocaine (and crack): Neurobiology. In: Lowinson JH, Ruiz P, Millman RB, Langrod JG, eds. Substance Abuse: A Comprehensive Textbook, 3d ed. Baltimore, Williams & Wilkins, 1997:166–181.
26. Hart CL, Jatlow P, Sevarino KA, McCance-Katz EF. Comparison of intravenous cocaethylene and cocaine in humans. Psychopharmacology (Berl) 2000;149:153–162.
27. McCance-Katz EF, Kosten TR, Jatlow P. Concurrent use of cocaine and alcohol is more potent and potentially more toxic than use of either alone: A multiple-dose study. Biol Psychiatry 1998;44:250–259.
28. Aigner TG, Balster RL. Choice behavior in rhesus monkeys: Cocaine versus food. Science 1978;201:534–535.
29. Stein MD. Medical consequences of substance abuse. Psychiatr Clin North Am 1999;22:351–370.
30. Harris D, Batki SL. Stimulant psychosis: Symptom profile and acute clinical course. Am J Addict 2000;9:28–37.
31. Volkow ND, Wang GJ, Fischman MW, et al. Relationship between subjective effects of cocaine and dopamine transporter occupancy. Nature 1997;386:827–830.
32. Gatley SJ, Volkow ND, Chen R, et al. Displacement of RTI-55 from the dopamine transporter by cocaine. Eur J Pharmacol 1996;296:145–151.
33. Mendelson JH, Mello NK. Management of cocaine abuse and dependence. N Engl J Med 1996;334:965–972.
34. King GR, Ellinwood EH. Amphetamines and other stimulants. In: Lowinson JH, Ruiz P, Millman RB, Langrod JG, eds. Substance Abuse: A Comprehensive Textbook, 3d ed. Baltimore, Williams & Wilkins, 1997:207–223.
35. Morgan J. Designer drugs. In: Lowinson JH, Ruiz P, Millman RB, Langrod JG, eds. Substance Abuse: A Comprehensive Textbook, 3d ed. Baltimore, Williams & Wilkins, 1997:264–269.
36. Miller NS, Gold MS. LSD and ecstasy: Pharmacology, phenomenology, and treatment. Psychiatr Ann 1994;24:131–133.
37. McCann UD, Ridenour A, Shaham Y, Ricaurte GA. Serotonin neurotoxicity after (+/−)3,4-methylenedioxymethamphetamine (MDMA; "ecstasy"): A controlled study in humans. Neuropsychopharmacology 1994;10:129–138.
38. Seiden LS, Sabol KE. Methamphetamine and methylenedioxymethamphetamine neurotoxicity: Possible mechanisms of cell destruction. NIDA Res Monogr 1996;163:251–276.
39. McCann UD, Szabo Z, Scheffel U, et al. Positron emission tomographic evidence of toxic effect of MDMA ("ecstasy") on brain serotonin neurons in human beings. Lancet 1998;352:1433–1437.
40. Bolla KI, McCann UD, Ricaurte GA. Memory impairment in abstinent MDMA ("ecstasy") users. Neurology 1998;51:1532–1537.
41. McCann UD, Mertl M, Eligulashvili V, Ricaurte GA. Cognitive performance in (+/−) 3,4-methylenedioxymethamphetamine (MDMA, "ecstasy") users: A controlled study. Psychopharmacology (Berl) 1999;143:417–425.
42. James RA, Dinan A. Hyperpyrexia associated with fatal paramethoxyamphetamine (PMA) abuse. Med Sci Law 1998;38:83–85.
43. Zukin SR, Sloboda Z, Javitt DC. Phencyclidine (PCP). In: Lowinson JH, Ruiz P, Millman RB, Langrod JG, eds. Substance Abuse: A Comprehensive Textbook, 3d ed. Baltimore, Williams & Wilkins, 1997:238–246.
44. Ghoneim MM, Hinrichs JV, Mewaldt SP, Petersen RC. Ketamine: Behavioral effects of subanesthetic doses. J Clin Psychopharmacol 1985;5: 70–77.
45. Controlled Substances Act (CSA), Title 21 U.S.C. 801 et seq.
46. Glennon RA. Classical hallucinogens: An introductory overview. NIDA Res Monogr 1994;146:4–32.
47. Pechnick RN, Ungerleider JT. Hallucinogens. In: Lowinson JH, Ruiz P, Millman RB, Langrod JG, eds. Substance Abuse: A Comprehensive Textbook, 3d ed. Baltimore, Williams & Wilkins, 1997:230–238.
48. Grinspoon L, Bakalar JB. Marihuana. In: Lowinson JH, Ruiz P, Millman RB, eds. Substance Abuse: A Comprehensive Textbook, 3d ed. Baltimore, Williams & Wilkins, 1997:199–206.
49. Lyons MJ, Toomey R, Meyer JM, et al. How do genes influence marijuana use? The role of subjective effects. Addiction 1997;92:409–417.
50. Tsuang MT, Lyons MJ, Eisen SA, et al. Genetic influences on DSM-III-R drug abuse and dependence: A study of 3372 twin pairs. Am J Med Genet 1996;67:473–477.
51. Sarafian TA, Magallanes JA, Shau H, et al. Oxidative stress produced by marijuana smoke: An adverse effect enhanced by cannabinoids. Am J Respir Cell Mol Biol 1999;20(6):1286–1293
52. Hendin H, Haas AP. The adaptive significance of chronic marijuana use for adolescents and adults. Adv Alcohol Subst Abuse 1985;4:99–115.
53. Klein TW, Lane B, Newton CA, Friedman H. The cannabinoid system and cytokine network. Proc Soc Exp Biol Med 2000;225:1–8.
54. Palmer SL, Khanolkar AD, Makriyannis A. Natural and synthetic endocannabinoids and their structure-activity relationships. Curr Pharm Des 2000;6:1381–1397.
55. Piomelli D, Giuffrida A, Calignano A, Rodriguez de Fonseca F. The endocannabinoid system as a target for therapeutic drugs. Trends Pharmacol Sci 2000;21(6):218–224
56. Rodriguez de Fonseca F, Carrera MRA, Navarro M, et al. Activation of corticotropin-releasing factor in the limbic system during cannabinoid withdrawal. Science 1997;276:2050–2054.

57. Hall W, Solowij N. Adverse effects of cannabis. Lancet 1998;352:1611–1616.
58. Sharp CW, Rosenberg NL. Inhalants. In: Lowinson JH, Ruiz P, Millman RB, Langrod JG, eds. Substance Abuse: A Comprehensive Textbook, 3d ed. Baltimore, Williams & Wilkins, 1997:246–264.
59. O'Brien CP. Drug addiction and drug abuse. In: Hardman JG, Limbird LE, eds: Goodman and Gilman's The Pharmacological Basis of Therapeutics, 9th ed. New York, McGraw-Hill, 1996:557–577.
60. Simon EJ. Opiates: Neurobiology. In: Lowinson JH, Ruiz P, Millman RB, Langrod JG, eds. Substance Abuse: A Comprehensive Textbook, 3d ed. Baltimore, Williams & Wilkins, 1997:148–158.
61. Dewey WL. Cannabinoid pharmacology. Pharmacol Rev 1986;38:151–178.
62. Weinbroum AA, Flaishon R, Sorkine P, et al. A risk-benefit assessment of flumazenil in the management of benzodiazepine overdose. Drug Saf 1997;17:181–196.
63. Reisine TR, Pasternak G. Opioid analgesics and antagonists. In: Hardman JG, Limbird LE, eds: Goodman and Gilman's The Pharmacological Basis of Therapeutics, 9th ed. New York, McGraw-Hill, 1996:521–555.
64. Ashton H. Guidelines for the rational use of benzodiazepines: When and what to use. Drugs 1994;48:25–40.
65. Jaffe JJ, Clifford CM, Ciraulo DA. Opiates: Clinical aspects. In: Lowinson JH, Ruiz P, Millman RB, Langrod JG, eds. Substance Abuse: A Comprehensive Textbook, 3d ed. Baltimore, Williams & Wilkins, 1997: 158–166.
66. Greenstein RA, Fudala PJ, O'Brien CP. Alternative pharmacotherapies for opiate addiction. In: Lowinson JH, Ruiz P, Millman RB, Langrod JG, eds. Substance Abuse: A Comprehensive Textbook, 3d ed. Baltimore, Williams & Wilkins, 1997:415–425.
67. Eissenberg T, Bigelow GE, Strain EC, et al. Dose-related efficacy of levomethadyl acetate for treatment of opioid dependence: A randomized clinical trial. JAMA 1997;277:1945–1951.
68. Kleber HD. Opioids: Detoxification. In: Galanter M, Kleber HD, eds. Textbook of Substance Abuse Treatment. Washington, American Psychiatric Press, 1994:191.
69. Strain EC, Stitzer ML, Liebson IA, Bigelow GE. Comparison of buprenorphine and methadone in the treatment of opioid dependence. Am J Psychiatry 1994;151:1025–1030.
70. O'Connor PG, Kosten TR. Rapid and ultrarapid opioid detoxification techniques. JAMA 1998;279:229–234.
71. Handelsman L, Rosenblum A, Palij M, et al. Bromocriptine for cocaine dependence: A controlled clinical trial. Am J Addict 1997;6:54–64.
72. Galanter M, Talbott D, Gallegos K, Rubenstone E. Combined Alcoholics Anonymous and professional care for addicted physicians. Am J Psychiatry 1990;147:64–68.
73. Beeder AB, Millman RB, Patients with psychopathology. In: Lowinson JH, Ruiz P, Millman RB, Langrod JG, eds. Substance Abuse: A Comprehensive Textbook, 3d ed. Baltimore, Williams & Wilkins, 1997:551–563.
74. Helzer JE, Pryzbeck TR. The co-occurrence of alcoholism with other psychiatric disorders in the general population and its impact on treatment. J Stud Alcohol 1988;49:219–224.
75. Miller NS, Millman RB, Keskinen S. Outcome at six and twelve months post inpatient treatment for cocaine and alcohol dependence. Adv Alcohol Subst Abuse 1990;9:101–120.

Appendix 66–1
Useful Drug Abuse Internet Sites

The following Internet sites are useful sources of information about drugs of abuse and the problems they cause. At the time of this writing, these sites were functional. However, Web addresses sometimes change, and it may be necessary to use one of the searching tools to find an updated address.

National Institute on Drug Abuse Capsules:
http://www.nida.nih.gov/NIDACapsules/ NCIndex.html
National Institute on Drug Abuse links:
http://www.nida.nih.gov/OtherResources.html
Drug Enforcement Administration publications:
http://www.usdoj.gov/dea/pubs/pblist.htm
Drug Enforcement Administration home page:
http://www.usdoj.gov/dea/index.htm
Higher Education Center for Alcohol and Other Drug Prevention:
http://www.edc.org/hec/
Partnership for a Drug-free America home page:
http://www.drugfreeamerica.org/legal.html
Partnership for a Drug-free America—Drug-free Resource Net:
http://www.drugfreeamerica.org/
National Clearinghouse for Alcohol and Drug Information—Research and Statistics:
http://www.health.org/survey.htm
Center for Substance Abuse Prevention (CSAP), Substance Abuse and Mental Health Services Administration (SAMHSA):
http://www.samhsa.gov/csap/CSAP.HTM
National Center on Addiction and Substance Abuse at Columbia University:
http://www.casacolumbia.org/
Office of National Drug Control Policy:
http://www1.whitehouse.gov/WH/EOP/ondcp/ html/ ondcp-plain.html
National Clearinghouse for Alcohol and Drug Information:
http://www.health.org/index.htm

67

SUBSTANCE-RELATED DISORDERS: ALCOHOL, NICOTINE, AND CAFFEINE

Paul L. Doering

Alcohol, nicotine, and caffeine are considered by most to be "socially acceptable" drugs, yet they impose an enormous social and economic cost on our society. More than 430,000 deaths each year are attributable to tobacco use, making tobacco the number one cause of death and disease in this country.[1] Smoking is responsible for 85% of all lung cancer deaths, approximately 80% of all chronic obstructive pulmonary disease deaths, and 30% of overall health disease deaths.[2]

Approximately 12.4 million persons in the United States report current heavy use of alcohol or alcohol abuse. Almost one-half of these persons meet *Diagnostic and Statistical Manual of Mental Disorders,* Fourth Edition. Text Revision (DSM-IV-TR) criteria for alcohol dependence, and almost 400,000 persons are in treatment for alcoholism at any one time.[3–5] Population-based surveys of current drinkers have found rates of 7% to 16% for alcohol abuse or dependence.[6] It has been estimated that as many as 40% of patients in emergency departments had consumed alcohol recently, and as many as 32% had alcohol levels of at least 80 mg/dL, the legal limit of intoxication in many states.[7]

An estimated 100,000 U.S. citizens die each year because of alcohol-related causes, including traffic collisions and cirrhosis of the liver. Direct and indirect health and social costs of alcoholism to the nation are estimated to be $166 billion annually.

Caffeine is currently the most widely used psychoactive substance in the world.[8] In the United States, more than 80% of adults regularly consume behaviorally active doses of caffeine.[9] Although research has shown that caffeine can cause a compulsive pattern of use, the prevalence of caffeine dependence and its clinical significance are difficult to determine.

The subjects of alcohol, tobacco, and caffeine abuse deserve much more attention than space permits in this chapter. Therefore, the information here should serve as a brief overview of these topics, and the reader desiring more details is urged to consult one or more of the many textbooks and articles devoted to these subjects.

ALCOHOL

EPIDEMIOLOGY OF ALCOHOL USE

Almost half (47.3%) of Americans ages 12 and older reported being current drinkers of alcohol in the 1999 National Household Survey of Drug Abuse (NHSDA).[3] This translates to an estimated 105 million people. Approximately one-fifth of persons 12 years of age and older (45 million people) participated in binge drinking, defined as having five or more drinks on the same occasion, at least once in the 30 days prior to the survey. In 1999, there were 12.4 million heavy drinkers, meaning that they drank five or more drinks on the same occasion on at least five different days in the past month.[3]

Among youths aged 12 to 17 years, an estimated 18.6% used alcohol in the month prior to the survey interview. The prevalence of current alcohol drinking increases with increasing age, from 3.9% among youths aged 12 to a peak of 66.6% for persons 21 years of age. In 1999, 54.0% of males (age 12 and older) were current drinkers compared with 41.1% of females. In contrast to the pattern for illicit drugs, the higher the level of educational attainment, the more likely was the current use of alcohol. In 1999, 74.0% of adults with college degrees were current drinkers compared with only 46.1% of those having less than a high school education.[3]

THE DISEASE MODEL OF ADDICTION AS APPLIED TO ALCOHOLISM

Individuals who are drug dependent frequently are regarded as constitutionally weak people who have brought their problems on themselves and deserve the consequences of their behavior. Even when the lay public and health care professionals acknowledge addiction as a disease process, it is often felt to be self-induced. The disease concept of addiction, using alcoholism as a model, states that addiction is a disease and that individuals who suffer from the disease do not choose to contract the disease any more than someone who suffers from heart disease or diabetes mellitus chooses to contract that illness. A *disease* is defined as "any deviation from or interruption of the normal structure or function of any part, organ, or system (or combination thereof) of the body that is manifested by a characteristic set of symptoms and signs and whose etiology, pathology, and prognosis may be known or unknown."[10] Alcoholism, which is discussed as a prototype, meets all the definitional criteria. Diagnostic criteria for alcoholism do not specify frequency of drinking or amount of alcohol consumed. The key determinant is whether drinking is compulsive, out of control, and consequential when one drinks.

Numerous biologic differences between alcoholics and normal individuals have been demonstrated, but discussions of the disease of alcoholism usually focus on three points. The first point involves interindividual differences in response to alcohol, based on the animal model. When a community of rats is offered two sources of water, one a solution of glucose and the other of alcohol, approximately 90% of the animals selectively choose glucose-water solution after testing both supplies. The remaining rats prefer alcohol. If the alcohol-preferring rats are separated from the remainder of the population, their offspring are significantly more likely to be alcohol-preferring.[11]

The experience of the animal studies led researchers to examine family trends in alcoholism and the possibility that alcoholism can be transmitted genetically. Data in human subjects suggest an association between a dopamine D_2-receptor gene and alcoholism,[12,13] although not all similar studies have replicated these results. More recent data suggest a similar genetic predisposition to polysubstance abuse.[12,13] A preliminary study in male veterans also showed an association of the D_2-receptor gene with cocaine dependence.[12,13] Although many researchers think it unlikely that there is a specific gene for addiction, it is possible that interactions among several genes combine in such a way as to be conducive to making a drug an effective reinforcer.[12,13]

The prevalence of alcoholism among the first-degree relatives of alcoholics (i.e., parents, siblings, children) is approximately 25% versus 8% in the adult population. Concordance for alcoholism among fraternal twins is approximately 31%, but among identical twins concordance is approximately 54%,[12,13] although data are conflicting. When children of alcoholic parents are separated at birth and placed in nonalcoholic homes, they remain three to five times more likely to become alcoholic than adoptees whose biologic parents are not alcoholic.[12,13] The opposite is also true—offspring of nonalcoholics adopted by alcoholics do not have elevated rates of alcohol problems.[12,13]

The difference in concordance between fraternal and identical twins and the greater likelihood of developing alcoholism among adoptees whose biologic parents are alcoholic argue for what some clinicians have called a *genetic predisposition,* which is the second focus point for the disease model of alcoholism. A genetically predisposed individual will not necessarily manifest alcoholic drinking behavior. As stated previously, a susceptible host and favorable conditions must combine for a disease process to occur. Sons of men with early-onset alcoholism appear especially predisposed to developing alcoholism.[12,13] Research into genetic influences on other forms of drug dependence is limited owing to their being less prevalent, a greater difficulty in recruiting subjects, lack of restriction of use to one class of drugs, and the changes in availability of illicit substances.

A third point regarding the disease of alcoholism regards possible biochemical abnormalities. Research findings are necessarily limited to animal trials and remain controversial. Behavioral genetics studies of drug self-administration in rats across different drugs and genotypes suggest that the drug-seeking behaviors maintained by alcohol, cocaine, and opiates may have some common biologic determinants.[12,13] Advances in techniques for analysis of brain electrophysiology suggest that alcoholics and their alcohol-naive offspring have similar electroencephalography (EEG) profiles.[12,13] If these findings are borne out with additional studies, it would support the concept of biologic differences between alcoholics and normal individuals that are innate rather than a consequence of exposure to alcohol. In addition, a family history of alcoholism has been shown to be associated with decreased subjective feelings of acute intoxication, less alcohol-induced anxiety, and fewer alcohol-induced decrements in psychomotor and cognitive test performance. EEGs done on this population of non-alcohol-dependent sons of alcoholics also showed less intense EEG alpha activity in response to alcohol challenge than did matched controls.[12,13] Other suggested biologic markers for alcoholism include differences in the activity of liver transaminase enzymes and platelet monoamine oxidase activity.

The belief that addiction is a self-induced disease or a constitutional weakness has been dismissed by clinicians in the addiction treatment field. Willpower and self-discipline cannot control genetics and possible biochemical abnormalities. Given that almost all the population will try alcohol and that over half drink alcohol regularly, the determination of who becomes alcoholic is based on more factors than environmental precipitants.

PHARMACOLOGY AND PHARMACOKINETICS OF ALCOHOL

ALCOHOL AS A DRUG

Alcohol is a central nervous system (CNS) depressant that shares many pharmacologic properties with the nonbenzodiazepine sedative-hypnotic drugs. It affects the CNS in a dose-dependent fashion, producing sedation that progresses to sleep, unconsciousness, coma, surgical anesthesia, and finally, fatal respiratory depression and cardiovascular collapse. Alcohol affects endogenous opiates and several neurotransmitter systems in the brain, including γ-aminobutyric acid (GABA), glutamine, and dopamine. Alcohol intake results in an increase in endogenous opioids,[14] and this may be responsible for the euphoria experienced with alcohol consumption. Currently, there are no clinically useful antagonists that can reverse all the pharmacologic effects of alcohol.

Alcohol is available in a variety of concentrations in various alcoholic beverages. There are approximately 14 g of alcohol in a 12-oz can of beer, 4 oz of nonfortified wine, or one shot (1.5 oz) of 80-proof whiskey. This amount will cause an increase in blood alcohol level of about 20–25 mg/dL in a healthy 70-kg male, although this varies with the time frame over which the alcohol is consumed, the type of alcoholic beverage, whether food is consumed along with it, and many patient variables. The lethal dose of alcohol in humans is variable, but deaths generally occur when blood alcohol levels are greater than 400–500 mg/dL.[15]

PHARMACOKINETICS

Absorption of alcohol begins in the stomach within 5 to 10 minutes of oral ingestion. The onset of clinical effects follows fairly rapidly. It is absorbed primarily from the duodenum but in smaller amounts from the stomach, esophagus, and mucous membranes. Peak serum concentrations of alcohol usually are achieved 30 to 90 minutes after finishing the last drink, although it is quite variable depending on the type of alcoholic beverage consumed, what and when the person last ate, and other factors.[15]

Over 90% of alcohol in the plasma is metabolized in the liver by three enzyme systems that operate within the hepatocyte. The remainder is excreted by the lungs and in urine and sweat. Alcohol is metabolized to acetaldehyde by alcohol dehydrogenase in the cell. In turn, acetaldehyde is metabolized to carbon dioxide and water by the enzyme aldehyde dehydrogenase. A second pathway for oxidation of alcohol uses catalase, an enzyme located in the peroxisomes and microsomes. The third enzyme system, the microsomal alcohol oxidase system, has a role in the oxidation of alcohol to acetaldehyde. These last two mechanisms are of lesser importance than the alcohol dehydrogenase-aldehyde dehydrogenase system.[15]

The metabolism of alcohol generally is said to follow zero-order pharmacokinetics.[16] This may in fact be an oversimplification because at very high or very low concentrations of alcohol the metabolism may follow first-order pharmacokinetics.[16] On average, the blood alcohol concentration is lowered from 15–22.2 mg/dL per hour in the nontolerant individual, assuming that the individual is in the postabsorptive state. Alcohol has a volume of distribution of 0.6–0.8 L/kg, representing the total body water.[15]

Acute Effects of Alcohol

At lower serum concentrations, euphoria and disinhibition may be noted. Slurred speech, altered perception of the environment, impaired judgment, ataxia, incoordination, nystagmus, and hyperreflexia may occur. As plasma levels increase or in different individuals, combative and destructive behavior may occur. With higher levels still, somnolence and respiratory depression may ensue. The typical effects on the body of various blood alcohol concentrations (BACs) are shown in Table 67–1, although effects vary from individual to individual.

TABLE 67–1. Specific Effects of Alcohol Related to the Blood Alcohol Concentration (BAC)

BAC (%)[a]	Effect
0.02–0.03	No loss of coordination, slight euphoria and loss of shyness. Depressant effects are not apparent.
0.04–0.06	Feeling of well-being, relaxation, lower inhibitions, sensation of warmth. Euphoria. Some minor impairment of reasoning and memory, lowering of caution.
0.07–0.09	Slight impairment of balance, speech, vision, reaction time, and hearing. Euphoria. Judgment and self-control are reduced, and caution, reason, and memory are impaired. It is illegal to operate a motor vehicle in some states at this level of intoxication.
0.10–0.125	Significant impairment of motor coordination and loss of good judgment. Speech may be slurred; balance, vision, reaction time, and hearing will be impaired. Euphoria. It is illegal to operate a motor vehicle at this level of intoxication.
0.13–0.15	Gross motor impairment and lack of physical control. Blurred vision and major loss of balance. Euphoria is reduced and dysphoria is beginning to appear.
0.16–0.20	Dysphoria (anxiety, restlessness) predominates, nausea may appear. The drinker has the appearance of a "sloppy drunk."
0.25	Needs assistance in walking; total mental confusion. Dysphoria with nausea and some vomiting.
0.30	Loss of consciousness.
≥ 0.40	Onset of coma, possible death due to respiratory arrest.

[a]Grams of ethyl alcohol per 100 mL of whole blood.

Alcohol Poisoning

If the BAC gets high enough, death becomes a very real possibility, especially with coadministration of other sedative-hypnotics. Acute alcohol poisoning usually occurs with rapid consumption of large quantities of alcoholic beverages because this type of drinking delivers a large bolus of alcohol to the gastrointestinal (GI) tract. Normally, one passes out before a toxic dose of alcohol can be ingested and/or the person vomits to rid the stomach of its toxic reservoir. With rapid drinking as described, the person may fall asleep or pass out without vomiting, allowing continued absorption from the GI tract until fatal BACs are achieved.

In the clinical setting, it is important to differentiate acute alcohol intoxication from certain other medical or surgical illnesses. Mental status changes may result from head trauma, and if the diagnosis is missed, the consequences could be disastrous. Appropriate diagnostic measures, such as computed tomography (CT), should be performed on any patient with deteriorating mental status, focal neurologic findings, failure to improve over time, new-onset seizures, or mental status out of proportion to the degree of intoxication.

Laboratory Studies

In the emergency room, a BAC should be ordered in any patient in whom alcohol ingestion is suspected, regardless of the presenting complaint. For clinical purposes, most laboratories report BAC in units of milligrams per deciliter. In legal cases, results are reported in percent (grams of ethyl alcohol per 100 mL of whole blood). For example, a whole blood alcohol level of 150 mg/dL reported in the hospital corresponds to 0.15% BAC obtained by law enforcement.

If the diagnosis is unclear, if the intoxication seems atypical, or when there is suspicion of multiple drug ingestions, a complete toxicologic screen to rule out the presence of other substances may be useful.

▶ TREATMENT: Alcohol-Related Disorders

ALCOHOL WITHDRAWAL

The *Diagnostic and Statistical Manual of Mental Disorders,* Fourth Edition, Text Revision (DSM-IV-TR) definition of alcohol withdrawal includes two main components.[4] The first component is a history of cessation or reduction in heavy and prolonged alcohol use. The second includes the presence of two or more of the symptoms of alcohol withdrawal: autonomic hyperactivity (sweating or tachycardia); increased hand tremor; insomnia; nausea or vomiting; transient tactile, visual, or auditory hallucinations; psychomotor agitation; anxiety; and tonic-clonic seizures. Signs and symptoms of alcohol withdrawal as well as acute alcohol intoxication are given in Table 67–2.

Goals for alcohol-dependent persons decreasing or discontinuing alcohol intake include (1) the prevention and treatment of withdrawal symptoms (including seizures and delirium tremens) and medical or psychiatric complications, (2) long-term abstinence after detoxification, and (3) entry into ongoing medical and alcohol-dependence treatment.

PHARMACOLOGIC THERAPY

A recent meta-analysis was performed to provide evidence based recommendations on the pharmacologic management of alcohol withdrawal.[17] Trials comparing different benzodiazepines demonstrated that all appear similarly efficacious in reducing signs and symptoms of withdrawal. However, there is some evidence that longer-acting agents may be more effective in preventing seizures. Longer-acting agents can pose a risk of excess sedation in selected groups, including the elderly and those with marked liver disease. Evidence shows, however, that longer-acting agents contribute to an overall smoother withdrawal course with fewer breakthrough or rebound symptoms.

TABLE 67–2. Signs and Symptoms of Alcohol Intoxication and Withdrawal

Intoxication	Withdrawal
Slurred speech	Tremor
Ataxia	Tachycardia
Nystagmus	Diaphoresis
Sedation	Labile blood pressure
Flushed face	Anxiety
Mood change	Nausea and vomiting
Irritability	Hallucinations
Euphoria	Seizures
Loquacity	Hyperthermia
Impaired attention	Delirium

Another consideration in the choice of benzodiazepine is their potential for abuse. Individuals with addictive disorders prefer certain agents over others. Agents with rapid onset of action, such as diazepam or alprazolam, demonstrate higher abuse potential because of their "reinforcing" effects. Those with slower onset of action, such as chlordiazepoxide, oxazepam, and halazepam, are less likely to be abused. This consideration may be relevant in an outpatient setting or for patients with a history of benzodiazepine or other substance abuse.[17]

Other agents have been shown to be better than placebo for reducing signs and symptoms of withdrawal, including chlormethiazole, an agent used in Europe.[17] Although barbiturates are used by approximately 10% of detoxification programs in the United States, no controlled trials with use of phenobarbital were identified for the meta-analysis.[17] Its use is, however, supported by uncontrolled studies. Unlike other barbiturates, phenobarbital has low abuse potential. It is long acting; can be administered reliably by oral, intramuscular, and intravenous routes; has well-documented anticonvulsant activity; and is inexpensive. However, the barbiturates (including phenobarbital) pose a greater risk of respiratory depression, particularly when combined with alcohol, and an overall lower safety profile than benzodiazepines when used in high doses.

Although phenothiazines, clonidine, and carbamazepine may reduce symptoms of alcohol withdrawal, no evidence supports their ability to prevent seizures or delirium tremens, and in fact, the phenothiazines may lower the seizure threshhold.[17] There is a small risk of excessive sedation, particularly in inadequately monitored patients, the elderly, or patients with significant liver disease. Other drugs used to treat symptoms of alcohol withdrawal include other barbiturates; alcohol itself; sympatholytics such as atenolol, thiamine, magnesium; and other neuroleptics such as haloperidol.

Treatment Regimens

Fixed-Schedule Therapy. Over the years, benzodiazepines given regularly at a fixed dosing interval have been considered the "gold standard" therapy for alcohol withdrawal. Chlordiazepoxide 50–100 mg orally every 6 hours for 1 day followed by 2 days at 25–50 mg every 6 hours is known to prevent delirium tremens and seizures.

The treatment guideline,[17] however, takes exception with this rigid approach, urging clinicians to allow for some degree of individualization within fixed-schedule therapy. Patients should be monitored and given additional medication when indicated by symptoms. This type of regimen is useful in patients with a history of seizures, patients with acute medical or surgical illness, or patients with a history of delirium tremens. It also may be preferable for pregnant women.[17]

Front Loading. *Front loading* refers to regimens in which frequent, high doses of medication are given to treat the early signs and symptoms of withdrawal. Diazepam is given in 20-mg doses every 2 hours until resolution of withdrawal symptoms. A total of 60 mg typically is required. Because of the long half-life of diazepam and its active metabolites, further doses are not required. This regimen also has been shown to decrease the incidence of seizures. Advantages of front loading are that medication administration and intensive monitoring are limited to the early symptomatic period of withdrawal.[17]

Symptom-Triggered Therapy. With symptom-triggered therapy, medication is given only when the patient has symptoms. This approach results in treatment that is shorter, potentially avoiding over-sedation and allowing the physician to focus on specific therapy for alcohol dependence.[17] A typical regimen would include diazepam 10–20 mg administered every hour when a structured assessment scale, such as the Clinical Institute Withdrawal Assessment–Alcohol, revised (CIWA-Ar), indicates that symptoms are moderate to severe.[18]

Treatment of Alcohol Withdrawal Seizures

Alcohol withdrawal seizures do not require treatment with an anticonvulsant drug unless they progress to status epilepticus because seizures usually end before diazepam or another drug can be administered.[19] Phenytoin, which is not cross-tolerant to alcohol, does not prevent or treat withdrawal seizures, and without an intravenous loading dose, therapeutic blood levels of phenytoin are not reached until acute withdrawal is complete. Patients experiencing seizures should be treated supportively. An increase in the dosage and slowing of the tapering schedule of the benzodiazepine used in detoxification or a single injection of a benzodiazepine may be necessary to prevent further seizure activity. Patients with a history of withdrawal seizures can be predicted to experience an especially severe withdrawal syndrome. In such patients, a higher initial dosage of a benzodiazepine drug and a slower tapering period of 7–10 days are advisable.

Treatment Settings

Alcohol withdrawal treatment can take place in hospitals, inpatient detoxification units, or outpatient settings. Inpatient treatment may be necessary when there are coexisting acute or chronic medical (including pregnancy), surgical, or psychiatric conditions that would complicate alcohol withdrawal. Only patients with mild to moderate symptoms should be considered for outpatient treatment, and it is a good idea to have a responsible, sober person available to help the patient monitor symptoms and administer medications. Patients with a strong craving for alcohol, those concurrently using other drugs, and those with a history of seizures or delirium tremens are not good candidates for outpatient treatment.

ALCOHOL DEPENDENCE

PHARMACOLOGIC MANAGEMENT

In the United States, disulfiram and naltrexone are the only two drugs specifically indicated for the treatment of alcohol dependence. Disulfiram acts as a deterrent for the resumption of drinking, and naltrexone is a competitive opioid antagonist that has been shown to reduce craving for alcohol. Other drugs, including nalmefene, acamprosate, various serotonergic agents (including selective serotonergic reuptake inhibitors), and lithium, also have been used either abroad or in the United States for off-label indications. Recently, an evidence-based review of the pharmacologic treatment of alcohol dependence was published.[20] Recommendations from this report will be incorporated into the discussion that follows.

Disulfiram

Disulfiram deters a patient from drinking by producing an aversive reaction if the patient drinks. In the absence of alcohol, disulfiram has minimal effects. It inhibits the liver enzyme aldehyde dehydrogenase in the biochemical pathway for alcohol metabolism, allowing acetaldehyde to accumulate. The resulting increase in acetaldehyde causes severe facial flushing, throbbing headache, nausea and vomiting, chest pain, palpitations, tachycardia, weakness, dizziness, blurred vision, confusion, and hypotension. Severe reactions including myocardial infarction, congestive heart failure, cardiac arrhythmia, respiratory depression, convulsions, and death can occur, particularly in vulnerable individuals. A *disulfiram reaction* can occur for up to 2 weeks after therapy has been discontinued, but the time of risk for occurrence of an aversive reaction is usually up to 4 to 7 days. The reaction can occur even from alcohol contained in mouthwashes, certain foodstuffs, and medicinals.[19]

Although disulfiram appeared to be effective in a series of small-scale studies, these were largely uncontrolled.[19] Other studies show conflicting results and generally indicate that factors such as compliance with other aspects of treatment may correlate better with abstinence than use of disulfiram.[19] A well-designed large-scale cooperative study of 605 male veterans treated for 1 year found 250 mg/day disulfiram to be no better than placebo or no pill in helping patients remain abstinent. The combined number of patients in the evidenced-based review of disulfiram was 1207. Authors of the review concluded that the studies provided only modest evidence that disulfiram reduces drinking frequencies without significantly enhancing abstinence rates.[20]

The disulfiram-alcohol interaction sometimes can be intense, causing serious problems for patients with cerebrovascular, cardiovascular, or severe pulmonary disease or chronic renal failure. The use of disulfiram in patients who may have occult vascular disease, such as those over 60 years of age and patients with diabetes, also should be avoided.[19] Vomiting during a disulfiram reaction can cause severe bleeding in a patient with esophageal varices, and for this reason, disulfiram is contraindicated in patients with cirrhosis with portal hypertension. Disulfiram can lower the seizure threshold and cause peripheral neuropathy and should be avoided in patients with these conditions. It has been linked to birth defects and therefore should not be used during pregnancy. Because disulfiram can cause drowsiness, it should be taken first on the weekend at bedtime and discontinued if the patient continues to be drowsy on awakening after 2–3 days of medication.

A rare but potentially fatal idiosyncratic hepatotoxicity can occur with disulfiram. As a result, baseline liver function tests should be obtained and the patient monitored for hepatotoxicity by symptoms and by repeating the liver function tests at 2 weeks, 3 months, 6 months, and then twice yearly thereafter.

The prescriber should wait at least 24 hours after the last drink before starting disulfiram, usually at a dose of 250 mg/day. At this dose there are fewer side effects than at 500 mg, although some research suggests that higher doses are needed to reliably produce an aversive reaction if the patient drinks.[19]

Naltrexone

Naltrexone, an opiate antagonist that has been available in the United States since 1984 for the treatment of opioid dependence, blocks the effects of exogenous opioids. In 1994 the Food and Drug Administration (FDA) approved it for use in the treatment of alcohol dependence. Naltrexone is thought to attenuate the reinforcing effects of alcohol,[20] and those who consume alcohol while taking naltrexone report feeling less intoxicated and having less craving for alcohol.[21,22]

The efficacy of naltrexone for use in alcohol dependence has been investigated in three placebo-controlled clinical trials.[23–25] In a combined analysis of the data from the 186 alcohol-dependent patients in the first two studies, patients randomized to receive 50 mg naltrexone daily for 12 weeks were more likely to remain abstinent and to avoid relapse to heavy drinking; 31% of placebo-treated patients remained abstinent compared with 54% of patients on naltrexone; 48% of placebo-treated patients avoided heavy drinking, whereas 75% of naltrexone-treated patients avoided drinking to excess successfully. Craving for alcohol also was significantly lower for patients on naltrexone.[21] In the third trial, end-of-study relapse rates for all patients were 53% and 35% for placebo- and naltrexone-treated patints, respectively. However, for compliant patients, the figures were 52% and 14%.[25]

Naltrexone should not be given to patients currently dependent on opiates because it can precipitate a severe withdrawal syndrome. Naltrexone has been shown to have dose-related hepatotoxicity, but this generally occurs at doses higher than those recommended for treatment of alcohol dependence. Nevertheless, it should be considered contraindicated in patients with hepatitis or liver failure, and liver function tests should be monitored monthly for the first 3 months and every 3 months thereafter.

Nausea is the most common side effect of naltrexone, occurring in about 10% of patients. Other side effects are headache, dizziness, nervousness, fatigue, insomnia, vomiting, anxiety, and somnolence.

Naltrexone should be given in a dose of 50 mg/day. This dose effectively blocks mu opioid receptors. Documentation is lacking to support routine use of higher doses.

Other Drugs

Acamprosate is a drug that has been studied extensively in Europe but is not currently available in the United States. Results with this drug have been consistently positive on reducing drinking frequency, with some evidence of enchanicing abstinence. Its future impact on U.S. practice is not yet clear.[26]

Nalmefene is a newer opioid antagonist that is structurally similar to naltrexone but with a number of potential pharmacologic advantages for the treatment of alcohol dependence, including no dose-dependent association with toxic effects to the liver, greater oral bioavailability, longer duration of antagonist action, and more competitive binding with opioid receptor subtypes that are thought to reinforce drinking. A double-blind, placebo-controlled trial[27] was conducted to evaluate the safety and efficacy of two doses of oral nalmefene for alcohol dependence. The 105 outpatient volunteers were abstinent for a mean of 2 weeks prior to random assignment to groups given placebo or 20 or 80 mg/day of nalmefene for 12 weeks. Results showed that significantly fewer patients treated with nalmefene than patients given placebo relapsed to heavy drinking through 12 weeks of treatment, with a significant treatment effect at the first weekly study visit. Outcomes did not differ between the groups given 20 and 80 mg nalmefene. The authors concluded that treatment with nalmefene was effective in preventing relapse to heavy drinking relative to placebo in alcohol-dependent outpatients and was accompanied by acceptable side effects. At the time this chapter was written, nalmefene was not available in the United States. Using the limited data on serotonergic agents in the evidence-based analysis,[20] these drugs were deemed not very promising, although most studies were confounded by high rates of comorbid mood disorders. Lithium lacks efficacy in the treatment of primary alcohol dependence.[20]

NICOTINE

Cigarette smoking is an enormous national health problem, and we, as health care professionals, are not doing an adequate job in helping people to quit. Only about one-half of the current smokers surveyed in studies conducted in the later 1980s and early 1990s reported that their doctors had ever advised them to quit smoking,[28,29] and only 3.6% of ex-smokers report that their physician helped them quit.[28] Other health care professionals did an even poorer job, with only 22% of dentists, 24% of nurses, and a pitiful 4% of pharmacists helping their patients to quit smoking.[30] The benefits of smoking cessation include a longer life and better health.[31]

EPIDEMIOLOGY OF TOBACCO USE

An estimated 66.8 million Americans reported current use of a tobacco product in 1999, a prevalence rate of 30.2% for the population 12 years of age and older.[3] Of the total population, 57.0 million (25.8% of the population) smoked cigarettes, 12.1 million (5.5% of the population) smoked cigars, 7.6 million (3.4% of the population) used smokeless tobacco, and 2.4 million (1.1% of the population) smoked tobacco in pipes.

Current cigarette smoking rates increase steadily by year of age, from 2.2% at age 12 to 43.5% at age 20. Overall, 14.9% of youths aged 12 to 17 years in 1999 smoked cigarettes currently. The rate of current cigarette use in the population aged 12 years and older was similar in 1999 (29.7%) to the rates estimated from 1994 through 1998. Among youths aged 12 to 17 years, the rate was 15.9% in 1999, not statistically different than in 1998 (18.2%) but significantly lower than the rate in 1997 (19.9%).[3]

ECONOMIC IMPACT OF SMOKING

The estimated direct cost of medical care for smoking-related illnesses in the United States in 1993 (the latest data available) was $50 billion.[32] Lost productivity caused by smoking cost the U.S. economy $47.2 billion in 1990, according to the Office of Technology Assessment. Adjusted for inflation, the total economic cost of smoking is more than $100 billion per year. These direct and indirect costs amount to $3.90 for each pack of cigarettes sold.[31]

HEALTH RISKS OF SMOKING

Each year more than 430,000 deaths, or 20% of the total deaths in the United States, are caused by smoking.[32] Cigarette smoking substantially increases the risk of (1) cardiovascular diseases such as stroke, sudden death, and heart attack, (2) nonmalignant respiratory diseases including emphysema, asthma, chronic bronchitis, and chronic obstructive pulmonary disease, (3) lung cancer, and (4) other cancers (e.g., mouth, pharynx, larynx, esophagus, stomach, pancreas, uterus, cervix, kidney, ureter, and bladder).

Exposure to environmental tobacco smoke (*passive exposure*) has been cited as the cause of 3000 lung cancer deaths and 35,000 to 40,000 heart disease deaths in the United States every year.[31] When children are exposed to environmental smoke, they have a higher risk of respiratory infection, asthma, and middle-ear infections than those who are not exposed. Sudden infant death syndrome occurs more often in infants whose mothers smoked during pregnancy than in offspring of nonsmoking mothers.[31] The harmful effects of smoking on reproduction and pregnancy include reduced fertility and fetal growth, as well as increased risk of ectopic pregnancy and spontaneous abortion.[31]

TABLE 67–3. Withdrawal Symptoms of Nicotine

Anxiety	Gastrointestinal disturbances
Craving for tobacco	Headache
Decreased blood pressure and heart rate	Hostility
	Increased appetite and weight gain
Depression	Increased skin temperature
Difficulty concentrating	Insomnia
Drowsiness	Restlessness
Frustration, irritability, impatience	

PHARMACOLOGY OF NICOTINE

Nicotine is a ganglionic cholinergic receptor agonist whose pharmacologic effects are highly dependent on dose. These effects include central and peripheral nervous system stimulation and depression, respiratory stimulation, skeletal muscle relaxation, catecholamine release by the adrenal medulla, peripheral vasoconstriction, and increased blood pressure, heart rate, cardiac output, and oxygen consumption.[33] Cigarette smoking or low doses of nicotine produce an increased alertness and increased cognitive functioning by stimulating the cerebral cortex. At higher doses, nicotine stimulates the "reward" center in the limbic system of the brain.[33]

Chronic nicotine ingestion may lead to physical and psychological dependence and tolerance to some of its pharmacologic effects. Abrupt smoking cessation in physically dependent smokers results in withdrawal symptoms, as shown in Table 67–3. Onset of these symptoms usually occurs within 24 hours and may last for days, weeks, or longer. The craving for tobacco may last for years.

Although some smokers do not develop physical or psychological dependence, most people who smoke 10–15 cigarettes daily for several weeks or longer do. Between 77% and 92% of smokers are addicted to nicotine in cigarettes.[32]

FDA'S ATTEMPTS TO CLASSIFY TOBACCO AS A DRUG

Over the years, the FDA has tried unsuccessfully to exert regulatory control over tobacco products. Culminating an exhaustive 2.5-year investigation of tobacco products, in 1996 President Clinton announced what was slated to be the final regulations of the FDA restricting the sale and promotion of cigarettes and smokeless tobacco.[34]

The Food Drug and Cosmetic Act (FDCA) defines a *drug* as any article (other than food) "intended to affect the structure or any function of the body."[35] With the emergence of a scientific consensus that the nicotine in cigarettes and smokeless tobacco causes and sustains addiction, the FDA felt confident that its regulatory authority over tobacco would be sustained. There was disclosure of thousands of pages of internal tobacco company documents that the FDA contends prove that the tobacco manufacturers know that nicotine causes significant pharmacologic effects, including addiction, and thus design their products to provide pharmacologically active doses of nicotine.[34]

These findings provided the basis for the FDA's assertion that cigarettes and smokeless tobacco are subject to FDA jurisdiction as products that contain a "drug" (nicotine) and a "device" (the cigarette itself) for delivering this drug to the body. According to the agency, nicotine exerts psychoactive effects on the brain that motivate repeated, compulsive use of the substance.

The tobacco industry went to court to have the regulations nullified. It argued that if the FDA had jurisdiction over tobacco as a drug, it also would have the authority (and probably the obligation) to take cigarettes off the market, as it has done with other unsafe drugs.[36] In 1997, FDA jurisdiction over tobacco was considered by the U.S. District Court of North Carolina. Judge William Osteen ruled for the FDA, finding that the FDA had acted appropriately under the FDCA when it classified nicotine as a drug and cigarettes as nicotine-delivery devices. The following year the U.S. Court of Appeals for the Fourth Circuit reversed this ruling in a two-to-one decision. The court noted that the reason the FDA chose to regulate cigarettes as a device rather than as a drug was that if cigarettes were drugs, the FDA would have to ban them; the FDA has more leeway with devices.

The FDA appealed the case to the U.S. Supreme Court. In a five-to-four decision, the Supreme Court affirmed the ruling of the appeals court that the FDA does not have jurisdiction over tobacco. The court stated, "Viewing the FDCA as a whole, it is evident that one of the Act's core objectives is to ensure that any product regulated by the FDA is 'safe' and 'effective' for its intended use. The Act generally requires the FDA to prevent the marketing of any drug or device where the 'potential for inflicting death or physical injury is not offset by the possibility of therapeutic benefit.'" The Court then reminded the FDA of its steadfast position that tobacco products are dangerous, and therefore, the logical consequence would be a mandatory ban on cigarettes if the FDA actually had jurisdiction. The Court found that a ban on tobacco products by the FDA would plainly contradict congressional policy, which has consistently been to take measures less severe than a ban in regard to tobacco regulation.

The Court described as "ironic" the FDA's position that cigarettes were "safe" when the agency also acknowledges that cigarettes kill 400,000 people annually. "The inescapable conclusion," the Court stated, "is that there is no room for tobacco products within the FDCA's regulatory scheme. If they cannot be used safely for any therapeutic purpose, and yet they cannot be banned, they simply do not fit." Congress is well aware of the dangers of smoking and has chosen not to ban cigarettes. The Court found that before an agency would be deemed to have the power to "regulate an industry constituting a significant part of the American economy," it would need much more explicit indications of that authority from Congress than congressional inaction in the face of the FDA's denials, for over 80 years, that it had jurisdiction over tobacco products.[36]

The debate as to who should regulate tobacco products rages on. Sentiment urging the FDA to regroup and try again to exert regulatory control over tobacco has been aired.[37] Others have called for the creation of a new federal agency whose authority would be to regulate tobacco products exclusively. The Tobacco Control Agency, the name suggested for this agency, would have the goals of: reducing smoking, developing and funding research, overseeing the development of a "safer cigarette," and testing cigarettes for compliance with its specifications, as well as requiring the disclosure of ingredients in cigarettes that might affect purchasing decisions.[37] Regardless of the proposal, any attempt to further regulate tobacco is sure to spark intense debate in Washington.

▶ TREATMENT: Nicotine Dependence

AGENCY FOR HEALTHCARE RESEARCH AND QUALITY CLINICAL PRACTICE GUIDELINE: TREATING TOBACCO USE AND DEPENDENCE

The Agency for Healthcare Research and Quality (AHRQ), the new name for the former Agency for Health Care Policy and Research (AHCPR), periodically convenes expert panels to develop clinical guidelines for health care practitioners when the need dictates. Because of the widespread prevalence of smoking-related illnesses, its related morbidity and mortality, and the economic burden imposed, AHCPR convened a panel of experts in 1994 to develop guidelines on the treatment of tobacco addiction. The AHCPR released its guideline for smoking cessation in 1996.[38] In June 2000, an updated version of the 1996 Smoking Cessation Clinical Practice Guideline was issued by AHRQ.[32]

The updated guideline was written because new, effective clinical treatments for tobacco dependence have been identified since 1994. The accelerating pace of tobacco research that prompted the update is reflected in the fact that 3000 articles on tobacco were identified as published between 1975 and 1994, contributing to the original guideline. Another 3000 were published between 1995 and 1999 and contributed to the updated guideline. These 6000 articles were screened and reviewed to identify a much smaller group of articles that served as the basis for guideline data analyses and panel opinion.[32] The updated guideline reflects new, effective clinical treatments of tobacco dependence. The new title of the guideline reflects the fact that all tobacco products, not just cigarettes, exact devastating costs to the nation's health and welfare. The report further highlights the fact that tobacco use results in true drug dependence, felt to be comparable with the dependence caused by opiates, amphetamines, and cocaine. For this reason, the reports make the irrefutable argument that chronic tobacco use warrants clinical intervention just as do other addictive disorders.

The guideline suggests strategies for providing appropriate treatments for every patient. The panel reminds us that effective treatments for tobacco dependence now exist and that every patient should receive at least minimal treatment every time he or she visits a clinician. The first step in this process, identification and assessment of tobacco use status, separates patients into three treatment categories:

1. Patients who use tobacco and are willing to quit should be treated using the 5 A's (ask, advise, assess, assist, and arrange).
2. Patients who use tobacco but are unwilling to quit at this time should be treated with the 5 R's of motivational intervention (relevance, risks, rewards, roadblocks, and repetition).
3. Patients who have quit using tobacco recently should be provided relapse-prevention treatment.

Figure 67–1 shows an overall approach to evaluating patients' needs and desires to quit smoking. Figure 67–2 is an algorithm for treating tobacco use.

KEY FINDINGS

The guideline identified a number of key findings that clinicians should use:

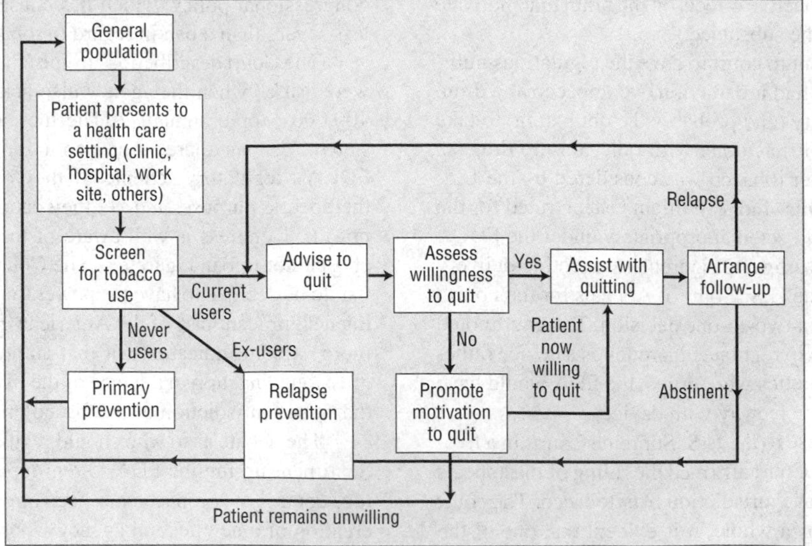

FIGURE 67–1. Model for treatment of tobacco use and dependence.

1. Tobacco dependence is a chronic condition that often requires repeated intervention. However, effective treatments exist that can produce long-term or even permanent abstinence.
2. Because effective tobacco dependence treatments are available, every patient who uses tobacco should be offered at least one of these treatments:
    - Patients willing to try to quit tobacco use should be provided with treatments that are identified as effective in the guideline.
    - Patients unwilling to try to quit tobacco use should be provided with a brief intervention that is designed to increase their motivation to quit.
3. It is essential that clinicians and health care delivery systems (including administrators, insurers, and purchasers) institutionalize the consistent identification, documentation, and treatment of every tobacco user who is seen in a health care setting.
4. Brief tobacco dependence treatment is effective, and every patient who uses tobacco should be offered at least brief treatment.
5. There is a strong dose-response relationship between the intensity of tobacco dependence counseling and its effectiveness. Treatments involving person-to-person contact (via individual, group, or proactive telephone counseling) are consistently effective, and their effectiveness increases with treatment intensity (e.g., minutes of contact).
6. Three types of counseling and behavioral therapies were found to be especially effective and should be used with all patients who are attempting tobacco cessation:
    - Provision of practical counseling (problem-solving/skills training).
    - Provision of social support as part of treatment (intratreatment social support).
    - Help in securing social support outside treatment (extratreatment social support).
7. Numerous effective pharmacotherapies for smoking cessation now exist. Except in the presence of contraindications, these should be used with all patients who are attempting to quit smoking. Five first-line

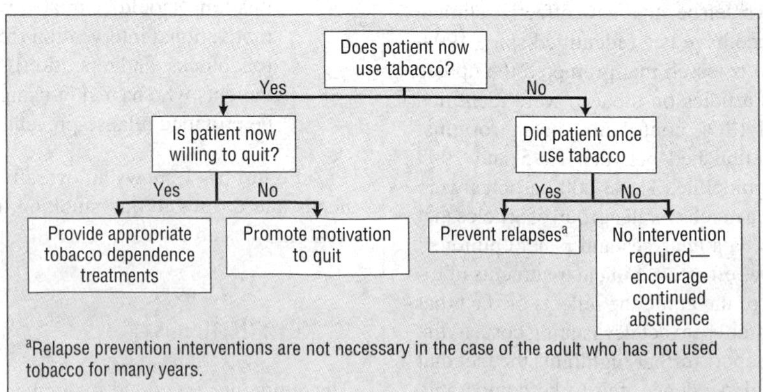

FIGURE 67–2. Algorithm for treating tobacco use.

pharmacotherapies were identified that reliably increase long-term smoking abstinence rates:

- Bupropion SR.
- Nicotine gum.
- Nicotine inhaler.
- Nicotine nasal spray.
- Nicotine patch.

Two second-line pharmacotherapies were identified as efficacious and may be considered by clinicians if first-line pharmacotherapies are not effective:

- Clonidine.
- Nortriptyline.

8. Tobacco dependence treatments are both clinically effective and cost-effective relative to other medical and disease-prevention interventions. As such, insurers and purchasers should ensure that

- All insurance plans include as a reimbursed benefit the counseling and pharmacotherapeutic treatments that are identified as effective in this guideline.
- Clinicians are reimbursed for providing tobacco dependence treatment just as they are reimbursed for treating other chronic conditions.

OTHER FACTORS IMPORTANT TO THE SUCCESS OF A SMOKING-CESSATION STRATEGY

The AHRQ expert panel emphasized the importance of the type and intensity of the contact with the counselor to the success of the intervention. When interventions last for more than 10 minutes, the increase in cessation rates is much better than when interventions do not involve contact with a professional. Group and individual counseling is more effective than no intervention in increasing abstinence rates, but self-help materials (e.g., handouts, pamphlets, brochures) are not. Interventions are more successful when they include social support and training in general problem-solving skills, stress management, and relapse prevention.[32] The number of treatment sessions offered is also important. Providing at least four to seven sessions significantly increased cessation rates, independent of the treatment's intensity.[32]

Comprehensive behavioral interventions are more effective in helping people quit smoking and remain abstinent, but less intensive treatments are beneficial as well. Even minimal contacts lasting less than 3 minutes and simple advice to quit are more successful than intervention involving no contact in increasing cessation rates.[32]

Counseling efficacy is further augmented by the addition of nicotine-replacement products. The cessation rates of nicotine patch users are approximately double the cessation rates of smokers who receive placebos, according to a metaanalysis review of the literature.[32] Although absolute quit rates have varied greatly, abstinence rates for the nicotine patch are estimated at 27% (ranging from 14%–69%) at the end of treatment and 22% (ranging from 13%–34%) at 6 months posttreatment.[32]

Although comprehensive programs are most effective, few smokers (10%–15%) seek formal assistance in quitting.[32] A health care professional who merely advises his or her patient to quit smoking is providing at least minimal assistance in the efforts.

PHARMACOLOGIC THERAPY FOR SMOKING CESSATION

All patients attempting to quit should be encouraged to use effective parmacotherapies for smoking cessation except in the presence of special circumstances. Long-term smoking-cessation pharmacotherapy should be considered as a strategy to reduce the likelihood of relapse. As with other chronic diseases, the most effective treatment of tobacco dependence requires the use of multiple modalities. Pharmacotherapy is a vital element of a multicomponent approach. The clinician should encourage all patients initiating a quit attempt to use one or a combination of efficacious pharmacotherapies, although pharmacotherapy use requires special consideration with some patient groups (e.g., those with medical contraindications, those smoking fewer than 10 cigarettes a day, pregnant/breast-feeding women, and adolescent smokers). The guideline panel identified five first-line medications (i.e., bupropion SR, nicotine gum, nicotine inhaler, nicotine nasal spray, and the nicotine patch) and two second-line medications (i.e., clonidine and nortriptyline) for smoking cessation. Each has been documented to increase significantly rates of long-term smoking abstinence. The role of pharmacotherapy is summarized in Table 67–4.

NICOTINE-REPLACEMENT THERAPY

The AHRQ guidelines recommend use of nicotine-replacement therapy (NRT) in the forms of transdermal nicotine patches, nicotine gum, nicotine sprays, and nicotine inhalers. The use of NRT is relatively safe, but it is not recommended for all smokers. Although cardiovascular disease is not an independent risk factor for acute myocardial events, NRT should be used with caution among particular cardiovascular patient groups: those in the immediate (within 2 weeks) post-myocardial infarction period, those with serious arrhythmias, and those with serious or worsening angina pectoris.[32]

Nicotine Gum

Thirteen studies met selection criteria for the panel's meta-analysis of nicotine gum.[32] Results of this analysis are shown in Table 67–5. Based on its meta-analysis, the panel recommends that patients should be encouraged to use these products. Clinicians should offer 4-mg rather than 2-mg nicotine gum to highly dependent smokers. As can be seen by the estimated odds ratio from this analysis, 2-mg nicotine gum improves long-term abstinence rates by approximately 30%–80% as compared with placebo. Furthermore, a close review of the literature suggests that the 4-mg gum is more efficacious than 2-mg gum as an aid to smoking cessation in highly dependent smokers. Nicotine gum is available in 2- and 4-mg (per piece) doses. The 2-mg gum is recommended for patients smoking less than 25 cigarettes per day, whereas the 4-mg gum is recommended for patients smoking 25 or more cigarettes per day. Generally, the gum should be used for up to 12 weeks with no more than 24 pieces per day. Clinicians should tailor the dosage and duration of therapy to fit the needs of each patient.

Nicotine gum currently is available exclusively as an over-the-counter medication and is packaged with important instructions on correct use, including chewing instructions. There is currently little evidence to suggest that combined use of the patch and gum increases abstinence beyond 24 weeks.

Gum should be chewed slowly until a peppery or minty taste emerges and then "parked" between cheek and gums to facilitate nicotine absorption through the oral mucosa. Gum should be chewed slowly and intermittently and parked for about 30 minutes or until

TABLE 67–4. Summary of Clinical Guidelines for Prescribing Pharmacotherapy for Smoking Cessation

Who should receive pharmacotherapy for smoking cessation?	All smokers trying to quit, except in the presence of special circumstances. Special consideration should be given before using pharmacotherapy with selected populations: those with medical contraindications, those smoking fewer than 10 cigarettes/day, pregnant/breast-feeding women, and adolescent smokers.
What are the first-line pharmacotherapies recommended in this guideline?	All five of the FDA-approved pharmacotherapies for smoking cessation are recommended, including bupropion SR, nicotine gum, nicotine inhaler, nicotine nasal spray, and the nicotine patch.
What factors should a clinician consider when choosing among the five first-line pharmacotherapies?	Because of the lack of sufficient data to rank order these five medications, choice of a specific first-line pharmacotherapy must be guided by factors such as clinician familiarity with the medications, contraindications for selected patients, patient preference, previous patient experience with a specific pharmacotherapy (positive or negative), and patient characteristics (e.g., history of depression, concerns about weight gain).
Are pharmacotherapeutic treatments appropriate for lighter smokers (e.g., 10–15 cigarettes/day)?	If pharmacotherapy is used with lighter smokers, clinicians should consider reducing the dose of first-line NRT pharmacotherapies. No adjustments are necessary when using bupropion SR.
What second-line pharmacotherapies are recommended in this guideline?	Clonidine and nortriptyline.
When should second-line agents be used for treating tobacco dependence?	Consider prescribing second-line agents for patients unable to use first-line medications because of contraindications or for patients for whom first-line medications are not helpful. Monitor patients for the known side effects of second-line agents.
Which pharmacotherapies should be considered with patients particularly concerned about weight gain?	Bupropion SR and nicotine-replacement therapies, in particular nicotine gum, have been shown to delay, but not prevent, weight gain.
Are there pharmacotherapies that should be especially considered in patients with a history of depression?	Bupropion SR and nortriptyline appear to be effective with this population.
Should nicotine replacement therapies be avoided in patients with a history of cardiovascular disease?	No. The nicotine patch in particular is safe and has been shown not to cause adverse cardiovascular effects.
May tobacco-dependence pharmacotherapies be used long term (e.g., 6 months or more)?	Yes. This approach may be helpful with smokers who report persistent withdrawal symptoms during the course of pharmacotherapy or who desire long-term therapy. A minority of individuals who successfully quit smoking use ad libitum NRT medications (gum, nasal spray, inhaler) long term. The use of these medications long term does not present a known health risk. Additionally, the FDA has approved the use of bupropion SR for long-term maintenance.
May pharmacotherapies ever be combined?	Yes. There is evidence that combining the nicotine patch with either nicotine gum or nicotine nasal spray increases long-term abstinence rates over those produced by a single form of NRT.

Reprinted from Ref. 42.

the taste dissipates. Acidic beverages (e.g., coffee, juices, soft drinks) interfere with the buccal absorption of nicotine, so eating and drinking anything except water should be avoided for 15 minutes before and during chewing. Patients often do not use enough gum to get the maximum benefit: They chew too few pieces per day, and they do not use the gum for a sufficient number of weeks. Instructions to chew the gum on a fixed schedule (at least one piece every 1–2 hours) for at least 1–3 months may be more beneficial than ad libitum use.

Nicotine Patch

According to the AHRQ guideline, the nicotine patch is an efficacious smoking-cessation treatment that patients should be encouraged to use. The panel included 27 studies in the meta-analysis comparing the nicotine patch with placebo. Results of this analysis are shown in Table 67–5. As can be seen from this analysis, the nicotine patch approximately doubles long-term abstinence rates over those produced by placebo interventions. The nicotine patch is available both as an over-the-counter medication and as a prescription medication. Treatment of 8 weeks or less has been shown to be as efficacious as longer treatment periods. The 16- and 24-hour patches are of comparable efficacy.[30] Clinicians should consider individualizing treatment based on specific patient characteristics, such as previous experience with the patch, amount smoked, degree of addictiveness, etc. Finally, clinicians should consider starting treatment on a lower patch dose in patients smoking 10 or fewer cigarettes per day.[32]

At the start of each day, the patient should place a new patch on a relatively hairless location, typically between the neck and waist. There are no restrictions on activity while using the patch. Patches should be applied as soon as the patient wakes on the quit day. With patients who experience sleep disruption, have the patient remove the 24-hour patch prior to bedtime or use the 16-hour patch.

Nicotine Nasal Spray

The AHRQ guideline concluded that nicotine nasal spray is an efficacious smoking-cessation treatment that patients should be encouraged to use.[32] Three studies met the selection criteria for inclusion in the

TABLE 67–5. Meta-analysis: Efficacy of and Estimated Abstinence Rates for Recommended Smoking-Cessation Pharmacotherapies

Pharmacotherapy	No. of Studies	No. of Arms	Estimated Odds Ratio (95% C.I.)	Estimated Abstinence Rate (95% C.I.)
Placebo versus Nicotine Gum	13			
Placebo		16	1.0	17.1
Nicotine gum		18	1.5 (1.3, 1.8)	23.7 (20.6, 26.7)
Placebo versus Nicotine Patch	27			
Placebo		28	1.0	10.0
Nicotine patch		32	1.9 (1.7, 2.2)	17.7 (16.0, 19.5)
Placebo versus Nicotine Nasal Spray	3			
Placebo		3	1.0	13.9
Nicotine nasal spray		3	2.7 (1.8, 4.1)	30.5 (21.8, 39.2)
Placebo versus Nicotine Inhaler	4			
Placebo		4	1.0	10.5
Nicotine inhaler		4	2.5 (1.7, 3.6)	22.8 (16.4, 29.2)
Placebo versus Bupropion SR	2			
Placebo		2	1.0	17.3
Bupropion SR		4	2.1 (1.5, 3.0)	30.5 (23.2, 37.8)
Placebo versus Clonidine	5			
Placebo		6	1.0	13.9
Clonidine		8	2.1 (1.4, 3.2)	25.6 (17.7, 33.6)
Placebo versus Nortriptyline	2			
Placebo		3	1.0	11.7
Nortriptyline		3	3.2 (1.8, 5.7)	30.1 (18.1, 41.6)

Adapted from Ref. 32.

meta-analysis comparing nicotine nasal spray with placebo. Results of this analysis also are shown in Table 67–5. As can be seen from this analysis, nicotine nasal spray more than doubles long-term abstinence rates when compared with a placebo spray. Nicotine nasal spray is available exclusively as a prescription medication. A dose of nicotine nasal spray consists of one 0.5-mg delivery to each nostril (1 mg total). Initial dosing should be one to two doses per hour, increasing as needed for symptom relief. Minimum recommended treatment is 8 doses per day, with a maximum limit of 40 doses per day (5 doses per hour). Each bottle contains approximately 100 doses. Recommended duration of therapy is 3 to 6 months. Patients should not sniff, swallow, or inhale through the nose while administering doses because this increases irritating effects. The spray is best delivered with the head tilted slightly back.[32]

Instructing Patients in the Use of NRT

Compliance with NRT improves when the patient is presented a clear rationale for its use and a realistic expectation about the response.[39] It should be explained to the patient that nicotine is responsible for addiction and that discontinuation of the nicotine causes craving for cigarettes, tension, irritability, sadness, problems with sleep, and difficulty concentrating. These are partly due to nicotine withdrawal. The patient should be told that using the patch results in less desire to smoke and provides an opportunity for a new nonsmoker to practice all the new nonsmoking skills without being burdened by craving. The patient should understand that with smoking, there are naturally peaks and valleys in the amount of nicotine in the bloodstream. With the patch there is a steady gradual rise in the blood nicotine concentration that levels off and remains constant for much of the day and then gradually decreases while the person is asleep. Maintaining an adequate blood level of nicotine lessens withdrawal symptoms.[39]

A similar rationale can be used if patients are using gum. It should be emphasized that NRT is not a "magic bullet" and that the use of coping skills is essential for abstinence. The patch or the gum only buys time by reducing withdrawal symptoms and giving individuals a chance to figure out alternatives that they can use in place of smoking in many different situations.[39]

Side Effects

Nicotine-replacement products have relatively few side effects. Nausea and light-headedness are possible signs of nicotine overdose that warrant a reduction of the nicotine dose.

The most frequent side effect with the nicotine patch is skin irritation related to the adhesive or the medium containing nicotine and not to the nicotine itself. About 50% of patients report skin irritation during the course of treatment with the patch.[30] The patch site can be rotated to diminish this problem. The use of over-the-counter hydrocortisone cream (1%) or triamcinolone cream (0.5%) is recommended as a local treatment for patch-related skin irritations. Switching to a different brand of patch also may alleviate the problem because different products use a different adhesive or medium. The gum can be used instead of the patch when the skin irritation is severe. Less than 5% of patients were forced to discontinue therapy because of skin reactions.[39]

About 23% of patients using the patch report sleep disturbances, but the insomnia is hard to differentiate from the sleeplessness that often accompanies withdrawal itself, especially during the first few weeks of quitting.

Duration

Those who commit to quitting smoking using the nicotine patch should be told to expect a minimum of 6–8 weeks of treatment. Using the therapy beyond 8 weeks is not associated with better success rates.[32] However, some patients will experience severe withdrawal even beyond 8 weeks, and these people may need to use the patch longer.

The duration of therapy with the gum should be at least 1 to 3 months on a fixed schedule rather than when one has the urge to smoke.[39] Studies have found, however, that 15%–20% of abstainers continue to use the gum for longer than 12 months.[32] Patients should be encouraged to stick with the patch and/or gum for the minimally acceptable duration of treatment.

Economic and Pharmacoeconomic Considerations

Most health insurers provide coverage for the chronic illnesses caused by smoking (e.g., chronic obstructive pulmonary disease, cancer, and myocardial infarction), yet few provide coverage for treating the nicotine addiction that caused those ailments.[30] For each life saved, smoking-cessation programs involving physician counseling cost an estimated $700–$2000.[40] Even after adding the cost of the nicotine patch to physician counseling, costs from the standpoint of a third-party payer range from $4390–$10,943 per quality-adjusted life year saved for males and $4955–$6983 per quality-adjusted life year saved for females (based on 15 minutes of physician counseling and 1–2 months of NRT).[41] Compared with the cost-effectiveness of other preventive treatments, these costs are actually small. For each life saved by treating mild hypertension, the cost ranges from $11,300–$24,408, and the preventive treatment of hypercholesterolemia is estimated to range from $65,511–$108,189 per year of life saved.[40] Thus smoking-cessation treatment is clearly more cost-effective in comparison. Treating tobacco dependence is particularly important economically in that it can prevent a variety of costly chronic diseases, including heart disease, cancer, and pulmonary disease. In fact, smoking-cessation treatment has been referred to as the "gold standard" of preventive interventions.[32]

It is important to note that smoking cessation is also cost-effective in special populations such as hospitalized patients and pregnant women. For hospitalized patients, successful tobacco abstinence not only reduces general medical costs in the short term but also reduces the number of future hospitalizations.[32] Smoking-cessation interventions for pregnant women are especially cost-effective because they result in fewer low-birth-weight babies and perinatal deaths; result in fewer physical, cognitive, and behavioral problems during infancy and childhood; and also yield important health benefits for the mother.[32]

The failure of a health plan to cover tobacco dependence treatment as an insured benefit could reduce access to these services and reduce the number of people seeking these services. It has been found that when smoking-cessation services are provided as a fully covered benefit by a health plan in contrast to a health plan that requires a significant copay, the overall use of cessation treatment increases and smoking prevalence within the health plan will decrease.[32] Moreover, the presence of prepaid or discounted prescription drug benefits increases patients' receipt of pharmacotherapy and smoking abstinence rates.[32]

BUPROPION

In 1997, the antidepressant drug bupropion, available since 1989 under the brand name Wellbutrin, was approved by the FDA in a sustained-release formulation (Zyban) for use as an aid in smoking cessation. Bupropion inhibits neuronal reuptake and potentiates the effects of norepinephrine and dopamine. Although its precise mechanism in smoking cessation is not well understood, dopamine has been associated with the rewarding effects of addictive substances. Withdrawal symptoms may be decreased by virtue of bupropion's inhibition of norepinephrine uptake. The AHRQ panel concluded that bupropion sustained release (SR) is an efficacious smoking-cessation treatment that patients should be encouraged to use.[32] Two large multicenter studies met selection criteria and were included in the meta-analysis comparing bupropion SR with placebo. Results of this analysis also are shown in Table 67–5. As can be seen from this analysis, the use of bupropion SR approximately doubles long-term abstinence rates when compared with placebo.

Bupropion is contraindicated in patients with a seizure disorder, a current or prior diagnosis of bulimia or anorexia nervosa, use of a monoamine oxidase (MAO) inhibitor within the previous 14 days, or in patients on another medication that contains bupropion. Bupropion SR can be used in combination with NRT. Bupropion SR is available exclusively as a prescription medication.

One study compared the effects of 100, 150, or 300 mg/day of bupropion SR or placebo for 7 weeks in 615 patients who visited the clinic each week for evaluation and counseling.[42] When the study was concluded, smoking-cessation rates were 19% with placebo and 28.8%, 38.6%, and 44.2% with the respective doses of the drug. The differences between the 150- and 300-mg doses and placebo were statistically significant. After 1 year, the respective rates were 12.4%, 19.6%, 22.9%, and 23.1%, indicating a fairly high rate of relapse in all groups.

Bupropion at a dose of 150 mg twice daily of sustained-release tablets was compared with the 21-mg nicotine patch separately and as combined therapy and with placebo in nearly 900 patients studied for 9 weeks. At the 10-week mark, smoking cessation had been accomplished in 20% of the placebo group, 32% of the group using the patch alone, 46% of the group using bupropion alone, and 51% of the group using combined therapy. All three active treatments were significantly better than placebo.[43] Unlike its use as an antidepressant, no seizures occurred with bupropion in smoking-cessation trials. Insomnia and dry mouth were the most frequent adverse effects. Other side effects noted in the trials were tremor, rash, and a few anaphylactoid reactions characterized by pruritus, urticaria, angioedema, and dyspnea. Insomnia also was reported.[43] For smoking cessation, the manufacturer recommends a dosage of 150 mg once daily for 3 days and then twice daily for 7–12 weeks or longer, with or without nicotine replacement. Patients are instructed to stop smoking during the second week of treatment and are encouraged to use counseling and support services along with the medication. For maintenance therapy, consider bupropion SR 150 mg twice daily for up to 6 months.[32]

SECOND-LINE MEDICATIONS

Second-line medications are pharmacotherapies for which there is evidence of efficacy for treating tobacco dependence, but they have a more limited role than first-line medications because (1) the FDA has not approved them for a tobacco-dependence treatment indication and (2) there are more concerns about potential side effects than exist with first-line medications.[30] Second-line treatments should be considered for use on a case-by-case basis after first-line treatments have been used or considered.

Clonidine

Clonidine is an efficacious smoking-cessation treatment. It may be used under a clinician's supervision as a second-line agent to treat tobacco dependence. Five studies met selection criteria and were included in the AHRQ panel's meta-analysis comparing clonidine with placebo. Results of this meta-analysis also are shown in Table 67–5. As can be seen, the use of clonidine approximately doubles abstinence rates when compared with a placebo. These studies varied the clonidine dose from 0.1–0.75 mg/day. The drug was delivered either transdermally or orally. It should be noted that abrupt discontinuation of clonidine can result in symptoms such as nervousness, agitation, headache, and tremor, accompanied or followed by a rapid rise in blood pressure and elevated catecholamine levels.

Because clonidine is used primarily as an antihypertensive medication and has not been approved by the FDA as a smoking-cessation medication, clinicians need to be aware of the specific warnings regarding this medication as well as its side-effect profile. Additionally, a specific dosing regimen for the use of clonidine has not been established. Because of the warnings associated with clonidine discontinuation, the variability in dosages used to test this medication, and a lack of FDA approval, the guideline panel chose to recommend clonidine as a second-line agent. Doses used in various clinical cessation trials have varied significantly from 0.15–0.75 mg/day orally to 0.10–0.20 mg/day transdermally without a clear dose-response relation to cessation. Initial dosing typically is 0.10 mg orally twice daily or 0.10 mg/day transdermally, increasing by 0.10 mg/day per week if needed. The dose duration also varied across the clinical trials, ranging from 3–10 weeks. Most commonly reported side effects include dry mouth, drowsiness, dizziness, sedation, and constipation. As an antihypertensive medication, clonidine can be expected to lower blood pressure in most patients. Therefore, clinicians may need to monitor blood pressure when using this medication.[30]

Nortriptyline

Nortriptyline is also considered to be efficacious as a second-line agent to treat tobacco dependence. Two studies were included in the AHRQ panel's metaanalysis comparing nortriptyline with placebo. Results of this metaanalysis also are shown in Table 67–5. As can be seen, the use of nortriptyline increases abstinence rates when compared with placebo.

Nortriptyline should be considered for smoking cessation under a clinician's direction with patients unable to use first-line medications because of contraindications or with patients who were unable to quit using first-line medications. Therapy is initiated 10–28 days before the quit date to allow nortriptyline to reach steady state at the target dose. Smoking-cessation trials have initiated treatment at a dose of 25 mg/day, increasing gradually to a target dose of 75–100 mg/day. Duration of treatment used in smoking-cessation trials has been approximately 12 weeks. Most commonly reported side effects include sedation, dry mouth, blurred vision, urinary retention, light-headedness, and shaky hands.

Trials have investigated the use of other antidepressants for smoking cessation, including other tricyclics and selective serotonin reuptake inhibitors. Because of a paucity of data, the AHRQ panel drew no conclusions about antidepressant therapy for smoking cessation except to recommend bupropion SR as a first-line agent and nortriptyline as a second-line agent.[32]

CAFFEINE

Caffeine is the most widely consumed, behaviorally active substance in the world.[44] *Caffeinism* is the term coined to describe the clinical syndrome produced by acute or chronic overuse of caffeine.[9] The syndrome usually is characterized by central nervous system (CNS) and peripheral manifestations, most notably anxiety, psychomotor alterations, sleep disturbances, mood changes, and psychophysiologic complaints. Table 67–6 summarizes typical manifestations of caffeine overuse syndrome.

As many as one in five adults consumes doses of caffeine generally considered large enough to cause clinical symptoms. Controlled double-blind studies demonstrate that caffeine has reinforcement properties in most people with a history of heavy prior use[45,46] and that this reinforcement is a function of dose and prior exposure.

Pharmacologically, the risk of developing some meaningful clinical manifestations becomes high when intake exceeds 500 mg/day. This places 20%–30% of North Americans at risk.[46] Recognizing that there are individual variations and accepting a conservative approach, these data suggest that perhaps 10%–20% of the North American adult population probably has meaningful clinical symptoms consistent with a diagnosis of caffeinism, a prevalence rate exceeding that of most other substances of abuse.

Caffeine has been proposed as a "model of drug abuse" despite the facts that its sale is largely unrestricted and that heavy consumption of caffeine-containing beverages is not considered to be drug abuse.

TABLE 67–6. Signs and Symptoms of Excessive Caffeine Intake

Restlessness	Gastrointestinal disturbances
Nervousness	Muscle twitching
Excitement	Rambling flow of thought or speech
Insomnia	Tachycardia or cardiac arrhythmia
Flushed face	Periods of inexhaustibility
Diuresis	Psychomotor agitation

A recent exhaustive review of caffeine dependence has focused on the potential for abuse of caffeine and the nature of tolerance and withdrawal and presents a symposia of current knowledge as to the site(s) and mechanism of action of caffeine.[45] A second comprehensive review of human and animal data on coffee and caffeine consumption and caffeine dependence, withdrawal, and reinforcement also has been published recently.[46] The information below represents a broad overview of these topics, and the reader interested in more detail is urged to consult these two reviews.[45,46]

EPIDEMIOLOGY OF CAFFEINE USE AND ABUSE

Caffeine is used by 80% of the population of the United States,[44] and its use can be problematic for some people. In a telephone survey[47] of 162 randomly selected caffeine users, researchers asked about generic DSM-IV-TR criteria for dependence, abuse, intoxication, and withdrawal pertaining to their caffeine use in the last year. The prevalence of endorsement of dependence items was 56% for strong desire or unsuccessful attempt to stop use, 50% for spending a great deal of time with the drug, 28% for using more than intended, 18% for withdrawal, 14% for using despite knowledge of harm, 8% for tolerance, and 1% for foregoing activities to use. Seven percent of users met DSM-IV-TR criteria for caffeine intoxication, and among those who had tried to stop caffeine permanently, 24% met DSM-IV-TR research criteria for caffeine withdrawal.

Average caffeine consumption in humans can range in different cultures and nations from 80–400 mg per person per day.[15] In the United States, caffeine consumption exceeds several billion kilograms annually. Per capita intake for the entire world's population approximated 70 mg/day. In the United States, this figure is considerably larger, at 210–238 mg.[46] The majority of caffeine users progress to a pattern of frequent or daily consumption. Approximately one-fourth eventually begin consuming large quantities, exceeding 500 mg/day, and conservatively, 10% of all adults then progress to develop the syndrome of caffeinism.[43] Mean daily consumption of caffeine in

American children is surprisingly high. The Framingham Children's Study[48] looked at the amounts of caffeine consumed each day by children between the ages of 6 and 10 years (mean 8.4 years for boys and 8.1 years for girls). Mean intake of caffeine was 16.0 ± 9.6 mg/day. Caffeineated soft drinks and chocolate furnished almost all the caffeine.

Caffeine is an added ingredient in approximately 70% of soft drinks consumed in the United States.[49] Although soft drink manufacturers' justification to regulatory agencies and the public for adding caffeine to soft drinks is that caffeine is a flavoring agent, in a recent study, only 8% of a group of regular cola soft drink consumers could detect the taste effect of the caffeine concentration found in most cola soft drinks. Thus soft drinks serve as a major source of caffeine intake without any apparent purpose beyond its stimulant effects.[49]

DIFFERENTIAL DIAGNOSIS

Caffeine intoxication is the only official diagnosis associated with caffeinism in the DSM-IV-TR. Caffeine-induced anxiety may manifest as restlessness, nervousness, excitement, insomnia, diuresis, flushing, gastrointestinal disturbance, muscle twitching, irritability, and jitteriness. If caffeine-induced insomnia requires specific treatment, caffeine-induced sleep disorder (DSM-IV-TR) is an appropriate diagnosis.[9,46]

Because caffeine consumption is so widespread and at times excessive, a thorough history of caffeine use should be included in the routine assessment of all new patients in primary care medical settings. In this manner, the practitioner can use the information gathered to uncover high levels of caffeine intake and then use the information to pinpoint the cause of clinical signs and symptoms typical of caffeinism. Clinical manifestations of caffeinism almost always will lessen in intensity or disappear completely within 1–2 weeks after removing the drug.[9]

PHARMACOLOGY OF CAFFEINE

Caffeine is rapidly and completely absorbed from the gastrointestinal tract,[9] reaching a peak blood level within 30–45 minutes of oral ingestion. It easily crosses the blood-brain barrier,[9] and levels achieved in the brain are proportional to the dose administered.

The half-life of caffeine in humans is approximately 3.5–5 hours. It is metabolized extensively according to a complex metabolic pathway occurring primarily in the liver.[9] Serious problems rarely result from overdoses of caffeine. In fact, the amount of caffeine needed to cause death in an average adult male is 5–10 g, the equivalent of 50–100 cups of regular brewed coffee.[9] Thus the risk of overdose from dietary sources of caffeine is virtually nonexistent.

Caffeine increases the heart rate and force of contraction. It also has a strong diuretic effect. The key factor promoting caffeine use and dosage increases may be the drug's reinforcing effect on pleasure and reward centers of the brain.[46] Caffeine's pharmacologic actions appear comparable (although less potent) in some aspects with those of other stimulants, such as amphetamines and cocaine. After years of uncertainty, it is apparent from both preclinical research and human studies that regular caffeine use does induce tolerance.[9,45,46]

CAFFEINE DEPENDENCE

Research[9,45,46] has shown that abstinence from caffeine induces a distinct withdrawal syndrome. Evidence for the existence of a caffeine dependence syndrome was presented by Strain and associates.[44] In a structured psychiatric interview, subjects self-identified as having problems with caffeine use were evaluated for features of a DSM-IV-TR diagnosis of drug dependence. Those judged as caffeine dependent manifested at least three of four criteria (i.e., tolerance, withdrawal, persistent desire, or unsuccessful attempt to reduce consumption and persistent use despite adverse psychological or physical consequences). Of 99 people screened, 27 were evaluated by means of a structured psychiatric interview modified from the diagnosis of caffeine dependence; 16 of those subjects (59%) met the criteria. In a second phase of the study, 11 of the 16 caffeine-dependent individuals participated in a 2-day double-blind crossover study of caffeine deprivation. Nine showed evidence of caffeine withdrawal during the placebo phase, a finding that validated one of the criteria for the diagnosis of dependence.

CAFFEINE WITHDRAWAL

The frequency of the caffeine withdrawal syndrome is not well known, but it may be common. Withdrawal can occur when individuals who previously have been consuming the drug on a regular basis suddenly discontinue their intake.[9] The syndrome can be characterized by the occurrence of headache, drowsiness, and fatigue. Sometimes the syndrome includes impaired psychomotor performance, difficulty concentrating, nausea, excessive yawning, and craving. These symptoms usually appear within 18–24 hours of discontinuation of intake, corresponding to the time required for the drug to leave the body.[9]

The caffeine-withdrawal headache is somewhat unique, starting with a sense of fullness in the head and progressing to throbbing and diffuse pain that is made worse by movement. The maximum intensity of the pain occurs 3–6 hours after beginning. Symptoms of caffeine withdrawal are summarized in Table 67–7.

In an effort to understand the relationship between caffeine dosing conditions and the emergence of withdrawal, Evans and Griffiths[50] performed a series of double-blind experiments in independent groups of healthy participants to assess the conditions under which withdrawal symptoms occur on cessation of low to moderate doses of caffeine. Their results show that significant caffeine-withdrawal symptoms can occur reliably when individuals are maintained on as little as 100 mg caffeine each day, and the severity of caffeine withdrawal is an increasing function of the caffeine maintenance dose. Administration of caffeine as a single daily dose produces physical dependence similar to that produced by three divided doses over the day, suggesting that the daily dose of caffeine consumed is more relevant to the development of caffeine dependence than the pattern of caffeine intake within the day. They showed that caffeine withdrawal occurs after as little as 3 consecutive days of caffeine exposure, with a somewhat increased severity of withdrawal observed after a week of caffeine exposure. Finally, when individuals were maintained on 300 mg caffeine per day, a substantial reduction in caffeine consumption or complete elimination is necessary for the manifestation of the full, classic withdrawal symptoms. This research provides the most complete parametric characterization of caffeine withdrawal to date.

When caffeine is reintroduced, relief of withdrawal symptoms tends to occur within 30–60 minutes. At present, this appears to be the most effective "treatment" for the caffeine-withdrawal syndrome.

TABLE 67–7. Signs and Symptoms of Caffeine Withdrawal

Headache	Difficulty concentrating
Drowsiness	Nausea
Fatigue	Excessive yawning
Impaired psychomotor performance	Craving

EFFECT ON SLEEP

Caffeine interferes with sleep in most nontolerant individuals.[9] Once tolerance has developed, people are much less likely to self-report sleep abnormalities, or they may sense that the insomnia has disappeared altogether. To illustrate, 53% of those consuming less than 250 mg/day agreed that caffeine before bedtime would prevent sleep compared with 43% of those consuming 250–749 mg/day and only 22% of those taking 750 mg/day or more.[9] Even though the higher-level consumers denied that caffeine interferes with their sleep, studies done in the sleep laboratory confirm that caffeine consumers do have greater sleep latency, more frequent awakenings, and altered sleep architecture and that these effects are dose-related.[9]

CAFFEINE-RELATED SOMATIC MANIFESTATIONS

Caffeine can cause other problems in addition to anxiety and nervousness. Users of high doses of caffeine often experience one or more of the following problems: urinary frequency and diuresis, headache, tachycardia, arrhythmias, tremulousness, diarrhea, gastrointestinal pain or discomfort, and light-headedness.[9] Less frequent symptoms include seeing "spots" in front of the eyes, "ringing" in the ears, a feeling of being unable to breathe, "tingling" in fingers and toes, and excessive perspiration. Caffeine also may precipitate a true panic attack.

COMORBID SUBSTANCE-RELATED DISORDERS

It is not uncommon for high users of caffeine to also be taking a variety of other psychoactive medications, mostly of the CNS depressant variety. Sedative-hypnotics and antianxiety agents are used significantly more often in those consuming high doses of caffeine than in those consuming low or moderate amounts. Approximately two-thirds of highest caffeine users reported using an antianxiety agent within the past month.[9] Similar effects on the brain reward pathways may help explain why excessive caffeine, alcohol, and tobacco use tend to occur in the same individuals.

▶ TREATMENT: Caffeinism

Caffeinism is treated by reducing or discontinuing the drug. It may be necessary to wean the patient off the drug because going "cold turkey" may produce such serious symptoms that the drug must be restarted. Decaffeinated beverages may be substituted slowly for the caffeinated type. Relapses are less likely to occur, however, when the drug is discontinued all at once, probably due to the considerable self-discipline required to continue weaning the drug when one knows that an increase in dose will cause the symptoms to abate.

It may be possible for some individuals simply to reduce their dosage of caffeine rather than discontinue it altogether. Others may be particularly sensitive to the drug, and they may not be able to handle even reduced intake of caffeine. Patients with cardiovascular disease, especially arrhythmias, should refrain totally, as should people with prior stroke or transient ischemic attacks. Peptic ulcer patients and those with bipolar mood disorder and schizophrenia should be encouraged to avoid caffeine altogether.

CONCLUSIONS

Use of alcohol, tobacco, and caffeine is so commonly accepted in our society that people take notice only when their use causes serious problems. When these problems do occur, the human and economic costs are enormous. Health professionals must be committed to helping people free themselves of the addictions that can occur with these common drugs.

REFERENCES

1. Perspectives in Disease Prevention and Health Promotion. Smoking-attributable mortality and years of potential life lost—United States, 1984. MMWR 1997:46:444–451.
2. Smoking and Health: A National Status Report, 2d ed. DHHS Publication No. (CDC) 87-8396. Rockville, MD, U.S. Department of Health and Human Services, 1990.
3. National Household Survey on Drug Abuse. Rockville, MD, U.S. Department of Health and Human Services, Substance Abuse and Mental Health Services Administration, 1999.
4. Diagnostic and Statistical Manual of Mental Disorders (DSM-IV-TR), 4th ed. (Text Revision). Washington, American Psychiatric Association, 2000:212–214.
5. National Institute on Drug Abuse and National Institute on Alcohol Abuse and Alcoholism: National Drug and Alcoholism Treatment Unit Survey (NDATUS), 1989: Main Findings Report. DHHS Publication No. (ADM) 91-1729. Rockville, MD, National Institute of Drug Abuse/National Institute on Alcohol Abuse and Alcoholism, 1990.
6. Fiellin DA, Reid MC, O'Connor PG. Outpatient management of patients with alcohol problems. Ann Intern Med 2000;133:815–827.
7. Holt S, Stewart IC, Dixon JMJ, et al. Alcohol and the emergency service patient. Br Med J 1983;28:638–640.
8. Gilbert RM. Caffeine consumption. In: Spiller GA, ed. The Methylxanthine Beverages and Foods: Chemistry, Consumption, and Health Effects. New York, Liss, 1984:185–213.
9. Greden JF, Walters A. Caffeine. In: Lowinson JH, Ruiz P, Millman RB, Langrod JG, eds. Substance Abuse: A Comprehensive Textbook. Baltimore, Williams & Wilkins, 1997:294–307.
10. Dorland's Illustrated Medical Dictionary, 28th ed. Philadelphia, Saunders, 1994:478.
11. McBride WJ, Li TK. Animal models of alcoholism: Neurobiology of high alcohol-drinking behavior in rodents. Crit Rev Neurobiol 1998;12: 339–369.
12. Anthenelli RM, Schuckit MA. Genetics. In: Lowinson JH, Ruiz P, Millman RB, Langrod JG, eds. Substance Abuse: A Comprehensive Textbook, 3d ed. Baltimore, Williams & Wilkins, 1997:41–51.
13. Schuckit MA. Genetics of the risk for alcoholism. Am J Addict 2000;9:103–112.
14. Valenzuela CF, Harris RA. Alcohol: Neurobiology. In: Lowinson JH, Ruiz P, Millman RB, Langrod JG, eds. Substance Abuse: A Comprehensive Textbook, 3d ed. Baltimore, Williams & Wilkins, 1997:119–142.
15. Baselt, RC. Ethanol. Disposition of Toxic Drugs and Chemicals in Man, 5th ed. Foster City, CA, Chemical Toxicology Institute, 2000:323–324.
16. Shoaf SE. Pharmacokinetics of intravenous alcohol: Two-compartment, dual Michaelis-Menten elimination. Alcohol Clin Exp Res 2000;24: 424–425.
17. Mayo-Smith MF. Pharmacological management of alcohol withdrawal. A meta-analysis and evidence-based practice guideline. JAMA 1997;278: 144–151.

18. Reoux JP, Miller K. Routine hospital alcohol detoxification practice compared to symptom triggered management with an objective withdrawal scale (CIWA-Ar). Am J Addict 2000;9:135–144.
19. Saitz R, O'Malley SS. Pharmacotherapies for alcohol abuse: Withdrawal and treatment. Med Clin North Am 1997;81:881–907.
20. Garbutt JC, West SL, Carey TS, et al. Pharmacological treatment of alcohol dependence: A review of the evidence. JAMA 1999;281(14):1318–1325.
21. O'Malley SS, Croop RS, Wroblewski JM, et al. Naltrexone in the treatment of alcohol dependence: A combined analysis of two trials. Psychiatr Ann 1995;25:681–685.
22. Volpicelli JR, Watson NT, King AC, et al. Effect of naltrexone on alcohol "high" in alcoholics. Am J Psychiatry 1995;152:613– 615.
23. O'Malley SS, Jaffe AJ, Chang G, et al. Naltrexone and coping skills therapy for alcohol dependence: A controlled study. Arch Gen Psychiatry 1992;49:881–887.
24. Volpicelli JR, Alterman AL, Hayashida M, et al. Naltrexone in the treatment of alcohol dependence. Arch Gen Psychiatry 1992;49:876–880.
25. Volpicelli JR, Rhines KC, Rhines JS, et al.. Naltrexone and alcohol dependence: Role of subject compliance. Arch Gen Psychiatry 1997;54: 737–742.
26. Whitworth AB, Fischer F, Lesch OM, et al. Comparison of acamprosate and placebo in long-term treatment of alcohol dependence. Lancet 1996;347:1438–1442.
27. Mason BJ, Salvato FR, Williams LD, et al. A double-blind, placebo-controlled study of oral nalmefene for alcohol dependence. Arch Gen Psychiatry 1999;56:719–724.
28. Frank E, Winkleby M, Altman D, et al. Predictors of physician's smoking cessation advice. JAMA 1991;266:3139–3144.
29. Glynn TJ, Manley MW, Solberg LI, et al. Creating and maintaining an optimal medical practice environment for treatment of nicotine addiction. In: Orleans C, Slade J, eds. Nicotine Addiction: Principles and Management. New York, Oxford University Press, 1993:162–181.
30. Marcus E, Emont SL, Corcoran RD, et al. Public attitudes about cigarette smoking: Results from the 1989 smoking activity volunteer executed survey. Public Health Rep 1994;109:124–134.
31. American Cancer Society. Cancer Facts and Figures. Atlanta, GA, American Cancer Society. Available at www3.cancer.org/cancerinfo; accessed March 12, 2001.
32. Fiore MC, Bailey WC, Cohen SJ, et al. Treating Tobacco Use and Dependence: Clinical Practice Guideline. Rockville, MD, U.S. Department of Health and Human Services, Public Health Service, June 2000.
33. McEvoy GK, ed. AHFS Drug Information—2000. Bethesda, MD, American Society of Health-System Pharmacists, 2000:1280.
34. Kessler DA, Barnett PS, Witt A, et al. The legal and scientific basis for FDA's assertion of jurisdiction over cigarettes and smokeless tobacco. JAMA 1997;277:405–409.
35. Title 21, United States Code 321(g)(1)(C), 321(h)(3).
36. Glantz LH, Annas GJ. Tobacco, the Food and Drug Administration, and Congress. N Engl J Med 2000;343:1802–1806.
37. Myers ML. Protecting the public health by strengthening the Food and Drug Administration's authority over tobacco products. N Engl J Med 2000;343:1806–1809.
38. Fiore MC, Wetter DW, Bailey WC, et al. Smoking Cessation Clinical Practice Guideline. AHCPR Publication No. 96–0692. Rockville, MD, Agency for Health Care Policy and Research, Public Health Service, U.S. Department of Health and Human Services, April 1996.
39. Tsoh JY, McClure JB, Skaar, KL, et al. Smoking cessation: 2. Components of effective intervention. Behav Med 1997;23:15–27.
40. Kaplan RM, Orleans, Perkins KA, et al. Marshaling the evidence for greater regulation and control of tobacco products: A call for action. Ann Behav Med 1995;17:3–14.
41. Fiscella K, Franks P. Cost-effectiveness of the transdermal nicotine patch as an adjunct to physicians' smoking cessation counseling. JAMA 1996;275:1247–1251.
42. Hurt RD, Sachs DP, Glover ED, et al. A comparison of sustained-release bupropion and placebo for smoking cessation. N Engl J Med 1997;337:1195–1202.
43. Jorenby DE, Leischow SJ, Nides MA, et al. A controlled trial of sustained-release bupropion, a nicotine patch, or both for smoking cessation. N Engl J Med 1999;340:685–691.
44. Strain EC, Mumford GK, Silverman K, et al. Caffeine dependence syndrome: Evidence from case histories and experimental evaluations. JAMA 1994;272:1043–1048.
45. Daly JW, Fredholm BB. Caffeine: An atypical drug of dependence. Drug Alcohol Depend 1998;51:199–206.
46. Nehlig A. Are we dependent upon coffee and caffeine? A review of human and animal data. Neurosci Biobehav Rev 1999;23:563–576.
47. Hughes JR, Oliveto AH, Liguori A, et al. Endorsement of DSM-IV dependence criteria among caffeine users. Drug Alcohol Depend 1998;52: 99–107.
48. Ellison RC, Singer MR, Moore LL, et al. Current caffeine intake of young children: amount and sources. Am Diet Assoc 1995;95:802–804.
49. Griffiths RR, Vernotica EM. Is caffeine a flavoring agent in cola soft drinks? Arch Fam Med 2000;9:727–734.
50. Evans SM, Griffiths RR. Caffeine withdrawal: A parametric analysis of caffeine dosing conditions. J Pharmacol Exp Ther 1999;289:285–294.

68

SCHIZOPHRENIA

M. Lynn Crismon and Peter G. Dorson

Schizophrenia is one of the most complex and challenging of psychiatric disorders. It represents a heterogeneous syndrome of disorganized and bizarre thoughts, delusions, hallucinations, inappropriate affect, and impaired psychosocial functioning. From the time that Kraepelin first described dementia praecox in 1896 until publication of the *Diagnostic and Statistical Manual of Mental Disorders,* 4th edition, Text Revised (DSM-IV-TR) in 2000, the description of this illness has continuously evolved.[1] Scientific advances that increase our knowledge of central nervous system (CNS) physiology and pathophysiology and genetics will likely improve our understanding of schizophrenia in the future.

EPIDEMIOLOGY

According to the Epidemiologic Catchment Area Study, the US lifetime prevalence of schizophrenia ranges from 0.6% to 1.9%, with an average of approximately 1%.[2] With only a few possible exceptions, the worldwide prevalence of schizophrenia is remarkably similar among all cultures. Schizophrenia most commonly has its onset in late adolescence or early adulthood and rarely occurs before adolescence or after the age of 40 years. Although the prevalence of schizophrenia is equal in males and females, the onset of illness tends to be earlier in males. Males most frequently have their first episode during their early twenties, whereas with females it is usually during their late twenties to early thirties.[1–3]

ETIOLOGY

Although the etiology of schizophrenia is unknown, research has demonstrated various abnormalities in brain structure and function. However, these changes are not consistent among all individuals with a diagnosis of schizophrenia, and much is yet to be learned about its pathogenesis. The cause of schizophrenia is likely multifactorial; that is, multiple pathophysiologic abnormalities may play a role in producing the similar but varying clinical phenotypes we refer to as schizophrenia.

A neurodevelopmental model has been evoked as a possible explanation for the etiology of schizophrenia. This model proposes that a genetic predisposition exists for schizophrenia and that an unknown *in utero* disturbance occurs, possibly in the second trimester of pregnancy. Evidence for this is provided by the abnormal neuronal migration demonstrated in most studies of schizophrenic brains. This "schizophrenic lesion" may result in abnormalities in cell shape, position, symmetry, connectivity, and functionally to the development of abnormal brain circuits.[3,4] Changes are consistent with a cell migration abnormality during the second trimester of pregnancy, and some studies associate upper respiratory infections during the second trimester of pregnancy with a higher incidence of schizophrenia.[5] Other studies show a relationship between obstetric complications or neonatal hypoxia and schizophrenia. Some studies also associate low birthweight (<2,500 g) with schizophrenia.[6] The resulting secondary "synaptic disorganization" associated with such insults is thought not to produce overt clinical manifestations of psychosis until adolescence or early adulthood because this is the corresponding time period of neuronal maturation.

Additional support for a developmental model is provided by the fact that although studies have shown decreased cortical thickness and increased ventricular size in many schizophrenics, this occurs in the absence of widespread gliosis. Gliosis, or the proliferation of glial cells, is thought to occur as a compensatory change in degenerative diseases of the brain. One hypothesis is that obstetric complications and hypoxia, in combination with a genetic predisposition, could activate a glutamatergic cascade that results in increased neuronal pruning. It is hypothesized that this genetic predisposition may be related to genes controlling *N*-methyl-D-aspartate (NMDA) receptor activity.[8] As a part of the normal neurodevelopmental process, pruning of dendrites occurs. In the normal individual, about 35% of dendrites are pruned by mid-adolescence as compared with their peak at about 2 years of age. Some studies associate abnormally high pruning with the development of schizophrenia. Furthermore, synaptic pruning predominantly involves glutamatergic dendrites. Hypoxia or other prenatal insult may result in a decreased number of basal neurons from which to start, and glutamatergic activation may exaggerate the pruning process. This is consistent with studies showing perinatal hypoxia being associated with earlier age of onset of schizophrenia.[6]

Numerous studies have shown neuropsychological abnormalities as early as 4 years of age in individuals who later develop schizophrenia. As compared with normal controls, one study found abnormalities in siblings, as well as the individual affected with schizophrenia. Impairment in reaching normal motor milestones, and abnormal movements in children as young as 8 months of age, have been associated with the development of schizophrenia. These findings indicate abnormalities in brain function long before the onset of psychotic symptomatology and provide empirical evidence for schizophrenia being a neurodevelopmental disorder.[6,8]

GENETICS

Although a specific abnormality has not been discovered, increasing evidence suggests a genetic basis for schizophrenia. Although the risk of developing schizophrenia is 0.6% to 1.9% in the general population, this increases to approximately 10% if a first-degree relative has the illness and to 3% if a second-degree relative has the illness.[1,9] If both parents have schizophrenia, the risk of producing a schizophrenic offspring increases to approximately 40%. Twin studies in dizygotic twins report that the risk of the second twin developing schizophrenia if one twin has the illness is between 12% and 14%. However, in monozygotic twins the risk increases to 48%.[9] Numerous adoption studies indicate that the risk for schizophrenia lies with the biologic parents, and change in the environment during the child's developmental stages does not alter this. If schizophrenia occurs in siblings, the onset of illness tends to occur at the same age in each, thus lessening the possibility of an environmental precipitant.

A search for a genetic linkage in schizophrenia has been difficult, and any genetic etiologies in schizophrenia are likely heterogeneous, but present with similar phenotypes. Potential loci have been identified on chromosomes 6, 8, 13, and 22.[10] If confirmed, these may only account for some cases of schizophrenia, but are more likely associated with a predisposition for the illness.[9,10]

PATHOPHYSIOLOGY

Computerized axial tomography (CAT) scans and magnetic resonance imaging (MRI) show increased ventricular size, particularly in the third and lateral ventricles, in subtypes of schizophrenics. Recent studies also show a small but definite decrease in brain size as compared to matched controls. These changes appear to be consistent with brain asymmetry, the ventricular enlargement being most pronounced in the left temporal horn, and the decreased cortical size being most obvious in the left temporal lobe.[11] These changes appear to correspond with changes in neuropsychological testing, and these patients may have poorer response with traditional antipsychotic medications.[8,11] Decreased cortical thickness reflects a decrease in the space between neurons (i.e., increased neuronal density) rather than a decrease in the number of neurons in the prefrontal lobe cortex.[3,4] This may result in a decreased number of axonal and dendritic communications between cells and, therefore, a loss of connectivity that could be important with respect to neuronal adaptivity and CNS homeostasis.[4] These changes are likely consistent with the evidence for abnormal neuronal pruning.[7]

NEUROTRANSMITTER CHANGES

Since the discovery of the role of dopamine (DA) as a neurotransmitter in 1958, and the observations that antipsychotic (AP) drugs are postsynaptic DA-receptor antagonists, there has been interest in a dopaminergic hypothesis for the pathophysiology of schizophrenia. However, these theories may be more appropriately oriented toward the treatment of psychosis with antipsychotics.

Four dopaminergic tracts are of primary interest (Table 68–1). The nigrostriatal tract originates with cell bodies from the A9 area in the substantia nigra and terminates with synapses in the caudate nucleus and putamen of the basal ganglia. The second tract, the mesolimbic pathway, projects from A10 in the midbrain ventral tegmentum to the cingulate gyrus and to limbic regions such as the amygdala, olfactory tubercle, and septal nuclei. The mesocortical tract extends from A10 to the prefrontal and frontal cortex. The tuberoinfundibular tract projects from the hypothalamus to the pituitary. Table 68–1 outlines the primary functional activity that is associated with each tract.[12]

Increasing evidence supports the presence of a DA-receptor defect in schizophrenia. Numerous positron emission tomography (PET) studies have shown regional brain abnormalities, including increased glucose metabolism in the caudate nucleus, and decreased blood flow and glucose metabolism in the frontal lobe and left temporal lobe.[3,4,13] This may indicate dopaminergic hyperactivity in the head of the caudate nucleus and dopaminergic hypofunction in the frontotemporal regions. PET studies using D_2-specific ligands provide data suggesting increased densities of D_2 receptors in the head of the caudate nucleus with decreased densities in the prefrontal cortex.[12,14] PET studies assessing D_1 function suggest that subpopulations of schizophrenics may have decreased densities of D_1 receptors in the caudate nucleus and the prefrontal cortex. Hypofrontality may be associated with lack of volition, one of the core negative symptoms seen in schizophrenia.[4,13] It is important to emphasize that it is unknown whether these changes represent a primary event or whether they are secondary processes related to other pathophysiologic abnormalities in schizophrenia. Because of the heterogeneity in the clinical presentation of schizophrenia, it has also been suggested that the DA hypothesis may be more applicable to "neuroleptic-responsive psychosis," with multiple different etiologies possibly being responsible for causing schizophrenia.[13]

Attempts have been made to develop relationships between these abnormal findings and behavioral symptoms present in schizophrenic patients. The positive symptoms are possibly more closely associated with receptor hyperactivity in the mesocaudate, whereas negative symptoms are most closely related to DA receptor hypofunction in the prefrontal cortex. Glutamatergic dysfunction has been suggested as being etiologic in schizophrenia. The glutamatergic system is one of the most widespread excitatory neurotransmitter systems in the brain. Alterations in its function, either hypo- or hyperactivity, can result in toxic neuronal reactions.[15] Dopaminergic innervation from the ventral striatum decreases the limbic system's inhibitory activity (perhaps through γ-aminobutyric acid [GABA] interneurons); thus, dopaminergic stimulation increases arousal. The corticostriatal glutamate pathways have the opposite effect, inhibiting dopaminergic function from the ventral striatum, therefore allowing the limbic system to have increased inhibitory activity. Descending glutamatergic tracts interact with dopaminergic tracts directly as well as through GABA interneurons. Glutamatergic deficiency produces symptoms

TABLE 68–1. Dopaminergic Tracts and Effects of Dopamine Antagonists

Dopamine Tract	Origin	Innervation	Function	Dopamine Antagonist Effect
Nigrostriatal	Substantia nigra (A9 area)	Caudate nucleus Putamen	Extrapyramidal system, movement	Movement disorders
Mesolimbic	Midbrain ventral tegmentum (A10 area)	Limbic areas (e.g., amygdala, olfactory tubercle, septal nuclei), Cingulate gyrus	Arousal, memory, stimulus processing, motivational behavior	Relief of psychosis
Mesocortical	Midbrain ventral tegmentum (A10 area)	Frontal and pre-frontal lobe cortex	Cognition, communication, social function, response to stress	Relief of psychosis Akathisia?
Tuberoinfundibular	Hypothalamus	Pituitary gland	Regulates prolactin release	Increased prolactin concentrations

similar to those of dopaminergic hyperactivity and possibly those seen in schizophrenia. Clinical support for this hypothesis comes from the fact that phencyclidine, a potent psychotomimetic, is a noncompetitive antagonist at the NMDA receptor, a major glutamate receptor. It is proposed that schizophrenia may involve some currently unknown *in utero* assault that leads to a developmental defect in NMDA receptor function—so-called NMDA hypofunction. This defect is proposed to have latent clinical expression with neuropsychological pathology from NMDA hypofunction not being seen until late adolescence or early adulthood. According to this theory, if NMDA hypofunction is accompanied by dopaminergic hyperactivity, then a DA antagonist responsive psychosis ensues. However, if DA hyperactivity is not present, then the symptoms are likely to be poorly responsive to typical antipsychotics.[16,17]

Serotonergic receptors are present on dopaminergic axons, and it is known that stimulation of these receptors will decrease DA release, at least in the striatum.[12] Although somewhat more diffuse, the distribution of serotonergic neurons is similar to that of dopaminergic neurons, thus allowing these two neurotransmitter systems to innervate the same areas. In fact, 5-hydroxytryptamine$_2$ (serotonin$_2$; 5-HT_2) receptors and D_4 receptors have been found to be colocalized in the cortex.[4] Schizophrenic patients with abnormal brain scans have higher whole-blood 5-HT concentrations, and these concentrations are correlated with increased ventricular size.[18] Atypical antipsychotics with potent 5-HT_2 receptor antagonist effects reverse worsening of symptomatology induced by 5-HT agonists in schizophrenic patients.[13]

The primary pathophysiologic abnormality in schizophrenia may occur in one of a number of different neurotransmitters (e.g., dopaminergic, glutamatergic, or serotonergic systems), with changes in other neurotransmitters occurring secondarily. For example, a primary defect resulting in abnormal presynaptic release of DA from the neuron and ineffective feedback mechanisms could lead to postsynaptic DA receptor hypersensitivity. The NMDA hypofunction model is another approach that could lead to dysregulation among neurotransmitter systems.

Schizophrenia is a complex disorder, and multiple etiologies may exist for the clinical syndrome we refer to as schizophrenia. Based on current knowledge, it is naive to think that any currently proposed etiology can adequately explain the genesis of this complex disease. Molecular research involving genetically determined subtle changes in G-proteins, protein metabolism, and other subcellular processes may well identify the biologic disturbances associated with schizophrenia.[19]

CLINICAL PRESENTATION

Schizophrenia is the most common functional psychosis, and there are as many clinical presentations of schizophrenia as there are individuals with the disorder. Despite numerous attempts to portray a stereotype in movies and on television, the stereotypic schizophrenic essentially does not exist. Moreover, schizophrenia does not mean "split personality." Schizophrenia is a chronic disorder of thought and affect with the individual having a significant disturbance in interpersonal relationships and ability to function in society on a daily basis.

The first psychotic episode may be sudden in onset with few premorbid symptoms, or commonly may be preceded by withdrawn, suspicious, peculiar behavior (schizoid). During the acute psychotic episodes, the patient loses touch with reality, and, in a sense, the brain creates a false reality to replace it. The patient experiences a variety of acute psychotic symptoms, including hallucinations (especially hearing voices), delusions (fixed false beliefs), ideas of influence (beliefs that one's actions are controlled by external influences), and so on. Thought processes are disconnected (loose associations), the patient may not be able to carry on logical conversation (alogia), and may have simultaneous, contradictory thoughts (ambivalence). The patient's affect may be flat (no emotional expression), or it may be inappropriate and labile. The patient is often withdrawn and inwardly directed (autism). Uncooperativeness, hostility, and verbal or physical aggression may be seen because of the patient's misperception of reality. Self-care skills are impaired, and the patient is frequently dirty, unkempt, and in general has poor hygiene. Sleep and appetite are often disturbed.

When the acute psychotic episode remits, the patient typically has residual features. This is an important point in differentiating schizophrenia from other psychotic disorders. Although residual symptoms and their severity vary, patients may have difficulty with anxiety management, suspiciousness, and lack of volition, motivation, insight, and judgment. Therefore, they often have difficulty living independently in the community. Because of poor anxiety management and suspiciousness, they are frequently withdrawn socially, and have difficulty forming close relationships with others. Most do not marry. In addition, impaired volition and motivation contribute to poor self-care skills and make it difficult for the schizophrenic patient to maintain employment. Schizophrenics frequently experience a lack of historicity, or difficulty in learning from their experiences. They may repeatedly make the same mistakes in social conduct and situations requiring judgment. They have difficulty understanding the importance of treatment, including medications, in maintaining their ability to function in society. Therefore, they tend to discontinue medications and other treatments, and this increases the risk of relapse and rehospitalization.

Although the course of the illness is variable, the long-term prognosis for many schizophrenic patients is poor. The disease is marked by intermittent acute psychotic episodes and impaired psychosocial functioning between acute episodes, with most of the deterioration in psychosocial functioning occurring within 5 years after the first psychotic episode.[20] By late life, the patient may appear "burned out," that is, the patient ceases to have acute psychotic episodes but residual symptoms, as previously described, persist. However, functional skills may actually improve as compared with earlier in the patient's life. In a subpopulation of patients, probably 5% to 15%, psychotic symptoms are nearly continuous, and response to typical antipsychotics poor.[21]

The DSM-IV-TR places a greater emphasis on the chronicity of schizophrenia and negative symptoms than do previous editions. Schizophrenia is a chronic disorder, and the patient's history must be carefully assessed for dysfunction that has persisted for longer than 6 months. After their first episode, schizophrenics rarely have a level of adaptive functioning as high as before the onset of the disorder. Table 68–2 summarizes the DSM-IV-TR criteria, and this reference should be consulted for a more detailed discussion of the differential diagnosis.[1]

The DSM-IV-TR[1] classifies the symptoms of schizophrenia into two categories, positive and negative. Recent research has identified a third separate symptom category, cognitive dysfunction (Table 68–3).[22] The areas of cognition found to be abnormal in schizophrenia include attention, working memory, and executive function.[8] Positive symptoms have traditionally attracted the most

TABLE 68–2. DSM-IV-TR Diagnostic Criteria for Schizophrenia

A. Characteristic symptoms: Two or more of the following, each persisting for a significant portion of at least a 1-month period:
   (1) delusions
   (2) hallucinations
   (3) disorganized speech
   (4) grossly disorganized or catatonic behavior
   (5) negative symptoms

   Note: Only one criterion A symptom is required if delusions are bizarre or if hallucinations consist of a voice keeping a running commentary on the person's behavior or two or more voices conversing with each other.

B. Social/occupational dysfunction: For a significant portion of the time since onset of the disorder, one or more major areas of functioning such as work, interpersonal relations, or self-care are significantly below the level prior to onset.

C. Duration: Continuous signs of the disorder for at least 6 months. This must include at least 1 month of symptoms fulfilling criterion A (unless successfully treated). This 6 months may include prodromal or residual symptoms.

D. Schizoaffective or mood disorder has been excluded.

E. Disorder is not due to a medical disorder or substance use.

F. If a history of a pervasive developmental disorder is present, there must be symptoms of hallucinations or delusions present for at least 1 month

Adapted from Ref. 1.

TABLE 68–3. Schizophrenia Symptom Clusters

Positive	Negative	Cognitive
Hallucinations	Affective flattening	Attention
Delusions	Alogia	Impaired working memory
	Anhedonia	Impaired executive function
	Avolition	

Refers. 2, 8, and 22.

attention and are the ones most affected by traditional AP drugs. However, negative symptoms and impairment in cognition are more closely associated with poor psychosocial function. This fact merits attention when one is examining pharmacologic options for treatment. Numerous authors have attempted to construct subtypes of schizophrenia, and it has been suggested that symptom complexes may correlate with prognosis, cognitive functioning, structural abnormalities in the brain, and response to AP drugs.[12] Negative symptoms may be more closely associated with prefrontal lobe dysfunction and positive symptoms with temporolimbic abnormalities. Many patients demonstrate both positive and negative symptoms. Andreasen and associates[8] found that patients with negative symptoms had more antecedent cognitive dysfunction, poor premorbid adjustment, low level of educational achievement, and a poorer overall prognosis.

▶ TREATMENT: Schizophrenia

DESIRED OUTCOME

Pharmacotherapy is the mainstay of treatment in schizophrenia, and it is essentially impossible in most patients to implement effective psychosocial rehabilitation programs in the absence of antipsychotic treatment. A pharmacotherapeutic treatment plan should be developed that delineates drug-related aspects of therapy. Because most deterioration in psychosocial functioning occurs within the first 5 years of the initial psychotic episode, treatment interventions should be particularly assertive during this period.[20] Explicit end points should be defined, including realistic goals of the target symptoms most likely to respond and the relative time course for response. Other goals include avoiding unwanted side effects, using the minimum effective dose, an emphasis on adequate time as a primary variable in determining response, and the limitation of augmentation medications to severely ill or nonresponsive patients.

NONPHARMACOLOGIC THERAPY

Psychosocial rehabilitation programs oriented toward improving patients' adaptive functioning are the mainstay of nondrug treatment for schizophrenia. These programs may include basic living skills, social skills training, basic education, work programs, and supported housing. In particular, programs aimed at employment and housing have been the more effective interventions and are considered "best practices" for persons with serious and persistent mental disorders. Programs that involve families in the care and lives of the patient have also been shown to decrease rehospitalizations and to improve functioning in the community. For particularly low-functioning patients, assertive intervention programs referred to as Active Community Treatment (ACT) are effective in improving patients' functional outcomes. ACT teams are available on a 24-hour basis and work in the patient's home and place of employment to provide comprehensive treatment, including medication, crisis intervention, daily living skills, and supported employment and housing.[22,23]

PHARMACOLOGIC THERAPY

ASSESSMENT PRIOR TO TREATMENT

The importance of initial assessment for accurate diagnosis cannot be underestimated in a patient presenting with acute psychosis. A thorough mental status examination, physical and neurologic examination, complete family and social history, and laboratory workup must be performed to confirm the diagnosis and exclude general medical or substance-induced causes of psychosis, such as acute or chronic drug ingestion. Laboratory tests, biologic markers, and commonly available brain imaging techniques do not assist in diagnosis or selection of medication. A pretreatment patient workup should include these areas of baseline studies: vital signs, complete blood count, electrolytes, hepatic function, renal function, cardiac function, thyroid function, and urine drug screen.

ANTIPSYCHOTIC MEDICATION CHOICES

Atypical Antipsychotics

Atypical antipsychotics (with the exception of clozapine) have become the agents of first choice in the treatment of schizophrenia, and most practice guidelines and consensus statements support this recommendation.[20,22–25] Depending on the dose of haloperidol used in comparative studies, controlled trials demonstrate that atypical APs such as olanzapine, risperidone, quetiapine, and ziprasidone have superior efficacy for the treatment of negative symptoms. Growing evidence also exists to support a positive effect of atypical APs on cognition. Whether these differences in negative symptom and cognition response are a result of differences in core efficacy or differences in side-effect profile is unknown. The major advantage of atypical antipsychotics may be in their side-effect profiles, as they generally have better overall tolerability than the traditional agents. To date, inadequate long-term maintenance treatment studies have been performed with atypical agents to adequately define the long-term clinical outcomes resulting from their widespread use. However, some experts believe that their use during the first 5 years of onset of the illness could help to prevent some of the deterioration associated with the disease.[20,24,25] However, adequate psychosocial rehabilitation programs must be used in conjunction with atypical antipsychotics if patients are to achieve their maximum functional capacity. Preliminary data on relapse rates and cost-effectiveness are presented in the section on pharmacoeconomics later in the chapter.

No universally accepted definition exists for an atypical AP. Common to all definitions, however, is the ability of the drug to produce antipsychotic response with few or no acutely occurring extrapyramidal side effects. Other attributes that have been ascribed to atypical APs include enhanced efficacy, particularly on negative symptoms and cognition; absence or near absence of tardive dyskinesia; and lack of effect on serum prolactin. To date, the only approved atypical AP that fulfills all of these criteria is clozapine, the prototypical agent.[26]

Risperidone fulfills the atypical criterion of having a low incidence of extrapyramidal side effects at low to moderate doses. In studies of randomly selected groups of schizophrenic patients in acute exacerbation, risperidone has proven efficacy and may be superior to haloperidol in treatment of negative symptoms. The mean optimal dose in parallel, fixed-dose studies was 4–6 mg daily. At doses greater than 6 mg daily, risperidone's profile is more similar to a typical AP.[24,25,27] Because risperidone appears to lose its atypical profile at higher doses, the lowest possible dose should be used in treatment. This may include gradual dose titration downward if patients do not respond initially, rather than upward titration as has been the traditional approach to dosing APs[24–26]

Olanzapine also has superior efficacy in treating negative symptoms, and a very low incidence of extrapyramidal side effects[24,25,28] The optimal dose range is 10–20 mg daily. Quetiapine does not appear to have as robust an effect on negative symptoms, but these results may be influenced by the lower haloperidol dose used in the comparative study.[29] Doses above 300 mg are necessary for optimal effects, with mean doses from clinical trials predicted to be between 350 and 450 mg/day. However, upward dose titration to 600 mg/day, or even to 800 mg/day is a common occurrence. From a clinical perspective, the optimal daily quetiapine dose appears unclear.

Ziprasidone in doses of 40–160 mg/day appears to have efficacy similar to other atypical agents; however, its side-effect profile does vary.[30] In particular, experience with ziprasidone's potential QTc prolongation during routine clinical use will ultimately decide whether ziprasidone is a first-line or alternate agent.[31,32] The side-effect profiles of individual atypical antipsychotics and individual patient characteristics should be used in deciding which drug to use in an individual patient. Information from the algorithm and the adverse effects sections should be utilized in arriving at this decision.

Traditional or Typical Antipsychotics

Because of side-effect profile and risk of tardive dyskinesia, traditional APs are less commonly prescribed today. All traditional APs are equal in efficacy when used in equipotent doses. Selection of medication should be based on the need to avoid certain side effects and concurrent medical or psychiatric disorders. No differences exist in efficacy between low- and high-potency typical APs; and high-potency drugs (e.g., haloperidol) are as effective in treating acute agitation as low-potency, highly sedating APs (e.g., chlorpromazine).

Previous patient or family history of response to an AP is helpful in the selection of an agent. Traditional dosage equivalents (expressed in "chlorpromazine equivalent dosages"—the equipotent dosage of any traditional AP compared with 100 mg of chlorpromazine) may assist in determining the effective dosage range if the need arises to treat a patient with a different traditional AP drug. However, because atypical APs differ in mechanism of action, the dose equivalents have little relevance when comparing dosages of atypical APs. Table 68–4 lists APs and their usual dosage ranges.

Pharmacotherapeutic Algorithm

Figure 68–1 outlines a suggested pharmacotherapeutic algorithm for schizophrenia.[24,25] Newer atypical APs are recommended as first-line treatment (i.e., stages 1, 2, and 3) because of their superior effect on negative symptoms and cognition, a lower incidence of acutely occurring extrapyramidal side effects, and growing evidence for a lower incidence of tardive dyskinesia. Although it is unclear how many newer atypical APs to try before proceeding to clozapine, because of safety concerns and the need for white blood cell (WBC) monitoring, it is generally recommended that patients be tried on multiple newer APs as monotherapy before proceeding to a trial of clozapine. The algorithm allows the clinician to skip stages if the individual clinical situation so dictates, and the important thing to remember is that "all roads lead to clozapine."[24,25] As new atypical APs reach the market, their placement in the algorithm needs to be evaluated. Unless clear evidence of superiority exists, Miller et al.[25] recommend that at least 40,000 patient exposures occur before positioning a newly approved medication in an algorithm. This allows minimal clinical experience with the new medication and the opportunity for uncommon, but perhaps severe, adverse reactions to potentially surface before deciding algorithm placement. Because of the lack of widespread clinical experience at the time of this writing, it is difficult to decide where ziprasidone best fits in the algorithm (i.e., first line or alternate agent). If the potential electrocardiogram (ECG) changes associated with ziprasidone have clinical significance, then it will become a reserve drug; however, if these turn out to be benign, then it will be a first-line agent.

If patient nonadherence is primarily because of AP side effects, then two different atypical AP trials are recommended before using a depot antipsychotic. If the patient has never received an adequate trial of a traditional AP, then a trial is recommended (stage 4) before

TABLE 68–4. Available Antipsychotics: Doses and Dosage Forms

Generic Name	Trade Name	Traditional Equivalent Dose (mg)[a]	Usual Dosage Range (mg/day)	Manufacturer's Maximum Dose (mg/day)	Dosage Forms[b]
Traditional Antipsychotics					
Chlorpromazine	Thorazine	100	100–800	2,000	T,L,LC,I,C-ER,S
Fluphenazine	Prolixin	2	2–20	40	T,L,LC,I
Haloperidol	Haldol	2	2–20	100	T,LC,I
Loxapine	Loxitane	10	10–80	250	C,LC
Molindone	Moban	10	10–100	225	T,LC
Mesoridazine	Serentil	50	50–400	500	T,LC,I
Perphenazine	Trilafon	10	10–64	64	T,LC,I
Thioridazine	Mellaril	100	100–800	800	T,LC
Thiothixene	Navane	4	4–40	60	C,LC
Trifluoperazine	Stelazine	5	5–40	80	T,LC,I
Atypical Antipsychotics					
Clozapine	Clozaril	NA	50–600	900	T
Olanzapine	Zyprexa	NA	10–20	20	T,I,O
Quetiapine	Seroquel	NA	250–600	800	T
Risperidone	Risperdal	NA	2–6	16	T,L
Ziprasidone	Geodon	NA	40–160	200	C

[a]NA. This parameter does not apply to atypical antipsychotics.
[b]C, capsule; ER or SR, extended or sustained release; I, injection; L, liquid solution, elixir, or suspension; LC, liquid concentrate; O, orally disintegrating tablets; R, rectal suppositories; T, tablet.

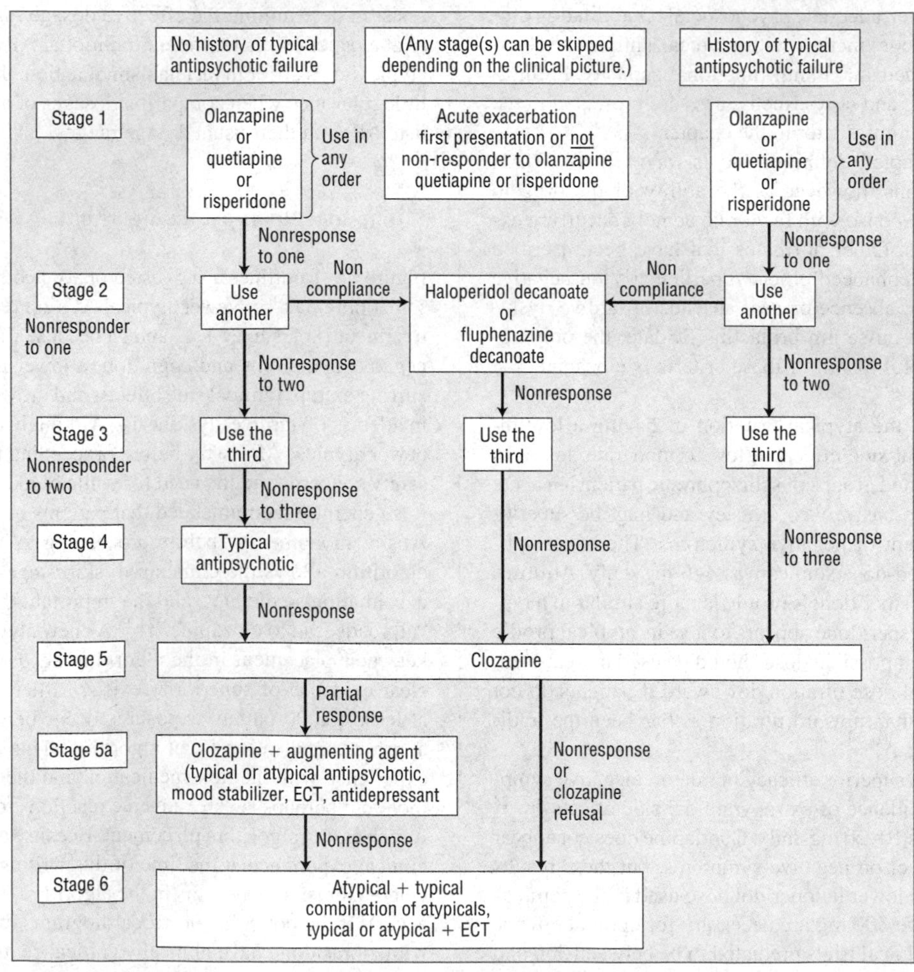

FIGURE 68–1. Texas Medication Algorithm Project algorithm for treatment of schizophrenia. Patient entry into the algorithm is determined by individual patient history and by clinical presentation. Algorithm stages can be skipped if clinically appropriate, and one may go back stages if indicated. In general, inadequately responding patients should not remain in stages 1 through 3 longer than 12 weeks. A patient may remain in stage 5 for 6 months, or longer. Ziprasidone is not placed in the algorithm because of inadequate clinical experience with it at the time of writing. Algorithm updates may be obtained at http://www.mhmr.state.tx.us/centraloffice/medicaldirector/tima.html[24,25] This algorithm figure is in the public domain and can be reproduced, with appropriate reference to the authors, without permission.

proceeding to clozapine at stage 5. The effects of a traditional AP in patients who have failed treatment only with atypical APs are unknown, and the risk of agranulocytosis with clozapine is significant enough that it is prudent to try a traditional AP in most patients before using clozapine.[22] It should be emphasized, however, that prolonged time periods should not occur before poorly responding patients receive the potential benefits of clozapine treatment. In general, a specific treatment stage prior to stage 5 (i.e., clozapine) should not last longer than 12 weeks in a poorly responding patient (see stabilization treatment).

Treatment algorithm recommendations after clozapine (stages 5a and 6) are based more on anecdotal experiences and clinical opinions than on empirical research.[24,25] These combination strategies are aimed at a small percentage of patients who have responded poorly to stages 1 through 5. These interventions should be implemented with careful evaluation of a patient's symptom response and discontinuation of the combination if improvement does not occur. See the later section on the treatment-resistant patient for a discussion of these strategy options.

PREDICTORS OF RESPONSE

Obtaining a thorough medication history is important, and previous AP treatment should help guide the selection of current drug therapy, in that either a good prior response favors the use of the same agent or a negative response should influence the selection of a dissimilar drug. Nonprescription and illicit drug use may influence psychiatric presentation and thus diagnosis or AP response. Amphetamine and other CNS stimulants, cocaine, corticosteroids, digitalis glycosides, indomethacin, marijuana, pentazocine, phencyclidine, and other drugs can induce psychosis in susceptible individuals or exacerbate psychosis in patients with preexisting psychiatric illness.[33] Schizophrenic patients who continue to abuse alcohol or drugs usually have poor response to medications and a poor prognosis. Alcohol, caffeine, and nicotine use potentially result in drug interactions.

Individual differences in patient response have been either proposed or identified, which may be clinically useful predictors of response.[34] Acute onset and short duration of illness, presence of acute stressors or precipitating factors, later age of onset, family history of affective illness, and good premorbid adjustment as reflected in stable interpersonal relationships or employment are all predictors of good response.[34]

Negative schizophrenic symptoms are less responsive to AP therapy. Although controversial, affective symptoms may correlate with an overall good response. However, other than these caveats, there are few data to support a relationship between drug response and schizophrenic subtypes. Neuropsychologic deficits related to cognition and neurologic soft signs may also correlate with poor AP response.[34]

A patient's subjective response within the first 48 hours after being administered a traditional AP may be associated with drug responsiveness.[35] An initial dysphoric response, demonstrated by stating a dislike of the medication, or feeling worse or zombie-like, combined with anxiety or akathisia-like symptoms, is associated with poor drug response, and likely, adverse effects. If continued on the same medication, the patient will likely be nonadherent.

The importance of developing a therapeutic alliance between the patient and the clinician cannot be underestimated. Patients who form positive therapeutic alliances are more likely to be adherent with all aspects of therapy, experience a better outcome at 2 years, and generally require smaller doses of AP medications.[22]

A certain minority of patients fail to benefit from AP therapy, and their psychosocial functioning may actually worsen. Unfortunately, there is no accepted method to identify these people before treatment.[34]

INITIAL TREATMENT

Initial dosing should follow the goals described in the pharmacotherapeutic treatment plan. The goals during the first 7 days should be decreased agitation, hostility, combativeness, anxiety, tension, aggression, and normalization of sleep and eating patterns. The usual recommendation is to initiate therapy and to titrate over the first few days to an average effective dose unless the patient's physiologic status or history indicates that this dose may result in unacceptable adverse effects.[36] Table 68–4 lists the usual dosage range, and an average dose is typically midrange. After a week on a stable dose, a modest dosage increase may be considered if the goals for week 1 have not been achieved (decreased agitation and uncooperativeness). If "cheeking" of medication is suspected, liquid formulations and orally disintegrating tablets of different APs are available (Table 68–4). If a patient has shown no improvement after 3 to 4 weeks at therapeutic doses, then an alternative AP should be considered; that is, moving to the next treatment stage in the algorithm (Fig. 68–1).[24,25]

Although some practitioners believe that larger daily doses are necessary in more severely symptomatic patients, fixed-dose studies of low versus high daily AP doses do not reveal any major differences in degree of symptom improvement, time to response, or length of hospitalization.[37] Some symptoms, such as agitation, tension, aggression, and increased motor activity, may respond more quickly, but side effects, especially extrapyramidal side effects, may be more common with higher doses. However, interindividual differences in dosage and patient response do occur. In partial but inadequate responders who are well tolerating the chosen AP, it may be reasonable to titrate above usual dose ranges, with the exception of thioridazine. However, this tactic should be time limited (i.e., 2 to 4 weeks), and if the patient does not achieve further improvement, the dose should either be decreased or an alternative treatment strategy tried.[24,25]

In general, rapid neuroleptization or the rapid titration of AP dosage is not indicated.[38] However, the intramuscular administration of an AP (e.g., haloperidol 2–5 mg IM) every 60 minutes on an as-needed basis can be used to assist in calming a severely agitated patient. Agitation can be manifested by loud, physically or verbally threatening behavior, motor hyperactivity, or physical aggression. Although this technique may assist in calming an acutely agitated, psychotic patient, it does not improve the extent of or time to remission, or the length of hospitalization. In the near future, parenteral forms of olanzapine and ziprasidone may be available.

Adjunctive benzodiazepines that are absorbed rapidly after intramuscular administration (e.g., lorazepam) are an alternative to intramuscular APs in the management of acute agitation or aggression. If the patient is receiving a reasonable daily dose of an AP (as previously described), the use of lorazepam 2 mg IM as needed in combination with the maintenance AP may actually be more effective in controlling agitation than using additional doses of the AP. In addition, it may assist in decreasing the overall AP dosage requirement, as well as the overall incidence of side effects, especially acute extrapyramidal side effects.

STABILIZATION THERAPY

Improvement is usually a slow but steady process over 6 to 12 weeks or longer. During the first 2 to 3 weeks, goals should include increased socialization and improvement in self-care habits and mood. Improvement in formal thought disorder should follow and may take an additional 6 to 8 weeks to respond. Early in the course of the illness symptoms may improve more rapidly than in individuals who are more chronically ill. In general, if a patient has not received a robust decrease in positive and negative symptoms within 12 weeks at adequate doses, then an alternate monotherapy AP in the algorithm should be considered. In a more chronically ill patient, symptoms may continue to improve for 3 to 6 months.

During acute stabilization, usual labeled doses of atypical APs are recommended (See Table 68–4); with traditional APs, a range of 300–1,000 mg of chlorpromazine equivalents daily is recommended.[36,38] An optimum dose of the chosen drug should be estimated in the initial treatment plan. If the patient begins to show adequate response before or at this dosage, then the patient should remain at this dosage as long as symptoms continue to improve. If necessary, dose titration may continue within the therapeutic range every week or two as long as the patient has no side effects.

Before changing medications in a poorly responding patient, the following should be considered: Were the initial target symptoms indicative of schizophrenia or did they represent manifestations of a different diagnosis, a long-standing behavioral problem, a substance abuse disorder, or a general medical condition? Is the patient adherent with pharmacotherapy? Are the symptoms poorly responsive to AP drugs (e.g., impaired insight or judgment, or fixed delusions)? How does the patient's current status compare with response during previous exacerbations? Would this patient potentially benefit from a change to a different treatment stage (see Fig. 68–1)? Does this patient qualify as a treatment-resistant schizophrenic patient?

The conclusion that a partially responding patient has achieved as much symptomatic improvement as possible is one that must be made with great care and after considering all possible treatment alternatives. However, treatment goals must be realistic. Medications are effective at decreasing many of the symptoms of schizophrenia (and are thus referred to as *palliative*), but they are not curative, and all symptoms may not abate. This being said, the treatment approach should be assertive. While one should expect none to minimal residual positive symptoms with effective treatment, it is still unclear what a realistic goal is with regard to maximum improvement in negative symptoms.

MAINTENANCE TREATMENT

Maintenance drug therapy prevents relapse, as shown in numerous double-blind studies. The average relapse rate after 1 year is 18% to 32% with active drug (including some nonadherent patients) versus 60% to 80% for placebo.[39]

After treatment of the first psychotic episode in a schizophrenic patient, medication should be continued for at least 12 months after remission.[39] Maintenance treatment in patients with multiple acute episodes is more difficult to define. However, it would appear that good medication responders should be treated for at least 5 years; then low-dose strategies or complete drug tapering and withdrawal may be considered to determine the need for continued treatment. When the need for continuous or lifetime pharmacotherapy is established, moderate doses are usually the most effective.[39]

Targeted medication administration based upon prodromal symptoms has been recommended as an alternative to continuous AP treatment in stabilized patients. However, studies show continuous medication to be more effective than targeted medication in preventing decompensation and in decreasing need for hospitalization, and in improving the extent and quality of employment.[40]

Antipsychotics should be tapered slowly before discontinuation. Abrupt discontinuation of APs, especially low-potency traditional APs and clozapine, can result in withdrawal symptoms, felt to be a manifestation of rebound cholinergic outflow. Insomnia, nightmares, headaches, gastrointestinal symptoms (e.g., abdominal cramps, stomach pain, nausea, vomiting, and diarrhea), restlessness, increased salivation, and sweating are reported. In general, when switching from one AP to another, the first AP should be tapered and discontinued over at least 1 to 2 weeks after the second AP is initiated. Tapering may need to occur more slowly with clozapine.

DEPOT ANTIPSYCHOTIC MEDICATIONS

Depot APs are recommended for patients who are unreliable in taking oral medication on a daily basis, and thus should not be used as first-line therapy. Before a depot AP is initiated, it should be determined whether the patient's medication nonadherence is because of side effects. If so, an alternative medication with a more favorable side-effect profile should be considered before a depot AP.

The patient's motivation for treatment is a major factor influencing outcome. Conversion from oral therapy to depot therapy is most successful in patients who have been stabilized on oral therapy. The ideal patient for depot therapy is the patient who does not like the daily reminder of oral medication or is unreliable in taking medications. Depot medications should not be used as "forced compliance" in uncooperative patients who refuse to consent to treatment.

Conversion from an oral AP to depot medication should start with stabilization on an oral dosage form of the same agent, or at least a short trial (3 to 7 days), to determine whether the patient tolerates the medication without significant side effects. For fluphenazine, the simplest conversion is the Stimmel method, which uses 1.2 times the oral daily dose for stabilized patients, rounding up to the nearest 12.5-mg interval, administered in weekly doses for the first 4 to 6 weeks; or 1.6 times the oral daily dose for more acutely ill patients.[41] Subsequently, fluphenazine decanoate may be administered once every 2 to 3 weeks. Oral fluphenazine may be overlapped for 1 week. For haloperidol, a factor of 10 to 15 times the oral daily dose is commonly recommended, rounding up to the nearest 50-mg interval, administered in a once-monthly dose with an oral haloperidol overlap for the first month. However, this may be inadequate in more clinically unstable patients. Ereshefsky et al.[42] performed an inpatient conversion study using the standard conversion from European trials (20 times the oral daily dose), but dividing the injection into consecutive doses of 100–200 mg every 3 to 7 days until the entire amount was given. With this method, oral medication overlap was unnecessary. The depot dose was decreased by 25% at the second and third months. The method was as safe as other methods, and had a lower relapse rate than the most commonly recommended guidelines. Preliminary data suggest that deviation from these conversion protocols may result in poor outcomes and increased adverse effects.[43]

Injection site reactions have been reported with the haloperidol decanoate 100 mg/mL preparation, consisting of painful pruritic swelling at the injection site.[44] Acute extrapyramidal side effects can be seen following injections with fluphenazine decanoate. Despite the fear of severe or persistent side effects occurring during depot therapy, research indicates that similar depot and oral doses result in a similar incidence of side effects. These issues appear less relevant if patients are stabilized on oral medication before conversion to an appropriate depot dose.

Depot APs should be administered by a deep, "Z-tract" intramuscular method, although there is some evidence that fluphenazine decanoate can be administered subcutaneously with similar results.

Depot preparations of selected atypical APs may be available in the near future.

METHODS TO ENHANCE PATIENT ADHERENCE

The chronic mentally ill may be nonadherent with medications based on denial of illness, lack of insight, grandiosity or paranoia, no perceived need for medication, perceived lack of input into choice of medication or dosage, side effects, misperceived "allergies," or the number of medications prescribed or doses received daily.[22] Education geared toward patients becoming more informed about their illness and the effectiveness and risks of treatment may help to increase adherence.[45] These programs should be staged so that patients initially receive basic information about their disorder and its symptoms and basic information about their medication and self-monitoring techniques. As the patient is capable of dealing with more complex information, more detailed information regarding schizophrenia, psychosocial treatments, and prognosis should be discussed. Patients and families should be taught self-monitoring techniques and when to report symptom exacerbation or medication side effects to the clinician.[22,45] Psychoeducation strategies should involve both individual counseling as well as group activities. Groups facilitated by trained individuals who have the illness may be more effective in enhancing awareness and acceptance of schizophrenia and necessary treatment than groups led only by professionals. Active involvement of family members further increases the likelihood of patient adherence with treatment. In addition to programs provided by community mental health centers, support groups operated by consumer groups such as local chapters of the National Alliance for the Mentally Ill are available in most metropolitan areas. In the hospital, self-medication administration often reinforces the patient's perception of their active role in their own treatment.

When patients miss outpatient appointments, active outreach interventions must be implemented to enhance patient engagement in treatment. These include both phone calls and home visits.[22,25,45,46]

MANAGEMENT OF THE TREATMENT-RESISTANT PATIENT

An official definition of "treatment resistance" does not exist.[21] In general, it reflects a patient who has had inadequate symptom response from multiple antipsychotic trials. Traditionally, treatment resistance has been defined as lack of improvement in positive symptoms, but it can be defined by poor improvement in negative symptoms, or even by medication intolerance. Between 10% and 30% of schizophrenic patients receive minimal symptomatic improvement with typical APs.[21,26,37] An additional group of patients (30% to 60%) has partial but inadequate improvement in symptoms or unacceptable side effects associated with AP use.[22]

Atypical Antipsychotics

Only clozapine has shown superiority over other APs in randomized clinical trials for the management of treatment resistant schizophrenia. Other atypical APs have either not been studied or evaluated in small open trials. In a classic study,[47] clozapine was effective in approximately 32% of treatment-resistant schizophrenic patients as compared to only 2% treated with a combination of chlorpromazine and benztropine. This study is considered a "classic" because not only did it prove the efficacy of clozapine in this population, but it also provided a definition for treatment-resistant schizophrenia. This definition includes treatment failures on three different traditional APs from at least two different chemical classes and a history of poor social functioning for the past 5 years.[47] It is significant that when using these criteria for treatment-resistance, almost no patients improved with trials of haloperidol and chlorpromazine. These criteria have been subsequently modified to require only two treatment failures, and would likely include both atypical and traditional APs. Other treatment candidates for clozapine include those patients who are neuroleptic intolerant and cannot tolerate even conservative doses of other APs.[26]

Symptomatic improvement with clozapine in the treatment-resistant patient often occurs slowly, and as many as 60% of patients may improve if clozapine is used for up to 6 months.[26] This, in combination with clozapine's adverse effects profile, provides sufficient information to conclude that clozapine is not a panacea for schizophrenia. However, as the only AP with proven efficacy in the treatment-resistant population, a therapeutic trial of clozapine is recommended at algorithm stage 5 for those patients who consent to its use and are willing to have the weekly to biweekly blood draws for WBCs. Polydipsia and hyponatremia (psychogenic water drinking) is a frequent problem among treatment-resistant patients, and clozapine reportedly decreases water drinking and increases serum sodium in such patients.[48]

Because of the risk of orthostatic hypotension, clozapine is usually titrated more slowly than other APs, particularly on an outpatient basis. If a 12.5-mg test dose does not produce hypotension, then clozapine 25 mg at bedtime is recommended, increased to 25 mg bid after 3 days, and then increased in 25–50 mg/day increments every 3 days until a dose of at least 300 mg/day is reached.[24] Because high doses are associated with significantly increased side effects, including seizures, a clozapine serum concentration is recommended before exceeding 600 mg/day. Although some clinicians add valproate when exceeding this dose to prevent the occurrence of seizures, no evidence supports this intervention, and it is more prudent to start valproate if a seizure occurs.

Augmentation and Combination Strategies

Little empirical evidence exists to guide treatment decisions for patients who do not respond to clozapine.[24,25] Numerous suggestions have been made regarding augmentation of clozapine or other atypical APs and using combinations of antipsychotics (see Fig. 68–1).[49]

Augmentation therapy involves the addition of a "non-AP" drug to an AP drug in a poorly or partially responsive patient, whereas combination treatment involves using two APs simultaneously. Theoretically, augmentation is based on the assumption that the mechanism of action of the augmentation agent will interact synergistically with the dopaminolytic to produce efficacy.[50] Several guidelines should be followed regarding augmentation: (a) augmentation should be used only in inadequately responding patients; (b) augmentation agents are rarely effective when used alone; (c) augmentation responders usually improve rapidly; and (d) if augmentation does not improve symptomatology, the augmenting agent should be discontinued.

Mood stabilizers are frequently used as an augmentation strategy, but with the exception of lithium, have not been widely evaluated. Lithium does not enhance antipsychotic effect, but may improve labile affect and agitated behavior in selected patients. Therefore, it may improve the overall clinical status in such patients.[22,37] Valproic acid and carbamazepine have also been used, and one small placebo-controlled trial supports added sympton improvement when valproate is used in combination with a traditional AP.[51] Enzyme induction with carbamazepine may cause a decrease in AP serum concentrations and potentially worsen psychotic symptoms in some patients.[37] Dosing of mood stabilizers in treatment-resistant schizophrenia is similar to their use in bipolar disorder[22] (see Chap. 70).

Serotonin (5-HT) reuptake inhibitors (SSRIs) have been used as augmentors with mixed reports. Consistently positive results have been reported when using SSRIs to treat obsessive-compulsive symptoms that worsen or arise during clozapine treatment.

Propranolol reportedly has an antiaggression effect when used in a variety of psychiatric disorders, but particularly in the organic aggressive syndrome. Although its efficacy is probably associated with its pharmacodynamic effects, concomitant use may increase AP serum concentrations of some APs as well.[37] It has been suggested that improvement with propranolol is primarily caused by a lessening of akathisia, and whether propranolol is effective as an augmenting agent in patients without symptoms of aggression or akathisia is unclear.[52] Patients should receive a test dose of 20 mg to evaluate tolerance, and if it is acceptable, initial propranolol dosing should be 20 mg three times daily. Dose increases should be in 60 mg/day increments, every 3 days. Patients should be monitored carefully for side effects related to β-adrenergic blockade. After the patient is β-blocked, the dose may be increased more rapidly as tolerated. Patients may need to be treated with adequate doses for 6 to 8 weeks in order to evaluate an antiaggression response. If appropriate response is not received with a daily dose of 800–1,000 mg, additional response is not usually achieved at higher doses.[53]

Combining a traditional AP with an atypical and combining different atypicals have been suggested as intervention strategies for treatment-resistant patients. These treatments are based upon the hypothesis that using antipsychotics with different mechanisms of action will result in greater efficacy than using any medication individually. Critics argue that combining a traditional AP with an atypical will negate the advantages of the atypical medications (e.g., less extrapyramidal side effects). Pharmacodynamically, it is not understood how combinations of APs would produce enhanced efficacy, and increased side effects is a possibility. Increased extrapyramidal side effects, elevated prolactin levels, and increased D_2 binding were demonstrated in one small study after addition of haloperidol 4 mg/day to stable doses of clozapine.[54] Although little empirical data exist to either support or refute the use of combination AP strategies, it is reasonable to cautiously try a time-limited combination trial in the treatment-resistant patient (stage 5a or 6 of the algorithm in Fig. 68–1).[24,25,49] As is evidenced in the treatment algorithm, this is usually indicated only after inadequate response to clozapine, or in a patient who refuses to give consent for clozapine treatment. Such combination treatment trials should be time limited (6 to 12 weeks) and the patient carefully evaluated with rating scales for changes in symptomatology. If no apparent improvement is observed, then one of the medications should be tapered and discontinued.[49]

ANTIPSYCHOTIC DRUG MECHANISM OF ACTION

The exact mechanism of action of antipsychotic medications is unknown. However, research has centered on their relative affinities to block the receptors of different neurotransmitters. Recent work has focused on the APs' relative affinities to block D_2 versus $5\text{-}HT_{2A}$ receptors. At least 60% to 65% occupation of D_2 receptors has traditionally been thought to be necessary to produce an effect on positive psychotic symptoms, whereas blockade of approximately $\geq$77% of D_2 receptors is associated with extrapyramidal side effects.[55] Traditional AP medications are dopaminergic antagonists, with high affinity for D_2 receptors. During chronic treatment with these agents, between 70% and 90% of D_2 receptors in the striatum are usually occupied. Thus, treatment with traditional APs frequently exceeds the threshold for production of extrapyramidal side effects. In contrast, during clozapine treatment only 38% to 63% of D_2 receptors are occupied. Even with doses as high as 900 mg daily, less than 70% of D_2 receptors are occupied.[56,57]

Newer atypical APs have variable D_2 binding. With low-dose risperidone (2–5 mg/day), D_2 binding ranges from 60% to 79%, but with doses greater than 6 mg daily, binding commonly exceeds the 77% threshold commonly associated with the development of extrapyramidal side effects. Risperidone 2 mg/day produces $5\text{-}HT_2$ binding greater than 70%, and with 4 mg/day it is nearly 100%.[55,56]

In the 10–20 mg/day dose range, olanzapine D_2 binding ranges from 71% to 80%, while at 30–40 mg/day, binding ranges from 83% to 88%. At 5 mg/day, $5\text{-}HT_{2A}$ receptors are near saturation of binding.[58] Thus, risperidone 6 mg and olanzapine 20 mg/day have similar D_2 binding, while both drugs have high $5\text{-}HT_{2A}$ occupancy even at the lower end of the usual therapeutic dose range.[56]

Quetiapine has the lowest D_2 binding. At clinical doses of 300–600 mg/day, D_2 binding ranges from 0% to 27%. Even at quetiapine 800 mg/day, only 30% of D_2 receptors are occupied. At these same daily doses, 45% to 90% of $5\text{-}HT_{2A}$ receptors are occupied. All of the binding data above are from studies that measured receptor binding at approximately 12 hours postdose. When quetiapine D_2 binding is examined 2 to 3 hours postdose, 58% and 64% of receptors were occupied with 400 mg and 450 mg, respectively. This finding led the investigators to conclude that transient blockade of dopamine receptors may be adequate to produce antipsychotic effect (and transient rise in serum prolactin concentrations), but long-term D_2 blockade is required for production of extrapyramidal side effects and sustained hyperprolactinemia. They further conclude that low D_2 binding, and thus atypicality, may be directly associated with how rapidly the AP disassociates from the D_2 receptor.[57,59] Kapur et al. also suggest that current APs can be classified into three different categories: (a) typical or traditional (high D_2 binding and low $5\text{-}HT_{2A}$ binding); (b) atypical (moderate to high D_2 binding and high $5\text{-}HT_2$ binding); and (c) atypical clozapine-like (low D_2 binding and high $5\text{-}HT_{2A}$ binding). The clinical significance of the differences between categories two and three are as yet unclear.[57,60]

At the time of this writing, there was no available information regarding receptor binding in humans with ziprasidone.

Multiple DA-receptor subtypes exist, with D_1 and D_2 being the best studied. Even with these two subtypes, their functioning has not been adequately elucidated. Although D_2 receptors are associated with traditional AP efficacy, D_1 receptors may serve as a permissive or modulating receptor for extrapyramidal side effects; some D_1 blockade as well as D_2 may be necessary to produce extrapyramidal side effects. For example, haloperidol has high D_2 affinity, but some D_1 binding, and produces a high incidence of extrapyramidal reactions, and clozapine, with rapid disassociation D_2 binding, greater D_1 and D_4 binding (relative to haloperidol) and high non-DA affinity, causes almost no extrapyramidal side effects.[60,61]

Traditional APs have effects on all four dopaminergic tracts (see Table 68–1). The primary therapeutic effects of traditional APs are thought to occur in the limbic system, including the ventral striatum, whereas extrapyramidal side effects are thought to be related to DA blockade in the dorsal striatum. Tolerance often develops to the acutely occurring extrapyramidal side effects within a few weeks, but tolerance to the AP effects appear to be less common, if not rare.

TABLE 68–5. Metabolism Pathways of Atypical Antipsychotics

Drug	Major Pathway(s)	Minor Pathway(s)
Clozapine	1A2	3A4, 2D6
Risperidone	2D6	
Olanzapine	1A2	3A4, 2D6, FMO3
Quetiapine	3A4	2D6
Ziprasidone	Aldehyde oxidase	3A4, 1A2

Traditional APs, to varying degrees, affect other neurotransmitter receptor systems, including blockade of muscarinic, α_1-adrenergic, and histaminic receptors. As a rule, the lower-potency APs, (such as chlorpromazine and thioridazine), are less specific for DA receptors and block other receptors as well.[12] These differences in affinity for nondopaminergic receptors are at least partially responsible for the varying side-effect profiles among AP agents. This offers a rational explanation for the side effects such as dry mouth, constipation, sinus tachycardia, and orthostatic hypotension, which are seen more commonly with the "low-potency" traditional APs.

Although recent research has largely focused on the ratio between 5-HT_{2A} blockade and D_2 blockade, atypical APs have varying effects upon multiple neurotransmitters. For example, clozapine has relative D_1 and D_4 selectivity and is an antagonist for 5-HT_2, 5-HT_6, and 5-HT_7 receptors. In rodents, clozapine and olanzapine also block NMDA antagonist neurotoxicity.[17] Ziprasidone differs from other atypical antipsychotics in being a significant agonist for 5-HT_{1A}, an antagonist for 5-HT_{1D} receptors, and an inhibitor of reuptake for norepinephrine and 5 HT.[62] As with the various mechanisms of other atypical APs, the clinical significance of these effects is unknown. However, these differences in pharmacodynamic profiles do point out that the atypical APs are not all alike, and that patients not obtaining an adequate clinical response (either efficacy or side effects), may have a superior response on an alternate atypical AP. Thus, serial atypical AP monotherapy trials should be tried in patients receiving a suboptimal clinical response (see treatment algorithm).

PHARMACOKINETICS

The APs are highly lipophilic and highly bound to membranes and plasma proteins. They distribute readily into most tissues with a high blood supply and may accumulate in tissues; therefore, they have large volumes of distribution.[63] Most APs are largely metabolized, primarily through the cytochrome P450 pathways in the liver, except for ziprasidone, which is largely metabolized by aldehyde oxidase. Table 68–5 outlines the metabolic pathways of selected APs. Most APs have fairly long elimination half-lives, most in the range of 20 to 40 hours. Thus, after dosage stabilization, most APs can be dosed once daily. Exceptions are quetiapine and ziprasidone, which have short half-lives (Table 68–6).[63,64]

Efforts to develop relationships between AP plasma concentration (Cp) and clinical response have been hampered by several factors, including the variable lag time between beginning AP treatment and symptom change, the subjective and relatively imprecise methods of measuring drug effect or symptom change in schizophrenia, and the presence of multiple metabolites. The most successful research assessing the relationship between AP Cp and response has been performed with haloperidol, fluphenazine, and clozapine, where therapeutic ranges have been suggested to be 3–15 ng/mL, 0.5–3 ng/mL, and >250–350 ng/mL respectively.

Early studies indicated that a clozapine plasma concentration greater than 350 ng/mL was associated with a greater probability of efficacy in treatment-resistant patients.[63,65] A recent study investigating the efficacy of three different fixed serum concentration ranges found both the 200–300 ng/mL and 350–450 ng/mL ranges to be predictive of response.[66] Furthermore, sedation increased with increasing serum concentrations. A 12-hour postdose clozapine serum concentration of at least 250 ng/mL is recommended if the patient is receiving divided clozapine doses, or 350 ng/mL if the patient is being dosed once daily. Whether increased symptom improvement occurs with continued dosage increases above these serum concentrations, and a potential maximum clozapine serum concentration, are poorly defined.

It is not cost-effective to monitor AP Cp routinely in all patients. Cp monitoring of the above three APs should be considered in patients who do not respond to reasonable doses within a 6 to 12 week period; in patients who develop unusual or severe adverse experiences; in patients who are taking concomitant medications that may cause drug interactions; in patients who have age or pathophysiologic changes suggesting a change in pharmacokinetics; or for assessment of patient adherence.[38]

The depot APs, fluphenazine decanoate (also available in an enanthate salt) and haloperidol decanoate, are esterified APs formulated in sesame seed oil for deep intramuscular injection. Their absorption from the muscle and metabolism to the free base is sufficiently

TABLE 68–6. Pharmacokinetic Parameters of Selected Antipsychotics

Drug	Bioavailability (%)	Half-Life (h)	Active Metabolites
Typical Antipsychotics			
Chlorpromazine	10–30	8–35	7-hydroxy, others
Fluphenazine	20–50	14–24	?
Fluphenazine decanoate		14.2 ± 2.2[a] days	
Haloperidol	40–70	12–36	Reduced haloperidol
Haloperidol decanoate		21 days	
Atypical Antipsychotics			
Clozapine	12–81	11–105	None with significant activity
Olanzapine	80	20–70	*N*-glucuronide; 2-OH-methyl; 4-*N*-oxide
Quetiapine	9 ± 4	6.88	7-OH-quetiapine
Risperidone	68	3–24	9-OH-risperidone
Ziprasidone	59	4–10	None

[a]Based upon multiple dose data. Single-dose data indicates half-life of 6 to 10 days.

Adapted from Refs. 41 and 63.

TABLE 68–7. Relative Side Effects Incidence of Commonly Used Antipsychotics

	Sedation	Extrapyramidal Side Effects	Anticholinergic	Orthostasis
Chlorpromazine	++++	+++	+++	++++
Clozapine	++++	±	++++	++++
Fluphenazine	+	++++	+	+
Haloperidol	+	++++	+	+
Loxapine	+++	+++	++	+++
Molindone	+	+++	++	++
Olanzapine	++	++	++	++
Perphenazine	++	+++	++	++
Quetiapine	++	+	+	++
Risperidone	+	++	+	++
Thioridazine	++++	+++	++++	++++
Trifluoperazine	++	+++	++	++
Thiothixene	+	++++	+	+
Ziprasidone	++	++	+	++

±, negligible; +, very low; ++, low; +++, moderate; ++++, high

slow to cause absorption to be the rate-limiting step in determining their respective, apparent half-lives.[41]

ADVERSE EFFECTS

Table 68–7 presents the relative incidence of common categories of AP side effects. The precise incidence of many of these side effects has not been systematically evaluated. Side effects are discussed with respect to organ system affected. Also, many of the side effects can be categorized by the neurotransmitter system affected, as listed in Table 68–8. A general approach to monitoring and assessing side effects requires prospective monitoring by clinicians, preferably using a thorough review of systems approach. Patient-oriented, self-rated, side-effect scales may also be helpful, because many schizophrenics do not readily complain of side effects, because of a lack of volition, a lack of perception of having input into their treatment, or poor understanding, or because of the actual interference of side effects themselves (e.g., sedation).

TABLE 68–8. Potential Adverse Effects by Receptor Blockade

Receptor Type	Adverse Effects
Histamine H_1	Sedation Weight gain Potentiation of CNS depressants
Muscarinic	Urinary retention Cognition and memory effects Sinus tachycardia Dry mouth Blurred vision Constipation
α_1-Adrenergic	Orthostatic hypotension Reflex tachycardia Potentiation of antihypertensives Sexual dysfunction
Dopamine D_2	Extrapyramidal side effects Prolactin elevation
Serotonin 5-HT_{2A}	Orthostatic hypotension Sedation
Serotonin 5-HT_{2C}	Weight gain

With the variety of APs currently available, using an alternative drug should be considered in patients who complain of poorly tolerated side effects. Because medication side effects are one of the primary predictors of patient nonadherence, the clinician should take advantage of the treatment options currently available in an attempt to improve patient outcomes. As new atypical APs become available, there is cause to reexamine the side effects and risks associated with different APs. As we learn more about relative side effect risk (e.g., acute extrapyramidal side effects, tardive dyskinesia, weight gain, glucose intolerance, QTc prolongation), then one must carefully consider which APs should be considered first-line treatment alternatives.

Autonomic Nervous System

Patients receiving APs, or APs in combination with anticholinergics (AChs), may experience ACh side effects (e.g., dry mouth, constipation, tachycardia, blurred vision, inhibition or impairment of ejaculation, urinary retention, impaired memory). Lower-potency agents are typical offenders, and the elderly are especially sensitive to these effects.[12,67] Of the atypical antipsychotics, clozapine and olanzapine have moderately high rates of anticholinergic effects. System-specific effects are discussed under the appropriate heading.

Dry mouth can be managed with increased intake of fluids, oral lubricants (Xerolube), ice chips, or use of sugarless chewing gum or hard candy. Constipation, caused by slowed peristaltic movement and decreased intestinal fluid content, should be closely monitored and treated, especially in the elderly. Paralytic ileus and necrolyzing colitis may also occur. Constipation can be treated with increases in fluid and dietary fiber intake, and exercise.

Central Nervous System

Extrapyramidal System.

DYSTONIA

Dystonia is defined as a state of abnormal tonicity, sometimes described simplistically as a severe "muscle spasm."[68] Dystonias may be dramatic, frightening, and painful. More accurately, they are prolonged tonic contractions, with a rapid onset, usually within 24 to 96 hours of dosage administration or dosage increase. They may

TABLE 68–9. Agents Used To Treat Extrapyramidal Side Effects

Generic Name	Equivalent Dose (mg)	Dosage Range (mg)
Antimuscarinics		
Benztropine[a]	1	1–8[b]
Biperiden[a]	2	2–8
Trihexyphenidyl	2	2–15
Anithistaminic		
Diphenhydramine[a]	50	50–400
Dopamine Agonist		
Amantadine	N/A	100–400
Benzodiazepines		
Lorazepam[a]	N/A	1–8
Diazepam	N/A	2–20
Clonazepam	N/A	2–8
β-Blockers		
Propranolol	N/A	20–160

[a]Injectable dosage form can be given intramuscularly for relief of acute dystonia.
[b]Dosage may be titrated to 12 mg with care; nonlinear pharmacokinetics have been demonstrated.

be life-threatening, as in the case of pharyngeal-laryngeal dystonias, and can contribute to patient nonadherence. Types of dystonic reactions include trismus, glossospasm, tongue protrusion, pharyngeal-laryngeal dystonia, blepharospasm, oculogyric crisis, torticollis, and retrocollis.

Two pathophysiologic theories for dystonia are proposed:[68] (a) DA release from presynaptic receptors transiently increases (increased synthesis and release) in compensatory response to DA blockade, and (b) heightened sensitivity of postsynaptic DA receptors (as brain AP concentration decreases), such that DA release has an enhanced effect. The actual mechanism may be a combination of these two theories.

Dystonic reactions occur primarily with traditional APs. Risk factors include younger patients (especially males), the use of high-potency agents, and high dosage. An overall incidence from the 1960s through the mid-1970s ranged from 2.3% to 10%, but as higher-potency traditional APs became more widely used, the rate increased to as high as 64%.

Pharmacotherapeutic treatment options are effective and straightforward, with the choice of intramuscular or intravenous AChs (Table 68–9) or benzodiazepines. Benztropine mesylate 2 mg or diphenhydramine 50 mg may be given intramuscularly or intravenously, with the options of diazepam 5–10 mg by slow intravenous push or lorazepam 1–2 mg intramuscularly. Relief is typically seen within 15 to 20 minutes of an intramuscular injection and within 5 minutes of intravenous administration. If no response is seen within 15 minutes of intravenous injection or within 30 minutes of intramuscular injection, repeat the dose. AP medication may be continued, with concomitant short term use of oral ACh agents.

In general, prophylactic ACh medications are not recommended routinely as prophylaxis with all traditional APs. However, prophylaxis is reasonable when using high-potency traditional APs (e.g., haloperidol or fluphenazine) in young men, and in patients with a history of dystonia.[69] Dystonias may also be minimized by the use of lower initial doses of traditional APs. The AChs are good choices for prophylaxis, whereas amantadine has not been proven effective for this purpose. The use of atypical APs to minimize the risk of dystonia is appropriate, particularly in patients with a history of dystonia, in patients at high risk, or in patients who express fear of dystonia.

AKATHISIA

Akathisia is defined as the inability to sit still and as being functionally motor restless. The most accurate diagnosis is made by combining subjective complaints with objective symptoms (pacing, shifting, shuffling, or tapping feet). Subjectively, patients may describe a feeling of inner restlessness or disquiet, a compulsion to move or remain in constant motion. Akathisia occurs in 20% to 40% of patients treated with high-potency traditional APs.[68] The majority of patients receiving traditional APs may actually experience akathisia, but the reported incidence reflects only patients who can verbalize their feelings or recognize akathisia as being different from psychosis. Akathisia is frequently accompanied by dysphoria. Detection of akathisia requires a high degree of interviewer sensitivity, and symptoms can be quantified by use of the Barnes Akathisia Scale.

The pathophysiology of akathisia is uncertain, but there are two current theories.[68] One theory states that mesocortical postsynaptic DA blockade leads to increased locomotor activity, unlike the cataleptic effect in the striatum. The alternate theory claims that akathisia is caused by DA antagonist-induced dysregulation of noradrenergic tracts that project from the locus ceruleus to the limbic system.[68]

Many treatments for akathisia, although accepted to be effective, are based on anecdotal data. Akathisia research is particularly difficult as the nature of the disorder is subjective. Treatment with ACh agents, usually considered the standard treatment for all acute extrapyramidal side effects, is disappointing for akathisia, but may be helpful in patients with concomitant pseudoparkinsonism.[68] Traditionally, reduction in AP dosage has been considered the best intervention; however, this may not be a realistic goal in an acutely psychotic patient. A logical alternative is to switch to an atypical antipsychotic or an AP previously used in the patient without adverse effect. However, akathisia may occasionally occur with atypical APs. Although head-to-head comparisons are not widely available, quetiapine and clozapine appear to have the lowest risk of producing akathisa.[25,56]

Diazepam 5 mg three times per day has been used for treatment of akathisia,[68] and β-blockers are being used with increasing frequency. Propranolol in doses up to 160 mg daily, nadolol in doses up to 80 mg daily, and metoprolol in β_2-selective doses of 100 mg daily or less were reported as effective.[70] The use of clonidine has also been investigated; a mean dose of 0.43 mg/day produced response in six patients, with maximum response within 24 to 48 hours of the previous dosage increase. Hypotension and sedation were the only observed side effects.

Preventive measures for akathisia include using the lowest possible traditional AP dose, or preferably, the use of atypical APs.

PSEUDOPARKINSONISM

Pseudoparkinsonism, an AP-induced extrapyramidal side effect, resembles idiopathic Parkinson's disease. A patient with pseudoparkinsonism may present with any of four cardinal symptoms: (a) akinesia, bradykinesia, or decreased motor activity including difficulty initiating movement as well as extreme slowness, mask-like facial expression, micrographia, slowed speech, and decreased arm swing; (b) tremor, known as pill-rolling type, predominant at rest, decreasing with movement, usually involving the fingers and hands, although it may be seen in the arms, legs, neck, head, and chin (it may often be activated in resting body parts by having the patient perform mechanical movements with one extremity); (c) cogwheel rigidity, seen as the patient's limbs yielding in jerky, ratchet-like fashion when passively moved by the examiner (a mild form may present as stiffness); and (d) postural abnormalities and instability manifested as stooped posture, difficulty in maintaining stability when changing body position, and a gait that ranges from slow and shuffling to festinating (a result of dysfunction in autonomic stability combined with a shift in the center of gravity due to the stooped posture). Accessory symptoms include the autonomic manifestations seborrhea, sialorrhea, and hyperhidrosis.[68] Fatigue and weakness may be noted, as well as speech abnormalities including dysphagia and dysarthria, and abnormal palmomental and glabellar reflexes. A variant of pseudoparkinsonism is rabbit syndrome, a perioral tremor.

The overall incidence ranges from 15.4% to 36%, depending on the traditional AP used. Akinesia alone can be seen in 59% of patients on high-potency agents. Other risk factors include increasing age and possibly female gender. The onset of symptoms is usually 1 to 2 weeks after initiation of AP therapy or dose increase.

The pathophysiology involves a relative deficiency of DA. Normal motor function is dependent on a balance between cholinergic and dopaminergic systems. AP blockade of postsynaptic DA receptors leads to a relative functional DA deficiency and cholinergic excess in the striatum resulting in motor abnormalities approximating those seen in Parkinson's disease.[68]

The efficacy of ACh medications in alleviating or attenuating pseudoparkinsonian symptoms is well established.[68] Benztropine is advantageous in that its longer half-life allows once to twice daily dosing. Typical dosing is 1–2 mg twice a day up to a usual maximum dosage of 8 mg daily, although some patients will continue to respond to doses up to 12 mg. Dosage titration should be slow, as benztropine displays nonlinear pharmacokinetics, and side effects may become unacceptable. Trihexyphenidyl (2–5 mg tid), diphenhydramine (25–50 mg tid), and biperiden (2 mg tid) usually require thrice-daily administration. Diphenhydramine produces more sedation than the other agents. Although it has been suggested that trihexyphenidyl is more likely to be abused, all of the anticholinergics have been abused for their euphoriant effects.[71] With all of these agents, symptoms typically begin to resolve within 3 to 4 days after initiation of treatment, but a minimum of at least 2 weeks of treatment is normally required for full response.

Amantadine is generally as efficacious for pseudoparkinsonism as AChs, with significantly less effect on memory function.[68] Amantadine has less potential than other DA agonists (bromocriptine and levodopa) for significant adverse effects. Its mechanism involves enhancement of dopaminergic tone in the striatum. Excessive doses may produce anxiety, agitation, and restlessness, as well as exacerbation of psychosis. Dosage adjustment is necessary with renal insufficiency.

The need for prophylactic use of these agents against pseudoparkinsonism is less convincing than with dystonias, and is unnecessary when using atypical APs.[68] The long-term treatment of pseudoparkinsonism with antiparkinsonian medication is controversial.[68] Most investigators believe that it is seldom necessary with maintenance AP therapy, whereas other investigators demonstrate a population of patients who have recurrence or worsening of pseudoparkinsonian symptoms upon discontinuation of ACh medication, even if the traditional AP is withdrawn gradually. An attempt should be made to taper and discontinue these agents 6 weeks to 3 months after symptoms resolve. If symptoms reappear, then switching to an atypical AP should be considered.

The risk of pseudoparkinsonism with atypical APs is extremely low. When risperidone is used in doses greater than 6 mg/day, the risk of pseudoparkinsonian symptoms approaches that with traditional agents. However, a head-to-head comparison of currently recommended risperidone doses (3–6 mg/day) found no difference in Parkinson symptoms between risperidone and olanzapine.[72] Quetiapine or clozapine are reasonable alternatives in a patient experiencing moderate to severe extrapyramidal side effects with other atypical APs.[24,25,68]

TARDIVE DYSKINESIA

Tardive dyskinesia is a syndrome characterized by abnormal involuntary movements occurring late in onset in relation to initiation of AP therapy. Tardive dyskinesia is sometimes irreversible and continues to be a controversial issue, clinically, legally, and ethically.

The classical description of tardive dyskinesia is the bucco-lingual-masticatory (BLM) syndrome, or orofacial movements. The onset of BLM movements is usually insidious. Typically, they are the first detectable signs of tardive dyskinesia, and begin with mild forward, backward, or lateral movements of the tongue. As the disorder progresses, more obvious or frank BLM movements appear, including tongue thrusting, rolling, or fly-catching movements, and chewing or lateral jaw movements. Tardive dyskinesia symptoms may interfere with the patient's ability to chew, speak, or swallow. Further complications include oral ulcerations, inability to wear dentures, and inflammation and loosening of mandibular joints. Eating difficulties and malnutrition may be primary physical complications of tardive dyskinesia. Weight loss may be seen in patients with esophageal or respiratory manifestations but not in those with truncal movements.

Facial movements include frequent blinking, brow arching, grimacing, upward deviation of the eyes, and lip smacking. Involvement of the extremities sometimes occurs, with the appearance of restless choreiform (irregular spasmodic) and distal athetosis (slow, writhing movement) of limbs including twisting, spreading, flexion (bending) and extension of fingers, toe tapping, and toe dorsiflexion (upward turning). Unusual posture, hyperextension, pelvic thrusting, axial hyperkinesia (excessive muscular activity of head and trunk), ballismus (jerking or shaking), exaggerated lordosis (bending backward), rocking, and swaying are occasionally observed. Among the more common differential diagnoses are withdrawal dyskinesias occurring after short-term use of APs, spontaneous orofacial dyskinesias in the elderly, orofacial dyskinesias in the edentulous, stereotypic movements in schizophrenics, Huntington's disease, and congenital torsion dystonia.

Orofacial movements are reported more commonly in older patients, whereas the truncal axial movements are classically reported in young adults. Movements may worsen with stress, decrease with sedation, and disappear during sleep. Concentration on motor tasks or attempts to suppress the movements voluntarily may actually increase them.

Early signs of tardive dyskinesia may be reversible, but if allowed to persist or if not detected in the early stages, they may be irreversible, even with drug discontinuation. When the AP dose is decreased or tapered and discontinued, there is often a worsening of abnormal movements and then possibly a slow improvement after months or years if the patient remains on lower doses or discontinues treatment.

There are no standardized criteria for the diagnosis of tardive dyskinesia. Abnormal involuntary movements can be detected early through physical assessment and the use of rating scales. Available rating scales include the Abnormal Involuntary Movement Scale (AIMS) and the Dyskinesia Identification System: Condensed User Scale (DISCUS).[68,73] Neither scale is diagnostic in itself.

The pathophysiology of tardive dyskinesia is complex and remains to be satisfactorily explained. The traditional theory is that postsynaptic D_2-receptor blockade in the nigrostriatum leads to hypersensitivity or D_2-receptor upregulation, and this effect has been shown in both animals and humans.[74] D_2 upregulation is generally considered in conjunction with a cholinergic dysfunction relative to dopaminergic activity or a classic DA/acetylcholine imbalance. These DA receptors are generally considered to have an inhibitory effect on acetylcholine function in the corpus striatum. DA function may be modulated by a negative feedback system involving two serial sets of GABA-mediated neurons. GABA output to the thalamus and motor cortex is reduced as a result, and this causes the movement disorder. Thus, tardive dyskinesia may represent an adaptive change to the loss of gating function usually produced by normal DA activity in extrapyramidal motor circuits. Deficiencies of this theory include: (a) it explains withdrawal dyskinesias or a transient movement disorder, but not persistent symptoms; (b) it does not explain concurrent tardive dyskinesia and parkinsonism in the same patient; (c) it does not account for the presence of presynaptic DA autoreceptors; and (d) postsynaptic receptor hypersensitivity usually develops soon after beginning APs, whereas tardive dyskinesia develops after prolonged use.[75] Lack of site specificity, degree or tightness of D_2 binding, and differential effects of APs on D_1 versus D_2 receptors may explain why traditional APs cause tardive dyskinesia while atypical APs have a significantly lower risk, and clozapine is associated with minimal or no risk of tardive dyskinesia. D_2 receptor antagonists' effects on decreasing GABA turnover and resulting GABA receptor hypersensitivity have also been theorized as a potential mechanism for tardive dyskinesia.[75]

Risk factors include increasing age; the occurrence of acute extrapyramidal side effects, poor AP drug response, diagnoses of organic mental disorder, diabetes mellitus, or mood disorders; and, possibly, female gender.[75,76] Duration of AP therapy, daily dosage, and possibly total cumulative dosage are probably the most significant risk factors. However, persistent dyskinesias occur with as little as 6 months of therapy. Overall morbidity and mortality are greater in tardive dyskinesia patients, and patients with tardive dyskinesia show a greater incidence of respiratory tract infections and cardiovascular illness.

With traditional APs, the reported incidence of tardive dyskinesia ranges from 0.5% to 62%.[75] Factors causing variation in epidemiologic studies are patient population characteristics, drug dosage, duration of therapy, varieties of methods used in the assessment of tardive dyskinesia, inadequacies in differentiating tardive dyskinesia from other movement disorders, and bias. In a study of first episode schizophrenia, the prevalence of persistent tardive dyskinesia was 19% after 4 years, and 26% after 6 years of drug exposure. Moreover, in elderly patients, the 3-year traditional AP treatment risk of tardive dyskinesia is 53%.[76]

AP dosage reduction may have a significant effect on outcome, if the patient can tolerate the reduction without return of psychotic symptoms.[75] Many patients with tardive dyskinesia are concerned about the possibility of worsening tardive dyskinesia symptoms if they are continued on medication. In one study, the syndrome remained stable over the years, and although a few patients worsened or only modest changes were seen, many patients improved on lower doses.[75] In another longitudinal study, remissions were seen in 25% of patients with tardive dyskinesia after 5 years of continued treatment.[77] However, an increased incidence of pseudoparkinsonism was seen in both of these studies.

Possibly only a small subgroup of patients with tardive dyskinesia will develop severe symptoms.[75] Although it is difficult to predict who will develop severe tardive dyskinesia, one sample of patients was characterized by a greater number of affective/schizoaffective patients; frequent eye blinking was a prodromal sign in 37%.[78]

Prevention is the single most important aspect of tardive dyskinesia, because treatment of the movements is difficult. Because of data suggesting a lower risk of tardive dyskinesia with atypical APs, these agents are considered treatments of first choice[79,80] (see Fig. 68–1). APs should be used only when they are indicated and they should be used at the minimum effective dose. When a patient is treated with APs for more than 3 months for an initial episode of illness, the need for continued treatment should be assessed. Regular neurologic examinations (AIMS or other scales) should be performed at baseline and at least quarterly to assess for early signs of tardive dyskinesia. At the first signs of tardive dyskinesia, the need for continuing AP treatment should be reassessed. In such situations, if the patient is taking a traditional AP and continuing treatment is indicated, the medication should be switched to an atypical AP. In nonpsychotic patients, traditional APs should only be used acutely to abort an aggressive behavior crisis, and always in combination with a behavioral treatment program.

There are no FDA-approved agents for treatment of tardive dyskinesia. Numerous drugs have been used, representing various strategies affecting CNS neurotransmission. Older strategies have been aimed at altering the DA, GABA, and cholinergic systems; these are reviewed elsewhere.[75]

α-Tocopherol (vitamin E) in daily doses of 1200–1600 IU has been used based on its antioxidant properties. Results from multiple short-term treatment studies have variously shown reduction in movements (usually patients with recent onset of tardive dyskinesia), or minor benefit in select patients, or no effect.[22,75,81] However, results from an unpublished study suggest that in patients treated with either vitamin E or placebo for as long as 1 year, both groups improved and there was no difference between vitamin E and placebo. No data exist regarding the use of prophylactic vitamin E to prevent the occurrence of tardive dyskinesia.

To date, there are no reports of tardive dyskinesia with clozapine monotherapy. Although introduced in the United States in 1990, it has been used in some European countries since the early 1970s. In two controlled trials lasting 22 to 52 weeks, it decreased abnormal involuntary movements by 50% or more.[75] Switching AP therapy to clozapine is a favored first-line pharmacotherapeutic strategy, particularly in patients with moderate to severe symptoms.[22,24,25] The atypical antipsychotics risperidone and olanzapine have rates of emergent dyskinesias significantly lower than with typical APs,[79,80] and these atypical APs may be considered as alternative treatments in patients with mild to moderate tardive dyskinesia.[75]

■ *Sedation and Cognition.* Sedation must be recognized as an AP side effect and not as an indication of therapeutic effect. It occurs more frequently with APs with antihistaminic properties. Chlorpromazine, thioridazine, mesoridazine, clozapine, olanzapine, and quetiapine are most frequently implicated. Administration of most or all of the daily dosage at bedtime (depending on the drug half-life) can decrease daytime sedation and in some patients eliminate the need for hypnotic agents. Sedation occurs early in treatment and may decrease over time. Oversedation plays a large role in cognitive, perceptual, and motor dysfunction.[82] With acute dosing, tasks requiring vigilance, attention, or motor behavior may be affected. However, the positive effects of medication are seen with chronic administration, evidenced by improvements in tasks involving visual-motor skills and attention. As compared with traditional agents, several studies have shown cognitive benefits of atypical antipsychotics. These positive effects on cognition are thought to be secondary to the atypical APs relative effects on prefrontal cortical functioning. Although atypical APs appear to have beneficial effects on cognition, as compared to traditional agents, this area has been inadequately investigated. It is not currently possible to compare atypical APs effects on cognition or to clearly evaluate the clinical significance of these differences.[62]

Seizures. APs lower the seizure threshold through GABA depletion, changes in CNS permeability leading to enhanced conduction of a discharge, disruption of DA-acetylcholine balance, or the activation of a latent seizure focus. There is an increased risk of drug-induced seizures in all patients treated with APs. However, this risk is greater if the following predisposing factors are present: preexisting seizure disorder, history of drug-induced seizure, abnormal electroencephalogram (EEG), and preexisting CNS pathology or head trauma. Seizures are more closely associated with the use of higher doses, rapid dosage increases, and upon initiation of treatment. When an isolated seizure occurs, a dosage decrease is first recommended; anticonvulsant therapy is not recommended. The highest potential seizure risk for an AP drug is with the use of chlorpromazine or clozapine, followed by trifluoperazine and perphenazine. Addition of lithium to a stable clozapine regimen has resulted in seizures in two reported cases.[83] If a change in AP therapy is required in the management of AP-induced seizures, atypical antipsychotics (other than clozapine), molindone, thioridazine, haloperidol, and fluphenazine are associated with the lowest potential.[84]

Thermoregulation. Poikilothermia, the body temperature adjusting to the ambient temperature, can be a serious side effect of AP therapy in temperature extremes.[85] Hyperpyrexia can be a danger in hot weather or during exercise. Inhibition of sweating, a result of ACh properties impairing the peripheral mechanisms of heat dissipation, can also contribute to this problem, which in its severest form can lead to heat stroke. Hypothermia is also a risk, particularly in the elderly. All patients receiving APs should be educated about these potential problems. Thermoregulatory problems are reportedly more common with the use of low-potency APs, and may occur with the more anticholinergic atypical antipsychotics.

Neuroleptic Malignant Syndrome. Neuroleptic malignant syndrome (NMS) occurs in 0.5% to 1% of patients receiving APs. NMS may occur more frequently in patients receiving high-potency, injectable, or depot APs, and in patients who are dehydrated, with physical exhaustion, or organic mental disorders.[86] NMS has been reported with atypical APs, including clozapine, as well as with typical AP.[26] However, the risk of NMS is lower with atypical than with traditional agents. The onset of symptoms varies from early in treatment to months later. It develops rapidly, over the course of 24 to 72 hours. NMS may occur after AP discontinuation, especially when depot agents are used. Possible mechanisms of NMS include disruption of the central thermoregulatory process or excess production of heat secondary to skeletal muscle contractions. The differential diagnosis includes heat stroke, lethal catatonia, anesthetic-associated malignant hyperthermia, ACh toxicity, and monoamine oxidase inhibitor (MAOI) drug interactions.

Cardinal signs and symptoms of NMS are body temperature exceeding 38°C (100.4°F), altered level of consciousness, autonomic dysfunction (tachycardia, labile blood pressure, diaphoresis, tachypnea, urinary or fecal incontinence), and rigidity. Laboratory evaluation, although considered nonspecific, frequently shows leukocytosis with or without left shift, increases in creatine kinase (CK), aspartate aminotransferase (AST), alanine aminotransferase (ALT), lactate dehydrogenase (LDH), and myoglobinuria.

Treatment should always begin with AP discontinuation and supportive care. The DA agonist bromocriptine, used in theory to reverse DA blockade, reduces rigidity, fever, or CK in up to 94% of patients, whereas the use of another DA agonist, amantadine, has been successfully used in up to 63% of patients.[87] Dantrolene has been used as a skeletal muscle relaxant, with effects on temperature, heart rate, respiratory rate, and CK in up to 81% of patients. AChs and benzodiazepines have been tried but appear to have little effect in most patients, and ACh use can complicate the clinical presentation with possible delirium. Wide recognition and rapid AP discontinuation has drastically reduced mortality from 20% fifteen years ago to 4% in the mid-1990s.

Many schizophrenics, despite having had NMS, will require future AP pharmacotherapy. Patient selection for rechallenge is important, as only those patients in need of reinstitution of APs should receive future trials. A review of AP rechallenges suggests that the risk of rechallenge is acceptable in most patients, provided there is careful monitoring, patient selection is appropriate, and the patient is observed for an extended period of time (2 weeks or more is suggested) without APs.[88] Neither patient-specific demographic variables nor AP agent used assist in predicting recurrence. In patients developing NMS on a traditional AP, an atypical AP should be used.

Psychiatric Side Effects. AP-induced akathisia, akinesia, and dysphoria may have unfortunate sequelae, resulting in what has been termed "behavioral toxicity."[35] Akathisia has resulted in impulsivity and, in extreme cases, violence and suicide. Akinesia, characterized by "diminished spontaneity," results in symptoms of apathy and withdrawal, often mistaken for the negative symptoms of schizophrenia; these patients may actually appear depressed on formal evaluation.

Delirium and psychosis are reported with larger doses of APs or combinations of AChs with APs. Chronic confusion and disorientation can occur in the elderly as a result of AP treatment.[67] Unfortunately, the link is not always made between initiation of AP therapy, and the patient may be misdiagnosed with an organic mental disorder. This clinical presentation, called a "pseudodementia," is easily reversible on discontinuation of the AP.

Exacerbation and new onset of obsessive-compulsive symptoms have been reported with clozapine, and has anecdotally been reported to improve with addition of an SSRI.[89]

Endocrine System. DA blockade in the tuberoinfundibular tract results in increased prolactin levels, because DA is the major prolactin-inhibiting factor. Galactorrhea may occur in up to 57% of women, and menstrual irregularities or amenorrhea in up to 97%. These effects may be dose related and are more common with the use of high-potency typical APs and risperidone. Gynecomastia and galactorrhea are reported in men as well. Tolerance does not appear to develop to these effects.[90] Switching to the atypical antipsychotics olanzapine, quetiapine, or ziprasidone, which have no appreciable sustained effect on prolactin, is the most reasonable treatment option. Bromocriptine in doses up to 15 mg daily, or amantadine in doses up to 300 mg daily, have also been used.

Weight gain is frequently reported in patients receiving APs.[91] Although the exact mechanism is uncertain, weight gain has been associated with antihistaminic effects, antimuscarinic effects, and blockade of 5-HT_{2C} receptors. However, dietary factors and activity levels may play a significant role in this population, as does renourishment after a period of poor self-care. Weight gain may be seen with most atypical antipsychotics. In particular, significant weight increases are associated with clozapine and olanzapine therapy in 40% or more of patients.[62,91] Risperidone and quetiapine may cause weight gain, but much less than that caused by clozapine or olanzapine. Utilizing a meta-analysis and a random effects model to predict weight gain after 10 weeks of treatment, Allison predicted the following mean weight increases with APs: clozapine, 4.45 kg; olanzapine,

4.15 kg; risperidone, 2.10 kg; haloperidol, 1.08 kg; and ziprasidone, 0.04 kg.[91] It remains to be seen whether these weight changes are also true in clinical practice.[91] Although ziprasidone is a potent 5-HT_{2C} antagonist, it has been suggested that its effects as a 5-HT_{1A} agonist counteract this effect and contribute to the reports of minimal weight gain.

Schizophrenics have a higher prevalence of type II diabetes than do the nonschizophrenic population. Beyond this, APs may adversely affect glucose levels, a consideration in diabetic patients. Clozapine and olanzapine can cause glucose dysregulation, the exacerbation of preexisting diabetes, and new onset diabetes. The extent to which these effects are related to weight increase is unclear.[62,92,93] A single-dose study has suggested that atypical APs impair glucose tolerance and increase insulin secretion, which would support a potential effect on glucose regulation independent of weight increase. A naturalistic study of patients taking clozapine found a 5-year rate of new-onset diabetes totaling 52%.[93] These effects appear uncommon with risperidone, and the risk with quetiapine and ziprasidone is currently unknown.[92] However, the relative risk of glucose dysregulation with various atypical APs and resulting sequelae have yet to be determined. Clozapine and olanzapine should be used with caution in patients with preexisting diabetes, and periodic measurement of weight and fasting glucose should be performed.

Cardiovascular System

Orthostatic Hypotension. Postural or orthostatic hypotension, defined as a greater than 20-mm Hg drop in systolic pressure, is caused by α-adrenergic blockade, which inhibits reflex vasoconstriction when rising to a sitting or standing position; this appears to be a combination of local vasodilatory effects and central inhibition of the vasomotor center, as well as sympatholysis leading to unopposed β-adrenergic effect.[85] Patients may experience light-headedness or syncope. Associated with lower potency traditional APs and atypical APs (especially on intramuscular or intravenous administration), orthostatic hypotension can occur in any patient, but diabetics, patients with preexisting cardiovascular disease, and the elderly seem particularly predisposed. For the mild case, patient education should address slow changes in posture to allow for adaptation or the use of support hose. For most patients, tolerance to this effect occurs within 2 to 3 months. If this does not occur, lower doses or a change to a AP with less α-blockade can be attempted.

Severe hypotensive episodes require more vigorous treatment. The patient should be placed in a Trendelenburg position. Volume expansion through intravenous fluids should be attempted before the use of pressor agents. Pure α-adrenergic pressor agents, such as phenylephrine (Neo-Synephrine) or metaraminol (Aramine), can be used, as well as norepinephrine (Levophed), which has α-agonist and β_1-adrenergic properties. Epinephrine (Adrenalin), a mixed α- and β-adrenergic agonist, should never be used because unopposed β-adrenergic stimulating effects will further lower a patient's blood pressure, potentially leading to cardiovascular collapse. Isoproterenol (Isuprel), which also has β-adrenergic stimulating effects, should also be avoided.

Electrocardiogram Changes. Low-potency typical agents, especially piperidine phenothiazines (such as thioridazine), clozapine, and ziprasidone, are more likely to cause ECG effects. ECG changes include increased heart rate (through sinus tachycardia from ACh effects, or reflex tachycardia from α-adrenergic blockade), flattened T waves, ST segment depression, and prolongation of QT and PR intervals. The most clinically important of these potential changes is prolongation of the QTc interval which has been associated with ventricular arrhythmias, including torsade de pointes syndrome. In a study submitted to the FDA,[31] thioridazine was shown to prolong the QTc interval on average about 20 msec longer than haloperidol, risperidone, olanzapine, or quetiapine.[62] The effect of thioridazine on QTc prolongation was dose related. For this reason, thioridazine and mesoridazine (an active metabolite of thioridazine) have received a black box warning in the FDA approved product labeling with regard to this effect. Torsade de pointes has been reported with thioridazine, which may be a cause of cardiac sudden death. Given the number of AP options currently available, there appear to be few reasons to use either thioridazine or mesoridazine. In the same study, ziprasidone prolonged the QTc interval about 10 msec longer than did haloperidol, risperidone, olanzapine, or quetiapine—about one half of the effect of thioridazine.[62] Furthermore, the ziprasidone effects were not dose related. Although the precise point at which QTc prolongation becomes clinically dangerous is unclear, it has been recommended to discontinue a medication associated with QTc prolongation if the interval consistently exceeds 500 msec.

Greater caution regarding AP choice and use is necessary in the elderly, in patients with preexisting cardiac disease, and in patients taking diuretics or medications that may prolong the QTc interval.[31,62,67] In patients older than 50 years of age, a pretreatment ECG is recommended, as are baseline serum potassium and magnesium levels. These factors should be considered when deciding whether to choose ziprasidone in a given patient.[64]

Lipid Changes. Clozapine therapy has been associated with elevations in serum triglycerides, but not cholesterol.[93] This has also been reported with olanzapine, but not yet with the other atypical APs. The clinical significance of these findings is unclear at present.[62]

Ophthalmologic Effects

Impairment in visual accommodation results from paresis of ciliary muscles, an ACh effect. Although bothersome, the effect is temporary in most cases. Photophobia may also result. Pilocarpine ophthalmic solution may be necessary in severe cases.[94]

Exacerbation of narrow-angle (angle closure) glaucoma can result from increases in intraocular pressure, another ACh effect. APs should be used with great caution in susceptible individuals.[94]

Opaque deposits in the cornea and lens occur with chronic phenothiazine treatment, most frequently with chlorpromazine. Although visual acuity is not usually affected, periodic slit-lamp ophthalmologic examinations are frequently recommended in patients receiving long-term treatment with phenothiazines. Because of cataract development and lenticular changes in animals, baseline and periodic eye exams are recommended in the product labeling for patients receiving quetiapine.[95] However, clinical experience with quetiapine since marketing has not supported a significant risk of cataracts.[24,25]

Retinitis pigmentosus can result from use of thioridazine doses greater than 800 mg daily. It is caused by melanin deposits, and can result in permanent visual impairment or blindness. There is no evidence that it is a function of cumulative dose.[94]

Hepatic System

Liver function test (LFT) abnormalities (elevated aminotransferases and alkaline phosphatase) are reported in up to 50% of patients on APs, and may occur without clinical symptoms.[96] This occurs most commonly in patients younger than 50 years of age and does not appear to be dose related. Mild LFT elevations are typically not significant, although they should be followed closely. If aminotransferases are greater than three times the upper limit of normal, AP therapy should be changed to a chemically unrelated AP.

Cholestatic hepatocanalicular jaundice can occur in up to 2% of patients receiving phenothiazines. It may be a hypersensitivity reaction, or a result of either the effects on bile composition or the direct toxic effect of a metabolite on biliary ductile hepatocytes impairing bile flow.[96] The onset is usually within the first 2 weeks of therapy, with prodromal symptoms of malaise, fatigue, fever, chills, arthralgias, myalgias, GI symptoms, and severe pruritus. Symptoms usually resolve without residual liver damage within 2 to 8 weeks upon discontinuation of the offending AP. Palliative treatment of pruritus with topical or oral antihistamines is frequently necessary. Resumption of AP therapy should be delayed as long as reasonably possible, and it should be done with a nonphenothiazine AP.

Genitourinary System

Urinary hesitancy and retention is reported with low-potency traditional APs and with clozapine. ACh effects cause smooth muscle slowing and paralyze the detrusor muscle of the bladder, requiring greater urine volume to evoke muscle contraction. Men with benign prostatic hypertrophy are especially prone to this effect.[67]

Urinary incontinence is felt by some to be unrelated to urinary retention. Instead, it may be mechanistically similar to a dystonic reaction. It is reported more frequently in older patients, especially women.[97]

The AP effects on sexual dysfunction can be frightening or devastating to most schizophrenics and can adversely affect compliance. Erectile dysfunction and impotence, considered an ACh effect, occurs in 25% to 60% of patients, most frequently with thioridazine. Although this can occur in a large number of untreated psychotic patients, it can be worsened by AP drugs. Anorgasmia and decreased libido in women have also been proposed to be ACh in nature. α-Adrenergic blockade is proposed to be the mechanism behind priapism and retarded and retrograde ejaculation. Again, thioridazine is the most frequently reported AP for these effects and is an α-blocker. Decreased libido may also be caused by sedation. In men, another possible, although not fully explored, mechanism of sexual dysfunction is decreased testosterone production secondary to hyperprolactinemia.[98] Although it is difficult to compare the prevalence of sexual dysfunction among the atypical agents, some authorities feel that those with less effect of prolactin secretion may cause less sexual dysfunction. In patients experiencing prolactin-related sexual dysfunction, changing to either olanzapine, quetiapine, or ziprasidone is a reasonable intervention.

Hematologic System

Transient leukopenia may occur during initial treatment with APs; however, it typically does not progress to clinically significant parameters.[99] If the WBC count is less than 3,000/mm^3, or if the absolute neutrophil count (ANC) is less than 1,000/mm^3, the AP should be discontinued, and the WBC monitored closely until it returns to normal. Agranulocytosis reportedly occurs in 0.01% of patients receiving APs, and with the traditional APs may occur more frequently with chlorpromazine and piperazine phenothiazines. The onset is usually within the first 8 weeks of therapy. Agranulocytosis may initially manifest clinically as a local infection, with sore throat, leukoplakia, erythema, and ulcerations of the pharynx. These symptoms in any patient receiving APs should signal the immediate need for a WBC. If either the WBC or ANC falls below these parameters, the drug should be discontinued immediately and the patient monitored closely for the development of secondary infections. There are also isolated, rare case reports of thrombocytopenia and eosinophilia.

Agranulocytosis is the clozapine-related adverse effect that significantly limits the clinical utility of this agent. Data on the incidence since the release of clozapine in February 1990, following stringent monitoring guidelines, reveal that the 1-year treatment risk of developing agranulocytosis with clozapine is approximately 0.8%, and the 18-month risk is 0.91%.[100] Increasing age and female gender are associated with greater risk. Based on available data, the time period for greatest risk appears to be between months 1 and 6 of treatment, and weekly WBC monitoring for the first 6 months of therapy is mandated in the FDA-approved product labeling.[101] After the first 6 months, the labeling allows the frequency of WBC monitoring to be decreased to every 2 weeks. If the total WBC count drops to less than 2,000/mm^3, or the ANC is less than 1,000/mm^3, clozapine should be discontinued and the patient monitored closely. Some clinicians have used the granulocyte colony stimulating factor filgrastim with hopes of improving the outcome by hastening resolution or decreasing morbidity. One case series that used filgrastim (starting dose of 300 μg/day SQ, increased by 300 μg/day until 900 μg/day is reached, and then continued until the agranulocytosis is resolved) demonstrated a decrease in time to resolution and decreased intensive care bed costs when compared to historical controls.[102] In cases of mild to moderate neutropenia (granulocytes between 2,000/mm^3 and 3,000/mm^3, or ANC between 1,000/mm^3 and 1,500/mm^3), which occurs in up to 2% of patients, clozapine should be discontinued with daily monitoring of complete blood counts until values return to normal.

Dermatologic System

Allergic reactions are rare and usually occur within 8 weeks of therapy, manifesting as maculopapular, erythematous, pruritic rashes that are evident on the face, neck, trunk, or extremities. Drug discontinuation and topical steroids are recommended.

Contact dermatitis, including the oral mucosa, may occur in patients or medical personnel. For patients, mixing the concentrate in a sufficient quantity of a nonacidic liquid and swallowing it quickly decreases problems in susceptible patients. Care should be taken in the handling and preparation of liquid traditional APs.

Phenothiazine structures can absorb ultraviolet light and energy, resulting in the formation of free radicals, which can have damaging effects on the skin. Erythema and severe sunburns can occur. Exposure to sunlight should be limited, and patients should be educated about the use of a maximally blocking sunscreen, hats, protective clothing, and sunglasses.[85]

Blue-gray or purplish skin coloration in areas exposed to sunlight occurs in patients receiving higher doses of low-potency phenothiazines during long-term administration, especially with chlorpromazine. It commonly occurs with concurrent corneal or lens pigmentation.

Sudden Death Syndromes

Although fewer sudden deaths occurred before AP use, it has been reported in schizophrenics before and after the advent of APs. Most theories emphasize a pharmacologic etiology. The most common theory is that ventricular arrhythmias progress to ventricular fibrillation and death. Another common hypothesis is that an impaired gag reflex from a laryngeal-pharyngeal dystonia leads to aspiration, hypoxia, and death, a syndrome known as "obstructive asphyxia" or "café coronary." Other potentially drug-related theories include hyperpyrexia, NMS, seizures, and toxic megacolon, whereas nondrug-related theories include acute exhaustive mania or Bell's mania, lethal catatonia, coronary artery disease, and the sequelae of alcohol and substance abuse.[103]

Miscellaneous Adverse Effects

A particularly curious and sometimes troubling side effect with clozapine is sialorrhea. Drooling, possibly adrenergic in etiology, occurs in the absence of pseudoparkinsonian symptoms.[104] Some cases respond to the addition of the α_2-adrenergic agonist clonidine, in doses of 0.1–0.2 mg.[105] It may also abate with benztropine therapy.

TOXICITY WITH OVERDOSE

Acute overdose with APs rarely results in serious symptomatology. Mild intoxication manifests as sedation, hypotension, and miosis, whereas with severe intoxication, agitation and delirium may typically progress to motor retardation, seizures, cardiac arrhythmias, respiratory arrest, and coma. Dystonias and pseudoparkinsonian symptoms also occur. Supportive measures, gastric lavage, and activated charcoal are recommended. Induction of emesis may be difficult because of effects on the chemoreceptor trigger zone, and dialysis is ineffective because of the degree of drug-protein binding. Phenytoin or sodium bicarbonate are useful in the treatment of quinidine-like cardiac conduction effects on the QRS or QTc intervals. Physostigmine is not generally recommended to reverse anticholinergic toxicity because of deleterious effects on arrhythmias and seizure threshold.[106]

USE IN PREGNANCY AND LACTATION

Currently available data assessing the risk of teratogenesis with AP agents are insufficient. Haloperidol was studied in the treatment of hyperemesis gravidarum without negative effect; it and other high-potency traditional agents appear to be preferred, but, unfortunately, this is primarily a result of a lack of published reports over decades of use. Case reports implicating limb malformations are rare, but should be considered in deciding on the need for first-trimester AP use. The risk of AP use must be weighed against the benefits of pharmacotherapy in patients who may be experiencing disorganized thoughts, delusions about change in body image or pregnancy, or who are unable to provide adequate prenatal care.[107] Other potential but largely unknown risks of APs throughout pregnancy are the incidence of behavioral teratogenicity on the neonate, receptor changes, perinatal effects (e.g., tonicity, strength, sucking), extrapyramidal side effects, jaundice, respiratory depression, and intestinal obstruction.

APs appear in breast milk with milk to plasma ratios of 0.5 to 1. Little is known about the effects of these drugs on the neonate. Although not contraindicated, the lowest dosage should be used in the mother, and the infant should be carefully monitored.

DRUG INTERACTIONS

Although drug interactions may occur through a variety of mechanisms, most occur because of pharmacodynamic or pharmacokinetic interactions. Common examples of pharmacodynamic interactions resulting in enhanced effect include the excess sedation that can occur when antipsychotics are used concomitantly with other medications that have sedative side effects (e.g., mood stabilizers, hypnotics, alcohol, antidepressants, anxiolytics, antihistamines). Additive antimuscarinic effects of antipsychotics used with other medications with antimuscarinic effects (e.g., antihistamines, antidepressants, antiparkinson agents) may result in urinary retention, constipation, blurred vision, or other anticholinergic side effects.[49] Both combined sedative and anticholinergic effects from multiple medications may result in impaired cognition, particularly in the elderly and patients predisposed to such problems.[62] Patients may be more likely to experience symptomatic orthostatic hypotension when an antipsychotic is used with other medications that cause orthostasis (e.g., antidepressants with α blockade, antihypertensive agents, diuretics). Although metoclopramide is a commonly prescribed medication for treating esophageal reflux, it is a DA antagonist, and patients are more likely to experience akathisia and other extrapyramidal side effects if it is used concomitantly with antipsychotics.[108] Although some SSRIs may interact with antipsychotics through enzyme inhibition, they may also interact through pharmacodynamic mechanisms. 5-HT_2 receptors are present on the presynaptic dopaminergic neuron, and their activation leads to decreased dopamine release from the presynaptic terminal. Increased availability of serotonin through SSRI effect may activate these receptors, decrease dopamine release, and add to the dopaminolytic effects of AP agents.[109] Thus, in the absence of enzyme inhibition, SSRIs may still precipitate akathisia or extrapyramidal side effects when added to a patient stabilized on an AP medication. A potentially more dangerous interaction may occur when medications that slow myocardial conduction (e.g., quinidine, procainamide, tricyclic antidepressants), and thus prolong the QTc interval, are used in combination with antipsychotics that significantly prolong the QTc interval, such as thioridazine, mesoridazine, or ziprasidone.[31,32,62,110] Medications that prolong the QTc interval should also be monitored carefully in patients taking concomitant diuretics.[64] These effects may all increase the risk of clinically significant side effects.

Although atypical antipsychotics may be affected to varying degrees by enzyme inhibitors and inducers, none of the available atypical APs have been shown to significantly affect the pharmacokinetics of other medications. Table 68–5 lists the pathways thought to be involved in the metabolism of atypical APs. Risperidone is metabolized by CYP 2D6 to its active metabolite, 9-OH-risperidone.[111,112] Because the metabolite is thought to have a pharmacodynamic profile similar to risperidone, inhibition or induction interactions are rarely clinically significant with risperidone. For example, if fluoxetine is added to risperidone, the increased concentration of risperidone is balanced by decreased concentrations of 9-OH-risperidone, leading to no net change in bioactive drug. However, as indicated above, SSRIs may also interact with antipsychotics through pharmacodynamic mechanisms.

After single-dose administration, the mean bioavailability of quetiapine is 9% with significant interindividual variation.[63] If a CYP 3A4 inhibitor (e.g., cimetidine, ketoconazole, nefazodone, grapefruit juice, erythromycin) is added to quetiapine, increased side effects (e.g., sedation, orthostasis) may occur. Fluoxetine may also decrease clearance of a medication such as quetiapine metabolized through CYP 3A4. However, with fluoxetine, it is the long-acting metabolite norfluoxetine, and not fluoxetine, that is the inhibitor of 3A4 metabolism. If an enzyme inducer such as carbamazepine or St. John's wort is added to quetiapine, then decreased AP effects may occur.[112,113]

Based upon current information, inhibitors of CYP 1A2 have the greatest potential for causing interactions with olanzapine.[112] Examples include cimetidine, fluvoxamine, and fluoroquinolone antibiotics (e.g., ciprofloxacin) to varying degrees. To date, however, no serious inhibition interactions have been reported with olanzapine, which may be a result of olanzapine's wide therapeutic index. Carbamazepine has been reported to increase olanzapine elimination by as much as 50%.[111] Cigarette smoking is a potent inducer of CYP 1A2, and one would expect lower mean olanzapine serum concentrations in smokers as compared to nonsmokers.

Because of the risk of seizures with higher clozapine tissue concentrations, inhibition interactions with clozapine are potentially significant. Fluvoxamine, in particular, has been reported to increase clozapine serum concentrations by an average of two- to threefold and up to fivefold.[114,115] Fluoxetine and erythromycin may increase clozapine serum concentrations in some patients, but to a lesser degree.[111] Mean clozapine serum concentrations are reported to be 32% lower in smokers as compared with nonsmokers.[111] Carbamazepine may also induce clozapine metabolism and lead to lower serum concentrations.[111]

A study with the potent CYP 3A4 inhibitor ketoconazole showed minimal effects on ziprasidone single-dose pharmacokinetics, with only a 33% mean increase in the ziprasidone area under the time versus concentration curve.[31,64] These results are consistent with data suggesting that aldehyde oxidase is the major metabolic pathway for ziprasidone, with only 30% to 35% being metabolized by CYP 3A4.[64,116]

Antidepressants are commonly used in combination with antipsychotics to treat depressive symptoms in individuals with schizophrenia. Different antidepressants have been reported to inhibit metabolism of different P450 pathways.[112] Table 68–10 summarizes the potential drug interactions between antidepressants and atypical antipsychotics. Potential enzyme inhibitor interactions with clozapine are the most clinically significant. Increased clozapine serum concentrations with a CYP 1A2 inhibitor such as fluvoxamine may precipitate seizures.[112] With the newer atypical antipsychotics, enzyme inhibitors are more likely to cause side effects such as increased sedation, orthostatic hypotension, or increased risk of akathisia and other extrapyramidal side effects.

PHARMACOECONOMIC CONSIDERATIONS

It is estimated that approximately 80% of individuals suffering their first schizophrenic break will have recurrent episodes and significant lifetime psychosocial dysfunction. In 1991 prices, the cost of schizophrenia in the United States was estimated to be $65 billion, with $19 billion of this in direct costs.[117] The public mental health care sector provides the majority of services for individuals with schizophrenia. Mental health care costs for schizophrenia represent disproportionate expenditures for crisis intervention and hospitalization as compared to comprehensive outpatient services oriented toward maintaining remission and improving psychosocial functioning. The minimal funding provided for efficient ambulatory mental health services further enhances the demand for hospitalization which diverts additional revenues that might be available for outpatient services. This has created a vicious revolving door cycle with respect to patient care and is one of the major challenges facing public mental health care.

The advent of more expensive atypical APs, accompanied by limited resources, has forced mental health care organizations to examine the outcomes and related economics of treating patients with the atypical agents as compared with the traditional, largely generic APs. Although medication costs are higher with atypical APs than with traditional agents, studies with different atypical APs have fairly consistently shown total mental health costs to be no higher or even lower when atypical APs are used.[118,119,120] Naturalistic studies show that clozapine's use in treatment-resistant patients is associated with a decrease in total patient care costs of nearly $10,000 per patient annually.[26] In a randomized controlled study evaluating clozapine versus haloperidol in patients with high hospital utilization, clozapine was somewhat more effective in decreasing Brief Psychiatric Rating Scale (BPRS) scores and better tolerated than haloperidol while having similar overall costs from a societal perspective.[121]

Of greater controversy is whether differences in cost-effectiveness exist among the atypical APs. Significant differences in acquisition cost among the atypical APs have produced controversy regarding formulary decisions in organized health care settings.[122] For example, although daily medication costs are significantly higher with olanzapine than with risperidone, one modeling study of a Medicaid database showed no significant difference in total Medicaid costs (i.e.,

TABLE 68–10. Antidepressant/Antipsychotic P450 Drug Interactions

INHIBITOR (Inhibits Substrate)	SUBSTRATE (Drug Metabolized by Pathway) 1A2	2D6	3A3/4
Bupropion (Wellbutrin)		Phenothiazines (some), Thioridazine, Clozapine,[a] Olanzapine[a]	
Citalopram (Celexa)		Phenothiazines, Thioridazine, Clozapine,[a] Olanzapine[a]	
Fluoxetine (Prozac)		**PHENOTHIAZINES,**[b] **THIORIDAZINE,** Clozapine,[a] Olanzapine[a]	**Clozapine, Quetiapine,** Ziprasidone
Fluvoxamine (Luvox)	**CLOZAPINE, THIORIDAZINE, HALOPERIDOL, OLANZAPINE, THIOTHIXENE**		**Clozapine, Quetiapine,** Ziprasidone
Nefazodone (Serzone)			**QUETIAPINE, Clozapine,** Ziprasidone
Paroxetine (Paxil)		**PHENOTHIAZINES, THIORIDAZINE,** Clozapine,[a] Olanzapine[a]	
Sertraline (Zoloft)		Phenothiazines, Thioridazine, Clozapine,[a] Olanzapine[a]	Clozapine, Quetiapine, Ziprasidone

[a]Indicates that this is a minor pathway for this substrate, and therefore, the possibility of a clinically significant interaction through this pathway is decreased.
[b]The inhibitor drug inhibits the metabolism of the substrate drug; therefore increasing the amount of substrate drug in the body, and the potential for side effects from the substrate drug. Boldface and capital letters reflect the relative potential for the interaction to be clinically significant; i.e., **HIGH, Moderate,** Low.

medications plus services) between olanzapine and risperidone when the two groups were controlled for severity of mental and medical illnesses.[123] Although this type study should not be taken as conclusive evidence, it does point out that multiple factors should be considered when determining the costs of a course of treatment with APs.

EVALUATION OF THERAPEUTIC OUTCOMES

Assessment of response has traditionally been done subjectively or empirically (a relative sense of how the clinician feels the patient is doing). A formal mental status examination (MSE) is used to structure the patient interview and focus on items related to appearance, mood, sensorium, intellectual functioning, and thought processes. However, the MSE is not specific for the measurement of drug response. Realistically, clinicians should be trained to use simple, standardized psychiatric rating scales to assist in objectively rating patients' drug responses.[24,25,62] The BPRS and the Positive and Negative Syndrome Scale (PANSS) were developed for use in clinical trials as research tools to quantify symptoms and improvement seen with AP treatment.[25] Objectively, the use of a numeric indicator (e.g., 20%, 30%, or 40% reduction in BPRS score) has been used to quantify overall symptom reduction and classify patients according to different degrees of response. However, these types of rating scales are too long and unwieldy to be routinely used within the time constraints of most clinical practices. Symptom scales used in clinical practice must be sufficiently brief to be used during an ordinary clinic visit (e.g., 15 to 30 minutes) while measuring both positive and negative symptoms, and being sufficiently representative of overall symptomatology. The Brief Positive and Negative Symptom Scale, developed by Miller et al., is an eight-item scale that meets such criteria.[24,25]

Similarly, the pharmacotherapeutic plan should include specific monitoring parameters for potential side effects. The plan should include the side effects to be monitored (e.g., extrapyramidal side effects, weight increase), how the potential side effect will be evaluated, and the frequency of assessment (e.g., daily, weekly).

Self-assessments can be a useful adjunct in treating the patient. Although the patient with schizophrenia may not always be accurate in evaluating symptom severity (in fact, just the opposite may occur), the use of patient self-assessments increases patient engagement in care and gives the clinician an opportunity to identify misconceptions the patient may have regarding symptoms associated with the illness, medication side effects, and the like.[45,124]

Traditionally, clinicians have often accepted partial symptom response in schizophrenia as success, and have not been aggressive in attempting to achieve greater symptomatic remission. In many respects the side-effect profile of traditional APs encouraged the acceptance of partial response and a tendency to not "rock the boat" in a patient with partial improvement. However, the advent of multiple different atypical APs with favorable side-effect profiles should encourage clinicians to be more assertive in attempting to achieve symptom remission. Furthermore, the systematic use and evaluation of augmentation and combination treatment strategies may be of value in more treatment-resistant patients (see Fig. 68–1).

CONCLUSIONS

Schizophrenia is a complex disease with multiple ramifications for patients and their families. Treatment issues remain clouded by the fact that the etiology of the illness is unknown. It is clear, however, that no single treatment modality is adequate to properly manage a patient with schizophrenia. APs are not a panacea and have multiple adverse effects in addition to the limitations of their efficacy. However, the advent of newer medications offers new treatment options in schizophrenia. When used within the context of multidisciplinary treatment, APs assist in keeping psychotic symptoms under control so that patients can appropriately participate in psychosocial rehabilitation programs. Scientific advances continue to expand our understanding of CNS physiology and the abnormalities present in schizophrenia. Advances in our understanding of the pathophysiology of schizophrenia should, in turn, result in the development of treatments which are more specific and more effective.

In practice, it is mandatory that clinicians appropriately use their expanding armamentarium. It is important that clinicians appreciate the pharmacodynamic basis for treatment interventions so that they can effectively design and implement rational pharmacotherapeutic regimens. Finally, it is critical that clinicians more objectively evaluate individual patient response to medication so that treatment can be optimized. With these strategies, the gap between practice and science can be narrowed and patients' lives benefited.

▶ PRINCIPLES OF PHARMACOTHERAPY

- A thorough patient evaluation (e.g., history, mental status exam, physical exam, laboratory analysis) should occur to establish a diagnosis of schizophrenia and to identify potential comorbidities, including substance abuse and general medical disorders.
- Patient care must occur in the context of a multidisciplinary mental health care environment that offers medication and comprehensive psychosocial treatment.
- Pharmacotherapy algorithms should emphasize monotherapies with optimal efficacy to side-effect ratios and progress to medications with greater side-effect risks and to combination regimens in treatment-resistant patients.
- Patients should have input into specific treatment choices for schizophrenia.
- Pharmacotherapy decisions should be guided by systematic monitoring of patient symptoms, preferably with the use of symptom rating scales.
- Adequate time on a given medication at a therapeutic dose is the most important variable in predicting medication response.
- Long-term maintenance antipsychotic treatment is necessary for the vast majority of patients with schizophrenia.
- Depot antipsychotic treatment should, in general, be reserved for patients who are unreliable in taking oral medications on a daily basis.
- Thorough patient and family psychoeducation should occur, including education about the illness, symptoms, prognosis, medication, psychosocial treatments, and methods to improve adaptive functioning.
- Nondrug treatment should be oriented toward psychosocial rehabilitation programs that improve adaptive functioning, including supported work and housing.

REFERENCES

1. Schizophrenia and other psychotic disorders. In: Diagnostic and Statistical Manual of Mental Disorders, 4th ed. (DSM-IV-TR). Washington, DC: American Psychiatric Association, 2000:297–319.
2. Kane JM. Schizophenia. N Engl J Med 1996;334:34–41.
3. Heckers S. Neuropathology of schizophrenia: Cortex, thalamus, basal ganglia, and neurotransmitter-specific projection systems. Schizophr Bull 1997;23:403–421.
4. Goldman-Rakic PS, Selemon LD. Functional and anatomical aspects of prefrontal pathology in schizophrenia. Schizophr Bull 1997;23:437–458.
5. Brown AS, Schaefer CA, Wyatt RJ, et al. Maternal exposure to respiratory infections and adult schizophrenia spectrum disorders: A prospective birth cohort study. Schizophr Bull 2000;26:287–96.
6. Seidman LJ, Buka SL Goldstein JM, et al. The relationship of prenatal and perinatal complications to cognitive functioning at age 7 in the New England cohorts of the national collaborative prenatal project. Schizophr Bull 2000;26:309–322.
7. Arnold SE. Neurodevelopmental abnormalities in schizophrenia: Insights from neuropathology. Dev Psychopathol 1999;11:439–456.
8. Andreasen NC. Schizophrenia: The fundamental questions. Brain Res Brain Res Rev 2000;31:106–112.
9. Kendler KS, Diehl SR. The genetics of schizophrenia: A current, genetic, epidemiologic perspective. In: Shore D, ed. Schizophrenia 1993. Rockville, MD, National Institute of Mental Health, 1993:87–111.
10. Mowry BJ, Nancauow DJ. Molecular genetics of schizophrenia. Clin Exp Pharmacol Physiol 2001;28:66–69.
11. Gur RE, Pearlson GD. Neuroimaging in schizophrenia research. In: Shore D, ed. Schizophrenia 1993. Rockville, MD, National Institute of Mental Health, 1993:163–179.
12. Ereshefsky L, Tran-Johnson TK, Watanabe MD. Pathophysiologic basis for schizophrenia and the efficacy of antipsychotics. Clin Pharm 1990;9:682–707.
13. Lieberman JA, Koreen AR. Neurochemistry and neuroendocrinology of schizophrenia: A selective review. In: Shore D, ed. Schizophrenia 1993. Rockville, MD, National Institute of Mental Health, 1993:197–255.
14. Gur RF. Functional brain-imaging studies in schizophrenia. In: Bloom FE, Kupfer DJ, eds. Psychopharmacology: The Fourth Generation of Progress. New York, Raven, 1995:1185–1192.
15. Henn FA. The NMDA receptor as a site for psychopathology. Primary or secondary role? Arch Gen Psychiatry 1995;52:1008–1010.
16. Olney JW, Farber NB. Response to commentaries and to the challenge of building a perfect theory to explain schizophrenia. Arch Gen Psychiatry 1995;52:1019–1024.
17. Olney JW, Farber NB. Glutamate receptor dysfunction and schizophrenia. Arch Gen Psychiatry 1995;52:998–1007.
18. Huttunen M. The evolution of the serotonin-dopamine antagonist concept. J Clin Psychopharmacol 1995;15(suppl 1):4S–10S.
19. Heritch AJ. Evidence for reduced and dysregulated turnover of dopamine in schizophrenia. Schizophr Bull 1990;16:605–615.
20. Lieberman JA. Atypical antipsychotic drugs as a first-line treatment of schizophrenia: A rationale and hypothesis. J Clin Psychiatry 1996; 57(suppl 11):68–71.
21. Kane JM. Treatment-resistant schizophrenic patients. J Clin Psychiatry 1996;57(suppl 9):35–40.
22. Herz MI, Work Group on Schizophrenia, American Psychiatric Association. Practice guideline for the treatment of patients with schizophrenia. Am J Psychiatry 1997;154(suppl 4):1–63.
23. Frances A, Docherty JP, Kahn DA, et al. Treatment of schizophrenia, 1999. The expert consensus guideline series. 1999;60(suppl 11):3–80.
24. Miller AL, Chiles JA, Chiles J, Crismon ML. TIMA procedural manual: Schizophrenia algorithm. Austin, TX, Texas Department of Mental Health and Mental Retardation, 2000. May be accessed at http://www.mhmr.state.tx.us/CentralOffice/MedicalDirector/timasczman.pdf
25. Miller AL, Chiles JA, Chiles JK, et al. The TMAP schizophrenia algorithms. J Clin Psychiatry 1999;60:649–657.
26. Meltzer HY. Atypical antipsychotic drugs. In: Bloom FE, Kupfer DJ, eds. Psychopharmacology: The Fourth Generation of Progress. New York, Raven, 1995:1277–1286.
27. Marder SR, Meibach RC, risperidone study group. Risperidone in the treatment of schizophrenia. Am J Psychiatry 1994;151:825–835.
28. Fulton B, Goa KL. Olanzapine. A review of its pharmacological properties and therapeutic efficacy in the management of schizophrenia and related psychoses. Drugs 1997;53:281–298.
29. Small JG, Hirsch SR, Arvanitis LA, et al. Quetiapine in patients with schizophrenia. A high- and low-dose double-blind comparison with placebo. Arch Gen Psychiatry 1997;54:549–557.
30. Daniel DG, Zimbroff DL Potkin SG, et al. Ziprasidone 80 mg/day and 160 mg/day in the acute exacerbation of schizophrenia and schizoaffective disorder: A 6-week placebo-controlled trial. Neuropsychopharmacology 1999;20:491–505.
31. Briefing document for Zeldox capsules (ziprasidone HCl). FDA Psychopharmacological Drugs Advisory Committee. New York, Pfizer Pharmaceuticals, July 19, 2000.
32. Gilcrest L. Advisory panel recommends approval of Pfizer's Zeldox for schizophrenia. Reuter Medical News, July 20, 2000.
33. Drugs that cause psychiatric symptoms. Med Lett Drugs Ther 1993; 35:65–70.
34. Awad AG. Drug therapy in schizophrenia: Variability of outcome and prediction of response. Can J Psychiatry 1989;34:711–720.
35. Van Putten T, Marder SR. Behavioral toxicity of anti-psychotic drugs. J Clin Psychiatry 1987;48(suppl 9):13–19.
36. Mossman D. A decision analysis approach to neuroleptic dosing: Insights from a mathematical model. J Clin Psychiatry 1997;58:66–73.
37. Wirshing WC, Marder SR, Van Putten T, Ames D. Acute treatment of schizophrenia. In: Bloom FE, Kupfer DJ, eds. Psychopharmacology: The Fourth Generation of Progress. New York, Raven, 1995:1259–1266.
38. Revised patient outcomes research team (PORT) recommendations. Personal communication. Anthony Lehman, Baltimore, MD, February 2001.
39. Csernansky JG, Newcomer JG. Maintenance drug treatment for schizophrenia. In: Bloom FE, Kupfer DJ, eds. Psychopharmacology: The Fourth Generation of Progress. New York, Raven, 1995:1267–1275.
40. Herz MI, Glazer WM, Mostert MA, et al. Intermittent vs maintenance medication in schizophrenia: Two-year results. Arch Gen Psychiatry 1991;48:333–339.
41. Ereshefsky L, Saklad SR, Jann MW, et al. Future of depot neuroleptic therapy: Pharmacokinetics and pharmacodynamic approaches. J Clin Psychiatry 1984;45:50.
42. Ereshefsky L, Toney G, Saklad SR, Seidel DR. A loading-dose strategy for converting from oral to depot haloperidol. Hosp Comm Psychiatry 1993;44:1155–1161.
43. Pabis DJ, Dorson PG, Crismon ML. Evaluation of inpatient depot antipsychotic prescribing. Ann Pharmacother 1996;30:1381–1386.
44. Hamann GL, Egan TM, Wells BG, et al. Injection site reactions after intramuscular administration of haloperidol decanoate 100 mg/mL. J Clin Psychiatry 1990;51:502–504.
45. Toprac MG, Rush AJ, Conner TM, et al. The Texas Medication Algorithm Project patient and family education program: A consumer-guided initiative. J Clin Psychiatry 2000;61:477–486.
46. Rush AJ, Crismon ML, Toprac MG, et al. Implementing guidelines and systems of care: Experiences with the Texas Medication Algorithm Project (TMAP). J Pract Psychiatry Behav Health 1999;5:75–86.
47. Kane J, Honigfeld G, Singer J, et al. Clozapine for the treatment-resistant schizophrenic: A double-blind comparison with chlorpromazine. Arch Gen Psychiatry 1988;45:789–796.
48. Spears NM, Leadbetter RA, Shutty MS. Clozapine treatment in polydipsia and intermittent hyponatremia. J Clin Psychiatry 1996;57:123–128.
49. Canales PL, Olsen J, Miller AL, Crismon ML. The role of antipsychotic polypharmacotherapy in the treatment of schizophrenia. CNS Drugs 1999;12:179–188.
50. Pickard D, Litman RE, Konicki PE, et al. Neurochemical and neural mechanisms of positive and negative symptoms in schizophrenia. In: Andreason NC, ed. Schizophrenia: Positive and Negative Symptoms and

Syndromes. Modern Problems in Pharmacopsychiatry. Basel, Karger, 1990;24:124–151.

51. Wassef AA, Dott SG, Harris A, et al. Randomized, placebo-controlled pilot study of divalproex sodium in the treatment of acute exacerbations of chronic schizophrenia. J Clin Psychopharmacol 2000;20:367–361.
52. Lipinski JF, Keck PE, McElroy SL. β-Adrenergic antagonists in psychosis: Is improvement due to treatment of neuroleptic-induced akathisia? J Clin Psychopharmacol 1988;8:409–416.
53. Yudolfsky SC, Silver JM, Hales RE. Pharmacologic management of aggression in the elderly. J Clin Psychiatry 1990;5(suppl 10):22–28.
54. Kapur S, Roy, P, Daskalakis J, Remington G. Increased dopamine D2 receptor occupancy and elevated prolactin level associated with addition of haloperidol to clozapine. Am J Psychiatry 2001;158:311–314.
55. Nyberg S, Eriksson B, Oxenstierna G, et al. Suggested minimal effective dose of risperidone based on PET-measured D2 and 5-HT2A receptor occupancy in schizophrenic patients. Am J Psychiatry 1999;156: 869–875.
56. Kapur S, Zipursky RB, Remington G. Clinical and theoretical implications of 5-HT2 and D2 receptor occupancy of clozapine, risperidone, and olanzapine in schizophrenia. Am J Psychiatry 1999;156:286–293.
57. Kapur S, Seaman S. Does fast dissociation from the dopamine D2 receptor explain the action of atypical antipsychotics: a new hypothesis. Am J Psychiatry 2001;158:360–396.
58. Kapur S, Zipursky RB, Remington G, Jones C. 5-HT2 and D2 receptor occupancy of olanzapine in schizophrenia: A PET investigation. Am J Psychiatry 1998;155:921–928.
59. Kapur S, Zipursky RB, Jones C, et al. A positron emission tomography study of quetiapine in schizophrenia: A preliminary finding of an antipsychotic effect with only transiently high dopamine D2 receptor occupancy. Arch Gen Psychiatry 2000;57:553–559.
60. Kapur S. A new framework for investigating antipsychotic action in humans: Lessons from PET imaging. Mol Psychiatry 1998;3:135–140.
61. Richelson E. Preclinical pharmacology of neuroleptics: Focus on new-generation compounds. J Clin Psychiatry 1996;57(suppl 11):4–11.
62. Miller AL, Dassori A, Ereshefsky L, Crismon ML. Recent issues and developments in antipsychotic use. In: Dunner DL, Rosenbaum JF, eds. Psychiatric Clinics of North America Annual Review of Drug Therapy 2001. Philadelphia, WB Saunders, 2001;8:209–235.
63. Ereshefsky L. Pharmacokinetics and drug interactions: Update for new antipsychotics. J Clin Psychiatry 1996;57(suppl 11):12–25.
64. Pfizer Inc. Ziprasidone (Geodon) package insert. New York, February 2001.
65. Perry PJ, Miller DD, Arndt SV, Cadoret RJ. Clozapine and norclozapine plasma concentrations and clinical response of treatment-refractory schizophrenic patients. Am J Psychiatry 1991;148:231–235.
66. VanderZwaag C, McGee M, McEvoy JP, et al. Response of patients with treatment-refractory schizophrenia to clozapine within three serum level ranges. Am J Psychiatry 1996;153:1579–1584.
67. Crismon ML. Psychotropic drugs in the elderly: Principles of use. Am Pharm 1990;NS30:57–63.
68. Holloman LC, Marder SR. Management of acute extrapyramidal effects induced by antipsychotic drugs. Am J Health Syst Pharm 1997;54: 2461–2477.
69. Arana GW, Goff DC, Baldessarini RJ, Keepers GA. Efficacy of ACh prophylaxis for neuroleptic-induced acute dystonia. Am J Psychiatry 1988;145:993–996.
70. Fleischhacker WW, Roth SD, Kane JM. The pharmacologic treatment of neuroleptic-induced akathisia. J Clin Psychopharmacol 1990;10: 12–21.
71. Wells BG, Marken PA, Rickman LA, et al. Characterizing anticholinergic abuse in community mental health. J Clin Psychopharmacol 1989;9: 431–435.
72. Conley RR, et al. Risperidone versus olanzapine in patients with schizophrenia and schizoaffective disorder. Atlanta, GA, Abstracts of the US Psychiatric and Mental Health Congress, November 11–14, 1999.
73. Sprague RL, Kalachnik JE. Reliability, validity, and a total score cutoff for the Dyskinesia Identification System Condensed User Scale (DISCUS) with mentally ill and mentally retarded populations. Psychopharmacol Bull 1991;27:51–58.
74. Silveresti CM, Seeman MV, Negrete JC, et al. Increased dopamine D2 receptor binding after long-term treatment with antipsychotics in humans: A clinical PET study. Psychopharmacology 2000;152:174–180.
75. Egan MF, Apud J, Wyatt RJ. Treatment of tardive dyskinesia. Schizophr Bull 1997;23:583–609.
76. Tandon R, Kasper S, Kane J, Juncos J. The scourge of extrapyramidal side effects: Have atypical antipsychotics solved the problem? J Clin Psychiatry 2000;61:955–962.
77. Chouinard G, Annable L, Mercier P, Ross-Chouinard A. A five-year follow-up study of tardive dyskinesia. Psychopharmacol Bull 1986;22:259–263.
78. Gardos G, Cole JO, Salomon M, Schniebolk S. Clinical forms of severe tardive dyskinesia. Am J Psychiatry 1987;144:895–902.
79. Chouinard G. Effects of risperidone in tardive dyskinesia: An analysis of the Canadian multicenter risperidone study. J Clin Psychopharmacol 1995;15(suppl 1):36S–44S.
80. Beasley CM, Dellva MA, Tamura RN, et al. Randomised double-blind comparison of the incidence of tardive dyskinesia in patients with schizophrenia during long-term treatment with olanzapine or haloperidol. Br J Psychiatry 1999;174:23–30.
81. Soares KV, McGrath JJ. Vitamin E for neuroleptic-induced tardive dyskinesia. Cochrane Database Syst Rev 2000;13(2):CD000209.
82. Cassens G, Inglis AK, Appelbaum PS, Gutheil TG. Neuroleptics: Effects on neuropsychological function in chronic schizophrenic patients. Schizophr Bull 1990;16:477–499.
83. Garcia G, Crismon ML, Dorson PG. Seizures in two patients after the addition of lithium to a clozapine regimen. J Clin Psychopharmacol 1994;14:426–428.
84. Lee JW, Crismon ML, Dorson PG. Seizure associated with olanzapine use. Ann Pharmacother 1999;33:554–556.
85. Simpson GM, Pi EH, Sramek JJ. Adverse effects of AP agents. Drugs 1981;21:138–151.
86. Guze BH, Baxter Jr LR. Neuroleptic malignant syndrome. N Engl J Med 1985;313:163–166.
87. Sakkas P, Davis JM, Hua J, et al. Pharmacotherapy of neuroleptic malignant syndrome. Psychiatr Ann 1991;21:157–164.
88. Wells AJ, Sommi RW, Crismon ML. Neuroleptic rechallenge after neuroleptic malignant syndrome: Case report and literature review. Drug Intell Clin Pharm 1988;22:475–480.
89. Levin Z, Hwang MY, Rotrosen J. The relationship between clozapine and obsessive-compulsive disorder. Comp Psychiatry 1996;37:74.
90. Zito JM, Sofair JB, Jaeger J. Self-reported neuroendocrine effects of APs in women: A pilot study. DICP 1990;24:176–180.
91. Allison DB, Mentore JL, Heo M, et al. Antipsychotic-induced weight gain: A comprehensive research synthesis. Am J Psychiatry 1999;156: 1686–1696.
92. Bettinger TL, Mendelson SC, Dorson PG, Crismon ML. Olanzapine-induced glucose dysregulation. Ann Pharmacother 2000;34:865–867.
93. Henderson DC, Cagliero E, Gray C, et al. Clozapine, diabetes mellitus, weight gain and lipid abnormalities: A five-year naturalistic study. Am J Psychiatry 2000;157:975–981.
94. Oshika T. Ocular adverse effects of neuropsychiatric agents: Incidence and management. Drug Saf 1995;12:256–263.
95. Zeneca Pharmaceuticals. Quetiapine (Seroquel) package insert. Wilmington, DE, September 2000.
96. Regal RE, Billi JE, Glazer HM. Phenothiazine-induced cholestatic jaundice. Clin Pharm 1987;6:787–794.
97. Nurnberg HG, Ambrosini PJ. Urinary incontinence in patients receiving neuroleptics. J Clin Psychiatry 1979;40:271–274.
98. Sullivan G, Lukoff D. Sexual side effects of AP medication: Evaluation and interventions. Hosp Community Psychiatry 1990;41:1238–1241.
99. Balon R, Berchou R. Hematologic side effects of psychotropic drugs. Psychosomatics 1986;27:119–120, 125–127.
100. Alvir JMJ, Lieberman JA, Safferman AZ, et al. Clozapine-induced agranulocytosis: Incidence and risk factors in the United States. N Engl J Med 1993;329:162–167.

101. Zhang M, Owen RR, Pope SK, Smith GR. Cost-effectiveness of clozapine monitoring after the first 6 months. Arch Gen Psychiatry 1996;53:954–958.
102. Gullion G, Yeh HS. Treatment of clozapine-induced agranulocytosis with recombinant granulocyte colony-stimulating factor. J Clin Psychiatry 1994;55:401–405.
103. Dorson PG, Crismon ML. CPZ accumulation and sudden death in a patient with renal insufficiency. Drug Intell Clin Pharm 1988;22:776–778.
104. Ereshefsky L, Watanabe MD, Tran-Johnson TK. Clozapine: An atypical antipsychotic agent. Clin Pharm 1989;8:691–709.
105. Grabowski J. Clonidine treatment of clozapine-induced hypersalivation. J Clin Psychopharmacol 1992;12:69–70.
106. Perry PJ, Alexander B, Liskow B. Psychotropic Drug Handbook, 7th ed. Washington, DC, American Psychiatric Press, 1997:1–129.
107. American Academy of Pediatrics Committee on Drugs. Use of psychoactive medication during pregnancy and possible effects on the fetus and newborn. Pediatrics 2000;105:880–887.
108. McEvoy GK, ed. AHFS Drug Information 2001. Bethesda, MD, American Society of Health-System Pharmacists, 2001:2830–2836.
109. Stoudemire A, Moran MG. Psychopharmacology in the medically ill patient. In: Schatzberg AF, Nemeroff CB, eds. Textbook of Psychopharmacology, 2nd ed. Washington, DC, American Psychiatric Press, 1998:931–959.
110. Hartigan-Go K, Bateman DN, Nyberg G, Martensson E, Thomas SH. Concentration-related pharmacodynamic effects of thioridazine and its metabolites in humans. Clin Pharmacol Ther 1996;60:543–553.
111. DeVane CL, Markowitz JS. Antipsychotics. In: Levy RH, Thummel KE, Trager WF, et al. Metabolic Drug Interactions. Philadelphia, Lippincott-William & Wilkins, 2000:245–258.
112. DeVane CL, Nemeroff CB. Psychotropic drug interactions 2000. TEN 2000;2(1):55–75.
113. Roby CA, Anderson GD, Kantor E, et al. St John's wort: Effect on CYP3A4 activity. Clin Pharmacol Ther 2000;67:451–457.
114. Chang WH, Augustin B, Lane HY, et al. *In vitro* and *in vivo* evaluation of drug-drug interaction between fluvoxamine and clozapine. Psychopharmacology 1999;145:91–98.
115. Wetzel H, Anghelescu I, Szegedi A, et al. Pharmacokinetic interactions of clozapine with selective serotonin reuptake inhibitors: Differential effects of fluvoxamine and paroxetine in a prospective study. J Clin Psychopharmacol 1998;18:2–9.
116. Prakash C, Kamel A, Cui D, et al. Identification of the major human liver cytochrome P450 isoform(s) responsible for the formation of the primary metabolites of ziprasidone and prediction of possible drug interactions. Br J Clin Pharmacol 2000;49(suppl 1):35S–42S.
117. Wyatt RJ, Henter I, Leary MC, et al. An economic evaluation of schizophrenia—1991. Psych Psych Epidemiol 1995;30(5):196–205.
118. Glazer WM. Formulary decisions and health economics. J Clin Psychiatry 1998;59(suppl 19):23–29.
119. Nightengale BS, Crumly JM, Liao J, et al. Economic outcomes of antipsychotic agents in a medicaid population: Traditional agents vs. risperidone. Psychopharm Bull 1998;34:373–82.
120. Almonds S, O'Donnell O. Cost analysis of the treatment of schizophrenia in the UK: A comparison of olanzapine and haloperidol. Pharmacoeconomics 1998;13:575–588.
121. Rosenheck R, Cramer J, Xu W, et al. A comparison of clozapine and haloperidol in hospitalized patients with refractory schizophrenia. N Engl J Med 1997;337:809–815.
122. Johnsrud M, Crismon ML, Thompson A, Grogg A. Risperidone and olanzapine utilization and expenditures within the Texas Medicaid program. Abstracts of the 2001 American Psychiatric Association Annual Meeting 2001;NR703:190.
123. Rascati KL, Johnsrud M, Crismon ML, et al. Olanzapine versus risperidone in the treatment of schizophrenia: A comparison of costs among Texas Medicaid patients. Abstracts of the 5th Annual Meeting of the International Society for Pharmacoeconomics and Outcomes Research. Value in Health 2001;5:PMH33. Value in Health 2001;4:151.
124. Chiles JA, Miller AL, Crismon ML, et al. The Texas Medication Algorithm project: Development and implementation of the schizophrenic algorithm. Psychiatr Serv 1999;50:69–74.

69

DEPRESSIVE DISORDERS

Judith C. Kando, Barbara G. Wells, and Peggy E. Hayes

Mood disorders (affective disorders) are among the most common mental disorders encountered in clinical practice and are divided into bipolar disorders and depressive disorders. The essential feature of these disorders is a major disturbance in mood. *Mood* is defined as a pervasive and sustained emotion that, in the extreme, markedly affects the person's perception of the world and ability to function adequately in society. A *mood disorder* occurs when a mood disturbance is combined with certain associated symptoms that impair the person's ability to function for a specific duration of time. Bipolar disorders (discussed in Chap. 70) refer to patients who have episodes of mania and/or hypomania usually alternating with episodes of depression.[1]

Patients with depressive disorders do not have episodes of mania or hypomania. Historically, various names (or classifications) have been used to describe depressive disorders, including *reactive, unipolar, psychotic and neurotic, exogenous and endogenous, agitated and retarded, primary and secondary,* and *involutional melancholia.*[2] Currently, the criteria listed in the *Diagnostic and Statistical Manual of Mental Disorders,* fourth edition, text revision (DSM-IV-TR), published by the American Psychiatric Association, are used to diagnose individuals with depressive disorders.[1] The use of these standardized criteria has greatly improved clinicians' ability to correctly diagnose and appropriately treat depressive disorders. Major depressive disorder and dysthymic disorder are two types of depressive disorders listed in the DSM-IV-TR. Dysthymic disorder is a chronic disturbance of mood involving depressed mood combined with at least two other symptoms such as appetite or sleep disturbance, low energy, low self-esteem, hopelessness, poor concentration, and indecisiveness. In addition, the patient has experienced a depressed mood more days than not for at least 2 years.[1] However, these symptoms are not of sufficient severity or duration to meet the specified criteria for major depression. This chapter focuses exclusively on the diagnosis and treatment of major depressive disorder.

Major depressive disorder is a common health problem of patients treated in primary care settings. Depression is associated with a high level of functional disability and increased use of outpatient medical services.[3,4] A 2-year follow-up study concluded that depressed patients have substantial and long-lasting impairments in social and physical functioning that equals or exceeds those of patients with chronic medical conditions.[5]

A frequent complication of depression is suicide. Approximately 15% of patients with unrecognized or inadequately treated depression commit suicide; this is approximately 30 times the rate of occurrence in nondepressed patients.[2,6] Although adequate treatment reduces the risk of suicide and improves functioning and well-being, studies conducted in primary care settings reported that even when depression is diagnosed accurately, few patients receive an adequate dose and duration of antidepressant treatment. The gap between research findings and clinical practice is especially wide in the management of depression.[3]

The introduction of effective antidepressant drugs with more favorable and distinctly different adverse event profiles and relatively greater safety in an overdose situation has enabled more patients to be managed successfully. Continuing developments in the management of depression and education of health care professionals will help to lessen the gap between research findings and clinical practice.

EPIDEMIOLOGY

The true prevalence of depressive disorders in the United States is unknown. Only 31% of depressed adults actually seek treatment.[7] The National Comorbidity Survey (NCS) reported that 17% of the population studied had a history of major depressive disorder in their lifetime, and more than 10% had an episode within the past 12 months.[8] Evidence from an earlier investigation supports increasing rates and a decreasing age of onset of depression in persons born after World War II, but a more recent evaluation found a stable current prevalence of depression when data from 1952 were compared with 1970.[9,10] There was a redistribution of occurrence of depression by sex and age, with a higher rate among younger women.[10]

Depression is two to three times as frequent in females as in males.[1,8] Although depression can occur at any age, adults 25 to 44 years of age experience the highest rates of major depression.[8] The estimated lifetime prevalence of major depression in individuals aged 65 to 80 recently was found to be 20.4% in women and 9.6% in men, decreasing with age.[7] Depressive disorders are common during adolescence, with comorbid substance abuse, suicide attempts, and deaths occurring frequently in these young patients.[11,12] Patients with depressive disorders frequently develop another psychiatric illness (comorbidity), especially anxiety disorders and alcoholism.[2,8]

Depressive disorders and suicide tend to cluster in families, and first-degree relatives of patients with depression are one and a half to three times more likely to develop depression than normal controls.[1,13,14] Approximately 8% to 18% of patients with major depression have at least one first-degree relative (father, mother, brother, or sister) with a history of depression compared with 5.6% of the first-degree relatives of a normal control group.[13,15] A recent twin study found that the heritability of liability to major depression was the same in men and women and equal to 39%, whereas the remaining 61% of the variance in liability was due to individual-specific environment.[15] Furthermore, the odds ratios for the occurrence of lifetime major depression in the second twin when the first twin already had developed major depression were 3.02 (females) and 3.29 (males) for monozygotic (identical) twins versus 1.59 (females) and 1.09 (males) for dizygotic twins.[15]

ETIOLOGY

The etiology of depressive disorders is too complex to be totally explained by a single social, developmental, or biologic theory. Several factors appear to work together to cause or precipitate depressive disorders. The symptoms reported by patients with major depression consistently reflect changes in brain monoamine neurotransmitters, specifically norepinephrine (NE), serotonin (5-HT), and dopamine (DA).[16–18] Although life is filled with unexpected events that cause pain (e.g., death of a loved one, loss of a job, major illness), not everyone becomes depressed. Most individuals adjust to life's challenges and suffer only mild, transient dysphoric feelings. However, other individuals exposed to these psychosocial stressors experience a major depressive episode. The initial episodes of depression, in contrast to later episodes, are more likely to be associated with stressful life events.[19] Certain factors (e.g., stressful events, medical illness, monoamine-depleting drugs) may place predisposed individuals, especially those with a family or personal history of depression, at high risk for developing a major depressive episode.[19]

PATHOPHYSIOLOGY

BIOGENIC AMINE HYPOTHESIS

The biogenic amine hypothesis came about as a result of several observations made in the early 1950s. One of these involved the antihypertensive drug reserpine. It was noted that reserpine depleted neuronal storage granules of NE, 5-HT, and DA and produced clinically significant depression in 15% or more of patients.[20] In addition, it was discovered that the hallucinogen lysergic acid diethylamide (LSD) blocked peripheral serotonin receptors. The conclusion was made that the mind-altering effects of LSD were secondary to similar effects on central serotonin.[18] However, this early hypothesis failed to explain the actual cause of depression. Although reuptake blockade or monoamine oxidase (MAO) inhibition occurs immediately on administration of an antidepressant, the clinical antidepressant effects generally are not observed until after 4 weeks of dosing.[21] Understanding the precise pathophysiology of depression requires further research, perhaps with a focus on the adaptive changes induced by antidepressants.[17]

PERMISSIVE HYPOTHESIS

In the early 1970s, Prange and colleagues put forth the "permissive hypothesis of affective illness" regarding the possible role of both NE and 5-HT in causing depression.[22] The theory states that decreased 5-HT levels permit the expression of the affective state, but the level of NE governs the type. Decreased NE levels cause depression, and elevated NE levels cause mania. According to this hypothesis, correcting the deficiency in 5-HT activity corrects the affective disease.

THEORIES OF POSTSYNAPTIC CHANGES IN RECEPTOR SENSITIVITY

A more perplexing aspect of the observed effects of antidepressants is the discrepancy between monoamine reuptake blockade (immediate) and any measurable improvement in depressive symptomatology (delayed). Accordingly, theories that focus on adaptive (or chronic) changes in amine receptor systems compared with acute changes emerged.

In the mid-1970s, it was recognized that chronic, but not acute, administration of antidepressants to animals caused desensitization of NE-stimulated cyclic AMP synthesis. In fact, for most antidepressants, downregulation of β-adrenergic receptors accompanies this desensitization.[23]

Studies of many antidepressants have demonstrated that either desensitization or downregulation of NE receptors corresponds to a clinically relevant time course for antidepressant effects.[16] Other studies have revealed downregulation of 5-HT_2 receptors following chronic administration of antidepressants.[24,25] Thus a theory based on postsynaptic changes in receptor sensitivity provides a cogent explanation of the delayed onset of activity of antidepressant drugs.[16]

DYSREGULATION HYPOTHESIS

The dysregulation hypothesis incorporates the diversity of antidepressant activity with the adaptive changes occurring in receptor sensitization over several weeks.[26] In this theory, emphasis is placed on a failure of homeostatic regulation of neurotransmitter systems rather than on absolute increases or decreases in their activities.[21,22] According to this hypothesis, effective antidepressant agents restore efficient regulation to the dysregulated neurotransmitter system.[26,27]

5-HT/NE LINK HYPOTHESIS

It is apparent that no single neurotransmitter theory of depression is adequate. The 5-HT/NE link hypothesis maintains that both the serotonergic and noradrenergic systems need to be functional for an antidepressant effect to be exerted.[17,24] The 5-HT/NE link hypothesis is also consistent with the rationale of the postsynaptic alteration theory of depression, which emphasizes the importance of β-adrenergic receptor downregulation for achieving an antidepressant effect.[23] Again, it has been proposed that both NE and 5-HT are necessary for homologous desensitization of central β-adrenergic receptors by antidepressants.[24]

ROLE OF DA IN DEPRESSION

Traditional explanations of the biologic basis of depressive disorders have focused largely on NE and 5-HT; however, most of the evidence that coalesced into the biogenic amine hypothesis of depression does not clearly distinguish between NE and DA.[28]

Several reviews suggest that elevation of DA neurotransmission in the nucleus accumbens may represent a final common pathway for at least part of the mechanism of action of antidepressant medications.[19,29] The mechanisms by which antidepressant drugs sensitize DA transmission remain unclear but may be mediated indirectly by primary actions at NE or 5-HT terminals.

The evidence supporting a dopaminergic mechanism of antidepressant action is entirely preclinical, and clinical studies evaluating the role of DA mechanisms in the action of classical antidepressants have not been conducted.[28]

The complexity of the interaction between 5-HT, NE, and possibly DA is gaining greater appreciation, but a more in-depth understanding of the precise mechanism is needed.

BIOLOGIC MARKERS

Investigators continue to search for biologic markers to assist in the diagnosis and treatment of depressed patients. Although no biologic marker has been discovered, several interesting biologic abnormalities are present in many depressed patients. Approximately 45% to 60% of patients with major depression have a neuroendocrine abnormality, including hypersecretion of cortisol, lack of cortisol suppression after dexamethasone administration [i.e., a positive dexamethasone suppression test (DST)], or an abnormal or diminished thyroid-stimulating hormone (TSH) response to the administration of thyrotropin-releasing hormone (TRH). The DST is the most specific measure of hypothalamic-pituitary-adrenal (HPA) axis overactivity. Dexamethasone administration suppresses adrenal corticosteroid production in normal subjects for 24 hours. Failure of dexamethasone to suppress plasma cortisol concentrations indicates overactivity or dysregulation of the HPA axis. Unfortunately, the high rate of false-positive and false-negative results limits the usefulness of testing for these markers and has lead to their relative lack of use in clinical practice.

Sleep studies in patients with major depression have identified several abnormalities that become more pronounced with advancing age. The onset of rapid eye movement (REM) sleep occurs sooner in depressed patients (decreased REM latency) than in the normal population. There also may be a decrease in slow-wave sleep, a shift of REM sleep activity to the first half of the night, increased disruption of sleep, and early morning awakening.[30] Sleep abnormalities occur in other psychiatric disorders and are not diagnostic for major depression.

CLINICAL PRESENTATION

When a patient presents with depressive symptoms, it is necessary to investigate the possibility of a medical, psychiatric, and/or drug-induced cause[31] (Table 69–1). Up to 25% of patients with chronic medical conditions (e.g., diabetes, myocardial infarction, carcinomas, stroke) will develop a major depressive episode during the course of their medical condition, and the depression often is not accurately diagnosed, especially in the elderly.[1,6]

All depressed patients, especially the elderly, should have a complete physical examination, mental status examination, and basic laboratory workup, including a complete blood count with differential, thyroid function tests, and electrolyte determinations, to identify any potential medical problems. A complete medication review should be performed because many drugs (e.g., propranolol[32]) may precipitate or worsen a depressive episode (see Table 69–1).

Major depressive disorder is characterized by one or more episodes of major depression. A major depressive episode is characterized by five or more of the symptoms described in Table 69–2. At least one of the symptoms is depressed mood (often an irritable mood in children or adolescents) or loss of interest or pleasure in nearly all activities.[1] The five symptoms must have been present nearly every day for at least 2 weeks and must represent a change from previous functioning. The clinician must consider presenting symptoms, their duration, and the patient's current level of social, occupational, or other important areas of functioning. Significant stressors or life events may trigger depression in some individuals but not others; and there may be an important precipitant at the beginning of the disorder.[1,19]

TABLE 69–2. DSM-IV-TR Criteria for Major Depressive Episode

A. Five (or more) of the following symptoms have been present during the same 2-week period and represent a change from previous functioning; at least one of the symptoms is either (1) depressed mood or (2) loss of interest or pleasure.

Note: Do not include symptoms that are clearly due to a general medical condition or mood-incongruent delusions or hallucinations.

1. Depressed mood most of the day nearly every day
2. Markedly diminished interest or pleasure in all, or almost all, activities most the day nearly every day
3. Significant weight loss when not dieting or weight gain (e.g., a change of more than 5% of body weight in a month), or decrease or increase in appetite nearly every day
4. Insomnia or hypersomnia nearly every day
5. Psychomotor agitation or retardation nearly every day (observable by others, not merely subjective feelings of restlessness or being slowed down)
6. Fatigue or loss of energy nearly every day
7. Feelings of worthlessness or excessive or inappropriate guilt (which may be delusional) nearly every day
8. Diminished ability to think or concentrate, or indecisiveness, nearly every day
9. Recurrent thoughts of death (not just fear of dying), recurrent suicidal ideation without a specific plan, or a suicide attempt or a specific plan for committing suicide

B. The symptoms cause clinically significant distress or impairment in social, occupational, or other important areas of functioning.

C. The symptoms are not due to the direct physiological effects of a substance (e.g., a drug of abuse, a medication) or a general medical condition (e.g., hypothyroidism).

D. The symptoms are not better accounted for by bereavement (i.e., after the loss of a loved one), the symptoms persist for longer than 2 months or are characterized by marked functional impairment, morbid preoccupation with worthlessness, suicidal ideation, psychotic symptoms, or psychomotor retardation.

Modified and reprinted with permission from the Diagnostic and Statistical Manual of Mental Disorders, 4th ed., text revision. Washington, DC. American Psychiatric Association, 2000.

TABLE 69–1. Common Medical Disorders, Psychiatric Disorders, and Drug Therapy Associated With Depression

Medical Disorders	Metabolic disorders	Anxiety disorders
Endocrine diseases	Electrolyte imbalance	Eating disorders
Hyperthyroidism	Hypokalemia	Schizophrenia
Hypothyroidism	Hyponatremia	**Drug Therapy**
Addison's disease	Hepatic encephalopathy	Alcohol
Cushing's disease	Cardiovascular disease	Antihypertensives
Deficiency states	Cerebral arteriosclerosis	Reserpine
Pernicious anemia	Congestive heart failure	Methyldopa
Wernicke's encephalopathy	Myocardial infarction	Propranolol hydrochloride
Severe anemia	Neurologic disorders	Guanethidine sulfate
Infections	Alzheimer's disease	Hydralazine hydrochloride
Encephalitis	Huntington's disease	Clonidine hydrochloride
Influenza	Multiple sclerosis	Diuretics
Mononucleosis	Parkinson's disease	**Hormonal Therapy**
Tuberculosis	Poststroke	Oral contraceptives
AIDS	Malignant disease	Steroids/ACTH
Collagen disorder	**Psychiatric Disorders**	**Acne Therapy**
Systemic lupus erythematosus	Alcoholism	Isotretinoin

Compiled from Ref. 31.

EMOTIONAL SYMPTOMS

Major depressive episode is characterized by a persistent, diminished ability to experience pleasure. A loss of interest and pleasure in usual activities, hobbies, or work is common. Patients appear sad or depressed, and they are often pessimistic and believe that nothing will help them feel better. Patients often weep or report crying spells. The presence of intense hopelessness and complete or near-total loss of interest and pleasure in usual activities may identify patients at risk for suicide.[33] Anxiety symptoms are present in almost 90% of depressed outpatients.

Patients often have guilt feelings that are unrealistic, and these may reach delusional proportions. Patients may feel that they deserve punishment and may view their present illness as a punishment. A depressed patient may hear voices (auditory hallucinations) saying that he or she is a bad person and that he or she should commit suicide. Depression with psychotic features may require hospitalization, especially if the patient becomes a danger to self or others.

PHYSICAL SYMPTOMS

Physical symptoms often motivate patients, especially the elderly, to seek medical attention. Chronic fatigue is a common complaint, with a decreased ability to perform normal, daily tasks. Fatigue often appears worse in the morning and does not improve with rest. Complaints of pain, especially headache, often accompany fatigue.

Sleep disturbances generally present as frequent early morning awakening (terminal insomnia), with difficulty returning to sleep. This may coexist with difficulty falling asleep (initial insomnia) and frequent nighttime awakening. Less frequently, depressed patients complain of increased sleep (hypersomnia), although they experience daytime exhaustion or fatigue.

Appetite disturbances, including complaints of decreased appetite, often result in substantial weight loss, especially in the elderly.[6] Some patients lose 2 lb or more per week without dieting. Other patients, especially in the ambulatory setting, may overeat and gain weight, although they actually may not enjoy eating. They may crave specific foods.

Some patients exhibit gastrointestinal complaints, others cardiovascular complaints, especially heart palpitations. Patients frequently present with a loss of sexual interest or libido.

INTELLECTUAL OR COGNITIVE SYMPTOMS

Intellectual or cognitive symptoms include a decreased ability to concentrate, slowed thinking, and a poor memory for recent events. Patients may appear confused and indecisive. Depression should be considered when cognitive symptoms are present in the elderly.[6]

PSYCHOMOTOR DISTURBANCES

Patients may appear noticeably slowed or retarded in physical movements, thought processes, and speech (psychomotor retardation). Conversely, depression may be accompanied by psychomotor agitation, manifesting as purposeless, restless motion (e.g., pacing, wringing of hands, outbursts of shouting).

SUICIDE RISK EVALUATION AND MANAGEMENT

Depressed patients should be assessed for suicidal thoughts. Widely held myths regarding suicide include the belief that people are more likely to commit suicide if they are asked about it, that people who attempt or talk about suicide are just looking for attention and are not serious, that suicidal people are crazy, and that most suicides are caused by a sudden traumatic event.

Factors that increase the risk for suicide include increasing age, being widowed, being unmarried, being unemployed, living alone, a history of a previous psychiatric admission, substance abuse, depression, feelings of hopelessness, prior attempts, family history of suicide, anniversary of a loss, presence of a serious medical problem, lack of a social support system, and refusal to seek help.[33] The presence of a very detailed plan with the intention and ability to carry it out indicates a high risk of suicide. Although women attempt suicide two to three times more often than men, men succeed about three times more frequently. Suicide is almost twice as common in the elderly as in the general population.[34] This appears to be a result of more determination, carefully planned acts, and fewer warning signs.[34] To assess the severity of suicidal thoughts, the clinician must be sensitive to hints of suicidal ideation, including a change in personality, a sudden decision to make a will or give away possessions, and any recent purchase of a gun or obtaining (or hoarding) a large supply of medications or other potentially toxic substances. It is important to remember that the risk of suicide in those recovering from major depression may increase as they develop the energy and capacity to act on a plan made earlier in a course of illness. It is not always possible to predict whether or when a depressed person will attempt suicide.

When suicidal intent is suspected, it is important to ask, "Are you thinking about harming or killing yourself?" If the risk is significant, the patient must be referred immediately to an appropriate health care professional.

▶ TREATMENT: Depressive Disorders

DESIRED OUTCOME

The goals of treatment of the acute depressive episode are to reduce the symptoms of depression and facilitate the patient's return to a premorbid level (before the onset of the illness) of functioning. Whether or not to hospitalize the patient is the first decision in the treatment plan. This decision is made in consideration of the patient's risk of suicide, physical state of health, social support system, and presence of a psychotic and/or catatonic depression.

GENERAL APPROACH TO TREATMENT

Studies comparing the efficacy of antidepressants have found that antidepressants are of equivalent efficacy in groups of patients when administered in comparable doses. Because one cannot predict which antidepressant will be the most effective in an individual patient, the initial choice is made empirically. Factors that often influence the choice of an antidepressant include the patient's past history of response, pharmacogenetics (the history of familial antidepressant response), the subtype of depression, the patient's concurrent medical history, the potential for drug-drug interactions, the adverse events profile, and drug cost.

Although the pathophysiology of major depression remains elusive, the clinician can now select from multiple drug therapies with different mechanisms of action.[35] Failure to respond to one antidepressant class or one antidepressant drug within a class does not predict a failed response to another drug class or another drug within the class.

Approximately 65% to 70% of patients with varying types of depression improve with drug therapy compared with 30% to 40% who improve with placebo. Melancholic depression appears to respond well to tricyclic antidepressants (TCAs), selective serotonin reuptake inhibitors (SSRIs), and electroconvulsive therapy (ECT).[35] Melancholic depression is characterized by a nearly complete absence of capacity for pleasure, diurnal mood swings (worse in the morning), early morning awakening, psychomotor disturbances, excessive guilt, and weight loss. A preferential response to MAO inhibitors has been reported in patients with atypical depression.[36] In atypical depression, two or more of the following are present: (1) weight gain or increase in appetite, (2) hypersomnia, (3) heavy feelings in arms or legs, and (4) interpersonal rejection sensitivity. Psychotically depressed individuals generally require either ECT or combination therapy with an antidepressant plus an antipsychotic agent.[37]

NONPHARMACOLOGIC THERAPY

In addition to pharmacologic interventions, psychotherapy should be employed whenever the patient is able and willing to participate. Psychotherapy alone is not recommended for the acute treatment of patients with severe and/or psychotic major depressive disorder. However, if the depressive episode is mild to moderate in severity, psychotherapy may be the first-line therapy.[38] The effects of psychotherapy and antidepressant medications are considered to be additive. Combined treatment may be advantageous for patients with partial responses to either treatment alone and for those with a chronic course of illness. However, for uncomplicated, nonchronic major depressive disorder, combined treatment may provide no unique advantage.[38] Although not well studied, cognitive therapy, behavioral therapy, and interpersonal psychotherapy appear to be equal in efficacy.[38] Maintenance psychotherapy as the sole treatment to prevent recurrence generally is not recommended. If there was a full response to combined medication and psychotherapy in the acute or continuation phases of treatment, medication may be all that is necessary in the maintenance phase of treatment to prevent a recurrence.[38]

Other means of treating depression include ECT and light therapy. ECT is a safe and very effective treatment for certain severe mental illnesses. Patients are candidates for ECT when a rapid response is needed, risks of other treatments outweigh potential benefits, there is a history of poor response to drugs and a good response to ECT, and the patient expresses a preference for ECT.[39] ECT is effective for all subtypes of major depressive disorder as well as other selected psychiatric illnesses.

A course of ECT generally consists of 6 to 12 treatments administered either unilaterally or bilaterally two to three times weekly. A rapid therapeutic response (10 to 14 days) has been reported. Although there are no absolute contraindications to the use of ECT, several conditions are associated with increased risk. These include increased intracranial pressure, cerebral lesions, recent myocardial infarction, recent intracerebral hemorrhage, bleeding, or otherwise unstable vascular condition. The use of an anesthetic as well as a nondepolarizing neuromuscular blocking agent decreases the morbidity associated with ECT.[39]

Adverse effects of ECT include cognitive dysfunction, cardiovascular dysfunction, prolonged apnea, treatment-emergent mania, headache, nausea, and muscle aches. Cognitive changes associated with ECT include confusion immediately after the seizure and retrograde and anterograde memory disturbance. Most cognitive disturbances are transient, but some patients may report permanent loss of memory of some events occurring over the months before, after, or during treatment.[39]

Relapse rates during the year immediately following ECT are high unless maintenance antidepressant medication is prescribed. ECT guidelines developed by the American Psychiatric Association include indications and contraindications for the appropriate use of ECT, procedures for obtaining informed consent, and issues in administering ECT.[39]

Some individuals experience depressive episodes during a particular season. This is referred to as *seasonal affective disorder* (SAD) and occurs most commonly in the winter, with remission in spring or summer.[40] Reduced environmental light may be the main precipitating factor of winter depression.[40] It has been theorized that there is a disturbance of the circadian rhythm caused by desynchronization between the solar clock and the human biologic clock during short photoperiods.[40] Bright-light therapy is used to resynchronize the disturbed rhythm.[41–43] The patient looks into a light box in the morning or evening for approximately 2 hours.[42] Some individuals will require antidepressant therapy in addition to light therapy or antidepressants for nonseasonal episodes of major depression.

The light therapy generally is well tolerated, with minor visual complaints being reported most frequently.[42] Consequently, anyone undergoing light therapy should receive baseline and periodic eye examinations.

Increasingly, people are turning to alternative forms of therapy, such as herbal medications. St. John's wort has been considered by many to be a new alternative treatment for depression.[44,45] Several evaluations have found that the active ingredient in St. John's wort, hypercium, is a safe and effective treatment for mild to moderate depression.[44,45] It has been compared with placebo, TCAs, and fluoxetine.[46,47] Side effects appear to be mild. St. John's wort is readily accessible as an over-the-counter medication. Although this may allow certain advantages such as reduced cost of therapy and self-treatment, it also has the potential to result in circumvention of the health care system. St. John's wort has been found to have several significant drug interactions with HIV medications (e.g., indinavir) and digoxin.[48] Perhaps most disconcerting is the fact that herbal medications are not regulated by the Food and Drug Administration (FDA), and the manufacturers are not required to adhere to good manufacturing practices. If St. John's wort is felt to be the treatment of choice in a particular patient, it should be administered under the guidance of a clinician trained in the treatment of depression. A single-source product should be used continuously from a reputable and trusted manufacturer.

PHARMACOLOGIC THERAPY

Antidepressants can be classified in several ways. One approach is by chemical structure, and another is by the presumed mechanism of antidepressant activity (Table 69–3). Although the link between the presumed mechanism of drug action and antidepressant

TABLE 69–3. Classification of Antidepressant Pharmacotherapy by Presumed Mechanism of Action

Mixed 5-HT/NE reuptake inhibitors	TCAs, venlafaxine
SSRIs	Fluoxetine, paroxetine, sertraline, fluvoxamine, citalopram
Selective norepinephrine reuptake inhibitors	Reboxetine[a]
Mixed serotonin effects	Trazodone, nefazodone
Mixed NE/DA reuptake inhibitors	Bupropion
Mixed serotonin/ norepinephrine effects	Mirtazapine
MAOIs	Phenelzine, tranylcypromine

[a]Has not yet received FDA approval.

response is tenuous, this classification has the advantage of being based on established pharmacology and clearly explains some of the adverse effects of the antidepressants. The knowledgeable clinician can use these facts to tailor treatment to individual patient needs and thereby optimize treatment outcome. Currently available antidepressants, their manufacturers, and initial dosages are shown in Table 69–4.

MIXED SEROTONIN AND NOREPINEPHRINE REUPTAKE INHIBITORS

Among the TCAs, amitriptyline and imipramine are the most extensively studied. Studies comparing the secondary amine TCAs (e.g., desipramine and nortriptyline) with the tertiary amine TCAs (e.g., amitriptyline and imipramine) found no clinically important difference in efficacy, but the secondary amines were more potent on a milligram-to-milligram basis.[49]

The TCAs are effective in treating all depressive subtypes, especially the severe melancholic subtype of major depressive disorder. All TCAs potentiate the activity of NE and 5-HT by blocking their reuptake. However, the potency and selectivity of TCAs for the inhibition of reuptake of NE and 5-HT vary greatly among these agents (Table 69–5). Because TCAs affect other receptor systems, anticholinergic, neurologic, and cardiovascular adverse events are reported frequently during TCA therapy.[49]

Venlafaxine, a structurally novel antidepressant, is a potent inhibitor of 5-HT and NE reuptake and a weak inhibitor of dopamine reuptake. Unlike the TCAs, it has virtually no affinity for muscarinic, histaminergic, and α_1-adrenergic receptors.[50]

Maprotiline and amoxapine are both inhibitors of NE reuptake, with less effect on 5-HT reuptake. Maprotiline is associated with a higher incidence of seizures than is imipramine or amitriptyline.[26] Amoxapine, while less sedating than some antidepressants, blocks cholinergic receptors, causing clinically significant anticholinergic effects.

SELECTIVE SEROTONIN REUPTAKE INHIBITORS

The impetus for the development of the SSRIs was the perceived need for antidepressants with an improved efficacy and adverse-effects profile compared with the traditional TCAs. There is a substantial body of knowledge to indicate that the efficacy of SSRIs is superior to placebo and equal to the TCAs in treating patients with major depression.[35] Patients who fail to respond to a TCA often respond to an SSRI, and vice versa. As a class, the SSRIs cause minimal to low anticholinergic effects.

SELECTIVE NOREPINEPHRINE REUPTAKE INHIBITORS

Reboxetine is a new selective NE reuptake inhibitor that is not available in the U.S. at this time. It has been found to be more effective than placebo and equal to imipramine and fluoxetine in the management of patients with depression.[51,52] In fact, a subanalysis of patients with severe depression found that reboxetine had superior efficacy when compared with fluoxetine.[52] Furthermore, reboxetine was found to be more effective in terms of social functioning in patients who achieved remission. These findings are preliminary and are being evaluated further.

TRIAZOLOPYRIDINES

Trazodone and nefazodone have dual actions on serotonergic neurons, acting as both a 5-HT_2 antagonist and 5-HT reuptake inhibitor.[53] They also appear to enhance 5-HT_{1A}-mediated neurotransmission. These drugs have negligible affinity for cholinergic and histaminergic receptors. Trazodone's use as an antidepressant agent has diminished greatly secondary to side effects (e.g., dizziness and sedation) and increased availability of alternative, better-tolerated agents. Nefazodone also has low affinity for α_1-adrenergic receptors. Similar to TCAs and SSRIs, the triazolopyridines are effective agents in treating major depression with no substantial evidence to support a unique spectrum of therapeutic activity.

AMINOKETONE

Bupropion, the only marketed aminoketone antidepressant, appears to have a unique mechanism of drug action.[54] It has no appreciable effect on the reuptake of NE or 5-HT, and its most potent neurochemical action is blockade of DA reuptake.

MIXED SEROTONIN-NOREPINEPHRINE EFFECTS

Mirtazapine, a TCA agent, enhances central noradrenergic and serotonergic activity through the antagonism of central presynaptic α_2-adrenergic autoreceptors and heteroreceptors.[55]

MONOAMINE OXIDASE INHIBITORS

The MAO inhibitors increase the concentrations of NE, 5-HT, and DA within the neuronal synapse through inhibition of the MAO enzyme. Studies of several MAO inhibitors have demonstrated that, similar to the TCAs, chronic therapy causes changes in receptor sensitivity (i.e., downregulation of β-adrenergic, α-adrenergic, and serotonergic receptors).[56,57]

Clinical features that predict preferential response to MAO inhibitors include mood reactivity, irritability, hypersomnia, hyperphagia, psychomotor agitation, hypersensitivity to rejection,[36] and the defining features of atypical depression.

The MAO inhibitors currently marketed in the United States are nonselective inhibitors of MAO A and MAO B. Phenelzine and tranylcypromine inhibit both these forms (isoenzymes) of MAO.

TABLE 69–4. Adult Dosages for Currently Available Antidepressant Medications[a]

Generic Name	Trade Name	Manufacturer	Suggested Therapeutic Plasma Concentration (ng/mL)	Initial Dose (mg/day)	Usual Dosage Range (mg/day)
Tricyclic Antidepressants					
Tertiary amines					
Amitriptyline	Elavil	Stuart	120–250[b]	50–75	100–300
	Endep	Roche			
	Generic	Various			
Clomipramine	Anafranil	Novartis		25	100–250
Doxepin	Adapin	Lotus Biochemical	110–250[b]	50–75	100–300
	Sinequan	Roerig			
	Generic	Various			
Imipramine	Tofranil	Novartis	200–300[b]	50–75	100–300
	Generic	Various			
Trimipramine	Surmontil	Wyeth-Ayerst		50–75	100–300
Secondary amines					
Desipramine	Norpramin	Marion Merrell Dow	125–300	50–75	100–300
	Generic	Various			
Nortriptyline	Pamelor	Novartis	50–150	25–50	50–150
	Generic	Various			
Protriptyline	Vivactil	Merck	70–240	10–20	15–60
Dibenzoxazepine					
Amoxapine	Asendin	Lederle	200–400[c]	50–150	100–400
	Generic	Various			
Tetracyclic					
Maprotiline	Ludiomil	Novartis	200–300[b]	50–75	100–225
	Generic	Various			
Mirtazapine	Remeron	Organon		15	15–45
Triazolopyridines					
Nefazodone	Serzone	Bristol-Myers Squibb		200	300–600
Trazodone	Desyrel	Apothecon		50–150	150–400
	Generic	Various			
Aminoketone					
Bupropion	Wellbutrin	Glaxo Wellcome	50–100	200	300–450
Monoamine Oxidase Inhibitors					
Phenelzine	Nardil	Parke-Davis		15	15–90
Tranlycypromine	Parnate	SmithKline Beecham		20	20–60
Selective Serotonin Reuptake Inhibitors					
Citalopram	Celexa	Forest		20	20–60
Fluoxetine	Prozac	Dista		10–20	10–80
Fluvoxamine	Luvox	Solvay		50	50–300
Paroxetine	Paxil	SmithKline Beecham		20	20–50
Sertraline	Zoloft	Roerig		50	100–200
Selective Norepinephrine Reuptake Inhibitor					
Reboxetine	Janssen			8	8–10
Serotonin/Norepinephrine Reuptake Inhibitor					
Venlafaxine	Effexor	Wyeth-Ayerst		75	75–375

[a]Doses listed are total daily doses; elderly patients are usually treated with approximately one-half of the dose listed.
[b]Parent drug plus demethylated metabolite.
[c]Parent drug plus hydroxymetabolite.
Compiled from Refs. 20, 23, 54, 63, 77, 79, and 84.

Moclobemide, an antidepressant marketed in Europe, is a selective and reversible inhibitor of MAO A. Clinical trials of moclobemide conducted in Europe have reported efficacy equal to TCAs and superior to placebo.[58]

ADVERSE EFFECTS

TCAs and Other Heterocyclics

The most commonly reported adverse effects of antidepressant therapy are summarized in Table 69–5. The TCAs affect several neurotransmitters and produce a wide range of pharmacologic actions, sometimes causing many unwanted adverse effects. The side effects most frequently associated with the TCAs (e.g., dry mouth, constipation, blurred vision, urinary retention, dizziness, tachycardia, memory impairment, and at higher doses, delirium) may result from blockade of cholinergic receptors.[56] These adverse effects often have an impact on patient tolerance and adherence, particularly in the elderly and those receiving long-term maintenance therapy. In general, anticholinergic effects and sedation are more severe during therapy with tertiary amine TCAs than with secondary amine TCAs.[59]

A common and potentially serious side effect of the TCAs is orthostatic hypotension, which has been attributed to the affinity of

TABLE 69–5. Relative Potencies of Norepinephrine and Serotonin Reuptake Blockade and Side-Effect Profile of Antidepressant Drugs

	Reuptake Antagonism		Anticholinergic Effects	Sedation	Orthostatic Hypotension	Seizures	Conduction Abnormalities
	Norepinephrine	*Serotonin*					
Tricyclic Antidepressants							
Tertiary amines							
Amitriptyline	++	++++	++++	++++	+++	+++	+++
Clomipramine	++	+++	++++	++++	++	++++	+++
Doxepin	++	++	+++	++++	++	+++	++
Imipramine	+++	+++	+++	+++	++++	+++	+++
Trimipramine	++	++	++++	++++	+++	+++	+++
Secondary amine							
Desipramine	++++	+	++	++	++	++	++
Nortriptyline	+++	++	++	++	+	++	++
Protriptyline	+++	++	++	+	++	++	+++
Dibenzoxazepine							
Amoxapine[a]	+++	++	+++	++	++	+++	++
Tetracyclics							
Maprotiline	+++	+	+++	+++	++	++++	++
Mirtazapine	0	0	+	++	++		+
Triazolopyridines							
Nefazodone	0	++	0	+++	+++	++	+
Trazodone	0	++	0	++++	+++	++	+
Aminoketone							
Bupropion	+	+	+	0	0	++++	+
Monoamine Oxidase Inhibitors							
Phenelzine	++	++	+	++	++	+	
Tranylcypromine	++	+	+	+	++	+	+
Selective Serotonin Reuptake Inhibitors							
Citalopram	0	++++	0	+	0	++	0
Fluoxetine	0	+++	0	0	0	++	0
Fluvoxamine	0	++++	0	0	0	++	0
Paroxetine	0	++++	+	+	0	++	0
Sertraline	0	++++	0	0	0	++	0
Selective Norepinephrine Reuptake Inhibitor							
Reboxetine	++++	0	+	0	+	0	0
Serotinin/Norepinephrine Reuptake Inhibitor							
Venlafaxine	++++	++++	+	+	0	++	+

++++ = High; +++ = moderate; ++ = low; + = very low; 0 = none.
[a]Also blocks dopamine receptors.
Compiled from Refs. 20, 23, 54, 63, 77, 84, and 87.

the TCAs for adrenergic receptors.[59] Orthostatic hypotension may be symptomatic, resulting in syncope, a particular concern when treating elderly patients due to the increased risk of falls and subsequent fractures.[60] Patients should be advised to rise slowly from a supine position, and prolonged bed rest should be avoided because of the deconditioning and a volume-contracting effect. Tilting the head of the bed upward can be helpful for some patients. Adequate fluid intake should be maintained, and blood pressure should be monitored both supine and standing. Antigravity support garments also can be helpful. Adequate ambulation and hydration along with proper drug selection, gradual dose increases, and patient education can minimize the risk of symptomatic orthostatic hypotension.

TCAs also cause cardiac conduction delays and may even induce heart block in patients with a preexisting conduction disease. TCA overdose can produce severe arrhythmias.[59] Due to these potential cardiovascular effects, caution should be exercised when prescribing these agents to patients with clinically significant cardiac disease. Other adverse effects that lead to patient noncompliance include weight gain, excessive perspiration, and sexual dysfunction.[59]

Abrupt withdrawal of TCAs is associated with symptoms suggestive of cholinergic rebound (e.g., dizziness, nausea, diarrhea, insomnia, and restlessness), especially if the daily dose exceeds 300 mg.[61,62]

Clomipramine is a tertiary amine TCA with 5-HT reuptake inhibiting properties. Although it is a commonly used antidepressant in Europe, in the United States it is approved only for the treatment of obsessive-compulsive disorder (see Chap. 72).

Amoxapine, the demethylated metabolite of loxapine, has intermediate sedative and anticholinergic potency.[61] Because of its postsynaptic receptor DA-blocking effects, its use may be associated with extrapyramidal side effects, including pseudoparkinsonism, dystonia, akathisia, and tardive dyskinesia.[26] Amoxapine offers no advantage over standard TCAs or other antidepressants.

Maprotiline, a tetracyclic drug, blocks reuptake of NE with little effect on 5-HT. It has intermediate sedative and anticholinergic effects and may cause less orthostatic hypotension than imipramine; however, an exanthematous rash occurs in approximately 4% of patients.[26] Maprotiline is also associated with a higher incidence of seizures than standard TCAs and is contraindicated in patients with a history of a seizure disorder.

Venlafaxine

The most commonly reported adverse effects with venlafaxine include nausea, constipation, somnolence, dry mouth, dizziness, nervousness, sweating, asthenia, abnormal ejaculation/orgasm, and anorexia.[50,63] These side effects are believed to be dose related. Venlafaxine may cause a dose-related increase in diastolic blood pressure, and baseline blood pressure is not a useful predictor of the occurrence of this phenomenon. Blood pressure should be monitored regularly during venlafaxine therapy, and dosage reduction or discontinuation may be necessary if sustained hypertension occurs.[63,64]

Selective Serotonin Reuptake Inhibitors

The SSRIs include fluoxetine, citalopram, sertraline, paroxetine, and fluvoxamine. Escitalopram, currently unavailable in the U.S., had a low rate of discontinuation due to side effects in clinical trials. In general, the SSRIs have a low affinity for histamine, α_1-adrenergic, and muscarinic receptors. They produce fewer anticholinergic and cardiovascular adverse effects than the TCAs, and they are not associated with weight gain.[65,66] The main adverse effects, which generally are mild and short lived, are gastrointestinal symptoms (i.e., nausea, vomiting, diarrhea), sexual dysfunction in both males and females, headache, insomnia, and fatigue.[66]

Although the SSRIs as a group are known to improve the anxiety symptoms associated with depression, a few patients experience an increase in anxiety symptoms or agitation early in treatment.

Selective Norephinephrine Reuptake Inhibitors

In clinical trials to date, reboxetine has been well tolerated. Side effects seen most frequently inlcude, dry mouth, constipation, hypotension, urinary hesitancy, and paresthesias. No significant effects on laboratory parameters, body weight, or vital signs were noted in short-term evaluations.[51,52]

Triazolopyridines

The adverse effect profile for trazodone and nefazodone is different from that of the other antidepressants. Trazodone and nefazodone have minimal anticholinergic effects and 5-HT agonist side effects but can cause orthostatic hypotension. Sedation, cognitive slowing, and dizziness are the most frequent dose-limiting side effects associated with trazodone.[49] Common adverse effects associated with nefazodone use include light-headedness, dizziness, orthostatic hypotension, somnolence, dry mouth, nausea, and asthenia.[53]

A rare but potentially serious adverse effect of trazodone is priapism, which is reported to occur in approximately 1 in 6000 male patients. Some cases have required surgical intervention (1 in 23,000), and permanent impotence may result.[67] There have been no reports of priapism associated with nefazodone use in men, but there is a published case report of nefazodone-induced clitoral priapism.[68]

Aminoketone

Adverse effects associated with bupropion include nausea, dizziness, tremor, insomnia, vomiting, constipation, dry mouth, and skin reactions. The occurrence of seizures in patients taking bupropion appears to be strongly associated with dose and may be increased by predisposing factors such as history of head trauma and central nervous system tumor. At daily doses of 450 mg (the ceiling dose) or less, the incidence of seizures is 0.4%.[69,70]

Mixed Serotonin-Norepinephrine Effects

The most common adverse effects reported in clinical trials in patients taking mirtazapine were somnolence, weight gain, dry mouth, and constipation. Both agranulocytosis and liver function test (LFT) elevations were noted in premarketing clinical trials. Two cases of agranulocytosis and one of neutropenia were reported. The incidence appears to be rare, and therefore, routine monitoring of blood indices is not recommended.[55] Additionally, LFT elevations were observed 1.4 times more frequently than with other antidepressants and 1.6 times more frequently than with placebo. No specific guidelines for LFT monitoring are recommended, but prescribers should consider obtaining baseline LFTs and monitoring these periodically throughout the course of therapy.[55]

MAO Inhibitors

The most common adverse effect of MAO inhibitors is postural hypotension; this is more likely to occur with phenelzine than with tranylcypromine.[56] Hypotensive reactions may be minimized through divided dosage scheduling. Anticholinergic side effects, especially dry mouth and constipation, are common but are mild compared with those associated with the TCAs.

Phenelzine, the most frequently prescribed MAO inhibitor, has mild to moderate sedating effects. Tranylcypromine may exert a stimulating effect, and insomnia may occur, so the last dose of the day should be administered in the early afternoon. Dose-related impotence and anorgasmia in males and orgasmic inhibition in females have been reported.[71,72] In addition, fever, myoclonic jerking, and brisk deep tendon reflexes may occur.[56,73]

Phenelzine, a hydrazine, has been associated with hepatocellular damage and weight gain. Tranylcypromine is a nonhydrazine MAO inhibitor and should be selected for patients with a history of liver disease if an MAO inhibitor is to be used.[56]

Hypertensive crisis, a potentially fatal but rare adverse reaction, may occur when MAO inhibitors are taken concurrently with certain foods, especially those high in tyramine (Table 69–6) or drugs (Table 69–7). Ten milligrams of tyramine can cause a marked pressor effect, and 25 mg can result in serious hypertensive crisis.[74] These incidents may culminate in cerebrovascular accident and death.[56] Symptoms of hypertensive crisis include occipital headache, stiff neck, nausea, vomiting, sweating, and sharply elevated blood pressure. In the past, hypertensive crises were treated with sublingual nifedipine, but recent reports of adverse events secondary to an uncontrollable fall in blood pressure and resulting rebound catecholamine release have lead to concerns over this practice.[75] Alternative agents, such as captopril, should be considered.[76]

Education of patients taking MAO inhibitors regarding dietary and medication restrictions is extremely important. Printed and verbal patient instructions should be provided. Patients unable to read and those with difficulty understanding or remembering medication instructions should not be given MAO inhibitors unless they have competent caregivers. Patients should be instructed regarding the necessity of consulting a health care professional before taking over-the-counter medications. Patients also should be informed of the symptoms of

TABLE 69–6. Dietary Restrictions for Patients Taking Monoamine Oxidase Inhibitors

Aged cheeses[a]
Sour cream[b]
Yogurt[b]
Cottage cheese[b]
American cheese[b]
Mild Swiss cheese[b]
Wine[c] (especially Chianti and sherry)
Beer
Herring[a] (pickled, salted, dry)
Sardines
Snails
Anchovies
Canned, aged, or processed meats
Monosodium glutamate
Liver (chicken or beef, more than 2 days old)
Fermented foods
Canned figs
Raisins
Pods of broad beans[a] (fava beans)
Yeast extract[a] and other yeast products
Meat extract (Marmite)
Soy sauce
Chocolate[d]
Coffee[d]
Ripe avocado
Sauerkraut
Licorice

[a]Clearly warrants absolute prohibition (e.g., English Stilton, blue, Camembert, cheddar).
[b]Up to 2 oz daily is acceptable.
[c]3 oz white wine or a single cocktail is acceptable.
[d]Up to 2 oz daily is acceptable: larger amounts of decaffeinated coffee are acceptable.

hypertensive crisis and be advised about what to do should those symptoms occur.

PHARMACOKINETICS

The pharmacokinetics of the antidepressants are summarized in Table 69–8. In general, the TCAs are absorbed rapidly after oral administration. Bioavailability is low (30% to 70% for most TCAs) as a result of the first-pass effect, which shows great interindividual variation.[77]

The TCAs have a large volume of distribution and concentrate in brain and cardiac tissue in laboratory animals. They are bound extensively and strongly to plasma albumin, erythrocytes, α_1-acid glycoprotein, and lipoprotein.[77]

The major metabolic pathways are demethylation, aromatic and aliphatic hydroxylation, and glucuronide conjugation. Enterohepatic cycling has been described.[77] Metabolism of TCAs appears to be linear within the usual dosage range. The elimination half-lives of the TCAs vary greatly among individual patients, and this may be determined genetically.[77]

The diversity of the SSRIs is evident not only in their chemical structures but also in their pharmacokinetic profiles. Fluoxetine has an elimination half-life of 2 to 3 days (4 to 5 days with multiple dosing). The single-dose half-life of norfluoxetine, the active metabolite, is 7 to 9 days. Paroxetine and sertraline have half-lives of approximately 24 hours. Unlike paroxetine, sertraline has an active metabolite, but the metabolite contributes minimally to the pharmacologic effects. Peak plasma concentrations of citalopram are observed within 2 to 4 hours after dosing, and the elimination half-life is about 30 hours. The SSRIs, with the exception of fluvoxamine and citalopram, are extensively bound to plasma proteins (94% to 99%). The SSRIs are extensively distributed to the tissues, and all, with the possible exception of citalopram, may have a nonlinear pattern of drug accumulation with long-term administration.[78]

Mirtazapine undergoes biotransformation via demethylation and hydroxylation followed by glucuronide conjugation.[55] The 1A2 and the 2D6 isoenzymes of the cytochrome P450 system may be responsible for the formation of the hydroxymetabolite, whereas the 3A4 isoenzyme may be responsible for the formation of the *N*-desmethyl and the *N*-oxide metabolite.[55] Although these metabolites are theoretically active, they are present at such low plasma concentrations as to contribute little to the overall pharmacologic profile of mirtazapine.

The elimination half-life of reboxetine is 13 hours. Reboxetine displays linear pharmacokinetics, with elimination being primarily renal. In addition, no inhibitory effects on the isoenyzmes of the cytochrome 450 system have been observed.[79]

Altered Pharmacokinetics

Factors reported to influence TCA plasma concentrations include disease states, genetics, age, cigarette smoking, and concurrent drug administration. Hepatic disease may reduce metabolic clearance of TCAs.[77] Renal failure does not alter nortriptyline metabolism, but the 10-hydroxy metabolite may accumulate and protein binding may be diminished, with resulting enhanced sensitivity to the drug.[77] Clinicians should be alert to the possibility of higher-than-expected plasma concentrations of some TCAs in the elderly. Because dose-related kinetics cannot be ruled out in the elderly, dosage adjustments based on plasma concentration monitoring may be difficult.

In cirrhotics, the half-lives of fluoxetine and norfluoxetine increased to 7.6 and 12 days, respectively.[78] Patients with hepatic impairment had a twofold increase in plasma concentrations of paroxetine.[80] Similarly, in patients with mild stable cirrhosis, the half-life of sertraline was 2.5 times greater than in patients without liver disease.[81] Patients with renal impairment had a two- to fourfold increase in paroxetine plasma concentrations compared with normal volunteers.[80] Plasma concentrations of SSRIs in the elderly are reported to be greater than in younger patients.[78]

TABLE 69–7. Medication Restrictions for Patients Taking Monoamine Oxidase Inhibitors

Amphetamines	Levodopa
Appetite suppressants	Local anesthetics containing sympathomimetic vasoconstrictors
Asthma inhalants	Meperidine
Buspirone	Methyldopa
Carbamazepine	Methylphenidate
Cocaine	Other antidepressants[a]
Cyclobenzaprine	Other MAOIs
Decongestants (topical and systemic)	Reserpine
Dextromethorphan	Rizatriptan
Dopamine	Stimulants
Ephedrine	Sumatriptan
Epinephrine	Sympathomimetics
Guanethidine	Tryptophan

[a]Tricyclic antidepressants may be used with caution by experienced clinicians in treatment-resistant populations.

TABLE 69–8. Pharmacokinetic Properties of Antidepressants

Generic Name	Elimination Half-life (h)[a]	Time of Peak Plasma Concentration (h)	Plasma Protein Binding (%)	% Bioavailable	Clinically Important Metabolites
Tricyclic Antidepressants					
Tertiary amines					
Amitriptyline	9–46	1–5	90–97	30–60	Nortriptyline; 10-hydroxynortriptyline
Clomipramine	20–24	2–6	97	36–62	
Doxepin	8–36	1–4	68–82	13–45	Desmethyldoxepin
Imipramine	6–34	1.5–3	63–96	22–77	2-Hydroxyimipramine; desipramine; 2-Hydroxydesipramine
Trimipramine	7–40	3	94–96	18–63	None
Secondary amines					
Desipramine	11–46	3–6	73–92	33–51	2-Hydroxydesipramine
Nortriptyline	16–88	3–12	87–95	46–70	10-Hydroxynortriptyline
Protriptyline	54–198	6–12	90–94	75–90	None
Dibenzoxazepine					
Amoxapine	8–30[b]	1–2	90	[c]	8-Hydroxyamoxapine
Tetracyclic					
Maprotiline	28–105	4–24	88	79–87	Desmethylmaprotiline
Mirtazapine	20–40	2	85	50	None known
Triazolopyridines					
Nefazodone	2–4	1	99	20	Meta-chlorophenylpiperazine; hydroxynefazodone; triazoledione
Trazodone	6–11	1–2	92	[c]	Meta-chlorophenylpiperazine
Aminoketone					
Bupropion	10–21	3	82–88	[c]	Bupropion threoamino alcohol; bupropion morpholinol
Monoamine Oxidase Inhibitors					
Phenelzine	1.5–4	[c]	[c]	[c]	
Tranylcypromine	1.5–3	[c]	[c]	[c]	
Selective Serotonin Reuptake Inhibitors					
Citalopram	33	2–4	80	≥80	Demethyl- and didemethylcitalopram
Fluoxetine	4–6 days[d]	4–8	94	95	Norfluoxetine
Fluvoxamine	15–26	2–8	77	53	None
Paroxetine	24–31	5–7	95		None
Sertraline	27	6–8	99	36[e]	*N*-Desmethylsertraline
Selective Norepinephrine Reuptake Inhibitor					
Reboxetine[f]	12–16	2	9	>60	
Serotonin/Norepinephrine Reuptake Inhibitor					
Venlafaxine	5	2	27–30		O-Desmethylvenlafaxine

[a]Biologic half-life in slowest phase of elimination.
[b]Amoxapine, 8 hours; 8-hydroxyamoxapine, 30 hours.
[c]No data available.
[d]4–6 days with chronic dosing; norfluoxetine, 4–16 days.
[e]Increases 30% to 40% when taken with food.
[f]Has not yet received FDA approval.

The area under the curve (AUC) of nefazodone and hydroxynefazodone is 25% greater in cirrhotics than in normal volunteers.[82] Patients with cirrhosis accumulate metabolites of bupropion to concentrations two to three times those in normal individuals.

Hepatic dysfunction did not alter the pharmacokinetics of reboxetine. Elderly patients and patients with severe renal impairment may need dose reduction.[79]

Plasma Concentration and Clinical Response

Studies in acutely depressed patients have demonstrated a correlation between antidepressant effect and plasma concentrations for some TCAs. The patient's clinical response, not plasma concentration, dictates dosage adjustments. Some patients with plasma concentrations outside the suggested therapeutic plasma concentration range respond, whereas others are nonresponsive regardless of their plasma concentration. See Table 69–4 for a listing of suggested therapeutic plasma concentration ranges.

For four TCAs (nortriptyline, desipramine, imipramine, and amitriptyline) there is more consistent evidence to support a minimal plasma concentration for clinical response. The best established therapeutic range is for nortriptyline.[83] Studies suggest a curvilinear plasma concentration-response relationship for nortriptyline, with a suggested therapeutic range of 50 to 150 ng/mL. Using logistic regression analysis of data from multiple published studies, it was found that within this range, 70% of patients with major depression responded versus only 29% of patients with plasma concentrations outside this range. Interestingly, the response rate generally was higher at the lower end of this range than at the upper limit.[83]

Using the same analysis, the therapeutic window for desipramine was 110 to 160 ng/mL. The remission rate was 50% within this range versus only 20% outside the range.[83] However, in the opinion of many clinicians, the data support a minimal threshold plasma concentration for clinical response, and a more commonly accepted range is 125 to 300 ng/mL.

Unfortunately, data for the tertiary amine TCAs are less convincing. Most investigators conclude that the desired plasma concentration range is defined by a plasma concentration below which patients are less likely to respond clinically and an upper plasma concentration limit that is associated with an increased risk for central nervous system and cardiac toxicity.

For the newer antidepressants, a correlation has not been established between plasma concentration and clinical response or adverse effects.

Plasma Concentration Monitoring

Because of interindividual variations in plasma concentrations achieved by a given dose, approximately 40% of patients receiving standard doses of TCAs may not obtain plasma concentrations within the desired therapeutic range.[84] Although plasma level monitoring is not performed routinely, some indications include inadequate response, relapse, serious or persistent adverse effects, use of higher than standard doses, suspected toxicity, elderly patients, pregnant patients, patients of African or Asian descent (because of slower metabolism), cardiac disease, suspected noncompliance, suspected pharmacokinetic drug interactions, and changing brands. Plasma concentration monitoring of TCAs, when used appropriately, can improve efficacy and minimize drug-related problems. Plasma concentrations should be obtained at steady state, usually after a minimum of 1 week at constant dosage. Sampling should be performed during the drug elimination phase, usually in the morning, 12 hours after the last dose. Samples collected in this manner are comparable for patients on once-, twice-, or thrice-daily regimens.[77]

DRUG INTERACTIONS

TCAs

Because the TCAs are metabolized in the liver through the cytochrome P450 system, they may interact with other drugs that modify hepatic enzyme activity or hepatic blood flow. TCAs are also extensively protein bound, which can cause drug interactions through displacement from protein-binding sites. Many commonly used medications can interact when given concurrently with TCAs. Pharmacokinetic and pharmacodynamic drug interactions involving TCAs are shown in Tables 69–9 and 69–10, respectively.

TCAs may reverse the hypotensive effects of certain sympatholytic antihypertensives (e.g., guanethidine, methyldopa, clonidine) because of inhibition of presynaptic uptake of the antihypertensive or desensitization of the α_2-adrenergic receptor.[85] Similarly, because of inhibition of presynaptic uptake, TCAs may increase the vasopressor response to direct-acting sympathomimetics such as phenylephrine, epinephrine, and NE. The vasopressor response to indirect-acting sympathomimetics such as ephedrine is decreased.[85] Adverse effects of any TCA would be additive with those of other drugs with similar pharmacologic effects (e.g., anticholinergic, sedative, or hypotensive drugs).[85]

TABLE 69–9. Pharmacokinetic Drug Interactions Involving Tricyclic Antidepressants

Elevates Plasma Concentrations of TCAs
Cimetidine
Diltiazem
Ethanol, acute ingestion
SSRIs
Haloperidol
Labetalol
Methylphenidate
Oral contraceptives
Phenothiazines
Propoxyphene
Quinidine
Verapamil
Lowers Plasma Concentrations of TCAs
Barbiturates
Carbamazepine
Ethanol, chronic ingestion
Phenytoin
Elevates Plasma Concentrations of Interacting Drug
Hydantoins
Oral anticoagulants
Lowers Plasma Concentrations of Interacting Drug
Levodopa

Compiled from Ref. 77.

Although MAO inhibitors and TCAs may be coadministered safely in refractory patients with apparent increased efficacy compared with monotherapy, severe reactions and fatalities have occurred. These reactions include hypertensive crises, hyperpyrexia, excitation, and convulsions, and they usually occur when TCAs are added to established MAO inhibitor therapy.[85]

SSRIs

Table 69–11 summarizes the drug interactions of non-TCA antidepressants. Drug-drug interactions may occur when an SSRI is coadministered with another drug metabolized through the cytochrome P450 system.[85] Two of the isoenzymes of the cytochrome P450 system, 2D6 and 3A4, are responsible for the metabolism of over 80% of currently marketed drugs.[86] The ability of an SSRI, or any antidepressant, to inhibit or induce the activity of these enzymes will be a significant contributory factor in determining its capability of causing a pharmacokinetic drug interaction when administered concomitantly.[86,87] See Table 69-12 for a comparison of the second- and third-generation antidepressant agents and their effects on the enzymes of the cytochrome P450 system.[86]

The long half-lives of fluoxetine (2 to 5 days in young healthy subjects) and of its active metabolite, norfluoxetine (7 to 9 days), ensure that, following discontinuation of the drug, active compounds persist in the body for weeks. The very slow elimination of fluoxetine makes it critical to ensure a 5-week washout after fluoxetine discontinuation before starting an MAO inhibitor.[86] For all other SSRIs, a 2-week washout is recommended. Serious and potentially fatal reactions may occur when any SSRI is coadministered with an MAO inhibitor, and coadministration is contraindicated.[85]

Patients prescribed concomitant phenytoin or carbamazepine with fluoxetine may have increased anticonvulsant plasma concentrations and symptoms of toxicity.[85] Markedly increased plasma

TABLE 69–10. Pharmacodynamic Drug Interactions Involving Tricyclic Antidepressants

Interacting Drug	Effect
Alcohol	Increased CNS depressant effects
Amphetamines	Increased effect of amphetamines
Androgens	Delusions, hostility
Anticholinergic agents	Excessive anticholinergic effects
Bepredil	Increased antiarrhythmic effect
Clonidine	Decreased antihypertensive efficacy
Disulfiram	Acute organic brain syndrome
Estrogens	Increased or decreased antidepressant response; increased toxicity
Guanadrel	Decreased antihypertensive efficacy
Guanethidine	Decreased antihypertensive efficacy
Insulin	Increased hypoglycemic effects
Lithium	Possible additive lowering of seizure threshold
Methyldopa	Decreased antihypertensive efficacy; tachycardia; CNS stimulation
Monoamine oxidase inhibitors	Increased therapeutic and possibly toxic effects of both drugs; hypertensive crisis; delirium; seizures; hyperpyrexia; serotonin syndrome
Oral hypoglycemics	Increased hypoglycemic effects
Phenytoin	Possible lowering of seizure threshold and reduced antidepressant response
Sedatives	Increased CNS depressant effects
Sympathomimetics	Increased pharmacologic effects of direct-acting sympathomimetics; decreased effects of indirect-acting sympathomimetics
Thyroid hormones	Increased therapeutic and possibly toxic effects of both drugs; CNS stimulation; tachycardia

Compiled from Ref. 77.

concentrations of TCAs with resulting symptoms of toxicity have been reported in patients taking fluoxetine.

Although no significant pharmacokinetic changes were present with the coadministration of warfarin and fluoxetine, altered anticoagulation effects, including bleeding, have been documented.[88] Similar findings have been noted with paroxetine and sertraline, and consequently, careful monitoring of prothrombin time is recommended when warfarin and an SSRI are administered concomitantly. The risk of using SSRIs in combination with other central nervous system active medications has not been evaluated systematically. Although coadministration appears relatively safe, caution should be used when prescribing an SSRI and other central nervous system active drug such as benzodiazepines.[65] There are case reports of elevated levels of TCAs when administered concomitantly with fluoxetine, sertraline, and paroxetine. In a patient on a stable dose of a TCA in whom therapy with an SSRI is being initiated, it is recommended that a blood level of the TCA be obtained. Therapy with the SSRI should be initiated carefully and conservatively. Consideration of a dose reduction of the TCA is appropriate for susceptible populations such as the elderly or those with cardiovascular disease.

Data to date suggest that citalopram may cause only moderate or no pharmacokinetic interactions when coadministered with TCAs. Coadministration of cimetidine reduced citalopram oral clearance by 29%, whereas the addition of fluvoxamine caused a significant increase in plasma concentrations of citalopram.[89] At this time, escitalopram is considered unlikely to be involved in clinically important pharmacokinetic interactions.

Newer Agents

Venlafaxine and its active metabolite, *O*-desmethylvenlafaxine, are only 30% protein bound, permitting coadministration with other highly protein bound drugs.[63] Venlafaxine did not cause any significant change in the pharmacokinetics of ethanol, diazepam, or lithium.[63] Venlafaxine is metabolized to its active metabolite by the cytochrome P450 2D6 isoenzyme, which is the source of the genetic polymorphism present in the metabolism of many antidepressants. Venlafaxine does not have an inhibitory effect on isoenzymes 1A2, 2C9, 2D6, or 3A4.[90] Although nefazodone is highly protein bound in vitro, nefazodone does not alter the in vitro protein binding of chlorpromazine, desipramine, diazepam, phenytoin, lidocaine, prazosin, propranolol, verapamil, or warfarin. However, it is unknown whether or not displacement of either nefazodone or other drugs occurs in vivo.[82] Triazolobenzodiazepines, such as triazolam and alprazolam, interacted significantly with nefazodone. When triazolam is coadministered with nefazodone, a 75% reduction in the dose of triazolam is recommended. If alprazolam is coadministered with nefazodone, a 50% dose reduction is recommended.[82] Astemizole is metabolized by the cytochrome P450 3A4 isoenzyme. Ketoconazole, erythromycin, and other inhibitors of 3A4 can block the metabolism of terfenadine and astemizole, resulting in an increased plasma concentration of parent drug. Increased plasma concentrations of terfenadine and astemizole are associated with QT prolongation and with rare cases of serious cardiovascular adverse events, including death. Nefazodone is an in vitro inhibitor of 3A4. Consequently, nefazodone should not be used concomitantly with astemizole.[82]

The concurrent use of mirtazapine and the MAO inhibitors should be avoided. In addition, 14 days should elapse between the discontinuation of an MAO inhibitor and the initiation of mirtazapine, and vice versa. Mirtazapine is metabolized by cytochrome P450 isoenzymes 1A2, 2D6, and 3A4. It is not yet known if medications that induce, inhibit, or serve as substrates for these isoenzymes will lead to significant drug interactions, since they have not yet been studied systematically.[55]

Reboxetine is 97% bound to plasma protein and therefore may have the potential to interact with other medications that are also highly plasma protein bound. One would predict few, if any, pharmacokinetic interactions with reboxetine, since investigations to date have found that it does not interfere with the activity of isoenzymes of the cytochrome P450 system and is primarily renally excreted.[79]

SPECIAL POPULATIONS

Elderly Patients

Depression in the elderly is a major public health problem. Many elderly depressed patients are undiagnosed or inadequately treated. Diagnosis is often missed or mistaken for another disorder, such as dementia. In the elderly depressed patient, depressed mood—the typical signature symptom of depression—may be less prominent than the other depressive symptoms such as loss of appetite, cognitive impairment, sleeplessness, anergia, and loss of interest in and enjoyment

TABLE 69–11. Drug Interactions of Non-TCA Antidepressants

Non-TCA	Interacting Drug/Drug Class	Effect
Dibenzoxazepine		
Amoxapine	Many of the drugs that interact with the TCAs	Similar response to that seen with TCA interaction
Tetracyclic		
Maprotiline	Many of the drugs that interact with the TCAs	Similar response to that seen with TCA interaction
Mirtazapine	MAOIs	Theoretically central serotonin syndrome could occur
Triazolopyridines		
Nefazodone	Alprazolam	Increased plasma concentrations of alprazolam
	Astemizole	Theoretically increased plasma concentrations of astemizole with potentially serious cardiovascular adverse effects
	Digoxin	Increased C_{max}, C_{min}, and AUC of digoxin by 29%, 27%, and 15%, respectively
	Haloperidol	Decreased clearance of haloperidol by 35%
	MAOIs	Hypertensive crisis; serotonin syndrome; delirium; coma; seizures; hyperpyrexia
	Propranolol	Decreased C_{max} and AUC of propranolol; increased C_{max}, C_{min}, and AUC of m-CCP metabolite of nefazodone
	Ritonavir	Increased AUC of ritonavir with potential for increased adverse events: headaches, dry mouth, nausea, somnolence, dizziness
	Terfenadine	Theoretically increased plasma concentrations of terfenadine with potentially serious cardiovascular adverse effects
	Triazolam	Increased plasma concentrations of triazolam; increased psychomotor impairment
Trazodone	CNS depressants	Increased CNS depression
	Digoxin	Increased serum concentrations of digoxin
	Ethanol	Additive impairment in motor skills
	Fluoxetine	Increased plasma concentrations of trazodone
	MAOIs	Theoretically central serotonin syndrome could occur
	Neuroleptics	Increased hypotension
	Phenytoin	Increased serum concentrations of phenytoin
	Tryptophan	Agitation, restlessness, poor concentration, nausea
	Warfarin	Decreased hypoprothrombinemic response
Aminoketone		
Bupropion	MAOIs	Increased toxicity of bupropion
	Medications that lower seizure threshold	Increased incidence of seizures
	Levodopa	Increased incidence of adverse experiences
	Ritonavir	Increased blood level of bupropion with increased risk of seizures
Selective Serotonin Reuptake Inhibitors		
Citalopram	Cimetidine	Reduced oral clearance of citalopram
	Fluvoxamine	Increased plasma concentrations of citalopram
	TCAs	Possible increased AUC of TCA
Fluoxetine	Alprazolam	Increased plasma concentrations and half-life of alprazolam; increased psychomotor impairment
	Anticoagulants	Possible increased risk of bleeding
	β-Adrenergic blockers	Increased metoprolol serum concentrations and bradycardia; possible heart block
	Buspirone	Decreased therapeutic response to buspirone
	Carbamazepine	Increased plasma concentrations of carbamazepine with symptoms of carbamazepine toxicity
	Dextromethorphan	Visual hallucinations (one patient only)
	Haloperidol	Increased haloperidol concentrations and increased extrapyramidal side effects
	Lithium	Neurotoxicity—confusion, ataxia, dizziness, tremor, absence seizures
	MAOIs	Severe or fatal reactions—confusion, nausea, double vision, hypomania, hypertension, tremor, serotonin syndrome
	Phenytoin	Increased plasma concentrations of phenytoin and symptoms of phenytoin toxicity

TABLE 69–11. (Continued)

Non-TCA	Interacting Drug/Drug Class	Effect
	TCAs	Markedly increased TCA plasma concentration with symptoms of TCA toxicity
	Terfenadine	Arrhythmias, shortness of breath, and orthostasis
	Trazodone	Headaches, dizziness, sedation
	Tryptophan	Agitation, restlessness, poor concentration, nausea
	Valproate	Increased valproate serum concentrations
Fluvoxamine	Alprazolam	Increased AUC of alprazolam by 96%, increased alprazolam half-life by 71%, and increased psychomotor impairment
	Astemizole	Theoretically increased plasma concentrations of astemizole with potentially serious cardiovascular effects
	β-Adrenergic blockers	Fivefold increase in propranolol serum concentration; bradycardia and hypotension with combined fluvoxamine and metoprolol
	Carbamazepine	Possible carbamazepine toxicity, although a controlled study did not support this
	Clozapine	Increased clozapine serum concentrations and increased risk for seizures and orthostatic hypotension
	Diazepam	Decreased clearance of diazepam and its active metabolite
	Diltiazem	Bradycardia
	Haloperidol	Increased haloperidol plasma concentrations
	Lithium	Increased serotonergic effects; seizures, nausea, tremor
	MAOIs	Potential for hypertensive crisis, serotonin syndrome, seizures, delirium
	Methadone	Increased methadone plasma concentrations with symptoms of methadone toxicity
	TCAs	Increased TCA plasma concentration
	Terfenadine	Theoretically increased plasma concentrations of terfenadine with potentially serious cardiovascular effects
	Theophylline	Increased serum concentrations of theophylline with symptoms of theophylline toxicity
	Tryptophan	Increased serotonergic effects and severe vomiting
	Warfarin	Increased hypoprothrombinemic response to warfarin
Paroxetine	Cimetidine	Increased paroxetine serum concentrations
	Desipramine	Increased plasma concentrations and half-life of desipramine
	MAOIs	Potential for hypertensive crisis, serotonin syndrome, seizures, delirium
	Warfarin	Possible increased risk for bleeding
Sertraline	Carbamazepine	Increased plasma concentrations of carbamazepine
	Diazepam	Small decrease in clearance of diazepam
	MAOIs	Serotonin syndrome, myoclonus, violent shaking
	TCAs	Increased plasma concentrations of secondary amine TCAs (desipramine, nortriptyline)
	Tolbutamide	Decreased clearance of tolbutamide (16%)
	Warfarin	Increased protime
Serotonin/Norepinephrine Reuptake Inhibitor		
Venlafaxine	Cimetidine	Reduced clearance of venlafaxine by 43%
		AUC and peak serum concentration of venlafaxine increased by 60%
	MAOIs	Potential for hypertensive crisis, serotonin syndrome, seizures, delirium

Compiled from Refs. 77, 85, 86.

of the normal pursuits of life.[91] Somatic complaints are quite frequent in elderly depressed patients.

Before initiating antidepressant treatment, the elderly patient should undergo a complete physical examination, including cardiovascular, cerebrovascular, ophthalmologic, gastrointestinal, and urinary systems.

Elderly depressed patients are often over- or undertreated. Overtreatment often occurs when age-related pharmacokinetic and pharmacodynamic factors are overlooked. Undertreatment often results from an overly conservative approach as a result of the patient's advanced age or concurrent medical problems. Plasma concentration monitoring for TCAs can be a useful tool for managing drug therapy in this patient population. A TCA would not be an appropriate first choice for a depressed patient with cardiac conduction delay. However, in the healthy elderly, cautious use of a secondary amine TCA (e.g., desipramine or nortriptyline) is indicated because of their defined therapeutic plasma concentration ranges, well established efficacy, and well-known adverse-effect profiles.[91]

The SSRIs are often selected as first-choice antidepressants in the elderly, and they may enable the clinician to avoid some of the more

TABLE 69–12. Newer Antidepressants and Cytochrome (CYP) P450 Enzyme Inhibitory Potential

Drug	CYP Enzyme 1A2	2C	2D6	3A4
Fluoxetine	0	++	++++(++++)[a]	++(++)[a]
Sertraline	0	++(++)[a]	+(++)[a]	+(+)[a]
Paroxetine	0	0	++++	0
Fluvoxamine	++++	++	0	++
Citalopram	0	0	0	+++
Nefazodone	0	0	0	++++
Venlafaxine	0	0	0	0
Bupropion	0	0	0	0
Mirtazapine	0	0	0	0
Reboxetine	0	0	0	0

[a]Inhibitory potential of major metabolite.
Taken from Ref. 78.

problematic adverse effects commonly associated with the TCAs (e.g., sedative, anticholinergic, and cardiovascular side effects). Nefazodone, bupropion, and venlafaxine are also often chosen because of their milder anticholinergic and less frequent cardiovascular side effects.[91]

Although phenelzine has been used safely and effectively in well-selected patients, the MAO inhibitors are usually reserved for treatment-resistant elderly patients because of the availability of newer, better-tolerated agents and the hypotensive side effects of the MAO inhibitors. Dietary and medication restrictions can also be a concern.[91]

Pediatric Patients

Accumulating evidence indicates that childhood depression occurs quite commonly. Symptoms of depression in the young may vary from accepted diagnostic criteria and include several nonspecific symptoms such as boredom, anxiety, failing adjustment, and sleep disturbance.[92]

Data collected under controlled conditions supporting the efficacy of antidepressants in children and adolescents are sparse. In the double-blind study by Preskorn and associates, imipramine was superior in efficacy to placebo only through the first 3 weeks of treatment.[93] Demonstration of efficacy in this population is confounded by the high placebo response rate. However, the TCAs and the SSRIs remain two viable treatment options. The SSRIs are better tolerated than the TCAs and are relatively safer in an overdose. Toxicity in overdose is important in the adolescent population, where suicide is a major concern.[94]

Antidepressant compounds are used to treat depressed children and adolescents because no other definitive therapies are available. Plasma concentration monitoring of TCAs is important to ensure safety. As in the adult population, plasma concentrations above 450 ng/mL are associated with increased risk of serious adverse effects including delirium, seizures, delayed cardiac conduction, and sudden death.[95]

Several cases of sudden death have been reported in children and adolescents taking desipramine. A baseline electrocardiogram (ECG) is recommended before initiating a TCA in children and adolescents, and many clinicians recommend an additional ECG when steady-state plasma concentrations are achieved.[95]

Although three antidepressants are FDA approved for use in children, none are approved for childhood depression. Imipramine is approved only for the treatment of enuresis, clomipramine for obsessive-compulsive disorder in children 12 years and older, and fluvoxamine for obsessive-compulsive disorder in children 8 years and older. Antidepressants should be initiated in this patient population at a dosage somewhat lower than in adults; however, adolescents usually require adult doses of TCAs, and 6 to 8 weeks may be required before an antidepressant response is evident. A typical regimen of imipramine is a starting dose of 1.5 mg/kg per day that is increased by 1.0 to 1.5 mg/kg every third day. The daily dose should not exceed 5 mg/kg.[96]

Several reviews have found that the SSRIs can be administered safely to pediatric patients (6 to 18 years of age). The dosing range and dosing titration as well as adverse effects were similar to that seen in adults.[97,98]

Pregnant and Lactating Patients

Approximately 10% of pregnant women develop serious depression. No major teratogenic effects have been identified with the SSRIs or TCAs.[99–101] Studies have been conducted evaluating birth anomalies, growth impairment, and behavioral teratogenicity. A metaanalysis of first-trimester exposure to TCAs found no significant association between exposure to TCAs and congenital malformations.[100] An additional evaluation compared birth defects in neonates exposed to fluoxetine and TCAs and women exposed to agents felt not to increase the baseline teratogenetic risk (such as penicillin or dental x-rays). Comparable rates of malformations were found across all three groups. However, a higher rate of miscarriages was seen in the fluoxetine and TCA group (13.5% and 12.2%, respectively) when compared with the control group (6.8%). This raised questions about the effect of depression, in addition to that of the antidepressant, on the rate of miscarriage.[101] Studies evaluating the development of children exposed prenatally to TCAs, fluoxetine, or nonteratogens found no differences in rates of prenatal complications, incidence of major malformations, and mean global IQ scores.

Some concern regarding the use of fluoxetine arose as a result of an evaluation of neonates where exposure to fluoxetine occurred before 25 weeks of gestation but not after (early exposure) versus exposure during the third trimester (late exposure) versus exposure to nonteratogens. Premature birth occurred in 14.3% of late-exposure neonates compared with 4.1% of infants born to the early-exposure group and 5.9% in the control group.[100] Additionally, birth weight, birth length, and maternal weight gain were less in the late-exposure group compared with the early-exposure and control groups. Evaluations to date do not support any teratogenic effects of fluoxetine but do raise questions regarding premature birth and fetal growth rate.[101]

If a TCA is withdrawn during pregnancy, it should be tapered gradually to avoid maternal or fetal withdrawal symptoms. If possible, drug tapering is usually begun 5 to 10 days before the estimated day of confinement.[101] Although the MAO inhibitors have demonstrated teratogenicity in animals, there are insufficient data in humans to permit firm conclusions. Similarly, there are inadequate data on the use of other antidepressants during pregnancy.

In summary, the risks and benefits of drug therapy during pregnancy always must be weighed, and concerns about the risks of untreated depression during pregnancy should be considered. These include the possibility of low birth weight secondary to poor maternal weight gain, suicidality, potential for hospitalization, potential for marital discord, inability to engage in appropriate obstetric care, and difficulty caring for other children.[38] Further evaluations of the new antidepressant agents are needed to fully understand the risk associated with their use at various stages of the gestational period. Additionally, the risks of not treating depression in a pregnant woman should not be minimized.

CLINICAL APPLICATION

A suggested algorithm for the management of depression is shown in Figure 69–1.

Dosing

Recommended initial doses and dosage ranges are shown in Table 69–4. The usual initial adult dose of most TCAs is 50 mg at bedtime, and the dose may be increased by 25 to 50 mg every third day. The recommended initial dose for the SSRIs is fluoxetine, 10 to 20 mg; paroxetine, 20 mg; sertraline, 50 mg; and citalopram, 20 mg.

Bupropion is usually initiated at 100 mg twice daily, and this dose may be increased to 100 mg three times daily after 3 days. Most patients will respond at 300 mg/day; however, an increase to 450 mg/day, given as 150 mg three times daily, may be considered in patients with no clinical response after several weeks of treatment at 300 mg/day. Additionally, a sustained-release formulation of bupropion is currently available and may be given as 200 mg twice a day in those individuals requiring higher dosages.

Typically, phenelzine is initiated at 15 mg in the morning and then increased by 15 mg every third day up to 60 mg/day. The dose should be given three times daily to minimize postural hypotension, with the last dose given in the early afternoon to lessen the likelihood of insomnia. Maintenance doses may be as low as 15 mg/day.

The usual starting dose of venlafaxine is 75 mg/day given in two or three divided doses and taken with food. Depending on tolerability, the dose is then increased to 150 mg/day. If needed, the dose

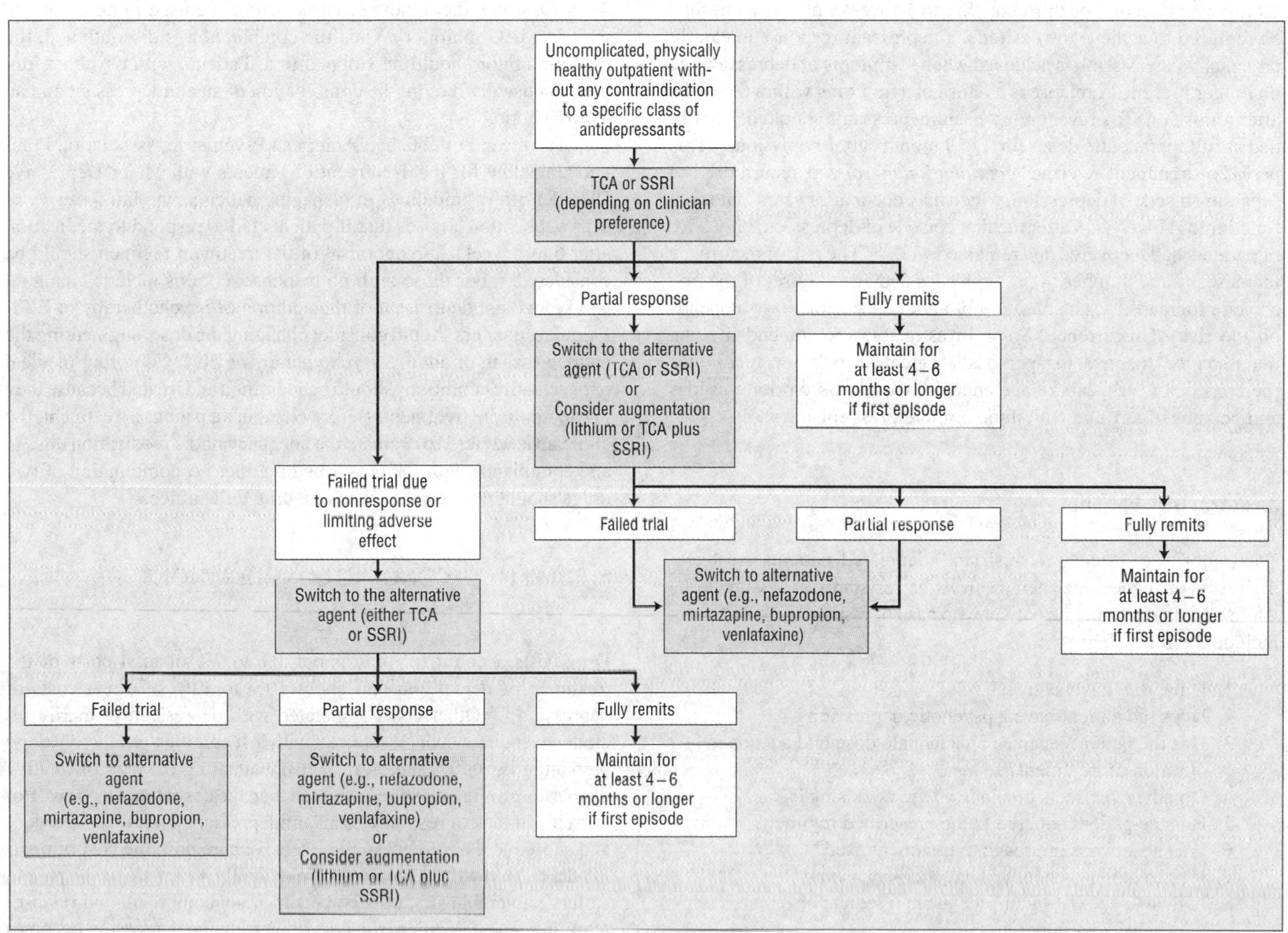

FIGURE 69–1. Algorithm for treatment of uncomplicated major depression.

may be further increased to 225 mg/day. Certain patients, including severely depressed patients, may need a dose up to 375 mg/day. A sustained-release formulation of venlafaxine is also available. The recommended starting dose is 75 mg/day administered with food. Dosage increases should occur in 75 mg/day increments with a maximum daily dose of 225 mg.

The starting dose of nefazodone is 100 mg given twice daily. Dose increases should occur in increments of 100 mg/day, on a twice-daily schedule, at intervals of no less than 1 week, with the usual effective dose range between 300 and 600 mg/day.

The recommended starting dose of mirtazapine is 15 mg/day administered in a single dose at bedtime. The maximum dose recommended is 45 mg/day. Dosage increases should occur every 1 to 2 weeks as indicated. Reboxetine dosing in clinical evaluations has ranged from 8 to 10 mg/day.[52]

Caution is urged when switching from one antidepressant to another. It is important to remember that 3 to 4 weeks is usually required before a mood-elevating response is seen. A 6-week trial at a maximum dosage is considered an adequate trial.[35] It is crucial to explain to the patient about the expected lag time before the onset of clinical response. Patients uneducated in this regard often fail to comply with their prescribed regimens.

In elderly patients, as a general rule, dosing is initiated at half the initial dose administered to younger adults, and the dose is increased at a slower rate. Thus desipramine or nortriptyline may be initiated at 10 to 25 mg/day or fluoxetine at 10 to 20 mg/day or alternatively 20 mg every second or third day. Six to 12 weeks of treatment may be required to achieve the desired antidepressant response in elderly patients.[32] A remission is achieved when symptoms of depression are no longer present. A relapse is a return of symptoms within 6 months after remission. To prevent relapse, antidepressants should be continued at full therapeutic doses for 4 to 9 months after remission.[35] This period of treatment is termed *continuation therapy*. A recurrence is a separate episode of depression, which may occur after years of normal functioning. Five years after the first episode of depression, only 25% of patients had recovered and remained well.[102] The risk of recurrence increases as the number of past episodes and age at onset of the first episode increase.[103] The duration of antidepressant therapy depends on the risk of recurrence. Some investigators recommend lifelong maintenance therapy for persons at greatest risk for recurrence (persons below 40 years of age and with two or more prior episodes and persons of any age with three or more prior episodes).[35]

Refractory Patients

The majority of "treatment resistant" depressed patients are likely the result of inadequate therapy (relative resistance).[35] Issues to be addressed in assessing the patient who has not responded to treatment include the following:

1. Is the diagnosis correct?
2. Does the patient have a psychotic depression?
3. Has the patient received an adequate dose and adequate duration of treatment?
4. Do adverse effects preclude adequate dosing?
5. Has the patient adhered to the prescribed regimen?
6. Was a stepwise approach to treatment used?
7. Was treatment outcome adequately measured?
8. Is there a coexisting or preexisting medical or psychiatric disorder?
9. Are there other factors that interfere with treatment?

When a patient has failed to respond, nondrug modalities including environmental manipulation, family counseling, cognitive therapy, or interpersonal psychotherapy are often beneficial.[35]

Three primary pharmacologic approaches are used when dealing with treatment nonresponse. The current antidepressant may be stopped and a trial with an unrelated agent initiated. For example, the patient may be switched from a TCA to an SSRI or an MAO inhibitor. Second, the current antidepressant can be augmented (potentiated) by the addition of lithium, liothyronine, or an anticonvulsant such as carbamazepine or valproic acid. A third approach to the treatment-resistant patient is to use concurrently two different classes of antidepressants (e.g., a TCA plus an MAO inhibitor).[35] As discussed previously, the combination of an SSRI and an MAO inhibitor should never be used.

There are accumulating data to support that 50% to 60% of previously treatment-resistant depressed patients respond to adequate doses of SSRIs. MAO inhibitors can be considered in the truly treatment-resistant population, especially for the patient with atypical features.[35]

Augmenting strategies, such as the addition of lithium to a TCA regimen, have been found to benefit some previously unresponsive patients. Several older trials support that addition of liothyronine to a TCA regimen may induce antidepressant response.[35]

Only a prescriber experienced in the use of such combinations should undertake concurrent use of a TCA and an MAO inhibitor. When this is undertaken, the MAO inhibitor is slowly added to the TCA. Desipramine is not recommended to be used in combination with an MAO inhibitor. When the combination is discontinued, the MAO inhibitor should be stopped first. Patients with psychotic depression usually require the combination of an antidepressant and an antipsychotic.[35]

The recently published American Psychiatric Association Practice Guideline for the Treatment of Patients with Major Depressive Disorder offers guidelines in managing patients who fail to respond. This publication advises that if patients fail to respond to medication after 6 to 8 weeks, a reappraisal of the treatment regimen should be considered.[35] For those with no response, options include changing to a second antidepressant or the addition of psychotherapy or ECT. Partial responders should consider changing the dose, augmenting the antidepressant, or adding psychotherapy or ECT. Comorbid medical or psychiatric conditions should be identified and treated because they may complicate treatment. Before changing a patient's treatment, the clinician is advised to evaluate the adequacy of the medication dosage and compliance with the prescribed regimen. A combination of two drugs should not be used when one drug will suffice.

PHARMACOECONOMIC CONSIDERATIONS

Drug costs account for only about 1% to 2% of total costs of the treatment of depression and about 10% to 12% of direct costs of depression.[104] Other costs associated with depression primarily include the indirect costs associated with lost earnings/productivity and premature death.[104] Therefore, when evaluating the cost of treating depression, more must be considered than the cost of medications. For example, if lack of response to an antidepressant leads to an overdose and subsequent treatment in the intensive care unit, the cost of treating depression will be increased dramatically. Likewise, if the patient suffers intolerable side effects, becomes noncompliant, and relapses requiring hospitalization, the cost of treating the depression becomes very expensive quite rapidly.

When SSRIs were introduced, many managed care organizations restricted these medications to those who had failed treatment with the TCAs or been unable to tolerate these agents, with the belief that the SSRIs represented a more expensive approach to the treatment of depression. Subsequent evaluations have shown that in fact the SSRIs represent a more economic approach to the treatment of depression when compared with TCAs when all treatment costs are considered.[105–108] The larger question seems to center around whether one SSRI is more economic than another. Initial findings suggest that fluoxetine may offer an overall cost advantage when compared with other SSRIs, but additional longer-term data are necessary before a final conclusion can be reached.[109]

A recent evaluation examined the cost-effectiveness of fluoxetine and nefazodone compared with TCAs in managed care settings.[110] This evaluation found that both nefazodone and fluoxetine were cost-effective when compared with imipramine, with nefazodone being slightly more cost-effective than fluoxetine.[110] These data further support the notion that a lower cost of drug therapy does not necessarily translate into an overall lesser cost for the treatment of depression.

Additional, longer-term studies in more diverse populations are necessary before judgments can be made regarding which of the newer antidepressant agents offers a cost advantage. It would be extremely useful if subpopulations and special populations (e.g., the elderly, those with comorbid substance abuse, those with comorbid anxiety disorders, and children) were studied and cost-effective agents in these subpopulations were identified. Also, the pharamacoeconomics of the medication management of depression in various health care environments such as public, private psychiatry, or primary care needs evaluation.[111]

EVALUATION OF THERAPEUTIC OUTCOMES

Several monitoring parameters, in addition to plasma concentrations, are useful in managing patients. Patients must be monitored for adverse effects, such as sedation, anticholinergic effects, and sexual dysfunction, and for remission of previously documented target symptoms. The presence of side effects does not necessarily indicate adequate dosage. In addition, changes in social and occupational functioning should be assessed. When TCAs are given concurrently with adrenergic neuronal blocking antihypertensives (e.g., guanethidine, methyldopa, clonidine), blood pressure should be monitored regularly. Patients receiving venlafaxine should have their blood pressure monitored at regular intervals. Patients older than 40 should receive a pretreatment electrocardiogram (ECG) before starting TCA therapy, and follow-up ECGs should be performed periodically. Patients should be monitored for the emergence of suicidal ideation after initiation of any antidepressant.

In addition to the clinical interview, psychometric rating instruments (e.g., patient-rated and clinician-rated scales) allow for rapid and reliable measurement of the nature and severity of depressive and associated symptoms (see Chap. 62). It is helpful to administer the rating scales prior to treatment, 6 to 8 weeks after initiation of therapy, and periodically thereafter. Interviewing a family member or friend (with the patient's permission) regarding symptoms and daily functioning also can assist in assessment of progress. It is recommended that patients be monitored closely for relapse or recurrence if the brand of antidepressant is changed. Patients should be monitored at more frequent intervals early in treatment. Monitoring is then continued at regular intervals throughout the continuation and maintenance phases of treatment. Regular monitoring also should be continued for several months after antidepressant therapy is discontinued.

CONCLUSIONS

Major depressive disorder remains one of the most commonly occurring mental illnesses in adults, and it is often undiagnosed and untreated. Pharmacologic intervention remains the cornerstone of antidepressant treatment. Antidepressant medications have a broad spectrum of neurochemical effects and influence a variety of receptors peripherally and centrally. Safe and effective use of antidepressants requires a thorough understanding of the pharmacology of these drugs and of the principles of monitoring efficacy and adverse effects. In addition, clinicians must have a thorough understanding of antidepressant drug interactions and other factors that may influence the pharmacokinetics of antidepressant drugs. Plasma concentration monitoring is unnecessary for most patients but can improve the outcome in some situations. The search for more effective antidepressants with more favorable adverse-effect profiles must continue.

▶ PRINCIPLES OF PHARMACOTHERAPY

- When evaluating a patient for the presence of depression, it is essential to rule out medical causes of depression and drug-induced depression.
- When determining if a patient has been nonresponsive to a particular pharmacotherapeutic intervention, it must be determined whether the patient has received an adequate dose for an adequate duration. If TCAs are being used, a serum level may be useful, especially in special populations such as the elderly and those with concurrent medications that may alter the pharmacokinetic profile of the TCAs.
- If the patient exhibits a partial response to a pharmacotherapeutic agent, augmentation therapy should be considered before the trial is abandoned and the patient is treated with an alternative therapeutic agent.
- When counseling patients with depression who are receiving pharmacotherapeutic interventions, the patient should be informed that adverse effects may occur immediately, while a resolution of symptoms may take 2 to 4 weeks.
- The efficacy of the regimen should be based on the resolution of the target signs and symptoms identified before treatment. Rating scales should be used whenever possible to evaluate and document response.
- Family members or a friend should be involved in the evaluation and assessment of response if feasible and with the patient's permission because the patient may not recognize the full extent of the signs and symptoms and their subsequent resolution.
- Whenever other medications are used concurrently with an antidepressant, evaluate the regimen for potential drug interactions, especially those involving the isoenzymes of the cytochrome P450 system.
- When evaluating response to an antidepressant agent, in addition to target signs and symptoms, consider

quality-of-life issues such as role, social functioning, and occupational functioning. In addition, the tolerability of the agent should be assessed because the occurrence of side effects may lead to noncompliance.

- An assessment of compliance should be made at every visit. Remember that accurate capsule or tablet counts do not mean the patient has consumed the medication or consumed it in the manner prescribed.

REFERENCES

1. American Psychiatric Association. Diagnostic and Statistical Manual of Mental Disorders, 4th ed., text revision (DSM-IV-TR). Washington, American Psychiatric Association, 2000:356.
2. Montgomery SA. Efficacy in the long-term treatment of depression. J Clin Psychiatry 1996;57(Suppl 2):24–30.
3. Katon W, Von Korff M, Lin E, et al. Collaborative management to achieve treatment guidelines: Impact on depression in primary care. JAMA 1995;273:1026–1031.
4. Wells KB, Sherbourne CD. Functioning and utility for current health of patients with depression or chronic medical conditions in managed primary care practices. Arch Gen Psychiatry 1999;56(101):897–904.
5. Hays RD, Wells KB, Sherbourne CD, et al. Functioning and well-being outcomes in patients with depression compared with chronic general medical illnesses. Arch Gen Psychiatry 1995;52:11–19.
6. Lebowitz BD, Pearson JL, Schneider LS, et al. Diagnosis and treatment of depression in late life: Consensus statement update. JAMA 1997;278:1186–1190.
7. Steffens DC, Skoog I, Norton MC, et al. Prevalence of depression and its treatment in an elderly population: The Cache County study. Arch Gen Psychiatry 2000;57(6):601–607.
8. Kessler RC, McGonagle KA, Zhao S, et al. Lifetime and 12-month prevalence of DSM-III-R psychiatric disorders in the United States: Results from the National Comorbidity Survey. Arch Gen Psychiatry 1994;51: 8–19.
9. Klerman GL, Weissman MM. Increasing rates of depression. JAMA 1989;261:2229–2235.
10. Murphy JM, Laird NM, Monso RR, et al. A 40-year perspective on the prevalence of depression: The Stirling County Study. Arch Gen Psychiatry 2000;57(3):209–215.
11. Kessler RC, Walters EE. Epidemiology of DSM-IIIR major depression and minor depression among adolescents and young adults in the National Comorbidity Survey. Depress Anxiety 1998;7(1):3–14.
12. Larsson B, Ivarsson T. Clinical characteristics of adolescent psychiatric inpatients who have attempted suicide. Eur Child Adolesc Psychiatry 1998;7(4):201–208.
13. Weissman MM, Gershon ES, Kidd KK, et al. Psychiatric disorders in the relatives of probands with affective disorder. Arch Gen Psychiatry 1984;41:13–21.
14. Warner V, Weissman MM, Mufson L, Wickramaratne PJ. Grandparents, parents, and grandchildren at high risk for depression: A three-generation study. J Am Acad Child Adolesc Psychiatry 1999;38(3):289–296.
15. Kendler KS, Prescott CA. A population based twin study of lifetime major depression in men and women. Arch Gen Psychiatry 1999;56(1): 39–44.
16. Stahl SM. Blue genes and the mechanism of action of antidepressants. J Clin Psychiatry 2000;61(3):164–165.
17. Delgado PL. Depression: The case for a monoamine deficiency. J Clin Psychiatry 2000;61(Suppl 6):7–11.
18. Hirschfield RM. History and the evolution of the monoamine hypothesis of depression. J Clin Psychiatry 2000;61(Suppl 6):4–6.
19. Kendler KS, Thornton LM, Gardner CO. Stressful life events and previous episodes in the etiology of major depression in women: An evaluation of the kindling hypothesis. Am J Psychiatry 2000;157(8):1243–1251.
20. Delgado PL, Moreno FA, Potter R, et al. Norepinephrine and serotonin in antidepressant action: Evidence from neurotransmitter depletion studies. In: Briley M, Montgomery SA, eds. Antidepressant Therapy at the Dawn of the Third Millennium. London, Marin Dunitz, 1997:141–163.
21. Baldessarini RJ. Drugs and the treatment of psychiatric disorders: II. Drugs used in the treatment of disorders of mood. In Gilman AG, Rall TW, et al. eds. Goodman and Gilman's The Pharmacologic Basis of Therapeutics, 8th ed. New York, Pergamon, 1990:404–435.
22. Prange AJ, Wilson IC, Lynn CW, et al. L-Tryptophan in mania. Arch Gen Psychiatry 1974;30:56–62.
23. Feighner JP. Mechanism of action of antidepressant medications. J Clin Psychiatry 1999;60(Suppl 4):4–11.
24. Frazer A. Pharmacology of antidepressants. J Clin Psychopharmacol 1997;17(2):2S–18S.
25. Stahl S. Basic psychopharmacology of antidepressants: 1. Antidepressants have seven distinct mechanisms of actions. J Clin Psychiatry 1998;59(Suppl 4):5–14.
26. Bryant SG, Brown CS. Current concepts in clinical therapeutics: Major affective disorders, part 1. Clin Pharm 1986;5:304–318.
27. Siever LJ, Davis KL. Overview: Toward a dysregulation hypothesis of depression. Am J Psychiatry 1985;142:1017–1031.
28. Willner P. Dopaminergic mechanisms in depression and mania. In: Bloom FE, Kupfer DJ, eds. Psychopharmacology: The Fourth Generation of Progress. New York, Raven, 1995:921–931.
29. Reddy PL, Khanna S, Subhash MN, et al. CSF amine metabolites in depression. Biol Psychiatry 1992;31:112–118.
30. Thase ME, Fasiczka AL, Berman SR, et al. Electroencephalographic sleep profiles before and after cognitive behavior therapy of depression. Arch Gen Psychiatry 1998;55(2):138–144.
31. Katon W, Sullivan MD. Depression and chronic medical illness. J Clin Psychiatry 1990;51(Suppl):3–11.
32. Thiessen BQ, Wallace SM, Blackburn JL, et al. Increased prescribing of antidepressants subsequent to beta-blocker therapy. Arch Intern Med 1990;150:2286–2290.
33. Malone KM, Oquendo MA, Haas GL, et al. Protective factors against suicidal acts in major depression: Reasons for living. Am J Psychiatry 2000;157(7):1084–1088.
34. Alexopoulois GS, Bruce HL, Hull J, et al. T. Clinical determinant of suicidal ideation and behavior in geriatric depression. Arch Gen Psychiatry 1999;56(11):1048–1053.
35. American Psychiatric Association. Practice guideline for the treatment of patients with major depressive disorder (revision). Am J Psychiatry 2000;157(Suppl):1–45.
36. Nierenberg AA, Alpert JE, Pava J, et al. Course and treatment of atypical depression. J Clin Psychiatry 1998;59(Suppl 1)18:5–9.
37. Rothschild AJ. Management of psychotic treatment-resistant depression. Psychiatr Clin North Am 1996;19(2):237–252.
38. Blackbum IM, Moore RG. Controlled acute and follow-up trial of cognitive therapy and pharmacotherapy in outpatients with recurrent depression. Br J Psychiatry 1997;171:328–334.
39. Klapheke MM. Electroconvulsive therapy consultation: an update. Convuls Ther 1997;13:227–241.
40. Partonen T, Partinen M. Light treatment for seasonal affective disorder: Theoretical considerations and clinical implications. Acta Psychiatr Scand 1994;377:41S–45S.
41. Partonen T, Lonnavist J. Seasonal affective disorder. Lancet 1998;352(9137):1369–1374.
42. Lafer B, Sachs GS, Labbate LA, et al. Side effects induced by bright light therapy. Am J Psychiatry 1994;151:1081–1083.
43. Labbate LA, Lafter B, Thibault A, Sachs GS. Phototherapy for seasonal affective disorder: A blind comparison of three different schedules. J Clin Psychiatry 1994;55:189–191.
44. Josey ES, Hackett RL. St. John's wort: A new alternative for depression? Int J Clin Pharmacol Ther 1999;37(3):111–119.
45. Gastor B, Holroyd J. St. John's wort for depression: A systematic review. Arch Intern Med 2000;160(2):152–156.

46. Shelton RC, Keller MB, Gelenberg A, et al. Effectiveness of St. John's wort in major depression: a randomized controlled trial. JAMA 2001;285:1978–1986.
47. Schrader E. Equivalence of St. John's wort extract (Ze 117) and fluoxetine: A randomized, controlled study in mild–moderate depression. Int Clin Psychopharmacol 2000;15(2):61–68.
48. McIntyre M. A review of the benefits, adverse events, drug interactions, and safety of St. John's wort (*Hypericum perforatum*): The implications with regard to the regulation of herbal medicines. J Altern Complement Med 2000;6(2):115–124.
49. Burke MJ, Preskorn SH. Short term treatment of mood disorders with standard antidepressants. In: Bloom FE, Kupfer DJ, eds. Psychopharmacology: The Fourth Generation of Progress. New York, Raven, 1995:1053–1065.
50. Ballenger JC. Clinical evaluation of venlafaxine. J Clin Psychopharmacol 1996;16(Suppl 2):29S–35S.
51. Berzewski H, Van Moffaert M, Gagiano CA. Efficacy and tolerability of reboxetine compared with imipramine in a double-blind study in patients suffering from major depressive episodes. Eur Neuropsychopharmacol 1997;7(Suppl 1):S37–S47.
52. Massana J, Moller HJ, Burrows GD, Montenegro RM. Reboxetine: A double-blind comparison with fluoxetine in major depressive disorder. Int Clin Psychopharmacol 1999;14(2):73–80.
53. Davis R, Whittington R, Bryson HM. Nefazodone: A review of its pharmacology and clinical efficacy in the management of major depression. Drugs 1997;53(4):608 636.
54. Horst WD, Preskorn SH, Mechanism of action and clinical characteristics of three atypical antidepressants: venlafaxine, nefazodone, bupropion. J Affect Disord 1998;51(3):237–254.
55. Gorman JM. Mirtazapine: Clinical overview. J Clin Psychiatry 1999;60(Suppl 17):9–13.
56. Bryant SG, Brown CS. Current concepts in clinical therapeutics: Major affective disorders, part 2. Clin Pharm 1986;5:385–395.
57. Peroutka SJ, Snyder SH. Long term antidepressant treatment decreases spiroperidol-labeled serotonin receptor binding. Science 1980;210: 88–90.
58. Hilton S, Jaber B, Ruch R. Moclobemide safety: Monitoring a newly developed product in the 1990s. J Clin Psychopharmacol 1995;15 (Suppl 2):76S–83S.
59. Settle ED Jr. Antidepressant drugs: disturbing and potentially dangerous adverse effects. J Clin Psychiatry 1998;59(Suppl 16):25–30.
60. Ray WA, Griffin MR, Schaffner W, et al. Psychotropic drug use and the risk of hip fracture. New Engl J Med 1987;316:363–369.
61. Haddad P. Antidepressant discontinuation reactions. In: Thompson C, chairperson. Discontinuation of antidepressant therapy: Emerging complications and their relevance [Academic Highlights]. J Clin Psychiatry 1998;59(10):541–548.
62. Moller HJ, Volz HP. Drug treatment of depression in the 1990s: An overview of achievements and future possibilities. Drugs 1996;52: 625–638.
63. Andrews JM, Ninan PT, Nemeroff CB. Venlafaxine: A novel antidepressant that has a dual mechanism of action. Depression 1996;4(2):48–56.
64. Feighner JP. Cardiovascular safety in depressed patients: Focus on venlafaxine. J Clin Psychiatry 1995;56(12):574–579.
65. Preskorn SH. Clinically relevant pharmacology of selective serotonin reuptake inhibitors: An overview with emphasis on pharmacokinetics and effects on oxidative drug metabolism. Clin Pharmacokinet 1997;32 (suppl 1):1–21.
66. Goldstein BJ, Goodnick PJ. Selective serotonin reuptake inhibitors in the treatment of affective disorders: III. Tolerability, safety and pharmacoeconomics. J Psychopharmacol 1998;12(3 Suppl B):S55–S87.
67. Aranoff GM. Trazodone associated with priapism. Lancet 1984;1:856.
68. Brodie-Meijer CC, Diemont Wl, Buijs PJ. Nefazodone-induced clitoral priapism. Int Clin Psychopharmacol 1999;14(4):257–258.
69. Johnston JA, Lineberry CG, Ascher JA. A 102 center prospective study of seizures in association with bupropion. J Clin Psychiatry 1991;52(11):450 456.
70. Nierenberg AA, Cole JO. Antidepressant adverse drug reactions. J Clin Psychiatry 1991;52(Suppl):40–47.
71. Rapp MS. Two cases of ejaculatory impairment related to phenelzine. Am J Psychiatry 1979;136:1200–1201.
72. Barton JL. Orgasmic inhibition by phenelzine. Am J Psychiatry 1979;136:1616–1617.
73. Rabkin JG, Quitkin FM, McGrath P, et al. Adverse reactions to monoamine oxidase inhibitors: II. Treatment correlates and clinical management. J Clin Psychopharmacol 1985;5:2–9.
74. Neil JF, Licata SM, May SJ, Himmelhock JM. Dietary noncompliance during treatment with tranylcypromine. J Clin Psychiatry 1979;40: 33–37.
75. Grossman E, Messerli FH, Grodzicki T, Kowey P. Should a moratorium be placed on sublingual nifedipine capsules given for hypertensive emergencies and pseudoemergencies? JAMA 1996;276:1328–1331.
76. Varon J, Marik PE. The diagnosis and management of hypertensive crises. Chest 2000;118:214–227.
77. Wells BG. Tricyclic antidepressants. In: Taylor WJ, Caviness MHD, eds. A Textbook for the Clinical Application of Therapeutic Drug Monitoring. Irving, TX, Abbott Laboratories, 1986:449–465.
78. DeVane CL. Metabolism and pharmacokinetics of the selective serotonin reuptake inhibitors. Cell Mol Neurobiol 1999;19(4):443–466.
79. Dostert P, Benedetti MS, Poggesi I. Review of the pharmacokinetics and metabolism of reboxetine, a selective noradrenaline inhibitor. Eur Neuropsychopharmacol 1997;7(Suppl 1):S23–S35.
80. Krastev Z, Terzivoanov D, Vlahov V, et al. The pharmacokinetics of paroxetine in patients with liver cirrhosis. Acta Psychiatry Scand 1989;350(Suppl):91–92.
81. Demolis JL, Angebaud P, Grange JD, et al. Influence of liver cirrhosis on sertraline pharmacokinetics. Br J Clin Pharmacol 1996;42(3):394 397.
82. Green DS, Barvhaiya RH. Clinical pharmacokinetics of nefazodone. Clin Pharmacokinet 1997;33(4):260–275.
83. Perry PJ, Pfohl BM, Holstad SC. The relationship between antidepressant response and tricyclic antidepressant plasma concentrations. Clin Pharmacokinet 1987;13:381–392.
84. Tricyclic antidepressants—Blood level measurements and clinical outcomes: An APA task force report. Am J Psychiatry 1985;142:155–162.
85. Hansten PD, Horn JR. Drug Interactions and Updates. Vancouver, WA, Applied Therapeutics, 1997:127–842.
86. Mitchell PB. Drug interactions of clinical significance with serotonin reuptake inhibitors. Drug Saf 1997;17(6):390–406.
87. DeVane CL. Differential pharmacology of newer antidepressants. J Clin Psychiatry 1998;59(Suppl 20):85–93.
88. Rosenbaum JR, Managing SSRI-drug interactions in clinical practice. Clin Pharmacokinetic 1995;29(Suppl 1):53–59.
89. Bezchlibnyk-Butler K, Alexksic I, Kennedy SH. Citalopram and drug interactions. J Psychiatry Neurosci 2000;25(3):241–254.
90. Ereshefsky L. Drug-drug interactions involving antidepressants: focus on venlafaxine. J Clin Psychopharmacol 1996;(3 Suppl 2):37S–50S.
91. Zisook S, Downs NS. Diagnosis and treatment of depression in late life. J Clin Psychiatry 1998;59(Suppl 4):80–91.
92. Cosgrave E, McGorry P, Allen N, Jackson H. Depression in young people: A growing challenge for primary care. Aust Fam Physician 2000;29(2):123–127.
93. Preskorn S, Weller E, Hughes C, et al. Depression in prepubertal children: DST nonsuppression predicts differential response to imipramine versus placebo. Psychopharmacol Bull 1987;23:128–133.
94. Larsson B, Ivarsson T. Clinical characteristics of adolescent psychiatric inpatients who have attempted suicide. Eur Child Adolesc Psychiatry 1998;7(4):201–208.
95. Leonard HL, Meyer HC, Swedo SE, et al. Electrocardiographic changes during desipramine and clomipramine treatment in children and adolescents. J Am Acad Child Adolesc Psychiatry 1995;34(11): 1460–1468.
96. Weller EB, Weller RA. Depressive disorders in children and adolescents. In: Garfinkel BD, Carlson GA, Weller EB, eds. Psychiatric Disorders in Children and Adolescents. Philadelphia, Saunders, 1990:17 19.

97. Hamilton JD, Bridge J. Outcome at 6 months for 50 adolescents with major depression treated in a health maintenance organization. J Am Acad Child Adolesc Psychiatry 1999;38(11):1340–1346.
98. Alderman J, Wolkow R, Chung M, Johnston HF. Sertraline treatment of children and adolescents with obsessive compulsive disorder or depression: Pharmacokinetics, tolerability, and efficacy. J Am Acad Child Adolesc Psychiatry 1998;37(4):386–394.
99. Altshuler LL, Cohen L, Szuba MP, et al. Pharmacologic management of psychiatric illness during pregnancy: Dilemmas and guidelines. Am J Psychiatry 1996;153:592–606.
100. Wisner KL, Gelenberg AJ, Leonard H, et al. Pharmacologic treatment of depression during pregnancy. JAMA 1999;282(13):1264–1269.
101. Baum AL, Misri S. Selective serotonin-reuptake inhibitors in pregnancy and lactation. Harvard Rev Psychiatry 1996;4:117–125.
102. Keller MB, Lavori PW, Mueller TI. Time to recovery, chronicity, and levels of psychopathology in major depression: A five year prospective follow up of 431 subjects. Arch Gen Psychiatry 1992;49:809–816.
103. Greden JF. Antidepressant maintenance medications: When to discontinue and how to stop. J Clin Psychiatry 1993;54(Suppl 8):39–45.
104. Smith W, Sherill A. A pharmacoeconomic study of the management of major depression: Patients in a TennCare HMO. Med Interface 1996;9(7):88–92.
105. Greenberg PE, Stiglin LE, Finkelstein LM, et al. The economic burden of depression in 1990. J Clin Psychiatry 1993;54:405–418.
106. Sclar DA, Robinson LM, Skaer TL, et al. Antidepressant pharmacotherapy: Economic outcomes in a health maintenance organization. Clin Ther 1994;16:715–730.
107. LePen C, Levy E, Ravily V, et al. The cost of treatment dropout in depression: A cost-benefit analysis of fluoxetine versus tricyclics. J Affective Disord 1994;31:1–18.
108. Skaer TL, Sclar DA. Robinson LM, et al. Economic evaluation of amitriptyline, desipramine, nortriptyline, and sertraline in the management of patients with depression. Curr Ther Res 1995;56: 556–567.
109. Sclar DA, Robinson LM, Skaer TL, et al. Antidepressant pharmacotherapy: Economic evaluation of fluoxetine, paroxetine, and sertraline in a health maintenance organization. J Int Med Res 1995;23: 395–412.
110. Revicki DA, Brown RE, Keller MB, et al. Cost-effectiveness of newer antidepressants compared with tricyclic antidepressants in managed care settings. J Clin Psychiatry 1997;58:47–58.
111. Conner TM, Crismon ML, Still DJ. A critical review of selected pharmacoeconomic analyses of antidepressant therapy. Ann Pharmacother 1999;33(3):364–372.

70
BIPOLAR DISORDER

Martha P. Fankhauser

Previously known as manic–depressive illness, bipolar disorder is a cyclic disorder with recurrent fluctuations in mood, energy, and behavior encompassing the extremes of human experiences. This disorder differs from recurrent major depression (or unipolar depression) in that a manic, hypomanic, or mixed episode occurs during the course of the illness. Bipolar disorder is an intriguing psychiatric disorder because it is genetically based, environmentally influenced, and widely varied in its clinical presentations.

EPIDEMIOLOGY

Epidemiologic studies report that the lifetime prevalence rate of a manic episode is 1.6% ± 0.3 for men and 1.7% ± 0.3 for women in the United States (approximately 4 million people).[1] The lifetime prevalence of bipolar I disorder (one or more manic or mixed episodes) is 0.4% to 1.6%; that for bipolar II disorder (recurrent major depressive episodes with hypomanic episodes) is 0.5% in community samples.[2,3] Bipolar I disorder occurs equally in men and women, whereas bipolar II disorder is more common in women.[2]

ETIOLOGY

The exact etiology of bipolar disorder is unknown, but it is believed to be based on genetic factors and caused by the dysregulation in the production or actions of neurotransmitters, hormones and cations, secondary messenger systems, neuroendocrine pathways, and biologic rhythms.

GENETIC FACTORS

Hereditary risk is an important determinant of who will develop bipolar disorder, but nongenetic factors (e.g., perinatal development, head trauma, environmental factors, stress) may be responsible for some cases. Bipolar disorder has a higher genetic risk than major depressive disorders.[4] Approximately 80% to 90% of patients with bipolar disorder have a biologic relative (e.g., parent, sibling, child) with a mood disorder (e.g., bipolar disorder, major depression, cyclothymia, dysthymia). First-degree relatives of these patients have a 15% to 35% risk of developing a mood disorder. Studies show a 78% to 80% concordance rate in monozygotic twins, compared with 20% in dizygotic twins.[5] The exact mechanism of genetic transmission is not known and may involve multifactorial inheritance. Linkage studies suggest that loci on 4, 6, 12, 18, 21, 22, and X chromosome may contribute to genetic susceptibility of bipolar disorder.[5,6]

SECONDARY MANIA

Several general medical or substance-related causes of mania have been identified (Table 70–1).[3] A complete medical and Many medication history and physical examination are necessary to rule out any organic causes. Laboratory testing may be warranted if the history or physical examination reveal any abnormalities (e.g., signs or symptoms of hypothyroidism). Medications known to cause mania, agitation, or insomnia should be discontinued.

PATHOPHYSIOLOGIC FACTORS

Many hypotheses have been proposed regarding the pathophysiology of mood disorders, including neurotransmitter, neuromodulator, signal transduction, neuroanatomic, and physiologic abnormalities.[4,7,8]

NEUROTRANSMITTER THEORIES

The most prominent and oldest hypotheses regarding mood disorders are those proposing an alteration in monoamine neurotransmitter concentrations in the central nervous system (CNS).[4,7,8] The monoamine hypothesis suggests an excess of catecholamines (primarily norepinephrine and dopamine) in mania and a functional deficit of neurotransmitters (primarily norepinephrine, dopamine, and/or serotonin [5-HT]) in depression. Norepinephrine, dopamine, and 5-HT are highly interdependent and interact with or modulate other neurotransmitter and hormone systems. The "permissive serotonin hypothesis" proposes that the central activity of 5-HT, which plays a critical role in modulating CNS activity (e.g., stabilization of the catecholamine system and inhibition of dopamine), is low in both mania and depression.[5] Lithium produces a subsensitivity of presynaptic inhibitory 5-HT_{1A} receptors that facilitates the release of 5-HT and increases postsynaptic 5-HT receptor activity.[9]

Dysregulation between neurotransmitter systems may produce a cyclic rhythm disturbance in the CNS.[4,7,8] Norepinephrine and dopamine dysregulation, for example, may play an important role in the development of mania. One hypothesis of the switch phenomenon from depression of mania involves the ratio of norepinephrine to dopamine. When norepinephrine activity decreases (as in depression), the dopamine activity predominates, and this may account for the switch to hypomania or mania. Increased dopaminergic activity may contribute to hyperactivity and psychosis associated with the severe stages of mania, and reduced dopamine activity may cause depression. Lithium inhibits the formation of dopamine, decreases the number of β-adrenergic receptors, and blocks dopamine and β-adrenergic receptor supersensitivity.[8,9] Lithium also blocks amphetamine-induced euphoric effects in humans and locomotor activity in animals.[9] Clonidine, an α_2-noradrenergic presynaptic agonist, limits norepinephrine release, and some clinicians have used it as an adjunctive agent for agitation and insomnia. Because of their antimania properties, antipsychotic medications that block dopamine activity (e.g., haloperidol, fluphenazine, olanzapine, risperidone) have are often used during the acute manic phase of the illness.[8] Antidepressants that augment norepinephrine, dopamine, and 5-HT activity have been used to treat bipolar depression; these agents may cause a switch to mania.

γ-Aminobutyric acid (GABA), the main inhibitory neurotransmitter in the CNS, is involved in the inhibition of norepinephrine and

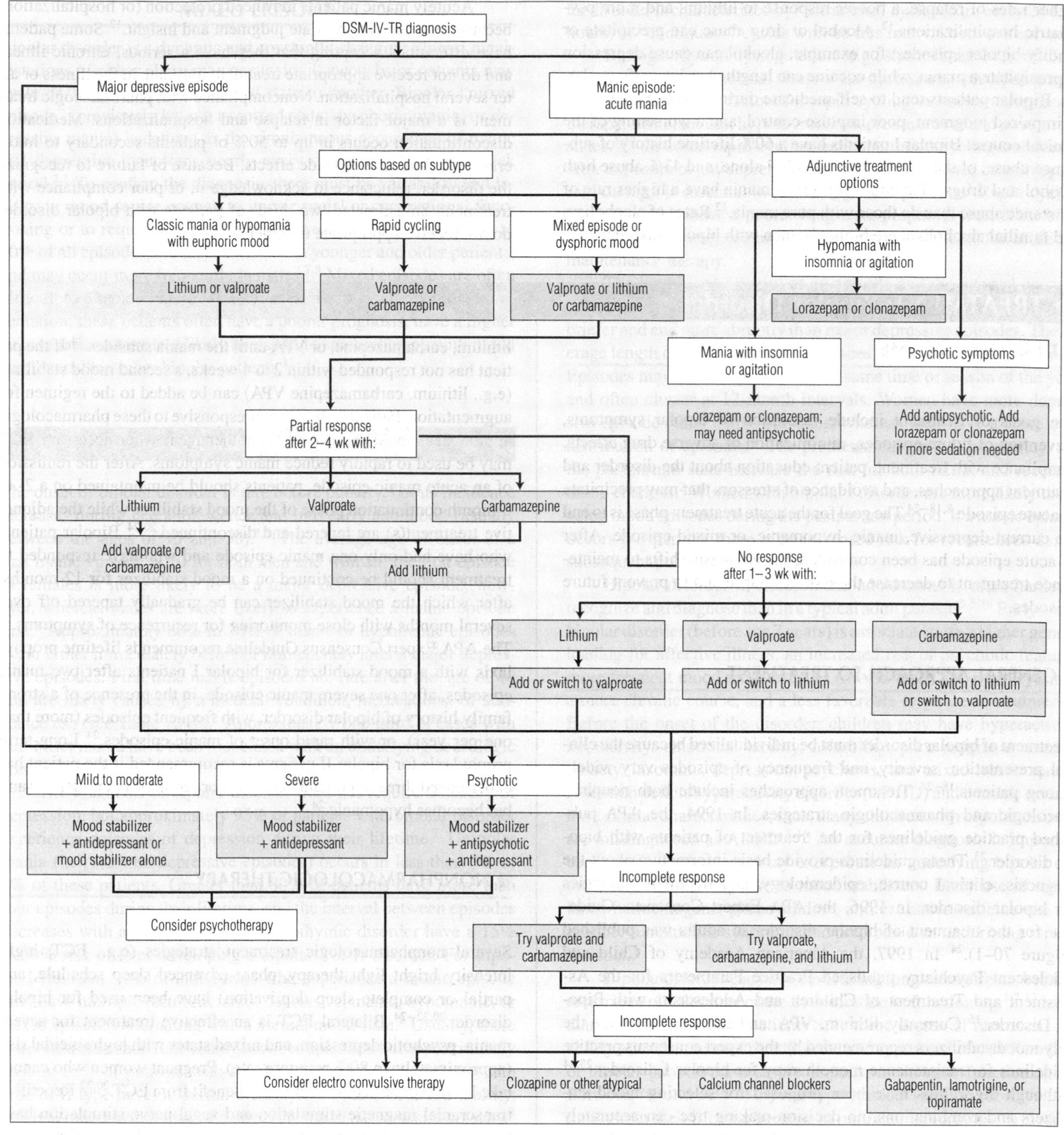

FIGURE 70–1. Algorithm for the treatment of disorder. *(Adapted from Ref. 24.)*

and Manic–Depressive Association (NDMDA) at 800–826–3632; National Alliance for the Mentally Ill (NAMI) at 800–950–6264; National Foundation for Depressive Illness (NFDI) at 800–248–4344; or National Mental Health Association (NMHA) at 800–969–6642.[24]

Patients (and family members) should be educated or counseled about (1) psychosocial or physical stressors that may precipitate an episode; (2) strategies on coping with stressful life events and using stress reduction techniques and problem-solving skills; (3) early recognition of the signs and symptoms of mania and depression and charting mood changes; (4) compliance with treatment recommendations; (5) development of crisis intervention plans; (6) importance of a stable sleep pattern, good nutrition, and regular exercise; (7) limitation of substances and drugs that can trigger mood episodes or affect the course of the illness; and (8) monitoring for adverse effects of medications and avoidance of drug–drug interactions.[12,24]

PHARMACOLOGIC THERAPY

DRUG TREATMENTS OF FIRST CHOICE

Lithium, the first mood stabilizer approved by the Food and Drug Administration (FDA), is effective for the acute and prophylactic treatment of bipolar disorder.[29] Although lithium is traditionally the drug of choice for bipolar disorder, anticonvulsants such as VPA and carbamazepine are accepted alternatives or adjuncts to lithium and may be more effective than lithium in several mood subtypes (e.g., mania with mixed or dysphoric features, rapid cycling, mania secondary to medical conditions).[11,18–24] Valproic acid is not FDA-approved, but divalproex sodium (DVPX) is converted to VPA in the stomach and is FDA-approved for the treatment of acute mania.[30] Carbamazepine is not FDA-approved for bipolar disorder.[25,31] Although carbamazepine and VPA are not FDA-approved for patients under age 18, and lithium is approved only for those aged 12 and older, these agents have been used in children for the treatment of bipolar disorder.[16] Further studies are needed to compare lithium, carbamazepine, VPA, and combination therapy in the acute and prophylactic treatment of severe mania, rapid or continuous cycling, and in mixed episodes.[8,18,28] Product information for carbamazepine, lithium, and VPA is found in Table 70–4, and information about alternative mood stabilizers is listed in Table 70–5. Table 70–6 includes recommendations for baseline and routine laboratory testing for patients receiving carbamazepine, lithium, and VPA.

Third-generation anticonvulsants such as gabapentin, lamotrigine, oxcarbazepine, and topiramate are not FDA-approved for bipolar disorder, but are being investigated as add-on therapies with standard mood stabilizers and as monotherapy for treatment-resistant bipolar disorders.[12,13,28,33–35] High potency benzodiazepines such as clonazepam and lorazepam are common alternatives to typical antipsychotics when patients are experiencing acute mania, agitation, and insomnia or cannot take mood stabilizers (e.g., during the first trimester of pregnancy).[22,28] Atypical antipsychotics such as clozapine, olanzapine, quetiapine, risperidone, and ziprasidone are demonstrating efficacy and fewer side effects than typical antipsychotics for the treatment of acute mania and agitation.[5,28] In 2000, the FDA approved olanzapine for the short-term treatment (i.e., fewer than 4 weeks) of acute manic episodes in bipolar I disorder.[36] Calcium channel antagonists (e.g., nimodipine, verapamil) are under investigation as mood stabilizers and may be considered alternative agents if a patient cannot tolerate lithium, carbamazepine or VPA or is nonresponsive to first-line approaches.[11,13,22,28,35]

TABLE 70–4. Names and Formulations of Mood Stabilizers

Generic Name	Brand Name	Formulations
Carbamazepine	Tegretol, Epitol	Tablet: 200 mg
	Tegretol	Chewable tablet: 100 mg Suspension: 100 mg/5 mL
	Tegretol-XR	Extended-release tablet: 100, 200, 400 mg
	Carbatrol	Extended-release capsule: 200, 300 mg
Lithium carbonate	Eskalith	Tablet: 300 mg Capsule: 300 mg
	Lithane	Capsule: 300 mg
	Lithotabs	Tablet: 300 mg
	Lithobid	Extended-release tablet: 300 mg
	Eskalith CR	Extended-release tablet: 450 mg
	Generic, Roxane	Tablet: 300 mg (scored) Capsule: 150, 300, 600 mg
Lithium citrate	Cibalith-S	8 mEq/5 mL
Valproic acid	Depakene	Capsule: 250 mg
Valproate sodium	Depakene	Syrup: 250 mg/5 mL
Divalproex sodium	Depakote	Enteric-coated tablet: 125, 250, 500 mg Sprinkle capsule: 125 mg
	Depakote ER	Enteric-coated, extended release tablet: 500 mg

TABLE 70–5. Product Formulations and Daily Dosage Range of Alternative Mood Stabilizers

Generic Name	Brand Name	Formulations	Daily Dose (mg/d)
Anticonvulsants			
Gabapentin	Neurontin	Capsule: 100, 300, 400, 600, 800 mg	900–3600
Lamotrigine	Lamictal	Tablet: 25, 100, 150, 200 mg Chewable tablet: 5, 25 mg	50–500
Topiramate	Topamax	Tablet: 25, 100, 200 mg Sprinkle capsule: 15, 25 mg	100–200
Antipsychotics			
Olanzapine	Zyprexa	Tablet: 2.5, 5, 7.5, 10, 20 mg	5–20
Risperidone	Risperdol	Tablet: 0.25, 0.5, 1, 2, 3, 4 mg Oral solution: 1 mg/mL	1–6
Benzodiazepines			
Clonazepam	Klonopin	Tablet: 0.5, 1, 2 mg	1.5–20
Lorazepam	Ativan	Tablet: 0.5, 1, 2 mg Oral solution: 2 mg/mL Injection: 2, 4 mg/mL	2–40
Calcium Channel Antagonists			
Nimodipine	Nimotop	Capsule: 30 mg	30–120
Verapamil	Verelan	Capsule: 120, 180, 240, 360 mg	80–480
	Calan, Isoptin	Film-coated tablet: 40, 80, 120 mg	
	Calan, Isoptin	Extended-release tablet: 120, 180, 240 mg	

TABLE 70–6. Baseline and Routine Laboratory Testing for Patients Treated With Mood Stabilizers

	Carbamazepine		Lithium		Valproate	
	Baseline	*Follow Up Every 6–12 mo*	*Baseline*	*Follow Up Every 6–12 mo*	*Baseline*	*Follow Up Every 6–12 mo*
Baseline Tests						
Complete physical exam	+	−	+	−	+	−
General chemistry screen	+	−	+	−	+	−
Urine toxicology for substance abuse	+	−	+	−	+	−
Recommended Tests for Mood Stabilizers						
Pregnancy test if needed	+	−	+	−	+	−
Cardiac: EKG	+[a]	−	+[a]	−		
Hematologic: CBC with differential	+	+[b]	+	+	+	+[b]
Platelet	+	+	−	−	+	+
Hepatic: liver enzymes	+	+[c]	−	−	+	+[c]
Metabolic	+	+	+	+	−	−
Serum electrolytes						
Total T_4, T_4 uptake, and TSH	+	+	+	+	−	−
Renal						
Serum creatinine	−	−	+[d]	+[d]	−	−
Urinalysis/osmolality/specific gravity	−	−	+	+[e]	−	−

[a]If > 40 yr or preexisting cardiac disease.
[b]CBZ and VPA: CBC monthly during first 2 months, then every 3–6 months; discontinue CBZ if platelets are < 100,000/mm^3 or WBC < 3, 000/mm^3.
[c]CBZ and VPA: LFTs monthly during first 2 months, then every 3–6 months; VPA: < 10 yr should have LFTs every 1–3 months.
[d]24-hour urine volume and creatinine clearance for impaired renal functioning every 3 months.
[e]if urine volume > 3 L/d.
EKG = electrocardiogram; CBC = complete blood count; TSH = thyroid-stimulating hormone; CBZ = carbamazepine; VPA = valproic acid; WBC = white blood cell count; LFT = liver function test.
Compiled from Refs. 8 and 24.

Lithium

In 1970, lithium carbonate was approved for the treatment of mania, and in 1974, it was approved for maintenance therapy for bipolar disorder.[29] Early placebo-controlled studies with lithium reported up to a 70% to 80% response rate in aborting an acute manic or hypomanic episode, but more recent studies suggest a more moderate effectiveness when compared to other agents.[18,37,38] In most comparison trials, lithium has better results in the treatment of acute mania than antipsychotics and carbamazepine, but its results are equivalent to those of VPA.[37] Monotherapy with lithium may be less effective for severe mania with psychotic features, mixed episodes, rapid or continuous cycling, alcohol and drug abuse, and in organic-induced mood states.[11,18,19,28,29,37]

It is estimated that at least 50% of lithium-treated patients may not have an adequate prophylactic response and that less than 40% of those with rapid-cycling or dysphoric mania respond to lithium.[5,11] Breakthrough mood episodes that resemble tolerance or refractoriness have been reported during lithium therapy.[28] Long-term lithium therapy may be more effective in patients with fewer prior episodes, with a history of euthymia or good functioning between episodes, and with a family history of bipolar illness with a positive response to lithium.[18,37] Patients maintained on "standard" serum concentrations of lithium (between 0.8 and 1.0 mEq/L) may have fewer relapses than patients maintained on lower serum concentrations (0.4 to 0.6 mEq/L). Approximately 20% to 40% of patients cannot tolerate the adverse effects or do not respond to lithium despite therapeutic plasma concentrations. Because lithium-induced hypothyroidism may contribute to rapid cycling, regular assessment of thyroid function and addition of thyroid hormone when levels are low may increase lithium's responsiveness.[29] Often, lithium therapy must be augmented with antidepressants, antipsychotics, benzodiazepines, or anticonvulsants during acute and maintenance therapy.[11,27,37]

Noncompliance with lithium therapy secondary to its side effects is a common problem during maintenance therapy.[37] Abrupt discontinuation of lithium prophylaxis may increase the risk of relapse, and rechallenge trials may show lithium to be less effective than before the abrupt discontinuation.[5,12,20,29,37] The exact cause of lithium discontinuation–induced refractoriness is not known, but may be related to inadequate dosing, noncompliance, difference in manic subtypes (e.g., rapid cycling, mixed affective states), comorbid substance abuse, and antidepressant-induced switches to mania.[12] If lithium is discontinued, a gradual tapering down of the dose by 300 mg/month has been recommended to reduce the risk of relapse.[20]

Divalproex Sodium, Sodium Valproate, or Valproic Acid

Originally utilized as an organic solvent,[5] VPA, or valproate, is a branched chain fatty acid. In the 1960s, VPA was discovered to have anticonvulsant properties (see Chapter 56) and later found to have antimigraine, mood-stabilizing, antianxiety, antipanic, and antiaggressive effects.[5,39] In 1995, the FDA approved the enteric-coated formulation DVPX for the acute treatment of mania. Several controlled studies have shown DVPX to be as effective as lithium in patients with pure mania, and DVPX may be more effective than lithium in certain subtypes of bipolar disorder (e.g., rapid cycling, mixed mania, secondary bipolar disorder, comorbid substance abuse).[5,8,11,12,38–41] Valproic acid is less effective in the treatment of acute depression than in the treatment of acute mania.[5,41] Uncontrolled studies report that VPA reduces or prevents recurrent manic, depressive, and mixed episodes.[5,41] Preliminary data suggest that VPA is safe and effective in children and adolescents with acute mania.[5]

Predictors of a positive response with VPA include rapid cycling, a high level of dysphoria or depression during the manic episode (mixed episode), concomitant panic attacks, mania associated with organic features (abnormal electroencephalogram [EEG]) or organic mental disorders, history of head trauma, and mental retardation.[5,18,19,40] Giving lithium, carbamazepine, antipsychotics, or benzodiazepines with VPA may augment its antimanic effects. Low-dose VPA (125 to 500 mg/d) has been reported to be effective in reducing mood cycling in bipolar II disorder and cyclothymia. Oral loading with DVPX, 20 mg/kg/d, may produce a rapid reduction in manic and psychotic symptoms (within 4 days) without causing major side effects, although there may be a lag time to obtain full antimanic efficacy.[12,42] Development of tolerance and loss of efficacy with VPA occurs in some patients after several years of treatment.[28]

Carbamazepine

A tricyclic compound, carbamazepine is marketed as an anticonvulsant and as an agent for paroxysmal pain syndromes, such as trigeminal neuralgia.[5] It has acute antimanic and prophylactic effects comparable with those of lithium and VPA in bipolar disorder.[5,11,12,18,20,21,28,41] Like antipsychotic agents, carbamazepine has a rapid onset of antimanic effects, and furthermore, its acute antimanic properties are more potent than its antidepressant effects.[5] Predictors of a positive response with carbamazepine include severe manic episodes, anxiety, dysphoria, schizoaffective or psychotic features, brain damage (abnormal EEG), early-onset manic episodes, and a negative family history for mood disorders.[18,19,28] There are some reports that carbamazepine may lose effectiveness over time (similar to lithium) and that patient with rapid-cycling bipolar disorder may not respond to carbamazepine monotherapy as well as they do to a combination of lithium and carbamazepine.[5,12,28,43]

ALTERNATE DRUG TREATMENTS

Antipsychotics

Psychotic symptoms may occur during a manic, mixed, or depressive episode and require an antipsychotic agent.[27,41] An acute manic episode may be treated with a mood stabilizer, an antipsychotic, or a combination of an antipsychotic and mood stabilizer for additive or synergistic effects.[5,8,20–22,24,44] Typical antipsychotic agents are effective in up to 70% of patients with acute mania, particularly those with psychosis and psychomotor agitation. Low-potency typical antipsychotics (chlorpromazine, thioridazine) are more sedating and cause more orthostatic hypotension, but have the advantage of causing fewer extrapyramidal side effects (EPS). The high-potency typical agents (haloperidol, fluphenazine) and moderate-potency; agents (perphenazine, thiothixene) cause less sedation and fewer blood pressure changes, but are more likely to cause EPS (akathisia may cause agitation). Depot antipsychotics (e.g., haloperidol and fluphenazine decanoate) may have a place in the maintenance of patients with treatment-resistant bipolar disorder.

Atypical antipsychotic agents that block D_2 and 5-HT_{2A} recptors (clozapine, olanzapine, quetiapine, risperidone, ziprasidone) cause fewer EPS and may be less likely to cause tardive dyskinesia than are typical agents.[5,27,41,45] Clozapine has antagonist properties at the 5-$HT_{1A,2C,3,6,7}$, $D_{1,2,4,5}$, $\alpha_{1,2}$-adrenergic, muscarinic $M_{1,2}$, and histamine H_1 receptors.[46] Clozapine monotherapy appears to have acute and long-term mood-stabilizing effects in refractory bipolar disorder, including conditions with mixed mania and rapid cycling,[27,41,46,47] but requires regular white blood cell monitoring for agranulocytosis.[46] Risperidone, a D_2 and 5-HT_{2A} antagonist, in combination with other mood-stabilizing agents, was effective in acute mania in several open-label trials and case reports/case series.[48–50] A double-blind clinical trial suggested that the efficacy of risperidone is equivalent to that of haloperidol and lithium in the management of acute mania.[51] Risperidone may have antidepressant properties, and it may induce mania in patients with bipolar disorder, especially those not receiving a concomitant mood stabilizer.[50] At dosages under 6 mg/d, risperiodone has few EPS; however, the incidence of EPS increases with higher dosages, and several cases of tardive dyskinesia have occurred.[45] Olanzapine, chemically and structurally similar to clozapine, has antagonist effects at the D_{1-4}, 5-HT $_{2A,2C,3,6}$, α_1-adrenergic, muscarinic M_1, and histamine H_1 receptors.[27,46] Although olanzapine has a lower incidence of EPS than risperidone, it may cause sedation, orthosatic hypotension, and weight gain.[36]

Patients with bipolar may be at increased risk of developing EPS, tardive dyskinesia, and depression from antipsychotic agents.[27,27,45] If antipsychotics are prescribed, the lowest possible dosage should be used. Once acute mania is controlled (usually within 7 to 28 days), the antipsychotic should be gradually tapered and discontinued, and the patient maintained on the mood stabilizer alone to avoid neurotoxicity, postmania depression, supersensitivity psychosis, EPS, and tardive dyskinesia.[27] Intermittent use of conventional antipsychotics has been associated with an increased risk of tardive dyskinesia in bipolar patients; therefore, antipsychotics should be used only in patients with psychotic symptoms.[22,45] The safety and efficacy of antipsychotics for the treatment of psychotic bipolar depression and as prophylactic agents in bipolar disorder is not known.[27,41]

Benzodiazepines

An alternative to antipsychotic therapy in acute mania is the use of anticonvulsant benzodiazepines that facilitate GABAergic transmission.[8,11,12,22] Clonazepam and lorazepam have been used in conjunction with lithium, VPA, and carbamazepine for agitation and insomnia during acute mania and added for the treatment of anxiety and insomnia during maintenance therapy.[11,12,20,28] Benzodiazepines cause minimal adverse effects compared to antipsychotics and, at higher doses, rapidly sedate agitated patients. They have efficacy in the treatment of acute mania or breakthrough mania, but no controlled studies have examined their use in prophylactic therapy.[12] Relative contraindications for long-term therapy with benzodiazepines are drug or alcohol abuse or dependency.[8] When no longer required, benzodiazepines should be gradually tapered over several weeks and discontinued to avoid withdrawal symptoms.

Antidepressants

Generally, it is not advisable to treat bipolar disorder with antidepressants since the depressive phase may last only a few weeks, and most agents take 2 to 4 weeks to exert their antidepressant effects.[12] Patients who have a history of mania after a depressive episode or who have frequent cycling should be treated cautiously with antidepressants.[8,20] Before the addition of an antidepressant, the patient should be on a therapeutic dosage or blood level of a primary mood stabilizer.[12] Using a smaller than usual dosage of antidepressant and a shorter course of treatment (compared to the treatment of major depression) may help to avoid switching the patient into a manic episode.[12] Once the depressive episode has resolved, the antidepressant should be gradually withdrawn, and the patient can be maintained on a mood-stabilizing agent.

Treatment algorithms such as the APA Expert Consensus Guideline recommend bupropion and selective serotonin reuptake inhibitors (SSRIs) as first-line antidepressants, and monoamine oxidase inhibitors (MAOIs) and venlafaxine as second-line agents, for the treatment of moderate or severe bipolar depression (see Chapter 69).[24] Bupropion has been recommended as the antidepressant of choice in patients with a high risk of developing mixed states or rapid cycling.[20,24] Tricyclic antidepressants (TCAs) should be avoided because of increased risks of inducing mania or rapid cycling.[12] Trazodone, a sedating antidepressant, is sometimes used as an adjunctive medication for insomnia.[24] Further clinical trials are necessary to evaluate the efficacy of nefazodone and mirtazapine in bipolar depression and to compare different classes of antidepressants for efficacy and risks of treatment-emergent mania.[12]

Clinicians have tried a variety of other treatments for depression, particularly in treatment-resistant cases. Lithium may be beneficial as an augmenting agent with standard antidepressants, but has only modest antidepressant effects when used alone.[24] If lithium monotherapy is not effective for the treatment of depression or rapid cycling, the addition of a second anticonvulsant mood stabilizer (e.g., carbamazepine, VPA) could be helpful.[12] Monotherapy with VPA has not been shown to be effective for the treatment of depression.[12] In preliminary studies, lamotrigine add-on or monotherapy showed improvement in treatment-refactory bipolar depression.[12] Alternative augmenting treatments for depression include estrogen replacement therapy for perimenopausal women, thyroid hormones, calcium channel blockers, atypical antipsychotics, dopamine agonists (e.g., pramipexole), phototherapy, and sleep deprivation.[12]

A psychotic depression can be treated with a mood stabilizer plus an antidepressant and antipsychotic agent or with ECT.[20,24] Electroconvulsive therapy remains the treatment of choice for a psychotic depression, during pregnancy, and for treatment-resistant depression and rapid cyclers.[12,53] The risk of ECT-induced mania may be higher with unilateral nondominant compared to bilateral ECT.[12] Acute neurotoxicity and delirium have been reported in patients receiving ECT with lithium (even at reduced dosages); therefore, lithium should be withdrawn and discontinued at least 2 days before ECT and should not be resumed until 2 to 3 days after the last ECT. Because carbamazepine, VPA, and benzodiazepines have anticonvulsant properties, these drugs should also be tapered down and discontinued prior to ECT.

Calcium Channel Antagonists

Verapamil, nifedipine, and nimodipine are alternative mood stabilizers if patients cannot be treated with lithium, carbamazepine, or VPA.[22] Preliminary data suggested that verapamil had acute antimanic effects, but subsequent open trials of verapamil in lithium-resistant mania, comparative studies with lithium, and a double-blind, placebo-controlled trial of verapamil in acute mania did not confirm this hypothesis.[22,54] Nifedipine (in combination with an antipsychotic) was reported to be effective in several treatment-refractory schizoaffective and bipolar manic patients.[5] Nimodipine may be more effective than verapamil or nifedipine in bipolar dosprder because of its anticonvulsant properties, high lipid solubility, and good penetration into the CNS.[5,11] Preliminary studies with nimodipine found it may be effective in ultra-rapid cycling patients and have augmenting effects when combined with lithium, carbamazepine, or other anticonvulsants.[12,28] The most common adverse effects of calcium channel antagonists are bradycardia and hypotension. The low teratogenic effects of these agents may make them preferable to standard mood stabilizers during pregnancy and breastfeeding.[5,22]

Alternative Anticonvulsants

Lamotrigine.

Approved as adjunct therapy for refractory partial seizures with or without generalization (see Chapter 56),[55] lamotrigine inhibits voltage-activated sodium channels that decrease the release of glutamate and aspartate and may potentiate the effects of dopamine and inhibit 5-HT_3 receptors.[10–13,55,56] According to case reports and open-label studies, lamotrigine has both antidepressant and mood-stabilizing effects in treatment-resistant bipolar I and II disorders; in rapid-cycling, dysphoric mania; and in mixed states; furthermore, it may have augmenting effects when combined with VPA or lithium.[33,56–66] A 4-week randomized, double-blind controlled trial showed lamotrigine (100 mg/d) to be as effective as lithium (800 mg/d) in acutely manic hospitalized patients.[67] When the efficacy and safety of lamotrigine was compared with that of olanzapine and lithium in a 4-week randomized controlled study; lamotrigine was found to have similar antimanic effects and good tolerability.[68] Two double-blind placebo-controlled studies with lamotrigine (50 and 200 mg/d) in depressed outpatients with bipolar I disorder demonstrated that monotherapy was effective and well tolerated in the treatment of bipolar depression.[69,70] A placebo-controlled study of lamotrigine (mean daily dosage, 274 mg ± 128 mg) and gabapentin (mean daily dosage, 3,987 mg ± 856 mg/d) reported that both agents were well tolerated, but that lamotrigine was more effective than gabapentin in patients with treatment-refractory bipolar and unipolar mood disorder.[71]

Generally, lamotrigine has fewer side effects if there is slow titration during the initiation of therapy.[13,22] Common adverse effects include nausea, headache, dizziness, ataxia, diplopia, drowsiness, tremor, and rash.[55] Approximately 10% of patients in premarketing clinical trials developed a maculopapular rash and required discontinuation of therapy.[55] Although most rashes are self-limiting and resolve with continued treatment, some cases have progressed to life-threatening conditions such as Stevens-Johnson syndrome.[55,56] The incidence of rash appears to be greatest with coadministration of VPA, with higher than recommended initial doses, and with rapid dose escalation.[55]

Gabapentin.

Although its structure is similar to that of GABA, gabapentin does not bind to the GABA receptor or interact with sodium or calcium channels in vitro.[13,22,72] The exact mechanism of action of gabapentin is unknown, but it has been shown to increase the activity of glutamic acid decarboxylase in vitro, increase GABA release and GABA turnover, and interfere with glutamate metabolism.[12,13,33,72,73] Already approved as an adjunct for partial or secondary generalized seizures (see Chapter 56), gabapentin is being investigated for the treatment of bipolar disorder, anxiety disorders, behavioral dyscontrol, cocaine dependence, neuropathic pain, movement disorders, and migraine prophylaxis.[13,74] Case reports, retrospective reviews, and open-label trials have shown that gabapentin has acute antimanic effects as an add-on to standard regimens of mood stabilizers.[13,33,34,73,75–82] Preliminary open-label studies suggest that gabapentin has efficacy in treating bipolar depression[78,83] and is useful as an augmenting agent for the maintenance phase of treatment.[84]

Gabapentin does not have an established therapeutic concentration range and does not require blood level monitoring.[12,13,33,72] It has several advantages: its side effects are mild and transient, it does not interfere with hepatic metabolism, and it does not interact significantly with other drugs. Gabapentin does cause somnolence, dizziness, ataxia, fatigue, blurred vision, diplopia, nystagmus, and tremor; titrating the dose up gradually, however, can minimize these effects. Less common adverse effects include weight increase, peripheral edema, dyspepsia, nervousness, anxiety, and hypomania.[13,72] When gabapentin is added for adjunctive therapy with other mood stabilizers, a slower titration may be necessary to minimize the potential for somnolence, fatigue, and dizziness.

Topiramate. An effective anticonvulsant in treating partial seizures with secondary generalizations (see Chapter 56), topiramate blocks voltage-activated sodium channels, enhances the activity of GABA at $GABA_A$ receptors by interacting with a nonbenzodiazepine receptor site, and blocks the ability of kainate to activate the kainate/AMPA subtype of glutamate receptors.[85–87] Several open-label nonrandomized studies have investigated the efficacy and tolerability of adding topiramate to standard mood stabilizers.[88–90] A trial in 58 patients with refractory bipolar disorder showed that topiramate (dosages of 25 to 400 mg/d, mean of 200 mg/d) was an effective add-on therapy (i.e., 62% of patients had marked or moderate improvement).[88] In a study with 18 bipolar and 2 schizoaffective patients who received adjunctive topiramate (100 to 300 mg/d), 60% of patients were responders, and all patients lost an average of 9.4 pounds by week 5.[89] A naturalistic study in 54 patients with bipolar disorder (who were either not responding or not tolerating standard mood-stabilizing agents) found that adjunctive topiramate (dosages of 25 to 1,200 mg/d) had acute antimanic and long-term anticycling effects.[90] Topiramate was associated with reduced appetite, a 6.2% weight reduction, and decreased body mass index after 1 year of treatment.

Topiramate has minimal drug interactions and does not require routine blood level monitoring.[85] The most common adverse effects associated with topiramate are dose-related (>200 mg/d) and are worse with rapid titration.[85] Treatment-emergent adverse effects reported in clinical trials include somnolence and fatigue, dizziness, ataxia, psychomotor slowing, difficulty with concentration, speech and language problems, nystagmus, abnormal vision, diplopia, tremor, nausea, dyspepsia, and anorexia.[85] If topiramate's titration is too rapid, anxiety, agitation, nervousness, and word-finding difficulties may occur.[86] Nephrolithiasis (primarily calcium phosphate renal stones) has been reported in 1.5% of patients in clinical trials.[85] Adequate daily hydration is essential to decrease the risk of stone formation. Weight loss of 1.6 to 6.5 kg has been reported during the first 3 months, although weight stabilizes after 15 to 18 months of treatment. Weight loss is generally found in women and in patients weighing more than 100 kg rather than those weighing less than 60 kg.[85,86]

Miscellaneous Anticonvulsants. Several anticonvulsants are being investigated in bipolar disorder because of their unique pharmacologic properties. One placebo-controlled study has indicated that phenytoin, a classic anticonvulsant with potent inhibition of voltage-activated sodium channels, has antimanic effects when combined with haloperidol.[91] Oxcarbazepine, a 10-keto analog of carbamazepine, blocks voltage-sensitive sodium channels, modulates voltage activated calcium currents, and increases potassium conductance.[32] Initial trials with patients who have bipolar disorder suggest that oxcarbazepine has mood-stabilizing effects similar to those of carbamazepine,[11,28] as well as the advantages of milder adverse effects, no autoinduction of liver enzymes, and fewer drug interactions.[32] Tiagabine, which has demonstrated antikindling properties, exerts its action by inhibiting GABA reuptake from the synaptic cleft.[92] A 14-day open-label trial in 8 acutely manic patients showed that tiagabine monotherapy did not have acute antimanic effects.[93] Other case reports suggest add-on tiagabine is effective in bipolar, schizoaffective, and refractory bipolar patients.[94,95] Zonisamide, a synthetic benzisoxazole derivative, is chemically classified as a sulfonamide and is structurally similar to 5-HT.[96] Zonisamide blocks voltage-sensitive sodium channels, reduces voltage-dependent T-type calcium currents without affecting L-type channels, and facilitates dopaminergic and serotonergic neurotransmission.[96] One open-label study of zonisamide in 15 bipolar patients during a manic episode showed that 80% had more than moderate improvement.[97]

Novel Agents

Several novel agents have been tried in bipolar disorder, but randomized, controlled trials are needed to determine their efficacy and safety.[98] High doses of levothyroxine sodium (0.15 to 0.4 mg/d) have been reported to have mood-stabilizing properties in rapid-cycling bipolar patients when combined with traditional mood-stabilizing agents. Physostigmine, a centrally acting cholinesterase inhibitor, and lecithin, a precursor for acetylcholine, have shown some potential in the treatment of acute mania. Psychostimulants such as methylphenidate and dextroamphetamine have been reported to decrease manic symptoms in some patients. Medications that decrease norepinephrine activity such as clonidine, an α_2-adrenergic presynaptic agonist, may help decrease manic symptoms when combined with mood-stabilizing agents. A dietary deficiency in omega-3 fatty acids (found in certain fish oils, and flaxseed oil that contains α-linolenic acid, a shorter chain omega-3 fatty acid) has been proposed as a potential cause of mood disorders.[99] Omega-3 fatty acids have been shown to suppress neuronal pathways and inhibit kindling processes by several mechanisms (e.g., inhibition of phosphatidylinositol and G-protein secondary messengers, blocking L-type calcium channels, and inhibition of PKC activity). Initial double-blind, placebo-controlled studies with high doses of omega-3 fatty acids reported some positive benefits in patients with bipolar disorder.[99,100]

COMBINATION THERAPIES

Although monotherapy is preferred for long-term maintenance, combinations of multiple drugs may be necessary for patients with mixed episodes, those who experience rapid cycling, or those with partial or no response to monotherapy.[23–25]

Lithium Combinations

The addition of VPA to lithium may have synergistic effects, and this combination is recommended as a first-line treatment in patients with treatment-refractory rapid cycling and mixed states.[25,26] Lithium plus VPA has demonstrated efficacy in maintenance therapy for bipolar I disorder.[26] Concomitant use of lithium and VPA appears to be well tolerated, but may increase the risk of sedation, weight gain, gastrointestinal complaints, and tremor.[25] The addition of carbamazepine to lithium monotherapy may also have synergistic effects and is an alternative choice for the rapid-cycling disorder, but the combination is not as popular because of the availability of newer anticonvulsants.[5,25] Neurotoxicity has been reported with concomitant use of lithium plus carbamazepine, particularly in patients with preexisting CNS disease.[25]

Combining lithium with calcium channel blockers is not recommended because of reports of neurotoxicity and severe bradycardia with verapamil and diltiazem.[25] Lithium is frequently combined with both traditional and atypical antipsychotics in euphoric acute mania with psychotic features.[25,27] Case reports of neurotoxicity (e.g., delirium, cerebellar dysfunction, extrapyramidal symptoms, severe tremors) have been reported in elderly patients who have bipolar disorder and in those who have preexisting encephalopathy and are receiving lithium and traditional antipsychotics.[25] Long-term combination therapy may also increase the risk of tardive dyskinesia. If antipsychotics are added to lithium, the antipsychotic dose should be low, and lithium levels should be maintained below 1.0 mEq/L.[25] Lithium has been combined with atypical antipsychotics such as clozapine, olanzapine, quetiapine, and risperidone, but further studies are necessary to determine if these agents cause neurotoxicity and additive side effects (e.g., sedation, weight gain).[25,27] Because of the risks of combining lithium with antipsychotios, it may be preferable to use benzodiazepines such as clonazepam and lorazepam, which have better tolerability and greater safety.[25] Long-term use of benzodiazepines should be avoided in patients with comorbid substance abuse. Initial reports of combining lithium with newer anticonvulsants such as gabapentin and lamotrigine suggest the combinations are safe and effective, but further studies are necessary.[25]

Valproic Acid Combinations

Combinations of VPA and carbamazepine may have synergistic effects, but the potential drug interactions make blood level monitoring of both agents essential. (For example, carbamazepine induces the metabolism of itself and VPA, while VPA may inhibit the metabolism of carbamazepine and displace it from protein-binding sites.[5,25]) Although VPA has been combined with traditional and atypical antipsychotics for patients with mixed state, rapid-cycling, or psychotic features, few data are available regarding its efficacy.[25] Clozapine and olanzapine may increase the risk of sedation and weight gain when combined with VPA. The combination of VPA and lamotrigine may be effective, but there is an increased risk of rashes, ataxia, tremor, sedation, and fatigue.[25] Because VPA can significantly increase the blood levels of lamotrigine, lower doses and gradual titration of lamotrigine are necessary to decrease the risk of dermatologic reactions.[25] Valproic acid plus gabapentin appears to be safe (with no drug interactions or major adverse reactions), but efficacy data are lacking.[25]

Carbamazepine Combinations

Some experts consider the combination of carbamazepine and a traditional antipsychotic to be a first-line treatment approach for euphoric acute mania with psychotic features.[25] The combination of carbamazepine with clozapine is not recommended, as both agents cause leukopenia, potentially increasing the risk of agranulocytosis.[5,25] Carbamazepine increases the hepatic metabolism of clozapine and other antipsychotic agents such as haloperidol, fluphenazine, and thiothixene; thus, dosage increases may be necessary. Combinations of calcium channel blockers with carbamazepine have a risk of causing neurotoxicity, and both verapamil and diltiazem can increase carbamazepine blood levels; thus, combination therapy should be closely monitored.[5,25] The combination of carbamazepine with nimodipine for treatment-refractory bipolar illness may have potential benefit.[12] Carbamazepine can increase the metabolism of other anticonvulsant agents such as lamotrigine, but has no significant interactions with gabapentin.[25]

SPECIAL POPULATIONS

Patients with comorbid medical conditions or concomitant substance abuse, those over 65 years of age, and pregnant patients may require different treatment approaches.[24] Recommendations for first-line and second-line mood stabilizers or alternative treatments for special populations are provided in Table 70–7. Approximately 20% to 50% of women with bipolar disorder relapse postpartum; therefore, prophylaxis with mood stabilizers is recommended immediately postpartum to decrease the risk of relapse.[101]

DRUG CLASS INFORMATION

Lithium

Pharmacology, Mechanism of Action, and Pharmacokinetics. Despite numerous investigations into the biologic and clinical properties of lithium, there is no unified theory for its mechanism of action.[8,9] Lithium is a monovalent cation and competes with other monovalent (sodium, potassium) and divalent cations (calcium, magnesium) in body tissues and at receptor sites. Neuropharmacologic effects of lithium include blockade of dopamine, β-adrenergic, and cholinergic receptor supersensitivity; decreases of β-adrenoceptor stimulation of adenylate cyclase; increase of 5-HT, aceytlcholine, and GABA function; and reduction of glutamate activity.[9] Lithium stabilizes postsynaptic-receptor sensitivity and has properties similar to those of calcium channel antagonists. Lithium decreases neurotransmitter activity by acting at the postsynaptic secondary messenger system; for example, it decreases neurotransmitter-coupled adenylate cyclase activity and AMP formation; inhibits receptor–G-protein coupling to muscarinic cholinergic and β-adrenergic receptors; and decreases phosphoinositide metabolism.[5,9] Finally, lithium inhibits the enzyme inositol-1-phosphatase within neurons that are linked to phosphatidylinositol and blocks cAMP stimulation by adrenergic agonists.

Lithium has unique pharmacokinetics because it is a monovalent cation. Lithium is rapidly absorbed, is widely distributed with no protein binding, is not metabolized, and is excreted unchanged in the urine and in other body fluids (Table 70–8).[102]

Adverse Effects. Approximately 35% to 93% of lithium-treated patients will experience adverse effects.[103] Side effects of lithium are divided into those that occur early in therapy but are generally innocuous and transient, those that occur with long-term therapy and are usually not dose-related, and toxic effects that occur with high serum concentrations.[24,102,103] Most adverse effects can be treated by lowering the dose, using sustained-release rather than immediate-release lithium products, and trying once daily dosage regimens.[29,103]

TABLE 70–7. Use of Mood Stabilizers in Special Populations

Condition	First Line	Second Line
Aggressive/violent patient	VPA or CBZ or lithium	VPA + lithium CBZ + lithium CBZ + VPA
Cardiac disease/heart failure	VPA	CBZ + lithium may worsen cardiac condition Calcium channel blockers
Drug abuse: alcohol or cocaine	VPA or lithium	CBZ VPA + lithium CBZ + lithium CBZ + VPA
Geriatric patients (in good health)	VPA or lithium	CBZ VPA + lithium CBZ + lithium CBZ + VPA
Liver disease	Lithium	Avoid CBZ + VPA Calcium channel blockers Antipsychotics
Renal disease	VPA or CBZ	VPA + CBZ Calcium channel blockers Antipsychotics
Neurologic disorder	VPA or CBZ	VPA + CBZ; lithium CBZ + lithium VPA + lithium Gabapentin, lamotrigine, topiramate
Pregnancy[a]	Antipsychotic, benzodiazepine, calcium channel antagonist or ECT; lithium may have fewer teratogenic effects than previously thought and may be considered during first trimester	Lithium or VPA after first trimester Clonazepam or CBZ used as third-line agents after first trimester Gabapentin, lamotrigine, topiramate

[a]All mood stabilizers (lithium, CBZ, VPA) have teratogenic risk; this risk is greater if the patient is on multiple agents; thus, monotherapy and lower serum levels are recommended. Gabapentin, lamotrigine, and topiramate have a class C pregnancy risk.
VPA = valproic acid; CBZ = carbamazepine; ECT = electroconvulsive therapy.
Compiled from Refs. 24 and 53.

TABLE 70–8. Pharmacokinetics of Mood Stabilizers

	Lithium	Valproate	Carbamazepine
GI tract absorption			
Regular release	Rapid; 95%–100%	Rapid; 100%	Slow and erratic; 85%–90%
Syrup/suspension/solution	Faster rate of absorption; 100%	Faster rate of absorption	Faster rate of absorption
Extended-release/enteric-coated tablets	Delayed absorption	Delayed absorption	NA
Time to reach peak serum concentrations	1–12 h	1–5 h (VPA), 3–5 h (DVPX)	1–5 h
Delay of absorption by food	Yes	Yes	Yes
Volume of distribution	0.7–1.0 L/kg 92 (free VPA) L/1.73 m²	11 (total)	1 L/kg
Crosses the placenta	Yes	Yes	Yes
Protein binding	No	90%–95%	70%–80%
Renal clearance	Yes; 10–40 mL/min	Yes	Yes
Metabolism	No	Hepatic oxidation and conjugation	Hepatic microsomal oxidation (P450 2D6/3A4)
Metabolites	No	Yes (inactive)	Yes (active) 10, 11 epoxide
Kinetics	First order	First order	First order (after initial enzyme induction phase)
Half-life ($t_{1/2}$)			
Adults (normal)	14–30 h	5–20 h	25–60 h (initial)
Adults (epilepsy)			30–40 h (initial)
After 3 weeks			12–20 h (due to autoinduction)
During mania	8–20 h		
Geriatric patients	Up to 36 h		
Reduced renal function	40–50 h		
Reduced liver function		$\uparrow t_{1/2}$	$\uparrow t_{1/2}$

GI = gastrointestinal; VPA = valproic acid; DVPX = divalproex sodium.
Compiled from Refs. 30, 31, and 102.

ACUTE SIDE EFFECTS

Taking the lithium with food, taking smaller doses with meals, changing to an extended-release product, or adding antacids or antidiarrheal agents can minimize the gastrointestinal side effects such as nausea and diarrhea that may occur early in treatment.[103] Muscle weakness and lethargy develop in about 30% of patients, but these symptoms are usually transient; lowering the daily dose, changing the dose from once daily to two or three times daily, or switching to extended-release products can minimize them.[103] Polydipsia with polyuria and nocturia occurs in up to 70% of patients initially; these side effects are usually mild and diminish with time. Patients with polydipsia may experience weight gain, probably because of increased consumption of high-calorie fluids or fluid retention. As many as 40% of patients complain of headache, memory impairment, mental confusion, a decreased ability to concentrate, and impaired fine motor performance. Impairment in cognitive functioning, loss of productivity, and loss of creativity during lithium treatment is a common reason for noncompliance.[103] A fine hand tremor may be evident in up to 50% of patients during the first week of lithium therapy, and this usually decreases in intensity with time. Stress, concomitant use of antidepressants or antipsychotics, caffeine, sympathomimetics, and impending toxicity may exacerbate the tremor.[103] Strategies to reduce the tremor include lowering the dose, dividing the dose to decrease peak serum concentrations, switching to an extended-release product, changing to a single bedtime dose, or adding a β-adrenergic antagonist (e.g., propranolol 20 to 120 mg/d, atenolol 50 mg/d, or metoprolol 20 to 80 mg/d).[8,103]

LATE-APPEARING SIDE EFFECTS

Lithium reduces the kidney's ability to concentrate urine and in some patients produces a nephrogenic diabetes insipidus.[102,103] The condition is associated with normal or elevated serum concentrations of antidiuretic hormone and does not respond to exogenous vasopressin. Characterized by low urine-specific gravity and a low osmolality polyuria (urine volumes >3 L/d), lithium-induced nephrogenic diabetes insipidus is treated with loop diuretics, thiazide diuretics, or triamterene.[103] Amiloride, a potassium-sparing diuretic, has weaker natriuretic effects than do thiazides and appears to be relatively safe with minimal effect on lithium clearance. Potassium supplements have been suggested as another treatment for lithium-induced polyuria.[5] Fluid restriction is not recommended because dehydration increases the risk of lithium toxicity. If edema occurs, treatment approaches include lowering sodium intake or using a diuretic (e.g., spironolactone); close monitoring for lithium toxicity is necessary because these treatments often increase lithium concentrations.[103]

Numerous studies have examined the issue of lithium-induced renal effects (e.g., glomerulosclerosis, tubular atrophy, interstitial nephritis, urinary casts). In general, lithium causes minimal nephrotoxicity if patients are maintained on the lowest effective dose, if adequate hydration is maintained, and if toxicity is avoided.[103] During long-term lithium therapy, there may be a slight decrease in glomerular filtration rate (GFR) that is related to normal aging processes. Because some patients receiving lithium therapy over time develop rising levels of serum creatinine, renal functioning should be monitored every 6 to 12 months.

Lithium is concentrated in the thyroid gland and interferes with thyroid hormone synthesis.[102] It blocks the release of thyroxine (T_4) and triiodothyronine (T_3) mediated by thyrotropin, inhibits the organification of iodine, decreases the sensitivity of cell surface receptors to thyroid-stimulating hormone (TSH), inhibits the peripheral conversion of T_4 to T_3, and stimulates the formation of antithyroid antibodies in some patients. Up to 30% of patients on maintenance lithium therapy develop transiently elevated TSH concentrations, and 5% to 15% of patients develop a goiter and/or hypothyroidism.[103] Lithium-induced hypothyroidism is not dose-related, is observed 10 times more frequently in women (particularly in those with rapid cycling), and usually occurs after at least 18 months of therapy.[8,103] Subclinical hypothyroidism (normal total and free T_4 with TSH > 6 mIU/mL) is indicative of insufficient thyroid functioning. Hypothyroidism does not require discontinuation of lithium, because exogenous thyroid hormone can be added to the regimen. If the TSH is greater than 5.0 mIU/mL, L-thyroxine (0.05 mg/d) can be added, with a TSH level measurement in 1 month, and increased up to 0.2 mg/d or higher (to achieve TSH > 0.1 and < 5.0 mIU/mL). When lithium is discontinued, the need for exogenous thyroid hormone should be reassessed, because hypothyroidism is almost always reversible.[103]

Lithium may cause a variety of benign and reversible cardiac effects, particularly T-wave flattening or inversion (in up to 30% of patients), atrioventricular block, and bradycardia.[5,102,103] Lithium rarely causes myocarditis, sinus node dysfunction, or sinoatrial block, but may aggravate ventricular arrhythmias and atrial premature contractions.[103] If a patient has significant preexisting cardiac disease, consultation with a cardiologist and an electrocardiograph is recommended before the initiation of lithium therapy.

Other late-appearing lithium side effects include benign reversible leukocytosis, weight gain, and a variety of dermatologic effects (e.g., acne and acneiform eruptions, alopecia, exacerbation of psoriasis, pruritic dermatitis, maculopapular rashes, folliculitis).[5,103] Perhaps related to changes in electrolyte and water homeostasis, to the consumption of high caloric beverages as a result of polydipsia, or to a decreased metabolic rate, 20% of patients gain more than 10 kg. Weight gain is a common reason for noncompliance and may be more common in women with lithium-induced hypothyroid and in those who are already overweight. Decreased libido, sexual dysfunction, dry mouth, alterations in taste, changes in glucose tolerance, hypercalcemia, and hyperparathyroidism have been reported.[103] Severe neurologic disturbances such as coarse hand tremors, ataxia, slurred speech, myasthenia gravis, EPS, pseudotumor cerebri, and papilledema are occasionally observed.

Toxicity. Lithium is an extremely toxic drug if accidentally or intentionally taken in overdose. Elderly patients are at increased risk of lithium toxicity because of decreases in renal blood flow, GFR, and total body water, plus they are more likely to be taking medications that increase lithium blood levels (e.g., thiazide diuretics, nonsteroidal anti-inflammatory drugs (NSAIDs), angiotensin-converting enzyme (ACE) inhibitors, verapamil, and β-blockers).[103,104] There are several situations that predispose patients to lithium toxicity: sodium restriction, dehydration, vomiting, diarrhea, and drug interactions that decrease lithium clearance. Heavy exercise, sauna baths, hot weather, and fever may promote sodium loss. Patients should be cautioned to maintain adequate sodium and fluid intake (2.5 to 3 quarts/d of fluids) and to avoid the excessive use of coffee, tea, cola, and other caffeine-containing beverages and alcohol.

Early signs of mild toxicity (1.2 to 1.5 mEq/L) include difficulty with memory and concentration, fine hand tremor, gastrointestinal upset, muscle weakness, and fatigue. Moderate to severe toxic side effects are usually observed at concentrations greater than 1.5 mEq/L. These include confusion, lethargy, ataxia, dysarthria, nystagmus, emesis, increased deep-tendon reflexes, coarse tremors, and muscle fasciculations. Above 3.0 mEq/L, the syndrome progresses with choreoathetosis, seizures, irreversible brain damage, respiratory complications, coma, and death.[103]

If severe lithium intoxication occurs (concentrations higher than 2.5 mEq/L when taken 12 hours after the last dose), lithium should be discontinued and gastric lavage started. The patient should be monitored for fluid balance, renal and electrolyte status, and neurologic changes.[8] When lithium concentrations are above 3.5 to 4.0 mEq/L, the serum concentration should be measured every 3 hours until it is below 1.0 mEq/L. If the concentration does not drop more than 10% every 3 hours or the lithium half-life is greater than 36 hours, intermittent hemodialysis (12 hours on and 12 hours off) should be started and continued until the lithium concentration is below 1.0 mEq/L when taken 12 hours after the last dialysis. Hemodialysis can increase lithium clearance by 50 mL/min and peritoneal dialysis by 15 mL/min; rebound increases in serum lithium concentrations may occur 5 to 8 hours after dialysis. Several reports of irreversible neurologic deficits with ataxia, deficits in memory, and kidney damage with reduced GFR have been reported with lithium intoxication.[103]

Teratogenicity. Infants whose mothers took lithium during the first trimester of pregnancy may have a lower incidence of cardiovascular defects (particularly Epstein's anomaly) than was previously thought.[53,103,105] Lithium has a category D pregnancy rating and is not recommended during pregnancy unless the benefits outweigh the risks. Lithium freely crosses the placenta and is found in equal concentrations in maternal and fetal blood. If lithium is used during pregnancy, it should be tapered down to the lowest effective dose to decrease the risk of relapse; it should be discontinued a few days prior to delivery to avoid a "floppy" infant syndrome.[53,103] Neonatal lithium effects include low Apgar scores, lethargy, hypotonia, bradycardia, cyanosis, shallow respiration, poor sucking, hypothyroidism, and nontoxic goiters.[5,53] Milk concentrations of lithium range from 30% to 50% of the mother's serum concentration, and serum concentrations in the nursing infant are 10% to 50% of the mother's; for these reasons, breastfeeding is discouraged.[5,53,106]

Drug Interactions. Several drug–drug interactions and cases of neurotoxicity have been reported with lithium (see Toxicity section).[102] Neurotoxicity may occur when lithium is combined with carbamazepine, diltiazem, losartan, methyldopa, metronidazole, phenytoin, and verapamil. Thiazide diuretics, NSAIDs, ACE inhibitors, and fluoxetine can elevate lithium levels, and neurotoxicity may occur. Analgesics such as acetaminophen or aspirin and loop diuretics are less likely to interfere with lithium clearance. Caffeine and theophylline may enhance the renal elimination of lithium. Because lithium has no effects on the hepatic metabolizing enzymes, it has fewer drug–drug interactions compared to carbamazepine and VPA.

Dosing and Administration. The recommended guidelines for baseline and routine laboratory testing for lithium are listed in Table 70–6. Information about dosing strategies and serum concentrations for the treatment of acute mania and for maintenance therapy are found in Table 70–9. Several dose prediction methods (e.g., a priori methods by Jermain, Pepin, and Zetin) have been developed to obtain therapeutic lithium concentrations more rapidly and with fewer blood level determinations.[107]

Lithium therapy is usually initiated with moderate doses (600 mg/d) for prophylaxis and higher doses (900 to 1,200 mg/d) for acute mania, using a two to three times a day dosing regimen. Immediate-release lithium preparation should be given in two or three divided daily doses, whereas the slow-release products (sustained- or controlled-release) may be given once or twice daily.[55] Divided dosing regimens and gradual titration of 300 to 600 mg/d every 2 to 3 days to target doses of 900 to 2,400 mg/d helps to minimize the early, dose-related side effects of nausea and tremor. Lower initial doses and a slower titration (e.g., increasing by 150 to 300 mg every 3 to 5 days)

TABLE 70–9. Dosing Strategies and Serum Concentrations of Mood Stabilizers

	Lithium	Valproate	Carbamazepine
Acute Mania			
Initial dosing	900 mg/d or 15 mg/kg/d in divided doses with meals	500–750 mg/d or 5–10 mg/kg/d in divided doses with meals; oral loading of 20 mg/kg/d with DVPX	100–200 mg bid with meals
Target dose	900–2400 mg/d; give bid or ≤ 1200 mg in single hs dose	1000–3000 mg/d or 20 60 mg/kg/d for mania; lower doses used for hypomania give bid or single hs dose	400–2400 mg/d or 10–15 mg/kg/d; give bid or if ≤ 1200 mg in single hs dose
Drug serum concentrations			
Adults	0.8–1.5 mEq/L	50–150 μg/mL (not well established)	4–15 μg/mL[a] (not well established)
Elderly/medically ill patients	0.6–0.8 mEq/L	40–75 μg/mL	4–8 μg/mL
Maintenance Therapy[b]			
Dose	600–1800 mg/d	15 45 mg/kg/d	400–1800 mg/d
Drug serum concentrations			
Adults	0.6–1.2 mEq/L	50–125 μg/mL	4–12 μg/mL
Elderly or medically ill patients	0.4–0.6 mEq/L	40–60 μg/mL	4–6 μg/mL

[a]CBZ serum levels decrease during the first 2–4 wk due to autoinduction of metabolism by the cytochrome P450 liver enzymes; higher doses of CBZ may be required to maintain adequate CBZ concentrations.

[b]There is no evidence that dosage reduction should be done for maintenance therapy of bipolar disorder, but lower doses are often tried when the patient is stabilized.

DVPX = divalproex sodium; CBZ = carbamazepine.

Compiled from Refs. 30, 31, and 102.

should be prescribed in the elderly and in clinical situations associated with an impairment of lithium excretion (e.g., concomitant diuretic therapy, low-salt diet, renal disease, dehydration, or decreased cardiac output).[104] A single dose at bedtime with extended-release products may be used in patients with polyuria because urine volume may be lower with the once-per-day schedule than with multiple doses per day. Currently, there is no therapeutic reference range for single-daily dosing with lithium. The 12-hour postdose value may be 12% to 33% higher with extended-release preparations and lower with regular-release tablets compared with divided dosage schedules.

The dose should be adjusted based on the steady-state serum concentration drawn 12 hours (± 30 minutes) after the last dose. A therapeutic trial (lithium serum concentrations of 0.6 to 1.2 mEq/L) should last a minimum of 4 to 6 weeks. Acutely manic patients should have a serum concentration of at least 0.8 mEq/L, and some patients may require serum concentrations of 1.2 to 1.5 mEq/L to achieve a therapeutic response. Although serum concentrations less than 0.6 mEq/L are associated with higher rates of relapse, some patients may do well at serum concentrations of 0.4 to 0.6 mEq/L.[29] For bipolar prophylaxis in elderly patients, serum concentrations of 0.4 to 0.8 mEq/L are usually effective.[104]

Therapeutic Drug Monitoring. When lithium is first started, determination of the non–steady-state serum concentration 12 hours after the last dose is recommended every 2 to 3 days in patients prone to toxicity (see Toxicity section). When the desired serum concentration has been achieved (after dosage adjustments), blood level monitoring should be done every 1 to 2 weeks for 2 months or until lithium concentrations are stabilized.[24] Acutely manic patients may have an increased lithium clearance; once the manic episode abates, the lithium blood levels may increase. Maintenance lithium serum concentrations are usually measured every 3 to 6 months, but can be adjusted to every 6 to 12 months for stabilized patients and every 1 to 2 months for patients with frequent mood episodes. Lithium level measurements are indicated 5 to 10 days after dosage changes, with the addition or deletion of drugs that affect lithium clearance, or with changes in renal functioning. Lithium levels should be monitored more frequently in the elderly, particularly when dosages are increased or if there are signs of toxicity.[104] Lithium clearance rates increase by 50% to 100% during pregnancy and return to normal postpartum; thus, lithium levels should be determined monthly during pregnancy and weekly the month before delivery. Lithium should be discontinued 2 to 3 days before delivery and restarted at prepregnancy doses a few days after delivery.[8]

Valproic Acid

Pharmacology, Mechanism of Action, and Pharmacokinetics. The exact mechanism of action of VPA is not known, but may be related to the inhibition of GABA metabolism, stimulation of GABA synthesis and release, increasing $GABA_B$ receptor density, and augmentation of the postsynaptic inhibitory effect of GABA.[5,39] Other pharmacologic properties of VPA include decreasing dopamine turnover, decreasing NMDA-mediated depolarization, and decreasing aspartate release.[5]

Valproate sodium is rapidly converted to VPA in the stomach, whereas DVPX sodium delayed-release tablets must pass into the small intestine to be converted to VPA.[30] Valproic acid is highly bound to albumin and other plasma proteins, and it is extensively metabolized in the liver.[5] A summary of the absorption, distribution, metabolism, and elimination data for VPA is found in Table 70–8.

Adverse Effects. The most frequent adverse effects with VPA are gastrointestinal complaints (nausea, indigestion, mild diarrhea, flatulence), tremor, and sedation.[5,30,39] The gastrointestinal complaints are usually transient, but giving the drug with food, using lower initial doses with gradual increases in doses, switching to DVPX, or adding an H_2-blocker such as ranitidine can minimize them.[5] Addition of a β-blocker may alleviate tremors, and giving the total daily dose at bedtime may minimize daytime sedation.[5] Other adverse effects of VPA include ataxia, lethargy, fine hand tremor, alopecia, changes in the texture or color of hair, pruritus, prolonged bleeding due to inhibition of platelet aggregation, transient increases in liver enzymes (transaminase and lactic dehydrogenase), hyperammonemia, and weight gain.[5,30] Valproate may chelate trace metals such as selenium or zinc, which contributes to hair loss; therefore, supplementation of selenium and zinc may help to manage hair thinning.[5,24]

Rare cases of agranulocytosis and hepatitis have been reported with VPA. Thrombocytopenia may occur at higher doses, and patients should be monitored for bleeding and bruising. Fatal necrotizing hepatitis is an idiosyncratic, non–dose-related adverse effect that occurs in 1 in 40,000 cases; all fatal cases were in children who were under the age of 10 and had severe seizure disorders that required; multiple anticonvulsants.[8,30] Children receiving VPA should be monitored for the signs and symptoms of hepatitis (nausea, vomiting, abdominal pain, malaise, lethargy, fever, and jaundice).[5] A life-threatening hemorrhagic pancreatitis has been reported in both children and adults receiving VPA.[30] Patients should be warned that nausea, vomiting, abdominal pain, and anorexia can be symptoms of pancreatitis and that prompt medical evaluation is required.[30] Polycystic ovary disease, menstrual abnormalities, hyperandrogenism, and peripheral insulin resistance have been reported in women taking VPA.[30]

Teratogenicity. Because VPA has been found to be teratogenic (Class D pregnancy rating), it is usually not recommended during the first trimester of pregnancy (1% to 5% risk of neural tube birth defects, primarily spina bifida).[30,53] Administration of folate may reduce the risk of neural tube defects, however, so the clinicians should discuss the risks versus the benefits of using VPA during pregnancy with patients who desire to become pregnant.[5] Valproic acid is excreted into human breast milk in low concentrations (from less than 1% to 10% of the mother's serum VPA level) and is considered to be compatible with breastfeeding.[30,53,106] One case report of thrombocytopenia and anemia from VPA exposure has been reported in a nursing infant.[106] If the mother receives VPA during breastfeeding, the infant should have routine blood level and laboratory monitoring like the mother.[53]

Drug Interactions. There are several complex interaction between VPA and others medications. It appears that VPA is a weak inhibitor of liver enzymes, it may displace other drugs that are highly protein-bound (e.g., warfarin), and it may be displaced from protein binding sites by aspirin.[5,12] The antiplatelet effects of VPA may potentiate the anticoagulant effects of warfarin and aspirin. In addition, VPA interferes with laboratory tests; (for example, it falsely elevates urine ketones and causes the results of thyroid function tests to be abnormal). The concomitant administration of VPA may increase the effects of other CNS depressants or anticonvulsants. In comparison to carbamazepine, VPA tends to increase serum concentrations of other anticonvulsants.[5] Valproic acid may displace carbamazepine from serum protein binding sites and inhibit the metabolism of carbamazepine-10,11-epoxide, thereby causing carbamazepine toxicity.[12] Hepatic metabolism induced by carbamazepine may decrease VPA serum concentrations.[30] Chlorpromazine, cimetidine, erythromycin, felbamate, and fluoxetine may inhibit liver metabolism of VPA and result in toxicity.[5] The combination of DVPX and lithium has been used for the maintenance treatment of bipolar I disorder, but may result in more adverse effects.[108]

Dosing and Administration. The initial starting dosage of VPA is 500 to 1,000 mg/d (5 to 10 mg/kg/d) in divided doses, and the dose is adjusted up by 250 to 500 mg every 1 to 3 days (based on clinical response and tolerability) to 1,000 to 3,000 mg/d (maximum of 60 mg/kg/d) (see Table 70–9).[24] Once an optimal dosage has been achieved, the total daily dose may be given at bedtime if tolerated.[5] Higher initial loading doses of DVPX (20 mg/kg/d or 1,200 to 1,500 mg/d in divided doses) have been used in acutely agitated manic patients, resulting in therapeutic serum levels within 5 days, and this may result in a more rapid onset of antimanic response.[42] Data from bipolar clinical trials indicated that patients with trough serum levels over 45 μg/mL during the first week of treatment responded earlier to VPA.[109] Although therapeutic serum concentrations have not been established for VPA in bipolar disorder, most clinicians use the anticonvulsant therapeutic range of 50 to 125 μg/mL taken 12 hours after the last dose. Patients with cyclothymia or mild bipolar II may have a therapeutic response to lower VPA doses and blood levels, whereas some patients with a more severe form of bipolar disorder may require up to 150 μg/mL.[11]

Therapeutic Drug Monitoring. Serum VPA levels are usually determined every 1 to 2 weeks during the first 2 months, and then every 3 to 6 months during maintenance therapy.[24] Recommended baseline and routine laboratory tests for VPA are listed in Table 70–6.

Carbamazepine

Pharmacology, Mechanism of Action, and Pharmacokinetics. Carbamazepine, a dibenzazepine derivative, is structurally related to TCAs.[5] The precise mechanism of action of carbamazepine in affective disorders remains to be elucidated.[11] It blocks the reuptake of norepinephrine, decreases the release of norepinephrine, increases acetylcholine in the striatum, decreases dopamine and GABA turnover, blocks calcium influx through the NMDA–glutamate receptor, and decreases the activity of adenylate cyclase. In animal models, carbamazepine is effective in inhibiting amygdala kindling in the temporal lobe stimulated by norepinephrine and dopamine. A summary of the absorption, distribution, metabolism, and elimination data for carbamazepine is found in Table 70–8 and in Chapter 56.

Adverse Effects. The most common adverse effects of carbamazepine involve CNS toxicity, which occurs in up to 60% of patients.[31] Neurologic side effects include drowsiness, dizziness, fatigue, clumsiness, ataxia, vertigo, blurred vision, diplopia, nystagmus, dysarthria, confusion, and headache. These side effects usually occur during the first few weeks of therapy, initiating therapy with low doses, gradually increasing the dose, or giving a larger bedtime dose may minimize these effects. Gastrointestinal side effects (nausea, vomiting, abdominal pain, diarrhea, constipation, anorexia) occur early in therapy in up to 15% of patients, but administering the drug with food or reducing the daily dose can minimize them.[31]

White blood cell counts (WBCs) decrease in 25% of patients and return to normal with carbamazepine discontinuation.[31] It is wise to monitor patients with low- or below normal pretreatment WBCs and neutrophil counts more closely because of their increased risks of developing leukopenia (e.g., every 2 weeks for the first 1 to 3 months of treatment). If leukopenia occurs (WBCs < 3,000/mm^3 or neutrophil counts < 1,000/mm^3), then the dose of carbamazepine should be decreased or discontinued. Carbamazepine may be restarted at lower doses when the counts return to normal ranges. Serious hematologic dyscrasias such as aplastic anemia are rare. Patients should be educated about the signs and symptoms of leukopenia (oral ulcers, sore throat, easy bruising, bleeding, fever).[5]

Other side effects of carbamazepine include hyponatremia, hypersensitivity and dermatologic reactions (e.g., pruritic and erythematous rashes, urticaria, photosensitivity reactions, a lupus erythematosus-like syndrome). Patients should be instructed to seek medical attention if they develop a rash, and carbamazepine should be discontinued because the rash can progress to exfoliative dermatitis or Stevens-Johnson syndrome, which are potentially life-threatening conditions.[5] When the rash is gone, a rechallenge with carbamazepine can be tried with prednisone cotreatment. If a second hypersensitivity rash occurs, the patient should not receive carbamazepine. A mild transient elevation of liver enzyme levels is common, but hepatitis and a significant increase in liver enzyme levels can occur.[31] Acute overdoses of carbamazepine are potentially lethal, and serum levels above 15 μg/mL are associated with ataxia, choreiform movements, seizures, and coma.

Teratogenicity. Although carbamazepine has a Class D pregnancy rating, it is considered a teratogenic agent that may cause craniofacial deformities, spina bifida (0.5% to 1%), and low birth weight.[5] Because the safe use of carbamazepine during pregnancy has not been established, caution should be used in prescribing carbamazepine during the first trimester of pregnancy. Carbamazepine is excreted in breast milk (the milk-to-maternal plasma ratio of carbamazepine is about 0.4).[31,106] There are two case reports of transient cholestatic hepatitis and jaundice in nursing infants.[31,53,106]

Drug Interactions. Carbamazepine induces the hepatic microsomal P450 enzymes (1A2, 3A4, 2C9/10, and 2D6), which increases the elimination rate of many commonly coprescribed agents, such as anticonvulsants, antidepressants, antipsychotics, benzodiazepines, warfarin, dicumarol, and theophylline.[5,31] Carbamazepine decreases the plasma levels and efficacy of oral contraceptives; thus, women who receive carbamazepine require higher dosage forms or alternative contraceptive methods.[12] Concomitant drug therapies that inhibit the CYP450 3A4 isoenzyme system may result in carbamazepine toxicity (e.g., cimetidine, diltiazem, erythromycin, fluoxetine, fluvoxamine, isoniazid, itraconazole, ketoconazole, nefazodone, propoxyphene, and verapamil).[12,31] When carbamazepine is combined with VPA, the carbamazepine dose should be reduced because VPA displaces carbamazepine from protein binding sites, thus increasing free levels.[5,12] Combining clozapine and carbamazepine is not recommended because of the possibility of bone marrow suppression with both agent.[5]

Dosing and Administration. During an acute manic episode, carbamazepine should be started at 200 to 400 mg/d in divided doses with meals and increased by 200 mg every 2 to 4 days up to 10 to 15 mg/kg/d.[31] If dose-related side effects (e.g., sedation, dizziness, ataxia, diplopia) occur during the first week of therapy, titrating the drug more slowly and giving a larger portion of the dose at bedtime may be required.[5] If there is no response after 2 weeks, then the dosage can be gradually increased to obtain serum concentrations between 4 and 12 μg/mL; some treatment-resistant patients may require serum concentrations up to 12 to 14 μg/mL. When patients are symptom-free, carbamazepine can be initiated with lower initial doses (e.g., 100 to 200 mg/d, increased by 100 to 200 mg/d every 3 to 5 days up to

600 to 1,200 mg/d). Carbamazepine should be withdrawn slowly to avoid precipitating the recurrence of bipolar symptoms.

There appears to be no significant correlation between carbamazepine serum concentration and degree of antimanic or antidepressant response.[12] The CSF level of its active 10,11-epoxide metabolite (carbamazepine-E) may correlate with degree of clinical improvement in bipolar patients.[5] Because CSF levels of carbamazepine-E are not monitored, most clinicians attempt to maintain serum concentrations of carbamazepine between 4 and 12 μg/mL.[12] During the first month of therapy, serum concentrations of carbamazepine may decrease (autoinduction of CYP450 3A4 hepatic oxidative enzymes that increase carbamazepine metabolism), and the dose may need to be increased to maintain therapeutic serum concentrations. Autoinduction of carbamazepine may begin by day 3 and can continue up to 30 days after the last dosage change.

Therapeutic Drug Monitoring. Carbamazepine serum levels are usually obtained every 1 to 2 weeks during the first 2 months, and then every 3 to 6 months during maintenance therapy.[24] Recommended baseline and routine laboratory tests for carbamazepine are listed in Table 70-6.

PHARMACOECONOMIC CONSIDERATIONS

Clinical studies suggest that there are significant differences in the onset of action and the tolerance to adverse effects for lithium, carbamazepine, VPA, and the newer anticonvulsants such as gabapentin, lamotrigine, and topiramate.[24,28] The mood stabilizers may have different efficacies for bipolar subtypes, and there are now recognized positive predictors for clinical response to treatment.[18–20,24,40] These factors have a potential impact on drug selection, response rates, noncompliance due to adverse effects, and treatment costs (outpatient and inpatient care).

A recent review of health economic studies found that the DVPX rapid loading dose method (20 mg/kg/d) was associated with shorter lengths of hospital stays, particularly in patients with rapid cycling or mixed states.[110,111] Other studies have reported cost savings for DVPX sodium and for the combination of carbamazepine and lithium over the cost of lithium alone.[111,112] Further studies are needed to compare the different mood stabilizers (monotherapy versus combination therapy), dosing regimens (standard titration versus oral loading), termination of therapy due to adverse effects, and total costs for treatment.

EVALUATION OF THERAPEUTIC OUTCOMES

The evaluation of therapeutic outcomes for bipolar disorder requires frequent laboratory monitoring and regular office visits (every 1 to 2 weeks for acute or frequent episodes or 1 to 3 months for stable patients with infrequent episodes).[23,24] Patients should be actively involved with their treatment and help to monitor target symptoms and adverse effects. Because some patients have a rapid onset or "switching" in episodes, they should be encouraged to call their physician (or mental health professional involved with their care) in order to receive prompt treatment. More frequent office visits, telephone calls, and intensive outpatient programs are first-line strategies to prevent hospitalization during the acute treatment phase of a manic or depressive episode.

CONCLUSIONS

Bipolar disorder has a diversity of manifestations, recurrences of mood states, and clinical subtypes that requires tailoring the pharmacotherapy to the individual patient. Different treatment approaches and a combination of mood stabilizers are often required, depending on the clinical state of the patient.[25] Bipolar disorder remains a challenge for clinicians because it is a constantly changing illness that requires close monitoring.

▶ PRINCIPLES OF PHARMACOTHERAPY

- Patients and family members should be educated about bipolar disorder (signs, symptoms, course, causes, outcomes) and treatments (nonpharmacologic and pharmacologic).
- The goal of therapy for bipolar disorder should be to minimize mood episodes, maximize compliance with therapy, improve the functioning of the patient, and limit adverse effects.
- Patients should be routinely assessed for signs and symptoms of mood episodes; compliance with pharmacotherapy; use of alcohol, substances of abuse, nicotine, and caffeine; concomitant medications that may interact with prescribed mood stabilizers; use of birth control methods during child-bearing years; suicidal ideation, intent, and plan; changes in energy level, sleep, appetite, weight, and libido; and adverse effects.
- Baseline and follow-up laboratory tests are required for some mood stabilizers (see Table 70–6, Baseline and Routine Laboratory Testing for Patients Treated With Mood Stabilizers). Drug level monitoring is required for lithium, carbamazepine, and VPA and should be obtained 12 hours postdose (preferably before the morning dose) and after steady-state serum concentrations are achieved (four to five times the $t_{1/2}$).
- Different mood episodes and subtypes of bipolar disorder respond differently to mood stabilizers (see Figure 70–1, Algorithm for the Treatment of Bipolar Disorder, and Table 70–7, Use of Mood Stabilizers in Special Populations).
- Adjunctive agents such as antidepressants, antipsychotics, and benzodiazepines are typically used in combination with mood stabilizers when the patient is experiencing an acute mood episode or when the condition is refractory to the mood-stabilizing agent alone. However, chronic use of these agents during maintenance therapy should be avoided.
- The combination of two or more mood stabilizers (e.g., lithium + carbamazepine, lithium + VPA, carbamazepine + VPA, lithium + carbamazepine + VPA) may be needed for patients who do not respond to monotherapy (e.g., refractory mood episodes, mixed states, rapid cycling).
- Alternative mood stabilizers (e.g., calcium channel blockers, atypical antipsychotics, and newer anticonvulsants such as gabapentin, lamotrigine, and topiramate) may be appropriate if the patient cannot tolerate lithium, carbamazepine, or VPA.
- Nonpharmacologic treatments such as ECT is effective for severe psychotic bipolar depression or acute mania when a rapid response is essential or when the use of medication is contraindicated.
- Lithium, carbamazepine, and VPA may have teratogenic risks and may cause adverse effects in the breastfed infant; thus, caution is advised when using these mood stabilizers during pregnancy and

breastfeeding. Using the lowest effective dose, discontinuing the agent during the first trimester, or using alternative mood stabilizers (e.g., atypical antipsychotics, calcium channel blockers, benzodiazepines, newer anticonvulsants) may be advisable in some patients.

- Maintenance (prophylaxis) therapy is based on the severity of the patient's disorder, the number of episodes, and risk of adverse effects. Patients who have experienced two or more episodes should receive lifelong therapy.

REFERENCES

1. Kessler RC, McGonagle KA, Zhao S, et al. Lifetime and 12-month prevalence of DSM-III-R psychiatric disorders in the United States: Results from the national comorbidity survey. Arch Gen Psychiatry 1994;51: 8–19.
2. American Psychiatric Association: *Diagnostic and Statistical Manual of Mental Disorders*, Fourth Edition, Text Revision. Washington, DC: American Psychiatric Association, 2000.
3. Schatzberg AF. Bipolar disorder: recent issues in diagnosis and classification. J Clin Psychiatry 1998;59[suppl 6]:13–19.
4. Nathan KI, Musselman DL, Schatzberg AF, Nemeroff CB. Biology of mood disorders. In: Schatzberg AF, Nemeroff CB, eds. Textbook of Psychopharmacology. Washington, DC: American Psychiatric Press, 1995:439–477.
5. Goodnick PJ, ed. Mania: Clinical and Research Perspectives. Washington, DC: American Psychiatric Press, 1990.
6. Pato CN, Kennedy JL, Bauer A, et al. Genetics of bipolar disorder. TEN 2000;2(4):33–41.
7. Goodwin FK, Jamison KR, eds. Manic-Depressive Illness. New York: Oxford University Press, 1990.
8. Janicak PG, Davis JM, Preskorn SH, Ayd FJ. Treatment with mood stabilizers. In: Janicak PG, Davis JM, Preskorn SH, Ayd FJ, eds. Principles and Practice of Psychotherapy, 2nd ed. Baltimore: Williams & Wilkins, 1997:403–473.
9. Lenex RH, Hahn CG. Overview of the mechanism of action of lithium in the brain: fifty-year update. J Clin Psychiatry 2000;61(suppl 9):5–15.
10. Meldrum BD. Update on the mechanism of action of antiepileptic drugs. Epilepsia 1996;37(suppl 6):S4–11.
11. Post RM, Ketter TA, Denicoff K, et al. The place of anticonvulsant therapy in bipolar illness. Psychopharmacology 1996;128:115–129.
12. Goldberg JF, Harrow M, eds. Bipolar Disorders: Clinical Course and Outcome. Washington, DC: American Psychiatric Press, 1999.
13. Botts SR, Raskind J. Gabapentin and lamotrigine in bipolar disorder. Am J Health-Syst Pharm 1999;56:1939–1944.
14. Resenick MM, Chaney KA, Chen J. G protein-mediated signal transduction as a target of antidepressant and antibipolar drug action: Evidence from model systems. J Clin Psychiatry 1996;57(suppl 13): 49–55.
15. Manji HK, Chen G, Hsiao JK, et al. Regulation of signal transduction pathways by mood-stabilizing agents: Implications for the delayed onset of therapeutic efficacy. J Clin Psychiatry 1996;57(suppl 13): 34–46.
16. Practice Parameters for the Assessment and Treatment of Children and Adolescents with Bipolar Disorder. J Am Acad Child Adolesc Psychiatry 1997;36:138–157.
17. Strakowski SM, McElroy SL, Keck PE, West SA. Suicidality among patients with mixed and manic bipolar disorder. Am J Psychiatry 1996;153:674–676.
18. Keck PE, McElroy SL. Outcome in the pharmacologic treatment of bipolar disorder. J Clin Psychopharmacol 1996;16(suppl 1):15S–23S.
19. Calabrese JR, Fatemi SH, Kujawa M, Woyshville MJ. Predictors of response to mood stabilizers. J Clin Psychopharmacol 1996;16(suppl 1): 24S–31S.
20. Sachs GS. Bipolar mood disorder: Practical strategies for acute and maintenance phase treatment. J Clin Psychopharmacol 1996;16(suppl 1): 32S–47S.
21. Bowden CL. Role of newer medications for bipolar disorder. J Clin Psychopharmacol 1996;16(suppl 1):48S–55S.
22. Dubovsky SL, Buzan RD. Novel alternatives and supplements to lithium and anticonvulsants for bipolar affective disorder. J Clin Psychiatry 1997;58:224–242.
23. Hirschfeld RMA, Clayton PJ, Cohen I, et al. Practice guideline for the treatment of patients with bipolar disorder. Am J Psychiatry 1994;151(suppl):1–31.
24. Frances A, Docherty JP, Kahn DA, et al. The expert consensus guideline series. Treatment of bipolar disorder. J Clin Psychiatry 1996;57(suppl 12):1–89.
25. Freeman MP, Stoll AI. Mood stabilizer combinations: a review of safety and efficacy. Am J Psychiatry 1998;155:12–21.
26. Solomon DA, Keitner GI, Ryan CE, et al. Lithium plus valproate as maintenance polypharmacy for patients with bipolar I disorder: a review. J Clin Psychopharmacol 1998;18:38–49.
27. Tohen M, Zarate CA. Antipsychotic agents and bipolar disorder. J Clin Psychiatry 1998;59(suppl 1):38–48.
28. Post RM, Frye MA, Denicoff KD, et al. Beyond lithium in the treatment of bipolar illness. Neuropsychopharmacology 1998;19:206–219.
29. Bowden CL. Key treatment studies of lithium in manic-depressive illness: efficacy and side effects. J Clin Psychiatry 1998;59(suppl 6): 13–19.
30. Depakote (divalproex sodium delayed-release) package insert. Abbott Park, IL: Abbott Laboratories; Revised July 31,2000.
31. Carbamazepine. In: McEvoy GK, Litvak K, Welsh OH et al. eds. AHFS Drug Information 2001. Bethesda, MD: American Society of Health-System Pharmacists, 2001:2085–2090.
32. Trileptal (oxcarbazepine) package insert. East Hanover, NJ: Novartis Pharmaceuticals; Revised January 2000.
33. Ferrier IN. Lamotrigine and gabapentin: alternatives in the treatment of bipolar disorder. Neuropsychobiology 1998;38:192–197.
34. Walden J, Normann C, Langosch J, et al. Differential treatment of bipolar disorder with old and new antiepileptic drugs. Neuropsychobiol 1998;38:181–184.
35. Post RM, Denicoff KD, Frye MA, et al. A history of the use of anticonvulsants as mood stabilizers in the last two decades of the 20th century. Neuropsychobiol 1998;38:152–166.
36. Zyprexa (olanzapine) package insert. Indianapolis, IN: Eli Lilly and Company; Revised March 17, 2000.
37. Bowden CL. Efficacy of lithium in mania and maintenance therapy of bipolar disorder. J Clin Psychiatry 2000;61(suppl 9):35–40.
38. Bowden CL, Brugger AM, Swann AC, et al. Efficacy of divalproex vs lithium and placebo in the treatment of mania. The Depakote Mania Study Group. JAMA 1994;271:918–924.
39. Guay DRP. The emerging role of valproate in bipolar disorder and other psychiatric disorders. Pharmacotherapy 1995;15:631–647.
40. Bowden CL. Predictors of response to divalproex and lithium. J Clin Psychiatry 1995;56(suppl 3):25–30.
41. Keck PE Jr, McElvoy SL, Strakowski SM. Anticonvulsants and antipsychotics in the treatment of bipolar disorder. J Clin Psychiatry 1998;59(suppl 6):74–81.
42. McElroy SL, Keck PE, Stanton SP, et al. A randomized comparison of divalproex oral loading versus haloperidol in the initial treatment of acute psychotic mania. J Clin Psychiatry 1996;57:142–146.
43. Denicoff KD, Smith-Jackson EE, Disney ER. et al. Comparative prophylactic efficacy of lithium, carbamazepine, and the combination in bipolar disorder. J Clin Psychiatry 1997;58:470–478.
44. McElroy SL, Keck PE, Strakowski SM. Mania, psychosis, and antipsychotics. J Clin Psychiatry 1996;57(suppl 3):14–26.
45. Kane J. Tardive dyskinesia in affective disorders. J Clin Psychiatry 1999;66(suppl 5):43–47.
46. Frye MA, Ketter TA, Altshuler LL, et al. Clozapine in bipolar disorder: treatment implications for other atypical antipsychotics. J Affect Disord 1998;48:91–104.
47. Calabrese JR, Kimmel SE, Woyshville MJ, et al. Clozapine for treatment-refractory mania. Am J Psychiatry 1996;153:759–764.

48. Tohen M, Zarate CA, Centorrino F, et al. Risperidone in the treatment of mania. J Clin Psychiatry 1996;57:249–253.
49. McIntyre R, Young LT, Hasey G, et al. Risperidone treatment of bipolar disorder. Can J Psychiatry 1997;42(1):88–90. Letter.
50. Ghaemi SN, Sach GS, Baldessano CF, et al. Acute treatment of bipolar disorder with adjunctive risperidone in outpatients. Can J Psychiatry 1997;42:196–199.
51. Segal J, Berk M, Brook S. Risperidone compared with both lithium and haloperidol in mania: a double-blind randomized controlled trial. Clin Neuropharmacol 1998;21(3):176–180.
52. Zarate CA Jr, Narendran R, Tohen M, et al. Clinical predictors of acute response with olanzapine in psychotic mood disorders. J Clin Psychiatry 1998;59:24–28.
53. Llewellyn A, Stowe ZN, Strader JR Jr. The use of lithium and management of women with bipolar disorder during pregnancy and lactation. J Clin Psychiatry 1998;59(suppl 6):57–64.
54. Janicak PG, Sharma RP, Pandey F, et al. Verapamil for the treatment of acute mania: a double-blind, placebo-controlled trial. Am J Psychiatry 1998;155:972–973.
55. Lamictal (lamotrigine) package insert. Research Triangle Park, NC: Glaxo Wellcome, Inc; February 1999.
56. Engle PM, Heck AM. Lamotrigine for the treatment of bipolar disorder. Ann Pharmacother 2000;34:258–262.
57. Sporn J, Sachs G. The anticonvulsant lamotrigine in treatment-resistant manic-depressive illness. J Clin Psychopharmacol 1997;17: 185–189.
58. Walden J, Hesslinger B, van Calker D, Berger M. Addition of lamotrigine to valproate may enhance efficacy in the treatment of bipolar affective disorder. Pharmacopsychiatry 1996;29:193–195.
59. Fatemi SH, Rapport DJ, Calabrese JR, et al. Lamotrigine in rapid-cycling bipolar disorder. J Clin Psychiatry 1997;58:522–527.
60. Kotler M, Matar MA. Lamotrigine in the treatment of resistant bipolar disorder. Clin Neuropharmacol 1998;2(1):65–67.
61. Calabrese JR, Bowder CL, McElroy SL, et al. Spectrum of activity of lamotrigine in the treatment of refractory bipolar disorder. Am J Psychiatry 1999;156:1019–1023.
62. Kusumaker V, Yatham LN. Lamotrigine treatment of rapid cycling bipolar disorder. Am J Psychiatry 1997;154:1171–1172.
63. Kusumaker V, Yatham LN. An open study of lamotrigine in refractory bipolar depression. Psychiatry Res 1997;72:145–148.
64. Bowden CL, Calabrese JR, McElroy SL, et al. The efficacy of lamotrigine in rapid cycling and nonrapid cycling patients with bipolar disorder. Biol Psychiatry 1999;45:3–8.
65. Calabrese JR, Rapport DJ, Shelton DM, et al. Clinical studies on the use of lamotrigine in bipolar disorder. Neuropsychobiol 1998;38:185–191.
66. Suppes T, Brown ES, McElroy SL, et al. Lamotrigine for the treatment of bipolar disorder: a clinical case series. J Affect Disord 1999;53(1):95–98.
67. Ichim L, Berk M, Brook S. Lamotrigine compared with lithium in mania: a double-blind randomized controlled trial. Ann Clin Psychiatry 2000;12(1)5–10.
68. Berk M. Lamotrigine and the treatment of mania in bipolar disorder. Eur Neuropsychopharmacol 1999;9(Suppl 4):S119–S123.
69. Calabrese JR, Bowder CL, Sach GS, et al. A double-blind placebo-controlled study of lamotrigine monotherapy in outpatients with bipolar I depression. J Clin Psychiatry 1999;60:79–88.
70. Bowden CL, Mitchell P, Suppes T. Lamotrigine in the treatment of bipolar depression. Eur Neuropsychopharmacol 1999;9(Suppl 4):S113–S117.
71. Frye MA, Ketter TA, Kimbrell TA, et al. A placebo controlled study of lamotrigine and gabapentin monotherapy in refractory mood disorders. J Clin Psychopharmacol 2000;20(16):607–614.
72. Neurontin (gabapentin) package insert. Morris Plains, NJ: Parke-Davis Pharmaceuticals; Revised February 1999.
73. Letterman L, Markowitz JS. Gabapentin: a review of published experience in the treatment of bipolar disorder and other psychiatric conditions. Pharmacotherapy 1999;19(5):565–572.
74. Magnes L. Nonepileptic uses of gabapentin. Epilepsia 1999;40(suppl 6):S66–S72.
75. Perugi G, Ruffolo G, Sartini S, et al. Clinical experience using adjunctive gabapentin in treatment-resistant bipolar mixed states. Pharmacopsychiatry 1999;32:136–141.
76. Erfurth A, Kammerer C, Grunze H, et al. An open label study of gabapentin in the treatment of acute mania. J Psychiatr Res 1998;43:261–264.
77. Knoll J, Stegman K, Suppes T. Clinical experience using gabapentin adjunctively in patients with a history of mania or hypomania. J Affect Disord 1998;49:229–233.
78. Young LT, Robb JC, Hasey GM, et al. Gabapentin as an adjunctive treatment in bipolar disorder. J Affect Disord 1999;55:73–77.
79. Cabras PL, Hardoy MJ, Hardoy MC, et al. Clinical experience with gabapentin in patients with bipolar or schizoaffective disorder: results of an open-label study. J Clin Psychiatry 1999;60:245–248.
80. Sokolsk KN, Green C, Maris DE, et al. Gabapentin as an adjunct to standard mood stabilizers in outpatients with mixed bipolar symptomatology. Ann Clin Psychiatry 1999;11(4)217–222.
81. Ghaemi SN, Katzow JJ, Desai SP, et al. Gabapentin treatment of mood disorders: a preliminary study. J Clin Psychiatry 1998;59(8):426–429.
82. McElroy SL, Soutullo CA, Keck PE Jr, et al. A pilot trial of adjunctive gabapentin in the treatment of bipolar disorder. Ann Clin Psychiatry 1997;9(2):99–103.
83. Young LT, Robb JC, Patelis-Siotis I, et al. Acute treatment of bipolar depression with gabapentin. Biol Psychiatry 1997;42:851–853.
84. Schaffer CB, Schaffer LC. Open maintenance treatment of bipolar disorder spectrum patients who responded to gabapentin augmentation in the acute phase of treatment. J Affect Disord 1999;55:237–240.
85. Topamax (topiramate) package insert. Raritan, NJ: Ortho-McNeil Pharmaceuticals; Revised May 2000.
86. Rosenfeld WE. Topiramate: a review of preclinical, pharmacokinetic, and clinical data. Clin Therapeutics 1997;19(6):1294–1308.
87. Markind JE. Topiramate: a new antiepileptic drug. Am J Health-Syst Pharm 1998;55:554–562.
88. Marcotte D. Use of topiramate: a new anti-epileptic as a mood stabilizer. J Affect Disord 1998;50:245–251.
89. Chengappa KNR, Rathmore D, Levine J, et al. Topiramate as add-on treatment for patients with bipolar mania. Bipolar Disord 1999;1:42–53.
90. McElroy SL, Suppes T, Keck PE Jr, et al. Open-label adjunctive topiramate in the treatment of bipolar disorders. Biol Psychiatry 2000;47:1025–1033.
91. Mischory A, Yaroslavsky Y, Bersudsky Y, et al. Phenytoin as an antimanic anticonvulsant: a controlled study. Am J Psychiatry 2000;157:463–465.
92. Suzdak PD, Jansen JA. A review of the preclinical pharmacology of tiagabine: a potent and selective anticonvulsant GABA uptake inhibitor. Epilepsia 1995;36:612–626.
93. Gunze H, Erfurth A, Marcuse A, et al. Tiagabine appears not be efficacious in the treatment of acute mania. J Clin Psychiatry 1999;60:759–762.
94. Schaffer LC, Schaffer CB. Tiagabine and the treatment of refractory bipolar disorder. Am J Psychiatry 1999;156(12):2014–2015. Letter.
95. Kaufman KR. Adjunctive tiagabine treatment of psychiatric disorders: three cases. Ann Clin Psychiatry 1998;10(4):181–184.
96. Zonegran (zonisamide) package insert. San Francisco, CA: Elan Pharmaceuticals; March 30, 2000.
97. Kanba S, Yagi G, Kamijimi K, et al. The first open study of zonisamide, a novel anticonvulsant shows efficacy in mania. Prog Neuro Psychopharmacol & Biol Psychiat 1994;18:707–715.
98. Milner KK, Amburgey ME, Cameron OG. Drug treatment of bipolar disorder. Formulary 1998;33:960–987.
99. Stoll AL, Lock CA, Marangell LB, et al. Omega-3 fatty acids and bipolar disorder: a review of prostaglandins, leukotrienes and essential fatty acids 1999;60(5&6):329–337.
100. Stoll AL, Severus WE, Freeman MP, et al. Omega-3 fatty acids in bipolar disorder: a preliminary double-blind, placebo-controlled trial. Arch Gen Psychiatry 1999;56:407–412.
101. Leibenluft E. Women with bipolar illness: Clinical and research issues. Am J Psychiatry 1996;153:163–173.

102. Lithium salts. In: McEvoy GK, Litvak K, Welsh OH, et al, eds. AHFS Drug Information 2001. Bethesda, MD: American Society of Health-System Pharmacists, 2001:2369–2377.
103. Dunner DL. Optimizing lithium treatment. J Clin Psychiatry 2000; 61(suppl 9):76–81.
104. Tueth MJ, Murphy TK, Evans DL. Special considerations: use of lithium in children and adolescents, and elderly patients. J Clin Psychiatry 1998;59(suppl 6):66–73.
105. Cohen LS, Friedman JM, Jefferson JW, et al. A reevaluation of risk of in utero exposure to lithium. JAMA 1994;271:146–150.
106. Chaudron LH, Jefferson JW. Mood stabilizers during breastfeeding: a review. J Clin Psychiatry 2000;61:79–90.
107. Wright R, Crismon ML. Comparison of three a priori methods and one empirical method in predicting lithium dosage requirements. Am J Health-Syst Pharm. 2000;57:1698–1702.
108. Solomon DA, Ryan CE, Keitner GI, et al. A pilot study of lithium carbonate plus divalproex sodium for the continuation and maintenance treatment of patients with bipolar I disorder. J Clin Psychiatry 1997;58:95–99.
109. Bowden CL, Janicak PG, Orsulak P, et al. Relation of serum valproate concentrations to response in mania. Am J Psychiatry 1996;153:765–770.
110. Keck PE, McElroy SL, Bennett JA. Health-economic implications of the onset of action of antimanic agents. J Clin Psychiatry 1996; 57(suppl 13):13–18.
111. Frye MA, Altshuler LL, Szuba MP, et al. The relationship between antimanic agent for treatment of classic or dysphoric mania and length of hospital stay. J Clin Psychiatry 1996;57:17–21.
112. Keck PE Jr, Nabulsi AA, Taylor JL, et al. A pharmacoeconomic model of divalproex vs lithium in the acute and prophylactic treatment of bipolar I disorder. J Clin Psychiatry 1996;57:213–222.

71

ANXIETY DISORDERS

Cynthia K. Kirkwood and Sarah T. Melton

Anxiety is an emotional state commonly caused by the perception of real or potential danger that threatens the security of an individual. Everyone experiences a certain amount of nervousness and apprehension when faced with a stressful situation. Usually the response is transient and contains a built-in control mechanism to return to a normal physiologic state.

If anxiety becomes excessive and out of proportion, it can produce uncomfortable and potentially incapacitating psychological and physical arousal. Some persons experience persistent, severe anxiety symptoms and possess irrational fears that significantly impair normal daily functioning. These persons often suffer from an anxiety disorder.[1]

Anxiety disorders are among the most frequent mental disorders encountered in clinical practice. One-fourth of the population will experience at least one anxiety disorder in their lifetime. Unfortunately, only 27% of patients with anxiety disorders receive professional treatment.[2]

Failure to diagnose and manage anxiety disorders results in negative outcomes—overuse of health care resources and increased morbidity and mortality.[3] Individuals with anxiety disorders develop cardiovascular, cerebrovascular, gastrointestinal, and respiratory disorders at a significantly higher rate than the general population.[4]

To treat anxiety appropriately, the clinician must make a reliable diagnosis. It is essential that the distinction between short-term symptoms of anxiety and anxiety disorders be understood. Common or situational anxiety is a normal response to a stressful situation. Although symptoms may be severe, they are temporary and usually last no more than 2 or 3 weeks. Although short-term, "as needed" treatment with an anxiolytic agent such as a benzodiazepine (BZ) is common and may provide some symptomatic relief, prolonged drug therapy is unnecessary.[5]

EPIDEMIOLOGY

According to the National Comorbidity Survey of noninstitutionalized persons aged 15 to 54 years, the 12-month prevalence rate for anxiety disorders averaged 17.2%, and the lifetime rate was 24.9%.[2] Social anxiety disorder (SAD) was the most common anxiety disorder, with a lifetime prevalence of 13.3% and 12-month rate of 7.9%.[7] The lifetime prevalence of generalized anxiety disorder (GAD) was 5.1%, panic disorder was 3.5%, and posttraumatic stress disorder (PTSD) was 7.8%.[2] Specific phobia has a lifetime prevalence rate of 11.3%; however, patients are not seriously impaired in terms of daily functioning, and few persons seek treatment.[1,2]

The annual economic burden of anxiety disorders in the United States was estimated to be $42.3 billion in 1990 ($1,542 dollars per sufferer). Nonpsychiatric medical treatment costs represented 54% of this figure ($23 billion), with expenses of $13.3 billion for psychiatric treatment, $4.1 billion for indirect workplace costs, and $1.2 billion in mortality costs. For anxious workers, 88% of the workplace costs result from lost productivity. All anxiety disorders are associated with impaired workplace performance, except specific phobia. Panic disorder and PTSD had the highest rates of health care service use.[6]

In general, anxiety disorders are a group of heterogeneous illnesses that develop before age 30 and are more common in women and those with a family history of anxiety and depression. Patients often develop another anxiety disorder, major depression, or substance abuse.[1,2] Anxiety disorders generally are chronic in nature, and although symptoms wax and wane over time, patients rarely are completely symptom-free.[1] Most patients with anxiety disorders can be treated effectively. However, long-term treatment may be required, and relapse after drug discontinuation is common.[7]

ETIOLOGY

The differential diagnosis of anxiety disorders includes medical and psychiatric illnesses and certain drugs. Evaluation of the anxious patient requires a complete physical and mental status examination, appropriate laboratory tests, a toxicologic screen, and a thorough knowledge of the patient's medical, psychiatric, and drug history.[7]

MEDICAL DISEASES ASSOCIATED WITH ANXIETY

Anxiety symptoms are an inherent part of the initial clinical presentation in several medical disorders, thus complicating the distinction between anxiety disorders and medical disorders.[7] If the anxiety symptoms are secondary to a medical illness, they usually will subside as the medical situation stabilizes. However, the knowledge that one has a physical illness may trigger anxious feelings and further complicate therapy.

Symptoms of anxiety frequently present in medical disorders include palpitations, tachycardia, chest pain or tightness, shortness of breath, and hyperventilation. Medical disorders most closely associated with anxiety are listed in Table 71–1.[7,8]

PSYCHIATRIC DISEASES ASSOCIATED WITH ANXIETY

Anxiety may be a concomitant symptom of several major psychiatric illnesses. Anxiety symptoms are extremely common in patients with mood disorders, schizophrenia, delirium, dementia, and substance use disorders. Most psychiatric patients will have two or more concurrent psychiatric disorders (comorbidity) within their lifetime.[2] To treat patients with anxiety disorders appropriately, it is important to assess and diagnose all comorbid psychiatric conditions adequately.

DRUG-INDUCED ANXIETY

The two major drug classes that cause anxiety symptoms are the central nervous system (CNS) stimulants and the depressants (Table 71–2). Anxiety occurs during the use of these drugs in a dose-dependent manner, but ingestion of minimal amounts may result in marked anxiety, including panic attacks, in some individuals.[9]

TABLE 71–1. Common Medical Disorders Associated with Anxiety Symptoms

Cardiovascular
Angina, arrhythmias, congestive heart failure, myocardial infarction, supraventricular tachycardia
Endocrine and Metabolic
Cushing's disease, hyperparathyroidism, hyperthyroidism, hypothyroidism, hypoglycemia, hyperkalemia, pheochromocytoma, vitamin B_{12} or folate deficiencies
Neurologic
CNS tumors, dementia, migraine, pain, Parkinson's disease, seizures, stroke, transient ischemic attacks
Respiratory System
Asthma, chronic obstructive lung disease, pulmonary embolus or infections
Others
Anemias, systemic lupus erythematosus

Compiled from Refs. 7 and 8.

Anxiety occurs occasionally during the use of CNS depressants, especially in children and the elderly; however, anxiety complaints are more common as complications of drug withdrawal after the abrupt discontinuation of these agents.[8]

PATHOPHYSIOLOGY

Data from biochemical and neuroimaging studies indicate that the modulation of normal and pathologic anxiety states is associated with multiple brain structures and abnormal function in several neurotransmitter systems, including norepinephrine (NE), γ-aminobutyric acid (GABA), and serotonin (5-HT). Current neuroanatomic models of fear and anxiety include several key brain structures. The amygdala, a temporal lobe structure, plays a critical role in the assessment of fear stimuli and response to danger.[10] The locus ceruleus (LC), located in the brainstem, is the primary NE-containing site in the brain, with widespread projections to areas responsible for implementing fear responses (e.g., vagus, lateral, and paraventricular hypothalamus). The hippocampus is integral in the consolidation of traumatic memory and, along with the entorhinal cortex, contextual fear conditioning (involved in chronic anxiety). The hypothalamus is the principal site for integrating neuroendocrine and autonomic responses to threat.[10] Imprinting of emotionally traumatic experiences is partially mediated by NE action on the β-receptors in the amygdala.[11]

NEUROCHEMICAL THEORIES

NORADRENERGIC MODEL

The basic premise of the noradrenergic theory is that the autonomic nervous system of anxious patients is hypersensitive and overreacts to various stimuli. Many anxious patients clearly display symptoms of peripheral autonomic hyperactivity.[10] In response to threat or fearful situations, the LC serves as an alarm center, activating NE release and stimulating the sympathetic and parasympathetic nervous systems. Chronic central noradrenergic overactivity downregulates α_2-adrenoreceptors in GAD and PTSD patients.[11,12] This receptor is hypersensitive in some patients with panic disorder.[10]

By administering drugs that have a relatively specific effect on the LC, researchers have further explored the NE theory of anxiety and panic disorder. Drugs with anxiogenic effects (e.g., yohimbine and isoproterenol) stimulate LC firing and increase noradrenergic activity. These agents often produce subjective feelings of anxiety and can precipitate a panic attack in those with panic disorder but not in normal volunteers or those with other psychiatric illnesses.[13,14] Drugs with anxiolytic or antipanic effects (e.g., BZs, antidepressants, clonidine) inhibit LC firing, decrease noradrenergic activity, and block the effects of anxiogenic drugs.[11]

TABLE 71–2. Drugs and Substances Associated with Anxiety Symptoms

CNS Stimulants
Amphetamines, caffeine, cocaine, ephedrine, methylphenidate
CNS Depressant Withdrawal
Alcohol, anxiolytics, barbiturates, narcotic agonists, sedative-hypnotics
Intoxication or Adverse Effect
Anticholinergics, anticonvulsants, antihistamines, antidepressants, antihypertensives, antiparkinsonian agents, antipsychotics (akathisia), bronchodilators, cycloserine, digoxin, dopamine, insulin, isoproterenol, nicotinic acid, oral contraceptives, over-the-counter sympathomimetics, steroids, thyroid preparations

Compiled from Refs. 1 and 8.

BENZODIAZEPINE RECEPTOR MODEL

The BZ receptor is functionally and structurally linked to the GABA type A ($GABA_A$) receptor and a chloride ion channel; this is referred to as the *GABA-BZ receptor complex.*[11] GABA, the major inhibitory neurotransmitter in the CNS, has a strong regulatory or inhibitory effect on the 5-HT, NE, and dopamine (DA) systems. When GABA binds to its receptor, the chloride ion channel opens and permits the influx of negatively charged chloride ions; this results in hyperpolarization of the cell membrane and causes a decrease in nerve cell excitability.[15]

The role of the GABA-BZ receptor complex in anxiety disorders has not been well characterized. Abnormal sensitivity to antagonism of the BZ receptor was demonstrated in both SAD and panic disorder patients.[12] In patients with GAD, downregulated central BZ receptors and low levels of peripheral lymphocyte and platelet BZ receptors that reverted to normal with treatment were reported.[16] Antidepressant potentiation of the $GABA_A$ modulatory effects of neurosteroids may contribute to their mechanism of action.[17] Abnormalities of GABA inhibition may lead to increased awareness or response to stress, as seen in PTSD.[18]

SEROTONIN MODEL

Although there is increasing evidence that the 5-HT system is altered in patients with anxiety disorders, definitive evidence that shows a clear abnormality in 5-HT function remains to be demonstrated. 5-HT is primarily an inhibitory neurotransmitter that is used by neurons originating in the raphe nuclei of the brain stem and projecting diffusely throughout the brain (e.g., cortex, amygdala, hippocampus, and limbic system). The diverse actions of 5-HT are regulated by at least 13 different receptor subtypes.[14] It is postulated that greater 5-HT activity reduces noradrenergic activity in the LC, inhibits defense/escape response via the periaqueductal gray region, and reduces hypothalamic release of corticotropin-releasing factor. The selective serotonin reuptake inhibitors (SSRIs) block the manifestations of panic.[14]

Low 5-HT activity may lead to a dysregulation of other neurotransmitters. NE and 5-HT systems are closely linked, and interactions between the two are reciprocal and vary. NE may act at presynaptic 5-HT terminals to decrease 5-HT release, and its activity at postsynaptic receptors can cause increased 5-HT release.[11] Stimulation of the postsynaptic 5-HT_2 receptors in the limbic system results in anxiety and avoidance behavior. Drugs with 5-HT_2 antagonist properties (e.g., trazodone, nefazodone, and mirtazapine) have potential anxiolytic effects.[17] Preliminary studies indicate that the 5-HT and $5HT_2$ antagonist *meta*-chlorphenylpiperazine (*m*-CPP) causes increased anxiety symptoms in GAD, SAD, and PTSD patients and panic attacks in some PTSD patients.[17,18]

Buspirone is a selective $5\text{-}HT_{1A}$ partial agonist that is effective for GAD but not for panic disorder. Because the selective $5\text{-}HT_{1A}$ partial agonists reduce serotonergic activity, GAD symptoms may reflect excessive 5-HT transmission or overactivity of the stimulatory 5-HT pathways. The role of 5-HT in panic disorder is unclear; however, 5-HT may play a role in the development of anticipatory anxiety.[13]

NEUROIMAGING STUDIES

Functional neuroimaging studies suggest that frontal and occipital brain areas are integral to the anxiety response. There is some evidence that patients with panic disorder have abnormal activation of the parahippocampal region and prefrontal cortex at rest. Panic anxiety is associated with activation of brain stem and basal ganglia (BG) areas.[13] In GAD patients, there is an abnormal increase in cortical activity and a decrease in BG activity. After BZ treatment, BG activity increases, and cortical activity is reduced.[13,16] Low striatal DA reuptake site density in positron-emission tomography (PET) studies in SAD patients suggest a dysfunction in the DA system.[12] Blood flow in the right dorsolateral prefrontal cortex and the left parietal cortex was increased in SAD but not in conditioned anxiety.[12] Neuroimaging studies have revealed decreased hippocampal volumes in patients with PTSD.[18]

CLINICAL PRESENTATION

The *Diagnostic and Statistical Manual of Mental Disorders*, Fourth Edition, Text Revision (DSM-IV-TR) classifies anxiety disorders into several categories[1] (Table 71–3). The characteristic features of these illnesses are anxiety and avoidance behavior. Obsessive-compulsive disorder is discussed in Chapter 72.

GENERALIZED ANXIETY DISORDER

The diagnostic criteria (Table 71–4) for GAD require persistent symptoms for at least 6 months.[1] The essential feature of GAD is unrealistic or excessive anxiety and worry about a number of events or activities.[1]

GAD has a gradual onset, usually in the early twenties, but may be precipitated in later life by severe psychological stressors. Most patients report onset of symptoms in childhood or adolescence. Stressful life events also may play a role in the persistence of symptoms. The course of the illness is chronic with multiple spontaneous exacerbations and remissions.[1,2] Patients report substantial interference with their lives and have a high probability of seeking treatment.[7] The majority of GAD patients eventually will develop another mental disorder.[2]

TABLE 71–3. DSM-IV-TR Classification of Anxiety Disorders

A. Generalized anxiety disorder
B. Panic disorder
  With agoraphobia
  Without agoraphobia
C. Agoraphobia without a history of panic disorder
D. Phobic disorders
  Social phobia (social anxiety disorder)
  Specific phobia
E. Obsessive-compulsive disorder
F. Posttraumatic stress disorder
G. Acute stress disorder

Compiled from Ref. 1. Reprinted with permission from the Diagnostic and Statistical Manual of Mental Disorders, Text Revision, Fourth Edition. Copyright 2000 American Psychiatric Association.

TABLE 71–4. DSM-IV-TR Diagnostic Criteria for Generalized Anxiety Disorder

A. Excessive anxiety and worry (apprehensive expectation), occurring more days than not for at least 6 months, about a number of events or activities (such as work or school performance).
B. The person finds it difficult to control worry.
C. Anxiety and worry, associated with three (or more) of the following six symptoms (with at least some symptoms present more days than not for the past 6 months):
  1. Restlessness or feeling keyed up or on edge
  2. Being easily fatigued
  3. Difficulty concentrating or mind going blank
  4. Irritability
  5. Muscle tension
  6. Sleep disturbance
D. Anxiety and worry, not confined to features of another psychiatric illness (e.g., having a panic attack, being embarrassed in public).
E. Constant worry causing significant distress, and significant impairment in social, occupational, or other important areas of functioning.
F. Excessive anxiety and worry, not caused by a drug substance (e.g., drugs of abuse or medications), or a general medical disorder, and not occurring exclusively as part of another psychiatric disorder (e.g., mood disorder).

Adapted and reprinted with permission from the Diagnostic and Statistical Manual of Mental Disorders, Text Revision, Fourth Edition. Copyright 2000 American Psychiatric Association.

PANIC DISORDER

Panic disorder begins as a series of unexpected (spontaneous) panic attacks involving an intense, terrifying fear similar to that caused by life-threatening danger. The unexpected panic attacks are followed by at least 1 month of persistent concern about having another panic attack, worry about the possible consequences of the panic attack, or a significant behavioral change related to the attacks.[1] During an attack, patients often describe an overwhelming sense of doom, a fear of dying or losing control, and numerous physical symptoms[1] (Table 71–5). Panic attacks usually last no more than 20 to 30 minutes,

TABLE 71–5. DSM-IV-TR Diagnostic Criteria for Panic Attack

A discrete period of intense fear or discomfort, in which at least four of the following symptoms developed abruptly and reached a peak within 10 minutes:

1. Palpitations or accelerated heart rate
2. Sweating
3. Trembling or shaking
4. Sensations of shortness of breath or smothering
5. Feeling of choking
6. Chest pain or discomfort
7. Nausea or abdominal distress
8. Feeling dizzy, unsteady, lightheaded, or faint
9. Derealization or depersonalization
10. Fear of losing control or going crazy
11. Fear of dying
12. Numbness or tingling sensations (paresthesias)
13. Chills or hot flushes

Adapted and reprinted with permission from the Diagnostic and Statistical Manual of Mental Disorders, Text Revision, Fourth Edition. Copyright 2000 American Psychiatric Association.

with the peak intensity of symptoms within the first 10 minutes. Often patients seek help at a physician's office or emergency department, only to have their symptoms resolve before or on arrival. Because panic symptoms mimic those present in several medical conditions, patients often are misdiagnosed, and multiple referrals are common.[1]

Secondary to the panic attacks, many patients eventually develop agoraphobia. Agoraphobia is anxiety about being in places or situations where escape might be difficult or where help might not be available in the event of a panic attack.[1] As a result, patients often avoid specific situations (e.g., crowded places, tunnels) where they fear a panic attack might occur.[1]

Panic disorder has an adverse impact on the patient's quality of life, including a significant degree of social and work impairment. Complications include depression (10% to 65% have major depressive disorder), alcohol abuse, and high use of health services and emergency rooms.[1] Patients with panic disorder have a high lifetime risk for suicide attempts compared with the general population.[19] The usual course is chronic but waxing and waning.

SOCIAL ANXIETY DISORDER

Symptoms in SAD persist for at least 6 months with the presence of significant distress or disability[1] (Table 71–6). SAD is characterized by an intense, irrational, and persistent fear of being negatively evaluated or scrutinized in a social or performance situation. Exposure to the feared social situation usually provokes an immediate situationally bound panic attack. The most common precipitating situations are speaking or eating in public, meeting new people, or writing in front of others. Blushing is the principal physical symptoms and distinguishes SAD from other anxiety disorders.[20] Other common physical symptoms include sweating, trembling, speech blocking, and difficulty using the toilet in public.[1]

TABLE 71–6. DSM-IV-TR Diagnostic Criteria for Social Anxiety Disorder

A. Marked, persistent fear of one or more social or performance situations in which the person is exposed to unfamiliar people or to possible scrutiny by others. The individual fears that he or she will act in a way (or show anxiety symptoms) that will be humiliating or embarrassing.
B. Exposure to the feared social situation provokes anxiety, which may take the form of a situationally bound or predisposed panic attack.
C. The person recognizes that the fear is excessive or unreasonable.
D. The feared social or performance situations are avoided or else are endured with intense anxiety or distress.
E. The avoidance, anxious anticipation, or distress in the feared social or performance situation(s) interferes significantly with the person's normal routine, occupational (academic) functioning or social activities or relationships, or there is marked distress about having the phobia.
F. In individuals under 18 years of age, the duration is at least six months.
G. Fear or avoidance is not caused by a drug substance (e.g., drugs of abuse or medication), or a general medical disorder, and not occurring exclusively as part of another psychiatric disorder (e.g., panic disorder).

Adapted and reprinted with permission from the Diagnostic and Statistical Manual of Mental Disorders, Text Revision, Fourth Edition. Copyright 2000 American Psychiatric Association.

SAD is subclassified into two types. In the generalized type, the individual fears social situations where embarrassment may occur. In the discrete subtype, fear is limited to one or two situations (i.e., performing, public speaking).[1] The mean age of onset of SAD is during the midteens.[1] SAD is chronic, and the severity of impairment fluctuates. The distinction between SAD and panic disorder is the rationale behind fear: Fear of anxiety symptoms is characteristic of panic disorder, whereas fear of embarrassment from social interaction typifies SAD.[1] The majority of SAD patients have a comorbid depressive, anxiety, or substance-abuse disorder.[20]

POSTTRAUMATIC STRESS DISORDER

Exposure to a traumatic event is required for a diagnosis of PTSD[1] (Table 71–7). The patient's response to trauma must include intense

TABLE 71–7. DSM-IV-TR Diagnostic Criteria for Posttraumatic Stress Disorder

A. Exposure to a traumatic event in which both of the following were present:
   1. The person experienced, witnessed or was confronted with an event(s) that involved actual or threatened death or serious injury, or a threat to the physical integrity of self or others.
   2. The person's response involved intense fear, helplessness, or horror.
B. The traumatic event is persistently reexperienced in one (or more) of the following ways:
   1. Recurrent and intrusive distressing recollections of the event (e.g., images, thoughts, or perceptions)
   2. Recurrent distressing dreams of the event
   3. Acting or feeling as if the traumatic event were recurring (e.g., a sense of reliving the experience, illusions, hallucinations, dissociative flashbacks)
   4. Physiologic reactivity on exposure to internal/external cues that symbolize an aspect of the traumatic event
C. Persistent avoidance of stimuli associated with the trauma and numbing of general responsiveness as indicated by at least three of the following:
   1. Efforts to avoid thoughts, feelings, or conversations associated with the trauma
   2. Efforts to avoid activities, places, or people that arouse recollections of the trauma
   3. Inability to recall an important aspect of the trauma
   4. Diminished interest or participation in significant activities
   5. Feeling of detachment or estrangement from others
   6. Restricted range of affect
   7. Sense of a foreshortened future (e.g., does not expect to have a career, marriage)
D. Persistent symptoms of increased arousal, as indicated by at least two of the following:
   1. Difficulty falling or staying asleep
   2. Irritability or outbursts of anger
   3. Difficulty concentrating
   4. Hypervigilance
   5. Exaggerated startle response
E. Duration of the disturbance (symptoms in criteria B, C, and D) is more than one month.
F. The disturbance causes clinically significant distress or impairment in social, occupational, or other important areas of functioning.

Adapted and reprinted with permission from the Diagnostic and Statistical Manual of Mental Disorders, Text Revision, Fourth Edition. Copyright 2000 American Psychiatric Association.

fear, helplessness, or horror. The resulting symptoms include persistent reexperiencing of the traumatic event, avoidance of stimuli associated with the trauma and numbing of general responsiveness, and persistent symptoms of hyperarousal. Symptoms from each category need to be present for greater than 1 month and cause significant distress or impairment. Most persons diagnosed with PTSD meet criteria for another mental disorder.[1] PTSD is a chronic, recurring condition highly associated with suicidal behavior.[20] Anxiety symptoms emerging within 1 month after exposure to a traumatic stressor are classified as acute stress disorder (ASD). Symptoms of ASD are experienced during or immediately after the trauma, last for at least 2 weeks, and resolve within 4 weeks.[1]

SPECIFIC PHOBIA

Specific phobia is marked and persistent fear of a circumscribed object or situation (e.g., storms, blood, bridges). Apart from contact with the feared object or situation, the patient is usually free of symptoms. Most persons simply avoid the feared object and adjust to certain restrictions on their activities.[1]

▶ TREATMENT: Generalized Anxiety Disorder

DESIRED OUTCOME

The goals of therapy in the acute management of GAD are to reduce the severity, duration, and frequency of the anxiety symptoms and to improve the patient's overall functioning. Long-term goals include prevention of anxiety symptoms and improved quality of life (QOL).

Once GAD is diagnosed, a patient-oriented treatment plan, which usually consists of both psychotherapy and drug therapy, is developed. The treatment plan depends on the patient's degree of emotional distress, age, medication history, medical status, and the potential outcomes of pharmacologic treatment. Clinical drug trials in outpatients with GAD indicate a high placebo response rate (50% to 60%), which suggests that some patients have a mild syndrome that may respond to psychotherapy alone.[5] Psychotherapy is the least invasive and safest treatment modality.[7] For patients experiencing anxiety symptoms severe enough to produce functional disability or discomfort, antianxiety medication is indicated.

NONPHARMACOLOGIC THERAPY

Nonpharmacologic treatment modalities in GAD include short-term counseling, stress management, psychotherapy, meditation, or exercise. Anxious patients should be instructed to avoid caffeine, nonprescription stimulants, and diet pills. Most GAD patients require psychological therapy, alone or in combination with antianxiety medication, to overcome fears and learn to improve coping abilities.[7] Consideration of the patient's clinical symptoms, personality, and life problems aids in the choice of psychological therapy. Cognitive therapy is the most effective psychological therapy in GAD patients. Supportive psychotherapy provides explanations and encouragement and allows formulation of strategies to manage anxiety-provoking situations effectively.

PHARMACOLOGIC THERAPY

The BZs are the most effective and safe medications for the amelioration of acute anxiety symptoms. All BZs are equally effective anxiolytics, and consideration of pharmacokinetic properties and the patient's clinical situation will assist in the selection of the most appropriate agent. Pharmacokinetic differences vary, and the clinician must monitor the patient's response to the initial treatment regimen. Because of the lack of dependency, antidepressants have emerged as the treatment of choice for the long-term management of anxiety. Buspirone, autonomic blocking agents, and hydroxyzine are additional anxiolytic options (Table 71–8). Because of the high risk of adverse effects and toxicity, barbiturates, antipsychotics, antipsychotic-antidepressant combinations, and antihistamines generally are not indicated in the treatment of GAD.[7] The BZs are more effective in treating the somatic/autonomic symptoms of GAD as opposed to the psychic symptoms (i.e., apprehension, worry), which are reduced by antidepressants.[17] Algorithms for the diagnosis, initial treatment with psychotherapy, and pharmacotherapy of GAD were published by Thompson.[22] Two other published algorithms discuss an approach for anxiety in primary care and management of anxiety disorders in patients with chemical dependency.[23,24] An algorithm for the pharmacologic management of GAD is shown in Figure 71–1.

TABLE 71–8. Nonbenzodiazepine Antianxiety Agents

Class/Generic Name	Brand Name	Manufacturer	Dosage Range (mg/day)[a]
Antidepressants			
Imipramine[b]	Tofranil	Novartis	50–200
Paroxetine	Paxil	GlaxoSmithKline	20–50
Trazodone[b]	Desyrel	Apothecon	200–400
Venlafaxine[c]	Effexor XR	Wyeth-Ayerst	75–225
Azapirones			
Buspirone[b,c]	BuSpar	Bristol-Myers Squibb	15–60[d]
Diphenylmethane			
Hydroxyzine[b,c]	Vistaril, Atarax	Pfizer, Roerig	200–400
β-Blockers			
Propranolol[b]	Inderal	Wyeth-Ayerst	80–160

[a]Elderly patients are usually treated with approximately one half of the dose listed.
[b]Available generically.
[c]FDA approved for anxiety.
[d]The dosage range in elderly patients appears to be the same but is not established.

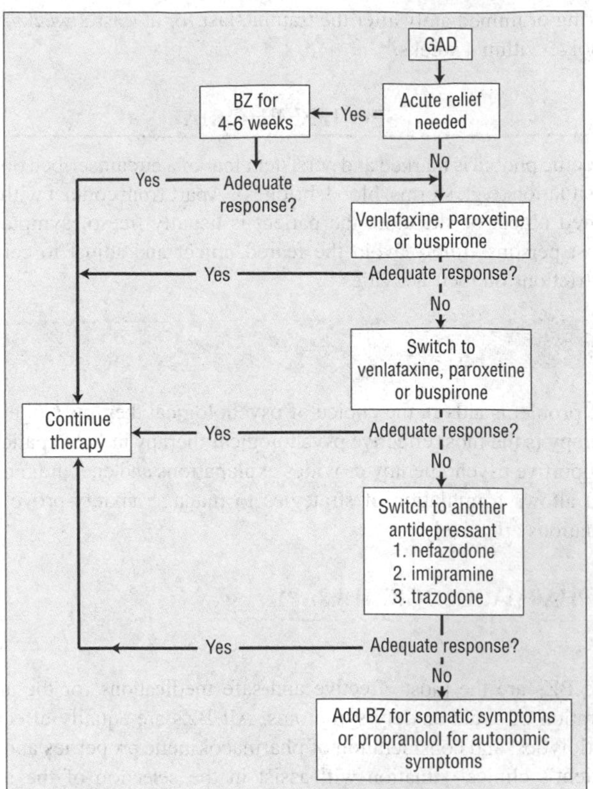

FIGURE 71–1. Algorithm for the management of generalized anxiety disorder. *(Adapted from Refs. 7 and 22.)*

BENZODIAZEPINE THERAPY

The BZs are the most frequently used drugs for treating GAD. Although all BZs possess anxiolytic properties, only 8 of the 15 currently marketed agents have Food and Drug Administration (FDA) approval for the treatment of GAD (Table 71–9). Estazolam, flurazepam, temazepam, quazepam, and triazolam are marketed as sedative-hypnotic agents. Clonazepam is marketed as an antipanic agent and anticonvulsant,[26] and midazolam is labeled for preoperative sedation. Alprazolam is indicated for the treatment of panic disorder with or without agoraphobia, as well as GAD.

Mechanism of Action

The BZ receptor model of anxiety (described in the pathophysiology section earlier) theorizes that BZs ameliorate anxiety through potentiation of the inhibitory activity of GABA.[11] The GABA–BZ receptor complex is composed of protein subunits arranged in a pentamer with a chloride ion channel in the center. BZs bind between the α_1 and γ subunits, whereas GABA binds between the α and β subunits.[15] When the BZ receptor is activated in the presence of GABA, the frequency of the chloride ion channels opening and the influx of chloride ions into the neuronal cell are increased. The resulting negatively charged hyperpolarized membrane prevents further depolarization by excitatory neurotransmitters. Other neurotransmitters (e.g., 5-HT, NE, DA) may be involved in BZ activity.

Pharmacokinetics

A wide difference in milligram potency exists between the BZ compounds; however, when dosage adjustments are made, all agents share similar anxiolytic and sedative-hypnotic activity.[27] Variations in lipid solubility between compounds may influence BZ pharmacokinetic properties. Differences in BZ pharmacokinetic and pharmacodynamic properties can assist the clinician in choosing an appropriate anxiolytic (Table 71–10). After a single dose, the onset, intensity, and duration of pharmacologic effects are important factors to consider when using BZs for the short-term, intermittent, or as-needed treatment of anxiety.

The primary determinant of a drug's onset of effect after a single oral dose is the rate of drug absorption. Because of high lipophilicity, diazepam and clorazepate are absorbed rapidly and distributed quickly into the CNS. Therefore, the onset of anxiolytic effect occurs within 30 to 60 minutes, which results in a rapid and intense relief of anxiety. High lipophilicity increases the extent of drug redistribution into the periphery, particularly adipose tissue, resulting in a shorter duration of effect after a single dose than indicated by single-dose elimination half-life studies.[28] Clinically, patients perceive a rapid onset of action, but some may experience an unpleasant feeling of drowsiness or loss of control. This "rush" may be euphoric and may contribute to an individual BZ's abuse potential. Chlordiazepoxide's onset of action is much slower because of decreased lipophilicity, slower absorption, and delayed passage into the CNS.

TABLE 71–9. Benzodiazepine Antianxiety Agents

Generic Name	Brand Name	Manufacturer	Approved Dosage Range (mg/day)[a]	Approximate Equivalent Dose (mg)
Alprazolam[b]	Xanax	Pharmacia & Upjohn	0.75–4 1.5–10[c]	0.5
Chlordiazepoxide[b]	Librium	ICN Pharmaceuticals	25–100	25
Clonazepam[b]	Klonopin	Roche	1–4[c]	0.25
Clorazepate[b]	Tranxene	Abbott	7.5–60	7.5
Diazepam[b]	Valium	Roche	2–40	5
Halazepam	Paxipam	Schering	20–160	20
Lorazepam[b]	Ativan	Wyeth-Ayerst	0.5–10	0.75–1
Oxazepam[b]	Serax	Faulding Pharmaceuticals	30–120	15

[a]Elderly patients are usually treated with approximately one-half of the dose listed.
[b]Available generically.
[c]Panic disorder dose.
Equivalent doses from Ref. 25.

TABLE 71–10. Pharmacokinetics of Benzodiazepine Antianxiety Agents

Generic Name	Time to Peak Plasma Level (h)	Elimination Half-Life, Parent (h)	Metabolic Pathway	Clinically Significant Metabolites	Protein Binding (%)
Alprazolam	1–2	12–15	Oxidation	—	80
Chlordiazepoxide	1–4	5–30	*N*-Dealkylation Oxidation	Desmethylchlordiazepoxide Demoxepam DMDZ[a]	96
Clonazepam	1–4	30–40	Nitroreduction	—	85
Clorazepate	1–2	Prodrug	Oxidation	DMDZ	97
Diazepam	0.5–2	20–80	Oxidation	DMDZ Oxazepam	98
Halazepam	1–3	14	Oxidation	DMDZ	97
Lorazepam	2–4	10–20	Conjugation	—	85
Oxazepam	2–4	5–20	Conjugation	—	97

[a]Desmethyldiazepam half-life 50–100 h.
Compiled from Ref. 28.

Compared with diazepam, lorazepam and oxazepam are relatively less lipophilic and have a slower onset of effect. These BZs have smaller volumes of distribution and a resulting longer duration of action.[28] Oxazepam absorption is slow, and peak levels are not obtained until 2 to 4 hours after a single dose; however, like lorazepam, oxazepam's anxiolytic effects are long lasting because extensive distribution does not occur.

Parenteral administration through the intramuscular route should be avoided with diazepam and chlordiazepoxide secondary to variability in the rate and extent of drug absorption. Intramuscular lorazepam provides rapid, reliable, and complete absorption; however, the preparation requires refrigeration.

After multiple dosing, the rate and extent of drug accumulation are functions of the drug's elimination half-life in relation to dosing intervals, clearance, and formation of active metabolites. Differences in clinical effects that occur during and after repeated dosages with the BZs are related in part to variability in metabolism and metabolite accumulation.[28]

The BZs undergo two primary metabolic processes, hepatic oxidation (catalyzed by cytochrome P450 3A4) and glucuronide conjugation. With the exception of lorazepam and oxazepam (which are conjugated only) and clonazepam (which undergoes nitroreduction), all BZs are oxidized first and then conjugated and excreted renally.[28,29] Diazepam's metabolism is also catalyzed by cytochrome P450 2C19.[29] Oxidation may be impaired in patients with liver disease, in the elderly, and in those who simultaneously use drugs that inhibit oxidation. Impaired oxidation results in higher levels of the parent drug and/or an active metabolite.

Many BZs are converted to desmethyldiazepam (DMDZ), an active metabolite with a long elimination half-life of about 100 hours[28] (see Table 71–10). DMDZ is further oxidized to oxazepam and then conjugated and excreted. After multiple dosing, accumulation of DMDZ is slow and extensive, providing a long-lasting antianxiety effect. If oxidation of DMDZ is impaired, the half-life is prolonged, and complications of drug accumulation (e.g., drowsiness) may result over time with repeated dosing.[30]

Clorazepate is a prodrug and possesses no anxiolytic effects until metabolism to DMDZ. Before absorption, clorazepate is metabolized rapidly in the stomach through a pH-dependent process under acidic conditions.

BZs with shorter half-lives (e.g., alprazolam, lorazepam, and oxazepam) reach steady-state plasma concentrations rapidly, and drug accumulation after repeated dosing is minimal. Oxazepam and lorazepam are not converted into active metabolites.[30]

BZ protein binding is extensive, especially for the long-elimination-half-life drugs. After a single dose of a long-elimination-half-life BZ, the expected duration of clinical activity may not parallel the drug's pharmacokinetic half-life because of drug redistribution.[28] After multiple dosing, drugs with long elimination half-lives and active metabolites may require 1 to 2 weeks to reach steady state.

Special Populations

In the elderly, secondary to a decreased capacity for oxidation and alterations in the volume of distribution, drug accumulation may result.[30] Patients with hepatic disease also are at risk for drug accumulation and subsequent complications. Therefore, intermediate- or short-acting BZs are preferred for chronic use in the elderly and those with liver disorders because of minimal accumulation and achievement of steady state within 1 to 3 days. BZs with long elimination half-lives may be dosed once a day at bedtime and may provide both hypnotic and daytime anxiolytic activity. Agents with shorter elimination half-lives should be administered in divided daily doses.

Adverse Events

The most common adverse events associated with BZ therapy involve CNS depression. This is manifested clinically as drowsiness, sedation, psychomotor impairment, and ataxia.[31] A transient mild drowsiness is experienced commonly by patients during the first few days of treatment; however, tolerance often develops. Disorientation, depression, confusion, irritability, aggression, and excitement have been reported.[31]

Impairment of memory and recall also may occur during BZ treatment. The memory loss induced by the BZs typically is limited to events occurring after drug ingestion (anterograde amnesia).[31] The anterograde amnesia is secondary to disordered consolidation processes that store information and is not impairment in the perception or retrieval of information.[32] BZs with high affinity for binding to the BZ receptor (e.g., lorazepam) appear to possess a higher potential for amnesia.

Abuse, Dependence, Withdrawal, and Tolerance

Two serious complications of BZ therapy are the potential for abuse and development of physical dependence. BZ abuse is rare in the general population of users; however, individuals with a history of multiple drug abuse (e.g., alcohol, sedatives) are at the greatest risk for becoming BZ abusers.[33]

Because of the chronicity of illness, persons with GAD and panic disorder are at high risk of developing BZ dependence.[33] BZ dependence is a physiologic phenomenon demonstrated by the appearance of a predictable abstinence syndrome (withdrawal symptoms) on abrupt discontinuation of therapy. Withdrawal symptoms may result because of the sudden dissociation of a BZ from its receptor site. After abrupt BZ discontinuation, an acute decrease in GABA neurotransmission results, producing a less inhibited CNS.[34]

Benzodiazepine Discontinuation

After BZ therapy is discontinued suddenly, several events can occur. Rebound symptoms represent an immediate but transient return of original symptoms having an increased intensity compared with baseline. Recurrence or relapse is the return of original symptoms with similar intensity as before treatment. About 25% of patients relapse within 4 weeks of BZ discontinuation, and 60% to 80% relapse within a year.[7] Withdrawal symptoms are the emergence of new symptoms and a worsening of preexisting symptoms after BZ discontinuation. Withdrawal symptoms may persist for days to weeks and resolve gradually over months.

Common symptoms of BZ withdrawal include anxiety, insomnia, restlessness, agitation, muscle tension, and irritability. Less frequently occurring symptoms are nausea, malaise, coryza, blurred vision, diaphoresis, nightmares, depression, hyperreflexia, and ataxia. Tinnitus, confusion, paranoid delusions, hallucinations, seizures, and psychosis occur rarely.[33] Seizures may occur with both therapeutic and high doses of short-elimination-half-life BZs, usually within 3 days of drug discontinuation. They may occur approximately 1 week after discontinuation of long-elimination-half-life agents. High BZ doses, a long duration of therapy, and concurrent ingestion of drugs that lower the seizure threshold are risk factors for withdrawal seizures.

The onset of withdrawal symptoms in patients ingesting BZs with short elimination half-lives occurs much earlier (within 24 to 48 hours) than in those taking BZs with long elimination half-lives (within 3 to 8 days).[33] Other factors associated with an increased incidence or severity of BZ withdrawal include high doses and long-term BZ therapy. Abrupt discontinuation of short-elimination-half-life BZs may produce a more severe withdrawal[34] than long-elimination-half-life agents.

Factors that increase the likelihood of BZ dependence include therapeutic doses for up to 3 to 6 weeks or for extended periods of time. Rebound symptoms are more intense after the ingestion of short-elimination-half-life BZs than long-elimination-half-life BZs. In patients who ingest BZs for more than 3 months, withdrawal symptoms are more likely and more severe; patients who experience withdrawal at this time usually do not wish to stop therapy.[33]

Several strategies to minimize the severity of BZ withdrawal include a 25% per week reduction in dosage until 50% of the dose is reached and then dosage reduction by one-eighth every 4 to 7 days. If BZ therapy exceeds 6 weeks, a slow dosage taper over several weeks is recommended. Tapering will not eliminate the emergence of withdrawal symptoms entirely but will prevent severe withdrawal. Slow drug taper is extremely important for the short-elimination-half-life drugs because some individuals have greater difficulty with discontinuation. Results of studies performed to evaluate the use of adjunctive carbamazepine, clonidine, and propranolol to attenuate BZ withdrawal were inconclusive.[34] Imipramine and valproate improved BZ taper success rates.[34] If patients experience difficulties, especially with the short-elimination-half-life agents, then substitution of a long-elimination-half-life BZ should be considered. Diazepam can be initiated as a loading dose (40% of daily consumption), followed by daily tapering of 10%. Clonazepam is an alternative agent. Phenobarbital could be used especially if the patient has mixed BZ and alcohol dependence.[33]

Although tolerance develops to the sedative, muscle relaxant, and anticonvulsant activities, the BZs do not appear to lose anxiolytic or antipanic efficacy.[7] The anxiolytic efficacy of BZs in long-term clinical trials (greater than 6 to 8 months of chronic use) has not been reported[17]; however, it is clear that some patients derive beneficial anxiolytic effects from chronic BZ ingestion.

Drug Interactions

Drug interactions with the BZs generally fall into two categories—pharmacodynamic and pharmacokinetic[29] (Table 71–11). Simultaneous use of alcohol and a BZ results in additive CNS depressant effects and lowers the therapeutic index of the BZ. In addition, concurrent use of a BZ and drugs with CNS depressant properties (e.g., narcotic agonists, antipsychotics, antihistamines) may potentiate the adverse sedative effects. When ingested alone in an overdose attempt, BZs are rarely life-threatening; however, the combination of BZs with alcohol or other CNS depressant agents is potentially fatal. SSRIs can inhibit BZ metabolism through inhibition of cytochrome P450 3A4 and 1A2 enzymes.[29] Nefazodone and fluvoxamine increased alprazolam concentrations; thus the alprazolam dose should be reduced by 50% when these agents are added.[29]

TABLE 71–11. Pharmacokinetic Drug Interactions with the Benzodiazepines

Drug	Effect
Alcohol (chronic)	Increased Cl of BZs
Carbamazepine	Decreased Cl of alprazolam
Cimetidine	Decreased Cl of alprazolam, diazepam, chlordiazepoxide, and clorazepate and increased $t_{1/2}$
Fluoxetine	Decreased Cl of alprazolam and diazepam
Fluvoxamine	Decreased Cl of alprazolam and prolonged $t_{1/2}$
Itraconazole	Potentially decreased Cl of alprazolam and diazepam
Ketaconazole	Potentially decreased Cl of alprazolam
Nefazodone	Decreased Cl of alprazolam, AUC doubled, and $t_{1/2}$ prolonged
Omeprazole	Decreased Cl of diazepam
Oral contraceptives	Increased free concentration of chlordiazepoxide and slightly decreased Cl; decreased Cl and increased $t_{1/2}$ of diazepam and alprazolam
Paroxetine	Decreased Cl of alprazolam
Phenobarbital	Increased Cl of clonazepam and reduced $t_{1/2}$
Phenytoin	Increased Cl of clonazepam and reduced $t_{1/2}$
Probenecid	Decreased Cl of lorazepam and prolonged $t_{1/2}$
Propranolol	Decreased Cl of diazepam and prolonged $t_{1/2}$
Rifampin	Increased metabolism of diazepam
Theophylline	Decreased alprazolam concentrations
Valproate	Decreased Cl of lorazepam

Key: AUC = area under the plasma concentration curve; Cl = clearance; $t_{1/2}$ = elimination half-life.
Compiled from Ref. 29.

Dosing and Administration

BZ dosage requirements vary widely among patients and must be individualized. Therapy should be initiated using low doses (e.g., diazepam 2 mg three times daily or its equivalent) and titrated upward to relieve anxiety symptoms and avoid adverse events. After an initial treatment response is achieved, agents with long elimination half-lives may be dosed at bedtime. Dosage adjustments should be made weekly. Three to 4 weeks of a daily dose of diazepam 40 mg (or its equivalent) constitutes an adequate clinical trial.[17]

The duration of BZ therapy should be monitored and generally should not exceed 4 to 6 months.[22] Intermittent therapy (3 to 4 weeks) is indicated in patients with recurring symptoms. Patients treated with BZs for less than 6 months have a higher relapse rate than those treated for more than 6 months[7]; thus a maintenance treatment of 6 months can benefit patients prone to relapse.[35] Individuals with persistent symptoms may require continuous treatment, but the risk of dependence must be weighed against the potential benefits.[5,36]

The elderly anxious patient requires additional monitoring when a BZ is prescribed. These patients have an enhanced sensitivity to BZs (both to therapeutic and CNS depressant effects) that may be related to pharmacokinetic alterations (e.g., decreased clearance).[30] The elderly are particularly susceptible to falls, sedation, impaired daytime functioning, and memory problems, which also may be enhanced by other drugs with CNS depressant effects. Thus dosages should be low and short-elimination-half-life agents prescribed.[30]

Patient education should include the anticipated length of drug therapy, potential side effects, and consequences of the ingestion of alcohol and other CNS depressants. Patients should understand that medications provide symptomatic relief but do not solve underlying psychological problems. Patients should be instructed not to decrease or discontinue BZ usage without contacting their physician.

BUSPIRONE THERAPY

Buspirone is a non-BZ anxiolytic that lacks anticonvulsant, muscle relaxant, hypnotic, motor impairment, and dependence properties. For the treatment of GAD with or without depressive symptoms, clinical trials found buspirone superior to placebo and as efficacious as BZs after 4 weeks.[37]

Mechanism of Action

Buspirone's anxiolytic mechanism of action is unknown; however, it does not interact with the GABA-BZ receptor complex or decrease noradrenergic neuron firing in the LC (it increases firing). Buspirone possesses activity as a 5-HT_{1A} partial agonist, binding to both pre- and postsynaptic receptors to increase 5-HT. Buspirone also increases DA concentrations through both dopamine agonist and DA_2 antagonist properties.[38]

Pharmacokinetics

After an oral dose, buspirone is absorbed rapidly and completely and undergoes extensive first-pass metabolism. Buspirone is 95% protein-bound. The mean elimination half-life is 2.5 hours. Buspirone is eliminated primarily by oxidative metabolism and is converted into both active and inactive metabolites.[39]

Adverse Events

A major advantage of buspirone is its lack of sedative properties. Adverse events include dizziness, nausea, headaches, nervousness, and dysphoria (especially with large single doses of 20 to 40 mg).[39]

Drug Interactions

Verapamil, diltiazem, itraconazole, and erythromycin increase buspirone levels. Rifampin caused a 10-fold reduction in buspirone levels. Buspirone reportedly increases cyclosporine and haloperidol levels and elevates blood pressure in patients taking a monoamine oxidase inhibitor (MAOI).[39]

Dosing and Administration

The recommended initial dose of buspirone is 7.5 mg two times daily with dosage increments of 5 mg/day every 2 to 3 days as needed.[39] The usual therapeutic dose of buspirone is 20 to 30 mg/day, with a maximum dose of 60 mg/day.[39] The onset of anxiolysis is not immediate, requiring a week or more before clinical effects occur; maximum therapeutic benefit may not be evident for 4 to 6 weeks.[39]

Buspirone is an agent of choice in the management of chronic, persistent anxiety.[40] It has minimal sedating properties and is not useful in clinical situations requiring immediate anxiolytic effects or for situations requiring as-needed anxiolytic therapy. Therefore, buspirone is an alternative for GAD patients who are unable to tolerate the sedative effects and psychomotor impairment of BZs, especially the elderly. Buspirone is not cross-tolerant with BZs and thus will not prevent or treat symptoms of BZ withdrawal.[40] When a patient is switched from a BZ to buspirone, the BZ should be tapered slowly before the buspirone is initiated. However, some clinicians advocate pretreatment with buspirone 20–40 mg/day for 2 to 4 weeks before initiating the BZ taper.[40]

Previous BZ therapy may lead to certain expectations of anxiolytic drug effects (immediate response and sedation) that buspirone does not demonstrate.[40] Therefore, patients who have received BZs should be advised of these differences at the outset of therapy. Buspirone is an appropriate choice for anxious patients with a history of alcohol or drug abuse because of its low potential for abuse.[24]

ADRENERGIC BLOCKING AGENTS

Propranolol and other β-blocking agents may be useful in patients with prominent cardiovascular symptoms of anxiety (e.g., palpitations or tremors). β-Blocking drugs are less effective anxiolytics than BZs,[41] and their usefulness may be restricted to anxiety patients whose physical symptoms, especially cardiovascular complaints, have not responded adequately to BZ therapy.

Although propranolol has a short elimination half-life (2 to 6 hours), β-blockade usually lasts for 8 to 12 hours after a single dose.[41] Propranolol 10 mg twice a day should be used initially and titrated gradually to anxiolytic response. Response is usually observed within 1 week of therapy. Emergence of adverse events (e.g., depression, fatigue) may limit the clinical usefulness of propranolol. On discontinuation, the dosage should be tapered to avoid rebound anxiety and cardiovascular effects.

ANTIDEPRESSANTS

Because of their adverse-events profile, antidepressants are considered first-line agents in the long-term management of GAD. The antianxiety response is delayed by 2 to 4 weeks. Venlafaxine extended release and paroxetine are FDA-approved antidepressants for GAD. Other agents include imipramine, nefazodone and paroxetine (see Table 71–8). The use of tricyclic antidepressants (TCAs) is limited by troublesome adverse events (e.g., sedation, orthostatic hypotension, anticholinergic effects, weight gain, and toxicity in overdose).[42]

Venlafaxine extended release alleviates anxiety in patients with and without comorbid depression. The reduction in psychic symptoms of anxiety and tension is not accompanied by significant reductions in somatic symptoms. Venlafaxine (dosed once daily) was effective at doses of 150 and 225 mg for 2 months in patients with GAD and conferred efficacy for 6 months.[43,44] The most common adverse events of venlafaxine were nausea, somnolence, and dry mouth.

Paroxetine was signicantly more effective than placebo at achieving response or remission after 2 months.[45] Nefazodone was effective in most patients in an open trial.[46] Antidepressants are alternatives for individuals with contraindications to BZ use or those with concomitant depressive symptoms.[40]

OTHER AGENTS

Studies have documented the efficacy of hydroxyzine (fixed dose of 50 mg/day), and case reports suggest that gabapentin may be effective.[46,47] Although the herbal preparation *Kava kava* was more effective than placebo for anxiety, many patients experience CNS effects (e.g., tremors, drowsiness, restlessness, headaches) and abdominal discomfort.[48]

PHARMACOECONOMIC CONSIDERATIONS

It is estimated that anxiety disorders account for 31.5% of the total costs of mental illness in the United States.[49] The social costs of anxiety disorders are reflected in increased rates of financial assistance, health care use, and substance abuse.[50] Physical disability was reported by 53% and occupational role disability was reported by 26% of GAD outpatients. The mean number of work days missed secondary to disability in the past month was 4.4 days.[51] These figures increase when GAD is comorbid with one or more other psychiatric disorders. GAD patients tend to use family practitioners and gastroenterologists more frequently than healthy controls.[52] Pharmacoeconomic analyses in the management of GAD have not been conducted.

EVALUATION OF THERAPEUTIC OUTCOMES

The goals of treatment and duration of therapy should be discussed with the patient at the beginning of therapy. Initially, anxious patients should be monitored twice weekly for a reduction in the frequency, duration, and severity of anxiety symptoms and improvement in occupational, social, and interpersonal functioning. The pharmacist should assess the patient for response to treatment by asking about the target symptoms of anxiety and emergence of adverse events. After achieving an optimal drug dosage, the patient can be evaluated monthly until drug discontinuation. Use of an objective measurement of anxiety symptoms (e.g., the Visual Analog Scale to rate the severity, frequency, and duration of symptoms) can assist in the evaluation of drug response.

▶ TREATMENT: Panic Disorder

DESIRED OUTCOME

Goals of therapy in panic disorder include a complete resolution of panic attacks, marked reduction in anticipatory anxiety and phobic avoidance, and maintenance of a clinical response that allows the patient to resume normal activities.[53] Despite treatment, only 49% of patients with panic disorder achieve full remission.[54]

Therapeutic options include a single pharmacologic agent, concurrent psychotherapy, or psychotherapy followed by pharmacotherapy. Most patients without situational avoidance will improve with pharmacotherapy alone; however, if avoidance is present, cognitive-behavioral therapy (CBT) typically is initiated concurrently. With all effective drug therapies, resolution of phobic avoidance tends to occur slowly, and many patients require concomitant CBT.

In the most comprehensive study to date, both imipramine and CBT alone were found to be equivalent in acute therapy for 3 months and during 6 months of maintenance therapy. Combined imipramine and CBT therapy was significantly better than CBT or imipramine alone for acute and maintenance therapy. At 6 months after discontinuation, only CBT alone maintained improvement (4% relapse) compared with a 25% relapse rate in patients treated with imipramine.[55]

NONPHARMACOLOGIC THERAPY

Patients should be educated to avoid substances that may precipitate panic attacks, including caffeine, drugs of abuse, and nonprescription stimulants.[1,56] CBT focuses on the correction of a patient's maladaptive thoughts and behaviors that initiate, perpetuate, or exacerbate panic symptoms.[56] Through CBT, the patient learns to decrease the fear and avoidance of internal and external signals associated with panic attacks. The cognitive restructuring and in vivo exposure (to feared stimuli) components of CBT target panic attacks and phobic-avoidance behavior.[56]

For patients who cannot or will not take medication, CBT alone is certainly indicated. CBT is associated with short-term improvement in 80% to 90% of patients and 6-month improvement in 75% of patients.[56] Combined fluvoxamine and exposure was superior to exposure alone in reducing phobic avoidance, and efficacy was maintained for 2 years.[57]

TABLE 71–12. Drugs Used in the Treatment of Panic Disorder

Class/Generic Name	Brand Name	Manufacturer	Starting Dose	Antipanic Dosage[a] Range (mg)
Serotonin reuptake inhibitors				
Citalopram	Celexa	Forest Labs	10 mg qd	20–60
Fluoxetine[b]	Prozac	Lilly	2.5–5 mg qd	20–40
Fluvoxamine[b]	Luvox	Solvay	25 mg qd	150–300
Paroxetine	Paxil	GlaxoSmithKline	10 mg qd	10–60[c]
Sertraline	Zoloft	Pfizer	12.5–25 mg qd	25–200[c]
Benzodiazepines				
Alprazolam[b]	Xanax	Pharmacia & Upjohn	0.25–0.5 mg tid	4–10[c]
Clonazepam[b]	Klonopin	Roche	0.25 mg tid	3–6[c]
Diazepam[b]	Valium	Roche	2–5 mg tid	30–40
Lorazepam[b]	Ativan	Wyeth-Ayerst	0.5–1 mg tid	3–4
Tricyclic antidepressants				
Clomipramine[b]	Anafranil	Tyco Healthcare	25 mg bid	75–200
Desipramine[b]	Norpramin	Aventis Pharmaceuticals	10–25 mg qd	150–300
Imipramine[b]	Tofranil	Tyco Healthcare	10–25 mg qd	150–300
Monoamine oxidase inhibitor				
Phenelzine	Nardil	Parke-Davis	15 mg bid	45–90

[a]Dosage used in clinical trials but not FDA-approved.
[b]Available generically.
[c]Dosage is FDA approved.

PHARMACOLOGIC THERAPY

Panic disorder is treated effectively with several drugs including the TCA imipramine, the BZs alprazolam and clonazepam, the MAOI phenelzine, and SSRIs[7,56] (Table 71–12). Alprazolam, clonazepam, sertraline, and paroxetine are approved for this indication. SSRIs are the first-line agents because of their improved tolerability[56,58]; however, these agents are expensive. In a meta-analysis of the pharmacotherapy of panic disorder, SSRIs and clomipramine had significantly greater effect sizes and improvement ratios than imipramine and alprazolam.[59] The American Psychiatric Association published a practice guideline for the treatment of panic disorder.[60] An algorithm for the pharmacologic therapy of panic disorder appears in Figure 71–2.

Except in instances in which rapid response is required (i.e., loss of a job), BZs are second-line agents. Because of the risk of dependency, BZs should be used only after several trials of antidepressants have failed.[60] Because of the emergence of depressive symptoms during BZ treatment, they should not be used as monotherapy in a patient who is clinically depressed or has a history of depression. In patients whose illness is complicated by a history of alcohol or drug abuse, BZs use should be avoided.[7,24] BZs often are used concomitantly (for 1 to 3 weeks) with antidepressants or CBT to stabilize initial symptoms to offset the delay in onset of effect of these treatments.[7,9,60]

ANTIDEPRESSANT THERAPY

Tricyclic Antidepressants

Imipramine is the most studied TCA, alleviating panic attacks in 75% of patients with panic disorder. Imipramine effectively blocks panic attacks within 3 to 5 weeks; however, maximal improvement (including antiphobic response) does not occur until 8 to 10 weeks.[60] The sequence of patient response is an initial decrease in the number of panic attacks, then diminution of anticipatory anxiety, followed by a reduction in phobic avoidance. Up to 40% of patients experience stimulant-like side effects, including anxiety, insomnia, jitteriness, and irritability.[56,60] These side effects often affect patient compliance significantly, prevent medication dosage increases, and interfere with the overall treatment outcome. Low initial doses and gradual dose titration can eliminate these unpleasant effects.[56]

Although imipramine and clomipramine are the most studied TCAs for panic disorder, desipramine and nortriptyline may be effective.[60,61] Problems with using TCAs in panic disorder are well documented and include stimulatory side effects, anticholinergic effects, orthostatic hypotension, delayed onset of antipanic effects, and toxicity in an overdose.[60] Approximately 25% of patients reportedly discontinue treatment because of side effects.[56] Weight gain is a problematic side effect associated with long-term therapy.[60]

Selective Serotonin Reuptake Inhibitors

Clinical studies indicate that all SSRIs are effective in panic disorder. The percentage of patients who become panic-free ranges between 60% to 80%.[60] The antipanic effect of SSRIs is delayed for 3 to 5 weeks, and some patients do not respond for 8 to 12 weeks.[60]

Typical antidepressant doses of SSRIs can cause side effects of insomnia, jitteriness, restlessness, and agitation and lead to drug discontinuation in panic patients. Transient gastrointestinal disturbances occur more frequently with SSRIs than with TCAs.[9] Thus low initial SSRI doses should be prescribed.[9,36] Sleep disturbances, headaches, and sexual dysfunction often are problematic.

Monoamine Oxidase Inhibitors

The majority of studies assessing the efficacy of MAOIs in treating panic disorder were poorly designed and lacked sufficient dosage and duration of treatment, adequate sample size, and valid ratings of panic attacks. The course of response mimics that of TCAs.[60] Side effects and dietary restrictions adversely affect patient acceptance.[10,60]

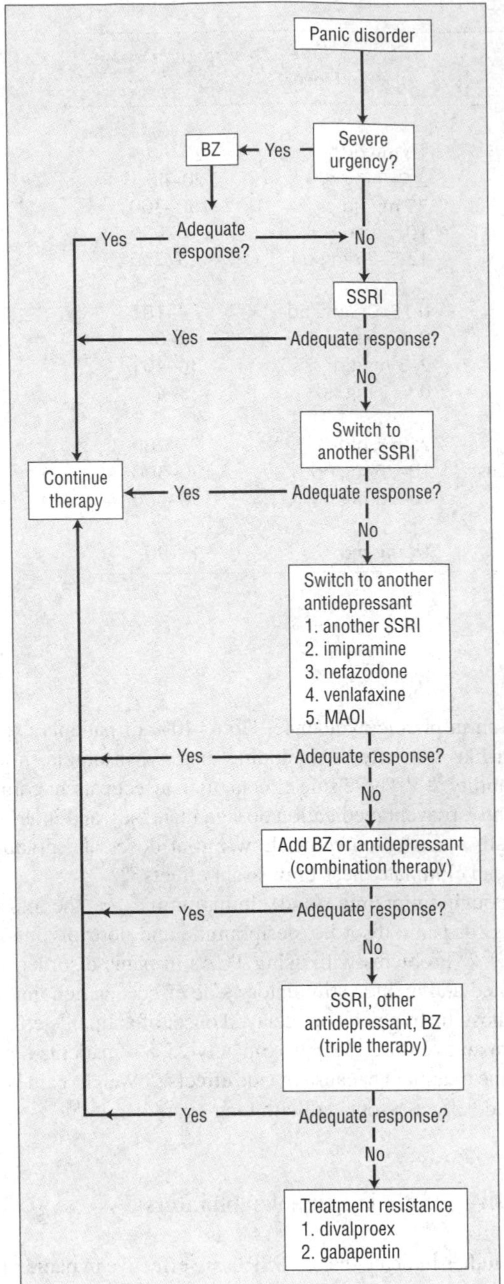

FIGURE 71–2. Algorithm for the management of panic disorder. *(Adapted from Refs. 9 and 58.)*

MAOIs are usually reserved for the most refractory or difficult patient.[56]

BENZODIAZEPINE THERAPY

Although BZs are effective antipanic agents, concerns over their use are prevalent. The development of dependency, interdose rebound anxiety, and the need for multiple daily dosing can limit their usefulness. The high-potency BZs clonazepam and alprazolam are used frequently.[56] Diazepam and lorazepam are possibly effective in treating panic disorder when taken in sufficiently high doses.[60] Therapeutic response to BZs occurs in 1 to 2 weeks, with further improvement occurring at weeks 4 to 6. It is estimated that 60% to 80% of panic disorder patients respond to BZs.[62] Alprazolam is an ideal agent for patients who need rapid relief. Patient acceptance of alprazolam usually is not a problem, and except for sedation, side effects are reported rarely. Relapse rates of 50% or higher are common despite slow drug tapering.[60]

OTHER AGENTS

Trazodone was effective in some patients, but bupropion was ineffective.[56] Venlafaxine, gabapentin, and nefazodone also may be effective.[63–65] The rate of use of alternative medicines in patients with panic disorder is high.[66]

TREATMENT RESISTANCE

Common reasons for treatment failures are comorbid psychiatric disorders, rapid dosage increases with resulting intolerable side effects, and underdosage.[56,60] All standard treatments should be tried before using augmentation strategies. The most common strategy used in patients with a partial response to one agent is to augment with low doses of another antipanic agent (e.g., TCA, BZ, or SSRI).[9] Limited data support the use of divalproex sodium as monotherapy in patients with concurrent mood swings.[67]

DOSING AND ADMINISTRATION

Acute Phase

The main goal of therapy in the acute phase is reduction of symptoms (e.g., resolution of panic attacks, reduction in anxiety and phobic fears, resumption of the patient's usual activities).[60] The duration of this phase is generally 1 to 3 months depending on the choice of medication. The guiding principle for using medication in panic disorder is to start low, use an adequate dose, and treat for an appropriate period of time. Side effects with the antidepressants, often from too high an initial dose, may prevent achievement of an optimal dosage, compromise treatment response, and contribute to patient noncompliance.

The duration of the acute phase with antidepressants is about 12 weeks.[60] Therapy should be altered if there is no response after 6 to 8 weeks of an adequate dose. When using imipramine, treatment should be initiated with 10 mg/day at bedtime and slowly increased by 10 mg every 2 to 4 days as tolerated to 75–100 mg/day and then increased by 25 mg every 2 to 4 days over a 2- to 4-week period.[56] Most patients require at least 150 mg/day of imipramine (or a combined imipramine-desipramine plasma concentration of 100–150 ng/mL).[56] If this dose is not effective, a higher dose (up to 300 mg/day) should be used.[9] Many patients with panic disorder are extremely sensitive to imipramine and experience an immediate stimulatory feeling or motor restlessness. The starting dose, therefore, is very conservative. Stimulatory side effects are transient and generally dissipate after several weeks of therapy.[9] Low daily doses of clomipramine (60 mg/day) were as effective but more tolerable than higher doses (150 mg/day).[61]

Low initial doses of SSRIs are recommended to avoid stimulatory side effects (e.g., insomnia, nervousness). Sertraline, initiated at 12.5 or 25 mg/day and titrated to 100–200 mg/day, is effective in panic disorder.[68] The starting dose of paroxetine is 10 mg, with dosage increases of 10 mg weekly; the target dose is 40 mg.[69] The starting dose of fluoxetine is 5 mg/day, with dosage increases every 2 or 3 days to a dosage range of 10–20 mg/day by the end of 2 weeks. Fluvoxamine 25–50 mg/day was increased to 150 mg/day in divided doses over 2 weeks in clinical trials (range, 100–300 mg/day).[70] Citalopram at doses of 20–60 mg reduced panic attacks and anxiety.[71]

The starting dose of phenelzine is 15 mg/day after the evening meal, increased by 15 mg/day every 3 to 4 days until 60 mg/day is reached. A dose of less than 45 mg/day is rarely effective. Dosages may be increased (up to 90 mg/day) if improvement is not achieved after 8 to 12 weeks. If a patient was on an antidepressant previously, it should be discontinued, and 2 weeks should lapse before phenelzine is started to prevent a potential drug interaction. Fluoxetine must be stopped 5 weeks before phenelzine (or another MAOI) can be started. Anticholinergic side effects are less severe with phenelzine than with TCAs, but orthostatic hypotension and insomnia are often more of a problem. After 3 weeks, most unpleasant side effects subside.

Hypertensive crisis following the ingestion of tyramine-containing foods or sympathomimetic drugs is the most serious, potentially life-threatening event encountered with phenelzine.[56] (See Chapter 69 for food and drug restrictions and side effects.) Patients should observe the food, drink, and drug restrictions for at least 24 hours before starting the first dose of phenelzine and for 2 weeks after stopping therapy.

The duration of the acute phase with BZs is approximately 1 month because response is rapid and occurs within 1 to 3 weeks. The starting dose of clonazepam is 0.25 mg twice a day, with dose increase to 1 mg by the third day of therapy. Further increases of dose (by 0.25 or 0.5 mg) every three days to 4 mg/day can be made if needed.[76] The starting dose of alprazolam is 0.25–0.5 mg three times daily, slowly increased over several weeks to reach an ideal dose. The duration of action may be as little as 4 to 6 hours with resulting "breakthrough" symptoms.[9] Most patients require 3–6 mg/day, and some need doses of 6–10 mg/day to obtain a full therapeutic (antipanic and antiphobic) response. Patients tolerate the initial side effects of alprazolam much better than those of imipramine or phenelzine. Because of its long half-life, clonazepam is an alternative to alprazolam if patients experience breakthrough panic symptoms at the end of a dosing interval.

Maintenance Phase and Discontinuation

The optimal length of therapy is unknown; however, the total duration of therapy appears to be 12 months before drug discontinuation over 4 to 6 months is attempted.[60,72] Successful maintenance with single weekly doses of fluoxetine has been described.[73] When medications are discontinued too early, a high rate of relapse occurs; thus longer periods of treatment are associated with more sustained response. Reinstitution of medication usually results in renewed clinical response.[60] In general, patients with more than two episodes should receive chronic therapy.[72]

Patients taking alprazolam, clonazepam, or imipramine for up to 8 months maintained antipanic efficacy without dosage increases. This indicates that tolerance does not develop to the antipanic effects of these agents.[31,71] The most important determinant of compliance with maintenance therapy is the tolerability of adverse events.[60] Some adverse events experienced short term become unbearable during long-term management (i.e., sexual dysfunction, weight gain). The major reason for imipramine discontinuation in long-term studies is weight gain, with a 35% dropout rate. The primary risk of long-term BZ use is the development of dependency and withdrawal reactions on discontinuation. Abuse of BZs usually is confined to patients with a personal or family history of substance or alcohol use.[34] Both TCAs and SSRIs can be associated with discontinuation symptoms.

Some patients receiving high-dose alprazolam (>4 mg/day) may have an extremely difficult time with drug taper, and the withdrawal schedule for all patients should be individualized. The taper phase is most successful when it is accomplished over a 4- to 6-month period.[34] Approximately 30% of the patients receiving high doses, even with slow taper, may experience transient, mild to moderate withdrawal symptoms (as discussed in the earlier section on BZs) and relapse of panic attacks. Adjunctive CBT reportedly facilitates BZ discontinuation.[36] Also, if a TCA is discontinued abruptly, a substantial number of patients will develop severe cholinergic rebound with upset stomach, nausea, vomiting, and abdominal cramping; thus TCAs should be reduced by 25 mg every 2 to 4 weeks.[56] The dose of phenelzine should be reduced by 15 mg every 2 to 4 weeks.

Patient education is essential. Patients should be informed regarding the lag time before a therapeutic response will occur and any problematic side effects. Many patients are reluctant to take medications for fear that drugs will worsen their illness or that they will become addicted. Adverse events are often perceived as a worsening of the illness and may contribute to noncompliance and prevent necessary medication increases. Patients receiving alprazolam or another BZ should be told not to decrease or discontinue therapy unless authorized by their physician.

PHARMACOECONOMIC CONSIDERATIONS

Patients with panic disorder have high rates of receiving welfare, disability benefits, and health care services. They also have impaired emotional and physical health status and experience poor marital and social functioning.[19] Fifty-three percent of patients reported occupational role disability, 34% indicated physical disability and a mean of 6.7 disability days during the past month.[51] Panic disorder patients had a higher rate of primary care and medical specialist visits (83%) than a healthy control group (36%) for 1 year.[52]

In the year after diagnosis, panic disorder patients reduced the use of general medical services by 94%, increased use of psychiatric services, and demonstrated marked improvement in productivity and well-being.[75] After 6 weeks of clonazepam, work productivity improved (from 71% to 88%), and personal happiness increased.[19] Measures of QOL improved with imipramine, clonazepam, and sertraline. Treatment with clomipramine, paroxetine, or fluoxetine improved work, social, and family responsibilities. Anxiety and phobic avoidance were significantly associated with QOL improvements but not reduction in the frequency of panic attacks, which is used most often as the measure of success in drug efficacy trials.[19]

EVALUATION OF THERAPEUTIC OUTCOMES

During the first 2 weeks of the acute phase of therapy, patients with panic disorder should be seen twice weekly to adjust medication doses based on improvement in panic symptoms and to monitor for adverse events. Once stabilized, the patient can be seen on a weekly basis until antipanic response is achieved. Subsequently, monthly visits should suffice. The patient should be counseled to maintain a diary to record the date, time, frequency, and duration of panic episodes and the severity of panic symptoms, anticipatory anxiety, and phobic avoidance. Treatment outcomes can be assessed by administering the seven-item Panic Disorder Severity Scale.[76] At scheduled visits, the clinician should inquire about the level of disability experienced by the patient. During drug discontinuation, the frequency of appointments should be increased to evaluate for emergence of withdrawal symptoms and monitor for relapse.

▶ TREATMENT: Social Anxiety Disorder

DESIRED OUTCOME

The goals of therapy in the management of SAD are to reduce the physiologic symptoms of anxiety and phobic avoidance of feared situations and increase participation in desired social activities.[77]

Early intervention helps to decrease impairment, the development of harmful coping strategies, and the onset of comorbid conditions.[77] Because SAD is associated with significant morbidity, patients should be treated aggressively once diagnosed. Therapeutic options include pharmacotherapy, psychological approaches, or a combination of the two.

NONPHARMACOLOGIC THERAPY

Nonpharmacologic treatments in SAD include CBT, exposure to feared situations, social skills training, and applied relaxation therapy.[77] Many patients respond to a combination of these therapies. Psychological treatment usually lasts several months and often is conducted in a group setting.

PHARMACOLOGIC THERAPY

SAD is effectively treated with SSRIs, MAOIs, BZs, β-blockers, and various other agents, but controlled trials are limited (Table 71–13). Paroxetine is the only medication approved for SAD. SSRIs are considered the first-line treatment because of their tolerability and efficacy.[20]

The patient's symptoms, prior treatments, comorbid conditions, and history of substance abuse direct treatment selections. Patients with comorbid depression or another anxiety disorder should be treated with an antidepressant. BZs and MAOIs should be avoided in patients with a history of alcohol or substance abuse.[24] Patients with discrete SAD may be treated on an as-needed basis with β-blockers. Generalized SAD requires daily medication over an extended period of time. The effect of long-term therapy can be assessed in terms of risks (e.g., sexual dysfunction) and benefits (e.g., decrease in anxiety, improved QOL) of therapy. An algorithm for the pharmacotherapy of generalized SAD appears in Figure 71–3.

ANTIDEPRESSANT THERAPY

Selective Serotonin Reuptake Inhibitors

SSRIs are considered the first-line agents for the treatment of SAD and should be used in patients with SAD who also have depression, other anxiety disorders, or substance abuse.[20] Controlled trials have demonstrated the efficacy of paroxetine,[78] fluvoxamine,[79] and sertraline[80] in SAD. Limited data suggest that citalopram and fluoxetine are also effective.[81,82]

Patients treated with paroxetine had improvement in anxiety and avoidance symptoms and a reduction of disability over a 12-week time period.[78] The rate of improvement ranged from 66% to 83%. Doses of paroxetine up to 50 mg/day were well tolerated, and side effects reported were similar to those seen in the treatment of depression (e.g., headache, somnolence, sexual dysfunction). The onset of effect was delayed and often not apparent for 4 to 8 weeks, with maximum benefit not observed until 12 weeks or longer.

Monamine Oxidase Inhibitors

Although effective in 77% of patients, phenelzine is a second-line agent for SAD because of tolerability and safety concerns.[83] Low-dose selegiline (10 mg/day), a specific monoamine oxidase B

TABLE 71–13. Drugs Used in the Treatment of Social Anxiety Disorder

Class/Generic Name	Brand Name	Manufacturer	Starting Dose	Dosage Range[a] (mg/day)
Selective serotonin reuptake inhibitors				
Citalopram	Celexa	Forest Labs	20 mg qd	20–40
Fluoxetine[c]	Prozac	Lilly	10–20 mg qd	10–60
Fluvoxamine[c]	Luvox	Solvay	25 mg bid	150–300
Paroxetine	Paxil	GlaxoSmithKline	10–20 mg qd	20–60[b]
Sertraline	Zoloft	Pfizer	25–50 mg qd	50–200
Benzodiazepines				
Alprazolam[c]	Xanax	Pharmacia & Upjohn	0.25 tid	1–6
Clonazepam[c]	Klonopin	Roche	0.25 mg bid	1–3
Monoamine oxidase inhibitors				
Phenelzine	Nardil	Parke-Davis	15 mg q pm	60–90
Selegiline[c]	Eldepryl	Somerset	5 mg bid	10
Other agents				
Buspirone[c]	Buspar	Bristol-Myers Squibb	10 mg bid	45–60
Gabapentin	Neurontin	Parke-Davis, Pfizer	100 mg tid	900–3600
Nefazodone	Serzone	Bristol-Myers Squibb	50 mg bid	200–600
Venlafaxine	Effexor	Wyeth-Ayerst	18.75 mg bid	50–150

[a]Dosage used in clinical trials but not FDA approved.
[b]Dosage is FDA approved.
[c]Available generically.
Compiled from Refs. 78–84, 86–88, 91–94.

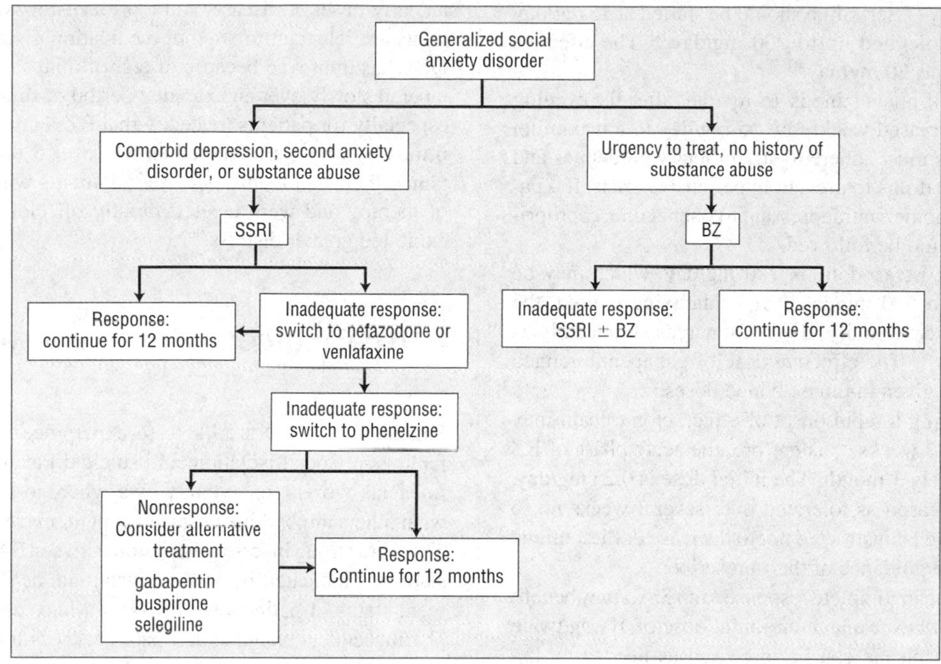

FIGURE 71–3. Algorithm for the pharmacotherapy of social anxiety disorder. *(Adapted from Refs. 20, 77, and 90.)*

inhibitor with minimal side effects, decreased symptoms of SAD in 32% of patients.[84]

Other Antidepressants

Open trials suggest that other 5-HT-potentiating medications may be effective in SAD.[20] After 2 months of treatment, imipramine showed only a 20% response rate. Most patients experienced side effects (e.g., light-headedness, rash, and sedation) to imipramine that interfered with their functioning.[85] In a 12-week trial of nefazodone, 70% of patients had moderate or marked improvement in social anxiety, avoidance, depression, and social functioning.[86] The majority of patients experienced side effects, including excessive fatigue or sedation. Venlafaxine was effective in patients who had failed or could not tolerate SSRI therapy.[87]

BENZODIAZEPINE THERAPY

The high-potency BZs alprazolam and clonazepam reduced anxiety symptoms in individuals with SAD.[88] Clonazepam improved fear and phobic avoidance, interpersonal sensitivity, fears of negative evaluation, and disability measures.[88] The use of clonazepam should be considered for patients who require a rapid onset of effect. Clonazepam is often prescribed in conjunction with an SSRI, psychotherapy, or both. Comorbid alcohol or substance abuse is a contraindication to the use of BZs. Because of the risk of dependency, BZs use should be reserved for use in patients at a low risk of substance abuse, those who need rapid treatment, or those who have not responded to other therapies.

β-BLOCKER THERAPY

Many of the problematic somatic features associated with SAD (e.g., rapid heart rate, sweating, blushing, tremor) are mediated by the β-adrenergic system. However, atenolol was not more effective than placebo in improving symptoms of generalized SAD over a 3-month period.[89] β-Blockers decrease the perception of anxiety by blunting the peripheral autonomic symptoms of arousal and often are used to decrease anxiety in performance-related situations. Patients with discrete SAD may benefit from administration of atenolol or propranolol on an as-needed basis 1 to 2 hours before a presentation or performance.[90]

OTHER AGENTS

Gabapentin, a nonbenzodiazepine GABA analog, was effective in a placebo-controlled trial over 14 weeks.[91] Adverse effects reported with gabapentin were dizziness and dry mouth. Although buspirone is not effective as monotherapy in SAD,[92] it may augment SSRIs.[93]

DOSING AND ADMINISTRATION

Acute Phase

The goal of therapy in the acute phase is to reduce physiologic symptoms of anxiety (e.g., tachycardia, flushing, and sweating) and begin to reduce social anxiety and phobic avoidance. The duration of this phase is 4 to 12 weeks, depending on the medication.

When using paroxetine, treatment should be initiated at 20 mg/day as a single daily dose administered in the morning with or without food. Patients should receive 20 mg/day for 2 to 4 weeks before the dose is increased slowly by 10 mg/day at weekly intervals as necessary to obtain a response.[20] Safety for paroxetine in SAD has been demonstrated in doses of up to 60 mg/day, but additional therapeutic benefits above 20 mg/day have not been shown.[94] Elderly patients and those with renal or hepatic impairment should begin paroxetine at 10 mg/day, and doses can be increased up to a maximum of 40 mg/day.

The starting dose for fluoxetine is 10 mg/day, which is then increased as tolerated and needed up to 60 mg/day.[82] If fluvoxamine is used, the initial dose is 50 mg/day, and it may be increased to a maximum of 300 mg/day.[79] Sertraline should be started at 25 mg/day and then increased as tolerated up to 200 mg/day.[80] The effective dosage for citalopram was 20 mg/day.[81]

The starting dose of phenelzine is 15 mg/day after the evening meal, and it may be increased weekly by 15 mg/day to a maximum of 90 mg/day.[83] Patients must adhere to strict dietary guidelines and avoid sympathomimetic drugs to prevent hypertensive crisis. If a patient is switched from another antidepressant to phenelzine, appropriate washout periods should be followed.

The initial dose of nefazodone is 100 mg/day, which may be increased as tolerated to 600 mg/day.[86] If venlafaxine is used, the initial dose is 18.75 mg twice daily. It is then increased gradually as tolerated to 150 mg/day.[87] The effective dose of gabapentin ranged from 900–3600 mg/day given in three divided doses.[91]

For patients requiring a rapid onset of effect, clonazepam may be effective within 1 to 2 weeks.[88] Therefore, the acute phase of BZ treatment is approximately 1 month. The initial dose is 0.25 mg/day, which then can be increased as tolerated over several weeks up to 3 mg/day. Patients should be instructed not to decrease or discontinue therapy unless under the guidance of their prescriber.

Patients who have an incomplete response to an SSRI may benefit from augmentation with buspirone at an initial dose of 10 mg twice daily.[93] The dose of buspirone can be increased as needed to 45–60 mg/day.

For patients with discrete SAD, 10–80 mg propranolol or 25–100 mg atenolol can be taken an hour before a performance situation.[90] It is recommended that the patient receive a test dose to assess tolerability.

Continuation Phase

The goals of therapy in the continuation phase are to extend the therapeutic benefits seen in the acute phase, especially the ability to participate in social activities and improvement in QOL. During this phase, the dose of medication that achieves maximum therapeutic benefit while minimizing adverse events is reached. This phase usually lasts 3 to 6 months.

Maintenance Phase and Discontinuation

There are minimal data on the long-term treatment of SAD. The relapse rate after discontinuation of acute paroxetine therapy was 63% within 12 weeks.[94] After improvement, at least a 1-year maintenance period is recommended.[20] This time period maintains improvement and decreases the rate of relapse.[20] Indications for long-term treatment include the presence of unresolved symptoms or comorbidity, an early onset of disease, and a prior history of relapse.[20] Many patients are reluctant to attempt medication discontinuation once their QOL has improved because of fear of relapse. Medication should be tapered slowly over an extended period of time (i.e., 4 to 12 weeks), especially for patients treated with a BZ. Patients on clonazepam for 6 months who were tapered slowly over 5 months generally maintained their treatment response.[95] Patients who received 11 months of therapy and were tapered rapidly off clonazepam over 3 weeks exhibited greater distress.[96]

PHARMACOECONOMIC CONSIDERATIONS

Patients with SAD are likely to experience functional impairment, feelings of social isolation, and suicidal ideation.[20] They report that financial barriers, uncertainty over where to go for help, and fear of what others might think or say prevent them from seeking treatment.[97] There is a strong inverse association between SAD and socioeconomic status, as indicated by lower educational achievement and employment status of patients with SAD.[20] Many patients may qualify for pharmaceutical manufacturer patient access-to-care programs to ease treatment costs.

Early intervention is important in the treatment of SAD, and pharmacotherapy can dramatically improve QOL. Patients treated with fluvoxamine and paroxetine showed a significantly greater improvement on work functioning, family life, and home functioning compared with placebo-treated patients.[78,79]

EVALUATION OF THERAPEUTIC OUTCOMES

During the acute phase of treatment, patients should be seen weekly while the dosage of medication is increased. Once the patient responds and the dosage is stabilized, monthly visits are appropriate. At each visit, the patient should be asked about adverse effects and improvement in symptoms. The patient should be instructed to keep a diary to record fear levels, physical symptoms, cognitions, and anxious behaviors to actual exposures to social situations.[78] The Liebowitz Social Anxiety Scale also may be used to monitor response.[20] The patient should be counseled about the gradual onset of medication effect and that the full therapeutic effect may not be achieved for 4 to 8 weeks. Patients should be told that long-term therapy will be required and that when therapy is discontinued, the dosage will need to be decreased gradually over 4 to 6 weeks.

▶ TREATMENT: Posttraumatic Stress Disorder

DESIRED OUTCOME

The goals of therapy in the management of PTSD are to decrease core symptoms, disability, and comorbidity and improve QOL and resilience to stress.[21] With the use of pharmacotherapy, many patients will improve substantially but retain some symptoms. Mild symptoms such as numbing or irritability linked to recollection of the trauma may persist.[21] Treatment regimens usually combine education, psychosocial support and/or treatment, and pharmacotherapy.[21]

NONPHARMACOLOGIC THERAPY

Psychotherapies for treating PTSD include anxiety management, CBT, exposure therapy, play therapy, and psychoeducation.[98] A focus on the traumatic event precipitating the PTSD is the mainstay of therapy. Many studies of patients undergoing CBT have included patients also receiving pharmacotherapy. By relieving the symptoms of PTSD with medicine, the patient may be able to more fully participate in psychotherapy.[21]

TABLE 71–14. Antidepressants Used in the Treatment of Posttraumatic Stress Disorder

Class/Generic Name	Brand Name	Manufacturer	Starting Dose	Dosage Range[a] (mg/day)
Selective serotonin reuptake inhibitors				
Fluoxetine[c]	Prozac	Lilly	10–20 mg qd	10–60
Fluvoxamine[c]	Luvox	Solvay	50 mg qd	100–250
Paroxetine	Paxil	GlaxoSmithKline	10–20 mg qd	20–60
Sertraline	Zoloft	Pfizer	25–50 mg qd	50–200[b]
Monoamine oxidase inhibitor				
Phenelzine	Nardil	Parke-Davis	15 mg q pm	45–75
Other antidepressants				
Bupropion[c]	Wellbutrin	Glaxo Wellcome	75 mg bid	150–400
Mirtazapine	Remeron	Organon	15 mg qhs	30–45
Nefazodone	Serzone	Bristol-Myers Squibb	50 mg bid	100–600
Trazodone[c]	Desyrel	Apothecon	50 mg qhs	150–400
Venlafaxine	Effexor XR	Wyeth-Ayerst	75 mg qd	75–225

[a]Dosage used in clinical trials but not FDA approved.
[b]Dosage is FDA approved.
[c]Available generically.
Compiled from Refs. 98–112.

Patients who have experienced trauma should be educated that they may experience anxiety, depression, nightmares, and even flashbacks as a normal reaction to the event.[21] Patients can be encouraged to talk and share their feelings with others they trust. Education to avoid excessive use of alcohol, nicotine, and other drugs during therapy is important.

PHARMACOLOGIC THERAPY

During the period of acute stress, the patient may require medication for sleep disturbance. If the patient has experienced four consecutive nights without sleep, a nonbenzodiazepine hypnotic can be prescribed (i.e., trazodone, zaleplon).[21] Few well-designed, controlled trials evaluating the pharmacotherapy of PTSD exist. The antidepressants (e.g., SSRIs, TCAs, MAOIs) have been studied the most (Table 71–14). Sertraline is the only medication approved for the treatment of PTSD. Medications evaluated as augmentation therapy include antiadrenergic drugs, anticonvulsants, anxiolytics, buspirone, and antipsychotics (Table 71–15). BZs use should be avoided in PTSD because they may worsen symptoms. An algorithm for the treatment of PTSD appears in Figure 71–4.

ANTIDEPRESSANT THERAPY

Selective Serotonin Reuptake Inhibitors

Sertraline was effective across a spectrum of PTSD-specific, global, and functional outcome measures in a controlled 12-week trial.[21] Approximately half the patients improved on symptom clusters of arousal and avoidance/numbing but not on reexperiencing/intrusion. Sertraline was effective in rape victims[100] and veterans in open trials.[101] All three PTSD symptom clusters were reduced by sertraline in patients with comorbid alcohol dependence.[102]

Fluoxetine, fluvoxamine, and paroxetine have also shown efficacy.[103–105] The SSRIs reduced the numbing symptoms of PTSD, whereas other medications have not. Adverse reactions reported in patients with PTSD treated with SSRIs include gastrointesinal symptoms, sexual dysfunction, insomnia, and agitation.[103–105] SSRIs are recommended as the first-line drug therapy for PTSD

TABLE 71–15. Drugs for Augmentation Used in the Treatment of Posttraumatic Stress Disorder

Class/Generic Name	Brand Name	Manufacturer	Starting Dose	Dosage Range[a] (mg/day)
Mood stabilizers				
Carbamazepine[b]	Tegretol	Novartis	100 mg bid	300–1200
Divalproex sodium	Depakote	Abbott	10 mg/kg/day in 2 doses	20–60 mg/kg/day
Gabapentin	Neurontin	Parke-Davis, Pfizer	100 mg tid	900–1200
Lamotrigine	Lamictal	Glaxo Wellcome	25 mg qd	50–500
Adrenergic agents				
Clonidine[b]	Catapres	Boehringer Ingelheim	0.05 mg bid	0.2–0.6
Guanfacine[b]	Tenex	Wyeth-Ayerst	1 mg qhs	1–3
Prazosin[b]	Minipress	Pfizer	1 mg qhs	2–10
Propranolol[b]	Inderal	Wyeth-Ayerst	10 mg bid	40–160
Other agents				
Buspirone[b]	Buspar	Bristol-Myers Squibb	10 mg bid	45–60
Risperidone	Risperdal	Janssen	0.5 mg qd	1–3

[a]Dosage used in clinical trials but not FDA approved.
[b]Available generically.
Compiled from Refs. 113–124.

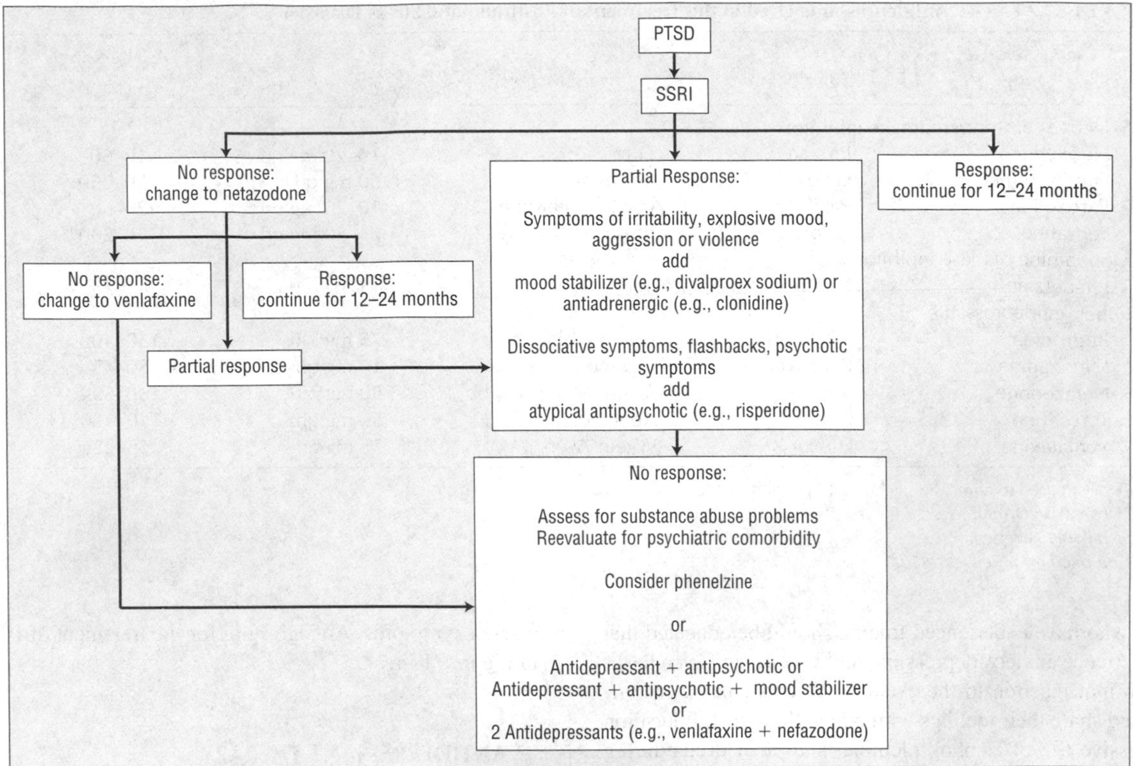

FIGURE 71–4. Algorithm for the pharmacotherapy of posttraumatic stress disorder. *(Adapted from Refs. 21, 98, 119, and 125.)*

because they assist patients in meeting treatment goals by decreasing symptoms and disability, increasing functioning, and treating comorbid conditions.[21,98]

Monoamine Oxidase Inhibitors

A review of MAOI and TCA trials in the treatment of PTSD concluded that the global efficacy of phenelzine (82%) exceed the global efficacy of TCAs (45%). The MAOIs decrease intrusive symptoms.[106] Phenelzine decreased insomnia, nightmares, and flashbacks and may be an alternative for patients who do not respond to SSRIs.

Other Antidepressants

Current guidelines recommend against using TCAs in the treatment of PTSD because they are associated with daytime drowsiness, toxicity in overdose, impaired reaction times, and increased risk of traffic accidents.[21,98] Nefazodone decreased all symptom clusters of PTSD, especially those of hyperarousal.[107] Depression, insomnia, nightmares, and anger also were improved. Patients who have failed therapy with other medications may respond to a trial of nefazodone.[108] Adverse effects from nefazodone were headache, dry mouth, diarrhea, and somnolence.[107,108] Trazodone and mirtazapine decreased some symptoms of PTSD.[109,110] The sedating effect of trazodone is used frequently to treat insomnia induced by SSRIs. Mirtazapine caused increased appetite, panic attacks, weight gain, sedation, and nausea in patients with PTSD.[110] Although bupropion decreased symptoms of depression and hyperarousal, most PTSD symptoms were unchanged.[111] Venlafaxine was effective in one patient who had failed therapy with serotonergic agents.[112]

ANTICONVULSANTS/MOOD STABILIZERS

Mood stabilizers may be used as augmentation therapy in cases of partial response to antidepressant therapy, especially those with prominent irritability or anger.[98] Anticonvulsants (thought to exert their mechanism, in part, through antikindling effects) have been effective in treating PTSD. The response rate for patients receiving lamotrigine was twice that of patients receiving placebo (50% and 25%, respectively).[113] The slow dosage escalation of lamotrigine, to avoid the development of a rash, however, may prolong the time required to reach an effective dose. Gabapentin, vigabatrin, divalproex sodium, and carbamazepine also were effective in open trials.[114–117] Potential drug interactions and adverse reactions, especially with divalproex sodium and carbamazepine, can complicate therapy. Lithium can be used adjunctively to manage irritability or mood swings.[118] Patients with PTSD and comorbid bipolar disorder should receive a mood stabilizer as first-line therapy.[98]

ANTIADRENERGIC THERAPY

Clonidine, guanfacine, propranolol, and prazosin decreased nightmares and startle response associated with PTSD by decreasing noradrenergic transmission.[119,120]

BUSPIRONE THERAPY

Buspirone improved all symptom clusters of PTSD, with the most benefit on hyperarousal symptoms.[121] Buspirone may be an effective augmenting agent for patients with incomplete response to antidepressants.[122]

ANTIPSYCHOTIC THERAPY

Risperidone, an atypical antipsychotic, decreased aggressive behavior, hyperarousal, vivid flashbacks, and nightmares in patients with PTSD.[123,124] Risperidone may be added to antidepressants and anticonvulsants in patients with psychosis, agitation, paranoia, or excessive hypervigilance.[21,98,119]

DOSAGE AND ADMINISTRATION

Acute Phase

PTSD symptoms respond slowly to pharmacotherapy, and some patients may never experience full resolution of symptoms. SSRIs should be started 3 weeks after exposure to a trauma in patients with no improvement in their acute stress response.[21] The initiation of an SSRI should be at a low dose with gradual titration upward to doses used to treat depression. An appropriate duration of antidepressant therapy is 8 weeks to determine response.[98]

The initial dose of sertraline is 25 mg given once daily with an increase to 50 mg/day after 1 week. The dose can be increased in weekly intervals by 50 mg/day up to a maximum dosage of 200 mg/day. Paroxetine may be initiated at 20 mg/day and increased by 10 mg/day in weekly intervals to a target dose of 40 mg/day and a maximum dosage of 60 mg/day. The initial dose of phenelzine is 15 mg given in the evening, and the dose is titrated to 45–60 mg/day. Dietary precautions must be followed and drug interactions carefully avoided to prevent hypertensive crisis. The dosing of other antidepressants is shown in Table 71–14.

If an anticonvulsant is used, the initial dose should be low, followed by slow titration. The doses for other agents used to augment therapy in PTSD are listed in Table 71–15.

Continuation Phase

Because patients may be undergoing psychotherapy, medication dosages often vary as the patient deals with past traumatic experiences. Symptoms continue to improve after the acute phase of therapy, and the maximal drug benefit (i.e., improvement of disability) may not be evident until after this time. Patients who do well on fluoxetine after 3 months of treatment generally continue to improve at follow-up at 15 months.[125] Clinical response at 3 months has been identified as a predictor of long-term outcome.[125]

Maintenance and Discontinuation

Patients with chronic PTSD who respond to medication should continue on the medication for 12 to 24 months.[98] Patients with residual symptoms should continue on medication for at least 24 months.[98] Some patients may continue on medication indefinitely. The decision on when to discontinue therapy is based on response to therapy, presence of ongoing stresses, and possible adverse effects.[98] The patient must be confident in the discontinuation plan and requires extra support throughout the process. Medication should be withdrawn and tapered slowly over a period of at least 1 month.[98] To lessen the likelihood of relapse in a patient with risk factors for relapse, medication should be tapered over a longer period of time (e.g., 6 to 12 weeks).[98]

PHARMACOECONOMIC CONSIDERATIONS

PTSD compares with depression in the level of disability it imposes on patients with the disorder.[21,119] Individuals fail to realize their potentials for career development, marriage, and education. Decreased productivity leads to a financial loss of greater than $3 billion per year.[21] This figure does not include economic loss associated with the failure of patients with PTSD to achieve their educational or career goals.[21,119] Treatment with effective pharmacotherapy can improve the QOL of these patients. Sertraline and fluoxetine improved measures of social and occupational functioning as well as the perception of improved QOL in patients with PTSD.[99,126]

EVALUATION OF THERAPEUTIC OUTCOMES

During the acute phase of therapy, patients should be seen weekly for a month and then every other week.[98] During months 3 to 6 of therapy, the patient can be seen monthly. In months 6 to 12 of therapy, visits can be extended to every 1 to 2 months. After a year of medication, the patient can be seen every 3 months. The patient should be asked about target symptoms of PTSD as well as other symptoms including sleep, anger outbursts, irritability, and disability.[98] The patient should maintain a diary to record the date and presence of symptoms of reexperiencing, avoidance behavior, hyperarousal, as well as comorbid conditions (e.g., panic attacks, obsessions and compulsions, suicidal ideation). A remission or good response in patients with PTSD is defined as a greater than 75% reduction in symptoms and response maintained for at least 3 months. Patients who have a 25% to 75% reduction in symptoms are considered partial responders. Patients who are nonresponsive to therapy have less than 25% reduction in symptoms.[98] Before deciding that a patient is not responsive to pharmacotherapy, the clinician should ensure that the medication trial has been adequate in both dose and duration.[98]

Many patients with PTSD are sensitive to the adverse effects of medications. They should be monitored carefully for adverse reactions that may delay the escalation of medication dosages or cause the patient distress. At each visit, the clinician should inquire about disability and QOL and thoroughly document the patient's response. When pharmacotherapy is discontinued, patients should be seen more frequently and monitored carefully for signs of relapse or medication withdrawal.

▶ TREATMENT: Specific phobia

Specific phobia is considered unresponsive to drug therapy, although highly responsive to behavioral therapy. The use of antidepressant medications may be detrimental in patients with specific phobias.

CONCLUSIONS

Theories about anxiety disorders have undergone major revisions over the past several years. Anxiety disorders are quite common, occurring in approximately 25% of the population during their lifetime. The proper management of anxiety disorders begins with the correct diagnosis; not all patients should receive antianxiety agents. Nonpharmacologic interventions often are effective alone or when combined with drug therapy.

There are several subtypes of anxiety disorders, and the diagnosis determines the type of drug and nonpharmacologic intervention selected. Although BZs remain the drugs of choice for situational anxiety, antidepressants have emerged as first-line therapy for GAD, SAD, and PTSD. The anxiolytic agents venlafaxine, paroxetine, or buspirone may be useful for patients who need chronic therapy for GAD or who cannot tolerate BZs. Antidepressants, including the SSRIs, and the BZs clonazepam and alprazolam are used extensively in patients with panic disorder. Research in the areas of SAD and PTSD has resulted in new pharmacologic treatment strategies.

▶ PRINCIPLES OF PHARMACOTHERAPY

- BZs are the drugs of choice for acute anxiety symptoms and antidepressants and buspirone are agents of choice for long-term management of GAD.
- BZs with short elimination half-lives are recommended for the elderly, for patients with hepatic disorders, and for those receiving drugs that impair oxidative metabolism.
- Antidepressants and buspirone have a lag time of 2 to 4 and 4 to 6 weeks, respectively, to achieve maximal antianxiety effects and do not have significant sedative, hypnotic, or muscle relaxant properties.
- Many patients with panic disorder are extremely sensitive to TCAs and SSRIs and experience an immediate stimulatory feeling that may compromise compliance.
- Because of its half-life, clonazepam is an alternative to alprazolam for patients with panic disorder having breakthrough panic symptoms at the end of a dosing interval.
- When monitoring the effectiveness of antidepressants in panic disorder, it is important to allow an adequate amount of time (10 to 12 weeks) to achieve full therapeutic response.
- The optimal duration of panic therapy is unknown, but at least 12 months is recommended, and some patients require chronic therapy.
- The SSRIs are considered first-line treatment for panic disorder, generalized SAD, and PTSD and should be used in patients who also have depression, other anxiety disorders, or a history of substance abuse.
- After treatment response in SAD, the patient should be continued on pharmacotherapy for at least 12 months before the medication is tapered slowly.
- Mood stabilizers may be helpful in patients with PTSD with prominent symptoms of irritability or anger. TCAs and BZs are not effective treatment options for PTSD.
- The symptoms of PTSD may respond slowly to pharmacotherapy, and an adequate initial antidepressant trial lasts at least 8 weeks; treatment duration is at least 12 to 24 months in length.

REFERENCES

1. American Psychiatric Association. Diagnostic and Statistical Manual of Mental Disorders, 4th ed, text revision (DSM-IV-TR). Washington, American Psychiatric Association, 2000:429–484.
2. Kessler RC, McGonagle KA, Zhao S, et al. Lifetime and 12-month prevalence of DSM-III-R psychiatric disorders in the United States: Results from the National Comorbidity Survey. Arch Gen Psychiatry 1994;51: 8–19.
3. Zajecka J. Importance of establishing the diagnosis of persistent anxiety. J Clin Psychiatry 1997;58(Suppl 3):9–13.
4. Bowen RC, Senthilselvan A, Barale A. Physical illness as an outcome of chronic anxiety disorders. Can J Psychiatry 2000;45:459–464.
5. Rickels K, Schwizer E. The spectrum of generalised anxiety in clinical practice: The role of short-term, intermittent treatment. Br J Psychiatry 1998;173(Suppl 34):49–54.
6. Greenberg PE, Sistsky T, Kessler RC, et al. The economic burden of anxiety disorders in the 1990s. J Clin Psychiatry 1999;60:427–435.
7. Gliatto MF. Generalized anxiety disorder. Am Fam Physician 2000; 62:1591–1600, 1602.
8. Marsh CM. Psychiatric presentations of medical illness. Psychiatr Clin North Am 1997;20:181–205.
9. DeVane CL. The place of selective serotonin reuptake inhibitors in panic disorder. Pharmacotherapy 1997;17:282–292.
10. Goddard AW, Charney DS. Toward an integrated neurobiology of panic disorder. J Clin Psychiatry 1997;58(Suppl 2):4–11.
11. Ninan PT. The functional anatomy, neurochemistry, and pharmacology of anxiety. J Clin Psychiatry 1999;60(Suppl 22):12–17.
12. Johnson MR, Lydiard RB. The neurobiology of anxiety disorders. Psychiatr Clin North Am 1995;18:681–725.
13. Gorman JM, Kent JM, Sullivan GM, Coplan JD. Neuroanatomical hypothesis of panic disorder, revised. Am J Psychiatry 2000;157:493–505.
14. Wisden W, Stephens DN. Towards better benzodiazepines. Nature 1999; 401:751–752.
15. Nutt DJ, Bell CJ, Malizia AL. Brain mechanisms of social anxiety disorder. J Clin Psychiatry 1998;59(Suppl 17):4–11.
16. Brawman-Mintzer O, Lydiard RB. Biologic basis of generalized anxiety disorder. J Clin Psychiatry 1997;58(Suppl 3):16–25.
17. Connor KM, Davidson JRT. Generalized anxiety disorder: Neurobiological and pharmacological perspectives. Biol Psychiatry 1998;44:1286–1294.
18. Nutt DJ. The psychobiology of posttraumatic stress disorder. J Clin Psychiatry 2000;61(Suppl 5):24–29.
19. Mendlowicz MV, Stein MB. Quality of life in individuals with anxiety disorders. Am J Psychiatry 2000;157:669–682.
20. Ballenger JC, Davidson JRT, Lecrubier Y, et al. Consensus statement on social anxiety disorder from the International Consensus Group on Depression and Anxiety. J Clin Psychiatry 1998;59(Suppl 17): 54–60.
21. Ballenger JC, Davidson JRT, Lecrubier Y, et al. Consensus statement on posttraumatic stress disorder from the International Consensus Group on Depression and Anxiety. J Clin Psychiatry 2000;61(Suppl 5):60–66.
22. Thompson PM. Generalized anxiety disorder treatment algorithm. Psychiatr Ann 1996;4:227–232.
23. Hales RE, Hilty DA, Wise MG. A treatment algorithm for the management of anxiety in primary care. J Clin Psychiatry 1997;58(Suppl 3): 76–80.
24. Osser DN, Renner JA, Bayog R. Algorthims for the pharmacotherapy of anxiety disorders in patients with chemical abuse and dependence. Psychiatr Ann 1999;29:285–299.
25. Shader, RI, Greenblatt DJ. Can you provide a table of equivalences for benzodiazepines and other marketed benzodiazepine agonists? J Clin Psychopharmacol 1997;17:331.
26. Klonopin package insert. Nutley, NJ, Roche Laboratories, June 1999.
27. Nelson J, Chouinard G. Guidelines for the clinical use of benzodiazepines: Pharmacokinetics, dependency, rebound and withdrawal. Can J Pharmacol 1999;6:69–83.

28. Bailey L, Ward M, Musa M. Clinical pharmacokinetics of benzodiazepines. J Clin Pharmacol 1994;34:804–811.
29. Tanaka E. Clinically significant pharmacokinetic drug interactions with benzodiazepines. J Clin Pharmacol Ther 1999;24:347–355.
30. Sheikh JI, Cassidy EL. Treatment of anxiety disorders in the elderly: Issues and strategies. J Anxiety Disord 2000;14:173–90.
31. Longo LP, Johnson B. Benzodiazepines: Side effects, abuse risk and alternatives (Addiction Part 1). Am Fam Physician 2000;61:2121–2128.
32. Möller H. Effectiveness and safety of benzodiazepines. J Clin Pharmacol 1999;19(Suppl 2):2S–11S.
33. Michelini S, Cassano GB, Frare F, Perugi G. Long-term use of benzodiazepines: Tolerance, dependence and clinical problems in anxiety and mood disorders. Pharmacopsychiatry 1996;29:127–134.
34. Rickels K, DeMartinis N, Rynn M, Mandos L. Pharmacologic strategies for discontinuing benzodiazepine treatment. J Clin Pharmacol 1999; 19(Suppl 2):12S–16S.
35. Mahe V, Balogh A. Long-term pharmacological treatment of generalized anxiety disorder. Int Clin Psychopharmacol 2000;15:99–105.
36. Lydiard RB, Brawman-Mintzer O, Ballenger JC. Recent developments in the psychopharmacology of anxiety disorders. J Consult Clin Psychol 1996;64:660–668.
37. Sramek JJ, Transman M, Suri A, et al. Efficacy of buspirone in generalized anxiety disorder with coexisting mild depressive symptoms. J Clin Psychiatry 1996;57:287–291.
38. Lechin F, van der Dijs B, Java H, et al. Effects of buspirone on plasma neurotransmitters in healthy subjects. J Neural Trans 1998;105:561–573.
39. Mahmood I, Sahajwalla C. Clinical pharmacokinetics and pharmacodynamics of buspirone, an anxiolytic drug. Clin Pharmacokinet 1999; 36:277–287.
40. Schweizer E, Rickels K. Strategies for treatment of generalized anxiety in the primary care setting. J Clin Psychiatry 1997;58(Suppl 3):27–31.
41. Morgan J, Tyrer P. Treating the somatic symptoms of anxiety. CNS Drugs 1994; Vol. 3:427–434.
42. Rickels K, Pollack MH, Sheehan DV, Haskins JT. Efficacy of extended-release venlafaxine in nondepressed outpatients with generalized anxiety disorder. Am J Psychiatry 2000;157:968–974.
43. Gelenberg AJ, Lydiard RB, Rudolph RL, et al. Efficacy of venlafaxine extended-release capsules in nondepressed outpatients with generalized anxiety disorder: A 6-month randomized controlled trial. JAMA 2000;283:3082–3088.
44. Rocca P, Fonzo V, Scotta M, et al. Paroxetine efficacy in the treatment of generalized anxiety disorder. Acta Psychiatr Scand 1997;95:444–450.
45. Pollack MH, Zaninelli R, Goddard A, et al. Paroxetine in the treatment of generalized anxiety disorder: Results of a placebo-controlled, flexible-dosage trial. J Clin Psychiatry 2001;62:350–357.
46. Ferreri M, Hantouche EG. Recent clinical trials of hydroxyzine in generalized anxiety disorder. Acta Psychiatr Scand 1998;98(Suppl 393): 102–108.
47. Letterman L, Markowitz JS. Gabapentin: A review of published experience in the treatment of bipolar disorder and other psychiatric conditions. Pharmacotherapy 1999;19:565–572.
48. Pittler MH, Ernst E. Efficacy of kava extract for treating anxiety: Systematic review and meta-analysis. J Clin Psychopharmacol 2000;20:84–89.
49. Rice DP, Miller LS. Health economics and cost implications of anxiety disorders and other mental disorders in the United States. Br J Psychiatry 1998:173(Suppl 34):4–9.
50. Leon AC, Portera L, Weissman MM. The social costs of anxiety disorders. Br J Psychiatry 1995;166(Suppl 27):19–22.
51. Ormel J, VonKorff M, Ustun TB, et al. Common mental disorders and disability across cultures: Results from the WHO collaborative study on psychological problems in general health care. JAMA 1994; 272:1741–1748.
52. Kennedy BL, Schwab JJ. Utilization of medical specialists by anxiety disorder patients. Psychosomatics 1997;38:109–112.
53. Starcevic V. Treatment goals for panic disorder. J Clin Psychopharmacol 1998;18(Suppl 2):19S–26S.
54. Keller MB, Yonkers KA, Warshaw MG, et al. Remission and relapse in subjects with panic disorder and panic disorder with agoraphobia: A prospective, short-interval naturalistic follow-up. J Nerv Ment Dis 1994;182:290–296.
55. Barlow DH, Gorman JM, Shear MK, Woods SW. Cognitive-behavioral therapy, imipramine, or their combination for panic disorder. JAMA 2000;283:2529–2536.
56. Saeed SA, Bruce TJ. Panic disorder: Effective treatment options. Am Fam Physician 1998;57:2405–2412.
57. de Beurs E, van Balkom AJ, van Dyck R, Lange A. Long-term outcome of pharmacological and psychological treatment of panic disorder with agoraphobia: A 2-year naturalistic follow-up. Acta Psychiatr Scand 1999;99:59–67.
58. Coplan JD, Pine DS, Papp LA, Gorman JM. An algorithm-oriented treatment approach for panic disorder. Psychiatr Ann 1996;26:192–201.
59. Boyer W. Serotonin uptake inhibitors are superior to imipramine and alprazolam in alleviating panic attacks: A meta-analysis. Int Clin Psychopharmacol 1995;10:45–49.
60. Gorman J, Shear K, Cowley D, et al. Practice guideline for the treatment of patients with panic disorder. Am J Psychiatry 1998;155(Suppl 5): 1–34.
61. Calliard V, Rouillon F, Viel JF, Markabi S, and the French University Antidepressant Group. Comparative effects of low and high doses of clomipramine and placebo in panic disorder: A double-blind controlled study. Acta Psychiatr Scand 1999;99:51–58.
62. Noyes R, Burrows GD, Reich JH, et al. Diazepam versus alprazolam for the treatment of panic disorder. J Clin Psychiatry 1996;57:349–355.
63. Papp LA, Coplan JD, Martinez JM, et al. Efficacy of open-label nefazodone treatment in patients with panic disorder. J Clin Psychopharmacol 2000;20:544–546.
64. Pollack MH, Worthington JJ, Otto MW, et al. Venlafaxine for panic disorder: Results from a double-blind, placebo-controlled study. Psychopharmacol Bull 1996;32:667–670.
65. Pande AC, Pollack MH, Crockatt J, et al. Placebo-controlled study of gabapentin in treatment of panic disorder. J Clin Psychopharmacol 2000;20:467–471.
66. Unutzer J, Klap R, Sturm R, et al. Mental disorders and the use of alternative medicine: Results from a national survey. Am J Psychiatry 2000;157:1851–1857.
67. Baetz M, Bowen RC. Efficacy of divalproex sodium in patients with panic disorder and mood instability who have not responded to conventional therapy. Can J Psychiatry 1998;43:73–77.
68. Pollack MH, Otto MW, Worthington JJ, et al. Sertraline in the treatment of panic disorder: A flexible-dose multicenter trial. Arch Gen Psychiatry 1998;55:1010–1016.
69. Ballenger JC, Wheadon DE, Steiner M, et al. Double-blind, fixed-dose, placebo-controlled study of paroxetine in the treatment of panic disorder. Am J Psychiatry 1998;155:36–42.
70. Hoehn-Saric R, McLeod DR, Hipsley PA. Effect of fluvoxamine on panic disorder. J Clin Psychopharmacol 1993;13:321–326.
71. Lepola UM, Wade AG, Leinonen EV, et al. A controlled, prospective, 1-year trial of citalopram in the treatment of panic disorder. J Clin Psychiatry 1998;59:528–534.
72. Sheehan DV. Current concepts in the treatment of panic disorder. J Clin Psychiatry 1999;60(Suppl 18):16–21.
73. Emmanuel NP, Ware MR, Brawn-Mintzer O, et al. Once-weekly dosing of fluoxetine in the maintenance of remission in panic disorder. J Clin Psychiatry 1999;60:299–301.
74. Moroz G, Rosenbaun JF. Efficacy, safety, and gradual discontinuation of clonazepam in panic disorder: A placebo-controlled, multicenter study using optimized dosages. J Clin Psychiatry 1999;60:604–612.
75. Salvador-Carulla L, Seguí J, Fernández-Cano P, Canet J. Costs and offset effect in panic disorder. Br J Psychiatry 1995;166(Suppl 27): 23–28.
76. Shear MK, Brown TA, Barlow DH, et al. The Multicenter Collaborative Panic Disorder Severity Scale. Am J Psychiatry 1997;154:1571–1574.
77. Fones CS, Manfro GG, Pollack MH. Social phobia: An update. Harvard Rev Psychiatry 1998;5:247–259.
78. Stein MB, Liebowitz MR, Lydiard RB, et al. Paroxetine treatment of generalized social phobia (social anxiety disorder): A randomized, controlled trial. JAMA 1998;280:708–713.

79. Stein MB, Fyer AJ, Davidson JRT, et al. Fluvoxamine treatment of social phobia (social anxiety disorder): A double-blind, placebo-controlled study. Am J Psychiatry 1999;156:756–760.
80. Katzelnick DJ, Kobak KA, Greist JH, et al. Sertraline for social phobia: A double-blind, placebo-controlled crossover study. Am J Psychiatry 1995;152:1368–1371.
81. Bouwer C, Stein DJ. Use of the selective serotonin reuptake inhibitor citalopram in the treatment of generalized social phobia. J Affect Disorder 1998;49:79–82.
82. Van Amerigen M, Mancini C, Streier DL. Fluoxetine efficacy in social phobia. J Clin Psychiatry 1993;54:27–32.
83. Heimberg RG, Liebowitz MR, Hope DA, et al. Cognitive behavioral group therapy versus phenelzine therapy for social phobia: 12-week outcome. Arch Gen Psychiatry 1998;55:1133–1141.
84. Simpson HB, Schneir FR, Marshall RD, et al. Low dose selegiline (L-Deprenyl) in social phobia. Depress Anxiety 1998;7:126–129.
85. Simpson HB, Schneir FR, Campeas RB, et al. Imipramine in the treatment of social phobia. J Clin Psychopharmacol 1998;18:132–135.
86. Van Amerigen M, Mancini C, Oakman JM. Nefazodone in social phobia. J Clin Psychiatry 1999;60:96–100.
87. Kelsey JE. Venlafaxine in social phobia. Psychopharmacol Bull 1995;31 (4):767–771.
88. Davidson JRT, Tupler LA, Potts NL. Treatment of social phobia with benzodiazepines. J Clin Psychiatry 1994;55(Suppl 3):28–32.
89. Turner SM, Beidel DC, Jacob RG. Social phobia: A comparison of behavior therapy and atenolol. J Consult Clin Psychol 1994;62(2):350–358.
90. Pollack MH. Social anxiety disorder: Designing a pharmacologic treatment strategy. J Clin Psychiatry 1999;60(Suppl 9):20–26.
91. Pande AC, Davidson JRT, Jefferson JW, et al. Treatment of social phobia with gabapentin: A placebo-controlled study. J Clin Psychopharmacol 1999;19:341–348.
92. van Vliet IM, den Boer JA, Westenberg HG, Pian KL. Clinical effects of buspirone in social phobia: A double-blind placebo-controlled study. J Clin Psychiatry 1997;58:164–168.
93. Van Amerigen M, Mancini C, Wilson C. Buspirone augmentation of selective serotonin reuptake inhibitors (SSRIs) in social phobia. J Affect Disord 1996;39:115–121.
94. Stein MB, Chartier MJ, Hazen AL, et al. Paroxetine in the treatment of generalized social phobia: Open-label treatment and double-blind placebo-controlled discontinuation. J Clin Psychopharmacol 1996;16: 218–222.
95. Sutherland SM, Tupler LA, Colkert JT, et al. A 2-year follow-up of social phobia: Status after a brief medication trial. J Nerv Mental Dis 1996;184:731–738.
96. Connor KM, Davidson JRT, Potts NL, et al. Discontinuation of clonazepam in the treatment of social phobia. J Clin Psychopharmacol 1998;18:373–378.
97. Olfson M, Guardino M, Struening E, et al. Barriers to the treatment of social anxiety. Am J Psychiatry 2000;157:521–527.
98. The Expert Consensus Guideline Series. Treatment of posttraumatic stress disorder. The Expert Consensus Panel for Posttraumatic Stress Disorder. J Clin Psychiatry 1999;60(Suppl 16):3–76.
99. Brady K, Pearlstein T, Asnis GM, et al. Efficacy and safety of sertraline treatment of posttraumatic stress disorder: A randomized controlled trial. JAMA 2000;283:1837–1844.
100. Rothbaum BO, Ninan PT, Thomas L. Sertraline in the treatment of rape victims with posttraumatic stress disorder. J Trauma Stress 1996;9(4): 865–871.
101. Kline NA, Dow BM, Brown SA, Matloff JL. Sertraline efficacy in depressed combat veterans with posttraumatic stress disorder. Am J Psychiatry 1994;151(4):621.
102. Brady KT, Sonne SC, Roberts JM. Sertraline treatment of comorbid posttraumatic stress disorder and alcohol dependence. J Clin Psychiatry 1995;56(11):502–505.
103. Connor KM, Sutherland SM, Tupler LA, et al. Fluoxetine in posttraumatic stress disorder. Br J Psychiatry 1999;175:17–22.
104. Marmar CR, Schoenfeld F, Weiss DS, et al. Open trial of fluvoxamine treatment for combat-related posttraumatic stress disorder. J Clin Psychiatry 1996;57(Suppl 8);66–72.
105. Marshall RD, Schneier FR, Fallon BA, et al. An open trial of paroxetine in patients with noncombat-related chronic posttraumatic stress disorder. J Clin Psychopharmacol 1998;18:10–18.
106. Southwick SM, Yehuda R, Giller CL, et al. Use of tricyclics and MAOIs in the treatment of PTSD: A quantitative review. In: Murburg MM, ed. Catecholamine function in PTSD: Emerging Concepts. Washington, American Psychiatric Press, 1994:293–305.
107. Hidalgo R, Hertzberg MA, Mellman T, et al. Nefazodone in posttraumatic stress disorder: Results from six open-label trials. Int Clin Psychopharmacol 1999;14:61–68.
108. Zisook S, Chentsova-Dutton YE, Smith-Vaniz A, et al. Nefazodone in patients with treatment-refractory posttraumatic stress disorder. J Clin Psychiatry 2000;61:203–208.
109. Hertzberg MA, Feldman ME, Beckham JC, et al. Trial of trazodone for posttraumatic stress disorder using a multiple baseline group design. J Clin Psychopharmacol 1996;16:294–298.
110. Connor KM, Davidson JRT, Weisler RH, Ahearn E. A pilot study of mirtazapine in post-traumatic stress disorder. Int Clin Psychopharmacol 1999;14:29–31.
111. Canive JM, Clark RD, Calais LA, et al. Bupropion treatment in veterans with posttraumatic stress disorder: An open study. J Clin Psychopharmacol 1998;18:379–383.
112. Hamner MB, Frueh BC. Response to venlafaxine in a previously antidepressant treatment-resistant combat veteran with post-traumatic stress disorder. Int Clin Psychopharmacol 1998;13(5):233–234.
113. Hertzberg MA, Butterfield MI, Feldman ME, et al. A preliminary study of lamotrigine for the treatment of posttraumatic stress disorder. Biol Psychiatry 1999;45:1226–1229.
114. Brannon N, Labbate L, Huber M. Gabapentin treatment for posttraumatic stress disorder. Can J Psychiatry 2000;45:84.
115. Macleod AD. Vigabatrin and posttraumatic stress disorder. J Clin Psychopharmacol 1996;16(2):190–191.
116. Clark RD, Canive JM, Calais LA, et al. Divalproex in posttraumatic stress disorder: An open-label clinical trial. J Trauma Stress 1999;12(2):395–401.
117. Looff D, Grimley P, Kuller F, et al. Carbamazepine for PTSD. J Am Acad Child Adolec Psychiatry 1995;34(6):703–704.
118. Forster PL, Schoenfeld FB, Marman CR, Lang AJ. Lithium for irritability in post-traumatic stress disorder. J Trauma Stress 1995;8(1):143–149.
119. Friedman MJ, Davidson JRT, Mellman TA, Southwick SM. Pharmacotherapy. In: Foa EB, Keane TM, Friedman MJ, eds. Effective treatments of PTSD. New York, Guilford Press, 2000:84–105.
120. Raskind MA, Dobie DJ, Kanter ED, et al. The α_1-adrenergic antagonist prazosin ameliorates combat trauma nightmares in veterans with PTSD: A report of 4 cases. J Clin Psychiatry 2000;61:129–133.
121. Duffy JD, Malloy PF. Efficacy of buspirone in the treatment of PTSD: An open trial. Ann Clin Psychiatry 1994;6:33–37.
122. Hamner M, Velmer H, Home D. Buspirone potentiation of antidepressants in the treatment of PTSD. Depress Anxiety 1997;5:137–139.
123. Monnelly E, Ciraulo DA. Risperidone effects on irritable aggression in posttraumatic stress disorder. J Clin Psychopharmacol 1999;19(4):377–378.
124. Krashin D, Oates EW. Risperidone as an adjunct therapy for posttraumatic stress disorder. Milit Med 1999;164:605–606.
125. Davidson JRT. Pharmacotherapy of posttraumatic stress disorder: Treatment options, long-term follow-up, and predictors of outcome. J Clin Psychiatry 2000;61(Suppl 5):52–56.
126. Malik ML, Connor KM, Sutherland SM, et al. Quality of life and PTSD: A pilot study assessing changes in SF-36 scores before and after treatment in a placebo-controlled trial of fluoxetine. J Trauma Stress 1999;12:387–393.

72

OBSESSIVE-COMPULSIVE DISORDER

Barbara G. Wells and Peggy E. Hayes

Although symptoms of obsessive-compulsive disorder (OCD) have been recognized for centuries and have remained virtually unchanged, OCD has only recently been the focus of extensive research. These investigations have greatly advanced our understanding of the epidemiology, etiology, and pharmacologic treatment of this disorder. Since the mid-1980s, the Food and Drug Administration (FDA) has approved five drugs, as effective for the treatment of OCD: clomipramine (Anafranil), fluoxetine (Prozac), fluvoxamine (Luvox), paroxetine (Paxil), and sertraline (Zoloft). Although OCD is officially classified as an anxiety disorder, it is presented as a separate illness because of its unique clinical presentation and treatment approach. OCD is the most disabling of the anxiety disorders and rarely remits without specific behavioral and pharmacologic interventions. Unfortunately, despite treatment the prognosis often remains poor, and many patients continue to suffer disabling symptoms and a lifelong disability.[1]

EPIDEMIOLOGY

The National Institute of Mental Health Epidemiologic Catchment Area Study (ECA) provides data regarding the prevalence of mental illness, including OCD. The ECA studies were extensive community surveys conducted from 1980 to 1984 in five areas across the United States. These studies estimated the prevalence of psychiatric illness among community populations and included persons not seeking psychiatric treatment.[2,3]

A most surprising finding was that OCD is approximately 50 times more common than previously reported by surveys conducted using clinical populations (or persons seeking treatment). The ECA studies found a lifetime prevalence of OCD ranging from 1.9% to 3.2% and a 1-year prevalence rate of 1.5% to 2.1%.[2] More recent data in children and adolescents suggest a lifetime prevalence of 1% to 2.3% and a 1-year prevalence of 0.7%. Prevalence rates appear to be similar in many different cultures around the world.[1]

OCD usually begins in late adolescence or early adulthood, but it may begin in childhood. Childhood-, adolescence-, and adult-onset OCD have a similar clinical presentation. In adults, the disorder is equally common in females and males, but in childhood-onset OCD, it is more common in boys than in girls.[1] Males tend to have an earlier modal age of onset (between ages 6 and 15 years for males vs ages 20 and 29 years for females). The onset is usually gradual with a chronic waxing and waning course.[1,3] OCD may have a familial component to its etiology.[4,5] Approximately 10% of first-degree relatives (mother, father, sibling) of patients with OCD have OCD, and another 8% have a subclinical form of the disorder. In a comparison group of first-degree relatives of normal subjects, there was a prevalence of only 2% for OCD and another 2% for the subclinical form.[4] When one twin has OCD, the concordance rate is higher for monozygotic twins than for dizygotic twins.[3,5]

PATHOPHYSIOLOGY

Although OCD occasionally begins following a brain injury, especially involving the basal ganglion (e.g., encephalitis or trauma), there is usually no neurologic precipitant. The most compelling evidence suggesting a biologic basis for OCD is the consistent successful treatment using selective and potent serotonin (5-HT) reuptake-blocking drugs. Treatment trials with drugs having other mechanisms of action have not been effective. The neurotransmitter 5-HT appears to play an important role in the pathogenesis of OCD.[6,7] Although studies of 5-HT function dominate research into the pathophysiology of OCD, a clear model of serotonergic dysfunction to explain the pathophysiology of OCD is lacking. (For example, is there a decrease or increase in serotonergic function, and what specific subtypes of 5-HT receptors are involved?)

SEROTONERGIC PROBES

Important evidence for an abnormality in 5-HT functioning comes from pharmacologic challenge studies that assess serotonergic responsiveness in OCD patients.[8,9] The most frequently used probe in studies of OCD has been *m*-chlorophenylpiperazine (m-CPP). A nonspecific postsynaptic 5-HT agonist and metabolite of the antidepressant trazodone, m-CPP produced very limited behavioral effects in normal volunteers. In untreated OCD patients, m-CPP produced a marked, but transient, increase in obsessions, depression, and anxiety symptoms.[3,5,8] These findings indicate an increased sensitivity to m-CPP in some untreated OCD patients. Treatment with clomipramine[3,5] and fluoxetine[8] abolished the pretreatment m-CPP-induced exacerbation of obsessive-compulsive symptoms. Several other 5-HT probes have been studied in OCD patients (metergoline, ipsapirone, L-tryptophan, fenfluramine). However, the serotonergic probes have been disappointing in their failure to identify a consistent 5-HT defect in OCD.[9]

BRAIN-IMAGING STUDIES

Structural brain-imaging studies with computed tomography and magnetic resonance imaging have not identified the presence of a clear lesion (structural pathology) in patients with OCD.[10,11] However, brain-imaging studies to assess the biochemical and physiologic function of the brain using single-photon emission computed tomography and positron emission tomography have produced consistent findings that identify three areas of increased/abnormal metabolic activity—the orbitofrontal cortex, cingulate cortex, and head of the caudate nucleus.[10,11] These areas may be involved in the pathophysiologic origin of OCD symptoms and may form a circuit that is "hyperactive" in OCD. However, these areas of increased metabolic activity may be merely compensating for areas of decreased brain activity. Successful pharmacologic treatment of OCD patients with increased metabolic activity in the caudate nucleus and the orbitofrontal cortex was associated with a return to normal metabolic functioning.

DOPAMINE MODEL

Because neurologic symptoms (tics) are part of the clinical presentation in some OCD patients, and because some patients have a family history of Tourette's syndrome, a disorder of dopamine (DA) dysfunction, DA dysregulation may contribute to some forms of OCD. The neurotransmitter DA is found in high concentrations in the caudate nucleus, an area believed to be "hyperactive" in OCD. OCD patients with tics often benefit from the addition of an antipsychotic to their treatment regimen.[3,12]

CLINICAL PRESENTATION

The Diagnostic and Statistical Manual of Mental Disorders, 4th edition, text revision (DSM-IV-TR) requires the presence of either obsessions and/or compulsions (although most patients have both) that are severe enough to cause marked distress, to be time-consuming (occupy more than 1 hour a day), and to cause significant impairment in social or occupational functioning (Table 72–1).[1] These individuals often recognize that their obsessions or compulsions are excessive or unreasonable. An obsession is a recurrent, persistent idea, thought, impulse, or image that is experienced as intrusive and inappropriate and produces marked anxiety. Common obsessions involve thoughts about contamination (such as a concern with germs, dirt, or toxic chemicals), repeated doubts (e.g., whether a door was left unlocked), and needing to have things in a particular order.[1,5] Individuals recognize obsessions as products of their own mind and attempt to ignore or suppress them. "No matter how hard I try, I cannot get this crazy thought out of my mind." An obsession produces a marked feeling of anxiety and is not simply excessive worry about a real life situation.[1,5]

TABLE 72–1. DSM-IV-TR Diagnostic Criteria for Obsessive-Compulsive Disorder

A. Either obsessions or compulsions:

Obsessions as defined by (1), (2), (3), and (4):

(1) Recurrent and persistent thoughts, impulses, or images that are experienced, *at some time during the disturbance,* as intrusive and *inappropriate and that cause marked anxiety or distress.*

(2) The thoughts, impulses, or images are not simply excessive worries about real-life problems.

(3) Attempts are made to ignore or suppress the thoughts, impulses, or images or to eliminate them.

(4) It is recognized that the obsessional thoughts, impulses, or images are a product of the person's own mind (not imposed from without).

Compulsions as defined by (1) and (2):

(1) Repetitive behaviors (e.g., hand washing, ordering, checking) or mental acts (e.g., praying, counting, repeating words silently) that the person feels driven to perform in response to an obsession, or according to certain rules.

(2) The behaviors or mental acts are aimed at preventing or reducing distress or preventing some dreaded event or situation; however, these behaviors or mental acts either are not connected in a realistic way with what they are designed to eliminate or they are clearly excessive.

B. The person has recognized that the obsessions or compulsions are excessive or unreasonable.*

C. The obsessions or compulsions cause marked distress, are time consuming (take more than 1 hour a day), or significantly interfere with the person's normal routine, occupational (or academic) functioning, or usual social activities or relationships.

D. If another Axis I disorder is present, the content of the obsessions or compulsions is not restricted to it (e.g., preoccupation with food in the presence of an eating disorder).

E. The disturbance is not due to the direct physiologic effects of a substance or a general medical condition.

*Does not apply to children.

Modified and reprinted with permission from the Diagnostic and Statistical Manual of Mental Disorders, 4th ed., Text Revision, Copyright 2000, American Psychiatric Association.

A compulsion is a repetitive, purposeful, intentional behavior or mental act usually performed in response to an obsession. The most common compulsions involve washing and cleaning, counting, checking, and requesting or demanding assurances. Compulsive behavior is not pleasurable and is designed to prevent discomfort or the occurrence of a dreaded event that is often unknown. For example, many patients are obsessed with feelings of doubt (e.g., whether a door was left unlocked), causing them marked distress, and leading to repetitive checking (or compulsive behaviors). These behaviors are usually performed according to certain rules or in a stereotyped fashion.[1,5]

The individual recognizes compulsions as senseless. Because patients recognize their behavior as silly, they become extremely adept at denying symptoms, disguising their rituals, and concealing their illness from friends and family members.[1,5]

In addition to primary symptoms, about 20% to 40% of patients have involuntary motor movements (e.g., facial tics and grimaces).[3,5] The overlap between Tourette's syndrome and OCD is well documented. Tourette's syndrome, a neurologic disorder that begins in childhood, is characterized by repetitive, involuntary, multiple motor and vocal tics.[13] Some OCD patients meet criteria for Tourette's syndrome, and some Tourette's patients have symptoms of OCD.[3,5]

Many patients experience disabling symptoms for several years before seeking treatment.[2,3] Typically, almost 7.5 years elapse between the onset of clinical symptoms and the first psychiatric visit.[2,3] Although the consequences of untreated OCD have not been systematically studied, OCD produces significant work and social disability. Depression and anxiety symptoms are also present in many patients with OCD, and depression often prompts patients to seek treatment.[1,3] The ECA study reported that approximately 50% of patients with OCD had another major psychiatric disorder (e.g., major depression, alcohol abuse or dependence, panic disorder, or schizophrenia). In most patients, OCD occurred first.[2,5] This means that certain illnesses (e.g., major depression, alcohol abuse, and panic disorder) might be consequences of untreated OCD or part of the natural course of OCD. Therefore, OCD patients seeking treatment commonly require treatment for a comorbid psychiatric disorder. OCD is a chronic disorder that for most patients continues throughout adult life.[1,5]

DIFFERENTIAL DIAGNOSIS

Patients with OCD are aware of the irrationality of their symptoms, are often ashamed to admit their symptoms, and are skilled at hiding them.[1–3,5] Therefore, most cases of OCD are not recognized by the primary care physician. Certain disorders have symptoms resembling OCD (known as OCD spectrum disorders), including trichotillomania (an urge to pull out one's hair), Tourette's syndrome, complex motor or vocal tics, eating disorders (15% of adult women with OCD had anorexia in adolescence), compulsive gambling, and compulsive sexual behaviors.[1,3] Patients with OCD often initially seek treatment from primary care physicians or dermatologists because of severe dermatitis from excessive washing.[3,5]

A distinction should be made between OCD and obsessive-compulsive personality disorder. Obsessions and compulsions are not present in obsessive-compulsive personality disorder. These individuals are preoccupied with orderliness, perfectionism, and control beginning early in childhood. Unlike individuals with OCD, those with obsessive-compulsive personality disorder do not view their behavior as irrational and do not wish to change, as they consider these personality features to be beneficial.[1,3,5]

▶ TREATMENT: Obsessive-Compulsive Disorder

DESIRED OUTCOME

A goal of treatment for OCD is to achieve as great a level of symptom reduction as possible while recognizing that a complete cure or elimination of all symptoms is unlikely.[14] An additional goal is to minimize adverse consequences on quality of life and to restore the patient to an optimal level of psychosocial and occupational functioning. However, most patients generally have symptom reduction far short of total symptom relief. Although several nondrug and drug therapies are superior to placebo, many patients continue to demonstrate significant symptomatology.

GENERAL APPROACH TO TREATMENT

In adolescents with OCD, cognitive-behavioral therapy (CBT) is generally selected first for milder OCD, but CBT plus a selective serotonin reuptake inhibitor (SSRI), such as fluoxetine, fluvoxamine, sertraline, or paroxetine, are selected for more severe OCD. In adults, CBT is selected first for milder OCD; CBT plus an SSRI or an SSRI alone is selected first for more severe OCD.[15] Clomipramine may be selected after two or three failed SSRI trials. Figure 72–1 presents an algorithm for the treatment of OCD.

NONPHARMACOLOGIC THERAPY

CBT is generally the treatment of choice for milder OCD in both adolescents and adults. For OCD, CBT involves exposure plus response prevention combined with cognitive therapy. When available, CBT should be offered to every OCD patient.[15] Two-thirds to three-fourths of patients who continue in therapy often respond,[16] but patients who agree to CBT must tolerate high levels of anxiety that often eventually cause them to discontinue therapy.[17] CBT should be added to the regimen when a patient has been a nonresponder or partial responder to a serotonin reuptake inhibitor (SRI) alone. SRIs include the SSRIs and clomipramine. CBT should be used alone if the patient is intolerant to side effects of medication, is pregnant, or has a medical condition that contraindicates medication.[15]

Exposure with response prevention is particularly helpful for contamination or other fears, symmetry rituals, counting/repeating, hoarding, and aggressive urges. Cognitive therapy is especially helpful for scrupulosity, moral guilt, and pathologic doubt. Thirteen to 20 sessions are typically required to treat uncomplicated OCD,[15] and an adequate trial is considered to be at least 20 hours.[18]

OCD patients with concomitant depression, psychosis, or mania are unlikely to respond to behavior therapy until these symptoms are well controlled with pharmacotherapy.[19] Eighty percent of patients will experience at least moderate improvement with combined treatment. Behavior therapy has little to offer the patient with severe obsessions who does not have compulsions (approximately 20% of OCD patients). In OCD patients who suffer from obsessive thoughts only (without compulsions), a trial of antiobsessional medication is a reasonable first choice.[19]

PHARMACOLOGIC THERAPY

MECHANISMS OF ACTION

Current evidence strongly indicates that 5-HT is important for the antiobsessional effects of medication. The SRIs inhibit 5-HT reuptake into the presynaptic neuron. Reuptake is the first and most important step in reducing 5-HT neurotransmission. Inhibiting reuptake of 5-HT makes more 5-HT available to postsynaptic receptors and reduces formation of the 5-HT metabolite, 5-hydroxyindoleacetic acid. Although other antidepressants, such as imipramine and amitriptyline, inhibit 5-HT reuptake, they are less potent and selective than the SRIs. Prolonged exposure to increased amounts of 5-HT following chronic antidepressant treatment (2–3 weeks) leads to altered responsiveness of postsynaptic 5-HT receptors or presynaptic autoregulatory receptors that may govern 5-HT release in specific brain regions.[14]

The most impressive and consistent evidence to support a role for 5-HT in treating OCD is that only potent 5-HT reuptake inhibitors appear to be consistently effective. Furthermore, an improvement in obsessional symptoms may correlate with plasma concentrations of clomipramine but not desmethylclomipramine, the metabolite of clomipramine with less selectivity for 5-HT reuptake inhibition. With clomipramine treatment, the decrease in obsessional symptoms correlates with a decrease in the concentration of 5-HIAA in cerebrospinal fluid, and a decrease in platelet 5-HT content.[14] The effectiveness of serotonergic agents in treating OCD lends support to the role of 5-HT in the etiology of OCD. However, because many patients fail to respond to these agents, the role of other neurotransmitter systems in the pathophysiology of OCD must continue to be explored.

GENERAL PRINCIPLES

For adults and adolescents with mild symptoms, CBT is generally selected as first-line treatment. Drug therapy is reserved for patients with moderate to severe symptoms. SRIs may be combined with CBT or used alone in adults with moderate to severe symptoms. An SSRI should be added when there has been no response or partial response to CBT alone. Generally, an SSRI is selected before clomipramine and whenever anticholinergic, cardiovascular, sexual, sedative, or weight gain side effects are a major concern. If one SSRI is ineffective, then another SSRI should be tried. Treatment resistance can be defined as failure to achieve at least a 25% reduction in baseline score on the Yale-Brown Obsessive Compulsive Scale (Y-BOCS). Clomipramine may be selected after two to three failed SSRI trials. Clomipramine may also be used to augment an SSRI in partially responsive or non responsive patients.[15]

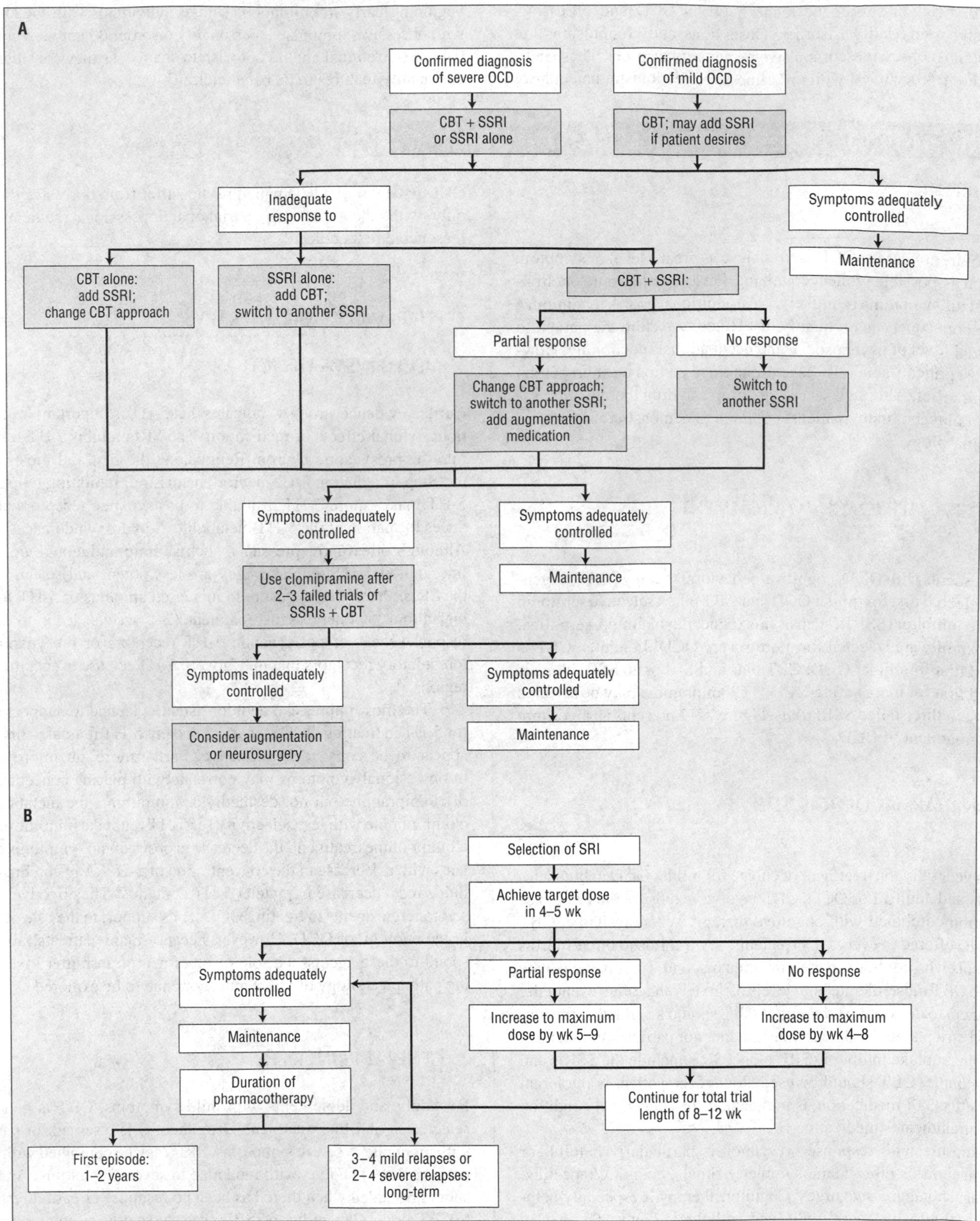

FIGURE 72–1. Algorithm for management of OCD in adults. **A.** Overall approach to treatment. **B.** Pharmacotherapeutic approach to treatment. (CBT, cognitive-behavioral therapy; SRI, serotonin reuptake inhibitor; SSRI, selective serotonin reuptake inhibitor.) *(Derived from Refs. 15 and 101.)*

COMORBID CONDITIONS

When OCD is complicated by comorbid illness, treatment strategies are individualized to the comorbid illness and to patient needs. In general, OCD in the pregnant patient is treated with CBT alone. OCD in a patient with cardiac or renal disease may be treated with CBT alone or CBT plus an SSRI. OCD in patients with Tourette's disorder may be treated with CBT plus a conventional antipsychotic and an SRI. OCD in the presence of attention-deficit hyperactivity disorder may be treated with CBT plus an SSRI and psychostimulant. OCD with panic disorder or social phobia may be treated with CBT and an SSRI. In a patient with OCD and major depression, CBT plus an SRI can be used, and the SRI should be started first for severe symptoms. CBT plus a mood stabilizer with or without an SRI may be used in patients with bipolar disorder. OCD may be treated with an SRI and antipsychotic in patients with comorbid schizophrenia.[15]

EFFICACY

The only medications consistently demonstrating efficacy in controlled clinical trials are the SRIs.[6,7,17,20–28] Overall, approximately 80% of patients who are compliant with drug and behavioral therapies have at least moderate improvement in symptoms.[29] Studies confirm the gradual improvement of obsessive and compulsive symptoms over a 4- to 10-week treatment period. For a review of the efficacy of drugs used to treat OCD, the reader is referred to Ellingrod's review.[30] It is unlikely that clinical trials will be able to demonstrate significant differences in efficacy between the SRIs, because 600–700 patients are probably required to show a statistically significant difference.[17]

In a 10-week randomized study of 31 patients treated with fluvoxamine, paroxetine, or citalopram, there was no significant difference in antiobsessional effects.[31] Another group found clomipramine to be as efficacious as fluoxetine or fluvoxamine in a one-on-one comparison.[32] A meta-analysis suggested that the efficacy of clomipramine was slightly superior to fluvoxamine, which was slightly superior to sertraline.[23] However, these data must be viewed with caution, because of varying methodologies between studies and differences in numbers of treatment-resistant patients and placebo responders. An additional meta-analysis supported the superiority of clomipramine over fluoxetine, fluvoxamine, and sertraline, but head-to-head double-blind comparisons would be the best evaluation of comparative efficacy.[7] Six of seven head-to-head comparisons of either fluoxetine, fluvoxamine, or paroxetine versus clomipramine found similar efficacy but a lower incidence of side effects with the SSRI.[33]

Although the FDA has not approved citalopram for treatment of OCD, evidence is accumulating to support its efficacy. Twenty-three children and adolescents with OCD were treated with citalopram (10–40 mg/day; modal dose, 40 mg/day) in an open trial design. More than 75% of patients showed a marked or moderate improvement.[34] In a double-blind, fixed-dose, placebo-controlled study, 401 patients were randomized to citalopram (20, 40, or 60 mg/day) or placebo. Both the Y-BOCs and the Clinical Global Impressions Scale scores were significantly more improved in the citalopram than in the placebo group at all three dosages. After 12 weeks of treatment, 63%, 54%, and 62% of patients taking citalopram 20 mg/day, 40 mg/day, and 60 mg/day were rated as "very much improved" or "much improved."[35]

Responders often experience only a 50% reduction in symptom severity. A patient showing partial response after 4–5 weeks of treatment may improve considerably if treatment is continued for several additional weeks. Approximately 60% to 70% of patients experience at least a moderate response to the SRIs as compared to 5% to 10% who respond to placebo.[6,17] Therefore, most patients continue to have symptoms severe enough to limit their functioning. Although this degree of improvement seems modest, patients usually find this improvement clearly preferable to their pretreatment condition and are often willing to tolerate substantial adverse effects to maintain partial symptom remission.

RELAPSE

Approximately 89% of 18 OCD patients chronically treated with clomipramine had a substantial recurrence of symptoms after a 7-week placebo period.[36] However, in a study of 35 OCD patients who discontinued fluoxetine after a good response, only 23% relapsed without medication during the first year.[37] Two years after discontinuation of therapy with clomipramine, fluvoxamine, or fluoxetine, relapse rates were 77% to 80%.[38] Behavior therapy that accompanies pharmacotherapy may not only increase the extent of symptom reduction, but may also enhance the persistence of improvement after drug therapy is discontinued.

PREDICTORS OF RESPONSE

Most investigators agree that factors failing to predict response to pharmacotherapy include severity of illness, presence of depression, duration of illness, type of symptoms (obsessions vs compulsions), dexamethasone resistance, reduced rapid-eye movement (REM) sleep latency, and platelet 5-HT measures.[14] However, Alarcon and associates[39] found that higher initial scores on the Y-BOCS were associated with poorer response to clomipramine. Furthermore, this group reported that the presence of cleaning rituals, such as washing or cleaning sinks, bathtubs, walls, and ovens, was a predictor of poor or modest response to clomipramine. An additional report found that the presence of panic or phobia with OCD is a positive predictor of response to clomipramine.[40] Good response to clomipramine was associated with a later age of OCD onset and certain early side effects (e.g., nervousness and erectile dysfunction).[41]

The SRIs may be more likely to be effective for pathologic doubt, mental rituals, and aggressive obsessions and urges than for slowness, hoarding, and tic-like symptoms.[15] Good response to fluoxetine was associated with early complaints of anxiety and reduced libido.[41] Response rates and overall improvement with fluoxetine is also associated with a history of remissions, no previous drug treatment, more severe OCD, or either low or high Hamilton Rating Scale for Depression scores.[42] The presence of hoarding obsessions and compulsions has been associated with poorer response to SSRIs.[43]

DOSING

Table 72–2 summarizes dosing guidelines. If there is inadequate response to an average SRI dose, then the dose should be pushed to the maximum dose within 4–9 weeks from the start of treatment. If there is an inadequate response after 4–6 weeks at the maximum dose, then another SRI should be tried. Eight to 13 weeks is considered an adequate trial before changing to another medication or augmenting with another agent.

MAINTENANCE

After patients have responded to the acute phase of treatment, treatment gains are maintained with maintenance phase strategies.

TABLE 72–2. Dosing of SRIs in Treatment of OCD

Generic Name	Usual Initial Daily Dose (mg)	Usual Daily Dosage Range (mg)	Average Target Daily Dose (mg)
Citalopram*	20	20–60	40
Clomipramine	10	100–250	150–200
Fluoxetine	20	20–80	40–60
Fluvoxamine	50	100–300	200
Paroxetine	20	20–60	40
Sertraline	50	75–200	150

*Not FDA-approved for treatment of OCD. Optimal dosing guidelines are not well established.
Modified from Ref. 15.

Monthly follow-up visits are recommended for at least 3 to 6 months, and a medication taper can be considered after 1 to 2 years of treatment. Medication should not be rapidly discontinued, and booster CBT sessions may reduce the risk of relapse when medication is withdrawn. Medication doses can be decreased by 25%, and then 2 months should lapse before again decreasing the dose, depending on response. Long-term or lifelong prophylactic maintenance medication is recommended after two to four severe relapses or three to four mild to moderate relapses.[15] Although the appropriate maintenance dose of the SRIs is unknown, it is notable that one investigator was successful in reducing the dose of clomipramine from a mean of 270 mg/day to 165 mg/day in the maintenance phase. Mundo and colleagues[44] studied patients successfully treated with clomipramine or fluvoxamine and reduced their doses by 33% to 66% for maintenance therapy. They found that maintenance therapy was successful with reduced dosages of the antiobsessional drug, with clear advantages for tolerability and compliance. However, study duration was only 102 days.[44]

SIDE EFFECTS

Most experts agree that the SSRIs are better tolerated than clomipramine. The SSRIs are less likely than clomipramine to cause cardiovascular, sedative, anticholinergic, and weight gain side effects. Clomipramine is less likely than the SSRIs to cause insomnia, akathisia, nausea, and diarrhea. Side effects may be more severe when larger doses are used and with faster dose escalation. Tolerance to adverse effects often develops over 6–8 weeks of treatment, and tolerance may be more likely to develop to nausea, diarrhea, sedation, diminished libido and/or orgasm, anxiety, restlessness, insomnia, and anticholinergic side effects than to akathisia.[15]

DRUG INTERACTIONS

SSRIs must not be given concurrently with monoamine oxidase inhibitors (MAOIs). It is usually recommended that 2 weeks elapse between administering an SSRI and an MAOI in either direction. However, 5 weeks should elapse after stopping fluoxetine before starting an MAOI, because of fluoxetine's long half-life of elimination. The concomitant use of an SSRI with sumatriptan warrants enhanced patient monitoring, as there are rare reports of mild to moderate symptoms suggestive of serotonin syndrome. Most patients tolerate this combination without incident.[45] SSRIs variably inhibit multiple components of the cytochrome P450 system that is responsible for metabolism of many psychotropic and other medications. Refer to Chap. 69 or the drug interaction literature for a more complete discussion of drug interactions involving the SRIs.

ALTERNATIVE PHARMACOLOGIC THERAPIES

Jenike and colleagues[46] conducted a 10-week, placebo-controlled trial in 64 patients with OCD, and found that only a subgroup of patients with symmetry or other atypical obsessions responded to therapy with phenelzine. Fluoxetine-treated patients (80 mg/day) improved significantly more than phenelzine-treated patients (60 mg/day) or placebo-treated patients. There was no efficacy of phenelzine overall or in a subgroup of patients with high levels of anxiety.[46] Based on limited data, the efficacy of MAOIs in OCD appears limited.

Benzodiazepines are rarely useful despite occasional case reports of response.[47] Limited evidence suggests that buspirone, a 5-HT_{1A} partial agonist, may occasionally be beneficial in the treatment of OCD.[48,49] These findings are preliminary, and further controlled studies with larger sample sizes are needed to assess whether buspirone is an effective agent in the treatment of OCD. Of 12 patients treated with St. John's wort (450 mg of hypericin 0.3%) in a 12-week open trial, 5 patients were "much" or "very much improved."[50]

SPECIAL POPULATIONS

Hepatic and Renal Disease

Clomipramine, fluoxetine, sertraline, paroxetine, fluvoxamine, and citalopram are extensively metabolized in the liver, and patients with significant liver disease should be prescribed these drugs cautiously and in lower doses than those used in healthy subjects. The pharmacokinetics of fluoxetine and fluvoxamine were similar in patients with renal failure and in healthy subjects; however, the manufacturer recommends starting with a lower dose in patients with renal impairment. The pharmacokinetics of sertraline is not altered in patients with significant renal dysfunction, and dosage adjustment is not necessary in these patients. Increased plasma concentrations of paroxetine occur in subjects with renal impairment. The initial dose of paroxetine should be reduced in patients with severe renal impairment, and upward titration should occur more slowly. No dosage adjustment is necessary for patients with mild to moderate renal impairment receiving citalopram.

Elderly Patients

There is little available information on treating OCD in the elderly. Case reports and anecdotal information suggest that the antiobsessional medications are likely to be equally effective in the elderly and in younger adults.[51,52] Selection of medication for an elderly person with OCD, however, should be based on history of response and adverse side-effect profile. Treatment should be initiated with low doses in elderly patients, and doses should be increased slowly, with vigilance for emergence of side effects. Some elderly patients may ultimately require doses similar to those used in younger adults, but doses must be individualized according to response and tolerance of side effects.

In elderly patients refractory to SSRIs, an augmentation strategy with minimal risk is to add buspirone to SSRI therapy. Buspirone has few side effects and appears to be a good choice for augmentation. On the other hand, clonazepam causes excessive sedation and may accumulate over time. It should not be prescribed as augmentation for the frail elderly or those with gait disturbances.[53]

Approximately 150 elderly patients received clomipramine in US clinical trials. Although no unusual age-related adverse effects were identified, age-related differences in efficacy or safety cannot be ruled out. This is especially true for elderly patients with coexisting diseases and those receiving concurrent drugs. Elderly patients receiving clomipramine may experience more sedation and anticholinergic adverse effects than younger adults.[6,54] Because of clomipramine's sedative and anticholinergic side effects, it is not usually chosen as first-line therapy for elderly OCD patients.

Plasma concentrations of fluoxetine are 127% higher in the elderly than in younger individuals receiving the same dose.[55] A lower or less frequent dosage should be considered for the elderly. The overall cardiovascular profile of fluoxetine appears quite favorable; however, Buff and associates[56] reported that atrial fibrillation and bradycardia developed in an 87-year-old woman shortly after fluoxetine was initiated. On fluoxetine rechallenge, these dysrhythmias recurred.

The multiple-dose elimination half-life of fluvoxamine was 17.4 and 25.9 hours in the elderly as compared to 13.6 and 15.6 hours in younger subjects at steady state for 50- and 100-mg doses, respectively.[57] The safety of fluvoxamine has not been adequately studied in the elderly and patients with cardiovascular disease. Dosage should be titrated slowly during initiation of fluvoxamine therapy in elderly patients.

Sertraline plasma clearance in elderly patients was approximately 40% lower than in a group of younger individuals. Clearance of desmethylsertraline was also decreased in elderly males, but not in elderly females. To date, the pattern of adverse reactions in the elderly appears to be similar to that in younger adults.

In a multiple-dose study in the elderly, paroxetine C_{min} concentrations were 70% to 80% greater than in nonelderly subjects. The manufacturer recommends that the initial dose be reduced in the elderly (10 mg/day). Doses should not exceed 40 mg/day. In worldwide premarketing trials, the adverse event profile was similar in elderly and nonelderly patients, but the patients in these studies were healthy.[58]

Citalopram half-life is increased in the elderly by 23% to 30%. Twenty mg is the recommended dose for most elderly patients, with titration to 40 mg/day only in nonresponders.

Children and Adolescents

Childhood and adult OCD appear to respond similarly to drug therapy. Data suggest that at least 50% of patients with childhood-onset OCD remain symptomatic as adults and have a chronic and debilitating course.[59]

Flament and colleagues[60] treated 19 children and adolescents with clomipramine in a 10-week, double-blind, placebo-controlled, crossover trial. Both this trial and a parallel group comparison[61] found clomipramine was significantly superior to placebo, and that 75% of patients had a moderate to marked improvement. In a double-blind, crossover study comparing clomipramine with desipramine, 48 children and adolescents completed the 10-week trial. Clomipramine was more effective than desipramine; however, desipramine was no more effective than placebo.[62] In both studies, clomipramine was well tolerated at doses of 3 mg/kg/day.

The SSRIs appear to be effective and well-tolerated in treatment of OCD in children. Of pharmacologic treatments, the SSRIs are generally considered first-choice agents. Sertraline, fluoxetine, and fluvoxamine are effective in children and adolescents. Treatment with an SSRI produces a favorable response in 75% of children and adolescents with OCD. A combination of SSRIs and CBT is preferred in most cases. In children, the most commonly described side effects of SSRI therapy include nausea, headache, tremor, gastrointestinal complaints, drowsiness, akathisia, insomnia, disinhibition, and agitation.[63] The reader is referred to a comprehensive review for details regarding clinical presentation, assessment, and treatment of OCD in children.[64]

Pregnant and Lactating Patients

In general, CBT alone should be used for pregnant patients except in cases where the risks of untreated OCD outweigh the risks of medication use in pregnancy (for example, a pregnant mother who will not eat because of contamination fears).[15] Women with a history of OCD should be informed that OCD may worsen during pregnancy and during the postpartum period. OCD symptoms may exacerbate during the first trimester, especially if pharmacotherapy is discontinued just before conception or early in pregnancy. Symptoms often improve during the second trimester and worsen during the third trimester.[65]

Data suggest that exposure to fluoxetine in the first trimester does not increase the risk of congenital malformations.[66,67] Transient withdrawal syndromes have been reported in infants exposed to imipramine and nortriptyline.[65] Prenatal clomipramine exposure has resulted in cases of infant hypothermia, respiratory acidosis, and seizures.[68,69]

If drug therapy during pregnancy is required, fluoxetine appears to be the safest choice. However, the neurobehavioral effects of prenatal exposure on the neonate and the child have not been fully elucidated. Clomipramine should probably be avoided during pregnancy.[65] Clonazepam may be considered for OCD symptoms in pregnant women with disabling anxiety, but with higher doses (2–5 mg) hypotonia, apnea, and failure to feed have been observed.[65]

In general, prescribing SSRIs during nursing is considered inadvisable. All SRIs are excreted into breast milk, and therefore, a decision must be made whether to discontinue nursing or discontinue drug therapy, weighing benefits against risks. With fluoxetine, one case of colic symptoms and unexplained high serum levels was reported in a breast-fed 5-week-old infant,[70] but several infants have been safely breast fed during maternal fluoxetine use.[71,72] Sertraline was undetectable in the plasma of a breast-fed infant whose mother was taking a dosage of 100 mg/day.[73] Paroxetine and fluvoxamine appear in milk in amounts similar to or less than fluoxetine,[74,75] but there is less clinical experience with their use during nursing.

SPECIFIC AGENTS

Clomipramine

The adverse effect profile of clomipramine is similar to the other tricyclic antidepressants (TCAs; refer to Chap. 69). The most frequently reported adverse effects are dry mouth, dizziness, tremor, fatigue, somnolence, constipation, and nausea. Other side effects include weight gain and sexual dysfunction, such as ejaculation failure, libido change, and impotence.

Because of the risk of seizures, the maximum daily dose should not exceed 250 mg, and caution should be used in prescribing clomipramine to patients with a history of seizures, alcoholism, or brain damage.[6,54] Similarly, caution should be used when prescribing clomipramine concomitantly with other drugs known to lower the seizure threshold.[54] Caution is also advised when prescribing clomipramine for patients with a history of liver disease, as rare reports of severe liver injury, some fatal, have been reported.[54]

Protein binding is approximately 97%, and the elimination half-life ranges from 31 to 37 hours. However, given reports of nonfirst-order elimination kinetics, these estimates should be viewed with caution.[76] Studies have reported that plasma clomipramine concentrations positively correlated with improvement in compulsions[77] and obsessions,[78] whereas plasma desmethylclomipramine levels were related to improvement in depression.[77] Mavissakalian and others[79] reported that plasma concentrations of clomipramine, but not desmethylclomipramine, correlated significantly with clinical response. Plasma concentrations of neither compound predicted response in children and adolescents. Clomipramine's drug-drug interactions are similar to those of the other TCAs. Refer to Chap. 69 for a review of these.

Clomipramine should be initiated at a dose of 25 mg/day (usually at bedtime) and gradually increased during the first 2 weeks to approximately 100 mg/day. Over the next several weeks, the dose may be increased gradually to a maximum of 250 mg/day. Initially, clomipramine should be administered in divided doses with meals to reduce gastrointestinal side effects, but after titration, the total daily dose may be given once daily at bedtime.[6,54] For maintenance therapy, many patients may have their dose reduced by 25% to 50%.

Fluoxetine

The most commonly reported fluoxetine-related side effects in OCD patients include nausea, headache, anxiety, sedation, insomnia, diarrhea, sexual dysfunction, and tremor.[80]

Absorption of fluoxetine is delayed when it is administered with food. It is approximately 95% bound to plasma proteins. With multiple daily dosing, the half-life of elimination of fluoxetine is 5.7 days, and that of norfluoxetine is reported to be 7 to 15 days.[81] No relationship has been established between plasma concentrations of fluoxetine or norfluoxetine and clinical response in treatment of OCD.[82]

Several fatal reactions have occurred with coadministration of MAOIs and fluoxetine. Therefore, MAOIs should not be administered until at least 5 weeks after discontinuation of fluoxetine. Fluoxetine is a potent inhibitor of CYP2D6 and CYP2C9, a moderate inhibitor of CYP3A3/4 and CYP2C19, and a weak inhibitor of CYP1A2.[83] The metabolism of both methylated and demethylated TCAs is impaired by fluoxetine. Therefore, the dose of a TCA should be reduced by 75% when fluoxetine is added, and 3 months should be allowed for a new steady-state TCA plasma concentration to be attained.[81] Multiple other drug-drug interactions have been associated with fluoxetine. Refer to Chap. 69 and the drug interaction literature for a more complete discussion.

The effective dose of fluoxetine in treating OCD is 20–80 mg/day. The manufacturer recommends an initial dose of fluoxetine of 20 mg/day given in the morning. An average target dose of 40–60 mg/day is recommended if there is insufficient response at the lower dose, and 80 mg/d is considered the maximum.[15] Doses greater than 20 mg/day may be administered once daily in the morning or on a twice-daily schedule (morning and noon).[80] Fixed-dose studies revealed no significant difference in efficacy between the 20-, 40-, and 60-mg doses, but individual patients may have a better response at the higher doses.

Fluvoxamine

The most commonly observed fluvoxamine-related adverse effects are insomnia, nausea, somnolence, fatigue, abnormal ejaculation, nervousness, dry mouth, tremor, anorexia, anorgasmia, sweating, and decreased libido.[57]

The half-life of elimination of the parent compound is 15 hours, and there are no known active metabolites. It is 77% plasma-protein bound. The pharmacokinetics of fluvoxamine are not affected by food intake.[84]

Fluvoxamine is a weak inhibitor of CYP2D6, and a potent inhibitor of CYP3A3/4, CYP1A2, CYP2C9, and CYP2C19.[83] Drug-drug interactions are reported between fluvoxamine and warfarin, theophylline, MAOIs, carbamazepine, alprazolam, propranolol, clozapine, phenytoin, TCAs, and selected other drugs. Coadministration of fluvoxamine with MAOIs should be avoided.[85] Refer to Chap. 69 and the drug interaction literature for a more complete discussion.

The recommended initial dose of fluvoxamine is 50 mg at bedtime. This dose should be increased in 50-mg increments every 4 to 7 days to an average target dose of 200 mg/day. The maximal dose is 300 mg/day. The manufacturer recommends that total daily doses of more than 100 mg be given in two divided doses. In many cases, a larger dose is given at bedtime.[57]

In children 8 to 17 years of age, the starting dose is 25 mg given at bedtime. This dose should be increased in 25-mg increments every 4 to 7 days as tolerated until maximum benefit is achieved, not to exceed 200 mg/day. Daily doses greater than 50 mg should be given in two divided doses. If divided doses are not equal, the larger dose should be given at bedtime.

Paroxetine

The most commonly observed side effects from paroxetine are nausea, somnolence, dry mouth, headache, dizziness, insomnia, weakness, and sexual dysfunction.[58] It is more likely to cause sedation than insomnia. The half-life of elimination of paroxetine is 24 hours, and it is metabolized to inactive metabolites. It is approximately 95% bound to plasma proteins.[58]

Paroxetine is a potent inhibitor of CYP2D6 and a weak inhibitor of CYP3A3/4 and CYP1A2.[83] Drug interactions may occur between paroxetine and tryptophan, MAOIs, warfarin, cimetidine, phenobarbital, phenytoin, TCAs, phenothiazines, type 1C antiarrhythmics, quinidine, and theophylline.[58] For a more complete discussion of paroxetine interactions, refer to Chap. 69.

The recommended initial dose of paroxetine is 20 mg/day, and the dose can be increased in 10-mg increments at intervals of at least 1 week. Once-daily administration is usually preferred (in the morning). The average target dose is 40–50 mg/day, and the maximal dose is 60 mg/day. Patients should be placed on the lowest effective dose for maintenance therapy.[58]

Sertraline

The adverse effects of sertraline are similar to the other SSRIs and include nausea, headache, diarrhea, insomnia, dry mouth, sexual dysfunction, and dizziness.[86]

The mean terminal elimination half-life of sertraline is about 26 hours. When administered with food, the area under the plasma concentration time curve is slightly increased, the C_{max} was 25% greater, and the T_{max} decreased from 8 hours to 5.5 hours. N-Desmethyl sertraline has an elimination half-life of 62 to 104 hours, but it is substantially less active than sertraline. Sertraline is 98% bound to plasma proteins.[86]

Sertraline is considered to have moderate potency as an inhibitor of CYP2D6, and to have low potency as an inhibitor of CYP3A3/4 and CYP1A2.[83] Sertraline was reported to cause a mean increase in prothrombin time of 8%. Cimetidine increased the sertraline area under the curve by 50%, the C_{max} by 24%, and the half-life by 26%. Sertraline caused a 32% decrease in diazepam clearance. Like other SSRIs, sertraline increases the plasma concentrations of TCAs, and should not be administered concurrently with the MAOIs. Sertraline also caused a 16% decrease in the clearance of tolbutamide.[86] For a more complete discussion of drug interactions associated with sertraline, refer to Chap. 69.

Dosage of sertraline is usually initiated at 50 mg/day. If the initial dose is ineffective, the dose may be increased at intervals of not less than 1 week up to a maximum of 200 mg/day. Sertraline may be administered as a once-daily dose in the morning or evening.[86] The dose-response curve for sertraline appears flat across doses of 50, 100, and 200 mg/day.

Citalopram

The FDA has not approved citopram for treatment of OCD. The adverse effects of citalopram in treatment of OCD are usually mild and transient and include nausea, vomiting, decreased sleep, increased dreaming, diminished sexual desire, and orgasmic dysfunction.[87]

The pharmacokinetics of citalopram are linear within the usual dosing range, and biotransformation is primarily hepatic, with a mean terminal half-life of approximately 35 hours. Parent drug and active metabolites, demethylcitalopram and didemethylcitalopram are about 80% bound to plasma proteins. The metabolites do not likely contribute significantly to efficacy.[88]

Citalopram is a weak inhibitor of CYP1A2, CYP2D6, and CYP2C19. Primary enzymes involved in the metabolism of citalopram are CYP3A4 and CYP2C19. Potent inhibitors of CYP3A4 (e.g., ketoconazole, itraconazole, and macrolide antibiotics) and potent inhibitors of CYP2C19 (e.g., omeprazole) might decrease the clearance of citalopram.[88]

Optimal dosing of citalopram in treatment of OCD has not been established. One study showed similar efficacy at 20 mg/day, 40 mg/day, and 60 mg/day.[35] In other studies, most patients took 40 or 60 mg/day.[87] Generally, patients should be initiated at 20 mg/day. Dose increases, if they occur, should be in increments of 20 mg at intervals of not less than 1 week.[88]

REFRACTORY PATIENTS

For most patients who respond to SRIs, the improvement is incom plete, and approximately 50% of patients are clinically unchanged after an adequate trial of SRIs.[89] If there is no response or partial response to CBT alone, an SRI should be added, and more intensive CBT can be undertaken. If there is no response or partial response to an SRI alone, CBT should be added, or another SRI can be tried. If there is no response to combined CBT and an SRI, then another SRI should be tried. If there is a partial response to combined CBT and SRI therapy, a switch to another SRI, more intensive CBT, or augmentation therapy can be initiated. After failing separate trials of two or three SSRIs and CBT, clomipramine should be tried. If there is no response or partial response to combined CBT and three SRI trials (one of which was clomipramine), then augmentation with another medication can be undertaken, and more intensive CBT can be tried.[15]

Although case reports of lithium report encouraging findings, in controlled studies of lithium augmentation of clomipramine and fluvoxamine, no clinically meaningful improvement was noted.[89] Clonazepam augmentation of fluoxetine therapy produced a 75% reduction in symptoms in a young man with childhood-onset severe OCD.[90]

Two open-label studies reported that addition of buspirone to ongoing fluoxetine treatment led to a greater reduction of obsessive and compulsive symptoms than did fluoxetine alone. Three separate controlled studies of the addition of buspirone to clomipramine, fluvoxamine, and fluoxetine failed to corroborate these initial reports.[89] Similarly, a double-blind study in 14 patients found that buspirone augmentation of clomipramine therapy was not associated with further improvement.[91] When buspirone is used as augmentation therapy, the initial dose is 5 mg three times daily, and the target dose should be 60–90 mg/day.[15]

One patient receiving clomipramine, 200 mg/day, was reported to improve with the addition of carbamazepine, dose escalating to 500 mg/day.[92] A previous report described successful carbamazepine augmentation of fluoxetine therapy in two patients with OCD and aggressive behavior.[93]

In 16 adult outpatients, in a randomized, open-label trial, citalopram (40 mg/day) plus clomipramine (150 mg/day) was more effective in refractory patients than was citalopram alone. These are preliminary findings that await confirmation in a larger, double-blind trial.[94]

The DA system may play a role in the pathobiology of Tourette's disorder. Furthermore, some forms of OCD, especially those comorbid with chronic tic disorders, may be associated with abnormal DA function.[95] Some investigators have studied SRI/DA receptor antagonist combination treatments in subgroups of OCD patients with SRI-resistant symptoms. However, DA receptor antagonists alone are not effective in the treatment of the core symptoms of OCD.

In an open-case series of 17 fluvoxamine nonresponders, 88% of patients with comorbid tic disorder diagnoses responded after pimozide was added, whereas only 22% of patients without these comorbid diagnoses responded.[12] The recommended initial dose of pimozide is 0.5 mg, and the target dose is 1–6 mg/day. Pimozide may cause cardiovascular problems and probably should not be used with clomipramine.[15] In a double-blind, placebo-controlled study, haloperidol or placebo was added to fluvoxamine in patients who had failed to respond to fluvoxamine monotherapy. Haloperidol was significantly more effective than placebo in reducing obsessive-compulsive symptoms. Furthermore, those with a concurrent chronic tic disorder demonstrated a preferential response to the fluvoxamine-haloperidol combination.[12] The recommended initial dose of haloperidol is 0.5 mg, and the target dose is 0.25–6 mg/day.[15] It is recommended that patients fail at least two trials of SRIs and clomipramine before haloperidol is tried because of the need for long-term treatment of this disorder and the risk of tardive dyskinesia and other movement disorders.[89]

Preliminary results from a 6-week, double-blind, placebo-controlled trial of low-dose risperidone (0.5–2 mg/day) added to an SRI in SRI-refractory OCD patients are encouraging. The authors report that treatment response was rapid and well-maintained.[89] An additional 8-week, open-label study reported that 50% of patients previously unresponsive to clomipramine responded after risperidone 3 mg/day was added.[96] The recommended initial dose of risperidone is 0.25 mg, and the target dose is 0.5–5 mg/day.[15] Thirty-six patients unresponsive to SRIs were given risperidone, up to 6 mg/day or placebo in a double-blind trial. Risperidone treatment resulted in a significant reduction in Y-BOCS scores.[97] Two open-label trials examined olanzapine augmentation. Nine patients who were partial responders to SSRIs were given olanzapine augmentation for a minimum of 8 weeks, in doses of 1.25–20 mg/day. Four patients experienced complete remission or major improvement. Three had partial remission.[98] Nine patients unresponsive to fluoxetine were given olanzapine in doses of 2–10 mg/day for 8 weeks. Three patients responded, but only one patient was "much improved."

PHARMACOECONOMIC CONSIDERATIONS

In 1990, the total cost to the US economy for OCD was $8 billion. This figure includes expenditures for direct costs ($2.1 billion) and indirect costs ($5.9 billion). Direct costs include costs of hospitalization, outpatient professional services, and medications. Indirect costs include costs associated with lost productivity, work loss, early retirement, and absenteeism. As OCD frequently has its onset in childhood or adolescence, loss of income over a lifetime is substantial. An estimated 2% of completed suicides in 1990 were attributable to OCD.[99] It is estimated that $2.2 billion is spent annually for inappropriate outpatient treatment, with 25% of survey respondents requiring hospitalization with average total hospital costs of $12,500. On average, a person with OCD loses 3 full years of wages over a lifetime.[100]

EVALUATION OF THERAPEUTIC OUTCOMES

OCD patients receiving pharmacotherapy should be monitored for target symptom response, adverse effects (including the emergence of suicidal ideas), and drug interactions. Symptom severity can be effectively monitored through periodic assessment using the Y-BOCS. For additional information on rating scales used to assess OCD patients, the reader is referred to Ellingrod's review.[30] In addition, changes in social and occupational functioning should be assessed. Regular monitoring should be assured for several months after OCD treatment is discontinued.

Patients older than 40 years of age should receive a pretreatment electrocardiogram (ECG) before starting clomipramine. In patients with a history of liver disease, baseline and periodic liver function tests are recommended when clomipramine is used. If clomipramine is given concurrently with sympatholytic antihypertensives, blood pressure should be regularly monitored. Although controversial, patients failing to respond to clomipramine may benefit once the dose is adjusted to bring the plasma concentration of clomipramine between 100 and 250 ng/mL. Patients taking clomipramine who develop fever and sore throat should have leukocyte and differential white blood counts assessed to evaluate for agranulocytosis.

CONCLUSIONS

OCD is a chronic and often profoundly disabling anxiety disorder with a lifetime prevalence rate of 2.5% in adults and 1% in children. Traditional psychotherapies have failed to offer significant benefit to OCD patients, but the effectiveness of both CBT and the SRIs is well established. These complementary treatments effect a substantial reduction in symptomatology in most patients. Although currently approved medications are far superior in efficacy compared with placebo, many responders continue to demonstrate disabling symptoms. Furthermore, the SRIs are associated with an adverse effect profile that is often problematic for a significant percentage of patients. A high rate of relapse is reported after medication discontinuation. Marked progress has been made in the treatment of this disorder over the last 10 years, and with continued research, the future holds still greater promise.

▶ PRINCIPLES OF PHARMACOTHERAPY

- When evaluating a person for OCD, remember that patients are often ashamed to admit their symptoms and are skilled at hiding them.
- In adults, CBT is selected first for milder OCD; CBT plus an SSRI or an SSRI alone is selected first for more severe OCD; when available, CBT should be offered to every OCD patient.
- Placebo-controlled trials confirm the efficacy of clomipramine, fluoxetine, fluvoxamine, sertraline, and paroxetine over a 4- to 10-week period.
- If one SSRI is ineffective, then another should be tried; clomipramine may be selected after two or three failed SSRI trials.
- Most successfully treated patients continue to have residual symptoms severe enough to limit functioning.
- Tolerance to SSRI adverse effects often develops over 6–8 weeks of treatment, and tolerance is more likely to develop to nausea, diarrhea, sedation, diminished libido and/or orgasm, anxiety, restlessness, insomnia, and anticholinergic side effects than to akathisia.
- Pharmacotherapy in elderly patients should be initiated with low doses, and doses should be increased slowly, with vigilance for emergence of side effects; some elderly patients will require doses similar to those used in younger adults.
- If there is no response or partial response to combined CBT and three separate SRI trials (one of which was clomipramine), then augmentation with another medication can be undertaken, and more intensive CBT can be tried.
- After successful treatment, a medication taper can be considered after 1 to 2 years of treatment. Long-term or lifelong prophylactic maintenance medication is recommended after two to four severe relapses or three to four mild to moderate relapses.

REFERENCES

1. American Psychiatric Association. Diagnostic and Statistical Manual of Mental Disorders, 4th ed, Text Revision (DSM-IV-TR). Washington, DC, American Psychiatric Press, 2000:417–423.
2. Karno M, Golding J, Sorenson S, Burnam A. The epidemiology of obsessive-compulsive disorder in five US communities. Arch Gen Psychiatry 1988;45:1094–1099.
3. Robertson MM, Yakeley J. Gilles de la Tourette syndrome and obsessive compulsive disorder. In: Fogel BS, Schiffer RB, eds. Neuropsychiatry. Baltimore, Williams & Wilkins, 1996:827–870.
4. Pauls DL, Alsobrook JP, Goodman W, et al. A family history of obsessive-compulsive disorder. Am J Psychiatry 1995;152:76–84.
5. Pato MT, Pato CN. Obsessive-compulsive disorder in adult life. In: Pato MT, Steketee G, eds. OCD Across the Life Cycle. Section III of Review of Psychiatry, vol 16. Washington, DC, American Psychiatric Press, 1997:30–55.
6. Clomipramine collaborative study group. Clomipramine in the treatment of patients with obsessive-compulsive disorder. Arch Gen Psychiatry 1991;48:730–738.

7. Greist JH, Jefferson JW, Kobah KA, et al. Efficacy and tolerability of serotonin transport inhibitors in obsessive-compulsive disorder. Arch Gen Psychiatry 1995;52:53–60.
8. Hollander E, DeCaria CM, Nitescu A, et al. Serotonergic function in obsessive-compulsive disorder: Behavioral and neuroendocrine responses to oral *m*-chlorophenylpiperazine and fenfluramine in patients and healthy volunteers. Arch Gen Psychiatry 1992;49:21–28.
9. Barr LC, Goodman WK, Price LH, et al. The serotonin hypothesis of obsessive compulsive disorder: Implications of pharmacologic challenge studies. J Clin Psychiatry 1992;53(suppl 4):17–28.
10. Insel TR. Toward a neuroanatomy of obsessive-compulsive disorder. Arch Gen Psychiatry 1992;49:739–744.
11. Baxter LR. Neuroimaging studies of human anxiety disorders: Cutting paths of knowledge through the field of neurotic phenomena. In: Bloom FE, Kupfer DJ, eds. Psychopharmacology: Fourth Generation of Progress. New York, Raven, 1995:1287–1300.
12. McDougle CJ, Goodman WK, Price LH. Dopamine antagonists in tic-related and psychotic spectrum obsessive compulsive disorder. J Clin Psychiatry 1994;55(suppl 3):24–31.
13. Hyde TM, Weinberger DR. Tourette's syndrome: A model neuropsychiatric disorder. JAMA 1995;273:489–501.
14. Insel TR. New pharmacologic approaches to obsessive compulsive disorder. J Clin Psychiatry 1990;51(suppl 10):47–51.
15. Expert Consensus Panel for Obsessive-Compulsive Disorder. Obsessive compulsive disorder executive summary: Recommendations for first-line treatments by clinical situation. J Clin Psychiatry 1997;58(suppl 4): 11–12.
16. Baer L. Behavior therapy for obsessive compulsive disorder in the office-based practice. J Clin Psychiatry 1993;54(suppl 6):10–15.
17. Rasmussen SA, Eisen JL, Pato MT. Current issues in the pharmacologic management of obsessive compulsive disorder. J Clin Psychiatry 1993;54(suppl 6):4–9.
18. Jenike MA, Rauch SL. Managing the patient with treatment-resistant obsessive compulsive disorder: Current strategies. J Clin Psychiatry 1994;55(suppl 3):11–17.
19. Jenike MA. Approaches to the patient with treatment-refractory obsessive compulsive disorder. J Clin Psychiatry 1990;51(suppl 2):15–21.
20. Mundo E, Bianchi L, Bellodi L. Efficacy of fluvoxamine, paroxetine, and citalopram in the treatment of obsessive-compulsive disorder: A single-blind study. J Clin Psychopharmacol 1997;17:267–271.
21. Greist J, Chouinard G, DuBoff E, et al. Double-blind comparison of three doses of sertraline and placebo in the treatment of outpatients with obsessive-compulsive disorder. Arch Gen Psychiatry 1995;52:289–295.
22. Flament MF, Bisserbe JC. Pharmacologic treatment of obsessive-compulsive disorder: Comparative studies. J Clin Psychiatry 1997; 58(suppl 12):18–22.
23. Jenike MA, Hyman S, Baer L, et al. A controlled trial of fluvoxamine in obsessive compulsive disorder: Implications for a serotonergic theory. Am J Psychiatry 1990;147:1209–1215.
24. Goodman WK, Price LH, Delgado PL, et al. Specificity of serotonin reuptake inhibitors in the treatment of obsessive-compulsive disorder: Comparison of fluvoxamine and desipramine. Arch Gen Psychiatry 1990;47:577–585.
25. Dominguez RA. Serotonergic antidepressants and their efficacy in obsessive compulsive disorder. J Clin Psychiatry 1992;53(suppl 10):56–59.
26. Jenike MA, Baer L, Summergrad P, et al. Sertraline in obsessive compulsive disorder: A double-blind comparison with placebo. Am J Psychiatry 1990;147:923–928.
27. Pigott TA, Pato MT, Bernstein SE, et al. Controlled comparisons of clomipramine and fluoxetine in the treatment of obsessive-compulsive disorder: Behavioral and biological results. Arch Gen Psychiatry 1990; 47:926–932.
28. Tamimi RR, Mavissakalian MR, Jones B, Olson S. Clomipramine versus fluvoxamine in obsessive-compulsive disorder. Ann Clin Psychiatry 1991;3:275–279.
29. Black DW. Obsessive-compulsive disorder and its relationship to other disorders. Resident Staff Physician 1997;43:64–76.
30. Ellingrod VL. Pharmacotherapy of primary obsessive-compulsive disorder. Pharmacotherapy 1998;18:936–960.
31. Mundo E, Bianchi L, Bellodi L. Efficacy of fluvoxamine, paroxetine, and citalopram in the treatment of obsessive-compulsive disorder: A single-blind study. J Clin Psychopharmacol 1997;17:267–271.
32. Flament MF, Bisserbe J-C. Pharmacologic treatment of obsessive-compulsive disorder: Comparative studies. J Clin Psychiatry 1997; 58(suppl 12):18–22.
33. Pigott TA, Seay SM. A review of the efficacy of selective serotonin reuptake inhibitors in obsessive-compulsive disorders. J Clin Psychiatry 1999;60:101–106.
34. Thomsen PH. Child and adolescent obsessive-compulsive disorder treated with citalopram: Findings from an open trial of 23 cases. J Child Adolesc Psycharmacol 1997;7:157–166.
35. Montgomery S, Kasper S, Bang-Hedegaard K, Lundbeck H. The SSRI citalopram is effective in the treatment of obsessive-compulsive disorder: Results from a double-blind, fixed-dose, placebo-controlled trial. Presented at the Annual Meeting of the American Psychiatric Association, Chicago, IL, May 13–18, 2000.
36. Pato MT, Zohar-Kadouch R, Zohar J, Murphy DL. Return of symptoms after discontinuation of clomipramine in patients with obsessive compulsive disorder. Am J Psychiatry 1988;145:1521–1525.
37. Fontaine R, Chouinard G. Fluoxetine in the long-term maintenance treatment of obsessive compulsive disorder. Psychiatr Ann 1989;19: 88–91.
38. Ravizza L, Barzega G, Billilno S, et al. Drug treatment of obsessive-compulsive disorder (OCD): Long-term trial with clomipramine and selective serotonin reuptake inhibitors (SSRIs). Psychopharmacol Bull 1996;32:167–173.
39. Alarcon RD, Libb JW, Spitler D. A predictive study of obsessive compulsive disorder response to clomipramine. J Clin Psychopharmacol 1993;13:210–213.
40. Austin LS, Lydiard B, Fossey MD. Panic and phobic disorders in patients with obsessive compulsive disorder. J Clin Psychiatry 1990;51: 45–48.
41. Ackerman DL, Greenland S, Bystritsky A. Side effects on predictors of drug-response in obsessive-compulsive disorder. J Clin Psychopharmacol 1999;19:459–465.
42. Ackerman DL, Greenland S, Bystritsky A. Clinical characteristics of response to fluoxetine treatment of obsessive-compulsive disorder. J Clin Psychopharmacol 1998;18:185–192.
43. Mataix-Cols D, Rauch SL, Manzo PA, et al. Use of factor-analyzed symptom dimensions to predict outcome with serotonin reuptake inhibitors and placebo in the treatment of obsessive-compulsive disorder. Am J Psychiatry 1999;156:1409–1416.
44. Mundo E, Bareggi SR, Pirola R, et al. Long-term pharmacotherapy of obsessive-compulsive disorder: A double-blind controlled study. J Clin Psychopharmacol 1997;17:4–10.
45. Gardner DM, Lynd LD. Sumatriptan contraindications and the serotonin syndrome. Ann Pharmacother 1998;32:33–38.
46. Jenike MA, Baer L, Minichiello WE, et al. Placebo-controlled trial of fluoxetine and phenelzine for obsessive-compulsive disorder. Am J Psychiatry 1997;154:1261–1264.
47. Hewlett WA, Vinogradov S, Agras WS. Clonazepam treatment of obsessions and compulsions. J Clin Psychiatry 1990;51:158–161.
48. Pato MT, Pigott TA, Hill JL, et al. Controlled comparison of buspirone and clomipramine in obsessive compulsive disorder. Am J Psychiatry 1991;148:127–129.
49. Jenike MA, Baer L. An open trial of buspirone in obsessive compulsive disorder. Am J Psychiatry 1988;145:1285–1286.
50. Taylor LVH, Kobak KA. An open-label trial of St. John's wort (*Hypericum perforatum*) in obsessive-compulsive disorder. J Clin Psychiatry 2000;61:575–578.
51. Sheikh JI, Salzman C. Anxiety in the elderly. Psychiatr Clin North Am 1995;18:871–883.
52. Stoudemire A, Moran MG. Psychopharmacologic treatment of anxiety in the medically ill elderly patient: Special considerations. J Clin Psychiatry 1993;54(suppl):27–33.

53. Pollard CA, Carmin CN, Ownby R. Obsessive-compulsive disorder in later life. In: Pato MT, Stekette G, eds. OCD Across the Life Cycle. Section III of Review of Psychiatry, vol 16. Washington, DC, American Psychiatric Press, 1997:63.
54. Ciba-Geigy. Anafranil package insert. Summit, NJ, 1998.
55. Preskorn SH. Recent pharmacologic advances in antidepressant therapy for the elderly. Am J Med 1993;94(suppl SA):2S–12S.
56. Buff DD, Brenner R, Kirtane SS, Gilboa R. Dysrhythmia associated with fluoxetine treatment in an elderly patient with cardiac disease. J Clin Psychiatry 1991;52:174–176.
57. Solvay Pharmaceuticals. Luvox package insert. Marietta, GA, 1998.
58. SmithKline Beecham Pharmaceuticals. Paxil package insert. Philadelphia, 1998.
59. Hollingsworth C, Tanguay P, Grossman L, et al. Long-term outcome of obsessive compulsive disorder in childhood. J Am Acad Child Psychiatry 1980;19:134–144.
60. Flament MF, Rapoport JL, Berg CJ, et al. Clomipramine treatment of childhood compulsive disorder. Arch Gen Psychiatry 1985;42: 977–983.
61. DeVaugh-Geiss J, Moroz G, Biederman J, et al. Clomipramine in child and adolescent obsessive-compulsive disorder: A multicenter trial. J Am Acad Child Adolesc Psychiatry 1992;31:45–49.
62. Leonard HL, Swedo S, Rapoport JL, et al. Treatment of obsessive compulsive disorder with clomipramine and desipramine in children and adolescents. Arch Gen Psychiatry 1989;46:1088–1092.
63. Thomsen PH. Obsessive-compulsive disorder: Pharmacologic treatment. Eur Child Adolesc Psychiatry 2000;9(suppl 1):176–184.
64. King RA, Leonard H, March J, et al. Practice parameters for the assessment and treatment of children and adolescents with obsessive-compulsive disorder. J Am Acad Child Adolesc Psychiatry 1998;37 (suppl 10):27S–45S.
65. Diaz SF, Grush LR, Sichel DA, Cohen LS. Obsessive-compulsive disorder in pregnancy and the puerperium. In: Pato MT, Steketee G, eds. OCD Across the Life Cycle. Section III of Review of Psychiatry, vol 16. Washington, DC, American Psychiatric Press, 1997:97–112.
66. Goldstein DJ. Effects of third trimester fluoxetine exposure on the newborn. J Clin Psychopharmacol 1995;15:417–420.
67. Pastuszak A, Schick-Poschetto B, Zuber C, et al. Pregnancy outcome following first trimester exposure to fluoxetine (Prozac). JAMA 1993; 269:2246–2248.
68. Ben Musa A, Smith CS. Neonatal effects of maternal clomipramine therapy (case report). Arch Dis Child 1979;54:405.
69. Schimmell MS, Katz EZ, Shaag Y, et al. Toxic neonatal effects following maternal clomipramine therapy. Clin Toxicol 1991;29:479–484.
70. Lester BM. Possible association between fluoxetine hydrochloride and colic in an infant. J Am Acad Child Adolesc Psychiatry 1993;32:1253–1255.
71. Burch KJ, Wells, BG. Fluoxetine/norfluoxetine concentrations in human milk. Pediatrics 1992;89:676–677.
72. Taddio A. Excretion of fluoxetine and its metabolite, norfluoxetine, in human breast milk. J Clin Pharmacol 1996;36:42–27.
73. Altshuler LL. Breast-feeding and sertraline: A 24-hour analysis. J Clin Psychiatry 1995;56:243–245.
74. Spigset O. Paroxetine levels in breast milk. J Clin Psychiatry 1996;57:29.
75. Wright S. Excretion of fluvoxamine in breast milk. Br J Clin Pharmacol 1991;31:209.
76. Jermain DM, Crismon LC. Pharmacotherapy of obsessive compulsive disorder. Pharmacotherapy 1990;10:175–198.
77. Stern RS, Marks IM, Mawson D, Luscombe DK. Clomipramine and exposure for compulsive rituals, I. Plasma levels, side effects, and outcome. Br J Psychiatry 1980;136:161–166.
78. Insel TR, Murphy DL, Cohen RM, et al. Obsessive compulsive disorder. Arch Gen Psychiatry 1983;40:605–612.
79. Mavissakalian MR, Jones B, Olson S, Perel JM. Clomipramine in obsessive compulsive disorder: Clinical response and plasma levels. J Clin Psychopharmacol 1990;10:261–268.
80. Dista Products. Prozac package insert. Indianapolis, 2000.
81. Van Harten J. Clinical pharmacokinetics of selective serotonin reuptake inhibitors. Clin Pharmacokinet 1993;24:203–220.
82. Koran LM, Cain JW, Dominguez RA, et al. Are fluoxetine plasma levels related to outcome in obsessive-compulsive disorder? Am J Psychiatry 1996;153:1450–1454.
83. Ereshefsky L, Riesenman C, Lam YWF. Serotonin selective reuptake inhibitor drug interactions and the cytochrome P450 system. J Clin Psychiatry 1996;57(suppl 8):17–25.
84. Finley PR. Selective serotonin reuptake inhibitors: Pharmacologic profiles and potential therapeutic distinctions. Ann Pharmacother 1994;28: 1359–1369.
85. Goodman WK, Ward H, Kablinger A, Murphy T. Fluvoxamine in the treatment of obsessive-compulsive disorder and related conditions. J Clin Psychiatry 1997;58(suppl 5):32–49.
86. Pfizer. Zoloft package insert. New York, 2000.
87. Koponen H, Lepola U, Leinonen E, et al. Citalopram in the treatment of obsessive-compulsive disorder: An open pilot study. Acta Psychiatr Scand 1997;96:343–346.
88. Forest Laboratories, Inc. Celexa package insert. St. Louis, MO, 2000.
89. McDougle CJ. Update on pharmacologic management of OCD: Agents and augmentation. J Clin Psychiatry 1997;58(suppl 12):11–17.
90. Leonard HL, Topol D, Bukstein O, et al. Clonazepam as an augmenting agent in the treatment of childhood-onset obsessive-compulsive disorder. J Am Acad Child Adolesc Psychiatry 1994;33:792–794.
91. Pigott TA, L'Heureux F, Hill JL, et al. A double-blind study of adjuvant buspirone hydrochloride in clomipramine-treated patients with obsessive-compulsive disorder. J Clin Psychopharmacol 1992;12:11–18.
92. Iwata Y, Kotani Y, Hoshino R, et al. Carbamazepine augmentation of clomipramine in the treatment of refractory obsessive-compulsive disorder. J Clin Psychiatry 2000;61:528–529.
93. Alarcon RD, Johnson BR, Lucas JP. Paranoid and aggressive behavior in two obsessive-compulsive adolescents treated with clomipramine. J Am Acad Child Adolesc Psychiatry 1991;30:999–1002.
94. Pallanti S, Quercioli L, Paiva RS, Koran LM. Citalopram for treatment-resistant obsessive-compulsive disorder. Eur Psychiatry 1999;14:101–106.
95. Goodman WK, McDougle CJ, Price LH, et al. Beyond the serotonin hypothesis: A role for dopamine in some forms of obsessive compulsive disorder? J Clin Psychiatry 1990;51:36–43.
96. Ravizza L. Therapeutic effect and safety of adjunctive risperidone in refractory obsessive-compulsive disorder (OCD). Psychopharmacol Bull 1996;32:677–682.
97. McDougle CJ, Epperson CN, Pelton GH, et al. A double-blind placebo-controlled study of risperidone addition in serotonin reuptake inhibitor-refractory obsessive-compulsive disorder. Arch Gen Psychiatry 2000;57:794–801.
98. Weiss EL, Potenza MN, McDougle CJ, et al. Olanzapine addition in obsessive-compulsive disorder refractory to selective serotonin reuptake inhibitors: An open-label case series. J Clin Psychiatry 1999;60:524–527.
99. Dupont R, Rice D, Shiraki S, et al. Economic costs of obsessive-compulsive disorder. Pharmacoeconomics 1995;2:102–109.
100. Hollander E, Kwon JH, Stein MB, et al. Obsessive-compulsive and spectrum disorders: Overview and quality of life issues. J Clin Psychiatry 1996;57(suppl 8):3–6.
101. American Pharmaceutical Association. Management of obsessive-compulsive disorder. In: APhA Guide to Drug Treatment Protocols: A Resource for Creating and Using Disease-specific Pathways. Washington, DC, American Pharmaceutical Association, 1997:OCDi–ii.

73

SLEEP DISORDERS

Judy L. Curtis and Donna M. Jermaine

Sleep is essential to human life, providing both emotional and physical restoration in ways not completely understood. Approximately one-third of our lives is spent sleeping, with a wide interindividual variability in the amount of sleep required per night (3–10 h/night).[1] About one-third of adults experience a sleep disorder in their lifetimes. Abnormalities in the normal physiology of sleep often cause three types of sleep problems: insomnia, excessive daytime sleepiness, and abnormal sleep behaviors.[2]

SLEEP PHYSIOLOGY

A circadian rhythm of sleep and waking is established shortly after birth and changes over the life cycle. Two oscillators with different period lengths control the circadian rhythm of sleep. One oscillator is located in the suprachiasmic nucleus (biologic clock), and the other occurs through neurobiologic mechanisms. Two peptides, delta-sleep-inducing peptide and factor S also appear to be involved in the biochemical regulation.[1] Synchronization of the sleep-wake cycle naturally lasts about 24.2 hours in an environment devoid of light cues. The 24-hour cycle imposed by the earth's rotation requires routinely occurring *zeitgebers,* or cues (e.g., clock, light, shower, breakfast time), to set the internal clock.[3]

NEUROCHEMISTRY

Sleep is a complex psychophysiologic phenomenon that ensues as wakefulness abates. Humans and most mammals have two major phases of sleep. These are non-rapid eye movement (NREM) sleep and rapid eye movement (REM) sleep. The reticular activating system is responsible for maintaining waking states or arousal. NREM is controlled by at least five different anatomic sites: basal forebrain, thalamus, hypothalamus, and dorsal raphe nucleus and nucleus tractus solitarius of the medulla. The midpons is necessary for REM sleep. Sleep is influenced by several neurotransmitters. Norepinephrine (NE)-containing neurons in the locus ceruleus are important in main taining normal sleep patterns. Increased firing of these neurons will result in a reduction of REM sleep and increased wakefulness. NE is involved in dreaming, and acetylcholine is involved in REM sleep. Serotonin is also involved in sleep regulation. Sleep is reduced when there are decreases in serotonin or destruction of the dorsal raphe nucleus in the brainstem, which contains most of the brain's serotonergic cell bodies. Serotonin is active during the nondreaming sleep. Dopamine has an alerting effect. Drugs that increase dopamine in the brain cause increased wakefulness; those which decrease dopamine cause sleepiness.[3,4] Other neurochemicals that influence sleep include histamine and neuropeptides (e.g., substance P and corticotropin-releasing factor) in the hypothalamus. These modulate neuronal activity during wakefulness.[4]

SLEEP CYCLE

Wakefulness is characterized by an electroencephalogram (EEG) of low voltage, fast activity, random eye movements and blinks, and a high muscle tone. NREM sleep is divided into four distinct stages. During NREM sleep, skeletal muscle tone and eye movements are low in comparison with wakefulness, and respiratory activity occurs at a slow, regular pace. Stage 1 sleep represents a transition between wakefulness and sleep that lasts between 0.5 and 7 min; the EEG reveals low-voltage (3- to 7-Hz), desynchronized activity. Stage 2 sleep is a low-voltage EEG with frequent "sleep spindles" (10- to 16-Hz spindle-shaped waves) and K-complexes (high-voltage spikes). Stages 3 and 4 are called *delta sleep* and consist of high-amplitude, slow waves.[5] stages 1 to 4 occur within 45 minutes of falling asleep. Most delta sleep occurs during the first half of the night.

REM sleep is characterized by the onset of low-voltage, mixed frequency EEG and bursts of bilaterally conjugate REMs.[5] During REM sleep, muscle tone is low, but autonomic functioning is highly variable.[3] Within 90 minutes of falling asleep, the first REM period commences and lasts only 5 to 7 minutes. The cycle lasts approximately 70 to 120 minutes and is repeated four to six times during the night.[5] REM periods lengthen progressively throughout the night.[3] A typical young adult spends approximately 75% of the night in NREM sleep and the remainder in REM sleep.[5] Dream reports occur in 80% to 90% of subjects if awakened during or at the end of an REM period.

In elderly individuals, the sleep pattern is altered, with a considerable decrease in delta sleep, REM sleep, and total sleep time.[5] Correspondingly, there is an increase in the number of awakenings and total time spent awake at night.[6] The contribution of daytime napping and specific sleep pathology (including sleep apnea and periodic leg movements) to this apparent decrease in sleep is unclear.

CLASSIFICATION

The Association of Sleep Disorders Center's International Classification of Sleep Disorders (ICSD) organizes more than 80 sleep disorders (based on pathophysiology) under the major headings of dyssomnias, parasomnias, medical/psychiatric sleep disorders, and proposed sleep disorders.[7] Similar to the ICSD, the *Diagnostic and Statistical Manual of Mental Disorders,* Fourth Edition, Text Revision (DSM-IV-TR), classifies sleep disorders based on presumed etiology into three major categories (Table 73–1) and requires a period of duration of 1 month before a sleep disorder is diagnosed.[8] Primary sleep disorders result from endogenous abnormalities in the sleep-wake timing or generating processes and are further classified as dyssomnias (abnormalities in the amount, timing, or quality of sleep) or parasomnias (abnormal behaviors associated with sleep). Sleep disorders secondary to

TABLE 73–1. DSM-IV Classification of Sleep Disorders

Primary Sleep Disorders
Dvssomnias
- Primary insomnia
- Primary hypersomnia
- Breathing-related sleep disorder
- Narcolepsy
- Circadian rhythm sleep disorder
  - Delayed sleep phase type
  - Jet lag type
  - Unspecified type
- Dyssomnias not otherwise specified

Parasomnias
- Nightmare disorder
- Sleep terror disorder
- Sleepwalking disorder
- Parasomnias not otherwise specified

Sleep Disorders Related to Another Mental Disorder
Insomnia related to another mental disorder
Hypersomnia related to another mental disorder
Other Sleep Disorders
Sleep disorder due to a general medical condition
Substance-induced sleep disorder

Adapted from Ref. 8.

another mental disorder, medical condition, or substance (concurrent use or discontinuation of a substance or a drug) are classified separately.

Polysomnography (PSG) measures multiple electrophysiologic parameters simultaneously during sleep and typically includes an EEG, electrooculogram (EOG), and electromyogram (EMG).[2] Two EOGs, one EEG, and one EMG are the minimal recordings used in scoring sleep stages.[9] Commonly measured objective parameters of sleep include sleep onset latency (amount of time to fall asleep), number of awakenings, number of stage shifts during the night, and first REM latency period. Other polysomnographic measures (e.g., oral and nasal airflow, respiratory effort, oxygen desaturation, periodic leg movements, gross motor activity, and nocturnal penile tumescence) also may be used to diagnose sleep disorders.[2,5]

INSOMNIA

Insomnia is a subjective complaint of difficulty falling asleep, maintaining sleep, or not feeling rested despite a sufficient opportunity to sleep.[8] A concurrent disturbance of daytime functioning (decreased concentration, fatigue) usually accompanies the sleep complaint. People with insomnia also have a higher use of medical services than those without insomnia.[1] Younger individuals usually complain of delays in sleep onset, whereas older patients complain of nocturnal awakening and shorter time periods of sleep.[8] The most important aspect in evaluating a sleep complaint is its duration. Transient (two to three nights) and short-term (<3 weeks) insomnia is not uncommon and usually is related to a precipitating factor, such as jet lag, stress, or illness. Long-term insomnia (>1 month) is considered chronic insomnia. The diagnosis requires difficulty in falling asleep or maintaining sleep. Further, impairment in functioning in social or occupational activities is also important for the diagnosis of insomnia. Medical conditions, psychiatric disorders, other sleep disorders, and disrupted sleep due to a medication must be ruled out for the diagnosis of insomnia.[1]

EPIDEMIOLOGY

Insomnia is the most prevalent sleep complaint in the general population.[2] A 1-year prevalence study of insomnia in the United States reported that one-third of individuals surveyed complained of insomnia, and 17% reported the symptoms to be serious.[1] Data from the National Institute of Mental Health Epidemiologic Catchment Area (ECA) study indicated that the 6-month prevalence of insomnia, defined as symptoms for 2 weeks, was 10.2%. Females; individuals who are unemployed, elderly, separated, or widowed; and those in the lower socioeconomic sector reported significantly higher rates of insomnia. Forty percent of those with insomnia had a concurrent psychiatric disorder (e.g., anxiety, depression, alcohol or substance abuse).[10]

Despite the widespread prevalence of insomnia, only 5% of individuals seek medical assistance for management.[11] Approximately 10% to 20% of insomniacs use nonprescription drugs or alcohol to alleviate symptoms. Of the 3% of the population who ingest hypnotics for insomnia, 11% report use exceeding 1 year.[12]

DIFFERENTIAL DIAGNOSIS

The causes of insomnia may be multidimensional and related to underlying situational stressors, medical or psychiatric illnesses, or medication use. Common identifiable causes of insomnia are listed in Table 73–2. Evaluation of transient insomnia should focus on possible acute stress, environmental disruptions (e.g., change in job, recent surgery, examinations), and drug-related causes. In patients with chronic sleep disturbances, a complete diagnostic evaluation should include physical and mental status examinations and routine laboratory tests (e.g., complete blood count with differential, liver function tests, thyroid function tests), as well as medication and substance abuse histories to rule out medical and psychiatric etiologies.

TABLE 73–2. Common Etiologies of Insomnia

Situational
Work or financial stress
Interpersonal conflicts
Major life events
Jet lag, shift work
Medical
Cardiovascular (angina, arrhythmias, heart failure)
Respiratory (asthma, sleep apnea)
Chronic pain
Endocrine disorders (diabetes, hyperthyroidism)
Gastrointestinal (gastroesophageal reflux, ulcers)
Neurologic (delirium, epilepsy, Parkinson's disease)
Pregnancy
Psychiatric
Mood disorders (depression, mania)
Anxiety disorders (generalized anxiety disorder, obsessive–compulsive disorder, panic disorder
Substance abuse (alcohol or sedative/hypnotic withdrawal)
Pharmacologically Induced
Anticonvulsants
Central adrenergic blockers
Diuretics
Selective serotonin reuptake inhibitors
Steroids
Stimulants

Compiled from Refs. 2 and 4.

▶ TREATMENT: Insomnia

Assessment of insomnia should include a history of the specific symptomatology, time course of onset, duration, frequency, daytime symptoms, sleep hygiene habits, and history of previous treatments. The therapeutic management of insomnia is determined by the duration of insomnia and may consist of a combination of general measures to improve sleep, psychotherapy, and pharmacotherapy. A treatment plan should be individualized based on the type of insomnia, severity of daytime impairment in functioning, patient age, and concurrent medical conditions. All unnecessary or high dosages of medications should be discontinued.[11] The expected duration of therapy and desired pharmacologic profile must be considered when choosing a hypnotic.

NONPHARMACOLOGIC THERAPY

General measures to improve insomnia are useful adjuncts to the specific treatment of identifiable etiologies. Cognitive, behavioral, and educational interventions include cognitive therapy, relaxation therapy (e.g., progressive muscle relaxation), stimulus-control therapy, light therapy, sleep deprivation, and sleep hygiene education. Between 70% and 80% of people with insomnia treated with nonpharmacologic methods will have a positive response.[12] Stimulus control, progressive muscle relaxation, and paradoxical intention meet the American Psychological Association (APA) criteria for empirically supported psychological treatment for insomnia. Three other treatment methods, sleep restriction, biofeedback, and multifaceted cognitive-behavior therapy, meet APA criteria for probable efficacious treatments. Sleep improvements with these methods show a sustained effect for at least 6 months after cessation of treatment.[12] Changes in sleep hygiene habits can improve the patient's sleep-wake routine and augment recovery from transient or short-term insomnia (Table 73–3). Patients with insomnia should avoid alcohol, stimulant, and nicotine use. Although alcohol enhances sleep onset, the subsequent sleep is disturbed and fragmented. Alcoholics frequently have insomnia for months to years after recovery.[4] Individuals with insomnia are sensitive to the arousal effects of mild stimulants and should avoid all caffeine-containing products and chocolate for at least 8 hours before bedtime.

TABLE 73–3. Nonpharmacologic Recommendations for Insomnia

Stimulus Control Procedures

1. Establish a regular time to wake up and to go to sleep (including weekends).
2. Sleep only as much as necessary to feel rested.
3. Go to bed only when sleepy. Avoid long periods of wakefulness in bed. Use the bed only for sleep or intimacy; do not read or watch television in bed.
4. Avoid trying to force sleep, if you do not fall asleep within 20–30 minutes, leave the bed and perform a relaxing activity (read, listen to music, watch television) until drowsy. Repeat this as often as necessary.
5. Avoid daytime naps.
6. Schedule worry time during the day. Do not take your troubles to bed.

Sleep Hygiene Recommendations

1. Exercise routinely (three to four times weekly), but not close to bedtime because this may cause arousal.
2. Create a comfortable sleep environment by avoiding temperature extremes, loud noises, and illuminated clocks.
3. Discontinue or reduce the use of alcohol, caffeine, and nicotine.
4. Avoid excessive fullness or hunger at bedtime.
5. Avoid drinking large quantities of liquids in the evening to prevent nighttime trips to the restroom.
6. Do something relaxing and enjoyable before bedtime.

Adapted from Ref. 31.

PHARMACOLOGIC THERAPY

NONBENZODIAZEPINE HYPNOTIC AGENTS

The benzodiazepines (BZs) largely replaced barbiturates (e.g., butalbital, pentobarbital, and secobarbital) because of the latter's propensity for the rapid development of tolerance, fatalities by overdose, development of physical and psychological dependence, withdrawal syndromes, and significant drug interactions.[5] Because of safety considerations, the barbiturates have few indications for use as hypnotics.[4]

Chloral hydrate therapy, which also offers no clinical advantage, may be complicated by gastrointestinal irritation, drug interactions, and fatalities in overdose. Chloral hydrate interacts with other sedatives, and the combination of chloral hydrate and alcohol has been termed a "Mickey Finn" or "knockout drops."[1]

The antidepressants (including amitriptyline, doxepin, and trazodone) are alternatives for patients with nonrestorative sleep who should not receive BZs.[13] From 1987 to 1996, use of antidepressants for sleep increased 146%.[14] Trazodone 50–100 mg is an effective hypnotic in patients with antidepressant-induced insomnia.[13]

Antihistamines are less effective than the BZs, and their use may be complicated by anticholinergic side effects.[1] Nonprescription sleep aids commonly contain antihistamines and analgesics. The amino acid L-tryptophan is no longer recommended for use as a hypnotic because of reports of eosinophilia-myalgia syndrome.[15]

Zolpidem, an imidazolpyridine chemically unrelated to BZs or barbiturates, acts selectively at the BZ_1 receptor and has minimal anxiolytic and no muscle relaxant or anticonvulsant effects. It is comparable in effectiveness to BZ hypnotics, reducing latency to sleep and increasing total sleep time and efficiency.[16] Zolpidem has little effect on sleep stages.[17] Zolpidem is metabolized by methyloxidation and hydroxylation to inactive metabolites. Its half-life is approximately 2.5 hours, and its duration of effect is 6 to 8 hours.

The most common adverse effects of zolpidem are drowsiness, amnesia, dizziness, headache, and gastrointestinal complaints.[16] Several cases of brief psychotic reactions have been reported in women.[18–20] Compared with BZs, zolpidem use is not associated with the development of tolerance or rebound insomnia after 35 days of continuous use.[21] Zolpidem also may have no significant effects on next-day psychomotor performance.[22] However, it is more expensive. The recommended daily dosage is 10 mg, but 5 mg is used in elderly patients and those with hepatic impairment. The dosage can be increased up to 20 mg nightly, but the incidence of adverse events is dose-related.[17]

Zaleplon is a recently approved hypnotic. It is a pyrazolopyrimidine and like zolpidem binds selectively to the BZ_1 receptor. Zaleplon has a rapid onset (maximal concentratons are reached between 0.9 and 1.5 hours), has a terminal half-life of about 1 hour, and is metabolized to inactive metabolites.[1,23] Zaleplon at doses of 5–20 mg has been shown to reduce sleep latency and at 20 mg to increase sleep duration when compared with placebo.[23] It does not appear to have significant rebound insomnia, withdrawal symptoms, daytime anxiety, sedation, or psychomotor impairment.[23,24]

Zaleplon does not significantly impair psychomotor performance, arousal, memory, or cognitive function the morning after administration. The most common side effects associated with zaleplon are dizziness, headache, and somnolence. Zaleplon may be an alternative for people who have trouble falling asleep. It can be used up to 4 to 5 hours before the individual has to get up due to its short half-life.[1,25] It is available in 5- and 10-mg capsules. The recommended dose is 10 mg for nonelderly adults and 5 mg for elderly people.[1]

Melatonin, a hormone released by the pineal gland at night, is available over the counter and is promoted as a sleep aid. It may be promising in neurologically devastated children and the elderly, as well as in individuals experiencing jet lag.[26,27] Marketed as a dietary supplement, no Food and Drug Administration (FDA) controls are imposed. Thus manufacturing and purity concerns should not be ignored.

Valerian is an herbal product that is used to promote sleep. German Commission E recommends its use for the management of restlessness and nervous disturbances of sleep. Its mechanism of action is not fully understood but may involve inhibition of the enzyme that breaks down γ-amino butyric acid (GABA). The recommended dose of valerian is 2–3 g given one to several times a day. It can be ingested as a tea. The dose of the tincture is 0.5–1 teaspoon. Again, as with melatonin, this product is not regulated by the FDA, and therefore, it is not subject to controls. Side effects appear to be similar to those of other sedatives; therefore, it is important that patients be warned not to drive or perform other tasks that require alertness. It should be avoided in pregnancy.[28]

BENZODIAZEPINE HYPNOTICS

In the United States, five BZs are marketed with a therapeutic indication for insomnia (Table 73–4); however, other BZs also are effective. BZs relieve insomnia by reducing the latency to sleep onset and number of awakenings and by increasing the total sleep time. BZs decrease the duration of stages 1 and 4 sleep and increase stage 2 sleep. Unlike the barbiturates, BZs do not decrease REM sleep to cause a severe REM rebound syndrome.[29]

Pharmacokinetics

BZ onset and duration of activity are the most important characteristics to be considered when choosing an agent. When used as a single dose, the extent of distribution and elimination half-life are important in predicting BZ duration of action. However, after multiple dosing, the elimination half-life and formation of active metabolites determine the extent of drug accumulation and resultant clinical effects.[30]

BZ pharmacokinetic properties are summarized in Table 73–4. The onset of action depends on the rate of absorption. Flurazepam and triazolam are absorbed rapidly. Temazepam is less lipophilic and has a slower onset of effect. Sedation after flurazepam, estazolam, and quazepam occurs within 1 to 2 hours after ingestion.[31]

Triazolam is redistributed quickly because of its high lipophilicity and thus has a short duration of effect.[30] Estazolam and temazepam are intermediate in their duration of action. The therapeutic effects of flurazepam and quazepam are long in comparison because of the active metabolites.

With the exception of temazepam, which is eliminated via conjugation, all BZ hypnotics are metabolized by hepatic microsomal oxidation and then undergo glucuronide conjugation. Oxidation may be inhibited in patients with impaired liver function, advanced age, or concurrent use of drugs that inhibit oxidation. Drugs that inhibit the cytochrome P450 3A4 enzyme (e.g., erythromycin, nefazodone, fluvoxamine, and ketoconazole) reduce the clearance of triazolam and increase its plasma concentrations.[32,33]

Triazolam (a short-elimination-half-life BZ), estazolam, and temazepam (intermediate-elimination-half-life BZs) lack clinically significant metabolites. Flurazepam and quazepam have long elimination half-lives. Flurazepam is metabolized rapidly to two short-acting metabolites, hydroxyethylflurazepam and flurazepam aldehyde. These metabolites contribute to sleep induction on the first night of therapy but are eliminated within 12 hours. *N*-Desalkylflurazepam (*N*-DAF) is an active metabolite that has a very long half-life and accumulates extensively during multiple dosing.[1] *N*-DAF accounts for most of flurazepam's pharmacologic effects. Quazepam and one of its metabolites, 2-oxoquazepam, have elimination half-lives of 39 hours. Quazepam's oxoquazepam metabolite is metabolized to *N*-DAF.[34] If oxidation of *N*-DAF is impaired, its half-life becomes prolonged, and complications of drug accumulation may result with repeated dosing; however, tolerance may develop to these effects.[30] *N*-DAF may be useful when daytime anxiety or early morning awakening are complaints, but daytime sedation and impaired psychomotor performance may complicate therapy.

Adverse Effects

High dosages of BZs with long or intermediate elimination half-lives have a greater potential for producing daytime sedation and

TABLE 73–4. Pharmacokinetics of Benzodiazepine Hypnotic Agents

Generic Name	t_{max} (h)[a]	Parent $t_{1/2}$ (h)	Daily Dose Range (mg)	Metabolic Pathway	Clinically Significant Metabolites
Estazolam	2	12–15	1–2	Oxidation	—
Flurazepam	1	8	15–30	Oxidation	Hydroxyethylflurazepam
					Flurazepam aldehyde
				N-dealkylation	*N*-DAF[b]
Quazepam	2	39	7.5–15	Oxidation	2-Oxo-quazepam
				N-dealkylation	*N*-DAF[b]
Temazepam	1.5	10–15	15–30	Conjugation	—
Triazolam	1	2	0.125–0.25	Oxidation	—

[a]Time to peak plasma concentration.
[b]*N*-desalkylflurazepam, mean half-life 47 to 100 hours.

performance impairment. These effects include excessive drowsiness, psychomotor incoordination, decreased concentration, and cognitive deficits. Tolerance to the central nervous system (CNS) carryover effects may develop with time. Rapidly eliminated BZs (i.e., triazolam) have less potential for producing daytime sedation.[1]

Tolerance to BZ hypnotic effect develops sooner with triazolam (after 2 weeks of continuous use) than with other BZ hypnotics.[1] The hypnotic efficacy of flurazepam, quazepam, and temazepam is maintained for 1 month of continuous nightly use.[1] Estazolam reportedly maintains the duration and quality of sleep at the maximum dosage (2 mg nightly) for up to 12 weeks.[35] Long-term use (>6 months) of BZs was associated with a low risk of abuse, side effects, and tolerance in patients with severe, chronic sleep disorders; however, efficacy has not been established.[36]

Anterograde amnesia is an impairment of memory and recall after drug ingestion reported to occur during BZ therapy. Anterograde amnesia occurs more frequently with triazolam than with temazepam[37]; however, anterograde amnesia has been reported with most BZs.[30] The lowest effective dosage should be used to avoid adverse effects on memory. When compared with temazepam, triazolam use was associated with a higher reported rate of confusion, bizarre behavior, agitation, and hallucinations. These CNS effects occurred with higher doses (68% of patients ingested 0.5–1.5 mg) and in older patients (mean of 63 years).[37] Because of the high incidence of CNS adverse effects, the United Kingdom suspended sales of triazolam in October 1991.[38] Controversy surrounding triazolam led the FDA to review the agent in 1990 and 1992. Triazolam was considered safe and effective, but caution was noted regarding possible memory problems.

Daytime anxiety and rebound insomnia are associated with the use of triazolam.[1] Rebound insomnia is characterized by increased wakefulness beyond baseline amounts that usually lasts for one to two nights after abrupt discontinuation of BZ hypnotics with short- or intermediate-elimination half-lives. Rebound insomnia occurs more frequently after high doses of triazolam, even when ingested intermittently.[39] The occurrence of rebound insomnia can be minimized by using the lowest effective dose and tapering the dose on discontinuation.[40]

The incidence of CNS side effects increases with age secondary to increased sensitivity to pharmacologic effects and prolonged BZ half-lives, which may increase the potential for drug accumulation. Prolonged sedation and cognitive and psychomotor impairment are concerns in the elderly. Short- and intermediate-elimination–half-life drugs are associated with fewer performance deficits; however, they may increase the chance of daytime anxiety in elderly patients. There is an association between falls and hip fractures and the use of long-elimination–half-life BZs; thus flurazepam and quazepam should be avoided in elderly patients.[6]

Guidelines

Hypnotic therapy is indicated in individuals with transient or short-term insomnia.[2] Patients should be counseled that sleep will return to normal when the precipitating stressor is eliminated and also be educated on strategies for stimulus control and good sleep hygiene (see Table 73–3). If the stressor is expected to last more than 1 week, intermittent hypnotic use (three or four nights per week) should be prescribed for no more than 3 weeks.

For patients with chronic insomnia, medical, psychiatric, and pharmacologic causes should be identified and managed.[1] If treatment of an underlying disorder fails to result in improvement, intermittent pharmacotherapy may be indicated. If the insomnia is psychophysiologic, several months of supervised hypnotic therapy may help alleviate anxiety and reestablish a regular sleep pattern on drug discontinuation; however, these patients require nonpharmacologic therapy as well.[12] Tolerance and dependence can be avoided by using hypnotics at the lowest possible dose, intermittently, and for the shortest duration possible. Patients should receive instruction on frequency of drug use and the expected duration of therapy to prevent development of dependence. Withdrawal symptoms can be diminished by tapering the dosage gradually. Patients should be counseled on rebound insomnia when BZ therapy is terminated.

Patients with difficulty initiating sleep and those who require daytime alertness should receive the short-acting BZ hypnotics or zaleplon. Those with difficulty maintaining sleep or early morning awakening may benefit from intermediate-elimination–half-life agents if daytime performance is required. Long-elimination–half-life BZs should be considered if management of daytime anxiety is required. There is no rationale for the concurrent use of two BZs to treat anxiety and insomnia.

BZ hypnotics should not be prescribed for individuals with sleep apnea, a history of substance abuse, or during pregnancy. Patients should be instructed to avoid alcohol; even alcohol on the day after ingestion of a long-elimination–half-life BZ can result in additive CNS impairment. Prescriptions for BZ hypnotics should be accompanied by printed information and verbal counseling on precautions.

SLEEP APNEA

Sleep-related respiratory abnormalities are diagnosed commonly in sleep laboratories using PSG. *Apnea* is defined as the cessation of airflow at the nose and mouth lasting at least 10 seconds. It is classified into two major categories: obstructive and central. Patients with sleep apnea have a high risk of morbidity and mortality.[41]

OBSTRUCTIVE SLEEP APNEA

Obstructive sleep apnea (OSA) is a potentially life-threatening condition characterized by repeated episodes of nocturnal breathing cessation with loud snoring and gasping, often reported by the bed partner.[42] OSA is estimated to occur in 1% to 9% of the population, predominantly in males.[2] OSA is caused by an occlusion of the upper airway (causes include obesity, polyps, enlarged tonsils, adenoids, or tongue) that occurs only during sleep.[42]

In OSA patients, airflow ceases while respiratory effort continues. The apneic episode is terminated by a reflex action to the fall in O_2 saturation that causes a brief miniarousal during which breathing resumes. Patients may be unaware of the miniarousals; however, the EEG clearly indicates activity that may cause fragmented sleep. Thus patients usually present with excessive daytime sleepiness. In severe cases, excessive somnolence may cause sleep attacks that can result in decrements in performance (leading, for example, to motor vehicle accidents). Additional daytime symptoms include morning headache, poor memory, and irritability.[42] Most individuals with OSA are overweight. Complications include arrhythmias, hypertension, cor pulmonale, and sudden death during somnolence.[42]

Treatment of OSA must be individualized and depends on the severity of the disordered breathing and the amount of sleep disruption.[43] Patients with severe apnea (>20 apneas/h on PSG and excessive daytime somnolence) and those with moderate apneas (5–20 apneas/h on PSG and excessive daytime sleepiness or other daytime symptoms) have shown significant improvement and reduction in mortality with treatment.[42] Nonpharmacologic measures are the treatments of choice. Weight loss may eliminate the apnea and reduce daytime hypersomnia[42]; however, improvement is only limited. Treatment of underlying causes of obstruction (e.g., tonsillectomy, nasal septal repair, nonsedating antihistamines for allergic rhinitis) may eliminate apneas during sleep. In patients with mild apnea and snoring with no daytime symptomatology, management may include avoidance of a supine sleep position.[43]

Nasal continuous positive airway pressure (CPAP) during sleep is the standard treatment for most patients with OSA.[42] CPAP elevates the pressure in the oropharyngeal space to maintain positive airway pressure during the respiratory cycle. Patient tolerance and compliance are the major limitations of CPAP. Although tracheostomy is an effective surgical procedure, it is reserved for use in treatment-resistant patients. Uvulopalatopharyngoplasty is a surgical procedure to enlarge the pharyngeal airspace that successfully reduces apnea in 50% of patients and snoring in 90%.[41,42] Upper airway resection also can be performed with new laser surgical techniques.[41]

The single most important pharmacologic intervention is the avoidance of all CNS depressants (i.e., alcohol, anxiolytics, hypnotics, narcotics, zolpidem).[41] Preliminary studies in chronic respiratory disorder patients suggest that zaleplon does not negatively affect respiratory function.[44] CNS depressant use is potentially lethal because it interferes with the brain's ability to produce the resumption of breathing. Drug therapy should be reserved for patients with mild forms of OSA and those who have failed other treatments. Protriptyline, in doses of 10–30 mg/d, reduces the frequency of apneas and increases O_2 saturation.[41] Protriptyline may be used for mild OSA without hypercapnia. The mechanism of action may be related to a decrease in REM sleep or an increase in the tonus of the musculature of the oropharynx. Anticholinergic side effects often complicate therapy.[43] Fluoxetine 20 mg/d was effective in reducing apneas in some patients.[44] Respiratory stimulants such as theophylline[46] and clonidine (in males)[47] also have been tried; however, efficacy is limited, and research has not documented long-term effectiveness. Medroxyprogesterone 60 mg has improved persons with sleep apnea and obesity-hypoventilation syndrome; however, controlled studies show no beneficial effects.[43]

CENTRAL SLEEP APNEA

Central sleep apnea (CSA) is characterized by repeated episodes of apnea caused by temporary loss of respiratory effort during somnolence. It accounts for less than 10% of all apneas. Hypercapnic patients usually present with morning headache and daytime somnolence, whereas nonhypercapnic patients complain of insomnia and nocturnal awakenings with shortness of breath or gasping. Although the majority of CSA cases are idiopathic, identifiable causes are nasal obstruction, autonomic system lesions (e.g., cervical cordotomy), neurologic diseases (e.g., poliomyelitis, encephalitis, myasthenia gravis), and congestive heart failure.[48] The primary treatment approach for the hypercapnic CSA patient is ventilatory support with O_2 and CPAP; acetazolamide, theophylline, and medroxyprogesterone have shown mixed results.[48] In refractory cases, diaphragmatic pacing, tracheostomy, or positive-pressure ventilation is helpful. In nonhypercapnic CSA patients, treatment may consist of BZs (triazolam or temazepam) to reduce arousals and acetazolamide, CPAP, and O_2 to stabilize breathing patterns.[48]

NARCOLEPSY

Narcolepsy is a chronic disease that typically begins before the age of 25 years. About 0.5% of the adult population has narcolepsy, with men and women being affected equally. There appears to be a genetic predetermination for narcolepsy, since 3% of patients have a first-degree relative with the disorder. An association has been made between narcolepsy and the human leukocyte antigens (HLAs) DQ6/DQB1*0602 and/or DR2/DRB1*1501.[50] Recent evidence suggests a second locus for HLA-associated narcolepsy on chromosome 4p13-q21.[49]

The essential feature of narcolepsy is excessive daytime sleepiness, with sleep attacks that may last up to 30 minutes. Individuals often complain of hypersomnia, fatigue, impaired performance, and disturbed nighttime sleep. Excessive daytime sleepiness occurs before the second decade of life, and the auxiliary symptoms (i.e., cataplexy, hypnagogic hallucinations, sleep paralysis) appear several years later.[49]

Cataplexy is an episode of sudden bilateral loss of muscle tone (generalized muscular weakness) resulting in the individual collapsing and often is precipitated by emotionally charged stimuli (e.g., laughter, anger, excitement). The individual remains conscious and the episode is brief, seconds to several minutes. Cataplexy occurs in 70% to 80% of people with narcolepsy. Sleep paralysis occurs when the individual is falling asleep or when waking. It is an episodic loss of voluntary muscle tone. The individual is awake but unable to move or speak. Hypnagogic (at the threshold of sleep) and hypnopompic (on awakening) hallucinations are brief, dreamlike experiences with more fragmentation and bizarre features than a typical dream.[49]

Sleep laboratory evaluation of the narcoleptic confirms the existence of excessive daytime sleepiness, disturbed nighttime sleep, and sleep-onset REM periods. The occurrence of sleep paralysis, cataplexy, and sleep-onset REM indicates that narcolepsy represents an abnormality in the regulatory mechanisms of REM sleep (possibly in the cholinergic system).[49]

▶ TREATMENT: Narcolepsy

Symptomatic management is both nonpharmacologic and pharmacologic. Counseling the patient and significant others is essential because family members often think that narcolepsy is voluntary and that the patient is lazy and nonproductive. Good sleep habits should be encouraged. If the patient's daily schedule allows, two or more brief daytime naps can be beneficial. Following a 15-minute nap, the patient may be refreshed for several hours. Support groups exist locally and nationally for people with narcolepsy.[51]

Pharmacologic treatment consists of the use of psychostimulants for excessive daytime sleepiness and antidepressants for cataplexy[49] (Table 73–5). Stimulants exert their effects by enhancing NE release from presynaptic neurons.[49] Modafinil's mechanism of action to promote wakefulness is unknown.[52] Methylphenidate, dextroamphetamine, and modafinil are approved by the FDA for use in narcolepsy. Amphetamines and methylphenidate have a fast onset of effect and durations of 3 to 4 and 6 to 10 hours, respectively. The dose may range from 5–60 mg/day, and divided daily doses are recommended; however, more expensive sustained-release formulations are available. Peak plasma concentrations of modafinil occur between 2 and 4 hours, and the drug's half-life is approximately

TABLE 73–5. Drugs Used to Treat Narcolepsy

Generic Name	Trade Name (Manufacturer)	Daily Dosage Range (mg)
Excessive Daytime Somnolence		
Dextroamphetamine	Dexadrine (SmithKline Beecham) generics (various)	5–60
Dextroamphetamine/amphetamine salts[a]	Adderall (Shire US)	5–60
Methamphetamine[b]	Desoxyn (Abbott)	5–15
Methylphenidate	Ritalin (Novartis), generics (various)	30–80
Modafinil	Provigil (Cephalon)	200–400
Pemoline	Cylert (Abbott)	37.5–112.5
Adjunct Agents for Cataplexy		
Imipramine	Tofranil (Novartis), generics (various)	50–250
Protriptyline	Vivactil (Merck), generics (various)	5–30
Nortriptyline	Aventyl (Lilly), Pamelor (Sandoz), generics (various)	50–200
Selegiline	Eldepryl (Somerset)	20–40
Gamma-hydroxybutyrate	(Orphan Medical)	60 mg/kg/night

[a]Dextroamphetamine sulfate, dextroamphetamine saccharate, amphetamine asparate, amphetamine sulfate.
[b]Not available in some states.
Compiled from Refs. 53 and 54.

15 hours. Modafinil's dose range is 200–400 mg/day given as a single dose. Preliminary evidence on modafinil suggests no evidence of tolerance, withdrawal symptoms after abrupt discontinuation, or risk of abuse.[53] Pemoline has a delayed onset of effect, but its duration is 8 to 10 hours; maximal effect may take several weeks. Pemoline's dose range is 18.75–112.5 mg/day. Liver function tests must be monitored (at 1 month and yearly) during pemoline therapy. Amphetamine use is associated with more likelihood of abuse and tolerance, especially when prescribed in high doses.[54] In one patient, bupropion 100 mg three times daily improved REM sleep propensity and sleepiness.[55]

The tricyclic antidepressants (TCAs), through blockade of NE and serotonin reuptake, are effective in reducing cataplexy and sleep paralysis. Imipramine, protriptyline, and nortriptyline are effective in approximately 80% of patients.[54] Selegiline improves hypersomnolence and cataplexy, presumably through REM suppression and increase in REM latency.[56,57] Tranylcypromine and codeine may improve cataplexy and increase daytime alertness.[58,59] γ-Hydroxybutyrate (GHB) is a therapeutic option without anticholinergic side effects.[60] GHB may decrease cataplexy episodes, sleep paralysis, hypnagogic hallucinations, and daytime sleepiness.

GUIDELINES

General principles of drug therapy for narcolepsy include using the lowest effective dose possible, employing gradual titration, and monitoring carefully for therapeutic and adverse events. The goal of therapy is to maximize alertness during normal waking hours or at selected times of the day. Scheduled naps can help to maintain wakefulness.[50] Naps should be encouraged instead of taking drugs. In addition, cataplexy may be treated on an as-needed basis in some patients. If the patient can predict the occurrence of cataplexy (associated with an anticipated specific stimulus), then a TCA can be ingested for only the day or two before and during the expected occurrence.

CIRCADIAN RHYTHM DISORDERS

The etiology of circadian rhythm disorders is a mismatch between an individual's biologic clock and the external time cues of the environment. Two commonly occurring circadian rhythm sleep disorders are jet lag and shift-work sleep problems.

JET LAG

Jet lag follows rapid travel over multiple time zones and results in varying degrees and durations of sleep onset or maintenance insomnia complaints and daytime sleepiness. Insomnia usually occurs every other night. Sleep disturbances last for 2 to 3 days but may prevail for 7 to 10 days if time zone changes are 8 to 12 hours. Compared with westward travel, eastward travel is associated with a longer duration of jet lag. Affected individuals also may suffer from decreased performance and alertness and gastrointestinal disturbances.[61]

Treatment of jet lag includes preventive measures and pharmacologic management. Jet lag can be avoided during coast-to-coast travel in the United States for durations of stay less than 7 days in a new time zone by adhering to the normal sleep-wake schedule from home. For longer lengths of stay, adjustment to a westbound time zone can be made by staying up and arising 1 to 2 hours later several days before the trip. Eastbound travelers also can adjust their schedule by retiring and arising earlier for several days before the trip.[61] Pharmacologic treatment of jet lag includes the use of short-acting BZs. Melatonin has been used investigationally to rapidly entrain the circadian rhythm.[4,61] Patients also should be instructed to avoid ingestion of alcohol.

SHIFT-WORK SLEEP PROBLEMS

Shift workers comprise approximately 20% of the workforce.[61] Working at night causes a misalignment in the sleep-wake cycle and circadian rhythms associated with a decrease in alertness, performance, and quality of daytime sleep. On nonworking nights, many night-shift workers experience insomnia.[61] Treatment may consist of recommending a daytime job, extending daytime sleep by sleeping in the afternoon, or scheduling a 2- to 3-hour afternoon nap on days off from work. Hypnotics may be useful.[62] Scheduled exposure to bright lights at night and darkness during the daytime improves psychological and behavioral adaptation to night work and daytime sleep.[63] Melatonin also has been used succesfully.[64]

DYSSOMNIAS NOT OTHERWISE SPECIFIED

A dyssomnia that is not primary, due to a general medical condition, or substance induced is categorized as *not otherwise specified.* Idiopathic restless legs syndrome and idiopathic periodic limb movements are examples.

RESTLESS LEGS SYNDROME

Restless legs syndrome (RLS), also known as *Ekbom's syndrome,* is a discomfort, not pain, verbalized as pins and needles, a crawling sensation, or cramping mainly in the calves but sometimes noted in the thighs or arms.[65] Males and females are equally affected, and RLS occurs most commonly in the elderly. Iron deficiency, pregnancy, and renal failure are associated with RLS. Caffeine, stress, or fatigue may worsen the symptoms. The diagnosis generally is made based on the clinical presentation.

The sensation generally is bilateral and occurs only during rest and inactivity and is relieved quickly by walking or moving the legs.[66] When the person tries to resume sleep, the discomfort returns, thus resulting in insomnia. Mild or intermittent symptoms generally require no treatment, but patients should be reassured that this is benign and chronic. Depression and suicidal ideation may occur in more severe cases.

BZs may be the first-line agents for less severe cases and in younger patients. Clonazepam, lorazepam, triazolam, and temazepam have been effective. Clonazepam 0.5–2.0 mg is the most studied.[31] Opiates, such as methadone 5–20 mg, codeine 30–120 mg, and oxycodone 2.5 mg, are very effective, but tolerance develops, and abuse potential is a concern because the condition is chronic. Other agents used include apomorphine infusion, amantadine, tramadol, magnesium, oxycodone, propoxyphene, gabapentin, bromocriptine, clonidine, and carbamazepine.[67–71] Tolerance may develop with any agent used; thus one approach is to alternate chemically unrelated agents weekly or biweekly.[66] Patients should take the agent early enough prior to bedtime to allow time for drug absorption.

In the most severe cases, levodopa and the dopamine agonists cabergoline, pergolide, pramipexole, and ropinirole may be considered.[65,66,72–75] Generally, the initial dose of levodopa is 50 mg 30 minutes before bedtime. This dose may be titrated, and most patients achieve benefit from levodopa 200 mg with carbidopa 50 mg.[76] However, rebound symptoms during the night and possibly during the day are noted. Dosing during the day or using the sustained-release product may alleviate rebound symptoms.

NOCTURNAL MYOCLONUS (PERIODIC LIMB MOVEMENTS)

Most patients with RLS also have periodic limb movements (PLMs), and approximately one-third of patients with PLMs have RLS.[65,66] However, the two disorders are distinct. Unlike RLS, PLMs is diagnosed in the sleep laboratory. A burst of muscle activity lasting 0.5 to 5 seconds is noted in the anterior tibialis EMG recording. Confirmation of diagnosis is at least 40 bursts in an 8-hour period of sleep.

PLMs are described as stereotypic, repetitive, periodic movements of the legs that occur every 20 to 40 seconds and last 10 minutes to several hours.[65,66] The movements generally involve the big toe, but the ankle, knee, and hip also may flex. PLMs occur during sleep. They may be terminated by a violent kick or other bodily movement. The person does not recognize the problem and notes only the daytime consequence of excessive daytime somnolence. Often the bed partner describes the person as a restless sleeper and notes that the bedcovers are in disarray. Renal failure is likely a predisposing condition to PLMs. BZ withdrawal and TCAs may precipitate the condition.

The treatment approach is similar to RLS. Milder cases do not require treatment. Clonazepam 0.5–2 mg is used frequently, as is baclofen 20–40 mg and opiates. TCAs generally worsen the problem; however, in one series, imipramine 25 mg improved symptoms in five patients.[31] Lamotrigine 100 mg also has improved symptoms.[77] The most severe cases are begun on levodopa or dopamine agonists. Alternating medications and allowing drug holidays may be helpful. Patients should take their medications early enough before bedtime to allow for drug absorption.

PARASOMNIAS

Parasomnias refer to a group of acute, episodic, physical phenomena that occur either exclusively during sleep or are exaggerated by sleep. Sleep walking (somnambulism) and sleep terrors are seen in children and may be considered normal to some degree at a certain age.[78] Somnambulism and sleep terrors occur most commonly from delta NREM sleep.[79] Somnambulism treatment consists primarily of protection from injury (e.g., putting safety latches on doors and windows, removing hazardous objects from bedrooms, and covering glass doors with heavy curtains). Theoretically, sleepwalking may be prevented by suppressing delta sleep. Although BZs suppress delta sleep, the risks of long-term, continuous exposure of a developing child to delta sleep suppressants is unknown. BZs, selective serotonin reuptake inhibitors (SSRIs), or TCAs may be beneficial in adults.[78] Sleep terrors treatment consists of counseling the parents to wait until the disorder is outgrown. As with somnambulism, sleep terrors occur during delta sleep; BZs may be useful in adults secondary to delta sleep suppression.[78]

Nightmares are an REM phenomenon associated with frequent, elaborate recall of frightening dream content (e.g., dreams of physical attacks and death). Treatment usually consists of psychological intervention. This may be as simple as a parent providing comfort and reassurance to a child with an occasional nightmare or as complex as intensive psychotherapy and use of cyproheptadine for an adult with frequent, highly disturbing nightmares.[80]

PHARMACOECONOMIC CONSIDERATIONS

Insomnia affects all three domains of quality of life: the ability to perform activities of daily living, emotional concerns, and interpersonal life.[81,82] Scores of patients with dyssomnias were compared with the general U.S. population norms using a health-related quality-of-life questionnaire. Results reflected significantly worse quality of life in persons with dyssomnias.[83] Direct costs of insomnia in 1995 were estimated to be \$13.9 billion.[84] Direct costs include the cost of health services and treatment. The estimated cost from absenteeism and sleep-related accidents is \$92.5 to \$107.5 billion per year. Indirect costs include absenteeism, decreased productivity, accidents, and increased morbidity (both psychiatric and nonpsychiatric) and mortality. Treatment of the sleep disorder is beneficial. For example, treatment with nasal CPAP for obstructive sleep apnea improved the number of years of expected good health by 5.5 quality-adjusted life years.[82]

Quality of life was severely impaired in shift workers, but hypnotic therapy markedly improved the disorder and quality of life.[62] Persons were once again able to enjoy their free time, and alertness was not affected by sedative use. Quality of life can be improved by smoking cessation, reductions in caffeine and alcohol intake, and reduction in intake of over-the-counter sleep aids. If the sleep disturbance is related to a side effect of an antidepressant, quality of life, compliance, and overall outcome can be improved by managing the side effect.[85]

EVALUATION OF THERAPEUTIC OUTCOMES

A decision analysis for dyssomnias is shown in Figure 73–1. Patients with short-term or chronic insomnia should be evaluated after 1 week of therapy to assess for drug effectiveness, adverse events, and adherence to nonpharmacologic recommendations. Patients should be instructed to maintain a daily sleep diary. The diary requires daily recording of bedtime, arising time, sleep onset latency, number and durations of awakenings, medication ingestion, naps, and an index of sleep quality.[86]

Individuals with sleep apnea treated with weight reduction and CPAP or drug therapy should be evaluated after 2 to 4 weeks of treatment for improvement in alertness and daytime symptoms (reduction in headache frequency and severity, improvement in memory, decreased irritability), and weight reduction. The bed partner can be consulted regarding reduced snoring and gasping episodes. A repeat PSG is indicated if the patient has not shown clinical improvement. Overall, the goals of therapy are to reduce the number of apneic episodes and improve O_2 saturation.

In people with narcolepsy, reduction in daytime sleepiness, cataplexy, hypnagogic and hypnopompic hallucinations, and sleep paralysis is monitored. Patients should be evaluated monthly until an optimal dose is achieved and then every 6 to 12 months to assess for the development of adverse drug events (e.g., mood changes, sleep disturbances, cardiovascular abnormalities). If symptoms increase during therapy, PSG should be performed.

Patients with RLS and/or PLMs should be evaluated monthly to monitor for excessive daytime somnolence, tolerance, efficacy, and adverse effects of the medications. Because the conditions are chronic, assessment should occur every 6 to 12 months and should include monitoring for depression because it is a frequent complication that should be treated.

CONCLUSIONS

Disturbances of sleep affect approximately one-third of the population. Effective management of sleep disturbances requires an accurate diagnosis. Treatment of sleep disorders includes both pharmacologic and nonpharmacologic modalities.

Identifiable causes of insomnia should be managed before pharmacologic therapy is considered. BZs are the preferable agents for the short-term treatment of insomnia; however, their use is

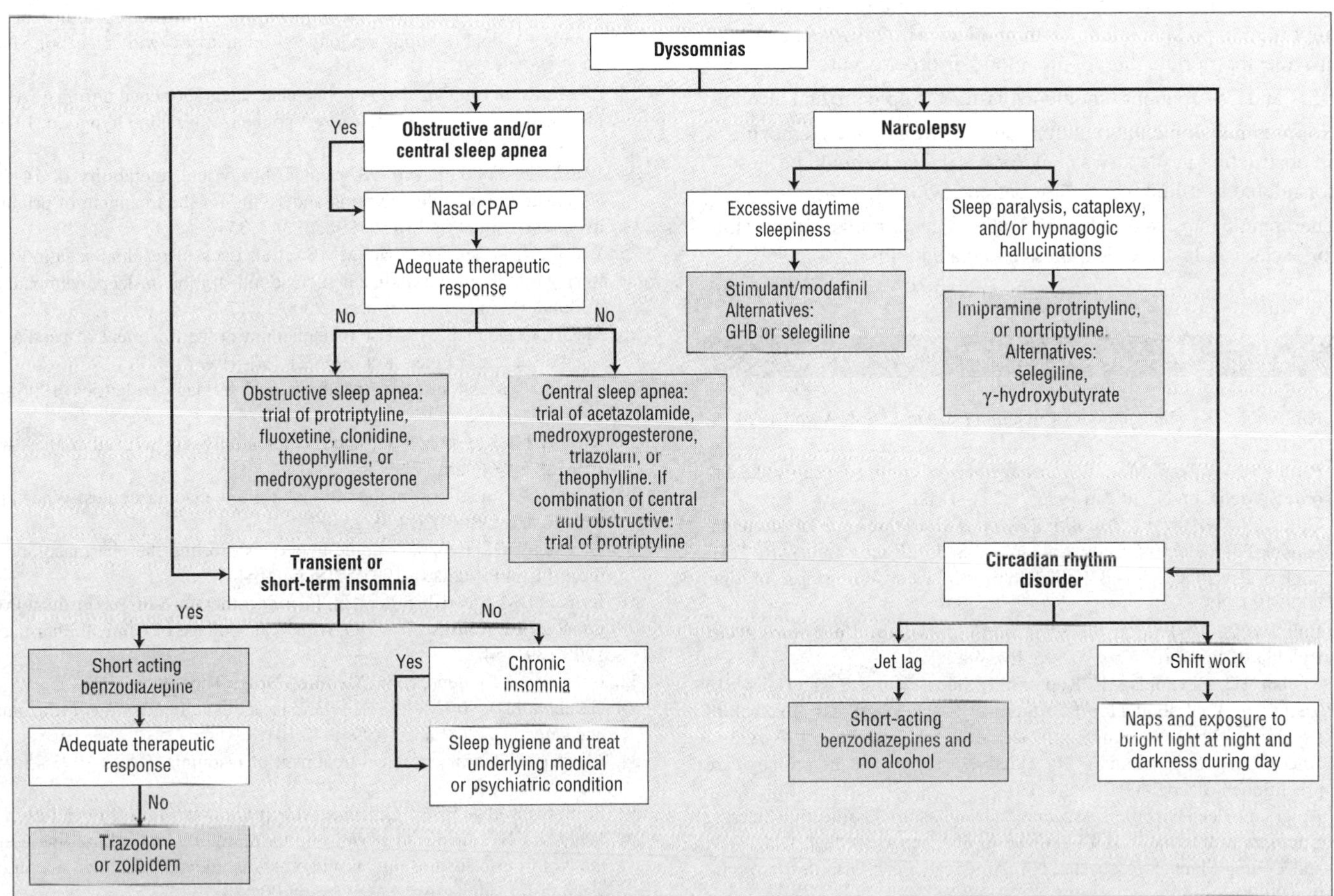

FIGURE 73–1. Algorithm for treatment of dyssomnias. (*Adapted and reprinted with permission from Jermain DM.* Sleep disorders. In Jann M. ed.: Pharmacotherapy self-assessment program. 2nd ed. Kansas City, MO. American College of Clinical Pharmacy, 1995:139–154.)

contraindicated in sleep apnea. Antidepressants are an alternative for insomnia, and they effectively manage sleep apnea and symptoms of narcolepsy. The psychostimulants and TCAs are effective treatments for patients with narcolepsy. Parasomnias and circadian rhythm disorders usually are managed nonpharmacologically. Mild cases of RLS and PLMs often are managed nonpharmacologically, but the more severe cases are treated with clonazepam, levodopa, or opiates.

▶ PRINCIPLES OF PHARMACOTHERAPY

- Insomnia for greater than 3 weeks should be suspected to be a symptom of a medical or psychiatric disorder.
- Common causes of insomnia include jet lag, significant psychosocial stress, excessive alcohol use, caffeine intake, and nicotine use.
- Sleep hygiene principles, such as relaxing before bedtime, exercising regularly, establishing a regular bedtime and wake up time, and discontinuing or reducing alcohol, caffeine, and nicotine, should be taught to patients with insomnia.
- BZ tolerance and dependence are avoided by using low-dose, intermittent therapy for the shortest possible duration.
- Long-acting BZs should be avoided in the elderly.
- Bedtime doses of antidepressants such as trazodone may be considered an alternative for patients experiencing insomnia.
- Monitoring mood symptoms of a patient experiencing a sleep disturbance after a significant loss or during a difficult time is important to prevent a long-term problem with insomnia and provide appropriate therapy if a mood disorder occurs.
- OSA and CSA patients should avoid BZs, zolpidem, and alcohol.
- Nonpharmacologic interventions such as weight loss, removing an obstruction in the airway, and/or nasal CPAP should be considered first-line therapy for patients with OSA.
- Therapeutic naps should be used rather than stimulants if possible for excessive daytime sleepiness associated with narcolepsy.

REFERENCES

1. Kirkwood CK. Management of insomnia. J Am Pharm Assoc 1999;39:688–696.
2. Farney RJ, Walker JM. Office management of common sleep-wake disorders. Med Clin North Am 1995;79:391–414.
3. Gillin CJ, Seifritz E, Zoltoski RK, et al. Basic science of sleep. In: Sadock BJ, Sadock VA, eds. Kaplan and Sadock's Comprehensive Textbook of Psychiatry, 7th ed. Philadelphia, Lippincott Williams & Wilkins, 2000:199–209.
4. Culebras A. Update on disorders of sleep and the sleep-wake cycle. Psychiatr Clin North Am 1992;15:467–489.
5. Neylan TC, Reynolds CF, Kupfer DJ. Sleep disorders. In: Hales RE, Yudofsky SC, Talbott JT, eds. American Psychiatric Press Textbook of Psychiatry, 2d ed. Washington, American Psychiatric Press, 1994:833.
6. Ancoli-Isreal S. Insomnia in the elderly: A review for the primary care practitioner. Sleep 2000;23:S23–S30.
7. American Sleep Disorders Association Diagnostic Classification Steering Committee. International Classification of Sleep Disorders: Diagnostic and Coding Manual. Rochester, NY, American Sleep Disorders Association, 1990:1.
8. American Psychiatric Association. Sleep disorders. In: Diagnostic and Statistical Manual of Mental Disorders, Text Revision, 4th ed. Washington, American Psychiatric Press, 2000:597.
9. Rechtschaffen A, Kales A. A Manual of Standardized Terminology, Techniques and Scoring System for Sleep Stages of Human Subjects. Public Health Service Publication No. 204. Washington, U.S. Government Printing Office, 1968:1.
10. Ford DE, Kamerow DB. Epidemiologic study of sleep disturbances and psychiatric disorders. JAMA 1989;262:1479–1484.
11. Dement WC. The proper use of sleeping pills in the primary care setting. J Clin Psychiatry 1992;53(Suppl 12):50–56. Walsh JK, Engelhardt CL. Trends in the pharmacologic treatment of insomnia. J Clin Psychiatry 1992;53(Suppl 12):10–17.
12. Morin CM, Hauri PF, Espie CA, et al. Nonpharmacologic treatment of chronic insomnia. Sleep 1999;22:1134–1156.
13. Nienberg AA, Alder LA, Peselow E, et al. Trazodone for antidepressant-associated insomnia. Am J Psychiatry 1994;151:1069–1072.
14. Walsh JK, Schweitzer PK. Ten-year trends in the pharmacological treatment of insomnia. Sleep 1999;22:371–375.
15. Hertzman PA, Blevins WL, Mayer J. Association of eosinophilia-myalgia syndrome with the ingestion of tryptophan. N Engl J Med 1990; 322:869–873.
16. Hoehns JD, Perry PJ. Zolpidem: A nonbenzodiazepine hypnotic for treatment of insomnia. Clin Pharm 1993;12:814–828.
17. Zolpidem for insomnia. Med Lett Drugs Ther 1993;35:35–36.
18. Ansseau M, Pichot W, Hansenne M, Gonzales-Moreno A. Psychotic reactions to zolpidem. Lancet 1992;339:809.
19. Markowitz JS, Brewerton TD. Zolpidem-induced psychosis. Ann Clin Psychiatry 1996;8:89–91.
20. Hoyler CL, Tekell JL, Silva JA. Zolpidem-induced agitation and disorganization. Gen Hosp Psychiatry 1996;18:452–453.
21. Scharf MB, Roth T, Vogel GW, Walsh JK. A multicenter, placebo-controlled study evaluating zolpidem in the treatment of chronic insomnia. J Clin Psychiatry 1994;55:192–199.
22. Roth T, Roehrs T, Vogel G. Zolpidem in the treatment of transient insomnia: A double-blind, randomized comparison with placebo. Sleep 1995;18:246–251.
23. Elie R, Ruther E, Farr Ik, et al. Sleep latency is shortened during 4 weeks of treatment with zaleplon, a novel nonbenzodiazepine hypnotic. J Clin Psychiatry 1999;60:536–544.
24. Walsh JK, Fry J, Erwin CS, et al. Efficacy and tolerability of 14-day administration of zaleplon 5 mg and 10 mg for the treatment of primary insomnia. Clin Drug Invest 1998;16:347–354.
25. Walsh JK, Pollak CP, Sharf MMB, et al. Lack of residual sedation following middle-of-the-night zaleplon administration in sleep maintenance insomnia. Clin Neuropharmacol 2000;23:17–21.
26. Jan JE, O'Donnell ME. Use of melatonin in the treatment of paediatric sleep disorders. J Pineal Res 1996;21:193–199.
27. Turow V. Melatonin for insomnia and jet lag. Pediatrics 1996;97:439.
28. Klepser TB, Kepser ME. Unsafe and potentially safe herbal therapies. Am J Health Syst Pharm 1999;56:125–138.
29. Ashton H. Guidelines for the rational use of benzodiazepines: When and what to use. Drugs 1994;48:25–40.
30. Greenblatt DJ. Benzodiazepine hypnotics: Sorting the pharmacokinetic facts. J Clin Psychiatry 1991;52(Suppl 9):4–10.
31. Jermain DM. Sleep disorders. In: Pharmacotherapy Self-Assessment Program, 2d ed. Kansas City, MO, American College of Clinical Pharmacy, 1995:139–154.
32. Nefazodone for depression. Med Lett Drugs Ther 1995;37:33–35.
33. Greenblatt DJ, von Moltke LL, Harmatz JS, et al. Interaction of triazolam and ketoconazole. Lancet 1995;345:191.
34. Maczaj M. Pharmacological treatment of insomnia. Drugs 1993;45:44–55.
35. ProSom package insert. Chicago, Abbott Laboratories, October 1991.
36. Schenck CH, Mahowald MW. Long-term, nightly benzodiazepine treatment of injurious parasomnias and other disorders of disrupted nocturnal sleep in 170 adults. Am J Med 1996;100:333–337.
37. Wysowski DK, Barash D. Adverse behavioral reactions attributed to triazolam in the Food and Drug Administration's spontaneous reporting system. Arch Intern Med 1991;151:2003–2008.

38. Ghaeli P, Dufresne RL, Stoukides CA. Triazolam treatment controversy. Ann Pharmacother 1994;28:1038–1040.
39. Kales A, Manfredi RL, Vgontzas AN, et al. Rebound insomnia after only brief and intermittent use of rapidly eliminated benzodiazepines. Clin Pharmacol Ther 1991;49:468–476.
40. Roehrs T, Vogel G, Roth T. Rebound insomnia: Its determinants and significance. Am J Med 1990;88(Suppl 3A):39–42.
41. Rapoport DM. Treatment of sleep apnea syndromes. Mt Sinai J Med 1994;61:123–130.
42. Brown LK. Sleep apnea syndromes: Overview and diagnostic approaches. Mt Sinai J Med 1994;61:99–112.
43. Kaplan J, Staats BA. Obstructive sleep apnea syndrome. Mayo Clin Proc 1990;65:1087–1094.
44. George CF. Perspectives on the management of insomnia in patients with chronic respiratory disorders. Sleep 2000;23:S31–S35.
45. Hanzeol DA, Proia NG, Hudgel DW. Response of obstructive sleep apnea to fluoxetine and protriptyline. Chest 1991;100:416–421.
46. Mulloy E, McNicholas WT. Theophylline in obstructive sleep apnea: A double-blind evaluation. Chest 1992;101:753–757.
47. Issa FG. Effect of clonidine in obstructive sleep apnea. Am Rev Respir Dis 1992;145:435–439.
48. Hanly PJ. Mechanisms and management of central sleep apnea. Lung 1992;170:1–17.
49. Aldrich MS. Narcolepsy. Neurology 1992;42(Suppl 6):34–43.
50. Nakayama J, Miura M, Honda M, et al. Linkage of human narcolepsy with HLA association to chromosome 4p13–q21. Genomics 2000;65;84–86.
51. Garma L, Murchand F. Nonpharmacological approaches to the treatment of narcolepsy. Sleep 1994;17:S97–S102.
52. U.S. Modafinil in Narcolepsy Multicenter Study Group. Randomized trial of modafinil as a treatment for the excessive daytime somnolence of narcolepsy. Neurology 2000;54:1166–1175.
53. U.S. Modafinil in Narcolepsy Multicenter Study Group. Randomized trial of modafinil for the treatment of pathological somnolence in narcolepsy. Ann Neruol 1998;43:88–97.
54. Standard of Practice Committee of the American Sleep Disorders Association. Practice parameters for the use of stimulants in the treatment of narcolepsy. Sleep 1994;17:348–351.
55. Rye DB, Dihenia B, Bliwise DL. Reversal of atypical depression, sleepiness, and REM-sleep propensity in narcolepsy with bupropion. Depress Anxiety 1998;7:92–95.
56. Mayer G, Meier KW, Hephata K. Selegiline hydrochloride treatment in narcolepsy: A double-blind, placebo-controlled study. Clin Neuropharmacol 1995;18:306–319.
57. Reinish LW, MacFarlane JG, Sandor P, Shapiro CM. REM changes in narcolepsy with selegiline. Sleep 1995;18:362–367.
58. Gernaat HBPE, Haffmans PMJ, Knegtering H, Birkenhager TK. Tranylcypromine in narcolepsy. Pharmacopsychiatry 1995;28:98–100.
59. Benbadis SR. Effective treatment of narcolepsy with codeine in a patient receiving hemodialysis. Pharmacotherapy 1996;16:463–465.
60. Scharf MB, Lai AA, Branigan B, et al. Pharmacokinetics of gammahydroxybutyrate (GHB) in narcoleptic patients. Sleep 1998;21:507–514.
61. Wagner DR. Circadian rhythm sleep disorders. In: Thorpy MJ, ed. Handbook of Sleep Disorders. New York, Dekker, 1990:493.
62. Puca FM, Perrucci S, Prudenzano MP, et al. Quality of life in shift work syndrome. Funct Neurol 1996;11:261–268.
63. Czeisler CA, Johnson MP, Duffy JF, et al. Exposure to bright light and darkness to treat physiologic maladaptation to night work. N Engl J Med 1990;322:1253–1259.
64. Skene DJ, Lockley W, Arendt J. Use of melatonin in the treatment of phase shift and sleep disorders. Adv Exp Med Biol 1999;467:79–84.
65. Ambrogetti A, Olson LG, Saunders NA. Disorders of movement and behaviour during sleep. Med J Aust 1991;155:336–340.
66. Krueger BR. Restless legs syndrome and periodic movements of sleep. Mayo Clin Proc 1990;65:999–1006.
67. Reuter I, Ellis CM, Ray Chaudhuri K, Nocturnal subcutaneous apomorphine infusion: I. Parkinson's disease and restless legs syndrome. Acta Neurol Scand 1999;100:163–167.
68. Evidente VG, Adler CH, Caviness JN, et al. Amantadine is beneficial in restless legs syndrome. Mov Disord 2000;15:324–327.
69. Lauerma H, Markkula J. Treatment of restless legs syndrome with tramadol: An open study. J Clin Psychiatry 1999;60:241–244.
70. Hornyak M, Voderholzer U, Hohagen F, et al. Magnesium therapy for periodic leg movements-related insomnia and restless legs syndrome: An open pilot study. Sleep 1998;21:501–505.
71. Chesson AL, Wise M, Davila D, et al. Practice parameters for the treatment of restless legs syndrome and periodic limb movements. Sleep 1999;22:961–968.
72. Stiasny K, Robbecke J, Schuler P, Oertel WH. Treatment of idiopathic restless legs syndrome (RLS) with the D_2-agonist cabergoline: An open clinical trial. Sleep 2000;23:349–354.
73. Wetter TC, Stiasny K, Winkelmann J, et al. A randomized controlled study of pergolide in patients with restless legs syndrome. Neurology 1999;52:944–950.
74. Montplaisir J, Nicolas A, Denesle R, Gomez-Mancilla B. Restless legs syndrome improved by pramipexole: A double-blind randomized trial. Neurology 1999;52: 938–943.
75. Ondo W. Ropinirole for restless legs syndrome. Mov Disord 1999;14: 138–140.
76. Becker PM, Jamieson AO, Brown WD. Dopaminergic agents in restless legs syndrome and periodic limb movements of sleep: Response and complications of extended treatment in 49 cases. Sleep 1993;16:713–716.
77. Staedt J, Stoppe G, Riemann H, et al. Lamotrigine in the treatment of nocturnal myoclonus syndrome (NMS): Two case reports. J Neural Transm 1996;103:355–361.
78. Mahowald MW, Schenck CH. NREM sleep parasomnias. Neurol Clin 1996;14:675–697.
79. Schenck CH, Mahowald MW. Parasomnias managing bizarre sleep-related behavior disorders. Postgrad Med 2000;107:145–156.
80. Schenck CH, Mahowald MW. REM sleep parasomnias. Neurol Clin 1996;14:697–720.
81. Idzikowski C. Impact of insomnia on health related quality of life. Pharmacoeconomics 1996;10:15–24.
82. Stoller MK. Economic effects of insomnia. Clin Ther 1994;16:873–897.
83. Wagner AK. Health related quality of life of people with dyssomnias. Presented at the American Society of Health System Pharmacists (ASHP) Annual Meeting, Philadelphia, 1995;52:FGF-3.
84. Walsh JK, Engelhardt CL. The direct economic costs of insomnia in the United States for 1995. Sleep 1999;22:S386–S393.
85. McElroy SL, Keck PE, Friedman LM. Minimizing and managing antidepressant side effects. J Clin Psychiatry 1995;56:49–55.
86. Morin CM. Insomnia: Psychological Assessment and Management. New York, Guilford Press, 1993:61.

74
DIABETES MELLITUS

Julie C. Oki and William L. Isley

Diabetes mellitus (DM) is a group of metabolic disorders characterized by hyperglycemia; associated with abnormalities in carbohydrate, fat and protein metabolism; and resulting in chronic complications including microvascular, macrovascular and neuropathic. Nearly 16 million Americans have DM, yet only about two-thirds of them have been diagnosed.[1] The economic burden of DM approximated 98 billion dollars in 1997 including direct medical and treatment costs as well as indirect costs attributed to disability and mortality.[1] DM is the leading cause of blindness in adults ages 20 to 74 years, and the leading contributor to development of end-stage renal disease. It also accounts for approximately 67,000 lower extremity amputations annually.[1] Finally, a cardiovascular event is responsible for 75% of deaths in individuals with type 2 DM.[1]

Although efforts to control hyperglycemia and associated symptoms are important, the major challenges in optimally managing the patient with DM are targeted at reducing or preventing complications, and improving life expectancy and quality of life. Research and drug development efforts over the past several decades have provided valuable information that apply directly to improving outcomes in patients with DM and have expanded the therapeutic armamentarium. Additionally, interventions to prevent disease in high-risk populations are under investigation.

EPIDEMIOLOGY

Type 1 DM usually develops in childhood or early adulthood, although some latent forms do occur. Type 1 DM accounts for up to 10% of all cases of DM and results from an autoimmune destruction of the pancreatic β-cell. This process is likely initiated by the exposure of a genetically susceptible individual to an environmental agent.[2] Candidate genes and environmental factors are reportedly prevalent in the general population but development of β-cell autoimmunity occurs in less than 10% of the population and progresses to diabetes mellitus in less than 1% of the population.[3]

The prevalence of β-cell autoimmunity appears proportional to the incidence of type 1 DM in various populations. For instance, the countries of Sweden, Sardinia, and Finland have the highest prevalence of islet cell antibody (3% to 4.5%) and are associated with the highest incidence of type 1 DM, 22 to 35 per 100,000.[4]

Preclinical β-cell autoimmunity precedes the diagnosis of type 1 DM by up to 9 to 13 years. Autoimmunity may remit in some perhaps less-susceptible persons, or can progress to β-cell failure in others. Obesity may also be a confounder as overlapping insulin resistance with β-cell dysfunction may result in the clinical manifestation of DM, with some persons requiring, and other persons not requiring, insulin therapy for management. Markers of autoimmunity have been detected in 14% to 33% of persons with type 2 DM in some populations and manifest with early failure of oral agents and insulin dependence. This type of DM has also been referred to as latent autoimmune diabetes in adults (LADA) or autoimmune DM in adults (AIDA).[4]

Type 2 DM is a heterogenous disorder of glucose metabolism. Type 2 DM accounts for as much as 90% of all cases of DM, and usually results from defects in insulin sensitivity and a relative defect in insulin secretion. The overall prevalence of type 2 DM in the United States is about 6.6% in persons age 20 to 74 years. However, there is likely one person undiagnosed for every two persons currently diagnosed with the disease.[5] One subset of type 2 DM, maturity-onset diabetes of youth (MODY), has an identifiable genetic defect in the glucokinase gene.[6] Additionally, other endocrine disorders, such as acromegaly and Cushing's syndrome, can be secondary causes of DM. See the section on other forms of diabetes mellitus later in this chapter for further discussion. These unusual etiologies, however, only account for 1% to 2% of the total cases of type 2 DM.

Multiple risk factors for the development of type 2 DM have been identified, including family history (i.e., parents or siblings with diabetes); obesity (i.e., $\geq$20% over ideal body weight, or body mass index (BMI) $\geq$27 kg/m^2; habitual physical inactivity; race or ethnicity (see list below); previously identified impaired glucose tolerance or impaired fasting glucose; hypertension ($\geq$140/90 mm Hg in adults); HDL cholesterol $\leq$35 mg/dL and/or a triglyceride level $\geq$250 mg/dL; history of gestational diabetes mellitus or delivery of a baby weighing >9 pounds; and polycystic ovary disease.[7] The prevalence of type 2 DM increases with age, is more common in women than in men in the United States, and varies widely among various racial and ethnic populations, being especially increased in some groups of Native Americans, Hispanic American, Asian American, African American, and Pacific Island people[4] (Figs. 74–1 and 74–2). While the prevalence of type 2 DM increases with age, the disorder is increasingly being recognized in adolescence. Much of the rise in adolescent type 2 DM is related to an increase in adiposity and sedentary lifestyle, in addition to an inheritable predisposition.[8] Most cases of type 2 DM do not have a well-known cause; therefore, it is uncertain whether it represents a few or many independent disorders manifesting as hyperglycemia.[9]

Gestational diabetes mellitus (GDM) complicates roughly 4% of all pregnancies in the United States.[10] Clinical recognition is important to reduce associated morbidity and mortality. Most women will return to a normoglycemia postpartum but 30% to 50% will develop DM or glucose intolerance later in life.

PATHOGENESIS, DIAGNOSIS, AND CLASSIFICATION

CLASSIFICATION

The American Diabetes Association Expert Committee on the Diagnosis and Classification of Diabetes Mellitus recommends the use of

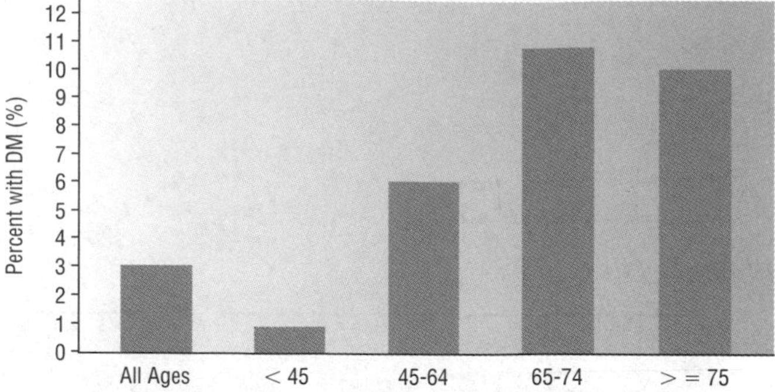

FIGURE 74–1. Percent of the population with diagnosed diabetes by age for the period 1991–1993. *(Adapted from National Institutes of Health. Diabetes in America, 2nd ed, 1995.)*

the terminology *type 1* (formerly insulin-dependent diabetes mellitus, IDDM, or juvenile onset) and *type 2* (formerly noninsulin-dependent diabetes mellitus, NIDDM, or adult onset) to represent the two major types of DM, and characterizes other forms as secondary, gestational, or with specified impairments of glucose tolerance (see Tables 74–1 and 74–2 for a more complete classification).[11]

DIAGNOSIS

In 1997, the Committee also redefined the diagnostic criteria for DM.[11] Table 74–3 summarizes the diagnostic criteria for diabetes mellitus. In general, the criteria requires that any one test consistent with the diagnosis of DM be confirmed with a second test, most often a fasting plasma glucose. Oral glucose tolerance tests (OGTT) are not routinely recommended but may be considered in an individual with a history of abnormal glucose tolerance or impaired fasting glucose in whom you highly suspect the presence of DM. Glycosylated hemoglobin (HbA1C) measurements are not sensitive enough to detect DM, but are the gold standard for long-term monitoring.

It is important to recognize that blood for plasma glucose should be drawn in a gray-top, sodium fluoride-containing tube, which inhibits red blood cell glycolysis. A serum glucose measurement (commonly obtained on multiphasic panels drawn in a red- or speckled-top tube) may yield significantly lower results than plasma glucose measurements potentially leading to a misclassification if used as an index for diagnosis. Capillary whole blood concentration is not recommended to diagnose diabetes mellitus.

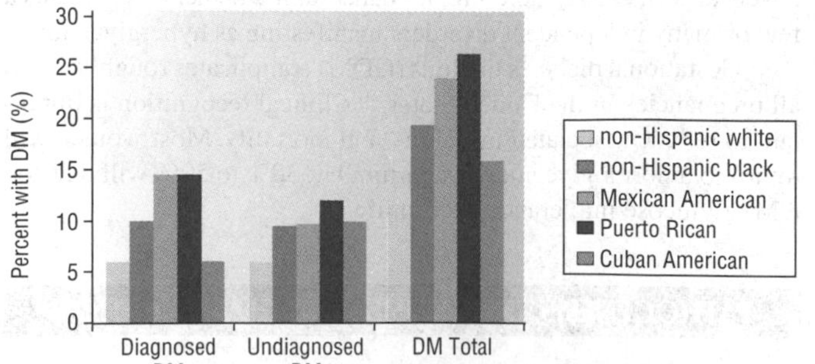

FIGURE 74–2. Prevalence of diabetes mellitus (ages 45 to 74 years) in US whites, blacks (1976–1980), and Latinos (1982–1984). *(Adapted from National Institutes of Health. Diabetes in America, 2nd ed, 1995.)*

TABLE 74–1. Classification of Diabetes Mellitus

Type 1
- Immune mediated
- Idiopathic

Type 2
- May range from predominantly insulin resistant to predominantly insulin deficient

Other specific types
- Genetic defects of β-cell function
- Genetic defects in insulin action
- Diseases of the endocrine pancreas
- Endocrinopathies
- Drug or chemical induced
- Infections
- Uncommon forms of immune-mediated diabetes
- Other genetic syndromes sometimes associated with diabetes

Gestational

SCREENING

Because of the low prevalence of type 1 DM and the acuteness of symptoms, screening for type 1 DM is not recommended.[12] Based on expert opinion, screening for type 2 DM should be performed in the health care setting every 3 years in all adults beginning at age 45 years.[13] Testing should be considered at an earlier age and more frequently in individuals with risk factors. The recommended screening test is fasting plasma glucose. OGTT (more costly, less convenient, less acceptance) can be performed alternatively or in addition to fasting plasma glucose when a high index of suspicion for the disease is present.[11]

Pregnant women should undergo risk assessment at their first prenatal visit and proceed with glucose testing (fasting or random plasma glucose) if at high risk (marked obesity, personal history of GDM, glycosuria, or a strong family history of diabetes mellitus).[10] If they meet diagnostic criteria for DM as noted above, no further testing is needed. In the absence of this, further testing is warranted in high-risk individuals as soon as is feasible. If glucose tolerance testing is negative, additional testing at 24 to 28 weeks is indicated in high-risk women. Women of average risk should also be assessed at 24 to 28 weeks.[10] Women at low risk for GDM (meeting all of the following: younger than 25 years of age, normal body weight, no family history of DM, no history of abnormal glucose metabolism or poor obstetric outcome, and not members of an ethnic/racial group with a high prevalence of diabetes) need not be screened according to the American Diabetes Association.[10] The World Health Organization still holds that all pregnant women should be screened regardless of relative risk.

Evaluation for GDM can be done in one of two ways. The one-step approach involves an OGTT only and may be cost-effective in high-risk patient populations. The two-step approach uses a screening test to measure plasma or serum glucose concentration 1-hour after a

TABLE 74–2. Categories of Glucose Tolerance

Fasting plasma glucose
- Normal: <110 mg/dL
- Impaired fasting glucose (IFG): ≥110 mg/dL and <126 mg/dL
- Diabetes mellitus: ≥126 mg/dL

Two-hour postload plasma glucose (oral glucose tolerance test)
- Normal: <140 mg/dL
- Impaired glucose tolerance (IGT): ≥140 mg/dL and <200 mg/dL
- Diabetes mellitus: ≥200 mg/dL

TABLE 74–3. Diagnostic Criteria for Diabetes Mellitus[a]

Symptoms of diabetes plus a random plasma glucose ≥200 mg/dL.[b]

or

Fasting plasma glucose ≥126 mg/dL.[c]

or

Two-hour plasma glucose ≥200 mg/dL during an oral glucose tolerance test (OGTT).[d]

[a]In the absence of unequivocal hyperglycemia with acute metabolic decompensation, these criteria should be confirmed by repeat testing on a different day. The third measure (OGTT) is not recommended for routine clinical use.
[b]Random is defined as any time of day without regard to time since last meal. The classic symptoms include polyuria, polydipsia, and unexplained weight loss.
[c]Fasting is defined as no caloric intake for at least 8 hours.
[d]The test should be performed as described by the World Health Organization, using a glucose load containing the equivalent of 75 g anhydrous glucose dissolved in water.

50-g oral glucose load (glucose challenge test [GCT]) and performs a diagnostic OGTT on the subset of women exceeding a glucose threshold of either >140 mg/dL (80% sensitive) or >130 mg/dL (90% sensitive). The diagnosis of GDM is based on a 75-g (not as well validated) or 100-g OGTT. Criteria for diagnosis of GDM based on OGTT are summarized in Table 74.4.

PATHOGENESIS

TYPE 1 DIABETES MELLITUS

Type 1 DM is characterized by an absolute deficiency of insulin. Most often this is the result of an immune-mediated destruction of pancreatic β-cells but rare unknown or idiopathic processes may contribute. What is evident are four main features: (a) a long preclinical period marked by the presence of immune markers when β-cell destruction is thought to occur; (b) hyperglycemia when 80% to 90% of β-cells are destroyed; (c) transient remission (so called, "honeymoon" phase); and (d) established disease with associated risks for complications and death. Unknown is whether there is one or more inciting factors (e.g., cow's milk, viral, dietary or other environmental exposure) that initiate the autoimmune process[2] (Fig. 74–3).

The autoimmune process is mediated by macrophages and T lymphocytes with circulating autoantibodies to various β-cell antigens. The most commonly detected antibody associated with type 1 DM is the islet cell antibody. The test for islet cell antibody, however, is difficult to standardize across laboratories. Other more readily measured circulating antibodies include insulin autoantibodies, antibodies directed against glutamic acid decarboxylase, antibodies against islet tyrosine phosphatase (IA2 and IA2β), and several others. More than 90% of newly diagnosed persons with type 1 DM have one or another of these antibodies, as will 3.5% to 4% of unaffected first-degree relatives. These antibodies are generally considered markers of disease rather than mediators of β-cell destruction. They have been used to identify individuals at risk for type 1 diabetes mellitus in evaluating disease prevention strategies. Other nonpancreatic autoimmune disorders are associated with type 1 DM, most commonly Hashimoto's thyroiditis, but the extent of organ involvement can be from no other organs to polyglandular failure.[14]

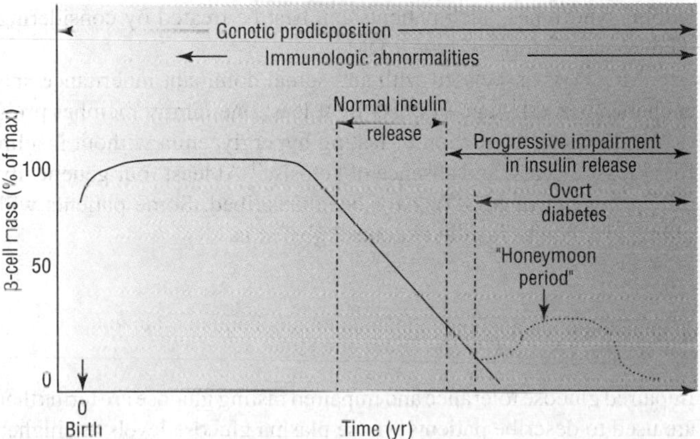

FIGURE 74–3. Scheme of the natural history of β-cell defect in type 1 diabetes mellitus. *(From ADA Medical Management of Type of 1 Diabetes, 3rd ed. 1998.)*

There are strong genetic linkages to the DQA and B genes and certain human leukocyte antigens (HLA) may be predisposing (DR3 and DR4) or protective (DRB1*04008-DQB1*0302 and DRB1*0411-DQB1*0302) on chromosome 6.[14] Other candidate gene regions have been identified on several other chromosomes as well. Because twin studies do not show 100% concordance, environmental factors such as infectious agents, chemical agents, and dietary agents are likely contributing factors in the expression of the disease.

TYPE 2 DIABETES MELLITUS

Type 2 DM is a heterogenous disorder characterized by the presence of both insulin resistance and relative insulin deficiency or β-cell dysfunction.[9] Insulin resistance manifests by an increase in lipolysis and free fatty acid production, increase in hepatic glucose production and decrease in skeletal muscle uptake of glucose. Free fatty acids indirectly lead to hyperglycemia by stimulating hepatic glucose production. β-Cell dysfunction is progressive and contributes to worsening blood glucose control with time.[15] Figure 74–4 summarizes a model of the progression of type 2 DM; from incipient glucose intolerance to fasting hyperglycemia to more progressive hyperglycemia with declining β-cell function. Most patients have both insulin resistance and some degree of insulin deficiency. (Lean, older African American patients may have insulin deficiency predominantly.) Insulin resistance per se is not the sine qua non for type 2 DM because many people with insulin resistance (particularly obese patients) do not develop glucose intolerance. Patients may have high insulin levels, but the insulin concentrations are inappropriately low for the level of glycemia.

Type 2 DM occurs when a diabetogenic lifestyle (excessive calories, inadequate caloric expenditure, and obesity) is superimposed upon a susceptible genotype. Weight gain associated with significant insulin resistance appears to vary between racial and ethnic groups. Overweight patients from the Indian subcontinent are mildly overweight by Western standards but may be very insulin resistant. The high prevalence of type 2 DM in Native American populations is usually associated with marked obesity.

The genetics of type 2 DM are not completely understood, but presumably this disease is related to multiple genes (with the exception of maturity onset diabetes of the young, discussed further below). Both pancreatic β-cell failure and insulin resistance may have genetic components.[16] There is also evidence of the effect of *in utero* environment on the future development of type 2 DM.[17]

In type 2 DM, increased cardiovascular risk appears to begin prior to the development of frank hyperglycemia, presumably because of the effects of insulin resistance. Stern and Haffner developed the "ticking clock" hypothesis of complications, asserting that the clock starts ticking for microvascular risk at the onset of hyperglycemia, while the clock starts ticking for macrovascular risk at some

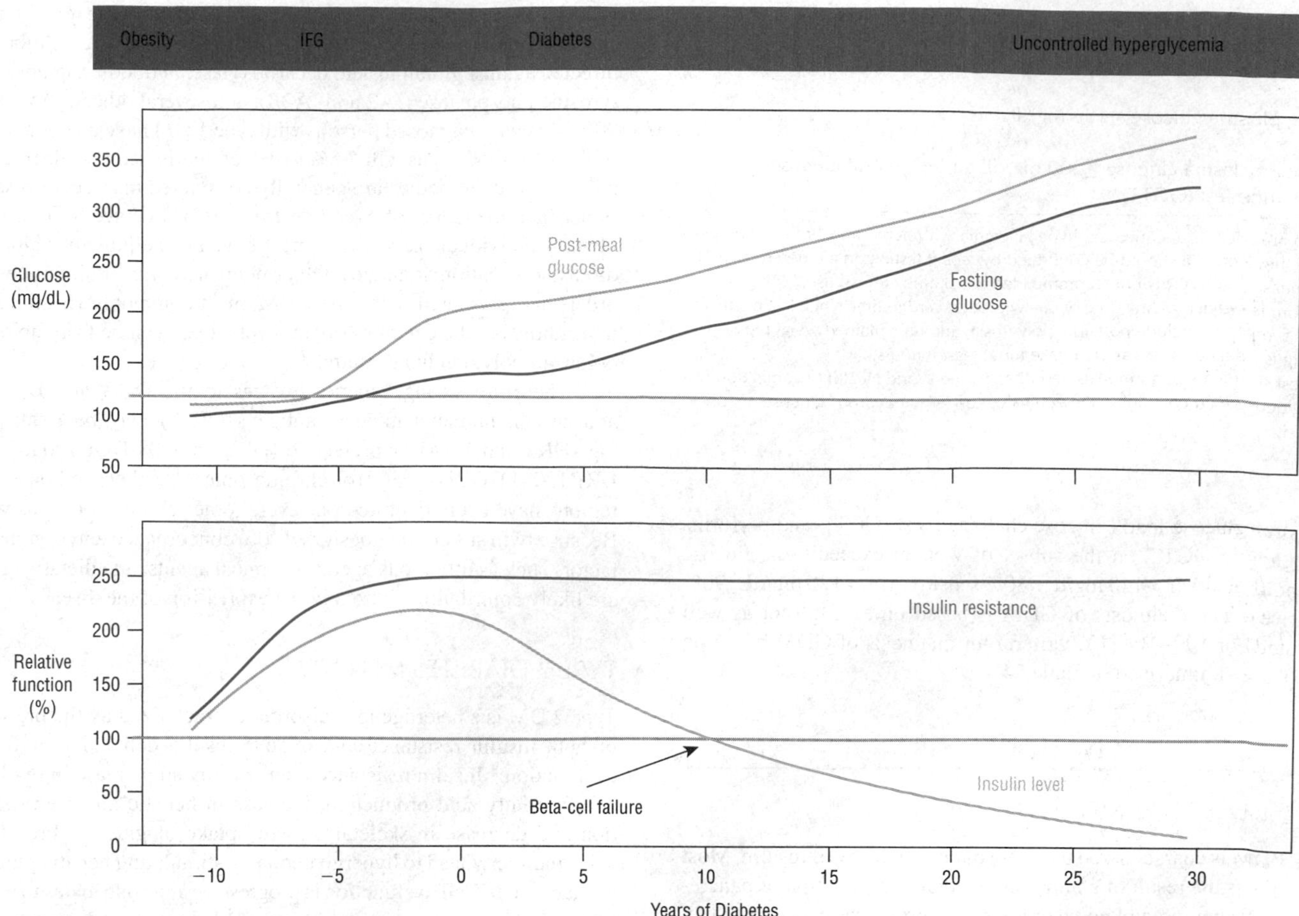

FIGURE 74–4. Natural history of type 2 diabetes. *IFG, impaired fasting glucose. *(Adapted from International Diabetes Center, Minneapolis, MN.)*

antecedent point, presumably with the onset of insulin resistance.[18] Insulin resistance is associated with a plethora of metabolic (small, dense low-density lipoprotein [LDL] particles; low high-density lipoprotein-cholesterol [HDL-C] levels; elevated remnant lipoproteins) and thrombotic (elevated type-1 plasminogen activator inhibitor [PAI-1], elevated fibrinogen) abnormalities. In dealing with the full scope of type 2 DM, we must extend our vision beyond simple glycemia to the full orb of "the insulin resistance syndrome," also known as "the metabolic syndrome," "the dysmetabolic syndrome," or "syndrome X."[19]

GESTATIONAL DIABETES MELLITUS

Gestational diabetes mellitus refers to the onset or initial recognition of glucose intolerance during pregnancy, usually in the second or third trimester.[10] It occurs in about 4% of all pregnancies. Patients with gestational diabetes have a 30% to 50% chance of ultimately developing DM, usually type 2 DM.

OTHER TYPES

Genetic defects of the β-cell or in insulin action pathways (insulin receptor mutations or postreceptor defects)[3] as well as disease of the exocrine pancreas (e.g., pancreatitis, pancreatic resection, or cystic fibrosis) are less common causes of DM.[11] Endocrinopathies producing insulin counterregulatory hormones excess (e.g., Cushing's syndrome—cortisol; acromegaly—growth hormone) may result in DM.[11] Certain medications, such as glucocorticoids, pentamidine, niacin, and α-interferon, may also lead to DM.[20]

The most recent classification by the American Diabetes Association also lists type 1 DM idiopathic to describe young patients (usually minorities) with intermittent insulin deficiency.[11] Such patients often are obese, have acanthosis nigricans, have a positive family history for type 2 DM, and lack the autoimmune markers of typical type 1 DM. With the exception of bouts of insulin deficiency manifested by diabetic ketoacidosis or hyperglycemic hyperosmolar nonketotic syndromes, such patients can best be treated by considering them to have a form of type 2 DM.

MODY is associated with autosomal dominant inheritance and is characterized by age of onset in at least one family member prior to age 25 years, correction of fasting hyperglycemia without insulin for at least 2 years, and absence of ketosis.[21] At least four genetically different types of MODY have been described. Some patients will ultimately require insulin to control glycemia.

IMPAIRED GLUCOSE TOLERANCE

Impaired glucose tolerance and impaired fasting glucose are terms that are used to describe patients whose plasma glucose levels are higher than normal but which are not diagnostic of DM[11] (see Table 74–2). Impaired glucose tolerance and impaired fasting glucose are risk factors for DM and cardiovascular disease, and are associated with the insulin-resistance syndrome. Although approximately 25% of these patients will develop DM, it is important not to categorize these patients as having DM until a definite diagnosis has been made because of social, insurance, and job implications for persons with DM.

The cut-points for fasting glucose measurements are based on the level of glycemia where retinopathy, a fairly pathognomic diabetic complication, appears. Fasting glucose measurements are not as predictive for indicating increased macrovascular risk. The World Health Organization's criteria for impaired glucose tolerance (i.e., fasting plasma glucose <140 mg/dL and 2 h post 75-g glucose load plasma glucose ≥140 mg/dL to <200 mg/dL with one intervening plasma glucose value ≥200 mg/dL) is a better predictor of increased macrovascular risk than the American Diabetes Association's current intermediate category of impaired fasting glucose. Presumably, patients with impaired fasting glucose are at increased risk for development of diabetes mellitus, but their risk for macrovascular disease does not appear to be as great as impaired glucose tolerance patients, which is about the same risk as patients with type 2 DM.

CLINICAL PRESENTATION

Autoimmune type 1 DM can occur at any age. Approximately 75% will develop the disorder before age 20 years, but the remaining 25%, including relatives of index patients, develop the disease as adults. Individuals with type 1 diabetes mellitus are often thin and are prone to develop diabetic ketoacidosis if insulin is withheld, or under conditions of severe stress with an excess of insulin counterregulatory hormones.[2] Twenty percent to 40% of patients with type 1 DM present with diabetic ketoacidosis after several days of polyuria, polydipsia, polyphagia, and weight loss. Occasionally, patients are diagnosed short of "metabolic bankruptcy" when they have blood tests drawn for other reasons or for early symptoms. Because newly diagnosed patients with type 1 DM often have a small amount of residual pancreatic β-cell function, they may enter a "honeymoon" phase when their blood glucose concentrations are relatively easy to control and small amounts of insulin are needed. Once this residual insulin secretion wanes, the patients are completely insulin deficient and have more labile glycemia.

Patients with type 2 DM often present without symptoms.[9] Other patients will present with advanced complications, particularly neuropathy. The diagnosis of type 2 diabetes mellitus should be entertained in obese patients; patients with a first-degree relative with type 2 diabetes mellitus; members of high-risk ethnic groups (African American, Hispanic American, Native American, Asian American, or Pacific Islander); women with a previous delivery of a large infant (>9 lb) or with a history of gestational diabetes mellitus; patients with hypertension; or patients with high triglycerides (≥250 mg/dL) or low HDL-C (≤35 mg/dL).[11] Because polycystic ovary disease is an insulin-resistant state, it is appropriate to screen women with this disorder for type 2 DM.[22]

▶ TREATMENT: Diabetes Mellitus

DESIRED OUTCOME

The primary goals of DM management are to reduce risk for microvascular and macrovascular disease complications, to ameliorate symptoms, to reduce mortality, and to improve quality of life.[23] Near-normal glycemia will reduce the risk for development of microvascular disease complications, but current evidence targets aggressive management of traditional cardiovascular risk factors (i.e., smoking cessation, treatment of dyslipidemia, intensive blood pressure control, and antiplatelet therapy) to reduce macrovascular disease odds.

Hyperglycemia not only increases risk for microvascular disease but contributes to poor wound healing, compromises white blood cell function, and leads to classic symptoms of DM: polyuria, polydipsia, polyphagia, and, in certain individuals, weight loss. Diabetic ketoacidosis and hyperosmolar hyperglycemic state are severe manifestations of poor diabetes control, invariably requiring hospitalization. Reducing potential for microvascular complications is targeted at adherence to therapeutic lifestyle intervention; that is, diet and exercise programs, and drug-therapy regimens, as well as at maintaining blood pressure as near normal as possible.

GENERAL APPROACH TO TREATMENT[23]

Appropriate care requires goal setting for glycemia, blood pressure, and lipid levels, regular complications monitoring, dietary and exercise modifications, medications, appropriate self-monitoring of blood glucose (SMBG), and laboratory assessment of the aforementioned parameters. Glucose control alone does not sufficiently reduce the aggregate of risk in persons with DM.

GLYCEMIC GOAL SETTING

Controlled clinical trials provide ample evidence that glycemic control is paramount in reducing microvascular complications in both type 1 DM[24] and type 2 DM.[25] Unless the risk outweighs the benefit (as in elderly patients, patients with advanced complications, and patients with other advanced disease), a HbA1C target of <7% is appropriate.[23] Further discussion of the major clinical trials appears below.

COMPLICATIONS MONITORING

The American Diabetes Association recommends initiation of complications monitoring at the time of diagnosis of diabetes mellitus.[23] Although controversial, current recommendations continue to advocate yearly dilated eye examinations. The feet should be examined at each visit, and a urine test for microalbumin once yearly is appropriate. Blood pressure should be assessed at every visit, and periodic assessment of lipid levels obtained.

SELF-MONITORING OF BLOOD GLUCOSE

The advent of SMBG in the early 1980s revolutionized the treatment of DM, enabling patients to know their blood glucose concentration at any moment easily and relatively inexpensively. Frequent SMBG is necessary to achieve near-normal blood glucose concentrations and to assess for hypoglycemia, particularly in patients with type 1 DM.[26] The more intense the insulin regimen is, the more intense the SMBG needs to be (four or more times daily in patients on multiple insulin injections per day). The utility and optimal frequency

TABLE 74–4. Criteria for Diagnosis of GDM*

	mg/dL
100-g glucose load	
Fasting	95
1-hour	180
2-hour	155
3-hour	140
75-g glucose load	
Fasting	95
1-hour	180
2-hour	155

*Two or more of the plasma concentrations must be met for diagnosis. The test should be done in the morning after an overnight fast of between 8 and 14 hours and after at least 3 days of unrestricted diet (≥150 g carbohydrate per day) and unlimited physical activity. The subject should remain seated and should not smoke during the test.

of SMBG for patients with type 2 DM is unresolved. Frequency of monitoring in type 2 DM should be sufficient to facilitate reaching glucose goals, but patients must be empowered to change their therapeutic regimen (lifestyle and medications) in response to test results, or no meaningful change is likely to be effected. The role of SMBG in improving glycemic control in type 2 DM patients is unproven.[27]

NONPHARMACOLOGIC THERAPY

DIET

Medical nutrition therapy is recommended for all persons with DM.[28] For underweight individuals with type 1 DM, the focus is on regulating insulin administration with a balanced diet to achieve and maintain a healthy body weight. Although still debated, in most situations, a high-carbohydrate (with modest simple sugar intake in the context of a mixed meal), low-fat (especially low in saturated fat), low-cholesterol diet is appropriate. Most patients with type 2 DM will additionally need caloric restriction. Rather than a set diabetic diet, advocate a diet using foods that are within the financial reach and cultural milieu of the patient. Bedtime and between meal snacks are not usually needed if pharmacologic management is appropriate.

ACTIVITY

In general, most patients with DM can benefit from increased activity.[29] Aerobic exercise improves insulin resistance and may improve glycemia markedly in some patients. The patient should choose an activity that she or he is likely to continue. Start exercise slowly in previously sedentary patients. Older patients, patients with long-standing disease, patients with multiple risk factors, and patients with previous evidence of atherosclerotic disease should have a cardiovascular evaluation, probably including an imaging study, prior to beginning a significant exercise regime.

TABLE 74–6. Classification of Lipids and Lipoprotein Levels in Adults

LDL Cholesterol (mg/dL)	Triglycerides (mg/dL)
Optimal <100	Normal <150
Near Optimal 100–129	Borderline 150–199
Borderline High 130–159	High 200–499
High 160–189	Very High ≥500
Very High ≥190	Total Cholesterol (mg/dL)
HDL Cholesterol (mg/dL)	Desirable <200
Low <40	Borderline High 200–239
High ≥60	High ≥240

Adapted from Ref. 86.

PHARMACOLOGIC THERAPY

Until 1995, there were only two classes of agents used in the management of DM: insulin (for type 1 and 2 DM) and sulfonylureas (for type 2 DM only). Both are categorized as hypoglycemics. With the exception of the short acting insulin secretogogues (mechanism of action similar to sulfonylurea), other oral therapies generally do not lower blood glucose concentrations below normal values unless given in combination with insulin or an insulin secretogogue. These may be better categorized as antihyperglycemic.

Since 1995, several classes of pharmacologic agents targeted to reduce hyperglycemia in type 2 DM have been developed. The therapeutic armamentarium for type 2 DM now consists of these classes of agents: sulfonylureas, meglitinides, biguanides, peroxisome proliferator-activated receptor γ (PPARγ) agonists (so-called thiazolidinediones or glitazones), and α-glucosidase inhibitors. In addition, insulin glargine, insulin aspart, and lispro insulin mixtures are available. Research into new routes of insulin delivery continue and may provide inhaled or oral insulin preparations in the future. This section reviews the pertinent pharmacology associated with these classes of medicine. The following section describes treatment strategies to employ these agents in managing patients with DM.

TABLE 74–5. Glycemic Goals of Therapy[a]

Biochemical Index	Nondiabetic	Goal	Action Suggested
Whole-blood (capillary)			
Preprandial glucose	<100 mg/dL	80–120 mg/dL	<80 or >140 mg/dL
Bedtime glucose	<110 mg/dL	100–140 mg/dL	<100 or >160 mg/dL
Plasma values			
Preprandial glucose	<110 mg/dL	90–130 mg/dL	<90 or >150 mg/dL
Bedtime glucose	<120 mg/dL	110–150	<110 or >180 mg/dL
HbA1c (%)[b]	<6	<7	>8

[a]Values for nonpregnant individuals. Action suggested depends on individual patient circumstances.
[b]HbA1c is referenced to range of 4% to 6% (mean 5%, standard deviation 0.5%).
Adapted from Ref. 23.

TABLE 74–7. Physiologic Effects of Insulin

	Anabolic Actions	Anticatabolic Actions
Liver	Glucose uptake Glycogen synthesis Lipogenesis	Inhibits gluconeogenesis Inhibits glycogenolysis Inhibits lipolysis
Muscle	Glucose uptake Glycogen synthesis Amino acid uptake Sustained protein synthesis	Inhibit glycogenolysis Inhibits proteolysis Inhibits fatty acid oxidation
Adipose Tissue	Glucose uptake Lipid synthesis Triglyceride uptake	Inhibits lipolysis

DRUG CLASS INFORMATION

Insulin

Pharmacology. The metabolic actions of insulin mimic its physiologic effects. In short, insulin is anabolic and anticatabolic. It plays a major role in protein, carbohydrate and fat metabolism. Table 74–7 summarizes insulin action. For a complete review of insulin action, the reader is referred to a standard physiology text.[30]

Characteristics. For practical purposes, insulins are categorized according to their strength, onset and duration of action, species source (human or animal), and purity. An additional category is the insulin analogs, where modification of the human insulin molecule has been made to impart alterations in pharmacokinetic and physicochemical properties. Table 74–8 summarizes available insulin preparations.

U-100 (100 units of insulin per milliliter) is the most common concentration of insulin used. U-500 (500 units of insulin per milliliter) is available for individuals requiring very large doses of insulin to reduce the number of injections required to deliver an adequate dose. For individuals requiring other concentrations (e.g., U-10), special diluents and empty sterile vials are available from the manufacturers to prepare appropriate dilutions.

Three types of insulin are available: pork, beef-pork mixture, and human insulin analogs. Beef insulin differs from human insulin by three amino acids, whereas pork insulin differs from human insulin by one amino acid. Beef insulin may be slightly more antigenic than pork insulin. Preparations of pure beef insulin are no longer available. Human insulin is derived from recombinant-DNA technology.

Recognizing the inconvenience of injecting short-acting insulins 30 minutes prior to a meal to achieve optimal postprandial glucose control and to mitigate delayed postmeal hypoglycemia from the prolonged duration of regular or semi-lente insulin, rapid-acting insulin analogs (e.g., lispro insulin and insulin aspart) were developed. Regular crystalline insulin self-associates into a hexameric structure. Regular insulin must dissociate into initially dimers, then monomers prior to absorption from the subcutaneous tissue. Lispro insulin (B-28 lysine, B-29 proline human insulin; monomeric) and insulin aspart (B-28 aspartic acid human insulin; mono- and dimeric) are more rapidly absorbed with shorter durations of effect compared to regular insulin.

Similar to problems with short-acting insulins, intermediate- and long-acting suspensions of insulin also have limitations in clinical practice. Variability in absorption, inconsistent suspension of the insulin by the patient or health care provider when drawing up a dose, inherent peak insulin action based on the pharmacokinetics of the products may all contribute to a labile glucose response, nocturnal hypoglycemia and fasting hyperglycemia. Altering the isoelectric point (pH value at which insulin is least soluble) to neutrality provides a solution of insulin which is soluble in acid but that will precipitate when injected into the body's neutral pH. Insulin glargine (A-21 glycine, B-30 a-arginine, B-30 b-arginine human insulin), a clear, colorless solution, was developed as a long-acting, "peakless" insulin analog.

Although insulin analogs have been developed to improve the pharmacokinetic characteristics of previously available insulin preparations, insulin analogs are modifications of human insulin and require assessment of their safety prior to approval. Considerations of relative antigenicity, insulin binding affinity, insulin response, and injection site reactions should be addressed in product development.

Purity of insulin refers to the amount of proinsulin and other impurities present in a given insulin product. Prior to 1980, most insulin contained enough impurities (300 to 10,000 ppm) to cause local reactions upon injection, as well as systemic adverse effects from antibody production. Modern technology has provided less-expensive techniques to purify insulin. As a result, all insulin products contain ≤10 ppm of proinsulin with purified preparations containing <1 ppm of proinsulin.

Pharmacokinetics. Regular crystalline insulin is a clear, colorless solution. Upon intravenous administration, the onset of regular insulin action is more immediate than with subcutaneous injection. The half-life of intravenous regular insulin is about 9 minutes. Therefore, when giving insulin by intravenous infusion, steady state is reached in roughly 45 minutes, or, conversely, the effect of a single intravenous dose is very short. Insulin is degraded in the liver, kidney, and muscle. Liver deactivation is 20% to 50% in a single passage. Approximately 15% to 20% of insulin metabolism occurs in the kidney. This may partially contribute to the lower insulin dosage requirements in patients with end-stage renal disease.

The most important fundamental concept related to insulin pharmacokinetics is the relative onset, peak and duration of effects from subcutaneous injections. Table 74–9 compares these properties of various insulin preparations by species. Note that animal source insulin has a slightly delayed onset, later peak and more prolonged duration of effect compared to similar types of human insulin. This should be considered when switching a patient from one source of insulin to another.

Efficacy. The efficacy of traditional insulins (e.g., regular, NPH, lente insulins) is unequivocal. With the advent of insulin analogs, efficacy is assessed similarly; effects on blood glucose, with additional considerations of whether they offer any unique advantages over traditional insulin in prespecified dosage regimens.

TABLE 74–8. Available Insulin Preparations

Brand Name	Manufacturer	Origin
Rapid Acting Insulins		
Humalog (insulin lispro)[1]	Lilly	Human (recombinant DNA)
Novolog (insulin aspart)	Novo-Nordisk	Human (recombinant DNA)
Short-Acting Insulins		
Regular Iletin I	Lilly	Beef-pork
Pork Regular Iletin II	Lilly	Pork
Regular purified pork insulin	Novo-Nordisk	Pork
Humulin R (regular)[1]	Lilly	Human (recombinant DNA)
Velosulin (regular, buffered)	Novo-Nordisk	Human (recombinant DNA)
Novolin R (regular)[2]	Novo-Nordisk	Human (recombinant DNA)
Intermediate-Acting Insulins		
NPH		
NPH Iletin I	Lilly	Beef-pork
Pork NPH Iletin II	Lilly	Pork
NPH purified pork	Novo-Nordisk	Pork
Humulin N[1]	Lilly	Human (recombinant DNA)
Novolin N[2]	Novo-Nordisk	Human (recombinant DNA)
Lente		
Lente Iletin I	Lilly	Beef-pork
Lente Iletin II	Lilly	Pork
Lente purified pork	Novo-Nordisk	Pork
Novolin L	Novo-Nordisk	Human (recombinant DNA)
Humulin L	Lilly	Human (recombinant DNA)
Lispro-Lispro protamine		
Humalog 75/25[3]	Lilly	Human (recombinant DNA)
Humalog 50/50[3]	Lilly	Human (recombinant DNA)
NPH-Regular Combinations		
Humulin 70/30[1]	Lilly	Human (recombinant DNA)
Novolin 70/30[2]	Novo-Nordisk	Human (recombinant DNA)
Humulin 50/50	Lilly	Human (recombinant DNA)
Long-acting insulins		
Humulin U (ultralente)	Lilly	Human (recombinant DNA)
Lantus (insulin glargine)	Aventis	Human (recombinant DNA)

[1] Available in cartridges for pens, in addition to vials.
[2] Available in prefilled disposable pens, in addition to cartridges and vials.
[3] Available in prefilled disposble pens only.

TABLE 74–9. Pharmacokinetics of Various Insulins Administered Subcutaneously

Type of Insulin	Onset (h)	Peak (h)	Effective Duration (h)	Maximum Duration (h)	Appearance
Animal					
Short acting					
Regular	0.5–2	3–4	4–6	6–10	Clear
Intermediate acting					
NPH	4–6	8–14	16–20	20–24	Cloudy
Lente	4–6	8–14	16–20	20–24	Cloudy
Human					
Rapid acting					
Aspart	0.5	1–2	3.5	NA	Clear
Lispro	<0.25	0.5–1.5	3–4	4–6	Clear
Short acting					
Regular	0.5–1.0	2–3	3–6	6–8	Clear
Intermediate acting					
NPH	2–4	6–10	10–16	14–18	Cloudy
Lente	3–4	6–12	12–18	16–20	Cloudy
Long acting					
Ultralente	6–10	10–16	18–20	20–24	Cloudy
Glargine	4	—	24	24+	Clear

Adapted from Ref. 64 and Novolog product label, June 7, 2000.

TABLE 74–10. Drugs Interfering with Glucose Tolerance

Drug	Effect on Glucose	Mechanism/Comment
Diazoxide	Increase	Decrease insulin secretion Decrease peripheral glucose use
Diuretics (thiazides)	Increase	Unclear
Glucocorticoids	Increase	Increase gluconeogenesis
Oral contraceptives	Increase	Unclear
Pentamidine	Decrease then increase	Toxic to β cells
Phenytoin	Increase	Decrease insulin secretion
β-Blockers	Increase or decrease	Decrease insulin secretion Decrease gluconeogenesis Decrease glycogenolysis
Streptozotocin	Increase	Toxic to β cells

Both insulin lispro and aspart have demonstrated better efficacy at lowering postprandial blood glucose than regular insulin in persons with type 1 DM and are generally considered more widely acceptable by patients (more convenient dosing). Insulin glargine has shown efficacy in reducing nocturnal hypoglycemia when given at bedtime, as compared to a regimen with NPH at bedtime in type 1 DM. Insulin glargine has also been assessed as noted below as an alternative to NPH in a bedtime dosage with oral agents administered during the day in type 2 DM.

ADVERSE EFFECTS

The most common adverse effect of insulin is hypoglycemia. In the Diabetes Control and Complications Study (DCCT)[24] the incidence of hypoglycemia and severe hypoglycemia (requiring assistance by another person) in type 1 DM was greater in the intensive insulin therapy group than in the standard, less-intense insulin-treated group. All patients receiving insulin therapy should be instructed on signs and symptoms of hypoglycemia and provided recommendations on how to manage it. Blood glucose monitoring is essential for those on insulin and is particularly of value in patients with hypoglycemia unawareness, a problem in which the usual counterregulatory response to a low blood glucose is blunted and sympathetic symptoms of hypoglycemia (e.g., tremulousness and tachycardia) are absent. The only symptom manifest in a person with hypoglycemia unawareness is neuroglycopenia (confusion, agitation, progressing to coma or seizures). It is best to avoid multiple episodes of hypoglycemia as this contributes to the development of hypoglycemia unawareness. Although oral administration of glucose (10–15 g) is the recommended treatment for hypoglycemia, individuals who have lost consciousness may require intravenous dextrose. When intravenous access cannot be established, intramuscular glucagon 1 g is the treatment of choice. For individuals suffering from hypoglycemic unawareness, glucagon should be prescribed and a person in close contact with the individual should be instructed on the preparation and administration of glucagon.

With human insulin and the more purified formulations of insulin the incidence of antibodies to insulin is reduced. Other hypersensitivity reactions are also lower in frequency but skin rash at the injection site still occasionally occurs. The lipodystrophies associated with insulin are still problematic. Lipohypertrophy results when insulin is injected into the same site and an increase in fat mass occurs at that site. Insulin absorption from a lipohypertrophy site is delayed and prolonged. This may contribute to changes in blood glucose control. Lipoatrophy is noted by a dimpling in the skin at the injection site. Lipoatrophy is caused by antibody formation at the site of injection leading to breakdown of fat at the injection site. Recommendations for management of lipoatrophy are to inject a more purified form of insulin or human insulin into the site. Lipoatrophy with lispro insulin administered by an insulin pump was recently reported.[31]

DRUG-DRUG INTERACTIONS

The most significant drug interactions with insulin are with agents that affect blood glucose metabolism. Table 74–10 lists commonly known drugs that affect blood glucose. Individuals receiving any of these agents in combination with insulin should monitor blood glucose to assess whether a change in the insulin regimen is warranted.

Dosing and Administration. The dose of insulin for any person with altered glucose metabolism must be individualized. In type 1 DM, the average daily requirement for insulin is 0.5 – 0.6 U/kg. During the honeymoon phase it may fall to 0.1–0.4 U/kg. During acute illness or with ketosis, states of relative insulin resistance, higher dosages are warranted—0.5 –1.0 U/kg. In type 2 DM, a dosage range of 0.7–2.5 U/kg is often required; the higher dosage is required for those patients with significant insulin resistance. Strategies on how to initiate and monitor insulin therapy are described in the therapeutics section below.

Sulfonylureas

Pharmacology. Sulfonylureas exert a hypoglycemic action by stimulating pancreatic secretion of insulin. Sulfonylureas bind to the pancreatic β-cell plasma membrane associated with the ATP-dependent K^+ channel. Upon binding, sulfonylureas close these channels causing depolarization of the membrane and opening of the voltage-dependent Ca^{2+} channels. An increase in intracellular calcium leads to an increase in insulin secretion.

CLASSIFICATION

Sulfonylureas are classified as first-generation and second-generation agents. The classification scheme is largely derived from differences in relative potency, relative potential for selective side effects and differences in binding to serum proteins (i.e., risk for protein-binding displacement drug interactions). First generation agents consist of acetohexamide, chlorpropamide, tolazamide, and tolbutamide. Each of these agents are lower in potency relative to second-generations drugs: glimepiride, glipizide, and glyburide (Table 74–11). It is important to recognize that all of the sulfonylureas are equally effective at lowering blood glucose when administered in equipotent doses.

Pharmacokinetics. All the sulfonylureas are metabolized in the liver; some to active, others to inactive metabolites (Table 74–11). Agents with active metabolites or parent drug that is renally excreted requires dosage adjustment or use with caution in patients with compromised renal function. The long duration of effect of chlorpropamide may be particularly problematic in elderly individuals whose renal function declines with age and, therefore, has great potential for accumulation resulting in severe and protracted hypoglycemia. Individuals at high risk for hypoglycemia (e.g., elderly individuals; those with renal insufficiency or advanced liver disease) should be given a short-acting agent such as tolbutamide or, in some instances, preferable treatment with insulin to minimize this risk.

Efficacy. As mentioned earlier, when given in equipotent doses, all the sulfonylureas are relatively equally effective at lowering blood glucose. On average, HbA1C will fall 1.5 to 2%. Individuals with a higher baseline HbA1C (higher average blood glucose) are likely to achieve greater reductions in HbA1C with sulfonylurea monotherapy, but still are unlikely to reach or sustain blood glucose goals in the target range.[25]

ADVERSE EFFECTS

The most common side effect of sulfonylureas is hypoglycemia. In addition to the high-risk individuals outlined above, those who skip meals, exercise vigorously, or who lose substantial amount of weight are also more likely to experience hypoglycemia.

Hyponatremia (serum sodium <129 mEq/L) is reportedly associated with tolbutamide, but it is most common with chlorpropamide and occurs in as many as 5% of individuals treated. An increase in antidiuretic hormone secretion is the mechanism for hyponatremia. Risk factors include age >60 years, female sex, and concomitant use of thiazide diuretics.

Weight gain is common with sulfonylureas. In essence, patients who are no longer glycosuric and who do not reduce caloric intake with improvement of blood glucose will store excess calories as fat. This is liken to achieving the weight the person may have been had DM not intervened.

Other notable, although much less common, adverse effects of sulfonylureas are skin rash, hemolytic anemia, gastrointestinal upset and cholestasis.

DRUG INTERACTIONS

Several drugs are thought to interact with sulfonylureas; Table 74–12 summarizes them by proposed mechanisms.[32] Additionally, other drugs known to alter blood glucose should be considered (Table 74–10).

DOSING AND ADMINISTRATION

The usual starting dose and maximum dose of sulfonylureas are summarized in Table 74–11. Lower dosages are recommended for most agents in elderly patients who may have compromised renal or hepatic function. Dosage can be titrated every 1 to 2 weeks (longer interval with chlorpropamide) to achieve glycemic goals. Some advocate initiating therapy with maximum dosage to more rapidly assess efficacy to a single-drug regimen.[33] The limitation with this study is that it only enrolled individuals with type 2 DM who did not become hypoglycemic after a run-in period of rapidly accelerating the dose of glyburide to maximum dosage.

Short Acting Secretogogues

Pharmacology. Similar to sulfonylureas, these secretogogues lowers glucose by binding to the sulfonylurea receptor, albeit, adjacent to the binding location of the sulfonylureas and stimulating pancreatic insulin secretion. Insulin release with repaglinide and nateglinide is glucose dependent and diminishes at low blood glucose concentrations. In the postabsorptive state or fasting condition, insulin secretion is minimal. This may reduce the potential for severe hypoglycemia.

Pharmacokinetics. Both repaglinide and nateglinide are rapidly absorbed after oral administration. Nateglinide is 98% bound to serum proteins, primarily albumin. Metabolism of nateglinide is by both cytochrome P450 isoenzymes CYP2C9 (70%) and CYP3A4 (30%). Nateglinide and its metabolites are rapidly and completely renally cleared with an estimated half-life of 1.5 hours. Repaglinide is predominantly metabolized by CYP3A4 with a half-life of about 1 hour. It is excreted in bile.

EFFICACY

Repaglinide[34] and nateglinide[35] produce more physiologic insulin release after a meal and better postprandial blood glucose lowering as compared to long-acting sulfonylureas. Whether this more physiologic insulin release will mean a difference in clinical outcomes remains to be seen. Their overall efficacy measured as reduction in HbA1C is 0.6% to 1%.

ADVERSE EFFECTS

The incidence of hypoglycemia is approximately 0.3%. Other side effects occur no more often than with placebo in controlled trials.

DRUG INTERACTIONS

Inducers or inhibitors of CYP3A4 may affect response to repaglinide or, less likely, to nateglinide. Nateglinide is also an inhibitor of CYP2C9. Drug interaction studies with these agents are limited.

DOSING AND ADMINISTRATION

Both repaglinide and nateglinide should be administered before each meal. Repaglinide is initiated at 0.5–2 mg with a maximum dose of 4 mg per meal (up to four meals a day or 16 mg/d). Nateglinide is 120 mg three times daily before each meal. The dose of nateglinide

TABLE 74–11. Oral Agents for Diabetes

Generic (Trade)	Equivalent Theapeutic Dose (mg)	Half-Life (h)	Duration (h)	Recommended Starting Dose: Nonelderly	Recommended Starting Dose: Elderly	Maximum Dose Per Day	Metabolism/ Elimination
Sulfonylureas (SU)							
First-generation SU							
Acetohexamide (Dymelor)	500	6	12–18	250 mg/d	125–250 mg/d	1.5 g	Metabolized in liver; metabolite potency is equal to or greater than that of parent compound; renally eliminated
Chlorpropamide (Diabinese)	250	35+	24–72	250 mg/d	100 mg/d	500 mg	Metabolized in liver; also excreted unchanged in urine
Tolazamide (Tolinase)	250	7	12–24	100–250 mg/d	100 mg/d	750–1000 mg	Metabolized in liver; metabolite less active than parent compound; renally eliminated
Tolbutamide (Orinase)	1000	7	6–12	1–2 g/d	500 mg/d to 500 mg bid	2–3 g	Metabolized in liver to inactive metabolites that are renally excreted
Second-generation SU							
Glimepiride (Amaryl)	2	4–6	18–28	1–2 mg/d	0.5–1 mg/d	8 mg	Metabolized in liver to inactive metabolites
Glipizide (Gluctrol, Glucotrol XL)	5–10	3	10–24	5 mg/d	2.5–5 mg/d	40 mg, 20 mg	Metabolized in liver to inactive metabolites; renally eliminated
Glyburide (DiaBeta, Micronase)	5	3	18–24	2.5 mg/d	1.25–2.5 mg/d	20 mg	Metabolized in liver; 50% of metabolites eliminated in urine, 50% in feces.
Glyburide, micronized (Glynase)	3	3	18–24	1.5–3 mg/d	1.5 mg/d	12 mg	Same as glyburide
Short-acting insulin secretogogues							
Nateglinide (Starlix)	NA	1	4	120 mg with meals	no adjustment	120 mg tid	Metabolized by CYP2C9 and 3A4 to weakly active metabolites that are renally eliminated
Repaglinide (Prandin)	NA	1–1.4	4	0.5–1 mg with meals	no adjustment	16 mg/d or 4 mg per meal up to 4 meals/d	Metabolized by CYP 3A4 to inactive metabolites which are excreted in bile
Biguanides							
Metformin (Glucophage)	NA	6.2	8–12	500 mg bid	assess renal function	2,550 mg	Renal elimination both filtration and secretion
α-Glucosidase inhibitors							
Acarbose (Precose)	NA	2.7–9	4–6	25–50 mg bid	no adjustment	300 mg	Eliminated in bile
Miglitol (Glyset)	NA		4–6	50 mg tid	no adjustment	300 mg	Eliminated renally
Thiazolidinediones							
Pioglitazone (Actos)	NA	3–7	24 (16–24 total)	15–30 mg	no adjustment	45 mg	Metabolized by CYP2C8 and 3A4 to active metabolites with longer half-lives than parent compound
Rosiglitazone (Avandia)	NA	3–4	12–24	2–4 mg/d or divided bid	no adjustment	8 mg	Metabolized by CYP2C8 and 2C9 to inactive metabolites that are renally cleared

can be lowered to 60 mg with each meal in patients who are near goal HbA1C when therapy is initiated. If a meal is skipped, the dose of these agents should also be skipped. No dosage adjustment in elderly patients is currently recommended, although data in elderly subjects is limited.

Biguanides

Pharmacology. Metformin is the only biguanide available. It reduces hepatic glucose production and has an additional effect to increase glucose utilization in the periphery (antihyperglycemic,

TABLE 74–12. Drug Interactions with Sulfonylureas

Interaction	Drugs
Displace sulfonylureas from protein binding	Clofibrate, phenylbutazone, salicylates, sulfonamides
Reduce hepatic sulfonylurea metabolism	Chloramphenicol, MAOIs, phenylbutazone
Decrease urinary excretion of sulfonylurea or metabolite	Allopurinol, probenecid

hepatic insulin sensitizers).[36] Metformin also may induce mild anorexia that facilitates glycemic control by minimizing weight gain or invariably promoting weight loss. Insulin must be present for metformin to work. Metformin favorably affects lipids, reducing fasting triglycerides by approximately 16%, LDL-C by approximately 8% and modestly increasing HDL-C by approximately 2%.

Pharmacokinetics. Metformin is well absorbed and has a volume of distribution that approximates body water. Elimination of metformin is by both renal tubular secretion and glomerular filtration. The average half-life of metformin is about 6 hours.

EFFICACY

Metformin was used in the United Kingdom Prospective Diabetes Study (UKPDS), reducing macrovascular disease endpoints in obese patients.[37] The results with concomitant sulfonylureas in a heterogeneous population (obese and nonobese) were conflicting, but, on balance, this drug improves macrovascular risk.[38]

ADVERSE EFFECTS

The most common adverse effects with metformin are nausea, vomiting, and diarrhea. Anorexia or a metallic taste are also frequently reported. These side effects are dose dependent and can be minimized by titrating the dose slowly and taking the medication with food. A new extended-release preparation of metformin (Glucophage XR)reduces gastrointestinal side effects and may be taken once daily, but may have a deleterious effect on lipids and may not have equal glycemic efficacy to immediate release metformin.[39]

Phenformin, another biguanide, was taken off the US market in 1977 because of its propensity to cause lactic acidosis (approximately 50% mortality).[40] Metformin has been used with minimal incidence of lactic acidosis as precautions for its use (avoid in patients with renal insufficiency, congestive heart failure requiring pharmacologic therapy, or conditions predisposing to hypoxemia or inherent lactic acidosis, and withhold prior to and until documentation of a normal creatinine postintravascular contrast dye studies) are widely recognized.

DRUG INTERACTIONS

Cimetidine competes for renal tubular secretion of metformin and concomitant administration leads to higher metformin serum concentrations, a risk for lactic acidosis. Other cationic drugs may interact similarly such as procainamide, digoxin, quinidine, trimethoprim and vancomycin.

DOSING AND ADMINISTRATION

Metformin can be initiated with immediate-release tablets at 500 mg twice a day with meals, or 850 mg once a day, and increased by 500 mg weekly or 850 mg every 2 weeks, to a total of 2,000 mg/d. The maximum recommended dose is 2,550 mg/d but one dose-finding study demonstrated no greater reduction in HbA1C beyond 2,000 mg/d.

Metformin XR can be initiated with 500 mg with the evening meal and increased by 500 mg weekly to a maximum dosage of 2,000 mg/d. If suboptimal glycemic control is achieved with once-daily administration of 2,000 mg/d, 1,000 mg bid with meals can be considered.

PPARγ Agonists

Pharmacology. Rosiglitazone and pioglitazone are two thiazolidinediones (glitazones). Glitazones are the first group of available agents targeted to activate PPARγ. Additional chemical entities with similar mechanism of action are in development. PPARγ agonists reduce insulin resistance in the periphery (sensitize muscle and fat to the actions of insulin) and possibly in the liver (insulin sensitizers, antihyperglycemics).[41] This is accomplished by activating PPARγ, a nuclear transcription factor that is important in fat cell differentiation and fatty acid metabolism. Insulin in significant quantities must be present for these actions.

Triglycerides generally decrease and HDL-C increases in patients using these drugs. However, LDL-C increases. The LDL-C increase appears to be with larger LDL particles that may be less atherogenic, but the clinical significance of this finding remains to be determined.

Pharmacokinetics

EFFICACY

Glycemic efficacy of these drugs is highly variable. The onset of action of these drugs is slow, taking 2 to 3 months to see full effect. Monotherapy is often ineffective unless the drugs are given very early in the course of disease when sufficient β-cell function and hyperinsulinemia are present.

Assessing the clinical trials used for approval of glitazones is often difficult because patients were usually withdrawn from previous therapy, had deterioration of glycemic control, and then were given study medication.[42] While the patients on active drug often had worse glycemia than baseline (before withdrawal of previous medications), the control achieved was usually better than placebo, so the therapeutic effect is deemed the difference in glycemia seen between study drug and placebo. The therapeutic relevance to clinic practice of such maneuvers is open to question.

ADVERSE EFFECTS

Edema and weight gain may be very problematic in patients taking glitazones with insulin or insulin secretagogues. Weight gains of >10 kg are not unusual. The patients with the best glycemic response often have the most weight gain. Fluid retention may induce or worsen congestive heart failure in patients with left ventricular compromise. Studies are presently underway to help define the safety of these agents in patients with known heart disease. Glitazones have not been tested in patients with New York Heart Association class III or IV heart failure. Although animal and in vitro studies suggest antiatherogenic activities of these drugs, it will be years before the results of clinical trials are available to prove that such a promise is actually fulfilled.

The newer glitazones (rosiglitazone and pioglitazone) do not appear to have the liver toxicity problems that led to the withdrawal from the market of the first drug in this class, troglitazone. However, liver function test monitoring is still recommended. Upon initiation of therapy with pioglitazone or rosiglitazone, baseline liver function tests (minimally AST and ALT) should be obtained, then repeated every other month for the first 12 months, then periodically thereafter. Neither drug should be instituted if the baseline AST or ALT exceeds 2.5 times the upper limit of normal. They should be discontinued if the AST or ALT exceed three times the upper limit of normal or if signs or symptoms evident of liver injury present.

DRUG INTERACTIONS

No significant drug interactions have yet been identified with rosiglitazone. Drugs that induce or inhibit CYP3A4 may accelerate or inhibit pioglitazone metabolism but to date, no clinically relevant interactions have been described.

DOSING AND ADMINISTRATION

Initial doses are 15–30 mg for pioglitazone and 2–4 mg/d for rosiglitazone. Maximum doses are 45 mg for pioglitazone and 8 mg/d for rosiglitazone. A slightly greater response may occur with rosiglitazone when dosages of 4 or 8 mg/d are divided in two.

α-Glucosidase Inhibitors

Pharmacology. α-Glucosidase inhibitors prevent the breakdown of sucrose and complex carbohydrates in the small intestine prolonging the absorption of carbohydrates.[43,44] The net effect from this action is to reduce postprandial blood glucose rise.

Pharmacokinetics. The action of (glucosidase inhibitors is limited to luminal side of the intestine. There is limited systemic absorption and the majority of these agents are eliminated in the feces.

EFFICACY

Postprandial glucose concentrations are reduced, while fasting glucose levels are relatively unchanged. Efficacy on glycemic control is modest (average reductions in HbA1C of 0.3% to 1%), affecting primarily postprandial glycemic excursions.

ADVERSE EFFECTS

Flatulence is a very common side effect and greatly limits their use. α Glucosidase inhibitors should be titrated slowly to reduce gastrointestinal intolerance. If a patient develops hypoglycemia while on an α-glucosidase inhibitor, oral glucose must be given (or parenteral glucose or glucagon) because the drug will inhibit the breakdown of more complex sugar molecules.

DOSING AND ADMINISTRATION

Dosage for both miglitol and acarbose are similar. Initiate with a very low dose (25–50 mg with one meal a day); increase very gradually (over months) to maximum of 50 mg tid for patients ≤60 kg or 100 mg tid for patients >60 kg.

PIVOTAL TRIALS

DIABETES CONTROL AND COMPLICATIONS TRIAL

Much of the last century in diabetes care was dominated by the debate over whether glycemic control actually was causative in complications of DM. Animal studies and some human studies suggested that the worse the glycemia the greater the risk of complications. But "the glucose hypothesis" was not ultimately accepted as proven until the publication of the DCCT in 1993. One thousand four hundred forty-one patients with type 1 DM were divided into two groups: those without complications (726 subjects, primary prevention), and those with early microvascular complications (715 subjects, secondary prevention). These two groups were then again divided into two groups, one randomized to receive conventional therapy (one or two shots of insulin daily and infrequent SMBG with no attempt to change therapy based on home blood glucose readings), and the other to receive intensive therapy (3+ injections of insulin daily or insulin pump, with frequent SMBG and alteration of insulin therapy based on SMBG results, plus frequent contact with a health professional). After 6.5 years mean followup with a difference in HbA1C between the two groups being ≈ 2% (≈ 9% vs ≈ 7%), retinopathy was decreased by 76% in the primary prevention cohort, with retinopathy progression reduced 54% in the secondary prevention group. Neuropathy was decreased by 60% in both groups combined. Microalbuminuria was decreased 39%, while macroproteinuria was reduced 54% with intensive therapy. Hypoglycemia was more common and weight gain greater with intensive therapy. A nonstatistically significant reduction in coronary events was seen in the intensively treated group as compared to the conventional group. The DCCT revolutionized therapy of DM, demanding that stricter glycemic control be the goal.

IMPLICATIONS OF THE UNITED KINGDOM PROSPECTIVE DIABETES STUDY

The UKPDS was a landmark study for the care of patients with type 2 DM, confirming the importance of glycemic control for reducing the risk of microvascular complications.[25] More than 5,000 patients with newly diagnosed type 2 DM were entered into the study. Patients were followed for an average of 10 years. The major portion of the study assessed "conventional therapy" (no drug therapy unless the patient was symptomatic or had fasting plasma glucose >270 mg/dL versus intensive therapy starting with either sulfonylureas or insulin, aimed at keeping the fasting plasma glucose <108 mg/dL. A subset of obese patients was studied using metformin as the primary therapeutic agent.

Significant findings from the study include:

1. Microvascular complications (predominantly the need for laser photocoagulation on retinal lesions) are reduced by 25% when median HbA1C is 7% as compared to 7.9%.[25]
2. A continuous relationship exists between glycemia and microvascular complications with a 35% reduction in

risk for each 1% decrement in HbA1C. No glycemic threshold for microvascular disease exists.[45]

3. Glycemic control has minimal effect on macrovascular disease risk.[25] Excess macrovascular risk appears to be related to conventional risk factors such as dyslipidemia and hypertension.[46]
4. Sulfonylureas and insulin therapy do not increase macrovascular disease risk.[25]
5. Metformin reduces macrovascular risk in obese patients.[37]
6. Vigorous blood pressure control reduces microvascular and macrovascular events.[46] There was no evidence for a threshold systolic blood pressure above 130 mm Hg for protection against complications. β-Blockers and angiotensin-converting enzyme inhibitors appear to be equally efficacious.[47]

THERAPEUTICS

TYPE 1 DIABETES MELLITUS

The choice of therapy for type 1 DM is simple: all patients need insulin. However, how that insulin is delivered to the patient is a matter of considerable practice difference among patients and clinicians. Historically, after the discovery of insulin by Banting and Best in 1921, frequent injections of regular insulin (initially the only insulin available) were given. Modifications of insulin led to longer-acting insulin suspensions and the use by many patients of one or two shots of longer-acting insulin each day. Because SMBG and HbA1C testing were not available at that time, patients and practitioners had no idea how well their patients blood glucose concentrations were controlled, other than a vague sense from an indirect method, measurement of glucose in the urine. While the renal threshold for glucose is relatively predictable in young healthy subjects, it is highly variable in older patients and patients with renal disease. The advent of SMBG and HbA1C testing in the 1980s revolutionized the care of diabetes, enabling patients and practitioners to directly access blood glucose for assessment, and enabling the patient to make instantaneous changes in the insulin regimen, if need be. Modern diabetes management would be impossible without these two tools.

Contemporary management of type 1 DM attempts to match carbohydrate intake with glucose-lowering processes, most commonly insulin, as well as with exercise. Diet is still "the cornerstone" of diabetes therapy, but unlike in previous years, attempts are made to allow the patient to live as normal a life as possible. Understanding the principles of glucose input and glucose egress from the blood will allow the practitioner and the patient great latitude in the management of patients with type 1 DM.

Simplistically speaking, one can break down normal insulin secretion into a relatively constant background level of insulin ("basal") for the fasting and postabsorptive period, and prandial spikes of insulin after eating ("bolus")(Fig. 74–5).[48] Insulin sensitivity and insulin secretion are not constant throughout the day, rendering the basal concept inaccurate, however, in most clinical situations; this approach provides a useful paradigm for understanding and applying insulin treatment for type 1 DM. The other basic principle to consider is that the timing of insulin onset, peak and duration of effect must match meal patterns and exercise schedules to achieve near normal blood glucose values throughout the day.

Historically, complexity of insulin regimens has usually been related to number of injections of insulin administered per day. This is a

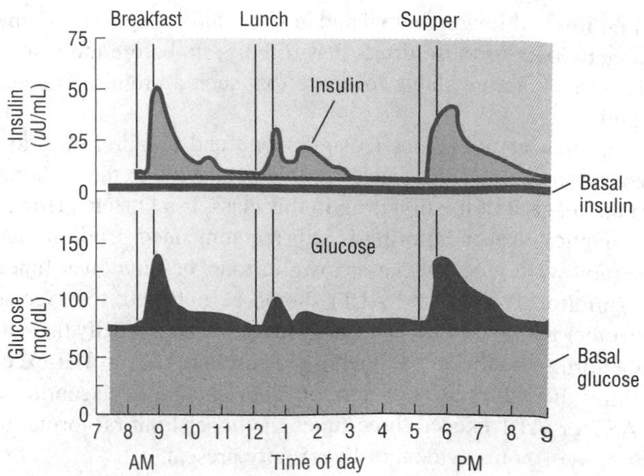

Intensive insulin therapy regimens

	7AM	11AM	5PM	HS
1. 2 doses, R + N or L	R + N or L		R + N or L	
2. 3 doses, R or rapid + N or L	R, Lis or A + N or L	R, Lis or A	R, Lis or A + N or L	
3. 4 doses, R or rapid acting + intermediate or ultralente	R, Lis or A + N, L or UL	R, Lis or A	R, Lis or A	N, L or UL
4. 4 doses, R or rapid acting + long acting	R, Lis or A	R, Lis or A	R, Lis or A	G
	← Adjusted Basal →			
5. CS-II pump	Bolus	Bolus	Bolus	

FIGURE 74–5. Relationship between insulin and glucose over the course of a day and how various insulin regimens could be given. A, aspart; CS-II, continuous subcutaneous insulin infusion; G, glargine; L, lente; Lis, lispro; N, NPH; R, regular; UL, ultralente.

reasonable classification. Clearly one injection of any insulin preparation daily will in no way mimic normal physiology, and therefore is unacceptable. Similarly, two injections of any insulin daily will fail to replicate normal insulin release patterns. Injection regimens that begin to approximate physiologic insulin release start with "split-mixed" injections of a morning dose of neutral protamine Hagedorn (NPH) and regular insulin before breakfast, and again before the evening meal. The presumption is made that the morning NPH insulin gives basal insulin for the day and covers the midday meal, the morning regular insulin covers breakfast, the evening NPH insulin gives basal insulin for the rest of the day, and the evening regular covers the evening meal. If patients are very compulsive about consistency of timing of their injections and meals and intake of carbohydrate, such a strategy may be somewhat successful. However, most patients are not sufficiently predictable in their schedule and food intake to allow "tight" glucose control with such an approach.

The first modification that is frequently made to such a regimen is the movement of the evening NPH to bedtime (now three total injections per day) because the fasting glucose in the morning is too high. This approach provides sufficient intensification of the insulin therapy for some patients. However, many patients need a more intense approach that also allows greater flexibility in their lifestyle.

The basal-bolus concept is an attempt to replicate normal insulin physiology with a combination of intermediate- or long-acting insulin to give the basal component and short-acting insulin to give the bolus component. Various strategies have been used for the former, including once or twice daily NPH, lente, or ultralente insulin, or once-daily insulin glargine. Most patients require two shots of all of the above insulins except insulin glargine. Also, all of the above insulins, with the exception of insulin glargine, have some degree of peak effect that must be considered in planning meals and activity. Insulin glargine is a feasible basal insulin supplement for most patients with type 1 DM. Of the long-acting insulin suspensions, twice daily ultralente is easiest to use.

The bolus insulin component is given before meals with either regular insulin, lispro insulin, or insulin aspart. The rapid onset of action and short time course of lispro insulin and insulin aspart more closely replicates normal physiology. This approach allows the patient to vary the amount of insulin injected, depending upon the preprandial SMBG level, the anticipated activity (upcoming exercise may reduce insulin requirement), and anticipated carbohydrate intake. Most patients will have a prescribed dose of insulin preprandially that they vary by use of a "sliding scale." This type of adjusted scale insulin is intended to optimize the insulin regimen. In light of the negative connotation of the term "sliding scale" (usually referring to giving insulin only after the blood glucose increases, rather than treating the underlying disorder), a better descriptor for the adjusted-dose insulin is variable-dose prandial insulin or insulin algorithm. Carbohydrate counting is a very effective tool for determining the amount insulin to be injected preprandially. Although general algorithms give rough guidelines, each patient will have to adjust the prescribed preprandial insulin dosage to achieve optimal glucose control.

As a rough estimate, patients may be begun on $\approx$ 0.6 U/kg/d with basal insulin 45% of total dose and prandial insulin 25% of total dose prebreakfast, 15% prelunch, and 15% presupper. Type 1 DM patients generally require between 0.5 and 1.0 U/kg/d. The need for significantly higher amounts of insulin suggests the presence of insulin antibodies or insulin resistance (coexistent endocrinopathy or type 2 DM).

Obviously insulin pump therapy (continuous subcutaneous insulin infusion [CSII], generally using lispro insulin to diminish aggregation) is the most sophisticated form of basal bolus insulin delivery system. Extensive discussion of this mode of therapy is beyond the scope of this text.[49] Nevertheless, the basic principles for implementation are the same. The one advantage of pump therapy is that the basal insulin dose may be varied, consistent with changes in insulin requirements throughout the day. In selected patients, this feature will allow greater glycemic control with CSII. However, insulin pumps require even greater attention to detail and frequency of SMBG than four injections daily. In appropriately selected patients willing to pay sufficient attention to detail of SMBG and insulin administration, CSII can be a very useful form of therapy.

Intensive therapy (basal bolus) to all adult patients with type 1 DM at the time of diagnosis is recommended to reinforce the importance of glycemic control from the outset rather than change strategies over time after lack of control. Occasional patients with an extended honeymoon period may need less intense therapy initially, but should be converted to basal bolus therapy as the onset of glycemic lability. For patients insisting on two injections daily, NPH and regular insulin (starting at 0.6 U/kg with two-thirds in the morning, two-thirds of morning dose as NPH, and one-half of evening dose as NPH) may be sufficient. Regardless of the regimen chosen, gross adjustments in the total insulin dose can be made based on HbA1C measurements and symptoms such as polyuria, polydipsia, and weight gain or loss. Finer insulin adjustments can be determined on the basis of the results of frequent SMBG.

All patients receiving insulin should have extensive education in the recognition and treatment of hypoglycemia. Yearly (or more often) questioning about the recognition of hypoglycemia is warranted. Documentation of frequency of hypoglycemia, particularly that requiring assistance of another person, visit to an emergent or urgent care facility, or hospitalization, should be recorded. In type 1 DM, the development of hypoglycemia unawareness is common. It may result from progression of disease with autonomic neuropathy. Loss of adrenergic warning signs in such a situation is a relative contraindication to intensive insulin therapy. More commonly, type 1 DM patients have loss of warning signs because of a presumed lower setpoint for release of counterregulatory hormones as a result of frequent episodes of hypoglycemia ("hypoglycemia begets hypoglycemia").[50] In such situations, more normal hypoglycemia awareness may be restored by reduction or redistribution of the insulin dose to eliminate significant hypoglycemic episodes.

Children and pubescent adolescents are relatively protected from microvascular complications and must be managed with consideration of what is practical. Therefore, it is not unreasonable to use less-intense management (two shots per day, premixed insulins) until the patient is postpubertal.[51]

Occasional patients have antibodies to injected insulin, but the significance of the antibodies is minimal.[52] Human insulin therapy has not totally eliminated insulin allergies, although most patients have a local reaction that will dissipate over time. If the allergic reaction does not improve or is systemic, insulin desensitization can be carried out.[53] Protocols for desensitization are available from major insulin manufacturers. While more common in the animal insulin era, lipohypertrophy is still seen in some patients with long-standing type 1 DM.[33] Such patients give their insulin injections in the same site to minimize discomfort. Because insulin absorption from an area of lipohypertrophy is unpredictable, avoidance of injections into these areas is mandatory.

Several common errors can occur in the therapy of patients with type 1 DM causing erratic glucose fluctuations:

1. Failure to take into account peaks of insulin action when using a peaking insulin and planning meals and/or activity. Eating should be planned around the peaks of the insulin.
2. Random rotation of insulin injection sites. There is sufficient variability of insulin absorption from site to site that this practice alone may cause wide glucose swings. The most consistent absorption of insulin is from the abdominal wall. We try to get our patients to take all their injections in the abdomen. If the patient is unable or unwilling to follow this advice, then systematic site rotation is the next preferable option. The patient always gives the insulin injection in the same region of the body the same time of the day each day. For instance, the arms are always used every morning. Needless to say, the patient would not inject in a limb and then go out and exercise that limb, increasing blood flow and insulin absorption.
3. Overinsulinization is a very common problem. The answer to all high blood glucose is not necessarily more insulin, as the patient may be insulinopenic, or may be "rebounding" from a previous low glucose and treating it with excessive amounts of carbohydrate. Fastidious SMBG, particularly during the night (or selected use of continuous glucose monitoring) will help sort this out. Also, practitioners sometimes do not adequately differentiate type 1 DM from type 2 DM when using insulin. Patients with type 1 DM are absolutely

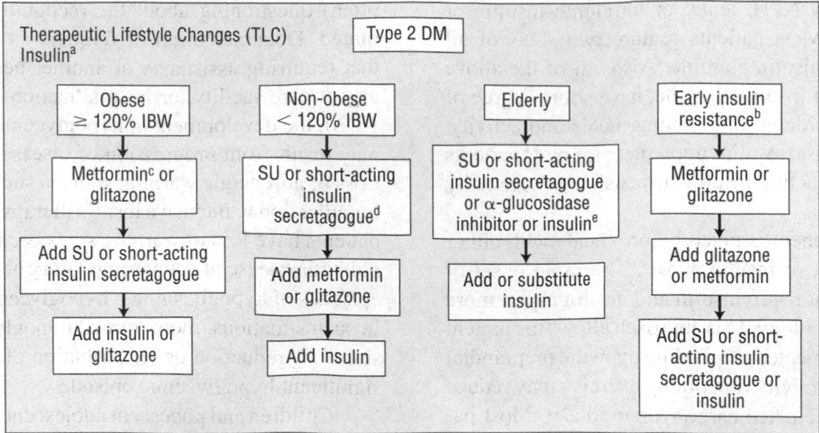

FIGURE 74–6. Algorithm for treating type 2 diabetes mellitus.

[a]TLC should be reinforced throughout treatment. At any point, particularly with severe metabolic decompensation, inulin may be used. Initial therapies with insulin may be more favorably accepted and instituted with a single bedtime injection of an intermediate- or long-acting insulin. See text for more details.

[b]Early insulin resistance refers to recognizing the disease when β-cell function is preserved. Although little evidence supports this, a meal-stimulated C-peptide response may assist in identifying these individuals.

[c]Metformin is preferred if there are no contraindications; the evidence from UKPDS supports it.

[d]In nonobese patients, metformin can be considered alternatively at this stage but because lean patients tend to have a relatively greater degree of β-cell dysfunction relative to insulin resistance, they may respond better to an insulin secretagogue.

[e]In elderly, the risk of hypoglycemia may be greater with SU than with short-acting insulin secretagogues, appropriately dosed insulin, or α-glucosidase inhibitors.

insulinopenic but have normal insulin sensitivity. Patients with type 2 DM have varying degrees of insulin resistance. Therefore, one unit change in the dose of insulin for a patient with type 1 DM may have a dramatic effect on glucose concentrations, whereas, in some patients with type 2 DM 10 to 20 times that amount of insulin may have little effect on glucose. Large changes in insulin dose in patients with type 1 DM are not usually indicated unless the patient's blood glucose control is very poor. Widely erratic SMBG results and/or weight gain often suggest overinsulinization.

4. When in doubt, always double-check the patient's technique for insulin dosing, insulin injection, and SMBG. Sometimes the simplest of errors results in miserable glycemic control.

TYPE 2 DIABETES MELLITUS

Pharmacotherapy for type 2 DM has changed dramatically in the last few years with the addition of several new drug classes and recommendations to achieve more stringent glycemic control. Symptomatic patients may initially require treatment with insulin to reduce glucose toxicity (which may reduce β-cell insulin secretion and worsen insulin resistance). Patients with HbA1C $\approx$ 7% or less are usually treated with therapeutic lifestyle measures. Those with HbA1C >7% but <8% are initially treated with single oral agents. Patients with higher initial HbA1C may benefit from initial therapy with two oral agents.

Depending on patient motivation and adherence to therapeutic lifestyle changes, most patients with HbA1C greater than 9% to 10% will likely require therapy with two or more agents to reach glycemic goals.

The best initial oral therapy for patients with type 2 DM is widely debated. Based on the results of the UKPDS and safety record, obese patients (>120% ideal body weight) should be started on metformin initially, titrated to at least $\approx$ 2,000 mg/d.[54] Near-normal weight patients may be treated with insulin secretagogues. Failure of initial therapy should result in addition rather than substitution (reserve substitution for intolerance to a drug due to side effects) of another class of drug. Initial combination therapy for patients with HbA1C >9% to 10% is not unreasonable, and an oral combination product (Glucovance) has been approved as a first-line treatment. Figure 74–6 is a therapeutic scheme used by the authors. Thiazolidinediones may be substituted in situations in which a patient is intolerant of, or has a contraindication to, metformin.

After a patient fails two drugs, adding a third class of oral agents (usually a thiazolidinedione) can be considered, though this triple therapy is not presently FDA approved. (Triple combination therapy with a sulfonylurea, metformin, and troglitazone was approved,[55] but troglitazone is no longer available for use.) An alternative is to add bedtime insulin, an intermediate-acting or long-acting insulin, to the initial oral agent used or two-drug combination.

Virtually all patients with type 2 DM ultimately become insulinopenic and will require insulin therapy. Insulin therapy for type 2 DM has changed dramatically in the last few years. Specifically, patients are often "transitioned" to insulin by using a bedtime injection of an intermediate- or long-acting insulin, using oral agents primarily for control during the day.[56,57] This strategy leads to less hyperinsulinemia during the day and is associated with less weight gain than the more-traditional insulin strategies. Because most patients are insulin resistant, insulin sensitizers are commonly used with insulin therapy. Patients with type 2 DM are usually well buffered against hypoglycemia. Patients should be monitored for hypoglycemia by asking about nocturnal sweating, palpitations, and nightmares, as well as SMBG. When bedtime insulin plus daytime oral medications fails, a conventional multiple daily-dose insulin regimen with or without an insulin sensitizer can be tried. Concerns and problems with insulin administration as addressed in the section on type 1 DM generally relate to the therapy of type 2 DM. However, patients with type 2 DM rarely have hypoglycemia unawareness and are better buffered against hypoglycemia. Also, the variability of insulin resistance means that insulin doses may range from 0.7 to 2.5 U/kg or more. Clearly, insulin therapy in patients with type 2 DM is empiric.

The availability of short-acting insulin secretagogues, very short-acting insulin, and α-glucosidase inhibitors, all of which target postprandial glycemia, has reminded practitioners that glycemic control is a function of fasting and preprandial glycemia and postprandial glycemic excursions.[58] Therefore, postprandial glucose measurements may need more emphasis. However, it remains to be seen whether targeting after-meal glucose excursions will have more of an effect on complications risk than more conventional strategies. α-Glucosidase inhibitors can be used as monotherapy in patients at risk for hypoglycemia, in patients manifesting primarily postprandial hyperglycemia, and in combination with virtually any other drug. In epidemiologic studies postglucose challenge glucose measurements are a better predictor of macrovascular disease risk.[59]

SPECIAL POPULATIONS

ADOLESCENT TYPE 2 DM[9]

Type 2 DM is increasing in adolescence. Obesity and physical inactivity seem to be particular culprits in the pathogenesis of this disease. Given the many years that the patient will have to live, extraordinary efforts should be expended in lifestyle modification measures in an attempt to ameliorate the glucose intolerance. Failing that strategy, the only labeled oral agent for use in children (10 to 16 years) is metformin. In adolescent females, the possibility of future pregnancy should be considered in the prescription of any drug regimen.

ELDERLY PATIENTS WITH DM

Elderly patients with newly diagnosed DM (almost always type 2 DM) present a different therapeutic calculus. Considering the risks of hypoglycemia in this population and the probable diminished long-term risk to develop microvascular complications, less-stringent glycemic goals should generally be set. Thinner, older patients may primarily be treated with shorter-acting insulin secretagogues or low-dose sulfonylureas (preferably not long-acting ones.) Risk for lactic acidosis increases with older age, making metformin therapy more problematic in octogenarians. Simple insulin regimens may be the easiest approach to glycemic control in elderly patients with newly diagnosed DM.

GESTATIONAL DM[11]

Gestational DM is diagnosed as previously described. Dietary therapy to minimize wide fluctuations in blood glucose is of paramount importance. Intensive educational efforts are usually necessary. Pregnant women without DM maintain plasma glucose concentrations between 50 and 130 mg/dL. Frequent SMBG is needed to tell whether dietary interventions are successful. If fasting plasma glucose is >105 mg/dL or if 2-hour postprandial glucose is >120 mg/dL on two or more occasions within a 2-week interval, insulin therapy is usually begun. One shot of NPH or a mixture of NPH and regular insulin in a 2:1 ratio given before breakfast may be adequate to reach glucose targets. Titration of insulin and switching to more complicated regimens is guided by SMBG results. In spite of the long-standing labeling of sulfonylureas as contraindicated in pregnancy, one recent randomized, open label, controlled trial evaluated the efficacy of glyburide as compared to insulin initiated after 11 weeks gestation.[60] Adequate control of blood glucose was achieved as compared to traditional insulin therapy with less hypoglycemia in the glyburide group. No evidence of any difference in complications, specifically, cord-serum insulin concentrations, incidence of macrosomia, caesarean delivery or neonatal hypoglycemia between regimens were noted. Glyburide was not detected in the cord serum of any infant. As the study limited enrollment beyond 11 weeks gestation, no conclusions regarding teratogenicity can be made from this study. The American Diabetes Association cites this study in a position paper and mentions its utility, but also warns that it is not a labeled use of the drug and suggests further studies are needed to establish its safety.[10] Patients with gestational DM should be evaluated at 6 weeks after delivery to ensure that normal glucose tolerance has returned. Because these patients' long-term risk for the development of DM is considerable, periodic assessment after that is warranted.

SECONDARY DIABETES

Secondary diabetes most commonly occurs due to exogenous corticosteroid administration. Such patients may respond to oral therapies, but often need insulin treatment. For most forms of secondary diabetes, insulin resistance is paramount, and treatment follows guidelines similar to that for patients with type 2 DM.

SPECIAL SITUATIONS

SICK DAYS

Acute self-limited illness rarely presents a major problem for patients with type 2 DM, but can be a significant challenge for insulinopenic type 1 DM patients.[61] While caloric intake generally declines, insulin sensitivity also decreases, meaning that it may take greater amounts of insulin to control blood glucose concentrations. Patients need to be adept at frequent SMBG, checking urine ketones, use of short-acting insulin (preferably lispro, in our experience), and understanding that sugar intake in this situation is not "bad" but may be necessary to "cover" the insulin therapy given to keep the patient out of diabetic ketoacidosis. We encourage patients to continue their usual insulin regimen and to use supplemental lispro based on SMBG results, with further additional insulin given if ketonuria develops. Sugar and electrolyte solutions, such as sports drinks, can be used to maintain hydration, to provide needed electrolytes if there is significant gastrointestinal or urinary losses, and to provide sugar to keep the patient from developing hypoglycemia because of the extra insulin that is usually needed. Most patients can be taught how to sufficiently manage sick days and avoid hospitalization.

DIABETIC KETOACIDOSIS AND HYPEROSMOLAR HYPERGLYCEMIC STATE[62]

Diabetic ketoacidosis and hyperosmolar hyperglycemic state are true diabetic emergencies. A comprehensive discussion of their treatment is beyond the scope of this book. Diabetic ketoacidosis is usually precipitated by the omitting of insulin in type 1 DM and intercurrent illness, particularly infection, in both type 1 DM and type 2 DM. Afflicted patients have a fluid deficit of several liters and a sodium and potassium deficit of several hundred milliequivalents. Restoration of intravascular volume acutely, followed by hypotonic saline, potassium supplements, and constant infusion insulin restore the patient's metabolic status relatively quickly. Bicarbonate administration is generally not needed and may be harmful. Treatment of the inciting medical condition is also important. Metabolic improvement is manifested by an increase in the serum bicarbonate or pH. Fluid administration alone will reduce the glucose concentration. Therefore, a fall in the blood glucose concentration should not be taken as evidence that the patient's metabolic status is improving. Rare patients will require larger amounts of insulin than those usually given (5–10 U/h). Constant infusion of a dose of insulin and the administration of intravenous glucose when the blood glucose level decreases to <250 mg/dL is preferable to titration of the insulin infusion based on the glucose level. The latter strategy may delay clearance of the ketosis and prolong treatment.

Hyperosmolar hyperglycemic state usually occurs in older patients with type 2 DM, at times undiagnosed, or in younger patients with prolonged hyperglycemia and dehydration or significant renal insufficiency. Infection or another medical illness is the usual precipitant. Fluid deficits are usually greater and blood glucose concentrations higher (at times >1,000 mg/dL) in these patients than in patients with diabetic ketoacidosis. Blood glucose levels should be lowered gradually with hypotonic fluids and low-dose insulin infusions. Mortality is high in this disorder.

HOSPITALIZATION FOR INTERCURRENT MEDICAL ILLNESS

Patients on oral agents may need transient therapy with insulin to achieve adequate glycemic control. In patients requiring insulin, receive scheduled doses of insulin with additional short-acting insulin. "Sliding-scale" insulin is to be discouraged, as it is notorious for not controlling glucose and for sometimes resulting in therapeutic misadventures with wide swings in the blood glucose as the patient "bounces" from hypoglycemia to hyperglycemia.[63] Recent work suggests improved outcomes in type 2 diabetes patients with acute myocardial infarctions[64] who receive constant intravenous insulin during the acute phase of the event to maintain near normal glucose concentrations. In the case of cardiac ischemia, the beneficial effects may be a result of reducing free fatty acids with insulin therapy. In patients treated with metformin, any illness leading to dehydration or hypoperfusion should lead to temporary discontinuation of the drug because of possible increased risk for lactic acidosis.

PERIOPERATIVE MANAGEMENT[65]

Surgical patients may experience worsening of glycemia for reasons similar to those listed above for intercurrent medical illness. Patients on oral agents may need transient therapy with insulin to control blood glucose. In patients requiring insulin, scheduled doses of insulin or continuous insulin infusions are preferred. For patients who can eat soon after surgery, the time-honored approach of giving one-half of the usual morning NPH insulin dose with dextrose 5% in water intravenously is acceptable, with resumption of scheduled insulin, perhaps at reduced doses, within the first day. For patients requiring more prolonged periods without oral nutrition and for major surgery, such as coronary artery bypass grafting and major abdominal surgery, constant infusion intravenous insulin is preferred. Metformin should be discontinued temporarily after any major surgery until it is clear that the patient is hemodynamically stable and normal renal function is documented.

REPRODUCTIVE-AGE WOMEN[66]

An increasing prevalence of DM has been noted in reproductive-age women. Prepregnancy planning is absolutely mandatory. Insulin is the only appropriate pharmacologic therapy for women contemplating pregnancy who were previously diagnosed with diabetes mellitus. Organogenesis is largely completed within 8 weeks, so good glycemic control should be obtained prior to conception. For women with diabetes mellitus controlled by lifestyle measures alone, conversion to insulin as soon as the pregnancy is confirmed is appropriate. For women with polycystic ovary disease who ovulate and become pregnant with insulin sensitizer therapy, conversion to insulin is mandatory as soon as pregnancy is confirmed.

PREGNANCY[67]

Insulin is the only acceptable pharmacologic therapy during pregnancy for women with diabetes mellitus in the United States. In Europe, metformin is sometimes used in pregnancy, but its use is eschewed in the United States. Patients previously treated with insulin may need intensification of their regimen to achieve therapeutic goals. Normal pregnancy is associated with a decrease in the blood glucose concentration as fuel is diverted to the fetus. Pregnant patients will be ingesting both meals and snacks daily. SMBG is generally intensified to try to reach glycemic targets and reduce fetal and maternal morbidity. Whether preprandial or postprandial glucose concentrations should be the target of therapy is hotly debated. Glucose targets during pregnancy are listed in Table 74–13. Ketosis should be avoided, requiring urine monitoring for ketones in the morning and if the blood sugar is >200 mg/dL.

SPECIAL TOPICS

LABORATORY MONITORING

HbA1C or glycosylated hemoglobin (GHb) measurements are not standardized nationally and are insensitive for detecting hyperglycemia. Whether HbA1C or GHb assays are superior for measuring glycemic control is debatable. HbA1C measurements are the "gold standard" for following long-term glycemic control for the previous 3 months.[68] Hemoglobinopathies can affect both measurements, increasing GHb measurements and decreasing HbA1C measurements performed by some methods. In some situations with shortened red blood cell survival, other strategies (measurement of fructosamine) are necessary to assess diabetes control.

TABLE 74–13. Blood Glucose Targets in Pregnancy

Time of day	mg/dL
Fasting	60–90
Premeal	60–105
Two hours after meal	60–120
0200 to 0600	60–100

The American Diabetes Association recommends a routine urinalysis at diagnosis in persons with type 2 DM as the initial screening for albuminuria. If positive, a 24-hour urine for quantitative assessment will assist in developing a treatment plan. When the urinalysis is negative for protein, a test to evaluate the presence of microalbumin is recommended.[69] In type 1 DM, microalbuminuria rarely occurs with short duration of disease or before puberty. Screening individuals with type 1 DM should begin with puberty and after 5 years' disease duration.

There are three methods for assessing microalbuminuria: (a) measure of urine albumin-to-creatinine ratio in a random spot collection (preferably the first morning void); (b) 24-hour timed collection; and (c) timed (e.g., 4-hour or 10-hour overnight) collection. Microalbuminuria on a spot urine specimen is defined as a ratio of 30–300 mg/g albumin/creatinine. On timed collections, microalbuminuria is defined as 30–300 mg/d or an albumin excretion rate of 20–200 μg/min. Because of wide intrapatient variability, persistence of microalbuminuria should be confirmed on at least two of three samples over 3 to 6 months. Additionally, when assessing urine protein or albumin, conditions that may cause transient elevations in urinary albumin excretion should be excluded. These conditions include short-term hyperglycemia, exercise, urinary tract infections marked hypertension, heart failure, and acute febrile illness.[69]

In type 2 DM, the presence of microalbuminuria is a strong risk factor for macrovascular disease and is frequently present at the time of diagnosis. Microalbuminuria may be a weaker predictor for future kidney disease in type 2 DM.

PREVENTION OF DM

Efforts to prevent type 1 DM with immunosuppressives[70] or insulin therapy[71] have been unsuccessful. A recently published lifestyle intervention trial done in Scandinavia showed a reduction in type 2 DM in treated patients as compared to controls.[72] The Diabetes Primary Prevention trial (DPP) in the United States is assessing the ability of lifestyle interventions or metformin to prevent the development of type 2 DM in high-risk individuals.[73] The thiazolidinedione troglitazone initially was used in this study, but in 1999, troglitazone was withdrawn after a participant taking the drug developed hepatic failure and ultimately died from complications.

PATIENT EDUCATION

It is not satisfactory to give patients with DM brief instructions with a few pamphlets and expect them to manage their disease adequately. Thinking that diabetes education is limited to one or two encounters is misguided; it is a lifetime exercise. Successful treatment of DM involves lifestyle changes for the patient (e.g., medical nutrition therapy, physical activity, self-monitoring of blood glucose and possibly of urine for ketones, and taking prescribed medications). Standards of diabetes self-management have been established and include a number of content areas listed in Table 74–14. The patient must be involved in the decision-making process and must learn as much about the disease and associated complications as possible. Emphasis should be placed on the evidence that indicates complications can be prevented or minimized with glycemic control and management of risk factors for cardiovascular disease. Recognition of the need for proper patient education to empower them into self-care has generated certification in diabetes education. Certified diabetes educators (CDEs) must document their patient education hours and sit for a certification examination that assesses the knowledge, tasks, and skills of an educator in order to become certified. An increasing number of nurses, pharmacists, dietitians, and physicians are becoming CDEs to document to the public that they meet a minimum standard for diabetes education and to fulfill quality initiatives in meeting guidelines for education recognition.[74]

TABLE 74–14. Content Areas of Instruction from the National Standards for Diabetes Self Management

Diabetes overview
Stress and psychosocial adjustment
Family involvement and social support
Nutrition
Exercise and activity
Medications
Monitoring and use of results
Relationships among nutrition, exercise, medication, and blood glucose monitoring
Prevention, detection, and treatment of acute complications
Prevention, detection, and treatment of chronic complications
Foot, skin, and dental care
Behavior change strategies, goal setting, risk factor reduction and problem solving
Preconception, pregnancy, and postpartum management
Use of health care systems and community resources

TREATMENT OF CONCOMITANT CONDITIONS AND COMPLICATIONS

RETINOPATHY[75]

Patients with established retinopathy should see an ophthalmologist every 6 to 12 months, or more often as necessary. Early background retinopathy may reverse with improved glycemic control. More advanced retinopathy will not regress with improved glycemia and may actually worsen with short-term improvements in glycemia. Studies are underway to determine whether medical therapy independent of glucose control will prevent the development of advanced retinopathy. Laser photocoagulation has markedly improved sight preservation in diabetic patients.

NEUROPATHY[76]

Peripheral neuropathy is the most common complication seen in type 2 DM patients in outpatient clinics. Paresthesias, numbness, or pain may be the predominant symptom. The feet are involved far more often than the hands. Improved glycemic control may alleviate some of the symptoms. Symptomatic therapy is empiric, including low-dose tricyclic antidepressants, anticonvulsants (phenytoin, gabapentin, and carbamazepine), topical capsaicin, and various pain medications, including nonsteroidal anti-inflammatory drugs.

Gastroparesis can be a severe and debilitating complication of DM. Improved glycemic control, discontinuation of medications which slow gastric motility, and the use of metoclopramide (preferably for only a few days at a time) or erythromycin may be helpful. Unfortunately, more efficacious medications have been found to have side effects that have kept them from long-term usage in DM patients. Gastric pacemakers as therapeutic hardware are presently under investigation for this complication.

Autonomic neuropathy may manifest as orthostatic hypotension. Such patients may require volume expanders or adrenergic agents. In severe cases, supine hypertension is extreme, mandating that the patient sleep in a sitting or semirecumbent position. The hallmark of diabetic diarrhea is its nocturnal occurrence. Diabetic diarrhea frequently responds to a 10- to 14-day course of an antibiotic such as doxycycline or metronidazole. In more unresponsive cases, octreotide may be useful. Cytopathy may benefit from cholinergic agents. Erectile dysfunction is often neuropathic and vasculogenic. Hypogonadism is a rare culprit in DM patients. Sildenafil is effective in about one-half of diabetic patients with impotence.

NEPHROPATHY[69]

Diabetes mellitus, and particularly type 2 DM, is the biggest contributor numerically to the development of end-stage renal disease in the United States. Glucose and blood pressure control are most important for the prevention of nephropathy, and blood pressure control is most important for retarding the progression of established nephropathy. Angiotensin-converting enzyme (ACE) inhibitors are the first recommended treatment modality. Recent studies also suggest a protective effect of angiotensin receptor blockers. Diuretics frequently are necessary due to the volume-expanded state of the patient. The National Kidney Foundation and Sixth Report of the Joint National Committee on Prevention, Detection, Evaluation, and Treatment of High Blood Pressure (JNC VI) recommend that patients with greater than 1 g proteinuria/d have their blood pressure goal be less than 125/75 mm Hg. This goal often is difficult to achieve.

PERIPHERAL VASCULAR DISEASE AND FOOT ULCERS

Claudication and nonhealing foot ulcers are common in type 2 DM patients.[77] Smoking cessation, correction of lipid abnormalities, and antiplatelet therapy are important strategies in treating claudicants. Pentoxifylline or cilostazol may be useful in selected patients. Revascularization is successful in selected patients. Local débridement and appropriate footwear and foot care are vitally important in the early treatment of foot lesions. In more advanced lesions, topical treatments may be of benefit. The role of hyperbaric oxygen therapy is controversial. Diabetic footcare is an excellent example of the adage, "an ounce of prevention is worth a pound of cure."

CORONARY HEART DISEASE

The risk for coronary heart disease (CHD) is two to four times greater in diabetic patients than in nondiabetic individuals. CHD is the major source of mortality in patients with DM. Recent studies suggest that multiple risk-factor intervention (lipids, hypertension, smoking cessation,[79] antiplatelet therapy)[80] will reduce the burden of excess macrovascular events. Epidemiologic data suggest that CHD prevention guidelines for type 2 DM apply equally to patients with type 1 DM.[81] β-Blocker therapy supplies an even greater protection from recurrent CHD events in diabetic patients than in nondiabetic subjects. Masking of hypoglycemic symptoms is a greater problem in type 1 DM patients than in those patients with type 2 DM. ACE inhibitors may have vascular protective effects, especially in DM patients.[82]

LIPIDS

The Scandinavian Simvastatin Survival Study (4S) showed 42% reduction in CHD events in diabetic patients with known CHD and very high LDL-C levels with simvastatin therapy (mean dose, 27 mg/d with LDL-C reduction approximately 35%).[83] Lesser degrees of risk reduction have been shown in other secondary prevention studies in patients treated with pravastatin with mild-to-moderate LDL-C elevation at baseline.[84] Primary prevention studies with statins have included only a small number of diabetic patients but suggest an effect on CHD event rates as well. The diabetic subgroup in the Veterans Administration HDL Intervention Trial (VA-HIT) of CHD patients with low HDL-C and low LDL-C showed approximately 22% reduction in CHD events in diabetic patients with known CHD when HDL-C was increased by approximately 6% by gemfibrozil.[85]

The new National Cholesterol Education Program (NCEP) Adult Treatment Panel III (ATP III)[86] guidelines classify the presence of DM as a CHD risk equivalent, and therefore recommend that LDL-C be lowered to <100 mg/dL. Unlike previous guidelines, more consideration is now given to HDL-C and triglycerides. The lipid classification scheme is given in Table 74–6. The primary target is the treatment of LDL-C. After the LDL-C goal is reached (usually with a statin), triglycerides are considered for pharmacologic management, assuming unresponsiveness to glycemic control efforts, weight management, and exercise. In such situations, a non-HDL-C goal is established (a surrogate for all apo B-containing particles). The non-HDL-C goal for patients with DM is <130 mg/dL. Niacin or a fibrate can be added to reach that goal if triglycerides are 201–499 mg/dL. Niacin or a fibrate can also be added if the LDL-C goal is reached but the patient has low HDL-C (<40 mg/dL). Patients with marked hypertriglyceridemia (≥500 mg/dL) are at risk for pancreatitis. Efforts to reduce triglycerides with glycemic control, elimination of other secondary causes (including medications), and drug therapy (fibrate and/or niacin) are effective treatment strategies.

HYPERTENSION

The role of hypertension in increasing microvascular and macrovascular risk in patients with DM has been confirmed in the UKPDS[46] and Hypertension Optimization Treatment (HOT)[87] trials. The American Diabetes Association recommends more aggressive goals for blood pressure (<130/80 mm Hg) in patients with DM and in patients with systolic hypertension (reduce systolic blood pressure to <160 mm Hg or by 20 mm Hg in patients with systolic blood pressure of 160–179 mm Hg).[23] The National Kidney Foundation suggests that the blood pressure goal be less than 130/80 mm Hg. In patients with greater than 1 g/d proteinuria and renal insufficiency, more aggressive therapy (<125/75 mm Hg) is advocated.[88] ACE inhibitors generally are recommended for initial therapy. Many patients require multiple agents. Diuretics or calcium channel blockers frequently are useful as second and third agents. Blood pressure goals are generally more difficult to achieve than glycemic goals or lipid goals in most diabetic patients.

TRANSPLANTATION[89]

Whole pancreas and islet cell transplantation are still relatively experimental procedures in patients with type 1 DM; those with end-stage renal disease also receiving kidney transplantation.

PHARMACOECONOMIC CONSIDERATIONS

As described in the introduction, the direct and indirect costs of DM are substantial. Much of the indirect costs are related to loss of productivity due to the significant morbidity (hospitalizations, loss of vision, lower extremity amputations, kidney failure, and cardiovascular events) associated with the disease. For a disease that affects only 5% to 6% of the population, it is responsible for 11% to 12% of health expenditures. With evidence from the DCCT and UKPDS to support intensive blood glucose control to reduce complications risk, the question of cost effectiveness comes into play.

An economic model based on the DCCT approximates that 120,000 persons in the U.S. would meet criteria for intensive intervention. The cost of implementing intensive therapy over the lifetime of the population is estimated at $4.0 billion dollars. The benefits of this strategy are net gains of 920,000 years of sight, 691,000 years free from end stage renal disease, and 678,000 years free from lower extremity amputations. The incremental cost per year of life gained is $28,661. This is well within the limits of a cost-effective strategy and compares favorably to treatment of high blood pressure or hypercholesterolemia.

Economic analysis of intensive therapy for type 2 DM is more complex. Outcomes must also factor in the burden of cardiovascular disease as the major cause of mortality. One model analyzed the health benefits and economics of treating type 2 DM with the goal of achieving normoglycemia but using outcomes based on the DCCT trial results. Accounting for the prevalence of cardiovascular disease in type 2 DM, an estimate of $16,002 incremental cost per quality-adjusted life-year gained was obtained. The limitation of this analysis is that while UKDPS did demonstrate an improvement in diabetes related outcomes, the overall efficacy on microvascular disease complications was not mirrored to the DCCT.

Two economic analyses were performed on data generated from the UKPDS, one assessing cost effectiveness of an intensive blood glucose control policy in type 2 DM and the other assessing improved blood pressure control in hypertensive patients with type 2 DM. In the first analysis, outcome was measured as the incremental cost per event-free year gained within the trial. Based on trial outcomes and assumptions, the incremental cost in the intensive treatment group per event-free year gained is $1366. While intensive treatment costs were higher, the cost per event-free year gained appears cost-effective. The second analysis showed the incremental cost per extra year free from microvascular and macrovascular endpoints from intensive blood pressure control in a standard clinical practice model to be $1498. The incremental cost per life year gained was estimated at $619, again demonstrating the cost effectiveness of intensive intervention.

EVALUATION OF THERAPEUTIC OUTCOMES

MONITORING OF THE PHARMACEUTICAL CARE PLAN

A comprehensive pharmaceutical care plan for the patient with DM will integrate considerations of goals to optimize blood glucose control and protocols to screen for, prevent or manage microvascular and macrovascular complications. In terms of standards of care for persons with DM, one can review the document published by the ADA that outlines initial and ongoing assessments for patients with DM22. For quality of care measures, one can refer to a document entitled, "Coordinated Performance Measurement for the Management of Adult Diabetes—A Consensus Statement" provided by The American Medical Association, The Joint Commission on Accreditation of Heathcare Organizations, and The National Committee for Quality Assurance. These two publications can provide guidance in development of a comprehensive clinical practice strategy that includes documentation to meet quality care initiatives.

The major performance measures will assess the ability to meet current standards of care. Recognizing the treatment goals for glycemia (HbA1c < 7%), lipids (LDL-C < 100 mg/dL; non-HDL-C < 130 mg/dL, TG < 200 mg/dL, and HDL-C > 45 mg/dL), and hypertension (minimally < 130/80 mm Hg; < 125/75 mm Hg if > 1 gm urine protein excretion in 24 hours) provide targets for monitoring and adjusting pharmacotherapy as discussed in various sections above. Glycemic control is paramount in managing type 1 or type 2 DM but, as readily identified from the above discussion, requires frequent assessment and adjustment in diet, exercise, and pharmacologic therapies. Minimally, HbA1c should be measured twice a year in patients meeting treatment goals on a stable therapeutic regimen. Quarterly assessments are recommended for those whose therapy has changed or who are not meeting glycemic goals. Fasting lipid profiles should be obtained as part of an initial assessment and thereafter at each follow-up visit if not at goal, annually if stable and at goal, or every two years if the lipid profile suggests low risk. Documenting regular frequency of foot exams (each visit), urine protein assessment (annually), dilated ophthalmologic exams (yearly, more frequently with identified abnormalities), and office visits for follow-up are also important. Annual administration of vaccines and routine assessment for and management of other cardiovascular risks (i.e. smoking and antiplatelet therapy) are components of preventive medicine strategies. The multiplicity of assessments for each patient visit are likely to be better facilitated utilizing an integrative computer program or standardized progress note forms, which assist the clinician in identifying whether the patient has met standards of care in the frequency of monitoring and achievement of defined targets of therapy.

▶ PRINCIPLES OF PHARMACOTHERAPY

- Diabetes mellitus is a group of metabolic disorders of fat, carbohydrate and protein metabolism that results from defects in insulin secretion, insulin action (sensitivity), or both.
- The two major classifications of diabetes mellitus are type 1 (insulin deficient) and type 2 (combined insulin resistance and relative deficiency in insulin secretion). They differ in clinical presentation, onset, etiology and progression of disease. Both are associated with microvascular and macrovascular disease complications.
- Goals of therapy in diabetes mellitus are directed at reducing symptoms of hyperglycemia, reducing the onset and progression of retinopathy, nephropathy and neuropathy complications, intensive therapy of associated cardiovascular risk factors, and improving quality and quantity of life.
- Intensive glycemic control (minimal HbA1C ≤7%) reduces risk for onset and progression of microvascular disease complications. In type 1 DM, this translates into multiple daily insulin injection regimens or use of an insulin pump. In type 2 DM, this translates into a need for multiple drug therapy (often including insulin), particularly as the disease progresses over time.
- Knowledge of the pharmacokinetics of insulin preparations, pharmacology of oral antidiabetic agents, patient's quantitative and qualitative meal patterns and activity level are essential to optimize blood glucose control while minimizing risks for

hypoglycemia and other adverse effects of pharmacologic therapies.

- Aggressive management of cardiovascular disease risk factors in type 2 DM is necessary to reduce the risk for adverse cardiovascular events or death. Smoking cessation, use of antiplatelet therapy as a primary prevention strategy, aggressive management of dyslipidemia minimally to goal LDL-C (<100 mg/dL) and secondarily to goal non-HDL-C (<130 mg/dL), and treatment of hypertension (again often requiring multiple drugs) minimally to <130/80 mm Hg are vital.
- Events that may alter response to therapy (i.e., illness, surgery, psychological stress) should be anticipated and managed prospectively when feasible.
- Patient education and ability to demonstrate self-care and adherence to therapeutic lifestyle and pharmacologic interventions are crucial to successful outcomes.
- Multidisciplinary teams of health care professions including physicians (primary care, endocrinologists, ophthalmologists, vascular surgeons), podiatrists, dietitians, nurses, pharmacists, social workers, behavioral health specialists, and certified diabetes educators are needed to optimize outcomes in persons with diabetes mellitus.

ADDENDUM

Since the initial completion of this chapter, three relevant updates have been reported.

- In August of 2001, the National Institutes of Health announced their unpublished findings from the Diabetes Prevention Program.[73] Individuals with impaired glucose tolerance reduced their risk for the development of type 2 diabetes mellitus by 58% with an intensive exercise and nutritional therapy intervention and by 31% with metformin treatment.[90]
- In September 2001, the American Association of Clinical Endocrinologists recommended in a white paper that the goal of blood glucose lowering in persons with diabetes mellitus should be an HbA1C of < 6.5%; that postprandial blood glucose targets should be defined as < 140 mg/dL and that high risk individuals for type 2 diabetes mellitus should be screened beginning at age 30 years.[91]
- Finally, on September 20, 2001, a series of clinical trials were published in the New England Journal of Medicine demonstrating the efficacy of angiotensin receptor blockers in preventing the clinical progression of renal disease in patients with type 2 diabetes mellitus.[92,93,94]

REFERENCES

1. American Diabetes Association. Diabetes facts and figures. Available at www.diabetes.org/main/application/commercewf?origin=*.jsp&event=link(B1). Accessed July 8, 2001.
2. Palmer JP Lernmark A. Pathophysiology of type I (insulin-dependent) diabetes. In: Porte D, Jr, Sherwin RS, eds. Ellenberg & Rifkin's Diabetes Mellitus, 5th ed. Stamford, CT, Appleton & Lange, 1997:455–486.
3. Raffel LJ, Scheuner MT, Rotter JI. Genetics of diabetes. In: Porte D Jr, Sherwin RS, eds. Ellenberg & Rifkin's Diabetes Mellitus, 5th ed. Stamford, CT, Appleton & Lange, 1997:401–454.
4. Bennett P, Rewers M, Knowler W. Epidemiology of diabetes mellitus. In: Porte D Jr, Sherwin RS, eds. Ellenberg & Rifkin's Diabetes Mellitus: Theory and Practice, 5th ed. New York, Elsevier Science, 1997:373–400.
5. American Diabetes Association. Diabetes facts and figures. Available at www.diabetes.org/main/applicatuib/commercewf?orig=*.jsp&event=link(B4_5). Accessed July 8, 2001.
6. Froguel P, Zouali H, Vionnet N, et al. Familial hyperglycemia due to mutations in glucokinase. Definition of a subtype of diabetes mellitus. N Engl J Med 1993;328:697–702.
7. Diabetes Care. Screening for diabetes. Diabetes Care 2001;24(suppl 1): S21–S24.
8. American Diabetes Association. Type 2 Diabetes in children and adolescents. Diabetes Care 2000;23:381–389.
9. Kahn SE, Porte D Jr. The pathophysiology of type II (non-insulin dependent) diabetes mellitus: Implications for treatment. In: Porte D Jr, Sherwin RS,eds. Ellenberg & Rifkin's Diabetes Mellitus, 5th ed. Stamford, CT, Appleton & Lange, 1997:487–512.
10. American Diabetes Association. Gestational diabetes mellitus. Diabetes Care 2001;24 Suppl 1:S77–S79.
11. American Diabetes Association. Report of the expert committee on the diagnosis and classification of diabetes mellitus. Diabetes Care 2001;24(suppl 1):S5–S19.
12. American Diabetes Association. Prevention of type 1 diabetes mellitus. Diabetes Care 2001;24(suppl 1):S117.
13. American Diabetes Association. Screening for type 2 diabetes. Diabetes Care 2001;24(suppl 1):S21–S24.
14. Janeway CA Jr. Immunology relevant to diabetes. In: Porte D Jr, Sherwin RS, eds. Ellenberg & Rifkin's Diabetes Mellitus, 5th ed. Stamford, CT, Appleton & Lange, 1997:287–300.
15. Turner RC, Cull CA, Frighi V: Glycemic control with diet, sulfonylurea, metformin, or insulin in patients with type 2 diabetes mellitus: Progressive requirement for multiple therapies (UKPDS 49). UK Prospective Diabetes Study (UKPDS) Group. JAMA 1999;281:2005–2012.
16. McCarthy M, Menzel S. The genetics of type 2 diabetes. Br J Clin Pharmacol 2001;51:195–199.
17. Barker DJ. The fetal origins of type 2 diabetes mellitus. Ann Intern Med 1999;130:322–324.
18. Haffner SM, Stern MP, Hazuda HP, Mitchell BD, Patterson JK. Cardiovascular risk factors in confirmed prediabetic individuals. Does the clock for coronary heart disease start ticking before the onset of clinical diabetes? JAMA 1990;263:2893–2898.
19. Reaven GM. Role of insulin resistance in human disease (syndrome X): An expanded definition. Annu Rev Med 1993;44:121–31.
20. Pandit MK, Burke J, Gustafson AB. Drug-induced disorders of glucose tolerance. Ann Intern Med 1993;118:529–539.
21. Fajans SS. Classification and diagnosis of diabetes. In: Porte D Jr, Sherwin RS, eds. Ellenberg & Rifkin's Diabetes Mellitus, 5th ed. Stamford, CT, Appleton & Lange, 1997:357–372.
22. Ehrmann DA, Barnes RB, Rosenfield RL. Prevalence of impaired glucose tolerance and diabetes in women with polycystic ovary syndrome. Diabetes Care 1999;22:141–146.
23. American Diabetes Association. Standards of medical care for patients with diabetes mellitus. Diabetes Care 2001;24(suppl1):S33–S43.
24. Diabetes Control and Complications Trial Research Group. The effect of intensive treatment of diabetes on the development and progression of long-term complications in insulin-dependent diabetes mellitus. N Engl J Med 1993;329:977–986.
25. UK Prospective Diabetes Study Group. Intensive blood-glucose control with sulphonylureas or insulin compared with conventional treatment and risk of complications in patients with type 2 diabetes (UKPDS 33). Lancet 1998;352:837–853.
26. American Diabetes Association. Self-monitoring of blood glucose. Diabetes Care 1994;17;81–86.
27. Kennedy L. Self-monitoring of blood glucose in type 2 diabetes: Time for evidence of efficacy. Diabetes Care 2001;24:977–978.
28. American Diabetes Association. Nutrition recommendations and principles for people with diabetes mellitus. Diabetes Care 2001;24(suppl 1): S44–S47.

29. American Diabetes Association. Diabetes mellitus and exercise. Diabetes Care 2001;24 (suppl 1):S51–S55.
30. Guyton AC, Hall JE, eds. Textbook of Medical Physiology, 10th ed. Philadelphia, WB Saunders, 2000:884–898.
31. Griffin ME, Feder A, Tamborlane WV. Lipoatrophy associated with lispro insulin in insulin pump therapy: an old complication, a new cause? Diabetes care 2001;24:174.
32. Gerich JE. Oral hypoglycemic agents. N Engl J Med 1989;321:1231–1245.
33. Stenman S, Mclander A, Groop PH, Groop LC. What is the benefit of increasing the sulfonylurea dose? Ann Intern Med 1993;118:169–172.
34. Landgraf R. Meglitinide analogues in the treatment of type 2 diabetes mellitus. Drugs Aging 2000;17:411–425.
35. Dunn CJ, Faulds D. Nateglinide. Drugs 2000;60:607–615.
36. Bailey CJ, Turner RC. Metformin. N Engl J Med 1996;334:574–579.
37. UK Prospective Diabetes Study (UKPDS) Group. Effect of intensive blood-glucose control with metformin on complications in overweight patients with type 2 diabetes (UKPDS 34). Lancet 1998;352:854–865.
38. UK Prospective Diabetes Study Group. UKPDS 28: A randomized trial of efficacy of early addition of metformin in sulfonylurea-treated type 2 diabetes. Diabetes Care 1998;21:87–92.
39. Bristol-Myers Squibb. Glucophage XR package insert. Princeton, NJ, January 2001.
40. Stacpoole PW. Metformin and lactic acidosis: Guilt by association? Diabetes Care 1998;21:1587–1588.
41. Lebovitz HE, Banerji MA. Insulin resistance and its treatment by thiazolidinediones. Recent Prog Horm Res 2001;56:265–294.
42. Gale EA. Lessons from the glitazones: A story of drug development. Lancet 2001;357:1870–1875.
43. Mooradian AD, Thurman JE. Drug therapy of postprandial hyperglycemia. Drugs 1999;57:19–29.
44. Campbell LK, Baker DE, Campbell RK. Miglitol: Assessment of its role in the treatment of patients with diabetes mellitus. Ann Pharmacother 2000;34:1291–1301.
45. Stratton IM, Adler AI, Neil HA. Association of glycaemia with macrovascular and microvascular complications of type 2 diabetes (UKPDS 35): Prospective observational study. BMJ 2000;321:405–412.
46. Adler AI, Stratton IM, Neil HA: Association of systolic blood pressure with macrovascular and microvascular complications of type 2 diabetes (UKPDS 36): Prospective observational study. BMJ 2000;321:412–419.
47. UK Prospective Diabetes Study Group. Efficacy of atenolol and captopril in reducing risk of macrovascular and microvascular complications in type 2 diabetes: UKPDS 39. BMJ 1998;317:713–720.
48. Strowig S, Raskin P. Intensive management of insulin-dependent diabetes mellitus. In: Porte D Jr, Sherwin RS, eds. Ellenberg & Rifkin's Diabetes Mellitus, 5th ed. Stamford, CT, Appleton & Lange, 1997:709–733.
49. Reynolds LR. Reemergence of insulin pump therapy in the 1990s. South Med J 2000;93:1157–1161.
50. Cryer PE. Hypoglycemia is the limiting factor in the management of diabetes. Diabetes Metab Res Rev 1999;15:42–46.
51. Rosenbloom AL, Schatz DA, Krischer JP, et al. Therapeutic controversy: Prevention and treatment of diabetes in children. J Clin Endocrinol Metab 2000;85:494–522.
52. Binder C, Brange J. Insulin chemistry and pharmacokinetics. In: Porte D Jr, Sherwin RS, eds., eds. Ellenberg & Rifkin's Diabetes Mellitus, 5th ed. Stamford, CT, Appleton & Lange, 1997:689–708.
53. American Diabetes Association. Medical management of type 1 diabetes mellitus, 3rd. ed. Kelly DB. Ed. Alexandria, VA: American Diabetes Association, 1998.
54. DeFronzo RA. Pharmacologic therapy for type 2 diabetes mellitus. Ann Intern Med 1999;131(4):281–303.
55. Yale JF, Valiquett TR, Ghazzi MN, et al. The effect of a thiazolidinedione drug, troglitazone, on glycemia in patients with type 2 diabetes mellitus poorly controlled with sulfonylurea and metformin. A multicenter, randomized, double-blind, placebo-controlled trial. Ann Intern Med 2001;134(Pt 1):737–745.
56. Shank ML, Del Prato S, DeFronzo RA. Bedtime insulin/daytime glipizide. Effective therapy for sulfonylurea failures in NIDDM. Diabetes 1995;44:165–172.
57. Yki-Jarvinen H, Ryysy L, Nikkila K. Comparison of bedtime insulin regimens in patients with type 2 diabetes mellitus. A randomized, controlled trial. Ann Intern Med 1999;130:389–396.
58. Bastyr EJ 3rd, Stuart CA, Brodows RG: Therapy focused on lowering postprandial glucose, not fasting glucose, may be superior for lowering HbA1C. IOEZ Study Group. Diabetes Care 2000;23:1236–1241.
59. Glucose tolerance and mortality: Comparison of WHO and American Diabetes Association diagnostic criteria. The DECODE study group. European Diabetes Epidemiology Group. Diabetes Epidemiology: Collaborative analysis of diagnostic criteria in Europe. Lancet 1999;354:617–621.
60. Langer O, Conway DL, Berkus MD, et al. A comparison of glyburide and insulin in women with gestational diabetes mellitus. N Engl J Med 2000;343:1134–1138.
61. Laffel L. Sick-day management in type 1 diabetes. Endocrinol Metab Clin North Am 2000;29:707–723.
62. American Diabetes Association. Hyperglycemic crises in patients with diabetes mellitus. Diabetes Care 2001;24(suppl 1):S83–S90.
63. Sawin CT. Action without benefit. The sliding scale of insulin use. Arch Intern Med 1997;157:489.
64. Malmberg K, Norhammar A, Wedel H: Glycometabolic state at admission: Important risk marker of mortality in conventionally treated patients with diabetes mellitus and acute myocardial infarction: Long-term results from the Diabetes and Insulin-Glucose Infusion in Acute Myocardial Infarction Circulation 1999;99:2626–2632.
65. Jacober SJ, Sowers JR. An update on perioperative management of diabetes. Arch Intern Med 1999;159:2405–2411.
66. American Diabetes Association. Preconception care of woman with diabetes. Diabetes Care 2001;24(suppl 1):S66–S68.
67. Ryan EA. Pregnancy in diabetes. Med Clin North Am 1998;82:823–845.
68. American Diabetes Association. Tests of glycemia in diabetes. Diabetes Care 2001;24(suppl 1):S80–S82.
69. American Diabetes Association. Diabetic nephropathy. Diabetes Care 2001;24(suppl 1):S69–S72.
70. Schernthaner G. Progress in the immunointervention of type 1 diabetes mellitus. Horm Metab Res 1995;27:547–554.
71. Kakka R, Koda-Kimble MA. Can insulin therapy delay or prevent insulin-dependent diabetes mellitus? Pharmacotherapy 1997;17:38–44.
72. Tuomilehto J, Lindstrom J, Eriksson JG, et al. Prevention of type 2 diabetes mellitus by changes in lifestyle among subjects with impaired glucose tolerance. N Engl J Med 2001;344:1343–1350.
73. The Diabetes Prevention Program. Design and methods for a clinical trial in the prevention of type 2 diabetes. Diabetes Care 1999;22(4):623–634.
74. Mensing C, Boucher J, Cypress M, et al. National standards for diabetes self-management education. Diabetes Care 2000;23:682–689.
75. American Diabetes Association. Diabetic retinopathy. Diabetes Care 2001;24(suppl1). S73–S76.
76. Vinik AI. Diabetic neuropathy: Pathogenesis and therapy. Am J Med 199;107(2B):27S–33S.
77. American Diabetes Association. Consensus development conference on diabetic foot wound care: 7–8 April 1999, Boston, Massachusetts. Diabetes Care 1999;22(8):1354–1360.
78. American Diabetes Association. Management of dyslipidemia in patients with diabetes. Diabetes Care 2001;24(suppl 1):S58–S61.
79. Haire-Joshu D, Glasgow RE, Tibbs TL. Smoking and diabetes (technical review). Diabetes Care 1999;22:1887–1898.
80. American Diabetes Association. Aspirin therapy. Diabetes Care 2001;24(suppl 1):S62–S63.
81. Orchard TJ, Forrest KY, Kuller LH, Becker DJ. Lipid and blood pressure treatment goals for type 1 diabetes: 10-Year incidence data from the Pittsburgh Epidemiology of Diabetes Complications Study. Diabetes Care 2001;24:1053–1059.
82. Heart Outcomes Prevention Evaluation Study Investigators. Effects of ramipril on cardiovascular and microvascular outcomes in people with

diabetes mellitus: Results of the HOPE study and MICRO-HOPE substudy. Lancet 2000;355:253–259.

83. Haffner SM, Alexander CM, Cook TJ. Reduced coronary events in simvastatin-treated patients with coronary heart disease and diabetes or impaired fasting glucose levels: Subgroup analyses in the Scandinavian Simvastatin Survival Study. Arch Intern Med 1999;159(22):2661–2667.
84. Goldberg RB, Mellies MJ, Sacks FM, et al. Cardiovascular events and their reduction with pravastatin in diabetic and glucose-intolerant myocardial infarction survivors with average cholesterol levels: Subgroup analyses in the cholesterol and recurrent events (CARE) trial. The Care Investigators. Circulation 1998;98:2513–2519.
85. Rubins HB, Robins SJ, Collins D, et al. Gemfibrozil for the secondary prevention of coronary heart disease in men with low levels of high-density lipoprotein cholesterol. Veterans Affairs High-Density Lipoprotein Cholesterol Intervention Trial Study Group. N Engl J Med 1999;341:410–418.
86. Executive Summary of The Third Report of The National Cholesterol Education Program (NCEP) Expert Panel on Detection, Evaluation, and Treatment of High Blood Cholesterol in Adults (Adult Treatment Panel III). JAMA 2001;285:2486–2497.
87. Hansson L, Zanchetti A, Carruthers SG. Effects of intensive blood-pressure lowering and low-dose aspirin in patients with hypertension: principal results of the Hypertension Optimal Treatment (HOT) randomised trial. HOT Study Group. Lancet 1998;351:1755–1762.
88. Bakris GL, Williams M, Dworkin L, et al. Preserving renal function in adults with hypertension and diabetes: A consensus approach. National Kidney Foundation Hypertension and Diabetes Executive Committees working Group. Am J Kidney Dis 2000;36:646–661.
89. Robertson RP, Davis C, Larsen J, et al. Pancreas and islet transplantation for patients with diabetes mellitus (technical review). Diabetes Care 2000;23:112–116.
90. American Association of Clinical Endocrinologists ACE Consensus conference on guidelines for glycemic control. Available at www.aace.com/pub/press/release/diabetesconsensuswhitepaper.php (accessed January 2, 2002).
91. National Institute of Diabetes and Digestive and Kidney Diseases (NIDDK). Clinical alert: diet and exercise dramatically delay type 2 diabetes; diabetes medication metformin also effective. Available at www.nlm.nih.gov/databases/alerts/diabetes01.html (accessed January 2, 2002).
92. Lewis Ej, Hunsicker LG, Clarke WR, et al. Renoprotective effect of the angiotensin-receptor antagonist irbesartan in patients with nephropathy due to type 2 diabetes. N Engl J Med 2001;345:851–860.
93. Brenner BM, Cooper ME deZeeuw D, et al. Effects of Losartan on renal and cardiovascular outcomes in patients with type 2 diabetes and nephropathy. N. Engl J Med 2001; 345:861–869.
94. Parving HH, Lehnert H, Brochner-Mortensen J, et al. N Engl J Med 2001;345:870–880.

75

THYROID DISORDERS

Charles A. Reasner, II, and Robert L. Talbert

Thyroid hormones affect the function of virtually every organ system. In the child, thyroid hormone is critical for normal growth and development. In the adult, the major role of thyroid hormone is to maintain metabolic stability. Substantial reservoirs of thyroid hormone in the thyroid gland and blood provide constant thyroid hormone availability. In addition, the hypothalamic-pituitary-thyroid axis is exquisitely sensitive to small changes in circulating thyroid hormone concentrations, and alterations in thyroid hormone secretion maintain peripheral free thyroid hormone levels within a narrow range. Patients seek medical attention for evaluation of symptoms owing to abnormal thyroid hormone levels or because of diffuse or nodular thyroid enlargement.

THYROID HORMONE PHYSIOLOGY

THYROID HORMONE SYNTHESIS

The thyroid hormones thyroxine (T_4) and triiodothyronine (T_3) are formed on thyroglobulin, a large glycoprotein synthesized within the thyroid cell (Fig. 75–1). Because of the unique tertiary structure of this glycoprotein, iodinated tyrosine residues present in thyroglobulin are able to bind together to form active thyroid hormones.[1,2]

IODIDE TRANSPORT AND ORGANIFICATION

Iodide is actively transported via a Na^+/I^- symporter from the extracellular space into the thyroid follicular cell against both electrical and biochemical gradients.[3] Structurally related anions such as SCN^- (thiocyanate), ClO_4^- (perchlorate), and TcO_4^- (pertechnetate) are competitive inhibitors of iodine transport.[4] In addition, bromine, fluorine, and lithium block iodide transport into the thyroid (Table 75–1). Inorganic iodide that enters the thyroid follicular cell is oxidized by thyroid peroxidase and is covalently bound (organified) to tyrosine residues of thyroglobulin (Fig. 75–2). It is interesting that although salivary glands and the gastric mucosa are able to actively transport iodide, they are unable to effectively incorporate iodide into proteins. Similarly, when tyrosine molecules are iodinated on proteins other than thyroglobulin, they lack the proper tertiary structure needed to allow the formation of active thyroid hormones.

IODOTYROSINE COUPLING

The iodinated tyrosine residues monoiodotyrosine (MIT) and diiodotyrosine (DIT) combine to form iodothyronines (Fig. 75–3). Thus, DIT and DIT combine to form T_4, whereas MIT and DIT constitute T_3. In addition to its role in iodine organification, the hemoprotein thyroid peroxidase also catalyses the formation of iodothyronines (coupling).

Iodine deficiency causes an increase in the ratio of MIT to DIT in thyroglobulin and leads to a relative increase in the production of T_3. Because T_3 is more potent than T_4, the increase in T_3 production in iodine-depleted areas may be beneficial. The thionamide drugs used to treat hyperthyroidism inhibit thyroid peroxidase and thus block thyroid hormone synthesis.

THYROID HORMONE SECRETION

Thyroglobulin is stored in the follicular lumen and must reenter the cell, where the process of proteolysis liberates thyroid hormone into the bloodstream. Thyroid follicles active in hormone synthesis are identified histologically by columnar epithelial cells lining follicular lumens, which are depleted of colloid. Inactive follicles are lined by cuboidal epithelial cells and are replete with colloid. Both iodide and lithium block the release of preformed thyroid hormone, through poorly understood mechanisms.

CHARACTERISTICS OF CIRCULATING THYROID HORMONES[5]

T_4 and T_3 are transported in the bloodstream by three proteins: thyroid-binding globulin (TBG), thyroid-binding prealbumin (TBPA), and albumin. It is estimated that 99.96% of T_4 and 99.5% of T_3 are bound to these proteins. Only the unbound (free) thyroid hormone is able to diffuse into the cell, elicit a biologic effect, and regulate thyroid-stimulating hormone (TSH) secretion from the pituitary.

Whereas T_4 is secreted solely from the thyroid gland, less than 20% of T_3 is produced in the thyroid. The majority of T_3 is formed from the breakdown of T_4 catalyzed by the enzyme 5′-monodeiodinase found in peripheral tissues. Because T_3 may be five times more active than T_4, the deiodinase enzymes play a pivotal role in determining overall metabolic activity. Three different 5′-monodeiodinase enzymes are present in the body.[6] Type I enzymes are present in peripheral tissues, whereas type II enzymes are found in the central nervous system, pituitary, and thyroid. Type III enzymes, found in the placenta, skin, and developing brain, inactivate T_4 and T_3.[5,74] The principal characteristics of these enzymes are listed in Table 75–2. T_4 may also be acted on by the enzyme 5′-monodeiodinase to form reverse T_3. Reverse T_3 has no known significant biologic activity. T_3 is removed from the body by deiodinative degradation and through the action of sulfotransferase enzyme systems to T_3 sulfate and 3,3-diiodothyronine sulfate.[8]

THYROTROPIN RECEPTORS[9]

The growth and function of the thyroid are stimulated by activation of the thyrotropin receptor by TSH. This receptor belongs to the family of G-protein-coupled receptors. The thyrotropin receptor is coupled to the α subunit of the stimulatory guanine-nucleotide-binding protein ($G_s\alpha$) activating adenylate cyclase and increasing the accumulation of cyclic adenosine monophosphate (AMP). This regulates the expression of thyroglobulin and thyroid peroxidase genes. A mutation in the receptor that results in chronic stimulation causes diffuse thyroid enlargement and hyperthyroidism (germ-line mutations) or autonomously functioning thyroid nodules (somatic mutation in an epithelial cell).[10] Conversely, thyrotropin resistance would result from point mutations, leading to abnormalities in the thyrotropin receptor-adenylate cyclase system.[9] Individuals with this abnormality have

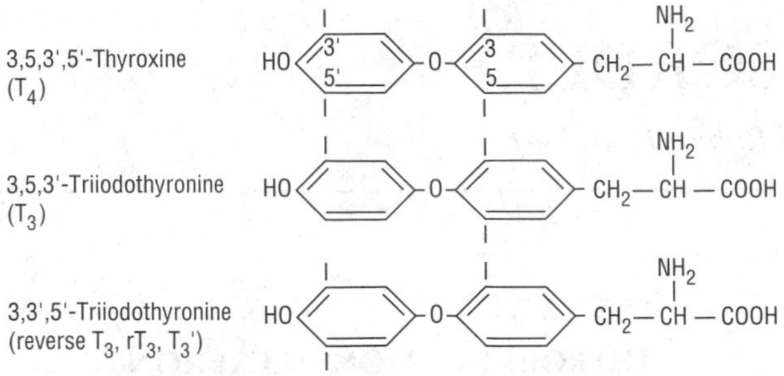

3,5,3',5'-Thyroxine (T_4)

3,5,3'-Triiodothyronine (T_3)

3,3',5'-Triiodothyronine (reverse T_3, rT_3, T_3')

FIGURE 75–1. Structure of thyroid hormones.

high levels of TSH but decreased thyroglobulin levels and a normal or small gland.

THYROID HORMONE RECEPTORS

Thyroid hormone receptors[11,12] regulate the transcription of target genes in the presence of physiologic concentrations of T_3. Thyroid receptors translocate from the cytoplasm to the nucleus and interact in the nucleus with T_3, target genes, and other proteins required for basal and T_3-dependent gene transcription. Thyroid receptors exist in multiple isoforms such as TRb2, TRb1, TRa1, and others in man and animals.

REGULATION OF THYROID HORMONE PRODUCTION

The production of thyroid hormone is regulated in two main ways. First, TSH secreted by the anterior pituitary regulates thyroid hormone. The secretion of TSH is itself under negative feedback control by the circulating level of free thyroid hormone and the positive influence of hypothalamic thyrotropin- releasing hormone (TRH). Second, extrathyroidal deiodination of T_4 to T_3 is regulated by a variety of factors including nutrition, nonthyroidal hormones, drugs, and illness.

THYROTOXICOSIS

Thyrotoxicosis[13] results when tissues are exposed to excessive levels of T_4, T_3, or both. Like many endocrine disorders, thyrotoxicosis occurs more frequently in women, with an estimated annual incidence of 3 per 1,000.

TABLE 75–1. Thyroid Hormone Synthesis and Secretion Inhibitors

Mechanism of Action	Substance
Blocks iodide transport into thyroid	Bromine Fluorine Lithium
Impairs organification and coupling of thyroid hormones	Thionamides Sulfonylureas Sulfonamide(?) Salicylamide(?) Antipyrine(?)
Inhibits thyroid hormone secretion	Iodide (large doses) Lithium

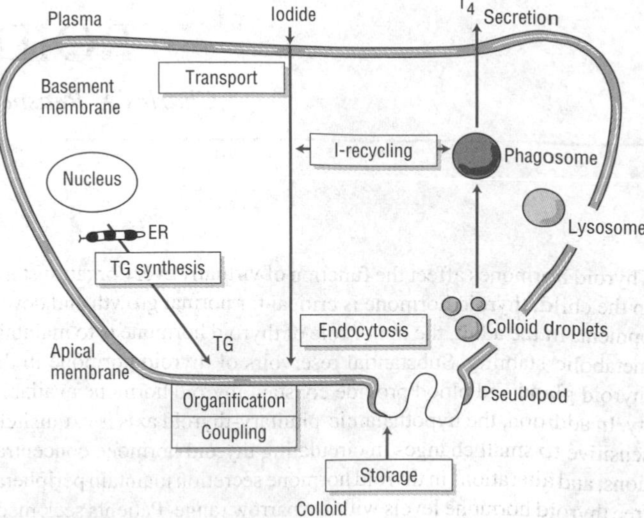

FIGURE 75–2. Thyroid hormone synthesis. Iodide is transported from the plasma, through the cell, to the apical membrane where it is organified and coupled to thyroglobulin (TG) synthesized within the thyroid cell. Hormone stored as colloid reenters the cell through endocytosis and moves back toward the basal membrane, where T_4 is secreted. Nonhormonal iodide is recycled.

CLINICAL PRESENTATION

The clinical manifestations of thyrotoxicosis include nervousness, emotional lability, easy fatigability, and heat intolerance. A cardinal sign is loss of weight concurrent with an increased appetite. In the elderly patient, and in the patient with very severe disease, anorexia may be present as well. The frequency of bowel movements may increase but frank diarrhea is unusual. Palpitations are a prominent and distressing symptom, particularly in the patient with preexisting heart disease. Proximal muscle weakness is common and is noted on climbing stairs or in getting up from a sitting position. Women may note their menses are becoming scanty and irregular.

A variety of physical signs may be elicited including warm, smooth, moist skin and unusually fine hair. Separation of the end of the fingernails from the nail beds (onycholysis) may be noted. Ocular signs that result from thyrotoxicosis include retraction of the eyelids

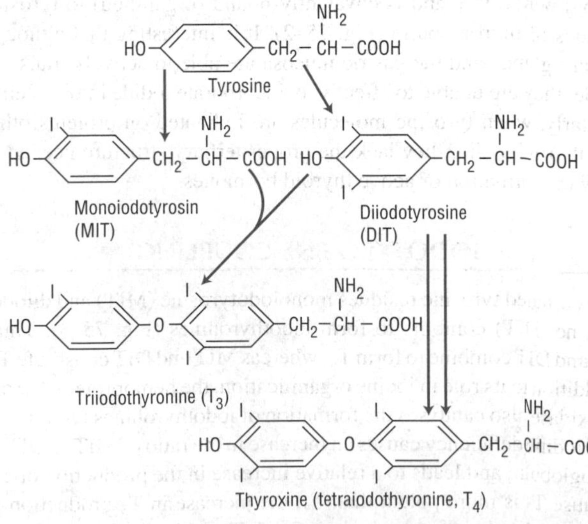

Tyrosine

Monoiodotyrosin (MIT)

Diiodotyrosine (DIT)

Triiodothyronine (T_3)

Thyroxine (tetraiodothyronine, T_4)

FIGURE 75–3. Scheme of coupling reactions. After tyrosine is iodinated to form MIT or DIT (organification of the iodine), MIT and DIT combine to form T_3, or two molecules of DIT form T_4.

TABLE 75–2. Properties of Iodothyronine 5′-Deiodinase Isoforms

Property	Type I	Type II	Type III
Effect of propylthiouracil	Increase	Decrease	Increase
Tissue localization	Thyroid, liver, kidney	Pituitary, thyroid, CNS, brown adipose tissue	Placenta, developing brain, skin
Preferred substrate	$rT_3 > T_4 > T_3$	$T_4 > T_3$	T_3 (sulfate) $> T_4$
Physiologic role	Extracellular T_3 production for peripheral tissue	Intracellular T_3 production, especially for brain in hypothyroidism or iodine deficiency	Inactivation of T_4 and T_3
Developmental expression	Expressed latest in development; predominant deiodinase in adult	Expressed second; especially high in brain and brown adipose tissue	Expressed first; high in developing brain; may be important for fetal thyroid hormone metabolism

rT_3, reverse T_3; PTU, propylthiouracil; T_3, triiodothyronine; T_4, thyroxine

and lagging of the upper lid behind the globe when the patient looks downward (lid lag). Physical signs of a hyperdynamic circulatory state are common and include tachycardia at rest, a widened pulse pressure, and a systolic ejection murmur. Gynecomastia is sometimes noted in men. Neuromuscular examination often reveals a fine tremor of the protruded tongue and outstretched hands. Deep-tendon reflexes are generally hyperactive.

DIFFERENTIAL DIAGNOSIS

Measurement of the radioactive iodine uptake (RAIU) is critical in the evaluation of the clinically thyrotoxic patient (Table 75–3). The normal 24-hour RAIU ranges from 10% to 30% with some regional variation owing to differences in iodine intake. An elevated RAIU indicates *true hyperthyroidism;* that is, the patient's thyroid gland is actively overproducing T_4, T_3, or both. Conversely, a low RAIU indicates the excess thyroid hormone is not a consequence of thyroid gland hyperfunction. The importance of differentiating true hyperthyroidism from other causes of thyrotoxicosis lies in the widely different prognosis and treatment of the diseases in these two categories. Therapy of thyrotoxicosis associated with thyroid hyperfunction is mainly directed at decreasing the rate of thyroid hormone synthesis, secretion, or both. Such measures are ineffective in treating thyrotoxicosis that is not the result of true hyperthyroidism, because hormone synthesis and regulated hormone secretion are already at a minimum.

TABLE 75–3. Differential Diagnosis of Thyrotoxicosis

Increased RAIU	Decreased RAIU
TSH-induced hyperthyroidism	Inflammatory thyroid disease
TSH-secreting tumors	Subacute thyroiditis
Selective pituitary resistance to T_4	Painless thyroid
Thyroid simulators other than TSH*	Ectopic thyroid tissue
TSAb (Graves' disease)	Struma ovarii
HCG (trophoblastic diseases)	Metastatic follicular carcinoma
Thyroid autonomy	Exogenous sources of thyroid hormone
Toxic adenoma	Medication
Multinodular goiter	Food

HCG, human chorionic gonadotropin; RAIU, radioactive iodine uptake; TSAb, thyroid-stimulating antibodies; TSH, thyroid-stimulating hormone.

*The RAIU may be decreased if the patient has been recently exposed to excess iodine.

Adapted from Ingbar SH, Braverman LE, Werner S. The Thyroid, 5th ed. Philadelphia, IB Lippincott, 1986, with permission.

CAUSES OF THYROTOXICOSIS ASSOCIATED WITH ELEVATED RAIU

TSH-INDUCED HYPERTHYROIDISM

To better understand these syndromes we must first review TSH biosynthesis and secretion. TSH is synthesized in the anterior pituitary as separate α- and β-subunit precursors. The α subunits from luteinizing hormone (LH), follicle-stimulating hormone (FSH), human chorionic gonadotropin (hCG), and TSH are similar, whereas the β subunits are unique and confer immunologic and biologic specificity. Free β subunits are devoid of receptor binding and biologic activity and require combination with an α subunit to express their activity. Criteria for the diagnosis of TSH-induced hyperthyroidism include (a) evidence of peripheral hypermetabolism; (b) diffuse thyroid gland enlargement; (c) elevated free thyroid hormone levels; and (d) elevated serum immunoreactive TSH concentrations. Because the pituitary gland is extremely sensitive to even minimal elevations of free T_4, a detectable TSH level in any thyrotoxic patient indicates the inappropriate production of TSH.

TSH-SECRETING PITUITARY ADENOMAS

TSH-secreting pituitary tumors[14,15] occur sporadically and release biologically active hormone that is unresponsive to normal feedback control. The mean age at diagnosis is around 40 years and women are more commonly diagnosed as having TSH-secreting pituitary tumors than are men (8:7). These tumors may cosecrete prolactin or growth hormone; therefore, the patients may present with amenorrhea/galactorrhea or signs of acromegaly. Most patients present with classic symptoms and signs of thyrotoxicosis. Visual-field defects may be present owing to impingement of the optic chiasm by the tumor. Tumor growth and worsening visual-field defects have been reported following treatment of thyrotoxicosis.

Diagnosis of a TSH-secreting adenoma should be made by demonstrating lack of TSH response to TRH stimulation, elevated α-subunit levels, and radiologic imaging. Note that MRI does not identify some small tumors. Moreover, 10% of "normal" individuals may have pituitary tumors noted on pituitary imaging.[16]

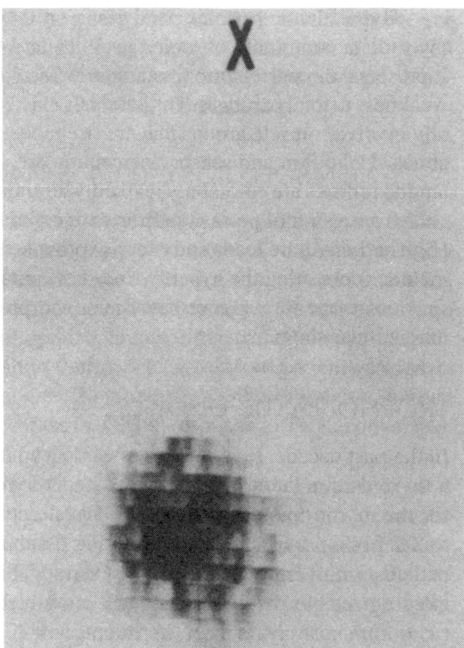

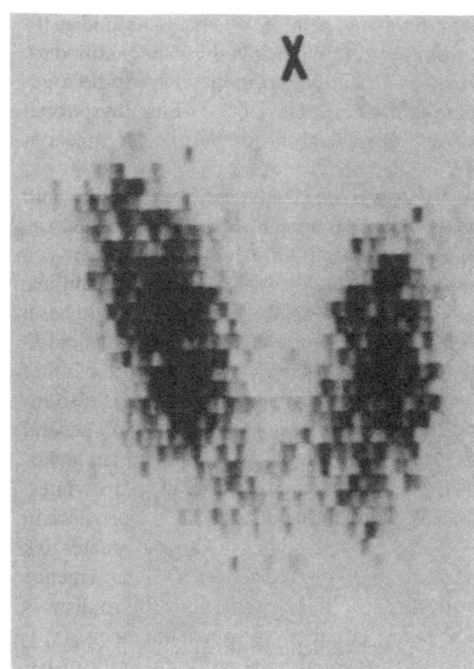

FIGURE 75–6. *Left*, autonomously functioning nodule is suppressing the remainder of thyroid gland. *Right*, previously suppressed lobes of thyroid gland are visualized 3 months after radioiodine treatment of hyperfunctioning nodule. The "X" is a marker for thyroid cartilage. *(From Becker KL, ed. Principles and Practice of Endocrinology and Metabolism. Philadelphia, Lippincott, 1990, with permission.)*

independent function may be documented by a failure of the autonomous nodule to decrease its iodine uptake during exogenous T_3 administration. RAI ablation, subtotal thyroidectomy, thionamides, and percutaneous ethanol injection are treatment options, but because thionamides do not halt the proliferative process in the nodule, definitive therapies are recommended. Because thyroid carcinoma is not a major consideration in an autonomously functioning thyroid nodule, observation is usually recommended for patients with autonomously functioning nodules who are euthyroid.

MULTINODULAR GOITERS

In multinodular goiters (Plummer's disease),[23] follicles with a very high degree of autonomous function coexist with normal or even nonfunctioning follicles. Thyrotoxicosis in a multinodular goiter occurs when the follicles with a high degree of autonomy generate enough thyroid hormone to exceed the needs of the patient. The pathogenesis of multinodular goiter is thought to be similar to toxic adenoma.[25] It is not surprising that this type of hyperthyroidism develops insidiously over a period of several years and predominantly affects older individuals with long-standing goiters. Often, elderly women present with subtle signs of hyperthyroidism that are superimposed on underlying heart disease. The patient's complaints of weight loss, depression, anxiety, and insomnia may be attributed to old age. Any unexplained chronic illness in an elderly patient presenting with a multinodular goiter calls for the exclusion of hidden thyrotoxicosis. Third-generation TSH assays and T_3 suppression testing may be useful in detecting subclinical hyperthyroidism.[26]

A thyroid scan will show patchy areas of autonomously functioning thyroid tissue. The preferred treatment for toxic multinodular goiter is radioactive iodine (RAI) or surgery. Surgery is usually selected for younger patients and patients in whom large goiters impinge on vital organs. Alternatively, percutaneous injection of 95% ethanol has also been used to destroy single or multinodular adenomas with a 5-year success rate approaching 80%.[24]

CAUSES OF THYROTOXICOSIS ASSOCIATED WITH SUPPRESSED RAIU

INFLAMMATORY THYROID DISEASE

Subacute Thyroiditis

Painful subacute (viral or de Quervain's) thyroiditis is believed to be caused by viral invasion of thyroid parenchyma. Typically, patients complain of severe pain in the thyroid region, which often extends to the ear on the affected side. With time, the pain may migrate from one side of the gland to the other. Low-grade fever is common. Systemic symptoms owing to thyrotoxicosis are present. On physical examination, the thyroid gland is firm and exquisitely tender. Signs of thyrotoxicosis are present.

Thyroid function tests typically run a triphasic course. Initially, serum thyroxine levels are elevated owing to release of preformed thyroid hormone from disrupted follicles. The 24-hour RAIU during this time is less than 2% owing to thyroid inflammation and TSH suppression by the elevated thyroxine level. As the disease progresses, intrathyroidal hormone stores are depleted and the patient may become mildly hypothyroid with an appropriately elevated TSH level. During the recovery phase, thyroid hormone stores are replenished and serum TSH elevation gradually returns to normal. Recovery is generally complete within 2 to 6 months. Most patients remain euthyroid and recurrences of painful thyroiditis are extremely rare. The patient with painful thyroiditis should be reassured that the disease is self-limited and is unlikely to recur. Thyrotoxic symptoms may be relieved with β-blockers. Aspirin (650 mg orally every 6 hours) usually relieves the pain. Occasionally, prednisone (20 mg orally three times a day) must be used to suppress the inflammatory process. Antithyroid drugs are not indicated because they do not decrease the release of preformed thyroid hormone.

Painless Thyroiditis

Since its description in 1975, painless (silent, lymphocytic, postpartum) thyroiditis has been recognized as a common cause of thyrotoxicosis and may represent as much as 15% of cases of thyrotoxicosis in North America. The etiology is not fully understood and may be heterogeneous. The triphasic course of this illness mimics that of painful thyroiditis. Most patients present with mild thyrotoxic symptoms. Lid retraction and lid lag are present, but exophthalmos is absent. The thyroid gland may be diffusely enlarged but thyroid tenderness is absent.

The 24-hour RAIU will be suppressed to less than 2% during the thyrotoxic phase of painless thyroiditis.[27,28] Antithyroglobulin and antimicrosomal antibody levels are elevated in more than 50% of patients. Painless thyroiditis frequently occurs during the immediate postpartum period, and individual patients may experience recurrence of the disease with subsequent pregnancies. Patients with mild hyperthyroidism and painless thyroiditis should be reassured that they have a self-limited disease. Adrenergic symptoms may be ameliorated with propranolol. Antithyroid drugs are not indicated because they do not decrease the release of preformed thyroid hormone.

ECTOPIC THYROID TISSUE

Struma Ovarii

Struma ovarii is a teratoid tumor of the ovary that is capable of making thyroid hormone. This extremely rare cause of thyrotoxicosis is suggested by the absence of thyroid enlargement in a thyrotoxic patient with a suppressed RAIU. The diagnosis is established by localizing functioning thyroid tissue in the ovary with whole-body radioactive iodine (^{131}I) scanning. Interestingly, struma ovarii without associated hyperthyroidism is much more common than struma ovarii associated with hyperthyroidism. Because the tissue is neoplastic and potentially malignant, combined surgical and radioiodine treatment of malignant struma ovarii for both monitoring and therapy of relapse is the recommended treatment.[29]

Follicular Cancer

In widely metastatic follicular carcinomas with relatively well-preserved function, sufficient thyroid hormone can be synthesized and secreted to produce thyrotoxicosis. In most instances, a previous diagnosis of thyroid malignancy has been made. The diagnosis can be confirmed by whole-body ^{131}I scanning. Treatment with ^{131}I is generally effective at ablating functioning thyroid metastases.

EXOGENOUS SOURCES OF THYROID HORMONE

Medication

The term *thyrotoxicosis factitia* denotes hyperthyroidism produced by the ingestion of exogenous thyroid hormone. Obesity is the most common nonthyroidal disorder for which thyroid hormone is used, but thyroid hormone has been used for almost every conceivable problem from menstrual irregularities and infertility to baldness. Because these patients do not benefit from treatment with thyroid hormone, the physician or patient may gradually increase the dose of hormone employed in an attempt to gain the desired effect. Obviously, thyrotoxicosis factitia can also occur when too large a dose of thyroid hormone is employed for conditions in which it is likely to be beneficial, such as hypothyroidism or nontoxic goiter. Rarely, thyrotoxicosis factitia is caused by the purposeful and secretive ingestion of thyroid hormone by disturbed patients (usually with a medical background) who wish to obtain attention or lose weight.

Thyrotoxicosis factitia should be suspected in a thyrotoxic patient without infiltrative ophthalmopathy or thyroid enlargement. The RAIU uptake is at low levels because the patient's thyroid gland function is suppressed by the exogenous thyroid hormone. Measurement of plasma thyroglobulin is a valuable laboratory aid in the diagnosis of thyrotoxicosis factitia. Thyroglobulin is normally secreted in small amounts by the thyroid gland; however, when thyroid hormone is taken orally, very low amounts of thyroglobulin are detectable in the plasma. In other entities characterized by a low RAIU, such as silent thyroiditis, leakage of preformed thyroid hormone results in elevated thyroglobulin levels. If a history of thyroid hormone ingestion is elicited or deduced, exogenous thyroid hormone should be withheld for between 4 and 6 weeks, and thyroid function tests should be repeated to document that the euthyroid state has been restored.[30]

Amiodarone may induce thyrotoxicosis (2% to 3% of patients) or hypothyroidism. Amiodarone contains 37.2% iodine by weight and approximately 6 mg/day of iodine is released for each 200 mg of amiodarone.[4,31] The recommended daily amount of iodine is 200 μg/day. Amiodarone interferes with type I 5′-deiodinase, leading to reduced conversion of T_4 to T_3, and iodide released from the drug owing to deiodination contributes to iodine excess, especially in iodine- deficient areas. Amiodarone also causes a destructive thyroiditis with loss of thyroglobulin and thyroid hormones. Iodine-induced thyroid dysfunction occurs primarily in patients with preexisting thyroid disease (Graves' disease, nodular goiter, Hashimoto's thyroiditis) known as type I, or in patients who have apparently normal thyroid glands (type II). The two types may be differentiated using color flow Doppler ultrasonography.[32] Type I amiodarone-induced hyperthyroidism responds well to thionamides, whereas type II may require glucocorticoids. An inflammatory process induced by amiodarone or iodine, which also leads to follicular cell damage and to subacute thyroiditis with leakage of thyroid hormones into the circulation, is associated with elevated interleukin-6 (IL-6) levels. The manifestations may be untypical symptoms such as ventricular tachycardia and exacerbation of underlying chronic obstructive pulmonary disease. Prednisone has been reported to normalize IL-6 and thyroid hormone values.[33] Iodinated glycerol improves some symptoms of chronic obstructive pulmonary disease but no objective measures of pulmonary function. This compound contains 15 mg of organic iodine per tablet or 25 mg/mL of solution. Thyroid dysfunction has been reported with this preparation, and patients with underlying thyroid disease need to be monitored carefully if iodinated glycerol is used.[34,35]

▶ TREATMENT: Hyperthyroidism

Three common treatment modalities are used in the management of hyperthyroidism: surgery, antithyroid medications, and RAI (Table 75–5). The overall therapeutic objectives are to eliminate the excess thyroid hormone and to minimize the symptoms and long-term consequences of hyperthyroidism. Therapy must be individualized based on the type and severity of hyperthyroidism, patient age and gender, existence of nonthyroidal conditions, and response to previous therapy.[13,36,37] Minimum clinical guidelines for the treatment of hyperthyroidism have been published by the American Thyroid Association.[38,39]

TABLE 75–5. Management of Hyperthyroidism

Modality	Maintenance Dose (mg/day)	Maximal Dose (mg/day)	Actions	Indications
Thiourea drugs			Inhibit thyroid synthesis (PTU also inhibits peripheral conversion of T_4 to T_3); may exert immunosuppressive actions	First-line therapy for Graves' hyperthyroidism; short-term therapy before ^{131}I or surgery
Propylthiouracil (PTH) 50-mg tablets	200–600	1200		
Methimazole (Tapazole) 5- and 10-mg tablets	10–60	120		
β-Adrenergic antagonists*			Ameliorate action of thyroid hormone in tissues	Adjunctive therapy; often therapy required for thyroiditis
Propranolol	80–160	480		
Nadolol	80–160	320		
Iodine-containing compounds			Inhibit T_4 and T_3 release	Preparation for surgery; thyrotoxic crisis
Lugol's solution	750	750		
Potassium iodide (SSKI)	10–300	400		
Miscellaneous				
Potassium perchlorate	NA	NA	Inhibits iodine transport	No routine indications
Lithium carbonate	NA	NA	Inhibits thyroid hormone synthesis and release	No routine indications
Glucocorticoids			Ameliorates actions of thyroid hormones in tissues; exerts immunosuppressive action (Graves' disease)	Severe subacute thyroiditis; thyrotoxic crisis
Radioactive Iodine (RAI, ^{131}I)	NA	2–10 mCi	Ablation of thyroid gland	First-line therapy for Graves' hyperthyroidism; treatment of choice for recurrent thyrotoxicosis; young adults to elderly; contraindicated in pregnancy, children, and active ophthalmopathy
Surgery	NA	NA	Removal of thyroid gland	Patients should be euthyroid prior to surgery; caution in elderly; cold iodine given prior to surgery

NA, not applicable; SSKI, saturated solution of potassium iodide.
*Not approved in the United States by the FDA for the treatment of thyrotoxicosis.

SURGERY

Surgical removal of the hypersecreting thyroid gland became feasible in 1923 when Plummer discovered that iodine reduced the gland's vascularity, making this definitive procedure possible. Traditional preparation of the patient for thyroidectomy includes propylthiouracil (PTU) or methimazole (MMI) until the patient is biochemically euthyroid (usually 6 to 8 weeks), followed by the addition of iodides (500 mg/day) for 10 to 14 days before surgery to decrease the vascularity of the gland. Levothyroxine may be added to maintain the euthyroid state while the thionamides are continued. Propranolol for several weeks preoperatively and 7 to 10 days after surgery has also been used to maintain a pulse rate of less than 90 beats/min. Combined pretreatment with propranolol and 10 to 14 days of potassium iodide also has been advocated.

The overall morbidity rate with surgery is 2.7%. Hyperthyroidism persists or recurs in 0.6% to 17.9% of patients after thyroidectomy for Graves' disease and is more common in children. The most common complications of surgery include hypothyroidism (up to about 49%), hypoparathyroidism (up to 3.9%), and vocal cord abnormalities (up to 5.4%). The frequent occurrence of hypothyroidism following surgery requires periodic followup for identification and treatment of these patients.[40–42]

PHARMACOLOGIC THERAPY

ANTITHYROID MEDICATIONS[43,44]

THIOUREA DRUGS

Two drugs within this category, PTU and MMI, are approved for the treatment of hyperthyroidism in the United States. They are classified as thioureylenes (thionamides), which incorporate a N—C—S = N group into their ring structures.

Mechanism of Action

PTU and MMI share several mechanisms to inhibit the biosynthesis of thyroid hormone.[43] First, these drugs serve as preferential substrates for the iodinating intermediate of thyroid peroxidase and divert iodine away from potential iodination sites in thyroglobulin. This prevents subsequent incorporation of iodine into iodotyrosines and, ultimately, into iodothyronine ("organification"). Second, they inhibit coupling of monoiodotyrosine and diiodotyrosine to form T_4 and T_3. The coupling reaction may be more sensitive to these drugs than the iodination reaction. Experimentally, these drugs exhibit immunosuppressive effects, although the clinical relevance of this finding is unclear. In patients with Graves' disease, antithyroid drug treatment has been associated with lower TSAb titers and restoration of normal suppressor T-cell function. However, perchlorate, which has a different mechanism of action, also decreases thyroid-stimulating antibodies, suggesting that normalization of the thyroid hormone level may itself improve the abnormal immune function. PTU inhibits the peripheral conversion of T_4 to T_3. This effect is acutely dose related and occurs within hours of PTU administration. MMI does not have this effect. Over time, depletion of stored hormone and lack of continuing synthesis of thyroid hormone results in the clinical effects of these drugs.

Pharmacokinetics

Both antithyroid drugs are well absorbed (80% to 95%) from the gastrointestinal tract, with peak serum concentrations about 1 hour after ingestion. The plasma half-life ranges of PTU and MMI are 1 to 2.5 hours and 6 to 9 hours, respectively, and are not appreciably affected by thyroid status. Urinary excretion is about 35% for PTU and less than 10% for MMI. These drugs are actively concentrated in the thyroid gland, which may account for the disparity between their relatively short plasma half-lives and the effectiveness of once-daily dosing regimens even with PTU. Approximately 60% to 80% of PTU is bound to plasma albumin, whereas MMI is not protein bound. Methimazole readily crosses the placenta and appears in breast milk. Older studies suggested that PTU crosses the placental membranes only one-tenth as well as MMI; however, these studies were done in the course of therapeutic abortion early in pregnancy. Newer studies show little difference between fetal concentrations of PTU and MMI and both are associated with elevated TSH in approximately 20% and low T_4 in approximately 7% of the fetuses.[45]

Dosing and Monitoring

PTU is available as 50-mg tablets and MMI as 5- and 10-mg tablets. MMI is approximately 10 times more potent than PTU. Initial therapy with PTU ranges from 300–600 mg daily, usually in three or four divided doses. MMI is given in three divided doses totaling 30–60 mg/day. Although the traditional recommendation is for divided doses, evidence exists that both drugs can be given as single daily doses.[38] Patients with severe hyperthyroidism may require larger initial doses, and some may respond better at these larger doses if the dose is divided. The maximal blocking doses of PTU and MMI are 1,200 and 120 mg daily, respectively. After the intrathyroidal pool of thyroid hormone is reduced and new hormone synthesis is sufficiently blocked, clinical improvement should ensue. Usually within 4 to 8 weeks of initiating therapy, symptoms are diminished and circulating thyroid hormone levels are returning to normal. At this time the tapering regimen can be started. Changes in dose for each drug should be made on a monthly basis, because the endogenously produced T_4 will reach a new "steady-state" concentration in this interval. Typical ranges of daily maintenance doses for PTU and MMI are 50–300 mg and 5–30 mg, respectively.

If the objective of therapy is to induce a long-term remission, the patient should remain on continuous antithyroid drug therapy for 12 to 24 months. Antithyroid drug therapy induces permanent remission rates of 10% to 98% with an overall average of about 40% to 50%.[46] This is much higher than the remission rate seen with propranolol alone, which is reported to range from 22% to 36%. Patient characteristics for a favorable outcome include patients older than 40 years of age; low ratio of T_4 to T_3 (<20); a small goiter (less than 50 g); short duration of disease (less than 6 months); no previous history of relapse with antithyroid drugs; duration of therapy 1 to 2 years or longer; and low TSAb titers at baseline or a reduction with treatment.[43] It is important that patients be followed every 6 to 12 months after remission occurs. If a relapse occurs, alternate therapy with RAI is preferred to a second course of antithyroid drugs. Relapses seem to plateau after about 5 years and eventually 5% to 20% of patients will develop spontaneous hypothyroidism.

Concurrent administration of thyroxine with thionamide therapy for thyrotoxicosis and subclinical hyperthyroidism may reduce autoantibodies directed toward the thyroid gland and improve the remission rate; however, these effects have not been consistently observed in all studies.[46,47] In a Japanese study, adjunctive treatment with thyroxine was associated with a 20-fold reduction in the recurrence rate of Graves' disease as compared to the recurrence rate seen in patients treated with antithyroid drugs alone. Attempts to reproduce these results in American and European patients with Graves' disease have failed to show any delay or reduction in the recurrence of Graves' disease with thyroxine administration.[48]

Adverse Effects

Minor adverse reactions to PTU and MMI have an overall incidence of 5% to 16% depending on the dose and the drug, whereas major adverse effects occur in 1.5% to 4.6% of patients receiving these drugs.[49,50] Pruritic maculopapular rashes (sometimes associated with vasculitis based on skin biopsy), arthralgias, and fevers occur in up to 5% of patients and may occur at greater frequency with higher doses and in children. Rashes often disappear spontaneously, but if persistent, may be managed with antihistamines.

Perhaps one of the most common side effects is a benign transient leukopenia characterized by a white blood cell (WBC) count of less than 4,000/mm.[3] This condition occurs in up to 12% of adults and 25% of children, and sometimes can be confused with mild leukopenia seen in Graves' disease. This mild leukopenia is not a harbinger of the more serious adverse effect of agranulocytosis, so therapy can usually be continued. If a *minor* adverse reaction occurs with one antithyroid drug, the alternate thiourea may be tried, but cross-sensitivity occurs in about 50% of patients.[43]

Agranulocytosis is the most serious adverse effect of thiourea drug therapy and is characterized by fever, malaise, gingivitis, oropharyngeal infection, and a granulocyte count less than 250/mm.[43] These drugs are concentrated in granulocytes and this reaction may represent a direct toxic effect rather than hypersensitivity. This toxic reaction has occurred with both thioureas, and the incidence varies from 0.5% to 6%. It is higher in patients older than 40 years of age who are receiving a methimazole dose greater than 40 mg/day or the equivalent dose of PTU, and is linked to HLA class II genes containing the DRB1*08032 allele.[51] Agranulocytosis almost always develops in the first 3 months of therapy. Because the onset is sudden, routine monitoring is not recommended. Colony-stimulating factors have been used with some success to restore cell counts to normal but it is unclear how effective this form of therapy is to routine supportive care.[52,53] Peripheral lymphocytes obtained from patients with PTU-induced agranulocytosis undergo transformation in the presence of other thioamides, suggesting that these severe reactions are immunologically mediated and patients should not receive other thionamides. Aplastic anemia has been reported with MMI and may be associated with an inhibitor to colony-forming units. Once antithyroid drugs are discontinued, clinical improvement is seen over several days to weeks. Patients should be counseled to discontinue therapy and contact their physician when flu-like symptoms such as fever, malaise, or sore throat develop.

Arthralgias and a lupus-like syndrome (sometimes in the absence of antinuclear antibodies) has been reported in 4% to 5% of patients. This generally occurs after 6 months of therapy. Uncommonly, polymyositis, presenting as proximal muscle weakness and elevated creatine phosphokinase, has been reported with PTU administration. Gastrointestinal intolerance is also reported to occur in 4% to 5% of patients. Hepatotoxicity, which usually occurs within the first 3 months of therapy, may be seen with both methimazole and PTU with a prevalence of about 1.3%.[50,54] In mice, MMI undergoes epoxidation of the C-4,5 double bond by P450 enzymes and, after being hydrolyzed, the resulting epoxide is decomposed to form *N*-methylthiourea, a proximate toxicant.[55] At moderate doses, some authors have found that initial enzyme elevations eventually normalize in most patients with continued therapy.[56] High doses of PTU are more likely to produce severe hepatitis and even death. Discontinuation of therapy usually results in complete resolution of hepatitis. Patients receiving interferon products for hepatitis C or other disorders may develop hyper- or hypothyroidism along with liver enzyme abnormalities.[57] Although older reports suggested that congenital skin defects (aplasia cutis) may be caused by methimazole and carbimazole, a recent registry review from the Netherlands could not find an association between maternal use of these drugs and skin defects.[58] Hypoprothrombinemia is a rare complication of thionamide therapy. Patients who have experienced a *major* adverse reaction to one thiourea drug should not be converted to the alternate drug because of cross-sensitivity.

IODIDES

Iodide was the first form of drug therapy for Graves' disease. Its mechanism of action is to acutely block thyroid hormone release, inhibit thyroid hormone biosynthesis by interfering with intrathyroidal iodide utilization (the Wolff-Chaikoff effect), and decrease the size and vascularity of the gland. This early inhibitory effect provides symptom improvement within 2 to 7 days of initiating therapy, and serum T_4 and T_3 concentrations may be reduced for a few weeks. Despite the reduced release of T_4 and T_3, thyroid hormone synthesis continues at an accelerated rate, resulting in a gland rich in stored hormones. The normal and hyperfunctioning thyroid soon escapes from this inhibitory effect within 1 to 2 weeks by decreasing the active transfer of iodide into the gland. Iodides are often used as adjunctive therapy to prepare a patient with Graves' disease for surgery, to acutely inhibit thyroid hormone release and quickly attain the euthyroid state in severely thyrotoxic patients with cardiac decompensation,[36] or to inhibit thyroid hormone release following radioactive iodine therapy. However, large doses of iodine may exacerbate hyperthyroidism or indeed precipitate hyperthyroidism in some previously euthyroid individuals (Jod-Basedow disease). This Jod-Basedow phenomenon is most common in iodine-deficient areas, particularly in patients with preexisting nontoxic goiter. Iodide is contraindicated in toxic multinodular goiter.

Potassium iodide is available either as a saturated solution (SSKI), which contains 38 mg of iodide per drop, or as Lugol's solution, which contains 6.3 mg of iodide per drop. The typical starting dose of SSKI is 3 to 10 drops daily (120–400 mg) in water or juice. There is no documented advantage to using doses in excess of 6–8 mg/day. When used to prepare a patient for surgery, it should be administered 7 to 14 days preoperatively. As an adjunct to RAI, SSKI should not be used before, but rather 3 to 7 days after RAI treatment so that the radioactive iodide can concentrate in the thyroid. The most frequent toxic effect with iodide therapy is hypersensitivity reactions (skin rashes, drug fever, rhinitis, conjunctivitis); salivary gland swelling; "iodism" (metallic taste, burning mouth and throat, sore teeth and gums, symptoms of a head cold, and sometimes stomach upset and diarrhea); and gynecomastia.

Other compounds containing organic iodide have also been used therapeutically for hyperthyroidism. These include various radiologic contrast media that share a triiodo- and monoaminobenzene ring with a propionic acid chain (e.g., iopanoic acid and sodium ipodate). The effect of these compounds is a result of the iodine content inhibiting thyroid hormone release, as well as competitive inhibition of 5′-monodeiodinase conversion related to their structures, which resemble thyroid analogs.[4]

ADRENERGIC BLOCKERS

Because many of the manifestations of hyperthyroidism are mediated by β-adrenergic receptors, β-blockers (especially propranolol) have been used widely to ameliorate thyrotoxic symptoms such as palpitations, anxiety, tremor, and heat intolerance. Although β-blockers are quite effective for symptom control, they have no effect on the urinary excretion of calcium, phosphorus, hydroxyproline, creatinine, or various amino acids, suggesting a lack of effect on peripheral thyrotoxicosis and protein metabolism. Furthermore, β-blockers neither reduce TSAb nor prevent thyroid storm. Propranolol and nadolol partially block the conversion of T_4 to T_3 but this contribution to the overall therapeutic effect is small in magnitude. Inhibition of conversion of T_4 to T_3 is mediated by D-propranolol, which is devoid of β-blocking activity, and L-propranolol, which is responsible for the antiadrenergic effects, has little effect on the conversion.

β-Blockers are usually used as adjunctive therapy with antithyroid drugs, RAI, or iodides when treating Graves' disease or toxic nodules; in preparation for surgery; or in thyroid storm. The only conditions for which β-blockers are primary therapy for thyrotoxicosis are thyroiditis and iodine-induced hyperthyroidism. The dose of propranolol required to relieve adrenergic symptoms is variable, but an initial dose of 20–40 mg four times daily is effective (heart rate less than 90 beats/min) for most patients. Younger or more severely toxic patients may require as much as 240–480 mg/day because there seems to be an increased clearance rate in these patients. β-Blockers are contraindicated in patients with congestive heart failure unless it is caused solely by tachycardia (high output) and in patients who have developed cardiomyopathy and heart failure. Nonselective agents and those lacking intrinsic sympathomimetic activity should be used with caution in patients with asthma, chronic obstructive lung disease, and diabetes mellitus (particularly insulin-dependent diabetes). Cardioselective and intrinsic sympathomimetic activity β-blockers may have a slight margin of safety in these situations. Other patients in whom contraindications exist are those with sinus bradycardia, those receiving monoamine oxidase inhibitors or tricyclic antidepressants, and those with spontaneous hypoglycemia. β-Blockers may also prolong gestation and labor during pregnancy. Other side effects include nausea, vomiting, anxiety, insomnia, light-headedness, bradycardia, and hematologic disturbances.

Antiadrenergic agents, such as centrally acting sympatholytics and calcium-channel antagonists, may have some role in the symptomatic treatment of hyperthyroidism. These drugs might be useful when contraindications to β-blockade exist. When compared to nadolol 40 mg twice daily, clonidine 150 μg twice daily reduced plasma catecholamines, whereas nadolol increased both epinephrine and norepinephrine after 1 week of treatment. Diltiazem 120 mg given every 8 hours reduced heart rate by 17%; fewer ventricular extrasystoles were noted after 10 days of therapy, and diltiazem has been shown to be comparable to propranolol in lowering heart rate and blood pressure.

RADIOACTIVE IODINE[19,59]

Although other radioisotopes have been used to ablate thyroid tissue, sodium iodide 131 (^{131}I) is considered to be the agent of choice for Graves' disease, toxic autonomous nodules, and toxic multinodular goiters. RAI is administered as a colorless and tasteless liquid that is well absorbed and concentrates in the thyroid. Sodium iodide 131 is a β-emitter with a tissue penetration of 2 mm and a half-life of 8 days. Other organs take up ^{131}I but the thyroid gland is the only organ in which organification of the absorbed iodine takes place. Initially, RAI disrupts hormone synthesis by incorporating into thyroid hormones and thyroglobulin. Over a period of weeks, follicles that have taken up RAI and surrounding follicles develop evidence of cellular necrosis, breakdown of follicles, development of bizarre cell forms, nuclear pyknosis, and destruction of small vessels within the gland, leading to edema and fibrosis of the interstitial tissue. Pregnancy is an absolute contraindication to the use of RAI.

β-Blockers may be given anytime without compromising RAI therapy, accounting for their role as a mainstay of adjunctive therapy to RAI treatment. If iodides are administered, they should be given 3 to 7 days *after* RAI to prevent interference with the uptake of RAI in the thyroid gland. Because thyroid hormone levels will transiently increase following RAI treatment owing to release of preformed thyroid hormone, patients with cardiac disease and elderly patients are often treated with thionamides prior to RAI ablation. Occasionally, in patients with underlying cardiac disease, it may be necessary to reinstitute antithyroid drug therapy following radioactive iodine ablation. The standard practice is to withdraw the thionamide 4 days prior to RAI treatment and to reinstitute it 4 days after therapy is concluded. Administering antithyroid drug therapy following RAI treatment may result in a higher rate of posttreatment recurrence or persistent hyperthyroidism.[59]

Corticosteroid administration will blunt and delay the rise in antibodies to the TSH receptor, thyroglobulin, and thyroid peroxidase while reducing T_3 and T_4 concentrations following RAI. Bartalena et al. found no progression in ophthalmopathy in patients receiving prednisone after RAI compared with methimazole (2% to 3% worsened) or no other treatment (5% with persistent worsening).[47,60] Theoretically, if shared thyroidal and orbital antigen is involved in the pathogenesis of Graves' ophthalmopathy, antigen released with RAI treatment could aggravate preexisting eye disease. Note also that thyroid ablation may decrease eye disease in the long-term by removing the source of antigen, but it is unclear whether RAI differs from surgery or thionamide for the risk of worsening eye disease.[61]

Destruction of the gland attenuates the hyperthyroid state, and hypothyroidism commonly occurs months to years following RAI. The goal of therapy is to destroy overactive thyroid cells, and a single dose of 4,000–8,000 rads results in a euthyroid state in 60% of patients at 6 months or less. The remaining 40% become euthyroid within 1 year, requiring two or more doses. It is advisable that a second dose of RAI be given 6 months after the first RAI treatment if the patient remains hyperthyroid. Variables that influence the outcome of RAI include gender (men are less likely to develop hypothyroidism), race (blacks are more resistant to ^{131}I), the size of the thyroid, severity of disease, and, perhaps, the level of TSAb. The acute, short-term side effects of ^{131}I therapy are minimal and include mild thyroidal tenderness and dysphagia. Concern over the development of thyroid carcinoma and leukemia and increased risk of mutations and congenital defects now appears to be unfounded because long-term followup studies have not revealed increased risk for these complications.[43,62] Although RAI is very effective in the treatment of hyperthyroidism, long-term followup from Great Britain suggests that among patients with hyperthyroidism treated with RAI, mortality from all causes and mortality resulting from cardiovascular and cerebrovascular disease and fracture are increased.[63]

A common approach to Graves' hyperthyroidism is to administer a single dose of 5–15 mCi (80–120 μCi/g of tissue).[43,59] Thyroid glands estimated to >80 g may require larger doses of RAI. Larger doses are likely to induce hypothyroidism and are seldom given outside the United States owing to the imposition of stringent safety restrictions. For example, in the United Kingdom, a nursery school teacher is advised to stay out of school for 3 weeks following a 15-mCi dose of ^{131}I.[64]

EVALUATION OF THERAPEUTIC OUTCOMES: HYPERTHYROIDISM

After therapy (surgery, thionamides, or RAI) for hyperthyroidism has been initiated, patients should be evaluated on a monthly basis until they reach an euthyroid condition. Clinical signs of continuing thyrotoxicosis (e.g., tachycardia, weight loss, heat intolerance) or the development of hypothyroidism (e.g., bradycardia, weight gain, lethargy) should be noted. β-Blockers may be used to control symptoms of thyrotoxicosis until the definitive treatment has returned the patient to a euthyroid state. After thyroxine replacement is initiated, the goal is to maintain both the free thyroxine level and the TSH concentration in the "normal range." After a stable dose of thyroxine is identified, the patient may be followed up every 6 to 12 months.

Finally, a common, potentially confusing clinical situation should be mentioned. Why are the TSH concentrations suppressed in some patients who are clinically hypothyroid and who have a low free T_4 level? In patients with long-standing hyperthyroidism, the pituitary thyrotrophs responsible for making TSH become atrophic. The average amount of time required for these cells to resume normal functioning is 6 to 8 weeks.[65] Therefore, if a thyrotoxic patient has his/her free T_4 concentration lowered rapidly, before the thyrotrophs resume normal function, a period of "transient central hypothyroidism" will be observed.

SPECIAL CONDITIONS

GRAVES' DISEASE AND PREGNANCY[66–68]

Inappropriate production of human chorionic gonadotropin (hCG) is a cause of abnormal thyroid function tests during the first half of pregnancy, and hCG can cause either subclinical (normal T_4, suppressed TSH) or overt hyperthyroidism. This is owing to the homology of hCG and TSH, as well as their receptors. Hyperthyroidism during pregnancy is almost solely caused by Graves' disease, with approximately 0.1% to 0.4% of pregnancies affected. Although the increased metabolic rate is usually well tolerated in pregnant women, two symptoms suggestive of hyperthyroidism during pregnancy are failure to gain weight despite good appetite and persistent tachycardia. There is no increase in maternal mortality or morbidity in well-controlled patients; however, postpartum thyroid storm has been reported in about

20% of untreated individuals. Fetal loss is also more common, owing to spontaneous abortion and premature delivery in untreated pregnant women. Transplacental passage of thyroid-stimulating antibodies may occur, causing fetal as well as neonatal hyperthyroidism.[69] An uncommon cause of hyperthyroidism is molar pregnancy; women present with a large for date uterus and evacuation of the uterus is the preferred management approach.[70–74]

Because RAI is contraindicated in pregnancy and surgery is usually not recommended (especially during the first trimester), antithyroid drug therapy is usually the treatment of choice. Methimazole readily crosses the placenta and appears in breast milk.

PTU is considered to be the drug of choice in pregnancy with the lowest possible doses used to maintain the maternal T_4 level in the high-normal range; however, as described earlier, there appears to be little difference between PTU and methimazole.[45] To prevent fetal goiter and suppression of fetal thyroid function, PTU is usually prescribed in daily doses of 300 mg or less and tapered to 50–150 mg daily after 4 to 6 weeks. PTU doses of less than 200 mg daily are unlikely to produce fetal goiter.[75] During the last trimester, TSAbs fall spontaneously, and some patients will go into remission so that antithyroid drug doses may be reduced. A rebound in maternal hyperthyroidism occurs in about 10% of women and may require more intensive treatment postpartum than in the last trimester of pregnancy.[69]

NEONATAL AND PEDIATRIC HYPERTHYROIDISM[76,77]

Following delivery, some babies will be hyperthyroid owing to placental transfer of TSAbs, which stimulates thyroid hormone production *in utero* and postpartum. This is likely if the maternal TSAb titers were quite high. The disease is usually expressed 7 to 10 days postpartum and treatment with antithyroid drugs (PTU 5–10 mg/kg/day or methimazole 0.5–1 mg/kg/day) may be needed for as long as 8 to 12 weeks until the antibody is cleared (IgG half-life is about 2 weeks). Iodide (potassium iodide 1 drop/d or Lugol's solution 1–3 drops/day) and sodium ipodate may be used for the first few days to acutely inhibit hormone release.

Childhood hyperthyroidism is usually managed with either PTU or methimazole. Long-term followup studies suggest that this form of therapy is quite acceptable, with 25% of a cohort experiencing remission every 2 years.[78]

THYROID STORM[79,80]

Thyroid storm is a life-threatening medical emergency characterized by severe thyrotoxicosis, high fever (often greater than 103°F/39.4°C), tachycardia, tachypnea, dehydration, delirium, coma, nausea, vomiting, and diarrhea. Precipitating factors for thyroid storm include infection, trauma, surgery, RAI treatment, and withdrawal from antithyroid drugs. It may occur at any age and has an average duration of 72 hours, although symptoms may persist up to 8 days if treatment is not aggressive. With aggressive treatment, the mortality rate has been lowered to 20%. The following therapeutic measures should be instituted promptly: (a) suppression of thyroid hormone formation and secretion; (b) antiadrenergic therapy; (c) administration of corticosteroids; and (d) treatment of associated complications or coexisting factors that may have precipitated the storm. Table 75–6 outlines the specific agents used in thyroid storm. PTU in large doses is the preferred thionamide because it interferes with the production of thyroid hormones and blocks the peripheral conversion of T_4 to T_3. If patients are unable to take medications orally, the tablets can be crushed into suspension and instilled by gastric tube. Iodides, which rapidly block the release of preformed thyroid hormone, should be administrated

TABLE 75–6. Drug Dosages Used in the Management of Thyroid Storm

Drug	Regimen
Propythiouracil	900–1,200 mg/day po in four or six divided doses
Methimazole	90–120 mg/day po in four or six divided doses
Sodium iodide	Up to 2 g/day IV in single or divided doses
Lugol's solution	5–10 drops tid in water or juice
Saturated solution of potassium iodide	1–2 drops tid in water or juice
Propranolol	40–80 mg every 6 h
Dexamethasone	5–20 mg/day po or IV in divided doses
Prednisone	25–100 mg/day po in divided doses
Methylprednisolone	20–80 mg/day IV in divided doses
Hydrocortisone	100–400 mg/day IV in divided doses

after PTU is initiated to inhibit iodide use by the overactive gland. If iodide is administered first, it could theoretically provide the substrate permitting the synthesis and storage of a large amount of thyroid hormone in the thyroid gland, which would prolong the duration of hyperthyroidism thereafter.

Antiadrenergic therapy with the short-acting agent esmolol may be used in the patient with pulmonary disease or at risk for cardiac failure because its effects may be rapidly reversed.[81] Corticosteroids are generally recommended, although there is no convincing evidence of adrenocortical insufficiency in thyroid storm, and the benefits derived from steroids may be owing to their antipyretic action and their effect of stabilizing blood pressure.[82] General supportive measures, including acetaminophen as an antipyretic (do not use aspirin or other nonsteroidal anti-inflammatory agents because they may displace bound thyroid hormone), fluid and electrolyte replacement, sedatives, digitalis, antiarrhythmics, insulin, and antibiotics, should be given as indicated. Plasmapheresis and peritoneal dialysis have been used to remove excess hormone when the patient has not responded to more conservative measures, although these measures do not always work.[83]

HYPOTHYROIDISM[63]

Hypothyroidism is defined as the clinical and biochemical syndrome resulting from decreased thyroid hormone production. Overt hypothyroidism occurs in 1.5% to 2% of women, and in 0.2% of men, and its incidence increases with age.[84–86] The vast majority of hypothyroid patients have thyroid gland failure (primary hypothyroidism). Pituitary failure is an uncommon cause of hypothyroidism but should be suspected in a patient with decreased levels of thyroxine and inappropriately normal or low TSH levels. Most patients with secondary hypothyroidism will have clinical signs of more generalized pituitary insufficiency such as abnormal menses and decreased libido, or evidence of a pituitary adenoma such as visual-field defects, galactorrhea, or acromegaloid features. Generalized (peripheral and central) resistance to thyroid hormone is extremely rare.

Thyroid hormone is essential for normal growth and development during embryonic life. Thyroid hormone deficiency during fetal and neonatal development results in mental retardation. In the child, thyroid hormone deficiency may manifest as growth retardation. In the adult, manifestations of hypothyroidism are varied and nonspecific. There is slowing of physical and mental activity as well as of cardiovascular, gastrointestinal, and neuromuscular function. Common symptoms of hypothyroidism include dry skin, cold intolerance, weight gain, constipation, and weakness. Complaints of lethargy and fatigue or loss of ambition and energy are also common but are less specific. Depression may result from untreated hypothyroidism.[87]

The most common signs of decreased levels of thyroid hormone include coarse skin and hair, cold or dry skin, periorbital puffiness, and bradycardia. Speech is often slow as well as hoarse. Reversible neurologic syndromes such as carpal tunnel syndrome, polyneuropathy, and cerebellar dysfunction may also occur. Muscle cramps, myalgia, and stiffness are frequent complaints of hypothyroid patients. Objective weakness is common, with proximal muscles being affected more than distal muscles. Slow relaxation of deep-tendon reflexes is common.

A rise in the TSH level is the first evidence of primary hypothyroidism. Many patients will have a T_4 level within the normal range (compensated hypothyroidism) and few, if any, symptoms of hypothyroidism. As the disease progresses the T_4 concentration will drop below the normal level. Interestingly, the T_3 concentration will often be maintained in the normal range in spite of a low T_4. The RAIU is not a useful test in the evaluation of a hypothyroid patient.

CAUSES OF HYPOTHYROIDISM

Table 75–7 outlines the causes of hypothyroidism.

CHRONIC AUTOIMMUNE THYROIDITIS

Autoimmune thyroiditis (Hashimoto's disease) is the most common cause of spontaneous hypothyroidism in the adult. Patients may present with either goitrous thyroid gland enlargement and mild hypothyroidism or with thyroid gland atrophy and more severe thyroid hormone deficiency. Both forms of autoimmune thyroiditis probably result from cell- and antibody-mediated thyroid injury. The bulk of evidence suggests that the presence of specific defects in suppressor T-lymphocyte function leads to the survival of a randomly mutating clone of helper T lymphocytes, which are directed against normally occurring antigens on the thyroid membrane. Once these T lymphocytes interact with thyroid membrane antigen, B lymphocytes are stimulated to produce thyroid antibodies.[88,89]

Antimicrosomal antibodies are present in virtually all patients with Hashimoto's thyroiditis and appear to be directed against the enzyme thyroid peroxidase, thyroglobulin, and other thyroid cell-membrane antigens. These antibodies are capable of fixing complement and inducing cytotoxic changes in thyroid cells. Antibodies that are capable of stimulating thyroid growth are also present in the goitrous variety of Hashimoto's disease; conversely, antibodies that inhibit the trophic effects of TSH are present in the atrophic type.[90]

TABLE 75–7. Causes of Hypothyroidism

Primary hypothyroidism
Hashimoto's disease
Iatrogenic hypothyroidism
Others
  Iodine deficiency
  Enzyme defects
  Thyroid hypoplasia
  Goitrogens
Secondary hypothyroidism
Pituitary disease
Hypothalamic disease

IATROGENIC HYPOTHYROIDISM

Iatrogenic hypothyroidism follows exposure to radiation (radioiodine or external radiation) or surgery. Hypothyroidism occurs within 3 months to a year after ^{131}I therapy in most patients treated for Graves' disease. Thereafter, it occurs at a rate of approximately 2.5% each year. External radiation therapy to the region of the thyroid using doses of greater than 2,500 rads for therapy of neck carcinoma also causes hypothyroidism. This effect is dose dependent, with more than 50% of patients developing hypothyroidism who have received more than 4,000 rads to the thyroid bed. Total thyroidectomy causes hypothyroidism within 1 month.

OTHER CAUSES OF PRIMARY HYPOTHYROIDISM

Iodine deficiency, enzymatic defects within the thyroid gland, thyroid hypoplasia, and maternal ingestion of goitrogens during fetal development may cause cretinism. Early recognition and treatment of the resultant thyroid hormone deficiency is essential for optimal mental development. Large-scale screening programs in North America, Europe, Japan, and Australia are now in place. The frequency of congenital hypothyroidism in North America and Europe is 1 per 3,500 to 4,000 live births. In the United States, there are racial differences in the incidence of congenital hypothyroidism, with whites being affected seven times as frequently as blacks.[91–94]

In the adult, iodine deficiency and goitrogens rarely cause hypothyroidism. Rarely, iodine ingestion in the form of expectorants can lead to hypothyroidism. In sensitive persons, the iodide blocks the synthesis of thyroid hormone, leading to an increased secretion of TSH, which causes thyroid enlargement.[43] Thus, both iodine excess and iodine deficiency can cause decreased secretion of thyroid hormone.

CAUSES OF SECONDARY HYPOTHYROIDISM

Pituitary Disease

TSH is required for normal thyroid secretion. Thyroid atrophy and decreased thyroid secretion follow pituitary failure. Pituitary insufficiency may be caused by destruction of thyrotrophs by either functioning or nonfunctioning pituitary tumors, surgical therapy, external pituitary radiation, postpartum pituitary necrosis (Sheehan's syndrome), infiltrative processes of the pituitary such as metastatic tumors, tuberculosis, histiocytosis, and autoimmune mechanisms. In all these situations, TSH deficiency most often occurs in association with other pituitary hormone deficiencies.

In most hypothyroid patients with pituitary disease, serum TSH concentrations are low or normal. A serum TSH concentration in the normal range is clearly inappropriate if the patient's T_4 is low.

Note that pituitary enlargement in hypothyroidism does not invariably indicate the presence of a primary pituitary tumor. Pituitary enlargement is seen in patients with severe primary hypothyroidism owing to compensatory hyperplasia and hypertrophy of the thyrotrophs. Serum TSH concentrations and pituitary enlargement decline during thyroid hormone replacement therapy, indicating that the TSH secretion is not autonomous. These patients are easily separated from patients with primary pituitary failure by measuring a TSH.

Hypothalamic Hypothyroidism

TRH deficiency also causes hypothyroidism. In both adults and children it may occur as a result of cranial irradiation, trauma, infiltrative diseases, or neoplastic diseases. Hypothalamic hypothyroidism is rare.

▶ TREATMENT: Hypothyroidism

PHARMACOLOGIC THERAPY

The goals of therapy are to restore normal thyroid hormone concentrations in tissue, provide symptomatic relief, prevent neurologic deficits in newborns and children, and reverse the biochemical abnormalities of hypothyroidism. Any of the commercially available thyroid preparations accomplish this goal (Table 75–8); however, levothyroxine (L-thyroxine) is considered to be the drug of choice. The thyroid preparations are either natural (i.e., desiccated thyroid, thyroglobulin) or synthetic (levothyroxine, liothyronine, liotrix) in origin. The availability of sensitive and specific assays for total and free hormone levels as well as TSH now allow more definitive dose titration to allow adequate replacement without inadvertent overdose. The response of TSH to TRH had been advocated by some for "fine-tuning" thyroid replacement, but this is not necessary if the sensitive immunoradiometric assays (IRMA) for TSH are used. The American Thyroid Association has published minimum clinical guidelines for the treatment of hypothyroidism.[39]

NATURAL THYROID HORMONES

Desiccated thyroid is derived from hog, beef, or sheep thyroid gland. The *United States Pharmacopeia,* 23rd edition, requires Thyroid USP to contain 38 μg (± 15%) of levothyroxine and 9 μg (± 10%) of liothyronine for each 65 mg (1 grain) of the labeled content of thyroglobulin. Thyroglobulin USP should contain 36 μg (± 15%) of levothyroxine and 12 μg (± 10%) of liothyronine for each 65 mg (1 grain) of the labeled content of thyroglobulin. Not all generic brands may be bioequivalent, and switching among brands in patients stabilized on one product should be discouraged. Thyroid USP, as an animal protein-derived product, may be antigenic in allergic or sensitive patients. Even though desiccated thyroid is inexpensive, its limitations preclude it from being considered as a drug of choice for hypothyroid patients. Thyroglobulin is a purified hog-gland extract but it has no clinical advantages and is not widely used.

SYNTHETIC THYROID HORMONES

Levothyroxine (T_4, L-thyroxine) is the drug of choice for thyroid replacement and suppressive therapy because it is chemically stable, relatively inexpensive, and free of antigenicity and has uniform potency. Because T_3 and not T_4 is the biologically more active form of thyroid hormone, levothyroxine administration results in a pool of thyroid hormone that is readily and consistently converted to T_3; in this regard levothyroxine may be thought of as a prohormone. The half-life of levothyroxine is approximately 7 days. This long half-life is responsible for a stable pool of prohormone and the need for only once-daily dosing with levothyroxine. Older studies with levothyroxine suggested that bioavailability was low and erratic; however, this product has been reformulated and the average bioavailability is now approximately 80%.[95–97] The bioavailability of Synthroid, Levoxine, and generic levothyroxine preparations were compared in a blinded, randomized, four-way crossover trial.[98] The study was sponsored by the manufacturers of Synthroid, who challenged the author's conclusions that the levothyroxine preparations are bioequivalent and should be interchangeable for the majority of patients. The time to maximal absorption is 2 hours, and this should be considered when T_4 and TSH concentrations are determined. Mucosal diseases such as sprue, diabetic diarrhea, and ileal bypass surgery may also reduce absorption. Cholestyramine, calcium carbonate, sucralfate, aluminum hydroxide,[99] ferrous sulfate,[100] soybean formula,[101] and dietary fiber supplements[102] may also impair the absorption of levothyroxine from the gastrointestinal tract. Drugs that increase

TABLE 75–8. Thyroid Preparations Used in the Treatment of Hypothyroidism

Drug/Dosage Form	Content	Relative Dose	Comments/Equivalency
Thyroid USP Armour Thyroid (T_4:T_3 ratio) 9.5 μg:2.25 μg, 19 μg:4.5 μg, 38 μg:9 μg, 57 μg:13.5 μg, 76 μg:18 μg, 114 μg:27 μg, 152 μg:36 μg, 190 μg:45 μg tablets	Desiccated beef or pork thyroid gland	1 grain (equivalent to 60 μg of T_4)	Unpredictable hormonal stability, inexpensive generic brands may not be bioequivalent
Thyroglobulin Proloid 32-mg, 65-mg, 100-mg, 130-mg, 200-mg tablets	Partially purified pork thyroglobulin	1 grain	Standardized biologically to give T_4:T_3 ratio of 2.5:1; more expensive than thyroid extract; no clinical advantage
Levothyroxine Synthroid, Levothroid and other generics 25-, 50-, 75-, 88-, 100-, 112-, 125-, 137-, 150-, 175-, 200-, 300-μg tablets; 200- and 500-μg/vial injection	Synthetic T_4	50–60 μg	Stable; predictable potency; generics are bioequivalent; when switching from natural thyroid to L-thyroxine, lower dose by 1/2 grain; variable absorption between products; $t_{1/2}$ = 7 d, so daily dosing; considered to be drug of choice
Liothyronine Cytomel 5-, 25-, and 50-μg tablets	Synthetic T_3	15–37.5 μg	Uniform absorption, rapid onset; $t_{1/2}$ = 1.5 d, monitor TSH assays
Liotrix Euthyroid, Thyrolar 1/4-, 1/2, 1-, 2-, and 3-strength tablets	Synthetic T_4:T_3 in 4:1 ratio	50–60 μg T_4 and 12.5–15 μg T_3	Stable; predictable; expensive; lacks therapeutic rationale because T_4 is converted to T_3 peripherally

nondeiodinative T_4 clearance include rifampin, carbamazepine, and possibly phenytoin. Selenium deficiency and amiodarone may block the conversion of T_4 to T_3.

Liothyronine (T_3) is chemically pure with known potency and has a shorter half-life of 1.5 days. Although it is widely used diagnostically in the T_3-suppression test, T_3 has some clinical disadvantages including a higher incidence of cardiac adverse effects, higher cost, and difficulty in monitoring with conventional laboratory tests. Liotrix is a combination of synthetic T_4 and T_3 in 4:1 ratio that attempts to mimic the natural hormonal secretion. It is chemically stable and pure and has a predictable potency. The major limitations to this product are high cost and lack of therapeutic rationale, because about 35% of T_4 is peripherally converted T_3.

Recently, a trial comparing levothyroxine alone to a combination of levothyroxine plus partial replacement with liothyronine (triiodothyronine) was published.[103] Patients received a regimen in which 50 μg of the usual dose of thyroxine was replaced by 12.5 μg of triiodothyronine. The order in which each patient received the two treatments was randomized. Biochemical, physiologic, and psychological tests were performed at the end of each treatment period. Although lower serum free and total thyroxine concentrations and higher serum total triiodothyronine concentrations after treatment with thyroxine plus triiodothyronine were noted, the TSH concentrations were not significantly different. Cognitive function was higher on some rating scales but neurophysiologic test scores were similar.

Dosing and Monitoring

During the mid-1980s the average dose of levothyroxine was about 160 μg/day. With the advent of more sensitive assay methods for TSH and the reformulation of levothyroxine, it is now apparent that many patients have been treated with excessive amounts of levothyroxine. More recent studies suggest that the average maintenance dose for most adults should be closer to about 110–120 μg/day. Indeed, as many as one-third of patients receiving levothyroxine 150 μg daily will be overreplaced. There is, however, a wide range of replacement doses, necessitating individualized therapy and appropriate monitoring to determine an adequate but not excessive dose.

The initial dose of levothyroxine is dependent on the patient's age, the presence of associated disorders, as well as the severity and duration of hypothyroidism.[104] In young patients with long-standing disease and in patients older than 45 years of age without known cardiac disease, therapy should be initiated with 50 μg daily of levothyroxine and increased to 100 μg daily after 1 month. The recommended initial daily dose for older patients or those with known cardiac disease is 25 μg/day titrated upward in increments of 25 μg at monthly intervals to prevent stress on the cardiovascular system. Some patients may experience an exacerbation of angina with higher doses of thyroid hormone. Although the TSH is very sensitive for under- or overreplacement, clinicians often fail to alter the dose of T_4 based on TSH clearly outside of the normal range.[105]

Patients with subclinical hypothyroidism (seen more commonly in the elderly, particularly in women) have no or few signs or symptoms, normal serum T_3 and T_4 concentrations, and an elevated basal TSH concentration.[86] The prevalence of this disorder is thought to be about 8%, but the reported range is quite wide.[106,107] Although the treatment of subclinical hypothyroidism is controversial, patients presenting with marked elevations in TSH (>10 mU/L) and high titers of TSAb or prior treatment with ^{131}I may be most likely to benefit from treatment.[108] Other patients who may improve with replacement include those with mild symptoms of hypothyroidism and depression. It should be noted that some studies find that only one of four treated patients experienced improvement.[107] Conservative treatment goals in this situation would be to maintain serum T_4 and T_3 levels in the normal range and reduce TSH to a value of 1.0 mU/L.

Once euthyroidism is attained, the daily maintenance dose of levothyroxine does not fluctuate greatly. As patients age, the dosing requirement may need to be reduced.[109] The ability to measure serum TSH concentrations has improved the accuracy with which thyroid hormone replacement can be monitored. Many clinicians now consider serum TSH concentration to be the most sensitive and specific monitoring parameter for adjustment of levothyroxine dose. Plasma TSH concentrations begin to fall within hours and are usually normalized within 2 weeks, but may take up to 6 weeks in some patients, depending on the baseline value. TSH and T_4 concentrations are both used to monitor therapy, and they should be checked every 6 weeks until an euthyroid state is achieved. Serum T_4 concentrations can be useful in detecting noncompliance, malabsorption, or changes in levothyroxine product bioequivalence. An elevated TSH concentration indicates insufficient replacement. The appropriate dose maintains the TSH concentration in the normal range.

In patients with hypothyroidism caused by hypothalamic or pituitary failure, alleviation of the clinical syndrome and restoration of serum T_4 to the normal range are the only criteria available for estimating the appropriate replacement dose of levothyroxine. Concurrent use of dopamine, dopaminergic agents (bromocriptine), somatostatin or somatostatin analogs (octreotide), and corticosteroids suppresses TSH concentrations and may confound the interpretation of this monitoring parameter.[110]

Thyroid-stimulating hormone suppressive levothyroxine therapy may also be given to patients with nodular thyroid disease and diffuse goiter, to patients with a history of thyroid irradiation, and to patients with thyroid cancer. The rationale for suppression therapy is to reduce TSH secretion, which promotes growth and function in abnormal thyroid tissue. In patients with solitary nodules who have not received radiation, TSH should be suppressed to 0.05–0.1 mU/L in premenopausal women and in men younger than 60 years old. A dose of levothyroxine of 100–150 μg/day is usually sufficient. In men older than 60 years of age and postmenopausal women, TSH levels should be reduced to 0.1–0.3 mU/L owing to the risk of more serious adverse effects in this population and reduced clearance of levothyroxine with advanced age. Levothyroxine may be given in nontoxic multinodular goiter to suppress the TSH to low-normal levels of 0.5–1.0 mU/L if the baseline TSH is >1.0 mU/L. Goiter size and thyroid volume may be reduced with suppression therapy. Diffuse goiter associated with autoimmune thyroiditis may also be treated with levothyroxine to reduce goiter size and thyroid volume. In patients with follicular or papillary thyroid cancer, current recommendations are to suppress the TSH to <0.02 mU/L. Doses of levothyroxine of up to 2.2–2.5 μg/kg may be needed to provide TSH levels of <0.02 mU/L in this population, and free T_4 levels T_3 are useful in detecting hyperthyroidism.[111]

Adverse Effects

Serious untoward effects are unusual if dosing is appropriate and the patient is carefully monitored during initial treatment. Levothyroxine replacement in athyreotic hypothyroid patients restores systolic and diastolic left ventricular performance within 2 weeks, and the use of levothyroxine may increase the frequency of atrial premature beats but not necessarily ventricular premature beats. Excessive doses of thyroid hormone may lead to heart failure, angina pectoris, and myocardial infarction; rarely, the latter may be caused by coronary artery spasm.[87,112–114] Allergic or idiosyncratic reactions can occur with the natural animal-derived products such as desiccated thyroid and thyroglobulin, but these are extremely rare with the synthetic products used today. The 0.05-mg Synthroid tablet is the least allergenic (owing to lack of dye and few excipients) and should be tried in the patient suspected to be allergic to thyroid hormone.

Hyperremodeling of cortical and trabecular bone because of hyperthyroidism leads to reduced bone density and may increase the risk of fracture. Compared to normal controls, excess exogenous thyroid hormone results in histomorphometric and biochemical changes similar to those observed in osteoporosis and untreated hyperthyroidism; however, at routinely used replacement doses, bone mineral density loss is less than with untreated hyperthyroidism and only slightly greater than in controls.[115–117] The risk for this complication of therapy seems to be related to the dose of levothyroxine, patient age, and gender. Markers for bone turnover include urinary cross-linked *N*-telopeptides pyridinoline of type I collagen, osteocalcin, and bone-specific alkaline phosphatase. When doses of levothyroxine are used to suppress TSH concentrations to below normal values (less than 0.3 mU/L) in postmenopausal women, this adverse effect is more likely to be seen. Cortical bone is affected to a greater degree than trabecular bone at suppressive doses of L-thyroxine.[92] In contrast, it appears to be much less likely in men and in premenopausal women. Maintaining the TSH between 0.7 and 1.5 mU/L with approximately 150 μg/day of levothyroxine does not alter bone mineral density in premenopausal women.[93]

SPECIAL CONDITIONS

MYXEDEMA COMA[118–120]

Myxedema coma is the end stage of long-standing, uncorrected hypothyroidism. Clinical features include hypothermia, advanced stages of hypothyroid symptoms, and altered sensorium ranging from delirium to coma. Mortality rates of 60% to 70% necessitate immediate and aggressive therapy with intravenous bolus thyroxine 300–500 μg. Glucocorticoid therapy with intravenous hydrocortisone 100 mg every 8 hours should be given until coexisting adrenal suppression is ruled out. Consciousness, lowered TSH concentrations, and normal vital signs are expected within 24 hours. Maintenance doses are typically 75–100 μg given intravenously until the patient stabilizes and oral therapy is begun. Supportive therapy must be instituted to maintain adequate ventilation, euglycemia, blood pressure, and body temperature. Any underlying disorder, such as sepsis, myocardial infarction, and the like obviously must be diagnosed and treated.

CONGENITAL HYPOTHYROIDISM[121–124]

In congenital hypothyroidism, full-maintenance therapy should be instituted early to improve the prognosis for mental and physical development. The average maintenance dose in infants and children depends on the age and weight of the child. Several studies demonstrate that aggressive therapy with levothyroxine is important for normal development and current recommendations are for initiation of therapy within 45 days of birth at a dose of 10–15 μg/kg/day.[121] This dose is used to keep T_4 concentrations at about 10 μg/dL within 30 days of starting therapy and is associated with improved IQs in treated infants. The dose is progressively decreased to a typical adult dose as the child ages, the adult dose being given in the age range of 11 to 20 years. *In utero* treatment of fetal goiter and hypothyroidism has been accomplished with the injection of thyroxine into the amniotic fluid.[125]

HYPOTHYROIDISM IN PREGNANCY[68,93,126–128]

Hypothyroidism during pregnancy leads to an increased rate of stillbirths and possibly lower psychological scores in infants born of women who received inadequate replacement during pregnancy.[129] Thyroid hormone is necessary for fetal growth and must come from the maternal side during the first 2 months of gestation. Although liothyronine may cross the placental membrane slightly better than levothyroxine, the latter is considered to be the drug of choice. The objective of treatment is to decrease TSH to 1 U/mL and to maintain free T_4 concentrations in the normal range. Based on elevated TSH levels during pregnancy, Delange[129] found that the mean dose of levothyroxine had to be increased by 36 μg/day to suppress TSH into the normal range. Increased production of binding proteins, a marginal decrease in free hormone concentration, modification of peripheral thyroid hormone metabolism, and increased thyroxin metabolism by the fetal-placental unit also contributes to increased thyroid hormone demand and the need for increased doses decreases after delivery.[67] Only approximately 20% of women need levothyroxine dose adjustment during pregnancy. After delivery the levothyroxine may need to be reduced based on T_3 concentrations and measurement of TSH.[130]

EFFECTS OF HYPOTHYROIDISM ON SELECTED MEDICATIONS

Hypothyroidism may affect the metabolism and clinical efficacy of several medications. Digitalis preparations have a decreased volume of distribution in the hypothyroid state, resulting in increased sensitivity to the digitalis effect. Therefore, many hypothyroid patients achieve a therapeutic effect at lower digitalis doses. Insulin degradation may be delayed in hypothyroidism, thereby requiring a lower insulin dose. Hypothyroidism delays the catabolism of clotting factors, and if a patient stabilized on warfarin is made euthyroid with levothyroxine, the patient may become excessively anticoagulated. Respiratory depressants such as barbiturates, phenothiazines, and opioid analgesics should be avoided because increased sensitivity may increase carbon dioxide retention and precipitate myxedema coma.

RECOMBINANT TSH IN THYROID CANCER[131,132]

Patients with previously treated thyroid carcinoma require lifelong monitoring for recurrent disease. Two diagnostic tests that play a central role in followup of these patients—radioiodine whole-body scanning and serum thyroglobulin measurement—are most accurate during TSH stimulation. Temporary discontinuation of thyroid hormone therapy was previously the sole effective approach for TSH-stimulated testing. However, hormone withdrawal was associated with the morbidity of hypothyroidism and occasional tumor progression. The introduction of recombinant TSH (rTSH)-stimulated testing offers an alternative therapy. Recent clinical trials show that the sensitivity of combined rTSH-stimulated radioiodine scanning and serum thyroglobulin measurement has equivalent sensitivity to testing after thyroid hormone withdrawal. Furthermore, measurement of the rTSH-stimulated thyroglobulin concentration is a more sensitive way to detect residual thyroid cancer or normal tissue than thyroglobulin measurement on thyroid hormone therapy alone.

NONTHYROIDAL ILLNESS

A wide variety of abnormalities of pituitary-thyroid function, serum thyroid hormone binding, and extrathyroidal thyroid hormone metabolism occur in patients with nonthyroidal illness. These abnormalities frequently result in decreased serum T_3 concentrations, and less often lead to a decreased serum T_4 concentration. Serum TSH concentrations are usually within the normal range. The presence of coexisting primary hypothyroidism can be recognized in patients who have other illnesses by an elevation in the TSH concentration.

The degree and extent of the abnormality in thyroid function generally correlates with the severity of the nonthyroidal illness. These conditions are frequently referred to as the "euthyroid sick syndrome." It is likely that these changes represent adaptive forms of hypothyroidism that serve to reduce the availability of thyroid hormones to lessen the impact of the nonthyroidal illness.[133]

Decreased serum T_3 concentrations occur in patients with both acute and chronic illnesses. The fundamental cause of decreased serum T_3 concentrations in these situations is decreased extrathyroidal conversion of T_4 to T_3. This reaction is normally mediated by T_4-5′-deiodinase. A circulating inhibitor of this enzyme, perhaps IL-6, is present in patients with nonthyroidal illness.[134] Serum total and free T_4 concentrations are usually normal. The serum reverse T_3 concentration is characteristically high because the same enzyme, 5′-deiodinase, that is necessary to convert T_4 to T_3 is necessary to convert reverse T_3 to its breakdown products. Acute respiratory infections and surgery acutely elevate IL-6, and T_3 concentration is inversely correlated.[135]

Low serum T_4 is seen in most critically ill patients. This change is caused by diminished serum T_4 binding resulting either from decrease serum concentrations of TBG, TBPA, albumin, or from inhibitors of T_4 binding. The free T_4 concentration is generally normal. This more severe degree of hypothyroidism, which occurs in severely ill patients, produces a greater reduction in thyroid hormone availability. The low serum T_4 concentrations in patients with nonthyroidal illness indicates a grave prognosis. In two studies, more than 60% of hospitalized patients with a low serum free-T_4 index died. T_4 or T_3 supplementation has been of no benefit in this situation, and in fact has increased morbidity.

To confuse matters, some patients with nonthyroidal illness have elevation of their serum T_4 concentration. Most commonly, this is seen in patients with psychiatric disorders during acute psychotic breaks. Thyroid hormone levels return to normal within 2 weeks after successful treatment of the underlying psychiatric disease. The occurrence of these abnormalities requires that care be taken in diagnosing hypothyroidism or hyperthyroidism in patients who have nonthyroidal illnesses.

GOITROUS THYROID DISEASE

Endemic goiter is the major thyroid disease throughout the world, affecting more than 200 million people. Many goitrous glands contain one or more nodules. The introduction of iodide supplementation has eliminated goiter as a major medical problem in developed countries, though it continues to be a problem in developing countries whose geographic position makes them more susceptible to iodide deficiency. In 1924, Marine postulated that periods of iodide deficiency resulted in cyclic hyperplasia and involution of thyroid follicular cells with eventual development of nodular hyperplasia.[136] This hypothesis is still used to explain goiter formation. Whatever the specific cause, the final common pathway appears to result from an inadequate thyroid hormone secretion with compensatory TSH secretion and eventual thyroid gland enlargement. The essential factor for the conversion of a hyperplastic iodine-deficiency goiter into a colloid goiter appears to be an acute reduction of TSH stimulation; therefore, any situation that would result in a cyclical increase and decrease in TSH secretion might eventually result in the production of a nodular goiter.

There has been an interest in the possibility that growth factors other than TSH play a role in the development of a goiter. Immunoglobulin fractions capable of stimulating thyroid growth have been found in patients with nontoxic goiter and Graves' disease. In these patients, thyroid growth-promoting immunoglobulin titers correlates with goiter size rather than with the thyroid hormone concentration.

Sporadic goiter is defined as a goiter occurring in a nonendemic goiter region. Although a number of known goitrogens and errors in thyroid hormone biosynthesis may cause goiter, the majority of cases of sporadic goiter have no known etiology.

Treatment of all goiters is a trial of thyroid hormone suppression in an effort to eliminate TSH as a possible stimulus for continued thyroid growth. Large, long-standing goiters seldom undergo significant reduction in size. If the patient is symptomatic (with dysphagia or dyspnea), or if there is a question of malignant thyroid involvement, surgery is recommended.

▶ PRINCIPLES OF PHARMACOTHERAPY

- The molecular biology of the thyroid hormones and their receptors has provided an in-depth understanding of the various mutations that give rise to hyper- and hypothyroidism.
- Thyrotoxicosis is most commonly caused by Graves' disease, which is an autoimmune disorder in which TSAb directed against the thyrotropin receptor elicits the same biologic response as TSH.
- Hyperthyroidism may be treated with antithyroid drugs such as PTU or MMI, RAI, or surgical removal of the thyroid gland; selection of the initial treatment approach is based on patient characteristics such as age, concurrent physiology (e.g., pregnancy) or comorbidities (e.g., chronic obstructive lung disease), and convenience.
- PTU and MMI reduce the synthesis of thyroid hormones and are similar in efficacy and adverse effects but their dosing range differs by 10-fold.
- Response to PTU and MMI is seen in 4 to 6 weeks with a maximal response in 4 to 6 months; treatment usually continues for 1 to 2 years and therapy is monitored by clinical signs and symptoms and by measuring the serum concentrations of TSH and free T_4.
- Many patients choose to have ablative therapy with ^{131}I rather than undergo repeated courses of PTU or MMI; most patients who receive RAI eventually become hypothyroid and require thyroid hormone supplementation.
- Surgery is typically performed in patients with large goiters that compress surrounding structures. Surgery should be done in high-volume centers to minimize complications.
- Adjunctive therapy with β-blockers controls the adrenergic symptoms of thyrotoxicosis but does not correct the underlying disorder; iodine may also be used adjunctively in preparation for surgery and acutely for thyroid storm.

- Hypothyroidism is most often caused by an autoimmune disorder known as Hashimoto's thyroiditis, and the drug of choice for replacement therapy is thyroxine (T_4).
- Monitoring of thyroxine replacement therapy is done by clinical signs and symptoms and by measuring the TSH (elevated for underreplacement) and free T_4 (below normal for underreplacement).

REFERENCES

1. Cavalieri RR. Iodine metabolism and thyroid physiology: Current concepts. Thyroid 1997;7:177–181.
2. Arvan P, Kim PS, Kuliawat R, et al. Intracellular protein transport to the thymocyte plasma membrane: Potential implications for thyroid physiology. Thyroid 1997;7:89–105.
3. De La Vieja A, Dohan O, Levy O, Carrasco N. Molecular analysis of the sodium/iodide symporter: Impact on thyroid and extrathyroid pathophysiology. Physiol Rev 2000;80:1083–105.
4. Wolf J. Perchlorate and the thyroid gland. Pharmacol Rev 1998;50:89–105.
5. Motomura K, Brent GA. Mechanisms of thyroid hormone action. Implications for the clinical manifestation of thyrotoxicosis. Endocrinol Metab Clin North Am 1998;27:1–23.
6. Salvatore D, Tu H, Harney JW, Larsen PR. Type 2 iodothyronine deiodinase is highly expressed in human thyroid. J Clin Invest 1996;98:962–968.
7. Salvatore D, Low SC, Berry M, et al. Type 3 iodothyronine deiodinase: Cloning, *in vitro* expression, and functional analysis of the placental selenoenzyme. J Clin Invest 1995;96:2421–2430.
8. LoPresti JS, Nicoloff JT. 3,5,3′-Triiodothyronine (T3) sulfate: A major metabolite in T3 metabolism in man. J Clin Endocrinol Metab 1994;78:688–692.
9. Paschke R, Ludgate M. The thyrotropin receptor in thyroid diseases. N Engl J Med 1997;337:1675–1681.
10. Leclere J, Bene MC, Aubert V, et al. Clinical consequences of activating germ-line mutations of TSH receptor, the concept of toxic hyperplasia. Horm Res 1997;47:158–162.
11. Brent GA. Thyroid hormone action: Down novel paths. Focus on "thyroid hormone induces activation of mitogen-activated protein kinase in cultured cells." Am J Physiol 1999;276:C1012–3.
12. Apriletti JW, Ribeiro RC, Wagner RL, et al. Molecular and structural biology of thyroid hormone receptors. Clin Exp Pharmacol Physiol Suppl 1998;25:S2–S11.
13. Kannan CR, Seshadri KG. Thyrotoxicosis. Dis Mon 1997;43:601–677.
14. Russo D, Arturi F, Chiefari E, Filetti S. Molecular insights into TSH receptor abnormality and thyroid disease. J Endocrinol Invest 1997;20:36–47.
15. Beck-Peccoz P, Brucker-Davis F, Persani L, Smallridge RC, Weintraub BD. Thyrotropin-secreting pituitary tumors. Endocr Rev 1996;17: 610–638.
16. Beck-Peccoz P, Persani L, Mantovani S, Cortelazzi D, Asteria C. Thyrotropin-secreting pituitary adenomas. Metabolism 1996;45:75–79.
17. Refetoff S. Resistance to thyroid hormone. Curr Ther Endocrinol Metab 1997;6:132–134.
18. Weetman AP. Graves' disease. N Engl J Med 2000;343:1236–1248.
19. Wartofsky L. Radioiodine therapy for Graves' disease: Case selection and restrictions recommended to patients in North America. Thyroid 1997;7:213–216.
20. Prummel MF, Wiersinga WM. Medical management of Graves' ophthalmopathy. Thyroid 1995;5:231–234.
21. Kodali VR, Jeffcote B, Clague RB. Thyrotoxic periodic paralysis: A case report and review of the literature. J Emerg Med 1999;17:43–45.
22. Fantz CR, Dagogo-Jack S, Ladenson JH, Gronowski AM. Thyroid function during pregnancy. Clin Chem 1999;45:2250–2258.
23. Siegel RD, Lee SL. Toxic nodular goiter. Toxic adenoma and toxic multinodular goiter. Endocrinol Metab Clin North Am 1998;27:151–168.
24. Mazzaferri EL. Evaluation and management of common thyroid disorders in women. Am J Obstet Gynecol 1997;176:507–514.
25. Tonacchera M, Pinchera A. Thyrotropin receptor polymorphisms and thyroid diseases. J Clin Endocrinol Metab 2000;85:2637–2639.
26. Koutras DA. Subclinical hyperthyroidism. Thyroid 1999;9:311–315.
27. Slatosky J, Shipton B, Wahba H. Thyroiditis: Differential diagnosis and management. Am Fam Physician 2000;61:1047–1052, 1054.
28. Kennedy JW, Caro JF. The ABCs of managing hyperthyroidism in the older patient. Geriatrics 1996;51:22–24, 27, 31–32.
29. Dardik RB, Dardik M, Westra W, Montz FJ. Malignant struma ovarii: Two case reports and a review of the literature. Gynecol Oncol 1999;73:447–451.
30. Braverman LE. Evaluation of thyroid status in patients with thyrotoxicosis. Clin Chem 1996;42:174–178.
31. Ross DS. Syndromes of thyrotoxicosis with low radioactive iodine uptake. Endocrinol Metab Clin North Am 1998;27:169–185.
32. Loh KC. Amiodarone-induced thyroid disorders: A clinical review. Postgrad Med J 2000;76:133–140.
33. Ajjan RA, Watson PF, Weetman AP. Cytokines and thyroid function. Adv Neuroimmunol 1996;6:359–386.
34. Wenzel KW. Disturbances of thyroid function tests by drugs. Acta Med Austriaca 1996;23:57–60.
35. Gittoes NJ, Franklyn JA. Drug-induced thyroid disorders. Drug Saf 1995;13:46–55.
36. Lazarus JH, Obuobie K. Thyroid disorders—An update. Postgrad Med J 2000;76:529–536.
37. Woeber KA. Update on the management of hyperthyroidism and hypothyroidism. Arch Fam Med 2000;9:743–747.
38. Franklyn JA. Management guidelines for hyperthyroidism. Baillieres Clin Endocrinol Metab 1997;11:561–571.
39. Singer PA, Cooper DS, Levy EG, et al. Treatment guidelines for patients with hyperthyroidism and hypothyroidism. Standards of Care Committee, American Thyroid Association. JAMA 1995;273:808–812.
40. Alsanea O, Clark OH. Treatment of Graves' disease: The advantages of surgery. Endocrinol Metab Clin North Am 2000;29:321–337.
41. Gough IR, Wilkinson D. Total thyroidectomy for management of thyroid disease. World J Surg 2000;24:962–965.
42. Witte J, Goretzki PE, Dotzenrath C, et al. Surgery for Graves' disease: Total versus subtotal thyroidectomy—Results of a prospective randomized trial. World J Surg 2000;24:1303–1311.
43. Cooper DS. Antithyroid drugs for the treatment of hyperthyroidism caused by Graves' disease. Endocrinol Metab Clin North Am 1998;27: 225–247.
44. Woeber KA. The year in review: The thyroid. Ann Intern Med 1999;131: 959–962.
45. Momotani N, Noh JY, Ishikawa N, Ito K. Effects of propylthiouracil and methimazole on fetal thyroid status in mothers with Graves' hyperthyroidism. J Endocrinol Metab 1997;82:3633–3636.
46. Raber W, Kmen E, Waldhausl W, Vierhapper H. Medical therapy of Graves' disease: Effect on remission rates of methimazole alone and in combination with triiodothyronine. Eur J Endocrinol 2000;142: 117–124.
47. Rittmaster RS, Abbott EC, Douglas R, et al. Effect of methimazole, with or without L-thyroxine, on remission rates in Graves' disease. J Clin Endocrinol Metab 1998;83:814–818.
48. McIver B, Rae P, Beckett G, Wilkinson E, Gold A, Toft A. Lack of effect of thyroxine in patients with Graves' hyperthyroidism who are treated with an antithyroid drug. N Engl J Med 1996;334:220–224.
49. Werner MC, Romaldini JH, Bromberg N, Werner RS, Farah CS. Adverse effects related to thionamide drugs and their dose regimen. Am J Med Sci 1989;297:216–219.
50. Bartalena L, Bogazzi F, Martino E. Adverse effects of thyroid hormone preparations and antithyroid drugs. Drug Saf 1996;15:53–63.
51. Tamai H, Sudo T, Kimura A, et al. Association between the DRB1*08032 histocompatibility antigen and methimazole-induced agranulocytosis in Japanese patients with Graves disease. Ann Intern Med 1996;124: 490–494.

52. Fukata S, Kuma K, Sugawara M. Granulocyte colony-stimulating factor (G-CSF) does not improve recovery from antithyroid drug-induced agranulocytosis: A prospective study. Thyroid 1999;9:29–31.
53. Tamai H, Mukuta T, Matsubayashi S, et al. Treatment of methimazole-induced agranulocytosis using recombinant human granulocyte colony-stimulating factor (rhG-CSF). J Clin Endocrinol Metab 1993;77:1356–1360.
54. Williams KV, Nayak S, Becker D, Reyes J, Burmeister LA. Fifty years of experience with propylthiouracil-associated hepatotoxicity: What have we learned? J Clin Endocrinol Metab 1997;82:1727–1733.
55. Mizutani T, Yoshida K, Murakami M, Shirai M, Kawazoe S. Evidence for the involvement of *N*-methylthiourea, a ring cleavage metabolite, in the hepatotoxicity of methimazole in glutathione-depleted mice: Structure-toxicity and metabolic studies. Chem Res Toxicol 2000;13:170–176.
56. Gurlek A, Cobankara V, Bayraktar M. Liver tests in hyperthyroidism: Effect of antithyroid therapy. J Clin Gastroenterol 1997;24:180–183.
57. Benelhadj S, Marcellin P, Castelnau C, et al. Incidence of dysthyroidism during interferon therapy in chronic hepatitis C. Horm Res 1997;48:209–214.
58. Van Dijke CP, Heydendael RJ, De Kleine MJ. Methimazole, carbimazole, and congenital skin defects. Ann Intern Med 1987;106:60–61.
59. Kaplan MM, Meier DA, Dworkin HJ. Treatment of hyperthyroidism with radioactive iodine. Endocrinol Metab Clin North Am 1998;27:205–223.
60. Bartalena L, Marcocci C, Bogazzi F, et al. Relation between therapy for hyperthyroidism and the course of Graves' ophthalmopathy. N Engl J Med 1998;338:73–78.
61. Tallstedt L, Lundell G. Radioiodine treatment, ablation, and ophthalmopathy: A balanced perspective. Thyroid 1997;7:241–245.
62. Franklyn JA, Maisonneuve P, Sheppard M, Betteridge J, Boyle P. Cancer incidence and mortality after radioiodine treatment for hyperthyroidism: A population-based cohort study. Lancet 1999;353:2111–2115.
63. Franklyn JA, Maisonneuve P, Sheppard MC, Betteridge J, Boyle P. Mortality after the treatment of hyperthyroidism with radioactive iodine. N Engl J Med 1998;338:712–718.
64. Franklyn JA. The management of hyperthyroidism. N Engl J Med 1994; 330:1731–1738.
65. Uy HL, Reasner CA, Samuels MH. Pattern of recovery of the hypothalamic-pituitary-thyroid axis following radioactive iodine therapy in patients with Graves' disease. Am J Med 1995;99:173–179.
66. Mestman JH. Hyperthyroidism in pregnancy. Endocrinol Metab Clin North Am 1998;27:127–149.
67. Glinoer D. What happens to the normal thyroid during pregnancy? Thyroid 1999;9:631–635.
68. Lazarus JH, Kokandi A. Thyroid disease in relation to pregnancy: A decade of change. Clin Endocrinol 2000;53:265–278.
69. Momotani N, Noh J, Ishikawa N, Ito K. Relationship between silent thyroiditis and recurrent Graves' disease in the postpartum period. J Clin Endocrinol Metab 1994;79:285–289.
70. Coukos G, Makrigiannakis A, Chung J, Randall TC, Rubin SC, Benjamin I. Complete hydatidiform mole. A disease with a changing profile. J Reprod Med 1999;44:698–704.
71. Ngowngarmratana S, Sunthornthepvarakul T, Kanchanawat S. Thyroid function and human chorionic gonadotropin in patients with hydatidiform mole. J Med Assoc Thai 1997;80:693–699.
72. Ayhan A, Tuncer ZS, Halilzade H, Kucukali T. Predictors of persistent disease in women with complete hydatidiform mole. J Reprod Med 1996;41:591–594.
73. Soto-Wright V, Bernstein M, Goldstein DP, Berkowitz RS. The changing clinical presentation of complete molar pregnancy. Obstet Gynecol 1995;86:775–779.
74. Goldstein DP, Berkowitz RS. Current management of complete and partial molar pregnancy. J Reprod Med 1994;39:139–146.
75. Momotani N, Yamashita R, Makino F, Noh JY, Ishikawa N, Ito K. Thyroid function in wholly breast-feeding infants whose mothers take high doses of propylthiouracil. Clin Endocrinol 2000;53:177–181.
76. Zimmerman D, Lteif AN. Thyrotoxicosis in children. Endocrinol Metab Clin North Am 1998;27:109–126.
77. Zimmerman D. Fetal and neonatal hyperthyroidism. Thyroid 1999;9:727–733.
78. Segni M, Leonardi E, Mazzoncini B, Pucarelli I, Pasquino AM. Special features of Graves' disease in early childhood. Thyroid 1999;9:871–877.
79. Dillmann WH. Thyroid storm. Curr Ther Endocrinol Metab 1997;6:81–85.
80. Ringel MD. Management of hypothyroidism and hyperthyroidism in the intensive care unit. Crit Care Clin 2001;17:59–74.
81. Knighton JD, Crosse MM. Anaesthetic management of childhood thyrotoxicosis and the use of esmolol. Anaesthesia 1997;52:67–70.
82. Burch HB, Wartofsky L. Life-threatening thyrotoxicosis. Thyroid storm. Endocrinol Metab Clin North Am 1993;22:263–277.
83. Samaras K, Marel GM. Failure of plasmapheresis, corticosteroids and thionamides to ameliorate a case of protracted amiodarone-induced thyroiditis. Clin Endocrinol 1996;45:365–368.
84. Wang C, Crapo LM. The epidemiology of thyroid disease and implications for screening. Endocrinol Metab Clin North Am 1997;26:189–218.
85. Arem R, Escalante D. Subclinical hypothyroidism: Epidemiology, diagnosis, and significance. Adv Intern Med 1996;41:213–250.
86. Adlin V. Subclinical hypothyroidism: Deciding when to treat. Am Fam Physician 1998;57:776–780.
87. Stagnaro-Green A. Recognizing, understanding, and treating postpartum thyroiditis. Endocrinol Metab Clin North Am 2000;29:417–430, ix.
88. Mukuta T, Yoshikawa N, Arreaza G, et al. Activation of T lymphocyte subsets by synthetic TSH receptor peptides and recombinant glutamate decarboxylase in autoimmune thyroid disease and insulin-dependent diabetes. J Clin Endocrinol Metab 1995;80:1264–1272.
89. Roura-Mir C, Catalfamo M, Sospedra M, Alcalde L, Pujol-Borrell R, Jaraquemada D. Single-cell analysis of intrathyroidal lymphocytes shows differential cytokine expression in Hashimoto's and Graves' disease. Eur J Immunol 1997;27:3290–3302.
90. Kasagi K, Kousaka T, Higuchi K, et al. Clinical significance of measurements of antithyroid antibodies in the diagnosis of Hashimoto's thyroiditis: Comparison with histological findings. Thyroid 1996;6:445–450.
91. Grant DB. Congenital hypothyroidism: Optimal management in the light of 15 years' experience of screening. Arch Dis Child 1995;72:85–89.
92. Glinoer D, Delange F. The potential repercussions of maternal, fetal, and neonatal hypothyroxinemia on the progeny. Thyroid 2000;10:871–887.
93. Mestman JH. Diagnosis and management of maternal and fetal thyroid disorders. Curr Opin Obstet Gynecol 1999;11:167–75.
94. Gruters A, Krude H, Biebermann H, Liesenkotter KP, Schoneberg T, Gudermann T. Alterations of neonatal thyroid function. Acta Paediatr Suppl 1999;88:17–22.
95. Blouin RA, Clifton GD, Adams MA, Foster TS, Flueck J. Biopharmaceutical comparison of two levothyroxine sodium products. Clin Pharm 1989;8:588–592.
96. Berg JA, Mayor GH. A study in normal human volunteers to compare the rate and extent of levothyroxine absorption from Synthroid and Levoxine. J Clin Pharmacol 1992;32:1135–1140.
97. Gottwald R, Lorkowski G, Petersen G, Schnitzler M, Lucker PW. Bioequivalence of two commercially available levothyroxine-Na preparations in athyreotic patients. Methods Find Exp Clin Pharmacol 1994;16:645–650.
98. Dong BJ, Hauck WW, Gambertoglio JG, et al. Bioequivalence of generic and brand-name levothyroxine products in the treatment of hypothyroidism. JAMA 1997;277:1205–1213.
99. Liel Y, Sperber AD, Shany S. Nonspecific intestinal adsorption of levothyroxine by aluminum hydroxide. Am J Med 1994;97:363–365.
100. Shakir KM, Chute JP, Aprill BS, Lazarus AA. Ferrous sulfate-induced increase in requirement for thyroxine in a patient with primary hypothyroidism. South Med J 1997;90:637–639.
101. Jabbar MA, Larrea J, Shaw RA. Abnormal thyroid function tests in infants with congenital hypothyroidism: The influence of soy-based formula. J Am Coll Nutr 1997;16:280–282.
102. Liel Y, Harman-Boehm I, Shany S. Evidence for a clinically important adverse effect of fiber-enriched diet on the bioavailability of levothyroxine in adult hypothyroid patients. J Clin Endocrinol Metab 1996;81:857–859.

103. Bunevicius R, Kazanavicius G, Zalinkevicius R, Prange AJ Jr. Effects of thyroxine as compared with thyroxine plus triiodothyronine in patients with hypothyroidism. N Engl J Med 1999;340:424–429.
104. Kabadi UM. Influence of age on optimal daily levothyroxine dosage in patients with primary hypothyroidism grouped according to etiology. South Med J 1997;90:920–924.
105. De Whalley P. Do abnormal thyroid stimulating hormone level values result in treatment changes? A study of patients on thyroxine in one general practice. Br J Gen Pract 1995;45:93–95.
106. Kabadi UM, Cech R. Normal thyroxine and elevated thyrotropin concentrations: Evolving hypothyroidism or persistent euthyroidism with reset thyrostat. J Endocrinol Invest 1997;20:319–326.
107. Jaeschke R, Guyatt G, Gerstein H, et al. Does treatment with L-thyroxine influence health status in middle-aged and older adults with subclinical hypothyroidism? J Gen Intern Med 1996;11:744–749.
108. Zulewski H, Muller B, Exer P, Miserez AR, Staub JJ. Estimation of tissue hypothyroidism by a new clinical score: Evaluation of patients with various grades of hypothyroidism and controls. J Clin Endocrinol Metab 1997;82:771–776.
109. Lindsay RS, Toft AD. Hypothyroidism. Lancet 1997;349:413–417.
110. Behnia M, Gharib H. Primary care diagnosis of thyroid disease. Hosp Pract (Off Ed) 1996;31:121–126, 131–134.
111. Taimela E, Koskinen P, Nuutila P, et al. Free thyroid hormones and a third-generation TSH assay in the detection of hyperthyroidism during long-term thyroxine treatment in thyroid carcinoma patients. Scand J Clin Lab Invest 1995;55:181–186.
112. Aronow WS. The heart and thyroid disease. Clin Geriatr Med 1995;11: 219–229.
113. Klemperer JD, Ojamaa K, Klein I. Thyroid hormone therapy in cardiovascular disease. Prog Cardiovasc Dis 1996;38:329–336.
114. Toft AD, Boon NA. Thyroid disease and the heart. Heart 2000;84:455–460.
115. Ross DS. Bone density is not reduced during the short-term administration of levothyroxine to postmenopausal women with subclinical hypothyroidism: A randomized, prospective study. Am J Med 1993;95: 385–388.
116. Greenspan SL, Greenspan FS. The effect of thyroid hormone on skeletal integrity. Ann Intern Med 1999;130:750–758.
117. Kung AW, Yeung SS. Prevention of bone loss induced by thyroxine suppressive therapy in postmenopausal women: The effect of calcium and calcitonin. J Clin Endocrinol Metab 1996;81:1232–1236.
118. Pittman CS, Zayed AA. Myxedema coma. Curr Ther Endocrinol Metab 1997;6:98–101.
119. Jordan RM. Myxedema coma. Pathophysiology, therapy, and factors affecting prognosis. Med Clin North Am 1995;79:185–194.
120. Wall CR. Myxedema coma: Diagnosis and treatment. Am Fam Physician 2000;62:2485–2490.
121. Anonymous. American Academy of Pediatrics AAP Section on Endocrinology and Committee on Genetics, and American Thyroid Association Committee on Public Health: Newborn screening for congenital hypothyroidism: Recommended guidelines. Pediatrics 1993;91:1203–1209.
122. Van Vliet G. Neonatal hypothyroidism: Treatment and outcome. Thyroid 1999;9:79–84.
123. LaFranchi S. Congenital hypothyroidism: Etiologies, diagnosis, and management. Thyroid 1999;9:735–740.
124. Macchia PE. Recent advances in understanding the molecular basis of primary congenital hypothyroidism. Mol Med Today 2000;6:36–42.
125. Bruner JP, Dellinger EH. Antenatal diagnosis and treatment of fetal hypothyroidism. A report of two cases. Fetal Diagn Ther 1997;12:200–204.
126. Roti E, Minelli R, Salvi M. Clinical review 80: Management of hyperthyroidism and hypothyroidism in the pregnant woman. J Clin Endocrinol Metab 1996;81:1679–1682.
127. Montoro MN. Management of hypothyroidism during pregnancy. Clin Obstet Gynecol 1997;40:65–80.
128. Atkins P, Cohen SB, Phillips BJ. Drug therapy for hyperthyroidism in pregnancy: Safety issues for mother and fetus. Drug Saf 2000;23:229–244.
129. Delange F. Neonatal screening for congenital hypothyroidism: Results and perspectives. Horm Res 1997;48:51–61.
130. Girling JC, de Swiet M. Thyroxine dosage during pregnancy in women with primary hypothyroidism. Br J Obstet Gynaecol 1992;99:368–370.
131. Ladenson PW. Strategies for thyrotropin use to monitor patients with treated thyroid carcinoma. Thyroid 1999;9:429–433.
132. Ladenson PW. Recombinant thyrotropin versus thyroid hormone withdrawal in evaluating patients with thyroid carcinoma. Semin Nucl Med 2000;30:98–106.
133. Chopra IJ. Clinical review 86: Euthyroid sick syndrome: Is it a misnomer? J Clin Endocrinol Metab 1997;82:329–334.
134. Yamazaki K, Yamada E, Kanaji Y, et al. Interleukin-6 (IL-6) inhibits thyroid function in the presence of soluble IL-6 receptor in cultured human thyroid follicles. Endocrinology 1996;137:4857–4863.
135. Murai H, Murakami S, Ishida K, Sugawara M. Elevated serum interleukin-6 and decreased thyroid hormone levels in postoperative patients and effects of IL-6 on thyroid cell function in vitro. Thyroid 1996;6:601–606.
136. Delange F. Screening for congenital hypothyroidism used as an indicator of the degree of iodine deficiency and of its control. Thyroid 1998;8:1185–1192.

76

ADRENAL GLAND DISORDERS

John G. Gums and Chris M. Terpening

The adrenal glands were first characterized by Eustachius in 1563 (Table 76–1). After Addison identified a case of adrenal insufficiency in a man, adrenal anatomy and physiology flourished. Most of the work done in the early and middle 1900s centered on the glucocorticoid cortisol. With the discovery of aldosterone by Simpson and Tait in 1952, adrenal pharmacology turned toward the mineralocorticoid. Conn[1] followed with his classical description of primary aldosteronism in 1955, and numerous clinicians and investigators have continued the discovery of the variety of disease processes promoted through the adrenal gland.

PHYSIOLOGY, ANATOMY, AND BIOCHEMISTRY

There are two adrenal glands located extraperitoneally to the upper poles of each kidney (Fig. 76–1). On average, each adrenal gland weighs 4 g and is 2 to 3 cm in width and 4 to 6 cm in length. The gland is fed by small arteries from the abdominal aorta and renal and phrenic arteries. Drainage of the adrenal gland occurs via the renal vein on the left and the inferior vena cava on the right.

The adrenal medulla occupies 10% of the total gland and is responsible for the secretion of catecholamines. The adrenal cortex accounts for the remaining 90% and is responsible for the secretion of three types of hormones (Fig. 76–2) from three separate zones.[2]

The zona glomerulosa, 15% of the total adrenal cortex, is responsible for mineralocorticoid production, of which aldosterone is the principal end product. Aldosterone maintains electrolyte and volume homeostasis by altering potassium and magnesium secretion and renal tubular sodium reabsorption. The zona fasiculata, the middle zone, makes up 60% of the cortex, is high in cholesterol, and is responsible for basal and stimulated glucocorticoid production. Glucocorticoids, mainly cortisol, are responsible for the regulation of fat, carbohydrate, and protein metabolism. The zona reticularis occupies 25% of the adrenal cortex and is responsible for all adrenal androgen production. The androgens testosterone and estradiol are the major end products and have influence within the reproductive system as well as affecting primary and secondary sex characteristics.

HORMONE PRODUCTION AND METABOLISM

Cortisol production is accomplished via two successive hydroxylations: the first at the 21 position by 21-hydroxylase (yielding 11-deoxycortisol) and the second at the 11 position by 11-hydroxylase, yielding cortisol or hydrocortisone.

Aldosterone is a by-product of the 21-hydroxylation of pregnenolone to form deoxycorticosterone. The oxidation of 18-hydroxycorticosterone to aldosterone is a unique feature of the zona glomerulosa, explaining why aldosterone is not affected during disease processes limited to the fasiculata and/or reticularis.

Androgens have a 19-carbon nucleus and serve as precursors to more potent analogs produced in the periphery. The adrenal gland can synthesize estradiol and estrone from testosterone and androstenedione, respectively; however, the quantities are extremely small. The rates of production for the various steroids produced by the adrenal gland are listed in Table 76–2.

Metabolism of glucocorticoids occurs in the liver and is responsible for converting inactive steroids to active metabolites, as well as deactivating the active steroids to less active or inactive metabolites. Most pharmaceutical steroid products are active; however, in the case of prednisone and cortisone, metabolism is necessary for the conversion to the active prednisolone and cortisol, respectively. Following metabolic conversion, glucocorticoids are excreted renally as less active or inactive metabolites.

After metabolism, glomerular filtration is primarily responsible for the elimination of endogenously produced glucocorticoids. The half-life of cortisol is 70 to 120 minutes; with aldosterone, the half-life is only 15 minutes because of an extremely high extraction ratio.

Metabolism and conversion of the various steroids can be altered by a variety of disease states and medicinal compounds. Drugs and diseases known to result in enhanced clearance of steroids include phenytoin, phenobarbital, rifampin, mitotane, aminoglutethimide, hyperthyroidism, and renal disease (dexamethasone only). Drugs and diseases known to result in reduced clearance of steroids include estrogens and estrogen-containing oral contraceptives, liver disease, age, pregnancy, hypothyroidism, anorexia nervosa, protein-calorie malnutrition, and renal disease (prednisolone only). Plasma glucocorticoids are bound to one of three plasma proteins in varying degrees. Corticosteroid-binding globulin (CBG), albumin, and α_1-glycoprotein are capable of binding glucocorticoids, with CBG being the principal binding protein.

The function of steroid binding is to serve as a reservoir of steroids in their inactive state. This binding may change the availability of glucocorticoids to receptor-activating sites. Therefore, a final but important variable in altered plasma concentration of free (active) steroids is concentration of plasma proteins.

REGULATION OF HORMONE SECRETION

The regulation of glucocorticoid secretion is accomplished by the pituitary hormone adrenocorticotropic hormone (ACTH). Under normal conditions, ACTH is released from the anterior pituitary in response to corticotropin-releasing hormone (CRH), which is secreted by the median eminence of the hypothalamus (Fig. 76–3).

Additionally, histochemical studies have demonstrated that certain neurotransmitters have the unique ability to stimulate production of CRH or ACTH directly. 5-Hydroxytryptamine (5-HT) and norepinephrine (NE) have both been shown to increase levels of ACTH. 5-HT causes a release of CRH through excitation of a cholinergic intervention. NE can cause direct stimulation of ACTH release, although this effect is still controversial. After release, ACTH stimulates the adrenal gland to release cortisol and to a lesser extent aldosterone and androgens. The rising cortisol concentration

TABLE 76–1. Landmarks in Adrenal Cortical History

Date	Discovery	Investigator
1563	Adrenal described	Eustachius
1855	Adrenal insufficiency in man	Addison
1856	Adrenalectomy fatal in dog	Brown
1895–1904	Discovery of epinephrine	Oliver
1910	Hypoglycemia of Addison's disease	Porges
1927	First active adrenal cortical extract	Hartman
1932	Life of patient with Addison's disease prolonged with salt	Loeb
1936	The "alarm reaction"	Selye
1938	Synthesis of deoxycorticosterone	Reichstein
1948	Partial synthesis of cortisone	Sarrett
1949	First anti-inflammatory use of cortisone	Hench/Kendall
1952	Discovery of aldosterone	Simpson/Tait
1955	Discovery of primary aldosteronism	Conn

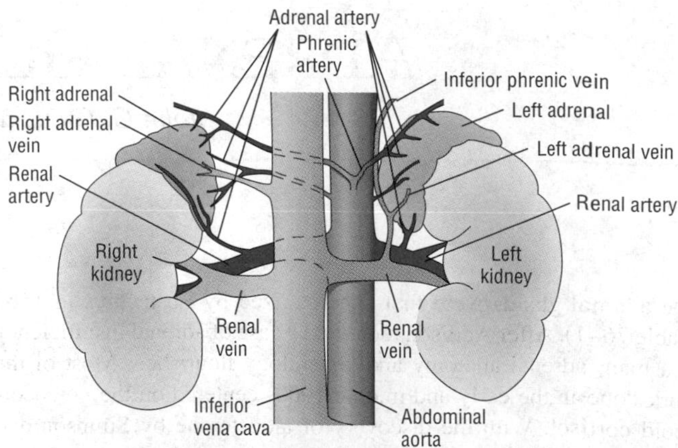

FIGURE 76–1. Anatomy of the adrenal gland.

inhibits the secretion of CRH and ACTH through a negative-feedback mechanism.

Regulation of adrenal androgens is accomplished in a manner similar to cortisol regulation. When plasma androgen reaches sufficient concentrations, production is terminated via a negative-feedback loop. Androgen release is increased during puberty and in women with hirsutism. Adrenal androgen release is decreased in fasting, anorexia nervosa, and aging.

Regulation of aldosterone secretion is considerably more complex. The renin-angiotensin system has the ability to respond to electrolyte and volume changes to increase or decrease aldosterone secretion. Renin production and subsequent aldosterone secretion are stimulated by blood pressure lowering, erect posture, salt depletion, β-adrenergic stimulation, and central nervous system excitation. Renin production is inhibited by salt loading, angiotensin II, vasopressin, potassium, calcium, blood pressure increases, and a variety of drugs. The conversion of renin substrate angiotensinogen to angiotensin I and subsequently to angiotensin II is the initial stimulus for aldosterone synthesis. Angiotensin II is acted on by aminopeptidase and converted to angiotensin III. Angiotensin II and III are both capable of stimulating the zona glomerulosa to secrete aldosterone. Following aldosterone secretion, increases in renal sodium and water retention as well as blood pressure are seen, thereby turning off the stimulus for renin release.

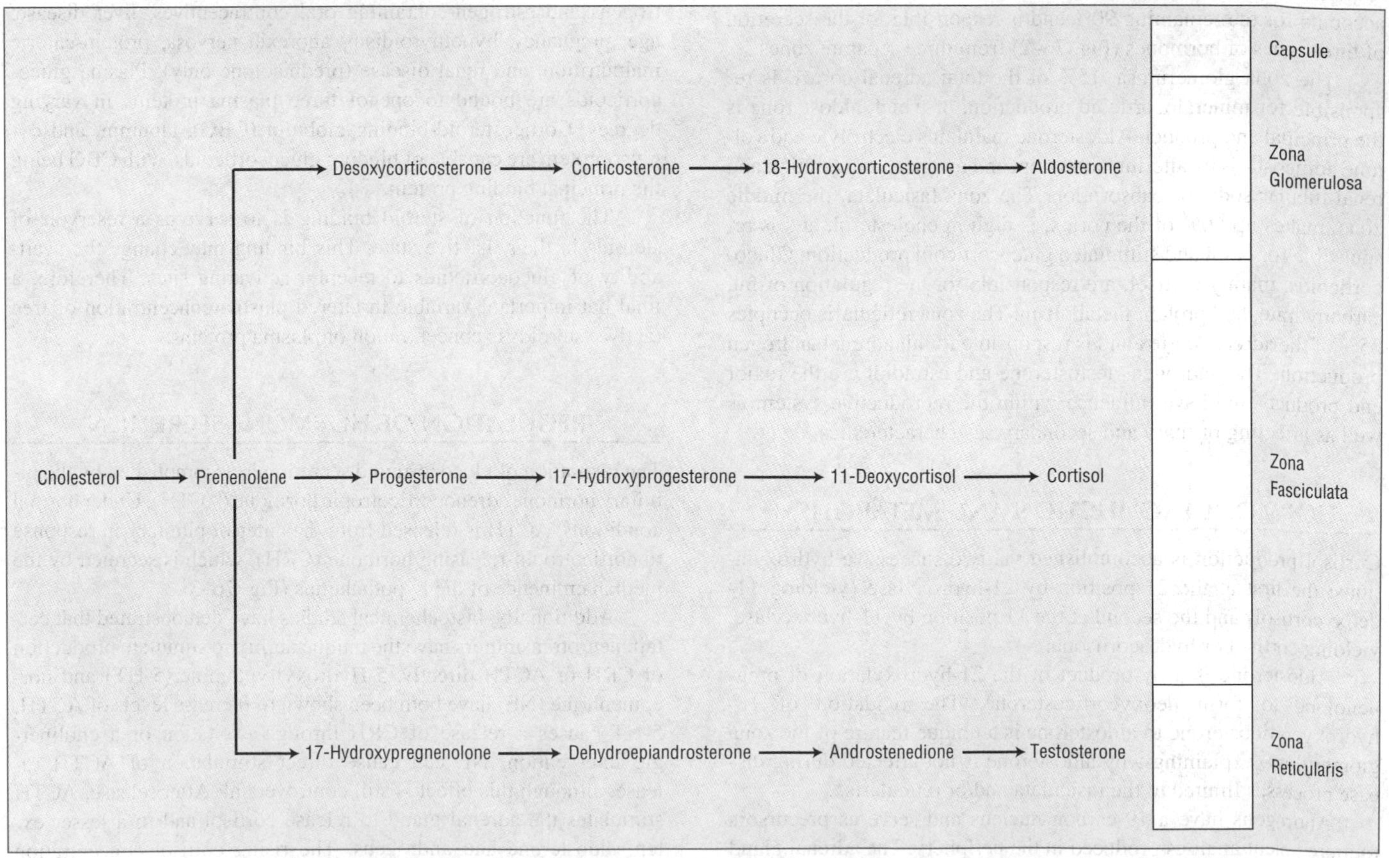

Capsule

Zona Glomerulosa: Desoxycorticosterone → Corticosterone → 18-Hydroxycorticosterone → Aldosterone

Zona Fasciculata: Cholesterol → Prenenolene → Progesterone → 17-Hydroxyprogesterone → 11-Deoxycortisol → Cortisol

Zona Reticularis: 17-Hydroxypregnenolone → Dehydroepiandrosterone → Androstenedione → Testosterone

FIGURE 76–2. Hormone synthetic pathways in relation to the zones of the adrenal gland.

TABLE 76–2. Rates of Adrenal Production and Plasma Concentrations of Various Steroids

Steroid	24-Hour Secretion (mg)	Plasma Concentration (ng/mL)
Aldosterone	0.15	0.15–0.17
Androstenedione	2.50 (female) 2.20 (male)	1.80 ± 0.21 (female) 1.14 ± 0.21 (male)
Corticosterone	1–4	2.4 ± 1.5 (female) 4.2 ± 2.2 (male)
Cortisol	8.0–25.0	20–140 (female) 40–180 (male)
11-Deoxycorticosterone	0.60	0.15–0.17
11-Deoxycortisol	0.40	0.95–2.50
Progesterone	0.0	0.20 ± 0.09 (female)[a] 11.8 ± 7.0 (female)[b] 0.18 ± 0.10 (male)
Testosterone	0.23 (female)	0.48 ± 0.14 (female) 5.59 ± 1.51 (male)

[a]Follicular phase of menstrual cycle.
[b]Luteal phase of menstrual cycle.

HYPERFUNCTION OF THE ADRENAL GLAND

CUSHING'S SYNDROME

In 1932, Cushing first described a syndrome of pituitary basophilism that attracted national attention. It was not until this time that patients with unexplained central obesity, cutaneous striae, osteoporosis, weakness, hypertension, diabetes mellitus, and congestion had a definite diagnosis. Cushing emphasized that the disease was of pituitary origin. Ten years later, Albright[3] focused his attention on the sugar hormone, which he believed originated from the adrenal cortex.

After development of a method for measuring urinary steroids, Daughaday discovered elevated steroids in the urine of Cushing's disease patients. Finally, the end product was identified, and Cushing's disease was correctly explained as an excess of cortisol in the plasma (hypercortisolism).

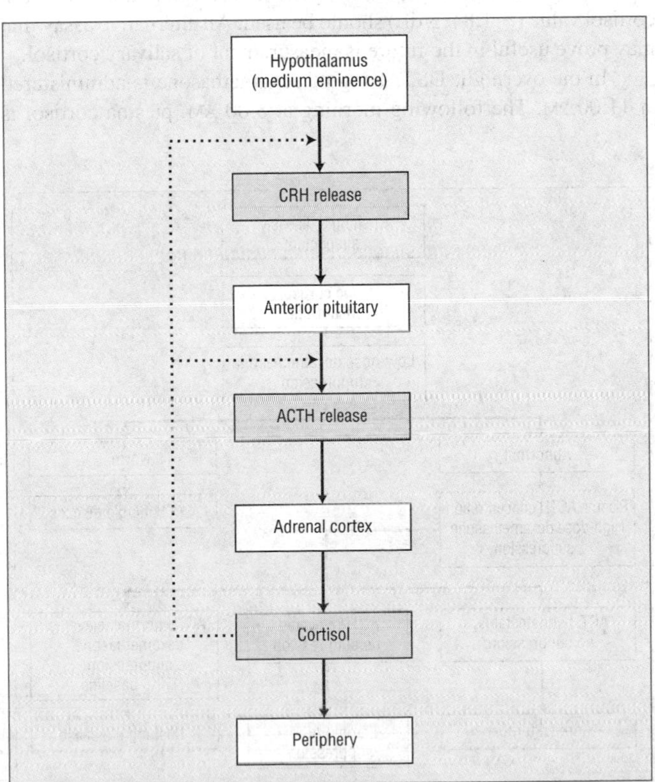

FIGURE 76–3. Regulation of cortisol secretion under normal conditions. CRH = corticotropin-releasing hormone; ACTH = adrenocorticotropic hormone.

ETIOLOGY

Cushing's syndrome results from the effects of supraphysiologic levels of glucocorticoids originating either from exogenous administration or from endogenous overproduction by the adrenal glands (ACTH-dependent) or by abnormal adrenocortical tissues (ACTH-independent). ACTH-dependent Cushing's syndrome is usually (~70% of Cushing's cases) caused by overproduction of ACTH by the pituitary gland, producing adrenal hyperplasia (Cushing's disease). Pituitary adenomas account for approximately 85% of these cases. Ectopic ACTH-secreting tumors and nonneoplastic corticotropin hypersecretion, possibly secondary to excess CRH production, are felt to be responsible for the remaining 12% of ACTH-dependent causes. Ectopic ACTH syndrome refers to excessive ACTH production resulting from a nonendocrine tumor, usually of the pancreas, thyroid, or lung. Small cell carcinoma of the lung will lead to ectopic ACTH secretion in 0.5% to 2% of cases. To distinguish between the various etiologies, a careful history and some pertinent laboratory work are required (Table 76–3).

The remaining 18% of Cushing's syndrome cases are ACTH-independent and are almost equally divided between adrenal adenomas and adrenal carcinomas, with rare cases caused by micronodular or macronodular hyperplasia.[4,5] The majority of adrenal cortex tumors are benign adenomas. Adrenal carcinoma is found more often in children than in adults with Cushing's syndrome.

CLINICAL PRESENTATION

The clinical symptoms most commonly seen with Cushing's syndrome are listed in Table 76–4.[5] The most common of these findings include central obesity and facial rounding. About 50% of patients will exhibit some peripheral obesity and fat accumulation. Facial plethora is caused by an underlying atrophy of the skin and connective tissue. Patients often are described as having moon facies with a buffalo hump. Fat accumulation in the dorsocervical area (buffalo hump) can be associated with any major weight gain, whereas increased supraclavicular fat pads are more specific for Cushing's syndrome.[5] Striae usually are present along the lower abdomen and take on a red to purple color.

Hypertension is seen in 75% to 85% of patients with Cushing's syndrome. Diastolic blood pressures greater than 119 mm Hg have been noted in over 20% of patients with Cushing's syndrome.[6] Hypertensive complications traditionally have been major contributors to the morbidity and mortality of Cushing's syndrome.

Gonadal dysfunction is common in patients with hypercortisolism. The abnormalities are principally the result of elevated levels of androgens in the females and cortisol in the males. Most common in females is amenorrhea, which is seen in up to 75% of females with the diagnosis. Excess androgen secretion is also responsible for the 80% of female patients who present with hirsutism.

Approximately 50% to 60% of patients will develop Cushing's-induced osteoporosis. Of these patients, 40% will present with back

TABLE 76–3. Various Etiologies of Cushing's Syndrome and Their Respective Differences

	Pituitary Dependent	Ectopic ACTH Syndrome	Adrenal Adenoma	Adrenal Carcinoma
Course	Slow	Rapid	Slow	Rapid
Symptoms	Mild to moderate	Atypical	Mild to moderate	Severe
Dominant sex/age	Female/male	Male	None noted	Children
Virilization	+	+	+	+++
Abdominal mass	0	0	0	++
Plasma ACTH concentration	Slightly elevated	High	0	0
Dexamethasone suppression test	≥50% suppression	No suppression	No suppression	No suppression
Iodocholesterol scan	Bilateral uptake	Bilateral uptake	Unilateral	None

pain, and about 20% of these will progress to compression fractures of the spine.

DIAGNOSIS

Diagnosis of Cushing's syndrome is relatively easy, but the differentiation between etiologies can be difficult[4,5,7] (Fig. 76–4). The diagnostic evaluation involves two steps. Initially, the presence of hypercortisolism must be established via the following tests: 24-hour urine free cortisol, midnight plasma cortisol, and/or the low-dose dexamethasone-suppression test (DST) (using 1 mg for the overnight test or 0.5 mg/6 h for the "classic" 2-day study). However, because these tests cannot determine the etiology of Cushing's syndrome, other tests and procedures subsequently will be employed. They may include any of the following: high-dose DST; plasma ACTH via immunoradiometric assay (IRMA) or radioimmunoassay (RIA); adrenal vein catheterization; metyrapone stimulation test; adrenal, chest, or abdominal computed tomography (CT); CRH stimulation test; inferior petrosal sinus sampling; and pituitary magnetic resonance imaging (MRI). Other possible tests and procedures include insulin-induced hypoglycemia, somatostatin receptor scintigraphy, the desmopression stimulation test, the naloxone CRH stimulation test, the loperamide test, the hexarelin stimulation test, and radionuclide imaging.[4–17] Table 76–5 summarizes some of the tests used to diagnose Cushing's syndrome.

Elevated urinary free cortisol (UFC) concentrations are highly suggestive of Cushing's syndrome. Normal reference values for UFC are 20 to 90 μg per 24-hour period. It is not unusual to detect a two- or threefold increase in urine cortisol in the patient with hyperfunction of the adrenal gland. Starvation, topical steroid application, hydration from water loading, and acute stress all are capable of elevating the UFC concentrations. Because other pathologic conditions can increase the amount of free cortisol, additional tests should be performed to confirm the diagnosis, or the diagnostic evaluation should be repeated when the acute stress has resolved. Of all urinary measures, UFC is the most useful for assessment of any patient with suspected Cushing's syndrome.[7]

The normal circadian rhythm of cortisol will demonstrate a 60% to 80% decline between 8:00 AM and 11:00 PM. This rhythm is lost in the Cushing's syndrome patient. Thus, while many patients with Cushing's syndrome will have serum cortisol values in the high-normal range if the serum is assayed in the morning, only 3.4% will have normal values if measured late at night.[7] Thus a midnight serum cortisol level of more than 7.5 μg/dL is a highly sensitive assay for Cushing's. However, this test requires that patients be admitted for more than 48 hours to avoid false-positive responses secondary to the stress of hospitalization. Also, if a patient is sleeping, a lower serum cortisol value (> 1.8 μg/dL) should be used. An alternative assay that may prove useful in the future is measurement of salivary cortisol.

In the overnight DST, 1 mg of dexamethasone is administered at 11:00 PM. The following morning at 8:00 AM, plasma cortisol is

TABLE 76–4. Clinical Features in Patients with Hypercortisolism

Feature	% Patients
Obesity	90
Hypertension	85
Facial plethora	84
Glucose intolerance	80
Menstrual dysfunction	76
Hirsutism	72
Striae	67
Myopathy	65
Muscular weakness	58
Osteoporosis	55
Psychiatric changes	55

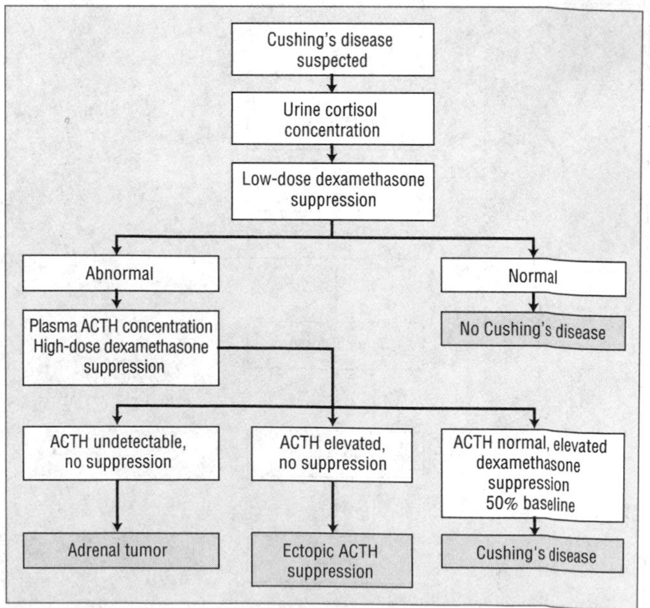

FIGURE 76–4. Algorithm for diagnosing Cushing's syndrome. ACTH = adrenocorticotropic hormone.

TABLE 76–5. Summary of Tests Used to Diagnose Cushing's Syndrome

Test	Normal	Hyperplasia	Adenoma	Carcinoma
Plasma				
Cortisol (μg/dL, AM/PM)	17/8	↑/↑↑	↑↑/↑↑	↑↑↑/↑↑↑
After low-dose DST	↓	↔	↔	↔
After high-dose DST	↓	↓/↔	↔	↔
ACTH (pg/mL)	10–80	↑↑	↓	↓
Urine				
Cortisol (μg/24 h)	20–90	↑↑	↑↑	↑↑↑

obtained for analysis. The Cushing's patient will not exhibit a suppressed cortisol concentration via the negative-feedback loop, and the morning cortisol concentration will be elevated (> 5 μg/dL).[5] The overnight DST is useful only as a screening tool for Cushing's syndrome because of a high sensitivity but a rather low specificity. Phenytoin, rifampin, phenobarbital, and other drugs that induce liver enzymes may cause an increase in the clearance rate of the dexamethasone, causing decreased levels leading to a falsely positive suppression test.[7] Plasma dexamethasone measured at the conclusion of this test can clarify results clouded by differences in metabolism from these drug interactions, individual variability, or patient noncompliance.

The first test used to determine the etiology of Cushing's syndrome is the plasma ACTH test. Plasma ACTH concentrations can be measured via RIA or IRMA.[7,16] In the ACTH-dependent Cushing's syndrome, ACTH may be normal or elevated. Very high levels of ACTH favor ectopic production. ACTH values are low in ACTH-independent (adrenal) Cushing's syndrome. ACTH levels may appear artificially low in some ectopic ACTH-producing tumors because ACTH can be secreted as an active prohormone that is not detected by the assay.

The high-dose DST operates under the same principle as the low-dose test.[5,7] The high-dose test has its main application in differentiating the adrenal hyperplasia patient from the patient with another form of hypercortisolism. The adrenal hyperplasia patient generally will demonstrate a 50% reduction in urinary steroids over baseline, whereas the others generally will not suppress. The high-dose test is based on the principle that patients with Cushing's syndrome not caused by adrenal tumors or ectopic ACTH production will suppress their hypothalamic-pituitary axis in the presence of glucocorticoids, but it takes much higher than normal doses. An overnight high-dose DST has been developed whereby the patient has a baseline serum cortisol drawn at 8:00 AM and 8 mg dexamethasone is taken at 11:00 PM. The next morning at 8:00 AM, another serum cortisol is drawn.[7,16] The high-dose test is most useful when the low-dose test and other diagnostic studies have confirmed the diagnosis of Cushing's syndrome. The high-dose DST has been studied in combination with ACTH and metapyrone testing and results in better specificity than either test alone.

Abnormal adrenal anatomy is effectively identified using high-resolution CT scanning and perhaps MRI. Nodules as small as 1 to 1.5 cm on the adrenal cortex are identified easily by CT scanning. With the use of thin-section scanning, nodules as small as 3 to 5 mm can be visualized.[7,18,19]

DIFFERENTIAL DIAGNOSIS

Although the diagnosis of Cushing's disease is not a difficult one, at times the clinician will need to differentiate it from syndromes that mimic Cushing's. Pseudo-Cushing's syndrome refers to a group of diseases that can mimic Cushing's disease. Patients with obesity, chronic alcoholism, depression, and acute illness of any type can cloud the diagnosis of Cushing's disease. Depressed patients, though mimicking the urinary steroid abnormalities of Cushing's disease, will not resemble a cushingoid patient in appearance. The chronic alcoholic will have his or her laboratory panel returned to baseline after he or she stops drinking. The obese patient often will have normal cortisol concentrations of both serum and urinary screening. Iatrogenic Cushing's syndrome, induced by glucocorticoid administration, often can be indistinguishable from Cushing's disease. A careful history and serum determination in a basal state can aid the clinician in making the diagnosis. If exogenous glucocorticoids are being taken, plasma cortisol levels may increase while corticosterone levels remain low.[7,20]

PITUITARY-DEPENDENT CUSHING'S DISEASE

The etiology of Cushing's disease of pituitary origin is unknown. A solitary adenoma is almost always the cause.[4] The tumor is usually a microadenoma (<1 cm in diameter), with macroadenomas being rare and corticotrophic hyperplasia and carcinomas being extremely rare.[5] A minority of cases may be caused by excessive ACTH secretion by nonneoplastic corticotropin cells. Currently, the optimal form of therapy uses the hypothalamic, pituitary, and adrenal glands as avenues for intervention.

▶ TREATMENT: Cushing's Syndrome

If left untreated, Cushing's syndrome is associated with a high percentage of morbidity and mortality owing to associated disorders such as diabetes mellitus, cardiovascular disease, and electrolyte abnormalities. These disorders limit the survival of the Cushing's disease patient to 4 to 5 years following initial diagnosis. The desired outcomes of treatment are to limit the morbidity and mortality and return the patient to a normal functional state by removing the source of hypercortisolism without causing any pituitary or adrenal deficiencies.

Once the etiology of the disease is identified, the treatment of choice for both ACTH-dependent and ACTH-independent Cushing's syndrome is surgical resection of any offending tumors.[21] However,

TABLE 76–6. Possible Treatment Plans in Cushing's Syndrome Based on Etiology

Etiology	Treatment				
			Dosing		
	Nondrug	Drug	*Initial*	*Usual*	*Max*
Ectopic ACTH syndrome	Surgery Chemotherapy Irradiation	Metyrapone (Metopirone), 250-mg tabs	1–1.5 g/d, divided q4–6h	1–6 g/d, divided q4–6h	6 g/d
		Aminoglutethimide (Cytadren), 250-mg tabs	0.5–1 g/d, divided 96 bid–qid ×2 weeks	1 g/d, divided q6	2 g/d
Pituitary dependent	Surgery Irradiation	Cyproheptadine (Periactin), 2 mg/5 mL syrup or 4-mg tabs	4 mg bid	24–32 mg/d, divided qid	32 mg/d
		Mitotane (Lysodren), 500-mg tabs	1–6 g/d, increased by 1–2 g/d q3–7d	9–10 g/d, divided tid–qid	16 g/d
		Metyrapone	See above	See above	See above
Adrenal adenoma	Surgery + postoperative replacement	Ketoconazole (Nizoral), 200-mg tabs	200 mg qd–bid	600–800 mg/d, divided bid	1200 mg/d
Adrenal carcinoma	Surgery	Mitotane	See above	See above	See above

many secondary treatment plans are available depending on the etiology of the disease[4,5,22] (Table 76–6).

PHARMACOLOGIC THERAPY

Pharmacotherapy of Cushing's syndrome[23,24] (dosing can be found in Table 76–6) can be divided into four categories based on the anatomic site of action of the agent: (1) steroidogenic inhibitors, (2) adrenolytic agents, (3) neuromodulators of ACTH release, and (4) glucocorticoid-receptor blocking agents.[22,25,26]

Steroidogenic inhibition may be accomplished with the following agents: metyrapone, aminoglutethimide, and ketoconazole. Either metyrapone or aminoglutethamide used alone has limited efficacy, with relapse occurring after discontinuation of therapy. Neither agent should be used after successful surgery. Their use should be restricted to the refractory patient who is not a surgical candidate. Combination therapy with these agents appears more effective than single-agent therapy and may cause fewer side effects.

Metyrapone (Metopirone, Novartis) inhibits 11-hydroxylase activity, resulting in cortisol-synthesis inhibition. Initially, patients may demonstrate an increase in plasma ACTH concentrations because of a sudden drop in cortisol. Metyrapone is biologically active following oral administration. Nausea, vomiting, vertigo, headache, dizziness, abdominal discomfort, and allergic rash have been reported following administration.[22,23]

Initially, aminoglutethimide (Cytadren, Novartis) was used to treat refractory forms of epilepsy, but it was later discovered to be a potent inhibitor of cortisol synthesis. Aminoglutethimide inhibits the conversion of cholesterol to pregnenolone early in the cortisol pathway.[22,27] Plasma cortisol concentrations are reduced by up to 50% following aminoglutethimide therapy. Side effects include severe sedation, nausea, ataxia, and skin rashes.[22,23,27] Most of these reactions are dose-dependent and limit the use of aminoglutethimide in most patients. Aminoglutethimide may decrease the anticoagulant effect of warfarin. Since aminoglutethimide can induce the metabolism of exogenous glucocorticoids, careful titration is required with steroid replacement.

Alone, aminoglutethimide is indicated for short-term use in inoperable Cushing's disease with ectopic ACTH syndrome as the suspected underlying etiology. Aminoglutethimide may be used in combination with metyrapone. Smaller doses of both drugs can be used, therefore minimizing the toxicity associated with either agent. The combination therapy appears effective for various etiologies of Cushing's disease and is useful in the inoperable patient.

The imidazole derivative antifungal ketoconazole[22,25,26] (Nizoral, Janssen) is highly effective in lowering cortisol in Cushing's disease, resulting in normal corticosteroid values in 84% of patients, with an additional 11% of patients reporting improvement. Patients can be maintained successfully for months to years on ketoconazole therapy. In addition to lowering serum cortisol levels, ketoconazole can cause gynecomastia and lower plasma testosterone values. All these effects are attributed to its inhibition of a variety of cytochrome P450 enzymes including 11-hydroxylase and 17-hydroxylase. The most common adverse effects are reversible elevation of hepatic transaminases, gynecomastia, and gastrointestinal upset.

The adrenolytic agent mitotane (*ortho-, para*-dichlorodiphenyldichloroethane, Lysodren, Bristol-Myers Squibb) is a cytotoxic drug that structurally resembles the insecticide chlorophenothane (DDT). Mitotane inhibits the 11-hydroxylation of 11-desoxycortisol and 11-desoxycorticosterone in the cortexs. The net result is a reduced synthesis of cortisol and corticosterone. It decreases cortisol secretion rate, plasma cortisol concentrations, urinary free cortisol, and plasma concentrations of the 17-substituted steroids.[23] This drug appears to selectively inhibit adrenocortical function without causing cellular destruction. Degeneration of cells within the zona fasiculata and reticularis occurs with resulting atrophy of the adrenal cortex. The zona glomerulosa is minimally affected during acute therapy but can become damaged following long-term treatment.

Because mitotane can severely reduce cortisol production, the patient should be hospitalized before initiating therapy. Mitotane should be continued as long as clinical benefits occur. Cortisol secretion rate, plasma cortisol concentration, urinary free cortisol, and urinary steroid production should be monitored to assess response to mitotane. If necessary, steriod replacement therapy can be given. Approximately 80% of mitotane-treated patients develop lethargy and somnolence, and other central nervous system adverse drug reactions occur in approximately 40% of patients. Furthermore, significant but reversible hypercholesterolemia can result from mitotane use.

Neuromodulatory agents include cyproheptadine, bromocriptine, valproic acid, and octreotide. None of the neuromodulatory agents has demonstrated consistent clinical efficacy in the treatment of Cushing's disease. The existence of a bromocriptine-responsive subset of patients remains controversial.[22]

Cyproheptadine (Periactin, Merck) can decrease ACTH secretion in the Cushing's disease patient. Morning plasma cortisol concentrations, as well as 24-hour urinary cortisol (free) concentrations, should be monitored. Side effects are minor and include sedation and hyperphagia. Cyproheptadine should be reserved for nonsurgical candidates who fail more conventional therapy. Because response rate is no more than 30%, patients should be followed closely for relapses.

Glucocorticoid receptor antagonism may be accomplished via RU-486 (mifepristone). RU-486 is a progesterone and glucocorticoid receptor antagonist that inhibits dexamethasone suppression and raises endogenous cortisol and ACTH values in normal subjects.[22,28] Limited clinical experience in Cushing's suggests that RU-486 is highly effective in reversing the manifestation of hypercortisolism. Because of its novel site of action as a receptor antagonist leading to higher cortisol and ACTH levels, the diagnosis of treatment-induced glucocorticoid insufficiency must rest on clinical signs only. The efficacy and long-term effects of RU-486 remain to be determined.

Spironolactone has been used for its competitive antagonism of aldosterone in the treatment of Cushing's syndrome. Spironolactone can provide symptomatic relief of the hypertension and hypokalemia often seen in Cushing's syndrome.

Close monitoring of 24-hour urinary free cortisol levels and serum cortisol levels is essential to monitor for adrenal insufficiency. Steroid secretion should be monitored with all these drugs and steroid replacement given as needed. Whatever the choice, pharmacologic therapy in pituitary-dependent disease is mainly centered around patient stabilization prior to surgery or in patients waiting for potential response to other therapies.

NONPHARMACOLOGIC THERAPY

SURGERY

During the last decade, the treatment of choice for Cushing's disease has been transsphenoidal resection of the pituitary microadenoma.[4,5,21] The advantages to this procedure include preservation of pituitary function, low complication rate, and high clinical improvement rate. The overall cure rate of histologically proven tumors approaches 90%.

Bilateral adrenalectomy surgery had been the mainstay of therapy for years. It is used now only in patients for whom transsphenoidal surgery and pituitary irradiation have failed or cannot be used.[5] Bilateral adrenalectomy rapidly reverses hypercortisolism. However, patients may develop Nelson's syndrome, which involves sella turcica enlargement and hyperpigmentation, caused by postoperative hypothalamic stimulation. Therefore, if bilateral adrenalectomy is used, it should be accompanied by some form of hypothalamic inhibition, such as cyproheptadine.

IRRADIATION

Irradiation (4000 to 5000 rads) of the pituitary has provided clinical improvement in approximately 50% of patients. Improvement is usually not seen until 6 to 12 months after therapy and can create pituitary-dependent hormone deficiencies. Most clinicians will reserve pituitary irradiation for the patient with a mild case of Cushing's disease or as an adjunct to another therapy.[29]

Adrenal Adenoma

Surgical resection of benign adrenal adenoma is associated with relatively few side effects and a high cure rate (95%). The contralateral gland in the patient with adrenal adenoma is usually atrophic. Therefore, steroid replacement is needed both perioperatively and postoperatively. Table 76–7 outlines an approach to steroid replacement for three separate routes of hydrocortisone. Therapy should be continued for 6 to 12 months following surgery. Before replacement therapy is discontinued, recovery of the adrenal axis may be assessed by administering ACTH and measuring cortisol response at 30 and 60 minutes. Cortisol levels should exceed 18 μg/dL before discontinuance of the exogenous steroids.[4]

Adrenal Carcinoma

Unlike the benign adenoma patient, patients with adrenal carcinoma have an unpredictable and unfavorable outcome with surgical resection.[5] Often, the complete tumor cannot be excised, leaving the patients with some degree of symptomatology and extra-adrenal involvement. Irradiation can be used if metastases are discovered. In the patient with adrenal carcinoma who is not a surgical candidate, the focus of treatment is on palliative pharmacologic intervention (e.g., mitotane).

Mitotane appears to be the drug of choice in inoperable functional and nonfunctional adrenal carcinoma. Tumor regression is seen in approximately 35% to 50% of the patients, with most regression occurring between the second and fourth months of therapy. Seventy-five percent of patients will exhibit a 30% fall in urinary steroids, with 50% of patients showing an improved clinical response after 5 months of treatment. Patient survival appears prolonged, although no adequate clinical trials are available to support this assumption.

TABLE 76–7. Alternative Steroid Replacement Regimens in the Adrenal Adenoma Patient

	Hydrocortisone Dose (mg)		
Time	*IV*	*IM*	*PO*
Operation day	300	50 before surgery and 50 after surgery	
Postoperative day 1	200	50 q12	
2	150	50 q12	
3	100	50 q12	
4		50 q12	25 q6
5		25 q12	25 q6[a]
7			25 q6
8–10			25 q8
11–20			25 q12
21+			20 at 8 AM 10 at 4 PM

[a]Add fludrocortisone 0.05–2.0 mg PO qd starting on postoperative day 5. Adjust dose based on blood pressure, body weight, and serum electrolytes.

TABLE 76–8. Potential Causes of Mineralocorticoid Excess

Primary Aldosteronism	
Aldosterone-producing adenoma (APA)	
Bilateral adrenal hyperplasia (BAH)	
Adrenal carcinoma	
Glucocorticoid-remediable hyperaldosteronism	
Secondary Aldosteronism	
Hypertensive	Nonhypertensive
Renal vascular hypertension	Sodium depletion
Renin-secreting tumors	Hemorrhage
Necrotizing vasculitis	Pregnancy
Estrogen therapy	Edema
	Bartter's syndrome
	Diuretic therapy
	Congestive heart failure

Metyrapone, aminoglutethimide, and ketoconazole may be given to attempt control of steroid hypersecretion. 5-Fluorouracil also has been used in combination therapy.

Ectopic Acth Syndrome

In the ectopic ACTH syndrome, multiple sites of tumors exist, and locating the ectopic site is essential but often difficult. Therefore, only approximately 10% of patients are cured following surgery, and the remaining 90% receive postoperative medication.

Pharmacologic management with metyrapone is effective and remains the agent of choice in the ectopic ACTH syndrome.[30] Aminoglutethimide and ketoconazole are alternative agents.[4,30,31] Mitotane has been tried in patients with ectopic ACTH syndrome; however, its side-effect profile generally limits its use. RU-486 (mifepristone) and the somatostatin analog octreotide have been reported to reduce the clinical signs of the ectopic ACTH syndrome.[26,30] Further evaluation of these agents is needed.

HYPERALDOSTERONISM

Excess aldosterone is categorized as either primary or secondary forms of hyperaldosterone[32–41] (Table 76–8).

Primary Aldosteronism

Etiology. Primary aldosteronism implies that the physiologic abnormality is within the adrenal cortex. The most common causes include a solitary adrenal adenoma (60%) or idiopathic adrenocortical hyperplasia (35% bilateral and 5% unilateral). Other rare causes include adrenal cortex carcinoma, primary adrenocortical hyperplasia, renin-responsive adrenocortical adenoma, and genetic mutations, such as in glucocorticoid-suppressible hyperaldosteronism.[34,35]

Clinical Presentation. The incidence of primary aldosteronism is disputed, with estimates ranging from approximately 0.5% to 9.5% of all hypertensive patients.[34,42] The disease is more common in women aged 30 to 50 years. Signs and symptoms may include arterial hypertension, muscle weakness, fatigue, tetany, parasthesia, paralysis, nocturnal polyuria, polydipsia, reduced glucose tolerance (25%), metabolic alkalosis, and headache, although many patients are asymptomatic. Hypokalemia (80% to 90%), suppressed renin activity, elevated plasma aldosterone concentrations, hypernatremia (>142 meq/L), hypomagnesemia, and an elevated bicarbonate concentration (>31 meq/L) are all common laboratory findings in primary aldosteronism.[35]

Diagnosis. The absolute diagnosis is relatively easy based on clinical findings and pertinent laboratory findings. However, as in Cushing's disease, the discovery of the underlying etiology is mandatory to ensure proper treatment. Table 76–9 lists the various abnormalities that must be ruled out when suspicion of hyperaldosteronism is high.

A serum potassium concentration of less than 3.5 mEq/L with a concurrent urinary potassium content greater than 30 mEq per 24 hours is suggestive of primary aldosteronism.[35] Normokalemia does not exclude the diagnosis of primary aldosteronism. Between 7% and 38% of patients with primary aldosteronism will have serum potassium concentrations greater than 3.6 mEq/L. The diagnosis of primary aldosteronism can be made with a plasma-aldosterone-to-plasma-renin-activity ratio (PA:PRA). A PA:PRA of greater than 30 with a plasma aldosterone value of greater than 20 ng/dL has been shown to be 90% sensitive and 91% specific.[39]

Differentiating between an aldosterone-producing adenoma (APA) and bilateral adrenal hyperplasia (BAH) is imperative to formulate a proper treatment plan. A majority of the adenomas are singular and small, less than 1 cm. The left adrenal gland is affected at a higher rate than the right. Patients with APA generally have more

TABLE 76–9. Differential Diagnosis of Primary Aldosteronism

Disease	Plasma Renin Concentration	Plasma Aldosterone Concentration	Blood Pressure
Primary aldosteronism	Low	High	High
Edematous disorders	High	High	Normal
Malignant hypertension	High	High	High
Congenital adrenal hyperplasia	Low	Low	High
Cushing's syndrome	Low to normal	Low to normal	High
Liddle's syndrome	Low	Low	High
Bartter's syndrome	High	High	Low to normal
Licorice ingestion	Low	Low	High
Low-renin essential hypertension	Low	Low to normal	High

severe hypertension, more profound hypokalemia, and higher plasma and urinary aldosterone levels compared with patients with BAH. CT scanning usually can detect most adenomas, although nonfunctional adenomas occasionally may cause confusion.

The underlying abnormality in BAH remains a mystery, but some investigators believe that a hormone factor stimulates the zona glomerulosa, resulting in increased sensitivity to angiotensin II.[34] In contrast to APA patients, patients with BAH are able to maintain control of the renin-angiotensin system, with little effect following doses of ACTH.

Therapeutic Management: BAH-Dependent Hyperaldosteronism. Spironolactone (Aldactone, Pharmacia), a competitive inhibitor of aldosterone, is the drug of choice in BAH-dependent hyperal- dosteronism.[35,36] Spironolactone inhibits aldosterone biosynthesis within the adrenal gland, making it extremely useful in overstimulated BAH patients. Spironolactone is available in oral form, with most patients responding to doses in the 25 to 400 mg/d range. The clinician should wait 4 to 8 weeks before reassessing the patient for urinary electrolytes and blood pressure control. Adverse effects of spironolactone include gastrointestional discomfort, impotence, gynecomastia, and menstrual irregularities. Additionally, because salicylates increase the renal secretion of canrenone, the active metabolite, patients should be advised to avoid concomitant therapy with salicylates. Because spironolactone blocks testosterone biosynthesis, it often is not used in men. The drug of choice in men and patients intolerant of spironolactone is amiloride (Midamor, Merck).[34,43] The usual dose is 5 mg twice a day up to 30 mg/d if necessary.

Second-line therapy often is required to control the blood pressure of patients with BAH. Agents useful as second-line choices include the calcium channel blockers, angiotensin-converting enzyme (ACE) inhibitors, and low-dose diuretics such as HCTZ.[35,43]

Therapeutic Management: APA-Dependent Hyperaldosteronism. The treatment of choice for APA-dependent aldosteronism remains laparoscopic resection of the adenoma.[44] If no primary lesion is found, resection of one and a half of the adrenal glands may be attempted, followed by supplemental spironolactone therapy.

Summary. The diagnosis of primary aldosteronism is made through the observation of elevated blood pressure, low serum potassium, high urinary potassium, elevated serum and urinary aldosterone, and an elevated PA:PRA (Fig. 76–5). Differentiating between the various etiologies is mandatory. Patients with adrenal adenomas can be distinguished from patients with hyperplasia by CT scan. Treatment

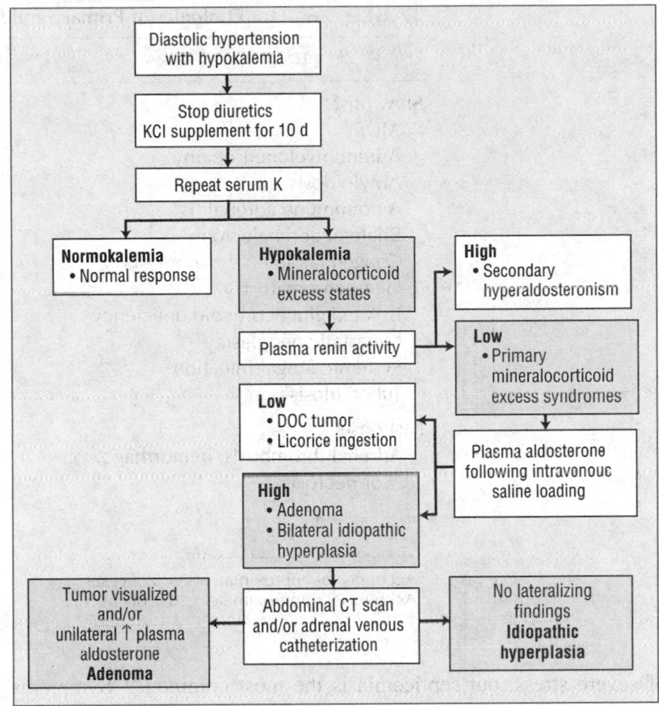

FIGURE 76–5. Algorithm for the diagnosis of primary aldosteronism.

depends on the etiology with surgical resection, well accepted as the treatment of choice in adenomas, and spironolactone or amiloride plus second-line agents in patients with hyperplasia.

Secondary Aldosteronism

Secondary hyperaldosteronism results from stimulation of the zona glomerulosa by an extra-adrenal factor, usually the renin-angiotensin system. Excessive potassium intake can create a physiologic increase in aldosterone, as can oral contraceptive use, pregnancy (10 times normal by third trimester), and menses. Congestive heart failure, cirrhosis, renal artery stenosis, and Bartter's syndrome also can lead to elevated aldosterone concentrations.

Treatment of secondary aldosteronism is dictated by etiology. Control or correction of the extra-adrenal stimulation of aldosterone secretion should resolve the disorder. Medical therapy with spironolactone is the mainstay of treatment until an exact etiology can be located.

HYPOFUNCTION OF THE ADRENAL GLAND

Primary adrenal insufficiency, or Addison's disease, involves the destruction of all regions of the adrenal cortex. Deficiencies arise in cortisol, aldosterone, and the various androgens.[45] Approximately 40% to 53% of patients with idiopathic primary adrenal insufficiency present with one or more clinical disorders involving multiple endocrine organs. The organs involved can include ovary, thyroid, pancreas, and parathyroid gland. This polyglandular failure syndrome is associated with the idiopathic etiology only and has not been seen with adrenal insufficiency associated with tuberculosis or other invasive diseases.

Secondary insufficiency most commonly results from exogenous steroid use, leading to suppression of the hypothalamic-pituitary axis and resulting in a deficiency of ACTH and low concentrations of androgen and cortisol. Chronic suppression also can result in atrophy of the anterior pituitary and hypothalamus, impairing recovery of function if the exogenous steroid is reduced. Secondary disease classically presents with normal concentrations of mineralocorticoids.

Approximately 90% of the adrenal cortex must be destroyed before adrenal insufficiency symptoms will occur.[46] Specific etiologies for both primary and secondary insufficiency are listed in Table 76–10. Symptoms common in patients with adrenal insufficiency include weakness, weight loss, increased pigmentation, hypotension, gastrointestinal symptoms, postural dizziness, and vitiligo.[45,47]

Adrenal hemorrhage can result from multiple etiologies, traumatic shock, coagulopathics, ischemic disorders, and other situations

TABLE 76–10. Etiologies of Primary and Secondary Adrenal Insufficiency

Primary Insufficiency	Secondary Insufficiency
Slow onset	
AIDS	Craniopharyngioma
Adrenomyeloneuropathy	Cure of Cushing's syndrome
Amyloidosis	Empty-sella syndrome
Autoimmune adrenalitis[a]	Tumors of the third ventricle
Bilateral adrenalectomy	Histiocytosis
Congenital adrenal hypoplasia	Hypothalamic tumors
Hemochromatosis	Hypopituitarism
Isolated glucocorticoid deficiency	Long-term corticosteroid administration
Metastatic neoplasia	Lymphocytic hypophysitis
Systemic fungal infection	Pituitary surgery, radiation, or tumor
Tuberculosis[b]	Sarcoidosis
Fast onset	
Adrenal thrombosis, hemorrhage, or necrosis	Postpartum pituitary necrosis
	Necrotic or bleeding pituitary macroadenoma
	Head trauma, lesions of the pituitary stalk
	Pituitary or adrenal surgery for Cushing's

[a]Accounts for approximately 70% of cases.
[b]Accounts for approximately 20% of cases.

of severe stress, but septicemia is the most common.[47] Symptoms include truncal pain, fever, shaking, chills, hypotension preceding shock, anorexia, headache, vertigo, vomiting, rash, psychiatric symptoms, abdominal rigidity or rebound, and death in 6 to 48 hours if not treated. The most common organisms found on autopsy are *Streptococcus pneumoniae, Staphylococcus,* and *Haemophilus influenzae.*

ADDISON'S DISEASE

Distinguishing Addison's disease from secondary insufficiency is difficult; however, the following guidelines may be helpful:

1. Hyperpigmentation usually is not seen in secondary adrenal insufficiency because of low amounts of melanocyte-stimulating hormone (MSH). Low amounts of MSH are present owing to a deficient pituitary secretion of ACTH and β-lipotropin, all of which are synthesized together in a common precursor peptide, pro-opiomelanocortin (POMC).
2. Aldosterone secretion usually is preserved in secondary insufficiency.
3. Weight loss, dehydration, hyponatremia, hyperkalemia, and elevated blood urea nitrogen are common in Addison's disease.
4. Addison's disease will have an abnormal response to the rapid ACTH stimulation test. Plasma ACTH levels are usually 400 to 2000 pg/mL in primary insufficiency versus normal to low (0 to 50 pg/mL; see Table 76–5) in secondary insufficiency. A normal cosyntropin stimulation test does not rule out secondary adrenal insufficiency.

The short cosyntropin stimulation test can be used to assess patients suspected of hypocortisolism. Patients are given 250 μg of synthetic ACTH intravenously or intramuscularly, with serum cortisol levels drawn at baseline and 30 to 60 minutes after the injection. An increase to a cortisol level of 20 μg/dL or greater rules out adrenal insufficiency. While this test remains the most commonly used method, in some patients with secondary adrenal insufficiency, this test will be normal. This result may be owing to the high dose of corticotropin given. Thus some clinicians suggest that higher cutoff values ($\geq$22 to 25 μg/dL) should be used.[48] Alternatively, studies have demonstrated that equivalent results can be seen using 1 μg cosyntropin. The normal response is 18 μg/dL or greater at baseline or 20 to 60 minutes after the injection. Other tests include the insulin hypoglycemia test, the metyrapone test, and the CRH stimulation test.[45,47,49]

Treatment of Addison's disease must include adequate patient education so that the patient is aware of treatment complications, expected outcome, missed doses, and drug side effects. The agents of choice are prednisone, hydrocortisone, and cortisone, with the treatment objective being the establishment of the lowest effective dose while mimicking the normal diurnal adrenal rhythm.[45] Usually, a twice-daily dosing schedule is adequate, with the dose used depending on the steroid chosen. A morning dose of cortisone (25 mg), hydrocortisone (20 mg), or prednisone (5 mg) followed by an evening dose of the same agent at 33% to 50% of the morning dose is usually sufficient to duplicate the normal circadian rhythm of cortisol production. To replace the mineralocorticoid loss, fludrocortisone acetate (Florinef, Apothecon) can be used. A dose of 0.05 to 0.2 mg by mouth once a day is adequate. If parenteral therapy is needed, 2 to 5 mg of deoxycorticosterone trimethylacetate in oil intramuscularly every 3 to 4 weeks can be used. The main reason for adding the mineralocorticoid is to minimize the development of hyperkalemia. Adverse effects must be monitored closely. Symptoms include gastric upset, edema, hypertension, hypokalemia, insomnia, excitability, and diabetes mellitus. In addition, patient weight, blood pressure, and electrocardiogram should be monitored regularly.[45,47]

The end point of therapy is difficult to assess in most patients, but a reduction in excess pigmentation is a good clinical marker. The development of features of Cushing's syndrome indicates excessive replacement. Treatment of secondary adrenal insufficiency is identical to primary disease treatment with the exception that mineralocorticoid replacement usually is not necessary. Patient education still should be stressed, with emphasis placed on establishing an alternate-day regimen.

ACUTE ADRENAL INSUFFICIENCY

Adrenal crisis, or Addisonian crisis, is characterized by an acute adrenocortical insufficiency. Adrenal crisis represents a true endocrine emergency. Anything that increases adrenal requirements dramatically can precipitate an adrenal crisis. Stressful situations, surgery, infection, and trauma all are potential triggering events, especially in the patient with some underlying adrenal or pituitary insufficiency. The most common cause of adrenal crisis is hypothalamic-pituitary-adrenal (HPA) axis suppression brought on by chronic use of exogenous glucocorticoids.

Early symptoms of acute adrenal insufficiency include myalgias, malaise, anorexia, weakness, and weight loss. As the situation continues, vomiting, fever, hypotension, and shock will develop. Hyponatremia, hypoglycemia, and hypercalcemia also may be present.

Treatment of adrenal crisis involves the administration of parenteral glucocorticoids. Hydrocortisone (Solu-cortef, Upjohn) is the agent of choice owing to its combined mineralocorticoid and glucocorticoid activity. Hydrocortisone is started at 100 mg intravenously through rapid infusion and followed by a continuos infusion or intermittent bolus of 100 mg every 6 to 8 hours. Intravenous administration is continued for 24 to 48 hours, at which time, if the patient is stable, oral hydrocortisone may be started at a dose of 50 mg every 8 hours for another 48 hours. Following oral maintenance therapy, a hydrocortisone taper is initiated until the dosage is 30 to 50 mg/d in divided doses. Fluid replacement often is required and may be accomplished with 5% dextrose and isotonic saline (D_5NS) at a rate to support blood pressure. If hyperkalemia is present after the hydrocortisone maintenance phase, additional mineralocorticoid usually is required. Fludrocortisone acetate in a dose of 0.1 mg by mouth daily is the agent of choice.

Patients with adrenal insufficiency should be instructed to carry a card or wear a bracelet or necklace, such as Medic Alert, that contains information about their condition. Patients also should have easy access to injectable hydrocortisone or glucocorticoid suppositories in case of an emergency or during times of physical stress, such as febrile illness or injury.[47]

HYPOALDOSTERONISM

Hypoaldosteronism is rare and usually is associated with low renin status, diabetes, complete heart block, or severe postural hypotension, or it may occur postoperatively following tumor removal.[2] Hypoaldosteronism may be part of a larger adrenal insufficiency or may be the only defect the patient has. In nonselective hypoaldosteronism, the etiology of the low aldosterone is most likely generalized adrenocortical insufficiency (see Addison's disease). In selective hypoaldosteronism, the etiology is usually a specific defect in the stimulation of adrenal aldosterone secretion (21-hydroxylase deficiency most common) or a defect in peripheral aldosterone action (decreased aldosterone receptors).

Laboratory analysis reveals low serum sodium and high serum potassium concentrations. Patients often will present with hyperchloremic metabolic acidosis. Because the deficiency is in the mineralocorticoid, replacement with fludrocortisone in a dose of 0.1 to 0.3 mg is usually effective. Patients should be followed for blood pressure response as well as electrolyte status.

CONGENITAL ADRENAL HYPERPLASIA

Because many enzyme systems are needed to complete the complex cholesterol-to-cortisol pathway, enzyme deficiencies may lead to disruptions of the normal cascade of events (see Fig. 76–2). This group of enzyme disorders is known as congenital adrenal hyperplasia mainly because of the resulting chronic adrenal gland stimulation that occurs following enzyme deficiency.[50,51] Any enzyme deficiency is capable of affecting any one or all three of the steroid pathways.[52] Therefore, treatment should be focused on replacement of the deficient hormone as well as cessation of chronic stimulation causing the hyperplasia. In Table 76–11, six of the most common enzyme deficiencies are briefly outlined.

ADRENAL VIRILISM

Virilism, excessive secretion of androgens from the adrenal gland, is seen more commonly in females, with hirsutism being the dominant feature. Women who present with hirsutism also may have voice deepening, increased muscle mass, menstrual abnormalities, clitoral enlargement, redistribution of body fat and loss of female body contour, breast atrophy, and hair recession and crown balding.[53] Although virilism may be easy to diagnose based on clinical symptoms, making the diagnosis on a biochemical basis is difficult. The most common etiology of virilism involves one of many possible congenital enzyme defects. Depending on the enzyme deficiency, accumulation of a variety of androgens, notably testosterone, can develop.

Treatment of virilism centers around suppression of the pituitary-adrenal axis with exogenous glucocorticoids. Choice of steroids is variable. In adults, the usual steroids used are dexamethasone (0.25 to 0.5 mg), prednisone (2.5 to 5.0 mg), or hydrocortisone (10 to 20 mg).[53] Antiandrogen use may allow lower steroid doses to be used.

HIRSUTISM

Hirsutism (hypertrichosis) is defined as more hair than is cosmetically acceptable. The majority of cases occur in women with some degree of excess androgen production, although certain drugs also may induce hirsutism. Examples of such drugs include minoxidil, phenytoin, cyclosporine, methyldopa, danazol, metoclopramide, phenothiazines, reserpine, and diazoxide. Androgen excess can be derived from either the ovaries or the adrenal glands, with a small fraction coming from pituitary disorders. Ovarian excess typically is associated with obesity and menstrual abnormalities. In the patient with hirsutism, congenital adrenal hyperplasia, adrenal tumors, and ovarian tumors should be ruled out.[53,54]

Cosmetic approaches generally are tried first, with laser photothermodestruction offering the greatest long-term success. Only when cosmetic surgery is ineffective should suppressive therapy be used. Glucocorticoids, such as dexamethasone, can be used if the androgen source is adrenal but may induce cushingoid symptoms even in doses of 0.5 mg/d. Oral contraceptives can be used in patients who require contraception concurrently. If oral contraceptives are used, a progestin with low androgen activity (norethynodrel or ethynodiol diacetate) should be employed.

Gonadotropin-releasing hormone may be an effective adjunct to oral contraceptives if the source of androgen is ovarian. Antiandrogens are often added to the more specific therapies. The most common

TABLE 76–11. Congenital Adrenal Hyperplasia (CAH)

Enzyme Deficiency (Disorder)	Symptoms	Lab Tests	Comments
20-Hydroxylase (nonvirilizing CAH)	Enlarged female genitalia and adrenal gland (due to cholesterol)	All steroids are low in blood and urine	Poor prognosis for infants
17-Hydroxylase (nonvirilizing CAH)	Hypertension usually present	Low concentrations of cortisol and estrogens	Mineralocorticoid replacement not necessary
21-Hydroxylase (virilizing CAH)	Pubertal irregularities (acne, early pubic hair, voice lowering, increased muscularity) Mature normally with replacement	High progesterone, renin, 17-hydroxyprogesterone and ACTH Low cortisol, sodium and aldosterone	Most common form of CAH (90% of total), incidence of 1/10,000 Monitor growth velocity, bone age, renin and 17-hydroxyprogesterone
11-Hydroxylase (virilizing CAH)	Hypertension, secondary to high deoxycortisol and virilism from androgen excess Mistaken for Cushing's, but no glucose intolerance	Low plasma cortisone and aldosterone High ACTH and MSH concentrations	Second most common form of CAH (9% of total), incidence of 1/100,000 Final step in biosynthesis of corticosterone and cortisol; found only in adrenal cortex
3-Hydroxysteroid dehydrogenase (mixed CAH)	Both cortisol and aldosterone deficiencies	Decreased aldosterone, cortisol, estrogens and androgens Increased pregnenolone and cholesterol	Defect effects both adrenals and gonads
18-Hydroxysteroid dehydrogenase (corticosterone methyloxidase deficiency)	Hypotension	Restricted to zona glomerulosa-sole aldosterone defect: hyponatremia, hyperkalemia, increased renin	Mineralocorticoid replacement without glucocorticoid replacement

include spironolactone, flutamide (Eulexin, Schering), and finasteride (Proscar, Merck), although none of these is FDA approved for the treatment of hirsutism. It can take 4 months for the antiandrogens to alleviate the hirsutism, and duration of therapy is unclear.[53,54]

PRINCIPLES OF GLUCOCORTICOID ADMINISTRATION

Originally, the term *glucocorticoid* was given to these agents to describe their glucose-regulating properties. However, carbohydrate metabolism is only one of a multitude of effects that steroids can exhibit. The activity produced is a function of the receptor activated (glucocorticoid versus mineralocorticoid) as well as the agent and dose prescribed.

The mechanism of glucocorticoids is complex and not fully known. The glucocorticoid enters the cell through passive diffusion and binds to its specific receptor. There are between 5000 and 100,000 receptors per cell. Steroids exhibit various binding affinities to the vast number of receptors in almost every tissue and therefore elicit a wide variety of biologic effects.

After binding to the receptor, there is a structural change that occurs in the receptor, known as *activation*. After activation, the receptor-steroid complex binds to DNA sites in the cell called *glucocorticoid regulatory elements* (GREs). This binding to the GREs stimulates or inhibits transcription of nearby genes.

The pharmacokinetics of the glucocorticoids varies with the agent given and the route of administration. In general, most steroids given by the oral route are well absorbed. Water-soluble agents are absorbed more rapidly following intramuscular injection than are lipid-soluble agents. Intravenous administration is recommended when a quick onset of action is needed. A summary of the steroids is provided in Table 76–12.

In addition to systemic steroids causing iatrogenic Cushing's syndrome, they also can lead to increased susceptibility to infection, osteoporosis, sodium retention with resulting edema, hypokalemia, hypomagnesemia, cataracts, peptic ulcer disease, seizures, and generalized suppression of the HPA axis. Long-term complications tend to be insidious and less likely to respond to steroid withdrawal.

Suppression of the HPA axis is a major concern whenever systemic steroids are tapered or withdrawn. Single doses of glucocorticoids can prevent the axis from responding to major stressors for several hours. In general, the longer the steroid is administered and the higher the dose used, the more suppression of the axis that occurs. However, the possibility of suppression occurs anytime the patient is exposed to supraphysiologic doses of a steroid.[49,55] Symptoms of steroid withdrawal resemble those seen in a patient with adrenocortical deficiency.

A number of recommendations for steroid tapering are available.[49,56,57] In general, patients who have been on long-term steroid therapy will need to be withdrawn gradually toward physiologic doses over months. On average, the normal adult produces approximately 20 to 30 mg cortisol per day, with the peak concentration occurring around 8:00 AM. As the steroid or steroid-equivalent dose approaches the 20- to 30-mg level, the taper should be slowed

TABLE 76–12. Relative Potencies of Glucocorticoids

Glucocorticoid	Anti-inflammatory Potency	Equivalent Potency (mg)	Approximate Half-life (min)	Sodium-Retaining Potency
Cortisone	0.8	25.0	30	2.0
Hydrocortisone	1.0	20.0	90	2.0
Prednisone	3.5	5.0	60	1.0
Prednisolone	4.0	5.0	200	1.0
Triamcinolone	5.0	4.0	300	0.0
Methylprednisolone	5.0	4.0	180	0.0
Betamethasone	25.0	0.6	100–300	0.0
Dexamethasone	30.0	0.75	100–300	0.0

and the patient checked for axis function. The primary mode to test HPA integrity is the ACTH test, either high or low dose. A normal ACTH test would indicate that daily steroid maintenance therapy is not needed. More recently, the use of exogenous human CRH was found to be nearly as useful in the assessment of pituitary-adrenal function.[58] Caution should be used to prevent disease exacerbation during the steroid taper to avoid the necessity of rebolusing the patient with another course of high-dose steroids. The dilemma of prolonged steroid administration is sometimes lessened by the use of an alternate-day therapy (ADT) regimen.[56,57] ADT theoretically minimizes the hypothalamic-pituitary suppression as well as some of the adverse effects seen with once-daily therapy. This can be especially important in the treatment of children and young adults, in whom growth suppression is a major concern. ADT is not recommended for initial management but rather in the management of the stabilized patient who needs long-term therapy. The patient will be exposed to "on" and "off" days, with the "on" day dose gradually increased with concurrent reduction in the "off" day dose over a period of 14 days. By the fourteenth day, the patient will be consuming medication only on the "on" day. It should be noted that not all patients will have equivalent disease control on ADT, and it should be avoided in certain indications.[57]

EVALUATION OF THERAPEUTIC OUTCOMES

Successful glucocorticoid therapy involves counseling the patient, monitoring the patient, and recognizing complications of therapy (Table 76–13). The risk-benefit ratio of glucocorticoid administration always should be considered, especially with concurrent disease states such as hypertension, diabetes mellitus, peptic ulcer disease, and uncontrolled systemic infections.

TABLE 76–13. Factors in Successful Glucocorticoid Therapy[59,60]

Monitoring	Glucose concentrations (serum and urine) Electrolytes (serum and urine) Ophthalmologic exams Stool tests for occult blood loss Growth and development (children and adolescents)
Counseling	Take with food to minimize gastrointestinal discomfort Never discontinue medication on your own; check with physician. Gradual dose reduction is usually necessary Carry or wear medical identification indicating that you are on long-term glucocorticoid therapy Dosage increases may be necessary at times of increased stress (surgery or emergency treatments) Be aware of potential side effects (i.e visual distrubances, bruising, delayed wound healing) What to do if you miss a dose. If your dosing schedule is: Every other day—Take as soon as possible if remembered that morning. If not remembered until later, skip that day. Take the next morning, then skip the following day. Every day—Take as soon as possible, but skip if almost time for the next dose. Never double doses.
Recognizing complications	Early in therapy and essentially unavoidable: insomnia, enhanced appetite, weight gain. Common in patients with underlying risk factors: hypertension, diabetes mellitus, peptic ulcer disease. Long-term intense treatment: Cushingoid habitus, hypothalamic-pituitary-adrenal suppression, impaired wound healing. Delayed and insidious: cataracts, atherosclerosis Rare and unpredictable: psychosis, glaucoma, pancreatitis

► PRINCIPLES OF PHARMACOTHERAPY

- CRH is secreted from the hypothalamus and stimulates the release of corticotropin (ACTH) from the anterior pituitary, which in turn stimulates glucocorticoid secretion from the adrenal cortex.
- Cushing's syndrome results from hypercortisolism originating either from exogenous administration or from endogenous overproduction by the adrenal glands or abnormal adrenocortical tissues.
- Surgery is the treatment of choice for both ACTH-dependent and ACTH-independent Cushing's syndrome, and pharmacologic treatment is reserved for use as adjunctive therapy or in refractory or inoperable disease.
- Pharmacologic agents for Cushing's syndrome can be divided into three categories: (a) steroidogenic inhibitors (mitotane, metyrapone, aminoglutethimide, ketoconazole), (b) neuromodulators of ACTH release (cyproheptadine, bromocriptine, valproic acid, octreotide), and (c) glucocorticoid-receptor blocking agents (mifepristone).
- Hyperaldosteronism is classified as excess aldosterone production from adrenal cortex (primary) or from stimulation of the zona glomerulosa by an extra-adrenal factor, usually the renin-angiotensin system.
- Primary aldosteronism is usually caused by an APA, which is treated with surgery, or bilateral adrenal hyperplasia, which is treatable with spironolactone or amiloride.
- Addison's disease (primary adrenal insufficiency) involves the loss of function of all regions of the adrenal cortex and a resulting deficiency in cortisol, aldosterone, and various androgens.
- Secondary adrenal insufficiency usually results from exogenous steroid use, leading to suppression of the hypothalamic-pituitary axis and decreased release of ACTH, resulting in low levels of androgens and cortisol.
- Virilism, the excessive secretion of androgens from the adrenal gland, is usually seen as hirsutism in females and is treated with glucocorticoid suppression of the pituitary-adrenal axis.
- Glucocorticoid suppression of the HPA axis occurs whenever a patient is exposed to supraphysiologic doses of a steroid and becomes a concern whenever the steroids are tapered or withdrawn.

REFERENCES

1. Conn JW. Primary aldosteronism, a new clinical syndrome. J Lab Clin Med 1955;45:6–17.
2. Orth DN, Kovacs WJ. The adrenal cortex. In: Wilson JD, Foster DW, Kronenberg HM, Larsen PR, eds. Williams' Textbook of Endocrinology. Philadelphia, Saunders, 1998:517–664.
3. Albright F. Cushing syndrome. Harvey Lect 1942–1943;38:123–186.
4. Neiman L, Cutler GB. Cushing's syndrome. In: Degroot LJ, ed. Endocrinology, 3d ed. Philadelphia, Saunders, 1995:1741–1769.
5. Orth DN. Cushing's syndrome. N Engl J Med 1995;332:791–803.
6. Danese RD, Aron DC. Cushing's syndrome and hypertension. Endocrinol Metab Clin North Am 1994;23:299–324.
7. Newell-Price J, Trainer P, Besser M, Grossman A. The diagnosis and differential diagnosis of Cushing's syndrome and pseudo-Cushing's states. Endoer Rev 1998;19:647–672.
8. Fiad TM, Kirby JM, Cunningham SK, McKenna TJ. The overnight single-dose metyrapone test is a simple and reliable index of the hypothalamic-pituitary-adrenal axis. Clin Endocrinol 1994;40:603–609.
9. de Herder WW, Krenning EP, Malchoff CD, et al. Somatostain receptor scintigraphy: Its value in tumor localization in patients with Cushing's syndrome caused by ectopic corticotropin or corticotropin-releasing hormone secretion. Am J Med 1994;96:305–312.
10. Malerbi DA, Liberman B, Corradini MC, et al. The desmopressin stimulation test in the differential diagnosis of Cushing's syndrome. Clin Endocrinol 1993;38:463–472.
11. Jackson RV, Hockings GI, Torpy DJ, et al. New diagnostic tests for Cushing's syndrome: Uses of naloxone, vasopressin and alprazolam. Clin Exp Pharmacol Physiol 1996;23:579–581.
12. Ambrosi B, Bochicchio D, Colombo P, Fadin C, Faglia G. Loperamide to diagnose Cushing's syndrome. JAMA 1993;270:2301–2302.
13. de Herder WW, Uitterlinden P, Pieterman H, et al. Pituitary tumour localization in patients with Cushing's disease by magnetic resonance imaging: Is there a place for petrosal sinus sampling? Clin Endocrinol 1994;40:87–92.
14. Snow K, Nai-Siang J, Kao P, Scheithauer BW. Biochemical evaluation of adrenal dysfunction: The laboratory perspective. Mayo Clin Proc 1992;67:1055–1065.
15. Avgerinos PC, Yanovski JA, Oldfield EW, et al. The metyrapone and dexamethasone suppression tests for the differential diagnosis of the adrenocorticotropin-dependent Cushing's syndrome: A comparison. Ann Intern Med 1994;121:318–327.
16. Findling JW, Raff H. Newer diagnostic techniques and problems in Cushing's disease. Endocrinol Metab Clin North Am 1999;28:191–210.
17. Arvat E, Giordano R, Ramunni J, et al. Adrenocorticotropin and cortisol hyperresponsiveness to hexarelin in patients with Cushing's disease bearing a pituitary microadenoma, but not in those with macroadenoma. J Clin Endocrinol Metab 1998;83:4207–4211.
18. Dunnick NR, Leight GS Jr, Roubidoux MA, et al. CT in the diagnosis of primary aldosteronism: Sensitivity in 29 patients. AJR 1993;160:321–324.
19. Shamma FN, Abrahams JJ. Imaging in endocrine disorders. J Reprod Med 1992;37:39–45.
20. Tsigos C, Crousus GP. Differential diagnosis and management of Cushing's syndrome. Annu Rev Med 1996;47:443–461.
21. Lamberts SWJ, van der Lely AJ, de Herder WW. Transsphenoidal adenomectomy is the treatment of choice in patients with Cushing's disease: Considerations concerning preoperative medical treatment and long-term follow up. J Clin Endocrinol Metab 1995;80:3111–3113.
22. Sonino N, Boscaro M. Medical therapy for Cushing's disease. Endocrinol Metab Clin North Am 1999;28:211–222.
23. McEvoy GK, ed. American Hospital Formulary Service (AHFS) Drug Information. American Society of Hospital Pharmacists, 2000:24–25, 113–119, 1022–1024, 2307–2309.
24. United States Pharmacopeial Convention, Inc. USPDI: Drug Information for the Health Care Professional, Vol. 1, 19th ed. Taunton, MA: Rand-McNally, 1999:67–69.
25. Engelhardt D. Steroid biosynthesis inhibitors in Cushing's syndrome. Clin Invest 1994;72:481–488.
26. Engelhardt D, Weber MM. Therapy of Cushing's syndrome with steroid biosynthesis inhibitors. J Steroid Biochem Mol Biol 1994;49:261–267.
27. Cocconi G. First generation aromatase inhibitors—Aminoglutethimide and testololactone. Breast Cancer Res Treat 1994;30:57–80.
28. Agarwal MK. The antiglucocorticoid action of mifepristone. Pharmacol Ther 1996;70:183–213.
29. Estrada J, Boronat M, Mielgo M, et al. The long-term outcome of pituitary irradiation after unsuccessful transsphenoidal surgery in Cushing's disease. N Engl J Med 1997;336:172–177.
30. Comi RJ, Gorden P. Long-term medical treatment of ectopic ACTH syndrome. South Med J 1998;91:1014–1018.

31. Winquist EW, Laskey J, Crump M, et al. Ketoconazole in the management of paraneoplastic Cushing's syndrome secondary to ectopic adrenocorticotropin production. J Clin Oncol 1995;13:157–164.
32. Bravo EL. Primary aldosteronism: Issues in diagnosis and management. Endocrinol Metab Clin North Am 1994;23:271–283.
33. Corry DB, Tuck ML. Secondary aldosteronism. Endocrinol Metab Clin North Am 1995;24:511–529.
34. Stewart PM. Mineralcorticoid hypertension. Lancet 1999;353:1341–1347.
35. Ganguly A. Primary aldosteronism. N Engl J Med 1998;339;1828–1834.
36. Holland OB. Primary aldosteronism. Semin Nephrol 1995;15:116–125.
37. Vallotton MB. Primary aldosteronism: I. Diagnosis of primary aldosteronism. Clin Endocrinol 1996;45:47–52.
38. Vallotton MB. Primary aldosteronism: II. Differential diagnosis of primary hyperaldosteronism and pseudoaldosteronism. Clin Endocrinol 1996;45:53–60.
39. Weinberger MH, Finebrg NS. The diagnosis of primary aldosteronism and separation of two major subtypes. Arch Intern Med 1993;153:2125–2129.
40. Torpy DJ, Stratakis CA, Chrousos GP. Hyper- and hypoaldosteronism. Vitam Horm 1999;57:177–216.
41. Young WF. Primary aldosteronism: A common and curable form of hypertension. Cardiol Rev 1999;7:207–214.
42. Fardella CE, Mosso L, Gomez-Sanchez C, et al. Primary hyperaldosteronism in essential hypertensives: Prevalence, biochemical profile, and molecular biology. J Clin Endocrinol Metab 2000;85:1863–1867.
43. Blumenfield JD, Sealey JE, Schlussel Y, et al. Diagnosis and treatment of primary hyperaldosteronism. Ann Intern Med 1994;121:877–885.
44. Gagner M, Pomp A, Heniford BT, et al. Laparoscopic adrenalectomy: Lessons learned from 100 consecutive procedures. Ann Surg 1997; 226:238–246.
45. Oelkers W. Adrenal insufficiency. N Engl J Med 1996;335:1206–1212.
46. Carey RM. The changing clinical spectrum of adrenal insufficiency. Ann Intern Med 1997;127:1103–1105.
47. Werbel SS, Ober KP. Acute adrenal insufficiency. Endocrinol Metab Clin North Am 1993;22:303–328.
48. Oelkers W. The role of high- and low-dose corticotropin tests in the diagnosis of secondary adrenal insufficiency. Eur J Endocrinol 1998;139:567–570.
49. Krasner AS. Glucocorticoid-induced adrenal insuffiency. JAMA 1999; 282:671–676.
50. Thorn GW. The adrenal cortex. Johns Hopkins Med J 1968;123:49–77.
51. Deaton MA, Glorioso JE, McLean DB. Congenital adrenal hyperplasia: Not really a zebra. Am Fam Physician 1999;59:1190–1196.
52. Kuttenn F, Couillin P, Girard F, et al. Late-onset adrenal hyperplasia in hirsutism. N Engl J Med 1985;313:224–231.
53. Rittmaster RS. Hirsutism. Lancet 1997;349:191–195.
54. Bergfeld WF. Hirsutism in women: effective therapy that is safe for long-term use. Postgrad Med 2000;107:93–104.
55. Henzen C, Suter A, Lerch E, et al. Suppression and recovery of adrenal response after short-term, high-dose glucocorticoid treatment. Lancet 2000;355:542–545.
56. Kountz DS, Clark CL. Safely withdrawing patients from chronic glucocorticoid therapy. Am Fam Physician 1997;55:521–552.
57. Baxter JD. Advances in glucocorticoid therapy. Adv Intern Med 2000; 45:317–349.
58. Schlaghecke R, Kornely E, Santen RT, et al. The effect of long-term glucocorticoid therapy on pituitary-adrenal responses to exogenous corticotropin-releasing hormone. N Engl J Med 1992;326:226 230.
59. United States Pharmacopeial Convention, Inc. USPDI: Advice for the Patient: Drug Information in Lay Language, Vol. 2, 19th ed. Taunton, MA: Rand-McNally 1999:612–616.
60. Barlow JE. Complications of therapy. In: Boumpas DT, moderator. Glucocorticoid therapy for immune mediated diseases: Basic and clinical correlates. Ann Intern Med 1993;119:1198–1208.

77

Pituitary Gland Disorders

Amy M. Heck, Jack A. Yanovski, and Karim Anton Calis

In the 1950s, Geoffrey Harris and his colleagues uncovered the physiologic importance of pituitary hormones and proposed the theory of neurohormonal regulation of the pituitary by the hypothalamus.[1] Today the pituitary gland is recognized for its essential role in body homeostasis, and for this reason, it is often referred to as the "master gland." The hypothalamus and the pituitary gland are closely connected, and together they provide a means of communication between the brain and many of the body's endocrine organs. The hypothalamus uses nervous input and metabolic signals from the body to control the secretion of pituitary hormones that regulate growth, thyroid function, adrenal activity, reproduction, lactation, and fluid balance.

ANATOMY AND PHYSIOLOGY

The hypothalamus (Fig. 77–1) is a small region at the base of the brain that receives autonomic nervous input from different areas of the body to regulate limbic functions such as motivation, emotion, sexual behavior, food and water intake, body temperature, cardiovascular function, respiratory function, and diurnal rhythms. In addition, the hypothalamus controls the release of hormones from the anterior and posterior regions of the pituitary gland. Neurons in the hypothalamus produce the vasopressin and oxytocin that are secreted by the posterior pituitary and make many hormone-releasing factors that stimulate or inhibit the release of trophic hormones from the anterior pituitary. At the base of the hypothalamus, a projection known as the median eminence is connected to the pituitary stalk. The median eminence is rich with nerve axons and blood vessels that provide both chemical and physical connections between the hypothalamus and the pituitary gland.

The pituitary gland, also referred to as the hypophysis, is located at the base of the brain in a cavity of the sphenoid bone known as the *sella turcica*. The pituitary is separated from the brain by an extension of the dura mater known as the *diaphragma sella* and is not in direct contact with cerebrospinal fluid. The pituitary is a very small gland, weighing between 0.4 g and 1 g in adults. It is divided into two distinct regions: the anterior lobe, or adenohypophysis, and the posterior lobe or the neurohypophysis (see Fig. 77–1).

The posterior pituitary gland secretes two major hormones: oxytocin and vasopressin (antidiuretic hormone) (Table 77–1). Oxytocin release from the posterior pituitary causes contraction of the smooth muscles in the breast during lactation and also plays a role in uterine contraction during parturition. Vasopressin is essential for proper fluid balance and acts on the renal collecting ducts to conserve water. Oxytocin and vasopressin are synthesized in the paraventricular and supraoptic nuclei of the hypothalamus. The posterior pituitary gland contains the terminal nerve endings of these two nuclei, as well as specialized secretory granules that release hormones in response to appropriate signals. Osmoreceptors located in the hypothalamus stimulate the supraoptic nuclei to release vasopressin in response to hyperosmotic extracellular fluid, and a negative-feedback control system exists to regulate fluid osmolarity. Suckling stimuli to the breast nipple cause nervous stimulation of the hypothalamus and release of oxytocin, which is responsible for milk ejection. It is important to note that loss of anterior pituitary function does not necessarily affect the release of vasopressin or oxytocin, because these hormones are actually synthesized in the hypothalamus.

Unlike the posterior pituitary, the release of anterior pituitary hormones is not regulated by direct nervous stimulation; instead, specific hypothalamic releasing and inhibitory hormones control it. The median eminence of the hypothalamus contains a large number of capillaries that converge to form a network of veins known as the hypothalamic-hypophysial portal circulation. Inhibiting and releasing hormones synthesized in the neurons of the hypothalamus reach the anterior pituitary via the hypothalamic-hypophysial portal vessels to control release of anterior pituitary hormones. Although there is a direct arterial blood supply to the anterior pituitary lobe, the hypothalamic-hypophysial portal vessels provide the primary blood supply (see Fig. 77–1). In contrast to the posterior pituitary, the anterior pituitary lobe is extremely vascular and has the highest rate of blood flow of all body organs.

The specialized secretory cells of the anterior pituitary lobe secrete six major polypeptide hormones (Table 77–1). These include growth hormone (GH) or somatotropin, adrenocorticotropic hormone (ACTH) or corticotropin, thyroid-stimulating hormone (TSH) or thyrotropin, prolactin (PRL), follicle-stimulating hormone (FSH), and luteinizing hormone (LH). The release of these hormones is regulated primarily by hypothalamic releasing and inhibiting hormones. Thyrotropin-releasing hormone (TRH) stimulates anterior pituitary release of TSH and prolactin, corticotropin-releasing hormone (CRH) stimulates anterior pituitary release of ACTH, growth hormone-releasing hormone (GHRH) stimulates anterior pituitary release of GH, and gonadotropin-releasing hormone (GnRH) stimulates anterior pituitary release of LH and FSH. Hypothalamic release of dopamine (prolactin inhibitory hormone) inhibits the release of prolactin. Prolactin differs from the other anterior lobe hormones in that an inhibiting factor, rather than a stimulating factor, from the hypothalamus is primarily responsible for controlling its release. Therefore, in the absence of hypothalamic input, an excess of prolactin is produced, whereas a deficiency state of other anterior pituitary hormones results.

Somatotropes comprise approximately one-third to one-half of the anterior pituitary lobe and secrete growth hormone. Growth hormone is essential for growth and development of all body cells and has important effects on carbohydrate and lipid metabolism. GH increases protein synthesis, hepatic glucose output, and lipolysis, while decreasing glucose utilization. The secretion of growth hormone is stimulated primarily by GHRH from the hypothalamus. The release of growth hormone is enhanced by ACTH, vasopressin (ADH), growth hormone-releasing peptide, sleep, exercise, physical or psychological stress, fasting, and a number of pharmacologic agents such as α-adrenergic agonists, β-adrenergic antagonists, dopamine agonists, and GABA agonists.[2] The hypothalamic hormone somatostatin is the most substantial inhibitor of growth hormone secretion. Other factors that inhibit growth-hormone secretion include postprandial hyperglycemia, elevated free fatty acids, elevated insulin-like growth

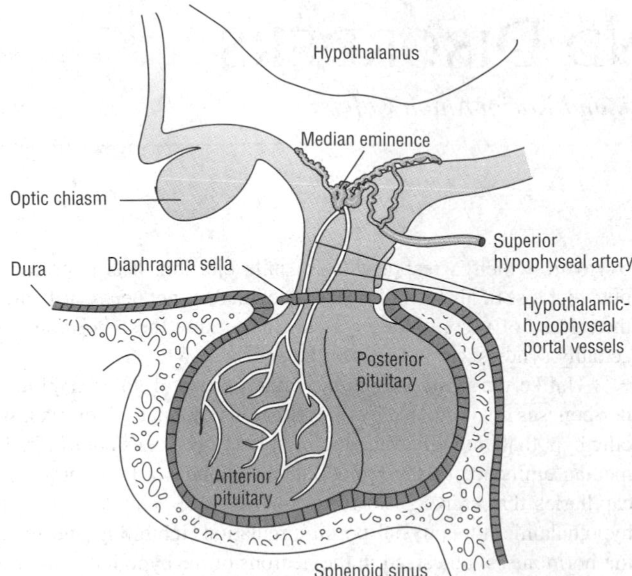

FIGURE 77–1. Illustration showing anatomic relationships of the pituitary gland to surrounding structures. *(From Kohler PO. Clinical Endocrinology. New York, John Wiley and Sons, 1986, p 12, Fig. 2–1 with permission.)*

factor-I (IGF-I, also known as somatomedin C), progesterone, and a number of pharmacologic agents including α-adrenergic antagonists, β-adrenergic agonists, serotonergic antagonists, dopamine antagonists, and chronic administration of glucocorticoids.[2]

Corticotropes, the second most abundant type of secretory cells found in the anterior pituitary, secrete ACTH. ACTH stimulates the adrenal cortex to release glucocorticoids, mineralocorticoids, and androgenic steroid hormones. Secretion of ACTH from the anterior pituitary is stimulated by CRH and is ultimately controlled by an internal diurnal rhythm, nervous input that leads to increased ACTH secretion following eating and physical or psychological stress, and a negative-feedback mechanism based on concentrations of circulating cortisol.

Thyrotropes secrete TSH, which stimulates the thyroid gland to synthesize thyroglobulin, thyroxine (T_4), and triiodothyronine (T_3). The secretion of TSH is stimulated by hypothalamic TRH and is regulated by negative feedback of elevated concentrations of circulating thyroxine and triiodothyronine. Thyrotropin secretion is inhibited by somatostatin and dopamine and can be stimulated by norepinephrine and serotonin.

Gonadotropes secrete both LH and FSH, which control the development and function of both male and female reproductive organs. FSH stimulates the growth of ovarian follicles and promotes testicular spermatogenesis. LH promotes sex-steroid production, produces ovulation in females, and maintains the function of testicular Leydig cells in males. Secretion of LH and FSH is regulated by hypothalamic release of GnRH. The release of LH and FSH is inhibited by negative feedback of sex steroids. FSH is also regulated by inhibin.

Lactotropes comprise approximately 15% to 20% of the normal pituitary and secrete prolactin. During pregnancy, the number of lactotropes can increase significantly because prolactin is needed for the formation of mammary tissue, production of milk, and lactation. The regulation of prolactin secretion by the nervous and endocrine systems is mainly inhibitory, and dopamine has been identified as the strongest inhibitor of prolactin secretion. Prolactin secretion is stimulated by TRH, vasoactive intestinal polypeptide (VIP), pregnancy, nursing, exercise, sleep, stress, and many pharmacologic agents, including dopamine antagonists, GABA agonists, histamine-2-receptor antagonists, estrogens, and opioids.[3]

Destruction of the pituitary gland may result in secondary hypothyroidism, hypogonadism, adrenal insufficiency, growth hormone deficiency, and hypoprolactinemia. The formation of certain types of pituitary tumors may result in pituitary hormone excess. Pituitary tumors may also physically compress the pituitary and prevent the release of the trophic hypothalamic factors that regulate pituitary hormones. In this chapter, the pathophysiology and role of pharmacotherapy in the treatment of acromegaly, short stature, hyperprolactinemia, and panhypopituitarism will be discussed.

ADRENOCORTICOTROPIC HORMONE

See Chap. 76.

THYROID-STIMULATING HORMONE

See Chap. 75.

LUTEINIZING HORMONE AND FOLLICLE-STIMULATING HORMONE

See Chap. 78.

VASOPRESSIN

See Chap. 51.

OXYTOCIN

See Chap. 78.

GROWTH HORMONE

Growth hormone has direct "anti-insulin" effects on lipid and carbohydrate metabolism. GH decreases utilization of glucose by peripheral tissues, increases lipolysis, and increases muscle mass. GH also stimulates gluconeogenesis in hepatocytes, impairs tissue glucose uptake, decreases insulin-receptor sensitivity, and impairs postreceptor insulin action. The growth-promoting effects of GH are largely mediated by insulin-like growth factors (IGF) also known as somatomedins. GH stimulates the formation of IGF-I in the liver, as well as in other peripheral tissues. This anabolic peptide acts as a direct stimulator of cell proliferation and growth. There are two types of insulin-like growth factors, IGF-I and IGF-II. IGF-I regulates growth to some extent before, and largely after, birth. In contrast, IGF-II is thought to primarily regulate growth *in utero*.[4] Growth hormone is secreted by the anterior pituitary in a pulsatile fashion with several short bursts that occur mostly at night. Because of the short half-life of growth hormone in the plasma (approximately 30 minutes), measurements of circulating GH concentrations throughout the waking hours are usually very low or undetectable. Daytime GH pulses are most likely to occur after meals, following exercise, or during periods of stress. The greatest amount of GH secretion occurs during the night within the first 1 to 2 hours of slow-wave sleep (stages III or IV). Secretion of growth hormone is lowest during infancy, increases slightly during childhood, reaches its peak during

TABLE 77–1. Regulation and Action of Pituitary Hormones

Hormone	Stimulation	Inhibition	Physiologic Effects
Anterior Pituitary Hormones			
Growth hormone (GH)	*Physiologic* GH-releasing hormone ACTH ADH GABA Norepinephrine Dopamine Serotonin Estrogen Sleep Stress Exercise *Pharmacologic* α-Adrenergic agonists (e.g., clonidine) β-Adrenergic antagonists (e.g., propranolol) Dopamine agonists (e.g., bromocriptine) GABA agonists (e.g., muscimol)	*Physiologic* Somatostatin Elevated IGF-I Growth hormone Progesterone Glucocorticoids Postprandial hyperglycemia Elevated free fatty acids *Pharmacologic* Dopamine antagonists (e.g., phenothiazines) α-Adrenergic antagonists (e.g., phentolamine) β-Adrenergic agonists (e.g., isoproterenol) Serotonin antagonists (e.g., methysergide)	Stimulates IGF-I production IGF-I and GH promote growth in all body tissues
Prolactin (PRL)	*Physiologic* TRH VIP Estrogen Serotonin Histamine Endogenous opioids Pregnancy and nursing *Pharmacologic* Dopamine antagonists (e.g., phenothiazines, haloperidol, methyldopa) Opiates Estrogens H_2-blockers (cimetidine) MAO inhibitors	*Physiologic* Dopamine GABA *Pharmacologic* Dopamine agonists (e.g., levodopa, bromocriptine, pergolide, cabergoline)	Lactation
Adrenocorticotropic hormone (ACTH)	CRH	Elevated cortisol	Glucocorticoid effects Pigmentation
Thyroid-stimulating hormone (TSH)	TRH Estrogens Norepinephrine Serotonin	Thyroxine Triiodothyronine Somatostatin Glucocorticoids Dopamine	Iodine uptake and thyroid hormone synthesis
Luteinizing hormone (LH)	*Physiologic* GnRH *Pharmacologic* Clomiphene	Estradiol Testosterone Fasting	Ovulation Maintains corpus luteum
Follicle-stimulating hormone (FSH)	*Physiologic* GnRH Menopause Ovarian disorders *Pharmacologic* Clomiphene	Estradiol Inhibin Fasting	Ovarian follicle development Stimulates estradiol and progesterone
Posterior Pituitary Hormones			
Vasopressin (ADH)	Hyperosmolality Volume depletion	Hypervolemia Hypoosmolality	Acts on renal collecting ducts to prevent diuresis
Oxytocin	Parturition Suckling		Uterine contraction Milk ejection

ADH, antidiuretic hormone; CRH, corticotropin-releasing hormone; GABA, γ-aminobutyric acid; GnRH, gonadotropin-releasing hormone; IGF-I, insulin-like growth factor; TRH, thyrotropin-releasing hormone; VIP, vasoactive intestinal peptide.

increased exercise capacity.[25–27] Octreotide also improves oxygen desaturation, sleep quality, and subjective symptoms of sleepiness in acromegalic patients suffering from sleep apnea.[28] Data from two major multicenter trials indicate that pituitary-tumor growth is halted during octreotide treatment, and a small number of patients actually experience tumor regression.[22,23] A more recent study determined that the growth of pituitary tumors during octreotide therapy is suppressed by approximately 83%.[29] The pharmacodynamic effects of octreotide LAR are similar to those of subcutaneously administered octreotide. Single, monthly doses of long-acting octreotide are at least as effective as daily doses of 300 or 600 μg of subcutaneous octreotide administered in divided doses three times daily in normalizing IGF-I levels and maintaining suppression of mean serum GH concentrations.[30]

Response to long-term therapy with octreotide is related to the presence and increased quantity of functioning somatostatin receptors located in the pituitary adenoma.[20,21] Identification of patients who will most likely respond to octreotide, prior to the initiation of therapy, is important when considering the high cost of this medication and the inconvenience of subcutaneous or intramuscular drug administration. Suppression of serum GH concentrations after a single 50-μg dose of octreotide has been used to predict a favorable long-term response (GH concentrations <1 μg/L after a standard OGTT in the presence of normal IGF-1 serum concentrations) to octreotide therapy.[20] Somatostatin-receptor imaging and serum GH concentrations after short-term (1 month) administration of octreotide appear to be even more accurate in predicting which patients will respond to long-term octreotide therapy than acute suppression of GH by a single dose of octreotide.[31]

The initial dose of octreotide for the treatment of acromegaly is 100 μg administered every 8 hours.[5,17,21] Some clinicians recommend a starting dose of 50 μg every 8 hours, then increasing the dose to 100 μg every 8 hours after 1 week, to improve the patient's tolerance of the adverse gastrointestinal effects.[11,20] The dose may be increased by increments of 50 μg every 1 to 2 weeks based on mean serum GH and IGF-I concentrations. Patients who experience a significant rise in GH prior to the end of the 8-hour dosing interval may benefit from decreasing the dosing interval to every 4 to 6 hours. Although doses as high as 1,500 μg per day have been used, doses above 600 μg daily generally do not offer additional benefits, and most patients are adequately managed with 100–200 μg three times daily.[20,22–24] Patients who are maintained on subcutaneous octreotide for at least 2 weeks and who show response to therapy, may be converted to the long-acting depot form of octreotide. The initial dose of octreotide LAR is 20 mg administered intramuscularly in the gluteal region every 28 days. Steady-state serum concentrations are not obtained until after 3 months of therapy. Therefore, dosage adjustments for octreotide LAR should not be considered until after this time. Some patients may require additional subcutaneous injections during the initial dose-titration phase in order to control symptoms. Octreotide LAR doses higher than 30 mg every 4 weeks have not been studied.

In an effort to provide continuous suppression of GH throughout a 24-hour period, several small studies have evaluated the use of continuous subcutaneous infusions or pulsatile subcutaneous infusions of octreotide via portable battery-powered pumps. Octreotide delivery in this manner results in improved suppression of serum GH and IGF-I concentrations with fewer adverse effects than do intermittent subcutaneous injections.[32]

Following subcutaneous injection, octreotide is rapidly absorbed, with peak serum concentrations occurring within 15 to 30 minutes. GH suppression lasts from 4 to 8 hours.[9,20] The elimination half-life of octreotide is approximately 90 minutes, and this is substantially longer than that of physiologic somatostatin, which has a half-life of only 3 minutes in the plasma.[14,20] Octreotide is extensively metabolized by the liver, and 32% of the drug is eliminated unchanged in the urine. Elderly patients may require lower doses of octreotide owing to decreased clearance of the drug and a prolonged elimination half-life. The pharmacokinetic properties of octreotide LAR are similar to those of subcutaneous octreotide following drug release from the depot microspheres.

The most common adverse effects of octreotide therapy are gastrointestinal disturbances such as diarrhea, nausea, abdominal cramps, malabsorption of fat, and flatulence.[5,11,14,17,20,21] These effects are dose dependent and can be seen within a few hours of the first octreotide injection. Gastrointestinal adverse effects occur in approximately 75% of patients, but usually subside within 10 to 14 days of continued treatment.[5,11,14,17,20,21] Octreotide has also been reported to cause injection-site pain (8%), clinically insignificant sinus bradycardia (15% to 20%), conduction abnormalities and arrhythmias (9%), and biochemical hypothyroidism (12%).[5,14,17] Because octreotide slows gastric emptying, long-term therapy may predispose patients to the development of gastritis and *Helicobacter pylori* infection.[33]

Octreotide also inhibits cholecystokinin release and gallbladder motility, predisposing patients to the development of cholelithiasis.[34–36] The development of gallstones is a long-term adverse effect of octreotide use and is largely dependent on geographic factors, dietary habits, and length of therapy.[5,11,14,17,20,21] Octreotide-induced gallstones are three times more common in China than in the United States and may be more prevalent in patients who ingest low-fat diets.[5] The incidence of gallstones in acromegalic patients receiving octreotide increases with length of therapy and has been reported to range from 20% to 50%.[5,11,21–24] Most patients, however, are asymptomatic, and the diagnosis of cholelithiasis is usually made following an ultrasonographic study that is not prompted by patient symptoms. It has been estimated that only 1% of patients will develop symptomatic gallstones during 1 year of octreotide treatment.[5,11,21] Because octreotide-induced gallstones are usually present without clinical symptoms, the latest U.S. Acromegaly Therapy Consensus Development Panel recommended that treatment of octreotide-induced gallstones be the same as that for gallstones in the general population.[5] Prophylactic cholecystectomy or medical therapy with ursodeoxycholic acid for acromegalic patients with asymptomatic gallstones is usually not recommended. However, limited data suggest that concomitant therapy with ursodeoxycholic acid may reverse the formation of sludge and gallstones in acromegalic patients receiving octreotide.[37]

The effect of octreotide on glucose metabolism in patients with acromegaly is multifactorial. Decreases in serum GH concentrations induced by octreotide should result in decreased hepatic gluconeogenesis and increased insulin-receptor sensitivity. However, octreotide also decreases insulin secretion and increases IGFBP-1, which is known to inhibit the insulin-like effects of IGF-I. In addition, octreotide delays the gastrointestinal absorption of glucose, which may further alter glucose metabolism in acromegalic patients. Small studies conducted in acromegalic patients with glucose intolerance have reported improvement in insulin sensitivity associated with octreotide therapy.[38,39] However, one study of 90 acromegalics reported that 11 (12%) patients developed impaired glucose tolerance and 16 (18%) patients developed frank diabetes mellitus while receiving octreotide.[40] In the same study, 27% of subjects who were diabetic at the beginning of the trial experienced an improvement in their glycemic control by the end of the 6-month study period.[40] Risk factors associated with worsening glucose tolerance included female gender and elevated baseline insulin values. Although octreotide appears to have a beneficial effect on glucose tolerance in most patients, glucose determinations should be obtained frequently in the early stages of octreotide therapy in all acromegalic patients. Although no clinical data are available, long-acting somatostatin analogs may theoretically improve glycemic control due to a more sustained drug release profile.

Octreotide has few significant drug-drug interactions. However, it can alter the absorption of some orally administered medications. Octreotide may substantially reduce serum concentrations of cyclosporine by decreasing its intestinal absorption, and the dosage of cyclosporine may need to be increased when these two medications are given concomitantly. Because octreotide has variable effects on glucose metabolism in patients with acromegaly, adjustments in the dose of insulin or oral antihyperglycemic agents may be needed. When bromocriptine and octreotide are administered concomitantly, the bioavailability of bromocriptine is increased by 40%.[41]

Bromocriptine and Octreotide Combination Therapy

Based on previous trials, octreotide is generally considered to be more effective than bromocriptine in reducing mean serum GH concentrations and normalizing IGF-I.[13,17,22,23] Several small studies suggest that combination therapy with octreotide and bromocriptine may be more beneficial than either drug alone.[14,41] Because of the potential for additive adverse effects while using both medications, combination therapy should be considered as a therapeutic option only for refractory patients who have not fully responded to either octreotide or bromocriptine therapy alone.

Pegvisomant

Pegvisomant is a new genetically engineered GH derivative that binds to GH receptors in the liver and inhibits IGF-1.[42] This investigational agent is different from other medications currently available for the management of acromegaly because it does not inhibit GH production; instead, it blocks the physiologic effects of GH on target tissues. Preliminary studies indicate that daily subcutaneous administration of 20 mg of pegvisomant to acromegalic patients for up to 12 weeks results in significant reductions in IGF-1 serum concentrations and clinical improvement in symptoms.[43] Adverse effects appear to be minimal, but there are theoretical concerns that blocking GH signaling may stimulate tumor growth in the long-term. Further study is needed to determine the long-term safety and efficacy of pegvisomant for the treatment of acromegaly.

PHARMACOECONOMIC CONSIDERATIONS

Cost-effectiveness comparisons of the various treatment options for patients with acromegaly have not been performed. Considering that approximately 40% of patients are not completely cured after transsphenoidal surgery, pharmacologic treatment often becomes necessary. Bromocriptine is considerably less expensive than octreotide. However, it is not effective in the majority of patients, and octreotide is often the only viable therapeutic option. Octreotide LAR offers a more convenient method of octreotide administration for acromegalic patients. Although this formulation is approximately twice the cost of subcutaneous octreotide, it may result in improved patient compliance, quality of life, and overall disease management. The drug therapy of choice in specific acromegalic patients should be determined by an individual's clinical response, suppression of serum GH concentrations, and normalization of IGF-I.[44]

CONCLUSIONS

Acromegaly is a chronic debilitating disease characterized by excess growth-hormone secretion most commonly caused by a GH-secreting pituitary adenoma. Transsphenoidal surgical resection of the adenoma is the treatment of choice for patients with acromegaly. Patients who are poor surgical candidates may receive radiation therapy or long-term pharmacologic therapy. Drug therapy options within the US for acromegaly are limited to dopamine agonists and the somatostatin analog octreotide. Dopamine agonists are generally not as effective as octreotide in suppressing GH concentrations or normalizing IGF-I values. However, a small subset of patients may respond to dopamine agonists, and these agents should be considered because of the potential cost advantages and convenience of oral administration. Octreotide has proved to be the most effective pharmacologic agent for the treatment of acromegaly and is typically administered by intermittent subcutaneous injections. Improved somatostatin analog delivery formulations, such as lanreotide and long-acting octreotide should improve patient compliance and quality of life.

GROWTH HORMONE DEFICIENCY

Short stature is a condition that is commonly defined by a physical height that is more than two standard deviations below the population mean and lower than the third percentile for height in a specific age group.[45–47] It is estimated that more than 1.8 million children in the United States can be characterized as having short stature.[47] Short stature is a very broad term describing a condition that may be the result of many different causes. A true lack of GH is among the least common causes and is known as growth-hormone-deficient (GHD) short stature. Absolute GH deficiency is a congenital disorder that can result from various genetic abnormalities such as GHRH deficiency, GH gene deletion, and developmental disorders, including pituitary aplasia or hypoplasia.[45,48] GH insufficiency is an acquired condition that can result secondary to hypothalamic or pituitary tumors, cranial irradiation, head trauma, pituitary infarction, and various types of central nervous system (CNS) infections. In addition, psychosocial deprivation, hypothyroidism, poorly controlled diabetes mellitus, treatment of precocious puberty with LHRH agonists, and pharmacologic agents such as glucocorticoids, methylphenidate, and dextroamphetamine may induce transient GH insufficiency.[45,48]

Short stature also occurs with several conditions that are not associated with a true GH deficiency or insufficiency. These conditions include intrauterine growth retardation; constitutional growth delay; malnutrition; malabsorption of nutrients associated with inflammatory bowel disease, celiac disease, and cystic fibrosis; chronic renal failure; skeletal and cartilage dysplasia; and genetic syndromes such as Turner's syndrome.[45,48] In addition, many children are diagnosed with idiopathic or normal variant short stature. These patients have heights that are significantly lower than the third percentile, but present with normal GH serum concentrations and no specific underlying explanation for short stature.[47,48]

Children with GHD short stature are usually born with an average birth weight. Decreases in growth velocity generally become evident between the age of 6 months and 3 years.[45,48] In contrast, GH insufficiency may arise at any age during growth and development.

GH-deficient or -insufficient children appear to be short and centrally obese with a prominent forehead and an immature face.[45] Because GH deficiency may be accompanied by the loss of other pituitary hormones, characteristics such as small genitalia, hypoglycemia, and hypothyroidism may also be noted.

Several factors must be considered in the diagnosis of GH deficiency or insufficiency. Standard epidemiologic growth charts developed by the National Center for Health Statistics (NCHS) are typically used to determine the percentile of anthropometric measurements such as height, weight, and head circumference. Pubertal stage is typically determined by using the Tanner method. The bone age is determined according to published standards, and growth velocity is calculated to determine the patient's height velocity percentile using standard growth-velocity charts.[45,48] Growth-hormone deficiency is rarely seen in the absence of delayed skeletal maturation and decreased growth velocity. In addition, several different provocative stimuli that induce GH secretion are used diagnostically to determine GH status. Common provocative pharmacologic GH stimuli include insulin-induced hypoglycemia, clonidine, L-dopa, arginine, glucagon, and growth hormone-releasing hormone.[46] A subnormal GH response is arbitrarily defined as a maximum GH serum concentration of <7 μg/L for 2 hours after administration of one of these agents.[46,49] Some centers use 10 μg/L as the maximum GH serum concentration to determine a subnormal GH response. The three generally accepted criteria for the definitive diagnosis of GH deficiency are a subnormal growth velocity, a delayed bone age, and a subnormal GH response to at least two provocative stimuli.[49] For prepubertal and early pubertal patients (Tanner stage less than III), priming with sex hormones is needed to improve specificity.[50] Some patients may exhibit clinical signs of GH deficiency, subnormal growth velocity, and delayed bone age, despite GH levels that are within normal limits after provocative testing. This makes diagnosis in this group of patients very difficult. Diagnosis based on GH stimulation tests becomes further complicated because of the paucity of data reporting the normal range of GH concentrations after provocative testing in healthy children and the fact that commercial GH assays currently available may not be equivalent.[46,49] One study comparing several different GH assays found a significant variation between measured GH serum concentrations.[49] Because of these limitations, careful consideration of multiple factors by a pediatric endocrinology specialist is required to diagnose growth-hormone deficiency correctly.

▶ TREATMENT: Growth Hormone Deficiency

PHARMACOLOGIC THERAPY

The treatment of growth-hormone deficiency with pituitary-derived human growth hormone was first reported in 1958.[51] The National Pituitary Agency was founded by the National Institutes of Health, in 1963, to coordinate the collection of human pituitary glands and to coordinate the purification of GH for administration to children with GHD. In 1985, three deaths linked to Creutzfeldt-Jakob disease (CJD) were identified in young individuals who were previously treated with human pituitary growth hormone.[52] In the United States, seven cases of CJD were reported in patients who had received human pituitary growth hormone prior to 1970.[52] Human pituitary growth hormone was withdrawn from the US market because of the strong likelihood that the CJD was transmitted through contaminated human pituitary-derived growth hormone. Shortly after the withdrawal of human pituitary growth hormone, the US Food and Drug Administration approved the first recombinant DNA-derived growth hormone for the treatment of GH insufficiency.[51] Prior to the introduction of recombinant growth hormone, the number of individuals who received treatment for GH insufficiency was relatively small owing to the limited availability of human pituitary tissue for GH extraction. Currently, with the widespread availability of recombinant growth-hormone products, a large number of children can receive growth hormone-replacement therapy at higher doses (Table 77–2). Unfortunately, human pituitary-derived growth hormone continues to be used today in some underdeveloped countries.

GH replacement therapy in children with documented GHD short stature produces a significant improvement in growth velocity within the first year of therapy.[49] This initial increase in growth velocity is often referred to as catch-up growth. Most of the initial studies evaluating the efficacy of GH therapy in GHD children were conducted for short periods of time in small numbers of patients, and, until recently, information about the long-term outcome of GH therapy was limited. Although growth velocity improves initially following GH therapy, the available data from patients receiving long-term growth hormone therapy suggest that final adult height is not substantially improved. The average final adult height typically reported in the literature is two standard deviations below the population mean.[53–55] Analysis of data compiled by the French National Register from 3,233 children with short stature who received growth hormone replacement therapy between 1973 and 1993, also reported a mean final height that was two standard deviations below the population mean after an average of 4 years of GH therapy.[56] Although these results are disappointing, it is important to note that a substantial percentage of patients included in these studies had initially received human pituitary growth hormone in relatively low doses because of its limited availability. In addition, current growth-hormone dosing regimens have changed with regard to frequency of administration, making these data difficult to apply to patients who are receiving GH-replacement therapy today. More recently, a study evaluating the adult height of children who received only recombinant-GH therapy with currently recommended dosing regimens suggests that current recombinant-GH therapy may have a greater impact on final adult height than previously reported.[57] Additionally, several studies suggest that initiation of GH therapy at an early chronologic age, prior to the onset of puberty, may be associated with a more favorable increase in final height.[55–57] Therefore, prompt diagnosis of growth hormone deficiency and initiation of replacement therapy with recombinant GH may be a crucial factor in optimizing the final adult height of children with GHD. Recombinant GH is currently considered the mainstay of therapy for the treatment of GHD short stature. However, additional well-controlled studies are needed to define the optimal use of GH therapy in patients with this disorder. A number of studies evaluating the effect of GH therapy on final adult height are ongoing.

Recombinant growth hormone has also been shown to increase short-term growth rate in patients with chronic renal insufficiency, Turner's syndrome, and Prader Willi syndrome, and is approved by the FDA for treatment of growth failure associated with these conditions.[49,51] GH is also FDA approved for the treatment of adult growth-hormone deficiency and AIDS wasting syndrome. Long-term GH therapy in growth-hormone deficient adults significantly

TABLE 77–2. Recombinant Growth Hormone Products

Product	Formulation	Recommended Dosing Regimen	FDA-Approved Indications
Protropin	Somatrem lyophilized powder for injection	Doses up to 0.1 mg/kg SQ 3 times weekly	Growth failure associated with chronic renal failure Growth hormone-deficient growth failure
Genotropin	Somatropin lyophilized powder for injection	0.16–0.24 mg/kg/wk SQ administered 6–7 times per week in divided doses	Growth failure associated with chronic renal failure Growth hormone-deficient growth failure
Norditropin	Somatropin lyophilized powder for injection	0.024–0.034 mg/kg SQ 6–7 times weekly	Growth failure associated with chronic renal failure Growth hormone-deficient growth failure
Nutropin	Somatropin lyophilized powder for injection	0.3 mg/kg/wk SQ or IM	Growth failure associated with chronic renal failure Growth hormone-deficient growth failure Short stature associated with Turner's syndrome
Nutropin AQ	Somatropin injection	0.3 mg/kg/wk SQ or IM	Growth failure associated with chronic renal failure Growth hormone-deficient growth failure Short stature associated with Turner's syndrome
Nutropin Depot	Somatropin lyophilized powder for injectable suspension	1.5–4.5 mg/kg SQ administered once or twice monthly	Long-term treatment of growth hormone-deficient growth failure
Humatrope	Somatrem lyophilized powder for injection	0.18–0.3 mg/kg/wk SQ or IM administered on 3 alternate days or 6 times per week in divided doses	Growth failure associated with chronic renal failure Growth hormone-deficient growth failure Adult-onset somatropin deficiency syndrome
Serostim	Somatrem lyophilized powder for injection	0.1 mg/kg SQ daily	AIDS wasting or cachexia
Saizen	Somatrem lyophilized powder for injection	0.06 mg/kg SQ or IM 3 times weekly	Growth failure associated with chronic renal failure Growth hormone-deficient growth failure

decreases body fat, increases muscle mass, and improves exercise capacity.[58] GH therapy in adults has been shown to improve cardiac risk profile, bone mineral density (BMD) and psychological well being.[59–61] In addition, GH is currently being investigated as an anabolic agent for certain catabolic states and for a variety of disorders, including infertility, obesity, and natural aging.[51]

The majority of short children in the United States do not have an identifiable medical cause for their condition, but with widespread availability of several recombinant-growth-hormone formulations, many children have received GH therapy regardless of the underlying etiology of their short stature. The use of recombinant-growth-hormone therapy in children with nongrowth hormone-deficient, or normal variant, short stature has been studied by several investigators.[62–65] Most of these studies indicate that these patients experience an improvement in short-term growth velocity, but improvements in final height have not been proven.[62–65] A subset of patients may maintain better growth with continued GH therapy, but the specific characteristics of this patient population remain to be determined.[62–64] The use of GH therapy in patients with non-growth hormone-deficient short stature is controversial. For example, although guidelines established for the use of growth hormone by the Lawson Wilkins Pediatric Endocrine Society do not consider GH to be a safe and effective treatment for non-GHD short stature,[49] a national survey of physicians revealed that a majority of pediatric endocrinologists regard GH therapy to be an appropriate treatment in certain patients with non-GHD short stature.[66] Additional long-term studies evaluating the efficacy and safety of GH therapy are needed to determine the role of GH therapy in non-GHD children.

Nine different recombinant-growth-hormone products are currently available for use in the United States. Somatrem (Protropin) was the first recombinant-GH product developed and used for the treatment of GH deficiency. This formulation contains the same 191 amino-acid sequence as human pituitary growth hormone with the exception of the terminal addition of a methionine amino-acid group. The remaining GH formulations (Genotropin, Norditropin, Nutropin, Nutropin AQ, *Nutropin Depot*, Humatrope, Serostim, and Saizen) contain somatropin. Somatropin is composed of the same amino acid sequence as human pituitary GH. Recombinant GH formulations must be administered by intramuscular or subcutaneous injection. Nutropin AQ is the only GH product that is available as a liquid formulation. The remaining products are formulated as lyophilized powders for injection, and patients must be instructed regarding proper reconstitution, storage, and administration. A newly formulated long-acting depot form of growth hormone, Nutropin Depot, is also available for once- or twice-monthly subcutaneous injection. This product may be particularly useful for patients who are noncompliant or who experience significant adverse effects from frequent injections. The potency of GH products is expressed as International Units per milligram (IU/mg) with 1 mg containing approximately 2.6 IU of growth hormone. Direct comparisons between the different recombinant growth-hormone products have not been published. Although some differences exist in recommended dosages, all GH products are generally considered to be equally efficacious. Usual recommended doses range from 0.15 to 0.3 mg/kg/wk.[43] Recombinant GH is usually administered subcutaneously in equal doses three to seven times per week depending on the specific GH product used.[48,49] Dosing regimens with greater frequency of administration provide more favorable short-term growth responses.[49] Growth hormone-replacement therapy should be initiated as early as possible after diagnosis of GH insufficiency and continued until a desirable height is reached or growth velocity has decreased to less than 2.5 cm per year after the pubertal growth spurt.

The bioavailability of recombinant GH is approximately 75% after subcutaneous administration and 60% after intramuscular administration. Following systemic administration, recombinant GH localizes to highly perfused organs, such as the kidney and liver, where it is metabolized to amino acids that then return to the systemic circulation. The elimination half-life of exogenous GH is approximately 3 to 5 hours.

Glucocorticoids may inhibit the growth-promoting effects of recombinant GH, and concomitant administration of androgens, estrogens, thyroid hormones, or anabolic steroids may accelerate epiphyseal closure and compromise final height.

Three large databases—the National Cooperative Growth Study (NCGS), the Kabi International Growth Study (KIGS), and the Australian OZGROW—were developed to collect postmarketing adverse effect data or reports associated with recombinant growth hormone. Development of these databases was prompted by the unexpected and tragic cases of CJD reported in patients treated with human pituitary growth hormone. These databases are maintained by pharmaceutical companies that manufacture GH products.[67] Recombinant GH is generally well tolerated in children, and adverse effects are relatively uncommon.[68,69] A small number of patients may complain of injection-site pain or arthralgias. Idiopathic intracranial hypertension (IIH), also known as pseudotumor cerebri, has been reported in a very small number of children receiving GH therapy. This condition usually develops within the first 8 to 12 weeks of treatment and presents with symptoms such as headache, blurred vision, diplopia, nausea, and vomiting.[67] The symptoms of IIH usually resolve after discontinuation of GH therapy, and long-term complications are rare. Cases of slipped capital femoral epiphysis (SCFE) have been reported in children with growth-hormone deficiency who are receiving GH therapy.[67] This condition is thought to occur as a result of the increased width of the femoral plate during GH treatment, but it has also been reported in GH-deficient children who are not receiving GH replacement. Patients with this condition typically complain of hip or knee pain. An orthopedic surgeon can manage SCFE, and GH therapy does not need to be withdrawn. Because growth hormone is known to cause decreased insulin sensitivity, hyperglycemia and diabetes mellitus may develop. A very small number of patients have developed frank diabetes mellitus during GH treatment, and all of these patients had specific predisposing risk factors for diabetes mellitus.[67–69] GH may promote the growth of various types of neoplasms and increase tumor recurrence rates in patients with a history of malignancy.[68,69] For this reason, GH should not be administered to patients with an active malignant tumor or a history of recurrent tumor growth. In 1988, a Japanese report indicated that children receiving GH therapy were twice as likely to develop leukemia as children who were not receiving the hormone.[70] A more recent analysis of all collected reports of leukemia associated with GH therapy determined that these children had other leukemia risk factors (Fanconi anemia, Bloom's syndrome, or a prior history of cancer).[71] GH therapy in children without these risk factors does not appear to predispose children to develop leukemia.[67–69] Finally, some patients may develop antibodies to recombinant GH. The development of antibodies during replacement therapy with recombinant-GH products has been reported to be relatively low, affecting approximately 15% to 20% of patients.[72,73] More importantly, the presence of GH antibodies does not adversely affect growth response and appears to be clinically insignificant except in patients with GH gene deletions.

Appropriate monitoring of GH therapy includes regular assessments of height, weight, growth velocity, serum alkaline phosphatase, and bone age every 6 to 12 months. Additional laboratory tests to monitor for potential adverse effects include serum glucose and thyroid function. The dose of GH will periodically need to be increased as weight increases in growing children.

GROWTH HORMONE-RELEASING HORMONE

The a synthetic GHRH product, known as sermorelin (Geref), is currently FDA-approved for the treatment of idiopathic growth-hormone deficiency in children. Sermorelin (GHRH (1-29)-NH_2) is composed of 29 amino-acid residues that are identical to the amino-terminal segment of human GHRH. Although not as effective as recombinant GH therapy, sermorelin does increase short-term growth velocity in children with idiopathic growth-hormone deficiency.[74,75] This product also increases growth velocity in children who have GH deficiency secondary to hypothalamic damage rather than pituitary abnormalities, as is observed with radiation-induced GH deficiency.[76] In most cases of radiation-induced GH deficiency, pituitary somatotropes are capable of secreting endogenous GH, and stimulation of these cells by exogenously administered GHRH may restore the natural pulsatile secretion of GH and result in increased growth rate.

The recommended dose of sermorelin is 0.03 mg/kg administered daily by subcutaneous injection. No serious adverse events have been identified. Pain at the site of injection is the most common adverse effect reported by patients receiving sermorelin therapy. Because normal pituitary function is needed for sermorelin to stimulate GH secretion, children should not receive GHRH therapy with sermorelin unless adequate capacity to secrete GH is documented by provocative GH-stimulation testing. Sermorelin may prove to be a beneficial therapeutic option in the treatment of various types of non-GHD short stature. However, owing to its mechanism of action, sermorelin does not have a role in the treatment of true GHD short stature.

FUTURE THERAPIES

A number of biosynthetic growth hormone-releasing peptides (GHRPs), including examorelin (Hexarelin), are currently under investigation for use in the treatment of various types of short stature.[77] Like synthetic GHRH, GHRP stimulates the secretion of GH. However, GHRPs act through different receptor mechanisms and can potentially be used synergistically with synthetic GHRH formulations. A significant advantage of GHRPs is that they are biologically active when administered intravenously, subcutaneously, nasally, and orally.[77–79] Small studies show that GHRPs are generally well tolerated, and short-term use in children with growth-hormone deficiency, normal-variant short stature, and idiopathic short stature results in increased growth velocity.[78,79] This new class of medications may offer significant therapeutic benefits in specific patient populations with short stature.

The use of IGF-I for the treatment of growth disorders associated with GH insensitivity is also currently under investigation. Because the growth-promoting effects of GH are primarily mediated by IGF-I, patients who are resistant to GH may benefit from IGF-I therapy. Growth-hormone resistance may result from hereditary abnormalities characterized by defective GH receptors, such as Laron-type dwarfism, or antibody formation to recombinant growth-hormone products. Several studies in a limited number of patients document increased growth in children with GH insensitivity receiving IGF-I.[51] The safety and efficacy of IGF-I are currently being studied in phase III clinical trials.

PHARMACOECONOMIC CONSIDERATIONS

The treatment of short stature with recombinant GH is very expensive. Despite the prohibitive cost, recombinant GH remains the mainstay of therapy for children with GHD short stature. However, treatment of non-GHD short stature with recombinant GH is not widely accepted. Although the benefits in final adult height reported in the literature are equivocal for those with non-GHD short stature, and are clearly less than ideal for those with GHD short stature, the increases in growth velocity, particularly in children with true GH deficiency, are associated with significant psychosocial benefits. Many clinicians believe that GH therapy can improve quality of life and should be made available to all children with short stature, regardless of whether or not they are GH deficient.[80] Until studies using recombinant GH more definitively demonstrate improvements in both final adult height and quality of life, the cost-effectiveness of GH, particularly for non-GHD short stature, remains uncertain.

CONCLUSIONS

Growth-hormone deficiency during childhood results in short stature. Replacement with recombinant GH is considered the mainstay of therapy for patients with GHD short stature, but its use for the treatment of non-GHD short stature remains controversial. Recombinant GH is safe for use in children and is associated with very few adverse effects. Although GH improves initial growth velocity, the long-term benefits with respect to final adult height remain to be determined. New therapeutic agents such as the synthetic growth hormone-releasing hormone sermorelin and other growth hormone-releasing peptides may provide benefits for patients with non-GHD short stature. Because growth-hormone regimens can be particularly demanding and inconvenient for patients, knowledge of the long-term benefits is critical to the development of rational, cost-effective treatments for patients with short stature.

PROLACTIN

PHYSIOLOGIC EFFECTS

Prolactin is secreted in a pulsatile fashion by the lactotroph cells of the anterior pituitary, with the highest peak concentrations observed during sleep.[3] The secretion of prolactin is regulated primarily by tonic hypothalamic inhibitory effects of dopamine. As described earlier in this chapter and listed in Table 77–1, many factors can affect prolactin secretion. During pregnancy, prolactin serum concentrations rise substantially above normal. All other conditions characterized by excess prolactin serum concentrations—known as hyperprolactinemia—are considered pathologic.

HYPERPROLACTINEMIA

Hyperprolactinemia is a state of persistent serum prolactin elevation. Prolactin concentrations greater than 20 μg/L observed on multiple occasions are generally considered indicative of hyperprolactinemia.[81,82] Hyperprolactinemia usually affects women of reproductive age and has been noted in 25% of women with secondary amenorrhea.[81,82] The incidence of hyperprolactinemia in the general population is reported to be less than 1%.[81]

Hyperprolactinemia has several etiologies. The most common causes are benign prolactin-secreting pituitary tumors, known as prolactinomas, and various medications. Prolactinomas are classified according to size. Prolactin-secreting microadenomas are less than 10 mm in diameter and often do not increase in size.[3,83,84] In contrast, macroadenomas are tumors with a diameter greater than 10 mm that continue to grow and can cause invasion of surrounding tissues.[3,83,84] In the presence of a prolactinoma, prolactin serum concentrations may remain normal or may be markedly elevated to thousands of micrograms per liter.

TABLE 77–3. Drug-Induced Hyperprolactinemia

Dopamine antagonists	Progestins
Phenothiazines	Gonadotropin-releasing-hormone analogs
Haloperidol	Benzodiazepines
Metoclopramide	Tricyclic antidepressants (clomipramine and nortriptyline)
Domperidone	Monoamine oxidase inhibitors
Prolactin Stimulators	H_2-Receptor antagonists (cimetidine)
Methyldopa	Opioids
Reserpine	**Other**
Serotonin reuptake inhibitors (SSRIs)	Verapamil
Dexfenfluramine	
Estrogens	

Any pharmacologic agent that antagonizes dopamine or increases the release of prolactin can induce hyperprolactinemia (Table 77–3). Serotonin is a strong stimulator of prolactin secretion, and serotonin-reuptake inhibitors (SSRIs) such as fluoxetine (Prozac), paroxetine (Paxil), sertraline (Zoloft), and fluvoxamine (Luvox) are the medications most frequently associated with hyperprolactinemia.[85] Prior to the increased use of SSRIs, antipsychotic medications with potent dopamine-receptor blockade, such as the phenothiazine derivatives and haloperidol (Haldol), were most often identified as the cause of drug-induced hyperprolactinemia.[3,86] Metoclopramide (Reglan) and domperidone, an antiemetic available in Europe, are potent dopamine-receptor antagonists reported to induce hyperprolactinemia.[85] Hormones such as estrogen and progesterone, commonly prescribed as oral contraceptives, can stimulate lactotroph growth to promote prolactin secretion and have been implicated in drug-induced hyperprolactinemia.[85] Although the exact mechanism of action remains to be determined, the calcium-channel-blocking agent verapamil (e.g., Calan, Isoptin) has been associated with cases of hyperprolactinemia.[3,85] Methyldopa (Aldomet) and reserpine, although not used frequently in clinical practice today, are antihypertensive agents that can stimulate prolactin secretion.[85] Prolactin concentrations may increase with the administration of gonadotropin-releasing hormone analogs such as leuprolide (Lupron) or goserelin (Zoladex).[85] Other medications rarely reported to cause hyperprolactinemia include H_2-receptor blocking agents, benzodiazepines, tricyclic antidepressants, dexfenfluramine, opioids, and monoamine oxidase inhibitors.[3,81,83,85] Prolactin levels do not typically rise to greater than 150 μg/L in cases of drug-induced hyperprolactinemia. Measurement of serum prolactin concentrations prior to the initiation of therapy with medications known to cause prolactin elevation may obviate the need for extensive examination of pituitary function and aid with the appropriate diagnosis of drug-induced hyperprolactinemia.

Less common etiologies include CNS lesions that physically compress the pituitary stalk and interrupt tonic hypothalamic dopamine secretion resulting in hyperprolactinemia.[81,83] Increased thyroid-releasing hormone (TRH) concentrations in hypothyroidism can stimulate prolactin secretion and cause hyperprolactinemia.[81,83] During conditions of renal or liver compromise, the clearance of prolactin is decreased, resulting in elevated prolactin concentrations.[81] Despite vigorous diagnostic effort, the cause of hyperprolactinemia cannot always be determined. This is known as idiopathic hyperprolactinemia and is most likely a result of the presence of very small tumors that are not detected by standard imaging techniques.[82] It should be noted that many physiologic factors, such as stress (including the stress of phlebotomy), sleep, exercise, coitus, and eating, can also induce transiently elevated prolactin levels.[3,82] This emphasizes the importance of obtaining multiple prolactin measurements to confirm the diagnosis. Ideally, after an intravenous line is placed in the patient's arm, the patient should rest in a supine position or in a chair for 2 hours before prolactin samples are collected.

Elevated prolactin serum concentrations inhibit gonadotropin secretion and sex-steroid synthesis.[82] Because prolactin concentrations higher than 60 μg/L are associated with anovulation, women with hyperprolactinemia typically present with menstrual irregularities such as oligomenorrhea or amenorrhea and infertility.[81–83] In addition, approximately 40% to 70% of women with hyperprolactinemia have galactorrhea.[82,83] Hyperprolactinemia in men, although rare, may cause decreased libido, erectile dysfunction, infertility, galactorrhea, or gynecomastia.[82,83] In the presence of a prolactin-secreting pituitary tumor, many patients with hyperprolactinemia may first present with headaches and visual-field disturbances that result from tumor compression of the optic chiasm.[83] The prolonged suppression of estrogen in premenopausal women with hyperprolactinemia leads to a decrease in bone mineral density and significant risk for the development of osteoporosis.[81,83] In addition, untreated hyperprolactinemia in women may increase the risk of ischemic heart disease.[83]

The diagnosis of hyperprolactinemia, as defined by multiple prolactin serum concentrations above 20 μg/L, is relatively simple. However, identifying the underlying cause of this abnormality may be more challenging. Patients with modest prolactin elevations should have multiple prolactin serum determinations to minimize the potential for detecting only transient increases in prolactin. A careful medication history is essential, and the presence of hypothyroidism, renal failure, or hepatic dysfunction should be evaluated. If the cause of hyperprolactinemia remains ambiguous, a CT scan or MRI study should be performed to determine the presence of a pituitary tumor.[81–83] If an underlying cause of elevated prolactin serum concentration is not determined, the hyperprolactinemia is considered to be idiopathic.

▶ TREATMENT: Hyperprolactinemia

The treatment of hyperprolactinemia depends on the underlying cause of the abnormality. In cases of drug-induced hyperprolactinemia, discontinuation of the offending medication and initiation of an appropriate therapeutic alternative usually normalizes serum prolactin concentrations.[85] In cases for which an appropriate therapeutic alternative does not exist, medical therapy with dopamine agonists is warranted. Sex-steroid replacement should also be considered.[85] Treatment options for the management of prolactinomas include clinical observation, medical therapy with dopamine agonists, radiation therapy, and transsphenoidal surgical removal of the tumor.[81–83,87] Because prolactin-secreting microadenomas are very small and typically do not increase in size, treatment of these tumors is primarily directed toward alleviating symptoms.[83,84,87] The goal of therapy is to normalize prolactin serum concentrations and reestablish gonadotropin secretion to restore fertility and reduce the risk of osteoporosis. In patients with asymptomatic elevations in serum prolactin, observation and close followup are appropriate.[81,82,84] Treatment goals are more aggressive in patients with prolactin-secreting macroadenomas because these tumors are larger and can cause invasion of local tissues with significant visual defects.[87] Therefore, in addition to normalizing prolactin concentrations, tumor shrinkage and correction of visual defects are primary goals of treatment.

Medical therapy with dopamine agonists is usually more effective than transsphenoidal surgery for both types of pituitary prolactinomas.[82–84,87] Postsurgical cure rates differ depending on tumor type and are reported to be approximately 70% for microprolactinomas and only 30% for macroprolactinomas.[3] In addition, long-term followup of patients with prior transsphenoidal surgical removal of prolactinomas indicates a relatively high recurrence rate (approximately 40%) within 5 years.[83] A 10-year followup of patients with microprolactinomas found a recurrence rate of only 27%.[88] This marked improvement in outcome has been largely attributed to advancements in neurosurgical techniques. Transsphenoidal surgery for the removal of prolactinomas is usually reserved for patients who are refractory to or who cannot tolerate therapy with dopamine agonists, and for patients with very large tumors that cause severe compression of adjacent tissues.[82,87] Radiation therapy may require several years for effective tumor shrinkage and reduction in serum prolactin concentrations and is usually used only in conjunction with surgery.[87,88]

PHARMACOLOGIC THERAPY

Medical therapy with dopamine agonists is very effective in normalizing prolactin serum concentrations, in restoring menstruation, and in reducing tumor size in approximately 70% to 100% of patients within 3 to 6 months of therapy.[84,87] Bromocriptine (Parlodel) has been the mainstay of therapy since the 1970s, and pergolide (Permax) has been used as an effective alternative in patients who are intolerant of the adverse effects associated with bromocriptine. Cabergoline (Dostinex) is a new long-acting dopamine agonist that offers the advantage of less-frequent dosing and it is replacing bromocriptine as the agent of choice for the medical management of prolactinomas.

BROMOCRIPTINE

Bromocriptine was the first D_2-receptor agonist to be used in the treatment of hyperprolactinemia and has been the mainstay of therapy for over 20 years. It inhibits the release of prolactin by directly stimulating postsynaptic dopamine receptors in the hypothalamus. Hypothalamic release of dopamine (prolactin inhibitory hormone) inhibits the release of prolactin. Decreases in serum prolactin concentrations occur within 2 hours of oral administration with maximal suppression occurring after 8 hours, and suppressive effects persisting for up to 24 hours. Medical therapy with bromocriptine normalizes prolactin serum concentrations, restores gonadotropin production, and shrinks tumor size in approximately 90% of patients with prolactinomas.[87,89]

For the management of hyperprolactinemia, bromocriptine therapy is typically initiated at 1.25–2.5 mg once daily at bedtime to minimize adverse effects.[81,82,87] The dose can be gradually increased by 1.25-mg increments every week to obtain desirable serum prolactin concentrations. Usual therapeutic doses of bromocriptine range from 2.5 to 15 mg per day, although some patients may require doses as high as 40 mg per day.[81,82] Bromocriptine is usually administered in two or three divided doses, but once-daily dosing is also effective.[90]

The most common adverse effects associated with bromocriptine therapy include central nervous system symptoms such as headache, lightheadedness, dizziness, nervousness, and fatigue. Gastrointestinal effects such as nausea, abdominal pain, and diarrhea are also common. Bromocriptine should be administered with food to decrease the incidence of adverse gastrointestinal effects. Although most of these adverse effects diminish with continued treatment, about 12% of patients will not tolerate the adverse effects associated with bromocriptine therapy.[90] Extended-release dosage forms of bromocriptine have been investigated to improve tolerability and compliance. These include a long-acting injectable form of bromocriptine (Parlodel LAR), which can be administered as monthly intramuscular injections in doses of 50–75 mg monthly, and a slow-release oral formulation (Parlodel SRO) that is given as a single daily dose of 5–15 mg. These formulations are as effective as immediate-release bromocriptine and may improve compliance.[91–93] Vaginal preparations of bromocriptine have also been studied in an effort to decrease the incidence of adverse effects associated with oral dosage forms.[94]

Because most patients with hyperprolactinemia are women with a principal complaint of infertility, the safety of bromocriptine in pregnancy must be considered. One report of more than 2,000 pregnancies in women who received bromocriptine during part or all of their gestation did not detect an increase in the risk for spontaneous abortion or incidence of congenital anomalies.[90] Although bromocriptine does not appear to be teratogenic, some clinicians discontinue therapy as soon as pregnancy is detected because the effects of *in utero* exposure to bromocriptine on gonadal function and fertility of the offspring remain to be determined.[84,87] In some patients with macroprolactinomas undergoing rapid tumor expansion, bromocriptine therapy must be continued throughout pregnancy.

PERGOLIDE

Pergolide (Permax) is a dopamine-receptor agonist with affinity for both D_1- and D_2-receptors. This agent is 10 to 1,000 times more potent than bromocriptine on a milligram per milligram basis. In the United States, pergolide is not FDA approved for the treatment of hyperprolactinemia and is most commonly prescribed for the treatment of parkinsonism. However, pergolide has been used for many years as a safe and effective alternative to bromocriptine in the management of patients with hyperprolactinemia and offers the advantage of once-daily dosing.[95,96]

For the treatment of hyperprolactinemia, pergolide therapy is initiated at a dose of 25 μg given once daily at bedtime. The average dose that achieves optimal suppression of prolactin serum concentrations is 50 μg per day given as a single dose.[95] Following oral administration, pergolide undergoes significant first-pass hepatic metabolism such that the parent compound is not detected in the serum. Pergolide has relatively high protein binding at 90%, and it is extensively metabolized by the liver into at least 10 different metabolites. It is not known whether these metabolites have significant pharmacologic effects in humans. Elimination is primarily renal with 55% of the dose excreted in the urine. Adverse effects of pergolide are similar to those of bromocriptine and include nausea, headache, vomiting, and dizziness in about 30% of patients. The use of pergolide during pregnancy has not been evaluated as extensively as has bromocriptine and should be avoided until additional data become available.

CABERGOLINE

Cabergoline (Dostinex) is a long-acting dopamine agonist with high selectivity and affinity for dopamine D_2-receptors. This agent is approved for the treatment of hyperprolactinemia and effectively reduces serum prolactin concentrations in 80% to 90% of hyperprolactinemic patients.[97–99] Cabergoline also effectively reduces tumor size in patients with both micro- and macroprolactinomas.[97,100] In a multicenter randomized trial comparing the efficacy of cabergoline and bromocriptine, serum prolactin levels were normalized in 83% of patients receiving cabergoline and in 58% of patients receiving bromocriptine after 6 months of therapy.[101] Cabergoline may also be effective in patients who are intolerant of or resistant to bromocriptine.[102]

Cabergoline is commercially available as 0.5-mg oral tablets. The initial dose of cabergoline for the treatment of hyperprolactinemia is 0.5 mg once weekly or in divided doses twice weekly. This dose may be increased by increments of 0.5 mg at 4-week intervals based on serum prolactin concentrations. The usual dose is 1–2 mg weekly; however, doses as high as 4.5 mg weekly have been used.[103] Recent studies have also evaluated the efficacy of a vaginal dosage form of cabergoline to reduce the adverse effects associated with oral therapy.[104]

Following oral administration, peak serum concentrations are obtained within 2 hours, and food does not affect absorption. Data from animal studies indicate that cabergoline is widely distributed to well-perfused organs, including the pituitary gland.[103] The elimination of cabergoline from the pituitary appears to be very slow; this rate may explain the long duration of action. Cabergoline is extensively metabolized in the liver by hydrolysis, and the dose should be reduced in patients with severe hepatic failure.[103] This drug is eliminated primarily in the feces, and the elimination half-life ranges from 79 to 155 hours in hyperprolactinemic patients.[103]

The most common adverse effects reported with the use of cabergoline are nausea, vomiting, headache, and dizziness.[97–100,103] These are similar to the adverse effects reported with bromocriptine and pergolide. However, in a large comparative study evaluating bromocriptine and cabergoline, fewer patients receiving cabergoline reported adverse effects than patients receiving bromocriptine, and only 3% of the patients in the cabergoline group withdrew from the study because of adverse effects, versus 12% of patients taking bromocriptine.[101] Other adverse events associated with the use of cabergoline include gastrointestinal complaints, drowsiness, fatigue, paresthesias, dyspnea, suffocation sensation, and epistaxis.[101,103] As with other dopamine agonists, adverse events usually occur early in therapy and subside with continued treatment. However, in one study 15% to 20% of patients receiving cabergoline experienced a recurrence of early symptoms or an onset of new symptoms after several weeks of treatment.[101] Mild to moderate decreases in blood pressure have been observed in up to 50% of patients taking cabergoline; however, the incidence of symptomatic orthostatic hypotension has not been significant.[97,98,101] Transient increases in serum alkaline phosphatase, bilirubin, and aminotransferases have been reported in small numbers of patients receiving cabergoline.[101] Pleuropulmonary disease has been reported with cabergoline, but only with larger doses used in the treatment of Parkinson's disease.[103]

The use of cabergoline in pregnancy has not been extensively studied. However, several case reports of women who received cabergoline therapy during the first and second trimesters of pregnancy have not documented an increased risk of spontaneous abortion, congenital abnormalities, or tubal pregnancy.[103] However, prospective data in large numbers of pregnancies is lacking. Owing to the long half-life and limited data on cabergoline use in pregnancy, most clinicians recommend that women receiving cabergoline therapy who plan to become pregnant should discontinue the medication 1 month before planned conception.

OTHER DOPAMINE AGONISTS

Other dopamine agonists that have been used in the treatment of hyperprolactinemia, but which are not commercially available in the United States, include lisuride, terguride, metergoline, dihydroergocristine, and quinagolide.[90] Quinagolide is a D_2-receptor agonist, used frequently in Europe, which is dosed once daily. Quinagolide is as effective as bromocriptine for the management of hyperprolactinemia and may also be effective in the treatment of patients who are resistant to or intolerant of bromocriptine.[90]

EVALUATION OF THERAPEUTIC OUTCOMES

Prolactin serum concentrations should be monitored every 3 to 4 weeks after the initiation of any dopamine-agonist therapy to assess efficacy and appropriately titrate medication dosage.[82] In addition, symptoms such as headache, visual disturbances, menstrual cycles in women, and sexual function in men should be evaluated to assess clinical response to therapy. Once prolactin concentrations have normalized and clinical symptoms of hyperprolactinemia have resolved with dopamine-agonist therapy, prolactin serum concentrations should be monitored every 6 to 12 months. In patients receiving long-term treatment, the medication can be discontinued every 5 years to determine whether remission has occurred.

PHARMACOECONOMIC CONSIDERATIONS

Medical therapy with dopamine agonists is more effective than either transsphenoidal surgery or radiation for the management of hyperprolactinemia, and bromocriptine is the mainstay of therapy. Because most patients receive therapy for long periods of time, the medical management of hyperprolactinemia may result in considerable costs. Although bromocriptine is frequently used to manage hyperprolactinemia, therapy with pergolide, which is equally effective, costs considerably less and offers the advantage of single-daily dosing. The cost of cabergoline therapy is approximately twice that of bromocriptine, and the costs associated with monitoring the response to therapy should be similar. However, cabergoline is more effective than bromocriptine and may offer additional advantages, such as a decreased incidence of adverse effects and improved patient compliance. Pharmacoeconomic studies are needed to assess whether the higher cost of cabergoline therapy is balanced by the potential added benefits.

CONCLUSIONS

Hyperprolactinemia is a common disorder that can have a significant impact on fertility. Hyperprolactinemia is most commonly caused by the presence of prolactin-secreting pituitary tumors and various medications that antagonize dopamine or increase the secretion of prolactin. Available treatment options for this disorder include medical therapy with dopamine agonists, radiation therapy, and transsphenoidal surgery. In most cases, medical therapy with dopamine agonists is considered the most effective treatment, and bromocriptine has been the mainstay of therapy. However, cabergoline appears to be better tolerated than bromocriptine and is at least as effective if not more effective than bromocriptine. For these reasons, cabergoline is replacing bromocriptine as the mainstay of medical therapy.

PANHYPOPITUITARISM

Panhypopituitarism is a condition of complete or partial loss of anterior and posterior pituitary function resulting in a complex disorder characterized by multiple pituitary-hormone deficiencies. Patients with panhypopituitarism may have ACTH deficiency, gonadotropin deficiency, growth-hormone deficiency, hypothyroidism, and hyperprolactinemia. Panhypopituitarism can be classified as either primary or secondary depending on the etiology. Primary panhypopituitarism involves an abnormality within the secretory cells of the pituitary, whereas secondary panhypopituitarism is caused by a lack of proper external stimulation needed for normal release of pituitary hormones. Some of the most common causes of panhypopituitarism include primary pituitary tumors, ischemic necrosis of the pituitary, surgical trauma, irradiation, and various types of CNS infections. Pharmacologic treatment of panhypopituitarism is essential and consists of replacement of specific pituitary hormone after careful assessment of individual deficiencies. This is accomplished by administration of glucocorticoids, thyroid-hormone preparations, and sex steroids. The administration of recombinant growth hormone may be also considered in growing children and, more recently, for GH-deficient adults. Patients with panhypopituitarism will need life-long replacement therapy and constant monitoring of multiple homeostatic functions.

▶ PRINCIPLES OF PHARMACOTHERAPY

- Drug therapy should be considered for acromegalic patients in whom surgery and irradiation are contraindicated, when rapid control of symptoms is indicated, or when other treatments fail to normalize GH concentrations. Dopamine agonists, such as bromocriptine, should be considered prior to initiating therapy with a somatostatin analog because of the potential cost advantages and convenience of oral administration.
- Octreotide (Sandostatin) suppresses mean serum GH concentrations to less than 5 μg/L and normalizes serum IGF-I concentrations in 50% to 60% of acromegalic patients. It halts tumor growth and is also effective in reducing the clinical signs and symptoms of acromegaly. The most common adverse effects of octreotide therapy include gastrointestinal disturbances such as diarrhea, nausea, abdominal cramps, malabsorption of fat, and flatulence, which occur in approximately 75% of patients

and usually subside within 10 to 14 days of continued treatment.

- Octreotide inhibits cholecystokinin release and gallbladder motility, predisposing acromegalic patients to the development of cholelithiasis. The incidence of gallstones in acromegalic patients receiving octreotide increases with length of therapy and has been reported to range from 20% to 50%. However, most patients are asymptomatic, and the diagnosis of cholelithiasis is usually made following routine ultrasonographic evaluation that is not prompted by patient symptoms. The treatment of octreotide-induced gallstones is the same as that for gallstones in the general population, and prophylactic cholecystectomy or medical therapy with ursodeoxycholic acid is usually not warranted.
- Recombinant GH is currently considered the mainstay of therapy for the treatment of children with GHD short stature. Prompt diagnosis of GHD and initiation of replacement therapy with recombinant GH is crucial in optimizing the final adult heights of children with GHD. The use of GH therapy in patients with non-GHD short stature is controversial.
- Nine different recombinant growth hormone products are currently available in the United States. The potency of GH products is expressed as International Units per milligram (IU/mg) with 1 mg containing approximately 2.6 IU of growth hormone. Although recommended dosages may vary, all GH products are generally considered to be equally efficacious.
- Pharmacologic agents that antagonize dopamine or that increase the release of prolactin can induce hyperprolactinemia. Medications commonly reported to induce hyperprolactinemia include SSRIs; phenothiazine derivatives; haloperidol (Haldol); metoclopramide (Reglan); domperidone, estrogens; progestins; verapamil (e.g., Calan, Isoptin); methyldopa (Aldomet); reserpine; gonadotropin-releasing hormone analogs; H_2-receptor antagonists; benzodiazepines; tricyclic antidepressants; dexfenfluramine; opioids; and monoamine oxidase inhibitors. Discontinuation of the offending medication and initiation of an appropriate therapeutic alternative usually normalizes serum prolactin concentrations. In cases for which an appropriate therapeutic alternative does not exist, medical therapy with dopamine agonists may be warranted. Sex-steroid replacement may also be considered.
- Medical therapy with dopamine agonists is usually more effective than transsphenoidal surgery for the treatment of pituitary prolactinomas. Bromocriptine (Parlodel) has been the mainstay of medical therapy since the 1970s. However, as many as 12% of patients do not tolerate the adverse effects associated with this medication. Pergolide (Permax), although not FDA approved for the treatment of hyperprolactinemia, has been used as a cost-effective alternative in patients who are intolerant of the adverse effects associated with bromocriptine.
- Cabergoline (Dostinex), a long-acting dopamine agonist, appears to be more effective than bromocriptine for the medical management of prolactinomas and offers the advantage of less-frequent dosing. Cabergoline may also be effective in patients who are intolerant of or resistant to bromocriptine.
- Pharmacologic treatment of panhypopituitarism consists of replacement of specific pituitary hormones such as glucocorticoids, thyroid-hormone preparations, sex steroids, and recombinant growth hormone where appropriate. Patients with panhypopituitarism will need life-long replacement therapy and constant monitoring of multiple homeostatic functions.

REFERENCES

1. Raisman G. An urge to explain the incomprehensible: Geoffrey Harris and the discovery of the neural control of the pituitary gland. Ann Rev Neurosci 1997;20:533–566.
2. Cuttler L. The regulation of growth hormone secretion. Endocrinol Metab Clin North Am 1996;25:541–571.
3. Molitch ME. Pathologic hyperprolactinemia. Endocrinol Metab Clin North Am 1992;21:877–901.
4. D'Ercole AJ. Insulin-like growth factors and their receptors in growth. Endocrinol Metab Clin North Am 1996;25:573–590.
5. Acromegaly Therapy Consensus Development Panel. Consensus statement: Benefits versus risks of medical therapy for acromegaly. Am J Med 1994;97:468–473.
6. Eugster EA, Pescovitz OH. Gigantism. J Clin Endocrinol Metab 1999;84(12):4379–4384.
7. Molitch ME. Clinical manifestations of acromegaly. Endocrinol Metab Clin North Am 1992;21:597–614.
8. Melmed S. Etiology of pituitary acromegaly. Endocrinol Metab Clin North Am 1992;21:539–551.
9. Melmed S, Ho K, Klibanski A, et al. Recent advances in pathogenesis, diagnosis, and management of acromegaly. J Clin Endocrinol Metab 1995;80:3395–3402.
10. Melmed S. Unwanted effects of growth hormone excess in the adult. J Pediatr Endocrinol Metab 1996;9(suppl 3):369–374.
11. Patel YC, Ezzat S, Chik CL, P, et al. Guidelines for the diagnosis and treatment of acromegaly: A Canadian perspective. Clin Invest Med 2000;23:172–187.
12. Giustina A, Barkan AL, Casanueva FF, et al. Criteria for cure of acromegaly: A consensus statement. J Clin Endocrinol Metab 2000;85: 526–529.
13. Orrego JJ, Barkan AL. Pituitary disorders. Drugs 2000;59:93–106.
14. Melmed S, Jackson I, Kleinberg D, Klibanski A. Current treatment guidelines for acromegaly. J Clin Endocrinol Metab 1998;83:2646–2652.
15. Fahlbusch R, Honegger J, Buchfelder M. Acromegaly—The place of the neurosurgeon. Metabolism 1996;45:65–66.
16. Giustina A, Zaltieri G, Negrini F, Wehrenberg WB. The pharmacological aspects of the treatment of acromegaly. Pharmacol Res 1996;34:247–268.
17. Jaffe CA, Barkan AL. Acromegaly recognition and treatment. Drugs 1994;47:425–445.
18. Abs R, Verhelst J, Maiter D, et al. Cabergoline in the treatment of acromegaly: A study of 64 patients. J Clin Endocrinol Metab 1998;83:374–378.
19. Colao A, Ferone D, Marzullo P, et al. Effect of different dopaminergic agents in the treatment of acromegaly. J Clin Endocrinol Metab 1997;82:518–523.
20. Lamberts S, Reubi JC, Krenning EP. Somatostatin analogs in the treatment of acromegaly. Endocrinol Metab Clin North Am 1992;21:737–752.
21. Lamberts SE, Van der Lely A, de Herder WW, Hofland LJ. Drug therapy: Octreotide. N Engl J Med 1996;334:246–254.
22. Vance ML, Harris AG. Long-term treatment of 189 acromegalic patients with the somatostatin analog octreotide. Results of the international multicenter acromegaly study group. Arch Intern Med 1991;151:1573–1578.
23. Ezzat S, Snyder PJ, Young WF, et al. Octreotide treatment of acromegaly: A randomized, multicenter study. Ann Intern Med 1992;117:211–218.
24. Newman CB, Melmed S, Snyder PJ, et al. Safety and efficacy of long-term octreotide therapy of acromegaly: Results of a multicenter trial in 103 patients—A clinical research center study. J Clin Endocrinol Metab 1995;80:2768–2775.
25. Merola B, Cittadini A, Colao A, et al. Chronic treatment with the somatostatin analog octreotide improves cardiac abnormalities in acromegaly. J Clin Endocrinol Metab 1993;77:790–793.
26. Padayatty SJ, Perrins EJ, Belchetz PE. Octreotide treatment increases exercise capacity in patients with acromegaly. Eur J Endocrinol 1996;134:554–559.

27. Giustina A, Boni E, Romanelli G. Cardiopulmonary performance during exercise in acromegaly, and the effects of acute suppression of growth hormone hypersecretion with octreotide. Am J Cardiol 1995;75:1042–1047.
28. Grunstein RR, Ho KKY, Sullivan CE. Effect of octreotide, a somatostatin analog, on sleep apnea in patients with acromegaly. Ann Intern Med 1994;121:478–483.
29. Thapar K, Kovacs KT, Stefaneanu L, et al. Antiproliferative effect of the somatostatin analogue octreotide on growth hormone-producing pituitary tumors: Results of a multicenter randomized trial. Mayo Clin Proc 1997;72:893–900.
30. Gillis JC, Noble S, Goa KL. Octreotide long-acting release (LAR): A review of its pharmacological properties and therapeutic use in the management of acromegaly. Drugs 1997;53:681–699.
31. Coloa A, Ferone D, Lastoria S, et al. Prediction of efficacy of octreotide therapy in patients with acromegaly. J Clin Endocrinol Metab 1996;81:2356–2362.
32. Harris AG, Kokoris SP, Ezzat S. Continuous versus intermittent subcutaneous infusion of octreotide in the treatment of acromegaly. J Clin Pharmacol 1995;35:59–71.
33. Anderson JV, Catnach S, Lowe DG, et al. Prevalence of gastritis in patients with acromegaly: Untreated and during treatment with octreotide. Clin Endocrinol 1992;37:227–232.
34. Eastman RC, Arakaki RF, Shawker T, et al. A prospective examination of octreotide-induced gall bladder changes in acromegaly. Clin Endocrinol 1992;36:265–269.
35. Ewins DL, Javaid A, Coskeran PB, et al. Assessment of gall bladder dynamics, cholecystokinin release and the development of gallstones during octreotide therapy for acromegaly. Q J Med 1992;300:295–306.
36. Stolk MFJ, van Erpecum KJ, Koppeschaar HPF, et al. Effect of octreotide on fasting gall bladder emptying, antroduodenal motility, and motilin release in acromegaly. Gut 1995;36:755–760.
37. Avila NA, Shawker TH Roach P, et al. Sonography of gallbladder abnormalities in acromegaly patients following octreotide and ursodiol therapy: Incidence and time course. J Clin Ultrasound 1998;26:289–294.
38. Ho KK, Jenkins AB, Furier SM, et al. Impact of octreotide, a long-acting somatostatin analogue, on glucose tolerance and insulin sensitivity in acromegaly. Clin Endocrinol 1992;36:271–279.
39. Sato K, Takamatsu K, Hashimoto K. Short-term effects of octreotide on glucose tolerance in patients with acromegaly. Endocr J 1995;42:739–745.
40. Koop BL, Harris AG, Ezzat S. Effect of octreotide on glucose tolerance in acromegaly. Eur J Endocrinol 1994;130:581–586.
41. Flogstad AK, Halse J, Grass P, et al. A comparison of octreotide, bromocriptine, or a combination of both drugs in acromegaly. J Clin Endocrinol Metab 1994;79:461–465.
42. Parkinson C, Trainer PJ. Pegvisomant: A growth hormone receptor antagonist for the treatment of acromegaly. Growth Horm IGF Res 2000;10:S119–S123.
43. Trainer PJ, Drake WM, Katznelson L, et al. Treatment of acromegaly with the growth hormone-receptor antagonist pegvisomant. N Engl J Med 2000;342:1171–1177.
44. Weekes LM, Ho KK, Seale JP. Treatment options in acromegaly: Benefits and costs. Pharmacoeconomics 1996;10:453–459.
45. Hindmarsh PC, Brook CGD. Short stature and growth hormone deficiency. Clin Endocrinol 1995;43:133–142.
46. Audi L, Granada ML, Carrascosa A. Growth hormone secretion assessment in the diagnosis of short stature. J Pediatr Endocrinol Metab 1996;9:313–324.
47. Hintz R. Growth hormone treatment of idiopathic short stature. Horm Res 1996;46:208–214.
48. Schwartz ID, Grunt JA. Growth, short stature, and the use of growth hormone: Considerations for the practicing pediatrician—An update. Curr Prob Pediatr 1997;27:14–40.
49. Lawson Wilkins Pediatric Endocrine Society Executive Committee. Guidelines for the use of growth hormone in children with short stature. A report by the drug and therapeutics committee of the Lawson Wilkins Pediatric Endocrine Society. J Pediatr 1995;127:857–867.
50. Marin G, Domene HM, Barnes KM, et al. The effects of estrogen priming and puberty on the growth hormone response to standardized treadmill exercise and arginine-insulin in normal girls and boys. J Clin Endocrinol Metab 1994;79:537–541.
51. Hintz R. Current and potential therapeutic uses of growth hormone and insulin-like growth factor-I. Endocrinol Metab Clin North Am 1996;25:759–773.
52. Fradkin JE, Schonberger LB, Mills JL, et al. Creutzfeldt-Jakob disease in pituitary growth hormone recipients in the United States. JAMA 1991;265:880–884.
53. Rikken B, Massa GG, Wit JM, and the Dutch Growth Hormone Working Group. Final height in a large cohort of Dutch patients with growth hormone deficiency treated with growth hormone. Horm Res 1995;43:136–137.
54. Chipman JJ, Hicks JR, Holcombe JH, Draper MW. Approaching final height in children treated for growth hormone deficiency. Horm Res 1995;43:129–131.
55. Serveri F. Final height in children with growth hormone deficiency. Horm Res 1995;43:138–140.
56. Coste J, Letrait M, Carel JC, et al. Long-term results of growth hormone treatment in France in children of short stature: Population, register-based study. BMJ 1997;315:708–713.
57. Blethen SL, Bapitista J, Kuntze J, et al. Adult height in growth hormone (GH)-deficient children treated with biosynthetic GH. J Clin Endocrinol Metab 1997;82:418–420.
58. Jorgensen JO, Thuesen L, Muller J, et al. Three years of growth hormone treatment in growth hormone-deficient adults: Near normalization of body composition and physical performance. Eur J Endocrinol 1994;130:224–228.
59. Cuneo RC, Judd S, Wallace JD, et al. The Australian multicenter trial of growth hormone (GH) treatment in GH-deficient adults. J Clin Endocrinol Metab 1998;83:107–116.
60. Kann P, Piepkorn B, Schehler B, et al. Effect of long-term treatment with GH on bone metabolism, bone mineral density and bone elasticity in GH-deficient adults. Clin Endocrinol 1998;48(5):561–568.
61. Wiren L, Bengtsson BA, Johannsson G. Beneficial effects of long-term GH replacement therapy on quality of life in adults with GH deficiency. Clin Endocrinol 1998;48:613–620.
62. Moore WV, Moore KC, Gifford R, et al. Long-term treatment with growth hormone of children with short stature and normal growth hormone secretion. J Pediatr 1992;120:702–708.
63. Loche S, Cambiaso P, Setzu S, et al. Final height after growth hormone therapy in non-growth-hormone-deficient children with short stature. J Pediatr 1994;125:196–200.
64. Wit J, Boersma B, DeMuinch Keizer-Schrama SM, et al. Long-term results of growth hormone therapy in children with short stature, subnormal growth rate and normal growth hormone response to secretagogues. Clin Endocrinol 1995;42:365–372.
65. Schmitt K, Blumel P, Walkhor T, et al. Short- and long-term (final height) data in children with normal variant short stature treated with growth hormone. Eur J Pediatr 1997;156:680–683.
66. Cuttler L, Silvers JB, Singh J, et al. Short stature and growth hormone therapy: A national study of physician recommendation patterns. JAMA 1996;276:531–537.
67. Blethen SL, MacGillivray MH. A risk-benefit assessment of growth hormone use in children. Drug Saf 1997;17:303–316.
68. Cowell CT, Dietsch S. Adverse events during growth hormone therapy. J Pediatr Endocrinol Metab 1995;8:243–252.
69. Blethen SL, Allen DB, Graves D, et al. Safety of recombinant deoxyribonucleic acid-derived growth hormone: The National Cooperative Growth Study experience. J Clin Endocrinol Metab 1996;81:1704–1710.
70. Wantanabe S, Tsunematsu Y, Fujimoto J, et al. Leukaemia in patients treated with growth hormone. Lancet 1988;1:1159–1160.
71. Stahnke N. Leukemia in growth-hormone-treated patients: An update. Horm Res 1992;38(suppl 1):56–62.

72. Rougeot C, Marchand P, Dray F, et al. Comparative study of biosynthetic human growth hormone immunogenicity in growth hormone deficient children. Horm Res 1991;35:76–81.
73. Pirazzoli P, Cacciari E, Mandini M, et al. Follow-up of antibodies to growth hormone in 210 growth hormone-deficient children treated with different commercial preparations. Acta Paediatr 1995;84:1233–1236.
74. Grunt JA, Schwartz ID, Buchanan C, et al. Effects of long-term growth hormone releasing hormone 1–29 in significantly short children. Acta Paediatr 1995;85:631–633.
75. Thorner M, Rochiccioli P, Colle M, et al. Once daily subcutaneous growth hormone-releasing hormone accelerates growth in growth-hormone deficient children during the first year of therapy. J Clin Endocrinol Metab 1996;81:1189–1196.
76. Ogilvy-Stuart AL, Stirling HF, Kelnart CJH, et al. Treatment of radiation-induced growth hormone deficiency with growth hormone-releasing hormone. Clin Endocrinol 1997;46:571–578.
77. Deghenghi R. Examorelin. Drugs Future 1996;21:366–368.
78. Pihoker C, Badger TM, Reynolds GH, et al. Treatment effects of intranasal growth hormone releasing peptide-2 in children with short stature. J Endocrinol 1997;155:79–86.
79. Bellone J, Ghizzoni L, Aimaretti G. Growth hormone-releasing effect of oral growth hormone-releasing peptide 6 (GHRP-6) administration in children with short stature. Eur J Endocrinol 1995;133:425–429.
80. American Academy of Pediatrics Committee on Drugs and Committee on Bioethics. Considerations related to the use of recombinant human growth hormone in children. Pediatrics 1997;99:122–129.
81. Kaye TB. Hyperprolactinemia. Causes, consequences, and treatment options. Postgrad Med 1996;99:265–268.
82. Biller BM, Luciano A, Crosignani PG, et al. Guidelines for the diagnosis and treatment of hyperprolactinemia. J Reprod Med 1999;44 (suppl 12):1075–1084.
83. Jones TH. The management of hyperprolactinaemia. Br J Hosp Med 1995;53:374–378.
84. Molitch ME. Medical treatment of prolactinomas. Endocrinol Metab Clin North Am 1999;28:143–169.
85. Davies PH. Drug-related hyperprolactinaemia. Adverse Drug React Toxicol Rev 1997;16:83–94.
86. Marken PA, Haykal RF, Fisher JN. Management of psychotropic-induced hyperprolactinemia. Clin Pharm 1992;11:851–856.
87. Colao A, Annunziato L, Lombardi G. Treatment of prolactinomas. Ann Med 1998;30:452–459.
88. Thomson JA, Davies DL, McLaren EH, et al. Ten-year follow-up of microprolactinomas treated by transsphenoidal surgery. BMJ 1994;309: 1409–1410.
89. Bevan JS, Bebster J, Burke CW, et al. Dopamine agonists and pituitary tumor shrinkage. Endocr Rev 1992;13:220–240.
90. Webster J. A comparative review of the tolerability profiles of dopamine agonists in the treatment of hyperprolactinaemia and inhibition of lactation. Drug Saf 1996;14:228–238.
91. Weingrill CO, Portes E, Mussio W, et al. Long-acting oral bromocriptine (Parlodel SRO) in the treatment of hyperprolactinemia. Fertil Steril 1992;57:331–335.
92. Tsagarakis S, Tsiganou E, Tzavara I, et al. Effectiveness of a long-acting injectable form of bromocriptine in patients with prolactin and growth hormone-secreting macroadenomas. Clin Endocrinol 1995;42:593–599.
93. Ciccarelli E, Grottoli S, Miola C, et al. Double-blind randomized study using oral or injectable bromocriptine in patients with hyperprolactinaemia. Clin Endocrinol 1994;40:193–198.
94. Dash RJ, Ajmani AK, Sialy R. Prolactin (PRL) response to oral or vaginal bromoergocriptine in hyperprolactinemic women. Horm Metab Res 1994;26:164.
95. Lamberts SWJ, Quik RFP. A comparison of the efficacy and safety of pergolide and bromocriptine in the treatment of hyperprolactinemia. J Clin Endocrinol Metab 1991;72:635–641.
96. Berezin M, Avidan D, Baron E. Long-term pergolide treatment of hyperprolactinemic patients previously unsuccessfully treated with dopaminergic drugs. Isr J Med Sci 1991;27:375–379.
97. Verhelst J, Abs R, Maiter D, et al. Cabergoline in the treatment of hyperprolactinemia: A study in 455 patients. J Clin Endocrinol Metab 1999;84:2518–2522.
98. Cannavo S, Curto L, Squadrito S, et al. Cabergoline: A first-choice treatment in patients with previously untreated prolactin-secreting pituitary adenoma. J Endocrinol Invest 1999;22:354–359.
99. Colao A, DiSarno A, Landi ML, et al. Macroprolactinoma shrinkage during cabergoline treatment is greater in naïve patients than in patients pretreated with other dopamine agonists: A prospective study in 110 patients. J Clin Endocrinal Metab 2000;85:2247–2252.
100. Ferrari CI, Abs R, Bevan JS, et al. Treatment of macroprolactinoma with cabergoline: A study of 85 patients. Clin Endocrinol 1997;46:409–413.
101. Webster J, Piscitelli G, Polli A, et al. A comparison of cabergoline and bromocriptine in the treatment of hyperprolactinemic amenorrhea. N Engl J Med 1994;331:904–909.
102. Delgrange E, Maiater D, Donckier J. Effects of the dopamine agonist cabergoline in patients with prolactinoma intolerant or resistant to bromocriptine. Eur J Endocrinol 1996;134:454–456.
103. Rains CP, Bryson HM, Fitton A. Cabergoline: A review of its pharmacological properties and therapeutic potential in the treatment of hyperprolactinaemia and inhibition of lactation. Drugs 1995;49:255–279.
104. Motta T, Colombo N, DeVincentiis S, et al. Vaginal cabergoline in the treatment of hyperprolactinemic patients intolerant to oral dopaminergics. Fertil Steril 1996;65:440–442.

78

PREGNANCY AND LACTATION: THERAPEUTIC CONSIDERATIONS

Denise L. Walbrandt Pigarelli and Connie K. Kraus

Drug use in pregnancy and lactation is a topic of frequent importance in practice, but it does not always receive much emphasis in formal training. Interestingly, the subject encompasses a dichotomous discussion of the benefits of drug therapy for the mother and the potential risks for the embryo/fetus. Drug use in pregnancy and lactation is a controversial area because of the medicolegal implications of therapy that may have a dual effect on mother and child.

Drugs do cross the placenta and enter into breast milk, and it is the duty of the clinician to promote safe drug use for both the pregnant and the nursing mother. The earliest interventions involve meeting pharmacologic needs prior to conception. During pregnancy, the use of interventions with demonstrated positive effects on fetal outcomes encourage the patient's active participation in preventive care. Acute care needs, whether common to women in general or due to the pregnancy, may arise. Likewise, a growing number of women begin pregnancies with a history of concomitant chronic illnesses. Treatment for these chronic conditions may need modification to ensure the best quality of care for the mother and the best outcome for the infant.

Pharmacotherapeutic issues also apply to selection of drugs during parturition and the postpartum period. Principles of drug use during lactation, although similar, are not the same as those applicable during pregnancy.

NATURAL COURSE OF PREGNANCY

PHYSIOLOGY

Because of the complexity of fertilization and subsequent pregnancy events, approximately 50% of embryos do not survive.[1] Most of these losses occur in the first 2 weeks after fertilization, and many women may not realize that they were pregnant. About 15% of the pregnancies that survive the first 2 weeks of gestation will be spontaneously lost later in the course of the pregnancy.[1]

Fertilization occurs when a sperm joins to an egg by attaching to a receptor on the outer protein layer of the egg, the zona pellucida. Immediately, the egg becomes unresponsive to other sperm. The attached sperm releases enzymes that cause the egg's chromosomes to mature and also allow the sperm to fully penetrate the zona pellucida and contact the egg's cell membrane. The membranes of the sperm and egg are then fused to create a new, single cell. Male and female chromosomes join in the new cell, fuse to create a single nucleus, and organize to set the stage for cell division.[1]

Fertilization usually occurs in the fallopian tube. Cell division continues for the first 2 days while the fertilized egg travels down the fallopian tube, reaching the uterine cavity on the third day.[1] Cell division continues for 2 to 3 more days in the uterine cavity before implantation begins.

Approximately 6 days after fertilization, the cell mass is termed a blastocyst. Human chorionic gonadotropin (hCG) is now produced in amounts that may be detected in commercial laboratories. The blastocyst sloughs the zona pellucida and rests directly on the endometrium, which responds to the denuded blastocyst by allowing it to begin to grow into the endometrial wall. After 6 days of this growth, the blastocyst lies implanted under the endometrium's surface and begins to receive nutrition from maternal blood.[1] It is now called an embryo.[2]

The embryonic period lasts from approximately 2 weeks after fertilization until 8 weeks after fertilization, when the conceptus is renamed a fetus. Most body structures are formed during the embryonic period, and they continue to grow and mature during the fetal period. The fetal period continues until the pregnancy reaches term, approximately 40 weeks after the last menstrual period.[2]

Gravidity refers to the number of times that a woman experiences pregnancy. A multiple birth is counted as a single pregnancy. Parity refers to the number of a woman's pregnancies that exceeded 20 weeks of gestation and also relates information regarding the outcome of each pregnancy. In sequence, the numbers reflect (1) term deliveries, (2) premature deliveries, (3) aborted and/or ectopic pregnancies, and (4) number of living children. A woman who has been pregnant four times; has experienced two term deliveries, one premature delivery, and one ectopic pregnancy; and has three living children would be designated by G_4P_{2113}.

PREGNANCY DATING

Approximately 280 days (about 40 weeks or 9 months) constitute the duration of a pregnancy; this time period extends from the first day of the last menstrual period to birth. Gestational age or menstrual age refers to the age of the embryo or fetus beginning with the first day of the last menstrual period, which is about 2 weeks prior to fertilization. To calculate an approximate pregnancy due date, the clinician adds 7 days to the first day of the last menstrual period and subtracts 3 months.[2]

For simple description purposes, pregnancy is divided into three periods of 3 calendar months, and each period of 3 months is called a trimester.

PREGNANCY SIGNS AND SYMPTOMS

The early symptoms of pregnancy include fatigue and increased frequency of urination.[3] At approximately 6 weeks' gestation, the pregnant woman may experience nausea and vomiting; this is commonly known as morning sickness, but may occur at any time of the day. Nausea and vomiting usually resolve at 12 to 18 weeks' gestation, but may persist into the second trimester as well.[3] Fetal movement is detected in the woman's lower abdomen at 16 to 20 weeks' of gestation.[3]

Signs of pregnancy may include sudden cessation of menses, changes in consistency of the cervical mucus, a bluish discoloration of the vaginal mucosa, increased skin pigmentation, and anatomic breast changes.[3]

MATERNAL PHARMACOKINETIC CHANGES IN PREGNANCY

During pregnancy, a woman's reduced gastrointestinal motility, increased gastric pH, and increased pulmonary alveolar drug uptake affect drug absorption.[4] Drug distribution in pregnancy may change because maternal plasma volume increases by 50%. Of the approximately 8-L increase in total body water during pregnancy, 40% is distributed to maternal compartments, and 60% is distributed to the amniotic fluid, placenta, and fetus.[4] Serum albumin levels fall during gestation from an average of 40 to 33 g/L at 40 to 41 weeks' gestation, resulting in a reduction in available binding sites for acidic drugs. However, plasma volume increases during pregnancy by 40% to 50%. The net impact on drug distribution is unaltered free drug serum concentration for many (but not all) drugs. Notable examples of drugs whose unbound fraction increases significantly during pregnancy include salicylic acid, sulfisoxazole, diazepam, valproic acid, and phenytoin.[4]

Pregnancy also affects drug elimination. The maternal hormones progesterone and estradiol affect hepatic drug metabolism in various ways; they enhance the hepatic metabolism for some drugs (e.g., phenytoin), while they inhibit this metabolism for others (e.g., theophylline).[4] In addition, the clearance of drugs excreted into the biliary system may slow because estrogen can cause cholestasis.[4] Renal drug clearance may be affected by an increased renal blood flow of 25% to 50% and an increased glomerular filtration rate of 50%.[4] Fortunately, these changes usually do not result in a clinically significant alteration that requires alteration of drug dosing.[4]

TRANSPLACENTAL DRUG TRANSFER

Although once thought to be a barrier to drug transfer, the placenta is fundamentally the organ of exchange for a number of substances, including drugs, between the mother and fetus.[5] The placenta functions fully for such transport by the fifth week after conception. Most drugs move across the membranes by passive diffusion, both to the fetus from the mother and from the fetus to the mother, as maternal serum levels decline. Such considerations as maternal dose, route of administration, maternal pharmacokinetic handling of the ingested substance, and maternal plasma protein binding may influence the actual amount of drug that reaches the fetus.[5] Characteristics of the ingested substance also influence the degree of transfer: high lipophilicity, low ionization, low maternal protein binding, and low molecular weight all enhance the degree of transfer.[5]

The degree to which exposure to a drug influences the embryo/fetus may also be a function of the timing of the exposure. It is generally thought that drug exposure during the embryonic period (the fifth through the tenth week of gestation) has the greatest potential influence on organ development.[5,6] Indeed, the most obvious teratogenic effects occur during this period.[5] Teratogenic effects may include loss of pregnancy, structural abnormalities, growth impairment, and functional loss.[6] However, more subtle changes in function or behavior may be associated with drug exposure at other times during pregnancy.[5]

DRUG SELECTION DURING PREGNANCY

Accounting for one-third of deaths of infants, congenital malformations occur in approximately 70 of 1000 births in North America and Europe.[7] It is estimated that 20% of congenital malformations originate from genetic or chromosomal abnormalities, and another 10% are due to environmental factors, only one of which is exposure to drugs. In the majority of cases, the cause of congenital abnormalities is unknown.

Teratogenicity is often defined broadly to include abnormal development of the embryo/fetus and, as noted earlier, can include loss of pregnancy, structural or long-term functional abnormalities, and abnormal uterine growth.[6] Adverse fetal drug effects are dependent on dosage, route of administration, concomitant exposure to other agents, and timing.[8,9] In terms of the timing of a drug exposure, there may be little effect during preimplantation (conception to 1 week postconception).[8] During organogenesis (2 to 8 weeks postconception), developing organs and organ systems may be quite vulnerable to drug effects. Exposure during the latter part of pregnancy may lead to functional and behavioral changes.

Of the many marketed drugs, only about 30 are associated with teratogenic effects.[9,10] Among these drugs are chemotherapeutic agents (e.g., methotrexate, cyclophosphamide); anticonvulsants (e.g., carbamazepine, phenytoin, valproic acid); sex hormones (e.g., androgens, diethylstilbestrol, danazol); warfarin; angiotensin-converting enzyme inhibitors, which may lead to renal failure in the neonate; anticholinergic drugs, which may lead to meconium ileus; oral hypoglycemic drugs, which may lead to neonatal hypoglycemia; antithyroid drugs, which may lead to fetal hypothyroidism; lithium; misoprostol; nonsteroidal anti-inflammatory agents, which may lead to constriction of the ductus arteriosus; psychoactive drugs, which may lead to withdrawal symptoms; retinoids (e.g., isotretinoin, etretinate); tetracyclines; and thalidomide.[9,10]

METHODS OF DETERMINING SAFETY OF DRUGS IN PREGNANCY

Although randomized, controlled trials form the basis for some of the most reliable assessments of drug safety, pregnant women are not usually eligible for participation in clinical trials. Other types of data are often used to estimate the risk associated with medication use during pregnancy, such as animal studies, case reports, case-control studies, prospective cohort studies, historical cohort studies, and voluntary reporting systems.

Although animal studies are a required component of drug testing, the extrapolation of the results of such testing to humans is not always accurate. One example is thalidomide, which was found to be safe in some animal models but proved to have teratogenic effects in human offspring.[9]

Case reports may be of limited value because an isolated occurrence of a birth defect in the infant of a woman who used a medication during her pregnancy may have occurred by chance.[9] The overall risk of congenital malformations from all causes is approximately 7%, but only a small part of this is likely due to drugs.[7] Because most pregnant women use drugs infrequently and the overall risk of drug-related teratogenic effects is low, it would take a very large number of exposures to appreciate an increased risk.[9] The few instances in which case reports have been helpful in establishing teratogenic risk were situations in which a drug was used infrequently, but was associated with a high rate of birth defects (isotretinoin), or it was used widely, but caused reproducible malformations (thalidomide).[10]

Case-control studies identify an outcome (congenital anomaly), match subjects with and without that outcome, and report how often there was exposure to a suspected agent.[9] The concern with this type of study is recall bias, because a woman with an affected pregnancy may be more likely to recall drugs used during the course of a pregnancy than would a woman who had a normal pregnancy outcome.

Cohort studies look at the intervention (use of a particular drug) in a group of persons and compare outcomes in a similar group of subjects without the intervention.[9] The fact that the study is prospective eliminates some of the problems with recall and bias. This approach has several potential disadvantages, however, such as the need for large numbers of participants, time, and potential loss to follow-up. Despite these disadvantages, cohort studies are often used for evaluating the effects of drug exposure on pregnancy outcomes.

An example of a cohort study was the Michigan Medicaid study, which consisted of data collected from 229,101 pregnancies over 7 years.[9] Similarly, in the PEGASUS project in Munich, Germany, a group of women were asked to prospectively record in a log book all use of medications, both prescribed and self-selected, throughout the course of pregnancy.[7,9] Information obtained through examination of the newborns and information learned about the pregnancies, such as maternal risk factors, will be linked with the drug utilization information. Other cohort studies have involved the development of teratology information services that pregnant women may contact for information about potential exposures during pregnancy and, in turn, be followed to assess the outcomes of the pregnancy.[9] In addition, some pharmaceutical companies have organized voluntary reporting systems for drugs used in pregnancy.[9] One such example is the Acyclovir in Pregnancy Registry.

RESOURCES

A commonly used source of information about drug safety in pregnancy is the category system of the Food and Drug Administration (FDA).[11] The categories for drug use in pregnancy range as follows:

A—Adequate, well-controlled studies in pregnant women have not shown an increased risk of fetal abnormalities.

B—Animal studies have revealed no evidence of harm to the fetus; however, there are no adequate and well-controlled studies in pregnant women.

or

Animal studies have shown an adverse effect, but adequate and well-controlled studies in pregnant women have failed to demonstrate a risk to the fetus.

C—Animal studies have shown an adverse effect and there are no adequate and well-controlled studies in pregnant women.

or

No animal studies have been conducted and there are no adequate and well-controlled studies in pregnant women.

D—Studies, adequate, well-controlled or observational, in pregnant women have demonstrated a risk to the fetus. However, the benefits of therapy may outweigh the potential risk.

X—Studies, adequate, well-controlled or observational, in animals or pregnant women have demonstrated positive evidence of fetal abnormalities. The use of the product is contraindicated in women who are or may become pregnant.

The FDA created these categories to provide therapeutic guidance regarding the risk versus benefit for drug use during pregnancy.[10] Some of the concerns with use of the FDA categories involve the difficulty of interpreting them and the difficulty of changing a drug's classification when new information becomes available.[10]

Another rating system, Teratogen Information System (TERIS), is also available.[8] This system was designed to assess the teratogenic risks of a drug and is developed based on expert opinion and literature review.[8]

GENERAL RECOMMENDATIONS FOR SELECTION OF MEDICATIONS IN PREGNANCY

Several principles may be helpful in selecting medications for use during pregnancy. The first is to consider using drugs that have been used for the longest periods of time with safety.[10] Table 78–1 illustrates selected drugs for a number of indications that are considered safe for use in pregnancy based on individual, large cohort studies, or meta-analyses of smaller studies.[10]

Whenever possible, the amount of drug administered should be at the lower end of the dosing range to minimize fetal exposure.[10] Finally, patients should be discouraged from self-medicating during pregnancy and encouraged to consult their provider for advice.

PRECONCEPTION PLANNING

There are approximately 4 million births in the United States each year.[12] Almost 50% of these pregnancies are unplanned.[13] In addition, many women may not seek health care for pregnancy until after the first trimester. Given the dynamic changes that occur during the first trimester, there is a growing effort to encourage preconception planning. Not only would such planning assist the prospective mother in identifying areas of risk for pregnancy, but also it would provide education and interventions to improve birth outcomes.

Several preconception interventions have been shown to improve pregnancy outcomes. One of these is the ingestion of folic acid to reduce the risk for neural tube defects,[12] which affect approximately 4000 pregnancies in the United States each year.[14,15] Of these pregnancies, one-third are spontaneously or electively aborted.[14] Controlled clinical trials have shown that folic acid supplementation prior to and during the early stages of pregnancy can reduce the incidence of neural tube defects by up to 50%.[14] Because the neural tube closes within the first 4 weeks of pregnancy and because so many pregnancies are unplanned and unrecognized until after this time, it is necessary to encourage women of childbearing potential either to consume folate-enriched foods or to use supplements prior to pregnancy.

The American Academy of Pediatrics Committee on Genetics endorses the recommendation from the U.S. Public Health Service is that all women of childbearing age should ingest 400 μg of folic acid daily to reduce the risk of neural tube defects in their potential offspring.[14] Because the consumption of foods naturally containing folic acid is variable from day to day and because folate from these sources is less well absorbed, it is suggested that women fulfill the daily requirement for folic acid through either folate-enriched foods or supplements.[15] Women who have had a pregnancy affected by a neural tube defect should receive 4000 μg (4 mg) of folic acid beginning 1 to 3 months prior to conception and continuing throughout the first trimester.[16] These higher doses of folic acid require the use of supplements.[14] Although folic acid supplementation may potentially mask the hematologic effects of vitamin B_{12} deficiency, but the risk of this occuring in otherwise healthy women has not been supported by clinical trials.[16] The evidence of a reduction in birth defects with supplementation of other vitamins and nutrients prior to and during pregnancy is weaker than that for supplementation of folic acid.[12]

Other preconception interventions with evidence of improving pregnancy outcomes include screening and immunization for rubella

TABLE 78–1. Selected Drugs That Can Be Used Safely During Pregnancy, According to Condition

Condition	Drugs of Choice	Alternative Drugs	Comments
Acne	Topical: erythromycin, clindamycin, benzoyl peroxide	Systemic: erythromycin, topical tretinoin (vitamin A acid)	Isotretinoin is contraindicated.
Allergic rhinitis	Topical: glucocorticoids, cromolyn, decongestants, xylometazoline, oxymetazoline, nephazoline, phenylephrine Systemic: diphenhydramine, dimenhydrinate, tripelennamine		
Constipation	Docusate sodium, calcium, glycerin, sorbitol, lactulose, mineral oil, magnesium hydroxide	Bisacodyl, phenolphthalein	
Cough	Diphenhydramine, codeine, dextromethorphan		
Depression	Tricyclic antidepressant drugs, fluoxetine	Lithium	When lithium is used in first trimester, fetal echocardiography and ultrasonography are recommended because of small risk of cardiovascular defects.
Diabetes	Insulin (human)		Hypoglycemic drugs should be avoided.
Headache			
Tension	Acetaminophen	Aspirin and nonsteroidal anti-inflammatory drugs, benzodiazepines	Aspirin and nonsteroidal anti-inflammatory drugs should be avoided in third trimester.
Migraine	Acetaminophen, codeine, dimenhydrinate	β-adrenergic receptor antagonists and tricyclic antidepressant drugs (for prophylaxis)	Limited experience with ergotamine has not revealed evidence of teratogenicity, but there is concern about potent vasoconstriction and uterine contraction.
Hypertension	Labetalol, methyldopa	β-adrenergic receptor antagonists, prazosin, hydralazine	Angiotensin-converting enzyme inhibitors should be avoided because of risk of severe neonatal renal insufficiency.
Hyperthyroidism	Propylthiouracil, methimazole	β-adrenergic receptor antagonists (for symptoms)	Surgery may be required; radioactive iodine should be avoided.
Mania (and bipolar affective disorder)	Lithium, chlorpromazine, haloperidol	For depressive episodes: tricyclic antidepressant drugs, fluoxetine, valproic acid	If lithium is used in first trimester, fetal echocardiography and ultrasonography are recommended because of small risk of cardiac anomalies; valproic acid may be given after neural tube closure is complete.
Nausea, vomiting, motion sickness	Diclectin (doxylamine plus pyridoxine)[a]	Chlorpromazine, metoclopramide (in third trimester), diphenhydramine, dimenhydrinate, meclizine, cyclizine	
Peptic ulcer disease	Antacids, magnesium hydroxide, aluminum hydroxide, calcium carbonate, ranitidine	Sucralfate, bismuth subsalicylate	
Pruritus	Topical: moisturizing creams or lotions, aluminum acetate, zinc oxide cream or ointment, calamine lotion, glucocorticoids Systemic: hydroxyzine, diphenhydramine, glucocorticoids	Topical: local anesthetics	
Thrombophlebitis, deep vein thrombosis	Heparin, antifibrinolytic drugs, streptokinase		Streptokinase is associated with a risk of bleeding; warfarin should be avoided.

[a]Not available in the United States.

From: Koren G, Pastuszak A, Ito S. Drug therapy: drugs in pregnancy. N Engl J Med 1998; 338(6): 1128-1137. *Adapted with permission, 2000 Copyright* © 1998 *Massachusetts Medical Society. All rights reserved.*

and varicella.[12] In addition, screening for and treatment of sexually transmitted diseases prior to pregnancy reduces risks.

Another important component of preconception and early pregnancy care involves the assessment and reduction of risks associated with the use of alcohol, tobacco, and other substances. Moderate or heavy use of alcohol (i.e., seven or more drinks per week, or five or more drinks on one occasion in the last month) is associated with potential adverse effects throughout pregnancy, but is particularly damaging during the early part of the first trimester when there may be a greater risk for spontaneous abortion and dysmorphologic changes in organ systems.[17,18] In addition, alcohol use has been linked to abnormal rates of growth and neurologic deficits.[17] One possible outcome of prenatal alcohol consumption, fetal alcohol syndrome, is regarded as a leading preventable cause of mental retardation in children. Many pregnant women are unaware of their pregnancy during the early part of the first trimester and may continue to use alcohol. As the preconception use of alcohol often indicates continued use of alcohol during pregnancy, it may be possible to screen for women at high risk for alcohol-related risks during pregnancy. Further, all women of childbearing age should be made aware that the rates of unplanned pregnancy are high and that the risks for alcohol-related, negative pregnancy outcomes are a function of sexual activity, ineffective contraceptive methods, and frequent use of alcohol. There has been no safe amount of alcohol identified for consumption by pregnant women; therefore, women who are considering pregnancy or are already pregnant should be encouraged to refrain from using alcohol.

It is estimated that 20% of pregnant women smoke during pregnancy.[19] The possible consequences of smoking during pregnancy include low birth weight, spontaneous abortion, preterm birth, premature detachment of the placenta, and fetal deformities.[19-22] Many of the defects associated with prenatal smoking may be related to hypoxia caused by carbon monoxide. One strategy to reduce the number of women who smoke during pregnancy is to encourage young women not to begin smoking. This approach is important, because the decline in rates of smoking among pregnant women is no different than the decline in rates among women in general, implying that the realization of pregnancy does not increase the number of women who stop smoking.[23] Behavioral therapy is suggested as first-line therapy to assist pregnant women in stopping smoking, as nicotine replacement products and other agents may carry some risk to the fetus.[20,24] If efforts to quit smoking without pharmacotherapeutic agents fail, it may be reasonable to consider use of nicotine replacement therapy or bupropion. Overall, the nicotine levels to which the fetus is exposed with patch or gum are lower than those anticipated with the use of cigarettes.[20]

Pregnant women may use other substances of abuse. For example, they may be using drugs like cocaine, alcohol, or tobacco concomitantly. Because of this, true differentiation of cocaine's effects on the developing fetus may be difficult. Cocaine exposure seems to be associated with changes in fetal growth, neurologic development, and behavior.[5] Other substances, such as opiates (heroin/methadone) may result in physical dependence and withdrawal in the infant.[5]

Finally, it is important to optimize control of maternal chronic illness in the preconception and early prenatal period. Fetal malformation and macrosomia have occurred in infants of women with type 1 diabetes, for example, particularly when euglycemia has not been achieved.[25] Several studies have suggested that optimal glycemic control early in pregnancy may be important to prevent birth defects. A study of women with diabetes who received standard prenatal care versus preconception care for diabetes demonstrated a reduction in hospitalizations and lengths of stay for both diabetic mothers and their infants.[26]

PREGNANCY-INFLUENCED ISSUES

GASTROINTESTINAL TRACT

Constipation occurs commonly in pregnancy. There may be many contributing factors, such as changes in dietary habits, fluid intake, and physical activity; delayed intestinal transit (most likely because of hormonal changes during pregnancy); and possibly obstruction.[27] Therapy for the constipation of pregnancy should be instituted first with non-drug modalities, such as education, physical exercise, biofeedback, and increased intake of dietary fiber and fluid. If additional therapy is warranted, the use of supplemental fiber and/or a stool softener such as docusate is appropriate. Milk of magnesia, magnesium citrate, lactulose, sorbitol, and bisacodyl are considered low-risk treatments for constipation in pregnancy, but should be reserved for occasional rather than routine use. Senna may also be used occasionally. Castor oil should be avoided in pregnancy because it can cause uterine contractions; mineral oil should be avoided in pregnancy because it can reduce the absorption of fat-soluble vitamins, such as vitamin K, and the decreased levels can lead to neonatal hemorrhage.[27]

Gastroesophageal reflux disease occurs in approximately 50% to 80% of pregnant women, and data reveal that decreased lower esophageal sphincter pressure (due to estrogen and progesterone causing smooth muscle relaxation) and increased intragastric pressure (due to the gravid uterus) are etiologic factors.[28] Therapy for gastroesophageal reflux disease in pregnancy includes lifestyle and dietary modifications (e.g., small, frequent meals; caffeine avoidance; food avoidance 3 hours before bedtime; elevation of the head of the bed) just as for nonpregnant patients, and pharmacologic therapy for pregnant patients who do not receive adequate relief from non-drug therapies.[29] Drug therapy for gastrointestinal reflux disease in pregnancy may be initiated with aluminum, calcium, or magnesium antacid preparations, although use of sodium bicarbonate should be avoided because of potential electrolyte and fluid abnormalities in the mother and fetus. Magnesium trisilicate should probably be avoided as well, because fetal renal, respiratory, cardiovascular, and muscular problems may occur with long-term, high-dose exposure. Sucralfate is another option for gastroesophageal reflux disease in pregnancy. Evidence also supports the use of cimetidine and ranitidine for this indication. Little literature is available regarding famotidine use in pregnancy, and no published information is available concerning nizatidine use in pregnancy. Combination antacids and nonprescription ranitidine have been shown in one small trial to be effective in patients unresponsive to antacids alone.[30] If a patient does not respond to histamine-2 receptor blockers, proton pump inhibitors are also a viable option for pregnant patients.[31,32]

The exact prevalence for hemorrhoids during pregnancy is unknown, but they may occur in as many as 40% to 50% of all pregnancies. Pathophysiologic causes of hemorrhoids during pregnancy may include constipation, venous dilation and engorgement due to pregnancy, and laxity of pelvic connective tissue because of hormones.[33] Therapy of hemorrhoids during pregnancy is generally conservative; high intake of dietary fiber, adequate oral fluid intake, and use of sitz baths are helpful.[33,34] Topical anesthetics may also be used. Other options for refractory hemorrhoids include sclerotherapy, photocoagulation, and surgery.

Nausea and vomiting affect 50% to 90% of pregnant women; however, hyperemesis gravidarum (i.e., severe nausea and vomiting requiring hospitalization for hydration and nutrition) occurs in only about 0.3% to 1%.[35] Possible, but not proved, causes of nausea and vomiting in pregnancy include elevated serum concentrations of hCG, abnormal autonomic nervous system function and resulting abnormal peristalsis, elevated serum concentrations of thyroid hormones, and psychological issues.[36] Although there is no scientific evidence to support the recommendation of dietary modifications, such as eating frequent small meals and avoiding fatty foods, many women find this approach helpful.[36,37] Other potentially helpful non-drug therapies include acupressure and psychotherapy.

Pharmacotherapy for nausea and vomiting in pregnancy includes drugs in the following categories: antihistamines, vitamins, anticholinergics, dopamine antagonists (including phenothiazines and metoclopramide), serotonin antagonists, prokinetic agents, and ginger.[36] Antihistamines (including doxylamine) have not been proved to be toxic during pregnancy and have shown efficacy in treating this disorder. Similarly, pyridoxine (vitamin B_6) and cyanocobalamin (vitamin B_{12}) have shown efficacy; the toxicity of these agents is not considered significant. The anticholinergic agents dicyclomine and scopolamine have not been shown to increase fetal malformation rates above those expected in the general population. Dicyclomine has no proved efficacy, and no randomized controlled trials exist that evaluate the effects of scopolamine for this disorder. Phenothiazines, with the exception of one study, have not been shown to increase the risk of fetal malformation, and this drug class has clearly demonstrated efficacy in treating nausea and vomiting in pregnancy. Metoclopramide has been used widely for nausea and vomiting in pregnancy, although no randomized clinical trials support its use; the drug has not been linked to an increased risk of malformations. Data evaluating the use of serotonin antagonists for pregnancy-induced nausea and vomiting are limited at this time. Ginger has no proved efficacy but is probably safe to use for nausea and vomiting in pregnancy.

GESTATIONAL DIABETES MELLITUS

About 4% of pregnant women develop gestational diabetes mellitus.[38] A woman who has risk factors for developing gestational diabetes mellitus (e.g., obesity, history of the condition, glycosuria, a strong family history of diabetes) should be screened for gestational diabetes mellitus at her first prenatal visit. If this screen is normal, she should have repeat testing between week 24 and week 28 of gestation. Pregnant women without these risk factors should undergo screening for gestational diabetes mellitus between week 24 and week 28 of gestation unless they are considered low risk. To be low risk, a woman must fulfill *all* of the following criteria: (1) age less than 25 years, (2) normal prepregnancy weight, (3) no known diabetes in first-degree relatives, (4) not a member of an ethnic group with a high prevalence of gestational diabetes mellitus, (5) no history of abnormal glucose tolerance, and (6) no history of abnormal obstetric outcome.

Screening for gestational diabetes mellitus utilizes the oral glucose challenge test. Initial screening involves measuring plasma glucose concentrations 1 hour after a 50-g oral glucose load; if the results are abnormal, a diagnostic 100-g oral glucose tolerance test should be completed. Of women with gestational diabetes mellitus, 80% will be identified if the glucose threshold value is more than140 mg/dL; 90% will be identified if the glucose threshold value is more than 130 mg/dL.[38]

First-line therapy for gestational diabetes mellitus includes nutritional and exercise interventions for all women and caloric restriction for obese women.[38] Daily self-monitoring of their blood glucose levels is necessary for all women with this condition. If nutritional and exercise interventions fail to result in a fasting whole blood glucose level equal to or less than 95 mg/dL and a 2-hour postprandial whole blood glucose level equal to or less than 120 mg/dL, insulin therapy with recombinant human insulin should be instituted;[38] glyburide may be considered after 11 weeks of gestation.[39] Women who require insulin therapy should also continue to monitor their glucose level postprandially. Goals for self-monitored blood glucose levels while on insulin therapy are as follows: preprandial plasma glucose level, 80–110 mg/dL; 1-hour postprandial plasma glucose level, less than 155 mg/dL; 2-hour postprandial plasma glucose level, less than 135 mg/dL.[40]

HYPERTENSION

In pregnancy, hypertension includes chronic hypertension, pregnancy-induced hypertension, gestational hypertension, and preeclampsia.[41] Preeclampsia is a condition consisting of hypertension, proteinuria (i.e., >300 mg in a 24-hour urine collection), and edema. Thrombocytopenia and abnormal liver function tests sometimes accompany preeclampsia.[42] The urine of pregnant patients should be tested for protein if (1) their blood pressure does not decrease by 10 to 20 mm Hg as expected during the second trimester, (2) their systolic pressure rises 30 mm Hg or their diastolic pressure rises 15 mm Hg over baseline, or (3) their blood pressure exceeds 140/90 mm Hg.[43]

Non-drug therapeutic approaches for hypertension in pregnancy have traditionally focused on activity restriction, psychosocial therapy, and biofeedback. In six studies of women with mildly elevated blood pressure, activity restriction had no effect on maternal or perinatal outcomes.[41] There have been no studies to evaluate activity restrictions in subjects with moderate to severe hypertension. Psychosocial support and biofeedback have not been found to have any clinically significant effects. Because of this lack of strong support for non-drug approaches, drug therapy should be initiated promptly in patients with hypertension in pregnancy.[41]

Because of its established efficacy and safety for mother and fetus, methyldopa is the first-line drug therapy for mild to moderate hypertension in pregnancy.[44,45] Alternatives include labetolol and other β-blockers, prazosin, nifedipine, isradipine, hydralazine, and clonidine.[10,41,44,45] The use of angiotensin-converting enzyme inhibitors is permissible in the first trimester, but should be discontinued after that time, if possible, because of associated renal toxicities in the fetus.[46,47] Diuretics should generally be avoided in pregnancy because they decrease plasma volume.[48] Severe hypertension in pregnancy may require multiple drug therapy or hospitalization for the intravenous (IV) administration of appropriate agents.

The cure for preeclampsia is delivery of the fetus if the pregnancy is at term. Preeclampsia may progress rapidly to eclampsia, a medical emergency, so weight, edema, and blood pressure must be studiously monitored in patients with preeclampsia. Infusions of hydralazine or labetolol for hypertension control and magnesium sulfate for seizure prevention are standard therapy for preeclampsia.[42]

Researchers have investigated the possible prevention of preeclampsia by means of calcium supplementation and/or antiplatelet agents (usually aspirin) in recent years. An evidence-based review suggests that calcium may be beneficial in women at high risk of developing preeclampsia and in those who have low dietary calcium intake.[49] Antiplatelet agents have small to moderate advantages for the prevention of preeclampsia, but the population of women most likely to benefit remains unknown.[50]

THYROID ABNORMALITIES

HCG may stimulate the thyroid gland because the structure of hCG is similar to that of thyrotropin.[51,52] Pregnant patients with excessive thyroid gland stimulation by this mechanism have gestational thyrotoxicosis.[51,52] Thyrotoxic patients usually present with vomiting, which can be severe; an increased serum level of free thyroxine; and a depressed thyrotropin level.[51,52] The degree of the thyroxine and thyrotropin abnormalities correlates with the severity of the vomiting, and no other findings are necessary to support the diagnosis of true thyrotoxicosis. Gestational thyrotoxicosis resolves with declining hCG concentrations at the completion of the first trimester.[52] Nausea and vomiting may be treated as for patients without this pseudohyperthyroid state.

VENOUS THROMBOEMBOLISM

Studies that cite the incidence of venous thromboembolism during and immediately after pregnancy are conflicting.[53] It is known, however, that women with hypercoagulable conditions and a history of venous thromboembolism before pregnancy have a higher risk of venous thromboembolism during pregnancy than do women without these prior problems. Therapy to prevent or treat venous thromboembolism during pregnancy must not include warfarin after the first 6 weeks of gestation because this drug may cause fetal bleeding, malformations of the nose, stippled epiphyses, or central nervous system anomalies.[53] Heparin is the drug of choice for prophylaxis or treatment of venous thrombolism during pregnancy. Low molecular weight heparins may present viable alternatives.[54]

ACUTE CARE ISSUES IN PREGNANCY

It is often necessary to address a wide range of acute care issues with pregnant women. For example, issues such as pain management and infectious diseases commonly arise during pregnancy.

HEADACHE

Women have a higher likelihood of experiencing tension and migraine headaches than do men. In fact, women are three times more likely than men to have migraine headaches.[55] The fluctuation of hormone levels during menstrual cycles, especially declining levels of estrogen, is often associated with migraine headaches.

The incidence of headache may actually decline during pregnancy, perhaps because of the consistently higher levels of circulating hormones. In one study, up to 48% of women with migraine and 28% of women with tension headache reported improvement in symptoms during pregnancy.[55] Some women have an increase in headache symptoms after delivery.

Acute care treatment for headache pain during pregnancy should include rest, reassurance, and ice applications.[8] If nonpharmacologic therapy for acute headache pain is not sufficient, the patient may receive acetaminophen and narcotic analgesics.[55] Nonsteroidal anti-inflammatory drugs (NSAIDs) and low-dose aspirin may also be considered, but should be avoided near term because of concerns about bleeding and early closure of the ductus arteriosus.[8] Sumatriptan is not considered suitable for use during pregnancy owing to concerns regarding vasoconstriction.[55]

Nausea and vomiting associated with migraine may be treated with metoclopramide.[8] For milder gastrointestinal symptoms, phosphorylated carbohydrate solution, doxylamine or pyridoxine may be helpful.[8] Medications such as trimethobenzamide, chlorpromazine, prochlorperazine, and promethazine are available for administration by non-oral routes, and they may be used for more severe vomiting.[8]

Preventive therapy for headache may be considered for women with frequent (three or four headaches per month) or incapacitating headaches. Propranolol has been used for this purpose.[8,55] Selective serotonin reuptake inhibitors, such as paroxetine, have also been used during pregnancy.[55]

PNEUMONIA

The incidence of pneumonia in pregnant women is the same as that in the general population, but the course of the illness in pregnancy is often more severe. Pneumonia has been reported as the third leading cause of death in pregnancy.[56] The increased morbidity and mortality rates during pregnancy may be due to alterations in the immune system (e.g., decreased lymphocyte production, changes in T-cell populations, decreased natural killer cell activity, reduced cytotoxic activity) and mechanical/anatomic changes.

Most cases of pneumonia that occur during pregnancy are bacterial; pneumococcus is the most common pathogen.[56] *Hemophilus influenzae* is the second most common isolate. Atypical bacteria such as *Mycoplasma, Chlamydia,* and *Legionella* are also seen. Less common are pneumonias caused by *Klebsiella* or *Staphylococcus aureus.* Clinical and laboratory evidence for the likely organism guide the treatment of bacterial pneumonias. Selection of antibiotic coverage is essentially the same as for the nonpregnant patient.

Influenza is the most common viral cause of pneumonia in pregnancy.[56] It tends to have a more virulent course during pregnancy and may be complicated by bacterial superinfections with *S. aureus, H. influenzae,* pneumococcus, and other gram-negative organisms.[56] In most cases, antiviral therapy will not be needed to treat pneumonia caused by influenza.

Pneumonia is a common complication of varicella infections during pregnancy.[56] It is estimated that 5% of women of childbearing age do not have immunity against varicella. Acyclovir in doses to 800 mg given orally five times daily for 10 days or 5–10 mg/kg given IV every 8 hours for severe cases have been recommended.[56] In addition, supportive measures such as the provision of supplemental oxygen, chest physiotherapy, bronchodilators, postural drainage, and fever control are beneficial.

Ideally, screening for varicella immunity takes place during preconception planning, and immunization is complete before conception. If a patient's history and titer show no immunity to varicella during early prenatal visits, the clinician should provide recommendations for avoidance of infection as well as recommendations for postpartum immunization. Pregnant women with risk factors for influenza infections should be offered immunization.[56]

URINARY TRACT INFECTION

With an estimated incidence of 8%,[57] urinary tract infections are common in pregnancy. The American College of Obstetricians and Gynecologists (ACOG) recommends a urine culture both at the initial prenatal visit and during the third trimester to screen pregnant women for such infections.[57] The U.S. Preventive Task Force recommends a urine culture between 12 and 16 weeks' gestation.[57] A urine culture is the preferred method for screening, as other methods, such as dipsticks that measure leukocytes and esterase, may fail to identify as many as 50% of patients with asymptomatic bacteriuria.

As with the general population, *Escherichia coli* is the principal infecting organism, present in 80% to 90% of infections. Other gram-negative rods, such as *Proteus mirabilis* and *Klebsiella pneumoniae,* also account for some infections. Urinary tract infections during pregnancy may occur as asymptomatic bacteriuria, acute cystitis, or pyelonephritis.

Asymptomatic bacteriuria may be present in up to 10% of pregnancies.[57] There is a 30% risk that untreated asymptomatic bacteriuria in pregnant women will progress to acute cystitis and a 50% risk that it will progress to pyelonephritis.[57] This rate of progression to symptomatic urinary tract infections is three to four times the rate in nonpregnant women.[58] The fact that there appears to be an increased risk for preterm delivery and low birth weight associated with asymptomatic bacteriuria underscores the need for screening and treatment in the pregnant population.[58,59]

Even though ampicillin and amoxicillin are considered safe medications for the treatment of asymptomatic bacteriuria during pregnancy, the incidence of *E. coli* resistance to these drugs may be up to 20% to 30%.[57,58] Nitrofurantoin is considered safe and effective for use in pregnancy; cephalexin is considered a good alternative. Sulfa-containing drugs may increase the risk for kernicterus in the newborn, and they should be avoided during the third trimester. Folate antagonists, such as trimethoprim, are relatively contraindicated during the first trimester of pregnancy. Fluoroquinolones and tetracyclines are contraindicated in pregnancy. The optimal duration of therapy for urinary tract infection during pregnancy has not been determined. Courses of 7 to 10 days are commonly used, but some studies have demonstrated that shorter courses may be sufficient.[57,58] A repeat culture to confirm cure is recommended.

Acute cystitis occurs in 0.3% to 1.3% of pregnancies.[58] In addition to having significant amounts of bacteria in the urine, women with acute cystitis complain of urinary frequency and pain.[57] The risks of low birth weight and preterm labor associated with acute cystitis have not been defined. Treatment for acute cystitis is the same as that described for asymptomatic bacteriuria.

Acute pyelonephritis complicates 1% to 2% of pregnancies,[58] sometimes leading to maternal sepsis and preterm labor and delivery.[57] Patients usually present with bacteriuria and systemic symptoms of fever, flank pain, nausea, and vomiting. Hospitalization is often necessary for pregnant women with pyelonephritis; there is a 2% risk that these patients will develop acute respiratory distress syndrome.[60] Inpatient therapy for pyelonephritis has included the IV administration of cephalosporins (e.g., cefazolin, ampicillin with gentamicin) or the intramuscular administration of ceftriaxone.[57] Outpatient antibiotic therapy for pyelonephritis may be considered if the woman is able to take medications orally and is not exhibiting symptoms of sepsis or preterm labor; cephalexin has been used for this purpose. The total duration of antibiotic therapy for acute pyelonephritis is 10 to 14 days.[58] This course may be followed by bedtime prophylaxis with nitrofurantoin for the duration of the pregnancy.[58]

SEXUALLY TRANSMITTED DISEASES

It is important to distinguish sexually transmitted diseases (STDs) that are bacterial in origin from those that are viral in origin because microbiologic cure is the usual endpoint of therapy for bacterial infections, whereas symptomatic control or delay in disease progression is the endpoint for viral illnesses. In addition, the concerns for pregnant women with STDs include intrauterine or perinatal transmission of the disease.[61] Those diseases that may be transmitted transplacentally, such as syphilis, ideally are discovered and treated early during the course of pregnancy. Diseases transmitted primarily during the birth process, such as *Chlamydia* infection, require identification prior to delivery so appropriate measures may be taken to decrease the likelihood of transmitting the infection to the newborn. Some genital infections may increase the likelihood of preterm labor and delivery (e.g., bacterial vaginosis in women), and these infections should be treated to decrease this risk.[61]

CHLAMYDIA INFECTIONS

Of the bacterial causes of STDs, *Chlamydia trachomatis* is the most likely responsible microorganism in the United States.[62] *Chlamydia* infections during pregnancy have been reported to be associated with premature rupture of membranes, preterm labor, and spontaneous abortion, although there is no scientific evidence to support these observations.[61] Transmission of *Chlamydia* at the time of delivery represents a risk of 10% to 20% for neonatal pneumonitis and 20% to 50% for conjunctivitis.[63] In addition, there is a risk of postpartum endometritis to the mother.

The current recommendation from the Centers for Disease Control (CDC) for the treatment of *Chlamydia* infection is erythromycin base, 500 mg four times daily for 7 days, or amoxicillin, 500 mg three times daily for 7 days, as preferred therapy.[61] Other agents that have been evaluated in pregnant women for evidence of microbiologic cure include clindamycin and azithromycin.[63]

Although erythromycin is considered a first-line therapy, failure rates of nearly 25% have been reported, primarily because of patients' inability to tolerate the medication.[62,64] Amoxicillin has superior microbiologic cure rates and is often better tolerated than erythromycin, but questions have been raised about whether amoxicillin provides long-term eradication of *Chlamydia* in the genital tract.[63,64] Like amoxicillin, azithromycin appears to have a higher rate of biologic cure than erythromycin does. Further, azitromycin has the advantage of single-dose therapy and lower rates of gastrointestinal side effects.[62,64] It is, however, more expensive than either erythromycin or amoxicillin and currently less studied.

GENITAL HERPES

Currently, 5% of women of childbearing age have clinically evident genital herpes, with 25% to 30% having subclinical infections.[65,66] The causative agent in most cases of genital herpes (approximately 85%) is herpes simplex virus-2 (HSV-2), but the incidence of transmission of herpes simplex virus-1 (HSV-1) is growing.[66] The risk of genital herpes in pregnancy comes from the risk of transmission of the virus to the neonate during birth. Approximately 45% of the time, neonatal infection is limited to eyes, skin, and mucous membranes.[65] Central nervous system transmission occurs in 35% of cases. Widely disseminated infection occurs approximately 20% of the time. With treatment, survival rates of 100%, 85%, and 20% are estimated with topical disease, central nervous system disease, and disseminated disease, respectively.[65] Mental retardation, seizures, and other central nervous system effects occur at rates of 5% in those with topical involvement, 65% in those with central nervous system disease, and 40% in survivors of disseminated disease.[65] HSV-1 neonatal infection most often involves the eyes, skin, and mucous membranes, while HSV-2 infections are more likely to lead to central nervous system involvement and disseminated disease.[67]

In 50% of cases where lesions are present at the time of delivery from a primary episode of herpes, neonatal infection will occur.[65] If the primary episode is asymptomatic, a 33% risk of infection exists. If a lesion is present during a recurrence, the risk of infection is 4%. If there is no evidence of recurrence at the time of delivery in a woman known to have genital herpes, the risk of transmission drops to 0.04%.[65]

The ACOG Committee on Practice Bulletins has recommended that antiviral therapy be given to pregnant women with primary HSV infections.[68] Although no antiviral has received FDA approval for use in pregnancy, acyclovir has been extensively used for treatment.[67] An acyclovir registry of 1129 pregnancies indicates no apparent adverse effects on infants with prenatal treatment.[65] Valacyclovir has been used for a shorter period of time than acyclovir, but also has not been associated with birth defects based on use recorded in a registry.[65] Famciclovir is another alternative, but has been less studied in pregnant women.

The ACOG recommends that women who have first-episode HSV infection or who have recurrent infections with active lesions at the time of delivery undergo cesarean section.[68] Antiviral therapy should be considered for women at or beyond 36 weeks' gestation if they are having a first-episode HSV infection. Antiviral therapy may also be considered for women at or beyond 36 weeks' gestation who are at risk for a recurrence of HSV infection. At the present time, it is not clear whether this therapy will reduce the need for cesarean section in women at risk for recurrence of HSV infection.

BACTERIAL VAGINOSIS

Although not an STD, bacterial vaginosis during pregnancy has recently been considered a possible cause of premature rupture of the membranes, preterm labor, and preterm birth.[61,63] It is found in 20% of pregnant women.[63]

Pregnant women with a history of preterm delivery should undergo screening for bacterial vaginosis early in the second trimester.[61] If the infection occurs, the recommended regimen for treatment is metronidazole, 250 mg three times daily for 7 days.[61] Historically, metronidazole was associated with possible teratogenic risk, but a meta-analysis of literature related to use of metronidazole in pregnancy failed to confirm any rationale for that concern.[61] The alternatives to the metronidazole regimen include a single 2-g dose of metronidazole or a course of clindamycin, 300 mg twice daily for 7 days.[61]

Women at low risk for preterm labor need not be screened for bacterial vaginosis, but symptomatic women may be treated with metronidazole, 250 mg three times daily for 7 days.[61] The two alternative regimens mentioned earlier are also appropriate alternatives for these patients; additionally, metronidazole gel 0.75%, one applicatorful administered vaginally twice daily for 5 days, has also been recommended for pregnant women who have symptomatic bacterial vaginosis without a history of preterm labor.[61]

CHRONIC ILLNESSES IN PREGNANCY

ALLERGIC RHINITIS, ASTHMA

The frequency and severity of symptoms determine the treatment of allergic rhinitis in the pregnant patient. If patients have seasonal symptoms only, the oral administration of antihistamines is appropriate.[69] Chlorpheniramine is a first-line recommendation, followed by tripelennamine.[69,70] Second-generation antihistamines (e.g., cetirizine, fexofenadine, loratadine) may be considered alternatives if the patient has significant sedation from the first-generation antihistamines and if the fetal organs have already formed. However, data regarding the use of second-generation antihistamines in pregnancy are minimal compared to the data for chlorpheniramine and tripelennamine. If pregnant patients have year-round symptoms of allergic rhinitis, nasal cromolyn is recommended as a first-line agent.[69,70] If cromolyn is ineffective, nasal beclomethasone is the second-line recommendation. Oral antihistamines, given orally, may be added to the regimen.[69]

Asthma is now considered the most common chronic disease in pregnancy and can cause a variety of negative pregnancy outcomes, such as preeclampsia, perinatal mortality, low birth weight, and congenital malformations.[69] It is essential to control asthma in the pregnant patient in order to minimize these adverse pregnancy outcomes. The goals of therapy for asthma in pregnant women are (1) complete asthma symptom control, (2) optimization of pulmonary function, (3) normalization of daily activity, (4) avoidance of asthma exacerbations, (5) minimization or elimination of the adverse effects of any medication taken, and (6) birth of a healthy baby.[71] The Working Group on Asthma and Pregnancy has recommended creating individualized asthma treatment plans that outline therapy options based on asthma symptoms.[70,71]

In addition to the medications recommended for the treatment of allergic rhinitis, other medications have been deemed safe and efficacious to use for asthma and related conditions in pregnancy. The orally inhaled anti-inflammatory agents (in order of preference) are cromolyn sodium and beclomethasone.[70] Prednisone may be used either as a burst with taper or alternate day therapy, if required. Inhaled β_2-agonists are the preferred agents for bronchodilation; theophylline is a second-line agent. For short-term nasal decongestant therapy, pseudoephedrine, given orally, or oxymetazoline, given intranasally (5 days or less), may be used.

DERMATOLOGIC CONDITIONS

The treatment of dermatologic conditions during pregnancy may often be delayed until after the delivery. Sometimes, however, it is necessary to implement treatment during the pregnancy. The major categories of medications utilized in dermatology are antiacne agents, antibiotics, antiviral agents, antihistamines, and antifungal agents.[72] Of all the dermatologic agents commonly used during pregnancy, only topical nystatin has been shown to have no fetal risk in controlled studies.[72] Recommended topical agents with minimal pregnancy risk include bacitracin, benzoyl peroxide, ciclopirox, clindamycin, erythromycin, metronidazole, mupirocin, permethrin, and terbinafine, among others. Topical corticosteroids are also thought to be safe for use in pregnancy. Systemic agents that may be safely used in pregnancy for dermatologic conditions include acyclovir, amoxicillin, azithromycin, brompheniramine maleate, cephalosporins, chlorpheniramine, cyproheptadine hydrochloride, dicloxacillin, diphenhydramine, erythromycin (except estolates), famciclovir, nystatin, penicillin, and valacyclovir. Lidocaine and lidocaine with epinephrine may safely be used topically during pregnancy.

DIABETES

The American Diabetes Association recommends that women with diabetes defer pregnancy until they have their condition under control with insulin and dietary interventions.[25] This recommendation is based upon knowledge of increased fetal loss and malformations resulting from suboptimally controlled diabetes.[40] In addition, it is known that type 1 diabetes patients are subject to increased risk of retinopathy during pregnancy and the first postpartum year.[73] Ophthalmologic examinations should be more frequent during this time.

Insulin is the drug treatment of choice for patients with both type 1 and type 2 diabetes during pregnancy.[25] However, it may be acceptable to use glyburide after the 11th week of gestation in patients with type 2 diabetes.[39] Medical nutrition therapy and supervised exercise programs should be continued throughout pregnancy as well. Goals for self-monitored blood glucose while on insulin therapy are as follows: preprandial plasma glucose level, 80–110 mg/dL; 1-hour postprandial plasma glucose level, less than 155 mg/dL; and 2-hour postprandial plasma glucose level less than 135 mg/dL.[40] These goals are the same as for gestational diabetes.

EPILEPSY

Maternal epilepsy is present in 0.5% of all pregnancies, and most infants born to affected mothers are healthy.[74] However, epilepsy may complicate pregnancy. For example, seizures may become more frequent because of the metabolic and hormonal changes in pregnancy, sleep deprivation and stress, and medication regimen adherence problems because of a perceived teratogenic risk of antiepileptic drug therapy.[74] In addition, free serum concentrations of the antiepileptic drug may change during pregnancy as a result of decreased drug absorption, increased volume of distribution, decreased protein binding because of hypoalbuminemia, increased hepatic drug metabolism, and increased renal drug clearance.[75] A woman's clinical condition rather than solely the free serum concentrations of antiepileptic drug should be the basis for any adjustments in dosage. Postpartum concentrations must also be monitored, as drug requirements will probably decrease as pregnancy-induced pharmacokinetic changes resolve.

Malformations occur in 5% to almost 10% of the offspring of women with epilepsy.[74,76,77] It is thought that genetics may play a small role in causing malformations in children whose parent(s) have epilepsy,[75] but the majority of congenital anomalies in these children are most likely due to antiepileptic drug therapy and inadequate folate intake. In the past few years, studies have confirmed that the risks of major congenital malformations are greatest with carbamazepine and valproate monotherapy, and the risk with valproate appears to be dose-related.[76–78] Combination regimens of antiepileptic drugs are also associated with higher malformation rates. However, the expected rates of malformations associated with other drug monotherapies and with combination therapies are inconsistent from report to report.

For the management of pregnant women with epilepsy, the American Academy of Neurology has recommended the use of antiepileptic drug monotherapy, if possible, and optimization of any drug therapy prior to conception.[79] Medication change exclusively to minimize teratogenic risk, such as the prior recommendation to switch to phenobarbital from other antiepileptic drugs, is *no longer* recommended. If drug withdrawal is planned, it should be attempted at least 6 months before conception is attempted. In addition, all women with epilepsy should take folic acid supplementation of at least 400 μg daily.[79] For women who remain on carbamazepine, divalproex sodium, or valproic acid, an α-fetoprotein check at 14 to 16 weeks' gestation and a level II ultrasound at 16 to 20 weeks' gestation are recommended to screen for neural tube defects.

HUMAN IMMUNODEFICIENCY VIRUS (HIV) INFECTION

Zidovudine is the mainstay of antiretroviral therapy and is recommended for use during pregnancy, labor and delivery, and the postpartum period.[80,81] During pregnancy, the continuation of any other antiretroviral therapies that the woman may be taking should be considered.[81] Additionally, inclusion of zidovudine is recommended after 14 weeks of gestation, whether it is added to the other agents or replaces another nucleoside analog. The current zidovudine dosing recommendation for adults (200 mg three times daily or 300 mg twice daily) can be used in the pregnant woman. Beginning 8 to 12 hours after birth, the infant should also receive zidovudine.[81]

HYPERTENSION

As noted earlier, blood pressure is expected to decrease by 10 to 20 mm Hg during the second trimester. Women who are diagnosed and treated for hypertension prior to pregnancy may be able to discontinue antihypertensive medications during the second trimester, but careful monitoring is essential because their blood pressure will undoubtedly rise again in the third trimester. The specific goal of antihypertensive therapy for pregnant women is uncertain, but there is concern for significant adverse fetal and maternal outcomes when the maternal blood pressure elevation is severe (≥170/90 mm Hg).[82] Mild hypertension in pregnancy (diastolic blood pressure of 90–99 mm Hg), moderate hypertension (diastolic blood pressure of 100–109 mm Hg), and severe hypertension (diastolic blood pressure of ≥110 mm Hg) all represent different risks to the fetus and mother, yet the absolute risks are not known.[41,82] When considering drug therapy in the treatment of hypertension during pregnancy, the clinician and patient must jointly assess the risks and benefits of any therapy. For women with severe hypertension, the benefits almost always outweigh the risks.

No evidence exists for superior efficacy of one agent versus another for blood pressure reduction during pregnancy.[82] Occasionally, it may be necessary to consider changing from one agent to another prior to or during pregnancy, such as switching from an angiotensin-converting enzyme inhibitor before beginning the second trimester of pregnancy in order to reduce teratogenic risk. However, some women may not tolerate medications other than those found to be efficacious prior to pregnancy, or the other drugs may not be as effective. In such cases, the risks and benefits of changing to a different agent solely for the purpose of avoiding teratogenicity must be considered carefully.

MENTAL HEALTH ISSUES: ANXIETY AND DEPRESSION

A pre-existing disorder, concerns associated with the pregnancy itself, or a combination of these issues may be responsible for anxiety and depression during pregnancy. Therapy should always involve psychotherapy, although medication may also be required. Oral clefting and cognitive and behavioral development problems have been associated with prenatal exposure to benzodiazepines, although the data do not clearly establish an incidence.[83] Whether tricyclic antidepressants or selective serotonin reuptake inhibitors (SSRIs) definitively cause developmental, cognitive, or behavioral toxicity in human fetuses is also unknown,[83,84] but recent cohort studies and meta-analyses have not demonstrated significant negative fetal outcomes with use of these agents during pregnancy.[84] The lowest possible dose of a medication should be used for the shortest possible time to minimize adverse fetal and maternal pregnancy outcomes.[83]

THYROID DISORDERS

Untreated hypothyroidism during pregnancy may result in significant cognitive and other neurologic deficits in the fetus. It also increases the risk of preeclampsia, premature birth, and low birth weight.[51,52,85] The causes of hypothyroidism during pregnancy include autoimmune diseases such as Hashimoto's thyroiditis, iodine deficiency (uncommon in the United States), and thyroid dysfunction following surgery or ablative therapy for Graves' disease.[52] Thyroid replacement therapy should be instituted if hypothyroidism is diagnosed during pregnancy; the goal is to attain free thyroxine index concentrations in the upper end of the normal range.[52] Women who receive thyroid replacement therapy prior to pregnancy can expect an increased dosage requirement of 25% to 50% during pregnancy. After delivery, maternal thyroid supplementation requirements decrease.

Hyperthyroidism during pregnancy may precipitate outcomes of fetal death, low birth weight,[51,52] malformations, and maternal heart failure.[52] Graves' disease is the most common cause of hyperthyroidism in pregnancy. Therapy for hyperthyroidism in pregnancy includes propylthiouracil, methimazole, or surgery. Propylthiouracil is the preferred agent because it crosses the placenta less readily and is less likely than methimazole to cause fetal malformations.[52] The goal of therapy for hyperthyroidism in pregnancy is to attain free thyroxine index concentrations in the upper end of the normal range and to attain nondetectable thyrotropin concentrations; this allows for minimization of the propylthiouracil dose. An additional factor that allows a reduction in the propylthiouracil dose is partial disease resolution as a result of the natural course of Graves' disease during pregnancy.

Within 3 to 6 months postpartum, women may experience either hypothyroidism or hyperthyroidism due to thyroiditis secondary to autoimmune factors.[52] The thyroiditis is usually self-limiting. This disorder is thought to occur in 2% to 16% of postpartum women.[52] If women are asymptomatic, despite the presence of either hypothyroidism or hyperthyroidism, treatment is not indicated.[52] Women who have hyperthyroid symptoms and are not breastfeeding should undergo radionuclide scanning to determine the cause of the disorder. If thyroiditis is suspected, only symptomatic treatment of hyperthyroid symptoms with β-blockers is indicated, although the patient should be monitored carefully because transient hypothyroidism may follow.[52] Women who have both symptoms and laboratory evidence of hypothyroidism should be treated with thyroxine therapy. Again, careful monitoring is required, as the condition usually resolves, and thyroxine therapy may be discontinued.

LABOR AND DELIVERY

Uterine activity during pregnancy and labor can be explained in terms of four phases—phase 0 (quiescence), phase 1 (activation), phase 2 (stimulation), and phase 3 (involution).[86] The transition from phase 0 to phase 1 may be explained as a loss of inhibition of uterine activity mediators, such as progesterone, prostacyclin, and others. Once activation has occurred, levels of oxytocin, prostaglandin E_2, and prostaglandin $F_{2\alpha}$ increase and are responsible for contractions of the uterus.

PRETERM LABOR

The leading cause of perinatal morbidity and mortality is preterm labor, defined as labor that occurs before 37 weeks' gestation.[86,87] It affects 7% to 10% of births in the United States. Risk factors for preterm labor include previous preterm delivery, infections (e.g., bacterial vaginosis, upper and lower urinary tract infections), maternal complicating factors (e.g., smoking, use of illicit drugs or alcohol), maternal age (i.e., <18 or >40 years), poverty, nonwhite race, premature rupture of membranes, multiple gestation, uterine functional causes (e.g., incompetent cervix, uterine septum), and fetal causes (e.g., congenital anomalies, growth retardation).[86,87]

There is no convincing evidence that routine cervical assessment or home monitoring of uterine activity improves outcomes.[86,87] Fetal fibronectin, an extracellular protein in cervical and vaginal secretions, has been found to be predictive of the risk of preterm delivery.[87] Its presence in the cervix or vagina after 20 to 24 weeks of gestation is unusual and is associated with a threefold increased risk of preterm delivery in women who present with contractions. Shorter cervical length, measured by transvaginal ultrasound, may also be predictive of risk.[87]

TOCOLYTIC THERAPY

The goal of tocolytic therapy is to postpone delivery long enough to reduce the incidence of problems associated with prematurity. Realistically, tocolytics do not reduce the actual number of premature deliveries, but they may allow sufficient time for the administration of antenatal corticosteroids to improve pulmonary maturity and for transportation of the mother to a facility equipped to deal with high risk deliveries.[88,89] Tocolytic drugs may prolong pregnancy from 48 hours up to 1 week.[88] There is presently no evidence that tocolytic therapy alone improves neonatal morbidity or mortality rates.[87]

Tocolytic therapy should not be used in cases of intrauterine infection, fetal distress, maternal hemodynamic instability, or vaginal bleeding.[86,87] Criteria for the initiation of therapy include regular contractions and cervical changes, although cervical dilation of greater than 3 cm may indicate that tocolytic therapy is less likely to be effective.[87]

The drugs most commonly used for acute tocolysis include magnesium sulfate, β-adrenergic agents, nonsteroidal anti-inflammatory agents, and non-dihydropyridine calcium channel blockers.[87] All of these agents are equivalent in efficacy, but differ in maternal and fetal side effect profiles.[86]

An infusion of magnesium sulfate is often used as a first-line agent.[86] Its mechanism of action is to suppress nerve impulses to the uterine smooth muscles by antagonizing intracellular calcium.[86,87] Although maternal side effects such as pulmonary edema occasionally occur, the treatment is considered safe. At toxic levels, hypotension, muscle paralysis, tetany, cardiac arrest, and respiratory depression may occur.[87]

β-Adrenergic agonists, such as terbutaline and ritodrine, are also commonly used in efforts to stop preterm labor. (Of the two, only ritodrine has FDA approval for this use.[86]) These drugs reduce intracellular calcium levels and reduce the sensitivity of the contractile unit to calcium.[86,87] Relative to the other agents, the β agonists have a higher incidence of maternal side effects, including hyperkalemia, arrhythmias, hyperglycemia, hypotension, and pulmonary edema.[86–88] Recommended terbutaline doses range from 250 μg to 500 μg, given subcutaneously, every 3 to 4 hours.[87] Ritodrine doses are 50–350 μg per minute, given IV.[87]

Nifedipine is associated with fewer side effects than magnesium or β-agonist therapy.[86] One of the concerns regarding the use of nifedipine is a potential negative effect on blood flow between the placenta and the uterus.[86] A common maternal side effect is hypotension.[87] Nifedipine is administered at 5–10 mg sublingually every 15 to 20 minutes (up to four doses) and 10–20 mg by mouth every 4 to 6 hours.[87]

Nonsteroidal anti-inflammatory agents, such as indomethacin, have also been used for tocolysis. The mechanism of action is to inhibit cervical prostaglandin activity.[87] The drug is first given rectally in a dose of 50–100 mg, followed by an oral dose of 25–50 mg every 6 hours.[87] Maternal side effects include nausea, heartburn, dizziness, and bleeding.[90] Serious neonatal complications, including necrotizing enterocolitis, intravascular hemorrhage, and patent ductus arteriosus have been reported in some studies.[86,90]

Because infection has been thought to play a role in the etiology of preterm labor, antibiotics have been used, in addition to tocolytics and corticosteroids, to improve the outcome of preterm labor.[91] Most studies of antibiotic use in preterm labor do not demonstrate a reduction in the incidence of preterm delivery, however.

After acute tocolysis has been achieved, continuation of tocolytic therapy is controversial. None of the agents currently used to treat women experiencing premature contractions has demonstrated efficacy for maintenance therapy.[92]

ANTENATAL CORTICOSTEROIDS

A number of clinical trials have demonstrated the benefit of administering antenatal corticosteroids for the prevention of respiratory distress syndrome, intraventricular hemorrhage, and death in infants delivered prematurely.[93] The current clinical recommendation is to administer beclomethasone, 12 mg given intramuscularly every 24 hours for two doses, or dexamethasone, 6 mg given intramuscularly every 12 hours for four doses, to pregnant women between 24 and 34 weeks' gestation who are at risk for preterm delivery within the next 7 days.[94] Benefits from antenatal corticosteroids are believed to begin within 24 hours and continue for up to 1 week.

It has become the practice to repeat the administration of corticosteroids if delivery has not occurred within 7 days.[93] In a retrospective review of outcomes of 710 infants born to mothers enrolled in the North American Thyrotropin-Releasing Hormone Trial,[93] it was found that repeat corticosteroid administration produced no overall improvement in outcomes for infants; however, there was an increase in mortality in the youngest gestational age infants, evidence of adrenal suppression, and a slight decrease in birth weight.[93] At the current time, the recommendation is that multiple doses of corticosteroids for fetal lung maturation not be given routinely, but their potential usefulness should be investigated in clinical trials.[94]

GROUP B *STREPTOCOCCUS* INFECTION

Infection with group B streptococci is associated with invasive disease in newborns and pregnant women.[95] Women colonized with group B *Streptococcus* during pregnancy have an increased risk of experiencing premature delivery and transmitting the bacteria to the infant during delivery.[96] Ten to thirty percent of pregnant women are colonized with group B *Streptococcus,* and approximately 1% to 2% of their infants have early-onset disease (i.e., symptoms occurring within the first 7 days of life).[95]

In 1990, it was estimated that the overall incidence of group B *Streptococcus* neonatal disease was approximately 1.8 per 1000 births, with early-onset infections accounting for 80% of the infections. Seventy-five percent of group B *Streptococcus* infections occur in full-term infants, with the other 25% occurring in premature infants.[95,96] The consequences of neonatal infections include bacteremia, pneumonia, and meningitis in the newborn. Antibiotics given at the onset of labor or with rupture of the membranes have decreased the transmission of bacteria to the neonate.[96]

In general, if a pregnant woman has previously delivered an infant with invasive group B *Streptococcus* disease, has had bacteriuria (i.e., presence of group B *Streptococcus*) during the current pregnancy, or seems likely to deliver at less than 37 weeks' gestation with unknown colonization, intrapartum antibiotics are recommended.[95] In 1996, the CDC promulgated recommendations utilizing two different strategies for the prevention of group B *Streptococcus* disease.[95] In the screening approach to prevention of group B *Streptococcus* disease, routine vaginal and rectal cultures should be done at 35 to 37 weeks' gestation. If the cultures are positive, intrapartum antibiotics are given. If negative, no antibiotics are given. If a women presents for delivery and no screening information is available, antibiotics are given for fever greater than or equal to 100.4°, for membrane rupture 18 hours or more earlier,[95] or if less than 37 weeks gestation. The second strategy involves a risk factor approach using the criteria for a woman presenting for delivery without screening information. The risk factor approach does not include universal screening in the third trimester.

Estimations in 1995 suggested that the risk-based strategy might decrease the incidence of early-onset disease by 41%; the screening technique, by up to 78%.[96] Continuous active surveillance of four areas of the United States demonstrated a 65% decline in early-onset disease subsequent to publication of the CDC recommendations. The incidence of group B *Streptococcus* infection declined from 1.7 in 1000 births in 1993 to 0.6 per 1000 in 1998.[97]

The currently recommended regimen for group B *Streptococcus* disease is penicillin G, 5 million U given IV, followed by 2.5 million U given every 4 hours until delivery.[95] Alternatively, ampicillin, 2 g given IV, followed by 1 g given every 4 hours has been suggested as an alternative.[95] The use of the narrower spectrum penicillin has been encouraged to reduce the risk that resistant organisms will develop.[96] For penicillin-allergic patients, clindamycin, 900 mg given IV every 8 hours, or erythromycin, 500 mg given IV every 6 hours until delivery, is suggested.[95] Increases in both erythromycin- and clindamycin-resistant isolates have been reported.[97,98]

CERVICAL RIPENING AND LABOR INDUCTION

For most of pregnancy, the cervix is closed and firm.[99] During the last few weeks of pregnancy, the cervix becomes softer and thinner to facilitate labor.[99] This process is likely mediated by hormonal changes, including final mediation by prostaglandins E_2 and $F_{2\alpha}$.[99,100]

Approximately 13% of pregnancies end by labor induction, stimulation of uterine contractions before natural labor begins.[100] The most common reason for labor induction is postmaturity (gestation greater than 42 weeks), but suspected fetal growth retardation, maternal hypertension, premature rupture of the membranes with no active labor in 4 hours, or social factors may also result in labor induction. Contraindications for induction include placenta previa, oblique or transverse lie, pelvic structure abnormality, prolapsed umbilical cord, or active genital herpes.[100,101] The primary concerns associated with induction of labor are that the labor may be ineffective or that side effects, such as uterine hyperstimulation, may adversely affect the infant, increasing the likelihood of cesarean section.[102]

Scoring systems to assess the likelihood of successful induction have been suggested. One system, the Bishop scoring system, assigns a value to several parameters, such as dilation, cervical effacement (thinning), cervical station (position of the fetal head), cervical consistency, and cervical position.[99] Higher scores have been associated with induction outcomes similar to those of spontaneous labor; lower scores may imply more difficulty in induction.[100] Subsequent investigators have determined that the degree of cervical dilation may be the best predictor of a successful vaginal delivery following labor induction.[99]

Nonpharmacologic methods for cervical ripening may range from less common procedures, such as nipple stimulation, to more commonly used methods, such as stripping of the membranes, amniotomy, or mechanical dilation with a balloon catheter.[99,100] Safe and inexpensive, membrane stripping is particularly of value when induction of labor is not urgent.[99] When done after 40 weeks' gestation, membrane stripping may decrease the need for further induction by

50%.[99] Balloon catheters are also inexpensive, reversible, and without systemic side effect.[99] If catheters are employed, augmentation with oxytocin is often necessary, ultimately increasing rates of cesarean section over catheter alone.[99]

Prostaglandin E_2 analogs (e.g., dinoprostone, Prepidil, Cervidil) are the most commonly used pharmacologic agents for cervical ripening.[100] Prepidil gel is administered intracervically in a dose of 500 μg.[100] This may be repeated after 6 hours, but no more than three doses should be given within 24 hours.[100] After administration, the patient should remain supine for 30 minutes. Contractions generally begin within 1 hour and peak within 4 hours.[100] A vaginal insert, Cervidil, contains 10 mg of dinoprostone with a slower, more constant release of medication than the gel.[99,100] The insert may be removed when labor begins or after a maximum of 24 hours.[99]

Misoprostol, a prostaglandin E_1 analog, is also used for cervical ripening and labor induction.[100] Although not FDA-approved for cervical ripening, misoprostol is an effective and inexpensive method. Intravaginally administered doses of 25 μg to 50 μg of the tablet for oral use may be administered every 4 to 6 hours, up to a maximum of six to eight doses.[100] Patients given misoprostol are less likely to need cesarean section or oxytocin.[100] Side effects, such as uterine hyperstimulation, are more often associated with use of misoprostol than with other methods of cervical ripening, however.[100,102] Misoprostol use has been associated with a shorter interval from induction to delivery than that associated with oxytocin.[99,102]

Oxytocin is the most commonly used agent for labor induction after cervical ripening because it is possible to titrate the dose. A solution of 10 mU/mL is used for infusion and may be delivered by either pulse or continuous infusion.[100] Controlling the rate of infusion avoids hypotension. Side effects associated with oxytocin include an antidiuretic effect, uterine hyperstimulation, and uterine rupture.[100] The fetal heart rate must be monitored with oxytocin therapy.

LABOR ANALGESIA

During the first phase of labor, pain is associated with uterine contractions; during the second phase, it is associated with perineal stretching.[103] Factors that may increase the pain associated with labor are first delivery, maternal immaturity, use of oxytocin, and history of dysmenorrhea. Conversely, regular exercise and organized preparation for childbirth may help decrease pain.[103]

NONPHARMACOLOGIC APPROACHES TO ANALGESIA

A number of nonpharmacologic strategies have been used to reduce the pain associated with childbirth. Controlled breathing (e.g., the Lamaze method), relaxation through biofeedback methods, massage, and the use of different body positions for labor may reduce sensation of pain.[103,104] Techniques such as hypnosis and acupuncture have also been used for labor, but they have had variable results and require trained personnel. Other strategies, such as use of transcutaneous electric nerve stimulation (TENS) and laboring in a bath of warm water (hydrotherapy) have been helpful in some cases.

PHARMACOLOGIC APPROACHES TO LABOR PAIN

The IV or intramuscular administration of narcotics is commonly used to treat the pain associated with labor. Agents commonly used include meperidine, morphine, and fentanyl.[103] Agents such as promethazine and hydroxyzine may be added to augment the effects of the narcotic agent. In comparison with epidural analgesia, the IV use of narcotics is less expensive, but usually thought to be less effective in controlling pain.[103,105]

Epidural analgesia involves introducing a catheter into the epidural space and administering a drug (e.g., bupivacaine, fentanyl) to provide pain relief during labor, especially during the first and second stages.[103,104] One potential complication of use of epidural analgesia may be puncture of the dura (less than 1% of cases), which may result in a severe postural headache.[103,104] Low back pain, hypotension, nausea, vomiting, itching, and urinary retention are less common side effects. Controversy exists regarding a possible association of epidural analgesia with extended labor and increased need for instrument-assisted delivery.[103]

Delivered directly to the intrathecal space, spinal analgesia offers the advantage of rapid control of pain.[103] Side effects are similar to those of epidural analgesia.[103] A combination of spinal and epidural analgesia may be used to allow rapid pain relief with the spinal component and mobility with the epidural agent.[103]

Finally, nerve blocks with anesthetic agents may be useful when spinal or epidural agents cannot be used.[103] Paracervical blocks may decrease pain associated with the first phase of labor. Potential side effects include decreased fetal heart rate and risk of fetal distress. A pudendal nerve block reduces pain resulting from perineal stretching during the second phase of labor. It may be used in conjunction with epidural analgesia to enhance pain relief.

POSTPARTUM ISSUES

DRUG USE DURING LACTATION

Medications enter breast milk via passive diffusion or active transport. Passive diffusion is the more common mode of drug movement into breast milk, and the concentration of drugs passing into milk via diffusion is directly proportional to the maternal serum concentration.[106] In addition, the pH of breast milk is slightly more acidic than is plasma, so medications that are weak bases, are poorly protein-bound, have higher lipid solubility, and tend to pass into breast milk.[106] Drugs that are lipophilic tend to concentrate in hind-milk, which contains a higher lipid content, rather than in fore-milk.[107] Hind-milk is usually released in the last few minutes of nursing, and fore-milk is released from the beginning until the last few minutes of the nursing session.

The milk:plasma ratio indicates the drug passage into breast milk from maternal plasma. A milk:plasma ratio of 1 indicates that the concentration of drug in breast milk is the same as the concentration in maternal plasma. When considering the ratio and maternal medication use, several factors should be assessed, such as variations in the ratio over time and the infant's ability to metabolize medication.[108] Finally, the amount of drug actually ingested by the infant may not achieve concentrations significant enough to produce an adverse effect.[106]

Other factors can also affect nursing infant exposure and response to maternal medications. For example, the infant's capacity to metabolize medications in the liver is decreased during the first 2 to 3 weeks of life.[107] Additionally, the glomerular filtration rate of a full-term newborn is only 30% to 40% of the adult's glomerular filtration rate; the infant's rate becomes normal between 2 and 12 months of life.[107]

Because breast milk is produced and secreted during nursing and immediately after a nursing session,[109] it is possible to implement strategies that minimize the infant's exposure to maternally ingested drugs. The ingestion of medication immediately prior to or immediately after a nursing session helps to minimize drug passage into breast milk because the drug is in the stage of absorption during the time that breast milk is being produced.[109] The use of short-acting medication forms also helps to minimize the amount of drug transmitted to an infant through breast milk.[109] Should a mother require a medication that is lipophilic, she may terminate nursing sessions prior to the ingestion of the hind-milk. Supplemental feeding may have to be provided to the infant under these circumstances.

According to the American Academy of Pediatrics, medications that are contraindicated in lactation include bromocriptine, cyclosporine, cyclophosphamide, doxorubicin, ergotamine, lithium, and methotrexate.[110] Other substances contraindicated in breastfeeding are drugs of abuse, including nicotine.[110]

MASTITIS

Usually caused by *Staphylococcus aureus,* a common bacterium found in an infant's mouth,[111] mastitis is a breast infection. Symptoms include swelling and tenderness of a wedge-shaped area of the breast. Therapy for mastitis includes antibiotic therapy for the mother (usually dicloxacillin or cephalexin) for 10 to 14 days, bedrest, adequate oral fluid intake, analgesia (acetaminophen is recommended), and frequent evacuation of the breast milk. Infants may continue to nurse as usual during treatment of mastitis.

POSTPARTUM DEPRESSION

Approximately 70% to 80% of women may experience a brief period of depression 72 to 96 hours after delivery;[112] this is often referred to as "baby blues." This depression will climax approximately 5 days after delivery and resolve by 10 days postpartum.[113] Lingering postpartum depression (i.e., postpartum major depression) has been reported to affect 10% to 20% of women. However, a recent report using the Edinburgh Postnatal Depression Scale showed that approximately 35% of subjects screened were depressed after delivery.[114] Postpartum major depression can manifest itself at any time up to 6 months after delivery.[112] The actual incidence of postpartum major depression obviously varies in reports and may be dependent upon the time after delivery that depression screening is conducted.

Both nondrug and drug options exist for the treatment of postpartum depression. Nondrug therapies include emotional support from family and friends, education about the condition, and psychotherapy. Bright light therapy (effective for seasonal affective disorder and nonseasonal depression) may also provide benefit.[115] Pharmacologic therapy for postpartum major depression should be considered if the symptoms are severe or persistent, because untreated depression may have negative effects on the mother's care of and relationship with the infant. Tricyclic antidepressants and SSRIs are efficacious for postpartum major depression and should be initiated at usual starting doses. After 2 weeks, the medication dosage may be increased if the woman's condition is unstable or has worsened.[113]

For the breastfeeding mother, there are additional concerns about the passage of a drug to the infant through breast milk. Antidepressant medications and their metabolites can be detected in the infants of breastfeeding mothers; however most infants exposed to these drugs experience few adverse effects.[113,116] It is recommended that pharmacologic therapy be administered for postpartum major depression, if necessary; that with informed consent, the selected medication be started at the lowest dose possible and titrated slowly; that the infant be monitored for possible adverse effects; and that the antidepressant dose be reduced if adverse effects are detected in the infant.[113]

RELACTATION

Declining serum prolactin concentrations cause a decrease in or cessation of lactation, and this can be problematic, as well as distressing, for mothers who desire to breastfeed their infants. Relactation is the process of increasing the breast milk supply for such women.[117] Lactation can also be induced in women who have not recently delivered a baby, such as adoptive mothers. The mainstay of therapy for this condition involves nipple stimulation, either by the infant's nursing or by pumping of the breast with a mechanical pump or the hand.[117] One small study showed that a substance in beer and nonalcoholic beer can stimulate prolactin secretion and, thus, increase milk production.[118]

Recommended pharmacologic therapy for relactation is metoclopramide; this drug should be used only if nondrug therapy is ineffective. The most commonly used dose is 10 mg taken orally three times daily,[117] and improvement in lactation may occur within 2 to 5 days of the initiation of metoclopramide therapy.[119] Breast milk production can be increased up to 100% or more in women who are 1 month postpartum or less; in mothers who are 8 to 12 weeks postpartum, milk production may be increased up to 40%.[117] Duration of therapy may range from 7 to 14 days.[117] Breast milk production may decrease after metoclopramide therapy is discontinued, but if lactation has been successfully established, it will continue. Adverse effects of metoclopramide are not expected in breastfed infants.[117]

Oxytoxin nasal spray, human growth hormone, and thyrotropin-releasing hormone are not recommended for use in relactation.[117]

CONCLUSION

Providing pharmacologic care to women during pregnancy can be rewarding and, at times, difficult. Many women perceive a high inherent risk of birth defects with drug exposure during pregnancy. This perception, linked with a high rate of unplanned pregnancy, may create anxiety because of drug exposure prior to discovery of a pregnancy. Pharmacists have an important role in collaborating with women and other health care providers to realistically evaluate the potential impact of drug or substance use on the outcome of a pregnancy. There are likewise many opportunities for pharmacists to participate in selection of drug therapy for acute care issues, as well as to optimize therapy for a chronic illness during the course of a pregnancy. In addition, pharmacists may be in a unique position to counsel pregnant women about the safe use of nonprescription medications.

The provision of drug information is an important responsibility of the pharmacist on the health care team caring for a pregnant woman. All those who provide health care for pregnant women should develop a list of medications generally considered safe for use in pregnancy. This formulary of agents generally consists of older drugs with an established favorable efficacy:risk ratio. When such a basic formulary is not sufficient, pharmacists can use their literature analysis skills to help interpret the significance of research findings and can share this information with patients and other health care colleagues.[120]

Additional resources include the reference texts *Drugs in Pregnancy and Lactation,*[121] *Drugs and Human Lactation,*[122] *Medications and Mothers Milk,*[123] and *Breastfeeding: A Guide for the Medical Profession.*[124]

REFERENCES

1. Namnoun AB, Hatcher RA. The menstrual cycle. In: Hatcher RA, Trussell J, Stewart F, et al., eds. Contraceptive Technology. 17th ed. New York: Ardent Media, 1998:69–76.

2. The morphological and functional development of the fetus. In: Cunningham FG, MacDonald PC, Gant NF, et al. Williams Obstetrics. 20th ed. Stamford, CT: Appleton & Lange, 1997:151–190.
3. Pernoll ML, Taylor CM. Normal pregnancy and prenatal care. In: DeCherney AH, Pernoll ML, eds. Current Obstetric Gynecologic Diagnosis and Treatment. 8th ed. Stamford, CT: Appleton & Lange, 1994:183–201.
4. Loebstein R, Lalkin A, Koren G. Pharmacokinetic changes during pregnancy and their clinical relevance. Clin Pharmacokinet 1997;33(5):328–343.
5. Wagner CL, Katikaneni LD, Cox TH, Ryan RM. The impact of prenatal drug exposure on the neonate. Obstet Gynecol Clin North Am 1998;25(1):169–194.
6. Larimore WL, Petrie KA. Drug use during pregnancy and lactation. Prim Care 2000;27(1):35–53.
7. Irl C, Hasford J, The PEGASUS Study Group. The PEGASUS project-a prospective cohort study for the investigation of drug use in pregnancy. Int J Clin Pharmacol Ther 1997;35(12):572–576.
8. Silberstein SD. Migraine and pregnancy. Neurol Clin 1997;15(1):209 231.
9. Irl C, Hasford J. Assessing the safety of drugs in pregnancy. Drug Saf 2000;22(3):169–177.
10. Koren G, Pastuszak A, Ito S. Drug therapy: drugs in pregnancy. N Engl J Med 1998;338(16):1128–1137.
11. Meadows M. Pregnancy and the drug dilemma. http://www.fda.gov/fdac/features/2001/301– prag. htm. (Accessed Nov 26, 2001).
12. Morrison EH. Periconception care. Prim Care 2000;27(1):1–12.
13. Allaire AD, Cefalo RC. Preconceptional health care model. Eur J Obstet Gynecol Reprod Biol 1998;78:163–168.
14. Committee on Genetics-American Academy of Pediatrics. Folic acid for the prevention of neural tube defects. Pediatrics 1999;104(2):325–327.
15. Botto LD, Moore CA, Khoury MJ, Erickson JD. Neural-tube defects. N Engl J Med 1999;341(20):1509–1519.
16. Iqbal MM. Prevention of neural tube defects by periconceptional use of folic acid. Pediatr Rev 2000;21(2):58–66.
17. Floyd RL, Ebrahim SH, Boyle CA. Preventing alcohol-exposed pregnancies among women of childbearing age: the necessity of a preconceptional approach. J Womens Health Gend Based Med 1999;8(6):733–736.
18. Floyd RL, Decoufle P, Hungerford DW. Alcohol use prior to pregnancy recognition. Am J Prev Med 1999;17(2):101–107.
19. Haustein KO. Cigarette smoking, nicotine and pregnancy. Int J Clin Pharmacol Ther 1999;37(9):417–427.
20. Okuyemi KS, Ahluwalia JS, Harris KJ. Pharmacotherapy of smoking cessation. Arch Fam Med 2000;9(3):270–281.
21. Shah NR, Bracken MB. A systematic review and meta-analysis of prospective studies on the association between maternal cigarette smoking and preterm delivery. Am J Obstet Gynecol 2000;182(2):465–472.
22. Ness RB, Grisso JA, Hirschinger N, et al. Cocaine and tobacco use and the risk of spontaneous abortion. N Engl J Med 1999;340(5):333–339.
23. Ebrahim SH, Floyd RL, Merritt RK, et al. Trends in pregnancy-related smoking rates in the United States, 1987–1996. JAMA 2000;283(3):361–366.
24. Hackman R, Kapur B, Koren G. Use of nicotine patch by pregnant women (Correspondence). 1999;341(22):1700.
25. Gold AE, Reilly R, Little J, Walker JD. The effect of glycemic control in the pre-conception period and early pregnancy on birth weight in women with IDDM. Diabetes Care 1998;21(4):535–538.
26. Herman WH, Janz NK, Becker MP, Charron-Prochownik D. Diabetes and pregnancy-preconception care, pregnancy outcomes, resource utilization and costs. J Reprod Med 1999;44:33–38.
27. Bonapace ES, Fisher RS. Constipation and diarrhea in pregnancy. Gastroenterol Clin North Am 1998;27(1):197–211.
28. Katz PO, Castell DO. Gastroesophageal reflux disease during pregnancy. Gastroenterol Clin North Am 1998;27(1):13–167.
29. Broussard CN, Richter JE. Treating gastroesophageal reflux disease during pregnancy and lactation. What are the safest therapy options? Drug Saf 1998;19(4):325–337.
30. Rayburn W, Liles E, Christensen H, Robinson M. Antacids vs. antacids plus non-prescription ranitidine for heartburn during pregnancy. Int J Gynaecol Obstet 1999;66:35–37.
31. Nielsen GL, Sorensen HT, Thulstrup AM, et al. The safety of proton pump inhibitors in pregnancy. Aliment Pharmacol Ther 1999;13:1085–1089.
32. Ruigomez A, Rodriguez LAG, Cattaruzzi C, et al. Use of cimetidine, omeprazole and ranitidine in pregnant women and pregnancy outcomes. Am J Epidemiol 1999;150:476–81.
33. Medich DS, Fazio VW. Hemorrhoids, anal fissure, and carcinoma of the colon, rectum and anus during pregnancy. Surg Clin North Am 1995;75(1):77–88.
34. Prenatal care. In: Cunningham FG, MacDonald PC, Gant NF, et al. Williams Obstetrics. 20th ed. Stamford, CT: Appleton & Lange, 1997: 227–250.
35. Culpepper-Morgan JA, Kreek MJ. Gastrointestinal disorders. In: Wallis LA, ed. Textbook of Women's Health. Philadelphia: Lippincott-Raven, 1998:393–404.
36. Mazzotta P, Magee LA. A risk-benefit assessment of pharmacological and nonpharmacological treatments for nausea and vomiting of pregnancy. Drugs 2000;59(4):781–800.
37. Lacroix R, Eason E, Melzack R. Nausea and vomiting during pregnancy: a prospective study of its frequency, intensity and patterns of change. Am J Obstet Gynecol 2000;182(2):931–937.
38. American Diabetes Association. Gestational diabetes mellitus. Diabetes Care 2000;23(suppl 1):S77–S79.
39. Langer O, Conway DL, Berkus MD, et al. A comparison of glyburide and insulin in women with gestational diabetes mellitus. N Engl J Med 2000;343(16):1134–1138.
40. American Diabetes Association. Preconception care of women with diabetes. Diabetes Care 2000;23(suppl 1):S65–S68.
41. Magee LA, Ornstein MP, van Dadelszen P. Fortnightly review: management of hypertension in pregnancy. BMJ 1999;318:1332–1335.
42. Cacciabaudo JM. Hypertension in women over the life phases. In: Wallis LA, ed. Textbook of Women's Health. Philadelphia: Lippincott-Raven, 1998:355–365.
43. United States Preventive Services Task Force. Guide to Clinical Preventive Services. 2nd ed. Baltimore: Williams & Wilkins, 1996:419–424.
44. Khedun SM, Moodley J, Naicker T, Maharaj B. Drug management of hypertensive disorders of pregnancy. Pharmacol Ther 1997;74(2):221–258.
45. National High Blood Pressure Education Working Group. Report on high blood pressure in pregnancy. Am J Obstet Gynecol 1990;163:1689–1712.
46. Burrows RF, Burrows EA. Assessing the teratogenic potential of angiotensin-converting enzyme inhibitors in pregnancy. Aust N Z J Obstet Gynaecol 1998;38(3):306–311.
47. Steffensen FH, Nielsen GL, Sorensen HT, et al. Pregnancy outcome with ACE-inhibitor use in early pregnancy. Lancet 1998;351(9102):596.
48. Kyle PM, Redman CWG: Comparative risk-benefit assessment of drugs used in the management of hypertension in pregnancy. Drug Saf 1992;7:223–234.
49. Atallah AN, Hofmeyr GJ, Dulcy L. Calcium supplementation during pregnancy for preventing hypertensive disorders and related problems (Cochrane Review). In: The Cochrane Library, Issue 3, 2000. Oxford: Update Software.
50. Knight M, Duley L, Henderson-Smart DJ, King JF. Antiplatelet agents for preventing and treating pre-eclampsia (Cochrane Review). In: The Cochrane Library, Issue 3, 2000. Oxford: Update Software.
51. Drake WM, Wood DR. Thyroid disease in pregnancy. Postgrad Med J 1998;74:583–586.
52. Mulder JE. Thyroid disease in women. Med Clin North Am 1998; 82(1):103–125.
53. Ginsberg JS. Thromboembolism and pregnancy. Thromb Haemost 1999; 82(2):620–625.
54. Chan WS, Ray JG. Low molecular weight heparin use during pregnancy: issues of safety and practicality. Obstet Gynecol Surv 1999;54(10):649–654.

55. Marcus DA. Focus on primary care diagnosis and management of headache in women. Obstet Gynecol Surv 1999;54(6):395–402.
56. Goodrum LA. Pneumonia in pregnancy. Semin Perinatol 1997;21(4): 276–283.
57. Delzell JE, Lefevre ML. Urinary tract infections during pregnancy. Am Fam Physician 2000;61:713–721.
58. Connolly A, Thorp JM. Urinary tract infections in pregnancy. Urol Clin North Am 1999;26(4):779–787.
59. Stapleton A, Stamm WE. Prevention of urinary tract infection. Infect Dis Clin North Am 1997;11(3):719–733.
60. Roberts JA. Management of pyelonephritis and upper urinary tract infections. Urol Clin North Am 1999;26(4):753–763.
61. Centers for Disease Control and Prevention. 1998 guidelines for the treatment of sexually transmitted diseases. MMWR Morb Mortal Wkly Rep 1998;47:1–116.
62. Adair CD, Gunter M, Stovall TG, et al. Chlamydia in pregnancy: a randomized trial of azithromycin and erythromycin. Obstet Gynecol 1998:91:165–168.
63. Brocklehurst P. Update on the treatment of sexually transmitted infections in pregnancy-1. Int J STD AIDS 1999;10:571–580.
64. Hueston WJ, Gunlikson Lenhart J. A decision analysis to guide antibiotic selection for chlamydia infections during pregnancy. Arch Fam Med 1997;6:551–555.
65. Scott LL. Prevention of perinatal herpes: prophylactic antiviral therapy? Clin Obstet Gynecol 1999;42(1):134–148.
66. Baker DA. The use of antiviral medications in the treatment of herpes simplex virus infections of women. Int J Fertil Womens Med 1999; 44(5):227–233.
67. Brown ZA. Genital herpes complicating pregnancy. Dermatol Clin 1998;16(4):805–810.
68. Preboth M. ACOG practice bulletin on management of herpes in pregnancy. Am Fam Physician 2000;61(2):556–557.
69. Schatz M, Petitti D. Antihistamines and pregnancy. Ann Allergy Asthma Immunol 1997;78:157–159.
70. National Asthma Education Program Report of the Working Group on Asthma and Pregnancy. Management of asthma during pregnancy. NIH Publication number 93–3279A, September 1993.
71. Luskin AT. An overview of the recommendations of the Working Group on Asthma and Pregnancy. J Allergy Clin Immunol 1999;103(2 part 2): S350–S353.
72. Reed BR. Dermatologic drugs, pregnancy, and lactation: a conservative guide. Arch Dermatol 1997;133:894–898.
73. The Diabetes Control and Complications Trial Research Group. Effect of pregnancy on microvascular complications in the diabetes control and complications trial. Diabetes Care 2000;23:1084–1091.
74. Schachter SC. Antiepileptic drug therapy: general treatment principles and application for special patient populations. Epilepsia 1999;40 (suppl 9):S20–S25.
75. Malone FD, D'Alton ME. Drugs in pregnancy: anticonvulsants. Semin Perinatol 1997;21(2):114–123.
76. Canger R, Battino D, Canevini MP, et al. Malformations in offspring of women with epilepsy: a prospective study. Epilepsia 1999;40(9):1231–1236.
77. Kaneko S, Battino D, Andermann E, et al. Congenital malformations due to antiepileptic drugs. Epilepsy Res 1999;33:145–158.
78. Samren EB, van Duijn CM, Christiaens L, et al. Antiepileptic drug regimens and major congenital abnormalities in the offspring. Ann Neurol 1999;46:739–746.
79. Practice parameter: management issues for women with epilepsy (summary statement). Report of the Quality Standards Subcommittee of the American Academy of Neurology. Neurology 1998;51(4):944–948.
80. Centers for Disease Control and Prevention. Report of the NIH panel to define principles of therapy of HIV infection and guidelines for the use of antiretroviral agents in HIV-infected adults and adolescents. MMWR Morb Mortal Wkly Rep 1998;47(RR-5): 59–65.
81. Centers for Disease Control and Prevention. Public health service task force recommendations for the use of antiretroviral drugs in pregnant women infected with HIV-1 for maternal health and for reducing perinatal HIV-1 transmission in the United States. www.hivatis.org (Accessed 2000 Sep 28).
82. Duley L, Henderson-Smart DJ. Drugs for rapid treatment of very high blood pressure during pregnancy (Cochrane Review). In: The Cochrane Library, Issue 2, 2000. Oxford: Update Software.
83. McGrath C, Buist A, Norman TR. Treatment of anxiety during pregnancy: effects of psychotropic drug treatment on the developing fetus. Drug Saf 1999;20(2):171–186.
84. Wisner KL, Gelenberg AJ, Leonard H, et al. Pharmacologic treatment of depression during pregnancy. JAMA 1999;282(13):1264–1269.
85. Haddow JE, Palomake GE, Allan WC, et al. Maternal thyroid deficiency during pregnancy and subsequent neuropsychological development of the child. N Engl J Med 1999;341:549–55.
86. Norwitz ER, Robinson JN, Challis JR. The control of labor. N Engl J Med 1999;341(9):660–666.
87. Weismiller DG. Preterm labor. Am Fam Physician 1999;59(3):593–602.
88. Hsieh C. The use of tocolytics in preterm labor. J Fam Pract 2000; 49(2):186.
89. Lam F, Elliot J, Jones SJ, et al. Clinical issues surrounding the use of terbutaline sulfate for preterm labor. Obstet Gynecol Surv 1998; 53(11):S85–S95.
90. Panter KR, Hannah ME, Amankwah KS, et al. The effect of indomethacin tocolysis in preterm labor on perinatal outcome: a randomised placebo-controlled trial. Br J Obstet Gynaecol 1999;106:467–473.
91. Chaim W, Maymon E, Mazor M. A review of the role of trials of the use of antibiotics in women with preterm labor and intact membranes. Arch Gynecol Obstet 1998; 261: 167–172.
92. Carr DB, Clark AL, Kernek K, Spinnato JA. Maintenance oral nifedipine for preterm labor: a randomized clinical trial. Am J Obstet Gynecol 1999; 181: 822–827.
93. Banks BA, Cnaan A, Morgan MA, et al. Multiple courses of antenatal corticosteroids and outcome of premature neonates. Am J Obstet Gynecol 1999;181(3):709–717.
94. Antenatal Corticosteroids Revisited: Repeat Courses. NIH Consensus Statement Online 2000 August 17–18; (cited 2000, Sept, 20); 17(2): 1–10.
95. Prevention of Perinatal Group B Streptococcal Disease: A Public Health Perspective. MMWR Online 1996; (cited 2000, August, 01); 45(RR-7); 1–24.
96. Schuchat A. Group B streptococcus. Lancet 1999:353:51–56.
97. Schrag SJ, Zywicki S, Farley MM, et al. Group B streptococcal disease in the era of intrapartum antibiotic prophylaxis. N Engl J Med 2000;342(1):15–20.
98. Morales WJ, Dickey SS, Bornick P, Lim DV. Change in antibiotic resistance of group B *Streptococcus:* impact on intrapartum managment. Am J Obstet Gynecol 1999;181:310–314.
99. Riskin-Mashiah, Wilkins I. Cervical ripening. Obstet Gynecol Clin North Am 1999;26(2):243–257.
100. Harman JH, Kim A. Current trends in cervical ripening and labor induction. Am Fam Physician 1999;60:477–484.
101. Chamberlain G, Zander L. Induction. BMJ 1999;318:995–998.
102. Hofmeyr GJ, Gulmezoglu AM, Alfirevic Z. Misoprostol for induction of labour: a systematic review. Br J Obstet Gynaecol 1999;106:798–803.
103. Stephens JB, Fenton LA, Fields SA. Obstetric analgesia. Prim Care 2000;27(1):203–221.
104. Findley I, Chamberlain G. Relief of pain. BMJ 1999;318:927–930.
105. Macario A, Scibetta WC, Navarro J, Riley E. Analgesia for labor pain. Anesthesiology 2000;92(3):841–850.
106. Loebstein R, Lalkin A, Koren G. Pharmacokinetic changes during pregnancy and their clinical relevance. Clin Pharmacokinet 1997;33: 328–343.
107. Yoshida K, Smith B, Kumar R. Psychotropic drugs in mothers' milk: a comprehensive review of assay methods, pharmacokinetics and of safety of breast-feeding. J Psychopharmacol 1999;13(1):64–80.
108. Ito S. Drug therapy: drug therapy for breast-feeding women. N Engl J Med 2000;343(2):118–126.
109. Rathmell JP, Viscomi CM, Ashburn MA. Management of nonobstetric pain during pregnancy and lactation. Anesth Analg 1997;85(5):1074–1087.

110. American Academy of Pediatrics, Committee on Drugs. The transfer of drugs and other chemicals into human milk. Pediatrics 1994;93:137–150.
111. Bedinghaus JM. Care of the breast and support of breast-feeding. Prim Care1997;24(1):147–160.
112. Duerbick NB, Reed KL. Pregnancy and lactation. In: Wallis LA, ed. Textbook of Women's Health. Philadelphia: Lippincott-Raven, 1998:663–674.
113. Epperson CN. Postpartum major depression: detection and treatment. Am Fam Physician 1999;59(8)2247–2254, 2259–2260.
114. Evins GG, Theofrastous JP, Galvin SL. Postpartum depression: a comparison of screening and routine clinical evaluation. Am J Obstet Gynecol 2000;182(5):1080–1082.
115. Corral M, Kuan A, Kostaras D. Bright light therapy's effect on postpartum depression. Am J Psychiatry 2000;157(2):303–304.
116. Schmidt K, Olesen OV, Jensen PN. Citalopram and breast-feeding: serum concentration and side effects in the infant. Biol Psychiatry 2000;47:164–165.
117. Anderson PO, Valdes V. Therapy consultation. Increasing breast milk supply. Clin Pharmacol Ther 1993;12:479–480.
118. Carlson HE, Wasser HL, Feidelberger RD. Beer-induced prolactin secretion: a clinical and laboratory study of the role of salsolinol. J Clin Endocrinol Metab 1985;60:673–677.
119. Smith GE. Metoclopramide-lactation promotion in partially or nonlactating patients (Drug Consult). In: Gelman CR, Rumack BH, Hess AJ, eds. DRUGDEX® System. Englewood, Colorado: MICROMEDEX, Inc. (Edition expires [12/2000]).
120. Gelman CR, Rumack BH, Hess AJ, eds. DRUGDEX® System. MICROMEDEX, Inc., Englewood, CO (Edition expires 12/2000).
121. Briggs GG, Freeman RK, Sumner JY. Drugs in Pregnancy and Lactation 5th ed. Baltimore, MD: Williams and Wilkins, 1998.
122. Bennet PN, Jensen AA, Drugs and Human Lactation: A Comprehensive Guide to the Content and Consequences of Drugs, Micronutrients, Radiopharmaceuticals, and Environmental and Occupational Chemicals in Human Milk. 2nd ed. New York, NY: Elsevier, 1996.
123. Hale T. Medications and Mothers' Milk 9th ed. Amarillo, TX: Pharmasoft Medical Publishing, 2000.
124. Lawrence RA, Lawrence RM. Breastfeeding: A Guide for the Medical Profession. 5th ed. St. Louis, MO: Mosby, 1998.

79

INFERTILITY

Cynthia L. Lieu and Tracey Yoshida

Infertility is the inability to conceive after 1 year of frequent contraception-free intercourse. Primary infertility occurs when the couple has never conceived a child, while secondary infertility occurs when a couple has previously conceived a child and is unable to achieve a subsequent pregnancy. The problem of infertility includes the inability to carry a pregnancy to live birth.

The majority of couples with infertility have specific contributing factors that can be addressed and treated with surgical repair and/or medical therapy. Medications can be administered to induce follicular development and ovulation, as sole therapy or in conjunction with intrauterine insemination (IUI) or assisted reproductive technology (ART) procedures. Although much publicized, only a small percentage of infertile couples require the use of ART procedures, which include *in vitro* fertilization and embryo transfer (IVF-ET), gamete intrafallopian transfer (GIFT), zygote intrafallopian transfer (ZIFT), and intracytoplasmic sperm injection (ICSI).

EPIDEMIOLOGY

In the United States, approximately 1 in 10 couples of reproductive age experiences some degree of infertility. The percentage of women who reported experiencing infertility increased from 8.4% (4.9 million) in 1988 to 10.2% (6.2 million) in 1995.[1] About 44% of these women sought medical services for infertility.

Factors that are contributing to the growing problem of infertility include an increased incidence of pelvic inflammatory disease and the decision of many women to delay childbearing until after the age of 35. Advances in reproductive endocrinology and technology are not only extending the age at which women can seek infertility treatments, but also they are allowing many couples the possibility of pregnancy when it had not been possible in the past.

Fecundability, the probability of conception during one menstrual cycle, is approximately 20% to 25% in young couples actively attempting to achieve pregnancy. The conception rate decreases as the age of the female partner and the duration of infertility increase.

ETIOLOGY AND PATHOPHYSIOLOGY

FEMALE REPRODUCTIVE PHYSIOLOGY

The menstrual cycle consists of two major phases, the follicular phase and the luteal phase, with ovulation separating the two. Day 1 of the cycle is the first day of menses. The follicular phase is from day 1 through ovulation, while the luteal phase is from ovulation until the beginning of the next cycle.

Hormonal relationships between the hypothalamus, pituitary, and ovaries influence the menstrual cycle (Fig. 79–1). The hypothalamus secretes gonadotropin-releasing hormone (GnRH) in pulsatile bursts every 60 to 90 minutes. Epinephrine and norepinephrine stimulate the release of GnRH, while dopamine, serotonin, and endogenous opioid peptides inhibit it.[2] In response to the GnRH bursts, the anterior pituitary secretes the gonadotropins, follicle-stimulating hormone (FSH) and luteinizing hormone (LH), in a pulsatile manner. Activin secreted by the granulosa cell also stimulates FSH release, while inhibin suppresses FSH secretion. In patients with hyperprolactinemia, the hypothalamic release of dopamine increases, inhibiting anterior pituitary prolactin release and suppressing the hypothalamic pulsatile secretion of GnRH.

During days 1 to 4 of the menstrual cycle, rising FSH levels cause the recruitment of a small group, or cohort, of follicles for continued growth and development.[3] Between days 5 and 7 of the cycle, one follicle becomes the dominant follicle, which will later rupture and release the oocyte during the cycle. The dominant follicle develops and secretes increasing amounts of estradiol and inhibin, which exert a negative feedback effect on hypothalamic secretion of GnRH and pituitary secretion of FSH, causing the remaining follicles in the cohort to cease development and undergo atresia.

Estradiol levels increase with follicular growth, stimulating the growth and development of the endometrial lining (preparing it for embryo implantation). Estrogen is also responsible for the production of adequate and good-quality cervical mucus. When the estradiol level remains elevated for a sustained period of time, the pituitary releases a midcycle LH surge. The LH surge stimulates the final stages of follicular maturation, ovulation (follicular rupture and extrusion of the oocyte) and luteinization of the granulosa cells to form the corpus luteum. Although their roles are not fully understood, prostaglandins are required for follicle rupture and expulsion of the oocyte, and the use of prostaglandin synthesis inhibitors interferes with ovulation. Ovulation occurs 34 to 36 hours after the onset of the LH surge and, on average, 10 to 16 hours after the LH peak.[3]

After ovulation, the oocyte is released and picked up by the fallopian tube, where it can be fertilized before traveling to the uterus for embryo implantation. Most conceptions occur when intercourse takes place from 2 days before ovulation to the day of ovulation.[4] Because the egg can be fertilized only within a 24-hour period and sperm survival is approximately 2 days, intercourse should occur every 48 hours within 48 hours of ovulation for optimal fecundity.[5]

After releasing the oocyte, the ruptured follicle develops into the corpus luteum. The function of the corpus luteum requires optimal preovulatory follicular development. The midcycle LH surge stimulates the synthesis and secretion of progesterone from the corpus luteum. Progesterone helps maintain the endometrial lining to sustain embryo implantation and maintain pregnancy, and also inhibits GnRH and gonadotropin release, preventing follicular development. If pregnancy occurs, human chorionic gonadotropin (hCG) from the placenta prevents regression of the corpus luteum and maintains steroid (progesterone and estrogen) production until approximately the ninth or tenth week of gestation, when placental steroidogenesis is well established. If fertilization of the oocyte or implantation does not occur, the corpus luteum degenerates and progesterone production declines. As the progesterone level decreases, endometrial shedding (menstruation) occurs, and a new cycle begins. At the end of the luteal

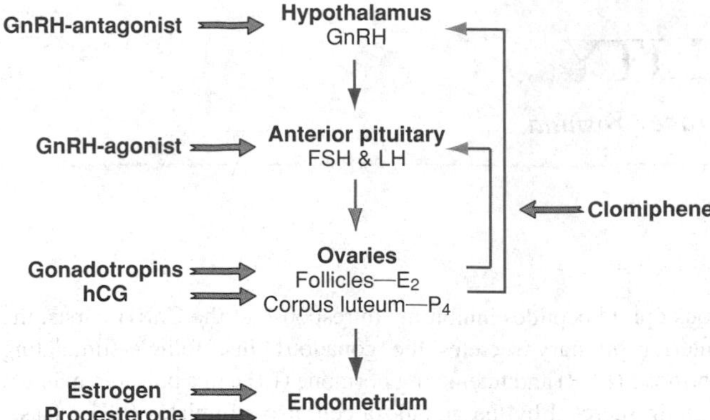

FIGURE 79–1. Hormonal relationships and sites of action of medications. GnRH = gonadotropin-releasing hormone; FSH = follicle-stimulating hormone; LH = luteinizing hormone; hCG = human chorionic gonadotropin.

phase, because of the demise of the corpus luteum and the subsequent decrease in estradiol production, FSH levels start to rise and begin follicular recruitment in the next cycle.

POTENTIAL CAUSES OF INFERTILITY

A successful full-term pregnancy is dependent on many factors, including proper fertilization, implantation in the uterus, and maintenance of the pregnancy. Factors that contribute to infertility can be classified as male factors, ovulatory factors, tubal factors, pelvic factors, uterine factors, immunologic factors, and infectious diseases. The incidence of these factors varies from study to study, according to the population evaluated. Often, multiple factors are responsible for infertility in a couple. When a complete infertility evaluation does not detect any abnormalities, the couple is said to have "unexplained" infertility or subfertility. Recurrent early pregnancy loss (at least two or three) may be due to genetic factors, endocrine abnormalities, anatomic defects, infections, or immunologic factors.

MALE INFERTILITY

The etiology of male infertility includes lifestyle factors, ejaculation problems, abnormalities of the semen, infection, structural abnormalities, or immunologic factors. Male infertility has also been associated with the presence of oxidative stress, due to an excess production of reactive oxygen species and/or a decrease in antioxidant defenses.[6] Treatment of the male partner may involve surgical repair or medical therapy. In addition, infertility caused by male factors can be treated by using IUI, with or without ovulation induction; donor sperm for insemination; or, in cases where severe sperm defects exist, ART with ICSI (i.e., the injection of a single sperm into the oocyte).

FEMALE INFERTILITY

Hypothalamic, pituitary, ovarian, adrenal, or other endocrinologic abnormalities may cause ovulatory dysfunction, which accounts for 30% to 35% of infertility cases. Polycystic ovary syndrome (PCOS), the most common ovarian cause of anovulation, encompasses a group of conditions that cause the ovaries to produce excessive androgens. A luteal phase defect, owing to inadequate corpus luteum function or progesterone production, may prevent the endometrium from sustaining embryo implantation and result in pregnancy loss.

Fallopian tube or pelvic abnormalities may interfere with ovum pickup and transport into the fallopian tube by the fimbria, fertilization, and transport of the ovum and sperm. Endometriosis may have mechanical effects, or it may cause endocrinologic or immunologic abnormalities that contribute to infertility. Uterine factors (e.g., congenital uterine anomalies, polyps, fibroids) rarely cause infertility, but have been associated with recurrent spontaneous abortion. Infections of the cervix and endometrium by *Mycoplasma, Chlamydia,* and *Ureaplasma* may contribute to infertility, pelvic inflammatory disease, and spontaneous abortion. The antigenic properties of sperm may also contribute to infertility.

CLINICAL PRESENTATION AND EVALUATION

The American Society for Reproductive Medicine (ASRM) recommends a formal evaluation after 12 or more months of infertility. An earlier evaluation and treatment is indicated if the woman (1) is over 35 years old; (2) has a history of oligomenorrhea/amenorrhea; (3) has known or suspected uterine/tubal disease or endometriosis, or (4) has a partner known to be subfertile.

Infertility is a problem of the couple, not just the male or the female. The standard infertility evaluation includes the medical and surgical history, as well as the physical examination of both partners; the semen analysis; an assessment of ovulation; the postcoital test; an evaluation of the fallopian tubes and uterus; and, if indicated, laparoscopy.[7] Additional tests can be performed if abnormalities are found during the initial evaluation.

The semen analysis focuses on fluid volume, sperm concentration, motility, and morphology. Because an abnormality is detected in the male partner in 40% to 50% of couples with infertility, the semen analysis should be done before an extensive evaluation and treatment of the female. Spermatogenesis takes approximately 90 days, and various medications and conditions can affect it (Table 79–1). Males whose semen shows abnormalities may undergo further evaluation, while semen cultures may rule out infections.

Ovulatory dysfunction can result in absence or irregularities of menses or luteal phase defects (disorders in progesterone production or effect). Inappropriate breast discharge may be due to increased prolactin secretion (Table 79–2).

Patients with PCOS may present with menstrual disorders (e.g., irregular, absent, or heavy menstrual periods), infertility, symptoms of hyperandrogenism (e.g., hirsutism, acne), and enlarged ovaries with multiple small cysts. Many PCOS patients have insulin resistance. Additional laboratory analysis often demonstrates elevated serum insulin levels, elevated LH levels, an elevated LH to FSH ratio, and a decreased level of hepatic sex hormone-binding globulin. Ovarian androgen production is increased, with elevated androgen levels that

TABLE 79–1. Factors That Can Impair Spermatogenesis

Alcohol	Cyclosporine
Allopurinol	Marijuana
Anabolic/androgenic steroids	Nicotine
Caffeine	Nitrofurantoin
Calcium channel blockers	Spironolactone
Chemotherapeutic agents	Sulfasalazine
Cimetidine	Tetracycline
Co-trimoxazole	Thermal exposure (fever, hot tubs, saunas)
Cocaine	
Colchicine	

Compiled from Refs. 5, 7, 8, 9, 10, and 11.

TABLE 79–2. Medications Associated with Hyperprolactinemia

Chlorpromazine
Cimetidine
Estrogen
Fluphenazine
Haloperidol
Medroxyprogesterone acetate
Methyldopa
Metoclopramide
Phenothiazine derivatives
Pimozide
Reserpine
Tricyclic antidepressants
Verapamil

Compiled from Refs. 12 and 13.

prevent normal follicular development, induce premature follicular atresia, and result in anovulation. These patients may eventually develop diabetes mellitus, dyslipidemia (e.g., low levels of high-density lipoprotein cholesterol, high triglyceride levels), hypertension, cardiovascular disease, and endometrial cancer.

The occurrence of pregnancy or the visualization or recovery of an ovum from the fallopian tube definitively documents ovulation. Tests used to assess ovulation indirectly are based on the physiologic changes associated with ovulation. For example, basal body temperature (BBT) charting or ovulation prediction kits make it possible to assess ovulation. Inadequate corpus luteum function and progesterone production may be diagnosed using the mid-luteal serum progesterone level, BBT charting, or endometrial biopsy.

Usually performed at the beginning of the infertility evaluation, BBT charting is a method of retrospectively and indirectly assessing ovulation. Table 79–3 lists key points for patient counseling about BBT measurement and charting. Progesterone production by the corpus luteum causes the BBT to rise during the luteal phase. Because ovulation occurs before the temperature rises, it is difficult to predict when it will occur. The BBT is useful to determine retrospectively if ovulation most likely occurred; occasionally, ovulation has not occurred even if a biphasic pattern was observed. Each episode of intercourse is marked on the temperature graph so that the physician can determine if the timing and frequency are adequate for conception, while significant events (e.g., lack of sleep, illness, medications taken) are marked on the graph to help the physician interpret the graph.

TABLE 79–3. Basal Body Temperature (BBT) Measurement and Charting

Use BBT thermometer (preferred) or normal fever thermometer.
Shake down thermometer, and place it at bedside before going to sleep at night.
Take first measurement on first day of menstrual period.
Take temperature for at least 5 minutes, each morning upon awakening, before any activity or getting out of bed.
Measure to nearest 0.1°F.
Chart temperatures on graph daily.
Temperature is lower before ovulation than after ovulation (biphasic pattern).
Nadir (at least 0.1°F lower than previous 6 days) signals approach of ovulation; rise of 0.4°F to 0.6°F between 2 consecutive days indicates that ovulation has occurred.
Mark chart with each episode of intercourse.
Mark chart when medications are taken, illness occurs, or changes in sleeping patterns occur.

TABLE 79–4. Using Ovulation Prediction Kits

Begin testing 3–4 days before expected day of ovulation (around day 10 of the menstrual cycle).
Test urine daily at the same time of day until color change is seen on test.
Have sexual intercourse within 24 hours of first positive test result and the following day.
Stop testing for the cycle after positive color change.
Read and follow instructions in each kit, because procedures vary among kits.
Watch or stopwatch with a second hand may be necessary for testing procedures.
Not all kits are equally effective in predicting time of ovulation.

Ovulation prediction kits detect the presence of LH in the urine and are used to estimate the time of ovulation or to schedule intercourse, IUI, or diagnostic tests (e.g., determination of mid-luteal serum progesterone level, endometrial biopsy, postcoital test). Table 79–4 lists key points for patient counseling on the use of ovulation prediction kits. As procedures vary among the different kits, patients should follow the instructions included with the kits carefully. Ideally, ovulation should occur within 24 hours after the ovulation prediction kit shows the first distinct color change. Unfortunately, ovulation prediction kits are not equally effective. Depending on the test used, ovulation may occur on the day that the urinary LH surge is detected, before the surge, or up to 4 days after the surge.[14]

The postcoital test is used to evaluate the quality of the midcycle cervical mucus and the sperm survival and motility in the cervical mucus. During the periovulatory period, the cervical mucus should be thin, clear, watery, very stretchable, and exhibit fern formation when dried on a glass slide.

The hysterosalpingogram allows the clinician to assess the uterine cavity for abnormalities and to evaluate fallopian tube patency. Use of the oil-soluble dye during the hysterosalpingogram is associated with an increased pregnancy rate following the procedure, compared with the use of water-soluble dye.[7]

Laparoscopy permits direct visualization of the pelvic cavity and is the only way to confirm the presence of endometriosis or adhesions. Patients with endometriosis may be asymptomatic, or they may present with infertility, dysmenorrhea, dyspareunia, or irregular menses. There is no correlation between the presence and severity of symptoms and the stage of endometriosis. The laparoscopy may be both diagnostic and therapeutic, as the clinician may perform surgical repairs, lysis of adhesions, or laser vaporization of endometriosis during the procedure.

Determinations of serum hormone levels are helpful in assessing ovarian reserve, monitoring the response to ovarian stimulation, predicting ovulation, and evaluating the possibility that other endocrine abnormalities are contributing to infertility. Estradiol and LH levels are used to monitor ovarian stimulation and predict ovulation. Total testosterone and dehydroepiandrosterone sulfate (DHEAS) levels are assessed in female patients who exhibit signs or symptoms of hyperandrogenism. Elevated prolactin levels or abnormal thyroid function may result in ovulatory dysfunction. Serum FSH, LH, and testosterone levels may be measured in males with abnormal results from the semen analysis.

The follicles produce estradiol, and serum levels rise throughout the follicular phase. Low serum estradiol levels indicate hypogonadism and correlate with failure to respond to clomiphene therapy. During ovarian stimulation with clomiphene or gonadotropin therapy, following serial estradiol levels allows the clinician to assess follicular development and estimate the time of ovulation. Rising estradiol levels from developing follicles result in a surge of LH before ovulation.

Serial serum LH levels or urinary LH testing (using ovulation prediction kits) make it possible to predict the timing of ovulation and to schedule intercourse and/or IUI in order to increase the probability of conception.

Elevated day 3 FSH levels indicate reduced ovarian reserve or ovarian failure, and they predict a poor response to ovarian stimulation and ART procedures. Although this condition is evident in women in their 40s, it can also occur in women in their 30s (premature ovarian failure). A small number of these patients are able to become pregnant using their own oocytes, but they often require extremely high doses of gonadotropin therapy or other variations from standard protocols to achieve pregnancy.

Serial ultrasound monitoring can be used to (1) assess follicular growth and development, (2) estimate the timing of ovulation, and (3) confirm ovulation. When patients are receiving medications for ovarian stimulation, ultrasound monitoring facilitates the assessment of their response to therapy and the adjustment of medication dosages. For patients undergoing ovulation induction, ultrasound monitoring may be performed to screen for potential ovarian cysts before the initiation of a cycle of medications. Ultrasound monitoring may be used to assess endometrial thickness at the time of ovulation; if the lining is too thin, implantation may not occur, and if the lining is too thick, there may be an increase in spontaneous pregnancy loss.[15]

▶ TREATMENT: Infertility

The goal of infertility therapy is to achieve a pregnancy that results in the birth of a healthy infant, while minimizing the stress, physical discomfort, financial costs, and risks (e.g., ovarian hyperstimulation syndrome, multiple gestations) associated with infertility treatment. The choice of treatment depends on the age of the female partner, duration of infertility, contributing factors to infertility, risks of treatment, and cost-effectiveness of the various therapies, given the situation of the couple. A general treatment algorithm for infertility is shown in Figure 79–2.

For a younger couple with unexplained infertility and a history of infertility for less than 2 years, the initial approach may be a 6- to 12-month period of expectant observation in which the couple uses timed intercourse in conjunction with BBT charting and/or ovulation prediction kits to increase the chance of conception. Cumulative pregnancy rates without treatment in couples with unexplained infertility range from 30% to 80% over 3 years of follow-up, depending on the age of the female and the duration of infertility.[16] If the couple does not achieve pregnancy in the 6- to 12-month period, the initiation of ovulation induction is appropriate.

General treatment algorithms for patients without tubal disease or severe male factor infertility begin with ovulation induction combined with IUI. Clomiphene citrate is used before gonadotropin therapy because it is less expensive, it is administered orally, and multiple follicles are less likely to develop. If clomiphene therapy is not successful, the next step is gonadotropin therapy. Couples who do not become pregnant using ovulation induction alone then undergo ART procedures. When the woman is more than 40 years of age, if there is no success after three cycles of ovulation induction with IUI, the couple should progress to ART procedures and consider the use of donor oocytes. For women of any age with blocked fallopian tubes, IVF appears to be more cost-effective than tubal surgery.[17]

For couples with significant male factor infertility, treatment begins with IUI with or without ovulation induction, then progresses to IVF with or without ICSI (depending on the severity of the sperm defect). With severe male factor infertility, insemination with donor sperm is more cost-effective than IVF with ICSI; however, it does not allow the male partner to provide genetic input. If the genetic input is desired, proceeding directly to IVF with ICSI may be preferred.[17]

The age of the female partner has a significant impact on the prognosis of the treatment of infertility. There is a significant reduction in success rates for women 35 to 39 years of age and a further reduction for women older than 40 years of age. The ovarian age, which reflects the decrease in the number of oocytes remaining, has been shown to be the most important age-related factor.[18] Patients with premature ovarian failure or postmenopausal women who receive a transfer of embryos derived from donor oocytes have a pregnancy rate similar to that seen with younger women.[19]

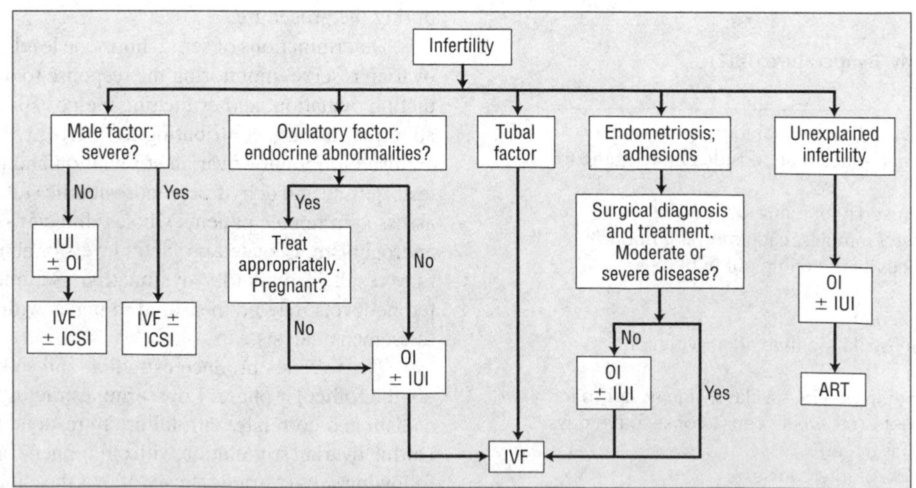

FIGURE 79–2. General treatment algorithm for infertility. IUI = intrauterine insemination; OI = ovulation induction; IVF = *in vitro* fertilization; ICSI = intracytoplasmic sperm injection; ART = assisted reproductive technology.

TABLE 79–5. Environmental Factors That Can Affect Fertility

2, 3, 7, 8-tetrachloro-p-dibenzodioxin
Alcohol
Chemical dusts
Chlorinated hydrocarbons
Cigarette smoking
Ethylene oxide
Heavy metals
Nitrous oxide
Organic solvents
Perchloroethylene
Pesticides
Radiant heat
"Recreational" drugs (e.g., marijuana, cocaine)
Solvent mixtures
Toluene

Compiled from Refs. 20, 21, and 22.

NONPHARMACOLOGIC THERAPY

Both women and men trying to conceive a child should be counseled to avoid medications, products, or activities that interfere with their ability to do so(Table 79–5). Obesity reduces pregnancy rates, so women with a body mass index greater than 30 should be advised to lose weight. In severely overweight women, weight reduction reduces insulin resistance; decreases insulin, leptin, LH, and androgen levels; decreases the abnormal LH to FSH ratio; and increases sex hormone-binding globulin levels.[23] Females should avoid excessive dieting and weight loss or overstrenuous exercise, however, because these activities can lead to menstrual and ovulatory abnormalities that impair fertility. Exposure to factors that affect sperm production or function can affect fertility for up to 15 weeks.[24] Females attempting conception should avoid prostaglandin synthetase inhibitors (e.g., nonsteroidal anti-inflammatory agents, aspirin) before or around the time of ovulation, as they may prevent the release of the oocyte.[25] Medications that can result in hyperprolactinemia or impair spermatogenesis (Table 79–2) should be avoided. Vaginal lubricants should be avoided because they can impair sperm motility and activity.

Females trying to become pregnant should be advised to eat a balanced diet and take folic acid (to reduce the risk of neural tube defects) and multivitamin supplementation. As oxidative stress is associated with male infertility, males with subfertility may benefit from antioxidant therapy (e.g., vitamins C and E, selenium), although beneficial amounts are not known and excessive amounts may be deleterious.[26,27]

INTRAUTERINE INSEMINATION (IUI)

For the IUI process, sperm are separated from the semen and the better quality sperm extracted for insemination. The sperm are injected transcervically into the uterus. IUI is performed after ovulation during a natural cycle or after ovulation induction with clomiphene or gonadotropin therapy. Most commonly, it is performed on the day following the urinary LH surge or approximately 36 hours after a single injection of hCG.

ASSISTED REPRODUCTIVE TECHNOLOGY (ART)

All techniques involving direct retrieval of oocytes from the ovary and manipulation of sperm and/or embryos to achieve pregnancy fall into the category of ART. These procedures include IVF-ET, GIFT, and ZIFT, and they account for less than 5% of infertility treatments.

With ART, more than one embryo is often transferred to the uterus to increase the likelihood of pregnancy.[28] The incidence of multiple gestations increases when larger numbers of embryos are transferred. Thus, ovulation induction and ART have significantly increased the number of multiple gestations and multiple births. Monitoring ovulation induction closely and limiting the number of embryos transferred can reduce the incidence of multiple gestations.

In Vitro Fertilization and Embryo Transfer (IVF-ET)

In IVF-ET, gonadotropins are administered to stimulate the development of multiple follicles, while serial measurements of serum estradiol levels and ovarian ultrasound monitoring are used to assess follicular growth and development. About 36 hours after hCG is administered to stimulate final follicular maturation, oocytes are retrieved and cultured with processed sperm (IVF). If the sperm count is significantly low or abnormal, ICSI is performed. Of all the treatments available for infertility, IVF is the only one that permits an assessment of fertilization. After the embryos are transferred into the uterus, progesterone supplementation is usually administered during the luteal phase to sustain the endometrium for the first trimester.

Gamete Intrafallopian Transfer (GIFT) and Zygote Intrafallopian Transfer (ZIFT)

For GIFT or ZIFT to occur, the woman must have at least one functional fallopian tube. Gametes or zygotes are transferred into the fallopian tubes during laparoscopy, allowing fertilization to occur *in vivo*. The transfer into the fallopian tube more closely simulates a natural cycle than does IVF, but it is more invasive and more expensive.

PHARMACOLOGIC THERAPY

Ovulation induction can be used in women with ovulatory disorders as a way to produce ovulation for a natural conception (intercourse) or as part of an insemination procedure. The agents that induce ovulation can also be used in a protocol for controlled ovarian hyperstimulation. The goal of controlled ovarian hyperstimulation is to produce multiple oocytes for an insemination cycle or for ART protocols. Some therapeutic agents augment the patient's natural endocrine process, while other agents take control of, and in some cases replace, the natural cycle.

CLOMIPHENE CITRATE

An orally active, nonsteroidal estrogen receptor modulator, clomiphene citrate (Clomid, Milophene, Serophene) inhibits the negative feedback response on the hypothalamus by bonding to estrogen receptors. This causes an increase in the release of FSH and LH, and a subsequent rise in their levels, promoting follicular growth and maturation. Enhancement of the natural hypothalamic-pituitary-ovarian axis is the primary mechanism of action, although pituitary and ovarian effects may occur.

The predominant indication for clomiphene citrate is for anovulatory or oligo-ovulatory infertility, including PCOS. It can also be useful in the treatment of unexplained infertility in ovulatory women and oligospermia in men. Clomiphene should be given only to women who have normal responses from the hypothalamus and pituitary to low estrogen levels. High FSH levels (greater than 30 mIU/mL) generally indicate absent or resistant follicles that will not respond well to clomiphene citrate.

Because there is a possible association between the dosage of clomiphene citrate and multiple birth, the dose should be low initially and then increased, if necessary, with each cycle. The recommended starting dosage is 50 mg/day for 5 days, beginning on day 5 of the cycle. Because women with PCOS may be ultrasensitive to the drug, the starting dose for these women may be lowered to 25 mg/day. Doses should be increased in a stepwise fashion in subsequent cycles to a maximum of 150 mg/day. If ovulation occurs, there is no advantage to increasing the dose. In fact, the antagonistic effects on estrogen receptors can affect endometrial proliferation and adversely affect implantation.

In view of the 5-day half-life of clomiphene, starting the regimen of clomiphene earlier in the cycle may avoid problems with implantation; several studies have demonstrated improved results when clomiphene begins earlier in the cycle.[29] Ovulation is expected 5 to 10 days after the last dose and is determined by urinary LH monitoring, plasma progesterone assay, vaginal ultrasound examination, or endometrial histology. Clomiphene citrate can elevate the BBT and lengthen the luteal phase, in addition to producing a triphasic pattern in the BBT. For these reasons, BBT monitoring of ovulation is not recommended in cycles in which clomiphene citrate is used. To ensure optimal timing for conception after ovulation, intercourse can be timed according to results of the ultrasound examination or ovulation prediction kits, or it should occur every other day for 1 week, beginning 4 to 5 days after the last day of clomiphene citrate administration.

A uterine ultrasound examination can be performed prior to the initiation of clomiphene citrate therapy to rule out the presence of ovarian cysts. Rates of multiple births have ranged from 5% to 12.3%, with the vast majority being twins. The antiestrogenic properties of clomiphene citrate cause reversible hot flashes in 11% of patients. Visual disturbances occur at an estimated rate of less than 2%. Blurring and spots or flushes (scintillating scotomata) are dose-related and are an indication to discontinue therapy. Although the drug may accentuate midcycle pain (mittelschmerz), abnormal ovarian enlargement or ovarian hyperstimulation syndrome are infrequent with normal doses of clomiphene citrate; however, they can occur with high or prolonged doses. Abdominal symptoms (e.g., discomfort, distention, bloating, abnormal uterine bleeding) occur in 5% to 6% of patients. Miscellaneous symptoms, including nausea, vomiting, breast tenderness, headache, and dizziness, occur in 1% to 2.5% of patients. The addition of estrogen alone or in combination with progesterone may increase pregnancy rates by improving abnormalities in the cervical mucus and endometrium that result from clomiphene citrate therapy.[30,31]

Of women whose only fertility problem is irregular or no ovulation, about 80% will ovulate, and 50% will become pregnant within 6 months of clomiphene citrate treatments. Therefore, the number of pregnancies achieved with clomiphene citrate is much lower than expected, even after successfully inducing ovulation. This may be due to the endometrial thinning and the production of hostile cervical mucus caused by the drug's antagonist effect on estrogen receptors. Clomiphene treatment for more than six consecutive cycles has not demonstrated an increase in pregnancy rates. If conception has not occurred within six ovulatory cycles, then alternative treatment should be considered.

TABLE 79–6. Gonadotropin Therapy

Medication	Contents	Route of Administration
Menotropins		
HMG (Pergonal, Humegon)	75 IU of FSH; 75 IU of LH 150 IU of FSH; 150 IU of LH	IM
hMG (Repronex)	75 IU of FSH; 75 IU of LH 150 IU of FSH; 150 IU of LH	IM, SC
Urofollitropins		
HP-FSH (Fertinex)	75 IU of FSH	SC
Recombinant products		
Follitropin-α (Gonal-F)	75 IU of FSH	SC
Follitropin-β (Follistim)	75 IU of FSH	SC

hMG = human menopausal gonadotropin; FSH = follicle-stimulating hormone; LH = luteinizing hormone; IM = intramuscular injection; SC = subcutaneous injection

GONADOTROPIN THERAPY

Women for whom clomiphene citrate therapy is not successful are candidates for more advanced methods of ovulation induction. Gonadotropin agents can produce ovulation for insemination or ART procedures. (Table 79–6) The ovaries must be able to respond normally to FSH and LH stimulation. Gonadotropins are relatively safe, when administered as ovulation-inducing drugs to properly selected patients, in correct dosages, and with appropriate monitoring. However, they are expensive, must be administered parenterally on a daily basis, and require more extensive monitoring than other methods. They are indicated only after a thorough infertility workup and careful counseling of the couple. *These agents should be prescribed and monitored only by individuals who are expert in their use.*

Human menopausal gonadotropin (hMG), also known as menotropin, comes from the urine of postmenopausal women; it contains both FSH and LH. Each vial of hMG should contain equal amounts of FSH and LH activity; however, radioimmunoassay suggests a dominance of FSH. In women who do not have primary ovarian failure, hMG produces ovarian follicular growth. Gonadotropins should not be used in women with primary ovarian failure as indicated by FSH levels greater than 30 mIU/mL.

Gonadotropins can also induce spermatogenesis in men who have primary or secondary pituitary hypofunction. Pretreatment with 5,000 IU of hCG is given three times a week until serum testosterone levels are within normal limits. This may take as long as 4 to 6 months. When testosterone levels are sufficient, hMG is given intramuscularly at a starting dose of 1 ampule (75 IU of FSH/75 IU of LH) three times a week with 2,000 IU of hCG given twice a week. If spermatogenesis is not sufficient after 4 months of treatment, the dose of hMG may be increased to two ampules three times a week.

Highly purified urofollitropin, like hMG, is extracted from the urine of postmenopausal women. It contains purified FSH and has minimal LH activity. Subcutaneous injection provides a benefit to patients by decreasing the pain associated with the intramuscular injection of hMG.

Products containing only FSH may be preferable to combination products such as hMG. Excessive LH during follicular development is thought to have a negative impact on the ovarian cycle by causing a rapid maturation in the preovulatory cells before they are aspirated for fertilization. This may not only affect oocyte quality, but also may be responsible for a reduced likelihood of fertilization, poor implantation, and increased risk of early spontaneous abortions. Purified FSH may be of particular benefit for women with PCOS who have an increased LH to FSH ratio and who have not become pregnant through clomiphene citrate therapy, in protocols not using GnRH agonists for pituitary desensitization[32] or women participating in ART programs. In protocols that include pituitary desensitization, a statistically significant difference in pregnancy rates between FSH therapy and hMG therapy has not been found.[32]

Naturally acquired gonadotropin products can contain batch-to-batch inconsistencies and have impurities that may affect their performance. In addition, the demand was quickly exceeding the supply of these naturally derived products. The development of recombinant FSH is an important advancement for ovulation induction. Two recombinant products, follitropin-α (Gonal F) and follitropin-β (Follistim), appear to have equal efficacy and to be well tolerated.[33] No serum anti-recombinant FSH antibodies have been detected. Adverse effects of recombinant FSH are similar to those of other FSH-containing products. Because recombinant FSH has almost no contamination (>99% FSH), it may be beneficial in women who have had dermatologic/allergic reactions to naturally derived gonadotropin agents.

A suggested initial dose of gonadotropins (based on FSH) is 75–150 IU/day, beginning on day 3 or 4 of the cycle. Once the serum estradiol concentration has risen steadily and is not excessive (<1,500 pg/mL), the patient continues to receive the same dosage until the serum concentration is between 500 and 2,000 pg/mL and one or two follicles have reached a diameter of 17 to 20 mm, as determined by ultrasound monitoring (exact criteria vary). The injections should be given at the same time each day and can be administered by the patient or her partner, if properly trained. Some regimens may involve twice a day dosing in patients with repeated implantation failures.[34] Generally, gonadotropin administration should not exceed 12 days, although a longer time may be required in poor responders. In some cases, clomiphene citrate is used in combination with gonadotropins, but it is questionable whether the pregnancy rate is enhanced.[35]

Adverse reactions associated with gonadotropins include febrile reactions, breast tenderness, abdominal pain, rash or swelling at the injection site, nausea, vomiting, diarrhea, and dermatologic symptoms. Ovarian hyperstimulation syndrome and multiple gestations are serious adverse reactions that can occur in ovulation induction and controlled ovarian stimulation protocols.

HUMAN CHORIONIC GONADOTROPIN (hCG)

In some cases, clomiphene citrate and other agents cause follicular maturation with an adequate rise in the follicular phase estradiol concentration, but ovulation fails to occur. If a lack of a midcycle gonadotropin surge is causing ovulation failure, treatment should include the exogenous administration of hCG (Pregnyl, Profasi), 5,000–10,000 IU given intramuscularly, 3 or 4 days after the last dose of clomiphene citrate or, if injectable gonadotropins are part of the regimen, when follicular diameter is 17 to 20 mm as determined by ultrasound examination.[36] The activity of hCG is essentially identical to that of LH, but it has a longer half-life (>24 hours versus 60 minutes). Hormonal monitoring and follicle ultrasound measurements help determine the appropriate timing of hCG administration to trigger ovulation. When insemination or ART procedures are not used, intercourse is advised the day after hCG administration and for the next 2 days. Recombinant hCG (Ovidrel), 250 μg given subcutaneously, was comparable to urinary hCG (5,000 IU) in inducing folliculogenesis, oocyte maturation, and luteinization after ovulation induction.[37]

Adverse effects associated with the administration of hCG include headache, irritability, restlessness, fatigue, edema, gynecomastia, and pain at the injection site. When it is necessary to use hCG for extended periods of time, as in male infertility, hCG-induced fluid retention may be problematic in patients with epilepsy, migraines, asthma, and cardiac or renal disease.

GONADOTROPIN-RELEASING HORMONE (GnRH)

When the process of GnRH stimulation is defective, the ultimate result is decreased ovarian estrogen production and anovulatory cycles. The pulsatile administration of GnRH replaces the faulty secretion of GnRH and more closely mimics the natural hormonal secretory pattern, including the pulsatile release of pituitary FSH and LH. In contrast, continuous stimulation with GnRH results in down-regulation of the normal FSH/LH response. GnRH therapy is effective in women with primary hypothalamic amenorrhea, hyperprolactinemia resistant to traditional therapy, and, to a lesser degree, PCOS.

Gonadorelin acetate (Lutrepulse) is a synthetic decapeptide with the identical amino acid sequence of endogenous GnRH. The average starting dose is 5 μg (range, 1–20 μg) administered via a portable programmable mini-pump for 21 days. The pulse interval may range from 60- to 120-minute intervals, with a 90-minute interval recommended most often. Women with PCOS who do not respond to clomiphene citrate alone may benefit from the addition of pulsatile GnRH, which can produce higher conception rates with minimal adverse events. The use of gonadorelin for ovulation induction more closely resembles the natural hormonal secretory pattern and requires minimal monitoring. However, it is not commonly used because of cost considerations.

Potential adverse effects with GnRH therapy are similar to those that occur with gonadotropin therapy, including ovarian hyperstimulation and increased risk for multiple gestations. The incidence of severe ovarian hyperstimulation syndrome is rare with gonadorelin, possibly because the pulsatile administration maintains the endogenous feedback mechanism. Other reactions such as inflammation, mild phlebitis, infection, and hematoma may occur as a result of IV administration.

GnRH AGONISTS

The administration of GnRH agonists causes a down-regulation of endogenous FSH and LH levels. Initially, GnRH agonists stimulate the release of pituitary gonadotropins; however, this effect diminishes with repeated dosing. The suppression of endogenous LH can decrease the number of oocytes released prematurely, improving oocyte quality and subsequently increasing pregnancy rates. The addition of a GnRH agonist to the treatment regimen for patients with PCOS has been associated with a reduced incidence of pregnancy loss and possible improvement in fertilization and cleavage rates.

GnRH agonists are administered via nasal spray (nafarelin, Synarel) or by subcutaneous injection (leuprolide, Lupron) daily for up to 3 weeks, starting in the luteal phase of the previous cycle (long protocol, most commonly used) or early in the follicular phase of a new cycle (short protocol). Administration beginning in the luteal phase effectively blocks endogenous gonadotropin secretion, especially the

LH surge. After a hypogonadotropic hypogonadal state is achieved, ovulation is induced through the administration of gonadotropins.

The initial stimulation effect of GnRH may cause vaginal bleeding, pelvic pain, and breast tenderness. With continued pituitary suppression, symptoms of estrogen deficiency occur, including hot flushes, headache, and vaginal dryness. When GnRH agonists are used in controlled ovarian stimulation, the addition of FSH prevents estrogen deficiency and, thus, minimizes side effects.

Ovarian cysts have been seen in approximately 15% of patients treated with GnRH agonists. They possibly result from the initial pituitary stimulation that causes the primordial follicles to grow, even though that growth halts with continued GnRH agonist pituitary suppression. Formation of ovarian cysts may require prolonged treatment with the GnRH agonist or surgical drainage before ovulation induction begins. Temporary impairment of perceived memory function, possibly related to rapid estrogen depletion, has been reported with GnRH agonists.[38]

GnRH ANTAGONISTS

To prevent a premature LH surge and premature ovulation, women undergoing controlled ovarian hyperstimulation may receive GnRH antagonists, ganirelix acetate (Antagon) and cetrorelix acetate (Cetrotide). Like GnRH agonists, GnRH antagonists suppress endogenous LH surges during ovarian stimulation. GnRH antagonists avoid the initial flare-up period seen with GnRH agonists, shortening the number of days necessary for LH suppression and allowing ovarian stimulation to begin within the spontaneous cycle.

In one study, Ganirelix, 0.25 mg/day administered subcutaneously, starting on day 7 and stopping after hCG was given, resulted in ongoing pregnancy rates of 37.1%.[39] Compared with leuprolide, it produces a similar pregnancy rate, with a shorter duration of therapy and fewer injections.[40]

The effect of GnRH analogs on pituitary and ovarian function is temporary and persists only as long as the administration of the analog continues. Hypothalamic-pituitary-ovarian function returns to baseline within 1 to 2 months after discontinuation of the GnRH analog.

ORAL CONTRACEPTIVES

The use of oral contraceptives prior to ovulation induction can improve the efficiency of ovarian down-regulation and allow flexibility in cycle scheduling. Pretreatment with oral contraceptives decreases early follicular phase androgen production, which may benefit initial follicular development. These changes in the follicular phase ovarian environment may improve folliculogenesis, oocyte quality, and cycle outcome. Oral contraceptives may also benefit women who are receiving GnRH agonists for the suppression of LH, because of their ability to decrease ovarian cyst formation (which can delay or cancel a stimulation cycle).[41,42]

ESTROGENS

Women may be given estrogen during the follicular phase to stimulate endometrial growth or to improve cervical mucus production. Estrogen is also used with progesterone to prepare the endometrium to receive a frozen-thawed embryo transfer or a donor oocyte-derived embryo transfer.

LUTEAL SUPPORT

In an assisted cycle, ovarian hyperstimulation and pituitary down-regulation with GnRH analogs shorten the luteal phase and cause abnormal decreases in serum progesterone and estrogen levels. Endometrial biopsies of women who have undergone controlled ovarian stimulation without embryo transfer have shown that more than 50% had endometrial development not suitable for implantation (e.g., delayed development of glandular features and advancement of stromal features). Although both hCG and progesterone have been used to provide luteal support in ART and donor programs, progesterone is more commonly used. Human chorionic gonadotropin is associated with an increased risk of ovarian hyperstimulation syndrome as a result of increased estradiol levels.

Progesterone in an oil suspension in doses ranging 50–100 mg is administered by intramuscular injection, beginning on the day of embryo transfer. The injections are usually given once or twice a day for long periods of time (10 to12 weeks) and can be very painful. Two vaginal preparations of progesterone, vaginal suppositories and a vaginal gel, can provide luteal support. The disadvantage of vaginal suppositories is that they produce unpleasant vaginal secretions as they melt, allowing progesterone to leak from the vagina. In addition, two to three times a day dosing is often necessary. A vaginal bioadhesive gel formulation containing 90 mg of micronized progesterone (Crinone) is approved for use in therapy for infertility. Patients using the progesterone gel may experience a globular discharge composed of the polymer and epithelial cells.

Intravaginal preparations produce lower progesterone plasma levels than those seen with intramuscular dosing. However, histologic, receptor, and ultrasonographic analyses show no significant differences in the effect on the endometrium between the two routes of administration.[43] This may be due to a "first-pass" uterine effect that allows for drug delivery to the uterus while minimizing systemic side effects.[44]

Natural progesterone is not well absorbed when given orally unless it is in a micronized form. A micronized oral progesterone formulation is available commercially (Prometrium); however, the Food and Drug Administration has not approved it for use in the treatment of infertility, and there is no information available on comparative trials with this product in ART protocols. There are case reports that it is being used in some infertility centers with success. Because the product's capsule contains peanut oil, its use is contraindicated in patients who are allergic to peanuts. Oral progesterone has a short half-life, necessitating two to three times a day dosing, and undergoes significant "first-pass" hepatic metabolism.

Progesterone is often dispensed with a warning against its use in pregnancy. Pharmacists should educate patients by informing them that these warnings are based on reports of congenital birth defects associated with the use of synthetic progestins commonly found in birth control pills. In addition, most reports are from the late 1970s and early 1980s, when progesterone doses were much higher than those used today. The use of natural progesterone in the treatment of infertility has not been associated with an increased risk of congenital malformations.

ALTERNATIVE AND MISCELLANEOUS AGENTS USED IN INFERTILITY TREATMENT

Many alternative agents have been tried to improve pregnancy rates in poor responders to the more traditional treatments. Low-dose aspirin

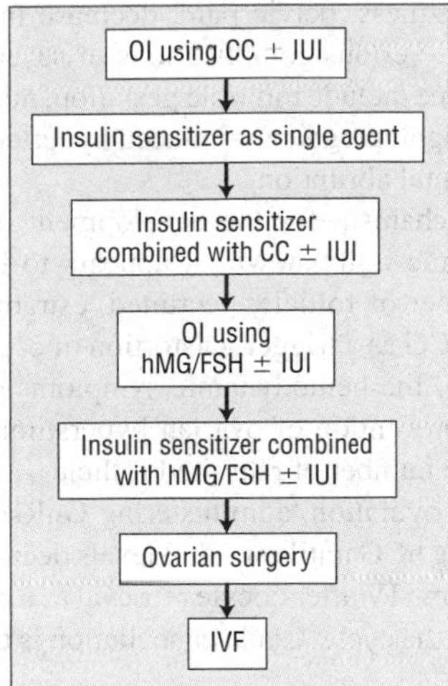

FIGURE 79–3. Ovulation induction in women with polycystic ovary syndrome (PCOS). OI = ovulation induction; CC = clomiphene citrate; IUI = intrauterine insemination; hMG/FSH = gonadotropin therapy with human menopausal gonadotropin and/or follicle-stimulating hormone; IVF = *in vitro* fertilization. *Adapted from ref. 48.*

has been used to increase ovarian and uterine blood flow velocity, which may improve ovarian response and implantation rates. Aspirin therapy can be a safe and inexpensive treatment for poor ovarian response in some patients.[45]

Impairments in insulin metabolism are a key component of PCOS, which is not corrected with the use of clomiphene citrate. Several reports have shown satisfactory reproductive outcomes with the oral administration of insulin-lowering agents in PCOS patients.[46] Reduction of insulin resistance and hyperinsulinemia reverses serum LH and androgen abnormalities; restores menstrual cycles and ovarian function; and also improves serum glucose, insulin, and lipid levels. Metformin (Glucophage), 500 mg three times daily, has been used successfully to restore menstrual cyclicity and ovulatory function in women with PCOS. Clomiphene may be added to metformin if patients fail to respond sufficiently to metformin alone.[47] Based on current data, metformin may be included in the step-wise approach to ovulation induction in women with PCOS (Fig. 79–3). Troglitazone has also been reported to increase ovulatory cycles,[49] but was withdrawn from the market because of liver toxicity. The ovulatory effects of two newer insulin sensitizers similar to troglitazone, rosiglitazone and pioglitazone, have not been extensively evaluated in the treatment of infertility caused by PCOS.

Abnormalities in the hypothalamic-pituitary control of ovarian hormone production can cause, among other things, a hostile cervical mucus. Because guaifenesin is relatively inexpensive and there have been no reports of detrimental effects during infertility treatments, it may be helpful in improving cervical mucus quality. Patients with abnormal results from a postcoital test and no defect in spermatogenesis or sperm quality may benefit from the administration of guaifenesin, 200 mg three times a day from day 5 of the cycle until ovulation. Patients who do not become pregnant despite marked improvement in mucus quality may have other associated fertility problems.

Dopamine agonists have been used in women whose infertility is related to hyperprolactinemia, with or without galactorrhea. They may reduce the size of prolactin-producing pituitary tumors and return serum prolactin concentrations to normal.[50] Normalizing the prolactin concentration restores central gonadotropin function. Bromocriptine, a semisynthetic ergotamine derivative, acts as a dopamine agonist to directly inhibit pituitary prolactin secretion. Cabergoline is a long-acting dopamine agonist with a high affinity for the dopamine-2 receptors. Cabergoline, which can be given just once or twice a week, is more effective in normalizing prolactin and restoring menses than bromocriptine, and it is significantly better tolerated. However, it is not yet recommended as first-line therapy for patients seeking treatment for infertility, because adequate safety data in pregnancy are not available.[51]

Bromocriptine treatment is usually initiated with a bedtime dose of 1.25 mg for 1 week and then titrated up based on serum prolactin concentrations. Doses greater than 15 mg/d are rare. Once ovulation begins to occur, bromocriptine should be taken during the follicular phase. Cabergoline is initiated at a dose of 0.25 mg twice weekly and titrated to a dose of 1 mg twice weekly based on serum prolactin concentrations. If pregnancy does not occur in a cycle as determined by a sensitive pregnancy test, the patient can stop taking the drug during the luteal phase and begin again after the next menses starts. If there is no objective indication that ovulation is occurring within 3 months, despite normal prolactin levels, then clomiphene citrate and/or gonadotropins should be used.

Nausea, headache, and dizziness are common side effects of bromocriptine. Psychiatric symptoms may occur in less than 1% of patients. Other complaints include orthostatic hypotension, nasal congestion, vomiting, constipation, and abdominal cramps. Slowing the dosage titration and taking the dose at bedtime with food can minimize the side effects from oral administration. There is no evidence of increased teratogenicity with the use of dopamine agonists, but barrier contraception is recommended until normal menstrual cycles are established.[51] If the only cause of infertility is chronic anovulation due to hyperprolactinemia, a 60% to 80% pregnancy rate can be achieved with this approach.[52] Bromocriptine is no longer used as nonspecific therapy for unexplained infertility.

Acupuncture has been demonstrated to benefit males with reduced sperm activity,[53] females with PCOS, and those whose infertility results from hormonal disturbances, anovulation, and uterine arterial blood flow impedance.[54]

With continued infertility, patients often look toward alternative or herbal products for a "cure." Bulletin boards in infertility sites on the Internet are full of suggestions about products to try and "success" stories involving a variety of products and treatments, including vitamins and Chinese herbs. There are very few scientific data to support the benefits of these agents in infertility therapy. Because of the lack of clinical data available, patients should weigh the potential benefits of these products with the potential risks, and they should not use such products without discussing it with their medical care provider.

TREATMENT FOR IMMUNOLOGIC DISORDERS

There is controversy regarding the validity and treatment of immunologic causes of infertility. The IV administration of immunoglobulin has been used to prevent the recurrent spontaneous abortion. Beginning in the follicular phase and continued every 3 to 4 weeks during the first 8 months of pregnancy, doses ranging from 200 to 250 mg/kg of immunoglobulin were given in one study.[55] Minor side effects associated with the infusion occurred. An ASRM Practice Committee Opinion Report states that the IV administration of immunoglobulin should be evaluated in a randomized trial and, until more information is obtained, its use in the management of recurrent spontaneous abortion should be considered an experimental treatment rather than a routine one.

Other treatments that have been used for immune disorders in infertility include daily low-dose aspirin, daily low-dose heparin, and steroids. Prolonged use of steroids may have significant adverse effects on both the mother and the fetus. Because of the bleeding risk associated with heparin and aspirin use, the risks and benefits of this approach to improving IVF success rates should be more fully determined before it becomes accepted as routine practice. There is a need for well-designed, prospective, randomized, placebo-controlled studies to determine the role of immunology in fertility, the effectiveness of proposed therapies, and the long-term consequences.

ADVERSE EVENTS ASSOCIATED WITH TREATMENT OF INFERTILITY

Most treatment protocols aim to induce multifollicular development; therefore, the main complications are ovarian hyperstimulation syndrome, and obstetric and postnatal complications as a result of multiple gestations. Clinical evidence does not indicate that hMG-hCG ovulation induction places fetuses at any greater risk of malformation than the normal population. However, fetal loss because of spontaneous abortion or premature delivery of multiple gestations is of concern.

OVARIAN HYPERSTIMULATION SYNDROME

The incidence of ovarian hyperstimulation syndrome is greater in protocols that use higher gonadotropin doses and GnRH analogs. In cycles that achieve serum estradiol levels higher than 6,000 pg/mL and/or involve the recruitment of more than 30 follicles, the incidence of ovarian hyperstimulation syndrome is as high as 80%. Fortunately, severe cases develop in less than 2% of assisted cycles.[56] Symptoms, such as bilateral ovarian enlargement and volume depletion caused by "third spacing" of fluids from the intravascular compartment, usually appear 3 to 10 days after ovulation or hCG injection. In severe cases, patients can develop electrolyte imbalances, renal impairment, pericardial effusions, adult respiratory distress syndrome, and thromboembolic phenomena. Patients should be advised to seek medical attention if they experience an increase in abdominal girth or weight gain, nausea or dizziness, pelvic pain, decrease in urine output, or shortness of breath. Serious complications of severe ovarian hyperstimulation syndrome include multiple gestation, miscarriage, prematurity, low birth weight, pregnancy-induced hypertension, gestational diabetes, and placental abruption.

The exact mechanism for the development of ovarian hyperstimulation syndrome is unknown. It appears to be at least partly related to the number of follicles recruited, estradiol level, and the administration of hCG as a trigger. Distortion of capillary permeability may account for the hemodynamic symptoms of the syndrome. Strategies for the prevention of ovarian hyperstimulation syndrome include limiting the number of recruited follicles, aspirating some of the follicles before ovulation, administering GnRH agonists instead of hCG, withholding hCG until estradiol levels decrease ("coasting"), administering albumin IV after oocyte retrieval as a prophylactic measure, and canceling the cycle. Cycle cancellation is the most common approach.[56]

Once severe ovarian hyperstimulation syndrome develops, treatment options are limited; they address primarily the major signs and symptoms. Osmotic diuresis and fluid resuscitation may help prevent renal failure. Ascites and effusions can be drained for symptomatic relief, and prophylactic anticoagulant therapy may be started. Patients at high risk for developing ovarian hyperstimulation syndrome, such as those with a history of PCOS or previous episodes of the syndrome, should undergo ovulation induction only with reduced doses and close monitoring.

OVARIAN CANCER

The relationship between ovarian cancer and treatment for infertility is controversial. Two hypotheses have been proposed. The first is that repeated ovulation increases the risk of a malignant transformation through disruption of the ovarian epithelium. The second is that the persistent stimulation of the ovary by pituitary gonadotropins increases the risk of ovarian cancer. Nulliparity[57] (i.e., never having children) and infertility itself, without exposure to fertility drugs, may be independent risk factors for ovarian cancer.[58,59] An association between fertility agents and the risk of breast and ovarian cancers has not been confirmed. More studies are needed to clarify the link between infertility treatment and ovarian cancer.

PHARMACOECONOMIC CONSIDERATIONS

In the United States, each individual state legislates insurance coverage. The type of coverage can vary considerably, with respect to the type and amount of treatments covered.[60,61] Many couples have limited or no health care coverage, and the high cost of infertility treatments places a burden on their life savings. Despite the significant cost implications, there have been very few analyses of the relative cost-effectiveness of infertility treatments in the United States.

Many issues are involved in the pharmacoeconomic considerations of infertility treatment. First of all, technological advances and new insights on infertility provide constantly changing treatment modalities. Second, nonstandardized treatment protocols and center-dependent success rates make comparisons for cost-effective analysis difficult. Next, the least expensive therapy may not always be the most effective. Finally, this type of analysis cannot take into account the emotional factors surrounding infertility and its treatment, or the indirect costs (e.g., time away from work) associated with treatment.

In one treatment center, IUI, clomiphene citrate with IUI, and hMG with IUI were shown to have similar costs per delivery. In addition, all these procedures were more cost-effective than IVF cycles.[16,62] Based on the finding that hMG with IUI is roughly one-third the cost of an IVF cycle, it has been suggested that most couples should have three to four attempts at hMG with IUI before resorting to IVF. Exceptions to this may be couples in which the woman is older than 38 or couples in which there is severe male factor infertility.[62]

In women more than 38 years old, it is more cost-effective to use donor oocytes; however, this does not take into account the emotional cost of not having a child with the mother's genetic input.[17] Similar issues arise concerning donor sperm. The use of ICSI for severe male factor infertility is more costly than the use of donor sperm. However, the pregnancy rates with donor insemination are significantly less than the pregnancy rates with ICSI, so it can take more cycles to establish a pregnancy. This not only increases indirect costs, but also affects emotional issues associated with treatment failure.

EVALUATION OF THERAPEUTIC OUTCOMES

Pharmacists are rarely involved in the therapeutic management of the patient with infertility. The treatment regimens, including drug and dose, are based on the patient's condition and response to follicular development and ovulation, which can vary from cycle to cycle even with the same medication and dosage. Most of the medications require monitoring by estradiol levels and ultrasound monitoring to ensure an adequate response and to avoid overstimulation of the ovaries.

The pharmacists' interaction with these patients is usually in the outpatient setting. The pharmacist should ensure that the patient understands the correct use of BBT measurements and ovulation prediction kits; the purpose of the medications used in the treatment of infertility; along with the method of administration, potential side effects, and the importance of being compliant with the prescribed administration and monitoring regimen. Patients should notify their physician if they experience an increase in abdominal girth, nausea, pelvic pain, decreased urine output, weight gain greater than 2.25 kg, dizziness, or shortness of breath.

It is important to recognize infertility's psychological and socioeconomic impact. Infertility is a major life crisis that is distressing for the couple. Emotional responses include feelings of loss, anxiety, depression, guilt, anger, bitterness, and frustration. Patients dealing with infertility feel out of control, and they often experience social isolation and strained interpersonal relationships. The financial burden and time commitment required for the evaluation and treatment processes can add to the stress of the couple. Psychological stress and depression can adversely affect reproductive function and IVF treatment outcome.[63,64] Other patients, support groups (e.g., RESOLVE), or mental health professionals can provide much needed emotional and/or psychological support for patients going through evaluation and treatment, as well as for those making decisions about whether to continue therapy. Personal stress management techniques (e.g., meditation, progressive muscle relaxation, imagery, autogenic training, yoga, cognitive restructuring) are important to maintain a balance with the patient's life and the evaluation and treatment process, and they may lead to increased pregnancy rates.[63]

▶ PRINCIPLES OF PHARMACOTHERAPY

- It is recommended that patients who do not conceive a child after 12 months of contraception-free intercourse seek evaluation and treatment for infertility; if the female partner is over 35 years of age or either partner has certain medical conditions or physical findings, seeking treatment after 6 months is indicated.
- Both the male and female partner must be evaluated to determine the cause(s) of infertility. Investigation of the male partner should be completed before beginning treatment of the female partner.
- The likely causes of infertility determine the treatment. More than one factor in one or both of the partners may contribute to the infertility.
- Some therapeutic agents used for induction of ovulation augment the patient's natural endocrine process (e.g., clomiphene citrate), while other agents take control of, and in some cases replace, the natural cycle (e.g., menotropins, gonadotropins).
- Clomiphene should be used at the lowest effective dose, because multiple births and adverse effects are dose-dependent.
- Clomiphene should not be used for more than 6 cycles because of the potential risk of ovarian cancer.
- Menotropins/gonadotropins are second-line therapeutic options because of cost, the high risk of multiple pregnancies, and ovarian hyperstimulation syndrome.
- Close daily monitoring by trained experts is *essential* when menotropins or gonadotropins are used, to minimize the risk of ovarian hyperstimulation and multiple gestation pregnancies.
- Ovarian hyperstimulation syndrome is a possible side effect of fertility drugs, but is rare with proper monitoring. Patients taking fertility drugs should be advised to notify their physician if they experience an increase in abdominal girth, nausea, pelvic pain, decreased urine output, weight gain of more than 2.25 kg, dizziness, or shortness of breath.
- Psychological support may be an important factor in improving outcome, because psychological stress and depression can adversely affect reproductive function and infertility treatment response.

REFERENCES

1. Chandra A, Stephen EH. Impaired fecundity in the United States: 1982–1995. Fam Plann Perspect 1998:30(1):34–42.
2. Carr BR. The ovary. In: Carr BR, Blackwell RE, eds. Textbook of Reproductive Medicine. Stamford, CT: Appleton & Lange, 1999:207–231.
3. Carr BR. The normal menstrual cycle: the coordinated events of the hypothalamic-pituitary-ovarian axis and the female reproductive tract. In: Carr BR, Blackwell RE, eds. Textbook of Reproductive Medicine. Stamford, CT: Appleton & Lange, 1999:233–243.
4. Wilcox AJ, Weinberg CR, Baird DD. Timing of sexual intercourse in relation to ovulation: effects on the probability of conception, survival of the pregnancy and sex of the baby. N Engl J Med 1995;333(23):1517–1521.
5. Spitz A, Kim ED, Lipshultz LI. Contemporary approach to the male infertility evaluation. Obstet Gynecol Clin North Am 2000;27(3):487–516.
6. Pasqualotto FF, Sharma RK, Kobayashi H, et al. Oxidative stress in normospermic men undergoing infertility evaluation. J Androl 2001;22(2):316–322.
7. Glatstein IZ, Harlow BL, Hornstein MD. Practice patterns among reproductive endocrinologists: further aspects of the infertility evaluation. Fertil Steril 1998;70(2):263–269.
8. Howards SS. Current concepts: treatment of male infertility. New Engl J Med 1995;332(5):312–317.
9. Hargreave TB, Mills JA. Investigating and managing infertility in general practice. BMJ 1998;316:1438–1441.
10. Sandlow JI. Shattering the myths about male infertility. Postgrad Med 2000;107(2):235–245.
11. Enders G. Clinical approaches to male infertility with a case report of possible nifedipine-induced sperm dysfunction. J Am Board Fam Pract 1997;10(2):131–136.
12. Zacur HA, Hutchison SM. Evaluation and therapy of hyperprolactinemia. In: Wallach EE, Zacur HA, eds. Reproductive Medicine and Surgery. St. Louis: Mosby, 1995:196–208.
13. Whitman-Elia GF, Windham NQ. Galactorrhea may be clue to serious problems: patients deserve a thorough workup. Postgrad Med 2000; 107(7):165–171.
14. Lieu CL, Keshishian K. Infertility: contributing factors, evaluation and assisted reproductive technology procedures. Part I. California Pharmacist Insights 1998;10(10):13–27.
15. Cedars M. Prediction, detection, and evaluation of ovulation. In: Keye WR, Chang RJ, Rebar RW, et al., eds. Infertility: Evaluation and Treatment. Philadelphia: WB Saunders, 1995:127–144.
16. Guzick DS, Sullivan MW, Adamson G, et al. Efficacy of treatment for unexplained infertility. Fertil Steril 1998;70(2):207–213.
17. Van Voorhis BJ, Stovall DW, Allen BD, et al. Cost-effective treatment of the infertile couple. Fertil Steril 1998;70(6):995–1005

18. The ESHRE Capri Workshop. Female infertility: treatment options for complicated cases. Hum Reprod 1997;12(6):1191–1196.
19. Centers for Disease Control and Prevention, American Society for Reproductive Medicine, Society for Assisted Reproductive Technology, RESOLVE. 1998 Assisted reproductive technology success rates: national summary and fertility clinic reports. U.S. Department of Health and Human Services, December 2000.
20. Hruska KS, Furth PA, Seifer DB, et al. Environmental factors in infertility. Clin Obstet Gynecol 2000;43(4):821–829.
21. Illions EH, Valley MT, Kaunitz AM. Infertility: a clinical guide for the internist. Med Clin North Am 1998;82(2):271–295.
22. Smith E, Hammonds-Ehlers M, Clark MK, et al. Occupational exposures and risk of female infertility. J Occup Environ Med 1997;39(2):138–146.
23. Butzow TL, Lehtovirta M, Siegberg R, et al. The decrease in luteinizing hormone secretion in response to weight reduction is inversely related to the severity of insulin resistance in overweight women. J Clin Endocrinol Metab 2000;85(9):3271–3275.
24. Silverberg KM. Evaluation of the couple with infertility in a managed care environment. Clin Obstet Gynecol 2000;43(4):844–853.
25. Mendonca LLF, Khamashta MA, Nelson-Piercy, et al. Non-steroidal anti-inflammatory drugs as a possible cause for reversible infertility. Rheumatology 2000;39:880–882.
26. Seibel MM. The role of nutrition and nutritional supplements in women's health. Fertil Steril 1999;72(4):579–591.
27. Wong WY, Thomas CMG, Merkus JMWM, et al. Male factor subfertility: possible causes and the impact of nutritional factors. Fertil Steril 2000;73(3):435–442.
28. Schieve LA, Peterson HB, Meikle SF, et al. Live-birth rates and multiple-birth risk using in vitro fertilization. JAMA 1999;282(19):1832–1838.
29. Biljan MM, Mahutte NG, Tulandi T, Tan SL. Prospective randomized double-blind trial of the correlation between time of administration and antiestrogenic effects of clomiphene citrate on reproductive end organs. Fertil Steril 1999;71(4):633–638.
30. Hurd WW, Randolph JF, Christman GM, et al. Luteal support with both estradiol and progesterone after clomiphene citrate stimulation for *in vitro* fertilization. Fertil Steril 1996;66(4):587–592.
31. Gerli S, Gholami H, Manna A, et al. Use of ethinyl estradiol to reverse the antiestrogenic effects of clomiphene citrate in patients undergoing intrauterine insemination: a comparative, randomized study. Fertil Steril 2000;73(1):85–89.
32. Agrawal R, Holmes JMA, Jacobs HS. Follicle-stimulating hormone or human menopausal gonadotropin for ovarian stimulation in in vitro fertilization cycles: a meta-analysis. Fertil Steril 2000;73(2):338–343
33. Prevost RR. Recombinant follicle-stimulating hormone: new biotechnology for infertility. Pharmacotherapy 1998;18(5):1001–1010.
34. Fox JH, Jackson KV, Rein MS, et al. A randomized clinical trial to evaluate the clinical effects of split- versus single-dose human menopausal gonadotropins in an assisted reproductive technology program. Fertil Steril 1996;65:598–602.
35. Ransom MX, Doughman NC, Garcia AJ. Menotropins alone are superior to a clomiphene citrate and menotropin combination for superovulation induction among clomiphene citrate failures. Fertil Steril 1996;65(6):1169–1174.
36. Carson DS, Bucci KK. Infertility in women: an update. J Am Pharm Assoc 1998;38(4):480–486.
37. Driscoll GL, Tyler JP, Hangan JT, et al. A prospective, randomized, controlled, double- blind, double-dummy comparison of recombinant and urinary HCG for inducing oocyte maturation and follicular luteinization in ovarian stimulation. Hum Reprod 2000;15(6):1305–1310.
38. Warnock JK, Bundren JC, Morris DW. Depressive symptoms associated with gonadotropin-releasing hormone agonists. Depress Anxiety 1998; 7(4):171–177.
39. Ganirelix Dose-Finding Study Group. A double-blind, randomized, dose-finding study to assess the efficacy of the gonadotropin-releasing hormone antagonist ganirelix (Org 37462) to prevent premature luteinizing hormone surges in women undergoing ovarian stimulation with recombinant follicle stimulating hormone (Puregon). Hum Reprod 1998;13(11): 3023–3031.
40. Fluker M, Grifo J, Leader A, et al. Efficacy and safety of ganirelix acetate versus leuprolide acetate in women undergoing controlled ovarian hyperstimulation. Fertil Steril 2001;75(1):38–45.
41. Biljan MM, Mahutte NG, Dean N, et al. Effects of pretreatment with oral contraceptive on the time required to achieve pituitary suppression with gonadotropin-releasing hormone analogues and on subsequent implantation and pregnancy rates. Fertil Steril 1998;70(6):1063–1069.
42. Biljan MM, Mahutte NG, Dean N, et al. Pretreatment with oral contraceptive is effective in reducing the incidence of functional ovarian cyst formation during pituitary suppression by gonadotropin-releasing hormone analogues. J Assist Reprod Genet 1998;15:599–604.
43. Gibbons WE, Toner JP, Hamacher P, Kolm P. Experience with a novel vaginal progesterone preparation in a donor oocyte program. Fertil Steril 1998;69(1):96–101.
44. Bulletti C, de Ziegler D, Flamigni C, et al. Targeted drug delivery in gynaecology: the first uterine pass effect. Hum Reprod 1997;12(5):1073–1079.
45. Rubinstein M, Marazzi A, de Fried EP. Low-dose aspirin treatment improves ovarian responsiveness, uterine and ovarian blood flow velocity, implantation, and pregnancy rates in patients undergoing in vitro fertilization: a prospective, randomized, double-blind placebo-controlled assay. Fertil Steril 1999;71(15):825–829.
46. Sills ES, Perloe M, Palermo GD. Correction of hyperinsulinemia in oligoovulatory women with clomiphene-resistant polycystic ovary syndrome: a review of therapeutic rationale and reproductive outcomes. Eur J Obstet Gynecol Reprod Biol 2000;91(2):135–141.
47. Nestler JE, Jakubowicz DJ, Evans WS, Pasquali R. Effects of metformin on spontaneous and clomiphene-induced ovulation in the polycystic ovary syndrome. N Engl J Med 1998;338(26):1876–1880.
48. Kim LH, Taylor AE, Barbieri RL. Insulin sensitizers and polycystic ovary syndrome: can a diabetes medication treat infertility? Fertil Steril 2000;73(6):1097–1098.
49. Hasegawa I, Murakawa H, Suzuki M, et al. Effect of troglitazone on endocrine and ovulatory performance in women with insulin resistance-related polycystic ovary syndrome. Fertil Steril 1999;71(2):323–327.
50. Paoletti AM, Cagnacci A, Depau GF, et al. The chronic administration of cabergoline normalizes androgen secretion and improves menstrual cyclicity in women with polycystic ovary syndrome. Fertil Steril 1996: 66(4);527–532.
51. Biller BM, Luciano A, Crosignani PG, et al. Guidelines for the diagnosis and treatment of hyperprolactinemia. J Reprod Med 1999;44(12 suppl): 1075–1084.
52. Crosignani PG. Management of hyperprolactinemia in infertility. J Reprod Med 1999;44(12 suppl):1116–1120.
53. Siterman S, Eltes F, Wolfson V, et al. Effect of acupuncture on sperm parameters of males suffering from subfertility related to low sperm quality. Arch Androl 1997;39(2):155–161.
54. Stener-Victorin E, Waldenstrom U, Tagnfors U, et al. Effects of electro-acupuncture on anovulation in women with polycystic ovary syndrome. Acta Obstet Gynecol Scand 2000;79(3):180–188.
55. Kiprov DD, Nachtigall RD, Weaver RC, et al. The use of intravenous immunoglobulin in recurrent pregnancy loss associated with combined alloimmune and autoimmune abnormalities. Am J Reprod Immunol 1996; 36:228–234.
56. Fluker MR, Hooper WM, Yuzpe AA. Withholding gonadotropins ("coasting") to minimize the risk of ovarian hyperstimulation during superovulation and *in vitro* fertilization-embryo transfer cycles. Fertil Steril 1999;71(2):294–301.
57. Rodriguez C, Tatham LM, Calle EE, et al. Infertility and risk of fatal ovarian cancer in a prospective cohort of US women. Cancer Causes Control 1998;9(6):645–651.
58. Mosgaard BJ, Lidegaard O, Kjaer SK, et al. Infertility, fertility drugs, and invasive ovarian cancer: a case-control study. Fertil Steril 1997;67(6): 1005–1012.

59. Venn A, Watson L, Bruinsma F, et al. Risk of cancer after use of fertility drugs with *in-vitro* fertilization. Lancet 1999; 354(9190):1586–1590.
60. Van Voorhis BJ, Sparks AE, Allen BD, et al. Cost-effectiveness of infertility treatments: a cohort study. Fertil Steril 1997;67(5):830–836.
61. Soules MR. Now that we have painted ourselves in a corner. Fertil Steril 1996;66(5):693–696.
62. Karande VD, Korn A, Morris R, et al. Prospective randomized trial comparing the outcome and cost of *in vitro* fertilization with that of a traditional treatment algorithm as first-line therapy for couples with infertility. Fertil Steril 1999;71(3):468–475.
63. Domar AD, Clapp D, Slawsby EA, et al. Impact of group psychological interventions on pregnancy rates in infertile women. Fertil Steril 2000; 73(4):805–811.
64. Csemiczky G, Landgren BM, Collins A. The influence of stress and state anxiety on the outcome of IVF-treatment: psychological and endocrinological assessment of Swedish women entering IVF-treatment. Acta Obstet Gynecol Scand 2000;79(2):113–118.

80

CONTRACEPTION

Lori M. Dickerson and Kathryn K. Bucci

A comprehension of the mechanisms involved in the hormonal regulation of the normal menstrual cycle is essential to understanding contraception and infertility in women (see Chapter 79, Infertility, for a review of the menstrual cycle). Contraception generally implies the prevention of pregnancy following sexual intercourse by inhibiting viable sperm from coming into contact with a mature ovum (i.e., methods that act as barriers or prevent ovulation) or by preventing a fertilized ovum from successfully implanting in the endometrium (i.e., mechanisms that create an unfavorable uterine environment).

Commonly used methods of reversible contraception include oral contraceptives, long-acting injectable or implantable progestins, condoms, spermicides, withdrawal, the diaphragm, periodic abstinence, and the intrauterine device. These methods differ in their relative effectiveness, safety, and patient acceptability.[1,2]

The actual effectiveness of any contraceptive method is difficult to determine because many factors affect contraceptive failure. A failure inherent in the proper use of the contraceptive alone is considered a method failure or perfect use failure. User failure or typical use failure takes into account the user's ability to follow directions correctly and consistently (Table 80–1).[1,2]

ORAL CONTRACEPTIVES

The most popular method of reversible contraception in the United States, oral contraceptives are highly effective (see Table 80–1).[1–3] When used correctly, their effectiveness approaches that of surgical sterilization.

COMPOSITION AND FORMULATIONS

The currently available oral contraceptives contain either a combination of a synthetic estrogen and synthetic progestin, or a progestin alone. Estrogens suppress follicle-stimulating hormone (FSH) and, thus, prevent the development of a dominant follicle. Estrogens also potentiate the action of the progestin component, which suppresses the luteinizing hormone (LH) surge. As a result, even if the estrogenic component does not adequately blunt follicular growth, the action of the progestin blocks ovulation. Estrogen also serves to stabilize the endometrial lining (bleeding cycle control), while the progestin contributes to other contraceptive effects on cervical mucus (thickened/impermeable) and the endometrium (involution/atrophy).[1–3]

The low-dose combination oral contraceptives that are currently available are modifications of the original products introduced in 1960; these modified products contain approximately three- to four-fold less estrogen and one-tenth the progestin dose found in the earlier pills.[4] Over the past decade, combination multiphasic (biphasic and triphasic) formulations have further lowered the total monthly hormonal dose without clearly demonstrating a significant clinical advantage.[1,2,4,5] Also introduced in 1960, the progestin only "minipills" (28 days of active hormone/cycle) are still available. Containing even lower doses of progestin than found in combination oral contraceptives and lacking the contribution of estrogen, minipills tend to be less effective than combination oral contraceptives with typical use and are generally reserved for women who must avoid estrogen.[5]

COMPONENTS

Two synthetic estrogens commonly used in oral contraceptives in the United States, ethinyl estradiol (EE) and mestranol, differ only by the presence of a methyl group attached to mestranol at the C-3 site. Mestranol, which must be converted by the liver to EE before it is pharmacologically active, is estimated to be 50% less potent than EE.[1,2,6]

Progestins currently used in oral contraceptives include ethynodiol diacetate, desogestrel, gestodene (not available in the United States), norgestimate, norethindrone, norethindrone acetate, norethynodrel, norgestrel, and norgestrel's active isomer levonorgestrel. Progestins vary in their progestational activity and differ with respect to inherent estrogenic, antiestrogenic, and androgenic effects.[1,2,6,7] Estrogenic and antiestrogenic properties are secondary to the extent of progestins' metabolism to estrogenic substances, whereas androgenic activity results from the structural similarity of the progestin to testosterone (receptor binding and activity) and the ability to affect free testosterone concentrations through impact on sex hormone-binding globulin, a major carrier protein for testosterone.[6,7]

Third-generation oral contraceptives contain newer progestins (e.g., norgestimate, desogestrel, gestodene). These progestins are potent progestational agents that appear to have no estrogenic effects and are less androgenic when compared to levonorgestrel on a weight basis. Unfortunately, clinical trials comparing the differences between oral contraceptives are few and sample size is small, so the actual relevance of these purported improvements in progestational selectivity and lower androgenic activity remains unknown.[3,4,8] Table 80–2 lists available oral contraceptive products by brand name and specifies hormonal composition.

CONSIDERATIONS WITH ORAL CONTRACEPTIVE USE

Oral contraceptives are highly effective and, when used properly, extremely safe.[4,9] Numerous noncontraceptive benefits, including relief from menstruation-related problems (e.g., decreased menstrual cramps, decreased ovulatory pain [mittelschmerz], decreased menstrual blood loss) and prevention of several diseases (e.g., ovarian and endometrial cancer, ovarian cysts, ectopic pregnancy, pelvic inflammatory disease, benign breast disease) have been attributed to the use of oral contraceptives (see Table 80–1). A complete medical history and physical examination should be obtained before a patient begins using an oral contraceptive, and the risks and precautions associated with oral contraceptive use warrant careful consideration.[1–4,6,9,10] The World Health Organization (WHO) has developed a graded list of precautions for clinicians to consider when they are providing oral contraceptives, and these precautions have replaced the traditional absolute and relative contraindications to the use of oral contraceptives.

TABLE 80–1. Comparison of Reversible Methods of Contraception

Method	Absolute Contraindications	Advantages	Disadvantages	Percent of Women With Pregnancy[a]	
				Lowest Expected	*Typical Use*
Episodic Contraceptive Methods					
Spermicides alone	Allergy to spermicide	Inexpensive No office visit required Some protection against STDs	High user failure rate Must be reapplied before each act of intercourse May cause local irritation in either partner May enhance HIV transmission	6.0	26.0
Condoms, male	Allergy to latex or rubber	Inexpensive Readily available No office visit required STD protection, including HIV (latex only)	High user failure rate Poor acceptance Possibility of breakage Efficacy decreased by oil-based lubricants Possible-allergic reactions to latex in either partner	3.0	14.0
Condoms, female (Reality)	Allergy to polyurethane History of toxic shock syndrome	Can be inserted just before intercourse or ahead of time; provides protection for 8 hours STD protection, including HIV	High user failure rate Dislike ring hanging outside vagina Cumbersome	5.0	21.0
Diaphragm with spermicide	Allergy to latex, rubber, or spermicide Recurrent UTIs History of toxic shock syndrome Abnormal gynecologic anatomy	Low cost Decreased incidence of cervical neoplasia Some protection against STDs Can be inserted for up to 6 hours before intercourse	High user failure rate Office visit required Decreased efficacy with increased frequency of intercourse Must be refitted after significant change in weight (+/−10 pounds) Increased incidence of vaginal yeast and UTIs Increased incidence of toxic shock syndrome Efficacy affected by oil-based lubricants Cervical Irritation	6.0	20.0
Cervical cap (Prentif)	Allergy to rubber or spermicide Recurrent UTIs History of toxic shock syndrome Abnormal gynecologic anatomy Abnormal Papanicolaou smear	Low cost Some protection against STDs Can be inserted just before or ahead of time; provides protection for 48 hours	High user failure rate Office visit required May be difficult for patient to use correctly Decreased efficacy with parity Cannot be used during menses Not possible for all patients	9.0	20.0
Sponge (Today)	Allergy to spermicide Recurrent UTIs History of toxic shock syndrome Abnormal gynecologic anatomy	Inexpensive Readily available No office visit required Some protection against STDs Can be inserted just before or ahead of time; provides protection for 24 hours	High user failure rate Problems removing the sponge due to vaginal dryness Cannot be used during menses	9.0	20.0
Hormonal Methods					
Oral contraceptives	Hepatic adenomas Thromboembolic disorders or history thereof Cerebrovascular or coronary artery disease	Decreased risk of PID, ovarian and endometrial cancer Improvement in endometriosis (probably) Fewer functional ovarian cysts (possibly)	Office visit required Increased risk of benign hepatocellular adenomas Mild increased risk of thromboembolism and stroke May elevate blood pressure	0.1	5.0

TABLE 80–1. (Continued)

Method	Absolute Contraindications	Advantages	Disadvantages	Percent of Women With Pregnancy[a]	
				Lowest Expected	*Typical Use*
	Known or suspected breast cancer Undiagnosed abnormal gynecologic bleeding Jaundice with pregnancy or previous pill use	Less salpingitis and ectopic pregnancy Prevention of benign breast disease (fibroadenoma and fibrocystic changes) Less rheumatoid arthritis (possibly) Increased bone density (possibly) Improvement in acne/hirsutism Significant improvement in menstruation-related problems: fewer cramps, less flow for fewer days, less iron deficiency anemia, more predictable menses, elimination of mittelschmerz, less dysmenorrhea and premenstrual syndrome	No protection against most STDs Estrogenic side effects (nausea, breast tenderness, fluid retention) Progestin side effects (acne, increased appetite, depression) Increased risk of myocardial infarction in older women, smokers		
Progestin-only oral contraceptives	Undiagnosed abnormal gynecologic bleeding	May be used by lactating women and women with cardiovascular risk Allows avoidance of estrogen-related side effects Protection against PID, iron deficiency anemia, and dysmenorrhea	Frequent spotting and amenorrhea Increased risk of ectopic pregnancy Must take every day at the same time	0.5	5.0
Progestin implants: levonorgestrel (Norplant and Norplant II,[b] Capronor)[b], 3 ketodesogestrel (Implanon[b]), nomegestrol acetate (uniplant[b])	Pregnancy Undiagnosed abnormal gynecologic bleeding Acute liver disease Benign or malignant liver tumors Known or suspected breast cancers Active thrombophlebitis or thromboembolic disease	Passive contraception Duration of efficacy varies; effective up to 5 years with Norplant in women <154 pounds Effects are quickly reversible Less menstrual cramping and mittelschmerz pain No suppression of lactation No metabolic disturbances Can be considered for use in women who have diabetes, hypertension, gall bladder disease, history of cardiovascular or thromboembolic disease and in women who are smokers or lactating	Requires outpatient surgical procedure Irregular menstrual bleeding, headaches, weight gain, acne Progestin side effects Local infection or bruising on insertion; removal may be difficult Expensive initially High discontinuation rate Unacceptable in patients using some anticonvulsants	0.05	0.05
Depo Provera	Pregnancy Undiagnosed abnormal gynecologic bleeding Known or suspected breast cancers Liver disease (relative contraindication) Severe depression (relative contraindication) Severe cardiovascular disease (relative contraindication)	Passive contraception No suppression of lactation No increased risk of thromboembolism May decrease seizure frequency Effective for 3 months Can be considered for use in women who have seizure disorders, diabetes, hypertension, gall bladder disease, history of cardiovascular or thromboembolic disease and in women who are smokers or lactating	Office visit required every 3 months Irregular menstrual bleeding, headache, weight gain, acne Delayed return of fertility Possible increased risk of breast cancer in younger users Decreased HDL Progestin side effects Decreased bone density in long-term users	0.3	0.3

TABLE 80–1. (Continued)

Method	Absolute Contraindications	Advantages	Disadvantages	Percent of Women With Pregnancy[a]: Lowest Expected	Percent of Women With Pregnancy[a]: Typical Use
Lunelle	Pregnancy Undiagnosed abnormal gynecologic bleeding Known or suspected breast cancers Thromboembolic disorders or history thereof Cerebrovascular or coronary artery disease Jaundice of pregnancy or with prior pill use	Effects quickly reversible Less menstrual cramping and mittelschmerz pain Less menstrual irregularity than other injectable or implantable methods	Office visit required monthly Progestin side effects Estrogen side effects	0.1	0.1
Intrauterine Devices (Hormonal and Nonhormonal)					
Copper-T 380A (ParaGard)	Multiple sexual partners or partner with multiple partners (high risk for STDs) History of PID or ectopic pregnancy, acute pelvic infection Abnormal uterine cavity/pelvic surgery/undiagnosed gynecologic bleeding Uterine or cervical cancer Wilson's disease Allergy to copper	Passive contraception Long-term contraception (can remain in place for up to 10 years) Less expensive per year and easier for some patients No delay in return of fertility after removal	Increased heavy bleeding Spotting between periods Increased cramping and dysmenorrhea Increased risk of ectopic pregnancy Office visit required Rarely, uterine perforation	0.6	0.8
Progesterone T (Progestasert)	Postpartum endometritis or infected abortion in previous 3 months Acute cervicitis or vaginitis (including BV) until infection controlled	Remains in place for 1 year Decreased cramping and dysmenorrhea Decrease in menstrual blood loss No delay in return of fertility after removal	Office visit required Must be changed each year Increased risk of ectopic pregnancy Rarely, uterine perforation	1.5	2.0
Levonorgestrel IUD[c]	Conditions associated with increased susceptibility to infections, including leukemia, AIDS, IV drug abuse, and corticosteroid use Valvular heart disease (relative contraindication) Nulliparity (relative contraindication) Genital actinomyces Wilson's disease Allergy to copper	Constant rate of hormone release for 5 years Possibly the single most effective reversible contraceptive method over 5-year period Decreased cramping, dysmenorrhea, menorrhagia Combines benefits of Norplant and Copper-T	Office visit required Irregular menstrual bleeding Rarely, uterine perforation	0.1	0.1

STD = sexually transmitted disease; HIV = human immunodeficiency virus; UTI = urinary tract infection; PID = pelvic inflammatory disease; HDL = high-density lipoprotein cholesterol; BV = bacterial vaginosis; AIDS = acquired immunodeficiency syndrome; IV = intravenous.

[a]Failure rates during first year of use, United States.

[b]Products in development.

[c]Products approved, but not yet available.

Compiled from Refs. 1, 2, 3, 6, 10, and 13.

TABLE 80–2. Composition of Commonly Prescribed Oral Contraceptives

Product	Composition				Spotting and BTB[a]
	Estrogen	μg[c]	Progestin	mg[c]	
50 μg Estrogen					
Necon 1/50, Nelova 1/50M, Norinyl 1+50, Ortho-Novum 1/50	Mestranol	50	Norethindrone	1	10.6
Norlestrin 1/50	E. estradiol	50	Nor. acetate	1	13.6
Norlestrin 2.5/50					
Ovcon-50	E. estradiol	50	Norethindrone	1	11.9
Ovral-28	E. estradiol	50	Norgestrel	0.5	4.5
Demulen 1/50, Zovia 1.50E	E. estradiol	50	Ethy. diacetate	1	13.9
Sub-50 μg Estrogen Monophasic					
Alesse, Levlite	E. estradiol	20	Levonorgestrel	0.1	26.5
Brevicon, Modicon, Necon 0.5/35, Nelova 0.5/35E	E. estradiol	35	Norethindrone	0.5	24.6
Demulen 1/35, Zovia 1/35E	E. estradiol	35	Ethy. diacetate	1	37.4
Desogen, Ortho-Cept	E. estradiol	30	Desogestrel	0.15	13.1
Levlen, Levora 0.15/30, Nordette	E. estradiol	30	Levonorgestrel	0.15	14.0
Loestrin 21 1/20[b]	E. estradiol	20	Nor. acetate	1	29.7
Loestrin 21 1.5/30[b]	E. estradiol	30	Nor. acetate	1.5	25.2
Lo-Ovral	E. estradiol	30	Norgestrel	0.3	9.6
Necon 1/35, Nelova 1/35E, Norinyl 1+35, Ortho-Novum 1/35	E. estradiol	35	Norethindrone	1	14.7
Ortho-Cyclen	E. estradiol	35	Norgestimate	0.25	14.3
Ovcon-35	E. estradiol	35	Norethindrone	0.4	11
Sub-50 μg Estrogen Multiphasic[b]					
Estrostep 21[b]	E. estradiol	20 (5)	Norethindrone	1 (5)	26.2
	E. estradiol	30 (7)	Norethindrone	1 (7)	
	E. estradiol	35 (9)	Norethindrone	1 (9)	
Jenest-28	E. estradiol	35 (7)	Norethindrone	0.5 (7)	17.3
	E. estradiol	35 (14)	Norethindrone	1 (14)	
Mircette	E. estradiol	20 (21)	Desogestrel	0.15 (21)	19.7
	E. estradiol	10 (5)			
Necon 10/11	E. estradiol	35 (10)	Norethindrone	0.5 (10)	17.6
Nelova 10/11	E. estradiol	35 (11)	Norethindrone	1 (11)	
Ortho-Novum 10/11					
Ortho-Novum 7/7/7	E. estradiol	35 (7)	Norethindrone	0.5 (7)	14.5
	E. estradiol	35 (7)	Norethindrone	0.75 (7)	
	E. estradiol	35 (7)	Norethindrone	1 (7)	
Ortho Tri-Cyclen	E. estradiol	35 (7)	Norgestimate	0.18 (7)	17.7
	E. estradiol	35 (7)	Norgestimate	0.215 (7)	
	E. estradiol	35 (7)	Norgestimate	0.25 (7)	
Tri Levlen, Triphasil	E. estradiol	30 (6)	Levonortestrel	0.05 (6)	15.1
Trivora-28	E. estradiol	40 (5)	Levonortestrel	0.075 (5)	
	E. estradiol	30 (10)	Levonortestrel	0.125 (10)	
Tri-Norinyl	E. estradiol	35 (7)	Norethindrone	0.5 (7)	25.5
	E. estradiol	35 (9)	Norethindrone	1 (9)	
	E. estradiol	35 (5)	Norethindrone	0.5 (5)	
Progestin Only					
Micronor/Nor-Q.D.	None	—	Norethindrone	0.35	42.3
Ovrette	None	—	Norgestrel	0.075	34.9

BTB = breakthrough bleeding; E = ethinyl estradiol; Nor. Acetate = norethindrone acetate; Ethy. Diacetate = ethynodiol diacetate.

[a]Reported prevalence of BTB and spotting in the third cycle of use. Information was submitted to the Food and Drug Administration by the manufacturer. These rates are derived from individual studies conducted by various investigators and, therefore, information should not be precisely compared.

[b]Also available with *iron*.

[c]Number in parentheses indicates the number of tablets (days) in each phase.

Compiled from Refs. 6 and 54.

Many patient-specific characteristics and concomitant disease states increase the patient's risk for adverse effects relating to oral contraceptive use (Table 80–3).[1,2,4,10–13]

WOMEN OVER 35 YEARS OF AGE

Generally, oral contraceptives are an acceptable form of birth control for nonsmoking women up to the time of menopause, with women over 35 using the lowest dose estrogen products.[1,2,6,13] An ex-smoker for at least 1 year can be regarded as a nonsmoker.[1] A recent case-controlled study of healthy, nonsmoking women over the age of 35 years indicated that the use of oral contraceptives increased the risk of myocardial infarction or stroke.[14,15] As women approach the perimenopausal stage, oral contraceptives will confer a benefit with respect to bone mineral density and vasomotor symptoms.[16,17] Women should switch from oral contraceptives to hormone replacement therapy between the ages of 50 and 55 years.[13,18]

SMOKING

Heavy smokers (>20 cigarettes per day) over the age of 35 should not use oral contraceptives containing estrogen; light smokers (<20 cigarettes per day) over the age of 35 should use them only with caution.[2,10,11,19] If smoking women use oral contraceptive agents, the 20-μg estrogen formulation should be used.[20,21] This extremely low dose oral contraceptive does not appear to have an impact on clotting factors and platelet activation, even in smokers.[22] Progestin-only pills are generally acceptable for women in whom an estrogen is contraindicated.[4,11] In smoking women older than 35 years, the risk of using oral contraceptives is likely to exceed the risk of pregnancy.[13]

HYPERTENSION

Combination oral contraceptives, even those containing less than 35 μg of estrogen, can cause small increases in blood pressure, although clinically significant increases are rare with low-dose agents.[1,2,11] If an oral contraceptive-related increase in blood pressure occurs, discontinuing the oral contraceptive usually restores blood pressure to pretreatment values within 3 to 6 months.[1,2] The use of low-dose oral contraceptives is acceptable in women with well controlled and monitored hypertension.[13] However, hypertensive women who have end-organ vascular disease (e.g., coronary artery disease, congestive heart failure, cerebrovascular disease) or who smoke should not use combination oral contraceptives.[13]

DIABETES

Oral contraceptives appear to affect carbohydrate and lipid metabolism, possibly through the progestin component.[2,11,23] With the exception of some levonorgestrel-containing products, formulations containing low doses of progestins do not significantly alter insulin, glucose, or glucagon release after a glucose load in healthy women or in those with a history of gestational diabetes.[2,23] The new progestins (e.g., desogestrel, norgestimate) are believed to have little, if any, effect on carbohydrate metabolism.[2,8] Studies of women with type 1 diabetes did not find any association between blood glucose control and the use of oral contraceptives.[24] In the Nurses' Health Study, women using oral contraceptives did not demonstrate any increased risk of developing type 2 diabetes.[25] Nonsmoking women with diabetes, but no associated vascular disease, can safely use oral contraceptives.[13] Diabetic women with vascular disease (e.g., hypertension, nephropathy, retinopathy, neuropathy) should not use oral contraceptives, however.[13]

DYSLIPIDEMIA

Generally, synthetic progestins adversely affect lipid metabolism by decreasing the level of high-density lipoprotein (HDL) and increasing the level of low-density lipoprotein (LDL). Estrogens tend to have more beneficial effects by increasing the removal of LDL from the circulation and increasing the level of HDL through increases in $ApoA_1$. Estrogens may also alter the composition of very low density lipoprotein (VLDL) and increase the level of triglycerides.[11] Most low-dose combination oral contraceptives, with the possible exception of monophasic levonorgestrel (0.150 mg) pills, have no significant impact on HDL, LDL, triglycerides, or total cholesterol.[1,7,11]

Although the lipid effects of oral contraceptives can theoretically influence cardiovascular risk, the mechanism of the increased incidence of cardiovascular disease in oral contraceptive users is believed to be secondary to thromboembolic and thrombotic changes, not atherosclerosis. Numerous epidemiologic studies have failed to find an association between the use of oral contraceptives and cardiovascular disease.[13,26] Women with controlled dyslipidemia can use low-dose oral contraceptives, although they need frequent monitoring by means of a fasting lipid panel after they begin using these agents.[13] Women with uncontrolled dyslipidemia (LDL > 160 mg/dL, HDL < 35 mg/dL, triglycerides >250 mg/dL) and additional risk factors (e.g., coronary artery disease, diabetes, hypertension, smoking, positive family history) should use an alternative method of contraception.[13]

THROMBOEMBOLISM

Estrogens play a dose-related role in the development of venous thrombosis and consequent pulmonary embolism, especially in women who smoke or have other underlying inherited conditions (e.g., deficiencies in antithrombin III, protein C, protein S levels; factor V Leiden mutation) or acquired conditions (e.g., immobility, trauma, surgery, certain malignancies) that predispose them to coagulation abnormalities.[1,2,27] Early observational studies reported the incidence of venous thromboembolism to be as high as 12 times greater in oral contraceptive users than in nonusers.[28] Recent reevaluation of these data suggest that although the association between non–third-generation oral contraceptive use and venous thromboembolism is valid, the risk is much less (less than threefold increase in relative risk) than originally thought.[6,29] In addition, the absolute risk is low (15 cases/100,000 woman-years). The increased risk of venous thromboembolism and pulmonary embolism appears to be limited to current users, with disappearance of the risk within 3 months after the use of the oral contraceptive ceases.[1,6,30] The 20-μg EE formulations do not appear to have an effect on clotting parameters, even in smokers, but whether these products lower the risk of thrombotic events has not been studied.[22,31]

European studies of third-generation oral contraceptives reported a possible relationship between these agents and the procoagulant effects of oral contraceptives. In early studies, researchers found that users of third-generation agents containing gestodene or desogestrel had a twofold greater risk of nonfatal venous thromboembolism than women using the older low-dose combination oral contraceptives.[5,32–34] More recent data have shown a small increase in the risk of venous thromboembolism, but do not establish a cause-and-effect relationship.[5,35–37] Some clinicians argue that this

TABLE 80–3. Precautions in the Provision of Combined Oral Contraceptives (OCs)

Precautions	Rationale/Discussion
World Health Organization Category #4: Refrain from providing combined oral contraceptives for women with the following diagnoses.	
• Deep vein thrombosis or pulmonary embolism, or a history thereof	• Estrogens promote blood clotting. Thromboembolic events related to known trauma or an intravenous needle are not necessarily a reason to avoid use of pills.
• Cerebrovascular accident (stroke), coronary artery or ischemic heart disease, or a history thereof	• Estrogens promote blood clotting.
• Structural heart disease, complicated by pulmonary hypertension, atrial fibrillation, or history of subacute bacterial endocarditis	• Estrogens promote blood clotting.
• Diabetes with nephropathy, retinopathy, neuropathy, or other vascular disease; diabetes of more than 20 years' duration	• Estrogens promote blood clotting.
• Breast cancer	• Breast cancer is a hormonally sensitive tumor. In theory, the hormones in OCs might cause some masses to grow.
• Pregnancy	• Current data do not show that hormonal contraceptives taken during pregnancy cause any significant risk of birth defects. However, hormonal contraceptives should not be given to pregnant women.
• Lactation (<6 weeks postpartum)	• There is some theoretical concern that the neonate may be at risk owing to exposure to steroid hormones during the first 6 weeks postpartum. OCs can diminish the volume of breast milk.
• Liver problems: benign hepatic adenoma or liver cancer, or a history thereof; active viral hepatitis; severe cirrhosis	• OCs are metabolized by the liver, and their use may adversely affect prognosis of existing disease.
• Headaches, including migraine (with aura), with focal neurologic symptoms	• Focal neurologic symptoms such as blurred vision, seeing flashing lights or zigzag lines, or trouble speaking or moving may be an indication of an increased risk of stroke.
• Major surgery with prolonged immobilization or any surgery on the legs	• Risk for deep vein thrombosis and pulmonary embolism is increased.
• Over 35 years old and currently a heavy smoker (20 or more cigarettes a day)	• Smoking increases the risk for cardiovascular disease.
• Hypertension, 160+ mmHg/100+ mmHg or with vascular disease	• Hypertension is an important risk factor for cardiovascular disease.
World Health Organization Category #3: Exercise caution if combined oral contraceptives are used or considered in the following situations and carefully monitor for adverse effects.	
• Postpartum <21 days	• There is some theoretical concern regarding the association between OC use up to 3 weeks postpartum and risk of thrombosis.
• Lactation (6 weeks to 6 months)	• In the first 6 months postpartum, use of OCs during breastfeeding diminishes the quantity of breast milk and may adversely affect the health of the infant.
• Undiagnosed abnormal vaginal/uterine bleeding	• Although OCs are often used to manage heavy bleeding, clinicians should be sure that the cause of the bleeding is known before prescribing OCs.
• Over 35 years of age and light smoker (fewer than 20 cigarettes/day)	• Smoking increases the risk for cardiovascular disease. All smokers should be warned of this risk and should be encouraged and advised to stop smoking.
• Past history of breast cancer, but no evidence of recurrence for 5 years	• Breast cancer is a hormonally sensitive tumor.
• Use of drugs that affect liver enzymes (rifampicin, rifabutin and griseofulvin); anticonvulsants (phenytoin, carbamazepine, barbiturates, topiramate, and primidone)	• OCs are metabolized by the liver. Drugs that affect liver enzymes could reduce the contraceptive effectiveness of OCs.
• Gallbladder disease: medically treated and current biliary tract disease and history of OC-related cholestasis	• Recent reports show that OCs may be weakly associated with the development of gallbladder disease. There is also concern that OCs may worsen existing gallbladder disease.
World Health Organization Category #2: Advantages generally outweigh theoretical or proven disadvantages and generally can be provided without restrictions in these conditions.	
• Severe headaches that definitely start after initiation of OCs; migraine headaches without focal neurologic symptoms (without aura)	• Migraine headaches with focal neurologic symptoms have been associated with an increased risk of stroke; any headaches clearly starting after initiation of pills may be related to pill use.
• Diabetes mellitus: gestational diabetes or diabetes without vascular disease	• Women with diabetes are at increased risk of heart disease and stroke, particularly if the woman smokes. Estrogens and progestins may slightly decrease glucose tolerance, but this is unlikely to happen with low-dose OCs.
• Major surgery without prolonged immobilization	• With the current low-dose pills, the problems associated with pill use and elective surgery have decreased.
• Sickle cell disease or sickle C disease	• Women with sickle cell disease are predisposed to occlusion of the microvasculature (because of abnormal, inflexible red blood cells). Studies of women with sickle cell disease have shown no significant differences between OC users and non-users with regard to coagulation studies, blood viscosity measurements, or incidence or severity of painful sickle cell crisis.
• Moderate blood pressure (140–159 mmHg/100–109 mmHg)	• Monitor blood pressure periodically. Hypertension is an important risk factor for cardiovascular disease.

TABLE 80–3. (Continued)

Precautions	Rationale/Discussion
• Undiagnosed breast mass	• Some clinicians and some clinical protocols suggest that women found to have a breast mass should not be provided combined OCs until cancer of the breast has been ruled out. Other clinicians are comfortable prescribing pills while the cause of the breast mass is being evaluated.
• Cervical cancer awaiting treatment and cervical intraepithelial neoplasia	• The risk of cervical cancer appears to be increased slightly in OC users. OC users may get Papanicolaou smears more regularly so that early dysplasia is more likely to be recognized. They also tend to have more sexual partners. Pill use may also alter susceptibility to infection with human papilloma virus a known risk factor for cancer of the cervix.
• Over 50 years of age	• Women over 50 are at increased risk for heart and cerebrovascular disease.
• Conditions likely to make it very difficult for a woman to take OCs consistently and correctly	• Mental retardation, major psychiatric illness, alcoholism, or other chemical abuse, and/or a history of repeatedly taking OCs or other medications incorrectly, make compliance with OC regimens difficult.
• Family history of hyperlipidemia	• Some types of hyperlipidemia increase a woman's risk for heart disease. Routine screening is not recommended by WHO because of the rarity of the conditions and the high cost of screening.
• Family history of death of a parent or sibling due to myocardial infarction before age 50	• Myocardial infarction in a mother or sister is especially significant and suggests a need for lipid evaluation.
World Health Organization Category #1: Do not restrict use of combined oral contraceptives for the following conditions.	
• Postpartum ≥21 days	
• Postabortion after first or second trimester or immediately after postseptic abortion	
• History of gestational diabetes	
• Varicose veins	
• Mild headaches	
• Irregular vaginal bleeding patterns, without or with heavy or prolonged bleeding and not anemia	
• Past history of pelvic inflammatory disease (PID)	
• Current or recent history of (within last 3 months) PID	
• Current or recent history of (within last 3 months) sexually transmitted infection (STI)	
• Vaginitis without purulent cervicitis	
• Increased risk of STI (i.e., multiple partners or partner who has multiple partners)	
• Infection with human immunodeficiency virus (HIV), high risk or HIV or acquired immunodeficiency syndrome (AIDS)	
• Benign breast disease	
• Family history of breast cancer	
• Cervical ectropion	
• Endometrial or ovarian cancer	
• Viral hepatitis carrier	
• Uterine fibroids	
• Past ectopic pregnancy	
• Obesity	
• Thyroid conditions: simple goiter, hyperthyroidism, hypothyroidism	
• Benign or malignant gestational trophoblastic disease	
• Iron deficiency anemia	
• Epilepsy	
• Schistosomiasis (uncomplicated or with fibrosis of the liver)	
• Malaria	
• Current use of antibiotics	
• Nulliparity or parity	
• Severe dysmenorrhea	
• *Tuberculosis, including pelvic*	
• Endometriosis	
• Benign ovarian tumors	
• Prior pelvic surgery	

Compiled from Refs. 2, 10, and 13.

difference reflects preferential prescribing of the newer, and perceived safer, progestin products for women at greater risk for venous thrombosis.[6,21,38,39] The Food and Drug Administration (FDA) has concluded that this evidence is not persuasive enough to support any changes in current prescribing patterns or to recommend discontinuation of third-generation oral contraceptives.[3,21]

Currently, oral contraceptives are contraindicated in any woman with a history of venous thromboembolism or pulmonary embolism (see Table 80–3). Women who develop thrombotic complications while taking a low-dose oral contraceptive should have an examination for an underlying coagulation disorder.[1,2,6,13] Some experts support the use of oral contraceptives in women with coagulation disorders *who have been properly anticoagulated,* citing the potential advantages of lowering the risk of fetal exposure to warfarin, bleeding corpus luteum cysts, and excessive blood loss during menses.[1,2,13]

CEREBROVASCULAR DISEASE

Both thrombotic and hemorrhagic stroke have been associated with the use of oral contraceptives. However, early studies used higher dose products and did not take into account independent risk factors for vascular disease (e.g., smoking, hypertension, advancing age). Recent studies evaluating low-dose oral contraceptives found the risk for stroke to be extremely low in healthy young women.[14,15,40,41] These results suggest that the effect of smoking in women less than 35 years old is minimal in the absence of hypertension and that hypertension may be the major risk factor for stroke.[6,42,43]

Cerebrovascular accidents are often preceded by persistent headaches (for weeks or months) and/or by temporary hemiparesis. Patients should be carefully screened and counseled to recognize warning signs of cerebrovascular accidents in order to decrease risk.

MIGRAINE HEADACHES

Women in their reproductive years frequently experience headaches, ranging in variety from tension headache to simple (without aura) and classic migraine (with aura).[13] Oral contraceptives usually decrease the frequency of migraine headaches, but they exacerbate symptoms in some women; headaches may even occur during the hormone-free interval (during menses). There is some evidence that migraine headaches are a risk factor for stroke and that classic migraine (with aura) may increase the risk of stroke more than simple migraine (without aura) does.[13,44] The absolute risk of stroke in women using oral contraceptives who experience simple migraines is relatively low, but the risk of stroke among those with classic migraines is still undetermined. Combination oral contraceptives may be used in young (<35 years of age), healthy, nonsmoking women with migraine headaches if they do not have focal neurologic signs.[13]

MYOCARDIAL INFARCTION

Generally, myocardial infarction in oral contraceptive users occurs primarily in those over 35 years of age who have additional risk factors for cardiovascular disease (e.g., smoking, diabetes, hypertension, obesity).[1,2,6] These risk factors, in particular smoking, appear to act synergistically with oral contraceptives to increase the risk of cardiovascular disease.[6] A large British study found a 21-fold increase in myocardial infarction among women who smoke more than 15 cigarettes daily, but no apparent increased risk in healthy, nonsmoking women, regardless of age.[45] Since the FDA lifted its restrictions on oral contraceptive use in healthy, nonsmoking women over 40 years of age in 1989, oral contraceptives containing 30 μg estrogen or less are being used more frequently in these women up to the age of menopause without evidence of significantly increased risk of cardiovascular events.[1,2,6,43] Recent data suggest that the use of low-dose oral contraceptives containing third-generation progestins may reduce the incidence of myocardial infarction to a rate that is similar to that of myocardial infarction in nonusers.[43,46] Therefore, healthy, nonsmoking women can safely use oral contraceptives without an increased risk of myocardial infarction. Women with a history of coronary artery disease, those who smoke and have other risk factors for myocardial infarction should not use combined oral contraceptives, but rather should use progestin-only or nonhormonal methods of contraception.[13]

CANCER

The risk for ovarian and endometrial cancer decreases by 40% to 50% with oral contraceptive use, and the beneficial effect is believed to persist for at least 15 years after the use ceases.[1,2,4,20,21] The relationship between oral contraceptives and other cancers is controversial. Oral contraceptives increase cervical ectopy, but the association with cervical cancer is unclear.

Worldwide epidemiologic data from 54 studies in 25 countries (many of which studied high-dose oral contraceptives) were recently reanalyzed to assess the relationship between the use of oral contraceptives and the risk of breast cancer.[47,48] Researchers concluded that women who began to use these agents before age 20 had a higher relative risk compared with users who began at later ages. They also found that women currently taking oral contraceptives and those within 10 years of ceasing to take them have a small increase in the risk of breast cancer, but these cancers were less clinically advanced than in women who had never used oral contraceptives.[13,47,48] Prospective U.S. data from the Nurses' Health Study cohort showed no overall relationship between the duration of oral contraceptive use and breast cancer, even in long-term users (>10 years), and researchers concluded that long-term past use, either overall or prior to a full-term pregnancy, did not increase the risk of breast cancer in women over 40 years of age.[49] It will take many years to discover what, if any, impact the low-dose oral contraceptives will have on breast cancer risk. The current recommendation is that a positive family history of breast cancer in a mother or sister, or both, or a history of benign breast disease should not be regarded as a contraindication to oral contraceptive use.[13]

SYSTEMIC LUPUS ERYTHEMATOSUS

The use of hormonal contraception is important in women with systemic lupus erythematosus, as the risk associated with pregnancy is high in this population. It has been thought that hormonal contraception may exacerbate the symptoms of systemic lupus erythematosus.[13,50] Retrospective studies have not found an association between combined oral contraceptives and disease flare-ups in these patients, but there does appear to be an association between deep vein thrombosis and oral contraceptive use in women with systemic lupus erythematosus and antiphospholipid antibodies.[13,50] Progestin-only contraceptives should be used in women with systemic lupus erythematosus and a history of vascular disease or antiphospholipid antibodies, and combination oral contraceptives should be avoided.[13,50]

CHOICE OF AN ORAL CONTRACEPTIVE

Before prescribing an oral contraceptive, the clinician must ask and answer several questions. Are there any precautions to consider in the

TABLE 80–4. Symptoms of a Serious or Potentially Serious Nature Associated With Oral Contraceptives (OCs)

Symptom	Possible Cause
Serious: OCs Should Be Stopped Immediately	
Loss of vision, proptosis, diplopia, papilledema	Retinal artery thrombosis
Unilateral numbness, weakness, or tingling	Hemorrhagic or thrombotic stroke
Severe pains in chest, left arm, or neck	Myocardial infarction
Hemoptysis	Pulmonary embolism
Severe pains, tenderness or swelling, warmth, or palpable cord in legs	Thrombophlebitis
Slurring of speech	Hemorrhagic or thrombotic stroke
Hepatic mass or tenderness	Liver neoplasm
Potentially Serious: OCs May Be Continued With Caution While Patient Is Being Evaluated	
Absence of menses	Pregnancy
Spotting or breakthrough bleeding	Cervical, endometrial, or vaginal cancer
Breast mass, pain, or swelling	Breast cancer
Right upper-quadrant pain	Cholecystitis, cholelithiasis, or liver neoplasm
Midepigastric pain	Thrombosis of abdominal artery or vein, myocardial infarction, or pulmonary embolism
Migraine (vascular or throbbing) headache	Vascular spasm which may precede thrombosis
Severe nonvascular headache	Hypertension, vascular spasm
Galactorrhea	Pituitary adenoma
Jaundice, pruritus	Cholestatic jaundice
Depression	Vitamin B_6 deficiency
Uterine size increase	Leiomyomata, adenomyosis, pregnancy

From Ref. 6, with permission.

use of oral contraceptives (see Table 80–3)? Does this form of contraception fit the patient's lifestyle, and will the patient be compliant? The clinician should discuss the advantages and disadvantages of all available forms of contraception with the patient to ensure that she can make an informed choice (see Table 80–1).

Progestin-only pills (minipills) tend to be less effective than combination oral contraceptives with typical use and are associated with irregular and unpredictable menstrual bleeding, as well as an increased frequency of functional ovarian cysts.[1,2,5,6] Irregular menstrual cycles indicate that ovulation has been inhibited; however, this is one of the most frequent reasons for the discontinuation of the minipill. Unlike combination oral contraceptives, minipills are always begun on the first day of menses and must be taken every day at approximately the same time to maintain contraceptive efficacy. In that minipills may not block ovulation (nearly 40% of women continue to ovulate normally), the risk of ectopic pregnancy is higher with their use than with the use of other hormonal contraceptives.

All combined oral contraceptives (monophasic and multiphasic) are similarly effective in preventing pregnancy (see Table 80–1). Although multiphasic pills have a lower total hormone dose per cycle, there is no convincing evidence that they provide any advantage or cause fewer side effects than monophasic pills. In addition, some women find monophasic pills to be simpler to take. A reasonable first choice of an oral contraceptive is a monophasic pill containing 30–35 μg of EE (see Table 80–2).[5,21] This strategy is based on evidence that the most serious side effects of combination oral contraceptives (i.e., thromboembolic events, stroke, myocardial infarction) result from excessive estrogen content.[1,2,6,21]

Products containing 20 μg of EE may cause less bloating and breast tenderness, and women over 40 years of age may prefer them. However, these low-estrogen oral contraceptives lead to more breakthrough bleeding and an increased risk of contraceptive failure if doses are missed.[2,5] Because all combined oral contraceptives raise sex hormone-binding globulin and decrease free testosterone levels, women may experience an improvement in acne symptoms.[51] Norgestimate-containing oral contraceptives have also been shown to improve acne symptoms, and Ortho Tri-Cyclen and Estrostep are specifically FDA-approved for this indication (see Table 80–2).[5,52,53]

Many symptoms occurring in the first cycle of oral contraceptive use (e.g., breakthrough bleeding and side effects related to estrogen excess) improve spontaneously by the second or third cycle of use as the body adjusts to the altered hormonal level.[1,6] Therefore, initial oral contraceptive use should be reevaluated during the first 3 to 6 months of therapy to determine if the patient is experiencing any adverse effects and if the patient wishes to continue medication.

If the patient complains of symptoms related to the use of the oral contraceptive, it is necessary to determine if the symptom indicates the presence or potential development of a serious illness (Tables 80–4 and 80–5).[2,6] Nearly all oral contraceptive-induced side effects parallel the symptoms and physiologic changes of pregnancy (hormone

TABLE 80–5. Which Symptoms May Be Warnings of Serious Trouble[a]

Five Signals	Possible Problem
Abdominal pain (severe)	Gallbladder disease, hepatic adenoma, blood clot, pancreatitis
Chest pain (severe), shortness of breath, or coughing up blood	Blood clot in lungs or myocardial infarction (heart attack)
Headaches (severe)	Stroke, hypertension, or migraine headache
Eye problems: blurred vision, flashing lights, or blindness	Stroke, hypertension, or temporary vascular problem of many possible sites
Severe leg pain (calf or thigh)	Blood clot in legs

[a]See your clinician if you have any of these problems, or if you develop depression, yellow jaundice, or a breast lump.
From Ref. 2, with permission.

excess) or the perimenopausal period (hormone deficiency). In some cases, symptoms relating to the hormonal imbalance may benefit from adjustments in the specific combination of estrogen and progestin, because progestins can contribute to estrogenic and antiestrogenic activity. However, the clinically significant differences between the low-dose oral contraceptives used today are difficult to distinguish. Several useful handbooks and articles are available to the practitioner in managing side effects associated with oral contraceptives.[1–3,6]

DRUG INTERACTIONS

The effectiveness of an oral contraceptive is sometimes limited by drug interactions that interfere with gastrointestinal absorption; increase intestinal motility by altering gut bacteriologic flora; and alter the metabolism, excretion, or binding of the oral contraceptive (Table 80–6).[2,3,5,6,13,21,54–56] The lower the dose of hormone in the oral contraceptive, the greater the risk that a drug interaction will compromise its efficacy. Women should be instructed to use a backup method of contraception (e.g., condoms) if there is a possibility of a drug interacting and altering the efficacy of the oral contraceptive.[2]

Women receiving anticonvulsants for a seizure disorder require special attention in regard to hormonal contraception. Giving a hormonal contraceptive concomitantly with phenobarbital, carbamazepine, or phenytoin reduces the contraceptive's efficacy, and many anticonvulsants (e.g., phenytoin) are known teratogens. The use of condoms in conjunction with high-estrogen oral contraceptives, injectable progestin-only contraceptives, or intrauterine devices may be considered for these women.[13]

PATIENT INSTRUCTIONS

Many women who take oral contraceptives are poorly informed about the proper use of these medications. The patient should first be given the patient package insert required to accompany all estrogen products and be instructed to read it carefully. The written information in the package insert should be supplemented with verbal information describing the way in which the medication works (primarily, by stopping the release of the egg from the ovary), both common and serious side effects, and the management of those side effects. Although there are often several transient self-limiting side effects (e.g., breast tenderness, bloating, breakthrough bleeding, spotting, nausea), the patient should be aware of the danger signals (see Table 80–5) that require immediate medical attention (see Table 80–4).[1,2,6] Also, the benefits and risks should be discussed in terms that the patient can understand, including the fact that oral contraceptives provide no physical barrier to the transmission of sexually transmitted diseases (STDs), including the human immunodeficiency virus (HIV). Detailed instructions for when to start taking the medication should be provided (either Sunday start or on the first day of the next menses). Patients should be told the importance of routine daily administration to ensure consistent plasma concentrations and improve compliance, and specific instructions should be given regarding what to do if a pill is not taken. Important drug interactions should be discussed.

The patient taking combination oral contraceptives should expect her menses to start within 1 to 3 days after taking the last active pill. She should start another pack of pills immediately after finishing a 28-day pack (no days between) or 1 week after finishing the previous 21-day pack, even if her menses is not completed.[1,2,6] The use of an additional contraceptive method is advisable while the patient is taking the first pack of pills (especially if she began 5 days or more after the start of her menses), if she misses more than one pill per cycle, or if she experiences severe diarrhea or vomiting for several days. Patients taking minipills should be advised to use a backup method for 48 hours if they are 3 or more hours late in taking their daily progestin dose.

DISCONTINUATION OF THE ORAL CONTRACEPTIVE, RETURN OF FERTILITY, AND BREASTFEEDING

Women who have used oral contraceptives may take longer to return to their baseline fertility than women who have used barrier contraception methods. Eventually, the percentage of women who conceive after discontinuing the use of oral contraceptives becomes the same as for barrier method users.[1,2,6]

Traditionally, women are counseled to allow two to three normal menstrual periods before becoming pregnant to permit the reestablishment of menses and ovulation.[1,2,6] However, in several large cohort and case-controlled studies, the infants conceived in the first month after an oral contraceptive was discontinued had no greater chance of being born with a birth defect than those born in the general population.[6]

It is acceptable to begin any method of hormonal contraception immediately after first- or second-trimester termination of pregnancy (spontaneous or induced). Following third-trimester childbirth, ovulation does not usually begin again for 3 weeks (even in a non-breastfeeding woman), and the risk of maternal thromboembolic disease is increased for approximately the same time period.[1,2,57,58] Ideally, therefore, estrogen-containing contraceptives are withheld until the third week after delivery, but progestin-only formulations can be initiated immediately.[1,2,21]

Because the hormones in oral contraceptives are excreted into breast milk, breastfeeding is generally regarded as a relative contraindication to oral contraceptive use. This contraindication was based on earlier formulations containing higher doses of hormones and probably does not apply to current formulations.[58] Another concern is that estrogens inhibit the action of prolactin in breast tissue receptors, resulting in decreased milk production and protein content.[2] Although this is not a particular problem in well-nourished breastfeeding women, many practitioners recommend progestin-only contraceptives because progestins do not diminish the amount of breast milk and provide highly effective contraception in breastfeeding women.[1,2,6,13]

EMERGENCY CONTRACEPTION

High doses of estrogens can cause almost immediate shedding of the endometrium and prevent implantation of the fertilized ovum.[2,59,60] Oral contraceptives in one-time high-doses are safe and effective as emergency contraception to prevent pregnancy after unprotected intercourse (e.g., condom breakage, diaphragm dislodging, sexual assault). The FDA has approved two hormonal contraceptive products (Preven and Plan B) specifically packaged for this use.

The Preven Emergency Contraceptive Kit contains four blue tablets, each containing 50 μg EE and 0.25 mg levonorgestrel (equivalent to four tablets of Ovral, also known as the Yuzpe regimen). The kit also contains a patient education booklet and a urine pregnancy test to determine if the woman is already pregnant. Plan B contains two white tablets, each containing 0.75 mg levonorgestrel (equivalent to two 20-tablet doses of Ovrette). The first dose of each of these regimens is to be taken within 72 hours of unprotected intercourse (although the sooner, the more effective); the second dose, 12 hours later.[2,60,61]

Despite the availability of the new products, it is still permissible to use regular contraceptives for emergency contraception. Specifically, the FDA has declared the following regimens safe and effective methods of emergency contraception: Ovral (2 tablets/dose); Nordette, Levlen, Levora, Lo/Ovral, Triphasil, Tri-Levlen, or Trivora

TABLE 80–6. Interactions of Oral Contraceptives (OCs) With Other Drugs

Interacting Drugs	Adverse Effects (Probable Mechanism)	Comments and Recommendation
Acetaminophen (Tylenol and others)	Possible decreased pain-relieving effect (increased metabolism)	Monitor pain-relieving response
Alcohol	Possible increased effect of alcohol	Use with caution
Ampicillin	Decreased contraceptive effect	Low but unpredictable incidence; use backup method of contraception
Anticoagulants (oral)	Decreased anticoagulant effect	Use with caution, monitor INR
Anticonvulsants (barbiturates, including phenobarbital and primidone; carbamazepine; felbamate; phenytoin; topiramate; vigabatrin)	Possible decreased contraceptive effect	Avoid simultaneous use; use alternative contraceptive (DMPA) for patients with seizure disorder
Antidepressants (Elavil, Norpramin, Tofranil, and others)	Possible increased antidepressant pharmacologic effect	Monitor for adverse effects
Benzodiazepine tranquilizers (Ativan, Librium, Serax, Tranxene, Valium, Xanax, and others)	Possible increased or decreased tranquilizer effects including psychomotor impairment	Use with caution; greatest impairment during drug-free week in oral contraceptive dosage
β-Blockers (Corgard, Inderal, Lopressor, Tenormin)	Possible increased β-blocker pharmacologic effect	Monitor cardiovascular status
Corticosteroids (cortisone)	Possible increased corticosteroid toxicity	Clinical significance not established
Griseofulvin (Fulvicin, Grifulvin V, and others)	Decreased contraceptive effect	Use backup method of contraception
Hypoglycemics (Tolbutamide, Diabinese, Orinase, Tolinase)	Possible decreased hypoglycemic effect	Monitor blood glucose
Methyldopa (Aldoclor, Aldomet, and others)	Possible decreased antihypertensive effect, especially with high-dose OCs	Monitor blood pressure
Non-nucleoside reverse transcriptase inhibitors (Sustiva, Viramune)	Decreased contraceptive effect (Viramune), possible decreased contraceptive effect (Sustiva)	Use alternative method of contraception
Phenytoin (Dilantin)	Decreased contraceptive effect, possible increased phenytoin effect	Use alternative contraceptive (DMPA); monitor phenytoin concentration
Pioglitazone (Actos)	Decreased contraceptive effect documented with previous thiazolidinedione, troglitazone (Rezulin); no documented interaction with rosiglitazone (Avandia); interaction with pioglitazone (Actos) not studied	Use alternative method of contraception
Protease inhibitors (Agenerase, Crixivan, Norvir, Viracept)	Decreased contraceptive effect (Agenerase, Norvir, Viracept), possible decreased contraceptive effect (Crixivan)	Use alternative method of contraception
Rifampin	Decreased contraceptive effect	Use backup method of contraception; use alternate method if planned concomitant use is long term
Sulfonamides	Decreased contraceptive effect	Use backup method of contraception
Tetracycline	Decreased contraceptive effect	Use backup method of contraception
Theophylline (Bronkotabs, Marax, Primatene, Quibron, Tedral, TheoDur, and others)	Decreased contraceptive effect, increased theophylline effect	Monitor theophylline concentration
Troleandomycin (TAO)	Jaundice (additive)	Avoid simultaneous use
Vitamin C	Increased serum concentration and possible increased adverse effects of estrogens with 1 g or more per day of vitamin C	Avoid high dose of vitamin C

INR = International Normalized Ratio; DMPA = depomedroxyprogesterone acetate.
Compiled from Refs. 2, 3, 5, 6, 13, 21, 53, and 54.

(4 tablets/dose); Alesse or Levlite (5 tablets/dose).[2] In addition, progestin-only pills can be used as emergency contraception, but a large number of tablets must be taken: Ovrette (20 tablets/dose).[2] When these regular contraceptives are used, the first dose should be taken within 72 hours of unprotected intercourse with a follow-up dose 12 hours after the first.[2]

The efficacy of any of the regimens for emergency contraception declines if they begin more than 72 hours after intercourse.[2] Treatment is totally ineffective by 7 days, when implantation usually occurs. Patients may experience nausea, vomiting, and breast tenderness with this regimen. Although some clinicians prescribe antiemetics prophylactically, others recommend simply repeating the dose if the patient vomits within an hour of taking the pills.

LONG-ACTING INJECTABLE AND IMPLANTABLE CONTRACEPTIVES

Steroids provide long-term contraception when injected or implanted into the skin. The most commonly used steroids for implantable contraception are progestins, either alone or in combination with estrogen.[1,2] Sustained progestin exposure blocks the LH surge, thus preventing ovulation; should ovulation occur, progestins reduce ovum motility in the fallopian tubes; and even if fertilization occurs, progestins thin the endometrium, reducing the chance of implantation. Progestins also thicken the cervical mucus, producing a barrier to sperm penetration. However, FSH is not intensely suppressed by progestin-only contraception; therefore, follicular growth and estrogen concentrations, although lower than normal at times, are maintained.

Women who particularly benefit from progestin-only methods, including minipills, are those who are breastfeeding, those who are intolerant to estrogens (i.e., have a history of estrogen-related headache, breast tenderness, nausea), those with concomitant medical conditions in which estrogen is not preferred (i.e., have a history of uncontrolled hypertension or dyslipidemia, history of venous thromboembolism, history of systemic lupus erythematosus); or those who smoke and are older than 35 years of age.[1,2] Pregnancy failure rates with long-acting progestin contraception are comparable to that of female sterilization. However, if pregnancy does occur while a woman is using one of the progestin-only methods, the risk of an ectopic pregnancy is greater than with other types of contraception. These long-acting methods of contraception do not offer protection from STDs, but the thickened cervical mucus may help prohibit the entry of bacteria into the upper pelvic region, thus preventing pelvic inflammatory disease (PID).

INJECTABLE PROGESTINS

Medroxyprogesterone acetate is similar in structure to naturally occurring progesterone. Depomedroxyprogesterone acetate (DMPA), 150 mg administered by deep intramuscular injection in the gluteal or deltoid muscle within 5 days after the onset of menstrual bleeding, inhibits ovulation for more than 3 months.[2,62] Although this injection may inhibit ovulation for up to 14 weeks, the dose should be repeated every 3 months (12 weeks) to ensure continuous contraception. The manufacturer recommends excluding pregnancy in women more than *1 week* late for repeat injection. Depo-Provera is available as a 150 mg/mL injection.[56]

DMPA can be used in lactating women, and it may increase the length of time that a woman can breastfeed.[2] Although DMPA is safe postpartum and no adverse effects have occurred in infants exposed to DMPA through breast milk, the manufacturer recommends initiating DMPA at 6 weeks postpartum in women who are breastfeeding. DMPA does not alter blood pressure or increase the risk of thromboembolic disorders. It may be used in women with seizure disorders; not only do anticonvulsant drugs have less effect on DMPA's efficacy, but also it may independently decrease the frequency of seizures.[2,63] Noncontraceptive benefits observed in women using DMPA include reducing the risk of anemia because less menstrual blood is lost and decreasing the incidence of menstrual cramps and pain at ovulation. The incidence of *Candida* vulvovaginitis, ectopic pregnancy, and PID, as well as endometrial and ovarian cancer, is decreased in women using DMPA for contraception compared with women using no contraception.

Return of fertility may be delayed after discontinuation of DMPA. The median time to conception from the first omitted dose is 10 months. Sixty-eight percent of women will be able to conceive within 12 months, 83% within 15 months, and 93% within 18 months of the last injection.[56]

Menstrual irregularities, including irregular unpredictable spotting or, more rarely, continuous heavy bleeding, are the most frequent adverse effects of DMPA. In some cases, bleeding may be severe enough to cause a significant drop in hemoglobin. Women who cannot tolerate prolonged bleeding may benefit from a short course of estrogen (e.g., 7 days of 2 mg estradiol or 1.25 mg conjugated estrogen given orally).[62] The incidence of irregular bleeding decreases from 30% in the first year to 10% thereafter (such that most women are amenorrheic after the first year). After 12 months of therapy, 57% of women report amenorrhea, with the incidence increasing to 68% after 2 years.[56]

Because estrogen concentrations may be lower than normal in women using DMPA, women can lose bone density. The clinical significance of this bone loss is unknown; it has not resulted in an increase in fracture rates.[62,64] Breast tenderness, weight gain, and depression occur less commonly (<5%). Weight gain averages 1 kg annually and may not resolve until 6 to 8 months after the last injection. Whether weight gain can be directly attributed to DMPA is debatable.[62,64] Minor alterations in total, LDL, and HDL cholesterol have been noted after DMPA exposure. A decrease in glucose tolerance has been observed in some patients. Clotting factors VII, VIII, IX, and X may be increased. The clinical significance of these minor alterations in metabolism is unknown.[56,62]

Although used in developing countries for decades, DMPA was not approved as a contraceptive in the U.S. market until 1992 because of a concern about a possible increased incidence of breast cancer. Overall, the risk of breast cancer in women who have used DMPA is not increased.[2,62] However, two studies suggest that the risk may be increased in some groups. One study from the WHO found a very slight increased risk in the first 4 years of use, but the risk did not increase with a longer duration of use.[65,66] Another study found a possible increased risk in women initiating use at an early age.[67] These studies suggest that if any effect exists at all, medroxyprogesterone may enhance the growth of already existing tumors. DMPA was approved for use in the United States as a contraceptive because worldwide data in millions of women showed benefit on maternal mortality and demonstrated other noncontraceptive benefits, outweighing any possible increased risk of breast cancer.

INJECTABLE ESTROGEN/PROGESTINS

Lunelle is a new once a month injectable contraceptive agent containing 5 mg of estradiol cypionate and 25 mg of medroxyprogesterone acetate.[68] Like Depo-Provera, it acts by suppressing ovulation. The addition of estrogen has minimal impact on contraceptive efficacy, but promotes regular bleeding patterns.[69] Lunelle is administered by an intramuscular injection, given every 23 to 32 days. Its efficacy is similar to that of other injectable/implantable contraceptives, and body weight does not appear to affect it.[69,70] It is a reversible form of contraception, and fertility returns as early as 1 month after discontinuation.[71]

Most women using Lunelle have regular monthly menstrual cycles, similar to women using nonhormonal contraceptive methods. Menstrual irregularities, such as breakthrough bleeding and spotting, are more common in the first three cycles of use, and less than 1% of women experience amenorrhea.[69] Other adverse events associated with Lunelle include headache, breast tenderness, weight gain, and acne. Precautions and drug interactions associated with Lunelle are similar to those for other estrogen- and progestin-containing contraceptive methods.

SUBDERMAL PROGESTIN IMPLANTS

Norplant, developed by the Population Council, became the first subdermal progestin implant approved for use in the United States in 1990.[2] The Norplant contraceptive system is currently a set of six implantable, nonbiodegradable, soft, silicone rubber capsules, each filled with 36 mg of crystalline levonorgestrel. Capsules are inserted just under the skin to provide continuous contraception for up to 5 years. Early clinical trials included implants with a hard capsule, but they resulted in higher contraceptive failure rates.[2] Because the cumulative pregnancy rate in all groups of women using Norplant significantly increases during the sixth year, Norplant should be replaced after 5 years. Even with the softer capsules currently available in the United States, failure rates may be unacceptable during the fourth and fifth years of use in women weighing more than 154 pounds. Replacement after 3 years in heavier women helps ensure effectiveness.[2,72]

A new system can be inserted immediately after removal of the old system. Removal of a Norplant system often becomes complicated as a result of poor insertion technique, broken capsules, or impedance by fibrous tissue. A "U" technique of Norplant removal using a 4-mm incision located parallel to the third and fourth implant appears to be an improvement over the manufacturer-recommended technique, especially for personnel who are not highly experienced in this procedure.[72,73] Norplant II, a levonorgestrel two-rod, 150-mg implant system that provides 3 years of contraception, may prove to be easier to insert and remove than the older system.[64,74] Other progestin implants, some of which are biodegradable, are under development.[74]

As with other progestin-only methods, the most common side effect of subdermal progestin implants is irregular menstrual bleeding. Approximately 60% to 70% of women using Norplant experience irregular bleeding during the first year after insertion. Prolonged bleeding can be treated with a short course of estrogen (e.g., 2 mg of estradiol or 1.25 mg of conjugated estrogen daily for 7 to 10 days).[1,2] Spotting and bleeding decrease in amount and duration with time, but adding several cycles of a low-dose combined oral contraceptive can resolve repeated monthly menstrual bleeding.[2] However, by the fifth year of use, regular bleeding cycles may resume in more than 60% of users. Regular cyclic bleeding in a woman who is using Norplant indicates return of ovulation and a higher risk of method failure.[72]

Fertility returns quickly after the removal of Norplant. Most women return to baseline ovulatory patterns within the first month after removal of the system. Other progesterone-related adverse effects that usually occur in the first year include headache (common), dizziness, breast tenderness, nervousness, nausea, acne, breast discharge, and weight gain. Because of the extremely low concentrations of levonorgestrel released from the Norplant system, drugs that significantly increase hepatic enzymes, including most antiepileptic medications (e.g., phenobarbital, carbamazepine, phenytoin) and rifampin, lower the efficacy of the contraceptive. Ovarian cysts may occur, but usually regress spontaneously within 1 month of detection.[1,2]

The noncontraceptive benefits of Norplant are similar to those of Depo-Provera, and no clinically significant adverse effects have been observed on carbohydrate metabolism in nondiabetic women, on bone density, on blood coagulation, or on lipid metabolism.[2,56,75,76]

PERIODIC ABSTINENCE

Highly motivated couples may use the abstinence (rhythm) method of contraception, avoiding sexual intercourse during the days of the menstrual cycle when conception is likely to occur. These women rely on physiologic changes, such as the basal body temperature and cervical mucus, during each cycle to determine the fertile period. The major reasons for the lack of acceptance are the relatively high pregnancy rates among users and the need to avoid intercourse for several days during each menstrual cycle. To overcome these drawbacks, many women use barrier methods or spermicides during the fertile period.[1,2]

BARRIER TECHNIQUES AND SPERMICIDES

The effectiveness of barrier methods and spermicides depends almost exclusively on a couple's motivation to use them consistently and correctly. These methods include the diaphragm, cervical cap, sponge, condom, and spermicides. Besides contraception, an advantage to using these methods is that they can reduce the rate of STD transmission.[1,2]

The diaphragm, a reusable dome-shaped rubber cap with a flexible rim that is inserted vaginally, fits over the cervix in order to decrease access of sperm to the ovum. The diaphragm is available in 11 sizes and requires a prescription from a physician who has fitted the patient for the correct size.[1,2] The effectiveness of the diaphragm depends on its function as a barrier and on the spermicidal cream or jelly placed in the diaphragm before insertion. The diaphragm may be inserted as long as 6 hours before intercourse and must be left in place for at least 6 hours after intercourse. If intercourse occurs more than once within 6 hours, the patient must not remove the diaphragm, but rather insert more spermicide and wear the diaphragm for 6 hours after subsequent acts of intercourse or use a condom. Contraindications to the diaphragm are listed in Table 80–1. Users of diaphragms appear to have a lower incidence of cervical neoplasia, which may be attributed to the adjunctive spermicide and the diaphragm's barrier effect against the human papilloma virus. Diaphragm use has also been associated with an increased incidence of urinary tract and yeast infections.

The Prentif cervical cap is a soft, deep, rubber cup with a firm round rim smaller than a diaphragm that fits over the cervix like a thimble.[1,2] Spermicide, used to fill the cap one-third full prior to insertion, is held in place against the cervix until the cap is removed. The cap remains effective for more than one episode (up to 48 hours) of intercourse without adding more spermicide; thus, it is less messy to use than a diaphragm. However, because of the limited number of sizes, it may not be possible to fit some women with this device. It is recommended that women not wear the cap for longer than 48 hours to reduce the risk of toxic shock syndrome.

The vaginal contraceptive sponge (Today) is pillow-shaped and contains 1 g of the spermicide nonoxynol-9.[2] It has a concave dimple on one side (to fit over the cervix and decrease the risk of dislodgement during intercourse) and a loop on the other side (to facilitate removal). After being moistened with tap water, the sponge is inserted into the vagina up to 6 hours before intercourse. The sponge provides protection for 24 hours, regardless of the frequency of intercourse during this time. After intercourse, the sponge must be left in place for at least 6 hours before removal. Sponges should not be left in place for more than 24 to 30 hours in order to reduce the risk of toxic shock syndrome. After use, sponges should be discarded (they are not effective for re-use). The sponge comes in one size and will soon be available over-the-counter. Production of the sponge was temporarily discontinued in 1995, but it is now being manufactured by a new company.[2,77]

Condoms are devices that create a mechanical barrier, preventing direct contact of the vagina with semen, genital lesions and discharges, and infectious secretions.[1,2] Most condoms made in the United States are made of latex rubber, which is impermeable to viruses; the small proportion (5%) made from young lamb intestine is not, however. Condoms are used worldwide as protection from STDs. When used in conjunction with any other barrier methods, their effectiveness theoretically approaches 95%. Spillage of semen or perforation and tearing of the condom can occur, but proper use minimizes these problems.[2,78] Mineral oil-based vaginal drug formulations (e.g., Cleocin vaginal cream, Premarin vaginal cream, Vagistat 1, Femstat, Monistat Vaginal suppositories), lotions, or lubricants can decrease the barrier strength of latex by 90% in just 60 seconds, thus making water-soluble lubricants preferable if they are to come in contact with latex condoms.[2]

The FDA approved a condom for women (Reality) in April 1993, and it appears to be as effective as the diaphragm in preventing pregnancy.[78] The female condom is a prelubricated, soft, loose-fitting polyurethane sheath, closed at one end, with flexible rings at both ends. Properly positioned, the ring at the closed end covers the cervix, and the sheath lines the walls of the vagina. The outer ring remains outside the vagina, covering the labia; this may make it more effective than the male condom in preventing transmission of diseases such as herpes because it protects the labia from contact with the base of the penis. The manufacturer reports a use-effective pregnancy rate of 26% per year, based on a 6-month follow-up study of 200 women.

Spermicides, most of which contain nonoxynol-9, are chemical surfactants that destroy sperm cell walls and offer some protection against STDs and cervical cancer.[2] They are available as foams, creams, suppositories, jellies, and film.[2] Spermicidal tablets or suppositories require 10 to 30 minutes to dissolve. Spermicides can cause local irritation in both men and women. Additional spermicide must be used each time intercourse is repeated.

INTRAUTERINE DEVICES

The low-grade intrauterine inflammation and increased prostaglandin formation caused by intrauterine devices (IUDs) appear to be primarily spermicidal, although interference with implantation is a backup mechanism. The IUD has several contraindications (see Table 80–1). The risk of PID among IUD users ranges from 1% to 2.5%. Because the increase in the risk of infection appears to be related to the introduction of bacteria into the genital tract during IUD insertion,[79] the risk is highest during the first 20 days after the procedure. Ideal patients for IUD use include parous, monogamous women who are not at risk for STDs or PID. Two IUDs are currently marketed in the United States; both are shaped like a T and are medicated, one with copper (ParaGard) and one with progesterone (Progestasert). A third IUD, one with levonorgestrel, is still in development.[2] ParaGard provides better contraceptive effectiveness than previous copper devices and can be left in place for 10 years. A disadvantage of Progestasert is that it must be replaced annually, but it has been associated with less blood loss during menstruation and less dysmenorrhea.

PHARMACOECONOMIC CONSIDERATIONS

More than half of all pregnancies in the United States are unintended.[1,2] Not all unintended pregnancies are unwanted; many are just "mis-timed." Nevertheless, the United States has a higher rate of induced abortions than most other industrialized Western nations. Whatever method is used, preventing unintended pregnancy is highly cost-effective. In regard to the acquisition cost of reversible contraception, spermicides alone are the least expensive method, followed by their use with condoms. Depo-Provera is slightly less expensive than Norplant and IUDs. Implantable and injectable methods carry a higher initial cost that can be prohibitive for some women, and the annual cost is greater if they are removed prior to their expiration. The diaphragm and cervical cap (with spermicide) are midrange in cost, with the female condom being slightly more expensive than the other female barrier methods. Oral contraceptives are the most expensive form of reversible contraception. These cost estimates are based on the assumption of 100 acts of intercourse annually. However, in regard to direct medical costs (i.e., method use, side effects, and unintended pregnancies) over 5 years, the copper IUD, vasectomy, Norplant, and Depo-Provera are the most cost-effective. Oral contraceptives are more cost-effective than methods with high failure rates (i.e., barrier methods, spermicides, withdrawal, and periodic abstinence), but even these methods are more cost-effective than no method.[80]

EVALUATION OF THERAPEUTIC OUTCOMES

Patients should receive both verbal and written instructions concerning the chosen method of contraception. Follow-up appointments can increase compliance, allow time for the patient to ask questions, and provide opportunities to address other health maintenance issues (self-breast examination, Papanicolaou smears, STD risk).[2]

At least annual blood pressure monitoring is recommended in all users of oral contraceptives. When a patient with a history of glucose intolerance or overt diabetes mellitus begins or discontinues the use of an oral contraceptive, it is necessary to monitor the glucose level closely for deterioration of the condition. Oral contraceptive users should receive at least annual (more frequent if they are at risk for STDs) cytology screening. Finally, the oral contraceptive users should undergo examination for clinical problems possibly relating to the oral contraceptive (e.g., breakthrough bleeding, amenorrhea, weight gain, acne).

Women using Norplant should be monitored for menstrual cycle disturbances, weight gain, local inflammation or infection at the implant site, acne, breast tenderness, headaches, and hair loss. Women using DMPA should be asked at 3-month follow-up visits about weight gain, any problems or concerns that they may have, menstrual cycle disturbances, and STD risks. Patients on DMPA should also be weighed and have their blood pressure checked and receive annual examinations (e.g., complete physical examination, Papanicolaou smear, mammogram) as indicated based on the patient's age.

CONCLUSIONS

Choosing a contraceptive method most suited to the patient's needs will significantly reduce the chance of unintended pregnancy. Typical use failure rates for some of the commonly used methods of reversible contraception are listed in Table 80–1. A medical and sexual history and a thorough physical examination are essential when evaluating the various available methods. Understanding the risks and precautions associated with the available methods is essential for both the patient and the prescriber (see Tables 80–1 and 80–3).

▶ PRINCIPLES OF PHARMACOTHERAPY

- The attitude of both the patient and the sexual partner toward various contraceptive methods, the effectiveness of the method, the reliability of the patient in using it correctly, and the patient's ability to pay must be carefully considered when selecting a contraceptive method.
- Patient-specific factors (e.g., frequency of intercourse, age, smoking status, concomitant diseases or conditions) that may prove to be a consideration or precaution for use of a specific method must be evaluated when selecting a contraceptive method.
- Side effects or difficulties using the chosen method should be carefully monitored and managed in consideration of patient-specific factors.
- The utility and satisfaction of the patient and partner(s) with a contraceptive method must be periodically reevaluated.
- Many practitioners recommend progestin-only contraceptives for breastfeeding women because progestins do not diminish the amount of breast milk and provide effective contraception.
- Accurate and timely counseling on the optimal use of the contraceptive method and strategies to minimize sexually transmitted diseases must be provided to all patients when contraceptive pharmacotherapy is initiated and on an ongoing basis.
- Certain oral contraceptives in high doses can be used as emergency contraception to prevent pregnancy after unprotected intercourse. Administration must occur within 72 hours of unprotected intercourse with a follow-up dose 12 hours after the first.

REFERENCES

1. Speroff L, Darnet P. A Clinical Guide for Contraception. 2nd ed. Baltimore: Williams & Wilkins, 1996:25–118, 129–174, 175–190, 229–262.
2. Hatcher RA, Trussel J, Stewart F, et al. Contraceptive Technology. 17th ed. New York: Ardent Media, 1998:211–248, 277–296, 325–356, 357–370, 405–466, 467–510, 511–544.
3. Cerel-Suhl SL, Yeager BF. Update on oral contraceptive pills. Am Fam Physician 1999;60(7):2073–2084.
4. Hormonal contraception. ACOG Technical Bull 1994;198:1–11.
5. Oral contraceptives. Med Lett Drugs Ther 2000;42(1078):42–44.
6. Dickey RP. Managing Contraceptive Pill Patients. 10th ed. Dallas, TX: Essential Medical Information Systems, 2000: 12–19, 48–62, 65–67, 72–76, 92–93, 108–113.
7. Carr BR. Uniqueness of oral contraceptive progestins. Contraception 1998;58:23S–27S.
8. Kaplan B. Desogestrel, norgestimate, and gestodene: the newer progestins. Ann Pharmacother 1995;29:736–42.
9. Colditz GA. Oral contraceptive use and mortality during 12 years of follow-up: the Nurses' Health Study. Ann Intern Med 1994;120:821–826.
10. World Health Organization. Improving access to quality care in family planning: medical eligibility criteria for contraceptive use. New York: World Health Organization, 1996.
11. Neinstein L. Contraception in women with special medical needs. Compr Ther 1998;24(5):229–250.
12. Corson SL. Contraception for women with health problems. Int J Fertil Menopausal Stud 1996;41:77–84.
13. ACOG Committee on Practice Bulletins-Gynecology. The use of hormonal contraception in women with coexisting medical conditions. ACOG Practice Bulletin, No. 18, July 2000.
14. Sidney S, Siscovick DS, Petitti DB, et al. Myocardial infarction and use of low-dose oral contraceptives: a pooled analysis of 2 US studies. Circulation 1998;98:1058–1063.
15. Schwartz SM, Petitti DB, Siscovick DS, et al. Stroke and use of low-dose oral contraceptives in young women: a pooled analysis of two US studies. Stroke 1998;29:2277–2284.
16. Gambacciani M, Spinetti A, Taponeco F, et al. Longitudinal evaluation of perimenopausal vertebral bone loss: effects of a low-dose oral contraceptive preparation on bone mineral density and metabolism. Obstet Gynecol 1994;83:392–396.
17. Casper RF, Dodin S, Ried RL. The effect of 20 mcg ethinyl estradiol/1 mg norethindrone acetate (Minestrin), a low-dose oral contraceptive, on vaginal bleeding patterns, hot flashes, and quality of life in symptomatic perimenopausal women. Menopause 1997;4:139–147.
18. Castracane VD, Gimpel T, Goldzieher JW. When is it safe to switch from oral contraceptives to hormonal replacement therapy? Contraception 1995;52:371–376.
19. Mosca L, Grundy SM, Judelson D, et al. AHA/ACC Scientific Statement. Guide to preventive cardiology for women. Circulation 1999;99:2480–2484.
20. Kaunitz AM. Oral contraceptive estrogen dose considerations. Contraception 1998;58:15S–21S.
21. Burkman RT, Shulman LP. Oral contraceptive practice guidelines. Contraception 1998;58:35S–43S.
22. Fruzzetti F, Ricci C, Fioretti P. Haemostasis profile in smoking and nonsmoking women taking low-dose oral contraceptives. Contraception 1994;49:579–592.
23. Godsland IF, Crook D. Update on the metabolic effects of steroidal contraceptives and their relationship to cardiovascular disease. Am J Obstet Gynecol 1994;170:1528–1536.
24. Garg SK, Chase HP, Marshall G, et al. Oral contraceptives and renal and retinal complications in young women with insulin-dependent diabetes mellitus. JAMA 1994;271:1099–1102.
25. Chasan-Taber L, Willett WC, Stampfer MJ, et al. A prospective study of oral contraceptives and NIDDM among US women. Diabetes Care 1997;20:330–335.
26. Chasan-Taber L, Stampfer MJ. Epidemiology of oral contraceptives and cardiovascular disease. Ann Intern Med 1998;128:467–477.
27. Bloemenkamp KWM, Rosendall FR, Helmerhorst FM, Vandenbroucke JP. Higher risk of venous thrombosis during early use of oral contraceptives in women with inherited clotting defects. Arch Intern Med 2000;160:49–52.
28. Helmrich SP, Rosenberg L, Kaufman DW, et al. Venous thromboembolism in relation to oral contraceptive use. Obstet Gynecol 1987;69:91–95.
29. Douketis JD, Ginsberg JS, Holbrook A, et al. A reevaluation of risk for venous thromboembolism with use of oral contraception and hormone replacement. Arch Intern Med 1997;157:1522–1530.
30. Grodstein F, Stampfer MJ, Goldhaber SZ, et al. Prospective study of exogenous hormone and risk of pulmonary embolism in women. Lancet 1996;348:983–987.
31. Basdevant A, Conrad J, Pelissier C, et al. Hemostatic and metabolic effects of lowering the ethinyl estradiol dose from 30 mcg to 20 mcg in oral contraceptives containing desogestrel. Contraception 1993;48:193–204.

32. Spitzer WO, Lewis MA, Heinemann LAJ, et al. Third generation oral contraceptives and risk of venous thromboembolic disorders: an international case-control study. BMJ 1996;312:83–88.
33. World Health Organization. WHO Collaborative Study of Cardiovascular Disease and Steroid Hormone Contraception. Venous thromboembolic disease and combined oral contraceptives: results of international multicentre case-control study. Lancet 1995;346:1589–1593.
34. Jick H, Jick SS, Gurewick V, et al. Risk of idiopathic cardiovascular death and nonfatal venous thromboembolism in women using oral contraceptives with differing progestagen components. Lancet 1995; 346:1589–1593.
35. Herings RMC, Urquhart J, Leufkens HGM. Venous thromboembolism among new users of different oral contraceptives. Lancet 1999;354:127–128.
36. Jick J, Bandenbroucke JP, Bloemenkamp KWM, et al. Incidence of venous thromboembolism in users of combined oral contraceptives. BMJ 2000;320:57.
37. Vandenbroucke JP, Helmerhorst FM, Rosendall FR, et al. Competing interests and controversy about third generation oral contraceptives. BMJ 2000;320:381.
38. Speroff L. Third-generation oral contraceptives and venous thrombosis. OB/GYN Clin Alert, June 1997; 11–12.
39. Lewis MA, Heinemann LAJ, MacRae KD, et al (Transnational Research Group on Oral Contraceptives and the Health of Young Women). The increased risk of venous thromboembolism and the use of third generation progestogens: role of bias in observational research. Contraception 1996;54:5–13.
40. Petitti DB, Sidney S, Bernstein A, et al. Stroke in users of low-dose oral contraceptives. N Engl J Med 1996;335:8–15.
41. Poulter NR, Chang CL, Farley TMM, et al. Haemorrhagic stroke, overall stroke risk, and combined oral contraceptives: results of an international, multicentre, case-control study. Lancet 1996;348: 498–510.
42. Speroff L. Low-dose oral contraceptives and stroke. OB/GYN Clin Alert 1996;13:49–51.
43. Consensus conference on combination oral contraceptives and cardiovascular disease. Fertil Steril 1999;71(6 suppl 3):1S–6S.
44. Chang CL, Donaghy M, Poulter N. Migraine and stroke in young women: a case-control study. The World Health Organisation Collaborative Study of Cardiovascular Disease and Steroid Hormone Contraception. BMJ 1999;318:13–18.
45. Croft P, Hannaford PC. Risk factors for acute myocardial infarction in women: evidence from the Royal College of General Practitioners' Oral Contraception Study. BMJ 1989;298:165–168.
46. Dunn N, Thorogood M, Faragher B, et al. Oral contraceptives and myocardial infarction: results of the MICA case-control study. BMJ 1999;12(318):1579–1583.
47. Collaborative Group on Hormonal Factors in Breast Cancer. Breast cancer and hormonal contraceptives: collaborative reanalysis of individual data on 53,297 women with breast cancer and 100,239 women without breast cancer from 54 epidemiological studies. Lancet 1996; 347:1713–1727.
48. Collaborative Group on Hormonal Factors in Breast Cancer. Breast cancer and hormonal contraceptives: Further results. Contraception 1996; 54(suppl 3):1S–106S.
49. Hankinson SE, Colditz GA, Manson JE, et al. A prospective study of oral contraceptive use and risk of breast cancer (Nurses' Health Study, United States). Cancer Causes and Control 1997;8:65–72.
50. Petri M, Robinson C. Oral contraceptives and systemic lupus erythematosus. Arthritis Rheum 1997;40:797–803.
51. Thorneycroft IH. Update on androgenicity. Am J Obstet Gynecol 1999;180:S28–S94.
52. Redmond GP, Olson WH, Lippman JS, et al. Norgestimate and ethinyl estradiol in the treatment of acne vulgaris: a randomized, placebo-controlled trial. Obstet Gynecol 1997;89(4):615–622.
53. Lucky AW, Henderson TA, Olson WH, et al. Effectiveness of norgestimate and ethinyl estradiol in treating moderate acne vulgaris. J Am Acad Dermatol 1997;37(5 Pt 1):746–754.
54. Weaver K, Glasier A. Interaction between broad-spectrum antibiotics and the combined oral contraceptive pill: a literature review. Contraception 1999;59:71–78.
55. Burroughs KE, Chambliss ML. Antibiotics and oral contraceptive failure. Arch Fam Med 2000;9:81–82.
56. Facts and Comparisons. St. Louis: Facts and Comparisons, 1999:234–245.
57. Gray RH, Campbell OM, Zacur HA, et al. Postpartum return of ovarian activity in nonbreastfeeding women monitored by urinary assays. J Clin Endocrinol Metab 1987;64:645–651.
58. American Academy of Pediatrics Committee on Drugs. The transfer of drugs and other chemicals into human milk. Pediatrics 1994;93(1):137–150.
59. Ovral as a "morning-after" contraceptive. Med Lett Drugs Ther 1989; 31:93–94.
60. An emergency contraceptive kit. Med Lett Drugs Ther 1998;40:102–103.
61. APhA Special Report. Emergency Contraception: The Pharmacist's Role. Washington, DC: American Pharmaceutical Association, 2000:1 21.
62. Kaunitz AM. Injectable depot medroxyprogesterone acetate contraception: an update for US clinicians. Int J Fertil Women's Med 1998;43: 73–83.
63. American Academy of Neurology. Practice parameter: management issues for women with epilepsy (summary statement). Neurology 1998; 51:944–948.
64. Kaunitz AM. Long-acting hormonal contraception: assessing impact on bone density, weight, and mood. Int J Fertil Women's Med 1999;44:110–117.
65. World Health Organization Collaborative Study of Neoplasia and Steroid Contraceptives. Breast cancer and depo-medroxyprogesterone acetate: a multinational study. Lancet 1991;44:419–430.
66. Bonhomme MG, Potts DM, Fortney JA, Allen MY. Safety of depot medroxyprogesterone acetate. Lancet 1991;338:942. Letter.
67. Paul C, Skett DCG, Spears GFS. Depo-medroxyprogesterone (Depo-Provera) and risk of breast cancer. BMJ 1989;299:759–762.
68. Kaunitz AM, Mishell DR. Lunelle monthly contraceptive injection (medroxyprogesterone acetate and estradiol cypionate injectable suspension): a contraceptive method for women in the US and worldwide. Contraception 1999;60:177–178.
69. Kaunitz AM, Garceau FJ, Cromie MA, and the Lunelle Study Group. Comparative safety, efficacy, and cycle control of Lunelle monthly contraceptive injection (medroxyprogesterone acetate and estradiol cypionate injectable suspension) and Ortho- Novum 7/7/7 oral contraceptive (norethindrone/ethinyl estradiol triphasic). Contraception 1999;60:179–187.
70. Rahimy MH, Cromie MA, Hopkins NK, Tong DM. Lunelle monthly contraceptive injection (medroxyprogesterone acetate and estradiol cypionate injectable suspension): effects on body weight and injection sites on pharmacokinetics. Contraception 1999;60:201–208.
71. Rahimy MH, Ryan KK. Lunelle monthly contraceptive injection (medroxyprogesterone acetate and estradiol cypionate injectable suspension): assessment of return of ovulation after three monthly injections in surgically sterile women. Contraception 1999;60:189–200.
72. Harrison PF, Rosenfield A. Research, introduction, and use: advancing from Norplant. Contraception1998;58:323–34.
73. Rosenberg MJ, Alvarez F, Barone MA, et al. A comparison of "U" and standard techniques for Norplant removal. Obstet Gynecol 1997;89:168–173.
74. Newton JR. New hormonal methods of contraception. Ballieres Clin Obstet Gynaecol 1996;10:87–101.
75. Diaz S, Reyes MV, Zepeda A, et al. Norplant implants and progesterone vaginal rings do not affect maternal bone turnover and density during lactation and after weaning. Hum Reprod 1999;11:2499–2505.
76. Suherman SK, Affandi B, Korver T. The effects of Implanon on lipid metabolism in comparison with Norplant. Contraception 1999;60:281–287.
77. Today Sponge product information. Allendale Pharmaceuticals, 1999.
78. Anon. The female condom. Med Lett Drugs Ther 1993;35:123–124.
79. Grimes DA. Intrauterine device and upper-genital-tract infection. Lancet 2000;356:1013–1019.
80. Trussel J, Leveque J, Koenig J, et al. The economic value of contraception: a comparison of 15 methods. Am J Public Health 1995;85:494–503.

[illegible]

[illegible] Weiss NS, Chetwynd KM, et al. [illegible] risk of acute myocardial infarction [illegible] 1997;[illegible]

Hennekens [illegible] Lancet 1995;[illegible]

[illegible]

81

MENSTRUATION-RELATED DISORDERS

Martha P. Fankhauser

Women commonly experience premenstrual, postpartum, and premenopausal mood and physical changes during their reproductive years.[1–3] *Dysmenorrhea,* painful cramps and backache at the onset of menses, is the most common menstrual problem in adolescents. *Premenstrual molimina* describes the mild physical symptoms of breast tenderness and bloating that occur premenstrually. *Premenstrual tension* or *premenstrual syndrome* (PMS) is the cyclic recurrence during the luteal phase of a combination of psychological, behavioral, and physical symptoms.[4] PMS refers to a group of menstruation-related disorders that occur during ovulatory menstrual cycles and resolve with menopause. A more severe subtype of PMS, called *late luteal phase dysphoric disorder* (LLPDD) and later renamed *premenstrual dysphoric disorder* (PMDD), is associated with significant mood and anxiety symptoms and an impairment in functioning.[5,6] *Maternity* or *baby blues* is characterized by a brief postpartum episode of tearfulness, emotional lability, anxiety, and sleep disturbance. Severe postpartum mood syndromes are called *postpartum depression* and *puerperal psychosis*.[3,7,8] The *perimenopausal phase* (or premenopause) reflects the time of transition to menopause and is associated with irregular menstrual cycles, a worsening of premenstrual symptoms (e.g., sleep disturbances, irritability, anxiety, depression, cognitive changes), and vasomotor complaints (hot flashes, night sweats).[9,10]

EPIDEMIOLOGY

More than 75% of women experience one or more physical or behavioral symptoms just before or during menses.[1,4,5] Common premenstrual symptoms include mood change, anxiety, sleep disturbances, change in appetite, poor concentration, fluid retention, breast tenderness, and various types of pain syndromes.[1,11] Point prevalence studies report that up to 50% of menstruating women have PMS, and 3% to 8% have symptoms severe enough to impair their daily functioning (i.e., PMDD).[1,4–6] PMS differs from PMDD in that the diagnosis of PMS requires no minimal number of symptoms and no functional impairment.[4]

The prevalence of dysmenorrhea (difficult and painful menstruation) increases from early to late adolescence and decreases after age 30 to 35 years. Approximately 40% to 50% of women have painful menstrual cramps, and up to 10% have impaired functioning for 1 to 3 days per month, such as missing work or school, because of pain.

Comorbid psychiatric disorders such as generalized anxiety disorder, panic disorder, social phobia, major depressive disorder, and dysthymia are common in women with PMDD.[12,13] Women with a history of major depressive disorder, bipolar disorder, postpartum depression, mood changes induced by oral contraceptives, and a family history of mood disorders or premenstrual depression have an increased risk for PMDD.[6] Compared with controls, women with PMDD are at higher risk for developing other affective disorders; have lower parity rates; and have higher rates of postpartum depression, past use of birth control pills, and alcohol and drug use.[2,14]

Women with PMDD and premenstrual irritability have an increased risk of experiencing depression during pregnancy and the postpartum period. Up to 70% of women with PMDD experience depressive symptoms, and 10% to 16% develop a major depression during pregnancy.[7,8] Maternity or baby blues, a common type of emotional disturbance, occurs in 50% to 80% of women; it typically peaks on the fourth or fifth day and remits within 2 weeks after delivery. A smaller percentage of women may experience feeling "high" (mild euphoria, increased energy) within the first few days after delivery and are more likely to become depressed later in the postpartum period. About 10% to 20% of women develop a nonpsychotic postpartum depression (a major depression that occurs anywhere from 24 hours to several months after delivery), and 0.1% to 0.2% experience puerperal psychosis.[3,7,8,15] As many as 60% of women with bipolar disorder have a relapse after childbirth. Risk factors for postpartum mood disorders include current stressful life events; a lack of social support; depressive symptoms during pregnancy; an unwanted pregnancy; a history of depression, bipolar disorder, postpartum depression, or premenstrual irritability; and a family history of mood disorders.[7,8,15]

Women experience menopause by their fifth decade. The menopausal transition (when hot flashes begin and there are changes in bleeding patterns) usually begins by the age of 47 years, and the last menses occurs around age 51.[2] It is estimated that as many as 80% of premenopausal women develop mood disturbances, and these individuals have higher prevalence rates of major depression (16% to 20%) during the climateric.[2] Perimenopausal women with a previous history of depression, PMDD, or postpartum depression are at increased risk of a recurrent depressive episode during the climateric.[2]

ETIOLOGY

Several biologic, cognitive, genetic, psychological, and social theories have been proposed for menstruation-related disorders, but there are no definite conclusions regarding the etiology.[2–4,9,16–18] Menstruation-related disorders are probably the result of a complex interaction between ovarian steroids and central neurotransmitters and neuropeptides.[4,5] The occurrence of physical and psychological symptoms associated with premenopause, the premenstrual or postpartum period, or with pregnancy is closely linked to the rise and fall of gonadotropins, ovarian hormones, serotonin (5-hydroxytryptamine or 5-HT), endorphins, and prostaglandins.[2,10,17,18] A genetic factor has been proposed for PMDD, because several twin studies have found higher concordance rates in monozygotic twins than in dizygotic twins.[4] Premenstrual and postpartum depression may also be genetically linked.[3]

During pregnancy and the postpartum period, hormonal changes are more extreme and sustained than they are in the normal menstrual cycle, thus, women are particularly vulnerable to the development or exacerbation of anxiety and mood disorders during these times.[15,17] It has been hypothesized that the dramatic drop in a woman's estrogen concentration after delivery may contribute to the onset of depressive symptoms, although there is no evidence for a single hormonal cause.[15,17] Postpartum thyroid dysfunction (e.g., antithyroid antibodies, hypothyroidism) may contribute to some cases of depression and can be treated with thyroid replacement.[15] Approximately 5% of postpartum women have transient hypothyroidism (sometimes preceded by hyperthyroidism) and may develop permanent thyroid dysfunction during the first year after delivery.[2]

Perimenopause, the 5 to 10 years preceding menopause, is associated with erratic ovarian function that causes change in the amount or the duration of menstrual flow, change in the length of the menstrual cycle, and skipped menstrual periods.[10] The number of ovarian follicles gradually diminishes during a woman's reproductive life, but by the fortieth year, the decline becomes more rapid; by menopause, only a few follicles remain. Menopause generally occurs between the ages of 47 and 53 years (average age of 51 years), and 90% of women experience menopause by age 55.[10] In natural menopause, the ovaries continue to secrete androgens, including testosterone and androstenedione, which can be converted to estrone, a weak estrogen. Surgical menopause occurs when the ovaries are removed and results in an abrupt and complete loss of the ovarian secretion of androgens, estrogens, and progesterone.

Because medical conditions, emotional/behavioral symptoms, and physiologic indices change during the menstrual cycle and can worsen premenstrually and postpartum, it is important to rule out other disorders that may contribute to mood fluctuations or pain syndromes (Table 81–1).[1,4,11,19–21] For example, dysmenorrhea may be "primary," which occurs during ovulatory cycles, or "secondary," which relates to pelvic pathology (e.g., infection caused by the placement of intrauterine devices, endometriosis, pelvic inflammatory disease, ovarian cyst, endometrial cancer, adhesions, and benign uterine tumors).

TABLE 81–1. Symptoms and Conditions That Change or Worsen Premenstrually

Medical Conditions	Emotional/Behavioral Changes
Acute porphyria	Aggression/anger/irritability/hostility
Adrenal disorders	Altered libido/sex drive
Allergies	Amotivation
Anemia	Anxiety/nervousness
Arthritis	Depression/feeling blue/crying
Asthma	Food cravings (sugar, carbohydrates, salty foods)
Chronic fatigue syndrome	Impulse control problems
Chronic pelvic pain	Obsessive-compulsive behaviors
Diabetes	Panic attacks
Dysmenorrhea	Poor concentration/memory impairment
Endometriosis	Psychosis/paranoia/hallucinations
Fibrocystic breast disease	Sleep changes (insomnia, hypersomnia)
Fibromyalgia	Suicidal ideation/tendencies
Genital herpes	**Physiologic Changes**
Hyperprolactinemia	Arteriolar responses to hormones and catecholamines
Hypoglycemia	Body temperature
Irritable bowel syndrome	Blood pressure and pulse
Migraine headaches	Gastrointestinal absorption
Multiple sclerosis	Gastrointestinal transit time
Polycystic ovarian disease	Hepatic metabolism
Seizures	Mucus cytology
Systemic lupus erythematosus	Renal clearance/elimination
Thyroid disorders	Respiration
Urticaria	Sodium retention
Physical Changes	Urinary excretion
Abdominal bloating	Weight
Acne	
Breast swelling/tenderness	
Cold sores	
Constipation	
Dizziness	
Fatigue	
Fluid retention/edema	
Headaches	
Hot flashes	
Muscle aches/pains	
Nausea/vomiting	
Palpitations	
Weight gain	

Compiled from Refs. 1, 11, 20, 21, and 27.

PATHOPHYSIOLOGY

The menstrual cycle is a rapidly changing biologic process that involves the hypothalamic-pituitary-ovarian axis with input from gonadotropin-releasing hormones (GnRHs), gonadotropins, ovarian hormones, neurotransmitters, and neuropeptides.[16,19,22–26] The hormonal feedback system that controls neuroendocrine balance is extremely complex and vulnerable to familial factors, psychosocial and environmental stresses, and circadian rhythms.[2,4,5]

HYPOTHALAMUS AND ANTERIOR PITUITARY HORMONES

The hypothalamic-pituitary-gonadal axis is responsible for the cyclic hormone secretion that regulates and controls ovulation and plays a role in mood disorders such as PMDD, postpartum depression, and perimenopausal depression.[10,25,26] The hypothalamus produces GnRH, a neurohormone that regulates the release of follicle-stimulating hormone (FSH) and luteinizing hormone (LH) from the anterior pituitary. The secretion of FSH and LH is under feedback control by estrogen.

At the beginning of the follicular phase when estrogen levels are low, FSH and LH levels begin to rise to stimulate ovarian follicular growth. As the follicle matures, it causes an increase in estrogen production. The rising estrogen levels precipitate a surge of LH secretion, which causes ovulation. After ovulation, the follicle becomes the corpus luteum (the luteal phase), which produces estrogen and progesterone. If fertilization does not occur, the corpus luteum degenerates, estrogen and progesterone levels decline, the uterine lining breaks down, and menstruation occurs. The decline in estrogen levels during the last few days of the luteal phase initiates the rise in FSH levels that marks the next menstrual cycle.

During the perimenopause phase, the number of ovarian follicles rapidly declines, and they become less responsive to FSH stimulation.[10] The reduction of estrogen secretion by the ovaries causes a rise in FSH and LH levels because of the loss of estrogen feedback inhibition at the hypothalamic-pituitary axis.

GONADOTROPIN-RELEASING HORMONES

To stimulate gonadotropin secretion and to cause ovulation, GnRH must be released in the correct amounts and at the right pulse rate.[27] Positive and negative feedback from neurotransmitters (including 5-HT, norepinephrine, epinephrine, dopamine, and endorphins) and LH, FSH, and ovarian hormones regulate the release of GnRH. Norepinephrine, epinephrine, and 5-HT promote GnRH secretion, whereas endogenous opiates decrease FSH and LH levels by inhibiting GnRH release from the hypothalamus. Continuous activation of GnRH pituitary receptors by GnRH agonists (GnRH-As) causes a desensitization of receptors, which stops gonadotropin secretion and shuts down the reproductive cycle.

PROLACTIN

In general, prolactin is secreted from the anterior pituitary during sleep in a pulsatile manner. Several physiologic factors influence the secretion of prolactin (e.g., stress, hypoglycemia, exercise, sleep). The prolactin level peaks in the middle of the menstrual cycle, during the luteal phase if ovulation occurs. Prolactin causes proliferation and differentiation of mammary tissues during pregnancy and milk production postpartum. Estrogens, 5-HT agonists (e.g., fenfluramine), and dopamine antagonists (e.g., antipsychotics) stimulate prolactin release, whereas 5-HT antagonists (e.g., cyproheptadine), dopamine agonists (e.g., bromocriptine), and antiestrogenic agents suppress prolactin release.[28] Changes in dopamine and prolactin activity may cause mania and psychotic symptoms prior to menses and during the postpartum period.

OVARIAN HORMONES

Gonadal hormones are the most potent peripherally generated chemical signals in the central nervous system that affect neurotransmitter synthesis, release, reuptake, and enzymatic inactivation.[26,29] The hypothesis that ovarian hormones are important for the pathophysiology of PMDD is supported by the fact that the onset and disappearance of symptoms are linked to ovulatory menstrual cycles, and by the fact that symptoms decline after drug-induced inhibition of ovulation, surgical ovariectomy, and menopause.[4,30]

ESTROGEN

Estrogen has significant effects on other neurotransmitters and neuromodulators (e.g., dopamine, norepinephrine, γ-aminobutyric acid [GABA], opioid, monoamine oxidase [MAO], and 5-HT).[17,26,29,31,32] For example, estrogen alters dopamine receptor sensitivity, increases dopamine turnover in the hypothalamus, increases norepinephrine synthesis, increases β-endorphin levels, inhibits MAO activity in platelets and the brain, enhances acetylcholine synthesis and neurotransmission, changes α_2 and β_2 receptor binding sensitivity, and increases 5-HT blood levels and receptor density.[9,10,28,29,31] Estrogen increases the availability of glutamate (an excitatory amino acid) and activates the excitatory N-methyl-D-aspartate (NMDA) pathway.[9] Overactivity of the NMDA neuronal impulses is associated with seizures (women have increased sensitivity for seizures during the follicular phase when there are preovulatory estrogen surges) and restless leg syndrome.[9] Estrogen has calcium channel-blocking properties and causes vascular muscle relaxation and increased blood flow.[9] Estrogens are involved in endometrial proliferation, bone growth, metabolic action (glucose and insulin), lipid metabolism (serum lipoprotein and triglycerides), and coagulability of blood. Estrogen causes sodium and water retention by increasing aldosterone levels.

Low estrogen levels in the brain have been implicated as a cause of menstruation-related mood disorders.[9,17,32–34] The premenstrual decline in ovarian function and the hypoestrogenic state may play a role in the pathogenesis of PMDD.[9] Some propose that abnormalities in the brain's reactions to normal variations in serum levels of ovarian hormones is a cause of menstruation-related and postpartum depression.[17] It has been proposed that the rate of decline in ovarian hormones during the late luteal and postpartum period is more important in causing depressive symptoms than are the absolute basal values.[17,28] Generally there is little difference in serum levels of estradiol or progesterone in women with PMDD compared with the levels in controls.[17,31] The rapid decline in estradiol and 5-HT levels and increases in prolactin levels immediately after delivery may contribute to postpartum mood changes.[3] A profound and prolonged postpartum estradiol deficiency state has been associated with both depression and psychosis.[9,15,17,34]

During the perimenopausal years, ovarian function becomes erratic and unpredictable, and hormone concentrations may fluctuate. Although estrogen levels tend to diminish during these years, they may increase up to two or three times normal at times and cause large fluctuations in hormone concentrations secondary to dysregulation of the hypothalamic-pituitary-ovarian axis.[9] Hypoestrogenic states may be responsible for hot flashes, night sweats, insomnia, vaginal dryness and atrophy, irritability, depression, anxiety, panic, and memory/cognitive impairment.[7,33] Continuous estrogen therapy (estrogen implants or transdermal application) has been effective in treating PMDD, postpartum depression and psychosis, and has mood-elevating effects in peri- and postmenopausal women.[10,17,34]

PROGESTERONE

Progestational agents, called progestins, increase MAO activity; reduce the production and receptor concentrations of 5-HT, dopamine, norepinephrine, and β-endorphins; and bind to $GABA_A$ benzodiazepine receptors.[9,29] Benzodiazepines and barbiturates are $GABA_A$ receptor agonists and produce sedation, fatigue, and depression.[9] High doses of synthetic progestins have sedative properties similar to those of benzodiazepines and barbiturates, and they may increase the seizure threshold. Women with PMS have lower levels of allopregnenolone and decreased $GABA_A$ receptor sensitivity than do controls.[35,36]

Early PMS research focused on a progesterone deficiency theory, but several studies have found no difference in progesterone levels during the menstrual cycle in women with or without PMS.[28] Progestins may cause breakthrough bleeding, amenorrhea, edema, nausea, cholestatic jaundice, rashes, thromboembolic disorders, drowsiness, sleep disturbances, and mental depression.[29] When progesterone is combined with estrogen for hormone replacement therapy, its antiestrogenic effects may reverse the benefits of estrogen therapy.[29,33]

TESTOSTERONE

During the reproductive years, the adrenal glands and ovaries produce androgens that are important as the substrate hormone for estrogen production.[37] Testosterone, the principal endogenous androgen, is important for sexual drive, energy level, mood, and bone mineralization. High androgen levels may increase irritability and aggression; androgenicity has been implicated in these symptoms in PMDD. Testosterone decreases MAO activity in platelets and the brain and decreases the metabolism of 5-HT, dopamine, and norepinephrine. Androgen deficiency in women may contribute to low libido, fatigue, decreased motivation, and lack of well-being.[32]

NEUROTRANSMITTERS AND NEUROPEPTIDES

The activity of neurotransmitters, neurohormones, and peptides (e.g., endogenous opiates, 5 HT, dopamine, norepinephrine, and GABA) parallels gonadal and ovarian hormonal fluctuations and functions in the feedback regulation of the ovulatory cycle.[1] Dysregulation of these systems may contribute to mood and anxiety disorders.

β-ENDORPHINS

Endogenous opiates are naturally occurring neuropeptides that play a role in gonadal and neurotransmitter activity (e.g., estrogen decreases β-endorphin levels, progesterone increases β-endorphin levels, and GnRH stimulates β-endorphin release).[28] β-Endorphins facilitate prolactin release and inhibit oxytocin, vasopressin, and LH release. Opiate antagonists increase LH release and decrease sexual drive and activity in humans.[28] The rapid decline in β-endorphin levels and decreases in GABA levels premenstrually may be related to fluctuations in progesterone. Levels of β-endorphins drop premenstrually (similar to an opiate-like withdrawal syndrome) and decrease at menopause.[13]

NOREPINEPHRINE

Dysregulation of the noradrenergic system has been proposed as a cause of depression and PMDD. Abnormal β_2-adrenergic receptor density, together with increased α_2-adrenergic binding sites, may be a trait factor in some women with PMDD.[37,38] Usually, women with PMDD report more current life stressors, and they have been reported to have elevated norepinephrine levels at rest and under mental stress when compared with controls.[39] Dysregulation of the stress response and increased norepinephrine activity may be responsible for anxiety symptoms, irritability, and insomnia reported in the luteal phase.

SEROTONIN

A serotonergic dysfunction has been proposed as the cause of premenstrual, postpartum, and climacteric dysphoria, irritability, carbohydrate craving, and sleep disturbances.[28,30,32,40] Estradiol has been reported to influence 5-HT activity (e.g., by altering platelet and synaptosomal 5-HT uptake, by down-regulating 5-HT_2 receptors, by causing diurnal changes in 5-HT activity).[4,17,32,41] Estrogen increases 5-HT activity and inhibits dopamine activity, whereas progesterone decreases 5-HT activity.[9,30] Estrogen replacement has been shown to significantly increase blood 5-HT levels in women with both natural and surgical menopause.[4]

Recent evidence suggests that 5-HT is pivotal in the pathogenesis of PMDD.[4,5] Compared to normal controls, women with PMDD have a blunted prolactin response to fenfluramine (a 5-HT-releasing agent).[42] Platelet uptake of 5-HT (a model for measuring serotonergic activity) and imipramine receptor binding in platelets have been reported to be decreased in patients with depression and during the week before menstruation among women with PMS.[5,43] Lower platelet content of 5-HT, lower whole blood 5-HT concentrations, lower levels of melatonin during the luteal phase, and a 5-HT_{1A} receptor subsensitivity have been reported in women with PMS compared with normal controls.[4,40] Lower levels of plasma-free tryptophan (a precursor of 5-HT) have been associated with postpartum depression and PMDD.[28] Dietary tryptophan depletion can aggravate depression, PMS, and postpartum depression, whereas dietary supplementation of 6 g/d premenstrually has been found to improve PMDD symptoms.[44]

MAO and catechol-o-methyltransferase (COMT) metabolize monoamines; in animal models, estradiol and testosterone decrease the activity of MAO and COMT, and progesterone increases it.[9,33] MAO inhibitors (MAOIs) and estrogen inhibit the MAO enzyme and prolong the activity of 5-HT, norepinephrine, and dopamine, which has antidepressant effects.[27,33] Tricyclic antidepressants block the reuptake of 5-HT and norepinephrine; selective serotonin reuptake inhibitors (SSRIs) block the reuptake of 5-HT into the presynaptic neuron, which increases the amount available for neurotransmission.

Antidepressants that augment 5-HT are effective in treating depression (e.g., PMDD, postpartum depression, climacteric depression, seasonal affective disorder), anxiety (e.g., panic disorder, social phobia, obsessive-compulsive disorder), and bulimia.[40,41] Buspirone, a 5-HT_{1A} agonist, is used to decrease anxiety symptoms. The strong relationship between premenstrual and postpartum depression, eating disorders, and anxiety disorders suggests that 5-HT plays an important role in menstruation-related disorders.[5,17,28,32,40]

γ-AMINOBUTYRIC ACID

GABA, a major inhibitory neurotransmitter, is linked with steroid activity: for example, $GABA_A$ receptors bind with progesterone and enhance LH secretion; $GABA_B$ receptors inhibit LH secretion.[26,28] Low GABA plasma levels and reduced $GABA_A$ receptor sensitivity have been reported in patients with depression and during the luteal phase in women with PMDD.[5,45] Benzodiazepines (agonists at the $GABA_A$/benzodiazepine receptor) have been used in the treatment of anxiety disorders, insomnia, and PMDD.

PROSTAGLANDINS

At menstruation, the shedding of the uterine lining releases arachidonate and stimulates prostaglandin synthesis. Prostaglandins occur in the menstrual fluid and cause uterine and gastrointestinal smooth muscle contraction. Prostaglandin inhibitors (e.g., nonsteroidal anti-inflammatory drugs [NSAIDs]) are effective in treating dysmenorrhea, headaches, and other pain syndromes. It has been suggested that a deficiency of prostaglandin E_1 (PGE_1) causes breast pain, on the rationale that low levels of PGE_1 may increase prolactin's effect on breast tissue and cause mastodynia.[46]

Cis-linolenic acid, an essential fatty acid contained in vegetable oils, is converted to γ-linolenic acid, the precursor to PGE_1. *Cis*-linolenic acid, magnesium, pyridoxine, zinc, and vitamin C are all involved in the synthesis of PGE_1. Products that promote the synthesis of PGE_1 (e.g., evening primrose oil, which contains γ-linolenic acid) have been used for breast pain.

VITAMIN OR MINERAL DEFICIENCY

A deficiency in vitamins, minerals, and other nutrients (e.g., calcium; magnesium; manganese; vitamins B, D, and E; linoleic acid; L-tryptophan) has been proposed as a cause of PMS. Pyridoxine (vitamin B_6) is a cofactor in the synthesis of dopamine and 5-HT; a coenzyme in the metabolism of protein, carbohydrate, and fat; and a contributor to the production of prostaglandins from essential fatty acids. A deficiency of pyridoxine decreases the synthesis of dopamine and 5-HT and may contribute to the development of depression.[47] Although pyridoxine is commonly used as a treatment for PMS, there is no evidence of pyridoxine deficiency in women with PMS.

Abnormalities in calcium or parathyroid hormone homeostasis may be a factor in depression.[47] Significant fluctuations in calcitonin, a calcium-regulating hormone, and low plasma calcium levels during the menstrual cycle may play a part in the etiology of PMS.[48,49] Estrogen regulates intestinal calcium absorption and metabolism, and parathyroid secretion.[49] Estrogen lowers the serum calcium level and acts as a calcium channel blocker, whereas progesterone can stimulate the influx of extracellular calcium into a cell.[9,49] Calcium influx into brain cells is involved with the release of many neurotransmitters. Calcium supplementation (1200 mg/day in two divided doses) has been shown to reduce PMS symptoms such as anxiety, depression, irritability, mood swings, headache, and cramps.[47–50]

Magnesium is part of many neuromuscular activities and cellular pathways that may affect PMS, and its levels fluctuate during the menstrual cycle.[49] Low intracellular magnesium levels have been reported in women with PMS compared with controls.[46] Low magnesium levels may cause a depletion of dopamine, resulting in increased prolactin concentrations. Dairy products and calcium can interfere with the gastrointestinal absorption of magnesium, but the significance of this is not known. Daily magnesium supplementation of 200 mg/day was reported to be helpful in reducing premenstrual fluid retention in women with PMS.[51]

CIRCADIAN RHYTHM DYSREGULATION

Some authorities have postulated that a circadian rhythm dysregulation is a link between mood disorders and the reproductive cycle.[2,18,52] Several studies have reported reduced and earlier secretion of nocturnal melatonin in women with PMDD.[53] The pineal gland secretes melatonin, a neurohormone and metabolite of 5-HT, under the influence of darkness, and the suprachiasmatic nuclei of the hypothalamus controls it through β-adrenergic receptors.[54] β-Adrenergic blockers such as propranolol suppress melatonin production and may cause insomnia, whereas tryptophan- and serotonin-augmenting agents increase melatonin levels.

Melatonin production is controlled by a circadian temperature rhythm and synchronized by the light-dark cycle. Bright light increases 5-HT levels during the day, and darkness promotes the synthesis of melatonin. The exposure to bright light in the evening suppresses not only the secretion of melatonin, but also the nocturnal drop in core body temperature.[54] The reduction in daytime sunlight, which increases melatonin secretion, may exacerbate PMS in the winter; this type of seasonal PMS may respond to phototherapy.[52] Early sleep deprivation may also help to correct circadian rhythm disturbances in PMDD.[55,56]

CLINICAL PRESENTATION

During their reproductive years, women are vulnerable to mood changes secondary to hormonal triggers associated with the premenstrual, pregnancy, postpartum, and perimenopause phases, as well as with exogenous hormone therapy.[2] Women have a lifetime prevalence of major depression two times higher than that of men, and women are more likely to experience atypical symptoms (e.g., increased appetite and weight gain, somatic symptoms, anxiety).[13,18,57,58] Approximately 50% of women with PMS complaints may have premenstrual exacerbation of an underlying anxiety or mood disorder.[1,12–14,58] Affective symptoms that are not confined to the luteal phase are likely related to a mood disorder such as dysthymia or major depression.[1] Premenstrual and postpartum exacerbation of several underlying disorders (i.e., anxiety, panic, depression, mania, bulimia, migraine headaches, asthma, arthritis, diabetes, endometriosis, and epilepsy) has been reported.[4,15,18,21]

PREMENSTRUAL SYNDROME

Although some women experience positive premenstrual changes, such as increased energy and productivity, the majority of women experience negative changes in mood, appetite, sleep, and energy.[1] Women with PMS usually rank anxiety, irritability, mood lability, and fatigue as the most distressing symptoms.[59] Common emotional and behavioral PMS symptoms include sadness, anhedonia, feelings of insecurity, low self-esteem, anger attacks, oversensitivity, crying episodes, decreased concentration, and food cravings. Physical changes (e.g., back pain, breast tenderness, headaches, water retention, and bloating sensations) may be better tolerated and cause less dysfunction than mood or behavioral changes do.[59]

PREMENSTRUAL DYSPHORIC DISORDER

PMDD is listed as an example of the category called Depressive Disorder Not Otherwise Specified in the *Diagnostic and Statistical Manual of Mental Disorders, Fourth Edition, Text Revision* (*DSM-IV-TR*).[6] In order to confirm a diagnosis of PMDD, women must chart symptoms for at least two cycles, using standardized prospective instruments (e.g., Prospective Record of the Impact and Severity of Menstruation [PRISM], the Calendar of Premenstrual Experiences [COPE], or Visual Analogue Scales [VAS] that rate symptom severity on a 100-mm scale).[4] The diagnosis of PMDD requires at least a 30% increase in symptom severity from the follicular to luteal phase.[4] At least five symptoms must occur premenstrually. At least one of the following symptoms must be present: depressed mood or hopelessness, tension or anxiety, affective lability [sudden mood swings], or irritability. In addition, the woman must experience any combination of the following: decreased interest in activities, difficulty concentrating, lack of energy, change in appetite (e.g., food craving), change in sleep, feeling out of control or overwhelmed, or other physical symptoms (e.g., breast tenderness, bloating).[6] The symptoms must occur regularly during the last week of the luteal phase and remit within a few days of the onset of menses in most menstrual cycles during the past year. The symptoms of PMDD must be severe enough to interfere markedly with school, work, usual activities, or relationships with others and be entirely absent for a least 1 week postmenses.[6]

The onset of PMDD typically occurs during the late teens to 20s (average age of onset, about 26 years), and the symptoms usually peak in the third or fourth decade.[2,14] PMDD may become more severe and refractory to initial treatments secondary to the decline in the ovarian production of estrogen that starts 10 years before menopause.[9] Severe PMDD may include episodes of psychosis, mania, and suicidal ideation, and it has resulted in marital discord, physical and verbal abuse of others, difficulties in parenting, criminal behavior, poor work or school performance, work absenteeism, social isolation, accidents, hospitalizations, suicide, and homicide.[1,14,28] If not treated, episodes of PMDD may progressively worsen and eventually result in a major depressive episode.[1,2,13,14,18,60]

POSTPARTUM DISORDERS

Postpartum psychiatric disorders are associated with marital conflict, impaired functioning, poor bonding with the infant, suicide, and infanticide.[3] Maternity blues is usually a benign and transient condition characterized by mood lability, depression, irritability, tearfulness, generalized anxiety, increased sensitivity to criticism, fatigue, and disruptions in sleep and appetite.[7,8] Postpartum depression usually occurs within 4 to 6 weeks of delivery, and the loss of energy, diminished concentration, and irritability that follows sleep deprivation may exacerbate it.[7] The signs and symptoms of postpartum depression are the same as those of a major depressive episode: suicide ideation, depressed mood, anhedonia, low energy, and guilty ruminations.[8] Puerperal psychosis can be manic in nature (e.g., agitation and restlessness, expansive or irritable mood, disorganized behavior, mood liability, insomnia) and occurs within the first 48 to 72 hours postpartum up to the first month after delivery.[8] Psychotic mothers may avoid their infant, have delusions or hallucinations about the baby, and are at risk for harming themselves and the baby. Most patients with puerperal psychosis require hospitalization and treatment with antipsychotics and/or mood stabilizers. Electroconvulsive therapy has been used for severe refractory mood and psychotic states.

PREMENOPAUSE

In the climacteric phase preceding menopause, women report more sleep disturbances, hot flashes, anxiety attacks, depression, irritability, short-term memory loss, and decreased libido.[9,10] Hot flashes may disrupt sleep, which can cause irritability, fatigue, and poor concentration.[2] Women with a past history of mood disorders, premenstrual and postpartum depression, and a lengthy and symptomatic menopause transition may be at risk for a major depressive episode.[2,10,29,57]

▶ TREATMENT: Menstruation-Related Disorders

The goals of treating menstruation-related disorders are to minimize symptoms and to improve functioning and well-being without causing adverse effects. It is recommended that the clinician follow a stepwise approach, beginning with nondrug therapies or the least toxic agent before resorting to experimental treatments. The weighing of risk versus benefit of pharmacologic interventions is important, because some medications cause significant adverse effects and may have teratogenic properties.[61–64] Little is known about the use of psychotropic medications during lactation; thus, the risk/benefit of exposing the infant to medications versus maternal mental health must be determined for each individual.[65]

GENERAL APPROACH

Before a diagnosis of a menstruation-related disorder is made, other medical or psychiatric conditions should be excluded (see Tables 81–1 and Table 81–2). Mood and anxiety disorders often first occur during childbearing years and may require standard pharmacologic treatment. (See Chapter 69 for a discussion of depressive disorders; Chapter 70, for bipolar disorders; and Chapter 71, for anxiety disorders.) Women with premenstrual symptoms should prospectively rate themselves daily for at least two menstrual cycles to determine baseline severity ratings so that treatments can be tailored to the most bothersome symptoms.[2,4] Women with severe PMDD (with impairment in functioning) may require immediate pharmacologic interventions. In general, five different treatment strategies are used for PMS and PMDD: (1) lifestyle changes to minimize precipitants, (2) physical and behavioral symptom relief, (3) modification of neurotransmitter/hormonal imbalances, (4) suppression of ovulation, and (5) removal of ovaries.

The use of psychotropic medications may be necessary during pregnancy and breastfeeding, depending on the severity of the disorder and the risk of relapse during the postpartum period.[15,61–63] Prophylactic antidepressants may be appropriate for women with a history of severe recurrent major depressive disorder, PMDD, and postpartum depression.[8] For women with a history of bipolar depression or puerperal psychosis, postpartum prophylaxis with a mood stabilizer such as lithium is recommended.[8] Prophylactic use of estradiol preparations may be an alternative approach to mood stabilizers for women with a history of severe postpartum depression or puerperal psychosis.[8]

Women in their 40s should be tested for estrogen and androgen deficiency, particularly if perimenopausal symptoms are present and if they complain of decreased libido and energy. An elevated serum FSH level (greater than 25 IU/L), in conjunction with a low free estradiol level (less than 40 pg/mL) measured on day 2 or 3 after the onset of menses, is suggestive of perimenopause. At menopause, FSH levels are usually higher than 40 IU/L, and estradiol levels are under 25 pg/mL. Middle-aged women with somatic and mood symptoms should undergo evaluation for perimenopausal depression. Estrogen replacement therapy can significantly reduce vasomotor symptoms; improve mood, sleep, and cognition; and decrease the risk of osteoporosis and cardiovascular disease.[9,29,33]

Hormonal fluctuations during the menstrual cycle, postpartum period, and peri- and postmenopause phase may cause differences in the pharmacokinetics and pharmacodynamics of drugs (e.g., changes in drug absorption, distribution, metabolism, and excretion). Thus, practitioners must be aware of gender differences when prescribing medications.[20,58]

NONPHARMACOLOGIC THERAPY

A wide variety of nonpharmacologic treatments are available for menstruation-related disorders. These should be tailored to the primary symptom complaints (or target symptoms) and tried first.[1,4,5,7,16,18,52,66,67] Nonpharmacologic treatments for menstruation-related disorders include (1) education about the symptoms, treatment approaches, and strategies to reduce target behaviors; (2) daily charting for two menstrual cycles to identify target symptoms; (3) reduction or discontinuation of alcohol, caffeine, nicotine, and drugs of abuse; (4) regular conditioning or aerobic exercise at least three times a week with an increase in the daily workout routine by 30 minutes during the premenstrual week; (4) bright, white morning and evening light for 1 week premenstrually for seasonal worsening of PMS; (5) regular, well-balanced, scheduled meals with adequate fiber, protein, carbohydrates, vitamins, calcium, and minerals; (6) reduced intake of salt, caffeine, fat, and simple sugars; (7) increased intake of phytoestrogen-rich foods (soybean products) and tryptophan-containing foods (fish, poultry, and dairy products); (8) adequate rest and a regular sleep cycle in a cool, dark room; (9) stress management, relaxation training, yoga, massages, biofeedback, and self-hypnosis; and (10) individual, group, or family therapy, cognitive behavioral therapy, support groups, and assertiveness training.

PHARMACOLOGIC THERAPY

There are no published consensus guidelines or algorithms for the pharmacologic treatment of premenstrual and postpartum mood disorders. Women with less severe PMS generally self-treat headaches

TABLE 81–2. Evaluation of Menstruation-Related Disorders

Type of Evaluation	Tests/Procedures/Assessments
Psychiatric evaluation	Past psychiatric history (particularly mood disorders and alcohol/substance abuse) History of symptoms; onset, duration, course, precipitation factors, previous treatments, and response Family history for premenstrual, postpartum, and perimenopausal mood disorders, treatment of other family members Rule out comorbid psychiatric disorders
Medical evaluation	Past and current history for endocrine and gynecologic disorders (dysmenorrhea, endometriosis, fibrocystic breast disease, thyroid abnormalities, abnormal Papanicolaou smear, irritable bowel syndrome) Physical and pelvic examinations Assess the presence and severity of common perimenopausal symptoms if >40 yrs • Vasomotor symptoms such as hot flashes or cold sweats • Sleep disturbances with frequency of awakenings • Decreased sexual desire and pleasure secondary to dysparcunia • Vaginal dryness • Memory difficulties, forgetfulness, wordfinding problems, difficulty concentrating
Laboratory tests	Chemistry panel, complete blood count with differential, and thyroid tests (to rule out anemia, hypothyroidism, or other disease states) Other tests: Follicle-stimulating hormone (FSH) ± estradiol measured day 2 or 3 of the menstrual cycle (to rule out estrogen deficiency if perimenopausal or symptoms of irregular bleeding or hot flashes) • Follicle-stimulating hormone (FSH) >25 IU/L and estradiol <40 pg/mL suggest perimenopause even if menstruation is regular Testosterone and sex hormone–binding globulin (SHBG) to rule out androgen deficiency • A low ratio of total testosterone to SHBG or a free testosterone level in the lower third of the normal range for women during their reproductive years suggests androgen deficiency Prolactin, to rule out cause of irregular menses or amenorrhea Vitamin B_6, B_{12}, folate, magnesium, and calcium, to rule out deficiences Bone density scan to rule out osteoporosis
Medication use	History of over-the-counter, herbal, and prescription medications (psychoactive agents, those that can induce psychiatric conditions); caffeine; alcohol; and substances/illicit drugs; oral or injectable hormonal contraceptives
Nutritional evaluation	Assessment of diet (protein, complex carbohydrates, phytoestrogens, salt, minerals, calcium, trace elements, vitamins) Well-balanced, regular meals
Exercise and sleep evaluation	Assessment of adequate and regular exercise and good sleep habits
Self premenstrual syndrome-rating for (PMS) and premenstrual dysphoric disorder (PMDD)	Two months of prospective daily rating of symptoms using a PMS rating scale.[a] Compare average ratings of two luteal phases to follicular phases (5–7 days postmenses and 5–7 days premenses); >30%–50% change in severity ratings required for PMDD plus a symptom-free week postmenses
Screening for postpartum mood disorders	Postpartum Depression Checklist (PDC); Edinburg Postnatal Depression Scale (EPDS)
Other evaluations	Daily basal body temperature to determine ovulation • Within 48 h of ovulation, a temperature spike of 0.3°C to 0.6°C (0.5°F to 1°F) occurs Morning and evening weights to monitor fluid retention

[a]Menstrual Distress Questionnaire (MDQ); PMS Diary (PMSD); Daily Rating Form (DRF); Premenstrual Assessment Form (PAF); Calendar of Premenstrual Experiences (COPE); Prospective Record of the Impact and Severity of Menstruation (PRISM); Visual Analogue Scale (VAS).
Complied from Refs. 1, 2, 7, 10, 11, and 118.

and cramps with aspirin, acetaminophen, and NSAIDs. Many women try exercise, dietary changes, and nutritional/herbal supplements as alternative "natural" therapies.[68] NSAIDs such as ibuprofen are the treatment of choice for dysmenorrhea and menstrual migraines. PMDD and postpartum depression are generally treated with 5-HT-augmenting antidepressants.[3,41] Fluoxetine, a 5-HT reuptake inhibitor, is the only medication currently approved by the Food and Drug Administration (FDA) to treat symptoms of PMDD, but other SSRIs are also effective. Although benzodiazepines may be useful in the treatment of acute anxiety and intermittent insomnia, these agents should be used only as adjuncts to antidepressants because they do not alleviate the core symptoms of depression.

For women with premenstrual exacerbation of an underlying depression, severe PMDD, postpartum depression, or climacteric depression, a 6- to 12-month course of an antidepressant is recommended. For PMDD and perimenopausal depression, some women benefit from continuous antidepressant dosing with an intermittent increase in dose prior to the onset of symptoms and a reduction in dose at the onset of menses.[27] Varying the antidepressant dosage and adding supplemental medications based on menstruation-related symptoms has empirically been shown to be helpful. It may be necessary to try several different treatments in order to find an acceptable therapy.

Perimenopausal symptoms usually respond to estrogen replacement therapy, along with 5-HT-augmenting antidepressants for severe mood or anxiety symptoms. The North American Menopause Society has recently published a consensus opinion and treatment algorithms for using hormone replacement therapy in postmenopausal women (see Chapter 83).[69] Menopausal depression should be treated with standard antidepressant therapy such as tricyclic antidepressants and SSRIs. Monotherapy with estrogen is generally not effective for menopausal depression, and progesterone may not only increase depressive symptoms, but also reduce the beneficial effects of estrogen.[2,17] Further studies are needed to determine if estrogen therapy can augment antidepressant medication in menopausal depression.[2,17,29,32,33]

A list of pharmacologic treatments used for menstruation-related symptoms appears in Table 81–3. An example of first-line and second-line treatment approaches for PMS/PMDD is shown in Table 81–4, and an algorithm for the treatment of PMDD is shown in Figure 81–1.

VITAMIN, MINERAL, HERBAL, NUTRITIONAL, AND HORMONAL THERAPIES

Daily supplementation of vitamins, minerals, and calcium, along with a well-balanced diet, is the first-line therapy for all menstruation-related disorders.[47] Adequate postpartum replacement of vitamins, minerals, and calcium is important to reduce deficiency states, particularly in women who breastfeed their infants. Over-the-counter (OTC) products that contain megadoses of vitamins, as well as minerals and trace elements, have been marketed for PMS without scientific testing. There are several brands of OTC products for PMS (e.g., a combination preparation of a mild diuretic, an analgesic, and an antihistamine), but no efficacy data are available for these products.

Vitamin B_6 is recommended for women taking oral contraceptives and estrogen therapy because estrogenic substances increase the demand for pyridoxine. Although pyridoxine has been reported to reduce the severity of premenstrual depression, fatigue, irritability, headache, and edema, controlled studies have provided little support for its efficacy in PMS.[46,47] A meta-analysis of PMS studies indicated that vitamin B_6 was not conclusively better than placebo, but that it did reduce depressive symptoms in women receiving oral contraceptives.[70] A double-blind placebo-controlled crossover study in which patients received 200 mg of magnesium plus 50 mg of vitamin B_6 revealed a synergistic effect in relieving anxiety-related symptoms (e.g., anxiety, irritability, nervous tension, mood swings) for one menstrual cycle, but overall there were no significant differences between individual treatments.[71] Vitamin B_6 has been reported to cause a reversible peripheral neuropathy with daily dosages of 200 mg or more.

Several PMS studies have reported that calcium reduces premenstrual mood changes, fluid retention, and pain.[48,49] Calcium supplementation (1200–1600 mg/day of elemental calcium in divided doses) may help prevent osteoporosis later in life, and it is a relatively safe and inexpensive treatment for PMS.[50] Daily or luteal administration of 200–360 mg/day of magnesium has been reported to improve some PMS symptoms and fluid retention compared with placebo treatment.[51]

Herbal products and nutritional supplements are promoted for PMS and menopause, but little is known about their dosing, efficacy, or safety.[72,73] Because the FDA does not regulate herbal preparations and dietary supplements, active ingredients may vary from brand to brand. St. John's wort (*Hypericum perforatum*), the most popular herbal remedy for depression, was reported to have efficacy in randomized controlled trials[72,73] and in one open-labeled PMS trial.[74] Several *in vitro* and human studies suggest that St. John's wort induces the hepatic cytochrome P450 system[72,75] and should not be combined with serotonin reuptake inhibitors because of the potential risk of a serotonin syndrome.[72,73]

Women with menstruation-related disorders may turn to alternative remedies that have not been proved effective.[11,73] Dong quai, which contains coumarin derivatives, is widely used in China for menstrual cramps and irregular menses. Chaste tree or chasteberry (*Vitex agnus castus*) has been used for PMS, mastodynia, and menstrual irregularities.[72,76] Black cohosh has been used for the treatment of dysmenorrhea and menopausal hot flashes,[72] and blue cohosh has been used for menstrual cramps and stimulation of menstrual flow. Valerian is an herbal sleep aid; chamomile is a sedative, antispasmodic, antipyretic, and anti-inflammatory agent; and kava is an agent used to treat anxiety and insomnia.[72,73] Products promoted for perimenopausal symptoms without scientific testing include dehydroepiandrosterone (DHEA), a steroid hormone produced by the adrenal glands and ovaries that is a precursor hormone for testosterone and estradiol passion flower for insomnia, pain, and climacteric complaints; wild yam root, which contains diosgenin, a precursor to progesterone; and phytoestrogens, plant-based hormones found in soybean food such as tofu and flax seeds that promote estrogenic effects.[72,77]

SYMPTOM-BASED APPROACHES

Dysmenorrhea and Cramps

NSAIDs inhibit prostaglandin synthesis and exhibit anti-inflammatory, analgesic, and antipyretic activity. Mefenamic acid has been reported to be effective in reducing menstrual pain, as well as breast tenderness, bloating, irritability, and depression.[78] NSAIDs such as ibuprofen, ketoprofen, and naproxen are also effective for dysmenorrhea and menstrual migraine. NSAIDs cause gastrointestinal side effects and are contraindicated in patients with aspirin sensitivity, peptic ulcer disease, gastritis, bleeding disorders, and renal insufficiency. For those who cannot tolerate NSAIDs, cyclooxygenase (COX)-2 inhibitors may be alternative agents in the treatment of dysmenorrhea. NSAIDs and COX-2 inhibitors should be prescribed for short-term use only and in the lowest effective dosages.

Headaches and Migraines

Approximately 60% of women complain of menstrual migraine attacks, and 8% to 14% experience migraines only premenstrually.[19,21] If migraines do not respond to NSAIDs or COX-2 inhibitors, 5-HT_{1D} agonists can be used for abortive migraine therapy; however, these agonists should not be combined with 5-HT-augmenting antidepressants such as SSRIs or MAOIs.[21] Ergotamines, analgesics, and antiemetics can provide symptomatic relief, if needed. Low-dose

TABLE 81–3. Pharmacologic Treatments for Menstruation-Related Disorders

Agent/Drug	Dose	Clinical Reason for Use
Vitamins and Minerals		
Pyridoxine	50–100 mg/day (>200 mg/day associated with risk of peripheral neuropathy)	A cofactor in the synthesis of DA and 5-HT; reduces depressive symptoms in women on OCs; little support for efficacy in PMS
Calcium (Ca)	1.2–2.5 g/day in divided doses for PMS; 1.0 g/day before menopause; 1.5 g/day after menopause	Intracellular Ca plays a role in cellular function; Ca supplementation reduces premenstrual mood changes, headache, and pain; helps to prevent osteoporosis (↑ bone loss as estrogen levels decline)
Magnesium (Mg)	50–100 mg bid; up to 360 mg/day in divided doses during luteal phase of PMS	Intracellular Mg plays an essential role in neuromuscular function and protein and carbohydrate enzyme systems; may reduce fluid retention in PMS
Vitamin E (α-tocopherol)	150–800 IU/day	A fat soluble vitamin that is involved in the functioning of many organs and systems; antioxidant effects; used to reduce breast tenderness and swelling; recommended for fibrocystic breast disease
OTC/Herbal Products		
Diphenhydramine	25–50 mg/day	Sedating antihistamine; used for sedative-hypnotic effects to induce sleep
Evening primrose oil	0.5–2 g bid during cycle or luteal phase	Contains γ-linolenic acid (a precursor to prostaglandin E_1); used for breast tenderness and pain; may not be effective based on placebo-controlled trials
Kava kava	90–100 mg dried kava extract tid	Herbal product used for anxiety, nervous tension, stress, agitation, and insomnia
Melatonin	0.1–2 mg hs	Metabolite of 5-HT; used as an OTC sleep-inducing agent for jet lag, sleep-wake cycle disorder, insomnia
Passion flower	4–8 g of herb (3–6 teaspoons) as a tea in divided doses	Herbal product used for anxiety, restlessness, nervousness, and insomnia
St. John's wort	300 mg (standardized to 0.3% hypericum) tid	Herbal product used for anxiety and mild to moderate depression; may have efficacy for premenstrual dysphoria
Valerian	400–900 mg hs (sleep aid); 330 mg extract tid (restlessness)	Herbal product used for anxiety, restlessness, nervousness, and insomnia
Diuretics		
Spironolactone	25–50 mg qday, bid on days 14–28	Synthetic steroid aldosterone antagonist with K^+-sparing effect
Hydrochlorothiazide	25–50 mg qday, bid on days 14–28	Diuretic that enhances the excretion of Na^+, Cl^-, K^+, and H_2O
Triamterene	50–100 mg qday, bid on days 14–28	K^+-sparing diuretic; structurally related to folic acid
NSAIDs		
Ibuprofen	200-400 mg q 4–6 h; or 600 mg bid	Prostaglandin inhibitor; reduces pain, swelling, headache, and cramping; start regular dosing 7–10 days prior to menses
Mefenamic acid	250–500 mg tid	See ibuprofen; not to exceed 7 days
Naproxen	500 mg, then 250–500 mg bid	See ibuprofen
Naproxen sodium	500 mg, then 275–550 mg bid	See ibuprofen
Hormones		
Estradiol		
Oral	0.5–2 mg/day	Used for perimenopause to decrease emotional and physical symptoms (i.e., vasomotor symptoms, atrophic vaginitis, osteoporosis); used with concomitant natural progesterone if uterus is present to ↓ risk of endometriosis; intermittent therapy for estrogen withdrawal headache; used for postpartum depression and psychosis (transdermal)
Transdermal	100- to 200-μg patch every 3 days during cycle	See oral estradiol
Progesterone		
Oral	100 mg/day and 200 mg/day on days 17–28	Combined with estrogen to reduce risk of endometriosis; natural progesterones recommended instead of synthetic; not recommended for monotherapy for PMS
Suppository	200–400 mg bid on days 17–28	See oral progesterone
Oral contraceptives	1 pill/day estrogen + progesterone; use monophasic or biphasic with low progesterone for PMDD	Suppresses the hypothalamic-pituitary system and prevents ovulation; regulates the menstrual cycle; used for the treatment of endometriosis or dysfunctional uterine bleeding

TABLE 81–3. (Continued)

Agent/Drug	Dose	Clinical Reason for Use
Testosterone		
Transdermal	150 μg/day patch twice weekly + estrogen therapy	Androgen therapy used for low libido, blunted motivation, fatigue; monitor for virilization and fluid retention
Methyltestosterone		
Oral	1.25 mg with esterified estrogens 0.625 mg/day or 2.5 with esterified estrogens 1.25 mg/day	See testosterone
Danazol	200–400 mg/day: onset of breast pain until first day of menses	Synthetic androgen with antiestrogen effects; used for mastalgia and to suppress ovarian function prior to ovariectomy
Gonadotropin-releasing hormone agonists		
Leuprolide	3.75–7.5 mg IM q 4 wk	Causes anovulation and drops estrogen levels to menopausal levels; add back estrogen + progestin may reverse hormone deficiency state; used for endometriosis and severe PMDD
Buserelin	400–900 μg/day intranasally	See leuprolide
Dopamine Agonist		
Bromocriptine	2.5 mg bid on days 10–28	DA agonist; ↓ prolactin and reduces breast swelling and pain; use only for severe mastodynia
Antidepressants		
Selective serotonin reuptake inhibitor (SSRI)		
Citalopram	20–40 mg/day; 10–20 mg/day luteal only	5-HT–augmenting agents with antidepressant and antianxiety effects; used for PMDD, postpartum depression, and perimenopausal depression; continuous dosing or intermittent luteal phase only dosing for PMDD
Fluoxetine	20–40 mg/day; 5–20 mg/day luteal only	
Fluvoxamine	50–200 mg/day; 25–50 mg/day luteal only	
Paroxetine	20–30 mg/day; 5–20 mg/day luteal only	
Sertraline	50–150 mg/day; 25–50 mg/day luteal only	
Serotonin-norepinephrine-dopamine reuptake inhibitor		
Venlafaxine	75–375 mg/day in divided doses	5-HT–, NE-, and DA-augmenting agent with antidepressant and antianxiety effects; may be effective for PMDD
Norepinephrine-dopamine reuptake inhibitor		
Bupropion	75 mg tid; 100–150 mg bid-tid	NE- and DA-augmenting agent with antidepressant effects; avoid in eating disorder patients due to potential seizure risk at >450 mg/day; may not be effective for PMDD
Tricyclic antidepressant (TCA)		
Amitriptyline	25–50 mg hs, prn sleep	Sedating TCA with high anticholinergic and antihistaminic effects; used for insomnia and migraine prophylaxis
Clomipramine	25–125 mg/day; 25–50 mg/day luteal only	5-HT > NE-augmenting agent with antidepressant and antianxiety effects; used for PMDD
Doxepin	25–50 mg hs	See amitriptyline; primarily used for insomnia
Nortriptyline	50–125 mg/day	Metabolite of amitriptyline with less anticholinergic and antihistaminic effects; used for PMDD
Serotonin antagonist		
Nefazodone	100–400 mg/day	5-HT_{2A} and α_1 antagonist with antidepressant and antiaxiety effects
Trazodone	150–400 mg/day in divided doses; 25–150 mg hs	See nefazodone; primarily used for insomnia
Antianxiety agents		
Alprazolam	0.25–4 mg/day in divided doses continuous or days 16–28	BZD that augments $GABA_A$ receptor; antianxiety effects; do not use in patients with a history of substance abuse; taper down by not more than 25%/day
Buspirone	15–60 mg/day in divided doses continuous or days 16–28	5-HT_{1A} agonist with antianxiety effects
Hypnotic Agents		
Temazepam	7.5–30 mg hs	BZD that augments $GABA_A$ receptor; marketed as a hypnotic agent; use prn only for insomnia
Zaleplon	5–20 mg hs	Non-BZD that binds at the $GABA_A$-BZD receptor; rapid hypnotic effect with no significant antianxiety effects; use prn only for insomnia
Zolpidem	5–10 mg hs	See zaleplon

OCs = oral contraceptives; DA = dopamine; 5-HT = 5-hydroxytryptamine; PMS = premenstrual syndrome; OTC = over-the-counter; NSAIDs-nonsteroidal anti-inflammatory drugs; PMDD = premenstrual dysphoric disorder; IM = intramuscular; NE = norepinephrine; BZD = benzodiazepine; GABA = γ-aminobutyric acid.
Compiled from Refs. 3, 4, 7, 11, 18, 47, 66, and 72.

TABLE 81–4. First- and Second-Line Treatment Approaches for Menstruation-Related Disorders

Disorder/Symptom	First-Line	Second-Line
Standard approaches for menstruation-related disorders	Counseling/education; charting of symptoms for 2 cycles; good nutrition/diet; aerobic exercise; good sleep hygiene; stress management	Eliminate caffeine, nicotine, alcohol, drugs of abuse
General mild symptoms (low energy, poor diet)	Multiple vitamins + minerals; 1.5 g/day calcium	Add pyridoxine, magnesium, vitamin E, zinc, herbal therapies
Dysmenorrhea	NSAIDs	Meclofenamic acid, mefenamic acid, COX-2 inhibitors
Migraine headaches	Mild-moderate: NSAIDs Severe: 5-HT_{1D} agonists for abortive therapy (do not combine with other 5-HT agents)	Prophylaxis with atenolol, propranolol; amitriptyline; verapamil; valproate; estradiol; or combination therapy
Bloating/edema	Mild: salt restriction Moderate: spironolactone	Amiloride, metolazone, hydrochlorothiazide, triamterene ± HCTZ
Breast pain/mastalgia	Stop caffeine Mild: Vitamin E; evening primrose oil	Moderate: bromocriptine Severe: danazol Last resort: leuprolide, other GnRH-As
Insomnia	Stop caffeine and nicotine Mild: kava, melatonin, passion flower, valerian Moderate: diphenhydramine, doxylamine	Moderate: amitriptyline, doxepin, imipramine, trazodone Severe: lorazepam, temazepam, zaleplon, zolpidem
Anxiety	Stop caffeine and nicotine; avoid stimulants; stress management; relaxation training	Mild: buspirone Moderate: SSRIs; nefazodone Severe: alprazolam, clonazepam, lorazepam (avoid if substance abuse)
Binge-eating/craving foods/weight gain	High protein diet; regular meals; aerobic exercise	SSRIs (intermittent for luteal phase exacerbation)
Depression/PMDD	Mild: St. John's wort Moderate: SSRIs Alternative: clomipramine, nefazodone, nortriptyline, venlafaxine	Moderate: OCs (monophasic or biphasic) Severe: danazol trial, then leuprolide (or other GnRH-As) ± estrogen add-back ± progesterone Last resort: bilateral ovariectomy ± estrogen add-back ± progesterone
Seasonal PMS/PMDD	Bright light therapy	SSRIs
Mood swings/irritability PMDD	Stop caffeine and nicotine Moderate: SSRIs (intermittent or continuous therapy) Severe: Increase SSRI dose during luteal phase	Severe: lithium, carbamazepine, valproate (risk of teratogenesis) Alternative: verapamil, gabapentin, lamotrigine, topiramate (investigational)
Postpartum blues	Watch closely for persistence >2 wks, psychoeducation, vitamin and calcium supplementation	Hypnotics for sleep (prn): zaleplon, zolpidem, temazepam, trazodone, TCAs
Postpartum depression	Rule out thyroiditis Antidepressants: SSRIs, venlafaxine, TCAs Hypnotics for sleep (prn): zaleplon, zolpidem, temazepam, trazodone, TCAs	Moderate: estradiol (transdermal) ± anxiolytics; combination with SSRIs Severe: ECT
Postpartum psychosis	Mood stabilizers (e.g., lithium) ± estradiol (transdermal) ± antipsychotics	Severe: ECT
Perimenopausal		
Hot flashes, day sweats, and night sweats	Dress in layers, avoid hot rooms and hot showers, sleep in a cool room, aerobic exercise	ERT/HRT, low dose OCs, clonidine, herbal preparations, dietary soy supplements
Vaginal dryness/ dyspareunia	Vaginal lubricants or moisturizers; regular sexual stimulation	ERT/HRT, vaginal estrogen creams, low-dose OCs, herbal preparations, dietary soy supplements
Decreased libido/low energy/fatigue	Avoid sedating medications, good nutrition/diet, aerobic exercise, good sleep hygiene	Moderate: bupropion (if depressed) Severe: testosterone (if low free testosterone) with concurrent estrogen replacement, DHEA
Depression/anxiety	SSRIs, venlafaxine	

COX-2 inhibitors – cyclooxygenase-2 inhibitors (celecoxib, rofecoxib)
DHEA – dehydroepiandrosterone
ECT – electroconvulsive therapy
ERT – estrogen replacement therapy
GnRH-As – gonadotropin-releasing hormone agonists (buserelin, goserelin, leuprolide, triptorelin)
HCTZ – hydrochlorothiazide
HRT – hormone replacement therapy
5-HT – serotonin
NSAIDs – nonsteroidal anti-inflammatory drugs (ibuprofen, ketoprofen, naproxen)
OCs – oral contraceptives
PMDD – premenstrual dysphoric disorder
PMS – premenstrual syndrome
PRN – as required
SSRIs – selective serotonin reuptake inhibitors (citalopram, fluoxetine, fluvoxamine, paroxetine, sertraline)
TCAs – tricyclic antidepressants (amitriptyline, clomipramine, imipramine, nortriptyline)
Compiled Refs. 1, 2, 3, 7, 8, 10, 15, 18, 66, 67, 72, and 105.

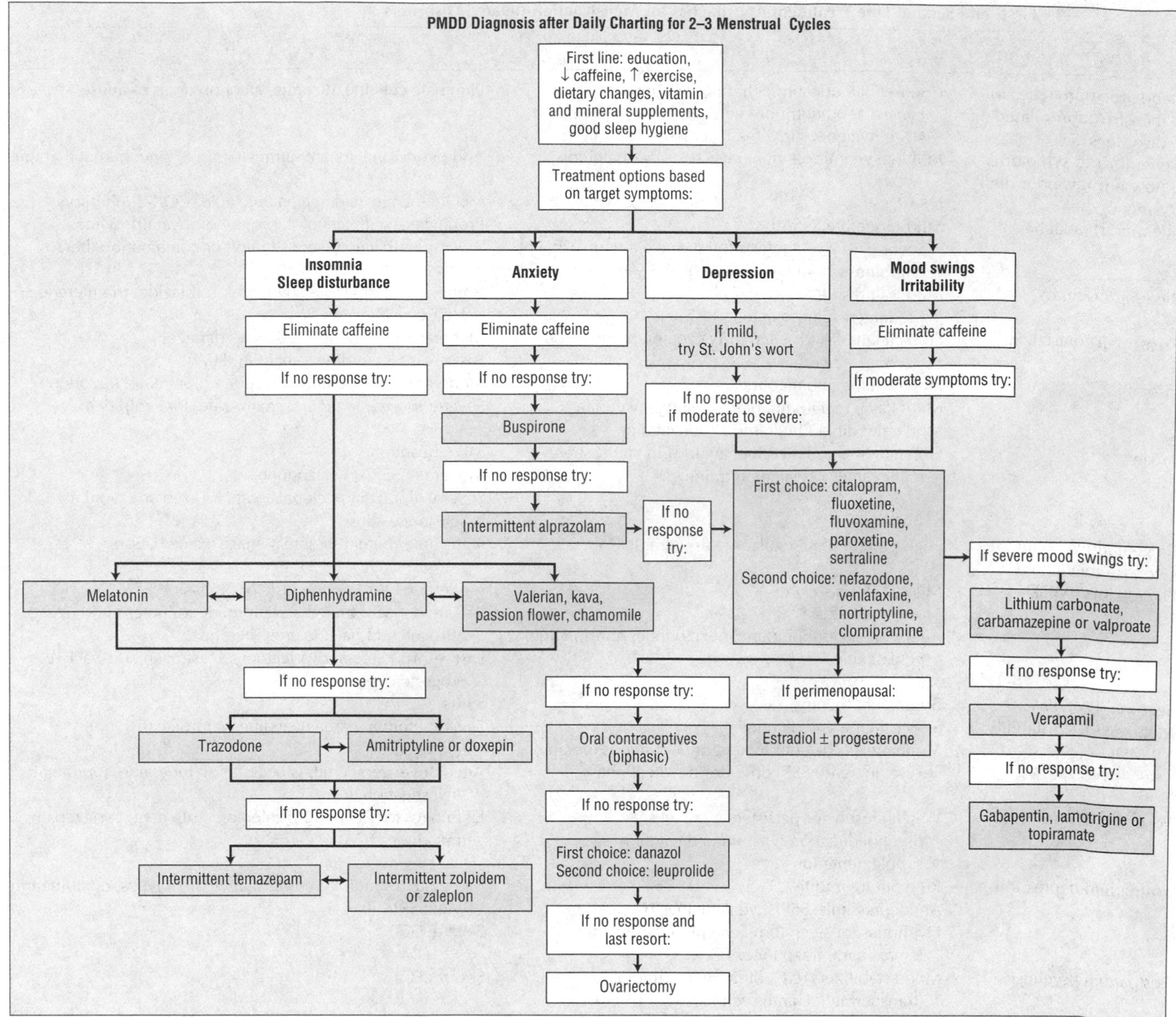

FIGURE 81–1. Algorithm for the treatment of premenstrual dysphoric disorder (PMDD).

intermittent estradiol therapy (oral or transdermal patch) started on days 24 to 26 and continued for 7 days through menstruation may help an "estrogen withdrawal" migraine.[21] If a women experiences a worsening of migraines with cyclic estradiol therapy, the dose can be lowered or changed to continuous oral or transdermal therapy.[19,21] Other prophylactic treatment approaches include the use of β-adrenergic blockers, calcium channel blockers, tricyclic antidepressants, or valproate. Agents that suppress ovulation, such as estrogen implants, danazol, and GnRH-As, have been used for menstrual migraines that are refractory to standard migraine therapies.[21]

Weight Gain and Bloating

Women with PMS commonly complain of bloating, swelling, and weight gain, despite little evidence that they actually retain fluid. Dietary salt restriction should be the first-line treatment. If sodium restriction is not effective and there is a documented weight gain of 5 pounds or more, diuretic therapy may be indicated. Spironolactone, an aldosterone antagonist with potassium-sparing properties, has been recommended for premenstrual weight gain and bloating.[4] Spironolactone has antiandrogenic effects, and women should not use it during pregnancy and lactation. Other diuretics (e.g., hydrochlorothiazide, metolazone, triamterene) have been used in treating premenstrual fluid retention.[18] Magnesium supplements have been reported to reduce premenstrual fluid retention after 2 months of treatment.[51]

Mastodynia

Vitamin E (α-tocopherol) decreases breast tenderness and swelling, and it is recommended for fibrocystic breast disease. Initial reports suggested that evening primrose oil, which contains the essential fatty acid γ-linolenic acid, reduces the severity of breast symptoms in PMS, but a meta-analysis of placebo-controlled studies concluded that it was not effective.[79] Although the oil may have little value in treating PMS, it is widely used as a nutritional supplement for breast tenderness.[11] The dopamine agonist, bromocriptine, has been used to inhibit prolactin secretion and reduce breast swelling, engorgement, and tenderness.[4,18] Antiestrogenic agents such as danazol and tamoxifen have been used to treat endometriosis and cystic mastitis. Danazol was reported to be highly effective for the relief of premenstrual mastalgia when given during the luteal phase only, but was less effective in treating the general symptoms of PMS.[80] Danazol should be reserved for the short-term treatment of breast pain or for the treatment of PMS that coexists with endometriosis and cystic mastitis resulting from androgenic and hypoestrogenic effects.[18]

Insomnia

Histamine$_1$ antagonists (e.g., diphenhydramine) and antidepressants with high histamine$_1$ blockade (doxepin, amitriptyline) have been used for acute sleep disturbances, but may cause anticholinergic side effects and daytime sedation. Trazodone, a 5-HT$_{2A}$ and α-adrenergic antagonist, has sedative properties at lower doses and may be useful to promote sleep. Trazodone has been used in combination with SSRIs, MAOIs, and bupropion as a hypnotic to reverse antidepressant-induced insomnia.

The chronic use of benzodiazepines is not recommended for insomnia because such use may lead to tolerance and physical dependence. If benzodiazepines are used for the acute treatment of insomnia, agents with shorter half-lives ($t_{1/2}$) should be used (e.g., lorazepam or temazepam). Ultra-short-acting hypnotic benzodiazepines (e.g., triazolam) are less likely to cause daytime sedation, but have an increased risk of causing anterograde amnesia, early morning insomnia, delirium, and withdrawal reactions. Zolpidem and zaleplon, nonbenzodiazepines that bind to the benzodiazepine$_1$ (omega$_1$) receptor subtype, are alternative agents for the treatment of premenstrual insomnia, but should be used only for short-term or intermittent therapy.

Melatonin has been used to regulate the sleep-wake cycle in the treatment of premenstrual and menopausal insomnia. It is not recommended during pregnancy and breastfeeding because of a lack of information about its safety.[54] Lower doses of melatonin (e.g., 0.1–1 mg hs) are effective in initiating sleep; higher doses may not improve the hypnotic effect.[54]

Anxiety

Before the advent of SSRIs, the treatment of PMS symptoms commonly included benzodiazepines. Compared with the SSRIs, the benzodiazepines have the advantage of acting quickly to reduce anxiety symptoms and promote sleep, but they also have the disadvantage of causing sedation, cognitive and motor impairment, tolerance, dependence, and withdrawal reactions. Alprazolam, a triazolobenzodiazepine marketed for the treatment of generalized anxiety and panic disorder, has been evaluated for the treatment of PMS in six double-blind, placebo controlled studies. Four of these studies reported that alprazolam was more effective than placebo in PMDD.[47] Intermittent dosing (e.g., 0.75–4 mg/day in divided doses 8 to 12 days before menses and gradually tapered down at menses by no more than 25%/day) and continuous dosing of alprazolam (e.g., 0.25 mg three times per day) reduced anxiety, irritability, tension, and feelings of being out of control in comparison to placebo. Because of the potential for dependency and worsening of mood, benzodiazepines should be used only for short-term treatment of menstruation-related mood disorders and should be avoided in dependency-prone patients.

Buspirone, a partial 5-HT$_{1A}$ agonist, has anxiolytic properties without causing sedation, cognitive impairment, or muscle relaxation. Buspirone is administered chronically for the treatment of anxiety, but some PMS studies used intermittent dosing (for 12 days before menstruation).[4,67] Not only does buspirone have minimal side effects, but also it has the advantage over benzodiazepines of not causing dependence or a withdrawal syndrome after abrupt discontinuation.

Depression

Serotonin deficiency or dysregulation (secondary to low levels of estradiol or high levels of MAO) during the premenstrual, postpartum, and premenopausal phase may be a cause of anxiety, depression, and irritability.[5,19,20,32,40,41] Initial studies using 5-HT-augmenting antidepressants (either continuous or intermittent dosing) reported positive benefits in reducing dysphoria, irritability, and tension in PMDD.[5,53,66] In addition, 5-HT antidepressants have been effective in reducing a premenstrual exacerbation of depression.[19] Nortriptyline and clomipramine, tricyclic antidepressants that inhibit the reuptake of 5-HT and norepinephrine, have been effective in the treatment of PMDD.[66,81] Nefazodone, a 5-HT$_{2A}$ antagonist with weak 5-HT reuptake inhibition, was reported to significantly improve PMS symptoms.[82] Venlafaxine, a 5-HT and norepinephrine reuptake inhibitor, may have efficacy in the treatment of PMDD.[14] L-tryptophan (the essential amino acid precursor for 5-HT) is currently not available as a dietary supplement, but it has been reported to be beneficial in PMDD.[44] Norepinephrine-augmenting antidepressants such as bupropion, desipramine, and maprotiline are generally less effective than serotonergic agents in the treatment of PMDD.[5,14,41,83–86]

Although several antidepressants have been shown to be effective for PMDD, serotonin reuptake inhibitors have a more favorable side effect profile and better efficacy data than other classes of antidepressants have.[14,41] Citalopram,[87] fluoxetine,[84,88–95] fluvoxamine,[96,97] paroxetine,[85,98] and sertraline,[83,86,99–103] have all been effective in PMDD placebo-controlled trials (60% to 90% efficacy rates with almost complete relief of symptoms). Although SSRIs take 3 weeks or more to relieve the symptoms of major depression, the agents work almost immediately to relieve premenstrual anxiety, depression, and irritability. SSRIs are generally well tolerated and effective in diminishing mood symptoms, irritability, food craving, overeating, and weight gain. The side effects of SSRIs, which are dose-related, are worse during the first few weeks of therapy (e.g., tiredness, sedation, upset stomach, nausea, decreased appetite, headache, dizziness, sweating, nervousness, insomnia, difficulty concentrating). A common long-term adverse effect of SSRIs is sexual dysfunction (e.g., decreased libido and delayed orgasm).[93] SSRIs have the advantage of not causing the significant weight gain, drowsiness, cardiovascular changes, and anticholinergic side effects that tricyclic antidepressants cause. Further, SSRIs appear to have minimal teratogenic risk when used in recommended doses during pregnancy.[61,63,64,104,105]

SSRIs may be effective in the treatment of PMDD at lower dosages than those required in major depression. Doses should be increased gradually if the agent's effectiveness erodes after several months of treatment.[53] If one SSRI is not effective or not tolerated, others should be tried until one is found to be effective. The intermittent administration of citalopram (10–30 mg/day) during the luteal phase has been reported to be more effective than continuous or semi-intermittent administration for PMDD.[87] A trial of intermittent luteal phase administration of clomipramine (25–75 mg/day)[81] and sertraline (50–100 mg/day)[102] reported a 1- to 2-day onset of effects. A study comparing full- or half-cycle sertraline treatment (50–150 mg/day) reported that both regimens were effective for PMS and that side effects were similar for both groups.[106] One study reported that women with PMDD who initially responded to full-cycle sertraline (100 mg/day) were successfully switched to half-cycle administration without a loss in efficacy.[103] With luteal phase administration, SSRIs may improve mood symptoms more than the physical discomforts. For postpartum and premenopausal depression, antidepressants are usually dosed daily at standard dosages for depression, although some women may respond to lower doses. Gender-related differences in the pharmacokinetics of antidepressants have been reported (e.g., higher plasma concentrations of amitriptyline, nortriptyline, clomipramine, imipramine, nefazodone, and sertraline in women).[19,20,58]

Mood Swings

Lithium carbonate, carbamazepine, and valproate are used as mood stabilizers and may be appropriate for women with predominant mood swings or those with a history of recurrent mood disorders.[18] Mood stabilizers should be used with caution during pregnancy because of their potential teratogenic effects. Lithium has numerous adverse effects (e.g., hypothyroidism) and requires routine blood level monitoring. Low-dose valproate (125–500 mg/day with mean serum levels of 32.5 μg/mL) was reported to decrease PMS symptoms and migraine headaches in a small study.[107] The usefulness of other investigational mood stabilizers such as verapamil, gabapentin, lamotrigine, and topiramate in the treatment of PMDD has not been evaluated.

HORMONAL THERAPIES

Progesterone

For many years, the administration of progesterone by vaginal suppositories during the luteal phase was a common hormonal treatment for PMS.[4] After several double-blind, placebo-controlled studies, it is now thought that progesterone is no better than placebo for treating PMS.[22,108] However, controversy still surrounds the form used (natural vs. synthetic), length of treatment (luteal phase vs. chronic therapy), and route of administration (oral, buccal/sublingual, vaginal, rectal, transdermal, topical, or implants).[22] An oral micronized form of natural progesterone is better absorbed and has advantages over synthetic progestins.[109] Progesterone may make some PMS symptoms worse (e.g., fatigue, depression, fluid retention, irritability, acne, increase in appetite), and it should be used with caution in certain medical conditions (e.g., migraine, seizure disorders, asthma, and cardiac or renal disease). Progestins are contraindicated in patients with thrombophlebitis and thromboembolic disorders. Because of its questionable efficacy and risk of adverse effects, progesterone-only therapy is not recommended as a treatment in PMS.

Estrogen

Estradiol, the active estrogen produced by the ovaries, is effective for menstrual migraines and for estrogen replacement therapy to control menopausal symptomatology. Estradiol implants and transdermal estradiol patches have been beneficial in reducing premenstrual symptoms.[4,9] The oral or transdermal administration of estradiol (combined with the cyclic or continuous administration of progesterone if the uterus is present) should be tried in perimenopausal women with significant premenstrual mood and physical symptoms. Given sublingually or transdermally, estradiol may be helpful for postpartum depression and psychosis.[8,17,34]

Chronic estradiol therapy suppresses ovulation and is more effective than oral conjugated estrogens.[4] Available products include a micronized and an ethinyl estradiol tablet; a cypionate and a valerate estradiol parenteral oil injection; a transdermal estradiol topical system; and a vaginal estradiol cream.[110] The transdermal estradiol patches may cause skin irritation and should be replaced at a new application site every 3 to 4 days. Because unopposed estrogen increases the risk for endometrial hyperplasia, intermittent or continuous progestin therapy (for 7 or more days of a cycle) is beneficial. Estradiol with intermittent progestin therapy (e.g., norethisterone 5 mg/day for 7 days each month to induce regular menses) may cause PMS-like side effects. Chronic estrogen-only therapy has certain risks (e.g., increasing risk of endometrial, ovarian, and breast cancer and gallbladder disease) and should not be administered during pregnancy.[29] Contraindications for using estrogens include breast cancer (relative contraindication), estrogen-dependent cancer, thrombophlebitis or thromboembolic disorders, undiagnosed abnormal uterine bleeding, and pregnancy.[29]

Estrogen-Progestin Combinations

Oral contraceptives cause anovulation and may reduce dysmenorrhea, depression, and irritability.[110] They can exacerbate PMS symptoms in approximately 30% of women, but some women may derive benefit. Biphasic or triphasic products have been used in PMS, but triphasic products may cause more mood swings.[28] A monophasic progesterone contraceptive agent may be given to inhibit hormone fluctuations, but may precipitate depressive symptoms.[19] Oral contraceptives high in progestin or progestin-only contraceptive agents may produce breakthrough bleeding and/or spotting, amenorrhea, acne, hirsutism, fatigue, and depression.[111] Pyridoxine replacement therapy, 50 mg/day, is recommended for women who become depressed while taking oral contraceptives. Because of the progestin effects, estrogen-progestin combinations have an increased risk of causing thrombophlebitis, pulmonary embolism, and cerebral thrombosis.

Testosterone

Testosterone replacement therapy, combined with estrogen replacement therapy, has been used in premenopausal and postmenopausal women to increase libido, decrease fatigue, and improve well-being.[37] Testosterone is available as methyltestosterone and in a combination product with esterified or conjugated estrogen, both to be given orally; in intramuscular injection, transdermal system, and implant forms (investigational); and as an oral, transdermal, and injectable estradiol and testosterone product.[112] Adverse effects of testosterone use in women include acne, edema, hirsutism, hoarseness, clitoral enlargement, menstrual irregularities, abnormal liver function tests, anxiety, mental depression, and insomnia.[112] Absolute contraindications include pregnancy and lactation. The lowest effective dose should be used, and patients should be monitored closely for virilization and fluid retention. Testosterone serum levels may need to be in the upper end of the normal range for ovulating women to restore libido.[37]

Gonadotropin-Releasing Hormone Agonists

Because of their down-regulation of pituitary gonadotropin secretion, GnRH-As (e.g., buserelin, goserelin, leuprolide, nafarelin, and triptorelin) cause a "medical ovariectomy" or "pseudomenopausal state."[4,113] The agents are used for the management of endometriosis and advanced breast cancer, as well as severe PMDD. GnRH-As can be administered subcutaneously, intranasally, by implants, or by intramuscular depot injections.[113] The initial administration of GnRH-As stimulates the release of FSH and LH from the pituitary, and then a down-regulation of the pituitary decreases ovarian stimulation to release estrogen and progesterone.[114] Initially, some women report a "flare" in PMS symptoms during the first few weeks of GnRH-As treatment, which is followed by a reduction in the physical and behavioral symptoms of PMS.[4] GnRH-As may improve cyclic mood changes and migraines during short-term therapy, but the chronic effects of suppressing ovarian hormone secretion could result in significant antiestrogen effects (osteoporosis and cardiovascular disease) and worsening of mood without low-dose hormone replacement therapy.[19]

GnRH-As therapy alone should not continue for longer than 6 months because of the risk of osteoporosis. The use of a combination of GnRH-As plus an "add-back" of estrogen/progestin may help to reverse antiestrogen and antiprogesterone effects, but may decrease the effectiveness of GnRH-As.[115] Low-dose GnRH-As therapy may be an option for PMS, but until the long-term safety is established, the agents should be used only for the most severe cases of PMS.[116]

SURGICAL THERAPY

Surgical ablation of the ovaries should be reserved as the last resort treatment for severe PMDD.[4] Before radical surgery, a 3- to 6-month trial of a GnRH-As or danazol is recommended to determine if anovulation is effective, because the ovariectomy is not reversible. A hysterectomy without an ovariectomy is not effective for PMS. A woman who has an ovariectomy without a hysterectomy needs both estrogen and progestin replacement therapy. Women who have both the ovariectomy and hysterectomy can receive continuous estradiol without intermittent progestin therapy because there is no risk for endometrial cancer.

PHARMACOECONOMIC CONSIDERATIONS

Few studies have prospectively documented the degree of functional impairment before or after specific treatments or have evaluated the pharmacoeconomic differences in treatments for premenstrual, postpartum, and perimenopausal disorders. Several PMDD studies have reported greater improvement in psychosocial functioning with sertraline than with desipramine or placebo, according to several rating scales (e.g., Daily Record of Severity of Problems, the Social Adjustment Scale, the Quality of Life Enjoyment and Satisfaction Questionnaire).[86,100,117] In all studies, the degree of functional impairment was substantial at baseline and similar to that seen in studies of major depression. The functional improvement correlated with the improvement in premenstrual symptoms and was evident by the second cycle of treatment.[118]

Untreated depression may contribute to the development of a chronic and refractory mood disorder that significantly impairs psychosocial functioning. More studies are needed because severe menstruation-related disorders are disabling; prompt diagnosis and efficacious treatments are essential to improve functioning, to reduce morbidity and mortality, and to decrease the negative impact on children and families.

EVALUATION OF THERAPEUTIC OUTCOMES

A trial of at least three menstrual cycles is needed to determine the treatment efficacy of one therapy and to adjust dosing before resorting to another therapy. Self-rating of PMS symptoms using a severity rating scale helps to monitor the efficacy of different treatment approaches.[1,118] The reduction of baseline premenstrual ratings (the average score for 5 to 7 days prior to menses) by 50% should be the minimum goal of therapy. Ideally, relief would be complete when premenstrual ratings are similar to postmenstrual ratings 5 to 7 days after the cessation of menses for several menstrual cycles.

Patients who are undergoing therapy for menstruation-related disorders should have a monthly examination by a clinician to assess efficacy, adverse effects, and adjust dosing, if needed. If first-line treatment approaches are not effective after several months, then alternative or combination therapies should be considered. For postpartum disorders, women should be monitored every 1 to 2 weeks to determine their response to treatments so that therapy can be adjusted or changed to alternative approaches, should it be required. Perimenopausal women should be monitored every 1 to 2 months to determine the effectiveness of treatment. Once a patient is stable and responding to the treatment plan, monitoring may be extended to every 3 to 6 months. Menopause is a health concern and should be monitored regularly because of the increased risk of osteoporosis, cardiovascular disease, and dementia. Throughout therapy, patients should be encouraged to eat well-balanced meals, to engage in regular exercise, to limit caffeine, to avoid drinking excessive alcohol or using drugs of abuse, to practice good sleep hygiene, and to take medications as prescribed to maximize treatment outcomes.

CONCLUSIONS

Menstruation-related disorders are very common and cause significant disability and impairment in functioning, if not properly treated. Therapeutic strategies should be individualized and targeted to the most distressing symptoms. If possible, medications should not be prescribed unless nonpharmacologic approaches have failed or unless symptoms disrupt the patient's functioning. The regular assessment and monitoring of menstruation-related disorders is necessary throughout the woman's reproductive years.

► PRINCIPLES OF PHARMACOTHERAPY

- A correct diagnosis of dysmenorrhea, premenstrual syndrome (PMS), premenstrual dysphoric disorder (PMDD), postpartum psychiatric disorders, and perimenopause is essential. An evaluation and careful workup should rule out other possible causes of the target symptoms.
- A stepwise treatment approach using safer agents first and reserving more toxic agents or combination therapies for refractory or severe symptoms is recommended for PMS and PMDD.

- Education, supportive therapy, regular exercise, dietary changes (e.g., limiting caffeine, salt, and alcohol), and good sleep hygiene are first-line approaches for all menstruation-related disorders.
- Nonsteroidal anti-inflammatory drugs (NSAIDs) are the treatment of choice for dysmenorrhea and menstrual headaches.
- Serotonin-augmenting agents (i.e., selective serotonin reuptake inhibitors [SSRIs]) are the most effective treatment for PMDD. SSRIs may be given intermittently during the luteal phase or continuously, although some women, if symptomatic, may require an increase in dose during the luteal phase.
- Combination therapies (e.g., hormonal agents plus antidepressants; NSAIDs plus antianxiety agents) may be needed if monotherapy is ineffective or if multiple symptoms are present for PMS and PMDD.
- Postpartum depression should be treated with antidepressants (and antipsychotics or mood stabilizers, if needed for psychosis). Electroconvulsive therapy should be considered for severe cases that involve psychosis or suicidality. Prophylaxis at the time of delivery is recommended for women with at least one previous postpartum depression.
- Perimenopausal women should be considered for hormone replacement therapy, because estrogen deficiency causes numerous health-related problems.
- After a 3-month trial of a pharmacologic agent, the risks versus the benefits of treatment should be evaluated, based on the severity of adverse effects and the efficacy of therapy for the menstrual disorder.

REFERENCES

1. Pearlstein T, Stone AB. Premenstrual syndrome. Psychiatr Clin N Am 1998;21(3):577–590.
2. Haynes P, Parry BL. Mood disorders and the reproductive cycle: affective disorders during the menopause and premenstrual dysphoric disorder. Psychopharmacol Bull 1998;34(3):313–318.
3. Suri R, Burt VK. The assessment and treatment of postpartum psychiatric disorders. J Pract Psychiatry Behav Health 1997;3:67–77.
4. Korzekwa MI, Steiner M. Premenstrual syndromes. Clin Obstet Gynecol 1997;40(3):564–576.
5. Steiner M, Pearlstein T. Premenstrual dysphoria and the serotonin system: pathophysiology and treatment. J Clin Psychiatry 2000;61(suppl 12):17–21.
6. American Psychiatric Association. Diagnostic and Statistical Manual of Mental Disorders. Fourth Edition, Text Revision. Washington, DC: American Psychiatric Press, 2000:771–774.
7. Llewellyn AM, Stowe ZN, Nemeroff CB. Depression during pregnancy and the puerperium. J Clin Psychiatry 1997;58(suppl 15):26–32.
8. Nonacs R, Cohen LS. Postpartum mood disorders: diagnosis and treatment guidelines. J Clin Psychiatry 1998;59(suppl 2):34–40.
9. Arpels JC. The female brain hypoestrogenic continuum from the premenstrual syndrome to menopause: a hypothesis and review of supporting data. J Reprod Med 1996;41:633–639.
10. Burt VK, Altshuler LL, Rasgon N. Depressive symptoms in the perimenopause: prevalence, assessment, and guidelines for treatment. Harvard Rev Psychiatry 1998;6(3):121–132.
11. Frye GM, Silverman SD. Is it premenstrual syndrome? Keys to focused diagnosis, therapies for multiple symptoms. Postgrad Med 2000; 107(5):151–159.
12. Yonkers KA. Anxiety symptoms and anxiety disorders: how are they related to premenstrual disorders? J Clin Psychiatry 1997;58(suppl 3): 62–67.
13. Yonkers KA. The association between premenopausal dysphoric disorder and other mood disorders. J Clin Psychiatry 1997;58(suppl 15):19–25.
14. Yonkers KA. Antidepressants in the treatment of premenstrual dysphoric disorder. J Clin Psychiatry 1997;58(suppl 14):4–10.
15. Altshuler LL, Hendrick V, Cohen LS. Course of mood and anxiety disorders during pregnancy and the postpartum period. J Clin Psychiatry 1998;59(suppl 2):29–33.
16. Halbreich U. Premenstrual syndromes: closing the 20th century chapters. Curr Opin Obstet Gynecol 1999;11:265–270.
17. Joffe H, Cohen LS. Estrogen, serotonin, and mood disturbance: Where is the therapeutic bridge? Biol Psychiatry 1998;44:798–811.
18. Parry BL. Psychobiology of premenstrual dysphoric disorder. Semin Reprod Endocrinol 1997;15(1):55–68.
19. Ensom MHH. Gender-based differences and menstrual cycle-related changes in specific diseases: implications for pharmacotherapy. Pharmacotherapy 2000;20(5):523–539.
20. Kashuba ADM, Nafziger AN. Physiological changes during the menstrual cycle and their effects on the pharmacokinetics and pharmacodynamics of drugs. Clin Pharmacokinet 1998;34(3):203–218.
21. Case AM, Reid RL. Effects of the menstrual cycle on medical disorders. Arch Intern Med 1998;158(13):1405–1412.
22. Freeman EW. Premenstrual syndrome: current perspectives on treatment and etiology. Curr Opin Obstet Gynecol 1997;9:147–153.
23. Mortola JF. Premenstrual syndrome—pathophysiologic considerations. N Engl J Med 1998;338(4):256–257.
24. Mortola JF. Premenstrual syndrome. Curr Ther Endocrinol Metab 1997; 6:251-256.
25. Korzekwa MI, Steiner M. Premenstrual syndromes. Clin Obstet Gynecol 1997;40:564–576.
26. Sundstrom I, Backstrom T, Wang M, et al. Premenstrual syndrome, neuroactive steroids and the brain. Gynecol Endocrinol 1999;13:206–220.
27. Jensvold MF. Nonpregnant reproductive-age women, part I. The menstrual cycle and psychopharmacology. In: Jensvold MF, Halbreich U, Hamilton JA, eds. Psychopharmacology and Women: Sex, Gender, and Hormones. Washington, DC: American Psychiatric Press, 1996:139–169.
28. Janowsky DS, Halbreich U, Rausch J. Association among ovarian hormones, other hormones, emotional disorders, and neurotransmitters. In: Jensvold MF, Halbreich U, Hamilton JA, eds. Psychopharmacology and Women: Sex, Gender, and Hormones. Washington, DC: American Psychiatric Press, 1996:85–106.
29. Stahl SM. Basic psychopharmacology of antidepressants, part 2: estrogen as an adjunct to antidepressant therapy. J Clin Psychiatry 1998;59(suppl 4):15–42.
30. Schmidt PJ, Nieman LK, Danaceau MA, et al. Differential behavioral effects of gonadal steroids in women with and in those without premenstrual syndrome. N Engl J Med 1998;338:209–216.
31. Archer JSM. Relationship between estrogen, serotonin, and depression. Menopause 1999;6:71–78.
32. Rubinow DR, Schmidt PJ, Roca CA. Estrogen-serotonin interactions: implications for affective regulation. Biol Psychiatry 1998;44:839–850.
33. Rodriguez MM, Grossberg GT. Estrogen as a psychotherapeutic agent. Clin Geriatr Med 1998;14(1):177–189.
34. Ahokas A, Aito M, Rimon R. Positive treatment effect of estradiol in postpartum psychosis: a pilot study. J Clin Psychiatry 2000;61:166–169.
35. Bicikova M, Dibbelt L, Hill M, et al. Allopregnenolone in women with premenstrual syndrome. Horm Metab Res 1998;30:227–230.
36. Sundstrom I, Andersson A, Nyberg S, et al. Patients with premenstrual syndrome have a different sensitivity to a neuroactive steroid during the menstrual cycle compared to control subjects. Neuroendocrinology 1998;67:126–138.
37. Davis SR. Androgen treatment in women. Med J Aust 1999;170:545–549.
38. Gurguis GNM, Yonkers KA, Phan SP, et al. Adrenergic receptors in premenstrual dysphoric disorder: I. Platelet α_2 receptors: G_i protein coupling, phase of menstrual cycle, and prediction of luteal phase symptom severity. Biol Psychiatry 1998;44:600–609.

39. Girdler SS, Pedersen CA, Straneva PA, et al. Dysregulation of cardiovascular and neuroendocrine responses to stress in premenstrual dysphoric disorder. Psychiatry Res 1998;81:163–178.
40. Severino SK. A focus on 5-hydroxytryptamine (serotonin) and psychopathology. In: Gold JH, Severino SK, eds. Premenstrual Dysphorias: Myths and Realities. Washington, DC: American Psychiatric Press, 1994:67–98.
41. Eriksson E. Serotonin reuptake inhibitors for the treatment of premenstrual dysphoria. Int Clin Psychopharmacol 1999;14(suppl 2):S27–S33.
42. FitzGerald M, Malone KM, Li S, et al. Blunted serotonin response to fenfluramine challenge in premenstrual dysphoric disorder. Am J Psychiatry 1997;154:556–558.
43. Halbreich U. Premenstrual dysphoric disorders: a diversified cluster of vulnerability traits to depression. Acta Psychiatr Scand 1997;95:169–176.
44. Steinberg S, Annable L, Young SN, et al. A placebo-controlled clinical trial of L-tryptophan in premenstrual dysphoria. Biol Psychiatry 1999;45:313–320.
45. Halbreich U, Petty F, Yonkers K, et al. Low plasma γ-aminobutyric acid levels during the late luteal phase of women with premenstrual dysphoric disorder. Am J Psychiatry 1996;153:718–720.
46. Chuong CJ, Dawson EB. Critical evaluation of nutritional factors in the pathophysiology and treatment of premenstrual syndrome. Clin Obstet Gynecol 1992;35:679–692.
47. Pearlstein T, Steiner M. Non-antidepressant treatment of premenstrual syndrome. J Clin Psychiatry 2000;61(suppl 12):22–27.
48. Thys-Jacobs S, Starkey P, Bernstein D, et al. Calcium carbonate and the premenstrual syndrome: effects on premenstrual and menstrual symptoms. Am J Obstet Gynecol 1998;179:444–452.
49. Thys-Jacobs S. Micronutrients and the premenstrual syndrome: the case for calcium. J Am Coll Nutr 2000;19(2):220–227.
50. Ward MW, Holimon TD. Calcium treatment for premenstrual syndrome. Ann Pharmacother 1999;33:1356–1358.
51. Walker AF, DeSouza MC, Vickers MF, et al. Magnesium supplementation alleviates premenstrual symptoms of fluid retention. J Women's Health 1998;7:1157–1165.
52. Parry BL, Berga SL, Mostofi N, et al. Plasma melatonin circadian rhythms during the menstrual cycle and after light therapy in premenstrual dysphoric disorder and normal control subjects. J Biol Rhythms 1997;12:47–64.
53. Gold JH, Premenstrual dysphoric disorder: an update. J Pract Psychiatry Behav Health 1999;5:209–215.
54. Avery D, Lenz M, Landis C. Guidelines for prescribing melatonin. Ann Med 1998;30:122–130.
55. Parry BL, Cover H, Mostofi N, et al. Early versus late partial sleep deprivation in patients with premenstrual dysphoric disorder and normal comparison subjects. Am J Psychiatry 1995;152:404–412.
56. Parry BL, Mostofi N, LeVeau B, et al. Sleep EEG studies during early and late partial sleep deprivation in premenstrual dysphoric disorder and normal control subjects. Psychiatry Res 1999;85:127–143.
57. Kornstein SG. Gender differences in depression: implications for treatment. J Clin Psychiatry 1997;58(suppl 15):12–18.
58. Frackiewicz EJ, Sramek JJ, Cutler NR. Gender differences in depression and antidepressant pharmacokinetics and adverse events. Ann Pharmacother 2000;34:80–88.
59. Bloch M, Schmidt PJ, Rubinow DR. Premenstrual syndrome: evidence for symptom stability across cycles. Am J Psychiatry 1997;154:1741–1746.
60. Roca CA, Schmidt PJ, Rubinow DR. A follow up study of premenstrual syndrome. J Clin Psychiatry 1999;60:763–766.
61. Altshuler LL, Cohen L, Szuba MP, et al. Pharmacologic management of psychiatric illness during pregnancy: dilemmas and guidelines. Am J Psychiatry 1996;153:592–606.
62. American Academy of Pediatrics Committee on Drugs. Use of psychoactive medication during pregnancy and possible effects on the fetus and newborn. Pediatrics 2000;105(4):880–887.
63. Cohen LS, Rosenbaum JF. Psychotropic drug use during pregnancy: weighing the risks. J Clin Psychiatry 1998;59(suppl 2):18–28.
64. Koren G, Pastuszak A, Itol S. Drugs in pregnancy. N Engl J Med 1998; 338(16):1128–1137.
65. Llewellyn A, Stowe ZN. Psychotropic medications in lactation. J Clin Psychiatry 1998;59(suppl 2):41–52.
66. Yonkers KA, Brown WA. Pharmacologic treatments for premenstrual dysphoric disorder. Psychiatry Ann 1996;26(9):586–589.
67. Pearlstein T. Nonpharmacologic treatment of premenstrual syndrome. Psychiatry Ann 1996;26(9):590–594.
68. Singh BB, Berman BM, Simpson RL, et al. Incidence of premenstrual syndrome and remedy usage: a national probability sample study. Altern Ther Health Med 1998;4(3):75–79.
69. A decision tree for the use of estrogen replacement therapy or hormone replacement therapy in postmenopausal women: Consensus Opinion of the North American Menopause Society. Menopause 2000;7:76–86.
70. Walker AF, DeSouza MC, Vickers MF, et al. Magnesium supplementation alleviates premenstrual symptoms of fluid retention. J Women's Health 1998;7:1157–1165.
71. De Souza MC, Walker AF, Robinson PA, et al. A synergistic effect of a daily supplement for 1 month of 200 mg magnesium plus 50 mg vitamin B_6 for the relief of anxiety-related premenstrual symptoms: a randomized, double-blind, crossover study. J Women's Health Gend Based Med 2000; 9(2):131–139.
72. Wong AHC, Smith M, Boon HS. Herbal remedies in psychiatric practice. Arch Gen Psychiatry 1998;55:1033–1044.
73. Klepser TB, Klepser ME. Unsafe and potentially safe herbal therapies. Am J Health Syst Pharm 1999;56:125–138.
74. Stevinson C, Ernest E. A pilot study of *Hypericum perforatum* for the treatment of premenstrual syndrome. Br J Obstet Gynaecol 2000;107: 870–876.
75. Ernst E. Second thoughts about safety of St. John's wort. Lancet 1999; 354:2014–2016.
76. Loch E-G, Selle H, Boblitz N. Treatment of premenstrual syndrome with a phytopharmaceutical formulation containing *Vitex agnus castus.* J Women's Health Gend Based Med 2000;9(3):315–320.
77. Brzezinski A, Adlercreutz H, Shaoul R, et al. Short-term effects of phytoestrogen-rich diet on postmenopausal women. Menopause 1997; 4:89–94.
78. Nonsteroidal anti-inflammatory agents. In: McEvoy GK, Litvak K, Welsh OH, et al., eds. AHFS Drug Information 2000. Bethesda, MD: American Society of Health-System Pharmacists, 2000:1771–1796.
79. Budeiri D, Li Wan Po A, Dornan JC. Is evening primrose oil of value in the treatment of premenstrual syndrome? Control Clin Trials 1996;17(1): 60–68.
80. O'Brien PMS, Abukhlil IEH. Randomized controlled trial of the management of premenstrual syndrome and premenstrual mastalgia using luteal phase-only danazol. Am J Obstet Gynecol 1999; 180:18–23.
81. Sundblad C, Hedberg MA, Ericksson E. Clomipramine administration during luteal phase reduces the symptoms of premenstrual syndrome: a placebo-controlled trial. Neuropsychopharmacology 1993;9:133–145.
82. Freeman EW, Rickels K, Sondheimer SJ, et al. Nefazodone in the treatment of premenstrual syndrome: a preliminary study. J Clin Psychopharmacol 1994;14:180–186.
83. Freeman EW, Rickels K, Sondheimer SJ, Wittmaack FM. Sertraline versus desipramine in the treatment of premenstrual syndrome: an open-label trial. J Clin Psychiatry 1996;57:7–11.
84. Pearlstein TB, Stone AB, Lund SA, et al. Comparison of fluoxetine, bupropion, and placebo in the treatment of premenstrual dysphoric disorder. J Clin Psychopharmacol 1997;17:261–266.
85. Eriksson E, Hedberg MA, Andersch B, et al. The serotonin reuptake inhibitor paroxetine is superior to the noradrenaline reuptake inhibitor maprotiline in the treatment of premenstrual syndrome. Neuropsychopharmacology 1995;12:167–176.
86. Freeman EW, Rickels K, Sondheimer SJ, et al. Differential response to antidepressants in women with premenstrual syndrome/premenstrual dysphoric disorder: a randomized controlled trial. Arch Gen Psychiatry 1999;56:932–939.
87. Wikander I, Sundblad C, Andersch B, et al. Citalopram in premenstrual dysphoria: Is intermittent treatment during luteal phases more

effective than continuous medication throughout the menstrual cycle? J Clin Psychopharmacol 1998;18:390–398.

88. Rickels K, Freeman EW, Sondheimer S, Albert J. Fluoxetine in the treatment of premenstrual syndrome. Curr Therapeutic Res 1990;48: 161–166.
89. Stone AB, Pearlstein TB, Brown WA. Fluoxetine in the treatment of late luteal phase dysphoric disorder. J Clin Psychiatry 1991;52:290–293.
90. Menkes DB, Taghavi, Mason PA, et al. Fluoxetine treatment of severe premenstrual syndrome. BMJ 1992;305:346–347.
91. Menkes DB, Taghavi, Mason PA, Howard RC. Fluoxetine's spectrum of action in premenstrual syndrome. Int Clin Psychopharmacol 1993;8: 95–102.
92. Wood SH, Mortola JF, Chan YF, et al. Treatment of premenstrual syndrome with fluoxetine: a double-blind, placebo-controlled, crossover study. Obstet Gynecol 1992;80:339–344.
93. Pearlstein TB, Stone AB. Long-term fluoxetine treatment of late luteal phase dysphoric disorder. J Clin Psychiatry 1994;5:332–335.
94. Steiner M, Steinberg S, Stewart D, et al. Fluoxetine in the treatment of premenstrual dysphoria. N Engl J Med 1995;332:1529–1534.
95. Su TP, Schmidt PJ, Danaceau MA, et al. Fluoxetine in the treatment of premenstrual dysphoria. Neuropsychopharmacology 1997;16:346–356.
96. Veeninga AT, Westenberg HGM, Weusten JTN. Fluvoxamine in the treatment of menstrually related mood disorders. Psychopharmacology 1990;102:414–416.
97. Freeman EW, Rickels K, Sondheimer SJ. Fluvoxamine for premenstrual dysphoric disorder: a pilot study. J Clin Psychiatry 1996;57(suppl 8): 56–59.
98. Yonkers KA, Gullion C, Williams A, et al. Paroxetine as a treatment for premenstrual dysphoric disorder. J Clin Psychopharmacol 1996;16:3–8.
99. Yonkers KA, Halbreich U, Freeman E, et al. Sertraline in the treatment of premenstrual dysphoric disorder. Psychopharmacol Bull 1996;32(1): 41–46.
100. Yonkers KA, Halbreich U, Freeman E, et al. Symptomatic improvement of premenstrual dysphoric disorder with sertraline treatment: a randomized controlled trial. JAMA 1997;278:983–988.
101. Young SA, Hurt PH, Benedek DM, et al. Treatment of premenstrual dysphoric disorder with sertraline during the luteal phase: a randomized, double-blind, placebo-controlled crossover trial. J Clin Psychiatry 1998;59:76–80.
102. Jermain DM, Preece CK, Sykes RL, et al. Luteal phase sertraline treatment for premenstrual dysphoric disorder: results of a double-blind, placebo-controlled, crossover study. Arch Fam Med 1999; 8:328–332.
103. Halbreich U, Smoller JW. Intermittent luteal phase sertraline treatment of dysphoric premenstrual syndrome. J Clin Psychiatry 1997;58;399–402.
104. Kulin NA, Pastuszak A, Sage SR, et al. Pregnancy outcome following material use of the new selective serotonin reuptake inhibitors: a prospective controlled multicenter study. JAMA 1998;279:609–610.
105. Wisner KL, Gelenberg AJ, Leonard H, et al. Pharmacologic treatment of depression during pregnancy. JAMA 1999;282:1264–1269.
106. Freeman EW, Rickels K, Arredondo F, et al. Full- or half-cycle treatment of severe premenstrual syndrome with a serotonergic antidepressant. J Clin Psychopharmacol 1999;19:3–8.
107. Jacobsen FM. Low-dose valproate: a new treatment for cyclothymia, mild rapid cycling disorders, and premenstrual syndrome. J Clin Psychiatry 1993;54:229–234.
108. Freeman EW, Rickels K, Sondheimer SJ, Polansky M. A double-blind trial of oral progesterone, alprazolam, and placebo in treatment of severe premenstrual syndrome. JAMA 1995;274:51–57.
109. McAuley JW, Kroboth FJ, Kroboth PD. Oral administration of micronized progesterone: a review and more experience. Pharmacotherapy 1996;16:453–457.
110. Estrogens. In: McEvoy GK, Litvak K, Welsh OH, et al., eds. AHFS Drug Information 2000. Bethesda, MD: American Society of Health-System Pharmacists, 2000:2790–2797.
111. Estrogen-progestin combinations. In: McEvoy GK, Litvak K, Welsh OH, et al., eds. AHFS Drug Information 2000. Bethesda, MD: American Society of Health-System Pharmacists, 2000:2776–2788.
112. Testosterone. In: McEvoy GK, Litvak K, Welsh OH, et al., eds. AHFS Drug Information 2000. Bethesda, MD: American Society of Health-System Pharmacists, 2000:2772–2776.
113. Leuprolide acetate. In: McEvoy GK, Litvak K, Welsh OH, et al., eds. AHFS Drug Information 2000. Bethesda, MD: American Society of Health-System Pharmacists, 2000:989–998.
114. Roca CA, Schmidt PJ, Bloch M, Rubinow DR. Implications of endocrine studies of premenstrual syndrome. Psychiatry Ann 1996;26:576–580.
115. Leather AT, Studd JWW, Watson NR, et al. The treatment of severe premenstrual syndrome with goserelin with and without "add-back" estrogen therapy: a placebo- controlled study. Gynecol Endocrinol 1999;13:48–55.
116. Sundstrom L, Nyberg S, Bixo M, et al. Treatment of premenstrual syndrome with gonadotropin-releasing hormone agonist in a low dose regimen. Acta Obstet Gynecol Scand 1999;8:891–899.
117. Pearlstein TB, Halbreich U, Batzar ED, et al. Psychosocial functioning in women with premenstrual dysphoric disorder before and after treatment with sertraline and placebo. J Clin Psychiatry 2000;61:101–109.
118. Thys-Jacobs S, Alvir JMJ, Fratarcangelo P. Comparative analysis of three PMS assessment instruments: the identification of premenstrual syndrome with core symptoms. Psychopharmacol Bull 1995;31:389–396.

82

ENDOMETRIOSIS

Cynthia L. Lieu

Endometriosis is a chronic, recurring disease that is defined by the presence of endometrial tissue (glands and stroma) outside of the uterine cavity, most commonly in the peritoneal cavity. Affecting as many as 10% of reproductive-age women, endometriosis is a major cause of chronic pelvic pain, dysmenorrhea, dyspareunia (painful intercourse), and infertility.

EPIDEMIOLOGY

Endometriosis is predominantly seen in women of reproductive age, but has been documented in females from 10.5 years to 76 years old.[1] Because laparoscopy or surgery is necessary to make a definitive diagnosis, the exact prevalence of endometriosis is unknown. Estimates range from 6% to 44%, but vary from 2.5% to 5.9% in fertile premenopausal women to 20% to 50% in infertile women.[2] The incidence is estimated to be 71% in women with pelvic pain, 84% in women with infertility and pelvic pain, and 45% to 50% in asymptomatic women who undergo laparoscopy.[3] Endometriosis affects 45% to 70% of adolescents with chronic pelvic pain and dysmenorrhea.[1] In the United States, endometriosis is the third leading cause of gynecologic-related hospitalizations and a leading cause of hysterectomy.[4] Approximately 4 per 1,000 women aged 15 to 64 years old are hospitalized with endometriosis each year, slightly more than those admitted with breast cancer.[5] Endometriosis has also been reported in men who receive high-dose estrogen therapy.[6]

ETIOLOGY

The etiology of endometriosis is uncertain. The most commonly accepted theory is transplantation of endometrial tissue from retrograde menstrual flow through the fallopian tubes, followed by implantation at ectopic sites. This theory is supported by the occurrence of endometrial lesions most commonly in the dependent portions of the pelvis and an increased likelihood of endometriosis in women with menstrual characteristics facilitating ectopic endometrial implantation.[5] Many more women experience retrograde menstruation than have endometriosis, suggesting that other mechanisms may play a role in the etiology. Other theories include metaplastic transformation of coelomic epithelium into functioning endometrial tissue, lymphatic and vascular spread to locations outside of the peritoneal cavity, iatrogenic mechanical transplantation, and deficient cell-mediated immunity (impairing clearance of endometriotic cells).[1,7] A genetic basis for endometriosis has been suggested by the increased prevalence in first-degree relatives of patients with endometriosis.[8] Endometriotic tissue has been found to express aromatase P450, resulting in higher local production of estrogen to maintain the growth and spread of the lesions.[3] Endometriosis may be the result of several mechanisms, with no single theory explaining all cases of the disease.

Risk factors for endometriosis include obstructed menstrual flow through the vagina, genital tract anomalies, and a family history.[7,9] Increased risk appears to be related to increased exposure to menstruation (Table 82–1). Increased time since the last pregnancy has also been linked to endometriosis. Factors that may decrease the risk of endometriosis include reduced menstrual cycling and suppression of estrogen by pregnancy, oral contraceptive (OC) use, and menopause. Personal habits that relate to decreased body estrogen levels, such as exercise and smoking, have been associated with a decreased risk for endometriosis, while patients with endometriosis tend to have more peripheral body fat and higher estrogen levels.[4] Exposure to environmental factors (e.g., chlorinated hydrocarbons, dioxin) has also been associated with endometriosis.[11]

PATHOPHYSIOLOGY

Endometriotic lesions contain estrogen and progesterone receptors. Symptoms are often related to their ability to respond to cyclic hormonal stimulation in women of reproductive age. Although most lesions are found in the pelvis (ovaries, anterior and posterior cul-de-sac, posterior surface of the broad ligament, uterosacral ligaments, fallopian tubes, peritoneum, pouch of Douglas, rectovaginal septum), they may also affect the adjacent bowels, bladder, and ureter.[3,10,12] Endometriosis has also been reported in pelvic lymph notes, pleural tissue, pulmonary parenchyma, bone, biceps muscle, peripheral nerves, brain, episiotomy scars after vaginal delivery, laparotomy scars after caesarean section, needle tracts after amniocentesis, and umbilical incisions after laparoscopic tubal ligation.[7] Endometriomas (endometrial cysts within the ovary) are the most typical lesions seen in patients with ovarian endometriosis.

Various immunologic abnormalities are demonstrated in patients with endometriosis (Table 82–2). It is not known whether they contribute to the formation of endometriotic lesions or are a result of the disease. Immunologic deficiencies may allow endometriotic tissue to implant and grow.

Pelvic pain may be secondary to inflammation, pressure, adhesions, neuronal involvement, and/or prostaglandin (PG) production. Increased macrophages and other peritoneal fluid inflammatory cells may release lysosomal enzymes, inducing tissue damage and pain.[13] Marked fibrosis and adhesions may result from acute or chronic inflammation resulting in tissue damage. Pain from adhesions may be a result of direct nerve damage (from tissue destruction and scar formation) or of devitalization and ischemia of parts of the internal pelvic organs (caused by damage to the blood supply). Pressure buildup within a fibrotic capsule surrounding endometriotic lesions during or after menses may result in menstrual pain. The pain may result from deep endometriosis involving the uterosacral ligament, the obturator, and femoral nerves. Increases in localized PG concentrations may sensitize pain receptors to chemical mediators and mechanical stimuli, or cause leukocytes to release lysosomal enzymes that cause tissue destruction and adhesion formation.

Infertility in patients with endometriosis may result from mechanical effects (interfering with ovum release and pickup), endocrine

TABLE 82–1. Factors Associated with Increased Risk for Endometriosis

Short menstrual cycle length (≤27 days)
Long menstrual flow duration (≥5–7 days)
Heavy flow
Significant cramping
Spotting before onset of menses
Early menarche
Late menopause
Delayed childbearing
Reduced parity

Compiled from Refs. 1, 4, 6, 9, and 10.

abnormalities, environmental changes within the fallopian tube or pelvis, or immune system deficiencies which could affect the oocytes or implantation[14] (Table 82–3). There is a progressive loss of ovarian reserve in women with stage III or IV endometriosis, independent of age.[17] Women with endometriosis who undergo *in vitro* fertilization (IVF) have a decreased number of oocytes retrieved, lower fertilization rates, and lower implantation rates, compared to those without the disease.

TABLE 82–3. Possible Contributing Causes of Endometriosis to Infertility

Pelvic adhesions
Fallopian tube dysfunction/obstruction
Limited fimbrial mobility
Pelvic distortion
Ovarian endometriosis (endometriomas)
Endocrine abnormalities
Ovulatory dysfunction, anovulation
Diminished ovarian reserve
Abnormalities in folliculogenesis
Luteinized unruptured follicle syndrome
Inadequate luteal function
Impaired steroidogenesis in preovulatory granulosa cells
Immunologic abnormalities in peritoneal fluid

Compiled from Refs. 15–19.

CLINICAL PRESENTATION

While symptoms facilitate the diagnosis of endometriosis, the severity of symptoms does not reliably correlate with the severity of disease. Many women with significant endometriosis are asymptomatic. Endometriotic lesions outside of the pelvic cavity may result in symptoms of a cyclic nature, associated with the menstrual cycle (Table 82–4). Patients often have symptoms for many years before a diagnosis is confirmed surgically. As long as ovarian tissues are functioning, endometriosis may exist during the entire reproductive life of the patient. Because of the decrease in estrogen production, there is a regression of endometriosis and associated symptoms in most patients after menopause.

Patients usually present with dysmenorrhea, dyspareunia, pelvic pain, or infertility. Dysmenorrhea is usually progressive, starting within 2 days of the onset of menstrual flow, continuing throughout menses and occasionally extending for several days afterwards.[9] The pain, often described as dull and aching, most often occurs in the lower abdomen and deep pelvis, bilaterally, radiating to the back and thighs. Dyspareunia is usually positional, worsening with deep penetration. It is usually associated with endometriosis affecting the uterosacral ligaments, deep pelvic implants, lesions of the rectovaginal septum, or a fixed retroverted uterus.[3]

Pelvic pain may be cyclic (occurring during or just before menses) or acyclic (occurring throughout the month). The pain increases in severity over time and can be incapacitating, causing the patient to stay in bed and not go to work or participate in normal daily activities. In patients with ovarian endometriosis, rupture or leakage of the cyst can produce acute abdominal pain.

Signs and symptoms of the disease can vary and there is no correlation between the site or number of endometriotic lesions with the type or severity of pain. Patients with severe symptoms may have minimal disease, while patients who are asymptomatic may have severe endometriosis.[12] Although there is a lack of correlation between pain and visible endometriosis, the degree of pain appears to be correlated with the depth of infiltration.[5] Hence, patients with severe pain often have deep implants surrounded by inflammatory tissue and fibrosis, whereas patients with infertility and minimal or no pain most often have superficial implants. Endometriosis should be suspected in a patient with infertility, when no other cause is apparent. The physical examination may be normal or abnormal. The exam may reveal an endometrioma, a fixed, retroverted uterus, uterosacral ligament abnormalities, lateral displacement of the cervix, or cervical stenosis.[1] Examination of the patient during menstruation increases the detection rate of endometriosis as compared to an examination not timed to the menstruation.[9]

TABLE 82–2. Immunologic Abnormalities Associated with Endometriosis

Increased concentrations of leukocytes (macrophages, T-helper lymphocytes, natural killer cells) in peritoneal fluid
Increased secretion of macrophage-derived growth factor from peritoneal macrophages
Increased concentrations of IL-1, TNF-α, IL-6, IL-8 in peritoneal fluid
Increased levels of IL-4 mRNA in mononuclear cells
Increased levels of IL-4 protein in peritoneal fluid and peripheral blood
Decreased levels of IL-2, IL-13, and γ-interferon in peritoneal fluid
Increased levels of transforming growth factor-β in peritoneal fluid
Decreased activity of natural killer cells
Decreased natural killer cell activity in peripheral blood mononuclear cells

Compiled from Ref. 7.

TABLE 82–4. Symptoms Associated with Extrapelvic Endometriosis

Site	Symptoms
Gastrointestinal tract	Dyschezia Hematochezia Cyclic bowel obstruction
Urinary tract	Hematuria Dysuria Flank pain
Surgical scars, umbilicus	Cyclic pain Tenderness Swelling
Lung	Hemoptysis Chest pain Shortness of breath
Peripheral nerves	Sciatica
Brain	Perimenstrual headaches Seizures

Compiled from Ref. 9.

Confirmation of the diagnosis by laparoscopic visualization and biopsy of lesions is recommended for patients with suspected endometriosis. Recognition of lesions requires an experienced surgeon, because of the variation in appearance and location. The characteristic lesion is the classic "chocolate cyst" of the ovary, indicative of an advanced stage of endometriosis. This is the result of a blood filled cavity within the endometrioma. However, endometriotic lesions have variable appearances, based on their location, size, and age. They can be red, blue, black, white, or nonpigmented. The red lesion is highly vascularized, the most active, and considered to be the first stage of endometriosis.[20] In adolescents, red lesions are found. With each menstrual cycle, there is shedding of the endometrial cells, then the lesion regrows until the next cycle. Repeated shedding induces an inflammatory reaction, resulting in scar formation and a change to a characteristic powder burn appearance. This black lesion is seen in patients with advanced endometriosis. White lesions, resulting from devascularization from the inflammatory process and subsequent fibrosis, are considered to be healed or inactive. Extensive adhesions may develop as the disease progresses, and lesions increase in number and size.

The American Society for Reproductive Medicine (ASRM) classifies pelvic endometriosis as Stage I (minimal), Stage II (mild), Stage III (moderate), or Stage IV (severe). Staging is based on points assigned for the severity of endometriosis and adhesions in the peritoneum, ovaries, and fallopian tubes observed during surgery (Table 82–5). Although a classification system should correlate symptom severity with physical findings and response to treatment, many researchers have found poor correlation between the stage of the disease with the severity of symptoms or the site of the lesions. Some investigators found that women with stage III and IV endometriosis have more severe dysmenorrhea and pelvic pain. It appears that the symptoms may correlate more with the site of the lesions and the degree of tissue infiltration than the stage of the disease. No classification system exists for extrapelvic endometriosis.

TABLE 82–5. Classification of Endometriosis

Stage (Severity)	Findings
I (minimal) and II (mild)	Scattered superficial implants on structures other than uterus, tubes, or ovaries No associated scarring or significant adhesions Rare or superficial implants on ovaries
III (moderate)	Multiple implants or small endometriomas ($\leq$2 cm) involving one or both ovaries Minimal peritubal or periovarian adhesions Scattered, scarred implants on other structures
IV (severe)	Large ovarian endometriomas Significant tubal or ovarian adhesions Tubal obstruction Obliteration of the cul-de sac Major uterosacral involvement Significant bowel or urinary tract disease

Compiled from Ref. 21.

Women with endometriosis have been found to have elevated levels of cancer antigen 125 (CA-125) in serum, menstrual effluent, and peritoneal fluid.[9] Because it is elevated in a number of other conditions, the test has poor reliability to be used as a screening test. In some women with endometriosis, it may be used to assess the severity of the disease and the response to surgical and medical treatment. Plasma levels are correlated with the total volume and depth of the endometriosis, but not the total surface area of endometriosis. Lower fertility rates may correlate with elevated postoperative CA-125 levels because of untreated disease.[22]

▶ TREATMENT: Endometriosis

DESIRED OUTCOME

The major goals of treatment of endometriosis are to alleviate pain and/or other symptoms associated with endometriosis, to minimize disease progression, and/or to restore or preserve reproductive function (Table 82–6).

GENERAL APPROACH TO TREATMENT

Currently available treatment options include medical therapy, surgical therapy, or a combination of surgical and medical therapy. The treatment chosen is dependent on the patient's age, severity of symptoms, duration of symptoms, type and extent of disease, desire for fertility, previous response to therapy, potential side effects of medical treatment, potential complications of surgery, and quality of life. Medical therapy alone is effective in treating symptoms of endometriosis, but not to eradicate lesions, prevent recurrence, or improve fertility. Surgical treatment may eradicate visible lesions, but postoperative medical therapy may be required to maintain symptom relief. The definitive treatment for endometriosis is hysterectomy; however, this is inappropriate for patients desiring pregnancy or future fertility.

TABLE 82–6. Goals of Treatment of Endometriosis

Eliminate/minimize pain associated with endometriosis
Eliminate/minimize other symptoms associated with endometriosis
Prevent disease progression
Prevent future pelvic disorders associated with advanced stages of endometriosis
Preserve/restore future reproductive function
Stop growth of endometriotic implants
Restore fertility—achieve pregnancy and live birth
Minimize/prevent complications/side effects of treatments
Minimize/prevent recurrence of endometriosis and/or symptoms
Minimize costs associated with disease or treatments

The optimum treatment regimen has not yet been established. Most of the published studies evaluating the treatment of endometriosis have been uncontrolled, poorly designed, or have small sample sizes. Recurrence of endometriosis is common, following both medical and surgical treatments.

For patients with signs and/or symptoms of endometriosis other than infertility, or those who fail to respond to empiric therapy with nonsteroidal anti-inflammatory agents (NSAIDs) and/or oral contraceptives (OCs), surgery is traditionally performed to evaluate and diagnose endometriosis. If ectopic lesions are visualized, they should be surgically treated. Postoperative medical therapy is usually initiated to treat remaining lesions. Recent reports recommend empiric gonadotropin-releasing hormone (GnRH) agonists instead of surgery in patients with clinically suspected endometriosis, if they fail to respond to NSAIDs and/or OCs. Figure 82–1 is a general treatment algorithm for endometriosis without infertility. Patients presenting

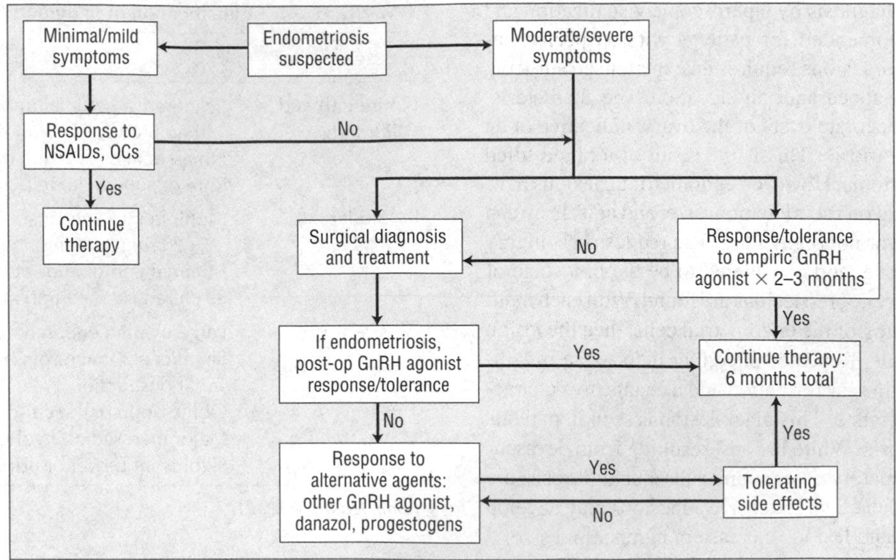

FIGURE 82–1. General treatment algorithm for endometriosis, without infertility. GnRH, gonadotropin-releasing hormone, NSAIDs, nonsteroidal anti-inflammatory agents; OCs, oral contraceptives; post-op, postoperative.

with infertility as the primary complaint may benefit from both surgical diagnosis and treatment and medical therapy (Fig. 82–2).

Hormonal therapy is designed to create a state of chronic anovulation to interrupt the cycle of stimulation and bleeding. As endometriotic lesions are responsive to estrogen, medical therapy is administered to induce either pseudopregnancy (e.g., by using continuous monophasic OCs or progestogens) or pseudomenopause (e.g., by using GnRH agonists) to inhibit or delay ectopic endometrial tissue growth.[3] Although the precise relationship between estradiol (E_2) levels and endometriotic lesion growth and symptoms is unknown, studies demonstrate some correlations (Table 82–7).

Until the development of GnRH agonists, danazol was the preferred therapy used to suppress estrogen; therefore, many subsequent trials compared GnRH agonists with danazol for efficacy.[24] OCs and progestogens have also been used to treat endometriosis symptoms.

In a review of randomized clinical trials, beneficial treatments for pain caused by endometriosis included hormonal treatments (e.g., danazol, medroxyprogesterone, GnRH agonists), combined ablation of endometrial deposits and uterine nerve, postoperative hormonal treatment, and cystectomy for ovarian endometrioma.[10] OC pills were considered likely to be beneficial for treating pain.

For patients with endometriosis-associated infertility, surgical eradication of endometrial lesions should occur during the diagnostic laparoscopy, as hormonal treatment alone and postoperative hormonal treatment do not improve fertility.[10,14] Postoperative hormonal treatment is not indicated for endometriosis-associated infertility (except with *in vitro* fertilization [IVF]) because of the delay in subsequent fertility therapy, the costs of treatment, and the potential side effects.[25] For those with minimal or mild disease, surgery is followed by expectant management for 6 months because long-term pregnancy rates in untreated women with minimal to mild endometriosis are high. If the patient does not achieve pregnancy, ovarian stimulation (using clomiphene or gonadotropins) with intrauterine insemination is used. IVF should be postponed for 2 to 3 years after surgery unless the female is 35 years of age or older, has failed other treatments, has prolonged infertility (>3 years), and/or has multiple-factor infertility. For those with moderate or severe disease, there may be no added benefit to using postsurgical medical treatment (except with IVF), and recurrence is likely to occur after completion of therapy in patients with severe endometriosis. Prolonged down-regulation with GnRH agonists before ovarian stimulation and IVF has a beneficial impact on oocyte number, pregnancy rate, and miscarriage rate, possibly because of improved folliculogenesis and oocyte quality.[26] Cystectomy for ovarian endometriomas should be performed before the use of assisted reproductive techniques, as their presence may interfere with

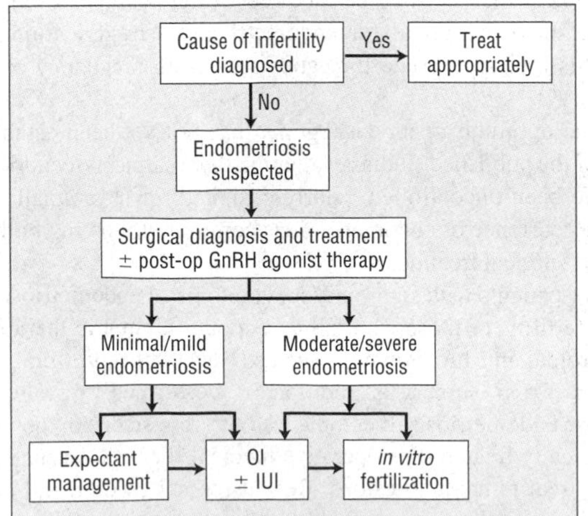

FIGURE 82–2. General treatment algorithm for endometriosis-associated infertility. GnRH, gonadotropin-releasing hormone; IUI, intrauterine insemination; OI, ovulation induction; Post-op, postoperative.

TABLE 82–7. Correlation of Estradiol (E_2) Concentrations with Lesions and Symptoms

E_2 Concentrations	Endometriotic Lesions	Consequences/Symptoms
10–20 pg/mL	Atrophy of lesions	Loss of bone minerals, vasomotor symptoms
30 pg/mL	Regression of lesions	
>40 pg/mL		Increased pain
>60 pg/mL	Growth of lesions	

Compiled from Ref. 23.

the techniques and response associated with IVF. Multiple IVF cycles may be required to achieve pregnancy in patients with endometriosis. Patients with milder disease have a higher pregnancy rate than patients with stage IV endometriosis.[18]

NONPHARMACOLOGIC THERAPY

SURGICAL THERAPY

The most common treatment for endometriosis is surgery. Surgical approaches to the management of endometriosis include laparoscopy or laparotomy, although laparoscopy is preferred. Laparotomy is used when the situation is too complex for a laparoscopic procedure. Surgery is required for diagnostic confirmation and for staging of endometriosis. Surgical treatment is indicated for patients with infertility, advanced lesions, endometriomas larger than 2–3 cm, extensive endometriosis, anatomic distortion of the pelvic structure, and adhesions.[3,12] It is also indicated for patients who fail medical therapy.

The goals of surgery are to relieve symptoms, restore fertility, remove endometrial lesions (if possible), and delay recurrence of the disease. Surgical treatments include resection or destruction of the visible lesions, ovarian cystectomies, lysis or resection of adhesions, and/or restoration of normal pelvic anatomy. Surgical techniques include excision of lesions, laser vaporization, endocoagulation, unipolar or bipolar electrocoagulation, presacral neurectomy, and/or laparoscopic uterosacral nerve ablation.[1,27] Potential complications of surgery include denervation of pelvic structures, damage to other pelvic structures, uterine prolapse, reduced fertility, and/or future formation of adhesions.[10]

Surgical treatment alone is not any better than medical therapy alone. Pain relief occurs in 70% to 100% of patients immediately following surgery.[1] Pain symptoms recur in 44% of patients within 1 year of treatment, and in 50% to 60% of patients within 2 years of the procedure.[28] Implants recur in 28% of patients within 18 months and in 40% within 9 years, while adhesions recur in 40% to 50% of patients.[1]

Although surgical treatment can be effective in reducing pain, it may fail to eradicate all endometriotic lesions. Because endometrial implants may not be readily visible or recognized by the surgeon (as a consequence of experience and expertise), medical treatment may be necessary to eliminate residual lesions postoperatively. GnRH agonists or combined therapy with danazol and medroxyprogesterone acetate (MPA) for 6 months after surgery significantly reduced pain and delayed recurrence of pain when compared with placebo.[10]

The presence of large endometriomas associated with severe adhesive disease may benefit from a short course of medical treatment before surgery to aid in surgical removal.[12] However, preoperative therapy may make it difficult for the surgeon to identify and resect small endometriotic lesions.

For patients desiring pregnancy or future fertility, surgery is conservative to preserve ovarian and reproductive function. For patients with mild or moderate endometriosis, destruction of implants improves fertility and pregnancy rates.[10] For patients with moderate or severe endometriosis, surgical therapy is necessary to eradicate endometriomas, resect lesions or adhesions that interfere with normal function, or restore normal pelvic anatomy, as medical treatment is ineffective in these cases.

The most definitive, effective method of treatment of endometriosis, and only possible cure, is a total abdominal hysterectomy and bilateral salpingo-oophorectomy, which abolishes estrogenic stimulation. This therapy is indicated for patients with severe persistent pelvic pain or recurrent disease resistant to other medical and surgical options, and who no longer desire fertility. If all functioning ovarian tissue is removed, it is associated with a minimal risk of recurrence. However, it is highly undesirable, because of the loss of fertility potential and complications associated with the lack of estrogen stimulation (e.g., osteoporosis, abnormalities in lipid profile). Endometriosis-related pain is eliminated in 90% of patients who have radical surgery.[29] Hormone replacement therapy (HRT) must be prescribed to young women who have this surgically induced menopause.

NUTRITIONAL THERAPY

Gastrointestinal (GI) symptoms related to endometriosis include epigastric pain, nausea, vomiting, early satiety, bloating and distention, and altered bowel habits that are worsened by eating and not relieved by a bowel movement. Often misdiagnosed as irritable bowel syndrome, these symptoms classically appear twice during the menstrual cycle: at ovulation, and just before and during menses. Fifty women with endometriosis and GI symptoms refractory to standard therapy were found to have ampulla of Vater-duodenal wall spasm, a dysfunction of the enteric nervous system.[30] Symptoms were significantly reduced after 8 weeks of treatment, consisting of dietary modifications (Table 82–8) and pharmacologic therapy with a γ-aminobutyric acid agonist (e.g., clonazepam 0.25 mg tid orally) to stabilize neural excitation of the enteric nervous system. It was speculated that hypersecretion of insulin resulted in the production of excessive pathway 2 prostaglandins (PGE_2 and $PGF_{2\alpha}$) that cause seizure activity of the enteric nerves.

PHARMACOLOGIC THERAPY

Because endometriotic lesions are hormonally sensitive, medications are used to relieve pain and to minimize progression of the condition by stopping growth and producing regression of ectopic lesions using hormonal suppression. Endometriosis is a chronic condition, and medical treatment does not eradicate the disease. There is a high

TABLE 82–8. Dietary Therapy for Endometriosis

Dietary Modifications	Reasons
Reduce or eliminate glycemic carbohydrates (e.g., rice, potatoes, pasta, carrots, corn, peas, beets, fruit juices)	Stimulus for insulin, which controls the eicosanoid system
Eliminate foods containing caffeine and tyramine (e.g., coffee, tea, colas, aged cheeses, ale, sherry, liquor, red meat, sausage, salami, pepperoni, bologna, Chinese pea pods, mixed Chinese vegetables)	Excitatory transmitters that stimulate nerves within the central nervous system and enteric nervous system
Add omega-3 (flax seed), omega-6, and omega-9 fatty acids	To balance the eicosanoid system and to control prostaglandin synthesis

Compiled from Ref. 30.

incidence of recurrence of symptoms and/or lesions after discontinuation of medical therapy. Because the various therapies are approximately equally effective, the medication chosen is based on safety, tolerability, cost, and desire for fertility.

Six months of continuous suppression of ovulation using danazol, MPA, OCs, or GnRH agonists were equally effective in reducing severe and moderate pain at 6 months (as compared to placebo).[10] The medical treatments have similar recurrence rates, but different side-effect profiles. In a comparison between GnRH agonists and danazol, women randomized to GnRH agonists were less likely to discontinue treatment, while adverse events were more frequent in women randomized to danazol.[24]

DRUG TREATMENTS OF FIRST CHOICE

For patients with suspected or documented endometriosis, GnRH agonists are currently considered the medical treatment of first choice, empirically or postoperatively. However, their use is limited by vasomotor symptoms and bone mineral density (BMD) loss caused by the hypoestrogenic state. Alternative therapies may be considered for patients who cannot tolerate the use of GnRH agonists or who require treatment for longer than 6 months, but their use may be limited by androgenic or progestogenic side effects or a negative impact on the lipid profile.

ALTERNATIVE DRUG TREATMENTS

For patients with minimal or mild symptoms, not immediately desiring pregnancy, and no abnormalities on pelvic examination, NSAIDs and OCs may be empirically used for the treatment of dysmenorrhea secondary to endometriosis because they are usually well tolerated and inexpensive. However, there is little information regarding the specific type of treatment used or the effectiveness of the therapy. In the only randomized controlled study of NSAIDs, naproxen sodium reduced menstrual pain completely or substantially more than placebo.[31] In patients who underwent laparoscopic treatment of moderate-to-severe endometriosis, postoperative administration of low-dose cyclic OCs was associated with a lower 12-month cumulative recurrence rate as compared to no treatment; however, there was no difference in the cumulative recurrence rate at 24 and 36 months after surgery.[32] OCs may also be administered following a treatment course of danazol or GnRH agonists to slow disease progression.

SPECIAL POPULATIONS

In adolescents, monophasic OCs administered in a continuous or cyclic manner is recommended after surgical treatment, due to the adverse effects on BMD associated with the GnRH agonists.[1] Evidence for the use of multiphasic products has not been established.

DRUG CLASS INFORMATION

Gonadotropin-Releasing Hormone Agonists

The GnRH agonists (synthetic derivatives of GnRH) are the most predictable form of medical therapy that inhibits estrogen production. They act by binding to pituitary gland receptors, resulting in an initial release of follicle-stimulating hormone (FSH) and leuteinizing hormone (LH) and increased ovarian estrogen production. Continuous or repeated administration of an agonist at nonphysiologic doses results in down-regulation of GnRH receptors, pituitary desensitization, and suppression of gonadotropin secretion. The result is eventual cessation of estrogen production by the ovaries and amenorrhea. With the hypoestrogenic environment, there is regression of endometriotic lesions and atrophy, resulting in an improvement of symptoms.

TABLE 82–9. GnRH Agonists Used for Endometriosis

Generic Name	Trade Name	Dosage and Administration
Goserelin acetate	Zoladex	3.6 mg every 28 days; subcutaneous pellet implant (anterior abdominal wall)
Leuprolide acetate	Lupron Depot	3.75 mg once a month; or 11.25 mg once every 3 months; intramuscular depot
Nafarelin acetate	Synarel	200–400 μg bid; intranasal spray

In a review of three placebo-controlled randomized clinical trials of GnRH agonists after surgery for endometriosis, patients who received 3 months of GnRH agonists had no difference in pain relief as compared to placebo. Patients with 6 months of therapy had significantly reduced pain scores and delayed pain recurrence by more than 12 months.[10] There was no difference in pregnancy rates or time to conception when compared to placebo.

The improvement or resolution of pain symptoms with GnRH agonists for the treatment of endometriosis is comparable to or better than treatment with danazol. GnRH agonists were associated with a more significant decrease in FSH after 4 weeks of treatment and a more significant decrease in mean serum E_2 concentration.[3] There was a 57% recurrence of symptoms within 6 months of the end of therapy. Patients with severe forms of the disease had a recurrence rate of 43.8%.

The GnRH agonists available in the United States are goserelin acetate, leuprolide acetate, and nafarelin acetate (Table 82–9). They are approved for administration for up to 6 months of therapy, limited by the side effects induced by chronic hypoestrogenism. The choice of the agonist used depends on the physician, the patient, and the route of administration. Although all GnRH agonists are effective in achieving hypoestrogenism, nafarelin results in slightly higher estrogen levels than leuprolide or goserelin.[33] In a comparison between nafarelin and leuprolide in women with severe symptoms of endometriosis, women receiving nafarelin had less bone mineral loss and fewer days with side effects of hot flushes and other hypoestrogenic symptoms, resulting in a more positive effect on quality of life.[34] A comparison between goserelin and nafarelin found no significant difference in the treatment results or side effects.[35]

At the beginning of GnRH agonist therapy, there is often a transient worsening of symptoms caused by the flare in gonadotropins and the resulting elevated estrogen levels. If therapy is started during the luteal phase of the menstrual cycle, this pain is diminished to a degree, and there is more rapid ovarian suppression.[13] Pain relief is initially noted after 1 to 2 months of therapy and continues during the 6 months of treatment. Six months after discontinuation of therapy, 59% of patients with dysmenorrhea and 88% of patients with dyspareunia remained free of symptoms.

GnRH agonists produce both subjective and objective improvement in patients with endometriosis. While they are not associated with androgenic or progestogenic side effects and do not have a negative impact on the lipid profile, therapy is limited by hypoestrogenic side effects. These include hot flushes, sweating, vaginal dryness,

TABLE 82–10. "Add-Back" Therapies Used with Gonadotropin-Releasing Hormone Agonists

Medroxyprogesterone acetate
Norethindrone
Transdermal 17β-estradiol
Conjugated equine estrogens
Estrogens in combination with progestins
Bisphosphonates (e.g., etidronate)
Progestins with bisphosphonates
Pulsatile parathyroid hormone

emotional instability, insomnia, and a reversible loss of BMD. Other side effects include depression, libido changes, headache, and fatigue. The long-term effects of hypoestrogenism, especially the loss of BMD leading to osteoporosis and deterioration in circulating lipoprotein levels, prevent the long-term use of GnRH agonists alone. While bone loss is documented with continued use of GnRH agonists for 6 months or more, there are varied results regarding the amount of bone loss recovered after discontinuation of therapy.[36]

Concurrent "add back" therapy to maintain the therapeutic response of the GnRH agonists, while minimizing potential adverse effects, has been evaluated. The goal of "add-back" therapy is to enhance compliance and potentially allow administration of GnRH agonist therapy for longer than 6 months, for patients in whom 6 months of therapy is inadequate. "Add-back" therapies investigated include combined estrogen and progesterone, progestins alone, and therapies aimed at reducing the hypoestrogenic bone loss (Table 82–10). "Add back" HRT, using combined estrogen and progesterone, is based on the estrogen threshold hypothesis that estrogen levels within certain concentrations can minimize adverse effects, such as vasomotor symptoms and bone loss, without stimulating the growth of endometriosis. Recurrence rates after discontinuation of GnRH agonists and "add-back" therapy are similar to rates after other medical treatments.[3] Disadvantages of "add-back" therapy may include administration of multiple medications and increased cost of combined therapies.

MPA or norethindrone, in combination with GnRH agonist therapy, both eliminate vasomotor symptoms and BMD loss. However, continuous administration of MPA appears to reverse the beneficial effects of GnRH agonists.[37] Norethindrone is effective, but high doses can lead to deterioration in lipid profiles.[33] The combination of estrogens and progestins is effective against vasomotor symptoms and preservation of BMD, but there is a danger of reversing the effect of the GnRH agonist on the endometriosis. Etidronate in combination with norethindrone effectively prevents bone loss and controls symptoms without adversely affecting the clinical efficacy of the GnRH agonist.

Although there was no difference in efficacy between goserelin acetate alone and goserelin plus low-dose transdermal 17β-estradiol (25 μg patches changed twice weekly) and MPA (5 mg), significantly fewer patients had hot flushes and loss of libido when treated with the combination therapy.[38] BMD loss at the lumbar spine was significantly lower in the HRT group but not completely prevented.

Goserelin (3.6 mg every 4 weeks) with oral continuous combined estradiol-norethisterone acetate "add-back" therapy daily for 24 weeks maintained BMD of the lumbar spine and diminished subjective side effects. This therapy also significantly reduced the number of endometriotic implants.[39] Goserelin alone resulted in a 5.02% decrease in the BMD of the lumbar spine.

In a randomized, double-blinded, placebo-controlled, multicenter study, goserelin alone (3.6 mg every 28 days) was compared to goserelin plus two doses (0.3 mg and 0.625 mg) of conjugated estrogens (Premarin) combined with 5 mg of MPA (Provera).[40] Although all three treatments were equally effective in relieving pelvic symptoms of endometriosis, HRT reduced the loss of BMD and the incidence of hot flushes and vaginal dryness associated with goserelin therapy.

There was no difference in the bone loss of the lumbar spine and hip associated with goserelin therapy for 6 to 24 months, with or without estradiol (2 mg/day) and norethisterone acetate (1 mg/day).[36] After 6 years of followup, recovery of BMD loss was not complete in either group of patients.

"Draw-back" therapy, consisting of pituitary desensitization using intranasal nafarelin 400 μg daily for 4 weeks, followed by a maintenance dose of 200 μg daily for 20 weeks, resulted in a decrease in hypoestrogenic symptoms and bone loss, when compared to 400 μg daily for 24 weeks.[23]

Danazol

A derivative of 17α-ethinyltestosterone, danazol was once the standard for treating endometriosis but adverse effects limited its use. Danazol suppresses pituitary gonadotropin (e.g., FSH, LH) secretion and inhibits ovarian steroidogenesis, resulting in anovulatory amenorrhea and a low estrogen state that does not support growth of endometriosis implants. Reduced sex hormone-binding globulin levels result in elevated free testosterone levels, which cause the androgenic side effects.[3] Danazol also has immunosuppressive properties, which may be beneficial due to the immunologic changes found in patients with endometriosis (Table 82–11).

Danazol results in regression of endometrial implants and symptomatic relief of pain. It is not effective in the treatment of ovarian endometriomas nor pain associated with adhesions, and does not improve fertility or prevent recurrence.[29] Therapy should be initiated during menses or after a negative pregnancy test to avoid fetal exposure associated with an early pregnancy. It is administered orally as 400–800 mg daily, in divided doses, for 6 months.

More than 80% of patients will have a noticeable reduction in symptoms within 2 months of beginning therapy, but approximately 50% of patients will have recurrence within 4 to 12 months after discontinuing therapy.[3] Pregnancy rates following treatment with danazol are similar to rates with expectant management; therefore, it is not indicated for patients with a primary complaint of infertility.

Bothersome side effects affect 85% of patients, and at least 10% of patients do not continue therapy.[3] Androgenic side effects include hirsutism, weight gain, fluid retention, decrease in breast size, oily skin and hair, acne, and voice changes; the deepening of the voice may be irreversible. Patients gain an average of 10 pounds during a course of therapy. Hypoestrogenic side effects include hot flushes, mood changes, and depression. Adverse changes in the lipid profile

TABLE 82–11. Immunosuppressive Activities Associated with Danazol Therapy in Patients with Endometriosis

Reduced serum levels of autoantibodies
Inhibited secretion of proinflammatory cytokines by monocytes
Reduced peripheral blood monocyte activation
Reduced number of macrophages that infiltrate the eutopic endometrium
Reduced peritoneal levels of proinflammatory cytokines produced by macrophages
Inhibited monocyte chemotactic protein-1 expression by endometrial cells

Compiled from Ref. 41.

include decreases in high-density lipoprotein (HDL) cholesterol and increases in low-density lipoprotein (LDL) cholesterol. Elevation of hepatic enzymes or jaundice has been reported with danazol, so periodic monitoring of liver function is recommended during therapy. Danazol is contraindicated during pregnancy, because it may cause external genitalia virilization of the female fetus. Although danazole induces amenorrhea, women should use barrier methods to prevent pregnancy during the entire course of therapy.

Progestogens

MPA is the most widely used progestogen for the treatment of endometriosis. Continuous use of progestogens results in a hypoestrogenic environment, reducing endometriotic implants similar to that seen with danazol.[29] Pain relief is comparable to that seen with danazol and superior to placebo, although dyspareunia is not effectively relieved. Side effects include breakthrough bleeding, weight gain, mood changes, fluid retention, and adverse effects on lipids. Some patients may experience delayed menstrual cycle recovery, with continued amenorrhea and anovulation; therefore, progestogens are not indicated for patients who desire immediate pregnancy.

Antiprogestins

Antiprogestins bind to progesterone receptors and demonstrate antiprogesterone and antiglucocorticoid activities. The first clinically available antiprogestin, mifepristone (also known as RU-486) has been shown to inhibit ovulation and disrupt endometrial integrity. For the treatment of endometriosis, a series of small studies have evaluated oral daily doses of 100 mg for 3 months, 50 mg for 6 months, and 5 mg for 6 months.[42] Although all three doses reduced pelvic pain and uterine cramping, a significant decrease in visible endometriotic lesions was seen only with the 50-mg dose. Both the 50-mg and 100-mg doses resulted in amenorrhea, whereas the 5-mg dose was associated with bleeding irregularities. Side effects from mifepristone included hot flushes, mild increase in liver transaminase levels, and depression. Unacceptable antiglucocorticoid effects (increased serum cortisol and adrenocorticotropic hormone levels) were associated with the 100-mg dosage regimen. Additional research with mifepristone is needed to determine the optimum dose and treatment regimen.

PHARMACOECONOMIC CONSIDERATIONS

Although not evaluated in studies, the costs associated with endometriosis involve not just the cost of the treatment(s); they also include lost productivity (incurring costs in the economy) and costs associated with a reduced quality of life.

Traditionally, surgical diagnosis and treatment of endometriosis has been performed prior to initiation of medical therapy for regression of lesions. However, recent reports indicate that primary therapy with a GnRH agonist is more cost-effective than surgery for the management of endometriosis and pelvic pain.[28]

Advantages of the surgical approach prior to medical therapy include the possibility of making a biopsy-proven diagnosis while lesions and adhesions can be surgically treated.[43] The efficacy of the surgery is highly dependent on the skill and experience of the surgeon to identify and remove or destroy all lesions. Disadvantages include the fact that the cause of pain may not be identified and that pain may recur postoperatively. Potential complications include bowel perforation, trauma to the major abdominal and pelvic vessels, anesthetic complications, and death.

After ruling out other potential causes of pelvic pain (e.g., ovarian cysts, myomas, cervical stenosis), the medical approach replaces the laparoscopy with empiric GnRH agonist treatment for 2 to 3 months. If there is no response to the agonist therapy, the patient then undergoes laparoscopy, and possible gastrointestinal, urologic, and psychologic evaluations.[43] Advantages of empiric medical treatment include avoidance of surgery and associated complications, the possibility of avoiding an invasive procedure (laparoscopy), and the ability to extend the course of medical therapy to 6 months if there is a response. The major disadvantage of the medical approach is recurrence of pain several years after completion of successful treatment, because anatomic abnormalities were not surgically corrected.

Empiric medical therapy can be significantly less expensive than surgery. Assuming a cost of $333 per month for leuprolide once a month, an initial 3-month course ($1,000) or a full 6-month course ($2,000), medical treatment is cost-effective as compared to a laparoscopic procedure (range of $5,000 to $10,000), without the risks associated with surgery.[43]

For patients with severe endometriosis, IVF may be more cost effective than surgical therapy before treatment of infertility.[44]

EVALUATION OF THERAPEUTIC OUTCOMES

Patients should be monitored for response to therapy, as demonstrated by alleviation of pain and other symptoms associated with endometriosis, and tolerance to side effects. Patients with endometriosis-associated infertility should be referred to a reproductive endocrinologist for complete evaluation and aggressive therapy to optimize pregnancy rates in a timely fashion.

If the patient does not respond to empiric therapy with NSAIDs or OCs, she should be advised to seek further evaluation and aggressive treatment by a physician with significant experience diagnosing and treating endometriosis. The patient should not have to deal with chronic severe endometriosis-related pain for years before being appropriately diagnosed and treated. Historically, patients have suffered with debilitating and painful symptoms for many years, seeing numerous physicians and having five or more laparoscopies, before a diagnosis of endometriosis was made or confirmed surgically (mean time to diagnosis of 9.28 years).[2]

Referral to a support group, such as the Endometriosis Association or the Endometriosis Research Center, may help the patient understand her condition and provide much needed support and/or recommendations to improve her quality of life.

▶ PRINCIPLES OF PHARMACOTHERAPY

- Endometriosis is a major cause of chronic pelvic pain, dysmenorrhea, dyspareunia, and infertility in females of reproductive age, including adolescents. Endometriosis should be suspected in a patient with infertility when no other cause is apparent.

- Although most endometriotic lesions are located in the pelvis, endometriosis should be suspected in patients with symptoms of a cyclic nature that are associated with the menstrual cycle.
- Although there is no correlation between the site or number of endometriotic lesions with the type or severity of pain, symptoms appears to be correlated with the site of the lesions and the degree of tissue infiltration.
- Surgery is essential for the diagnosis and staging of endometriosis, although all lesions may not be detected because of their appearance and inexperience of the surgeon.
- Treatment options for endometriosis are dependent on the patient's age, severity of symptoms, duration of symptoms, type and extent of disease, desire for fertility, previous response to therapy, potential side effects of medical treatment, potential complications of surgery, and quality of life.
- Patients who fail to respond to empiric therapy with NSAIDs and/or OCs should be evaluated by a physician to diagnose endometriosis and/or to rule out other potential causes of the symptoms.
- Medical therapy is designed to interrupt the cycle of stimulation and bleeding associated with endometriotic lesions.
- Patients with endometriosis-related infertility require surgical treatment, as medical treatment alone does not improve fertility.
- Despite resolution of symptoms and regression/removal of lesions with medical and/or surgical treatment, recurrence of endometriosis is common.
- The most definitive treatment of endometriosis is a total abdominal hysterectomy and bilateral salpingo-oophorectomy, but it is associated with the loss of fertility potential and complications associated with the lack of estrogen stimulation.

REFERENCES

1. Propst AM, Laufer MR. Endometriosis in adolescents; incidence, diagnosis and treatment. J Reprod Med 1999;44:751–758.
2. Thomas EJ. The clinician's view of endometriosis. Int J Gynecol Obstet 1999;64(suppl 1):S1–S3.
3. Minjarez DA. Update on the medical treatment of endometriosis. Obstet Gynecol Clin North Am 2000;27(3):641–651.
4. Eskenazi B, Warner ML. Epidemiology of endometriosis. Obstet Gynecol Clin North Am 1997;24(2):235–258.
5. Speroff L, Glass RH, Kase NG. Clinical Gynecologic Endocrinology and Infertility, 6th ed. Philadelphia, PA, Lippincott, Williams & Wilkins, 1999.
6. Oral E, Arici A. Pathogenesis of endometriosis. Obstet Gynecol Clin North Am 1997;24(2):219–233.
7. Witz CA. Current concepts in the pathogenesis of endometriosis. Clin Obstet Gynecol 1999;42(3):566–585.
8. Hadfield RM, Mardon HJ, Barlow DH, et al. Endometriosis in monozygotic twins. Fertil Steril 1997;68(5):941–942.
9. Duleba AJ. Diagnosis of endometriosis. Obstet Gynecol Clin North Am 1997;24(2):331–346.
10. Farquhar CM. Endometriosis. BMJ 2000;320(7247):1449–1452.
11. Hruska KS, Furth PA, Seifer DB, et al. Environmental factors in infertility. Clin Obstet Gynecol 2000;43(4):821–829.
12. Moghissi KS. Medical treatment of endometriosis. Clin Obstet Gynecol 1999;42(3):620–632.
13. Daftary G, Olive DL. Endometriosis and adenomyosis in pelvic pain. Infert Reprod Med Clin North Am 1999;10(4):685–700.
14. Ledger WL. Endometriosis and infertility: An integrated approach. Int J Gynecol Obstet 1999;64(suppl 1):S33–S40.
15. Burns WN, Schenken RS. Pathophysiology of endometriosis-associated infertility. Clin Obstet Gynecol 1999;42(3):586–610.
16. Gutmann JN. Endometriosis and ovulation induction. Infert Reprod Med Clin North Am 2000;11(3):369–383.
17. Hock DL, Sharafi K, Dagostino L, et al. Contribution of diminished ovarian reserve to hypofertility associated with endometriosis. J Reprod Med 2001;46(1):7–10.
18. Schenken RS. Modern concepts of endometriosis. J Reprod Med 1998; 43:269–275.
19. Zreik TG, Olive DL. Pathophysiology: The biologic principles of disease. Obstet Gynecol Clin North Am 1997;24(2):259–268.
20. Nisolle M, Donnez J. Peritoneal endometriosis, ovarian endometriosis, and adenomyotic nodules of the rectovaginal septum are three different entities. Fertil Steril 1997;68(4):585–596.
21. Lessey BA. Medical management of endometriosis and infertility. Fertil Steril 2000;73(6):1089–1096.
22. Kwok A, Lam A, Ford R. Deeply infiltrating endometriosis: Implications, diagnosis, and management. Obstet Gynecol Surv 2001;56(3):168–177.
23. Tahara M, Tetsu M, Yokoi T, et al. Treatment of endometriosis with a decreasing dosage of a gonadotropin-releasing hormone agonist (nafarelin): A pilot study with low-dose agonist therapy ("draw-back" therapy). Fertil Steril 2000;73(4):799–804.
24. Farquhar C, Sutton C. The evidence for the management of endometriosis. Curr Opin Obstet Gynecol 1998;10:321–332.
25. Buyalos RP, Agarwal SK. Endometriosis-associated infertility. Curr Opin Obstet Gynecol 2000;12;377–381.
26. Dokras A, Olive DL. Endometriosis and assisted reproductive technologies. Clin Obstet Gynecol 1999;42(3):687–698.
27. Schlaff WD. Extending the treatment boundaries: Zoladex and add-back. Int J Gynecol Obstet 1999;64(suppl 1):S25–S31.
28. Winkel CA. A cost-effective approach to the management of endometriosis. Curr Opin Obstet Gynecol 2000;12:317–320.
29. Donnez J. Today's treatments: Medical, surgical and in partnership. Int J Gynecol Obstet 1999;64(suppl 1):S5–S13.
30. Mathias JR, Franklin R, Quast DC, et al. Relation of endometriosis and neuromuscular disease of the gastrointestinal tract: New insights. Fertil Steril 1998;70(1):81–88.
31. Barlow D. Today's treatments: How do you choose? Int J Gynecol Obstet 1999;64(suppl 1):S15–S21.
32. Muzii L, Marana R, Caruana P, et al. Postoperative administration of monophasic combined oral contraceptives after laparoscopic treatment of ovarian endometriomas: A prospective, randomized trial. Am J Obstet Gynecol 2000;183(3):588–592.
33. Kettel LM, Hummel WP. Modern medical management of endometriosis. Obstet Gynecol Clin North Am 1997;24(2):361–373.
34. Zhao SZ, Kellerman LA, Francisco CA, et al. Impact of nafarelin and leuprolide for endometriosis on quality of life and subjective clinical measures. J Reprod Med 1999;44:1000–1006.
35. Bergqvist A. A comparative study of the acceptability and effect of goserelin and nafarelin on endometriosis. Gynecol Endocrinol 2000;14(6): 425–432.
36. Pierce SJ, Gazvani MR, Farquharson RG. Long-term use of gonadotropin-releasing hormone analogs and hormone replacement therapy in the management of endometriosis: A randomized trial with a 6-year follow-up. Fertil Steril 2000;74(5):964–968.
37. Surrey E. Steroidal and nonsteroidal "add-back" therapy: Extending safety and efficacy of gonadotropin releasing hormone agonists in the gynecology patients. Fertil Steril 1995;64:673–685.
38. Howell R, Edmonds DK, Dowsett M, et al. Gonadotropin releasing hormone analogue (goserelin) plus hormone replacement therapy for the treatment of endometriosis. A randomized control trial. Fertil Steril 1995;64:474–481.

39. Franke HR, van de Weijer PH, Pennings TM, et al. Gonadotropin-releasing hormone agonist plus "add-back" hormone replacement therapy for treatment of endometriosis: A prospective, randomized, placebo-controlled, double-blind trial. Fertil Steril 2000;74(3):534–539.
40. Moghissi KS, Schlaff WD, Olive D, et al. Goserelin acetate (Zoladex) with or without hormone replacement therapy for the treatment of endometriosis. Fertil Steril 1998;69(6):1056–1062.
41. Boucher A, Lemay A, Akoum A. Effect of hormonal agents on monocyte chemotactic protein-1 expression by endometrial epithelial cells of women with endometriosis. Fertil Steril 2000;74(5):969–975.
42. Kettel LM, Murphy AA, Morales AJ, et al. Preliminary report on the treatment of endometriosis with low-dose mifepristone (RU-486). Am J Obstet Gynecol 1998;178(6):1151–1156.
43. Barbieri RL, Primary gonadotropin-releasing hormone agonist therapy for suspected endometriosis: A nonsurgical approach to the diagnosis and treatment of chronic pelvic pain. Am J Managed Care 1999;5(suppl): S291–S298.
44. Philips Z, Barraza-Llorens M, Posnett J. Evaluation of the relative cost-effectiveness of treatments for infertility in the UK. Hum Reprod 2000;15 (1):95–106.

83

HORMONE REPLACEMENT THERAPY

Sophia N. Kalantaridou, Susan R. Davis, and Karim Anton Calis

Menopause is the permanent cessation of menses following the loss of ovarian follicular activity.[1] The term *menopause* is derived from the Greek words, *menas* (month) and *pausis* (cessation). Menopause is a physiologic event in a woman's life that, by definition, occurs after 12 consecutive months of amenorrhea[2]—so the time of the final menses is determined retrospectively. Women who have undergone hysterectomy have to rely on their symptoms to estimate the actual time of menopause.

The median age at the onset of menopause in the United States is 51 years,[3] while the average life expectancy for women is 79.7 years.[4] Thus, American women can expect to be postmenopausal for more than one-third of their lives. Clinically, menopause is important because the decline of sex steroids in approximately two-thirds of women results in symptoms that adversely affect quality of life and increase the risk for osteoporosis and possibly coronary heart disease.

Although the age at menarche has steadily declined throughout the centuries, probably a result of improved nutrition, the age at menopause onset appears to have been relatively stable. However, on average, cigarette smokers experience menopause 2 years earlier than nonsmokers.[3] Women who have undergone hysterectomy are also more likely to have an earlier menopause despite preservation of their ovaries. Approximately 1% of women develop ovarian failure before the age of 40 years (premature menopause or premature ovarian failure).[5]

Morbidity and mortality attributed to sex-steroid deficiency may be modified by the use of hormone replacement therapy (HRT). HRT use is associated with increased life expectancy in postmenopausal women.[6]

The proposed benefits of estrogen replacement therapy include prevention and treatment of bone loss, protection against urogenital atrophy, preservation of cognitive function, and possibly prevention of cardiovascular disease and dementia.

There is also epidemiologic evidence to suggest that women who use estrogen replacement therapy may be at reduced risk for carcinoma of the colon, oral bone loss, tooth loss with increasing age, and possibly macular degeneration. These apparent long-term health benefits are in addition to estrogen's recognized role in alleviating the well-known symptoms of the menopausal transition (i.e., hot flashes and night sweats). Nonetheless, the advantages of HRT must be weighed against potential risks, including thrombosis and the increased incidence of breast cancer observed in epidemiologic studies of postmenopausal estrogen use.[7]

MENOPAUSE AND POSTMENOPAUSAL HORMONE REPLACEMENT

PHYSIOLOGY

Characteristics of the human menstrual cycle throughout reproductive life have been well described.[8] A woman is born with approximately 400,000 primordial follicles in her ovaries. During a normal reproductive life span, she ovulates less than 1,000 times. The vast majority of follicles undergo atresia.

The hypothalamic-pituitary-ovarian axis dynamically controls reproductive physiology throughout the reproductive years. The pituitary is regulated by pulsatile secretion of gonadotropin-releasing hormone (GnRH) from the hypothalamus. Follicle stimulating hormone (FSH) and luteinizing hormone (LH), produced by the pituitary in response to GnRH, regulate ovarian function. These gonadotropins are also influenced by negative feedback from the sex steroids estradiol and progesterone. Ovarian follicular activity is reflected by the circulating concentrations of sex steroids and peptide hormones (such as inhibin and activin). The sex steroids include estradiol, produced by the dominant follicle; progesterone, produced by the corpus luteum after the maturation of the dominant ovarian follicle; and androgens, primarily testosterone and androstenedione, secreted by the ovarian stroma. Sex steroids are important for the healthy functioning of many organs, including the cardiovascular system, bones, brain, skin, and the reproductive and urogenital tracts. They act primarily by regulating gene expression.

Pathophysiologic changes associated with menopause are caused by the loss of ovarian follicular activity.[1] Ovarian primordial follicle numbers decrease with advancing age, and at the time of the menopause, few follicles remain in the ovary. Hence, the postmenopausal ovary is no longer the primary site of estradiol or progesterone synthesis. The postmenopausal ovary secretes primarily androstenedione and testosterone. In contrast to the acute fall in circulating estrogen at the time of menopause, the decline in circulating androgens commences in the decade leading up to the average age of natural menopause, and closely parallels increasing age.[9] Androgens are secreted by both the ovaries and the adrenal glands. Following menopause, direct ovarian androgen secretion appears to account for as much as 50% of testosterone production, with the adrenal gland being a less important source. Hypertrophy of the ovarian stroma may develop after menopause, probably secondary to high LH concentrations, thereby resulting in increased ovarian testosterone production. Alternatively, the ovaries may become fibrotic and a poor source of sex steroids.

No endocrine event clearly signals the time just prior to final menses.[10] Nonetheless, as women age, a progressive rise in circulating FSH[11] and a concomitant decline in ovarian inhibin[10] are observed. In women who continue to experience menstrual bleeding, FSH determinations on day 2 or 3 of the menstrual cycle are considered elevated when concentrations exceed 10–12 mIU/mL, an indication of diminished ovarian reserve. Clear elevations in serum FSH are seen in women around the age of 40.[10] When ovarian function has ceased, serum FSH concentrations are greater than 40 mIU/mL.

The perimenopause is the period immediately prior to the menopause and the first year after menopause. The menopausal transition is the period of time when the endocrinologic, biologic, and clinical features of the approaching menopause commence.[10] The menopausal transition usually begins approximately 4 years prior to menopause and is characterized by menstrual cycle irregularity caused by increased frequency of anovulatory cycles. Women in the perimenopausal years are more likely to seek medical consultation than are premenopausal or postmenopausal women. Vasomotor symptoms (hot flashes and night sweats), psychological symptoms (anxiety, mood swings, and depression), and disturbances of sexuality are markedly increased in the perimenopause. Menopause is characterized by a 10- to 15-fold increase in circulating FSH concentrations as compared to concentrations of FSH in the follicular phase of the cycle, a four- to fivefold increase in LH, and a more than 90% decrease in circulating estradiol concentrations.[10] During the perimenopause, FSH concentrations may rise to the postmenopausal range during some cycles, but return to premenopausal levels during subsequent cycles. Thus, high concentrations of FSH should not be used to diagnose menopause in perimenopausal women. However, vasomotor symptoms in perimenopausal women may require treatment despite the presence of menstrual bleeding. Abnormal thyroid function and other conditions that may cause similar symptomatology first should be excluded. Dysfunctional uterine bleeding may occur during the perimenopausal years because of anovulatory cycles, but other gynecologic causes also should be considered. Treatment options for dysfunctional uterine bleeding include progestins or low-dose oral contraceptives.

An observational study of more than 9,000 postmenopausal women examined the relationship between endogenous estrogens and bone mineral density,[12] bone loss,[13] fractures,[14] and breast cancer.[15] Women with detectable serum estradiol concentrations (5–25 pg/mL) had a 6% to 7% higher bone mineral density at the total hip and spine as compared to women with undetectable levels (<5 pg/mL).[12] They also had significantly less bone loss at the hip than women with undetectable levels.[13] Women with undetectable serum estradiol concentrations had a relative risk of 2.5 for subsequent hip and vertebral fractures.[14] However, women with the highest estradiol serum concentrations had the greatest risk of developing breast cancer.[15]

CLINICAL PRESENTATION OF MENOPAUSE

Vasomotor symptoms, hot flashes, and night sweats are common symptoms of estrogen withdrawal. Mild vasomotor symptoms can often be alleviated by lifestyle modification, reduction in the intake of caffeine and hot beverages, exercise, and other general good-health practices. However, for those experiencing significant vasomotor symptoms, no therapy has been shown to be as effective as estrogen replacement in alleviating hot flashes. Vaginal dryness is also directly related to estrogen insufficiency, but some women can find adequate relief from nonestrogenic vaginal creams. Most women with significant vaginal dryness, however, require local or systemic estrogen therapy to replenish moisture.

Although some would accept a range of other symptoms to be typical of estrogen deficiency (e.g., mood swings, depression, insomnia, migraines, formication, arthralgia, myalgia, urinary frequency), the relationship between these symptoms and the absolute decline in estrogen is more controversial. Many women, nonetheless, experience relief of such symptoms with estrogen replacement therapy.

▶ TREATMENT: Menopause

The goals of HRT are to enhance the quality of life, to treat menopausal symptoms, and to reduce morbidity and mortality associated with sex-steroid deficiency. Postmenopausal HRT is a subject of major interest in the field of women's health. Therapy directed at menopausal symptoms, such as hot flashes, is often short-term. However, therapy directed at other HRT indications, such as osteoporosis prevention or treatment, should be long-term. Pharmacologic therapies for menopause are predominantly hormonal. In women with an intact uterus, HRT consists of an estrogen plus a progestin given as cyclic or continuous-combined regimens. Scheduled withdrawal bleeding occurs with cyclic HRT, whereas no bleeding occurs with continuous-combined therapy. In women who have undergone hysterectomy, estrogen replacement therapy (ERT) is given unopposed by a progestin.

Treatment of menopausal symptoms can be effectively managed in some patients with lifestyle modification, including exercise, weight control, smoking cessation, and a healthful diet. More recently, however, dietary supplements and other nonpharmacologic therapies have been promoted as the "natural" alternatives to HRT. To date, there is little to support the use of such nonprescription products, which include various herbal remedies and soy-based supplements.

NONPHARMACOLOGIC THERAPY: PHYTOESTROGENS

Phytoestrogens are plant compounds with estrogen-like biologic activity[16] and relatively weak estrogen-receptor binding properties. Epidemiologic studies suggest that consumption of a phytoestrogen-rich diet, as seen in traditional Asiatic societies, is associated with a lower risk of breast cancer and cardiovascular disease. However, none of these studies have taken into account other lifestyle variations or genetic differences between the populations studied.

The biologic potencies of phytoestrogens vary, and the majority of these compounds are nonsteroidal in structure and less potent than the synthetic estrogens. There are three main classes of phytoestrogens: isoflavones, lignans, and coumestans, all of which are found in plants or their seeds.[16] The most commonly studied phytoestrogen is the isoflavone class. Genistein and daidzein are the most abundant active components of isoflavones. Of note, the concentration of isoflavones per gram of soy protein varies considerably among preparations.

Also, a single plant often contains more than one class of phytoestrogen. Common food sources of phytoestrogens include soybeans (isoflavones), cereals and oilseeds such as flaxseed (lignans), and alfalfa sprouts (coumestans). After consumption of plant lignans and isoflavones, complex enzymatic metabolic conversions occur in the gastrointestinal tract, resulting in the formation of heterocyclic phenols whose chemical structure resembles that of the estrogens.[16]

Several studies have shown improved vaginal symptoms and cytology maturation index with phytoestrogen supplementation.[17–19] In most published studies, the phytoestrogen supplement administered exceeded the estimated daily intake reported for Japanese women by at least twofold. Current data suggest that phytoestrogen supplementation as soy or linseed is no more effective than wheat placebo in relieving hot flashes in postmenopausal women. There is no evidence that phytoestrogens ameliorate other symptoms that characterize the menopause transition, such as anxiety, depression, arthralgia, myalgia, or headache, which comprise a large part of the Kupperman Index of menopausal symptoms. In fact, with soy supplementation the Kupperman Index does not change.[20]

Phytoestrogens decrease low-density lipoprotein (LDL) cholesterol and triglyceride concentrations, with no significant change in HDL cholesterol concentrations.[21] Furthermore, phytoestrogens have the ability to inhibit LDL oxidation and normalize vascular reactivity in estrogen-deprived primates.[22] In addition, bone density may be improved by phytoestrogens.[22] Common adverse effects include constipation, bloating, and nausea.[20]

With respect to breast cancer, published data are both conflicting and confusing. Two studies, one conducted in Singaporean women[23] and another in Chinese women,[24] did not show any risk reduction in postmenopausal women in association with high dietary soy intake.

In the setting of estrogen-receptor-positive breast cancer, exogenous phytoestrogens may stimulate breast cancer cell growth when consumed in low-to-moderate concentrations (i.e., an amount obtainable from a supplemented diet).[25] Concern also exists regarding adverse effects that may occur when women take excessive amounts of phytoestrogens. At present, multiple studies suggest that phytoestrogen supplements offer no benefit in menopausal symptom relief and may potentially exacerbate the disease in women with estrogen-receptor-positive breast cancer.

There is increasing evidence from cell-line studies that phytoestrogens interfere with the effect of tamoxifen on breast cancer cells.[26] Thus, for women taking tamoxifen, phytoestrogen supplementation cannot be routinely recommended.

Data from cell-line studies also suggest that low phytoestrogen intake has little or no effect on estrogen-receptor-negative breast cancer cells, but very high concentrations may inhibit cancer cell growth.[27] The latter effect, however, has not been well studied and may require large doses of phytoestrogen that are not clinically feasible.

To date, much of the rationale for phytoestrogen use in treating menopause is derived from observational studies. Larger, long-term studies are needed to document the effects of phytoestrogens on the breast, bone, and endometrium. Furthermore, differences among classes of phytoestrogens must be identified clearly, including dosing and biologic activity, before phytoestrogens can be considered an alternative to conventional HRT in postmenopausal women.

PHARMACOLOGIC THERAPY: HORMONAL REGIMENS

ESTROGEN AND PROGESTIN TREATMENT

Estrogens

Estrogens are naturally occurring hormones or synthetic steroidal or nonsteroidal compounds with estrogenic activity. Various systemically administered estrogens (typically oral and transdermal) are suitable for replacement therapy (Table 83–1). Estrogens can be administered orally, transdermally (patches, creams, or gels), intravaginally (creams, tablets, rings), intramuscularly, or in the form of subcutaneously implanted pellets. An intranasal estradiol spray is available overseas and soon also will be available in the United States. The choice of estrogen delivery (product, route, and method) should be determined in consultation with the patient to ensure acceptability and enhance compliance. In general, the oral and transdermal routes are the most frequently used, with oral CEE (conjugated equine estrogens) being the most popular estrogen in the United States. There is no evidence that one estrogen compound is more effective than another in relieving menopausal symptoms, preventing cardiovascular disease, or preventing or treating osteoporosis.

TABLE 83–1. Systemic Estrogen Products Available in the United States

Estrogen	Dosage Strength
Oral estrogens	
Conjugated equine estrogens	0.3, 0.625, 0.9, 1.25, 2.5 mg
Esterified estrogens	0.3, 0.625, 1.25, 2.5 mg
Estropipate (piperazine estrone sulfate)	0.625, 1.25, 2.5, 5 mg
Ethinyl estradiol	0.02, 0.05 mg
Micronized estradiol	0.5, 1, 2 mg
Transdermal estrogens	
17β-Estradiol	25, 37.5, 50, 75, 100 μg

Oral Estrogen Administration. Oral CEE has been available for more than 50 years. CEE is prepared from the urine of pregnant mares and is composed of estrone sulfate (50% to 60%) and multiple other equine estrogens such as equilin and 17α-dihydroequilin.[28]

Estradiol is the predominant and most active form of endogenous estrogens. A micronized form of estradiol (produced by a technique that yields extremely small particles of the pure hormone) is readily absorbed from the small intestines.[28] When given orally, estradiol is metabolized by the intestinal mucosa and the liver during the first hepatic passage, and only 10% reaches the circulation as free estradiol. Gut and liver metabolism convert a large proportion of estradiol to the less-potent estrone. Thus, measurement of serum estradiol is not useful for monitoring oral estrogen replacement. The principal metabolites of micronized estradiol are estrone and estrone sulfate. Administration of estradiol via the oral route results in estrone concentrations that are three to six times those of estradiol. Ethinyl estradiol is a highly potent semisynthetic estrogen that has similar activity following administration by the oral or parenteral routes.

Orally administered estrogens stimulate the synthesis of hepatic proteins and increase the circulating concentrations of sex hormone-binding globulin, which, in turn, may compromise the bioavailability of androgens and estrogens.

Parenteral estrogen administration bypasses the gastrointestinal tract and thereby avoids the first-pass liver metabolism. Parenteral routes of estrogen delivery result in a more physiologic estradiol-to-estrone ratio (estradiol > estrone) as seen in the normal premenopausal state. Women with elevated triglyceride concentrations or significant liver function abnormalities may benefit from parenteral therapy. Parenteral estrogen therapy also is less likely to affect sex hormone-binding globulin as compared to oral therapy.

Transdermal administration shares the advantages of other parenteral estrogen routes. Transdermal systems have the added advantage of delivering estradiol to the general venous circulation at a continuous rate. Reactions at the application site occur in about 10% of women who use reservoir (alcohol-based) patches. The newer matrix systems (estrogen in adhesive) are generally better tolerated, and only 5% of women experience skin reactions.[29] The incidence of skin irritation diminishes when the application site is rotated. Topical anti-inflammatory products can be applied for managing the skin rashes.

Percutaneous gel or cream preparations are convenient, but variability in drug absorption is common. This form of estrogen is used for systemic therapy and has been available in France for over 20 years.

Estradiol pellets (implants) containing pure crystalline 17 β-estradiol have been available for more than 50 years. They are inserted subcutaneously into the anterior abdominal wall or buttock. Pellets are difficult to remove and may continue to release estradiol for a long time after insertion. Implantation should not be repeated until serum estradiol concentrations have fallen to values similar to those at the mid-follicular phase of the menstrual cycle. Estradiol pellets have gained little popularity in the United States.

TABLE 83–2. Standard Estrogen Doses for Preventing Bone Loss[30–34]

Estrogen	Dose
Conjugated equine estrogens	0.625 mg given orally once daily
Esterified estrogens	0.625 mg given orally once daily
Estradiol valerate	2 mg given orally once daily
Estropipate (piperazine estrone sulfate)	1.5 mg given orally once daily
Ethinyl estradiol	5 μg given orally once daily
Micronized 17β-estradiol	2 mg given orally once daily
Transdermal 17β-estradiol	50 μg/24 h transdermally (applied once or twice weekly)
Implanted 17β-estradiol	50 mg pellets implanted subcutaneously every 6 months
Percutaneous 17β-estradiol	1 mg in the form of cream or gel applied daily

Intranasal 17β-estradiol spray, which enables single-daily or twice-daily dosing, also has been developed for use in postmenopausal women.

Vaginal creams, tablets, and rings are used for the treatment of urogenital atrophy. However, this treatment has more than a local effect. Nonetheless, at low doses, local application can reverse atrophic vaginal changes and avoid significant systemic absorption. Vaginal rings are a sustained-delivery system composed of a biologically inert liquid polymer matrix with pure crystalline estradiol that can maintain adequate estradiol concentrations.

Typically, the initial dose of ERT is the minimally effective dose necessary to relieve vasomotor symptoms and prevent bone loss.[30] The standard dose of estrogen previously believed to be effective in maintaining bone mass is equivalent to 0.625 mg of conjugated equine estrogen (Table 83–2).[30–34]

However, new evidence indicates that lower doses of estrogen are effective in controlling postmenopausal symptoms[35] and reducing bone loss.[36] A low dose of oral conjugated equine estrogens (0.3 mg/day) is equivalent to a daily transdermal dose of 25 μg of estradiol or 1 mg of oral micronized estradiol.[37] If adverse effects such as breast tenderness occur with standard doses, lowering the dose may resolve the problem and improve patient compliance. Alternatively, if vasomotor symptoms are not adequately controlled with a lower-dose regimen, increasing the estrogen dose may be a reasonable option.

ADVERSE EFFECTS

Common adverse effects of estrogen include nausea, headache, breast tenderness, and heavy bleeding. Initiating therapy with low doses of estrogen often will minimize breast tenderness, unscheduled bleeding, and other potential adverse effects. Transdermal estrogen is less likely than oral estrogen to cause nausea and headache. Also, transdermal estrogen is associated with a lower incidence of breast tenderness and deep vein thrombosis than oral estrogen.[38] Changing from one estrogen regimen to another can in many cases alleviate certain adverse effects.

Progestins

Because of the increased risk of endometrial hyperplasia and endometrial cancer with estrogen monotherapy (unopposed estrogen), women who have not undergone hysterectomy should be concurrently treated with a progestin in addition to the estrogen. Progestins reduce nuclear estradiol receptor concentrations, suppress DNA synthesis, and decrease estrogen bioavailability by increasing the activity of endometrial 17-hydroxysteroid dehydrogenase, an enzyme responsible for the conversion of estradiol to estrone.[39]

TABLE 83–3. Progestin Doses for Preventing Endometrial Hyperplasia

Progestin	Standard Oral Dose
Dydrogesterone	10–20 mg for 12 to 14 days per calendar month
Medroxyprogesterone acetate	5–10 mg for 12 to 14 days per calendar month or 2.5 mg daily continuously throughout calendar month
Micronized progesterone	200 mg for 12 to 14 days per calendar month
Norethisterone	0.7–1 mg for 12 to 14 days per calendar month
Norethindrone acetate	5 mg for 12 to 14 days per calendar month (0.14 mg or 0.25 mg is used in continuous regimens administered transdermally)
Norgestrel	0.15 mg for 12 to 14 days per calendar month
Levonorgestrel	150 μg for 12 to 14 days per calendar month

Several progestin regimens designed to prevent endometrial hyperplasia are available (Table 83–3). Progestins must be taken for a sufficient period of time during each cycle. A minimum of 12 to 14 days of progestin therapy each month is required for complete protection against estrogen-induced endometrial hyperplasia.[40] It should be noted that even use of low-dose estrogen, including some vaginal preparations, requires progestin coadministration for endometrial protection in women with an intact uterus.[41] However, rarely is there a need for progestin administration in women who have undergone hysterectomy.

Progestins can be used in combination with estrogen in a cyclical fashion for 12 to 14 days of the month (sequential HRT) or daily throughout the month (continuous combined HRT). Sequential HRT results in scheduled vaginal withdrawal bleeding, although in older women this is often scant or altogether absent. Continuous combined HRT ultimately results in endometrial atrophy and the absence of vaginal bleeding. Various HRT regimens which combine an estrogen and a progestin are available (Table 83–4).

The first generation of progestins included the C-19 androgenic progestins norethisterone, norgestrel, and levonorgestrel. More recent preparations have included the C-21 progestins dydrogesterone and medroxyprogesterone acetate (MPA), which are less androgenic. Micronized progesterone has also become available for use in postmenopausal women. The most commonly used oral progestins are MPA, micronized progesterone, and norethisterone acetate. The latter also can now be administered transdermally in the form of a combined estrogen-progestin patch. MPA (5–10 mg) remains the most commonly used progestin in the United States, but the Postmenopausal Estrogen/Progestin Interventions (PEPI) trial showed micronized progesterone (200 mg) to be an effective alternative to MPA.[40] A randomized, double-blind, placebo-controlled crossover study found that the addition of cyclic MPA (10 mg/day for 14 days) to transdermal estrogen therapy (100 μg) did not produce any consistent adverse physical or psychological effects in women, regardless of their previous premenstrual syndrome history.[42] In addition, another double-blind, placebo-controlled crossover study revealed that MPA given alone

TABLE 83–4. Common Postmenopausal Hormone Replacement Therapy Regimens

Regimen	Estrogen Dose	Progestin Dose
Oral conjugated equine estrogens plus medroxyprogesterone acetate	0.625 mg	5 mg for 14 days per 28-day cycle (cyclical regimen)
Oral conjugated equine estrogens plus medroxyprogesterone acetate	0.625 mg	2.5 mg or 5 mg (continuous regimen)
Oral ethinyl estradiol plus norethindrone	5 μg	1 mg (continuous regimen)
Oral estradiol plus norgestimate	1 mg	0.09 mg (continuous regimen)
Transdermal estradiol and norethindrone acetate	50 μg/24 h	140 μg/24 h or 250 μg/24 h (continuous regimen)

(10 mg/day on days 16 to 25 of each month) does not cause adverse symptoms in postmenopausal women.[43]

Adverse Effects. Common adverse effects of progestins include irritability, depression, and headache. Changing from a cyclic to a continuous regimen, or changing from one progestin to another, may decrease the incidence or severity of these untoward effects.

Adverse effects of progestins are difficult to evaluate and can vary with the agent administered. Some women experience "premenstrual-like" symptoms, such as mood swings, bloating, fluid retention, and sleep disturbance. New methods and routes of progestin delivery (e.g., parenterally by an intranasal spray or locally by an intrauterine device that releases levonorgestrel or a progesterone-containing bioadhesive vaginal gel) may be associated with fewer adverse effects. Women who are unable to tolerate a progestin may be given unopposed estrogen if they are informed of the significant increased risk for endometrial cancer and have endometrial biopsy annually or whenever vaginal bleeding occurs.

Methods of Estrogen and Progestin Administration

Cyclic Estrogen/Progestin Treatment. Estrogen is typically administered continuously (daily). A progestin is coadministered with the estrogen for at least 12 to 14 days of a 28-day cycle.[40] The progestin causes scheduled withdrawal bleeding in approximately 90% of women. With this regimen, bleeding usually begins 1 to 2 days after the last progestin dose.[21] Occasionally, however, bleeding can begin during the latter phase of progestin administration. Women who receive a cyclic HRT regimen should undergo a baseline pelvic examination. Endometrial biopsy should be considered if bleeding occurs at any time other than the expected time of withdrawal bleeding or when heavier or more prolonged withdrawal bleeding occurs.[44]

Endovaginal ultrasonography also has been used in the evaluation of abnormal uterine bleeding in women receiving HRT. However, there is no universal agreement that endovaginal ultrasonography is adequate to exclude endometrial pathology.[34]

Continuous-Combined Estrogen/Progestin Treatment. For many women, the scheduled withdrawal bleeding is one of the main reasons for avoiding or discontinuing HRT. Because there is no physiologic need for bleeding, HRT regimens that reduce or prevent monthly bleeding have been developed. Continuous-combined estrogen/progestin administration is intended to prevent the endometrial proliferative effect of estrogen and to result in endometrial atrophy. However, initially it causes unpredictable spotting or bleeding, which usually resolves within 6 to 12 months. Decreasing the estrogen dose or increasing the progestin dose usually decreases or stops the spotting. Occasionally, a drug-free period of 1 or 2 weeks may be useful to stop the bleeding.

Women who have recently undergone menopause have a higher risk for excessive, unpredictable bleeding while receiving continuous therapy; thus, this regimen is best reserved for women who are at least 2 years postmenopause.

Women who are given continuous HRT should undergo a baseline pelvic examination. Endometrial evaluation must be considered when irregular bleeding persists for more than 6 months after initiating therapy.[44]

Continuous-combined HRT is more acceptable than traditional cyclic therapy. In a study using oral HRT,[46] 93% of women who took oral continuous-combined hormone therapy were compliant after 1 year of treatment, and 73% were still compliant after 2 years of treatment. This is compared with 66% and 49%, respectively, for women on cyclic therapy. The acceptance of continuous-combined regimens using continuous parenteral estrogen along with an oral progestin is similar to that of continuous-combined oral hormone therapy.[47]

ANDROGENS

The therapeutic use of testosterone in women, although controversial, is becoming more widespread.[48] Nonetheless, data to support this practice are limited, as only a few randomized trials have been conducted. There is a cluster of symptoms that appear to characterize androgen deficiency in women: loss of sexual desire; diminished well-being; loss of energy; and, over time, decreased bone mass and reduced muscle strength.[40] There is substantial evidence that androgen replacement, usually in the form of testosterone, is effective in alleviating these physical and psychological symptoms of androgen insufficiency. Symptoms are more pronounced in women who have undergone surgical menopause because of the abrupt cessation of testosterone production by the ovaries. Following oophorectomy, testosterone and androstenedione serum concentrations decrease by about 50%. Testosterone replacement therapy is accepted for women who have undergone surgical menopause, but should also be considered for naturally menopausal women and those who have experienced premature ovarian failure.

In women, androgens may act directly via the androgen receptor or indirectly after conversion to estrogen. Androgens are the precursor hormones for estrogen production in the ovaries, as well as in extragonadal sites, including bone, adipose tissue, and the brain.

Although estrogen replacement improves vaginal dryness, vasomotor symptoms, and general well being, it has minimal effect on libido. Estrogen combined with androgen significantly improves sexual activity, satisfaction, and pleasure more than that reported with estrogen monotherapy. Androgen replacement appears to be effective and safe when given in doses that achieve circulating androgen serum concentrations near the physiologic range for young women of reproductive age. The goal is to produce beneficial effects on well being and quality of life without incurring undesirable virilizing adverse effects.[48] Nonetheless, oral testosterone therapy can decrease high-density lipoprotein cholesterol and apolipoprotein A1, and can also lower triglycerides.[49] The addition of methyltestosterone to esterified estrogen in cynomologus monkeys does not negate the coronary artery vasodilator effect of estrogen.[50] Furthermore, exogenous testosterone therapy increases the brachial artery flow-mediated vasodilation and the vasodilation induced by glyceryl trinitrate in postmenopausal women stabilized on HRT.[51]

There are no data regarding the effects of exogenous androgen therapy on the incidence of breast cancer. However, androgen receptors are found in approximately 50% of mammary tumors and their presence is associated with longer survival in women with operable breast cancer.[48]

Testosterone is available as oral methyltestosterone in the United States and as testosterone implants in the United Kingdom. Of the available oral preparations, methyltestosterone in combination with esterified estrogen (either 0.625 mg esterified estrogen plus 1.25 mg methyltestosterone or 1.25 mg esterified estrogen plus 2.5 mg methyltestosterone) is the most widely studied.

Relative contraindications to testosterone therapy include moderate to severe acne, clinical hirsutism, and androgenic alopecia. Absolute contraindications to androgen replacement include pregnancy or lactation and known or suspected androgen-dependent neoplasia.

Adverse effects from excessive dosage include virilization, fluid retention, and potentially adverse lipoprotein lipid effects, which are more likely with oral administration.

Testosterone replacement for women is now available in a variety of formulations (Table 83–5).[48] The recent development of a transdermal testosterone matrix patch, specifically for use in women, may provide a new option for women requiring testosterone replacement.[52,53] Testosterone replacement should not be administered to postmenopausal women who are not receiving concurrent estrogen replacement.

SELECTIVE ESTROGEN-RECEPTOR MODULATORS

Recent advances in the molecular pharmacology of estrogen and estrogen receptors have resulted in the development of selective estrogen-receptor modulators (SERMs). The SERMs, a new type of nonhormonal therapy, bind to estrogen receptors and function as tissue-specific estrogen antagonists or agonists. SERMs are compounds that act like estrogens in some target tissues, while antagonizing their effects in others. The ideal SERM would protect against coronary artery disease, osteoporosis, and dementia. It would further decrease the incidence of breast, endometrial, and colorectal cancer without exacerbating menopausal symptoms or increasing the risk of venous thromboembolism or gallbladder disease. To date, no SERM meets these ideals. Tamoxifen, the first-generation SERM, has estrogen antagonist activity on the breast and estrogen-like agonist activity on the bone and the endometrium.[54] The second generation of SERMs, most notably raloxifene (a nonsteroidal benzothiophene derivative), recently became available for the treatment of osteoporosis.[55,56] Raloxifene decreases bone loss in recently menopausal women without affecting the endometrium and has estrogen-like actions on lipid metabolism. Although the effects of raloxifene on coagulation and fibrinolysis parameters have been reported to differ from those of estrogen,[57] the actual clinical rates of thromboembolic events are somewhat similar. The Multiple Outcomes of Raloxifene Evaluation (MORE) study, a multicenter randomized, blinded, placebo-controlled trial, showed that raloxifene increases bone mineral density in the spine and femoral neck, and reduces the risk of vertebral fractures.[58] More importantly, the same study suggested that raloxifene use is associated with a lower incidence of breast cancer compared to placebo.[59] Nonetheless, raloxifene use increases the risk of venous thromboembolism to a degree similar to that of oral estrogen.[58] In contrast to estrogens, raloxifene is not indicated for the treatment of hot flashes.[60] Raloxifene generally is well tolerated; however, it is associated with a slight increase in leg cramps and may exacerbate hot flashes.[55]

TIBOLONE

Tibolone is a gonadomimetic synthetic steroid in the norpregnane family with combined estrogenic, progestogenic, and androgenic activity.[61] It has several active metabolites, including a $\Delta 4$-isomer, and 3α-OH and 3β-OH compounds.[61] The $\Delta 4$-isomer metabolite confers significant progestogenic and androgenic properties. Tibolone has beneficial effects on mood, libido, and bone density, and improves menopausal symptoms and vaginal atrophy. In addition, it causes endometrial atrophy and, therefore, does not usually cause withdrawal bleeding when used in women who have had amenorrhea for at least 1 year. Tibolone is not recommended during perimenopause because it may cause irregular bleeding. Its use is associated with a low rate of bleeding, ranging from 10% to 15% during the initial months of treatment to about 4% after 6 months of treatment.[28]

Little is known about the long-term effects of tibolone on breast cancer and cardiovascular disease. It reduces concentrations of total

TABLE 83–5. Androgen Replacement Regimens Used for Women

Regimen	Dose	Frequency	Route
Methyltestosterone (in combination with esterified estrogen)	1.25–2.5 mg	Daily	Oral
Mixed testosterone esters	50–100 mg	Every 4 to 6 weeks	Intramuscular
Testosterone pellets	50 mg	Every 6 months	Subcutaneous (implanted)
Transdermal testosterone system*	150 μg/24 h	Every 3 to 4 days	Transdermal patch
Nandrolone decanoate	50 mg	Every 8 to 12 weeks	Intramuscular

*Undergoing clinical trials.

cholesterol, triglycerides, and lipoprotein (a). However, tibolone significantly decreases HDL cholesterol, and thus it may increase overall cardiovascular risk.[28] Further studies are necessary to identify the true risk/benefit ratio of tibolone with respect to its overall effect on coronary artery disease and breast cancer. The major adverse effects of tibolone include weight gain and bloating.

TREATMENT CONSIDERATIONS AND PATIENT ASSESSMENT

Contraindications

HRT is contraindicated in women with endometrial cancer, breast cancer, undiagnosed vaginal bleeding, recent vascular thrombosis, or active liver disease.[62]

Relative contraindications include uterine leiomyoma, migraine headaches, and seizure disorder.[21] In addition, oral estrogen should be avoided in women with hypertriglyceridemia, liver disease, and gallbladder disease. For these women, transdermal administration is a safer approach.

HRT Adverse Effects

The main reasons for discontinuing HRT are side effects such as bleeding, breast tenderness, bloating, and "premenstrual-like symptoms." Reducing the dose or changing the regimen or the route of administration can minimize these effects.

Pretreatment Assessment

The initial visit of a perimenopausal or postmenopausal woman is the most appropriate time to obtain a complete medical history, perform a physical examination, and educate the patient.[21] The risks and benefits of HRT should be discussed with the patient so that she can make a rational decision about whether to use HRT. Medical history should include determination of a personal or family history of thrombotic problems. The physical examination should include a complete cardiovascular exam, clinical assessment of thyroid status, and breast and pelvic examinations. Papanicolaou cervical cytologic examination and screening mammography negative for malignancy are required before initiating HRT. Thyroid function tests, lipoprotein lipid profile, and iron studies should also be performed at the discretion of the physician.

BENEFITS OF HRT

Immediate HRT Benefits: Relief of Menopausal Symptoms

Hot Flashes. Vasomotor symptoms, hot flashes, and night sweats are the symptoms of estrogen withdrawal. Hot flashes are the classic sign of menopause and the major clinical complaint of American women during the perimenopausal and early menopausal years. Hot flashes are a sensation of warmth, frequently accompanied by skin flushing and perspiration.[29] A chill may follow as the core body temperature drops. Hot flashes may occur in women of any age who experience acute estrogen withdrawal. They can be occasional or frequent, last from seconds to an hour, and are characterized by symptoms ranging from mild warmth to profuse sweating. For some women hot flashes are a minor nuisance, but for others it can be a disturbing symptom that disrupts their sense of well being and causes problems in their social and professional lives. They usually occur spontaneously but are often increased in frequency or severity in hot or humid weather or after ingestion of caffeine, alcohol, or spicy foods.[63]

Hot flashes occur in up to 75% of menopausal women, and the prevalence is higher in the first two postmenopausal years. Women who have undergone surgical menopause tend to have more intense menopausal symptoms than those who experience a natural menopause.

Without treatment, hot flashes typically disappear within 1 to 2 years, but in some untreated women they continue for more than 20 years.[38] Women experiencing mild vasomotor symptoms often experience relief by lifestyle modification, reduction in intake of caffeine and hot beverages, exercise, and other good general health practices. However, no therapy has been shown to be as effective as estrogen replacement in alleviating significant vasomotor symptoms. Estrogens diminish hot flashes in most women, and there is a dose-dependent relation between estrogen administration and suppression of hot flashes.

Alternatives to estrogen for treatment of hot flashes include selective serotonin reuptake inhibitors such as venlafaxine, methyldopa, clonidine, medroxyprogesterone acetate, and megestrol acetate. Venlafaxine, a potent inhibitor of neuronal serotonin and norepinephrine reuptake, significantly reduces vasomotor symptoms at doses of 37.5–150 mg/day.[64] This drug is considered by some to be a first-line therapy for the treatment of hot flashes in women for whom HRT is contraindicated.[64] Nutritional supplements that contain soy protein may ameliorate hot flashes. To date, randomized, placebo-controlled trials have not established the efficacy of herbal remedies, homeopathic treatments, or acupuncture for the prevention or treatment of hot flashes.

Vaginal Atrophy. Estrogen receptors have been demonstrated in the lower genitourinary tract, and at least 50% of postmenopausal women suffer symptoms of urogenital atrophy caused by estrogen deficiency.[65] Atrophy of the vaginal mucosa results in vaginal dryness and dyspareunia. Lower urinary tract symptoms include urethritis, recurrent urinary tract infection, and urinary urgency and frequency. Most women with significant vaginal dryness because of vaginal atrophy require the use of local or systemic estrogen therapy for symptom relief. Such treatment also reduces the risk of recurrent urinary tract infections, possibly by modifying the vaginal flora.[7] Urinary incontinence, which becomes more prevalent with increasing age, is not usually improved by estrogen therapy.

Vaginal administration of low-dose estrogen provides an alternative approach to urogenital atrophy that is safe and acceptable. Concomitant progestin therapy is unnecessary if women are using low-dose micronized 17β-estradiol. However, the regular use of conjugated equine estrogen vaginal creams by women with an intact uterus requires intermittent progestin challenges (i.e., for 10 days every 12 weeks). This is an important caveat because vaginal atrophy requires long-term estrogen treatment.[7]

Long-Term Goals of HRT

Osteoporosis Prevention. Menopause is accompanied by accelerated bone loss, and the central role of estrogen deficiency in postmenopausal osteoporosis is well established. Estrogen deficiency results in bone loss through its actions in accelerating bone turnover and uncoupling bone formation from resorption. In fact, annual decrements in bone mass of 3% to 5% are common in the years soon after the menopause, and 0.5% to 1% decrements are seen after 65 years of age.[66] Observational studies suggest that ERT reduces the risk of spinal fracture by about 50% and of hip fracture by 30%.[38] The reduction in fracture risk is greatest with higher estrogen doses and prolonged duration of use.[67] Estrogen replacement reduces bone turnover and increases bone density in postmenopausal women of all ages. Nonetheless, the protective effect persists as long as the treatment is maintained. With cessation of therapy, postmenopausal bone loss resumes at the same rate as that in untreated women. Ten years after HRT discontinuation, bone density and fracture risk were similar in women who had used ERT and those who had not.[68] The ability of estrogen therapy to increase bone mass is enhanced by added androgens, calcium supplementation, and exercise. General protective measures, such as adequate calcium intake, regular weight-bearing exercise, and the avoidance of detrimental lifestyle habits such as smoking and alcohol abuse are appropriate for all women. Also, adequate exposure to sunlight is believed to protect against vitamin D deficiency, but many Western women are deficient in this vitamin. A determination of serum 25-hydroxy-vitamin D should be obtained in all women found to have osteoporosis.

Osteoporosis is a serious age-related disease that affects millions of women throughout the world. It is defined as a systemic skeletal disease characterized by low bone mass and microarchitectural deterioration with subsequent increase in bone fragility and susceptibility to fracture.[69] Low bone density is the most important risk factor for osteoporosis.

According to the World Health Organization (WHO), a woman with bone mineral density greater than 2.5 standard deviations below the mean peak density has osteoporosis.[70] Bone mass measurement accurately determines the bone density in the spine and the hip. The current "gold standard" method of bone density testing is dual-energy x-ray absorptiometry (DXA).[71]

Osteoporosis affects approximately 28 million Americans and bears an economic burden of $14 billion per year.[72] It results in approximately 1.5 million fractures in the United States each year. The annual fracture rate in women who are approximately 65 years of age is 1% to 2%, whereas in women who are approximately 75 years of age it is 6% to 10%.[70] Furthermore, morbidity and mortality are significantly increased after an osteoporotic fracture. Of all the fractures that are a consequence of osteoporosis (vertebral, hip, and wrist), hip fracture is the most serious. During the first year after an osteoporotic hip fracture, mortality is estimated at 23% and increases with age.[73]

Currently, the management of osteoporosis incorporates efforts both for prevention and treatment (see Chap. 90). There are several agents approved by the US Food and Drug Administration (FDA) for the prevention and treatment of postmenopausal bone loss: estrogen (for prevention and treatment), alendronate (5 mg daily for prevention; 10 mg daily for treatment), raloxifene (for prevention), and calcitonin (for treatment).[72] Estrogen, however, is the treatment of choice. Natural and synthetic estrogens exert a positive effect on bone mineral density in a dose-dependent fashion, independent of age and mode of administration.[74] Treatment can begin several years after the menopause without loss of efficacy in reducing fracture risk.[67,68]

The decision, however, to start and continue hormone therapy is greatly influenced by the clinician's awareness of bone density evaluations and their clinical utility.[75] The National Osteoporosis Foundation (NOF) recommends routine bone-density testing for all women 65 years of age or older and for younger women who have clinical risk factors and who have met criteria for treatment based on T-scores.[76] The clinical risk factors emphasized by the NOF are (a) personal history of low-trauma fracture after age 45, (b) a family history of osteoporosis, (c) current cigarette smoking, and (d) low body weight.[76] Other risk factors, such as the use of glucocorticoids, are also important. NOF recommends intervention with pharmacologic agents for osteoporosis for all women with T-scores of −2.0 and below and for women with T-scores of −1.5 to −2.0 who also have risk factors.[76] The age at which treatment should be initiated has not been established clearly. A recent cross-sectional study suggests that women starting HRT later in life achieve a similar degree of bone preservation as those who start at the time of menopause.[68] On the other hand, in the study of osteoporotic fractures, significant protection from hip fracture was found only among women who began HRT within 5 years after menopause—and not among women who began later.[77]

An 8-year prospective study suggested that HRT has a more pronounced effect on the axial bone mass than that of the peripheral skeleton.[78] This is most likely a result of the relatively high turnover in vertebral bodies, consisting mainly of trabecular bone, as compared to the predominantly cortical femur bones. The standard bone-sparing daily estrogen dose is equivalent to 0.625 mg of conjugated equine estrogen (Table 83–2).[30–34]

The PEPI trial illustrates the favorable effects of estrogen on bone following the onset of menopause.[79] This randomized, double-blinded, placebo-controlled trial studied 875 healthy postmenopausal women between the ages of 45 and 64 years. They were randomized to one of the following treatments in 28-day cycles: (a) placebo; (b) 0.625 mg of conjugated equine estrogen continuously plus 10 mg of medroxyprogesterone acetate for 12 days; (c) 0.625 mg of conjugated equine estrogen plus 2.5 mg of medroxyprogesterone acetate continuously; or (d) 0.625 mg of conjugated equine estrogen continuously plus 200 mg of micronized progesterone for 12 days.[79] Overall, women assigned to HRT, regardless of the regimen, had significantly higher bone mineral density in both the hip and the spine at the 36-month evaluation compared with those assigned to placebo.[79] Active HRT resulted in mean total increases ranging from 3.5% to 5% in spinal bone mineral density and approximately 1.7% in hip bone mineral density.[79]

The recommended daily intake of elemental calcium is 1,000 mg for premenopausal women and postmenopausal women who are taking estrogen replacement, and 1,500 mg for postmenopausal women who are not taking estrogen replacement.[80] To achieve this amount of calcium, most women require supplementation to their dietary intake.

Even low doses of estrogen may increase bone mass when they are supplemented with adequate calcium intake. A recent randomized controlled study showed that 0.3 mg of esterified estrogen administered along with adequate calcium (1,000 mg/day of elemental calcium) prevented bone loss in postmenopausal women.[36] Furthermore, for elderly women, continuous low-dose HRT combined with adequate calcium and vitamin D prevented bone loss.[81] A 25 μg/day estradiol transdermal system is now approved for osteoporosis prevention as well as for treating menopausal symptoms.

ANDROGEN REPLACEMENT

Androgen receptors have been demonstrated in human osteoblast-like cell lines, and androgens have been shown to directly stimulate bone cell proliferation and differentiation. Total and bioavailable serum testosterone are the greatest predictors of bone mineral density and bone loss in premenopausal, perimenopausal, and postmenopausal women.[82] A double-blinded, randomized, placebo-controlled study showed that esterified estrogen alone (1.25 mg daily) prevented spinal bone mineral loss, whereas the same dose of estrogen plus 2.5 mg of methyltestosterone significantly increased the spinal bone mineral density.[49] A similar conclusion was reached after postmenopausal women were treated with 50-mg estradiol implants or 50-mg estradiol implants along with 50-mg testosterone implants.[83] Bone density in women receiving the combination of estrogen and testosterone increased sooner and to a greater degree than in those who received estrogen alone.[83] Estrogen monotherapy decreases bone resorption in postmenopausal women, whereas the combined estrogen-androgen regimen increases bone formation.[84] Nonetheless, prospective data confirming a reduction in fracture rate with androgen replacement are lacking, and specific guidelines cannot be given for this indication until additional data regarding safety and efficacy are available.

OTHER AGENTS

For women at high risk for osteoporosis who have contraindications for HRT, alternative regimens include raloxifene, the bisphosphonates, and calcitonin. The FDA has approved raloxifene (60 mg daily) for postmenopausal osteoporosis. The MORE study showed that raloxifene substantially decreases the vertebral fracture risk in postmenopausal women (relative risk using 60 mg of raloxifene daily is 0.7; relative risk using 120 mg of raloxifene daily is 0.5).[58] This study also showed that the frequency of vertebral fractures was reduced both in women who had preexisting fractures and those who did not. However, the risk of nonvertebral fracture for raloxifene versus placebo did not differ significantly.[58] Regardless, clinical trials have shown greater effects on bone mineral density with ERT than with raloxifene.[85]

The bisphosphonates are also useful alternatives to HRT. Bisphosphonates are analogs of pyrophosphate that inhibit bone resorption. Drugs in this class include alendronate, etidronate, pamidronate, risedronate, and tiludronate. Alendronate is the first biphosphonate approved by the FDA for treatment of osteoporosis.[86] Alendronate has no known impact on the incidence of cardiovascular disease or breast or endometrial cancer. It should be noted that estrogen administration along with bisphosphonates produces greater gains in bone density than either agent alone.[87,88]

Treatment with salmon calcitonin results in increased spinal bone density,[89] but this effect is less than that seen with estrogen or the biphosphonates. Nasal calcitonin (200 IU daily) also has been shown to reduce the risk of new vertebral fractures in postmenopausal women with osteoporosis.[89]

Cardiovascular Disease Prevention. A large number of observational studies suggest a reduction in risk for cardiovascular disease (CVD) associated with the use of HRT in postmenopausal women. Meta-analyses estimate the average risk reduction to be about 30%.[90] Estrogen replacement therapy has been shown to positively influence many risk factors for cardiovascular disease, mainly by favorably altering the blood lipid profile.[91] The route of administration of estrogen, however, influences its effects on serum lipids. Transdermally administered estrogen has less of an effect on serum lipid concentrations than does orally administered estrogen. However, estrogen-induced alterations in serum lipids account for only one-third of the observed clinical benefits of estrogens.[92] Direct actions of estrogen on blood vessels, including improved endothelial function, contribute substantially to the cardiovascular protective effects of estrogen.[92] The beneficial effect of estrogen on vascular endothelial function may occur via the promotion of nitric oxide release, which results in vasodilation, reduced release of endothelin, inhibition of adhesion-molecule expression, and increased endothelial proliferation and migration to areas of injury.[44] Estrogen alters serum lipid concentrations, coagulation and fibrinolytic systems, antioxidant systems, and the production of other vasoactive molecules that can influence the development of vascular disease.[92] Despite this biologic plausibility and supporting evidence from epidemiologic studies, data from prospective randomized clinical trials are lacking. Thus, recommendations regarding the use of HRT for the prevention of CVD must await data from ongoing randomized trials. Postmenopausal HRT may be beneficial in women who have not yet developed coronary artery disease[93,94] but not in women with established CVD.[95]

CVD is the leading cause of death in women in the United States, and the incidence of CVD gradually increases in postmenopausal women. Adherence to a healthful lifestyle (cessation of smoking, regular exercise, healthy diet, and body mass index less than 25) may prevent the onset of CVD in postmenopausal women.[96,97] Nonetheless, menopause is associated with many negative effects on CVD risk factors in women. Analysis of data from the Nurses' Health Study,[98] a prospective cohort study, showed that women who have undergone a bilateral oophorectomy had double the risk of coronary artery disease as compared to those who had not undergone premature surgical menopause. This same study showed that the women most likely to benefit from HRT are those with the greatest cardiovascular risk, and that HRT users with coronary risk factors have the greatest reduction in mortality (relative risk 0.51).[6] Newer data from the Nurses' Health Study showed that postmenopausal estrogen use substantially decreases the risk for major coronary events in women without previous heart disease.[93] In this study, current use of hormone therapy was associated with an age-adjusted relative risk of 0.54 for major coronary events.[93] Among women taking HRT, the risk for coronary events was similarly reduced in those currently taking 0.625 mg of CEE daily and those taking 0.3 mg of CEE daily as compared to those who never used estrogens.[93] Also, the reduction in risk for CVD was similar among women taking oral CEE alone (relative risk 0.55) and those taking estrogen plus progestin (relative risk 0.64).[93] However, the risk for stroke was statistically increased among women taking 0.625 mg or more of conjugated estrogen daily and among women taking estrogen plus a progestin.[93] This is intriguing, because most risk factors for coronary disease are also risk factors for stroke.[99] Some have hypothesized that HRT may have mixed effects, causing thrombotic events while at the same time improving the lipoprotein lipid profile.[99] Accordingly, such prothrombic activity might have an adverse effect on the cerebrovascular circulation, thereby resulting in increased incidence of stroke. Another surprising finding from the Nurses' Health Study was that longer duration of hormone use was associated with less coronary benefit than short duration of hormone use. The relative risk for a major coronary event increased from 0.4 for less than 1 year of current use to 0.7 for 10 or more years.[99]

The PEPI trial evaluated cardiovascular disease risk factors in a large, prospective randomized trial and found that estrogen decreases serum total cholesterol and LDL cholesterol concentrations, increases serum high-density lipoprotein (HDL) cholesterol and triglycerides, and decreases serum Lp(a) lipoprotein.[100] Furthermore, when given orally to hypercholesterolemic women, estrogen replacement significantly lowers LDL and total cholesterol.[101,102] It should be noted that a comparison of estrogen with simvastatin suggests that simvastatin is better at lowering LDL-cholesterol, whereas estrogen is better at raising HDL cholesterol.[102]

The PEPI trial confirmed that HRT does not increase blood pressure. This trial compared several progestin regimens and found that HRT regimens including micronized progesterone attenuate the beneficial effects of estrogen to a lesser degree than those containing medroxyprogesterone acetate.[100] Also, studies conducted in ovariectomized rhesus monkeys treated with estradiol, natural progesterone, and medroxyprogesterone acetate have shown a direct effect of estrogen and progesterone on coronary artery reactivity.[103] In untreated animals, coronary artery vascular muscle cells were hyperreactive, but this hyperreactivity was abolished by treatment *in vivo* with physiologic concentrations of estrogen alone or in combination with progesterone. However, the addition of medroxyprogesterone acetate negated the effects of estrogen.[103]

Raloxifene has effects on serum lipid concentrations that are similar to but less pronounced than those of estrogen; however, raloxifene may lower serum Lp(a) lipoprotein concentrations more.[57] Furthermore, although raloxifene lowers serum LDL cholesterol concentrations, it does not increase HDL cholesterol and has no significant effect on triglycerides.[104] Its role in the secondary prevention of CHD in postmenopausal women is unknown but is currently being evaluated in a large, randomized, prospective trial—the Raloxifene Use for the Heart (RUTH) study.[105]

The studies of intermediate outcomes were put in perspective by the results of a secondary prevention trial of CVD. No effect was seen with HRT in postmenopausal women with established CVD in the Heart and Estrogen/Progestin Replacement Study (HERS),[95] a randomized, placebo-controlled trial that evaluated whether the use of estrogen and medroxyprogesterone acetate can reduce the number of nonfatal myocardial infarctions and cardiovascular events. Women were randomized to receive either combined estrogen-progestin (0.625 mg/day of conjugated equine estrogen and 2.5 mg/day of medroxyprogesterone acetate) or placebo.[95] Although women assigned to HRT had favorable changes in lipids, there were no significant differences in any cardiovascular outcome at the end of this 4-year study.[95] The group receiving HRT experienced more cardiovascular events than the placebo group in year 1, but fewer cardiovascular events in years 4 and 5.[95] Thus, for women with a history of coronary artery disease, the HERS study suggests that HRT should not be administered for cardioprotection alone. Nonetheless, the HERS study had some design limitations: women were already medicated with cardioprotective drugs, were able to commence statins during the study (more women on placebo than active treatment did so), and were allowed to change therapy during the study (analysis was based on "intention to treat").[7]

On the other hand, most observational studies showing cardioprotection in HRT users may present selection bias because generally only relatively healthy women are given HRT.[106] This was not true of HERS, a study in which participants were older (mean age 66.7 years) and had preexisting heart conditions. Finally, estrogen users in observational studies are more likely to be long-term users, whereas the participants in HERS were short-term users.[107]

A recent 3-year, randomized, controlled trial showed that neither estrogen alone (0.625 mg of CEE per day) nor estrogen plus progestin (0.625 mg of CEE plus 2.5 mg of medroxyprogesterone acetate per day) affected the progression of coronary atherosclerosis in women with established coronary artery disease.[108] However, the investigators did not undertake any dynamic measurements such as response to acetylcholine, which is known to be improved with estrogen, but rather a static measurement of arterial diameter. Hence, these findings are of limited clinical value. Also, in this study as in HERS, HRT was initiated late in life (an average of 23 years after the cessation of menses). Thus, HRT may not protect against secondary events when initiated many years after the menopause.

Additional randomized, controlled trials are underway to answer some of the questions raised by HERS regarding risk/benefit issues concerning HRT. One of these trials, the Women's Health Initiative (WHI), sponsored by the National Institutes of Health, includes approximately 27,000 women free of coronary disease who were randomly assigned to receive estrogen plus a progestin or placebo if they had a uterus, or estrogen or placebo if they did not. The results of this study are expected in 2005 and hopefully will give more definitive answers about the use of HRT in postmenopausal women. The trial completed enrollment and is now several years into a planned 9-year study period. Preliminary findings from the WHI trial were presented in the form of a press release: "Women in WHI who were taking hormones (estrogen and progestin or estrogen alone) had somewhat more cardiovascular events (heart attacks, strokes, and blood clots in the legs and lungs) than those taking placebo. The actual number of women having any one of these events was very small (less than 1 percent). The increase did not meet statistical criteria for stopping the trial and, therefore, may have occurred by chance."[109]

Thus far, published studies have not resolved the question of whether HRT can prevent CVD. The long-term trials of HRT for the primary prevention of CVD that are currently underway, including the WHI, will provide the answer to the question of whether HRT prevents CVD and whether the potential benefits exceed the associated risks.[110]

OTHER POTENTIAL EFFECTS OF HRT

Mood, Cognition, and Alzheimer's Disease

Most studies show that clinical depression is not more common during menopause than at other times of life. However, a recent study suggests that estrogen use is associated with a significant improvement in mood in depressed perimenopausal women.[111] In addition, some epidemiologic studies indicate that estrogen use is associated with better performance on both verbal and visual memory testing in later life.[112] Several reports suggest that ERT may have a beneficial effect on cognition and might reduce the risk of dementia. Nonetheless, a recent review regarding the effects of HRT on cognition in postmenopausal women suggested that the improvement in cognition observed in perimenopausal women appears to be related to overall menopausal symptom improvement, with no appreciable benefits in women who are asymptomatic.[113]

Several observational studies have suggested that ERT may be protective against Alzheimer's disease (see Chap. 65). One longitudinal study of 1,124 elderly women initially free of Alzheimer's disease, Parkinson's disease, or stroke, found that estrogen use was significantly related both to a later age of onset and to a reduction in the relative risk of Alzheimer's disease. In this study, the overall relative risk of Alzheimer's disease among ERT users was 0.40.[114] Also, the duration of ERT use is associated with a progressive reduction in the incidence of Alzheimer's disease.[115] Biologic mechanisms for some of these effects include activation of the cholinergic system, antioxidant action, neurotrophic stimulation, and anti-amyloidogenic properties. However, controlled studies show that short-term estrogen therapy does not improve symptoms in most women with Alzheimer's disease.[116–118] Perhaps the ability to observe the beneficial effects of HRT may depend on the timing of the intervention. It should be noted that at present there are no published long-term, prospective, randomized, controlled studies that show beneficial effects of estrogen on the incidence or progression of Alzheimer's disease. Until such data are available, the long-term use of ERT to protect against Alzheimer's disease cannot be recommended.

Colon Cancer

Colorectal cancer is the fourth most common cancer and the second leading cause of cancer death in the United States (see Chap. 127).

Accumulating evidence suggests that HRT may decrease the risk for colorectal cancer. In the Nurses' Health Study, the risk for colorectal cancer was decreased among women currently receiving HRT.[119] Furthermore, a meta-analysis of 18 epidemiologic studies confirmed that current HRT use may reduce the risk of colorectal cancer.[120]

However, the relationship between postmenopausal HRT and reduction of risk of colon cancer should still be viewed with caution, as this apparent risk reduction is from observational studies and has not been confirmed by prospective, randomized trials.

Other

Several studies have demonstrated a relationship between tooth loss and alveolar residual ridge resorption and systemic osteoporosis. Nearly 32% of US women between the ages of 65 and 69 years do not have any teeth. Both the Nurses' Health Study[121] and the Leisure World Study[122] found that current use of HRT was associated with a reduction in risk of tooth loss.

A recent population-based study suggested that HRT given for one or more years is associated with a decreased risk of peripheral arterial disease among postmenopausal women.[123] The role of HRT in peripheral arterial disease prevention, however, is unknown.

The PEPI trial showed that oral HRT with 0.625 mg of CEE slightly decreased both fasting insulin and glucose concentrations.[124] However, after oral glucose challenge, glucose concentrations were increased.[124] HRT appears to have a beneficial effect on fasting glucose among women with elevated fasting insulin concentrations. The addition of micronized progesterone or medroxyprogesterone acetate, however, had little impact on glucose and insulin serum concentrations.[124]

A meta-analysis of randomized controlled trials showed that unopposed estrogen, or estrogen combined with a progestin, has no effect on body weight, suggesting that HRT does not cause weight gain in excess of that normally observed at the time of menopause.[125]

RISKS OF HRT

Breast Cancer

A major concern of postmenopausal women is that HRT increases breast cancer risk. The lifetime risk of developing breast cancer in the United States is approximately one in eight women,[126] and the greatest incidence occurs in women over the age of 60 years (see Chap. 125).

A collaborative reanalysis of data from 51 studies evaluating over 52,000 women with breast cancer and 108,000 controls showed that the risk of breast cancer increases with long-term estrogen use.[127] The most significant finding in this study was that women who had a body mass index greater than the upper limit of normal ($\geq$25 kg/m^2) had no increase in breast cancer risk with HRT use.[127] Schairer et al. reported a similar observation.[128]

No significant increase in breast cancer risk was observed for women using HRT for less than 5 years.[127] For women who used HRT with or without a progestin for more than 5 years (median of 11 years), a relative risk of 1.35 was reported. Furthermore, although the increased relative risk was highly significant ($P < 0.0001$), the excess number of women with breast cancer after estrogen use was small. In those who used HRT for 5, 10, or 15 years, the excess number of women with breast cancer was 1 to 3, 3 to 9, and 5 to 20 cases, respectively per 1,000 women who began estrogen use between the ages of 50 and 70 years.[127] Also, the rate of increase in breast cancer risk in a woman using HRT after menopause (2.3% per year) was similar to that for a woman with delayed menopause (2.8% per year).[127] Therefore, postmenopausal HRT appears to mimic the prolongation of ovarian sex-steroid production seen in women with delayed menopause. In addition, 5 years after discontinuing HRT, the risk of breast cancer was no longer increased.[127]

According to the Nurses' Health Study, after 5 years of HRT there is an increase of two cases of breast cancer in 1,000 women, and after 10 years, there was an increase of six cases in 1,000 women.[129] In this study, the overall adjusted relative risk for women using estrogen alone and estrogen plus a progestin was 1.32 and 1.41, respectively, as compared to those who had never taken hormones.[129] Also, the Iowa Women's Health Study showed that exposure to HRT is associated with an increased risk of breast cancer that has a favorable prognosis.[130]

In an observational study of over 400,000 women, Willis et al.[131] reported that, after 9 years of follow up, use of HRT was associated with a significantly decreased risk of fatal breast cancer. A similar reduction in overall mortality from breast cancer among current users of HRT was also evident in the Nurses' Health Study.[6]

A study of the effects of HRT in women with a family history of breast cancer found that those who were current users had approximately the same increased relative risk compared to those who did not have a family history.[132] The overall mortality for women with a family history of breast cancer from all causes was significantly reduced among HRT users.[132] These data suggest that HRT use in women with a family history of breast cancer is not associated with a significantly increased incidence of the disease. Moreover, HRT use in such individuals is associated with significantly reduced overall mortality.[132]

Sex-steroid deficiency during menopause results in lipomatous involution of the breast that is reflected by decreased mammographic breast density and markedly improved radiotransparency of breast tissue. Thus, mammographic changes indicating breast cancer can be recognized more easily and earlier after the menopause. Conversely, postmenopausal HRT results in increased mammographic breast density,[133] and increased density on mammography has been associated with higher breast cancer risk.[134]

In the normal premenopausal breast, during the follicular phase of the cycle, estrogen interacts with estrogen receptors to induce gene expression and proliferation.[39] In the luteal phase of the cycle, progesterone interacts with progesterone receptors to enhance the proliferative and glandular effects.[39] With corpus luteum regression and the onset of menses, programmed cell death occurs in breast tissue. Therefore, during each menstrual cycle, events leading to growth and differentiation of breast epithelium followed by involution are observed.[39] Epidemiologic studies suggest that the addition of a progestin to estrogen may further increase the breast cancer risk beyond that associated with estrogen alone.[128,135] Furthermore, greater breast epithelial cell proliferation and breast epithelial cell density has been observed in women taking estrogen plus progestin, as compared to those women taking estrogen alone.[136]

Of note, raloxifene does not increase breast density after 2 years of treatment.[137] To the contrary, results from the MORE study suggest that raloxifene use may be protective, with an overall reduction in breast cancer risk of 78%, as compared to placebo.[59]

Endometrial Cancer

The major proven risk associated with estrogen replacement is stimulation of cell mitosis and proliferation in the endometrium leading to endometrial hyperplasia (a premalignant lesion) and cancer.[39] In the PEPI trial, 62% of women who took 0.625 mg of unopposed conjugated estrogen had some form of hyperplasia at 36 months compared to 2% of those who took placebo.[40] In contrast, the development of endometrial hyperplasia did not differ between any of the combination HRT regimens and placebo.[40] This study confirms the safety of the 200-mg cyclical micronized progesterone, the 10-mg cyclical MPA, and the 2.5-mg continuous MPA.[40]

The effects of long-term HRT on the risk of developing endometrial cancer were evaluated in a case-control study.[138] Unopposed estrogen replacement was associated with a significant increase in the overall risk for developing endometrial cancer ($P < 0.0001$).[138] The overall risk per 5 years of unopposed estrogen use was 2.17. The sequential addition of progestin to estrogen for at least 10 days of the treatment cycle, or continuous combined estrogen/progestin, did not increase the risk of endometrial cancer.[138]

Unopposed moderate- or high-dose estrogen therapy is associated with a significant increase in the incidence of endometrial cancer, and longer durations of exposure increase this risk.[139] With unopposed ERT, the risk of endometrial cancer increases within 2 years.[39] The excess risk increases with dose and duration of estrogen (10 years of unopposed estrogen increases the risk 10-fold), is apparent within 2 years of the start of treatment, and persists for many years after estrogen replacement is discontinued.

Estrogen-induced endometrial cancer is usually of a low stage and grade at the time of diagnosis,[38] and it can almost entirely be prevented by progestin coadministration. Also, lower doses of estrogen may be associated with a lower risk of endometrial hyperplasia.[36] Raloxifene does not result in endometrial hyperplasia, has no effect on endometrial thickness, is not associated with polyp formation, and has virtually no proliferative effect on the endometrium.[140] Therefore, raloxifene does not cause vaginal bleeding, spotting, or discharge.[141] Long-term studies, however, are required to determine whether raloxifene use reduces the risk of endometrial cancer.

Ovarian Cancer

Lifetime risk of ovarian cancer is low (1.7%). Epidemiologic studies of the association between HRT and ovarian cancer have yielded inconsistent results. A recent prospective cohort study of more than 40,000 postmenopausal women suggests that women receiving combination estrogen/progestin therapy are not at increased risk for ovarian cancer, even after long-term use.[142] However, it appears that women receiving long-term unopposed estrogen (for 10 years or more) may be at an increased risk for ovarian cancer.[142,143] Additional large, controlled studies are needed to confirm these findings.

Venous Thromboembolism

Venous thromboembolism, including thrombosis of the deep veins of the legs and embolism to the pulmonary arteries, is uncommon in the general population. The absolute risk of venous thromboembolism in non-HRT users is approximately 1 in 10,000 women.[144] However, a recent study showed that this risk is increased 3.6-fold in women who use HRT.[144] Nonetheless, lower doses of estrogen are associated with a decreased risk for thromboembolism as compared to higher doses.[144]

In the HERS study, deep-venous thrombotic events and pulmonary embolic events were reported more frequently among HRT users.[145] However, these women had established cardiovascular disease and thus were at higher risk for these events.

Risk factors predisposing for venous thromboembolism in women receiving HRT were examined in the PEPI trial, and only low baseline fibrinogen concentrations were associated with increased risk.[146] The authors suggest that the significantly lower fibrinogen concentrations observed among women who subsequently developed venous thromboembolic events may be an indicator of a specific, but as yet undefined, coagulopathy that is magnified in the presence of exogenous hormones.[146] Currently, there is no indication for thrombophilia screening before initiating HRT. However, HRT should be avoided in women at high risk for thromboembolic events.

Gallbladder Disease

Gallbladder disease is a commonly cited complication of oral estrogen use.[147] The Nurses' Health Study showed that the age-adjusted relative risk of cholecystectomy is 2.2 for women currently taking 0.625 mg of CEE.[147] In this study, the risk of cholecystectomy increased with duration of HRT use and did not resolve after discontinuation.[147] Transdermal estrogen is an alternative to oral therapy for women at high risk for cholelithiasis.

INDIVIDUALIZING HRT

Clinicians should discuss HRT with all postmenopausal women. Menopause is a natural life event, not a disease. The decision to take HRT must be individualized and based on several parameters, including menopausal symptoms, osteoporosis risk, coronary artery disease risk, breast cancer risk, and thromboembolism risk. Furthermore, pharmacologic methods to reduce the risks of cardiovascular disease and bone loss that do not involve the use of HRT should be addressed.

HRT has bone-preserving and possibly cardioprotective effects, and the benefits of HRT may outweigh the risks for most postmenopausal women because many more women die from coronary heart disease or hip fracture than from breast cancer. To provide patient-specific information on the risks and benefits of HRT, Col et al.[148] developed a decision-analytic Markov state transition model to compare the following four clinical strategies: (a) conservative care (i.e., no treatment); (b) HRT; (c) alendronate therapy; and (d) raloxifene therapy. The decision model simulates the natural history of healthy, white, 50-year-old postmenopausal women receiving each treatment strategy. According to this model, for women at average risk for CVD, breast cancer, and hip fracture, HRT increased life expectancy more than either raloxifene or alendronate therapy (gain in life expectancy of 8 months versus 5 months and 1 month, respectively).[148] Women at high risk for CVD (multiple risk factors) should benefit most from HRT, with gains in life expectancy exceeding 3 years. However, no single therapeutic choice was consistently better or worse than the other for all women, and gains in life expectancy depended on each woman's individual risk profile. Thus, women at lowest risk for hip fracture and CVD would not benefit substantially from any of these treatments.[148] The gain in life expectancy from HRT was greater among women at high risk for CVD, whereas the gain from raloxifene was greater among women at high risk for breast cancer.[148] The gain in life expectancy from alendronate therapy was less than 3 months for most women.

To further simplify decision making, Col et al. developed a partition diagram that identifies the optimal treatment according to a

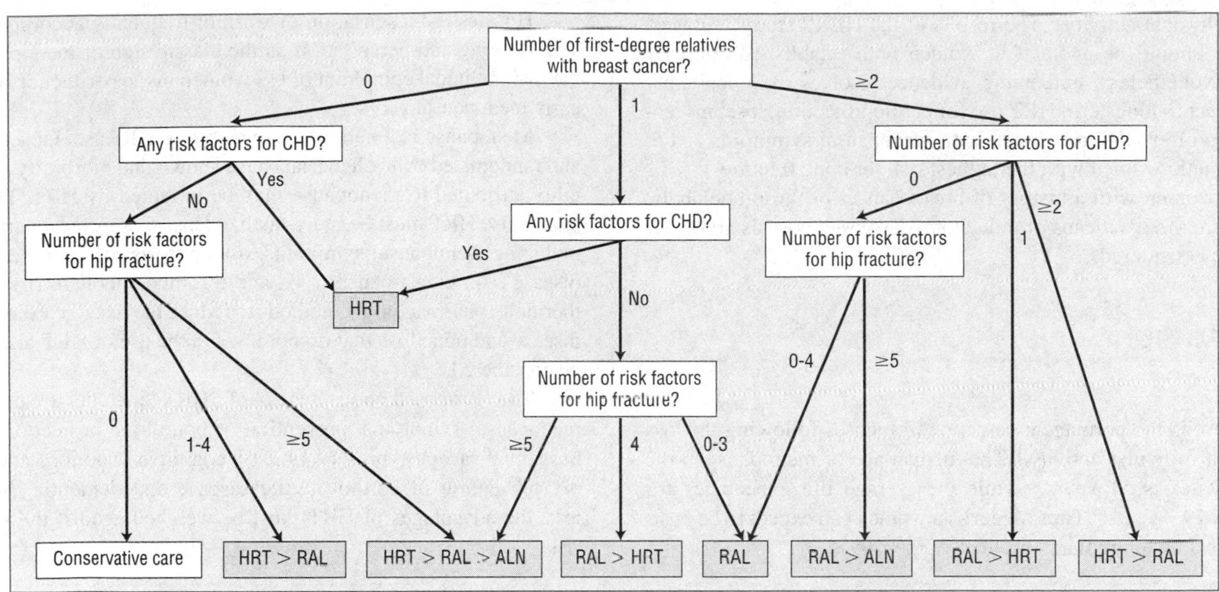

FIGURE 83–1. Optimal treatment according to individual risk factor profile. Preferred therapy for 50-year-old women with different levels of risk for hip fracture, coronary heart disease (CHD), and breast cancer. Each shaded rectangle depicts treatments associated with a gain in life expectancy of 6 months or more compared with conservative care. Rectangles with multiple treatments indicate that all listed choices are associated with gains of 6 months or more, listed from highest to lowest gain. ALN, alendronate sodium therapy, HRT, hormone replacement therapy; RAL, raloxifene hydrochloride therapy. *(Reprinted with permission from Arch Intern Med 1999;159:1458–1466.)*

woman's risk-factor profile, using a gain in life expectancy of 6 months as a threshold (Fig. 83–1).[148]

EVALUATION OF THERAPEUTIC OUTCOMES

After the patient begins HRT, a brief followup visit 6 weeks later may be useful to discuss patient concerns about HRT and to evaluate the patient for symptom relief, adverse effects, and patterns of withdrawal bleeding. Additional followup should be determined based on the patient's initial response to therapy and the need for any modification of the regimen.

Women receiving HRT should undergo annual monitoring, including a medical history and physical examination, pelvic examination, blood pressure measurement, and routine breast cancer and endometrial cancer surveillance as indicated.[44]

Although bone densitometry has been shown to predict fractures, at present there are no guidelines for follow-up bone mineral density testing. However, in women with significant bone loss, repeat testing should be performed as clinically indicated.

PHARMACOECONOMIC CONSIDERATIONS

A prospective study showed that patients' willingness to pay for HRT greatly exceeds the costs associated with mild and severe menopausal symptoms, indicating that HRT is considered economically advantageous by women.[149] Women can achieve major improvement in their quality of life from using HRT and are prepared to sacrifice a proportion of their income to achieve the desired effects.

Estrogens and progestins used for postmenopausal hormone therapy are among the most commonly prescribed medications in the United States. A double-blinded, randomized trial of estrogens alone or estrogens plus progestins found no difference in quality of life between the two groups.[150] Nonetheless, only a fraction of women ever fill their HRT prescriptions, and only 25% to 40% continue to take postmenopausal hormone therapy for more than 1 year.[151] Furthermore, only 5% to 6% take HRT for more than 5 years.[152] This may be a result of women's attitudes toward HRT, fear of cancer, lack of adequate information, or adverse effects associated with HRT.

A recent US population-based study showed that sociodemographic factors were more strongly associated with use of HRT than were clinical factors.[153] Furthermore, use of HRT was more common among women in the South and West regions than in the Northeast.[153] In addition, use of HRT was more common among college graduates.[153] Also, women who have undergone hysterectomy use HRT more frequently than do women with an intact uterus (58.7% vs 19.6%).[153]

The cost of HRT can vary depending on the route and method of delivery. Transdermal preparations are about twice as expensive as their equivalent oral preparations.[154] Raloxifene adversely affects hot flashes. Given that the main use of HRT is for the treatment of hot flashes, it seems unlikely that raloxifene would be an alternative for most current HRT users. Raloxifene is likely to be used for women who may be considered for non-HRT osteoporosis treatments such as the biphosphonates.[154] Thus, raloxifene may be more cost effective if it is given to older women who are at the highest risk of fracture. The average wholesale price of raloxifene is approximately $2.00/day as compared to $0.50/day for oral estrogen and $0.65/day for oral estrogen plus a progestin.[85]

Women with coronary risk factors (e.g., hypertension, lipid abnormalities, family history of heart disease) may benefit from HRT even if they have a family history of breast cancer.[148] However, modifications of cardiac risk factors by other means can also be considered in this group (e.g., dietary or pharmacologic lipid lowering, antioxidants, aspirin, physical activity). The results of the HERS study[95] suggest that HRT should be avoided in women with established coronary disease. Nonetheless, until more evidence resolves the uncertainty with respect to long-term HRT use for cardioprotection, it seems reasonable to offer HRT to women with menopausal symptoms and to asymptomatic women with the highest risk for bone fracture.

For women with a history of breast cancer or thromboembolic disease, alternative means of reducing risk of osteoporosis and CVD should be considered.

CONCLUSIONS

Menopause is the permanent cessation of menses following the loss of ovarian follicular activity.[1] The median age of menopause in the United States is 51 years,[3] while the average life expectancy for women is 79.7 years.[4] Thus, American women can expect to be postmenopausal for more than one-third of their lives.

Hot flashes, a sensation of warmth frequently accompanied by skin flushing and perspiration, is the classic sign of menopause and the major clinical complaint of US women in the perimenopausal and early menopausal years.

Menopause is a natural life event, not a disease. Observational and randomized controlled trials have shown that morbidity and mortality attributed to menopause may be modified by HRT. The decision to use HRT must be individualized based on several parameters, including menopausal symptoms, osteoporosis risk, coronary artery disease risk, breast cancer risk, and thromboembolism risk.[148] Furthermore, pharmacologic methods to reduce the risk of cardiovascular disease and bone loss that do not involve the use of HRT also should be considered.

The proposed advantages of HRT include treatment of menopausal symptoms, prevention of bone loss, protection against urogenital atrophy, preservation of cognitive function, and possibly prevention of cardiovascular disease and dementia. Nonetheless, the advantages of HRT must be weighed against the potential risk.[7]

PREMATURE OVARIAN FAILURE AND PREMENOPAUSAL HORMONE REPLACEMENT

PATHOPHYSIOLOGY

Premature ovarian failure (POF) is a condition characterized by sex-steroid deficiency, amenorrhea, and infertility in women younger than 40 years of age. Premature ovarian failure is not an early natural menopause. Normal menopause results from ovarian follicle depletion, whereas POF is characterized by intermittent ovarian function in one-half of affected women.[155] These women produce estrogen intermittently and may ovulate despite the presence of high gonadotropin concentrations.[156] Pregnancies have occurred in 5% to 10% of women after the diagnosis of POF—even in women with no follicles observed on ovarian biopsy.

Premature ovarian failure may occur on the basis of ovarian follicle dysfunction or ovarian follicle depletion[155–161] and may present as either primary amenorrhea (absence of menses in a girl who has reached the age of 16) or secondary amenorrhea (cessation of menses in a woman previously menstruating for 6 months or more) (Table 83–6).

TABLE 83–6. Etiology of Premature Ovarian Failure[155–161]

Idiopathic: karyotypically normal spontaneous premature ovarian failure
Autoimmunity: (a) isolated autoimmune premature ovarian failure or (b) as a component of an autoimmune polyglandular syndrome in association with Addison's disease, hypothyroidism, hypoparathyroidism, or mucocutaneous candidiasis
Iatrogenic: chemotherapy, radiation
X-chromosome abnormalities
Gonadotropin and gonadotropin-receptor abnormalities: signal defects
Enzyme deficiencies: cholesterol desmolase, 17α-hydroxylase, 17–20 desmolase
Galactosemia
Blepharophimosis, ptosis, and epicantus inversus syndrome type 1: rare autosomal dominant syndrome in which premature ovarian failure is the predominant syndrome
Perrault's syndrome: familial autosomal recessive premature ovarian failure in association with deafness

In most cases, the etiology cannot be identified. In the majority of patients, ovarian failure develops after the establishment of regular menses. Young women with POF who develop ovarian dysfunction before they achieve peak adult bone mass, sustain sex-steroid deficiency for more years than do naturally menopausal women. This deficiency can result in a significantly higher risk for osteoporosis[162] and cardiovascular disease.[163] Approximately 67% of women with spontaneous POF have significant bone loss despite taking standard HRT.[162] Importantly, a survey of more than 19,000 women between the ages of 25 and 100 years suggests that ovarian failure occurring before 40 years of age is associated with significantly increased mortality, with the age-adjusted odds ratio for all-cause mortality being 2.14 (95% CI, 1.15–3.99).[164]

CLINICAL PRESENTATION

There is no characteristic menstrual pattern or history that precedes POF. Approximately 50% of patients with this condition have a history of oligomenorrhea or dysfunctional uterine bleeding (prodromal premature ovarian failure), and about 25% develop amenorrhea acutely. Some patients develop amenorrhea postpartum, while others experience it after discontinuing oral contraceptives. Primary amenorrhea is not associated with symptoms of estrogen deficiency. In cases of secondary amenorrhea, symptoms may include hot flashes, night sweats, fatigue, and mood changes. Prodromal POF may present with hot flashes even in women who menstruate regularly. Incomplete development of secondary sex characteristics may occur in women with primary amenorrhea, whereas these characteristics are typically normal in women with secondary amenorrhea. In general, women with POF have normal fertility before the disorder develops.

Approximately 50% of women with POF have been found to have documented ovarian follicle function.[155] Nonetheless, in most cases, the follicles do not function normally. In contrast to normal controls, women with POF have a poor correlation between follicle diameter and serum estradiol concentrations, but nearly 20% of these women ovulate intermittently. Inappropriate luteinization of graafian follicles appears to be a major pathophysiologic mechanism impairing follicle function in young women with spontaneous POF.[155]

Premature ovarian failure is defined by the presence of at least 4 months of amenorrhea and at least two serum FSH concentrations measuring greater than 40 mIU/mL (obtained at least 1 month apart) in women younger than 40 years of age. A complete history should be taken regarding other factors that can affect ovarian function such as prior ovarian surgery, chemotherapy, radiation, and autoimmune disorders. In patients with primary amenorrhea, particular attention should be paid to breast and pubic hair development according to Tanner stages. Short stature, stigmata of Turner's syndrome, and other dysmorphic features of gonadal dysgenesis should be considered. Ideally, a pelvic examination should be performed, but this is not always clinically appropriate. Alternatively, transabdominal ultrasonography can be performed in primary amenorrhea to confirm the presence of normal anatomic structures. In the majority of cases, physical examination is completely normal. A karyotype should be performed in all patients experiencing premature ovarian failure. Women with ovarian failure and a karyotype containing a Y chromosome should undergo bilateral gonadectomy because there is a substantial risk for gonadal germ-cell neoplasia.[165] Ovarian biopsy and antiovarian antibody testing are investigational procedures with no proven clinical benefit in POF. As clinically indicated, the workup should include tests for the diagnosis of other possible associated autoimmune disorders such as hypothyroidism, diabetes mellitus, and Addison's disease.

Young women find the diagnosis of POF particularly traumatic and frequently need extensive emotional and psychological support. While most of these women will in fact be infertile, it is important to emphasize that POF can be transient and that spontaneous pregnancies have occurred even years after diagnosis.

▶ TREATMENT: Premature Ovarian Failure

Postmenopausal women who take HRT prolong their exposure to estrogen beyond the average age of completion of their reproductive phase. In contrast, women with POF need exogenous sex steroids to compensate for the decreased production by their ovaries. It is worthwhile noting that 47% of young women with POF have significantly reduced bone mineral density within 1.5 years of their diagnosis despite taking standard HRT.[162] Several reasons may explain this finding. Significant bone loss may occur in the years preceding the development of overt ovarian failure (i.e., during the prodromal phase of premature ovarian failure). Bone loss in the decade preceding natural menopause is significantly related to reductions in circulating total and free testosterone concentrations—not estradiol.[82] The goal of therapy in young women with POF is to provide a hormone replacement regimen that maintains bone mass as effectively as the normal, functioning ovary. This usually requires the administration of estrogen at a dose greater than the standard dose given to older women experiencing natural menopause. Estrogen *underdosing* in women with POF may be a significant contributing factor to the reduced bone mineral density. Another important factor that may contribute to bone loss is the delay in diagnosis. It is not uncommon for young women with POF to experience several years of amenorrhea without sex-hormone replacement, thereby resulting in significant bone loss during this interval of estrogen deficiency.

PHARMACOLOGIC THERAPY: HORMONAL REGIMENS

Optimal HRT depends on whether the patient has primary or secondary amenorrhea. Young women with primary amenorrhea in whom secondary sex characteristics have failed to develop should initially be exposed to very low doses of estrogen in an attempt to mimic the gradual pubertal maturation process. A typical regimen is as follows: 0.3 mg of CEE unopposed (i.e., no progestin) daily for 6 months with incremental dose increases at 6-month intervals until the required maintenance dose is achieved. Gradual dose escalation often results in optimal breast development and allows time for the young woman to adjust psychologically to her physical maturation. Cyclical progestin therapy, given 12 to 14 days per month, should be instituted toward the end of the second year of treatment.

Women with secondary amenorrhea who have been estrogen deficient for 12 months or longer should also initially be given low dose estrogen replacement to avoid adverse effects such as mastalgia and nausea. However, the dose can be titrated up to maintenance levels over a 6-month period, and progestin therapy can be instituted concomitantly. Women with a brief history of secondary amenorrhea are less likely to experience undesired effects from HRT if they are given a reduced dose for the first month of therapy followed by a full dose from the second month onward.

An estrogen dose equivalent to at least 1.25 mg of CEE (or 100 μg of transdermal estradiol) is needed to achieve adequate estrogen replacement in young women. A progestin should be given for 12 to 14 days per calendar month to prevent endometrial hyperplasia (Table 83–7). Estrogens given in usual replacement doses do not suppress spontaneous follicular activity or ovulation. Because women with POF can have spontaneous pregnancies, hormone replacement should produce regular, predictable menstrual flow patterns (i.e., only cyclic regimens should be used). If these patients miss an expected menses, they should be tested for pregnancy and should discontinue HRT.

Androgen replacement should also be considered for women with premature ovarian failure experiencing persistent fatigue, poor well being, and low libido despite adequate estrogen replacement. In these young women, testosterone replacement may be important for the development and maintenance of normal muscle mass and preservation of bone mineral content. An ongoing study at the National Institutes of Health is evaluating the effectiveness of long-term testosterone supplementation, in addition to standard hormone replacement, in protecting women with POF from bone loss. This study employs a transdermal system that delivers the equivalent of the normal daily ovarian testosterone production (150 μg/day).

Importantly, all women with POF should understand that HRT must be continued at least until the average age of natural menopause and that long-term followup is necessary.

EVALUATION OF THERAPEUTIC OUTCOMES

Young women with POF should be monitored annually for their response to treatment, and their compliance with HRT should be regularly assessed. These patients also should be evaluated continuously for the presence of signs and symptoms of associated autoimmune endocrine disorders, such as hypothyroidism, adrenal insufficiency, and diabetes mellitus. Baseline bone mineral density testing should be performed in all women with POF. Mammography should be performed annually after the age of 40 years in accordance with accepted guidelines. Additional mammography screening in premenopausal

TABLE 83–7. Premenopausal Hormone Replacement Therapy for Young Women With Premature Ovarian Failure

Regimen	Dose	Frequency	Route
Estrogen replacement			
Conjugated equine estrogen	1.25 mg	Daily	Oral
Piperazine estrone sulfate	2.5 mg	Daily	Oral
Micronized 17β-estradiol	4 mg	Daily	Oral
Transdermal estrogen system	100 μg/24 h	Once or twice weekly	Transdermal (patch)
Progestin replacement			
Medroxyprogesterone acetate	10 mg	12–14 days*	Oral
Dydrogesterone	20 mg	12–14 days*	Oral
Norethindrone	1 mg	12–14 days*	Oral
Norethisterone acetate	10 mg	12–14 days*	Oral
Micronized progestrerone	200 mg	12–14 days*	Oral
Transdermal norethindrone	250 μg/24 h	12–14 days*	Transdermal

*Per calendar month.

women younger than age 40 years who are receiving physiologic HRT is not warranted. Other tests should be performed as clinically indicated.

CONCLUSIONS

Approximately 1% of women spontaneously develop ovarian failure before the age of 40 years.[5] Premature ovarian failure is not an early natural menopause. Most affected women produce estrogen intermittently and may ovulate despite the presence of high gonadotropin concentrations.[156] However, these women sustain sex-steroid deficiency for more years than do naturally menopausal women. This results in a significantly higher risk for osteoporosis[162] and cardiovascular disease.[163]

Women with POF need exogenous sex steroids to compensate for the decreased production by their ovaries. Thus, premenopausal HRT is required at least until these women reach the age of "natural menopause."

The goal of therapy is to provide a hormone replacement regimen that maintains bone mass as effectively as the normal, functioning ovary. This usually requires the administration of estrogen at a dose greater than the standard dose given to older women experiencing natural menopause.

Because women with POF can have spontaneous pregnancies, the HRT should produce regular, predictable menstrual flow patterns. If these patients miss an expected menses, they should be tested for pregnancy and promptly discontinue the HRT.

Annual followup should include assessment of HRT compliance and evaluation for signs and symptoms of associated endocrine disorders.[156]

▶ PRINCIPLES OF PHARMACOTHERAPY

- The major indication for short-term perimenopausal HRT is the relief of menopausal symptoms (hot flashes, night sweats, and vaginal atrophy) and improvement in quality of life. The severity of menopausal symptoms varies significantly between women.
- Absolute contraindications for HRT include endometrial cancer, breast cancer, undiagnosed vaginal bleeding, recent vascular thrombosis, or active liver disease.
- Unless contraindicated, HRT is the treatment of choice for osteoporosis prevention and treatment. Long-term HRT prevents bone loss and reduces fracture risk.
- The use of long-term HRT for cardiovascular disease prevention remains controversial. HRT may offer the benefit of primary prevention of cardiovascular disease, but its use for secondary prevention is not recommended.
- Individual patient evaluation is essential to determine the appropriateness of long-term estrogen therapy. The benefits and risks of HRT should be reassessed annually in light of new patient information and emerging data from large, randomized trials.
- HRT may increase the risk of breast cancer, but the associated risk is small.
- Young women with premature ovarian failure need exogenous sex steroids to compensate for the decreased production by their ovaries. Thus, premenopausal HRT for these young women is required at least until they reach the age of "natural menopause."
- Women with premature ovarian failure require larger doses of estrogen than those used in postmenopausal HRT regimens.

REFERENCES

1. Richardson SJ, Senikas JF, Nelson JF. Follicular depletion during the menopausal transition: Evidence for accelerated loss and ultimate exhaustion. J Clin Endocrinol Metab 1987;65:1231–1237.
2. World Health Organization. Research on the Menopause in the 1990s. Report of a WHO Scientific Group. WHO Technical Report Series No. 866, 1996.
3. Bromberger JT, Matthews KA, Kuller LH, et al. Prospective study of the determinants of age at menopause. Am J Epidemiol 1997;145:124–133.

4. Annual Report of the Board of Trustees of the Federal Old Age and Survivors Insurance and Disability Insurance Trust Funds. Washington, DC, US Government Printing Office, 1995, Report No. Tb1 II.D2.
5. Coulam CB, Adamson SC, Annegers JF. Incidence of premature ovarian failure. Obstet Gynecol 1986;67:604–606.
6. Grodstein F, Stampfer MJ, Colditz GA, et al. Postmenopausal hormone therapy and mortality. N Engl J Med 1997;336:1769–1775.
7. Davis SR. Hormone replacement therapy: Indications, benefits and risks. Aust Fam Physician 1999;28:437–445.
8. Treloar AE, Boynton RE, Behn BG, Brown BW. Variation of the human menstrual cycle through reproductive life. Int J Fertil 1967;12:77–126.
9. Zumoff B, Strain GW, Miller LK, Rosner W. Twenty-four-hour mean plasma testosterone concentration declines with age in normal premenopausal women. J Clin Endocrinol Metab 1995;80:1429–1430.
10. Burger HG. The endocrinology of the menopause. J Steroid Biochem Mol Biol 1999;69:31–35.
11. Lee SJ, Lenton EA, Sexton L, Cooke ID. The effect of age on the cyclical patterns of plasma LH, FSH, oestradiol and progesterone in women with regular menstrual cycles. Hum Reprod 1988;3:851–855.
12. Ettinger B, Pressman A, Sklarin P, et al. Associations between low concentrations of serum estradiol, bone density, and fractures among elderly women: The study of osteoporotic fractures. J Clin Endocrinol Metab 1998;83:2239–2243.
13. Stone K, Bauer DC, Black DM, et al. Hormonal predictors of bone loss in elderly women: A prospective study. J Bone Miner Res 1998;13: 1167–1174.
14. Cummings SR, Browner WS, Bauer D. Endogenous hormones and the risk of hip and vertebral fractures among older women. N Engl J Med 1998;339:733–738.
15. Cauley JA, Lucas FL, Kuller LH, et al. Elevated serum estradiol and testosterone concentrations are associated with a high risk for breast cancer. Ann Intern Med 1999;130:270–277.
16. Murkies AL, Wilcox G, Davis SR. Phytoestrogens: Clinical review. J Clin Endocrinol Metab 1998;83:297–303.
17. Wilcox G, Wahlqvist M, Burger HG, Medley G. Oestrogenic effects of plant foods in postmenopausal women. BMJ 1990;301:905–906.
18. Dalais FS, Rice GE, Wahlqvist ML, et al. Effects of dietary phytoestrogens in postmenopausal women. Climacteric 1998;1:124–129.
19. Brzezinski A, Adlercreutz H, Shaoul R, et al. Short-term effects of phytoestrogen-rich diet on postmenopausal women. Menopause 1997;4:89–94.
20. Albertazzi P, Pansini F, Bonaccorsi G, et al. The effect of dietary soy supplementation on hot flushes. Obstet Gynecol 1998;91:6–11.
21. McNagny SE. Prescribing hormone replacement therapy for menopausal symptoms. Ann Intern Med 1999;131:605–616.
22. Wroblewski-Lissin L, Cooke JP. Phytoestrogens and cardiovascular health. J Am Coll Cardiol 2000;35:1403–1410.
23. Lee HP, Gourley L, Duffy SW, et al. Dietary effects on breast-cancer risk in Singapore. Lancet 1991;337:1197–2000.
24. Yuan JM, Wang QS, Ross RK, et al. Diet and breast cancer in Shangai and Tianjin, China. Br J Cancer 1995;71:1353–1358.
25. Wang TT, Sathyamoorthy N, Phang JM. Molecular effects of genistein on estrogen receptor mediated pathways. Carcinogenesis 1996;17: 271–275.
26. Schwartz JA, Liu G, Brook SC. Genistein-mediated attenuation of tamoxifen-induced antagonism from estrogen receptor-regulator genes. Biochem Biophys Res Commun 1998;253:38–43.
27. Wang C, Kurzer MS. Phytoestrogen concentrations determines effects on DNA synthesis in human breast cancer cells. Nutr Cancer 1997;28: 236–247.
28. Sturdee DW. Newer HRT regimens. Br J Obstet Gynaecol 1997; 104:1109–1115.
29. Greendale GA, Lee NP, Arriola ER. The menopause. Lancet 1999; 353:571–580.
30. Lindsay R, Hart DM, Clark DM. The minimum effective dose of estrogen for postmenopausal bone loss. Obstet Gynecol 1984;63:759–763.
31. Mashcak CA, Lobo RA, Dozono-Takano R, et al. Comparison of pharmacodynamic properties of various estrogen formulations. Am J Obstet Gynecol 1982;144:511–518.
32. Horsman A, Jones M, Francis R, Nordin C. The effect of estrogen dose on postmenopausal bone loss. N Engl J Med 1983;309:1405–1407.
33. Field CS, Ory SJ, Wahner HW, et al. Preventive effects of transdermal 17β-estradiol on osteoporotic changes after surgical menopause: A two-year placebo-controlled trial. Am J Obstet Gynecol 1993;168:114–121.
34. Genant HK, Baylink DJ, Gallagher JC, et al. Effects of estrone sulphate on postmenopausal bone loss. Obstet Gynecol 1990;76:579–584.
35. Utia WH, Burry KA, Archer DF, Gallagher JC, The Esclim Study Group, et al. Efficacy and safety of low, standard and high dosages of an estradiol transdermal system (Esclim) compared with placebo on vasomotor symptoms in highly symptomatic menopausal patients. Am J Obstet Gynecol 1999;181:71–79.
36. Genant HK, Lucas J, Weiss S, et al. Low-dose esterified estrogen therapy: Effects on bone, plasma estradiol concentrations, endometrium, and lipid concentrations. Estratab/Osteoporosis Study Group. Arch Intern Med 1997;157:2609–2615.
37. Schneider HPG, Gallagher JC. Moderation of the daily dose of HRT: Benefits for patients. Maturitas 1999;33(suppl):25–29.
38. Barrett-Connor E. Hormone replacement therapy. BMJ 1998;317: 457–461.
39. Casper RF. Estrogen with interrupted progestin HRT: A review of experimental and clinical studies. Maturitas 2000;34:97–108.
40. The Writing Group for the Postmenopausal Estrogen/Progestin Interventions (PEPI) Trial. Effects of hormone replacement therapy on endometrial histology in postmenopausal women. JAMA 1996;275:370–375.
41. Cushing KL, Weiss NS, Voight LF, et al. Risk of endometrial cancer in relation to use of low-dose, unopposed estrogens. Obstet Gynecol 1998;91:35–39.
42. Kirkham C, Hahn PM, Van Vugt DA, et al. A randomized double-blind, placebo-controlled, crossover trial to assess the side effects of medroxyprogesterone acetate in hormone replacement therapy. Obstet Gynecol 1991;78:93–97.
43. Prior JC, Alojado N, McKay DW, et al. No adverse effects of medroxyprogesterone treatment without estrogen in postmenopausal women: Double-blind, placebo-controlled, crossover trial. Obstet Gynecol 1994;83:24–28.
44. NAMS Consensus Opinion. A decision tree for the use of estrogen replacement therapy or hormone replacement therapy in postmenopausal women: Consensus opinion of the North American Menopause Society. Menopause 2000;7:76–86.
45. Archer DF, Lobo RA, Land HF, Pickar JH. A comparative study of transvaginal uterine ultrasound and endometrial biopsy for evaluating the endometrium of postmenopausal women taking hormone replacement therapy. Menopause 1999;6:201–208.
46. Doren M, Reuther G, Minne HW, Schneider HPG. Superior compliance and efficacy of continuous combined oral estrogen-progestogen therapy in postmenopausal women. Am J Obstet Gynecol 1995;173:1446–1451.
47. Grey AR, Cundy TF, Reid IR. Continuous combined oestrogen/progestin therapy is well tolerated and increases bone density at the hip and spine in postmenopausal osteoporosis. Clin Endocrinol 1994;40:671–677.
48. Davis S. Androgen replacement in women: A commentary. J Clin Endocrinol Metab 1999;84:1886–1891.
49. Watts NB, Notelovitz T, Timmons MC, et al. Comparison of oral estrogens and estrogens plus androgens on bone mineral density, menopausal symptoms, and lipid-lipoprotein profiles in surgical menopause. Obstet Gynecol 1995;85:529–537.
50. Honore EK, Williams JK, Adams MR, et al. Methyltestosterone does not diminish the beneficial effects of estrogen replacement therapy on coronary artery reactivity in cynomolgus monkeys. Menopause 1996;3: 23–26.
51. Worboys S, Kotsopoulos D, Teede H, et al. Evidence that parenteral testosterone therapy may improve endothelium-dependent and -independent vasodilation in postmenopausal women already receiving estrogen. J Clin Endocrinol Metab 2001;86:158–161.
52. Shifren JL, Braunstein GD, Simon JA, et al. Transdermal testosterone treatment in women with impaired sexual function after oophorectomy. N Engl J Med 2000;343:682–688.
53. Kalantaridou SN, Calis KA, Godoy H, et al. Transdermal testosterone replacement for young women with spontaneous premature ovarian failure:

A pilot study. Abstract No. 2322 from the Endocrine Society 82nd Annual Meeting. June 21–24, 2000, Toronto, Canada.
54. Burger HG. Selective oestrogen receptor modulators. Horm Res 2000; 53(suppl 3):25–29.
55. Delmas PD, Bjarnason NH, Mitlak BH, et al. Effects of raloxifene on bone mineral density, serum cholesterol concentrations, and uterine endometrium in postmenopausal women. N Engl J Med 1997;337: 1641–1647.
56. Bryant HU, Dere WH. Selective estrogen receptor modulators: An alternative to hormone replacement therapy. Proc Soc Exp Biol Med 1998; 217:45–52.
57. Walsh BW, Kuller LH, Wild RA, et al. Effects of raloxifene on serum lipids and coagulation factors in healthy postmenopausal women. JAMA 1998;279:1445–1451.
58. Ettinger B, Black DM, Mitlak BH, et al. Reduction of vertebral fracture risk in postmenopausal women with osteoporosis treated with raloxifene: Results from a 3-year randomized clinical trial. Multiple Outcomes of Raloxifene Evaluation (MORE) investigators. JAMA 1999;282: 637–645.
59. Cummings SR, Eckert S, Krueger KA, et al. The effect of raloxifene on risk on breast cancer in postmenopausal women—Results from the MORE randomized trial. JAMA 1999;281:2189–2197.
60. Cohen FJ, Lu Y. Characterization of hot flashes reported by healthy postmenopausal women receiving raloxifene or placebo during osteoporosis prevention trials. Maturitas 2000;34:65–73.
61. Moore RA. Livial: A review of clinical studies. Br J Obstet Gynaecol 1999;106(suppl):1–21.
62. American College of Obstetrics and Gynecology. Hormone replacement therapy technical bulletin (No. 166). Washington, DC, American College of Obstetrics and Gynecology, 1992.
63. Hammond CB. Menopause and hormone replacement therapy: An overview. Obstet Gynecol 1996;87(suppl):2–15.
64. Loprinzi CL, Kugler JW, Sloan JA, et al. Venlafaxine in management of hot flashes in survivors of breast cancer: A randomized controlled trial. Lancet 2000;356:2059–2063.
65. Bachmann GA. A new option for managing urogenital atrophy in postmenopausal women. Cont Obstet Gynecol 1997;42:13–28.
66. Greenspan SL, Maitland LA, Myers ER, et al. Femoral bone loss progresses with age: A longitudinal study in women over age 65. J Bone Miner Res 1994;9:1959–1965.
67. Michaelsson K, Baron JA, Farahmand BY, et al. for the Swedish Hip Fracture Study Group. Hormone replacement therapy and risk for hip fracture: Population-based case-control study. BMJ 1998;316:1858–1863.
68. Schneider DL, Barrett-Connor EL, Morton DJ. Timing of postmenopausal estrogen for optimal bone mineral density. The Rancho Bernardo Study. JAMA 1997;277:543–547.
69. Consensus Development Conference. Prophylaxis and treatment of osteoporosis. Am J Med 1993;94:646–650.
70. Seeman E. Osteoporosis: Trials and tribulations. Am J Med 1997; 103(suppl):74–87.
71. Bracker MD, Watts NB. How to get the most out of bone densitometry. Postgrad Med 1998;104:77–86.
72. Watts NB. Postmenopausal osteoporosis. Obstet Gynecol Surv 1999; 54:532–538.
73. Ray WA, Griffin MR, Baught DK. Mortality following hip fracture before and after implementation of the prospective payment system. Arch Intern Med 1990;150:2109–2114.
74. Doren M, Samsioe G. Prevention of postmenopausal osteoporosis with oestrogen replacement therapy and associated compounds: Update on clinical trials since 1995. Hum Reprod Update 2000;6:419–426.
75. Rozenberg S, Kroll M, Vandromme J, et al. Effect of bone density evaluation on hormone replacement therapy prescription. Maturitas 1996;24:57–61.
76. National Osteoporosis Foundation. Physician's guide to prevention and treatment of osteoporosis. Belle Mead, NJ, Excerpta Medica, 1998.
77. Cauley JA, Seeley DG, Ensrud K, et al. for the Study of Osteoporotic Fractures Research Group. 1995 Estrogen replacement therapy and fractures in older women. Ann Intern Med 1995;122:9–16.
78. Eiken P, Nielsen SP, Kolthoff N. Effects on bone mass after eight years of hormone replacement therapy. Br J Obstet Gynaecol 1997;104:702–707.
79. The Writing Group for the Postmenopausal Estrogen/Progestin Interventions (PEPI) Trial. Effects of hormone therapy on bone mineral density. Results from the Postmenopausal Estrogen/Progestin Interventions (PEPI) Trial. JAMA 1996;276:1389–1396.
80. NIH Consensus Conference. Optimal calcium intake. NIH Consensus Development Panel on Optimal Calcium Intake. JAMA 1994;272: 1942–1948.
81. Recker RR, Davies KM, Dowd RM, Heaney RP. The effect of low-dose continuous estrogen and progesterone therapy with calcium and vitamin D on bone in elderly women. A randomized controlled trial. Ann Intern Med 1999;130:897–904.
82. Slemenda C, Longcope C, Peacock M, et al. Sex steroids, bone mass and bone loss: A prospective study of pre-, peri-, and postmenopausal women. J Clin Invest 1996;97:14–21.
83. Davis SR, McCloud P, Strauss BJG, Burger H. Testosterone enhances estradiol's effects on postmenopausal bone density and sexuality. Maturitas 1995;21:227–236.
84. Raisz LG, Witta B, Artis A, et al. Comparison of the effects of estrogen alone and estrogen plus androgen on biochemical markers of bone formation and resorption in postmenopausal women. J Clin Endocrinol Metab 1995;81:37–43.
85. Umland EM, Rinaldi C, Parks SM, Boyce EG. The impact of estrogen replacement therapy and raloxifene on osteoporosis, cardiovascular disease, and gynecologic cancers. Ann Pharmacother 1999;33:1315–1328.
86. Hosking D, Chilvers CED, Christiansen C, et al. for the Early Postmenopausal Intervention Cohort Study Group. Prevention of bone loss with alendronate in postmenopausal women under 60 years of age. N Engl J Med 1998;338:485–492.
87. Lindsay R, Cosman F, Lobo RA, et al. Addition of alendronate to ongoing hormone replacement therapy in the treatment of osteoporosis: A randomized controlled clinical trial. J Clin Endocrinol Metab 1999;84:3076–3081.
88. Wimalawansa SJ. A four-year randomized controlled trial of hormone replacement and bisphosphonate, alone or in combination, in women with postmenopausal osteoporosis. Am J Med 1998;104:219–226.
89. Chesnut CH, Silverman S, Andriano K, et al. A randomized trial of nasal spray salmon calcitonin in postmenopausal women with established osteoporosis: The prevent recurrence of osteoporotic fractures study. PROOF Study Group. Am J Med 2000;109:267–276.
90. Barrett-Connor E, Grady D. Hormone replacement therapy, heart disease and other considerations. Annu Rev Public Health 1998;19:55–72.
91. Mosca L. The role of hormone replacement therapy in the prevention of postmenopausal heart disease. Arch Intern Med 2000;160:2263–2272.
92. Mendelsohn ME, Karas RH. The protective effects of estrogen on the cardiovascular system. N Engl J Med 1999;340:1801–1811.
93. Grodstein F, Manson JE, Colditz GA, et al. A prospective observational study of postmenopausal hormone therapy and primary prevention of cardiovascular disease. Ann Intern Med 2000;133:933–941.
94. Barrett-Connor E, Stuenkel C. Hormones and heart disease in women: Heart and Estrogen/Progestin Replacement Study in perspective. J Clin Endocrinol Metab 1999;84:1848–1853.
95. Hulley S, Grady D, Bush T, et al. Randomized trial of estrogen plus progestin for secondary prevention of coronary heart disease in postmenopausal women. JAMA 1998;280:605–613.
96. Hu FB, Stampfer MJ, Manson JE, et al. Trends in the incidence of coronary heart disease and changes in diet and lifestyle in women. N Engl J Med 2000;343:530–537.
97. Stampfer MJ, Hu FB, Manson JE, et al. Primary prevention of coronary heart disease in women through diet and lifestyle. N Engl J Med 2000;343:16–22.
98. Stampfer MJ, Colditz GA, Willett WC, et al. Postmenopausal estrogen therapy and cardiovascular disease: Ten years follow-up from the Nurses Health Study. N Engl J Med 1991;325:756–762.
99. Grady D, Hulley SB. Hormones to prevent coronary disease in women: When are observational studies adequate evidence? Ann Intern Med 2000;133:999–1001.

100. The Writing Group for the Postmenopausal Estrogen/Progestin Interventions (PEPI) Trial. Effects of estrogen or estrogen/progestin regimens on heart disease risk factors in postmenopausal women. JAMA 1995;273:199–208.
101. Davidson MH, Testolin LM, Maki KC, et al. A comparison of estrogen replacement, pravastatin, and combined treatment for the management of hypercholesterolemia in postmenopausal women. Arch Intern Med 1997;157:1186–1192.
102. Darling GM, Johns JA, McCloud PI, Davis SR. Estrogen and progestin compared with simvastatin for hypercholesterolemia in postmenopausal women. N Engl J Med 1997;337:595–601.
103. Minshall RD, Stanckzyk FZ, Miyagawa K, et al. Ovarian steroid protection against coronary artery hyperreactivity in rhesus monkeys. J Clin Endocrinol Metab 1998;83:649–659.
104. Johnston CC Jr, Bjarnason NH, Cohen FJ, et al. Long-term effects of raloxifene on bone mineral density, bone turnover, and serum lipid concentrations in early postmenopausal women: Three-year data from two double-blind, randomized, placebo-controlled trials. Arch Intern Med 2000;160:3444–3450.
105. Barrett-Connor E, Wenger NK, Grady D, et al. Hormone and nonhormone therapy for the maintenance of postmenopausal health: The need for randomized controlled trials of estrogen and raloxifene. J Womens Health 1998;7:839–847.
106. Grodstein F, Stampfer MJ, Manson JE, et al. Postmenopausal estrogen and progestin use and the risk for cardiovascular disease. N Engl J Med 1996;335:453–461.
107. Bush TL. Preserving cardiovascular benefits of hormone replacement therapy. J Reprod Med 2000;45:259–272.
108. Herrington DM, Reboussin DM, Brosnihan KB, et al. Effects of estrogen replacement on the progression of coronary-artery atherosclerosis. N Engl J Med 2000;343:522–529.
109. Lenfant C. Preliminary trends in the Women's Health Initiative. Bethesda, MD, National Heart, Lung, and Blood Institute Communications office, April 3, 2000. Press release.
110. Rossouw JE. Hormone replacement therapy and cardiovascular disease. Curr Opin Lipidol 1999;10:429–434.
111. Schmidt PJ, Nieman L, Danaceau MA, et al. Estrogen replacement in perimenopause-related depression: A preliminary report. Am J Obstet Gynecol 2000;183:414–420.
112. Sano M. Understanding the role of estrogen on cognition and dementia. J Neural Transm Suppl 2000;59:223–229.
113. Yaffe K, Sawaya G, Lieberburg I, Grady D. Estrogen therapy in postmenopausal women: Effects on cognitive function and dementia. JAMA 1998;279:688–695.
114. Tang MX, Jacobs D, Stern Y, et al. Effect of estrogen during menopause on risk and age at onset of Alzheimer's disease. Lancet 1996;348: 429–432.
115. Paganini-Hill A, Henderson VW. Estrogen replacement therapy and risk of Alzheimer disease. Arch Intern Med 1996;22:13–17.
116. Mulnard RA, Cotman CW, Kawas C, et al. Estrogen replacement therapy for treatment of mild to moderate Alzheimer disease. A randomized controlled trial. Alzheimer's Disease Cooperative Study. JAMA 2000;283:1007–1015.
117. Wang PN, Liao SQ, Liu RS, et al. Effects of estrogen on cognition, mood and cerebral blood flow in AD: A controlled study. Neurology 2000;54:2061–2066.
118. Henderson VW, Paganini-Hill A, Miller BL, et al. Estrogen for Alzheimer's disease in women: Randomized, double-blind, placebo-controlled trial. Neurology 2000;54:295–301.
119. Grodstein F, Martinez ME, Platz EA, et al. Postmenopausal hormone use and risk for colorectal cancer and adenoma. Ann Intern Med 1998;128:705–712.
120. Grodstein F, Newcomb PA, Stampfer MJ. Postmenopausal hormone therapy and the risk of colorectal cancer: A review and meta-analysis. Am J Med 1999;106:574–582.
121. Grodstein F, Colditz GA, Stampfer MJ. Post-menopausal hormone use and tooth loss: A prospective study. J Am Dent Assoc 1996;127:370–377.
122. Paganini-Hill A. The benefits of estrogen replacement therapy on oral health. The Leisure World Cohort. Arch Intern Med 1995;155: 2325–2329.
123. Westendorp IC, in't Veld BA, Grobbee DE, et al. Hormone replacement therapy and peripheral arterial disease: The Rotterdam study. Arch Intern Med 2000;160:2498–2502.
124. Espeland MA, Hogan PE, Fineberg SE, et al. for the PEPI investigators. Effect of postmenopausal hormone therapy on glucose and insulin concentrations. Diabetes Care 1998;21:1589–1595.
125. Norman RJ, Flight IH, Rees MC. Oestrogen and progestogen hormone replacement therapy for perimenopausal and post-menopausal women: Weight and body fat distribution. Cochrane Database Syst Rev 2000;CD001018.
126. Swanson GM. Breast cancer risk estimation. A translational statistic for communication to the public. J Natl Cancer Inst 1993;85:848–849.
127. Collaborative Group on Hormonal Factors in Breast Cancer. Breast cancer and hormone replacement therapy: Collaborative reanalysis of data from epidemiological studies of 52,705 women with breast cancer and 108,411 women without breast cancer. Lancet 1997;350:1047–1059.
128. Schairer C, Lubin J, Troisi R, et al. Menopausal estrogen and estrogen-progestin replacement therapy and breast cancer risk. JAMA 2000;283:485–491.
129. Colditz GA, Hankinson BSS, Hunter DD, et al. The use of estrogens and progestins and the risk of breast cancer in postmenopausal women. N Engl J Med 1995;332:1589–1593.
130. Gapstur SM, Morrow M, Sellers TA. Hormone replacement therapy and risk of breast cancer with a favorable histology. JAMA 1999;281: 2091–2097.
131. Willis DB, Callee EE, Miracle-McMahill HL, Heath CW Jr. Estrogen replacement therapy and risk of fatal breast cancer in a prospective cohort of postmenopausal women in the United States. Cancer Causes Control 1996;7:449–457.
132. Sellers TA, Mink PJ, Cerhan JR, et al. The role of hormone replacement therapy in the risk of breast cancer and total mortality in women with a family history of breast cancer. Ann Intern Med 1997;127:973–980.
133. Greendale GA, Reboussin BA, Sie A, et al. for the Postmenopausal Estrogen/Progestin Interventions (PEPI) investigators. Effects of estrogen and estrogen-progestin on mammographic parenchymal density. Ann Intern Med 1999;130:262–269.
134. Boyd NF, Byng JW, Jong RA, et al. Quantitative classification of mammographic densities and breast cancer risk: Results from the Canadian National Breast Cancer Screening Study. J Natl Cancer Inst 1995;87:670–675.
135. Ross RK, Paganini-Hill A, Wan PC, Pike MC. Effect of hormone replacement therapy on breast cancer risk: Estrogen versus estrogen plus progestin. J Natl Cancer Inst 2000;92:328–332.
136. Hofseth LJ, Raafat AM, Osuch JR, et al. Hormone replacement therapy with estrogen or estrogen plus medroxyprogesterone acetate is associated with increased epithelial proliferation in the normal postmenopausal breast. J Clin Endocrinol Metab 1999;84:4559–4565.
137. Freedman M, Martin JS, O'Gorman J, et al. Digitized mammography: A clinical trial of postmenopausal women randomly assigned to receive raloxifene, estrogen, or placebo. J Natl Cancer Inst 2001;93:51–56.
138. Pike MC, Peters RK, Cozen W, et al. Estrogen-progestin replacement therapy and endometrial cancer. J Natl Cancer Inst 1997;89:1110–1116.
139. Lethaby A, Farquhar C, Sarkis A, et al. Hormone replacement therapy in postmenopausal women: Endometrial hyperplasia and irregular bleeding. Cochrane Database Syst Rev 2000;CD000402.
140. Goldstein SR, Scheele WH, Rajagopalan SK, et al. A 12-month comparative study of raloxifene, estrogen, and placebo on the postmenopausal endometrium. Obstet Gynecol 2000;95.95–103.
141. Cohen FJ, Watts S, Shah A, et al. Uterine effects of 3-year raloxifene therapy in postmenopausal women younger than age 60. Obstet Gynecol 2000;95:104–110.
142. Lacey JV, Mink PJ, Schatzkin A, et al. Ovarian cancer and hormone replacement therapy in a prospective cohort study. Abstract presented at

the Annual Meeting of the American Association for Cancer Research, New Orleans, Louisiana, 2001.

143. Rodriguez C, Patel AV, Calle EE, et al. Estrogen replacement therapy and ovarian cancer mortality in a large prospective study of US women. JAMA 2001;285:1460–1465.
144. Jick H, Derby LE, Myers MW, et al. Risk of hospital admission for idiopathic venous thromboembolism among users of postmenopausal oestrogens. Lancet 1996;348:981–983.
145. Grady D, Wenger NK, Herrington D, et al. for the Heart and Estrogen/Progestin Replacement Study Research Group. Postmenopausal hormone therapy increases risk for venous thromboembolic disease. Ann Intern Med 2000;132:689–696.
146. Whiteman MK, Cui Y, Flaws JA, et al. Low fibrinogen concentration: A predisposing factor for venous thromboembolic events with hormone replacement therapy. Am J Hematol 1999;61:271–273.
147. Grodstein F, Colditz GA, Stampfer MJ. Postmenopausal hormone use and cholecystectomy in a large prospective study. Obstet Gynecol 1994;83:5–11.
148. Col NF, Pauker SG, Goldberg RJ, et al. Individualizing therapy to prevent long-term consequences of estrogen deficiency in postmenopausal women. Arch Intern Med 1999;159:1458–1466.
149. Zethraeus N, Johannesson M, Henriksson P, Strand RT. The impact of hormone replacement therapy on quality of life and willingness to pay. Br J Obstet Gynaecol 1997;104:1191–1195.
150. Medical Research Council. Randomized comparison of estrogen versus estrogen plus progestogen hormone replacement therapy in women with hysterectomy. BMJ 1996;312:473–478.
151. Ettinger B, Pressman A. Continuation of postmenopausal hormone replacement therapy in a large health maintenance organization: Transdermal matrix versus oral estrogen therapy. Am J Manag Care 1999;7:779–785.
152. Avis NE, McKinlay SM. The Massachusetts Women's Health Study: An epidemiologic investigation of the menopause. J Am Med Womens Assoc 1995;50:45–50.
153. Keating NL, Cleary PD, Rossi AS, et al. Use of hormone replacement therapy by postmenopausal women in the United States. Ann Intern Med 1999;130:545–553.
154. Torgerson DJ, Reid DM. The pharmacoeconomics of hormone replacement therapy. Pharmacoeconomics 1999;16:9–16.
155. Nelson LM, Anasti JN, Kimzey LM, et al. Development of luteinized graafian follicles in patients with karyotypically normal spontaneous premature ovarian failure. J Clin Endocrinol Metab 1994;79:1470–1475.
156. Kalantaridou SN, Davis SR, Nelson LM. Premature ovarian failure. Endocrinol Metab Clin North Am 1998;27:989–1006.
157. Kalantaridou SN, Braddock DT, Patronas NJ, Nelson LM. Treatment of autoimmune premature ovarian failure. Hum Reprod 1999;14:1777–1782.
158. The Finish-German APECED consortium. An autoimmune disease, APECED, caused by mutations in a novel gene featuring two PHD-type zinc-finger domains. Nat Genet 1997;17:399–403.
159. Kalantaridou SN, Chrousos GP. Molecular defects causing ovarian dysfunction. Ann N Y Acad Sci 2000;900:40–45.
160. Zlotogora J, Sagi M, Cohen T. The blepharophimosis, ptosis, and epicanthus inversus syndrome: Delineation of two types. Am J Hum Genet 1983;35:1020–1027.
161. Nishi Y, Hamamoto K, Kajiyama M, et al. The Perrault syndrome: Clinical report and review. Am J Med Genet 1988;31:623–629.
162. Anasti JN, Kalantaridou SN, Kimzey LM, et al. Bone loss in young women with karyotypically normal spontaneous premature ovarian failure. Obstet Gynecol 1998;91:12–15.
163. Van Der Schouw YT, Van Der Graaf Y, Steyerberg EW, et al. Age at menopause as a risk for cardiovascular mortality. Lancet 1996;347:714–717.
164. Snowdon DA, Kane RL, Beeson WL, et al. Is early natural menopause a biologic marker of health and aging? Am J Public Health 1989;79:709–714.
165. Davis SR. Premature ovarian failure. Maturitas 1996;28:1–8.

84
ERECTILE DYSFUNCTION

Mary Lee

Erectile dysfunction is a common disorder of men older than 40 years of age. Many factors predispose to the development of erectile dysfunction, including arteriosclerosis, diabetes mellitus, hypertension, and concurrent medications.

In general, if the underlying cause of erectile dysfunction can be identified and reversed, then sexual dysfunction can be ameliorated. However, in many patients, this is not possible. Use of vacuum erection devices, disease-specific treatments, or surgery may be indicated.

Several definitions of erectile dysfunction exist. However, the National Institutes of Health Consensus Development Panel on Impotence defines erectile dysfunction as the failure to achieve a penile erection suitable for sexual intercourse.[1] Patients may refer to it as impotence.

Erectile dysfunction must be distinguished from disorders of libido, ejaculatory disorders, or infertility, which are caused by different pathophysiologic mechanisms and are treated with alternative agents (Table 84–1). However, a patient may suffer from one or more disorders of sexual dysfunction. For example, an elderly man may have primary hypogonadism, and as a result, have decreased libido. Erectile dysfunction may develop secondary to the decrease in sexual drive. In such patients, diagnosis of sexual disorders is a key to initiating the most appropriate treatment.

This chapter reviews the indications, mechanism, dosing regimen, and adverse effects of common modes of treatment for erectile dysfunction.

EPIDEMIOLOGY

The incidence of erectile dysfunction is low in men younger than 40 years of age, but it increases as men age.[2–4] The Massachusetts Male Aging Study, a cross-sectional survey of a random sample of 1,290 men in the Boston area, was conducted during the period 1987–1989. It reported an overall prevalence of 52% for any degree of erectile dysfunction in men aged 40 to 70 years, with a 40% prevalence in men aged 40 years, and a 67% prevalence in men aged 70 years.[1,2]

Although erectile dysfunction is sometimes assumed to be a symptom of the aging process in men, it is unclear whether the incidence is directly related to increasing patient age. Erectile dysfunction is more likely to result from concurrent medical conditions of the patient (e.g., hypertension, arteriosclerosis, hyperlipidemia, diabetes mellitus, psychiatric disorders) or from medications that patients may be taking for these diseases.[2–4] For example, up to 50% of patients with diabetes mellitus develop erectile dysfunction, and medications such as β-blockers are associated with a high incidence of erectile dysfunction.

PHYSIOLOGY OF A NORMAL PENILE ERECTION

A normal penile erection requires the full functioning of several physiologic systems: vascular, nervous, and hormonal. The patient must also be psychologically receptive to sexual stimuli.

VASCULAR SYSTEM

The penis comprises two corpora cavernosa on the dorsal side and one corpus spongiosum on the ventral side. The corpus spongiosum surrounds the urethra and forms the glans penis. The corpora are composed of multiple, interconnected sinuses, which can fill with blood to produce an erection. The corpora are encased by the tunica albuginea, a fibrous tissue membrane, which has limited distensibility. In the flaccid state, arterial flow into and venous outflow from the corpora are balanced. During the erectile phase, arterial blood flow increases and blood fills the sinusoids within the corpora, which causes penile swelling and elongation. The erection is prolonged by a decrease in venous outflow from the corpora, which is caused by compression of subtunical venules by the swollen corpora (Fig. 84–1).

Arterial flow into the corpora is enhanced by acetylcholine-mediated vasodilation. Acetylcholine does not directly enhance arterial flow to the corpora or increase sinusoidal filling of the corporal tissue. Rather, acetylcholine is a co-neurotransmitter, which works along with other nonpeptidinergic intracellular neurotransmitters—including cyclic guanosine monophosphate (cGMP), cyclic adenosine monophosphate (cAMP), or vasoactive intestinal polypeptide—to produce vasodilation.

Acetylcholine probably works through two different pathways to produce an erection. In one pathway, acetylcholine, in the presence of sexual stimulation to genital tissue, enhances the production of nitric oxide by endothelial cells and nonadrenergic-noncholinergic (NANC) neurons. Nitric oxide enhances the activity of guanylate cyclase enzyme, which increases the conversion of cyclic guanosine triphosphate to cGMP. cGMP decreases intracellular calcium concentrations in smooth-muscle cells of penile arteries and cavernosal sinuses. As a result, smooth-muscle relaxation occurs, which enhances arterial blood flow to and blood filling of the corpora.[5] An erection results (Fig. 84–2).

In an alternative pathway, acetylcholine stimulates a smooth-muscle cell-membrane receptor to enhance the activity of adenyl cyclase. Adenyl cyclase increases the conversion of cyclic adenosine triphosphate (cATP) to cyclic adenosine monophosphate (cAMP), a

TABLE 84–1. Types of Sexual Dysfunction in Men

Type of Dysfunction	Definition
Decreased libido	Decreased sexual drive or desire.
Increased libido	Precocious puberty. Inappropriate and excessive sexual drive or desire.
Erectile dysfunction (impotence)	Failure to achieve a penile erection suitable for sexual intercourse.
Delayed ejaculation	Commonly referred to as "dry sex." Ejaculation is delayed or absent.
Retrograde ejaculation	Ejaculate passes retrograde into the bladder, instead of toward the anterior urethra (antegrade) and out of the penis.
Infertility	Sperm are insufficient in number or have inadequate motility and fail to fertilize the ovum.

potent muscle relaxant. Similar to cGMP, cAMP decreases intracellular calcium concentrations to produce smooth-muscle relaxation in cells of the arteries and cavernosal sinuses. Arterial blood flow to and blood filling of the corpora are enhanced, and a penile erection results (Fig. 84–2).[5]

NERVOUS SYSTEM AND PSYCHOGENIC STIMULI

Some erections are mediated by a sacral nerve reflex arc (e.g., erections can occur while the patient is sleeping). However, in the presence of sensory sexual stimulation, erections are mediated by the central nervous system. That is, when a patient sees an attractive partner, hears sweet words, smells a particular scent, tastes or touches a pleasant object, this can result in an erection. In this case, the patient's brain processes this information and the nervous impulse is carried down the spinal cord to peripheral cholinergic nerves, which innervate the vascular supply to the corpora, resulting in an erection.

The medial preoptic area of the hypothalamus is thought to be that portion of the brain responsible for integrating external stimuli. Here dopamine exerts a proerectogenic effect, whereas, α_2-adrenergic stimulation causes the penis to become and/or remain flaccid. Nerve impulses, after moving down the spinal cord, travel to the penis by efferent peripheral nerves, including inhibitory sympathetic neurons (T_{11}–L_2), proerectogenic parasympathetic neurons (S_2–S_4), and proerectogenic somatic neurons (S_2–S_4).

Acetylcholine produces an erection by working along with other coneurotransmitters, including cGMP and cAMP, as described earlier. Thus, an erection is *initiated* by the action of nerves, *maintained* by arterial blood filling of the corpora, and *sustained* by occlusion of venous outflow from the corpora.

Detumescence, or the progression of an erect penis to a flaccid state, results from the actions of norepinephrine, which contracts vascular smooth muscle to decrease arterial inflow to the corpora and contraction of sinusoidal tissue in the corpora. As a result, venous outflow from the corpora increases.

HORMONAL SYSTEM

Testosterone stimulates libido or sexual drive in males. Within the normal physiologic serum concentration range (normal, 300–1,100 ng/dL), sexual drive is normal. Patients with serum testosterone levels below the normal range may complain of loss of energy, loss of muscle strength, depressive mood, and decreased libido.

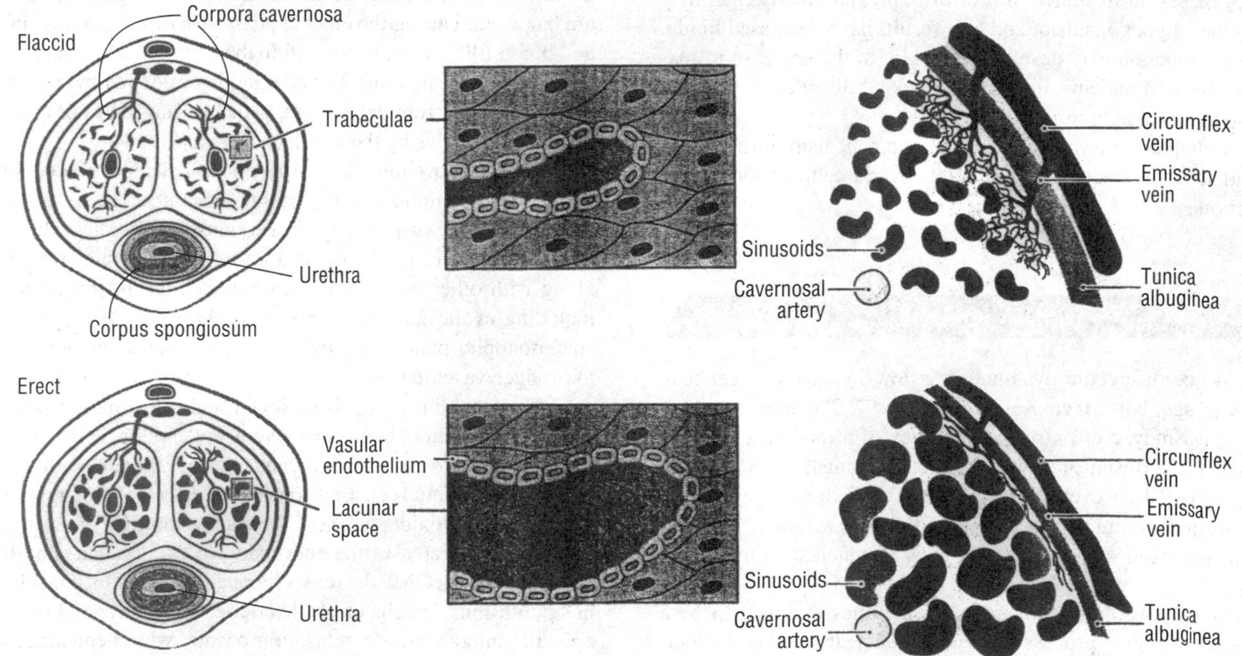

FIGURE 84–1. Microanatomy of and vascular changes in the penis in flaccid and erect states. In the flaccid state, arterial flow into and venous outflow from the corpora are balanced. During the erectile phase, arterial blood flow increases and blood fills the sinusoids within the corpora, which causes penile swelling and elongation. The erection is prolonged by a decrease in venous outflow from the corpora, which is caused by compression of subtunical venules by the swollen corpora. *(Adapted from Korenman SG. Insights into erectile dysfunction: A practical approach. Am J Med 1998;105:135–144.)*

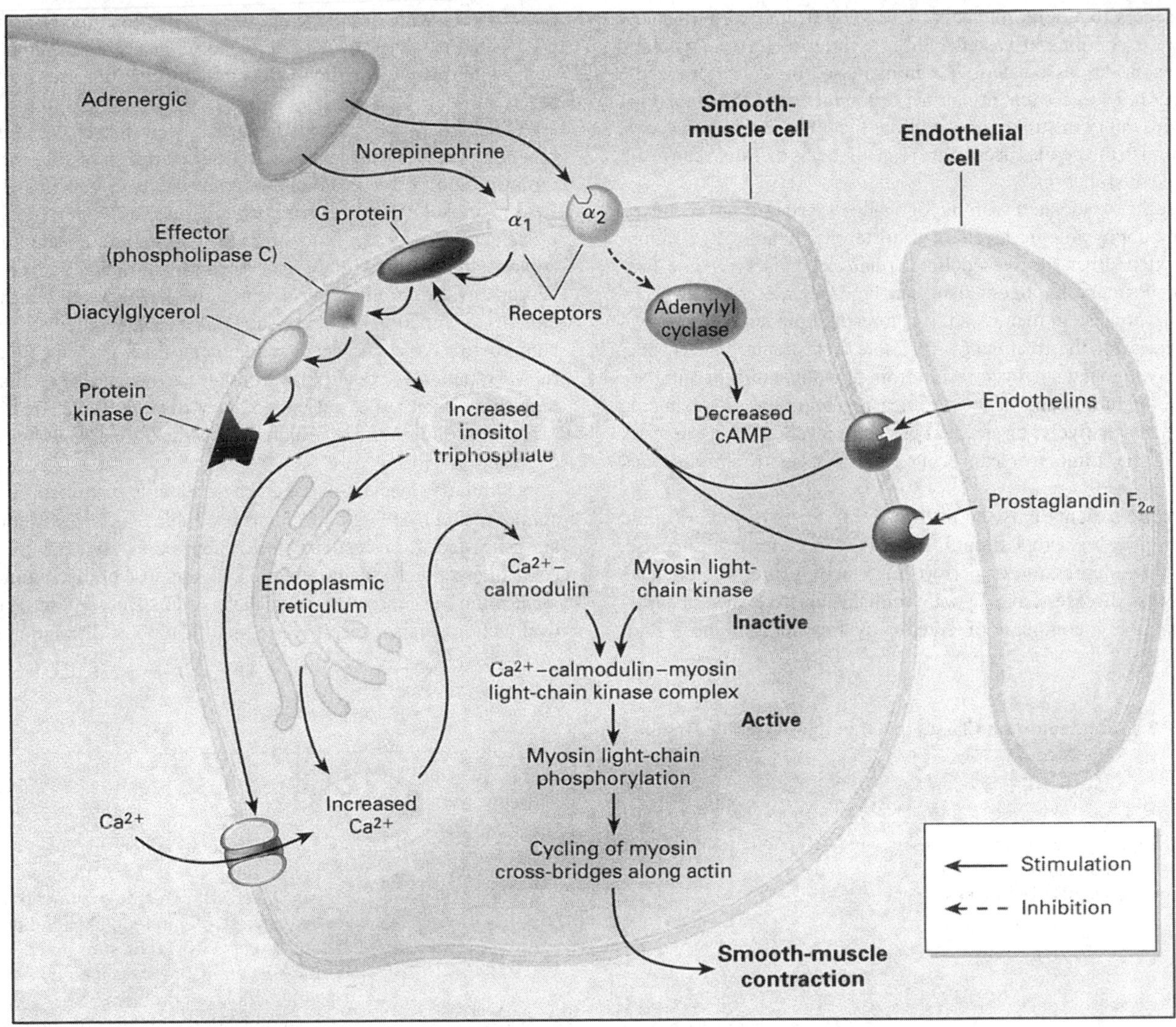

FIGURE 84–2. Molecular mechanism of penile smooth muscle relaxation. cAMP and cGMP, the intracellular second messengers mediating smooth-muscle relaxation, activate their specific protein kinases, which phosphorylate certain proteins to cause opening of potassium channels, closing of calcium channels, and sequestration of intracellular calcium by the endoplasmic reticulum. The resultant fall in intracellular calcium leads to smooth muscle relaxation. Sildenafil inhibits the action of phosphodiesterase (PDE) type 5, thus increasing the intracellular concentration of cGMP. Papaverine is a nonspecific inhibitor. GTP, guanosine triphosphate; eNOS, endothelial nitric oxide synthetase. *(Adapted with permission from Lue T. Erectile dysfunction. N Engl J Med 2000;342:1804–1805.)*

When libido is decreased, a patient may not develop erections, but the relationship with serum testosterone levels is a complicated one. Approximately one-third of men older than 50 years of age have hypogonadism. But patients with normal serum testosterone levels may have erectile dysfunction, and patients with subnormal serum testosterone levels may have normal sexual function.[6]

PATHOPHYSIOLOGY

Erectile dysfunction can result from any single abnormality or combination of abnormalities of the four systems necessary for a normal penile erection. Thus, any disease or drug therapy for that disease that interferes with the vascular, nervous, or hormonal systems, or with perception of psychogenic stimuli necessary for a normal penile erection, can produce erectile dysfunction. Vascular, neurologic, or hormonal etiologies of erectile dysfunction are collectively referred to as *organic erectile dysfunction*. Patients in the last category have *psychogenic erectile dysfunction*. Erectile dysfunction can result from primary or secondary disorders of these systems. In some cases, if the underlying disorder is corrected, the patient's erectile dysfunction is ameliorated or cured. However, in other patients, the cause of erectile dysfunction is multifactorial, and for this reason, it is not easily cured.

Diseases that compromise vascular flow to the corpora cavernosum (e.g., peripheral vascular disease, arteriosclerosis, essential hypertension) are associated with an increased incidence of erectile dysfunction. Diseases that impair nerve conduction to the brain (e.g., spinal cord injury or stroke) or conditions that impair peripheral nerve conduction to the penile vasculature (e.g., diabetes mellitus) can result in erectile dysfunction.

Diseases associated with hypogonadism, primary or secondary, result in subphysiologic levels of testosterone, which cause diminished sexual drive (decreased libido) and secondary erectile dysfunction. Primary hypogonadism can be associated with the normal aging process in men. Also, it can result from surgical removal of the testes for the treatment of prostate or testicular cancer. Secondary hypogonadism may result from hypothalamic or pituitary disorders of luteinizing hormone releasing hormone or luteinizing hormone, respectively; or elevated prolactin levels, which can result from pituitary tumors or can occur in patients with chronic renal failure.

Finally, patients must be in the "right" mental frame of mind to be receptive to sexual stimuli. Patients who suffer from malaise, have reactive depression or performance anxiety, are sedated, have Alzheimer's disease, have hypothyroidism, or have mental disorders commonly complain of erectile dysfunction. In most studies, patients with psychogenic erectile dysfunction generally exhibit a higher response rate to various interventions than do patients with organic erectile dysfunction, as their disease is often less severe.

Social habits of patients have also been linked to erectile dysfunction. The vasoconstrictor effect of cigarette smoking may compromise blood flow to the corpora and decrease cavernosal filling. Heavy smokers with erectile dysfunction may experience an improvement of erectile function if they discontinue smoking. Excessive ethanol intake may lead to androgen deficiency, peripheral neuropathy, or chronic liver disease, all of which can contribute to erectile dysfunction. Patients should be screened for these social habits before the start of specific treatments for erectile dysfunction. If relevant, patients should be appropriately educated about discontinuing these habits to avoid unnecessary treatments for erectile dysfunction and to optimize response to medical treatments for erectile dysfunction.

Similarly, medications may cause erectile dysfunction through similar pathophysiologic mechanisms (Table 84–2).[7–13] Medications are estimated to be responsible for approximately 10% to 25% of cases of erectile dysfunction. Reducing the dose or discontinuing the medication can generally reverse the problem. But sometimes erectile dysfunction persists despite dose modification or discontinuation of

TABLE 84–2. Medication Classes that Can Cause Erectile Dysfunction[7]

Drug Class	Proposed Mechanism By Which Drug Causes Erectile Dysfunction	Special Notes
Anticholinergic agents: antihistamines, antiparkinsonian agents, tricyclic antidepressants, phenothiazines	Anticholinergic activity	• Second-generation nonsedating antihistamines (e.g., loratadine) are not associated with erectile dysfunction. • Selective serotonin reuptake inhibitor antidepressants can be substituted for tricyclic antidepressants if erectile dysfunction is a problem.[8,9] • Phenothiazines with less anticholinergic effect (e.g., chlorpromazine) can be substituted in some patients if erectile dysfunction is a problem.
Dopamine agonists (e.g., metoclopramide, phenothiazines)	Inhibit prolactin inhibitory factor, thereby increasing prolactin levels	Increased prolactin levels are associated with blocking testosterone production from the testes. Depressed libido results.
Estrogens, antiandrogens (e.g., luteinizing hormone-releasing hormone superagonists, digoxin, spironolactone, ketoconazole, cimetidine)	Suppress testosterone-mediated stimulation of libido	In the face of a decreased libido, a secondary erectile dysfunction develops.
Central nervous system depressants (e.g., barbiturates, narcotics, benzodiazepines, short-term use of large doses of alcohol)	Suppress perception of psychogenic stimuli	
Agents that decrease penile blood flow (e.g., diuretics, peripheral, β-adrenergic antagonists, or central sympatholytics (methyldopa, clonidine, guanethidine)[10,11]	Reduce arteriolar flow to corpora	• Any diuretic that produces a significant decrease in intravascular volume can decrease penile arteriolar flow.[12,13] • Safer antihypertensives include angiotensin-converting enzyme inhibitors, postsynaptic α_1-adrenergic antagonists (terazosin, doxazosin), calcium-channel blockers, and angiotensin II receptor antagonists.

the causative agent. This is because the underlying disease—and not just the medication to treat the disease—is contributing to the disorder. An excellent review of medication-induced erectile dysfunction is available.[7]

CLINICAL PRESENTATION

Erectile dysfunction can affect men emotionally in several ways. Some patients may become depressed, develop performance anxiety, or suffer from embarrassment. Such events can lead to marital difficulties and avoidance of sexual intimacy. If a patient suspects that his medications may be causing erectile dysfunction, he may refuse to continue treatments.

A patient with erectile dysfunction is often too embarrassed to see a physician voluntarily for this problem. It is common for the patient to be brought to the physician by his wife, who becomes frustrated, depressed, or concerned about the quality of their marital life. Thus, patients with erectile dysfunction benefit from education about the disease, professional counseling, and, when necessary, specific treatment for the disease.

DIAGNOSIS

With the availability of effective medications in the late 1990s, diagnostic evaluation of erectile dysfunction became streamlined, as the identification of the precise cause of the dysfunction was less critical. However, a diagnostic work up is justified to identify any reversible or treatable underlying causes of erectile dysfunction. Key assessments include a thorough description of the severity of the erectile dysfunction, a complete medical history, a review of concurrent medications, a physical examination, and selected clinical laboratory tests.[14]

To assess the severity of the erectile dysfunction, the patient should be asked about onset and frequency. For this purpose, physicians and other primary care professionals sometimes use a standardized questionnaire, such as the International Index of Erectile Dysfunction. It includes 15 questions about the quality of erectile dysfunction and sexual intercourse (Fig. 84–3).[14] The physician should carefully assess the patient's expectations and motivations for erectile function to ensure that they are reasonable.

A complete medical history should be obtained to identify concurrent medical illnesses that are risk factors for organic or psychogenic erectile dysfunction. If these underlying diseases are not optimally responding to treatment, this should be addressed before specific treatment for erectile dysfunction is initiated. Also, if the patient smokes cigarettes, drinks excessive amounts of ethanol, or uses recreational drugs, these social habits should be discontinued before specific treatment for erectile dysfunction is started.

The patient should provide a complete listing of prescription and over-the-counter medications for review. The physician and pharmacist should assess this list and identify drugs that may be contributing to erectile dysfunction. If possible, a causative drug should be discontinued or the dose should be reduced to minimize the adverse reaction in the patient.

A physical examination of the patient should include a check for signs of hypogonadism, including gynecomastia, small testicles, and decreased body hair. The penis should also be evaluated for diseases associated with penile curvature (e.g, Peyronie's disease), which are also associated with erectile dysfunction. Femoral and lower extremity pulses should be assessed to provide an indication of vascular supply to the genitals. Anal sphincter tone and other genital reflexes should be checked to provide an indication of the integrity of the nerve supply to the penis.

Selected laboratory tests should be obtained to check for the presence of underlying diseases that could cause erectile dysfunction. These include a serum blood glucose, serum lipid profile, and serum thyroxine (T_4) level. Serum testosterone level should be checked in patients older than 50 years of age and in younger patients who complain of decreased sexual drive. Serum testosterone levels follow a circadian pattern of secretion, with the highest levels occurring during the morning hours. To interpret serum testosterone levels properly, serum samples should be obtained in the mornings. At least two serial serum testosterone levels are needed to confirm the presence of hypogonadism.[15]

▶ TREATMENT: Erectile Dysfunction

MANAGEMENT OPTIONS

The goal of treatment is an improvement in the quantity and quality of penile erections suitable for intercourse. Simple as this may sound, health care providers need to ensure that patients have reasonable expectations for any therapies that are initiated. Furthermore, only patients with erectile dysfunction should be treated. Patients who have normal sexual function should not seek—or be encouraged to seek—treatment in an effort to enhance sexual function or enable increased activity.

GENERAL APPROACH TO TREATMENT

The first step in clinical management of erectile dysfunction is to identify and, if possible, to reverse underlying causes. As previously mentioned, risk factors for erectile dysfunction, including hypertension, diabetes mellitus, smoking, or chronic ethanol abuse, should be addressed and minimized to the degree possible. Patients should be counseled to initiate measures to promote heart-healthy living styles, including a regimen of physical fitness, weight loss to achieve a normal body mass index, low-cholesterol diets, and smoking cessation, when relevant. In some cases, these types of interventions are sufficient to restore erectile function. However, if erectile dysfunction fails to respond to these measures, specific treatment is indicated.

For patients with psychogenic erectile dysfunction, psychotherapy may be used as monotherapy, or as an adjunct to specific treatments for the disorder. To enhance the relevance of psychotherapy, both the patient and his partner should be included in the counseling sessions. Also, treatment should be individualized and should address those immediate factors that may be causing performance anxiety or depression, rather than the remote, deep-seated reasons for psychologic disorders.[16] The effectiveness of psychotherapy is generally low, and long-term psychotherapy is often necessary.

Questions	Response options
1. How often were you able to get an erection during sexual activity? 2. When you had erections with sexual stimulation, how often were your erections hard enough for penetration?	0 = No sexual activity 1 = Almost never/never 2 = A few times (much less than half the time) 3 = Sometimes (about half the time) 4 = Most times (much more than half the time) 5 = Almost always/always
3. When you attempted sexual intercourse, how often were you able to penetrate (enter) your partner? 4. During sexual intercourse, how often were you able to maintain your erection after you had penetrated (entered) your partner?	0 = Did not attempt intercourse 1 = Almost never/never 2 = A few times (much less than half the time) 3 = Sometimes (about half the time) 4 = Most times (much more than half the time) 5 = Almost always/always
5. During sexual intercourse, how difficult was it to maintain your erection to completion of intercourse?	0 = Did not attempt intercourse 1 = Extremely difficult 2 = Very difficult 3 = Difficult 4 = Slightly difficult 5 = Not difficult
6. How many times have you attempted sexual intercourse?	0 = No attempts 1 = One to two attempts 2 = Three to four attempts 3 = Five to six attempts 4 = Seven to ten attempts 5 = Eleven plus attempts
7. When you attempted sexual intercourse, how often was it satisfactory for you?	0 = Did not attempt intercourse 1 = Almost never/never 2 = A few times (much less than half the time) 3 = Sometimes (about half the time) 4 = Most times (much more than half the time) 5 = Almost always/always
8. How much have you enjoyed sexual intercourse?	0 = No intercourse 1 = No enjoyment 2 = Not very enjoyable 3 = Fairly enjoyable 4 = Highly enjoyable 5 = Very highly enjoyable
9. When you had sexual stimulation or intercourse, how often did you ejaculate? 10. When you had sexual stimulation or intercourse, how often did you have the feeling of orgasm or climax?	0 = No sexual stimulation/intercourse 1 = Almost never/never 2 = A few times (much less than half the time) 3 = Sometimes (about half the time) 4 = Most times (much more than half the time) 5 = Almost always/always
11. How often have you felt sexual desire?	1 = Almost never/ never 2 = A few times (much less than half the time) 3 = Sometimes (about half the time) 4 = Most times (much more than half the time) 5 = Almost always/always
12. How would you rate your level of sexual desire?	1 = Very low/none at all 2 = Low 3 = Moderate 4 = High 5 = Very high
13. How satisfied have you been with your overall sex life? 14. How satisfied have you been with your sexual relationship with your partner?	1 = Very dissatisfied 2 = Moderately dissatisfied 3 = About equally satisfied and dissatisfied 4 = Moderately satisfied 5 = Very satisfied
15. How do you rate your confidence that you can get and keep an erection?	1 = Very low 2 = Low 3 = Moderate 4 = High 5 = Very high

FIGURE 84–3. International Index of Erectile Function Questionnaire. All questions are preceded by the phrase, "Over the past 4 weeks." *(Reprinted with permission from Kirby R, Carson C, Goldstein I. Erectile Dysfunction, A Clinical Guide. Oxford, England, ISIS Medical Media, 1999:30–31).*

TABLE 84–3. Dosing Regimens for Selected Drug Treatments for Erectile Dysfunction

Route of Administration	Generic Name (Brand Name)	Dosage Form	Common Dosing Regimen
Oral	Yohimbine (Aphrodyne, Yocon, Yohimex)	5.4-mg tablet or capsule	5.4 mg tid
	Sildenafil (Viagra)	25-mg, 50-mg, 100-mg tablets	25–100 mg 1 hour before intercourse
	Apomorphine (Uprima)[a]	sublingual tablets	
	Methyltestosterone (Oreton, Android)	10-mg, 25-mg tablets and capsules	10–40 mg daily
	Fluoxymesterone (Halotestin)	2-mg, 5-mg, 10-mg tablets	5–20 mg daily
	Trazodone (Desyrel)[b]	50-mg, 100-mg, 150-mg, 300-mg tablet	50–150 mg daily
	Phentolamine (Spontane, Vasomax)[a]	oral or buccal tablets	
Topical	Testosterone patch (Testoderm)	4 mg/patch, 6 mg/patch	4–6 mg/d; apply to scrotum
	Testosterone patch (Testoderm-TTS)	4 mg/patch, 6 mg/patch	4–6 mg/d; apply to arm, buttock, back
	Testosterone patch (Androderm)	2.5 mg/patch	2.5–5 mg/d; apply to arm, back, abdomen, thigh
	Testosterone gel (Androgel 1%)	5 g/pkt, 10 g/pkt	5–10 g/d; apply to shoulders, upper arms, abdomen
Intramuscular	Testosterone cypionate (Depo-Testosterone)	100 mg/mL, 200 mg/mL	200–400 mg every 2 to 4 weeks
	Testosterone enanthate (Delatestryl)	100 mg/mL, 200 mg/mL	200–400 mg every 2 to 4 weeks
	Testosterone propionate	100 mg/mL	25–50 mg two to three times a week
Intraurethral	Alprostadil (Muse)	125-μg, 250-μg, 500-μg, 1,000-μg pellets	125–1,000 μg 5 to 10 minutes before intercourse
Intracavernosal	Alprostadil (Caverject)	5 μg, 10 μg, 20 μg injection	2.5–60 μg 5 to 10 minutes before intercourse
	Alprostadil (Edex)	5 μg, 20 μg, 20 μg, 40 μg injection	2.5–60 μg 5 to 10 minutes before intercourse
	Papaverine[b]	30 mg/mL injection	Variable, usually used in combination[c]
	Phentolamine[b]	2.5 mg/mL injection	Variable, usually used in combination[c]

[a]Not yet commercially available at the time this chapter was written.
[b]Not FDA-approved for this use.
[c]See Table 84–5.

Specific treatments for erectile dysfunction include medical devices, pharmacologic treatments, and surgery. The ideal treatment for this disorder should have a fast onset, be effective, be convenient to administer, be cost-effective, have a low incidence of serious adverse effects, and be free of serious drug interactions. Currently, no treatment for erectile dysfunction is ideal (Table 84–3). The least invasive therapy is the vacuum erection medical device, and it is associated with the fewest serious adverse effects. The most invasive is surgical implantation of a penile prosthesis, and it is associated with the most serious adverse effects. Generally, when choosing among treatment approaches, those which are least invasive are chosen first, while more invasive therapies are reserved for patients who fail to respond to first-line agents. A sample algorithm that guides selection of treatment is shown in Fig. 84–4.

VACUUM ERECTION DEVICES

A vacuum erection device (VED) has three parts: a pump to generate a negative vacuum pressure; a cylinder, which is closed at one end and into which the penis is inserted; and tubing to connect the pump to the cylinder. The patient inserts his penis into the cylinder, which is then pushed up flush against his lower abdomen to create a vacuum chamber. Then, the patient activates the pump to produce a vacuum pressure, which draws arteriolar blood into the corpora cavernosa. To prolong the erection, the patient may also use constriction bands or tension rings, which are placed at the base of the penis, to keep the arteriolar blood in and to reduce venous outflow from the penis. With the assistance of loading cones to protect the glans, these bands or rings can be rolled over the glans penis and up the shaft. Alternatively, they can be first threaded onto the plastic cylinder before the penis is inserted. Once the penis is erect, the band or ring can be rolled off the cylinder onto the base of the penis (Fig. 84–5).

The VED's onset of action is comparatively slow (30 minutes), which requires that both the patient and his sexual partner be patient. For this reason, VEDs appear to work best in older patients who are married or have stable sexual relationships. In this group, VEDs are considered first-line therapy, and the overall satisfaction rate is 60% to 80%.[17–19]

VEDs may also be used as second-line therapy in patients who fail oral or injectable drug treatments for erectile dysfunction. The

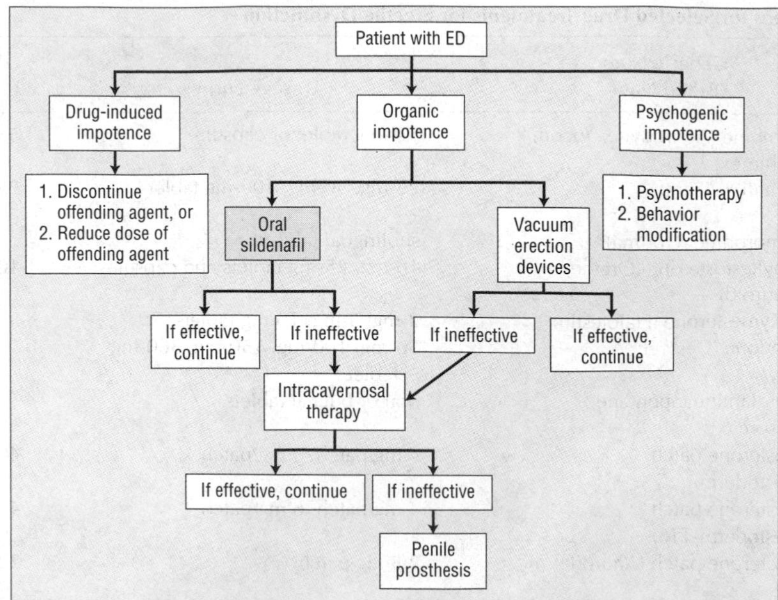

FIGURE 84–4. Algorithm for selecting treatment for erectile dysfunction (ED).

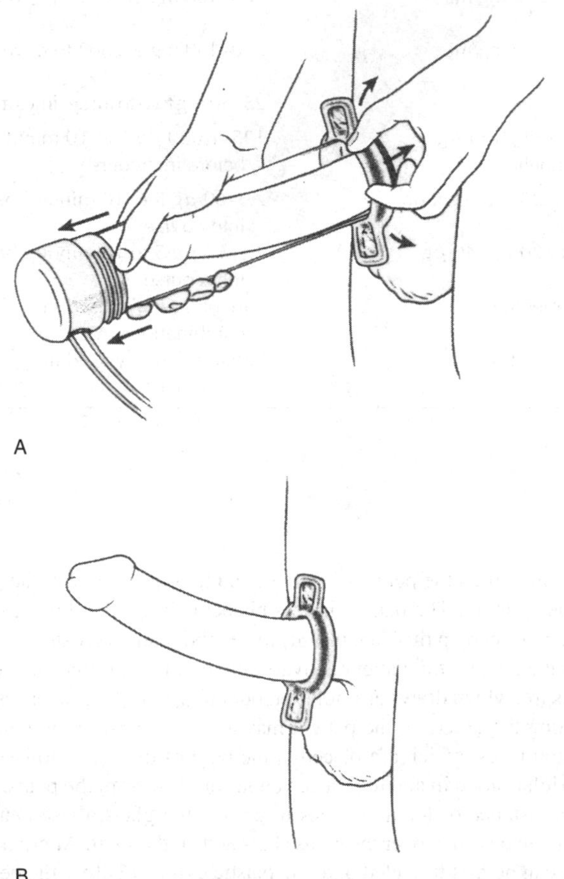

FIGURE 84–5. Technique for using a vacuum erection device with tension band or rubber constriction ring. **A,** The patient inserts his penis into the cylinder, which is then pushed up flush against his lower abdomen to create a vacuum chamber. Then, the patient activates the pump to produce a vacuum pressure, which draws arteriolar blood into the corpora cavernosa. **B,** To prolong the erection, the patient may also use constriction bands or tension rings, which are placed at the base of the penis, to keep the arteriolar blood in and reduce venous outflow from the penis. *(Reprinted with permission from Kirby R, Carson C, Goldstein I. Erectile Dysfunction, A Clinical Guide. Oxford, England, ISIS Medical Media, 1999:52.)*

combination of VED with intracavernosal[20] or intraurethral[21] alprostadil is associated with a higher rate of efficacy than use of the VED alone. As a result, combination therapy may sometimes be attempted before surgery is considered in the patient who fails VED monotherapy.

VEDs are available with manual or battery-operated pumps. The latter offer greater convenience, particularly in patients with arthritis of the hands, who find the pumps to be too difficult and tiring to operate. The American Urological Association recommends the use of commercially available VEDs by prescription only.[22]

Pain or injury from VEDs most often are caused by the rubber rings or tension bands used to sustain an erection. Because these rings trap blood in the corpora, and reduce arteriolar flow into the penis, the penile shaft may feel cold and numb. If the rings or bands are applied for longer than 30 to 60 minutes, the penile shaft may turn bluish and hurt. Patients may complain that a hinge-like erection is produced in that the penis pivots on the rubber ring or tension band. Patients may also sometimes fail to ejaculate.

VEDs are contraindicated in patients with sickle cell disease. These patients are prone to priapism, which can be exacerbated by the use of rubber rings or tension bands with VEDs. The devices should also be used cautiously in patients on oral anticoagulants. This is also because warfarin, through a poorly understood and idiosyncratic mechanism, can cause priapism.

SILDENAFIL

MECHANISM

Sildenafil (Viagra) is a phosphodiesterase isoenzyme type 5 inhibitor, which decreases catabolism of cGMP, a vasodilatory neurotransmitter in the corporal tissue. Cyclic GMP is normally produced during sexual stimulation; sildenafil therefore only produces an erection when the man is stimulated after taking the medication. In this situation, nitric oxide, released by neurons or endothelial cells, enhances the activity of guanylate cyclase, the enzyme responsible for the conversion of guanylate triphosphate to cGMP (Fig. 84–6).[23]

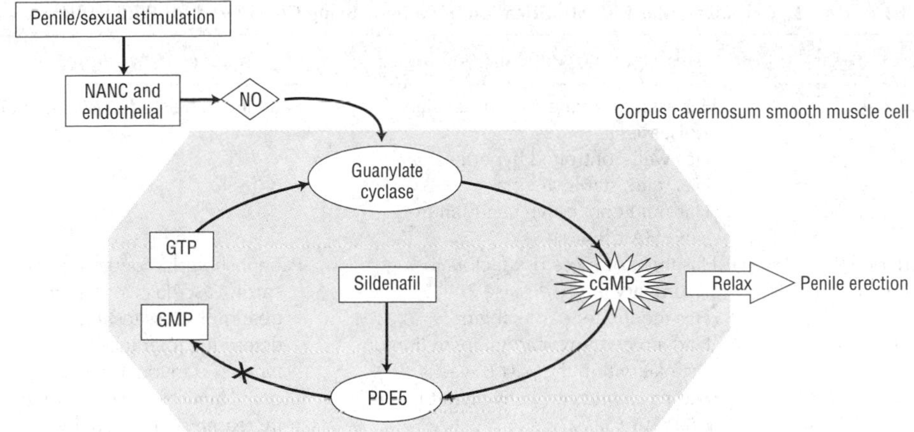

FIGURE 84–6. Nitric oxide (NO)-cyclic guanosine monophosphate (cGMP) mechanism of penile erection and the NO-enhancing effect of the phosphodiesterase type 5 (PDE5) inhibitor sildenafil. GTP, guanosine triphosphate; NANC, nonadrenergic noncholinergic neurons. *(Reprinted with permission from Zusman RM. Cardiovascular data on sildenafil citrate. Am J Cardiol 1999;83(5A):2C.)*

Sildenafil is highly selective for the phosphodiesterase isoenzyme type 5 found in genital tissue. However, phosphodiesterase isoenzyme type-5 is also found in peripheral vascular tissue, tracheal smooth muscle, and platelets. Sildenafil's inhibition of phosphodiesterase in these nongenital tissues can produce adverse effects.

EFFICACY

Because of its apparent effectiveness, convenient route of administration, and comparatively low incidence of serious adverse effects, sildenafil is considered a first-line therapy, particularly in younger patients.

In doses of 25–100 mg, sildenafil produces satisfactory erections in 56% to 82% of patients. Its effectiveness appears to be dose-related. That is, as the dose increases, a greater percentage of patients report a positive clinical response with an improved quality of penile erections.[24–27] Approximately 30% to 40% of patients fail to respond to sildenafil.

Sildenafil has proven effective in patients with all three types of organic erectile dysfunction (vascular, neurologic, or hormonal etiologies).[24,26] Although patients with an intact peripheral nerve supply to the corpora appear to respond better than those with peripheral neurologic deficits, sildenafil has been reported to be effective in patients who have undergone radical prostatectomy[27] and those with spinal cord injury.[28] This is probably because sildenafil's actions are mediated by locally acting neurotransmitters.

Sildenafil should not be used in patients with normal erectile function. Also, according to FDA-approved labeling, sildenafil should not be used in combination with other forms of therapy for erectile dysfunction.

PHARMACOKINETICS

Sildenafil has an initial onset of 30 minutes and a peak onset of 1 hour, if taken on an empty stomach. A fatty meal delays the peak onset by about 1 hour. Therefore, patients should be instructed to take the medication on an empty stomach 30 to 60 minutes prior to sexual intercourse. For some patients, the onset of sildenafil may be perceived to be slow, which is the rationale for the company to be investigating a dosage form, which may be more quickly absorbed by mouth.

The absolute oral bioavailability of sildenafil is approximately 40%. It is hepatically catabolized by the P450 microsomal isoenzymes 3A4 (major route) and 2C9 (minor route). The *N*-desmethyl metabolite is pharmacologically active, with 50% of the parent drug's potency. Sildenafil and its active metabolite are highly protein bound (96% for sildenafil). The plasma half-life of sildenafil is 4 hours. Approximately 80% of sildenafil and its metabolites are excreted in stool, and approximately 13% is excreted in the urine. In patients with hepatic impairment or severe renal dysfunction, the initial dose of sildenafil should be reduced to 25 mg.[23]

DOSING

The usual oral dose of sildenafil is 50 mg. The dose may be increased to 100 mg to improve treatment response. The ideal dose should produce an erection suitable for intercourse that lasts no more than 1 hour. A particular dose of sildenafil should be tried at least three times before the dose is increased.

A lower starting dose of 25 mg is recommended in patients who have difficulty metabolizing sildenafil or clearing it and its metabolites. This includes elderly patients (over age 65), patients with liver cirrhosis or severe renal disease (creatinine clearance less than or equal to 30 mL/min), and patients taking drugs known to inhibit the hepatic catabolism of sildenafil through their action on the cytochrome P450 isoenzyme 3A4 (e.g., cimetidine, erythromycin, clarithromycin, ketoconazole, or itraconazole). Patients should be advised to take no more than what is prescribed and to use only one dose per day. Doses greater than 100 mg have not consistently produced improved erectile responses.[23]

ADVERSE EFFECTS

Most adverse effects of sildenafil are mild or moderate and self-limited, rarely requiring treatment discontinuation. In usual doses, the most common adverse effect of sildenafil is headache (16% of patients).[23] Sildenafil may also cause facial flushing (10%), dyspepsia (7%), nasal congestion (4%), and dizziness (2%), all of which result from inhibition of phosphodiesterase isoenzyme type 5 in extragenital tissues.[23]

TABLE 84–4. Cardiovascular Risk Stratification of Patients Being Considered for Sildenafil[29–33]

Risk Category	Description of Patients' Conditions	Management Approach
Low Risk	Has asymptomatic cardiovascular disease Has well-controlled hypertension Has mild, stable angina Has mild congestive heart failure (NYHA Class 1)*	Patient can be started on sildenafil.
Moderate Risk	Has three or more risk factors for coronary artery disease Has moderate, stable angina Had a recent myocardial infarction or stroke within the past 6 weeks Has moderate congestive heart failure (NYHA Class 2)[a]	Patient should undergo a complete cardiovascular workup and treadmill stress testing to determine tolerance to increased myocardial energy consumption associated with increased sexual activity.
High Risk	Has unstable or symptomatic angina, despite treatment Has poorly controlled hypertension Has severe congestive heart failure (NYHA Class III or IV)* Had a recent myocardial infarction or stroke within 2 weeks Has moderate or severe valvular heart disease	Sildenafil is contraindicated

[a]NYHA, New York Heart Association. See Chap. 13.

Sildenafil produces an 8–10-mm decrease in systolic and a 5–6-mm decrease in diastolic blood pressure starting about 1 hour after a dose and lasting for 4 hours. Although most patients are asymptomatic as a result of these blood pressure changes, some patients, particularly those taking multiple antihypertensives or nitrates, or those with baseline hypotension, may develop adverse effects as a consequence of these peripheral vascular effects.[23,29]

In 1998, following the marketing of sildenafil in the United States, 123 sildenafil-associated deaths were reported. About 67% of these patients died of myocardial infarction or cardiac arrest, and 36% of these patients developed cardiovascular symptoms within 5 hours of sildenafil administration. Interestingly, nitrates were administered to less than 20% of these patients.

The American College of Cardiology and American Heart Association attempted to determine whether the deaths were caused by sildenafil, drug interactions with sildenafil, or underlying cardiovascular disease of the patient that could have been worsened by increased sexual activity. While their findings were not conclusive, these recommendations were made (Table 84–4):[30–33]

- Patients should be prescribed sildenafil only when medically indicated.
- Patients with stable ischemic heart disease and who are not taking nitrates can probably be treated safely with sildenafil.[30,31]
- Patients at moderate risk of major cardiovascular events after sexual intercourse should undergo formal cardiovascular testing for myocardial ischemia by using a treadmill test.
- If the patient suffers from hypotension or develops significant electrocardiographic changes with treadmill testing, then sildenafil should be avoided.
- If the patient is able to tolerate treadmill testing, sildenafil 25 mg can be initiated cautiously in the office.
- If hypotension develops, then sildenafil should not be continued.
- Patients at high risk of major cardiovascular events after sexual intercourse should not be prescribed sildenafil.

Sildenafil causes increased sensitivity to light, blurred vision, or loss of blue-green color discrimination in 3% to 10% of patients. This results from the agent's inhibition of phosphodiesterase type 6 in the retina, particularly at doses larger than 100 mg.[34,35] Although no long-term ocular adverse effects have been reported with sildenafil, caution is recommended or sildenafil is contraindicated in patients at risk of ophthalmologic problems (e.g., retinitis pigmentosa, a genetic disease associated with phosphodiesterase deficiency). Also, pilots who use blue and green lights to guide airplanes during landing should not use sildenafil around the times they will be flying.

Sildenafil inhibits phosphodiesterase isoenzyme type 5 in platelets, which theoretically could inhibit platelet aggregation. Although sildenafil has not caused bleeding in healthy subjects, it should be used cautiously in patients taking aspirin or other antiplatelet agents and in patients with bleeding tendencies.

DRUG INTERACTIONS

Patients taking organic nitrates by any route of administration may develop severe hypotension if these products are used with sildenafil. This is a result of two major factors: (a) organic nitrates on their own will produce hypotension, and (b) organic nitrates supply extra nitric oxide, which can stimulate the activity of guanylate cyclase and increase tissue levels of cGMP. For this reason, nitrates (e.g., isosorbide dinitrate, isosorbide mononitrate, or nitroglycerin) are contraindicated within 24 hours of administration of sildenafil.[29,30]

If severe hypotension occurs, the patient should be placed in a Trendelenburg position and aggressive fluid administration should be initiated. If severe hypotension continues, parenteral α-adrenergic agonists (e.g., dopamine, levarterenol, epinephrine) should be cautiously administered.

Interestingly, dietary sources of nitrates, nitrites, or L-arginine (a precursor for nitrates) do not interact with sildenafil. This is because these dietary sources do not increase circulating levels of nitric oxide in humans.[29]

Sildenafil does not appear to interact with antihypertensive medications. In one retrospective analysis of patients taking sildenafil in combination with β-adrenergic blocking agents, α-adrenergic blocking agents, diuretics, angiotensin-converting enzyme inhibitors, or calcium-channel blockers, the incidence of hypotension was similar to that reported in patients taking sildenafil alone.[36]

The hepatic metabolism of sildenafil may be inhibited by P450 hepatic microsomal enzyme inhibitors of CYP 3A4, including cimetidine, erythromycin, clarithromycin, ketoconazole, and itraconazole. In these patients, the starting dose of sildenafil should be no larger than 25 mg. However, the clinical importance of elevated levels of sildenafil as a result of these drug interactions is unclear.[23,33] Only one recent case report described a patient who developed severe hypotension with the combination of sildenafil and ritonavir.[37]

TESTOSTERONE REPLACEMENT REGIMENS

MECHANISM

Testosterone replacement regimens supply exogenous testosterone and restore serum testosterone levels to the normal range (300–1,100 ng/dL). In so doing, testosterone replacement regimens correct symptoms of hypogonadism, which include malaise, loss of muscle strength, depressed mood, and decreased libido. Testosterone can directly stimulate androgen receptors in the central nervous system and is thought to be responsible for maintaining normal sexual drive. Alternatively, testosterone can be converted peripherally to dihydrotestosterone by 5α-reductase enzyme, which is abundant in the prostate, skin, and genital tissues. Dihydrotestosterone can stimulate intracellular receptors in other target tissues, including the prostate. This can lead to enhanced growth of the prostate.

INDICATIONS

Testosterone replacement regimens are indicated in symptomatic patients with primary or secondary hypogonadism, as confirmed by the presence of a decreased libido and low serum concentrations of testosterone.[38] Simultaneous serum luteinizing hormone (LH) levels help to distinguish patients with primary hypogonadism, who have elevated LH levels, from those with secondary hypogonadism, who have decreased LH levels.

Testosterone replacement regimens should never be administered to men with normal serum testosterone levels.

EFFICACY

Testosterone replacement regimens restore muscle strength and sexual drive and improve mood in patients with hypogonadism. Improvements are generally observed within days or weeks of the start of testosterone replacement. Administration of testosterone will correct the serum testosterone level to the normal range. No additional benefit has been demonstrated for large doses of testosterone, which increase the serum testosterone level from the low end to the upper end of the normal range, or to the above-normal range.[6] Testosterone replacement regimens do not directly correct erectile dysfunction; instead, they improve libido, thereby correcting secondary erectile dysfunction.

Testosterone replacement regimens can be administered orally, parenterally, and topically (Table 84–3). Injectable testosterone replacement regimens are preferred for treatment of symptomatic patients with primary or secondary hypogonadism because they are effective, inexpensive, and not associated with the bioavailability problems or hepatotoxic adverse effects of oral androgens.[5,38] Although convenient for the patient, testosterone patches and gel are much more expensive than other forms of androgen replacement; therefore, they should be reserved for those patients who refuse injectable testosterone.[39]

PHARMACOKINETICS

Natural testosterone has poor oral bioavailability because of extensive first-pass hepatic metabolism, and large doses must therefore be taken. To improve oral bioavailability, alkylated derivatives were formulated. Of these, methyltestosterone and fluoxymesterone have improved oral bioavailability, are more resistant to hepatic catabolism, and can be taken in smaller daily doses, which are potentially safer. However, oral alkylated derivatives of testosterone agents are associated with a higher incidence of serious hepatotoxicity, and therefore, are not preferred for management of sexual dysfunction.

Several testosterone esters have been formulated for intramuscular injection with different durations of action (Table 84–3). The shorter-acting testosterone propionate, which requires dosing three times a week, has largely been replaced with testosterone cypionate or enanthate. The latter formulations offer greater convenience as they can be dosed every 2, 4, or 6 weeks in most patients. Both testosterone cypionate and enanthate produce suprapharmacologic patterns of serum testosterone during the dosing interval, in that the peak level exceeds normal physiologic levels for a portion of the dosing interval. Before the next dose, the serum level may decrease to a level below normal physiologic levels. This unnatural pattern of serum testosterone vacillation may be associated with some of the mood swings that occur in some patients.

Topical testosterone replacement regimens can be delivered as once-daily patches or gel. Testosterone patches increase serum testosterone levels into the normal range in 2 to 6 hours. Serum testosterone levels return to baseline 24 hours after patch administration. However, unlike oral or injectable supplements, topical testosterone products produce physiologic patterns of serum testosterone levels throughout the day. The clinical importance of this biochemical effect is unknown.[40] Testosterone patches 4 mg or 6 mg are applied every 24 hours. To mimic the normal diurnal pattern of testosterone secretion, the patch should be applied once daily in the morning upon arising.

The original Testoderm brand patch was formulated for scrotal application. Scrotal skin is thinner and has a richer vascular supply than does the skin on the arms or thighs. Therefore, application of Testoderm patches produced excellent absorption of the hormone. However, the patch could fall off when the scrotum became damp or moist, when the patient exercised, or if the scrotum was excessively hairy.

For improved convenience, the Androderm or Testoderm TTS patches were formulated for application to the arms, buttocks, or back; Androderm can also be applied to the thighs. The addition of absorption enhancers and different adhesives has been linked to a higher incidence of contact dermatitis with Androderm patches, as compared to the original Testoderm scrotal patch.[41] The testosterone gel 1% formulation (Androgel) is applied in much larger doses—5 or

10 g each day—to the skin of the shoulders, upper arms, or abdomen. The hormone is absorbed quickly, within 30 minutes, but it may take several hours for complete absorption of the dose. For this reason, the patient should be reminded to wait at least 5 to 6 hours after application before showering. To prevent inadvertent transfer of testosterone gel to others, the patient should thoroughly wash his hands with soap and water after administration of a dose.

DOSING

Table 84–3 lists the usual doses for testosterone replacement regimens. An adequate treatment trial with a particular dose is considered to be 2 to 3 months. Thus, a dose should not be increased until the patient has used one particular dose for at least this time period.

Before initiating any testosterone replacement regimen in patients 40 years of age or older, the patient should be screened for the presence of benign prostatic hyperplasia and prostate cancer. Both of these diseases are testosterone-dependent conditions and may be worsened by the exogenous administration of testosterone. If the patient has benign prostatic hyperplasia, testosterone replacement may be initiated cautiously. However, if the patient develops bothersome voiding symptoms, he will require specific intervention for benign prostatic hyperplasia, if testosterone supplementation is to be continued. If the patient is found to have prostate cancer, this is a contraindication to androgen supplementation.

ADVERSE EFFECTS

Testosterone replacement regimens can cause sodium retention, which can cause weight gain, or exacerbate hypertension, congestive heart failure, and edema. Gynecomastia can also occur as a result of conversion of testosterone to estrogen in peripheral tissues. This has most often been reported in patients with liver cirrhosis.

Deleterious serum lipoprotein changes have also been reported, including decreasing HDL-cholesterol levels. However, no cases of cardiovascular disease have been reported with testosterone replacement regimens. Large doses of testosterone can stimulate erythropoiesis, and polycythemia may result. In one retrospective study of 45 elderly men receiving testosterone enanthate or testosterone cypionate intramuscularly every 2 weeks, 24% of the patients developed polycythemia, which required phlebotomy or a temporary cessation of hormone therapy.[42] Thus, patients on long-term testosterone replacement regimens must undergo clinical laboratory testing for serum testosterone, a lipid profile, and a hematocrit every 6 to 12 months.[42] Repeated serum testosterone levels that exceed the normal range require a dosage reduction or increased interval between drug doses. An abnormal lipid profile may require lifestyle and dietary modification, and if necessary, antihyperlipidemic drug therapy. If the hematocrit exceeds 55%, the testosterone replacement regimen should be withheld temporarily.

Exogenous testosterone may also exacerbate benign prostatic hyperplasia or enhance the growth of prostate cancer. For this reason, patients should be monitored for urinary voiding difficulty and should have an annual digital rectal examination and clinical laboratory test for prostate specific antigen. If prostate cancer is present, testosterone replacement regimens must be discontinued.

Oral testosterone replacement regimens have caused hepatotoxicity, which has ranged from mild elevations of hepatic transaminases to serious liver diseases, including peliosis hepatis (hemorrhagic liver cysts), hepatocellular and intrahepatic cholestasis, and benign or malignant tumors. For this reason, parenteral testosterone replacement regimens are preferred.

Topical testosterone patches may cause contact dermatitis, which responds well to topical corticosteroids.

ALPROSTADIL

MECHANISM

Alprostadil, also known as prostaglandin E_1, stimulates adenyl cyclase. This enzyme stimulates smooth-muscle cell-membrane receptors to increase production of cAMP, a neurotransmitter that causes smooth-muscle relaxation of the arterial blood vessels to the corpora and sinusoidal tissues in the corpora. This results in enhanced blood flow to and blood filling of the corpora (Fig. 84–1).

Alprostadil is commercially available as an intracavernosal injection (Caverject, Edex) and as an intraurethral insert (Muse).

INDICATIONS

Both commercially available formulations of alprostadil are FDA-approved as monotherapy for the management of erectile dysfunction. Alprostadil is more effective by the intracavernosal route than by the intraurethral route.[43–45]

The enhanced efficacy of intracavernosal injection of alprostadil may be related to the excellent bioavailability of the drug when injected directly into the corpora cavernosum. High local tissue concentrations are achieved following intracavernosal injection. In contrast, intraurethral alprostadil doses generally are several hundred times larger than intracavernosal doses. Intraurethral alprostadil must be absorbed from the urethra, through the corpus spongiosum, and into the corpus cavernosum, where it exerts its full proerectogenic effect.

Although many other agents, including papaverine and phentolamine, have been used off-label for intracavernosal therapy, alprostadil is preferentially prescribed. This is because the FDA has approved intracavernosal alprostadil for erectile dysfunction, and because it has a low potential for causing prolonged erections and priapism, which can result from stasis of blood in the corpora. This pooled blood can produce a local inflammatory reaction and a subsequent fibrotic reaction, and permanent erectile dysfunction can be the long-term consequence.

In addition, the metabolism of alprostadil affords it greater safety, as compared to other vasoactive, proerectogenic agents. Alprostadil is rapidly catabolized to inactive metabolites by enzymes within corporal tissue. Also, any alprostadil that escapes local tissue catabolism is rapidly metabolized by the lungs.[5,46,47]

Both formulations of alprostadil are considered more invasive than VEDs or sildenafil. For this reason, intracavernosal alprostadil is generally prescribed after patients fail to respond to or cannot use VEDs and sildenafil. Intracavernosal alprostadil is preferred over intraurethral alprostadil because the former is more effective than the latter. Also, intracavernosal alprostadil may be preferred in patients with diabetes mellitus who are accustomed to injectable drug therapy and may suffer from peripheral neuropathies, which decreases the patient's perception of pain upon injection. Intraurethral alprostadil is generally reserved as a treatment of last resort for patients who fail other less invasive and more effective forms of therapy and also refuse surgery.

INTRACAVERNOSAL ALPROSTADIL

EFFICACY

In various controlled and uncontrolled studies, the overall efficacy of intracavernosal alprostadil is 70% to 90%.[5,46,47] In a large parallel design, double-blind, multicenter study, Linet et al.[46] documented three relevant characteristics of intracavernosal alprostadil:

1. The effectiveness of alprostadil is dose related over the range of 2.5–20 μg. The mean duration of erection is directly related to the dose of alprostadil administered and range from 12 to 44 minutes.
2. The lowest effective dose appeared to be 2.5 μg. The median effective dose ranged from 3 μg to 5 μg. A higher percentage of patients with psychogenic and neurogenic erectile dysfunction responded to alprostadil and at a lower dose when compared to patients with vasculogenic erectile dysfunction.
3. Tolerance does not appear to develop with continued use of intracavernosal alprostadil at home.

Although intracavernosal alprostadil is highly effective, a high proportion of patients elect to discontinue its use. Depending on the study and the length of observation, 30% to 50% of patients voluntarily discontinue therapy usually during the first 6 to 12 months. Common reasons for this include lack of perceived effectiveness; inconvenience of administration; an unnatural, nonspontaneous erection; needle phobia; loss of interest; and cost of therapy.[5,49–51]

Approximately one-third of patients will not respond to usual doses of intracavernosal alprostadil. In these patients, intracavernosal alprostadil has been used successfully along with VEDs. Such combination therapy may be tried in patients before transitioning to more invasive surgical procedures.[20] Alternatively, intracavernosal injections can be tried that use synergistic combinations of vasoactive agents that act by different mechanisms. Table 84–5 lists examples of such mixtures. Intracavernosal drug combinations typically produce an erection that lasts longer than an erection produced by monotherapy with any one of the agents in the mixture. In addition, because of the low dosage of each agent in the combination, fewer systemic and local fibrotic adverse effects develop, compared with high-dose monotherapy. For example, when used in low dose combination regimens, papaverine is less likely to induce hypotension and liver dysfunction, and phentolamine is less likely to induce tachycardia and hypotension.

PHARMACOKINETICS

Intracavernosal injection should be into one corpus cavernosum only. From this injection site, the drug will reach the other corpus cavernosum through vascular communications between the two corpora. Alprostadil acts rapidly. The onset is 5 to 15 minutes. The duration is directly related to the dose, and within the usual dosage range of 2.5–20 μg, the duration of the erection is less than 1 hour. Local enzymes in the corpora cavernosum quickly metabolize alprostadil. Any alprostadil that escapes into the systemic circulation is deactivated on first passage through the lungs. Hence, the plasma half-life of alprostadil is approximately 1 minute. Also, dose modification is not necessary in patients with renal or hepatic diseases.

DOSING

The usual dose of intracavernosal alprostadil is 10–20 μg, with a maximum recommended dose of 60 μg. Doses greater than 60 μg have not produced any greater improvement in penile erection, but they may cause prolonged erections lasting more than 1 hour or systemic hypotension.[5,46–48] The dose should be administered 5 to 10 minutes before intercourse. The manufacturer recommends that patients be slowly titrated up to the minimally effective dosage. Under a physician's supervision, patients should be started with a 1.25-μg dose, and then increased by 1.25–2.50-μg increments at 30-minute intervals up to the lowest dose that produces a firm erection for 1 hour and does not produce adverse effects. In clinical practice, this is rarely done because it is time-consuming. Instead, many physicians start the patient on 10 μg and move quickly up the dosage range to identify the best dose for the patient. To avoid adverse effects patients should receive no more than one injection per day and not more than three injections per week.[47]

Intracavernosal injections should be performed using a 0.5-inch, 27- or 30-gauge needle. Also, a tuberculin syringe or a syringe prefilled with diluent as supplied by the manufacturer should be used to ensure precise measurement of doses. Patients with needle phobia, poor vision, or poor manual dexterity can use commercially available autoinjectors (e.g., PenInject) to facilitate the administration of intracavernosal alprostadil.

Intracavernosal injections require that the patient or his sexual partner practice good aseptic technique (to avoid infection), and optimally have good manual skills and visual ability. Also, the patient should not fear needles. When practicing self-injection, the patient

TABLE 84–5. Combination Intracavernosal Injection Regimens

Reference No.	Papaverine Concentration (mg/mL)[a]	Phentolamine Concentration (mg/mL)[a]	Alprostadil Concentration (μg/mL)[a]	Atropine Concentration (mg/mL)[a]
50	20	0.67	67	
52	5		5	
53	30	0.5		
54	7.5		5	
54	7.5	0.005		
55	9	0.5		
55	4.5	0.25	5	
56	12.1	1.01	10.1	0.15
57	30	1.5	10	
57	30	1.0		
57	30	2.0	20	

[a]Concentration of each drug is expressed as the amount of medication per milliliter of the final formulation.

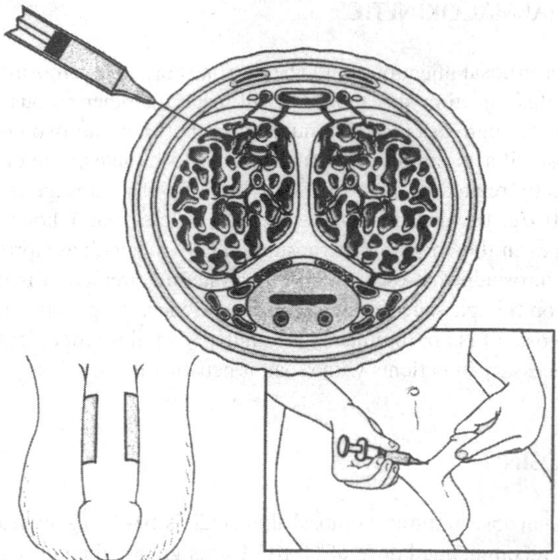

FIGURE 84–7. Technique for administration of intracavernosal injections. *(Reprinted with permission from Kirby R, Carson C, Goldstein I. Erectile Dysfunction, A Clinical Guide. Oxford, England, ISIS Medical Media, 1999:58.)*

should use one hand to firmly hold the glans penis against his thigh to expose the lateral surface of the shaft. The injection should be made at right angles into one of the lateral surfaces of the proximal third of the penis. The injection should never be made into the dorsal or ventral surface of the penis. This will prevent inadvertent injection of the drug into arteries on the dorsal surface or the urethra on the ventral surface, respectively. After the injection, the penis should be massaged to help distribute the drug into the opposite corpus cavernosum. Injection sites should be rotated with each dose. Finally, manual pressure should be applied to the injection site for 5 minutes to reduce the likelihood of hematoma formation (Fig. 84–7).[47] A protocol for teaching proper technique based on the "see it done, then do it yourself" has been published and is an excellent resource.[58]

Once the optimal dosage of intracavernosal alprostadil is established, the patient should return for routine medical followup every 3 to 6 months. Some patients may subsequently require dosage adjustment, and this is largely attributed to worsening of the underlying disease that is contributing to the erectile dysfunction.[51,57]

ADVERSE EFFECTS

Intracavernosal alprostadil is most commonly associated with local adverse effects, which occur most often during the first year of therapy. However, it is believed that improved administration technique with continued use accounts for the lower frequency of adverse effects during subsequent treatment periods.

Intracavernosal injections are associated with several local adverse effects. Cavernosal plaques or areas of fibrosis at injection sites form in approximately 2% to 12% of patients. When these occur, the patient should suspend further injections until the plaques resolve.[59] The concern about these plaques is that these may cause penile curvature, similar to Peyronie's disease, which make sexual intercourse difficult to impossible. The cause for corporal fibrosis and plaque formation is unknown. This adverse effect may be caused by poor injection technique[60,61] or by alprostadil itself. Although patients have developed corporal fibrosis, alprostadil may be less likely to cause this adverse effect as compared to other intracavernosal drug combinations, such as phentolamine or papaverine. This may be because alprostadil inhibits the action of endothelial-derived transforming growth factor-β_1, thereby preventing development of fibrotic tissue.[62] Unlike cavernosal fibrosis associated with large doses and repeated administration of papaverine, penile scarring secondary to alprostadil appears to be unpredictable.

Alprostadil causes penile pain in approximately 10% to 44% of patients.[47,63–65] This has been described as a burning discomfort or dull pain near the injection site or during the erection, which generally does not persist after the penis becomes flaccid. The pain is usually mild, generally does not require discontinuation of therapy, and often abates even with continued treatment. However, 2% to 5% of patients require discontinuation of alprostadil because of severe pain. The pain may be managed by oral analgesics (e.g., acetaminophen), if necessary. One investigator has recommended adding procaine to intracavernosal alprostadil, but this may mask the signs of more serious adverse effects of the drug or of penile injury during intercourse, and it is not recommended.[63] The mechanism of this adverse reaction is poorly understood. Alprostadil may intrinsically produce pain.[65] Also, this may be a result of the pH of the parenteral solution. Alprostadil is acidic and the commercially available Caverject formulation is buffered with a sodium citrate, a weak base, to reduce pain on injection.[64]

Priapism, a prolonged, painful erection lasting more than 1 hour, occurs in 1% to 15% of treated patients.[47] It most often occurs during the dose titration period and is rare thereafter. Blood sludging in the corpora can lead to tissue hypoxia and cavernosal fibrosis and scarring, particularly if priapism develops. The risk for this is greatest for erections that persist beyond 4 hours. Patients are advised to seek medical attention immediately when drug-induced erections last more than 1 hour, as this is considered a urologic emergency. Its management includes supportive care, including analgesics for pain and sedatives for anxiety. In addition, needle aspiration of sludged blood in the corpora or intracavernosal injection of α-adrenergic agonists has been used. These procedures facilitate venous drainage of the corpora, allowing the venous outflow to "catch up" with arterial inflow.

Corporal aspiration entails insertion of a large-bore needle into the corporal bodies to drain accumulated blood followed by irrigation of the corpora with physiologic saline solution. This procedure is typically done at the bedside, and the patient receives local anesthetic before the procedure.

α-Adrenergic agonists have been administered as intracavernosal injections or as irrigating solutions.[65] Phenylephrine is the preferred agent because it has potent α-adrenergic vasoconstrictor effect and no β-adrenergic stimulatory effects, which can produce unwanted tachycardia.[65] The likelihood of prolonged erections with intracavernosal alprostadil is dose-related. Therefore, to prevent this adverse effect, the lowest effective dose should be used and the dose should be titrated to ensure that the duration of the erection is no more than 1 hour.[48]

Other local adverse effects include injection site hematomas and bruising. These are largely the result of unskillful injection techniques. To minimize the risk of injection site hematomas, patients should be advised to apply pressure to the injection site for 5 minutes following each dose. Similarly, infection at the injection site has been reported. Meticulous aseptic technique is recommended to avoid this complication.

Intracavernosal alprostadil rarely causes systemic adverse effects, owing to the agent's local action and rapid metabolism by the lungs. However, large doses greater than 20 μg are associated with dizziness and hypotension in some patients. This is one reason why such large doses are not commonly used.

Intracavernosal injection therapy should be used cautiously in patients at risk of priapism, which includes patients with sickle cell disease or lymphoproliferative disorders. It should also be used cautiously in patients who may develop bleeding complications secondary to injections, including patients with thrombocytopenia or those on anticoagulants. It should also be used cautiously in patients who may use poor quality injection technique, including patients with psychiatric disorders, obese patients (who may not be able to reach or see the penile injection site), patients who are blind, and patients with severe arthritis.[48]

INTRAURETHRAL ALPROSTADIL

EFFICACY

Intraurethral alprostadil inserts are marketed as Muse, a medicated urethral system for erection, which is composed of a pellet inside a prefilled urethral applicator. Multiple studies show alprostadil to have an overall effectiveness rate of 43% to 60%,[43–45] as compared to 70% to 90% for intracavernosal alprostadil. Its decreased effectiveness and inconvenient administration method have resulted in this product being considered a second-line treatment option for patients with erectile dysfunction. However, some patients respond to intraurethral alprostadil even when intracavernosal alprostadil did not work for them.[67]

To improve treatment response to intraurethral alprostadil, it has been combined with an adjustable penile constriction band.[68]

PHARMACOKINETICS

Following intraurethral installation, alprostadil is absorbed quickly through the urethra, into the corpus spongiosum, and into the corpora cavernosum. As much as 90% of each dose is absorbed by the urethra and corpus spongiosum in less than 10 minutes, with peak absorption occurring in 20 to 25 minutes. It is estimated that approximately 20% of each dose is delivered to the corpora cavernosum. As with intracavernosal injections of alprostadil, any drug absorbed into the systemic circulation is rapidly metabolized on first pass through the lungs.

The onset after intraurethral insertion is similar to that of intracavernosal injection, 5 to 10 minutes.

DOSING

The usual dose for intraurethral alprostadil is 125 1,000 μg. The dose should be administered 5 to 10 minutes before sexual intercourse. Not more than one dose per day is recommended. Before administration, the patient should be advised to empty his bladder, voiding completely.

Similar to intracavernosal injection treatments, intraurethral insertion of alprostadil requires good manual and visual skills to minimize the risk of urethral injuries. Intraurethral alprostadil is supplied in a prefilled intraurethral applicator. With one hand the patient holds the glans penis, and with the other hand, the patient inserts the intraurethral applicator 0.5-inch into the urethra. The drug pellet is then pushed into the urethra. The penis should then be massaged to enhance drug absorption (Fig. 84–8).

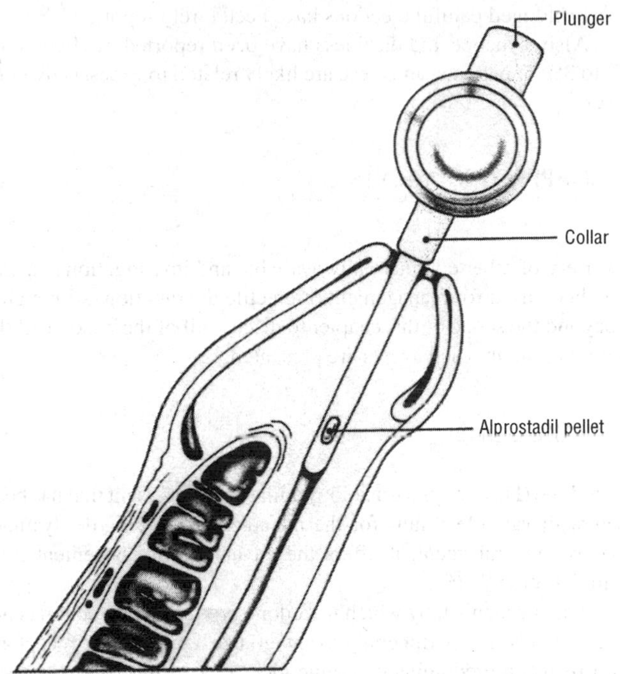

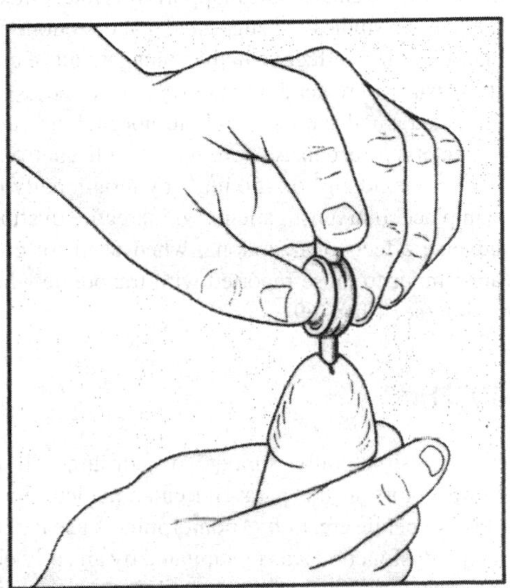

FIGURE 84–8. Technique for administration of intraurethral alprostadil with a Muse applicator. *(Reprinted with permission from Kirby R, Carson C, Goldstein I. Erectile Dysfunction, A Clinical Guide. Oxford, England, ISIS Medical Media, 1999:62.)*

ADVERSE EFFECTS

The urethra can be injured because of improper administration technique. Injuries can lead to urethral stricture and difficulty in voiding. Patients should receive complete education about optimal administration procedures before the start of treatment.

Urethral pain has been reported in 24% to 32% of patients. Usually it is mild and does not require discontinuation of treatment. Female sexual partners may experience vaginal burning, itching, or pain, which is probably related to transfer of alprostadil from the man's urethra to the woman's vagina during intercourse. However, the resumption of sexual intercourse could also produce such symptoms.

Prolonged painful erections have been rarely reported.[5,45,47]

Also, syncope and dizziness have been reported rarely, in only 2% to 3% of patients, and these are likely related to excessively large doses.

UNAPPROVED AGENTS

A variety of other commercially available and investigational agents have been used for management of erectile dysfunction. Although it is beyond the scope of this chapter to discuss all of them, some of the more commonly used agents are presented.

TRAZODONE

Trazodone (Desyrel) is a triazolopyridine antidepressant that has been used with variable results for the management of erectile dysfunction. As an oral agent, it offers the advantage of convenient drug administration.[69–72]

The mechanism by which trazodone produces an erection is not clear. It likely acts peripherally to antagonize α-adrenergic receptors. As a result, a predominant cholinergic effect results, which causes peripheral arteriolar vasodilation and relaxation of cavernosal tissues, which enhances blood filling of the corpora. Intracavernosal injection of trazodone in experimental studies supports this likely mechanism.[69]

Although initial studies[70,71] suggested that trazodone 50–200 mg by mouth daily might be effective in the management of erectile dysfunction, these trials were generally poorly controlled, were nonrandomized, included small samples, and did not include validated objectives parameters of response. More recent well-controlled studies show that trazodone 50 mg[8] or 150 mg[72] by mouth daily is no more effective than placebo in most patients with erectile dysfunction.

The adverse effects of trazodone, when used for erectile dysfunction, are similar to those reported with trazodone when used to treat depression (see Chap. 69).

APOMORPHINE

Apomorphine is structurally similar to morphine. It stimulates dopamine-2 receptors in the paraventricular nucleus in the brain, which produces a penile erection. Apomorphine's use in the management of erectile dysfunction was precipitated by an early observation of its proerectogenic effects in patients with Parkinson's disease.[73]

Although published clinical trials of apomorphine are limited,[74] premarketing data submitted to FDA to document the efficacy of apomorphine for treatment of erectile dysfunction shows that in the presence of sexual stimulation and in a dose-related fashion, apomorphine 2, 3, and 4 mg improves the quality of penile erections (maintains penile erections firm enough for sexual intercourse) in approximately 42% to 67% of patients. Although the efficacy is less than sildenafil, apomorphine does compare favorably.[74,75]

Sublingual administration of apomorphine is associated with a fast onset of approximately 10 to 25 minutes and bypasses first-pass hepatic metabolism of the drug. The faster onset of apomorphine is viewed as a significant advantage when compared to sildenafil; therefore, apomorphine, if approved by FDA, will be marketed for sublingual administration only. Food does not affect absorption of sublingual apomorphine.

The recommended doses of apomorphine are likely to be 2, 3, or 4 mg sublingually. It can be taken as frequently as every 8 hours. Patients should take a sip of water to moisten the mouth and then place a tablet under the tongue.

The most common adverse effect of sublingual apomorphine is dose-related nausea, which occurs in up to 3% and 21% of patients receiving the 2 mg and 4 mg doses, respectively. Patients receiving larger doses appear to develop tolerance to the gastrointestinal adverse effects to apomorphine as long as a slow titration up to the full dose is used. Headache (2% to 21%), dizziness (4% to 14%), sweating (2% to 10%), somnolence (0% to 15%), and yawning (5% to 14%) have also been reported. These usually do not require discontinuation of treatment. If the patient feels dizzy or faint, the patient should be advised to lie flat with legs slightly elevated. As a precaution, the manufacturer will likely recommend that the patient not perform hazardous tasks, such as driving a car, for 2 hours following a dose of apomorphine.[75] Dizziness is thought to be a vasovagal reaction to apomorphine, not the result of an arrhythmogenic effect or a direct myocardial depressant effect.

Large doses of apomorphine may produce fainting if combined with ethanol. Patients should limit ethanol intake to no more than two glasses of beer or wine in the 6-hour period before administration of apomorphine.

In patients taking long-acting nitrates, a small percentage of patients may experience a 5-mm Hg or 10-mm Hg drop in systolic and diastolic blood pressures, respectively. Although concomitant use is not contraindicated, caution is recommended.[76] If dizziness develops, the patient should be instructed to lie down.

To date, no hypotensive reactions have occurred in patients taking apomorphine and commonly used antihypertensives, including diuretics, angiotensin-converting enzyme inhibitors, β-blockers, calcium-channel blockers, or α-adrenergic antagonists.[75,76]

Apomorphine should be avoided in patients who have had serious allergic reactions to morphine.

In summary, apomorphine has a faster onset than sildenafil, which allows greater spontaneity in one's sex life. It should prove to be a useful treatment alternative to sildenafil, particularly in those patients who cannot tolerate the hypotensive adverse effects of the sildenafil. Also, it may be an alternative treatment for patients taking concurrent nitrates. However, its mechanism of action is less selective than that of sildenafil, and apomorphine may therefore produce a wider array of adverse effects.[75] Apomorphine is not currently marketed in the United States. If approved by FDA, its brand name will be Uprima.

YOHIMBINE

Yohimbine, a tree-bark derivative also known as yohimbe, is commercially available from multiple manufacturers. It is widely used by consumers as an aphrodisiac to improve sexual drive. This can be explained by yohimbine's α_2-adrenergic blocking effects in the central nervous system, which increase catecholamines and improve mood. However, some investigators believe that yohimbine has proerectogenic effects. Although controversial, several mechanisms have been postulated. Yohimbine may reduce peripheral α-adrenergic tone, thereby permitting a predominant cholinergic tone. This could result in a vasodilatory response.[5]

The usual oral dose is 5.4 mg three times a day.

A controlled clinical trial has shown high-dose yohimbine (100 mg daily) to be no more effective than placebo.[77] Based on a meta-analysis of published studies that came to the same conclusion, the American Urological Association has cautioned against the use of yohimbine.[22] In addition, yohimbine can cause many systemic adverse effects, including anxiety, insomnia, tachycardia, and hypertension.

PAPAVERINE

Papaverine inhibits cavernosal phosphodiesterase enzyme, thereby decreasing metabolic catabolism of cAMP in cavernosal tissue. As a result of the enhanced tissue levels of cAMP, smooth-muscle relaxation occurs. Cavernosal sinusoids fill with blood and a penile erection results.[5,78]

Papaverine is not FDA-approved for erectile dysfunction, and intracavernosal papaverine monotherapy is not commonly used for management of erectile dysfunction. This is largely because large doses are required, and these produce adverse effects when the drug is absorbed systemically (priapism [35%], corporal fibrosis [35%], hypotension, and hepatotoxicity [less than 2%]).[51,79,80] But the commercially available product has been used in extemporaneous formulations in combination with phentolamine or with phentolamine and alprostadil. A variety of formulas have been used, but few comparisons of them have been published. At this time, no one mixture has been proven better than other mixtures (Table 84–5).

A portion of each papaverine dose is systemically absorbed, and its prolonged plasma half-life of 1 hour contributes to adverse effects. By combining smaller doses of papaverine with other vasoactive agents, combination formulations are considered to be safer and associated with the potential for fewer serious adverse effects.[79,80]

The usual dose of papaverine is 7.5–60 mg when used as a single agent for intracavernosal injection. When used in combination, the dose decreases to 0.5–20 mg (Table 84–5).

If treated with papaverine, patients with a history of underlying liver disease or alcohol abuse should have liver function tests routinely checked at baseline and every 6 to 12 months during continued treatment.[79]

PHENTOLAMINE

Phentolamine is a competitive nonselective α-adrenergic blocking agent. It reduces peripheral adrenergic tone and enhances cholinergic tone. As a result, it improves cavernosal filling and is pro-erectogenic.

Phentolamine has most often been administered as an intracavernosal injection. Monotherapy has been avoided as large doses would be required for an erection, and at these doses, systemic hypotensive adverse effects would be prevalent. Most often, phentolamine has been used in combination with other vasoactive agents for intracavernosal administration. A ratio of 30 mg papaverine and 0.5–1.0 mg phentolamine is typical, and the usual dose ranges from 0.1 mL to 1.0 mL of the mixture. Such a mixture promotes local effects of phentolamine and minimizes systemic hypotensive adverse effects (Table 84–5).[5]

Hypotension is the most common adverse effect of intracavernosal phentolamine. It is more common and more severe with large doses or in patients with poor injection technique who have injected into a vein (rather than the cavernosa). Prolonged erections have also been reported in patients who used excessive doses of combination intracavernosal therapy.

Oral phentolamine (Spontane, Vasomax) is undergoing investigation for erectile dysfunction in the United States. Such a product would offer a more convenient method of administration. However, preliminary studies in small groups of patients suggest that its efficacy may be in the range of 37% to 50%, less than that of sildenafil.[81,82]

OTHER TREATMENTS FOR ERECTILE DYSFUNCTION

Several other medications have been suggested as possibly effective in patients with erectile dysfunction (Table 84–6). Because no well-controlled, comparative studies have been performed on these regimens, they cannot be recommended at this time.

PENILE PROSTHESES

Surgical insertion of a penile prosthesis is the most invasive treatment for erectile dysfunction. It is reserved for those patients who fail to respond to or who are not candidates for less invasive oral or injectable treatments.

Prosthesis insertion requires anesthesia and skilled urologists. Two prostheses are widely used: malleable and inflatable. Malleable

TABLE 84–6. Other Medications Used for Erectile Dysfunction

Agent	Proposed Mechanism	Reference No.
Nitroglycerin, topical	Peripheral vasodilator, probably increases cGMP	83–85
Aminophylline, topical	Phosphodiesterase inhibitor, probably increases cGMP	86
Moxisylyte (also known as thymoxamine)	α-Adrenergic antagonist, probably allows a peripheral cholinergic predominant tone	87
Minoxidil, topical	Peripheral vasodilator	85
Bromocriptine	Reduces elevated prolactin levels, which can cause decreased libido	5
Pentoxifylline	Improves red blood cell flow through arterioles	88
Zinc	Corrects zinc deficiency, which has been linked to erectile dysfunction in patients with chronic renal failure	89
Vasoactive intestinal polypeptide	Increases cAMP synthesis	90, 91

prostheses consist of two bendable rods that are inserted into the corpora cavernosa. The patient appears to have a permanent erection after the procedure; the patient is able to bend the penis into position at the time of intercourse.

The inflatable prosthesis has several parts, including two inflatable rods and a pump-reservoir mechanism. When activated, the device pumps saline solution from the reservoir into the rods, causing inflation. The inflatable prosthesis produces a more natural erection, in that the patient only develops an erection when the device is activated. Some newer advances in inflatable prosthesis technology have resulted in devices with the pump, reservoir, and rods all in one unit, and these can be placed during shorter surgical procedures and are less likely to malfunction (Fig. 84–9).

Penile prostheses provide penile rigidity suitable for vaginal intercourse and are associated with a greater than 90% patient satisfaction rate. The surgical success rate after insertion is 82% to 98%.[5,92]

After a prosthesis is inserted, the corporal tissue is destroyed and the patient will no longer respond to oral or intracavernosal vasoactive therapies for erectile dysfunction or VEDs. Therefore, surgical intervention should be viewed as a treatment modality of last resort for patients who do not respond to or cannot tolerate other less-invasive forms of therapy.

Penile prostheses are not recommended for patients with psychogenic ED unless a full psychiatric examination is performed and it shows that the patient can use the devices safely.

Adverse effects of prosthesis insertion can occur early or late after the surgical procedure. The most common early complication is infection. Meticulous surgical technique and prophylactic antibiotics are routinely employed to minimize this problem. Late complications include mechanical failure of the prosthesis, particularly when inflatable prostheses have been inserted. With improved technology, the mechanical failure rate has decreased to 5%.[5] Other late complications include erosion of the rods through the penis or late-onset infection. Although some salvage procedures have been devised, in many cases, the prosthesis may require removal.

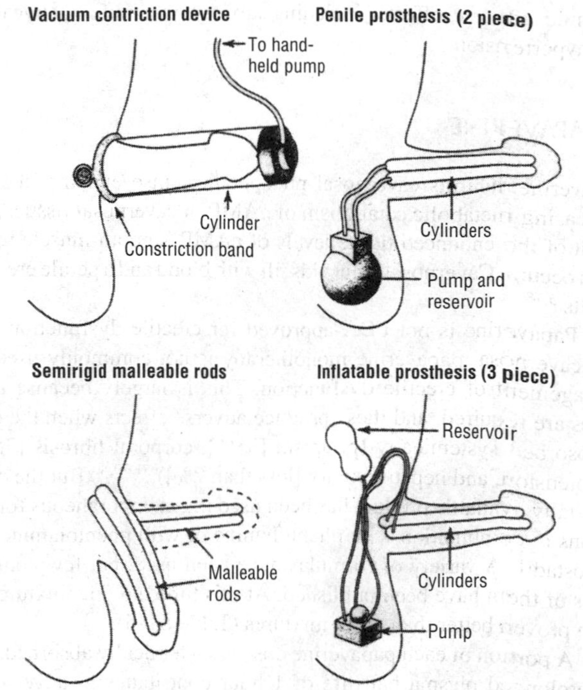

FIGURE 84–9. Devices and prostheses for surgical implantation in patients with erectile dysfunction. *(Adapted with permission from Wagner G, de Tegada IS. Update on male erectile dysfunction. BMJ 1998;316:681.)*

EVALUATION OF THERAPEUTIC OUTCOMES

The primary therapeutic outcomes of specific treatments for erectile dysfunction include (a) improvement in the quantity and quality of penile erections suitable for intercourse and (b) avoidance of adverse drug reactions and drug interactions.

To assess the improvement in the quantity and quality of penile erections suitable for intercourse after treatment, the physician should conduct a thorough pretreatment assessment of the patient and his sexual partner to determine the severity and duration of the patient's erectile dysfunction and to identify treatments that have been tried but failed. Some physicians also conduct a baseline quality of life assessment using a standardized instrument, such as the International Index of Erectile Dysfunction.[14]

After the patient has completed a clinical trial period of 1 to 3 weeks with a specific treatment for erectile dysfunction, the physician should repeat these assessments to determine whether the quality and quantity of penile erections suitable for intercourse has improved. It should be noted that a patient's level of satisfaction is highly individualized depending on his lifestyle and expectations. Therefore, a patient who has successful intercourse once a week might be completely satisfied; whereas another patient might judge this to be unsatisfactory. Patients with unrealistic expectations in this regard need to be identified and counseled by their physicians to avoid adverse effects of excessive use of proerectogenic agents.

Failure to improve the quality and quantity of penile erections suitable for intercourse after an appropriate clinical trial period with a specific treatment for erectile dysfunction occurs in a significant percentage of patients, as previously described. In this case, physicians generally take these steps in this order:

1. Ensure that the patient has been prescribed a maximum tolerated dose of a specific treatment before discarding it as ineffective.
2. Switch to another drug, usually with a greater potential for adverse effects and complications than the first drug initiated (see Fig. 84–4).
3. Reserve surgical treatment for patients who fail to respond to drug treatment.

CONCLUSIONS

Erectile dysfunction is a common disorder of aging men. Its incidence is higher in patients with underlying medical disorders that compromise the vascular, neurologic, hormonal, or psychogenic systems necessary for a normal penile erection. Medications are common causes of erectile dysfunction. By correcting the underlying etiology, erectile dysfunction can be reversed without the use of specific treatments.

When treatments for erectile dysfunction are needed, the least invasive forms of treatment should be used first, as they produce the lowest incidence of serious adverse effects. VEDs or sildenafil are therefore considered first-line treatments. If these fail, intracavernosal alprostadil injection therapy can be initiated. If this fails, the patient can be tried on a combination of intracavernosal alprostadil plus VED, combination intracavernosal therapy, or intraurethral alprostadil. If this fails, the patient may require insertion of a penile prosthesis.

Selection of initial treatment requires consideration of the efficacy of a regimen, convenience of the route of administration, rapidity of onset and adequacy of duration of action, adverse effects, and cost of therapy. Some insurance companies do not reimburse for drug treatments for erectile dysfunction; therefore, cost may be an important issue for some patients.

Pharmacists should be careful to counsel patients appropriately when dispensing medications for erectile dysfunction so that patients can optimize their response to treatment and avoid adverse effects. In addition, pharmacists should be familiar with those medications that commonly cause erectile dysfunction so that they can properly advise prescribers about modifications in medication regimens that may ameliorate or eliminate erectile dysfunction and the need to initiate specific drug treatments for erectile dysfunction.

Pharmacists who counsel patients about drug therapies for erectile dysfunction should take the initiative to provide relevant information. Advice should be clear and simple. Patient confidentiality and privacy, which are extremely important to men with erectile dysfunction, should be maintained at all times.

▶ PRINCIPLES OF PHARMACOTHERAPY

- The incidence of erectile dysfunction is low in men less than 40. It increases as men age, likely a result of concurrent and common medical conditions that impair the vascular, neurologic, psychogenic, and hormonal systems necessary for a normal penile erection.
- Many commonly used drugs have sympatholytic, anticholinergic, sedative, or antiandrogenic effects that may exacerbate or contribute to the development of erectile dysfunction. Pharmacists should be familiar with these agents and be prepared to make recommendations to physicians to minimize the effect of these drugs on a patient's erectile function.
- Specific treatments for erectile dysfunction include medical devices, pharmacologic treatments, psychotherapy, and surgery.
- The ideal treatment should have a fast onset, be effective, be convenient to administer, be cost-effective, have a low incidence of serious adverse effects, and be free of serious drug interactions. Currently, no ideal treatment for erectile dysfunction exists.
- Specific treatment is first initiated with least invasive forms of treatment, including vacuum erection devices and sildenafil, followed by intracavernosal injections or intraurethral inserts, and finally by surgical insertion of a penile prosthesis.
- Vacuum erection devices have a slow onset of action (30 minutes) and therefore are most effective in elderly couples in a stable relationship.
- Although sildenafil is convenient and effective in patients with a variety of causes for erectile dysfunction, it fails in 30% to 40% of patients. Also, sildenafil is contraindicated in patients taking any form of nitrate, including topical nitrates.
- Testosterone supplementation can improve erectile function in patients who have decreased libido secondary to primary or secondary hypogonadism. Testosterone supplementation should not be used in patients with erectile dysfunction who have normal serum testosterone levels.
- Although intracavernosal alprostadil injections are effective in patients with a variety of causes for erectile dysfunction, it fails in one-third of patients. Also, it should be used cautiously in patients at risk of priapism, which includes patients with sickle cell disease or lymphoproliferative disorders.

REFERENCES

1. NIH Consensus Development Panel on Impotence. Impotence. JAMA 1993;270:83–90.
2. Feldman HA, Goldstein I, Hatzichristou DG, Krane RJ, McKinlay JB. Impotence and its medical and psychosocial correlates: results of the Massachusetts Male Aging Study. J Urol 1994;151:54–61.
3. Laumann EO, Paik A, Rosen RC. Sexual dysfunction in the United States prevalence and predictors. JAMA 1999;281:537–544.
4. Melman A, Gingell JC. The epidemiology and pathophysiology of erectile dysfunction. J Urol 1999;161:5–11.
5. Lue TF. Erectile dysfunction. N Engl J Med 2000;342:1802–1813.
6. Buena F, Swerdloff RS, Steiner BS, et al. Sexual function does not change when serum testosterone levels are pharmacologically varied within the normal male range. Fertil Steril 1993;59:1118–1123.
7. Keene LC, Davies P. Drug-related erectile dysfunction. Adverse Drug React Toxicol Rev 1999;18:5–24.
8. Costabile RA, Spevak M. Oral trazodone is not effective therapy for erectile dysfunction: A double-blind, placebo controlled trial. J Urol 1999; 161:1819–1822.
9. Hollander E, McCarley A. Yohimbine treatment of sexual side effects induced by serotonin reuptake blockers. J Clin Psychol 1992;53:207–209.
10. Weiss RJ. Effects of antihypertensive agents on sexual function. Am Fam Physician 1991;44:2075–2082.
11. Barksdale JD, Gardner SF. The impact of first-line antihypertensive drugs on erectile dysfunction. Pharmacotherapy 1999;19:573–581.
12. TOMHS Study Group. Long-term effects on sexual function of five antihypertensive drugs and nutritional hygienic treatment in hypertensive men and women. Treatment of mild hypertension study (TOMHS). Hypertension 1997;29:8–14.
13. Morley JE, Kaiser FE. Impotence in elderly men. Drugs Aging 1992;2: 330–334.
14. Lue TF. Erectile dysfunction: Problems and challenges. J Urol 1993;149: 1256–1257.
15. Buvat J, Lemaire A. Endocrine screening in 1,022 men with erectile dysfunction: Clinical significance and cost-effective strategy. J Urol 1997; 158:1764–1767.
16. Masters WH, Johnson VE. Human Sexual Inadequacy. Boston, Little, Brown, 1970.
17. Witherington R. Vacuum constriction device for management of erectile impotence. J Urol 1989;141;320–324.
18. Soderdahl DW, Thrasher JB, Hansberry KL. Intracavernosal drug-induced erection therapy versus external vacuum devices in the treatment of erectile dysfunction. Br J Urol 1997;79:952–957.
19. Korenman SG. New insights into erectile dysfunction: A practical approach. Am J Med 1998;105:135–144.
20. Chen J, Godschalk MF, Katz PG, Mulligan T. Combining intracavernous injection and external vacuum as treatment for erectile dysfunction. J Urol 1995;153:1476–1477.
21. John H, Lehmann K, Hauri D. Intraurethral prostaglandin improves quality of vacuum erection therapy. Eur Urol 1996;29:224–226.
22. Montague DK, Barada JH, Belker AM, et al. Clinical guidelines panel on erectile dysfunction: Summary report on the treatment of organic erectile dysfunction. J Urol 1996;156:2007–2011.
23. Langtry HD, Markham A. Sildenafil a review of its use in erectile dysfunction. Drugs 1999;57:967–989.
24. Goldstein I, Lue TF, Padma-Nathan H, et al. Oral sildenafil in the treatment of erectile dysfunction. N Engl J Med 1998;338:1397–1404.
25. Jarow JP, Burnett AL, Geringer AM. Clinical efficacy of sildenafil citrate based on etiology and response to prior treatment. J Urol 1999;162:722–725.

26. Rendell MS, Rajfer J, Wicker PA, Smith MD for the Sildenafil Diabetes Study Group. Sildenafil for the treatment of erectile dysfunction in men with diabetes. JAMA 1999;281:421–426.
27. Derry FA, Dinsmore WW, Fraser M, et al. Efficacy and safety of oral sildenafil (Viagra) in men with erectile dysfunction caused by spinal cord injury. Neurology 1998;51:1629–1633.
28. Zippe CD, Kedia A, Kedia K, Nelson DR, Agarwal S. Treatment of erectile dysfunction after radical prostatectomy with sildenafil citrate (Viagra). Urology 1998;52:963–966.
29. Cheitlin MD, Hutter AM, Brindis RG, et al. Use of sildenafil (Viagra) in patients with cardiovascular disease. Circulation 1999;99:168–177.
30. Conte CR, Pepine CJ, Sweeny M. Efficacy and safety of sildenafil citrate in the treatment of erectile dysfunction in patients with ischemic heart disease. Am J Cardiol 1999;83:29C–34C.
31. Herrmann HC, Chang G, Klugherz BD, Mahoney PD. Hemodynamic effects of sildenafil in men with severe coronary artery disease. N Engl J Med 2000;342:1622–1626.
32. Kloner RA, Jarow JP. Erectile dysfunction and sildenafil citrate and cardiologists. Am J Cardiol 1999;83:576–582.
33. Carson CC (program chair). Experience and Progress in the Management of Erectile Dysfunction (symposium). April 28, 2000, University of North Carolina, Chapel Hill, North Carolina.
34. Marmor MF, Kessler R. Sildenafil (Viagra) and ophthalmology. Surv Ophthalmol 1999;44;153–162.
35. Vobig MAM, Klotz T, Staak M, Bartz-Schmidt KU, Englemann U, Walter P. Retinal side effects of sildenafil. Lancet 1999;353:375–376.
36. Zusman RM, Morales A, Glasser DB, Osterloh IH. Overall cardiovascular profile of sildenafil citrate. Am J Cardiol 1999;83:35C–44C.
37. Hall MCS, Ahmad S. Interaction with sildenafil and HIV-1 combination therapy. Lancet 1999;353:2071–2072.
38. Lund BC, Bever-Stille KA, Perry PPJ. Testosterone and andropause: The feasibility of testosterone replacement therapy in elderly men. Pharmacotherapy 1999;19:951–956.
39. Anonymous. Testosterone patches for hypogonadism. Med Lett Drugs Ther 1996;38:49–50.
40. Cunningham GR, Cordero E, Thomby JI. Testosterone replacement with transdermal therapeutic systems. JAMA 1989;261:2525–2530.
41. Jordan WP. Allergy and topical irritation associated with transdermal testosterone administration: A comparison of scrotal and nonscrotal transdermal systems. Am J Contact Dermatol 1997;8:108–113.
42. Hajjar RR, Kaiser FE, Morley JE. Outcomes of long-term testosterone replacement in older hypogonadal males: A retrospective analysis. J Clin Endocrinol Metab 1997;82:3793–3796.
43. Porst H. Transurethral alprostadil with MUSE (medicated urethral system for erection) vs intracavernous alprostadil—A comparative study in 103 patients with erectile dysfunction. Int J Impot Res 1997;9:187–192.
44. Fulgham PF, Cochran JS, Denman JL, et al. Disappointing initial results with transurethral alprostadil for erectile dysfunction in a urology practice setting. J Urol 1998;160:2041–2046.
45. Padma-Nathan H, Hellstrom WJG, Kaiser FE, et al. Treatment of men with erectile dysfunction with transurethral alprostadil. N Engl J Med 1997;336:1–7.
46. Linet OI, Ogring FG for the Alprostadil Study Group. Efficacy and safety of intracavernosal alprostadil in men with erectile dysfunction. N Engl J Med 1996;334:873–877.
47. Meinhardt W, Kropman RF, Vermeij P. Comparative tolerability and efficacy of treatments for impotence. Drug Saf 1999;20:133–146.
48. Stackl W, Hasun R, Marberger M. The use of prostaglandin E1 for diagnosis and treatment of erectile dysfunction. J Urol 1990;8:84–86.
49. Mulhall JP, Jahoda AE, Cairney M, et al. The causes of patient dropout from penile self-injection therapy for impotence. J Urol 1999;162:1291–1294.
50. De la Taile A, Delmas V, Amar E, Boccon-Gibod L. Reasons of dropout from short- and long-term self-injection therapy for impotence. Eur Urol 1999;35:312–317.
51. Rowland DL, Boedhoe HSM, Dohle G, Slob AK. Intracavernosal self-injection therapy in men with erectile dysfunction: Satisfaction and attrition in 119 patients. Int J Impot Res 1999;11:145–151.
52. Zaher TF. Papaverine plus prostaglandin E1 versus prostaglandin E1 alone for intracorporal injection therapy. Int Urol Nephrol 1998;30:193–196.
53. Gasser TC, Roach RM, Larsen EH, Madsen PO, Bruskewitz RC. Intracavernous self-injection with phentolamine and papaverine for the treatment of impotence. J Urol 1987;137:678–680.
54. Floth A, Schramek P. Intracavernous injection of prostaglandin E1 in combination with papaverine: enhanced effectiveness in comparison with papaverine plus phentolamine and prostaglandin E1 alone. J Urol 1999; 145:56–59.
55. Shenfeld O, Hanani J, Shalhav A, Vardi Y, Goldwasser B. Papaverine-phentolamine and prostaglandin E1 versus papaverine-phentolamine alone for intracorporeal injection therapy: A clinical double-blind study. J Urol 1995;154:1017–1019.
56. Montorsi F, Guazzoni G, Bergamaschi F, Ferini-Strambi L, Barbieri L, Rigatti P. Four-drug intracavernous therapy for impotence due to corporal veno-occlusive dysfunction. J Urol 1993;140:1291–1295.
57. Garcia-Reboll L, Mulhall JP, Goldstein I. Drugs for the treatment of impotence. Drugs Aging 1997;11:140–151.
58. Broderick GA. Intracavernous pharmacotherapy. Urol Clin North Am 1996;23:111–126.
59. Chew KK, Stuckey BGA, Earle CM, Dhaliwal SS, Keough EJ. Penile fibrosis in intracavernosal prostaglandin E1 injection therapy for erectile dysfunction. Int J Impot Res 1997;9:225–229.
60. Chen RN, Laken MM, Montague DK, Ausmundson S. Penile scarring with intracavernosal injection therapy using prostaglandin E1: A risk factor analysis. J Urol 1996;155:138–140.
61. The European Alprostadil Study Group. The long-term safety of alprostadil (prostaglandin-E1) in patients with erectile dysfunction. Br J Urol 1998;82:538–543.
62. Saenz de Tejada I, Moreland RB. Physiology of erection, pathophysiology of impotence and implications of PGE1 in the control of collagen synthesis in the corpus cavernosum. In: Goldstein I, Lue TF, eds. The Role of Alprostadil in the Diagnosis and Treatment of Erectile Dysfunction. Princeton, Excerpta Medica, 1993:3–16.
63. Schramek P, Plas EG, Hubner WA, Pfluger H. Intracavernous injection of prostaglandin E1 plus procaine in the treatment of erectile dysfunction. J Urol 1994;152:1108–1110.
64. Moriel EZ, Rajfer J. Sodium bicarbonate alleviates penile pain induced by intracavernous injections for erectile dysfunction. J Urol 1993;149:1299–1300.
65. Chen J, Godschalk MF, Katz PG, Mulligan T. Incidence of penile pain after injection of a new formulation of prostaglandin E1. J Urol 1995;154:77–79.
66. Lee M, Cannon B, Sharifi R. Chart for preparation of dilutions of alpha-adrenergic agonists for intracavernous use in treatment of priapism. J Urol 1995;153:1182–1183.
67. Engel JD, McVary KT. Transurethral alprostadil as therapy for patients who withdrew from or failed prior intracavernous injection therapy. Urology 1998;51:687–692.
68. Lewis RW. Combined use of transurethral alprostadil and an adjustable penile constriction band in men with erectile dysfunction: results from a multicenter clinical trial. J Urol 1998;159(suppl):237. Abstract.
69. Azadzoi KM, Payton T, Krane RJ, Goldstein I. Effects of intracavernosal trazodone hydrochloride: Animal and human studies. J Urol 1990: 144:1277–1282.
70. Montorsi F, Strambi LF, Guazzoni G, et al. Effect of yohimbine-trazodone on psychogenic impotence: A randomized double-blind, placebo-controlled study. Urology 1995;44:732–736.
71. Lance R, Albo M, Costabile RA, Steers WD. Oral trazodone as empirical therapy for erectile dysfunction: A retrospective review. Urology 1995;46:117–120.
72. Meinhardt W, Schmitz PIM, Kropman RF, et al. Trazodone, a double-blind trial for treatment of erectile dysfunction. Int J Impot Res 1997;9:163–165.
73. O'Sullivan JD, Hughes AJ. Apomorphine-induced penile erections in Parkinson's disease. Move Disord. 1998;13:536–639.
74. Heaton JPW, Morales A, Adams MA, Johnston B, El-Rashidy R. Recovery of erectile dysfunction by the oral administration of apomorphine. Urology 1995;45:200–206.

75. TAP Pharmaceuticals. Premarketing material submitted to the FDA, 1999.
76. Fagan TC, Buttler S, Marbury T, et al. Cardiovascular safety of sublingual apomorphine in patients on stable doses or oral antihypertensive agents and nitrates. Am J Cardiol 2001;88:760–766.
77. Teloken C, Rhoden EL, Sogari P, Dambros M, Souto CAV. Therapeutic effects of high-dose yohimbine hydrochloride on organic erectile dysfunction. J Urol 1998;159:122–124.
78. Fallon B. Intracavernous injection therapy for male erectile dysfunction. Urol Clin North Am 1995;22:833–845.
79. Brown SL, Haas CA, Koehler M, Bodner DR, Seftel AD. Hepatotoxicity related to intracavernous pharmacotherapy with papaverine. Urology 1998;52:844–847.
80. Nehra A, Barrett DM, Moreland RB. Pharmacotherapeutic advances in the treatment of erectile dysfunction. Mayo Clin Proc 1999;74:709–721.
81. Goldstein I and the Vasomax Study Group. Efficacy and safety of oral phentolamine (Vasomax) for the treatment of men with erectile dysfunction. J Urol 1998;159(suppl):240. Abstract.
82. Zorgniotti AW. Experience with buccal phentolamine mesylate for impotence. Int J Impot Res 1994;6:37–41.
83. Claes H, Baert L. Transcutaneous nitroglycerin therapy in the treatment of impotence. Urol Int 1989;44:309–312.
84. Gramkow J, Lendorf A, Zhu J, Meyhoff HH. Transcutaneous nitroglycerine in the treatment of erectile dysfunction: A placebo-controlled trial. Int J Impot Res 1999;11:35–39.
85. Cavallini G. Minoxidil versus nitroglycerin: A prospective double-blind controlled trial in transcutaneous erection facilitation for organic impotence. J Urol 1991;146:50–53.
86. Gomaa A, et al. Topical treatment of erectile dysfunction: A randomized double-blind placebo-controlled trial of cream containing aminophylline, isosorbide dinitrate, and codergocrine mesylate. BMJ 1996;312:1512–1525.
87. Costa P, Sarrazin B, Bressolle F, Colson MH, Bondil P, Saudubray F. Efficacy and side effects of intracavernous injections of moxisylyte in impotent patients: A dose-finding study versus placebo. J Urol 1993;149:301–305.
88. Korenman SG, Viosca SP. Treatment of vasculogenic sexual dysfunction with pentoxifylline. J Am Geriatr Soc 1993;41:363–366.
89. Antoniou LD, Sudhaker T, Shaihoub RJ, Smith JC. Reversal of uremic impotence by zinc. Lancet 1977;2:895–898.
90. Gerstenberg TC, Metz P, Ottsesen B, Fahrenkrug J. Intracavernosal self-injection with vasoactive intestinal polypeptide and phentolamine in the management of erectile dysfunction. J Urol 1992;147:1277–1279.
91. Sandhu D, Curless E, Dean J, Hackett G, Liu S, Savage D, Oakes R, Frentz G. A double-blind, placebo-controlled study of intracavernosal vasoactive intestinal polypeptide and phentolamine mesylate in a novel auto-injector for the treatment of non-psychogenic erectile dysfunction. Int J Impot Res 1999;11:91–97.
92. Pearl RM, McGhee RD. Penile revascularization in the treatment of vasculogenic impotence. Plast Reconstruct Surg 1987;80:2–84.

85

Management of Benign Prostatic Hyperplasia

Mary Lee

Benign prostatic hyperplasia (BPH) is the most common benign neoplasm of American men. A nearly ubiquitous condition among elderly men, BPH is of major societal concern, given the large number of men affected, the long-term nature of the condition, and the health care costs associated with it.

This chapter discusses BPH and its available treatments: "watchful waiting," finasteride, α-adrenergic antagonists, and surgery.

EPIDEMIOLOGY

About 80% of elderly men develop microscopic evidence of pathologic changes associated with BPH, according to the results of autopsy studies. About one-half of the patients with microscopic changes develop an enlarged prostate gland or increased tone of the muscular component of the prostate gland, and as a result have difficulty emptying the contents of the urinary bladder. About one-half of symptomatic patients eventually require treatment.

The peak incidence of clinical BPH occurs at 63 to 65 years of age. Symptomatic disease is uncommon in men younger than 50 years of age, but some urinary-voiding symptoms are present by the time men turn 60 years of age. The Boston Area Normative Aging Study estimated that the cumulative incidence of clinical BPH was 78% in patients at age 80 years.[1] Similarly, the Baltimore Longitudinal Study of Aging projected that approximately 60% of men of at least 60 years of age would develop clinical BPH.[2]

NORMAL PROSTATE PHYSIOLOGY

Located anterior to the rectum, the prostate is a small heart-shaped, chestnut-sized gland located below the urinary bladder. It surrounds the proximal urethra like a doughnut.

Round, soft, symmetric, and mobile on palpation, a normal prostate gland in an adult man weighs 4–20 g. Physical examination of the prostate must be done by digital rectal examination. That is, the prostate is manually palpated by inserting a finger into the rectum. Thus, the prostate is "felt" through the rectal mucosa.

The prostate has two major functions: (a) To secrete fluids that make up a portion of the ejaculate volume; and (b) to provide secretions with possible antibacterial effect related to their high concentrations of zinc.

At birth, the prostate is pea-sized and weighs approximately 1 g. The prostate stays that size until the boy reaches puberty. At that time, the prostate undergoes its first growth spurt, growing to its normal adult size by the time the young man is 25 to 30 years of age. The prostate remains this size until the patient reaches age 40, when a second growth spurt begins and continues until the man is 70 to 80. During this period, the prostate can double or triple in size. At surgery, patients with severely symptomatic BPH have prostates as large as 50–80 g.

The prostate gland comprises three types of tissue: epithelial tissue, stromal tissue, and the capsule. Epithelial tissue, also known as glandular tissue, produces ejaculate secretions. These secretions are delivered into the urethra.

Stromal tissue, also known as smooth muscle tissue, is embedded with α_1-adrenergic receptors. Stimulation of these receptors by norepinephrine causes smooth muscle contraction, which results in an extrinsic compression of the urethra, reduction of the urethral lumen, and decreased urinary bladder emptying. The normal prostate is composed of a higher amount of stromal tissue than epithelial tissue, as reflected by a stromal-to-epithelial tissue ratio of 2:1. This ratio is further exaggerated to 5:1 in patients with BPH, which has implications for drug treatment selection.

The capsule, or outer shell of the prostate, is composed of fibrous connective tissue and smooth muscle, which is also embedded with α_1-adrenergic receptors. When stimulated with norepinephrine, the capsule also contracts around the urethra (Fig. 85–1).

Testosterone is the principal testicular androgen in males, whereas androstenedione is the principal adrenal androgen. These two hormones are responsible for penile and scrotal enlargement, increased muscle mass, and maintenance of the normal male libido. These androgens are converted by 5α-reductase to dihydrotestosterone (DHT), an active metabolite. Two types of 5α-reductase exist. Type I enzyme is localized to hair follicles, frontal scalp, liver, and skin. DHT produced at these target tissues causes acne, increased body and facial hair, and male pattern baldness. Type II enzyme is localized in the prostate, genital tissue, and scalp. In these target tissues, DHT causes prostate enlargement and prostate growth (Table 85–1).[3]

In prostate cells, DHT has greater affinity for intraprostatic androgen receptors than does testosterone, forming a more stable complex with the androgen receptor. Thus, it is considered a more potent androgen. It is largely responsible for the normal growth of the prostate during the first growth spurt, as well as the development of BPH during the second growth spurt.[3]

Estrogen, a product of peripheral metabolism of androgens, is believed to stimulate the growth of the stromal portion of the prostate gland. Estrogens are produced when testosterone and androstenedione are converted by aromatase enzymes in adipose tissues. In addition, estrogens may induce the androgen receptor.[4] As men age, the ratio of serum levels of testosterone to estrogen decreases as a result of a decline in testosterone production by the testes and also increased adipose tissue conversion of androgen to estrogen.

PATHOPHYSIOLOGY

While the precise pathophysiologic mechanisms that cause BPH remain unclear, the role of intraprostatic DHT and type II 5α-reductase

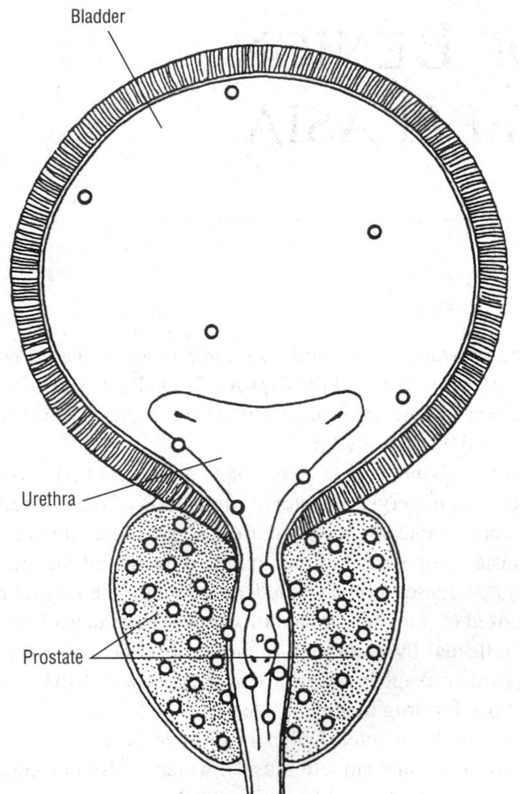

FIGURE 85–1. Representation of the anatomy of and α-adrenergic receptor distribution in the prostate, urethra, and bladder. *(Reproduced with permission from the Western Medical Journal 1994;161:501.)*

in the development of BPH is evidenced by several observations:

- BPH does not develop in men who were castrated before puberty.
- Castration causes an enlarged prostate to shrink.
- Patients with type II 5α-reductase enzyme deficiency do not develop BPH.
- Administration of testosterone to orchiectomized dogs of advanced age produces BPH.

The pathogenesis of BPH is often described as resulting from both static and dynamic factors. Static factors relate to anatomic enlargement of the prostate gland, which produces a block at the bladder neck and thereby obstructs urinary outflow. Enlargement of the gland depends on androgen stimulation of epithelial tissue and estrogen stimulation of stromal tissue in the prostate. Dynamic factors relate to excessive α-adrenergic tone of the stromal component of the prostate gland, which results in contraction of the prostate gland around the urethra, narrowing the urethral lumen.

Symptoms of BPH disease may result from static and/or dynamic factors, and this reality must be recognized when drug therapy is considered. For instance, patients may present with obstructive voiding symptoms but have prostates of normal size. In these patients, dynamic factors are likely responsible for the symptoms. But in patients with enlarged prostate glands, static and dynamic factors are likely working in concert to produce the observed symptoms.

Static factors may be accentuated by environmental factors. Patients who are stressed or in pain may experience an exacerbation of voiding difficulty. In these situations, excessive α-adrenergic tone may precipitate excessive contraction of prostatic stromal tissue. When the stressful event resolves, voiding symptoms often disappear.[5]

MEDICATION-RELATED SYMPTOMS

Medications in several pharmacologic categories should be avoided in patients with BPH as they may exacerbate symptoms. Testosterone replacement regimens, used to treat primary or secondary hypogonadism, deliver additional substrate that can be metabolized to DHT by the prostate. α-Adrenergic agonists, used as oral or intranasal decongestants (e.g., pseudoephedrine, ephedrine, phenylephrine), can stimulate α-adrenergic receptors in the prostate, resulting in muscle contraction. By decreasing the caliber of the urethral lumen, bladder emptying may be compromised.

Also, drugs with significant anticholinergic adverse effects (e.g, antihistamines, phenothiazines, tricyclic antidepressants, or anticholinergic drugs used as antispasmodics or to treat Parkinson's disease) may decrease urinary bladder detrusor muscle contractility. For patients with BPH, who have a narrowed urethral lumen, the loss of effective detrusor contraction could result in acute urinary retention. Diuretics, particularly large doses, can produce polyuria, which may present as urinary frequency similar to that experienced in patients with BPH.

CLINICAL PRESENTATION

Patients with BPH can present with a variety of symptoms and signs of disease. All symptoms of BPH can be divided into two categories: obstructive and irritative.

TABLE 85–1. Characteristics of 5α-Reductase Isoenzymes in Various Target Tissues

Characteristics	Type I	Type II
Localized sites	Scalp, skin (all over the body), and liver	Prostate, scalp, liver, genital skin
Clinical manifestations of the presence of the hormone	Acne; increased body and facial hair	Male pattern baldness; BPH; virilization of the fetus
Clinical manifestations of the absence of the hormone	Unknown at this time	Involution of the prostate, ambiguous genitalia in newborns even though the patient is genetically a male (also referred to as pseudohermaphroditism)
Inhibited by finasteride	+	+++

Obstructive symptoms, also known as prostatism or bladder outlet obstruction, result when dynamic and/or static factors reduce bladder emptying. The force of the urinary stream becomes diminished, urinary flow rate decreases, and bladder emptying is incomplete or takes a longer time. Patients report urinary hesitancy and straining and a weak urine stream. Urine dribbles out of their penis, and their bladder always feels full even after they have voided. Some patients state that they need to press on their bladder to force urine out. In severe cases, patients may go into urinary retention when bladder emptying is not possible. In these cases, suprapubic pain can result from bladder overdistension.

About 50% to 80% of patients have irritative voiding symptoms, which typically occur late in the disease course. Irritative voiding symptoms result from long-standing obstruction at the bladder neck. To compensate, the bladder muscle undergoes hypertrophy so that it can generate a greater contractile force to force urine past the anatomic obstruction at the bladder neck. Although initially helpful, decompensation eventually occurs, and the hypertrophied bladder muscle is no longer able to generate adequate contractile force, as it becomes hypersensitive and ineffective in storing urine. As a result, small amounts of urine irritate the bladder and initiate a bladder emptying response. Patients complain of urinary frequency and urgency. Bedwetting or clothes wetting occur. Patients report waking up every 1 to 2 hours at night to void, which significantly reduces quality of life.

Symptoms of BPH vary over time. Symptoms may improve, remain stable, or worsen spontaneously. Thus, BPH is not necessarily a progressive disease; in fact, some patients experience symptom regression. Between one-third and two-thirds of men with mild disease stabilize or improve without treatment over 2.5 to 5.0 years.[5,6] However, other patients experience a slow progression of disease.

Another characteristic of BPH is that some men suffer from silent prostatism. While they have obstructive or irritative voiding symptoms, they adapt to them and do not voluntarily complain about them. Such patients do not present for medical treatment until complications of BPH disease arise.

Complications of untreated BPH include:

- Chronic renal failure from long-standing bladder outlet obstruction
- Gross hematuria when tissue growth exceeds the blood supply
- Overflow urinary incontinence or unstable bladder
- Recurrent urinary tract infection that results from urinary stasis
- Bladder diverticula
- Bladder stones

All of these complications can be potentially serious or, in the elderly patient, life-threatening. Approximately 20% of patients with symptomatic BPH require treatment because of disease complications.[4] Symptoms, signs, and complications of BPH (e.g., both obstructive and irritative voiding symptoms, decreasing peak urinary flow rate, and acute urinary retention) generally worsen in severity over time, with symptom severity greatest in older men. Prostate size also increases with age, at a rate approximating 0.6 g/y. Older men with prostates greater than 40 g were three times as likely to have severe symptoms or suffer from acute urinary retention.[7,8]

DIAGNOSTIC EVALUATION

Because the common obstructive and irritative voiding symptoms associated with BPH are not unique to the disease and can be presenting symptoms of other genitourinary tract disorders, including prostate or bladder cancer, neurogenic bladder, prostatic calculi, or urinary tract infection, the patient presenting with signs and symptoms of BPH must be thoroughly evaluated.

A careful medical history should be taken to ensure that a complete listing of symptoms is collected, as well as to identify concomitant disorders that may be contributing to voiding symptoms. This history should be followed by a thorough medication history, including all prescription and nonprescription medications as well as dietary supplements the patient is taking. Any drugs that could be causing the patient's symptoms should be identified. If possible, the suspected drugs should be discontinued or the dosing regimen modified to ameliorate the voiding symptoms.

The patient should also undergo a physical examination, including a digital rectal examination, although the size of the prostate gland does not always correspond to symptoms. BPH usually presents as an enlarged, soft, smooth, symmetric gland, greater than 20 g in size. Some patients have only a slightly enlarged gland and yet have bothersome or even serious voiding difficulties, usually the result of dynamic factors. Other patients have an intravesical enlargement of the prostate gland (i.e., the gland grows into the urinary bladder and produces a ball-valve blockage of the bladder neck). This type of prostate enlargement is not palpable on manual examination.

The patient's perception of the severity of BPH symptoms guides development of a therapeutic plan. To evaluate perceptions objectively, validated instruments, such as the American Urological Association (AUA) Symptom Index, are commonly used. Using the AUA index, the patient rates the "bothersomeness" of seven obstructive and irritative voiding symptoms.[2,7,9]

Objective measures of bladder emptying include peak and average urinary flow rate (normal is at least 10–15 mL/sec). This is determined using a uroflowmeter, which literally checks the rate of urine flow out of the bladder. This is a quick noninvasive outpatient procedure in which the patient's urinary flow is clocked during voiding. A low urinary flow rate implies failure of bladder emptying, but the degree of bladder outlet obstruction correlates poorly with peak urinary flow rate.

Another objective measure is postvoid residual urine volume (normal is 0 mL). This is a simple outpatient procedure and is determined after the patient has attempted to empty his bladder. A straight catheter is inserted to drain any urine remaining in the bladder. A high postvoid residual (PVR) urine volume (more than 25–30 mL) also implies failure of bladder emptying and a predisposition for urinary tract infections. Because there is a weak correlation among voiding symptoms, prostate size, and urinary flow rate, most physicians use a combination of measures—including the patient's assessment of symptoms along with objective evaluation of urinary outflow and presence of complications of BPH—to determine the need for treatment.

Clinical laboratory tests can also be helpful in evaluating the patient with possible BPH. Elevated serum blood urea nitrogen (BUN) and creatinine values can indicate development of renal insufficiency caused by long-standing bladder outlet obstruction. Abnormal urinalysis results may be caused by hematuria or urinary tract infection, which can cause voiding symptoms. Prostate-specific antigen (PSA) is used in combination with digital rectal examination of the prostate to screen for prostate cancer, which can also cause voiding difficulty.

Many other tests can be performed if additional information is needed to assess the severity of BPH disease or assist in the preoperative assessment of the patient, including a voiding cystometrogram, transrectal ultrasound of the prostate, intravenous pyelogram, renal ultrasound, and prostate biopsy.[3]

▶ TREATMENT: Benign Prostatic Hyperplasia

As a disease of symptoms, BPH is treated by relieving manifestations that are bothering the patient.[9] Patients are usually stratified into three severity groups for assessing the need for treatment (Table 85–2). However, recent literature about the natural history of BPH and the significant risk of disease complications suggests that physicians should also consider prevention of serious complications of BPH as a goal of treatment in selected patients. This is a controversial topic, which is complicated by many issues, including the variable costs of treatment options, the inability to clearly identify patients who experience spontaneous regression or disease stabilization from those in whom symptoms progress, and the potential benefit that may occur in a comparatively small number of treated patients.

Management options include watchful waiting, drug treatment, or surgical intervention. The most definitive recommendation for BPH treatment is the Clinical Practice Guideline on BPH: Diagnosis and Treatment published by the Agency for Healthcare Research and Quality (AHRQ; formerly the Agency for Health Care Policy and Research), a unit within the US Department of Health and Human Services (Fig. 85–2).[9]

NONPHARMACOLOGIC THERAPY

Patients with mild disease are asymptomatic or have mildly bothersome symptoms and have no complications of BPH disease. In these patients, no specific treatment is indicated. These patients can be managed with "watchful waiting," which entails having the patient return for reassessment at regular 3- to 6-month intervals.

At each return visit, the patient should complete a standardized, validated survey tool to assess severity of symptoms. A digital rectal examination, urinary flow rate, postvoid residual urine volume, and routine laboratory tests (BUN and serum creatinine) should be obtained. Watchful waiting also includes thorough patient education about the disease and behavior modification to avoid practices that exacerbate voiding symptoms. Behavior modification includes fluid restriction close to bedtime and frequent emptying of the bladder (to avoid overflow incontinence and urgency).

TABLE 85–2. Categories of BPH Disease Severity Based on Symptoms and Signs

Disease Severity	AUA Symptom Score	Typical Symptoms and Signs
Mild	≤ 7	Asymptomatic Peak urinary flow rate < 10 mL/sec Postvoid residual urine volume > 25–50 mL Increased BUN and serum creatinine
Moderate	8–19	All of the above signs plus obstructive voiding symptoms and irritative voiding symptoms (signs of detrusor instability)
Severe	≥ 20	All of the above plus one or more complications of BPH

If symptoms progress to moderate severity, the patient should be offered specific treatment. In these patients, watchful waiting delays—but does not decrease—the need for prostatectomy. In symptomatic patients, watchful waiting can lead to intractable urinary retention, increased postvoid residual urine volumes, and significant voiding symptoms. Therefore, watchful waiting is not recommended for symptomatic patients.[10] For patients with BPH of moderate severity, treatment options include drug therapy and surgery.

Patients with severe symptoms or serious complications of BPH should be offered surgical correction (i.e., prostatectomy). Drug therapy is considered an interim measure in such patients, as it likely only delays worsening of complications and the need for surgical intervention.[3,10]

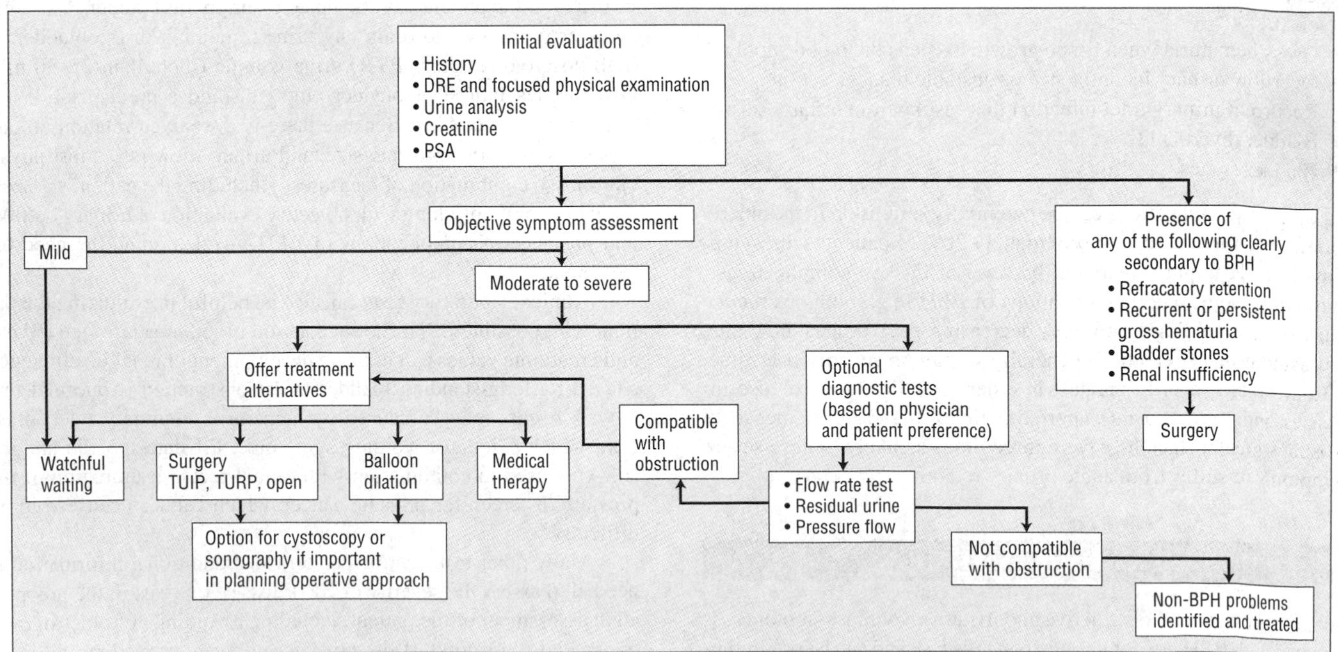

FIGURE 85–2. Management algorithm for benign prostatic hyperplasia. Reprinted from the AHRQ guidelines.[9]

TABLE 85–3. Summary of Medical Treatment Options for BPH

Category	Mechanism	Drug (Brand name)	Daily dose
Reduces static factor	Blocks 5α-reductase enzyme	Finasteride (Proscar)	5 mg by mouth daily
	Blocks dihydrotestosterone at its intracellular receptor	Bicalutamide (Casodex)	50 mg by mouth daily
		Flutamide (Eulexin)	100–250 mg by mouth three times daily
	Blocks pituitary release of luteinizing hormone	Leuprolide (Lupron)	7.5 mg intramuscularly monthly or 22.5 mg intramuscularly every 3 months
		Nafarelin	400 μg subcutaneously daily
	Blocks pituitary release of luteinizing hormone and blocks androgen receptor	Megestrol acetate	40–250 mg by mouth three times daily
Reduces dynamic factor	Blocks α_1-adrenergic receptors in prostatic stromal tissue	Prazosin (Minipress)	2 mg by mouth two to three times daily
		Terazosin (Hytrin)	1–10 mg by mouth daily
		Doxazosin (Cardura)	1–12 mg by mouth daily
	Blocks α_{1A} receptors in the prostate	Tamsulosin (Flomax)	0.4–0.8 mg by mouth daily

PHARMACOLOGIC THERAPY

Drug therapy for BPH can be categorized into two groups: agents that interfere with testosterone's stimulatory effect on prostate gland enlargement (reducing the static factor), and agents that relax prostatic smooth muscle (reducing the dynamic factor; Table 85–3). Of the agents that interfere with testosterone's stimulatory effect on prostate gland size, the only agent approved by the US Food and Drug Administration (FDA) is finasteride. Other agents that interfere with androgen stimulation of the prostate have not been popular in the United States because of the many adverse effects associated with their use. Leuprolide and goserelin produce decreased libido, erectile dysfunction, gynecomastia, and hot flashes. Bicalutamide and flutamide produce nausea, diarrhea, and hepatotoxicity.

Of the agents that relax prostatic smooth muscle, second- and third-generation α_1-adrenergic antagonists have been most widely used. These agents relax the intrinsic sphincter and prostatic smooth muscle, thereby enhancing urinary outflow from the bladder. α_1-Adrenergic antagonists do not reduce prostate size.

Selection of a particular agent for a patient should be determined on a case-by-case basis after a patient-provider discussion of risks and benefits of various treatments. The AHRQ guidelines include a summary balance sheet that is a useful tool for primary care providers to use in explaining to patients risks and benefits of various treatment options.[3,6,9] With drug therapy for BPH, patients must understand that the benefits continue only as long as the medication is taken.

Drug therapy should be initiated with a single agent, usually with an α_1-adrenergic antagonist.[11] Adding finasteride to a failing α_1-adrenergic antagonist regimen offers no benefit, except possibly in patients with prostate glands whose size exceeds 40–50 g.[12] If a therapeutic dose regimen of an α_1-adrenergic antagonist fails, surgery is recommended.

In patients unable to tolerate the adverse effects of full doses of α_1-adrenergic antagonists, finasteride should be initiated. Patients who fail to respond to finasteride have two options: combination treatment with an α_1-adrenergic antagonist plus finasteride or surgery. Recent literature suggests that combination treatment with terazosin and finasteride is more effective than finasteride alone—but only as effective as terazosin alone. If a patient fails the combination of terazosin and finasteride, the patient should undergo surgical correction.[12]

Finally, health care providers must remember that, for BPH, treatment is dictated by quality of life concerns, not medical factors. The AHRQ guideline is clear: "In choosing treatment for a disease such as BPH, which principally affects the quality rather than the quantity of life, and where the optimal decision may be dictated by personal values rather than scientific evidence, different patients may have different opinions concerning the benefits and harms of direct outcomes."[9]

FINASTERIDE

Finasteride competitively inhibits type II 5α-reductase in the prostate cell, scalp, and genital skin. The agent decreases serum DHT levels by 70%. Finasteride is indicated for management of moderate to severe BPH disease. In patients with severe disease, this agent generally must be used with urethral catheterization because of its slow onset.

Ideal patients for finasteride therapy are those with enlarged prostate glands of at least 50–60 g in size.[11] Finasteride may also be preferred in patients with BPH and certain cardiac disorders. Those with conditions such as uncontrolled arrhythmias or poorly controlled angina and patients taking multiple antihypertensive agents cannot take second-generation α_1-adrenergic antagonists (e.g., prazosin, terazosin, doxazosin) because of the risk of hypotensive adverse effects or complications from hypotensive adverse effects.

Finasteride reduces prostate size by 25%, increases peak urinary flow rate by 1.6–2.0 mL/sec, improves voiding symptoms in approximately 30% of treated patients, and produces very few serious adverse effects. It appears to be most effective in patients with significantly enlarged prostates of 40–50 g or more. Compared to α_1-adrenergic antagonists, finasteride has several disadvantages. Finasteride has a delayed onset of action; an adequate clinical trial is 6 to 12 months. In addition, the percentage of patients who experience objective improvement is less with finasteride than with α-adrenergic antagonists. Finally, finasteride is more expensive than α_1-adrenergic antagonists. Therefore, some physicians consider finasteride to be a second-choice agent for treatment of BPH.[13–28]

Finasteride is well absorbed from the gastrointestinal tract (95%), and its absorption is unaffected by food. Peak serum concentrations are reached 1 to 2 hours after the dose. Finasteride is highly protein bound. The liver extensively metabolizes finasteride to inactive metabolites, which are largely excreted in stool. The plasma half-life is 4.7 to 7.1 hours, but its biologic half-life is probably longer, because decreased serum DHT levels persist for up to 2 weeks after finasteride dosing is stopped.[13,29]

For BPH, finasteride is given in doses of 5 mg by mouth daily for at least 6 to 12 months.[13,30,31] The dose can be taken with meals or on an empty stomach, and no dosage adjustment is needed in patients with renal dysfunction. Although no dosage reduction is recommended in patients with hepatic insufficiency, patients should be monitored carefully. Maximal reductions in prostate volume or symptom improvement may not be evident until 12 months, but noticeable changes from baseline should occur after 6 months of continuous treatment. No clinically relevant drug interactions have been reported with finasteride.

Patients must continue to take finasteride as long as they respond. Upon discontinuation of finasteride, prostate size and voiding symptoms generally return to baseline.

Finasteride has few adverse effects. Ejaculation disorders (dry sex or delayed ejaculation) have been reported in 3% to 15% of treated patients. A possible result of decreased prostatic secretion, and therefore of ejaculate volume, these disorders are reversible with discontinuation of finasteride.

Erectile dysfunction is also reported, and it may be secondary to ejaculation disorders. But because elderly men with BPH commonly develop erectile dysfunction as they age, develop concurrent medical illnesses, and take medications, finasteride therapy may not be the cause of erectile dysfunction.

Other minor adverse effects include nausea, abdominal pain, asthenia, dizziness, flatulence, headache, rash, muscle weakness, and gynecomastia.

Finasteride is in FDA pregnancy category X, which means that it is contraindicated in pregnant females. Exposure of the fetus to finasteride may produce pseudohermaphrodite offspring with ambiguous genitalia, similar to those of patients with a rare genetic deficiency of type II 5α-reductase. Because of this teratogenic effect, women who are pregnant or seeking to become pregnant should not handle finasteride tablets and should not have contact with semen from finasteride-treated men. Women pharmacists of childbearing age should handle this product with rubber gloves if there is any chance that they are pregnant.

Normal doses of finasteride reduce serum PSA levels by 50%. For this reason, PSA levels must be measured before treatment begins, and the patient should have a digital rectal examination. After 6 months of therapy, the patient should have a repeat PSA. If the level does not decline by 50% and the patient has adhered to finasteride therapy, he should be evaluated for prostate cancer. Annually thereafter, the patient should have a PSA assay and digital rectal examination, and patients with any rise in PSA levels should by evaluated for prostate cancer.[16,32]

α-ADRENERGIC ANTAGONISTS

Three generations of α-adrenergic antagonists have been used to treat BPH through their relaxation of smooth muscle in the prostate and bladder neck.[33–45] Because of their dose-limiting adverse effects on the heart (tachycardia and arrhythmias), first-generation agents such as phenoxybenzamine have been replaced by the second-generation postsynaptic α_1-adrenergic antagonists and third-generation uroselective postsynaptic α_{1A}-adrenergic antagonists.[33,34]

The second- and third-generation α-adrenergic antagonists are considered to be equally effective for BPH. These agents generally increase urinary flow rates by 2–3 mL/sec in 60% to 70% of treated patients, and reduce postvoid residual urine volume. They have no effect on decreasing prostate volume. Terazosin and tamsulosin produce durable responses for 3 to 4 years.[43,44] Finally, α-adrenergic antagonists do not reduce PSA levels, preserving the utility of this prostate cancer marker in this high-risk population.[45]

Second-generation agents include prazosin, terazosin, and doxazosin. These differ in terms of duration of action and dosing schedule. Whereas prazosin requires dosing two to three times a day, terazosin and doxazosin offer more convenient once-daily dosing. However, all three agents antagonize peripheral vascular α_1-adrenergic receptors, in addition to those in the prostate. As a result, first-dose syncope, orthostatic hypotension, and dizziness are characteristic adverse effects. Also, additive blood pressure lowering effects commonly occur when these agents are used along with antihypertensive agents, which limits use of these agents in some patients.

Tamsulosin is the only third-generation α_{1A}-adrenergic antagonist available in the US market. It represents an advance over second-generation agents in that it is selective for prostatic α_{1A} receptors, which comprise approximately 70% of the adrenergic receptors in the prostate gland.[35,36] Blockade of these receptors results in smooth muscle relaxation of the prostate and bladder neck without causing peripheral vascular smooth muscle relaxation. Tamsulosin has low affinity for vascular α_{1B} receptors, which explains why hypotension is not a common adverse effect and why the agent has not been studied for as a therapy for hypertension.

Tamsulosin's selectivity for α_{1A} receptors has multiple implications. Dose titration is unnecessary; therefore, patients can begin therapy with the lowest maintenance dose, 0.4 mg orally once a day. Patients can be instructed to take the dose anytime during the day, unlike terazosin[46,47] and doxazosin,[48–51] which should be taken at bedtime. The onset of peak action is quicker, in the range of 2 weeks, because no dosage titration is necessary. No decreases in blood pressure or increases in heart rate have been reported in normotensive patients, subgroups of patients with well-controlled hypertension, or those with uncontrolled hypertension.[37,38] Thus, tamsulosin allows initiation of treatment with a therapeutic dose that is not limited by cardiovascular adverse effects, unlike terazosin and doxazosin.[52–63] Finally, the addition of tamsulosin to selected antihypertensive regimens of patients does not result in potentiation of the hypotensive effect of furosemide, enalapril, nifedipine, and atenolol.[39]

Therefore, tamsulosin represents a good choice particularly when patients cannot tolerate hypotension, or when the titration would be too complicated for the patient or produce an unacceptable delay in onset for a particular patient.

Although not supported by controlled clinical trials, terazosin also may be preferred in patients with both moderate symptoms of BPH and hypercholesterolemia, because it reduces total cholesterol and serum triglycerides.

TABLE 85–4. Dosing Schedule of α-Adrenergic Antagonists in Patients with BPH

Drug	Half-life (h)	Usual Daily Dosage	Time to Peak Effect on BPH Symptoms*
Prazosin (Minipress)	2–3	2–10 mg in two to three divided doses	2–4 weeks
Terazosin (Hytrin)	12	1–10 mg as a single dose; max 20 mg	2–4 weeks
Doxazosin (Cardura)	19–22	1–4 mg as a single dose; max 12 mg	2–4 weeks
Tamsulosin (Flomax)	14–15	0.4–0.8 mg as a single dose	1 day

*Time to peak effect on BPH symptoms is dependent on the titration period to full therapeutic doses.

This table is adapted with permission from Lee M, Sharifi R. Benign prostatic hyperplasia: Diagnosis and treatment guideline. Ann Pharmacother *1997;31: 481–486.*

A summary of the usual and starting doses of α-adrenergic antagonists is included in Table 85–4. Tamsulosin is commercially available as a controlled-release oral tablet.

When using second-generation α-adrenergic antagonists, slow titration up to a therapeutic maintenance dose is necessary to minimize orthostatic hypotension and first-dose syncope. Conservatively, dosage increases should be done in an orderly stepwise process, with dosage increases occurring at 2- to 7-day intervals, depending on the patient's response to the medication. A faster titration schedule can be used as long as the patient does not develop orthostatic hypotension or dizziness. Two sample titration schedules for terazosin are described here:

- Schedule 1: Slow titration

  Days 1–3: 1 mg at bedtime
  Days 4–14: 2 mg at bedtime
  Weeks 2–6: 5 mg at bedtime
  Weeks 7 and on: 10 mg at bedtime

- Schedule 2: Quicker titration

  Days 1–3: 1 mg at bedtime
  Days 4–14: 2 mg at bedtime
  Weeks 2–3: 5 mg at bedtime
  Weeks 4 and on: 10 mg at bedtime

Patients should continue taking the drug as long as they continue to respond to it. If BPH symptoms worsen, the patients should see his physician for a dosage increase or discuss an alternative form of treatment.

No dosage adjustments are recommended for α-adrenergic antagonists in patients with renal failure. Because these drugs are hepatically catabolized, the lowest effective dose should be used in patients with hepatic dysfunction, and patients should be monitored carefully for adverse effects. No specific dosing guidelines are yet available in this patient population.[60]

Approximately 10% to 12% of patients discontinue second-generation α_1-adrenergic antagonists because of adverse effects, especially those affecting the cardiovascular system (e.g., syncope, dizziness, and hypotension).[42,61]

Patients who tolerate hypotension poorly should avoid second-generation α_1-adrenergic antagonists. This includes patients with poorly controlled angina, serious cardiac arrhythmias, patients with reduced circulating volume, and patients on multiple antihypertensives.[62] These patients are candidates for tamsulosin[56,62] or finasteride, if drug therapy is deemed necessary.

Tiredness and asthenia, retrograde ejaculation, flu-like symptoms, and nasal congestion are the most common adverse effects of tamsulosin. These adverse effects are unavoidable, but by properly educating the patient, they should not lead to discontinuation of treatment.

Caution is needed when cimetidine is used with tamsulosin or other α-adrenergic antagonists, as a drug-drug interaction leads to decreased metabolism of the latter agents.[63]

SURGICAL INTERVENTION

The gold standard for treatment of patients with moderate or severe symptoms of BPH and all patients with complications of BPH is prostatectomy performed either transurethrally or suprapubically.[10,64,65] Surgical removal of the prostate offers the highest rate of symptom improvement, but it also has the highest complication rate.

With transurethral prostatectomy (TURP), an endoscopic resectoscope inserted through the urethra is used to remove the inside core of the prostate. This enlarges the urethral opening at the bladder neck. TURP is performed only in men with smaller prostates (<50 g), so that the resection can be completed in less than 1 hour. Often performed as outpatient surgery, this procedure produces on average a peak urinary flow increase of 125% and improvement of voiding symptoms by almost 90% in approximately 90% of patients.[5] A very common complication of TURP is retrograde ejaculation, occurring in up to 75% of patients. Significant bleeding, urinary incontinence, and erectile dysfunction occur in smaller but important numbers of patients (2% to 15%). Approximately 12% to 15% of patients require second surgeries within 8 years.[64]

Men with larger prostates require an open surgical procedure or open prostatectomy. This necessitates hospitalization for at least a few days, anesthesia, and a longer recuperation time. Adverse effects of open prostatectomy include bleeding, urinary and soft tissue infection, retrograde ejaculation in 77% of patients, erectile dysfunction in 16% to 33% of patients, and urinary incontinence in 2% of patients. The reoperation rate is 3% to 5% at 10 years.[64]

Prostatectomy is ineffective for relieving irritative voiding symptoms of BPH because prostatectomy does not affect the detrusor muscle of the bladder.[65] These patients may respond to oral anticholinergic agents (e.g., oxybutynin, L-hyoscyamine), which improve bladder compliance and decrease detrusor muscle irritability, as discussed in Chap. 86.

A new trend in surgical treatment is use of less invasive or minimally invasive outpatient surgical procedures to remove excessive prostate tissue.[5] These procedures characteristically are short (lasting minutes), have a lower potential to produce adverse effects, are less expensive than continuous drug therapy lasting years, and may be particularly useful in debilitated patients.

Of the procedures available, only transurethral incision of the prostate (TUIP) has been thoroughly evaluated. This procedure is ideal for patients with moderate or severe BPH symptoms who have an enlarged prostate gland less than 30 g in size. TUIP is as effective as TURP, but requires less operation time, causes less blood loss, and produces fewer adverse effects.[66,67] TUIP involves making two to three incisions at the bladder neck to widen the opening. These incisions are made using an endoscopic resectoscope.

PHYTOTHERAPY

Although phytotherapy is widely used in Europe for the management of BPH,[68] the published data on herbal agents are largely inconclusive and conflicting. Studies often lack placebo controls, which is essential in assessing treatments for BPH because spontaneous regression of symptoms can occur. Furthermore, as these agents are marketed under the Dietary Supplements Health and Education Act, their efficacy, safety, and quality are not regulated by the FDA.

For these reasons, herbal products—including saw palmetto berry (*Serenoa repens*),[69–72] stinging nettle (*Urtica dioica*),[73] and African plum (*Pygeum africanum*)[74]—are not recommended for BPH. An excellent review on phytotherapy for BPH has been published.[68]

EVALUATION OF THERAPEUTIC OUTCOMES

The primary therapeutic outcome of BPH therapy is restoration of adequate urinary flow without adverse effects. As a disease in which therapy is directed at those symptoms the patient finds most bothersome, assessment of outcomes likewise depends on how the patient perceives the effectiveness and acceptability of therapy. Use of a validated, standardized instrument—such as the AUA Symptom Index or International Prostate Symptom Score—for assessing patient quality of life is critically important in this process.[2,7,9]

In patients being treated with pharmacotherapy, objective measures of bladder emptying are also useful at an appropriate time after drug therapy begins (6 to 12 months for finasteride, earlier with α-adrenergic antagonists). These include the uroflowmeter and postvoid residual urine volume, as described in the Diagnostic Evaluation section of this chapter.

Key laboratory tests to monitor on an ongoing basis are serum BUN and creatinine and the urinalysis. Because this patient population is at high risk for prostate cancer, annually PSA should be measured and a digital rectal examination performed. For patients taking finasteride, PSA must be compared with baseline and 6-month responses, as described in the Finasteride section above.

SUMMARY

A nearly ubiquitous disease of aging men, symptomatic BPH requires medical attention to preserve patient quality of life and avoid complications, many of which can be life-threatening in this patient population. In men who have no or minor symptoms, "watchful waiting" is the therapeutic option of choice, as BPH remains stable or even regresses in about one-half of these men.

For those with moderate to severe symptoms but no complications, pharmacotherapy is indicated. An α_1-adrenergic antagonist is the agent of first choice. Second-generation adrenergic blockers—including prazosin, terazosin, or doxazosin—are useful, but they cause more cardiovascular adverse effects than does tamsulosin. If patients fail adrenergic-blockade therapy, surgery is indicated.

In patients who have complications of BPH (chronic renal failure, gross hematuria, overflow urinary incontinence, recurrent urinary tract infections, bladder diverticula, or bladder stones), surgery is required. Although it has more adverse complications than does pharmacotherapy or watchful waiting, surgery is considered the gold standard in treating BPH.

▶ PRINCIPLES OF PHARMACOTHERAPY

- Although BPH is rare in men younger than 50 years of age, it is very common in men 60 years of age and older as a result of hormone-driven growth in size of the prostate. It commonly results from both static factors (gradual enlargement of the prostate) and dynamic factors (exposure to agents or situations that constrict the gland's smooth muscle).
- While most men have hyperplasia of the prostate, only about 50% of men have symptoms. Thus, when symptoms occur, other causes—including medications such as antihistamines, phenothiazines, tricyclic antidepressants, or anticholinergic agents—should be ruled out during the BPH diagnostic workup.
- Specific treatments for BPH include watchful waiting, drug therapy, and surgery.
- No therapy is needed for men with no or few symptoms. They should be managed with watchful waiting, which includes return visits at 3- to 6-month intervals for reassessment.
- If symptoms progress to moderate severity, drug therapy or surgery is indicated, as waiting longer will not avoid the need for prostatectomy. Drug therapy is an interim measure, as worsening of patient symptoms is likely, eventually leading to intractable urinary retention, increased postvoid residual urine volumes, and significant voiding problems in some patients.
- Drug therapy can be directed at static or dynamic factors. Finasteride, by interfering with testosterone's stimulatory effect on prostate gland enlargement, affects static factors. The α_1-adrenergic antagonists, by relaxing prostatic smooth muscle, address dynamic factors.
- The drugs of choice are the α_1-adrenergic antagonists. Older second-generation α-adrenergic antagonists (prazosin, terazosin, or doxazosin) are equally effective but can cause problematic adverse cardiovascular effects (hypotension, dizziness). In patients who cannot tolerate hypotensive effects of α_1-adrenergic agents, the third-generation agent tamsulosin is a good alternative.
- Finasteride is useful primarily in patients with large prostates who wish to avoid surgery or cannot tolerate the side effects of α_1-adrenergic antagonists.
- Surgery is the gold standard of treatment, as it is the only intervention that relieves symptoms in the greatest number of men with BPH. However, the two most widely used techniques are

associated with the highest rates of complications, including problems such as retrograde ejaculation and erectile dysfunction.

- Although widely used in Europe for BPH, phytotherapy should be avoided. Studies of these herbal medicines are inconclusive, and the purity of available products is questionable.

ACKNOWLEDGMENT

Some portions of this chapter were adapted with permission from Lee M. Health issues in the elderly male. In: Pharmacotherapy Self-Assessment Program Module 6 Respiratory and Endocrinology, 3rd ed. Kansas City, MO, American College of Clinical Pharmacy, 1999:181–207.

REFERENCES

1. Glynn RJ, Campion EW, Bouchard GR, Silbert JE. The development of benign prostatic hyperplasia among volunteers in the normative aging study. Am J Epidemiol 1985;131:79–90.
2. Roehrborn CG. The Agency for Health Care Policy and Research Clinical guidelines for the diagnosis and treatment of BPH. Urol Clin North Am 1995;22:445–453.
3. McConnell JD. Benign prostatic hyperplasia: Treatment guidelines and patient classification. Br J Urol 1995;76(5):29–46.
4. Walsh PC. The role of estrogen/androgen synergism in the pathogenesis of benign prostatic hyperplasia. J Urol 1988:139:826.
5. Tammela T. Benign prostatic hyperplasia: Practical treatment guidelines. Drugs Aging 1997;10:349–366.
6. Barry MJ. Epidemiology and natural history of benign prostatic hyperplasia. Urol Clin North Am 1990;17:495–507.
7. Girman C, Panser L, Chute C, et al. Natural history of prostatism: Urinary flow rates in a community-based study. J Urol 1993;150:887–892.
8. Chute CG, Panser LA, Girman CJ, et al. The prevalence of prostatism: A population-based survey of urinary symptoms. J Urol 1993;150:85–89.
9. S Department of Health and Human Services Public Health Service Agency for Health Care Policy and Research. Clinical practice guideline number 8. Benign prostatic hyperplasia: Diagnosis and treatment. Rockville, MD, US Department of Health and Human Service, 1994: 1–215.
10. Wasson JH, Reda DJ, Bruskewitz RC, Elinson J, Keller AM, Henderson WG for the Veterans Affairs Cooperative Study Group on Transurethral Resection of the Prostate. A comparison of transurethral surgery with watchful waiting for moderate symptoms of benign prostatic hyperplasia. N Engl J Med 1995;332:75–79.
11. Roehrborn CG. Meta-analysis of randomized clinical trials of finasteride. Urology 1998;51(suppl 4a):46–49.
12. Lepor H, Williford WO, Barry MJ, et al. for the Veterans Affairs Cooperative Studies Benign Prostatic Hyperplasia Study Group. The efficacy of terazosin, finasteride, or both in benign prostatic hyperplasia. N Engl J Med 1996;335:533–539.
13. Gormley GJ, Stoner E, Bruskewitz RC, Imperato-McGinley J, Walsh P, McConnell JD. The effect of finasteride in men with benign prostatic hyperplasia. N Engl J Med 1992;327:1185–1192.
14. Moore E, Bracken B, Bremner W, et al. Proscar: Five-year experience. Eur Urol 1995;28:305–309.
15. Hudson PB, Boake R, Trachtenberg J, et al. and the North American Finasteride Study Group. Efficacy of finasteride is maintained in patients with benign prostatic hyperplasia treated for five years. Urology 1999;53: 690–695.
16. Ekman P for the Scandinavian Finasteride Study Group. Maximum efficacy of finasteride is obtained within 6 months and maintained over six years. Eur Urol 1998;33:312–317.
17. Boyle P, Gould AL, Roehrborn CG. Prostate volume predicts outcome of treatment of benign prostatic hyperplasia with finasteride: Meta-analysis of randomized clinical trials. Urology 1996;48:398–405.
18. McConnell JD, Bruskewitz R, Walsh P, et al. for the Finasteride Long-Term Efficacy and Safety Study Group. The effect of finasteride on the risk of acute urinary retention and the need for surgical treatment among men with benign prostatic hyperplasia. N Engl J Med 1998;338: 557–563.
19. Drach GW, Layton TN, Binard WJ. Male peak urinary flow rate: Relationship to volume voided and age. J Urol 1979;122:210–214.
20. Wasson JH. Finasteride to prevent morbidity from benign prostatic hyperplasia. N Engl J Med 1998;338:612–613.
21. Lepor H for the Tamsulosin Research Group. Long-term efficacy and safety of terazosin in patients with benign prostatic hyperplasia. Urology 1995;45:406–413.
22. Lieber MM. Pharmacologic therapy of prostatism. Mayo Clin Proc 1998;73:590–596.
23. Nickel JC. Long-term implications of medical therapy on benign prostatic hyperplasia end points. Urology 1998;51(suppl 4a):50–57.
24. Andersen JT, Ekman P, Wolf H, et al. Can finasteride reverse the progress of benign prostatic hyperplasia and risk of prostatectomy? Urology 1991;38(S):4–8.
25. Andersen JT, Nickel JC, Marshall VR, Schulman CC, Boyle P. Finasteride significantly reduces acute urinary retention and need for surgery in patients with symptomatic benign prostatic hyperplasia. Urology 1997;49:839–845.
26. Andersen JT, Ekman P, Wolf H and the Scandinavian Benign Prostatic Hyperplasia Study Group. Can finasteride reverse the progress of benign prostatic hyperplasia? A two-year placebo-controlled study. Urology 1995;46:631–637.
27. Nickel JC, Fradet Y, Boake RC and the Prospect Study Group. Efficacy and safety of finasteride therapy for benign prostatic hyperplasia, results of a 2-year randomized controlled trial (the Prospect Study). CMAJ 1996;155:1251–1259.
28. Marberger MJ on behalf of the Prowess Study Group. Long-term effects of finasteride in patients with benign prostatic hyperplasia: A double-blind, placebo-controlled, multicenter study. Urology 1998;51:677–686.
29. Rittmaster RS. Finasteride. N Engl J Med 1994;330:120–125.
30. Stoner E and members of the Finasteride Study Group. Three-year safety and efficacy data on the use of finasteride in treatment of benign prostatic hyperplasia. Urology 1994;43:284–294.
31. Kaufman KD, Gormley GI, Binkowitz B, Jacobsen CA, Bruno K. Finasteride Male Pattern Baldness Study Group. The effects of oral finasteride on scalp hair growth in men with male pattern baldness. Endocr Soc Ann Meet Prog Abstr 1995;77:325. Abstract.
32. Pannek J, Marks LS, Pearson JD, et al. Influence of finasteride on free and total serum prostate specific antigen levels in men with benign prostatic hyperplasia. J Urol 1998;159:449–453.
33. Caine P, Perlberg S, Shapiro A. Phenoxybenzamine for benign prostatic obstruction. Urology 1981;17:542–546.
34. Abrams P, Shah PJR, Stone R, Choa RG. Bladder outlet obstruction treated with phenoxybenzamine. Br J Urol 1982;54:527–530.
35. Chapple CR, Burt RP, Andersson PO, Greengrass P, Wyllie M, Marshall I. α-1-Adrenoceptor subtypes in the human prostate. Br J Urol 1994;74:585–589.
36. Chapple CR. Pharmacotherapy for benign prostatic hyperplasia—The potential for α1-adrenoceptor subtype-specific blockade. Br J Urol 1998; 81(suppl):34–47.
37. Chapple CR, Wyndaele JJ, Nordling J, Boeminghaus F, Ypma AFGVM, Abrams P on behalf of the European Tamsulosin Study Group. Tamsulosin, the first prostate selective alpha-1A-adrenoreceptor antagonist. Eur Urol 1996;29:155–167.

38. Lowe FC. Coadministration of tamsulosin and three antihypertensive agents in patients with benign prostatic hyperplasia: Pharmacodynamic effect. Clin Ther 1997;19:730–742.
39. DeMey C. Cardiovascular effects of alpha-blockers used for the treatment of symptomatic BPH: Impact on safety and well being. Eur Urol 1998;34(suppl 2):18–28.
40. Siegal D, Lopez J. Trends in antihypertensive drug use in the US. Do the JNC-V recommendations affect prescribing? JAMA 1997;278:1745–1748.
41. Suzuki H. Treatment of benign prostatic hyperplasia and hypertension in elderly hypertensive patients. Br J Urol 1998;81(suppl 1):51–55.
42. Tewari A, Narayan P. Alpha-adrenergic blocking drugs in the management of benign prostatic hyperplasia: Interactions with antihypertensive therapy. Urology 1999;53(suppl 3A):14–20.
43. Lepor H for the Terazosin Research Group. Long-term efficacy and safety of terazosin in patients with benign prostatic hyperplasia. Urology 1995;45:406–413.
44. Schulman CC, Lock TMTW, Buzelin JM and the European Tamsulosin Study Group. Tamsulosin: 3-Year followup of efficacy and safety in 516 patients with LUTS suggestive of BPO. J Urology 1998;159:256. Abstract #983.
45. Roehrborn CG, Oesterling JE, Olson PJ, Padley RJ for the HYCAT Investigator Group. Serial prostate-specific antigen measurements in men with clinically benign prostatic hyperplasia during a 12-month placebo-controlled study with terazosin. Urology 1997;50:556–561.
46. Lepor H, Auerbach S, Puras-Baez A, et al. A randomized placebo-controlled multicenter study of the efficacy and safety of terazosin in the treatment of benign prostatic hyperplasia. J Urol 1992;148:1467–1474.
47. Lloyd SN, Buckley JF, Chilton CP. Terazosin in the treatment of benign prostatic hyperplasia: A multicenter, placebo-controlled trial. Br J Urol 1992;70:17–21.
48. MacDiarmid SA, Emery RT, Ferguson SF, McGuirt-Franklin R, McIntyre WJ, Johnson DE. A randomized double-blind study assessing 4 versus 8 mg doxazosin for benign prostatic hyperplasia. J Urol 1999;162:1629–1632.
49. Chapple CR. Selective α1-adrenoceptor antagonists in benign prostatic hyperplasia: Rationale and clinical experience. Eur Urol 1996;29:129–144.
50. Janknegt RA, Chapple CR. Efficacy and safety of the alpha-1-blocker doxazosin in the treatment of benign prostatic hyperplasia. Eur Urol 1993;24:319–326.
51. Lepor H. Alpha blockade for the treatment of benign prostatic hyperplasia. Urol Clin North Am 1995;22:375–386.
52. Michel MC, Bressel HU, Mehlburger L, Goepel M. Tamsulosin: Real life clinical experience in 19,365 patients. Eur Urol 1998;34(suppl 2):37–45.
53. Narayan P, Tewari A and members of the United States 93–01 Study Group. A second phase III multicenter placebo controlled study of 2 dosages of modified release tamsulosin in patients with symptoms of benign prostatic hyperplasia. J Urol 1998;160:1701–1706.
54. Schulman CC, Cortvriend J, Jonas U, Lock TMTW, Vaage S, Speakman MJ on behalf of the European Tamsulosin Study Group. Tamsulosin, the first prostate-selective alpha 1A-adrenoreceptor antagonist. Analysis of a multinational, multicentre, open-label study assessing the long-term efficacy and safety in patients with benign prostatic obstruction (symptomatic BPH). Eur Urol 1996;29:145–154.
55. Lepor H for the Tamsulosin Investigator Group. Long-term evaluation of tamsulosin in benign prostatic hyperplasia: Placebo-controlled double-blind extension of phase III trial. Urology 1998;51:901–906.
56. Lee E, Lee C. Clinical comparison of selective and non-selective α1-adrenoreceptor antagonists in benign prostatic hyperplasia: Studies on tamsulosin in a fixed dose and terazosin in increasing doses. Br J Urol 1997;80:606–611.
57. Lepor H for the Tamsulosin Investigator Group. Phase III multicenter placebo-controlled study of tamsulosin in benign prostatic hyperplasia. Urology 1998;51:892–900.
58. Chapple CR, Wyndaele JJ, Nordling J, Boeminghaus F, Ypma AFGVM, Abrams P on behalf of the European Tamsulosin Study Group. Tamsulosin, the first prostate selective α_{1A}-adrenoceptor antagonist. Eur Urol 1996;20:155–167.
59. Fulton B, Wagstaff AJ, Sorkin EM. Doxazosin. Drugs 1995;49:295–320.
60. Wilde MI, McTavish D. Tamsulosin. Drugs 1996;52:883–898.
61. Kaplan SA, D'Alisera PM. Tolerability of α-blockade with doxazosin as a therapeutic option for symptomatic benign prostatic hyperplasia in the elderly patient: A pooled analysis of seven double-blind, placebo-controlled studies. J Gerontol 1998;53A:M201–M206.
62. DeMey C, Michel MC, McEwen J, Moreland T. A double-blind comparison of terazosin and tamsulosin on their differential effects on ambulatory blood pressure and nocturnal orthostatic stress testing. Eur Urol 1998;33:481–488.
63. Anonymous. Tamsulosin for benign prostatic hyperplasia. Med Lett 1997;39:96.
64. Roos NP, Ramsey EW. A population based study of prostatectomy: Outcomes associated with different surgical procedures. J Urol 1987;37:1184–1187.
65. Kuo HC, Chang SC, Hsu T. Predictive factors for successful surgical outcome of benign prostatic hypertrophy. Eur Urol 1993;24:12–16.
66. Hellstrom P, Lukkarinen O, Kontturi M. Bladder neck incision or transurethral electroresection for the treatment of urinary obstruction caused by small prostate? A randomized urodynamic study. Scan J Urol Nephrol 1986;20:187–192.
67. Christensen MM, Aagaard J, Madsen PO. Transurethral resection versus transurethral incision of the prostate: A prospective randomized study. Urol Clin North Am 1990;17:621–630.
68. Lowe FC, Fagelman E. Phytotherapy in the treatment of benign prostatic hyperplasia: An update. Urology 1999;53:671–678.
69. Lowe FC. Saw palmetto berry in the treatment of benign prostatic hyperplasia. Clin Res Reg Affairs 1997;14:53–66.
70. Plosker G, Grogden RM. Serenoa repens (Permixon)—A review of its pharmacology and therapeutic efficacy in benign prostatic hyperplasia. Drug Aging 1996;9:379–395.
71. Marks LS, Tyler VE. Saw palmetto extract: Newest (and oldest) treatment alternative for men with symptomatic benign prostatic hyperplasia. Urology 1999;53:457–461.
72. Wilt TJ, Ishani A, Stark G, MacDonald R, Lau J, Mulrow C. Saw palmetto extracts for treatment of benign prostatic hyperplasia. JAMA 1998;280:1604–1609.
73. Wagner H, Flachsbarth H, Vogel G. A new antiprostatic principal of stinging nettle (*Urtica dioica*) roots. Phytomed 1994;1:213–224.
74. Andro MC, Riffaud JP. *Pygeum africanum* extract for the treatment of patients with benign prostatic hyperplasia: A review of 25 years of published experience. Curr Ther Res 1995;56:796–817.

86

URINARY INCONTINENCE

Eric S. Rovner, Jean Wyman, Thomas Lackner, and David Guay

Urinary incontinence (UI) is defined as a condition wherein the *involuntary* loss of urine causes a social or hygienic problem and is objectively demonstrable. UI is a very common and yet underreported condition. Compared with continent controls, patients with UI have an overall poorer quality of life. Patients with UI may have depression as a result of the perceived lack of self-control, loss of independence, and lack of self-esteem, and they often curtail their activities for fear of an "accident." UI may have serious medical and economic ramifications for untreated or undertreated patients, including skin breakdown, infection, rashes, and worsening of decubitus ulcers.

This chapter highlights the epidemiology, etiology, pathophysiology, and treatment of stress, urge, and overflow UI in men and women.

EPIDEMIOLOGY

Determining the true prevalence of UI is difficult because of problems with definition, reporting bias, and other methodologic issues.[1] Epidemiologic studies have not historically used a standard definition of the condition nor a standard methodology for data recording, with some studies including "postvoid dribbling," while other studies specify "urinary leakage causing a social or hygienic problem." Nevertheless, the number of people suffering with UI is certainly great, and the impact of this condition is substantial, crossing all racial, ethnic, and geographic boundaries.

One of the earliest comprehensive epidemiologic studies on UI was conducted by Diokno and colleagues using a standardized survey questionnaire.[2] The Medical, Epidemiologic, and Social Aspects of Aging (MESA) survey found that the prevalence of UI in noninstitutionalized women 60 years of age and older was approximately 38%. Almost one-third of those surveyed noted urine loss at least once weekly and 16% noted UI daily.

The condition can affect people of all age groups but the peak incidence of UI, at least in women, seems to occur either around the age of menopause or during the elderly years. In the United States, chronic UI is one of the most common reasons cited for institutionalization of the elderly, and the condition is frequently encountered in the nursing home setting.[3]

Some studies report a higher incidence of UI overall in white populations[4,5] as compared to African Americans, but differences in access to health care as well as cultural attitudes and mores may contribute to these differences.

Consistent across all studies in unselected, noninstitutionalized populations, is the fact that UI is at least half as common in men as in women.[6,7] Overall, the prevalence of UI in men has been recently estimated to be about 9%.[8] Unlike in women, UI clearly correlates with men's ages, with the prevalence of UI in men increasing with age across most studies and the highest prevalence recorded in the oldest patient cohorts.[8]

ETIOLOGY AND PATHOPHYSIOLOGY

ANATOMY

The lower urinary tract consists of the bladder, urethra, urinary or urethral sphincter, and the surrounding musculofascial structures including connective tissue, nerves, and blood vessels. The urinary bladder is a hollow organ composed almost entirely of smooth muscle and connective tissue located deep in the bony pelvis in men and women. The urethra is a hollow tube that acts as a conduit for urine flow out of the bladder. The urinary or urethral sphincter is a combination of smooth and striated muscle within and surrounding the most proximal portion of the urethra adjacent to the bladder in both men and women. This is a functional but not anatomic sphincter that includes a portion of the bladder neck or outlet as well as the proximal urethra.

URINARY CONTINENCE

To prevent incontinence during the bladder filling/storage phase of the micturition cycle, the urethra, or, more accurately, the urethral sphincter, must maintain adequate resistance to the flow of urine from the bladder at all times until voluntary voiding is initiated. Urethral resistance or closure is maintained to a large degree by the functional urinary sphincter, a combination of smooth and striated muscles within and external to the urethra. Variable contributions to urethral resistance may also come from the urethral mucosa, submucosal spongy tissue, and the overall length of the urethra. During bladder filling/storage, the bladder accommodates increasing volumes of urine flowing in from the upper urinary tract without a significant increase in bladder (intravesical) pressure. In addition, bladder or detrusor smooth muscle activity is normally suppressed during the filling phase by centrally mediated neural reflexes. Normal bladder emptying occurs with a decrease in urethral resistance concomitant with a volitional bladder contraction. The bladder contraction occurs in a coordinated fashion resulting in a rise in intravesical pressure. The rise in intravesical pressure should be of adequate magnitude and duration to empty the bladder to completion. A decrease in urethral resistance and funneling of the bladder outlet results in opening of the functional urinary sphincter and urine flow into the urethra until the bladder is emptied completely.

The primary motor input to the detrusor muscle of the bladder is along the pelvic nerves emanating from spinal cord segments S2–S4. Parasympathetic impulses travel to the bladder along the efferent fibers of the pelvic nerves. The impulses are passed through ganglia situated in the bladder wall before reaching their target. Acetylcholine appears to be the primary neurotransmitter at the neuromuscular junction in the human lower urinary tract. Both volitional and involuntary contractions of the detrusor muscle are mediated by activation of postsynaptic muscarinic receptors by acetylcholine. Of the five known subtypes of muscarinic receptors, bladder smooth-muscle cholinergic receptors are mainly of the M-2 variety. However, M-3 receptors are responsible for both the emptying contraction of a normal micturition, as well as involuntary bladder contractions, which may result in UI.[9] Thus, most pharmacologic antimuscarinic therapy is primarily anti-M-3 based (see below discussion).

The bladder and urethra normally operate in unison during the bladder-filling-and-storage phase, as well as the bladder-emptying phase of the micturition cycle. The smooth and striated muscles of the bladder and urethra are organized during the micturition cycle by a number of reflexes coordinated at the pontine micturition center in the midbrain. Disturbances in the neural regulation of micturition at any level (brain, spinal cord, or pelvic nerves) often lead to characteristic changes in lower urinary tract function that may result in UI.

MECHANISMS OF URINARY INCONTINENCE

Simply stated, UI may occur only as a result of abnormalities of the urethra (including the bladder outlet and urinary sphincter) or the bladder or from a combination of abnormalities of both structures.[10] Abnormalities may result in either overfunction or underfunction of the bladder and/or urethra with the resulting development of UI. While this simple classification scheme excludes extremely rare causes of UI such as congenital ectopic ureters and urinary fistulas, it is useful in gaining a working understanding of the condition.

URETHRAL UNDERACTIVITY (STRESS URINARY INCONTINENCE)

Some patients characteristically note UI during activities such as exercise, running, lifting, coughing, and sneezing. This implies that the compromised urethral sphincter is no longer able to resist the flow of urine from the bladder during periods of physical activity. In essence, increases in intra-abdominal pressure during physical activity are transmitted to the bladder (an intra-abdominal organ), compressing it and forcing urine through the sphincter.

This type of UI is known as stress urinary incontinence (SUI). Although the exact etiology of urethral underactivity and SUI in the woman is incompletely understood, clearly identifiable risk factors include pregnancy, childbirth, menopause, cognitive impairment, obesity, and age.[11,12] The prevalence of SUI in women appears to peak during or after the onset of menopause. This implies that hormonal factors are important in maintaining continence.

In men, SUI is most commonly the result of prior lower urinary tract surgery or injury with resulting compromise of the sphincter mechanism within and external to the urethra. Radical prostate surgery for treatment of adenocarcinoma of the prostate is probably the most common setting in which surgical manipulation leads to UI. Transurethral resection of the prostate (TURP) for benign prostatic hyperplasia (BPH; see Chap. 85) may also lead to SUI in men.

BLADDER OVERACTIVITY (URGE URINARY INCONTINENCE)

Bladder overactivity—including bladder filling and urinary storage characterized by involuntary bladder contractions—is termed urge urinary incontinence (UUI). Symptoms of bladder overactivity occur because the detrusor muscle is overactive and contracts inappropriately during the filling phase.

The symptoms caused by the overactive bladder are typically urinary frequency, urgency, and urge incontinence. Frequency is defined as emptying the bladder more often than eight times per day and experiencing urgency as a sudden, strong desire to urinate. People suffering from bladder overactivity typically have to empty their bladders frequently and when they experience a sensation of urgency, they may leak urine if they are unable to reach the toilet quickly or if the sensation of urgency is very strong.

The amount of urine lost may be large, as the bladder may empty completely. Sleep may be disturbed, as the need to void may be experienced during the night. Nighttime frequency (nocturia) and nocturnal incontinence (enuresis) are often particularly disruptive.

Most patients with overactive bladder and UUI have no identifiable underlying etiology. In fact, the most common cause of bladder overactivity and UUI is "idiopathic." Clearly identifiable risk factors for UUI include normal aging, neurologic disease (including stroke, Parkinson's disease, multiple sclerosis, and spinal cord injury), and bladder outlet obstruction (i.e., prostatism).

The mechanism for bladder overactivity must be either neurogenic or myogenic. The neurogenic hypothesis ascribes the overactive bladder and UUI to disease-related changes within the central or peripheral nervous system.[13] The myogenic hypothesis states that overactive bladder and UUI result from changes within the smooth muscle of the bladder wall itself.[14] Precipitating factors such as bladder outlet obstruction can cause a partial denervation of smooth muscle, leading to a state of decreased responsiveness to activation of intrinsic nerves but supersensitivity to contractile agonists and direct electrical activation.[15] However, in practice, UUI is difficult to categorize as either neurogenic or myogenic in origin, as conditions often seem to be interconnected and complementary.

URETHRAL OVERACTIVITY AND/OR BLADDER UNDERACTIVITY (OVERFLOW INCONTINENCE)

Overflow incontinence, the result of urethral overactivity and bladder underactivity, is an important but rare type of UI in both men and women. Overflow incontinence results when the bladder is filled to capacity at all times but is unable to empty, causing urine to leak from a distended bladder past a normal outlet and sphincter.

In the setting of urethral overactivity, the resistance to the flow of urine during volitional voiding is increased resulting in functional or anatomic obstruction and incomplete bladder emptying. Common causes of urethral overactivity in men include BPH and prostate cancer. In women, urethral overactivity is rare, but may result from cystocele formation, or surgical overcorrection (iatrogenic obstruction) following anti-incontinence surgery. In both sexes, overflow UI may be associated with systemic neurologic dysfunction or diseases, such as spinal cord injury or multiple sclerosis.

Bladder underactivity may also result in overflow incontinence. Under certain circumstances, the detrusor muscle of the bladder may become progressively weakened and eventually lose the ability to voluntarily contract. In the absence of adequate contractility, the bladder is unable to empty completely, and large volumes of residual urine are left after micturition. Both myogenic and neurogenic factors have been implicated in producing the impaired contractility seen in this condition.

MIXED INCONTINENCE AND OTHER TYPES OF URINARY INCONTINENCE

Various types of UI may coexist in the same patient. The combination of bladder overactivity and urethral underactivity is termed *mixed incontinence*. This is often a difficult diagnosis to make because of the often-confusing array of presenting symptoms. Bladder overactivity may also coexist with impaired bladder contractility. This is most common in the elderly and is termed detrusor hyperactivity with impaired contractility.[16]

Functional incontinence is not caused by bladder- or urethra-specific factors. Rather, in patients with conditions such as dementia, cognitive or mobility deficits are linked to UI more than is any extrinsic or intrinsic deficit of the lower urinary tract. Another example of functional incontinence occurs in the postoperative orthopedic surgery patient. Following extensive orthopedic reconstructions such as total hip arthroplasty, patients are often immobile secondary to pain or traction. The treatment of this type of UI may involve only placing a urinal or commode at the bedside that allows for simplified access to toileting.

Finally, many localized or systemic illnesses may also result in UI because of their effects on the lower urinary tract or the surrounding structures, including:

Dementia/delirium
Depression
Urinary tract infection (cystitis)
Postmenopausal atrophic urethritis or vaginitis
Diabetes
Neurologic disease (e.g., cerebrovascular accident, Parkinson's disease, multiple sclerosis, spinal cord injury)
Pelvic malignancy
Constipation
Congenital malformations

Many commonly used medications may also aggravate existing voiding dysfunction and UI (Table 86–1).

CLINICAL PRESENTATION

UI may present in a number of ways, depending on the underlying pathophysiology. A complete medical history, including an assessment of symptoms and a physical examination, is essential in correctly classifying the type of incontinence and thereby assuring appropriate therapy.

TABLE 86–1. Medications Influencing Lower Urinary Tract Function

Medication	Effect
Diuretics	Polyuria, frequency, urgency
α-Receptor antagonists	Urethral relaxation and SUI in women
α-Receptor agonists	Urethral constriction and urinary retention in men
Calcium-channel blockers	Urinary retention
Narcotic analgesics	Urinary retention from impaired contractility
Sedative hypnotics	Mixed incontinence caused by delirium, immobility
Antipsychotics	Anticholinergic effects and urinary retention
Anticholinergics	Urinary retention
Antidepressants, tricyclic	Anticholinergic effects, α-agonist effects
Alcohol	Polyuria, frequency, urgency, sedation, delirium
Angiotensin-converting enzyme inhibitors (ACEI)	Cough as a result of ACEI may aggravate SUI by increasing intra-abdominal pressure

URINE LEAKAGE

UI represents a spectrum of severity in terms of both volume of leakage and degree of bother to the patient. Considering also patient discomfort in talking about urine leakage, the clinician must probe during the patient interview to determine accurately the precise nature of the problem.

The use of absorbent products such as panty liners, pads, or diapers is an obvious point to discuss, but the clinician must keep in mind that their use varies among patients. The number and type of pads may not relate to the amount or type of incontinence, as their use is a function of personal preference and hygiene. A high number of absorbent pads may be used every day by a patient with severe, high-volume UI, or alternatively, by a fastidiously hygienic patient with low-volume leakage who simply changes pads often to avoid a sense of wetness or odor. Nevertheless, a large number of pads that are described by the patient as "soaked" is indicative of high-volume urine loss.

Regardless of the volume of urine loss, the desire to seek evaluation and therapy for UI in all patients is almost always elective and contingent on the degree of bother to the individual patient. As with use of absorbent products, patients differ in the amount of urine loss they will tolerate before considering the condition bothersome enough to seek medical assistance.

SYMPTOMS

Under the best of circumstances, UI is difficult to categorize based on symptoms alone (Table 86–2).[17] In a study of patients who appeared to have SUI based on symptoms and patient history, urodynamics showed that only 72% of patients had SUI as the sole cause of incontinence.[18]

Patients with urethral underactivity or SUI characteristically complain of urinary leakage with physical activity. Volume of leakage

TABLE 86–2. Differentiating Bladder Overactivity from Urethral Underactivity

Symptoms	Bladder Overactivity	Urethral Underactivity
Urgency (strong, sudden desire to void)	Yes	Sometimes
Frequency with urgency	Yes	Rarely
Leaking during physical activity (e.g., coughing, sneezing, lifting)	No	Yes
Amount of urinary leakage with *each episode* of incontinence	Large if present	Usually small
Ability to reach the toilet in time following an urge to void	No or just barely	Yes
Nocturnal incontinence (presence of wet pads or undergarments in bed)	Yes	Rare
Nocturia (waking to pass urine at night)	Usually	Seldom

Adapted from Ref. 17.

is proportional to the level of activity. They will often leak urine during periods of exercise, coughing, sneezing, lifting, or even when rising from a seated to a standing position. Patients with pure SUI will not have leakage when physically inactive, especially when they are supine. Often, they will have little or no UI at night, will not awaken to void during the night (nocturia), will not wet their bed, and often do not even wear absorbent products at bedtime. Urinary urgency and frequency may be associated with SUI, either as a separate component caused by bladder overactivity (mixed incontinence), or as a compensatory mechanism wherein the patient with SUI learns to toilet frequently to avoid large volume urine loss during physical activity.

Typical symptoms of bladder overactivity include frequency, urgency, and urge incontinence. Nocturia and nocturnal incontinence are often present. Patients will often wear protection both day and night. Urinary frequency can be affected by a number of factors unrelated to bladder overactivity, including excessive fluid intake (polydipsia) and bladder hypersensitivity states such as interstitial cystitis and urinary tract infection, and these should be ruled out. In some patients, bladder overactivity may manifest as UI without awareness in the absence of a sense of urinary urgency or frequency. Urinary urgency, a sensation of impending micturition, requires intact sensory input from the lower urinary tract. In patients with spinal cord injury, sensory neuropathies, and other neurologic diseases, a diminished ability to perceive or process sensory input from the lower urinary tract may result in bladder overactivity and UI without urgency or urinary frequency. When the bladder contraction occurs without warning and sensation is absent, the condition is referred to as reflex incontinence.

Patients with overflow incontinence may present with considerable obstructive urinary symptoms, including lower abdominal fullness, hesitancy, and straining to void, decreased force of urinary stream, interrupted stream, and a vague sense of incomplete bladder emptying. These patients may also have a significant component of urinary frequency and urgency. In patients with acute urinary retention and overflow incontinence, lower abdominal pain may also be present. Although these symptoms are not specific for overflow incontinence, they may warrant further investigation including an assessment of postvoid residual urine volume.

SIGNS

A presenting complaint of UI mandates a directed physical examination and a brief neurologic assessment. This should ideally include an abdominal examination to exclude a distended bladder, a neurologic assessment of the perineum and lower extremities, a pelvic exam in women (looking especially for evidence of prolapse or hormonal deficiency), and a genital and prostate examination in men.

SUI can usually be objectively demonstrated by having the patient cough or strain during the examination and observing the urethral meatus. In women, SUI may be associated with varying degrees of vaginal prolapse including cystourethrocele (bladder and urethral prolapse), enterocele (small bowel prolapse), rectocele (rectal prolapse), and uterine prolapse. These conditions may have important implications for therapy.

Perineal skin maceration, erythema, breakdown, and ulceration may be indicative of chronic, severe UI. Patients with chronic incontinence may also manifest fungal infections of the skin of the perineum and upper thighs.

In both sexes, digital rectal examination provides an opportunity to check ambient rectal tone, the integrity of the sacral reflex arc (e.g., anal wink), as well as assess the patient's ability to perform a voluntary pelvic floor muscle contraction (i.e., "Kegel" exercise), which may be an important factor in deciding on appropriate therapy. In men, a digital examination of the prostate assesses for the presence of prostate cancer, inflammation, and benign enlargement.

A cursory neurologic examination includes an assessment of reflexes, rectal tone, and sensory or motor deficits in the lower extremities, which might be indicative of systemic or localized neurologic disease. As noted previously, neurologic diseases have the potential to affect bladder and sphincter function and thus may have significant implications in the incontinent patient.

PRIOR MEDICAL OR SURGICAL ILLNESS

UI may present in the setting of concurrent, seemingly unrelated illnesses. New-onset UI may be the initial manifestation of certain systemic illnesses such as diabetes mellitus, metastatic malignancies, multiple sclerosis, and other neurologic illnesses. Central nervous system disease, or injury above the level of the pons, generally results in symptoms of bladder overactivity and UUI. Spinal cord injury or disease may manifest as bladder overactivity and UUI or as overflow incontinence, depending on the spinal level and completeness of the injury or disease.

Medications may have wide-ranging effects on lower urinary tract function (Table 86–1). A thorough inquiry into the use of new medications in the setting of recent-onset UI may show a relationship.

Acute UI manifest in the immediate postoperative setting may be secondary to a number of factors, including surgical manipulation and immobility, and to a number of medications, including analgesics. In the postoperative setting, acute urinary retention and overflow incontinence is not uncommonly related to the administration of anesthetic agents and/or narcotic analgesics in the perioperative period. These agents may have profound effects on bladder contractility that are completely reversible once the agents are metabolized and excreted.

Prior surgery may have effects on lower urinary tract function. UI following prostate surgery in men is very suggestive of injury to the sphincter and resultant SUI. Pelvic surgery for benign and malignant conditions may result in denervation or injury to the lower urinary tract. This includes bowel surgery and gynecologic procedures. For example, new-onset total UI following gynecologic surgery for uterine fibroids suggests the possibility of intraoperative bladder injury and subsequent development of a postoperative vesicovaginal fistula. Radiation therapy to the pelvis for malignant disease (e.g., prostate cancer or cervical cancer) may result in injury to the bladder or urethra and subsequent UI.

In women, UI may be related to several gynecologic factors, including childbirth, hormonal status, and prior gynecologic surgery. Pregnancy and childbirth, particularly vaginal delivery, is associated with SUI and pelvic prolapse. Significant SUI in the nulliparous women is rather uncommon. UI that becomes progressive at or around menopause suggests a hormonal component potentially responsive to estrogen-replacement therapy.

Finally, UI may present in the setting of other significant pelvic floor disorders, signs, and symptoms. Constipation, diarrhea, fecal incontinence, dyspareunia, sexual dysfunction, and pelvic pain may be related to UI. A history of gross hematuria in the setting of UI mandates further urologic investigation, including radiologic imaging of the upper urinary tract and cystoscopy. Acute dysuria with or without hematuria in the setting of UI suggests cystitis. A urinalysis and urine culture should be performed in these patients.

▶ TREATMENT: Urinary Incontinence

NONPHARMACOLOGIC TREATMENT

Nonpharmacologic treatment of UI constitutes the chief form of incontinence management at a primary care level. For patients in whom pharmacologic or surgical management is inappropriate or undesired, nondrug approaches are the only option. This would include patients who are not medically fit for surgery or those who plan future pregnancies (as these may adversely affect long-term surgical outcomes); those with overflow incontinence who cannot be managed with surgery or drug therapy; those with comorbid conditions that place them at high risk for adverse effects from drug therapy; those who are delaying surgery or do not want to undergo surgery; and those with mild to moderate symptoms who do not want to take medication.

For additional information on nonpharmacologic interventions for UI, readers are referred to comprehensive literature reviews and consensus opinions of treatment guidelines on nonpharmacologic interventions by multidisciplinary experts.[19,20] Table 86–3 summarizes the basic nondrug approaches.

Behavioral interventions are the first line of treatment for SUI, UUI, and mixed UI.[19,21–23] These include lifestyle modifications, scheduling regimens, and pelvic floor muscle rehabilitation (Table 86–3). Because the key to the success with any type of behavioral intervention is the motivation of the patient or caregiver, these individuals must be active participants in developing a treatment plan. Regular follow-up is needed to help motivate patients and caregivers, and to monitor treatment outcomes.

PHARMACOLOGIC TREATMENT

URGE URINARY INCONTINENCE

Pharmacotherapy is useful when UUI symptoms are not adequately controlled with behavioral therapies, particularly in patients with a low functional bladder capacity. In many cases, the combined use of pharmacotherapy with behavioral therapy produces a better response than either intervention alone.

Proven to be the most effective agents in suppressing premature detrusor contractions, enhancing bladder storage, and relieving UUI symptoms and complications, anticholinergic/antispasmodic drugs constitute the pharmacotherapy of first choice for UUI (Tables 86–4 and 86–5).[19,24–39] Drugs with anticholinergic activity act by antagonizing muscarinic cholinergic receptors, through which efferent parasympathetic nerve impulses evoke detrusor contraction. In addition, women with mixed UI or UUI plus urethritis or vaginitis may benefit from topical or systemic estrogen (alone or in combination with an anticholinergic drug).

Immediate-Release Oxybutynin

Even though about one-fourth of patients discontinue therapy because of its nonurinary antimuscarinic effects, oxybutynin immediate-release (IR) remains the drug of first choice for UUI and the "gold standard" against which other drugs are compared. In addition to these antimuscarinic effects (e.g., dry mouth, constipation, vision impairment, confusion, cognitive dysfunction, tachycardia), oxybutynin IR is associated with orthostatic hypotension secondary to α-adrenergic receptor blockade as well as sedation and weight gain from histamine H_1-receptor blockade.[19,25,30,40–43] Furthermore, adverse effects jeopardize medication adherence and can prevent dose escalation to that needed for optimal benefit.

The high incidence of adverse effects to oxybutynin IR may, at least in part, be explained by transient high peak serum concentrations (C_{max}) and the area under the plasma concentration-versus-time curve (AUC) that are twofold higher in elderly patients than in younger adults after both single and multiple doses.[44] Oxybutynin IR is best tolerated when the dose is gradually escalated from no more than 2.5 mg twice daily to 2.5 mg three times daily after 1 month, then further increased in increments of 2.5 mg/day every 1 to 2 months until the desired response or the maximum recommended or tolerated dose is attained. The optimal response usually requires no more than 5 mg three times daily (Table 86–4).[25,45]

Adverse effects of oxybutynin IR can sometimes be managed by a dose reduction if this does not significantly compromise drug efficacy. Dry mouth can be relieved by the use of sugarless hard candy, gum, or a saliva substitute. Constipation can be minimized by increasing the intake of water, dietary fiber, physical activity such as walking, or laxative therapy. The need for multiple daily dosing of oxybutynin IR can further jeopardize adherence, especially in elderly people who generally take multiple medications and are more likely to be cognitively impaired.

Extended-Release Oxybutynin

Because of problems with oxybutynin IR, oxybutynin extended-release (XL) was developed. It can be considered an alternative for the first-line therapy of UUI (Table 86–5).

Oxybutynin XL (Ditropan XL, Alza) is an extended-release formulation of oxybutynin.[46] Its extended-release system consists of an osmotically active bilayer core (comprising a drug layer and a push layer containing osmotically active components) surrounded by a semipermeable membrane. Throughout the gastrointestinal tract, water permeates through the rate-controlling membrane into the tablet core, causing the drug to go into suspension and the push layer to expand, pushing the suspended drug out through an orifice.[30] Following oral administration, oxybutynin XL is completely absorbed, and neither the rate nor extent of absorption are significantly affected by administration with food.

Unlike oxybutynin IR, oxybutynin XL delivers a controlled amount of oxybutynin chloride continuously throughout the gastrointestinal tract over a 24-hour time period, reducing first-pass metabolism by cytochrome P450 (CYP450) isozyme 3A4, which is present in higher concentrations in the upper portion of the small intestine than the lower gastrointestinal tract.[46,47] This results in relative bioavailabilities of oxybutynin and its active *N*-desethyloxybutynin metabolite of 153% and 69%, respectively, for oxybutynin XL and oxybutynin IR.[48] The greater ratio of parent drug to active metabolite after oxybutynin XL administration, and probably less importantly lower C_{max}, are believed to be the reasons for fewer dose/concentration-dependent adverse effects and better patient tolerance with the XL preparation as compared to oxybutynin IR.[49] The elimination of oxybutynin XL is not known to be altered in patients with renal or hepatic impairment or in geriatric patients (up to 78 years of age).[46] The absence of an effect of advanced age on oxybutynin XL pharmacokinetics is unexpected since the clearance of oxybutynin IR is significantly lower in elderly individuals.

TABLE 86–3. Nonpharmacologic Management of Urinary Incontinence

Intervention	Description	Patient Characteristics
Lifestyle Modifications	Self-management strategies targeted toward reducing or eliminating risk factors that cause or exacerbate urinary incontinence	Smoking cessation for patients with cough-induced stress incontinence; weight reduction for obese patients with stress incontinence; good bowel hygiene for patients with constipation; caffeine reduction, selected dietary and fluid modifications for patients with urge incontinence (e.g., eliminate aspartame, spicy foods, citrus fruits, carbonated beverages)
Scheduling Regimens		
Timed voiding	Toileting on a fixed schedule whose interval does not change, typically q2h during waking hours	Used for stress, urge, and mixed incontinence in patients with cognitive or physical impairments; also used in patients without impairments who have infrequent voiding patterns
Habit retraining	Scheduled toiletings with adjustments of voiding intervals (longer or shorter) based on patient's voiding pattern	Used for stress, urge, and mixed incontinence in institutionalized or homebound patients with cognitive or physical impairments; may also be used in patients who have diuretic-induced incontinence
Patterned urge response toileting (PURT)	A specialized type of habit training that involves the use of an electronic monitoring device to identify the timing of incontinent episodes	Used for stress, urge, and mixed incontinence in institutionalized and homebound elderly populations
Prompted voiding	Scheduled toiletings that require prompts to void from a caregiver, typically q2h; patient assisted in toileting only if response is positive; used in conjunction with operant conditioning techniques for rewarding patients for maintaining continence and appropriate toileting	Used for stress, urge, and mixed incontinence in patients who are functionally able to use toilet or toilet substitute, able to feel urge sensation, and able to request toileting assistance appropriately; primarily used in institutional settings or in homebound patients with an available caregiver
Bladder training	Scheduled toiletings with progressive voiding intervals; includes teaching of urge control strategies using relaxation and distraction techniques, self-monitoring, and use of reinforcement techniques; sometimes combined with drug therapy	Used for stress, urge, and mixed incontinence in patients who are cognitively intact, able to toilet, and motivated to comply with training program
Pelvic Floor Muscle Rehabilitation		
Pelvic floor muscle exercises (e.g., Kegel exercises)	Regular practice of pelvic floor muscle contractions; may involve use of pelvic floor muscle contraction for urge inhibition	Used for stress, urge, and mixed incontinence in patients who can correctly contract their pelvic floor muscles without use of accessory muscles; requires a cognitively intact and highly motivated patient
Vaginal weight training	Active retention of increasing vaginal weights; typically used in combination with pelvic floor muscle exercises at least twice a day	Women with stress incontinence who are cognitively intact, can correctly contract pelvic floor muscles, able to stand, and who have sufficient vaginal vault and introitus to retain cone and are highly motivated; contraindicated in patients with moderate to severe pelvic organ prolapse
Biofeedback	Use of electronic or mechanical instruments to display visual or auditory information about neuromuscular or bladder activity; used to teach correct pelvic floor muscle contraction and/or urge inhibition	Used for stress, urge, and mixed incontinence in patients who are able to understand analog or digital signals, who are motivated, and who have the capability to learn voluntary control through observation
Nonimplantable electrical stimulation	Application of electrical current to sacral and pudendal afferent fibers through vaginal, anal, or surface electrodes; used to inhibit bladder overactivity and to improve awareness, contractility, and efficiency of pelvic muscle contraction	Used for stress, urge, and mixed incontinence in patients who are highly motivated; contraindicated in patients with diminished sensory perception, moderate or severe pelvic organ prolapse; urinary retention, history of cardiac arrhythmia, or demand cardiac pacemaker
Extracorporeal magnetic innervation	Pulsed magnetic stimulation to pelvic floor musculature causing depolarization of motor neurons, thus inducing pelvic floor muscle contraction; stimulation is provided	Initially tested in women with stress incontinence; contraindicated in patients with demand cardiac pacemakers, or with metallic joint replacements;

TABLE 86–3. (Continued)

Intervention	Description	Patient Characteristics
	through a specially designed chair that contains a device for producing a pulsing magnetic field (e.g., Neotonus, Inc., Marietta, GA)	may be useful treatment option when other approaches fail or are not feasible
Anti-Incontinence Devices		
Intravaginal support device (pessaries and bladder neck support prostheses)	Pessaries and other intravaginal devices designed to support the bladder neck, relieve minor pelvic organ prolapse, and change pressure transmission to the urethra (e.g., Introl device, Johnson & Johnson Medical, Arlington, TX; Coloplast AS, Espergarde, Denmark)	Used for female stress incontinence; in postmenopausal women, estrogen replacement is typically prescribed to prevent ulceration and breakdown of vaginal tissue; requires good manual dexterity to manipulate device
External occlusive device	Small, single-use device that covers the urethral meatus which is removed for voiding in women (e.g., FemAssist, Insight Medical, Boston; CapSure, Bard Urological, Covington, GA); a penile clamp (e.g., Cunningham clamp) is available for men	Used for female and male stress incontinence; used in cognitively intact patients with good manual dexterity
Intraurethral occlusive device (urethral plug)	Small, single-use device that is worn in the urethra to provide mechanical obstruction to prevent urine leakage; removed for voiding (e.g., FemSoft Insert, Rochester Med. Corp., Stewartville, MN)	Used for female stress incontinence patients who are cognitively intact with good manual dexterity; contraindicated with primary urge incontinence, urinary tract infection, urethral stricture, and any anatomic or pathologic condition making catheter passage difficult
Complex valved catheter (investigational)	Intraurethral occlusive device that has a unidirectional valve that can be opened to permit voiding and resealed; may be left indwelling over longer period of time than intraurethral occlusive devices but requires a clinician to insert and remove; several devices are currently undergoing testing	Female stress incontinence and overflow incontinence
Supportive Interventions		
Toileting substitutes and other environmental modifications	Urinals, bedside commodes, elevated toilet seats	Used for patients with mobility impairments that make it difficult to reach a toilet in a timely fashion
Physical therapy	Gait and/or strength training	Used for frail elderly patients with mobility impairments that make it difficult to reach a toilet in a timely fashion
Absorbent products	Variety of reusable and disposable pads and pant systems; some products contain a polymer that absorbs urine and wicks away from the body	Used for all types of incontinence
External collection devices (men only)	Condom catheter with leg bag	Used in men with urge, stress, and overflow incontinence and in those with functional impairments
Catheters	Disposable, intermittent catheters and indwelling urethral and suprapubic catheters	Used for overflow incontinence; also used in patients who are bed bound or with significant mobility impairments and severe incontinence, those with terminal illness, and those with sacral pressure ulcers until healing occurs

Controlled studies have demonstrated that oxybutynin XL is significantly more effective than placebo and equally effective as oxybutynin IR in reducing the mean number of UI episodes, restoring continence, decreasing the number of micturitions per day, and increasing urine volume voided per micturition (Table 86–5).[29,30,40–42,50–52]

In short-term studies of up to 12 weeks, oxybutynin XL was better tolerated than oxybutynin IR, with approximately 7% of patients discontinuing treatment because of adverse effects (as compared to approximately 27% taking oxybutynin IR).[19,25,30,40,41,45,46] The rate and severity of adverse effects did not differ significantly between elderly persons 65 years of age and older and younger adults with the XL preparation. A 12-week study demonstrated the superiority of oxybutynin XL over tolterodine IR in reducing the mean number of weekly incontinent episodes and micturitions.[38]

Oxybutynin XL, available only in a tablet formulation, is administered once daily, with or without food, and should not be crushed or chewed (Table 86–4). Like oxybutynin IR, the dosage does not require adjustment in patients of advanced age, or in patients with renal or hepatic impairment. However, treatment should still be initiated at the smallest recommended dosage in elderly people (5 mg once daily).[31,46] The maximum benefit of oxybutynin XL may not be realized for up to 4 weeks after starting therapy or after dose escalation. No known clinically relevant drug-drug interactions with either oxybutynin XL or oxybutynin IR have been identified. However, other drugs with anticholinergic activity may increase overall anticholinergic

TABLE 86–4. Pharmacotherapeutic Options in Patients with Urinary Incontinence

Type	Drug Class	Drug Therapy (Dose)	Comments
Overactive bladder	Anticholinergic agents/antispasmodics	Oxybutynin IR (2.5–5 mg bid, tid, or qid), oxybutynin XL (5–30 mg qd), tolterodine IR (1–2 mg bid), tolterodine LA (2–4 mg qd) propantheline (15 mg tid + 60 mg HS up to 60 mg qid) on an empty stomach	Anticholinergics are the first-line drug therapy (oxybutynin or tolterodine are preferred).
	Tricyclic antidepressants	Imipramine, doxepin, nortriptyline, desipramine (25–100 mg HS)	TCAs are generally reserved for patients with an additional indication (e.g., depression, neuralgia)
	Estrogen (only in women with urethritis or vaginitis)	Conjugated estrogen 0.5 g vaginal cream 3 times per week for up to 8 months. Repeat course if symptom recurrence. Or use estradiol vaginal insert/ring [2 mg (1 ring)] and replace after 90 days if needed. If ineffective, start systemic therapy with oral conjugated estrogens (0.3–0.625 mg/day) orally immediately after food to decrease nausea.	Marginally effective. Few adverse effects with cream and vaginal insert Progestin (e.g., medroxyprogesterone 2.5–10 mg/day) with systemic estrogen if patient has intact uterus
Stress	α-Adrenergic agonists	Pseudoephedrine (15–60 mg tid) with food, water, or milk	Pseudoephedrine is first-line therapy for women with no contraindication (notably hypertension). Phenylpropanolamine was the preferred agent until its removal from the US market in 2000.
	Estrogen	See estrogens (above). Topical route preferred	Considered a somewhat less-effective alternative to pseudoephedrine. Combined pseudoephedrine and estrogen is only slightly more effective than pseudoephedrine alone in postmenopausal women.
	Imipramine	25–100 mg HS	Imipramine is an optional therapy when first-line therapy is inadequate.
Overflow (atonic bladder)	Cholinomimetics	Bethanechol (25–50 mg tid or qid) on an empty stomach	Avoid use if patient has asthma or heart disease. Short-term use only. Never give IV or IM because of life-threatening cardiovascular and gastrointestinal reactions.

bid, twice daily; HS, at bedtime; IM, intramuscular; IR, immediate-release; IV, intravenous; qid, 4 times daily; TCAs, tricyclic antidepressants; tid, thrice daily; XL, extended-release; LA, long-acting.

TABLE 86–5. Efficacy of First-Choice Drugs for Bladder Overactivity in Placebo-Controlled Trials[a]

Drug (reference no.)	Decreased Incontinence Episodes	Restored Continence	Decreased Frequency of Micturitions	Increased Volume per Void
Oxybutynin IR[19,25–28]	24–52	16–67	−2–63	9–24
Oxybutynin XL[30,31]	47	37	1	13
Tolterodine[26,27,32–38]	16–33	9	4–19	11–20
Tolterodine LA[39]	23	NR	6	14

IR, immediate-release; XL, extended-release; NR, not reported.

[a]All values constitute mean or median drug effect (drug response minus placebo response in percent), predominantly using pooled data from multiple independent studies.

effects (i.e., produce a pharmacodynamic interaction), as would be expected.[46]

Tolterodine

Tolterodine (Detrol, Pharmacia) is a competitive muscarinic receptor antagonist that can be considered first-line therapy of UI in patients with symptoms of urinary frequency, urgency, or urge incontinence (Tables 86–4 and 86–5).[32]

Controlled studies demonstrate that tolterodine is significantly more effective than placebo and as effective as oxybutynin IR in decreasing the mean daily number of micturitions and the mean volume voided per micturition (Table 86–5).[26,33–37] However, while two controlled trials showed significant decreases in the mean number of incontinence episodes per 24 hours as compared to placebo, most studies have not and the manufacturer's product information does not claim a significant improvement in this symptom (Table 86–5).[27,33–37] The only controlled study of tolterodine's ability to restore urinary continence reported an insignificant effect rate of 9% over placebo.[33]

In a controlled study of 1,529 adult outpatients with urinary frequency and UUI, tolterodine LA, an extended-release formulation of tolterodine tartrate, decreased significantly the mean number of weekly incontinence episodes (23%) over placebo and 7% more than the immediate-release formulation. Patient withdrawal rates did not differ significantly between the two treatments, but dry mouth was observed significantly less often in patients taking the LA formulation than among those patients receiving the IR product.[39]

A major consideration in using tolterodine is its pharmacokinetics, specifically its metabolism. The agent is predominantly eliminated by hepatic metabolism that exhibits genetic polymorphism.[32] The principal metabolic pathway in extensive metabolizers involves oxidation of the parent drug by CYP450 isozyme 2D6 to the active 5-hydroxymethyl metabolite (DD01), followed by further oxidation and dealkylation.

In poor metabolizers who lack the CYP450 isozyme 2D6 (approximately 7% of the US population), a number of drug interactions are theoretically possible but have not been shown to be clinically important. The principal metabolic pathway involves CYP450 isozyme 3A4, with dealkylation of the amino group, oxidation to a dealkylated hydroxy metabolite, and further oxidation to a dealkylated acid metabolite that undergoes glucuronidation. Because tolterodine is metabolized by CYP450 isozyme 3A4, its elimination may be impaired by inhibitors of this isozyme (e.g., fluoxetine, sertraline, fluvoxamine, macrolide antibiotics, imidazoles, grapefruit juice). Fluoxetine, an inhibitor of CYP450 isozymes 2D6 and 3A4, decreases the metabolism of tolterodine to DD01, resulting in a nearly fivefold increase in the tolterodine AUC with a 52% increase in the C_{max} and a 20% decrease in the AUC of norfluoxetine.[53] Whether tolterodine significantly alters the pharmacokinetics of drugs metabolized by CYP450 isozyme 2D6 is unknown, so caution is advised with concurrent use of these agents.

Although one of two Phase I pharmacokinetic studies comparing healthy elderly volunteers (aged 64 to 80 years) with healthy volunteers younger than 40 years of age found no difference in pharmacokinetic parameters between the groups, the other study noted that the mean serum concentrations of tolterodine and DD01 were 20% and 50% greater in elderly volunteers than in young healthy volunteers, respectively. Despite possibly altered pharmacokinetics in elderly individuals, no differences in the incidence and severity of adverse effects between these age groups have been noted in clinical trials, and, therefore, no dosage adjustment is recommended on the basis of age alone.[32]

Tolterodine elimination is diminished in patients with impaired hepatic function. Patients with hepatic cirrhosis who are extensive metabolizers exhibit a higher mean AUC of DD01, serum tolterodine and DD01 concentrations, and a longer terminal disposition half-life of tolterodine and DD01 than do healthy subjects who are extensive metabolizers. The tolterodine AUC was higher in cirrhotic patients who were poor metabolizers than in healthy poor metabolizers.[32] If the use of tolterodine cannot be avoided in patients with hepatic impairment or in those receiving inhibitors of CYP450 isozyme 3A4, and possibly CYP450 isozyme 2D6, the initial dose should be reduced by 50% to tolterodine IR 1 mg twice daily or tolterodine LA 2 mg once daily (Table 86–4).[32] No formal tolterodine dosage recommendation is possible based on available information for individuals who have hepatic impairment and are taking a CYP450 isozyme 3A4 inhibitor; intuitively, the initial dose should not exceed 1 mg twice daily (IR) or 2 mg once daily (LA).

The elimination of tolterodine has not been evaluated in patients with impaired renal function and, therefore, the drug should be used more cautiously in such individuals (i.e., starting dose of the IR product of 1 mg twice daily with gradual dose escalation as needed to a maximum of 2 mg twice daily, or a starting dose of the LA formulation of 2 mg once daily with gradual dose escalation as needed to 4 mg once daily).[32]

Tolterodine is better tolerated than oxybutynin IR, with about 8% of patients discontinuing treatment (compared with approximately 27% of individuals taking oxybutynin IR).[17,25,27,33,34,36,40,54] The most common adverse effects of tolterodine are dry mouth, dyspepsia, headache, constipation, and dry eyes.[32]

Tolterodine, available only as a tablet formulation, is administered with or without food, and should not be crushed or chewed. The maximum benefit from tolterodine may not be realized for up to 8 weeks after starting therapy or dose escalation.

Other Agents

Other drugs for treating UUI are less effective, no safer, or have not been adequately studied (Table 86–5).[19,55]

Tricyclic antidepressants (TCA) are generally no more effective than oxybutynin IR and exhibit a high incidence of bothersome and serious adverse effects (e.g., orthostatic hypotension, cardiac conduction abnormalities, dizziness, confusion, life-threatening in overdose situations). Therefore, their use should be limited to individuals with an additional medical indication for the TCA (e.g., depression, neuropathic pain); to patients with mixed UI (because of their effect of decreasing bladder contractility and increasing outlet resistance); and possibly to those with nocturnal incontinence associated with altered sleep patterns.[19,55–58] Because of the lower incidence of adverse effects, the TCAs desipramine and nortriptyline may be preferred over imipramine and doxepin. However, because of their lower anticholinergic activity, they may also not be as effective.

Propantheline, another possible treatment, has a high incidence of adverse effects and is only modestly effective for UUI.[59–62] When used, propantheline appears to be best tolerated at a dose of no more than 15 mg three times daily plus 60 mg at bedtime.[59]

Flavoxate, a tertiary amine that relaxes smooth muscle *in vitro*, is not recommended for treating UUI because four controlled trials have revealed that it is no more effective than placebo.[19]

Dicyclomine hydrochloride, an anticholinergic agent that relaxes smooth muscle, produced minimal benefit and bothersome adverse effects in two small studies.[64,65]

Hyoscyamine, an anticholinergic and antispasmodic drug, has also been suggested for treating UUI but data are insufficient to recommend its use.[19]

Catheterization Combined with Medications

Patients with UUI and a postvoid residual (PVR) urine volume exceeding 100 mL (or 20% of total bladder volume) should be treated by intermittent self-catheterization along with frequent voiding between catheterizations to maintain a bladder volume of less than 400 mL. Patients with smaller bladder volumes generally do not need to be catheterized.

If intermittent catheterization is not possible, surgical placement of a suprapubic catheter may be necessary. The use of a chronic indwelling catheter should be avoided because of the increased occurrence of urinary tract infections and nephrolithiasis.

Patients who are able to maintain bladder volumes of less than 400 mL with catheterization, or who do not need to catheterize, may experience symptom relief with oxybutynin IR, oxybutynin XL, or tolterodine IR or LA, as these relax the detrusor muscle and enhance bladder storage. Patients with UUI and symptoms of retention who have achieved the target bladder volume may benefit from an α_1-receptor antagonist that relaxes the internal bladder sphincter. Bethanechol, a cholinergic agonist that stimulates bladder contractions, may also be useful. However, it causes numerous bothersome (e.g., muscle and abdominal cramping and diarrhea) and potentially life-threatening adverse effects and should not be used in patients with asthma or heart disease.[19]

URETHRAL UNDERACTIVITY

Urethral underactivity, or SUI, may be aggravated by agents with α-receptor blocking activity, including prazosin, terazosin, doxazosin, methyldopa, clonidine, guanfacine, guanadrel, and labetalol. The goal of therapy is to improve the urethral closure mechanism by either stimulating α-adrenergic receptors in the smooth muscle of the bladder neck and proximal urethra or enhancing the supportive structures underlying the urethral epithelium.

Estrogens

Local and systemic estrogens have been considered the mainstays of pharmacologic management of SUI since the 1940s. Estrogens are believed to work via several mechanisms, including enhancement of the proliferation of urethral epithelium, local circulation, and numbers and/or sensitivity of urogenital α-adrenergic receptors.[66]

Open trials support the use of a variety of estrogens in the management of SUI: transdermal estradiol,[67] conjugated estrogen vaginal cream,[68–70] Estring,[71] oral-conjugated estrogen,[72] oral quinestradol,[73,74] oral estriol,[75–77] intramuscular estrogens,[78] estriol vaginal suppositories,[79] and oral estradiol.[77] Variable effects of estrogen treatment on urodynamic parameters, such as maximum urethral closure pressure, functional urethral length, and pressure transmission ratio, have been noted in these studies.

Unfortunately, results of four placebo-controlled comparative trials have not been as favorable, finding no significant clinical or urodynamic effects for oral estrogen as compared with placebo (Table 86–4).[80–83] Systemic estrogen therapy is associated with numerous adverse effects, including mastodynia, uterine bleeding, and nausea.[55] If estrogens are to be used in the treatment of SUI, only topical products should be administered unless other benefits of estrogen therapy (e.g., bone, cardiovascular, or cognitive) are desired.

α-Adrenergic Agonists

Numerous open trials have supported the use of a variety of α-receptor agonists in SUI, including ephedrine,[84] norfenefrine,[85,86] phenylpropanolamine,[87,88] and midodrine.[89] Phenylpropanolamine was withdrawn from the US market in late 2000 because of a risk of stroke in women using the agent.[90,91] Some patients may have leftover supplies of this agent or obtain it from international sources. If so, those with the contraindications listed below—especially coronary artery disease and/or cardiac arrhythmias—should be warned against self-treatment with this or other α-adrenergic agonists.

Placebo-controlled comparative trials with phenylpropanolamine,[92,93] norfenefrine,[94] and norephedrine[95] support the modest efficacy of these agents in mild or moderate SUI. These agents have been found to variably affect maximum urethral closure pressure and functional urethral length.

Adverse effects include hypertension, headache, dry mouth, nausea, insomnia, and restlessness.[55] Contraindications to α-receptor agonist use include the presence of hypertension, tachyarrhythmias, coronary artery disease, myocardial infarction, cor pulmonale, hyperthyroidism, renal failure, and narrow-angle glaucoma.

Usual doses are ephedrine 25–50 mg four times daily (25 twice daily in elders) and pseudoephedrine 60 mg three times daily (15–30 mg three times daily in elders; Table 86–4).

Several studies have evaluated whether the clinical and urodynamic effects of combination estrogen-α-receptor agonist therapy exceed those of the individual therapies in SUI.[96–100] In general, combination therapy has resulted in somewhat superior clinical and urodynamic responses compared with monotherapy, including severity of complaints, amount of urine lost per episode, number of daily voluntary micturitions, number of leakage episodes per day, patient preference, pad use, maximum urethral closure pressure, functional urethral length, and pressure transmission ratio.

Other Agents

Insufficient data are available to support the use of agents other than estrogens or α-receptor agonists in the management of SUI. Two open trials have supported the use of imipramine,[101,102] and one supported the use of propranolol.[78,103]

OVERFLOW INCONTINENCE

Overflow incontinence secondary to benign or malignant prostatic hyperplasia may be amenable to pharmacotherapy. For management of malignant prostatic disease, the reader is referred to Chap. 128. The pharmacotherapy of BPH is described in Chap. 85.

SURGICAL TREATMENT

Only rarely does surgery play a role in the initial management of UI.[104] In the absence of secondary complications from UI (e.g., skin breakdown, infection), the decision to surgically treat *symptomatic* UI should be based on the premise that the degree of bother or lifestyle compromise to the patient is great enough to warrant an *elective* operation and that nonoperative therapy is either undesired or has been ineffective.

Successful application of surgery depends most on defining the underlying abnormalities responsible for UI (bladder versus urethra, underactivity versus overactivity). Once the underlying factor or factors are clear, other considerations come into play: renal function, sexual function, severity of the leakage, history of prior abdominal or pelvic surgery, the presence of concurrent abdominal or pelvic pathology requiring surgical correction, and finally, the patient's suitability for, and willingness to accept the risks of, surgery.

When patients with uncomplicated SUI become dissatisfied with the initial management approaches of pelvic floor exercises, medications, and/or behavioral modification,[104] surgical treatment assumes the primary role.

Surgical correction of female SUI (urethral underactivity) is directed toward either: (a) repositioning the urethra and/or creating a backboard of support, or otherwise stabilizing the urethra and bladder neck in a well-supported retropubic ("intra-abdominal") position that is receptive to changes in intraabdominal pressure; or (b) creating coaptation and/or compression or otherwise augmenting the urethral resistance provided by the intrinsic sphincteric unit, with (i.e., sling) or without (i.e., periurethral injectables) urethral and bladder neck support.

In men, SUI may be treated surgically with collagen or the artificial urinary sphincter. The vast majority of collagen injections in men are performed in a retrograde fashion under direct vision through a cystoscope. However, a transabdominal, transvesical, suprapubic "antegrade" approach has also been used.[105]

The artificial urinary sphincter is generally considered to be the "gold standard" for the treatment of male SUI. Placement of this manually operated silicone device has been associated with very high long-term success and satisfaction rates.[106]

Most patients with UUI are managed nonsurgically with a combination of behavioral modification, pelvic floor exercise, and pharmacologic therapy. Only rarely is surgery applied to the problem of UUI.[105] When employed, surgery may involve bladder denervation, implantation of a sacral nerve stimulator, or augmentation (enlargement) cystoplasty.

Currently there are no effective surgical treatments for bladder underactivity. After an appropriate evaluation is performed for reversible causes, the most effective management for this condition is intermittent self-catheterization performed by the patient or a caregiver three or four times per day. Alternative methods of management that are less satisfactory are indwelling urethral or suprapubic catheters and urinary diversion.

Urethral overactivity is most commonly caused by anatomic obstruction. Anatomic obstruction in men is most often caused by benign prostatic enlargement, which is discussed in Chap. 85.

Rarely, bladder outlet obstruction may be caused by a functional obstruction at the level of the bladder neck. Hypertrophy of the smooth muscle fibers at the level of the bladder neck in men and women may result in obstruction to the flow of urine. In those patients who fail pharmacologic therapy with α-receptor antagonists, endoscopic incision using the cystoscope is highly effective in treating this very uncommon condition.

EVALUATION OF THERAPEUTIC OUTCOMES

In the long-term management of UI, the patient-specific clinical signs/symptoms of most distress ("bother") to the individual need to be monitored. Use of a daily diary may be very useful in this regard. Some of the survey instruments used in incontinence research can be modified for use in clinical monitoring. In addition, quantitating the use of ancillary supplies such as pads may be useful. The goal of therapy is to minimize those signs/symptoms of most "bother" to the patient as well as the use of pads and other ancillary supplies/devices. Total elimination of UI signs/symptoms may not be possible, and patients and practitioners need to establish realistic goal(s) of therapy. As the therapies for UI frequently have nuisance adverse effects, such as anticholinergic effects like xerostomia, xerophthalmia, and constipation that may compromise regimen adherence, the presence and severity of adverse effects need to be carefully elicited at each healthcare practitioner visit. Emergence of adverse effects may necessitate drug dosage adjustment or use of alternative strategies (e.g., chewing sugarless gum or sucking on hard sugarless candy or use of saliva substitutes in xerostomia) or even drug discontinuation.

▶ PRINCIPLES OF PHARMACOTHERAPY

- Accurate diagnosis and classification of UI type is critical to the selection of appropriate pharmacotherapy (Table 86–4).
- Patient-specific treatment goal(s) should be identified, frequently necessitating reaching a balance between efficacy and tolerability of drug therapy. Treatment goals are not static and may change over time.
- Patient characteristics such as age, comorbidities, and ability to adhere to the prescribed regimen may also influence the choice of therapy.
- Achievement of the therapeutic goals requires careful dose titration.
- If the therapeutic goals are not achieved, a second agent may be added or a switch to an alternative single agent can be made.
- When pharmacotherapy is initiated, the patient must understand and agree with the plan of therapy. Adherence must be continuously reinforced.
- When evaluating a patient for UI, it is essential to rule out drug-induced or drug-aggravated incontinence.
- Anticholinergic agents should be considered the therapy-of-choice for bladder overactivity (UUI).
- Mixed urinary incontinence (especially UUI with SUI) is not infrequently found and may necessitate combination drug therapy.
- Nonpharmacologic therapy should be continued even if pharmacotherapy must be initiated.

REFERENCES

1. Arnold EP, Burgio K, Diokno AC, et al. Epidemiology and natural history of urinary incontinence (UI). In: Abrams P, Khoury S, Wein AJ, eds. Incontinence. Plymouth, U.K.: Plymbridge Distributors, 1999:199–226.
2. Diokno AC, Brock BM, Brown MB, et al. Prevalence of urinary incontinence and other urological symptoms in the noninstitutionalized elderly. J Urol 1986;136:1022–1025.

3. Ouslander JG, Kane RL, Abrass IB. Urinary incontinence in elderly nursing home patients. JAMA 1982;248:1194–1198.
4. Bump RC. Racial comparisons and contrasts in urinary incontinence and pelvic organ prolapse. Obstet Gynecol 1993;81:421–425.
5. Burgio KL, Matthews KA, Engel BT. Prevalence, incidence and correlates of urinary incontinence in healthy, middle-aged women. J Urol 1991;146:1255–1259.
6. Fliegner JR, Glenning PP. Seven years experience in the evaluation and management of patients with urge incontinence of urine. Aust N Z J Obstet Gynecol 1979;19:42–44.
7. Breakwell SL, Walker SN. Differences in physical health, social interaction and personal adjustment between continent and incontinent homebound aged women. J Community Health Nurs 1988;5:19–31.
8. Malmsten UG, Milsom I, Molander U, Norlen LJ. Urinary incontinence and lower urinary tract symptoms: An epidemiological study of men aged 45–99 years. J Urol 1997;158:1733–37.
9. Andersson K-E. The overactive bladder: Pharmacologic basis of drug treatment. Urology 1997;50(6A suppl):74–84.
10. Blaivas JG, Heritz DM. Classification, diagnostic evaluation and treatment overview. In: Blaivas JG, ed. Topics in Clinical Urology—Evaluation and Treatment of Urinary Incontinence. New York, Igaku-Shoin, 1996:22–45.
11. Kuh D, Cardozo L, Hardy R: Urinary incontinence in middle-aged women: Childhood enuresis and other lifetime risk factors in a British prospective cohort. J Epidemiol Community Health 1999;53(8): 453–458.
12. Groutz A, Gordon D, Keidar R, Lessing JB, Wolman I, David MP, Chen B. Stress urinary incontinence: Prevalence among nulliparous compared with primiparous and grand multiparous premenopausal women. Neurourol Urodyn 1999;18(5):419–425.
13. deGroat WC. A neurologic basis for the overactive bladder. Urology 1997;50(6A suppl):36–52.
14. Brading AF. A myogenic basis for the overactive bladder. Urology 1997;50(6A suppl):57–67.
15. Turner WH, Brading AF. Smooth muscle of the bladder in the normal and the diseased state: Pathology, diagnosis and treatment. Pharmacol Ther 1997;75:77–110.
16. Resnick NM, Yalla S. Detrusor hyperactivity with impaired contractile function. An unrecognized but common cause of incontinence in the elderly patient. JAMA 1987:257:3076–3081.
17. Rovner ES, Wein AJ. Today's treatment of overactive bladder and urge incontinence. Womens Health Prim Care 2000;3:179–192.
18. James M, Jackson S, Shepard A, Abrams P. Pure stress leakage symptomatology: Is it safe to discount detrusor instability? Br J Obstet Gynaecol 1999;106:1255–1258.
19. Fantl JA, Newman DK, Colling J, et al. Urinary incontinence in adults: Acute and chronic management. Clinical practice guideline, No. 2, 1996 Update. Rockville, MD, Agency for Health Care Policy and Research, 1996.
20. Abrams P, Khoury S, Wein A, eds. Incontinence. Proceedings from the First International Consultation on Incontinence. Plymouth. UK. Health Publication, 1999.
21. Wilson PD, Bo K, Bourcier A, et al. Conservative management in women. In: Abrams P, Khoury S, Wein A, eds. Incontinence. Proceedings from the First International Consultation on Incontinence. Plymouth, UK, Health Publication, 1999:579–636.
22. Fonda D, Benvenuti F, Castleden M, et al. Management of incontinence in older people. In: Abrams P, Khoury S, Wein A, eds. Incontinence. Proceedings from the First International Consultation on Incontinence. Plymouth, UK, Health Publication, 1999:731–774.
23. Kondo A, Hedlund H, Siroky M, et al. Conservative management in men. In: Abrams P, Khoury S, Wein A, eds. Incontinence. Proceedings from the First International Consultation on Incontinence. Plymouth, UK, Health Publication, 1999:669–690.
24. Ouslander JG, Schnelle JF, Uman G, et al. Does oxybutynin add to the effectiveness of prompted voiding for urinary incontinence among nursing home residents? A placebo-controlled trial. J Am Geriatr Soc 1995;43:610–617.
25. Burgio KL, Locher JL, Goode PS, et al. Behavioral vs drug treatment for urge urinary incontinence in older women: A randomized controlled trial. JAMA 1998;280:1995–2000.
26. Drutz HP, Appell RA, Gleason D, Klimberg I, Radomski S. Clinical efficacy and safety of tolterodine compared to oxybutynin and placebo in patients with overactive bladder. Int Urogynecol 1999;10:283–289.
27. Abrams P, Freeman R, Anderstrom C, Mattiasson A. Tolterodine, a new antimuscarinic agent: As effective but better tolerated than oxybutynin in patients with an overactive bladder. Br J Urol 1998;81:801–810.
28. Tapp AJ, Cardozo LD, Versi E, Cooper D. The treatment of detrusor instability in post-menopausal women with oxybutynin chloride: A double blind placebo controlled study. Br J Obstet Gynaecol 1990;97:1063–1064.
29. Riva D, Casolati E. Oxybutynin chloride in the treatment of female idiopathic bladder instability. Clin Exp Obstet Gynecol 1984;11:37–42.
30. Schmidt RA, The Oxybutynin XL Study Group. Efficacy of controlled-release, once-a-day oxybutynin chloride for urge urinary incontinence. Jerusalem, International Continence Society, Sept. 14–17, 1998:188.
31. ALZA Corporation. Ditropan XL (oxybutynin chloride) extended-release tablets. Data on file. Palo Alto, CA, 1999.
32. Pharmacia & Upjohn. Detrol (tolterodine) package insert, Kalamazoo, MI, March 1998.
33. Pharmacia & Upjohn. Detrol (tolterodine). Data on file. Kalamazoo, MI, 1998.
34. Appell RA. Clinical efficacy and safety of tolterodine in the treatment of overactive bladder: A pooled analysis. Urology 1997;50(suppl 6A): 90–96.
35. Chancellor M, Freedman S, Mitcheson HD, Antoci J, Primus G, Wein A. Tolterodine, an effective and well tolerated treatment for urge incontinence and other overactive bladder symptoms. Clin Drug Invest 2000;19:83–91.
36. Rentzhog L, Stanton SL, Cardozo L, Nelson E, Fall M, Abrams P. Efficacy and safety of tolterodine in patients with detrusor instability: A dose-ranging study. Br J Urol 1998;81:42–48.
37. Millard R, Tuttle J, Moore K, et al. Clinical efficacy and safety of tolterodine compared to placebo in detrusor overactivity. J Urol 1999;161: 1551–1555.
38. Appell RA, Sand P, Dmochowski R, et al. Prospective randomized controlled trial of extended-release oxybutynin chloride and tolterodine tartrate in the treatment of overactive bladder: Results of the OBJECT study. Mayo Clin Proc 2001;76:358–363.
39. Van Kerrebroeck P, Kreder K, Jonas U, et al. Tolterodine once daily: Superior efficacy and tolerability in the treatment of the overactive bladder. Urology 2001;57:414–421.
40. Nilsson CG, Lukkari E, Haarala M, Kivela A, Hakonen T, Kiilholma P. Comparison of a 10-mg controlled release oxybutynin tablet with a 5-mg oxybutynin tablet in urge incontinent patients. Neurourol Urodyn 1997;16:533–542.
41. Birns J, Malone Lee JG, and the Oxybutynin CR Study Group. Controlled-release oxybutynin maintains efficacy with a 43% reduction in side effects compared with conventional oxybutynin treatment. Neurourol Urodyn 1997;16:429–430.
42. Anderson RU, Mobley D, Blank B, et al. Once daily controlled versus immediate-release oxybutynin chloride for urge urinary incontinence. OROS Oxybutynin Study Group. J Urol 1999;161:1809–1812.
43. Katz IR, Sands LP, Bilker E, et al. Identification of medications that cause cognitive impairment in older people: The case of oxybutynin chloride. J Am Geriatr Soc 1998;46:8–13.
44. Hughes KM, Lang JCT, Lazare R, et al. Measurement of oxybutynin and its *N*-desethyl metabolite in plasma and its application to pharmacokinetic studies in young, elderly and frail elderly volunteers. Xenobiotica 1992;22:859–869.
45. Amarenco G, Marquis P, McCarthy C, Richard F. Efficacy of oxybutynin on health related quality of life (HRQL) in 1701 women suffering from urinary urge incontinence (UUI). Eur Urol 1998;33(suppl 1):32–38.
46. ALZA Corporation. Ditropan XL (oxybutynin chloride) extended-release tablets package insert. Palo Alto, CA, 1999.

47. Paine MF, Khalighi M, Fisher JM, et al. Characterisation of interintestinal and intraintestinal variations in human CYP3A-dependent metabolism. J Pharmacol Exp Ther 1997;283:1552–1562.
48. Gupta SK, Sathyan G. Pharmacokinetics of an oral once-a-day controlled-release oxybutynin formulation compared with immediate-release oxybutynin. J Clin Pharmacol 1999;39:289–296.
49. Buyse G, Waldeck K, Ver C, Bjork H, Casaer P, Andersson K-E. Intravesical oxybutynin for neurogenic bladder: Less systemic side effects due to reduced first-pass metabolism. J Urol 1998;160:892–896.
50. Gleason DM, Susset J, White C. Evaluation of a new once-daily formulation of oxybutynin for the treatment of urinary urge incontinence. Urology 1999;54:420–423.
51. Susset JG, Gleason DM, White CF, et al. Open-label safety and dose conversion/determination of once-daily OROS oxybutynin chloride for urge urinary incontinence. J Urol 1998;159(suppl):36.
52. Moore KH, Hay DM, Imrie AE, Watson A, Goldstein M. Oxybutynin hydrochloride (3 mg) in the treatment of women with idiopathic detrusor instability. Br J Urol 1990;66:479–485.
53. Michalets EL. Update: Clinically significant cytochrome P-450 drug interactions. Pharmacotherapy 1998;18:84–112.
54. Jonas U, Hofner K, Madersbacher H. Efficacy and safety of two doses of tolterodine versus placebo in patients with detrusor overactivity and symptoms of frequency, urge incontinence, and urgency: Urodynamic evaluation. World J Urol 1997;15:144–151.
55. Owens RG, Karram MM. Comparative tolerability of drug therapies used to treat incontinence and enuresis. Drug Saf 1998;2:123–139.
56. Milner G, Hills NF. A double-blind assessment of antidepressants in the treatment of 212 enuretic patients. Med J Aust 1968;1:943–947.
57. Castleden CM, George CF, Renwick AG, Asher MJ. Imipramine—A possible alternative to current therapy for urinary incontinence in the elderly. J Urol 1981;125:318–320.
58. Lose G, Jorgenson L, Thuriedborg P. Doxepin in the treatment of female detrusor overactivity: A randomized double-blind crossover study. J Urol 1989;142:1042–1026.
59. Deguecker J. Drug treatment of urinary incontinence in the elderly: Controlled trial with vasopressin and propantheline bromide. Geront Clinica 1965;7:311–317.
60. Zorzitto ML, Jewett MAS, Fernie GR, et al. Effectiveness of propantheline bromide in the treatment of geriatric patients with detrusor instability. Neurourol Urodyn 1986;5:133–140.
61. Blaivas JG, Labib AB, Michalik SJ, Zayed AAH. Cystometric response to propantheline in detrusor hyperreflexia: Therapeutic implications. J Urol 1980;124:259–262.
62. Holmes DM, Montz FJ, Stanton SL. Oxybutynin versus propantheline in the management of detrusor instability: A patient-regulated variable dose trial. Br J Obstet Gynaecol 1989;96:607–612.
63. Thuroff JW, Bunke B, Ebner A, et al. Randomized, double-blind, multicentre trial on treatment of frequency, urgency and incontinence related to detrusor hyperactivity: Oxybutynin versus propantheline versus placebo. J Urol 1991;145:813–817.
64. Beck RP, Arnusch D, King C. Results in treating 210 patients with detrusor overactivity incontinence of urine. Am J Obstet Gynecol 1976;125:593–596.
65. Castleden CM, Duffin HM, Millar AW. Dicyclomine hydrochloride in detrusor instability: A controlled clinical pilot study. J Clin Exp Gerontol 1987;9:265–270.
66. Schreiter F, Fuchs P, Stockamp K. Estrogenic sensitivity of α-receptors in the urethral musculature. Urol Int 1976;31:13–19.
67. Makinen JI, Pitkanen YA, Salmi TA, Gronroos M, Rinne R, Paakkari I. Transdermal estrogen for female stress urinary incontinence in postmenopause. Maturitas 1995;22:233–238.
68. Bergman A, Karram MM, Bhatia NN. Changes in urethral cytology following estrogen administration. Gynecol Obstet Invest 1990;29:211–213.
69. Hilton P, Stanton SL. The use of intravaginal oestrogen cream in genuine stress incontinence. Br J Obstet Gynecol 1983;90:940–944.
70. Bhatia NN, Bergman A, Karram MM. Effects of estrogen on urethral function in women with urinary incontinence. Am J Obstet Gynecol 1989;160:176–181.
71. Ouslander JG, Cooper E, Godley D. Estrogen treatment for incontinence in frail older women. J Am Geriatr Soc 1999;47:1383–1384. Letter.
72. Sartori MGF, Baracat EC, Girao MJBC, Goncalves WJ, Sartori JP, Rodrigues de Lima G. Menopause genuine stress urinary incontinence treated with conjugated estrogens plus progestogens. Int J Gynecol Obstet 1995;49:165–169.
73. Jameson RM. The medical treatment of stress incontinence. Br J Clin Prac 1969;23:457–459.
74. Musiani U. A partially successful attempt at medical treatment of urinary-stress incontinence in women. Urol Int 1972;27:405–410.
75. Faber P, Heidenreich J. Treatment of stress incontinence with estrogen in postmenopausal women. Urol Int 1977;32:221–223.
76. Molander U, Milsom I, Ekelund P, Arvidsson L, Ericksson O. A health care program for the investigation and treatment of elderly women with urinary incontinence and related urogenital symptoms. Acta Obstet Gynecol Scand 1991;70:137–142.
77. Rud T. The effects of estrogens and gestagens on the urethral pressure profile in urinary continent and stress incontinent women. Acta Obstet Gynecol Scand 1980;59:265–270.
78. Salmon UJ, Walter RI, Geist SH. The use of estrogens in the treatment of dysuria and incontinence in postmenopausal women. Am J Obstet Gynecol 1941;42:845–851.
79. Iosif CS. Effects of protracted administration of estriol on the lower genitourinary tract in postmenopausal women. Arch Gynecol Obstet 1992;251:115–120.
80. Samsioe G, Jansson I, Mellstrom D, Svanborg A. Occurrence, nature, and treatment of urinary incontinence in a 70-year-old female population. Maturitas 1985;7:335–342.
81. Wilson PD, Faragher B, Butler B, Bu'Lock D, Robinson EL, Brown ADG. Treatment with oral piperazine oestrone sulphate for genuine stress incontinence in postmenopausal women. Br J Obstet Gynecol 1987;94:568–574.
82. Jackson S, Shepherd A, Brookes S, Abrams P. The effect of oestrogen supplementation on post-menopausal urinary stress incontinence: A double-blind placebo-controlled trial. Br J Obstet Gynecol 1999;106:711–718.
83. Jackson S, Shepherd A, Abrams P. Does oestrogen supplementation improve the symptoms of postmenopausal urinary stress incontinence? Neurourol Urodyn 1997;16:350–351. Abstract.
84. Diokno AC, Taub M. Ephedrine in treatment of urinary incontinence. J Urol 1975;5:624–625.
85. Diernaes E, Rix P, Sorensen T, Alexander N. Norfenefrine in the treatment of female stress incontinence assessed by one-hour pad weighing test. Urol Int 1989;44:28–31.
86. Lose G, Lindholm P. Clinical and urodynamic effects of norfenefrine in women with stress incontinence. Urol Int 1984;39:298–302.
87. Awad SA, Downie JW, Kiruluta HG. Alpha-adrenergic agents in urinary disorders of the proximal urethra. Part I. Sphincteric incontinence. Br J Urol 1978;50:332–335.
88. Stewart BH, Banowsky LHW, Montague DK. Stress incontinence: Conservative therapy with sympathomimetic drugs. J Urol 1976;115:558–559.
89. Jonas D. Treatment of female stress incontinence with midodrine: A preliminary report. J Urol 1977;118:980–982.
90. Kernan WN, Viscoli CM, Brass LM, et al. Phenylpropanolamine and the risk of hemorrhagic stroke. N Engl J Med 2000;343:1826–1832.
91. Fleming GA. The FDA, regulation, and the risk of stroke. N Engl J Med 2000;343:1886–1887. Editorial.
92. Collste L, Lindskog M. Phenylpropanolamine in treatment of female stress urinary incontinence. Urology 1987;30:398–403.
93. Fossberg E, Beisland HO, Lundgren RA. Stress incontinence in females: Treatment with phenylpropanolamine. Urol Int 1983;38:293–299.
94. Lose G, Rix P, Diernaes E, Alexander N. Norfenefrine in the treatment of female stress incontinence. Urol Int 1988;43:11–15.
95. Ek A, Andersson K-E, Gullberg B, Ulmsten U. The effects of long-term treatment with norephedrine on stress incontinence and urethral closure pressure profile. Scand J Urol Nephrol 1978;12:105–110.

96. Ahlstrom K, Sandahl B, Sjoberg B, Ulmsten U, Stormby N, Lindskog M. Effect of combined treatment with phenylpropanolamine and estriol, compared with estriol treatment alone, in postmenopausal women with stress urinary incontinence. Gynecol Obstet Invest 1990;30:37–43.
97. Kinn A-C, Lindskog M. Estrogens and phenylpropanolamine in combination for stress urinary incontinence in postmenopausal women. Urology 1988;32:273–280.
98. Ek A, Andersson K-E, Gullberg B, Ulmsten U. Effects of oestradiol and combined norephedrine and oestradiol treatment on female stress incontinence. Zbl Gynakol 1980;102:839–844.
99. Kiesswetter H, Hennrich F, Englisch M. Clinical and urodynamic assessment of pharmacologic therapy of stress incontinence. Urol Int 1983;38:58–63.
100. Beisland HO, Fossberg E, Moer A, Sander S. Urethral sphincteric insufficiency in postmenopausal females: Treatment with phenylpropanolamine and estriol separately and in combination. Urol Int 1984;39:211–216.
101. Lin H-H, Sheu B-C, Lo M-C, Huang S-C. Comparison of treatment outcomes of imipramine for female genuine stress incontinence. Br J Obstet Gynecol 1999;106:1089–1092.
102. Gilja I, Radej M, Kovacic M, Parazajder J. Conservative treatment of female stress incontinence with imipramine. J Urol 1984;132:909–911.
103. Gleason DM, Reilly RJ, Bottaccini MR, Pierce MJ. The urethral continence zone and its relation to stress incontinence. J Urol 1974;112:81–88.
104. Urinary Incontinence Guideline Panel. Urinary Incontinence in Adults: Clinical Practice Guideline. AHCPR Pub. No. 92–0038. Rockville, MD, Agency for Health Care Policy and Research., Public Health Service, U.S. Department of Health and Human Services, March 1992.
105. Klutke CG, Tiemann DD, Nadler RB, Andriole GL. Early results with antegrade collagen injection for post-radical prostatectomy stress urinary incontinence. J Urol 1996;156:1703–1706.
106. Litwillwer SE, Kim KB, Fone PD, DeVere White RW, Stone AR. Post-prostatectomy incontinence and the artificial urinary sphincter: A long-term study of patient satisfaction and criteria for success. J Urol 1996;156:1975–1980.

87

FUNCTION AND EVALUATION OF THE IMMUNE SYSTEM

Philip D. Hall and Janet L. Karlix

Knowledge of the immune system has expanded rapidly over the past decade, enabling a better understanding of normal immune system function as well as an identification of the role of immune system dysfunction in a multitude of disease states. To evaluate the immune system adequately in disease processes, it is vital to understand normal immune function and to recognize immune dysfunction. This chapter presents first an overview of the immune system and then a discussion of the evaluation of immune function in the clinical setting. The term *immune system* encompasses a wide range of components, including mechanical immunodefenses, soluble mediators, and cellular and humoral immune responses. Cells involved in the immune response from granulocytes to antigen-presenting cells to lymphocytes develop from a common pluripotent stem cell. Please refer to Chap. 98 for a review of normal hematopoiesis. The section illustrating immune function also will focus on laboratory examinations commonly available in clinical settings or likely to be available in the near future.

The immune system primarily serves to protect the body against infectious pathogens. To accomplish this task, the immune system exhibits specificity, memory, mobility, and replicability. *Specificity* indicates that the immune system can distinguish between non-cross-reacting antigens. *Memory* allows a quicker and more vigorous response to a subsequent pathogenic invasion. Because elements of the immune system are *mobile,* local reactions may provide systemic protection. All cellular components of the immune system can *replicate,* allowing the immune response to be amplified.[1] In addition, the immune response normally distinguishes "self" from "nonself" to prevent damage to the host. This discrimination between self and nonself is done by the adaptive or specific arm of the immune response. The immune system commonly is separated into two functional divisions: innate (nonspecific) and adaptive (specific)[2] (Table 87–1). Despite this simple separation, these divisions interact heavily.

The *innate* arm provides the first line of defense against pathogens. One of the most frequently overlooked methods of host defense is the body's ability to provide a physical and chemical defense against invading pathogens. The skin, the largest organ of the body, has the primary role of providing this physical defense. Alterations in the skin, such as burns or abrasions, allow an easier route of entry for pathogens. The gastrointestinal tract also plays an important role in providing a physical defense against pathogenic invasion. The low pH of the stomach (pH 1–2) kills many organisms. The constant sloughing of intestinal cells also limits systemic infection because infected cells are replaced frequently. Drugs, such as cell cycle-specific antineoplastic agents, that disrupt the sloughing process leave the patient at an increased risk of infection. Likewise, the respiratory tract has its forms of physical defense, the cilia lining the epithelium of the lungs helping to repel inhaled organisms. Mucus that coats the epithelial cells serves in part to prevent microorganisms from adhering to cell surfaces. The combination of cilia, mucus, and coughing provides a natural barrier to invasion via the respiratory tract. Other examples of mechanical or nonspecific defenses include normal urine flow, lysozymes in tears and saliva, and the normal flora in the throat, the lower gastrointestinal tract, and the genitourinary tract. It is these physical and chemical defenses that often form the first line of defense against infectious pathogens. It is well known that conditions or devices that allow microorganisms to transgress these normal barriers predispose patients to infections. As such, patients with a substantial loss of the skin from a burn or those requiring mechanical ventilation, bladder catheterization, or central venous access are at increased risk of infection.

THE IMMUNE RESPONSE

When an infectious pathogen eludes the physical defenses of the body, an immune response involving both soluble mediators and leukocytes is then generated against the pathogen.

INNATE RESPONSE

Innate immunity is present from birth and involves the stimulation of cells that nonspecifically recognize foreign invaders and destroy them. The innate leukocytes are monocytes, macrophages, neutrophils, basophils, mast cells, and eosinophils. All except basophils act as phagocytes, whereas mast cells and basophils secrete inflammatory mediators when stimulated. The phagocytes recognize, internalize, and destroy invading pathogens. These cells use either opsonin-dependent or opsonin-independent phagocytosis. For opsonin-dependent phagocytosis, complement or antibodies coat infectious pathogens in a process termed *opsonization,* and then the antibody or complement binds to the receptors on the innate leukocyte (Fig. 87–1), thereby activating the phagocytic process. For opsonin-independent phagocytosis, receptors on phagocytes (e.g., macrophage scavenger receptors or macrophage mannose receptors) directly recognize ligands (e.g., lipoteichoic acid from gram-positive organisms, lipopolysaccharide from gram-negative organisms, or mannoses) on the surfaces of infectious pathogens[3] (see Fig. 87–1).

The granulocytes of the body include neutrophils, eosinophils, and basophils. The cytoplasmic granules of these cells often contain inflammatory mediators or digestive enzymes. Neutrophils are polymorphonuclear cells, often denoted as PMNs for this reason, which serve as the primary human defense against pathogenic bacteria and comprise the majority of leukocytes in the bloodstream. Neutrophils respond to chemotactic factors, such as interleukin (IL)-8 and C3a and

TABLE 87–1. Functional Divisions of the Immune System

	Innate	Adaptive
Physical barriers	Skin and mucous membranes	None
Specificity	None	Yes
Memory	No	Yes
Soluble factors	Lysozymes, complement, acute-phase proteins	Antibodies, cytokines
Cells	Neutrophils, monocytes, macrophages, NK[a] cells, eosinophils	B-lymphocytes, T-lymphocytes

[a]NK = natural killer.
From Ref. 42, with permission.

C5a, breakdown products of complement, that are released from infected or inflamed tissue. Neutrophils migrate to sites of infection in a process termed *chemotaxis,* whereupon they recognize, adhere to, and phagocytize pathogens. Neutrophils can only recognize pathogens coated with either complement or immunoglobulin (Ig) G (antibody) via the complement and antibody receptors located on the surface of the neutrophil. Once bound, the neutrophil then releases its granular contents into vacuoles and generates the release of oxidative metabolites, thereby killing engulfed pathogens.[4]

Eosinophils are also granulocytic cells but have a minor role in combating bacterial infections. Patients with drug-induced neutropenia or other neutrophil deficiency states are not protected against microbial pathogens by eosinophils. However, eosinophils play a major role against non-phagocytable multicellular pathogens, such as parasites. After activation via high-affinity receptor for IgE (i.e., Fcϵ), granule exocytosis releases the granule contents (e.g., major basic protein) into the microenvironment to lyse the parasite. Eosinophils recognize pathogens coated by complement or IgE, a subclass of antibody. Because of their ability to bind IgE, eosinophils contribute to the pathogenesis of allergic disorders (i.e., asthma).[5]

Macrophages and monocytes are mononuclear cells also capable of phagocytosis. These cells also have the ability to release soluble factors with inflammatory properties. Monocytes are found within the bloodstream, whereas macrophages are found in the tissues. Tissue macrophages are believed to arise from the migration of monocytes. Macrophages differ from monocytes by possessing an increased number of Fc and complement receptors. Macrophages are found within specific tissues such as the liver, spleen, gastrointestinal tract, lymph nodes, brain, and others. These specific types of macrophages are often called *histiocytes* or are referred to by a specialized name depending on the site where they are found (e.g., Kupffer cells in the liver, osteoclasts in the bone, microglial cells in the central nervous system, etc.). The term *reticuloendothelial system* (RES) was used commonly to refer to macrophages found in reticular connective tissue; however, the preferred nomenclature is now the *mononuclear phagocyte system.*[6]

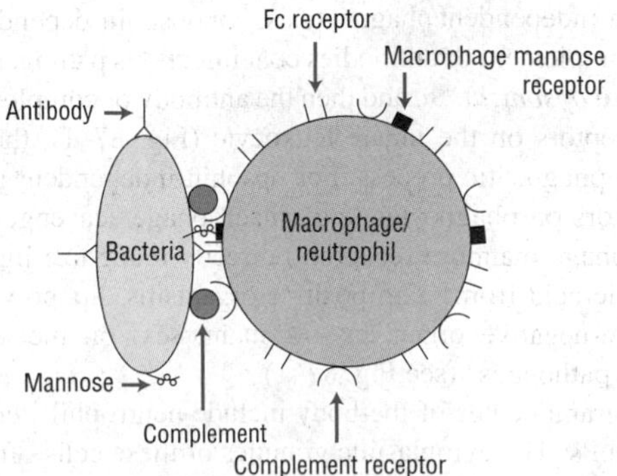

FIGURE 87–1. Phagocytosis of bacteria by macrophages and neutrophils. Macrophages and neutrophils recognize bacteria opsonized (coated) with antibody or complement. On the surface of the macrophages and neutrophils reside receptors for the antibody (Fc receptor) and complement (CR1, CR3, CR4). In addition, macrophages can directly recognize the large number of mannoses in the carbohydrates on the surface of bacteria via the macrophage mannose receptor.

Despite the first description of dendritic cells, Langerhans cells, occurring in 1868, our understanding of the biologic function of dendritic cells did not improve dramatically until the last decade. Before encountering a pathogen, most dendritic cells are in an immature/resting state with limited ability to activate T-lymphocytes; however, they express numerous receptors (e.g., Fc receptors of IgG and IgE and macrophage mannose receptor) to capture antigen. After taking up antigen, they dramatically increase their expression of major histocompatibility complex (MHC) class II, B7, CD40, and adhesion molecules. Dendritic cells then begin to migrate through the tissues toward lymphoid organs (e.g., spleen and lymph nodes) to present antigen to T-lymphocytes.[7]

In addition to phagocytosing pathogens, macrophages and dendritic cells act as antigen-presenting cells (APCs) to stimulate the adaptive (specific) system. Macrophages and dendritic cells internalize the organism, digest it into small peptide fragments, and then combine these antigenic fragments together with MHC proteins. Once the APC has formed the antigen-MHC complex, the APC places the complex on its surface. This surface complex is recognized by the T-cell receptor on the surface of a T-lymphocyte. Recognition of the antigen-MHC complex by the T-cell receptor is the first step in activation of

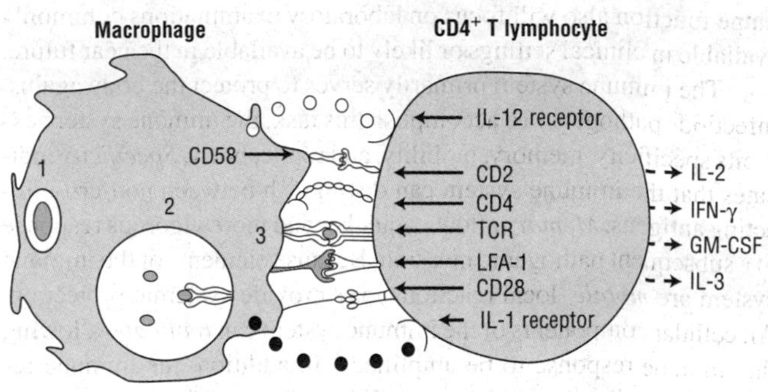

FIGURE 87–2. Macrophage presentation to CD4+ T lymphocytes. After phagocytosis of the bacteria by the macrophage (1), the bacteria is digested into small peptides and becomes associated with MHC class II within the endosome (2). Finally the MHC class II plus antigen is expressed on the surface of the macrophage (3). CD4+ T lymphocyte activation requires the T-lymphocyte receptor (TCR) to recognize the antigenic peptide plus MHC class II as well as the B7-CD28 interaction. IL-1 and IL-12 secreted by the macrophage also activates the T lymphocyte. The CD2-CD58 and LFA-1-ICAM-1 (adhesion molecules) interaction allows for adherence between the T lymphocyte and macrophage. Upon activation, CD4+ lymphocytes secrete numerous cytokines to up-regulate the immune response (IL-2, IFN-γ) and growth factors (IL-3, GM-CSF).

the T-lymphocyte (Fig. 87–2). Other cells, B-lymphocytes and mast cells, can act as APCs.[1,2,8]

Mast cells and basophils act primarily by releasing inflammatory mediators. Mast cells are tissue cells predominately associated with IgE-mediated inflammation. They are especially abundant in the skin, lungs, and nasal mucosa. Granules within the mast cells contain large amounts of preformed mediators that include histamine, heparin, serotonin, etc. Mast cells can phagocytize, destroy, and present bacteria to other immune cells. Basophils are similar to mast cells because they contain granules filled with histamine; however, they typically are found circulating in the blood and are not found in connective tissue. Like mast cells, basophils also express high-affinity IgE Fc receptors. IgE-mediated anaphylaxis [type I hypersensitivity (see Chap. 89)] is caused by the stimulation of mast cell and/or basophil degranulation, the release of preformed mediators, by allergen binding to IgE bound on the surface of mast cells or basophils.[9]

Soluble mediators of innate immunity include complement and C-reactive protein (CRP). The complement system consists of more than 30 proteins in the plasma and on cell surfaces that play a key role in immune defense. The four major functions of the complement system include (1) the ability to lyse certain microorganisms and cells, (2) the ability to stimulate the chemotaxis of phagocytic cells, (3) the ability to coat or opsonize foreign pathogens, which allows phagocytosis of the pathogen by leukocytes expressing complement receptors, and (4) the clearance of immune complexes. Complement factors (C3a, C5a) act as chemotaxis factors for phagocytic cells.[1,10]

Two different pathways stimulate the complement cascade. In the classic pathway, antibody binding to its target antigen or CRP binding to bacteria or fungi activates the first component of complement (C1), thereby initiating the complement cascade. Mannose-binding protein, an acute-phase reactant, binds to mannose-rich glycoconjugates on microorganisms and also can activate the classic pathway. The alternative complement pathway does not require the presence of a specific complement-fixing antibody but is stimulated directly by microbial cell walls. Patients with hereditary deficiencies of complement have recurrent bacterial infections.[1,10]

ADAPTIVE RESPONSE

In order to amplify the immune response, activation of the adaptive immune system is required. The adaptive immune response differs from the innate immune response in two critical areas: specificity and memory. T- and B-lymphocytes comprise the cells of the adaptive response. These cells have surface receptors specific for the invading organism. In a manner that uses genetic rearrangement of their DNA, it is estimated that lymphocytes have the ability to recognize over 10^{16} different types of antigens. Generally, the body will employ both the innate and adaptive immune responses to kill foreign pathogens.[1]

The adaptive immune response can be divided into two major arms: humoral or cellular-mediated. The B-lymphocytes and plasma cells, activated B-lymphocytes that secrete antibody, comprise the humoral arm of the adaptive immune response. The humoral response is so denoted because it was found that the factors that provided the immune protection could be found in the humor or serum. The cell-mediated arm is mediated by T-lymphocytes. The immune protection provided by these cells could not be transferred by serum alone. Rather, it is essential to actually have T-lymphocytes present; thus the term *cell-mediated immunity*. T-lymphocytes are specially tailored to defend against infections that are intracellular, such as virally infected cells, whereas B-lymphocytes secrete antibodies that can neutralize pathogens prior to their entry into host cells.

T-lymphocytes do not recognize intact antigen. T-lymphocytes recognize processed antigen in association with the MHC. APCs (e.g., macrophages, dendritic cells, Kupffer cells) phagocytize the pathogen, break down the pathogen, and then express peptide fragments of the processed antigen in association with the MHC on their surfaces. T-lymphocytes express a specific antigen receptor, T-cell receptor (TCR). The TCR is comprised of two chains, with each chain having a variable and a constant region. The variation of the amino acid sequence within the variable domain of TCR gives the cell its unique antigen specificity. Linked to the TCR is a complex of single chains known as the *CD3 complex*.[1,11]

Naive T-lymphocytes, cells that have not been exposed previously to antigen specific for their TCR, require two signals for activation. The first signal of activation involves the T-lymphocyte recognizing both the processed antigen and the MHC molecule complex. The second signal involves the interaction of the B7-1 (CD80) or B7-2 (CD86) molecule on the APC with the CD28 molecule on the surface of the T-lymphocyte (see Fig. 87–2). Without the second signal, the T-lymphocyte becomes *anergic* or *inactive*. Memory T-lymphocytes are less dependent on the second signal than are naive T-lymphocytes. CD28 is expressed on both resting and activated T-lymphocytes, whereas CTLA-4, a second ligand for B7 on T-lymphocytes, is expressed only on activated T-lymphocytes. CTLA-4 binding B7 transduces a negative signal, so its function may be to terminate T-lymphocyte activation.[12] After the two activation signals, a message is sent through the TCR to the CD3 complex into the cell. Then a calcium influx occurs with subsequent activation of the T lymphocyte. Activated $CD4^+$ T lymphocytes release various soluble factors (e.g., IL-2) to stimulate T-lymphocytes and other cells of the immune system (see Fig. 87–2) and to express high-affinity IL-2 receptor. Autocrine stimulation by IL-2 leads to the proliferation of the activated T-lymphocyte.

Cell surface markers or functional activity delineate T-lymphocyte populations. All T-lymphocytes express the CD3 protein. Typically, T-lymphocytes are further divided into helper cells ($CD4^+$), suppressor cells ($CD8^+$), and cytotoxic cells ($CD8^+$). Each of the subclasses appears to play a distinct role in the cell-mediated immune response. The primary role of $CD4^+$ cells is to stimulate other cells in the immune response. Based on surface markers, two subgroups of $CD4^+$ T-lymphocytes have been identified: helper/inducer ($CD4^+$, $CD29^+$) and helper/suppressor ($CD4^+$, $CD45RA^+$). The helper/inducer subtype amplifies the immune response and $CD8^+$ cytotoxic cells.[13] The helper/suppressor induces $CD8^+$ suppressor cells.[14] Functionally, $CD4^+$ cells can be divided into Th1 and Th2. This functional system was first described in mice. Th1 cells secrete IL-2 and γ-interferon and stimulate $CD8^+$ cytotoxic cells, whereas Th2 cells secrete IL-4, IL-5, and IL-10 and stimulate B-lymphocyte production of antibody.[15] This functional classification of $CD4^+$ T-lymphocytes is not as distinct in humans as in mice but has been well described in several disease states. For example, patients infected with human immunodeficiency virus (HIV) exhibit a shift from the normally predominant Th1 subclass to the Th2 subclass.[16]

$CD8^+$ suppressor cells downregulate the immune response once the pathogen has been destroyed. Obviously, continued activation of the immune response may not be beneficial to the host. Downregulation of autoreactive cells also may occur to prevent autoimmune disease. $CD8^+$ cytotoxic cells are instrumental in killing cells recognized as foreign, such as those which have become infected by a virus. These cells also play an important beneficial role in the eradication of tumor cells but also are responsible for rejection of transplanted organs. $CD8^+$ T-lymphocytes recognize antigen in association with MHC class I.

To fully activate the $CD8^+$ cytotoxic T-lymphocyte requires $CD4^+$ T-lymphocyte activation, namely, the Th1 subset, and its subsequent secretion of IL-2 (Fig. 87–3*A*). This model of $CD8^+$

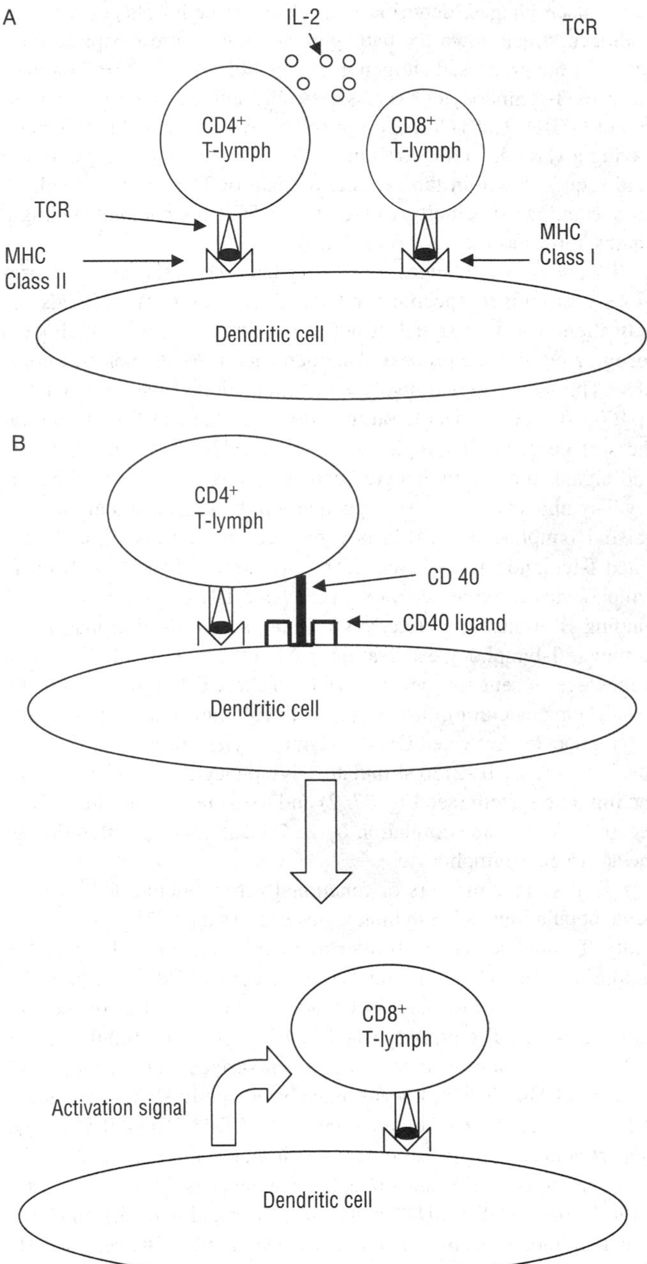

FIGURE 87–3. In the classic model of CD8+ T-lymphocyte activation (*A*), the CD4+ and CD8+ T-lymphocytes recognize antigen on the same dendritic cell. In the presence of IL-2 from the activated CD4+ T-lymphocyte and the recognition of antigen in association with MHC class I, the CD8+ T-lymphocyte becomes activated. In the new model (*B*), activated CD4+ T-lymphocytes activate dendritic cells via CD40 ligand binding to CD40. The activated dendritic cell then migrates through the tissues to present antigen to CD8+ T-lymphocytes. If recognition via the TCR on the CD8+ T-lymphocyte occurs, the dendritic cell can fully activate the CD8+ T-lymphocyte without the presence of CD4+ T-lymphocytes.

cytotoxic T-lymphocyte activation requires the close proximity of two rare-antigen-specific T-lymphocytes. In addition, some CD8+ cytotoxic T-lymphocyte responses can occur in the absence of CD4+ T-lymphocytes. New data suggest that CD4+ T-lymphocytes can activate/prime APCs through CD40. This interaction primes the APC (e.g., dendritic cell) to fully activate CD8+ cytotoxic T-lymphocytes[17] (see Fig. 87–3*B*).

Unlike neutrophils and macrophages, cytotoxic T-lymphocytes are unable to ingest their targets, so they destroy target cells by two different mechanisms: the perforin system and the Fas ligand pathway. After recognition by the cytotoxic T-lymphocyte, cytoplasmic granules containing perforins and granzymes are oriented rapidly toward the target cell, and the contents of the granules are released into the intracellular space. Like the membrane attack complex formed after complement activation, perforins form a pore in the target-cell membrane. Besides a direct cytotoxic effect on the target cell, the pores produced by perforins allow the granzymes to penetrate into the target cell to induce apoptosis. The second mechanism of cytotoxicity involves binding of the Fas ligand on the cytotoxic T-lymphocyte to the Fas receptor on the target cell. The Fas ligand is predominately expressed on CD8+ cytotoxic T-lymphocytes and natural killer (NK) cells, and its expression increases after activation. After killing by either mechanism, the cytotoxic T-lymphocyte detaches from the target cell and attacks other targets.[18]

B-lymphocytes recognize antigen via its associated antibody or immunoglobulin located on the surface of the cell. The antibody on the surface can recognize an intact pathogen, such as bacteria, and present antigen to T-lymphocytes (i.e., acting as an APC). However, the major function of B-lymphocytes is to produce antibody to bind to the invading pathogen, a process that first entails activation of the lymphocyte. The activation of B-lymphocyte also requires two steps: (1) recognition of antigen by the surface immunoglobulin and (2) the presence of B-lymphocyte growth factors (IL-4, -5, and -6) secreted by activated CD4+ T-lymphocytes. Once activated, the B-lymphocyte becomes a plasma cell, a differentiated cell capable of producing and secreting large quantities of antibody. A fraction of activated B-lymphocytes do not differentiate into plasma cells but rather form a pool of memory cells. The memory cells will respond to subsequent encounters with the pathogen and allow for a quicker and more vigorous response to the pathogen. Some B-lymphocytes can become activated without help from T-lymphocytes, but these responses generally are weak and do not invoke memory.[1,11]

When binding of a specific antigen to the surface immunoglobulin receptor of B-lymphocytes occurs, the B-lymphocyte matures into a plasma cell and produces large quantities of antibody that have the ability to bind to the inciting antigen. The secreted antibodies may be of five different isotypes. On primary exposure to the pathogen, the plasma cell will secrete IgM, but there is a switch to predominately IgG during the first exposure. On second exposure, the memory B-lymphocytes predominately will produce IgG. Isotype switching from IgM to IgG, IgA, or IgE is controlled by T-lymphocytes. Table 87–2 illustrates normal serum concentrations for the five different isotypes.[19]

An antibody or immunoglobulin is a glycoprotein comprised of two different chains, heavy and light (Fig. 87–4). The basic structure of every immunoglobulin consists of four peptide chains: two identical heavy chains and two identical light chains held together by disulfide bonds. The basic structure of the antibody is a Y-shaped figure. Each arm of the Y is formed by the linkage of the end of the light chain to its heavy-chain partner. These arms contain the portions described as the fragments of antigen binding (Fab fragment). The stem of the Y contains the heavy chains that comprise the fragment crystallizable (Fc fragment) portion of the antibody. It is within the Fc portion that complement is activated once the antibody has bound its target. Likewise, it is the Fc portion of the antibody that is recognized by Fc receptors on the surface of phagocytes (see Fig. 87–1). The amino acid composition of the same isotype is homogeneous except in the variable regions of the light (V_L) and heavy chains (V_H). The

TABLE 87–2. Five Immunoglobulin Classes in Humans and Their Characteristics

	IgG	IgA	IgM	IgD	IgE[a]
Serum conc. (mg/dL)	600–1200	140–260	70–120	0.3–30	0.002–0.2
Serum half-life (days)	23	6	5	3	2
Antibacterial lysis	+	+	+++	?	?
Antiviral activity	+	+++	+	?	?
Complement fixation	+	0	++++	0	0
Placental transfer	Yes	No	No	No	No
Location	Serum, amniotic fluid	Serum, colostrum, GI and respiratory tracts, saliva, tears	Serum	Serum, membrane receptor on B-lymphocytes	Serum

[a]IgE is involved in allergic response and parasitic infections; also measured in IU/mL, with a normal concentration range of 1–150 IU/mL.

variation in amino acid composition of the variable region gives the antibody its unique specificity (see Fig. 87–4).

IgG, the most prevalent of the antibody classes, comprises approximately 80% of serum antibody. IgG is usually the second isotype of antibody to be produced in an initial humoral immune response. IgG is the only isotype of antibody that can cross the placenta. Therefore, early maternal humoral protection of neonates is due primarily to maternal IgG that crossed the placenta in utero.

Four different subclasses of IgG have been described: IgG_1, IgG_2, IgG_3, and IgG_4. These subclasses differ slightly in their constant amino acid sequences. IgG_1 constitutes the majority (60%) of the subclasses. It appears that different subclasses recognize different types of antigen. IgG_1 and IgG_3 are responsible principally for recognition of protein antigens, whereas IgG_2 and IgG_4 commonly bind to carbohydrate antigens.[20] Other differences in the subclasses are the ability to activate complement, with IgG_3 and IgG_1 being the most efficient and IgG_4 unable to activate complement.

IgM can be found on the surface of B-lymphocytes as a monomeric Y-shaped structure. IgM, secreted from plasma cells, is a pentamer in which five of the monomers are joined together by a

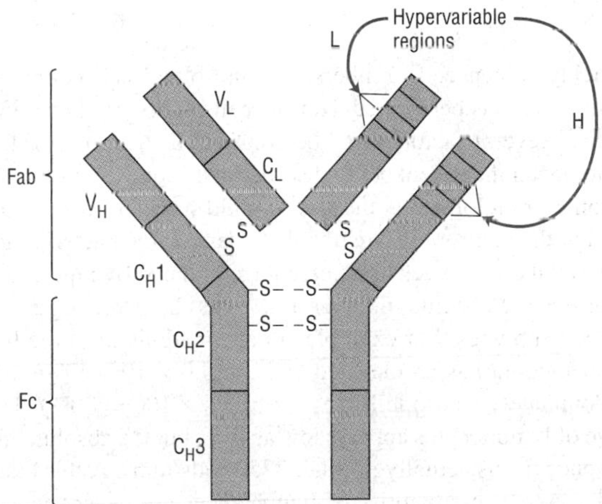

FIGURE 87–4. IgG molecule. Prototype of immunoglobulin molecule showing heavy (H) and light (L) chains, each with constant (C) and variable (V) regions, each of which has a hypervariable region. Antigen combines with antibody in the cavity formed by the hypervariable ends of H and L chains. These two chains are joined by disulfide bonds (S–S). Light chains consist of one variable (V_L) and one constant (C_L) region, whereas heavy chains consist of one variable (V_H) and three or four constant regions (C_H1 through C_H3), but IgE has an additional C_H4 region. Light chains and V_H and C_H1 make up the Fab region. The COOH ends of the molecules are in the constant regions, and the NH_2 ends of the molecules are in the variable regions. *(Reprinted with permission from JAMA 1992;268(20):2790–2796. Copyright © 1992, American Medical Association.)*

joining chain (J-chain). IgM is the first class of antibody to be produced on initial exposure to an antigen. Because the pentameric form of IgM has no Fc portions exposed, phagocytic cells cannot bind pathogens opsonized by IgM. However, IgM is an excellent activator of complement cascade by the classic pathway.

IgA is found primarily in the fluid secretions of the body, tears, saliva, and nasal fluids, as well as the gastrointestinal and respiratory tracts. IgA functions by preventing pathogens from adhering to and infecting the epithelial cells at these sites. IgA is also secreted in a nursing mother's breast milk, as are IgG and IgM in lower concentrations. In bodily secretions, IgA is in a dimeric form in which two monomers are held together by a J-chain and secretory chain.

IgD is the least understood isotype. IgD is found on the surfaces of B-lymphocytes at different stages of maturation and may be involved in the differentiation of these cells. The main function of circulating IgD has not yet been determined.

IgE is the least common of the serum antibody isotypes. Most of the IgE in the body is bound to the IgE Fc receptors on mast cells. When the IgE on the surface of mast cells binds antigen, it causes the release of various inflammatory substances (e.g., histamine) from the mast cell. The overall effect is the stimulation of inflammation. Asthma and hay fever are a few examples of allergic reactions due primarily to antigen binding to IgE.

NK cells, often referred to as *large granular lymphocytes*, are defined functionally by their ability to lyse target cells without prior sensitization and without restriction by the MHC. Resting NK cells express the intermediate-affinity IL-2 receptor, CD122. On exposure to IL-2, NK cells exhibit greater cytotoxic activity against a wide variety of tumors. NK cells recognize target cells by two mechanisms. First, NK cells express an IgG Fc receptor, CD16, that allows recognition of IgG-coated cells. Second, NK cells express killer-activating and killer-inhibiting receptors. The killer-activating receptors recognize multiple targets on normal cells; however, the binding of MHC class I to the killer-inhibitor receptor blocks release of perforins and granzymes. Therefore, cells (e.g., tumor cells and virally infected cells) that downregulate MHC class I expression are susceptible to NK cell cytolysis. NK cells play an important role in surveillance against tumors and virally infected host cells and in the regulation of hematopoiesis.[1,21]

MAJOR HISTOCOMPATIBILITY COMPLEX

The MHC, an association of genes found on chromosome 6 in humans, is also known as the *HLA complex*. The genes from this complex encode for molecules that play a pivotal role in immune recognition and response. The MHC complex is divided into three different classes: I, II, and III. The molecules encoded by class I HLA genes include HLA-A, HLA-B, and HLA-C antigens. These molecules can be found on all nucleated cells within the body as well as on platelets. Class I antigens are not found on mature red blood cells. Molecules encoded by class II HLA genes include HLA-DP, HLA-DQ, and HLA-DR molecules. The expression of these molecules is more restricted and can be found primarily on APCs such as macrophages, dendritic cells, B-lymphocytes, etc. The class III HLA antigens encode for soluble factors, complement, and tumor necrosis factors.

In order for a $CD4^+$ T-lymphocyte to become activated, it must recognize the antigenic peptide in association with MHC class II (see Fig. 87–2). $CD8^+$ T-lymphocytes recognize antigenic peptide in association with class I molecules. Class I molecules generally contain endogenous peptides from within the cell such as viruses, whereas class II molecules contain exogenous peptides from antigen that has been phagocytosized such as bacteria (see Fig. 87–2). For it to destroy a virally infected cell, a $CD8^+$ cytotoxic T-lymphocyte requires two steps. First, its TCR must recognize the antigenic fragment such as a viral protein in association with MHC class I. The second step involves the costimulatory step of B7-CD28 binding. Because any cell can become infected, it is advantageous that the $CD8^+$ cytotoxic T-lymphocyte recognizes the MHC class I molecule that is expressed on all cells except red blood cells. The ability of the MHC class I to present endogenous peptides allows the $CD8^+$ cytotoxic T-lymphocytes to constantly screen cells for infection.[22]

CYTOKINES

Research has shown that many of the cytokines have a broad spectrum of effects depending on their concentration, the presence of other factors, and the target cell. Cytokines orchestrate the complex homeostasis of cells and tissues by acting in both an autocrine and a paracrine fashion. For example, activated $CD4^+$ T-lymphocytes secrete IL-2 to activate itself as well as $CD8^+$ T-lymphocytes and NK cells. Cytokines, soluble factors released or secreted by cells, affect the activity of other cells or the secreting cell itself. Cytokines also can be membrane-bound (e.g., IL-1α) and require direct cell-to-cell contact. It is also important to remember that in vivo cytokines do not act alone but in combination with other cytokines. For example, activated $CD4^+$ T-lymphocytes secrete both IL-2 and interferon-γ that are synergistic in activating NK cells. As shown in Table 87–3, cytokines are broadly classified as regulatory or hematopoietic growth factors.[11,23–28] It should be remembered that this classification does not describe all their activities. Granulocyte-macrophage colony-stimulating factor (GM-CSF) released by activated T-lymphocytes acts as a hematopoietic growth factor but also activates granulocytes and macrophages to phagocytize foreign pathogens.

The division of the immune system into the two functional groups does not imply that the divisions do not interact. In order to generate a vigorous immune response, both soluble mediators (e.g., complement, antibody, and cytokines) and cells (e.g., neutrophils, macrophages, T-lymphocytes, and B-lymphocytes) are needed. Generally, the innate system will respond first. Macrophages and neutrophils in the tissues will recognize the opsonized pathogen (see Fig. 87–1). In order to amplify the immune response, the macrophages will present antigen to $CD4^+$ T-lymphocytes (see Fig. 87–2). The activated $CD4^+$ T-lymphocytes will then secrete cytokines to activate B-lymphocytes, $CD8^+$ T-lymphocytes, NK cells, macrophages, and neutrophils. The next section of this chapter will look at evaluating the immune system.

EVALUATION OF COMPONENTS OF THE IMMUNE SYSTEM

Assessment of a patient's immune function requires consideration of multiple components, including mechanical defenses, cell phenotypes and numbers, and soluble components. Recent developments in biotechnology have allowed extraordinary progress in characterization of immune function. Despite the technological advances, careful patient evaluations are required to properly identify patients with compromised immune systems. Specific methods for assessment of patient immune status are discussed below.

MECHANICAL AND NONSPECIFIC IMMUNODEFENSES

As discussed earlier, the mechanical aspects of host defense are extremely important in protection from infection; therefore, assessment of mechanical defenses is critical. Much of the assessment of mechanical immunodefense is accomplished by recognition of situations where it is compromised. Careful patient examination usually reveals the extent of compromise, and laboratory tests generally are not necessary for evaluation of this component. To evaluate the extent of compromise in mechanical immunodefenses, the clinician should examine the patient carefully and identify the specific types of risks present. Specific examples of altered mechanical defenses are listed in Table 87–4.

CELLULAR ASPECTS OF IMMUNE FUNCTION

A major aspect of the assessment of immune function relates to the cells of the immune system. Assessment of cells in the clinical setting includes determination of cell number, cell type, and/or function. Generally, quantification of the cell types and numbers is performed first because of its rapid turn-around and correlation with the clinical picture.

QUANTIFICATION

To quickly screen cell numbers, a white blood cell count (WBC) with differential is performed. Normal cell counts are shown in Table 87–5.[29,30] Several factors must be considered. A normal cell count does not mean that a leukocyte disorder does not exist. For example, in chronic granulomatous disease, a child has a normal neutrophil count, but the neutrophils are unable to destroy the bacteria. Second, a differential comes back as a percentage of the WBC; therefore, one must assess the absolute number as well as the percentage of white blood cell subtypes. For example, a patient admitted to the hospital with pneumonia has an elevated WBC (15.0×10^3 cells/mm^3) that is predominately neutrophils (segs + bands $\times$ 100 = 80%). The percentage of lymphocytes appears low at 15%, but the absolute number of lymphocytes is actually normal, 2250 cells/mm^3. A third factor to consider is that the majority of lymphocytes are in secondary lymphoid organs (e.g., lymph nodes and spleen), and changes in peripheral blood lymphocytes do not always mirror changes in the secondary lymphoid organs.[31] Additionally, most granulocytes, macrophages, and mast cells are in the tissues, not the bloodstream.

The numbers of granulocytes (i.e., neutrophils, basophils, and eosinophils) and monocytes generally are assessed by a WBC with differential. It has long been recognized that the lower the absolute neutrophil count, the greater is the risk of infection. Drugs (e.g., chemotherapy) and diseases (e.g., collagen-vascular disorders) may lower the neutrophil count and make the patient more susceptible to

TABLE 87–3. Cytokines

Cytokines	Sources	Principal Effects
Regulatory		
IL-1	Macrophages, fibroblasts, endothelial cells	Activation of T- and B-lymphocytes, hematopoietic growth factor, and induction of inflammatory events
IL-2	$CD4^+$ T-lymphs (Th1 subset)	Activation of T-lymphs, B-lymphs, and NK cells
IL-4	$CD4^+$ T-lymphs (Th2 subset), mast cells	B- and T-lymph growth factor, activation of macrophages, promotes IgE production, proliferation of bone marrow precursors
IL-5	$CD4^+$ T-lymphs (Th2 subset), mast cells	Activation of B-lymphs and eosinophils, promotes IgE production
IL-6	$CD4^+$ T-lymphs (Th2 subset), macrophages, mast cells, fibroblasts	T- and B-lymph growth factor, hematopoietic growth factor, augments inflammation
IL-8	T-lymphs, monocytes, endothelial cells, fibroblasts	Neutrophil and T-lymph chemotaxis
IL-10	T- and B-lymphs, macrophages	Cytokine synthesis inhibitory factor, growth of mast cells
IL-12	Macrophages, neutrophils, dendritic and Langerhans cells	Induce Th1, cells, ⇑ NK cell activity, ⇑ generation of cytotoxic T-lymphs
IL-13	Activated T-lymphs	Proliferation of B-lymphs, suppression of proinflammatory cytokines, directs IgE isotype switching
IL-14	T-lymphs	Induces B-lymph proliferation, inhibits secretion of Igs
IL-15	Macrophages, fibroblasts, epithelial cells	T-lymph proliferation
IL-16	$CD8^+$ T-lymphs, epithelial cells	Chemoattractant for $CD4^+$ T-lymphs and eosinophils; stimulation of secondary cytokine secretion from and proliferation of $CD4^+$ T-lymphs
TNF-α	Macrophages, NK cells, T-lymphs, B lymphs, mast cells	Activation of neutrophils, endothelial cells, lymphs and liver cells to produce acute-phase proteins
TNF-β	T-lymphs	Tumoricidal
IFN-α	Monocytes, other cells	Antiviral, activation of NK cells and macrophages, up-regulation MHC class I
IFN-γ	T-lymphs, NK cells	Activation of macrophages, NK cells, up-regulation of MHC classes I and II
Hematopoietic growth factors		
IL-3	T-lymphs	Maturation and differentiation of hematopoietic and mast cells
IL-7	Bone marrow stromal cells	Lymphopoietin
IL-9	T-lymphs	Maturation and proliferation of T-lymphs and mast cells
IL-11	BM stromal cells	Maturation of B-lymphs and megakaryocytes
G-CSF	Macrophages, endothelial cells, fibroblasts	Maturation and activation of neutrophils
GM-CSF	T-lymphs, macrophages, endothelial cells, fibroblasts	Maturation and activation of granulocytes, monocytes-macrophages, and eosinophils
M-CSF	Macrophages, endothelial cells, fibroblasts	Maturation and activation of monocytes/macrophages
Erythropoietin	Kidney, liver	Maturation of RBCs
Stem cell factor	Bone marrow stromal cells, hepatocytes	Activation of mast cells, early-acting growth factor for myeloid and lymphoid precursors
c-MPL ligand	Bone marrow stromal cells, liver, kidney	Lineage-specific growth factor for megakaryocytes (platelets)
FLT3 ligand	Bone marrow stromal cells	Early-acting growth factor; maturation of dendritic cells

infections. Patients with a neutrophil count below 1500 cells/mm^3 are considered to have neutropenia. Functional analysis of these cell types is rarely done in routine clinical practice. Patients with functional deficits in these cell types generally are referred to tertiary medical centers for evaluation and treatment.

A routine WBC with differential can determine the total lymphocyte count. Total lymphocyte count has been used as a measure of nutritional status because it changes rapidly with nutrient loss or repletion. This is a relatively gross measure of a patient's immune status, although it has been correlated with patient outcome and risk of infection. Quantification of specific lymphocyte subsets is also important in certain clinical situations.

The availability of monoclonal antibodies against lymphocyte cell surface markers (CDs) and the invention of flow cytometry have allowed specific quantification of lymphocyte subsets. These evaluations are valuable for assessment of patients with immune-deficiency states such as acquired immunodeficiency syndrome (AIDS) and leukemias, as well as for patients who have received organ transplants. They allow the detection of specific lymphocyte subsets such as $CD4^+$ and $CD8^+$ T-lymphocytes. Quantification of $CD3^+$ and $CD4^+$ cells is

TABLE 87–4. Examples of Alteration in Mechanical Immunodefenses That Result in Impaired Immune Status

Reduced gastric pH
Achlorhydria
Use of histamine-2 blockers and proton pump inhibitors
Patients with acquired immunodeficiency syndrome (AIDS)
Break in skin barrier
Burns
Surgical incision
Penetrating trauma
Vascular access devices
Impaired mucociliary function of the lungs
Smoking
Impaired esophageal or epiglottal function
Endotracheal intubation
Stroke
Recumbent position
Altered urine flow
Urinary stones
Anatomic deformities obstructing flow
Bladder catheter
Anatomic alterations of the heart resulting in turbulent blood flow and endocarditis

used to monitor OKT3 immunosuppression and in the clinical management of AIDS patients, respectively.

The principle underlying the determination of lymphocyte subsets is a characteristic cell surface marker (cluster designation, or CD) that distinguishes one subset from another. The CD is usually a protein or glycoprotein on the surface of the cell. Cells can be detected by monoclonal antibodies that bind to the specific CDs such as CD4 or CD8. The monoclonal antibodies have been bound to substances such as fluorescein or phycoerythrin dyes that fluoresce green or red, respectively, when exposed to light of a certain wavelength. This fluorescence then allows detection and enumeration of the lymphocyte subsets by a flow cytometer. The flow cytometer analyzes individual cells to determine their fluorescence (presence or absence of surface-bound antibody) as well as light scatter (to determine cell size). Flow cytometry can be used for leukocyte phenotyping, tumor cell phenotyping, and some types of DNA analysis. Some of the more common CD antigens and their respective cellular distribution are listed in Table 87–6.[32]

TABLE 87–5. Leukocytes in Adults

Cell	Absolute Count (Range)[a]	Percent (Range)
White blood cells	7.5 (4.5–11.0)	100
Neutrophils	4.5 (2.3–7.7)	60 (50–70)
Eosinophils	0.2 (0.0–0.45)	3 (0–5)
Basophils	0.04 (0.0–0.2)	1 (0–2)
Monocytes	0.3 (0.0–0.8)	4 (0–10)
Lymphocytes	2.1 (1.6–2.4)	32 (28–39)
T-lymphocytes	1.4 (1.1–1.7)	72 (67–76)[b]
CD4+	0.8 (0.7–1.1)	42 (38–46)[b]
CD8+	0.7 (0.5–0.9)	35 (31–40)[b]
B-lymphocytes	0.3 (0.2–0.4)	13 (11–16)[b]
NK cells	0.3 (0.2–0.4)	14 (10–19)[b]
CD4:CD8 ratio	1.2 (1.0–1.5)	

[a]Times 10^3 cells/mm^3.

[b]Percentage of lymphocyte subpopulations expressed as percentage of total lymphocyte population.

TABLE 87–6. Cluster of Differentiation (CD) Guide: Characterization of Human Leukocyte Antigens

CD	Predominant Cellular Distribution
CD1	Thymocytes, Langerhans cells
CD3	T-lymphocytes
CD4	Helper T-lymphocytes, monocytes, macrophages
CD5	T-lymphocytes, B-lymphocyte subset
CD8	Cytotoxic/suppressor T-lymphocytes, NK[a] cells
CD14	Monocytes, neutrophils
CD20	B-lymphocytes
CD25	Activated T-lymphocytes, B-lymphocytes, IL-2 receptor alpha chain (Tac)
CD29	CD4+ T-lymphocyte subset (helper/inducer)
CD33	Myeloid progenitor cells
CD34	Hematopoietic progenitor cells that include the stem cell
CD45RA	CD4+ T-lymphocyte subset (helper/suppressor), B-lymphocytes, NK cells
CD56	NK cells

[a]NK = natural killer.

FUNCTIONAL EVALUATION OF IMMUNE RESPONSE

IN VIVO

The most common in vivo assay of lymphocyte function is the delayed hypersensitivity skin test. This test specifically evaluates the presence of delayed-type hypersensitivity or memory T-lymphocytes. By injecting a small amount of test material, antigen to which the patient has been exposed previously, into the patient's skin, a visual assessment can be made of the patient's ability to react to the antigen.

When an antigen to which a normal patient has previously been exposed previously is injected into the skin, the area of the injection becomes infiltrated with lymphocytes within a few hours. In the next stage, additional lymphocytes and phagocytes (e.g., macrophages and neutrophils) infiltrate. The maximal intensity of the inflammatory reaction is 24 to 72 hours. This reaction is often referred to as *type IV hypersensitivity* (i.e., cell-mediated; see Chap. 89). In type I hypersensitivity, a positive skin reaction is evident usually within 15 minutes and always within 24 hours. Type I hypersensitivity involves the release of histamine from basophils and mast cells when antigen binds to the IgE on the surface of these cells.

There are a number of reasons that a patient will not react to an antigen injected intradermally. Most commonly, the patient may not have had a previous exposure to the antigen. Nonresponsiveness may occur from anergy, dysfunction of cell-mediated immunity, due to immunosuppression from drugs (e.g., corticosteroids, cyclosporine, etc.) or disease (e.g., AIDS, cancer, etc.). A small subset of patients may be genetically unresponsive to the antigen.

A delayed hypersensitivity skin test can be performed by two methods. In one method, the patient can be administered a dose of antigen at a time sufficiently preceding the skin test that the immune response can develop. Then the skin test with the same antigen is applied and extent of reactivity measured. The most common method is to administer a panel of five or six recall antigens. The most common antigens are *Candida*, coccidiodin, mumps, *Trichophyton*, and purified protein derivative of tuberculin (PPD). More than 90% of the population will show a positive reaction to two or more of these antigens. After injection of the recall antigens, the patient should be observed carefully for the occurrence of immediate reactions. Measurements in millimeters of induration and erythema at the site of injection should be taken 24, 48 and 72 hours after injection. A reaction is considered positive if the diameter of induration and erythema is 5 mm or greater. Reaction to even a single antigen indicates a functioning cell-mediated immunity. The degree of sensitivity relates to the area of induration.[32]

The accepted indications for delayed hypersensitivity skin testing include evaluation of immune disorders and chronic diseases that cause cellular immune dysfunction (e.g., uremia, cancer, AIDS, etc.), exposure to infectious pathogens (e.g., *Mycobacterium tuberculosis*), evaluation of nutritional status (because malnutrition can result in cellular immune deficit), and in some cases, assessment of immune senescence.

In vivo assessment of B-lymphocyte function involves immunizing the patient with a protein (e.g., tetanus toxoid) and a polysaccharide (e.g., Pneumovax) antigen to quantitate antibody response after immunization. After 2 to 3 weeks, the patient's serum is tested for antibodies specific for the immunized antigen. This test measures B-lymphocyte responsiveness to the inoculated antigens but is reserved for patients who are suspected to have impaired B-lymphocyte function.[32]

IN VITRO

There are a number of specific lymphocyte functional assays, but most of these assays are used in the research setting. Many of these assays are performed at most tertiary-care medical centers. One of these tests is the lymphocyte proliferation assay. In this assay, lymphocytes are obtained from a patient's peripheral blood and cultured in vitro. The cells are exposed to nonspecific mitogens such as pokeweed mitogen, phytohemagglutin or concanavalin A. Then the cells are incubated in growth media containing tritium-labeled [^{3}H]thymidine, a DNA precursor. In the presence of the mitogens, normal lymphocytes will be stimulated to proliferate. Proliferation results in incorporation of [^{3}H]thymidine, which can be measured on a β-scintillation counter. The patient sample would be compared with normal, healthy controls. Patients with immune deficiencies (e.g., AIDS, cancer, etc.) have fewer active or less active lymphocytes, as detected by this test.

A modification of the lymphocyte proliferation assay is used in allogeneic bone marrow transplantation to evaluate how closely a donor and host are "matched" in order to predict a patient's risk for graft-versus-host disease. A mixed-lymphocyte culture (MLC) assesses the potential of the donor cells to attack the host cells, graft-versus-host disease (see Chap. 134). In this test, donor cells and host cells are incubated in vitro. The host lymphocytes are irradiated prior to the incubation so that they cannot proliferate. In vitro, [^{3}H]thymidine is provided to the cells, and uptake is measured. The degree of uptake is related to proliferation of donor lymphocytes. If the cells are well matched, proliferation is minimal. If the cells are mismatched, proliferation will be noted, and the level of proliferation will be predictive of the potential extent of graft-versus-host disease.

In addition to the test just described, a number of other tests have been devised to evaluate the function of CD8$^+$ T-lymphocytes, NK cells, and monocytes-macrophages. Although these evaluations are not performed commonly, they may be helpful in some specific diseases. A thorough discussion of these tests is available.[33]

HUMORAL ASPECTS OF IMMUNE FUNCTION

The humoral components of the immune system (e.g., immunoglobulins, complement, and cytokines) are often assessed. Assays of humoral components may be either quantitative to determine the absolute concentration of the factor or qualitative to determine the function of the component.

IMMUNOGLOBULINS

The most common evaluation of immunoglobulins is the estimation of total immunoglobulin. This is obtained by subtracting the albumin concentration from the total protein concentration. This difference gives a gross estimation of the total immunoglobulin concentration. Actual determination of the total immunoglobulin concentration is done by serum protein electrophoresis (SPEP). Five separate zones are detected by this method: albumin, α_1-globulin, α_2-globulin, β-globulin, and γ-globulin. The γ-globulin fraction contains the five isotypes of immunoglobulin (i.e., IgG, IgA, IgM, IgE, and IgD). A normal total immunoglobulin or γ-globulin concentration ranges from 0.8 to 1.6 g/dL. This test is used to determine if patients have hypogammaglobulinemia (i.e., primary and secondary immunodeficiencies), a monoclonal peak (e.g., multiple myeloma or Waldenstrom's macroglobulinemia), or a polyclonal hypergammaglobulinemia (e.g., chronic inflammatory conditions such as systemic lupus erythematosus and chronic active hepatitis). Total immunoglobulin or γ-globulin concentrations cannot be used to measure antigen-specific antibodies or specific isotypes.

In a patient suspected of having humoral immune deficiency or B-lymphocyte failure (i.e., primary and secondary immunodeficiency), specific immunoglobulin isotypes in the plasma should be measured. These usually are determined by radial immunodiffusion or by rate nephelometry. Table 87–2 lists the normal concentrations of the different isotypes.

There are many indications for the measurement of antigen-specific antibody. Some common indications are listed in Table 87–7. The most common methods to perform these measurements include enzyme-linked immunosorbent assay (ELISA), radioimmunoassay (RIA), and radioallergosorbent test (RAST). The most common reason to measure antigen-specific antibody is to determine whether or

TABLE 87–7. Potential Indications for Measurement of Antigen-specific Antibody

Environmental or drug allergy
Exposure to or infection with bacteria
Streptococci (ASO titer)
Staphylococcus aureus (teichoic acid antibody)
Neisseria gonorrhoeae
Legionella pneumophila
Exposure to or infection with viruses
Human immunodeficiency virus
Cytomegalovirus
Epstein-Barr virus
Hepatitis A, B, or C
Rubella
Exposure to or infection with other pathogens
Syphilis
Lyme disease
Typhoid
Chlamydia
Immune disorders
Rheumatoid factor antibody, rheumatoid arthritis
Anti-nuclear antibodies, systemic lupus erythematosus
Platelet-associated IgG, idiopathic thrombocytopenia
Blood typing and crossmatching
Transplantation
HLA antibodies

not a patient has been exposed to an infectious agent. Generally, IgM antibodies directed against the pathogen indicate an active infection, whereas IgG antibodies directed against the pathogen indicates prior exposure. For example, in hepatitis A and cytomegalovirus infections, the presence of the IgM antibody against the virus supports the diagnosis of an active infection, whereas the presence of the IgG antibody signifies immunity to the virus. Initially, plasma cells produce IgM in response to an infection, but memory B-lymphocytes produce IgG. Therefore, IgG concentrations will go up in a second exposure, but IgM antibodies will be present during an active infection and shortly after recovery from the infection. Other uses of antigen-specific antibody include determining if a patient has had exposure and is likely to be protected from further infection (e.g., rubella virus) or to indicate adequate response to vaccination (e.g., hepatitis B).

Antigen-specific IgE is commonly measured in patients with allergies. Because the presence of antigen-specific IgE is related to clinical allergy, measurement of these antibodies can be helpful in diagnosing allergies and determining offending substances. A standard method for determination of allergen-specific IgE is the RAST. The basic technique involves adding the antigen of interest that is bound to beads or disks to the patient's serum. After precipitation and several washings, the antibody bound to the beads or disks is isolated. Finally, a radiolabeled antibody that binds to IgE is added. After further washings, the radiolabeled antibody bound to IgE, which is bound to the antigen on the beads or disks, is counted on a gamma counter.

Antigen skin testing is the preferred method to determine the presence of allergen-specific IgE. When it is produced, IgE binds to high-affinity IgE Fc receptors on basophils or mast cells. Contact of an allergen with the specific IgE on the basophil or mast cell surface causes activation of these cells and the release of inflammatory mediators (e.g., histamine). When this occurs systemically, it can cause anaphylaxis. When it occurs in a confined area such as the skin, erythema and induration are observed within a few minutes of allergen injection. This is the principle used for detection of penicillin allergy, as well as for environmental or food allergies. A positive skin reaction (5 mm or greater of induration) within 15 to 20 minutes is indicative of the presence of allergen-specific IgE.

IgG SUBCLASSES

There are four subclasses of IgG: IgG_1, IgG_2, IgG_3, and IgG_4 that make up 65%, 20%, 10%, and 5% of total plasma IgG, respectively. Concentrations of the subclasses are often measured in patients with primary and secondary immunodeficiencies. IgG_2 and IgG_4 deficiencies are associated with chronic infections. IgG_4 deficiencies are also associated with autoimmune disorders. ELISA can be performed to determine the IgG subclasses.

COMPLEMENT SYSTEM

The complement system consists of a group of over 30 different proteins involved in lysing and opsonizing invading pathogens as well as serving as chemotactic factors. Numbers following the letter C (e.g., C1, C2) name the various proteins of the complement system. A global assessment of the complement system is the CH_{50}. The CH_{50}, the total hemolytic complement test, measures the ability of the patient's entire classic complement system to lyse sheep red blood cells opsonized with antibody. This test does not provide an indication of the function of any specific complement component but is used as a screening test for any complement system defects. If a defect is found, individual complement proteins can then be evaluated by functional or immunochemical methods. Assessment of the complement system is important in patients suspected of having humoral immune deficiencies (i.e., recurrent infections).

Several disease states can alter complement concentrations. Systemic lupus erythematosus, rheumatoid arthritis with vasculitis, poststreptococcal glomerulonephritis, gram-negative infections, and subacute bacterial endocarditis are associated with a decrease in CH_{50} assay and various components of the complement system. The liver is the primary source of several components of the complement system (i.e., C2, C3, C4, and factors B and D); therefore, in liver failure, a decrease in complement levels is observed. Inherited complement deficiencies have been described in patients with systemic lupus erythematosus, recurrent gonococcal and meningococcal infections, Raynaud's phenomenon, and hereditary angioedema.[10,32]

CYTOKINES

Scientists have identified and cloned many of the various natural cytokines within the body responsible for altering immune function. Methods to detect levels of these cytokines within the blood have been developed. For nearly all the currently identified cytokines, commercial kits are available to measure endogenous and exogenously administered cytokines. ELISA and RIA are the most common methods to measure cytokines. ELISAs and RIAs are easy to run but measure immunoreactivity, not biologic activity. Bioassays measure biologic activity but are cumbersome and extremely variable. Therefore, most researchers prefer ELISAs and RIAs.[34,35]

We are still at the very early stages of interpreting the clinical relevance of endogenous cytokine concentrations. Not only is the immune system affected by cytokines such as IL-1, IL-6, and tumor necrosis factor α, but other systems (e.g., skeletal, endocrine, and central nervous system) are also affected. Measurement of cytokine concentrations may be important in evaluation of the immune system as well as other systems.

When administering cytokines in therapeutic trials, we may change not only the concentration of that particular cytokine but also the concentration of other cytokines. Several studies have demonstrated that the systemic administration of GM-CSF to patients increases concentrations not only of GM-CSF but also of tumor necrosis factor α, IL-6, macrophage colony-stimulating factor, and erythropoietin.[36,37] Secondary endogenous cytokine release should be taken into account when monitoring cytokine concentrations.

In the future, tissue concentrations as well as blood concentrations may be measured. For example, while many centers currently measure cyclosporine concentrations to estimate the potential for immunosuppressive effects, it may be more advantageous to monitor IL-2 concentrations. One of the primary actions of cyclosporine is the inhibition of IL-2 production. Furthermore, perhaps it would be beneficial to measure tissue concentrations of IL-2 in the transplanted organ to get a better estimate of the state of immunologic suppression.

SOLUBLE RECEPTORS AND RECEPTOR ANTAGONISTS

In addition to T-lymphocyte activation, important regulators in the pathophysiology of the inflammatory response are cytokine inhibitors. Two types of cytokine inhibitors have been described: (1) receptor-binding antagonists and (2) cytokine-binding proteins.[38]

The best characterized receptor-binding antagonist is the IL-1 receptor antagonist (IL-1RA). IL-1RA blocks the binding of IL-1 to its receptor by competing for the same binding site, but IL-1RA does not possess agonist activity.[39] Currently, IL-1RA is being investigated in several inflammatory conditions (e.g., rheumatoid arthritis). In an inflammatory response, there is a delicate balance of IL-1 and IL-1RA, with an excess of IL-1 leading to disease progression. It is estimated that only 5% of IL-1 receptors need to be bound by IL-1 to stimulate the cell.[40] This requires an excess of IL-1RA to block IL-1's activity and to modify the disease process. Preliminary results from clinical trials of IL-1RA in rheumatoid arthritis are encouraging.

Cytokine-binding proteins bind the cytokine before it is able to reach its target receptor. The cytokine-binding proteins may act to inhibit the cytokine's activity by preventing the cytokine from binding to its receptor, or the cytokine-binding protein also may serve as binding proteins that protects the cytokine from degradation.[38] The best characterized cytokine-binding proteins are soluble cytokine receptors. Several soluble cytokine receptors have been described both in vitro and in vivo, soluble IL-2 receptor (sIL-2R), sIL-4R, sIL-6R, sIL-7R, sIFN-γR, and soluble tumor necrosis factor receptors (sTNFRs).

Like IL-1, tumor necrosis factor α (TNF-α) plays a central role in the inflammatory response by increasing the expression of adhesion molecules in the tissues and stimulating production of proinflammatory cytokines (e.g., IL-2 and IL-8), prostaglandins, and nitric oxide. sTNFRs exist in two forms, 55 kDa (type I, sTNFRI) and 75 kDa (type II, sTNFRII). sTNFRs act primarily as inhibitors of tumor necrosis factor by preventing tumor necrosis factor from binding to the membrane-bound TNFRs.[41] Therapeutically, both monoclonal antibodies against tumor necrosis factor (e.g., infliximab) and sTNFRs (e.g., etanercept) have been evaluated in clinical trials to immunomodulate tumor necrosis factor. Both infliximab and etanercept are approved by the Food and Drug Administration (FDA) for the treatment of rheumatoid arthritis. Our better understanding of soluble receptors and receptor antagonists allows us to better mimic natural mechanisms for minimizing the toxicity of administering cytokines (e.g., IL-1, IL-2, TNF-α, etc.) as well as immunomodulation of various diseases (e.g., solid-organ transplant rejection, collagen-vascular disorders, sepsis, etc.).

SUMMARY

Our understanding of the immune system has increased dramatically over the last decade. An immune response encompasses dynamic events involving both immunologic cells (e.g., phagocytes and lymphocytes) and soluble mediators (e.g., complement, cytokines, and antibodies). A better understanding of the normal immune response allows us to investigate the pathophysiology of diseases where the immune response is inappropriate. All clinicians need a basic understanding of the immune system and a familiarity with parameters to monitor immune system function in order to refine the development of immunologic treatments for diseases ranging from diabetes mellitus to collagen-vascular disorders to cancer.

REFERENCES

1. Delves PJ, Roitt IM. The immune system (first of two parts). N Engl J Med 2000;343:37–49.
2. Male D, Roitt I. Introduction to the immune system. In: Roitt I, Brostoff J, Male D, eds. Immunology, 5th ed. London, Mosby, 1997: 1–12.
3. Medzhitov R, Janeway C. Innate immunity. N Engl J Med 2000; 343:338–344.
4. Lehrer RI, Ganz T, Selsted MF, et al. Neutrophils and host defense. Ann Intern Med 1988;109:127–142.
5. Weller PF. The immunobiology of eosinophils. N Engl J Med 1991; 324:1110–1118.
6. Seljelid R, Eskeland T. The biology of macrophages. Eur J Haematol 1993;51:267–275.
7. Banchereau J, Steinman RM. Dendritic cells and the control of immunity. Nature 1998;392:245–252.
8. Klein J, Sato A. The HLA system (first of two parts). N Engl J Med 2000;343:702–709.
9. Costa JJ, Weller PF, Galli SJ. The cells of the allergic response, mast cells, basophils, and eosinophils. JAMA 1997;278:1815–1822.
10. Walport MJ. Complement (two parts). N Engl J Med 2001;344:1058–1066, 1140–1144.
11. Delves PJ, Roitt IM. The immune system (second of two parts). N Engl J Med 2000;343;108–117.
12. Reiser H, Stadecker MJ. Costimulatory B7 molecules in the pathogenesis of infectious and autoimmune diseases. N Engl J Med 1996;335:1369–1377.
13. Morimoto C, Letvin NL, Boyd W, et al. The isolation and characterization of human helper inducer T-cell subset. J Immunol 1985;134:3762–3769.
14. Morimoto C, Letvin NL, Distaso JA, et al. The isolation and characterization of human suppressor inducer T-cell subset. J Immunol 1985; 134:1508–1515.
15. Romagnani S. Human Th1 and Th2 subsets: Regulation of differentiation and role in protection and immunopathology. Int Arch Allergy Immunol 1992;98:279–285.
16. Clerici M, Hakim F, Venzon DJ, et al. Changes in interleukin-2 and interleukin-4 production in asymptomatic, human immunodeficiency virus-seropositive individuals. J Clin Invest 1993;91:759–765.
17. Lanzavecchia A. Licence to kill. Nature 1998;393:413–414.
18. Liu CC, Young LHY, Young JDE. Lymphocyte-mediated cytolysis and disease. N Engl J Med 1996;335:1651–1659.
19. Feldmann M. Cell cooperation in the antibody response. In: Roitt I, Brostoff J, Male D, eds. Immunology, 5th ed. London, Mosby, 1997: 139–155.
20. Heiner DC. IgG subclass composition of intravenous immunoglobulin preparations: Clinical relevance. Rev Infect Dis 1986;8(Suppl 4):S391–395.
21. Lanier LL. NK cell receptors. Annu Rev Immunol 1998;16:359–393.
22. Klein J, Sato A. The HLA system (first of two parts). N Engl J Med 2000;343:702–709.
23. Basic components. In: Chapel H, Haeney M, eds. Essentials of Clinical Immunology. London, Blackwell Scientific Publications, 1993:1–32.
24. Oppenheim JJ, Ruscetti FW, Faltynek C. Cytokines. In: Stites DP, Terr A, eds. Basic and Clinical Immunology. Norwalk, CT, Appleton and Lange, 1991: 78–100.
25. Du XX, Williams DA. Interleukin-11: A multifunctional growth factor derived from the hematopoietic microenviroment. Blood 1994;83:2023–2030.
26. Zurawski G, de Vries JE. Interleukin-13: An interleukin 4-like cytokine that acts on monocytes and B cells, but not on T cells. Immunol Today 1994;15:19–26.
27. Trinchieri G. Function and clinical use of interleukin-12. Curr Opinion Hematol 1997;4:59–66.
28. Kennedy MK, Park LS. Characterization of interleukin-15 (IL-15) and the IL-15 receptor complex. J Clin Immunol 1996;16:134–43.
29. Hannet I, Erkeller-Yuksel F, Lydyard P, et al. Developmental and maturational changes in human blood lymphocyte subpopulations. Immunol Today 1992;13:215–218.
30. Bakerman S. White blood count and differential. In: Bakerman S, ed. ABCs of Interpretive Laboratory Data. Greenville, NC, Interpretive Laboratory Data, Inc., 1984: 444–447.
31. Westermann J, Pabst R. Lymphocyte subsets in the blood: A diagnostic window on the lymphoid system? Immunol Today 1990;11:406–410.
32. Fleisher TA, Tomar RH. Introduction to diagnostic laboratory immunology. JAMA 1997;278:1823–1834.
33. Rose NR, Friedman H, Fahey JL, eds. Manual of Clinical Laboratory Immunology, 3d ed. Washington, American Society of Microbiology, 1986: Chaps. 43–46.

34. Van Brunt J. Assaying cytokines. Biotechnology 1991;9:439–441.
35. Rabinowitz J, Petros WP, Peters WP. Cytokine kinetics: Clinical pharmacology studies complementing recombinant growth factor trials. Cancer Bull 1994;46:40–47.
36. Rabinowitz J, Petros WP, Stuart A, Peters WP. Characterization of endogenous cytokine concentrations after high-dose chemotherapy with autologous bone marrow support. Blood 1993;81:2452–2459.
37. Stehle B, Weiss C, Ho A, Hunstein W. Serum levels of tumor necrosis factor alpha in patients treated with granulocyte-macrophage colony stimulating factor. Blood 1990;75:1895–1896.
38. Heaney ML, Golde DW. Soluble cytokine receptors. Blood 1996;87:847–857.
39. Dinarello CA. The role of the interleukin-1 receptor antagonist in blocking inflammation mediated by interleukin-1. N Engl J Med 2000;343:732–734.
40. Eisenberg SP, Evans RJ, Arend WP, Verderber E. Primary structure and functional expression from complementary DNA of a human interleukin-1 receptor antagonist. Nature 1990;343:341–346.
41. Dinarello CA. Proinflammatory cytokines. Chest 2000;118:503–508.
42. Hall PD. Immunomodulation with intravenous immunoglobulin. Pharmacotherapy 1993;13:564–573.

88

Systemic Lupus Erythematosus and Other Collagen-Vascular Diseases

Jeffrey C. Delafuente

The collagen-vascular diseases are a heterogeneous group of diseases that can involve the musculoskeletal system, integument, and blood vessels. Each collagen-vascular disease has its own set of diagnostic criteria, although diagnosis can be difficult because of overlapping and nonspecific clinical presentations. The etiology of the various collagen-vascular diseases is often unknown, although the immune system usually is involved in mediation of disease. Therefore, pharmacotherapy usually includes anti-inflammatory agents with or without immunosuppressive drugs.

Although the prevalence of other collagen-vascular diseases may be greater than that of systemic lupus erythematosus (SLE) (e.g., polymyalgia rheumatica), SLE is discussed most extensively in this chapter because it is a major collagen-vascular disease with numerous clinical manifestations, its pharmacotherapy can be complex, and a plethora of data are available on the therapy of SLE. Since all the diseases discussed in this chapter have an immune-mediated pathogenesis, the therapeutic principles of SLE can be applied to other autoimmune collagen-vascular diseases. The collagen-vascular diseases discussed include systemic sclerosis, polymyositis/dermatomyositis, polymyalgia rheumatica, and systemic vasculitis; these were chosen because they are seen in general practice.

SYSTEMIC LUPUS ERYTHEMATOSUS

SLE is a fluctuating multisystem disease with a diversity of clinical presentations. Abnormal immunologic function and formation of antibodies against "self" antigens underlie the pathogenesis of SLE.

The term *lupus erythemateux* was first used in 1851 by Cazenave, a Frenchman who described an illness in a patient with manifestations occurring in the skin. It is not surprising that SLE was first recognized as a skin disorder because cutaneous manifestations constitute one of the most common clinical features of the disease. Further descriptions by Kaposi in 1872 and Osler in 1895 led to the concept of a multisystem disease as it became recognized that patients developed complications in other organ systems.[1,2]

The hallmark of SLE is the development of autoantibodies to cellular nuclear components that leads to a chronic inflammatory autoimmune disease. Recognition of SLE as an autoimmune disease of multisystemic nature led the American College of Rheumatology (ACR) to develop criteria for identifying lupus patients (Table 88–1). These criteria were developed in 1971, revised in 1982, and modified slightly in 1997. The criteria do not include all the clinical manifestations of the disease and are used primarily for distinguishing SLE from other collagen-vascular diseases.[3] If 4 or more of the 11 criteria are documented at any time in a patient's medical history, the diagnosis of SLE can be made with about 95% specificity and 85% sensitivity.[4] Although these criteria may be helpful, diagnosis requires additional serologic, immunopathologic, and clinical evaluations.

EPIDEMIOLOGY

The incidence of SLE in the United States is estimated to be 2 to 8 per 100,000 persons per year, with a prevalence between 20 and 60 cases per 100,000 persons.[5] International studies report similar ranges.[6,7] The disease occurs predominantly in women, with a reported female-to-male ratio approaching 10:1. This predominance is seen mostly in the 15- to 64-year age group.[6,7] The reported incidence in blacks in the United States is higher than in whites, including an earlier peak incidence in black females compared with white females.[5,6] Although the most typical SLE patient is a young adult woman, the disease can occur in people of any age or race and either gender.

ETIOLOGY

The etiology of abnormal autoantibody production and development of SLE is still unknown. Genetic, environmental, and hormonal factors all may play a role in loss of "self" tolerance and expression of disease. A popular theory is that autoimmune disease, such as SLE, develops in genetically susceptible individuals after exposure to a triggering agent, possibly something in the environment.[5,8]

Genetic analysis shows that at least three or four genes are required in the expression of lupus in humans.[9] Family and twin studies indicate a genetic predisposition for the development of SLE. For example, there is a 3- to 10-fold increase in SLE in monozygotic twins compared with dizygotic twins.[10] The risk in dizygotic twins is the same as that in first-degree relatives. Evidence indicates that major histocompatibility complex (MHC) genes, such as the human leukocyte antigen (HLA) genes, may be important in lupus. However, non-MHC-linked genes, such as complement receptor genes and immunoglobulin receptor genes, also may contribute to disease susceptibility.[11] Environmental agents that may have a role in induction or activation of SLE include sunlight (i.e., ultraviolet light), drugs, chemicals such as hydrazine and aromatic amines (found in hair dyes), foods, and infection with viruses or bacteria.[8,12] A number of viruses have been implicated as causative agents in genetically susceptible people, but much of the evidence is circumstantial.[13] Additionally, androgen may inhibit and estrogen enhance the expression of autoimmunity, and elevated circulating prolactin levels have been associated with lupus in males and females.[5,14]

PATHOPHYSIOLOGY

SLE represents a clinical syndrome rather than a discrete disease with a unique pathogenesis.[15] SLE has a large spectrum of symptoms and organ-system involvement. A major event in the development of SLE is excessive and abnormal autoantibody production and the formation of immune complexes. Patients may develop autoantibodies against multiple nuclear, cytoplasmic, and surface components of multiple

TABLE 88–1. Revised Criteria for Classification of Systemic Lupus Erythematosus[a]

Criterion	Definition
Malar rash	Fixed erythema, flat or raised, over the malar eminences, tending to spare the nasolabial folds
Discoid rash	Erythematous raised patches with adherent keratotic scaling and follicular plugging; atrophic scarring may occur in older lesions
Photosensitivity	Skin rash as a result of unusual reaction to sunlight, by patient history or physician observations
Oral ulcers	Oral or nasopharyngeal ulceration, usually painless, observed by a physician
Arthritis	Nonerosive arthritis involving two or more peripheral joints, characterized by tenderness, swelling, or effusion
Serositis	Pleuritis—convincing history of pleuritic pain or rub heard by a physician or evidence of pleural effusion or Pericarditis—documented by ECG or rub or evidence of pericardial effusion
Renal disorder	Persistent proteinuria greater than 0.5 g/day or greater than 3+ if quantitation not performed or Cellular casts—may be red cell, hemoglobin, granular, tubular, or mixed
Neurologic	Seizures—in the absence of offending drugs or known metabolic derangements, e.g., uremia, ketoacidosis, or electrolyte imbalance or Psychosis—in the absence of offending drugs or known metabolic derangements, e.g., uremia, ketoacidosis, or electrolyte imbalance
Hematologic disorder	Hemolytic anemia—with reticulocytosis or Leukopenia—fewer than 4000/mm^3 total on two or more occasions or Lymphopenia—fewer than 1500/mm^3 on two or more occasions or Thrombocytopenia—fewer than 100,000/mm^3 in the absence of offending drugs
Immunologic disorder	Anti-DNA; antibody to native DNA in abnormal titer or Anti-Sm; presence of antibody to Sm nuclear antigen or Positive finding of antiphospholipid antibodies based on (1) an abnormal serum level of IgG or IgM anticardiolipin antibodies, (2) a positive test result for lupus anticoagulant using a standard method, or (3) a false-positive serologic test for syphilis known to be positive for at least 6 months and confirmed by *Treponema pallidum* immobilization or fluorescent treponemal antibody absorption test.
Antinuclear	An abnormal titer of antinuclear antibody by immunofluorescence or an antibody equivalent assay at any point in time and in the absence of drugs known to be associated with drug-induced lupus syndrome

[a]The proposed classification is based on 11 criteria. For the purpose of identifying patients in clinical studies, a person shall be said to have systemic lupus erythematosus if any 4 or more of the 11 criteria are present, serially or simultaneously, during any interval of observation. *From Tan EM, Cohen AS, Fries JF, et al. The 1982 revised criteria for the classification of systemic lupus erythematosus. Arthritis Rheum 1982;25:1274; and Hochberg MC. Updating the American College of Rheumatology Revised Criteria for the Classification of Systemic Lupus Erythematosus. Arthritis Rheum 1997;40;1725, with permission.*

types of cells in multiple organ systems; this fact underlines the multisystemic nature of the disease.

Excessive autoantibody production results from hyperactive B-lymphocytes and Th2 helper lymphocytes. Multiple mechanisms may be involved in the development of hyperactive lymphocytes, including impairment of immune regulatory processes involving T-lymphocytes (suppressor T cells), cytokines (e.g., interleukins, interferon-γ, tumor necrosis factor α, transforming growth factor β), and natural killer cells. Many autoantibodies are directed against nuclear constituents of the cell and are called collectively *antinuclear antibodies*. Several antinuclear antibodies are important because their presence or absence may aid in the diagnostic and clinical evaluation of patients with SLE. The SLE patient usually has more than one antigen-specific antinuclear antibody in his or her serum and tissues.[16] These are antibodies against such nuclear constituents as double-stranded, or native, DNA (dsDNA), single-stranded or denatured DNA (ssDNA), and RNA. Four RNA-associated antigens frequently occurring in SLE are the Smith (Sm) antigen, ribonuclear

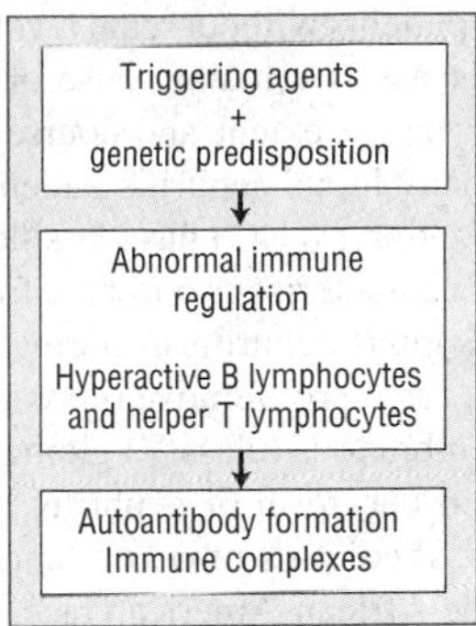

FIGURE 88–1. Pathogenesis of systemic lupus erythematosus. Environmental factors, such as infectious organisms, drugs, and chemicals, serve as triggering agents in genetically susceptible individuals to induce a state of immune dysregulation. These abnormal immune responses lead to hyperactive T helper lymphocyte and B lymphocyte function. Suppressor T lymphocyte function, cytokine production, and other immune regulatory mechanisms also are abnormal, and fail to downregulate autoantibody formation from hyperactive B lymphocytes. The autoantibodies formed from this immune dysregulation become pathogenic and form immune complexes that lead to damage of host tissue.

protein (RNP), Ro (SS-A) antigen, and La (SS-B) antigen. Histone, a basic component of chromatin and nucleosomes, is another important nuclear component against which antinuclear antibodies are formed in lupus patients.[2,17] Antibodies to Ro, La, Sm, or RNP antigens plus antibodies to dsDNA will detect most patients with SLE.[18]

Antibodies also may be directed against the phospholipid moiety of the prothrombin activator complex (lupus anticoagulant) and against cardiolipin. The lupus anticoagulant and anticardiolipin antibodies constitute the two main types in a group of autoantibodies called *antiphospholipid antibodies*.

Tissue damage ensues from inflammatory reactions most likely caused from immune-complex formation, complement activation, and lymphocyte and macrophage activation. An overview of the pathogenesis[19] of SLE is illustrated in Fig. 88–1.

TABLE 88–2. Clinical Signs and Symptoms of SLE and Incidence[20,21]

Sign/Symptom	Incidence (%)
Musculoskeletal	
Arthritis and arthralgia	42–79
Consitutional	
Fatigue	80–100
Fever	41–86
Weight loss	31–71
Mucocutaneous	55–85
Butterfly rash	10–61
Photosensitivity	11–58
Raynaud's phenomenon	10–34
Discoid lesions	9–29
Central nervous system	12–75
Psychosis	5–52
Seizures	6–26
Pulmonary	
Pleuritis	31–57
Pleural effusion	12–40
Cardiovascular	
Pericarditis	2–48
Myocarditis	8–40
Heart murmur	12–44
ECG changes	34–70
Renal	31–65
Gastrointestinal	
Nausea	7–53
Abdominal pain	8–34
Bowel hemorrhage (vasculitis)	1–6
Hepatomegaly	25
Splenomegaly	10–20
Hematologic	
Anemia	30–78
Leukopenia	35–66
Thrombocytopenia	7–30
Lymphadenopathy	10–59

CLINICAL PRESENTATION

As mentioned previously, SLE is a multisystem disease. Table 88–2 lists many of the signs and symptoms and incidences[20,21] in patients with SLE. Although certain of these may be more common than others, each patient presents differently, and the course of the disease is highly unpredictable. Furthermore, SLE is not static, and most patients have fluctuations or flare-ups during the course of the disease.

Nonspecific signs and symptoms such as fatigue, fever, anorexia, and weight loss are seen frequently in patients with active disease. Musculoskeletal involvement (e.g., arthralgia, myalgia, arthritis) is very common in SLE,[20,21] with arthritis and arthralgia frequently the chief complaint on initial presentation of the disease.[21] Joint involvement tends to be symmetric and may affect multiple sites. Objective evidence of musculoskeletal disease often is missing, although a few patients may present with deforming arthritis or subcutaneous nodules.

Manifestations in the skin and mucous membranes are nearly as common as those involving the musculoskeletal system.[20,21] The most well known of these is the butterfly rash, which occurs over the bridge of the nose and the malar eminences. The classic butterfly rash is seen in approximately one-half of patients and often is observed after sun exposure. In fact, photosensitivity is common to many SLE patients who present with cutaneous manifestations. Skin lesions characteristic of discoid lupus occur in 10% to 20% of patients with SLE and may occur without other clinical or serologic evidence of lupus.[20] Some individuals are said to develop *subacute cutaneous lupus erythematosus,* the nature of whose lesions falls between discoid (one type of *chronic cutaneous lupus erythematosus*) and the butterfly rash (an example of *acute cutaneous lupus erythematosus*).[22] Other cutaneous manifestations include vasculitis (which may be ulcerative), livedo reticularis, periungual erythema, Raynaud's phenomenon, and alopecia.

Another common source of symptomatology in SLE is the pulmonary system, with manifestations such as pleurisy, coughing, and dyspnea. Pleurisy may present as pleuritic pain, a pleural rub, or a pleural effusion that usually is exudative in nature. Lupus pneumonitis may present acutely with fever, dyspnea, tachypnea, cough, rales, and patchy infiltrates or chronically with interstitial fibrosis. Lupus pneumonitis is an uncommon manifestation of SLE and has a poor prognosis.[20,22]

Cardiac manifestations of SLE often present as pericarditis, myocarditis, electrocardiographic (ECG) changes, or valvular heart disease, including the classic cardiac lesion of Libman-Sacks endocarditis (nonbacterial verrucous endocarditis).[20,23] Coronary artery disease is occurring with increasing frequency as the life expectancy of SLE patients increases.[24] It is thought that the development of heart disease in these patients is multifactorial. Hypertension, obesity, and hyperlipidemia are common in patients with SLE. Corticosteroid therapy and underlying renal disease may be contributing factors in the development of these cardiac risk factors.[23]

Neuropsychiatric manifestations of SLE may present in a diversity of ways, including psychosis, depression, seizure, stroke, peripheral neuropathy, cognitive impairment, and others. Overt psychosis is seen in up to 12% of patients with SLE, and severe depression is thought to be related to the disease rather than to a reactive depression.[20]

Symptoms associated with gastrointestinal manifestations often are nonspecific for lupus and include dyspepsia, abdominal pain, nausea, and difficulty swallowing. Mesenteric vasculitis may be problematic, particularly if arterial perforations occur. Hepatomegaly may present in some patients, although liver dysfunction is not characteristic of lupus. Pancreatitis also may be present.[20]

HEMATOLOGIC MANIFESTATIONS

Anemia is found in many patients with SLE. It is usually an anemia of chronic inflammation, with a mild normochromic, normocytic smear and low serum iron but adequate iron stores. Some patients may develop a hemolytic anemia with a positive Coombs' test. Leukopenia, usually mild, is present in approximately half of SLE patients. Both granulocytes and lymphocytes may be affected, but there is usually a larger decrease in the amount of circulating granulocytes. The absolute number of both T-lymphocytes and B-lymphocytes decreases. Thrombocytopenia may occur in SLE and usually is caused by antiplatelet antibodies, resulting in phagocytosis by macrophages in the spleen, liver, lymph nodes, and bone marrow.[20,23]

Another significant finding associated with SLE is the presence of antiphospholipid antibodies such as the lupus anticoagulant (LA) and anticardiolipin antibodies. Although the LA is directed against the prothrombin activator complex and implies potential bleeding complications, this is not the case. In fact, the presence of LA, anticardiolipin, or other antiphospholipid antibodies may be associated with thrombosis, neurologic disease, thrombocytopenia, and fetal loss.[25,26] Thrombotic events occur in more than 10% of patients with SLE.[25] Not all patients with antiphospholipid syndrome have lupus. If a patient has no concomitant autoimmune disease, the syndrome is *primary*. If a patient has accompanying SLE, the syndrome is *secondary*.[27]

LUPUS NEPHRITIS

Clinical evidence of renal involvement, such as a rising serum creatinine or proteinuria level, generally is associated with a poorer outcome compared with patients without renal involvement. Progression to end-stage renal disease is a major cause of morbidity and mortality in SLE. However, the extent and course of renal disease are quite variable, and many lupus nephritis patients do very well. The World Health Organization (WHO) has classified lupus nephritis on the basis of histologic characteristics observed following renal biopsy. This system identifies lupus nephritis as normal (class I), mesangial, (classes IIA and IIB), focal proliferative (class III), diffuse proliferative (class IV), or membranous (class V) glomerulonephritis.[2] Many patients progress from one form of nephritis to another during the course of the disease. Predictors of poorer outcome in proliferative lupus nephritis include African-American race, increased serum creatinine level, poor initial response to immunosuppressive drugs, hypertension, and persistent nephrotic syndrome.[28]

DIAGNOSIS

As mentioned earlier, the diagnostic criteria listed in Table 88–1 should not be the primary means for diagnosing SLE, although many of the criteria may be valuable in the diagnostic process. Epidemiologic characteristics, clinical signs and symptoms, and common laboratory abnormalities are all used in diagnosing SLE.

Once the disease is suspected, serologic tests may be helpful in making the diagnosis. A serologic test used extensively to aid in the diagnosis of SLE is the fluorescent antinuclear antibody (ANA) test. Nearly all SLE patients are ANA-positive, but other diseases also can be associated with a positive test (Table 88–3); however, in other diseases, many of the positive ANA tests are of a lower titer. The pattern of immunofluorescence of the ANA test also may be of diagnostic value (see Table 88–3), with a peripheral (also called *rim*) pattern being specific for SLE. Detecting antibodies to specific nuclear constituents also may be useful diagnostically. Antibodies to native DNA (dsDNA) and to Sm antigen are quite specific for and are considered diagnostic of SLE.[18,29]

PROGNOSIS

In earlier years, SLE was associated with a poor prognosis. For example, the classic report of patients diagnosed between 1949 and 1953 showed a 4-year survival rate of 51%.[30] Today, probably as a result of improved treatment and improved diagnostic techniques that allow earlier diagnosis, the 10- and 20-year survival rates approach 90% and 70%, respectively.[14,31]

Prior to the 1970s, renal disease used to be the leading cause of death in patients with SLE. However, with the ability to better manage patients with kidney disease (e.g., dialysis), infection and coronary artery disease have replaced renal disease as the most common cause of death from SLE.[14,22,28]

TABLE 88–3. Antinuclear Antibody Test: Patterns, Antigens, and Specificities

Pattern	Antigen	Disease
Peripheral	dsDNA	SLE
Speckled	Acidic nuclear protein	Rheumatoid arthritis
	Ribonucleoprotein	SLE
	Extractable nuclear antigen	Scleroderma
		Mixed connective tissue disease
Homogeneous	dsDNA, ssDNA	Rheumatoid arthritis
	Histones	SLE, drug-induced lupus
Nucleolar	Nucleolar RNA	Progressive systemic sclerosis

ds = double-stranded; ss = single-stranded.

▶ TREATMENT: Systemic Lupus Erythematosus

Desired treatment outcomes for the patient with SLE are twofold: (1) management of symptoms and induction of remission during times of disease flare and (2) maintenance of remission for as long as possible between disease flares. An approach to the management of the patient with SLE is outlined in Fig. 88–2. Because of the variability in clinical presentation of disease, treatment will vary accordingly and should be highly individualized. Optimal care of the patient with SLE will offer education and support services in addition to the nonpharmacologic and pharmacologic treatments discussed below. Numerous lupus organizations exist throughout the world and can be located by contacting the Lupus Foundation of America[32] (*http://www.lupus.org*), the Arthritis Foundation[33] (*http://www.arthritis.org*), and Lupus Canada[34] (*http://www.lupuscanada.org*).

NONPHARMACOLOGIC THERAPY

Several nonpharmacologic measures can be employed to manage symptoms and help maintain remission. Fatigue is a common symptom in patients with lupus.[31] A balanced routine of rest and exercise, while avoiding overexertion, is essential in managing fatigue.[35] Avoidance of smoking may be particularly important because hydrazines in tobacco smoke may be an environmental trigger of lupus.[8,35] No specific dietary measures are known to affect the clinical course of lupus definitively. However, fish-oil derivatives might prevent miscarriages in pregnant women with antiphospholipid antibodies,[35] but alfalfa sprouts should be avoided because they contain the amino acid L-canavanine, which is thought to alter T- and B-cell responses and may exacerbate lupus.[8,35] Many patients with SLE will need to limit exposure to sunlight and use sunscreens to block the possible exacerbating effects of ultraviolet light. The amount of sunlight exposure limitation should be individualized.

PHARMACOLOGIC THERAPY

Drug therapy for SLE is often designed to suppress the immune response and inflammation. Table 88–4 lists common agents and doses used to control SLE. In general, the choice of drug therapy depends on the extent and severity of disease. Table 88–5 describes selected monitoring parameters and adverse events for many of the drugs used to treat collagen-vascular diseases.

NONSTEROIDAL ANTI-INFLAMMATORY DRUGS

As discussed earlier, signs and symptoms such as fever, arthritis, and serositis are among the most common in patients with active disease. Therefore, in many patients with mild disease, initial treatment with a nonsteroidal anti-inflammatory drug (NSAID) is a logical choice. The choice of NSAIDs in SLE is empirical. The dose used should be adequate to provide anti-inflammatory effects, although low-dose aspirin may be useful in the management of patients with antiphospholipid syndrome.[25]

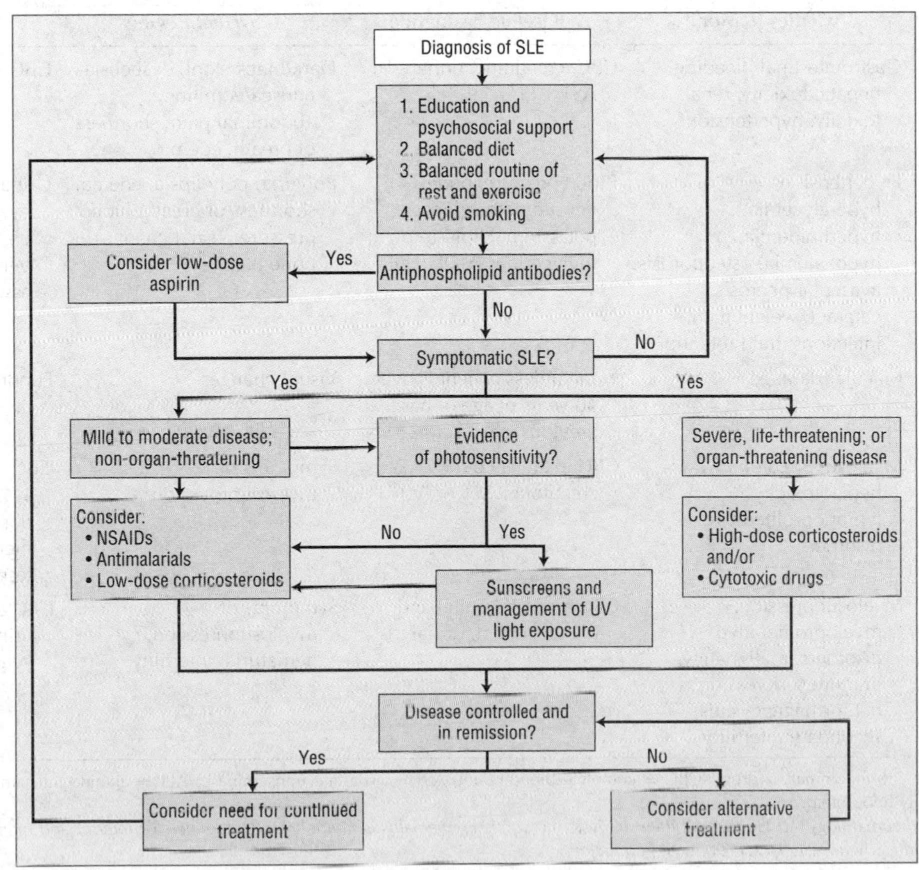

FIGURE 88–2. General approach to the management of SLE.

TABLE 88–4. Drug Treatment of Systemic Lupus Erythematosus

Drug Class	Drug and Dose	Indication
NSAID	Various agents Anti-inflammatory dose	Mild disease: fever, arthritis, skin rash, serositis
Antimalarial	Hydroxychloroquine, 200–400 mg PO daily Chloroquine, 250–500 mg PO daily	Mild disease: arthritis, skin rash, serositis
Corticosteroid	Prednisone 1–2 mg/kg/day PO (or equivalent)	Initial control of severe disease
	<1 mg/kg/day (or equivalent)	Control of mild disease or maintenance after disease suppression with higher doses
	Methylprednisolone, 500–1000 mg IV daily × 3–6 day	Life-threatening disease
Cytotoxic	Cyclophosphamide, 0.5–1.0 g/m^2 IV monthly for 6 months; then every 3 months for 2 to 3 years Azathioprine, up to 4 mg/kg/day PO Cyclophosphamide, up to 3 mg/kg/day PO	Most commonly used in severe lupus nephritis; may be necessary for other severe disease mainifestations

TABLE 88–5. Monitoring Adverse Effects of Drugs Commonly Used in SLE

Drug	Toxicities to Monitor	Baseline Evaluation	Monitoring	
			System Review	*Laboratory*
Salicylates, NSAIDs	Gastrointestinal bleeding, hepatic toxicity, renal toxicity, hypertension	CBC, creatinine, urinalysis, AST, ALT	Dark/black stool, dyspepsia, nausea/vomiting, abdominal pain, shortness of breath, edema	CBC yearly, creatinine yearly
Corticosteroids	Hypertension, hyperglycemia, hyperlipidemia, hypokalemia, osteoporosis, avascular necrosis, cataract, weight gain, infections, fluid retention	Blood pressure, bone densitometry, glucose, potassium, cholesterol, triglycerides (HDL, LDL)	Polyuria, polydipsia, edema, shortness of breath, blood pressure, visual changes, bone pain	Urinary dipstick for glucose every 3–6 months, total cholesterol yearly, bone densitometry yearly to assess osteoporosis
Hydroxychloroquine	Macular damage	None unless patient is over 40 years of age or has previous eye disease	Visual changes	Funduscopic and visual fields every 6–12 months
Azathioprine	Myelosuppression, hepatotoxicity, lymphoproliferative disorders	CBC, platelet count, creatinine, AST or ALT	Symptoms of myelosuppression	CBC and platelet count every 1–2 weeks with changes in dose (every 1–3 months thereafter), AST yearly, Pap test at regular intervals
Cyclophosphamide	Myelosuppression, myeloproliferative disorders, malignancy, immunosuppression, hemorrhagic cystitis, secondary infertility	CBC and differential and platelet count, urinalysis	Symptoms of myelosuppression, hematuria, infertility	CBC and urinalysis monthly, urine cytology and Pap test yearly for life

Key: NSAIDs = nonsteroidal anti-inflammatory drugs; CBC = complete blood count; AST = aspartate transaminase; ALT = alanine transaminase; HDL = high-density lipoprotein; LDL = low-density lipoprotein.

From American College of Rheumatology Ad Hoc Committee on Systemic Lupus Erythematosus Guidelines. Guidelines for referral and management of systemic lupus erythematosus in adults. Arthritis Rheum 1999;42:1790, with permission.

Patients with SLE taking NSAIDs may experience a decline in renal function because of drug effects and not the underlying disease. Prostaglandins may be important mediators of renal hemodynamics in patients with SLE, possibly increasing susceptibility to the renal sequelae of prostaglandin inhibition.[26] This may be particularly important for patients with nephritis. Awareness of this effect is important because declining renal function may be attributed mistakenly to progression of lupus nephritis. There also exist reports of an association between aseptic meningitis in SLE patients and the use of NSAIDs.[4,26]

ANTIMALARIAL DRUGS

Antimalarial agents such as chloroquine and hydroxychloroquine have been used successfully in the management of discoid lupus and SLE. A few controlled trials provide evidence for the role of antimalarial therapy in controlling disease exacerbations and as steroid-sparing agents.[36–38] In general, the manifestations of SLE that can be managed with antimalarials are cutaneous manifestations, arthralgia, pleuritis, mild pericardial inflammation, fatigue, cognitive dysfunction, and mild anemia and leukopenia.[39] Because these drugs are not effective immediately, they are best used in long-term management. Response to chloroquine occurs in 1 month, whereas the maximal effect of hydroxychloroquine may not occur for 3 to 6 months.[26] Hydroxychloroquine probably is safer than chloroquine and is considered the antimalarial of first choice.

The mechanism of action of the antimalarial drugs is uncertain. It has been proposed that antimalarials interfere with T-lymphocyte activation.[26] Other effects of antimalarials that may benefit patients with SLE include inhibition of cytokines, decreased sensitivity to ultraviolet light, anti-inflammatory activity, antiplatelet effects, and antihyperlipidemic activity.[39]

Dosage and duration of therapy depend on patient response, tolerance of side effects, and development of retinal toxicity, which is a potentially irreversible adverse reaction associated with long-term therapy, especially with chloroquine. Current recommended doses of antimalarials in SLE are hydroxychloroquine 200–400 mg daily and chloroquine 250–500 mg daily. After 1 or 2 years of treatment, gradual tapering of dosage can be attempted. Some patients may require only one or two tablets per week to suppress cutaneous manifestations.[40]

Side effects of these drugs include central nervous system effects (e.g., headache, nervousness, insomnia, and others), dermatitis, pigmentary changes of the skin and hair, gastrointestinal disturbance (e.g., nausea), flulike symptoms, and reversible cycloplegia resulting from deposition of the drug in the cornea. Retinal toxicity is uncommon when the currently recommended doses are used and is least common with hydroxychloroquine[26]; however, because of the possibility of permanent damage associated with the retinopathy, an ophthalmologic evaluation should be done at baseline and every 3 months when chloroquine is used and every 6 to 12 months when hydroxychloroquine is used. If retinal abnormalities are noted, antimalarial therapy should be discontinued or the dose reduced.[26]

CORTICOSTEROIDS

Corticosteroid therapy is commonplace in therapeutic regimens for SLE. Although evidence for improved survival with corticosteroid therapy is inadequate, these agents are known to be effective for suppressing the clinical expression of disease and are considered by many to be a major factor in the improved prognosis in recent years. Although most controlled trials of corticosteroid therapy have been conducted in patients with severe lupus nephritis, evidence suggests that corticosteroids are also effective in the management of severe cases of central nervous system disease, pneumonitis, polyserositis, vasculitis, thrombocytopenia, and other clinical manifestations.[26]

A patient with the diagnosis of SLE does not automatically require corticosteroid therapy. Mild disease with such manifestations as fever, arthralgia, pleuritis, or skin manifestations may respond adequately to NSAIDs or antimalarials, but patients with clinical manifestations that are more serious or unresponsive to other drugs may require corticosteroids. Some patients with chronic or subacute cutaneous lupus erythematosus may benefit from topical or intralesional administration of corticosteroids.[41]

The goal of treatment when using corticosteroids in SLE is to suppress and maintain suppression of active disease with the lowest dose possible. In patients with mild disease, low-dose therapy (prednisone 15–20 mg daily) is adequate, but in patients with more severe disease (severe hemolytic anemia or cardiac involvement), higher doses, such as prednisone 1–2 mg/kg daily, may be required. Once adequate suppression of disease is achieved, the dose should be tapered to the minimum amount required for continued disease suppression. When analyzing the need to treat with corticosteroids, the clinician should consider other conditions that may increase the risk of corticosteroid therapy, such as infection, hypertension, atherosclerotic disease, diabetes, obesity, osteoporosis, and psychiatric disease.[4,26]

Steroid pulse therapy is the administration of short-term, high-dose intravenous corticosteroids with the goal of inducing remission in SLE patients with serious, life-threatening disease, such as diffuse proliferative glomerulonephritis, central nervous system involvement, or hemolytic disease. A standard pulse regimen consists of intravenous methylprednisolone 500–1000 mg for 3 to 6 consecutive days. Pulse therapy usually is followed by high-dose prednisone (40–60 mg/day) therapy that is tapered rapidly to low-dose maintenance therapy.[26] Potential advantages of pulse therapy over high-dose oral steroids include a quicker response and avoidance of side effects associated with the longer duration of therapy required with oral steroids. Although generally well tolerated, methylprednisolone pulse therapy may result in significant adverse effects, including infection, gastrointestinal disturbances, rapid increases in blood pressure, arrhythmias, seizures, and sudden death. Furthermore, there are insufficient data from controlled clinical trials to clearly define the role of pulse steroids in the management of SLE. Thus pulse therapy represents an alternative mode of treatment for patients with life-threatening disease or disease unresponsive to other pharmacotherapy.

CYTOTOXIC DRUGS

A considerable amount of literature exists describing the use of cytotoxic and immunosuppressive drugs in SLE, although few of these are reports of controlled clinical trials. Included in this category are the alkylating agent cyclophosphamide and the antimetabolite azathioprine. These agents, usually used in combination with corticosteroids, have been the mainstays of immunosuppressive therapy. Although both are known to suppress and stabilize extrarenal disease activity, much of the evaluation of these agents has focused on lupus nephritis, a major factor associated with morbidity and mortality in SLE.

Evidence supporting the use of cyclophosphamide in lupus nephritis has been collected over the last several decades. Controlled clinical trials have shown that cyclophosphamide improved the long-term outcomes in lupus nephritis.[42] Based on controlled trials, combination prednisone and cyclophosphamide has become standard treatment for focal and diffuse proliferative lupus nephritis (WHO class III/IV) and is superior to prednisone alone.[15] There are no studies examining cyclophosphamide in earlier stages of nephritis (WHO class II/III), and therefore, corticosteroids remain the treatment of choice for these less severe forms of nephritis.[42] A meta-analysis of clinical trials revealed that pulse intravenous cyclophosphamide plus prednisone was more effective at increasing patient survival and renal function than prednisone only.[43] Cyclophosphamide plus corticosteroids preserves renal function and decreases the risk of developing end-stage renal failure requiring dialysis and renal transplantation.[15] Intermittent pulse administration of intravenous cyclophosphamide is preferred over daily oral therapies because of reduced adverse effects. However, pulse cyclophosphamide plus prednisone is not always effective. Other cytotoxic combinations have been examined, but none has been found to be significantly better than any other at reducing the risk of death or renal failure.[15]

When used in combination with corticosteroids, cyclophosphamide is dosed at 1–3 mg/kg for oral therapy and 0.5–1.0 g/m^2 of body surface area for intravenous therapy. The most common route of cyclophosphamide administration is intravenous, although there is no evidence that this is better than oral administration.[42] Likewise, there is no evidence to suggest the optimal duration of treatment. Based on empirical experience, cyclophosphamide generally is dosed monthly for 6 months and then every 3 months for a period of 1 year after the nephritis is in remission.[28,42] Of course, cyclophosphamide therapy is not without risk. Serious toxic effects include suppression of hematopoiesis, opportunistic infections, bladder complications (e.g., hemorrhagic cystitis and cancer), sterility, and teratogenesis. White blood cell counts must be monitored during cyclophosphamide therapy, and if the nadir is less than 1500/mm^3, the dose must be adjusted to keep the white cell count above 1500/mm^3. Nausea and vomiting associated with cyclophosphamide can be controlled with oral ondansetron plus dexamethasone.[42]

Azathioprine has not been studied as extensively as cyclophosphamide for lupus nephritis. Additionally, azathioprine is only slightly more effective than prednisone alone.[28] Azathioprine may find usefulness in treating early-onset and less severe nephritis.[28] Azathioprine is given orally in doses up to 3 mg/kg per day, often in combination with corticosteroids for severe disease.[26] Azathioprine generally is less toxic than cyclophosphamide, but adverse reactions may be serious and include suppression of hematopoiesis, opportunistic infections, cancer, hepatotoxicity, pulmonary fibrosis, pancreatitis, and teratogenesis.

Some investigations have indicated variable rates of success using intravenous cyclophosphamide for lupus nephritis.[44,45] Cyclophosphamide often is administered intravenously in intermittent pulse doses to minimize toxicity. To decrease the risk of bladder toxicity, patients should be well hydrated with oral or intravenous fluids, and urinary output should be monitored. Mesna may be used to prevent hemorrhagic cystitis. Mesna is administered as a bolus of 25 mg/kg 30 minutes before cyclophosphamide therapy and 3, 6, and 9 hours after thereapy.[29]

Cyclophosphamide may be of benefit to some patients with other serious, refractory manifestations of lupus, including neuropsychiatric manifestations.[46,47] Reports of the use of other cytotoxic drugs for lupus in recent years include methotrexate[48,49] and mechlorethamine (nitrogen mustard).[50]

Cytotoxic therapy is useful in combination with corticosteroids, allowing for lower steroid doses and improved efficacy compared with steroids alone. However, cytotoxic therapy must be monitored closely for adverse effects, and maximum response may take 6 months or longer in some patients. No data from controlled trials are available to support the combination of two or more cytotoxic agents; however, this approach has been used in patients refractory to standard therapies.[15,42]

ALTERNATIVE AND EXPERIMENTAL TREATMENTS

As the pathogenesis of SLE continues to be elucidated, new and promising treatments are being developed. Several alternative treatments reportedly successful in managing various manifestations of SLE are listed in Table 88–6. However, the pharmacotherapist should be aware that many of these are reports of uncontrolled trials. Furthermore, in addition to reports of success, the literature contains reports

TABLE 88–6. Alternative and Experimental Treatments for SLE

Treatment	Symptom	Reference
Plasmapheresis	Multiple severe symptoms—nephritis, CNS, thrombocytopenia, anemia, leukopenia	51
Cyclosporine	Nephritis	52
	Multiple symptoms—anemia, leukopenia, thrombocytopenia, nephritis	53
Immune globulin	Multiple symptoms—anemia, thrombocytopenia, nephritis	54, 55
Thromboxane A_2 synthetase inhibitor	Nephritis	56, 57
Prostaglandin E_1	Nephritis	58
	Cutaneous vasculitis, peripheral neuropathy	59
Ultraviolet-A1 irradiation	Multiple symptoms—rash	60
Monoclonal antibodies	Nephritis	61, 62
Dihydroepiandrosterone (DHEA)	Multiple symptoms	63
Bromocriptine	Multiple symptoms—fatigue, rash, Raynaud's, arthritis/arthralgia	64
Danazol	Thrombocytopenia, hemolytic anemia	65

of unsuccessful or controversial treatments for many of these therapies (e.g., plasmapheresis or immune globulin for lupus nephritis). A number of newer agents are being examined and include antibodies to various immune cell surface antigens, ablative chemotherapy with stem cell transplantation, thalidomide, cladaribine, fludarabine, mycophenolate mofetil, and combination chemotherapies.[15,66]

SPECIAL POPULATIONS

PREGNANCY AND SLE

Pregnancy in SLE patients has been associated with exacerbation of disease during pregnancy, exacerbation during the early postpartum period, a greater incidence of spontaneous abortion, and a greater chance of developing preeclampsia or pregnancy-induced hypertension (particularly in patients with nephritis).

Exacerbation of lupus during pregnancy seems to be less likely if the disease is in remission at conception.[67] Disease exacerbations can be managed aggressively with corticosteroids, if needed, with little concern about harm to the fetus.[68] The decision to use other classes of drug therapy to control disease exacerbation should be highly individualized, although hydroxychloroquine or NSAIDs probably can be used safely, if needed.[68] In fact, it may be safer to continue hydroxychloroquine during pregnancy than to discontinue the drug.[69] The decision to use cytotoxic drugs during pregnancy should be made with extreme caution because of potential harmful effects (e.g., teratogenesis, fetal loss) to the fetus, particularly during the first trimester. Azathioprine may be the safest of the cytotoxic drugs if needed during pregnancy.[68]

Antiphospholipid antibodies may be associated with a greater likelihood of spontaneous abortion. Corticosteroids, aspirin, and heparin, alone and in various combinations, have been used to try to improve fetal outcome.[70] Fetal survival increases with all these therapies, and none has been shown superior.[26] The optimal treatment regimen for pregnant patients with antiphospholipid antibodies is yet to be determined, although it has been recommended that women with prior fetal loss after the first trimester receive low-dose aspirin.[71] Additionally, women with a history of preeclampsia or nephritis with or without a history of hypertension should be considered for low-dose aspirin.[71] Although there is an increased chance of a high-risk pregnancy in women with SLE, appropriate planning and disease management will result in a high likelihood of a successful pregnancy and a healthy child.

ANTIPHOSPHOLIPID SYNDROME AND THROMBOSIS

As mentioned earlier, the presence of antiphospholipid antibodies may result in several clinical manifestations including thrombosis. There is no agreement on prophylaxis of patients with antiphospholipid antibodies but without a history of thromboembolism.[25] In such patients, low-dose aspirin (100–325 mg/day) may be used prophylactically, although efficacy has not been established.[25] Patients with an acute thrombotic event should receive standard treatment with anticoagulants (e.g., heparin). Follow-up treatment with warfarin to prevent recurrence may require an INR of 3 or greater in patients with antiphospholipid syndrome.[72] However, currently, there is no consensus on the intensity of anticoagulation or duration of secondary prophylaxis.[27]

DRUG-INDUCED LUPUS

One of the earliest descriptions of a drug-induced SLE-like syndrome was reported in 1945 and was associated with the use of sulfadiazine.[73] Today, procainamide and hydralazine are associated most commonly with drug-induced lupus (DIL), although numerous other drugs have been implicated[74] (Table 88–7). A consensus on diagnostic criteria for DIL does not exist, and many reported cases do not satisfy the 1982 revised ACR criteria for identification of SLE patients.[74] It has been suggested that DIL should be suspected in patients with no history of idiopathic lupus who develop ANAs and at least one clinical feature of SLE and whose symptoms resolve following drug discontinuation.[74]

The epidemiologic characteristics of DIL are different from those of idiopathic SLE. In general, patients with procainamide- or hydralazine-induced lupus develop the disease much later in life compared with idiopathic SLE probably because the majority of people who use these drugs are older. Other observations include a greater percentage of white patients and an absence of female predominance when compared with idiopathic SLE.[73,74]

Patients of the slow acetylator phenotype may have a greater risk for developing DIL, particularly with procainamide and hydralazine.[73,74] In DIL, the development of a positive ANA test occurs more rapidly and symptoms present more often with a slow acetylator phenotype.[73] Procainamide-induced lupus can present as early as 1 month or as late as 12 years after starting therapy. Hydralazine-induced lupus is related to dose and appears in patients receiving 100 mg/day or more.[74]

Musculoskeletal symptoms are the most common clinical manifestations, whereas renal and central nervous system involvement is much less common compared with idiopathic SLE.[73] Pleuropulmonary manifestations are also common, particularly in procainamide-induced disease. Fever is also common in DIL.[73,74]

A positive ANA test is found in nearly all procainamide- or hydralazine-induced cases.[73,74] The immunofluorescence pattern usually is homogeneous, and antibodies are primarily against ssDNA and not dsDNA as in idiopathic SLE. Antibodies to Sm antigen are absent in DIL.[73] Antihistone antibodies are associated with DIL but are not

TABLE 88–7. Medications Implicated in Drug-Induced Lupus

Acebutolol	Leuprolide	Phenylbutazone
Aminoglutethimide	Levodopa	Phenytoin
Atenolol	Lithium	Prazosin
Captopril	Lovastatin	Primidone
Carbamazepine	Mephenytoin	**Procainamide**
Chlorpromazine[a]	Methimazole	Promethazine
Chlorprothixene	**Methyldopa**	Propylthiouracil
Clonidine	Methysergide	Psoralen
Danazol	Metrizamide	**Quinidine**
Diclofenac	Minoxidil	Spironolactone
Disopyramide	Nalidixic acid	Streptomycin
Ethosuximide	Nitrofurantoin	Sulindac
Gold salts	Nomifensine	Sulfasalazine
Griseofulvin	Oral contraceptives	Tetracycline
Hydralazine	*p*-Aminosalicylate	Thioridazine
Ibuprofen	**Penicillamine**	Timolol
Interferon (α,γ)	Penicillin	Tolazamide
Isoniazid	Perphenazine	Tolmetin
Labetalol	Phenelzine	Trimethadione

[a]Drugs in boldface represent those with best evidence of association.
Adapted from Yung RL, Richardson BC. Drug-induced lupus, Rheum Dis Clin North Am 1994;20:62, with permission.

POLYMYALGIA RHEUMATICA

CLINICAL MANIFESTATIONS

Polymyalgia rheumatica (PMR) is characterized by aching and morning stiffness of the neck, shoulder, and pelvic girdle musculature and torso. Stiffness is greatest following periods of inactivity, such as sleeping. Pain and morning stiffness may last from 1 to 6 hours. Fatigue, anorexia, and low-grade fever are common signs and symptoms. The erythrocyte sedimentation rate (ESR) generally is more than 40 mm/h and often is more than 100 mm/h. Some patients go from exhibiting no symptoms to overt clinical manifestations overnight, whereas others have a gradual onset of symptoms over a number of weeks. The etiology is unknown. There is a close association between PMR and temporal arteritis or giant cell arteritis. Some researchers suggest that these disease entities are variants of the same disorder. PMR occurs primarily in individuals older than 50 years of age, with a mean age onset of approximately 70 years.[88]

▶ TREATMENT: Polymyalgia Rheumatica

The treatment of choice for PMR is prednisone at a dose of 10–20 mg/day. This therapy is so effective that if improvement does not occur within a week, another diagnosis should be considered. The ESR should decrease by 2 weeks and be normal after 4 weeks of therapy. The prednisone should be tapered beginning several weeks following control of symptoms. The rate of tapering is based on clinical response. A taper of 2.5 mg/day at 2- to 4-week intervals to 5–10 mg/day followed by a slower tapering of 1 mg/day at monthly intervals has been suggested.[88,89] The lowest dose of prednisone that controls symptoms should be used for maintenance, which is usually between 7 and 15 mg/day. Maintaining the ESR in the normal range is a good monitoring parameter. For elderly patients, the normal ESR may be slightly higher than that usually given as a reference value by the clinical laboratory. PMR is a self-limited disease, and patients usually continue maintenance therapy for 2 to 5 years. Patients may experience a relapse when the prednisone is discontinued and may require prednisone therapy for up to 15 years.[90] Every-other-day prednisone has not been as successful as daily therapy. Methotrexate has been tried in patients refractory to prednisone, but it does not improve the disease activity or allow for a prednisone dose reduction.[91]

PMR-associated temporal arteritis and giant cell arteritis require aggressive therapy with high-dose corticosteroids such as prednisone at a dose of 40–60 mg/day or higher. These forms of arteritis can cause permanent loss of vision if not treated promptly. Patients should be educated to seek immediate medical care for possibly related symptoms such as jaw pain on chewing, temporal headache, visual changes, or mental status changes.

SYSTEMIC VASCULITIS

CLINICAL MANIFESTATIONS

Clinical manifestations of vasculitis are heterogeneous and are due to inflammation and damage to blood vessels. Vasculitis can be primary, as in Wegener's granulomatosis and polyarteritis nodosa, or secondary from other diseases, such as rheumatoid arthritis or SLE. Immune complexes can develop at the site of the vessel damage, or circulating immune complexes can be deposited in the vessel wall. The immune complexes can then activate the humoral immune system, leading to inflammation and damage. Cellular-mediated immunity also may be involved in some vasculitides.[92] There are numerous forms of vasculitis, and there is currently no universally accepted scheme to classify them. Table 88–8 lists some systemic vasculitis syndromes. Vasculitides are very heterogeneous, which has limited large clinical trials from being conducted. Small studies and anecdotal experiences often guide therapeutic decision making.[93]

TABLE 88–8. Classification of Systemic Vasculitis Syndromes

Hypersensitivity vasculitis
Due to exogenous agents
Drugs
Infection
Henoch–Schönlein purpura
Serum sickness-like reactions
Due to endogenous agents
Autoimmune disease
Malignancy
Systemic connective tissue diseases
Cryoglobulinemia
Systemic necrotizing vasculitis
Polyarteritis nodosa
Polyangiitis overlap syndrome
Allergic granulomatosis
Wegener's granulomatosis
Giant cell arteritis
Temporal arteritis
Takayasu's arteritis
Thromboangiitis obliterans (Buerger's disease)

▶ TREATMENT: Systemic Vasculitis

There are few controlled trials of pharmacologic treatments for the various forms of vasculitis. Treatment is guided by the severity, prognosis, and response of the vasculitis. For example, a drug-induced hypersensitivity vasculitis resulting in a rash may require only that the drug be discontinued. At the other end of the spectrum, Wegener's granulomatosis is a fatal vasculitis if not treated aggressively with corticosteroids, often in combination with cyclophosphamide. Each type of vasculitis has its recommended therapeutic protocol, which usually includes the use of anti-inflammatory agents and immunosuppressive agents either alone or in combination.

EVALUATION OF THERAPEUTIC OUTCOMES

The diversity of clinical features and disease severity associated with the collagen-vascular diseases leads to a number of possible clinical outcomes with a broad range of desired therapeutic outcomes. Achieving desired therapeutic outcomes for most of the collagen-vascular diseases is highly variable. Currently, it is not possible to predict which patients will have a satisfactory therapeutic response and which will have unrelenting progressive disease. These diseases often have fluctuating courses, necessitating frequent changes in drug therapy and drug doses.

Evaluation of drug therapy of several of the collagen-vascular diseases often only requires monitoring for resolution of symptoms such as rash or muscle pain. However, patients with life-threatening disease receiving aggressive pharmacotherapy may require intensive monitoring and evaluation of therapy. For example, the patient receiving cytotoxic drug therapy for severe lupus nephritis requires close monitoring of laboratory indices of renal function as well as monitoring of symptomatology and laboratory indices for possible bone marrow suppression, infection, cystitis, or other undesired therapeutic outcomes.

Evaluation of therapeutic outcomes also should include an awareness of the possibility of drug therapy mimicking signs and symptoms of disease, such as the lupus patient receiving NSAID therapy and presenting with renal insufficiency or the patient with PM receiving prednisone and presenting with an exacerbation of muscle weakness.

As patients live longer, as is the case with SLE, outcome measures other than mortality will be needed to assess the effect of treatment. Clinicians and researchers working with lupus patients have developed and continue to refine some of these alternative outcome measures. Three important domains for assessing lupus patients include disease activity, accumulated damage, and quality of life.[94] Several instruments useful for assessing patients with SLE are listed in Table 88–9.[94] Pharmacotherapists can expect to see increased use of these and similar instruments for assessment of treatment outcomes in patients with SLE.

CONCLUSION

SLE is a disease that affects multiple organ systems and consists of abnormal immunologic function and the development of autoantibodies. The disease is quite variable in clinical presentation and progression. The cause of lupus is unknown, although several factors (e.g., genetics, environment, and hormones) may predispose an individual to the development of the disease. Although SLE was once thought to be rapidly fatal, today nearly 90% of patients survive 10 years.

Drug therapy is nonspecific and is aimed at suppressing the inflammation and abnormal immune response associated with active disease. Clinical trials with various agents often have been inadequate and contradictory, and the therapeutic management of lupus is not optimal. Nevertheless, drug therapy of recent years probably has contributed significantly to the improved survival of these patients. As the understanding of SLE progresses and advances in biotechnology occur, we can expect to see the development of more specific and optimal treatment and further improvement in survival.

Each of the collagen-vascular diseases has its own recommended form of therapy. For most of these diseases, there are few well-controlled clinical trials evaluating pharmacotherapy. Treatment of most of these diseases requires anti-inflammatory or immunosuppressive drugs. Monitoring therapeutic outcomes is essential because drugs and drug doses may need to be modified frequently.

▶ PRINCIPLES OF PHARMACOTHERAPY

- SLE can have a tremendous psychological impact on patients in addition to its physiologic effects. Therefore, education and support services are essential for optimal management on diagnosis of lupus.
- Nonspecific symptoms, especially fatigue, present frequently in SLE patients and often are debilitating. Therefore, a balanced routine of rest, exercise, and diet is an essential component of treatment.
- Because of the fluctuating, diverse presentation of SLE and other collagen-vascular diseases, pharmacologic and nonpharmacologic treatment should be highly individualized.
- Drug therapy options for patients with mild to moderate manifestations of SLE should include NSAIDs, antimalarials, and low-dose corticosteroids.
- Drug therapy options for patients with severe manifestations of SLE should include high-dose corticosteroids and cytotoxic drugs (usually cyclophosphamide).
- Monitoring therapeutic outcomes is critical because the drugs used to treat collagen-vascular diseases frequently cause severe adverse events, and the disease process can fluctuate between spontaneous remissions and disease exacerbations.

TABLE 88–9. Instruments Used for Assessing Outcome Measures in Patients with SLE

Outcome Domain	Instrument
Disease activity	Systemic Lupus Activity Measure (SLAM)
	Systemic Lupus Erythematosus Activity Index (SLEDAI)
	British Isles Lupus Activity Group (BILAG)
Accumulated damage	Systemic Lupus International Collaborating Clinics/American College of Rheumatology (SLICC/ACR) Damage Index
Quality of life	Health Assessment Questionnaire (HAQ) Functional Ability Index
	Medical Outcome Survey Short Form (MOS SF-20) and (MOS SF-36)

REFERENCES

1. Benedek TG. Historical background of discoid and systemic lupus erythematosus. In: Wallace DJ. Hahn BH, eds. Dubois' Lupus Erythematosus, 5th ed. Baltimore, Williams & Wilkins, 1997: 3–16.
2. Kotzin BL, O'Dell JR. Systemic lupus erythematosus. In: Frank MM, Austen KF, Claman HN, Unanue ER, eds. Samter's Immunologic Diseases, 5th ed. Boston, Little, Brown, 1995: 667–697.
3. Tan EM, Cohen AS, Fries JF, et al. The 1982 revised criteria for the classification of systemic lupus erythematosus. Arthritis Rheum 1982;25: 1271–1277.
4. Hochberg MC, for the Diagnostic and Therapeutic Criteria Committee of the American College of Rheumatology. Updating the American College of Rheumatology revised criteria for the classification of systemic lupus erythematosus (Letter). Arthritis Rheum 1997;40:1725.
5. Cooper GS, Dooley MA, Treadwell EL, et al. Hormonal, environmental, and infectious risk factors for developing systemic lupus erythematosus. Arthritis Rheum 1998;41:1714–1724.
6. McCarty DJ, Manzi S, Medsger TA. Incidence of systemic lupus erythematosus. Arthritis Rheum 1995;38:1260–1270.
7. Hochberg MC. The epidemiology of systemic lupus erythematosus. In: Wallace DJ, Hahn BH, eds. Dubois' Lupus Erythematosus, 5th ed. Baltimore, Williams & Wilkins, 1997: 49–65.
8. Mongey AB, Hess EV. The role of environment in systemic lupus erythematosus and associated disorders. In: Wallace DJ, Hahn BH, eds. Dubois' Lupus Erythematosus, 5th ed. Baltimore, Williams & Wilkins, 1997: 31–47.
9. Winchester RJ. Systemic lupus erythematosus: Pathogenesis. In: Koopman WJ, ed. Arthritis and Allied Conditions: A Textbook of Rheumatology, 13th ed. Baltimore, Williams & Wilkins, 1997: 1361–1391.
10. Hahn BH. Pathogenesis of systemic lupus erythematosus. In: Kelley WN, Harris ED, Ruddy S, Sledge CB, eds. Textbook of Rheumatology, 5th ed. Philadelphia, Saunders, 1997: 1015–1027.
11. Vyse TJ, Kotzin BL. Genetic basis of systemic lupus erythematosus. Curr Opin Immunol 1996;8:843–851.
12. Hess EV. Environmental lupus syndromes. Br J Rheum 1995;34:597–599.
13. Denman AM. Systemic lupus erythematosus: Is a viral aetiology a credible hypothesis? J Infect 2000;40:229–233.
14. Mills JA. Systemic lupus erythematosus. N Engl J Med 1994;330:1871–1879.
15. Balow JE, Boumpas DT, Austin HA III. New prospects for treatment of lupus nephritis. Semin Nephrol 2000;20:32–39.
16. Olhoffer IH, Peng SL, Craft J. Revisiting autoantibody profiles in systemic lupus erythematosus. J Rheumatol 1997;24:297–302.
17. Harley JB. Autoantibodies in systemic lupus erythematosus. In: Koopman WJ, ed. Arthritis and Allied Conditions: A Textbook of Rheumatology, 13th ed. Baltimore, Williams & Wilkins, 1997: 1347–1360.
18. Egner W. The use of laboratory tests in the diagnosis of SLE. J Clin Pathol 2000;53:424–432.
19. Hahn BH. An overview of the pathogenesis of systemic lupus erythematosus. In: Wallace DJ, Hahn BH, eds. Dubois' Lupus Erythematosus, 5th ed. Baltimore, Williams & Wilkins, 1997: 69–75.
20. Lahita RG. Clinical presentation of systemic lupus erythematosus. In: Kelley WN, Harris ED, Ruddy S, Sledge CB, eds. Textbook of Rheumatology, 5th ed. Philadelphia, Saunders, 1997: 1028–1039.
21. Wallace DJ. The clinical presentation of systemic lupus erythematosus. In: Wallace DJ, Hahn BH, eds. Dubois' Lupus Erythematosus, 5th ed. Baltimore, Williams & Wilkins, 1997: 627–633.
22. Boumpas DT, Fessler BJ, Austin HA III, et al. Systemic lupus erythematosus: Emerging concepts. 2. Dermatologic and joint disease, the antiphospholipid antibody syndrome, pregnancy and hormonal therapy, morbidity and mortality, and pathogenesis. Ann Intern Med 1995;123:42–53.
23. Boumpas DT, Austin HA III, Fessler BJ, et al. Systemic lupus erythematosus: Emerging concepts. 1. Renal, neuropsychiatric, cardiovascular, pulmonary, and hematologic disease. Ann Intern Med 1995;122:940–950.
24. Manzi S, Meilahn EN, Rairie JE, et al. Age-specific incidence rates of myocardial infarction and angina in women with systemic lupus erythematosus: Comparison with the Framingham Study. Am J Epidemiol 1997;145:408–415.
25. Wahl DG, Bounameaux H, de Moerlosse P, Sarasin FP. Prophylactic antithrombotic therapy for patients with systemic lupus erythematosus with or without antiphospholipid antibodies: Do the benefits outweigh the risks? Arch Intern Med 2000;160:2042–2048.
26. Hahn BH. Management of systemic lupus erythematosus. In: Kelley WN, Harris ED, Ruddy S, Sledge CB, eds. Textbook of Rheumatology, 5th ed. Philadelphia, Saunders, 1997: 1040–1056.
27. Lockshin MD. Answers to the antiphospholipid-antibody syndrome? N Engl J Med 1995;332:1025–1027.
28. Austin HA, Balow JE. Treatment of lupus nephritis. Semin Nephrol 2000;20:265–276.
29. Pisetsky DS, Gilkeson G, St. Clair EW. Systemic lupus erythematosus: Diagnosis and treatment. Med Clin North Am 1997;81:113–129.
30. Merrell M, Shulman LE. Determination of prognosis in chronic disease, illustrated by systemic lupus erythematosus. J Chron Dis 1955;1:12–32.
31. Urowitz MB, Gladman DD. How to improve morbidity and mortality in systemic lupus erythematosus. Rheumatology 2000;39:238–244.
32. Lupus Foundation of America, Inc., 1300 Picard Drive, Suite 200, Rockville, MD, 301-670-9292 or 800-558-0121.
33. Arthritis Foundation, 1330 West Peachtree Street, Atlanta, GA, 404-872-7100.
34. Lupus Canada, Box 64034 5512-4 ST NW, Calgary, Alberta, Canada T2K 6J1, 800-661-1468.
35. Wallace DJ. Principles of therapy and local measures. In: Wallace DJ, Hahn BH, eds. Dubois' Lupus Erythematosus, 5th ed. Baltimore, Williams & Wilkins, 1997: 1099–1108.
36. The Canadian Hydroxychloroquine Study Group. A randomized study of the effect of withdrawing hydroxychloroquine sulfate in systemic lupus erythematosus. N Engl J Med 1991;324:150–154.
37. Williams HJ, Egger MJ, Singer JZ, et al. Comparison of hydroxychloroquine and placebo in the treatment of the arthropathy of mild systemic lupus erythematosus. J Rheumatol 1994;21:1457–1462.
38. Meinao IM, Sato EI, Andrade LE, et al. Controlled trial with chloroquine diphosphate in systemic lupus erythematosus. Lupus 1996;5:237–241.
39. Wallace DJ. Antimalarial agents and lupus. Rheum Dis Clin North Am 1994;20:243–263.
40. Wallace DJ. Antimalarial therapies. In: Wallace DJ, Hahn BH, eds. Dubois' Lupus Erythematosus, 5th ed. Baltimore, Williams & Wilkins, 1997: 1117–1139.
41. Redford TW, Small RE. Update on pharmacotherapy of systemic lupus erythematosus. Am J Health Syst Pharm 1995;52:2686–2695.
42. Ortmann RA, Klippel JH. Update on cyclophosphamide for systemic lupus erythematosus. Rheum Dis Clin North Am 2000;26:363–375.
43. Bansal VK, Beto JA. Treatment of lupus nephritis: A meta-analysis of clinical trials. Am J Kidney Dis 1997;29:193–199.
44. Valeri A, Radhakrishnan J, Estes D, et al. Intravenous pulse cyclophosphamide treatment of severe lupus nephritis: A prospective five-year study. Clin Nephrol 1994;42:71–78.
45. Martinelli R, Pereira LJC, Santos ES, Rocha H. Clinical effects of intermittent, intravenous cyclophosphamide in severe systemic lupus erythematosus. Nephron 1996;74:313–317.
46. Neuwelt CM, Lacks S, Kaye BR, et al. Role of intravenous cyclophosphamide in the treatment of severe neuropsychiatric systemic lupus erythematosus. Am J Med 1995;98:32–41.
47. Ramos PC, Mendez MJ, Ames PRJ, et al. Pulse cyclophosphamide in the treatment of neuropsychiatric systemic lupus erythematosus. Clin Exp Rheumatol 1996;14:295–299.
48. Walz LeBlanc BA, Dagenasis P, Urowitz MB, Gladman DD. Methotrexate in systemic lupus erythematosus. J Rheumatol 1994;21:836–838.
49. Wise CM, Vuyyuru S, Roberts WN. Methotrexate in nonrenal lupus and undifferentiated connective tissue disease: A review of 36 patients. J Rheumatol 1996;23:1005–1010.
50. Wallace DJ, Metzger AL. Successful use of nitrogen mustard for cyclophosphamide resistant diffuse proliferative lupus glomerulonephritis: Report of 2 cases (Letter). J Rheumatol 1995;22;801–802.

51. Euler HH, Schroeder JO, Harten P, et al. Treatment-free remission in severe systemic lupus erythematosus following synchronization of plasmapheresis with subsequent pulse cyclophosphamide. Arthritis Rheum 1994;37:1784–1794.
52. Radhakrishnan J, Kunis CL, D'Agati V, Appel GB. Cyclosporine treatment of lupus membranous nephropathy. Clin Nephrol 1994;42:147–154.
53. Caccavo D, Lagana B, Mitterhofer AP. Long-term treatment of systemic lupus erythematosus with cyclosporin A. Arthritis Rheum 1997;40:27–35.
54. Francioni C, Galeazzi M, Fioravanti A, et al. Long term IV Ig treatment in systemic lupus eyrthematosus. Clin Exp Rheumatol 1994;12:163–168.
55. Schroeder JO, Zcuner RA, Euler HH, Loffler H. High-dose intravenous immunoglobulins in systemic lupus erythematosus: Clinical and serological results of a pilot study. J Rheumatol 1996;23:71–75.
56. Yoshida T, Kameda H, Ichikawa Y, et al. Improvement of renal function with a selective thromboxane A_2 synthetase inhibitor, DP-1904, in lupus nephritis. J Rheumatol 1996;23:1719–1724.
57. Pierucci A, Simonetti BM, Pecci G, et al. Improvement of renal function with selective thromboxane antagonism in lupus nephritis. N Engl J Med 1989;320:421–425.
58. Lin CY. Improvement in steroid and immunosuppressive drug resistant lupus nephritis by intraveous prostaglandin E_1 therapy. Nephron 1990;55:258–264.
59. Yoshikawa Y, Mizutani H, Shimizu M. Systemic lupus erythematosus with ischemic peripheral neuropathy and lupus anticoagulant: Response to intravenous prostaglandin E1. Cutis 1996;58:393–396.
60. McGrath H. Ultraviolet-A_1 irradiation decreases clinical disease activity and autoantibodies in patients with systemic lupus erythematosus. Clin Exp Rheumatol 1994;12:129–135.
61. Stafford FJ, Fleisher TA, Lee G, et al. A pilot study of anti-CD5 ricin A chain immunoconjugate in systemic lupus erythematosus. J Rheumatol 1994;21:2068–2070.
62. Wacholtz MC, Lipsky PE. Treatment of lupus nephritis with CD5 Plus, an immunoconjugate of an anti-CD5 monoclonal antibody and ricin A chain. Arthritis Rheum 1992;35:837–839.
63. Van Vollenhoven RF, Engleman EG, McGuire JL. Dehydroepiandrosterone in systemic lupus erythematosus: Results of double-blind, placebo-controlled, randomized clinical trial. Arthritis Rheum 1995;38:1826–1831.
64. McMurray RW, Weidensaul D, Allen SH, Walker SE. Efficacy of bromocriptine in an open label therapeutic trial for systemic lupus erythematosus. J Rheumatol 1995;22:2084–2091.
65. Cervera H, Jara LJ, Pizarro S, et al. Danazol for systemic lupus erythematosus with refractory autoimmune thrombocytopenia or Evans' syndrome. J Rheumatol 1995;22:1867–1871.
66. Strand V. New therapies for systemic lupus erythematosus. Rheum Dis Clin North Am 2000;26:389–406.
67. Hayslett JP. The effect of systemic lupus erythematosus on pregnancy and pregnancy outcome. Am J Reprod Immunol 1992;28:199–204.
68. Khamashta MA, Ruiz-Irastorza G, Hughes GR. Systemic lupus erythematosus flares during pregnancy. Rheum Dis Clin North Am 1997,23. 15–30.
69. Parke A, West B. Hydroxychloroquine in pregnant patients with systemic lupus erythematosus. J Rheumatol 1996;23:1715–1718.
70. Petri M. Systemic lupus erythematosus and pregnancy. Rheum Dis Clin North Am 1994;20:87–118.
71. Brennecke SP, Brown MA, Crowther CA, et al. Aspirin and prevention of preeclampsia. Aust NZ J Obstet Gynaecol 1995;35:38–41.
72. Khamashta MA, Cuadrado MJ, Mujic F, et al. The management of thrombosis in the antiphospholipid-antibody syndrome. N Engl J Med 1995; 332:993–997.
73. Price EJ, Venables PJW. Drug-induced lupus. Drug Saf 1995;12:283–290.
74. Yung RL, Richardson BC. Drug-induced lupus. Rheum Dis Clin North Am 1994;20:61–86.
75. Clarke AE, Petri MA, Manzi S, et al. An international perspective on the well-being and health care costs for patients with systemic lupus erythematosus. J Rheumatol 1999;26:1500–1511.
76. Clarke AE, Bloch DA, Danoff DS, Esdaile JM. Decreasing costs and improving outcomes in systemic lupus erythematosus: Using regression trees to develop health policy. J Rheumatol 1994;21:2246–2253.
77. Lacaille D, Clarke AE, Bloch DA, et al. The impact of disease activity, treatment and disease severity on short term costs of systemic lupus erythematosus. J Rheumatol 1994;21:448–453.
78. McInnes PM, Schuttinga J, Sanslone WR, et al. The economic impact of treatment of severe lupus nephritis with prednisone and intravenous cyclophosphamide. Arthritis Rheum 1994;37:1000–1006.
79. Yarboro CH, Wesley R, Amantea MA, et al. Modified oral ondansetron regimen for cyclophosphamide-induced emesis in lupus nephritis. Ann Pharmacother 1996;30:752–755.
80. Wigley FM. Systemic sclerosis: Clinical features. In: Klippel JH, Dieppe PA, eds. Rheumatology, 2d ed. Philadelphia, Mosby 1998: 9.1–9.14.
81. Medsger TA, Steen VD. Classification, prognosis. In: Clements PH, Furst DE, eds. Systemic Sclerosis. Baltimore, Williams & Wilkins, 1996: 51–64.
82. Seibold JR, Furst DE, Clements PJ. Treatment of systemic sclerosis by disease modifying drugs. In: Clements PH, Furst DE, eds. Systemic Sclerosis. Baltimore, Williams & Wilkins, 1996: 535–548.
83. Steen VD. Organ involvement: renal. In: Clements PH, Furst DE, eds. Systemic Sclerosis. Baltimore, Williams & Wilkins, 1996: 425–440.
84. Dalakas MC. Immunopathogenesis of inflammatory myopathies. Ann Neurol 1995;37(Suppl 1):S74–86.
85. Targoff IN. Diagnosis and treatment of polymyositis and dermatomyositis. Compr Ther 1990;16:16–24.
86. Ghate J, Katsambas A, Augerinou G, Jorizzo JL. A therapeutic update on dermatomyositis/polymyositis. Int J Dermatol 2000;39:81–87.
87. Dalakas MC. Update on the use of intravenous immune globulin in the treatment of patients with inflammatory muscle disease. J Clin Immunol 1995;15(Suppl 6):70S–75S.
88. Epperly TD, Moore KE, Harrover JD. Polymyalgia rheumatica and temporal arteritis. Am Fam Physician 2000;62:789–796, 801.
89. Evans JM, Hunder GG. Polymyalgia rheumatica and giant cell arteritis. Rheum Dis Clin North Am 2000;26:493–515.
90. Brooks RC, McGee SR. Diagnostic dilemmas in polymyalgia rheumatica. Arch Intern Med 1997;157:162–168.
91. Feinberg HL, Sherman JD, Schrepferman CG, et al. The use of methotrexate in polymyalgia rheumatica. J Rheumatol 1996;23:1550–1552.
92. Gay RM Jr, Ball GV. Vasculitis. In: Koopman WJ, ed: Arthritis and Allied Conditions: A Textbook of Rheumatology, 13th ed. Baltimore, Williams & Wilkins, 1997: 1491–1524.
93. Jayne D. Evidence-based treatment of systemic vasculitis. Rheumatology 2000;39:585–595.
94. Gladman DD, Urowitz MB, Fortin P, et al. Systemic lupus international collaborating clinics conference on assessment of lupus flare and quality of life measures in SLE. J Rheumatol 1996;23:1953–1955

89

ALLERGIC AND PSEUDOALLERGIC DRUG REACTIONS

Joseph T. DiPiro, Dennis R. Ownby, and Lauren S. Schlesselman

Allergic drug reactions are adverse medication effects that involve immunologic mechanisms. Adverse drug effects not proven to be immune mediated but resembling allergic reactions in their clinical presentation are referred to as *allergic-like* or *pseudoallergic reactions*.[1]

Allergic reactions are responsible for up to 5% of reactions to medications among hospitalized patients.[2–5] The true frequency of allergic drug reactions is difficult to determine because many reactions may not be reported and others may be difficult to distinguish from nonallergic adverse events. Dermatologic reactions represent the most frequently recognized and reported form of allergic drug reactions.

MECHANISMS OF ALLERGIC DRUG REACTIONS

Drugs can cause allergic reactions by a variety of immunologic mechanisms. Although some reactions are relatively well defined, the majority are due to mechanisms that are either unknown or poorly understood.[6]

The following criteria suggest that a drug reaction may be immunologically mediated[7]: (1) The reaction occurs in a small percentage of patients receiving the drug, (2) the observed reaction does not resemble the drug's pharmacologic effect, (3) the type of manifestation is similar to that seen with other allergic reactions (e.g., anaphylaxis, urticaria, serum sickness), (4) there is a lag time between first exposure of the drug and reaction, (5) the reaction is reproduced even by minute doses of the drug, (6) the reaction is reproduced by agents with similar chemical structures, (7) eosinophilia is present, and (8) the reaction resolves after the drug has been discontinued. Exceptions to each of these criteria are observed commonly.

Many allergic reactions can be classified into one of four immunopathologic categories: types I, II, III, and IV[8,9] (Table 89–1 and Fig. 89–1). Some drug reactions suspected of being immunologically mediated are considered possibly allergic. Examples include drug-associated skin eruptions, drug fever, drug-induced hepatitis, and interstitial nephritis. Other drug reactions can be classified as *pseudoallergic* or *idiosyncratic*. Examples include anaphylactoid (anaphylaxis-like) reactions to radiocontrast media, sulfite sensitivity, and reactions to local anesthetics.

EFFECTORS OF ALLERGIC DRUG REACTIONS

Allergic drug reactions can involve most of the major components of the immune system, including the cellular elements, immunoglobulins, complement, and cytokines. Most immunoglobulin isotypes have been implicated in immunologically mediated drug reactions. Immunoglobulin E (IgE) bound to basophils or mast cells mediates immediate (anaphylactic-type) reactions. IgG or IgM antibodies also may be involved in allergic reactions, resulting in destruction of cells and tissues.

CELLULAR ELEMENTS

A variety of cells may be involved in immunologic drug reactions. Basophils, mast cells, eosinophils, and lymphocytes are involved most frequently. Platelets and vascular endothelial cells are also important because they also can release a number of inflammatory mediators. Most cells of the body, including nerve cells, can become involved directly or indirectly in allergic drug reactions.[10]

MEDIATORS OF ALLERGIC REACTIONS[11]

The release of a number of preformed, pharmacologically active chemical mediators [e.g., histamine, serotonin, eosinophil chemotactic factor (ECF-A), neutrophil chemotactic factor (NCF-A), and bradykinin-generating factor, also known as basophil kalikrein of anaphylaxis (BK-A)] are triggered by antigen cross-linking IgE molecules on the surface of circulating basophils and tissue mast cells. Newly generated mediators include platelet-activating factor (PAF) and arachidonic acid metabolites (e.g., prostaglandins, thromboxanes, leukotrienes). Each of these mediators is discussed in the following sections.

Histamine is a low-molecular-weight amine compound formed by decarboxylation of histidine and stored in basophil and mast cell granules. The release of histamine from these cells is triggered by antigen cross-linking IgE bound to specific receptors on the surface membranes of mast cells and basophils. The tissue effects of histamine are evident within 1 to 2 minutes, but it is rapidly metabolized within 10 to 15 minutes. The major effects of histamine on target tissues include increased capillary permeability, contraction of bronchial and vascular smooth muscle, and hypersecretion of mucous glands.

Serotonin is also a low-molecular-weight amine stored in and released from platelets and mast cells with effects similar to histamine. It may cause vasoconstriction or vasodilatation in some animal species but has no proven role in human anaphylaxis. Eosinophil chemotactic factor(s) are a group of preformed cellular tetrapeptides and dodecapeptides released by stimulated mast cells. They attract eosinophils to inflammatory sites and participate in phagocytosis. Neutrophil chemotactic factor is a high molecular-weight protein that enhances neutrophil migration to areas of mast cell activation. Bradykinin-generating factor is a series of proteases that activate Hageman factor, resulting in the production of kinins, including bradykinin, which is more potent than histamine on a molar basis in causing vascular permeability and contraction of smooth muscle.

PAF is a glyceride-derived substance that is released by mast cells, alveolar macrophages, neutrophils, platelets, and other cells but not by basophils. It has potent bronchoconstrictor effects and also causes platelet aggregation and lysis. It attracts neutrophils and causes their activation. Also, PAF enhances vascular permeability and can cause pain, pruritus, and erythema.

TABLE 89–1. Classification of Allergic Drug Reactions

Type	Descriptor	Characteristics	Typical Onset	Drug Causes
I	Anaphylactic (IgE mediated)	Allergen binds to IgE on basophils or mast cells resulting in release of inflammatory mediators	Within 30 min	Penicillin immediate reaction Blood products Polypeptide hormones Vaccines Dextran
II	Cytotoxic	Cell destruction occurs because of cell-associated antigen that initiates cytolysis by antigen-specific antibody (IgG or IgM). Most often involves blood elements.	Typically 5–12 h	Penicillin, quinidine, phenylbutazone, thiouracils, sulfonamides, methyldopa
III	Immune complex	Antigen–antibody complexes form and deposit on blood vessel walls and activate complement. Result is a serum-sickness-like syndrome.	3–8 h	May be caused by penicillins, sulfonamides, radiocontrast agents, hydantoins
IV	Cell mediated (delayed)	Antigens cause activation of lymphocytes, which release inflammatory mediators.	24–48 h	Tuberculin reaction

The leukotrienes (LTs) are metabolites of arachidonic acid produced through the 5-lipoxygenase pathway that have potent effects on bronchial and vascular smooth muscle. Three important leukotrienes, LTC_4, LTD_4, and LTE_4, are produced by basophils or mast cells. These three substances are also referred to as *cystinyl leukotrienes* and in older literature as *slow-reacting substances of anaphylaxis* (SRS-A). The LTs have more potent and longer-lasting bronchoconstrictor effects than histamine and also can increase vascular permeability and cause arteriolar vasoconstriction followed by vasodilatation. Their effects are slower in onset but longer lasting than those of histamine. Another product, LTB_4, is a potent chemoattractant, particularly for neutrophils. It is also produced by neutrophils, macrophages, and monocytes.

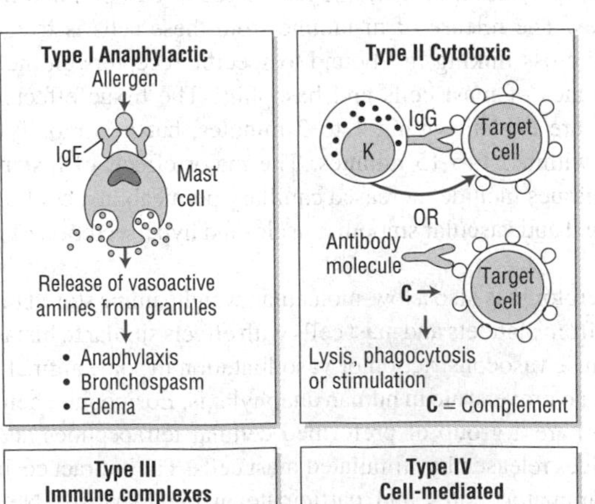

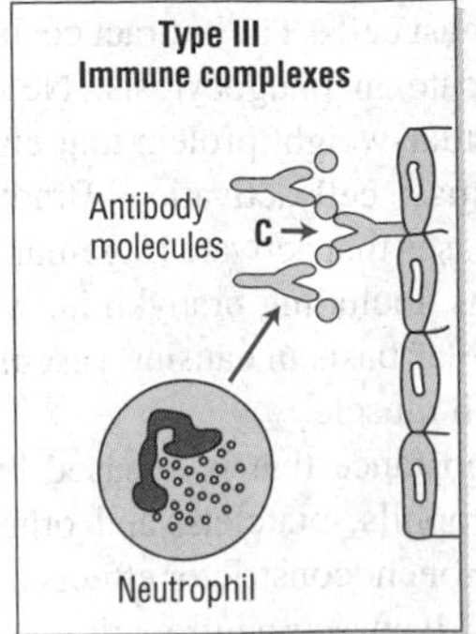

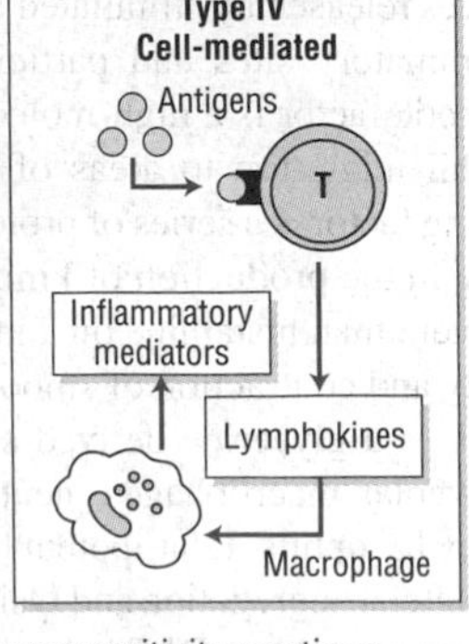

FIGURE 89–1. Types of hypersensitivity reactions.

Prostaglandins (PGs) and thromboxanes are metabolites of arachidonic acid produced through the cyclooxygenase pathway. Some prostaglandins have vasoconstrictive and/or bronchodilatory properties, whereas others are vasodilatory (e.g., PGD_2) and/or bronchoconstrictive (e.g., $PGF_{2\alpha}$). PGD_2 is the major prostaglandin product of mast cells. It is a potent inhibitor of platelet aggregation. Thromboxanes cause platelet aggregation and are important regulators of coagulation.

The complement system consists of approximately 20 plasma proteins and is involved in hypersensitivity through a variety of immunologic responses, including enhancement of phagocytosis (opsonization of target cells), cell lysis, and generation of anaphylatoxins (C3a, C4a, and C5a), which can cause non-IgE-mediated activation of mast cells and release of inflammatory mediators.

CLASSIFICATION OF IMMUNOPATHOLOGIC DRUG REACTIONS

Immunologic mechanisms have been identified for some drug reactions. Many can be classified into one of four immunopathologic reactions, as described below. In general, small-molecular-weight compounds (<10,000 MW) are not immunogenic. Most drugs are less than 1000 MW. To become immunogenic, these small compounds must first combine with carrier proteins in plasma or tissue. The combination of the drug bound to a carrier protein can be recognized as foreign, leading to an immune response. The more likely a drug is bound to a protein, the greater is the risk that it will produce an allergic reaction. Penicillin G (356 MW) is an example of a drug that binds covalently to serum proteins through amide or disulfide linkages. For drugs such as the sulfonamides, the parent compound first must be converted to a metabolite before it can combine with the macromolecule. The species that combines with the carrier macromolecule is referred to as a *hapten* or an *incomplete antigen*. Some macromolecular drugs such as insulin are referred to as *complete antigens* because they are large enough to initiate an immune response without binding to another protein.

TYPE I

Type I reactions require the presence of IgE specific for the drug antigen or other allergen. IgE specific for the drug allergen is produced on initial exposure to the antigen, and then it binds to basophils and mast cells. On repeat exposure to the antigen, two or more IgE molecules on the basophil or mast cell surface may bind to one multivalent antigen molecule (referred to as *cross-linking;* see Fig. 89–1) initiating an activation of the cell. Activation causes the extracellular release of granules with preformed inflammatory mediators including histamine, serotonin, heparin, proteases (tryptase in the mast cell), bradykinin-generating factor, eosinophil chemotactic factors, and neutrophil chemotactic factor, as well as generation of newly formed mediators, as previously discussed, such as LTs, prostaglandins, thromboxanes, and PAF, among others.

Generation of a type I reaction can be evident as an immediate hypersensitivity reaction, or anaphylaxis. Immediate reactions may be limited to single organs, typically in the nasal mucosa (rhinitis), respiratory tract (acute asthma), skin, or gastrointestinal tract, or can involve multiple organs simultaneously, termed *analphylaxis*.

TYPE II

Type II immunopathologic reactions involve destruction of host cells (usually blood cells) through cytotoxic antibodies by one of two mechanisms (see Fig. 89–1). First, the drug binds to the cell as a hapten (e.g., the platelet or red blood cell). Antibodies (IgG or IgM) specific for the bound drug or to a component of the cell surface that has been altered by the drug then bind, initiating a cytolytic reaction. The cell destruction may be mediated by complement or by phagocytic cells that have Fc receptors on their surfaces. Activation of complement near the cell surface can result in loss of cell membrane integrity and cell death. Alternatively, neutrophils, monocytes, or macrophages may bind to the cell coated with antibody bound by IgG Fc receptors on the attacking cell surface, resulting in phagocytosis of the target cell. The process of enhancement of phagocytosis by antibody-covered cell surfaces is referred to as *opsonization.* In addition, cell-bound IgG may direct the nonphagocytic action of T cells or natural killer cells, which results in cell destruction by a process called *antibody-dependent cellular cytotoxicity* (ADCC). This process can proceed in a nonspecific fashion as T cells bind to the target cell through IgG Fc receptors on the T-cell surface. Contact is necessary between the target and effector cells.

Cells commonly affected by these types of reactions include erythrocytes, leukocytes, and platelets, resulting in hemolytic anemia, agranulocytosis, or thrombocytopenia, respectively. This process may be initiated by drugs such as penicillin, quinidine, quinine, phenacetin, cephalosporins, and sulfonamides, among others.

Another type of reaction that may affect the formed elements in blood is the "innocent bystander" reaction. With this type of reaction, antigen-antibody complexes formed in blood adhere nonspecifically to cells. Complement is then activated, resulting in cell lysis.

TYPE III

Type III immunologic reactions are caused by antigen-antibody complexes that are formed in blood. The complexes form with drug allergen and antibody in varying ratios and may deposit in tissues, resulting in local or disseminated inflammatory reactions. Antigen-antibody complex formation can result in platelet aggregation, complement activation, or macrophage activation. Chemotactic substances such as C4a are also produced, and they cause the influx of neutrophils and result in the release of a number of toxic substances from the neutrophil (e.g., proteinases, collagenases, kinin-generating enzymes, and reactive oxygen and nitrogen substances), which can cause local tissue destruction.

Platelet aggregation also may occur as a result of immune-complex formation, resulting in the formation of microthrombi and the release of vasoactive mediators. Also, insoluble complexes may be phagocytized by macrophages and activate these cells.

The formation of antigen-antibody complexes can lead to clinical syndromes such as the Arthus reaction. In this model, a high level of preformed specific IgG antibody combines with antigen to produce a localized edematous, erythematous reaction within 5 to 8 hours. The reaction involves local formation of insoluble antigen-antibody complexes, complement activation with anaphylatoxin release, mast cell degranulation, and influx of polymorphonuclear cells.

TYPE IV

Type IV immunopathologic reactions are mediated by T cells and involve delayed hypersensitivity. Type IV reactions require memory T cells specific for the antigen in question. On exposure to the antigen, the T cells become activated and produce an inflammatory response. Although these reactions may be associated with adverse effects (e.g., contact dermatitis), they also may be useful for diagnostic purposes. Examples of the latter include the purified protein derivative (PPD) antigen from *Mycobacterium tuberculosis* used in the tuberculin skin test and other recall skin test antigens, such as mumps. After intradermal injection, these antigens produce a local reaction (erythema and induration) within 48 to 72 hours. Delayed contact hypersensitivity also can be caused by a wide variety of chemicals and drugs.

OTHER ALLERGIC REACTIONS

The mechanisms of many allergic reactions are not known, although they are believed to be immune mediated. Perhaps most common are the delayed dermatologic reactions that occur with a variety of drugs (especially penicillins and sulfonamides). These reactions may be evident as macropapular, morbilliform, or erythematous rashes; exfoliative dermatitis; photosensitivity reactions; or eczema. These reactions often cause pruritus, urticaria, and angioedema.

Other serious dermatologic syndromes may be the result of immunologic reactions. These include Stevens-Johnson syndrome, characterized by rash, erythema multiforme with mucous membrane involvement, and toxic epidermal necrolysis (widespread blister formation in the epidermis), which are referred to as *febrile mucocutaneous syndromes*. Drugs commonly associated with these syndromes include the penicillins, sulfonamides, and anticonvulsants such as phenytoin and phenobarbital, as well as a number of other agents. Drug-induced fever also may involve immunologic mechanisms. Other general types of reactions believed to be immune mediated include hepatic drug reactions (cholestatic or hepatocellular) and pulmonary reactions, e.g., interstitial pneumonitis, which has been associated with nitrofurantoin.

ANAPHYLACTOID REACTIONS

A number of substances can produce an anaphylactoid (anaphylaxis-like) reaction that is similar to anaphylaxis in clinical signs and symptoms. The substances causing these reactions can produce the direct release of inflammatory mediators from cells by a pharmacologic effect rather than through cell-bound IgE. These reactions are sometimes referred to as *pseudoallergic*, but not all pseudoallergic reactions are anaphylactoid. Drugs that can produce anaphylactoid reactions include vancomycin (most common), opiates, iodinated radiocontrast agents, amphotericin, and D-tubocurarine. A number of other agents (including aspirin) may produce anaphylactoid reactions by altering the metabolism of inflammatory mediators such as prostaglandins or kinins.

CLINICAL MANIFESTATIONS OF ALLERGIC AND ALLERGIC-LIKE REACTIONS

ANAPHYLAXIS

Anaphylaxis is an acute, life-threatening allergic reaction involving multiple organ systems.[12,13] From 1.2% to 15% of the U.S. population may be at risk of anaphylactic reactions.[14] Although many drugs may cause anaphylaxis (or anaphylactoid) reactions, those reported most commonly are aspirin and other nonsteroidal anti-inflammatory drugs, penicillins, and insulins.[15] The manifestations of anaphylaxis may include signs and symptoms referable to the skin, gastrointestinal tract, respiratory tract, and cardiovascular system. Patients may experience adverse effects involving any combination of these systems. Common dermatologic manifestations include urticaria, angioedema, and pruritus.[15] Gastrointestinal manifestations include nausea, abdominal pain, vomiting, and diarrhea. With respiratory tract involvement, the patient may experience dyspnea or wheezing. The major cardiovascular manifestations include hypotension, tachycardia, and arrhythmias.

Anaphylactic reactions generally begin within 30 minutes but almost always within 2 hours after exposure to the inciting allergen. The risk of fatal anaphylaxis is greatest within the first few hours. After apparent recovery, anaphylaxis may recur 6 to 8 hours after antigen exposure. Because of the possibility of these late-phase reactions, patients should be observed for at least 12 hours after an anaphylactic reaction. Fatal anaphylaxis most often results from asphyxia due to airway obstruction either at the larynx or within the lungs. Cardiovascular collapse may occur as a result of asphyxia in some cases, whereas in others cases cardiovascular collapse may be the dominant manifestation.

SERUM SICKNESS

Serum sickness is a clinical syndrome resulting from the effects of soluble circulating immune complexes that form under conditions of antigen excess. The reaction commonly results from the use of heterologous antisera containing foreign (donor) antigens such as equine serum in the form of antitoxins or antivenins. The onset of serum sickness usually occurs 7 to 14 days after antigen administration. Fever, malaise, and lymphadenopathy are the most common clinical manifestations. Arthralgias, urticaria, and morbilliform skin eruption also may be present. Although often associated with administration of heterologous antisera, serum sickness also may be caused by drugs, including sulfonamides, hydantoins, penicillins, and cephalosporins (especially cefaclor). In addition, immune-complex-mediated systemic lupus erythematosus-like syndrome has been attributed to reactions from drugs such as hydralazine, procainamide, isoniazid, and phenytoin.

DRUG FEVER

Fever may occur in response to an inflammatory process or develop as a manifestation of a drug reaction. Drug fever occurs in as many as 10% of hospital inpatients.[16] A large number of drugs have been reported to cause fever, including methyldopa, procainamide, phenytoin, barbiturates, quinidine, and a variety of antibiotics. These drugs may affect the central nervous system directly to alter temperature regulation or stimulate the release of endogenous pyrogens (e.g., interleukin-1 and tumor necrosis factor) from white blood cells. Drugs also may cause fever as a result of their pharmacologic effects on tissues, e.g., fever resulting from massive tumor cell destruction caused by chemotherapy. However, the mechanism of drug fever remains unknown for agents such as amphotericin B and radiographic contrast agents.

The temperature pattern of drug-induced fever is quite variable. It may be low grade and continuous or spiking and intermittent. A temporal relationship between drug administration and occurrence of fever has been noted for some medications. Generally, withdrawal of the causative agent results in prompt defervescence as soon as the drug is completely metabolized. Fever usually recurs on readministration of the causative agent.

DRUG-INDUCED AUTOIMMUNITY

Autoimmune diseases have been associated with drugs and may involve a variety of tissues and organs. A commonly recognized drug-related autoimmune disorder is systemic lupus erythematosus (SLE) induced by procainamide, hydralazine, or isoniazid. Other drugs associated with SLE include methyldopa, β-adrenergic blockers, penicillamine, quinidine, interferon-γ, and sulfasalazine.[17] The most common clinical manifestations include arthralgias, myalgias, and polyarthritis. Facial rash, ulcers, and alopecia occur less frequently. Renal or pulmonary involvement also may occur. These reactions typically develop several months after beginning the drug and generally resolve soon after it is discontinued.[18]

Other syndromes believed to involve autoimmune mechanisms include drug-induced hemolytic anemia due to methyldopa, renal interstitial nephritis produced by methicillin, and hepatitis caused by phenytoin and halothane. Interstitial nephritis is characterized by fever, rash, and eosinophilia associated with proteinuria and hematuria. Hepatic damage due to drugs generally is manifested as either hepatocellular necrosis or cholestatic hepatitis. Drug-induced hepatitis has been associated with phenothiazines, sulfonamides, halothane, phenytoin, and isoniazid (see Chap. 38). Hepatocellular destruction is evidenced by elevations in serum transaminases. Hepatomegaly and jaundice sometimes may be evident. Cholestasis may be manifested by jaundice and elevations in serum alkaline phosphatase and sometimes by rash, fever, and eosinophilia.

VASCULITIS

Vasculitis is a clinicopathologic process characterized by inflammation and necrosis of blood vessels. The vasculitic process may be limited to the skin or may involve multiple organs, including the liver or kidney, joints, or central nervous system. Characteristically, cutaneous vasculitis is manifested by purpuric lesions that vary in size and number. Vasculitis also may be manifested as papules, nodules, ulcerations, or vesiculobullous lesions, generally occurring on the lower extremities, but the upper extremities, including the hands, also may be involved. Drugs associated with vasculitis include allopurinol, β-lactam antibiotics, sulfonamides, thiazide diuretics, and phenytoin.

DERMATOLOGIC REACTIONS

A wide variety of dermatologic drug reactions have been reported to have an immunologic basis.[19] As noted previously, cutaneous reactions are the most common manifestations of allergic drug reactions.

TABLE 89–2. Top 10 Drugs or Agents Reported to Cause Skin Reactions

	Reactions per 1000 Recipients
Amoxicillin	51.4
Trimethoprim-sulfamethoxazole	33.8
Ampicillin	33.2
Iopodate	27.8
Blood	21.6
Cephalosporins	21.1
Erythromycin	20.4
Dihydralazine hydrochloride	19.1
Penicillin G	18.5
Cyanocobalamin	17.9

Adapted from Ref. 19.

Although most dermatologic reactions are mild and resolve promptly after discontinuing the drug, some may progress to serious or even life-threatening reactions (e.g., toxic epidermal necrolysis or Stevens-Johnson syndrome). Cutaneous adverse reactions were reported to occur in 2.7% of hospitalized patients.[20] Serious dermatologic drug reactions are estimated to occur in 1.9 cases per 1 million people per year and can have a mortality rate as high as 40%.[21,22] Table 89–2 lists drugs and agents most commonly associated with cutaneous reactions.[23] Antimicrobials are implicated most frequently. In a report of almost 6000 children, about 12% developed rashes with cefaclor compared with 7.4% with penicillins and 8.5% with sulfonamides.[24] The clinical presentation of dermatologic drug reactions is discussed in more detail in Chapter 108.

RESPIRATORY REACTIONS

Drugs also may produce upper or lower respiratory tract reactions, including rhinitis and asthma. Respiratory tract manifestations may result from direct injury to the airways or may occur as a component of a systemic reaction (e.g., anaphylaxis). Asthma may be induced by aspirin and other nonsteroidal anti-inflammatory agents, as discussed in the following paragraphs, or by sulfites used as preservatives in foods and medications. Other pulmonary drug reactions believed to be immunologic include acute infiltrative and chronic fibrotic pulmonary reactions. The latter is often caused by antineoplastic agents such as bleomycin. For a more detailed discussion of drug-induced pulmonary disease, see Chapter 29.

HEMATOLOGIC REACTIONS

Most formed elements and soluble components of the hematopoietic system may be affected by immunologic drug reactions. Eosinophilia is a common manifestation of drug hypersensitivity and may be the only presenting sign. Hemolytic anemia may result from hypersensitivity to drugs. Other hematologic reactions include thrombocytopenia, granulocytopenia, and agranulocytosis. For a detailed discussion of hematologic drug reactions, see Chapter 102.

FACTORS RELATED TO THE OCCURRENCE OR SEVERITY OF ALLERGIC DRUG REACTIONS

A number of factors influence the likelihood of allergic drug reactions. Among these are the dose of the allergen, the route of exposure, and the sensitivity of the individual as determined by age, genetics, or environmental factors. For many drugs, the severity of a reaction is determined by the dose and the duration of exposure. A relatively larger dose or longer duration of treatment encourages development of drug sensitivity. The route of administration also influences drug sensitivity. The topical route of drug administration appears to be the most likely to sensitize and predispose to drug reactions. The oral route is the safest, and the parenteral route is the most hazardous for administration of drugs in sensitive individuals. There are relatively few reported cases of immediate hypersensitivity-associated deaths with oral β-lactam antimicrobials. Although intravenous administration is more likely to result in severe immediate reactions in a sensitized individual, it may be the least likely route for initially inducing sensitivity. One possible explanation is that intravenous administration results in systemic drug exposure for the shortest period of time.

Individual host factors are also important in determining drug sensitivity. There may be a genetic predisposition for some types of allergic reactions. Slow acetylators of procainamide and hydralazine are at increased risk for SLE.

Drug allergies appear to develop with equal frequency in atopic and nonatopic individuals.[6] In addition, patients with a history of drug allergy appear to be at increased risk of adverse reactions to other pharmacologic agents. Age seems to be related to the risk of allergic reactions because they occur less frequently in children. This may be related to immaturity of the immune system or decreased exposure. The presence of concurrent diseases predisposes to drug reactions. Examples include the morbilliform rash that occurs after ampicillin administration to patients with infectious mononucleosis and the reactions that occur with trimethoprim-sulfamethoxazole in acquired immunodeficiency syndrome (AIDS) patients.

DRUGS COMMONLY CAUSING ALLERGIC OR ALLERGIC-LIKE DRUG REACTIONS

β-LACTAM ANTIMICROBIALS

Allergic reactions to penicillin occur in 0.7% to 8% of treatment courses but was as high as 15% in one retrospective report of hospitalized patients treated with penicillin.[25,26] While most patients reporting penicillin allergy do not have allergy, a reported history is associated with a higher likelihood of positive skin test reactivity.[28] The most common reactions to penicillin include urticaria, pruritus, and angioedema. All four of the major types of hypersensitivity reactions have been reported with penicillin, as well as some reactions that do not fit into these categories. A wide variety of idiopathic reactions occurs, e.g., maculopapular eruptions, eosinophilia, Stevens-Johnson syndrome, and exfoliative dermatitis. Maculopapular rash occurs in about 2% of treatment courses of penicillin and in 5.2% to 9.5% with ampicillin. The incidence of ampicillin rash increases to 69% to 100% of patients with Epstein-Barr virus infection, cytomegalovirus infection, or acute lymphocytic leukemia.

Some aspects of the mechanism of penicillin immunogenicity have been determined. Because benzylpenicillin is a relatively small molecule (MW 356), it must combine with macromolecules (presumably proteins) to elicit an immune response. Penicillin may bind covalently to the lysine residues of proteins such as albumin through an amide linkage involving the β-lactam ring (Fig. 89–2). This is the penicilloyl-protein conjugate and is referred to as the *major antigenic determinant*. In addition, a number of other penicillin metabolites may bind covalently to proteins. These are referred to as *minor antigenic determinants*. The terms *major* and *minor* refer to the relative

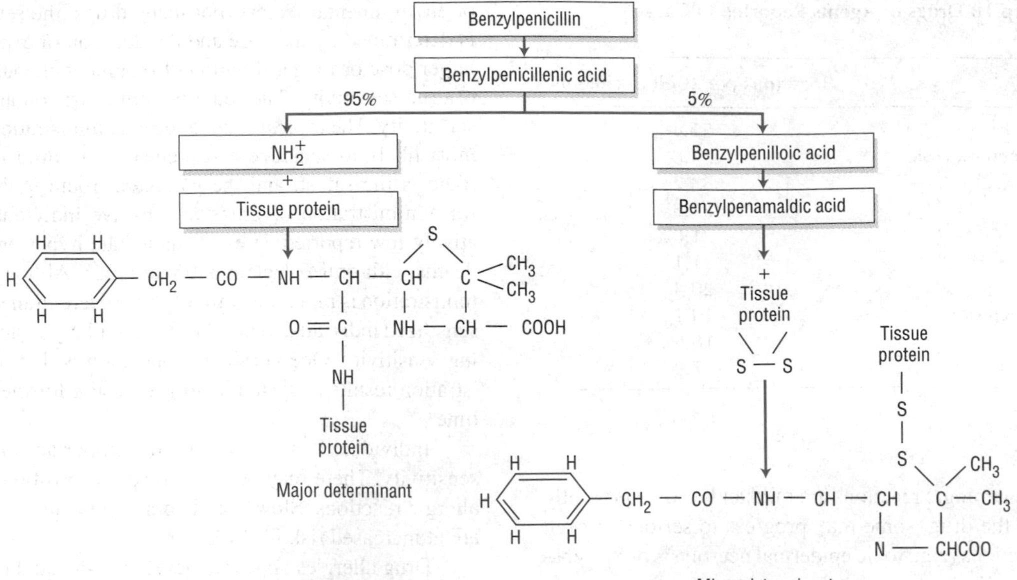

FIGURE 89–2. Formation of the benzyl penicilloyl hapten–protein complex.

proportions of these conjugates that are formed and not to the clinical severity of the reactions generated. In fact, the minor antigenic determinants are more likely to cause anaphylactic reactions. The humoral immune response to penicillin has been well studied. From one report of 60 patients who received 3 g or more per day of penicillin for at least 10 days, 38% had detectable IgG response to benzylpenicilloyl groups and 18% had detectable IgE response.[27] Immediate hypersensitivity reactions may be mediated by IgE for minor as well as major determinants.

Patients who are allergic to penicillins also may be sensitive to other β-lactams.[28] The exact incidence of cross-reactivity between cephalosporins and penicillins is not known, although it is believed to be low.[29]

Most allergists would not administer cephalosporins to patients who had history of hives from penicillin, although some studies have suggested that there is little risk of an allergic response to a cephalosporin even in a person with a positive skin test to penicillin.[30–33] The postmarketing surveillance report by Anne and Reisman states that there has been no increase in allergic reactions to second- and third-generation cephalosporins in patients with histories of penicillin allergy.[33] Results of skin testing with cephalosporins have not been thought to be reliable because the mechanism of cephalosporin sensitivity has not been defined clearly. One study from France has suggested that skin tests are predictive with a number of β-lactam antibiotics, but this study only performed oral challenges on skin test-negative children.[32] At present, patients with positive penicillin skin tests are advised not to receive cephalosporins if they can be avoided. Patients who have experienced only mild cutaneous reactions, such as maculopapular rashes, may receive cephalosporins with caution.

Other new β-lactam derivatives (e.g., monobactams and carbapenems) have been studied for potential cross-reactivity with penicillins. In vitro and in vivo studies have demonstrated that the monobactam aztreonam only weakly cross-reacts with penicillin and that it may be administered safely to most patients who are penicillin-allergic.[34,35] In contrast, there appears to be considerable cross-reactivity between imipenem (a carbapenem) and penicillin. Therefore, imipenem (and other carbapenems) should not be administered to patients who have positive penicillin skin tests.

RADIOCONTRAST MEDIA

Radiocontrast agents frequently cause allergic-like reactions because these agents are used commonly in medical practice. Between 5% and 10% of patients receiving radiocontrast agents experience some type of adverse reaction. Of the variety of reactions reported, approximately 1% are urticarial and 0.25% dypnea, and severe reactions occur as infrequently as 0.01%. In addition, radiocontrast agents may cause dose-dependent toxic reactions that can cause cardiovascular effects, arrhythmias, changes in renal blood flow, diuresis, or proteinuria.[36,37] The older, high-osmolar agents that are now used less commonly have a greater frequency of reactions compared with the newer, low-osmolar agents.

The mechanism of reactions to radiocontrast agents is not clearly understood. Allergic-like reactions are not IgE mediated. Potential mechanisms of reactivity include the activation of complement directly by the radiocontrast agents.[39] Also, the older, high-osmolar radiocontrast agents can activate mast cells and basophils directly (IgE-independent mechanism), resulting in the release of inflammatory mediators.[40] The low-osmolar contrast agents appear to result in fewer anaphylactoid reactions. In a report of 800 intravascular procedures, the frequency of immediate generalized reactions to high-osmolar radiocontrast agents was 9.1%. This contrasted with a frequency of 0.5% in 181 intravascular procedures using low-osmolar agents in patients who previously had experienced an immediate generalized reaction with high-osmolar agents.[41] The relative risk of having a reaction to a lower-osmolarity, nonionic agent is estimated to be at least five times lower than with conventional agents.[37]

Patients at risk of reactions to radiocontrast agents are difficult to identify. History is helpful, because a patient who has experienced previous reactions is more likely to experience subsequent reactions. The risk of allergic reactions to radiocontrast media is greater in women and in patients with a history of atopy or asthma.[37,38] Despite a common misconception, a seafood allergy does not predispose to radiocontrast media reactions. Neither skin tests nor oral tests are useful for predicting reactions to these agents. Some regimens have been recommended to prevent reactions in patients who have experienced them previously. One pretreatment regimen includes the administration of prednisone 50 mg orally 13, 7, and 1 hours before the procedure, diphenhydramine 50 mg orally or intramuscularly 1 hour before the procedure, and ephedrine 25 mg orally 1 hour before.[42] The ephedrine should be omitted if the patient has angina, arrhythmia, or hypertension. Guidelines have been published for treatment of acute reactions to contrast media and may include adrenergic agents such as epinephrine, fluid replacement, diphenhydramine, H_2-receptor antagonist, and systemic corticosteroids.[36,43]

INSULIN

Insulin is capable of producing allergic reactions through a variety of immunologic mechanisms. A protein molecule, insulin is a complete antigen. Allergic reactions have been reported with beef, pork, and recombinant human insulin, although the frequency of reactions with human insulin appears low. Reactions to insulin may involve the insulin molecule itself or other substances that have been added to insulin (e.g., protamine). The majority of patients have anti-insulin antibodies after a few months of therapy.

Insulin reactions may be limited to the site of injection, or they may produce systemic reactions. Local reactions present most often as a wheal and flare at the injection site and may occur immediately after injection or up to 8 to 12 hours later. Generally, these reactions are mild, do not require treatment, and resolve with continued insulin administration. If a patient does not tolerate the local reaction well, antihistamines may be given or a different insulin source (or product of higher purity) may be substituted. Rarely, systemic reactions to insulin (e.g., urticaria or anaphylaxis) occur. IgE-mediated reactions to insulin allergy appear to be declining with greater use of human insulins.[44] Skin testing with various products can aid in selecting the type of insulin least likely to cause a systemic reaction. Human insulin appears to be least allergenic but occasionally may cause reactions. In some patients, insulin desensitization may be indicated.

ASPIRIN AND NONSTEROIDAL ANTI-INFLAMMATORY DRUGS

Aspirin and other nonsteroidal anti-inflammatory drugs (NSAIDs) produce characteristic reactions in susceptible patients.[45,46] The two general types of reactions to aspirin are urticaria/angioedema and rhinosinusitis/asthma. Approximately 1% of the population exposed to NSAIDs experiences urticaria or angioedema, whereas about 0.5% experiences rhinosinusitis/asthma.[47,48]

The rhinosinusitis/asthma syndrome typically develops in middle-aged patients who are nonatopic and have no history of aspirin intolerance. Generally, it progresses from rhinitis to sinusitis with nasal polyps and steroid-dependent asthma. It is uncommon in children and young adults. However, children with asthma may be aspirin-sensitive. In retrospective studies, 1.9% to 5.6% of asthmatics are aspirin-sensitive,[49] whereas up to 40% of steroid-dependent asthmatics may be aspirin-sensitive.[50] In aspirin-sensitive asthmatics, administration of aspirin and NSAIDs may provoke an asthmatic attack. Ketorolac can cause severe, life-threatening bronchospasm in aspirin-sensitive asthmatics.[52] The mechanism of aspirin sensitivity is not completely understood. One suspected mechanism of aspirin and NSAID sensitivity is cyclooxygenase blockade, which may facilitate production of alternative arachidonic acid metabolites (e.g., LTs). This is supported by the observation that the reaction occurs with other NSAIDs but infrequently with acetaminophen or salicylates. It is possible that aspirin and NSAIDs may stimulate mast cells directly to release inflammatory mediators. Also, subjects with aspirin-induced asthma have a marked increase in airway responsiveness to LTs.[52]

In patients with asthma or those suspected of being sensitive to aspirin, an oral challenge can be performed. This should be performed with great caution in a hospital setting with resuscitation equipment at hand. For patients known to be aspirin-sensitive, the major preventive measure is avoidance. Other agents reported to be cross-reactive with aspirin include tartrazine dye, indomethacin, and phenylbutazone.

NSAIDs also have been associated with pulmonary infiltrates and eosinophilia (PIE) syndrome. This syndrome is associated with fever, cough, dyspnea, infiltrates on chest roentgenogram, and a peripheral eosinophilia that develop 2 to 6 weeks after initiating treatment. PIE syndrome occurs more frequently for naproxen compared with other NSAIDs and is noted to resolve rapidly after discontinuation of the offending agent.[53]

SULFONAMIDES

Sulfonamide drugs are a common cause of allergic reactions. These agents are included in a number of drug classes, including antimicrobials, diuretics, oral hypoglycemics, and carbonic anhydrase inhibitors. Although immediate reactions can occur, sulfonamides typically cause delayed cutaneous reactions, often beginning with fever and then followed by a rash (e.g., morbilliform eruptions, erythema multiforme, or less frequently, toxic epidermal necrolysis).[54] Other reactions to sulfonamides may include mucocutaneous, gastrointestinal, hepatic, renal, or hematologic complications, which may be fatal. It is believed that sulfonamide reactions are immune-mediated and involve the production of reactive metabolites (hydroxylamines).[55]

Trimethoprim-sulfamethoxazole (TMP-SMZ) is used frequently for preventive or active treatment of *Pneumocystis carinii* pneumonia in patients with the acquired immunodeficiency syndrome (AIDS). Adverse reactions to TMP-SMZ have been observed to occur much more frequently in these patients compared with those without AIDS. Adverse effects to TMP-SMZ occur in 50% to 80% of AIDS patients compared with 10% of other immunocompromised patients.[56] TMP-SMZ was associated with an adverse-event rate of 26.3 per 100 person-years and hypersensitivity events at 22 per 100 person-years. Adverse-event rate was related to lower $CD4^+$ cell count. When CD4+ cell count was less than 100, the adverse drug event rate was 31 per 100 person-years.[57]

EXCIPIENTS

Pharmaceutical products contain a number of "inert" additives (e.g., dyes, fillers, buffers, stabilizers) in addition to the therapeutic ingredient. These ingredients are not always inert and may cause adverse effects, including allergic reactions.

TARTRAZINE

The azo dye tartrazine (FD&C yellow no. 5) is associated with anaphylactoid reactions, acute bronchospasm, urticaria, rhinitis, and contact dermatitis. Although the immunologic mechanisms are unclear, approximately 10% of aspirin-sensitive asthmatics are also intolerant to tartrazine,[58–60] suggesting a role for tartrazine as a cyclooxygenase inhibitor. As little as 0.85 μg or as much as 25 mg of tartrazine has provoked positive responses.[58]

SULFITES

Sulfites (including sulfur dioxide, sodium sulfite, sodium and potassium bisulfite, and sodium and potassium metabisulfite) are used commonly as antioxidants in pharmaceutical products and some foods. Over 250 cases of adverse reactions associated with ingestion of sulfites (usually in foods) have been reported to the Food and Drug Administration (FDA),[61] including wheezing, dyspnea, chest tightness, urticaria, angioedema, flushing, weakness, nausea, anaphylaxis, and death. Although the FDA has banned the use of sulfites in fresh fruits and vegetables, they were not banned in drug products because of the lack of a suitable substitute.

IgE-mediated and nonimmunologic sulfite hypersensitivity has been demonstrated in children with a history of chronic asthma. Adverse reactions to sulfite-preserved injectables, such as gentamicin, metoclopramide, and doxycycline, have been reported. In contrast to reactions caused by foods, these reactions do not occur more frequently in steroid-dependent asthmatics and do not always coincide with a positive oral sulfite challenge.[62] Blunted bronchodilation may be observed in asthmatics following inhalation of sulfite-containing nebulizer solutions. Although many nebulizer solutions contain sulfites, metered-dose inhalers do not. Many aqueous epinephrine products also contain sulfites. The FDA labeling states that in emergency situations when sulfite-free preparations are not available, sulfite-containing epinephrine should not be withheld from a sulfite-intolerant individual because small subcutaneous doses of sulfites are usually well tolerated. However, an increased risk of anaphylaxis exists after subcutaneous injection in rare patients with a positive oral challenge to 5 to 10 mg of sulfite.

PARABENS

Parabens (including methyl-, ethyl-, propyl-, and butylparaben) are used widely in pharmaceutical products as a biocidal agent. The majority of allergic reactions to parabens are observed after topical exposure. Delayed hypersensitivity contact dermatitis occurs more often in individuals with preexisting dermatitis.[58] Immediate hypersensitivity after parenteral administration is rare. Although these agents are chemically related to benzoic acid and *p*-aminobenzoic acid, the evidence for cross-sensitivity is lacking.[58]

LATEX AS AN ALLERGEN

Although not a drug, latex is now identified as a cause of allergic reactions in patients and health care workers. A diagnosis of latex allergy requires identification of latex-specific IgE and symptoms consistent with IgE-mediated reactions.[63] Latex-allergic individuals can have any of the symptoms seen in persons allergic to other allergens, but the most common are dyspnea, bronchospasm, anxiety, urticaria, flushing, and anaphylaxis.

Reactions due to dry-rubber latex products (e.g., vial stoppers, syringe plungers, and injection ports) are less frequent than to natural-rubber products (e.g., medical gloves, condoms, and catheters).[64] Several latex proteins (e.g., rubber elongation factor, prenyltransferase, and hevein) have been implicated in the IgE-mediated reactions.[63] Cross-sensitivity has been documented in individuals allergic to various foods, including bananas, kiwi, chestnut, papaya, plums, avocados, and peaches.

Although the prevalence of latex allergy among the general population remains less than 1%, high-risk individuals have been identified, including spina bifida patients, patients having undergone recurrent surgical procedures, and health care professionals.[63] Increased exposure to latex may account for the increased incidence of latex-specific IgE found among these individuals. Atopic individuals within these groups may be at an even greater risk.

The frequency of latex allergy among patients with neural tube defects ranges from 12% to 65%.[65] These patients undergo frequent catheterization, enemas, and bowel disempactions, allowing for increased exposure to latex-containing medical supplies.

Because of the ubiquity of latex-containing supplies within the medical setting, patients undergoing recurrent surgical procedures experience increased exposure to latex. Latex is absorbed readily through internal tissue during invasive procedures. Patients undergoing urologic procedures involving instrumentation of the bladder appear to have a greater risk of developing latex sensitivity.

With the institution of universal precautions as a means to avoid occupational hazards of blood-borne pathogens, the use of protective gloves became standard practice. The appearance of latex allergy as a serious medical problem has been associated with these practices. An estimated 5% to 15% of health care professionals are allergic to latex.[63]

Patient and health care provider education is crucial to decrease latex exposure through environment modification. Health care providers should be alerted to high-risk groups. Lists of latex-containing medications and devices, along with reasonable substitutes, are necessary in high-risk environments, including pharmacies, nursing homes, and surgical suites.

PACLITAXEL AND CARBOPLATIN

Chemotherapy agents are implicated in hypersensitivity reactions in 5% to 15% of patients who receive them.[66] The combination regimen of paclitaxel and carboplatin frequently is responsible for producing hypersensitivity reactions. Each agent precipitates a distinct reaction, allowing for differentiation between causative factors.

During early phase I trials, hypersensitivity reactions were observed when paclitaxel was administered rapidly.[67] The reaction, typically occurring shortly after initiation of the first dose, is due to Cremophor, the polyoxyethylated castor oil vehicle for paclitaxel.[68] Severe reactions are characterized by dyspnea, bronchospasm, urticaria, and hypotension. Minor reactions include flushing and rashes. In patients receiving a 3-hour infusion, the incidence of severe reactions is reduced to 1.3%, and the incidence of minor reactions is 42%.[69] To reduce the risk of hypersensitivity reaction, patients are routinely premedicated with steroids and H_1 receptor and H_2 receptor antagonists. Therapy usually can be resumed the same day in patients experiencing minor reactions. Even patients experiencing life-threatening reactions can be retreated successfully following desensitization.

Carboplatin hypersensitivity develops after six or more courses of carboplatin or its parent compound, cisplatin.[70] Reactions typically develop shortly after completing the infusion or up to 3 days after therapy.[71] Symptoms of severe reaction include tachycardia, dyspnea, facial swelling, rigors, and hypotension. Mild reactions include itching, erythema, and facial flushing. Desensitization with carboplatin usually is not successful due to previous prolonged exposure.

LAMOTRIGINE

Lamotrigine produces a hypersensitivity reaction similar to aromatic anticonvulsants. Symptoms include onset of fever within 2 to 6 weeks of initiation of therapy, followed by skin eruptions, lymphadenopathy, and internal organ involvement. The majority of skin eruptions present as an exanthematous rash. A small number of patients develop Stevens-Johnson syndrome or toxic epidermal necrolysis. Organ damage manifests primarily as hepatitis, eosinophilia, disseminated intravascular coagulopathy, and nephritis. Concomitant use of valproate significantly increases the risk of hypersensitivity due to reduced lamotrigine metabolism, leading to a prolonged elimination half-life.[72]

▶ TREATMENT: Allergic Reactions

The basic principles for management of allergic reactions to drugs or biologic agents include (1) discontinuation of the medication or agent when possible, (2) treatment of the adverse clinical signs and symptoms, and (3) substitution, if necessary, of another agent.[1]

Identification of patients at high risk for allergic drug reactions requires a careful history and, where appropriate, performance of specific tests to evaluate sensitivity.[73] One of the most helpful tests to evaluate risk is the allergen skin test. For some drugs, skin testing can demonstrate the presence of drug-specific IgE and predict a relatively high risk of immediate hypersensitivity reactions. Note that skin testing does not predict the risk of delayed or most dermatologic reactions.

A higher proportion of patients report an "allergic reaction" to penicillin than actually experience a reaction. However, patients with a history of penicillin allergy are recognized to have a four- to sixfold greater risk of subsequent reactions.[25] In addition, a negative history of penicillin allergy does not eliminate the risk of immediate reactions because many serious and even fatal allergic reactions to β-lactam antibiotics occur in patients who have no history of penicillin allergy.[25]

Skin testing can reduce the uncertainty of penicillin sensitivity and should be performed in all patients who have a history of penicillin allergy and require treatment with these agents. Testing for the major penicillin determinant is accomplished with penicilloyl-polylysine (PPL; Pre-Pen, Kremers-Urban). If this agent is used alone, patients reacting only to minor determinants will be missed. At present, there is no commercially available product that can be used to test for most of the minor determinants. Benzylpenicillin (at a concentration of 10,000 U/mL) has been used; however, some reactive patients still will be missed. Penicillin skin testing can facilitate the safe use of penicillin in 90% of patients with a history of penicillin allergy.[74] The procedure for performing penicillin skin testing is presented in Table 89–3.

The National Institute of Allergy and Infectious Diseases reported a collaborative trial to test the predictive value of skin testing with major and minor penicillin derivatives.[75] The frequency of IgE-mediated reactions was 1.2% and 0% (568 patients) with a positive and negative history of penicillin allergy, respectively, in subjects who were all skin test-negative. Of skin test-positive patients who received penicillin, 22% experienced immediate or accelerated penicillin allergy. Of skin test-positive patients, 84% had dermal reactions to skin testing with the major determinant (benzylpenicilloyl octalysine), whereas 16% reacted only to an experimental minor determinant mixture of benzylpenicillin, benzylpenicilloate, and benzylpenicilloyl-*N*-propylamine.

Immediate hypersensitivity reactions to penicillin are rare after a properly performed negative skin test when both major and minor determinants are used. Dermatologic reactions occur in 1% of skin test-negative patients.[25] A negative penicillin skin test indicates that the risk of life-threatening reactions is extremely low with administration of penicillin or other β-lactams. Occasionally, patients may experience systemic reactions after skin testing. Also, certain types of patients (e.g., those with dermatographism or taking antihistamines) may be unsuitable for skin testing because a false-positive or false-negative test may result. Penicillin is the only drug for which the predictive value of skin testing has been well established. The value of skin testing for evaluating the risk of adverse reactions to other drugs is largely unknown.

ANAPHYLAXIS

Anaphylaxis requires prompt treatment to minimize the risk of serious morbidity or death. On presentation, attention should be given first to stopping the likely offending agent, if possible, and restoring

TABLE 89–3. Procedure for Performing Penicillin Skin Testing

A. Percutaneous (prick) skin testing

Materials	Volume
Pre-Pen 6 × 10^6M	1 drop
Penicillin G 10,000 U/mL	1 drop
β-Lactam drug 3 mg/mL	1 drop
0.03% albumin-saline control	1 drop
Histamine control (1 mg/mL)	1 drop

1. Place a drop of each test material on the volar surface of the forearm.
2. Prick the skin with a sharp needle inserted through the drop at a 45° angle gently tenting the skin in an upward motion.
3. Interpret skin responses after 15 minutes.
4. A wheal at least 2 × 2 mm with erythema is considered positive.
5. If the prick test is nonreactive, proceed to the intradermal test.
6. If the histamine control is nonreactive, the test is considered uninterpretable.

B. Intradermal skin testing

Materials	Volume
Pre-Pen 6 × 10^6M	0.02 mL
Penicillin G 10,000 U/mL	0.02 mL
β-Lactam drug 3 mg/mL	0.02 mL
0.03% albumin-saline control	0.02 mL
Histamine control (0.1 mg/mL)	0.02 mL

1. Inject 0.02–0.03 mL of each test material intradermally (amount sufficient to produce a small bleb).
2. Interpret skin responses after 15 minutes.
3. A wheal at least 6 × 6 mm with erythema and at least 3 mm greater than the negative control is considered positive.
4. If the histamine control is nonreactive, the test is considered uninterpretable.

Antihistamines may blunt the response and cause false-negative reactions.

From Sullivan TJ. Current Therapy in Allergy. St Louis, Mosby, 1985:57–61.

TABLE 89–4. Treatment of Anaphylaxis

1. Place patient in recumbent position and elevate extremities.
2. Monitor vital signs often (or continuously if possible).
3. Apply tourniquet proximal to site of antigen injection; remove every 10–15 min.
4. Administer epinephrine 1:1000 into nonoccluded site: 0.3–0.5 mL subcutaneously or intramuscularly in adults and 0.01 mL/kg subcutaneously or intramuscularly in children.
5. Administer aqueous epinephrine 1:1000 into site of antigen injection; 0.15–0.25 mL subcutaneously in adults and 0.005 mL/kg subcutaneously in children.
6. Establish and maintain airway with oropharyngeal airway device, endotracheal intubation, transtracheal catheterization, or cricothyrotomy.
7. Administer oxygen at 6–10 L/min.
8. Institute rapid fluid replacement with 0.9% sodium chloride, lactated Ringer's, or colloid solution (e.g., 5% albumin or 4% hetastarch).
9. For hypotension in adults, administer norepinephrine, 32 μg/min (use 8 mg in 500 mL dextrose 5%) with the rate adjusted to maintain low-normal blood pressure. Alternatively, administer dopamine at 2–10 μg/kg/min intravenously.
10. If refractory hypotension is present, administer cimetidine 300 mg or ranitidine 50 mg, intravenously over 3–5 min.
11. If bronchospasm is present, administer aminophylline 6 mg/kg intravenously over 20 min.
12. Administer hydrocortisone sodium succinate 100 mg intravenously (push) and 100 mg intravenously in saline every 2–4 h to block the late-phase reaction.
13. Administer diphenhydramine 1–2 mg/kg intravenously (up to 50 mg) over 3 min to block histamine-1 receptors.
14. For adults taking a β-adrenergic blocker, administer atropine (0.5 mg intravenously) every 5 min until heart rate is greater than 60 beats/min, or isoproterenol 2–20 μg/min intravenously titrated to heart rate of 60 beats/min, or glucagon 0.5 mg/kg intravenously (push) followed by 0.07 mg/kg/h continuously intravenously.

From Weiss ME, Adkinson NF, Clin Allergy 1988;18:515–540.

respiratory and cardiovascular function. A protocol for the treatment of anaphylaxis is presented in Table 89–4. Epinephrine is administered as primary treatment to counteract bronchoconstriction and vasodilatation. Epinephrine should be administered intramuscularly. If blood pressure is not restored by epinephrine, crystalloids should be administered intravenously to restore intravascular volume. Typically, 1 L of 0.9% sodium chloride or lactated Ringer's solution will be administered over 10 to 15 minutes. This may be repeated if the patient is still believed to be volume-depleted. Intravenous fluids should be given early in the course in an attempt to prevent shock. A maintenance intravenous fluid will then be initiated. An immediate priority is establishment and maintenance of an airway. This should be achieved by the use of endotracheal intubation if necessary. When a patient with anaphylaxis is hypotensive, vasopressors also will be needed in addition to crystalloids. Norepinephrine is the vasoconstrictor agent of choice for treatment of anaphylactic shock, although dopamine also may be useful.

A number of other agents may be required for treatment of anaphylactic reactions. Corticosteroids (hydrocortisone sodium succinate intravenously) are recommended to prevent the late-phase reaction. Aminophylline may be used as adjunctive therapy for bronchospasm. Histamine (H_1) receptor blockers (such as diphenhydramine) may be administered to reduce some of the symptoms associated with anaphylaxis; however, these agents are not effective as primary therapy. H_2 receptor blockers such as cimetidine have been used for treatment of refractory hypotension,[76] although routine use is controversial.

DESENSITIZATION

For some patients allergic to penicillin, no reasonable alternatives exist, and penicillin therapy may be necessary for treatment of severe, life-threatening infection. In this situation, penicillin desensitization should be considered. Desensitization can reduce the risk of anaphylaxis but does not influence the likelihood of other types of reactions such as exfoliative dermatitis or Stevens-Johnson syndrome.

Penicillin desensitization should be performed in a hospital setting where resuscitation equipment is readily available by a physician experienced in the risks and management of severe allergic reactions. The potential risks and benefits should be discussed with the patient. Prior to initiating the protocol, the patient should be stabilized and fluid, pulmonary, and cardiovascular function optimized. The use of premedicants (antihistamines or corticosteroids) is controversial because these agents may mask the early signs of acute reactions and do not reliably reduce the severity of acute reactions. About one-third of patients who have undergone desensitization experience mild, transient allergic reaction either during the desensitization procedure or during penicillin therapy.[25] Patients who can take oral medication should undergo desensitization with oral penicillin. Protocols for oral and intravenous penicillin desensitization[77,78] are presented in Tables 89–5 and 89–6. It is important that once the desensitization protocol is

TABLE 89–5. Protocol for Oral Desensitization

	Phenoxymethyl Penicillin			
Step[a]	*Concentration (U/mL)*	*Volume (mL)*	*Dose (U)*	*Cumulative Dose (U)*
1	1000	0.1	100	100
2	1000	0.2	200	300
3	1000	0.4	400	700
4	1000	0.8	800	1500
5	1000	1.6	1600	3100
6	1000	3.2	3200	6300
7	1000	6.4	6400	12,700
8	10,000	1.2	12,000	24,700
9	10,000	2.4	24,000	48,700
10	10,000	4.8	48,000	96,700
11	80,000	1.0	80,000	176,700
12	80,000	2.0	160,000	336,700
13	80,000	4.0	320,000	656,700
14	80,000	8.0	640,000	1,296,700
Observe for 30 min				
15	500,000	0.25	125,000	
16	500,000	0.5	250,000	
17	500,000	1.0	500,000	
18	500,000	2.25	1,125,000	

[a]The interval between steps is 15 min.
From Ref. 78.

TABLE 89–6. Parenterai Desensitization Protocol

Injection No.	Benzylpenicillin Concentration (U)	Volume (mL)	(Route)
1[a,b]	100	0.1	ID
2	100	0.2	SC
3	100	0.4	SC
4	100	0.8	SC
5[b]	1000	0.1	ID
6	1000	0.3	SC
7	1000	0.6	SC
8[b]	10,000	0.1	ID
9	10,000	0.2	SC
10	10,000	0.4	SC
11	10,000	0.8	SC
12[b]	100,000	0.1	ID
13	100,000	0.3	SC
14	100,000	0.6	SC
15[b]	1,000,000	0.1	ID
16	1,000,000	0.2	SC
17	1,000,000	0.2	IM
18	1,000,000	0.4	IM
19	Continuous IV infusion at 1,000,000 U/h		

[a]Administer doses at intervals of not less than 20 min.
[b]Observe and record skin wheal-and-flare response.
From Ref. 78.

begun it not be interrupted except for severe reactions. Antihistamines or epinephrine may be administered to treat reactions. In addition, if the patient completes the desensitization regimen and then undergoes penicillin treatment, a lapse between doses of as little as 24 hours can allow for reemergence of sensitivity.

Desensitization of TMP-SMZ can be achieved within 2 days in most AIDS patients.[79] This can be accompanied by use of the following schedule of doses (milligrams of sulfamethoxazole-trimethoprim): day 1: 9 A.M., 4 and 0.8; 11 A.M., 8 and 1.6; 1 P.M., 20 and 4; 5 P.M., 40 and 8; day 2: 9 A.M., 80 and 16; 3 P.M., 160 and 32; 9 P.M., 200 and 40; day 3: 9 A.M., 400 and 80 and 400 and 80 daily thereafter.

Skin tests often become negative during and shortly after desensitization. The mechanism by which desensitization is protective is unclear. It does not seem to be that penicillin-specific IgE is neutralized or that IgG as "blocking antibody" is produced. One possible explanation is that basophils and mast cells attain some degree of tolerance on exposure to the antigen.

▶ PRINCIPLES OF PHARMACOTHERAPY

- Allergic reactions are responsible for up to 5% of reactions to medications among hospitalized patients.
- The following criteria suggest that a drug reaction may be immunologically mediated: (1) The reaction occurs in a small percentage of patients receiving the drug, (2) the observed reaction does not resemble the drug's pharmacologic effect, (3) the type of manifestation is similar to that seen with other allergic reactions (anaphylaxis, urticaria, serum sickness), (4) there is a lag time between first exposure of the drug and reaction, (5) the reaction is reproduced even by minute doses of the drug, (6) the reaction is reproduced by agents with similar chemical structures, (7) eosinophilia is present, and (8) the reaction resolves after the drug has been discontinued. Exceptions to each of these criteria are observed commonly.
- Factors that influence the likelihood of allergic drug reactions are the dose of the allergen, the route of exposure, and the sensitivity of the individual as determined by age, genetics, or environmental factors. For many drugs, the severity of a reaction is determined by the dose and duration of exposure.
- Anaphylaxis is an acute, life-threatening allergic reaction involving multiple organ systems that generally begins within 30 minutes but almost always within 2 hours after exposure to the inciting allergen. Anaphylaxis requires prompt treatment to restore respiratory and cardiovascular function. Epinephrine is administered as primary treatment to counteract bronchoconstriction and vasodilatation. Intravenous fluids should be administered to restore intravascular volume.
- Patients with a history of a reaction to penicillin are advised not to receive cephalosporins if they can be avoided.
- Bewteen 5% and 10% of patients receiving radiocontrast agents experience some type of adverse reaction. Low-osmolar contrast agents appear to result in fewer anaphylactoid reactions.
- The two general types of reactions to aspirin are urticaria/angioedema (1% of the population) and rhinosinusitis/asthma (0.5%). Aspirin-sensitive patients also may be sensitive to other NSAIDs.
- Adverse reactions to TMP-SMZ have been observed to occur much more frequently in AIDS patients compared with those without AIDS (50% to 80% of AIDS patients compared with 10% in other immunocompromised patients).
- The basic principles of management of allergic reactions to drugs or biologic agents include (1) discontinuation of the medication or agent when possible, (2) treatment of the adverse clinical signs and symptoms, and (3) substitution, if necessary, of another agent.
- One of the most helpful tests to evaluate risk of penicillin allergy is the skin test. Skin testing can demonstrate the presence of penicillin-specific IgE and predict a relatively high risk of immediate hypersensitivity reactions. Skin testing does not predict the risk of delayed or most dermatologic reactions.

REFERENCES

1. Anderson JA. Allergic reactions to drugs and biologic agents. JAMA 1992;268:2845–2857.
2. Parker CW. Drug allergy (a review in three parts). N Engl J Med 1975;292:511, 732, 957.
3. Jick H. Adverse drug reactions: The magnitude of the problem. J Allergy Clin Immunol 1984;74:555.
4. DeWeck AI. Drugs as allergens. J Allergy Clin Immunol 1986;78:1047.
5. Stafford CT. Adverse drug reactions. Med Times 1988;116:31–42.
6. Borish L, Tilles SA. Immune mechanisms of drug allergy. Immunol Clin North Am 1998;18:717–729.

7. DeSwarte RD. Drug allergy. In: Patterson R, ed. Allergic Diseases, 4th ed. Philadelphia, Lippincott, 1993.
8. Roitt I, Brastoff J, Male D. Immunology, 4th ed. London, Mosby, 1996.
9. Anonymous. Disease management of drug hypersensitivity: a practical approach. Ann Allerg Asthma Immunol 1999;83:665–700.
10. Schwartz LB, Austen KF. The mast cell and mediators of immediate hypersensitivity: In: Samter M, Talmage DW, Frank MM, et al., eds. Immunologic Diseases, 5th ed. Boston, Little, Brown, 1995.
11. Serafin WF, Austen KF. Mediators of immediate hypersensitivity reactions. N Engl J Med 1987;317:30–34.
12. Stafford CT. Life-threatening allergic reactions. Postgrad Med 1989;86: 235–241.
13. Bochner BS, Lichtenstein LM. Anaphylaxis. N Engl J Med 1991;324: 1785–1790.
14. Neuqut AI, Ghatak AT, Miller RL. Anaphylaxis in the United States: An investigation into its epidemiology. Ann Intern Med 2001;161:15–21.
15. Kemp SF, Lockey RF, Wolf BL, Lieberman P. Anaphylaxis: A review of 266 cases. Arch Intern Med 1995;155:1749–1754.
16. Johnson DH, Cuhna BA. Drug fever. Infect Dis Clin North Am 1996; 10:85–91.
17. Prince EJ, Venables PJ. Drug-induced lupus. Drug Safety 1995;12:283–290.
18. Rich MW. Drug-induced lupus: The list of culprits grows. Postgrad Med 1996;100:299–302.
19. Roujeau JC, Stern RS. Severe adverse cutaneous reactions to drugs. N Engl J Med 1994;331:1272–1285.
20. Hunziker T, Kunzi U, Braunschweig S, et al. Comprehensive hospital drug monitoring: Adverse drug reactions—A 20-year survey. Allergy 1997;52:388–393.
21. Mockenhaupt M, Schopf E. Epidemiology of drug-induced severe skin reactions. Semin Cutan Med Surg 1996;15:236–243.
22. Stern RS, Steinberg LA. Epidemiology of adverse cutaneous reactions to drugs. Dermatoepidemiology 1995;13:681–688.
23. Bigby M, Jick S, Jick H, et al. Drug-induced cutaneous reactions: A report from the Boston Collaborative Drug Surveillance Program on 15,438 consecutive inpatients, 1975 to 1982. JAMA 1986;256:3359–3363.
24. Ibia EO, Schwartz RH, Wiederman BL. Antibiotic rashes in children: A survey in a private practice setting. Arch Dermatol 2000;136:849–854.
25. Weiss ME, Adkinson NF. Immediate hypersensitivity reactions to penicillin and related antibiotics. Clin Allergy 1988;18:515–540.
26. Lee CE, Zembower TR, Fotis MA, et al. The incidence of antimicrobial allergies in hospitalized patients. Arch Intern Med 2000;160:2819–2822.
27. Adkinson NF. Risk factors for drug allergy. J Allergy Clin Immunol 1984; 74:567–572.
28. Baldo BA. Penicillins and cephalosporins as allergens: Structural aspects of recognition and cross-reactions. Clin Exp Allergy 1999;29:744–749.
29. Salkind AR, Cuddy PG, Foxworth JW. Is this patient allergic to penicillin? An evidence-based analysis of the likelihood of penicillin allergy. JAMA 2001;285:2498–2505.
30. Anne S, Reisman RE. Risk of administering cephalosporin antibiotics to patients with histories of penicillin allergy. Ann Allergy Asthma Immunol 1995;74:167–170.
31. Wickern GM, Nish WA, Bitner AS, Freeman TM. Allergy to β-lactams: A survey of current practices. J Allerg Clin Immunol 1994;94:725–731.
32. Ponvert C, Le Clainche L, de Blic J, et al. Allergy to β-lactam antibiotics in children. Pediatrics 1999;104:45.
33. Anne S, Reisman RE. Risk of administering cephalosporin antibiotics to patients with histories of penicillin allergy. Ann Allergy Asthma Immunol 1995;74:167–170.
34. Saxon A, Beall GN, Rohr AS, et al. Immediate hypersensitivity reactions to β-lactam antibiotics. Ann Intern Med 1987;107:204–215.
35. Kishiyama JL, Adelman DC. The cross-reactivity of β-lactam antibiotics. Drug Safety 1994;10:318–327.
36. Bush WH, Swanson DP. Acute reactions to intravascular contrast media: Types, risk factors, recognition, and specific treatment. Am J Radiol 1991;157:1153–1161.
37. Lang DM, Alpeen MB, Visitainer PF, et al. Gender risk for anaphylactoid reaction to radiographic contrast media. J Allergy Clin Immunol 1995;95:813.
38. Murphy KJ, Brunberg JA, Cohan RH. Adverse reactions to gadolinium contrast media. AJR 1996;167:847–849.
39. Marshall GD, Lieberman PL. Anaphylactoid reactions to radiocontrast agents. Immunol Allerg Clin North Am 1998;18:799–807.
40. Banks JA, Kagey-Sobotka A, Lichtenstein LM, et al. Spontaneous histamine release after exposure to hyperosmolar solutions. J Allergy Clin Immunol 1986;78:51.
41. Greenberger PA, Patterson R. The prevention of immediate generalized reactions to radiocontrast media in high-risk patients. J Allergy Clin Immunol 1991;87:867–872.
42. Greenberger PA. Contrast media reaction. J Allergy Clin Immunol 1984;74:600.
43. Cohan RH, Leder RA, Ellis JH. Treatment of adverse reactions to radiographic contrast media in adults. Radiol Clin North Am 1996;34:1055–1076.
44. Patterson R, Roberts M, Grammer LC. Insulin allergy: Re-evaluation after two decades. Ann Allergy 1990;64:459–462.
45. Samter M, Stevenson DD. Reactions to aspirin and aspirin-like drugs. In: Samter M, Talmage DW, Frank MM, et al., eds. Immunologic Diseases, 5th ed. Boston, Little, Brown, 1995.
46. Stevenson DD. Diagnosis, prevention and treatment of adverse reactions to aspirin and non-steroidal anti-inflammatory drugs. J Allergy Clin Immunol 1984;74:617.
47. Chafee FH, Settipane GA. Aspirin intolerance: I. Frequency in an allergic population. J Allergy Clin Immunol 1974;53:193.
48. MacDonald JR, Mathison DA, Stevenson DD. Aspirin intolerance in asthma: Detection by oral challenge. J Allergy Clin Immunol 1972;50: 198.
49. Falliers CJ. Aspirin and subtypes of asthma risk factor analysis. J Allergy Clin Immunol 1973;52:141.
50. Kowalski M. Aspirin sensitive rhinosinusitis and asthma. Allergy Proc 1995;16:77–80.
51. Vicks SD, Dean JR, Tenholder MF. Ketorolac induced respiratory failure in an aspirin-sensitive asthmatic. Immunol Allergy Pract 1991;13:23–25.
52. Lee TH. Mechanisms of aspirin sensitivity. Am Rev Respir Dis 1992;145:S34–S36.
53. Goodwin SD, Glenny RW. Nonsteroidal anti-inflammatory drug-associated pulmonary infiltrates with eosinophilia. Arch Intern Med 1992;152:1521–1524.
54. Anonymous. Serious adverse reactions with sulfonamides. FDA Drug Bull 1984;14:5–6.
55. Reider MJ, Uetrecht J, Shear NH, et al. Diagnosis of sulfonamide hypersensitivity reactions by in vitro "rechallenge" with hydroxylamine metabolites. Ann Intern Med 1989;110:286–289.
56. Santomauro JT, Stover DE. *Pneumocystis carinii* pneumonia. Med Clin North Am 1997;81:299–318.
57. Moore RD, Fortgang I, Keruly J, Chaisson RE. Adverse events from drug therapy for human immunodeficiency virus disease. Am J Med 1996;101:34–40.
58. Weiner M, Bernstein IL. Adverse Reactions to Drug Formulation Agents: A Handbook of Excipients. New York, Marcel Dekker, 1989.
59. American Academy of Pediatrics Committee on Drugs. "Inactive" ingredients in pharmaceutical products. Pediatrics 1985;76:635–642.
60. Lockey SD. Hypersensitivity to tartrazine (FD&C yellow no. 5) and other dyes and additives present in foods and pharmaceutical products. Ann Allergy 1977;38:206–210.
61. Stevenson DD, Simon RA. Sensitivity to ingested metabisulfites in asthmatic subjects. J Allergy Clin Immunol 1981;68:26–32.
62. Smolinski SC. Review of parenteral sulfide reactions. J Toxicol Clin Toxicol 1992;30:597–606.
63. Poley GE, Slater JE. Latex allergy. J Allerg Clin Immunol 2000;105:1054–1062.
64. Senst BL, Johnson RA. Latex allergy. Am J Health Syst Pharm 1997;54:1071–1075.

65. Steelman WM. Latex allergy precautions: A research-based protocol. Nurs Clin North Am 1995;30:475–493.
66. Weiss RB. Hypersensitivity reactions. Semin Oncol 1992;19:458–477.
67. Bookman MA, Kloth DD, Kover PE, et al. Intravenous prophylaxis for paclitaxel-related hypersensitivity reactions. Semin Oncol 1997;24:S19-13–S19-15.
68. Lorenz W, Reimann HJ, Schmal A, et al. Histamine release in dogs by Cremophor EL and its derivatives: Oxethylated oleic acid is the most effective constituent. Agents Actions 1977;7:63–67.
69. Eisenhauer EA, ten Bokkel Huinink WW, Swenerton KD, et al. European-Canadian randomized trial of paclitaxel in relapsed ovarian cancer: High-dose versus low-dose and long versus short infusion. J Clin Oncol 1994;12:2654–2666.
70. Hendrick AM, Simmons D, Cantwell BMJ. Allergic reactions to carboplatin. Ann Oncol 1992;3:239–240.
71. Markman M, Kennedy A, Webster K, et al. Clinical features of hypersensitivity reactions to carboplatin. J Clin Oncol 1999;17:1141–1145.
72. Schlienger RG, Knowles SR, Shear NH. Lamotrigine-associated anticonvulsant hypersensitivity syndrome. Neurology 1998;51:1172–1175.
73. Weiss ME, Adkinson NF. Diagnostic testing for drug hypersensitivity. Immunol Allerg Clin North Am 1998;18:731–734.
74. Gadde J, Spence M, Wheeler B, Adkinson NF. Clinical experience with penicillin skin testing in a large inner-city STD clinic. JAMA 1993;270:2456–2463.
75. Sogn DD, Evans R, Shepherd GM, et al. Results of the National Institute of Allergy and Infectious Diseases collaborative clinical trial to test the predictive value of skin testing with major and minor penicillin derivatives in hospitalized patients. Arch Intern Med 1992;152:1025–1032.
76. Yarbrough JA, Moffitt JE, Brown DA, et al. Cimetidine in the treatment of refractory anaphylaxis. Ann Allergy 1989;63:235–238.
77. Sullivan TJ. Current Therapy in Allergy. St. Louis, Mosby, 1985: 57–61
78. Weiss ME, Adkinson NF. Immediate hypersensitivity reaction to penicillin and related antibiotics. Clin Allergy 1988;18:515–540.
79. Caumes E, Guermonprez G, Lecomte C, et al. Efficacy and safety of desensitization with sulfamethoxazole and trimethoprim in 48 previously hypersensitive patients infected with human immunodeficiency virus. Arch Dermatol 1997;133:465–469.

90
OSTEOPOROSIS AND OSTEOMALACIA

Mary Beth O'Connell and Mary Elizabeth Elliott

Osteoporosis is a major public health problem for both men and women. Low bone density, the hallmark of osteoporosis, contributes to fracture risk. Osteoporotic fractures are associated with pain, kyphosis, disability, and increased mortality. Osteomalacia, or deficient bone mineralization, is less common but also leads to skeletal muscle weakness, fractures, and other complications. This chapter reviews bone physiology, pathophysiology, and assessment and offers nonpharmacologic and pharmacologic management strategies for these skeletal diseases.

PHYSIOLOGY

NORMAL FUNCTION OF BONE

The skeleton provides structural support, is a reservoir of calcium and other ions, and protects vital organs and the hematopoietic system. A constant ionic environment is critical for life. To preserve ion homeostasis, bone resorption and loss will occur.

TYPES AND COMPOSITION OF BONE

About one-fifth of the human skeleton is trabecular bone, a meshwork of vertical and horizontal struts (Table 90–1). Cortical or compact bone is formed in layers (lamellae). Trabecular bone has a greater surface area and is in close contact with cells in the marrow cavity that affect bone turnover. Because of this, trabecular bone is more metabolically active than cortical bone.

Bone is a highly ordered three-dimensional structural composite of organic matrix and crystalline mineral ideally suited to meet the mechanical demands placed on it. The organic matrix is primarily protein (90% type I collagen) and cells (osteoclasts, osteoblasts, and osteocytes). The mineral, apatite, is mainly calcium and phosphate. Bone contains 99% of the body's calcium and 85% of its phosphorus.[1]

BONE REMODELING AND HORMONAL CONTROL

The mature skeleton undergoes constant remodeling throughout life. Annually, about 4% of cortical bone and about 28% of trabecular bone are remodeled.[2] Remodeling repairs microfractures, adapts bone to weight bearing, and provides access to mineral stores. Remodeling is performed by teams of osteoclasts and osteoblasts, termed *basic multicellular units* (BMUs). Osteoclasts resorb bone, and osteoblasts fill in osteoid that is subsequently mineralized. Osteoclasts are derived from the macrophage/monocyte line, whereas osteoblasts arise from fibroblast precursors. In resorbing cortical bone, osteoclasts create 100- to 200-μm tunnels through Haversian canals. In trabecular bone, 60- to 70-μm pits (Howship lacunae) are excavated. Resorption takes 3 to 4 weeks, with formation and mineralization taking 3 to 4 months.[3] In young adulthood, formation equals resorption. Aging, menopause, and certain diseases and drugs create an imbalance between formation and resorption, resulting in bone loss.

Steps in remodeling are resorption, reversal, formation, and quiescence (Fig. 90–1). Mechanisms that trigger resorption are under intense investigation. At any given time, 90% of bone surfaces are covered by osteoblastic lining cells. Within bone, osteocytes ("retired" osteoblasts) may act as mechanosensors, reacting to strain and sensing fatigue damage.[2,4] Osteocytes communicate with lining cells through long cytoplasmic processes (Fig. 90–2). A homing signal, originating in osteocytes and communicated by lining cells, is thought to summon osteoclast precursors to initiate resorption.

Osteoblasts regulate osteoclastic activity (Fig. 90–3). Osteoblasts secrete macrophage/monocyte colony-stimulating factor (M-CSF), also called *colony-stimulating factor 1,* to promote differentiation of osteoclast precursors. Osteoblasts also secrete a ligand that binds to a receptor on osteoclast precursors, promoting differentiation and maturation. This receptor is receptor activator of nuclear factor κB (RANK), and the ligand is RANKL. Another key player, osteoprotegerin (OPG), is a "decoy" receptor released from osteoblasts. OPG competes with RANK, preventing osteoclastic differentiation. At a given point, the balance between OPG and RANKL regulates osteoclastic activity and thus resorption. Regulation of osteoblast secretion of M-CSF, RANKL, and OPG is complex, involving parathyroid hormone (PTH), 1α,25–dihydroxyvitamin D (calcitriol), leptin, estrogen, and other agents[5,6] (see Fig. 90–3).

During resorption, osteoclasts attach to bone by an integrin, $\alpha V\beta 3$. An area with a leak-proof seal is created under the osteoclast's ruffled border. Protons are pumped into the area to dissolve bone (see Fig. 90–3). Proteins are digested by cathepsin K, a protease unique to bone. When excavation is complete, osteoclasts undergo apoptosis or move to a new section.

In reversal, osteoclasts depart and osteoblasts arrive at the resorption site.[5] Osteoblast differentiation is regulated primarily through transcription factor *cbfa–1*.[7] Factors released from resorbed bone [transforming growth factor β (TGF-β) and platelet-derived growth factor (PDGF)], insulin-like growth factor 1 (IGF-1), and other factors promote bone formation. During formation, osteoblasts fill the cavity with osteoid (see Fig. 90–1). Mineralization begins when the osteoid layer is about 20 μm thick. Osteoblasts release vesicles that provide calcium and phosphate, block mineralization inhibitors, and provide nuclei for crystallization, thus promoting mineralization.[8] Quiescence, when newly formed bone is covered with lining cells, follows mineralization.

Bone mineral density (BMD) reflects the balance between resorption and formation. Peak BMD is attained between the ages of 20 and 35 in men and women.[9] Some 60% to 70% of the variance in peak BMD may be attributed to genetic differences. Polymorphisms of collagen type 1, vitamin D receptor, estrogen receptor, and other genes are being investigated as contributors to this variance.

TABLE 90–1. Bone Composition

Bone	Percent Cortical Bone	Percent Trabecular Bone
Total body	80	20
Midradius	95	5
Distal radius	30–50	30–50
Femur neck	75	25
Trochanter	50	50
Lumbar spine	40	60

Antiresorptive agents have profound effects on osteoblast and osteoclast function (e.g., estrogen increases OPG and tilts the balance toward less resorption; bisphosphonates promote osteoclast apoptosis and inhibit resorption). Research will provide new pharmacologic interventions. These may include anabolic agents (PTH or analogues), effectors of the OPG/RANK/RANKL pathway (OPG mimics), and osteoclast inhibitors (apoptotic agents or antagonists of integrins, hydrogen ion secretion, or cathepsin K).

VITAMIN D METABOLISM AND REGULATION OF SERUM CALCIUM AND PHOSPHATE

Vitamin D maintains calcium homeostasis and indirectly supports mineralization by promoting calcium absorption (Fig. 90–4). Vitamin D_3 (cholecalciferol) is made in sun-exposed skin from 7-dehydrocholesterol. A few foods and fortified milk contain vitamin D_3 or vitamin D_2 (ergocalciferol, a plant product). In this chapter, vitamin D_3 and D_2 will be termed *vitamin D* because they work similarly. Vitamin D undergoes hepatic conversion to 25-hydroxyvitamin D (calcidiol). PTH stimulates renal conversion of 25-hydroxyvitamin D to the active form, 1α,25-dihydroxyvitamin D (calcitriol, or 1,25-dihydroxycholecalciferol). Decreased serum calcium concentrations lead to increased serum levels of PTH, which elevates calcitriol levels (see Fig. 90–4). Calcitriol promotes intestinal calcium absorption, and calcitriol and PTH work together to release calcium from bone to restore homeostasis.[10]

Phosphorus is less tightly regulated than calcium. Excess phosphorus is ingested and absorbed ordinarily. The kidneys excrete the excess, with the renal set point defining serum phosphorus levels. PTH affects the set point and decreases phosphorus reabsorption.

OSTEOPOROSIS

Osteoporosis is "characterized by low bone mass and microarchitectural deterioration of bone tissue leading to enhanced bone fragility and a consequent increase in fracture risk."[11] Bone loss results when resorption exceeds formation. The World Health Organization (WHO) classifies bone mass based on T scores. For an individual's BMD, a *T score* is the number of standard deviations away from the mean BMD for the young normal population. Normal bone mass is a T score greater than −1, osteopenia is a T score of −1 to −2.5, and at a T score of less than −2.5, the patient has osteoporosis.[12] Clinically, osteoporosis is categorized as postmenopausal, age-related, or secondary. Postmenopausal osteoporosis affects primarily trabecular bone in the decade after menopause, with predominantly vertebral and distal forearm fractures. Age-related osteoporosis results from bone loss that begins shortly after peak bone mass is obtained, affects both cortical and trabecular bone, and increases vertebral, hip, and forearm fractures. Secondary osteoporosis is caused by certain medications or diseases and affects both types of bone.

EPIDEMIOLOGY

Applying WHO BMD classifications to femoral BMD data from the Third National Health and Nutrition Examination Survey (NHANES III, conducted in 1988–1994), the respective osteopenia and osteoporosis prevalences are as follows in several subgroups of Americans[13]:

- Non-Hispanic white women: 52% and 20%
- Mexican-American women: 49% and 10%
- Non-Hispanic black women: 35% and 5%
- Men of all races: 47% and 6%, using the mean young male BMD
- Men of all races: 33% and 4%, using the mean young female BMD

Osteoporosis increases with age. The percentage of women with osteoporosis is 15% for ages 50 to 59, 22% for ages 60 to 69, 39% for ages 70 to 80, and 70% for those 80 years of age and older.[14] Osteoporosis prevalences for white female nursing home residents were 64% for ages 65 to 74, 71% for ages 75 to 85, and 86% for ages older than 85 years.[15] Although low BMD contributes to fracture risk, those with a normal BMD can fracture, and some with osteoporosis do not.

Approximately 1.5 million fractures secondary to osteoporosis are reported each year in the United States: 700,000 vertebral fractures, 250,000 hip fractures, 250,000 wrist fractures, and 300,000 other limb fractures.[16] The lifetime risks of a 50-year-old woman experiencing fractures are 15% for the spine, 14% for the wrist, 14% for the hip, and 31% for other fractures.[11] The lifetime risk of a 50-year-old African-American women experiencing a hip fracture is 6%, for a white man 5% to 6%, and for an African-American man 3%. Fractures increase with age and lower BMD.

ETIOLOGY AND RISK FACTORS

Multiple genetic, medical, social, and environmental factors affect the risk of developing osteoporosis, falling, or fracturing a bone (Table 90–2). The magnitude and significance of these risk factors vary by gender, ethnicity, and age.[17–20] Risk-factor models, however, explain only 20% to 34% of BMD variance.[21] Future models with genetic factors may account for more variance.

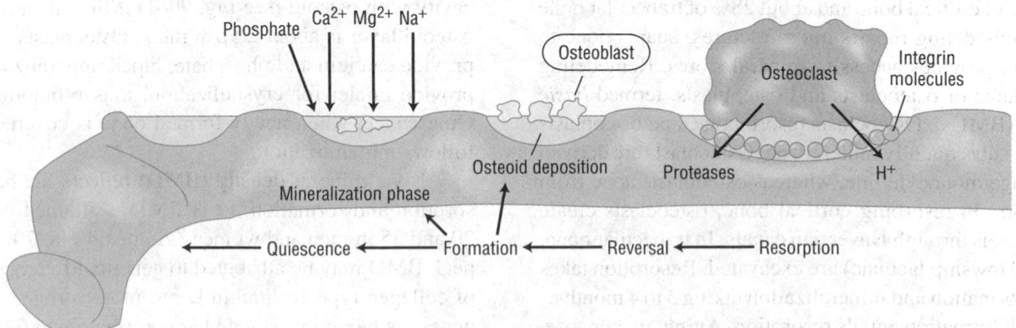

FIGURE 90–1. Steps in bone remodeling: resorption, reversal, formation, and quiescence. See text for details.

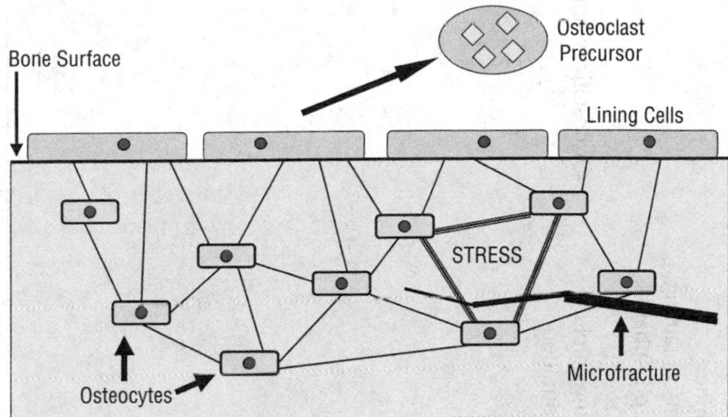

FIGURE 90–2. Relationship between forces in bone and the remodeling/resorption response. Osteocytes act as mechanosensors within the mineralized matrix, detecting stress, strain, and microfractures. Osteocytes communicate with each other and with lining cells on the bone surface through cytoplasmic processes. Osteocytes respond to the environment and can trigger resorption when appropriate, such as for a microfracture or with a change in weight bearing. Osteocytes communicate with the lining cells, which send out a homing signal to summon osteoclasts to the area. If a microfracture is being repaired, there may be no net loss of bone as the excavated bone is replaced. With a dramatic decrease in weight bearing (such as immobilization from being bed-bound), there will be net loss as the bones are reset to a lower load.

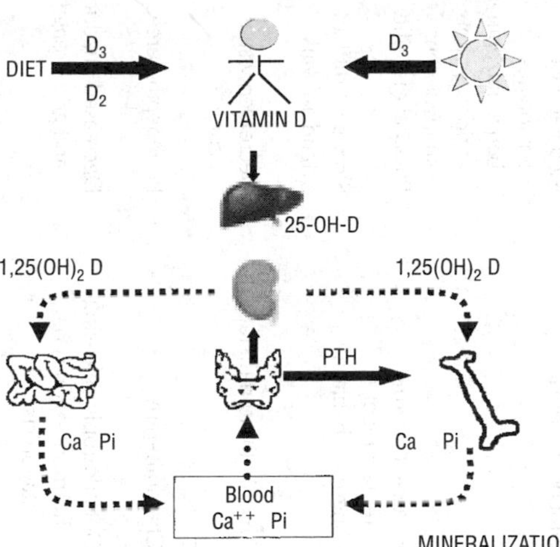

FIGURE 90–4. Effects of vitamin D and PTH on calcium balance. Vitamin D_3 is produced in sunlit skin. Vitamin D_3 (cholecalciferol) or vitamin D_2 (ergocalciferol) are present in a few foods, including fortified milk. Vitamin D is converted in the liver to 25-OH vitamin D. Maintenance of adequate calcium and phosphorus concentrations is required for normal physiology and bone mineralization. Decreased serum calcium triggers release of PTH, in turn increasing 1,25-(OH)$_2$ vitamin D (calcitriol). Calcitriol enhances intestinal calcium and phosphorus absorption and, in concert with PTH, releases calcium from bone to restore calcium balance.

PATHOPHYSIOLOGY

POSTMENOPAUSAL OSTEOPOROSIS

A few years after peak BMD is achieved, usually in young adulthood, bone loss begins. The rate of loss accelerates at menopause. Approximately 10% to 25% of bone is lost in the decade after menopause.

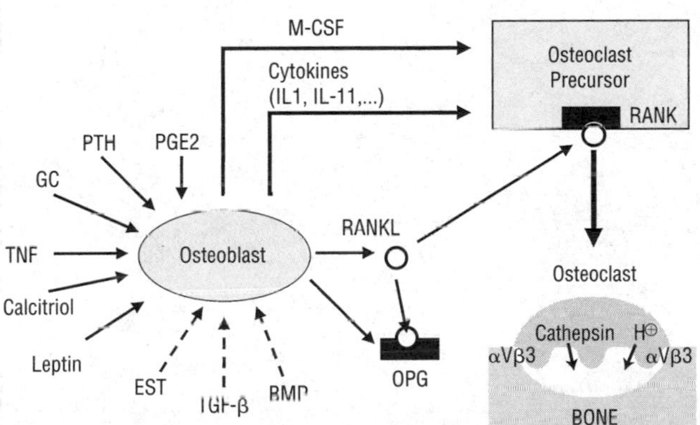

FIGURE 90–3. Control of osteoclastic bone resorption by osteoblasts. Most factors that stimulate osteoclast differentiation and maturation work through the osteoblast and the OPG/RANK/RANKL pathway, considered the "final common pathway" affecting the osteoclast. On the right is an osteoclast precursor. It has a receptor, RANK, and the osteoclast is activated on RANK occupation with RANKL (RANK ligand) (*black open circle*). Osteoblasts secrete RANKL. However, osteoblasts also secrete a "decoy receptor" called OPG that binds RANKL and antagonizes the RANK/RANKL system. Whether osteoclast maturation and resorption occur depends on this competition between the osteoclast RANK receptor and OPG for RANKL. At the left, an osteoblast receives input from endocrine and local effectors. The solid lines represent agents (PTH, TNF, calcitriol, and others) that stimulate osteoclastic activity and cause bone resorption working through osteoblasts to stimulate the RANKL pathway. Dashed lines represent factors (estrogen and other agents) that will "tone down" the RANK system and minimize resorption. During resorption (*lower right*), the osteoclast binds to the bone surface through a protein or integrin termed $\alpha V\beta 3$. Protons pumped into the area and the cathepsin K protease degrade bone. When excavation is complete, osteoclasts move out and osteoblasts move in to form new bone.

After the first 7 to 10 years of menopause, bone loss in women slows to 8% to 12% per decade.[22]

Estrogen deficiency increases bone resorption more than formation. This appears to depend on tumor necrosis factor (TNF), interleukin-1 (IL-1), interleukin-11, interleukin-6, M-CSF, and prostaglandin E_2, which stimulate osteoclastic activity through the OPG/RANK/RANKL system[3,6] (see Fig. 90–3). Reduced TGF-β, associated with estrogen loss, enhances osteoclast action through decreased apoptosis. Osteocytes also may play a role. Normally, with more weight-bearing, osteocytes trigger increased BMD. With menopause, osteocyte apoptosis blunts this response.[4,5] With resetting of the mechanostat set point at menopause, increased loading is required to maintain bone.[4] After menopause, some estrogen is still synthesized in adipose tissue. Women with the highest estrogen concentrations after menopause had the lowest fracture risk.[23]

AGE-RELATED OSTEOPOROSIS

With aging, bone is lost. Age-related bone loss in men is 3% to 4% per decade after peak BMD is attained,[24] which is less than the 8% to 12% per decade loss by women 10 years after menopause.[22] Bone resorption increases with age, but changes in bone formation are not observed consistently. Increased apoptosis of osteocytes may decrease responses to mechanical strain and hinder bone repair.[4] Cortical porosity from years of remodeling and decreased trabecular connectivity, particularly of horizontal struts, promotes microarchitectural deterioration of bone not always reflected in BMD. Aging also increases fracture risk in other ways that are independent of BMD. Comorbid conditions, cognitive impairment, medications, and deconditioning can increase falls. Four to six percent of falls lead to fracture, one-quarter of them hip fractures.[25]

Inadequate calcium, vitamin D, and nutritional intake contribute to bone loss and fractures. Vitamin D insufficiency results from poor sun exposure, decreased cutaneous production, insufficient dietary intake, and decreased absorption.[10] Calcium and vitamin D insufficiency promotes secondary hyperparathyroidism and associated bone loss[26] (see Fig. 90–4).

TABLE 90–2. Risk Factors Associated with Osteoporosis, Falls, and Hip Fractures

Genetic	Lifestyle	Diet	Obstetric and Gynecology History	Chronic Illnesses	Medications	Fall-Related Conditions
Female sex	Minimal exercise	Low calcium intake any time in life	Late menarche	Low bone mineral density	Glucocorticoids	Medications: anxiolytics, benzodiazepines, antidepressants, antihypertensives
White or Asian ethnicity	Sedentary	Lactose intolerance	Early natural menopause	History of fragility fracture	Excessive thyroid replacement	Physical disability
Family history of osteoporosis or fractures	Smoking	High caffeine intake	Surgical menopause	Falls	Long-term heparin	Slow gait, difficult tandem walk
Small body frame (tall, thin, low body mass index)	Excessive alcohol	High phosphorous intake	Oophorectomy without replacement therapy	Hyperthyroidism	Chronic lithium therapy	Decreased visual acuity
Older age	Minimal sun exposure		Nulliparity	Cushing's syndrome	Chemotherapy	Poor depth perception
		Weight loss greater than 10% after age 50	Amenorrhea associated with anorexia nervosa, medications, or excessive exercise	Multiple myeloma or metastatic cancer to the bone	Gonadotropin-releasing hormone agonist or antagonists	Decreased quadriceps and grip strength
		Anorexia nervosa		Diabetes	Anticonvulsants	Inability to rise from a chair
		Long-term parenteral nutrition		Altered GI or hepatobiliary function	Drugs altering calcium absorption: tetracycline, phenothiazine derivatives, cyclosporine, aluminum-containing antacids, phosphate binders	Use of walking aids
				Arthritis	Drugs altering calcium elimination: loop diuretics	Orthostatic hypotension
				Cognitive impairment		
				Poor self-rated health		
				Gastric surgery		
				Stroke		
				Posttransplantation		
				Poor depth perception		
				Poor contrast sensitivity		
				Tachycardia at rest		
				Occult osteogenesis imperfecta		
				Mastocytosis		
				Prolactinoma		
				Hemolytic anemia, *hemochromatosis*, thalassemia		
				Ankylosing spondylitis		

OSTEOPOROSIS IN MEN

Osteoporosis and fractures are less common in men because their peak BMD is 20% to 40% higher than women's, they lose less bone after the peak, they have a shorter life expectancy than women, they experience fewer falls, and they have a gradual versus distinct cessation of hormone production. Men's bones also have a mechanical advantage because their larger diameter makes them more fracture-resistant.

Age-related bone loss in men is 3% to 4% per decade after peak BMD is attained.[27] Although fewer men than women have osteoporosis, men suffer 25% of all hip fractures and are more likely than women to die within 1 year of fracture.[9] Male osteoporosis remains an underappreciated problem.

Hypogonadism—secondary to age-related decreases in testosterone and increased sex hormone–binding globulin (SHBG) or from endocrine dysfunction or androgen ablation—can cause bone loss. Estrogen, synthesized from testosterone by the enzyme aromatase, appears more important than testosterone in men for bone maintenance, with greater bone density seen in men with higher estradiol levels.[28] Secondary causes often contribute to male osteoporosis. Other fracture risk factors are listed in Table 90–2.

DRUG-INDUCED OSTEOPOROSIS

Several medications can cause bone loss: systemic glucocorticoids (see the section "Glucocorticoid-Induced Osteoporosis" below),[29–31] excessive thyroid replacement, some antiepileptic drugs, and long-term heparin use. Adjustment of thyroid dose to normalize thyroid-stimulating hormone (TSH) is appropriate and can help avoid bone loss.

Some anticonvulsants affect vitamin D metabolism and can lead to osteomalacia. This is seen ordinarily only in those who are on multiple anticonvulsants, are institutionalized, or have multiple comorbidities (see the section "Osteomalacia" below).[10]

Heparin therapy in excess of 15,000 to 30,000 units daily for greater than 3 to 6 months is associated with bone loss and vertebral fractures. Low-molecular-weight heparins such as enoxaparin pose less risk of bone loss.

CLINICAL PRESENTATION

The usual presentation of osteoporosis is shortened stature; kyphosis; lordosis; vertebra, hip, or forearm fracture; and/or bone pain. Many patients are unaware that they have osteoporosis and only present after fracture. Fractures can occur after bending, lifting, or falling or independent of any activity. Vertebral fractures are the most common. Multiple vertebral fractures may lead to dorsal kyphosis and exaggerated cervical lordosis, frequently referred to as *dowager's* or *widow's hump*. Subsequent chest wall changes can lead to pulmonary and cardiovascular complications. Collapsed vertebrae rarely lead to spinal cord compression. Recurrent fractures are common. Depression and lower self-esteem can result from pain and physical changes.

FRACTURE OUTCOMES

Fractures can be devastating. While acute fracture pain usually resolves in 2 to 3 months, chronic fracture pain can occur, manifested as a deep, dull, nagging pain near the fracture site. Up to 67% of hip fracture patients have not regained their prefracture function 1 year after hip fracture.[11] About 50% of women will spend some time in a nursing home after a hip fracture, and 14% of them have stays longer than 1 year. Between 12% and 36% of hip fracture patients die within 1 year following the fracture.

PATIENT ASSESSMENT

Patient assessment should include history of nontraumatic adult fractures, nontraumatic adult fractures in first-degree relatives, comorbidities, diet, surgery, menstrual history, physical activity, falls, prior and current medications, and smoking and alcohol history. A complete physical examination and laboratory analysis to rule out secondary causes and to assess kyphosis (dowager's hump) and back pain is needed. Lateral spine radiographs to detect vertebral fractures are reasonable with new or severe back pain. For patients with osteoporosis but no risk factors, secondary causes (see Table 90–2) should be sought. Surveys and questionnaires are used in research, but a convenient universal tool for clinical practice is not available yet. A risk factor checklist can be developed from Table 90–2.

RADIOLOGIC AND ULTRASOUND QUANTIFICATION OF BONE LOSS

BMD is the best predictor of fracture risk. For every 1 standard deviation (SD) below mean young-adult BMD (a decrease in T score by 1 unit), the risk of fracture increases about twofold. Measurement of central (hip and spine) BMD with dual energy x-ray absorptiometry (DXA) is the "gold standard" for osteoporosis diagnosis. DXA is accurate, efficient, and uses minimal radiation. Quantitative computed tomography (QCT) measures trabecular and cortical bone separately but is impractical for routine use. Measurements at peripheral sites (forearm, heel, and phalanges) with single energy x-ray absorptiometry (SXA), ultrasound, or DXA are used for screening purposes. Portable units can be used in a pharmacy or clinic. Although peripheral measures are predictive of fractures, their predictive accuracy is less than that of hip BMD.

Peripheral bone measurements can be helpful as a screening tool because if bone density is low at one site, it is likely to be low at others. This correlation is not perfect because some individuals will have a normal T score at one site and osteopenia or even osteoporosis at another.[32] These discrepancies may result from different rates of bone loss at different sites with aging. Differences also depend on the instrument used and the normal reference population against which the T score is calculated. Consensus does not exist regarding what peripheral T score should be used as a threshold for obtaining a central DXA measurement.

With passage of the Bone Mass Measurement Act in 1998, Medicare patients became eligible for BMD testing. The Health Care Financing Administration regulations provide reimbursement to providers for BMD measurement for patients with estrogen deficiency and clinical risk for osteoporosis, those with vertebral abnormalities or primary hyperparathyroidism, and those on long-term glucocorticoid therapy (>7.5 mg prednisone per day for >3 months) or Food and Drug Administration (FDA)–approved osteoporosis therapy.[33]

Knowledge of low BMD encourages prevention and leads to positive lifestyle changes.[34]

BIOCHEMICAL AND BIOPSY EVALUATION

Biochemical evaluation for the osteoporotic patient should include a complete blood count, chemistry panel (including calcium-corrected albumin, phosphorus, and alkaline phosphatase), and 25-hydroxyvitamin D concentration.[35,36] When no cause is apparent, specialized tests are warranted, guided by clinical suspicion. Hyperparathyroidism is associated with a serum PTH level that is inappropriately elevated relative to serum ionized calcium. Measurement of TSH, with free T_4 and free T_3 determinations as necessary, can be used to rule out hyperthyroidism. Urinary or serum cortisol concentrations can detect Cushing's syndrome. Celiac sprue (gluten sensitivity) with poor nutritional and/or low vitamin D status is detectable with antibody tests. Serum protein electrophoresis can rule out myeloma. Renal tubular acidosis causes bone loss and would be suspected from reduced bicarbonate and/or associated abnormalities such as high plasma chloride or abnormal (usually low) potassium. Twenty-four hour urine calcium (or urine calcium-creatinine ratio) can be measured to assess hypercalciuria. Sometimes it is used to assess calcium absorption, although its utility and accuracy are questionable. Genetic testing is not commonly performed but is likely to increase.

Biochemical markers of bone turnover are used in clinical trials and are marketed heavily. Markers of bone resorption include *C*-terminal or *N*-terminal telopeptides and deoxypyridinoline. Bone formation markers include bone-specific alkaline phosphatase, osteocalcin, and *C*-terminal and *N*-terminal procollagen extension peptides. Significant debate, however, continues regarding clinical utility of markers. Markers may prove useful in predicting fracture risk, monitoring of therapy, or increasing patient adherence.[37]

Bone biopsy is rarely useful for osteoporosis but can rule out suspected secondary causes, such as osteomalacia.

▶ PREVENTION AND TREATMENT: Osteoporosis

In patients at risk of developing osteoporosis, the goals of prevention are to achieve optimal peak bone mass and to minimize further bone loss. Osteoporosis prevention ideally begins early in life, when children, adolescents, and young adults can increase peak bone mass. Goals of treatment are to minimize bone loss and to decrease falls and fractures. Pain control may be needed acutely after fracture and chronically for severe osteoporosis.

NONPHARMACOLOGIC PREVENTION AND TREATMENT

Figure 90–5 provides an osteoporosis management algorithm that incorporates both nonpharmacologic and pharmacologic approaches (see guideline section below). In this section, nondrug interventions—diet, social habits, and exercise—are detailed.

DIET CHANGES

For all individuals, a well-balanced diet with adequate calcium and vitamin D (Table 90–3) is essential for healthy bones.[38] Dairy products account for most dietary calcium intake, since calcium in fruits and vegetables is not well absorbed. Most Americans, especially older people, ingest insufficient calcium. In evaluating the patient, a practical approach is to count calcium contributions from certain key foods: milk, yogurt, cheese, ice cream, cottage cheese, and fortified orange juice (Table 90–4). If adequate intakes cannot be achieved with these foods and other readily identifiable sources, calcium supplements are needed (Table 90–5).

Few unfortified foods contain substantial amounts of vitamin D. In the United States, milk is fortified with 400 IU/quart of vitamin D. Children and young adults produce most of their vitamin D from casual exposure to sunlight. Between 5 and 15 minutes of daily exposure (without sunscreen) generally is sufficient, except during winter months in cooler climates. Vitamin D insufficiency can result when traditional or religious garments that minimize skin exposure are worn. Older adults have vitamin D insufficiency because they spend little time outdoors, have reduced cutaneous synthetic capacity, and do not consume sufficient vitamin D in their diets.[10] Vitamin D supplements are needed in these situations.

Caffeine modestly increases calcium excretion and has been linked to increased fracture risk in elderly women. However, in a clinical study, effects on BMD were small, seen only at the hip, and not observed in younger women.[39] Any effect caffeine has can be offset by increased calcium intake.[40]

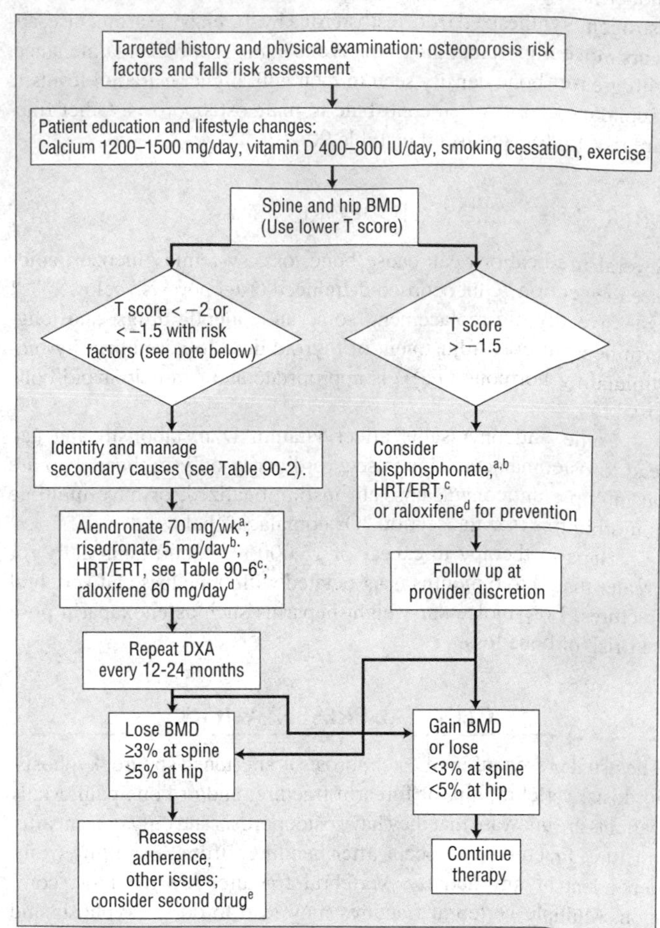

FIGURE 90–5. Algorithm for osteoporosis management.

[a]Contraindications to alendronate include hypocalcemia; esophageal abnormalities which delay esophageal emptying, such as achalasia or strictures; inability to stand or sit upright for 30 min. Do not give if creatinine clearance <35 mL/min.

[b]Contraindications to risedronate include hypocalcemia; inability to stand or sit upright for 30 min. Precaution is recommended for those with renal impairment.

[c]Contraindications to HRT/ERT include include estrogen-dependent tumors, undiagnosed uterine bleeding, increased risk of thromboembolic events. Pelvic/pap and mammogram prior to initiation of HRT/ERT with periodic reassessment generally advisable.

[d]Contraindications to raloxifene include active thromboembolic disorders. Not for use in premenopausal women.

[e]Nasal calcitonin 200 IU/day if other medications not tolerated.

Note: Guidelines released while this text was in production recommend treatment for women with T scores < −2.5; with low-trauma fractures and low BMD; or with T scores > −1.5 with risk factors.[138]

TABLE 90–3. Daily Calcium and Vitamin D Requirements

	Adequate Calcium Intake	Adequate Vitamin D Intake
Infant		
Birth–6 mos.	210 mg	200 IU
6 mos.–1 yr	270 mg	200 IU
Children		
1–3 yrs	500 mg	200 IU
4–8 yrs	800 mg	200 IU
9–13 yrs	1300 mg	200 IU
Adolescents		
14–18 yrs	1300 mg	200 IU
Adults		
19–50 yrs	1000 mg	200 IU
51–70 yrs	1200 mg	400 IU
≥71 yrs	1200 mg	600 IU

From Ref. 38.

Dietary phosphorus does not interfere with calcium absorption.[41]

Teenagers who drink excessive amounts of carbonated beverages have an increased fracture risk.[42] This may be a "milk displacement" effect (by drinking soft drinks, the person does not drink enough milk), but it is troubling because of widespread use of carbonated beverages.

Excessive vitamin A intake, of more than 1.5 mg daily, may also increase fracture risk, based on studies in Sweden, where vitamin A supplements are used commonly.[43]

Low vitamin K status may be linked with osteoporosis. The bone matrix protein osteocalcin requires vitamin K–dependent γ-carboxylation. In hip fracture patients, low vitamin K and elevated undercarboxylated osteocalcin were found.[44] Supplements are not recommended currently.

The Framingham Study showed increased bone loss with the lowest protein intake.[45] Increased nutritional intake is associated with increased bone density, and improved protein intake is associated with better outcomes in hip fracture patients.

TABLE 90–4. Dietary Sources of Calcium

Food	Serving Size	Calcium Content (mg)
Whole milk	1 cup	291
Skim milk	1 cup	302
Ice cream	1 cup	200
Yogurt (low-fat)	1 cup	345–415
American cheese	1 oz	150
Cheddar cheese	1 oz	211
Cottage cheese (low-fat)	1 cup	154
Swiss cheese	1 oz	250
Cheese pizza	1 slice	150
Fortified orange juice	1 cup	350
Sardines	3 oz	372
Salmon with bones	3 oz	167
Bokchoy	1/2 cup	126
Broccoli	1 cup	100–136
Collards, raw	1/2 cup	179
Figs, dried	5 medium	126
Soybeans	1 cup	131
Spinach	1/2 cup	113
Tofu	4 oz	106
Turnip greens	1/2 cup	126

SOCIAL HABIT CHANGES

Smoking increases hip fracture risk and is associated with decreased BMD, earlier menopause, thinness, altered estrogen metabolism, increased PTH levels, and decreased vitamin D status. Smoking cessation improves BMD.[46]

Alcohol use has been associated with low BMD and fracture in some but not all studies. In a study of 30,000 people, increased hip fracture risk was seen in men drinking more than 27 drinks weekly. For women, the association was less clear.[47] Although lower levels of alcohol intake have not been proven unequivocally to affect BMD, moderation should be encouraged. Alcohol use is clearly associated with increased risk of falls.

EXERCISE

Bone mass and structure change in response to the stress and strain a person puts on them.[48] Long-term exercise (over a period of years) during youth increases a person's peak BMD, and lifelong physical activity increases BMD. Although short-term exercise increases BMD, continued activity appears necessary to maintain benefit.[49] Exercise also enhances calcium and estrogen therapy.[48] In addition to effects on bone, physical activity reduces fracture risk likely related to reduced falls and improvements in balance, posture, flexibility, range of motion, muscle strength, and endurance.

Physical activity should be encouraged for patients with osteoporosis as tolerated. Before starting an exercise program for an elderly patient or one with severe osteoporosis, a medical examination is recommended. Referral to a physical therapist is often helpful.

Excessive exercise can produce amenorrhea with consequent bone loss and increased fracture risk.[50]

PHARMACOLOGIC PREVENTION AND TREATMENT

Nonpharmacologic interventions generally are not sufficient to prevent osteoporosis in older patients or to treat existing bone depletion, making drug therapy necessary. Table 90–6 describes the over-the-counter and prescription medications available for osteoporosis. At this time, controversy continues over whether the drug of choice for postmenopausal osteoporosis is hormonal therapy or a bisphosphonate, as discussed below. This choice depends on patient and prescriber characteristics and preferences. Organizations have outlined differing approaches, and these provide an overview into the nuances of prevention and treatment of osteoporosis and osteopenia.

TREATMENT GUIDELINES

A National Institutes of Health (NIH) osteoporosis consensus development panel concluded in 2000 that calcium, vitamin D, bisphosphonates, hormone-replacement therapy (HRT), and selective estrogen receptor modulators (SERMs) are useful for increasing BMD and preventing fractures (only vertebral data were available for HRT and SERMs).[51] Phytoestrogens increase BMD in animals. Nasal calcitonin increased spine BMD, but the only study to demonstrate decreased vertebral fractures had several shortcomings. Greater emphasis should be placed on medications with proven fracture prevention, especially hip fracture prevention, since BMD is only a surrogate marker. The NIH panel recommended calcium and vitamin D as

TABLE 90–5. Calcium Product Selection[a]

Product	Calcium Content	Calcium (mg)
Calcium carbonate	40%	
Trade name and generic		200–600
Generic suspension		500/5 mL
Titralac liquid		400/5 mL
Titralac chewable		168
Extra strength		300
Tums chewable		200
E-X		300
Ultra		500
Other chewable brands		168–500
Viactiv chews		500
Mylanta soothing lozenges		240
Cal Carb-HD powder		2.4 g per 7-g packet
Calcium carbonate with Vitamin D[b]		
Generic + Vit D (125 IU)		600
Calcilyte + Vit D (200 IU)[c]		500
Calel-D + Vit D (200 IU)		500
Caltrate + Vit D (125 IU)		600
OsCal + Vit D (125 IU)		500
Calcium citrate	24%	
Generic		240
Citracal		200
Citracal Liquitab[c]		500
Citracal + Vit D (200 IU)[b]		316
Calcium phosphate tribasic	39%	
Posture		600
Posture-D (125 IU)[b]		600
Dical-D chewable wafers + Vit D 200 IU		232

[a]Only calcium products with 500 to 600 mg per tablet or with an alternative dosage form (i.e., chewable, liquid, dissolvable tablet) are listed.
[b]When using a combination product, determine if total vitamin D ingestion is needed and adequate based on the person's age or needs. Multivitamins usually contain 400 IU vitamin D.
[c]Tablet for solution.

important prerequisites for therapy. Without sufficient calcium and vitamin D, other treatments cannot improve bone architecture.

The North American Menopause Society Consensus conference in 1999 recommended HRT (estrogen-progestin combination therapy) or estrogen-replacement therapy (ERT) for postmenopausal women under 65 years of age with a femoral T score below −2 with no risk factors or below −1.5 with risk factors.[52] For women 65 years of age or older, the conference recommended HRT/ERT for those with prevalent fractures or T scores of −2.5 or lower. BMD testing every 3 to 5 years was recommended to assess individuals not on therapy. Other therapies (e.g., raloxifene, bisphosphonates, calcitonin, calcium, and vitamin D) were recommended for woman unable or unwilling to take HRT.

The American College of Preventive Medicine 1999 report on HRT concluded that insufficient evidence existed to recommend HRT for all postmenopausal women.[53] Women with coronary risk factors may benefit from HRT, in concert with risk modification. HRT should be avoided or used cautiously in women with heart disease, and HRT should be avoided in women with a history of breast cancer or thromboembolic disease. This group suggested that indefinite HRT use was warranted, with periodic review of the decision to continue therapy as further evidence accumulates.

The 1998 National Osteoporosis Foundation Guidelines recommend HRT, alendronate, or calcitonin for women with a vertebral fracture.[54] Women 65 years of age or older should be offered hip bone density measurement and provided therapy depending on T score and risk factors. Postmenopausal women younger than 65 years of age and without risk factors should exercise, stop smoking, receive adequate calcium and vitamin D, and consider BMD testing. For women unwilling to be treated, BMD testing is not recommended, but positive lifestyle changes should be encouraged. Raloxifene and risedronate are not included because they were investigational when these guidelines were prepared in 1998.

The 1998 International Committee for Osteoporosis Clinical Guidelines recommended alendronate or HRT for all postmenopausal women with a fracture (alternatives were cyclic etidronate or intranasal calcitonin).[11] For women concerned about osteoporosis, treatment should be provided for those with T scores below −2.5, prevention with HRT if acceptable (alternatives were alendronate or raloxifene) for those with T scores of −1 to −2.5, and prevention with adequate vitamin D and calcium for those with T scores greater than −1 and for women with no risks and concerns.

Based on a Markov model, a woman's risk for hip fracture, coronary artery disease, and breast cancer dictates strategies for osteoporosis prevention.[55] For a woman with low risk for all three conditions, conservative care is preferred. For women at risk for heart disease, HRT would be preferred and would increase life expectancy by 20 to 29 months. For women at risk for breast cancer but not heart disease,

TABLE 90–6. Osteoporosis Prevention and Treatment Medications

Drug	Dose	Kinetics	Adverse Effects
Calcium	200–1500 mg/day See Tables 90–3 and 90–5 Divided doses	Absorption: predominantly active transport with some passive diffusion, fractional absorption 28–60%, fecal elimination for the unabsorbed and renal elimination for the absorbed calcium	Constipation, gas, rare kidney stones
Vitamin D_2 or D_3	200–800 IU/day; if malabsorption or multiple anticonvulsants, may require higher doses (4000 IU daily or more)	Metabolism to inactive products in the kidney	Hypercalcemia, hypercalciuria, (weakness, headache, somnolence, nausea, cardiac rhythm disturbance; other symptoms can accompany hypercalcemia)
	For vitamin D deficiency, 50,000 IU once weekly or once monthly can be used; monitor serum calcium		
Bisphosphonates			
Alendronate (Fosamax)	5 mg daily for prevention, 10 mg daily or 70 mg weekly for treatment	Poorly absorbed, 1–5%; Renal elimination; avoid alendronate if Cl_{Cr} is less than 35 ml/min	Nausea; dyspepsia; abdominal pain; diarrhea; esophageal, gastric, or duodenal irritation, perforation, ulceration, or bleeding
Risedronate (Actonel)	5 mg daily, 30–35 mg weekly investigational	Risedronate should be used cautiously in patients with renal impairment	
Estrogens, oral		Metabolism	Common: Vaginal bleeding or spotting, breast enlargement and tenderness, fluid retention, increased weight, increased triglycerides. Uncommon: facial hair growth, bloating, nausea, vomiting, leg pain, headache, migraine, increase/decrease in sexual desire, dizziness, mood changes, endometrial cancer with unopposed therapy
Conjugated estrogens (Premarin)	0.3, 0.625, 0.9, 1.25, 2.5 mg		
Synthetic conjugated estrogens (Cenestin)	0.625, 0.9 mg		
Micronized estradiol (Estrace, generics)	0.5, 1, 2 mg		
Esterified estrogens (Estratab, Menest)	0.3, 0.625, 1.25, 2.5 mg		
Ethinyl estradiol (Estinyl)	0.02, 0.05, 0.5 mg		
Estropipate (Ogen, Ortho-Est, generic)	0.625, 1.25, 2.5, 5 mg		
Estrogens, estradiol patch			Rare: Thromboembolism, skin darkening, acne, rash, loss of hair, blurred vision, breast secretions, stomach pain, jaundice, gallbladder attack
Estraderm	0.05, 0.1 mg/24 h		
Alora	0.05, 0.075, 0.1 mg/24 h		
Climara	0.025, 0.05, 0.075, 0.1 mg/24 h		
Esclim	0.025, 0.0375, 0.05, 0.075, 0.1 mg/24 h		
Vivelle/Vivelle-Dot	0.0375, 0.05, 0.075, 0.1 mg/24 h		

(*Continued*)

TABLE 90–6. Osteoporosis Prevention and Treatment Medications (*Continued*)

Drug	Dose	Kinetics	Adverse Effects
Progestins		Metabolism	Withdrawal bleeding and spotting, breast tenderness and enlargement, bloating, edema, abdominal cramps, anxiety, irritability, depression, mood changes, acne
Medroxyprogesterone (Provera, generics)	2.5–5 mg daily or 5–10 mg 12–14 days/month		
Micronized progesterone (Prometrium)	100 mg daily		
Norethindrone acetate			
Trimegestone (investigational)	0.7–1 mg		
HRT, oral		Metabolism	Per estrogen and progestin
Prempro	0.625 mg conjugated estrogens and 2.5 or 5 mg medroxyprogesterone daily		
Premphase	0.625 mg conjugated estrogens daily and 5 mg medroxyprogesterone for 14 days		
Femhrt 1/5	5 μg ethinyl estradiol and 1 mg norethindrone acetate		
Activella (pending)	1 mg estradiol and 0.5 mg norethindrone acetate		
HRT, patch			
Combipatch	0.05 mg estradiol and 0.14 or 0.25 mg norethindrone acetate		
SERM			
Raloxifene (Evista)	60 mg daily	Hepatic metabolism; highly protein bound	Hot flushes, leg cramps, thromboembolic events
Testosterone		Hepatic metabolism. Highly protein bound, to SHBG.	Local skin irritation, injection-site discomfort, Reverses ERT induced HDL increases, hirsutism, acne, hoarseness, liver function abnormalities, erythrocytosis, exacerbation of benign prostatic hypertrophy; avoid if h/o prostate cancer or elevated PSA
Methyltestosterone (for women)	1.25–2.5 mg (combined with estradiol)		
Testosterone (for men)			
Patch Androderm	5-mg skin patch/day		
Testoderm-TTS	5-mg skin patch/day		
Testoderm	4 or 6-mg scrotal patch/day		
Injection	Testosterone enanthate 50–400 mg IM q 2–4 weeks		
Gel (Andro-gel)	1% gel: 50 mg topically per day		
Calcitonin (Miacalcin)	Intranasal: 200 IU daily, alternating nares IM or SC: 100 IU/day	Renal metabolism; 3% nasal availability	Intranasal formulation: rhinitis, epistaxis, and nasal irritation Subcutaneous administration: GI symptoms, injection-site pain, and flushing

raloxifene would be preferred and would increase life expectancy by 8 to 10 months. Alendronate would be chosen for women who cannot or will not use HRT or raloxifene, and it would increase life expectancy by 1 to 3 months. In women at high risk for hip fracture over a 10-year period, the number needed to treat would be 213 to 227 with HRT, raloxifene, or alendronate.

Some investigators suggest that reliance on HRT is overemphasized and that other agents are underused.[56,57] They base their opinion on the lack of long-term protection from short-term HRT use, lack of studies showing that HRT prevents hip fracture, and the observation that some women continue to lose bone while on HRT.

More definitive answers about ERT and HRT will come from the Women's Health Initiative (WHI) clinical trial begun in 1993, which enrolled 10,000 women of ages 50 to 79 for a 10-year study. WHI is evaluating the effects of ERT/HRT, low-fat diets, calcium plus vitamin D supplementation, and counseling programs on cardiovascular disease, cancer, and fractures.

ANTIRESORPTIVE MEDICATIONS

Calcium

With calcium deficiency and even slight hypocalcemia, PTH levels rise and the PTH–vitamin D axis promotes bone resorption to regain calcium homeostasis (see Fig. 90–4). To prevent secondary hyperparathyroidism and bone destruction, adequate calcium should be ingested[38] (see Table 90–3).

Clinical Effectiveness. A total of 35 randomized, controlled trials, calcium balance studies, and bone metabolic studies document that higher calcium intake prevents or reduces bone loss in adults.[58] In 15 studies that included children, higher calcium intakes were associated with larger increases in BMD. Calcium is less effective during the first 5 years after menopause, when estrogen deficiency is the predominant cause of accelerated bone loss. Calcium's effects are augmented when combined with other antiresorptive therapies or exercise. The combination of calcium and vitamin D decreases nonvertebral, vertebral, and hip fractures.[11]

Calcium Administration. Most children and adults ingest insufficient calcium and require supplements. Individuals with certain characteristics or conditions—such as lactose intolerance, nondairy vegetarianism, malnutrition, low-fat diets, glucocorticoid therapy, and antiresorptive therapy—require evaluation for calcium supplementation.

Calcium carbonate is the salt of choice because it contains the highest concentration of elemental calcium and is the least expensive (see Table 90–5). Calcium carbonate tablets should be ingested with meals to enhance absorption from increased acid secretion. Calcium citrate absorption is acid-independent and need not be taken with meals. The fraction of calcium absorbed decreases with dose, so divided doses (500–600 mg or less) are recommended.

Disintegration and dissolution rates vary significantly between products and lots. Products with good disintegration and dissolution rates and lead contents of less than 1 μg/day should be recommended. For populations at risk, children, pregnant or lactating women, and renal failure patients using calcium as a phosphate binder, lead intakes are suggested to be less than 1–6 μg/day.

Diuretics

Thiazide diuretics increase urinary calcium reabsorption. A 10-year study of 83,728 women demonstrated fewer fractures among patients currently taking thiazides.[59] Prescribing thiazide diuretics solely for osteoporosis is not recommended but is a reasonable choice for patients with osteoporosis who require a diuretic.

Vitamin D and Metabolites

Vitamin D deficiency is extremely common in the elderly, especially long-term care residents. Vitamin D deficiency results from insufficient intake, decreased sun exposure, or decreased cutaneous production. Reduced renal synthesis of calcitriol can also occur because of age or liver or kidney dysfunction.

Clinical Effectiveness. Vitamin D 400 IU/d given to elderly women improved femur and spine BMD.[11] Combined calcium and vitamin D (700–800 IU/d) supplementation reduced nonvertebral fractures in community dwellers and nursing home residents.[11] Reduced vertebral fractures were demonstrated with calcitriol 0.25 μg twice daily for 3 years, but the study was criticized on several grounds, e.g., counting "new" vertebral fractures on the same vertebra with each new decrease in vertebral height.[60] Calcitriol is not approved for osteoporosis treatment. Doxercalciferol (1α–hydroxyvitamin D_2) is under investigation for osteoporosis treatment.

Vitamin D Administration. Given the low cost and safety of vitamin D, no patient should be deficient in this vitamin (see Table 90–3).[38] Most multivitamin tablets contain 400 IU vitamin D, and combination calcium–vitamin D products contain 100–200 IU per dose (see Table 90–5). For seniors, one multivitamin tablet daily (two tablets daily for those over 70 years old) should be adequate to ensure sufficient vitamin D intake.

In patients with vitamin D deficiency, oral vitamin D 50,000 IU once weekly for 8 weeks is useful, with periodic serum calcium and 25-hydroxyvitamin D monitoring. Once the person is replete, one to two multivitamin tablets daily should suffice for maintaining serum concentrations. In the nursing home, vitamin D 50,000 IU orally once a month is reasonable.[10]

In patients with severe hepatic disease, low serum levels of 25-hydroxyvitamin D may result from poor fat absorption. Vitamin D supplementation to achieve 20–45 ng/mL of 25-hydroxyvitamin D is reasonable.[36] When vitamin D is not absorbed (e.g., gluten-sensitive sprue), 25-hydroxyvitamin D (calcidiol) administration can be considered.

With renal dysfunction, calcitriol (1,25-dihydroxyvitamin D) is used. This drug requires careful titration and serum calcium and creatinine level monitoring because of its hypercalcemic potential and the limited calciuric ability of the dysfunctional kidney.

Bisphosphonates

Bisphosphonates adsorb to bone apatite and are incorporated permanently into bone. Osteoclasts are unable to adhere to bone surfaces containing bisphosphonates. The estimated terminal half-lives of bisphosphonates are similar to bone turnover (1–10 years). Relative potencies are 1 for etidronate, 10 for clodronate, 100 for pamidronate, 100–1000 for alendronate, 1000–10,000 for risedronate and ibandronate, and 10,000+ for zoledronate.[61] Etidronate and clodronate also inhibit bone mineralization, which can cause osteomalacia. At the time this chapter was prepared, alendronate and risedronate were FDA-approved for prevention and treatment of postmenopausal and glucocorticoid-induced osteoporosis, and alendronate was approved for osteoporosis in men.

Clinical Effectiveness. Of the antiresorptive agents, bisphosphonates provide the greatest BMD increases. The effect is dose-dependent. Respective BMD changes after alendronate 10 mg[62,63] and risedronate 5 mg[64] were lumbar spine 5.4% to 6%, 5.4%; femoral neck 2.9%, 1.6%; and trochanter 4.4% to 5.9%, 3.3%. BMD increases are greatest in the first year of therapy[61] and continue for at least 7 years of therapy. After discontinuation, BMD is maintained or decreases slowly but remains higher than that of nonusers.[11] BMD increases are seen in women,[62–64] men,[65] elderly patients,[61] and patients taking glucocorticoids.[29,31] Combination therapy with ERT/HRT produces greater BMD increases than either medication alone.[63] Reductions in vertebral,[61,64] nonvertebral,[64] and hip fractures[61,66] have been demonstrated.

Intermittent administration also has been evaluated. Seven years of intermittent cyclic etidronate (3-month cycles of 400 mg/d for 2 weeks and then calcium and vitamin D for 11 weeks) continuously increased vertebral BMD and decreased vertebral fracture rate.[67] Intermittent cyclic etidronate evaluated for up to 4 years had an additive effect with HRT on vertebral and hip BMD, with no reported osteomalacia, whereas 33% of those on etidronate alone had osteomalacia.[68] Various other intermittent dosing strategies—including ibandronate intravenous bolus every 3 months, pamidronate infusions every 2 to 3 months, and intramuscular clodronate every 1 to 2 weeks—are being studied. Alternative delivery systems, such as transdermal zoledronate, also are under investigation.[61]

Bisphosphonate Administration. Bisphosphonates must be administered very carefully to avoid serious gastrointestinal adverse effects and at the same time optimize the agents' poor bioavailability. All bisphosphonates are poorly absorbed (1% to 5%), with food, beverages, and calcium significantly decreasing absorption. Therefore, these medications should be taken 30 to 120 minutes before breakfast with a full glass of water (not coffee, juice, mineral water, or milk). The patient should remain in an upright position for at least 30 minutes. Calcium and, when needed, vitamin D also should be used but administered at different times.

Patient adherence to therapy may be increased with once-weekly bisphosphonate administration, and the patient is exposed to the agent much less often. In addition, since the rate of turnover of the cells lining the gastrointestinal tract is about 5 days, any cells damaged during exposure in a given week likely would be replaced before the next week's dose is taken. Several regimens of bisphosphonates have been studied, including once-weekly alendronate 70 mg[62] and risedronate 30–35 mg.[69] Once-weekly alendronate administration achieves similar BMD results, has similar gastrointestinal adverse effects, and does not impair mineralization compared with daily doses of 10 mg.[62]

The most common bisphosphonate adverse effects, i.e., nausea, abdominal pain, and dyspepsia, occur in, respectively, 11%, 14%, and 18% of women taking alendronate 10 mg, similar to the percentages of women taking placebo in clinical trials complaining of those side effects.[70] Gastrointestinal event rates were higher in the alendronate–nonsteroidal anti-inflammatory drug (NSAID) group but not significantly different from the placebo–NSAID group. Increased perforations, ulcerations, and bleeding (PUB) have been seen in the oldest women in studies, but the frequencies were not significantly different from events for similarly aged women in the placebo group. PUB can result when administration directions are not followed or when bisphosphonates are prescribed for patients with contraindications. Patients should be encouraged to discuss gastrointestinal complaints with a health care provider.

Risedronate, a pyridinyl bisphosphonate, may have fewer gastrointestinal effects than alendronate, an amino bisphosphonate, but long-term comparisons are not yet available.

Estrogen and Hormonal Therapy

ERT has been investigated for osteoporosis therapy for many years. Combination estrogen-progestin therapy (termed HRT) is used only in women with an intact uterus to prevent and potentially protect them from endometrial cancer. ERT and HRT increase BMD in all age groups, but a paucity of data exists about fracture prevention. Combined with conflicting evidence about the utility of ERT/HRT in cardiovascular disease prevention and with women's fears about developing estrogen-dependent breast cancer, use of ERT and HRT for prevention and treatment of osteoporosis continues to be controversial. Estrogen and other hormone products are FDA-approved for osteoporosis prevention but not for treatment.

Estrogen receptors exist on osteoblasts, osteoclasts, macrophage cells, intestinal cells, and many other tissues. Estrogens decrease osteoclast recruitment and activity, inhibit PTH peripherally, increase calcitriol concentrations and intestinal calcium absorption, and decrease renal calcium excretion. Estrogens decrease cytokine levels and decrease the activity of the OPG/RANK/RANKL pathway, inhibiting bone resorption. Response to estrogen deficiency and replacement may be related to estrogen receptor (alleles *P, X, p,* and *x*) and vitamin D receptor (alleles *B* and *b*) polymorphism, with larger decreases with deficiency and smaller increases to therapy seen with genotypes *xx, PP,* and *bb*.[71]

Clinical Effectiveness

BONE DENSITY AND FRACTURES

Pooled results from prevention studies showed that ERT/HRT increased lumbar spine BMD by 4.9% in the first year and by 7.0% in the second year, femoral neck BMD by 2.3% in the first year, and forearm BMD by 3% in the first year and 5% in the second year.[51] In treatment trials, ERT/HRT increased lumbar spine BMD by 7% and forearm BMD by 3.3%. Most gains were seen within the first few years of treatment, with slight increases or a plateau thereafter. Both younger and older postmenopausal women achieve increased BMD with ERT/HRT and experience accelerated bone loss with discontinuation.[11] Progestins added to ERT resulted in no change or a slight increase in BMD.[72] BMD effects are increased when ERT/HRT is combined with alendronate.[63]

A dose of 0.625 mg conjugated equine estrogens (CEEs) or equivalent often provides an acceptable balance between BMD increases and adverse reactions. However, lower doses, such as 0.025 mg transdermal estradiol,[73] 0.3 mg CEE with 2.5 mg medroxyprogesterone acetate,[74] and 0.3 mg esterified estrogens[75] also produce significant BMD changes. Oral and transdermal estrogens at equivalent doses and continuous or cyclic ERT/HRT administration have similar BMD effects. ERT implants and intrauterine impregnated devices and creams can yield therapeutic hormone concentrations and also have shown positive effects. In an elderly cohort, current continuous ERT use (mean 20 years) started near menopause was associated with the highest BMD at four different skeletal sites.[76] However, BMD in women with current continuous use for about

9 years starting after age 60 was slightly less than but not significantly different from that in continuous users. Both groups produced greater responses than for those who had used ERT previously for up to 10 years, started therapy later in life and received therapy for a short time, and never used ERT.

ERT/HRT decreased vertebral fractures in a few clinical trials. Vertebral fractures were decreased by up to 61% and nonspine fractures by 30% to 40%.[77] Observational studies suggested but could not prove that ERT/HRT decreased hip fractures. Relative risk-odds ratios for hip fractures in current users were 0.18 to 0.84, with not all differences being significant.[11,56,57,77] In the Study of Osteoporotic Fractures, only women older than age 75 years with current ERT use had significantly fewer hip fractures compared with women aged 65 to 75 years.[77] In contrast, ERT was associated with fewer hip fractures in black women younger than age 75 years.[78] A meta-analysis of published osteoporosis nonvertebral fracture studies found a 35% reduction in nonvertebral fractures in women under age 60 years, with the reduction closer to 50% for hip and wrist fractures; however, a 12% nonsignificant reduction occurred in women over 60 years of age.[79] Protection is diminished after HRT has been discontinued for at least 5 years.[11,56]

CARDIOVASCULAR DISEASE AND LIPIDS

The decision to use ERT/HRT is influenced by extraskeletal benefits. The mechanisms by which ERT/HRT might prevent cardiovascular disease include favorable lipid alterations; decreased vascular tone; preserved endothelial function; decreased fibrinogen and plasminogen activator inhibitor type 1, antithrombin III, and thromboxane A_2 formation; increased factor VII and protein C; decreased fasting glucose and insulin; and increased prostacyclin I_2, blood flow, stroke volume, and antioxidant activity.[80] Mean percentage changes from seven clinical trials after CEEs were 0.2% to 8% decrease in total cholesterol, 7% to 19% increase in high-density lipoprotein (HDL) cholesterol, 0.3% to 20% decrease in low-density lipoprotein (LDL) cholesterol, and 8% to 39% increase in triglycerides.[81] ERT also decreases apolipoprotein B and lipoprotein (a) and increases apolipoprotein A–1. Similar effects are seen with other oral estrogens. The lipid effect can be less and occur later with transdermal products. ERT's positive lipid effect is only maintained while on therapy. Progestins and androgens minimize or eliminate the positive ERT lipid effects, but they minimize or eliminate the increase in triglycerides. HRT produced a smaller rise in HDL cholesterol,[82] but LDL cholesterol, triglyceride, and apolipoprotein A–1 and B changes were similar to changes with ERT.[83] The combination of CEEs with pravastatin produced a greater decrease in LDL cholesterol, no further effect on HDL cholesterol, and reversal of the triglyceride increase seen with CEEs alone.[84]

Based on the observational Nurses' Health Study, both HRT and ERT were associated with decreased risk for major coronary artery disease.[85] A 35% to 50% reduction in morbidity and mortality from coronary artery disease has been documented in ERT/HRT epidemiology studies.[53,80]

Secondary prevention with ERT/HRT is not recommended. The Heart and Estrogen/Progestin Replacement Study (HERS) randomized 2763 postmenopausal women under 80 years of age with coronary artery disease to receive either 0.625 mg CEE plus 2.5 mg medroxyprogesterone acetate daily or placebo for an average follow-up period of 4.1 years. HRT did not prevent nonfatal myocardial infarction or development of coronary artery disease.[86] Events increased the first year; women on HRT had fewer cardiovascular events than did the placebo group after 4 or 5 years of therapy, but the difference failed to reach statistical significance. HRT lowered LDL cholesterol and increased HDL cholesterol. More definitive answers will be provided by the WHI study when its results become available.

OTHER BENEFITS

Other potential benefits of ERT have been validated to varying degrees. ERT can decrease urge and stress incontinence, vaginal atrophy, dyspareunia, urinary tract infections, and tooth loss and can slow the aging of skin. Many women experience more energy and a positive mood, but the opposite also can be experienced, especially when progestins are added. Although cerebral blood flow may be increased, the effect on stroke incidence is minimal to negligible. Effects on cognitive functions from cohorts or patients with Alzheimer's disease are variable and inconclusive.

ERT/HRT Administration

ABSOLUTE CONTRAINDICATIONS

ERT/HRT contraindications include active or suspected estrogen-dependent cancer, abnormal vaginal bleeding, severe liver disease, and active vascular thrombosis. Relative contraindications include migraine headaches, history of thromboembolic disease (especially during pregnancy or with past oral contraceptive use), hypertriglyceridemia, uterine fibroids, endometriosis, gallbladder disease, strong family history of breast cancer, and chronic hepatic dysfunction.

PRODUCTS, DOSES, AND ROUTES

The suggested daily ERT doses for osteoporosis prevention are CEE 0.625 mg, ethinyl estradiol 0.02 mg, estropipate 0.625 mg, esterified estrogens 0.625 mg, micronized estradiol 1 mg, 17-β-estradiol 2 mg, estrone sulfate 1.5 mg, and transdermal estradiol 0.05 mg/day. Vaginal administration from creams or rings results in significant systemic absorption, but these formulations are not approved for osteoporosis. ERT products are not considered interchangeable. Each product produces different estradiol and estrone concentrations. Estradiol is the predominant endogenous estrogen before menopause, whereas estrone is the predominant endogenous estrogen after menopause. Oral estradiol is converted via the first-pass effect to estrone, whereas transdermal estradiol bypasses the liver and produces higher estradiol concentrations. The major and minor components of CEEs and other combination estrogen products may have beneficial effects.

ERT is usually administered continuously with continuous or cyclic progestin. Continuous HRT therapy is used most commonly because 60% to 80% of women will be amenorrheic 6 to 12 months after starting therapy and fewer women will develop endometrial hyperplasia.[87] Until that time, unpredictable spotting and bleeding can occur. If amenorrhea does not develop after 10 to 12 months, the patient should be evaluated. A predictable bleeding pattern with cyclic therapy may be preferred by some women with unpredictable bleeding. Continuous ERT alone is used for women with a hysterectomy. If unopposed estrogen is used for women with an intact uterus, 85% of the women will be amenorrheic, but all women should have annual endometrial biopsies.

Continuous medroxyprogesterone 2.5–5 mg, micronized progesterone 100 mg daily, norethindrone acetate 0.5–1 mg orally or 0.14–0.25 mg transdermally, or cyclic medroxyprogesterone 5–10 mg for 12 to 14 days every month can be used. Daily administration improves adherence and promotes amenorrhea. With the continuous medroxyprogesterone regimen, the percentage of women with amenorrhea is 55% to 92% at 6 months and 75% to 100% at 1 year.[87] Progestin implants, gels and intrauterine devices, and biweekly[88] or quarterly[89] progestin administration are under investigation. Investigational medroxyprogesterone 10 mg for 14 days every 3 months produced a longer and sometimes heavier and/or unscheduled menses that occurred less frequently but was preferred over the monthly cyclic regimen. The combination patch with estradiol 0.05 mg and norethindrone acetate 0.14 or 0.25 mg has been approved for treatment of vasomotor symptoms of menopause, vaginal atrophy, and hypoestrogenic conditions and is being investigated for osteoporosis.

ERT Adverse Effects. The risks of ERT/HRT must be discussed with all women (Table 90–6). Use of unopposed ERT is associated with up to a 9.5-fold increase in endometrial carcinoma, with the risk rising with longer duration.[90] Concomitant progestin therapy for at least 12 to 14 days a month usually eliminates this risk and may even be protective.[11] ERT/HRT can cause benign increased breast density on mammography. Generally, the relative risk values for breast cancer are between 1.1 and 1.5, with the risk increasing slightly with longer duration (at least 15–20 years) and the addition of a progestin.[90] The Nurses' Health Study revealed a relative risk for breast cancer of 1.4 for HRT and 1.3 for CEEs and other estrogens.[90] Risk returns to baseline in past users.

Small studies have reported menopausal symptom relief and BMD increases with ERT for women in breast cancer remission, most of whom have had no recurrence.[91] Of note, women who develop breast cancer while on ERT/HRT generally have longer survival, although effect wanes after 12 years.[92] Proposed theories include better access to health care, more preventive health behaviors, earlier detection with better survival rates, and less cardiovascular disease and mortality. Cohort studies do not find an association between ERT/HRT and ovarian cancer, but case-control studies report odds ratios between 1.2 and 1.6.[90] Better definition of this risk awaits WHI results.

Adverse effects (see Table 90–6) may decrease over time. During cyclic therapy, vaginal bleeding should be evaluated if it occurs on days 1 to 9 or 16 to 31 if progestin is given for the first 10 days. For the continuous regimen, vaginal bleeding should be evaluated if it is heavier than premenopausal periods, lasts for more than 10 days, occurs more than once a month, or persists after 10 months of therapy. Breast tenderness can be decreased through use of a more supportive bra or an exercise bra and by wearing the bra to bed. Lower estrogen dose, estrogen break, different progestin, decreased caffeine, or a short course of hydrochlorothiazide can also most commonly decrease breast tenderness.

If migraines occur, a transdermal estrogen product may eliminate this side effect. HRT taken at bedtime or with food can minimize nausea. If bloating occurs, a different progestin or low-dose hydrochlorothiazide may help. In patients with mood changes, the clinician may switch to a different progestin, decrease the intermittent dose, or use a continuous low-dose regimen. A 2.5-fold increase in cholelithiasis is seen with ERT/HRT.

Although the rate of venous thromboembolic events (VTEs) is two to three times that of nonusers, the incidence is low, with 2 to 3 cases per 10,000 women per year.[93] The highest VTE incidence was within 1 year of ERT/HRT initiation.

Progestins are more likely responsible for breast density changes and discomfort, acne, fluid retention, and psychological side effects and should be altered before estrogen therapy is changed to resolve these adverse effects.

ERT/HRT ADHERENCE AND PERSISTENCE

Low ERT/HRT adherence and persistence (continuing to take medications over time) are important issues for pharmacists and other health care professionals to address because only 54% of women continue this therapy past the first year. In addition, ethnic differences exist for HRT prescribing, with white women prescribed these agents most frequently.[94] Women who use ERT/HRT generally are better educated, practice other preventive health behaviors, and have higher socioeconomic status, better insurance coverage, and greater access to health care than do women in general. Therapy is stopped most often because of a perceived lack of effect or because of adverse drug effects.[95] Women who have never used ERT/HRT perceive hormones to be harmful, not beneficial, or not natural, and these misperceptions must be dealt with for therapy to be successful.

For ERT/HRT to be effective in preventing or treating osteoporosis, women must be educated about the long-term effects and development of tolerance to adverse reactions. Dosage manipulation can decrease or eliminate some adverse events. BMD measurement can influence a woman's decision to use HRT.[34]

Selective Estrogen Receptor Modulators

Raloxifene was the first SERM approved for prevention and treatment of postmenopausal osteoporosis. Investigational SERMs include toremifene, droloxifene, lasofoxifene, and idoxifene. Raloxifene is a reasonable choice for osteoporosis prevention or treatment for the woman who cannot or should not take estrogen (e.g., because of concern about breast cancer risk). For the woman with severe osteoporosis, for whom fracture risk reduction is paramount, a bisphosphonate is likely a better choice.

Clinical Effectiveness. Raloxifene increases spine and hip BMD by 2% to 3%.[96] It decreased vertebral fractures in osteoporotic women, but it is not proven to reduce hip fractures.[97] Raloxifene increases hip BMD similarly to estrogen, but estrogen increases spine BMD more than does raloxifene.

Raloxifene acts as an antagonist in uterine and breast tissue. Because of this, it does not increase the risk of endometrial carcinoma, as do estrogen and tamoxifen. It decreased invasive breast cancer by 76% in one study.[98] It is not approved for breast cancer prevention or treatment, but it is being compared with tamoxifen in a prevention trial for women who have increased breast cancer risk (in the Study of Tamoxifen and Raloxifene [STAR] trial).

Raloxifene decreases total and LDL cholesterol but does not change HDL cholesterol.[96] Whether raloxifene decreases cardiovascular risk awaits the results of the prevention trial mentioned above.

Raloxifene Administration. Raloxifene 60 mg daily is used for both prevention and treatment of postmenopausal osteoporosis. Raloxifene use is associated with a threefold increased risk of VTEs, similar to the risk with estrogen. Raloxifene is contraindicated for those with active thromboembolic disease. The thromboembolic risk of raloxifene should be considered for patients with compromised ambulation status. Other adverse effects include hot flushes and leg cramps.

Oral Contraceptives

Oral contraceptive use (ethinyl estradiol 20–40 μg) increased BMD, especially in trabecular bone, in nine studies and produced no change in four studies in pre-, peri-, and postmenopausal women.[99] In some epidemiology studies evaluating older, higher-dose oral contraceptives, a positive BMD effect that increased with duration was seen. Oral contraceptives may be marginally beneficial in women who are amenorrheic secondary to intense exercise, anorexia nervosa, or perimenopause.[99] Safety of oral contraceptives in older women needs further study. Variable BMD effects are seen with depot medroxyprogesterone acetate, which may vary by patient age and duration of use.[100]

Phytoestrogens

Plants such as black cohosh, dong quai, ginseng, licorice, and wild Mexican yams are thought to contain phytoestrogens and to be helpful for menopausal symptoms.[101] The isoflavone class of phytoestrogens (genistein, diadzein) may have weak estrogenic and antiestrogenic activity. Soybeans and soy flour, not soy oils and soy lecithin, contain high quantities of isoflavones. In the only human study, 90 mg but not 56 mg per day of isoflavones increased spinal BMD, but neither increased total-body or proximal femur BMD.

Ipriflavone 200 mg three times daily, a synthetic isoflavone partially metabolized to diadzein, has shown modest to no increases in BMD.[101,102] Ipriflavone is available in health food stores. Of concern is the subclinical lymphocytopenia produced in some women taking ipriflavone. Nineteen percent of these women's lymphocyte counts did not return to normal after 2 years off therapy.[102] Therefore, its use should be discouraged.

Testosterone and Anabolic Steroids

Methyltestosterone 1.25 or 2.5 mg oral and testosterone implants 50 mg every 3 months and patches (both investigational) are being coadministered with ERT/HRT in women with depression or with decreased libido, sexual function, or energy level or after oophorectomy. Concomitant methyltestosterone or testosterone therapy generally produced greater BMD effects than ERT alone.[103] Daily 10% dehydroepiandrosterone cream increased BMD in older women.

Although anabolic steroids enhance osteoblast activity, in clinical trials their effect is predominantly decreased resorption, which may be secondary to increased muscle mass and strength. BMD changes are generally small, and most women develop adverse reactions.

Tibolone

Tibolone, a weak estrogen, progesterone, and androgen agonist, relieves hot flushes and does not cause endometrial proliferation. In postmenopausal women, tibolone increased spine and hip BMD by 6.9% and 4.5%, respectively, after 2 years.[104] Effects on fractures, cardiovascular disease, and breast and uterine cancer are unknown. Currently used in Europe, tibolone is not FDA-approved for use in the United States.

Calcitonin

Calcitonin is released from the thyroid gland when serum calcium is elevated. Pharmacologic doses decrease resorption. Calcitonin is indicated for osteoporosis treatment for women at least 5 years past menopause. The agent is also used in men, although it is not approved for this indication. Because it is less effective than other osteoporosis medications, calcitonin is used most often for patients with fracture pain or for whom other therapy is unsuitable.

Clinical Effectiveness. The largest calcitonin study randomized 1255 osteoporotic women, most with prevalent vertebral fractures, to receive nasal calcitonin at 100, 200, or 400 IU/d or placebo for up to 5 years (PROOF study).[105] The 200-IU regimen increased spine BMD and reduced new vertebral fractures by 36%. A dose-response relationship did not exist, and 59% of patients dropped out of the study. Calcitonin does not consistently affect hip BMD and does not decrease hip fractures.

Calcitonin may provide pain relief to some patients with acute fractures, but this effect has not been studied thoroughly.

Calcitonin Administration. Salmon calcitonin is used clinically because it is more potent and longer lasting than the mammalian form. The intranasal dose is 200 IU daily, alternating nares. Subcutaneous administration at 100 IU/d is available but used rarely.

Nasal calcitonin may cause rhinitis, epistaxis, and nasal irritation. Subcutaneous administration can produce gastrointestinal symptoms, injection-site pain, and flushing.

Investigational Antiresorption Agents

OPG, a competitive inhibitor of the OPG/RANK/RANKL system, blocks osteoclastic differentiation and has been effective in animals. Administration of OPG, a large protein, will pose problems. Agents to enhance endogenous OPG, decrease RANKL production, or block RANKL binding to RANK are being developed. Blocking RANK signal transduction through Jun NH_2-terminal kinase (JNK), NF-κB, or TNF receptor-associated factor (TRAF) adapter molecules are other possibilities.[3]

Agents to block osteoclast attachment or bone matrix degradation are under consideration. These include antagonists of the $\alpha V\beta_3$ integrin receptor, inhibitors of cathepsin K, and osteoclast-selective H^+-ATPase inhibitors to prevent acidification of resorption lacunae.

Older agents being considered include strontium[106] and NSAIDs. Although a link between NSAIDs and decreased fractures was suggested, a study of 750,000 patients showed similar fracture risk for regular and incidental NSAID users.[107]

INVESTIGATIONAL BONE-FORMATION THERAPY

Parathyroid Hormone

Although PTH can increase bone resorption, PTH (1–84) and its amino terminal fragment (1–34) are anabolic if used once daily. The anabolic activity may result from decreased osteoblast apoptosis and increased bone formation from the longer-lived osteoblasts.

In a major study of PTH (1–34), 20-μg doses produced similar effectiveness and fewer side effects than 40-μg doses.[108] In 1637 patients with prior vertebral fractures, 14% of those receiving placebo had new vertebral fractures compared with 5% and 4% of those on, respectively, 20- and 40-μg doses of PTH (1–34). Compared with placebo, BMD increased by 9 and 13 more percentage points in the lumbar spine and 3 and 6 more percentage points in the femur among those taking the two respective PTH (1–34) doses. Side effects were minor (occasional nausea and headache) but occurred more often with the higher dose of PTH (1–34).

Subcutaneous daily PTH also has been studied in combination with estrogen, where the combination increased hip and spine BMD and decreased fractures in postmenopausal women more than with estrogen alone.[109] Administration of PTH (1–34) reversed corticosteroid-induced osteoporosis.[110] Intermittent PTH (1–34) also improved BMD in men with idiopathic osteoporosis.[111]

Given the expense and inconvenience of daily subcutaneous injections, PTH (1–34), if approved, may be targeted toward those with prior vertebral fractures who are at high risk of fractures.

HMG-CoA Reductase Inhibitors

In searching for agents to increase bone formation through bone morphogenetic proteins, 3-hydroxymethyl-4-glutaryl CoA reductase inhibitors (statins) were discovered to increase bone density dramatically in animal models.[3] Interest in the potential skeletal benefits of statins was heightened by the discovery that aminobisphosphonates also affect cholesterol biosynthesis, although at a different step than statins.

Observational studies have linked statin use with decreased fracture risk.[112] Data from the WHI, however, did not confirm skeletal benefit.[113] Further, a large case-control study did not demonstrate reduction in fracture risk for statin-treated patients.[114,115]

Growth Hormones and Factors

Growth hormone (GH) and IGF-1 play important roles in bone turnover and remodeling.[116] Further, serum concentrations of both GH and IFG-1 decline with advancing age, and decreased IGF-1 has been observed in osteoporotic individuals. Neither GH or IGF-1, however, has been demonstrated to consistently improve bone density. In addition, these agents have effects on multiple tissues other than bone.[3] Adverse effects reported for GH and for IGF-1 include alterations in glucose utilization and peripheral edema.

Fluoride

Fluoride increases osteoblastic activity and bone formation. This may occur through intracellular signaling pathways involving tyrosine phosphatases and MAP kinases. However, despite 30 years of clinical study, antifracture efficacy of fluoride remains doubtful, and fluoride may increase bone fragility. In one study, men and women given fluoride monophosphate and women given lower-dose slow-release sodium fluoride had fewer vertebral fractures. However, these findings were not validated in two other studies. Further, a meta-analysis determined that fluoride lacked antifracture efficacy.[117] Fluoride is currently not recommended for therapy. However, this may change pending the FDA's decision on the sustained-release product.

VERTEBROPLASTY AND KYPHOPLASTY

Vertebroplasty and kyphoplasty are surgical procedures in which cement is instilled into vertebral bodies to strengthen and stabilize spinal fractures and relieve pain. The degree of pain relief and the long-term benefits and complications of the procedures await further study.

SPECIAL POPULATIONS

WOMEN WITH AMENORRHEA

Women with amenorrhea—secondary to conditions such as excessive exercise or anorexia nervosa—lose bone because of estrogen deficiency. Higher fracture risk in anorexia nervosa also may result from smaller bone size. Although oral contraceptives have been used for these individuals, HRT may be marginally effective.[118] Lost bone may only be partially regained. Factors other than estrogen, such as overall nutritional status, likely play a role.

MEN

Some men with osteoporosis possess clearly identifiable risk factors (e.g., very advanced age, low body weight, tobacco or alcohol abuse, or prednisone use). In others, further investigation for secondary causes is warranted (see "Patient Assessment" above). Measurement of free or total testosterone also can help assess the etiology of the bone problems.

Management of male osteoporosis until recently had been modeled after guidelines for women. Lifestyle changes—improved exercise, diet, and if needed smoking and/or alcohol cessation (see Fig. 90–5)—represent the cornerstone of current recommendations for therapy in men. Alendronate, now FDA-approved for men, has proven vertebral fracture efficacy, and for men with low BMD or established osteoporosis, it is the drug of first choice.[65] Osteoporosis due to secondary causes should be managed with antiresorptive therapy as necessary.

For the man with symptomatic hypogonadism (i.e., decreased libido, diminished energy, or erectile dysfunction) and a normal prostate examination and serum level of prostate-specific antigen, testosterone can be considered and may improve BMD in those who tolerate the therapy. Testosterone patches (5 mg daily), intramuscular injections (50–400 mg every 2 to 4 weeks), or 1% gel are available. Transdermal or injected testosterone treatment increases bone density in men. Testosterone replacement must be considered carefully, especially in the elderly, who are at higher risk of prostate cancer and benign prostatic hypertrophy (BPH). Adverse effects of testosterone therapy include local skin reactions to topical formulations, exacerbation or unmasking of BPH or prostate carcinoma, erythrocytosis, decreased HDL cholesterol, and aggressive behavior.[119]

ELDERLY PATIENTS

In elderly patients, prevention of falls assumes great importance in eliminating fractures secondary to osteoporosis. Exercises to improve muscle strength, gait, balance, and flexibility should be performed. The need for ambulation assistive devices (e.g., canes, walkers) and assistance with transferring from various positions or for toileting should be reviewed. Vision should be assessed, with appropriate corrective lenses and/or surgery as needed.

The home environment should be reevaluated to minimize falls. Loose rugs and extension cords should be eliminated, grab bars mounted in the bathroom, handrails installed on stairs, nonskid tape placed in bathtubs, and adequate lighting ensured.

A patient's medication profile should be reviewed for use of medications that have been linked with falls: NSAIDs, psychotropic, sedative-hypnotic, antidepressant, antihypertensive, and diuretic medications. Sedative-hypnotic agents should be discontinued or switched to short-acting agents, and all benzodiazepines should be eliminated. When benzodiazepines are used, seniors are especially vulnerable to falls and hip fractures immediately after therapy begins and after 1 month of continuous therapy. Both long- and short-acting benzodiazepines, antidepressants, antipsychotics, and other psychoactive medications are not safe.[120] Other central nervous system medications also should be eliminated or changed if altered balance or confusion result. Diuretics should be given early in the day to prevent nocturnal voiding. Orthostatic blood pressure changes should be evaluated. Patients should be warned about medications that contribute to orthostasis and should be warned about abrupt postural changes. The use of hip protectors may decrease fractures after falls,[121] but most patients do not like wearing them.

Adequate amounts of calcium and vitamin D should be obtained through diet or supplements (see Table 90–3). For elderly persons with severe osteoporosis, a 25-hydroxyvitamin D level should be determined after beginning vitamin D supplementation to ensure adequacy. Smoking cessation and exercise begun late in life still have positive bone effects.

Estrogens decrease bone loss and are associated with decreased risk of hip and spine fractures. Elderly patients have a greater incidence of ERT/HRT associated breast enlargement and tenderness, which decreases over time. Lower doses (0.3 mg CEE or equivalent) may be effective in the elderly.[73–75] Starting hormones at a lower dose and increasing them later to 0.625 mg CEE or equivalent as needed may decrease adverse effects, increase acceptance and adherence, and prevent bone loss.

For elderly women with significant bone loss or fracture history and no personal or family history of cardiovascular or Alzheimer's disease, bisphosphonates may be preferred over ERT/HRT. Esophageal dysfunction should be ruled out, and the patient's ability to adhere to the complex administration process must be ensured before beginning therapy. Once-weekly dosing of these agents would be desirable to minimize gastrointestinal exposure to bisphosphonates. Patients with renal impairment (<35 mL/min) should not be given alendronate. Risedronate should be used cautiously in patients with renal impairment.

Nasal calcitonin may decrease osteoporotic bone pain in the elderly. If it is effective, narcotic and NSAID doses can be decreased or eliminated as pain subsides.

TRANSPLANT RECIPIENTS

In organ and bone marrow transplant recipients, bone loss can result from use of several medications before, during, and after transplantation: glucocorticoids, loop diuretics, aluminum-containing phosphate binders, cyclosporine, and tacrolimus (the latter two based on animal data).[122] Other factors also can lead to osteoporosis in these patients, including hyperparathyroidism, hypogonadism, hypovitaminosis D, decreased calcium intake or absorption, hepatic congestion, prerenal azotemia, cystic fibrosis, and impaired osteoblast function. The greatest bone loss and highest fracture incidence are seen within 6 to 12 months after transplant.

Before transplant, BMD should be measured and vitamin D and gonadal status assessed. Therapy guidelines and lifestyle changes should be followed (see Fig. 90–5) and hypogonadism corrected for those with low BMD. Prevention and treatment efforts should continue after transplant.

Bisphosphonates should not be used in graft recipients with creatinine clearances of less than 30 mL/min or in pediatric transplant recipients. Glucocorticoid doses should be reduced as quickly as possible. Estrogen enhances hepatic metabolism of cyclosporine. Since ovulation and testosterone production may increase after transplant, hormone supplementation may not be needed thereafter. Calcitriol may be needed instead of vitamin D_2 or D_3 depending on the severity of renal or liver dysfunction. A multidisciplinary clinic may be best suited to identify and ensure appropriate therapy for transplant recipients.[123]

PATIENTS TAKING PROTEASE INHIBITORS

In a study of HIV-positive men who were taking protease inhibitors, lumbar spine BMD was lower than in healthy controls and men with HIV who were not taking these drugs.[124] Osteoblast and osteoclast recruitment and function were compromised to varying degrees by indinavir and ritonavir, indicating the possibility that these medications produce unfavorable bone changes over time. BMD measurements may be warranted in patients taking protease inhibitors and therapies instituted as clinically indicated.

PATIENTS WITH ARTHRITIS

Patients with rheumatoid arthritis also develop osteoporosis at additional locations, the juxtaarticular and bone erosion sites. OPG ligand is produced in rheumatoid synovium.

Glucocorticoid use also contributes to bone loss in patients with rheumatoid arthritis, and it should be managed as outlined below (see "Glucocorticoid-Induced Osteoporosis" and ACR guidelines[30]). Otherwise, treatment is similar to current recommendations for both women and men. Investigational agents are being explored to alter the OPG/RANK/RANKL system.

PATIENTS WITH CYSTIC FIBROSIS

Adults with cystic fibrosis had average T scores of −1.5 to −2.5, and children with cystic fibrosis had Z scores of −0.3 to −2.8 (compared with an age-matched control group).[125] Patients with cystic fibrosis are shorter, develop kyphosis (hump back), and have vertebral fracture rates of 0.05 to 4.3 per 100 person-years.

In these patients, osteoporosis may result from vitamin D deficiency, glucocorticoid use, calcium malabsorption, hypogonadism, inactivity, increased cytokines, and lung transplantation. Prevention and treatment efforts usually include adequate calcium and vitamin D (800–1000 IU/d) intake, correction of hypogonadism, exercise, potential use of GH in short children, and reductions in glucocorticoid dose and use. Until the safety of bisphosphonates is determined in children, they are not recommended.

PHARMACOECONOMIC CONSIDERATIONS

Annual direct costs for osteoporotic fractures were estimated to be \$15.2 billion (in 1998 dollars), with a tripling expected by 2040.[11,51] Estimates of health care costs for women age 45 and older indicated that 6.9% of direct medical expenditures are for osteoporosis, with half of these expenses borne by Medicare. Direct costs in the year following hip fracture are from \$16,000 to \$36,000 per fracture. Indirect costs of hip fracture, including quality of life, may add another \$20,000 per fracture.[11,126] Appreciation of these costs has established osteoporosis as a public health priority.

The estimated cost for each quality-adjusted life year (QALY) for treating women with T scores below −2 is \$51 to \$8447, varying by age, with the lowest cost for the oldest women.[127] This analysis assumed that drug treatment would cost $300 per year and that each hip fracture results in $30,000 of medical costs. The NOF estimated that for women with average fracture risks, age-specific costs of osteoporosis prevention or treatment per QALY were $13,794 for the 50-year-old, $6884 for the 60-year-old, $2924 for the 70-year-old, and $949 for the 80-year-old. These figures assumed that treatment decreased fracture risk by one-third and that treatment costs were $500 per year. To put these pharmacoeconomic figures into perspective, the average cost per QALY saved was $2800 for Papanicolaou smears done every 3 years after age 65, $34,000 for lovastatin for men aged 45 to 54 with cholesterol levels of 300 mg/dL or higher, $32,000 for hypertension treatment for those aged 40 and older with diastolic blood pressures of 95 to 104 mm Hg, and $62,000 for annual mammography for women 40 to 49 years of age.[128] The NOF, based on its economic analysis, indicated that treatment would be appropriate for postmenopausal women with T scores of less than −2 and in those with T scores below −1.5 who also have certain risk factors.

Key pharmacoeconomic issues are the human and economic burden from an expanding elderly population, development of new, more effective, but potentially more expensive medications, enhanced screening and identification of patients at risk, and targeting of high-risk populations.

EVALUATION OF THERAPEUTIC OUTCOMES

Persons receiving prevention or treatment with ERT/HRT, bisphosphonates, or calcitonin should be examined at least annually. For women on ERT/HRT, this visit includes an annual breast and pelvic examination, mammography, and Papanicolaou smear. Excessive bleeding should be evaluated with an endometrial biopsy, transvaginal ultrasonography, or a dilatation and curettage if needed. Medication adherence and tolerance should be evaluated at each physician or primary care visit and by the pharmacist.

After 6 to 12 months of antiresorptive therapy, effects on BMD can be detected. In clinical practice, measurements are conducted every 12 to 36 months, with Medicare reimbursing only for repeat exams after 23 months. The American Association of Clinical Endocrinologists' guidelines recommend BMD measurement every 2 to 3 years if baseline BMD T score is less than −1.5.[129] For prevention programs, BMD should be assessed every 1 to 2 years until stabilized and then every 2 to 3 years thereafter. For treatment programs, BMD should be measured every year for 3 years. If stable, BMD measurement can be done every 2 years; otherwise, annual BMD determinations should be continued until stable. Since many women with decreased BMD within the first year of therapy show gain in the second year,[130] results for medication usage may require 2 years of evaluation.

Controversy exists about the clinical utility of monitoring therapy with biochemical markers of bone turnover.

GLUCOCORTICOID-INDUCED OSTEOPOROSIS

The incidence of osteoporosis induced by use of glucocorticoid agents such as prednisone is unknown, but fracture incidence for those on systemic glucocorticoids is estimated at 30% to 50%.[29] Although bone loss is continuous throughout steroid therapy, the greatest loss is experienced during the first 6 to 12 months.[29,30] Trabecular bone (ribs, vertebrae, and pelvis) is affected more than cortical bone. Women, men, and children are susceptible. Oral doses of greater than 7.5 mg of prednisone or equivalent[29,30] and inhaled doses of greater than 800–1200 μg of beclomethasone, 800–1000 μg of budesonide, 750 μg of fluticasone, and 1000 μg of flunisolide[31] generally are required for significant bone loss, but loss and fractures can occur with lower doses.

PATHOPHYSIOLOGY

Glucocorticoids decrease muscle strength and bone formation and increase bone resorption.[29,30] Glucocorticoids can decrease calcium absorption and increase renal calcium excretion, contributing to secondary hyperparathyroidism. Glucocorticoid effects on vitamin D are variable. Differentiation, replication, and life span of osteoblasts is reduced, as is osteoid synthesis. Osteoblasts change in their sensitivity to prostaglandins, PTH, cytokines, growth factors, and calcitriol. Changes at the pituitary and gonadal level decrease synthesis of estrogen and testosterone. Myopathy can decrease mobility and lead to further bone loss.

DIAGNOSIS

Measurement of 24-hour urinary calcium excretion may be helpful in assessing calcium balance and need for calcium supplementation, diuretic therapy, and medication adjustment. If malnutrition or other metabolic problems are suspected, 25-OH vitamin D can be measured. Bone turnover markers are altered but do not always correlate with BMD changes. All abnormal laboratory values should be evaluated to rule out other causes for bone loss.

X-ray examination can indicate steroid-induced osteoporosis. Vertical and horizontal trabeculae tend to be equally thin and translucent. Pseudocallus formations occur in large numbers around stress fractures. These findings are not seen with postmenopausal or senile osteoporosis. The ACR Task Force on Osteoporosis Guidelines recommend hip BMD measurements for all patients beginning therapy with or on glucocorticoids and spine BMD measurements for patients age 60 and older.[30]

▶ PREVENTION AND TREATMENT: Glucocorticoid-Induced Osteoporosis

The best means of preventing glucocorticoid-induced osteoporosis is to discontinue the offending agent. If this is not possible, glucocorticoid exposure should be minimized by using the lowest possible dose for the shortest duration. Alternate-day therapy does not eliminate bone loss; the effects of pulse (intermittent) therapy are controversial. Inhaled steroids have less effect on bone than does oral therapy. Secondary causes of osteoporosis should be treated appropriately.

All patients receiving pulse or continuous glucocorticoids should adopt lifestyle changes (i.e., stop smoking, increase exercise, decrease caffeine, phosphate, and alcohol intake, and prevent falls) and ingest adequate amounts of calcium and vitamin D. According to the ACR guidelines, calcium intakes should be 800 mg for children between 1 and 5 years of age, 1200 mg for children 6 and 10 years of age, and 1500 mg for other patients.[30] All children should receive 400 IU and adults 800 IU vitamin D per day. Thiazide diuretics have been recommended for patients with greater than 300 mg of calcium excreted in the urine over 24 hours, but this recommendation is controversial.

HRT should be offered to all women on steroids. Oral contraceptives with an equivalent of 50 μg of estradiol should be given to premenopausal or perimenopausal women with menstrual irregularities or amenorrhea. Testosterone should be considered for men with low testosterone concentrations.

If therapy continues for more than 3 months, antiresorptive therapy should be used. Based on a meta-analysis of available studies, bisphosphonates produce greater bone density increases than do calcitonin, fluoride, and vitamin D.[29] Spine and hip BMD are increased and vertebral fractures are decreased with alendronate, risedronate, and cyclic etidronate. The ACR does not recommend bisphosphonates for younger patients until their long-term effects are better defined. Women wishing to conceive should not use bisphosphonates.

All patients should receive follow-up BMD measurements within 1 year and then every 2 years. If bone loss is greater than 3% to 5% per year, additional medications are needed. Therapy is continued up to 3 years after steroid discontinuation in patients with low bone mass.

OSTEOMALACIA

Osteomalacia is characterized by defective mineralization of the organic matrix of bone. Defective mineralization in the infant or child produces rickets, with characteristic skeletal deformities and decreased growth of long bones. In the adult, the syndrome is referred to as *osteomalacia.*

EPIDEMIOLOGY

The incidence of osteomalacia is not known precisely but is lower in the United States because milk is supplemented with vitamin D. Many elderly people, especially those housebound or in institutions, have inadequate vitamin D levels and are at increased risk for osteomalacia. Osteomalacia can be insidious and coexist with osteoporosis, which can be the first skeletal manifestation of osteomalacia. Osteomalacia is more prevalent in countries with little sun exposure and minimal dietary supplementation and where traditional clothing that covers most of the skin is worn. Dark-skinned individuals synthesize less vitamin D cutaneously.

PATHOPHYSIOLOGY

Pathogenetic mechanisms leading to osteomalacia include low serum calcium or phosphorus, chronic acidosis, hypophosphatasia, abnormal bone matrix, and drug-induced mineralization defects. The most common cause is vitamin D deficiency secondary to inadequate intake, decreased sun exposure, or malabsorption.[131]

Renal disease is associated with decreased 25-OH vitamin D 1α-hydroxylase, with consequently decreased calcitriol and poor calcium absorption. In vitamin D–dependent rickets type 1 (pseudo-vitamin D–deficient rickets), a genetic defect exists in 25-OH vitamin D 1α-hydroxylase. Vitamin D–dependent rickets type II (hereditary vitamin D–resistant rickets) results from defects in the vitamin D receptor or its activity.[132] In vitamin D–resistant rickets (hereditary hypophosphatemic rickets), renal phosphate reabsorption is defective, and 25-OH vitamin D 1α-hydroxylase activity is inadequate.[133] The etiology is unclear, but a genetic defect in the *PHEX* gene may allow inappropriate activity of an undefined inhibitor of phosphate reabsorption that also lowers serum calcitriol levels. Pancreatitis, chronic hepatobiliary disease, Crohn's disease, gastrectomy, and celiac sprue are also risk factors for vitamin D deficiency.

Other chronic disorders cause osteomalacia. Phosphate depletion from low dietary intake, phosphate-binding antacids, and oncogenic osteomalacia (potentially phosphaturic effect) can cause osteomalacia. Hypophosphatasia is an inborn error of metabolism in which deficient activity of alkaline phosphatase causes impaired mineralization of bone matrix. Acidosis from renal dysfunction, distal renal tubular acidosis, hypergammaglobulinemic states (e.g., multiple myeloma), and drugs (e.g., chemotherapy) compromises bone mineralization. Renal tubular disorders secondary to Fanconi's syndrome, hereditary diseases (e.g., Wilson's disease, a defect in copper metabolism), acquired disease (e.g., myeloma), and toxins (e.g., lead) cause osteomalacia to varying degrees. Chronic wastage of phosphorus and/or calcium limits mineralization, which may be further compromised by acidosis and secondary hyperparathyroidism.

DRUG-INDUCED OSTEOMALACIA

Patients receiving anticonvulsants, particularly phenytoin, phenobarbital, or carbamazepine, may develop osteomalacia.[134] Although this adverse effect is often cited, minimal evidence exists for osteomalacia in adults living in the community receiving monotherapy. Anticonvulsant-associated osteomalacia is usually seen in patients living in an institution or those receiving multiple anticonvulsant drugs. The mechanism is not clear but may involve induction of the hepatic microsomal cytochrome P450 system and increased vitamin D metabolism. Vitamin D requirements of patients receiving anticonvulsant medications may be increased. Rifampin also can cause osteomalacia through increased metabolism of vitamin D.

Defective mineralization can result from continuous or intermittent etidronate treatment or sodium fluoride. Aluminum also can be absorbed and accumulate in patients with severe renal impairment or in patients undergoing hemodialysis.

CLINICAL PRESENTATION

Adult osteomalacia often has an insidious presentation. The underlying disorder may be more apparent than skeletal defects (e.g., diarrhea in sprue). Diffuse skeletal pain, bony tenderness, and proximal muscle weakness may occur. Pain on movement and muscle weakness may result in a characteristic waddling gait. Hypophosphatemia and secondary hyperparathyroidism may contribute to these symptoms. Tetany can result from sufficiently depressed serum ionized calcium.

Skeletal deformities (infrequent in adults) include bowing, pigeon chest, scoliosis, kyphosis, and shortening of the spine. Typical findings on x-ray films include osteopenia and pseudofractures (Looser's zones), more commonly seen in the pelvic rami or upper femora.

Various etiologies produce differing biochemical pictures. Determination of serum content of calcium (albumin corrected), phosphorus, alkaline phosphatase, urea nitrogen, creatinine, PTH, 25-OH vitamin D, and calcitriol, as well as urinary calcium and creatinine, can help in determining the cause, deciding on treatment, and monitoring efficacy therapy. Definitive diagnosis is by bone biopsy.

▶ PREVENTION AND TREATMENT: Osteomalacia

Treatment of osteomalacia depends on the underlying cause. Management may be difficult and may require a renal, bone, or endocrine specialist.

With disordered vitamin D metabolism caused by anticonvulsants or rifampin, supplemental vitamin D (4000 IU/d) can be effective.[134]

Treatment of osteomalacia from vitamin D deficiency is vitamin D therapy, with dose depending on severity. Supplements of 800–4000 IU/d or 50,000 IU weekly for 8 weeks may be necessary. For sprue, a gluten-free diet is necessary. With intestinal malabsorption, high oral doses (50,000–100,000 IU/d) or daily intramuscular injections of 10,000 IU vitamin D may be required. Sun exposure also can be useful. Serum calcium and 25-OH vitamin D monitoring is necessary with high vitamin D doses.[131]

Renal disease with deficient calcitriol synthesis can be treated with calcitriol, with careful monitoring of serum calcium and creatinine. This compound has a 6-hour half-life and a rapid onset of action. Patients with renal dysfunction should decrease oral phosphate ingestion, use a phosphate binder, and avoid aluminum-containing antacids.[135]

Vitamin D–dependent rickets type I can be treated with calcitriol (0.25–1 μg/day) to achieve physiologic levels. Vitamin D–dependent rickets type II can be treated with high vitamin D doses or calcitriol if necessary. Often, maintenance of serum calcitriol above the physiologic level is required, with doses of calcitriol up to 30–60 μg/day.[132]

For vitamin D–resistant rickets, patients can be treated with calcitriol and phosphate supplements.[133]

For oncogenic osteomalacia, tumor resection is best. Otherwise, pharmacologic doses of calcitriol (1.5–3 μg/day) and phosphate supplementation may help.[136]

For osteomalacia with renal tubular acidosis, acidosis is corrected with oral bicarbonate. For osteomalacia from Fanconi's syndrome, treatment depends on the underlying disorder but often includes phosphate supplements and vitamin D analogues.[137]

No established treatment exists for hypophosphatasia. Intramedullary rods can help prevent fractures. Bone marrow transplant is being considered.

CONCLUSION

Osteoporosis can be prevented or minimized through an active lifestyle and a healthy diet throughout life. Postmenopausal estrogen deficiency, aging, and various diseases and medications can lead to osteoporosis. Currently, bone resorption can be decreased, but new strong bone cannot be created. Thus prevention is the key. Prevention of osteoporosis includes smoking cessation, exercise, adequate calcium and vitamin D intake, and ERT/HRT. Depending on bone density, bisphosphonates also can be used. Treatment relies on preventing further bone loss with calcium and vitamin D supplementation, bisphosphonates, ERT/HRT, and nasal calcitonin; preventing falls and fractures; and controlling pain. Pharmacists can play a major role in preventing and treating osteoporosis, resolving medication-related problems, ensuring adherence and persistence with drug therapy, and encouraging patients to make positive lifestyle changes.

Osteomalacia is a disease of decreased bone mineralization with multiple etiologies involving calcium, phosphorus, or vitamin D homeostasis. Eliminating or treating the underlying cause is the first step. In most cases, pharmacologic doses of vitamin D or treatment with calcitriol is required, in addition to treating underlying causes. Depending on etiology, other vitamin D analogues or other modalities are used.

▶ PRINCIPLES OF PHARMACOTHERAPY

- Osteoporosis prevention begins at birth and continues throughout life. Everyone should ingest adequate amounts of calcium and vitamin D, exercise regularly, and not smoke.
- To ensure adequate calcium intakes, most Americans will need supplementation with 500 mg of elemental calcium once or twice a day.
- Most elderly patients require vitamin D supplementation of 400–800 IU/day, which can be achieved with one to two multivitamin tablets.
- Bone density testing can enable diagnosis of osteoporosis and influence prevention and treatment decisions.
- Alendronate and risedronate can be used for osteoporosis prevention and treatment. They produce the greatest increases in BMD and have documented hip and vertebral fracture prevention.
- ERT (HRT for women with an intact uterus) decreases bone loss and vertebral fractures. Use begins either at menopause or after age 65 and is potentially continued for life. ERT/HRT improves postmenopausal symptoms and may have other benefits.
- Nasal calcitonin can be used to treat osteoporosis when other therapies are not tolerated.
- Male osteoporosis is often secondary to specific diseases and drugs and responds well to bisphosphonate therapy.
- Pharmacists and other primary care providers should educate patients on osteoporosis prevention/treatment and the use of their medications. These professionals can counsel patients regarding adverse effects with ERT/HRT and bisphosphonates and can help improve adherence to and persistence with pharmacotherapy.
- Pharmacists can provide information to patients and clinicians on risks and management strategies associated with glucocorticoid-induced osteoporosis.
- Osteomalacia, although less common than osteoporosis, can be insidious and can coexist with osteoporosis. It should be considered in those who are likely to be vitamin D deficient, such as housebound or institutionalized seniors.

REFERENCES

1. Glimcher MJ. The nature of the mineral phase in bone: Biological and clinical implications. In: Avioli LV, Krane SM, eds. Metabolic Bone

Disease and Clinically Related Disorders. San Diego, Academic Press, 1998: 23–50.
2. Manolagas SC. Corticosteroids and fractures: A close encounter of the third cell kind. J Bone Miner Res 2000;15:1001–1005.
3. Rodan GA, Martin TJ. Therapeutic approaches to bone diseases. Science 2000;289:1508–1514.
4. Martin RB. Toward a unifying theory of bone remodeling. Bone 2000; 26:1–6.
5. Teitelbaum SL. Bone reabsorption by osteoclasts. Science 2000;289: 1504–1508.
6. Hofbauer LC, Khosla S, Dunstan CR, et al. The roles of osteoprotegerin and osteoprotegerin ligand in the paracrine regulation of bone reabsorption. J Bone Miner Res 2000;15:2–12.
7. Ducy P, Schinke T, Karsenty G. The osteoblast: A sophisticated fibroblast under central surveillance. Science 2000;289:1501–1504.
8. Lian JB, Stein GS, Canalis E, et al. Bone formation: Osteoblast lineage cells, growth factors, matrix proteins, and the mineralization process. In: Favus MJ, ed. Primer on the Metabolic Bone Diseases and Disorders of Mineral Metabolism. Philadelphia, Lippincott Williams & Wilkins, 1999: 14–29.
9. Anderson FH, Cooper C. Hip and vertebral fractures. In: Orwoll ES, ed. Osteoporosis in Men: The Effects of Gender on Skeletal Health. San Diego, Academic Press, 1999: 29–49.
10. Holick MF. Sunlight dilemma: Risk of skin cancer or bone disease and muscle weakness. Lancet 2001;357:4–6.
11. National Osteoporosis Foundation. Osteoporosis: Review of the evidence for prevention, diagnosis and treatment and cost-effectiveness analysis. Osteoporos Int 1998;8(Suppl 4):1–88.
12. Meunier PJ, Delmas PD, Eastell R, et al. Diagnosis and treatment of osteoporosis in postmenopausal women: Clinical guidelines. Clin Ther 1999;21:1025–1044.
13. Looker AC, Orwoll ES, Johnston CC, et al. Prevalence of low femoral bone density in older U.S. adults from NHANES III. J Bone Miner Res 1997;12:1761–1768.
14. Kanis JA, WHO group. Assessment of fracture risk and its application to screening for postmenopausal osteoporosis: Synopsis of a WHO report. Osteoporos Int 1994;4:368–381.
15. Zimmerman SI, Girman CJ, Buie VC, et al. The prevalence of osteoporosis in nursing home residents. Osteoporos Int 1999;9:151–157.
16. Riggs BL, Melton LJ. The worldwide problem of osteoporosis: Insights afforded by epidemiology. Bone 1995;17:505S–511S.
17. Cummings SR, Nevitt MC, Browner WS, et al. Risk factors for hip fracture in white women. N Engl J Med 1995;332:767–773.
18. Bohannon AD, Hanlon JT, Landerman R, Gold DT. Association of race and other potential risk factors with nonvertebral fractures in community-dwelling elderly women. Am J Epidemiol 1999;149:1002–1009.
19. Lau EMC, Cooper C. The epidemiology of osteoporosis: The Oriental perspective in a world context. Clin Orthop 1996;323:65–74.
20. Kanis J, Johnell O, Gullberg B, et al. Risk factors for hip fracture in men from southern Europe: The MEDOS Study. Osteoporos Int 1999;9: 45–54.
21. Melton LJ. Epidemiology of spinal osteoporosis. Spine 1997;22(24S): 2S–11S.
22. Hannan MT, Felson DT, Dawson-Hughes B, et al. Risk factors for longitudinal bone loss in elderly men and women: The Framingham Osteoporosis Study. J Bone Miner Res 2000;15:710–720.
23. Ettinger B, Pressman A, Sklarin P, et al. Associations between low levels of serum estradiol, bone density, and fractures among elderly women: The study of osteoporotic fractures. J Clin Endocrinol Metab 1998;83:2239–2243.
24. Heaney RP. Pathophysiology of osteoporosis. Endocrinol Metab Clin North Am 1998;27:255–265.
25. King MB. Tinetti ME. Falls in community-dwelling older persons. J Am Geriatr Soc 1995;43:1146–1154.
26. McKenna MJ. Freaney R. Secondary hyperparathyroidism in the elderly: Means to defining hypovitaminosis D. Osteoporos Int 1998;8(Suppl 2): S3–S6.
27. Melton LJ. Epidemiology of fractures. In: Orwoll ES, ed. Osteoporosis in Men: The Effects of Gender on Skeletal Health. San Diego, Academic Press, 1999: 1–13.
28. Amin S, Zhang Y, Sawin CT, et al. Association of hypogonadism and estradiol levels with bone mineral density in elderly men from the Framingham study. Ann Intern Med 2000;133:951–963.
29. Adachi JD, Olszynski WP, Hanley DA, et al. Management of corticosteroid-induced osteoporosis. Semin Arthritis Rheum 2000; 29:228–251.
30. American College of Rheumatology Task Force on Osteoporosis Guidelines. Recommendations for the prevention and treatment of glucocorticoid-induced osteoporosis. Arthritis Rheum 1996;39:1791–1801.
31. Goldstein MF, Fallon JJ, Harning R. Chronic glucocorticoid therapy-induced osteoporosis in patients with obstructive lung disease. Chest 1999;116:1733–1749.
32. Faulkner KG, von Stetten E, Miller P. Discordance in patient classification using T-scores. J Clin Densitom 1999;2:343–350.
33. Miller PD, Zapalowski C, Kulak CAM, Bilezikian JP. Bone densitometry: the best way to detect osteoporosis and to monitor therapy. J Clin Endocrinol Metab 1999;84:1867–1871.
34. Jamal SA, Ridout R, Chase C, et al. Bone mineral density testing and osteoporosis education improve lifestyle behaviors in premenopausal women: A prospective study. J Bone Miner Res 1999;14:2143–2149.
35. Sklarin PM, Shoback DM, Langman CB. History and physical examination. In: Favus MJ, ed. Primer on the Metabolic Bone Diseases and Disorders of Mineral Metabolism. Philadelphia, Lippincott Williams & Wilkins, 1999: 113–115.
36. Holick MF, Adams JS. Vitamin D metabolism and biological function. In: Avioli LV, Krane SM, eds. Metabolic Bone Disease and Clinically Related Disorders. San Diego, Academic Press, 1998: 123–164.
37. Riggs BL. Are biochemical markers for bone turnover clinically useful for monitoring therapy in individual osteoporotic patients? Bone 2000;26:551–552.
38. Institute of Medicine. Dietary Reference Intakes for Calcium, Phosphorus, Magnesium, Vitamin D, and Fluoride. Washington, National Academy Press, 1997.
39. Cooper C, Atkinson EJ, Wahner HW, et al. Is caffeine consumption a risk factor for osteoporosis? J Bone Miner Res 1992;7:465–471.
40. Barger-Lux MJ, Heaney RP. Caffeine and the calcium economy revisited. Osteoporosis Int 1995;5(2):97–102.
41. Heaney RP. Dietary protein and phosphorus do not affect calcium absorption. Am J Clin Nutr 2000;72:758–761.
42. Wyshak G. Teenaged girls, carbonated beverage consumption, and bone fractures. Arch Pediatr Adolesc Med 2000;154:610–613.
43. Melhus H, Michaelsson K, Kindmark A, et al. Excessive dietary intake of vitamin A is associated with reduced bone mineral density and increased risk for hip fracture. Ann Intern Med 1998;129:770–778.
44. Binkley NC, Suttie JW. Vitamin K nutrition and osteoporosis. J Nutr 1995;25:1812–1821.
45. Hannan MT, Tucker KL Dawson-Hughes B, et al. Effect of dietary protein on bone loss in elderly men and women: The Framingham Osteoporosis Study. J Bone Miner Res 2000;15:2504.
46. Cornuz J, Feskanich D, Willett WC, Colditz GA. Smoking, smoking cessation, and risk of hip fracture in women. Am J Med 1999;106:311–314.
47. Hoidrup S, Gronback M, Gottschau A, et al. Alcohol intake, beverage preference, and risk of hip fracture in men and women: Copenhagen Centre for Prospective Population Studies. Am J Epidemiol 1999;149:993–1001.
48. Dalsky GP. Effect of exercise on bone: Permissive influence of estrogen and calcium. Med Sci Sports Exerc 1990;22:281–285.
49. Winters KE, Snow CM. Detraining reverses positive effects of exercise on the musculoskeletal system in premenopausal women. J Bone Miner Res 2000;15:2495–2503.
50. Cumming DC. Exercise-associated amenorrhea, low bone density, and estrogen replacement therapy. Arch Intern Med 1996;156:2193–2195.

51. NIH Consensus Development Panel on Osteoporosis Prevention, Diagnosis, and Therapy. Osteoporosis prevention, diagnosis and therapy. JAMA 2001;285:785–795.
52. North American Menopause Society. A decision tree for the use of estrogen replacement therapy or hormone replacement therapy in postmenopausal women: Consensus opinion of the North American Menopause Society. Menopause 2000;7:76–86.
53. Nawaz H, Katz DL. American College of Preventive Medicine practice policy statement: Perimenopausal and postmenopausal hormone replacement therapy. Am J Prevent Med 1999;17:250–254.
54. Heinemann DF. Osteoporosis: An overview of the National Osteoporosis Foundation clinical practice guide. Geriatrics 2000;55(5):31–36.
55. Col NF, Pauker SG, Goldberg RJ, et al. Individualizing therapy to prevent long-term consequences of estrogen deficiency in postmenopausal women. Arch Intern Med 1999;159:1458–1466.
56. Reginster J-Y, Bruyere O, Audran M, et al. Do estrogens effectively prevent osteoporosis-related fractures? Calcif Tissue Int 2000;67:191–194.
57. Orwoll ES, Nelson HD. Does estrogen adequately protect postmenopausal women against osteoporosis: An iconoclastic perspective (Commentary). J Clin Endocrinol Metab 1999;84:1872–1874.
58. Heaney RP. Calcium, dairy products and osteoporosis. J Am Coll Nutr 2000;19:83S–99S.
59. Feskanich D, Willett WC, Stampfer MJ, Colditz GA. A prospective study of thiazide use and fractures in women. Osteoporos Int 1997;7:79–84.
60. Gillespie WJ, Henry DA, O'Connell DL, Robertson J. Vitamin D and vitamin D analogues for preventing fractures associated with involutional and postmenopausal osteoporosis. Cochrane Collaboration Volume 2000(4).
61. Watts NB. Treatment of osteoporosis with bisphosphonates. Endocrinol Metab Clin North Am 1998;27:419–439.
62. Schnitzer T, Bone HG, Crepaldi G, et al. Therapeutic equivalence of alendronate 70 mg once-weekly and alendronate 10 mg daily in the treatment of osteoporosis. Aging Clin Exp Res 2000;12:1–12.
63. Bone HG, Greenspan SL, McKeever C, et al. Alendronate and estrogen effects in postmenopausal women with low bone mineral density. J Clin Endocrinol Metab 2000;85:720–726.
64. Harris ST, Watts NB, Genant HK, et al. Effects of risedronate treatment on vertebral and nonvertebral fractures in women with postmenopausal osteoporosis: A randomized controlled trial. JAMA 1999;282:1344–1352.
65. Orwoll E, Ettinger M, Weiss S, et al. Alendronate for the treatment of osteoporosis in men. New Engl J Med 2000;343:604–610.
66. McClung MR, Geusens P, Miller PD, et al. Effect of risedronate on the risk of hip fracture in elderly women. N Engl J Med 2001;344:333–340.
67. Miller PD, Watts NB, Licata AA, et al. Cyclical etidronate in the treatment of postmenopausal osteoporosis: Efficacy and safety after seven years of treatment. Am J Med 1997;103:468–476.
68. Wimalawansa SJ. Combined therapy with estrogen and etidronate has an additive effect on bone mineral density in the hip and vertebrae: Four-year randomized study. Am J Med 1995;99:36–42.
69. Delaney MF, Fowler L, Hurwitz S, et al. Bone density changes in response to once weekly risedronate (Abstract). J Bone Miner Res. 2000;15 (Suppl 1):M394.
70. Bauer DC, Black D, Ensrud K, et al. Upper gastrointestinal tract safety profile of alendronate. Arch Intern Med 2000;160:517–525.
71. Deng H-W, Li J, Li J-L, et al. Change of bone mass in postmenopausal Caucasian women with and without hormone replacement therapy is associated with vitamin D receptor and estrogen receptor genotypes. Hum Genet 1998;103:576–585.
72. Writing Group for the PEPI Trial. Effects of hormone therapy on bone mineral density: Results from the postmenopausal estrogen/progestin interventions (PEPI) trial. JAMA 1996;276:1389–1396.
73. Weiss SR, Ellman H, Dolker M. A randomized controlled trial of four doses of transdermal estradiol for preventing postmenopausal bone loss. Obstet Gynecol 1999;94:330–336.
74. Recker RR, Davies KM, Dowd RM, Heaney RP. The effect of low-dose continuous estrogen and progesterone therapy with calcium and vitamin D on bone in elderly women: A randomized, controlled trial. Ann Intern Med 1999;130:897–904.
75. Genant HK, Lucas J, Weiss S, et al. Low-dose esterified estrogen therapy: Effects on bone, plasma estradiol concentrations, endometrium, and lipid levels. Arch Intern Med 1997;157:2609–2615.
76. Schneider DL, Barrett-Connor EL, Morton DJ. Timing of postmenopausal estrogen for optimal bone mineral density: The Rancho Bernardo Study. JAMA 1997;277:543–547.
77. Umland EM, Rinaldi C, Parks SM, Boyce EG. The impact of estrogen replacement therapy and raloxifene on osteoporosis, cardiovascular disease, and gynecologic cancers. Ann Pharmacother 1999;33:1315–1328.
78. Grisso JA, Kelsey JL, Strom BL, et al. Risk factors for hip fracture in black women. N Engl J Med 1994;330:1555–1559.
79. Torgerson DJ, Bell-Syer SEM. Hormone replacement therapy and prevention of nonvertebral fractures: A meta-analysis of randomized trials. JAMA 2001;285:2891–2897.
80. Kardos A, Casadei B. Hormone replacement therapy and ischemic heart disease among postmenopausal women. J Cardiovasc Risk 1999;6:105–112.
81. Pickar JH, Thorneycroft I, Whitehead M. Effects of hormone replacement therapy on the endometrium and lipid parameters: A review of randomized clinical trials, 1985–1995. Am J Obstet Gynecol 1998;178:1087–1099.
82. Writing Group for the PEPI Trial. Effects of estrogen or estrogen/progestin regimens on heart disease risk factors in postmenopausal women: The Postmenopausal Estrogen/Progestin Interventions (PEPI) trial. JAMA 1995;273:199–208.
83. Folsom AR, McGovern PG, Nabulsi AA, et al. Changes in plasma lipids and lipoproteins associated with starting or stopping postmenopausal hormone replacement therapy. Am Heart J 1996;132:952–958.
84. Davidson MH, Testolin LM, Maki, KC, et al. A comparison of estrogen replacement, pravastatin, and combined treatment for the management of hypercholesterolemia in postmenopausal women. Arch Intern Med 1997;157:1186–1192.
85. Grodstein F, Stampfer MJ, Manson JE, et al. Postmenopausal estrogen and progestin use and the risk of cardiovascular disease. N Engl J Med 1996;335:453–461.
86. Hulley S, Grady D, Bush T, et al. Randomized trial of estrogen plus progestin for secondary prevention of coronary heart disease in postmenopausal women. JAMA 1998;280:605–613.
87. Udoff L, Langenberg P, Adashi EY. Combined continuous hormone replacement therapy: A critical review. Obstet Gynecol 1995;86:306–316.
88. Cano A, Tarin JJ, Duenas JL. Two-year prospective, randomized trial comparing an innovative twice-a-week progestin regimen with a continuous combined regimen as postmenopausal hormone therapy. Fertil Steril 1999;71:129–136.
89. Ettinger B, Selby J, Citron JT, et al. Cyclic hormone replacement therapy using quarterly progestin. Obstet Gynecol 1994;103(Suppl 13):693–700.
90. Tavani A, La Vecchia C. The adverse effects of hormone replacement therapy. Drugs Aging 1999;14:347–357.
91. Speroff L. Postmenopausal hormone therapy and breast cancer. Obstet Gynecol 1996;87:44S–54S.
92. Schairer C, Gail M, Byrne C et al. Estrogen replacement therapy and breast cancer survival in a large screening study. J Natl Cancer Inst 1999;91:264–270.
93. Gutthann SP, Rodriguez LAG, Castellsague J, Oliart AD. Hormone replacement therapy and risk of venous thromboembolism: Population based case-control study. Br Med J 1997;314:796–800.
94. Brown AF, Perez-Stable EJ, Whitaker EE, et al. Ethnic differences in hormone replacement prescribing patterns. J Gen Intern Med 1999;14:663–669.
95. Faulkner DL, Young C, Hutchins D, McCollam JS. Patient noncompliance with hormone replacement therapy: A nationwide estimate using a large prescription claims database. Menopause 1998;5:226–229.
96. Johnston CC, Bjarnason NH, Cohen FJ, et al. Long-term effects of raloxifene on bone mineral density, bone turnover, and serum lipid levels in early postmenopausal women: Three-year data from two double-blind,

randomized, placebo-controlled trials. Ann Intern Med 2000;160:3444–3450.
97. Ettinger B, Black DM, Mitlak BH, et al. Reduction of vertebral fracture risk in postmenopausal women with osteoporosis treated with raloxifene: Results from a 3-year randomized clinical trial. Multiple Outcomes of Raloxifene Evaluation (MORE) investigators. JAMA 1999;282:637–645.
98. Cummings SR, Eckert S, Krueger KA, et al. The effect of raloxifene on risk of breast cancer in postmenopausal women: Results from the MORE randomized trial. Multiple Outcomes of Raloxifene Evaluation (MORE) investigators. JAMA 1999;281:2189–2197.
99. Kuohong W, Borgatta L, Stubblefield P. Low-dose oral contraceptives and bone mineral density: An evidence-based analysis. Contraception 2000;61:77–82.
100. Bahamondes L, Perrotti M, Castro S, et al. Forearm bone density in users of Depo-Provera as a contraceptive method. Fertil Steril 1999;71:849–852.
101. Umland EM, Cauffield JS, Kirk JK, Thomason TE. Phytoestrogens as therapeutic alternatives to traditional hormone replacement in postmenopausal women. Pharmacotherapy 2000;20:981–990.
102. Alexandersen P, Toussaint A, Christiansen C, et al. Ipriflavone in the treatment of postmenopausal osteoporosis: A randomized controlled trial. JAMA. 2001;285:1482–1488.
103. Shoupe D. Androgens and bone: Clinical implications for menopausal women. Am J Obstet Gynecol 1999;180:S329–S333.
104. Moore RA. Livial: A review of clinical studies. Br J Obstet Gynaecol 1999;106(Suppl 19):1–21.
105. Chesnut CH, Silverman S, Andriano K. A randomized trial of nasal spray salmon calcitonin in postmenopausal women with established osteoporosis: The Prevent Recurrence of Osteoporotic Fractures Study. Am J Med 2000;109:267–276.
106. Boivin G, Deloffre P, Perrat B, et al. Strontium distribution and interactions with bone mineral in monkey iliac bone after strontium salt (S12911) administration. J Bone Miner Res 1996;11:1302–1311.
107. van Staa TP, Leufkens HGM, Cooper C. Use of nonsteroidal anti-inflammatory drugs and risk of fractures. Bone 2000;27:563–568.
108. Neer RM, Arnaud CD, Zanchetta JR, et al. Effect of parathyroid hormone (1–34) on fractures and bone mineral density in postmenopausal women with osteoporosis. N Engl J Med 2001;344:1434–1441.
109. Lindsay R, Nieves J, Formica C, et al. Randomised controlled study of effect of parathyroid hormone on vertebral bone mass and fracture incidence among postmenopausal women on oestrogen with osteoporosis. Lancet 1997;350:550–555.
110. Lane NE, Sanchez S, Modin GW, et al. Parathyroid hormone treatment can reverse corticosteroid-induced osteoporosis: Results of a randomized controlled clinical trial. J Clin Invest 1998;102:1627–1633.
111. Kurland ES, Cosman F, McMahon DJ, et al. Parathyroid hormone as a therapy for idiopathic osteoporosis in men: Effects on bone mineral density and bone markers. J Clin Endocrinol Metab 2000;85:3069–3076.
112. Meier CR, Schlienger RG, Kraenzlin ME, et al. HMG-CoA reductase inhibitors and the risk of fractures. JAMA 2000,283:3205–3210.
113. LaCroix AZ, Cauley JA, Jackson R, et al. Does statin use reduce risk of fracture in postmenopausal women? Results from the Women's Health Initiative Observational Study (WHI-OS) (Abstract). J Bone Miner Res 2000;15(Suppl 1):1066.
114. van Staa TP, Wegman S, de Vries F, et al. Use of statins and risk of fractures. JAMA 2001;285:1850–1855.
115. Hennessy S, Strom BL. Statins and fracture risk. JAMA 2001;285:1888–1889.
116. Boonen S, Mohan S, Dequeker J, et al. Downregulation of the serum stimulatory components of the insulin-like growth factor (IGF) system [IGF-I, IGF-II, IGF binding protein (BP)-3, and IGFBP-5] in age-related (type II) femoral neck osteoporosis. J Bone Miner Res 1999;14:2150–2158.
117. Haguenauer D, V Welch V, Shea B, et al. Fluoride for treating osteoporosis. Cochrane Collaboration 2000(4).
118. Klibanski A, Biller BM, Schoenfeld DA, et al. The effects of estrogen administration on trabecular bone loss in young women with anorexia nervosa. J Clin Endocrinol Metab 1995;80:898–904.
119. Francis RM. The effects of testosterone on osteoporosis in men. Clin Endocrinol 1999;50:411–414.
120. Wang PS, Bohn RL, Glynn RJ, et al. Hazardous benzodiazepine regimens in the elderly: Effects of half-life, dosage, and duration on risk of hip fracture. Am J Psychiatry 2001;158:892–898.
121. Kannus P, Parkkari J, Niemi S, et al. Prevention of hip fracture in elderly people with use of a hip protector. N Engl J Med 2000;343:1506–1513.
122. Rodino MA, Shane E. Osteoporosis after organ transplantation. Am J Med 1998;104:459–469.
123. Joy MS, Neyhart CD, Dooley MA. Pharmacy practice insights: A multidisciplinary renal clinic for corticosteroids-induced bone disease. Pharmacotherapy 2000;20:206–216.
124. Wang MWH, Teitelbaum SL, Tebas P, et al. HIV protease inhibitors cause osteoporosis (Abstract M196). J Bone Miner Res 2000;15(Suppl):S503.
125. Ott SM, Aitken ML. Osteoporosis in patients with cystic fibrosis. Clin Chest Med 1998;19:555–567.
126. Tosteson A. The economic impact of osteoporosis. In: Osteoporosis Prevention, Diagnosis, and Therapy. NIH Consensus Statement No. 111, Bethesda, MD, 2000;17(1):1–36.
127. Epstein RS, Feng W, Hirsch LJ, Kelly M. Intervention thresholds for the treatment of osteoporosis: Comparison of different approaches to decision making. Osteoporosis Int 1998;8(Suppl 1):S22–S27.
128. Tengs TO, Adams ME, Pliskin JS, et al. Five-hundred life-saving interventions and their cost-effectiveness. Risk Analysis 1995;15:369–390.
129. Osteoporosis Task Force. AACE clinical practice guidelines for the prevention and treatment of postmenopausal osteoporosis. J Fla Med Assoc 1996;83:552–566.
130. Cummings SR, Palermo L, Browner W, et al. Monitoring osteoporosis therapy with bone densitometry: Misleading changes and regression to the mean. JAMA 2000;283:1318–1321.
131. Klein GL. Nutritional rickets and osteomalacia. In: Favus MJ, ed. Primer on the Metabolic Bone Diseases and Disorders of Mineral Metabolism. Philadelphia, Lippincott Williams & Wilkins, 1999:315–319.
132. Liberman UA, Marx SJ. Vitamin D–dependent rickets. In: Favus MJ, ed. Primer on the Metabolic Bone Diseases and Disorders of Mineral Metabolism. Philadelphia, Lippincott Williams & Wilkins, 1999:323–328.
133. Glorieux FH. Hypophosphatemic vitamin D–resistant rickets. In: Favus MJ, ed. Primer on the Metabolic Bone Diseases and Disorders of Mineral Metabolism. Philadelphia, Lippincott Williams & Wilkins, 1999:328–331.
134. Bikle DD. Drug-induced osteomalacia. In: Favus MJ, ed. Primer on the Metabolic Bone Diseases and Disorders of Mineral Metabolism. Philadelphia, Lippincott Williams & Wilkins, 1999:343–347.
135. Goodman WG, Coburn JW, Slatopolsky E, Salusdy IB. Renal osteodystrophy in adults and children. In: Favus MJ, ed. Primer on the Metabolic Bone Diseases and Disorders of Mineral Metabolism. Philadelphia, Lippincott Williams & Wilkins, 1999:347–363.
136. Drezner MK. Tumor-induced osteomalacia. In: Favus MJ, ed. Primer on the Metabolic Bone Diseases and Disorders of Mineral Metabolism. Philadelphia, Lippincott Williams & Wilkins, 1999:331–337.
137. Chesney RW. Fanconi syndrome and renal tubular acidosis. In: Favus MJ, ed. Primer on the Metabolic Bone Diseases and Disorders of Mineral Metabolism. Philadelphia, Lippincott Williams & Wilkins, 1999:340–343.
138. Hodgson SF, Watts NB, Bilezikian JP, et al. American Association of Clinical Endocrinologists 2001 medical guidelines for clinical practice for the prevention and management of postmenopausal osteoporosis. Endocr Pract 2001;7:293–312.

91

RHEUMATOID ARTHRITIS

Arthur A. Schuna

Rheumatoid arthritis is the most common systemic inflammatory disease characterized by symmetrical joint involvement. Extraarticular involvement including rheumatoid nodules, vasculitis, eye inflammation, neurologic dysfunction, cardiopulmonary disease, lymphadenopathy, and splenomegaly are manifestations of the disease. Although the usual disease course is chronic, some patients will enter a remission spontaneously.

EPIDEMIOLOGY

Rheumatoid arthritis is estimated to have a prevalence of 1% to 2% and does not have any racial predilections. It can occur at any age, with increasing prevalence up to the seventh decade of life. The disease is three times more common in women. In people aged 15 to 45 years, women predominate by a ratio of 6:1; the sex ratio is approximately equal among patients in the first decade of life and in those more than 60 years old.

Epidemiologic data suggest that a genetic predisposition and exposure to unknown environmental factors may be necessary for expression of the disease. The major histocompatibility complex (MHC) molecules, located on T-lymphocytes, appear to have an important role in most patients with rheumatoid arthritis. These molecules can be characterized using human lymphocyte antigen (HLA) typing. A majority of patients with rheumatoid arthritis have HLA-DR4, HLA-DR1, or both antigens found in the MHC region. Although the MHC region is important, it is not the sole determinant, because patients can have the disease without these HLA types. Rheumatoid arthritis is six times more common among dizygotic twins and nontwin children of parents with rheumatoid factor-positive, erosive rheumatoid arthritis when compared with children whose parents do not have the disease. If one of a pair of monozygotic twins is affected, the other twin has a 30 times greater risk of developing the disease.[1,2]

PATHOPHYSIOLOGY

Chronic inflammation of the synovial tissue lining the joint capsule results in the proliferation of this tissue. The inflamed, proliferating synovium characteristic of rheumatoid arthritis is called *pannus* (Fig. 91–1). This pannus invades the cartilage and eventually the bone surface, producing erosions of bone and cartilage and leading to destruction of the joint. The factors that initiate the inflammatory process are unknown.

The immune system is a complex network of checks and balances designed to discriminate self from nonself (foreign) tissues. It helps rid the body of infectious agents, tumor cells, and products associated with the breakdown of cells. In rheumatoid arthritis this system no longer can differentiate self from nonself tissues and attacks the synovial tissue and other connective tissues.

The immune system has both humoral and cell-mediated functions (Fig. 91–2). The humoral component is necessary for the formation of antibodies. These antibodies are produced by plasma cells. Most patients with rheumatoid arthritis form antibodies called *rheumatoid factors*. Rheumatoid factors have not been identified as pathogenic, nor does the quantity of these circulating antibodies always correlate with disease activity. Seropositive patients tend to have a more aggressive course of their illness than do seronegative patients. Immunoglobulins can activate the complement system. The complement system amplifies the immune response by encouraging chemotaxis, phagocytosis, and the release of lymphokines by mononuclear cells which are then presented to T-lymphocytes. The processed antigen is recognized by MHC proteins on the lymphocyte, which activates it to stimulate the production of T and B cells. The proinflammatory cytokines tumor necrosis factor (TNF) and interleukin-1 (IL-1) appear to be key substances in the initiation and continuance of rheumatoid inflammation. Lymphocytes may be either B cells (derived from bone marrow) or T cells (derived from thymus tissue). T cells may be either T-helper (which promote inflammation) or T-suppressor cells (which attenuate the inflammatory response). Activated T cells produce cytotoxins, which are directly toxic to tissues, and cytokines, which stimulate further activation of inflammatory processes and attract cells to areas of inflammation. Macrophages are stimulated to release prostaglandins and cytotoxins. Activated B cells produce plasma cells, which form antibodies. These antibodies in combination with complement result in the accumulation of polymorphonuclear leukocytes (PMNs). These PMNs release cytotoxins, oxygen free radicals, and hydroxyl radicals that promote cellular damage to synovium and bone. Patients with rheumatoid arthritis appear to have an excessive amount of T-helper cell activity in synovial tissues.

Vasoactive substances also play a role in the inflammatory process. Histamine, kinins, and prostaglandins are released at the site of inflammation. These substances increase both blood flow to the site of inflammation and the permeability of blood vessels. These substances cause the edema, warmth, erythema, and pain associated with inflamed joints and also make it easier for granulocytes to pass from blood vessels to the site of inflammation.

The end results of the chronic inflammatory changes are variable. Loss of cartilage may result in a loss of the joint space. The formation of chronic granulation or scar tissue can lead to loss of joint motion or bony fusion (called *ankylosis*). Laxity of tendon structures can result in a loss of support to the affected joint, leading to instability or subluxation. Tendon contractures also may occur, leading to chronic deformity.[2–4]

CLINICAL PRESENTATION

The symptoms of rheumatoid arthritis usually develop insidiously over the course of several weeks to months. Prodromal symptoms include fatigue, weakness, low-grade fever, loss of appetite, and joint pain. Stiffness and muscle aches (myalgias) may precede the development of joint swelling (synovitis). Fatigue may be more of a problem in the afternoon. During disease flares, the onset of fatigue begins earlier in the day and subsides as disease activity lessens. Most commonly, joint involvement tends to be symmetrical; however, early in

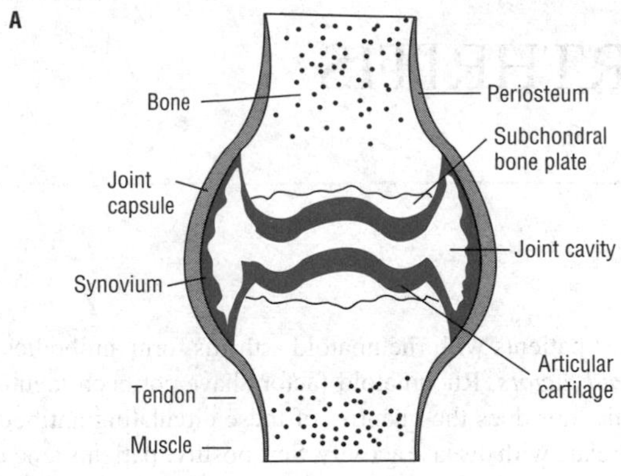

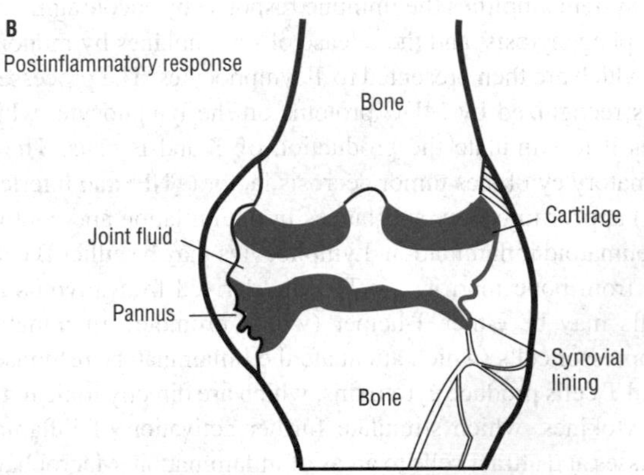

FIGURE 91–1. (*A*) Schematic diagram of a normal diarthrodial joint. (*B*) Schematic diagram of a knee joint with active rheumatoid arthritis showing pannus invading and destroying the cartilage and bone. *(Reproduced from the Arthritis Foundation Allied Health Professions Teaching Slide Collection, Copyright © 1980, with permission.)*

the disease some patients present with an asymmetrical pattern involving one or a few joints that eventually develops into the more classic presentation. About 20% of patients develop an abrupt onset of their illness with fevers, polyarthritis, and constitutional symptoms (e.g., depression, anxiety, fatigue, anorexia, and weight loss).[1,2] No single test or physical finding can be used to make the diagnosis of rheumatoid arthritis, but criteria have been developed to aid in its diagnosis (Table 91–1).

JOINT INVOLVEMENT

The joints affected most frequently by rheumatoid arthritis are the small joints of the hands, wrists, and feet (Fig. 91–3). In addition, elbows, shoulders, hips, knees, and ankles may be involved. Patients usually experience joint stiffness that typically is worse in the morning. The duration of stiffness tends to be correlated directly with disease activity, usually exceeds 30 minutes, and may persist all day. Chronic inflammation with lack of an adequate exercise program results in loss of range of motion, atrophy of muscles, weakness, and deformity. A functional classification scale may be used to indicate a patient's degree of impairment (Table 91–2).

On examination, the swelling of the joints may be visible or may be apparent only by palpation. The swelling feels soft and spongy because it is caused by proliferation of soft tissues or fluid accumulation within the joint capsule. The swollen joint may appear erythematous and feel warmer than nearby skin surfaces, especially early in the course of the disease. In contrast, the swelling associated with osteoarthritis usually is bony (caused by osteophytes) and infrequently is associated with signs of inflammation.

Involvement of the hands and wrists is common in rheumatoid arthritis. Hand involvement is manifested by pain, swelling, tenderness, and grip weakness during the acute phase and by subluxation, instability, deformity, and muscle atrophy in the chronic phase of the disease. Functional difficulties with clasp, grasp, and pinch alter both

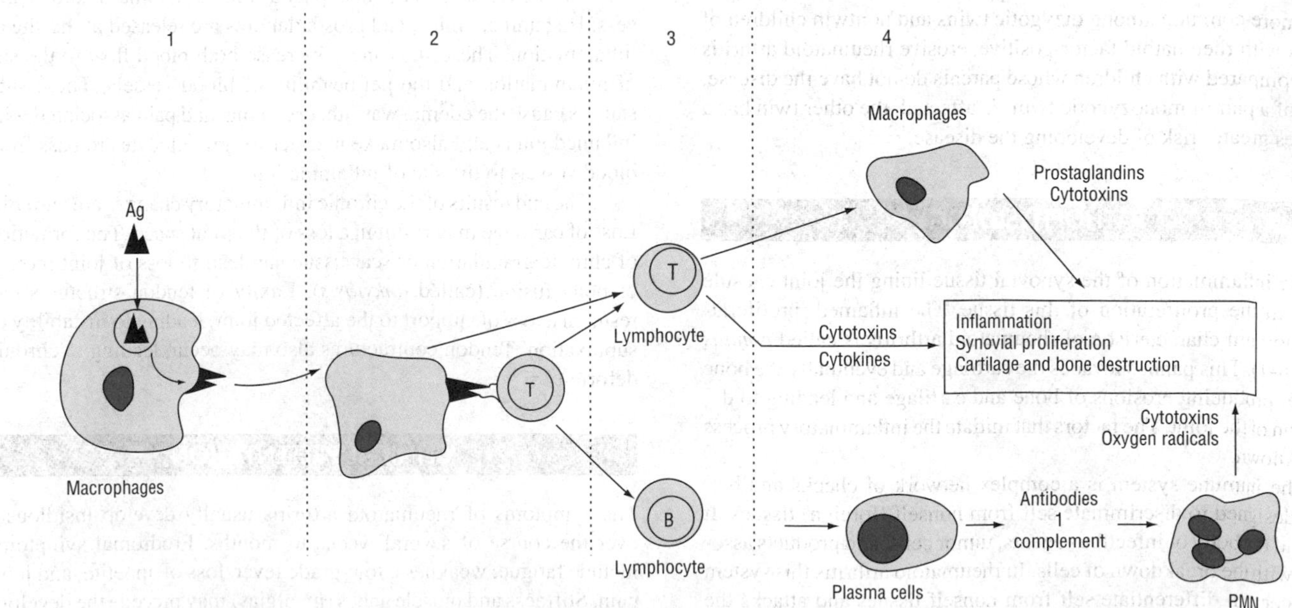

FIGURE 91–2. Pathogenesis of the inflammatory response. Phase 1: Antigen-presenting cell phagocytizes antigen. Phase 2: Antigen is presented to a T-lymphocyte. The T-lymphocyte attaches to antigen at the MHC portion of cell wall causing activation. Phase 3: An activated T cell stimulates T- and B-lymphocyte production, promoting inflammation. Phase 4: Activated T cells and macrophages release factors that promote tissue destruction, increase blood flow, and result in cellular invasion of synovial tissue and joint fluid. Ag = antigen; PMN = polymorphonuclear leukocyte.

TABLE 91–1. American Rheumatism Association Criteria for Classification of Rheumatoid Arthritis—1987 Revision

Criteria[a]	Definition
1. Morning stiffness	Morning stiffness in and around the joints lasting at least 1 hour before maximal improvement.
2. Arthritis of three or more joint areas	At least three joint areas simultaneously have soft tissue swelling or fluid (not bony overgrowth alone) observed by a physician. The 14 possible joint areas are (right or left): PIP, MCP, wrist, elbow, knee, ankle, and MTP joints.[b]
3. Arthritis of hand joints	At least one joint area swollen as above in wrist, MCP, or PIP joint.
4. Symmetrical arthritis	Simultaneous involvement of the same joint areas (as in 2) on both sides of the body (bilateral involvement of PIP, MCP, or MTP joints is acceptable without absolute symmetry).
5. Rheumatoid nodules	Subcutaneous nodules, over bony prominences, or extensor surfaces, or in juxtaarticular regions, observed by a physician.
6. Serum rheumatoid factor	Demonstration of abnormal amounts of serum rheumatoid factor by any method that has been positive in less than 5% of normal control subjects.
7. Radiographic changes	Radiographic changes typical of rheumatoid arthritis on posteroanterior hand and wrist x-rays, which must include erosions or unequivocal bony decalcification localized to or most marked adjacent to the involved joints (osteoarthritis changes alone do not qualify).

[a]For classification purposes, a patient is said to have rheumatoid arthritis if he or she has satisfied at least four of these seven criteria. Criteria 1 through 4 must be present for at least 6 weeks. Patients with two clinical diagnoses are not excluded. Designation as classic, definite, or probable rheumatoid arthritis is not to be made.
[b]PIP = proximal interphalangeal; MCP = metacarpophalangeal; MTP = metatarsophalangeal.

strength and fine motor movement. These difficulties can affect the activities of daily living (ADLs) necessary for self-care. Tenosynovitis involving the flexor tendons of the hands can result in restriction of motion or locking of digits in a flexed position. Tenosynovitis of the extensor tendons of the hand may result in pain, swelling, and spontaneous rupture with loss of function.

Deformity of the hand may be seen with chronic inflammation. Subluxations of the wrists and metacarpophalangeal (MCP) joints may be seen. The thumbs may develop flexion at the MCP joint and hyperextension of the interphalangeal (IP) joint, which may make pinch grip difficult. Involvement of tendons in the hands can result in either hyperextension at the proximal interphalangeal (PIP) joint and flexion of the distal interphalangeal (DIP) joint (called a *swan-neck deformity;* see Fig. 91–4) or flexion at PIP joint with hyperextension of the DIP joint (called a *boutonniere deformity;* see Fig. 91–5). Ulnar deviation of the fingers also may occur as a result of tendon abnormalities associated with rheumatoid arthritis (Fig. 91–6).

Wrist involvement can result in joint-space narrowing, collapse, and subluxation leading to grip weakness. Destruction of the cartilage at the radioulnar joint results in pain with rotational movement of

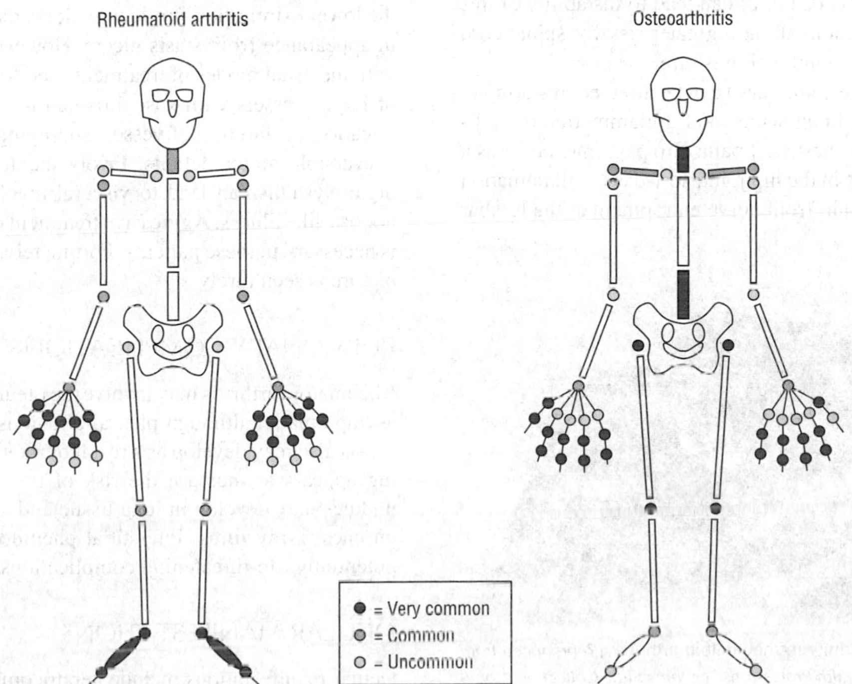

FIGURE 91–3. Patterns of joint involvement in rheumatoid arthritis and osteoarthritis.

TABLE 91–2. Functional Classifications of Rheumatoid Arthritis

Class I	Capable of all activities without handicap
Class II	Able to conduct normal activities despite handicap of discomfort or limited mobility of one or more joints
Class III	Functional capacity only adequate to perform a few of the normal duties of usual occupation
Class IV	Bed or confined to wheelchair, capable of little or no self-care

the forearm. Carpal tunnel syndrome is caused by entrapment of the median nerve by inflamed synovium. This results in pain and tingling in the fingers and grip weakness.

Swelling at the elbow is most evident at the radiohumeral joint. Shoulder pain may result from involvement of the joint itself or from tendon inflammation (tendinitis) or inflammation of the bursa (bursitis) near the deltoid muscle.

The knee also can be involved, with loss of cartilage, instability, and joint pain. Synovitis of the knee may cause the formation of a cyst behind the knee called a *popliteal* or *Baker's cyst*. These cysts may become painful as they get tense, or they may rupture, producing a clinical picture similar to thrombophlebitis secondary to the release of inflammatory components into the area of the calf muscle. Chronic joint pain leads to muscle atrophy, which can result in a laxity of the ligamentous structures that support the knee, causing instability. Maintenance of an adequate range of motion of the knee is essential to normal gait.

Foot and ankle involvement in rheumatoid arthritis is common. The metatarsophalangeal (MTP) joints are involved commonly in rheumatoid arthritis, making walking difficult. Subluxation of the metatarsal heads leads to "cock-up" toe deformities. Subluxation also may cause a flexion deformity at the PIP joint of the toe, leading to pressure necrosis of the skin over the joint secondary to irritation caused by shoes. Hallux valgus (lateral deviation of the digit) and bunion or callus formation may occur at the great toe (Fig. 91–7). A widening of the foot occurs commonly with long-standing disease.

Involvement of the spine usually occurs in the cervical vertebrae; lumbar vertebral involvement is rare. Involvement of the first and second cervical vertebrae (C1–C2) can lead to instability of this joint. Patients with this problem are at a greater risk for spinal cord compression, although this complication is rare.

The temporomandibular joint (jaw) can be affected, resulting in malocclusion and difficulty in chewing food. Inflammation of cartilage in the chest can lead to chest wall pain. Hip pain may occur as a result of destructive changes in the hip joint, soft-tissue inflammation (e.g., bursitis), or referred pain from nerve entrapment at the lumbar vertebrae.

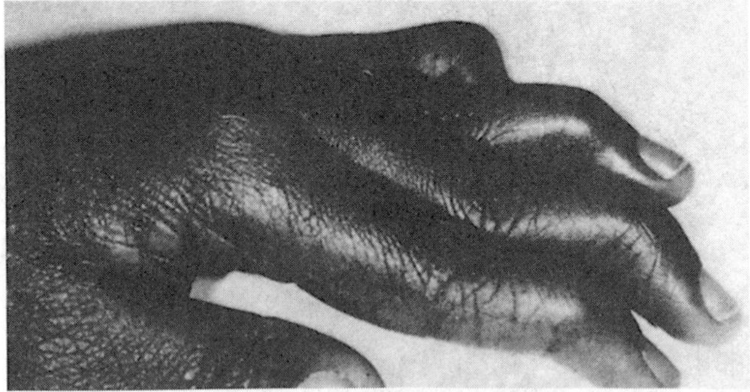

FIGURE 91–4. Swan-neck deformity in rheumatoid arthritis. *(Reproduced from the Arthritis Foundation Allied Health Professions Teaching Slide Collection, Copyright ©1980, with permission.)*

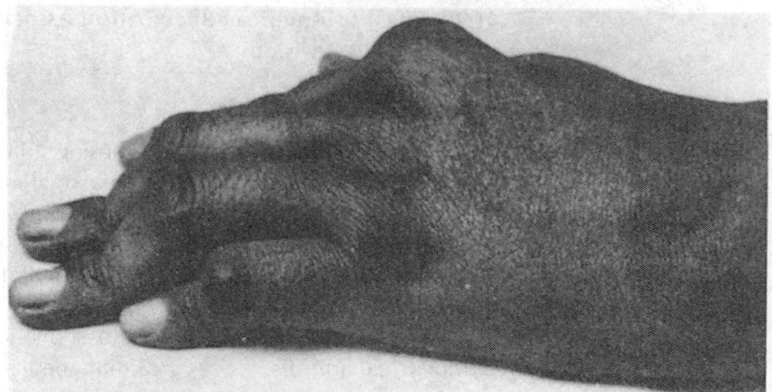

FIGURE 91–5. Boutonniere deformity in rheumatoid arthritis. *(Reproduced from the Arthritis Foundation Allied Health Professions Teaching Slide Collection, Copyright ©1980, with permission.)*

EXTRAARTICULAR INVOLVEMENT

RHEUMATOID NODULES

Rheumatoid nodules occur in 20% of patients with rheumatoid arthritis. These nodules are seen most commonly on the extensor surfaces of the elbows, forearms, and hands but also may be seen on the feet and at other pressure points. They also may develop in the lung or pleural lining of the lung and, rarely, in the meninges. Rheumatoid nodules usually are asymptomatic and do not require any special intervention. Nodules are observed more commonly in patients with erosive disease.[5]

VASCULITIS

Vasculitis usually is seen in patients with long-standing rheumatoid arthritis. Vasculitis may result in a wide variety of clinical presentations. Invasion of blood vessel walls by inflammatory cells results in an obliteration of the vessel, producing infarction of tissue distal to the area of involvement. Most commonly, small-vessel vasculitis produces infarcts near the ends of the fingers or toes, especially around the nail beds. These infarcts are usually of little consequence.

Vasculitis also may cause the breakdown of skin, especially in the lower extremities, producing ulcers that may be indistinguishable in appearance from stasis ulcers. However, these ulcers do not heal with the usual modes of treatment used for stasis ulcers. Involvement of larger vessels with vasculitis can result in life-threatening complications. Infarction of vessels supplying blood to nerves can cause irreversible motor deficits. Involvement of vessels supplying other organ systems can lead to visceral involvement and a polyarteritis nodosa-like illness. Aggressive treatment of the inflammatory process is necessary in these patients. Fortunately, the more serious vasculitic picture is seen rarely.

PULMONARY COMPLICATIONS

Rheumatoid arthritis may involve the pleura of the lung, which is often asymptomatic, although pleural effusions may result. Pulmonary fibrosis also may develop as a result of rheumatoid involvement; smoking appears to increase the risk of this complication. Rheumatoid nodules may develop in lung tissue and appear similar to neoplasms on chest x-ray films. Interstitial pneumonitis and arteritis are rare, potentially life-threatening complications of rheumatoid arthritis.

OCULAR MANIFESTATIONS

Ocular manifestations include keratoconjunctivitis sicca and inflammation of the sclera, episclera, and cornea. Atrophy of the lacrimal

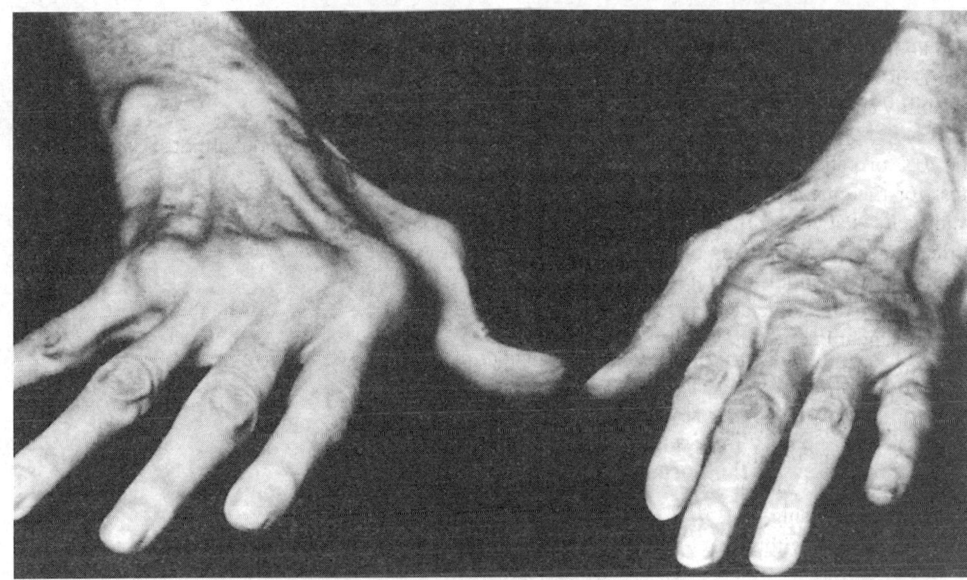

FIGURE 91–6. Ulnar deviation of the fingers of the right hand. *(Reproduced from the Arthritis Foundation Allied Health Professions Teaching Slide Collection, Copyright ©1980, with permission.)*

duct may result in a decrease in tear formation, causing dry and itchy eyes, termed *keratoconjunctivitis sicca*. When this is observed in association with rheumatoid arthritis, it is referred to as *Sjögren's syndrome*. Artificial tears may be used to relieve symptoms. Inflammation of the superficial layers of the sclera (episcleritis) is generally self-limiting. Involvement of deeper tissues (scleritis) usually results in a more serious, painful, and chronic inflammation. Rheumatoid nodules may develop on the sclera.

CARDIAC INVOLVEMENT

The heart is sometimes affected by rheumatoid arthritis, but only rarely are the changes symptomatic. Pericarditis may occur, resulting in the accumulation of fluid. Although many patients show evidence of previous pericarditis at autopsy, the development of clinically evident pericarditis with tamponade is a rare complication. Cardiac conduction abnormalities and aortic valve incompetence, caused by aortic root dilatation, may occur. Myocarditis is a rare complication of rheumatoid arthritis.

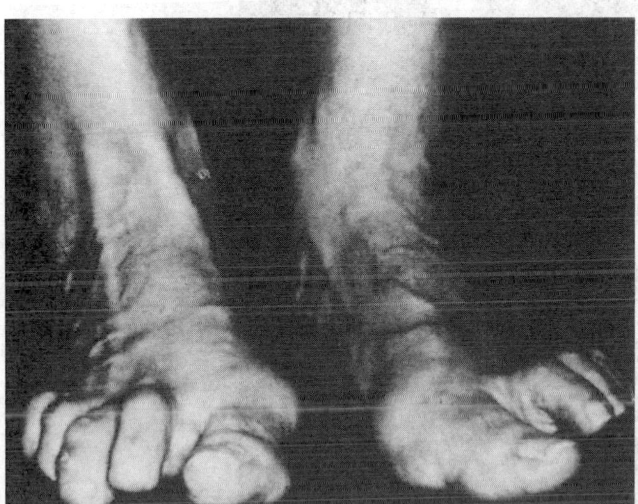

FIGURE 91–7. Foot involvement of rheumatoid arthritis with hallux valgus deformity of the first digit and hammer-toe deformity of second through fifth digits bilaterally. *(Reproduced from the Arthritis Foundation Allied Health Professions Teaching Slide Collection, Copyright ©1980, with permission.)*

FELTY'S SYNDROME

Rheumatoid arthritis in association with splenomegaly and neutropenia is known as *Felty's syndrome*. Thrombocytopenia also may be a manifestation of the syndrome. Patients with Felty's syndrome and severe leukopenia are more susceptible to infection. The decrease in granulocytes appears to be mediated by the immune system because splenectomy does not result in improvement of the patient.[5]

OTHER COMPLICATIONS

Lymphadenopathy may occur in patients with rheumatoid arthritis, particularly in nodes proximal to more actively involved joints. Renal involvement is rare but can be associated with treatment, including nonsteroidal anti-inflammatory drugs (NSAIDs), gold salts, and penicillamine. Amyloidosis is a rare complication of long-standing rheumatoid arthritis. It appears to be more common in Europe than in the United States.

LABORATORY FINDINGS

Hematologic tests often reveal a mild to moderate anemia with normocytic, normochromic indices. The hematocrit may fall as low as 30%. The anemia is usually inversely related to inflammatory disease activity and is referred to as an *anemia of chronic disease*. This type of anemia does not respond to iron therapy and can present a diagnostic dilemma because NSAIDs may induce gastritis and chronic blood loss leading to iron-deficiency anemia. Laboratory tests useful in differentiating these anemias include stool guaiac (or other stool tests for occult blood), serum iron/iron-binding capacity ratio (decreased in iron deficiency), and mean corpuscular volume (more likely to be decreased in iron deficiency). Other causes of anemia also must be considered in the differential diagnosis (see Chap. 99).

Thrombocytosis is another common hematologic finding with active rheumatoid arthritis. Platelet counts rise and fall in direct correlation with disease activity in many patients. Thrombocytopenia may result from toxicity of gold salts, penicillamine, or immunosuppressive therapy. Thrombocytopenia also may be observed in Felty's syndrome or vasculitis.

Although leukopenia is associated with Felty's syndrome, it also may result from toxicity of gold, penicillamine, and immunosuppressive drugs. Leukocytosis is seen commonly as a result of corticosteroid treatment.

The erythrocyte sedimentation rate (ESR) is usually elevated in patients with rheumatoid arthritis and other inflammatory diseases. This test is very nonspecific, and although the ESR usually falls as patients respond to therapy, there is a large variability among patients in response to treatment.

Rheumatoid factor is present in 60% to 70% of patients with rheumatoid arthritis. The usual laboratory test for rheumatoid factor is an antibody specific for IgM rheumatoid factor. Patients with rheumatoid arthritis and a negative test for rheumatoid factor may have IgG or IgA rheumatoid factors, but tests for these are not routinely available. Rheumatoid factor tests may be reported positive at a specific serum dilution. Serum is diluted to a standard series of dilutions; the greatest dilution that yields a positive test result will be reported (e.g., rheumatoid factor positive at 1:640). Some laboratories quantify rheumatoid factor rather than using titers. Higher dilutional titers or serum concentrations of rheumatoid factors usually indicate a more severe disease, but like the ESR, the large interpatient variability makes this test difficult to use as a means of assessing patient progress. Rheumatoid factor may be positive in patients without rheumatoid arthritis (Table 91–3).

TABLE 91–3. Diseases Associated with a Positive Rheumatoid Factor

Rheumatic diseases
Rheumatoid arthritis
Sjögren's syndrome (with or without arthritis)
Systemic lupus erythematosus
Progressive systemic sclerosis
Polymyositis/dermatomyositis
Infectious diseases
Bacterial endocarditis
Tuberculosis
Syphilis
Infectious mononucleosis
Infectious hepatitis
Leprosy
Other causes
Aging
Interstitial pulmonary fibrosis
Cirrhosis of the liver
Chronic active hepatitis
Sarcoidosis

Antinuclear antibodies (ANAs) are detected in 25% of patients with rheumatoid arthritis. These antibodies usually have a diffuse pattern of immunofluorescence. Tests for antibodies to double-stranded DNA (usually positive in systemic lupus erythematosus) are negative. Serum complement is usually normal, although complement concentrations of joint fluid often are depressed from consumption secondary to the inflammatory process. In patients with vasculitis, serum complement concentrations may be low.

Synovial fluid usually is turbid because of the large number of leukocytes in inflammatory fluid. White cell counts of 5000 to 50,000/mm^3 are not uncommon in inflamed joints. The fluid is usually less viscous than that in normal joints or in fluid associated with osteoarthritis. Glucose concentrations of joint fluid are normal or low compared with those in serum drawn at the same time as synovial aspirates. The decrease is not as profound as the decrease associated with joint infection or systemic lupus erythematosus.

Radiologic manifestations of rheumatoid arthritis include soft-tissue swelling and osteoporosis near the joint (periarticular osteoporosis). Erosions tend to occur later in the course of the disease and usually are seen first in the MCP and PIP joints of the hands and the MTP joints of the feet. Erosions usually are seen first at the margin of the joint near the interface of the head of the bone with the synovial tissue (Fig. 91–8).

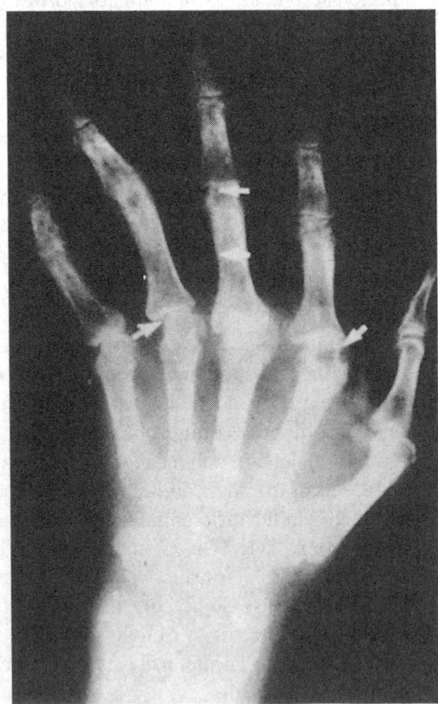

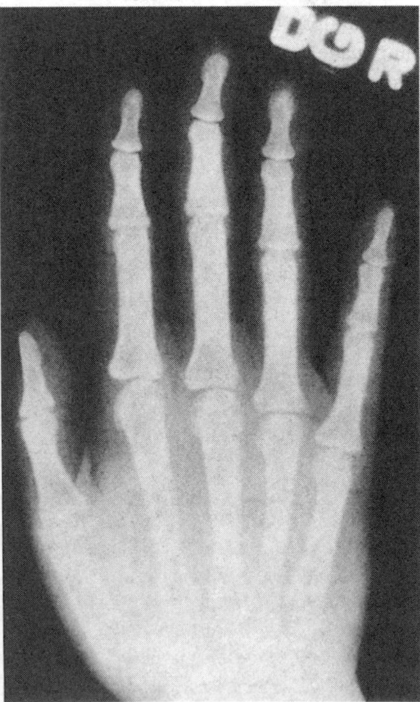

FIGURE 91–8. Radiograph of normal hand (*right*) and hand with rheumatoid arthritis (*left*) with joint-space narrowing, periarticular osteoporosis, and erosions (*see arrows*). *(Reproduced from the Arthritis Foundation Allied Health Professions Teaching Slide Collection, Copyright ©1980, with permission.)*

SERONEGATIVE INFLAMMATORY ARTHRITIS

Although rheumatoid arthritis may have a negative rheumatoid factor titer, a number of other systemic inflammatory arthritic conditions exist including psoriatic arthritis, ankylosing spondylitis and arthritis associated with inflammatory bowel disease. These conditions often tend to be less aggressive than those typically seen with rheumatoid arthritis. Detailed discussion about these conditions is beyond the scope of this chapter, but further information may be found elsewhere.[2] Management principles are similar to those for rheumatoid arthritis.

▶ TREATMENT: Rheumatoid Arthritis

DESIRED OUTCOME

The primary objective is to improve or maintain functional status, thereby improving quality of life. Treatment of rheumatoid arthritis is a multifaceted approach that includes pharmacologic and nonpharmacologic therapies. Recent emphasis has been placed on aggressive treatment early in the disease course. The ultimate goal is to achieve complete disease remission, although this goal is seldom achieved. Additional goals of treatment include controlling disease activity and joint pain, maintaining the ability to function in daily activities or work, improving the quality of life, and slowing destructive joint changes.

NONPHARMACOLOGIC THERAPY

Rest, occupational therapy, physical therapy, use of assistive devices, weight reduction, and surgery are the most useful types of nonpharmacologic therapy used in patients with rheumatoid arthritis. Rest is an essential component of a nonpharmacologic treatment plan. It relieves stress on inflamed joints and prevents further joint destruction. Rest also aids in alleviation of pain. Too much rest and immobility, however, may lead to decreased range of motion and, ultimately, muscle atrophy and contractures.

Occupational and physical therapy can provide the patient with skills and exercises necessary to increase or maintain mobility. These disciplines also may provide patients with supportive and adaptive devices such as canes, walkers, and splints.

Other nonpharmacologic therapeutic options include weight loss and surgery. Weight reduction helps to alleviate inflamed joint stress. This should be instituted and monitored with close supervision of a health care professional. Tenosynovectomy, tendon repair, and joint replacements are surgical options for patients with rheumatoid arthritis. Such management usually is reserved for patients with severe disease.[6,7]

PHARMACOLOGIC THERAPY

Figure 91–9 presents a treatment algorithm for rheumatoid arthritis. This figure reflects a more aggressive treatment approach than has been suggested previously. Prevention of destructive disease is the basis for this treatment strategy. Many rheumatologists believe early introduction of disease-modifying antirheumatic drugs (DMARDs) results in a more favorable outcome. DMARDs include methotrexate, gold, hydroxychloroquine, sulfasalazine, penicillamine, leflunomide, and azathioprine. Biologic agents including etanercept and infliximab have the potential to modify outcomes, but when these agents should be used in relation to other therapies remains to be determined. It has been suggested that they be considered only after patients have failed other DMARDs, including at least methotrexate at doses equal to 25 mg weekly.[8] Some factors identified as predictors for poor outcome include early age of disease onset, high-titer rheumatoid factor, elevated ESR, and swelling of more than 20 joints.

NSAIDs alone do not prevent joint erosions seen in rheumatoid arthritis, possibly because of the limited role prostaglandins play in the inflammatory cascade (see Fig. 91–2). Used as primary therapy, NSAIDs should be given on a scheduled basis in anti-inflammatory doses. This approach should be used only in patients with milder disease and should not be tried for more than 3 months as monotherapy unless the patient demonstrates a satisfactory response. When used

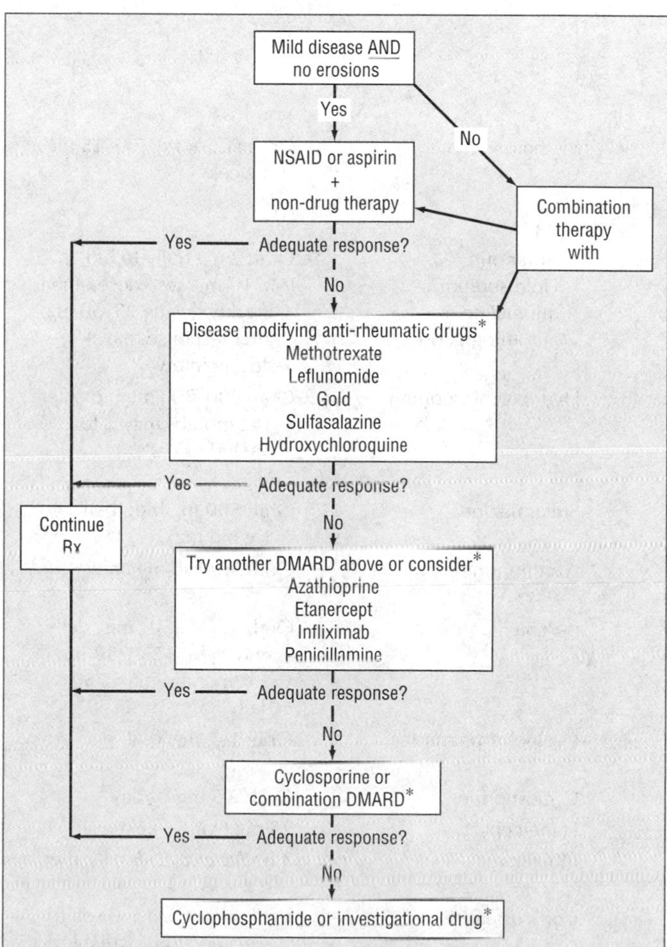

FIGURE 91–9. Algorithm for treatment of rheumatoid arthritis. *Corticosteroids may be necessary for patients with severe inflammatory disease in any of these phases to enable the patient to be more functional while awaiting the beneficial effects of therapy or in patients with partial responses to therapy.

in combination with DMARDs, NSAIDs may be used as adjunctive therapy for symptomatic control. In some patients, as-needed dosing may be adequate.

DMARDs or biologic agents should be used in all patients except those with limited disease or those with class IV disease in whom little reversibility of disease is expected. Of the DMARDs, methotrexate appears to have the best long-term outcome. It is less likely to be discontinued than other DMARDs for reasons of toxicity or lack of efficacy. Gold, hydroxychloroquine, sulfasalazine, azathioprine, or penicillamine should be considered in patients who have contraindications or are refractory to methotrexate (although their long-term usefulness appears to be only about 30% to 40% because of either loss of effect or toxicity). Leflunomide appears to have similar efficacy with methotrexate, although long-term direct comparative studies are lacking.

The biologic agents etanercept and infliximab are options for patients who fail treatment with other DMARDs. Infliximab should be given in combination with methotrexate to prevent development of antibodies that may reduce drug efficacy or induce allergic reactions.

Combination therapy with two or more DMARDs may be effective when single-DMARD treatment is unsuccessful.[9–12] The combinations of cyclosporine plus methotrexate and methotrexate plus sulfasalazine and hydroxychloroquine have been shown to be particularly effective.[11]

Corticosteroids can be used in various ways. They are valuable in controlling symptoms before the onset of action of DMARDs. A burst of corticosteroids can be used in acute flares. Continuous low doses may be adjuncts when DMARDs do not provide adequate disease control. Corticosteroids may be injected into joints and soft tissues to control local inflammation. Steroids seldom should be used as monotherapy because of their high risk of toxicity with chronic use, particularly in high doses. In addition, there are no data to suggest that they alter the disease course. NSAIDs and DMARDs have steroid-sparing properties that permit reductions of steroid doses.

For monitoring parameters and dosing guidelines for DMARDs and NSAIDs used in rheumatoid arthritis, see Tables 91–4 and 91–5.[13–21]

TABLE 91–4. Usual Doses and Laboratory Monitoring Parameters for Antirheumatic Drugs

Drug	Usual Dose	Initial	Maintenance
NSAIDs	See Table 91–6	S_{Cr} or BUN, CBC q 2–4 weeks after starting therapy x 1–2 months Salicylates: serum salicylate levels if therapeutic dose and no response	Same as initial plus stool guaiac q 6–12 months
Methotrexate	Oral, SC, or IM: 7.5–15 mg q week	Baseline: AST, ALT, alk phos, alb, t. bili, hep B & C studies, CBC w/plt, S_{Cr}	CBC w/plt, AST, alb q 1–2 months
Gold			
Auranofin	Oral: 3 mg daily to bid	Baseline: UA, CBC w/plt	Same as initial q 1–2 months
Gold sodium thiomalate or aurothioglucose	IM: 10-mg test dose, then weekly dosing 25–50 mg, after response may ↑ dosing interval	Baseline and until stable: UA, CBC w/plt preinjection	Same as initial every other dose
Hydroxychloroquine	Oral: 200–300 mg bid; after 1–2 months may ↓ to 200 mg bid or daily	Baseline: color fundus photography and automated central perimetric analysis	Ophthalmoscopy q 9–12 months and Amsler grid at home q 2 weeks
Sulfasalazine	Oral: 500 mg bid; then ↑ to 1 g bid max.	Baseline: CBC w/plt, then q week × 1 month	Same as initial q 1–2 months
Azathioprine	Oral: 50–150 mg daily	CBC w/plt, AST q 2 weeks × 1–2 months	Same as initial q 1–2 months
D-Penicillamine	Oral: 125–250 mg daily; may ↑ by 125–250 mg q 1–2 months, max. 750 mg daily	Baseline: UA, CBC w/plt, then q week × 1 month	Same as initial q 1–2 months, but q 2 weeks if dose change
Cyclophosphamide	Oral: 1–2 mg/kg/day	UA, CBC w/plt q week x 1 month	Same as initial q 2–4 weeks
Cyclosporine	Oral: 2.5 mg/kg/day	S_{Cr}, blood pressure q month	Same as initial
Etanercept	25 mg twice weekly	None	None
Infliximab	3 mg/kg at 0, 2, 6 wks, then q 8 wks	None	None
Corticosteroids	Oral, IV, IM, IA, and soft tissue injections: variable	Glucose, blood pressure q 3–6 months	Same as initial plus bone density studies q 12 months

Key: alb = albumin; alk phos = alkaline phosphatase; ALT = alanine aminotransferase; AST = aspartate aminotransferase; BUN = blood urea nitrogen; CBC = complete blood count; hep = hepatitis; IA = intraarticular; IM = intramuscular; IV = intravenous; plt = platelet; q = every; S_{Cr} = serum creatinine; SC = subcutaneous; t. bili = total bilirubin; UA = urinalysis.

TABLE 91–5. Clinical Monitoring of Drug Therapy in Rheumatoid Arthritis

Drug	Toxicities Requiring Monitoring	Symptoms to Inquire About[a]
NSAIDs and salicylates	GI ulceration and bleeding, renal damage	Blood in stool, black stool, dyspepsia, nausea/vomiting, weakness, dizziness, abdominal pain, edema, weight gain, shortness of breath (SOB)
Corticosteroids	Hypertension, hyperglycemia, osteoporosis[b]	Blood pressure if available, polyuria, polydipsia, edema, SOB, visual changes, weight gain, headaches, broken bones or bone pain
Azathioprine	Myelosuppression, hepatotoxicity, lymphoproliferative disorders	Symptoms of myelosuppression (extreme fatigue, easy bleeding or bruising, infection), jaundice
Gold (intramuscular or oral)	Myelosuppression, proteinuria, rash, stomatitis	Symptoms of myelosuppression, edema, rash, oral ulcers, diarrhea
Hydroxychloroquine	Macular damage, rash, diarrhea	Visual changes including a decrease in night or peripheral vision, rash, diarrhea
Methotrexate	Myelosuppression, hepatic fibrosis, cirrhosis, pulmonary infiltrates or fibrosis, stomatitis, rash	Symptoms of myelosuppression, SOB, nausea/vomiting, lymph node swelling, coughing, mouth sores, diarrhea, jaundice
Penicillamine	Myelosuppression, proteinuria, stomatitis, rash, dysgeusia	Symptoms of myelosuppression, edema, rash, diarrhea, altered taste perception, oral ulcers
Sulfasalazine	Myelosuppression, rash	Symptoms of myelosuppression, photosensitivity, rash, nausea/vomiting
Etanercept	Local injection-site reactions, infection	Symptoms of infection
Infliximab	Immune reactions, infection	Postinfusion reactions, symptoms of infection

[a]Altered immune function increases infection, which should be considered particularly in patients taking azathioprine, methotrexate, and corticosteroids or other drugs as a symptom of myelosuppression.
[b]Osteoporosis is not likely to manifest early in treatment, but all patients should be taking appropriate steps to prevent bone loss.
From American College of Rheumatology Ad Hoc Committee on Clinical Guidelines. Guidelines for monitoring drug therapy in rheumatoid arthritis. Arthritis Rheum 1996;39:723–731.

NONSTEROIDAL ANTI-INFLAMMATORY DRUGS

NSAIDs generally are accepted as first-line therapy for the symptomatic treatment of mild rheumatoid arthritis (Table 91–6). NSAIDs possess both analgesic and anti-inflammatory properties and reduce stiffness associated with rheumatoid arthritis. NSAIDs mainly inhibit prostaglandin synthesis, which is only a small portion of the inflammatory cascade (see Fig. 91–2). NSAIDs alone will not prevent joint erosions, and most rheumatologists advocate early combination therapy with DMARDs except in very minimal disease.[16] Cyclooxygenase-2 (COX-2)-specific NSAIDs have a better gastrointestinal safety profile and similar therapeutic efficacy as conventional NSAIDs.[22,23] For discussion of the mechanism of action, adverse effects, and drug interactions, see the anti-inflammatory drugs section of Chapter 92.

METHOTREXATE

Methotrexate (MTX) is now considered the DMARD of choice by many rheumatologists for treating rheumatoid arthritis. In psoriatic arthritis it not only treats the joint symptoms but also improves the skin disease for most patients. MTX is contraindicated in pregnant and nursing women. It is also contraindicated in patients with chronic liver disease, immunodeficiency, pleural or peritoneal effusions, leukopenia, thrombocytopenia, preexisting blood disorders, and a creatinine clearance of less than 40 mL/min.

Absorption of MTX is variable and averages about 70% of an oral dose. MTX is 35% to 50% bound to albumin; it may be displaced by highly protein-bound drugs such as NSAIDs, but the clinical importance of this interaction is not known. MTX is extensively metabolized intracellularly to polyglutamated derivatives. It is excreted by the kidney, 80% unchanged, by glomerular filtration and active transport. Some MTX may be reabsorbed, but this transport process may be saturated even with low doses, resulting in increased renal clearance.

MTX inhibits cytokine production, inhibits purine biosynthesis, and may stimulate release of adenosine, all of which may lead to its anti-inflammatory properties. The drug has a fairly rapid onset of action; results may be seen as early as 2 to 3 weeks after starting therapy. Some 45% to 67% of patients remain on MTX therapy in studies ranging from 5 to 7 years.[24–26] MTX may be given intramuscularly, subcutaneously, or orally. Doses greater than 15 mg per week generally are given parenterally because of decreased oral bioavailability of larger doses.

The toxicities of MTX therapy are mainly gastrointestinal, hematologic, pulmonary, and hepatic. Stomatitis occurs in 3% to 10% of patients and may be painful or painless. Diarrhea, nausea, and vomiting may occur in up to 10% of patients. The most common hematologic toxicity is thrombocytopenia in 1% to 3% of patients. Leukopenia also may occur, but in a smaller number of patients. Although pulmonary fibrosis and pneumonitis can be severe adverse effects, they are rare.

Elevated liver enzymes may occur in up to 15% of patients; cirrhosis is rare. Liver function tests, aspartate aminotransferase (AST) or alanine aminotransferase (ALT), should be performed periodically. MTX should be discontinued if these test values show sustained results greater than twice the upper limits of normal. An albumin blood level also should be checked periodically as a sign of liver toxicity because some patients may not have liver inflammation manifested by AST or ALT elevation. Liver biopsy is now recommended before beginning MTX therapy only for patients with a history of excessive alcohol use, ongoing hepatitis B or C infection, or recurring elevation of aspartate aminotransferase. Biopsies during MTX therapy are recommended only for patients who develop consistently abnormal liver function tests.[27]

Since the drug is teratogenic, patients should use contraception to avoid pregnancy and discontinue the drug if conception is planned.

TABLE 91–6. Dosage Regimens and Durations of Antiplatelet Effect for Nonsteroidal Anti-Inflammatory Drugs

Drug	Recommended Anti-Inflammatory Total Daily Dosage		Dosing Schedule	Approximate Duration of Antiplatelet Effect
	Adult	*Children*		
Aspirin	2.6–5.2 g	60–100 mg/kg	qid	14 days
Celecoxib	200–400 mg	—	Daily–bid	None
Diclofenac	150–200 mg	—	tid to qid Extended release, bid	5–10 h
Diflunisal	0.5–1.5 g	—	bid	2–7 days
Etodolac	0.2–1.2 g (max. 20 mg/kg)	—	tid to qid	36 h
Fenoprofen	0.9–3.0 g	—	qid	15–24 h
Flurbiprofen	200–300 mg	—	bid to qid	24–48 h
Ibuprofen	1.2–3.2 g	20–40 mg/kg	tid to qid	5–10 h
Indomethacin	50–200 mg	2–4 mg/kg (max. 200 mg)	bid to qid Extended release, daily	24–48 h
Ketoprofen	150–300 mg	—	tid to qid Extended release, daily	5–10 h
Meclofenamate	200–400 mg	—	tid to qid	24–48 h
Meloxicam	7.5–15 mg	—	Daily	None generally but monitor
Nabumetone	1–2 g	—	Daily to bid	4–7 days
Naproxen	0.5–1.0 g	10 mg/kg	bid Extended release, daily	4 days
Naproxen sodium	0.55–1.1 g	—	bid	4 days
Nonacetylated salicylates	1.2–4.8 g	—	bid to 6×/day	None
Oxaprozin	0.6–1.8 g (max. 26 mg/kg)	—	Daily to tid	8–10 days
Piroxicam	10–20 mg	—	Daily	7–20 days
Rofecoxib	12.5–50 mg	—	Daily	None
Sulindac	300–400 mg	—	bid	4 days
Tolmetin	0.6–1.8 g	15–30 mg/kg	tid to qid	8–16 h

Because it is a folic acid antagonist, MTX can induce a folic acid deficiency. This deficiency is thought to be partly responsible for MTX toxicity, and supplementation with folic acid has been shown to alleviate some adverse effects. Addition of folic acid to an MTX regimen for rheumatoid arthritis does not compromise drug efficacy.[28–32]

LEFLUNOMIDE

Leflunomide is a DMARD that inhibits pyrimidine synthesis, leading to an inhibition of lymphocyte proliferation and modulation of inflammation. It is given as a loading dose of 100 mg daily for 3 days, followed by a maintenance dose of 20 mg daily. Lower doses may be used if patients have gastrointestinal intolerance, complain of hair loss, or have other signs of dose-related toxicity. The loading dose allows the patient to achieve a therapeutic response usually within the first month. The long elimination half-life of the drug (14–16 days) would require the patient to take the drug for months to achieve steady state without a loading dose.

Leflunomide has efficacy similar to MTX for treating rheumatoid arthritis. The drug may cause liver toxicity and is contraindicated in patients with pre-existing liver disease. Patients taking the drug should have ALT monitored monthly initially and periodically thereafter as long as they continue treatment.

The drug is teratogenic, and appropriate contraceptive measures are recommended to avoid pregnancy for all sexually active male and female patients taking the leflunomide. If conception is desired, leflunomide must be discontinued. Because leflunomide undergoes enterohepatic circulation, the drug takes many months to drop to a plasma concentration considered safe during pregnancy ($<0.02\ \mu g/mL$). Cholestyramine may be used to rapidly clear the drug from plasma. Unlike many DMARDs, leflunomide does not produce bone marrow toxicity, so blood cell monitoring is not necessary.[33–36]

GOLD

Gold is available as oral (auranofin) or intramuscular (aurothioglucose or gold sodium thiomalate) dosage forms. The antirheumatic effects of oral or injectable gold may be delayed for 3 to 6 months. Auranofin is poorly absorbed from the gastrointestinal tract, and the extent of distribution to various body compartments is unknown. Urinary excretion accounts for approximately 60% of the drug absorbed. Aurothioglucose and gold sodium thiomalate are absorbed rapidly after intramuscular injection, although aurothioglucose may be absorbed more slowly because it is an oil suspension. Injectable gold is 85% to 95% protein bound. Metabolism of parenteral gold is unknown, but the compounds probably are not degraded to elemental gold. Urinary elimination averages 70%. Both drugs are cleared very slowly from the body; they can be detected in the urine 12 to 15 months after drug discontinuation in patients who have received cumulative doses of 1 g with auranofin or aurothioglucose.

Toxicities of gold compounds are similar whether taken orally or parenterally. Metallic taste can be a harbinger of other adverse effects. Dermatologic effects such as skin rash and stomatitis require discontinuation of gold therapy; patients may be rechallenged with gold after resolution of these side effects if they are not severe. Renal toxicity manifests as proteinuria or hematuria; hematologic toxicity presents as anemia, leukopenia, or thrombocytopenia. These toxicities are reversible if the drug is discontinued. Gastrointestinal events such as nausea, vomiting, and diarrhea resolve with time or dosage decrease and are more common with auranofin. Injectable gold preparations, particularly gold sodium thiomalate, may cause nitrotoid reactions that may involve flushing, palpitations, hypotension, tachycardia, headache, or blurred vision. Such reactions are self-limiting and usually respond to change of gold salt.

Patients may experience increased joint symptoms for 1 to 2 days after an injection. This is referred to as a *postinjection disease flare*. If the flare is severe, therapy must be changed.[16,17]

HYDROXYCHLOROQUINE

The pharmacokinetics of hydroxychloroquine (HCQ) are poorly understood. It is well absorbed orally and widely distributed to body tissues. HCQ is partially metabolized in the liver and is excreted by the kidney. The onset of action of HCQ may be delayed up to 6 weeks, but the drug is considered a therapeutic failure only when 6 months of therapy without a response has elapsed.

The main advantage of HCQ is the lack of myelosuppressive, hepatic, and renal toxicities that may be seen with other DMARDs, which simplifies monitoring. Short-term toxicities of HCQ include gastrointestinal effects such as nausea, vomiting, and diarrhea, which can be managed by taking doses with food. Ocular toxicity includes accommodation defects, benign corneal deposits, blurred vision, scotomas (small areas of decreased or absent vision in the visual field), and night blindness. Although the risk of true retinopathy with HCQ approaches zero, preretinopathy may occur in 2.7% of patients. All patients must understand the importance of adhering to HCQ monitoring guidelines, as delineated in Table 91–5. Any visual change must be reported immediately. Dermatologic toxicities include rash, alopecia, and increased skin pigmentation; neurologic adverse effects such as headache, vertigo, and insomnia usually are mild.[16,37,38]

SULFASALAZINE

Sulfasalazine, a prodrug, is cleaved by bacteria in the colon into sulfapyridine and 5-aminosalicylic acid (5-ASA). It is believed that the sulfapyridine moiety is responsible for the agent's antirheumatic properties, although the exact mechanism of action is not known. Once the colonic bacteria have cleaved sulfasalazine, sulfapyridine and 5-ASA are absorbed rapidly from the gastrointestinal tract. Sulfapyridine distributes rapidly throughout the body, but higher concentrations are found in certain tissues such as serous fluid, liver, and intestines. Both sulfasalazine and its metabolites are excreted in the urine. Antirheumatic effects should be seen in 1 to 2 months.

Use of sulfasalazine is often limited by its adverse effects. Gastrointestinal adverse effects such as nausea, vomiting, diarrhea, and anorexia are the most common. These can be minimized by initiating therapy with low doses and titrating gradually to higher doses, dividing the dose more evenly throughout the day, or using enteric-coated preparations. Rash, urticaria, and serum sickness-like reactions can be managed with antihistamines and, if indicated, corticosteroids. If a hypersensitivity reaction occurs, therapy should be stopped immediately and another DMARD substituted. Sulfasalazine has been associated with leukopenia, alopecia, stomatitis, and elevated hepatic enzymes. It also may cause the patient's urine and skin to turn a yellow-orange color.

Sulfasalazine's absorption can be decreased when antibiotics are used that destroy the colonic bacteria. Sulfasalazine also binds iron supplements in the gastrointestinal tract that can lead to a decreased absorption of sulfasalazine. The administration of these two agents should be separated temporally to avoid this interaction. Sulfasalazine can potentiate warfarin's effects by displacing it from protein-binding sites. Close monitoring of the patient's international normalized ratio (INR) is indicated.[39–41]

AZATHIOPRINE

Azathioprine is a purine analogue that is converted biologically to 6-mercaptopurine and is believed to interfere with DNA and RNA synthesis. Azathioprine is absorbed rapidly after oral dosing and is approximately 30% bound to plasma proteins. The major route of elimination is renal, and doses should be reduced by 25% for patients with creatinine clearances (Cl_{Cr}) of 10–50 mL/min and by 50% for a CL_{Cr} of less than 10 mL/min.

Antirheumatic effects can be seen within 3 to 4 weeks. If no response is seen after 12 weeks at maximal dosages, azathioprine should be discontinued.

The major adverse effect associated with azathioprine use is reversible bone marrow suppression (e.g., leukopenia, macrocytic anemia, pancytopenia, and thrombocytopenia) that appears to be dose-related. When this occurs, it is common practice to stop the drug temporarily until the marrow recovers. Therapy may be reinstituted at a 25% dose reduction. Other adverse effects include gastrointestinal intolerance, oncogenic potential, stomatitis, infections, drug fever, and hepatotoxicity. Allopurinol inhibits xanthine oxidase, which decreases the metabolism of 6-mercaptopurine and increases the likelihood of myelosuppression. If the two agents must be used together, azathioprine should be reduced to approximately 30% of the usual dose.[16,42]

D-PENICILLAMINE

The pharmacokinetics of D-penicillamine (DP), a heavy metal chelating agent, are not well known. The drug is absorbed quickly from the gastrointestinal tract, but food, antacids, and iron will decrease the amount absorbed. The extent of distribution to body tissues is unknown. DP is metabolized in the liver and excreted mainly as inactive disulfide metabolites in the urine and feces.

Therapeutic effects may be delayed 1 to 3 months after starting therapy. Most clinical responses are seen within 6 months. Early adverse effects of DP include a pruritic, erythematous skin rash, metallic taste, and hypogeusia (decreased taste sensation). Hypogeusia may last 2 to 3 months and resolves without intervention. A rash or metallic taste occurring after 6 months of therapy with DP requires the drug to be decreased or withheld. It may be reinstituted at a lower dose. Stomatitis, which may be painful or painless, usually improves with a decrease in DP dose. Nausea, vomiting, anorexia, and dyspepsia may occur and are managed by dosage reduction. DP may induce glomerular nephritis, which manifests as proteinuria and hematuria. Other autoimmune diseases include polymyositis, Goodpasture's syndrome, myasthenia gravis, systemic lupus erythematosus, and pemphigus. If any of these develop, DP must be discontinued. Although autoimmune diseases are rare, they are the primary reason most clinicians reserve DP for patients with rheumatoid arthritis who are resistant to other therapies.[43]

CYCLOSPORINE

Cyclosporine (CSA) may be considered for treating rheumatoid arthritis in patients who fail more conventional therapies. It is a potent modulator of the immune system that reduces the production of cytokines involved in T-cell activation as well as having direct effects on B cells, macrophages, bone, and cartilage cells. Its absorption is variable and incomplete, and the drug has a large volume of distribution (about 13 L/kg). CSA undergoes hepatic metabolism and has many metabolites; one or more of these may have pharmacologic action. The principal route of elimination is biliary; less than 10% is excreted in the urine.

The onset of action of CSA appears to be 1 to 3 months. Clinically important toxicities of CSA 1–10 mg/kg per day include hypertension, hyperglycemia, nephrotoxicity, tremor, gastrointestinal intolerance, hirsutism, and gingival hyperplasia. Hypertension and nephrotoxicity appear to be reversible after CSA is discontinued.

Because drug therapy for rheumatoid arthritis is long term (perhaps lifelong) and commonly is administered to older adults, the current recommendation is to reserve CSA for patients refractory to or intolerant of other DMARDs. The drug should be avoided in patients with current or past malignancy, uncontrolled hypertension, renal dysfunction, immunodeficiency, low white blood cell or platelet count (unless secondary to Felty's syndrome), or liver function test results greater than twice the upper limits of normal. It should be used cautiously in patients 65 years of age or older and in those with controlled hypertension, pre-malignant conditions, active infection, pregnancy, or lactation. Also, patients taking antiepileptic drugs, ketoconazole, fluconazole, trimethoprim, erythromycin, verapamil, diltiazem, or NSAIDs or who are concurrently using or previously used alkylating agents such as cyclophosphamide should use CSA with caution.[44–46]

BIOLOGIC AGENTS

Etanercept

Etanercept is a fusion protein consisting of two p75 soluble TNF receptors linked to an Fc fragment of human IgG_1. The drug binds to TNF, making it biologically inactive and preventing it from interacting with the cell-surface TNF receptors and thereby activating cells.

The drug is given by subcutaneous injection, 25 mg twice weekly, usually through self-injections or administration by a family caregiver. Aside from local injection-site reactions, adverse effects are rare. There have been case reports of pancytopenia and neurologic demyelinating syndromes that have prompted Food and Drug Administration (FDA) warnings, but the incidence of these complications is not known at this time. No laboratory monitoring is required.

Since TNF is important in helping the body fight infection, there is concern that etanercept may predispose patients to serious infection. For this reason, the drug should be avoided in patients with preexisting infection or in those at high risk for developing infection. Those who develop infections while taking etanercept should have their treatment discontinued temporarily.

Most clinical trials have used etanercept in patients who failed DMARDs. Response was seen in 60% to 75% of patients. The drug also has been shown to be useful in juvenile rheumatoid arthritis, for which it is approved by the FDA, and psoriatic arthritis. It has been shown in clinical trials to slow erosive disease progression to a greater degree than oral methotrexate therapy.[16,17,47–51]

Infliximab

Infliximab is a chimeric antibody combining portions of mouse and human IgG_1. An anti-TNF antibody was created by exposing mice to human TNF. The binding portion of that antibody was fused to a human constant-region IgG_1 to reduce the antigenicity of the foreign protein. This antibody, when injected in humans, binds to TNF and prevents its interaction with TNF receptors on inflammatory cells.

Infliximab is given by intravenous infusion at a dose of 3 mg/kg at 0, 2, and 6 weeks and then every 8 weeks. To prevent the formation of antibodies to this foreign protein, MTX should be given orally in doses typically used to treat rheumatoid arthritis for as long as the patient continues on the drug.

The drug may increase risk of infection, with upper respiratory infections being the most common. An acute infusion reaction with symptoms including fever, chills, pruritus, and rash may occur within 1 to 2 hours after giving the drug. Autoantibodies and lupus-like syndrome also have been reported. In clinical trials, the combination of methotrexate plus infliximab halted progression of joint damage in patients and was superior to MTX monotherapy.[16,17,47,48,52]

CORTICOSTEROIDS

Corticosteroids are used in rheumatoid arthritis for their anti-inflammatory and immunosuppressive properties. They interfere with antigen presentation to T-lymphocytes, inhibit prostaglandin and leukotriene synthesis, and inhibit neutrophil and monocyte superoxide radical generation. Corticosteroids also impair migration and cause redistribution of monocytes, lymphocytes, and neutrophils, thus blunting the inflammatory and autoimmune responses.

Oral corticosteroids are absorbed rapidly and completely from the gastrointestinal tract. They are metabolized and inactivated primarily by the liver and excreted in the urine. The elimination half-life of most corticosteroids is sufficiently long that once-daily dosing is possible.

Oral corticosteroids can be used in several ways. They can be used in bridging therapy, continuous low-dose therapy, and short-term high-dose bursts to control flares. Oral steroids (e.g., prednisone, methylprednisolone) can be used to control pain and synovitis while DMARDs are taking effect. This is termed *bridging therapy* and is often used in patients with debilitating symptoms when DMARD therapy is initiated. Patients with difficult-to-control disease may be placed on low-dose, long-term corticosteroid therapy to control their symptoms. Prednisone doses below 7.5 mg daily are well tolerated but are not devoid of the long-term adverse effects associated with corticosteroids. The lowest dose of corticosteroid that controls symptoms should be used to reduce adverse effects. Alternate-day dosing of low-dose oral corticosteroids usually is ineffective in rheumatoid arthritis; symptoms usually flare on days without medication. High-dose corticosteroid bursts often are used to suppress disease flares. High doses are sustained for several days until symptoms are controlled, followed by a taper to the lowest effective dose.

Corticosteroids also may be delivered by injection. The intramuscular route is preferable in patients with compliance problems, since a depot effect is achieved. Depot forms of corticosteroids include triamcinolone acetonide, triamcinolone hexacetonide, and methylprednisolone acetate. This provides the patient with 2 to 8 weeks of symptomatic control. The depot effect provides a physiologic taper, avoiding hypothalamic-pituitary axis (HPA) suppression. It should be noted that the onset of effect via this route may be delayed by several days. Intravenous corticosteroids may be used to provide the patient with large amounts of drug during a steroid burst to control severe symptoms. Intra-articular injections of depot forms of corticosteroids can be useful in treating synovitis and pain when a small number of joints are affected. The onset and duration of symptomatic relief are similar to those of intramuscular injection. The intraarticular route often is preferred because it is associated with the fewest number of systemic adverse effects. If efficacious, intra-articular injections may be repeated every 3 months. No one joint should be injected more than two to three times per year because of the risk of accelerated joint destruction and atrophy of tendons. Soft tissues such as tendons and bursae also may be injected. This may help control the pain and inflammation associated with these structures. The onset and duration of symptomatic relief are similar to those of intramuscular and intra-articular injections.

Adverse effects are the major limitations to the long-term use of corticosteroids. They include HPA suppression, Cushing's syndrome, osteoporosis, myopathies, glaucoma, cataracts, gastritis, hypertension, hirsutism, electrolyte imbalances, glucose intolerance, skin atrophy, and increased susceptibility to infections. To minimize these effects, use the lowest effective corticosteroid dose and limit the duration of use. Patients on long-term therapy should be given calcium and vitamin D (and estrogen supplements for postmenopausal women) to minimize bone loss. Alendronate, etidronate, or calcitonin may be necessary in patients with evidence of clinically important bone loss. There is no evidence that corticosteroids alone increase the risk of gastrointestinal ulcerations, even though they have been implicated often. Therefore, gastrointestinal protective measures usually are not indicated.[53–55]

INTERLEUKIN-1 RECEPTOR ANTAGONIST

Interleukin-1 receptor antagonist (IL-1ra; anakinra; kineret) is a naturally occurring anti-inflammatory cytokine that was nearing approval in the United States when this chapter was prepared. By binding to IL-1 receptors on target cells, it prevents the interaction between IL-1 and the cell.

IL-1 is very important in the pathogenesis of rheumatoid arthritis. It stimulates release of chemotactic factors and adhesion molecules, and these promote migration of inflammatory leukocytes to tissues. It also causes release of factors known to dilate blood vessels and direct cytotoxins that produce connective tissue damage.

In a double-blind, placebo-controlled trial, IL-1ra 150 mg given by daily subcutaneous injection had a response rate of 43% compared with 27% for placebo-treated patients. Less radiographic progression of joint damage was noted in those receiving IL-1ra. Injection-site reactions were the most common adverse effect noted.[56,57]

MISCELLANEOUS THERAPIES

Minocycline has been shown to have antirheumatic activity and may be of benefit in some patients. The mechanism of action is not known. When to use this antimicrobial agent in the management of rheumatoid arthritis remains to be determined.[58]

Although cyclophosphamide has been used in the past for severe rheumatoid arthritis when vasculitis is present, the benefit in most cases is outweighed by potential risks. Of primary concern is the oncogenic potential, but hematologic complications as well as risks associated with immunosupression also have limited its usefulness.[42]

PHARMACOECONOMIC CONSIDERATIONS

The total cost of treating a patient with rheumatoid arthritis is estimated to be between $5000 and $7300 annually (1991 dollars). Of this, drugs account for roughly 10% of the total, excluding monitoring costs. These costs are approximately three times the cost of medical care for patients of similar age and gender without rheumatoid arthritis. However, if biologic agents such as etanercept or infliximab are used, the cost of this drug therapy alone may be as much as $12,000. The costs must be balanced against the high cost of disability on earning potential in these patients. Men with rheumatoid arthritis have average annual wages 50% lower than those of similar age without rheumatoid arthritis. In women with the disease, average annual wages are only 25% of those without. The costs of disability make treatment worth the price if disability can be prevented or delayed and patients can continue to function as productive members of society.[59]

EVALUATION OF THERAPEUTIC OUTCOMES

The evaluation of therapeutic outcomes is based primarily on improvements of clinical signs and symptoms of rheumatoid arthritis. Clinical signs of improvement include a reduction in joint swelling, decreased warmth over actively involved joints, and decreased tenderness to joint palpation. Improvement in rheumatoid arthritis symptoms includes reduction in perceived joint pain and morning stiffness, longer time to onset of afternoon fatigue, and improvement in ability to perform ADLs.

Joint radiographs may be of some benefit in assessing the progression of the disease and should show little or no evidence of disease progression if treatment is effective.

Laboratory monitoring is of little value in monitoring individual patient response to therapy. Monitoring of toxicity of drugs is shown in Tables 91–4 and 91–5. Routine monitoring of patients is essential to the safe use of these drugs. In addition, patients should be questioned about symptoms of the adverse effects outlined in the drug section of this chapter.

CONCLUSION

Rheumatoid arthritis is the most common inflammatory arthritis, affecting approximately 1% of the population. The disease is characterized by symmetrical swelling and stiffness of the involved joints. The stiffness is usually more prominent in the morning. Extra-articular features of rheumatoid arthritis include rheumatoid nodules, vasculitis, and ocular, cardiac, and pulmonary complications. The course of the disease is highly variable. Treatment is aimed at relieving pain and inflammation and maintaining and preserving joint function. The initial drug treatment in patients with mild disease is either aspirin or NSAIDs. Nondrug therapy, including exercise and adequate rest periods, should be used early in the course of treatment. One of the DMARDs such as MTX, gold, or HCQ may be added to NSAID therapy in patients with inadequate response to initial treatment or those with more active disease. Sulfasalazine, penicillamine, and azathioprine may be effective in patients failing to respond to or having serious toxicity to other DMARDs. Combination DMARDs or biologicals may be considered in those who fail adequate trials of single-agent therapy. Corticosteroids are a useful adjunct for treatment, but because of adverse effects, they should be used in the lowest possible dose for the shortest possible treatment interval.

▶ PRINCIPLES OF PHARMACOTHERAPY

- Consider multiple drug regimens, including NSAIDs and DMARDs with or without corticosteroids in all but the mildest forms of rheumatoid arthritis.
- NSAIDs as monotherapy should be given a trial of no greater than 3 months before considering adding a DMARD in patients who do not achieve adequate response to NSAID alone. If adequate response is achieved with a DMARD, an NSAID use can be used "as needed" in many patients.
- Corticosteroids can be used in these three situations: early in treatment to provide symptomatic relief while waiting for a DMARD to work, in low doses chronically for patients who fail to get an adequate response from a DMARD, and in bursts to treat acute flairs of disease.
- When DMARDs used singly are ineffective, combination therapy or biologic agents such as etanercept or infliximab may be used to induce a response.
- Pharmacotherapy is only part of the therapeutic regimen that should include physical therapy, exercise, and rest. Assistive devices and orthopedic surgery also may be necessary in some patients.
- Patients require careful monitoring for toxicity and therapeutic benefit for the duration of treatment.

REFERENCES

1. Harris ED. The clinical features of rheumatoid arthritis. In: Kelly WN, Harris ED, Ruddy S, Sledge CB, eds. Textbook of Rheumatology, 5th ed. Philadelphia, Saunders, 1997: 898–932.
2. Schumacher HR, Klippel JH, Koopman WJ, eds. Primer of the Rheumatic Diseases, 11th ed. Atlanta, The Arthritis Foundation, 1998.
3. Firestein GS. Etiology and pathogenesis of rheumatoid arthritis. In: Kelley WN, Harris ED, Ruddy S, Sledge CB, eds. Textbook of Rheumatology, 5th ed. Philadelphia, Saunders, 1997.
4. Weyand CM, Goronzy JJ. Pathogenesis of rheumatoid arthritis. Med Clin North Am 1997;81:29–55.
5. Hard ER. Extraarticular manifestations of rheumatoid arthritis. Semin Arthritis Rheum 1979;8:151–176.
6. American College of Rheumatology Ad Hoc Committee on Clinical Guidelines. Guidelines for the management of rheumatoid arthritis. Arthritis Rheum 1996;39:713–722.
7. Harris ED. The treatment of rheumatoid arthritis. In: Kelley WN, Harris ED, Ruddy S, Sledge CB, eds. Textbook of Rheumatology, 5th ed. Philadelphia, Saunders, 1997:933–950.
8. Smolen JS, Breedveld FC, Burmester GR, et al. Consensus statement on the initiation and continuation of tumor necrosis factor blocking therapies in rheumatoid arthritis. N Engl J Med 2000;59:504–505.
9. O'Dell JR, Haire CE, Erickson N, et al. Treatment of rheumatoid arthritis with methotrexate alone, sulfasalazine and hydroxychloroquine, or a combination of all three medications. N Engl J Med 1996;334: 1287–1291.
10. Cash JM, Wilder RL. Refractory rheumatoid arthritis: therapeutic options. Rheum Disease Clinics North Am 1995;21:1–18.
11. Verhoeven AC, Boers M, Tugwell P. Combination therapy in rheumatoid arthritis: Updated systematic review. Br J Rheumatol 1998;37:612–619.
12. Pincus T, O'Dell JR, Kremer JM. Combination therapy with multiple disease-modifying antirheumatic drugs in rheumatoid arthritis: A preventive strategy. Ann Intern Med 1999;131:768–774.
13. Luqmani R, Gordon C, Bacon C. Clinical pharmacology and modification of autoimmunity and inflammation in rheumatoid disease. Drugs 1994;47:259–285.
14. Jain R, Lipsky PE. Treatment of rheumatoid arthritis. Med Clin North Am 1997;81:57–83.
15. American College of Rheumatology Ad Hoc Committee on Clinical Guidelines. Guidelines for monitoring drug therapy in rheumatoid arthritis. Arthritis Rheum 1996;39:723–731.
16. Anonymous. Drugs for rheumatoid arthritis. Med Lett Drugs Ther 2000;42:57–64.
17. Schuna AA. Update on treatment of rheumatoid arthritis. J Am Pharm Assoc 1998;38:728–737.
18. Schuna AA, Megeff C. New approaches in the treatment of rheumatoid arthritis. Am J Health Syst Pharm 2000;57:225–237.
19. Li E, Brooks P, Conaghan PG. Disease-modifying antirheumatic drugs. Curr Opin Rheumatol 1998;10:159–168.
20. Cash JM, Klippel JH. Second-line therapy for rheumatoid arthritis. N Engl J Med 1994;330:1368–1375.
21. Conaghan PG, Brooks P. Disease-modifying antirheumatic drugs including methotrexate, gold, antimalarials, and penicillamine. Curr Opin Rheumatol 1995;7:167–173.
22. Langman MJ, Jensen DM, Watson DJ, et al. Adverse upper gastrointestinal effects of rofecoxib compared with NSAIDs. JAMA 1999;282:1929–1933.
23. Silverstein FE, Faich G, Goldstein JL, et al. Gastrointestinal toxicity with celecoxib versus nonsteroidal anti-inflammatory drugs for osteoarthritis and rheumatoid arthritis. JAMA 2000;284:1247–1255.
24. Pincus T, Marcum SB, Callahan LF. Long-term drug therapy for rheumatoid arthritis in seven rheumatology private practices: II. Second line drugs and prednisone. J Rheumatol 1992;19:1885–1894.
25. Jessop JD, O'Sullivan MM, Lewis PA, et al. A long-term 5-year randomized controlled trial of hydroxychloroquine, sodium aurothiomalate, auranofin and penicillamine in the treatment of patients with rheumatoid arthritis. Br J Rheumatol 1998;37:992–1002.
26. Wolfe F, Hawley DJ, Cathey MA. Termination of slow acting antirheumatic therapy in rheumatoid arthritis: A 14-year prospective evaluation of 1017 consecutive starts. J Rheumatol 1990;17:994–1002.
27. Kremer JM, Alarcon GS, Lightfoot RW Jr, et al. Methotrexate for rheumatoid arthritis: Suggested guidelines for monitoring liver toxicity. Arthritis Rheum 1994;37:316–328.
28. Morgan SL, Baggott JE, Vaughn WH, et al. The effect of folic acid supplementation on the toxicity of low-dose methotrexate in patients with rheumatoid arthritis. Arthritis Rheum 1990;33:9–18.
29. Schnabel A, Gross WL. Low-dose methotrexate in rheumatic diseases: Efficacy, side effects and risk factors for sided effects. Semin Arthritis Rheum 1996;39:310–327.
30. Barnworth B, Labat L, Moride Y, Schaeverbeke T. Methotrexate in rheumatoid arthritis: An update. Drugs 1994;47:25–50.
31. Kremer JM. Methotrexate and emerging therapies. Rheum Dis Clin North Am 1998;24:651–658.
32. O'Dell JR. Methotrexate use in rheumatoid arthritis. Rheum Dis Clin North Am 1997;23:779–796.
33. Prakash A, Jarvis B. Leflunomide: A review of its use in active rheumatoid arthritis. Drugs 1999;58:1137–1164.
34. Smolen JS, Kalden JR, Scott DL, et al. Efficacy and safety of leflunomide compared with placebo and sulphasalazine in active rheumatoid arthritis: A double-blind, randomised, multicentre trial. European Leflunomide Study Group. Lancet 1999;353:259–266.
35. Sharp JT, Strand V, Leung H, et al. Treatment with leflunomide slows radiographic progression of rheumatoid arthritis: Results from three randomized trials of leflunomide in patients with active rheumatoid arthritis. Leflunomide Rheumatoid Arthritis Group. Arthritis Rheum 2000;43: 495–505.
36. Strand V, Cohen S, Schiff M, et al. Treatment of active rheumatoid arthritis with leflunomide compared with placebo and methotrexate.

Leflunomide Rheumatoid Arthritis Investigators Group. Arch Intern Med 1999;159:2542–2550.
37. Levy GD, Munz SJ, Paschal J, et al. Incidence of hydroxychloroquine retinopathy in 1207 patients in a large multicenter outpatient practice. Arthritis Rheum 1997;40:1482–1486.
38. Block JA. Hydroxychloroquine and retinal safety. Lancet 1998;351:771.
39. Rains CP, Noble S, Faulds D. Sulfasalazine: A review of its pharmacological properties and therapeutic efficacy in the treatment of rheumatoid arthritis. Drugs 1995;50:137–156.
40. Weinblatt ME, Reda D, Henderson W, et al. Sulfasalazine treatment for rheumatoid arthritis: A metaanalysis of 15 randomized trials. J Rheumatol 1999;26:2123–2130.
41. Box SA, Pullar T. Sulphasalazine in the treatment of rheumatoid arthritis. Br J Rheumatol 1997;36:382–386.
42. Gaffney K, Scott DG. Azathioprine and cyclophosphamide in the treatment of rheumatoid arthritis. Br J Rheumatol 1998;37:824–836.
43. Munro R, Capell HA. Penicillamine. Br J Rheumatol 1997;36:104–109.
44. Horton S, Resman-Targoff BH, Thompson DF. Use of cyclosporine in rheumatoid arthritis. Ann Pharmacother 1993;27:44–46.
45. Richardson C, Emery P. Clinical use of cyclosporine in rheumatoid arthritis. Drugs. 1995;50(Suppl 1):26–36.
46. Tugwell P. International consensus recommendations on cyclosporine use in rheumatoid arthritis. Drugs 1995;50(Suppl 1):48–56.
47. Moreland LW, Heck LW Jr, Koopman WJ. Biologic agents for treating rheumatoid arthritis. Arthritis Rheum 1997;40:397–409.
48. Maini RN, Taylor PC. Anticytokine therapy for rheumatoid arthritis. Annu Rev Med 2000;51:207–229.
49. Jarvis B, Faulds D. Etanercept: A review of its use in rheumatoid arthritis. Drugs 1999;57:945–966.
50. Lovell DJ, Giannini EH, Reiff A, et al. Etanercept in children with polyarticular juvenile rheumatoid arthritis. N Engl J Med 2000;342:763–769.
51. Bathon JM, Martin RW, Flieschmann RM, et al. A comparison of etanercept and methotrexate in patients with early rheumatoid arthritis. N Engl J Med 2000;343:1586–1593.
52. Lipsky PE, van der Heijde DMFM, St. Clair EW, et al. Infliximab and methotrexate in the treatment of rheumatoid arthritis. N Engl J Med 2000;343:1594–1602.
53. Kirwan JR and the Arthritis and Rheumatism Council Low-Dose Glucocorticoid Study Group. The effect of glucocorticoids on joint destruction in rheumatoid arthritis. N Engl J Med 1995;333:142–146.
54. Moeser PJ. Corticosteroid therapy for rheumatoid arthritis: Benefits and limitations. Postgrad Med 1991;90:175–182.
55. Caldwell JR, Furst DE. The efficacy and safety of low-dose corticosteroids for rheumatoid arthritis. Semin Arthritis Rheumatol 1991;21:1–11.
56. Bresnihan B, Alvaro-Garcia JM, Cobby M, et al. Treatment of rheumatoid arthritis with recombinant human interleukin-1 receptor antagonist. Arthritis Rheum 1998;41:2196–2204.
57. Jiang Y, Genant HK, Watt I, et al. A multicenter, double-blind, dose-ranging, randomized, placebo-controlled study of recombinant human interleukin-1 receptor antagonist in patients with rheumatoid arthritis. Arthritis Rheum 2000;43:1001–1009.
58. Trentham DE, Dynesius-Trentham RA. Antibiotic therapy for rheumatoid arthritis: Scientific and anecdotal appraisals. Rheum Dis Clin North Am 1995;21:817–834.
59. Pincus T. Underestimated long-term medical and economic consequences of rheumatoid arthritis. Drugs 1995;50(Suppl 1)1:1–14.

92

OSTEOARTHRITIS

Larry E. Boh and Mary Elizabeth Elliott

Osteoarthritis (OA) is the most common joint disease, affecting nearly 50% of those over 65 years of age and almost all individuals over age 75.[1] Public health implications of OA are substantial, in that it ranks second only to cardiovascular diseases in causing severe chronic disability.[1–4] Concern about the human and economic costs of this disease have prompted exciting recent advances concerning etiology and treatment.

OA affects primarily the weight-bearing joints of the axial and peripheral skeleton, causing pain, limitation of motion, deformity, and progressive disability. Other names for OA include *osteoarthrosis, degenerative joint disease* (DJD), and *hypertrophic arthritis,* but these terms have shortcomings. OA implies lack of inflammation and excess materials in the joint, DJD suggests a wearing out of the joint, and hypertrophic arthritis describes the overgrowth of bone and cartilage that is only one aspect of OA.

The term *osteoarthritis* best reflects degenerative changes that occur in cartilage, a metabolically dynamic tissue, and the associated bone. OA is characterized by increased destruction and subsequent proliferation of cartilage and bone. The regenerated articular surfaces do not possess the same qualities and architecture as the original joint, and overgrowth of cartilage and bone leads to pain, decreased or altered motion, crepitus, and possibly local inflammation.[5–9] The pain of OA typically is worsened with use and relieved with rest. Morning stiffness of short duration and "gelling" of the joints after inactivity are also common.

The inflammation associated with OA is usually mild or localized, in contrast to that of rheumatoid arthritis or other inflammatory disease. As such, the major goals of OA therapy are to alleviate pain and other symptoms, minimize disability, and educate the patient.[8,9] Nonpharmacologic therapy is the foundation of OA management. It includes patient education, strengthening and range-of-motion exercises, use of assistive devices, joint protection, and weight loss as necessary. Pharmacologic therapy is based on treatment with nonopioid analgesics such as acetaminophen, followed by nonsteroidal anti-inflammatory drugs (NSAIDs), often at analgesic doses, inhibitors specific for the cyclooxygenase-2 (COX-2) enzyme when indicated, and topical analgesic creams containing capsaicin or methylsalicylate. Opioid analgesics and intraarticular glucocorticoid injections are best limited to those with specific clinical features or lack of response to other therapies. New therapeutic approaches are being developed based on recent information on chondrocyte metabolism and control of proteases that contribute to cartilage destruction.

EPIDEMIOLOGY

OA is the most prevalent of the rheumatic diseases, responsible for enormous disability and loss of productivity.[1,10–15] Prevalence increases with age, and radiographic data show that OA at some skeletal site occurs in the majority of people older than 65 years of age and in nearly everyone over 75 years of age.[1,10] Despite intense epidemiologic study, the exact prevalence of OA is unknown owing to the uncertainties and variations of diagnostic definition and reporting mechanisms.[10,13] Another confounder is that many patients with radiographically apparent OA do not have symptoms that lead them to medical care.

PREVALENCE BY AGE, SEX, AND RACE

In the United States, the most frequently cited series of prevalence data is reported by the National Centers for Health Statistics (NCHS).[4] These are the National Health Interview Survey (NHIS) and the National Health and Nutrition Examination Survey (NHANES), based on probability samples of the U.S. civilian, noninstitutionalized population over age 20. Using this information, an estimated 15.8 million adults, or 12% of those between 25 and 74 years of age, have signs and symptoms of OA. Prevalence of OA increases with age. In those younger than age 45, about one-fifth had OA of the hands or feet in the most recent survey; for those aged 75 to 79 years, 85% and 51% had OA in the hands and feet, respectively. OA of the knee occurred in less than 0.1% of those aged 25 to 34 years but in 10% to 20% for those aged 65 to 74 years. OA severity also increases with age. For those between 65 and 74 years of age, 33% had moderate to severe knee OA, and 50% had moderate to severe hip OA. The National Arthritis Data Workgroup, using NHANES and other data, has projected that by the year 2020, 18.2% of Americans (59.4 million people) will be affected by OA.[4]

In the United States, men and women are about equally affected by OA, but older women are twice as likely as men to have OA of the knee and hands.[1,11,12] Women are also more likely to have inflammatory OA involving the proximal and distal joints of the hands, giving rise to the formation of Bouchard's and Heberden's nodes, respectively.[1] One study, based on 6585 randomly selected individuals in a Dutch village, confirmed the increased prevalence and severity of OA by sex.[14] In those aged 65 to 70 years, 75% of women but less than 60% of men had OA of the distal intraphalangeal joint (Fig. 92–1).

Racial, ethnic, and urban-rural differences in OA prevalence are difficult to establish because of variations in sampling procedures and diagnostic criteria. Knee OA appears to be twice as prevalent in black as opposed to white women.[4] Chinese, East Indian, and Native American people have lower incidences of hip OA than do Caucasians.[10] These differences, possibly related to lifestyle, occupation, and genetic variation, underscore the variety of factors to consider in evaluating prevalence data.

INCIDENCE

The overall incidence of hip or knee OA was approximately 200 per 100,000 person-years in a large population-based study.[15] The incidence of hip OA was greater in women than in men, whereas the rate for knee disease did not differ between genders. Rates for knee and hip OA increase with age in men but plateau in postmenopausal women. Based on these population data, one-half million symptomatic cases of idiopathic OA are estimated to occur annually in the U.S. white population.[15]

A

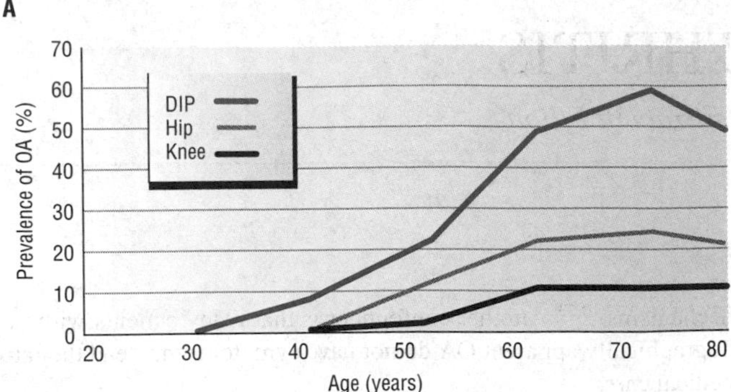

B

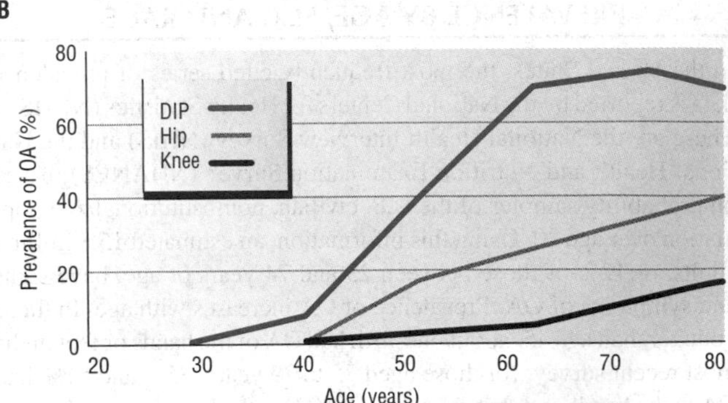

FIGURE 92–1. Prevalence of radiologic OA of the hip, knee, and DIP joints. (*A*) Men. (*B*) Women. *(Adapted from van Saase JL, van Romunde LK, Cats A, et al. Epidemiology of osteoarthritis: Zoetermeer survey. Comparison of radiological osteoarthritis in a Dutch population with that in 10 other populations. Ann Rheum Dis 1989;48:271–280.)*

RISK FACTORS

OBESITY

Increased body weight is strongly associated with hip and knee OA but also is associated with hand OA.[1,11,13,16–18] Obesity often precedes OA, contributing to its development rather than resulting from decreased activity in those with OA. In the Framingham Study, those in the highest quintile of body mass at the beginning of 36 years of follow-up had a relative risk for developing knee OA of 1.5 for men and 2.1 for women. For severe knee OA, these values were 1.9 for men and 3.2 for women. In a study of 1108 men followed for 36 years, body mass indices of men in their twenties were associated with later development of OA.[19] A twin study in women showed that for every additional kilogram of body mass, the risk of later developing OA increased by 9% to 13%.[20] In obese persons without OA, weight loss of even 5 kg decreased by one-half their risk of later developing knee OA.[16] In addition to being a risk factor for OA, obesity is also a predictor for the necessity of prosthetic surgery for OA.[21]

OCCUPATION, SPORTS, AND TRAUMA

Those participating in activities involving repetitive motion or injury are at increased risk for developing OA. Workers exposed to repetitive stress of the hands or lower limbs are at higher risk for OA of the stressed joints.[6,17,22] Lower extremity OA in some professional sports is also increased, likely secondary to repetitive motion, trauma to the joint, loss of ligament integrity, or damage to the meniscus. Risk for OA depends on the type and intensity of physical activity. Framingham Study results showed that heavy physical activity increases knee OA risk, especially in the obese, whereas moderate or light activity does not.[23]

Interestingly, long-distance runners are not at higher risk of developing OA.[24] Age at injury does matter because older individuals who damage ligaments tend to develop OA more rapidly than the young person when similarly injured.

Finally, there are interesting inverse associations between quadriceps strength and knee OA and disability. Quadriceps weakness, once thought to result from disuse atrophy in OA patients, may precede and even contribute to the development of OA, possibly through decreased knee stability.[25,26]

GENETIC FACTORS

Heredity plays a role with some osteoarthritis.[10,17] Heberden's nodes are 10 times more prevalent in women than in men, with twofold higher risk if the woman's mother had them. Genetic links also have been forged with OA of the first metatarsophalangeal joint and with generalized OA. Premature development of OA is associated with a defect in type II procollagen.[1,27] The discovery of a genetic link between the cartilage matrix and OA may shed light on disease development and has the potential to aid in screening and treatment strategies in certain groups of patients.

OSTEOPOROSIS

An inverse correlation between OA and osteoporosis has been demonstrated, and both men and women with OA have increased bone mineral density at numerous skeletal sites.[6,17,28–30] This relationship may derive from the influence of body weight on both disease states because heavy individuals have higher bone density as well as increased risk of OA. Despite their lower risk of osteoporosis, individuals with OA are not protected against fracture. OA patients tend to be less posturally stable and more likely to fall, so despite the higher bone density, their fracture rates are similar to those of patients without OA.[10,29,30]

PATHOPHYSIOLOGY

In OA, cartilage and the associated joint are affected. Improved understanding of articular cartilage physiology has transcended the wear-and-tear theory of OA. Some changes in the OA joint may reflect compensatory processes to maintain function in the face of ongoing joint destruction.[1,5,6,31–34] As such, the pathogenesis of OA involves not only biomechanical forces but also inflammatory, biochemical, and immunologic factors.

Before discussing these factors, a review of OA classification and diagnostic criteria is warranted. OA falls into two major etiologic classes. *Primary (idiopathic) OA,* the most common, has no identifiable cause. Subclasses of primary are *localized OA,* involving one or two sites, and *generalized OA,* affecting three or more sites. *Erosive arthritis* is used to describe disease when underlying bone is affected. *Secondary OA* is that associated with a known cause[31,35,36] (Table 92–1). These include trauma, metabolic or endocrine disorders, and congenital factors.

To aid uniform reporting of rheumatic diseases, a classification scheme and criteria for OA of the hip, knee, and hand were devised by the American College of Rheumatology (ACR).[8,9,37] Criteria include subjective and objective factors, including pain, bony changes on examination, erythrocyte sedimentation rate (ESR), and radiographic features consistent with OA. For hip OA, a patient must have hip pain

TABLE 92–1. Classification of Osteoarthritis

Primary (Idiopathic)	Secondary
Localized	Trauma—acute/chronic
Generalized	Underlying joint disorder
	Local (fracture/infection)
	Diffuse (rheumatoid arthritis)
Erosive	Systemic metabolic or endocrine disorders
	Wilson's disease
	Acromegaly
	Hyperparathyroidism
	Hemochromatosis
	Paget's disease
	Diabetes mellitus
	Obesity
	Crystal deposition disease
	Basic calcium phosphate crystal disease
	Calcium pyrophosphate dihydrate
	Hydroxyapatite
	Other calcium-containing crystals
	Monosodium urate monohydrate
	Neuropathic disorders
	Intra-articular corticosteroid overuse
	Avascular necrosis
	Bone dysplasia

Compiled from Refs. 31, 35, and 36.

plus two of the following: ESR of less than 20 mm/h, radiographic femoral or acetabular osteophytes, or radiographic joint space narrowing. For knee OA, a patient must have knee pain and radiographic osteophytes plus one of the following: age greater than 50 years, morning stiffness of 30 minutes or less duration, or crepitus on motion.

To understand the pathophysiology of OA, familiarity with the normal joint is essential. To this end, a review of the biochemistry and function of normal cartilage and of the diarthrodial joint is provided. Excellent detailed reviews of cartilage and bone biochemistry and function are available.[5–7,31,33,34]

NORMAL CARTILAGE

FUNCTION

In the diarthrodial joint (Fig. 92–2), cartilage provides a low-friction surface covering the concave and convex ends of the bone. Cartilage has viscoelastic properties that provide lubrication with motion, shock absorbency during rapid movements, and load support. Its major features are to (1) enable movement within the required range of motion, (2) distribute a load across joint tissues, thereby preventing damage, and (3) stabilize the joint during use. It is avascular, aneural, and alymphatic with a calcified base over a thin layer of cortical bone, the subchondral plate. Cartilage is easily compressed, losing up to 40% of its original height when a load is applied. Compression increases the area of contact and disperses force more evenly to underlying bone. Because cartilage is thin (2–5 mm), loading energy is transmitted from it to bone, tendons, ligaments, and muscle surrounding the joint.

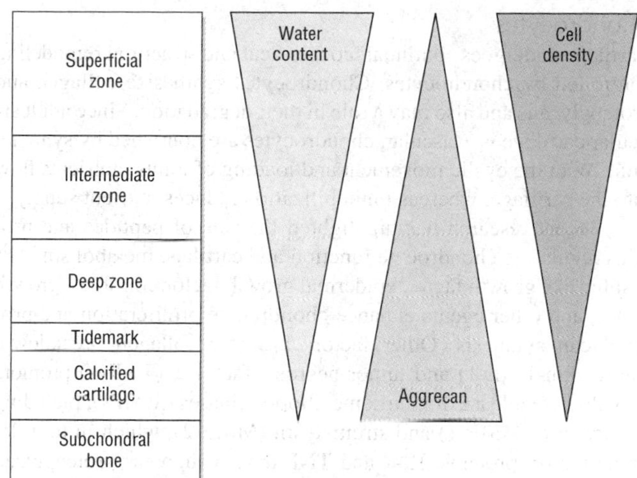

FIGURE 92–3. Structure and composition of articular cartilage by zone. *(Adapted from Refs. 5 and 6.)*

STRUCTURE AND BIOCHEMICAL COMPOSITION OF CARTILAGE

Articular cartilage is a hydrated (75% to 80% water), complex extracellular matrix (ECM) with a small number of chondrocytes (<5%). The remaining 20% to 25% of matrix contains three types of molecules: collagens, large aggregates of proteoglycans, and noncollagenous proteins. Cartilage has four zones: a superficial or tangential zone, an intermediate or transitional zone, the deep or radial zone, and the calcified cartilage zone located below the tidemark and above subchondral bone. Zones differ by chondrocyte content, collagen organization, and heterogeneity of proteoglycan components (Fig. 92–3). Within the basal zone, perpendicular type II collagen fibers anchor cartilage to subchondral bone. At the superficial zone, densely packed collagen fibers running parallel to the surface provide a low-shear surface and contribute to smooth working of the joint.

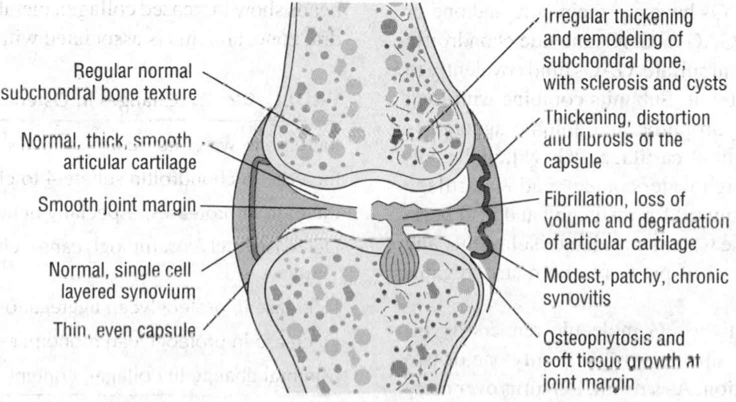

FIGURE 92–2. Characteristics of OA in the diarthrodial joint (right).

Chondrocytes

Cartilage undergoes continual biochemical and structural remodeling controlled by chondrocytes. Chondrocytes synthesize collagen and proteoglycans and also play a role in their degradation. Since adult articular cartilage is avascular, chondrocytes are nourished by synovial fluid. With the cyclic movement and loading of joints, nutrients flow into the cartilage, whereas immobilization reduces nutrient supply.

Recent research has highlighted the role of peptides and proteins regulating chondrocyte function and cartilage metabolism.[5,6,32] Insulin-like growth factor, epidermal growth factor, fibroblast growth factor, and other agents enhance chondrocyte proliferation and proteoglycan synthesis. Other factors promote collagen breakdown. Interleukin-1 (IL-1) and tumor necrosis factor α (TNF-α) promote chondrocyte release of matrix metalloproteinases (MMPs), including collagenase (MMP-1) and stromelysin (MMP-2), which in turn degrade matrix proteins. IL-1 and TNF-α also suppress proteoglycan and collagen synthesis in the ECM.[5,6,32]

There is intense interest in discovering how growth factors regulate chondrocyte function and enhance articular cartilage repair. When reviewing interesting discoveries in this field, one must be cautious about applying findings from one tissue to another, extrapolating in vitro to in vivo data, and developing therapeutic agents to target one factor. Because the actions of growth factors and cytokines have multiple complex roles in the regulation of articular cartilage, they should be viewed more as messengers, effectors, or signaling agents.[6,31,32]

Biomechanical factors, including load and strain, also affect chondrocyte function. In some studies, joint loading markedly increased proteoglycan synthesis.[6] Further examination of interactions among biomechanical, biochemical, and cellular events in cartilage may provide important insights into OA.

Collagen

Five types of collagen (II, IX, X, XI, and VI) are located in cartilage. Type II collagen comprises 90% to 95% of the total collagen in articular cartilage.[5,6,31] Type VI appears to attach chondrocytes to the matrix. Type IX collagen, a proteoglycan, may link matrix molecules together. The cross-linked network of type II collagen fibrils with other ECM proteins provides tensile strength and maintains cartilage volume and shape. Orientation of collagen fibers is critical: Superficial fibers are parallel to the surface, reducing friction and allowing forces to be dissipated; basal layer collagen fibers are perpendicular to the surface to anchor cartilage to the calcified zone or subchondral bony endplate.

Proteoglycans

The cartilage matrix is comprised of large proteoglycan (PG) aggregates within a collagen network. PGs have a protein core and one or more glycosaminoglycan chains (GAGs). GAGs include chondroitin sulfate, keratan sulfate, and dermatan sulfate. GAGs bind covalently to the protein core, forming a PG subunit. Subunits combine with long hyaluronate molecules to form hydrophilic and anionic aggregates that maintain the high water content of cartilage. PGs within the collagen network, coupled with the high water content, endow cartilage with the viscoelastic properties required for resiliency and load bearing. Under pressure, the PGs release water and enhance solute flux and chondrocyte nutrition; with removal of pressure, the matrix regains water.

The structural complexity of the PG molecule renders it vulnerable to degradation by MMPs, since cleavage of only one or two peptide bonds can destroy its function. As a result, PG turns over more rapidly than collagen. When protease degradation of PGs has been induced experimentally, cartilage has maintained its shape but lost its elasticity.[5,6]

With degradation of the ECM, collagen and PG fragments are released into the synovial fluid, eventually reaching the blood and urine. Methods to identify and quantitate these fragments are being sought as potential aids in diagnosis or monitoring of disease and also may provide insights into metabolic changes in OA.

OSTEOARTHRITIC CARTILAGE

BIOCHEMICAL CHANGES

Numerous compositional differences have been noted between cartilage in OA and in normal individuals (Table 92–2). Early in OA, cartilage water content increases. The resulting cartilage is thicker but is less able to resist mechanical forces. These changes are poorly understood but may reflect a damaged collagen fiber network unable to properly constrain PGs, with the result that PGs gain water.[5,6,31] In addition, with more severe disease, cartilage PG content decreases, possibly through the action of MMPs.

Changes in GAG composition also occur, with decreased keratan sulfate and an increased ratio of chondroitin-4-sulfate to chondroitin-6-sulfate. These changes may interfere with proper collagen-PG interaction in cartilage. Increased collagen synthesis and altered distribution and diameter of the fibers are seen, but collagen content does not appear to change until severe disease is present.[5,6,31]

Earlier theories suggested that cartilage was passively eroded in OA, but in fact, there is increased metabolic activity, suggesting a reparative response to damage.[5,6,31] Despite the increased matrix synthesis controlled by the chondrocytes, there continues to be a loss of PG, reflecting a net loss as degradation proceeds faster than synthesis.

Destruction of cartilage occurs in two ways. For the intrinsic pathway, chondrocytes themselves degrade the cartilaginous matrix. The extrinsic pathway involves inflamed synovium, pannus, and inflammatory cells. Intense research efforts are directed toward understanding the roles of MMPs and other collagen-degrading enzymes. MMPs are zinc-containing proteinases falling into five related subgroups. MMPs normally are held in check by tissue inhibitors of metalloproteinases (TIMPs), but substances that activate MMPs also exist and are elaborated by chondrocytes.[38,39] Imbalance between MMPs and TIMPs in synovial fluid or local tissues can lead to proteolysis of the ECM, promoting osteoarthritic changes. Recent work showed that cartilage from osteoarthritic human joints exhibited increased collagen-degrading activity colocalized with increased levels of MMP mRNA.[40]

In addition to abnormal cartilage turnover in OA, collagen metabolism in bone is also increased. Osteoarthritic human femoral heads show increased collagen metabolism, especially in the subchondral zone, and this is associated with increased MMP-2 (stromelysin)

TABLE 92–2. Changes in Osteoarthritic Cartilage

Increase in water content
Increase in chondroitin sulfate-4 to chondroitin sulfate-6 ratio
Increase in proteases, especially neutral metalloproteinases
Decrease in glycosaminoglycans—chondroitin sulfate and keratan sulfate
Decrease in proteoglycan aggregation
Decrease in proteoglycan monomer size
Minimal change in collagen content

Compiled from Refs. 5, 6, and 31.

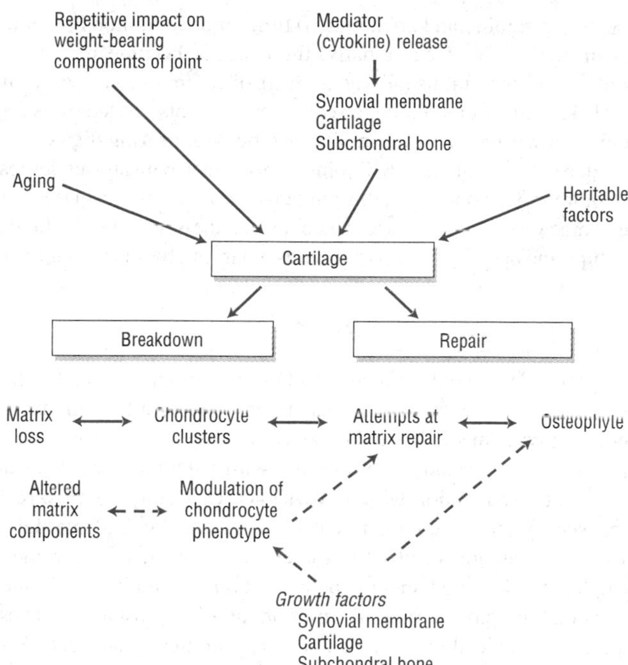

FIGURE 92–4. Factors contributing to the development of osteoarthritis. *(From Hamerman D. The biology of osteoarthritis. N Engl J Med.1989;320:1322–1330, with permission.)*

activity. This highly localized increased bone collagen metabolism may relate to changes in joint structure, thereby contributing to disease progression in OA.[41]

In summary, the slow progressive changes in OA consist of an increase in water content, loss of PG, and reduction of PG aggregates of cartilage. This results in failure of the cartilage to repair itself. Alterations in bone can occur in association with cartilage destruction. The series of pathologic changes results in loss of cartilage, structural changes in bone, and ultimately, severe pain. An overview of the development of OA is shown in Fig. 92–4.

PATHOLOGIC CHANGES

Pathologic changes in bone and cartilage accompany the biochemical changes just described. Intermediate- and late-stage changes in OA are characterized in humans, and animal models have provided insight into early events in OA. Changes are similar for weight-bearing compared with non-weight-bearing joints and for idiopathic OA compared with secondary OA. The following changes are observed in cartilage[5,6,31,33,34]:

1. Initial thickening of articular cartilage as ECM is damaged and water content increases
2. Proliferation of chondrocytes and increase in ECM anabolic and catabolic activity secondary to tissue damage or alterations in ECM structure
3. Decline in response of chrondrocytes to stabilize or restore tissue, resulting in progressive cartilage loss
4. Possible moderate inflammation of the joint synovial lining
5. Fibrillation or splitting of the noncalcified cartilage, likely related to the biochemical changes described earlier (This exposes the underlying bone, which ultimately may lead to microfractures of the subchondral bone.)

As cartilage is destroyed, subchondral bone undergoes pathologic changes, particularly for those areas especially lacking of protective cartilage. Below the superficial layer, increased osteoblast and osteoclast activity associated with osteolytic foci is seen. Exposed bone may contain fibrous or chondroid tissue, presumably reflecting reactive bone resorption and vascular changes. With continued progression of OA, cartilage is eroded completely, leaving denuded subchondral bone to become dense, smooth, and glistening (eburnation). A more brittle, stiffer bone results, with decreased weight-bearing ability and development of sclerosis and microfractures.[5,6,31,33,34] Microfractures lead to callus and osteoid production. New bone formation at the joint margins, away from the area of cartilage destruction, is referred to as *osteophytes.* An interesting observation is that osteophytes can occur in the absence of cartilage destruction, and conversely, cartilage destruction can occur in the absence of osteophytes. Osteophytes may be an attempt to stabilize joints rather than a destructive aspect of OA.

The joint capsule and synovium also show pathologic changes in OA. Inflammation, such as synovitis, occurs and may result from release of inflammatory mediators from chondrocytes, such as prostaglandins.[5,6,31,33,34] Inflammation is localized to the affected joint, in contrast to that seen in rheumatoid or other inflammatory arthritides.

SIGNS AND SYMPTOMS

The clinical presentation of OA (Table 92–3) depends on duration and severity of disease and the number of joints affected. The predominant symptom is a localized, deep, aching pain associated with the affected joint. If more than one joint is involved or if systemic symptoms are present, another form of arthritis or connective tissue disease should be considered. However, many patients with pathologically or radiographically documented OA are asymptomatic.[42]

Early in OA, pain accompanies joint activity and decreases with rest. With progression, pain occurs with minimal activity or at rest. Pain is not related to the destruction of cartilage, which lacks pain fibers. Rather, the pain arises from the activation of nociceptive nerve endings by the mechanical and chemical irritants related to joint pathology.[43] Sources of OA pain can be related to the periosteum, increased intraosseous pressure, microfracture, and damage to ligaments, synovium, and meniscus.[43] Pain caused by bursitis, tendonitis, or muscular pain may complicate the clinical presentation and requires an accurate diagnosis. OA patients report changes in OA symptoms with certain weather conditions.

Joints most affected in primary OA are the distal interphalangeal (DIP) and proximal interphalangeal (PIP) joints of the hand, the first carpometacarpal (CMC) joint, knees, hips, cervical and lumbar spine, and the first metatarsophalangeal (MTP) joint of the toe. Limitation of motion, stiffness, crepitus, and deformities may occur. Limitation of motion is related to loss of articular surfaces, muscle spasms, capsular contracture, and mechanical blockage secondary to osteophytosis. Patients also may register decreased range of motion of an affected joint by describing limitations in activities of daily living. A sense of weakness or instability (the joint "gives way") is also reported by patients with lower extremity involvement.

Joint stiffness, typically less than 30 minutes, commonly accompanies OA, unlike the longer stiffness associated with rheumatoid arthritis. Stiffness resolves with motion and is described as a "gelling phenomenon." Crepitus is a crackling or grating sound heard with joint movement, caused by irregularity of joint surfaces. Joint enlargement is related to bony proliferation or to thickening of the

TABLE 92–3. Clinical Presentation of Osteoarthritis

Age
Usually elderly
Sex
Age <45 more common in men
Age >45 more common in women (hands)
Symptoms
Pain
Deep, aching
Pain on motion
Early in disease—pain with use
Late in disease—pain at rest
Stiffness
Rarely exceeds 15 min; related to weather
Localized to involved joints
Limited joint motion
Instability of weight-bearing joints
Crepitus, crackling
Signs/Physical Examination
Monoarticular or oligoarticular; asymmetrical involvement
Joints frequently involved
Hands—DIP, PIP, first carpometacarpal joint
Foot—first metatarsophalangeal joint
Hips, knees, cervical spine, lumbar spine
Observations on Joint Examination
Bony proliferation or occasional synovitis
Local tenderness
Crepitus
Muscle atrophy
Limited motion with passive/active movement
Effusions
Characteristics of Synovial Fluid
High viscocity
Mild leukocytosis (<2000 WBC/mm^3)
Laboratory Values
No specific test
ESR, hematologic survey, chemistry survey are normal
No systemic manifestations

DIP = distal interphalangeal; PIP = proximal interphalangeal; ESR = erythrocyte sedimentation rate.
Compiled from Refs. 7, 17, 32, and 35.

synovium and joint capsule. The presence of a warm, red, tender joint may suggest an inflammatory type of synovitis.

Joint deformity may be present in the later stages of OA as a result of subluxation, collapse of subchondral bone, formation of bone cysts, or bony overgrowths. Patient descriptions of joint swelling require close clinical inspection to separate synovial thickening (inflammation) from the bony proliferation observed in OA.

PHYSICAL EXAMINATION

Examination of the affected joints reveals tenderness, crepitus, and possible joint enlargement.[17,35,37] Physical examination findings in OA, in contrast to that for rheumatoid arthritis, are shown in Fig. 91–3.

HANDS

OA of the hand mainly affects the DIP, PIP, and first CMC joints. Heberden's and Bouchard's nodes are bony enlargements (osteophytes) of the DIP and PIP joints, respectively. Heberden's nodes usually develop slowly, are painless, appear on lateral and medial aspects of the joint, and are about 10 times more common in women than in men.[17,35,37] Occasionally, these nodes become red, warm, swollen, and painful, usually as a result of trauma or use. A strong female hereditary predominance can often be demonstrated by asking the patient whether her own mother had bony-appearing digits.

In patients with first CMC joint involvement, pain and tenderness are common. Osteophytes at this joint give the radial aspect of the hand the characteristic square appearance termed the *shelf sign*. Difficulty pinching and opening the tops of bottles or jars is a frequent complaint.

KNEES

The knee is commonly affected in OA. It is important to localize the symptoms because the joint has three separate articulations: the patellofemoral, medial, and lateral compartments. Pain related to climbing stairs typically is associated with patellofemoral joint involvement. Presentation with a bowlegged deformity (genu varum) is caused by medial compartment involvement; knock-knee deformity (genu valgum) results from lateral compartment involvement. Symptoms of knee OA include pain, tenderness, crepitation, limited extension with passive or active motion, and joint instability. These symptoms may lead to decreased activity and muscle atrophy. Transient joint effusions also may occur. The synovial fluid typically is noninflammatory (white blood cell count < 2000/mm^3 with normal protein).

HIPS

Hip OA is common in the elderly. The symptoms are associated with three patterns of hip joint involvement: superolateral, medial pole, and concentric. Hip OA is associated with buttock or groin pain with weight bearing, standing, or walking. Stiffness is common, especially after inactivity, and joint motion may be limited. Pain located on the outside of the hip typically is bursitis and should not be confused with hip OA.

SPINE

Degenerative changes result from involvement of the intervertebral disks, vertebral bodies, or posterior apophyseal articulations. In the spine, L3 and L4 involvement is most common. If there is nerve root compression, this is associated with pain, paresthesias, loss of reflexes, and muscle weakness in the distribution of the affected nerve root.

FEET AND OTHER JOINTS

Involvement of the feet is limited primarily to the first MTP joint. Pain, tenderness, and stiffness are the predominant symptoms.

Other joints not commonly involved include the shoulder, elbow, and acromioclavicular, sternoclavicular, and temporomandibular joints.

LABORATORY FINDINGS

No specific clinical laboratory abnormalities occur in *primary* OA.[17,35,37] ESR, routine chemistry studies, complete hematologic profiles, and urinalysis generally are normal. The ESR may be slightly elevated in patients with generalized or erosive inflammatory OA. The rheumatoid factor test is negative. Analysis of synovial fluid reveals fluid with high viscosity. A mild leukocytosis (<2000 white blood cells/mm^3) with predominantly mononuclear cells can be seen. If secondary OA is suspected, specific laboratory tests can help identify the cause.

RADIOLOGIC EVALUATION

Radiologic evaluation is an absolute necessity in the diagnosis of OA.[17,35,37] Radiographic changes are often absent in early, mild OA. With disease progression and loss of cartilage, there can be joint space narrowing, subchondral bony sclerosis, and development of marginal osteophytes and cysts. In late OA, subluxation and deformity can occur. Osteopenia and joint erosions are uncommon except in erosive OA. Published radiographic grading scale criteria are available for clinical trial assessments, but standardization of criteria is essential to ensure reproducibility.[37,42]

Technetium-99m studies often can detect changes in early OA when plain radiographs may not show differences. Newer techniques—computed tomography, magnetic resonance imaging, and ultrasound—have been used but are not suitable for routine use in OA.[17,31,32,37,42] Joint arthroscopic examination can confirm a diagnosis or establish the extent of OA in a particular joint but is rarely needed for an OA diagnosis.

DIAGNOSIS

The diagnosis of OA is critically dependent on patient history, clinical examination of the affected joint(s), and radiologic findings. The major diagnostic goals are (1) to distinguish patients with OA from other connective tissue diseases that may involve DIP joints, such as psoriatic arthritis or Reiter's syndrome, and (2) to identify patients with secondary OA. Diagnosis is relatively straightforward, but a complete examination of all clinical information is necessary before an accurate diagnosis be made. The ACR has published algorithms for the classification of patients with OA of the hands, knees, and hips.[8,9,37] These criteria serve as useful guidelines both for clinical practice and for clinical trial outcomes.

PROGNOSIS

The prognosis for patients with primary OA is variable and depends on the joint involved. If a weight-bearing joint or the spine is involved, considerable morbidity and disability are possible. In the case of secondary OA, the prognosis depends on the underlying cause. Available treatment of the cause may prevent further progression but does not reverse joint changes already present.

▶ TREATMENT: Osteoarthritis

DESIRED OUTCOME

Management of the patient with OA begins with a diagnosis based on a careful history, clinical examination, radiologic findings, and an assessment of the extent of joint involvement. Treatment should be tailored to the individual. It always includes patient education and can include, as necessary, physical and occupational therapy, weight management, drug therapy, and surgery. Goals are (1) to educate the patient, caregivers, and relatives, (2) to relieve pain and stiffness, (3) to maintain or improve joint mobility, (4) to limit functional impairment, and (5) to maintain or improve quality of life.[44]

GENERAL APPROACH TO TREATMENT

Treatment for the OA patient depends on the distribution and severity of joint involvement, comorbid disease states, concomitant medications, and allergies (Fig. 92–5). Management for all individuals with OA should begin with patient education, with physical and occupational therapy, and with weight loss and assistive devices as needed.

Since drugs do not change disease course, they are targeted toward symptoms. For most patients, there will not be a significant inflammatory component, and pharmacologic treatment is intended for pain relief, in contrast to anti-inflammatory therapy for those with rheumatoid arthritis. Scheduled acetaminophen, up to 4 g/d, should be tried initially. If this is ineffective, low-dose NSAIDs can be tried, with specific COX-2 inhibitors preferable for some patients. Short-term use of opioid analgesics, with or without acetaminophen or NSAIDs, can be effective for flares, but long-term opioid use is discouraged. Application of capsaicin or methyl salicylate topical creams over specific joints can be used in combination with oral acetaminophen or NSAIDs for added pain relief.

For those with knee effusions, joint aspiration followed by glucocorticoid injection can relieve pain. Caution is required in this approach because of the risk for infection. It is limited to three or four injections per year because of the risk of cartilage destruction.[9] Intraarticular (IA) injections of hyaluronate can be tried, but this is not a proven therapy. If symptoms are intractable, or if there is functional joint impairment, an orthopedic surgeon can be consulted.

Finally, for patients interested in clinical trials, investigational strategies with oral doxycycline, matrix metalloproteinase inhibitors (MMPIs), intramuscular injection of pentosan polysulfate and polysulfated glycosaminoglycans, or cartilage transplants may be considered.

NONPHARMACOLOGIC THERAPY

The first step in OA treatment is patient education about OA, about the extent of the patient's disease, the prognosis, and what is to be done. Education is paramount, in that OA is often seen as a "wear and tear" disease, an inevitable consequence of aging for which nothing helps. Even worse, patients may resort to the use of alternative but unproven medications or quackery. Patients should be warned about these and encouraged to access information from local or national units of the Arthritis Foundation (Atlanta, Georgia) or at *http://www.arthritis.org*. The Arthritis Foundation provides literature about OA and OA medications, as well as information about local clinics and agencies offering physical and economic assistance. The Arthritis Foundation also sponsors support groups and public education programs.

The benefits of patient education have been highlighted in a variety of programs, including those using monthly telephone contact between trained volunteers and individuals with OA.[45–47] Volunteers speak with patients about symptoms, function, drugs, and clinic visits, with the result of improved pain and functional status at low cost. Likewise, OA patients participating in the Arthritis Foundation's

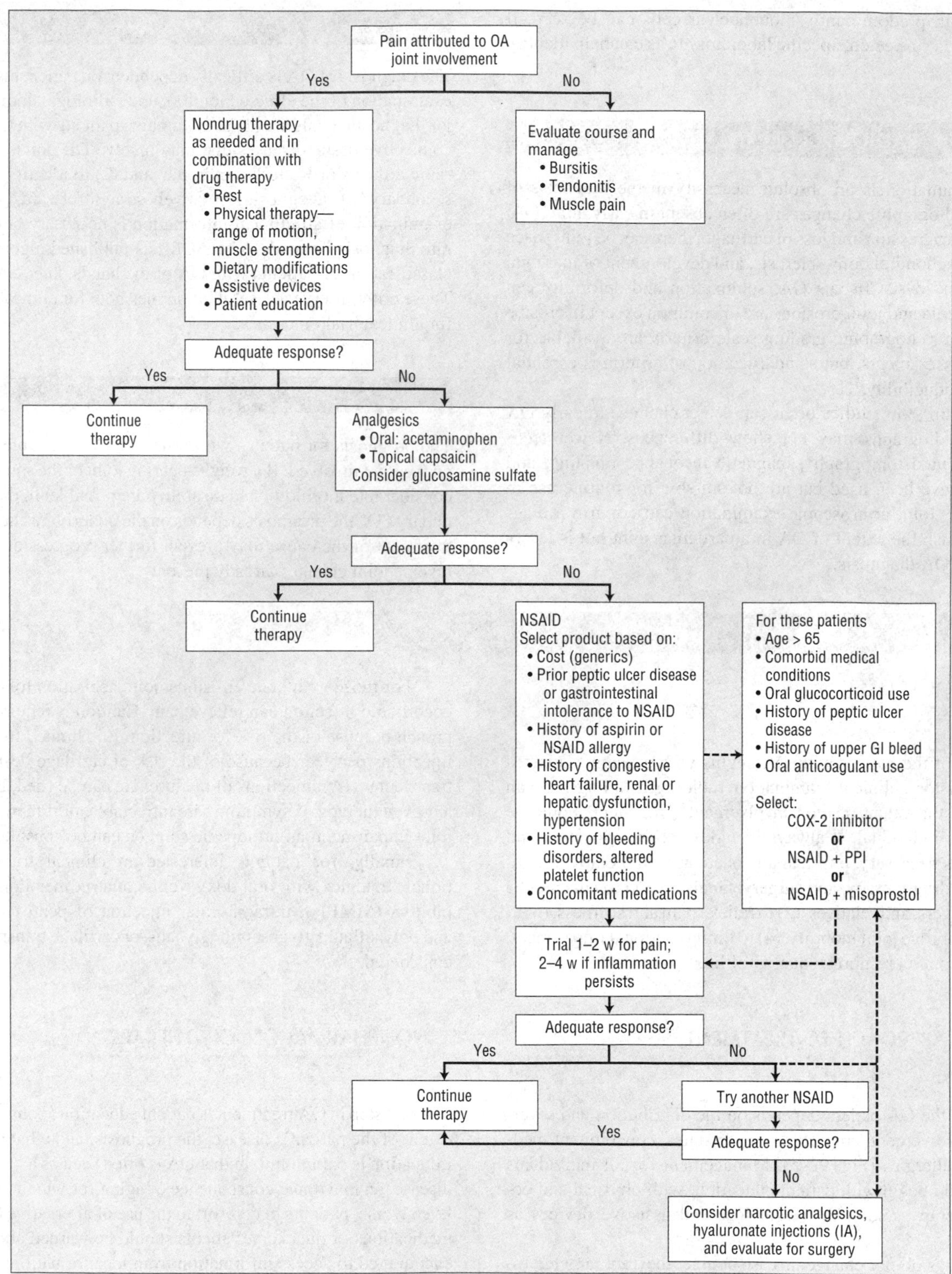

FIGURE 92–5. Treatment for OA.

Self-Management Program reported decreases in joint pain and OA-related clinic visits and increased physical activity and quality of life.[48]

DIET

Dietary counseling for the overweight OA patient is warranted given the clear association between obesity and OA. Excess weight increases the biomechanical load on weight-bearing joints[49] and can contract the muscles that span and stabilize joints. Weight loss is associated with decreased symptoms and decreased disability,[50–52] but controlled studies are needed to confirm benefits. Although dietary intervention for overweight OA patients is reasonable, weight loss usually requires a motivated patient and a structured weight-loss program.

GLUCOSAMINE AND CHONDROITIN

OA has proven to be a disease whose symptoms can be alleviated but whose progress has been impossible to stop. Because of this, clinicians were very interested to learn in early 2001 that the dietary supplement glucosamine had shown evidence in clinical studies of providing disease-modifying therapy in patients with OA. If these findings are confirmed as glucosamine becomes used more widely, it would be the first such agent identified for OA. In one clinical trial, joint space in patients' knees decreased significantly among those taking placebo, according to baseline and posttherapy x-ray films. However, among patients taking glucosamine sulfate 1500 mg once daily for 3 years, joint space decreased slightly but not significantly so. Symptoms improved in those taking glucosamine but worsened among patients taking placebo.[53,54]

In practice, glucosamine is often combined with the shark cartilage derivative chondroitin sulfate. Interest in these two agents was spurred initially by anecdotal reports of patient benefit, by the fact that these substances stimulate proteoglycan synthesis from articular cartilage in vitro, by their use in veterinary medicine, and because they appear to be well tolerated. At this point, the relative contribution of chondroitin is uncertain, and it is the more expensive component of the dual therapy. A metaanalysis concluded that the combination probably has "some degree of efficacy" for treatment of OA.[55]

In addition, glucosamine and chondroitin are marketed in the United States as dietary supplements, and neither the products nor their purity is regulated effectively by the Food and Drug Administration (FDA).

PHYSICAL AND OCCUPATIONAL THERAPY

Physical therapy—with heat or cold treatments and an exercise program—helps to maintain and restore joint range of motion and reduce pain and muscle spasms. Warm baths or warm water soaks may decrease pain and stiffness. Heating pads should be used with caution, especially in the elderly, and patients should be warned not to fall asleep on the heat source or to lie on it for more than brief periods to minimize the risk of burns. Exercise programs for OA can strengthen muscles and improve joint function and motion.[56] Isometric exercise is preferred over isotonic exercises because the latter can aggravate the affected joint. Quadriceps strengthening and exercise programs can improve physical functioning and can decrease disability, pain, and analgesic use.[57–60] Exercises should be taught and then observed before the patient exercises at home. Exercises should be performed three to four times daily. If severe pain develops with exercise, the patient should be instructed to decrease the number of repetitions.

The decision about whether to encourage walking should be made carefully on an individual basis. With weak or deconditioned muscles, the load is transmitted excessively to the joints, so weight-bearing activities can exacerbate symptoms. However, avoidance of activity by those with hip or knee OA leads to further deconditioning. A program of patient education, muscle stretching and strengthening, and supervised walking can improve physical function and decrease pain in patients with knee OA.[16] Guidelines for exercises in OA can be obtained from the Arthritis Foundation.[59]

Referral to the physical therapist (PT) and occupational therapist (OT) is especially helpful for patients with functional disabilities. The PT can assess muscle strength and joint stability and can recommend exercises and appropriate use of heat. The PT also can provide assistive and orthotic devices, such as canes, walkers, braces, heel cups, and insoles for use in exercise or for daily activities. The OT can provide guidance in joint protection, energy conservation, and use of assistive devices such as splints. Selection of appropriate activities and assistive devices is highly patient specific and requires that the patient be instructed carefully in their use.

SURGERY

Surgery can be recommended for OA patients with severe pain unresponsive to conservative therapy or that causes substantial functional disability and interference with lifestyle.[61,62] For patients with mild disease of the knee, an osteotomy will correct the misalignment of genu varum or genu valgum. Joint debridement can be used to remove free cartilage fragments, eliminate locking, and reduce pain. However, the ACR regards this as unproven therapy because of a lack of well-controlled studies. If osteophytes are large, removal may increase range of motion. For advanced disease, a partial or total arthroplasty can relieve pain and possibly improve motion, especially with hip surgery. Indications for total hip replacement were developed by a National Institutes of Health (NIH) consensus development conference,[61] and indications for total-knee replacement were summarized based on three consensus groups of orthopedic surgeons.[62] Arthrodesis (joint fusion) can reduce pain but will restrict motion. Restorative approaches involve soft tissue grafts, penetration of subchondral bone, cell transplantation, and use of growth factors or artificial matrices.[63] The cartilage that is formed does not duplicate normal articular cartilage in its composition, structure, or mechanical properties. Cartilage-restoration approaches are investigational, and results regarding pain control and joint function have been mixed.

PHARMACOLOGIC THERAPY

Drug therapy in OA is targeted at relief of pain. OA is seen commonly in older individuals who have other medical conditions, and OA treatment is often long term. As such, a conservative approach to drug treatment, focusing on the needs of the individual patient, is warranted (see Fig. 92–5). For mild or moderate pain, topical analgesics or simple oral analgesics can be used. If these measures fail, or if there is inflammation, NSAIDs may be useful. Even when drug therapy is initiated, appropriate nondrug therapies should be continued and reinforced because these are the cornerstone of OA management and may provide as much relief as drug therapy.

ANALGESICS

Osteoarthritic pain can arise from several sites. Pain can result from osteophyte growth with stretching of the periosteum, microfractures, synovitis, and damage to ligaments and meniscus.[43] Cartilage itself contains few nerve endings and thus is not a direct source of pain.

The oral analgesic of choice is acetaminophen, 325–650 mg four times daily, with a maximum dose of 4 g/d. In the case of acetaminophen failure, nonaspirin NSAIDs are used most often next, and aspirin is not specifically recommended for use in OA.[44]

However, aspirin continues to prove useful for some OA patients, and the discussion here will focus on basic concepts regarding aspirin use in inflammatory arthritis. To counter inflammation, the dose of aspirin needs to be at least 3.6 g/d. Although serum concentration monitoring is not routine with analgesic doses, pharmacokinetic considerations may warrant monitoring of serum salicylate concentrations when anti-inflammatory doses are used or when questions of efficacy or toxicity arise.

Elimination of salicylate is by zero-order kinetics, so the serum half-lives range from 2 hours for analgesic doses to more than 20 hours for anti-inflammatory doses. Aspirin is highly protein-bound, so increasing doses result in higher free-drug levels as binding sites saturate. Low serum albumin, increasing age, and concomitant use of highly protein-bound drugs can increase salicylate toxicity. Another variable affecting aspirin pharmacokinetics is urinary pH, since an alkaline urine promotes salicylate excretion. Therapeutic salicylate concentrations range from 15 to 25 mg/dL, whereas tinnitus can occur with levels above 30 mg/dL. A number of acetylated and nonacetylated salicylate products exist (Table 92–4), and several factors should be considered in selecting a product.

First, salicylates can cause adverse gastrointestinal effects ranging from mild discomfort to gastric ulcers with severe complications.[64,65] To minimize gastrointestinal upset, salicylates should be taken with food or milk. Enteric-coated products cause less gastric mucosal injury compared with buffered or plain aspirin,[65] but these should not be taken with antacids or milk, which can alter the coating. Nonacetylated salicylates also produce less gastrointestinal irritation and bleeding than does aspirin.[66]

Second, the decreased platelet aggregation observed with aspirin is not seen with the nonacetylated salicylate products.[66] As such, nonacetylated salicylates are safer alternatives in patient with a bleeding disorders or who are scheduled for surgery.

Third, some patients are aspirin-intolerant.[67] Aspirin ingestion can trigger two types of reactions. Type A is characterized by bronchoconstriction, vasomotor rhinitis, nasal polyps, and/or laryngeal

TABLE 92–4. Medications Commonly Used in the Treatment of Osteoarthritis

Medication	Dosage and Frequency	Maximum Dosage (mg/d)
Oral Analgesics		
Acetaminophen	325–650 mg every 4–6 hours or 1 g 3–4 times/day	4000
Tramadol	50–100 mg every 4–6 hours	400
Topical Analgesics		
Capsaicin 0.025% or 0.075%	Apply to affected joint 3–4 times per day	—
Nutritional supplements		
Glucosamine sulfate	500 mg 3 times/day or 1500 mg once daily	1500
Nonsteroidal Anti-inflammatory Drugs (NSAIDs)		
Carboxylic acids		
Acetylated salicylates		
Aspirin, plain, buffered, or enteric-coated	325–650 mg every 4–6 hours for pain. Anti-inflammatory doses start at 3600 mg/day in divided doses	3600[a]
Nonacetylated salicylates		
Salsalate	500–1000 mg 2–3 times a day	3000[a]
Diflunisal	500–1000 mg 2 times a day	1500
Choline salicylate[b]	500–1000 mg 2–3 times a day	3000[a]
Choline magnesium salicylate	500–1000 mg 2–3 times a day	3000[a]
Acetic acids		
Etodolac	800–1200 mg/day in divided doses	1200
Diclofenac	100–150 mg/day in divided doses	200
Indomethacin	25 mg 2–3 times a day; 75 mg SR once daily	200; 150
Ketorolac[c]	10 mg every 4–6 hours	40
Nabumetone[d]	500–1000 mg 1–2 times a day	2000
Propionic acids		
Fenoprofen	300–600 mg 3–4 times a day	3200
Flurbiprofen	200–300 mg/day in 2–4 divided doses	300
Ibuprofen	1200–3200 mg/day in 3–4 divided doses	3200
Ketoprofen	150–300 mg/day in 3–4 divided doses	300
Naproxen	250–500 mg twice a day	1500
Naproxen sodium	275–550 mg twice a day	1375
Oxaprozin	600–1200 mg daily	1800
Fenamates		
Meclofenamate	200–400 mg/day in 3–4 divided doses	400
Mefenamic acid[e]	250 mg every 6 hours	1000
Oxicams		
Piroxicam	10–20 mg daily	20
Meloxicam	7.5 mg daily	15
Coxibs		
Celecoxib	100 mg twice daily or 200 mg daily	200 (400 for RA)
Rofecoxib	12.5–25 mg daily	25 (50 for dysmenorrheic pain)

[a]Monitor serum salicylate levels over 3–3.6 g/day.
[b]Only available as a liquid; 870 mg salicylate/5 mL.
[c]Not approved for treatment of OA for more than 5 days.
[d]Nonorganic acid but metabolite is an acetic acid.
[e]Not approved for treatment of OA.

edema. This occurs in 2% to 4% of asthmatic patients, with cross-sensitivity to other NSAIDs (although a nonacetylated salicylate may be tolerated). Type B is associated with urticaria and angioedema, reactions generally occurring with other salicylates.[67] Other toxic responses to aspirin products include impaired renal function and increases in serum transaminases.

Another factor to consider in product selection is cost. Nonacetylated products are considerably more expensive than plain aspirin.

The ACR recommends the simple analgesic acetaminophen as first-line drug therapy for pain management in OA.[44] Comparable relief of mild to moderate OA pain has been demonstrated for acetaminophen at 2.6–4 g/d, compared with aspirin 650 mg four times daily, ibuprofen at 1200 or 2400 mg daily, naproxen 750 mg/d, and other NSAIDs.[44] However, other studies have reported that patients experienced better pain control with NSAIDs and that NSAIDs may be superior for severe OA pain.[68,69] A metaanalysis of knee OA trials noted that NSAID-treated patients had greater pain relief than those taking analgesics.[68] Other work showed that OA patients preferred NSAIDs to acetaminophen.[69] These differences may reflect the need by some OA patients for anti-inflammatory action, which acetaminophen does not possess. Given the overall merits of acetaminophen concerning efficacy, toxicity, and cost, however, the ACR recommends an initial trial with acetaminophen for OA patients requiring drug therapy.

Although acetaminophen is one of the safest analgesics, its use still carries some risks.[70,71] Rare but potentially fatal hepatotoxicity with overdose is well documented. It should be used with caution in patients with liver disease and avoided in those who chronically abuse alcohol. Although acetaminophen use has been weakly associated with the occurrence of end-stage renal disease, it poses less renal risk than do the NSAIDs, and the National Kidney Foundation recommends acetaminophen as the drug of choice for those with impaired renal function. However, the National Kidney Foundation discourages long-term consumption of acetaminophen and recommends it use only when the patient is supervised by a physician. The National Kidney Foundation also strongly discourages the use of over-the-counter combination analgesic products because this is associated with increased prevalence of renal failure. Finally, patients should be warned about the potential toxicity when they inadvertently ingest more than the recommended dose when using both nonprescription and prescription products containing acetaminophen.

Topical products can be used alone or in combination with oral analgesics or NSAIDs. Capsaicin, isolated from hot peppers, releases and ultimately depletes substance P from afferent nociceptive nerve fibers. Substance P has been implicated in the transmission of pain in arthritis, and capsaicin cream has been shown in four controlled studies to provide pain relief in OA when applied over affected joints.[72,73] To be effective, capsaicin must be used regularly, and it may take several weeks to work. It is well tolerated, except that some patients experience a temporary burning sensation at the site of application. Patients should be warned not to get the cream in their eyes or mouth and to wash their hands after application. Although use is recommended four times a day, tapering the regimen to twice-daily application may enhance long-term adherence and still provide adequate pain relief.[73]

Other analgesics that can be used include tramadol, a centrally acting analgesic, or stronger narcotics such as codeine. These agents often are reserved for patients who have failed single- or multiple-agent therapy with simple analgesics, topical agents, or NSAIDs. Propoxyphene is not more effective than safer analgesics and likely overprescribed, especially in the elderly.[73] Tramadol or other narcotic agents should be reserved for short-term use for severe pain. Ideally, limited quantities should be prescribed, with only one or two refills, to minimize abuse potential and to promote ongoing assessment of OA symptoms. If pain is intolerable and limits activities of daily living, a surgical referral often is preferable to continued reliance on narcotics.

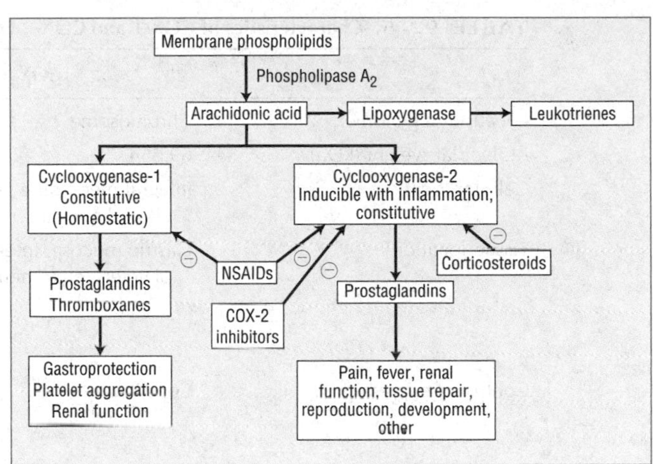

FIGURE 92–6. Pathway of synthesis of prostaglandins and leukotrienes. COX-1 and COX-2 are cyclooxygenase 1 and 2 enzymes. *(Adapted from Refs. 75, 77–79).*

NONSTEROIDAL ANTI-INFLAMMATORY DRUGS

NSAIDs have analgesic properties at lower doses and anti-inflammatory effects at higher doses. NSAIDs from a variety of chemical classes are available (see Table 92–4), and more are in development, particularly COX-2–specific inhibitors.[74–76] All NSAIDs display comparable analgesic and anti-inflammatory efficacy and are similarly beneficial in OA, although individual patient response differs among NSAIDs. Although the mechanism of action of NSAIDs is incompletely understood, blockade of prostaglandin synthesis through inhibition of cyclooxygenase (both COX-1 and COX-2 enzymes) constitutes an important part of NSAID action[75,77] (Fig. 92–6). Given the similar efficacy of nonspecific NSAIDs and COX-2–specific inhibitors, toxicity and cost considerations will play major roles in determining the place in therapy of these extremely widely used agents. It is thus worth understanding how COX-1 and COX-2 enzymes are affected differently by drugs, and in particular, it is worth examining the "COX-2 paradigm"[75,76] to understand differences in toxicity of NSAIDs and COX-2 inhibitors and to understand possible oversimplications in this paradigm.

Prostanoids and the COX-2 Paradigm

Table 92–5 depicts basic facts about cyclooxygenase (COX) enzymes and their inhibition.[75–80] Crucial for the presently marketed COX-2–specific inhibitors is their extremely high specificity, since they have several hundred-fold higher potency against COX-2 than COX-1, exerting virtually no COX-1 activity at therapeutically achievable concentrations. Various experimental systems have been used to assess the COX-2 versus COX-1 selectivity of various NSAIDs, including purified recombinant enzyme, transfected cells, and whole-blood assays, but these systems are not in complete agreement. One of the best methods may be the whole-blood assay, where synthesis of thromboxane from platelets is used to assess COX-1 activity and production of prostaglandin E_2 (PGE_2) in response to lipopolysaccharide addition to measure COX-2.[75]

The basis for selectivity of NSAIDs has been studied intensively.[74,79] Nonspecific NSAIDs penetrate the enzyme active site

TABLE 92–5. Characteristics of COX-1 and COX-2 Enzymes

	COX-1 Enzyme	COX-2 Enzyme
Location in genome	Chromosome 9	Chromosome 1
Molecular weight (kDa)	69,054	69,093
Cellular location	Integral membrane protein in ER and nuclear envelope	Integral membrane protein in ER and nuclear envelope
Tissue location	Gastric mucosa, intestine, kidney, platelets, endothelial cells, other	Macrophages, fibroblasts, chondrocytes, epithelial cells, endothelial cells, synoviocytes, CNS, bone, kidney, reproductive tract, other
Control of expression	Constitutive	Rapidly inducible: inflammation, IL-1, TNF TGF-β mitogens, lipopolysaccharides Constitutive in some tissues
Effect of glucocorticoids	Unaffected	Inhibited (transcriptional level)
Enzymologic function	Arachidonic acid → PGG_2 → PGH_2. (PGH_2 → final products [PGs, PGI_2, TX] depends on tissue)	Arachidonic acid → PGG_2 → PGH_2 PGH_2 → final products (PGs, PGI_2) depends on tissue
Biologic function	Gastrointestinal mucosal integrity, platelet aggregation; renal function; other	Inflammation, development, renal function, reproduction, bone metabolism, other
Kinetics of inhibition by NSAIDs	Immediate, competitive inhibition (strong for COX-1 inhibitors, weak for COX-2 inhibitors)[a]	COX-2 inhibitors: noncompetitive (irreversible?), time-dependent COX-I inhibitors: competitive, immediate

[a]Aspirin inhibition is irreversible.
Compiled from Refs. 75–84.

for both COX-1 and COX-2 and block entry of the enzyme's usual substrate, arachidonic acid. COX-2 inhibitors are much more potent at inhibiting COX-2; they interact with a side pocket within the active site of COX-2, a site missing from COX-1, a feature not exploited by nonspecific NSAIDs. Moreover, COX-2 inhibitors undergo a time-dependent process producing extremely tight binding within the COX-2 active site. This high-affinity—possibly irreversible—binding to COX-2 provides excellent COX-2 inhibition at concentrations with virtually no effect on COX-1. This enzymologic specificity has propelled COX-2–specific inhibitor drugs into a favorable marketing position.

The COX-2 enzyme is not normally expressed in most body tissues, but it is induced rapidly by inflammatory mediators, local injury, and a wide variety of stimuli, including interleukins, interferon, and tumor necrosis factor[77] (see Fig. 92–6 and Table 92–5). COX-1 products perform "housekeeping" or routine and beneficial homeostatic functions such as generation of gastroprotective prostaglandins to promote gastric blood flow and bicarbonate generation. COX-1 is expressed constitutively in gastric mucosa, vascular endothelial cells, platelets, and renal collecting tubules, so COX-1–generated prostaglandins also participate in hemostasis and renal hemodynamic balance. According to the COX-2 paradigm, COX-1 blockade (as with nonspecific NSAIDs) is undesirable and can lead to gastrointestinal ulcers, increased bleeding risk, and compromised renal function in susceptible individuals. Specific COX-2 inhibition is considered desirable for the potential lack of such toxicities while exerting anti-inflammatory and analgesic effects.

Although this paradigm has merit, several issues and observations regarding COX enzymes and NSAIDs require further scrutiny and could carry implications for COX-2 inhibitor safety.[74–86] These observations and issues include the following:

1. Gastroprotection by COX-1 and gastropathy via COX-1 blockade may not be as simple as originally thought. Knockout mice lacking COX-1 do not develop spontaneous gastropathy, but they do develop ulcers when given nonspecific NSAIDs.
2. COX-2 activity in the gastric mucosa may be helpful in some situations. COX-2 is induced with gastric injury and is seen at the rim of ulcers in humans, and COX-2 inhibitors retard ulcer healing in animals and angiogenesis in experimental systems.
3. COX-2 activity may be beneficial in renal function. COX-2 has some constitutive expression in the kidney, and its intrarenal distribution and its upregulation in salt depletion suggest that it helps regulate renal hemodynamics in some situations.
4. COX-2 inhibitor's analgesic mechanism may not be as simple as sometimes viewed because COX-2 inhibitors reduce pain even in noninflammatory conditions.
5. There may be a tendency to overprescribe COX-2 inhibitors, especially in patients who are frail, if the potential toxicities of these agents are unappreciated.
6. Given that aspirin blocks the COX-1 enzyme, the GI safety advantage of COX-2–specific inhibitors may be blunted by the concomitant use of aspirin, even at low doses.
7. Concern has arisen about possible cardiac toxicities of the available COX-2 inhibitors. Patients taking rofecoxib had more thrombotic events than did patients taking naproxen. However, in the Vioxx Gastrointestinal Outcomes Research Study (VIGOR), the antiplatelet effects of naproxen confuse the issue, since it is not

clear whether the cardiac differences resulted from a rofecoxib toxicity, a naproxen benefit, or both. Patients taking rofecoxib also had significantly more adverse events related to hypertension and congestive heart failure.[85,86]

Despite these complexities, good and mounting evidence indicates that COX-2–specific inhibitors relieve pain in many OA patients with a lower risk of GI adverse events than nonspecific NSAIDs. COX-2 inhibitors, members of the "coxib" class newly created by the World Health Organization (WHO),[83] have become extremely widely used over a short period of time. These agents continue to be studied intensely not only for their efficacy and toxicity profile in rheumatic disease but also for exciting potential applications such as the prevention of Alzheimer's disease and colorectal cancer.

Pharmacokinetic and Efficacy Considerations for NSAID Use

Prescription-strength NSAIDs generally are used in patients with OA after treatment with acetaminophen or aspirin proves ineffective or is not tolerated or in patients with inflammation. Selection of an NSAID depends on the prescriber's experience, medication cost, patient preference, toxicities, and adherence issues. All NSAIDs have analgesic and anti-inflammatory effects similar to aspirin, with fewer gastrointestinal complaints.[66,74,87] This last characteristic is advantageous, but most NSAIDs are much more expensive than aspirin, unless generic products such as ibuprofen or naproxen are used.

The various NSAIDs exhibit several pharmacokinetic similarities, the most clinically important difference being serum half-life ranging from 1 hour for tolmetin to 50 hours for piroxicam.[66,77] NSAIDs have high oral availability, are highly protein-bound, and are absorbed as active drugs (except for sulindac and nabumetone, which require hepatic conversion for activity). Elimination of NSAIDs largely depends on hepatic inactivation, with a small fraction of active drug being renally excreted. NSAIDs penetrate joint fluid and achieve levels of approximately 60% of average plasma concentration; this may account for the extended efficacy even of NSAIDs with a short serum half-life.[66,77] Analgesic effects begin in 1 to 2 hours and last up to 24 hours, whereas anti-inflammatory effects may develop over 2 to 3 weeks. Therapeutic drug monitoring for NSAIDs has not yet proven useful.

Patient response to NSAIDs is highly variable, in that a given patient may respond well to one NSAID but poorly to a chemically related NSAID.[66] A recent systematic review of studies of NSAIDs for OA found no evidence to support a definitive ranking of NSAID efficacy.[88] The prescriber often relies on personal experience in choosing an NSAID. To assess efficacy in the individual patient, a trial that is adequate in time (2–3 weeks) and dose (either anti-inflammatory or analgesic) is needed. If the first trial fails, another NSAID in the same or another chemical class can be tried and so on until an effective agent is found. Patients must understand this approach, appreciate the necessity of adherence to medication therapy throughout this process, and actively participate in assessment of drug efficacy. Combination of an NSAID with another NSAID or aspirin increases adverse effects without providing additional benefit.[64–66]

Recent work with COX-2–specific inhibitors showed that these agents are effective in OA to a similar extent as older NSAIDs. For example, in a 1-year study of rofecoxib, 748 subjects randomized to this drug at 12.5 or 25 mg daily or to diclofenac 50 mg three times daily showed similar improvement in pain and in the patient's and physician's global assessments, although the latter two measures showed a slight superiority of diclofenac.[89] In a 12-week trial of 1003 subjects with knee OA, celecoxib at 100 or 200 mg twice daily was more effective than placebo and was comparable with naproxen 500 mg twice daily for improvement in pain, physical functioning, and joint stiffness.[90]

Gastrointestinal Effects of NSAIDs

The most common adverse effects of NSAIDs involve the gastrointestinal tract, and gastrointestinal intolerance contributes to many treatment failures.[64,65,82,91] Minor complaints—nausea, dyspepsia, anorexia, abdominal pain, flatulence, and diarrhea—affect 10% to 60% of patients. To minimize these symptoms, NSAIDs should be taken with food or milk, except in the case of enteric-coated products, which should *not* be taken with milk or antacids.

All NSAIDs have the potential to cause gastrointestinal bleeding through direct or indirect (systemic) mechanisms.[64,65,82,91] Most NSAIDs (except nabumetone and the COX-2 inhibitors celecoxib and rofecoxib) are weak acids that are uncharged in the stomach. Unionized NSAIDs enter gastric mucosal cells, release hydrogen ions intracellularly, and are concentrated ("ion trapped") within cells, killing some and producing the detrimental local effects. Gastric mucosal damage also can be triggered systemically through NSAID inhibition of gastroprotective prostaglandins.

Much effort has been directed toward quantifying the risk of gastrointestinal adverse events with NSAID use and in identifying those for whom NSAID therapy is most risky. The true incidence of adverse gastrointestinal effects is difficult to determine because of variability in the symptoms assessed, differences in the populations studied, the time course and extent of NSAID use, and concurrent medications.[87] An added difficulty is the poor correlation between gastrointestinal ulceration and gastrointestinal symptoms, where 50% of dyspeptic patients have a normal-appearing mucosa and 40% of asymptomatic persons have endoscopic evidence of erosive gastritis.[64] Fecal occult blood is an unreliable predictor of complications.[64–66] Patient-specific factors can identify those at increased risk for NSAID-induced ulcers and ulcer complications[44] (see Fig. 92–5).

Two issues are helpful in considering agents to combat NSAID-induced mucosal injury. One is whether gastric or duodenal mucosa is protected. The second is outcome, where serious ulcer complications are more clinically relevant but require larger studies than those assessing endoscopically evident ulceration. Although NSAID use is associated with injury throughout the gastrointestinal tract, the most common sites are the gastric and duodenal mucosae.[64,65] The incidence of gastric ulcers with NSAID use is approximately 11% to 13% and that for duodenal ulcers is 7% to 10%, but incidence figures depend on the definition and size of ulcers counted (3 versus 5 mm) and other variables.[82,91–93] Serious gastrointestinal complications associated with NSAID use are perforations, gastric outlet obstruction, and gastrointestinal bleeding. Such complications occur in 1.5% to 4% of patients per year. Although this represents a small percentage of patients, NSAID use is so widespread that even small percentages translate into substantial morbidity and mortality. In addition, the risk increases to 9% per year for patients of advanced age with a history of peptic ulcer or gastrointestinal bleeding and cardiovascular disease.[92] An estimated 16,500 deaths per year are associated with NSAID use in rheumatoid arthritis or OA patients.[82]

H_2-receptor antagonists (H_2RAs) prevent NSAID induced *duodenal* ulcer lesions but not *gastric* ulcers.[65,91] High-dose H_2RAs may prevent gastric ulcers, but concerns about design of the study preclude definitive conclusions. At present, the value of H_2RAs appears to be limited to preventing NSAID-induced duodenal ulcers.[44,93]

Only misoprostol has demonstrated protection against both gastric and duodenal NSAID-induced ulcers and, most important, their associated complications.[92,94,95] Furthermore, misoprostol does not interfere with the anti-inflammatory effects of the NSAIDs. Unfortunately, misoprostol therapy causes frequent diarrhea and abdominal cramps. Because of its abortifacient properties, misoprostol is contraindicated in pregnancy (unless it is being used with mifepristone for medical abortion) and in women of child-bearing age who are not maintaining adequate contraception. It must be dispensed in its original container, which carries a warning for these individuals. Misoprostol is also available in a combination product with diclofenac, which bears the same restrictions as misoprostol alone.

Other agents have been evaluated in attempts to prevent NSAID-induced gastropathy. Sucralfate was less effective than misoprostol in preventing NSAID-induced gastric ulcers, but data on duodenal ulcer prevention are limited, and no data on reduction of complication rate are available.[94] Omeprazole has been compared with misoprostol and has been compared with ranitidine for healing NSAID-induced gastric and duodenal ulcers and for preventing further gastric or duodenal ulcer formation. Omeprazole was modestly more effective than either misoprostol or ranitidine in promoting healing and preventing recurrence of both gastric and duodenal ulcers.[96,97] Omeprazole also was more effective at improving patient's quality of life and promoting symptom relief, especially compared with misosprostol. However, this study had several limitations and confounders regarding the rate of ulcer occurrence and patient status regarding *Helicobacter pylori* status and prednisone use. Also, ulcer complications were not addressed, although a reduction was presumed by analogy with the effect of misosprostol to reduce both ulcers and complications.[92]

Gastrointestinal Effects of COX-2 Inhibitors

For OA patients at high risk for gastrointestinal complications who need an NSAID, the ACR recommendations include either a COX-2–selective NSAID or a nonspecific NSAID in combination with either a proton pump inhibitor or misoprostol. The potential of COX-2 inhibitors to relieve OA pain with reduced gastrointestinal and other toxicities provided the major impetus for development of these drugs.

It is too early to determine precisely what advantage coxibs will enjoy in widespread clinical practice, but several lines of evidence indicate that they will live up to their promise of reduced gastrointestinal toxicity. First, a study of 25 NSAIDs with varying COX-1/COX-2 selectivity demonstrated that NSAIDs that were least potent against COX-1 had the smallest effects on prostaglandin synthesis in samples of human gastric mucosa. Unfortunately, this study did not include celecoxib or rofecoxib, but these findings are consistent with the concept that an NSAID virtually devoid of COX-1 activity would not interfere with gastric prostaglandin synthesis.[98]

Second, studies of both rofecoxib and celecoxib using endoscopy to assess appearance of gastric ulcers demonstrated little or no increase in ulcers with these agents. In one study that assessed the effect of celecoxib on gastric ulcers, 1,149 patients with rheumatoid arthritis were randomized to receive placebo or celecoxib 100, 200, or 400 mg bid or naproxen 500 mg bid. The incidence of endoscopically determined gastroduodenal ulcers after 12 weeks was significantly higher with naproxen (26%) than with any celecoxib dose (6%, 4%, and 8%, respectively) and placebo (4%).[99]

Similar results were recorded in a study of OA patients. For rofecoxib, 775 OA patients were randomized to receive rofecoxib 25 or 50 mg daily, ibuprofen 800 mg three times daily, or placebo. Endoscopically defined ulcers at 12 and 24 weeks were fewer with either rofecoxib dose than with ibuprofen. In a planned combined analysis including a total of 1517 patients, ulcer incidence at 12 weeks was similar with placebo and the two rofecoxib doses.[100]

Finally, COX-2–specific inhibitors have caused fewer serious gastrointestinal events or ulcer complications than nonspecific NSAIDs. These findings are important because there is not a proven consistent correlation between the appearance of endoscopically observed gastric ulcers and serious gastrointestinal adverse effects. Serious gastrointestinal events are commonly defined as perforations, gastric outlet obstruction, or bleeding, but studies do not always include exactly these categories or report separate types of events.

It is daunting to carry out studies large enough to discern differences between groups for relatively rare events. In one review, eight double-blind studies where patients were randomized to receive rofecoxib at 12.5, 25, or 50 mg daily, another NSAID (ibuprofen, diclofenac, or nabumetone), or placebo were combined and examined.[101] The analysis showed that there was a modestly but significantly lower risk of the combined gastrointestinal events of perforations, symptomatic ulcers, and gastrointestinal bleeding for rofecoxib compared with nonspecific NSAIDs, although the combined event rate was higher for rofecoxib than for placebo. This analysis did not report these gastrointestinal events separately, it did not report gastric outlet obstruction, and it did include "symptomatic gastrointestinal ulcers" in the combined end point. It is thus unclear if rofecoxib carried less risk of perforations, obstructions, and gastrointestinal bleeding, separately or combined. As far as could be determined, patients taking aspirin were excluded from the studies reviewed in this analysis.

A more recent study randomized 8076 rheumatoid arthritis patients to receive rofecoxib 50 mg daily or naproxen 500 mg bid, and patients taking aspirin were excluded. Those randomized to rofecoxib experienced a 50% lower risk of gastrointestinal events, defined as perforations, bleeding, obstruction, or symptomatic gastroduodenal ulcers.[102]

Celecoxib's gastrointestinal toxicity profile also has been studied in a randomized, double-blind fashion. A comparison was made for celecoxib 400 mg twice daily (a higher dose than generally used clinically) versus other NSAIDs at standard dose. Celecoxib use was associated with a reduced incidence for the combined end point of symptomatic ulcers and ulcer complications (perforations, gastric outlet obstruction, or bleeding).[103] The group taking celecoxib as a whole did not exhibit a significant decrease in ulcer complications as defined earlier, nor was a reduction seen for those taking celecoxib with aspirin. For patients not taking aspirin, ulcer complications decreased significantly. In a pooled analysis of 14 randomized, controlled trials comparing celecoxib, comparative NSAID, or placebo for periods of 2 to 24 weeks, ulcer complications (bleeding, perforation, or gastric outlet obstruction) were evaluated. Few gastrointestinal complications were identified overall, but significantly fewer occurred with celecoxib (0 of 1864 subjects for placebo, 2 of 6376 for celecoxib, and 9 of 2768 for other NSAIDs).[104]

Most studies of COX-2 inhibitors have reported on the occurrence of minor gastrointestinal side effects or dyspepsia or subject withdrawal due to gastrointestinal adverse effects. Despite substantial reduction in ulcers and serious gastrointestinal effects seen with COX-2 inhibitors, only slight or very modest differences in overall gastrointestinal complaints have been found between COX-2 inhibitors and nonspecific NSAIDs.[90,100,101,103]

Three conclusions can be drawn from these studies on COX-2 inhibitors and gastrointestinal toxicity:

1. Although use of COX-2 inhibitors is associated with fewer serious gastrointestinal adverse events than

nonspecific NSAIDs, further study and postmarketing surveillance are necessary to watch closely for such events in actual clinical practice, especially for patients at high risk.

2. Even with COX-2 inhibitors, as for nonspecific NSAIDs, patient-reported dyspepsia, endoscopic ulcerations, and serious gastrointestinal complications do not correlate well.
3. Given that even 30 mg aspirin is sufficient to suppress gastric prostaglandin production,[77] coupled with the uncertain gastrointestinal safety benefit for a COX-2 inhibitor over a nonspecific NSAID for patients taking aspirin, it is unclear how large an advantage COX-2 inhibitors will provide for patients concurrently taking aspirin for cardioprotection.

Other Toxicities Associated with NSAIDs

NSAID use is associated with renal nephropathies, including acute renal insufficiency, tubulointerstitial nephropathy, hyperkalemia, and renal papillary necrosis.[105] Clinical findings in NSAID-induced renal syndromes include increased serum creatinine and blood urea nitrogen, hyperkalemia, elevated blood pressure, peripheral edema, and weight gain. Mechanisms of NSAID injury include direct toxicity and renal dysfunction mediated through prostaglandin inhibition. Local generation of prostaglandins promotes compensatory vasodilatation of renal blood vessels to preserve renal function, especially in the face of volume contraction or diminished cardiac output, so some patients are more prone to NSAID-induced renal injury than others (Fig. 92–7). At high risk are patients with severe heart disease (including congestive heart failure), severe hepatic disease, nephrotic syndrome, chronic renal disease, advanced age, or volume depletion secondary to comorbid disease or diuretic therapy.[105] Sulindac and nonacetylated salicylates may be less likely to cause renal insufficiency, but close monitoring is advisable for high-risk patients taking any NSAID, with monitoring of serum creatinine at baseline and within a few days (for NSAIDs with short half-lives) to a week (for agents with longer half-lives) after drug initiation.

COX-2–specific inhibitors carry the potential for renal toxicity because COX-2 activity has been demonstrated in a variety of sites in human and animal kidneys and is upregulated in salt-depleted states[105,106] (see Fig. 92–7). The effect on glomerular filtration rate of short-term treatment of subjects with COX-2 inhibitors has been

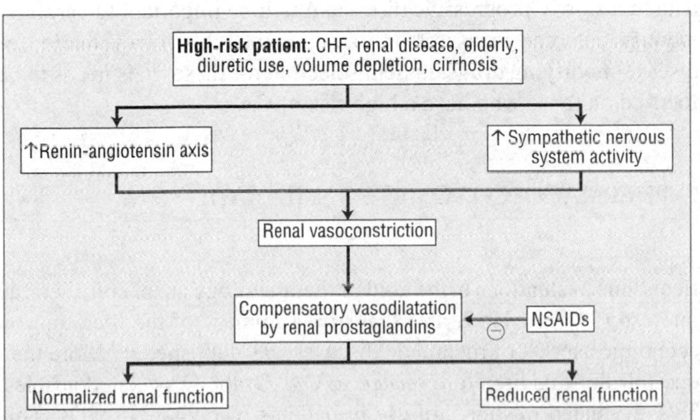

FIGURE 92–7. Mechanisms implicated in NSAID-induced renal injury. *(Adapted from Ref. 105.)*

transient and/or less than the effects of traditional NSAIDs. However, COX-2 inhibitors decrease urinary prostaglandins similarly to other NSAIDs, and COX-2 inhibitors cause sodium and potassium retention. Whether coxibs possess any practical advantages regarding renal toxicity compared with other NSAIDs is uncertain. Until or unless this is demonstrated, coxibs should be prescribed with the same caution as other NSAIDs in patients at increased risk for renal dysfunction.

Although all NSAIDs can cause drug-induced hepatitis, this is not common. NSAIDs most frequently implicated include diclofenac and sulindac.[107] Patient monitoring should include baseline liver studies consisting of the transaminases, aspartate aminotransferase (AST) and alanine aminotransferase (ALT), with therapy stopped if these values exceed two to three times the upper limit of normal.

Other toxic effects of NSAIDs include hypersensitivity reactions, rash, and central nervous system complaints of drowsiness, dizziness, headaches, depression, confusion, and tinnitus.[66,77] Although NSAIDs generally should be avoided in patients with asthma who are aspirin-intolerant, preliminary evidence suggests that COX-2–specific inhibitors may not pose as great a risk.[108] Celecoxib is a sulfonamide and is thus contraindicated for those with sulfa allergies.

All nonspecific NSAIDs inhibit COX-1–dependent thromboxane production in platelets and thus increase bleeding risk. Aspirin inhibition is irreversible, and bleeding time normalizes after 5 to 7 days as new platelets enter the circulation. Other nonspecific NSAIDs inhibit thromboxane formation reversibly, with normalization of platelet function 1 to 3 days after the drug is stopped. The nonacetylated salicylate products and nabumetone, which have partial COX-2 selectivity, may be preferable to nonspecific NSAIDs.[66,74,77] COX-2 specific inhibitors do not block thromboxane synthesis and should pose even less bleeding risk. A study using blood obtained from subjects treated with supratherapeutic doses of celecoxib (600 mg twice daily) and regular doses of naproxen (500 mg twice daily) showed the expected substantial decrease in platelet aggregation and thromboxane production with naproxen but no effect with celecoxib.[109] Although one would expect COX-2 inhibitors to carry a greatly decreased risk of serious bleeding events, further clinical experience is necessary to bear this out.

Finally, NSAIDs should be used cautiously during pregnancy because of the risk to the fetus posed by the bleeding problems associated with any NSAID that affects COX-1.[110] In late pregnancy, all NSAIDs should be avoided because of the risk of premature closure of the ductus arteriosus. Both celecoxib and rofecoxib fall into the FDA's pregnancy category C.

Important drug interactions with NSAIDs can be pharmacokinetic or pharmacodynamic in origin and have been reviewed.[77,80,111] The most potentially serious interactions include the use of NSAIDs with lithium, warfarin, oral hypoglycemics, methotrexate, antihypertensives, angiotensin-converting enzyme (ACE) inhibitors, β-blockers, and diuretics. Anticipation and careful monitoring often can prevent serious events when these drugs are considered. Patient use of over-the-counter (OTC) NSAIDs and H_2RAs also should be assessed because a combination of NSAIDs may increase the risk of gastrointestinal toxicity, leading to self-medication with an OTC H_2RA product.

Celecoxib does not appear to inhibit cytochrome P450 2C9, 2C19, or 3A4.[80] However, given its metabolism by CYP2C9, a potential for interactions exists if celecoxib is taken with CYP2C9 inhibitors. Because warfarin and celecoxib are metabolized by CYP2C9, and since postmarketing warfarin-celecoxib interactions have been noted, patients receiving both medications should be followed closely.[80]

In vitro evidence shows inhibition of CYP2D6 by celecoxib, so a potential for interactions exists for drugs metabolized by CYP2D6. In clinical studies, increased celecoxib levels were seen with fluconazole administration, and celecoxib appears to increase lithium levels. No clinically significant interactions have been documented with methotrexate, glyburide, ketoconazole, phenytoin, or tolbutamide.

Rofecoxib is metabolized in the liver, primarily by cytosolic rather than microsomal enzymes, with little renal excretion of unchanged drug. Rofecoxib is not recommended for patients with moderate to severe hepatic impairment. Based on clinical studies, potentially interacting drugs include methotrexate (MTX) and warfarin. Rofecoxib at 75 mg daily modestly increased MTX concentrations and at 50 mg daily modestly elevated the international normalized ratios (INRs) of warfarin patients. Given that other NSAIDs can increase lithium, increased care is advisable for patients receiving any NSAID and lithium. Additionally, rifampin can decrease rofecoxib concentrations. Clinically significant interactions were not observed when rofecoxib was administered with cimetidine, digoxin, oral contraceptives, or ketoconazole. As for other NSAIDs and as discussed under renal effects, caution must be used when certain patients are treated with COX-2 inhibitors. These agents may decrease the antihypertensive effects of ACE inhibitors and may interfere with the natriuretic effect of diuretics by affecting renal prostaglandin production.[80]

A continuing controversy is whether NSAIDs help or hinder progression of OA.[66,74,112] Animal studies demonstrated that salicylates and some NSAIDs suppressed PG biosynthesis in articular cartilage, whereas diclofenac and piroxicam stimulated PG synthesis. Limited human data suggest a twofold risk for progression of knee OA if indomethacin therapy is continued.[112] Although the study had limitations, and further clinical trial data are needed in humans, the findings clearly raise some interesting issues concerning selection of NSAIDs and duration of therapy. This appears to be another reason to consider starting therapy with acetaminophen.

CORTICOSTEROIDS

Systemic corticosteroid therapy is not recommended in OA, given the lack of proven benefit and the well-known adverse effects with long-term use.[7–9] Intraarticular glucocorticoid injections can provide relief when local inflammation or joint effusion exists, but large responses to placebo injections make demonstration of benefit difficult.[7–9,44,113] Aspiration of the effusion and injection of glucocorticoid are carried out aseptically, and examination of aspirate to rule out infection is recommended. After injection, the patient should minimize activity and stress on the joint for several days.

Intraarticular glucocorticoids should be used infrequently, i.e., at 4- to 6-month intervals for a given joint and with no more than three to four injections per year. Corticosteroid injection into the ligaments or pericapsular areas can bring relief and is associated with less risk compared with the intraarticular route.

HYALURONATE INJECTIONS

Agents containing hyaluronic acid (HA) (sodium hyaluronate) are available for intra-articular injection for treatment of knee AO.[114] High-molecular-weight HA is an important constituent of normal cartilage, with viscoelastic properties providing lubrication with motion and shock absorbency during rapid movements. Endogenous HA also may have anti-inflammatory effects. Because the concentration and molecular size of synovial HA decrease in OA, administration of exogenous HA products has been studied, with the theory that this could reconstitute synovial fluid and reduce symptoms. Injections temporarily increase viscosity, but this effect is transient and modest. Although HA injections were reported to decrease pain, many studies were short term and poorly controlled, and placebo injections also often reduced reported OA pain dramatically.[114]

HA products are injected once weekly, using aseptic technique, for either 3 or 5 weeks. Injections are well tolerated, although there can be pain with injection and local skin reactions, including rash, ecchymoses, and pruritus.

These products may be beneficial for those unresponsive to other therapy, but further study and clinical use are needed to determine their ultimate place in therapy. These agents are expensive because the treatment includes both drug costs and administration costs.

DISEASE-MODIFYING DRUGS

Disease-modifying drugs are targeted not at pain relief but at preventing, retarding, or reversing damage to articular cartilage.[115] Most products have been tested in animal models, and limited human data are available.

Heparinoid products contain glycosaminoglycans, such as Rumalon (glycosaminoglycan peptide complex from bovine trachea or bronchial cartilage) or Arteparon (chondroitin-4-sulfate and chondroitin-6-sulfate, from extracts of calf cartilage and bone marrow). These compounds appear to stimulate cartilage synthesis but also may inhibit degradative enzymes in articular cartilage. However, concerns include reports of bleeding attributed to the heparinoid structure of the GAGs and anaphylaxis associated with the antigenic proteins in the compounds.[115]

Agents such as sodium pentosan polysulfate and calcium pentosan polysulfate have been studied in animal models and in vitro. Such agents may affect expression of MMPs and reduce OA symptoms in animals, but the clinical potential of these agents remains unclear.[116] Other approaches are based on affecting chondrocyte function or inhibiting cytokines that contribute to cartilage degradation.

Pharmacologic agents that could mimic TIMPs in theory would decrease cartilage destruction. Some studies have explored the use of tetracycline or doxycycline, which appear to inhibit the degradative MMPs.[32,115,117,118] Synthetic TIMP mimics are also being investigated.[119]

Despite the excitement surrounding these new approaches, they should be considered experimental because few data are from controlled human studies. Ongoing clinical trials have begun with some of these therapies. To provide the most accurate interpretation of the data in a slowly progressive disease, it will be important to carefully identify outcome measures and assessment tools for evaluation of disease-modifying drugs. Patient selection for these trials needs to be focused on those who have a high risk of OA.[115]

PHARMACOECONOMIC CONSIDERATIONS

Economic evaluations in the field of rheumatology are of considerable interest.[120–122] In 1997, an exhaustive summary of the literature on economic aspects of rheumatic diseases was published.[120] More than one-third of this literature related to OA. Of the OA-related articles, 38% evaluated misoprostol use in patients receiving NSAIDs. This interest was not surprising, given the high economic cost of using misoprostol for ulcer prevention.

Subsequently, an analysis of the cost-effectiveness of misoprostol was reported,[120] based on data from a study of RA patients taking NSAIDs.[92] Misoprostol was shown to be cost-effective if reserved for high-risk patients. The cost of avoiding one serious gastrointestinal complication would be $94,766 if all NSAID patients were given misoprostol but only $4101 if misoprostol were limited to high-risk patients. This work is consistent with the concept of selecting high-risk patients for prophylactic therapy. COX-2 inhibitors are recommended by ACR guidelines for those at high risk of adverse gastrointestinal events, and efforts have begun to address cost-effectiveness of COX-2 inhibitor use. For those without risk factors, an estimated 500 patients would need treatment with a COX-2 inhibitor, costing $400,000, to avoid the one serious gastrointestinal complication expected with a nonspecific NSAID. For high-risk individuals, however, the number needed to treat would drop to only 40, costing $30,000.[123] With evidence of increased gastrointestinal safety and with huge patient demand, COX-2 inhibitors are used heavily. Better estimates of risk and cost-effectiveness may provide more exact answers regarding which individuals will most benefit and at what cost or savings.

To provide some perspective on patient-care costs, a 1997 report on more than 10,000 OA patients followed in a managed-care setting showed that the mean annual cost of care per patient was $543, with hospital costs accounting for 46%, medications 32%, and ambulatory care 22%.[124] The 46% figure is understandable because although few patients were hospitalized, each in-patient stay was costly. Other pharmacoeconomic considerations for OA involve the selection of therapy for the initial treatment of patients with OA. Use of a simple OTC analgesic (acetaminophen) as initial therapy has greatly reduced medication costs in comparison with the use of NSAIDs, many of which had been by prescription only. NSAID costs range from $20 to $100 per month depending on the medication, daily dose, and regimen selected. Although this can be viewed as a reduction in the cost of prescription medications, cost shifting to "out of pocket" expense greatly affects those on fixed incomes. Many elderly patients, most likely to need OA drugs, have little or no prescription reimbursement. Careful attention to this cost shifting to OTC products—acetaminophen or NSAIDs—needs to be given for all patients receiving therapy for OA.

NSAIDs as a chemical category of analgesics and anti-inflammatory agents have been considered therapeutically equivalent, at least until the development of the coxib class. This does not imply that the agents are therapeutically interchangeable. Patient response to these agents is highly individualized. When starting therapy, it is often useful to consider the cost of the product and its generic availability among factors for product selection. Both these factors are of importance to patients on fixed incomes and those on limited budgets, as well as for the health care system costs.

EVALUATION OF THERAPEUTIC OUTCOMES

Pharmacotherapy monitoring in OA is patient-specific, focusing on the degree and extent of joint involvement, patient age, concomitant medications and comorbidities, and the nondrug and drug therapy selected. To monitor efficacy, the patient's baseline pain can be assessed with a visual analogue scale, and range of motion for affected joints can be assessed with flexion, extension, abduction, or adduction. Depending on the joint affected, measurement of grip strength and 50-ft walking time can help assess hand or hip/knee OA, respectively. Baseline radiographs can document the extent of joint involvement and may be repeated when symptoms worsen. Other measures include the clinician's global assessment based on the patient's history of activities and limitations caused by OA as well as documentation of analgesic or NSAID use. Lastly, disease-specific quality of life (QOL) questionnaires for arthritis are valuable in assessing clinical response to interventions.[125–127]

Establishment of monitoring parameters for adverse effects depends on the therapeutic regimen. Often the direct approach is best. Patients should be asked first if they are having any "problems" with their medications rather than listing a series of adverse effects. This can be followed with more direct questions relating to the most common adverse effects associated with the respective medication. With most NSAIDs, symptoms of abdominal pain, heartburn, nausea, or change in stool color provide valuable clues to identify gastrointestinal complaints. Patients also should be monitored for any signs of skin rash, headaches, drowsiness, weight gain, or alterations in blood pressure. Baseline serum creatinine determinations, hematology profiles, and serum transaminases with repeat levels as needed are useful in identifying specific toxicities to the kidney, liver, gastrointestinal tract, or bone marrow.

CONCLUSION

OA is a very common, slowly progressive disorder that affects diarthrodial joints. It is characterized by progressive deterioration of articular cartilage resulting in the loss of cartilage and formation of osteophytes. Clinical manifestations occur late in life and include gradual onset of joint pain, stiffness, and limitation of motion. The primary treatment goals are to reduce pain, maintain function, and prevent further destruction. An individualized approach based on nondrug modalities such as education, rest, exercise, and weight loss as needed, with the addition of drug therapy, can succeed in meeting these goals. Recommended drug treatment starts with acetaminophen 4 g/d or less and topical analgesics as needed. If acetaminophen is ineffective, NSAIDs, preferably at analgesic doses, may be used. NSAIDs are generally well tolerated but, because of wide use, contribute to many serious adverse events. Individuals at increased risk for toxicity, especially for gastrointestinal or cardiovascular/renal events, deserve special attention. Experimental therapy aimed at preventing the progression of OA requires further clinical investigation before entering widespread clinical use.

▶ PRINCIPLES OF PHARMACOTHERAPY

- The most common form of arthritis is OA. It affects individuals in the middle to later years of life, with women more commonly affected than men after age 45 years.
- OA is primarily a disease of cartilage that reflects a failure of the chondrocyte to maintain proper balance between cartilage formation and destruction.
- The most common symptom associated with OA is pain, which leads to decreased function and motion.
- Patients have bony proliferation of affected joints that should be differentiated from the swelling of rheumatoid or inflammatory arthritis.
- OA is not a systemic disease like rheumatoid arthritis. The joint distribution often involves the knees, hips, and hands, although other joints also can be affected.
- Nonpharmacologic therapy is the foundation of the pharmaceutical care plan. It should be initiated prior to or

simultaneously with initiation of simple analgesics such as acetaminophen (≤4 g/day).

- Glucosamine, alone or with chondroitin sulfate, warrants further study for its potential to relieve OA symptoms and possibly slow disease progression.
- Failure with simple analgesics warrants trial with an NSAID in low doses, with anti-inflammatory doses considered for those with inflammation.
- NSAIDs are associated with gastrointestinal, renal, liver, or central nervous system toxicity. The appropriate monitoring with complete blood count, serum creatinine, and hepatic transaminase levels is valuable in detecting potential toxicity. COX-2 specific inhibitors appear to carry less bleeding risk, but there is no assurance that these agents will carry less renal risk than other NSAIDs.
- Prevention of NSAID-induced gastrointestinal toxicity includes using enteric-coated products or nonacetylated salicylates. The use of misoprostol has shown to be effective in reducing both gastric and duodenal ulcers and the associated complications. H_2RAs are effective in preventing duodenal ulcers but not gastric ulcers; sucralfate appears equal to placebo; and omeprazole may have comparable effects to misoprostol, although reductions in complications have not been studied.
- COX-2–specific inhibitors can be used for individuals at high risk of gastrointestinal toxicity and appear to pose less gastrointestinal risk than other NSAIDs. Further experience with these new agents is necessary, particularly with regard to their effects on the renal and cardiovascular systems.
- OA is a chronic, usually progressive disease. New therapies are being studied that may prevent further joint progression, thereby limiting or delaying the need for surgery.

REFERENCES

1. Fife RS. Epidemiology, pathology and pathogenesis. In: Klippel JH, ed. Primer on the Rheumatic Diseases, 11th ed. Atlanta, Arthritis Foundation, 1997: 216–217.
2. Yelin E, Callahan LF. The economic cost and social and psychological impact of muscloskeletal conditions. Arthritis Rheum 1995;38:1351–1362.
3. Loeser RF. Aging and the etiopathogenesis and treatment of osteoarthritis. Rheum Dis Clin North Am 2000;26:547–567.
4. Lawrence RC, Helmick CG, Arnett FC, et al. Estimates of the prevalence of arthritis and selected musculoskeletal disorders in the United States. Arthritis Rheum 1998;41:778–799.
5. Buckwalter JA, Mankin HJ. Articular cartilage: I. Tissue design and chondrocyte-matrix interactions. J Bone Joint Surg 1997;79A:600–611.
6. Buckwalter JA, Mankin HJ. Articular cartilage: II. Degeneration and osteoarthrosis, repair, regeneration, and transplantation. J Bone Joint Surg 1997;79A:612–632.
7. Hochberg MC. Clinical features and treatment. In: Klippel JH, ed. Primer on the Rheumatic Diseases, 11th ed. Atlanta, Arthritis Foundation, 1997: 218–221.
8. Hochberg MC, Altman RD, Brandt KD, et al. Guidelines for the medical management of osteoarthritis: I. Osteoarthritis of the hip. Arthritis Rheum 1995;38:1535–1540.
9. Hochberg MC, Altman RD, Brandt KD, et al. Guidelines for the medical management of osteoarthritis: II. Osteoarthritis of the knee. Arthritis Rheum 1995;38:1541–1546.
10. Lawrence RC, Hochberg MC, Kelsey JL, et al. Estimates of the prevalence of selected arthritic and musculoskeletal diseases in the United States. J Rheumatol 1989;16:427–441.
11. Felson DT, Anderson JJ, Naimark A, et al. The prevalence of chondrocalcinosis in the elderly and its association with knee osteoarthritis: The Framingham study. J Rheumatol 1989;16:1241–1245.
12. Spector TD, Hochberg MC. Methodological problems in the epidemiological study of osteoarthritis. Ann Rheum Dis 1994;53:143–146.
13. Davis MA, Ettinger WH, Neuhaus JM, et al. Knee osteoarthritis and physical functioning: Evidence from the NHANEWSI epidemiologic follow-up study. J Rheumatol 1991;18:591–598.
14. Van Saase JL, Van Romunde LK, Cats A, et al. Epidemiology of osteoarthritis: Zoetermeer survey. Comparison of radiological osteoarthritis in a Dutch population with that in 10 other populations. Ann Rheum Dis 1989;48:271–280.
15. Cooper C. Osteoarthritis: Epidemiology. In: Klippel JH, Dieppe PA, eds. Rheumatology. London, Mosby–Year Book, 1994:3.1–3.4.
16. Felson DT, Zhang Y, Anthony JM, et al. Weight loss reduces the risk for symptomatic knee osteoarthritis in women. Ann Intern Med 1992; 117:535–539.
17. Solomon L. Clinical features of osteoarthritis. In: Kelly WN, Harris ED, Ruddy S, Sledge CB, eds. Textbook of Rheumatology, 5th ed. Philadelphia, Saunders, 1997:1383–1393.
18. Carman WJ, Sowers M, Hawthorne VM, et al. Obesity as a risk factor for osteoarthritis of the hand and wrist: A prospective study. Am J Epidemiol 1994;139:119–129.
19. Gelber AC, Hochberg MC, Mead LA, et al. Body mass index in young men and the risk of subsequent knee and hip osteoarthritis. Am J Med 1999;107:542–548.
20. Cicuttini FM, Baker JR, Spector TD. The association of obesity with osteoarthritis of the hand and knee in women: A twin study. J Rheumatol 1996;23:1221–1226.
21. Sandmark H, Hogstedt C, Lewold S, et al. Osteoarthritis of the knee in men and women in association with overweight, smoking, and hormone therapy. Ann Rheum Dis 1999;58:151–155.
22. Bergenudd H, Lindgarde F, Nilsson B. Prevalence and co-incidence of degenerative changes of the hands and feet in middle age and their relationship to occupational workload, intelligence and social background. Clin Orthop 1989;239:306–310.
23. McAlindon TE, Wilson PWF, Aliabadi P, et al. Level of physical activity and the risk of radiographic and symptomatic knee osteoarthritis in the elderly: The Framingham study. Am J Med 1999;106:151–157.
24. Lane NE, Bloch DA, Hubert HB, et al. Running, osteoarthritis, and bone density: Initial 2-year longitudinal study. Am J Med 1990;88:453–459.
25. O'Reilly SC, Jones A, Muir KR, et al. Quadriceps weakness in knee osteoarthritis: The effect on pain and disability. Ann Rheum Dis 1988; 557:588–594.
26. Hurley MV. The role of muscle weakness in the pathogenesis of osteoarthritis. Rheum Dis Clin North Am 1999;25:283–298.
27. Eye DR, Weis MA, Moskowitz RW. Cartilage expression of a type II collagen mutation in an inherited form of osteoarthritis associated with a mild chondrodysplasia. J Clin Invest 1991;87:357–361.
28. Hannan MT, Anderson JJ, Zhang Y, et al. Bone mineral density and knee osteoarthritis in elderly men and women: The Framingham study. Arthritis Rheum 1993;12:1671–1680.
29. Stewart A, Black AJ. Bone mineral density in osteoarthritis. Curr Opin Rheumatol 2000;13:464–467.
30. Jones G, Nguyen T, Sambrook PN, et al. Osteoarthritis, bone density, postural stability, and osteoporotic fractures: A population based study. J Rheumatol 1995;22:921–925.
31. Mankin HJ, Brandt KD. Pathogenesis of osteoarthritis. In: Kelly WN, Harris ED, Ruddy S, Sledge CB, eds. Textbook of Rheumatology, 5th ed. Philadelphia, Saunders, 1997: 1369–1382.
32. Kraus VB. Pathogenesis and treatment of osteoarthritis. Med Clin North Am 1997;81:85–112.
33. Buckwalter JA, Glimcher MJ, Cooper RR, et al. Bone biology: I. Structure, blood supply, cells, matrix, and mineralization. J Bone J Surg Am 1995;77A:1256–1275.
34. Buckwalter JA, Glimcher MJ, Cooper RR, et al. Bone biology: II. Formation, form, modeling, remodeling, and regulation of cell function. J Bone J Surg Am 1995;77A:1276–1288.

35. Dieppe P. Osteoarthritis: Clinical features and diagnostic problems. In: Klippel JH, Dieppe PA, eds. Rheumatology. London, Mosby–Year Book, 1994: 1–16.
36. Mankin HJ, Brandt KD, Shulman LE. Workshop on the etiopathogenesis of osteoarthritis. J Rheumatol 1986;13:1130–1134.
37. Mazzuca S. Plain radiography in the evaluation of knee osteoarthritis. Curr Opin Rheumatol 1997;9:263–267.
38. Yoshihara Y, Nakamura H, Obata K, et al. Matrix metalloproteinases and tissue inhibitors of metalloproteinases in synovial fluids from patients with rheumatoid arthritis or osteoarthritis. Ann Rheum Dis 2000;59: 455–461.
39. Towle CA, Wright M, Hecht AC, et al. A matrix metalloproteinase proenzyme activator produced by articular cartilage. Biochem Biophys Res Commun 1998;247:324–331.
40. Freemont AJ, Byers RJ, Taiwo YO, et al. In situ zymographic localisation of type II collagen degrading activity in osteoarthritic human articular cartilage. Ann Rheum Dis 1999;58:357–365.
41. Mansell JP, Bailey AJ. Abnormal cancellous bone collagen metabolism in osteoarthritis. J Clin Invest 1998;101:1596–1603.
42. Ravaud P, Dougados M. Radiographic assessment in osteoarthritis. J Rheumatol 1997;24:786–791.
43. Creamer P. Osteoarthritis pain and its treatment. Curr Opin Rheumatol 2000;12:450–455.
44. ACR Subcommittee on Osteoarthritis Guidelines. Recommendations for the medical management of osteoarthritis of the hip and knee: 2000 Update. Arthritis Rheum 2000;43:1905–1915.
45. Rene J, Weinberger M, Mazzuca SA, et al. Reduction of joint pain in patients with knee osteoarthritis who have received monthly telephone calls from lay personnel and whose medical treatment regimens have remained stable. Arthritis Rheum 1992;35:511–515.
46. Kovar PA, Allegrante JP, MacKenzie CR, et al. Supervised fitness walking in patients with osteoarthritis of the knee. Ann Intern Med 1992;116:529–534.
47. Weinberger M, Tierney WM, Cowper PA, et al. Cost-effectiveness of increased telephone contact for patients with osteoarthritis: A randomized, controlled trial. Arthritis Rheum 1993;36:243–246.
48. Superio-Cabuslay E, Ward MM, Long KR. Patient education interventions in osteoarthritis and rheumatoid arthritis: A meta-analytic comparison with nonsteroidal anti-inflammatory drug treatment. Arthritis Care Res 1996;9:292–301.
49. Nevitt MC, Lane N. Body weight and osteoarthritis. Am J Med 1999; 197:632–633.
50. Williams RA, Foulshen BM. Weight reduction in osteoarthritis using phentermine. Practitioner 1981;225:231–232.
51. Martin K, Nicklas BJ, Bunyard LB, et al. Weight loss and walking improve symptoms of knee osteoarthritis in overweight women with knee pain. Arthritis Rheum 1998;10(S):225.
52. Felson DT, Zhang Y, Anthony JM, et al. Weight loss reduces the risk for symptomatic knee osteoarthritis in women. Ann Intern Med 1992;116:535–539.
53. Reginster JY, Deroisy R, Rovati LC, et al. Long-term effects of glucosamine sulphate on osteoarthritis progression: A randomised, placebo-controlled clinical trial. Lancet 2001;357:251–256.
54. McAlindon T. Glucosamine for osteoarthritis: Dawn of a new era? (Editorial). Lancet 2001;357:247–248.
55. McAlindon TE, LaValley MP, Gulin JP, et al. Glucosamine and chondroitin for treatment of osteoarthritis: A systematic quality assessment and meta-analysis. JAMA 2000;283(11):1469–1475.
56. Puett DW, Griffin MR. Published trials of nonmedicinal and noninvasive therapies for hip and knee osteoarthritis. Ann Intern Med 1994;121:133–140.
57. Ettinger WH Jr, Burns R, Messier SP, et al. A randomized trial comparing aerobic exercise and resistance exercise with a health education program in older adults with knee osteoarthritis: The Fitness Arthritis and Seniors Trial (FAST). JAMA 1997;277:25–31.
58. Van Baar Me, Dekker J, Oostendorp RAB, et al. The effectiveness of exercise therapy in patients with osteoarthritis of the hip or knee: a randomized clinical trial. J Rheumatol 1998;25:2432–2439.
59. Baker K, McAlindon T. Exercise for knee osteoarthritis. Curr Opin Rheumatol 2000;12:456–463.
60. O'Reilly SC, Muir KR, Doherty M. Effectiveness of home exercise on pain and disability from osteoarthritis of the knee: A randomised controlled trial. Ann Rheum Dis 1999;58(1):15–19.
61. NIH. Total hip replacement. NIH Consensus Statement 1994;12:1–31.
62. Dieppe P, Basler H-D, Chard J, et al. Knee replacement surgery for osteoarthritis: Effectiveness, practice variations, indications and possible determinants of utilization. Rheumatology 1999;38:73–38.
63. LaPrade RF, Swiontkowski MF. New horizons in the treatment of osteoarthritis of the knee. JAMA 1999;281:876–878.
64. Hollander D. Gastrointestinal complications of nonsteroidal anti-inflammatory drugs: Prophylactic and therapeutic strategies. Am J Med 1994;96:274–281.
65. Lichtenstein DR, Syngal S, Wolfe MM. Nonsteroidal anti inflammatory drugs and the gastrointestinal tract. Arthritis Rheum 1995;1:5–18.
66. Furst DE. Are there differences among nonsteroidal anti-inflammatory drugs? Arthritis Rheum 1994;1:1–9.
67. Morassut P, Yang W, Karsh J. Aspirin intolerance. Semin Arthritis Rheum 1989;19:22–30.
68. Eccles M, Freemantle N, Mason J, for the North of England Non-Steroidal Anti-Inflammatory Drug Guideline Development Group. North of England Evidence Based Guideline Development Project: Summary guideline for nonsteroidal anti-inflammatory drugs versus basic analgesia in treating the pain of degenerative arthritis. Br Med J 1998;317:526–530.
69. Pincus T, Swearingen C, Cummins P, et al. Preference for nonsteroidal anti-inflammatory drugs versus acetaminophen and concomitant use of both types of drugs in patients with osteoarthritis. J Rheumatol 2000; 27(4):1020–1027.
70. Henrich WL, Agodoa LE, Barrett B, et al. Analgesics and the kidney: Summary recommendations to the Scientific Advisory Board of the National Kidney Foundation from an ad hoc committee of the National Kidney Foundation. Am J Kidney Dis 1996;27:162–165.
71. Whitcomb DC, Block GD. Association of acetaminophen hepatotoxicity with fasting and ethanol use. JAMA 1994;272:1845–1850.
72. Altman RD, Aven A, Holmburg CE, et al. Capsaicin cream 0.025% as monotherapy for osteoarthritis: A double-blind study. Semin Arthritis Rheum 1994;23(Suppl 3):25–39.
73. Schnitzer TJ. Non-NSAID pharmacologic treatment options for the management of chronic pain. Am J Med 1998;105(1B):45S–52S.
74. Simon LS. Biologic effects of nonsteroidal anti-inflammatory drugs. Curr Opin Rheumatol 1997;9:178–182.
75. Hawkey CJ. COX-2 inhibitors. Lancet 1999;353:307–314.
76. Mandell BF. COX 2-selective NSAIDs: Biology, promises, and concerns. Cleve Clin J Med 1999;66:285–292.
77. Pepper GA. Nonsteroidal anti-inflammatory drugs: New perspectives on a familiar drug class. Rheumatology. 2000;35.223–244.
78. Golden BD, Abramson SB. Selective cyclooxygenase-2 inhibitors. Rheum Dis Clin North Am. 1999;25:359–378.
79. Garavito RM, DeWitt DL. The cyclooxygenase isoforms: Structural insights into the conversion of arachidonic acid to prostaglandins. Biochim Biophys Acta1999;1441:278–287.
80. Kaplan-Machlis B, Klostermeyer BS. The cyclooxygenase-2 inhibitors: Safety and effectiveness. Ann Pharmacother 1999;33:979–988.
81. Jones MK, Wang H, Peskar BM, et al. Inhibition of angiogenesis by nonsteroidal anti-inflammatory drugs: Insight into mechanisms and implications for cancer growth and ulcer healing. Nature Med 1999;5:1418–1423.
82. Wolfe MM, Lichenstein DR, Singh G. Medical progress: Gastrointestinal toxicity of nonsteroidal anti-inflammatory drugs. N Engl J Med 1999;340:1888–1899.
83. Lichtenstein DR, Wolfe MM. COX-2-selective NSAIDs: New and improved? JAMA 2000;284:1297–1299.
84. Crofford LJ, Lipsky PE, Brooks P, et al. Basic biology and clinical application of specific cyclooxygenase-2 inhibitors Arthritis Rheum 2000;43:4–13.

85. Mukherjee D, Nissen SE, Topol EJ. Risk of cardiovascular events associated with selective COX-2 inhibitors. JAMA 2001;286:954–959.
86. Anonymous. FD&C Report: Pink Sheet, Feb. 12, 2001, pp 3–8.
87. Miwa LJ, Jones JK, Pathiyal A, et al. Value of epidemiologic studies in determining the true incidence of adverse events: The nonsteroidal anti-inflammatory drug story. Arch Intern Med 1997;157:2129–2136.
88. Towheed T, Shea B, Wells G, et al. Analgesia and nonaspirin, nonsteroidal anti-inflammatory drugs of osteoarthritis of the hip. Cochrane Library 2000(3).
89. Cannon GW, Caldwell JR, Holt P, et al. Rofecoxib, a specific inhibitor of cyclooxygenase 2, with clinical efficacy comparable with that of diclofenac sodium: Results of a one-year, randomized, clinical trial in patients with osteoarthritis of the knee and hip. Arthritis Rheum 2000;43:978–987.
90. Bensen WG, Fiechtner JJ, McMillen JI, et al. Treatment of osteoarthritis with celecoxib, a cyclooxygenase-2 inhibitor: A randomized controlled trial. Mayo Clin Proc 1999;74:1095–1105.
91. Wallace JL. Nonsteroidal anti-inflammatory drugs and gastroenteropathy: The second hundred years. Gastroenterology 1997;112:1000–1016.
92. Silverstein FE, Graham DY, Senior JR, et al. Misoprostol reduces serious gastrointestinal complications in patients with rheumatoid arthritis receiving nonsteroidal anti-inflammatory drugs. Ann Intern Med 1995;123:241–249.
93. Hudson N, Taha AS, Russell RI, et al. Famotidine for healing and maintenance in nonsteroidal anti-inflammatory drug-associated gastroduodenal ulceration. Gastroenterology 1997;112:1817–1822.
94. Agrawal NM, Roth S, Graham DY, et al. Misoprostol compared with sucralfate in the prevention of nonsteroidal anti-inflammatory drug-induced gastric ulcer: A randomized, controlled trial. Ann Intern Med 1991;115:195–200.
95. Graham DY, White RH, Moreland LW, et al. Duodenal and gastric ulcer prevention with misoprostol in arthritis patients taking NSAIDs. Ann Intern Med 1993;119:257–262.
96. Yeomans ND, Tulassay Z, Juhasz L, et al. A comparison of omeprazole with ranitidine for ulcers associated with nonsteroidal anti-inflammatory drugs. N Engl J Med 1998;338:719–726.
97. Hawkey CJ, Karrasch JA, Szczepanski L, et al. Omeprazole compared with misoprostol for ulcer associated with nonsteroidal anti-inflammatory drugs. N Engl J Med 1998;338:727–734.
98. Cryer B, Feldman M. Cyclooxygenase-1 and cyclooxygenase-2 selectivity of widely used nonsteroidal anti-inflammatory drugs. Am J Med 1998;104:413–421.
99. Simon LS, Weaver AL, Graham DY, et al. Anti-inflammatory and upper gastrointestinal effects of celecoxib in rheumatoid arthritis: A randomized controlled trial. JAMA 1999;282:1921–1928.
100. Hawkey C, Laine L, Simon T, et al, for the Rofecoxib Osteoarthritis Endoscopy Multinational Study Group. Comparison of the effect of rofecoxib (a cyclooxygenase 2 inhibitor), ibuprofen, and placebo on the gastroduodenal mucosa of patients with osteoarthritis. Arthritis Rheum 2000;43:370–377.
101. Langman JM, Jensen DM, Watson DJ, et al. Adverse upper gastrointestinal effects of rofecoxib compared with NSAIDs. JAMA 1999;282:1929–1933.
102. Bombardier C, Laine L, Reicin A, et al. Comparison of upper gastrointestinal toxicity of rofecoxib and naproxen in patients with rheumatoid arthritis. N Engl J Med. 2000;343:1520–1528.
103. Silverstein FE, Faich G, Goldstein JL, et al. Gastrointestinal toxicity with celecoxib vs nonsteroidal anti-inflammatory drugs for osteoarthritis and rheumatoid arthritis: The CLASS study. A randomized, controlled trial. JAMA 2000;284:1247–1255.
104. Goldstein JL, Silverstein FE, Agrawal NM, et al. Reduced risk of upper gastrointestinal ulcer complications with celecoxib, a novel COX-2 inhibitor. Am Gastroenterol 2000;95:1681–1690.
105. Whelton A. Nephrotoxicity of nonsteroidal anti-inflammatory drugs: Physiologic foundations and clinical implications. Am J Med 1999;106 (5B):13S–24S.
106. Rossat J, Maillard M, Nussberger J, et al. Renal effects of selective cyclooxygenase-2 inhibition in normotensive salt-depleted subjects. Clin Pharmacol Ther 1999;66:76–84.
107. Rodriguez LA, Williams R, Derby LE, et al. Acute liver injury associated with nonsteroidal anti-inflammatory drugs and the role of risk factors. Arch Intern Med 1994;154:311–316.
108. Dahlen B, Szczeklik A, Murray JJ. Celecoxib in patients with asthma and aspirin intolerance. N Engl J Med 2001;344:142.
109. Leese PT, Hubbard RC, Karim A, et al. Effects of celecoxib, a novel cyclooxygenase-2 inhibitor, on platelet function in healthy adults: A randomized, controlled trial. J Clin Pharmacol 2000;40:124–132.
110. Roubenoff R, Hoyt J, Petri M, et al. Effects of anti-inflammatory and immunosuppressive drugs on pregnancy and fertility. Semin Arthritis Rheum 1988;18:88–110.
111. Johnson AG, Seideman P, Day RO. Adverse drug interactions with nonsteroidal anti-inflammatory drugs (NSAIDs): Recognition, management and avoidance. Drug Safety 1993;8:99–127.
112. Brandt KD. Should nonsteroidal anti-inflammatory drugs be used to treat osteoarthritis? Rheum Dis Clin North Am 1993;19:29–45.
113. Rehman Q, Lane NE. Getting control of osteoarthritis pain: An update on treatment options. Postgrad Med 1999;106:127–134.
114. Brandt KD, Smith GN Jr., Simon LS. Intraarticular injection of hyaluronan as treatment of knee osteoarthritis: What is the evidence? Arthritis Rheum 2000;43:1192–1203.
115. Brandt KD. Toward pharmacologic modification of joint damage in osteoarthritis. Ann Intern Med 1995;122:874–875.
116. Ghosh P. The pathobiology of osteoarthritis and the rationale for the use of pentosan polysulfate for its treatment. Semin Arthritis Rheum 1999;28:211–267.
117. Yu LP, Smith GN, Brandt KD, et al. Reduction of the severity of canine osteoarthritis by prophylactic treatment with oral doxycycline. Arthritis Rheum 1992;35:1150–1159.
118. Smith GN Jr, Yu LP Jr, Brandt KD, et al. Oral administration of doxycycline reduces collagenase and gelatinase activities in extracts of human osteoarthritic cartilage. J Rheumatol 1998;25:532–535.
119. Dahlberg L, Billinghurst RC, Manner P, et al. Selective enhancement of collagenase-mediated cleavage of resident type II collagen in cultured osteoarthritic cartilage and arrest with a synthetic inhibitor that spares collagenase 1 (matrix metalloproteinase 1). Arthritis Rheum 2000;43:673–682.
120. Ferraz MB, Maetzel A, Bombardier C. A summary of economic evaluations published in the field of rheumatology and related disciplines. Arthritis Rheum 1997;40:1587–1593.
121. Gabriel SE, Crowson CS, Campion ME, et al. Indirect and nonmedical costs among people with rheumatoid arthritis and osteoarthritis compared with nonarthritic controls. J Rheumatol 1997;24:43–48.
122. Maetzel A, Ferraz MB, Bombardier C. The cost-effectiveness of misoprostol in preventing serious gastrointestinal events associated with the use of nonsteroidal anti-inflammatory drugs. Arthritis Rheum 1998;41:16–25.
123. Peterson WL, Cryer B. COX-1-sparing NSAIDs: Is the enthusiasm justified? JAMA 1999;282:1961–1963.
124. Lanes SF, Lanza LL, Radensky PW, et al. Resource utilization and cost of care for rheumatoid arthritis and osteoarthritis in a managed care setting: the importance of drug and surgery costs. Arthritis Rheum 1997; 40:1475–1481.
125. Dougados M. Clinical assessment of osteoarthritis in clinical trials. Curr Opin Rheumatol 1995;7:87–91.
126. Gill TM, Geinstein AR. A critical appraisal of the quality of quality-of-life measurements. JAMA 1994;272:619–626.
127. Wilson IB, Cleary PD. Linking clinical variables with health-related quality of life: A conceptual model of patient outcomes. JAMA 1995; 273:59–65.

93

GOUT AND HYPERURICEMIA

David W. Hawkins and Daniel W. Rahn

The term *gout* describes a disease spectrum including hyperuricemia, recurrent attacks of acute arthritis associated with monosodium urate crystals in leukocytes found in synovial fluid, deposits of monosodium urate crystals in tissues (tophi), interstitial renal disease, and uric acid nephrolithiasis.[1]

Hyperuricemia may be an asymptomatic condition with an increased serum uric acid as the only apparent abnormality. Statistically, hyperuricemia is defined as a serum urate concentrations greater than 2 standard deviations above the population mean. However, for determination of the risk for gout, hyperuricemia is defined as a supersaturated urate concentration.[2] By this definition, a urate concentration greater than 7.0 mg/dL is abnormal and is associated with an increased risk for gout. This corresponds to a measured value greater than 7.5 mg/dL by most autoanalyzers.

EPIDEMIOLOGY

Population studies have shown that serum urate concentration (and consequently the risk of gout) correlates with age, serum creatinine level, blood urea nitrogen level, male gender, blood pressure, body weight, and alcohol intake. Serum urate concentrations are normally distributed with slight skewing toward higher values. Mean values are 6.8 mg/dL for men and 6.0 mg/dL for women.

There is a direct correlation between the serum uric acid concentration and both the incidence and prevalence of gout. The incidence of gout varies from 20 to 35 per 100,000 persons, with an overall prevalence of 1.6 to 13.6 per thousand. Prevalence increases with age, especially in men.[1] Men are affected by gout approximately 10 times more often than women. Although no genetic marker has been isolated for gout, the familial nature of gout strongly suggests an interaction between genetic and environmental factors.

ETIOLOGY AND PATHOPHYSIOLOGY

In humans, uric acid is the end product of the degradation of purines. Uric acid serves no known physiologic purpose and therefore is regarded as a waste product. In lower animals, the enzyme uricase breaks down uric acid to the more soluble allantoin, and thus uric acid does not accumulate. Gout occurs exclusively in humans in whom a miscible pool of uric acid exists. Under normal conditions, the amount of cumulated uric acid is about 1200 mg in men and about 600 mg in women. The size of the urate pool is increased severalfold in individuals with gout. This excess accumulation may result from either overproduction or underexcretion.

OVERPRODUCTION OF URIC ACID

The purines from which uric acid is produced originate from three sources: dietary purine, conversion of tissue nucleic acid to purine nucleotides, and de novo synthesis of purine bases. The purines derived from these three sources enter a common metabolic pathway leading to the production of either nucleic acid or uric acid. Under normal circumstances, uric acid may accumulate excessively if production exceeds excretion. The average human produces about 600 to 800 mg of uric acid each day.

Several enzyme systems regulate purine metabolism. Abnormalities in these regulatory systems can result in overproduction of uric acid. Uric acid also may be overproduced as a consequence of increased breakdown of tissue nucleic acids, as with myeloproliferative and lymphoproliferative disorders. Dietary purines play an unimportant role in the generation of hyperuricemia in the absence of some derangement in purine metabolism or elimination.

Two enzyme abnormalities resulting in an overproduction of uric acid have been well described (Fig. 93–1). The first is an increase in the activity of phosphoribosyl pyrophosphate (PRPP) synthetase, which leads to an increased concentration of PRPP. PRPP is a key determinant of purine synthesis and thus uric acid production. The second is a deficiency of hypoxanthine-guanine phosphoribosyl transferase (HGPRT).

HGPRT is responsible for the conversion of guanine to guanylic acid and hypoxanthine to inosinic acid. These two conversions require PRPP as the cosubstrate and are important reutilization reactions involved in the synthesis of nucleic acids. A deficiency in the HGPRT enzyme leads to increased metabolism of guanine and hypoxanthine to uric acid and more PRPP to interact with glutamine in the first step of the purine pathway.[3] Complete absence of HGPRT results in the childhood Lesch-Nyhan syndrome, characterized by choreoathetosis, spasticity, mental retardation, and markedly excessive production of uric acid. A partial deficiency of the enzyme may be responsible for marked hyperuricemia in otherwise normal, healthy individuals.

UNDEREXCRETION OF URIC ACID

Uric acid does not accumulate as long as uric acid production is balanced with elimination. Uric acid is eliminated in two ways. About two-thirds of the uric acid produced each day is excreted in the urine. The rest is eliminated through the gastrointestinal tract after enzymatic degradation by colonic bacteria.

A decline in the urinary excretion of uric acid to a level below the rate of production leads to hyperuricemia and an increased miscible pool of sodium urate. Almost all the urate in plasma is freely filtered across the glomerulus. The concentration of uric acid appearing in the urine is determined by multiple renal tubular transport processes in addition to the filtered load. Evidence favors a four-component model including glomerular filtration, tubular reabsorption, tubular secretion, and postsecretory reabsorption.[2]

Approximately 90% of filtered uric acid is reabsorbed in the proximal tubule, probably by both active and passive transport mechanisms. There is a close linkage between proximal tubular sodium reabsorption and uric acid reabsorption, so states that enhance sodium reabsorption (e.g., dehydration) also lead to increased uric acid reabsorption. The exact site of tubular secretion of uric acid has not been

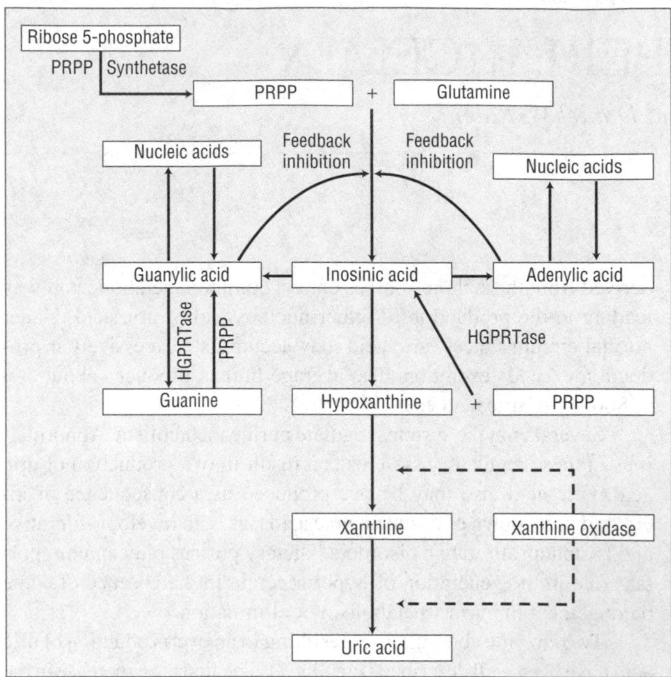

FIGURE 93–1. Purine metabolism.

determined; this too appears to involve an active transport process. Postsecretory reabsorption occurs somewhere distal to the secretory site.

Factors that decrease uric acid clearance or increase its production will result in an increase in serum urate concentration. Some of these factors are listed in Table 93–1. Drugs that decrease renal clearance of uric acid through modification of filtered load or one of the tubular transport processes are listed in Table 93–2.

The pathophysiologic approach to the evaluation of hyperuricemia requires determining whether the patient is overproducing or underexcreting uric acid. This can be accomplished by placing the patient on a purine-free diet for 3 to 5 days and then measuring the amount of uric acid excreted in the urine in 24 hours. Normal individuals produce 600 to 800 mg of uric acid daily and excrete less than 600 mg in urine. Individuals who excrete more than 600 mg on a purine-free diet may be considered overproducers. Hyperuricemic individuals who excrete less than 600 mg of uric acid per 24 hours on a purine-free diet may be classified as underexcretors of uric acid. It is very difficult in clinical practice, however, to maintain someone on a purine-free diet for several days. On a regular diet, excretion of greater than 1000 mg per 24 hours reflects overproduction; less than this is probably normal.

TABLE 93–1. Conditions Associated with Hyperuricemia

Primary gout	Obesity
Diabetic ketoacidosis	Sarcoidosis
Myeloproliferative disorders	Congestive heart failure
Lactic acidosis	Renal dysfunction
Lymphoproliferative disorders	Down syndrome
Starvation	Lead toxicity
Chronic hemolytic anemia	Hyperparathyroidism
Toxemia of pregnancy	Acute alcoholism
Pernicious anemia	Hypoparathyroidism
Glycogen storage disease type 1	Acromegaly
Psoriasis	Hypothyroidism

TABLE 93–2. Drugs Capable of Inducing Hyperuricemia and Gout

Diuretics	Ethanol	Ethambutol
Nicotinic acid	Pyrazinamide	Cytotoxic drugs
Salicylates (<2 g/d)	Levodopa	Cyclosporine

CLINICAL PRESENTATION

Gout is a disease manifested by acute attacks of arthritis, nephrolithiasis, gouty nephropathy, and aggregated deposits of sodium urate (tophi) in cartilage, tendons, synovial membranes, and elsewhere.

ACUTE GOUTY ARTHRITIS

Acute attacks of gouty arthritis are characterized by rapid onset of excruciating pain, swelling, and inflammation. The attack typically is monoarticular at first, most often affecting the first metatarsophalangeal (MTP) joint (great toe) and then, in order of frequency, the insteps, ankles, heels, knees, wrists, fingers, and elbows. In one-half of initial attacks, the first MTP joint is affected. Of gouty patients, 90% experience attacks in the great toe at some point in their disease.

The predilection of acute gout for peripheral joints of the lower extremity is probably related to the low temperature of these joints combined with high intraarticular urate concentration. Synovial effusions are postulated to occur transiently in weight-bearing joints in the course of a day with routine activity. At night, water is reabsorbed from the joint space, leaving behind a supersaturated solution of monosodium urate, which can precipitate attacks of acute arthritis. Attacks generally begin at night with the patient awakening from sleep in excruciating pain.

The development of crystal-induced inflammation involves a number of chemical mediators causing vasodilation, increased vascular permeability, and chemotactic activity for polymorphonuclear leukocytes.[4] Phagocytosis of urate crystals by the leukocytes results in rapid lysis of cells and a discharge of proteolytic enzymes into the cytoplasm. The ensuing inflammatory reaction is associated with intense joint pain, erythema, warmth, and swelling. Fever is common, as is leukocytosis. Untreated attacks may last from 3 to 14 days before spontaneous recovery.

Although acute attacks of gouty arthritis may occur without apparent provocation, a number of conditions may precipitate an attack. These include stress, trauma, alcohol ingestion, infection, surgery, rapid lowering of serum uric acid by ingestion of uric acid-lowering agents, and ingestion of certain drugs known to elevate serum uric acid concentrations. The diagnosis is best accomplished by aspiration of synovial fluid from the affected joint and identification of intracellular crystals of monosodium urate monohydrate in synovial fluid leukocytes. Other crystal-induced arthropathies that may resemble gout on clinical presentation are caused by calcium pyrophosphate dihydrate crystals (pseudogout) and calcium hydroxyapatite crystals, which are associated with calcific periarthritis, tendinitis, and arthritis.[5,6]

URIC ACID NEPHROLITHIASIS

Nephrolithiasis occurs in 10% to 25% of patients with gout.[7] Factors that predispose individuals to uric acid nephrolithiasis include excessive urinary excretion of uric acid, an acidic urine, and a highly concentrated urine. The risk of renal calculi approaches 50% in individuals whose renal excretion of uric acid exceeds 1100 mg/d. In addition to pure uric acid stones, hyperuricosuric individuals are at increased risk for mixed uric acid–calcium oxalate stones and pure calcium oxalate stones. Uric acid stones are usually small, round, and radiolucent. Uric acid stones containing calcium are radiopaque.[7]

Uric acid has a pK_a of 5.5. Therefore, when the urine is acidic, uric acid exists primarily in the un-ionized, less soluble form. At a urine pH of 5.0, urine is saturated at a uric acid level of 15 mg/dL. When the urine pH is 7.0, the solubility of uric acid in urine is increased to 200 mg/dL.[8] In patients with uric acid nephrolithiasis, urinary pH typically is less than 6.0 and frequently less than 5.5. When an acidic urine is saturated with uric acid, spontaneous precipitation of stones may occur.

GOUTY NEPHROPATHY

There are two types of gouty nephropathy: acute uric acid nephropathy and chronic urate nephropathy.[9] In acute uric acid nephropathy, acute renal failure occurs as a result of blockage of urine flow secondary to massive precipitation of uric acid crystals in the collecting ducts and ureters. This syndrome is a well-recognized complication in patients with myeloproliferative or lymphoproliferative disorders and is a result of massive malignant cell turnover, particularly after initiation of chemotherapy.

Chronic urate nephropathy is caused by the long-term deposition of urate crystals in the renal parenchyma. Microtophi may form, with a surrounding giant cell inflammatory reaction. A decrease in the kidney's ability to concentrate urine and the presence of proteinuria may be the earliest pathophysiologic disturbances. Hypertension and nephrosclerosis are common associated findings. Although renal failure occurs in a higher percentage of gouty patients than expected, it is not clear that hyperuricemia per se has a harmful effect on the kidney. The chronic renal impairment seen in individuals with gout may result largely from the co-occurrence of hypertension, diabetes mellitus, and atherosclerosis.

TOPHACEOUS GOUT

Tophi (urate deposits) are uncommon in the general population of gouty subjects and are a late complication of hyperuricemia. The most common sites of tophaceous deposits in patients with recurrent acute gouty arthritis are the base of the great toe, helix of the ear, olecranon bursae, Achilles tendon, knees, wrists, and hands.[2] Eventually, even the hips, shoulders, and spine may be affected. In addition to causing obvious deformities, tophi may damage surrounding soft tissue, cause joint destruction and pain, and even lead to nerve compression syndromes including carpal tunnel syndrome.

▶ TREATMENT: Gout and Hyperuricemia

The goals in the treatment of gout are to terminate the acute attack, prevent recurrent attacks of gouty arthritis, and prevent complications associated with chronic deposition of urate crystals in tissues.[10] Patients should be advised to reduce their dietary intake of saturated fats and meats high in purines (e.g., organ meats).[11]

ACUTE GOUTY ARTHRITIS

Acute attacks of gouty arthritis may be treated successfully with colchicine or any of a variety of nonsteroidal anti-inflammatory drugs (NSAIDs) (Fig. 93–2).

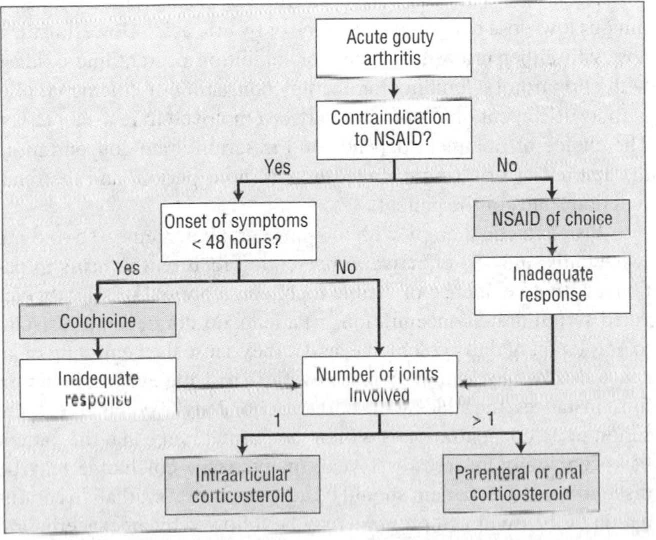

FIGURE 93–2. Treatment algorithm for acute gouty arthritis.

Colchicine can be given orally or parenterally. Unless contraindications exist or the patient has renal insufficiency, the usual oral dose is 1 mg initially, followed by 0.5 mg every 2 hours until the joint symptoms subside, until the patient develops abdominal discomfort or diarrhea, or until a total dose of 8 mg has been administered.[12] About 75% to 95% of patients with acute gouty arthritis respond favorably to colchicine when ingestion of the drug is begun within 24 to 48 hours of the onset of joint symptoms.[13] If the initiation of colchicine is delayed longer than 48 hours after the onset of acute symptoms, the probability of success with the drug diminishes substantially.

The major problem associated with the use of oral colchicine is that it causes gastrointestinal side effects in 50% to 80% of patients before the relief of the attack.

This high incidence of gastrointestinal side effects may be circumvented by administering colchicine intravenously. Except in patients with renal insufficiency, the initial intravenous dose of colchicine is 2 mg. If relief is not obtained, an additional 1-mg dose may be given at 6 and 12 hours to a total dose of 4 mg for a specific attack. The colchicine should be diluted with 20 mL normal saline before administration to minimize sclerosis of the vein. The intravenous administration of colchicine eliminates most of the gastrointestinal symptoms associated with the oral dose but subjects the patient to the risk of local extravasation, which can cause inflammation in and necrosis of the surrounding tissue. Very small, difficult-to-inject veins and renal impairment represent relative contraindications to intravenous colchicine therapy.

Because of the risk of bone marrow toxicity, colchicine should be discontinued for 7 days following initial therapy with either oral or intravenous administration. Colchicine should not be used intravenously in individuals who are neutropenic, have severe renal impairment (a creatinine clearance of less than 10 mL/min), or have combined renal and hepatic insufficiency. The dose should be decreased by 50% in individuals with renal insufficiency (a creatine clearance of

10–50 mL/min) and limited to a total dose of 2 mg in patients receiving oral maintenance colchicine.[14]

Indomethacin is as effective as colchicine in the treatment of acute gouty arthritis. Because acute gastrointestinal toxicity occurs far less frequently with indomethacin than with colchicine, it is preferred. Side effects unique to indomethacin include headache and dizziness. All NSAIDs have been implicated in the cause of gastric ulceration and bleeding, but with short-term therapy, this is not likely.

For treatment of acute gouty arthritis, indomethacin may be begun with a relatively large dose for the first 24 to 48 hours and then tapered over 3 to 4 days to minimize the risk of recurrent attacks. For example, 75 mg of indomethacin should be given initially, followed by 50 mg every 6 hours for 2 days and then 50 mg every 8 hours for 1 or 2 days.

A number of other NSAIDs (e.g., naproxen, fenoprofen, ibuprofen, and piroxicam) are also effective in relieving the inflammation of acute gout. There is no evidence that any given NSAID is superior to all the others in the management of acute gout.[15] All NSAIDs should be used with caution in individuals with a history of acid peptic disease, heart failure, chronic renal failure, or coronary artery disease.

Corticosteroids may be used to treat acute attacks of gouty arthritis, but they are reserved primarily for resistant cases or for patients with a contraindication to colchicine and NSAID therapy.[15] Doses of 40–80 USP units of adrenocorticotropic hormone gel are given intramuscularly every 6 to 8 hours for 2 to 3 days, and then the doses are reduced in stepwise fashion and discontinued. Intraarticular administration of triamcinolone hexacetonide in a dose of 20–40 mg may be useful in treating acute gout limited to a single joint. Prednisone may be administered orally in doses of 30–60 mg for 3 to 5 days in patients with multiple-joint involvement. Because rebound attacks may occur on steroid withdrawal, the dose should be tapered gradually by 5-mg decreases over 10 to 14 days and discontinued.

NEPHROLITHIASIS

The medical management of uric acid nephrolithiasis includes hydration sufficient to maintain a urine volume of 2 to 3 L/d, alkalinization of urine, avoidance of purine-rich foods, moderation of protein intake, and reduction of urinary uric acid excretion.

Maintenance of a 24-hour urine volume of 2 to 3 L with an adequate intake of fluids is desirable for all gouty patients but especially for those with excessive (>1.0 g/day) uric acid excretion. Alkalinizing agents should be used with the objective of making the urine less acidic. Urine pH should be maintained at 6.0 to 6.5. In this pH range, up to 85% of uric acid will be in the form of the soluble urate ion.

Reduction of urine acidity can be accomplished by the administration of sodium bicarbonate or Shohl's solution (40 g citric acid and 98 g sodium citrate per liter). With the former, 2–6 g/day is given in equally divided doses at 6- to 8-hour intervals. A dose of 20–60 mL of Shohl's solution per day, given in three or four divided doses, provides an equivalent amount of alkali. If use of a sodium salt is contraindicated, potassium citrate may be used instead.

One must keep in mind that older patients with uric acid kidney stones also may have hypertension, congestive heart failure, or renal insufficiency and obviously should not be exposed to overload with alkalinizing sodium salts or unlimited fluid intake. Acetazolamide, a carbonic anhydrase inhibitor, produces rapid and effective urinary alkalinization and sometimes is used in conjunction with alkali therapy. When a 250-mg dose of acetazolamide is given at bedtime, the excretion of an acidic urine in the early morning hours is avoided. The usual tachyphylaxis (rapid tolerance) to this drug is obviated by a daily repletion dose of bicarbonate.

Since the advent of allopurinol, a low-purine, low-protein diet in the patient with uric acid lithiasis is no longer as critical as it once was; however, it is still advisable to instruct the patient to avoid foods rich in purine and to limit protein to no more than 90 g/day. Such a diet is still palatable and reduces appreciably the amount of uric acid in the urine.

The mainstay of drug therapy for recurrent uric acid lithiasis is allopurinol. It is effective in reducing both serum and urinary uric acid levels, thus preventing the formation of calculi. Allopurinol is also recommended as prophylactic treatment in patients who will receive cytotoxic agents for the treatment of lymphoma or leukemia. The marked increase in uric acid production associated with cytolysis of a neoplasm predisposes a patient to the development of uric acid nephrolithiasis.

PROPHYLACTIC THERAPY

After the first attack of acute gouty arthritis or after the passage of the first renal stone, a decision to institute prophylactic therapy must be entertained. If the first episode was mild and responded promptly to treatment, the patient's serum urate concentration was elevated only minimally, and the 24-hour urinary uric acid excretion was not excessive (<1000 mg/24 hours on a regular diet), then prophylactic treatment can be withheld. Some patients never have a second attack or a second stone. Others may not experience a second gouty episode for 5 to 10 years. A wait-and-see attitude, therefore, seems justified in patients who meet these conditions.[5]

On the other hand, if the patient had a severe attack of gouty arthritis, a complicated course of uric acid lithiasis, a substantially elevated serum uric acid (>10.0 mg/dL), or a 24-hour urinary excretion of uric acid of more than 1000 mg, then prophylactic treatment should be instituted immediately after resolution of the acute episode. Prophylactic therapy is also appropriate for patients with frequent attacks (more than two or three per year) of gouty arthritis even if the serum uric acid concentration is normal or only minimally elevated.

Recurrences of acute gouty arthritis may be prevented with continuous low-dose daily oral colchicine or by uric acid—lowering therapy with either uricosuric agents or inhibition of xanthine oxidase with allopurinol. Combination therapy consisting of colchicine plus a uricosuric agent or allopurinol may be employed in resistant cases. The choice of treatment depends on the serum urate concentration, the amount of uric acid excreted in a 24-hour period, and the renal function status of the patient.

Prophylactic therapy with low-dose oral colchicine, 0.5–0.6 mg twice daily, may be effective in preventing recurrent arthritis in patients with no evidence of visible tophi and a normal or slightly elevated serum urate concentration.[12] Patients do not become resistant to or tolerant of daily colchicine, and if they sense the beginning of an acute attack, they should increase the dose to 1 mg every 2 hours; in most instances, the attack will abort after 1 or 2 mg of colchicine. If the serum urate concentration is within the normal range and the patient has been symptom-free for 1 year, maintenance colchicine may be discontinued. The patient should be advised, however, that discontinuation of the treatment program may be followed by an exacerbation of acute gouty arthritis.

Patients with a history of recurrent acute gouty arthritis and a significantly elevated serum uric acid concentration probably are best managed with uric acid–lowering therapy. Colchicine at a dose of 0.5 mg twice daily should be administered during the first 6 to 12 months of antihyperuricemic therapy to minimize the risk of acute attacks that may occur during initiation of uric acid–lowering therapy. The therapeutic objective of antihyperuricemic therapy is to reduce the serum urate concentration below 6 mg/dL, well below the saturation point.

Reduction of the serum urate concentration can be accomplished pharmacologically by increasing the renal excretion of uric acid or by decreasing its synthesis. The drugs used most widely to increase uric acid excretion are probenecid and sulfinpyrazone. Several other uricosuric drugs are available in Europe, but they have not been approved for use in the United States.

URICOSURIC DRUGS

Uricosuric drugs increase the renal clearance of uric acid by inhibiting the renal tubular reabsorption of uric acid. Therapy with uricosuric drugs should be started at a low dose to avoid marked uricosuria and possible stone formation. The maintenance of adequate urine flow and alkalinization of the urine with sodium bicarbonate or Shohl's solution during the first several days of uricosuric therapy further diminish the possibility of uric acid stone formation. Probenecid is given initially at a dose of 250 mg twice a day for 1 to 2 weeks and then 500 mg twice a day for 2 weeks. Thereafter, the daily dose is increased by 500-mg increments every 1 to 2 weeks until satisfactory control is achieved or a maximum dose of 2.0 g is reached. The initial dose of sulfinpyrazone is 50 mg twice a day for 3 to 4 days and then 100 mg twice a day, increasing the daily dose by 100-mg increments each week up to 800 mg/day.

The major side effects associated with uricosuric therapy are gastrointestinal irritation, rash and hypersensitivity, precipitation of acute gouty arthritis, and stone formation. These drugs are contraindicated in patients who are allergic to them and in patients with impaired renal function (a creatinine clearance below 50 mL/min); for such patients, allopurinol should be used.

XANTHINE OXIDASE INHIBITOR

Currently, allopurinol is the only drug approved for use in inhibiting uric acid synthesis. Both allopurinol and its major metabolite, oxypurinol, are xanthine oxidase inhibitors and thus impair the conversion of hypoxanthine to xanthine and xanthine to uric acid. Allopurinol also lowers the intracellular concentration of PRPP. Because of the long half-life of its metabolite, allopurinol can be given once daily. An oral daily dose of 300 mg usually is sufficient. Occasionally, as much as 600–800 mg/day may be necessary.

Allopurinol is the antihyperuricemic drug of choice in patients with a history of urinary stones or impaired renal function, in patients who have lymphoproliferative or myeloproliferative disorders and need pretreatment with a xanthine oxidase inhibitor before initiation of cytotoxic therapy to protect against acute uric acid nephropathy, and in patients with gout who are overproducers of uric acid. The major side effects of allopurinol are skin rash, leukopenia, occasional gastrointestinal toxicity, and increased frequency of acute gouty attacks with the initiation of therapy.

ASYMPTOMATIC HYPERURICEMIA

Questions are often raised regarding the indications for drug therapy for asymptomatic hyperuricemia. The purported benefits from treatment include prevention of acute gouty arthritis, tophi formation, nephrolithiasis, and chronic urate nephropathy. The first three complications are easily controlled should they develop; therefore, antihyperuricemic therapy is not warranted to prevent these conditions. The prevention of urate nephropathy might be a stronger indication because it is irreversible even with proper treatment. Available data indicate, however, that gouty nephropathy is extremely rare in the absence of clinical gout, and evidence that elevation of uric acid by itself may cause renal disease is weak and inconclusive.[16,17] As discussed previously, renal impairment is very rare in the absence of concurrent hypertension and atherosclerosis. In addition, it is unclear whether uric acid—lowering therapy protects renal function in such individuals. Available data thus do not justify therapy for most patients with asymptomatic hyperuricemia.

PHARMACOECONOMIC CONSIDERATIONS

Assuming no treatment of asymptomatic hyperuricemia, pharmacoeconomic considerations apply only to the management of the acute and chronic clinical manifestations of gout.

In a cost-effectiveness analysis in patients with nontophaceous recurrent gouty arthritis, urate-lowering therapy was found to reduce costs if patients experienced two or more recurrent attacks per year.[18] Generic allopurinol was associated with a lower incremental cost-effectiveness ratio than were either probenecid or sulfinpyrazone.

In the case of chronic tophaceous gout, a need to continue long-term therapy with a urate-lowering drug clearly exists. Allopurinol generally is less expensive than uricosuric therapy and may be more effective. Comparative trials are lacking. For severe cases, combination therapy may be indicated. Many clinicians will add colchicine to the regimen to reduce the likelihood of precipitating acute gouty arthritis, but this does not appear to be a cost-effective measure.

CONCLUSION

Hyperuricemia may lead to acute arthritis, chronic gout, or kidney stones or remain asymptomatic. Asymptomatic hyperuricemia need not be treated, especially if the serum urate concentration remains below 10 mg/dL.

Acute gouty arthritis requires either colchicine or an NSAID to treat the underlying inflammatory condition. The management of uric acid kidney stones includes hydration and alkalinization of the urine. Prevention of recurrent gouty arthritis or recurrent nephrolithiasis and treatment of chronic gout require hypouricemic therapy with either a uricosuric drug or allopurinol. Allopurinol is the hypouricemic drug of choice in patients with a history of uric acid stones or renal insufficiency and in patients known to be overproducers of uric acid.

▶ PRINCIPLES OF PHARMACOTHERAPY

- Asymptomatic hyperuricemia discovered incidentally requires no therapy.
- Acute gouty arthritis may be treated effectively with short courses of high-dose nonacetylated NSAIDs or colchicine.
- Individuals with contraindications to NSAIDs (e.g., active peptic ulcer disease, renal impairment, heart failure, or history of hypersensitivity) or individuals who cannot ingest medications orally may be treated with intravenous corticosteroids or intraarticular corticosteroids.
- Intravenous colchicine is rapidly effective but cannot be administered to individuals with renal impairment or extrahepatic biliary obstruction. A single intravenous dose should not exceed 2–3 mg, with a cumulative total dose not exceeding 4–5 mg per episode.
- Recurrent attacks of gouty arthritis can be prevented effectively through administration of uric acid–lowering therapy.
- Treatment with urate-lowering drugs is considered cost-effective for acute gouty arthritis in patients having two or more attacks of gout per year.
- When allopurinol is used, start with a low dose (100 mg/d) after the acute attack has settled, and adjust the dose every 4 weeks until the goal is reached (serum urate of <6 mg/dL). Give colchicine (0.5 mg twice daily) during the first 3 months of therapy, and stop allopurinol if rash develops or liver function tests become abnormal.
- Uricosuric agents should be avoided in patients with renal impairment (a creatinine clearance below 50 mL/min), a history of renal calculi, and overproduction of uric acid.
- Uric acid nephrolithiasis should be treated with adequate hydration (2–3 L/day), a daytime urine-alkalinizing agent, and a 250-mg bedtime dose of acetazolamide.
- Individuals with tophaceous deposits have a large uric acid pool and benefit from allopurinol adminstration.

REFERENCES

1. Kelley WN, Worthman RL. Gout and hyperuricemia. In: Kelley WN, Harris EP, Ruddy S, Sledge CB, eds. Textbook of Rheumatology. Philadelphia, Saunders, 1997: 1313–1351.
2. Levinson DJ, Becker MA. Clinical gout and the pathogenesis of hyperuricemia. In: Koopman WJ, ed. Arthritis and Allied Conditions, 13th ed. Baltimore, Williams & Wilkins, 1997: 2041–2071.
3. Wilson JM, Young AB, Kelley WN. Hypoxanthine-guanine phosphoribosyltransferase deficiency. N Engl J Med 1983;309:900–910.
4. Beutler A, Schumacher HR. Gout and "pseudogout": When are arthritis symptoms caused by crystal deposition? Postgrad Med 1994;95:103–116.
5. McGill NW. Gout and other crystal arthropathies. Med J Aust 1997;166: 33–38.
6. Schumacher HR. Crystal-reduced arthritis: An overview. Am J Med 1996; 100(Suppl 2A):46S–52S.
7. Yu T. Nephrolithiasis in patients with gout. Postgrad Med 1978;63: 164–170.
8. Worthman RL. Management of hyperuricemia. In: Koopman WJ, ed. Arthritis and Allied Conditions, 13th ed. Baltimore, Williams & Wilkins, 1997: 2073–2083.
9. Klineberg JR. Role of the kidneys in the pathogenesis of gout. Postgrad Med 1978;63:145–150.
10. Star VL, Hochberg MC. Prevention and management of gout. Drugs 1993;45:212–222.
11. Davis JC. A practical approach to gout: Current management of an "old" disease. Postgrad Med 1999;106:115–123.
12. Emmerson BT. The management of gout. N Engl J Med 1996;334:445–451.
13. Tan N, Lertratanakul Y, Barr WG. Acute gouty arthritis. Postgrad Med 1993;94:73–87.
14. Evans TI, Wheeler MT, Small RE, et al. A comprehensive investigation of inpatient intravenous colchicine use shows more education is needed. J Rheumatol 1996;23:143–148.
15. Conaghan PG, Day RO. Management and prevention of gout: Risks and benefits of drugs used. Curr Ther 1995;(Apr):75–80.
16. Dykman D, Simon EE, Avioli W. Hyperuricemia and uric acid nephropathy. Arch Intern Med 1987;147:1341–1345.
17. Harris MD, Siegel LB, Alloway JA. Gout and hyperuricemia. Am Fam Physician 1999;59:925–934.
18. Ferrgz MB, O'Brien B. A cost effectiveness analysis of urate lowering drugs in nontophaceous recurrent gouty arthritis. J Rheumatol 1995;22: 908–914.

94

GLAUCOMA

Timothy S. Lesar

The glaucomas are a group of ocular disorders involving optic neuropathy characterized by changes in the optic nerve head (optic disk) and loss of visual sensitivity and field. Increased intraocular pressure (IOP), a traditional diagnostic criterion for glaucoma, is thought to play an important role in the pathogenesis of glaucoma but is no longer a diagnostic criterion for glaucoma. Two major types of glaucoma have been identified: open angle and closed angle. Open-angle glaucoma accounts for the great majority of cases. Either type may be a primary inherited disorder, congenital, or secondary to disease, trauma, or drugs. Both primary and secondary glaucomas may be caused by a combination of open-angle and closed-angle mechanisms (Table 94–1). Glaucoma affects up to 2.5 million individuals in the United States and 66.8 million individuals worldwide, of which 135,00 in the United States and 6.7 million worldwide will have bilateral blindness as a result. The prevalence rate varies with age, race, diagnostic criteria, and other factors. Overall, in the United States, open-angle glaucoma occurs in 1.5% of the population over 30 years of age, 1.3% of whites and 3.5% of blacks. The incidence of open-angle glaucoma increases with increasing age. The incidence of the disease in patients 80 years of age is 3% in whites and 5% to 8% in blacks.

The incidence of closed-angle glaucoma also varies by ethnic group, with higher incidence in individuals of Eskimo, Chinese, and Asian-Indian descent. Incidence rates of 1% to 4% have been reported in these populations.[1,2] This chapter reviews the pathophysiology, clinical findings, and drug therapy of glaucoma.

PATHOPHYSIOLOGY

MECHANISM OF OPTIC NEUROPATHY

OPEN-ANGLE GLAUCOMA

The specific cause of glaucomatous optic neuropathy is presently unknown. Previously, increased IOP was considered to be the sole cause of the visual damage; however, it is now recognized that IOP is only one of many factors associated with the development and progression of glaucoma. Increased susceptibility of the optic nerve to retinal ischemia, a reduced or dysregulated blood flow, excitotoxicity, autoimmune reactions, and other abnormal physiologic processes are likely additional contributory factors.

Indeed, open-angle glaucoma may represent a number of distinct diseases or conditions that simply manifest the same symptoms. Susceptibility to visual loss at a given IOP varies considerably; some patients do not demonstrate damage at high IOPs, whereas other patients have progressive visual-field loss despite an IOP in the "normal" range (normal-tension glaucoma).

Although IOP poorly predicts which patients will have visual-field loss, the risk of visual-field loss clearly increases with increasing IOP within any range. Reduction of IOP, no matter what the level of pretreatment IOP, slows or prevents progression of visual-field loss and optic disk changes in most patients.

The mechanism by which an IOP too great for the susceptibility of a given eye increases the risk for nerve damage remains controversial. Multiple mechanisms are likely to be operative in a spectrum of combinations to produce the death of optic nerve ganglion cells observed in glaucoma. Pressure-sensitive astrocytes and other cells in the optic disk supportive structure matrix may produce changes and remodeling of the disk, resulting in axonal death. Vasogenic theories suggest that optic nerve damage results from insufficient blood flow to the retina secondary to the increased perfusion pressure required in the eye, dysregulated perfusion, or vessel wall abnormalities and results in degeneration of axonal fibers of the retina. Another theory suggests that the IOP may disrupt axoplasmal flow at the optic disk.

Recently, focus on the mechanisms of the retinal ganglion cell apoptosis and the role of excessive glutamate and nitric oxide found in glaucoma patients has broadened the focus of drug therapy research to include evaluation of agents that act as neuroprotectants. Such agents may be particularly useful in patients with normal-pressure glaucoma, in whom pressure-independent factors may play a relatively larger role in disease progression. These agents would target risk factors and underlying pathophysiologic mechanisms of disease other than IOP.[1–14]

CLOSED-ANGLE GLAUCOMA

The role of increased IOP in closed-angle glaucoma (CAG) is more clear. In CAG, a physical blockage of trabecular meshwork is present. In many cases, single or multiple episodes of excessively high IOP (>40 mm Hg) result in optic neuropathy. Very high IOP (>60 mm Hg) may result in permanent loss of visual field within a matter hours to days. One type of CAG, known as "creeping" angle closure, occurs in patients with narrow angles and may result in continuously increased IOP in ranges more similar to primary open-angle glaucoma (POAG), and similar to POAG, individuals differ in the degree and rapidity of visual loss from any given elevated IOP.[1]

AQUEOUS HUMOR DYNAMICS AND IOP

Presently, the drug therapy of glaucoma is designed to reduce IOP, even if it is in the normal range, thereby reducing the risk of progression of visual loss. An understanding of IOP and aqueous humor dynamics will assist the reader in understanding the drug therapy of glaucoma.[1–2,15–17]

Aqueous humor is formed in the ciliary body (Figs. 94–1 and 94–2) through both filtration and secretion. Because ultrafiltration depends on pressure gradients, blood pressure and IOP changes influence aqueous humor formation. Osmotic gradients produced by active secretion of sodium and bicarbonate and possibly other solutes such

TABLE 94–1. General Classification of Glaucoma

- I. Primary glaucoma
  - A. Open angle
  - B. Angle closure
    - 1. With pupillary block
    - 2. Without pupillary block
- II. Secondary glaucoma
  - A. Open angle
    - 1. Pretrabecular
    - 2. Trabecular
    - 3. Posttrabecular
  - B. Angle closure
    - 1. Without pupillary block
    - 2. With pupillary block
- III. Congenital glaucoma

as ascorbate from the ciliary body epithelial cells into the aqueous humor result in movement of water from the pool of stromal ultrafiltrate into the posterior chamber, forming the aqueous humor. Carbonic anhydrase (primarily isoenzyme type II), α- and β-adrenergic receptors, and sodium- and potassium-activated ATPases are found on the ciliary body epithelium and appear to be involved in this secretion of the solutes sodium and bicarbonate.

Receptor systems controlling aqueous inflow have not been elucidated fully. Pharmacologic studies suggest that β-adrenergic agents increase inflow, whereas α_2-adrenergic-, α-adrenergic-blocking, β-adrenergic-blocking, dopamine-blocking, carbonic anhydrase–inhibiting, and adenylate cyclase–stimulating agents decrease aqueous inflow. Aqueous humor produced by the ciliary body is secreted into the posterior chamber at a rate of approximately 2 to 3 μL/min. The pressure in the posterior chamber produced by the constant inflow pushes the aqueous humor between the iris and lens and through the pupil into the anterior chamber of the eye[1,2,15–19] (see Fig. 94–2).

Aqueous humor in the anterior chamber leaves the eye by two routes: (1) filtration through the trabecular meshwork to Schlemm's canal (80% to 85%) and (2) traversal of the anterior face of the iris and absorption into iris blood vessels (uveoscleral outflow). Cholinergic agents such as pilocarpine increase outflow by physically pulling open the meshwork pores secondary to ciliary muscle contraction. The uveoscleral outflow of aqueous humor is also increased by prostaglandin $F_{2\alpha}$ analogues, and β- and α_2-adrenergic agonists. Constant inflow of aqueous humor from the ciliary body and resistance to outflow result in an IOP great enough to produce an outflow rate equal to the inflow rate (see Fig. 94–2).

The median IOP measured in large populations is 15.5 ± 2.5 mm Hg; however, the distribution of pressures around the mean is skewed to the right (toward higher readings). IOP is not constant and changes with pulse, blood pressure, forced expiration or coughing, neck compression, and posture. IOP is measured by tonometry: indentation tonometry, applanation tonometry, or a noncontact method using an air pulse. These methods may result in slightly different pressure readings. IOPs consistently greater than 21 mm Hg are found in 5% to 8% of the general population. The incidence increases with age such that "abnormal" (i.e., >22 mm Hg) IOP is found in 15% of those 70 to 75 years of age. Intermittently very high IOP (>40 mm Hg) is found in patients with CAG. The increased IOP in all types of glaucoma results from the decreased facility for aqueous humor outflow through the trabecular meshwork. Aqueous humor production in POAG is normal.[1,2,15–17]

IOP demonstrates considerable circadian variation primarily because of changes in the rate of aqueous humor formation. This circadian variation results in a minimum IOP at approximately 6 p.m. and a maximum IOP at awakening. The circadian IOP variation is usually

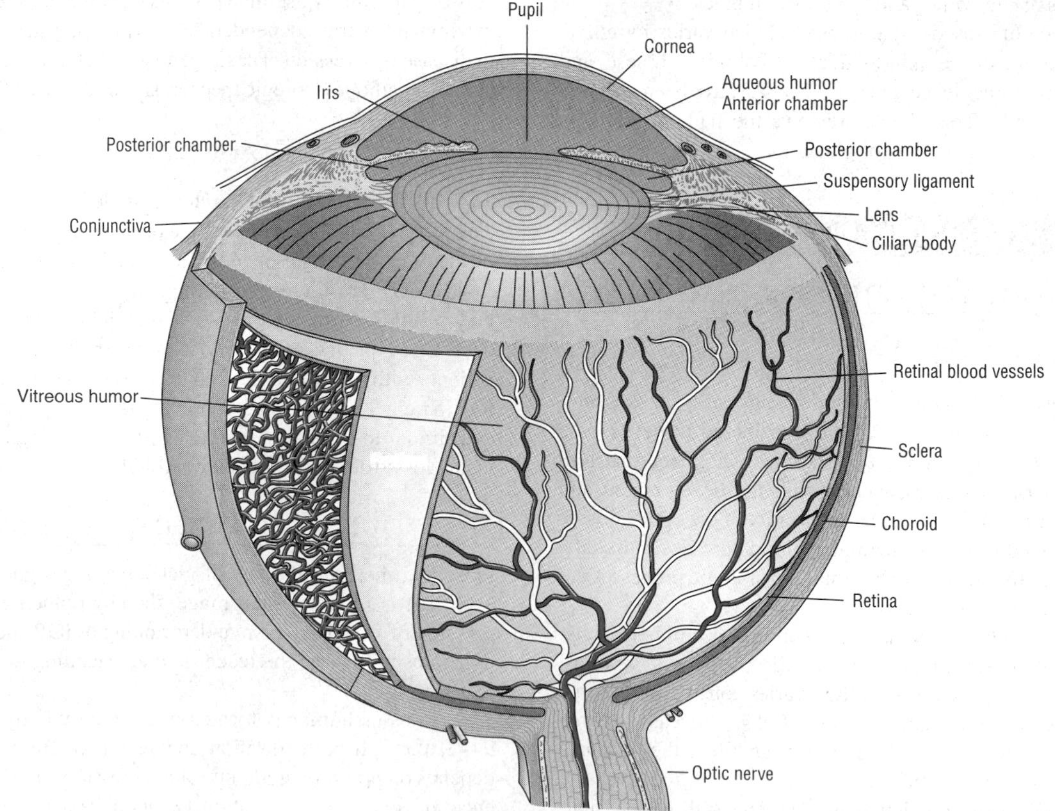

FIGURE 94–1. Anatomy of the eye.

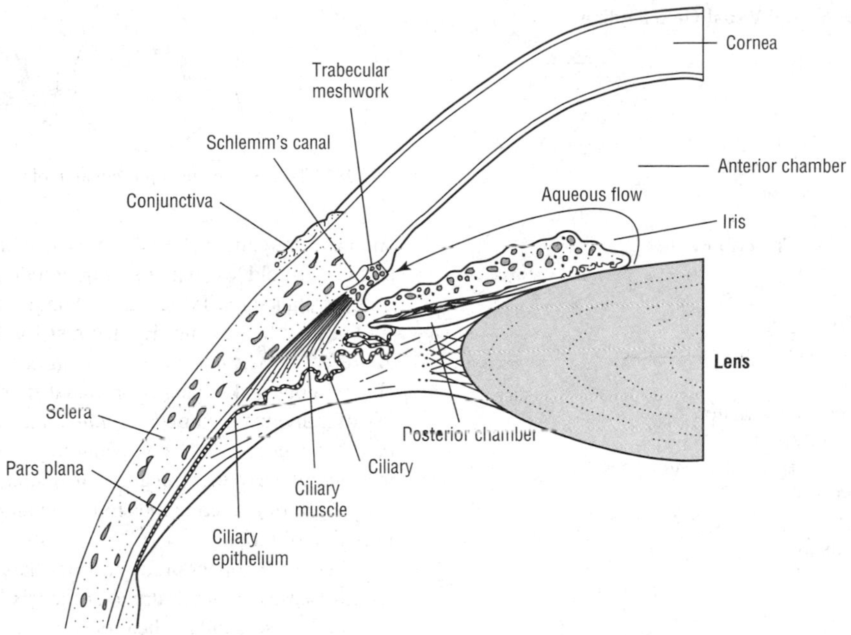

FIGURE 94–2. Anterior chamber of the eye and aqueous humor flow.

less than 3 to 4 mm Hg; however, it may be greater in patients with glaucoma. This circadian variation and the poor relationship of IOP with visual loss make measurement of IOP a poor screening test for glaucoma.

Although increased IOP within any range is associated with a higher risk of glaucomatous damage, it is both an insensitive and nonspecific diagnostic and monitoring tool. Of individuals with IOP between 21 and 30 mm Hg, only 0.5% to 1% per year will develop optic disk changes and visual-field loss (i.e., glaucoma) over 5 to 15 years. However, more subtle retinal damage—such as alteration of color vision, decreased contrast sensitivity, and peripheral acuity—occurs in a higher percentage of patients with IOPs greater than 21 mm Hg, and the incidence of visual-field defects increases to as high as 28% in individuals with IOPs above 30 mm Hg. For a given abnormal IOP, the incidence of glaucoma increases with age. In patients with preexisting optic nerve damage, the worse the existing damage, the more sensitive the eye is to a given IOP. On the other hand, as many as 20% to 30% of patients with glaucomatous visual-field loss have an IOP of less than 21 mm Hg (called *normal-tension glaucoma,* referring to the normal IOP). Thus the absolute IOP is a poor predictor of optic nerve damage and therefore outcome of drug therapy. More direct measurements of therapeutic outcome such as optic disk examination and visual-field evaluation also must be used as monitors of drug therapy.[1,2,15–22]

OPTIC DISK AND VISUAL FIELDS

The optic disk is the portion of the optic nerve ophthalmoscopically visible as it leaves the eye. It consists of approximately one million retinal ganglion nerve cell axons, blood vessels, and supporting connective tissue structures (lamina cribosa). The small depression within the disc is termed the *cup* (Fig. 94–3). A normal physiologic cup does not extend below the retinal surface and has a diameter of less than one-third that of the disk (cup-to-disk ratio <0.33). The common alterations of the optic disk found in glaucoma are listed in Table 94–2. These disk changes result from optic nerve degeneration and death and remodeling of the supporting structures. As the nerve axons die, the cup becomes larger in relation to the whole disk. A loss of retinal nerve fiber layer visibility is seen in the majority of glaucoma patients with detectable visual-field loss. This pattern of changes is consistent with visual-field losses and loss of visual sensitivity seen in glaucoma.[1,2,15–17]

Determination of visual field allows assessment of optic nerve damage and is a primary monitoring parameter in treatment. However, visual-field changes lag behind optic disk changes, and a loss of 20% of axons usually is required before detectable visual-field defects are noted. The peripheral visual field is measured using a visual-field instrument called a *perimeter.* Characteristic visual-field loss occurs in glaucoma (Fig. 94–4; see also Table 94–2), but loss of central visual acuity usually does not occur until late in the disease. Other indicators such as color vision changes and contrast sensitivity may allow earlier and more sensitive detection of glaucomatous changes.[1,2]

GENETICS

A number of major gene loci associated with POAG have been identified. How mutations in any of these genes result in increased IOP with

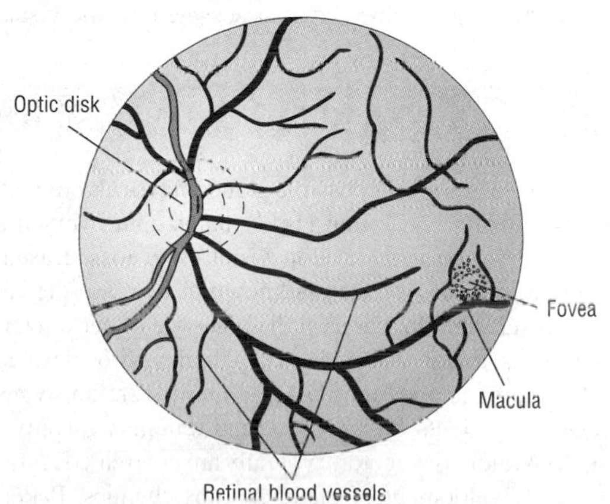

FIGURE 94–3. Normal fundus of the eye and optic disk and cup.

TABLE 94–2. Optic and Visual-Field Findings in Glaucoma

Optic Disk Findings
Cup-to-disk ratio > 0.5
Progressive increase in cup size
Cup-to-disk ratio asymmetry > 0.2
Vertical elongation of the cup
Excavation of the cup
Increases exposure of lamina cribosa
Pallor of the cup
Splinter hemorrhages
Cupping to edge of disk
Notching of the cup (usually superior or inferior)

Visual-Field Findings
General peripheral field constriction
Isolated scotomas (blind spots)
Nasal visual-field depression ("nasal step")
Enlargement of blind spot
Large, arclike scotomas
Reduced contrast sensitivity
Reduced peripheral acuity
Altered color vision

loss of visual field has not been elucidated. One gene, *glc1a,* codes for the trabecular meshwork–induced glucocorticoid response protein (TIGR), also called *protein myocilin,* in the trabecular meshwork. Improved understanding of the genetic origins of POAG hopefully will lead to new diagnostic tools and therapies that target the underlying causes of the disease.[1,2,21]

OPEN-ANGLE GLAUCOMA

SYMPTOMS AND DIAGNOSIS

POAG is a bilateral, genetically determined disorder constituting 60% to 70% of all glaucomas and 90% to 95% of primary glaucomas. POAG manifests as optic nerve degeneration characterized by disk changes and visual-field loss (see Table 94–2). An increased IOP is not required for diagnosis of POAG. POAG is a chronic, slowly progressive disease found primarily in individuals older than 50 years, although it may occur earlier. Symptoms do not present until substantial visual-field constriction occurs. Central visual acuity typically is maintained, even in the late stages of the disease. POAG is a bilateral disease; however, one eye may have greater progression of disease than the other. Detection and diagnosis involve evaluation of the optic disk and retinal nerve fiber layer, assessment of the visual fields,

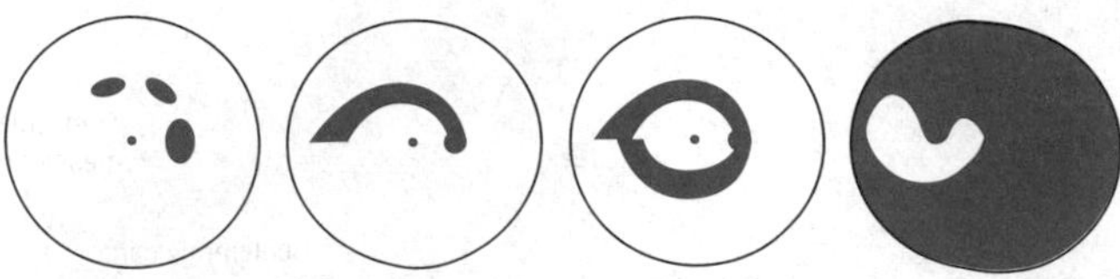

FIGURE 94–4. Schematic representation of the progression of visual-field loss.

and measurement of IOP. The presence of characteristic disk changes and visual-field loss with or without increased IOP confirms the diagnosis of glaucoma. Typical disk changes and field loss occurring at an IOP of less than 21 mm Hg account for 20% to 30% of patients and are referred to as *normal-tension glaucoma.* Elevated IOP (>21 mm Hg) without disk changes or visual-field loss is observed in 5% to 7% of individuals (known as *glaucoma suspects*) and is referred to as *ocular hypertension.* New technologies such as retinal tomography may allow early identification of ocular hypertension patients with early signs of glaucomatous retinal changes, thus allowing for earlier initiation of therapy.[1,2,15–17]

Secondary open-angle glaucoma has many causes, including systemic diseases, trauma, surgery, rubeosis, lens changes, ocular inflammatory diseases, and medications. A system for classifying secondary glaucomas into pretrabecular, trabecular, and posttrabecular forms has been proposed. This classification allows drug therapy to be chosen on the basis of the pathogenic mechanism involved. In pretrabecular forms, a normal meshwork is covered that does not permit aqueous humor outflow. Trabecular forms of secondary glaucoma result from either an alteration of meshwork or an accumulation of material in the intertrabecular spaces. The posttrabecular forms result primarily from disorders causing increased episcleral venous blood pressure.[1,2,15–17]

PROGNOSIS

In most cases of POAG, the overall prognosis is excellent when POAG is discovered early and treated adequately. Even patients with advanced visual-field loss can have continued visual-field loss reduced if the IOP is maintained at low enough pressures (often <10–12 mm Hg). Progression of visual-field loss still occurs in 8% to 20% of patients despite reaching standard therapy IOP goals. However, in untreated patients or in those failing to achieve target IOP reduction, up to 80% have continued visual-field loss. Estimates of progression to bilateral blindness in treated patients range from 4% to 22%. Thus the keys to medical treatment of POAG are an effective, well-tolerated drug regimen, close monitoring of therapy, and adherence. Medications will control IOP successfully in 60% to 80% of patients over a 5-year period. Availability of newer, highly effective, well-tolerated agents may improve the prognosis further.[1,2,15–17,20–24]

▶ TREATMENT: Ocular Hypertension

Treatment of the patient with possible glaucoma (ocular hypertension, i.e., patients with IOP >22 mm Hg) remains controversial because only 0.5% to 1% per year develop visual-field loss. Based on the presence or absence of risk factors known to increase the chance of developing visual-field loss and on the presence of certain individual traits, therapy is initiated in selected patients with elevated IOPs. These risk factors include high IOP (>30 mm Hg), family history of glaucoma, black patients, high myopia, and patients with only one eye.

Patients without risk factors typically are not treated and are monitored for the development of glaucomatous changes. Patients with significant risk factors usually will be treated with a well-tolerated topical agent such as a β-blocking agent, brimonidine, a topical carbonic anhydrase inhibitor (CAI), or prostaglandin analogue depending on individual patient characteristics. Optimally, therapy is initiated in one eye to assess efficacy and tolerance. Use of second- or third-line agents (e.g., pilocarpine, epinephrine, or apraclonidine) when first-line agents fail to reduce IOP depends on risk-benefit assessment of each patient.

The cost, inconvenience, and frequent side effects of combination therapies, anticholinesterase inhibitors, and oral CAIs result in an unfavorable risk-benefit ratio in patients with possible glaucoma, and such therapies are thus indicated only in high-risk patients.

The goal of therapy is to lower the IOP to a level associated with a decreased risk of optic nerve damage—usually a 25% to 30% decrease, but greater decreases may be required in high-risk patients or those with higher initial IOPs. Drug therapy should be monitored by measurement of IOP, examination of the optic disk, assessment of the visual fields, and evaluation of the patient for drug side effects and adherence to therapy. Patients who are unresponsive to or intolerant of a drug should be switched to an alternative agent rather than given an additional drug. Many clinicians prefer to discontinue all medications in patients failing to respond adequately to simple topical therapy, closely monitor for development of disk changes or visual-field loss, and treat again when such changes occur.[1,2,15–17]

▶ TREATMENT: Open-Angle Glaucoma

All patients with elevated IOP and characteristic optic disk changes and/or visual-field defects not due to other factors (i.e., glaucoma by definition) should be treated. Recent findings that one in five patients with "normal" IOP and glaucomatous retinal nerve findings (i.e., normal-tension glaucoma) do not have progression of visual-field loss if left untreated have prompted recommendations to monitor normal-tension glaucoma patients without immediate threat of loss of central vision and treat only when progression is documented. Some controversy exists as to whether the initial therapy of glaucoma should be surgical trabeculectomy (filtering procedure), argon laser trabeculectomy, or medical therapy.[1,2,15,16] Presently, drug therapy remains the most common initial treatment modality.

Drug therapy of patients with documented glaucomatous change with either elevated or normal IOP is initiated in a stepwise manner (Fig. 94–5) starting with lower concentrations of a single well-tolerated topical agent. The goal of therapy is to prevent further visual loss. A "target" IOP is chosen based on a patient baseline IOP and the amount of existing visual-field loss. Typically, an initial target IOP reduction of 30% is desired. Greater reductions may be desired in patients with very high baseline IOPs or advanced visual-field loss. Patients with normal baseline IOPs (normal-tension glaucoma) may have target IOPs of less than 10 to 12 mm Hg.

PHARMACOTHERAPEUTIC APPROACH

Usually a β-blocker is used if no contraindications exist because this class of drugs has a long history of successful use, providing a combination of clinical efficacy and tolerability. The newer agents brimonidine, prostaglandin analogues, and topical CAIs are also considered suitable first-line therapy or alternative initial therapy in patients with contraindications to or other concerns with β-blockers (see Fig. 94–5). Pilocarpine, epinephrine (or dipivefrin), and apraclonidine are used commonly as second-line therapies because of their increased frequency of adverse effects.

Therapy optimally is started as a single agent in one eye (except in patients with very high IOP or advanced visual-field loss) to evaluate drug efficacy and tolerance. Monitoring of therapy should be individualized: IOP should be measured and the optic disk should be visualized initially every 2 to 4 weeks and then every 1 to 6 months when stabilized, and the visual field should be measured every 3 to 12 months (more frequently after any change in drug therapy).

Patients always should be questioned regarding adherence to and tolerance of prescribed therapy. Initial IOP response does not predict long-term IOP control, requiring regular monitoring of IOP. Using more than one drop per dose does not improve response but increases the likelihood of side effects and the cost of therapy. When using more than one medication, apply drops at least 5 to 10 minutes apart to provide optimal ocular contact for each agent.

The value of an agent to which the patient has shown a loss of IOP control following an initial response can be measured by discontinuing the medication completely and determining if an increase in IOP occurs. Patients responding to but intolerant of initial therapy may be switched to another drug or to an alternative dosage form of the same medication. For patients failing to respond to the highest tolerated concentrations of an initial drug, a switch to an alternative agent after 1 day of concurrent therapy—or, if only a partial response occurs, addition of another topical drug to be used in combination—should be considered. A number of drugs or drug combinations may need to be tried before an effective and well-tolerated regimen is identified. Because of the frequency of side effects, carbachol, topical cholinesterase inhibitors, and oral CAIs are considered last-line agents to be used in patients who fail less toxic combination topical therapy.

NONPHARMACOLOGIC THERAPY: LASER AND SURGICAL PROCEDURES

When drug therapy fails, is not tolerated, or is excessively complicated, surgical procedures such as argon laser trabeculoplasty (ALT) or a surgical trabeculectomy (filtering procedure) to produce aqueous humor drainage paths may be performed to improve outflow. Laser trabeculoplasty is usually an intermediate step between drug therapy and trabeculectomy. Procedures with higher complication rates, such as those involving placement of draining tubes or destruction of the ciliary body (cyclodestruction), may be required when other methods fail[1,2,25] (see Fig. 94–3).

Surgical methods for reduction of IOP involve the creation of a channel through which aqueous humor can flow from the anterior chamber to the subconjunctival space (filtering bleb), where it is reabsorbed by the vasculature. A major reason for failure of the procedure is healing and scarring of the sight.

Modification of the healing process to maintain patency is possible with the use of antiproliferative agents. The antiproliferative agents 5-fluorouracil (5-FU) and mitomycin are used in patients undergoing glaucoma filtering surgery to improve success rates by reducing the inflammatory response and fibroblast proliferation. Although used most commonly in patients with increased risk for sub optimal surgical outcome (after cataract surgery and previous failed filtering procedure), use of these agents also improves success in low-risk patients.[26–28]

EVALUATION OF THERAPEUTIC OUTCOMES

The ultimate goal of drug therapy in the glaucoma patient is to preserve visual function through reduction of IOP to a level at which no

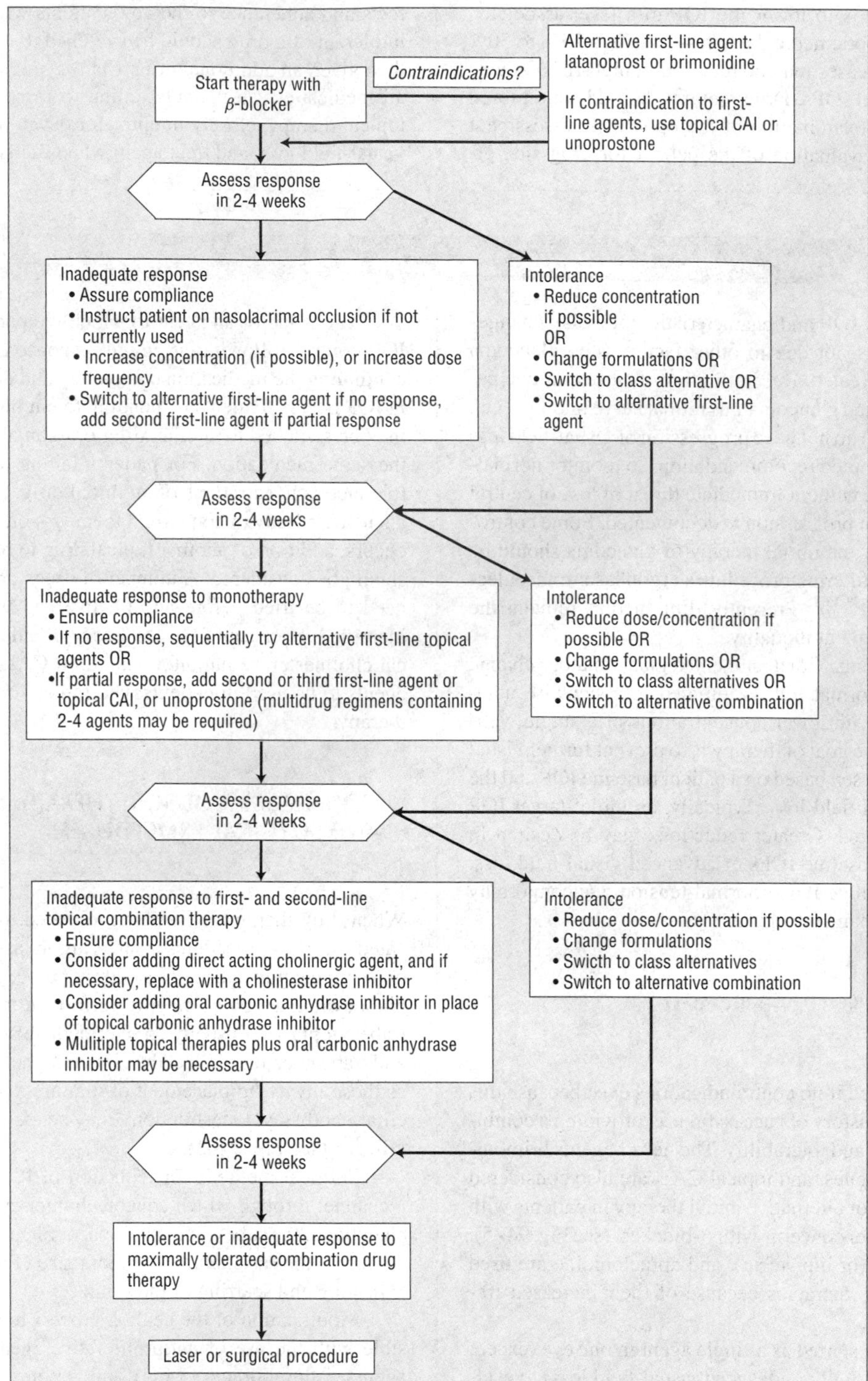

FIGURE 94–5. Algorithm for the pharmacotherapy of open-angle glaucoma.

further optic nerve damage occurs. Because of the poor relationship between IOP and optic nerve damage, no specific target IOP exists. Indeed, drugs used to treat glaucoma agents may act in part to halt visual-field loss through mechanisms separate from or in addition to IOP reduction, such as improvements in retinal or choroidal blood flow. Often a 25% to 30% reduction is desired, but greater reductions (40% to 50%) may be desired in patients with initially high IOPs. For patients with glaucoma, an IOP of less than 21 mm Hg generally is desired, with progressively lower target pressures desired for greater levels of glaucomatous damage. Even lower IOPs (possibly even below 10 mm Hg) are required in patients with very advanced disease, those showing continued damage at higher IOPs, and those with normal-tension glaucoma and pretreatment pressures in the low to middle teens. The IOP considered acceptable for a patient is often a balance of desired IOP and acceptable treatment-related toxicity and patient quality of life.

PATIENT EDUCATION

An important consideration in patients failing to respond to drug therapy is adherence. Poor adherence or nonadherence occurs in 25% to 60% of glaucoma patients. A large percentage of patients also fail to use topical ophthalmic drugs correctly. Patients should be taught the following procedure:

- Wash and dry the hands; shake the bottle if it contains a suspension.
- With a forefinger, pull down the outer portion of the lower eyelid to form a "pocket" to receive the drop.
- Grasp the dropper bottle between the thumb and fingers with the hand braced against the cheek or nose and the head held upward.
- Place the dropper over the eye while looking at the tip of the bottle; then look up and place a single drop in the eye.
- The lids should be closed (but not squeezed or rubbed) for 1 to 3 minutes after instillation. This increases the ocular availability of the drug.
- Recap bottle and store as instructed.

Note that many patients are physically unable to administer their own eyedrops without assistance. Nasolacrimal occlusion (NLO) also should be used to improve ocular bioavailability and reduce systemic absorption.[1,2,15–17,29,30] The patient induces NLO for 1 to 3 minutes by closing the eyes and placing the index finger over the nasolacrimal drainage system in the inner corner of the eye. This maneuver, as well as eyelid closure itself, decreases punctal drainage of drug, thereby decreasing the amount of drug available for systemic absorption from the nasopharyngeal mucosa. The use of NLO may improve drug response significantly, reduce side effects, and allow less frequent dose intervals and the use of lower drug concentrations.

Use of more than one drop per dose increases costs, does not improve response significantly, and may increase side effects. When two drugs are to be administered, instillations should be separated by at least 3 to 5 minutes (preferably 10 minutes) to prevent the drug administered first from being washed out. The patient should be taught not to touch the dropper bottle tip with eye, hands, or any surface.

Adherence to glaucoma therapy commonly is inadequate, and it always should be considered as a possible cause of drug therapy failure. Assessment of adherence by health care providers generally is poor, so all patients should be encouraged continually to administer prescribed therapy diligently as instructed. To improve adherence, the patient, family, and care providers should be fully informed of the expectations of therapy and the need to continue therapy despite a lack of symptoms. Possible side effects of the medication and ways to reduce them should be discussed. Adherence will be improved by good communication, close monitoring, and use of well-tolerated and convenient drug regimens.[1,2,15–17]

CLOSED-ANGLE GLAUCOMA

Primary CAG accounts for 5% or less of primary glaucomas; however, when CAG occurs, it may need to be treated as an emergency to avoid visual loss. CAG results from mechanical blockage of the (usually normal) trabecular meshwork by the peripheral iris. Partial or complete blockage of the meshwork occurs intermittently, resulting in extreme fluctuations between normal IOP with no symptoms and very high IOP with symptoms of acute CAG. Between attacks of CAG, the IOP is usually normal unless the patient has concomitant open-angle glaucoma or nonreversible blockage of the meshwork with synechiae ("creeping" angle closure) that develops over time in the narrow-angle eye. Primary CAG occurs in patients with inherited shallow anterior chambers, which produce a narrow angle between the cornea and iris or tight contact between the iris and lens (pupillary block). The presence of a narrow angle is determined by visualization of the angle by gonioscopy. Other tests for CAG involve provocation of an angle closure-induced IOP increase. These tests attempt to produce angle closure through mydriasis (dark-room test, mydriasis test) or gravity (prone test) and measure any increase in IOP resulting from the provocative test.

Two major types of classic, reversible primary CAG have been described: CAG with pupillary block and CAG without pupillary block. CAG with pupillary block results when the iris is in firm contact with the lens. This produces a relative block of aqueous flow through the pupil to the anterior chamber, resulting in a bowing forward of the iris, which blocks the trabecular meshwork. CAG with pupillary block occurs most commonly when the pupil is in middilation. In this position, the combination of pupillary block and relaxed iris allows the greatest bowing of the iris; however, angle closure may occur during miosis or mydriasis.

CAG without pupillary block occurs in patients with an abnormality called a *plateau iris*. The iris root in this case is inserted anteriorly, very close to the trabecular meshwork. Mydriasis causes the peripheral iris to bunch up and block the meshwork. The mydriasis produced by anticholinergic drugs or any other drug results in precipitation of both types of CAG glaucoma, whereas drug-induced miosis may produce pupillary block.

Patients with untreated CAG typically experience intermittent nonsymptomatic or prodromal symptoms brought on by precipitating events. The symptoms include blurred or hazy vision with halos around lights, caused by a hazy, edematous cornea, and occasionally headache.

Increased IOP during such prodromal episodes is not great enough or long enough to produce the other symptoms of a full-blown attack. Such prodromal attacks last 1 to 2 hours, at which time pupillary block is broken by further mydriasis or miosis or miosis occurs in patients with plateau iris. Acute CAG produces the symptoms associated with a cloudy, edematous cornea, ocular pain or discomfort, nausea, vomiting, abdominal pain, and diaphoresis. On examination, the patient is found to have a closed-angle, narrow anterior chamber, hyperemic conjunctiva and an edematous and hyperemic optic disk. The rate at which IOP increases may be a determinant of when full-blown symptoms occur. Visual fields demonstrate generalized constriction. In prolonged attacks, total loss of vision may occur if the IOP is high enough. Tonometry reveals IOPs as high as 40 to 90 mm Hg. Patients who have developed synechiae blocking the trabecular meshwork may have elevated IOP chronically with intermittent very high IOP when angle closure occurs.

The goal of initial therapy for acute CAG with high IOP is rapid reduction of the IOP to preserve vision and to avoid surgical or laser iridectomy on a hypertensive, congested eye. Iridectomy is the definitive treatment of CAG; it produces a hole in the iris that permits aqueous humor flow to move directly from the posterior chamber to the anterior chamber. Drug therapy of an acute attack typically involves administration of pilocarpine, hyperosmotic agents, and a secretory inhibitor (β-blocker, α_2-agonist, prostaglandin $F_{2\alpha}$ analog, or a topical or systemic CAI). With miosis produced by pilocarpine, the peripheral iris is pulled away from the meshwork. Although traditionally the drug of choice, the use of pilocarpine as initial therapy is controversial. Miotics may worsen angle closure by increasing pupillary block and producing anterior movement of the lens because of drug-induced accommodation.

At IOPs greater than 60 mm Hg, the iris may be ischemic and unresponsive to miotics; as the pressure drops and the iris responds, miosis occurs. During this time, the tendency to use excessive amounts of pilocarpine must be avoided. The dose of pilocarpine commonly used is a 1% or 2% solution instilled every 5 minutes for two or three doses and then every 4 to 6 hours. However, many practitioners withhold application of pilocarpine until the IOP has been reduced by other agents and then apply a single drop of 1% to 2% pilocarpine to produce miosis. In either case, the unaffected contralateral eye should be treated with the miotic every 6 hours to prevent development of angle closure. An osmotic agent also commonly is administered because these drugs produce the most rapid decrease in IOP. Oral glycerin 1–2 g/kg can be used if an oral agent is tolerated; if not, intravenous mannitol 1–2 g/kg should be used. Osmotic agents reduce IOP by withdrawing water from the eye secondary to the osmotic gradient between the blood and the eyes. These drugs are among the first-line agents in the short-term treatment of CAG or other forms of acute very high IOP elevations. Topical corticosteroids often are used to reduce the ocular inflammation and reduce the development of synechiae in CAG eyes. In classic CAG, once the IOP is controlled, pilocarpine may be given every 6 hours until iridectomy is performed. Patients failing therapy altogether will require an emergency iridectomy. Peripheral iridectomy essentially "cures" primary CAG without significant synechiae. Long-term drug therapy is not used unless IOP remains high due to the presence of synechiae blocking the trabecular meshwork or concurrent POAG. In such cases, the pharmacotherapeutic approach is essentially identical to that for the POAG patient, or laser or surgical procedures are performed.[1,2]

DRUG-INDUCED GLAUCOMA

A number of medications have been associated with increased IOP or carry labeling that cautions against use of the medication in glaucoma patients. The potential for a medication to produce or worsen glaucoma depends on the type of glaucoma and whether or not the patient is treated adequately.

Patients with treated, controlled POAG are at minimal risk of induction of an increase in IOP by systemic medications with anticholinergic properties or vasodilators; however, in patients with untreated glaucoma or uncontrolled POAG, the potential of these medications to increase IOP should be considered. Topical anticholinergic agents used to produce mydriasis may result in an increase in IOP. Potent anticholinergic agents such as atropine or homatropine are most likely to increase IOP. Weaker anticholinergics, such as tropicamide, that produce less cycloplegia are less likely to increase IOP and are favored, along with phenylephrine, when mydriasis is desired in POAG patients. Inhaled, nasal, topical, or systemic glucocorticoids may increase IOP in both normal individuals and patients with POAG.

Patients with POAG appear to be particularly susceptible to glucocorticoid-induced increases in IOP. Glucocorticoids reduce the facility of aqueous humor outflow through the trabecular meshwork. The decreased facility of outflow appears to result from the accumulation of extracellular material blocking the trabecular channels. The potential of a glucocorticoid to increase IOP is related to its

TABLE 94–3. Drugs That May Induce or Potentiate Increased IOP

Open-Angle Glaucoma
Ophthalmic corticosteroids (high risk)
Systemic corticosteroids
Nasal/inhaled corticosteroids
Fenoldapam
Ophthalmic anticholinergics
Succinylcholine
Vasodilators (low risk)
Cimetidine (low risk)

Closed-Angle Glaucoma
Topical anticholinergics
Topical sympathomimetics
Systemic anticholinbergics
Heterocyclic antidepressants
Low-potency phenothiazines
Antihistamines
Ipratropium
Benzodiazepines (low risk)
Theophylline (low risk)
Vasodilators (low risk)
Systemic sympathomimetics (low risk)
CNS stimulants (low risk)
Tetracyclines (low risk)
Carbonic anhydrase inhibitors (low risk)
Monoamine oxidase inhibitors (low risk)
Topical cholinergics (low risk)

anti-inflammatory potency and intraocular penetration. Thus patients should be treated with the lowest potency and dose and for the shortest time possible when steroids are indicated.

In patients predisposed to CAG (i.e., narrow anterior chambers), angle closure may be produced by any drug that causes mydriasis (e.g., anticholinergics) or swelling of the lens (e.g., sulfa compounds). The topical use of anticholinergics or sympathomimetic agents most likely will result in angle closure. Systemic and inhaled anticholinergic and sympathomimetic agents also must be used with caution in such patients. As discussed previously, potent miotic agents such as echothiophate may produce angle closure by increasing pupillary block. Drugs associated with potentiation of glaucoma are listed in Table 94–3.

PHARMACOLOGIC AGENTS USED IN GLAUCOMA

β-BLOCKING DRUGS

The topical β-blocking agents are the most commonly used antiglaucoma medications. β-Blockers lower IOP by 20% to 30% with a minimum of local ocular side effects. These are commonly the agents of first choice in treating POAG if no contraindications exist.[1,2,15–17] The β-blocking agents produce ocular hypotensive effects by decreasing the production of aqueous humor by the ciliary body without producing substantial effects on aqueous humor outflow facility. The mechanism by which β-blockers decrease aqueous humor inflow remains controversial, but it is most frequently attributed to β_2-adrenergic receptor blockade in the ciliary body.

Five ophthalmic β-blockers are presently available: timolol, levobunolol, metipranolol, carteolol, and betaxolol. Timolol, levobunolol, and metipranolol are nonspecific β-blocking agents, whereas betaxolol is a relatively β_1-selective agent. Carteolol is a nonspecific blocker with intrinsic sympathomimetic activity (ISA). Despite differences in potency, selectivity, lipophilicity, and ISA, the five agents reduce IOP to a similar degree, although betaxolol has been reported to produce somewhat less lowering of IOP than timolol and levobunolol. However, visual outcomes may be similar, possibly due to a more favorable effect of betaxolol on retinal blood flow compared with nonspecific β-blockers.[32] Levobunolol may be more effective than timolol and betaxolol in reducing post-cataract surgery IOP increases. Levobunolol solution is more effective in controlling IOP than other agents when given as aqueous solutions on a once-daily schedule (up to 70% of patients). Timolol in the form of a gel-forming solution (Timolol XE, Merck, West Point, PA) provides equivalent IOP control with once-daily administration when compared with an equal concentration of the aqueous solution administered twice daily. The choice of a specific β-blocking agent generally is based on differences in side-effect potential, individual patient response, and cost.

Local side effects with β-blockers usually are tolerable, although stinging on application occurs commonly, particularly with betaxolol solution (less with betaxolol suspension) and metipranolol. Other local effects include dry eyes, corneal anesthesia, blepharitis, blurred vision, and rarely, conjunctivitis, uveitis, and keratitis. Some local reactions may be a result of preservatives used in the commercially available products. Switching from one agent to another or switching the type of formulation may improve tolerance in patients experiencing local side effects.

Systemic effects are the most important adverse effects of β-blockers. Drug absorbed systematically may produce decreased heart rate, reduced blood pressure, negative inotropic effects, conduction defects, bronchospasm, central nervous system effects, and alteration of serum lipids and may block the symptoms of hypoglycemia. The β_1-specific agents betaxolol and possibly carteolol (due to ISA) are less likely to produce the systemic side effects caused by β-adrenergic blockade, such as the cardiac effects and bronchospasm, but a real risk still exists. The use of timolol as a gel-forming liquid or betaxolol as a suspension allows administration of less drug per day and therefore reduces the chance for systemic side effects compared with the aqueous solutions.

Because of their systemic side effects, all ophthalmic β-blockers should be used with caution in patients with pulmonary diseases, sinus bradycardia, second- or third-degree heart block, congestive heart failure, atherosclerosis, diabetes, and myasthenia gravis, as well as in patients receiving oral β-blocker therapy. Use of NLO technique during administration will reduce the risk or severity of systemic side effects as well as optimize response. Overall, β-adrenergic blocking agents are well tolerated by patients, and most potential problems can be avoided by appropriate patient evaluation, drug choice, and monitoring of drug therapy. In patients failing or having an inadequate response to single-drug therapy with a β-blocking agent, the addition of a CAI, parasympathomimetic agent, prostaglandin analogues, or an α_2-adrenergic receptor agonist usually will result in additional IOP reduction. Epinephrine or dipivefrin added to a β-blocking agent (particularly nonspecific β-blockers) usually results in only minimal additional IOP reduction.[1–3,12–14,18,19,29–31]

α_2-ADRENERGIC AGONISTS

Brimonidine and the less lipid-soluble and less receptor-selective apraclonidine are α_2-adrenergic agonists structurally similar to clonidine. Apraclonidine is indicated (brimonidine is also effective) for prevention or control of postoperative or post-laser treatment increases in IOP, and both are indicated in the treatment of open-angle glaucoma. Brimonidine is considered a first-line or adjunctive agent in the therapy of POAG, and apraclonidine is seen as a second-line or adjunctive therapy.

Both these agents are also useful in short-term management of acute CAG. α_2-Agonists reduce IOP by decreasing the rate of aqueous humor production (some increase in uveoscleral outflow also occurs with brimonidine). The drugs reduce IOP by 18% to 27% at peak (2 to 5 hours) and by 10% at 8 to 12 hours. Comparative trials demonstrate a reduction in IOP similar to that obtained with 0.5% timolol. Use of apraclonidine 0.5% or brimonidine 0.2% every 8 to 12 hours appears to provide maximum IOP-lowering effects in long-term use. Use of NLO may improve response and allow the longer dosing frequency (i.e., every 12 hours).

Some patients have demonstrated a loss of IOP control with use of apraclonidine for periods greater than 1 to 2 months; however, many patients demonstrate long-term IOP control. A similar loss of IOP control has not been found with brimonidine. Confirmation of continuing IOP-lowering effects of α_2 agonists is required for all patients using the class for prolonged periods. Combinations of α_2-agonists with β-blockers, prostaglandin analogues, or CAIs produces additional IOP reduction.

Local adverse effects occur frequently with apraclonidine and brimonidine. An allergic-type reaction characterized by lid edema, eye discomfort, foreign-object sensation, itching, and hyperemia occurs in approximately 30% of patients with apraclonidine. Brimonidine produces this adverse effect in up to 8% of patients. This reaction commonly necessitates drug discontinuation. Systemic side effects may be somewhat greater with brimonidine than with apraclonidine and include dizziness and somnolence, dry mouth, and a reduction in blood pressure and pulse. α_2-Agonists should be used with caution in patients with cardiovascular diseases, renal compromise, cerebrovascular disease, and diabetes, as well as in those taking antihypertensives and other cardiovascular drugs, monoamine oxidase inhibitors, and tricyclic antidepressants. In terms of overall efficacy and tolerability, brimonidine approximates that achieved with β-blockers.[1–2,15–17,29,30]

PROSTAGLANDIN $F_{2\alpha}$ ANALOGS

The prostaglandin $F_{2\alpha}$ analogs latanoprost, travoprost, and brimatoprost, and the docosonoid unoprostone reduce IOP by increasing the uveoscleral outflow of aqueous humor. Some differences in receptor sites and mechanisms of action may exist between the two classes because additional IOP reduction occurs when they are used in combination.

Reduction in IOP with once-daily doses of prostaglandin $F_{2\alpha}$ analogs (a 25% to 35% reduction) is similar to or greater than that seen with timolol 0.5% twice daily. In addition, nocturnal control of IOP is improved compared with timolol. Interestingly, administration of prostaglandin $F_{2\alpha}$ analogs twice daily may reduce the IOP control compared with single daily dosing. The drugs are also more effective when given at nighttime compared with administration in the morning.

Unoprostone 0.15% reduces IOP somewhat less than prostaglandin $F_{2\alpha}$ analogs and requires twice-daily administration. Prostaglandin $F_{2\alpha}$ analogs and unoprostone are well tolerated and produce fewer systemic side effects than timolol. Local ocular tolerance generally is good with ocular reactions such as punctate corneal erosions and conjunctival hyperemia occurs. Local intolerance occurs in 10% to 25% of patients with these agents.

With prostaglandin $F_{2\alpha}$ analogs, altered iris pigmentation occurs in 15% to 30% of patients, particularly those with mixed-color irises (blue-brown, green-brown, blue gray-brown, or yellow-brown eyes), which become more brown in color over 3 to 12 months. The frequency of iris pigmentation changes increases with corresponding increases in the duration of treatment. The long-term consequences of this pigment change are unknown. Hypertrichosis and increased eyelash pigmentation also have been reported. Unoprostone also has been associated with increased pigmentation.

These agents have been associated with uveitis, and caution is recommended in patients with ocular inflammatory conditions. Cystoid macular edema also has been reported with latanoprost. Cases of worsening of herpetic keratitis have been reported.

Prostaglandin analogs can be used in combination with other antiglaucoma agents for additional IOP control due to their unique mechanism of action. Given its excellent efficacy and side-effect profile, prostaglandin $F_{2\alpha}$ analogs provide an alternative monotherapy or adjunctive therapy in patients not responding to or tolerating other agents. Some glaucoma experts have advocated the use of prostaglandin $F_{2\alpha}$ analogs as first-line therapy in POAG. Studies of long-term tolerance, efficacy, and the implications of iris pigmentation changes are needed to clearly define the place of prostaglandin $F_{2\alpha}$ analogs in glaucoma therapy. The present role of unoprostone is as a second-line agent.[17–19,29,30,33,34]

CARBONIC ANHYDRASE INHIBITORS

TOPICAL AGENTS

CAIs reduce IOP by decreasing ciliary body aqueous humor secretion. CAIs appear to inhibit aqueous production by blocking active secretion of sodium and bicarbonate ions from the ciliary body to the aqueous humor.[1–3,24] Topical CAIs such as dorzolamide and brinzolamide are well tolerated and are indicated for monotherapy or adjunctive therapy of open-angle glaucoma and ocular hypertension. Relatively specific inhibitors of carbonic anhydrase enzyme II such as dorzolamide and brinzolamide reduce IOP by 15% to 26%.

Topical CAIs generally are well tolerated. Local side effects include transient burning and stinging, ocular discomfort and transient blurred vision, tearing, and rarely, conjunctivitis, lid reactions, and photophobia. A superficial punctate keratitis occurs in 10% to 15% of patients. Brinzolamide produces somewhat fewer local side effects than dorzolamide. Systemic side effects are unusual despite the accumulation of drug in red blood cells (RBCs). Because of their favorable side-effect profile, topical CAIs provide a useful alternative agent for monotherapy or adjunctive therapy in patients with inadequate response to or those unable to use other agents. The drugs may add additional IOP reduction in patients using other single or multiple topical agents. The usual dose of topical CAI is one drop every 8 to 12 hours. Administration every 12 hours produces somewhat less IOP reduction than administration every 8 hours. Use of NLO should optimize response to CAI given at any interval.[1,2,15–19,29,30,35]

SYSTEMIC AGENTS

Systemic CAIs are indicated in patients failing to respond to or tolerate maximum topical therapy. Systemic and topical CAIs should not be used in combination because no data exist concerning improved IOP reduction, and the risk for systemic side effects is increased. Oral CAIs reduce aqueous humor inflow by 40% to 60% and IOP by 25% to 40%. The available systemic CAIs (see Table 94–4) produce equivalent IOP reduction but differ in potency, side effects, dosage forms, and duration of action. Despite their excellent effects on elevated IOP of any etiology, the systemic CAIs frequently produce intolerable side effects. As a result, CAIs are considered third-line agents in the treatment of POAG.

On average, only 30% to 60% of patients are able to tolerate CAI therapy for prolonged periods. Intolerance to CAI therapy results most commonly from a symptom complex attributable to systemic acidosis and including malaise, fatigue, anorexia, nausea, weight loss, altered taste, depression, and decreased libido. Other side effects include renal calculi, increased uric acid, blood dyscrasias, diuresis, and myopia. Elderly patients do not tolerate CAIs as well as younger patients. The three available CAIs produce the same spectrum of side effects; however, the drugs differ in the frequency and severity of the side effects listed. Acetazolamide (standard or sustained-release capsules) and methazolamide are considered the best-tolerated CAIs.

CAIs should be used with caution in patients with sulfa allergies, sickle-cell disease, respiratory acidosis, pulmonary disorders, renal calculi, electrolyte imbalance, hepatic disease, renal disease, diabetes mellitus, or Addison's disease. Concurrent use of a CAI and a diuretic may rapidly produce hypokalemia. High-dose salicylate therapy may increase the acidosis produced by CAIs, whereas the acidosis produced by CAIs may increase the toxicity of salicylates.[1–2,15–19,29,30]

PARASYMPATHOMIMETIC AGENTS

The parasympathomimetic (cholinergic) agents reduce IOP by increasing aqueous humor trabecular outflow. The increase in outflow is a result of physically pulling open the trabecular meshwork secondary to ciliary muscle contraction, thereby reducing resistance to outflow. These agents reduce uveoscleral outflow.

Pilocarpine, the parasympathomimetic agent of choice in POAG, is available as an ophthalmic solution, an ocular insert, and a hydrophilic polymer gel (see Table 94–4). Pilocarpine produces similar (20% to 30%) reductions in IOP as seen with β-blocking agents. Pilocarpine in POAG or "glaucoma suspects" is initiated as 0.5% or 1% solution, one drop three to four times daily. The use of NLO improves response and reduces the need for an every-6-hour dosing frequency. Use of one drop of 2% pilocarpine every 6 to 12 hours and NLO provides optimal response in many patients. Both drug concentration and frequency may be increased if IOP reduction is inadequate. Patients with darkly pigmented eyes frequently require higher concentrations of pilocarpine than patients with lightly pigmented eyes. Concentrations of pilocarpine above 4% rarely improve IOP control in patients other than those with darkly pigmented eyes.

Pilocarpine 4% gel (Pilocarpine HS) once daily is equivalent to treatment with pilocarpine solution 4% four times daily or timolol 0.5% twice daily. When using every-24-hour dosing of pilocarpine gel, the adequacy of IOP control late in the dosing interval should be confirmed.

The pilocarpine Ocusert is a solid, elliptical, sustained-release device designed for placement in the conjunctival sac and delivery of pilocarpine over a 7-day period. The Ocusert should be placed in the eye at bedtime so that early side effects occur during sleep. The advantages of the Ocusert are convenience of weekly placement, possibly improved control of diurnal IOP increases, and decreased frequency of side effects. The disadvantages include a "burst" release of drug on insertion, increased cost, discomfort, undetected loss of the device, and increased dexterity required for unit placement.

Ocular side effects of pilocarpine include miosis, which decreases night vision and vision in patients with central cataracts. Constriction of the visual field occurs secondary to miosis and should be considered when evaluating visual-field changes in a glaucoma patient. Pilocarpine ciliary muscle contraction produces accommodative spasm, particularly in young patients still able to accommodate

TABLE 94–4. Topical Drugs Used in the Treatment of Open-Angle Glaucoma

Drug	Pharmacologic Properties	Common Brand Names	Dose Form	Strength (%)	Usual Dose[a]	Mechanism of Action
β-Adrenergic Blocking Agents						
Betaxolol	Relative β_1-selective	Betoptic Betoptic-S	Solution Suspension	0.5 0.25	1 drop bid 1 drop bid	All reduce aqueous production of ciliary body
Carteolol	Nonselective, ISA[b]	Ocupress	Solution	1	1 drop bid	
Levobunolol	Nonselective	Betagan	Solution	0.25, 0.5	1 drop bid	
Metipranolol	Nonselective	Optipranolol	Solution	0.3	1 drop bid	
Timolol	Nonselective	Timoptic, Betimol Timoptic XE	Solution Gelling solution	0.25, 0.5 0.25, 0.5	1 drop qd–bid[a] 1 drop qd[a]	
Nonspecific Adrenergic Agonists						
Epinephrine	Nonselective α, β agonists	Epinal (borate salt) Glaucon, Epifrin (HCl)	Solution Solution	0.5 0.5, 1, 2	1 drop bid 1 drop bid	Increased aqueous humor outflow
Dipivefrin	Prodrug	Propine	Solution	0.1	1 drop bid	
α_2-Adrenergic Agonists						
Apraclonidine	Specific α_2-agonists	Iopidine	Solution	0.5	1 drop bid–tid[a]	Both reduce aqueous humor production; brimonidine known to also increase uveoscleral outflow
Brimonidine		Alphagan P	Solution	0.15	1 drop bid–tid[a]	
Cholinergic Agonists						
Direct acting						
Carbachol	Irreversible	Carboptic, Isopto Carbachol	Solution	0.75, 1.5, 2.25,3	1 drop bid–tid[a]	All increase aqueous humor outflow through trabecular meshwork
Pilocarpine	Irreversible	Isopto-Carpine, Pilocar Pilopine HS Ocusert-Pilo	Solution Gel Solid insert	0.25, 0.5, 1,2, 4, 6, 8, 10 4 20 & 40 μg/h	1 drop bid–tid[a] 1 drop qid Every 24 h at HS Once weekly	
Cholinesterase inhibitors						
Demecarium	Reversible	Humorsol	Solution	0.125, 0.25	Bid–q3 days	
Echothiophate		Phospholine iodide	Solution	0.03, 0.06, 0.125, 0.25	Qd–bid	
Physostigmine		Eserine	Ointment	0.25	Bid–tid	
Carbonic Anhydrase Inhibitors						
Topical						
Brinzolamide	Carbonic anhydrase type II inhibition	Azopt	Suspension	1	Bid–tid[a]	All reduce aqueous humor production of ciliary body
Dorzolamide		Trusopt	Solution	2	Bid–tid[a]	
Systemic						
Acetazolamide		Diamox Diamox Sequels	Tablet Injection Capsule	125 mg, 250 mg 500 mg/vial 500 mg	125–250 mg bid–qid 250–500 mg 500 mg bid	
Dichlorphenamide		Daranide	Tablet	50 mg	25–50 mg qd–tid	
Methazolamide		Neptazane	Tablet	25 mg, 50 mg	25–50 mg bid–tid	
Prostaglandin Analogs						
Latanoprost	Prostaglandin $F_{2\alpha}$ analog	Xalatan	Solution	0.005%	1 drop q p.m.	Increases aqueous uveoscleral outflow
Brimatoprost		Lumigan	Solution	0.03%	1 drop q p.m.	
Travoprost		Travatan	Solution	0.004%	1 drop q p.m.	
Unoprostone		Rescula	Solution	0.15%	1 drop bid	

(Continued)

TABLE 94–4. (Continued)

Drug	Pharmacologic Properties	Common Brand Names	Dose Form	Strength (%)	Usual Dose[a]	Mechanism of Action
Combinations						
Timolol-dorzolamide		Cosopt	Solution	Timolol 0.5% Dorzolamide 2%	1 drop twice daily	
Epinephrine-pilocarpine		E-Pilo	Solution	Epinephrine Pilocarpine	1 drop bid–qid	

[a]Use of nasolacrimal occlusion will increase number of patients successfully treated with longer dosage intervals.
[b]ISI-intrinsic sympathomimetic activity.

(prepresbyopic). Pilocarpine also may produce frontal headache, browache, periorbital pain, eyelid twitching, and conjunctival irritation or injection early in therapy, which tends to decrease in severity over 3 to 5 weeks of continued therapy.

Cholinergics produce a breakdown of the blood–aqueous humor barrier and may result in a worsening of an ocular inflammatory reaction or condition. Systemic cholinergic side effects of pilocarpine—such as diaphoresis, nausea, vomiting, diarrhea, cramping, urinary frequency, bronchospasm, and heart block—are rare but may be seen in patients using high concentrations (6% to 8%) or with overzealous use in treatment of acute angle closure. Other side effects associated with direct-acting miotics include retinal tears or detachment, allergic reaction, permanent miosis, cataracts, precipitation of CAG, and rarely, miotic cysts of the pupillary margin.

Carbachol is a potent direct-acting miotic agent; its duration of action is longer than that of pilocarpine (8 to 10 hours) because of resistance to hydrolysis by cholinesterases. This drug also may act as a weak inhibitor of cholinesterase. Patients with an inadequate response to or intolerance of pilocarpine as a result of ocular irritation or allergy frequently do well on carbachol. The ocular and systemic side effects of carbachol are similar to but more frequent, constant, and severe than those of pilocarpine.[1,2,15–17,29,30]

The cholinesterase inhibitors used most commonly in the treatment of POAG are the long-acting, relatively irreversible agents demecarium, echothiophate, and (see Table 94–4). These agents are potent inhibitors of pseudocholinesterase, but they also inhibit true cholinesterase. Because of the serious ocular and systemic toxic effects of these agents, the cholinesterase inhibitors are reserved primarily for patients not responding to or intolerant of other therapy. Because of their cataractogenic properties, many ophthalmologists will use these agents only in patients without lenses (aphakia) or those with artificial lenses (pseudophakia). The ocular and periocular parasympathomimetic side effects are more common and more severe than with pilocarpine or carbachol.

In addition to the parasympathomimetic effects, the cholinesterase inhibitors may produce severe fibrinous iritis (particularly with the irreversible inhibitors), synechiae, iritic cysts, conjunctival thickening, and occlusion of the nasolacrimal ducts. Cataracts occur at high frequency with the use of cholinesterase inhibitors, particularly echothiophate, after about 10 to 18 months of therapy. The incidence of cataracts appears to increase with increasing concentration, with up to 60% of patients developing cataracts at higher concentrations. The inhibition of systemic pseudocholinesterase by these agents decreases the rate of succinylcholine hydrolysis, resulting in prolonged muscle paralysis. Cholinesterase inhibitors should be discontinued at least 2 weeks before procedures in which succinylcholine is to be used.

The role of cholinesterase inhibitors in glaucoma is limited by the frequency and potential toxicity of these agents. In phakic patients, cholinesterase inhibitors should be administered only if intolerance or failure results with other antiglaucoma medications. Cholinesterase inhibitors have been shown to provide additional IOP lowering effects when used with β-blockers, CAIs, and sympathomimetic (adrenergic) agents. As with all agents for glaucoma, therapy should be initiated with lower concentrations of these agents. A once-daily administration frequency should be used in most patients unless very high IOP is present.

Use of NLO likely will improve response and reduce systemic side effects and should be done by all patients administering cholinesterase inhibitors. The cholinesterase inhibitors should be used with caution in patients with asthma, retinal detachments, narrow angles, bradycardia, hypotension, heart failure, Down's syndrome, epilepsy, parkinsonism, peptic ulcer, and ocular inflammation, as well as in those receiving cholinesterase inhibitor therapy for myasthenia gravis or exposure to carbamate or organophosphate insecticides and pesticides.[1–2,15–17,29,30]

EPINEPHRINE AND DIPIVEFRIN

The mechanism of action by which epinephrine lowers IOP has not been fully elucidated; however, a β_2-receptor-mediated increase in outflow facility through the trabecular meshwork and the uveoscleral route appears to be the primary mechanism. Compared with β-blockers or miotics, epinephrine and dipivefrin reduce IOP less. Epinephrine used in combination with parasympathetic agents, prostaglandin $F_{2\alpha}$ analogs, or CAIs results in additional IOP lowering. Epinephrine plus betaxolol may result in greater IOP reduction than when it is used in combination with nonspecific β-blockers.

Epinephrine is available as epinephrine hydrochloride, epinephrine bitartrate, and epinephryl borate solutions. Epinephryl borate and epinephrine hydrochloride are labeled as the concentration of epinephrine base; however, epinephrine bitartrate 2% is equivalent to epinephrine base 1.1%. The various salts of epinephrine produce equivalent IOP-lowering effects and adverse reactions. Patients with minor ocular irritation from one salt of epinephrine occasionally may benefit from use of another salt because of differences in pH of the commercial solutions. Use of the prodrug dipivefrin allows use of lower concentrations secondary to improved intraocular absorption (10- to 15-fold). The 0.1% dipivefrin produces equivalent IOP reduction to 1% to 2% epinephrine. Dipivefrin therefore may be tolerated by patients unable to tolerate epinephrine solutions, and it is often chosen over other epinephrine products when this class of drugs is indicated.

A factor limiting the usefulness of epinephrine is the high frequency of local ocular side effects. Tearing, burning, ocular discomfort, browache, conjunctival hyperemia, punctate keratopathy, allergic blepharoconjunctivitis, rare loss of eyelashes, stenosis of the nasolacrimal duct, and blurred vision may occur. Prolonged use (>1 year) may result in deposition of pigment (adrenochrome) in the conjunctiva and cornea. Pigment also may deposit in soft contact lenses, turning them black. These side effects occur less frequently with dipivefrin. Epinephrine may produce mydriasis (particularly when combined with a β-blocker) and may precipitate acute CAG in patients with narrow anterior chambers. A transient increase in IOP may occur with initial therapy, particularly in patients not using other antiglaucoma medications. A relative contraindication to the use of epinephrine (and dipivefrin) is aphakia (i.e., after cataract removal) or lens dislocation because of the development of degeneration of the macular portion of the retina. The edema is dose-dependent and disappears with drug discontinuation.

Systemic side effects of epinephrine include headache, faintness, increased blood pressure, tachycardia, arrhythmias, tremor, pallor, anxiety, and increased perspiration. Epinephrine should be used with caution in patients with cardiovascular diseases, cerebrovascular diseases, aphakia, CAG, hyperthyroidism, and diabetes mellitus, as well as in patients undergoing anesthesia with halogenated hydrocarbon anesthetics. Using NLO with epinephrine and dipivefrin will improve therapeutic response and reduce risk of systemic side effects.[1–2,15–17,29,30]

FUTURE DRUG THERAPIES

New agents, improved formulations, and novel approaches to the reduction of IOP and other methods of prevention of glaucomatous visual-field loss hopefully will provide more effective and better-tolerated therapies.

Agents that act through mechanisms other than IOP reduction are likely to be part glaucoma therapy in the future. Such agents may act as either "retinal nerve protectants," inhibitors of apoptotic cell death, blockers of nitric oxide synthetase, blockers of excitotoxicity factors, growth factor supplementation, or through regulation of retinal blood flow.[3–19]

CONCLUSION

The glaucomas are a group of primary and secondary diseases, the management of which presents a considerable challenge to the pharmacotherapist. Successful therapy requires rational use of antiglaucoma medications by the clinician and patient adherence to the selected regimen, combined with conscientious monitoring for side effects and disease progression. The reward for successful therapy is considerable: the maintenance of vision. The overview of the clinical findings, pathology, and drug therapy presented in this chapter provides the clinician with the fundamentals necessary to understand and treat glaucoma.

▶ PRINCIPLES OF PHARMACOTHERAPY

- The objective of treating POAG is to reduce IOP.
- Effective glaucoma therapy stops or reduces progression of visual-field loss in most patients.
- Factors in addition to IOP determine progression of visual loss or therapeutic success.
- Each patient needs an effective, well-tolerated, and convenient drug regimen for treating glaucoma.
- Initial drug choice should be based on a match of patient and drug characteristics.
- Local adverse events are common with topical glaucoma medications.
- Topical glaucoma medications have the potential to produce significant adverse systemic effects.
- Patient and family education is necessary to ensure adherence and successful outcomes in glaucoma treatment.

REFERENCES

1. Coleman AL. Glaucoma. Lancet 1999;354:1803–1810.
2. Infield DA, O'Shea J. Glaucoma: Diagnosis and management. Postgrad Med J 1998:74:709–715.
3. Khaw PT, Cordiero MF. Towards better treatment of glaucoma. Br Med J 2000;320(7250):1619–1620.
4. Dreyer FB, Lipton SA. New perspectives in glaucoma. JAMA 1999; 281:306–308.
5. Stewart WC. Perspectives in the medical treatment of glaucoma. Curr Opin Ophthalmol 1999;10(2):99–108.
6. Chung HS, Harris A, Evans DW, et al. Vascular aspects in the pathophysiology of glaucomatous optic neuropathy. Surv Ophthalmol 1999;43 (Suppl 1):S43–50.
7. Ritch R. Neuroprotection: Is it already applicable to glaucoma therapy? Curr Opin Ophthalmol 2000;11(2):78–84.
8. Weinreb RN, Levin LA. Is neuroprotection a viable therapy for glaucoma? Arch Ophthalmol 1999;117(11):1540–1544.
9. Schwartz M, Yoles E. Neuroprotection: A new treatment modality for glaucoma? Curr Opin Ophthalmol 2000;11(2):107–111.
10. Vorwerk CK, Gorla MS, Dreyer EB. An experimental basis for implicating excitotoxicity in glaucomatous optic neuropathy. Surv Ophthalmol 1999;43(Suppl 1):S142–150.
11. Neufeld AH. Nitric oxide: A potential mediator of retinal ganglion cell damage in glaucoma. Surv Ophthalmol 1999;43(Suppl 1):S129–135.
12. Osborne NN, Ugarte M, Chao M, et al. Neuroprotection in relation to retinal ischemia and relevance to glaucoma. Surv Ophthalmol 1999;43 (Suppl 1):S102–128.
13. Kaufman PL, Gabelt BT, Cynader M. Introductory comments on neuroprotection. Surv Ophthalmol 1999;43(Suppl 1):S89–90.
14. Yu DY, Su EN, Cringle SJ, et al. Systemic and ocular vascular roles of the antiglaucoma agents beta-adrenergic antagonists and Ca^{2+} entry blockers. Surv Ophthalmol 1999;43(Suppl 1):S214–222.
15. Alward WL. Medical management of glaucoma. N Engl J Med 1998; 339(18):1298–1307.
16. King A, Migdal C. Clinical management of glaucoma. J R Soc Med 2000; 93(4):175–177.
17. Hoyng PF, van Beek LM. Pharmacological therapy for glaucoma: A review. Drugs 2000;59(3):411–434.
18. Kooner KS. New agents in glaucoma therapy. Int Ophthalmol Clin 1999; 39(3):1–15.
19. Kaufman PL, Gabelt B, Tian B, Liu X. Advances in glaucoma diagnosis and therapy for the next millennium: New drugs for trabecular and uveoscleral outflow. Semin Ophthalmol 1999;14(3):130–143.
20. Caprioli J. The treatment of normal-tension glaucoma. Am J Ophthalmol 1998;126(4):578–581.
21. Kamal D, Hitchings R. Normal-tension glaucoma: A practical approach. Br J Ophthalmol 1998;82(7):835–840.
22. Drance SM. The Collaborative Normal-Tension Glaucoma Study and some of its lessons. Can J Ophthalmol 1999;34:1–6.
23. Hattenhauer MG, Johnson DH, Ing HH. The probability of blindness from open angle glaucoma. Ophthalmology 1998;105:2099–2104.
24. Quigley HA. Proportion of those with open angle glaucoma who become blind. Ophthalmology 1999;106:2039–2041.
25. Cooper. Surgical management off the glaucomas. Aust NZ J Ophthalmol 1999;27:350–352.

26. Cordeiro MF, Siriwardena D, Chang L, Khaw PT. Wound healing modulation after glaucoma surgery. Curr Opin Ophthalmol 2000;11(2):121–126.
27. Donohue EK, Cioffi GA. Glaucoma surgery: Are there new perspectives in perioperative pharmacology? Curr Opin Ophthalmol 1999;10(2):93–98.
28. Loon SC, Chew PT. A major review of antimetabolites in glaucoma therapy. Ophthalmologica 1999;213(4):234–245.
29. Schuman JS. Antiglaucoma medications: A review of safety and tolerability issues related to their use. Clin Ther 2000;22(2):167–208.
30. Vogel R, Strahlman E, Rittenhouse KD. Adverse events associated with commonly used glaucoma drugs. Int Ophthalmol Clin 1999;39(2):107–124.
31. Stewart WC, Garrison PM. Beta-blocker-induced complications and patients with glaucoma. Arch Intern Med 1998;158:221–226.
32. Drance SM. Introductory comments on potential differences between beta-blockers in the treatment of open-angle glaucoma. Surv Ophthalmol 1999;43(Suppl 1):S173–175.
33. Eisenberg DL, Camras CB. A preliminary risk-benefit assessment of latanoprost and unoprostone in open-angle glaucoma and ocular hypertension. Drug Safety 1999;20(6):505–514.
34. Linden C, Alm A. Prostaglandin analogues in the treatment of glaucoma. Drugs Aging 1999;14(5):387–398.
35. Naskar R, Vorwerk CK, Dreyer EB. Saving the nerve from glaucoma: Memantine to caspaces. Semin Ophthalmol 1999;14(3):152–158.

95

ALLERGIC RHINITIS

J. Russell May

Rhinitis is inflammation of the nasal mucous membrane. Allergic rhinitis is caused by mucous membrane exposure to inhaled allergenic materials that elicit a specific response mediated by immunoglobulin E (IgE). It is characterized by sneezing, nasal itching, and watery rhinorrhea, often associated with nasal congestion. Itching of the throat, eyes, and ears frequently accompanies allergic rhinitis.

Two types of allergic rhinitis exist. Seasonal allergic rhinitis, commonly known as *hay fever,* occurs in response to specific allergens present at predictable times of the year—during the spring and/or fall blooming seasons. Seasonal allergens include pollen from trees, grasses, and weeds, and these typically cause more acute symptoms. Perennial allergic rhinitis is a year-round disease caused by nonseasonal allergens, such as house dust mites, animal dander, and molds. It typically results in subtle, chronic symptoms. Unfortunately, some patients have a combination of these two types of allergic rhinitis, with symptoms year round that are exacerbated further seasonally.

EPIDEMIOLOGY AND ETIOLOGY

Allergic rhinitis is one of the most common medical disorders found in humans. An estimated 20% to 25% of the American population is affected, with some believing the percentage to be much higher.[1] It ranks as the sixth most prevalent chronic illness in the United States.[2] Patients are limited in their ability to carry out normal daily functions: Their concentration is impaired, sleep is disturbed, social interaction is limited, and emotional well-being is affected.[3]

In addition, the impact of allergic rhinitis goes well beyond these minor inconveniences. Allergic rhinitis is associated with several serious medical conditions, including asthma, sinusitis, otitis media, nasal polyposis, respiratory infections, and orthodontic malocclusions.[1]

PREDISPOSING FACTORS

Allergic rhinitis has a strong genetic predisposition. A family history of allergic rhinitis, atopic dermatitis, or asthma suggests that rhinitis is allergic. Likewise, a personal history of other atopic diseases (e.g., atopic dermatitis as an infant) predisposes to the development of allergic rhinitis later in life.[4,5] The risk of developing allergic rhinitis is approximately 30% for children with one atopic parent and approaches 50% for those with two allergic parents.[2] Peak incidence occurs in childhood and adolescence, with approximately 70% of patients developing symptoms by the age of 30 years.[6]

Allergen exposure is another predisposing factor. For allergic rhinitis to occur, an individual must be exposed to a protein that elicits the allergic response in that individual. Many potential sufferers never develop symptoms because they never come into contact with the allergen that would produce symptoms in them.

For reasons that are unclear, positive skin tests indicating allergen sensitization have been observed more frequently in people in higher socioeconomic classes and in people who live in suburban areas (compared with those living in more crowded and polluted inner-city areas). The degree of pollen exposure may be a larger contributing pathogenic factor in inducing sensitization than air pollution.[7] However, once symptoms have started, they can be exacerbated by various nonspecific irritants, such as cigarette smoke, strong odors, air pollution, and climatic changes.

ALLERGENS

Allergens that produce seasonal rhinitis are the protein components of airborne pollen grains from a variety of trees, grasses, and weeds. Ragweed and grass pollen are the most common offenders in the United States; however, this changes with the geographic region. In general, tree pollens cause symptoms in the spring, grass pollens cause symptoms in the late spring to summer, and weed pollens are the culprits in the late summer to early fall. Patients who are hypersensitive to all three may have overlapping problem periods that can lead to a misdiagnosis of perennial rhinitis. Flowering plants that depend on insect pollination usually do not cause allergic rhinitis.

To complicate matters further, the antigenic components of many grasses—including fescue, Kentucky bluegrass, orchard, redtop, and timothy—are similar, resulting in cross-allergenicity. Fortunately, the trees that produce many of the offending airborne pollens produce antigenically distinct pollens. These trees include ash, beech, birch, cedar, hickory, maple, oak, poplar, and sycamore.

Mold spores are also important allergens. Spores are present year round; however, mold growth on decaying vegetation increases seasonally. Thus mold spores can be responsible for both perennial and seasonal allergies.

Indoor allergens usually are present perennially; most important among these are house dust mite fecal proteins, animal dander, cockroaches, and certain mold species.

PHYSIOLOGY AND PATHOPHYSIOLOGY

NASAL PHYSIOLOGY

Knowledge of nasal physiology aids in the understanding of allergic rhinitis. The nose performs three "air conditioning" functions to prepare incoming gases and their contents for the lungs. During the fraction of a second that air is in the nose, it is heated, humidified, and cleaned. The cleaning process plays a role in the development of allergic rhinitis. As the air passes through the nose, the turbulence throws particulate matter against a mucous blanket. The rhythmic movements of the nasal cilia cause the mucous blanket to move posteriorly at approximately 9 mm/min, where it is eventually swallowed; therefore, foreign particles are removed via the gastrointestinal tract and do not reach the lungs.

The vascular tissue in the nose is erectile. Stimulation of sympathetic fibers causes vasoconstriction, reduction in erectile tissue size, and airway widening. Parasympathetic stimulation causes vasodilatation, increase in erectile tissue size, and airway narrowing.

Located in the nasal mucosa are the mast cells, which participate in the regulation of nasal patency by releasing such mediators as histamine. These are described below.

IMMUNE RESPONSE TO ALLERGENS

Allergic reactions in the nose are mediated by antigen-antibody responses during which allergens interact with specific IgE molecules bound to nasal mast cells and basophils. In allergic people, these cells are increased in both number and reactivity. During inhalation, airborne allergens enter the nose and are processed by lymphocytes, which produce antigen-specific IgE, thereby sensitizing genetically predisposed hosts to those agents. Upon nasal reexposure, IgE bound to mast cells interacts with airborne allergen, triggering release of inflammatory mediators (Fig. 95–1).[8]

Both immediate and late-phase reactions are observed after allergen exposure. The immediate reaction occurs within minutes, resulting in the rapid release of preformed mediators and newly generated mediators from the arachidonic acid cascade as the mast cell membrane is disturbed (Table 95–1).[9] These mediators of immediate hypersensitivity include histamine, leukotrienes (LTs) C_4, LT D_4,

TABLE 95–1. Mast Cell Mediators

Mediator	Effect
Preformed and Rapidly Released	
Histamine	Stimulates irritant receptors Pruritus Vascular permeability Mucosal permeability Smooth muscle contraction
Neutrophil chemotactic factor	Influx of inflammatory cells
Eosinophil chemotactic factor	Influx of inflammatory cells
Kinins	Vascular permeability
N-α-tosyl L-arginine methyl esterase	Vascular permeability
Newly Generated	
Leukotrienes	Smooth muscle contraction Vascular permeability Mucus secretion Chemotaxis Mucus secretion Neutrophil chemotaxis
Thromboxanes	Smooth muscle spasm
Platelet-activating factor	Mucus secretion Airway permeability Chemotaxis Vascular permeability
Granule Matrix Contents	
Heparin	Anti-inflammatory
Tryptase	Protein hydrolysis
Kallikrein	Protein hydrolysis

LT E_4, prostaglandin D_2, tryptase, and kinins.[10,11] In addition, the mast cell has been found to be a source of several cytokines that probably are relevant to the chronicity of the mucosal inflammation that characterizes allergic rhinitis.[12] The physiologic responses to these inflammatory mediators include vasodilatation, increased vascular permeability, and production of nasal secretions.[10,13] Histamine, the most important mediator, causes vascular engorgement, leading to nasal congestion, direct stimulation of mucus secretion, and increased glandular secretion.

Four to eight hours after the initial exposure to an allergen, a late-phase reaction occurs in 50% of allergic rhinitis patients.[14] This response, thought to be due to cytokines released primarily by mast cells and thymus-derived helper lymphocytes, is characterized by profound infiltration and activation of migrating cells. This inflammatory response likely is responsible for the persistent, chronic symptoms of allergic rhinitis, including nasal congestion. The inflamed mucosae become hyperresponsive, a state characterized by exacerbation of nasal symptoms when the patient is exposed to nonspecific or irritant triggers. Subsequent exposure to lower doses of the same allergen produces repeated or persistent nasal symptoms in such a "primed" host.

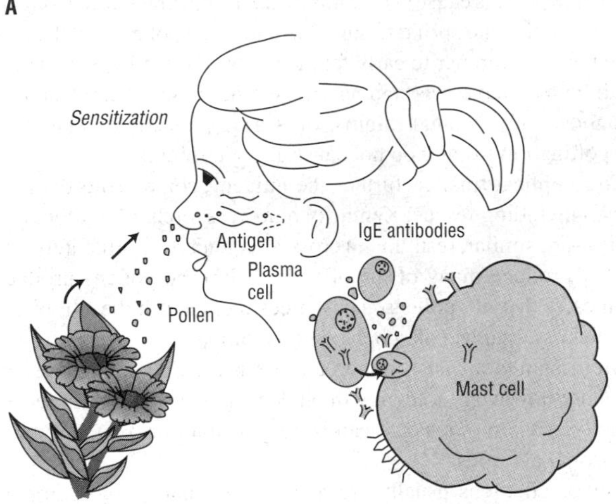

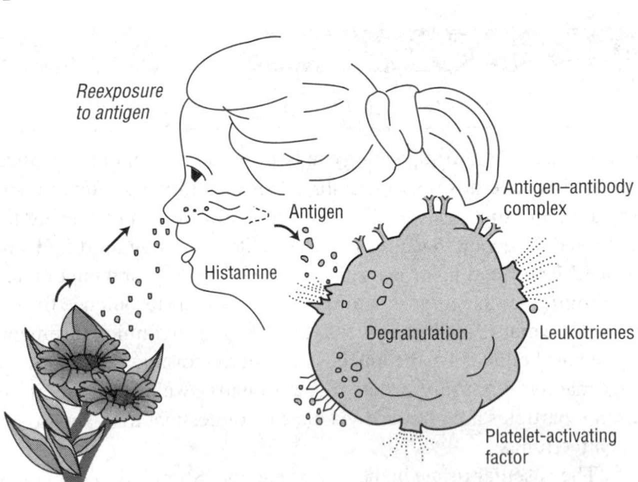

FIGURE 95–1. Allergen sensitization and the allergic response. ***A.*** Exposure to antigen stimulates IgE production and sensitization of mast cells with antigen-specific IgE antibodies. ***B.*** Subsequent exposure to the same antigen produces an allergic reaction when mast cell mediators are released.

CLINICAL PRESENTATION

SYMPTOMS AND DIAGNOSIS

The patient with allergic rhinitis typically complains of clear rhinorrhea, paroxysms of sneezing, nasal congestion, postnasal drip, and pruritic eyes, ears, nose, or palate. Symptoms of allergic conjunctivitis are associated more frequently with seasonal than perennial allergic rhinitis, since a majority of the perennial allergens, such as dust mites and molds, are indoors, where air velocity is too low for substantial deposition of allergenic particles on the conjunctivae.

Symptoms secondary to the late-phase reaction, predominantly nasal congestion, begin 3 to 5 hours after antigen exposure and peak at 12 to 24 hours. Subsequent symptoms, both allergic and irritant, are elicited more easily because of the priming effect. For instance, a ragweed-sensitive patient, when exposed to ragweed pollen out of season, responds with modest symptoms and may be very tolerant of irritants such as air pollution or tobacco smoke. During the ragweed season, however, when the nasal mucosa is already inflamed, exposure to small doses of pollen or to irritants to which the patient is usually tolerant elicits a more severe response.

Allergic rhinitis is differentiated from other causes of rhinitis by a thorough history, physical examination, and certain diagnostic tests. The medical history consists of a careful description of symptoms, environmental factors and exposures, results of previous therapy, use of other medications, previous nasal injuries, previous nasal or sinus surgery, family history, and the presence of other medical problems. Identification of specific causative allergens may be difficult. For example, a reaction induced by mowing the lawn may not be caused by grass pollens but by the disturbance of various weeds, molds, or other plants in the lawn. With perennial allergic rhinitis, the cause-effect relationship is less clear, making the diagnosis more difficult, especially with such covert allergens as house dust mites and molds.

Physical examination may reveal allergic shiners, a transverse nasal crease caused by repeated rubbing of the nose, and adenoidal breathing. Pale, bluish, edematous nasal turbinates coated with thin, clear secretions are characteristic. Tearing, conjunctival injection and edema, and periorbital swelling may be present.

Nasal scrapings will provide a representative sample of cells infiltrating the nasal mucosa and can be helpful in supporting the diagnosis.[15] Microscopic examination of the nasal smear from an allergic individual typically will show numerous eosinophils. The blood eosinophil count may be elevated in allergic rhinitis, but it is nonspecific and has limited usefulness.[16]

The preceding diagnostic evaluation is supported by determination of the presence or absence of specific IgE allergen skin testing or in vitro assays [e.g., radioallergosorbent test (RAST)]. Two different methods of skin testing are available. The epicutaneous test, also known as the *scratch* or *prick test,* is performed by making a superficial wound in the outermost layer of skin. A drop of antigen is placed in the wound and allowed to diffuse into the underlying skin. The intradermal test is performed by injecting 0.01–0.05 mL of diluted allergen between the layers of skin. With each procedure, a positive test produces a wheal and flare reaction within 15 to 30 minutes. The epicutaneous prick test is the fastest and least expensive screening tool; intradermal tests should be reserved for patients who give negative prick tests but who are suspected of having an allergic etiology for common symptoms.[17]

The variability in potency and stability of skin testing extracts led to the development of standardized extracts, which have a defined potency and are labeled with a common unit, the bioequivalent allergy unit (BAU).[18] This measure provides the allergist with guidance in selecting common safe and effective doses for diagnostic tests as well as for treatment. Skin test results may vary depending on the anatomic site, method of skin testing, or even time of day at which the test is performed.[17] Also, the concurrent use of antihistamines or sympathomimetic agents may alter the test response. Numerous allergens are available for testing, including extracts of tree, grass, and weed pollens and molds, foods, and other miscellaneous inhalants. Selection should be based on patient history.

RAST is an assay for measurement of specific IgE. Because it is expensive and less sensitive than skin tests, its use is rarely justified in clinical practice.[19] Such in vitro testing may be useful when appropriate specific skin test extracts are not available, when negative controls produce a wheal reaction, when antihistamine therapy cannot be discounted, or in the presence of dermatographia.[20] Total IgE levels are elevated in only 30% to 40% of allergic rhinitis patients, and it is also elevated in some nonallergic conditions, thus limiting its diagnostic usefulness.[16,20]

COMPLICATIONS

Not only is allergic rhinitis aggravating, it also frequently leads to further complications, particularly if the patient does not receive adequate treatment. Symptoms of untreated rhinitis may lead to inability to sleep, chronic malaise, fatigue, and poor work or school efficiency. Patients often are plagued by loss of smell or taste, with sinusitis or polyps underlying many cases of allergy-related hyposmia.[21,22] Postnasal drip with cough also can be bothersome.

The role of allergic rhinitis in the development of acute otitis media or chronic middle ear effusion remains controversial. Children with allergic rhinitis appear to be at greater risk of these conditions because of nasal obstruction, insufflation of nasal secretions into the middle ear via eustachian tube obstruction, and negative middle ear pressure.[23] Hearing problems in children related to middle ear effusion may lead to delayed development of language in young children or school problems in older children.[24]

Structural facial and dental problems can result from chronic allergic rhinitis.[25,26] The chronic edema and venous stasis may contribute to the development of a high-arched, V-shaped palate. Mouth breathing caused by nasal obstruction can be responsible for dental malocclusion and orthodontic problems. Constant upward rubbing of the nose (*allergic salute*) can cause a permanent transverse crease across the lower nose; nasal congestion leads to venous pooling and dark circles under the eyes known as *allergic shiners*.

Allergic rhinitis is clearly a risk factor for asthma, with approximately 90% of asthmatics younger than 16 years of age having allergies.[16] Asthma is more common in those with perennial than seasonal allergic rhinitis, and it is less likely to be "outgrown" when associated with allergic rhinitis.[27]

Recurrent and chronic sinusitis (most often nonbacterial) are relatively common complications of allergic rhinitis. However, the hypersecretion associated with the inflammatory process, coupled with nasal obstruction, leads to stasis of secretions in the sinuses, offering ideal breeding grounds for bacteria. Nasal polyps are less common but nonetheless bothersome; they require specific therapy but may improve with management of the underlying allergic state. Epistaxis also can be a problem; it is related to mucosal hyperemia and inflammation.

► TREATMENT: Allergic Rhinitis

DESIRED OUTCOME

The therapeutic goal for patients with allergic rhinitis is to minimize or prevent symptoms. This goal should be accomplished with no or minimal, tolerable drug side effects with reasonable medication expense. The patient should be able to maintain a normal lifestyle, including participating in outdoor activities, yard work, and playing with pets as desired.

TABLE 95–2. Pharmacotherapeutic Options

Medication Class	Symptoms Controlled	Comments
Antihistamines		
Systemic	Sneezing, rhinorrhea, itching, conjunctivitis	For seasonal allergic rhinitis, begin treatment before allergen exposure. Older, less expensive agents should be tried first. If sedation is a problem, move to nonsedating choices. For perennial allergic rhinitis, use as an alternative to or in combination with an intranasal steroid.
Ophthalmic	Conjunctivitis	Logical addition to nasal steroids if ocular symptoms are present.
Intranasal	Sneezing, rhinorrhea, nasal pruritus	Option for seasonal allergic rhinitis. Warn patients of potential drowsiness.
Decongestants		
Systemic	Nasal congestion	Only needed when nasal congestion is present.
Topical	Nasal congestion	Only needed when nasal congestion is present. Do not exceed 3–5 days.
Intranasal Corticosteroids	Sneezing, rhinorrhea, itching, nasal congestion	For seasonal allergic rhinitis, an option when congestion is present. Must begin therapy before allergen exposure. Excellent choice for perennial rhinitis.
Mast Cell Stabilizers	See Comments	Prevents symptoms; therefore, for seasonal allergic rhinitis, use before offending allergen's season starts. For perennial rhinitis, improvement may not be seen for up to 1 month.
Intranasal Anticholinergics	Rhinorrhea	Reserve for use when above therapies fail or cannot be tolerated.

GENERAL APPROACH TO TREATMENT

Once the causative allergens and the specific symptoms are identified, management consists of three possible approaches: (1) allergen avoidance, (2) pharmacotherapy for prevention or treatment of symptoms, and (3) specific immunotherapy. The pharmacotherapy for symptoms approach includes several options that are based on patient-specific information (Table 95–2).

AVOIDANCE

Avoidance of offending allergens is the most direct method of preventing allergic rhinitis, but it is often the most difficult to accomplish, especially for perennial allergens. Mold growth can be reduced by maintaining household humidity below 50% and removing obvious growth with bleach or disinfectant. Patients sensitive to animals will benefit most by removing pets from the home; however, most animal lovers are reluctant to comply with this approach. Cats may be more of a problem than dogs. Cat allergen is so prevalent that 25% of cat-free houses contained detectable cat allergen in one survey.[28] Species differences may exist with dogs such that a person may be allergic to one dog but not another.

Efforts to eliminate dust mites should be rigorous, particularly in the bedroom. Exposure to dust mites can be reduced by encasing mattresses and pillows with impermeable covers and washing bed linens in hot water.[29] Washable area rugs are preferable to wall-to-wall carpeting. Acaricide treatment of carpets has been shown to denature the dust mite allergen. Atopic infants who are exposed to high levels of dust mites are at increased risk for developing asthma.[30] Environmental control of these allergens may be helpful in forestalling further rhinitis and preventing later asthma.

Older central air-filtration systems for houses were expensive and minimally effective. High-efficiency particulate air (HEPA) filters have minimal effect on the heavy mite allergens but are effective in removing lightweight particulates, including pollens, mold spores, and cat allergen, thus reducing allergic respiratory symptoms.[31]

Patients with seasonal allergic rhinitis should keep windows closed and minimize time spent outdoors during pollen seasons. Use of fans that direct outside air into the house should be avoided. Filter masks can be worn while gardening or mowing the lawn.

When avoidance is impractical, is unacceptable to the patient, or produces only a partial response, pharmacotherapeutic approaches can be used to prevent and treat allergic rhinitis.

PHARMACOLOGIC THERAPY

First-line therapeutic modalities for treating allergic rhinitis are directed at relief of symptoms. Antihistamines and decongestants (both oral and topical) generally are used first in treating allergic rhinitis with medications. Knowledge of pathophysiology and the inflammatory state has led to prophylactic therapy for more severe disease using agents such as cromolyn and topical steroids. However, in attempting to assess the evidence supporting any particular therapy, clinicians have difficulty interpreting the medical literature for a variety of reasons, including lack of uniformity in the research methodologies, inappropriate drug controls, and failure to identify types of rhinitis in study subjects (perennial versus seasonal and allergic versus nonallergic).

ANTIHISTAMINES

Histamine H_1-receptor antagonists are competitive antagonists to histamine. They bind to H_1 receptors without activating them, preventing histamine binding and action.[32] Newer antihistamines also may inhibit mediator release; however, the exact mechanism is not understood. Antihistamines are available in oral, ophthalmic, and intranasal dosage forms.

Antihistamines are more effective in preventing the actions of histamines than in reversing these actions once they have taken place. Reversal of symptoms is, at least in part, caused by the anticholinergic properties of these drugs. This activity is responsible for the drying

TABLE 95–3. **Relative Adverse Effect Profiles of Antihistamines**

Medication	Relative Sedative Effect	Relative Anticholinergic Effect
Alkylamine Class		
Brompheniramine maleate	Low	Moderate
Chlorpheniramine maleate	Low	Moderate
Dexchlorpheniramine maleate	Low	Moderate
Ethanolamine Class		
Carbinoxamine maleate	High	High
Clemastine fumarate	Moderate	High
Diphenhydramine hydrochloride	High	High
Ethylenediamine Class		
Pyrilamine maleate	Low	Low to none
Tripelennamine hydrochloride	Moderate	Low to none
Phenothiazine Class		
Promethazine hydrochloride	High	High
Piperidine Class		
Azatadine maleate	Moderate	Moderate
Cyproheptadine hydrochloride	Low	Moderate
Phenindamine tartrate	Low to none	Moderate
"Nonsedating" Peripherally Selective Class		
Cetirizine	Low to moderate	Low to none
Fexofenadine	Low to none	Low to none
Loratadine	Low to none	Low to none

effect of antihistamines, which reduces the problem of nasal, salivary, and lacrimal gland hypersecretion. Antihistamines antagonize capillary permeability, wheal-and-flare formation, and itching.

In general, the antihistamines are well absorbed, have large volumes of distribution, and are metabolized by the liver. Serum half-lives vary considerably between patients.[32] Also, the therapeutic effects of these agents are more prolonged than might be predicted by their half-lives.

Drowsiness is usually the chief complaint of patients who take antihistamines. It can interfere with a patient's ability to drive a car or operate machinery and may interfere with the patient's ability to function adequately at the workplace. The sedative effects of antihistamines vary from class to class. Table 95–3 lists common antihistamines and their relative potential for causing sedation. The table also gives the agents' relative anticholinergic effects.

The sedative effects of antihistamines can be useful in patients who suffer from sleeplessness caused by the symptoms of allergic rhinitis. In these patients, a bedtime dose may prove beneficial. The mechanism for sedation is not well understood, but its central effect depends on the drugs' ability to cross the blood-brain barrier. Most older antihistamines are lipid-soluble and cross this barrier easily.

The newer, highly selective peripheral histamine H_1-receptor antagonists have little or no central or autonomic nervous system effects. The term *nonsedating antihistamines* has been used to describe the agents in this class, especially fexofenadine and loratadine, although sedation is one of the more common patient complaints with these agents. Cetirizine also acts peripherally, but its sedation rate is greater than the two agents.

The nonsedating agents should not be substituted automatically for older agents. Many patients respond to and tolerate the older agents quite well. Because many of the older agents are available generically, they are much less expensive. Average wholesale price of many of the generically available agents is less than $5 for a 30-day supply, compared with more than $50 for some of the nonsedating agents.

Anticholinergic (drying) effects lend to the agents' therapeutic efficacy, but they also cause most adverse effects. Dry mouth, difficulty in voiding urine, constipation, and potential cardiovascular effects may be troublesome. Table 95–3 lists several antihistamines and their relative anticholinergic effects. Keep in mind that the differences may be small. Patients with a predisposition to urinary retention (e.g., elderly men and those on concurrent anticholinergic therapy) should use antihistamines with caution. Caution also should be used in patients with increased intraocular pressure, hyperthyroidism, and cardiovascular disease.

Other adverse effects of antihistamines include loss of appetite, nausea, vomiting, and epigastric distress.

Antihistamines are more effective when taken approximately 1 to 2 hours before anticipated exposure to the offending allergen. If tolerance develops to the therapeutic effect, a change to an agent in a different chemical class may be effective.

Patients should be counseled about the proper use of antihistamines. Adverse effects, especially drowsiness, should be emphasized. Patients should be warned against taking other central nervous system depressants, including the use of alcohol. Patients should be told *not* to take a double dose when a dose is missed. Taking the antihistamine with meals or at least a full glass of water will help prevent the gastrointestinal side effects (e.g., nausea, vomiting, and epigastric distress). Patients should check with their pharmacists and read labels before taking nonprescription medications. Many cold products and sleep aids contain antihistamines. Patients should be instructed not to use more than one antihistamine at a time. Table 95–4 lists the recommended dosages of the commonly prescribed agents.

For seasonal allergic rhinitis, an intranasal antihistamine, azelastine, is available. Patient satisfaction is high with this agent because it rapidly relieves symptoms. However, patients should be warned of its potential for drowsiness. The systemic availability of this product is approximately 40%.[33]

Allergic conjunctivitis, often associated with allergic rhinitis, can be treated with an ophthalmic antihistamine such as levocabastine. Systemic antihistamines usually are effective for allergic conjunctivitis, making the ocular product unnecessary. However, levocabastine is a logical addition to nasal steroids when ocular symptoms occur.

TABLE 95–4. Oral Dosages of Commonly Prescribed Antihistamines and Decongestants

Medication	Dosage and Interval	
	Adults	*Children*
Antihistamines		
Chlorpheniramine maleate, plain	4 mg every 6 h	6–12 yr: 2 mg every 6 h 2–6 yr: 1 mg every 6 h
Chlorpheniramine maleate, sustained release	8–12 mg daily at bedtime or 8–12 mg every 8 h	6–12 yr: 8 mg at bedtime <6 yr: Not recommended
Diphenhydramine hydrochloride	25–50 mg every 8 h	5 mg/kg/day divided every 8 h (up to 25 mg per dose)
Clemastine fumarate	1.34 mg twice daily to 2.68 mg three times daily	Not recommended
Loratadine	10 mg once daily	10 mg once daily
Fexofenadine	60 mg twice daily	6–11 yr: 30 mg twice daily
Cetirizine	5–10 mg once daily	>6 yr: 5 mg once daily
Decongestants		
Pseudoephedrine	60 mg every 4–6 h 120 mg every 12 h for sustained release	6–12 yr: 30 mg every 4–6 h 2–5 yr: 15 mg every 4–6 h
Ephedrine sulfate	25–50 mg every 4 h	2–3 mg/kg/day divided every 4 h (up to 25 mg every 4 h)

DECONGESTANTS

Topical and systemic decongestants are sympathomimetic agents that act on adrenergic receptors in the nasal mucosa, producing vasoconstriction. Decongestants shrink swollen mucosa and improve ventilation. When nasal congestion is part of the clinical picture, decongestants work well in combination with antihistamines.

Topical Decongestants

Topical decongestants are applied directly to swollen nasal mucosa via drops or sprays. Table 95–5 lists the common topical decongestants and their duration of action. The use of these agents results in little or no systemic absorption.

Because these agents are extremely effective and are available to patients over the counter (OTC), they are widely used. However, prolonged use of these agents (for more than 3 to 5 days) can result in a condition known as *rhinitis medicamentosa,* or *rebound vasodilation,* with associated congestion. Patients who develop this condition use more spray more often with less response. While the methods used to treat this "addiction" have not been studied formally, several are used commonly. Abrupt cessation works, but it is difficult because of rebound congestion that may leave the patient congested for several days or weeks. Sleeping may become difficult. Nasal steroids have been used successfully, but they take several days to work. Weaning the patient off topical decongestants can be accomplished by decreasing the dosing frequency or the concentration over several weeks. Combining the weaning process with nasal steroids may prove useful.

Other side effects of topical decongestants include burning, stinging, sneezing, and dryness of the nasal mucosa.

Patients should be counseled on the use of topical decongestants to prevent rhinitis medicamentosa. Patients should be instructed to use as small a dose as possible as infrequently as possible and only when absolutely necessary (e.g., at bedtime to aid in falling asleep). Duration of therapy always should be limited to 3 to 5 days.

TABLE 95–5. Duration of Action of Topical Decongestants

Medication	Duration (h)
Short Acting	
Phenylephrine hydrochloride	Up to 4
Intermediate Acting	
Naphazoline hydrochloride	4–6
Tetrahydrozoline hydrochloride	
Long Acting	
Oxymetazoline hydrochloride	Up to 12
Xylometazoline hydrochloride	

Systemic Decongestants

Oral decongestants are not as effective on an immediate basis as the topical agents, but they may last longer and cause less local irritation. Also, rhinitis medicamentosa is not a problem with older agents. The most commonly used agents are pseudoephedrine and ephedrine. The pharmacokinetic variables for these agents are summarized in Table 95–6.

Pseudoephedrine appears to be the safest systemic decongestant. Doses of 180 mg have been shown to produce no measurable change in blood pressure or heart rate.[34] In higher doses (210–240 mg), pseudoephedrine has raised both blood pressure and heart rate.[35] Both

TABLE 95–6. Pharmacokinetic Variables of Systemic Decongestants

Medication	Half-Life (h)	Mechanism of Metabolism or Elimination
Pseudoephedrine	3–8	Partially metabolized; majority excreted unchanged in urine
Ephedrine	3–6	Majority excreted unchanged in urine

pseudoephedrine and ephedrine can cause mild central nervous system stimulation, even at therapeutic doses.

Table 95–4 lists the usual doses for pseudoephedrine and ephedrine. Because most of the studies on the effect of decongestants on blood pressure were performed in normotensive patients, hypertensive patients should, unless absolutely necessary, avoid these drugs, especially ephedrine. Severe hypertensive reactions can occur with any of these agents when given concomitantly with monoamine oxidase inhibitors.[36]

COMBINATION PRODUCTS

Numerous products combine an antihistamine with a decongestant. The combination is rational because of the different mechanisms of action. Both older and nonsedating antihistamines are available in such combinations. As mentioned previously, patients should read labels to avoid therapeutic duplication.

NASAL STEROIDS

Nasal steroids are an excellent choice for treating perennial rhinitis, and these can be useful in seasonal rhinitis, especially if dosed in advance of symptoms. Nasal steroids appear to be effective with minimal side effects. In one consensus report, nasal steroids are recommended as initial therapy, along with avoidance of allergens in seasonal allergic rhinitis and perennial rhinitis.[37]

Multiple mechanisms are involved with the effects of nasal steroids on the nasal mucosa: reducing inflammation by blocking mediator release, suppressing neutrophil chemotaxis, reducing intracellular edema, causing mild vasoconstriction, and inhibiting mast cell–mediated late-phase reactions.[38] Table 95–7 lists the available nasal steroids and their usual doses.

TABLE 95–7. Dosage of Nasal Steroids

Medication	Dosage and Interval
Beclomethasone dipropionate	>12 yr: 1 inhalation (42 μg) per nostril 2–4 times a day (maximum, 336 μg/day) 6–12 yr: 1 inhalation per nostril 3 times per day
Beclomethasone dipropionate, monohydrate	>12 yr.: 1–2 inhalations once daily 6–12 yr: 1 inhalation per nostril (42 μg) twice daily to start
Budesonide	>6 yr: 2 sprays (64 μg) per nostril in A.M. and P.M., or 4 sprays per nostril in A.M. (maximum, 256 μg)
Flunisolide	Adults: 2 sprays (50 μg) per nostril twice daily (maximum, 400 μg) Children: 1 spray per nostril 3 times a day
Fluticasone	Adults: 2 sprays (100 μg) per nostril once daily; after a few days decrease to 1 spray per nostril Children >4 yr and adolescents: 1 spray per nostril once daily (maximum, 200 μg/day)
Mometasone furoate	>12 yr: 2 sprays (100 μg) per nostril once daily
Triamcinolone acetonide	>12 yr: 2 sprays (110 μg) per nostril once daily (maximum, 440 μg/day)

Topical steroids produce only minor side effects, most commonly sneezing, stinging, headache, and epistaxis. Suppression of the hypothalamic-pituitary-adrenal axis has not been a problem with therapeutic doses. Local infections with *Candida albicans* have occurred rarely.

The therapeutic benefits of topical steroids are not immediate. Patients need to understand this to ensure cooperation and continuation of therapy. Some patients notice improvement in a few days, but peak responses may not be observed for 2 to 3 weeks. Once a response is achieved the dosage may be reduced. Blocked nasal passages should be cleared with a decongestant before administration to ensure adequate penetration of the spray. Patients should be advised to avoid sneezing or blowing their nose for at least 10 minutes after administration. Topical steroids should not be used in patients with nasal septum ulcers or recent nasal surgery or trauma.

OTHER INHALANT MEDICATIONS

Cromolyn sodium and ipratropium bromide offer two additional approaches for treating allergic rhinitis. Cromolyn sodium is a mast cell stabilizer. Increased interest in this product has resulted from it becoming available OTC. Ipratropium bromide is an anticholinergic agent useful in perennial allergic rhinitis.

Cromolyn sodium nasal spray is used for the symptomatic prevention and treatment of allergic rhinitis. It has the property of preventing antigen-triggered mast cell degranulation and release of the mediators of allergic reactions, including histamine. Cromolyn sodium has no direct antihistaminic, anticholinergic, or anti-inflammatory properties. Similar to topical steroids, the most common side effects—sneezing and nasal stinging—result from local irritation. The dose in adults and children older than 6 years of age is one spray in each nostril three to four times per day at regular intervals. Cromolyn sodium must cover the entire nasal lining; therefore, patients should be instructed to clear nasal passages before administration. Inhaling through the nose during administration aids in this process.

For seasonal rhinitis, treatment with cromolyn sodium should be initiated just before the usual start of the offending allergen's season and continued throughout the season. In perennial rhinitis, the effects may not be seen for 2 to 4 weeks; therefore, antihistamines or decongestants may be needed during this initial phase of therapy. As cromolyn sodium begins to work, the need for these medications should decrease.

Ipratropium nasal spray is an anticholinergic agent that exhibits antisecretory properties when applied locally. It provides symptomatic relief of rhinorrhea associated with allergic rhinitis. The 0.03% solution is given as two sprays (42 μg) two to three times daily. The optimal dose should be determined based on the specific patient's symptoms and response. Adverse effects are mild, with the most common being headache, nosebleeds, and nasal dryness.

IMMUNOTHERAPY

The first report of the successful use of grass pollen extract injections to treat allergic rhinitis was published in 1911 by Noon.[39] The therapy was first called *desensitization;* however, this did not seem appropriate because skin reactivity remained. The name was later changed to *hyposensitization*. While this term is still used today, *immunotherapy* is used more commonly.

Immunotherapy is the slow, gradual process of injecting increasing doses of antigens responsible for eliciting allergic symptoms in a patient with the hope of increasing tolerance to the allergen when natural exposure occurs. Several immunologic changes have been documented resulting from immunotherapy that likely result in its effectiveness[40]: diminished IgE production, increased IgG production, changes in T-lymphocytes, reduced inflammatory mediator release from sensitized cells, and diminished tissue responsiveness.

Immunotherapy is expensive, has significant potential risks, and requires a major time commitment from the patient. For these reasons, it should be considered only in a select group of patients. Candidates for immunotherapy should have a strong history of severe symptoms unsuccessfully controlled by avoidance and pharmacotherapy. Patients who have been unable to tolerate the adverse effects of properly managed drug therapy also should be considered. Patients must be committed to the necessary regular office visits required to complete this long course of therapy.

The selection of antigens should be based on patient history and skin test results. Numerous régimens for administration of selected allergens have been suggested. In general, very dilute solutions are given one to two times per week. The concentration is increased until the maximum tolerated dose is achieved. This maintenance dose is continued every 2 to 6 weeks, depending on clinical response. Best results usually are obtained when injections are given year round rather than seasonally.

Adverse reactions can occur with immunotherapy and range from mild to life-threatening. Among the most common are mild local reactions, consisting of induration and swelling at the site of the injection. Other more serious reactions (e.g., generalized urticaria, bronchospasm, laryngospasm, vascular collapse) occur rarely; deaths can result from anaphylactic reactions. Severe reactions are treated with epinephrine, antihistamines, and systemic corticosteroids.

Several patient types have been identified as poor candidates for immunotherapy, including: patients with any medical condition that would compromise the ability to tolerate an anaphylactic-type reaction, patients with impaired immune systems, and patients with a history of nonadherence to therapy.[40]

PHARMACOECONOMIC CONSIDERATIONS

The economic impact of allergic rhinitis is enormous. When looking at both prescription and nonprescription drug expenditures, the estimated annual medication cost in the United States is $2.3 billion ($56 for prescription drugs and $56 for OTC drugs per patient per year).[41] Because the majority of these patients visited a physician, an additional $1.1 billion must be added to account for physician billing. Indirect costs related to missed school or workdays and loss of productivity may approach the amount for the direct costs.[42]

The most cost-effective choice will be an individualized decision. Seasonal allergic rhinitis patients who see improvement and can tolerate OTC and/or generic antihistamines will experience the least impact on out-of-pocket medical and drug expenses. If these are not effective, the economic picture becomes more complicated. Choices should follow the logical path based on symptoms, tolerance, and efficacy, as described earlier in this chapter.

EVALUATION OF THERAPEUTIC OUTCOMES

With allergic rhinitis, the major outcomes issues include the effect of the disease on a patient's life, the efficacy and tolerability of treatment, and patient satisfaction. Consideration must be given to how the condition is affecting the patient's job or school performance, family and social interactions, and other aspects of quality of life. The drug therapy should prevent or minimize symptoms with minimal or no side effects. The patient should not have difficulty obtaining needed medication for financial or other reasons. Patients should be questioned about their satisfaction with the management of their allergic rhinitis. The management should result in minimal disruption to their lives.

Both the Medical Outcomes Study 36-Item Short Form Health Survey (SF-36) and the Rhinoconjunctivitis Quality of Life Questionnaire have been used to evaluate outcomes of treatment for seasonal and perennial allergic rhinitis.[43–45] These tools go beyond measuring improvement in symptoms and include such items as sleep quality, nonallergic symptoms (e.g., fatigue, poor concentration, and others), emotions, and participation in a variety of activities. How well each of the current treatment modalities performs and how they compare in improving patient outcomes remain to be determined.

Currently, the therapeutic goal for patients with allergic rhinitis is to minimize or prevent symptoms. Evaluation of success is accomplished primarily through the discussions with the patient in which both relief of symptoms and tolerance of drug therapy must be discussed.

▶ PRINCIPLES OF PHARMACOTHERAPY

- Allergic rhinitis is one of the most common diseases in people. Treatment is justified in most cases because of the potential for complications.
- In allergic rhinitis, patients must be thoroughly knowledgeable about the proper timing and administration of prophylactic regimens.
- If the patient cannot tolerate or is unable to remain compliant with the chosen drug regimen, alternatives should be discussed and mutually selected.
- Therapeutic modalities include avoidance of allergens and pharmacologic management with antihistamines, topical and systemic decongestants, topical steroids, cromolyn sodium, and immunotherapy.
- Patient counseling regarding the proper selection and use of an available drug therapy is crucial to successful management of allergic rhinitis.
- The pharmaceutical care plan for the allergic rhinitis patient would include the following:
  - Develop a professional relationship with the patient so that he or she sees the pharmacist as a major resource in the treatment of their allergic rhinitis.
  - Take responsibility to identify, resolve, and prevent any of the drug-related problems related to the patient's care.
  - Participate in physical assessment of the patient's symptoms and triage patients when necessary.
  - Discuss and agree on therapeutic end points for allergic rhinitis, including the patient's acceptable level of symptom relief, onset of symptom relief expectations, and seasonal starts and stops.

- Discuss adverse drug reaction self-monitoring and prevention based on treatment selection.
- Assess patient attitude toward adherence to and persistence with oral, ocular, intranasal, or immunologic therapies.
- Ensure proper match of treatment to symptoms and intervene with prescriber if necessary.
- Conduct seasonal or annual review with patient.
- Establish positive relationship with prescribers to ensure that they understand your role in the care of the allergic rhinitis patient.

REFERENCES

1. Spector SL. Supplement: New insights into allergic rhinitis: Quality of life, associated airway diseases, and antihistamine potency. Overview of comorbid associations of allergic rhinitis. J Allergy Clin Immunol 1997;99(2):S773–780.
2. Naclerio R. Allergic rhinitis. N Engl J Med 1991;325:860–869.
3. Juniper E, Guyatt G, Andersson B, Ferrie P. Comparison of powder and aerosolized budesonide in perennial rhinitis: Validation of rhinitis quality of life questionaire. Ann Allergy 1993;70:225–230.
4. Weeke E. Epidemiology of allergic diseases in children. Rhinology 1992; 13(Suppl):5–12.
5. Sibbald B, Rink E. Epidemiology of seasonal and perennial rhinitis: Clinical presentation and medical history. Thorax 1991;46:895–901.
6. Evans R. Epidemiology and natural history of asthma, allergic rhinitis, and atopic dermatitis. In: Middleton E Jr, Reed CE, Ellis EF, et al., eds. Allergy: Principles and Practice, 4th ed. St. Louis, Mosby–Year Book, 1993: 1109–1136.
7. Crimi P, Boidi M, Minale P, et al. Differences in prevalence of allergic sensitization in urban and rural school children. Ann Allergy Asthma Immunnol. 1999;83:252–256.
8. Gomez E, Corrado O, Baldwin D, et al. Direct in vivo evidence for mast cell degranulation during allergen-induced reactions in man. J Allergy Clin Immunol 1986;78:637–645.
9. Naclerio R, Togias A. The nasal allergic reaction: Observations on the role of histamine. Clin Exp Allergy 1991;21(Suppl 2):13–19.
10. Raphael G, Baraniuk J, Kaliner M. How and why the nose runs. J Allergy Clin Immunol 1991;87:457–467.
11. White M, Kaliner M. Mediators of allergic rhinitis. J Allergy Clin Immunol 1992;90:699–704.
12. Bradding P, Iain H, Wilson S, et al. Immunolocalization of cytokines in the nasal mucosa of normal and perennial rhinitic subjects. J Immunol 1993;151:3853–3865.
13. Mygind N. Glucocorticosteroids and rhinitis. Allergy 1993;48:476–490.
14. Clark RR, Baroody FM. What drives the symptoms of allergic rhinitis? J Respir Dis 1998;19:S6–15.
15. Romero J, Scadding G. Eosinophilia in nasal secretions compared to skin prick and nasal challenge in the diagnosis of nasal allergy. Rhinology 1992;30:169–175.
16. Kalliner M, Lemanske R. Rhinitis and asthma. JAMA 1992;268:2807–2829.
17. Turkeltaub P. Skin testing. In: Creticos PS, ed. Immunotherapy: A Practical Guide to Current Procedures, Vol. 2. Milwaukee, American Academy of Allergy and Immunology, 1994: 2–11.
18. Turkeltaub P. Standardized extracts in practice. In: Creticos PS, ed. Immunotherapy: A Practical Guide to Current Procedures, Vol. 4. Milwaukee, American Academy of Allergy and Immunology, 1994. 4.
19. Badhwar A, Druce H. Allergic rhinitis. Med Clin North Am 1992;76: 789–803.
20. International rhinitis management working group. International consensus report on the diagnosis and management of rhinitis. Allergy 1994;49:1–34.
21. Cowart B, Flynn-Rodden K, McGeady S, Lowry L. Hyposmia in allergic rhinitis. J Allergy Clin Immunol 1993;91:747–751.
22. Apter A, Mott A, Cain W, et al. Olfactory loss and allergic rhinitis (clinical conference). J Allergy Clin Immunol 1992;90:670–680.
23. Ziering RW, Klein GI. Allergic rhinitis: Measures to control the misery. Postgrad Med 1992;91:225–232.
24. Nuss R, Berman S. Medical management of persistent middle ear effusion. Am J Asthma Allergy Pediatr 1990;4:17–22.
25. Trask G, Shapiro G, Shapiro P. The effects of perennial allergic rhinitis on dental and skeletal development: A comparison of sibling pairs. Am J Orthodont Dentofac Orthoped 1987;92:286–293.
26. Shapiro G, Shapiro P. Nasal airway obstruction and facial development. Clin Rev Allergy 1984;2:225–236.
27. Verdiani P, Di CS, Baronti A. Different prevalence and degree of nonspecific bronchial hyperreactivity between seasonal and perennial rhinitis. J Allergy Clin Immunol 1990;86:576–582.
28. Ferguson BJ. Allergic rhinitis: Recognizing signs, symptoms and triggering allergens. Postgrad Med 1997;101:110–116.
29. Colloff M, Ayres J, Carswell F, et al. The control of allergens of dust mites and domestic pets: A position paper. Clin Exp Allergy 1992;22 (Suppl 2):1–28.
30. Sporik S, Holgate S, Platts-Mills T. Exposure to house dust mite allergen and the development of asthma in childhood: A prospective study. N Engl J Med 1990;323:502.
31. Reisman R, Mauriello P, Davis G, et al. A double-blind study of the effectiveness of a high efficiency particulate air (HEPA) filter in the treatment of patients with perennial allergic rhinitis and asthma. J Allergy Clin Immunol 1990;85:1050–1057.
32. Simons FE, Simons KJ. The pharmacology and use of H_1-receptor antagonist drugs. N Engl J Med 1994;330:1663–1670.
33. Astelin product information. Wallace Laboratories, Cranbury, NJ, 1997.
34. Empey DE, Young GA, Letley E, et al. Dose response study of the nasal decongestant and cardiovascular effects of pseudoephedrine. Br J Clin Pharmacol 1980;9:351–358.
35. Drew CDM, Knight GT, Hughes DTD, et al. Comparison of the effects of D-(−)-ephedrine and L-(+)-pseudoephedrine on the cardiovascular and respiratory systems in man. Br J Clin Pharmacol 1978;6: 221–225.
36. Drug interaction facts. In: Tatro DS, ed. Facts and Comparisons. Facts and Comparisons, St. Louis, 1999.679.
37. International Rhinitis Management Working Group. International consensus report on the diagnosis and management of rhinitis. Allergy 1994;49(Suppl 19):1–34.
38. Quintiliani R. Hypersensitivity and adverse reactions associated with the use of newer intranasal corticosteroids for allergic rhinitis. Curr Ther Res 1996;57:478–488.
39. Noon L. Prophylactic inoculation against hayfever. Lancet 1911;1:1572–1573.
40. Schoenwetter WF. Safe allergen immunotherapy. Postgrad Med 1996; 100:123–135.
41. Storms W, Meltzer EO, Nathan RA, Selner JC. The economic impact of allergic rhinitis. J Allergy Clin Immunol 1997;99:S820–S824.
42. Rossoff LJ, Stempel DA, Alam R, et al. The health and economic impact of allergic rhinitis. Am J Manage Care 1997;3:S8–S18.
43. Bousquet J, Duchateau J, Pignat JC, et al. Improvement of quality of life by treatment with cetirizine in patients with perennial allergic rhinitis as determined by a French version of the SF-36 questionnaire. J Allergy Clin Immunol 1996;98:309–316.
44. Meltzer EO, Nathan RA, Selner JC, Storms W. Quality of life and rhinitic symptoms: Results of a nationwide survey with the SF-36 and RQLQ questionnaires. J Allergy Clin Immunol 1997;99:S815–S819.
45. Harvey RP, Comer C, Sanders B, et al. Model for outcomes assessment of antihistamine use for seasonal allergic rhinitis. J Allergy Clin Immunol 1996;97:1233–1241.

[illegible] Cancer [illegible] Charles [illegible]

[illegible]

- [illegible] a [illegible] or [illegible] diagnostic tool.
- [illegible] toward adherence to and persistence [illegible] contribute to [illegible] symptoms and [illegible] years.
- [illegible] to improve [illegible] prescriptions to optimize [illegible] in the care of [illegible]

[illegible]

[illegible]
[illegible] 2000;[illegible]
Marcus [illegible] (1993) [illegible] in [illegible] 1993 [illegible] 236–240
[illegible]
[illegible] 1993;[illegible] 293–298.
8. [illegible]

96

ACNE AND PSORIASIS

Nital M. Patel, Silvia S. Elias, and Nina H. Cheigh

Nearly 2000 different skin disorders are readily visible and brought to the attention of health care practitioners daily. Patients may be screened to identify dermatologic disorders, identify drug-induced causes of dermatoses, initiate drug therapy (considering vehicle and active ingredients), and monitor for therapeutic effect, adverse reactions, and patient compliance. Some references for nondermatologists are *Primary Care Dermatology*[1] and *Color Atlas and Synopsis of Clinical Dermatology*.[2]

The clinical approach to solving dermatologic problems involves analysis, assessment, and establishment and initiation of a treatment plan followed by careful drug monitoring (Table 96–1). This algorithm is similar to problem-solving approaches in other specialties, but major differences include the development of an objective database by physical examination of lesions on the integument and mucous membranes as well as description of the dermatoses in specific, brief, concise, and uniform terminology. Important aspects of the physical examination of skin and definitions of lesion types are presented. This is designed to assist in identification of common dermatologic disorders and appropriate treatment regimens. Examination of the skin should include observations on color and consistency of lesions, anatomic localization and distribution, configuration, size, border, and other superficial characteristics.

LESION CHARACTERISTICS

COLOR

Lesion color, attributed to a variety of causes, is of major diagnostic importance. The consistency of color also should be noted. Some lesions have consistent color throughout, whereas others may vary in color from the border to an area of central clearing or may demonstrate multiple colors and hues (Table 96–2).

DISTRIBUTION

Distribution of lesions may be helpful in determining a diagnosis (Figs. 96–1 and 96–2). Lesions may be localized to an anatomic area or generalized over the body surface. Lesions limited to specific anatomic regions such as light-exposed areas or body-fold areas (intertriginous) should be differentiated.

CONFIGURATION

Configuration is also essential to diagnosis and may be defined as the relationship of one lesion to another or how lesions are grouped (Table 96–3). Lesion size can be approximated in centimeters or using familiar objects (e.g., 5 cm or the size of a dime); borders should be categorized as demarcated (sharply circumscribed) or diffuse (ill defined). Superficial characteristics such as elevations or depressions in skin, changes in texture, presence of moisture or dried exudate, and firmness also should be noted. Usually, the characteristics of a lesion are communicated in a few singular terms describing the morphologic type of lesion. Description of lesion type, along with color, distribution, size, and configuration, is the most accepted method of communicating what is noted by physical assessment. Use of uniform terminology aids in diagnosis and allows others to visualize the lesions.

ACNE

Acne vulgaris, the most common skin disease, affects 80% of the population between the ages of 12 and 25 years.[3] Although acne is generally self-limiting, it can persist for years and can result in disfigurement and scarring and have profound psychological effects on patients.[3–6] It is important for the health care professional to play a major role in educating patients on causes of acne, recommending treatment regimens, and counseling on proper medication use.

DIAGNOSIS

Generally, the diagnosis of acne vulgaris consists of a finding that includes a mixture of lesions of acne (e.g., comedones, pustules, papules, nodules, and cysts) on the face, back, or chest. Although there is no precise definition for acne, most practitioners consider the presence of 5 to 10 comedones to be diagnostic. Other dermatologic conditions, such as folliculitis, acne rosacea, and other various acneform disorders, sometimes may be confused with acne vulgaris.

CLINICAL MANIFESTATIONS

Acne is found primarily on the face and, to a lesser degree, on the upper back, chest, and shoulders. Lesions can vary morphologically and are classified primarily as either inflammatory or noninflammatory. The clinical presentation of acne can range from a mild comedonal form to severe inflammatory necrotic acne of the face, chest, and back. Formation of the primary lesion, the comedo, may be thought of simplistically as plugging of the pilosebaceous follicle. In acne, the follicular canal widens, and an increase in cell production is seen.[3] Sebum mixes with excess loose cells in the follicular canal to form a keratinous plug. The resulting lesion appears as a "blackhead," or open comedo. The brown or black color is not a result of dirt accumulation but that of melanin.[3] Inflammation or trauma to the follicle may lead to formation of a whitehead," or closed comedo. If the follicular wall is damaged or ruptured, the contents of the follicle may extrude into

TABLE 96–1. An Approach to Solving the Dermatologic Problems of Patients

Knowledge Base	Action	Patient Database
Dermatologic manifestations	Analyze the problem	Subjective data Objective data
Therapeutic end points Risk versus benefit Pharmaceutic and pharmacokinetic considerations Drug/disease/lab interactions	Assess the problem Establish optimal treatment plan for the patient	
Monitoring parameters	Monitor the patient Therapeutic effect Adverse effects Compliance	

TABLE 96–2. Examples of Lesional Color Variation

Lesion Description	Color	Pathophysiologic Mechanism	Precipitating Factor(s)
Hyperpigmented	Darkened areas	Melanin deposition	Pregnancy, sunlight, oral contraceptives
Hypopigmented	Lightened	Lack of melanin	Autoimmune phenomena
Jaundiced	Yellowish	Increased bilirubin or carotene	Hepatitis
Cyanotic	Bluish	Excess reduced hemoglobin	Hypoxia
	Reddish blue	Capillary stasis	Increased red blood cells
Erythematous	Red	Dilation of blood vessels	Inflammation, sunburn
Violaceous	Purple	Aging lesion, formerly erythematous	Bruising trauma

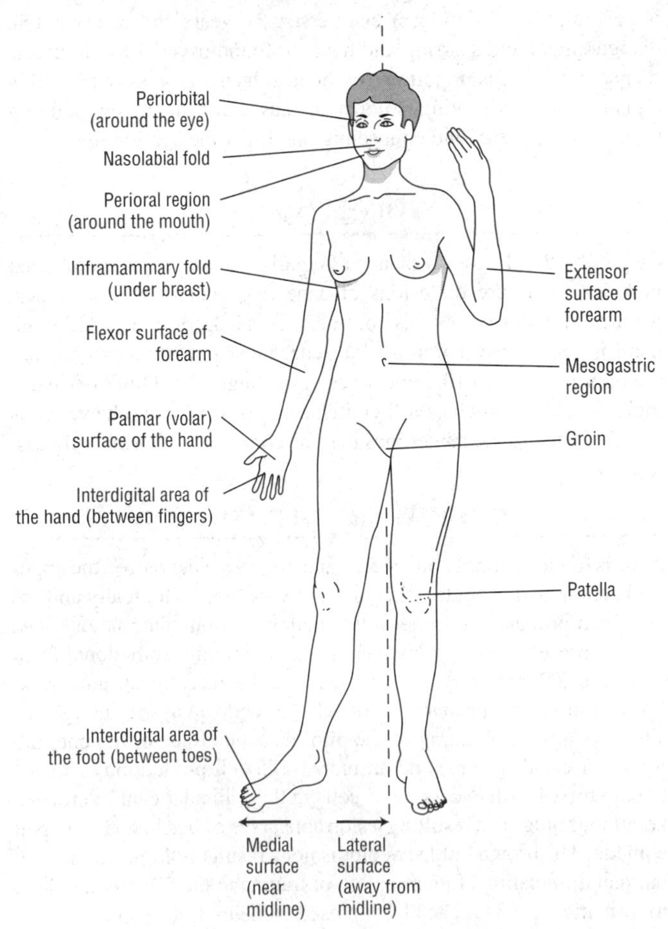

FIGURE 96–1. Anterior (ventral) surfaces of the body.

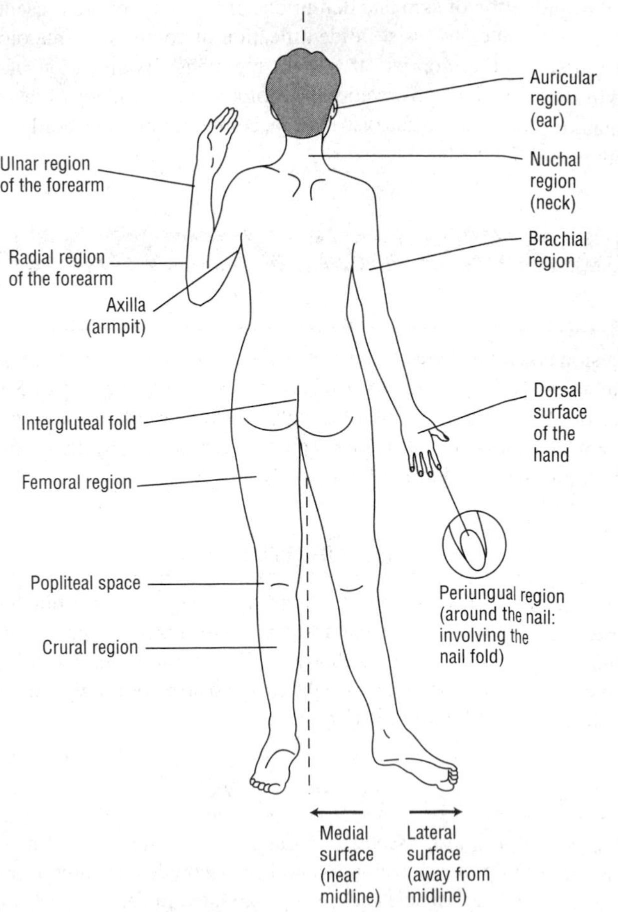

FIGURE 96–2. Posterior (dorsal) surfaces of the body.

TABLE 96–3. Examples of Lesional Configuration

Type	Description
Clustered	Grouped lesions
Linear	Straight line
Annular	Circular
Polycyclic	Two or more adjacent, circular lesions
Serpiginous	Snake-like with wavy borders
Geographic	Irregular map-like borders

dermis and present clinically as a pustule. Closed comedones are of clinical importance because they may presage larger, inflammatory lesions.[3]

Acne lesions may take months to heal completely, and fibrosis associated with healing may lead to permanent scarring. Most forms of adolescent acne are self-limiting, but more severe forms may be persistent and require aggressive treatment.

PATHOPHYSIOLOGY

Although an exact cause of acne is unknown, the pathogenesis of acne is multifactorial, and thus treatment is directed at these factors (Table 96–4). Pathogenic theories of acne development include the roles of androgens, sebum production, *Propionibacterium acnes,* and follicle growth.[3,5,6] Sebaceous glands, normally found on the face, chest, back, and shoulders, develop at puberty in response to androgen stimulation. Sebum produced in these glands is transported through ducts to the canal and onto the surface of the skin. The follicular canal also contains fine vellus hair, keratinous material, and bacteria (primarily *P. acnes*). Acne formation is believed to be caused by a derangement in the structure or function of normal sebaceous follicles (Fig. 96–3).

ANDROGENS

Increased androgen activity at puberty triggers growth of sebaceous glands and enhanced production of sebum. Although testosterone is the most potent androgen, its metabolites and weaker androgens (e.g., androstenedione, dehydroepiandrosterone, and dehydroepiandrosterone sulfate) are increased in acne patients and also may stimulate sebaceous gland activity.[3] Skin, hair follicles, and sebaceous glands

TABLE 96–4. Major Pathophysiologic Features of Acne and Responsive Pharmacotherapeutic Agents

Feature	Systemic Drug	Topical Drug
Sebum production/ secretion	Estrogens Antiandrogens Spironolactone Isotretinoin	None established
Abnormal desquamation of follicular epithelium	Isotretinoin Antibiotics	Tretinoin Salicylic acid Adapalene Tazarotene
Propionibacterium acnes proliferation	Tetracycline Minocycline Doxycycline Erythromycin Clindamycin Cotrimoxazole Isotretinoin	Erythromycin Clindamycin Benzoyl peroxide Azelaic acid Dapsone
Inflammation	Corticosteroids Isotretinoin Nonsteroidal anti-inflammatory agents	Metronidazole Intralesional corticosteroids Sulfur Adapalene Azelaic acid Dapsone

metabolize androgens to active dihydrotestosterone, and acne-prone areas of skin demonstrate increased metabolic activity.[3]

SEBUM PRODUCTION

Sebum is produced in the sebaceous glands and consists of glycerides, wax esters, squalene, and cholesterol. The glyceride component of sebum is converted to free fatty acids and glycerol by lipases, products of *P. acnes.*[3] Free fatty acids may irritate the follicular wall and cause increased cell turnover and inflammation. Recently, glycerol has been identified as a substrate for *P. acnes,* whereas free fatty acids may function as a measure of *P. acnes* activity and viability.[3] Although patients with acne have been shown to have increased sebum production, there is variation among patients with acne, indicating that this disease is not solely related to sebaceous gland activity.[3]

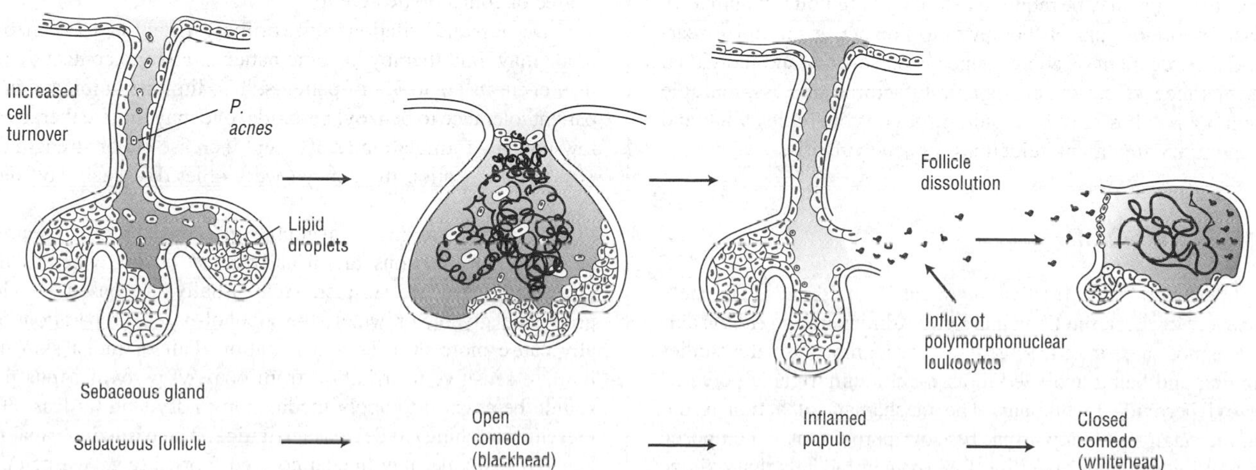

FIGURE 96–3. Cross-sectional view of the sebaceous follicle.

FOLLICLE ACTIVITY

The primary change in acne is an alteration in the pattern of keratinization within the follicle. Abnormal alterations in the follicle wall and its cell growth have been noted histologically in association with acne.[3] Increased production of loosely adherent keratin cells has been correlated with obstruction of the follicles seen in comedo formation. It is unknown whether this abnormality is inherent or secondary to irritation and other factors.

BACTERIA

P. acnes, a resident anaerobic organism, proliferates in the environment created by the mixture of excessive sebum and follicular cells and may lead to inflammation.[3] Although *P. acnes* counts typically are higher in patients with acne, the pathogenic role of this organism is not that of a simple infection. *P. acnes* may be considered antigenic and capable of causing increased antibody formation (IgG and IgM), leading to an inflammatory response.[3] Immune-complex-mediated complement activation as a result of *P. acnes* may lead to vascular leakage, mast cell degranulation, and leukocyte chemotaxis.[8] Levels of antibodies to *P. acnes* are higher in patients with severe forms of acne than in normal controls. *P. acnes* may activate the complement cascade via both classic and alternate pathways and produce direct tissue damage.[3] Also, chemotactic factors may be secreted by *P. acnes,* diffuse through the follicle wall, and activate neutrophil chemotaxis and complement. Hydrolytic enzymes released by complement activation may damage the follicle wall and lead to more severe, inflammatory acne. Neutrophils are an important factor in severe inflammatory acne, and patients may demonstrate neutrophil defects of either very high or low chemotaxis as well as impaired phagocytosis. *P. acnes* also may evoke a cell-medicated immune response.[3] Although the exact cause of acne is unclear, its pathogenesis involves various factors that are apparently interrelated (Fig. 96–4).

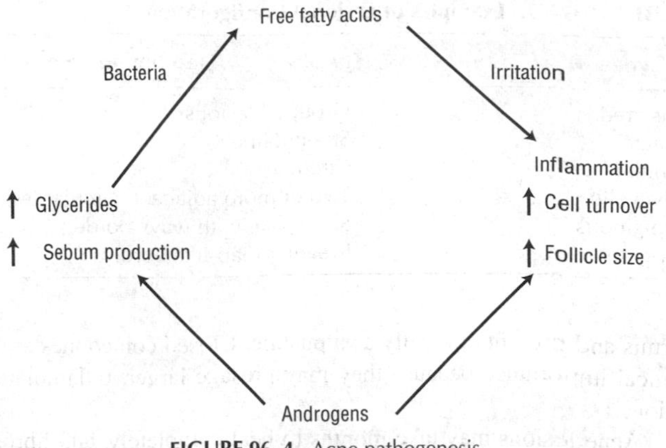

FIGURE 96–4. Acne pathogenesis.

PATIENT ASSESSMENT

In assessing a patient with acne, an indepth drug and medical history should be obtained to determine if there are any exacerbating factors that can be eliminated (Table 96–5).

TABLE 96–5. Examples of Components to Patient History for Acne

Onset and duration of acne	All current and recent topical and systemic medications
Family history	All topical products such as soaps, moisturizers, astringents, and cosmetics
Exacerbating factors	Environmental and occupational exposures to chemicals and toxins
Previous history of antiacne agents with efficacy and adverse effect data	Allergies (food, drug, environmental)

▶ TREATMENT: Acne Vulgaris

TOPICAL PHARMACOLOGIC THERAPY

Aggressive therapy may be required to modify or inhibit inflammatory acne. An important goal of therapy is to prevent or minimize scarring, and the treatment of choice depends on severity and individual patient tolerance. Because acne is a multifactorial process, multiple treatment approaches may be required for control. Tables 96–6 and 96–7 summarize treatment guidelines for acne vulgaris.

BENZOYL PEROXIDE

Benzoyl peroxide is an effective treatment for mild and moderately severe acne. However, the Food and Drug Administration (FDA) currently does not categorize it as generally recognized as safe; studies are ongoing and being analyzed to assess the tumorigenic potential of benzoyl peroxide in humans. The mechanism of action is uncertain, although it is known that benzoyl peroxide is decomposed on the skin by cysteine, liberating free oxygen radicals that oxidize bacterial proteins.[8] Daily application of 10% benzoyl peroxide for 2 weeks can reduce free fatty acid levels by 50% and *P. acnes* levels by 98%.[8] Benzoyl peroxide increases the sloughing rate of epithelial cells, loosens the follicular plug structure, and thus possesses some degree of comedolytic activity.[9]

Dryness and irritation from a primary irritant such as benzoyl peroxide may limit therapy in some patients; allergic contact dermatitis may occur in 1% to 3% of patients.[10] To limit irritation and increase patient tolerance to benzoyl peroxide, one may initiate therapy with a low-potency formulation (2.5%) and increase either strength (5% to 10%) or application frequency (every other day, each day, and then twice a day).

Benzoyl peroxide is available in soaps, lotions, creams, and gels. Gel formulations are usually most potent, whereas the lotions and soaps are weaker. Gels usually are based on alcohol, propylene glycol, or water; the alcohol-based preparations generally cause more dryness and irritation. Fair or moist skin usually is more sensitive to irritation from benzoyl peroxide; thus patients should be advised to apply medication to dry skin (at least 30 minutes after washing) to decrease irritation. The oxidizing capability of benzoyl peroxide may bleach colored fabrics (e.g., washcloths and pillowcases).

TABLE 96–6. Topical Acne Treatment Guidelines

Active Ingredient	Formulation	Strength (%)	Regimen	Potential Side Effects
Benzoyl peroxide	Soaps, lotions creams, gels	2.5–10	Initially every other day, or daily, then twice daily	Irritation based on form/strength Bleaching/staining of clothing
Tretinoin	Creams, gels, solution, microsphere gel, liquid polymer	0.025–0.05	Initially every other day or daily	Moderate erythema, burning, stinging, pruritus Concomitant use of other irritants increases likelihood of undue irritation
Sulfur/resorcinol/ salicylic acid	Creams, lotions, gels, soaps	0.5–10 in various combinations	Daily	
Clindamycin	Solution, gel, lotion	1	Twice daily	Drying, gastrointestinal effects (Pseudomembranous colitis)
Tetracycline	Solution	2.2	Twice daily	Burning and stinging following application, skin discoloration
Erythromycin	Solution, powder, gel	1.5–2	Twice daily	Drying, erythema
Adapalene	Gel, lotion, cream, solution	0.03–0.1	Daily	Moderate erythema, drying, stinging, burning, pruritus
Azelaic acid	Cream	20	Twice daily	Mild, transient, local erythema, burning, pruritus
Tazarotene	Gel, Cream	0.1	Daily or twice daily	Moderate erythema, burning, stinging, pruritus

SULFUR, RESORCINOL, AND SALICYLIC ACID

Sulfur, resorcinol, and salicylic acid are keratolytic and mildly antibacterial. The term *keratolytic* refers to the effect of solubilization of the intracellular cement of keratin cells in the stratum corneum. Although evidence for efficacy in the treatment of acne is conflicting, each agent has been classified as safe and effective by an advisory review panel of the FDA. Combinations of these agents often are considered synergistic (e.g., sulfur and resorcinol, salicylic acid and benzoyl peroxide). Keratolytic products, in the concentration allowed, may be less irritating than benzoyl peroxide and tretinoin; however, they are not considered effective comedolytic agents, as are benzoyl peroxide and tretinoin. Disadvantages of these agents include the odor created by hydrogen sulfide on reaction of sulfur with the skin, the brown scale from use of resorcinol, and the remote possibility of salicylism from repeated use of sufficient concentrations of salicylic acid on highly permeable (inflamed and/or abraded) skin.

TOPICAL ANTIBACTERIAL PRODUCTS

Topical antibacterials other than benzoyl peroxide and salicylic acid (e.g., clindamycin, erythromycin, and tetracycline) have been used effectively to treat acne by concentrating local antimicrobial activity

TABLE 96–7. Oral Acne Treatment Guidelines

Active Ingredient	Formulation	Strength (mg)	Regimen	Potential Side Effects
Tetracycline	Tablets, capsules	250–500	1 g/day initially, if no response in 2–3 weeks or severe acne, 2–3 g/day Maintenance 125–500 mg/day	Gastrointestinal upset, photoreactivity, drug and food interactions
Minocycline	Tablets, capsules, suspension	50–100	100 mg twice daily	CNS effects (dizziness, drowsiness) Discoloration of skin
Doxycycline	Tablets, capsules, suspension, syrup	50–100	50–100 mg twice daily	Discoloration, gastrointestinal upset (esophagitis), photoreactivity
Erythromycin	Tablets as various salts	250–500	1 g/day as base, if no response in 2–3 weeks or severe acne, 2–3 g/day. Maintenance 250–500 mg/day	Gastrointestinal upset, cutaneous reactions, drug interactions
Clindamycin	Capsules	75, 150, 300	300–450 mg/day	Diarrhea, pseudomembranous colitis
Isotretinoin	Capsules	10, 20, 40	0.5–1 mg/kg/day in two divided doses Maximum of 2 mg/kg/day	Cheilitis, erythema, dryness, gastrointestinal effects, teratogenicity

in the skin and subsequently decreasing the risk of systemic toxicity. Many clinical trials that compare the efficacy of topical versus systemic antibacterials are difficult to evaluate because formulations may have been prepared extemporaneously or different vehicles were used.[11,12]

Although it does not necessarily correlate with clinical response, inhibition of *P. acnes* is accomplished most effectively by clindamycin. In one study, in vivo topical clindamycin significantly reduced the numbers of *P. acnes,* whereas topical erythromycin and tetracycline did not.[13] Reduction of the percentage of free fatty acids in sebum has been noted with the use of topical tetracycline and erythromycin.[13]

A topical preparation of erythromycin plus zinc has been reported to be significantly better than 500 mg/d oral tetracycline in reducing overall acne severity and papule lesion counts.[14] In a randomized, double-blind study of 122 patients with acne vulgaris, a 4% erythromycin and zinc combination lotion was more effective than 2% erythromycin lotion. The higher concentration of erythromycin may have been more effective, or the zinc acetate complex may have enhanced the penetration of erythromycin into the pilosebaceous unit.[15]

Disadvantages of topical antibiotic dosage forms include occasional irritation and stinging on application. Although tetracyclines are the most frequently prescribed oral antibiotics for acne, they are not frequently prescribed topical antibiotics. On the skin, tetracycline photoxidizes to produce a visible yellow tinting.[13] Though rare, diarrhea and pseudomembranous colitis may occur from the use of topical clindamycin.[16,17] Antimicrobial resistance from widespread use of topical antibiotics for acne has been postulated but not substantiated as a clinically significant problem.[13]

AZELAIC ACID

Azelaic acid is a naturally occurring substance that interferes with DNA synthesis in some of the bacteria associated with acne vulgaris.[18] Inhibition of thioredoxin reductase by azelaic acid provides a rationale for this property.[19] Azelaic acid also demonstrates a potential anti-inflammatory role. In a series of investigations using 20% azelaic acid cream as a therapy for acne, it was found that the treatment, compared with vehicle, significantly reduced inflammatory lesions at 1 month and noninflammatory lesions at 2 months.[20] In an open study of 100 unselected patients of either gender, the attained rates of improvement indicate that topical 20% azelaic acid cream can be considered an effective therapy.[21] Although uncommon, mild transient erythema, burning, and pruritus are the most frequently reported side effects. Azelaic acid is not a primary irritant and is generally well tolerated by acne patients. It is distinct, in that it is antibacterial, has comedolytic activity, and is not a primary irritant. Because of its combined activity, topical azelaic acid offers a twice-daily cost-effective single-product option for the treatment of mild to moderate acne.

TRETINOIN

Tretinoin, a topical vitamin A analog, is a comedolytic agent that increases cell turnover in the follicular wall and decreases cohesiveness of cells, leading to extrusion of existing comedones and inhibition of the formation of new comedones.[22] Tretinoin also decreases the number of cell layers in the stratum corneum from 14 to 5.[8] A "flare" of acne may appear suddenly after initiation of treatment, followed by clinical clearing in about 8 to 12 weeks.[8] Irritation, erythema, and peeling often limit successful therapy, and allergic contact dermatitis has been reported in a few patients, although not as frequently as with benzoyl peroxide.[22] Tolerance to irritation may be managed by titrating strength and frequency of application. Tretinoin is currently available in 0.05% solution (most irritating), 0.01% and 0.025% gels, and 0.025%, 0.05%, and 0.1% creams (least irritating). Treatment initiation with 0.025% cream usually is recommended for mild acne in people with easily irritated and nonoily skin, 0.01% gel for moderate acne in easily irritated skin with oily complexion, and 0.025% gel for moderate acne with nonsensitive and oily skin. Two newer reformulations of tretinoin, Retin-A Micro and Avita, have been introduced. Although Retin-A Micro contains a microsphere vehicle consisting of porous beads, Avita contains a liquid-polymer vehicle. These newer reformulations are less irritating than standard vehicles for tretinoin.

Once control is established, therapy should be continued at the lowest effective concentration and at the maximum effective interval sufficient to minimize acne exacerbations.[23] Concomitant use of an antibacterial agent with tretinoin can decrease keratinization, inhibit *P. acnes,* and decrease inflammation. In addition, both benzoyl peroxide and tretinoin have shown additive or synergistic effects in the treatment of inflammatory acne.[23,24] A combination of benzoyl peroxide each morning and tretinoin at bedtime may enhance efficacy and be less irritating than either agent used alone.[24] When using tretinoin, patients should be advised to apply the medication to dry skin approximately 30 minutes after washing to minimize erythema and irritation. Slowly increasing application frequency from every other day, to daily, and then twice daily may increase tolerance to tretinoin. Increased sensitivity to sun exposure, wind, cold, and other irritants also has been evident in patients using tretinoin.

ADAPALENE

Adapalene, available as 0.1% aqueous gel or as an alcoholic solution, is a retinoid-mimetic compound used for treatment of mild to moderate acne.[5,25] Adapalene has been shown to have selective affinity for retinoic acid receptor (RAR) subtypes RAR-γ and RAR-β found in the epidermis.[5,25] It also has comedolytic and anti-inflammatory effects.[25] Vehicle-controlled and comparative studies have demonstrated the utility of adapalene in the treatment of acne.[25–27] Adapalene 0.1% gel produced a greater reduction in total lesion counts than tretinoin 0.025% gel at week 12, and it was significantly better tolerated, resulting in less erythema, pruritus, burning, stinging, and peeling.[27] Thus adapalene 0.1% gel can be used as an alternative to tretinoin 0.025% gel in patients with mild to moderate acne with better patient tolerability.[26,27]

TAZAROTENE

Tazarotene, a prodrug, is a synthetic acetylenic retinoid that is converted to an active metabolite, tazarotenic acid, following topical application. This new-generation retinoid also selectively binds to RARs and can alter expression of genes involved in cell proliferation, cell differentiation, and inflammation.[5] Tazarotene 0.1% and 0.05% gel have been shown to be more effective than vehicle in the treatment of acne vulgaris.[27] The 0.1% gel was slightly more effective than the 0.05% gel in decreasing lesion counts. Dose-related adverse effects included erythema, pruritus, stinging, and burning.[27] Although effective for the treatment of acne, as currently formulated and used, this product is similar to tretinoin gel in its primary irritant effects on the face in the treatment of acne.

DAPSONE

Topical dapsone is in clinical development for acne because it demonstrates both antibacterial and anti-inflammatory activity.

SYSTEMIC PHARMACOLOGIC THERAPY

ORAL ANTIBACTERIAL AGENTS

Few well-controlled, double-blind studies have been conducted on the efficacy of oral antibiotics in acne. Nevertheless, oral antibiotics are considered effective and relatively safe for inflammatory acne.[13,28] Tetracycline (and derivatives), erythromycin, clindamycin, and cotrimoxazole can significantly decrease the percentage of free fatty acids in skin surface lipids and also decrease numbers of *P. acnes.*[13] Tetracycline exhibits additional activity by reducing the amount of keratin in sebaceous follicles and by inhibiting chemotaxis, phagocytosis, complement activation (by the alternate pathway), and cell-mediated immunity.[13] Tetracycline also appears to have an affinity for inflammatory cells and bacteria, resulting in higher drug concentrations in areas of inflamed skin.[13] Drawbacks to the use of tetracycline include a drug-food interaction with dairy products, photosensitivity, gastrointestinal disturbances, hepatotoxicity, and predisposition to superinfections (vaginal candidiasis). In refractory cases, minocycline or doxycycline may be effective because of greater lipid solubility and enhanced penetration into tissue and sebaceous follicles.[29] Minocycline has been used as long-term therapy for acne vulgaris. Disadvantages of minocycline include vestibular toxicity, discoloration of skin and visceral tissues, and drug-induced lupus erythematosus.[29,30]

Clindamycin use for acne is limited by diarrhea and risk of pseudomembranous colitis. Erythromycin has a somewhat safer adverse-effect profile when compared with tetracycline; however, efficacy profiles are similar.[13,31]

Although cotrimoxazole may be effective in tetracycline-resistant acne, it should perhaps be reserved for refractory cases to minimize risk of resistance.[13,32] Another consideration in the use of oral antibiotics for acne is a potential interaction with oral contraceptives. Ampicillin and tetracycline decrease intestinal flora necessary for hydrolysis of conjugated ethinyl estradiol excreted into bile; thus enterohepatic recirculation is interrupted, and active estrogen is reduced.[33] The clinical importance of this interaction is not well established, but several pregnancies have been reported with concurrent use of ampicillin or tetracycline and oral contraceptives.[33] Women taking oral contraceptives (especially agents containing less than 50 μg estrogen) should be informed of the potential for this interaction, especially before initiation of long-term oral antibiotics.[34]

ORAL CONTRACEPTIVES

Androgen levels correlate with sebum production and may affect the development of acne.[35] Based on this evidence, alteration of androgen levels represents a potential hormonal treatment for acne in women.[35] The combination of norgestimate and ethinyl estradiol has been shown to increase sex hormone binding globulin (SHBG), causing a decrease in unbound, biologically active androgens such as free testosterone.[35,37] In January 1997, the FDA approved Ortho Tri-Cyclen for use as antiacne therapy.[7] This triphasic combination oral contraceptive, containing a fixed dose of ethinyl estradiol 0.035 mg and increasing doses of norgestimate 0.180, 0.215, and 0.250 mg, was studied in two multicenter, randomized, double-blind, placebo-controlled trials that concluded that oral contraceptives containing 0.035 mg ethinyl estradiol along with a triphasic dose of norgestimate can be an effective treatment alternative for moderate acne in women.[36,37]

ANTIANDROGENS AND OTHER HORMONAL THERAPIES

Androgen receptor blockers, such as spironolactone, flutamide, and cyproterone acetate, have been studied.[36] The most widely used agent in this group is cyproterone acetate (not available in the United States). Other drugs that can reduce androgen levels include gonadotropin-releasing hormone agonists, 5-α-reductase inhibitors, and corticosteroids.[36]

ISOTRETINOIN

Isotretinoin is a compound that affects most of the etiologic factors involved in inflammatory acne including (1) decreased sebum production and change in sebum composition, (2) inhibition of *P. acnes* growth within follicles, (3) inhibition of inflammation, and (4) altered patterns of keratinization within follicles (decreased size and increased differentiation).[38,39] Oral isotretinoin is indicated for patients with severe recalcitrant nodular or inflammatory acne unresponsive to conventional therapies. In a recent survey of dermatologists, it was concluded that for patients with moderate or mild acne who respond with less than 50% improvement after 6 months of conventional therapies, oral isotretinoin should be considered for therapeutic use.[40] After a 16-week course, isotretinoin produces a greater than 70% success rate followed by a prolonged remission of more than 20 months.[41]

Isotretinoin dosing guidelines range from 0.5 to 1.0 mg/kg per day, but the cumulative dose taken by patients during a treatment course may be the major factor influencing long-term outcome.[42] Optimal results generally have occurred when *cumulative* doses have attained a range of 120 to 150 mg/kg.[42] Although the costs of therapy with isotretinoin are greater in the first year, it has been demonstrated that isotretinoin can be more cost-effective than long-term antibiotic treatment.[43]

Adverse effects from isotretinoin are numerous, frequent, and often dose-related.[44,45] About 90% of patients receiving isotretinoin therapy suffer from mucocutaneous effects. Drying of the mucosae of the mouth, nose, and eyes is the most common problem, with relatively rare involvement of the genitoanal mucosae. Cheilitis and skin desquamation occurs in over 80% of patients receiving therapy. Less frequently, the conjunctiva and nasal mucosa are affected. Systemic side effects mostly involve arthralgias and muscle stiffness, occurring in 15% of patients. These muscle and joint pains, including complaints of backache, may be attributed to catabolic effects on mesenchymal tissues of cartilage, connective tissue, and bone. Disturbances in lipid metabolism also may occur, resulting in hypertriglyceridemia in more than 25% of patients.[42,44,45]

An increase in creatinine phosphokinase and blood glucose, as well as photosensitivity, pseudotumor cerebri, and excess granulation tissue, has occurred during use of isotretinoin.[41] The incidence of teratogenicity after maternal exposure to isotretinoin is high and well documented.[46] Of 16 case reports of adverse pregnancy outcomes in women exposed to isotretinoin, 9 were spontaneous abortions and

7 were babies with major birth defects (i.e., hydrocephalus, small or partially occluded external auditory canals, and cardiac abnormalities). Although five normal pregnancies were reported, the timing of exposure to isotretinoin was uncertain.

EVALUATION OF THERAPEUTIC OUTCOMES

Contrary to popular belief, environmental factors such as diet, lack of appropriate hygiene, certain hairstyles, and early cosmetic use do not necessarily play a role in acne formation.[7] Although various etiologic theories exist, acne is primarily due to an alteration in the pattern of keratinization within the follicle.[3,7] In most patients, therapy should be directed at correcting abnormal follicular keratinization and inhibition of *P. acnes* to control inflammatory acne. Systemic therapy should be reserved for patients who do not respond to topical therapy or who are at risk for scarring. Mild inflammatory acne, which consists of scattered small papules or pustules, tends to develop in teenage and young-adult women. Treatment with once- or twice-daily application of a topical antibacterial in combination with a comedolytic agent is recommended.[3] Agents that combine both activities include azelaic acid and benzoyl peroxide.

In patients with moderate severity (inflammatory lesions on the face and trunk), the combination of a topical comedolytic agent applied once or twice daily with either a topical or a systemic antibiotic is appropriate. A possible alternative for women unresponsive to typical therapies is hormonal therapy with estrogen or an antiandrogen.[3] Patients with nodular lesions and significant scarring potential are candidates for systemic isotretinoin therapy if conventional treatments have failed.

Concepts of therapy should be conveyed to the patient, and the importance of compliance and prevention of new acne activity should be emphasized. Achievement of clinical response by any given therapeutic regimen may require 6 to 8 weeks. Patients also may notice an "exacerbation" of acne after initiation of topical comedolytic therapy. Follicular plugging may take approximately 4 weeks to evolve into an inflammatory lesion; therefore, new follicular plugging should be significantly less likely to occur by 2 months of effective therapy. For topical agents, all acne-prone areas should be treated because the purpose of therapy is to prevent or minimize the formation of new lesions[8] and to minimize the risk of scarring, a permanent end point for moderate to severe disease.

PSORIASIS

Psoriasis is a common chronic disease characterized by recurrent exacerbations and remissions of thickened, erythematous, and scaling plaques. It is universal in occurrence and affects approximately 2% of the U.S. population.[47] This debilitating disease occurs in all racial groups but more frequently in whites. It is equally common in males and females.[48] The mean age of onset is 27 years, with approximately 50% of cases occurring in the most productive years between the ages 20 and 60 years; however, the age of onset is widely variable from infancy to old age.[49] About 80% of patients are affected by the most common form, stable plaque psoriasis, which covers up to 20% of the body surface (mean body surface area of involvement is about 7%).

PATHOPHYSIOLOGY

The exact cause of psoriasis is unknown. A validated, adequate animal model using human skin explants has been developed. In immunodeficient mice, it was established that psoriasis may be caused primarily by immunocytes inducing secondary activation and disordered growth of keratinocytes and vascular endothelium.[50] There are several hypotheses regarding the pathophysiology of psoriasis (Table 96–8).

TABLE 96–8. Pathophysiologic Aspects of Psoriasis

Defects in epidermal cell cycle
Disruption in arachidonic acid metabolism
Genetics
Exogenous trigger factors
Climate
Stress
Infection
Trauma
Drugs
Immunologic mechanisms

DEFECTS IN EPIDERMAL CELL CYCLE

The search for an inherent skin defect as a pathogenic mechanism for psoriasis has provided numerous hypotheses. Psoriatic epidermal cells proliferate at a rate sevenfold faster than normal epidermal cells.[3,51,52] The germinative cell population increases in psoriatic skin, and duration of the cell cycle is calculated at 37.5 hours (versus 300 hours in normal skin).[52] Lesion-free skin in psoriatic patients generally is considered to be involved because epidermal proliferation is elevated in apparently normal skin of psoriatic patients.[53]

DISRUPTION IN ARACHIDONIC ACID METABOLISM

Other abnormalities found in psoriatic skin include evidence of increased metabolic activity and increased cGMP, DNA, RNA, IgG, and C3.[52,53] In psoriatic lesions, arachidonic acid levels are 30 times normal, 12-L-hydroxy-5,8,10,14-eicosatetraenoic acid (HETE) levels are 80 times normal, and prostaglandin E_2 levels are 50% higher than normal. Glucocorticoids normalize levels of arachidonic acid and HETE by inhibition of phospholipase A, and these activities may be partly responsible for regression of psoriatic lesions.[52]

GENETICS

There is a significant genetic component in psoriasis, but the exact mode of inheritance is uncertain.[54] Approximately 36% of patients with psoriasis have at least one immediate relative with the disorder.[49] Monozygotic twins have a higher concordance for psoriasis than do dizygotic twins.[49] Studies of histocompatibility antigens in psoriatic patients indicate statistically significant associations on the B, C, and D loci, more specifically, HLA-B13, HLA-B17, and HLA-B37.[53,55] The most significant association is with HLA-Cw6, where the relative likelihood for developing psoriasis is 9 to 15 times normal. In addition, the HLA-B13 and HLA-B17 loci appear to be linked with the gene that expresses HLA-Cw6.[53]

EXOGENOUS TRIGGER FACTORS

Factors such as climate, stress, infection, trauma, and drugs may aggravate psoriasis. Warm seasons and sunlight reportedly improve psoriasis in 80% of patients, whereas 90% report worsening in cold weather. In addition, stress worsens psoriasis in 30% to 40% of patients; however, the exact role stress plays in exacerbation of psoriasis is uncertain.

Infection has been identified retrospectively as a common precipitating factor in psoriasis. A review of 245 cases of psoriatic children indicates that 25% had initial onset of the disease after clinically documented infections, whereas 54% had exacerbation during a 2- to 3-week interval after an upper respiratory infection.[56] Another study indicates that exacerbation of psoriasis is common 1 to 2 weeks after acute streptococcal infection.[57]

Lesions may occur at the site of injury to normal-appearing skin (Koebner response). The incidence is variable, ranging up to 76% of patients in retrospective studies and 51% in prospective studies.[53] The Koebner response may be induced by a variety of traumatic causes including rubbing, venipuncture, bites, surgery, and pressure. The mechanism for development of the Koebner response is unknown and is not unique to psoriasis. The length of time between injury and lesion development, although variable, is usually a few days to weeks. Lithium carbonate and β-adrenergic-blocking agents are among the most commonly noted drugs to exacerbate psoriasis.[58,59]

CLINICAL PRESENTATION

The clinical appearance of psoriasis, although not scarring, may be cosmetically disfiguring, especially for patients with severe disease. In general, psoriatic lesions are characterized by sharply demarcated, erythematous papules and plaques often covered with silver-white fine scales. Initial lesions are usually small papules that enlarge over time and coalesce into plaques, sometimes as serpiginous or geographic forms. If the fine scale is removed, a salmon-pink lesion is exposed, perhaps with punctate bleeding from prominent dermal capillaries (Auspitz sign).

TABLE 96–9. Psoriatic Patient Assessment

Onset and duration of psoriasis
Family history
Exacerbating factors
Previous history of antipsoriasis agents with efficacy and side-effect data
All current and recent topical and systemic medications
Environmental and occupational exposure to chemicals and toxins
Allergies (food, drug, environmental)

The appearance of psoriatic lesions also varies depending on the area of the body affected and the variant type of psoriasis. Scalp psoriasis ranges from diffuse scaling on an erythematous scalp to thickened plaques with exudation, microabscesses, and fissures. Trunk, back, arm, and leg lesions may be generalized, scattered, discrete, guttate (droplike) lesions or large plaques. Palms, soles, face, and genitalia may be involved as well. Affected nails often are pitted and associated with subungual keratotic material. Yellow spots under the nail plate also may be seen.

Psoriatic arthritis is a distinct clinical entity in which both psoriatic lesions and inflammatory "arthritis" occur. Classically, distal interphalangeal joints and adjacent nails are involved, but knees, elbows, wrists, and ankles also may be involved. Skin lesions usually precede joint involvement, although the reverse may occur, or skin lesions and joint disease may occur simultaneously. The clinical appearance of psoriasis sometimes may be confused with numerous other dermatologic diseases; thus the differential diagnosis is important, and histopathology is often useful.

PATIENT ASSESSMENT

Evaluation and education of the psoriatic patient are of great importance because of the myriad drug therapy options available as nonprescription and prescription products (Table 96–9).

▶ TREATMENT: Psoriasis

Although the exact cause of psoriasis is unknown, in a majority of patients, treatment approaches are usually reliable and offer good clinical control. Psoriasis is often a lifelong relapsing and remitting disease, so modes of therapy should be selected with long-term consequences in mind. Major factors for consideration include the extent and site of disease involvement and the age of the patient. The goal of therapy is to achieve resolution of lesions, but partial clearing is acceptable at times using regimens with decreased toxicity and increased patient acceptability. Drug treatments for psoriasis are listed in Table 96–10. Treatment guidelines are listed in Tables 96–11 and 96–12.

TOPICAL PHARMACOLOGIC THERAPY

EMOLLIENTS AND KERATOLYTICS

Moisturizers or emollients hydrate the stratum corneum (after application of an occlusive oily film) and minimize evaporation of water from the stratum corneum.[59] Hydration causes the stratum corneum to swell and flatten the surface contour. Moisturizers may decrease the binding forces within the horny layer, enhance desquamation, and eliminate scaling.[60] Moisturizers also may increase pliability of the skin, have antipruritic activity, and possess mild vasoconstrictor activity. Moisturizers often need to be applied several times a day to achieve a beneficial response. Adverse effects include folliculitis and allergic or irritant contact dermatitis.

Keratolytics are used to remove scale, smooth the skin, and decrease hyperkeratosis.[60] Salicylic acid, the most frequently used

TABLE 96–10. Examples of Drug Treatments for Psoriasis

Topical	Systemic
Emollients and keratolytics	Ultraviolet A and oral psoralens (systemic PUVA)
Corticosteroids	Methotrexate
Coal tar	Sulfasalazine
Anthralin	Cyclosporine
Calcipotriene	Tacrolimus
Tazarotene	Acitretin
Ultraviolet A and topical psoralens (topical PUVA)	Mycophenolate mofetil
	Methotrexate

TABLE 96–11. Topical Psoriasis Treatment Guidelines

Active Ingredient	Formulation	Strength (%)	Regimen	Potential Side Effects
Emollients	Lotions, creams, ointments	N/A	Three to four times daily	Folliculitis, contact dermatitis
Salicylic acid (keratolytic)	Gels, lotions	2–10	Two to three times daily	Can be irritating Has resulted in salicylism
Coal tar	Creams, gels, lotions, ointments, solutions	1–48.5	Apply in evening, allowing to remain through the night	Messy and burdensome Can be irritating Photoreactions
Anthralin	Creams, ointments	0.1–1	Usually in the evening, allowing to remain through the night. Short contact regimens have also been used	Stains skin and clothing Can be irritating
Calcipotriene	Ointment, solution, cream	0.005	Apply twice daily, no more than 100 g/wk, for up to 8 days	Burning and stinging in 10% of patients
Corticosteroids	Creams, lotions, ointments, solutions	Variable potency	Two to four times daily for maintenance; may use occlusion at night	Local tissue atrophy, striae, epidermal thinning, glucocorticoid systemic effects
Methoxsalen	Lotion	≤1	Soak or apply to area prior to UVA therapy	Photoreaction, exaggerated burning

keratolytic agent, generally is applied in concentrations of 2% to 10%. A possible mechanism of salicylic acid keratolysis is that it causes a decrease in corneocyte-to-corneocyte cohesion in the abnormal horny layer of psoriatic skin. Lower concentrations of salicylic acid exhibit a keratin-dispersing effect, whereas concentrations of 5% or higher have a corneolytic (exfoliative) action.[61] Although salicylic acid may enhance percutaneous penetration of some drugs, it also produces local irritation.[60] Application of salicylic acid to large, inflamed areas of skin is capable of inducing salicylism with symptoms of nausea, vomiting, tinnitus, or hyperventilation.[62]

COAL TAR

Although tar derivatives have been used to treat skin diseases for two millennia, relatively little is known about their composition or mechanism of action.[63] Tars are derived from wood such as pine or juniper, shale (ichthammol), and bituminous coal (coal tar). In recent years, wood and shale tars have fallen out of use because they possess relatively less efficacy than coal tar.[63] Coal tar contains numerous hydrocarbon compounds formed from distillation of bituminous coal.[63] When applied to normal skin, coal tar causes predominantly transient epidermal hyperplasia during the first 2 weeks of therapy followed by a cytostatic effect with epidermal thinning.[64] There is additional evidence that ultraviolet B light–activated coal tar photoadducts with epidermal DNA and inhibits DNA synthesis. This normalized epidermal replication rate leads to reduction in plaque elevation.[65,66]

Coal tar is an effective treatment for psoriasis; however, it is a burdensome, time-consuming treatment with disadvantages that include unpleasant odor, ability to stain skin and clothing, ability to reversibly darken or alter light hair colors, and ability to tarnish silver in jewelry. Coal tar usually is applied topically to lesions (often at bedtime) but also may be used in bath water and as a shampoo. Short-contact treatment allows for application of tar just 2 hours before light treatment and avoids overnight applications that may interfere with sleep.

Risk of carcinogenicity is a concern with the long-term use of topical coal tar. Crude coal tar contains numerous polynuclear aromatic hydrocarbons that are known carcinogens. Retrospective studies

TABLE 96–12. Oral Psoriasis Treatment Guidelines

Active Ingredient	Formulation	Strength	Regimen	Potential Side Effects
Sulfasalazine	Suspension, tablets	250 mg/5 mL, 500 mg	3–4 g/day	Gastrointestinal upset
Methoxsalen	Capsules	10 mg	Dosed on a mg/kg 2 hours before UVA exposure	Burns, erythema, gastrointestinal upset, CNS effects, ocular damage
Methotrexate	Tablets, injection	2.5 mg; 20–25 mg/mL	2.5–5 mg every 12 hours for three doses every week	Anemia, leukopenia, thrombo-cytopenia, gastrointestinal upset
Acitretin	Capsules	10 mg, 25 mg	25–50 mg daily	Dry mouth and lips, eye irritation, arthralgia, monitor liver function tests
Cyclosporine	Capsules, solution	25 mg, 100 mg, 100 mg/mL	3–4 mg/kg/day in two divided doses; may increase to 5 mg/kg/day in one month if no response	Nephrotoxicity, gastrointestinal upset, hypertension, tremor, monitor liver function tests
Tacrolimus	Capsules	1 mg/5 mg	0.15 mg/kg twice daily, titrate based on side effects	Nephrotoxicity, gastrointestinal upset

of psoriatic patients treated with crude coal tar have not indicated any increase in cancer cases compared with controls[63]; however, there are cases indicating a higher rate of cutaneous carcinoma in patients exposed to tar and ultraviolet B light. Controlled studies are lacking to assess the carcinogenicity risk associated with clinical use of crude and refined coal tars.

TOPICAL CORTICOSTERIODS

Topical corticosteroids play an important *adjunctive* role in the treatment of psoriasis by decreasing erythema, pruritus, and scaling. The mechanism of action for topical corticosteroid efficacy in psoriasis is uncertain. Steroid receptors have been identified in the skin, and synthesis and mitosis of DNA in epidermal cells have been halted by topical corticosteroids in hairless mice.[67,68] However, humans mount a tachyphylactic response to topical corticosteroid antimitotic effect after only 72 hours of treatment. Topical corticosteroids appear to inhibit phospholipase A, lowering amounts of arachidonic acid, prostaglandins, and leukotrienes in the skin.[69] Coupled with local vasoconstriction, these agents are useful to reduce erythema and pruritus, but as antipsoriatic agents they are best used adjunctively with a product that specifically functions to normalize epidermal hyperproliferation.

A wide variety of topical corticosteroids are available in various potencies and vehicles as described in USP-DI.[70]

1. Products with a *low-potency* ranking have a modest anti-inflammatory effect and are safest for long-term application. These products are also the safest products for use on the face and intertriginous areas, in infants and young children, and with occlusion.
2. Products with a *medium-potency* ranking are used in moderate inflammatory dermatoses. Examples of conditions for which these products are used frequently include chronic eczematous dermatoses such as hand eczema and atopic eczema. Medium-potency preparations may be used on the face and intertriginous areas for limited periods of time.
3. *High-potency* preparations are used in severe inflammatory dermatoses. Examples of conditions for which these products are used frequently include more severe eczematous dermatoses, lichen simplex chronicus, and psoriasis. They are used for intermediate duration of treatment or for longer periods in areas with thickened skin secondary to chronic conditions. High-potency preparations also may be used on the face and intertriginous areas but only for short periods of time.
4. *Very high-potency* products are used primarily as an alternative to systemic adrenocorticoid therapy when local areas are involved. Examples of conditions for which very high-potency products are used frequently include thick, chronic lesions caused by psoriasis, lichen simplex chronicus, and discoid lupus erythematosus. There is a high likelihood of skin atrophy with the use of very high-potency preparations. They are used for only short periods of time and on relatively small surface areas. Generally, occlusive dressings should not be used with these products.

The choice of corticosteroid and vehicle depends on severity and extent of involvement, the anatomic region of the body to be treated, and the anticipated duration of treatment. Topical corticosteroids are available in ointments, creams, lotions, gels, sprays, shampoos, mousses, and impregnated adhesive tapes.

An ointment is considered the most clinically effective dosage form in psoriasis treatment because it consists of an oily phase that is occlusive and conveys a hydrating effect as well as enhancement of penetration of the corticosteroid into the dermis by its lipophilicity.[71] Ointments are not suited for use in areas such as the axilla, groin, or other intertriginous areas where maceration and folliculitis may develop secondary to the occlusive effect. Creams typically are emulsified products with an aqueous phase and are preferred occasionally by patients as more cosmetically desirable. They may be used in intertriginous areas even though their lower oil content makes them more drying than ointments.

In severe, acute forms of psoriasis and other inflammatory dermatoses, a patient may be instructed to apply a high-potency topical steroid every 2 hours for 24 to 48 hours, followed by gradual tapering down of applications to the rate of three or four times a day. For maintenance, application one to two times a day conveys cost-effective and nearly maximal vasoconstriction. Adverse reactions are not uncommon. Local tissue atrophy, degeneration, and striae are manifestations of corticosteroid effect on collagen synthesis and fibroblast growth. If detected early, atrophy and striae may be reversible on drug discontinuation, but in numerous cases of prolonged therapy with high-potency agents, these changes may be long-lasting. Thinning of the epidermis may result in visibly distended capillaries (telangiectasias) and purpura. Acneform eruptions and masking of symptoms of bacterial or fungal skin infections also have been reported with topical corticosteroid use.

Systemic consequences of topical corticosteroid use include risk of suppression of the hypothalamic-pituitary-adrenal axis, hyperglycemia, and development of cushingoid features. Avoidance of prolonged therapy with high-potency agents minimizes the risk of these side effects. Tachyphylaxis and rebound flare of psoriasis after abrupt cessation of topical corticosteroid therapy also can occur. With proper monitoring, topical corticosteroids are a safe and effective adjunctive approach to psoriasis treatment.

ANTHRALIN

Anthralin, an anthrone derivative of chrysarobin (from the South American araroba tree), is used topically to treat psoriasis.[72] Although anthralin (under the name dithranol) has been used for 70 years in Great Britain, it has only recently been used extensively in the United States. Anthralin appears to inhibit DNA synthesis by intercalation between DNA strands.[73] Another possible mechanism is that anthralin may decrease epidermal proliferation by mitochondrial inhibition. Irritation and inflammation are common with anthralin therapy and, to some degree, may correlate with clinical efficacy.[72,74] Other hypotheses support the role of anthralin-generated free radicals in producing both antipsoriatic effects and irritation.[75]

Inflammation, irritation, and staining of skin and clothing (via oxidation and binding to keratins) are often therapy-limiting effects. Fortunately, anthralin exerts its clinical effects at low cellular concentrations; therefore, short-contact therapy regimens (application for 20 minutes) have been found effective with decreased side effects.[76] Titrating the strength of anthralin gradually from a low concentration (0.1% to 0.25%) to a higher concentration (0.5% to 1%) may minimize irritation.

Anthralin traditionally was formulated in stiff paste bases to provide adherence to plaques. More recently, cream formulations have been developed that are more cosmetically appealing and appear to be as effective clinically. The patient must apply anthralin products only to affected areas of skin because contact with uninvolved skin may result in excessive and unwanted irritation and staining, which usually disappears within 1 to 2 weeks of discontinuation. Staining of affected plaques is a sign of resolution because cell turnover has been slowed enough to take up the stain.[73] Despite the demonstrated efficacy of anthralin, some patients will not tolerate local irritation and staining.

CALCIPOTRIENE

Calcipotriene, a synthetic 1,25-dihydroxyvitamin D_3 analog, is used in the treatment of mild to moderate plaque psoriasis.[77] Calcipotriene binds to receptors in epidermal keratinocytes, resulting in the inhibition of cell proliferation and induction of cell differentiation.[78] Calcium metabolism may be altered by the application of calcipotriene, even with restricted use according to FDA labeling. Hypercalcemia has been reported with application of calcipotriene.[77,79,80] The long-term effects of altered calcium homeostasis are unknown. Calcipotriene has been evaluated in several open-label or randomized, double-blind controlled studies and has been shown to be effective in improving or clearing psoriatic plaques.[79,81–83] On average, improvement was seen within 2 weeks of treatment, with approximately 70% of the patients demonstrating marked improvement after 8 weeks of therapy. Adverse effects include lesional and perilesional irritation, occurring in approximately 10% of treated patients and consisting of mild burning and stinging. Irritant dermatitis occurs more commonly on the face.[77,84] Dry skin, peeling, rash, and worsening of psoriasis also have been reported.

TAZAROTENE

Tazarotene, a synthetic retinoid, is a prodrug that exerts its pharmacologic activity when hydrolyzed to its active metabolite, tazarotenic acid. Although this metabolite has similar pharmacologic actions to other retinoids, it has been shown to have specific affinity for the retinoic acid receptors RAR-γ and RAR-β, which enhance gene expression.[88] Tazarotene appears to affect the primary pathogenic factors involved in psoriasis: abnormal differentiation, hyperproliferation of the keratinocyte, and inflammation.[88,89] It has been evaluated for use in large, multicenter, vehicle-controlled trials. Treatment with 0.1% gel resulted in substantial reduction in the severity of erythema, scaling, and plaque elevation with 12-week therapies. In these studies, the 0.1% gel was somewhat more efficacious, but the 0.05% formulation was associated with less irritation.[88,89] Predominant treatment-related adverse effects were mild to moderate pruritus, burning/stinging, or erythema. These local reactions have been shown to be dose- and frequency-related.[90–92] Application of the gel to eczematous skin or to more than 20% of body surface area is not recommended because this may lead to extensive systemic absorption.[90] Based on the results of these clinical trials, tazarotene 0.05% and 0.1% gels, applied once daily, are effective for the treatment of mild to moderate plaque psoriasis.[88,90,91]

SYSTEMIC PHARMACOLOGIC THERAPY

ACITRETIN

Acitretin, a retinoic acid analog, is the active metabolite of etretinate and has demonstrated clinical effects similar to etretinate. Acitretin is indicated for the treatment of severe psoriasis, including erythrodermic and generalized pustular types, and is expected to replace etretinate, although some cases of patients responding to etretinate and not acitretin exist.[85] Although the mechanism for treatment in patients with severe psoriasis is not clearly defined, it has shown significant clearing when administered. The initial recommended dose is 25 or 50 mg, with therapy being continued until lesions have resolved.

As with other retinoids, acitretin is associated with side effects such as hypervitaminosis A (i.e., dry lips/cheilitis, dry mouth, dry nose, dry eyes/conjunctivitis, dry skin, pruritus, scaling, and hair loss). Other systemic side effects include hepatotoxicity, skeletal changes, hypercholesterolemia, and hypertriglyceridemia. To counteract hyperlipidemic effects, gemfibrozil has been studied for concomitant use with acitretin.[86] In addition, acitretin is a known teratogen and thus is contraindicated in females who are pregnant or who plan pregnancy within the 3 years following drug discontinuation. Acitretin is eliminated more rapidly, and thus only a short period of contraception following treatment has been suggested as compared with etretinate.[87] A major drawback is that acitretin metabolizes to some degree to etretinate, which in turn poses the original hazard identified with etretinate use (prolonged retention in the host).

CYCLOSPORINE

Systemically administered cyclosporine demonstrates immunosuppressive activity by inhibiting an early step of T-cell activation and also has anti-inflammatory activity by inhibiting the release of inflammatory mediators from mast cells, basophils, and polymorphonuclear cells.[93] Given these mechanisms, cyclosporine has been evaluated for use in the treatment of both cutaneous and articular manifestations of psoriasis.[93–96] An oral microemulsion formulation of cyclosporine (Neoral) has shown a better pharmacokinetic profile, resulting in a more consistent and predictable rate of absorption.[96]

Adverse effects of cyclosporine include hypertension, paresthesia, hypertrichosis, gingival hyperplasia, and renal dysfunction.[93,97] Recent evaluation of 30 psoriatic patients receiving long-term cyclosporine therapy indicated a need for renal biopsies or change of treatment after 2 years because all biopsies demonstrated features consistent with cyclosporine-related nephropathy.[97] A 1-year multicenter trial investigated the efficacy and safety of intermittent use of the immunosuppressant in the microemulsion form. Patients received three courses of therapy, with a maximum 12-week duration per course, but significant increases in serum creatinine were still found.[98] Lower maintenance doses of cyclosporine also have been studied to alleviate or prolong progression to cyclosporine-induced nephropathy.[99]

TACROLIMUS

Tacrolimus, an immunosuppressant indicated for organ allograft rejection, has been found to be efficacious as an immunomodulator in the treatment of recalcitrant psoriasis on the basis of psoriasis as a T-cell-mediated disease.[100–102] In a double-blind, placebo-controlled trial, patients receiving tacrolimus at oral doses of 0.05 mg/kg per day (increased up to 0.15 mg/kg per day as needed) resulted in efficacious treatment of recalcitrant plaque-type psoriasis.[102] Frequently reported adverse effects included diarrhea, paresthesia, and insomnia. Other toxicities, including renal insufficiency, also have been reported. As a topical agent, tacrolimus was approved on February 2001, in the United States, for the treatment of atopic dermatitis; however, trials establishing efficacy of topical tacrolimus in psoriasis are lacking to date.

MYCOPHENOLATE MOFETIL

Therapy with oral mycophenolic acid, a weak organic acid, was investigated in the 1970s for the treatment of moderate to severe psoriasis. Its ability to inhibit purine biosynthesis and show immunosuppressive activity was demonstrated by several multicenter, double-blind, placebo-controlled studies. Recent introduction of mycophenolate mofetil, a morpholinoester of mycophenolic acid, has recreated interest in its antipsoriatic properties. Commonly reported side effects include genitourinary symptoms (e.g., urgency, frequency, and dysuria), hematologic effects (including anemia, neutropenia, and thrombocytopenia), and an increased incidence of viral and bacterial infections. Oral mycophenolate mofetil, as well as topical mycophenolic acid, may undergo further clinical studies to determine usefulness in the treatment of patients with severe psoriasis.[103]

SULFASALAZINE

Oral sulfasalazine (3–4 g/day for 8 weeks) has been reported to be an effective therapy for plaque-type psoriasis in some patients.[104] When used as a single agent in the treatment of psoriasis, it is not as effective as is therapy with methotrexate, psoralens plus ultraviolet A light (PUVA), or etretinate. One possible advantage of sulfasalazine therapy compared with other systemic treatments is its lower incidence of severe side effects.[104]

BIOLOGIC THERAPY

Psoriasis is currently a major focus for biologic therapy due to the immunologic component of psoriasis. The primary biologic agents that are being developed for use in psoriasis are immunomodulating agents. Although there are no FDA-approved biologic agents for psoriasis, they are emerging as an important treatment approach.[105]

COMBINATION THERAPY

SYSTEMIC THERAPY: PHOTOCHEMOTHERAPY—ORAL AND TOPICAL PSORALEN AND LONG-WAVE ULTRAVIOLET A LIGHT

The use of PUVA has been studied since the early 1970s and was approved by the FDA in 1982. Efficacy studies indicated that control of psoriasis occurred in nearly 90% of patients.[106]

Psoralens react with nucleic acids and intercalate between base pairs. When DNA is irradiated with long-wave ultraviolet light (320 to 400 nm, ultraviolet A), the psoralens covalently bind to pyrimidine bases, forming a cross-link.[107] PUVA also may affect immune responses in the skin and circulating lymphocytes, as demonstrated by a decreased ability to mount delayed hypersensitivity responses to contact sensitizers and increased risk of cutaneous cancer in treated patients.[108,109]

Candidates for PUVA therapy usually have severe, incapacitating psoriasis unresponsive to topical therapies and are without history of photosensitivity, skin cancers, cataracts, or x-ray therapy of the skin. Methoxsalen [8-methoxypsoralen (8-MOP)] is usually dosed at 0.6 to 0.8 mg/kg and is given 2 hours before exposure to ultraviolet A. Serum methoxsalen concentrations usually peak within 0.5 to 2 hours of ingestion; however, a large interindividual and intraindividual variation in absorption may complicate titration of effective therapy.[110] Dosing of ultraviolet A is determined by patient skin type and history of previous response to ultraviolet radiation.

TOPICAL PSORALENS

The use of PUVA has been proven to be beneficial for psoriasis.[110–114] Several studies involving plaque psoriasis, comparing oral and bath-water delivery of 8-MOP, have found that the bath-water form was as effective, required reduced amounts of ultraviolet A and was associated with fewer side effects.[114,116] Recently, local bath-PUVA therapy also has been studied in the management of chronic palmoplantar eczema.[119]

EVALUATION OF THERAPEUTIC OUTCOMES

Psoriasis is a relatively common hyperproliferative epidermal disorder for which several effective therapeutic modalities control rather than cure the condition. Recognition of the pathogenic factors associated with psoriasis, selection of an appropriate treatment regimen, and monitoring for adverse effects as well as disease progression often lead to a satisfactory outcome. Concepts of therapy should be conveyed adequately to the patient, and the importance of compliance should be emphasized.

Achievement of clinical efficacy by any given therapeutic regimen requires days to weeks. Initial dramatic response may be achieved with some agents such as tazarotene and/or corticosteroids; however, sustained benefit with pharmacologically specific antipsoriatic therapy usually requires a range of about 2 to 8 weeks for noticeable response with most other therapies. Positive response to therapy is noted as normalization of involved areas of skin as measured by reduced erythema and scaling as well as reduction of plaque elevation.

As with most pharmacotherapy choices, risk-benefit issues are of great importance in treating an epidermal-based disorder that may be seriously debilitating to the patient. The purpose of pharmacotherapy in this disorder is often to keep or establish the patient functional in his or her social and job environments as well as to preserve emotional and physical health.

Rational dermatologic therapy must be principled in the pathogenesis of the disorder. Major advances in recent years have allowed a better understanding of disease mechanisms and have produced a high level of interest in the development of pharmacotherapeutic approaches to treatment. Common skin disorders such as acne and psoriasis are excellent clinical models for demonstrating broad areas of pharmacologic intervention and therapeutic benefit. For many other common dermatologic disorders, these same principles apply.

▶ PRINCIPLES OF PHARMACOTHERAPY

- The pathogenesis of acne is multifactorial, including androgen-stimulated sebum production, follicular abnormalities, and bacterial (*P. acnes*) action on sebum to create breakdown products that produce inflammation.

- Contrary to popular belief, diet, hygiene, cosmetic use, and certain hairstyles do not necessarily play a role in the development of acne.
- In mild inflammatory acne, topical treatment with once- to twice-daily application of an antibacterial agent as well as a comedolytic agent is recommended.
- Acne patients with scarring potential and those not responding to topical therapy may use the combination of a topical comedolytic agent with a systemic antibiotic.
- Acne patients with nodular lesions and scarring potential are candidates for systemic isotretinoin therapy.
- The clinical response in acne is delayed and is not fairly assessed, regardless of therapeutic regimen, until 6 to 8 weeks of therapy.
- Since topical agents are disease-preventive, all acne-prone areas should be treated to prevent or minimize the formation of new lesions and to minimize the risk of scarring.
- Exogenous factors such as climate, stress, infection, trauma, and drugs may aggravate or trigger psoriasis in an individual who is otherwise genetically predisposed to expression of the disease.
- Warm seasons and sunlight improve psoriasis in 80% of patients, whereas a majority report worsening with cold or hot temperature extremes.
- Adjunctive topical therapies include psoriasis emollients, keratolytics, and corticosteroids.
- A positive response to psoriasis therapy is noted as "normalization" of involved areas measured by reduced erythema and scaling as well as reduction of plaque elevation.
- The risk-benefit ratio is an important consideration in the treatment of psoriasis, and the goal is to maintain a functional status for the patient.
- Disease-modifying therapies for psoriasis include topical calcipotriene and tazarotene, light-source treatments such as coal tar plus ultraviolet B and PUVA, and systemic treatments such as methotrexate, hydroxyurea, cyclosporine, and acitretin.

REFERENCES

1. Arndt KA, Wintroub BU, Robinson JK, et al., eds. Primary Care Dermatology. Philadelphia, Saunders, 1997.
2. Fitzpatrick TB, Johnson RA, Wolff K, et al. Color Atlas and Synopsis of Clinical Dermatology Common and Serious Diseases, 4th ed. New York, McGraw-Hill, 2001.
3. Leyden JJ. Therapy for acne vulgaris. N Engl J Med 1997;336:1176–1162.
4. Morgan M, McCreedy R, Simpson J, et al. Dermatology quality of life scales: A measure of the impact of skin diseases. Br J Dermatol 1997; 136:202–206.
5. Thiboutot DM. Acne: An overview of clinical research findings. Dermatol Clin 1997;15:97–109.
6. Layton AM, Seukeran D, Cunliffe WJ. Scarred for life? Dermatology 1997;195(Suppl 1):15–21.
7. Landow K. Dispelling myths about acne. Postgrad Med 1997;102:94–112.
8. Arndt KA, ed. Acne. In: Manual of Dermatologic Therapeutics, 5th ed. Boston, Little, Brown, 1995: 3–15.
9. Melski JW, Arndt KA. Topical therapy for acne. N Engl J Med 1980;302: 503–506.
10. Eaglstein WH. Allergic contact dermatitis to benzoyl peroxide. Arch Dermatol 1968;97:527.
11. Franz TJ. On the bioavailability of topical formulations of clindamycin hydrochloride. J Am Acad Dermatol 1983;9:66–73.
12. Eady EA, Holland KT, Cunliffe NJ. Should topical antibiotics be used for the treatment of acne vulgaris? Br J Dermatol 1982;107: 235–246.
13. Eady EA, Holland KT, Cunliffe WJ. The use of antibiotics in acne therapy: Oral or topical administration? J Antimicrob Chemother 1982;10:89–117.
14. Schachner L, Eaglstein W, Kittles C, Mertz P. Topical erythromycin and zinc therapy for acne. J Am Acad Dermatol 1990;22:253–260.
15. Habbema L, Koopmans B, Menke HE, et al. A 4% erythromycin and zinc combination (Zineryt) versus 2% erythromycin (Eryderm) in acne vulgaris: A randomized double-blind comparative study. Br J Dermatol 1989;121:497–502.
16. Becker LE, Bergstresser PR, Whiting DA, et al. Topical clindamycin therapy for acne vulgaris. Arch Dermatol 1981;117:482–485.
17. Parry MF, Rha CK. Pseudomembranous colitis caused by topical clindamycin phosphate. Arch Dermatol 1986;122:583–594.
18. Mackrides PS, Shaughnessy AF. Azelaic acid therapy for acne. Am Fam Physician 1996;54:2457–2459.
19. Schallreuter KU, Wood JW. A possible mechanism of action for azelaic acid in the human epidermis. Arch Dermatol Res 1989;202:168–171.
20. Cunliffe WJ, Holland KT. Clinical and laboratory studies on treatment with 20% azelaic acid cream for acne. Acta Derm Venereol (Stockh) 1989;143(Suppl):31–34.
21. Cavicchini S, Caputo R. Long-term treatment of acne with 20% azelaic acid cream. Acta Derm Venereol (Stockh) 1989;143(Suppl):40–44.
22. Thomas JR III, Doya JA. The therapeutic uses of topical vitamin A acid. J Am Acad Dermatol 1981;4:505–513.
23. Berson DS, Shalita AR. The treatment of acne: The role of combination therapies. J Am Acad Dermatol 1995;32:S31–S41.
24. Hurwitz S. The combined effect of vitamin A acid and benzoyl peroxide in the treatment of acne. Cutis 1976;17:585–590.
25. Brogden RN, Goa KL. Adapalene: A review of its pharmacological properties and clinical potential in the management of mild to moderate acne. Drugs 1997;53:511–519.
26. Shalita A, Weiss J, Chalker D, et al. A comparison of the efficacy and safety of adapalene gel 0.01% and tretinoin gel 0.025% in the treatment of acne vulgaris: A multicenter trial. J Am Acad Dermatol 1996;34:482–485.
27. Shalita A, Chalker D, Griffith R, et al. Double-blind study of AGN 190168, a new retinoid gel, in the topical treatment of acne vulgaris. J Invest Dermatol 1993;100:542.
28. Ad Hoc Committee on the Use of Antibiotics in Dermatology. Systemic antibiotics for treatment of acne vulgaris: Efficacy and safety. Arch Dermatol 1975;111:1630–1636.
29. Jonas M, Cunha BA. Minocycline. Ther Drug Monit 1982;4:137–145.
30. Shapiro LE, Knowles SR, Shear NH. Comparative safety of tetracycline, minocycline, and doxycycline. Arch Dermatol 1997;133:1224–1230.
31. Gammon WR, Meyer C, Lantis S, et al. Comparative efficacy of oral erythromycin versus oral tetracycline in the treatment of acne vulgaris. J Am Acad Dermatol 1986;14:183–186.
32. Nordin K, Hallander H, Fredriksson T, Rylander C. A clinical and bacteriological evaluation of the effect of sulphamethoxazole-trimethoprim in acne vulgaris resistant to prior therapy with tetracyclines. Dermatologica 1978;157:245–253.
33. Hansten PD, Horn JR. Inhibition of oral contraceptive efficacy. Drug Interact Newslett 1985;5:7–10.
34. Miller DM, Helms SE, Brodell RT. A practical approach to antibiotic treatment in women taking oral contraceptives. J Am Acad Dermatol 1994;30:1008–1011.
35. Lucky AW, Henderson TA, Olson WH, et al. Effectiveness of norgestimate and ethinyl estradiol in treating moderate acne vulgaris. J Am Acad Dermatol 1997;37:746–754.
36. Shaw JC. Antiandrogen and hormonal treatment of acne. Dermatol Clin 1996;14:803–811.
37. Redmond GP, Olson WH, Lippman JS, et al. Norgestimate and ethinyl estradiol in the treatment of acne vulgaris: A randomized, placebo-controlled trial. Obstet Gynecol 1997;89:615–622.

38. Rumsfield JA, West DP, Tse CST, et al. Isotretinoin in severe, recalcitrant cystic acne: A review. Drug Intell Clin Pharm 1983;17:329–333.
39. Saurat JH. Oral isotretinoin: Where now, where next? Dermatology 1997;195(Suppl 1):1–3.
40. Ortonne JP. Oral isotretinoin treatment policy: Do we all agree? Dermatology 1997;195(Suppl 1):34–37.
41. Shalita AR, Cunningham WJ, Leyden JJ, et al. Isotretinoin treatment of acne and related disorders: An update. J Am Acad Dermatol 1983;9: 629–638.
42. Meigel WN. How safe is oral isotretinoin? Dermatology 1997;195 (Suppl 1):22–28.
43. Newton JN. How cost-effective is oral isotretinoin? Dermatology 1997; 195(Suppl 1):10–14.
44. Gilchrest BA. Retinoid pharmacology and skin. In: Mukhtar H, ed, Pharmacology of the Skin. Boca Raton, CRC Press, 1995:167–181.
45. Goulden V, Cunliffe WJ. The long-term experience with isotretinoin treatment of acne. In: Dahl MV, Lynch PJ, eds. Current Opinion in Dermatology. Philadelphia, Current Science, 1995:231–234.
46. Adverse effects with isotretinoin. FDA Drug Bull 1983;13:21–23.
47. Krueger GG, Bergstresser PR, Lowe NJ, et al. Psoriasis. J Am Acad Dermatol 1984;11:937–947.
48. Watson W. Psoriasis: Epidemiology and genetics. Dermatol Clin 1984;2: 363–371.
49. Farber EM, Nail ML. The natural history of psoriasis in 5600 patients. Dermatologica 1974;148:1–18.
50. Wrone-Smith T, Nickoloff BJ. Dermal injection of immunocytes induces psoriasis. J Clin Invest 1996;98:1878–1887.
51. Weinstein GD, McCullough JL, Ross PA. Cell kinetic basis for pathophysiology of psoriasis. J Invest Dermatol 1985;85:579–583.
52. Baden HP. Biology of the epidermis and pathophysiology of psoriasis and certain ichthyosiform dermatoses. In: Soter NA, Baden HP, eds. Pathophysiology of Dermatologic Diseases. New York, McGraw-Hill, 1984:101–126.
53. Krueger GG. Psoriasis: Current concepts of its etiology and pathogenesis. In: Dobson RL, Thiers BH, eds. Yearbook of Dermatology. Chicago, Year Book, 1981.
54. Elder JT. Cytokine and genetic regulation of psoriasis. In: Callen JP, ed. Advances in Dermatology, Vol. 10. St. Louis, Mosby–Year Book, 1995: 99–134.
55. Russell TJ, Schultes LM, Kuban DJ. Histocompatibility (HLA) antigens associated with psoriasis. New Engl J Med 1972;287:738–740.
56. Nyfors A, Lemholt K. Psoriasis in children: A short review and a survey of 245 cases. Br J Dermatol 1975;92:437–442.
57. Whyte HJ, Baughman RD. Acute guttate psoriasis and streptococcal infection. Arch Dermatol 1964;89:350–356.
58. Skoven I, Thormann J. Lithium compound treatment and psoriasis. Arch Dermatol 1979;117:1185–1187.
59. Neumann HAM, van Joost T. Adverse reactions of the skin to metoprolol and other beta-adrenoreceptor-blocking agents. Dermatologica 1981; 162:330–335.
60. Marks R. Topical therapy for psoriasis: General principles. Dermatol Clin 1984;2:383–388.
61. Weirich EG. Dermatopharmacology of salicylic acid: I. Range of dermatotherapeutic effects of salicylic acid. Br Med J 1979;1:661.
62. Davies MG, Briffa DV, Greaves MW. Systemic toxicity from topically applied salicylic acid. Br Med J 1979;1:661.
63. Lin AN, Moses K. Tar revisited. Int J Dermatol 1985;24:216–218.
64. Polano MK. Topical Skin Therapeutics. London, Churchill-Livingstone, 1984:95.
65. Lavker RM, Grove GL, Kligman AM. The atrophogenic effect of crude coal tar on human epidermis. Br J Dermatol 1981;105:77–82.
66. Lowe NJ, Breeding J, Wortzman MS. The pharmacological variability of crude coal tar. Br J Dermatol 1982;107:475–479.
67. Cornell RC, Stoughton RB. The use of topical steroids in psoriasis. Dermatol Clin 1984;2:397–409.
68. Cornell RC. Topical glucocorticoids in dermatology. In: Dahl MV, Lynch PJ, eds. Current Opinion in Dermatology, 2d ed. Philadelphia, Current Science, 1995.193–197.
69. Hammarstrom S, Hamberg M, Duell EA, et al. Glucocorticoid in inflammatory proliferative skin disease reduces arachidonic and hydroxyeicosatetraenoic acids. Science 1977;197:994–996.
70. Corticosteroids (topical). In: United States Pharmacopeia Drug Information (USP-DI), Vol 1, 21st ed. Taunton, MA, 2001:1012–1013.
71. Burdick KH, Haleblian JK, Poulsen BJ, Cobner SE. Corticosteroid ointments: Comparison by two human bioassays. Curr Ther Res 1973;15: 233–242.
72. Ashton RE, Andre P, Lowe NJ, Whitefield M. Anthralin: Historical and current perspectives. J Am Acad Dermatol 1983;9:173–192.
73. Swanbeck G, Thyresson N. Interaction between dithranol and nucleic acids. Acta Derm Venereol (Stockh) 1965;45:344–348.
74. Barr RM, Misch KJ, Hensby CN, et al. Arachidonic acid and prostaglandin levels in dithranol erythema: Time course study. Br J Clin Pharmacol 1983;16:715–717.
75. Finnen MJ, Lawrence CM, Shuster S. Inhibition of dithranol inflammation by free-radical scavengers. Lancet 1984;2:1129–1130.
76. Gorsulowsky DC, Voorhees JJ, Ellis CN. Anthralin therapy for psoriasis: A new look at an old compound. Arch Dermatol 1985;121:1509–1511.
77. Kirsner RS, Federman D. Treatment of psoriasis: Role of calcipotriene. Am Fam Physician 1995;52:137–239.
78. Berth-Jones J, Fletcher A, Hutchinson PE. Epidermal cytokeratin and immunocyte responses during treatment of psoriasis with calcipotriol. In: Norma AW, Bouillon R, Thomasset M, eds. Vitamin D: Gene Regulation, Structure-Function Analysis and Clinical Application. Berlin, de Gruyter, 1991:424.
79. Cunliffe WJ, Claudy A, Faiross G, et al. A multicenter comparative study of calcipotriol and betamethasone 17-valerate in patients with psoriasis vulgaris. J Am Acad Dermatol 1992;26:736–743.
80. De Jong EM, van de Kerkhof PM. Simultaneous assessment of inflammation and epidermal proliferation in psoriatic plaques during long-term treatment with the vitamin D analogue MC 903: Modulations and interrelations. Br J Dermatol 1991;124:221–229.
81. Kragballe K, Fogh K. Treatment of psoriasis by the topical application of the novel cholecalciferol analogue calcipotriol (MC 903). Arch Dermatol 1989;125:1647–1652.
82. Kragballe K, Gjertsen BT, DeHoope D, et al. Double-blind, right/left comparison of calcipotriol and betamethasone valerate in treatment of psoriasis vulgaris. Lancet 1991;337:193–196.
83. Berth-Jones J, Chu AC, Dodd WAH, et al. A multicenter parallel-group comparison of calcipotriol ointment and short contact dithranol therapy in chronic plaque psoriasis. Br J Dermatol 1992;127:266–271.
84. Fisher DA. Allergic contact dermatitis to propylene glycol in calcipotriene ointment. Cutis 1997;60:43–44.
85. Bleiker TO, Bourke JF, Graham-Brown RAC, et al. Etretinate may work where acitretin fails. Br J Dermatol 1997;136:368–370.
86. Vahlquist C, Olsson AG, Lindholm A, et al. Effects of gemfibrozil on hyperlipidemia in acitretin-treated patients: Results of a double-blind cross-over study. Acta Derm Venereol (Stockh) 1995;75:377–380.
87. Lambert WE, Meyer E, DeLeenheer AP, et al. Pharmacokinetics of acitretin. Acta Derm Venereol (Stockh) 1994;186:122–123.
88. Duvic M, Nagpal S, Asano AT, et al. Molecular mechanisms of tazarotene action in psoriasis. J Am Acad Dermatol 1997;37:S18–S24.
89. Chandraratna RAS. Tazarotene: The first receptor-selective topical retinoid for the treatment of psoriasis. J Am Acad Dermatol 1997;37: S12–S17.
90. Weinstein GD, Krueger GG, Lowe NJ, et al. Tazarotene gel, a new retinoid, for topical therapy of psoriasis: Vehicle-controlled study of safety, efficacy, and duration of therapeutic effect. J Am Acad Dermatol 1997;37:85–92.
91. Weinstein GD. Tazarotene gel: Efficacy and safety in plaque psoriasis. J Am Acad Dermatol 1997;37:S33–S38.
92. Marks R. Clinical safety of tazarotene in the treatment of plaque psoriasis. J Am Acad Dermatol 1997;37:S25–S32.
93. Olivieri I, Salvarani C, Cantini F, et al. Therapy with cyclosporine in psoriatic arthritis. Semin Arthritis Rheum 1997;27:36–43.

94. Tourne L, Durez P, Van Vooren JP, et al. Alleviation of HIV-associated psoriasis and psoriatic arthritis with cyclosporine. J Am Acad Dermatol 1997;37:501–502.
95. Jones G, Crotty M, Brooks P. Psoriatic Arthritis Meta-analysis Study Group. Psoriatic arthritis: A qualitative overview of therapeutic options. Br J Rheumatol 1997;36:95–99.
96. Erkko P, Granlund H, Nuutinen M, et al. Comparison of cyclosporin A pharmacokinetics of a new microemulsion formulation and standard oral preparation in patients with psoriasis. Br J Dermatol 1997;136: 82–88.
97. Zachariae H, Kragballe K, Hansen HE, et al. Renal biopsy findings in long-term cyclosporin treatment of psoriasis. Br J Dermatol 1997;136: 531–535.
98. Berth-Jones J, Henderson CA, Munro CS, et al. Treatment of psoriasis with intermittent short course cyclosporin (Neoral): A multicentre study. Br J Dermatol 1997;136:527–530.
99. Shupack J, Abel E, Bauer E, et al. Cyclosporine as maintenance therapy in patients with severe psoriasis. J Am Acad Dermatol 1997;36:423–432.
100. Thompson AW, Carroll PB, McCauley J, et al. FK506: A novel immunosuppressant for treatment of autoimmune disease. Springer Semin Immunopathol 1993;14:323–344.
101. Jegasothy BV, Ackerman CD, Todo S, et al. Tacrolimus (FK 506): A new therapeutic agent for severe recalcitrant psoriasis. Arch Dermatol 1992; 128:781–785.
102. European FK 506 Multicentre Psoriasis Study Group. Systemic tacrolimus (FK 506) is effective for the treatment of psoriasis in a double-blind, placebo-controlled study. Arch Dermatol 1996;132:419–423.
103. Kitchin JE, Pomeranz MK, Pak G, et al. Rediscovering mycophenolic acid: A review of its mechanism, side effects and potential uses. J Am Acad Dermatol 1997;37:445–449.
104. Gupta AK, Ellis CN, Siegel MT, et al. Sulfasalazine improves psoriasis. Arch Dermatol 1990;126:487–493.
105. Gordon KB, West DP. Biologic therapy in dermatology. In: Wolverton SE, ed. Comprehensive Dermatologic Drug Therapy, 1st ed. Philadelphia, Saunders, 2001:928–942.
106. Bickers DR. Position paper: PUVA therapy. J Am Acad Dermatol 1983;8: 265–270.
107. Cole RS. Light-induced crosslinking of DNA in the presence of a furocoumarin (psoralen). Biochem Biophys Acta 1970;217:30–39.
108. Thorvaldsen J, Volden G. PUVA-induced diminution of contact allergic and irritant skin reactions. Clin Exp Dermatol 1980;5:43–46.
109. Elmets CA, Bergstresser PR. Ultraviolet radiation effects on immune processes. Photochem Photobiol 1982;36:715–719.
110. Goldstein DP, Carter DM, Ljunggren B, Burkholder J. Minimal phototoxic doses and 8-MOP plasma levels in PUVA patients. J Invest Dermatol 1982;78:429–433.
111. Fischer T, Alsins J. Treatment of psoriasis with trioxsalen baths and dysprosium lamps. Acta Derm Venereol (Stockh) 1976;56:383–390.
112. Salo OP, Lassus A, Taskinen J. Trioxsalen bath plus UVA treatment of psoriasis. Acta Derm Venereol (Stockh) 1981;61:551–554.
113. Berne B, Fischer T, Michealsson G, Noren P. An 8-year follow-up of 149 psoriasis patients. Photodermatology 1984;1:18–22.
114. Turjanmaa K, Salo H, Reunala T. Comparison of trioxsalen bath and oral methoxsalen PUVA in psoriasis. Acta Derm Venereol (Stockh) 1985;65:86–88.
115. Lowe NJ, Weingarten D, Bourget T, et al. PUVA therapy for psoriasis: Comparison of oral and bath-water delivery of 8-methoxypsoralen. J Am Acad Dermatol 1986;14:754–760.
116. David M, Lowe NJ, Halder RM, Borok M. Serum 8-methoxypsoralen (8-MOP) concentrations after bath water delivery of 8-MOP plus UVA. J Am Acad Dermatol 1990;23:931–932.
117. Schempp CM, Muller H, Czech W, et al. Treatment of chronic palmoplantar eczema with local bath-PUVA therapy. J Am Acad Dermatol 1997;36:733–737.

97
DRUG-INDUCED SKIN REACTIONS

Silvia S. Elias, Nital M. Patel, and Nina H. Cheigh

Cutaneous drug reactions occur in approximately 2% to 3% of medical inpatients, and skin rash is a frequent reason for patient visits to physicians.[1,2] Establishment of a relationship between medication use and subsequent development of cutaneous reactions, however, is often difficult. Unfortunately, mechanisms underlying adverse drug reactions are poorly understood, and few diagnostic tests are available to properly establish cause and effect. Patients with drug-induced reactions often are taking more than one drug, making detection of the causative agent difficult. The picture is further complicated because small doses of a drug may evoke severe reactions even if that agent previously was well tolerated.[3]

DRUG HISTORY

A thorough and organized approach is essential to proper diagnosis of a drug-induced skin reaction. Patient evaluation should include (1) a comprehensive drug history, (2) awareness of various clinical manifestations of drug allergy and cutaneous reactions, (3) awareness of factors that favor development of allergic reactions to drugs, and (4) awareness of the immunologic and nonimmunologic mechanisms involved in cutaneous reactions to drugs.[4–6]

A patient may experience a skin reaction while on multiple drugs. Most authorities advise that the first drug(s) to consider is(are) that initiated within the week preceding the reaction. This short temporal relationship does not hold for all drugs [e.g., onset perhaps 2 weeks after discontinuation of semisynthetic penicillins, onset after perhaps 6 months for β-blocker-induced psoriasiform eruptions, onset after 2 months to perhaps 5 years for some forms of drug-induced systemic lupus erythematosus (SLE)].[7] Each drug should be considered individually as a potential cause. Adverse drug reactions can be classified into two categories: types A and B[8] (Table 97–1). Type A reactions, accounting for 80% of reported adverse drug reactions, are produced by known pharmacologic drug actions and usually are dose-dependent and predictable to some extent. Reactions classified as type B generally are uncommon and unpredictable.

A Guide to Drug Eruptions[9] is updated at 4- to 5-year intervals and is a useful source of confirmed and tabulated information on drug-induced skin reactions. Other useful resources include *Drug Eruption Reference Manual 2001*[10] and *Cutaneous Drug Reactions,*[11] which cites over 6500 references and is categorized by drug name and skin disorder. With an increased number of drugs undergoing shorter premarketing phases, a greater number and variety of skin reactions are expected to occur during postmarketing surveillance. The pharmacist plays an important role in identifying and reporting possible drug induced skin reactions and in monitoring or preventing recurrence.

DIAGNOSIS

Although several in vitro and in vivo tests have been used to diagnose drug allergy, the availability and reliability of these tests are limited.[12–14] The in vitro radioallergosorbent test (RAST) may be used to detect IgE or IgG antibodies and has produced reasonably reliable results in detecting penicillin allergy. The modified Coombs test and bacteriophage inhibition test have even higher sensitivity for detecting IgG and IgE antibodies, although more elaborate laboratory resources are required. The lymphocyte transformation test is an in vitro test for diagnosis of both immediate and delayed drug reactions, but results depend on the drug and type of skin eruption.[9]

Patch testing, useful in assessing allergic and irritant contact dermatitis, has limited to no utility for other types of skin reactions such as delayed hypersensitivity reactions and fixed-drug eruptions.[9] Scratch or prick testing with drugs and/or metabolites may be useful in immediate-type reactions, but there are practical limitations to this method. Dechallenge-rechallenge continues to be regarded as the most definitive method for ascertaining drug-induced reactions. However, it is often not an option if a patient has experienced a potentially life-threatening reaction or if the suspected agent cannot be discontinued. In some cases, rechallenge may not result in the same reaction, which further clouds the picture. Symptoms of an allergic drug reaction usually have an acute onset, may last several minutes to months, or may occur periodically throughout an exposure period. An accurate description of the characteristics of a cutaneous drug reaction should be obtained. Although drug hypersensitivity is impossible to predict, certain drug and host factors increase the likelihood of a reaction.

CLINICAL PRESENTATION

Drug allergy is more frequent in older individuals[15] and may be related to immune-response capability and to increased exposure to drugs. Individual genetic factors also may predispose an individual to drug allergy, and variability in drug metabolism, immune response, tissue receptor sites, and elaboration of immunologic mediators may all play a role.[16] In addition, a previous history of allergic drug reactions may increase the likelihood of developing a new allergic reaction. Hepatic and renal disorders may alter drug biotransformation and increase the likelihood of an allergic response.[17]

To induce an immune response (i.e., hypersensitivity reaction), the drug or its metabolite must act as or form a complete antigen. For example, proteins contained in sera, vaccines, biologicals, and allergens may act as complete antigens; however, many drugs are small molecules and must bind with larger molecules to create a complete antigen. Haptens are often drugs capable of such binding. Once a complete antigen is formed, the immune system reacts to neutralize, destroy, or eliminate it from the host.

The route of administration may influence drug allergy. For example, topical application of drugs has the greatest propensity to induce allergy, followed by the intravenous route and the oral route. Although not strictly dose-related, such factors as the number of drugs, the dose of drug, and the duration of therapy may influence the likelihood of developing a hypersensitivity reaction.

The host's ability to react to antigenic material is the basis for specific immune reactions. The ultimate physiologic role of the

TABLE 97–1. Classification of Adverse Drug Reactions

Type A: Common and Predictable Adverse Reactions
- I. Effects of overdosage
- II. Immediate or delayed adverse effects
- III. Secondary or indirect effects
  - A. Related to drug alone
  - B. Related to both disease and drug
- IV. Interactions between/among drugs

Type B: Uncommon and Unpredictable Reactions
- I. Intolerance
- II. Idiosyncratic reaction
- III. Hypersensitivity reactions

Compiled from Ref. 8.

immune system is to differentiate "self" from "nonself" and eliminate foreign materials from the body. The type of immunologic mediation of hypersensitivity may determine the category of reaction and thus the clinical presentation of drug-induced skin disorders. For a discussion of allergic drug reaction mechanisms, see Chapter 89.

Because any drug may induce cutaneous reactivity, a complete review of drug-induced skin reactions is not practical; however, for common cutaneous drug reactions, their clinical course, possible mechanisms, etiologies, and management are described in the next sections. Maculopapular reactions and urticaria occur most often. The clinical type and frequency of cutaneous reactions to drugs for a series of 225 patients are listed in Table 97–2.[17]

MACULOPAPULAR ERUPTIONS

CLINICAL PRESENTATION

Maculopapular eruptions are the most common drug-induced skin reactions. Lesions are somewhat nonspecific but may be measles-like in their clinical manifestations in that they resemble viral exanthems and may be called *morbilliform, scarlatiniform,* or *rubelliform eruptions*. These reactions often start on the trunk or in areas of pressure or trauma and frequently are symmetrical. Individual lesions may be flat or raised and vary in size from a few millimeters to large, confluent areas. In some cases, vesicles also may be present. Mild fever and involvement of mucous membranes or palms and soles, though less frequent, also may occur.[18,19]

The course of a maculopapular eruption is classified as an *early* or *late* reaction. Individual patient responses may vary, with reactions occurring between the first day of exposure to 2 weeks or more after therapy. In the early reaction, the eruption usually appears within hours or up to 3 days after drug administration to previously sensitized patients. The late reaction appears most commonly at about 9 days but with wide variability after drug exposure.[18,19] Maculopapular rashes generally do not persist for prolonged periods, although recurrence may present as more serious and extensive exfoliative skin reactions.[13] Occasionally, eruptions decrease or disappear even with continued medication use and may not always recur with drug rechallenge.[18] Although the penicillins have been well documented as a cause of drug-induced maculopapular eruption, many other drugs have been associated with maculopapular eruptions[9,20,21] (Table 97–3).

TABLE 97–2. Type and Frequency of Cutaneous Drug Reactions

Eruption Type	Total no. (%)	Verified by Provocation no. (%)
Fixed-drug eruption	77 (34.2)	51 (66.2)
Exanthematous eruption	71 (31.6)	47 (66.2)
Urticaria/angioedema	45 (20.0)	26 (57.8)
Gold dermatitis	15 (6.7)	0 (0)
Purpuric eruption	5 (2.2)	0 (0)
Erythema multiforme	4 (1.8)	2 (50.0)
Toxic epidermal necrolysis	3 (1.3)	0 (0)
Stevens–Johnson syndrome	2 (0.9)	1 (50.0)
Exfoliative dermatitis	2 (0.9)	1 (50.0)
Systemic lupus erythematosus–like eruption	1 (0.4)	0 (0)
TOTAL	225 (100.0)	128 (56.9)

Compiled from Ref. 17.

TABLE 97–3. Selected Drugs Associated with Maculopapular Eruptions

Allopurinol	Nitrofurantoin
Azithromycin	Ofloxacin
Barbiturates	Penicillamine
Benzodiazepines	Penicillins
Captopril	Phenothiazines
Carbamazepine	Phenylbutazone
Chloramphenicol	Phenytoin
Ciprofloxacin	Piroxicam
Enalapril	Pyrazolon derivatives
Erythromycin	Rifampin
Ethionamide	Sertraline
Etoposide	Streptomycin
Gold salts	Sulfonamides (includes sulfonylureas and thiazides)
Hydantoin derivatives	Sulindac
Ibuprofen	Tetracyclines
Indomethacin	Tolmentin
Isoniazid	
Nelfinavir	

Compiled from Refs. 8, 9, and 20–24.

PATHOGENESIS

Although the variable and unpredictable course of these eruptions makes classification of the reaction difficult, some maculopapular reactions are possibly due to cell-mediated immune response. This has been suggested by skin testing, lymphocyte transformation, and macrophage migration inhibition tests.[13,19] Humoral immune-complex mechanisms also have been suggested.[13]

▶ TREATMENT: Maculopapular Eruptions

Generally, maculopapular reactions fade within a few days after discontinuation of the offending agent, and thus patient history and temporal relation to drug exposure often may be major diagnostic clues. Patients usually receive palliative treatment with tepid or cool water baths or compresses. Systemic antihistamines may be added for pruritus. Severe reactions may be treated with a short-term course of a systemic corticosteroid.[6]

URTICARIA, ANGIOEDEMA, AND ANAPHYLAXIS

CLINICAL PRESENTATION

Urticarial reactions are the second most common cutaneous manifestation of drug allergy. Lesions consist of raised, well-defined, pruritic, erythematous wheals (hives) that are highly variable in size and number. Urticarial lesions may manifest as a single focus at the site of an injection or may appear as a large, generalized eruption with numerous lesions extending over the chest or trunk. These lesions are unique in that they are evanescent or transient, disappearing within a matter of hours; however, new ones may continue to appear until the offending agent is eliminated from the system. Urticaria also occasionally can be accompanied by vesicle formation.

Typically, the course of drug-induced urticaria is acute, occurring within 12 to 36 hours and resolving within 1 to 3 days of exposure. Chronic urticaria usually has been present at least 6 weeks and has a more prolonged, sometimes relatively indefinite course. Other symptoms that may accompany urticaria in late reactions include fever, lymphadenopathy, joint swelling, and arthralgias. In some cases, urticaria may be the first manifestation of anaphylaxis, thus indicating close monitoring for any swelling around the lips or tongue or for tightness of breath. Anaphylactic syndrome is characterized by the acute onset of skin and mucosal lesions and progression to gastrointestinal symptoms, peripheral vascular collapse, and shock. Urticarial reactions can be caused by food, allergens, infection, temperature changes, and drugs[9,20,21,25] (Table 97–4).

PATHOGENESIS

Immunologically, urticarial lesions are caused by IgE-dependent circulating immune complexes. Mast cells and basophils play a central role in the pathogenesis of these immediate reactions by their affinity for IgE. Various drugs or foreign substances do not require an allergic mechanism to liberate histamine and can produce urticaria. Certain amines may displace histamine from intracellular storage sites, whereas other drugs directly degranulate mast cells through complement or arachidonic acid–dependent pathways.[9,18,28] Examples of nonimmunologic drugs that cause histamine release include acetylsalicylic acid, atropine, opiates, quinine, thiamine, pilocarpine, iodinated radiocontrast dyes, and nonsteroidal anti-inflammatory drugs. Because immunologic and nonimmunologic reactions are indistinguishable clinically, differential diagnosis can be made by immunologic investigations.[9,13,19]

TABLE 97–4. Selected Drugs Associated with Urticaria, Angioedema, and Anaphylaxis

Acetylsalicylic acid	Insulin	Opiates
Amitriptyline	Interleukin-2	Penicillins
Bisacodyl	Iodinated radiocontrast media	Ranitidine
Celecoxib	Mannitol	Rofecoxib
Cyclophosphamide	Mesna	Senna
Filgrastim	Metoclopramide	Sulfonamides
Gold	Naproxen	Sulindac
Heparin	Nizatidine	Tolmentin
Ibuprofen	Omeprazole	
Indomethacin		

Compiled from Refs. 9, 20, 21, 25, and 26.

▶ TREATMENT: Urticaria, Angioedema, and Anaphylaxis

The primary treatment of urticaria involves identification of the offending agent and subsequent discontinuation. Because urticaria is mediated by histamine, various antihistamines such as diphenhydramine, chlorpheniramine, hydroxyzine and its active metabolite, cetirizine, as well as newer, less sedating agents, have been used. Doxepin exhibits affinity for both H_1 and H_2 receptors and has been shown to be effective in those unresponsive to conventional antihistamines.[28,29] Topical doxepin 5% cream also has been evaluated but does not appear to be as effective and has potential for systemic absorption and sensitization.[29] Other topical agents other than mild antipruritic agents are not very useful, and classic topical antihistamines (such as diphenhydramine) are best avoided because of their high incidence of contact sensitization.[28,30]

FIXED-DRUG ERUPTIONS

CLINICAL PRESENTATION

A typical fixed-drug reaction, presenting as an erythematous or hyperpigmented round or oval lesion, is distinctive in behavior and appearance. Lesions may range in size from a few millimeters to nearly 20 cm in diameter.[9] These lesions usually change color from a pale red to a dusky red or violaceous hue over a brief period of time. A gray-brown hyperpigmented spot persists and deepens in color with each exposure to the medication. Although lesions can occur on any part of the skin or mucosal membranes, there seems to be a preference for the oral mucosa and genitalia.[19,31] Often patients complain of pruritus and a painful burning sensation. An important characteristic of this disease is recurrence of the eruption (within 30 minutes to 8 hours) in the exact location as the previous reaction on reexposure, hence the term *fixed-drug eruption*.[31]

PATHOGENESIS

The pathogenesis of this cutaneous reaction is still not well understood. Typically, a single drug is responsible for the reaction, although some patients react to chemically related compounds.[31] The sole cause of fixed-drug reactions is thought to be due to drugs or chemicals[9,21,25] (Table 97–5). Diagnosis typically is confirmed by histology.[9,31] Histopathologic examinations suggest that there is a lymphocyte-mediated attack on epidermal cells that leads to the lichenoid tissue injury.[32]

TABLE 97–5. Selected Drugs Associated with Fixed-Drug Eruptions

Barbiturates	Gold	Phenylbutazone
Carbamazepine	Griseofulvin	Quinidine
Dapsone	Hydralazine	Sulfasalazine
Digoxin	Hydroxyurea	Sulfonamides
Dimenhydrinate	Ibuprofen	Sulindac
Diphenhydramine	Ipecac	Tetracyclines
Disulfiram	Metronidazole	Trimethoprim
Epinephrine	Phenolphthalein	
Erythromycin	Phenothiazines	

Compiled from Refs. 9, 21, 23, and 25.

▶ TREATMENT: Fixed-Drug Reactions

Systemic corticosteroids and antihistamines often are used, but they typically have minimal or no apparent effect on the course of fixed-drug eruptions.[31] The offending drug should be removed and not readministered because the reaction may extend to additional areas of skin and mucous membranes and also may progress to formation of bullous lesions in some patients.[9] Conservative measures are useful occasionally, including cool water compresses during the short acute phase and perhaps bleaching creams for hyperpigmentation in the chronic phase.[19,31,32]

PHOTOSENSITIVITY

CLINICAL PRESENTATION

Photosensitivity is a broad term used to describe adverse reactions to light energy. Sun- and drug-induced photoreactions are more common due to increased use of tanning booths and increased number of photosensitizing chemicals in cosmetics and drugs[9,13,19,20,25,33] (Table 97–6). Clinically, these reactions appear very similar to a sunburn and can include erythema, edema, papules, and plaquelike perhaps urticarial lesions, sometimes with vesicle formation. The hallmark of photosensitivity eruptions is appearance on areas of skin that receive the greatest exposure to sunlight (the tops of the ears, nose, cheeks, lateral and lower posterior surfaces of the neck, extensor surfaces of the forearms, and dorsa of the hands).[9] In some cases, the eruption can occur on non-sun-exposed areas and become generalized over the body.[34] Chronically, reactions may become hyperpigmented or hypopigmented, perhaps atrophic, and with yellowish papules as well as telangiectasias.

PATHOGENESIS

Photosensitivity is a phenomenon that can be further subgrouped into *phototoxic* reactions and *photoallergic* reactions. Phototoxicity, a nonimmunologic reaction, resembles a sunburn and appears to be dose-dependent.[25] It occurs secondary to ingestion or topical application of an agent that potentiates solar energy. The drug acts as a chromophore and absorbs ultraviolet light (potentially ultraviolet A and/or ultraviolet B), causing damage to adjacent tissue. Clinically, patients respond with erythema, pain, and possibly frank blistering within 30 minutes to several hours after exposure. Most of the damage is present on exposed skin only. Histologically, dermal edema, dyskeratosis, and necrosis of keratinocytes can be seen.[33]

A photoallergic reaction is less common and involves an immunologic mechanism; thus there is a delay between exposure to the drug and the onset of eruption.[20,25] The presumed mechanism is that of a type IV cell-mediated hypersensitivity response. It is postulated that ultraviolet light (ultraviolet A and B are both capable of having active spectra, depending on the drug) reacts with the drug or metabolite in the skin to produce a hapten. This hapten combines with a tissue antigen to form a complete antigen, eliciting an allergic response on subsequent exposure.[9] Once sensitization is achieved, minimal amounts of drug usually are needed to produce a reaction.[9] The initial eruption, a papulovesicular eczematous dermatitis, occurs from 1 to 14 days after exposure. Histopathologic findings are similar to those of contact dermatitis.[9,33]

TABLE 97–6. Selected Drugs Associated with Photosensitivity Reactions

Amiodarone	Phenylbutazone
Barbiturates	Piroxicam
Benzodiazepines	Promethazine
Carbamazepine	Protryptyline
Chlorothiazide	Psoralens
Chlorpromazine	Quinidine
Dacarbazine	Simvastatin
5-Fluorouracil	Sulfonamides
Furosemide	Sulfonylureas
Ketoprofen	Sulindac
Mitomycin C	Tetracyclines
Naproxen	Thiazides
Oral contraceptives	

Compiled from Refs. 9, 13, 19, 20, 25, 33, and 39.

▶ TREATMENT: Photosensitivity

Appropriate treatment of photosensitivity depends on the type of reaction. Managing patients with phototoxic reactions parallels that of routine burn care and avoidance of agents that may cause phototoxicity. Systemic and topical antihistamines and corticosteroids have been shown to be ineffective.[33] For patients with acute photoallergic reactions, topical corticosteroids and antihistamines can be used for symptomatic relief. Prednisone, starting at 1 mg/kg per day and tapered over 3 weeks, can be effective for highly symptomatic individuals. In both scenarios, avoidance of sunlight and appropriate use of sunscreens that block ultraviolet A and B are indicated.[19,33,35,36]

ALOPECIA

CLINICAL PRESENTATION

Alopecia, most commonly affecting the scalp, is characterized by localized or generalized hair loss. Drug-induced hair loss usually presents as a diffuse, nonscarring alopecia that is reversible after drug discontinuation. Because of other causes of alopecia—such as infections, thyroid disease, anemia, and trauma—diagnosis of drug-induced hair loss may be difficult.[25] Selected offending agents are included in Table 97–7.[20,25,37,38]

TABLE 97–7. Selected Drugs Associated with Alopecia

Anticonvulsants	Hydroxyurea
Busulfan	Interferon-α
Carbamazepine	Isotretinoin
Clofibrate	Methotrexate
Colchicine	Mitoxantrone
Cyclophosphamide	Oral contraceptives
Doxorubicin	Propranolol
Ethionamide	Tricyclic antidepressants
Etretinate	Valproate sodium
Filgrastim	Vitamin A, high dose
Heparin	Warfarin
Hydantoin derivatives	

Compiled from Refs. 20, 25, 37, and 38.

PATHOGENESIS

Drug-induced alopecia results from damage to proliferating cells in the anagen (actively growing) hair follicle. This results in a thin, fragile hair shaft that breaks even with minor trauma.[37] Certain agents, such as thioamides, used to treat hyperthyroidism, cause a dose-dependent hair loss and also change the texture of hair to dry, brittle, and lusterless.[9] In women on oral contraceptive therapy, sufficient progesterone stimulation via androgenic effects may cause reversible alopecia.[40]

▶ TREATMENT: Alopecia

Management of drug-induced alopecia depends on the etiology of the hair loss. Most cases are reversible on discontinuation of the drug. To best determine a particular drug cause, hair regrowth with drug discontinuation and reexacerbation of the problem on reexposure should be observed. In some patients receiving chemotherapy, a scalp-cooling method has been evaluated to induce vasoconstriction of blood vessels, thus resulting in decreased drug levels to hair follicles. The efficacy of this treatment has been highly variable.[37] Other methods of treatment include topical minoxidil and oral finasteride.[20]

VASCULITIS

CLINICAL PRESENTATION

Vasculitis is characterized by inflammation and damage of blood vessels that may affect various organ systems. It commonly appears on the lower extremities or pressure-dependent areas of the skin as erythematous or violaceous lesions. Lesions, ranging in size from a pinpoint to several centimeters, often are macular but may be palpable with variable morphology.[41] Urticarial lesions may coexist with purpura, and in severe cases, development of vesicular, bullous, hemorrhagic, ulcerating, or necrotic lesions may be seen. Lesions may persist for weeks and in some cases become yellow to brown during resolution.[41] Systemic symptoms such as burning, stinging, malaise, arthralgias, and fever also may be present. Other manifestations, such as involvement of the liver, kidney, brain, and joints, also may be present. Some drug causes of vasculitis are listed in Table 97–8.[9,13,18]

TABLE 97–8. Selected Drugs Associated with Vasculitis

Allopurinol	Indomethacin	Quinine
Anticoagulants	Penicillins	Rituximab
Cimetidine	Phenylbutazone	Sulfonamides
Fluoxetine	Phenytoin	Thiazides
Hydralazine	Piroxicam	
Ibuprofen	Propylthiouracil	

Compiled from Refs. 9, 13, 18, and 42.

PATHOGENESIS

Although it is difficult to pinpoint the etiology of most vasculitides, it is possible that free antigen is present in circulating blood. Complexation with IgE antibodies and the resulting release of histamine leads to increased vascular permeability and allows immune complexes from the circulation to migrate to target tissue, fix complement, and lyse cells.

▶ TREATMENT: Vasculitis

Palliative treatment with bed rest and compression of lesions may promote healing. Oral corticosteroids, cyclophosphamide, plasmapheresis, indomethacin, dapsone, colchicine, and aspirin also have been used in treatment.[41]

HYPERPIGMENTATION

DRUGS THAT MAY CAUSE PIGMENTARY CHANGES

Changes in skin color may be caused by the drug itself, disturbances in melanin formation, or both.[34] Drugs known to induce pigmentary changes include hydantoins, metals[9,36] (Table 97–9), antimalarials, phenothiazines, oral contraceptives, tetracyclines, chemotherapeutic agents (Table 97–10), and amiodarone.[43,44]

ANTICONVULSANTS

Anticonvulsants, such as phenytoin, phenobarbital, and carbamazepine, have been reported to produce a brown patchy hyperpigmentation on light-exposed areas.[9] Individuals who take these

TABLE 97–9. Heavy Metal–Induced Hyperpigmentation

Agent	Color	Region Involved	Special Features
Mercury	Gray-brown, slate green	Skin folds (topical), gingival pigmentation (systemic)	Caused by deposition of metallic granules and increased melanin production; formerly used in bleaching agents.
Silver	Slate gray, blue-gray	Sun-exposed areas, mucosa, sclerae, nails	Silver granule deposition that activates melanin production; occurs months to years after ingestion.
Bismuth	Blue gray	Skin, conjunctiva, oral and vaginal mucosa, black line along gingival margin	Deposition of metallic granules or interaction with bacteria in mouth; more common with parenteral use.
Arsenic	Brown, bronze	Trunk, "raindrop"-shaped hyperkeratotic papulonodular lesions; palms, soles	Activates enzymes that form melanin and deposit in skin; used systemically for psoriasis and as a health tonic; pigmentation appears 1–20 years after exposure.
Gold	Blue-gray	Periorbital, generalized chrysiasis, sun-exposed areas	Caused by deposition of metallic particles in epidermis; occurs months to years after exposure and is permanent.

Compiled from Refs. 9 and 43.

TABLE 97–14. Selected Drugs Associated with Drug-Induced SLE

Most Common	Good Evidence	
Hydralazine	Atenolol	Minocycline
Procainamide	Carbamazepine	Penicillamine
Quinidine	Chlorpromazine	Phenytoin
	Isoniazid	Sulfasalazine
	Methyldopa	Thiazides

Compiled from Refs. 11, 19, 21, 44, 46, 66, and 67.

can be subdivided into four types[11]:

1. Induction of SLE in patients who have never had SLE.
2. Aggravation of SLE, usually systemic.
3. Induction of cutaneous discoid or subacute lupus erythematosus.
4. Induction of serologic changes only: Antinuclear antibodies are of a different type—lupus erythematosus cells.

Selected drugs implicated in inducing lupus are listed in Table 97–14.[11,19,21,44,46,66,67]

PATHOGENESIS

Autoantibody responses in idiopathic and drug-induced lupus are similar in that both are characterized by antinuclear antibodies. However, titers of anti-double stranded DNA can be seen in idiopathic lupus, whereas this is found rarely (<1%) in drug-induced lupus. In addition, antihistone antibody occurs in a higher percentage of patients with drug-induced lupus.[67]

▶ TREATMENT: Drug-Induced SLE

Withdrawal of the offending medication is the mainstay of treatment for drug-induced lupus. Symptomatic treatment, such as nonsteroidal anti-inflammatory agents for arthralgias, also may be helpful. In patients with cutaneous or systemic manifestations, corticosteroids and/or immunosuppressants may be administered.[65]

ANTICOAGULANT-INDUCED SKIN NECROSIS AND PURPLE TOE SYNDROME

Although anticoagulants such as heparin and warfarin are commonly used medicines, an estimated 0.01% to 0.1% of patients receiving anticoagulant therapy develop skin necrosis.[68]

WARFARIN

CLINICAL PRESENTATION

Of patients with reported warfarin-induced skin necrosis, 85% are female, whereas the purple toe syndrome occurs predominately in males. Skin necrosis generally occurs between the third and tenth day of treatment. Patients typically complain of a sudden onset of cold or painful sensation, followed by well-demarcated erythematous lesions that usually progress to purpuric and hemorrhagic areas. These lesions occur in areas of subcutaneous fatty tissue and commonly involve the breasts, thighs, buttocks, and penis. Histologically, skin necrosis due to warfarin presents very specifically with hemorrhage and breakdown of precapillary arterioles.[69]

The purple toe syndrome is a rare complication of warfarin therapy. Most lesions typically develop 3 to 8 weeks after initiation of anticoagulation and are characterized by the sudden appearance of bilateral violaceous discoloration on the toes and sides of the feet. The affected area is cold and tender to touch, although some patients have reported a burning sensation. Most patients who develop warfarin-induced skin necrosis have been receiving anticoagulation for venous thrombosis, whereas those who develop purple toe syndrome typically have been receiving anticoagulation in association with atrial fibrillation or chronic heart failure.[68,70]

PATHOGENESIS

Patients receiving excessive initial doses of warfarin, thus causing a severe and rapid depression of factor VII and protein C, have presented with skin necrosis attributed to a hypercoagulable state.[68,69] Other mechanisms, including cytokines such as tumor necrosis factor (TNF) and direct toxicity to epithelial cells by warfarin, have been proposed. Finally, immunologically mediated hypersensitivity also has been considered.[71]

▶ TREATMENT: Warfarin-Induced Skin Necrosis

Rapid reversal with vitamin K can be initiated if skin necrosis is discovered early in anticoagulant therapy. Intravenous anticoagulation with heparin should be initiated while warfarin is discontinued. Since most indications for warfarin require long-term treatment, reinitiation of warfarin at lower doses has been well documented. Interestingly, a majority of patients previously affected with skin necrosis are not likely to redevelop lesions on reinitiation of anticoagulant therapy.[68–70] Approximately 50% of patients require surgical intervention, such as debridement, skin grafting, and amputation.[70] Other immediate treatments such as vasodilation, steroids, vitamin C, and sympathetic nerve blocks have been evaluated without documented success.[69]

HEPARIN

CLINICAL PRESENTATION

The frequency of heparin-induced skin necrosis is extremely low and clinically indistinguishable from warfarin-induced skin necrosis. Lesions typically involve the abdominal wall, upper and lower extremities, and hands. Generally occurring within 5 to 10 days of initiation of therapy, heparin-induced skin necrosis can occur regardless of the route of administration.[68] Case reports of low-molecular-weight heparins inducing skin necrosis also have been documented.[72]

PATHOGENESIS

In contrast to warfarin-induced skin necrosis, patients who have developed heparin-induced necrosis do not have deficiencies in the coagulation pathways. Heparin-induced thrombocytopenia has been postulated as a possible etiologic factor. In addition, although the significance of the association is unknown, greater than 80% of reported patients had comorbid conditions such as hypertension, diabetes mellitus, malignancy, and connective tissue disorders.[68]

▶ TREATMENT: Heparin-Induced Skin Necrosis

Immediate cessation of the offending agent is required because heparin-induced skin necrosis is associated with high mortality. The risk of redevelopment of skin necrosis due to reinstitution of heparin therapy has not been evaluated; thus the risk is unknown.[68]

NEUTROPHILIC ECCRINE HIDRADENITIS

CLINICAL PRESENTATION

Neutrophilic eccrine hidradenitis (NEH) is an inflammatory dermatosis that primarily affects eccrine glands and is seen most commonly in patients undergoing chemotherapy. Erythematous macules, papules, plaques, and nodules are clinical manifestations, whereas the neutrophilic infiltrate of eccrine glands and degeneration of these cells are seen histologically.[73] In some cases, fever has been the presenting symptom; thus infection must be ruled out.

PATHOGENESIS

There are three described mechanisms of NEH: (1) a cutaneous manifestation of acute myelogenous leukemia, (2) a toxic effect of cytarabine, and (3) a neutrophilic dermatosis within a spectrum.[73] Chemotherapeutic agents capable of concentrating in the eccrine sweat glands depend on the partition coefficient and dissociation constant of the drug. The drug concentrates in sweat and causes local cutaneous reactions secondary to inflammation and destruction of sweat glands. Some drugs associated with NEH are listed in Table 97–15.[73–75]

▶ TREATMENT: Neutrophilic Eccrine Hidradenitis

Typically, clinical manifestations of neutrophilic eccrine hidradenitis resolve within 1 to 4 weeks without treatment. Systemic corticosteroids may be useful in patients with fever and symptomatic lesions, but preferably with no evidence of infection.[74]

TABLE 97–15. Selected Drugs Associated with Neutrophilic Eccrine Hidradenitis

Acetaminophen	Doxorubicin
Bleomycin	Lomustine
Chlorambucil	Mitoxantrone
Cyclophosphamide	Zidovudine
Cytarabine	

Compiled from Refs. 73–75.

SEVERE SKIN REACTIONS

For several decades, the nomenclature and classification of severe, sometimes life-threatening skin reactions have been much debated. There is disagreement whether erythema multiforme (EM), Stevens-Johnson syndrome (SJS), and toxic epidermal necrolysis (TEN) are distinctive diseases or are all within a single *erythema multiforme spectrum*.[76–78] A consensus classification was proposed by an international group of dermatologists that is based on the patterns of skin lesions and on the extent of epidermal detachment (Table 97–16).[76]

ERYTHEMA MULTIFORME AND STEVENS-JOHNSON SYNDROME

CLINICAL PRESENTATION

EM is an acute cutaneous reaction of variable morphology that evolves and changes over time. Typically, the hands, feet, face, limbs, and mucous membranes are the sites affected, with possible nonspecific prodromal symptoms such as an upper respiratory infection. Initially, a round 1- to 10-cm erythematous macule may appear that becomes edematous and papular over time.[79] These lesions may enlarge into plaques or form an erythematous periphery, while the center clears, becoming cyanotic or purpuric and forming an "iris" or target lesion.[80] Lesions begin to resolve in 4 to 5 days, with complete healing in 2 to 4 weeks, although new lesions can continue to appear during this period.[79] In addition, postinflammatory hyperpigmentation can occur without healing.

SJS is considered a severe variant of EM with extensive mucosal and conjunctival edema, erosions, high fever, myalgias, vomiting, diarrhea, and arthralgias. Skin lesions may be severe with large bullae and areas of denudation. The onset of these lesions is variable, but healing usually occurs within 6 weeks. Complications include

TABLE 97–16. Classification of Severe Skin Reactions

Type	Lesions	Epidermal Detachment
Bullous erythema multiforme	Localized typical lesions, or raised atypical targets, primarily on extremites	<10% of body surface area
Stevens–Johnson syndrome (SJS)	Purpuric macules or flat atypical targets on trunk	<10% of body surface area
SJS/Toxic epidermal necrolysis (TEN) overlap	Widespread purpuric macules or flat atypical targets	10%–30% of body surface area
TEN with maculae	Purpuric macules or flat atypical targets	>30% of body surface area
TEN on large erythema	Large epidermal sheets without purpuric macules or target lesions	>10% of body surface area

Compiled from Ref. 76.

TABLE 97–17. Selected Drugs Associated with Erythema Multiforme/Stevens-Johnson Syndrome

Acetaminophen	Macrolides	Propranolol
Allopurinol	Methazolamide	Quinolones
Carbamazepine	Penicillins	Sulfadiazine
Cephalosporins	Phenobarbital	Sulfonamides
Cotrimoxazole	Phenylbutazone	Thiazides
Ibuprofen	Phenytoin	Valproic acid

Compiled from Refs. 77, 82, 86, 87, 91, and 95.

TABLE 97–18. Selected Drugs Associated with Toxic Epidermal Necrolysis

Acetaminophen	Indomethacin	Ranitidine
Allopurinol	Lamotrigine	Sulfonamides
Barbiturates	Macrolides	Sulindac
Carbamazepine	Penicillins	Tetracyclines
Chloramphenicol	Phenylbutazone	Tolmetin
Ibuprofen	Phenytoin	Valproic acid
Imidazole antifungal agents (e.g., ketoconazole)	Quinine	
	Quinolones	

Compiled from Refs. 87 and 90–96.

keratitis, conjunctival scarring, blindness, pneumonia, dehydration, and esophagitis.[79]

PATHOGENESIS

Although various etiologic factors have been identified, the exact pathogenesis remains unknown. There is evidence that indicates that both an immune-complex mechanism and cell-mediated immune reactivity may be involved.[77] Another theory suggests that cytotoxic T cells release TNF-α , causing keratinocyte degeneration.[77] Further, it also has been proposed that patients with EM SJS are phenotypically slow acetylators of drugs.[77,80] Identification of the etiologic factor is also difficult because EM may be precipitated by a wide variety of factors. Although various medications (Table 97–17) and herpes simplex virus (HSV) are the most frequent causes of EM, there are other precipitating causes such as bacteria, fungi, vaccines, and other diseases.[78–81]

Diagnosis of EM is based primarily on history, clinical appearance, and histology. Histopathologically, it has been shown that eosinophils were present more commonly in EM/SJS than in other severe diseases, such as TEN.[83] Often, prodromal symptoms are treated with antibiotics; thus etiology (i.e., virus, bacteria, or drug) is difficult to clarify.

▶ TREATMENT: Erythema Multiforme and Stevens–Johnson Syndrome

Because mild forms of EM are self-limiting, symptomatic therapy such as antihistamines for pruritus, tap water compresses for blisters and necrosis, and half-strength hydrogen peroxide gargles for oral lesions may be instituted. Careful monitoring for progression to more severe forms or development of complications is essential. The efficacy of using systemic corticosteroids for severe EM and SJS is not clearly defined.[84–86] Typically, EM resolves within 2 to 3 weeks, but recurrences are common, especially if the EM is due to recurrent HSV infections.[81] Interestingly, concurrent intracranial radiation and phenytoin apparently lead to an increased risk of SJS. Additional reactive metabolites as a result of combined radiation and phenytoin may be responsible for this unusual drug reaction.[82]

TOXIC EPIDERMAL NECROLYSIS

CLINICAL PRESENTATION

TEN is a severe reaction of the skin characterized by erythema and extensive detachment of the epidermis (necrolysis). Although it is a rare disease, TEN is associated with a relatively high mortality rate.[77,87] Typically, there is a prodromal state with nonspecific symptoms such as fever, cough, sore throat, pyrexia, and myalgia, followed by an acute onset of cutaneous manifestations occurring within 1 to 3 days. The eruption may present in various forms, often as a macular lesion with a burning sensation that becomes widespread over the body. The lesions may form large flaccid bullae within the erythema or progress directly to massive detachment of the epidermis. At this point, the epidermis is easily sloughed by light mechanical pressure, with outer coverings of ruptured bullae clinging to underlying tissue. This appearance of a sheetlike loss of epidermis is most characteristic of TEN. Because lesions may appear on any area of skin (e.g., palms, soles, mouth, throat, nose, trachea, eyelids, conjunctiva, cornea, and vagina), the picture may be similar to a second-degree burn or scald. Although virtually the entire skin surface may be involved with close to 100% of the epidermis, the hairy areas of the scalp seem not to be affected.[87]

Complications are numerous and include fluid and electrolyte imbalance from the loss of epidermis, septicemia, corneal ulcerations, and conjunctivitis. Systemic involvement is also common and may be due to the same process that destroys the epidermis.[87] Internal manifestations include dysphagia, gastrointestinal ulceration, hepatocellular damage, pneumonia, nephritis, and myocardial damage. Normocytic anemia, leukopenia, granulocytopenia, and neutropenia also are commonly present.[87–89]

PATHOGENESIS

Pathogenic mechanisms responsible for TEN are attributed to defective control of keratinocyte apoptosis, mediated by a cell surface death receptor F_{as} and its ligand, CD95L.[89] The onset of TEN after drug exposure suggests an immunologic-mediated reaction.[87,88] A TEN-like eruption has occurred in patients with a graft-versus-host reaction after bone marrow transplant or blood transfusion.[80,89] Although there is no reliable test to prove correlations, drugs are the main cause of TEN (Table 97–18).[87,90–94] Other reported causes include bacterial, viral, and fungal infections, as well as chemicals, immunizations, and malignancies.[90–96]

The prognosis for TEN depends on the patient's age, extent of skin involvement, concurrent diseases, and complications.[13] Mortality is estimated at about 3% within the first 3 to 4 days of the acute episode.[13,87] After the acute episode, the epidermis may regenerate within 2 to 3 weeks, with complete healing usually in less than 6 weeks.

▶ TREATMENT: Toxic Epidermal Necrolysis

Management of TEN must include immediate identification and withdrawal of the precipitating factor. The principles of symptomatic treatments are essentially the same as for burn patients.[87] Therapy includes IVIG[90] and fluid and electrolyte maintenance, treatment or prevention of infections, prevention of ocular complications, and aggressive nutritional support.

Although the empirical use of systemic corticosteroid therapy is well documented, it is controversial because of a lack of well-controlled studies.[84,85] Some clinicians advocate corticosteroid use only within the first 48 to 72 hours of onset to prevent progression of complications[91]; others attribute delayed morbidity to systemic steroid use.[88] Other treatment modalities include plasmapheresis, cyclosporine, and cyclophosphamide.[87]

REFERENCES

1. Shapiro S, Slone D, Siskind V, et al. Drug rash with ampicillin and other penicillins. Lancet 1969;2:969–972.
2. Johnson M, Johnson KG, Engel A. Prevalence, morbidity, and cost of dermatologic diseases. J Am Acad Dermatol 1984;11:930–936.
3. Baer RL, Witten VM, eds. Drug eruptions. In: Yearbook of Dermatology 1960–1961 Series. Chicago, Year Book, 1961:9–37.
4. Witte K, West DP. Immunology of adverse reactions to drugs. Pharmacotherapy 1982;2:54–65.
5. Witte KW, West DP. Immunology of adverse reactions to antimicrobial agents. In: Jeljaszewicz J, Pulverer G, eds. Antimicrobial Agents and Immunity. London, Academic Press, 1986:217–249.
6. Arndt KA. Drug eruptions, allergic. In: Arndt KA, ed. Manual of Dermatologic Therapeutics, 5th ed. Boston, Little, Brown, 1995:60–63.
7. Bruinsma W. Drug monitoring in dermatology. Int J Dermatol 1986;25:166–168.
8. DeShazo RD, Kemp SF. Allergic reactions to drugs and biologic agents. JAMA 1997;278:1895–1906.
9. Bruinsma W. A Guide to Drug Eruptions, 6th ed. Oosthuizen, Netherlands, De Zwaluw, 1995.
10. Litt JZ. Drug eruption reference manual 2001. New York, Parthenon Publishing Group, 2001.
11. Zurcher K, Krebs A, eds. Cutaneous drug reactions: An integral synopsis of today's systemic drugs. Basel, Switzerland, Karger, 1992.
12. Merk HF, Mukhtar H, Hertl M. Drug-induced skin disorders. In: Mukhtar H, ed. Pharmacology of the Skin. Boca Raton, CRC Press, 1992:151–166.
13. Schulz KH. Cutaneous manifestations of drug allergy. In: De Weck AL, Bundgaard H, eds. Allergic Reactions to Drugs. Berlin, Springer-Verlag, 1983:135–162.
14. Roujeau JC, Stern RS. Severe adverse cutaneous reactions to drugs. N Engl J Med 1994;331:1272–1285.
15. Nelson HS. Allergic reactions to drugs. Adv Asthma Allergy 1976;3:18–35.
16. Sullivan TJ. Drug allergy. In: Middleton E Jr, Reed CE, Ellis EF, et al., eds. Allergy Principles and Practice. St. Louis, Mosby–Year Book, 1993:1726–1746.
17. Alanko K, Stubb S, Kauppinen K. Cutaneous drug reactions: Clinical types and causative agents. Acta Derm Venereol (Stockh) 1989;69:223–226.
18. Wintroub BU, Stern R. Cutaneous drug reactions: Pathogenesis and clinical classification. J Am Acad Dermatol 1985;13:167–179.
19. Merk HF, Hertl M. Immunologic mechanisms of cutaneous drug reactions. Semin Cutan Med Surg 1996;15:228–235.
20. Prussick R. Adverse cutaneous reactions to chemotherapeutic agents and cytokine therapy. Semin Cutan Med Surg 1996;15:267–276.
21. Gruppo Italiano Studi Epidemiologici in Dermatologica. Cutaneous reactions to alimentary tract medications: Results of a seven-year surveillance program and review of the literature. Dermatology 1996;193:11–16.
22. Schissel DJ, Singer D, David-Bajar K. Azithromycin eruption in infectious mononucleosis: a proposed mechanism of interaction. Cutis 2000; 65:163–166.
23. Fortuny C, Vicente MA, Medina MM, et al. Rash as a side effect of nelfinavir in children. AIDS 2000;14:335–336.
24. Fernandes B, Brites M, Goncalo M, et al. Maculopapular eruption from sertraline with positive patch tests. Contact Dermatitis 2000;42:287.
25. Garnis-Jones S. Dermatologic side effects of psychopharmacologic agents. Dermatol Clin 1996;14:503–507.
26. Crouch TE, Stafford CT. Urticaria associated with COX-2 inhibitors. Ann Allergy Asthma Immunol 2000;84:140.
27. Saenz de San Pedro B, Quiralte J, Florido JF. Fixed drug eruption caused by dimenhydrinate. Allergy 2000;55:297.
28. Greene SL, Reed CE, Schroeter AL. Double-blind crossover study comparing doxepin with diphenhydramine for the treatment of chronic urticaria. J Am Acad Dermatol 1985;12:669–675.
29. Smith PF, Corelli RL. Doxepin in the management of pruritus associated with allergic cutaneous reactions. Ann Pharmacother 1997;31:633–634.
30. Yaffe SJ, Bierman CW, Cann HM, et al. Antihistamines in topical preparations. Pediatrics 1973;51:299–301.
31. Korkij W, Soltani K. Fixed drug eruption. Arch Dermatol 1984;120: 520–524.
32. Shiohara T, Nickoloff BJ, Sagawa Y, et al. Fixed drug eruption: Expression of epidermal keratinocyte intercellular adhesion molecule-1. Arch Dermatol 1989;125:1371–1376.
33. Wolverton SE. Update on cutaneous reactions. In: James WD, Cockerell CJ, eds. Comprehensive Dermatologic Drug Therapy. St. Louis, Mosby–Year Book, 1997:65–83.
34. Epstein JH, Wintroub BU. Photosensitivity due to drugs. Drugs 1985;30: 42–57.
35. Mammen L, Schmidt CP. Photosensitivity reactions: A case report involving NSAIDs. Am Fam Physician 1995;52:575–578.
36. Robison HN, Morison WL, Hood AF. Thiazide diuretic therapy and chronic photosensitivity. Arch Dermatol 1985;121:522–524.
37. Dawber RBR, Ebling FJG, Wojnarowska FT. Disorders of hair, alopecia of chemical origin. In: Champion RH, Burton JL, Ebling FJG, eds. Textbook of Dermatology, 5th ed. Oxford, Blackwell, 1992:2582–2584.
38. Brodin MB. Drug-related alopecia. Dermatol Clin 1987;5:571–579.
39. Drugs that cause photosensitivity. Med Lett 1986;28:51–52.
40. Jelinek JE. Cutaneous side effects of oral contraceptives. Arch Dermatol 1970;101:181–186.
41. Mackel SE. Treatment of vasculitis. Med Clin North Am 1982;6:941–954.
42. Dereure O, Navarro R, Rossi J-F, et al. Rituximab-induced vasculitis. Dermatology 2001;203:83–84.
43. Granstein RD, Sober AJ. Drug and heavy metal-induced hyperpigmentation. J Am Acad Dermatol 1981;5:1–18.
44. Shapiro LE, Knowles SR, Shear NH. Comparative safety of tetracycline, minocycline, and doxycycline. Arch Dermatol 1997;133:1224–1230.
45. Moller H. Pigmentary disturbances due to drugs. Acta Derm Venereol (Stockh) 1966;46:423–431.
46. Knowles SR, Shapiro L, Shear NH. Serious adverse reactions induced by minocycline: Report of 13 patients and review of the literature. Arch Dermatol 1996;132:934–939.
47. Basler RSW. Minocycline-related hyperpigmentation. Arch Dermatol 1985;121:606–608.
48. Job CK, Yoder L, Jacobson RR, Hastings RC. Skin pigmentation from clofazimine therapy in leprosy patients: A reappraisal. J Am Acad Dermatol 1990;23:236–241.
49. Masur H, Tuazon C, Gill V, et al. Effect of combined clofazimine and ansamycin therapy on *Mycobacterium avium–Mycobacterium intracellulare* bacteremia in patients with AIDS. J Infect Dis 1987;155:127–129.
50. Crovato F, Levi L. Clofazimine in the treatment of annular lupus erythematosus. Arch Dermatol 1981;117:249–250.
51. Michaelson G, Molin L, Ohman S, et al. Clofazimine, a new agent for the treatment of pyoderma gangrenosum. Arch Dermatol 1976;112:344–349.
52. Trimble JW, Mendelson DS, Fetter BF, et al. Cutaneous pigmentation secondary to amiodarone therapy. Arch Dermatol 1983;119:914–918.
53. Huff JC, Weston WL, Tonnesen MG. Erythema multiforme: A critical review of characteristics, diagnostic criteria, and causes. J Am Acad Dermatol 1983;8:763–775.

54. Roujeau JC, Bioulac-Sage P, Bourseau C, et al. Acute generalized exanthematous pustulosis. Arch Dermatol 1991;127:1333–1338.
55. Lazarov A, Livni E, Halevy S. Generalized pustular drug eruptions: Confirmation by in vitro tests. J Eur Acad Dermatol Venereol 1998;10:36–41.
56. Shapiro LE, Shear NH. Mechanisms of drug reactions: The metabolic track. Semin Cutan Med Surg 1996;15:217–227.
57. Beylot C, Doutre MS, Beylot-Barry M. Acute generalized exanthematous pustulosis. Semin Cutan Med Surg 1996;15:244–249.
58. Knowles S, Gupta AK, Shear NH. The spectrum of cutaneous reactions associated with diltiazem: Three cases and a review of the literature. J Am Acad Dermatol 1998;38:201–206.
59. Cannavo SP, Borgia F, Guarneri F, et al. Acute generalized exanthematous pustulosis following use of ticlopidine. Br J Dermatol 2000;142:577–578.
60. Brouard MC, Prins C, Mach-Pascual S, et al. Acute generalized exanthematous pustulosis associated with STI571 in a patient with chronic myeloid leukemia. Dermatology 2001;203:57–59.
61. Thédenat B, Loche F, Albes B, et al. Acute generalized exanthematosus pustulosis with photodistribution pattern induced by sertraline. Dermatology 2001;203:87–88.
62. Bocquet H, Bagot M, Roujeau JC. Drug-induced pseudolymphoma and drug hypersensitivity syndrome (drug rash with eosinophilia and systemic symptoms: DRESS). Semin Cutan Med Surg 1996;15:250–257.
63. Callot V, Roujeau JC, Bagot M, et al. Drug-induced pseudolymphoma and hypersensitivity syndrome. Arch Dermatol 1996;132:1315–1321.
64. Milionis HJ, Skopelitou A, Elisaf MS. Hypersensitivity syndrome caused by amitriptyline administration. Postgrad Med J 2000;76:361–363.
65. Rich MW. Drug-induced lupus: The list of culprits grows. Postgrad Med 1996;100:299–307.
66. McGuiness M, Frye RA, Deng JS. Atenolol-induced lupus erythematosus. J Am Acad Dermatol 1997;37:298–299.
67. Yung RL, Johnson KJ, Richardson BC. New concepts in the pathogenesis of drug-induced lupus. Lab Invest 1996;73:746–759.
68. Sallah S, Thomas DP, Roberts HR. Warfarin and heparin-induced skin necrosis and the purple toe syndrome: Infrequent complications of anticoagulant treatment. Thromb Haemost 1997;78:785–790.
69. DeFranzo AJ, Marasco P, Argenta LC. Warfarin-induced necrosis of the skin. Ann Plast Surg 1995;34:203–208.
70. Jillella AP, Lutcher CL. Reinstituting warfarin in patients who develop warfarin skin necrosis. Am J Hematol 1996;52:117–119.
71. Hermes B, Haas N, Henz BM. Immunopathological events of adverse cutaneous reactions to coumarin and heparin. Acta Derm Venereol (Stockh) 1997;77:35–38.
72. Tonn ME, Schaiff RA, Kollef MH. Enoxaparin-associated dermal necrosis: A consequence of cross-reactivity with heparin-mediated antibodies. Ann Pharmacother 1997;31:323–326.
73. Beutner KR, Packman CH, Markowitch W. Neutrophilic eccrine hidradenitis associated with Hodgkin's disease and chemotherapy. Arch Dermatol 1986;122:809–811.
74. Bernstein EF, Spielvogel RL, Topolsky DL. Recurrent neutrophilic eccrine hidradenitis. Br J Dermatol 1992;127:529–533.
75. Susser W, Witaker-Worth D, Grant-Kels J, et al. Mucocutaneous reactions to chemotherapy. J Am Acad Dermatol 1999;40:367–398.
76. Bastuji-Garin S, Rzany B, Stern RS, et al. Clinical classification of cases of toxic epidermal necrolysis, Stevens-Johnson syndrome, and erythema multiforme. Arch Dermatol 1993;129:92–96.
77. Mockenhaupt M, Schopf E. Epidemiology of drug-induced severe skin reactions. Semin Cutan Med Surg 1996;15:236–243.
78. Assier H, Bastuji-Garin S, Revuz J, et al. Erythema multiforme with mucous membrane involvement and Stevens-Johnson syndrome are clinically different disorders with distinct causes. Arch Dermatol 1995;131:539–543.
79. Huff JC, Weston WL, Tonnesen MG. Erythema multiforme: A critical review of characteristics, diagnostic criteria, and causes. J Am Acad Dermatol 1983;763–775.
80. Fitzpatrick TB, Elsen AZ, Wolff K, et al. Erythema multiforme. In: Fitzpatrick TB, et al, eds. Dermatology in General Medicine, 3d ed. New York, McGraw-Hill, 1987:555–563.
81. Choy AC, Yarnold PR, Brown JE, et al. Virus induced erythema multiforme and Stevens-Johnson syndrome. Allergy Proc 1995;16:157–161.
82. Micali G, Linthicum K, Han NH, West DP. Increased risk of erythema multiforme major when anticonvulsant and radiation therapies are combined. Pharmacotherapy 1999;19:223–227.
83. Rzany B, Hering O, Mockenhaupt M, et al. Histopathological and epidemiological characteristics of patients with erythema exudativum multiforme major, Stevens-Johnson syndrome and toxic epidermal necrolysis. Br J Dermatol 1996;135:6–11.
84. Barton P, Flowers F. Controversies in the management of erythema multiforme and toxic epidermal necrolysis. In: Dahl MV, Lynch PJ, eds. Current Opinion in Dermatology, 2d ed. Philadelphia, Current Science, 1995.
85. Duarte AM, Pruksachatkunakorn C, Schachner LA. Life-threatening dermatoses in pediatric dermatology. In: Callen JP, ed. Advances in Dermatology, Vol. 10. St. Louis, Mosby–Year Book, 1995:329–371.
86. Cheriyan S, Patterson R, Greenberger PA, et al. The outcome of Stevens-Johnson syndrome treated with corticosteroids. Allergy Proc 1995;16:151–155.
87. Revuz JE, Roujeau JC. Advances in toxic epidermal necrolysis. Semin Cutan Med Surg 1996;15:258–266.
88. Westly ED, Wechsler HL. Toxic epidermal necrolysis. Arch Dermatol 1984;120:721–726.
89. Goeens J, Song M, Fondu P. Haematological disturbances and immune mechanisms in toxic epidermal necrolysis. Br J Dermatol 1986;114:255–259.
90. Chaffin JJ, Davis SM. Suspected lamotrigine-induced toxic epidermal necrolysis. Ann Pharmacother 1997;31:720–723.
91. Roujeau JC, Kelly JP, Naldi L, et al. Medication use and the risk of Stevens-Johnson syndrome or toxic epidermal necrolysis. N Engl J Med 1995;333:1600–1607.
92. Halevi A, Ben-Amitai D, Garty BZ. Toxic epidermal necrolysis associated with acetaminophen ingestion. Ann Pharmacother 2000;34:32–34.
93. Velez A, Moreno J-C. Second case of ranitidine-related toxic epidermal necrolysis in a patient with idiopathic thrombocytopenic purpura. J Am Acad Dermatol 2000;42:305.
94. Fritsch P, Sidroff A. Drug-induced Stevens-Johnson syndrome/toxic epidermal necrolysis. Am J Clin Dermatol 2000;6:349–360.
95. Shirato S, Kagaya F, Suzuki Y, et al. Stevens-Johnson syndrome induced by methazolamide treatment. Arch Ophthalmol 1997;115:550–553.
96. Stella M, Cassano P, Bollero D, et al. Toxic epidermal necrolysis treated with intravenous high-dose immunoglobulins: Our experience. Dermatology 2001;203:45–49.

98
HEMATOPOIESIS

William P. Petros and Gwynn D. Long

Hematopoiesis is defined as the formation and maturation of blood cells and their derivatives. There is a tremendous daily turnover rate of cells in this system, with more than 6 billion cells produced per kilogram of body weight every 24 hours.[1] These accelerated processes result in vastly exaggerated and rapid responses to the slightest perturbation.

In humans, hematopoiesis takes place primarily in the bone marrow. Hematopoietic cells were among the first to be evaluated for their biologic functions and pattern of maturation, and recent identification of the protein molecules (cytokines) that seem to regulate this system has yielded an extraordinary amount of new information regarding its control. The process of continual hematopoietic cell production is complicated, involving interactions between immature cells, the surrounding microenvironment, and cytokines.

HEMATOPOETIC SYSTEM

The hematopoietic system consists of three primary cell components: leukocytes, platelets, and erythrocytes. The first group encompasses a functionally diverse group of cells that includes neutrophils, eosinophils, basophils, monocytes/macrophages, lymphocytes, and plasma cells. Typical concentrations of mature hematopoietic cells found in the peripheral blood of adults are shown in Table 98–1.

LEUKOCYTES

NEUTROPHILS (SEGS AND BANDS)

The major functions of neutrophils (also known as polymorphonuclear leukocytes) are to prevent pathogenic microorganism invasion and to localize and kill these microorganisms if they do invade the body. These effects are mediated by a series of events, including migration to the site (chemotaxis), recognition/attachment to the invader, phagocytosis, lysosomal fusion, degranulation, and local generation of oxidants (respiratory burst) and degrading enzymes (Fig. 98–1).[2] A neutrophil is attracted to the site of infection by chemotactic factors. Once migration to the site has occurred, the neutrophil ingests the opsonized microorganism. (Opsonization is the process whereby antibody and complement coat the microorganism, allowing for increased neutrophil recognition.) Following ingestion or phagocytosis, the cytoplasmic granules within the neutrophil fuse with the phagosome or phagocytosed microorganism, thereby initiating degranulation and release of enzymes. These degrading enzymes kill the microorganism through oxygen reduction. Secretion of these enzymes may also result in localized host-tissue injury. The actions of cytokines such as granulocyte colony-stimulating factor (G-CSF) and granulocyte-macrophage colony-stimulating factor (GM-CSF) may intensify neutrophil activity.[3]

EOSINOPHILS

Although eosinophils are less efficient than neutrophils, they elicit similar effector functions. Eosinophil activity is directed primarily against large invaders, such as helminths and other parasites that cannot be phagocytized. During an allergic reaction, activated mast cells secrete chemicals that attract and stimulate eosinophils, which in turn produce substances that neutralize or degrade the reaction products of mast cells. Unfortunately, the eosinophil constituents may also damage normal tissue and cause secondary histamine release. High concentrations of eosinophils for prolonged periods may result in damage to the cardiac and central nervous systems, with possible pulmonary and dermatologic involvement.[4]

BASOPHILS AND MAST CELLS

Through a massive release of their granule contents upon stimulation, basophils and mast cells function as mediators of inflammatory processes. The released chemicals include heparin, histamine, and other substances. The mediator may be vasoactive, bronchoconstrictive, and/or chemotactic (attractive) for eosinophils.[5,6]

MONOCYTES/MACROPHAGES

Derived from the granulocyte-monocyte colony-forming unit, monocytes are peripheral cells in transit from the bone marrow to tissues. Once in the tissues, under the influence of local factors, monocytes become macrophages. Macrophages exist in the liver (Kupffer's cells), spleen, lymph nodes, microglial (CNS) cells, skin (Langerhans cells), and bone.

Monocytes and macrophages perform a variety of functions, including initiation of immune responses for recognition by lymphocytes, regulation of immune response intensity, phagocytosis of foreign invaders, tumor cytotoxicity, degradation of cellular debris, and secretion of peptide molecules called monokines (a subclassification of cytokines).[7] Examples of monokines include interferons, tumor necrosis factor, and interleukin-1. Monokines and other cytokines regulate the activity of these cells.

LYMPHOCYTES

The primary functions of lymphocytes are to control and be the effector cells for the immune system. Many of these cells also are important synthetic sites for various cytokines. Lymphocytes can be functionally divided into cells that display cell-mediated immunity (T cells) and those that are responsible for humoral immunity (B cells; Table 98–2). Several different T-cell subtypes are found in peripheral blood. These include the cytotoxic suppressor T cells (CD8), which attack intracellular pathogens and regulate the size and duration of

TABLE 98–1. Average (Normal Range) Adult Blood Cell Concentrations

White cell count ($\times 10^9$/L)		7.8 (4.4–11.3)
Red cell count ($\times 10^{12}$/L)	Male	5.21 (4.52–5.90)
	Female	4.60 (4.10–5.10)
Hemoglobin[a] (mg/dL)	Male	15.7 (14.0–17.5)
	Female	13.8 (12.3–15.3)
Hematocrit	Male	0.46 (0.42–0.50)
	Female	0.40 (0.36–0.45)
Mean corpuscular volume (fL/red cell)		88.0 (80.0–96.1)
Platelet count ($\times 10^9$/L)		311 (172–450)

[a]May be 0.5–1.0 mg/dL lower in black patients.

TABLE 98–2. Lymphocyte-Mediated Immune Function

Cellular Immunity (T Cells)
1. Provides resistance against intracellular pathogens such as viruses, protozoa, fungi, and bacteria
2. Mediates allogeneic transplant rejection
3. Responsible for contact dermatitis
4. Provides autologous reaction to tumor cells

Humoral Immunity (B Cells)
1. Serves as major component of allergic reactions and other autoimmune diseases
2. Aids in eradication of encapsulated bacteria
3. Inactivates circulating toxins
4. May play role in antitumor reactions

the immune response, as well as helper T cells (CD4). The latter cells are responsible for delayed hypersensitivity, stimulation of B-cell differentiation (maturation), and antibody production, in addition to regulation of inflammatory reactions. B lymphocytes ultimately become plasma cells, which produce immunoglobulin specific for an antigen attached to the cell's surface.

Null cells are a separate subset of lymphocytes that lack surface markers of B or T origin. These cells, also referred to as large granular lymphocytes (LGLs), are thought to perform functions such as direct cytotoxicity to foreign entities, and they act either alone (natural killer cells) or in concert with immunoglobulin (antibody-dependent cellular cytotoxicity).[8,9] (Further details regarding lymphocytes are found in Chapter 87, Immune System.)

PLATELETS

There are several mechanisms by which platelets (thrombocytes) interact to facilitate blood coagulation. These include localization of the thrombus; provision of a specific receptor site for clotting factors, as well as the necessary phospholipid surface for the conversion of prothrombin to thrombin; and protection of thrombin from antithrombin. The process begins with a vascular injury that causes platelets to adhere to the exposed collagen fibers of the damaged wall as blood flows out. These events require the presence of other plasma proteins, namely, von Willebrand factor. Platelets then aggregate through a process that is calcium-dependent. Following aggregation, various platelet mediators are released (thromboxane, serotonin, platelet

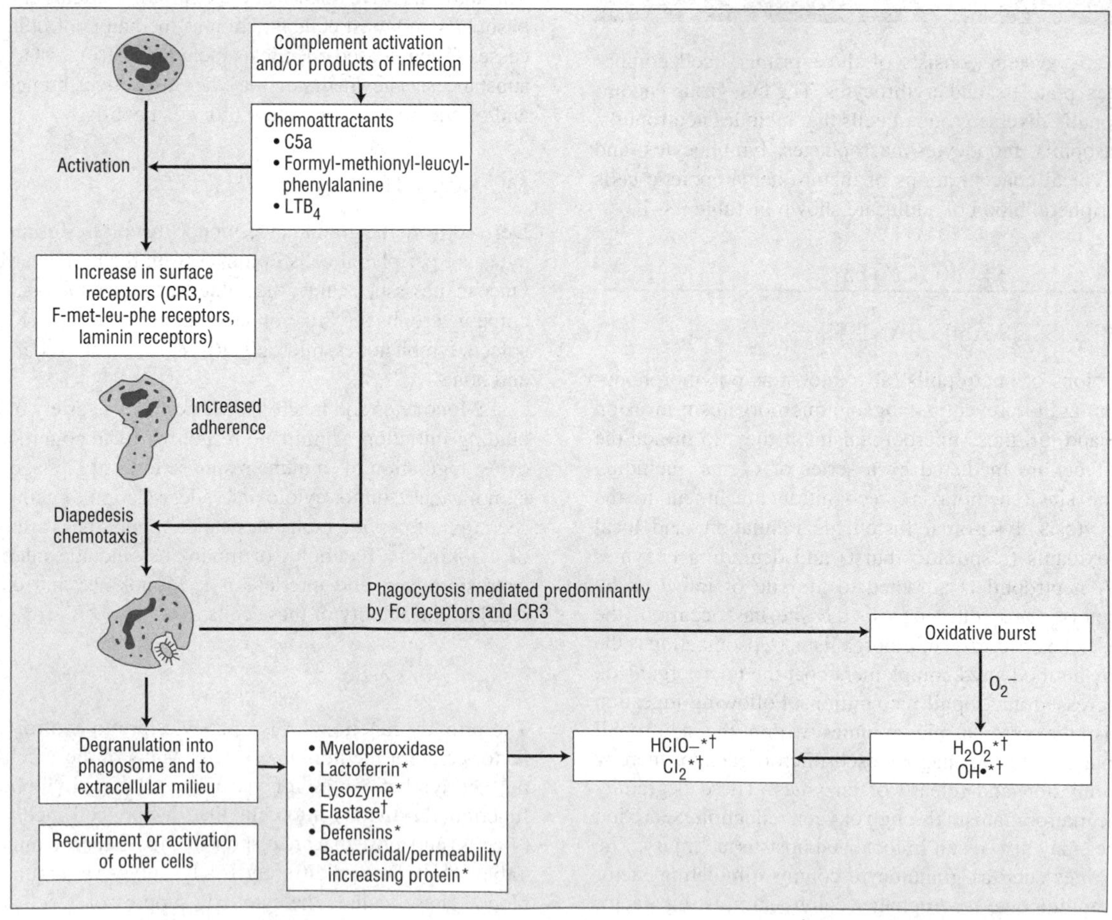

FIGURE 98–1. Neutrophil responses to infection or inflammation. *Microbicidal; †Damage to host tissues.

factor V), resulting in the formation of an irreversible platelet aggregate with subsequent formation of a stable fibrin cross-linked clot.[10,11]

ERYTHROCYTES

The primary function of the erythrocyte is to carry oxygen from the lungs to the peripheral tissues. Its optimal design enables efficient oxygen transport via the hemoglobin molecule. The general metabolic state of the patient and local factors control oxygen release.

HEMATOPOIETIC STRUCTURE AND COMPARTMENTS

Embryonic development of hematopoietic tissue occurs in the yolk sac mesenchyme, with fetal transition occurring in the liver and spleen. Very immature hematopoietic cells can also appear in umbilical cord blood, but not many are evident in the peripheral blood of adults.[12] The ultimate location of immature hematopoietic cells is in the bone marrow. The average adult has approximately 1.7 L of bone marrow, which provides an optimal environment for the development and proliferation of hematopoietic cells. The hematopoietic bone marrow is located primarily in the central portion of the pelvis, ribs, vertebrae, skull, and femora/humeri epiphyses. The anatomic structure of the bone marrow is characterized by the central venous marrow sinus, which is linked by coarse vascular sinusoids that intertwine a reticulin mesh where the cells are suspended. Thus, hematopoiesis occurs in the extravascular marrow spaces, which also contain endothelial cells, fibroblasts, macrophages, and adipocytes, collectively termed bone marrow stroma.[13] Stromal cells are thought to be important hematopoietic components, providing growth factors, collagen, and cell adhesion proteins.[14] When these cells are combined with accessory cells (lymphocytes/monocytes) and cytokines, the mixture is referred to as the hematopoietic microenvironment. Egress of more mature cells from the bone marrow occurs through the endothelial cell barrier. Release of cells such as neutrophils may be stimulated by complement, steroids, or endotoxin. Immature (progenitor) cells that may ultimately become any one of the blood cellular components can be mobilized from the bone marrow into peripheral blood by the administration of a cytotoxic chemotherapy drug (e.g., cyclophosphamide)[15] or a colony-stimulating factor (G-CSF or GM-CSF).[16] This process is commonly referred to as "priming" the bone marrow for peripheral blood progenitor or stem cell transplantation (see Chapter 134).

The least mature hematopoietic cell, accounting for only a fraction of a percentage of bone marrow cells, is referred to as the stem cell. Because these cells have the unique potential to ultimately become any of the mature hematopoietic cells, they are termed pluripotent. Importantly, they have self-renewal capacity (Fig. 98–2).[17] Extensive research has been conducted describing the morphologic and immunologic characteristics indicative of the earliest stem cell, but investigators have yet to arrive at a consensus model. Only a small percentage of these cells is likely to be dividing at any one time, and thus most are dormant in the cell cycle. Stem cell renewal and differentiation occur within the bone marrow under the influence of the marrow microenvironment. Stromal endothelial cells, fibroblasts, and fat cells (adipocytes) are necessary to support stem cell proliferation and division by providing anchorage for adhesion and secreting various hematopoietic growth factors necessary for differentiation. It is the characteristics of the local microenvironment (cellular matrix and growth factor concentrations) that influence the differentiation of a particular hematopoietic lineage, favoring it over another.

The next step in hematopoietic cell differentiation is thought to be represented by committed pluripotent stem cells that can still differentiate into any cell line (red blood cells [RBCs], white blood cells [WBCs], platelets); however, they have a limited capacity for self-renewal (see Fig. 98–2).

Cells that differentiate can proceed to either myeloid or lymphoid cell precursors (oligopotent progenitors). These cells may ultimately become B or T lymphocytes in the case of lymphoid cells. Myeloid progenitors may become granulocytes, erythrocytes, macrophages, or megakaryocytes as displayed in Figure 98–2. Nomenclature for immature hematopoietic cells often uses terms developed during *in vitro* experiments of cell proliferation. Thus, the term *burst-forming unit* (BFU) or *colony-forming unit* (CFU) is added to the suffix of the cell lines ultimately produced by the specific cell.

Leukocytes found in the peripheral blood can generally be classified into neutrophils (most frequently occurring blood leukocyte subdivided into the more mature segs and less mature bands), lymphocytes, monocytes, eosinophils, basophils, and the tissue derivative

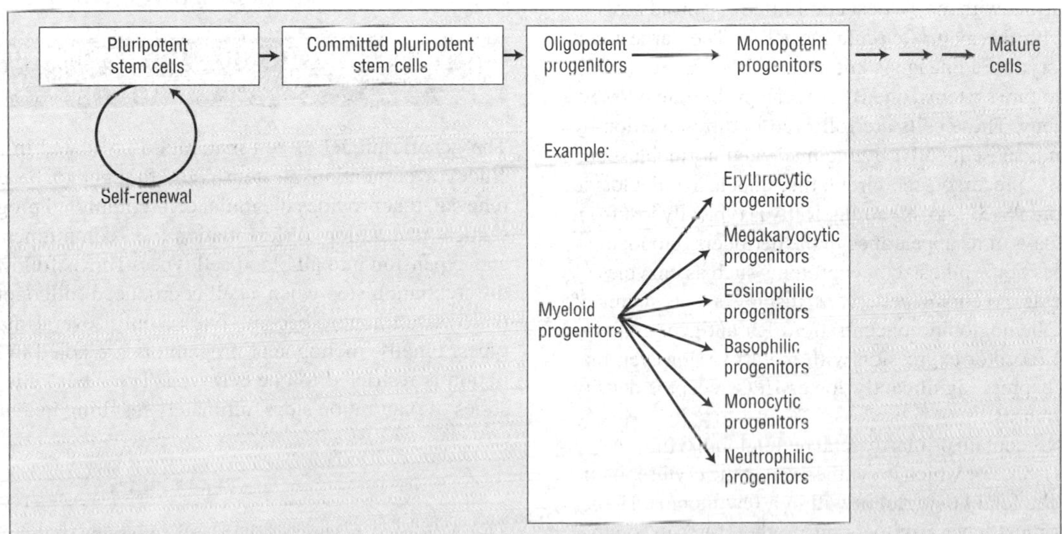

FIGURE 98–2. Rudimentary model of hematopoiesis displaying the basic steps a cell may take from its inception as a stem cell in the bone marrow, through stages in which it can become multiple (oligopotent) or only one specific (monopotent) type of mature blood cell.

of basophils, the mast cell. Immature neutrophils such as metamyelocytes are rarely seen in peripheral blood. Strictly speaking, the group of cells referred to as granulocytes includes neutrophils, eosinophils, and basophils, although common use tends to include only the neutrophils. The terminally differentiated leukocytes, which are usually not seen in blood, include the macrophage or histiocyte (derived from monocytes) and plasma cells (derived from B lymphocytes).

Most of the body's neutrophils and neutrophilic precursors reside in the bone marrow (approximately 9 billion cells) in contrast to the circulation (approximately 700 million). Similarly, only 1% of the eosinophils in the body are found in peripheral blood, whereas the skin, lungs, and gastrointestinal tract are the preferred sites of residence.[4] There is no marrow reserve pool of monocytes. Neutrophil development in the bone marrow begins with the stem cell and proceeds through intermediate precursors, such as the myeloblast, promyelocyte, myelocyte, and metamyelocyte.

Only a small fraction of the total body pool of lymphocytes resides in the blood. Immature T cells are evident in the circulation on their way to full maturation in the thymus. Mature B lymphocytes express surface immunoglobulin, which functions as an antigen receptor. Most of these cells migrate from the bone marrow to areas such as the lymph nodes (dense collections of lymphocytes, plasma cells, and macrophages that are supplied by postcapillary venules and drained by a system of efferent lymphatics) and spleen, where antigenic stimulation results in specific immunoglobulin production.[13] Approximately 75% of blood lymphocytes are T cells; 15%, null cells; and 10%, B cells. Various antigens expressed on the lymphocyte surface, depending on the degree of cell maturity and function, are termed clusters of differentiation (CD).

Progenitor cells that give rise to platelets are referred to as colony-forming unit megakaryocyte (CFU-MK). Megakaryocytes account for only 0.05% to 0.02% of marrow cells. Morphologic changes in both the cytoplasm and nucleus accompany the maturation of megakaryocytes. At differing stages of maturation, therefore, it is possible to see granules, organelles, and increasing segmentation of the nucleus. Cells in this lineage progress through three stages of development: commitment, proliferation, and differentiation, similar to that of leukocytes.[18,19]

The term *erythron* has been used to describe collectively the erythropoietic cellular pathway, composed of all cells involved in erythropoiesis, starting with the earliest committed erythroid progenitor and ending with the mature circulating RBC. The earliest cell committed to the erythroid lineage is known as a BFU-E (erythroid). Through *in vitro* culture systems, one BFU-E can proliferate into several hundred progeny. These cells are followed in differentiation by the CFU-E cell and, subsequently, by the nucleated normoblast and the immediate RBC precursor, the circulating anuclear reticulocyte as outlined in Figure 98–3. The remaining RNA is typically lost from the RBC within 2 days of its appearance in the peripheral blood; thus, the mature cell does not synthesize new proteins such as enzymes.[20]

The erythrocyte precursor cell types display a continuum of changes in shape, hemoglobin concentration, Rh antigen, and erythropoietin (EPO) receptor expression with maturity. However, mature erythrocytes express significantly lower EPO receptor density than do proerythroblasts.[21]

Neonatal RBCs contain primarily fetal hemoglobin (HbF). Adult hemoglobin (HbA), 85% of which is synthesized in the erythropoietic marrow, replaces the fetal hemoglobin within a few months. Heme-synthesizing cells must have a mitochondria; therefore, its synthesis cannot occur in the mature erythrocyte. Genetic alterations in hemoglobin structure may dramatically alter the stability or solubility of the hemoglobin and also cell confirmation. The characteristic

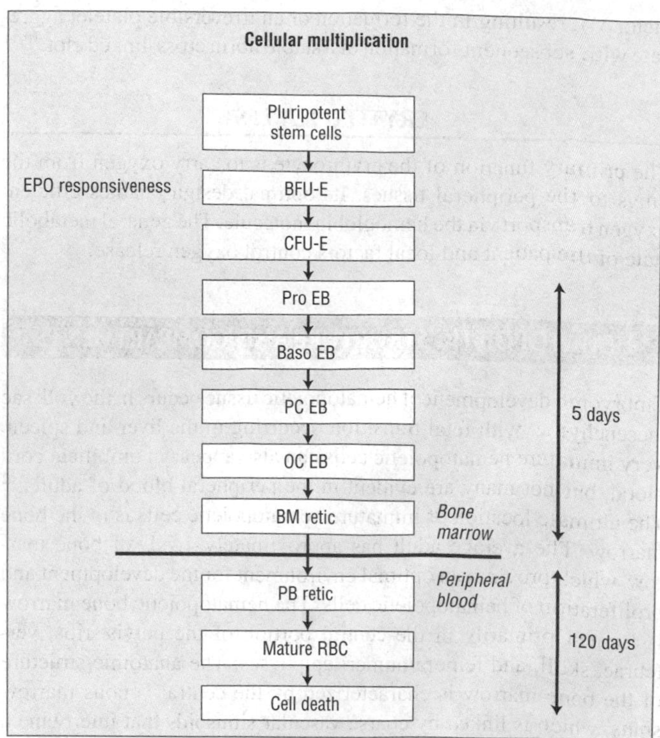

FIGURE 98–3. Proposed differentiation pattern of cells into mature erythrocytes with identification of various immature cell types. In addition, the cells that may be stimulated by the cytokine erythropoietin (EPO) are identified. BFU = burst-forming unit; E = erythroid; CFU = colony-forming unit; EB = erythroblast; PC = polychromatophilic; OC = orthochromatophilic; BM = bone marrow; retic = reticulocyte; PB = peripheral blood; RBC = red blood cell.

biconcave-disk shape of the normal RBC is approximately $8 \times 2\ \mu$m. Pathologic alterations in plasma lipids may affect the outer phospholipid membrane of the RBC, thus changing the cell's shape and survival. Blood types are characterized by the antigenic structure of the external surface of the cell membrane. The interactions of antibodies with RBC surface antigens affect the membrane function, integrity, and phagocytosis of the cells.

NATURAL REGULATION OF CELL PROLIFERATION AND DIFFERENTIATION

The generic model of cell maturation presented in Figure 98–2 includes a population of stem cells, thought to be capable of self-renewal, that provides the initial cell (committed progenitor) for subsequent maturation, differentiation (i.e., commitment to a cell line), and expansion into all blood cell types. This is followed by an initial differentiation step when a cell is produced (oligopotent progenitor) that will ultimately become one of only several mature blood cell types. Finally, monopotent progenitors are noted in which differentiation is restricted to one cell type. The latter cells then undergo a series of maturation steps, ultimately resulting in a mature cell.

STEM CELLS

The action of a stem cell in self-renewing rather than differentiating and the selection of lineage by a multipotential progenitor cell during the differentiation process are thought to be stochastic (random) events. Conversely, the survival and proliferation of the

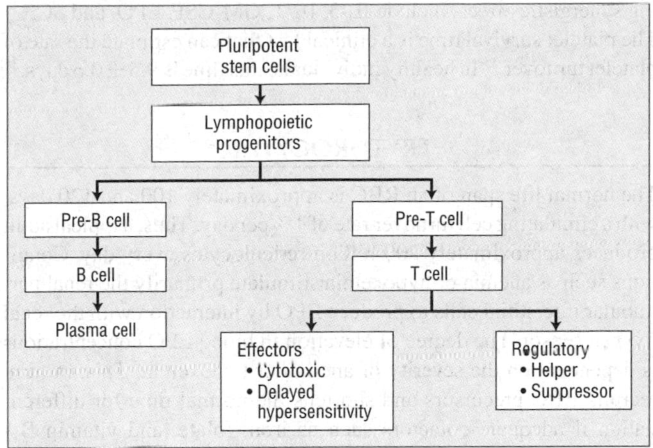

FIGURE 98–4. Pattern of lymphocyte maturation and differentiation into T and B cells. The plasma cell is a factory for antibodies, whereas the T cells have both effector and regulatory functions on the immune system.

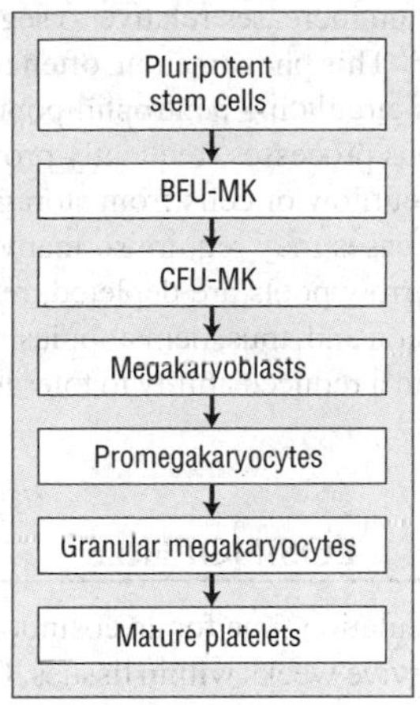

FIGURE 98–6. Maturation steps of megakaryocyte precursors prior to becoming mature platelets. BFU = burst-forming unit; MK = megakaryocyte; CFU = colony-forming unit.

subsequent progenitor cells are thought to be regulated by the group of cytokines referred to as colony-stimulating factors (also known as CSFs, hematopoietins, hematopoietic cytokines, or hematopoietic growth factors).[22] Receptors for a variety of CSFs are present on the surface of stem cells, which agrees with *in vitro* studies demonstrating stimulatory activity for cytokines such as stem cell factor (SCF), IL-6, G-CSF, IL-11, IL-12, and leukemia inhibitory factor when present in combinations. Whether or not the therapeutic use of a CSF that is thought to act primarily on more mature cells will exhaust (deplete) the stem cell pool over the course of multiple cycles of therapy is under active debate and study.[23] Proposed "cascades" of hematopoiesis are represented in Figures 98–3 through 98–6. Inserted within some figures are the suspected sites in the process where CSFs are thought to interact by promoting the production, proliferation, and survival of hematopoietic cells. These schema are simple representations of a system of complex interactions between stimulatory and inhibitory cytokines that may not be adequately described by the *in vitro* models used thus far to define them. (Details regarding the clinical pharmacology of individual CSFs are presented in Chapter 124.)

Immature bone marrow precursor cells such as the myeloblast (first recognizable cell of granulocytic differentiation), promyelocyte, myelocyte, and erythroblast are thought to be capable of replication. This is in contrast to most mature hematopoietic cells, which are incapable of division. Exceptions to the latter statement include monocytes, macrophages, and tissue mast cells. Evaluation of reasons for a change in hematopoietic cellular concentration over time must be conducted with a thorough knowledge of the mechanisms of both cellular production and destruction.

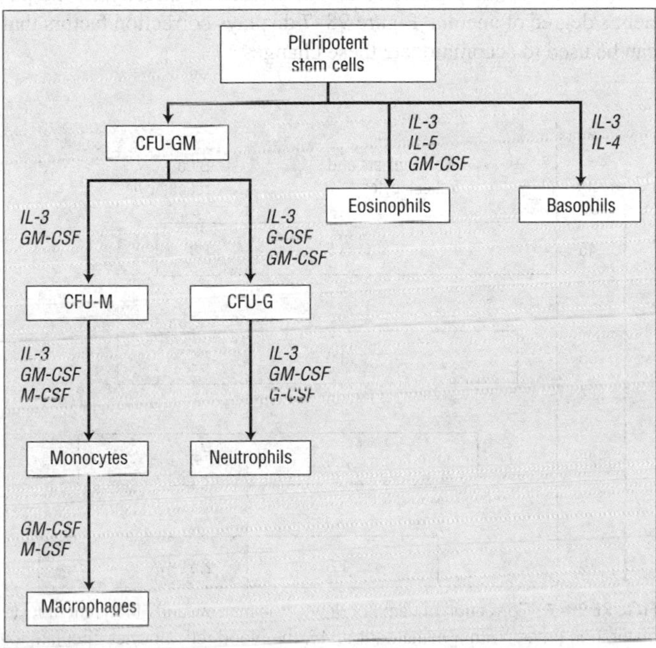

FIGURE 98–5. Maturation of precursor cells into granulocytes and macrophages, including some intermediate precursor cells (CFU-GM, G, and M). The colony-stimulating factors (CSFs) that affect the more terminal (mature) pathways are also shown. (CSFs that regulate immature cell types are not displayed.) CFU = colony-forming unit; G = granulocyte; M = monocyte.

NEUTROPHILS

Blood neutrophils are in constant exchange with an equal number of "marginated" cells. The latter are stuck to the walls of vessels in the peripheral blood, liver, lungs, and spleen. Therefore, demargination or the opposite, increased adhesion, can dramatically change the peripheral neutrophil concentration, even though cell production remains constant. A variety of stimuli can result in demargination, including infection, exercise, epinephrine, corticosteroids, and sickle cell anemia.[24] Conversely, transient neutropenia can occur via stimulation of margination by conditions such as malaria, some viral infections, and onset of hemodialysis.[25]

Normally, it takes 14 days for neutrophil production and differentiation in the bone marrow. It is believed that G-CSF, GM-CSF, and IL-3 are important regulatory molecules of neutrophil production (see Fig. 98–5). A healthy adult will produce approximately 1.6 billion neutrophils per kilogram body weight per day.[26] As blood neutrophils are totally replaced at least twice in each 24-hour period, the average circulation time for any one cell is approximately 6 to 12 hours. Most of this removal is thought to be for effector functions in the tissues and not simply an elimination process.

The total number of noncirculating (i.e., storage) neutrophils is more than 15 times the number in blood. Absolute storage cell numbers are subject to alteration by prior exposure to chemotherapy or deficiency in cofactors required for their synthesis (e.g., folate). When conditions call for an acute increase in blood neutrophils, the pattern of cells thus changes to one more similar to that in the marrow (i.e., band concentration increases relative to seg concentration; normal ratio <0.1–0.3).[27] This phenomenon, often referred to as a "shift to the left," denotes a circulating neutrophil population made of less mature cells. Infectious processes frequently provoke such a shift, as well as an increased outflow of cells from storage forms in the bone marrow, but extreme cases may require so many granulocytes at the infection site that marrow pools are depleted, resulting in neutropenia. Cytokine expression and, thus, hematopoiesis may be impaired in the elderly, resulting in a reduced ability to tolerate myelosuppressive chemotherapy.[28]

EOSINOPHILS

The typical blood circulation time for an eosinophil is approximately 6 hours, but it may survive weeks within tissues. Cytokines thought to be important in eosinophil production or function include IL-1, IL-3, GM-CSF, G-CSF, and, perhaps most important, IL-5. Corticosteroids cause a transient margination of eosinophils and inhibit release of mature cells from the bone marrow.[4]

MONOCYTES AND MACROPHAGES

Both macrophages and T lymphocytes secrete cytokines that stimulate monocytopoiesis.[29] Examples of cytokines that act on relatively mature monocytes include M-CSF and GM-CSF. Blood monocytes have a shorter marrow transit time than neutrophils (6 vs. 13 days, respectively), and there is no monocyte reserve in the marrow.[27] The peripheral blood turnover of these cells is much slower (circulation half-life 3 days) than for neutrophils; similarly, tissue macrophages are thought to be very long-lived. Macrophages may be able to produce their own progeny as well as attract additional monocytes for differentiation in the local environment.

LYMPHOCYTES

Immature T cells produced in the bone marrow ultimately migrate to the thymus, where they both expand and mature into immunologically competent cells (see Fig. 98–4). A variety of cytokines, including IL-2, IL-4, and IL-7, facilitate lymphopoiesis, whereas others such as transforming growth factor-β may decelerate this process.[30] T lymphocytes are probably the longest lived hematopoietic cell, as there is experimental evidence that the life span of some is greater than 10 years.

The term *lymphokine* is used to describe cytokines secreated by T cells. Lymphokines such as IL-2 are important in both activation and proliferation of the immune response, while monokines are also important regulators of lymphocyte development. T and B lymphocytes have important interactions with each other in both lymphocyte development and activation, which seem necessary for immunocompetence. There is some evidence for age-associated reductions in circulating helper and suppressor T cells and B cells.[31]

PLATELETS

Thrombopoiesis is the term used to describe the process of platelet production. The bone marrow manufactures 40,000 platelets/μL of blood each day. Proliferation and differentiation of platelet precursors are thought to be primarily influenced by cytokines such as IL-6, IL-11, leukemia inhibitory factor, and perhaps most specifically, by thrombopoietin (megakaryocyte growth and development factor; see Fig. 98–6).[32,33] Other hematopoietins that may act in concert, producing synergistic effects include IL-3, IL-1, GM-CSF, EPO, and SCF.[34] The platelet survival time is a clinical test that can estimate the rate of platelet turnover.[35] In healthy individuals, this time is 9.5 ± 0.6 days.[36]

ERYTHROCYTES

The normal life span of an RBC is approximately 100 and 120 days, with a circulating cell turnover rate of 1% per day. Thus, a typical adult produces approximately 200 billion reticulocytes every day. Conditions such as anemia or hypoxemia stimulate primarily the renal peritubular interstitial cells to produce EPO by interaction with the renal oxygen sensor. The degree of elevation in blood EPO concentrations is dependent on the severity of anemia or hypoxemia. This, in turn, recruits RBC precursors and shortens the normal time for differentiation if adequate cofactors such as iron, folate, and vitamin B_{12} are present. Although the overall time for differentiation is shortened (as is the duration of time that a reticulocyte spends in the marrow), the RBC's blood maturation time is lengthened. The increase in EPO concentrations is relatively quick (within hours), but the effects on marrow transpire over several days. The ultimate increase in RBC mass occurs at an even slower pace, generally over weeks to months (see Fig. 98–3). Multiple other endogenous cytokines are also thought to play a role in either stimulating or inhibiting erythropoiesis by acting on the early progenitors. These include GM-CSF, G-CSF, IL-1, IL-3, IL-6, IL-9, SCF, and some stromal proteins.[21]

Adequate production of RBCs for a degree of anemia is best assessed by evaluation of the number of circulating reticulocytes. Although the normal range is approximately 0.4% to 1.7% of the RBCs, this percentage would obviously be higher in anemic patients with adequate productive capacity. The calculation of a corrected reticulocyte count involves multiplying the percent circulating reticulocytes by the hemoglobin concentration and dividing the result by the normal hemoglobin level expected for a healthy patient with similar characteristics. Additional correction accounts for the increased life span of reticulocytes in the peripheral blood, depending directly on the patient's degree of anemia. Figure 98–7 displays correction factors that can be used to accommodate these changes.[37]

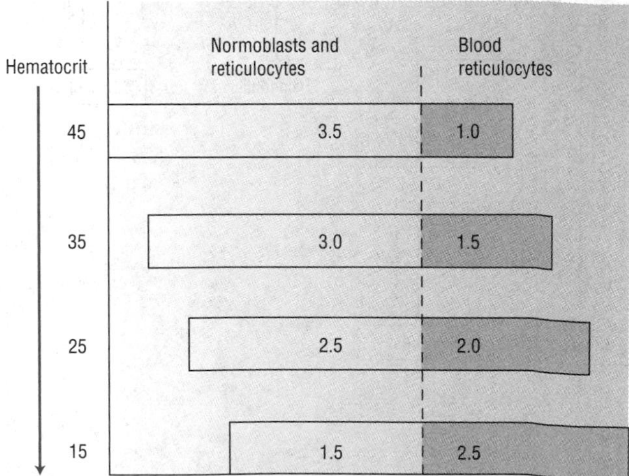

FIGURE 98–7. Correction of hematocrit with the marrow and blood reticulocyte maturation times. With a hematocrit of 45, the blood reticulocytes circulate for 1 day, whereas reduction in hematocrit to 15 results in a 2.5-day circulation time. The numbers found under the blood reticulocyte concentrations can be used as a correction factor in evaluation of reticulocyte concentrations. *(From Hillman RS, Finch CA. Red Cell Manual. Philadelphia, FA Davis, 1992, p. 59. Reprinted with permission.)*

Direct assessment of erythropoiesis in the bone marrow can be performed by estimating the myeloid to erythroid (M/E) cell ratio from a marrow aspirate. The range of the normal adult ratio is 3:1 to 5:1, but changes in erythroid or myeloid production can obviously influence the ratio. RBCs lose flexibility with age and eventually undergo lysis or are phagocytized and removed by the monocyte-macrophage system (primarily via the spleen). Accelerated red cell destruction can be grossly quantitated by determining increases in plasma concentrations of bilirubin and lactate dehydrogenase (LDH).[37]

Although clinical laboratories measure RBC concentrations with excellent accuracy, the most useful tool for assessment of the blood's oxygen-carrying capacity is the hemoglobin concentration because of the variability in RBC size. The average RBC and hemoglobin concentrations in healthy adult male and female patients are approximately 5.21 and 4.60 $\times$ $10^6/mm^3$, respectively, and 15.7 and 13.8 g/dL, respectively. Variations in normal concentrations will also be evident, depending on age, menstruation status, race, environmental factors, and pregnancy.[38]

DISEASE-ASSOCIATED HEMATOPOIETIC CHANGES

NEUTROPHILS

The usual definition of neutropenia is an absolute neutrophil count below $1,800/mm^3$ in white patients, $1,400/mm^3$ in black patients, and $1,500/mm^3$ for children 1 month to 10 years old. Clinical manifestations of neutropenia (i.e., infection) are not typically evident without other cofactors until the concentration drops below $1,000/mm^3$.[39] Accompanying factors that may influence the risk of infection for a particular patient include skin and mucous membrane integrity; vascular tissue supply; nutritional status; and lymphocytopenia, monocytopenia, or hypogammaglobinemia. Persistent agranulocytosis (less than $500/mm^3$ or no measurable neutrophils) is almost uniformly fatal without the use of supportive antibiotics.

Disorders resulting in defective granulopoiesis can be subdivided into those that result in marrow aplasia or diseases that replace the normal neutrophilic component. (See Chapter 102 for drug-induced neutropenia.) Diseases associated with granulopoietic suppression include viral infection, tuberculosis, anorexia, autoimmune diseases (e.g., systemic lupus erythematosus), Felty's syndrome (rheumatoid arthritis/splenomegaly/leukopenia), myelodysplastic syndromes, and leukemias.[39,40] A congenital form of severely defective neutrophil production (Kostmann's syndrome) has been described that is possibly a result of defective regulation of the late-acting hemopoietin G-CSF.[41] Patients with the rare disorder of cyclic neutropenia display periodic wide fluctuations in the WBCs at approximately 3 week intervals that last for 3 to 6 days. Other forms of chronic neutropenias may occur with adequate marrow stores and can be relatively benign in symptomatology.

Neutrophilia is typically defined as an absolute neutrophil count greater than 7.5 $\times$ 10^9 cells/L of blood and is sometimes referred to as a leukemoid reaction, if extreme.[24] Acute neutrophilia may be a result of emotional or physical stimuli (e.g., exercise, seizures, labor, pain, temperature changes), infections, inflammation or tissue necrosis, or drugs or toxins (e.g., CSFs, epinephrine, corticosteroids, lithium, vaccines, endotoxin). Chronic causes of increased neutrophilia include persistent infections, inflammation, malignancies, drugs, metabolic or endocrine disorders, cigarette smoking, hereditary or congenital abnormalities, and myeloproliferative diseases such as polycythemis vera.[24]

EOSINOPHILS

Eosinophilia (absolute count greater than $700/mm^3$) may result from neoplastic processes, parasitic or fungal infections, gastrointestinal disorders, malignancies, dermatitis, granulomatous disorders (e.g., sarcoidosis, Wegener's disease), or collagen-vascular diseases in addition to the more typical cause, allergic reactions.[42] One mechanism that may be common to several of these etiologic factors is antigenic stimulation of T cells, which produce a cytokine (IL-5) that mediates eosinophil proliferation.[43] Infections may cause eosinopenia; however, its significance is not thought to be of concern in that setting.

BASOPHILS

Basophilia occurs frequently in patients with myeloproliferative disorders and in association with inflammatory reactions and diseases. Viral infections, iron deficiency, or lung cancer can sometimes increase basophil counts. Mastocytosis is usually evident only on analysis of tissue or bone marrow mast cells. Causes include hypersensitivity reactions, malignancy, osteoporosis, and chronic liver or renal disease.

MONOCYTES

Monocytosis ($>0.8 \times 10^9$ cells/L of blood) occurs with some infections (e.g., tuberculosis, histoplasmosis, toxoplasmosis, bacterial endocarditis, salmonellosis), collagen-vascular diseases (rheumatoid arthritis, systematic lupus erythematosus), gastrointestinal disorders (ulcerative colitis, alcoholic liver disease), leukemias, and up to 60% of nonhematologic malignancies, whereas abnormally low monocyte concentrations occur in patients with hairy cell leukemia or aplastic anemia.[44]

LYMPHOCYTES

Significant reductions in lymphocyte concentration ($<1 \times 10^9$ cells/L of blood) can be evident without apparent cause or in a variety of diseases, including acute inflammatory disorders, severe uremia, immune deficiency diseases such as systemic lupus erythematosus, chronic infections such as tuberculosis or human immunodeficiency virus (HIV) infection, malignancies, and connective tissue diseases.[45] Lymphocytosis ($>4 \times 10^9$ cells/L) may occur with mononucleosis, pertussis, measles, or chickenpox, and in lymphoid malignancies. A progressive increase in mature lymphocytes may be indicative of chronic lumphocytic leukemia. Increased levels of atypical lymphocytes may occur in patients with infections. (e.g., mononucleosis, hepatitis, cytomegalovirus,), allergic reactions, or lymphomas.[46]

PLATELETS

Both qualitative and quantitative platelet disorders have important pathophysiologic consequences. Thrombocytopenia, defined as a platelet count less than 150,000 cells/mm^3, may result from a defect in production, increased sequestration, or accelerated destruction.[47]

Certain stimuli may damage the marrow by reducing the number of megakaryocytes available. Drugs, chemicals, radiation, and infection are among the potential causes of marrow injury. Diseases that produce general bone marrow failure or those that invade the bone marrow may result in thrombocytopenia. Examples of the latter include cancers such as leukemia, lymphoma, myelofibrosis, myelodysplasia, and metastatic solid tumors (breast and prostate cancer) and infections such as those caused by mycobacterium. Suboptimal platelet production may also result from defects in maturation seen with vitamin B_{12} and/or folate deficiency or in congenital syndromes.[48]

Alteration in platelet distribution may also result in thrombocytopenia. Splenomegaly is the most frequent cause of increased platelet sequestration.

Owing to its accelerated destruction of platelets, idiopathic thrombocytopenic purpura (ITP) is a common cause of thrombocytopenia. Antiplatelet antibodies combine with platelets in ITP, thus sensitizing them to removal by the immune system. Accelerated platelet destruction can also occur in patients with connective tissue disorders. Approximately 14% of patients with systemic lupus erythematosus experience thrombocytopenia similar to ITP.

ERYTHROCYTES

Suboptimal erythropoiesis can be classified by changes in the size of RBCs noted on examination of the peripheral blood. Because the excretory and endocrine functions of the kidney usually mirror each other, renal dysfunction can lead to anemia by reduction in EPO production, resulting in a normochromic, normocytic pattern. Other causes of insufficient erythropoiesis include replacement of bone marrow by fibrosis, solid tumors, or leukemia, as well as defects in erythroid maturation. Relative deficiencies in the cofactors required for heme-RBC synthesis such as iron, folate, and vitamin B_{12} may also be important contributors. Structurally, RBC macrocytosis denotes defects in the maturation of the nucleus, whereas microcytosis is indicative of cytoplasmic defects (reduced hemoglobin synthesis). (A detailed description regarding the pathogenesis and treatment of anemic disorders is found in Chapter 99.)

Exaggerated erythropoiesis with increased RBC mass (polycythemia) can be mistaken for a reduction in plasma volume. Symptoms are not always immediately evident, but may progress to reduced tissue oxygenation, thrombosis, and congestive heart failure. The most common cause is hypoxia; alternative causes can be grouped according to their ability to stimulate EPO production. EPO (or a similar cytokine) may be produced in response to genetic alterations or a variety of malignancies, including angioblastoma, hepatomas, and hypernephroma.[49] Polycythemia vera, a malignancy of the bone marrow stem cells, results in an increased sensitivity of RBC precursors to stimulation by EPO and is accompanied in many patients by thrombocytosis and leukocytosis.

CLINICAL USES OF HEMATOPOIETIC CELLS

HEMATOPOIETIC STEM CELL TRANSPLANTATION

High-dose chemotherapy with or without irradiation is beneficial in the treatment of a number of malignant diseases (see Chapter 134). The dose of chemotherapy that can be administered, however, is limited by hematopoietic toxicity that can result in prolonged periods of pancytopenia with the attendant risks of serious infection and bleeding. The infusion (transplantation) of bone marrow following the high-dose therapy can overcome this hematopoietic toxicity, resulting in subsequent repopulation of the bone marrow and recovery of hematopoiesis. Bone marrow transplantation (BMT) involves the removal of bone marrow from the donor, administration of intensive doses of chemotherapy (with or without irradiation) to the recipient, and infusion of the donor bone marrow (stem cells) to the recipient. If the donor and recipient are the same individual (i.e., the patient serves as his or her own donor), the procedure is termed autologous bone marrow transplantation. If the marrow comes from another individual, the procedure is termed allogeneic bone marrow transplantation. Most allogeneic donors are HLA-matched siblings, but the use of alternative donors such as HLA-matched related volunteer donors or umbilical cord blood cells is increasing.

Allogeneic transplantation is complicated by the immune recognition of host tissues by donor T lymphocytes, resulting in a syndrome called graft-versus-host disease. Because immune recognition of tumor cells also occurs (graft-versus-tumor effect), the relapse rates associated with allogeneic transplants are lower than those associated with autologous transplants for similar disease stages. Allogeneic transplantation is used more commonly for diseases primarily involving the bone marrow, such as acute and chronic leukemias, aplastic anemia, thalassemia, and severe combined immunodeficiency.

Autologous transplantation is more commonly used in lymphoma and Hodgkin's disease and selected solid tumors such as breast cancer, ovarian cancer, and germ cell tumors. A number of laboratory techniques are evolving to allow the bone marrow harvested for autologous transplantation to expand in the laboratory prior to infusion and to cleanse the marrow of potential malignant cell contamination.

Small numbers of hematopoietic progenitor (stem) cells capable of reconstituting hematopoiesis circulate in the blood under normal circumstances.[50] Commonly referred to as peripheral blood progenitor cells (PBPCs), these circulating progenitor cells increase in number during recovery from myelosuppressive chemotherapy or after treatment with cytokines such as G-CSF or GM-CSF.[16,51] These cells can be collected by a process called leukapheresis and stored for reinfusion following high-dose chemotherapy. Hematopoietic recovery is generally more rapid following rescue with PBPCs as compared with rescue with bone marrow. Potential tumor cell contamination may also be less with PBPC transplants. The use of PBPCs has essentially replaced the use of autologous bone marrow, and allogeneic transplants of PBPCs are becoming more common.

Cytokine-mobilized PBPC transplants from allogeneic donors have recently been shown to result in more rapid white cell and platelet engraftment and shorter hospital stays than bone marrow transplants.[52] The incidence of acute graft-versus-host disease is not increased, but there is a significant increase in the incidence of chronic graft-versus-host disease with PBPC. Relapse rates and overall survival rates are similar.

Only about one-third of patients who would otherwise be eligible for allogeneic bone marrow transplantation have HLA-matched related donors. One alternative is the use of closely HLA-matched, unrelated donor marrow. The National Marrow Donor Program (NMDP) is a registry of volunteer marrow donors now containing more than 4 million members. By coordinating the activities of a network of donor, collection, and transplant centers, the NMDP facilitates the identification of potential donors and the procurement of marrow. Unrelated donor marrow transplants are associated with an increased incidence of graft-versus-host disease compared to related donor transplants; however, recent advances in tissue typing and donor matching and graft-versus-host disease prophylaxis have resulted in comparable overall survival rates for many diseases.

Grafts of PBPCs from unrelated donors are also increasingly used for transplantation. The cells are collected by leukapheresis and spare the donor from potential complications related to general or spinal anesthesia and pain associated with bone marrow harvest. Unrelated PBPC transplants are associated with more rapid engraftment compared to unrelated BMT with no increase in graft-versus-host disease or relapse rates.[53]

Many patients do not have HLA-matched family members or unrelated donors in the marrow registries. An alternative for these patients is the use of human umbilical cord blood, which contains hematopoietic stem cells capable of reconstituting bone marrow function following high-dose chemotherapy.[54] An almost unlimited number of cord blood donors is potentially available, because the cord and its associated blood are commonly discarded following delivery. There are cord blood banks in which cord blood cells are HLA-typed, cryopreserved, and made available for transplantation for appropriate recipients. To date, the majority of cord blood progenitor cell transplantations performed have been in children because of the relatively small number of cells available from a cord blood unit, although the number of cord blood transplantations performed in adults is increasing. Laboratory methods to expand the number of progenitor cells in cord blood units are under investigation. Cord blood transplants are thought to lead to less graft-versus-host disease than transplants from matched unrelated bone marrow donors with similar degrees of matching, and they may prove to be an important source of progenitor cells for transplantation in the near future.

The application of allogeneic transplantation has been limited to younger patients without comorbid conditions secondary to the toxicity of the myeloablative preparative regimen and the allogeneic bone marrow graft. Recently, a number of centers have reported successful allogeneic engraftment following nonmyeloablative, immunosuppressive conditioning regimens.[55,56] The goal of this approach is to establish donor hematopoiesis and a graft-versus-tumor effect while minimizing toxicity. These transplants can be offered to older patients and to patients with disorders that may be responsive to immune-based therapy, but not to the high-dose regimens previously used with allogeneic transplantation, such as renal cell carcinoma and melanoma.

ADOPTIVE IMMUNOTHERAPY

Experiments involving the administration of immune system cells for the purpose of cancer treatment (adoptive immunotherapy) have been conducted for well over a decade; however, the clinical benefit has only recently been substantiated. As described earlier, nonspecific, total depletion of donor T cells following high-dose chemotherapy and stem cell re-infusion produces fewer graft versus-host effects, but attenuated anticancer responses. However, it has been shown that careful attention to the T-cell dose and timing of infusion may maximize the potential for beneficial immunologic responses and minimize graft-versus-host effects. It has been found that the administration of allogeneic donor lymphocyte infusions to patients with leukemia relapse following stem cell transplantation has anticancer efficacy in diseases such as chronic myelogenous leukemia (65% complete response), acute nonlymphocytic leukemia or myelodysplastic syndrome (25% complete response).[57] Some of these remissions have prolonged durability. The complications of donor lymphocyte infusions include the obvious risk of graft-versus-host disease, but the condition does not develop in all patients who have clinical benefit. This mode of therapy can also result in marrow aplasia for approximately 20% of patients; it is self-limiting or treatable with G-CSF in most cases, however.

GENE THERAPY

Hematopoietic progenitor cells are the focus of intense research in gene therapy. The self-renewal capacity of these cells makes them an obvious target for delivering corrective genetic information for a variety of both hematologic and metabolic inherited disorders, such as sickle cell anemia, thalassemia, immunodeficiency syndromes, and glycogen storage diseases.

TRANSFUSION AND BLOOD PRODUCT SUPPORT

Advances in blood banking and transfusion support have been critical to the improved outcome of therapy for patients with hematologic and malignant diseases. Platelet transfusions are indicated for the prevention and treatment of bleeding. In general, prophylactic platelet transfusions are not indicated for platelet counts above 10,000 cells/mm^3 unless the patient is febrile or actively bleeding. Pletelets are available as pooled random donor concentrates obtained from RBC donations (six to eight donors per transfusion) or single-donor platelets collected by apheresis. The use of ABO-compatible platelets and leukocyte filters has been shown to decrease the development of alloimmunization and refractoriness to platelet transfusions and is cost-effective. Leukocyte filters also decrease the risk of transmission of cytomegalovirus and febrile transfusion reactions. Packed RBC transfusions are indicated to keep hemoglobin levels greater than 7–8 g/dL to maintain adequate oxygen-carrying capacity. Each unit of packed RBCs should increase the hemoglobin level by approximately 1g/dL unless active blood loss is evident. RBCs should also be filtered to reduce the risk of nonhemolytic, febrile transfusion reactions. Patients who are candidates for bone marrow transplantation should receive blood products that have been irradiated with 2,500 cGy to prevent transfusion-associated graft-versus-host disease.

Fresh-frozen plasma contains the components of the coagulation system and is indicated for the replacement of deficient coagulation factors II, V, VII, X, XI, and XIII. Factors VIII and IX deficiencies are treated with specific factor concentrates. Fresh-frozen plasma is also used for the rapid reversal of warfarin anticoagulation and in the treatment of disseminated intravascular coagulation. Thrombotic thrombocytopenic purpura is treated by means of a therapeutic plasma exchange with fresh-frozen plasma as the replacement fluid. Cryoprecipitate, which contains factor VIII, von Willebrand's factor, and fibrinogen, is indicated for the treatment of von Willebrand's disease that does not respond to desmopressin acetate and for fibrinogen replacement (see Chapter 100).

The IV administration of immunoglobin (Ig) has been used in a variety of hematologic disorders, but for most of these situations, it is still considered experimental or indicated only when other therapeutic options have been exhausted. Patients with deficient immunoglobin production (e.g., agammaglobinemia, hypogammaglobulinemia) or function (e.g., chronic lymphocytic leukemia, multiple myeloma, children with HIV) may benefit from this therapy with the goal of raising the IgG level such that there is less chance for bacterial infection (<500 mg/dL). This approach has other pharmacologic properties as well, including blockade of Fc receptors, modification of complement activation, and modulation of the immune response by anti-idiotypic antibodies.[58] It is also beneficial for patients with ITP who are at high bleeding risk or need higher platelet counts prior to surgery.[59] Post-transplant prophylaxis (approximately 3 months) with Ig given IV is also sometimes used in patients receiving allogeneic hematopoietic stem cell transplantation for prevention of bacterial sepsis and acute graft-versus-host disease. The IV treatment with Ig may benefit patients whose platelet counts do not increase substantially despite transfusions, owing to the formation of alloantibodies.

REFERENCES

1. Erslev AJ, Lichtman MA. Structure and function of the marrow. In: Williams WJ, Beutler E, Erslev AJ, Lichtman MA, eds. Hematology. 4th ed. New York: McGraw-Hill, 1990:37.
2. Lehrer RI, Ganz T, Selsted ME, et al. Neutrophils in human diseases. N Engl J Med 1987;317:687–694.

3. Lieschke GJ, Burgess AW. Granulocyte colony-stimulating factor and granulocyte-macrophage colony-stimulating factor. N Engl J Med 1992; 327:28–35.
4. Weller PF. The immunobiology of eosinophils. N Engl J Med 1991; 324:1110–1118.
5. Kitamura Y, Kasugai T, Arizono N, Matsuda H. Development of mast cells and basophils: processes and regulation mechanisms. Am J Med Sci 1993;306:185–191.
6. Galli SJ, Dvorak AM, Dvorak HF. Morphology, biochemistry, and function of basophils and mast cells. In: Williams WJ, Beutler E, Erslev AJ, Lichtman MA, eds. Hematology, 4th ed. New York: McGraw-Hill, 1990:840.
7. Johnston RB. Monocytes and macrophages. N Engl J Med 1988;318:747–752.
8. Kipps TJ, Carson DA. Functions of B lymphocytes and plasma cells in immunoglobulin production. In: Williams WJ, Beutler E, Erslev AJ, Lichtman MA, eds. Hematology, 4th ed. New York: McGraw-Hill, 1990: 932.
9. Kipps TJ, Carson DA. Functions of T lymphocytes: T-cell receptors for antigen. In: Williams WJ, Beutler E, Erslev AJ, Lichtman MA, eds. Hematology, 4th ed. New York: McGraw-Hill, 1990:939.
10. Thompson AR, Harker LA. Manual of Hemostasis and Thrombosis, 3rd ed. Philadelphia: FA Davis, 1983:47.
11. Mustard JF, Packham MA, Kinlough-Rathbone RL. Platelets, blood flow, and the vessel wall. Circulation 1990;81(suppl 1):I40–I41.
12. Gordon MY. Physiological mechanisms in BMT and haematopoiesis-revisited. Bone Marrow Transplant 1993;11:193–197.
13. Weiss LP. Functional organization of the hematopoietic tissues. In: Hoffman R, Benz EJ, Shattil SJ, et al., eds. Hematology—Basic Principles and Practice. New York: Churchill Livingstone, 1991:82.
14. Greenberger J. The hematopoietic microenvironment. Crit Rev Oncol Hematol 1991;11:65–84.
15. To LB, Shepperd KM, Haylock DN, et al. Single high doses of cyclophosphamide enable the collection of high numbers of hematopoietic stem cells from the peripheral blood. Exp Hematol 1990;18:442–447.
16. Peters WP, Rosner G, Ross M, et al. Comparative effects of granulocyte-macrophage colony-stimulating factor (GM-CSF) and granulocyte colony-stimulating (G-CSF) factor on priming peripheral blood progenitor cells for use with autologous bone marrow after high-dose chemotherapy. Blood 1993;81:1709–1719.
17. Spangrude GJ, Heimfeld S, Wessman IL. Purification and characterization of mouse hematopoietic stem cells. Science 1988;241:58–62.
18. Williams N, Levine RF. The origin, development and regulation of megakaryocytes. Br J Hematol 1982;52:173–180.
19. Hoffman R. Regulation of megakaryocytopoiesis. Blood 1989;74:1196–1212.
20. Papayannopoulou T, Abkowitz J. Biology of erythropoiesis, erythroid differentiation, and maturation. In: Hoffman R, Benz EJ, Shattil SJ, et al., eds. Hematology—Basic Principles and Practice. New York: Churchill Livingstone, 1991:252.
21. McGuire MJ, Spivak JL. Erythropoiesis. In: Anderson KC, Ness PM, eds. Scientific Basis of Transfusion Medicine—Implications for Clinical Practice. Philadelphia: WB Saunders, 1994:1.
22. Ogawa M. Differentiation and proliferation of hematopoietic stem cells. Blood 1993;81:2844–2853.
23. Moore MAS. Does stem cell exhaustion result from combining hematopoietic growth factors with chemotherapy? If so, how do we prevent it? Blood 1992;80:3–7.
24. Dale DC. Neutrophilia. In: Williams WJ, Beutler E, Erslev AJ, Lichtman MA, eds. Hematology, 4th ed. New York: McGraw-Hill, 1990:816.
25. Coates T, Baehner R. Leukocytosis and leukopenia. In: Hoffman R, Benz EJ, Shattil SJ, et al., eds. Hematology—Basic Principles and Practice. New York: Churchill Livingstone, 1991:552.
26. Gabrilove J. Granulopoiesis. In: Anderson KC, Ness PM, eds. Scientific Basis of Transfusion Medicine—Implications for Clinical Practice. Philadelphia: WB Saunders, 1994:17.
27. Boggs DR, Winkelstein A. White Cell Manual. Philadelphia: FA Davis; 1983:29.
28. Rothstein G. Hematopoiesis in the aged: a model of hematopoietic dysregulation? Blood 1993;82:2601–2604.
29. Bagby GC, Segal GM. Growth factors and the control of hematopoiesis. In: Hoffman R, Benz EJ, Shattil SJ, et al., eds. Hematology—Basic Principles and Practice. New York: Churchill Livingstone, 1991:97.
30. Jordan SC. Cytokines and lymphocytes. In: Kunkel SL, Remick DG, eds. Cytokines in Health and Disease. New York: Marcel Dekker, 1992: 309.
31. Yamashiki M, Nishimura A, Kosaka Y, James SP. Two-color analysis of peripheral lymphocyte surface antigens in inherently healthy adults. J Clin Lab Anal 1994;8:22–26.
32. Du XX, Williams DA. Interleukin-11: a multifunctional growth factor derived from the hematopoietic microenvironment. Blood 1994;83: 2023–2030.
33. Metcalf D. Thrombopoietin—at last. Nature 1994;369:519–520.
34. Gordon MS, Hoffman R. Growth factors affecting human thrombocytopoiesis: potential agents for the treatment of thrombocytopenia. Blood 1992;80:302–307.
35. Shulman NR, Jordan JV Jr. Platelet kinetics. In: Colman RW, Hirsh J, Marder VJ, Saltzman EW, eds. Hemostasis and Thrombosis. Basic Principles and Clinical Practice, 2nd ed. Philadelphia: JP Lippincott, 1987:341–351.
36. Harker LA, Finch CA. Thrombokinetics in man. J Clin Invest 1969; 48:963–974.
37. Hillman RS, Finch CA. Red Cell Manual. Philadelphia: FA Davis, 1992:59.
38. Glassman AB. Anemia: diagnosis and clinical considerations. In: Harmening DM, ed. Clinical Hematology and Fundamentals of Hemostasis, 2nd ed. Philadelphia: FA Davis, 1992:54.
39. Lichtman MA. Classification and clinical manifestations of neutrophil disorders. In: Williams WJ, Beutler E, Erslev AJ, Lichtman MA, eds. Hematology, 4th ed. New York: McGraw-Hill, 1990:802.
40. Malech HL, Gallin JI. Neutrophils in human disease. N Engl J Med 1987;317:687–694.
41. Dong F, Hoefsloot LH, Schelen AM, et al. Identification of a nonsense mutation in the G-CSF receptor in severe congenital neutropenia. Proc Natl Acad Sci 1994;91:4480–4484.
42. Boggs DR, Winkelstein A. White Cell Manual, 4th ed. Philadelphia: FA Davis, 1983:54.
43. Sanderson CJ. Interleukin-5, eosinophils and disease. Blood 1992; 79:3101–3109.
44. Lichtman MA. Classification and clinical manifestations of disorders of monocytes and macrophages. In: Williams WJ, Beutler E, Erslev AJ, Lichtman MA, eds. Hematology, 4th ed. New York: McGraw-Hill, 1990:879.
45. Williams WJ. Lymphocytopenia. In: Williams WJ, Beutler E, Erslev AJ, Lichtman MA, eds. Hematology, 4th ed. New York: McGraw-Hill, 1990:964.
46. Williams WJ. Lymphocytosis. In: Williams WJ, Beutler E, Erslev AJ, Lichtman MA, eds. Hematology, 4th ed. New York: McGraw-Hill, 1990:963.
47. Rutherford CJ, Frenkel EP. Thrombocytopenia: issues in diagnosis and therapy. Med Clin North Am 1994;78:555–575.
48. Williams WJ. Classification and clinical manifestations of disorders of hemostasis. In: Williams WJ, Beutler E, Erslev AJ, Lichtman MA, eds. Hematology, 4th ed. New York: McGraw-Hill, 1990:1338.
49. Tabbara IA. Erythropoietin biology and clinical applications. Arch Intern Med 1993;153:298–304.
50. Kessinger A, Armitage JO, Landmark JD, et al. Autologous peripheral hematopoietic stem cell transplantation restores hematopoietic function following marrow ablative therapy. Blood 1988;71:723–727.
51. To LB, Shepperd KM, Haylock DN, et al. Single high doses of cyclophosphamide enable the collection of high numbers of hematopoietic cells from the peripheral blood. Exp Hematol 1990;18:442–447.

52. Champlin RE, Schmitz N, Horowitz MM, et al. Blood stem cells compared with bone marrow as a source of hematopoietic cells for allogeneic transplantation. Blood 2000;95:3702–3709.
53. Ringden O, Remberger M, Runde V, et al. Peripheral blood stem cell transplantation from unrelated donors: a comparison with marrow transplantation. Blood 1999;94:455–464.
54. Auerbach AD, Liu Q, Ghosh R, et al. Prenatal identification of potential donors for umbilical cord blood transplantation for Fanconi anemia. Transfusion 1990;30:682–687.
55. Slavin S, Nagler A, Naparstek E, et al. Nonmyeloablative stem cell transplantation and cell therapy as an alternative to conventional bone marrow transplantation with lethal cytoreduction for the treatment of malignant and nonmalignant hematologic diseases. Blood 1998;91:756–763.
56. Khouri IF, Keating M, Korbing M, et al. Transplant-lite: induction of graft-versus-malignancy using fludrabine-based nonablative chemotherapy and allogeneic blood progenitor-cell transplantation as treatment for lymphoid malignancies. J Clin Oncol 1999;16:2817–2824.
57. Baron F, Beguin Y. Adoptive immunotherapy with donor lymphocyte infusions after allogeneic HPC transplantation. Transfusion 2000;40:468–476.
58. Otten A, Bossuyt PMM, Vermeulen M, Brand A. Intravenous immunoglobulin treatment in hematological diseases. Eur J Haematol 1998;60:73–85.
59. George JN, Woolf SH, Gary E, et al. Idiopathic thrombocytopenic purpura: a practice guideline developed by explicit methods for the American Society of Hematology. Blood 1996;88:3–40.

99

ANEMIAS

Tracey A. Waddelow and Thomas T. Sproat

Anemias are a group of diseases characterized by a decrease in either hemoglobin or red blood cells (RBCs) that reduces the oxygen-carrying capacity of blood. Anemias can result from inadequate RBC production or an accelerated loss of RBC mass, or they can be a manifestation of a host of systemic disorders such as infection, chronic renal disease, or malignancy. Because they are often a sign of underlying pathology, a rapid diagnosis of the cause of the anemia is essential.

Anemias can be classified on the basis of the morphology of the RBCs, etiology, or pathophysiology. Table 99–1 gives some examples of anemias in these classifications. Iron deficiency anemia (IDA), anemia of chronic disease (ACD), and anemias associated with acute bleeding account for about 75% of all anemias.[1] The remaining anemias are the result of such conditions as bone marrow damage, decreased erythropoiesis, and hemolysis.

MATURATION AND DEVELOPMENT OF RBCs

In adults, RBCs are formed in the marrow of the vertebrae, ribs, sternum, clavicle, pelvic (iliac) crest, and the proximal epiphyses of the long bones. In children, most bone marrow space is hematopoietically active to meet increased RBC requirements.

In normal RBC formation, an undifferentiated progenitor cell, a pluripotent stem cell, yields an erythroid burst–forming unit. Erythropoietin (EPO) and cytokines such as IL-3 and granulocyte-macrophage colony-stimulating factor (GM-CSF) stimulate this cell to form an erythroid colony–forming unit (CFU-E) in the marrow. The CFU-E is very sensitive to EPO and produces proerythroblasts. Subsequent divisions yield basophilic erythroblasts, polychromatic erythroblasts, pyknotic erythroblasts, reticulocytes, and finally an erythrocyte. During this process, the nucleus becomes smaller with each division, finally disappearing in the normal erythrocyte (Fig. 99–1). Hemoglobin and iron are incorporated into the gradually maturing RBC, which is released from the marrow into the circulating blood as a reticulocyte. The maturation process takes about 1 week; several days are then necessary for the reticulocyte to lose its nucleus and become an erythrocyte.

STIMULATION OF ERYTHROPOIESIS

The hormone EPO, 90% of which is produced by the kidneys, initiates the production of RBCs. A decrease in tissue oxygen concentration signals the kidneys to increase the production and release of EPO into the plasma, which (1) stimulates stem cells to differentiate into proerythroblasts, (2) increases the rate of mitosis, (3) increases the release of reticulocytes from the marrow, and (4) induces hemoglobin formation. Accelerated hemoglobin synthesis makes it possible to achieve the critical hemoglobin concentration necessary for RBC maturity more rapidly, and a feedback mechanism stops further RBC nucleic acid synthesis, causing an earlier release of reticulocytes. Early appearance of reticulocytes, in larger quantities, in the peripheral circulation (reticulocytosis) is another indication that RBC production is being stimulated.

SYNTHESIS OF HEMOGLOBIN

Hemoglobin consists of a protein component with two α- and two β-chains; each chain is linked to a heme group consisting of a porphyrin ring structure with an iron atom chelated at its center, which is capable of binding oxygen. The hemoglobin formed in an adult is composed of 96% hemoglobin A (two α- and two β-chains), 3% hemoglobin A_2 (two α- and two δ-chains), and 1% fetal hemoglobin (two α- and two γ-chains). These polypeptide chains are attached to and folded around each heme structure, giving hemoglobin its unique tetrahedron shape.

The initial step in the synthesis of heme from the substrate succinyl CoA and glycine requires the presence of pyridoxine phosphate (vitamin B_6) as a catalyst. Following its synthesis in the cytoplasmic mitochondria of the RBC, heme diffuses into the extramitochondrial space, combines with the completed α- and β-chains, and forms hemoglobin.

Under normal conditions, the body produces approximately 6.25 g of hemoglobin daily. Maximal output of hemoglobin in the event of a hemolytic disease has been estimated at about 40 g daily. Consequently, if the bone marrow functions at maximal capacity, the normal RBC survival time of 120 days can decrease to 18 to 20 days before an anemia develops. When hemolytic destruction of RBCs exceeds marrow production capacity and anemia develops, the hemoglobin value decreases to a steady-state level at which production is equal to destruction. Hemoglobin values in these hemolytic anemias, such as sickle cell anemia, will remain stable unless other factors further shorten the RBC life span.

The affinity of hemoglobin for oxygen is influenced by three intracellular components and by temperature. Increasing hydrogen ion concentration (decreasing pH), carbon dioxide, and 2,3-bisphosphoglycerate (2,3-BPG), together with increased temperature, all enhance the ability of hemoglobin to release oxygen into tissue by decreasing oxygen affinity.

BODY IRON

The body of the average adult male contains about 3.8 g of iron; that of the female, about 2.3 g of iron. Approximately 80% of the iron exists in the form of hemoglobin. Another 13% exists as myoglobin, while a similar percentage exists as a combination of ferritin and hemosiderin. Because inorganic iron is quite toxic, the body has an intricate system for iron absorption, transport, storage, assimilation, and elimination.

ABSORPTION OF IRON

The normal daily Western diet contains approximately 12 to 15 mg of iron, mainly in the ferric (Fe^{3+}) nonabsorbed form. After being

TABLE 99–1. Classification Systems for Anemias

- I. Morphology
  - Macrocytic anemias
    - Megaloblastic anemias
      - Vitamin B_{12} deficiency
      - Folic acid deficiency anemia
  - Microcytic, hypochromic anemias
    - Iron deficiency anemia
    - Genetic anomaly
      - Sickle cell anemia
      - Thalassemia
      - Other hemoglobinopathies (abnormal hemoglobins)
  - Normocytic anemias
    - Recent blood loss
    - Hemolysis
    - Bone marrow failure
    - Anemias of chronic disease
    - Renal failure
    - Endocrine disorders
    - Myeloplastic anemias
- II. Etiology
  - Deficiency
    - Iron
    - Vitamin B_{12}
    - Folic acid
    - Pyridoxine
  - Central—caused by impaired bone marrow function
    - Anemia of chronic disease
    - Anemia of the elderly
    - Malignant bone marrow disorders
  - Peripheral
    - Bleeding (hemorrhage)
    - Hemolysis (hemolytic anemias)
- III. Pathophysiology
  - Excessive blood loss
    - Recent hemorrhage
    - Trauma
    - Peptic ulcer
    - Gastritis
    - Hemorrhoids
  - Chronic hemorrhage
    - Vaginal bleeding
    - Peptic ulcer
    - Intestinal parasites
    - Aspirin and other nonsteroidal anti-inflammatory agents
  - Excessive RBC destruction
    - Extracorpuscular (outside the cell) factors
      - RBC antibodies
      - Drugs
      - Physical trauma to RBC (artificial valves)
      - Excessive sequestration in the spleen
    - Intracorpuscular factor
      - Heredity
      - Disorders of hemoglobin synthesis
  - Inadequate production of mature RBCs
    - Deficiency of nutrients (B_{12}, folic acid, iron, protein)
    - Deficiency of erythroblasts
      - Aplastic anemia
      - Isolated (often transient) erythroblastopenia
      - Folic acid antagonists
      - Antibodies
    - Conditions with infiltration of bone marrow
      - Lymphoma
      - Leukemia
      - Myelofibrosis
      - Carcinoma
    - Endocrine abnormalities
      - Hypothyroidism
      - Adrenal insufficiency
      - Pituitary insufficiency
    - Chronic renal disease
    - Chronic inflammatory disease
      - Granulomatous diseases
      - Collagen-vascular diseases
    - Hepatic disease

RBC = red blood cell.

ionized by stomach acid and then reduced to the ferrous state (Fe^{2+}), this iron is absorbed primarily in the duodenum and, to a smaller extent, in the jejunum via intestinal mucosal cell uptake. Subsequently, it is transferred across the cell into the plasma.[2] The average intake of iron from this diet is about 6 mg per 1,000 calories (about 10 to 30 mg of iron per day).[3]

Daily requirements for iron are 1 mg in adult males and postmenopausal females, and 1.5 to 3 mg in menstruating females. This 1- to 3-mg amount represents about 5% to 10% of daily dietary intake. Children and pregnant women have increased iron needs. Children require more iron because of growth-related increases in blood volume, and pregnant women have an increased iron demand brought about by fetal development. As much as 8 to 12 mg daily can be absorbed if iron requirements increase sufficiently. Iron overload does not occur, however, because only the amount of iron lost per day is absorbed.

Heme iron, found in meat, fish, and poultry, is about three times more absorbable than the nonheme iron found in vegetables and dietary supplements. Gastric acid and other dietary components such as ascorbic acid increase the absorption of nonheme iron. Dietary components that form insoluble complexes or chelates with iron (phytates, tannates, and phosphates) decrease absorption.[4] Phytates, a natural component of grains, brans, and some other vegetables, can form stable, poorly absorbed complexes and partially explain the increased prevalence of IDA in poorer countries, where grains and vegetables compose a disproportionate part of the normal diet and the more readily absorbed heme iron is lacking in their diet. Finally, because gastric acid improves iron absorption, patients who have undergone a gastrectomy or have achlorhydria will have decreased iron absorption. The amount of iron absorbed from food depends on the body stores, the rate of RBC production, the type of iron provided in the diet, and any other substances present that may enhance or inhibit iron absorption.

INCORPORATION OF IRON INTO HEME

A specific plasma transport protein called transferrin delivers iron to the bone marrow for incorporation into the RBC hemoglobin molecule. Transferrin enters cells by binding to transferrin receptors; these circulate and then attach to cells needing iron. Conversely, there are fewer transferrin receptors on the surface of cells not currently needing iron, thus preventing iron-replete cells from receiving excess iron.[5]

Circulating transferrin is normally about 30% saturated with iron. Transferrin delivers extra iron to other body storage sites, such as the liver, marrow, and spleen, for later use. This iron is stored within macrophages as ferritin or hemosiderin. Ferritin consists of a ferric hydroxyphosphate core surrounded by a protein shell called apoferritin. Hemosiderin can be described as compacted ferritin molecules with an even greater iron/protein shell ratio; physiologically, it is a more stable, but less available, form of storage iron.

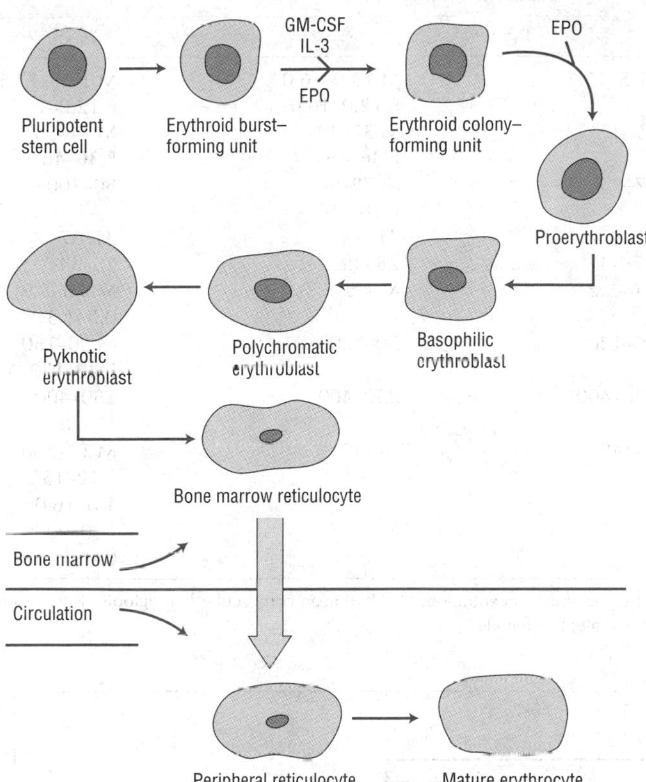

FIGURE 99–1. Erythrocyte maturation sequence. EPO = erythropoietin; GM-CSF = granulocyte-macrophage colony-stimulating factor; IL-3 = interleukin-3.

NORMAL DESTRUCTION OF RBCs

Phagocytic breakdown destroys older blood cells, primarily in the spleen but also in the marrow (Fig. 99–2). Amino acids from the globin chains return to an amino acid pool; heme oxygenase acts on the porphyrin heme structure to form biliverdin and to release its iron. Iron returns to the iron pool to be reused while biliverdin is further catabolized to bilirubin. Then the bilirubin is released into the plasma, where it binds to albumin, and is transported to the liver for glucuronide conjugation and excretion via bile. If the liver is unable to perform the conjugation, as seen with intrinsic liver disease or over saturation of conjugation enzymes by excessive cell hemolysis, the result would be an elevated indirect (unconjugated) bilirubin laboratory value. Should there be an obstruction in the biliary excretion pathway for the already conjugated bilirubin, an elevated direct bilirubin would result. Comparison of direct and indirect bilirubin values helps to determine if the defect in bilirubin clearance occurs before or after bilirubin enters the liver.

The hemoglobin in RBCs, which is destroyed by intravascular hemolysis, becomes attached to haptoglobin and is carried back to the marrow for processing in the normal manner.

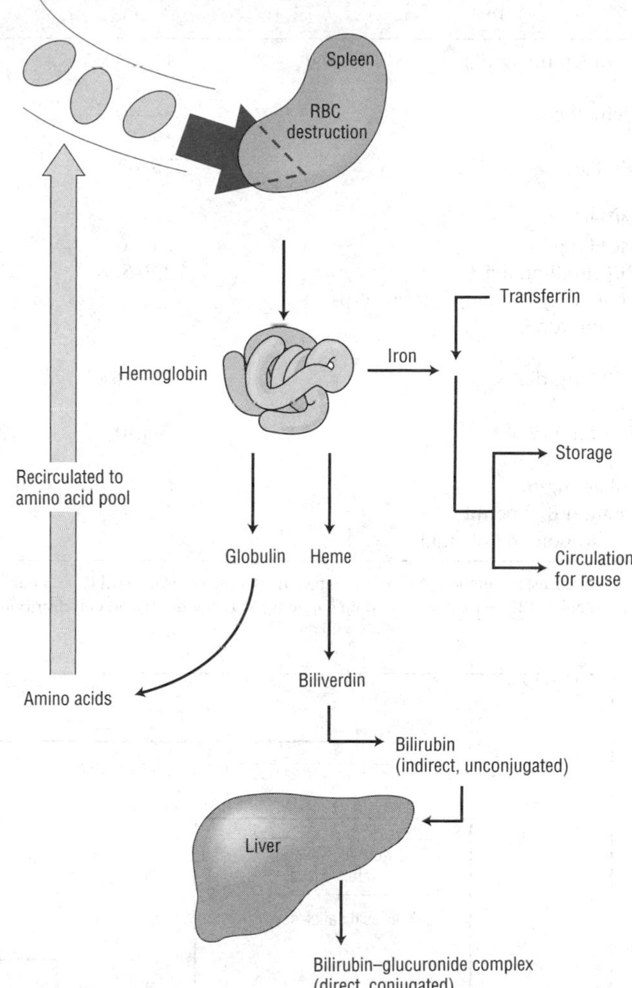

FIGURE 99–2. Destruction of red blood cells (RBCs).

DIAGNOSIS OF ANEMIA

GENERAL PRESENTATION

The presenting signs and symptoms of anemias depend on the rate of development of the anemia, the age of the patient, and the cardiovascular status of the patient. Anemia of recent onset is most likely to present with cardiorespiratory symptoms such as tachycardia, lightheadedness, and breathlessness, whereas if the onset is more chronic in nature, the presenting symptoms may include fatigue, weakness, headache, vertigo, faintness, sensitivity to cold, pallor, and loss of skin tone. These symptoms represent the manifestation of an illness, not a specific disease. Signs and symptoms of other primary hematologic diseases such as lymphadenopathy, hepatosplenomegaly, or bone tenderness, should be noted, if present.

LABORATORY EVALUATION

The initial evaluation of anemia involves a complete blood cell count, including RBC indices; a reticulocyte index; examination of a peripheral blood smear; and examination of a stool sample for occult blood. The results from the preliminary evaluation determine the need for other studies. Table 99–2 shows normal hematologic values. By definition, anemia is present in adults if the hematocrit is less than 41% or the hemoglobin is less than 13.5 g/dL in males and less than 12 g/dL in females.

Figure 99–3 provides a broad, general algorithm for the diagnosis of anemias based on laboratory data. There are many exceptions and additions to this algorithm, but it can serve as a guide to the typical presentation of the most common types and causes of anemia.

HEMOGLOBIN

Values given for hemoglobin represent the amount of hemoglobin per volume of whole blood. The higher values seen in males are due to

TABLE 99–2. Normal Hematologic Values

Test	Reference Range (yr)			
	2–6	*6–12*	*12–18*	*18–49*
Hemoglobin (g/dL)	11.5–15.5	11.5–15.5	M 13.0–16.0 F 12.0–16.0	M 13.5–17.5 F 12.0–16.0
Hematocrit (%)	34–40	35–45	M 37–49 F 36–46	M 41–53 F 36–46
MCV (fL)	75–87	77–95	M 78–98 F 78–102	80–100
MCHC (%)	—	31–37	31–37	31–37
MCH (pg)	24–30	25–33	25–35	26–34
RBC (million/mm^3)	3.9–5.3	4.0–5.2	M 4.5–5.3	M 4.5–5.9
Reticulocyte count, absolute (%)				0.5–1.5
Serum iron (μg/dL)		50–120	50–120	M 50–160 F 40–150
TIBC (μg/dL)	250–400	250–400	250–400	250–400
RDW (%)				11–16
Ferritin (ng/mL)	7–140	7–140	7–140	M 15–200 F 12–150
Folate (ng/mL)				1.8–16.0[a]
Vitamin B_{12} (pg/mL)				100–900[a]
Erythropoietin (mU/mL)				0–19

[a]Varies by assay method. MCV = mean corpuscular volume; MCHC = mean corpuscular hemoglobin concentration; MCH = mean corpuscular hemoglobin; RBC = red blood cell; TIBC = total iron-binding capacity; RDW = red blood cell distribution width; M = male; F = female.

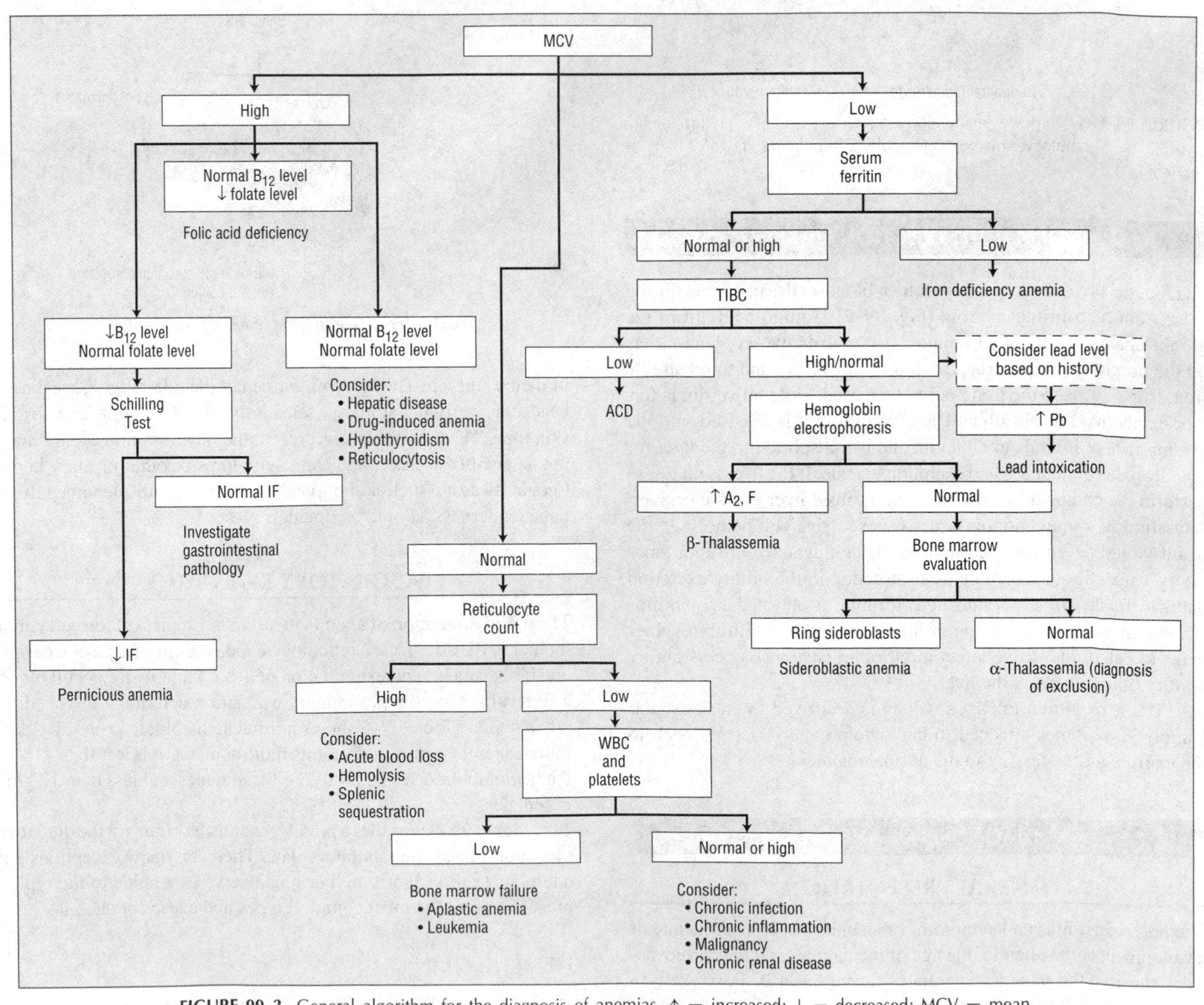

FIGURE 99–3. General algorithm for the diagnosis of anemias. ↑ = increased; ↓ = decreased; MCV = mean corpuscular volume; IF = intrinsic factor; TIBC = total iron-binding capacity; ACD = anemia of chronic disease; Pb = lead; A_2 = hemoglobin A_2; F = hemoglobin F; WBC = white blood cells.

stimulation of RBC production by androgenic steroids and, to a lesser extent, to the decrease in hemoglobin in females caused by the loss of blood during menstruation. The level of hemoglobin can be used as a very rough estimate of the oxygen-carrying capacity of blood. It can be reduced because of a decreased quantity of hemoglobin per RBC or because of a decreased actual number of RBCs.

HEMATOCRIT

Expressed as a percentage, hematocrit (Hct) is the actual volume of RBCs in a unit volume of whole blood. In general, it is about three times the hemoglobin value. An alteration in this ratio may occur with abnormal cell size or shape and often indicates pathology. A low hematocrit indicates a reduction in either the number or the size of RBCs, or an increase in plasma volume.

RBC COUNT

An actual count of red cells per unit of blood, the RBC count is an indirect estimate of the hemoglobin content of the blood.

RBC INDICES

In 1934, Maxwell Wintrobe introduced indices to describe the size and hemoglobin content of the RBCs. These Wintrobe indices are calculated from the hemoglobin, hematocrit, and RBC count.

Mean Corpuscular Volume (Hct/RBC Count)

Mean corpuscular volume (MCV) represents the average volume of RBCs. Cells are said to be macrocytic if they are larger than normal, microcytic if they are smaller than normal, and normocytic if their size falls within normal limits. Folic acid and vitamin B_{12} deficiency anemias yield macrocytic morphology, whereas iron deficiency and thalassemia are examples of microcytic anemias. A falsely elevated MCV occurs with reticulocytosis because reticulocytes are larger than erythrocytes. The MCV is also falsely elevated in the presence of cold agglutinins and hyperglycemia.

Mean Corpuscular Hemoglobin (Hgb/RBC Count)

The percent volume of hemoglobin in an RBC is the mean corpuscular hemoglobin (MCH). Two morphologic changes, microcytosis or hypochromia, can reduce the MCH. A microcytic cell contains less hemoglobin because it is a smaller cell, whereas a hypochromic cell has a low MCH because of the decreased amount of hemoglobin present in a normocytic cell. Cells can be both microcytic and hypochromic, as seen with IDA, and the MCH alone cannot distinguish between microcytosis and hypochromia. The most common cause of an elevated MCH is macrocytosis (e.g., folate deficiency). A falsely elevated MCH occurs in patients with hyperlipidemia.

Mean Corpuscular Hemoglobin Concentration (Hgb/Hct)

The weight of hemoglobin per volume of cells is the average corpuscular hemoglobin concentration (MCHC). Because the MCHC is independent of cell size, it is more useful than the MCH in distinguishing between microcytosis and hypochromia. A low MCHC always indicates hypochromia; a microcyte with a normal hemoglobin concentration will have a low MCH, but a normal MCHC. Patients with hyperlipidemia have a falsely elevated MCHC. It is routinely low in IDA, but it can also be decreased in other hemoglobin synthesis disorders.

TOTAL RETICULOCYTE COUNT

Although an indirect assessment, the total reticulocyte count is an indication of new RBC production. In a normal situation, 1% of RBCs are replaced daily; this represents a reticulocyte count of 1%. The reticulocyte count in normocytic anemia can differentiate hypoproliferative marrow from a compensatory marrow response to an anemia. Occasionally, a patient's hematocrit decreases while the absolute number of reticulocytes remains the same, resulting in a falsely elevated reticulocyte percentage. For example, if a patient's hematocrit decreases by 50% (e.g., from 50% to 25%), the corresponding reticulocyte percentage doubles. Expressing the reticulocyte count as an absolute number corrects this problem; multiplying the percentage of reticulocytes (expressed as a decimal) by the total RBC count makes this possible. Multiplying the reticulocyte percentage by the patient's hematocrit and then dividing the product by an average normal hematocrit (for men or women) also produces a corrected percentage of reticulocytes.

RED BLOOD CELL DISTRIBUTION WIDTH (RDW)

The higher the RBC distribution width, the more variable the size of the RBCs. The distribution width increases in early IDA (often prior to changes in other parameters), but this change is not specific for this disease. The distribution width can also be helpful in the diagnosis of a mixed anemia. A patient can have a normal MCV, yet have a wide RBC distribution width. This would indicate presence of microcytes and macrocytes, which would yield a "normal" average RBC size.

SERUM IRON

The level of serum iron is the concentration of iron bound to transferrin. Normally, transferrin is about one-third bound (saturated) to iron. Unfortunately, the serum iron level of many patients with IDA remains within the lower limits of normal, giving a false-negative test result. There is also a 20% to 30% diurnal variation in serum iron levels (it is best to draw blood levels in the morning), as well as a 20% to 25% day-to-day variation among individuals.[6] Consequently, as a diagnostic tool, serum iron levels are best interpreted in conjunction with the total iron-binding capacity (TIBC). The serum iron level decreases with IDA and ACD, and it increases with hemolytic anemias and iron overload.

TOTAL IRON-BINDING CAPACITY

An indirect measurement of the iron-binding capacity of serum transferrin, the TIBC evaluation is performed by adding an excess of iron to plasma to saturate all transferrin with iron. The excess (unbound) iron is then removed, and the serum iron concentration is determined. Unlike the serum iron level, the TIBC is remarkably constant. The finding of a low serum iron level and a high TIBC indicates IDA. Patients with infection, malignancy, and uremia may have a decreased TIBC and a decreased serum iron level, findings that are consistent with the diagnosis of ACD.

PERCENTAGE TRANSFERRIN SATURATION

The ratio of the serum iron level to the TIBC indicates transferrin saturation. It is expressed as a percentage, that is,

$$\text{Transferrin saturation} = (\text{Serum iron}/\text{TIBC}) \times 100$$

Normally transferrin is 20–50% saturated with iron. In IDA, transferrin saturation of only 15% or lower is commonly seen.

SERUM FERRITIN

The concentration of ferritin (storage iron) in the serum is proportional to total iron stores and, consequently, is a reliable indicator of body iron stores. Low serum ferritin levels are virtually diagnostic of IDA, as they decrease only in association with IDA. In contrast, serum iron levels may decrease both in IDA and in ACD.

FOLIC ACID

The results of folic acid measurements may vary, depending on the assay method used. Decreased serum folic acid levels indicate a folate deficiency megaloblastic anemia that may coexist with a vitamin B_{12} deficiency anemia. An erythrocyte folic acid level is less volatile than serum levels; it is slow to decrease in an acute process such as drug-induced folic acid deficiency and slow to increase with oral folic acid replacement. The clinical utility of determining the erythrocyte folic acid level is questionable, however, and the procedure should be reserved for cases in which the clinician suspects folic acid depletion and the serum folic acid may be falsely elevated or depleted.

VITAMIN B_{12}

The level of vitamin B_{12} (cyanocobolamine) may vary according to the assay method used. Low levels indicate vitamin B_{12} deficiency anemia.

SCHILLING TEST

The purpose of the Schilling test is to diagnose vitamin B_{12} deficiency anemia caused by a B_{12} absorption defect resulting from a lack of intrinsic factor (pernicious anemia). The patient first receives an oral dose of radiolabeled vitamin B_{12}. Two hours later, the patient receives a large intramuscular dose of nonlabeled vitamin B_{12} to saturate plasma transport proteins. Any excess vitamin B_{12} that is not taken up by the transport proteins or stored in the liver will be excreted in the urine. A 24-hour urine collection is then measured for radioactivity. If sufficient gastrointestinal intrinsic factor is being produced, the B_{12} will be absorbed.

Normally, more than 7% of the absorbed radiolabeled B_{12} appears in the urine over 24 hours. Patients with pernicious anemia excrete less than 7% of the original oral radiolabeled dose. If oral absorption is impaired (less than 7% excreted), part II of this test is conducted 5 to 7 days after part I. The second stage of the Schilling test differentiates inadequate secretion of intrinsic factor by the stomach from an abnormality in absorption by the ileum. Radiolabeled vitamin B_{12} is administered orally with a sufficient amount of intrinsic factor. Results within the normal range (i.e., >10%) indicate that the defect is in the production of intrinsic factor as opposed to other causes of vitamin B_{12} deficiency, such as dietary deficiency or small bowel pathology.

If the results in part II are still low, then the third stage of the test is conducted. The patient is given tetracycline, 250 mg four times daily for 10 days. Tetracycline reduces the intestinal bacteria in blind loop syndrome. Blind loops occur when a segment of the intestine is blocked off from the rest of the intestinal tract such that nothing can pass through. The loops are subject to bacterial overgrowth that may lead to malabsorption. If the excretion of radiolabeled vitamin B_{12} improves after the tetracycline, then there is a malabsorptive syndrome related to the intestinal bacteria.

COOMBS TEST

Antiglobulin tests, also called Coombs tests, indicate hemolytic anemia caused by an immune response. A direct Coombs test detects antibodies bound to erythrocytes, whereas an indirect Coombs test measures antibodies present in the serum. A positive finding in a direct antiglobulin test is usually indicative of immune hemolysis.

ERYTHROPOIETIN LEVELS

Healthy individuals require 10–30 mU/mL of EPO to maintain normal hemoglobin and hematocrit concentrations. Endogenous EPO levels can increase up to 100- to 1,000-fold during hypoxia or anemia. This marked increase does not occur in patients with end-stage renal disease, patients receiving chemotherapy, and patients with acquired immunodeficiency syndrome (AIDS), especially those taking azidothymidine (AZT). These patients will have an erythropoietin response that is insufficient to correct their anemia.

SPECIFIC ANEMIAS

ANEMIAS CAUSED BY ABNORMAL HEMOGLOBIN SYNTHESIS

A defect in hemoglobin synthesis, as well as acquired defects in EPO precursor cell metabolism, may cause changes in iron incorporation, producing a cell with an excess of nonheme iron within the cytoplasm. Called sideroblasts, these cells cause sideroblastic anemia, which is usually microcytic. Sideroblastic anemia can be congenital (hereditary, sex-linked in males) or acquired. The acquired forms can be either primary or secondary to drugs, toxins (e.g., lead, alcohol), or other disease states. Hypocupremia has long been associated with sideroblastosis. Excess zinc intake causes sideroblastic anemia by binding preferentially to copper, impairing copper absorption and leading to hypocupremia.[7] Primary acquired sideroblastic anemia is usually classified as a myelodysplastic syndrome and may eventually transform into acute myeloblastic leukemia in some patients.

Other hereditary defects in heme synthesis can lead to an overproduction of heme precursors, resulting in porphyria. The most common form, acute intermittent porphyria (AIP), results from a hereditary (autosomal dominant) partial deficiency in the enzyme uroporphyrinogen I synthetase, which is responsible for converting porphobilinogen to uroporphyrinogen. This deficiency inhibits the normal feedback mechanism of porphyrin synthesis, leading to an excess production of heme intermediate pigments uroporphyrin I and coproporphyrin I. These products can be detected in abnormal amounts in urine and feces to confirm the diagnosis of AIP.

Neuropsychiatric, neuromuscular, and autonomic dysfunction and intense abdominal pain characterize AIP. In the liver, this enzyme deficiency results in the increased inducibility of abnormal heme intermediates by certain drugs. Drugs and agents known to induce hepatic cytochrome P450 or to increase hepatic heme turnover are theoretically capable of precipitating porphyria. Barbiturates,[8] estrogens,[9] alcohol,[10] and heavy metals such as lead have been documented to induce porphyria in genetically susceptible people.

Genetic expression of an abnormal amino acid substitution in either the α- or β-globin chains can lead to a variety of hemoglobinopathies causing hemolytic diseases such as sickle cell anemia and thalassemia (see Chapter 101, Sickle Cell Anemia). Four genes control α-chain production, and two genes regulate β-chain production. Thalassemias result when these genes are defective. If three or four α-genes or both β-genes are not functioning properly, a major thalassemia, which is often incompatible with life, develops. Fortunately, thalassemia minor (trait) is more common. The trait results from deficiencies in one or two α-genes or one β-gene. For example, if α-genes are affected, normal β-chains would accumulate in the cell and damage the membrane. This cell would then be prematurely cleared from the circulation, exacerbating the anemia. Surviving cells have inadequate hemoglobin and are microcytic and hypochromic.

Thalassemia is most commonly seen in patients of Asian, Mediterranean, or African descent; it is frequently asymptomatic, requiring no treatment. It is important to distinguish thalassemia from IDA to avoid inappropriate iron therapy. Although both are microcytic, the MCV tends to be much lower with thalassemia than with IDA. Also, target cells may be seen on the peripheral smear in patients with thalassemia. Finally, in contrast to patients with IDA, ferritin levels are normal or increased in patients with thalassemia. Hundreds of these abnormal hemoglobin diseases exist and are best diagnosed by hemoglobin electrophoresis.

HEMOCHROMATOSIS (IRON OVERLOAD)

Hereditary hemochromatosis is an autosomal recessive disease caused by a gene mutation on chromosome 6 designated HFE. The majority of patients with hereditary hemochromatosis have a mutation called C282Y, which leads to a decrease in transferrin-mediated uptake of iron from the blood to the crypt cells and a corresponding increase in iron absorption from the intestine.[11] These patients can absorb up to three times as much iron from their diets as normal individuals. As a result, iron deposition in the form of hemosiderin occurs in various tissues, such as the liver, pancreas, heart, adrenals, testes, pituitary, and kidneys. This deposition causes a variety of conditions in multiple organ systems, including cirrhosis and various forms of heart disease, arthropathy, diabetes mellitus, and portal hypertension. Hemochromatosis patients are also more susceptible to infections with microorganisms such as *Vibrio vulnificus, Listeria monocytogenes, Yersinia enterocolitica, Salmonella enteritidis, Klebsiella pneumoniae, Escherichia coli,* mucor species. Typically, hemochromatosis is not diagnosed until the 5th decade of life.

Secondary or acquired hemochromatosis results from some abnormality other than a primary increase in intestinal iron absorption. Possible causes of secondary hemochromatosis include excess medicinal or dietary iron or repeated blood transfusions.[12] Marked increases in transferrin saturation (>50% in premenopausal women and >60% in men and postmenopausal women) are suggestive of this disease and warrant further evaluation of ferritin levels and liver biopsy. This disease is rare, with a prevalence of less than 0.1%.[13]

▶ TREATMENT: Hemochromatosis (Iron Overload)

Early diagnosis with periodic prophylactic phlebotomy employed early in the disease can ameliorate late-stage disease complications. Each 0.5 L of blood contains 200–250 mg of iron. The usual phlebotomy schedule is 1 unit weekly until the patient is mildly hypoferritinemic (the length of time for weekly phlebotomy varies and can be up to 2 to 3 years), then every 2 to 4 months as needed to keep the ferritin level below 50 μg/L. If treatment begins early, the life expectancy and quality of life are normal in these patients. When phlebotomy starts later, treatment can ameliorate the symptoms of liver pain and enlargement and painful joints, but the endocrine changes are largely irreversible.

The use of an iron chelator, deferoxamine, is useful in acute iron intoxications or in iron overload caused by multiple RBC transfusions. The usual dose is 40–50 mg/kg/day infused intravenously (IV) at 15 mg/kg/h or 20–40 mg/kg/day as a subcutaneous infusion over 8 to 12 hours. A fixed 2-g dose of deferoxamine infused at 15 mg/kg/h is also used after each unit of RBCs. If the creatinine clearance rate is less than 10 mL/min, the dose should be reduced by 50%. Rapid infusion can produce hypotension and shock. It is important to monitor the patient's urine until it is no longer pink; the loss of the pink color is an indicator that the dose of deferoxamine is adequate. These patients also need dietary counseling to limit their intake of iron through red meat, alcohol, and vitamin C, which can aid iron absorption.

IRON DEFICIENCY ANEMIA

PATHOPHYSIOLOGY

Over 500 million people worldwide have iron deficiency anemia (IDA). While not a lethal condition, IDA is associated with increased risks of infections, diminished work productivity, and developmental delays. Causes differ widely between developed and underdeveloped countries. The most common causes of IDA in undeveloped countries are malnutrition and hookworms. In more industrialized nations, the risks for developing IDA are largely related to dietary factors. Diets limited in meat or fresh fruits and vegetables or diets high in substances that form complexes with iron may result in IDA. Other causes of IDA include chronic illnesses, inflammatory conditions like rheumatoid arthritis, and malabsorptive syndromes. Situations that increase the demand for iron are blood donations, endurance sports, menstruation, pregnancy and lactation, infancy, and adolescence.[14] At diagnosis, the cause of IDA must be considered a consequence of blood loss until ruled out. More than 50% of adults with IDA have some form of gastrointestinal bleeding. Blood loss may occur as a result of many disorders, including trauma, angiodysplasia, hemorrhoids, peptic ulcers, gastritis, gastrointestinal malignancies, diverticular disease, copious menstrual flow, nose bleeds, or postpartum bleeding. Occult blood loss from a single gastrointestinal lesion has been shown to be a frequent cause of "idiopathic" IDA.[15] Less common causes include hemoglobinuria and iron sequestration of pulmonary hemosiderosis.

Diseases contributing to the development of IDA include rheumatoid arthritis (with chronic aspirin ingestion), various malignancies, and renal disease. With IDA, the possibility of a multifactorial cause must always be considered. Other possible causes of hypochromic, microcytic anemia include ACD, thalassemia (especially thalassemia minor), sideroblastic anemia, and heavy metal (mostly lead) poisoning (see Fig. 99–3).

SIGNS AND SYMPTOMS

Patients with IDA may be asymptomatic, or they may have vague, general signs and symptoms associated with other anemias: easy fatigability, tachycardia, palpitations, tachypnea on exertion. Other manifestations of IDA include koilonychia (spooning of the nails), angular stomatitis and glossitis, smooth tongue, brittle nails, cheilosis, dysphagia due to esophageal webs (Plummer-Vinson syndrome), and pica, a craving for substances such as clay, ice, or cornstarch. These symptoms usually do not appear until the hemoglobin concentration falls below 8 or 9 g/dL of whole blood. In April of 1998, the Centers for Disease Control (CDC) published revised recommendations to prevent and control iron deficiency in the United States, focusing on children and women of childbearing age.[16]

LABORATORY MANIFESTATIONS

Generally, abnormal laboratory findings in patients with IDA include low serum iron and ferritin levels and a high TIBC. In the early stages of IDA, the RBC size is not changed. Low concentrations of ferritin (10–12 g/L) are the earliest and most sensitive indications of iron deficiency. The disadvantage of using this parameter to evaluate iron stores is the fact that renal or liver disease, malignancies, infection, or inflammatory processes may elevate the measured values to greater than 50 g/L and these values may not correlate with iron stores in the bone marrow.[17] The hemoglobin, hematocrit, and RBC indices usually remain normal.

In the later stages of IDA, the hemoglobin and hematocrit fall below normal values, and a microcytic, hypochromic anemia develops. Microcytosis may precede hypochromia as erythropoiesis is programmed to maintain normal hemoglobin concentration in deference to cell size. As a consequence, even slightly abnormal hemoglobin and hematocrit levels may indicate significant depletion of iron stores and should not be ignored.

As noted earlier, transferrin saturation (i.e., serum iron level divided by the TIBC) is also useful in assessing IDA. Low values (below 15%) likely indicate IDA, although low serum transferrin saturation values may also be present in inflammatory disorders. Fortunately, the TIBC usually helps to differentiate the diagnosis in these patients: a TIBC greater than 400 g% suggests IDA, whereas values below 200 g% usually represent inflammatory disease. With continued progression of IDA, anisocytosis occurs (variations in RBC size) and poikilocytosis (variations in RBC shape) develop. The blood smear of a patient with severe IDA can contain hypochromic cells, target cells, pencil-shaped cells, and occasional nucleated RBCs.

The level of free erythrocyte protoporphyrin can also be used in the diagnosis of IDA. Iron normally binds with protoporphyrin to form heme; therefore, a low serum iron level elevates the serum concentration of protoporphyrin not bound to iron. This test is very helpful in distinguishing between iron deficiency and thalassemia minor, because values are normal in patients with thalassemia and elevated in patients with IDA. Unfortunately, free erythrocyte protoporphyrin is also elevated in inflammatory disorders and lead poisoning, which makes it less effective in distinguishing IDA in patients who may have these other two conditions.

Finally, in rare cases, a bone marrow examination can be performed to assess bone marrow iron stores. Documentation of decreased hemosiderin can confirm the diagnosis of IDA.

▶ TREATMENT: Iron Deficiency Anemia

DIETARY SUPPLEMENTATION AND THERAPEUTIC IRON PREPARATIONS

Treatment of IDA usually consists of dietary supplementation and administration of therapeutic iron preparations. Iron absorption varies greatly with different foods. Iron is poorly absorbed from vegetables, grain products, dairy products, and eggs; it is best absorbed from meat, fish, and poultry. Substitution of meat for eggs, milk, or cheese in a mixed meal has been shown to quadruple the absorption of iron from the entire meal.[18] Beverages have also been shown to affect iron absorption. For example, orange juice doubles the absorption of iron from an entire meal, whereas tea or milk reduces absorption to less than one-half.[19,20] It is recommended that meat, orange juice, and other ascorbic acid–rich foods be included in meals and that if milk and tea are used, they be consumed in moderation between meals.

In most cases of IDA, the oral administration of iron therapy with soluble ferrous iron salts is appropriate. Iron is best absorbed in the reduced ferrous form, with maximal absorption occurring in the duodenum primarily because the acid medium of the stomach and mucopolysaccharide chelator substances that prevent the iron from precipitating maintain the iron in a soluble form. In the alkaline environment of the small intestines, iron tends to form insoluble complexes that are unavailable for absorption. Based on these considerations, the preferred iron preparation is a non–enteric-coated ferrous salt. Slow-release or sustained-release iron preparations do not undergo sufficient dissolution until reaching the small intestines, which significantly reduces iron absorption and can attenuate the hematinic effects.[21,22]

The dose depends on the patient's ability to tolerate the administered iron. In patients with IDA, it is generally recommended that approximately 200 mg elemental iron be administered daily, usually in two or three divided doses to maximize tolerability.[23] Table 99–3 shows the percent elemental iron of commonly available iron salts. Note that ferrous sulfate is also available as an exsiccated form that contains approximately 30% elemental iron as compared to the nonexsiccated form that is only 20% elemental iron. The percentage of iron absorbed progressively decreases as the dose increases, but the absolute amount absorbed increases. Because food interferes with the absorption of iron, it should preferably be administered 1 hour or more before meals. Many patients must take their iron with food because they experience nausea and diarrhea when iron is administered on an empty stomach. Giving smaller amounts of iron with each administration may minimize these adverse effects. Although some forms of iron are combined with ascorbic acid or antacids, these combinations do not enhance absorption from iron preparations when given orally on an empty stomach. Gradually introducing the iron formulation and escalating the dose with food can improve compliance with oral iron therapy.

Therapeutic doses of iron should increase hemoglobin values by 1 g per week. As the hemoglobin level approaches normal, the rate of

TABLE 99–3. Oral Iron Products

Salt	Amount of Elemental Iron Provided
Ferrous sulfate	60–65 mg/300- or 325-mg tablet
Ferrous sulfate exsiccated	65 mg/200-mg tablet
Ferrous gluconate	37–39 mg/300 or 325 mg tablet
Ferrous fumarate	33 mg/100 mg tablet
Polysaccharide-iron complex	150 mg/capsule 50 mg/tablet

increase slows progressively. A hemoglobin response of less than 2 g over a 3-week period is unacceptable and warrants further evaluation. Reticulocytosis occurs within 7 to 10 days after the initiation of iron therapy. If the patient does not develop reticulocytosis, it is necessary to reevaluate the diagnosis or therapy.

Iron therapy should continue for a period sufficient for complete restoration of iron stores. The time interval required to accomplish this goal varies, although at least 3 to 6 months of therapy is usually necessary.[24] Patients with negative iron balances caused by bleeding may require iron replacement therapy for only a month after correction of the underlying lesion, whereas patients with recurrent negative balances may require long-term treatment. This latter group may require as little as 30–60 mg of elemental iron daily.

Adverse reactions to therapeutic doses of iron are primarily gastrointestinal in nature and consist of discoloration of feces (dark), constipation or diarrhea, nausea, and vomiting. Failure to develop at least some of these symptoms, even mildly, may indicate noncompliance. If these side effects become intolerable, the dose may be taken with meals or the total daily dose may be decreased to 110–120 mg elemental iron. As noted, however, the administration of iron with meals reduces the amount of iron absorbed by more than one-half.

Failure to respond to appropriate treatment regimens necessitates reevaluation of the patient's condition. Common causes of treatment failure include noncompliance with therapy, misdiagnosis, presence of a concomitant anemia-inducing disease, malabsorption, and blood loss equal to the rate of production. Malabsorption can be ruled out by the iron test in which plasma iron levels are determined at half-hour intervals for 2 hours following the administration of 50 mg of elemental iron as liquid ferrous sulfate. If plasma iron levels increase by more than 50 μg during this time, absorption is satisfactory.

PARENTERAL IRON THERAPY

When there is evidence of iron malabsorption or intolerance of orally administered iron or when long-term noncompliance is a problem, parenteral iron therapy may be necessary. Patients with significant blood loss who refuse transfusions and in whom oral iron therapy is not possible may also require parenteral iron therapy. Patients receiving chronic hemodialysis or chronic ambulatory peritoneal dialysis and need parenteral iron therapy commonly receive EPO in conjunction with the iron.

Iron dextran, a complex of ferric hydroxide and dextran containing 50 mg of iron/mL, may be given intramuscularly or IV. Methods of IV administration include multiple slow injections of undiluted iron dextran solution or an infusion of a diluted preparation. This latter method is often referred to as total dose infusion. The intramuscular administration of iron dextran should take place via Z-tract (a technique to handle intramuscular injections of irritating substances with minimal tracking of the medication through surrounding tissues) to minimize staining of the skin. Because each intramuscular dose is limited to 2 mL (100 mg of iron), multiple injections are often required. Problems with intramuscular administration include patient discomfort, sterile abscesses, tissue necrosis, or atrophy. In addition, up to 30% of an administered dose remains physiologically unavailable. For these reasons, the IV route is the preferred route of administration.

Equations for calculating the appropriate dose in patients with IDA and patients with anemia secondary to blood loss can be found in Table 99–4. When given by IV administration, the dose should not exceed 50 mg of iron per minute (1 mL/min). The manufacturer suggests no more than 100 mg of iron dextran be administered daily.

TABLE 99–4. Equations for Calculating Doses of Iron Dextran

In patients with iron deficiency anemia:

Adults + children over 15 kg

$$\text{Dose (mL)} = 0.0442\,(\text{desired Hgb} - \text{observed Hgb}) \times \text{LBW} + (0.26 \times \text{LBW})$$

$$\text{LBW males} = 50\text{ kg} + (2.3 \times \text{inches over 5 ft})$$

$$\text{LBW females} = 45.5\text{ kg} + (2.3 \times \text{inches over 5 ft})$$

Children 5–15 kg

$$\text{Dose (mL)} = 0.0442\,(\text{desired Hgb} - \text{observed Hgb}) \times W + (0.26 \times W)$$

Hgb = hemoglobin
mL = milliliter
W = Weight
LBW = lean body weight

In patients with anemia secondary to blood loss (hemorrhagic diathesis or long-term dialysis):

$$\text{mg of iron} = \text{blood loss} \times \text{hematocrit}$$

where blood loss is in milliliters and hematocrit is expressed as a decimal fraction.

However, numerous reports have been made in which the total dose of iron dextran needed was administered as a single dose by IV infusion.[25,26] Although not approved by the Food and Drug Administration (FDA), this method is efficacious and convenient.

If the patient receives the total dose required to correct the anemia in a single dose, there is an increased possibility of adverse reactions such as arthralgias, myalgias, flushing, malaise, and fever. Other adverse reactions include staining of the skin, pain at the injection site, allergic reactions, and rarely, anaphylaxis. Patients most likely to experience adverse effects with iron dextran include individuals with a history of allergies, asthma, or an inflammatory disease. Patients with preexisting immune-mediated diseases such as active rheumatoid arthritis or systemic lupus erythematosus are considered at high risk for adverse reactions because of their hyperreactive immune response capabilities. It is suggested that all patients considered for an iron dextran injection receive a test dose of 25 mg intramuscularly or IV, or a 5- to 10-minute infusion of the diluted solution. Patients should then be observed for more than 1 hour for untoward reactions. Patients receiving total dose infusions can have the remaining solution infused during the next 2 to 6 hours if no adverse effects occur.

Newer iron products are becoming available for parenteral administration. Sodium ferric gluconate is available in the United States and appears to produce fewer anaphylactic reactions than does iron dextran, although it still requires the use of a test dose prior to therapy.[27,28] Iron sucrose has been evaluated in 23 patients with documented sensitivity to iron dextran.[29] All patients were undergoing hemodialysis and had either mild or severe reactions to iron dextran. They were given 100 mg of iron sucrose IV in 10 consecutive dialysis sessions, and their vital signs and adverse effects were compared with those in 3 dialysis sessions without iron infusions. Patients were not given test doses. There were increases in hemoglobin level, hematocrit, transferrin saturation, and ferritin level; a decrease in the TIBC; and no serious adverse drug reaction for the total of 223 doses of iron sucrose.

Iron dextran must be processed by macrophages for the iron to be biologically available. The absorption and metabolism characteristics vary with the route and amount of drug given. Absorption of an intramuscular dose of iron dextran occurs in two phases. During the first 72 hours, iron dextran is absorbed primarily through the lymphatics into the left superior vena cava. A smaller amount is absorbed directly through the intramuscular capillary network into the blood.[24] A second, slower phase involves uptake of the iron dextran complex by macrophages, with subsequent transport through the lymphatics into the blood. About 60% of an intramuscular dose of iron dextran is absorbed after 3 days, and up to 90% is absorbed within 3 weeks.[30] The remainder is absorbed slowly over several months or longer.

When iron dextran is given IV, the iron is taken up immediately by the reticuloendothelial system.[31] Small to intermediate IV doses (50–500 mg of elemental iron) can be cleared from the plasma within 3 days of administration. In contrast, larger IV doses of iron dextran (500 mg of elemental iron) are processed by the reticuloendothelial system at a constant rate of 10–20 mg/h.[32] Doses this large are associated with increased plasma concentrations of iron dextran for as long as 3 weeks.

Once iron is absorbed into the blood, cells of the reticuloendothelial system (i.e., macrophages) phagocytize the iron dextran complex and cleave the dextran moiety, making free iron available to the body as circulating iron, transferrin-bound iron, or storage iron (ferritin and hemosiderin). Iron dextran can remain within these cells for many months.

When large amounts of parenteral iron are administered, either by total dose infusion or by multiple intramuscular or IV doses, the patient's iron status should be closely monitored. Hemoglobin and hematocrit should be measured weekly, and serum iron and ferritin levels should be measured at least every month.

TRANSFUSIONS

Another form of treatment of IDA involves blood transfusions. This form of therapy requires extreme caution when cardiovascular compromise exists, however. Once the hematocrit value falls below 30%, the oxygen-carrying capacity in older patients drops precipitously, predisposing them to ischemia. Tachycardia, angina, ischemic patterns on electrocardiogram (ECG), cerebrovascular insufficiency, postural hypotension, and prerenal azotemia are strong indications for transfusions to maintain the hematocrit above 30%. An exception to this treatment option relates to the patient who has developed low hematocrit values over extended time periods. These patients often demonstrate cardiac compromise after transfusion despite hematocrits in the 20s. Therapy in these patients should consist of iron therapy, followed by transfusion only if necessary.

MEGALOBLASTIC ANEMIAS

Megaloblastosis results from interference in folic acid– and vitamin B_{12}–interdependent nucleic acid synthesis in the immature erythrocyte. The rate of RNA and cytoplasm production exceeds the rate of DNA production. The maturation process is retarded, resulting in an abnormally large cell. Synthesis of the RNA and DNA necessary for cell division depends on a series of reactions catalyzed by vitamin B_{12} and folic acid. As shown in Figure 99–4, dietary folates are absorbed in this process and converted (A) to 5-methyl tetrahydrofolate, which is then converted via a B_{12}-dependent reaction (B) to tetrahydrofolate (C). After gaining a carbon, tetrahydrofolate is converted to a folate cofactor (D), 5, 10-methylene tetrahydrofolate, used by thymidylate synthetase enzyme (E) in the biosynthesis of nucleic acids. The 5,10-methylene tetrahydrofolate cofactor is converted to dihydrofolate (F) during biosynthesis. Normally, dihydrofolate reductase enzyme reduces dihydrofolate back to tetrahydrofolate (C), which can again pick up a carbon and be recycled to produce more 5,10-methylene tetrahydrofolate (D).

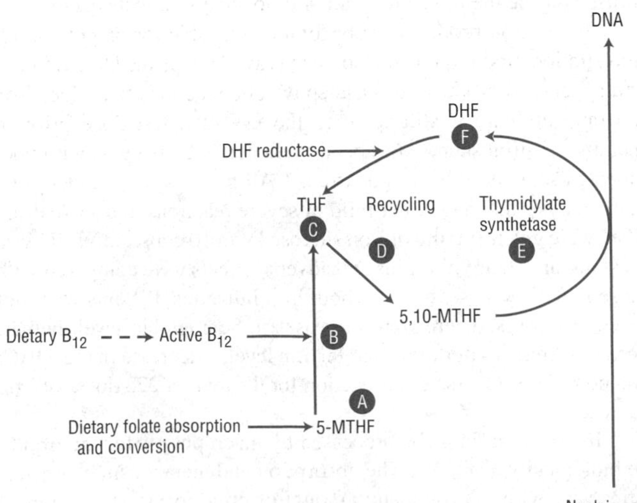

FIGURE 99–4. Drug-induced megaloblastosis. DHF = dihydrofolate; THF = tetrahydrofolate; 5-MTHF = 5-methyl THF; 5,10-METHF = 5,10-methylene THF.

VITAMIN B_{12} DEFICIENCY ANEMIA

ETIOLOGY AND PATHOPHYSIOLOGY

Adult-onset pernicious anemia has an estimated annual incidence of 100 per 1 million population, and it is slightly more common in women. There is a sharp increase in incidence with advancing age, suggesting that it is a consequence of gastric epithelial aging.

Vitamin B_{12} is necessary for DNA synthesis, is important in metabolic reactions involving folic acid, and is essential in maintaining the integrity of the neurologic system. It is a water-soluble vitamin obtained by ingestion of primarily meat and dairy products. Body stores of vitamin B_{12} range from 2 to 5 mg, with daily requirements being approximately 1 to 5 μg. The average daily diet contains more than 20 μg of B_{12}; it would take 1,360 days (3 to 4 years) for a B_{12} deficiency to develop in a person deprived of vitamin B_{12}.

The three major causes of vitamin B_{12} deficiency are inadequate intake, decreased absorption, and inadequate utilization. Inadequate dietary consumption of vitamin B_{12} is rare. It usually occurs only in patients who are strict vegetarians, because body stores are large and meats and vegetables are readily available sources of this nutrient.

Decreased absorption of vitamin B_{12} is seen in patients with a deficiency of intrinsic factor and can be diagnosed with the Schilling test. The condition is rarely diagnosed in patients whose age is less than 35. A decrease in the production of intrinsic factor results in acquired pernicious anemia, while dysfunction of the intrinsic factor causes congenital pernicious anemia. Vitamin B_{12} deficiency may also result from overgrowth of bacteria in the bowel that use vitamin B_{12} or from injury or removal of ileal receptor sites where vitamin B_{12} and the intrinsic factor complex are absorbed. Blind loop syndrome, fish tapeworm infestations, intestinal resections, tropical sprue, gastrectomy, surgical resection of the ileus, pancreatic insufficiency, regional enteritis, and Crohn's disease may all contribute to the development of vitamin B_{12} deficiency.[33]

In portal blood, vitamin B_{12} is bound to the transport protein, transcobolamin II, which rapidly delivers the vitamin to sites of utilization and storage. In persons with a transcobolamin II deficiency, vitamin B_{12} cannot be transported from the blood to utilization and storage sites. Consequently, the patient has a normal vitamin B_{12} level, but clinical evidence of frank B_{12} deficiency.

SIGNS AND SYMPTOMS

As in most forms of anemia, symptoms appear when the body can no longer tolerate the increased cardiac output stimulated by the anemia. Clinically, patients with vitamin B_{12} deficiency may be pale and mildly icteric, and they may develop gastric mucosal atrophy, followed by neuropsychiatric abnormalities as a result of combined degeneration of the spinal cord and brain. The most frequently reported neurologic symptoms are paresthesias and ataxia. Other reported symptoms include glossitis, diminished vibratory sensation in the lower extremities, muscle weakness, dysphagia, anorexia, irritability, dementia, and psychosis.[34]

LABORATORY FINDINGS

In macrocytic anemias, the MCV is usually elevated to 110–140 fL, but some vitamin B_{12}–deficient patients may have a normal MCV. Mild leukopenia and thrombocytopenia may be present. A peripheral blood smear demonstrates macrocytosis accompanied by hypersegmented polymorphonuclear leukocytes (one of the earliest and most specific indications of this disease), oval macrocytes, anisocytosis, and poikilocytosis. Serum lactate dehydrogenase (LDH) and indirect bilirubin levels may be elevated as a result of hemolysis or ineffective erythropoiesis. Serum iron concentrations and transferrin saturation are usually elevated, although iron levels may be low in 21% to 33% of patients with pernicious anemia.[35] Other laboratory findings include a low reticulocyte count, low serum vitamin B_{12} level (<100 pg/mL), and low hematocrit (sometimes as low as 10% to15%).[35] The bone marrow shows marked erythroid hyperplasia and megaloblastic changes in the cells of erythroid lineage.

Screening of all patients with a suspected low vitamin B_{12} level is advisable. Vitamin B_{12} values below 150 pg/mL in a patient with macrocytosis, hypersegmented polymorphonuclear leukocytes, peripheral neuropathy, or dementia is diagnostic of B_{12} deficiency, even though the Schilling test results may be normal. About one-third of patients with pernicious anemia will not demonstrate macrocytosis if their condition is complicated by iron deficiency, thalassemia, or a predominant neurologic involvement.

Vitamin B_{12} values of 200–300 pg/mL are suggestive of depletion, and the patient should undergo repeated testing in 1 to 3 months. If this value is less than 200 pg/mL, a Shilling test should be performed. In patients with normal findings on the Schilling test, vitamin B_{12} should be administered orally and continued until the vitamin B_{12} level is greater than 300 pg/mL. Patients who have abnormal findings on the Schilling test or who do not respond to oral therapy must receive vitamin B_{12} intramuscularly.[36]

When evaluating low serum vitamin B_{12} levels, it is important to rule out other causes besides dietary deprivation and malabsorption. For example, levels may be falsely low in patients receiving antibiotics, anticonvulsants, cytotoxic agents, oral contraceptives, and high-dose vitamin C. In addition, conditions that can result in falsely low vitamin B_{12} levels include multiple myeloma, malignancy, aplastic anemia, and transcobalamin I deficiency; gastrectomy, the third trimester of pregnancy, and radioisotope diagnostic studies have also been associated with falsely low vitamin B_{12} levels. Additional laboratory abnormalities that may be present in patients with vitamin B_{12} deficiency include parietal cell antibodies, serum intrinsic factor–blocking antibody, and elevated serum levels of both homocysteine and methylmalonic acid.

▶ TREATMENT: Vitamin B_{12} Deficiency Anemia

In the rare cases of nutritional deficiency, the oral or IV administration of vitamin B_{12} is beneficial. The oral administration of vitamin B_{12} (cobalamin) can also be used effectively to treat pernicious anemia, but in much larger doses than those used to treat B_{12} deficiency. Cobalamin can be absorbed by both an intrinsic factor–dependent and intrinsic factor–independent route. The independent route is less effective, however, and requires large doses of vitamin B_{12} to provide adequate absorption.[37] Cyanocobalamin absorption rate studies have confirmed observed clinical responses to oral doses of 1,000 μg/day. The mean absorption rate in patients with pernicious anemia is 1.2% across a wide range of doses.[38]

A commonly used initial parenteral vitamin B_{12} regimen consists of daily injections of 800–1,000 μg of cyanocobalamin or hydroxycobalamin for 1 to 2 weeks. This initial 2-week therapy should saturate vitamin B_{12} stores in the body and resolve clinical manifestations of the deficiency. The dosage can then be decreased to 100–1,000 μg once weekly until the hemoglobin and hematocrit are normal. Thereafter, monthly injections of 100–1,000 μg for life should be administered.[33]

Most patients respond rapidly to vitamin B_{12} therapy. Bone marrow becomes normoblastic after 24 hours, reticulocytosis is evident within a few days, the hemoglobin begins to rise after the first week, and the leukocyte and platelet counts normalize after about 7 days. Failure to observe these findings usually indicates an incorrect diagnosis or other factors contributing to the anemia, such as iron deficiency or thalassemia trait. The neuropsychiatric signs and symptoms can be reversible if they are of less than 6 months' duration, but they may be permanent if they have been present for an extended period of time. Demands for iron may be greater during the initiation of therapy as a result of increased erythropoiesis.[39]

Potential adverse effects associated with vitamin B_{12}–induced reticulocytosis include hyperuricemia and hypokalemia. Rebound thrombocytosis may precipitate thrombotic events. Another side effect of vitamin B_{12} therapy is sodium retention. This effect is more likely to occur in the patient with compromised cardiovascular status because of an expansion of the intravascular volume secondary to the sudden increase in the production of RBCs.

FOLIC ACID DEFICIENCY ANEMIA

ETIOLOGY AND PATHOPHYSIOLOGY

Folic acid is a heat-labile vitamin necessary for the production of nucleic acids, proteins, amino acids, purines, and thymine—hence, DNA and RNA. Because humans are unable to synthesize total daily folate requirements, they depend on a dietary source of this vitamin. Major dietary sources of folate include fresh, green, leafy vegetables and fruits, especially citrus fruits, yeast, and mushrooms, and such animal organs as liver and kidney. Even though body demands for folate are high, owing to high rates of RBC synthesis and turnover, the minimum daily requirement is 50 to 100 μg. The body stores approximately 10 to 20 mg folate; therefore, cessation of dietary folate intake would result in the depletion of all body stores within a few months. Folic acid deficiency results in the development of large functionally immature erythrocytes termed megaloblasts.

Major causes of folic acid deficiency include inadequate intake, decreased absorption, hyperutilization, and inadequate utilization. Folic acid deficiency is associated with poor eating habits; thus, it is common in elderly patients, alcoholics, food faddists, the poverty stricken, and those who are chronically ill or in demented states. The absorption of folic acid may decrease in patients who have malabsorption syndromes such as nontropical and tropical sprue or in those who have received certain drugs. Celiac disease is a common cause of folate malabsorption, but other conditions such as Crohn's disease and extensive small bowel resection can also reduce absorption.[21] Alcoholism often results in a diet deficient in folic acid; alcohol also interferes with folic acid absorption, interferes with folic acid utilization at the cellular level, and decreases hepatic stores of folic acid.

Hyperutilization of folic acid may occur when the rate of cellular division is increased. Examples include pregnancy; hemolytic anemia; myelofibrosis; malignancy; chronic inflammatory disorders such as Crohn's disease, rheumatoid arthritis, or psoriasis; long-term dialysis; and growth spurts seen in adolescence and infancy. This is primarily of importance when the daily intake of folate is borderline, resulting in inadequate replacement of folate stores.

Several drugs (e.g., sulfasalazine, trimethoprim-sulfamethoxazole, methotrexate) have been reported to cause a folic acid deficiency megaloblastic anemia either by interfering with folate absorption or by inhibiting the dihydrofolate reductase enzyme necessary for conversion of dihydrofolate to its active tetrahydrofolate form (see Chapter 102).

Although phenytoin may induce a megaloblastic anemia, folic acid supplementation in these patients may decrease phenytoin's anticonvulsant activity by increasing the metabolism of phenytoin.[40] Therefore, routine supplementation is not recommended, but close monitoring for this potential interaction is advised.

SIGNS AND SYMPTOMS

Symptoms associated with folate deficiency are similar to those seen in patients with vitamin B_{12} deficiency. The major difference between these two disease entities is the relative absence of neurologic manifestations in folate deficiency megaloblastic anemia. Symptoms have an insidious onset that often precludes early diagnosis.

LABORATORY FINDINGS

Laboratory changes associated with folate deficiency megaloblastic anemia are similar to those seen in vitamin B_{12} deficiency anemia, except that the vitamin B_{12} level is normal. Decreases occur in the serum folate level (<3 ng/mL) and the RBC folate level (<150 ng/mL). Because serum folate levels are quite sensitive to short-term changes in folate balance, the erythrocyte folate level is a better indicator of true tissue folate stores. Erythrocyte folate levels are established during erythrocyte formation and persist throughout the life span of the cell, making this test less sensitive to daily folate variations.

▶ TREATMENT: Folic Acid Deficiency Anemia

Therapy for folic acid deficiency consists of the administration of exogenous folic acid. For replenishment of folate stores, it is generally recommended that therapy begin orally with 1–5 mg daily. Even in patients with documented absorption problems, 1 mg daily is usually sufficient. Therapy should continue for approximately 4 months, which is a sufficient amount of time for all folate-deficient RBCs to be cleared from the circulation. Once the cause of the deficiency is corrected, therapy can usually be discontinued.

Long-term folate administration may be necessary in chronic hemolytic states, refractory malabsorption syndromes, and myelofibrosis. It is also recommended that patients with a folic acid deficiency be placed on diets containing foods high in folates. For patients with cardiovascular problems, the approach is the same as that for vitamin B_{12} deficiency anemia. Low-dose folate therapy (500 μg daily) may be administered when anticonvulsant drugs produce a megaloblastic anemia and may make it unnecessary to cease administering the anticonvulsant.

Although megaloblastic anemia during pregnancy is rare, the most common cause is folate deficiency. The condition usually manifests itself as an underweight, premature infant and suboptimal health for the mother. Prophylactic folate therapy during pregnancy in women with poor diets, multiple pregnancies, and thalassemia minor may be a useful preventive measure. The recommended dose is 200–300 μg daily. Folic acid supplementation (800–1,000 μg daily) prior to conception and during pregnancy reduces the incidence of neural tube defects in the general population.[41] Higher doses (4 mg daily) reduce the incidence of neural tube defects in the children of patients who have given birth to previous offspring with these disorders.[42] Finally, it has been suggested that supplementation with 10 mg of folic acid daily may reduce the incidence of cleft lip.[43] It is clearly essential that women in their childbearing years maintain adequate folic acid intake.

Symptomatic improvement, as evidenced by increased alertness, appetite, and cooperation, often takes place early during a course of treatment. Reticulocytosis occurs within 2 to 3 days and peaks within 5 to 8 days after beginning therapy. Hematocrit begins to rise within 2 weeks of beginning therapy and should reach normal levels within 2 months. The MCV initially increases because of an increase in reticulocytes, but then gradually decreases to normal.

ANEMIA OF CHRONIC DISEASE

PATHOPHYSIOLOGY

Anemia of chronic disease is a hypoproliferative anemia that has traditionally been associated with infectious, inflammatory, hepatic diseases, or neoplastic diseases lasting more than 1 or 2 months.[44,45] Pathologically, the RBCs have a shortened life span, and the bone marrow's capacity to respond to EPO is inadequate to maintain normal hemoglobin concentration. The cause of this defect is still not certain, but appears to involve a block in the release of iron from the reticuloendothelial cells of the marrow. Various cytokines, such as IL 1, γ-interferon, and tumor necrosis factor released during these illnesses may inhibit the production or action of EPO, or the production of RBCs.[46]

LABORATORY FINDINGS

Examination of the bone marrow reveals an abundance of iron, so it appears that the release mechanism for this iron is the central defect. Patients with ACD usually have a decreased serum iron level, but unlike those with IDA, their serum ferritin level is normal or increased and their iron-binding capacity decreased. Generally, ACD is normocytic and can be severe; hematocrits as low as 25% have been reported in 20% of patients.[47] The diagnosis is usually one of exclusion, with particular emphasis on the possibility of IDA as the primary anemia or as a coexistent anemia with ACD because of chronic disease–associated conditions (e.g., gastrointestinal blood loss from aspirin, other nonsteroidal anti-inflammatory agents, or steroids) or malignancy-associated bleeding. Although usually referred to as ACD, it can occur in conditions with fairly rapid onset of several weeks, such as a pneumonia. It can also coexist with anemia of renal disease and IDA. Table 99–5 lists common diseases associated with ACD.

TABLE 99–5. Diseases Causing Anemia of Chronic Disease

Common Causes
Chronic Infections
Tuberculosis
Other chronic lung infections
Human immunodeficiency virus
Subacute bacterial endocarditis
Osteomyelitis
Chronic urinary tract infections
Chronic inflammation
Rheumatoid arthritis
Systemic lupus erythematosus
Rheumatoid (collagen-vascular) diseases
Inflammatory osteoarthritis
Gout
Chronic inflammatory liver diseases
Malignancies
Carcinoma
Lymphoma
Leukemia
Multiple myeloma
Less Common Causes
Alcoholic liver disease
Congestive heart failure
Thrombophlebitis
Chronic obstructive lung disease
Ischemic heart disease

SIGNS AND SYMPTOMS

As with the other forms of anemia, fatigue, breathlessness, swollen feet, chest pains, and decreased mental acuity are among the signs and symptoms of ACD. The practitioner should maintain a high index of suspicion in any patient with known chronic disease. ACD may coexist with IDA and folic acid deficiency, as many of these patients will have reduced dietary intake or gastrointestinal blood loss.

▶ TREATMENT: Anemia of Chronic Disease

The treatment of ACD is somewhat less specific than the treatment of other anemias. Recovery from the anemia usually occurs with resolution of the underlying process. During inflammation, iron therapy is ineffective by either the oral or parenteral route. Transfusions of RBCs are effective, but should be limited to situations in which oxygen transport is inadequate because of concomitant medical problems. The hemoglobin level indicating the need for an RBC transfusion varies from 8 to 10 g/dL, based on factors such as cost, convenience, and risk of infectious complications.

Exogenous EPO (recombinant human EPO or epoetin alfa) has been used to stimulate erythropoiesis in patients with chronic disease. These patients have a relative EPO deficiency, in which EPO levels are not as elevated as they should be for the degree of anemia that exists. They also have a relatively impaired response to epoetin alfa. In one study of 221 patients with anemia and chronic lymphocytic leukemia, epoetin alfa given at a dosage of 150 units/kg three times weekly increased the hematocrit by nearly 6% as compared with 1.5% in the placebo group.[48] Of the epoetin alfa patients, 30% achieved a hematocrit higher than 38%, as compared to only 5% in the placebo group. Patients who reached a hematocrit of 38% reported a significant improvement in energy level, self-rated health, physical function, and social function.

Several other studies of epoetin alfa in patients with non-Hodgkin's lymphoma and multiple myeloma also showed that 45% to 65% of patients responded to epoetin alfa (increase in hemoglobin by more than 2 g/dL), as compared with a 0% to 21% response rate in the study control arms. The proportion of patients who required transfusions also decreased by 50% as compared with placebo. Doses of 150 units/kg given subcutaneously three times weekly are effective, and increasing the dose to 300 units/kg produced a response in another 25% of patients.[49–52]

Two large trials involving more than 3,000 patients with non-myeloid malignancies undergoing chemotherapy reported on the use of epoetin alfa.[53,54] Both trials found that epoetin alfa therapy improved quality-of-life indicators independent of tumor response and that it significantly increased hemoglobin levels and decreased the need for transfusions. Although doses in these two studies were given subcutaneously three times weekly, Gabrilove and colleagues have reported equivalent responses with less frequent administration (i.e., epoetin alfa, 40,000 units given subcutaneously in one weekly dose).[55]

Epoetin alfa therapy may have other clinical benefits as well. In a randomized study of 375 patients with solid tumors or hematologic malignancies, patients who received epoetin alfa had fewer transfusion requirements, an improved quality of life, and, surprisingly, a longer median survival (17 months vs. 11 months) as compared with patients who received a placebo.[56] Longer follow-up is needed to confirm the survival benefit observed in the preliminary analysis.

Most patients tolerate epoetin alfa therapy well. Iron deficiency can occur in patients treated with epoetin alfa, however, and close monitoring of iron levels is necessary during epoetin alfa therapy. Oral iron supplementation should be given if transferrin saturation drops to 20% or the serum ferritin level drops below 100 μ/L. Some patients develop "functional" iron deficiency, in which the iron stores are normal, but the supply of iron to the erythroid marrow is less than that needed to support the demand for RBCs. Many practitioners, therefore, routinely supplement epoetin alfa therapy with oral iron therapy. The hypertension commonly seen in end-stage renal disease patients on epoetin alfa is far less common in patients with cancer or AIDS. More common toxicities of epoetin alfa are fever, bone pain, and fatigue.

ANEMIA OF CHRONIC RENAL FAILURE

Patients with chronic renal failure have normochromic, normocytic anemia for several reasons. Decreased EPO production by the kidneys is the primary mechanism of severe anemia associated with end-stage renal disease.[57] The uremic environment of chronic renal failure decreases the life span of RBCs, creating an increased demand for RBCs that decreased serum erythropoietin levels often cannot supply.[58] An increased demand for folic acid for new RBC production, coupled with the body's limited folic acid stores, can lead to a folic acid deficiency anemia. Finally, many patients with chronic renal failure become iron-deficient because of blood and iron loss from hemodialysis.[59] (See Chapter 43, Acute Renal Failure.)

▶ TREATMENT: Anemia of Chronic Renal Failure

Patients with chronic renal failure are unable to produce appropriate levels of EPO, and many of these patients are transfusion-dependent. Owing to the inherent risks associated with repeated transfusions (e.g., febrile reactions, iron overload, hepatitis, AIDS, rejection of future transplants), epoetin alfa has become the mainstay in the management of anemia associated with renal failure.

The goal of epoetin alfa therapy is to raise the hematocrit to a target level as close to 36% as possible. Starting doses of epoetin are 50–100 units/kg, administered three times weekly. Doses should be reduced as the hematocrit approaches 36%. The dose of epoetin alfa should then be individualized to maintain the hematocrit within the range of 30% to 36%. There are considerable interpatient half-life variations for this product, and its use may require individual regimens for optimum therapeutic value.

Epoetin alfa may be administered IV or subcutaneously. The subcutaneous route provides more sustained epoetin alfa concentrations, which are more advantageous than the peak and trough levels achieved with IV bolus administration. This suggests that the amount of time that the levels remain above baseline EPO concentrations may be most important in determining hematopoietic response.[60]

The major side effect encountered with epoetin alfa therapy for chronic renal failure is an elevation of diastolic blood pressure. Approximately 30% to 47% of patients receiving this product experience this effect, which is thought to occur as a consequence of an increase in peripheral vascular resistance. It is estimated that 25% of these patients will experience an increase greater than 10 mm Hg, thus producing or aggravating existing hypertension and often requiring adjustments in blood pressure medications.[61] No evidence exists that this blood pressure change is related to a direct pressor effect of epoetin alfa. It appears that the major risk factor for the development of hypertension is the severity of the anemia, not the rate of rise of hematocrit with therapy.

One major reason for a patient's failure to respond to epoetin alfa therapy is the depletion of iron stores. Iron deficiency arises during this therapy primarily because raising hematocrit levels requires a massive transfer of iron from storage areas to RBCs for the manufacture of new hemoglobin. Other causes of iron deficiency include blood loss secondary to bleeding, retention of blood in dialyzer and tubing, or laboratory test phlebotomy. Chronic renal failure patients with transferrin saturations of at least 20% and serum ferritin levels below 100 ng/mL are probably candidates for concurrent iron therapy.[62] The agent of choice for prevention of iron storage deficiency is ferrous sulfate, 325 mg at bedtime. As with any IDA, if a patient does not respond to oral iron supplementation, parenteral iron therapy is indicated. Fortunately, most patients respond appropriately to oral iron therapy.

ANEMIA IN THE ELDERLY AND PEDIATRIC POPULATIONS

One of the most common clinical problems observed in the elderly is anemia.[63] Although it is often assumed that anemia is an inevitable part of the aging process, studies in healthy elderly populations demonstrate that this is not necessarily true.[64] What is observed in these patients is a progressive decrease in bone marrow reserve with age and a decrease in hormonal response to hematologic stress.[61] Although hemoglobin levels usually remain normal, the diminished marrow reserve leaves the elderly patient more susceptible to other causes of anemia. For example, such patients may develop multiple minor and often unrecognized diseases that negatively affect erythropoiesis.[65] One often overlooked major factor that may contribute to anemia in the older population is nutritional status. Anemia is rarely encountered in affluent and healthy elderly communities.[66] Cross-sectional studies demonstrate a higher prevalence of anemia in low socioeconomic populations, as well as a high prevalence of other nutritional deficiencies. Thus, nutritional deficiencies not usually severe enough to affect the hematopoietic system in the younger population may account for anemia in the aged.

In contrast to anemias in adults, which tend to be manifestations of some broader underlying pathology,[67] anemias in the pediatric population are more often due to a primary hematologic abnormality such as a hypoplastic or hemolytic anemia. The age of the child can yield some clues to the etiology of the anemia. In neonates, blood loss and hemolysis are common causes of anemia. Owing to the increased survival rate among premature infants, more children are born with decreased iron stores. Dietary deficiency of iron in the first 6 to 12 months of life is less common today, however, because of the increased use of iron supplementation during breastfeeding and use of iron-fortified formulas. Iron deficiency becomes more prominent

TABLE 99–6. Common Classes of Hemolytic Anemias

Intrinsic (intracorpuscular; usually genetically inherited)
Membrane defect
Spherocytosis and elliptocytosis
Hemoglobin defect
Sickle cell anemia
Thalassemia syndrome
Metabolic defect
Glucose-6-phosphate dehydrogenase (G6PD) deficiency
Many other enzyme deficiencies
Extrinsic
Membrane defect
Autoimmune hemolytic anemias
Oxidants, may cause unstable hemoglobin to clump

when children change to regular diets. Adolescents are also prone to IDA, especially those who participate in faddish diets. Many more children are attending daycare centers at an earlier age, which is resulting in a higher incidence of anemia due to frequent infections and acute inflammation. Also, as more children in the United States are born to parents of Asian and African backgrounds, the incidence of hemoglobin-related disorders has increased.[68]

HEMOLYTIC ANEMIA

PATHOPHYSIOLOGY

Hemolytic anemia results from decreased survival time of RBCs secondary to destruction in the spleen or circulation. The severity of hemolytic anemia varies with the mechanism. Hemolysis may be mild, chronic, compensated, and lifelong or acute, severe, and life-threatening.

The normal 120-day life span of an RBC comes from its inherent flexibility in passing through the microvasculature and spleen without disruption of the cell membrane or sequestration and phagocytosis by reticuloendothelial cells. Hemolysis, as defined by an RBC life span of less than 120 days, results from one of three primary defects: (1) membrane defects, (2) alterations in hemoglobin solubility or stability, and (3) changes in intracellular metabolic processes. These changes in membrane integrity, hemoglobin stability, and cell metabolism can be intrinsic or extrinsic in origin. Intrinsic defects are intracorpuscular changes and are often genetically determined; extrinsic defects, or extracorpuscular changes, are usually the cause of acquired hemolytic anemia. Acquired disorders result mainly from a direct effect on the membrane and less often from alterations in hemoglobin or metabolism. Table 99–6 lists examples of the different classes of hemolytic anemias.

Causes of hemolytic anemia in the younger patient differ from those in the elderly patient. Most younger patients exhibit congenital disease, whereas older patients most often experience autoimmune hemolytic anemia. A positive result in a Coombs test is diagnostic in the latter group.

Hereditary spherocytosis is the most common inherited disorder of the RBC membrane. In this disorder, RBCs lose their flexible biconcave characteristics and become tight spheres. These altered cells can still deliver oxygen to body cells, but when these rigid cells enter the splenic microcirculation, they cannot pass through the pores lining the sinusoids of the spleen; consequently, they become trapped in the splenic pulp, where they are eventually destroyed by the reticuloendothelial cells. Patients with hereditary spherocytosis are at risk of developing cholelithiasis or cholecystitis, pigment bile stones, mild jaundice, and splenomegaly. The treatment of choice for hereditary spherocytosis is folate supplementation and splenectomy. Although the spherocytosis persists, the hemolysis is no longer a problem once the spleen has been removed.

Alterations in hemoglobin's solubility or stability, as seen with sickle cell anemia and the thalassemias, cause cell deformations leading to hemolysis (see Chapter 101, Sickle Cell Anemia).

Finally, alterations in cell metabolism (enzymopathies) lead to hemolytic disease by changing cell dimensions and hemoglobin solubility. The two major metabolic pathways necessary for normal RBC metabolism are the hexose monophosphate shunt pathway, with its associated enzyme systems, and the Embden–Myerhof pathway of anaerobic glycolysis. The former is responsible primarily for maintaining hemoglobin in the reduced state and thus preventing the formation of methemoglobin, while the latter metabolizes glucose to lactic acid, which leads to adenosine triphosphate formation.

The most common metabolic abnormality resulting in a hemolytic syndrome is glucose-6-phosphate dehydrogenase (G6PD) deficiency in the hexose monophosphate shunt pathway. Hemoglobin is oxidized to methemoglobin and then to sulfhemoglobin. Heinz bodies of denatured hemoglobin form, resulting in damage to the RBC membrane. Hemolysis results from the action of the spleen and reticuloendothelial system on these damaged cells. The disease more typically occurs in whites of Mediterranean descent on exposure to oxidant drugs (e.g., sulfamethoxazole, dapsone) and chemicals or with infection.

LABORATORY FINDINGS

Hemolytic anemias tend to be normocytic and normochromic (see Fig. 99–3). An increased reticulocyte count is evidence of an attempt to maintain RBC mass. A peripheral blood smear may reveal sickle cells, target cells, spherocytes, elliptocytes, and fragmented RBCs. Decreased haptoglobin is seen, caused by increased hemoglobin-haptoglobin complex formation. LDH increases secondary to release from RBCs; however, this is a very nonspecific enzyme. Hemoglobinuria may result, and an increase in indirect bilirubin often occurs.

▶ TREATMENT: Hemolytic Anemia

Therapy for hemolytic anemia consists of managing the underlying cause of the anemia. Clearly, avoidance of precipitating oxidant medications and chemicals in patients with G6PD deficiency is essential. Currently, there is no specific therapy that compensates for this enzyme deficiency. Steroids and other immunosuppressive agents have been used for management of autoimmune hemolytic anemias. In some instances, a splenectomy is indicated in an attempt to reduce RBC destruction.

▶ PRINCIPLES OF PHARMACOTHERAPY

- Anemias are a group of diseases characterized by a decrease in either the hemoglobin or the volume of red blood cells (RBCs), which results in decreased oxygen-carrying capacity of blood.
- Anemias are often a sign of underlying pathology; a rapid diagnosis of the cause of the anemia is essential.
- Patients with acute-onset anemias are most likely to present with tachycardia, light-headedness, and dyspnea; those with chronic anemia often present with weakness, fatigue, headache,

vertigo, faintness, sensitivity to cold, pallor, and loss of skin tone.

- Defects in hemoglobin synthesis can result in a wide variety of disorders, including sideroblastic anemia (excessive nonheme iron in RBCs), acute intermittent porphyria (enzyme deficiency leading to neuromuscular symptoms), and thalassemia (dysfunction of genes controlling globulin chain production).
- Iron deficiency anemia (IDA) is characterized by decreased levels of ferritin (most sensitive marker) and serum iron, as well as decreased transferritin saturation; the hemoglobin and hematocrit fall late in the disease. Total iron-binding capacity (TIBC) is increased. RBC morphology includes anisocytosis, hypochromia, and microcytosis. Most patients with IDA are adequately treated with oral ferrous sulfate therapy, although parenteral iron therapy is necessary in selected patient populations.
- Vitamin B_{12} deficiency can be due to inadequate intake, decreased absorption, and inadequate utilization. Anemia caused by a lack of intrinsic factor, resulting in decreased vitamin B_{12} absorption, is called pernicious anemia. Vitamin B_{12} deficiency is manifested as a macrocytic anemia with hypersegmented polymorphonuclear leukocytes and oval macrocytes. Usually, vitamin B_{12} levels and the reticulocyte count are low. Neurologic symptoms may also be present. Oral replacement is appropriate for dietary deficiency, but most patients with intrinsic factor deficiency or other absorption problems require parenteral replenishment.
- Folic acid deficiency is also manifested as a macrocytic anemia. It results from inadequate intake, decreased absorption, hyperutilization, or inadequate utilization. Treatment consists of the oral administration of folic acid, even in patients with absorption problems. Adequate folic acid intake is essential in women of childbearing years to decrease the incidence of neural tube defects in their children.
- Anemia of chronic disease (ACD) is a diagnosis of exclusion. It results from chronic inflammation, infection, or malignancy, and it can occur as early as 1 to 2 months after the onset of these processes. The serum iron level is usually decreased, but in contrast to IDA, the serum ferritin concentration is normal or increased, and TIBC is usually decreased. Treatment is aimed at correcting the underlying pathology.
- Patients with chronic renal failure have several reasons to be anemic. The primary mechanism is decreased erythropoietin production. The administration of epoetin alfa is now the standard of care for management of anemia associated with chronic renal failure. Iron supplementation may also be necessary in some patients.
- Hemolytic anemia results in decreased survival time of RBCs secondary to destruction in the spleen or in the circulation. There are many causes of hemolytic anemia. Hemolytic anemias are normocytic and normochromic. An increased reticulocyte count, together with higher levels of lactate dehydrogenase and indirect bilirubin, is seen. A peripheral blood smear may reveal sickle cells, target cells, spherocytes, elliptocytes, and fragmented RBCs. Haptoglobin is decreased. As with ACD, treatment is directed toward correcting or controlling the underlying pathology.

REFERENCES

1. Bergin JJ. Evaluation of anemia. Postgrad Med J 1985;77:253–269.
2. Charlton RW, Bothwell TH. Iron absorption. Ann Rev Med 1983;34: 55–68.
3. Committee on Iron Deficiency of the AMA Council on Foods and Nutrition. Iron deficiency in the United States. JAMA 1968;203:407.
4. Hallberg L, Rossander L, Skanberg A-B. Phytates and the inhibitory effect of bran on iron absorption in man. Am J Clin Nutr 1987;45:965–988.
5. Cook JD, Skikne BS, Baynes RD. Serum transferrin receptor. Ann Rev Med 1993;44:63–74.
6. Long R. Diurnal variation of serum iron in normal individuals. Clin Chem 1978;24:842–847.
7. Ramadurai J, Shapiro C, Kozloff M, Telfer M. Zinc abuse and sideroblastic anemia. Am J Hematol 1993;42:227–228.
8. Hryhorczuk DO, Hogan MM. Variegate porphyria and heavy metal poisoning from ingestion of moonshine. South Med J 1983;76:1027–1031.
9. McKenzie AW, Acharya U. Oestrogen-induced familial porphyria. Br J Dermatol 1975;92:707–709.
10. Doss M, Baumann H, Sixel F. Alcohol in acute porphyria. Lancet 1982; 1:1307. Letter.
11. Andrews NC. Disorders of iron metabolism. N Engl J Med 1999;341: 1986–1995.
12. Kirking MH. Treatment of chronic iron overload. Clin Pharm 1991;10: 775–783.
13. Edwards CQ, Griffen LM, Goldgar D, et al. Prevalence of hemochromatosis among 11,065 presumably healthy blood donors. N Engl J Med 1988;318:1355–1362.
14. Marx JJM. Iron deficiency in developed countries: prevalance, influence of lifestyle factors and hazards of prevention. Eur J Clin Nutr 1997;51:491–494.
15. Rockey DC, Cello JP. Evaluation of the gastrointestinal tract in patients with iron-deficiency anemia. N Engl J Med 1993;329:1691–1695.
16. Recommendations to prevent and control iron deficiency in the United States. MMWR 1998;47:1–36.
17. Beissner RS, Trowbridge AA. Clinical assessment of anemia. Postgrad Med 1986;80:83–95.
18. Cok JD. Food iron absorption in human subjects—III. Comparison of the effect of animal proteins on non-heme iron absorption. Am J Clin Nutr 1976;29:859–867.
19. Dallman PR, Siimes MA, Stekel A. Iron deficiency in infancy and childhood. Am J Clin Nutr 1980;6:86–118.
20. Monsen ER, Hallberg L, Layrisse M. Estimation of available dietary iron. Am J Clin Nutr 1978;31:134–141.
21. McGrath K. Treatment of anaemia caused by iron, vitamin B_{12} or folate deficiency. Med J Aust 1989;151:693–697.
22. Beutler E. The common anemias. JAMA 1988;259:2433–2437.
23. Dallman PR. Iron deficiency: diagnosis and treatment. West J Med 1981; 134:496–505.
24. Beresford CR, Goldberg L, Smith JP. Local effects and mechanism of absorption of iron preparations administered intramuscularly. Br J Pharmacol 1957;12:107–114.
25. Auerbach M, Witt D, Toler W, et al. Clinical use of the total dose intravenous infusion of iron dextran. J Lab Clin Med 1988;111:566–570.
26. Halpin TC, Bertino JS, Rothstein FC. Iron-deficiency anemia in childhood inflammatory bowel disease: treatment with intravenous iron-dextran. JPEN J Parenter Enteral Nutr1982;6:9–11.
27. Faich G, Strobos J. Sodium ferric gluconate complex in sucrose: safer intravenous iron therapy than iron dextrans. Am J Kidney Dis 1999;33: 464–470.
28. Matzke GR. Intravenous iron supplementation in end-stage renal disease patients. Am J Kidney Dis 1999;33:595–597.
29. Van Wyck DB, Cavallo G, Spinowitz BS, et al. Safety and efficacy of iron sucrose in patients sensitive to iron dextran: North American clinical trial. Am J Kidney Dis 2000;36:88–97.
30. Will G. The absorption, distribution and utilization of intramuscularly administered iron-dextran: a radioisotope study. Br J Haematol 1968;14:395–406.
31. Grime AJ, Hutt MSR. Metabolism of 59Fe-dextran complex in human subjects. Br J Med 1957;2:1074–1077.
32. Henderson PA, Hillman RS. Characteristics of iron dextran utilization in man. Blood 1969;34:357–375.
33. Clementz GL, Schade SG. The spectrum of vitamin B_{12} deficiency. Am Fam Physician 1990;41:150–162.

34. Healton EB, Savage DG, Brust JC. Neurologic aspects of cobalamin deficiency. Medicine 1991;70:229–245.
35. Christensen DJ. Diagnosis of anemia: clues to greater precision. Postgrad Med J 1983;73:293–297, 300.
36. McRae TD, Freedman ML. Why vitamin B_{12} deficiency should be managed aggressively. Geriatrics 1989;44:70–79.
37. Doscherholmer A, Hager PS, Liu M. A dual mechanism of vitamin B_{12} plasma absorption. J Clin Invest 1957;36:1551–1557.
38. Berlin H, Berlin R, Brante G. Oral treatment of pernicious anemia with high doses of vitamin B_{12} without intrinsic factor. Acta Med Scand 1968;184:247–258.
39. Carmel R, Weiner JM, Johnson CS. Iron deficiency occurs frequently in patients with pernicious anemia. JAMA 1987;257:1081–1083.
40. MacCosbe PE, Toomey K. Interaction of phenytoin and folic acid. Clin Pharm 1983;2:362–369.
41. Cziezel AE, Dudas I. Prevention of the first occurrence of neural tube defects by periconceptual vitamin supplementation. N Engl J Med 1992;327:1832.
42. MRC Vitamin Study Research Group. Prevention of neural tube defects. Results of the Medical Research Council Vitamin Study. Lancet 1991;338:131.
43. Tobarova M. Periconceptual supplementation with vitamins and folic acid to prevent recurrence of cleft lip. Lancet 1982;2:217.
44. Lee GR. The anemia of chronic disease. Semin Hematol 1983;20: 465–479.
45. Samson D. The anaemia of chronic disorders. Postgrad Med J 1983;59: 543–550.
46. Means RT, Krantz SB. Progress in understanding the pathogenesis of the anemia of chronic disease. Blood 1992;80;1639–1647.
47. Cash JM, Sears DA. The anemia of chronic disease: spectrum of associated diseases in a series of unselected hospitalized patients. Am J Med 1989;87:638–644.
48. Rose E, Rai K, Revicki D, et al. Clinical and health status assessments in anemic chronic lymphocytic leukemia (CLL) patients treated with epoetin alfa (EPO). Blood 1994;84:526a.
49. Osterborg A, Boogaerts MC, Cimino R, et al. Recombinant human erythropoietin in transfusion-dependent anemic patients with multiple myeloma and non-Hodgkin's lymphoma: a randomized trial. Blood 1996; 87:2675–2682.
50. Cazzola M, Messinger D, Battistel V, et al. Recombinant human erythropoietin in the anemia associated with multiple myeloma or non-Hodgkin's lymphoma: dose finding and identification of predictors of response. Blood 1995;86:4446–4453.
51. Garton JP, Gertz MA, Witzig TE, et al. Epoetin alfa for the treatment of the anemia of multiple myeloma. Arch Intern Med 1995;155:2069–2074.
52. Dammacco F, Silvestris F, Castoldi GL, et al. The effectiveness and tolerability of epoetin alfa in patients with multiple myeloma refractory to chemotherapy. Int J Clin Lab Res 1998;28:127–134.
53. Glaspy J, Bukowski R, Steinberg D, et al. Impact of therapy with epoetin alfa on clinical outcomes in patients with nonmyeloid malignancies during cancer chemotherapy in community oncology practice. J Clin Oncol 1997;15:1218–1234.
54. Demetri GD, Kris M, Wade J, et al. Quality-of-life benefit in chemotherapy patients treated with epoetin alfa is independent of disease response or tumor type: results from a prospective community oncology study. J Clin Oncol 1998;16:3412–3425.
55. Gabrilove JL, Cleeland CS, Livingston RB, et al. Clinical evaluation of once-weekly dosing of epoetin alfa in chemotherapy patients: improvements in hemoglobin and quality of life are similar to three-times-weekly dosing. J Clin Oncol 2001;19:2875–2882.
56. Littlewood TJ, Bajetta E, Nortier JWR, et al. Effects of epoetin alfa on hematologic parameters and quality of life in cancer patients receiving nonplatinum chemotherapy: results of a randomized, double-blind, placebo-controlled trial. J Clin Oncol 2001;19:2865–2874.
57. Paganini EP. Overview of anemia associated with chronic renal disease: primary and secondary mechanisms. Semin Nephrol 1989;9:3–8.
58. Shaw AB. Haemolysis in chronic renal failure. Br Med J 1967;2:213–216.
59. Van Wyck DB. Iron deficiency in patients with dialysis-associated anemia during erythropoietin replacement therapy: strategies for assessment and management. Semin Nephrol 1989;9:21–24.
60. Eschbach JW, Adamson JW. Recombinant human erythropoietin: implications for nephrology. Am J Kidney Dis 1988;11:203–209.
61. Lipschitz DA, Udupa KB, Milton KY, Thompson CO. Effect of age on hematopoiesis in man. Blood 1984;63:502–509.
62. Adamson JW, Eschback JW. Treatment of the anemia of chronic renal failure with recombinant human erythropoietin. Ann Rev Med 1990;41: 349–360.
63. Guyatt GH, Patterson C, Ali M. Diagnosis of iron deficiency anemia in the elderly. Am J Med 1990;88:205–209.
64. Baldwin JG, Lichtenstein LS. Longitudinal study of hemoglobin and hematocrit in the elderly. Blood 1986;68(5, suppl 1):52a.
65. Mansouri A, Lipschitz DA. Anemia in the elderly patient. Med Clin North Am 1992;76:619–630.
66. Gary PJ, Goodwin JS, Hunt WE. Iron status and anemia in the elderly: new findings and a review of previous studies. J Am Geriatr Soc 1983;31: 389–399.
67. Berliner N, Duffy TP, Abelson HT. Approach to the adult and child with anemia. In: Hoffman R, Benz EJ, Shattil SJ, et al., eds. Hematology: Basic Principles and Practice. 2nd ed. New York: Churchill Livingstone, 1995:468–483.
68. Graham EA. The changing face of anemia in infancy. Pediatr Rev 1994; 15:175–183.

100

COAGULATION DISORDERS

Betsy Bickert and Janet L. Kwiatkowski

REGULATION OF HEMOSTASIS

A series of complex actions and reactions of procoagulant and anticoagulant events regulate hemostasis and thrombosis.[1,2] The exact mechanisms that precisely regulate the balance between clot formation and lysis are not completely understood. The physiologic interaction and regulation involves four major components of the normal hemostatic system: (1) the vessel wall, (2) platelets, (3) the coagulation system, and (4) the fibrinolytic system.

COMPONENTS OF THE HEMOSTATIC SYSTEM

VESSEL WALL AND PLATELETS

The blood vessel and circulating platelets play central roles in primary hemostasis. The involvement of the vessel wall includes vasoconstriction, formation of platelet plugs, and regulation of coagulation and fib rinolysis following endothelial injury (Fig. 100–1). Platelet response to vascular injury includes four phases: (1) adhesion, (2) secretion, (3) aggregation, and (4) elaboration of procoagulant activity. The formation of a platelet plug proceeds through the sequence of platelet adhesion to exposed subendothelial connective tissue structures; platelet aggregation following secretion of adenosine diphosphate, thromboxane A2, thrombin, and other granule contents; contribution of platelet coagulant activity to the coagulation process, which stabilizes the plug with a fibrin mesh; and retraction of the platelet mass to provide a dense thrombus.[1]

The endothelial cell, especially its surface, is intimately involved in the balance between clotting and bleeding. These cells secrete von Willebrand factor and anticoagulant proteins, such as tissue plasminogen activator. Prostaglandins, such as prostacyclin, inhibit platelet aggregation, whereas thromboxane A_2, which is released by platelets, promotes aggregation. Thrombomodulin on the surface of the cell reacts with thrombin to activate proteins C and S, which inhibit the plasma cascade of coagulation factors. There is a dynamic balance of fibrinolysis and fibrin formation, both of which interact with platelets at the cell surface to keep the blood in fluid phase and prevent bleeding at the same time.[1,2]

COAGULATION SYSTEM

Twelve plasma proteins are considered coagulation factors (Table 100–1). It is convenient to divide the coagulation factors into three groups on the basis of biochemical properties. These groups include vitamin K-dependent factors (II, VII, IX, and X), contact activation factors (XI, XII, prekallikrein, and high molecular weight kininogen), and thrombin-sensitive factors (V, VIII, XIII, and fibrinogen).

Coagulation factors circulate as inactive precursors (zymogens). Coagulation of blood entails a cascading series of proteolytic reactions. At each step, a clotting factor undergoes limited proteolysis and becomes an active protease (designated by a lowercase "a," as in Xa). This clotting factor enzyme activates the next clotting factor until ultimately an insoluble fibrin clot has formed.

Clotting begins at either an intrinsic or an extrinsic pathway, with subsequent factor interactions converging at the common pathway (see Fig. 100–1). Both pathways can be activated when normal components of the vascular endothelium come into contact with blood. Tissue factor resides in many organs (i.e., brain, lungs, kidneys, and liver) extrinsic to blood, and can initiate the extrinsic clotting pathway by activating factor VII. Factor VIIa, calcium, tissue thromboplastin, and factor X form a lipoprotein complex that results in activation of factor X. After this step, the extrinsic system enters the common pathway along with the intrinsic pathway.

In the intrinsic pathway, all the protein factors necessary for coagulation are present in the circulating blood. Contact of circulating factor XII with subendothelial membrane initiates the intrinsic pathway. This activation phase involves several other factors, such as high molecular weight kininogen and prekallikrein. Factor XIIa, with cofactor high molecular weight kininogen, activates factor IX to factor IXa. Factor VIIIa, factor IXa, calcium, and platelet phospholipid activate factor X. Factor Xa, Va, calcium, and platelet phospholipid convert prothrombin to thrombin. A fibrin clot is formed after thrombin converts fibrinogen to fibrin.

Because thrombin has a central role in coagulation, its generation is the focus of two important regulatory systems. In one such system, antithrombin forms complexes with thrombin and inactivates thrombin, as well as several other serine proteases (e.g., IXa, Xa, XIa, XIIa). Patients with a hereditary or acquired deficiency of antithrombin have a high incidence of recurrent thromboembolic disease. Heparin enhances the inhibitory capacity of antithrombin and is present on the surface of endothelial cells. The second system involves thrombin's activation of protein C, which exerts an inhibitory influence on clot formation.[1] Protein C and its cofactor, protein S, are vitamin K-dependent proteins that inactivate factors V and VIII of the coagulation cascade (see Fig. 100–1).

FIBRINOLYSIS

The coagulation and fibrinolytic systems serve two interrelated and opposing functions. The formation of a fibrin clot occurs as a result of the coagulation system, whereas the fibrinolytic system dissolves the polymerized clot and restores blood flow. As a regulatory mechanism in clot formation, the fibrinolytic system contributes to the localized repair of damaged endothelium. Plasminogen is incorporated into the clot formation by binding to fibrin. Plasminogen activators (tissue-type plasminogen activator and urokinase-like plasminogen activator) are released in response to thrombin or venous stasis. Plasminogen is converted to plasmin, which enzymatically digests fibrin, dissolves the clot, and releases a number of fibrin degradation products (FDPs). The interaction between plasminogen activators, plasminogen, and fibrin restricts the fibrinolytic activity to the site of the clot. Plasminogen activator inhibitor type 1 (PAI-1) and α_2-plasmin inhibitor inactivate plasmin to prevent systemic fibrinolysis.[1]

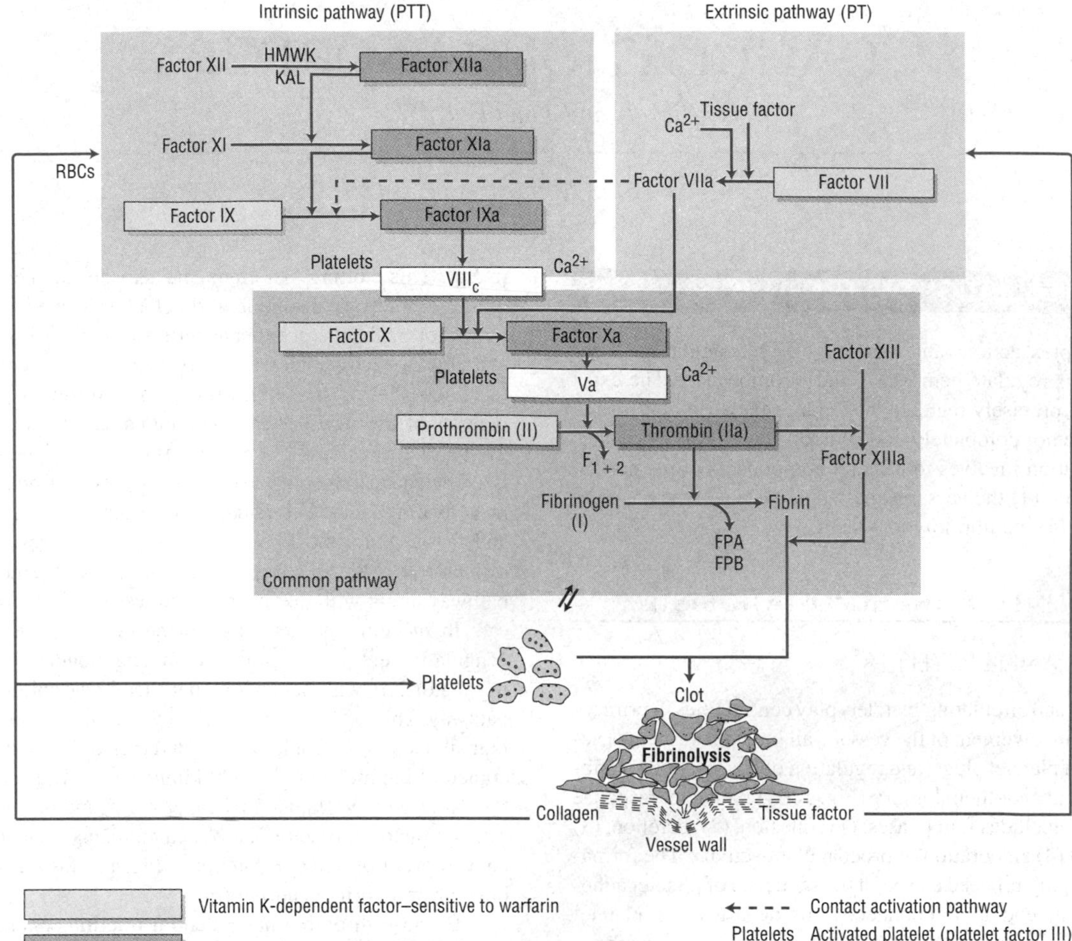

FIGURE 100–1. Schema of the hemostatic system, showing interaction of vessel wall, platelets, coagulation pathways, and fibrinolytic system. Important features of the coagulation pathways include the contact activation phase, vitamin K-dependent factors (affected by warfarin), the activated serine proteases that are inhibited by heparin: antithrombin, and the role of platelets and calcium. Factors VIIIc and Va are nonenzymatic cofactors that are inactivated by protein C. The protime (PT) measures the function of the extrinsic and common pathways; the activated partial thromboplastin time (APTT) measures the function of the intrinsic and common pathways. HMWK = high molecular weight kininogen; KAL = kallikrein; RBCs = red blood cells. *(Adapted from Ref. 100.)*

TABLE 100–1. Blood Coagulation Factors

Factor[a]	Synonym	Biologic Half-Life	Blood Product Source
I	Fibrinogen	100–150 h	Cryoprecipitate (200–300 mg/bag)
II	Prothrombin	50–80 h	FFP, PCC
V	Proaccelerin	24 h	FFP
VII	Proconvertin	6 h	Recombinant VIIa, FFP, PCC
VIII	Antihemophilic factor	12 h	FFP, PCC, factor concentrates, cryoprecipitate
IX	Christmas factor	24 h	FFP, PCC, factor concentrates
X	Stuart-Power factor	25–60 h	FFP, PCC
XI	Plasma thromboplastin antecedent	40–80 h	FFP,
XII	Hageman factor	50–70 h	
XIII	Fibrin-stabilizing factor	150 h	FFP, cryoprecipitate

[a]Coagulation factors are numbered with Roman numerals in order of their discovery. Factor III (tissue factor) and factor IV (calcium ions) have been omitted. There is no factor VI. PCC = prothrombin complex concentrate; FFP = fresh-frozen plasma.

TABLE 100–2. Laboratory Procedures

Procedure	Identifies	Causes of Prolonged Value	Clinical Manifestations
Bleeding time	Platelet function: adhesion, aggregation, and release	Thrombocytopenia Inherited qualitative platelet defects von Willebrand disease Uremia Collagen defects Antiplatelet drugs Factor V deficiency Afibrinogenemia	Bleeding from the gums Easy bruising Bleeding following surgery or tooth extraction Nose bleeds
Prothrombin time (PT)	Factors of common pathway: I, II, V, X Factors of extrinsic pathway: VII	Newborn Vitamin K deficiency Inherited factor deficiencies Warfarin Liver disease Lupus anticoagulant Afibrinogenemia	Bleeding: uterine surgery, childbirth, trauma Bleeding in newborn: umbilical cord, intracranial, gastrointestinal
Activated partial thromboplastin time (aPTT)	Factors of contact phase: HMWK, XII, prekallikrein Factors of intrinsic pathway: VIII, IX, XI Factors of common pathway: I, II, V, X	Inherited factor deficiencies Lupus anticoagulant Heparin therapy Liver disease Afibrinogenemia von Willebrand disease	Increased incidence of thrombotic disease with lupus anticoagulant Joint and muscle bleeding with factor deficiencies Mucosal bleeding with von Willebrand disease
Thrombin time (TT)	Fibrinogen Inhibitors of fibrin aggregation	Afibrinogenemia Heparin therapy	Life-long hemorrhagic disease

HMWK = high molecular weight kininogen.

LABORATORY TESTS

A detailed clinical history, a physical examination, and the results of a few laboratory tests can establish the initial diagnosis of coagulation disorders.[1–3] The most common screening tests include determinations of bleeding time, prothrombin time (PT), activated partial thromboplastin time (aPTT), and thrombin time, together with a platelet count. The results of these standard laboratory procedures can distinguish bleeding disorders caused by defects in the intrinsic, extrinsic, and common coagulation pathways or alterations in the number of functioning platelets (see Fig. 100–1). Specific assays of individual coagulation factors and platelet function tests can be performed after abnormalities are identified by initial screening tests. Simple tests that are available in most clinical settings are summarized in Table 100–2.

BLEEDING TIME

The measurement of a bleeding time assesses platelet number and function and capillary integrity. Bleeding time measures the length of time to the cessation of bleeding following a standardized skin cut.[1,3] The bleeding time is prolonged with thrombocytopenia. It is also prolonged with qualitative abnormalities of platelet function. These include inherited platelet disorders such as Glanzmann thrombasthenia and Bernard-Soulier syndrome. Medications that interfere with platelet function, such as aspirin, also cause a prolonged bleeding time. Renal failure, fibrinogen disorders, and collagen defects such as Ehlers-Danlos syndrome can also cause prolongation of the bleeding time.

PROTHROMBIN TIME

The PT assesses the function of the extrinsic and common pathways of the coagulation system.[1] In particular, the test measures the activity of the vitamin K-dependent factors II, VII, and X. The prothrombin time reflects the time required for fibrin strands to appear after the addition of tissue thromboplastin to a patient's plasma. Thus, it yields evidence about the current synthetic capacity of the liver, the adequacy of vitamin K absorption, and the inhibition of clotting factor synthesis by warfarin.

ACTIVATED PARTIAL THROMBOPLASTIN TIME

The activated partial thromboplastin time (aPTT) measures the activity of the intrinsic and common pathways.[1] The aPTT is the time required for a fibrin clot to form after partial thromboplastin, calcium, and an activating agent are added to the patient's plasma. This measure is widely used for monitoring heparin therapy.

THROMBIN TIME

As a measure of the time to convert fibrinogen to fibrin, the thrombin time is affected by quantitative and qualitative abnormalities of fibrinogen and the presence of thrombin inhibitors or FDPs.[3] The thrombin time measures the time required for the formation and the appearance of the fibrin clot after thrombin is added to plasma. It is commonly used to monitor the effect of systemic fibrinolytic therapy and can be modified for monitoring heparin therapy.

CONGENITAL COAGULATION DISORDERS

HEMOPHILIA

Hemophilia is a bleeding disorder that results from a congenital deficiency in a plasma coagulation protein. Hemophilia A (classic hemophilia) is caused by a deficiency of factor VIII, while hemophilia B (Christmas disease) is caused by a deficiency of factor IX. The incidence of hemophilia A is approximately 1 in 5,000 male births.[4–6] Hemophilia B occurs less commonly, with only one-fourth the incidence of hemophilia A.[5,6] There are no significant racial differences in the incidence of hemophilia.

Thirty percent of severe hemophilia patients have a negative family history, presumably representing a spontaneous mutation. Both hemophilia A and hemophilia B are recessive, X-linked diseases; that is, the defective gene is located on the X chromosome. In general, the disease affects only males, while females are carriers. Affected males have the abnormal allele on their X chromosome and no matching allele on their Y chromosome. Thus, their sons would be normal (assuming the mother is not a carrier), and their daughters would be obligatory carriers. Female carriers have one normal allele and, therefore, do not usually have a bleeding tendency. Sons of a female carrier and a normal male have a 50% chance of being hemophiliacs, whereas daughters have a 50% chance of being carriers. Thus, there is a "skipped generation" mode of inheritance in which the female carriers, who are the children of hemophiliacs, do not express the disease, but can pass it on to the next male generation.

Hemophilia has been observed in a small number of females as when a hemophiliac marries a female carrier. Female carriers can rarely exhibit a hemophilia phenotype when the normal X chromosome becomes excessively inactivated through a process called lyonization. Hemophilia can also occur in female patients who have only one X chromosome, as in Turner's syndrome.[7]

In 1984, researchers isolated and cloned the human factor VIII gene.[8] It is a large gene, consisting of 186 kilobases (kb).[5,9] More than 500 different mutations in the factor VIII gene, including point mutations, deletions, and insertions, have been described.[5,6] Deletions and nonsense mutations are often associated with the more severe forms of factor VIII deficiency, because no functional factor VIII is produced. In 1993, researchers identified an inversion in the factor VIII gene at intron 22 that accounts for about 45% of severe hemophilia A gene abnormalities.[10] This discovery has greatly simplified carrier detection and prenatal diagnosis for families with this gene mutation.

The factor IX gene, cloned and sequenced in 1982, consists of only 34 kb and thus is significantly smaller than the factor VIII gene.[5] Unlike the factor VIII gene in patients with severe hemophilia A, the factor IX gene in patients with hemophilia B has no predominant mutation. Direct gene mutation analysis is simpler in hemophilia B because of the smaller gene size, and to date more than 600 different mutations are known.[8] The majority of these mutations are single base pair substitutions. Approximately 3% of factor IX gene mutations are deletions or complex rearrangements. Because these mutations are associated with a severe phenotype they are of prognostic significance.[8]

Hemophilia B Leyden is a rare variant in which factor IX levels are initially low, but rise at puberty. This phenotype results from a mutation in the promoter region of the gene that is apparently ameliorated by the action of testosterone.[5,11] The identification of this genotype is clinically important, because it confers a better prognosis.

CLINICAL PRESENTATION

The characteristic bleeding manifestations of hemophilia include ecchymoses, bleeding into joint spaces (hemarthroses), muscle hemorrhages, and excessive bleeding after surgery or trauma. The severity of clinical bleeding usually correlates with the degree of deficiency of factor VIII or factor IX. Factor VIII and factor IX activity levels generally are measured in units (U/mL) with 1 U/mL representing 100% of the factor found in 1 mL of normal plasma. Normal plasma levels range from 0.5–1.5 U/mL.[5] Patients with less than 0.01 U/mL (1%) of either factor are classified as severe hemophiliacs; those with 0.01–0.05 U/mL (1%–5%) are moderate hemophiliacs, and those with greater than 0.05 U/mL (5%) are mild hemophiliacs (Table 100–3). Patients with severe disease often experience frequent spontaneous hemorrhages and joint space bleeding, while those with moderate disease have excessive bleeding following trauma and rarely experience spontaneous hemarthroses. Patients with mild hemophilia may have so few symptoms that their condition is undiagnosed for many years and usually have excessive bleeding only after significant trauma or surgery. Occasionally, those with severe disease (less than 1% factor activity) may not display a severe phenotype; conversely, some with milder forms of the disease may have more severe bleeding symptomatology. The majority of patients with hemophilia present with clinical manifestations after the age of 1 year, when they begin to walk and increase their risk of bleeding.

The most common bleeding problem in patients with hemophilia is a joint hemorrhage, which most frequently occurs in the elbow or the knee.[12] Hemarthroses may be spontaneous. The patient experiences joint pain, swelling, erythema, and decreased range of motion.

TABLE 100–3. Laboratory and Clinical Manifestations of Hemophilia

	Severe	Moderate	Mild
Factor VIII/IX activity level[a]	<0.01 U/mL	0.01–0.05 U/mL	>0.05 U/mL
% of patients with hemophilia A	70%	15%	15%
% of patients with hemophilia B	50%	30%	20%
Bleeding manifestations			
Age at onset	≤1 yr	1–2 yr	2 yr–adult
Neonatal symptoms			
PCB	Usual	Usual	Rare
ICH	Occasional	Uncommon	Rare
Muscle/joint hemorrhage	Spontaneous	Minor trauma	Major trauma
CNS hemorrhage	High risk	Moderate risk	Rare
Postsurgical hemorrhage (without prophylaxis)	Frank bleeding, severe	Wound bleeding, common	Wound bleeding, with factor < 0.3 U/mL
Oral hemorrhage following trauma, tooth extraction	Usual	Common	Common

[a]Normal range of factor VIII/IX activity level is 0.5–1.5 U/mL (50%–150%). 1 U/mL corresponds to 100% of the factor found in 1 mL of normal plasma. PCB = postcircumcisional bleeding; ICH = intracranial hemorrhage; CNS = central nervous system.

Adapted from Ref. 5 with permission.

Because repeated joint hemorrhages can lead to chronic, disabling arthropathies, these bleeding episodes warrant aggressive treatment. The regular administration of prophylactic factor replacement can reduce or prevent joint bleeding and chronic damage.[5]

Intramuscular hemorrhages are also a hallmark of hemophilic bleeding. Presenting signs may be vague, such as pain with motion of the affected muscle or with swelling. Sequelae may include life-threatening blood loss, especially with bleeding in the thigh or iliopsoas muscle, and compression of nerves or blood vessels.

Mouth bleeding can occur after minor trauma, such as a torn frenulum, or after dental extractions. Hematuria is another common problem in hemophilia. Because spontaneous gastrointestinal bleeding is uncommon, it is necessary to seek an underlying cause (e.g., an ulcer or a polyp) when such bleeding does occur.

Bleeding into the central nervous system, one of the most serious bleeding complications of hemophilia, can occur either spontaneously or following head trauma. Bleeding into the tongue, pharynx, or retropharynx is another serious area of bleeding which can result in airway obstruction.

DIAGNOSIS

The diagnosis of hemophilia should be considered in any male with unusual bleeding. A family history of bleeding is also helpful in the diagnosis, but only 20% to 30% of patients have an affected family member.[5,13] Brothers of patients with hemophilia should be screened; sisters should have carrier testing.

Screening tests usually reveal a prolonged aPTT with a normal PT, platelet count, and bleeding time. An isolated prolonged aPTT suggests a deficiency of a factor in the intrinsic coagulation pathway (factors VIII, IX, XI, and XII). Other causes of a prolonged aPTT are listed in Table 100–2. Specific factor assays must then be performed to determine the type and level of factor deficiency. Because patients with von Willebrand disease also have low levels of factor VIII, tests for this disorder should be performed in all patients with a factor VIII deficiency.

Recent advances in molecular genetic analysis have greatly improved the accuracy of carrier status evaluation. Thus, female relatives of patients with hemophilia who are at risk of being carriers for the disorder should be tested. Additionally, the appropriate factor level should be assayed in female carriers to identify those with levels less than 0.3 U/mL (30%) who might themselves be at risk of bleeding.

Patients with severe hemophilia A should be tested for the common factor VIII gene inversion. If the patient has this mutation, family members should undergo testing to determine if they also have the mutation and, thus, are carriers. In those patients with hemophilia A who lack the inversion mutation, other methods of determining the carrier status of their family members are available.[14] Techniques for determining carrier status in families with hemophilia B are similar, although no predominant mutation like the factor VIII inversion has been found. The smaller size of the factor IX gene facilitates direct DNA mutational analysis.[14]

Hemophilia can be diagnosed prenatally by chorionic villus sampling in the 10th to 11th gestational week or by amniocentesis after 15 weeks' gestation.[5,15] Fetal blood can be sampled and assayed directly for factor VIII levels by the 18th to 20th week of gestation.[5,15] This procedure is less useful for diagnosing factor IX deficiency, because factor IX levels are physiologically low in fetuses and infants.[5,16]

▶ TREATMENT: Hemophilia

The comprehensive care of hemophilia requires a multitude of medical and paramedical personnel.[5,9] The patient is best managed in specialized centers with trained personnel and appropriate laboratory, radiologic, and pharmaceutical services. The health care team includes hematologists, orthopedic surgeons, nurses, physical therapists, dentists, genetic counselors, psychologists, and social workers.

Patients with hemophilia should receive routine immunizations, including immunization against hepatitis B. Hepatitis A vaccine is also recommended for patients with hemophilia because of the risk (although small) of transmitting the causative agent through factor concentrates.[17] The use of a small-gauge needle can prevent excessive bleeding. Some health care providers advocate giving immunizations subcutaneously rather than intramuscularly to decrease the risk of hematoma formation.

A few special considerations apply to the perinatal care of male infants of hemophilia carriers. Intracranial or extracranial hemorrhage has been estimated to occur in about 3.5% of newborns with hemophilia.[18] There is no clear consensus on the optimal mode of delivery or the use of prophylactic factor replacement in male infants of hemophilia carriers.[18,19] Circumcision should be postponed until a diagnosis of hemophilia is excluded. Factor levels can be assayed from cord blood samples or from peripheral venipuncture. Arterial puncture should be avoided because of the risk of hematoma formation.

Intravenous (IV) factor replacement therapy to treat or prevent bleeding is the mainstay of treatment for hemophilia. It is common for families to learn how to treat patients with factor concentrate at home. Parents may learn to infuse factor for younger children, and older children and adult patients may learn self-administration. Home health care nursing support may also be helpful, particularly for the youngest patients in whom venous access may be difficult. Administration of factor at home is more convenient for families and allows for earlier treatment of acute bleeding episodes. Serious bleeding episodes always require medical evaluation, however.

HISTORY OF HEMOPHILIA TREATMENT

Therapy for hemophilia has undergone dramatic advances over the past few decades. Forty years ago, the administration of fresh-frozen plasma was the only available treatment. The introduction of cryoprecipitate in the early 1960s allowed more specific therapy for hemophilia A.[5,6,9] Intermediate-purity factor VIII and IX concentrates became available in the 1970s.[5,6] Plasma-derived factor concentrates are made from the donations of thousands of people. Contamination of plasma pools with hepatitis B, hepatitis C, and human immunodeficiency virus (HIV) during the late 1970s and early 1980s resulted in transmission to the majority of patients with severe hemophilia. Since the mid-1980s, plasma-derived concentrates have been manufactured using a variety of virus-inactivating techniques including dry heat, pasteurization, and treatment with chemicals (e.g., solvent-detergent mixtures).[6,9] Since 1986, there has been no transmission of HIV through factor concentrates to patients with hemophilia in the United States.[5,6,9] Protein purification, introduced in the 1990s, produced high-purity concentrates with increased amounts of factor VIII or factor IX relative to the product's total protein content. Recombinant factor VIII and then factor IX also became available.[5,9] Finally,

TABLE 100–4. Factor Concentrates

Brand Name	Product Type	Viral Inactivation or Exclusion Method	Other Contents
Factor VIII Concentrates			
Alphanate	Plasma	Solvent detergent	albumin, heparin, vWF
Hemophil M	Plasma	Solvent detergent, monoclonal Ab	albumin
Humate P	Plasma	Pasteurization	albumin, vWF
Koate-HP	Plasma	Solvent detergent	albumin, heparin, vWF
Method M	Plasma	Solvent detergent, monoclonal Ab	albumin
Monarc M	Plasma	Solvent detergent	
Monoclate P	Plasma	Pasteurization, monoclonal Ab	albumin
Profilnate OSD	Plasma	Solvent detergent	
Bioclate	Recombinant	None	albumin
Helixate FS	Recombinant	Solvent detergent	albumin (fermentation only)
Kogenate FS	Recombinant	Solvent detergent	albumin (fermentation only)
Recombinate	Recombinant	None	albumin
ReFacto	Recombinant	None	
Factor IX Concentrates			
AlphaNine SD	Plasma	Solvent detergent	heparin
Mononine	Plasma	Monoclonal Ab, ultrafiltration	heparin
Benefix	Recombinant	None	
APCC			
Autoplex T	Plasma	Dry heat	Heparin, IIa, VIIa, VIIIa, IXa, Xa
FEIBA	Plasma	Vapor heat	IIa, VIIa, VIIIa, IXa, Xa
PCC			
Bebulin VH	Plasma	Vapor heat	Heparin, II, VII, VIII, IX, X
Hemonyne	Plasma	Dry heat	II, VII, VIII, IX, X
Konyne 80	Plasma	Dry heat	II, VII, VIII, IX, X
Profilnine SD	Plasma	Solvent detergent	II, VII, VIII, IX, X
Proplex T	Plasma	Dry heat	Heparin, II, VII, VIII, IX, X
Other			
NovoSeven	Recombinant VII	None	
Hyate C	Porcine VIII	Freeze-dried	

APCC = activated prothrombin complex concentrate; PCC = prothrombin activated complex concentrate; vWF = von Willebrand factor.

gene therapy for the treatment of hemophilia is now in the early stages of clinical trials.

HEMOPHILIA A

Table 100–4 summarizes the factor VIII products currently available in the United States. The majority of patients are treated with high-purity products. In general, products that have the lowest risk of transmitting infectious disease should be used.

RECOMBINANT FACTOR VIII

Derived from cultured Chinese hamster ovary cells or baby hamster kidney cells transfected with the human factor VIII gene,[20] recombinant factor VIII is produced from DNA technology. Because it is not derived from blood donations, the risk of transmitting infections through the administration of recombinant factor VIII is low. For this reason, recombinant products are generally favored over plasma-derived products. First-generation recombinant factor VIII products contain human albumin as a stabilizing protein, however.[6] These products, therefore, have a theoretical risk of transmitting human infection, although hepatitis and HIV infection have never been reported with their use.[5] Second-generation recombinant factor VIII products that lack human protein as a stabilizer (although it may be included in the culture process) are now available.

Clinical trials have demonstrated that recombinant factor VIII products result in equal or better patient recovery rates (immediate post-infusion factor VIII levels) and have comparable effectiveness to the plasma-derived products.[20–22] In children, recombinant factor VIII has been shown to produce a better response and recovery rate than plasma-derived product.[23] The risk of developing an inhibitory antibody to factor VIII with the use of recombinant factor VIII is 20%–25%.[20] Although there were initial concerns of an increased risk of inhibitor development with recombinant products, it now appears that the difference is attributable to more frequent inhibitor screening in the recombinant product trials with the detection of transient inhibitors that might otherwise have been missed.[21]

PLASMA-DERIVED FACTOR VIII PRODUCTS

Several different plasma-derived factor VIII products are available (see Table 100–4). These products are produced from the plasma of thousands of donors and, therefore, potentially can transmit infection. Donor screening, viral reduction through purification steps, and viral inactivation procedures (e.g., dry heat, pasteurization, solvent-detergent treatment) have all resulted in a safer product.[13] No cases of HIV transmission from factor concentrates have been reported since 1986.[5] However, there have been isolated reports of hepatitis C infection with the use of plasma-derived products.[5] Additionally, there have been outbreaks of hepatitis A virus associated with plasma-derived products, likely because solvent-detergent treatment does not inactivate this non-enveloped virus.[17] Parvovirus has also been reported to be transmitted in plasma-derived factor VIII products.[13] Finally, there remains concern about the possibility for infection with as yet unidentified viruses that currently used methods would not inactivate.

Factor VIII concentrates can be classified according to their level of purity, which refers to the specific activity of factor VIII in the product. Cryoprecipitate is a low-purity product, containing a specific factor VIII activity level of less than 5 U/mg of protein.[5] Intermediate-purity products have a specific activity of factor VIII of 1–10 U/mg of protein, while high-purity products have a specific activity of 50–1,000 U/mg of protein.[5] Ultrahigh-purity plasma-derived products are prepared using monoclonal antibody purification steps and have a specific activity of 3,000 U/mg of protein prior to the addition of albumin as a stabilizer.

Cryoprecipitate, which contains factor VIII, factor XIII, fibrinogen, and von Willebrand factor, also can be used to treat factor VIII deficiency. However, because this product currently does not undergo a viral inactivation process, it is no longer considered a primary form of treatment in countries where factor VIII concentrates are available. Cryoprecipitate contains approximately 80–120 U of factor VIII per unit, and the volume is calculated to achieve the desired factor VIII correction.[12,24]

FACTOR VIII CONCENTRATE REPLACEMENT

Appropriate dosing of factor VIII concentrate depends on several considerations, including the half-life of the infused factor, the patient's body weight, and the volume of distribution. Whether or not the patient has developed an inhibitory antibody to factor VIII and the titer of this antibody also influence treatment. Recovery studies, which measure the immediate post-infusion factor level, and survival studies, which assess the half-life of the factor, can establish individual pharmacokinetics. The location and magnitude of the bleeding episode determine the percent correction to target, as well as the duration of treatment. Serious or life-threatening bleeding requires peak factor levels of greater than 0.75–1 U/mL (75%–100%), while less severe bleeding may be treated with a goal of 0.3–0.5 U/mL (30%–50%) peak plasma levels. Table 100–5 provides general guidelines for the management of bleeding in different locations.

TABLE 100–5. Guidelines for Factor Replacement Therapy for Hemorrhage in Hemophilia A and B

Site of Hemorrhage	Hemostatic Factor Level (% of normal)	Factor Dosing		Comment
		Hemophilia A	*Hemophilia B**	
Joint	30%–50%, minimum	20–40 U/kg qd PRN	30–40 U/kg qod PRN	Rest/immobilization/physical therapy rehabilitation following bleed. Several doses may be necessary to prevent or treat target joint.
Muscle	40%–50%, minimum	20–40 U/kg qd PRN	40–60 U/kg qod PRN	Calf/forearm bleed is limb threatening, significant blood loss with femoral/retroperitoneal bleed.
Oral mucosa	Initially 50%; then antifibrinolytic coverage usually suffices	25 U/kg	50 U/kg	Antifibrinolytic therapy is critical. Do not use with PCCs or APCCs.
Epistaxis	Initially 80%–100%; then 30% until healing occurs	40–50 U/kg; then 30–40 U/kg qd	80–100 U/kg; then 70–80 U/kg qod	Local measures: pressure/packing/cautery useful for severe or recurrent bleed.
Gastrointestinal	Initially 100%; then 30% until healing occurs	40–50 U/kg; then 30–40 U/kg qd	80–100 U/kg; then 70–80 U/kg qod	Lesion is usually found; endoscopy highly recommended. Antifibrinolytic therapy may be useful.
Genitourinary	Initially 100%; then 30% until healing occurs	40–50 U/kg; then 30–40 U/kg qd	80–100 U/kg; then 70–80 U/kg qod	Evaluate for stones or urinary tract infection. Lesion usually not found. Prednisone 1–2 mg/kg/d × 5–7d may be useful.
Central nervous system	Initially 100%; then 50%–100% for 10–14 d	50 U/kg; then 25 U/kg q12h *or* CI	100 U/kg, then 50 U/kg q24h CI of HPPs may be possible	Anticonvulsants frequently used preventively, neurologic follow-up. Lumbar puncture requires prophylactic factor coverage.
Trauma or surgery	Initially 100%; then 50% until wound healing begins; then 30% until wound healing complete	50 U/kg; then dose q12h *or* by CI	100 U/kg; then dose q24h *or* as above	Perioperative and postoperative management plan must be in place preoperatively; evaluation for inhibitors crucial prior to elective surgery.

PCCs = prothrombin complex concentrates; APCCs = activated prothrombin complex concentrates; CI = continuous infusion; HPPs = high-purity products.
From Ref. 5 with permission.
*Higher doses may be required if recombinant factor concentrate is used.

Factor VIII is a large molecule that remains in the intravascular space. Therefore, the plasma volume, approximately 50 mL/kg, can be used to estimate the volume of distribution.[12,25] In general, each unit of factor VIII concentrate infused per kilogram of body weight yields a 2% rise in plasma factor VIII levels. The following equation may be used to calculate an initial dose of factor VIII:

$$\text{Factor VIII (units)} = (\text{Desired level} - \text{Baseline level}) \times 0.5 \times (\text{Weight in kilograms})$$

The baseline level is usually omitted from the equation because it is negligible compared to the desired level. The half-life of factor VIII ranges from 8–15 hours.[25] It is generally necessary to administer half of the initial dose approximately every 12 hours to sustain the desired level of factor VIII. A single treatment may be adequate for minor bleeding such as mouth bleeding or slight muscle hemorrhages. Because of the potential for long-term joint damage with hemarthroses, however, 2 or 3 days of treatment are often recommended for these bleeds. Serious bleeding episodes may require maintaining 70%–100% factor activity for a week or longer. As previously mentioned, factor VIII dosing depends on several variables and each case must be considered individually. Individual pharmacokinetics may help guide treatment, particularly for serious bleeding episodes.

Alternatively, factor VIII may be administered as a continuous infusion when prolonged treatment is required, such as in the perioperative period or for serious bleeding episodes. Infusion rates ranging from 1.5–6 U/kg/h have been reported to maintain factor VIII levels of 100%.[26] The administration of factor concentrate via continuous infusion may reduce factor requirements by 20%–50%.[26] A gradual decrease in factor VIII clearance during the first 5–6 days of treatment contributes to the lower factor concentrate requirements.[27] Daily factor level monitoring can help determine the appropriate rate of infusion.

The administration of factor VIII concentrate via continuous infusion has been shown to be safe and effective, and it may be more convenient than bolus therapy for hospitalized patients.[27] When continuous infusion is used for surgery, supplemental bolus infusion doses may be required in the immediate perioperative period to maintain adequate factor VIII levels.[27] The advantages of continuous infusion include the maintenance of a steady-state plasma level, with avoidance of potentially subtherapeutic trough levels, and a reduction in cost associated with decreased factor requirements. A potential side effect with continuous infusion is thrombophlebitis at the delivery site. Concomitant infusion of saline[27] or the addition of heparin (2–5 U/mL) to the infusion bag can minimize this risk.[26,27] Bacterial contamination of the concentrate is another theoretical concern. However, studies have shown that the products can remain sterile for greater than a week if prepared and kept under appropriate conditions.[26] Finally, concerns about the stability of the formulations appear to be unwarranted in that most of the high-purity factor VIII concentrates have been shown to remain stable for at least 7 days after reconstitution.[26]

OTHER PHARMACOLOGIC THERAPY

In patients with mild factor VIII deficiency, treatment with 1-desamino-8-D-arginine vasopressin (desmopressin acetate, DDAVP) is often adequate for minor bleeding episodes. A synthetic analog of the antidiuretic hormone vasopressin, DDAVP causes release of factor VIII from endogenous storage sites. The recommended dose of DDAVP is 0.3 μg/kg diluted in 30–50 mL of normal saline and infused IV over 15–30 minutes.[5,12] In those that are responsive, this results in an average threefold (range two- to tenfold) increase in factor VIII levels within 30–60 minutes.[5,12,28,29] The infusion of DDAVP may be repeated daily for up to 2–3 days. Tachyphylaxis with an attenuated response may develop after that, and factor concentrate therapy may be necessary if the patient requires further treatment. Factor levels should be measured to ensure that an adequate response has been achieved. Treatment with DDAVP will not result in hemostasis for patients who have severe hemophilia and for those who are only marginally responsive. Also, it should not be used as primary therapy for life-threatening bleeding episodes such as intracranial hemorrhage.[12]

DDAVP may be administered intranasally via a concentrated nasal spray.[30] It effectively increases factor VIII levels, but its peak effect occurs 60–90 minutes after administration, somewhat longer than with DDAVP administered IV.[5,29] The dosage is one spray (150 μg) for children who weigh less than 50 kg and two sprays (300 μg) for those who weigh more than 50 kg.[29] The nasal spray may serve as an alternative to the IV formulation, especially in patients with mild bleeding episodes.

Very few adverse effects are associated with DDAVP. The most commonly observed side effect is facial flushing.[31] Side effects less frequently reported include mild headaches, increased heart rate, and decreased blood pressure. Thrombosis is a rare complication associated with DDAVP.[5] Because of its antidiuretic effects, DDAVP also has the potential to cause water retention, which may lead to severe hyponatremia. This may be a particular problem in children less than 1 to 2 years old in whom hyponatremic seizures have been reported.[5,28] Therefore, DDAVP use should be avoided in this age group.[5,12] Mild fluid restriction and monitoring of urine output is also recommended with DDAVP administration.[5,12]

Antifibrinolytic therapy inhibits clot lysis and therefore is a useful adjunctive therapy in the treatment of hemophilia. These antifibrinolytic agents are particularly beneficial in the treatment of oral bleeding because of the high concentration of fibrinolytic enzymes present in saliva. Two currently available antifibrinolytics are aminocaproic acid and tranexamic acid. Aminocaproic acid is given at a dosage of 100 mg/kg (maximum 5 g) every 6 hours and may be administered orally or IV.[5] The dosage of tranexamic acid is 25 mg/kg (maximum 1.5 g) orally every 8 hours or 10 mg/kg (maximum 1 g) IV every 8 hours.[5,32]

HEMOPHILIA B

Therapeutic options for hemophilia B have improved greatly over the past several years, first with the production of monoclonal antibody-purified plasma-derived products and then with the licensure of recombinant factor IX. Products that are currently available in the United States for treatment of hemophilia B are listed in Table 100–4.

RECOMBINANT FACTOR IX

First marketed in the United States in 1996,[5,6] recombinant factor IX is produced in Chinese hamster ovary cells transfected with the factor IX gene. Blood and plasma products are not used to produce recombinant factor IX nor to stabilize the final product; thus, recombinant factor IX has an excellent viral safety profile.[33] Clinical trials have shown the product to be safe and efficacious in the treatment of acute bleeding episodes and in the management of bleeding associated with surgical procedures.[34] Although the half-life of recombinant factor IX is similar to that of the plasma-derived products, recovery is approximately 28% lower.[34] As a result, doses of recombinant factor IX concentrate must be higher than those of plasma-derived products to achieve equivalent plasma levels. Because individual pharmacokinetics may vary, recovery and survival studies should be performed to determine optimal treatment. Recombinant factor IX is often considered the treatment of choice for hemophilia B, particularly for children.

PLASMA-DERIVED FACTOR IX PRODUCTS

High-purity factor IX plasma concentrates have been available in the United States since the early 1990s.[28] These products are derived from plasma through biochemical purification and monoclonal immunoaffinity techniques. Other viral inactivation measures, such as solvent-detergent or chemical treatment, are also employed.

Before the high-purity products were approved for use, hemophilia B had been treated with factor IX concentrates that also contained other vitamin K-dependent proteins (factors II, VII, and X), known as prothrombin complex concentrates (PCCs). These products contain small amounts of activated factors generated during processing, and their use has been associated with thrombotic complications, including deep venous thrombosis, pulmonary embolism, myocardial infarction, and disseminated intravascular coagulation (DIC).[35,36] The risk of such complications is highest in patients who are receiving high or repetitive doses of PCCs, in those who have liver disease, in neonates, and in patients who have experienced crush injuries or who are undergoing major surgery.[28,36] Concomitant use of PCCs and antifibrinolytics should be avoided because of the risk of thrombosis.

Owing to the lower purity of PCCs and their thrombogenic potential, these products are not first-line treatment for hemophilia B, although they are still used in the treatment of patients with hemophilia A or B who have developed inhibitory antibodies against factor VIII or factor IX, respectively. High-purity factor IX concentrates have excellent efficacy in the treatment of bleeding episodes and in the control of bleeding associated with surgical procedures.[37,38] Their viral safety profile has also been reported to be excellent,[38] and the risk of thromboembolic complications is low.[5]

FACTOR IX CONCENTRATE REPLACEMENT

Factor IX is a relatively small protein. Unlike factor VIII, it is not limited to the intravascular space, but also passes into the extravascular compartment. This results in a volume of distribution that is twice that of factor VIII.[12] In general, for plasma-derived factor IX concentrates, each unit of factor IX infused per kilogram of body weight yields a 1% rise in the plasma level of factor IX. The following equation can be used to calculate the initial dose:

$$\text{Plasma-derived factor IX (units)} = (\text{Desired level} - \text{Baseline level}) \times (\text{Weight in kilograms})$$

As with the similar calculation for factor VIII dosing, the baseline level term can be omitted from the formula. Because the recovery of recombinant factor IX is approximately 20% lower than that of the plasma-derived products, the following adjustment is made:

$$\text{Recombinant factor IX (units)} = (\text{Desired level} - \text{Baseline level}) \times 1.2 \times (\text{Weight in kilograms})$$

A recovery study to determine optimal dosing is recommended for patients who receive recombinant factor IX because of the wide interpatient variability.

Because the half-life of factor IX is approximately 24 hours, dosing can be less frequent than with factor VIII. Table 100–5 provides general guidelines for dosing factor IX, based on the site and severity of the bleeding episode. As with factor VIII replacement therapy, individual pharmacokinetics may vary, and monitoring the patient's factor IX levels helps optimize therapy.

PROPHYLACTIC REPLACEMENT THERAPY

Traditional therapy for hemophilia has been given on demand, as the bleeding episode occurs. However, recurrent joint bleeding can damage the joint and lead to the development of severe physical disability. Thus, it would be preferable to prevent bleeding episodes and avoid the resultant damage. Known as prophylactic factor replacement therapy, this approach entails the regular infusion of concentrate to maintain the deficient factor at a minimum of 0.01 U/mL (1%).

In effect, this prophylactic replacement therapy converts severe hemophilia into a milder form of the disease. The rationale behind it is that patients with moderate hemophilia rarely experience spontaneous hemarthroses, and they have a much lower incidence of chronic arthropathy. Patients with hemophilia A usually require 25–40 U of factor VIII per kilogram of body weight given every other day or three times a week.[39] For hemophilia B, the usual dosage is 25–40 U/kg of factor IX given twice instead of three times weekly because of the longer half-life of factor IX.[5,40]

Primary prophylaxis is regular replacement therapy started at a young age (usually before the patient is 2 years old), prior to the onset of joint bleeding.[39] The results of primary prophylaxis have been very promising. In the Swedish experience, children who began prophylaxis at 1 to 2 years of age experienced almost no bleeding episodes and had normal joint examinations and radiographs over a 5-year period.[39–41] Secondary prophylaxis begins after significant joint bleeding has already occurred. It is associated with a significant reduction in the number of joint bleeding episodes, as well as some clinical improvement.[42–44] Patients receiving prophylaxis had better orthopedic outcomes than patients whose treatment consisted of the on-demand administration of factor replacement concentrates.[43] However, radiographic evidence of joint disease rarely improves and often progresses despite the institution of secondary prophylaxis.[5,44] Therefore, it may not be possible to avoid chronic arthropathy when prophylaxis is initiated after significant joint bleeding has already occurred; this supports a need for earlier intervention.

Prophylactic replacement therapy is now in widespread use in Europe. Although the Medical and Scientific Advisory Council of the National Hemophilia Foundation of the United States has recommended primary prophylaxis beginning at 1 to 2 years of age for children with severe hemophilia,[5] this therapeutic approach has not yet been widely accepted in the United States. There are several disadvantages associated with prophylactic regimens that may be responsible for this lack of acceptance. Perhaps most important is the increased cost of prophylactic replacement therapy. Factor requirements have been estimated to be at least threefold higher with prophylactic regimens than with treatment on demand.[39,45] The use of individual pharmacokinetics to titrate dosage may help to lessen costs.[39] Other issues to consider are the inconvenience to families and the possible difficulties with compliance. Central venous lines may be necessary for the frequent administration of factor concentrates, particularly in children less than 3 to 5 years old, the age targeted for initiation of primary prophylaxis regimens. Potential complications include surgical risks, infection, and catheter-related deep venous thrombosis.[46,47]

Catheter-related sepsis is a frequent problem, reported to occur in up to 50% of patients with hemophilia who have central lines.[46,47] Finally, there are concerns that the routine use of primary prophylaxis may overtreat some patients with severe hemophilia who would not have displayed a severe clinical phenotype. Prospective, randomized studies and more formal cost-effectiveness analyses are needed to determine the relative benefits and optimal timing of prophylactic factor replacement therapy.

TREATMENT OF INHIBITORS IN HEMOPHILIA

Neutralizing antibodies to factor VIII and IX, known as inhibitors, develop in a subset of patients with hemophilia, challenging the management of these patients. The development of inhibitors is probably the most common serious complication of factor replacement therapy. The reported incidence of inhibitor development has varied considerably, depending on the population studied, the study design, the method of detection, and the frequency and duration of testing. Inhibitor formation has been reported to occur in 6% to 52% of patients with factor VIII deficiency.[48] The reported prevalence of inhibitors is much lower in hemophilia B, occurring in only 1% to 4% of patients.[49]

Most inhibitors develop in childhood, often after relatively few exposure days.[49] Patients with severe hemophilia are much more likely to develop inhibitors than those with milder forms of the disease.[28] A possible explanation is that the low levels of factor produced in patients with mild and moderate hemophilia may induce immune tolerance in these individuals. In contrast, factor levels are undetectable in patients with severe hemophilia, and infused factor VIII, regarded as a foreign protein, may provoke an antibody response. Similarly, in patients with severe hemophilia, there is a higher rate of inhibitor development (23% to 40%) in those with mutations that result in undetectable plasma factor VIII levels.[51] The rate of inhibitor development is lower (3% to 13%) in patients with missense mutations and small deletions when circulating, albeit abnormal, protein is present.[50,51] The rate of inhibitor formation varies even among patients with identical mutations, which suggests that host factors modify the risk. One possibility is that HLA genotype may influence the risk of inhibitor formation.[48,51]

Inhibitors are usually immunoglobulin of the IgG subclass that are directed against the factor coagulant portion of the complex. The presence of an inhibitor is suspected when there is a decreased clinical response to factor replacement. It may also be discovered incidentally on routine laboratory screening. Inhibitors are measured with the Bethesda assay, and titers are reported in Bethesda units (BU). One BU is the amount of inhibitor needed to inactivate half of the factor VIII or factor IX in a mixture of inhibitor-containing plasma and pooled normal plasma.[49] Patients with inhibitors to factor VIII or factor IX are divided into two groups: low responders, who have low levels of inhibitors (<10 BU/mL) and generally have little or no rise in antibody titers after exposure to the factor, and high responders, who have higher inhibitor levels (>10 BU/mL) and develop an increase in antibody titer after exposure (anamnestic response).[49]

The inhibitor titer, the site and magnitude of bleeding, and the patient's past response to therapy determine the approach to treatment. For patients with a low titer of inhibitors, administering high doses of the specific factor can often control bleeding episodes. Two to three times the usual replacement dose and more frequent dosing intervals are often necessary to overcome the antibody. Factor level monitoring and clinical assessments help in evaluating the adequacy of treatment. Additional supportive measures, such as immobilization and the administration of antifibrinolytics, should be employed, where appropriate.

In the presence of a high titer of inhibitors, it may be impossible to administer enough factor VIII or factor IX to neutralize the antibody and achieve a hemostatic plasma level. Therefore, the approach to treatment of bleeding episodes in these patients is to use agents that bypass the factor to which the antibody is directed. The mainstay of treatment for both hemophilia A and hemophilia B and a high titer inhibitor has been the use of PCCs that contain the vitamin K-dependent factors II, VII, IX, and X or activated PCCs.[28] The usual dosage is 50–100 U/kg administered every 12 to 24 hours, depending on the severity of the bleeding episode.[49] The maximum dose should not exceed 200 U/kg/day. As previously mentioned, there is a risk of serious thrombotic complications associated with the use of PCCs and activated PCCs. Additionally, because these products contain small amounts of factor VIII and larger amounts of factor IX, they can stimulate an anamnestic response in patients with hemophilia A and, more commonly, in those with hemophilia B.[35] Patients with factor IX inhibitors may occasionally develop severe allergic reactions in response to infusion of factor IX–containing products; therefore, it is wise to monitor these patients closely.[52]

A new bypassing agent, recombinant factor VIIa, is thought to be hemostatically active only at the site of tissue injury where tissue factor is present; thus, the risk of systemic thrombotic events associated with this agent is minimal.[53] Additionally, because recombinant VIIa is not a plasma-derived product, both viral transmission and anamnestic responses to factor VIII or factor IX are unlikely.[35] The initial dose for bleeding episodes is 90–120 μg/kg.[28,53] A drawback is the product's short half-life, which necessitates dosing every 2 hours. The continuous infusion of recombinant factor VIIa, which may be more convenient and cost-effective, has been successful.[54,55] Recombinant factor VIIa appears to be efficacious in controlling bleeding episodes and in managing hemophilia during surgical procedures.[53] Patients treated with bypassing agents must be monitored clinically, because there are no laboratory tests that directly measure the effectiveness of the treatment.

Porcine factor VIII is an alternative therapeutic option for patients who have hemophilia A and inhibitors. In general, porcine factor VIII is most useful when the inhibitor titer is less than 50 BU.[25,49] The recommended initial dose is 50–100 U/kg for those with inhibitor titers less than 50 BU.[25] The rationale is that porcine factor VIII is enough like human factor VIII to participate in the coagulation cascade, yet most factor VIII inhibitors have absent or only weak neutralizing activity against nonhuman factor VIII. However, cross-reactivity with porcine factor VIII does occur, and there is also the potential for developing a high titer of antibody against porcine factor VIII. Although the rise in antibody titer is generally lower than that seen with the administration of human factor VIII,[49] anamnestic responses may occur and can limit future use.[35] Other potential side effects include severe allergic reactions and thrombocytopenia.[25,35,49] Because of these limitations, porcine factor VIII is usually indicated only after recombinant factor VIIa and PCC have failed or when hemorrhages are severe.[49] An advantage to porcine factor VIII is that treatment response may be monitored with factor VIII levels.

The ideal therapy for patients with hemophilia and inhibitors is to eradicate the inhibitor so that future treatment with factor VIII or factor IX concentrates is possible. Immune tolerance therapy, which involves the regular infusion of high doses of the factor to which the antibody is directed, may accomplish this eradication. A variety of different dosing regimens, ranging from 25 U/kg every other day to more than 200 U/kg every day have been employed. Some treatment protocols include adjunctive immunomodulatory therapy, such as the

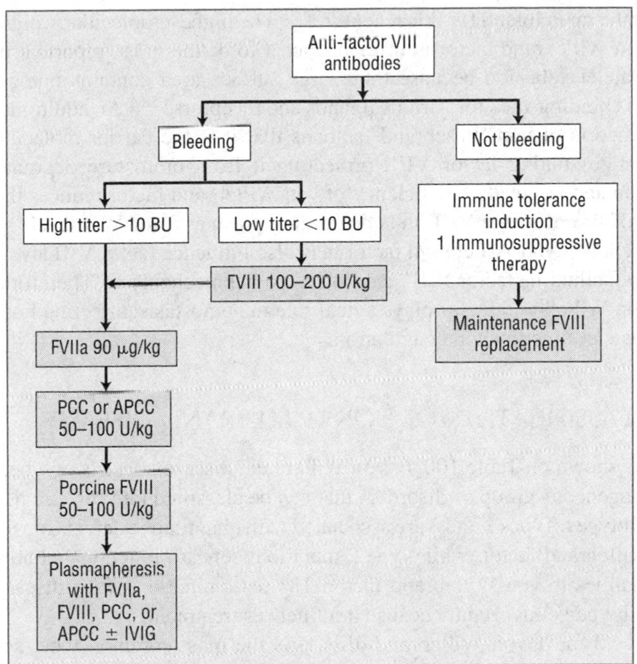

FIGURE 100–2. Treatment algorithm for the management of patients with hemophilia A and factor VIII inhibitors. BU = Bethesda unit; PCC = prothrombin complex concentrate; APCC = activated prothrombin complex concentrate, IVIG = intravenous immune globulin.
*Factor VII a may be used instead, particularly for major bleeding.

administration of cyclophosphamide, prednisone, and intravenous immune globulin.[56] The overall response rate is approximately 60% to 80%, and it is best in patients with low inhibitor titers and those in whom the inhibitor has recently developed.[5,57,58] Weeks to years of therapy may be required to eradicate the antibody. Unfortunately, immune tolerance therapy is costly, takes a great deal of time, and often requires the placement of a central venous catheter.[5] Once achieved, however, immune tolerance facilitates the management of bleeding episodes with specific factor replacement therapy.

Figure 100–2 summarizes the therapeutic options in the management of hemophilia A patients with inhibitors. The same algorithm can be applied to the management of hemophilia B patients, except that factor IX should be substituted for factor VIII. The use of porcine factor VIII is not indicated for the inhibitors in hemophilia B.

GENE THERAPY IN HEMOPHILIA

The use of gene therapy for hemophilia A and B is currently under investigation. A number of different viral and nonviral vectors have been used to transfer the recombinant factor gene to human cells, such as liver and muscle cells.[59,60] Even low levels of factor expression through gene therapy should reduce bleeding episodes in patients with severe hemophilia, a rationale for gene therapy similar to that for prophylactic factor replacement. Furthermore, given that there is a broad range of physiologically normal factor levels, very tight regulation of gene expression is not necessary. The safety and efficacy of this approach to treatment remain to be determined. Potential benefits to gene therapy include patient convenience, viral safety, and decreased cost. Possible drawbacks to gene therapy include a risk of inhibitor formation, tumorigenesis related to integration of the viral vector, and concerns about long-term gene expression.[61,62]

PAIN MANAGEMENT IN HEMOPHILIA

Pain, both acute and chronic, can be a common occurrence for patients with hemophilia. The likely cause of acute pain is bleeding, and control of the bleeding episode should ease the pain. Chronic pain may be the result of permanent joint changes. Surgical intervention may help to alleviate the pain, as may an intensive physical therapy program.[63] The intra-articular administration of dexamethasone may also be useful.[64] Acetaminophen may be used, although narcotic analgesia may be required for more severe pain. In general, patients with hemophilia should avoid the use of aspirin and other nonsteroidal anti-inflammatory drugs (NSAIDs), which impair platelet function and increase the risk of bleeding. Pharmacists may play an important role in educating patients about the myriad of over-the-counter medications that contain aspirin and about the bleeding risks associated with NSAIDS. Cyclooxygenase-2 (COX 2) inhibitors have less antiplatelet activity and may be an option for pain management.

SURGERY IN HEMOPHILIA

The goal of treatment of the patient with hemophilia undergoing a surgical procedure is to maintain factor levels of at least 0.5 to 0.7 U/mL (50% to 70%) during surgery and in the postoperative periods in order to prevent excessive bleeding.[12] Intermittent dosing or continuous infusion factor replacement may accomplish this goal. Before surgery, factor concentrate is usually infused to obtain a plasma level of 1 U/mL (100%). Replacement therapy is continued to maintain plasma levels greater than 0.5 U/mL (50%) for 5 to 7 days or longer, depending on the type of surgery.[12] Preoperative evaluation for elective procedures should include the measurement of an inhibitor titer and assessment of the recovery and half-life of infused factor in the patient. Elective surgery should not proceed unless therapeutic plasma levels can be obtained.

EVALUATION OF THERAPEUTIC OUTCOMES

The main goal in the treatment of hemophilia is to control and prevent bleeding episodes and their long-term sequelae, such as chronic arthropathies. Pharmacologic and nonpharmacologic interventions should be aimed at achieving this goal. Treatment response can be monitored through clinical parameters, such as cessation of bleeding and resolution of symptoms. It may also be useful to determine plasma factor levels, particularly for severe bleeding episodes. Home therapy for the administration of factor concentrates is common among these patients, because this approach can lead to earlier treatment and more independence for the patient. Diaries in which the patient documents symptoms, the dose of factor replacement, adjuvant therapies used, and treatment response can help the caregiver evaluate the success of home therapy. Monitoring the number and type of bleeding episodes and measuring trough plasma factor levels makes it possible to evaluate the adequacy of prophylactic regimens. Physical examination with evaluation of joint range of motion and radiographs of target joints indicates the long-term success of preventing and treating arthropathies.

Clinicians should check for the development of inhibitors, especially in patients with severe disease and exposure to factor concentrates, at least yearly and with any suspicion of poor treatment response. The development of inhibitors challenges the management and control of bleeding episodes. A full understanding of the clinical situation and the titer of the inhibitor is mandatory to address all treatment options for each patient. Because there is no laboratory test to measure the effectiveness of therapy in this scenario, close clinical monitoring for worsening or resolution of the symptoms is essential to optimize the outcome.

VON WILLEBRAND DISEASE

The most common congenital bleeding disorder, von Willebrand disease has a prevalence of 1% to 2%.[65–67] It refers to a family of disorders caused by a quantitative and/or qualitative defect of von Willebrand factor, a glycoprotein that plays a role in both platelet aggregation and coagulation. Unlike hemophilia, von Willebrand disease has an autosomal inheritance pattern, resulting in an equal frequency of disease in males and females.

The gene for von Willebrand factor is located on chromosome 22 and is 178 kb in length.[66] Transcription and translation produce a large primary product that subsequently undergoes complex modifications, resulting in von Willebrand factor multimers of various sizes with molecular weights ranging from 500 to 20,000 kd.[66] Von Willebrand factor is synthesized in megakaryocytes and endothelial cells. Megakaryocyte-derived von Willebrand factor is made up mostly of low molecular weight multimers, is stored in the α granules of platelets, and is released following platelet activation.[66] The von Willebrand factor produced in endothelial cells is stored in the Weibel-Palade bodies and consists predominantly of high molecular weight forms.[30] The contents of Weibel-Palade bodies are secreted via a pathway regulated by physiologic stimuli, such as thrombin or plasmin, in response to endothelial injury.[30,31,65] Low molecular weight von Willebrand factor multimers are also secreted continually by endothelial cells.

Von Willebrand factor is important for both primary and secondary hemostasis. In response to vascular injury, it promotes platelet adhesion by interacting with the glycoprotein Ib receptor on platelets.[30,31] It can also facilitate platelet aggregation by binding to the platelet glycoprotein IIb/IIIa receptor, although fibrinogen is the main ligand for this receptor.[30,31] The highest molecular weight von Willebrand factor multimers appear to be the most important in platelet adhesion because their large surface area contains numerous binding sites for various ligands and receptors.[65,66] An additional function of von Willebrand factor is that it is the carrier molecule for circulating factor VIII, protecting it from premature degradation and removal. A deficiency of von Willebrand factor reduces the half-life of factor VIII, thus decreasing plasma factor VIII levels as well.[31,65] Von Willebrand factor may also influence factor VIII levels by facilitating factor VIII secretion and other mechanisms. Therefore, von Willebrand factor plays a dual role in hemostasis, affecting both platelet function and coagulation.

CLASSIFICATION OF VON WILLEBRAND DISEASE

As shown on Table 100–6, von Willebrand disease consists of a heterogeneous group of disorders that can be classified into three major subtypes. Types 1 and 3 are associated with quantitative defects in von Willebrand factor, while type 2 mutations refer to functional abnormalities in von Willebrand factor. The determination of the disease subtype is important, because it influences treatment.

Type 1 von Willebrand disease is the most common type, accounting for 70% to 80% of cases.[66,67] It is characterized by a mild to moderate reduction in the level of von Willebrand factor (although its multimeric structure is normal) and a similar reduction in the level of factor VIII. It is usually inherited in an autosomal dominant fashion with variable penetrance and expression.[66,67] Bleeding symptoms are often only very mild to moderate.[65,66]

Type 2 von Willebrand disease, diagnosed in 15% to 20% of affected patients, is characterized by a qualitative abnormality of von Willebrand factor.[66,67] Bleeding manifestations may be more severe than with type 1 disease. Inheritance is most often autosomal dominant, but may be recessive.[66,67] Type 2 von Willebrand disease may be further subdivided into four variants. Type 2A is the most frequent subtype and is characterized by a reduced von Willebrand factor–platelet interaction and an absence of high and intermediate molecular weight factor multimers. Type 2B is a less common variant in which there is an abnormal von Willebrand factor that has an increased affinity for the platelet glycoprotein Ib receptor. This is associated with variable degrees of thrombocytopenia. In addition, there are usually no high molecular weight forms of von Willebrand factor.[66] Type 2M arises from a qualitative defect in von Willebrand factor that impairs its interaction with platelets; it is similar to type 2A, except that there is

TABLE 100–6. Revised Classification of von Willebrand Disease

Revised Type	Defect	Previous Type
1	Partial quantitative	I, I platelet normal, I platelet low, IA, I-1, I-2, I-3
2A	Qualitative; decreased platelet-dependent function associated with the absence of high molecular weight vWF multimers	IIA, IIA-1, IIA-2, IIA-3, IB, I platelet discordant, IIC, IID, IIE, IIF, IIG, IIH, II-I
2B	Qualitative; increased affinity for platelet glycoprotein Ib; reduction of high molecular weight vWF multimers	IIB, I New York, Malmö
2M	Qualitative decreased platelet-dependent function not caused by the absence of high molecular weight vWF multimers	B, Vincenza, IC, ID
2N	Decreased affinity of factor VIII	Normandy, defective binding factor VIII
3	Quantitative; complete deficiency of vWF	III

vWF = von Willebrand factor.

Adapted from Ref. 101, with permission.

no measurable reduction in the high molecular weight multimers.[68] Finally, type 2N von Willebrand disease (Normandy) is a rare form of the disease in which von Willebrand factor has a markedly reduced affinity for factor VIII. This leads to a moderate to severe reduction of factor VIII plasma levels with normal von Willebrand factor levels.[30,68]

Type 3 von Willebrand disease refers to a severe quantitative variant of the disease in which von Willebrand factor is nearly undetectable and factor VIII levels are very low. It is often inherited in an autosomal recessive fashion.[30,68] The clinical phenotype is severe, reflecting major deficits in primary hemostasis and coagulation. There is also a platelet-type pseudo von Willebrand disease in which von Willebrand factor is normal, but there is a defect in the platelet glycoprotein Ib receptor that causes an increased affinity for von Willebrand factor.[67] As a result, it is phenotypically similar to type 2B disease, but should be distinguished from it because the treatment is different.

Acquired von Willebrand disease is a rare bleeding disorder that is similar to the congenital form of the disease. It has been reported primarily in association with autoimmune disorders, such as systemic lupus erythematosus, lymphoproliferative disorders, endocrine disorders, congenital cardiac defects, and neoplastic disease.[67,69] Certain medications also have been associated with acquired von Willebrand disease, including valproic acid, dextran, and ciprofloxacin.[69] Bleeding manifestations vary from mild to severe, and the condition often resolves with treatment of the underlying disease. In the acquired disease, von Willebrand factor appears to be synthesized in normal amounts, but then rapidly removed from plasma by anti-von Willebrand factor antibodies, adsorption to tumor cells, or other mechanisms.[67,69]

CLINICAL PRESENTATION

The clinical manifestations of von Willebrand disease are variable, and many patients are either asymptomatic or exhibit minimal bleeding symptoms. Those who are symptomatic usually present with the mucocutaneous bleeding that is typical of platelet disorders. Common bleeding manifestations include recurrent epistaxis, gingival bleeding with minor manipulation, and bruising.[31] Menorrhagia is also a frequent problem, reported to occur in 40% to 78% of affected women.[65,70] Bleeding may be prolonged with minor surgery, particularly with surgeries involving mucosal surfaces (e.g., tonsillectomy and dental extractions). Muscle and joint bleeding, the hallmark of hemophilia, is rarely seen in von Willebrand disease and is usually limited to patients with severe disease and very low levels of factor VIII.

DIAGNOSIS

When a patient has a lifelong history of mucocutaneous bleeding and a family history of abnormal bleeding, the clinician should suspect von Willebrand disease. Several different laboratory tests are helpful in diagnosing the hemostatic abnormality. Initial screening tests include determinations of PT, aPTT, and bleeding time, as well as a platelet count. The PT is normal, whereas the aPTT may be prolonged in relation to the reduction in plasma factor VIII levels. The platelet count is usually normal, although thrombocytopenia is common in type 2B and platelet-type pseudo von Willebrand disease. The bleeding time, which measures platelet function, is often prolonged, but may be normal in patients with milder forms of the disease.

Specific laboratory tests to investigate the possible presence of von Willebrand disease include measurement of von Willebrand factor antigen (vWF:Ag) level, factor VIII assay, determination of ristocetin cofactor activity, and von Willebrand factor multimer analysis. Plasma concentrations of von Willebrand factor increase with cigarette smoking, exercise, pregnancy, and infection, as well as with the use of certain medications, such as corticosteroids, birth control pills, and DDAVP.[68] Repeated test measurements may be necessary to make the diagnosis because of physiologic variations in plasma levels.

Electroimmunoassay, immunoradiometric assay, or enyzme-linked immunosorbent assay (ELISA) can be used to quantify vWF:Ag.[67] Because vWF:Ag levels are known to vary with different ABO blood types,[71] interpretation requires reference to values specific for the patient's blood type. The vWF:Ag level is usually low in types 1 and 2 von Willebrand disease and virtually absent in type 3 disease. Factor VIII levels are normal or mildly decreased in patients with type 1 or 2 disease and very low (< 10%) in those with type 3 disease.[67] Ristocetin, an antibiotic that causes platelet aggregation in the presence of functional von Willebrand factor, is used to measure von Willebrand factor activity. The assay is performed by mixing platelet-free patient plasma, normal formalin-fixed platelets, and ristocetin, and then quantitating the extent of platelet agglutination. Ristocetin cofactor activity is usually reduced in parallel to vWF:Ag levels in types 1 and 3, and decreased to a greater extent than vWF:Ag in type 2 disease (except type 2B).[67] Ristocetin-induced platelet agglutination is useful to further distinguish type 2B disease, as a low concentration of ristocetin induces excessive aggregation in type 2B disease.

Von Willebrand factor multimers can be analyzed by separating them by size on an agarose gel. All multimer sizes are present in type 1 disease, while a reduction in intermediate and high molecular weight multimers is characteristic of type 2 disease. Type 3 patients lack all types of von Willebrand factor multimers. A summary of the laboratory findings in the various types of von Willebrand disease is provided in Table 100–7.

TABLE 100–7. Typical Laboratory Findings in von Willebrand Disease Variants

	von Willebrand Disease Variants					
	1	*2A*	*2B*	*2M*	*2N*	*3*
Factor VIII	↓	↓	↓ or N	↓ or N	↓↓	↓↓
vWF:Ag	↓	↓	N or ↓	↓	↓ or N	ND
vWF:Rcof	↓	↓↓	↓↓	↓↓	↓ or N	ND
RIPA	↓ or N	↓	↑	↓ or N	↓ or N	↓↓
vWF multimers in plasma	N	Largest and intermediate absent	Largest absent	N	N	All absent

N = normal; Ag = antigen; Rcof = ristocetin cofactor activity; RIPA = ristocetin-induced agglutination; ND = not detected; vWF = von Willebrand factor.
Adapted from Ref. 101 with permission.

▶ TREATMENT: von Willebrand Disease

The specific type of von Willebrand disease, as well as the location and severity of bleeding, determine the approach to treatment. Local measures, including pressure, ice, and topical thrombin, can often control superficial bleeding. Systemic treatment is used for bleeding that cannot be controlled in this manner and for the prevention of bleeding with surgery. The goal of systemic therapy is to correct the platelet adhesion and coagulation defects. This may be accomplished by stimulating the release of endogenous von Willebrand factor or by administering products that contain von Willebrand factor and factor VIII. General guidelines for the treatment of von Willebrand disease are shown in Figure 100–3.

REPLACEMENT THERAPY

The treatment of choice for patients with types 2B, 2M, and 3 von Willebrand disease and for patients with type 1 or type 2A von Willebrand disease who are unresponsive to DDAVP is replacement therapy with plasma-derived von Willebrand factor-containing products.[30,72] Several virus-inactivated, intermediate- or high-purity factor VIII concentrates contain sufficient amounts of functional von Willebrand factor.[30,73] Ultrahigh-purity (monoclonal antibody-derived) plasma-derived products and recombinant factor VIII products contain only negligible amounts of von Willebrand factor and are inadequate for the treatment of von Willebrand disease. A very high-purity plasma-derived von Willebrand factor concentrate and a recombinant von Willebrand factor product are currently in clinical trials.[30] Because these von Willebrand factor concentrates do not contain appreciable factor VIII, concomitant administration of a factor VIII-containing product may be necessary for patients with severe disease and low levels of factor VIII.[30] Cryoprecipitate contains approximately 80–100 U of von Willebrand factor per unit, and it was the mainstay of therapy for von Willebrand disease in the past.[24,72] However, because cryoprecipitate is not virally inactivated, it is seldom used as first-line treatment. General guidelines for the dosing of replacement therapy in patients with von Willebrand disease unresponsive to DDAVP are provided in Table 100–8.

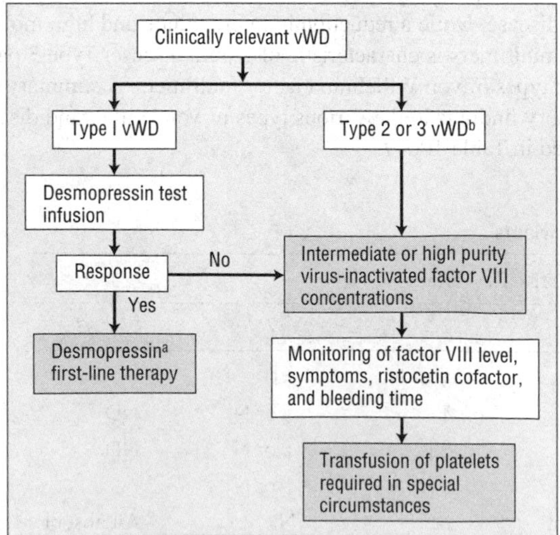

FIGURE 100–3. Guidelines for the treatment of von Willebrand disease (vWD). [a]Factor VIII concentrate should be used for life-threatening bleeding. [b]Some patients with type 2 vWD may respond to desmopressin.

OTHER PHARMACOLOGIC THERAPY

A synthetic analog of vasopressin, DDAVP stimulates the endothelial cell release of von Willebrand factor and factor VIII by incompletely understood mechanisms.[29] It is effective for patients with von Willebrand disease who have adequate endogenous stores of functional von Willebrand factor. This group includes most patients with type 1 disease and some patients with type 2A disease. Conversely, DDAVP is not appropriate for patients with type 3 disease, who lack stores of von Willebrand factor. DDAVP also is not usually recommended for the treatment of type 2B disease, because the release of additional abnormal von Willebrand factor may exacerbate thrombocytopenia.[66] However, DDAVP has been reported to be beneficial in some patients with type 2B disease.[72] If DDAVP is used for type 2B disease, close monitoring is necessary.

The dose of DDAVP for von Willebrand disease is identical to that used in the treatment of mild factor VIII deficiency, 0.3 μg/kg given IV over 15 to 30 minutes. In general, patients with von Willebrand disease have a better response to DDAVP than those with hemophilia, with an average three- to fivefold rise in von Willebrand factor and factor VIII levels.[29] The response to DDAVP in a given patient is usually consistent, and a trial of DDAVP should establish if the medication is likely to be effective for the individual. DDAVP is preferable to the use of plasma-derived products for patients who have an adequate response because DDAVP does not carry a risk of viral transmission. An added benefit is that DDAVP is substantially less costly than the plasma-derived products. (For a discussion of the side effects of DDAVP, see the section on the treatment of hemophilia A.)

DDAVP can be administered every 12 to 24 hours, but the response diminishes with repeated treatment. Beyond three to four doses, DDAVP is often no longer effective, and alternative replacement therapy may be necessary if prolonged treatment is required. Laboratory monitoring, including vWF:Ag measurements, factor VIII assays, ristocetin cofactor activity assessments, and clinical examinations, will help determine the adequacy of treatment.

TABLE 100–8. Replacement Therapy in von Willebrand Disease[a]

Condition	Therapy
Major surgery	Maintenance of factor VIII level ≥50% for 1 week Prolonged treatment in type 3 patients (>7 days)
Minor surgery	Maintenance of factor VIII level ≥50% for 1–3 days Maintenance of factor VIII level >20%–30% for additional 4–7 days
Dental extraction	Single infusion to achieve factor VIII level >50%; antifibrinolytics
Spontaneous or post-traumatic bleeding	Usually, single infusion or 20–40 U/kg

[a]The yield of factor VIII after first infusion is similar to that observed in hemophilia A (about 2% increment over baseline amount for every 1 U/kg of factor VIII infused). *Adapted from Ref. 31 with permission.*

The intranasal administration of DDAVP, at the same dosage as that used in mild factor VIII deficiency, can be useful in the treatment of mild bleeding episodes. One or two doses administered at the start of menses may be helpful in controlling menorrhagia.[30,65] Oral contraceptives may be very effective in controlling this symptom as well.[30,65,72] Inhibitors of the fibrinolytic system may be of special value in those tissues rich in plasminogen activators, such as the mouth, especially with tooth extractions.[32] These agents should be avoided in urinary tract bleeding, however, because of the risk of thrombosis and obstruction.[30,72] Like patients with hemophilia, those with von Willebrand disease should be encouraged to avoid NSAIDs because of their effects on platelet function.

OTHER CONGENITAL FACTOR DEFICIENCIES

In addition to deficiencies in factors VIII and IX, congenital deficiencies in fibrinogen; in factors II, V, VII, X, XI, XII, XIII; as well as combinations of factor deficiencies, have been reported.[74] Contact factor abnormalities, including deficiencies in factor XII and prekallikrein, prolong the aPTT, but do not lead to any bleeding diathesis. It is important to identify these disorders so that treatment is not inappropriate. The only contact factor deficiency associated with bleeding symptoms is factor XI deficiency. Also known as hemophilia C, this deficiency is particularly common in people of Ashkenazi Jewish descent.[75,76] Bleeding does not usually occur spontaneously, but there may be excessive bleeding after trauma or surgery. Most other deficiencies are inherited as autosomal recessive disorders and are rare. Some patients with abnormal molecules, such as fibrinogen, may have an increased tendency to develop thromboembolic disease. Most of these deficiencies are treated with fresh-frozen plasma, although newer specific concentrates are becoming available. Cryoprecipitate, which is rich in fibrinogen, may be used to treat patients with fibrinogen deficiency or dysfunctional fibrinogen (dysfibrinogenemias).

COMPLICATIONS OF REPLACEMENT THERAPY

Transmission of blood-borne viruses is always a concern when blood and blood-derived products are used. The infection of a large number of hemophiliac patients with hepatitis viruses and HIV during the 1980s prompted the development of virucidal methods to inactivate infectious agents.[5,6,9] All currently available plasma-derived factor concentrates come from screened donors and undergo viral inactivation procedures in an effort to reduce the risk of viral transmission. Heat treatment, which includes dry and wet heat, is one method of viral inactivation. Wet heat is applied while the concentrate is in suspension or in solution (pasteurization) and appears to be more effective than dry heat.[5,6,9] Other methods of viral inactivation include chemical (solvent-detergent) and affinity chromatography with monoclonal antibodies. Solvent-detergent treatment inactivates lipid-coated viruses such as HIV and hepatitis B and C; however, it is not effective against nonenveloped viruses, including hepatitis A.[5,6,77,78] Outbreaks of hepatitis A associated with factor concentrates have occurred.[17,77,78] Another nonenveloped virus that has been identified in plasma-derived products, parvovirus B19,[13] may be particularly important for patients with hemophilia and HIV infection because it can cause chronic anemia in patients with immune deficiency.[77]

Other complications associated with factor administration include allergic reactions, fever, chills, urticaria, and nausea. PCCs and activated PCCs also have the potential to cause thromboembolic complications, including deep vein thrombosis, pulmonary embolism, myocardial infarction, and DIC, likely related to the presence of activated vitamin K-dependent factors.[35,36,79] Antifibrinolytics should be avoided in patients receiving PCCs or activated PCCs to avoid thrombotic complications.[35]

Porcine factor VIII, used in the treatment of patients with inhibitors to factor VIII, is not known to transmit human viruses. However, allergic-type reactions (e.g., fever, chills, skin rashes, nausea, headaches) have been reported.[35,49] Patients who experience these reactions may be treated with hydrocortisone and/or diphenhydramine. Thrombocytopenia is another potential complication of porcine factor VIII use.[35,49]

Recombinant factor VIII has a low risk of viral transmission. Adverse effects of these products include metallic taste, mild dizziness, mild rash, burning at the infusion site, and a small drop in blood pressure.[80]

PHARMACOECONOMIC CONSIDERATIONS

Treatment of severe hemophilia is often expensive, with a substantial portion of the cost related to the pricing of factor concentrates.[81] The highly purified plasma-derived products and recombinant factor concentrates are considerably more expensive than the low- and intermediate-purity products. However, the viral safety of recombinant products must be weighed against the added cost. Recombinant products are often used, particularly for children with hemophilia. With prophylactic factor replacement regimens to prevent chronic arthropathy more widespread, factor usage and cost of treatment has greatly increased over that for on-demand therapy.[45,82] The positive impact on patient lifestyle must be weighed against the drawbacks of cost, the potential need for permanent venous access, and patient compliance. Finally, the use of immune tolerance therapy is associated with extremely high factor usage and cost, but with the potential benefit of eradicating an inhibitor. A formal cost-benefit analysis has suggested that this therapy may be cost-effective over the patient's lifetime.[81]

As noted earlier, the optimal management of von Willebrand disease starts with adequate identification of the patient's disease type. DDAVP is considerably less expensive than plasma-derived factor VIII concentrates.[29] It should be the treatment of choice for all patients responsive to the test dose because of its viral safety, reduced cost, and ease of administration.

ACQUIRED COAGULATION DISORDERS

DISSEMINATED INTRAVASCULAR COAGULATION

The systemic activation of coagulation that results from DIC leads to clot formation in the microvasculature, often with compensatory bleeding owing to consumption of coagulation factors and platelets. Although the causes for DIC can be diverse, the pathophysiology leading to DIC is the same once the triggering event occurs (Fig. 100–4). An overwhelming insult leads to the formation of thrombin and plasmin beyond the control of the regulatory systems. Once thrombin is formed, it leads to the cleavage of fibrinopeptide A and B from fibrinogen, leaving a fibrin monomer. The monomer polymerizes into a clot, leading to microvascular and macrovascular thrombosis while consuming platelets by trapping them in the clots. Thrombosis will ultimately decrease blood flow to multiple

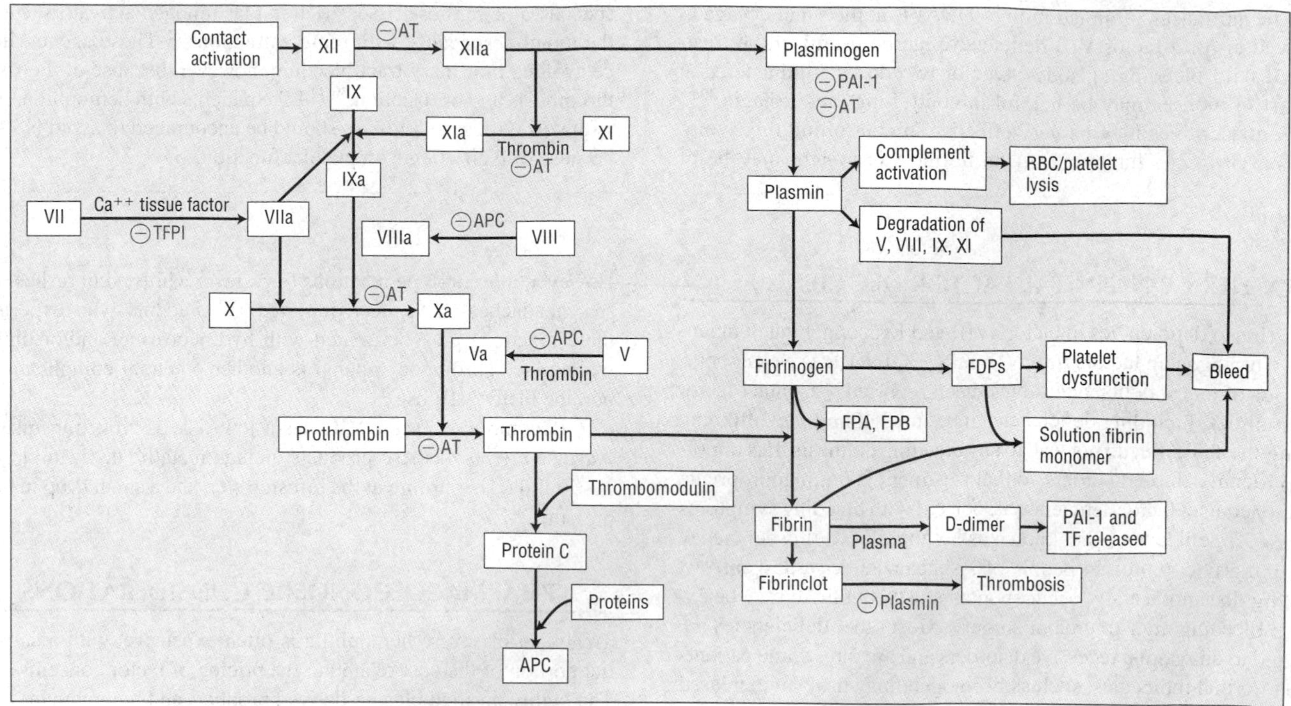

FIGURE 100–4. Pathophysiology of disseminated intravascular coagulation. APC = activated protein C; AT = antithrombin; PAI-1 = plasminogen activator inhibitor type 1; TFPI = tissue factor pathway inhibitor; FPA, FPB = fibrinopeptides A and B; RBC = red blood cell; FDP = fibrin degradation products.

organs, leading to organ damage. Plasmin cleaves fibrinogen into fibrin(ogen) degradation products (FDP), which can combine with the fibrin monomer before polymerization. The monomer becomes a soluble fibrin monomer, impairing hemostasis and leading to hemorrhage. Also, some of the FDPs may adhere to platelets, causing platelet dysfunction that may contribute to clinically significant hemorrhage. In addition, plasmin is a proteolytic enzyme that can degrade factors V, VIII, IX, XI, and other plasma proteins. Circulation of plasmin can activate the complement system, leading to red blood cell and platelet lysis. The activated complement system also increases vascular permeability that can cause hypotension and shock.[83]

Complicating this process is an intricate web of feedback systems. Thrombin induces activation of factors V and XI while it also activates protein C that inhibits the activation of the same. Antithrombin is a serine protease that mediates the antithrombotic effect of heparin. It also inhibits the activation of thrombin, plasmin, and factors IXa, Xa, XIa, and XIIa.[84]

Acute DIC is characterized by a rapid and extensive depletion of coagulation factors and inhibitors, as well as excessive fibrinolysis in an attempt to compensate for microvascular clotting. Normally, a balanced dynamic process of clotting and fibrinolysis operates to prevent organ dysfunction, bleeding, or clotting. In acute DIC, excessive intravascular coagulation overcomes the normal inhibitory processes. In subacute or chronic DIC, the balance between depletion and synthesis of coagulation factors in the circulation may make the diagnosis difficult, as patients may be asymptomatic, bleeding, and/or forming thromboses.

In summary, bleeding problems observed during DIC can be the product of the consumption of coagulation factors during clotting, the depletion or dysfunction of platelets, interference in fibrin formation by FDPs, and lysis of clots by plasmin. In parallel with the bleeding process, thrombosis is occurring, and the extent of microvascular obstruction will determine the degree of organ damage.

CLINICAL PRESENTATION

Acute DIC occurs secondary to many clinical conditions as listed in Table 100–9. Thirty percent to 50% of patients with gram-negative sepsis may develop DIC. It also may occur in association with infections with gram-positive organisms, fungi, and viruses.[85] Women in the late stages of pregnancy complicated by placental abruption or placenta previa, a dead fetus, or amniotic fluid embolism have a greater than 50% incidence of acute DIC.[85] Patients who have severe hypotension, who require prolonged surgery, or who suffer tissue injury such as burns or heat stroke may experience DIC.

Subacute and chronic DIC is more commonly associated with malignancies, especially solid tumors. Mucin-producing carcinomas, such as prostate cancer, may be associated with chronic DIC.[86,87] Acute promyelocytic leukemia (APML) is almost always linked to a unique form of DIC that most commonly presents as bleeding caused by a severe hyperfibrinolytic state along with an activated coagulation system.[86] In addition, vascular disorders (e.g., giant hemangioendotheliomas) and chronic liver disease have been associated with chronic DIC.

DIAGNOSIS

In any of the previously mentioned clinical situations, DIC should be suspected when a patient has signs or symptoms of bleeding, clotting, or both. It should also be considered if the patient develops bleeding from many sites, including oozing from IV lines or from the sites of invasive procedures. DIC should be suspected if the patient develops

TABLE 100–9. Conditions Associated With Disseminated Intravascular Coagulation

Cardiovascular	Pulmonary
Acute myocardial infarction	Adult respiratory distress syndrome
Aortic aneurysm	Empyema
Aortic balloons	Hyaline membrane disease
Giant hemangiomas	Pulmonary embolism
Peripheral vascular disease	Pulmonary infarction
Postcardiac arrest	**Tissue Injury**
Prosthetic devices	Burns
Infectious	Crush-injuries
Arbovirus	Extensive surgery
Aspergillus	Head trauma
Candida albicans	Multiple trauma
Cytomegalovirus	**Miscellaneous**
Ebola virus	Acid/base imbalance
Gram-negative bacteria	Acute liver failure
Gram-positive bacteria	Amphetamines
Herpesvirus	Anaphylaxis
Histoplasma	Autoimmune diseases
Influenza	Cholestasis
Kala-azar	Chronic inflammatory diseases
Malaria	Collagen vascular disease
Mycobacteria	Extracorporeal circulation
Mycoplasma	Extracorporeal membrane oxygenation
Paramyxoviruses	Fat embolism
Rocky Mountain spotted fever	Heat stroke
Rubella	Hemorrhagic telangiectasia
Typhoid	Hepatitis
Varicella	Leukemia
Variola	Lightning strikes
Intravascular hemolysis	Near-drowning
Hemolytic transfusion reaction	Organic solvent poisoning
Minor hemolysis	Paroxysmal nocturnal hemoglobinuria
Massive transfusion	Peritoneovenous shunts
Newborn	Renal vascular disorders
Birth asphyxia	Severe anoxia
Hypothermia	Snake bite
Meconium or amnotic fluid aspiration	Solid tumors
Necrotizing enterocolitis	Transplant rejection
Respiratory distress syndrome	
Shock	
Obstetrics	
Abortion	
Amniotic fluid embolism	
Fatty liver of pregnancy	
Placental abruption	
Preeclampsia	
Retained fetus syndrome	

peripheral cyanosis of the extremities, purpura and petechiae, or hemorrhagic bullae in the appropriate clinical setting.[83]

The basis for a diagnosis of DIC is a combination of laboratory test results in the setting of a known causative clinical disorder.[83,85] The relative importance of any particular laboratory test is controversial. Routine tests of blood coagulation, including prothrombin time and aPTT, should be done. The PT and aPTT are usually prolonged. Occasionally, both times may be decreased rather than increased.[83] The thrombin time is usually prolonged, because of the absolute decrease in fibrinogen as well as the presence of FDPs, which inhibit the conversion of fibrinogen to fibrin.[87] Liver disease may cause a decreased synthesis of coagulation factors, and the subsequent abnormal laboratory results can be difficult to differentiate from DIC.

Increased levels of FDPs are not specific to DIC, but elevated levels occur in 85% to 100% of patients with DIC.[83] Because FDPs are metabolized in the liver and excreted by the kidney, organ damage may increase the level of FDPs.[88] However, an increased FDP level may be helpful in identifying compensated DIC, as it may be the only abnormal laboratory result. D-dimer is formed when plasmin digests cross-linked fibrin; thus, the level of D-dimer is a more specific measure of FDPs and should be elevated only in DIC.[89]

Fibrinogen levels and platelet counts are usually decreased in patients with DIC. Fifty percent of patients have schistocytes (red blood cell fragments) in fulminant DIC.[83] Unfortunately, these findings may also be evident in patients with severe liver disease with hypersplenism. Depressed antithrombin, protein C, and protein S levels are seen in most patients. Severe initial decreases in antithrombin levels occur in septic DIC. Activity levels below 50% to 60% correlate with poor outcome.[84]

Thrombin cleaves fibrinopeptides A and B from fibrinogen; thus, the levels of fibrinopeptides A and B should be elevated in patients with DIC. Initial studies have shown a good correlation between an elevated level of fibrinopeptide A and DIC, but other inflammatory conditions such as systemic lupus erythematosus, infections, and thrombosis may also result in elevated levels, thus decreasing the specificity of this test.

Factor VIII and V levels should be decreased in DIC, but results of these tests may be quite variable because of the systemic activation of the coagulation system. The most specific findings of DIC are a low platelet count associated with an elevated D-dimer level and depressed antithrombin and fibrinogen levels. Other molecular markers may have a greater correlation to DIC, but are not yet widely available.

▶ TREATMENT: Disseminated Intravascular Coagulation

If unrecognized and left untreated, DIC may lead to death as a result of hemorrhage and/or thrombosis. Because of the different mechanisms and clinical manifestations that can occur with DIC, however, there is some controversy regarding optimal treatment. Even so, there is a consensus that the most important step in the treatment of DIC is treatment of the underlying disease.[83,85,87,89] In a pregnant woman with placental abruption or retained placenta in whom the disease is self-limited, delivery of the fetus with the products of conception usually returns hemostasis to normal. In those patients who have overwhelming sepsis or shock, antibiotics and treatment of hypotension are the mainstays of therapy. In patients who are receiving maximum treatment for the underlying condition, but in whom the process is worsening or in whom bleeding develops, additional treatments may be used.

The efficacy of transfusing fresh-frozen plasma or platelets has not been proven in randomized clinical trials, but is rational for patients who are bleeding or require invasive procedures.[85] Fresh-frozen plasma replaces clotting factors, fibrinogen, protein S, protein C, and antithrombin. If hypofibrinogenemia is severe, cryoprecipitate may be useful as a concentrated source of fibrinogen. Although it has been argued that replacement of coagulation factors "adds fuel to the fire," in practice this does not appear to make the situation worse, and it frequently improves hemostasis.

Trials of antithrombin concentrate in the treatment of DIC from various causes show some beneficial effect on improving DIC score, decreasing duration of DIC, or improving end-organ function.[84,85] A meta-analysis of a number of well-designed studies demonstrated a trend toward decreased mortality (from 56% to 44%).[85] In addition to variable efficacy, antithrombin is an expensive product with only intermittent availability. Therefore, restricting its use to patients at high risk for morbidity and mortality should be considered.

Anticoagulation is controversial in patients with DIC.[83,85,87,89] The main pathogenic factor of DIC is considered to be the generation of intravascular thrombin. Interference of thrombin activity by an agent such as heparin appears to be a logical therapeutic step. The main advantage of heparin is that it can prevent further thrombosis and consumption of hemostatic factors; it has no influence on an already established microthrombus within the vasculature. Because the major complication of heparin therapy is bleeding, some experts argue against its use in patients with an existing bleeding disorder. There are numerous anecdotal reports of improvement in individual patients, but controlled clinical studies are lacking. Heparin has not been shown to reduce morbidity or mortality in uncontrolled series.[85,87] Heparin rarely restores the coagulopathy to normal, although both the deficiency of coagulation factors and the thrombocytopenia may improve. If the patient does not respond to the replacement of coagulation factors, the administration of heparin, followed by factor replacement, may improve the coagulopathy; the rationale is that most patients with DIC are deficient in antithrombin, which affects the ability of the heparin-antithrombin complex to inhibit thrombin.

Heparin is given subcutaneously or as a continuous IV infusion. The dosage of heparin for DIC is controversial, ranging anywhere from full-dose to low-dose heparin.[85,87,89] Full-dose heparin in adults requires that 5,000 U be administered as an IV bolus, followed by a continuous infusion at 1,000 U/h or according to a weight-based heparin-dosing regimen. Some experts advocate using low-dose heparin, such as an infusion of 500 U/h in adults, and adjusting the dose based on clinical and laboratory data. Low-dose heparin given subcutaneously has been used with success. Monitoring of heparin therapy is difficult because the aPTT is often elevated before the initiation of heparin therapy. Therefore, it is best to follow D-dimer and fibrinogen levels.

Anticoagulation is contraindicated in patients with life-threatening or serious bleeding (e.g., intracranial, retroperitoneal, pericardial). Patients with symptomatic thromboemboli, extensive fibrin deposition, persistent coagulation abnormalities despite replacement of hemostatic factors, solid tumors, or chronic DIC may benefit from heparin therapy.[85,86] Historically, an infusion of low-dose heparin, 7.5 U/kg/h, has been used in patients with APML, along with the administration of platelets, fresh-frozen plasma, and cryoprecipitate.[86] The availability of differentiation agents may decrease or prevent the need for anticoagulation of these patients.[89] Patients with solid tumors who are symptomatic from a thrombosis should receive an infusion of heparin, 15 U/kg/h. Once asymptomatic, the heparin administration can become subcutaneous.

In two uncontrolled trials, patients tolerated the use of low molecular weight heparin well, and this approach showed a possible beneficial outcome.[85] A randomized, double-blind study compared the efficacy of dalteparin with that of low-dose heparin. Dalteparin was more effective at improving bleeding symptoms, but there was no difference in mortality.[85]

Antifibrinolytics, such as aminocaproic acid, have been used in patients in whom the dominant clinical picture is one of excessive fibrinolysis.[85] Because aminocaproic acid can increase fibrin deposition, many experts believe that it is contraindicated more often than not. In patients with chronic liver disease who manifest dominant fibrinolysis, attempts to inhibit the fibrinolytic system have generally been unsuccessful. Patients with APML may benefit from an antifibrinolytic, as hyperfibrinolysis is the dominant clinical feature of their condition. Tranexamic acid and aminocaproic acid have shown benefits in patients with APML.[85]

Critically ill patients may develop vitamin K deficiency. In addition, patients with DIC may consume vitamin K and may need supplementation to replenish stores.[87] Other treatment modalities may include the use of protein C concentrate; lepirudin; anti-tissue factor antibody; recombinant tissue factor pathway inhibitor (TFPI); thrombomodulin; or thrombin inhibitors such as dermatan sulphate, anti-plasminogen activator inhibitor type 1, and dithiocarbamates.[85,89–92]

EVALUATION OF THERAPEUTIC OUTCOMES

The management of DIC is surrounded by controversy, and the optimal approach to these patients is still to be determined. Diagnosis and treatment of the underlying disease should be the goal in all cases. Determining, if possible, the dominant process (i.e., hemorrhage vs. thrombosis) can help focus the treatment approach correctly. This is often impossible, however, so clinicians institute replacement therapy of the deficient clotting factors and attempt to control the clotting problems with agents such as heparin.

Risk versus benefit, as well as any contraindications, should be considered at the start of any given therapy for each patient. Monitoring therapy for DIC with laboratory tests can be difficult, because the underlying process can cause a variety of laboratory abnormalities. For example, monitoring the effect of heparin by using the aPTT can be a complex task, especially when the patient has an abnormal baseline aPTT; in this case, monitoring fibrinogen and D-dimer may be more useful in detecting any need to adjust therapy. In addition, it is important to combine laboratory parameters with clinical assessment to make rational treatment adjustments. Aggressive hemodynamic stabilization and other supportive measures to prevent organ failure are also important in the overall management and prognosis of patients with DIC.

VITAMIN K DEFICIENCY

Vitamin K is a cofactor for the activation of factors II, VII, IX, and X.[93] When vitamin K deficiency occurs, the inactive precursors of these coagulation factors that do not bind calcium accumulate in the plasma. Vitamin K is also necessary for the active forms of protein C and S, which inhibit the activated factor V and VIII molecules. In most clinical situations, vitamin K deficiency causes a bleeding diathesis as a result of the marked deficiency of factors II, VII, IX, and X.

Vitamin K is a fat-soluble vitamin. Vitamin K_1, phytonadione, is found in green vegetables. Bacteria in the large intestine produce vitamin K_2, the menaquinones, which require bile salts to be solubilized and absorbed.[93] Vitamin K_3, the menadiones, are synthetic, water-soluble vitamin K compounds.[95]

HEMORRHAGIC DISEASE OF THE NEWBORN

Newborns are vitamin K-deficient at birth, although not completely; some maternal vitamin K crosses the placenta.[94] The level may continue to fall during the neonatal period because the infant's gut has not had sufficient time to undergo bacterial colonization. Breast milk contains a low vitamin K content in comparison to infant formulas and therefore breastfed infants are more vulnerable to developing vitamin K deficiency. In addition, the plasma concentrations of the vitamin K-dependent factors are physiologically low in infants.[16] Vitamin K deficiency in neonates can cause hemorrhagic disease of the newborn (HDN) with bleeding manifestations including bleeding from the umbilical cord or the gastrointestinal tract and intracranial hemorrhage.[94]

Early HDN, at birth, is usually the result of maternal ingestion of anticonvulsants, warfarin, rifampin, or isoniazid. Treating these women prior to delivery with vitamin K may decrease the incidence of HDN among their offspring.[94] Classic HDN usually appears during the first week of life, and it results from the lack of prophylactic vitamin K. Risk factors identified for late HDN, which occurs at 4 to 6 weeks, include cholestatic liver disease, exclusive breastfeeding, and failure to give adequate vitamin K at birth.[94] The use of oral vitamin K at birth is also associated with a higher incidence of late HDN. It has been suggested that the intramuscular route of administration allows the vitamin K to act as a depot preparation and may explain the lower rate of late HDN with this route.[94]

The levels of vitamin K-dependent coagulation factors are low at birth. Without adequate vitamin K, these levels may fall even further. In this situation, the PT and the aPTT are prolonged, but the thrombin time, fibrinogen level, and platelet count are normal. Most infants achieve adult levels by 3 months of age if intramuscular phytonadione was received at birth.[94]

In the United States, infants usually receive 1 mg of phytonadione intramuscularly at birth for prophylaxis. Most infants build up vitamin K_1 and K_2 stores in the liver during the first month of life. The speed of repletion is dependent on the amount of milk or formula received. Menadiol, vitamin K_3, has been associated with hepatotoxicity, aplastic anemia, hyperbilirubinemia, and kernicterus in neonates and should be avoided.[95] Fresh-frozen plasma is used to treat hemorrhages.

MALABSORPTION

Patients may become vitamin K-deficient because of poor nutrition or malabsorption.[95] A careful dietary history is important in this regard. Broad-spectrum antibiotics may sterilize the large intestine and prevent vitamin K_2 production.[96]

Vitamin K absorption is dependent on both bile acids and pancreatic enzymes to create micelles.[97] Malabsorption resulting from diseases of the small intestine or pancreas—such as cystic fibrosis, Crohn's disease, ulcerative colitis, cholestatic liver disease, celiac disease, amyloidosis, Whipple's disease, and short-bowel syndrome—may cause abnormal development in children, weight loss, muscle wasting, steatorrhea, vitamin deficiencies, and anemia. Significant malabsorption can occur even without the symptoms of diarrhea or steatorrhea.

Patients with malabsorption or obstructive jaundice may require the parenteral administration of vitamin K. Phytonadione, 10 mg weekly, is usually sufficient in adults. Menadiol may be an alternative in adults as it does not require bile salts for absorption, but diffusion occurs in the distal portion of the small intestine and colon.

▶ TREATMENT: Vitamin K Deficiency

Phytonadione or menadiol are used to treat vitamin K deficiency. The dose, frequency, and duration of vitamin K depend on the severity of the deficiency and the patient's response.[95] The dose of vitamin K ranges from 1 to 25 mg and may be administered orally, intramuscularly, subcutaneously, or IV. After an oral dose of vitamin K_1, the blood coagulation factors increase within 6 to 12 hours. When administered parenterally, the PT may take 12 to 24 hours to normalize, although improvement usually occurs within 1 to 2 hours. Failure to correct the PT after 48 hours should raise suspicion about the etiology of the coagulation abnormality (e.g., liver disease).

The appropriate route of administration is dependent on the severity, as well as the cause, of the vitamin K deficiency. For instance, in patients with severe hypoprothrombinemia, it is best to avoid the intramuscular route because of the risk of forming a hematoma. Because of the rare anaphylactic reaction associated with the IV route of administration, this route is often restricted to patients who are thrombocytopenic or unable to absorb the drug via the gastrointestinal tract. Vitamin K can be administered subcutaneously to those patients without IV access. Bleeding patients should receive fresh-frozen plasma as a source of vitamin K-dependent factors to ensure immediate correction. Adults on long-term total parenteral nutrition (TPN) should have 10 mg of vitamin K added to the TPN solution weekly. Pediatric TPN patients receive it daily in the multivitamin additive.

LIVER DISEASE

Bleeding disorders can be associated with liver disease.[1] The degree of coagulopathy correlates with the degree of hepatocellular disease. The liver synthesizes the majority of blood coagulation factors (e.g., fibrinogen and factors II, VII, IX, X, XII, XIII, and V) and inhibitors of coagulation (e.g., antithrombin, protein C and S). The ability of the liver to clear activated clotting factors and their degradation products is reduced with liver failure.[96] Primary fibrinolysis occurs due to a decline in the level of the inhibitors of plasmin activation.[1] Decreased platelet count and function are fairly common findings in liver disease. The development of DIC may potentially worsen the coagulopathy.

The PT, the aPTT, and the thrombin time are useful in screening for a deficiency of liver-dependent factors. The PT is sensitive to deficiencies in the vitamin K-dependent factors. The aPTT helps to determine deficiencies in factor IX, as well as some other factors. The thrombin time is helpful in detecting hypofibrinogenemia, dysfibrinogenemia, and the presence of FDPs that interfere with fibrin polymerization. Because defects in polymerization may occur before severe hypofibrinogemia, this may be an indication of the degree of liver dysfunction. The level of D-dimer should be normal unless DIC is present.

Factor V is synthesized by hepatic cells, but is not dependent on vitamin K. Therefore, it may be useful in distinguishing vitamin

K deficiency from liver disease. Deficiency of antithrombin occurs with severe hepatocellular disease and may contribute to the development of DIC. In acute hepatic failure, the level of plasminogen may be low, reflecting decreased synthesis or increased catabolism associated with DIC. The level of factor VIII is usually elevated in liver disease, whereas it is decreased in DIC.[96]

▶ TREATMENT: Liver Disease

Treatment of the coagulopathy associated with liver disease is recommended for overt bleeding or for the correction of coagulation parameters (e.g., PT, aPTT) prior to an invasive procedure. Major bleeding may occur with normal coagulation parameters secondary to esophageal varices or peptic ulcer disease. To ensure that vitamin K deficiency is not contributing to the abnormalities, adults may receive 10 mg of vitamin K for one or several days.

When a patient bleeds in association with a coagulopathy, replacement therapy with platelets and fresh-frozen plasma may decrease bleeding. Fresh-frozen plasma supplies all the missing coagulation factors, but fluid overload may be a serious problem. If fluid overload becomes an issue, plasma exchange may be considered. If the patient has ascites, the half-life of many of these factors is decreased, and it is difficult to correct the coagulopathy. PCCs can be given, but there is an increased risk of precipitating intravascular coagulation and causing DIC if it is not already present. In general, the use of these concentrates is not recommended. Only when the administration of fresh-frozen plasma does not correct the coagulopathy and the patient continues to have serious bleeding should PCCs be considered.

The use of heparin and antifibrinolytic drugs is controversial. The administration of aminocaproic acid may be successful, especially with mucosal bleeding. Heparin has not been demonstrated to improve survival in acute liver failure and may exacerbate bleeding.[96] In the few clinical studies that have been done, neither controlled nor uncontrolled trials have shown any definite benefit with heparin in severe acute hepatic necrosis.

Antithrombin concentrates have been evaluated in fulminant liver failure. They had no benefit on mortality, clinical complications, or coagulation laboratory findings.[96] Desmopressin may decrease the bleeding time and the International Normalized Ratio in chronic liver disease.[96] The administration of recombinant factor VIIa has successfully corrected coagulation parameters in patients with liver disease.[98,99]

▶ PRINCIPLES OF PHARMACOTHERAPY

- Hemophilia A and B are inherited bleeding disorders resulting from a congenital deficiency in factors VIII and IX, respectively.
- The goal of therapy for hemophilia is to arrest bleeding when it occurs and to prevent bleeding episodes and their long-term complications.
- Factor concentrates (either plasma-derived or recombinant technology products) have largely replaced the use of blood products like cryoprecipitate. The dosage and duration of these depend on the site and severity of bleeding.
- In mild cases of hemophilia A, 1-desamino-8-D-arginine vasopressin (DDAVP) sometimes can be used.
- DDAVP is often the agent of choice for the treatment of type 1 and type 2A von Willebrand disease.
- Plasma-derived factor VIII concentrates are used in the treatment of patients with type 3 von Willebrand disease, those with some subtypes of type 2 von Willebrand disease, and those who are not responsive to DDAVP.
- The optimal approach for patients with disseminated intravascular coagulation remains to be determined. The goal of treatment is to diagnose and treat the underlying disease.
- Prophylactic use of vitamin K_1 can effectively prevent hemorrhagic disease of the newborn.

REFERENCES

1. Kottke-Marchant K. Laboratory diagnosis of hemorrhagic and thrombotic disorders. Hematol Oncol Clin North Am 1994;8:809–853.
2. Bick RL, Murano G. Physiology of hemostasis. Clin Lab Med 1994; 14:677–707.
3. DeMott WR, Coagulation. In: Jacobs DS, DeMott WR, Grady HJ, eds. Laboratory Test Handbook.Cleveland, OH: Lexi-Comp, 1996:225–270.
4. Soucie JM, Evatt B, Jackson D, et al. Occurrence of hemophilia in the United States. Am J Hematol 1998;59:288–294.
5. DiMichele D, Neufeld EJ. Hemophilia: a new approach to an old disease. Hematol Oncol Clin North Am 1998;12(6):1315–1344.
6. Mannucci PM, Tuddenham GD. The hemophilias: progress and problems. Semin Hematol 1999;36 (4, suppl 7):104–117.
7. Chuansumrit A, Sasanakul W, Goodeve A, et al. Inversion of intron 22 of the factor VIII gene in a girl with severe hemophilia A and Turner's syndrome. Thromb Haemost 1999;82(4):1379.
8. Lillicrap D. Molecular diagnosis of inherited bleeding disorders and thrombophilia. Semin Hematol 1999;36(4):340–351.
9. Hoyer LW. Hemophilia A. N Engl J Med 1994;330(1):38–47.
10. Lakich D, Kazazian H, Antonarakis SE, Gitschier J. Inversions disrupting the factor VIII gene are a common cause of severe hemophilia A. Nat Genet 1993;5(3):236–241.
11. Crossley M, Ludwig M, Stowell KM, et al. Recovery from hemophilia B Leyden: an androgen-responsive element in the factor IX promoter. Science 1992;257(5068):377–379.
12. Furie B, Limentani SA, Rosenfield CG. A practical guide to the evaluation and treatment of hemophilia. Blood 1994;84(1):3–9.
13. Cohen AJ. Treatment of inherited coagulation disorders. Am J Med 1995;99:675–682.
14. Goodeve AC. Advances in carrier detection in haemophilia. Haemophilia 1998;4(4):358–364.
15. Tedgard U. Carrier testing and prenatal diagnosis of haemophilia-utilisation and psychological consequences. Haemophilia 1998;4:365–369.
16. Andrew M. Developmental hemostasis: relevance to hemostatic problems during childhood. Semin Thromb Hemost 1995;21(4):341–356.
17. Richardson LC, Evatt BL. Risk of hepatitis A infection in persons with hemophilia receiving plasma-derived products. Transfus Med Rev 2000;14(1):64–73.

18. Kulkarni R, Lusher JM. Intracranial and extracranial hemorrhages in newborns with hemophilia: a review of the literature. J Pediatr Hematol Oncol 1999;21(4):289–295.
19. Kulkarni R, Lusher JM, Henry RC, Kallen DJ. Current practices regarding newborn intracranial haemorrhage and obstetrical care and mode of delivery of pregnant haemophilia carriers: a survey of obstetricians, neonatologists and haematologists in the United States, on behalf of the National Hemophilia Foundation's Medical and Scientific Advisory Council. Haemophilia 1999;5(6):410–415.
20. Bray GL, Gomperts ED, Courter S, et al. A multicenter study of recombinant factor VIII (Recombinate): safety, efficacy, and inhibitor risk in previously untreated patients with hemophilia A. The Recombinate Study Group. Blood 1994;83(9):2428–2435.
21. Schwartz RS, Abildgaard CF, Aledort LM, et al. Human recombinant DNA-derived antihemophilic factor (factor VIII) in the treatment of hemophilia A. Recombinant Factor VIII Study Group. N Engl J Med 1990;323(26):1800–1805.
22. Lusher JM, Arkin S, Abildgaard CF, et al. Recombinant factor VIII for the treatment of previously untreated patients with hemophilia A: safety, efficacy, and development of inhibitors. Kogenate Previously Untreated Patient Study Group. N Engl J Med 1993;328(7): 453–459.
23. Kelly KM, Butler RB, Farace L, et al. Superior in vivo response of recombinant factor VIII concentrate in children with hemophilia A. 1997;130(4):537–540.
24. Fresh-Frozen Plasma, Cryoprecipitate, and Platelets Administration Practice Guidelines Development Task Force of the College of American Pathologists. Practice parameters for the use of fresh-frozen plasma, cryoprecipitate, and platelets. JAMA 1994;271:777–781.
25. Shord SS, Lindley CM. Coagulation products and their uses. Am J Health Syst Pharm 2000;57:1403–1420.
26. Varon D, Martinowitz U. Continuous infusion therapy in haemophilia. Haemophilia 1998;4:431–435.
27. Hay CRM, Doughty HI, Savidge GF. Continuous infusion of factor VIII for surgery and major bleeding episodes. Blood Coagul Fibrinolysis 1996;7(suppl 1):S15–S19.
28. Lusher JM. Transfusion therapy in congenital coagulopathies. Hematol Oncol Clin North Am 1994;8(6):1167–1180.
29. Mannucci PM. Desmopressin (DDAVP) in the treatment of bleeding disorders: the first 20 years. Blood 1997;90(7):2515–2521.
30. Phillips MD, Santhouse A. von Willebrand disease: recent advances in pathophysiology and treatment. Am J Med Sci 1998;316(2):77–86.
31. Castaman G, Rodeghiero F. Current management of von Willebrand disease. Drugs 1995;50(4):602–614.
32. Mannucci PM. Hemostatic drugs. N Engl J Med 1998;339(4):245–253.
33. Adamson S, Charlebois T, O'Connell B, Foster W. Viral safety of recombinant factor IX. 1998;35(2 suppl 2):22–27.
34. White G, Shapiro A, Ragni M, et al. Clinical evaluation of recombinant factor IX. 1998;35(2 suppl 2):33–38.
35. Green D. Complications associated with the treatment of haemophiliacs with inhibitors. Haemophilia 1999;5(suppl 3):11–17.
36. Kohler M. Thrombogenicity of prothrombin complex concentrates. Thromb Res 1999;95(4 suppl 1):S13–S17.
37. Goldsmith JC, Kasper CK, Blatt PM, et al. Coagulation factor IX: successful surgical experience with a purified factor IX concentrate. Am J Hematol 1992;40:210–215.
38. Shapiro AD, Ragni MV, Lusher JM, et al. Safety and efficacy of monoclonal antibody purified factor IX concentrate in previously untreated patients with hemophilia B. Thromb Haemost 1996;75(1):30–35.
39. Ljung RC. Prophylactic infusion regimens in the management of hemophilia. Thromb Haemost 1999;82(2):525–530.
40. Lofqvist T, Nilsson IM, Berntorp E, Petterson H. Haemophilia prophylaxis in young patients: a long-term follow-up. J Intern Med 1997;241:395–400.
41. Lusher JM. Prophylaxis in children with hemophilia: is it the optimal treatment? Thromb Haemost 1997;78(1):726–729.
42. Liesner RJ, Khair K, Hann IM. The impact of prophylactic treatment on children with severe haemophilia. 1996;92.973–978.
43. Aledort LH, Haschmeyer RH, Petterson H. A longitudinal study of orthopaedic outcomes for severe factor-VIII-deficient haemophiliacs. The Orthopedic Outcome Study Group. J Intern Med 1994;236(4):391–399.
44. Manco-Johnson MJ, Nuss R, Geraghty S, Funk S. A prophylactic program in the United States: experience and issues. Semin Hematol 1994;31(2, suppl 2):10–12.
45. Smith PS, Teutsch SM, Shaffer PA, et al. Episodic versus prophylactic infusions for hemophilia A: a cost-effectiveness analysis. J Pediatr 1996;129(3):424–431.
46. Bollard CM, Teague LR, Berry EW, Ockelford PA. The use of central venous catheters (portacaths) in children with haemophilia. Haemophilia 2000;6(2):66–70.
47. Blanchette VS, Al-Musa A, Stain A, et al. Central venous access devices in children with hemophilia: an update. Blood Coagul Fibrinolysis 1997;8 (suppl 1):S11–S14.
48. Vermylen J. How do some haemophiliacs develop inhibitors? Haemophilia 1998;4(4):538–542.
49. Manno CS. Treatment options for bleeding episodes in patients undergoing immune tolerance therapy. Haemophilia 1999;5(suppl 3):33–41.
50. Tuddenham EG, McVey JH. The genetic basis of inhibitor development in haemophilia A. Haemophilia 1998;4(4):543–545.
51. Hay CRM. Why do inhibitors arise in patients with haemophilia A? Br J Haematol 1999;105:584–590.
52. Warrier I, Ewenstein BM, Koerper MA, et al. Factor IX inhibitors and anaphylaxis in hemophilia B. J Pediatr Hematol Oncol 1997;19(1): 23–27.
53. Hedner U. Treatment of patients with factor VIII and factor IX inhibitors with a special focus on the use of recombinant factor VIIa. Thromb Haemost 1999;82(2):531–539.
54. Schulman S, Group r-C. Safety, efficacy and lessons from continuous infusion with rFVIIa. Haemophilia 1998;4:564–567.
55. Chuansumrit A, Isarangkura P, Angchaisurksiri P, et al. Controlling acute bleeding episodes with recombinant factor VIIa in haemophiliacs with inhibitor: continuous infusion and bolus injection. Haemophilia 2000;6:61–65.
56. DiMichele DM. Immune tolerance: a synopsis of the international experience. Haemophilia 1998;4:568–573.
57. Nilsson IM. Immune tolerance. Semin Hematol 1994;31(2 suppl 4): 44–48.
58. Mariani G, Scheibel E, Nogao T, et al. Immunetolerance as treatment of alloantibodies to factor VIII in hemophilia. The International Registry of Immunetolerance Protocols. Semin Hematol 1994;31(2 suppl 4):62–64.
59. Connelly S, Kaleko M. Gene therapy for hemophilia A. Thromb Haemost 1997;78(1):31–36.
60. Eisensmith RC, Woo SLC. Viral vector-mediated gene therapy for hemophilia B. Thromb Haemost 1997;78(1):24–30.
61. Kay MA, High K. Gene therapy for the hemophilias. Proc Natl Acad Sci U S A 1999;96:9973–9975.
62. Lusher JM. Gene therapy for hemophilia A and B: patient selection and follow-up, requirements for a cure. Thromb Haemost 1999;82(2):572–575.
63. Beeton K, Cornwell J, Alltree J. Muscle rehabilitation in haemophilia. Haemophilia 1998;4(4):532–537.
64. Fernandez-Palazzi F, Caviglia HA, Salazar JR, et al. Intraarticular dexamethasone in advanced chronic synovitis in hemophilia. Clin Orthop Rel Res 1997;343:25–29.
65. Werner EJ. Von Willebrand disease in children and adolescents. Pediatr Clin North Am 1996;43(3):683–707.
66. Schneppenheim R, Thomas KB, Sutor AH. Von Willebrand disease in childhood. 1995;21(3):261–275.
67. Federici AB. Diagnosis of von Willebrand disease. Haemophilia 1998;4.654–660.
68. Batlle J, Torea J, Rendal E, Fernandez MF. The problem of diagnosing von Willebrand disease. J Intern Med 1997;242(suppl 740):121–128.
69. Nitu-Whalley IC, Lee CA. Acquired von Willebrand syndrome-report of 10 cases and review of the literature. Haemophilia 1999;5(5):318–326.
70. Kouides PA. Females with von Willebrand disease: 72 years as the silent majority. Haemophilia 1998;4:665–676.

71. Gill JC, Endres-Brooks J, Bauer PJ, et al. The effect of ABO blood group on the diagnosis of von Willebrand disease. Blood 1987;69(6): 1691–1695.
72. Mannucci PM. Treatment of von Willebrand disease. Haemophilia 1998; 4:661–664.
73. Menache D, Aronson DL. New treatments of von Willebrand disease: plasma derived von Willebrand factor concentrates. Thromb Haemost 1997;78(1):566–570.
74. Bolton-Maggs PHB. The rarer inherited coagulation disorders: a review. Blood Rev 1995;9:65–76.
75. Seligsohn U. Factor XI deficiency. Thromb Haemost 1993;70(1):68–71.
76. Bolton-Maggs PH. The management of factor XI deficiency. Haemophilia 1998;4(4):683–688.
77. Ludlam CA. Viral safety of plasma-derived factor VIII and IX concentrates. Blood Coagul Fibrinolysis 1997;8(suppl 1):S19–S23.
78. Giangrande PL. Hepatitis in haemophilia. Br J Haematol 1998;103(1): 1–9.
79. Kohler M, Hellstern P, Lechler E, et al. Thromboembolic complications associated with the use of prothrombin complex and factor IX concentrates. Thromb Haemost 1998;80(3):399–402.
80. Bray GL, Gomperts ED, Courter S, et al. A multicenter study of recombinant factor VIII (Recombinate): safety, efficacy, and inhibitor risk in previously untreated patients with hemophilia A. The Recombinate Study Group. Blood 1994;83(9):2428–2435.
81. Colowick AB, Bohn RL, Avorn J, Ewenstein BM. Immune tolerance induction in hemophilia patients with inhibitors: costly can be cheaper. Blood 2000;96:1698–1702.
82. Miners AH, Sabin CA, Tolley KH, Lee CA. Assessing the effectiveness and cost-effectiveness of prophylaxis against bleeding in patients with severe haemophilia and severe von Willebrand disease. J Intern Med 1998;244(6):515–522.
83. Bick RL. Disseminated intravascular coagulation: pathophysiological mechanisms and manifestations. Semin Thromb Hemost 1998;24:3–18.
84. Bucur SZ, Levy JH, Despotis GJ, et al. Uses of antithrombin III concentrate in congenital and acquired deficiency states. Transfusion 1998;38:481–497.
85. Levi M, de Jonge E, van der Poll T, ten Cate H. Disseminated intravascular coagulation. Thromb Haemost 1999;82(2):695–705.
86. Arkel YS. Thrombosis and cancer. Semin Oncol 2000;27:362–374.
87. Baglin T. Disseminated intravascular coagulation: diagnosis and treatment. BMJ 1996;312:683–687.
88. Muller-Berghaus G, ten Cate H, Levi M. Disseminated intravascular coagulation: clinical spectrum and established as well as new diagnostic approaches. Thromb Haemost 1999;82:706–712.
89. Carey MJ, Rodgers GM. Disseminated intravascular coagulation: clinical and laboratory aspects. Am J Hematol 1998;59:65–73.
90. Cofrancesco E, Boschetti C, Leonardi P, et al. Dermatan sulphate for the treatment of disseminated intravascular coagulation (DIC) in acute leukaemia: a randomized, heparin-controlled pilot study. Thromb Res 1994;74:65–75.
91. Maruyama I. Recombinant thrombomodulin and activated Protein C in the treatment of disseminated intravascular coagulation. Thromb Haemost 1999;82:718–721.
92. Pernerstorfer T, Hollenstein U, Hansen JB, et al. Lepirudin blunts endotoxin-induced coagulation activation. Blood 2000;95:1729–1734.
93. Vermeer C, Schurgers LG. A comprehensive review of vitamin K and vitamin K antagonists. Hematol Oncol Clin North Am 2000;14:339–353.
94. Zipursky A. Prevention of vitamin K deficiency bleeding in newborns. Br J Haematol 1999;104:430–437.
95. Marcus R, Coulston AM. Fat-soluble vitamins: vitamins A, K, and E. In:Hardman JG, Limbird LE, Molinoff PB, et al., eds. Goodman and Gilman's The Pharmacological Basis of Therapeutics. New York: McGraw-Hill, 1996:1573–1590.
96. Pereira SP, Langley PG, Williams R. The management of abnormalities of hemostasis in acute liver failure. Semin Liver Dis 1996;16(4):403–414.
97. Sokol RJ. Fat-soluble vitamins and their importance in patients with cholestatic liver diseases. Gastroenterol Clin North Am 1994;23:673–705.
98. Bernstein DE, Jeffers L, Erhardtsen E, et al. Recombinant factor VIIa corrects prothrombin time in cirrhotic patients: a preliminary study. Gastroenterol 1997;113:1930–1937.
99. Kalicinski P, Kaminski A, Drewniak T, et al. Quick correction of hemostasis in two patients with fulminant liver failure undergoing liver transplantation by recombinant activated factor VII. Transpl Proceed 1999;31:378–379.
100. Stead RB. Regulation of hemostasis. In: Goldhaber SZ, ed. Pulmonary Embolism and Deep Vein Thrombosis. : Philadelphia: Saunders, 1985:28–40.
101. Ewenstein BM. von Willebrand disease. Annu Rev Med 1997;48: 525–542.

101
SICKLE CELL ANEMIA

Clarence E. Curry, Jr., and Eula D. Beasley

Although Herrick has generally been credited with the discovery of sickle cell anemia (SCA),[1] Konotey-Ahulu has presented evidence that Ghanaians had recognized the problem in Africa long before Herrick's 1910 description appeared in the medical literature.[2] Such information suggests that SCA is not a distinctly modern problem, as once thought. Since the time of Herrick's description, SCA has been well characterized through advances of molecular biology and related disciplines, such as protein chemistry.

It was Nobel laureate Linus Pauling and his coworkers who, by means of moving boundary electrophoresis, found that hemoglobin from a patient with SCA had mobility different from that of hemoglobin from a normal adult.[3] As a result, the hemoglobin of SCA patients was referred to as sickle hemoglobin or hemoglobin S (Hb-S) and the hemoglobin of normal individuals, hemoglobin A (Hb-A). The door had been opened for greater exploration of this condition, leading to better treatment options.

EPIDEMIOLOGY

It is a common misconception that sickle hemoglobin is found only in people of African heritage. To the contrary, it also occurs in people from a wide geographic area, including the Mediterranean region, parts of Greece and Italy, as well as India, Iran, and Turkey. Serjeant has noted that sickle hemoglobin is becoming more common in the United Kingdom, France, the Netherlands, Belgium, and Germany.[4] Those in Central America and South America are also affected.

Hb-S is the most frequently reported sickle gene among the black population in the United States, where the frequency of sickle cell trait is about 8% and that of sickle cell disease (SCD) is about 1 in 400. Hemoglobin C (Hb-C) appears primarily in the inhabitants of west and northern Africa or in descendants of people from this area, with the highest frequency in northern Ghana.[5] Hb-C has a frequency of about 3% in the U.S. population. Other abnormal hemoglobins seen in various areas are hemoglobin E (Sri Lanka, Malaysia, Thailand, Cambodia, Laos, Burma, Indonesia, Vietnam, and the Philippines) and hemoglobin D (India, Pakistan, Afghanistan, and Iran). Of all the sickle hemoglobin genes, Hb-S is the most common.

For years, it has appeared that the sickle cell trait offered a degree of protection against malarial infection. Abnormal red blood cells (RBCs) are less easily parasitized by *Plasmodium falciparum* than are normal RBCs. Consequently, reports have suggested that persons who are heterozygous for the sickle gene (trait) have a selective advantage in regions (tropical areas) where malaria is hyperendemic. The advantage that individuals with the trait have over those with normal hemoglobin now appears to be a limited one, occurring during the early childhood years before the child has developed a substantial degree of acquired immunity from his or her own antibody production.[5]

Patients with SCA have inherited two genes for the S hemoglobin. Figure 101–1 illustrates the genetic profiles possible for the offspring of parents with normal hemoglobin, sickle cell trait, and SCA. A person with entirely normal hemoglobin is designated AA. A person with the sickle cell trait is designated AS. A person with SCA is represented as SS. When one parent has normal hemoglobin and the other carries the sickle cell trait (example one), the children may have either normal hemoglobin or sickle cell trait. No child from this union will have SCA. When both parents carry the trait (example two), there is a 50% chance that their child will carry sickle cell trait, a 25% chance that the child will have SCA, and a 25% chance that the child will have normal hemoglobin. If one parent has SCA and the other parent has normal hemoglobin (example three), all offspring will carry the trait. Offspring from the union of one parent with SCA and the other with sickle cell trait have a 50% chance of having SCA and a 50% chance of carrying sickle cell trait (example four). The union of two persons with SCA, if able to produce offspring, would produce only children with SCA.

ETIOLOGY

The biochemical defect that leads to the development of Hb-S involves the substitution of valine for glutamic acid as the sixth amino acid in the β-polypeptide chain. Another abnormal hemoglobin commonly included in the SCD group, Hb-C is produced by the substitution of lysine for glutamic acid as the sixth amino acid in the β-chain (Fig. 101–2).

Because the α-chains of Hb-S, Hb-A, and Hb-C are structurally identical, the chemical difference in the β-chain explains sickling and its related sequelae. When deoxygenated, both Hb-S and Hb-A have similar physical properties in dilute solutions. In concentrated solutions, however, deoxygenated Hb-S is insoluble and forms a gel, whereas deoxygenated Hb-A remains soluble. This solubility difference represents the physiochemical basis for sickling.

Although SCA is a form of SCD in which both abnormal genes code for formation of Hb-S, the term *sickle cell disease* does not necessarily mean that the patient is homozygous for hemoglobin S (Hb-SS). Varying degrees of anemia may also be present in other variants of SCD. As previously noted, a person who carries sickle cell trait has one normal gene (A) and one abnormal gene (S, C, D). Such a person does not belong in the SCD group. A person with a genotype of AS is often referred to as a heterozygote. The heterozygous states can be pathologic, especially sickle-C and sickle-thalassemia. β-Thalassemia is often found in conjunction with Hb-S. β^+-Thalassemia usually has a milder course than β^0-thalassemia; the predicament of patients with the latter condition is similar to that of the homozygous SS patient. In addition, several haplotypes characterize the β^s-gene, resulting in differing clinical and hematologic courses. Included among these types are the three most commonly found in the United States: the Central Africa Republic (CAR) haplotype, characterized by severe disease; the Atlantic West African Senegal (SEN) haplotype, characterized by mild disease; and the Central West African Benin (BEN) haplotype, characterized by a course intermediate to that of the other two haplotypes. Although there are a number of other haplotypes seen around the world, the remaining major types include Saudi Arabian (Saudi)

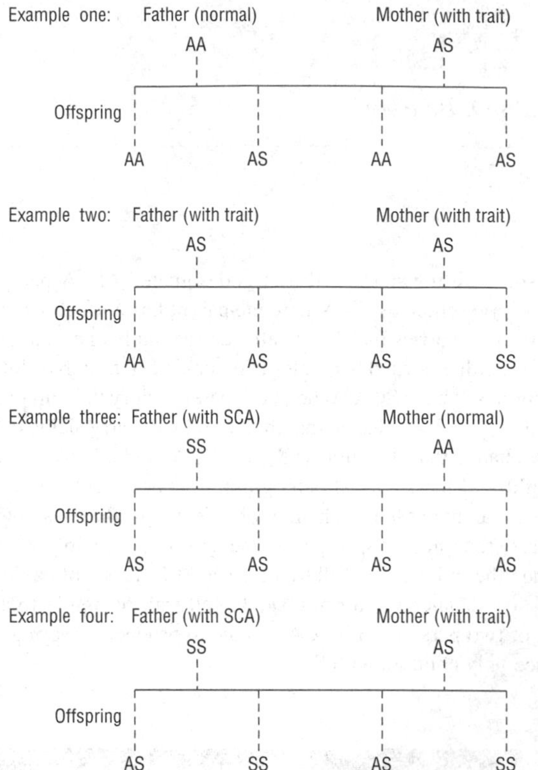

FIGURE 101–1. Inheritance scheme for the sickle gene. A = hemoglobin A (normal), and S = hemoglobin S (sickle hemoglobin).

and Cameroon (CAM). Both of these types usually follow milder courses of illness.[6]

PATHOPHYSIOLOGY

In the pathogenesis of SCD, three known problems are primarily responsible for various clinical manifestations: impaired circulation, destruction of RBCs, and stasis of blood flow. These three problems probably relate directly to two major disturbances involving RBCs. First, damage to the membrane of the RBCs containing Hb-S may cause these cells to lose potassium and water, leading to a dehydrated state that enhances the formation of sickled forms. After continual repetitions of this process, the RBC membrane probably retains greater quantities of calcium and develops a more rigid form, that of an irreversibly sickled cell (ISC).

Second, there is an alteration of the flow properties of RBCs containing polymerized Hb-S. The polymerization process results from the β-chain substitution of valine for glutamic acid.[7,8] Polymerization allows deoxygenated hemoglobin molecules to exist as a semisolid gel. Small changes in the mean corpuscular hemoglobin concentration (MCHC) affect this process. Temperature, pH, and the oxygen affinity of the RBCs contribute to the deoxygenation process. Because these cells have more difficulty deforming themselves than normal cells, they remain more rigid, retarding their flow, particularly through the microcirculation. The tendency toward vaso-occlusion is under the influence of a complex set of interactions between endothelial cells, sickle cells and various plasma components.[9] The presence of sickled RBCs increases blood viscosity and encourages sludging in the capillaries and small venous vessels. Such obstructive events lead to local tissue hypoxia, which tends to accentuate the pathologic process. The cycle of sickling and unsickling that occurs in response to variations in oxygen tension results in damage to the cell membrane. It leads to the loss of membrane flexibility and to the production of the ISC. Membranes of ISCs are permanently deformed, regardless of the oxygenation state of the hemoglobin within the cell.

The normal life span of an RBC is 120 days. The typical sickled cell survives for about 10 to 20 days. Intravascular destruction of sickle cells may occur at an accelerated rate. The stresses of circulation, including the circulation of rigid deoxygenated cells, and repetitive sickle-unsickle cycles are likely to lead to cell fragmentation.

It has been known for a number of years that some cells of patients with SCD contain increased amounts of hemoglobin F (Hb-F), or fetal hemoglobin. The primary hemoglobin present in the fetus from mid to late gestation, Hb-F binds oxygen more tightly than does Hb-A. Fetal hemoglobin does not appear to participate in the gelling of deoxygenated Hb-S, and RBCs that contain Hb-F sickle less readily than cells with Hb-S. In contrast, ISCs exhibit a lower concentration of Hb-F and a higher MCHC. ISCs are also smaller than other RBCs of patients with SCA. Increased levels of fetal hemoglobin moderate or even ameliorate the disease in some patients, thereby producing more benign forms of SCA.

The pathogenesis of a number of the clinical manifestations associated with SCD is not easily attributed directly to the sickling phenomenon. Other factors may be responsible. For example, there may be early signs of impaired reticuloendothelial function in SCA as a result of functional asplenia, defined as the loss of splenic function with an intact spleen. Patients with functional asplenia have increased susceptibility to infection by encapsulated organisms (particularly pneumococcal disease) and to disseminated intravascular coagulation (DIC). These patients may also have deficient opsonization.

A

Hb-A

Position	1	2	3	4	5	6*	7
β-chain	valine–	histidine–	leucine–	threonine–	proline–	glutamate–	glutamate

B

Hb-S

Position	1	2	3	4	5	6*	7
β-chain	valine–	histidine–	leucine–	threonine–	proline–	valine–	glutamate

C

Hb-C

Position	1	2	3	4	5	6*	7
β-chain	valine–	histidine–	leucine–	threonine–	proline–	lysine–	glutamate

FIGURE 101–2. The sixth-position (*) amino acid in the β chain differentiates **(A)** Hb-A from **(B)** Hb-S and **(C)** Hb-C.

CLINICAL PRESENTATION

In patients who are homozygous for Hb-S, anemia usually appears from 4 to 6 months after birth. Symptoms are delayed because the infant's RBCs contain mainly Hb-F, and fetal hemoglobin's oxygen-carrying ability and its lesser propensity to engage in sickling prevents the development of early clinical symptoms. (Sufficient quantities of Hb-S are present at birth to allow a diagnosis to be made by hemoglobin electrophoresis, however.) As RBC turnover occurs during those early months, cells containing Hb-S gradually replace those containing Hb-F, which typically leads to attacks of pain frequently accompanied by fever. Pneumonia and splenomegaly are also common findings. Many patients initially present with pain and swelling of the hands and feet, commonly referred to as "hand-and-foot syndrome" or dactylitis.

Many states have established newborn screening programs for SCA and other hemoglobinopathies along the lines of the long-standing phenylketonuria (PKU) screening programs.[10] Newborn screening is an important strategy, because it affords clinicians the opportunity to apply earlier preventive and therapeutic methods. However, the commonly used tests (e.g., Sickledex, Sickleprep) do not differentiate between patients who have the sickle cell trait and those who have SCD. Making this distinction requires hemoglobin electrophoresis, isoelectric focusing, high-performance liquid chromatography, or DNA analysis.[8] In addition, high levels of Hb-F may interfere with the screening assay. Alternatively, direct analysis of DNA obtained from amniotic fluid can provide a prenatal diagnosis.

Persons with sickle cell trait are usually asymptomatic, although some clinical signs and symptoms have occasionally been associated with sickle cell trait. Impairment of renal function, which probably arises from the sickling of RBCs, tends to result in dilute urine. Patients with such an impairment may be at some risk of dehydration during periods in which the body normally conserves water, as in hot and dry weather. Hematuria has also been noted and probably also relates to sickling within the kidney. Although some persons with sickle cell trait may experience abnormalities under certain conditions, these instances are not routine, and trait carriers are not considered to have clinical disease.

The usual clinical signs and symptoms associated with SCA include chronic anemia, fever and pallor, arthralgia, scleral icterus, abdominal pain, weakness, anorexia, fatigue, enlargement of liver and heart, and hematuria. Infants may show an enlargement of the spleen. In the typical patient with SCA, the hemoglobin level is reduced and the reticulocyte count increased. The platelet and leukocyte counts are usually higher than normal, and the peripheral blood smear demonstrates sickle forms. In contrast, the clinical presentation of patients with hemoglobin SC disease (Hb-C disease) is characterized primarily by mild anemia (hemoglobin levels above 9 g/dL), infrequent episodes of pain, persistence of splenomegaly into adult life, and excessive target cells in the peripheral blood smear.

Patients with SCD experience delayed growth and sexual maturation. Both height and weight are usually below average. Fertility problems tend to occur more often, and some menstrual abnormalities are more prevalent in female SCD patients than in normal women.[5,11] Other typical physical characteristics include a protuberant abdomen with exaggerated lumbar lordosis, usually an asthenic appearance with rather long extremities and tapered fingers, and frequently a barrel-shaped chest. One report indicates that, despite abnormal test results for bone age, zinc concentrations, and somatomedin c levels, no correlation could be established with growth status. As a result, it was concluded that nutritional factors alone could not explain poor growth in SCD patients.[12]

The previously high mortality rate of early childhood has been reduced for patients with SCD, while life expectancy for these patients has risen to 48 years and 42 years, for females and males respectively.[13,14]

SICKLE CELL CRISIS

Chronic hemolytic anemia in the SCD patient is periodically interrupted by crises, particularly in childhood. Patients with Hb-SS disease experience crises more often than do patients with Hb-C disease or some other variants. Although fever, infections, dehydration, hypoxia, acidosis, and sudden temperature alterations can precipitate crises, multiple factors are often at work in bringing about a crisis. The time between crises is called the steady-state period, and patients not in crisis are said to be in the steady state.[2]

TABLE 101–1. Manifestations of Sickle Cell Disease: Crises and Complications

Crisis	Characteristic
Aplastic	Bone marrow failure
Hemolytic	Massive hemolysis
Splenic sequestration	Sequestration of red blood cells
Vaso-occlusive	Infarction/pain
Organ System	**Complication**
Pulmonary	Acute chest syndrome
Neurologic	Various, including cerebrovascular accident
Dermatologic	Chronic ulcers
Cardiovascular	Hypertrophy
Genitourinary	Priapism, hematuria, hyposthenuria
Skeletal	Aseptic necrosis, osteomyelitis
Ocular	Retinal problems
Hepatic	Cholelithiasis

TYPES OF SICKLE CELL CRISES

Four types of crises are generally described clinically (Table 101–1).

APLASTIC CRISIS

Generally, aplastic crisis occurs in patients under the age of 18; it is characterized by a decrease in the reticulocyte count and a rapidly developing severe anemia. The bone marrow is hypoplastic. There may be associated pain. The crisis is thought to be caused by a viral infection, particularly B19 parvovirus.[15]

HEMOLYTIC CRISIS

Patients with a hemolytic crisis show a rate of hemolysis even greater than that usually present. Hemoglobin and RBC levels fall, often without a change in the number of reticulocytes and with a hyperplastic bone marrow. Pain and fever may accompany this crisis. An increase in the icteric state is usually evident. Care should be taken to avoid confusing this condition with glucose-6-phosphate dehydrogenase (G6PD) deficiency, particularly during a febrile episode when antipyretics are used.

SEQUESTRATION CRISIS

A sudden massive enlargement of the spleen and liver, resulting from the sequestration by these organs of blood from the reticuloendothelial system, characterizes a sequestration crisis. There is a dramatic fall in hematocrit and hemoglobin concentration, with no evidence of marrow failure or accelerated hemolysis. The trapping of the sickled RBCs by the spleen also leads to a drop in circulating blood volume, which can result in hypotension and shock. The condition is most often seen in infants and children, as their spleens are intact and have not undergone multiple infarctions and fibrosis. Because repeated infarctions lead to autosplenectomy as the disease progresses, the incidence of this type of crisis declines as adolescence approaches. These crises can cause sudden death in young children. They are rarely seen in adult Hb-SS patients, but may be seen in adult Hb-SC or sickle cell thalassemia patients.[11]

VASO-OCCLUSIVE (INFARCTIVE) CRISIS

The most common type of crisis is the vaso-occlusive crisis, which is usually characterized by pain affecting the involved areas, without other changes in hemoglobin or other laboratory values. Laboratory changes that may be seen include leukocytosis, increased serum levels of fibrinogen, and decreased serum pH and bicarbonate level.

Manifestations of Crises

Early death has been associated with the number of pain episodes in patients who have SCD and are older than 20 years. One study found that adult patients with three or more episodes of pain per year had a higher death rate than those with fewer than three episodes per year.[16] Several factors precipitate painful crises, including dehydration, muscular exertion, emotional upset, and changes in climate. The following are the commonly observed manifestations:

Sickle cell dactylitis (hand-and-foot syndrome). In this condition, which occurs in infancy and early childhood, the dorsal aspects of the hands and feet, as well as the fingers and toes, swell. Erythema accompanies the swelling. The episodes are painful, but there usually is no permanent damage. Children most likely to develop severe SCD later in life are those who experience dactylitis, along with severe anemia and noninfectious leukocytosis, during the first 2 years of life.[17]

Involvement of joints and extremities. Areas of infarction over the long bones or in the periarticular tissues of the larger joints may cause this form of crisis. The pain often mimics that of rheumatic fever and may migrate from one site to another. Mild temperature elevations may be noted.

Abdominal involvement. Pain may simulate an acute abdominal process, suggesting the need for surgical intervention. The episodes, which may be severe and episodic, are usually related to areas of infarction in abdominal structures. The pain may be severe and episodic in nature. Although the usual duration is about 3 to 4 days, courses are occasionally protracted. Low-grade fever is often present.

Hepatic involvement. Some degree of hyperbilirubinemia is common in SCD. A rise in the serum bilirubin level well beyond the steady-state value, associated with right upper quadrant pain, is characteristic of hepatic involvement in a sickle cell crisis. Widespread intrahepatic sickling may occur, leading to hepatocellular necrosis and swelling. Such an extensive occurrence can be fatal, so it is important to identify these severe obstructive jaundice processes, as well as episodes of cholelithiasis, as early as possible. Hepatic crises are seen more often in older patients.

Pulmonary involvement. Lung infarctions occur in both children and adults with SCD. Children seem to have pulmonary episodes most often because of infection. It can sometimes be very difficult to distinguish between infection and infarction; indeed, both may be present. Infection is usually caused by pneumococci; infarction is often related to embolization from sickled RBCs or pieces of necrotic bone marrow tissue.

COMPLICATIONS

Acute chest syndrome (ACS) is the leading cause of death among patients with Hb-S disease. It is characterized by cough, dyspnea, chest pain, fever, pulmonary infiltration, and an equivocal response to antibiotic therapy.[18] The Cooperative Study of Sickle Cell Disease (CSSCD) showed an increased hematocrit as a major risk factor for adults in the development of ACS.[19] As many as one-half of patients with SCD develop ACS at least once.[20] Pulmonary infarcts often involve the lower lobes of the lungs and are a frequent cause of pleural effusions. Pneumonia occurs most often in the middle and upper lobes. These pulmonary manifestations can and do occur in the absence of bone, joint, or abdominal pain.

There has long been disagreement over the predominant cause of ACS. The National Acute Chest Syndrome Study Group recently reported that patients with ACS experienced hypoxia, decreased hemoglobin values, or progressive multilobar pneumonia, and it appeared to be precipitated by fat embolism and infection, particularly community-acquired pneumonia. Older patients and those having neurologic symptoms seem at greater risk for progressing to respiratory failure.[21]

A syndrome characterized by damage to one or more organs simultaneously can also occur, particularly in patients with high hematocrit. The onset may be due to arterial hypoxia, as may be seen in ACS. Sudden syncope may be the only predisposing event, and symptoms seem to result from the insufficient perfusion of one or more organs.[22]

Neurologic abnormalities can occur in both adults and children. Vaso-occlusive processes occasionally lead to cerebral vascular occlusion that manifests itself as the signs and symptoms of stroke, such as drowsiness, paralysis, transitory or permanent blindness, aphasia, visual disturbances, spinal cord infarction, and convulsions. The onset is usually sudden, but occasionally may be gradual. Milder symptoms may occur as a result of vascular stasis. Some patients recover rapidly and completely, while others are left with permanent neurologic deficits. In addition, some patients who have SCA with no prior history of stroke have been found to have changes on magnetic resonance imaging (MRI) of the brain that suggests infarction or ischemia. These "silent infarcts" have been reported to occur in up to 17% to 18% of Hb-SS patients.[23]

Chronic leg ulcers can become a difficult problem and a common finding in many young adults with SCA. The inner aspect of the lower leg just above the ankle is the site most often affected. Ulcers are often seen after trauma or infection. They are usually slow to heal, taking several weeks to a year.

Cholelithiasis is a common occurrence in the SCD patient. It is seen more frequently and at a younger age among these patients than in the general population. It is the result of the chronic hemolysis that results in increased bilirubin production. Cholecystitis, exemplified by pain in the right iliac fossa, can be confused with abdominal pain crises.[24]

As with any anemia, cardiovascular abnormalities, including cardiac enlargement and various murmurs, can occur in patients with SCD. Patients complain of various degrees of exertional dyspnea, tachycardia, and palpitation owing to the decreased oxygen-carrying capacity of the system. Effects are most prominent in Hb-SS disease.

Sickling in the sinusoids of the penis can cause priapism, a very painful complication that develops in certain male patients with SCD. The sickling produces a sustained painful erection that may last several hours or several days. Impotence has been reported after repeated episodes. An interesting syndrome, called the ASPEN (Association of Sickle Cell Disease, Priapism, Exchange Transfusion and Neurological Events) syndrome, has occurred in some patients with priapism after partial exchange transfusion to treat the condition.[25] The syndrome is characterized by severe headache and other neurologic symptoms, ranging from seizures to obtundation that requires ventilation.

Destructive bone and joint problems are frequently evident. Aseptic necrosis, particularly of the femoral or humeral heads, causes permanent damage and disability. This problem arises both in patients with Hb-SS disease and in heterozygous patients. Patients with SCD also have an increased incidence of osteomyelitis; the organism most often responsible is *Salmonella*.

Ocular problems occur in the form of transient monocular blindness, visual field defects from retinal hemorrhage, retinal detachment, vitreous hemorrhage, venous microaneurysms, and neovascularization in the adult. Patients with Hb-SC disease are most likely to suffer from these disorders.

Renal complications include unilateral hematuria and hyposthenuria. Death from renal disease is unusual among younger patients, but does occur among older patients with SCD.

Finally, pregnancy introduces an increased risk for the mother with SCD and for the fetus. However, these risks are not so great as to prohibit continuation of the pregnancy. The anemia of SCD may lead to intrauterine growth retardation. Preterm labor and premature delivery are common occurrences in mothers with SCD, and the risk of spontaneous abortion is increased. The incidence of preeclampsia is also higher than in mothers who do not have SCD. The periodicity of past pain crisis is predictive of the likely events during pregnancy, although some patients may experience increased frequency of pain crisis during pregnancy. The presentation of such patients is similar to that of nonpregnant patients—severe localized or generalized pain, low-grade fever, and mild leukocytosis.[26]

▶ TREATMENT: Sickle Cell Disease

Although a cure for SCD has been elusive, appropriate, comprehensive care can have a positive impact on both longevity and general quality of life. This care includes the use of traditional prophylactic and symptomatic general supportive care, as well as the judicious use of newer, more specific therapies aimed at altering hematologic capacity and function.

Treatment for patients with SCA involves the use of general measures to meet the unique demands for increased erythropoiesis. Additional interventions may be aimed at preventing or treating complications of the disease. When crises occur, the type and severity of the crisis determine the appropriate therapeutic plan. A treatment overview is shown in Table 101–2.

GENERAL MANAGEMENT

FOLIC ACID

Patients with SCD have an increased demand for folic acid because of accelerated erythropoiesis. Low serum folate levels are common. Megaloblastic changes have been reported, but the actual incidence of megaloblastic anemia in association with SCD is unknown. Although folic acid supplementation is not clearly essential, the standard of care is to provide folic acid supplementation. A dose of 1 mg/day is most commonly used.

TABLE 101–2. Treatment of Sickle Cell Disease

General Preventive Measures		
Intervention	***Population***	***Comments***
Folic acid	All patients	
Pneumococcal vaccine	All patients	Administration in childhood recommended.
Penicillin prophylaxis	Children less than 5 years	Penicillin-allergic patients excluded. Asplenic children older than 5 years may require continuous therapy.
Haemophilus influenzae vaccine	All children	
Hydroxyurea	Adult patients with frequent painful episodes, severe symptomatic anemia, history of chest syndrome, or severe vaso-occlusive complications	Further study needed on safety and efficacy in children.
Transfusion therapy	Pediatric patients who have had strokes	May be useful in selected adult patients.
Crises		
Crisis	***Treatment***	***Comment***
Aplastic crisis	Supportive treatment	Blood transfusion if anemia is severe
Hemolytic crisis	Supportive treatment	
Sequestration crisis	Whole blood transfusion, empiric broad-spectrum antibiotics	Splenectomy in life-threatening or recurring cases.
Vaso-occlusive crisis	Hydration and analgesics	Avoid overhydration.

mean of 7.2% to a mean of 21%, and there was a marked decrease in the number of days of hospitalization in the five responding patients who were treated for 6 months or longer. The drug regimen was well tolerated. An increase in the blood urea nitrogen (BUN) level was frequently recorded during the infusion, likely because of the conversion of arginine to urea. The levels, however, decreased within a few hours after the drug administration.[40]

There is now renewed interest in the possible use of 5-aza-2-deoxycytidine to stimulate fetal hemoglobin production. Virtually abandoned in the past because of concerns regarding the cytotoxicity of 5-azacytidine, this derivative has now been studied in a small number of patients with SCD who did not respond to hydroxyurea. In one study, 5-aza-2-deoxycytidine was studied in eight adult patients, five of whom had failed to respond to hydroxyurea and two of whom had experienced only a transient increase in fetal hemoglobin level following treatment with hydroxyurea. The remaining patient had never received hydroxyurea. In this phase I/II study, 5-aza-2-deoxycytidine resulted in an increase in fetal hemoglobin in all patients. In the seven hydroxyurea nonresponders, fetal hemoglobin, which had only increased from 2.28% to 2.6% with hydroxyurea use, increased to 12.7% with 5-aza-2-deoxycytidine use. As the only drug-related side effect noted was transient neutropenia, this drug may have a role in treating patients who fail to respond to hydroxyurea. Additional studies are under way.[41]

Clotrimazole causes a decrease in cell density by blocking cation transport channels in the erythrocyte membrane. The decrease seen, however, is less than that demonstrated with hydroxyurea therapy. It is unclear whether this agent will be clinically useful in the treatment of SCA.[9]

Poloxamer 188 (Flocor), a purified poloxamer, is an investigational agent given IV to improve blood flow and restore oxygen delivery. The drug is under study for use in sickle cell crises. Its properties have been described as rheologic, cytoprotective, antiadhesive, and antithrombotic. Patients receiving poloxamer 188 have experienced briefer painful episodes, have had fewer analgesic requirements, and have spent less time in hospitals. Poloxamer 188 clinical trials are still in progress.[42]

PENTOXIFYLLINE

A xanthine derivative, pentoxifylline increases RBC deformity and inhibits platelet aggregation. One study that used a pentoxifylline regimen of 400 mg given orally three times per day showed a significant decrease in the number and severity of painful crises in patients receiving the drug.[43] Not all studies, however, have reported positive results. Sherer and Glover found that although several case reports and studies have noted either a decrease in the number or the severity of vaso-occlusive episodes in patients receiving pentoxifylline, these studies generally lacked appropriate scientific design or size to make definitive conclusions.[44] The routine use of pentoxifylline in patients with SCD is not recommended, but this agent may present an option for patients who cannot tolerate proven therapeutic approaches such as hydroxyurea.[44]

ERYTHROPOIETIN

Because erythropoietin therapy has been used in only a limited number of patients with SCD and the clinical results have been inconsistent, its routine use in these patients cannot be recommended.[45] One study of erythropoietin in combination with hydroxyurea suggests that there may be a role for erythropoietin therapy in patients who do not respond to hydroxyurea alone. In this study, a dose of 400 U/kg/wk was given for 3 to 4 weeks in conjunction with hydroxyurea therapy. Results, however, were not conclusive.[46] More studies are necessary to determine the role, if any, for erythropoietin therapy in SCD patients.

TRANSFUSION THERAPY

In some patients with SCD, transfusion therapy may be beneficial in treating the life-threatening complications of their disease. For example, transfusions are often required for sudden severe anemia in pediatric patients experiencing sequestration crises. Blood transfusions may also be needed during aplastic crisis if the anemia is severe. Patients experiencing ACS may also require transfusions.[9] The use of transfusions in SCD patients undergoing surgery with general anesthesia has reduced the risk of postoperative complications. Other patients in whom transfusions may be useful include patients with complicated obstetric problems, refractory leg ulcers, or refractory and protracted painful episodes. Transfusions may also be useful in patients with severe priapism if they are given early in the episode.[9]

Transfusions help to prevent stroke recurrence in children. Repeated transfusions in children with SCA reduce the stroke recurrence rate from approximately 50% to about 10% over 3 years. The goal of transfusions is to achieve and maintain an Hb-S concentration of less than 30% of total hemoglobin for 3 to 5 years. After 4 years of therapy, many clinicians give transfusions less frequently and allow the Hb-S concentration to rise to 50% of total hemoglobin.[9]

Prophylactic transfusions to prevent stroke altogether may also be beneficial. In one trial, prophylactic transfusions significantly reduced the incidence of stroke over a 2-year period in children 2 to 16 years of age. Stroke occurrence rate was reduced from 16% in patients receiving standard care to 2% in those who received prophylactic transfusions.[47]

Although the benefits of transfusion therapy are relatively clear in some clinical situations, the usefulness of this therapy in other situations remains controversial. The risks of transfusion therapy must be weighed against possible benefits. The risks associated with transfusion therapy include sensitization to the blood received, for example. Alloimmunization occurs in 18% to 36% of SCD patients who receive blood transfusions. The use of leukocyte-reduced RBC transfusions or HLA-matched units in chronically transfused patients may reduce the risk of alloimmunization.[48] Transfusion-related infections also remain a concern. Routine blood screening and immunization with hepatitis B vaccine have reduced the risk of infection. Presently, hepatitis C is considered the most serious risk associated with transfusion therapy, with an infection rate of approximately 1 in every 100,000 transfusions. The risk of contracting acquired immunodeficiency syndrome (AIDS) from blood transfusions, while still of concern, has decreased with routine blood screening. The risk of human immunodeficiency virus (HIV) transmission is now approximately 1 in every 500,000 units of exposed blood [48] Iron accumulation is another complication of transfusions. Chelation therapy may be successful in treating this complication, although compliance to prescribed chelation regimens is generally not optimal.[9]

Unique to the population with SCD is a constellation of features that may occur in response to blood transfusion; this is often referred to as the sickle cell hemolytic transfusion reaction syndrome.[49] This syndrome includes manifestations of an acute or delayed transfusion reaction. During the hemolytic reaction, the patient develops symptoms suggestive of a pain crisis, or symptoms worsen if the patient is already in crisis. There may be a significant decrease in the patient's absolute reticulocyte count compared to his or her usual value. The patient may also develop an anemia post-transfusion that is more severe than previously observed because of the rapid drop in hemoglobin and hematocrit during hemolysis, accompanied by a suppression of erythropoiesis. Alloantibodies and autoantibodies that formed as a result of past transfusions can serve as a trigger, causing a return of symptoms in the post-recovery period. Subsequent transfusions may further worsen the clinical situation by exacerbating the anemia. There may be no serologic explanation for the hemolytic transfusion reaction. Recovery, as evidenced by reticulocytosis with a gradual increase in the hemoglobin level, may occur only after the withholding of further transfusions. Although some patients tolerate further transfusions after recovery, others may experience a recurrence of the hemolytic transfusion reaction.[34]

HEMATOPOIETIC STEM CELL TRANSPLANTATION

In some patients with SCD, hematopoietic stem cell transplantation has been curative. The procedure, however, has a treatment-related mortality rate of about 10%. With the availability of present supportive care that allows many patients to live into their 50s, it can be difficult to identify patients for whom transplantation is warranted. The best candidates for transplantation are SCD patients who are younger than 16 years of age; have severe complications such as refractory pain, stroke, or recurrent ACS; and have an HLA-matched donor. Only 1 in 100 SCD patients meet these criteria.[9]

An interim report of a U.S. multicenter trial of bone marrow transplantation in 50 patients with SCD showed a 94% survival rate and an 84% event-free survival, results that are similar to those previously reported from European studies. All of the patients in the study were less than 16 years of age, had symptomatic SCD, and had an HLA-identical sibling donor. The follow-up period for these patients ranged from 38 to 95 months (median 57.9 months). Two patients died from chronic graft-versus-host disease, and one died of intracranial hemorrhage. Of the 47 surviving patients, 5 experienced graft rejection and recurrent SCD. These rejections occurred a median of 5.1 months after transplantation. Based on this interim data, it appears that a stable engraftment of donor cells can eradicate or arrest the clinical manifestations of SCD.[50] The risks associated with transplantation, however, must be carefully considered. Efforts to decrease post-transplant risk of seizure or intracranial bleeding include prophylactic anticonvulsant therapy, aggressive platelet support, and stringent patient selection.[51]

TREATMENT OF COMPLICATIONS

PRIAPISM

Stuttering priapism, episodes that last a few minutes to 2 hours, resolve spontaneously. Severe episodes, lasting more than 2 to 3 hours, generally require medical attention. The initial goals of treatment are to provide appropriate analgesic therapy and to reduce anxiety. Morphine and hydroxyzine may be useful in achieving these goals. Hydration should also be initiated. Both ice packs and hot baths have been used in the treatment of priapism. The use of ice packs, however, may be painful. Heat may be beneficial by increasing blood flow and improving venous outflow, but it may not be effective in patients with infarctive priapism. Although transfusions have been given to these patients, the usefulness of this therapeutic intervention is not established.[52]

Clinicians have used both vasoconstrictors and vasodilators in the treatment of priapism. Vasoconstrictors, such as phenylephrine or epinephrine, are thought to work by forcing blood out of the corpus cavernosum into the venous return. Epinephrine use has been associated with increases in heart rate and blood pressure.[52] In one prospective study, aspiration followed by intrapenile irrigation with epinephrine was effective and well tolerated.[53] In this study, as much blood as possible was aspirated from the corpus cavernosum, and the area was irrigated with a 1:1,000,000 solution of epinephrine. The procedure resolved the priapism in 37 of the 39 occasions in which it was used. The therapy was well tolerated with no serious immediate or long-term side effects. On two occasions, a small intrapenile hematoma formed after treatment.

Vasodilators, such as terbutaline and hydralazine, induce relaxation of the smooth muscle of the vasculature. It is suggested that this relaxation allows oxygenated arterial blood to enter the corpus cavernosum. This arterial blood displaces or washes out the damaged sickle cells that are stagnant in the corpus cavernosum.[52] Terbutaline has been used to treat priapism, but it has not been formally studied in patients with SCA.[54,55]

Exchange transfusions have had mixed success in the treatment of priapism, and they have been associated with severe neurologic syndromes. Surgical interventions used in severe refractory priapism have included a variety of shunt procedures. Although these surgical procedures have been successful in some cases, they have a high failure rate, and complications frequently ensue. Complications have included skin sloughing, cellulitis, and urethral fistulas.[53]

Mantadakis and colleagues reported the successful use of pseudoephedrine (30 mg/day given orally at bedtime) in SCD patients to decrease the number of recurrent episodes of priapism.[53] There have been no controlled studies on the use of pseudoephedrine, however. Hormonal therapy has also been administered in an effort to decrease the production or action of testosterone. There are limited data on the successful use of gonadotropin-releasing hormone analogs.[56,57] Hydroxyurea therapy may be useful in preventing recurrent episodes of priapism.[58]

ACUTE CHEST SYNDROME

Patients with ACS should use incentive spirometry frequently (e.g., at least every 2 hours). In incentive spirometry, the patient tries to take long, slow, deep breaths. A visual indicator on the spirometer indicates when the patient achieves the targeted flow rate or volume. In addition to spirometry, proper management of pain is important. The goal is to provide relief while avoiding analgesic-induced hypoventilation. Appropriate fluid therapy should avoid overhydration, which may exacerbate respiratory distress.[59] Early use of broad-spectrum antibiotics is also recommended. Studies indicate that infection is common with ACS and may involve gram-positive, gram-negative, or atypical bacteria.[60] Oxygen therapy is appropriate for patients who are hypoxic or in acute distress. Transfusions are often used in the treatment of acute lung disease. Hydroxyurea therapy, chronic transfusions, and hematopoietic stem cell transplantation may be of use in preventing recurrences of ACS in selected patients.[59] The use of nitrous oxide inhalation also merits further study.[20,61]

MANAGEMENT OF CRISES

Aplastic Crisis

Treatment of aplastic crisis is primarily supportive. The patient may need blood transfusions if anemia is severe. In addition, the patient should be receiving folic acid supplementation, because folic acid deficiency has been implicated as a cause of aplastic crisis. Although it is possible that a bacterial infection may precipitate aplastic crisis, it is more likely that a virus, probably a parvovirus, is the precipitating factor.[62,63] Consequently, antibiotic therapy generally is not warranted with aplastic crisis.

Hemolytic Crisis

There is no specific treatment for hemolytic crisis. Treatment is supportive and may include blood transfusions.

Sequestration Crisis

Splenic sequestration crisis is a major cause of mortality in young patients with SCD. The sequestration of RBCs in the spleen may result in a rapid drop of hematocrit, leading to hypovolemia, shock, and death. Treatment includes whole-blood transfusion to correct hypovolemia. Broad-spectrum antibiotic therapy, which includes coverage for pneumococci and *H. influenzae*, may also be beneficial, because infection may precipitate crises.

The indications for splenectomy are controversial. Splenic sequestration crises tend to recur, however, and prompt splenectomy remains a treatment option. Splenectomy is probably indicated, even after a single sequestration crisis, if that event is life-threatening. Repetitive episodes, even if less serious, also may merit a splenectomy. For children less than 2 years of age, chronic blood transfusions have been recommended to prevent sequestration and to permit a delay of splenectomy until the age of 2, when the risk of postsplenectomy septicemia becomes less.[10,64]

Vaso-Occlusive Crisis

Hydration and analgesia are the mainstays of treatment for vaso-occlusive (painful) crises. Fluid replacement at a rate of 3 to 4 L/day has been recommended for adults. This can be given either IV or orally, if feasible.[36] It is not clear which specific fluid should be used for IV hydration. Some clinicians recommend the use of dextrose 5% in water or dextrose 5% with 1/4 normal saline. The administration of free water may reverse the movement of free water out of the RBC and, therefore, decrease intracellular hemoglobin concentrations. The rate of polymerization of sickle hemoglobin increases as the intracellular hemoglobin concentration increases. Patients with documented hyponatremia should receive fluids with increased sodium concentrations. Overly aggressive hydration, particularly with sodium-containing fluids, may lead to volume overload, ACS, and heart failure.[20]

The American Pain Society has provided guidance in the treatment of pain in sickle cell crisis (Table 101–4).[65] There is great variability in the frequency and severity of acute pain episodes associated with SCD. Thus, the pain should be assessed and analgesic therapy tailored for each patient. Aggressive therapy to relieve pain and enable the patient to attain maximum functional ability should be initiated.

TABLE 101–4. Pain Management for Patients with Sickle Cell Disease

- Assess pain to confirm it is related to sickle cell disease.
- Initiate aggressive therapy to relieve pain and enable maximum functional ability.
- Treat based on characteristics of pain.

Mild to Moderate Pain

Use nonsteroidal anti-inflammatory drugs or acetaminophen if not contraindicated. If pain persists, add an opioid. If pain unrelieved, increase opioid strength or dose.

Moderate to Severe Pain

Use opioids with or without nonsteroidal anti-inflammatory drugs (NSAIDs) and adjuvant medications. Select opioid formulation based on typical duration of painful episode (less than 24-h duration: formulations with short duration of action; episodes lasting several days: sustained release opioids with short-acting opioids as needed for breakthrough pain or until sustained release product reaches steady state).

Severe Pain/Acute Episode

Select medication and loading dose based on history of analgesic use, if applicable. Administer opioid intravenously if possible. Titrate to pain relief. Order opioid on a scheduled basis to maintain relief around the clock (ATC). Use a rescue dose for breakthrough pain (one-fourth to one-half of one ATC dose.) Consider use of adjuvant medications (e.g., anti-inflammatory agents, antihistamines) to enhance efficacy. Consider use of patient-controlled analgesia (PCA) in patients with prior history of good pain control using PCA, after satisfactory pain relief achieved with aggressive opioid titration schedule, if pain is inadequately controlled with bolus titration, or if too frequent dosing is required for maintenance of relief.

- Use nonpharmacologic interventions as appropriate based on a comprehensive assessment.
  Behavioral (e.g., relaxation, deep breathing, behavior modification)
  Psychological (e.g., distraction, social support)
  Physical (e.g., hydration, heat, massage, physical therapy)

Adapted from Ref. 65 with permission.

Treatment of mild to moderate pain should include the use of nonsteroidal anti-inflammatory drugs (NSAIDs) or acetaminophen, unless there are contraindications to their use. If mild to moderate pain persists, an opioid should be added.

Persistent or moderate to severe pain should be treated by increasing the opioid strength or dose. The characteristics and expected duration of pain should determine the choice of opioid. Pain that is generally of short duration (less than 24 hours) should be treated with opioids or opioid formulations with a short duration of action. These agents also offer fast onset of action. Patients in whom pain persists for several days should be treated with sustained-release opioid preparations. In these patients, short-acting opioids should be used for breakthrough pain. Commonly used opioids include morphine, hydromorphone, codeine, oxycodone, hydrocodone, and methadone. Meperidine use should be reserved for very brief treatment courses in patients for whom it has previously been effective or in patients who are allergic to or cannot tolerate other opioids. The accumulation of normeperidine, a metabolite, can cause central nervous system side effects, ranging from dysphoria to seizures. Therefore, it is recommended that meperidine not be used for more than 48 hours at doses greater than 600 mg in 24 hours. Its use is contraindicated in patients with impaired renal function because normeperidine is excreted through the kidneys.[65]

Severe pain should be treated aggressively until the pain is tolerable. Both prior history and current assessment are important considerations. If the patient has been on long-term opioid therapy at home, tolerance may have developed. In these cases, the pain of acute crises can be treated with a different potent opioid or a larger dose of the same medication. The IV route of administration is preferred for severe pain. The analgesics should be titrated to relief. Analgesics should be administered around the clock rather than as needed to maintain relief, although an as-needed dose for breakthrough pain should be prescribed. Effective combination therapy may enhance analgesic efficacy while decreasing side effects. For example, anti-inflammatory agents and antihistamines can be combined with opioids.[65] Although hospitalization is necessary for severe crisis, milder cases may be treated on an outpatient basis with rest, hydration, warmth, and the oral administration of analgesics.

Because infection can precipitate crises, an infectious etiology should be ruled out in presenting patients. Appropriate empiric therapy should be initiated in patients with high fever or patients who are critically ill.

PHARMACOECONOMIC CONSIDERATIONS

Targeted screening of African Americans has been shown to be cost-effective. The incremental cost-effectiveness ratio of targeted screening (versus no screening) is $6,709 per life year gained and of universal screening (versus targeted screening) is $30,760 per life year gained. Universal screening may provide for a certain degree of cost-effectiveness since targeted screening, is associated with variable delivery rates and may not adequately cover the entirety of the population potentially having the disease.[66]

Although drugs are one of the most important factors in payment and reimbursement decisions regarding SCD, the overall cost of hospital-related care for SCD is considerable.[67] A 1996 national estimate places the cost per patient at $6,300 per hospitalization. Newer therapies, such as the administration of hydroxyurea and the transplantation of hematopoietic stem cells, are especially costly. The cost of a year of hydroxyurea therapy has been estimated to be $3,000, while the cost of a hematopoietic stem cell transplantation is estimated to range between $100,000 and $200,000.[68]

Two studies conducted in Illinois and South Carolina have shown that a small number of patients consume a disproportionate amount of care as a result of severe illness.[69,70] The South Carolina study also reported that predictors of costly hospitalizations included living at a distance from the hospital and having an admission diagnosis of painful respiration.[70] A primary care approach that takes advantage of the opportunities to care for patients with SCD by using telemedicine offers the promise of improved access to care for patients living some distance from the hospital and, possibly, may reduce costs.[71] Undoubtedly, the number of high-use patients reported in these studies, when multiplied by the number of SCD patients around the United States, suggests that it will be necessary to spend much more per capita than the recurrent cost of new therapies like hydroxyurea or the one-time cost plus follow-up costs of transplantation.[68] These therapies, although expensive, may keep patients out of emergency and inpatient beds, improving the cost-effectiveness of those therapies over a patient's lifetime. Of course, it is presumed that therapy, if successful, will also improve the patient's quality of life.

EVALUATION OF THERAPEUTIC OUTCOME

In the long-term management of the patient with SCA, folic acid can help to prevent folate deficiency and megaloblastic changes. Folate levels and MCV values should be monitored. Evaluation of the efficacy of prophylactic immunizations and antibiotics involves monitoring for the occurrence of pneumococcal or *Haemophilus* infections. When infections do occur, appropriate antibiotic therapy should be initiated and the patient monitored for laboratory and clinical improvement.

The efficacy of gelation inhibitors such as hydroxyurea can best be assessed in terms of the decrease in number, severity, and duration of sickle cell pain crises. Fetal hemoglobin concentrations or MCV values may also provide some indication of the patient's response to therapy. When painful crises do occur, the evaluation of the effectiveness of analgesics depends mainly on the subjective assessments made by the patient and health care practitioners. Adequate hydration is important in the resolution of painful crisis. However, caution should be exercised to avoid overhydration, especially in patients predisposed to complications from this therapy (e.g., those with impaired renal function or cardiac dysfunction). The success of blood transfusions post-stroke can be measured by clinical progression or the occurrence of subsequent strokes.

CONCLUSION

The goals of the general management of SCA are to decrease the number of sickle cell crises, to decrease the complications arising from the disease, and to improve the overall quality of the patient's life. The general care of SCA patients still includes folate administration and appropriate immunization. Gelation inhibitors, especially hydroxyurea, may decrease the frequency and severity of painful episodes. Continued studies on other possible agents that may reduce crises or reverse organ damage are warranted.

▶ PRINCIPLES OF PHARMACOTHERAPY

- Sickle cell disease is an inherited disorder caused by a defect in the gene for hemoglobin.
- Patients may have one defective gene (sickle cell trait) or two defective genes (sickle cell disease).
- Although most often seen in persons of African ancestry, other ethnic groups are affected.
- Sickle cell disease may cause various kinds of crises, growth retardation, myocardial infarction, aseptic necrosis of joints, and cholelithiasis.
- Folate administration is recommended for patients with sickle cell disease because of the demands of accelerated erythropoiesis.
- Patients with sickle cell disease should receive the pneumococcal vaccine and *Haemophilus influenzae* type b vaccine to decrease their risk of developing infections by encapsulated organisms.
- Blood transfusions, which increase the percentage of normal hemoglobin, have been shown to be beneficial in decreasing the occurrence of stroke in children with sickle cell disease.
- Hydroxyurea has been shown to decrease the incidence of painful crises when given prophylactically to patients with sickle cell disease. However, the patient population that receives hydroxyurea should be carefully selected and monitored.
- Fluid replacement, at a rate of 3–4 L/day, is recommended in treating vaso-occlusive crises. Overhydration should be avoided.

- Analgesic options include the parenteral or oral administration of opioids, nonsteroidal anti-inflammatory agents, and acetaminophen. The patient characteristics and the severity of the crisis should determine the choice of agent and regimen.

REFERENCES

1. Herrick JB. Peculiar elongated and sickle-shaped red blood corpuscles in cases of severe anemia. Arch Intern Med 1910;6:517–521.
2. Konotey-Ahulu FID. The sickle cell diseases: clinical manifestations including the "sickle cell." Arch Intern Med 1974;133:611–619.
3. Pauling L, Itano HA, Singer SJ, et al. Sickle cell anemia: a molecular disease. Science 1949;110:543–548.
4. Serjeant GR. Geography and the clinical picture of sickle cell disease: an overview. Ann N Y Acad Sci 1989;565:109–119.
5. Serjeant GR. Sickle Cell Disease. 2nd ed. New York: Oxford Medical Publications, 1992.
6. Powars DR. Beta-s-gene-cluster haplotypes in sickle cell. Hematol Oncol Clin North Am 1991;5:476–447, 485–486.
7. Bunn HF. Pathogenesis and treatment of sickle cell disease. N Engl J Med 1997;337:762–769.
8. Serjeant GR. Sickle cell disease. Lancet 1997;350(9079):725–730.
9. Steinberg MH. Management of sickle cell disease. N Engl J Med 1999;340:1021–1030.
10. Buchanan GR. Sickle cell disease: recent advances. Curr Probl Pediatr 1993;23:219–229.
11. Embury SH, Vichinsky EP. Sickle cell disease. In: Hoffman R, Benz EJ, Shattil SJ, et al., eds. Hematology: Basic Principles and Practices. 3rd ed. New York: Churchill Livingstone, 2000:510–554.
12. Finan AC, Elmer MA, Sasanow SR, et al. Nutritional factors and growth in children with sickle cell disease. Am J Dis Child 1988;142:237–240.
13. Davis H, Schoendorf KC, Gergen PJ, Moore RM Jr. National trends in the mortality of children with sickle cell disease, 1968 through 1992. Am J Public Health 1997;87:1317.
14. Platt OS, Brambilla DJ, Rosse WF, et al. Mortality in sickle cell disease: life expectancy and risk factors for early death. N Engl J Med 1994;330:1639.
15. Ohene-Frempong K. Sickle cell disease. In: Burg FD, Ingelfinger JR, Wald ER, Polin RA, eds. Gellis and Kagan's Current Pediatric Therapy 16. Philadelphia: WB Saunders, 1999:696.
16. Platt OS, Thorington BD, Brambilla DJ, et al. Pain in sickle cell disease: rates and risk factors. N Engl J Med 1994;325:11–16.
17. Miller ST, Sleeper LA, Pegelow CH, et al. Prediction of adverse outcomes in children with sickle cell disease. N Engl J Med 2000;342:83–89.
18. Sprinkle RH, Cole T, Smith S, et al. Acute chest syndrome in children with sickle cell disease. J Pediatr Hematol Oncol 1986;8:105–110.
19. Castro O, Brambilla DJ, Thorington B, et al. The acute chest syndrome in sickle cell disease: incidence and risk factors. The Cooperative Study of Sickle Cell Disease. Blood 1994;84:643–649.
20. Gladwin MT, Rodgers GP. Pathogenesis and treatment of acute chest syndrome of sickle-cell anemia. Lancet 2000;355 (9214):1476–1478.
21. Vichinsky EP, Neumayr LD, Earles AN, et al. Causes and outcomes of the acute chest syndrome in sickle cell disease. National Acute Chest Syndrome Study Group. N Engl J Med 2000;342:1855–1865.
22. Hassell KL, Eckman JR, Lane PA. Acute multiorgan failure syndrome: a potentially catastrophic complication of severe sickle cell pain episodes. Am J Med 1994;96:155–162.
23. Kinney TR, Slepper LA, Wang WC, et al. Silent cerebral infarcts in sickle cell anemia: a risk factor analysis. Pediatrics 1999;103:640–645.
24. Lachman BS, Lazerson J, Starshak RJ, et al. The prevalence of cholelithiasis in sickle cell disease as diagnosed by ultrasound and cholecystography. Pediatrics 1979;64:601–603.
25. Siegel JF, Rich MA, Brock WA. Association of sickle cell disease, priapism, exchange transfusion, and neurological events: ASPEN syndrome. J Urol 1993;150:1480–1482.
26. Eckman JR, Koshy M. Sickle cell disease and pregnancy. Hematology 2000. American Society of Hematology. www.hematology.org/education/educationbook.cfm#32.
27. Committee on Infectious Diseases, 1999–2000. Technical report: prevention of pneumococcal infections, including the use of pneumococcal conjugate and polysaccharide vaccines and antibiotic prophylaxis. Pediatrics 2000;106:367–376.
28. CDC Recommendations and Reports. Preventing pneumococcal disease among infants and young children. MMWR Morb Mortal Wkly Rep 2000; 49:1–38.
29. El-Hazmi MAF, Bahakim HM, Al-Swailem AM, et al. Symptom-free intervals in sicklers: does pneumococcal vaccination and penicillin prophylaxis have a role? J Trop Pediatr 1990;36:56–62.
30. Agil A, Sadrzadeh SM. Hydroxyurea protects against oxidative damage. Redox Rep 2000;5(1):29–34.
31. Charache S, Terrin ML, Moore RD, et al. Effect of hydroxyurea on the frequency of painful crises in sickle cell anemia. N Engl J Med 1995;332: 1317–1322.
32. Wilson S. Acute leukemia in a patient with sickle cell anemia treated with hydroxyurea. Ann Intern Med 2000;133:925–926.
33. Claster S, Vichinsky E. First report of reversal of organ dysfunction in sickle cell anemia by the use of hydroxyurea: splenic regeneration. Blood 1996;88:1951–1953.
34. Rosse WF, Narla M, Petz LD, Steinberg MH. New views of sickle cell disease pathophysiology and treatment. Hematology 2000. American Society of Hematology. www.hematology.org/education/hematology00.cfm.
35. Droxia product labeling. PDR Electronic Library. Montvale, NJ: Medical Economics Company, 2000.
36. Steinberg MH. Review: sickle cell disease—present and future treatment. Am J Med Sci 1996;312:166–174.
37. Jayabose S, Tugal O, Sadoval C, et al. Clinical and hematologic effects of hydroxyurea in children with sickle cell anemia. J Pediatr 1996;120:559–565.
38. Rogers ZR. Hydroxyurea therapy for diverse pediatric populations with sickle-cell disease. Semin Hematol 1997;34(3 suppl 3):42–47.
39. Kinney TR, Helms RW, O'Branski EE, et al. Safety of hydroxyurea in children with sickle cell anemia: results of the HUG-KIDS study, a phase I/II trial. Blood 1999;94:1550–1554.
40. Atweh GF, Sutton M, Nassif I. Sustained induction of fetal hemoglobin by pulse butyrate therapy in sickle cell disease. Blood 1999;93:1790–1797.
41. Koshy M, Dorn L, Bressler L, et al. 2-deoxy 5-azacytidine and fetal hemoglobin induction in sickle cell anemia. Blood 2000:96:2379–2384.
42. Platt A, Eckman J. Sickle Cell Research: Web Update—August 1999. www.emory.edu/PEDS/SICKLE/Reserch.htm (Accessed 2000 August 30).
43. Ambrus JL. Stiff red cell syndrome: a review of the treatment of sickle cell disease with pentoxifylline. J Med 1993;24:1–9.
44. Sherer JT, Glover, PH. Pentoxifylline for sickle cell disease. Ann Pharmacother 2000;34:1070–1074.
45. Charache S. Experimental therapy. Hematol Oncol Clin North Am 1996; 10:1373–1382.
46. El-Hazmi MA, al-Momen A, Kandaswany S, et al. On the use of hydroxyurea/erythropoietin combination therapy for sickle cell anemia. Acta Haematol 1995:94(3):128–134.
47. Adams RJ, McKie VC, Hsu L, et al. Prevention of a first stroke by transfusions in children with sickle cell anemia and abnormal results of transcranial Doppler ultrasonography. N Engl J Med 1998;339: 5–11.
48. Vichinsky EP. Current issues with blood transfusions in sickle cell disease. Semin Hematol 2001;38(suppl 1):14–22.
49. Petz LD, Calhoun L, Shulman IA, et al. The sickle cell hemolytic transfusion reaction syndrome. Transfusion 1997;37:382–392.
50. Walters MC, Storb R, Patience M, et al. Impact of bone marrow transplantation for symptomatic sickle cell disease: an interim report. Blood 2000;95:1918–1924.
51. Reed W, Vichinsky EP. New considerations in the treatment of sickle cell disease. Annu Rev Med 1998;49:461–474.

52. Powars DR, Johnson CS. Priapism. Hematol Oncol Clin North Am 1996; 10:1363–1372.
53. Mantadakis E, Ewalt DH, Cavender JD, et al. Outpatient penile aspiration and epinephrine irrigation for young patients with sickle cell anemia and prolonged priapism. Blood 2000;95:78–82.
54. Shanta TR, Finnerty DP, Rodriguez AL. Treatment of persistent penile erection and priapism using terbutaline. J Urol 1989;141:1427–1429.
55. Shanta TR. Intraoperative management of penile erection by using terbutaline. Anesthesiology 1989;70:707–709.
56. Levine LA, Guss SP, Gonadotropin-releasing hormone analogues in the treatment of sickle cell anemia-associated priapism. J Urol 1993;150: 475–477.
57. Steinberg J, Eyre RC. Management of recurrent priapism with epinephrine self-injection and gonadotropin-releasing hormone analogue. J Urol 1995; 153:152–153.
58. Al Jamia AH, Al Dabbous TA. Hydroxyurea in the treatment of sickle cell associated priapism. J Urol 1998;159:1642.
59. Vichinsky E, Styles L. Pulmonary complications. Hematol Oncol Clin North Am 1996;10:1275–1286.
60. Dover GT, Vichinsky EP, Serjeant GR, Eckman JR. Update in the treatment of sickle cell anemia: issues in supportive care and new strategies. www.hematology.org/education/hematology99.html Accessed 2000 September 21.
61. Sullivan KJ, Goodwin SR, Evangelist J, et al. Nitrous oxide successfully used to treat acute chest syndrome of sickle cell disease in a young adolescent. Crit Care Med 1999;7:2563–2568.
62. Rao SP, Miller ST, Cohen BJ. Transient aplastic crisis in patients with sickle cell disease: B19 parvovirus studies during a 7-year period. Am J Dis Child 1992;146:1328–30.
63. Mallouh AA, Qudah A. An epidemic of aplastic crisis caused by human parvovirus B19. Pediatr Infect Dis J 1995;14:31–34.
64. Evans JPM. Practical management of sickle cell disease. Arch Dis Child 1989;64:1748–1751.
65. American Pain Society. Guideline for the management of acute and chronic pain in sickle cell disease. Glenview, IL: 1999.
66. Panepinto JA, Magid D, Rewers MJ, Lane PA. Universal versus targeted screening of infants for sickle cell disease: a cost-effectiveness analysis. J Pediatr 2000;136(2):201–208.
67. Davis H, Moore RM, Gergen PJ. Cost of hospitalizations associated with sickle cell disease in the United States. Public Health Rep 1997;112:40–43.
68. Shechter AN. Sickle cell disease expenditures and outcomes. Public Health Rep 1997;112:38–39.
69. Woods K, Karrison T, Koshy M, et al. Hospital utilization patterns and costs for sickle cell patients in Illinois. Public Health Rep 1997;112: 44–51.
70. Nietert PJ, Abboud MR, Zoller JS, Silverstein MD. Costs, charges and reimbursements for persons with sickle cell disease. J Pediatr Hematol Oncol 1999;21(5):389–396.
71. Woods K, Kutlar A, Grigsby RK , et al. Primary care delivery for sickle cell patients in rural Georgia using telemedicine. Telemed J 1998;(4):353–361.

102

DRUG-INDUCED HEMATOLOGIC DISORDERS

Kenneth P. Klinker, J. William Harbilas, and Thomas E. Johns

Hematologic disorders have long been a potential risk of modern pharmacotherapy. Granulocytopenia (agranulocytosis) was reported in association with one of medicine's early therapeutic agents, sulphanilamide, in 1938.[1] Some agents cause predictable hematologic disease (e.g., antineoplastics), but others induce idiosyncratic reactions not directly related to the drugs' pharmacology. Such drug-induced hematologic disorders may include aplastic anemia, agranulocytosis, megaloblastic anemia, thrombocytopenia, and hemolytic anemia.[2]

By most reports, idiosyncratic drug-induced hematologic disorders are rare. Relatively few epidemiologic studies have addressed the actual incidence of these adverse reactions. A recent report from The Netherlands estimated the incidence of drug-associated agranulocytosis as 1.6 to 2.5 cases per million inhabitants per year.[3] Similar results were found in epidemiologic studies in Thailand.[4,5] Older data from a study conducted in Europe and Israel estimated the incidences of aplastic anemia and agranulocytosis to be 0.5 and 3.1 cases per million per year, respectively.[6]

Although rare, drug-induced hematologic disorders are important because they are associated with significant morbidity and mortality. An epidemiologic study held in the United States estimated that 4,490 deaths in 1984 were attributable to blood dyscrasias from all causes. Aplastic anemia was the leading cause of death, followed by thrombocytopenia, agranulocytosis, and hemolytic anemia.[7] Like most other adverse drug reactions, drug-induced hematologic disorders are more common in the elderly than in the young; the risk of death also appears to be greater with increasing age. The risk of agranulocytosis has been reported to be higher in women than in men.[4]

Because of the seriousness of drug-induced hematologic disorders, it is necessary to track the development of these disorders in order to predict their occurrence and to estimate their incidence. Reporting during postmarketing surveillance of a drug is the most common method of establishing the incidence of adverse drug reactions. The MedWatch program supported by the Food and Drug Administration is one such program.[8] Many facilities have similar drug-reporting programs to follow adverse drug reaction trends and to determine whether an association between a drug and an adverse drug reaction is causal or coincidental. In the case of drug-induced hematologic disorders, these programs can enable practitioners to confirm that an adverse event is indeed the result of drug therapy rather than one of many other potential causes; general guidelines are readily available.[9,10] Because drug-induced blood disorders are dangerous, rechallenging a patient with a suspected agent in an attempt to confirm a diagnosis may not be ethical. *In vitro* studies with the offending agent and cells or plasma from the patient's blood have been described to determine causality.[11] These methods are often expensive, however, and require facilities and expertise that are not generally available. One study demonstrated that only 19% of the cases with suspected drug-induced agranulocytosis could be documented by *in vitro* testing.[12]

The rarity and seriousness of drug-induced hematologic disorders make it extremely important that clinicians be able to evaluate suspect drugs quickly and to interrupt therapy when necessary. Throughout the past decades, lists of drugs that have been associated with adverse events have been developed to help clinicians identify possible causes of adverse events. Unfortunately, these lists are comprehensive and include commonly used drugs, making it difficult to elicit the root cause of any abnormality. It is imperative that clinicians use a rational approach in determining causality and identifying the agents that definitely cause the reaction. Focusing on the issue, performing a high-quality investigation, developing appropriate criteria, using levels of evidence to grade the response, and having a quantifiable summary can all help to ensure the validity of the findings. A systematic approach to evaluate the information available in the literature also helps the clinician to focus and intervene on the cause of the disorder.

The understanding of drug-induced hematologic disorders requires a basic understanding of hematopoiesis (see Chap. 98, Hematopoiesis). The pluripotential hematopoietic stem cells in the bone marrow, which have the ability to self-reproduce, maintain the blood. These pluripotential hematopoietic stem cells are further differentiated to intermediate precursor cells, which are also called "progenitor cells" or "colony-forming cells." Committed to a particular cell line, these intermediate stem cells differentiate into colonies of each type of blood cell in response to a particular colony-stimulating factor (Fig. 102–1).

Drug-induced hematologic disorders can affect any cell line, including white blood cells (WBCs), red blood cells (RBCs), and platelets. When a drug causes decreases in all three cell lines accompanied by a hypoplastic bone marrow, the result is termed drug-induced aplastic anemia. The decrease in WBC count alone by a medication is termed drug-induced agranulocytosis. Drugs can affect RBCs by causing a number of different anemias, including drug-induced immune hemolytic anemia, drug-induced oxidative hemolytic anemia, or drug-induced megaloblastic anemia. A drug-induced decrease in platelet count is termed drug-induced thrombocytopenia.

DRUG-INDUCED APLASTIC ANEMIA

Ehrlich first described aplastic anemia in 1888 following an episode of failed hematopoiesis identified during the autopsy of a pregnant women.[13] Since then, there have been 500 to 2500 cases reported annually, with up to 33% diagnosed in patients greater than 60 years of age.[13] A number of variables can incite immune destruction of the bone marrow, the most common are drugs, chemicals, toxins, viruses, and radiation.

Drug-induced aplastic anemia is classified as an acquired form of the disorder and accounts for 7% to 86% of cases of aplastic anemia.[14] It is considered the most serious drug-induced blood dyscrasia because of the associated high mortality rate, often exceeding 50% of treated cases.[15] It is characterized by pancytopenia (presence of anemia, neutropenia, and thrombocytopenia) with a hypocellular or "fatty" bone marrow and no gross evidence of increased peripheral blood cell destruction.[2] A diagnosis of aplastic anemia can be

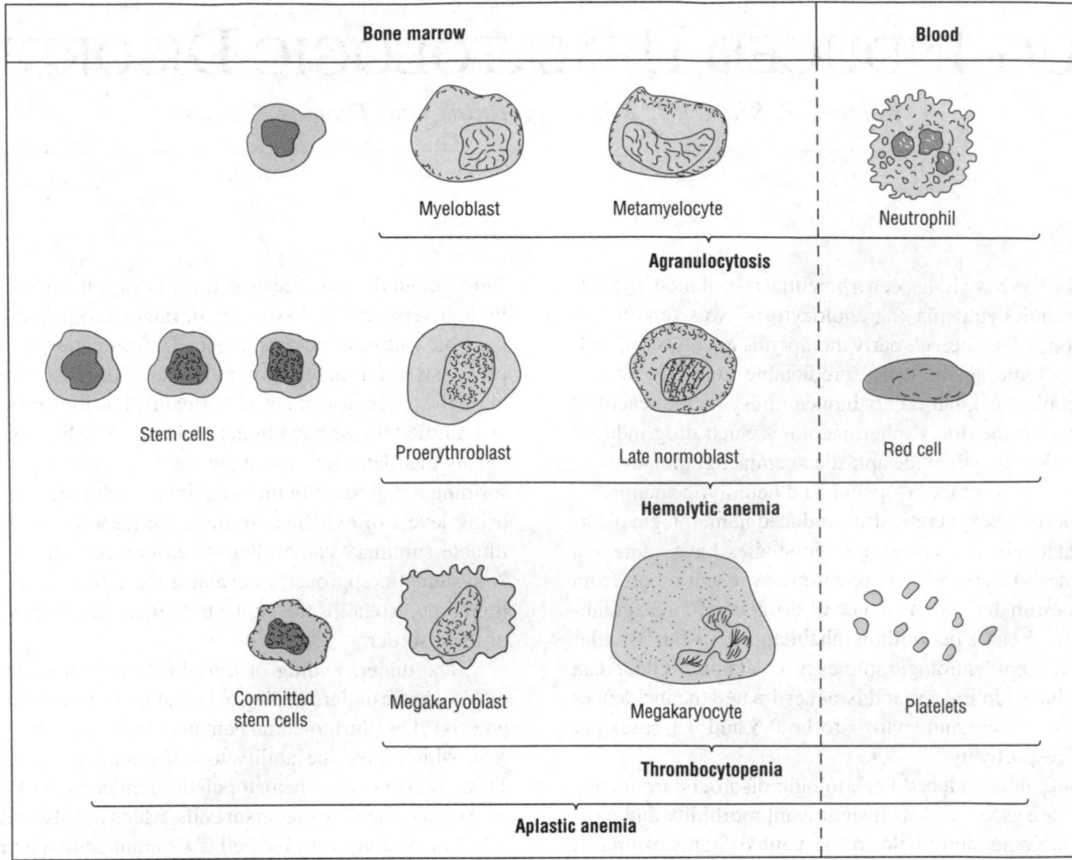

FIGURE 102–1. Differentiation of the stem cell to committed cell lines, illustrating the origins of various drug-induced hematologic disorders.

made by the presence of two of the following criteria: a WBC count of 3,500/μL or less, a platelet count of 55,000/μL or less, or a hemoglobin value of 10 g/dL or less with a reticulocyte count of 30,000/μL or less.[15] Severe aplastic anemia is defined by at least two of the following three peripheral blood findings: neutrophil count of less than 500/μL, platelet count of less than 20,000/μL, and anemia with a corrected reticulocyte index of less than 1%.[15,16] The prognosis is extremely poor if the neutrophil count declines to less than 200/μL.[17] A bone marrow aspirate and biopsy are required to exclude other causes of pancytopenia, including neoplastic infiltration or significant myelofibrosis.[18] There must also be no history of iatrogenic exposure to cytotoxic chemotherapy that is known to cause transient bone marrow suppression or to intensive radiation.

The onset of drug-induced aplastic anemia is variable and insidious. Symptoms appear on the average about 6.5 weeks after the initiation of the offending agent,[19] sometimes after the drug has been discontinued. Clinical features of drug-induced aplastic anemia depend on the degree to which each cell line is suppressed, similar to idiopathic disease. Symptoms of anemia include pallor, fatigue, and weakness, while fever, chills, pharyngitis, or other infection may characterize neutropenia. Thrombocytopenia, often the initial clue to diagnosis, is manifested by easy bruisability, petechiae, and bleeding.

The incidence of drug-induced aplastic anemia is estimated at 0.5 to 7.8 cases per 1 million population per year.[6,20,21] Higher rates of occurrence have been seen in patients taking such drugs as indomethacin, penicillamine, and gold compounds.[15] Table 102–1 lists drugs that have been associated with drug-induced aplastic anemia.

The cause of drug-induced aplastic anemia is damage to the pluripotential hematopoietic stem cells, before their differentiation to committed stem cells. This damage effectively reduces the normal levels of circulating erythrocytes, neutrophils, and platelets. Three mechanisms have been proposed as causes of damage to the pluripotential hematopoietic stem cells.[19,22] The most common proposed mechanism is direct, dose-dependent drug toxicity. This type of injury leads to transient marrow failure secondary to direct suppression of proliferating cell lines, and hematopoietic suppression continues with dose escalation. Most often caused by chemotherapy or radiotherapy, this injury is frequently iatrogenic. The second mechanism is idiosyncratic and operates through toxic metabolites. Further, individual variations in the pharmacokinetics of the suspected agent or a hypersensitivity of the stem cells to the destructive effects of the implicated drug may increase the potential for apoptosis. The third mechanism is a drug- or metabolite-induced immune reaction specific to the stem cell population. It is proposed that immunologically mediated, tissue-specific organ destruction occurs following exposure to an inciting antigen

TABLE 102–1. Drugs Associated with Aplastic Anemia

Acetazolamide	Felbamate	Phenothiazines
Aspirin	Furosemide	Phenytoin
Captopril	Gold salts	Propylthiouracil
Carbamazepine	Indomethacin	Quinacrine
Chloramphenicol	Interferon-α	Quinidine
Chloroquine	Methimazole	Sulfonamides
Chlorothiazide	Oxyphenbutazone	Sulfonylureas
Chlorpromazine	Penicillamine	Sulindac
Dapsone	Pentoxifylline	Ticlopidine
Diclofenac	Phenobarbital	

(drug) that activates cells and cytokines of the immune system, leading to the death of stem cells.[22] There is little evidence that drug-induced aplastic anemia results from the destruction of the microenvironment of the bone marrow.[18]

The antineoplastic agents exemplify the dose-dependent mechanism for the development of aplastic anemia. Many of these agents have the ability to suppress one or more cell lines in a reversible manner. The degree of suppression and the cell line involved depends on the nature of the particular drug and its potential for inhibiting marrow proliferation. Chloramphenicol, an antimicrobial agent, also causes a bone marrow depression that is dose-dependent and reversible. In this reaction, chloramphenicol affects primarily the erythroid cell line due to an injury of the mitochondria, resulting in inhibition of protein synthesis with a subsequent reduction in reticulocytes and hematocrit.[23]

Idiosyncratic drug-induced aplastic anemia secondary to direct toxicity may be characterized by dose independence, a latent period prior to the onset of anemia, and continuance of the marrow injury following drug discontinuation.[24] Drugs that cause aplastic anemia in a minority of patients suggest an abnormal metabolism or excretion. Chloramphenicol, already known to cause a dose-dependent reaction, is the prototype drug for the idiosyncratic mechanism, with an approximate incidence of 1 case per 20,000 patients treated;[17] however, the overall incidence has fallen with decreased use of this agent.[24] The idiosyncratic mechanism is believed to result from abnormal metabolism of chloramphenicol. The nitrobenzene ring on chloramphenicol is thought to be reduced to form a nitroso group on the chloramphenicol molecule.[23] The nitroso group may then interact with DNA in the stem cell, causing damage to the chromosomes and, eventually, cell death. Other investigators have hypothesized that bacteria from the gastrointestinal tract may metabolize chloramphenicol to marrow-toxic metabolites.[25] There appears to be no relationship between the dose-dependent and idiosyncratic reactions seen with chloramphenicol.

Other drugs thought to induce aplastic anemia through toxic metabolites include phenytoin and carbamazepine. Investigators have theorized that metabolites from phenytoin and carbamazepine bind covalently to macromolecules in the cell and then cause cell death either by exerting a direct toxic effect on the stem cell or by causing the death of lymphocytes involved in regulating hematopoiesis.[26]

Of the three potential mechanisms, the most common cause of drug-induced aplastic anemia is the development of an immune reaction. Early laboratory observations revealed that the removal of T lymphocytes from samples of patients with aplastic anemia improved *in vitro* colony formation.[27] Further, overproduction of cytokines (e.g., tumor necrosis factor, interferon-γ) from activated T lymphocytes appears to be responsible for hematopoietic failure, as well as for the initiation of apoptosis.[28] Clinical evidence supporting this hypothesis revolves around improved hematopoiesis in patients who receive a conditioning regimen with antithymocyte globulin and cyclophosphamide prior to allogeneic bone marrow transplantation (BMT).[29] After the initiation of immunosuppressive therapy, bone marrow concentrations of interferon-γ decreased, while all cell lines improved.[30] Inciting agents (i.e., drugs) are suspected to affect the function of suppressor T cells, which could inhibit stem cell production.[19]

Inconsistencies in the identification of antibodies to medication have made it difficult to implicate drugs as the main determinant for the development of hematologic disease. Rather, clinical history and exposure history determine the assignment of causality. Additional supporting evidence for an immunologic basis as a mechanism of aplastic anemia comes from a prospective, randomized, placebo-controlled trial evaluating the efficacy of antilymphocyte globulin and methylprednisolone, with or without cyclosporine in patients with severe aplastic anemia.[31] The primary response variable was an improvement in blood counts (i.e., platelets, erythrocytes, and leukocytes) at 3 months. Patients receiving therapy with antilymphocyte globulin, methylprednisolone, and cyclosporine had a response rate of 65% versus a response rate of 39% in the group not receiving cyclosporine. This finding lends support to the fact that patients receiving aggressive immunotherapy are more likely to recover from a hematologic disorder and further implicates immunomodulation as a cause of disease.

Genetic predisposition may also influence the development of drug-induced aplastic anemia. Studies in animals and a case report of chloramphenicol-induced aplastic anemia in identical twins suggest a genetic predisposition to the development of drug-induced aplastic anemia.[18,23] Further, pharmacogenetic research into genotypes of the cytochrome P450 system that focuses on patients who may be slow or normal metabolizers of drugs may increase the clinician's ability to predict the development of aplastic anemia. Initial case-control studies have not had the power necessary to identify a statistical difference between controls and cases, but continued research may provide evidence to altered metabolism in this population.[32]

▶ TREATMENT: Drug-Induced Aplastic Anemia

Because of an extremely high mortality rate among patients with this disorder, it is imperative that drug-induced aplastic anemia be diagnosed quickly and therapy initiated immediately. It must be emphasized that prognosis, response to therapy, and management of drug-induced aplastic anemia is similar to that of idiopathic disease.[33] The goals of therapy are to improve peripheral blood counts so that patients do not require transfusions and are not at risk for opportunistic infections.

As with all cases of drug-induced hematologic disorders, the first step is to remove the suspected offending agent. Early withdrawal of the agent may allow for reversal of the aplastic anemia.[17] The next step is to provide adequate supportive care, including symptomatic treatment of infection and transfusion support with erythrocytes and platelets. Appropriate supportive care is essential, as the major causes of mortality in patients with aplastic anemia are infections and bleeding. A recent study showed that 62% of deaths were due to infections, consisting mostly of bacterial and fungal pathogens.[34] Current treatment guidelines do not include chemoprophylaxis, except in patients undergoing BMT. Therefore, in patients receiving immunotherapy, fever of unknown origin should be aggressively managed.

A recent retrospective analysis reviewing the outcomes of patients who underwent allogeneic BMT for severe aplastic anemia between 1978 and 1991 showed an 89% response rate (including complete and partial responses).[35] The 15-year survival rate for complete and partial responders to BMT was 75% and 64%, respectively. Improvement in supportive care, prevention of graft versus host disease, and improved engraftment have further enhanced survival benefits. Considerations in deciding to treat patients with BMT are the availability of a donor, the age of the patient, the absolute neutrophil count, and the number of transfusions received prior to transplantation.[35]

An alternative to BMT is immunosuppressive therapy. Current options for this approach include antithymocyte globulin, antilymphocyte globulin, cyclosporine, and glucocorticoids. Antithymocyte globulin is a polyclonal immunoglobulin that disrupts cell-mediated immune responses and may have some immunostimulatory effects.[36] Antithymocyte globulin monotherapy may achieve response rates up to 50% of patients.[37] Recommended dosing of antithymocyte globulin has varied from 40 mg/kg/day for 4 days to 15–20 mg/kg/day for 8 to 14 days. Shorter, more intense regimens are preferred, as they are associated with fewer adverse events (i.e., serum sickness).[38] Corticosteroids (i.e., methylprednisolone) have long been used in conjunction with antithymocyte globulin for the management of drug-induced aplastic anemia, but their efficacy is questionable.[17] They have minimal effects on hematopoiesis, although they benefit patients by decreasing the incidence of serum sickness. Methylprednisolone dosing is 1 mg/kg/day for 4 weeks. Cyclosporine blocks T-lymphocyte proliferation and function through alterations in IL-2 concentrations. Cyclosporine dosing has varied from 4–6 mg/kg/day to 10–12 mg/kg/day with response rates equivalent to those of antithymocyte globulin monotherapy. Recommended dosing of cyclosporine is 5 mg/kg/day and titrated to a target blood concentration of 500 ng/mL. Adverse effects of cyclosporine include hypertension, renal failure, tremor, electrolyte abnormalities, and opportunistic infections.

The optimal immunosuppressive regimen is a combination of antithymocyte globulin, glucocorticoids, and cyclosporine. Three-year survival rates can approach 90%,[31,39] which is comparable to that for BMT and makes immunosuppressive therapy a plausible option for patients who are elderly (age >50 years), those who lack an eligible donor, and those who have less severe disease. A recent study evaluating immunosuppressive therapy in the elderly revealed a 6-year survival rate of 50%.[40] These data provide additional support for the aggressive management of all patients with aplastic anemia, regardless of age. Long-term complications of immunosuppressive therapy include relapse and conversion to other stem cell disorders (e.g., myelodysplastic syndrome, acute myelogenous leukemia, paroxysmal nocturnal hemoglobinuria), which have occurred with relatively high incidence.[17,35]

Granulocyte colony-stimulating factor (G-CSF),[41] granulocyte-macrophage colony-stimulating factor (GM-CSF),[42] and IL-1[43] have also been investigated in the treatment of aplastic anemia. G-CSF, in combination with aggressive immunotherapy, may improve trilineage hematopoietic reconstitution, but it is unclear whether current data support a positive effect on outcomes (i.e., infectious complications and improved survival).[41] Therefore, prospective evaluations are required to further delineate the role of G-CSF in aplastic anemia. If long-term bone marrow suppression continues after initial treatment with optimal immunosuppression, the only viable option at present is allogeneic BMT. Otherwise, aggressive immunosuppressive therapy plays a distinct role in treating patients with drug-induced aplastic anemia and provides a viable alternative to patients ineligible for BMT.

DRUG-INDUCED AGRANULOCYTOSIS

It is possible to define drug-induced agranulocytosis as a drug-mediated reduction in the number of mature myeloid cells in the blood (granulocytes and immature granulocytes [bands]) to a total count of 500/μL or less. Symptoms of agranulocytosis include sore throat, fever, malaise, weakness, and chills. It occurs more frequently in females than in males,[44] with an overall estimated incidence of 1.6 to 3.4 million persons per year.[3,15] The overall mortality rate in agranulocytosis is 16%; the rate increases among patients with agranulocytosis when they develop bacteremia or renal failure.[45] The symptoms can appear rapidly, within 7 to 14 days after the initiation of the offending agent. In contrast, patients with phenothiazine-induced agranulocytosis can be asymptomatic at the time of diagnosis, probably because they have a milder form of the disorder.[46] In the large majority of cases, drug-induced agranulocytosis will resolve over time.[46] Table 102–2 provides a list of medications that have been associated with drug-induced agranulocytosis.

A number of different mechanisms may lead to drug-induced agranulocytosis. Initially, it was thought that drugs affected only the mature granulocytes, causing a "maturation arrest." In recent years, however, studies have demonstrated that drugs may have a toxic effect on the myeloid colony-forming unit in the bone marrow (either a direct toxic effect or an antibody-mediated effect);[47,48] this may be the most frequent mechanism of drug-induced agranulocytosis.[44]

Drug-induced agranulocytosis can be classified into three types.[49] The type I reaction is immune-mediated and involves the drug or drug metabolite, antibodies, and neutrophils. A type II reaction is associated with accumulated drug toxicity in hypersensitive individuals. The final type, type III, results from a combination of both immune and toxic mechanisms.

It has been postulated that drug-induced immune agranulocytosis (type I) develops by one of four different mechanisms.[50] The first mechanism involves drug adsorption on the membrane of the neutrophil. The drug-membrane complex then acts as a hapten to stimulate antibody formation. The antibodies produced attach to the drug-membrane complex, causing WBC destruction through complement activation and removal by the phagocytic system (Fig.102–2). This hapten-type reaction is often seen when drugs, such as the penicillin derivatives, are given in large doses. The dose at which this immune-mediated reaction occurs is higher than 150 mg/kg/day with the majority of penicillin derivatives, but has occurred at lower doses.[48,51,52]

The second mechanism of immune-mediated agranulocytosis is called the "innocent bystander phenomenon." In this reaction, the drug combines with a drug-specific antibody. The complex is

TABLE 102–2. Drugs Associated with Agranulocytosis

Acetaminophen	Flucytosine	Penicillamine
Acetazolamide	Fosphenytoin	Pentazocine
Allopurinol	Furosemide	Phenothiazines
p-Aminosalicylic acid	Ganciclovir	Phenytoin
Benzodiazepines	Gentamicin	Primidone
β-Lactam antibiotics	Gold salts	Procainamide
Brompheniramine	Griseofulvin	Propranolol
Captopril	Hydralazine	Propylthiouracil
Carbamazepine	Hydroxychloroquine	Pyrimethamine
Chloramphenicol	Imipenem–cilastatin	Quinine
Chloropropamide	Imipramine	Rifampin
Cimetidine	Isoniazid	Streptomycin
Clindamycin	Levodopa	Sulfonamides
Clomipramine	Lincomycin	Sulfonylureas
Clozapine	Meprobamate	Thiazide diuretics
Colchicine	Methazolamide	Ticlopidine
Dapsone	Methimazole	Tocainide
Desipramine	Methyldopa	Tolbutamide
Doxycycline	Metronidazole	Vancomycin
Ethacrynic acid	Nitrofurantoin	Zidovudine
Ethosuximide	NSAIDs	

NSAIDs = nonsteroidal anti-inflammatory drugs.

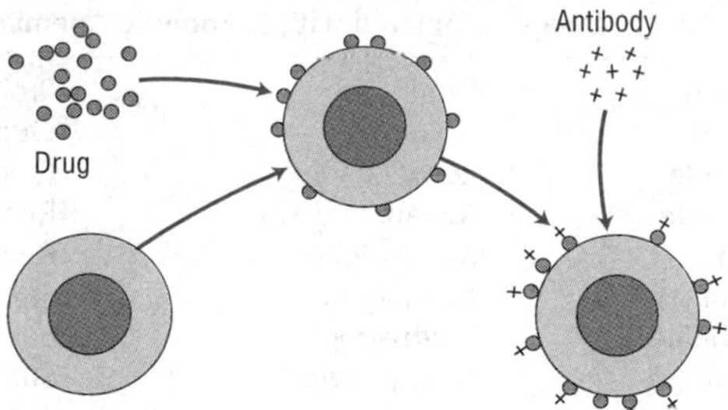

FIGURE 102–2. Drug adsorption mechanism. The drug binds to the membrane of the blood cell. Antibodies are formed to the drug-membrane complex (a hapten). The antibodies then attach to the complex, and cell toxicity occurs. *From Petz LD. Drug-induced haemolytic anaemia. Ballieres Clin Haematol 1980:91:455–482. With permission.*

nonspecifically adsorbed to the neutrophil membrane, resulting in complement activation. The activated complement then destroys the cell (Fig. 102–3). Quinidine has been associated with this type of reaction.

Functioning in a manner somewhat similar to that of the second mechanism, the third mechanism of immune response involves a protein carrier that combines with the drug and then attaches to the cell membrane. This, in turn, causes antibody formation. The antibodies attach to the drug protein carrier–membrane complex and activate complement. The cells are then cleared by the phagocytic system (Fig. 102–4).

The final mechanism for an immune-mediated reaction is the production of autoantibodies to a "spoiled membrane." The offending drug alters the neutrophil membrane, which induces the formation of autoantibodies (antibodies that attach directly to the neutrophil). Their attachment to the neutrophil causes cellular destruction by the phagocytic system.

The onset of symptoms associated with immune-mediated mechanisms is rapid, occurring in 7 to 15 days of drug exposure. In the case of penicillin-induced agranulocytosis, the patient can often begin taking penicillin again, at a lower dosage, after the neutropenia has resolved without any relapse of drug-induced agranulocytosis.[51,52] Because of the rapid onset of symptoms and the dose-related phenomenon, a second mechanism (type II) could possibly be involved with penicillin-induced agranulocytosis. This mechanism involves an accumulation of drug to toxic concentrations in hypersensitive individuals. Researchers have shown with *in vitro* cell cultures that penicillin derivatives in high concentrations inhibit the growth of

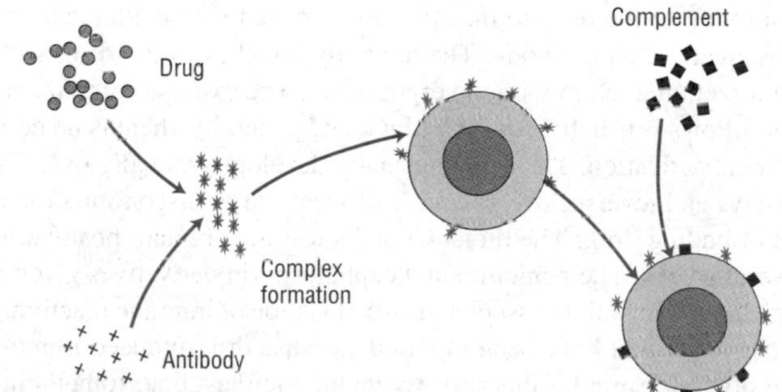

FIGURE 102–3. Innocent bystander mechanism. The drug induces antibody formation. The antibodies and drug form a complex in the serum, and the complex nonspecifically binds to the cell membrane. Complement is activated, and the cell is lysed. *From Petz LD. Drug-induced haemolytic anaemia. Ballicres Clin Haematol 1980:91:455–482. With permission.*

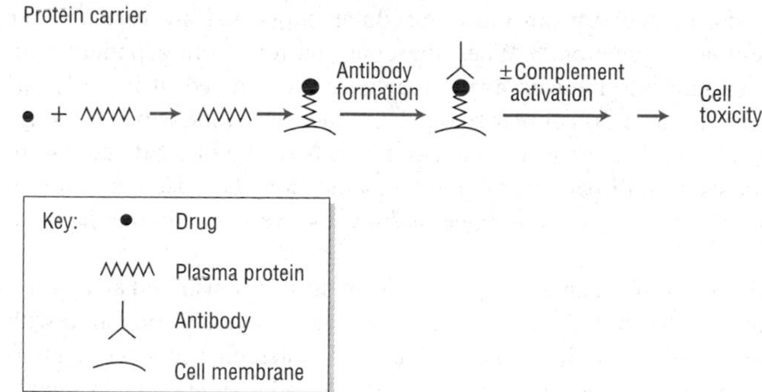

FIGURE 102–4. Protein carrier mechanism. The drug combines with a plasma protein. The complex then attaches to the cell membrane, and antibody formation is stimulated. Antibodies later attach to the complex and activate complement. The cell is lysed then by the complement. *From Ref. 50, with permission.*

myeloid colony-forming units in patients recovering from drug-induced agranulocytosis.[53] Penicillin derivatives, therefore, may suppress WBCs by several mechanisms.

Antithyroid medications such as propylthiouracil and methimazole produce agranulocytosis in about 0.3% to 0.6% of patients.[54,55] The mechanism by which antithyroid agents cause agranulocytosis is unknown, but antibodies to granulocytes have been demonstrated.[56,57] In a study by Cooper and coworkers,[54] agranulocytosis occurred more frequently in older patients (> 40 years old), and it appeared within 2 months after the initiation of therapy. The investigators also reported a possible dose relationship with methimazole.[54] For patients receiving less than 30 mg/day of methimazole, no agranulocytosis occurred, but in patients receiving higher doses, neutropenia was evident.[54] There appeared to be no dose relationship with conventional doses of propylthiouracil. However, another study demonstrated no relationship between age or dose in the incidence of thionamide-induced agranulocytosis.[58]

Ticlopidine is an antiplatelet agent indicated for the treatment of cerebrovascular disease and the prevention of reocclusion associated with stent placement. It produces agranulocytosis in approximately 2.4% of patients,[59] reportedly by inhibiting myeloid colony growth.[60] This evidence supports a potential direct toxic effect of ticlopidine on the bone marrow. In addition, ticlopidine is associated with an increase in concentrations of prostaglandin E_1, a known myelosuppressant.[61] Other factors association with the development of agranulocytosis include poor medullary reserve and age. Agranulocytosis occurs within 1–3 months from the initiation of therapy. Removal of the agent is the best treatment option, with counts returning to normal within 2 to 4 weeks.

The phenothiazines as a group are known to cause a type II drug-induced agranulocytosis. The onset of phenothiazine-induced agranulocytosis is approximately 2 to 15 weeks after the initiation of therapy.[50] Although, there is one report of acute agranulocytosis in a child who accidentally ingested a large quantity of chlorpromazine.[47] Usually, patients have ingested 10–20 g of a phenothiazine before the onset of neutropenia. Phenothiazine-induced agranulocytosis occurs most frequently in females older than 50 years of age.[46] The mechanism by which phenothiazines cause the drug-induced agranulocytosis has been studied primarily with chlorpromazine,[46] which is thought to affect cells in the cell cycle phase that manufactures enzymes needed for DNA synthesis (G_1 phase) or the phase in which cells are resting and not committed to cell division (G_0 phase).[46] The antipsychotic agents are known to precipitate proteins and may coprecipitate polynucleotides so they can no longer participate in nucleic acid synthesis. Chlorpromazine also increases the loss of macromolecules from the intracellular pools that are essential for cellular replication.[46] When the bone marrow from a patient with phenothiazine-induced agranulocytosis is examined, it initially appears to have no cellularity (aplastic), but over time it becomes hyperplastic. It is believed that toxic effects of the phenothiazines are not seen in all patients taking the medications because the majority of patients have enough bone marrow reserve to overcome the toxic effects.[46]

Clozapine, an antipsychotic agent, has demonstrated an approximately 10-fold higher incidence of agranulocytosis compared with other antipsychotics.[62] The incidence of clozapine-induced agranulocytosis increases with age and occurs more frequently in female patients.[63] There appear to be no dose-related effects with clozapine-induced agranulocytosis.[63] The agranulocytosis is reversible if detected early in therapy; therefore, close monitoring of the WBC count is warranted. An *in vitro* study has suggested that the formation of a free radical metabolite may be responsible for clozapine-induced agranulocytosis.[64] The resulting oxidative stress caused by this metabolite may cause cytotoxicity or an immune reaction.[64]

▶ TREATMENT: Drug-Induced Agranulocytosis

The primary treatment of drug-induced agranulocytosis is the removal of the offending drug. Following discontinuation of the drug, most cases of neutropenia resolve over time, and only symptomatic treatment (e.g., antimicrobials for infections) is necessary. Sargramostim (GM-CSF) and filgrastim (G-CSF) have been used to shorten the duration of neutropenia with varying degrees of success. A recent review of 118 cases of nonchemotherapy-induced agranulocytosis treated with colony-stimulating factors revealed a decrease in the duration of neutropenia with a trend toward improved mortality, especially in patients with granulocyte counts of less than 100 cells/μL.[65] The time to recovery of the granulocyte count ranged from 3 to 15 days.[66–69]

DRUG-INDUCED HEMOLYTIC ANEMIA

Following their release from the bone marrow, normal RBCs have 120 days before they are removed by phagocytic cells of the spleen and liver. The process of destroying RBCs prematurely is referred to as hemolysis, which can occur either because of defects in the RBCs themselves or because of abnormal changes in the intravascular environment. Drugs can promote hemolysis by both processes.

The causes of drug-induced hemolytic anemia can be divided into two categories: immune or metabolic. Those in the first category may operate much like the process that leads to immune-regulated agranulocytosis, or they may suppress regulator cells, which allows the production of autoantibodies. The second category involves the induction of hemolysis by metabolic abnormalities in the RBCs. Patients with drug-induced hemolytic anemia can present with signs of intravascular or extravascular hemolysis. Intravascular hemolysis, the lysis of RBCs in the circulation, can result from trauma, complement fixation to the RBC, or exogenous toxic factors. Extravascular hemolysis refers to the ingestion of RBCs by macrophages in the spleen and liver, a process that requires the existence of surface abnormalities on RBCs, such as bound immunoglobulin.[70] The onset of drug-induced hemolytic anemia is variable and depends on the drug and mechanism of the hemolysis. Table 102–3 provides a list of drugs that have been associated with drug-induced hemolytic anemia.

TABLE 102–3. Drugs Associated with Hemolytic Anemia

ACE inhibitors	Isoniazid	Procainamide
Acetaminophen	Levodopa	Quinidine
Acetazolamide	Levofloxacin	Quinine
Acetohexamide	Mefanamic acid	Rifabutin
Amprenavir	Metaxolone	Rifampin
β-Lactam antibiotics	Methadone	Streptomycin
Dimenhydrinate	Methyldopa	Sulfonamides
Flurbiprofen	Methysergide	Sulfonyureas
Gatifloxacin	Nomifensine	Tacrolimus
Grepafloxacin	NSAIDs	Tetracycline
Hydralazine	Omeprazole	Ticlopidine
Hydrochlorothiazide	p-Aminosalicylic acid	Tolbutamide
Imipenem–cilastatin	Phenazopyridine	Tolmetin
Indinavir	Probenecid	Triamterene

ACE = angiotensin-converting enzyme; NSAIDs = nonsteroidal anti-inflammatory drugs.

DRUG-INDUCED IMMUNE HEMOLYTIC ANEMIA

A laboratory test called the direct Coombs test (or direct anti-human globulin test), which identifies foreign immunoglobulins either in the patient's serum or on the RBCs themselves, is the best means to identify drug-induced immune hemolytic anemia. The Coombs test begins with the antiglobulin serum, which is produced by injecting rabbits with preparations of human complement, Fc fragments, or immunoglobulins. The rabbits produce antibodies that are foreign to human immunoglobulins and complement. The direct Coombs test involves combining the patient's RBCs with the antiglobulin serum. If the patient's RBCs are coated with antibody or complement (as a result of a drug-induced process), the antibodies in the serum (produced by the rabbit) will attach to the Fc regions of the autoimmune globulins on two separate RBCs, creating a lattice formation called agglutination.[71] This agglutination is considered positive for the presence of IgG or complement on the cell surfaces.

An indirect Coombs test can identify antibodies in a patient's serum. This test is performed by combining the patient's serum with normal RBCs, then subjecting them to the direct Coombs test. Antibodies that have attached to the normal RBCs will be identified. This process is important in blood bank procedures.

The mechanisms that have been proposed to explain how drugs can induce immune hemolytic anemia are similar to the mechanisms that produce drug-induced agranulocytosis. The first mechanism is the adsorption of the drug to the RBC membrane to form a hapten and, subsequently, an antibody. The antibody attaches to the drug without direct interaction with the erythrocyte. The extravascular anemia that follows is usually caused by IgG, and generally, there is no complement activation. The anemia usually develops gradually over 7 to 10 days and reverses over a couple of weeks after discontinuation of the offending drug. The direct Coombs test may remain positive for several weeks. The penicillin and cephalosporin derivatives given in high doses are mainly associated with this type of immune reaction.[72] Other drugs that have been reported to cause drug-induced immune hemolytic anemia by this process include tetracycline, tolbutamide and semi-synthetic penicillins.[72] Streptomycin is also associated with this type of reaction and is associated with activation of the complement system.[73]

Like drug-induced agranulocytosis, immune hemolytic anemia has been associated with the formation of immune complexes in a reaction formally known as the "innocent bystander phenomenon." Quinidine and phenacetin are the prototype drugs of this reaction, but many other drugs have been implicated, including quinine and several sulfonamides. Drugs that induce this reaction form a "neoantigen" with a specific alloantigen on the RBC. This neoantigen, in turn, forms complexes with drug-specific antibodies (IgG or IgM) that adhere to the RBC membrane. Complement then lyses the RBC membrane.[72] Interestingly, the trimolecular complex is attached very loosely to the RBC.[72] As soon as complement is activated, the complex can detach and move on to other RBCs, and to leukocytes or platelets. Because of this low affinity, only a small amount of drug is needed to cause the reaction, and the direct Coombs test is positive for complement only. RBCs are essentially victims or "innocent bystanders" of the immunologic reaction. This type of mechanism is associated with acute intravascular hemolysis that can be severe, sometimes leading to hemoglobinuria and renal failure. Following discontinuation and clearance of the drug from the circulation, the direct Coombs test will be negative.

A third type of immune-mediated mechanism has occurred with cephalosporin derivatives. The cephalosporins can combine with nonspecific proteins, including albumin, IgG, IgA, and fibrinogen, and adhere to the RBC; when this happens, a Coombs test will have a positive result. The binding is not immunologic in origin, and hemolytic anemia has not been associated with this reaction (Fig. 102–5). However, the nonspecific binding of antibodies to the RBC membrane can cause difficulties in cross-matching patients for blood transfusions.[72]

The fourth mechanism is the best described. Methyldopa, like a few other drugs, is known to induce true autoantibodies to RBCs; the antibodies can be identified without the presence of the offending drug or its metabolites. About 20% of patients receiving methyldopa have a positive finding on Coombs test, but less than 1% of these patients experience hemolysis. The result of a Coombs test usually becomes positive 3 to 6 months after the beginning of therapy, but hemolysis develops from 4 to 6 months to more than 2 years after the start of therapy. After the withdrawal of the drug, results of the Coombs test can remain positive for many months.[73]

The mechanism by which methyldopa induces antibody production is not completely known, but there are several hypotheses. One suggests that methyldopa inhibits suppressor T-lymphocyte function, resulting in uncontrolled autoantibody formation by B cells.[74] More recent data, however, have not supported this concept.[75] Another hypothesis suggests that the offending drug may bind to immature RBCs, altering the membrane antigens and inducing autoantibodies.[76]

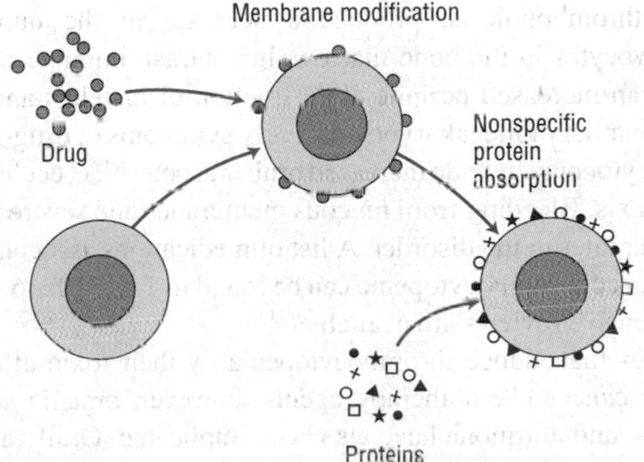

FIGURE 102–5. Nonspecific binding of proteins mechanism. The drug combines with the cell membrane, which, in turn, causes a nonspecific binding of serum protein. This reaction is seen primarily with the cephalosporins, and no cell lysis or toxicity occurs. *From Petz LD. Drug-induced haemolytic anaemia. Ballieres Clin Haematol 1980:91:455–482. With permission.*

Overall, however, the reason that only some patients develop autoantibodies, and that only some of those have hemolytic disease, is not known. In an effort to explain why patients may have a positive result from a Coombs test and no hemolysis, Kelton demonstrated that methyldopa impairs the ability of these patients to remove antibody-sensitized cells.[77] In Coombs-positive patients receiving methyldopa, patients with impairment of the reticuloendothelial system could not clear the RBCs coated with autoantibodies from their bloodstream, and therefore hemolysis did not occur. Patients with hemolysis had no impairment of the reticuloendothelial system. Procainamide has also been reported to cause a positive result on the direct anti-human globulin test and hemolytic anemia.[78] Other drugs that have been reported to cause autoimmune hemolytic anemia include levodopa, mefanamic acid, and diclofenac.[76]

DRUG-INDUCED OXIDATIVE HEMOLYTIC ANEMIA

A hereditary condition, drug-induced oxidative hemolytic anemia most often accompanies a glucose-6-phosphate dehydrogenase (G6PD) enzyme deficiency, but it can occur because of other enzyme defects (NADPH methemoglobin reductase or GSH peroxidase). A G6PD deficiency is a disorder of the hexose monophosphate shunt, which is responsible for producing NADPH in erythrocytes, which in turn keeps glutathione in a reduced state. Reduced glutathione is a substrate for glutathione peroxidase, an enzyme that removes peroxide from erythrocytes, thus protecting them from oxidative stress.[79] Without reduced glutathione, oxidative drugs may oxidize the sulfhydryl groups of hemoglobin, removing them prematurely from the circulation (i.e., causing hemolysis).

A G6PD deficiency is the most common of all enzyme defects, affecting millions of people. Because the G6PD gene is located on the X chromosome, the disorder is consequently inherited via a sex-linked mode. There are many G6PD variants, but the most common types occur in American and African blacks (about 10% to 11%), people from Mediterranean areas (e.g., Greeks, Sardinians, and Khurdic and Sephardic Jews), and Asians.[73,79] The Mediterranean variety tends to be more severe, and those with this defect also may experience hemolysis from the ingestion of fava beans ("favism").[79]

The degree of hemolysis depends on the severity of the enzyme deficiency and the amount of oxidative stress. However, the dose required for hemolysis to occur is often less than prescribed quantities of the suspected agent.[80] Although severe hemolysis is rare.[80] Any drug that places oxidative stress on the RBC will cause drug-induced oxidative hemolytic anemia. There was one case of drug-induced oxidative hemolytic anemia that occurred in a child when dapsone (an oxidizing agent) was transferred through the breast milk of the mother, who was taking the drug.[81] For a list of agents associated with drug-induced oxidative hemolytic anemia refer to Table 102–4.

TABLE 102–4. Drugs Associated with Oxidative Hemolysis

Ascorbic acid	Hydroxychloroquine	Primaquine
Benzocaine	Menadiol	Salazosulfapyridine
Chloramphenicol	Methylene blue	Sulfacetamide
Chloroquine	Nalidixic acid	Sulfamethoxazole
Dapsone	Nitrofurantoin	Sulfanilamide
Diazoxide	Nitrofurazone	Sulfapyridine
Furazolindone	Phenazopyridine	

▶ TREATMENT: Drug-Induced Hemolytic Anemia

TREATMENT OF DRUG-INDUCED IMMUNE HEMOLYTIC ANEMIA

The severity of drug-induced immune hemolytic anemia is usually a function of the rate of hemolysis. Hemolytic anemia caused by drugs via the hapten/adsorption and autoimmune mechanisms tend to be slower in onset and mild to moderate in severity. Conversely, hemolysis prompted via the neoantigen mechanism (innocent bystander) phenomenon may have a sudden onset, lead to severe hemolysis, and result in renal failure. The treatment of drug-induced immune hemolytic anemia includes the removal of the offending agent and supportive care. Glucocorticoids are usually unnecessary, and practitioners have questioned their efficacy.[76] The IV administration of immunoglobulins has been used in severe cases of immune hemolytic anemia, but are not standard therapy.[82]

TREATMENT OF DRUG-INDUCED OXIDATIVE HEMOLYTIC ANEMIA

Removal of the offending drug is the primary treatment for drug-induced oxidative hemolytic anemia. No other therapy is usually necessary, as most cases of drug-induced oxidative hemolytic anemia are mild in severity. Patients with these enzyme deficiencies should be advised to avoid medication capable of inducing the hemolysis.

DRUG-INDUCED MEGALOBLASTIC ANEMIA

In drug-induced megaloblastic anemia, the development of RBC precursors called megaloblasts in the bone marrow is abnormal. Deficiencies in either B_{12} or folate are responsible for the impaired proliferation and maturation of hematopoietic cells, resulting in cell arrest and subsequent sequestration. Examination of peripheral blood shows a rise in the mean corpuscular hemoglobin concentration. These megaloblastic changes are due to the direct or indirect effects of the drug on DNA synthesis. Some patients may have a normal-appearing cell line, and diagnosis must be made through alterations in B_{12} and folate concentrations. The abnormality can be seen in any portion of the replication process, including DNA assembly, base precursor metabolism, or RNA synthesis.[83]

The antimetabolite chemotherapeutic agents, because of their pharmacologic action on DNA replication, are most frequently associated with drug-induced megaloblastic anemia. Methotrexate, an irreversible inhibitor of dihydrofolate reductase, causes megaloblastic anemia in 3% to 9% of patients.[84] Dihydrofolate reductase is an enzyme responsible for generating tetrahydrofolate, an essential factor in making deoxythymidine triphosphate, which is necessary for DNA synthesis. Other drugs such as cotrimoxazole, phenytoin, or the barbiturates have also been implicated in megaloblastic anemia. Cotrimoxazole, for example, has been reported to cause drug-induced megaloblastic anemia with both low and high doses,[85,86] particularly in patients with a partial B_{12} or folate deficiency.[83] Because the drug's affinity for human dihydrofolate reductase is low, patients with adequate stores of these vitamins are probably at low risk of developing drug-induced megaloblastic anemia if they are taking cotrimoxazole. It has been postulated that phenytoin, primidone, and phenobarbital cause drug-induced megaloblastic anemia by either inhibiting folate absorption or by increasing folate catabolism. In both instances, the patient develops a relative deficiency of folate. Table 102–5 provides a list of drugs that have been suggested as causative factors in drug-induced megaloblastic anemia.

TABLE 102–5. Drugs Associated with Megaloblastic Anemia

p-Aminosalicylate	Hydroxyurea	Phenytoin
Azathioprine	6-Mercaptopurine	Primidone
Chloramphenicol	Metformin	Pyrimethamine
Colchicine	Methotrexate	Sulfasalazine
Cyclophosphamide	Neomycin	Triamterene
Cytarabine	Nitrofurantoin	Trimethoprim
5-Fluorodeoxyuridine	Oral contraceptives	Vinblastine
5-Fluorouracil	Phenobarbital	

▶ TREATMENT: Drug-Induced Megaloblastic Anemia

When drug-induced megaloblastic anemia is related to chemotherapy, no real therapeutic option is available, and the anemia becomes an accepted side effect of therapy. If drug-induced megaloblastic anemia results from cotrimoxazole, a trial course of folinic acid, 5–10 mg up to four times a day, may correct the anemia.[85,86] Folic acid supplementation of 1 mg every day often corrects the drug-induced megaloblastic anemia produced by either phenytoin or phenobarbital, but some clinicians suggest that supplementation of folic acid may decrease the effectiveness of the antiepileptic medications.[87]

DRUG-INDUCED THROMBOCYTOPENIA

Thrombocytopenia is defined as a platelet count below 150,000/μL. There are three types of drug-induced thrombocytopenia: direct toxicity reactions, hapten-type immune reactions, and innocent bystander-type immune reactions. Direct toxicity reactions, resulting in suppressed thrombopoiesis, produce a decrease in the number of megakaryocytes in the bone marrow. In contrast, immune reactions result in an increased peripheral destruction of platelets and an increased number of megakaryocytes. Early symptoms of drug-induced thrombocytopenia include increased bruising, petechiae, ecchymoses, and epistaxis. Bleeding from mucous membranes and severe purpura can appear later in the disorder. A list of medications associated with drug-induced thrombocytopenia can be found in Table 102–6. Several comprehensive reviews are available.[88,89]

Drugs that induce thrombocytopenia by their toxic effects are primarily cancer chemotherapy agents; however, organic solvents, pesticides, and amrinone have also been implicated. Orally administered amrinone has been shown to cause thrombocytopenia in up to 18.6% of patients.[90] The only commercially available formulation of amrinone in the United States is to be given IV, and it is associated with a 2% to 4% incidence of thrombocytopenia, possibly reflecting the short-term nature of IV administration compared to the oral route. Although investigators have demonstrated an amrinone-dependent

TABLE 102–6. Drugs Associated with Thrombocytopenia

Abciximab	Ethambutol	Nalidixic acid
Acetaminophen	Fluconazole	Nitroglycerin
Amiodarone	Furosemide	Novobiocin
Aminoglutethimide	Glibenclamide	Oxprenolol
Aminosalicylic acid	Gold salts	Oxyphenbutazone
Amphotericin B	Haloperidol	Oxytetracycline
Ampicillin	Heparin	Penicillin
Amrinone	Hydrochlorothiazide	Piperacillin
Aspirin	Ibuprofen	Piroxicam
Captopril	Indinavir	Procainamide
Carbamazepine	Indomethacin	Quinidine
Cephalothin	Interferon-α	Quinine
Chlorothiazide	Iopanoic acid	Ranitidine
Chlorpromazine	Isoniazid	Rifampin
Chlorpropamide	Levamisole	Sirolimus
Cimetidine	Linezolid	Sulfonamide antibiotics
Danazol	Lithium	Sulindac
Diatrizoate	Low molecular	Tolmetin
Diazepam	weight heparin	Trimethoprim
Diazoxide	Meclofenamate	Valproic acid
Diclofenac	Methicillin	Vancomycin
Diethylstilbestrol	Methyldopa	
Digoxin	Minoxidil	

antibody, it is believed that because of the rapid onset, the dose-related response, and the absence of amnestic effect, a non-immune-mediated peripheral destruction of platelets may be responsible for the thrombocytopenia.[90] Additional data suggest that this toxic effect may be due to the amrinone metabolite, N-acetylamrinone.[91]

In the majority of patients, drug-induced thrombocytopenia develops through an immunologic mechanism. The agents most commonly implicated are quinine, quinidine, gold salts, sulfonamide antibiotics, and heparin.[89] Study of these agents has revealed extensive information regarding the mechanism of drug-induced immune thrombocytopenia. In hapten-type reactions, the offending drug binds to certain platelet glycoproteins, most commonly Ib/IX, V, and IIb/IIIa.[92] Antibodies are generated that bind to these drug-bound glycoprotein epitopes. After the binding of drug-dependent antibodies to the platelet surface, lysis occurs through complement activation or through clearance from the circulation by macrophages.

Hapten-mediated immune thrombocytopenia usually occurs at least 7 days after the initiation of the drug, although it may occur much sooner if the exposure is actually a reexposure to a previously administered drug. It occurs frequently in patients receiving large doses of the medication (e.g., penicillin derivatives > 150 mg/kg).[93,94] The recovery period, once the suspected drug is discontinued, is often short in duration.[95]

Rare cases of acute profound thrombocytopenia (i.e., platelet count less than 20,000/μL) have been reported with the glycoprotein IIb/IIIa receptor antagonist abciximab.[96–98] Although the mechanism is unknown, it is thought that abciximab binding to the glycoprotein IIb/IIIa receptor may induce the expression of ligand-induced binding sites. These new binding sites may react with antibodies, leading to an increased clearance of platelets.[98,99] In a report that does not support this immunologic hypothesis, Peter and associates describe a patient with demonstrated platelet activation and subsequent thrombocytopenia.[100] In clinical trials with abciximab plus heparin, the incidence of thrombocytopenia with platelet count less than 50,000/μL ranged from 1.3% to 1.6%. In comparison, patients who received placebo plus heparin, thrombocytopenia ranged from 0.3% to 0.7%.[98] Published case reports indicate that the incidence of acute profound thrombocytopenia with abciximab is less than 1% and that nadir platelet counts of 1,000–4,000/μL occurred from 2 to 31 hours following bolus infusion.[98] This time course contrasts with that of other hapten-type thrombocytopenias; the decrease in platelet count can occur within hours of first drug exposure.

Because abciximab is co-administered with heparin, it is important to distinguish between abciximab-induced and heparin-induced thrombocytopenia. Performing a heparin-induced platelet aggregation study is helpful in making this differentiation. Pseudothrombocytopenia, defined as *in vitro* platelet aggregation in blood anticoagulated with ethylene-diamine-tetra-acetic acid (EDTA), is clinically insignificant, but it must also be differentiated from thrombocytopenia induced by abciximab. In this case, microscopic examination of a peripheral blood smear, along with repeated platelet counts in citrate-anticoagulated blood samples, makes the distinction possible.[101]

Heparin can cause at least two types of thrombocytopenia.[102] The first is a mild, reversible, non-immune-mediated reaction that occurs 2 to 4 days after the initiation of therapy. The platelet count slowly returns to normal following an initial decline, despite continued heparin therapy. This benign condition is thought to result from weak activation of platelets, leading to sequestration.[102] No major sequelae develop from this type of heparin-induced thrombocytopenia.

The second type of heparin-induced thrombocytopenia is severe and may be associated with a platelet count below 100,000/μL and thrombosis.[102,103] The platelet count generally begins to decline 5 to 10 days after the start of heparin therapy (sooner in patients previously treated with heparin). Thrombocytopenia and thrombosis may develop with low-dose heparin,[102,104] heparin-coated catheters,[105] or even heparin flushes. Historically, the reaction was thought to be mediated by the formation of antibodies to the platelet-heparin complex. Recent evidence suggests a complex interaction between heparin, platelet factor 4 (PF4), platelet membrane Fc receptors, and possibly heparin-like molecules on the surface of endothelial cells (Fig. 102–6). Circulating heparin reacts with PF4 to produce a complex that is seen as an antigen. Antibodies, predominantly IgG, react with this heparin-PF4 conjugate to form immune complexes that bind to Fc receptors on the platelet membrane. Platelet activation and aggregation occur, with subsequent release of more circulating PF4 to interact with heparin and bind to heparin-like molecules on the surface of endothelial cells. This interaction between PF4 and endothelial cells leads to antibody binding and increases the risk of thrombosis.[106] The incidence of heparin-induced thrombocytopenia with thrombosis has been reported to be three to four times higher with heparin from bovine sources than with heparin from porcine sources,[107,108] but several studies have demonstrated no differences between animal sources of heparin.[108–111] Several types of assays are available to aid in the diagnosis of heparin-induced thrombocytopenia, including platelet activation assays, platelet aggregation studies, and enzyme-linked immunosorbent assay methods, each with varying sensitivities and specificities.[112]

Low molecular weight heparins bind less well to PF4 than unfractionated heparin does and would, therefore, seem less likely to produce thrombocytopenia. In a study designed to examine the incidence of heparin-induced thrombocytopenia in patients receiving prophylaxis for venous thromboembolism following hip surgery, it was found that thrombocytopenia occurred in 2.7% of patients treated with unfractionated heparin compared to 0% of patients treated with low molecular weight heparin. Interestingly, 2.2% of those who received low molecular weight heparin developed heparin-dependent antibodies.[113] Therefore, low molecular weight heparin should not be expected to eliminate the risk of thrombocytopenia. Caution should be observed in interpreting these data, however; low molecular weight heparin should not be considered an alternative to

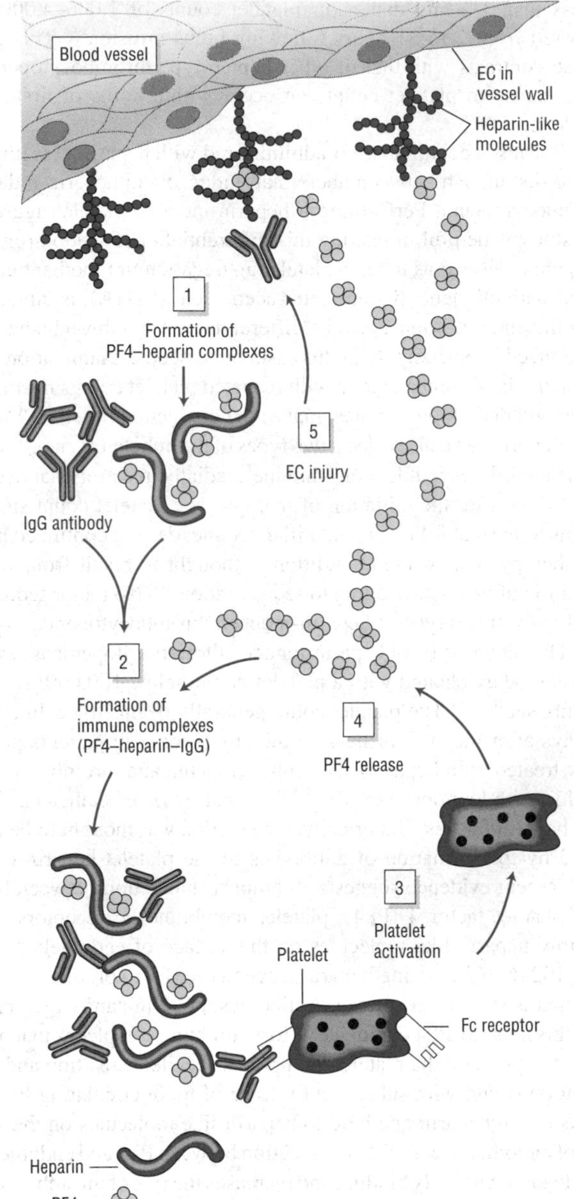

FIGURE 102–6. Proposed explanation for the presence of both thrombocytopenia and thrombosis in heparin-sensitive patients who are treated with heparin. Injected heparin reacts with platelet factor 4 (PF4), which is normally present on the surface of endothelial cells (ECs) or released in small quantities from circulating platelets, to form PF4-heparin complexes (1). Specific IgG antibodies react with these conjugates to form immune complexes (2) that bind to Fc receptors on circulating platelets. Fc-mediated platelet activation (3) releases PF4 from α-granules in platelets (4). Newly released PF4 binds to additional heparin, and the antibody forms more immune complexes, establishing a cycle of platelet activation. PF4 released in excess of the amount that can be neutralized by available heparin binds to heparin-like molecules (glycosaminoglycans) on the surface of ECs to provide targets for antibody binding. This process leads to immune-mediated EC injury (5) and heightens the risk of thrombosis and disseminated intravascular coagulation. *From Ref. 106, with permission.*

unfractionated heparin in patients with heparin-induced thrombocytopenia because of the potential for cross-reactivity with heparin-dependent antibodies. In patients with heparin-dependent antibodies, *in vitro* cross-reactivity of unfractionated heparin with the heparinoid, danaparoid sodium, has been demonstrated to occur in 19.6% to 40% of patients and 25.5% to 100% of those receiving low molecular weight heparins.[113,114] The clinical relevance of this *in vitro* cross-reactivity to danaparoid has yet to be determined.

The thrombocytopenia induced by gold salts is related to antibody formation to platelets.[115,116] The incidence of gold-induced thrombocytopenia ranges from 1% to 3%, and the condition often has an abrupt and severe onset.[115] The autoantibody formed to the platelet appears to be associated with the HLA antigens, which are located on the platelet membrane and on a number of other different cells in the body.[115,116] An interaction between the gold salts and the HLA antigens causes the platelets to be recognized as nonself, thus inducing destruction of the platelets. The most commonly reported HLA antigen associated with induction of the autoantibodies is DR-3, but DR-4 may also interact with the antibodies.[115–117] The exact mechanism by which gold causes the formation of the autoantibody to regulated DR-3 and DR-4 antigens has not been elucidated. In addition to gold, autoantibodies have been identified for α-methlydopa.[88]

The third mechanism described for drug-induced thrombocytopenia is the innocent bystander-type immune response. The most commonly implicated drug is quinidine, and the drug-induced thrombocytopenia is frequently related to higher doses of the drug.[118] Quinidine may also form a hapten with the platelet membrane to produce thrombocytopenia.[119]

▶ TREATMENT: Drug-Induced Thrombocytopenia

The primary treatment of drug-induced thrombocytopenia is removal of the offending drug and symptomatic treatment of the patient. The use of corticosteroid therapy in the treatment of drug-induced thrombocytopenia is controversial, although some authors recommend it in severe symptomatic cases.[120] In gold salt–induced thrombocytopenia, however, some investigators believe prednisone in a dose of 60 mg daily is beneficial in correcting the thrombocytopenia.[115]

In the case of heparin-induced thrombocytopenia with thrombosis, all forms of heparin must be discontinued, including heparin flushes, and anticoagulation with danaparoid, argatroban, or the recombinant hirudin, lepirudin initiated.[121,122] These agents should also be considered for the treatment of patients who have acute heparin-induced thrombocytopenia without thombosis because of the increased risk of thrombosis occurring in these patients. Because of the increased risk of venous limb gangrene, warfarin should not be used alone to treat acute heparin-induced thrombocytopenia complicated by deep vein thrombosis.[122] Ancrod, a defibrinogenating snake venom, is no longer recommended as a treatment for heparin-induced thrombocytopenia because of its inability to achieve rapid anticoagulation, its potential to cause venous limb gangrene when co-administered with warfarin, and its reduced efficacy compared to that of danaparoid.[122] The relatively high risk of continued thrombocytopenia with thrombosis is a contraindication for the use of low molecular weight heparin in the treatment of acute heparin-induced thrombocytopenia.[122] Abciximab-induced acute profound thrombocytopenia is effectively treated with platelet transfusion, if clinically indicated.[92]

▶ PRINCIPLES OF PHARMACOTHERAPY

- Drug-induced hematologic disorders are, in general, rare adverse effects associated with drug therapy.

- Drug-induced hematologic disorders are more common in women and the elderly; the risk of death also appears greater with increasing age.
- Reporting during postmarketing surveillance of a drug is usually the method by which the incidence of rare adverse drug reactions is established.
- The most common drug-induced hematologic disorders include aplastic anemia, agranulocytosis, megaloblastic anemia, thrombocytopenia, and hemolytic anemia.
- Drug-induced hematologic disorders range from mild reductions in affected cell lines to life-threatening reactions associated with significant morbidity and mortality.
- The mechanisms of drug-induced hematologic disorders are thought to be the result of direct toxicity or an immune reaction.
- Clinicians should be cognizant of agents with the potential of causing hematologic disorders and educate prescribers and patients accordingly.
- Frequent laboratory monitoring may be warranted for agents commonly demonstrating severe hematologic reactions.
- The primary treatment of drug-induced hematologic disorders is removal of the drug in question and symptomatic support of the patient.
- Because drug-induced blood disorders are dangerous, rechallenging a patient with a suspected agent in an attempt to confirm a diagnosis may not be ethical.

REFERENCES

1. Johnston FD. Granulocytopenia following the administration of sulphanilamide compounds. Lancet 1938;2:1044–1047.
2. Council for International Organizations of Medical Sciences. Standardization of definitions and criteria of assessment of adverse drug reactions: drug-induced cytopenia. Int J Clin Pharmacol Toxicol 1990;29:75–81.
3. van der Klauw MM, Goudsmit R, Halie MR. A population-based case cohort study of drug-associated agranulocytosis. Arch Intern Med 1999;159:369–374.
4. Shapiro S, Surapol I, Kaufman DW, et al. Agranulocytosis in Bangkok, Thailand: a predominantly drug-induced disease with an unusually low incidence. Am J Trop Med Hyg 1999;60:573–577.
5. Issaragrisil S, Sriratamasaatavorn C, Piankijaagum A. Incidence of aplastic anemia in Bangkok. Blood 1991;77:2166–2168.
6. Patton WN, Duffull SB. Idiosyncratic drug-induced haematologic abnormalities. Drug Saf 1994;11:445–462.
7. Hine LK, Gerstman BB, Wise RP, Song YT. Mortality resulting from blood dyscrasia in the United States. Am J Med 1990;88:151–153.
8. Kessler DA. Introducing MEDWatch: a new approach to reporting medication and device adverse effects and product problems. JAMA 1993;269:2765–2768.
9. ASHP reports. ASHP guidelines on adverse drug reaction monitoring or reporting. Am J Hosp Pharm 1989;46:336–337.
10. Rieder MJ. *In-vivo* and *in-vitro* testing for adverse drug reactions. Pediatr Clin North Am 1997;44:93–111.
11. Parent-Mussin DM, Sensebe L, Leqlise MC, et al. Relevance of *in-vitro* studies of drug-induced agranulocytosis: report of 14 cases. Drug Saf 1993;9:463–469.
12. Claas FHJ. Drug-induced immune granulocytopenia. Baillieres Clin Immunol Allergy 1987;1:357–368.
13. Gale RP, Champlin RE, Feig SA, et al. Aplastic anemia: biology and treatment. UCLA conference. Ann Intern Med 1981;95:477–494.
14. Heimpel H. Epidemiology and etiology of aplastic anemia. In: Schrezenmeier H, et al., eds. Aplastic Anemia: Pathophysiology and Treatment. Cambridge, UK: Cambridge University Press, 2000:97–116.
15. International Agranulocytosis and Aplastic Anemia Study. Risk of agranulocytosis and aplastic anemia: a first report of their relation to drug use with special reference to analgesics. JAMA 1986;256:1749–1757.
16. Camitta BM, Thomas ED, Nathan DG. A prospective study of androgens and bone marrow transplantation for treatment of severe aplastic anemia. Blood 1979;53:504–514.
17. Shadduck RK. Aplastic anemia. In: Williams WJ, et al., eds. Hematology. 5th ed. New York: McGraw-Hill, 1995:238–251.
18. Vincent PC. *In vitro* evidence of drug action in aplastic anemia. Blood 1984;49:3–12.
19. Heimpel H, Heit W. Drug-induced aplastic anemia: clinical aspects. Clin Haematol 1980;9:641–662.
20. Modan B, Segal S, Shani M, et al. Aplastic anemia in Israel: evaluation of the etiological role of chloramphenicol on a community wide basis. Am J Med Sci 1975;270:441–445.
21. Lubran MM. Hematologic side effects of drugs. Ann Clin Lab Sci 1989;19:114–121.
22. Young NS, Maciejewski J. The pathophysiology of acquired aplastic anemia. N Engl J Med 1997;336:1365–1372.
23. Yunis AA, Miller AM, Salem Z, et al. Chloramphenicol toxicity: pathogenetic mechanisms and the role of the p-NO_2 in aplastic anemia. Clin Toxicol 1980;17:359–373.
24. Malkin D, Koren G, Saunders EF. Drug-induced aplastic anemia pathogenesis and clinical aspects. Am J Pediatr Hematol Oncol 1990;12:402–410.
25. Jimenez JJ, Arimura GK, Abou-Khalil WH, et al. Chloramphenicol-induced bone marrow injury: possible role of bacterial metabolites of chloramphenicol. Blood 1987;70:1180–1185.
26. Gerson WT, Fine DG, Spielberg SP, et al. Anticonvulsant-induced aplastic anemia: increased susceptibility to toxic drug metabolites *in vitro*. Blood 1983;61:889–893.
27. Kagan WA, Ascensao JA, Pahwa RN, et al. Aplastic anemia: presence in human bone marrow of cells that suppress myelopoiesis. Proc Natl Acad Sci U S A 1985;82:188–192.
28. Selleri C, Sato T, Anderson S, et al. Interferon-γ and tumor necrosis factor-α suppress both early and late stages of hematopoiesis and induce programmed cell death. J Cell Physiol 1995;165:538–546.
29. Mathe G, Amiel JL, Schwarzenberg L, et al. Bone marrow graft in man after conditioning by antilymphocytic serum. BMJ 1970;2:131–136.
30. Platanias L, Gascon P, Bielory L, et al. Lymphocyte phenotype and lymphokines following anti-lymphocyte globulin therapy in patients with aplastic anemia. Br J Haematol 1987;66:437–443.
31. Frickhofen N, Kaltwasser J, Schrezenmeier H, et al. Treatment of aplastic anemia with antilymphocyte globulin and methylprednisolone with or without cyclosporine. N Engl J Med 1991;324:1297–1304.
32. Marsh JC, Chowdry J, Parry-Jones N, et al. Study of the association between cytochromes P450 2D6 and 2E1 genotypes and the risk of drug and chemical induced idiosyncratic aplastic anemia. Br J Haemotol 1999;104:266–270.
33. Marin-Fernandez P. Clinical presentation, natural course, and prognostic factors. In: Schrezenmeier H, et al., eds. Aplastic Anemia: Pathophysiology and Treatment. Cambridge, UK: Cambridge University Press, 2000:117–133.
34. Weinberger M, Elattar I, Marshall D, et al. Patterns of infection in patients with aplastic anemia and the emergence of *Aspergillus* as a major cause of death. Medicine 1992;71(1):24–43.
35. Doney K, Leisenring W, Storb R, et al. Primary treatment of acquired aplastic anemia: outcomes with bone marrow transplantation and immunosuppressive therapy. Ann Intern Med 1997;126:107–115.
36. Colby C, Stoukides CA, Spitzer TR. Antithymocyte immunoglobulin in severe aplastic anemia and bone marrow transplantation. Ann Pharmacother 1996;30:1164–1174.
37. Young N, Speck B. Antithymocyte and antilymphocyte globulins: clinical trials and mechanism of action. In: Young S, et al., eds. Aplastic Anemia. Stem Cell Biology and Advances in Treatment. New York: Alan R Liss, 1984:221–226.
38. Tichelli A, Schrezenmeier H, Bacigalupo A. Immunosuppressive treatment of aplastic anemia. In: Schrezenmeier H, et al., eds. Aplastic

Anemia: Pathophysiology and Treatment. Cambridge, UK: Cambridge University Press, 2000:154–196.

39. Bacigalupo A, Broccia G, Codra G, et al. Antilymphocyte globulin, cyclosporin, and granulocyte colony-stimulating factor in patients with acquired severe aplastic anemia (SAA): a pilot study of the EBMT SAA Working Party. Blood 1995;85:1348–1353.
40. Tichelli A, Socie G, Henry-Amar M, et al. Effectiveness of immunosuppressive therapy in older patients with aplastic anemia. Ann Intern Med 1999;130:193–201.
41. Schrezenmeier H. Role of cytokines in the treatment of aplastic anemia. In: Schrezenmeier H, et al., eds. Aplastic Anemia: Pathophysiology and Treatment. Cambridge, UK: Cambridge University Press, 2000: 197–229.
42. Antin JH, Smith BR, Holmes W, et al. Phase I/II study of recombinant human granulocyte-macrophage colony-stimulating factor in aplastic anemia and myelodysplastic syndrome. Blood 1988;72:705–713.
43. Walsh CE, Liu JM, Anderson SM, et al. A trial of recombinant human interleukin-I in patients with severe refractory aplastic anaemia. Br J Haematol 1992;80:106–110.
44. Heit W, Heimpel H, Fischer A, et al. Drug-induced agranulocytosis: evidence for the commitment of bone marrow haematopoiesis. Scand J Haematol 1985;35:459–468.
45. Julia A, Olona M, Bueno J, et al. Drug-induced agranulocytosis: prognostic factors in a series of 168 episodes. Br J Haematol 1991;79:366–371.
46. Pisciotta V. Drug-induced agranulocytosis. Drugs 1978;15:132–143.
47. Burckart GJ, Snidow J, Bruce W. Neutropenia following acute chlorpromazine ingestion. Clin Toxicol 1981;18:797–801.
48. Neftel KA, Muller MR, Hauser SD, et al. More on penicillin-induced leukopenia. N Engl J Med 1983;308:901.
49. Heit WF. Hematologic effects of antipyretic analgesics: drug-induced agranulocytosis. Am J Med 1983;75:65–68.
50. Young GA, Vincent PC. Drug-induced agranulocytosis. Baillieres Clin Haematol 1980;9:483–504.
51. Kirkwood CF, Smith LL, Rustagi PK, et al. Neutropenia associated with beta-lactam antibiotics. Clin Pharm 1983;2:569–578.
52. Homayouni H, Gross PA, Setia V, et al. Leukopenia due to penicillin and cephalosporin homologues. Arch Intern Med 1979;139:827–828.
53. Neftel KA, Hauser SP, Muller MR. Inhibition of granulopoiesis *in vivo* and *in vitro* by beta-lactam antibiotics. J Infect Dis 1985;152:90–98.
54. Cooper DS, Goldmiriz D, Lewin AA, et al. Agranulocytosis associated with antithyroid drug. Ann Intern Med 1983;98:26–29.
55. Tajiri J, Noguchi S, Murakami T, et al. Antithyroid drug-induced agranulocytosis: the usefulness of routine white blood cell count monitoring. Arch Intern Med 1990;150:621–624.
56. Toth AL, Mant MJ, Shivji S, et al. Propylthiouracil-induced agranulocytosis: an unusual presentation and a possible mechanism. Am J Med 1988;85:725–727.
57. McIntyre PA, Laleli YR, Hodkinson BA, et al. Evidence for antileukocyte antibodies as a mechanism for drug-induced agranulocytosis. Trans Assoc Am Phys 1971;84:217–225.
58. Werner MC, Romaldini JH, Bromberg N, et al. Adverse effects related to thionamide drugs regimen. Am J Med Sci 1989;297:216–219.
59. Hass WK, Easton JD, Adams HP, et al. for the Ticlopidine Aspirin Study Group. A randomized trial comparing ticlopidine hydrochloride with aspirin for the prevention of stroke in high-risk patients. N Engl J Med 1989;321:501–507.
60. Quaglino D, Venturoni L, Cretara G, et al. Reversible bone marrow suppression primarily involving granulopoiesis following the use of ticlopidine. Haematologica 1982;67:940–941.
61. Resegotti L, Pistone MA, Testa D, et al. Bone marrow culture in patients treated with ticlopidine. Nouv Rev Fr Hematol 1985;27:19–22.
62. Krupp, P, Barnes P. Leponex-associated granulocytopenia: a review of the situation. Psychopharmacology 1989;99(Suppl):S118–21.
63. Alvir JM, Lieberman JA, Safferman AZ, et al. Clozapine-induced agranulocytosis: incidence and risk factors in the United States. N Engl J Med 1993;329:162–167.
64. Fischer V, Haar JA, Greiner L, et al. Possible role of free radical formation in clozapine (Clozaril) induced agranulocytosis. Mol Pharmacol 1991;40:846–853.
65. Beauchesne MF, Shalansky SJ. Nonchemotherapy drug-induced agranulocytosis: a review of 118 patients treated with colony-stimulating factors. Pharmacotherapy 1999;19(3):299–305.
66. Teitelbaum AH, Bell AJ, Brown SL. Filgrastim (r-metHuG-CSF) reversal of drug-induced agranulocytosis. Am J Med 1993;95:245–246.
67. Nielsen H. Recombinant human granulocyte colony-stimulating factor (rhG-CSF): Filgrastim treatment of clozapine-induced agranulocytosis. J Intern Med 1993;234:529–531.
68. Bjorkholm M, Pisa P, Arver S, Beran M. Haematologic effects of granulocyte-macrophage colony-stimulating in a patient with thiamazole-induced agranulocytosis. J Intern Med 1992;232:443–445.
69. Nand S, Bayer R, Prinz R. Granulocyte-macrophage colony-stimulating factor for the treatment of drug induced agranulocytosis. Am J Hematol 1991;37:267–269.
70. Tabbara IA. Hemolytic anemias: diagnosis and management. Med Clin North Am 1992;76:649–669.
71. McKenzie SB. Hemolytic anemias due to extrinsic factors. In: Balado D, ed. Textbook of Hematology, 2nd ed. Baltimore: Williams & Willkins, 1996:245–257.
72. Thomas AT. Autoimmune hemolytic anemias. In: Lee RG, et al., eds. Wintrobe's Clinical Hematology, 10th ed. Baltimore: Williams & Wilkins, 1999:1233–1263.
73. Jandl JH. Immunohemolytic anemias. In: Strangis JT, ed. Blood, Textbook of Hematology, 2nd ed. Boston: Little, Brown, 1996:421–518.
74. Kirtland HH, Mohler DN, Horwitz DA. Methyldopa inhibition of suppressor-lymphocyte function: a proposed cause of autoimmune hemolytic anemia. N Engl J Med 1980;302:825–832.
75. Garratty G, Arndt P, Prince HE, Schulman IA. The effect of methyldopa and procainamide on suppressor cell autoantibody production. Br J Haematol 1993;84:310.
76. Packman CH, Leddy JP. Drug-related immune hemolytic anemia. In: Williams WJ, et al., eds. Hematology, 5th ed. New York: McGraw-Hill, 1995:691–697.
77. Kelton JG. Impaired reticuloendothelial function in patients treated with methyldopa. N Engl J Med 1985;313:596–600.
78. Kleinman S, Nelson R, Smith L, et al. Positive direct antiglobulin tests and immune hemolytic anemia in patients receiving procainamide. N Engl J Med 1984;311:809–812.
79. Beutler E. G6PD deficiency. Blood 1994;84:3613–3636.
80. Gordan-Smith EC. Drug-induced oxidative hemolysis. Clin Haematol 1980;9:557–586.
81. Sanders SW, Zone JJ, Foltz RR, et al. Hemolytic anemia induced by dapsone transmitted through breast milk. Ann Intern Med 1981;96:465–466.
82. Flores G, Cunningham-Rundles C, Newland AC, et al. Efficacy of intravenous immunoglobin in the treatment of autoimmune hemolytic anemia: results in 73 patients. Am J Hematol 1993;44:237–242.
83. Scott JM, Weir DG. Drug-induced megaloblastic change. Clin Haematol 1980;9:587–605.
84. Weinblatt ME. Toxicity of low dose methotrexate in rheumatoid arthritis. J Rheumatol 1985;12 (suppl 12):S35–S39.
85. Magee F, O'Sullivan H, McCann SR. Megaloblastosis and low-dose trimethoprim-sulfamethoxazole. Ann Intern Med 1981;95: 657.
86. Kobrinsky NL, Ramsay NK. Acute megaloblastic anemia induced by high-dose trimethoprim-sulfamethoxazole. Ann Intern Med 1981;94: 780–781.
87. Rivey MP, Schotteluis DD, Berg MJ. Phenytoin-folic acid: a review. Drug Intell Clin Pharm 1984;18:292–301.
88. George JN, Raskob GE, Rizvi R, et al. Drug-induced thrombocytopenia: a systematic review of published case reports. Ann Intern Med 1998;129:886–890.

89. George JN, El-Harake MA, Aster RH. Thrombocytopenia due to enhanced platelet destruction by immunologic mechanisms. In: Beutler E, Lichtman MA, Coller BS, Kipps TJ, eds. Williams Hematology. 5th ed. New York: McGraw-Hill, 1995:1315–1355.
90. Ansell J, Tiarks C, McCue J, et al. Amrinone-induced thrombocytopenia. Arch Intern Med 1984;144:949–952.
91. Ross MP, Allen-Webb EM, Pappas JB, et al. Amrinone-associated thrombocytopenia: pharmacokinetic analysis. Clin Pharmacol Ther 1993;53:661–667.
92. Kiefel V. Differential diagnosis of acute thrombocytopenia. In: Warkentin TE, Greinacher A, eds. Heparin-induced Thrombocytopenia. New York: Marcel Dekker, 2000:17–41.
93. Murphy MF, Riordant T, Minchinton RM, et al. Demonstration of an immune-mediated mechanism of penicillin-induced neutropenia and thrombocytopenia. Br J Haematol 1983;55:155–160
94. Salamon DJ, Nusbacher J, Stroupe T, et al. Red cell and platelet-bound IgG penicillin antibodies in a patient with thrombocytopenia. Transfusion 1984;24:395–398.
95. Miescher PA, Graf J. Drug-induced thrombocytopenia. Clin Haematol 1980;9:505–519.
96. Berkowitz SD, Harrington RA, Rund MM, et al. Acute profound thrombocytopenia after c7E3 Fab (abciximab) therapy. Circulation 1997;95:809–913.
97. Joseph T, Marco J, Gregorini L. Acute profound thrombocytopenia after abciximab therapy during coronary angioplasty. Clin Cardiol 1998;21:851–852.
98. Jubelirer SJ, Koenig BA, Bates MC. Acute profound thrombocytopenia following c7E3 Fab (abciximab) therapy: case reports, review of the literature and implications for therapy. Am J Hematol 1999;61:205–208.
99. Cines DB. Glycoprotein IIb/IIIa antagonists: potential induction and detection of drug-dependent antiplatelet antibodies. Am Heart J 1998; 135:S152–S159.
100. Peter K, Straub A, Kohler B, et al. Platelet activation as a potential mechanism of GP IIb/IIIa inhibitor-induced thrombocytopenia. Am J Cardiol 1999;84:519–524.
101. Stiegler H, Fischer Y, Steiner S, et al. Sudden onset of EDTA-dependent pseudothrombocytopenia after therapy with the glycoprotein IIb/IIIa antagonists c7E3 Fab. Ann Hematol 2000;79:161–164.
102. Johnson RA, Lazarus KH, Henry DH. Heparin-induced thrombocytopenia prospective study. Am J Hematol 1984;17:349–353.
103. Cines DB, Kaywin P, Bina M, et al. Heparin-associated thrombocytopenia. N Engl J Med 1980;303:788–795.
104. Cheng TC. Thrombocytopenia associated with minidose heparin therapy. Postgrad Med 1981;70:73–78.
105. Laster JL, Nichols WK, Silver D. Thrombocytopenia associated with heparin-coated catheters in patients with heparin-associated antiplatelet antibodies. Arch Intern Med 1989;149:2285–2287.
106. Aster RH. Heparin-induced thrombocytopenia and thrombosis. N Engl J Med 1995;332:1374–1376.
107. King DJ, Kelton JG. Heparin-associated thrombocytopenia. Ann Intern Med 1984;100:535–540.
108. Bell WR, Royall RM. Heparin-associated thrombocytopenia: a comparison of three heparin preparations. N Engl J Med 1980;303:902–907.
109. Green D, Martin GJ, Shoichet SH, et al. Thrombocytopenia in a prospective, randomized, double-blind trial of bovine and porcine heparin. Am J Med Sci 1984;288:60–64.
110. Rao AK, White GC, Sherman L, et al. Low incidence of thrombocytopenia with porcine mucosal heparin: a prospective multicenter study. Arch Intern Med 1989;149:1285–1288.
111. Bailey RT, Ursick JA, Heim KL, et al. Heparin-associated thrombocytopenia: a prospective comparison of bovine lung heparin, manufactured by a new process, and porcine intestinal heparin. Drug Intell Clin Pharm 1986;20:374–378.
112. Warkentin TE, Barkin RL. Newer strategies for the treatment of heparin-induced thrombocytopenia. Pharmacotherapy 1999;19:181–195.
113. Warkentin TE, Levine MN, Hirsh J, et al. Heparin-induced thrombocytopenia in patients treated with low-molecular-weight heparin or unfractionated heparin. N Engl J Med 1995;332:1330–1335.
114. Kikta MJ, Keller MP, Humphrey PV, et al. Can low molecular weight heparins and heparinoids be safely given to patients with heparin-induced thrombocytopenia syndrome? Surgery 1993;114:705–710.
115. Armstrong RD, Faith A, Panayi GS, et al. Gold-induced thrombocytopenia: detection of anti-platelet antibody. Clin Rheumatol 1983;2:183–188.
116. Adachi JD, Bensen WG, Singal DP, et al. Gold induced thrombocytopenia: platelet associated IgG and HLA typing in three patients. J Rheumatol 1984;11:355–357.
117. Coblyn JS, Weinblatt M, Holdsworth D, et al. Gold-induced thrombocytopenia: a clinical and immunogenic study of twenty-three patients. Ann Intern Med 1981;95:178–181.
118. Kelton JG, Meltzer D, Moore J, et al. Drug-induced thrombocytopenia is associated with increased binding of IgG to platelets both *in vivo* and *in vitro*. Blood 1981;58:524–529.
119. Chong BH, Berndt MC, Koutts J, et al. Quinidine-induced thrombocytopenia and leukopenia: demonstration and characterization of distinct antiplatelets and antileukocyte antibodies. Blood 1983;62:1218–1223.
120. Pedersen-Bjergaard U, Andersen M, Hansen PB. Drug-induced thrombocytopenia: clinical data on 309 cases and the effect of corticosteroid therapy. Eur J Clin Pharmacol 1997;52:183–189.
121. Chong BH, Ismdil F, Cade J, et al. Heparin-induced thrombocytopenia: studies with a new low molecular weight heparinoid, Org 10172. Blood 1989;73:1592–1596.
122. Hirsch J, Warkentin TE, Raschke R, et al. Heparin: mechanism of action, pharmacokinetics, dosing considerations, monitoring, efficacy, and safety. Chest 1998;114:489S–510S.

103 LABORATORY TESTS TO DIRECT ANTIMICROBIAL PHARMACOTHERAPY

Michael J. Rybak and Jeffrey R. Aeschlimann

Appropriate antimicrobial pharmacotherapy for a given infectious disease requires knowledge of the infecting pathogen, host characteristics, and the drug's expected activity against the pathogen. The most fundamental aspect of therapy starts with an appropriate diagnosis. A vast array of laboratory tests is available to assist the clinician in verifying the presence of infection and for monitoring the response to therapy. Although useful, these tests are subject to interpretation and cannot be substituted for sound clinical judgment. Organism susceptibility to a given group of antimicrobials is key to determining the patient's therapy. Host characteristics, however, such as immune status, infection-site location, and body organ function, play a significant role in selecting the most appropriate antimicrobial for a given individual.[1] This chapter reviews the routinely used laboratory tests that are used to assist in the diagnosis and treatment of infection.

LABORATORY TESTS CONFIRMING THE PRESENCE OF INFECTION

NONSPECIFIC TESTS

A variety of tests are used by the clinician to determine whether a patient has an infection. Although no single test can prove a patient is infected, when used in combination with clinical findings, tests are helpful to establish the diagnosis of infection. Because many tests are nonspecific, there are often factors other than infection that can cause a test to be reported as positive when no infection exists. Therefore, the importance of careful interpretation and sound clinical judgment cannot be overemphasized. This chapter reviews the commonly employed tests and their interpretation and application for the diagnosis and management of infection.

WHITE BLOOD CELL COUNT AND DIFFERENTIAL

The major role of the white blood cell (WBC) is to defend the body against invading organisms such as bacteria, viruses, and fungi. The normal range of the WBC is 4,500–10,000 cells/mm^3. WBCs are usually elevated in response to infection. The WBC count can become elevated in response to a number of noninfectious causes including stress, inflammatory conditions such as rheumatoid arthritis, and leukemia, or in response to certain drugs (e.g., corticosteroids).

White blood cells are divided into two groups: the granulocytes, which have prominent cytoplasmic granules, and the agranulocytes, which lack granules. Polymorphonuclear granulocytes or neutrophils (PMNs) are made up of neutrophils, basophils, and eosinophils. The two other classes of WBCs are the monocytes and lymphocytes. Neutrophils are the most common type of WBCs in the blood, comprising approximately 70% of the total WBC count. In response to infection, they leave the bloodstream and enter the tissue to interact with and phagocytize offending pathogens. Mature neutrophils are sometimes referred to as *segs* because of their segmented nucleus, which usually consists of two to five lobes. Immature neutrophils lack this segmented feature and are referred to as *bands*. During an acute infection, immature neutrophils, such as bands (single-lobed nucleus), are released from the bone marrow into the bloodstream at an increased rate, and the percentage of bands (usually $\leq 5\%$) may increase in relationship to mature cells. The change in the ratio of mature to immature cells is often referred to as a *shift to the left* because of the way the cells were counted by hand with a microscope and charted from immature to mature cells.

Leukocytosis is a normal host defense to infection and is an important adjunct to antimicrobial therapy. Unfortunately, bacterial infection is a common complication of neutropenia from cancer chemotherapy. These patients are incapable of increasing their WBCs in response to infection. In fact, susceptibility to infection in these patients is highly dependent on their WBC status. Patients with neutrophil counts of less than 500 cells/mm^3 are at high risk for the development of bacterial or fungal infections. The absence of leukocytosis also occurs in the elderly and in severe cases of sepsis.[2]

Lymphocytes comprise 15% to 40% of all white cells and are of central importance to the immune system. Two functional types of lymphocytes are the T cell, which is involved in cell-mediated immunity, and the B cell, which produces antibodies involved in humoral immunity. Lymphocytosis is frequently associated with acute viral infections such as Epstein-Barr virus infection (mononucleosis) and cytomegalovirus and rarely with unusual bacterial infections (i.e., *Brucella* spp. infections).

T lymphocytes are characterized on the basis of function (type 1 or type 2) and on the basis of surface antigen. Most type 1 and type 2 T cells carry a T4 (CD4) marker that recognizes class II major histocompatibility complex (MHC) antigens and most cytoxic T cells carry a T8 (CD8) marker, which recognizes class I MHC antigens. A severe deficiency of CD4 cells is associated with human immunodeficiency virus (HIV). Malignancies may also adversely affect cellular immunity. Patients with Hodgkin's disease and other types of lymphoma exhibit defective cell-mediated immunity that predisposes them to a variety of infections, notably fungal diseases and infections by the *Listeria* species. Drug treatment with cytotoxic chemotherapy and corticosteroids may also have profound deleterious effects on cell-mediated immunity.[4] Defects in cell-mediated immune function can be demonstrated by a variety of simple laboratory tests, including quantification of lymphocytes on a routine complete blood cell

Cell type	Cellular function
Macrophage/monocyte	Antigen presenting cell Surveillance of antigens
Neurophils	Defense against bacteria and fungus
Eosinophils	Defense against parasite Response against allergic reactions
Basophil	Allergic response
B lymphocyte	Antibody production Antigen presenting cell
T lymphocytes	Cellular immunity against virus and tumors Regulation of the immune system

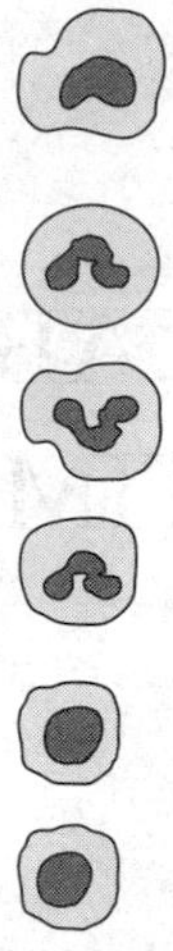

FIGURE 103–1. Various cell types and their biological function.

count and skin testing for anergy. A more detailed investigation includes quantitative measurements of CD4+ and CD8+ cells. Monocytosis is less frequently correlated with acute bacterial infection, although its presence has been associated with the response of certain infections (e.g., tuberculosis) to chemotherapy. Eosinophilia may result from parasitic infection. Figure 103–1 describes a number of cell types and their biologic function.

OTHER TESTS

There are a variety of nonspecific laboratory tests that are useful to support the diagnosis of infection. The inflammatory process initiated by an infection sets up a complex of host responses. Activation of complements, such as C3a and C5a, initiates inflammation and sets off a cascade of changes and the subsequent release of mediators, all of which can be measured and monitored. Serum complement concentrations, particularly C3, are usually consumed as part of the host defense mechanism and are subsequently reduced during the early stages of an acute infectious process. Acute-phase reactants, such as the erythrocyte sedimentation rate (ESR) and the C-reactive protein, are elevated in the presence of an inflammatory process but do not confirm the presence of infection, because they are often elevated in noninfectious conditions, such as collagen vascular diseases and arthritis. Large elevations in ESR are associated with infections such as endocarditis, osteomyelitis, and intra-abdominal infections.[5]

Changes in endothelial membranes and the presence of a foreign pathogen and its endotoxins cause certain cytokines, such as the interleukins (IL) IL-1, IL-6, IL-8, and tumor necrosis factor (TNF)-α to be produced by macrophages or lymphocytes. Fluctuations in cytokine levels occur during the course of an infection, which may be useful in staging and monitoring the response to therapy. Although abnormally high levels of TNF have been associated with a variety of noninfectious causes, spiked elevations in TNF are found in patients with serious infections, such as sepsis. Studies of the relationship of circulating mediators to patient outcome have determined the value of endotoxin and cytokine measurements in patients with sepsis. Although the combination of elevations in endotoxin and individual cytokines has correlated well with the mortality rate, measurement of IL-6 was by far the best individual cytokine that predicted patient outcome.[6] Direct and rapid measurement of endotoxin and cytokines at the bedside may be available in the future to assist clinicians in diagnosing, staging, and monitoring serious infections, such as sepsis.[7]

LABORATORY IDENTIFICATION OF PATHOGENS

COLONIZATION VERSUS INFECTION

Pathogens are organisms that are capable of damaging host tissues and that elicit specific host responses and symptoms that are consistent with an infectious process. These organisms are transferred from patient to patient, vector to patient (animals, insects, and so on), environment to patient (e.g., hospital settings), or are derived from the patient's own flora. On the other hand, the human body contains a vast variety of microorganisms that colonize body systems and make up the so-called "normal" flora. These organisms occur naturally in the tissues of the host and provide some benefits, including defense by occupying space, competing for essential nutrients, stimulating cross-protective antibodies, and suppressing the growth of potentially pathogenic bacteria and fungi (Table 103–1).

Organisms that comprise the normal flora can become pathogenic when host defenses become impaired, or if they are translocated to other body sites during trauma. The identification of an organism considered to be normal flora in a wound or otherwise sterile body cavity or fluid often becomes a dilemma for the clinician in deciding whether or not a patient is infected and whether or not the patient requires treatment. Such is the case with *Staphylococcus epidermidis* when it is identified in the blood of a hospitalized patient. *S. epidermidis* is considered normal skin flora and commonly colonizes intravenous catheters. In these conditions, the identification of the organism must be taken in light of the patient circumstances (signs and symptoms, laboratory indices supporting infection) and the probability of the organism being responsible for the infection. Often, the simple removal of the catheter may eliminate the organism from the bloodstream, thereby preventing misdiagnosis and unnecessary application of antimicrobials.[8]

DIRECT EXAMINATION

Direct examination of tissue or body fluids believed to be infected can provide simple, rapid information to the clinician. Microscopic examination of wet mount specimen preparations can provide valuable information regarding potential pathogens. Applications of this procedure with or without staining preparations include direct examination of sputum, bronchial aspirates, scrapings of mucosal lesions, and urinary sediment. The Gram stain is one of the first identification

TABLE 103–1. Examples of Normal Bacterial Flora

	Gram-Positive		Gram-Negative		
	Cocci	*Rods*	*Cocci*	*Rods*	Other
Skin	*Staphylococcus* spp. (e.g., *S. epidermidis*) *Streptococcus* spp.	*Corynebacterium* spp. *Propionibacterium* spp.		Enteric bacilli (some sites) *Acinetobacter* spp. (Coccobacilli)	
Oropharynx	Streptococci—Viridans group Micrococcus	*Corynebacterium* spp.	Neisseria	*Haemophilus* spp.	Spirochetes
Gastrointenstinal tract	*Enterococcus* spp. *Peptostreptococcus* spp.	*Lactobacillus, Clostridium*		*Bacteroides* spp. Enteric bacilli (*E. coli, Klebsiella* spp.)	
Genital tract	*Streptococcus* spp. *Staphylococcus* spp.	*Lactobacillus* *Corynebacterium* spp.		*Enterobacteriaceae* *Prevotella* spp.	*Mycoplasma*

tests run on a specimen brought to the laboratory. For this procedure, crystal violet is applied as the primary stain with iodine added to enhance the staining process and to form a crystal violet-iodine complex. Alcohol decolorization is the next step in the procedure. Gram-negative cells are decolorized by the addition of alcohol, and they take in a red color when counterstained by safranin. Gram-positive cells are not decolorized by alcohol and retain the crystal violet color and appear purple. Gram staining in conjunction with microscopic examination may provide a presumptive diagnosis and some indication of the organism's characteristics (gram-positive, gram-negative, gram-variable, bacillus, or cocci). This is extremely useful information for the selection of empiric antibiotic therapy.

Gram stains are routinely performed on cerebral spinal fluid in cases of suspected meningitis, on urethral smears for venereal diseases, and on abscess or effusion specimens. They are helpful in identifying organisms, which may not grow on culture and which would otherwise be missed. Although Gram stains of sputum are routinely performed when respiratory tract infections are suspected, there is controversy regarding the usefulness of this test because the sputum is often contaminated with mixed or normal flora. The predominance of one particular organism, the overall number of organisms present, the amount of PMNs present, and the presence or absence of a significant amount of squamous epithelial cells (< 10 per low-power field) may improve the significance of the sputum Gram stain specimen.[9] Figure 103–2 lists some common infecting pathogens grouped according to Gram stain and other characteristics.

A variety of other staining techniques are used to identify pathogens. In particular, staining procedures are used for those pathogens that are best identified microscopically because of their poor growth characteristics in the laboratory setting. The best examples of these are the Ziehl-Neelsen stain for acid-fast bacilli, which is used for the identification of mycobacteria, and the India ink, potassium hydroxide (KOH), and Giemsa stains, which are useful for detecting certain fungi.[9]

CULTURES

Isolation of the etiologic agent by culture is the most definitive method available for the diagnosis and eventual treatment of infection. Although suspicion of a specific pathogen or group of pathogens is helpful to the laboratory for the selection of specific cultivating media, the more common procedure for the laboratory is to screen for the presence of any potential pathogen. After receipt of a clinical specimen, the laboratory will inoculate the specimen in a variety of artificial media. Some culture media are designed to differentiate various organisms on the basis of biochemical characteristics or to select specific organisms on the basis of resistance to certain antimicrobials. Other media are commonly employed for the isolation of more fastidious organisms, such as *Listeria, Legionella,* mycobacteria, or *Chlamydia*. Cultures for viruses are more difficult to perform and are primarily undertaken by larger institutions or outside laboratories because of the technical expense and time involved in processing samples.

When a culture is obtained, careful attention must be taken to ensure that specimens are appropriately collected and transported to the laboratory. Every effort should be made to avoid contamination with normal flora and to ensure that the specimen is placed in the appropriate transport media. Culture specimens should be transported to the laboratory as soon as possible because organisms may perish from prolonged exposure to air or drying. This is especially important for swab specimen preparations. Transport media may not be ideal for all organisms. Specimens that contain fastidious organisms or anaerobes require special transport media and should be immediately forwarded to the laboratory for processing. Last, the source of the specimen should be clearly recorded and forwarded along with the culture to the laboratory. This process will aid the laboratory in differentiating true pathogens from the expected, normal flora, and it will help in the selection of the appropriate culture media.

Detection of microorganisms in the bloodstream by standard culturing techniques is difficult because of the inherently low yield of organisms diluted by blood, humoral factors with bactericidal activity, and the potential of antimicrobial pretreatment affecting organism growth. Newer automated systems employing the use of media-containing culture bottles and innovative organism detection techniques have improved this situation. Most blood collection bottles dilute the blood specimen 1:10 with growth media to neutralize the bactericidal properties of blood and antimicrobials. The addition of a polyanionic anticoagulant abolishes the effect of complement and antiphagocytic activity in the specimen. Some laboratories also add β-lactamase to their blood collection bottles. Antibiotic-binding resin bottles, such as Bactec 16 B, are also commercially available.

Rapid detection of bacteria or fungi within a few hours of specimen collection is now possible by the use of automated culturing systems, such as Bactec (Becton Dickinson Diagnostic Instruments, Sparks, MD), that use bottles of growth media containing a fluorescent sensor to monitor culture bottles for the presence of CO_2 every 10 minutes as a by-product of microorganism growth. Computers monitoring the system alert laboratory personnel of positive culture results by both audible and visual alarms. Once detected, a battery

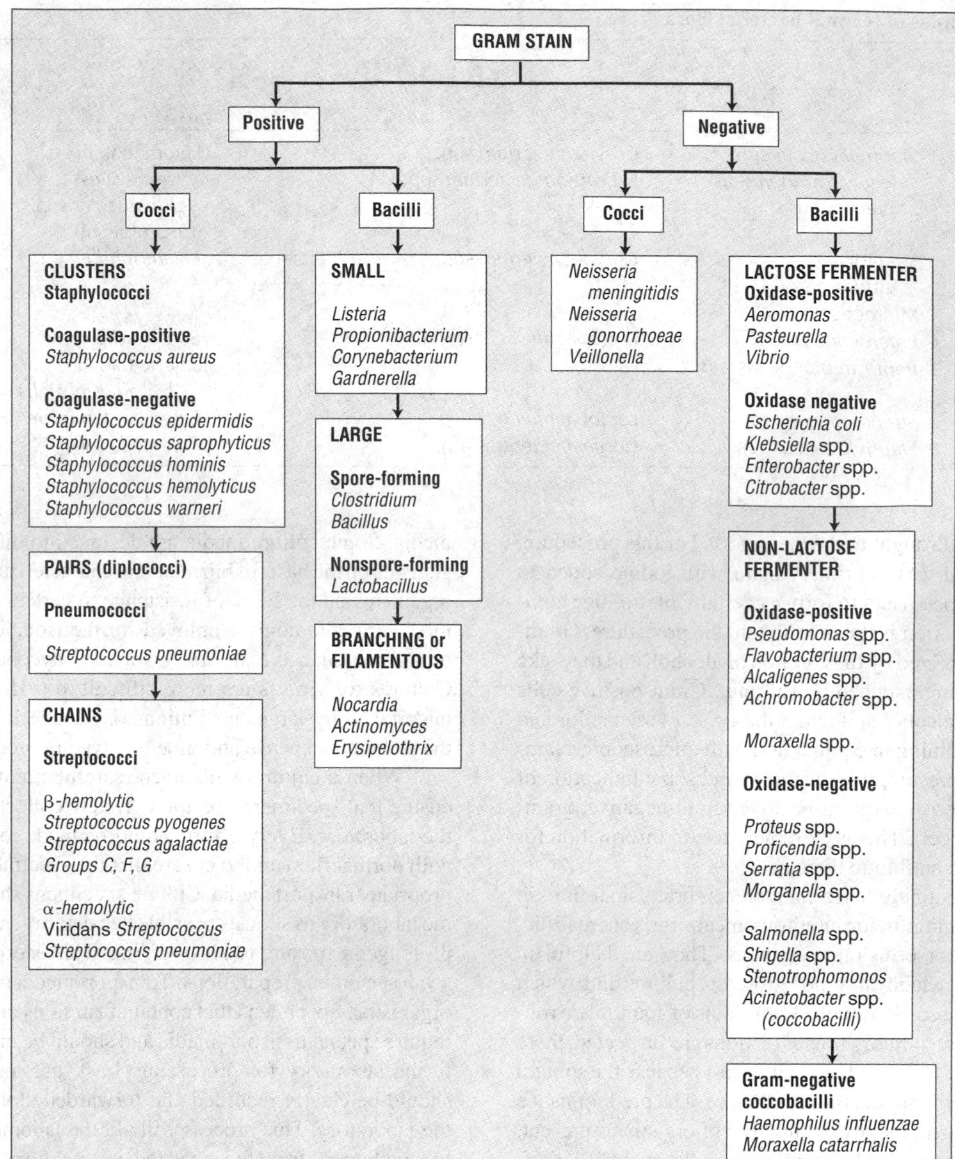

FIGURE 103–2. Important bacterial pathogens classified according to Gram stain and morphologic characteristics.

of testing can be performed rapidly that shortens the reporting time and that enables clinicians to obtain preliminary information about the organism.[10,11]

The initial identity of the organism can be determined by a variety of testing procedures. General schemes differentiate organisms into primary groups, such as gram-positive and gram-negative bacteria. This can be accomplished by simple Gram staining, as previously described, by evaluating organism growth patterns on selective media, and by testing for the presence or absence of specific enzymes and chemical characteristics, such as hemolytic and fermentation properties. For example, a nonlactose-fermenting, gram-negative bacilli that is oxidase positive may suggest *Pseudomonas aeruginosa* as opposed to a variety of other potential gram-negative organisms. This preliminary information, which is readily obtainable from the laboratory, may greatly assist the clinician in choosing the appropriate empiric therapy.

Definitive identification of organisms requires more complex testing procedures and devices that can further differentiate the organism on the basis of specific fermentation and biochemical reactive properties. Commercially available automated systems can inoculate the test organism into a series of panels containing a variety of test media, sugars, and other reagents. The system can then photometrically determine the results and compare the findings to a library of organism characteristics to produce a definitive identification.

Viral agents may be detected by direct observation of inoculated culture cells for cytopathic effects or by detection of antigens after incubation by immunofluorescent methods. The culture method is most useful for organisms such as cytomegalovirus (CMV) or herpes simplex virus, because these viral agents are rapidly propagated in culture cells, making them easily detected.

DIAGNOSIS OF INFECTION USING IMMUNOLOGIC AND MOLECULAR METHODS

ANTIBODY AND ANTIGEN DETECTION

The use of immunologic methods for the diagnosis and monitoring of human-host immune response to infection has become an indispensable laboratory tool. This is especially important in the detection of microorganisms, such as bacteria, fungi, and viruses, which would otherwise elude detection or severely delay results from conventional culturing techniques. These methods have the advantage of a rapid turnaround time and an acceptable level of sensitivity and specificity. Some tests (e.g., identification of group A streptococci) are simple to use, can be performed conveniently in the physician's office, and may often be used to decide whether antibiotics should be administered for a suspected upper respiratory infection.

The primary immunologic methods involve the detection and quantification of antibodies directed against a specific pathogen or its components (i.e., surface proteins of HIV, such as p24 antigen). The commercial availability of specific monoclonal antibodies in a variety of testing formats has led to an increased use of these methods for direct pathogen detection. Although pathogen antigenic proteins may be increased and, therefore, easily detected during acute infection, detection of past or asymptomatic infection may be difficult because of undetectable levels of antigen and, therefore, low antibody titers. Continued advancement in test sensitivity (the capability to detect a true positive state) and specificity (the capability to detect a negative state), as well as the use of amplification techniques, will likely improve these tests in the near future. Antibody or antigen detection may be accomplished by a variety of techniques, including immunofluorescence, which has been routinely used for the detection of cytomegalovirus, respiratory syncytial virus, varicella-zoster virus, *Treponema pallidum* (syphilis), *Borrelia burgdorferi* (Lyme's disease), and *Chlamydia trachomatis*. Latex agglutination is useful for detecting meningococcal capsular antigens in cerebral spinal fluid of patients suspected of having bacterial meningitis and as an aid in the diagnosis of *Legionella pneumophila*. Enzyme-linked immunosorbent assay (ELISA) is a commonly employed method for detecting HIV, herpes simplex virus, respiratory syncytial virus, pneumococcal serum antibody, *Neisseria gonorrhoeae*, and *Haemophilus pylori*.[12]

MOLECULAR TECHNIQUES FOR THE DETECTION OF MICROORGANISMS

HYBRIDIZATION DNA PROBES

Highly sensitive and specific molecular methods are now available for the rapid detection and identification of a variety of pathogens. The two primary molecular techniques commonly used are nucleic acid hybridization, which involves the binding of a specific DNA or RNA probe to its target or DNA amplification schemes. Probe-based methods require the extraction of DNA or RNA from a clinical specimen (body fluid, tissue, WBC) or directly from a microorganism culture. The extract is then tested for the presence of pathogen DNA or RNA using a probe that contains a specific oligonucleic acid-based sequence for the organism. For example, a probe with a sequence of ACTGTT would bind to the complementary organism nucleic acid sequence of TGACAA. Because the probe is labeled with a signal-emitting molecule (radiolabeled, colorimetric, or chemoluminescent), a match would be detected. The primary means for detection involves the use of separation of the organism DNA into specific fragments (gel electrophoresis), the mixing of the DNA fragments with the labeled probe (hybridization), transfer and fixation of the mixture to specialized paper or nylon membranes (Southern or Northern blotting), and transfer to radiographic or photographic film for processing. These techniques have been used for many years and are fairly standardized methods for the detection of a variety of organisms.[13]

Hybridization probes are useful for a variety of diagnostic and clinical applications, including the direct examination of organisms in tissue, which enables the evaluation and documentation of organism infestation, location, distribution, and host response. The use of hybridization probes is particularly helpful for the detection of slow-growing organisms, such as *Mycobacterium tuberculosis, N. gonorrhoeae,* and certain species of fungi. This technique is also used to document the presence or absence of antimicrobial-resistant genes in a cell culture and to track the spread of resistant microorganisms in hospital and outpatient settings.

Although widely employed, the use of hybridization probes is often limited by their lack of sensitivity. Probe amplification methods are available that improve the sensitivity of these assays. The principle of these probe amplification schemes is to boost the probe's signal-emitting molecule to make it more easily detected. The most advanced signal amplification system available is the branched DNA (bDNA) probe system (Chiron Corp., Emeryville, CA). This system uses multiple probes and multiple signal-emitting molecules (reporters). The target-binding probe contains two hybridization regions. One region is complementary to the target, and the other region is capable of binding with the bDNA amplification multimer. The amplification multimer binds multiple reporter molecules (as many as 3,000), which provides a significant boost in the probe's signal. Branched DNA probe systems are being developed for rapid detection of hepatitis B and C, HIV-1, and CMV. Because of the system's high specificity and quantitative ability, bDNA probe assays may be useful for therapeutic monitoring, such as in the case of monitoring the response to antiretroviral therapy in acquired immunodeficiency syndrome (AIDS).[14]

NUCLEIC ACID AMPLIFICATION METHODS

Nucleic acid amplification methods are now considered a standard laboratory tool. They have had a tremendous impact on the diagnosis and treatment of infectious diseases. These highly sensitive methods have the capability to detect and quantitate minute amounts of target nucleic acid in a rapid manner. The polymerase chain reaction (PCR) is based on the capability of a DNA polymerase to copy and elongate a targeted strand of DNA. This is accomplished by the use of short oligonucleotide primers (20 to 25 nucleotides long) that correspond to the DNA targeted to be expanded. After an excess of primers and heat-stable DNA, polymerases are added to the targeted DNA mixture, and the targeted DNA is denatured and separated by a process of cycling hot and cool temperatures. The heat-stable DNA polymerase elongates the primers on the two separate strands of DNA, thereby generating two new strands of targeted DNA. The process of cycling is typically repeated 20 to 35 times. Each cycle doubles the amount of DNA originally present at the start of the cycle, thereby exponentially increasing the overall number of DNA copies. In theory, more than 1 million copies of the original DNA can be generated from as few as 20 cycles.

Although this amplification technique is very sensitive and has tremendous application potential, it is not without problems. The powerful amplification procedure may yield false-positive results when samples are contaminated by nucleic acid left over from previously amplified DNA. Other problems include primer artifact formation and nonspecific hybridization of primers to DNA samples. Several modifications to the original PCR technology have been made over the years to improve the sensitivity and application potential for PCR, including the use of multiple sets of amplification primers; the amplification of two or more target DNA sequences simultaneously; PCR amplification of RNA by converting targeted RNA with reverse transcriptase to complementary DNA templates, which are then suitable for DNA amplification by traditional PCR techniques; and the use of thermostable DNA polymerase.

The cost-benefit ratio of PCR as compared to traditional microbiologic methods must be evaluated. Molecular amplification schemes such as PCR are likely to find early acceptance in situations in which rapid turnaround time is essential to improve patient diagnosis and outcome, for eaxample, for the isolation and detection of fastidious or slow-growing organisms such as *M. tuberculosis* and *B. burgdorferi*. Another potential application for this technology is the early detection of multidrug-resistant organisms. Amplification of resistant gene markers would aid in rapid selection of the most appropriate therapy in the treatment of organisms in which days or weeks are traditionally required for culturing and determining basic susceptibility. Examples fitting this description include the rapid detection of isoniazid and rifampin gene markers for *M. tuberculosis,* early detection of the *mec* gene responsible for methicillin resistance in *S. aureus,* and identification of resistant genes responsible for production of β-lactamase capable of destroying specific cephalosporins.[14,15]

EVALUATION OF THE PHARMACODYNAMIC PROPERTIES OF ANTIMICROBIALS

The laboratory evaluation of antimicrobial susceptibility is an important component of the pharmacotherapeutic management of infectious diseases. With the rapid increases in antimicrobial resistance in bacteria, fungi, and viruses, the integration of susceptibility data into empiric treatment choices and subsequent regimen modifications is becoming even more crucial. As well, analysis of organism susceptibility profiles is a mandatory step for many cost-containment strategies, such as antimicrobial streamlining programs or intravenous-to-oral switch protocols.[16]

Although most susceptibility tests used are well characterized and standardized by the National Committee for Clinical Laboratory Standards (NCCLS), there still is much controversy concerning methods, interpretation, and integration of the results into the management of the patient.[17] Often, susceptibility reporting methods can make the pharmacodynamic optimization of antimicrobial therapy potentially difficult. Nevertheless, many investigations show that the general susceptibility profile of an infecting organism can correlate with both clinical and microbiologic responses to therapy.

Most standardized and well-accepted test methods evaluate the susceptibility of aerobic, nonfastidious bacteria. In recent years, substantial progress has been made in the development of sensitive, specific, and reproducible tests for anaerobes, yeasts, mycobacteria, and viruses. As technology continues to advance testing methods, more rapid and accurate procurement of results should help to aid the clinician in the diagnosis and treatment of all infectious diseases. These systems are often very expensive, but the pharmacotherapist can play an important role in the collaborative assessment of the impact of these tests on the overall costs and quality of care for the patient with infection. The discussion of these tests in the upcoming sections suggests potential areas in which pharmacoeconomic evaluation is useful.

MINIMAL INHIBITORY CONCENTRATION

The minimal inhibitory concentration (MIC) is the lowest antimicrobial concentration that prevents visible growth of an organism after 24 hours of incubation in a specified growth medium. The MIC allows for quantitative determination of *in vitro* antibacterial activity. Classically, MIC testing via the macrotube method involves the use of liquid growth medium (broth), doubling serial dilutions of antimicrobials in test tubes, and a standard inoculum of bacteria (1–5 × 10^5 colony-forming units [CFU]/mL). The tubes (1–2 mL) are incubated at ≈35°C (95°F) for 18–24 hours and then examined for visible bacterial growth (Fig. 103–3). Although macrodilution MIC testing is laborious and supply intensive, it does enable a large inoculum of bacteria to be tested, which can help to detect small numbers of resistant subpopulations or the presence of inducible resistance.[18]

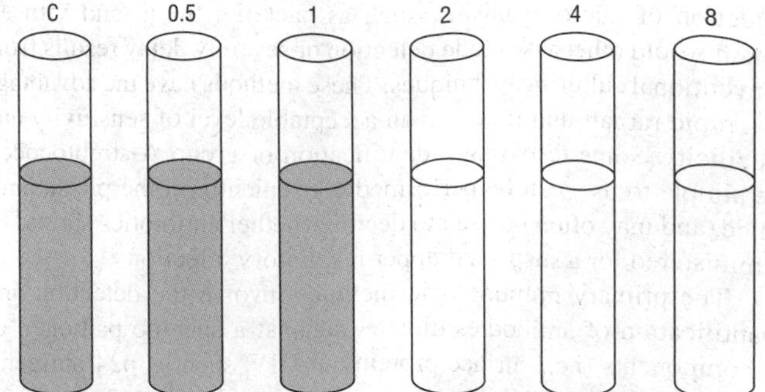

FIGURE 103–3. Macrotube minimal inhibitory concentration (MIC) determination. The growth control (C), 0.5-mg/L, and 1-mg/L tubes are visibly turbid, indicating bacterial growth. The MIC is read as the first clear test tube (2 mg/L).

The use of 96-well microtiter plates enabled the increased use of broth-dilution MIC testing in the clinical laboratory, as it significantly reduced the amount of labor and media needed. Volumes of 100–200 μL or less of media are used, and multichannel pipets, automated systems, or both can allow for the rapid preparation of numerous tests (Fig. 103–4). The microdilution MIC test method is the most commonly used method in the clinical microbiology laboratory.[19]

Although microdilution MIC testing is a vast improvement over macrodilution MIC testing, it still has important shortcomings, including decreased flexibility of the antimicrobial test panels (especially with premade or premanufactured trays), as well as a decrease in the sensitivity to detect some forms of antimicrobial resistance as compared to the macrodilution method. Although the preparation of several serial twofold drug dilutions and inoculation with bacteria are time-consuming, expensive, and infeasible for most clinical

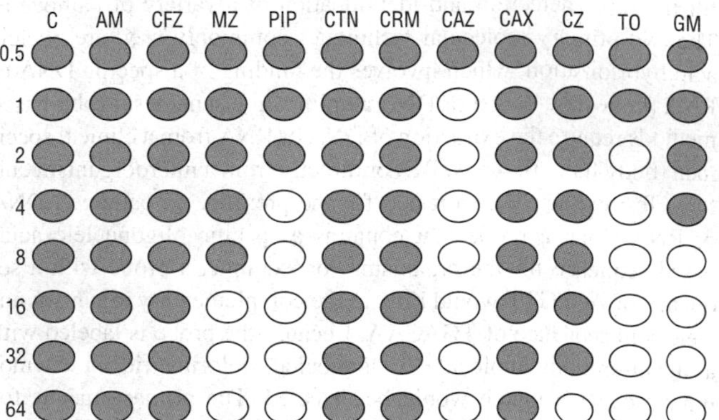

FIGURE 103–4. A prepared microtiter minimal inhibitory concentration (MIC) tray (96 wells). The tray provides a range of MICs from 0.5 mg/h to 64 mg/L. The panel represents antibiotics commonly tested against gram-negative pathogens. This tray indicates that the organism is resistant to ampicillin (AM), cefazolin (CFZ), cefotetan (CTN), cefuroxime (CRM), ceftriaxone (CAX), and gentamicin (GM). The isolate is sensitive to mezlocillin (MZ), piperacillin (PIP), ceftazidime (CAZ), and tobramycin (TO). The isolate would be considered intermediately susceptible to ceftizoxime (CZ).

laboratories, these problems are minimized by the automation of computer-assisted testing systems.

The MIC can also be determined using solid agar. For the agar dilution MIC determination, the antimicrobial is added to the molten agar just prior to its solidification to make the desired test concentration. After the agar has hardened, suspensions of test bacteria are applied to the agar. As with broth MIC methods, the agar MIC is the lowest concentration that prevents the visible growth of the organism after an overnight incubation period. Although agar dilution MICs were once considered the standard susceptibility test for certain slow-growing organisms such as *M. tuberculosis,* their use is declining in most clinical labs with the advent of more rapid and less cumbersome contemporary susceptibility testing methods (PCR, radiometric, or fluorometric tests).

LIMITATIONS AND PROBLEMS WITH MIC TESTING

Although the MIC is the most rigorously tested and standardized *in vitro* test of antimicrobial activity, it is not problem-free. Some of these problems are academic in nature, whereas others can have important implications for the everyday management of patients with serious infections.

It is important to remember that the MIC does not represent equivalent antimicrobial activity against all bacteria present in an infection. Some bacteria may be more or less susceptible, and inadequate exposure to the antimicrobial *in vivo* could potentially select for more resistant subpopulations, negatively impacting the clinical response to infection. Many times, resistance may not be detected using the inocula tested *in vitro* but may be present *in vivo,* where a much higher inoculum increases the chances for spontaneously resistant mutants.[20]

Many factors can influence the *in vitro* MIC value obtained and its relevance to the *in vivo* situation. The bacterial growth medium used and cation content can significantly affect the activity of many drugs. For example, aminoglycosides are less active against *P. aeruginosa* in a medium supplemented with physiologic concentrations of magnesium and calcium (standardized method) than in a medium without these cations.[17] MIC values of antibiotics highly bound to plasma proteins are often significantly higher in a medium containing human serum, but testing of these drugs in a serum-supplemented medium has not gained widespread acceptance. The bacterial inoculum significantly affects the MIC of some drugs against certain organisms. This is particularly true for most β-lactam antibiotics and gram-negative bacilli, where a 100-fold increase in the size of an inoculum can increase the β-lactam's MIC to such an extent as to make a susceptible organism at a lower inoculum become resistant. Fortunately, standardized guidelines for testing and quality assurance procedures proposed by the NCCLS attempt to minimize the impact of these problems and are followed by most clinical and research laboratories.[21,22]

With the multitude of factors (e.g., mechanical errors, organism growth characteristics) that could affect the interpretation of *in vitro* MIC testing and its application to treatment of infections, it is impressive that correlations between susceptibility and clinical outcomes have been observed. Not all patients infected with susceptible organisms, however, will have an adequate clinical or microbiologic response. In these situations of paradoxic antimicrobial therapy failure, the potential confounders mentioned earlier should be considered as possibly being related to observed failure. Data are accumulating that indicate that the combination of *in vitro* susceptibility parameters, such as the MIC, with *in vivo* antimicrobial pharmacokinetic parameters (pharmacodynamic parameters) can result in a better prediction of therapeutic response than organism susceptibility alone.

DISK DIFFUSION ASSAY

The disk diffusion assay method for susceptibility testing (Kirby-Bauer method) was developed in the 1960s by Bauer and coworkers to reduce the labor needed for tube dilution susceptibility testing, and it still is one of the most reliable methods for evaluating qualitative antimicrobial susceptibilities in the clinical laboratory.[23] Up to 12 antibiotic-impregnated disks are placed on an agar plate previously streaked with a standard suspension of bacteria ($1–2 \times 10^8$ CFU/mL). The drug diffuses in a concentration gradient from the disk out into the agar. The plate is incubated (18–24 hours at 35°C [95°F]), and bacterial growth occurs only in areas in which the drug concentrations are below those required to cause inhibition. The diameters of the zones of inhibition are measured via calipers or automated scanners and compared to standard interpretive zone sizes to determine susceptibility, intermediate susceptibility, or resistance to the antimicrobials tested (Fig. 103–5). Because factors such as agar composition, incubation temperature, bacterial inoculum, and antibiotic paper disk composition can influence results, standards for test conditions and interpretive zone sizes are defined by the NCCLS. Because the relationships between MIC and zone size are not always perfect (i.e., some organisms with higher MICs may have large zone sizes as compared to other organisms with similar MICs), breakpoint zone size values are chosen that minimize the possibilities of a major classification error (i.e., a resistant organism being reported as susceptible).

The Kirby-Bauer method is simple to perform, easy to interpret, and flexible with respect to which antimicrobial agents to test. Until the development of automated systems, Kirby-Bauer testing was by far the most common method for susceptibility testing in the clinical microbiology laboratory. A survey of clinical microbiology laboratories indicated that only 27% of laboratories perform disk diffusion as the primary susceptibility test versus 73% for microdilution, automated testing systems, or both—a near reversal of the percentages that were observed in 1983.[19,22]

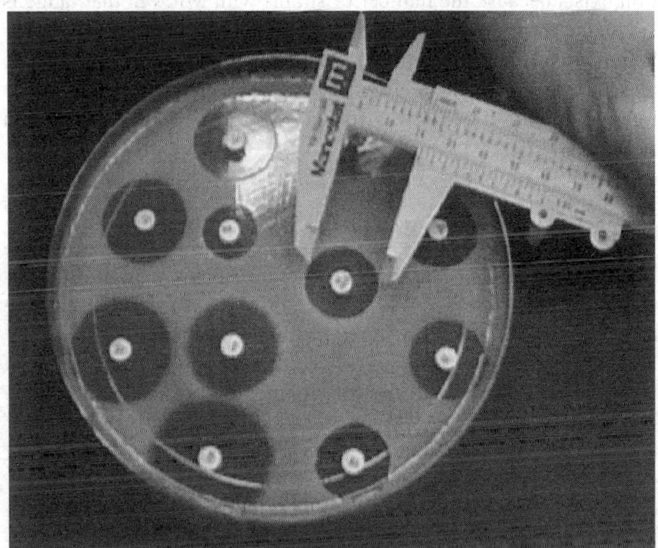

FIGURE 103–5. Disk diffusion susceptibility test. Antibiotic impregnated disks are placed on the surface of a plate previously inoculated with the test organism. The plate is incubated for 18 hours and the subsequent zones of inhibition are measured. The zone size correlates to the sensitivity of the organism. The larger the zone size, the more sensitive the organism to the specific antibiotic. On the basis of predetermined zone breakpoints, organisms may be classified as susceptible, resistant, or intermediately susceptible to the antibiotic.

DETERMINATION AND INTERPRETATION OF QUALITATIVE AND QUANTITATIVE SUSCEPTIBILITIES

Despite many *in vitro*, animal, and human studies that show correlations between quantitative MICs and clinical outcomes, MIC data often are qualitatively expressed by deeming an organism as either susceptible, intermediate to moderately susceptible, or resistant to the given antimicrobial agent.[22] This simplification allows quicker and easier interpretation of susceptibility data by noninfectious disease practitioners who might not be able to interpret, or may have no need for, the MIC value.

Many factors are considered when determining these qualitative susceptibility classifications. Pharmacokinetic properties, such as the peak serum concentration, elimination half-life, and degree of protein binding, are included, as well as the MIC frequency distribution.[17] The establishment of a breakpoint in an area of common MIC values is undesirable, because a substantial fluctuation in the susceptibility classifications of organisms would occur because of the inherent twofold variability observed during serial dilution MIC testing. The clinical and bacteriologic responses observed for an antimicrobial agent against different strains of bacteria with various MIC values help to support the clinical relevance of the breakpoints chosen. Most often, the consideration of these factors results in a susceptibility breakpoint of between one-sixteenth to one-fourth of the achievable peak serum concentration.[24]

Pathogens classified as susceptible to an antibiotic are those with the lowest MICs, and they are the most likely to be eradicated during therapy of infections using typical drug doses. Conversely, resistant organisms are bacteria with significantly higher MICs that will cause a less-than-optimal clinical response, even at the highest doses. Organisms that are moderately sensitive or that are intermediately susceptible are less clearly defined; these organisms appear to be less likely to be effectively treated as compared to a susceptible strain. Treatment of organisms in this range may be successful when maximum doses of a drug are used or when the drug is known to be concentrated in the infected body site. In some cases, the intermediate classification exists because the number of strains with MICs in that range is small and their susceptibility is really indeterminate (i.e., the organism may be either susceptible or resistant). Finally, the intermediate classification serves as a buffer zone to avoid major changes in the interpretation of the MIC value because of the twofold variability in testing.

ISSUES WITH QUALITATIVE SUSCEPTIBILITY TESTING

There are concerns that the "user-friendly" breakpoint susceptibility system (susceptible, intermediate, or resistant) oversimplify the decision-making processes in the treatment of infectious diseases.[17] Determination of breakpoint concentrations often does not factor in the impressive alterations in pharmacokinetics in critically ill patients. For example, a critically ill patient may fail antimicrobial therapy of a susceptible organism at the usual doses. If serum concentrations or concentrations at the site of infection were assayed (not commonly done), one might discover suboptimal concentrations, possibly related to poor tissue perfusion. Likewise, a patient with severe vascular insufficiency and a diabetic foot infection may fail a course of therapy with normal doses of an antimicrobial and a susceptible organism because of inadequate drug delivery. Some investigators have shown that different outcomes can be achieved for susceptible organisms with different MIC values[25,26] and that substantial (although not acceptable) rates of clinical or microbiologic cure can occur for infections caused by resistant organisms.[27] These reports emphasize that susceptibility does not unequivocally correlate with clinical success and that resistant organisms do not always equate with impending clinical failure.

Similarities in the spectrum of activity for classes of antibiotics have led to the concept of "class testing." Thus, cephalothin susceptibility results are extrapolated to other first-generation cephalosporins, such as cephalexin or cefazolin. Likewise, susceptibility to an antibiotic that typically has minimal activity usually ensures that other more potent agents in its class will have activity as well. Many gram-negative organisms, however, have developed extended-spectrum β-lactamases (ESBLs) that often have different activity against members of the same drug class. These developments limit the utility of class testing to reduce susceptibility testing workload. In the setting of an inadequately responding infection with a common ESBL-producing organism, the pathogen may be susceptible to a class antibiotic (if used) but resistant to the antimicrobial agent being administered to the patient.

OTHER SUSCEPTIBILITY TESTS

EPSILOMETER TEST

The Epsilometer test (E-test; AB Biodisk, Solna, Sweden) is a relatively new development in susceptibility testing that combines the quantitative benefits of microtiter MIC testing with the ease of agar diffusion testing. A plastic strip impregnated with a known, prefixed concentration gradient of antibiotic is placed on an agar plate streaked with a suspension of known bacterial inoculum. The drug instantly diffuses from the plastic strip to form an effective concentration gradient within the agar. After overnight incubation, elliptical zones of inhibition are formed; the point where the bottom of the ellipse crosses the plastic strip is correlated to a printed MIC value on the strip (Fig. 103–6).

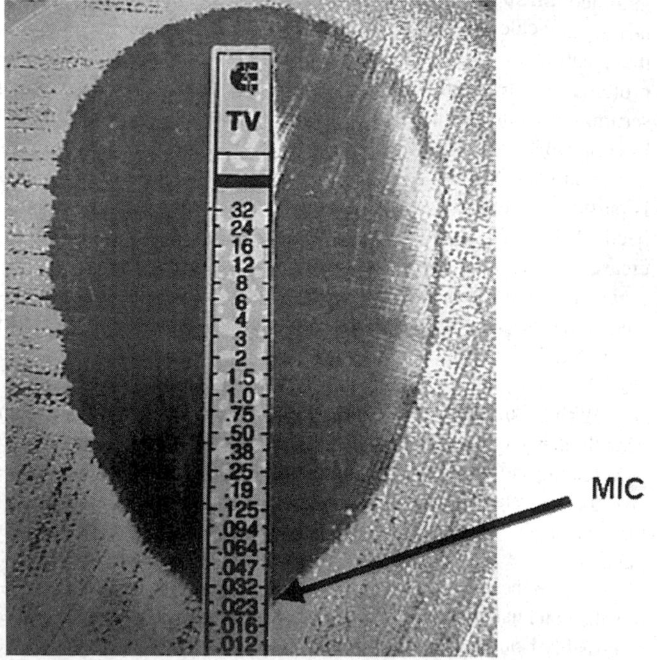

FIGURE 103–6. Photograph of E-strip susceptibility test. The minimal inhibitory concentration (MIC) is determined from the point where the zone of inhibition intersects with the numerical scale. (Photograph courtesy of Anti-Infective Research Laboratory, Wayne State University, Detroit, MI.)

Many investigators have analyzed the E-test's correlation with standard susceptibility methods and assessed its potential clinical use. In general, values obtained with E-test methods are comparable or even more consistent and accurate than standard methods. In fact, the E-test method is the recommended method for susceptibility testing of *Streptococcus pneumoniae*. In addition, good correlation with more laborious agar or broth dilution methods is documented for other fastidious or difficult-to-test organisms, such as *Haemophilus influenzae,* anaerobes, *Bartonella, Flavobacterium, Legionella,* and nutritionally variant streptococci.[28–30] The widespread clinical use of the E-test is limited, however, because of the excessive costs of the test strips in relation to the benefits gained from their use.

SPIRAL GRADIENT MINIMAL INHIBITORY CONCENTRATION DETERMINATIONS

The spiral gradient MIC is performed using an apparatus that applies a sample of antimicrobial spirally from the center of an agar plate to its periphery. Because of the exponential deposition of the sample, an antimicrobial gradient is formed. Bacterial inocula are streaked radially on the plate, and the distance of growth toward the center is measured after proper incubation. The distance of growth is measured and correlated with a MIC based on predetermined drug concentrations at various distances.[17] This method is useful for the testing of anaerobic bacteria and for testing in the research setting, but as with the E-test, its clinical use is limited because of its prohibitively high costs of operation.[18,30]

AUTOMATED MICROBIAL SUSCEPTIBILITY TESTING

Various degrees of automation have been applied to susceptibility testing. Early advances included automated preparation of microtiter trays, instrument-assisted readers, and computer-assisted result databases.[18] Although these improvements helped to decrease preparation and interpretation times, these methods still required an 18- to 24-hour lag period for bacterial growth to evaluate susceptibility. The availability and increased use of rapid automated susceptibility tests began in the 1980s, and continues to increase. In 1991, approximately 15% of clinical microbiology laboratories reported using rapid automated test systems.

Rapid antimicrobial susceptibility systems often incorporate the use of microprocessors, robotics, and microcomputers to produce results in as few as 3 hours.[19] Also, these systems allow for rapid identification of organisms through the use of biochemical test batteries. There are two rapid susceptibility test systems in common use in clinical microbiology laboratories. The Vitek system (bioMerieux Vitek, Hazelwood, MO) uses technology originally developed for use in spacecraft to identify and test organisms rapidly for antimicrobial susceptibility.[19] This system uses small plastic reagent "cards" (see Fig. 103–7) that contain 30 or 45 wells for the testing of various antimicrobials or indicator chemicals. Bacterial test suspensions (25 μL total, providing $\approx 2 \times 10^5$ CFU/well) enter the wells by capillary diffusion and growth is monitored automatically via photometric assessment of turbidity every hour for up to 15 hours. When the growth control reaches a specified turbidity level, growth curves for all wells are calculated and compared to the growth control curve for slope normalization. Computerized linear regression and the use of best-fit line coefficients produce an algorithm-derived MIC. The clinical laboratory can control the results output generated (qualitative, quantitative, or both).

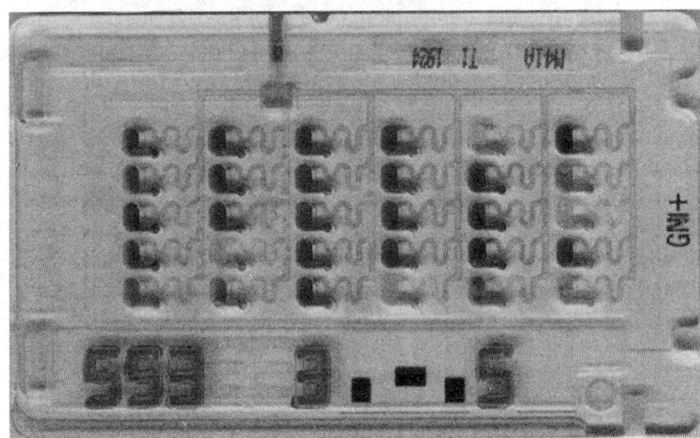

FIGURE 103–7. Vitek system for bacterial susceptibility testing.

The MicroScanWalkAway system (Baxter Diagnostics, Inc., Microscan Division, West Sacramento, CA) is a rapid test system that uses fluorogenic substrate hydrolysis as an indicator of bacterial growth.[19] This system uses standard microdilution test trays and a computer-controlled incubator and reader unit that can perform robotic manipulations, such as reagent addition and tray rotation, to allow for spectrophotometric or fluorometric growth assessments. Bacterial inocula ($\approx 6 \times 10^4$ CFU/well for gram-negative organisms and $\approx 10^5$ CFU/well for gram-positive organisms) are added to the wells, and growth is detected by the production of fluorophores from hydrolysis of amidomethylcoumarin or methyl umbelliferyl fluorogenic substrates. Although this method is a more sensitive assessment of growth as compared to turbidity, its indirect nature allows for the possibility of bacterial growth without hydrolysis of the fluorophores; this occurrence is rare, however. As with the Vitek system, growth curves are generated and algorithms applied for the determination of MICs; output is via computer or video display.

With integration and mergers being commonplace in health care systems around the country, an adequate correlation between susceptibility results obtained from these different systems is important to enable different institutions to compare data reliably. A good correlation between the Vitek and MicroScan WalkAway systems has been shown, with acceptable rates for the categories "very major" and "major discrepancies" shown between the two systems.[31] Both the Vitek and WalkAway systems contain information management systems that allow for the storage and rapid retrieval of susceptibility data. Both systems are also capable of producing chartable patient data reports, antibiograms, and epidemiologic reports. Importantly, these systems can be interfaced with other clinical information systems, such as the pharmacy, infection control, or other laboratory data systems, which may improve clinical outcomes.[32,33]

APPLICATION OF RAPID AUTOMATED SUSCEPTIBILITY TESTING AND IMPACT ON CLINICAL OUTCOMES

Although rapid systems are widely used, there are only minimal data to suggest that they can have an appreciable impact on patient care and outcomes. Rapid testing was associated with a higher likelihood of more appropriate antimicrobial therapy and a change to a more appropriate or less costly therapy in a cohort of 226 patients with bacteremia.[34] Doern and colleagues reported that the use of rapid systems allowed for modification of antimicrobial therapy 24 hours sooner in a group of patients with bacteremia.[35] These investigators also reported that rapid tests helped to decrease the time to provision of susceptibility and identification results by ≈12 hours as compared to a procedure simulating the "usual" methods.[36] A significantly lower, infection-related mortality rate was seen in the rapid test group (7%) versus the usual-method group (12.7%). Statistically fewer microbiology tests, blood cultures, and other laboratory or clinical tests associated with infections were performed in the rapid group, and mean antimicrobial costs per patient were nearly $300 less than with the usual-method group. The mean cost of hospitalization was approximately $4,000 less for the rapid group versus the usual-method group.

PROBLEMS WITH RAPID AUTOMATED SUSCEPTIBILITY SYSTEMS

There are some disadvantages and pitfalls associated with rapid susceptibility systems. Antibiotic test panels or cards are premanufactured in a limited number of combinations, and the number of antibiotics tested per panel is limited; more than one test card may be necessary for some institutions. Compared to the Kirby-Bauer method, flexibility to modify the antimicrobial test battery is extremely compromised. The substantial initial capital investment for rapid systems, as well as the added and continual costs for disposable trays and maintenance could obviate the cost savings from the decreased manual labor, while producing similar workloads, as compared to traditional agar dilution testing.[18,37,39]

The growth of fastidious or anaerobic bacteria is such that rapid systems cannot be reliably used; because of this, numerous test methods must be available in the clinical laboratory for the different potential pathogens isolated from clinical specimens. Another potential problem with rapid testing is the unreliable detection of important resistance mechanisms, such as type-1 inducible or chromosomally mediated (derepressed) β-lactamase resistance in *Serratia, Pseudomonas, Enterobacter,* indole-positive *Proteus* and *Providencia,* and *Morganella* species.[20,21] Inducible resistance requires a longer period for detection than that used in rapid systems, whereas derepressed mutants often occur naturally, but at rates of 1 in 10^{6-7} organisms, which is lower than the number of bacteria tested. Initially, rapid systems also had problems detecting methicillin-resistant *Staphylococcus aureus* (MRSA), but improvements in the media used and in the computerized analysis have substantially improved the ability to detect MRSA.[38] Still, very heterogeneous MRSA (such as 1 MRSA in 10^{6-8} organisms) may not be detected because of the low inoculum that is used.[20] Regardless of improvements in the rapid systems, it is still recommended to verify the presence of methicillin resistance by other standard and accepted methods.

ADVANCES IN SUSCEPTIBILITY TESTING FOR MYCOBACTERIA, FUNGI, AND VIRUSES

Impressive advances have been made in the past decade in the areas of mycobacterial, fungal, and viral susceptibility testing. The use of radiometric techniques, such as the Bactec system (Becton Dickinson Diagnostic Instruments, Sparks, MD), has revolutionized the analysis of antimicrobial susceptibility in *M. tuberculosis.* Radiometric susceptibility testing involves the incubation of *M. tuberculosis* in liquid media containing ^{14}C-labeled growth substrate. As organisms grow, respiration causes the release of ^{14}C, which is then detected. The growth indices for antimicrobial-containing bottles are compared to those of a control bottle with the calculation of a MIC. The use of this method, coupled with the rapid processing of samples, has reduced the time to susceptibility result generation to ≈2.5 weeks.[40]

Antimicrobial susceptibility testing for *Mycobacterium avium* complex (MAC) is less standardized because of its intrinsic antimicrobial resistance and different colony variants with differing susceptibilities, among other factors. The broth radiometric method for quantitative MIC determination thus far appears to be the most consistent and reproducible method, and it has been advocated for use by leading experts in mycobacteriology.[41] Although data are limited, there appears to be a correlation between *in vitro* susceptibility profiles and clinical response to MAC infection, especially for the macrolide antimicrobials.[41,42] In the future, the use of molecular probes for mycobacterial resistance genes will most likely become a standard for rapid susceptibility determinations, especially in light of the increasing problems with antimicrobial resistance in mycobacteria. Probes or PCR techniques for the *katG* gene, which is needed in order to cause isoniazid (INH) susceptibility, and the *rpoB* gene, which alters the β-subunit of RNA polymerase causing rifampin resistance, have been evaluated in the research laboratory and hold promise for eventual clinical application.[40]

There has been a rapid increase in the prevalence of fungal infections in the past two decades. An increase in the use of antifungal agents and, not surprisingly, an increase in the detection of antifungal resistance has followed.[43] For many years, no standardized susceptibility tests were available, and there was no way to assess correlations between *in vitro* tests and clinical outcome. Since then, an NCCLS task force has issued guidelines for both macro- and microdilution susceptibility tests that produce a greater than 90% inter- and intralaboratory reproducibility.[44] Although routine antifungal testing is not recommended, periodic batch testing for antibiograms and surveillance of resistance or testing of patients with oropharyngeal candidiasis refractory to therapy may be warranted.[43–45]

Published studies show an acceptable correlation of more rapid and less cumbersome test methods, such as microdilution, E-test, and disk diffusion (for fluconazole) with standard macrodilution testing. More importantly, clinical studies show the correlation of these *in vitro* tests for fluconazole susceptibility with outcomes in HIV and AIDS patients with oropharyngeal candidiasis and cryptococcal meningitis.[43–46] There are much less or a complete lack of data correlating susceptibility and clinical outcome for other azoles, amphotericin B, filamentous fungi (such as *Aspergillus fumigatus*), immunosuppressed patients without HIV or AIDS, or for patients with candidemia or deep-seated infections.[45] Future research should further define the relationships for these antifungals and organisms.

FUTURE METHODS FOR EVALUATION OF ANTIMICROBIAL ACTIVITY

There are many innovative methods under investigation to provide both qualitative and quantitative assessments of antimicrobial activity. Flow cytometry, a method commonly used to assess human cell lines for abnormalities, has also been studied for its use in bacterial cell analysis. Flow cytometry has the potential to analyze the cellular diversity that is present in bacterial cultures, as well as the gross morphologic effects of antimicrobials on these cells. It also has the potential advantages of (a) rapid determination of susceptibility (one to two cell growth cycles as quick as 10 minutes for some organisms); (b) better quantification of the subinhibitory and postantibiotic effects of antimicrobials; (c) the ability to investigate cellular changes related to the mechanism of antimicrobial action; and (d) the ability to evaluate the effects of both concentration and time on cellular changes.[47]

DETECTION OF RESISTANCE FACTORS

There are a number of direct resistance detection methods in use. β-Lactamase production can be rapidly and easily detected in the clinical laboratory with the use of nitrocephin disks. Nitrocephin is a chromogenic cephalosporin derivative that changes color upon hydrolysis by β-lactamase. Colonies from a growing bacterial culture can be touched to a disk, with the results of β-lactamase production noted in a few minutes. Although rapid and reliable, this method is limited to the assessment of strains of staphylococci, enterococci, *H. influenzae*, *M. catarrhalis*, and *N. gonorrhoeae*. The nitrocephin disk also cannot detect β-lactam resistance caused by altered penicillin-binding proteins (PBPs) or by some of the newer ESBLs.[18]

In general, the detection of ESBLs can be difficult. As many as 29% to 75% of strains known to possess ESBL will appear sensitive to cefotaxime or ceftazidime by disk diffusion. This may be a function of test insensitivity, or it may also be related to the breakpoint values being set too high.[20] A double-disk diffusion assay using a β-lactamase inhibitor, such as clavulanate, and various cephalosporins has been shown to more accurately detect the presence of ESBLs (Fig. 103–8). The use of PCR or DNA probes for detection of β-lactamases is limited to the research setting, because they lack sufficient sensitivity and specificity for routine use in the clinical setting. In the years to come, these molecular biologic techniques should become more refined and more prominent.

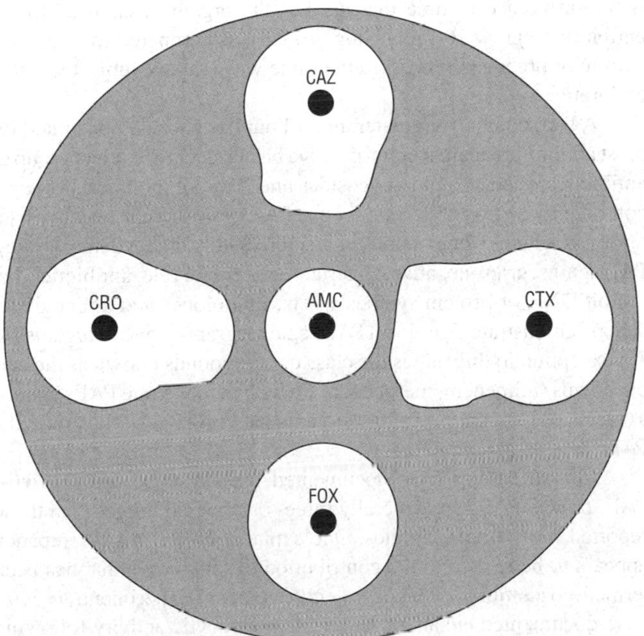

FIGURE 103–8. Double-disk diffusion test for detection of extended-spectrum β-lactamases (ESBLs). The cephalosporins ceftazidime (CAZ), cefotaxime (CTX), cefoxitin (FOX), and ceftriaxone (CRO) are placed on the outside of an agar plate. The disk in the center contains amoxicillin and clavulanate (AMC). The extension in zones observed for ceftazidime, cefotaxime, and ceftriaxone is caused by the clavulanate restoration or augmentation of activity and indicates the presence of ESBL. The cefoxitin zone size is unchanged, indicating that the ESBL present does not hydrolyze this drug.[6]

Detection of methicillin resistance in *Staphylococcus* is difficult because of the heterogeneous expression of the phenotype. Not all bacteria in a given population will express methicillin resistance (even though they may have the genetic ability to do so); in some cases, only 1 in 10^{4-6} cells may express the resistance phenotype.[39] Methicillin resistance is the result of the *mecA* gene, which encodes for an altered PBP (PBP 2a′) with low binding affinity for β-lactams. Screening via oxacillin disks or by oxacillin-containing agar (6 g/mL) were once considered the gold standard for resistance detection prior to the development of PCR and DNA probes specific for *mecA*. The *mecA* PCR test is available for clinical use, is 99% sensitive and specific, and allows for the rapid (within 6 hours) determination of the presence of methicillin resistance. In theory, the presence of a single copy of *mecA* in a clinical isolate could be detected. Many laboratories, however, do not yet use the *mecA* PCR probe because of its high costs. The use of this test could potentially increase, if it can allow for the more rapid discontinuation of empiric vancomycin therapy, especially in hospitals where methicillin resistance is high. In such situations, the cost of the test could be far outweighed by lower antimicrobial costs and the potential for decreased vancomycin resistance.

The detection of decreased vancomycin susceptibility in staphylococci has become more important with the recent isolation of vancomycin-intermediate *Staphylococcus aureus* (VISA) and the increased prevalence of vancomycin-resistant enterococci (VRE). The vancomycin screening agar method (Brain-Heart Infusion agar containing 6 mg/L of vancomycin) appears to be an inexpensive and reliable way to detect vancomycin resistance for both of these problem pathogens.[86] With this test, the growth of any colonies from a sample (10^5–10^6 cfu) of the test organism after 24 hours of incubation indicates the presence of organisms with decreased vancomycin susceptibility (VISA) or vancomycin resistance (VRE). Most MIC methods used in the clinical laboratory that incorporate at least a 16-hour incubation period also appear to reliably detect strains of VISA.[87]

SPECIAL *IN VITRO* TESTS OF ANTIMICROBIAL ACTIVITY

MINIMAL BACTERICIDAL CONCENTRATION

As previously mentioned, the MIC is the most widely used laboratory parameter for making decisions on antimicrobial therapy. In some circumstances (e.g., meningitis, endocarditis), however, where bactericidal activity may be more predictive of a favorable infection outcome, it may be of more value to determine the bactericidal activity of a select group of antibiotics. The minimal bactericidal concentration (MBC) is performed in conjunction with the broth microtiter MIC test. After the MIC is determined, aliquots of fluid from the microtiter wells that demonstrate no visible growth are plated onto antibiotic-free agar plates and incubated overnight for a period of 24 hours. The MBC is defined as the lowest concentration of drug that kills 99.9% (a 3-$\log_{10}$ cfu/mL reduction) of the initial organism density.[21] The MIC often approximates the MBC for certain antibiotic classes such as the aminoglycosides and the quinolones. This, however, cannot be assumed for β-lactam antibiotics and glycopeptides. For some bacteria, the MBC may exceed the MIC substantially, which may overestimate the potential *in vivo* response. When the MBC exceeds the MIC by ≥32 times, the organism is said to be tolerant of the antimicrobial. The phenomenon of tolerance has been documented to occur with β-lactams and glycopeptides against staphylococci, streptococci, and enterococci. The mechanism for tolerance is poorly understood but is thought to be related to the release, use, and production of an enzyme known as autolysin. Autolysin may aid in the destruction of the bacterial cell wall and may be triggered by the interaction of cell wall active antibiotics and their target site, such as PBPs. The clinical significance of tolerance, however, is unknown at this time.[48,49]

TIMED-KILL CURVES

Timed-kill curve experiments are not routinely performed in the clinical laboratory but provide important additional data on the effect of antimicrobial concentration on the rate and extent of bacterial killing. For timed-kill curve testing, a standard quantified inoculum of bacteria (6 $\log_{10}$ cfu/mL) is placed in a test tube containing liquid growth media. The bacterial suspension is then exposed to desired concentrations of antimicrobial. The mixture is incubated and samples are removed at regular intervals to determine the number of living cells at the given time points. The viable count is plotted versus time to construct the timed-kill profile of the antimicrobial. By standard convention, the tested concentration of antimicrobial is considered to be bactericidal if it causes at least a 3-$\log_{10}$ cfu/mL reduction in viable inoculum.[50]

EFFECT OF CONCENTRATION ON ANTIMICROBIAL KILLING ACTIVITY

The relationship between concentration and antimicrobial killing activity has been documented for most antibiotic classes. Although all antibiotics appear to demonstrate an initial increase in killing activity as a function of antibiotic concentrations that approach or slightly exceed the MIC, a continued linear relationship between antibiotic killing and concentration is not demonstrated for all antibiotics. For example, the β-lactam and glycopeptide antibiotics do not achieve a greater rate of killing once the concentration has exceeded four to five times the MIC. These antibiotics are said to exhibit concentration-independent effects. On the other hand, aminoglycosides and quinolone antibiotics continue to demonstrate increased bactericidal effects as a function of concentration many times above the MIC of the microorganisms in a linear fashion.

The principles of concentration-dependent and independent killing are demonstrated in Fig. 103–9. In these timed-kill curve experiments, *Pseudomonas aeruginosa* was exposed *in vitro* to tobramycin, ciprofloxacin, and ticarcillin at concentrations below and above the MIC of the organisms.[51] Both tobramycin and ciprofloxacin demonstrate concentration-dependent killing activity, achieving greater killing with increasing increments of concentration. Ticarcillin's maximal killing activity, however, is achieved at four times the MIC. Information regarding the effect of antimicrobial concentration on organism killing is important to determine the most appropriate dosage and administration schemes (such as continuous infusion for concentration-independent effects versus intermittent dosing for concentration-dependent effects) to ensure the optimal outcome for each class of antimicrobial.

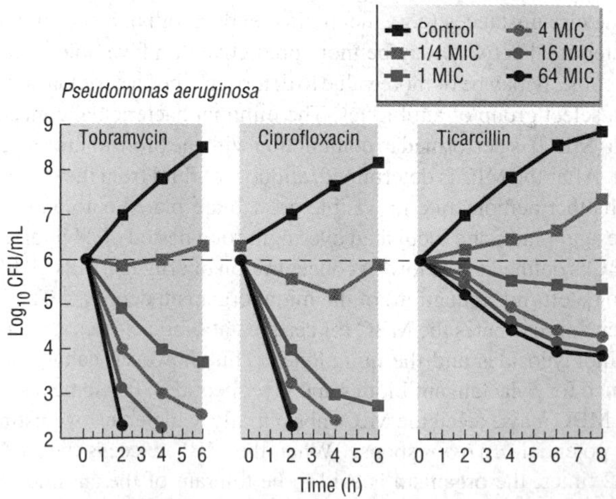

FIGURE 103–9. Killing curves depicting the effect of concentration on antibiotic bactericidal activity. CFU, colony-forming units; MIC, minimal inhibitory concentration. 0.25–64 times the MIC; the organism tested was *P. aeruginosa* ATCC 27853.[51]

POSTANTIBIOTIC EFFECT

The postantibiotic effect (PAE) is the persistent suppression of organism growth (usually measured in hours) after exposure and removal of an antibiotic. Some of the earliest experiments examined the PAE of penicillin on streptococci and staphylococci. The PAE secondary to penicillin against streptococci may be caused by irreversible binding of penicillin to a targeted PBP in the organism's cell wall. The regeneration of new PBPs is necessary for the streptococci to resume normal growth. In general, the PAE experiment is performed by exposing a fixed inoculum of organism to a set concentration of antibiotic (usually some multiple of the MIC). The antibiotic is then removed either by inactivation (such would be the case when a β-lactam is inactivated by the use of β-lactamase) or removal by binding the antibiotic to a resin, centrifugation of the mixture (and removal of the supernatant containing the antibiotic) with resuspension of the organism in an antibiotic-free growth medium or dilution of the antibiotic (1,000-fold dilution with antibiotic-free medium) to a concentration that is far below the MIC of the organism. The PAE is the difference in time that it takes the organism exposed to the antibiotic to grow 10-fold (1-log growth), as compared to a separate culture of organism processed the same way and not subjected to the antibiotic.[52]

A PAE equal to or greater than 1 hour has been demonstrated for most antibiotics against gram-positive bacteria. Only a select group of antibiotics, such as aminoglycosides and fluoroquinolones, however, consistently demonstrate a significant PAE against gram-negative bacteria. β-Lactams, for example, characteristically do not demonstrate a PAE against gram-negative bacteria. As a general rule, antibiotics that inhibit DNA or protein synthesis (e.g., quinolones and aminoglycosides) demonstrate significant PAEs against gram-negative organisms. An exception to this rule is the class of compounds known as the carbapenems (imipenem, meropenem), which demonstrate PAEs against a select group of gram-negative organisms. Fig. 103–10 illustrates the PAE for several compounds.

Animal studies have documented the existence of an *in vivo* PAE. *In vivo* PAEs are generally three- or fourfold longer than those reported from *in vitro* studies. One explanation for this discrepancy appears to be related to the contribution of leukocytes that has been termed postantibiotic leukocyte enhancement. Experiments *in vitro* have documented enhanced leukocyte phagocytic activity following antibiotic exposure.[53,54]

ANTIMICROBIAL COMBINATION TESTING

Antimicrobial combination therapy is often required to treat infections depending on the degree of severity, type of pathogen, or specific infection type. Examples of infections that may require combination therapy include empiric treatment of serious infection before the pathogen or antibiotic susceptibility is known, treatment of infections

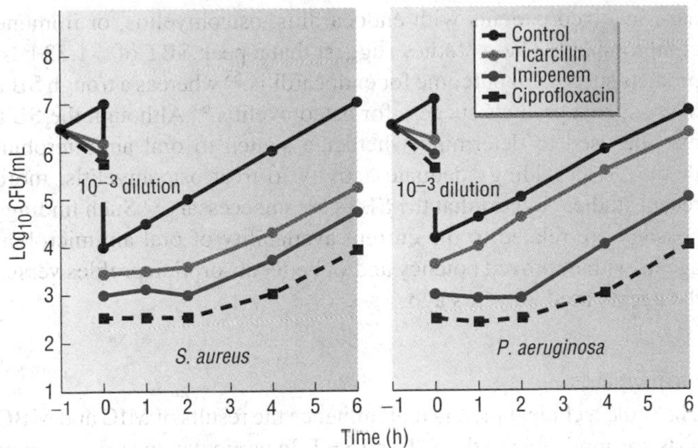

FIGURE 103–10. Postantibiotic effect. In this experiment, a fixed inocula of *S. aureus* and *P. aeruginosa* are exposed to ticarcillin, imipenem, and ciprofloxacin at a set concentration of four times the MIC. The organism and the antibiotic is then diluted 1,000-fold to a point where the antibiotic concentration is far below the MIC of the organism. Growth suppression of *S. aureus* following exposure to these three drugs (PAE) occurs for approximately 2 hours. Growth suppression of *P. aeruginosa*, however, is only demonstrated for imipenem and ciprofloxacin. The β-lactam ticarcillin has no effect on the growth of *P. aeruginosa.*[51,52]

in neutropenic patients, enterococcal endocarditis, and treatment of bacteremia, sepsis, or pneumonia caused by *P. aeruginosa*. The combination of antibiotics from different classes may result in activity that is significantly greater than the sum of activity of either agent alone. When this occurs, the combination is said to demonstrate synergy. If the combination of two or more antibiotics results in an effect that is worse than either agent alone, the combination is said to be antagonistic. Results that are neither synergistic or antagonistic (in between) are said to be indifferent or additive.[55]

Although there is little debate that the combination of a β-lactam and an aminoglycoside is required for treatment of enterococcal endocarditis, the concept of combination therapy is not universally accepted for the treatment of all infections. For example, there is ongoing debate as to whether the combination of a broad-spectrum β-lactam and an aminoglycoside or the β-lactam alone is most appropriate for the empiric treatment of febrile neutropenic patients.[56,57] Although *in vitro* antagonism has been demonstrated for several combinations (penicillin plus tetracycline, chloramphenicol and an aminoglycoside, fluoroquinolones and rifampin), *in vivo* antagonism has been demonstrated infrequently.

There are two primary methods that are used in the laboratory to determine the effect of combination antibiotic therapy. The first method is the fractional inhibitory concentration (FIC or "checkerboard" method). The FIC is performed in a similar manner as the microtiter broth MIC except that it tests two antibiotics on the same microtiter plate. Twofold serial fold dilutions (high to low) of one antibiotic are made in one direction on the plate (e.g., from right to left) while dilutions of the second antibiotic are made from another direction on the same plate (e.g., from top to bottom). This method produces all possible combinations of twofold concentration dilutions for the two drugs being tested. The test bacteria are added to all wells at a standard inoculum and the test results are read in a similar fashion as the MIC test after appropriate incubation. The FIC is expressed mathematically by calculation of the FIC index. The FIC index is calculated as:

$$FIC_{index} = \frac{A}{MIC_A} + \frac{B}{MIC_B}$$

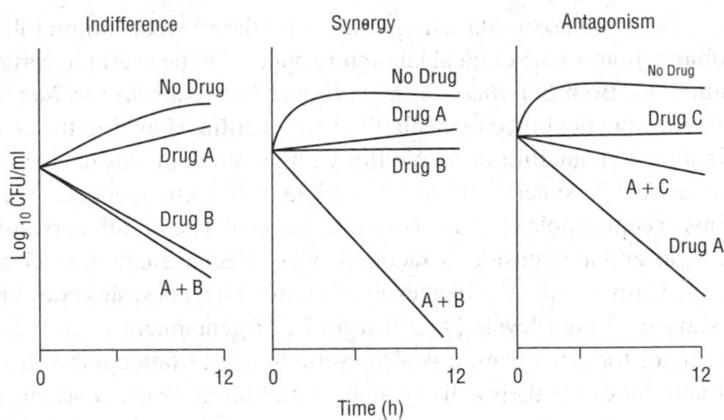

FIGURE 103–11. Timed-kill curve illustrating indifference, synergy, and antagonism.

where *A* or *B* is the lowest concentration of the drug that is inhibitory in the presence of the second drug, and the MIC is the minimal inhibitory concentration of each drug tested alone. Synergism by the checkerboard method is defined as an FIC index of ≤ 0.5, indifference is defined as an FIC index of > 0.5–4.0, and antagonism is defined as an FIC index of > 4.0.[58]

The second most common method to determine the effects of antibiotic combinations is the timed-kill curve method. The experiments are similar to the timed-kill curve methods described earlier except that two antibiotics are tested in the same tube at fixed concentration fractions of the MIC for each drug. In this method, synergism is defined as a 100-fold decrease in organism cfu/mL at 24 hours for the combination as compared to the most potent antibiotic tested alone. Antagonism is defined as an increase in organism count (≥ 100-fold) at 24 hours[58] (Fig. 103–11).

OTHER METHODS

Other methods for testing combination antibiotic therapy include the double-disk diffusion test and the double E-test methods. The double-disk diffusion method is performed by placing two different antibiotic-impregnated paper disks onto a solid agar medium plate containing the test organism. The disks are placed in proximity to each other in a way that their zones of inhibition would not be expected to overlap. A synergistic or additive effect is observed when there is an extension of the zones of inhibition between the two drugs.[59] The E-test method is similar to what has been previously described except that two antibiotic E-test strips are crossed at the individual MIC of each antibiotic. Similar to the disk-diffusion method, an extension of the zone of inhibition from either antibiotic alone is considered additive or synergistic.[60]

LIMITATIONS

Unfortunately, none of the procedures for testing the effects of antimicrobial combination have been adequately examined to determine whether the results of these tests are predictive of clinical outcome. In addition, these tests have limitations. For example, the FIC method is plagued by reproducibility problems. Also, it can only evaluate the inhibitory effects of the two antibiotics, and assessments are made only at one time point (18 or 24 hours). The timed-kill curve method is labor intensive, lacks the ability to detect additive effects using current definitions, often is only evaluated at the 24-hour time point, and has no concentration standards at which the antibiotics are to be tested. Finally, there is a lack of correlation between these two methods for detecting synergism.[61]

Despite these limitations, prediction of the effect of antimicrobial combinations in the clinical laboratory appears to be useful in certain situations. Both *Enterococcus faecalis* and *Enterococcus faecium* are inhibited but not killed by penicillin or ampicillin. However, the combination of penicillin or ampicillin with an aminoglycoside such as gentamicin is synergistic and bactericidal. For enterococcal infections except simple cystitis, the combination of a penicillin derivative plus an aminoglycoside is recommended. Because enterococci are intrinsically resistant to low levels of aminoglycosides, susceptibility testing with high levels ($\geq$ 500 μg/mL) of gentamicin is used as a predictor for synergism. It is also useful to test certain combinations of antibiotics for their activity against multidrug-resistant strains of bacteria isolated from patients. In these settings, it is hoped that the resistance to one or both of the test antibiotics will be reduced through a synergistic interaction between the two antibiotics.[61]

LABORATORY MONITORING OF ANTIMICROBIAL THERAPY

An understanding of antimicrobial agent disposition *in vivo* is important for the selection of therapy and for the monitoring of clinical or bacteriologic responses. The clinician needs to recognize the concentrations expected in the bloodstream, as well as the expected delivery of the antimicrobial to the sites where infection can occur. Combining this knowledge with knowledge of expected activity against the infecting organism constitutes a pharmacodynamic approach to the treatment of infections.

Serum concentration monitoring is the most common method used to individualize antimicrobial therapy. The therapeutic window is, however, quite large for most antimicrobial agents, and exact toxic or therapeutic ranges are not well defined. In this context, therapeutic monitoring often is not justified. The clinical benefits of adjusting concentrations to hypothetically "correct" values are unknown, especially in light of the additional costs that concentration monitoring adds to the therapy. There are some antimicrobials for which proper monitoring appears to be justified based on either toxicity or efficacy.

METHODS OF ANTIBIOTIC ASSAY

SERUM BACTERICIDAL TITER

Serum inhibitory titers (SITs) and serum bactericidal titers (SBTs) are sometimes used to monitor the antimicrobial therapy of certain serious infections such as osteomyelitis and endocarditis. SITs and SBTs are determined in a similar manner as microdilution MICs and MBCs, but dilutions of the patient's serum are used instead of known concentrations of antimicrobial. Patient serum that is collected near the expected peak, midpoint, and/or trough concentration of the antimicrobial dose may be used. The highest twofold dilution of the sample that inhibits the visible growth of the patient's infecting organism is the SIT, while the highest dilution that kills 99.9% of the original bacterial inoculum is the SBT. The values for the SIT and SBT are expressed as the number of twofold serial dilutions relative to the original sample (e.g., SIT = 1:32, SBT = 1:8).

Although standards have been developed for the performance of the SIT/SBT in clinical labs, they are rarely used currently. This may be because the SBTs needed to optimize clinical outcome in all infections are not clear and/or the data that they provide does little to alter the standard therapy. Most clinical investigations of the SBT have involved patients with endocarditis, osteomyelitis, or immune compromise.[62] These studies suggest that a peak SBT of >1:32 best predicts successful outcome for endocarditis,[63] whereas a trough SBT of >1:2 best predicts success for osteomyelitis.[64] Although the SBT may be used to determine whether a switch to oral antimicrobial therapy is providing adequate activity to treat osteomyelitis, more recent studies suggest that the SBTs are unnecessary.[65] Such findings possibly are related to the current availability of oral antimicrobial agents with improved potency and/or better absorption profiles versus the agents used 20 years ago.

Limitations

The same technical factors that influence the results of MIC and MBC tests are applicable to the SIT and SBT. In particular, the use of serum versus broth for making dilutions of the sample may be important, particularly for highly protein-bound drugs. These and other issues related to the performance and interpretation of the SBT necessitate standardization to make the test of greater clinical value.[62]

MICROBIOLOGIC ASSAY

Bioassay of antimicrobial agents is performed by several methods. The most commonly employed method is a modification of the disk-diffusion technique used for determining antibiotic susceptibility. Paper disks are placed onto, or wells are punched into, the surface of an agar containing bacteria that are known to be highly susceptible to the agent to be assayed. A fixed volume (usually 10 μL) of known concentration of the drug to be assayed or sampled is placed on the disks or in the wells. The measured zone of inhibition and the logarithm of drug concentration are plotted; the drug concentration in unknown samples is determined from measurement of the zone size surrounding disks spotted with unknown concentrations of drug. Advantages of this method include its relative ease of performance and low cost for equipment. Disadvantages include possible interference by other antibiotics present in the sample, lack of precision, and slow turnaround time (usually 24 to 48 hours).

FLUORESCENCE POLARIZATION IMMUNOASSAY

The fluorescence polarization immunoassay (FPIA) technique involves the application of the principles of fluorescence when molecules are exposed to light. A fluorescein-labeled drug and antibody directed against the drug are added in constant amounts to samples or standards. The antibody-fluorescein-labeled drug complex results in a change in the fluorescence polarization. When the fluorescein-labeled drug complexes with the antibody, a quantifiable change in the fluorescence polarization occurs. When a sample containing nonfluorescein-labeled drug (i.e., a patient's serum sample) is mixed with the standard mixture, competition for antibody binding occurs. This competitive binding results in a decrease in the binding-related fluorescence polarization. Comparison of the change caused by the patient sample to changes caused by standard concentrations determines the specific drug concentration in the patient sample.

In the clinical laboratory setting, FPIA is the most commonly used assay method for the determination of aminoglycoside and vancomycin serum concentrations. Advantages of this technique include automation through the use of the TDx system (Abbott Laboratories, North Chicago, IL). Disadvantages include the expense for reagents and the cost for the purchase of the automated system.

RADIOIMMUNOASSAY

Radioimmunoassay (RIA) uses radiolabeled drug and antibody directed against the specific drug to help determine the concentration contained in an unknown sample. Similar to FPIA, radiolabeled antibiotic and unlabeled antibiotic (in a patient's serum sample) are equilibrated with the antibody. The amount of free radiolabeled drug is measured and compared to values obtained with standard concentrations in order to determine the concentration in the patient sample. Although the RIA has good sensitivity and specificity, its main disadvantage is the expense and hassle of disposal of the radioactive waste generated during the test.

HIGH-PRESSURE LIQUID CHROMATOGRAPHY

In the high-pressure liquid chromatography (HPLC) technique, separation of different molecular species is accomplished by passing a mobile solvent phase over a stationary phase. Drugs with a polarity similar to that of the stationary phase are retained for a time on the chromatography column and then released. These temporarily retained substances are detected using ultraviolet, fluorescence, electrochemical, or radiometric methods. The detector response is proportional to the amount of molecules seen; standard curves containing known drug concentrations are related to the detector response, usually recorded as peak area or peak height. Advantages include a rapid turnaround time, precision, and an ability to detect metabolites. Disadvantages include the cost of instruments and the expertise required.

TIMING OF COLLECTION OF SERUM SAMPLES

Peak and/or trough concentrations are monitored for only a select few antimicrobials in the current clinical setting. As with all serum drug-concentration monitoring, the samples should be collected so as to provide the most meaningful data for pharmacokinetic analyses. When possible, all samples should be obtained after steady state is achieved, but this may not always be possible because true steady state may not occur in critically ill patients with altered hemodynamics, kidney, and/or liver function.

The timing of the peak concentration is more critical than the trough concentration. Specifically, the peak concentration should be obtained only after the distribution phase is completed in order to prevent overestimation of the volume of distribution when first-order pharmacokinetic calculations are performed. Because the distribution phase may differ between different antibiotics (e.g., aminoglycosides and vancomycin), or even between different dosage regimens of the same antibiotic (e.g., "traditional" vs "extended-interval" aminoglycoside dosing),[66] the clinician should plan sample collection times accordingly. Regardless of the specific sample timing considerations, it is always crucial to meticulously record the complete antimicrobial dosing history prior to sample collection in order to ensure proper interpretation.

SPECIFIC AGENTS

The aminoglycosides and vancomycin are the most commonly monitored antimicrobials in the clinical setting. Although the monitoring of these agents has been extensively studied, this practice has been challenged recently, especially for vancomycin. A summary of the recommendations for serum concentration monitoring of these agents is shown in Table 103–2.

AMINOGLYCOSIDES

The influence of serum aminoglycoside levels on clinical response in gram-negative infection has been reported in several studies, but one review concluded that the widely disseminated therapeutic ranges for serum levels were poorly supported by these data.[67,68] Controversy also surrounds the relationship between serum aminoglycoside concentrations and the development of nephrotoxicity and ototoxicity.

TABLE 103–2. Suggested Therapeutic Serum Concentrations for Selected Antimicrobial Agents

		Target Concentrations	
Drug	**Time of Collection**	*(mg/L)*	*Comments*
Aminoglycosides[70,71]	Peak (1 h after the start of a 15- to 45-min infusion)	< 5	Urinary tract infections
Traditional dosage regimens			
Gentamicin		> 5	Bacteremia
Tobramycin		> 6	Bacterial pneumonia
		> 12	Endocarditis caused by *Pseudomonas aeruginosa*
	Trough	< 2–3	High trough concentrations are most likely a result and not a cause of nephrotoxicity
Amikacin	Peak	> 15	Urinary tract infections
		> 20	Bacteremia
		> 24	Bacterial pneumonia, other serious infections
	Trough	< 9–10	See comments regarding trough gentamicin/tobramycin concentrations
Single daily dosage regimens[76]			
Gentamicin	8 h postdose	1.5–6	Concentrations above this range associated with nephrotoxicity in one study with netilmicin
Netilmicin			
Tobramycin			
Vancomycin[80,81]	Peak (1–2 h after a 30- to 60-min infusion)	20–50	Recommendations should be considered tentative, as definitive data are not available
	Trough	< 10	Therapeutic monitoring is probably not necessary for most patients

Early studies suggested that trough concentrations exceeding 2–4 mg/L for gentamicin and tobramycin and 10 mg/L for amikacin predisposed patients to nephrotoxicity. More recent analyses of several patient variables concluded that these other patient factors may be more important and that the development of ototoxicity and nephrotoxicity is more closely related to the total exposure and duration of therapy.[72] Although the clinical benefit of specific levels still remains unproved, the ranges listed in Table 103–2 can be applied based on controlled studies.

Newer regimens of "once-daily" or "extended-interval" aminoglycoside administration have gained widespread acceptance for use in the clinical setting.[70,71] These regimens attempt to exploit the pharmacodynamics of these agents to maximize activity (concentration-dependent bacterial killing, postantibiotic effect, and reduced adaptive resistance), while also attempting to minimize drug toxicity by minimizing exposure of target organs to the drug. Although a plethora of prospective studies have been performed that evaluate once-daily aminoglycoside dosing, much controversy still exists.[71–73] Most studies show either equal rates of efficacy and toxicity or a trend toward improved efficacy and reduced toxicity for extended interval dosage regimens. Many meta-analyses have also been performed on these study data.[74] However, because the studies are heterogeneous and because they possess many weaknesses, most meta-analyses have subsequently inherited these scientific study flaws.[73,75] Additional prospective studies are needed, but they will most likely be plagued by the inherent obstacles of clinical study design and implementation, as well as by a lack of funding because of the generic availability of aminoglycosides.

The doses employed for extended interval dosing are typically 5–7 mg/kg/day, although the dose and/or interval may be adjusted based on renal function or observed serum concentrations.[76–78] Traditional methods of serum concentration monitoring (peak and trough concentrations) are uninformative for once-daily dosing, because concentrations 24 hours after a dose should be undetectable even in patients with mild renal dysfunction. Pharmacokinetic monitoring of extended interval aminoglycosides should be accomplished by obtaining a peak sample at least 1 hour after the infusion to allow for the extended distribution phase with higher doses followed by a mid-dose sample taken 6 to 12 hours after the dose.[66] A single-point, nomogram-based dosing method using mid-dose serum samples has also been evaluated and is used widely in the clinical setting.[77]

VANCOMYCIN

Convincing data do not exist to correlate vancomycin concentrations with efficacy and/or toxicity. Although IV vancomycin had been associated with oto- and nephrotoxicity in humans, most reports occurred with older and less-pure formulations, as well as with extremely high concentrations that are uncommonly encountered currently.[79] Indeed, studies in animals reveal that it is not ototoxic and only minimally nephrotoxic. The "red man" syndrome reported with IV vancomycin also has not been correlated with serum concentrations, but may occur more frequently with infusions less than 2 hours in duration.[80]

Most methods of empiric vancomycin dosing provide peak concentrations between 20 mg/L and 50 mg/L and trough concentrations of 5–20 mg/L. Because vancomycin appears to possess a time-dependent killing activity profile it has been recommended that the time above the organism's MIC should extend for the entire dosing interval. However, some limited data suggest that a specific vancomycin AUC/MIC may be an important parameter for successful outcome in some patients. In addition, *in vitro* pharmacodynamic evaluations of VISA suggest that AUC/MIC for vancomycin is important when the MIC approaches 4 mg/L. Further research in this area is important to confirm these relationships. Since the majority of currently clinical isolates have MICs ≤ 2 mg/L, current dosing recommendations and minimal monitoring is feasible for most patients. In patients not responding to traditional therapy, organism susceptibility should be checked and changes to the dosing regimen should be considered.[79,81–84]

INTEGRATION OF MINIMAL INHIBITORY CONCENTRATION AND SERUM CONCENTRATION DATA

A considerable advance in our understanding of the role of drug pharmacokinetics and pharmacodynamics in the effective treatment of infectious diseases has occurred. Integration of MIC information with antimicrobial pharmacokinetic data has led to the design of regimens that achieve target levels of exposure based on organism susceptibility and the antimicrobial properties of the drug against the particular organism.

For example, a better response is predicted for a given dose of an antimicrobial with concentration-dependent killing activity against an organism with a lower MIC versus a higher MIC, even if both organisms are considered susceptible. The pharmacodynamic principles behind this are a maximization of the peak (maximum) serum concentration (Cpmax)-to-MIC ratio and are illustrated in Fig. 103–12. The clinical applicability of this principle could be to modify either the dosage of the current aminoglycoside used to achieve the suggested Cpmax:MIC ratio of $\geq 10:1$, or to switch to a different aminoglycoside that allows for better optimization of this ratio (such as a switch from gentamicin to tobramycin for an organism

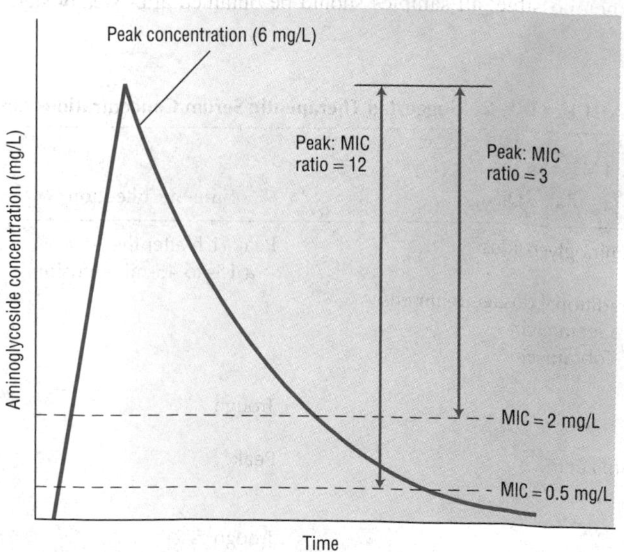

FIGURE 103–12. Illustration of the concept of peak concentration to the minimal inhibitory concentration (MIC) ratio for aminoglycosides. The MIC for the given organism to gentamicin is 2 mg/L, whereas the tobramycin MIC is 0.5 mg/L. Administration of gentamicin would result in a suboptimal peak: MIC ratio (< 10), which could increase the chances for development of resistance or an inadequate response. Administration of tobramycin would result in a peak:MIC ratio of 12, which should improve efficacy. Note that modification of the gentamicin regimen to produce peak serum concentrations of ≥ 20 mg/L (as commonly done with once-daily administration) would also result in a peak:MIC ratio of ≥ 10.

with lower tobramycin MIC). The clinical validity of this concept has been shown in studies of susceptible organisms with aminoglycosides and fluoroquinolones.[25,26]

The ratio of overall *in vivo* exposure to an antimicrobial, measured by the area under the plasma concentration versus time curve (AUC) to an organism's susceptibility (the AUC:MIC ratio), is another pharmacodynamic parameter proposed to be used for dosage optimization.[85] For seriously ill patients, a breakpoint AUC:MIC ratio of $\geq$ 125 was associated with clinical response, while breakpoint AUC:MIC ratios of $\geq$ 125 and $\geq$ 250 were associated with stepwise decreases in the time to eradicate the infecting organism.[85]

For β-lactam antimicrobial efficacy, the achievement of concentrations above an organism's MIC for a critical amount of time (time > MIC) appears to be the most important pharmacodynamic parameter.[22,27] The Cpmax:MIC ratio does not appear to be as crucial a factor for response, although the AUC:MIC ratio has also been suggested as a predictor for β-lactam treatment outcome.[22] In the setting of otitis media, for example, a time > MIC of approximately 40% to 50% appears to correlate with rates of response greater than 90%.[27]

Most of the data on pharmacodynamic optimization has been generated in controlled clinical settings. Evaluation of the best and most efficient ways to apply these data to everyday clinical practice is ongoing, and it should result in either the expansion of monitoring for certain antimicrobials or the proposal of nomograms that allow for rapid drug and dose selections that enhance the likelihood for optimal therapy based on the type of infection, patient-specific parameters, and local antimicrobial susceptibility patterns. Such possibilities present exciting opportunities for the pharmacotherapy specialist to become directly involved in the development of multidisciplinary protocols that could improve care for patients with infections in all health care settings.

▶ PRINCIPLES OF PHARMACOTHERAPY

- The pharmacotherapist needs to understand and properly use clinical laboratory tests to help confirm the presence of infection and to acquire knowledge about the host's characteristics (such as immune status).
- Familiarity with normal host flora and typical pathogens will help decide whether a patient is truly infected or merely colonized.
- The development of molecular testing systems has improved our ability to diagnose infection and determine the antimicrobial susceptibilities for numerous fastidious or slow-growing pathogens, such as mycobacteria and viruses.
- Although highly standardized, *in vitro* antimicrobial susceptibility testing has limitations and often cannot truly mimic the conditions found at the site of an infection. This may have implications for discordance between *in vitro* susceptibility results and *in vivo* response to therapy.
- Integration of quantitative *in vitro* susceptibility test results with the pharmacokinetic and pharmacodynamic properties of antimicrobials by the pharmacotherapist can impact the care of patients with infections positively.
- Rapid automated susceptibility test systems appear to improve therapeutic outcomes of patients with infection, especially when linked to other relevant clinical information systems.
- Although not routinely performed in the clinical setting, laboratory tests that determine an antimicrobial's pharmacodynamic properties, such as the effect of concentration, the postantibiotic effect, and the effect of combination antimicrobials are important to consider in the understanding and application of therapy to patients with infection.

REFERENCES

1. Sanders CC. A problem with antimicrobial susceptibility tests. ASM News 1991;57:187–190.
2. Bodey GP. Quantitative relationship between circulating leukocytes and infection in patients with acute leukemia. Ann Intern Med 1966;64: 328–340.
3. Rouse BT, Horohov DW. Immunosuppression in viral infection. Rev Infect Dis 1986;8:850–873.
4. Boumpas DT, Paliogianni F, Anastassiou ED, et al. Glucocortico-steroid action on the immune system: Molecular and cellular aspects. Clin Exp Rheumatol 1991;9:413–423.
5. Sox HC, Liang MH. The erythrocyte sedimentation rate: Guidelines for rational use. Ann Intern Med 1986;104:515–523.
6. Casey LC, Balk RA, Bone RC. Plasma cytokine levels correlate with survival in patients with the sepsis syndrome. Ann Intern Med 1993;15: 771–778.
7. Bone RC, Larson CB. Gram-negative urinary tract infections and the development of SIRS. J Crit Illness 1996;11(suppl):S20–S29.
8. Herwaldt LA, Geiss M, Kao C, Pfaller MA. The positive predictive value of isolating coagulase-negative staphylococci from blood cultures. Clin Infect Dis 1996;22:14–20.
9. Chapin K. Clinical microscopy. In: Murray PR, Baroon EJ, Pfaller MA, et al., eds. Manual of Clinical Microbiology, 6th ed. Washington, DC, ASM Press, 1995:33–51.
10. Forbes BA, Granato PA. Processing specimens for bacteria. In: Murray PR, Baroon EJ, Pfaller MA, et al., eds. Manual of Clinical Microbiology, 6th ed. Washington DC, ASM Press, 1995:265–281.
11. Smith-Elekes S, Weinstein MP. Blood cultures. Infect Dis Clin North Am 1993;7:221–234.
12. Herrmann JE. Immunoassays for the diagnosis of infectious diseases. In: Rose NE, de Marario EC, Folds JD, et al., eds. Manual of Clinical Laboratory Immunology, 5th ed. Washington, DC, ASM Press, 1997: 130–157.
13. Tenover F. DNA hybridization techniques and their application to the diagnosis of infectious diseases. Infect Dis Clin North Am 1993;7: 171–181.
14. Podzorski RP, Persing DH. Molecular detection and identification of microorganisms. In: Rose NE, de Marario EC, Folds JD, et al., eds. Manual of Clinical Laboratory Immunology, 5th ed. Washington, DC, ASM Press, 1997:130–157.
15. Rosenthal N. Tools of the trade-recombinant DNA. N Engl J Med 1994,331:315–317.
16. Hitt CM, Nightingale CH, Quintiliani R, Nicolau DP. Streamlining antimicrobial therapy for lower respiratory tract infections. Clin Infect Dis 1997;24(suppl 2):S231–S237.
17. Ackerman BH, Dello Buono FA. *In vitro* testing of antibiotics. Pharmacotherapy 1996;16(2):201–221.
18. Jorgensen J. Antimicrobial susceptibility testing of bacteria that grow aerobically. Infect Dis Clin North Am 1993;7:393–409.
19. Ferraro MJ. Automated antimicrobial susceptibility testing: What the infectious diseases subspecialist needs to know. Curr Clin Topics Infect Dis 1995;145:103–119.
20. Sanders CC, Thomson KS, Bradford PA. Problems with detection of β-lactam resistance among nonfastidious gram-negative bacilli. Infect Dis Clin North Am 1993;7:411–424.
21. National Committee for Clinical Laboratory Standards (NCCLS). Methods for Dilution Antimicrobial Susceptibility Tests for Bacteria that Grow Aerobically, 3rd ed, approved standard. NCCLS document M7-A3 (ISBN 1-56238-209-8). NCCLS, 771 East Lancaster Avenue, Villanova, PA, 19085, 1993.

22. Craig WA. Qualitative susceptibility tests versus quantitative MIC tests. Diagn Microbiol Infect Dis 1993;16:231–236.
23. Bauer AW, Kirby MM, Sherris JC, et al. Antibiotic susceptibility testing by a standardized, single-disk method. Am J Clin Pathol 1966;45: 493–496.
24. Hessen MT, Kaye D. Principles of selection and use of antimicrobial agents. Infect Dis Clin North Am 1995;9:531–545.
25. Moore RD, Lietman PS, Smith CR. Clinical response to aminoglycoside therapy: Importance of peak concentration to minimal inhibitory concentration. J Infect Dis 1987;155:93–99.
26. Peloquin CA, Cumbo TJ, Nix DE, et al. Evaluation of intravenous ciprofloxacin in patients with nosocomial lower respiratory tract infections. Arch Intern Med 1989;149:2269–2273.
27. Craig WA. The future—Can we learn from the past? Diagn Microbiol Infect Dis 1997;27:49–53.
28. Hsueh PR, Chang JC, Teng LJ, et al. Comparison of E-test and agar dilution method for antimicrobial susceptibility testing of *Flavobacterium* isolates. J Clin Micro 1997;35:1021–1023.
29. Wolfson C, Branley J, Gottlieb T. The E-test for antimicrobial susceptibility testing of *Bartonella henselae*. J Antimicrob Chemother 1996;38: 963–968.
30. Olsson-Liljequist B, Nord CE. Methods for susceptibility testing of anaerobic bacteria. Clin Infect Dis 1994;18(suppl 4):S293–S296.
31. Rittenhouse SF, Miller LA, Utrup LJ, Poupard JA. Evaluation of 500 gram-negative isolates to determine the number of major susceptibility interpretation discrepancies between the Vitek and Microscan Walkaway for 9 antimicrobial agents. Diagn Microbiol Infect Dis 1996;26: 1–6.
32. Evans RS, Classen DC, Pestotnik SL, et al. Improving empiric antibiotic selection using computer decision support. Arch Intern Med 1994;154:878–884.
33. Pestotnik SL, Classen DC, Evans RS, Burke JP. Implementing antibiotic practice guidelines through computer-assisted decision support: Clinical and financial outcomes. Ann Intern Med 1996;124:884–890.
34. Trenholme GM, Kaplan RL, Karakusis PH, et al. Clinical impact of rapid identification and susceptibility testing of bacterial blood culture isolates. J Clin Microbiol 1989;27:1342–1345.
35. Doern GV, Scott DR, Rashad AL. Clinical impact of rapid antimicrobial susceptibility testing of blood culture isolates. Antimicrob Agents Chemother 1982;21:1023–1024.
36. Doern GV, Vautour R, Gaudet M, Levy B. Clinical impact of rapid *in vitro* susceptibility testing and bacterial identification. J Clin Microbiol 1994;32:1757–1762.
37. Granato P. The impact of same-day versus traditional overnight testing. Diagn Microbiol Infect Dis 1993;16:237–243.
38. Chambers H. Detection of methicillin-resistant staphylococci. Infect Dis Clin North Am 1993;7:425–433.
39. Berke I, Tierno P. Comparison of efficacy and cost-effectiveness of BIOMIC VIDEO and Vitek antimicrobial susceptibility test systems for use in the clinical microbiology laboratory. J Clin Microbiol 1996;34:1980–1984.
40. Inderlied CB. Antimycobacterial susceptibility testing: Present practices and future trends. Eur J Clin Microbiol Infect Dis 1994;13: 980–993.
41. Heifets L. Susceptibility testing of *Mycobacterium avium* complex isolates. Antimicrob Agents Chemother 1996;40:1759–1767.
42. Sison JP, Yao Y, Kemper CA, et al. Treatment of *Mycobacterium avium* complex infection: Do the results of *in vitro* susceptibility tests predict therapeutic outcome in humans? J Infect Dis 1996;173:677–683.
43. Pfaller MA, Rex JH, Rinaldi MG. Antifungal susceptibility testing: Technical advances and potential clinical applications. Clin Infect Dis 1997;24:776–784.
44. Rex JH, Pfaller MA, Galgiani JN, et al. Development of interpretive breakpoints for antifungal susceptibility testing: Conceptual framework and analysis of *in vitro-in vivo* correlation data for fluconazole, itraconazole, and candidal infections. Clin Infect Dis 1997;24:235–247.
45. Ghannoum MA. Is antifungal susceptibility testing useful in guiding fluconazole therapy? Clin Infect Dis 1996;22(suppl 2):S161–S165.
46. Witt MD, Lewis RJ, Larsen RA, et al. Identification of patients with acute AIDS-associated cryptococcal meningitis who can be effectively treated with fluconazole: The role of antifungal susceptibility testing. Clin Infect Dis 1996;22:322–328.
47. Pore RS. Antibiotic susceptibility testing by flow cytometry. J Antimicrob Chemother 1994;34:613–627.
48. Voorn GP, Kuyvenhoven J, Goessens WHF, et al. Role of tolerance in treatment and prophylaxis of experimental *Staphylococcus aureus* endocarditis with vancomycin, teicoplanin, and daptomycin. Antimicrob Agents Chemother 1994;38:487–493.
49. Handwerger S, Tomasz A. Antibiotic tolerance among clinical isolates of bacteria. Rev Infect Dis 1985;7:368–386.
50. Amsterdam D. Susceptibility testing of antimicrobials in liquid media. In: Lorian V, ed. Antibiotics in Laboratory Medicine, 4th ed. Baltimore, Williams & Wilkins, 1996:52–111.
51. Craig WA, Ebert SC. Killing and regrowth of bacteria *in vitro:* A review. Scand J Infect Dis Suppl 1991;74:63–70.
52. Craig WA, Gudmundsson S. Postantibiotic effect. In: Lorian V, ed. Antibiotics in Laboratory Medicine, 4th ed. Baltimore, Williams & Wilkins, 1996:296–329.
53. McDonald PJ, Hakendorf P, Pruul H. Postantibiotic leukocyte enhancement: Increased susceptibility of bacteria pretreated with antibiotics to activity of leukocytes. Rev Infect Dis 1981;3:38–44.
54. Craig WA. Post-antibiotic effects in experimental infection models: Relationship to *in vitro* phenomena and to treatment of infections in man. J Antimicrob Chemother 1993;31(suppl D):149–158.
55. Rybak MJ, McGrath BJ. Combination antimicrobial therapy for bacterial infections: Guidelines for the clinician. Drugs 1996;52:390–405.
56. De Jongh CA, Joshi JH, Newman KA, et al. Antibiotic synergism and response in gram-negative bacteremia in granulocytopenic cancer patients. Am J Med 1986;80:96–100.
57. Ramphal R, Gucalp R, Rotstein C, et al. Clinical experience with single agent and combination regimens in the management of infection in the febrile neutropenic patient. Am J Med 1996;100:(suppl 6A): 83S–89S.
58. Elipoulos G, Moellering RC Jr. Antimicrobial combinations. In: Lorian V, ed. Antibiotics in Laboratory Medicine, 4th ed. Baltimore, Williams & Wilkins, 1996:330–397.
59. Moeller O, Holmgren J. A paper disc technique for studying antibacterial synergism. Acta Pathol Microbiol Scand 1969;76:141–145.
60. White RL, Burgess DS, Manduru M, Bosso JA. Comparison of three different *in vitro* methods of detecting synergy: Time-kill, checkerboard, and E test. Antimicrob Agents Chemother 1996;40:1914–1918.
61. Cappelletty DM, Rybak MJ. Comparison of methodologies for synergism testing of drug combinations against resistant strains of *Pseudomonas aeruginosa*. Antimicrob Agents Chemother 1996;40:677–683.
62. Vosti K. Serum bactericidal test: past, present, and future use in the management of patients with infections. Curr Clin Topics Infect Dis 1989;10:43–55.
63. Weinstein MP, Stratton CW, Acklery A, et al. Multicenter collaborative evaluation of a standardized serum bactericidal test as a prognostic indicator in infective endocarditis. Am J Med 1985;78:262–269.
64. Weinstein MP, Stratton CW, Hawley HB, Acklery A, Reller LB. Multicenter collaborative evaluation of a standardized serum bactericidal test as a predictor of therapeutic efficacy in acute and chronic osteomyelitis. Am J Med 1987;83:218–222.
65. Peltola H, Unkila-Kallio L, Kallio MJT, and the Finnish Study Group. Simplified treatment of acute staphylococcal osteomyelitis of childhood. Pediatrics 1997;99:846–850.
66. Demczar DJ, Nafziger AN, and Bertino JS. Pharmacokinetics of gentamicin at traditional versus high doses: Implications for once-daily dosing. Antimicrob Agents Chemother 1997;41:1115–1119.
67. Moore RD, Smith CR, Lietman PS. The association of aminoglycoside plasma levels with mortality in patients with gram-negative bacteremia. J Infect Dis 1984;149:443–448.
68. McCormack JP, Jewesson PJ. A critical reevaluation of the "therapeutic range" of aminoglycosides. Clin Infect Dis 1992;14:320–339.

69. Bertino JS, Booker LA, Franck PA, et al. Incidence of and significant risk factors for aminoglycoside-associated nephrotoxicity in patients dosed by using individualized pharmacokinetic monitoring. J Infect Dis 1993;167:173–179.
70. Bates RD, Nahata MC. Once-daily administration of aminoglycosides. Ann Pharmacother 1994;28:757–766.
71. Rotschafer JC, Rybak MJ. Single daily dosing of aminoglycosides: A commentary. Ann Pharmacother 1994;28:797–801.
72. Blaser J, Konig C, Simmen H-P, Thurnheer U. Monitoring serum concentrations for once-daily netilmicin dosing regimens. J Antimicrob Chemother 1994;33:341–348.
73. Bertino JS, Rotschafer JC. Single daily dosing of aminoglycosides—A concept whose time has not yet come. Clin Infect Dis 1997;24:820–823. Editorial response.
74. Ali MZ, Goetz MB. A meta-analysis of the relative efficacy and toxicity of single daily dosing versus multiple daily dosing of aminoglycosides. Clin Infect Dis 1997;24:796–809.
75. Gilbert DN. Meta analyses are no longer required for determining the efficacy of single daily dosing of aminoglycosides. Clin Infect Dis 1997;24:816–819. Editorial response.
76. Gilbert DN, Lee BL, Dworkin RJ, et al. A randomized comparison of the safety and efficacy of once-daily gentamicin or thrice-daily gentamicin in combination with ticarcillin-clavulanate. Am J Med 1998;105: 182–191.
77. Nicolau DP, Freeman CD, Belliveau PP, et al. Experience with a once-daily aminoglycoside program administered to 2,184 adult patients. Antimicrob Agents Chemother 1995;39(3):650–655.
78. Rybak MJ, Abate BJ, Kang SL, et al. Prospective evaluation of the effect of an aminoglycoside dosing regimen on rates of observed nephrotoxicity and ototoxicity. Antimicrob Agents Chemother 1999;43:1549–1555.
79. Cantu TG, Yamanaka-Yuen NA, Lietman PS. Serum vancomycin concentrations: Reappraisal of their clinical value. Clin Infect Dis 1994;18: 533–543.
80. Healy DP, Sahai JV, Fuller SH, et al. Vancomycin-induced histamine release and "red man syndrome: Comparison of 1- and 2-hour infusions. Antimicrob Agents Chemother 1990;34:550–554.
81. Moellering RC Jr. monitoring serum vancomycin levels: Climbing the mountain because it is there? Clin Infect Dis 1994;18:544–546. Editorial.
82. Karam CM, McKinnon PS, Neuhauser MM, et al. Outcome assessment of minimizing vancomycin monitoring and dosing adjustments. Pharmacotherapy 1999;19:257–266.
83. Moise PA, Forrest A, Bhavnani SM, et al. Area under the inhibitory curve and a pneumonia scoring system for predicting outcomes of vancomycin therapy for respiratory infections by *Staphylococcus aureus*. Am J Health Syst Pharm 2000;57:S4–S9.
84. Aeschlimann JR, Allen GP, Hershberger E, Rybak MJ. Activities of LY333328 and vancomycin administered alone or in combination with gentamicin against three strains of vancomycin-intermediate *Staphylococcus aureus* in an in vitro pharamacodynamic infection model. Antimicrob Agents Chemother 2000;44:2991–2998.
85. Forrest A, Nix DE, Ballow CH, et al. Pharmacodynamics of intravenous ciprofloxacin in seriously ill patients. Antimicrob Agents Chemother 1993;37:1073–1081.
86. Jorgensen JH and Ferraro MJ. Antimicrobial susceptibility testing: Special needs for fastidious organisms and difficult-to-detect resistance mechanisms. Clin Infect Dis 2000;30:799–808.
87. Tenover FC, Lancaster MV, Hill BC, et al. Characterization of staphylococci with reduced susceptibilities to vancomycin and other glycopeptides. J Clin Microbiol 1998;36:1020–1027.

104

ANTIMICROBIAL REGIMEN SELECTION

Betty J. Abate and Steven L. Barriere

Choosing an antimicrobial agent to treat infections is far more complicated than matching a drug to a known or suspected pathogen.[1] Most clinicians generally follow a systematic approach to select an antimicrobial regimen (Table 104–1). Problems arise when this systematic approach is replaced by prescribing broad-spectrum therapy to cover as many organisms as possible. Consequences of not using the systematic approach include the use of more expensive and potentially more toxic agents, which may, in turn, lead to widespread resistance and difficult to treat superinfections. Another abuse of antimicrobial agents is administration when they are not needed. An example of this is prescribing antibacterials for self-limited, clinical conditions that are most likely viral in origin.

Initial selection of antimicrobial therapy is nearly always empiric, which is the initiation of antimicrobials, sometimes prior to documentation of the presence of infection, and before the offending organism is identified. Infectious diseases are generally acute, and a delay in antimicrobial therapy may result in serious morbidity or even mortality. An example is the rapidly lethal nature of various forms of meningitis. Thus, empiric antimicrobial therapy selection is based on information gathered from the patient's history and physical examination and results of Gram stains or of rapidly performed tests on specimens from the infected site. This information, combined with knowledge of the most likely offending organism(s) and an institution's local susceptibility patterns, should result in a rational selection of antibiotics to treat the patient.

This chapter outlines a systematic approach for the selection of antimicrobial therapeutic regimens. The principles for selection of prophylactic antimicrobial regimens are discussed in Chap. 121.

CONFIRMING THE PRESENCE OF INFECTION

FEVER

The presence of a temperature greater than the expected 98.6°F (37°C) "normal" body temperature is considered a hallmark of infectious diseases. Body temperature is controlled in the hypothalamus. In addition, the circadian rhythm, a built-in temperature cycle, is also operational. The daily temperature rhythm may vary for each individual. In a healthy person, the internal thermostat is set between the morning low temperature and the afternoon peak as controlled by the circadian rhythm. During fever, the hypothalamus is reset at a higher temperature level.[2]

Fever is defined as a controlled elevation of body temperature above the normal range. The average normal body temperature range taken orally is 98.0°F to 98.6°F (36.7°C to 37.0°C). Body temperatures obtained rectally are generally 1.0°F (0.6°C) higher, and axillary temperatures are 1.0°F (0.6°C) lower than oral temperatures, respectively. Skin temperatures are also less than the oral temperature but may vary depending on the specific measurement method. Fever can be a manifestation of disease states other than infection. Collagen vascular (autoimmune) disorders and several malignancies may have fever as a manifestation. Fever of unknown or undetermined origin is a diagnostic dilemma and is reviewed extensively elsewhere.[3]

Many drugs have been identified as causes of fever.[4] Drug-induced fever is defined as persistent fever in the absence of infection or other underlying condition. The fever must coincide temporally with the administration of the offending agent and disappear promptly upon its withdrawal, after which the temperature remains normal. Possible mechanisms of drug-induced fever are either a hypersensitivity reaction or development of antigen (drug)-antibody complexes that result in the stimulation of macrophages and release of interleukin-1 (IL-1). Although this is not a common drug effect (accounting for no more than 5% of all drug reactions), it should be suspected when obvious reasons for fever are not present. Almost any medication can produce fever, but certain ones appear to be responsible more often than others. These include β-lactam antibiotics, anticonvulsants, and a variety of other medications, including allopurinol, hydralazine, nitrofurantoin, sulfonamides and related compounds, phenothiazines, and methyldopa.[4]

Noninfectious etiologies of fever may be referred to as false-positives. Although these certainly may confuse the clinician, even more troublesome are false-negatives: the absence of fever in a patient with signs and symptoms consistent with an infectious disease. Careful questioning of the patient or family should be done to assess the ingestion of any medication that can mask fever. These include aspirin, acetaminophen, nonsteroidal anti-inflammatory agents, and corticosteroids. The use of antipyretics should be discouraged during the treatment of infection unless absolutely necessary because they may mask a poor therapeutic response. Moreover, elevated body temperature, unless very high (>105°F/40.5°C), is not harmful and may be beneficial as previously noted.[2]

SIGNS AND SYMPTOMS

WHITE BLOOD CELL COUNT

Most infections result in elevated white blood cell (WBC) counts (leukocytosis) because of the increased production and mobilization of granulocytes (neutrophils, basophils, eosinophils), lymphocytes, or both to ingest and destroy invading microbes. The generally accepted range of normal values for WBC counts is between 4,000 and 10,000 cells/mm^3. Values above or below this range hold important prognostic and diagnostic value.

Bacterial infections are associated with elevated granulocyte counts, often with immature forms (band neutrophils) seen in peripheral blood smears (left-shift). Mature neutrophils are also referred to as segmented neutrophils or polymorphonuclear leukocytes (PMNs). The presence of immature forms is an indication of an increased bone marrow response to the infection. With infection, peripheral WBC counts may be very high, but they are rarely higher than 30,000–40,000 cells/mm^3. Because leukocytosis indicates the normal host

TABLE 104–1. Systematic Approach for Selection of Antimicrobials

Confirm the presence of infection
- Careful history and physical
- Signs and symptoms
- Predisposing factors

Identification of the pathogen (Chap. 103)
- Collection of infected material
- Stains
- Serologies
- Culture and sensitivity

Selection of presumptive therapy considering every infected site
- Host factors
- Drug factors

Monitor therapeutic response
- Clinical assessment
- Laboratory tests
- Assessment of therapeutic failure

response to infection, low leukocyte counts after the onset of infection indicate an abnormal response and are generally associated with a poor prognosis of bacterial infection.

The most common granulocyte defect is neutropenia, a decrease in absolute numbers of circulating neutrophils. A thorough description of the consequences of neutropenia is discussed in Chap. 120. Relative lymphocytosis, even with normal or slightly elevated total WBC counts, is generally associated with tuberculosis and viral or fungal infections. Increases of monocytes may be associated with tuberculosis or lymphoma and increases in eosinophils may be associated with allergic reactions to drugs or metazoan infections. Many types of infections may be accompanied by a completely normal WBC count and differential.

LOCAL SIGNS

The classic signs of pain and inflammation may be manifested by swelling, erythema, tenderness, and purulent drainage. Unfortunately, these are only visibly apparent if the infection is superficial or in a bone or joint. The manifestations of inflammation in deep-seated infections, such as meningitis, pneumonia, endocarditis, and urinary tract infection, must be ascertained by examining tissues or fluids. For example, the presence of neutrophils in spinal fluid, lung secretions (sputum), and urine is highly suggestive of a bacterial infection.

Symptoms referable to an organ system must be carefully sought out, for they not only help in establishing the presence of infection, but also aid in narrowing the list of potential pathogens. For example, a febrile patient with complaints of flank pain and dysuria may well have pyelonephritis. In this situation, enteric gram-negative bacilli, especially *Escherichia coli,* are the predominant pathogens. If a febrile patient has no symptoms referable to an organ system, however, but only constitutional complaints, the list of possible infectious diseases is quite long.[3] A febrile individual with cough and sputum production probably has a pulmonary infection. What is not so evident, however, is the etiologic organism in this situation, because it may be caused by bacteria, mycobacteria, viruses, chlamydia, or mycoplasmas.[5] In this situation, attention to the patient's history and background disease states is important. Even more important is a careful examination of the infected material (in this case sputum) to try and ascertain the identity of the pathogen.

IDENTIFICATION OF THE PATHOGEN

MICROBIOLOGY ISSUES

Infected body materials must be sampled, if at all possible or practical, before institution of any antimicrobial therapy for two reasons. First, a Gram stain of the material may rapidly reveal bacteria, or an acid-fast stain may detect mycobacteria or actinomycetes. Second, a delay in obtaining infected fluids or tissues until after antimicrobial therapy is started may result in false-negative culture results or alterations in the cellular and chemical composition of infected fluids. This is particularly true in patients with urinary tract infections, meningitis, and septic arthritis.[6]

Blood cultures should nearly always be performed in the acutely ill, febrile patient. Blood culture collection is usually timed to sharp elevations in temperature, suggesting the possibility of microorganisms or microbial antigens in the bloodstream. Ideally, blood should be obtained from peripheral sites as two sets (one set consists of an aerobic bottle and one set of an anaerobic bottle) from two different sites approximately 1 hour apart. In selected infections, bacteremia is qualitatively continuous (e.g., endocarditis), so cultures may be obtained at any time.[7]

In addition to the infected materials produced by the patient (e.g., blood, sputum, urine, stool, wound, or sinus drainage), other less-accessible fluids or tissues must be obtained based on localized signs or symptoms (e.g., spinal fluid in meningitis, joint fluid in arthritis). Abscesses and cellulitic areas should also be aspirated.

INTERPRETING RESULTS

After positive Gram stain, culture results, or both are obtained, the clinician must be cautious in determining whether the organism recovered is a true pathogen, a contaminant, or a part of the normally expected flora (see Chap. 103) from the site of specimen collection. This latter consideration is especially problematic with cultures obtained from the skin, oropharynx, nose, ears, eyes, throat, and perineum. These surfaces are heavily colonized with a wide variety of bacteria, some of which may be pathogenic in certain settings. For example, coagulase-negative staphylococci are found in cultures of all the aforementioned sites, yet are seldom regarded as pathogens unless recovered from blood, venous access catheters, or prosthetic devices.

Importantly, cultures of specimens from purportedly infected sites, which are obtained by sampling from or through one of these contaminated areas, may contain significant numbers of the normal flora. In the case of urine cultures, the urinalysis should be used in combination with culture results to assess the presence of WBCs, nitrite, and leukocyte esterase that help confirm infection as opposed to colonization.

Particularly problematic are expectorated sputum specimens that must be carefully evaluated by the determination of the presence of squamous epithelial cells and leukocytes.[5] A predominance of epithelial cells in sputum specimens casts doubt on the pathogenic role of any bacteria recovered, especially when multiple types of organisms are seen on Gram stain. In contrast, the discovery of leukocytes in large numbers with one predominant type of organism is a more reliable indicator of a valid collection. In general, however, sputum evaluation has poor sensitivity and specificity as a diagnostic test.[5]

Caution must also be used in the evaluation of positive culture results from normally sterile sites (e.g., blood, cerebrospinal fluid, or joint fluid). The recovery of bacteria normally found on the skin in large quantities (e.g., coagulase-negative staphylococci, diphtheroids) from one of these sites may be a result of contamination of the specimen rather than a true infection. These organisms may be pathogenic in certain settings.

Gram-staining techniques, culture methods, and serologic identification, as well as susceptibility testing, are discussed in detail in Chap. 103. Emphasis must be placed on the proper collection and handling of specimens and careful assessment of Gram stain or other test results in guiding the clinician toward appropriate selection of initial antimicrobial therapy.[8]

SELECTION OF PRESUMPTIVE THERAPY

To select rational antimicrobial therapy for a given clinical situation, a variety of factors must be considered. These include the severity and acuity of the disease, host factors, factors related to the drugs used, and the necessity for using multiple agents. In addition, there are generally accepted drugs of choice for the treatment of most pathogens (see Appendix 104–1).

Drugs of choice are compiled from a variety of sources and are intended as guidelines rather than as specific rules for antimicrobial use. These choices are influenced by local antimicrobial susceptibility data rather than information published by other institutions or national compilations. Each institution usually publishes an annual summary of antibiotic susceptibilities (antibiogram) for organisms cultured from patients. Antibiograms contain both the number of isolates for common species and the percentage susceptible to the antibiotics tested. To further guide empiric antibiotic therapy, some hospitals publish unit-specific antibiograms in unique patient care areas, such as intensive care units or burn units.

Susceptibility of bacteria may differ substantially among hospitals within a community. For example, the prevalence of methicillin-resistant *Staphylococcus aureus* (MRSA) in some centers is quite high, whereas in other centers, the problem may be nonexistent. This particular situation will influence the selection of therapy for possible *S. aureus* infection where either a β-lactam compound or vancomycin would be the choices. The problem of differing susceptibilities is not only limited to gram-positive bacteria but also to gram-negative organisms, and all drug classes are affected.

Empiric therapy is directed at organisms that are known to cause the infection in question. These organisms for different sites of infection are discussed in Chaps. 105 to 123. To define the most likely infecting organisms, a careful history and physical examination must be performed. Place of acquisition of infection should be determined, for example, the home (community-acquired), nursing home environment, or hospital-acquired (nosocomial). Nursing home patients may be exposed to potentially more resistant organisms because they are often surrounded by ill patients who may be receiving antibiotics. Other important questions to ask infected patients regarding the history of the present illness include:

1. Are any other people sick at home, especially children?
2. Are any unusual pets kept in the home such as pigeons?
3. Where are you employed (that is, are they exposed to contaminated meat or infectious biohazards)?
4. Has there been any recent travel, for example, to endemic areas of fungal infections or developing countries?

HOST FACTORS

Several host factors should be considered when evaluating a patient for antimicrobial therapy. The most important factors are drug allergies, age, pregnancy, genetic or metabolic abnormalities, renal and hepatic function, site of infection, concomitant drug therapy, and underlying disease states.

ALLERGY

Allergy to an antimicrobial agent generally precludes its use. Careful assessment of allergy histories must be performed because many patients confuse common adverse drug effects, such as gastrointestinal (GI) disturbance, with true allergic reactions.[9] Among the most commonly cited antimicrobial allergies are those to penicillin, penicillin-related compounds, or both. In the absence of complete penicillin skin testing capabilities, a rule of thumb for giving cephalosporins to patients allergic to penicillin is to avoid giving them to patients who give a good history for immediate or accelerated reactions (anaphylaxis, laryngospasm) and to give them under close supervision in patients with a history of delayed reactions, such as a rash.[10] If gram-negative infection is suspected or documented, therapy with a monobactam may be appropriate, because cross-reactivity with other β-lactams is virtually nil.[11]

AGE

The patient's age is an important factor, both in trying to identify the likely etiologic agent and in assessing the patient's ability to detoxify or eliminate the drug(s) to be used. The best example of an age determinant of organisms is in bacterial meningitis where the pathogens differ as the patient grows from the neonatal period, through infancy and childhood, and into adulthood.[12]

In the case of the neonate, hepatic and liver function is not well developed. The use of chloramphenicol can lead to shock and cardiovascular collapse (gray baby syndrome) caused by the inability of the newborn's liver to metabolize and detoxify the drug.[13] Serum concentrations of chloramphenicol must be monitored to ensure that concentrations of the drug do not exceed 20 to 25 μg/mL. Neonates (especially when premature) may develop kernicterus when given sulfonamides. This results from displacement of bilirubin from serum albumin.[14] Additional special drug considerations for pediatric patients include low frequency of adverse effects and compliance enhancing features (e.g., absorption not affected by food, once- to twice-daily dosing, and good taste).[15,16]

The major physiologic change in persons greater than 65 years is a decline in functioning nephrons that in turn results in decreased renal function.[17] This is usually manifested by an increased incidence of side effects caused by antimicrobials that are renally eliminated. For example, renal toxicity caused by aminoglycosides may be apparent much sooner during therapy than in younger patients. Oral absorption is also decreased in the elderly; in most cases, however, this has not proven clinically significant. Furthermore, in many cases, no identifiable cause of adverse drug effects can be determined other than "old age," thus, increased monitoring is always warranted in the elderly.

PREGNANCY

During pregnancy, not only is the fetus at risk for drug teratogenicity (see Chap. 78), but also the pharmacokinetic disposition of certain drugs may be altered.[18] Penicillins, cephalosporins, and aminoglycosides are cleared from the peripheral circulation more rapidly during pregnancy. This is probably a result of marked increases in intravascular volume, glomerular filtration rate, and hepatic and metabolic activities, especially during late pregnancy. The net result is that maternal serum antimicrobial concentrations may be as much as 50% lower during this period than in the nonpregnant state. Increased dosages of certain compounds may be necessary to achieve therapeutic levels during late pregnancy.

METABOLIC ABNORMALITIES

Inherited or acquired metabolic abnormalities will influence the therapy of infectious diseases in a variety of ways. For example, patients with impaired peripheral vascular flow may not absorb drugs given by intramuscular injection. In addition, certain metabolic states may predispose patients to enhanced drug toxicity. For example, patients who are phenotypically slow acetylators of isoniazid are at greater risk for peripheral neuropathy.[19] Patients with severe deficiency of glucose-6-phosphate dehydrogenase (G6PD) may develop significant hemolysis when exposed to drugs, such as sulfonamides, nitrofurantoin, nalidixic acid, antimalarials, dapsone, and, perhaps, chloramphenicol.[20] Although mild deficiencies are found in blacks, the more severe forms of the disease are generally confined to persons of eastern Mediterranean origin.

ORGAN DYSFUNCTION

Patients with diminished renal or hepatic function, or both, will accumulate certain drugs unless the dosage is adjusted.[21,22] Recommendations for dosing antibiotics in liver dysfunction are not as formalized as guidelines for renal dysfunction.[22] Antibiotics that should be adjusted in severe liver disease include chloramphenicol, clindamycin, erythromycin, metronidazole, and rifampin. Significant accumulation may occur when both liver and renal dysfunction are present for these drugs: cefotaxime, nafcillin, piperacillin, and sulfamethoxazole.

CONCOMITANT DRUGS

Any concomitant therapy the patient is receiving may influence the selection of drug therapy, the dosage, and monitoring. For example, administration of isoniazid to a patient who is also receiving phenytoin may result in phenytoin toxicity. This is caused by an inhibition of phenytoin metabolism by isoniazid. Furthermore, drugs that possess similar adverse-effect profiles may increase the risk for effects, for example, two drugs that cause nephrotoxicity or neutropenia. Lists of potentially severe drug-drug interactions are provided in Tables 104–2 and 104–3.

CONCOMITANT DISEASE STATES

Concomitant disease states may influence the selection of therapy. Certain diseases will predispose patients to a particular infectious disease or will alter the type of infecting organism. For example, patients with diabetes mellitus and the resulting peripheral vascular disease often develop infections of the lower extremity soft tissue. Moreover, the alterations in peripheral blood flow associated with the disease, and perhaps altered immunity, make such infections more difficult to treat than in nondiabetics. Patients with chronic lung disease or cystic fibrosis develop frequent pulmonary infections, which may be caused by somewhat different microorganisms than are found in otherwise normal hosts.

Patients with immunosuppressive diseases, such as malignancies or acquired immunologic deficiencies, are highly predisposed to infections, and the types of organisms may be vastly different from what would be expected (Chap. 120). For example, patients undergoing chemotherapy for acute forms of leukemia are often profoundly granulocytopenic and are predisposed to infections caused by bacteria and fungi.[23] Patients with the acquired immunodeficiency syndrome (AIDS) often become infected with an enormous variety of organisms (Chap. 123).[24]

Many factors predisposing to infection are related to disruption of the host's integumentary barriers. For example, trauma, burns, and iatrogenic wounds induced in surgery may lead to a substantial risk of infection, depending on the severity and location of the injury or disruption. For a complete discussion of the various risks involved in surgical procedures see Chap. 121.

DRUG FACTORS

PHARMACOKINETIC AND PHARMACODYNAMIC CONSIDERATIONS

Integration of both pharmacokinetic and pharmacodynamic properties of an agent is important when choosing antimicrobial therapy to ensure efficacy and to prevent resistance.[25] Early researchers relied solely on pharmacokinetic properties such as area under the drug concentration curve (AUC), maximum observed concentration (peak) and drug half-life to optimize therapy. Pharmacodynamics is the study of the relationship between drug concentration and the effects on the microorganism (see Chap. 103). Researchers now realize the important relationship between both kinetic and dynamic parameters that has resulted in new measurements such as AUC/minimal inhibitory concentration (MIC) ratio, peak/MIC ratio, and time (T) the concentration is above MIC (T > MIC).

Aminoglycosides exhibit concentration-dependent bactericidal effects.[25] An example of integration of kinetics and dynamics is the use of high-dose, once-daily aminoglycosides. For these regimens, the drug is given as a single large daily dose to maximize peak/MIC ratio. Aminoglycosides also possess a post-antibiotic effect (persistent suppression of organism growth after concentrations fall below the MIC) that appears to contribute to the success of high-dose, once-daily administration.[26] Fluoroquinolones exhibit concentration-dependent killing activity but optimal killing appears to be characterized by the AUC/MIC ratio.[27,28]

β-Lactams and vancomycin display time-dependent bactericidal effects. Killing activity is only marginally enhanced if drug concentration exceeds the MIC. Therefore, the important kinetic and dynamic relationship for these antimicrobials is the duration that drug concentrations exceed the MIC (T > MIC). Effective dosing regimens require serum drug concentrations to exceed the MIC for at least 40% to 50% of the dosing interval.[25] Frequent small doses or a continuous infusion of β-lactams appear to be correlated with a good outcome.[29]

The ability of bacteriostatic antimicrobial agents to eradicate infections is reliant upon host immune function and a post-antibiotic effect. Examples include clindamycin, macrolides, and tetracyclines.[25]

TISSUE PENETRATION

The importance of tissue penetration varies with site of infection. Some of the difficulties interpreting data include a lack of correlation with clinical outcomes and poor understanding of whether the antimicrobial agents are present in a biologically active form.[30] An example of the former problem is the recognized efficacy of drugs with low biliary fluid concentrations in the treatment of cholecystitis, cholangitis, or both, and the absence of the enhanced efficacy of drugs whose primary route of elimination is biliary excretion of active drug. An example of the latter difficulty is with penetration to

TABLE 104–2. Major Drug Interactions with Antimicrobials

Antimicrobial	Other Agent(s)	Mechanism of Action/Effect	Clinical Management
Aminoglycosides	Neuromuscular blocking agents	Additive adverse effects	Avoid
	Nephrotoxins (N) or ototoxins (O) (e.g., amphotericin B (N) cisplatin (N/O), cyclosporine (N), furosemide (O), NSAIDs (N), radio contrast (N), vancomycin (N))	Additive adverse effects	Monitor aminoglycoside SDC and renal function
Amphotericin B	Nephrotoxins (e.g., aminoglycosides, cidofovir, cyclosporine, foscarnet, pentamidine)	Additive adverse effects	Monitor renal function
Azoles	See Chap. 119		
Chloramphenicol	Phenytoin, tolbutamide, ethanol	Decreased metabolism of other agents	Monitor phenytoin SDC, blood glucose
Foscarnet	Pentamidine IV	Increased risk of severe nephrotoxicity/hypocalcemia	Monitor renal function/ serum calcium
Isoniazid	Carbamazepine, phenytoin	Decreased metabolism of other agents (nausea, vomiting, nystagmus, ataxia)	Monitor drug SDC
Macrolides/azalides	Digoxin	Decreased digoxin bioavailability and metabolism	Monitor digoxin SDC; avoid if possible
	Theophylline	Decreased metabolism of theophylline	Monitor theophylline SDC
Metronidazole (also cefmandole, moxalactam, cefperazone)	Ethanol (drugs containing ethanol)	Disulfiram-like reaction	Avoid
Penicillins and cephalosporins	Probenecid, aspirin	Blocked excretion of β-lactams	Use if prolonged high concentration of β-lactam desirable
Ciprofloxacin/ norfloxacin	Theophylline	Decreased metabolism of theophylline	Montior theophylline
Moxifloxacin	Amiodarone, procainamide	Increased Q-T interval	Avoid
Sparfloxacin/ Gatifloxacin	Antiarrhythmics	Increased Q-T interval	Avoid
Quinolones	Multivalent cations (antacids, iron, sucralfate, zinc, vitamins, dairy, citric acid) didanosine	Decreased absorption of quinolone	Separate by 2 hours
Rifampin	Azoles, cyclosporine, methadone propranolol, protease inhibitors (PI), oral contraceptives, tacrolimus, warfarin	Increased metabolism of other agent	Avoid if possible
Sulfonamides	Sulfonylureas, phenytoin, warfarin	Decreased metabolism of other agent	Monitor blood glucose, SDC, PT
Tetracyclines	Antacids, iron, calcium, sucralfate	Decreased absorption of tetracycline	Separate by 2 hours
	Digoxin	Decreased digoxin bioavailability and metabolism	Monitor digoxin SDC; avoid if possible

Azalides: clarithromycin and azithromycin
Azoles: fluconazole, itraconazole, and ketoconazole
Macrolide: erythromycin
Protease inhibitors: aprenavir, indinavir, lopinavir/ritonavir, nelfinavir, ritonavir, and saquinavir
Quinolones: ciprofloxacin, gatifloxacin, levofloxacin, lomefloxacin, norfloxacin, ofloxacin, sparfloxacin
SDC: serum drug concentrations

deep infections, such as abscesses, where various factors, such as acid pH, WBC products, and various enzymes, may inactivate even high concentrations of certain drugs.

The central nervous system (CNS) is one body site where antimicrobial penetration is relatively well defined and correlations with clinical outcomes are established.[31] Cerebrospinal fluid (CSF) concentrations of antimicrobial agents necessary to cure bacterial meningitis have been defined, and drugs that do not reach significant concentrations in the CSF should either be avoided or instilled directly if feasible.

Caution must be taken in selecting an antimicrobial agent for clinical use on the basis of tissue or fluid penetration. Body fluids where drug concentration data are clinically relevant include CSF, urine, synovial fluid, and peritoneal fluid. Apart from these areas, more attention should be paid to clinical efficacy, antimicrobial spectrum, toxicity, and cost than to comparative data on penetration into a given body site.

The proper route of administration for an antimicrobial is dependent on the site of infection. Parenteral therapy is warranted when patients have positive blood cultures (except possibly in the case of pyelonephritis) or are being treated for meningitis or febrile neutropenia. Severe pneumonia is often initially treated with intravenous antibiotics and switched to oral therapy as clinical improvement is evident.[5,32,33] Patients treated in the ambulatory

TABLE 104–3. Major Drug Interactions with Antiretroviral (AR) Agents

Antiretroviral	Other Agent(s)	Mechanism of Action/Effect	Clinical Management
Groups of antiretrovirals with similar drug interactions:			
PI[a]/ Delavirdine/ Efavirenz	Ergot alkaloids midazolam/triazolam/alprazolam	Decreased metabolism of other agents	Avoid
	Phenobarbital/phenytoin/ carbamazepine	Increased metabolism of AR Decreased metabolism of anticonvulsants	Monitor anticonvulsant SDC
PI[a]/ Delavirdine	Lovastatin/simvastatin	Decreased metabolism of statin drug	Avoid
	Rifabutin	Increased metabolism of AR Decreased metabolism of rifabutin	Avoid
	Rifampin	Increased metabolism of AR	Avoid
	Sildenafil	Decreased metabolism of sildenafil	Max dose of sildenafil 25 mg/48 h
PI[a]/ Nevirapine	Oral contraceptives (OC)	Increased metabolism of OC	Use alternative method
Individual agents in alphabetical order by generic name:			
Delavirdine[b]	Antacids/didanosine	Decreased absorption of delavirdine	Separate by 1 h
	Clarithromycin	Decreased metabolism of clarithromycin	Dose adjust in renal faiulre
	Dapsone/warfarin/quinidine Dihydropyridine Ca++ channel antagonists	Decreased metabolism of the other agent	Monitor warfarin/ avoid others
	H_2 blockers/proton pump inhibitors	Decreased absorption of delavirdine	Avoid
	Indinavir	Increased metabolism of indinavir	Indinavir 1,000 mg tid
	Ketoconazole	Decreased metabolism of delavirdine	Avoid
Didanosine	Allopurinol	Decreased metabolism of didanosine	Avoid
	Drugs requiring low pH; dapsone, indinavir, itra/ketoconazole pyrimethamine tetracyclines/quinolones	Decreased absorption of the other agent	Separate by 2 h For quinolones: 6 h before or 2 h after
	Methadone	Decreased didanosine SDC	Increase didanosine
	Ritonavir	Formulation incompatibility	Separate by 2.5 h
Efavirenz[b]	Clarithromycin	Decreased clarithromycin SDC	Avoid: use azithromycin
	Indinavir	Increased metabolism of indinavir	Indinavir 1,000 mg tid
	Rifabutin	Increased metabolism of rifabutin	Rifabutin 450 mg qd
Indinavir[b]	Delavirdine/efavirenz/nevirapine	Increased metabolism of indinavir	Indinavir 1,000 mg tid
	Itra/ketoconazole/	Decreased metabolism of indinavir	Indinavir 600 mg tid
Nevirapine[b]	Indinavir	Increased metabolism of indinavir	Indinavir 1,000 mg tid
	Methadone/opiates/warfarin	Increased metabolism of other agents	Titrate to response/monitor warfarin
	Phenobarbital/phenytoin/ carbamazepine	Unknown	Monitor anticonvulsant SC
	Ketoconazole/ Rifampin/ Tacrolimus	Increased metabolism of other agents	Avoid
Ritonavir[b]	Amiodarone/flecainide propafenone/quinidine Ca++ channel antagonists	Decreased metabolism of other agents	Avoid
	Clarithromycin	Decreased metabolism of clarithromycin	Dose adjust in renal failure
	Didanosine	Formulation incompatibility	Separate by 2.5 h
	Despiramine	Decreased metabolism of desipramine	Reduce dose of despiramine
	Ketoconazole	Decreased metabolism of ketoconazole	Max dose of ketoconazole 200 mg qd
	Meperidine/methadone	Increased metabolism of other drug	Titrate to response
	Theophylline	Increased metabolism of theophylline	Monitor theophylline
	Warfarin	Increased metabolism of warfarin	Monitor warfarin
Zidovudine	Ribavirin	Ribavirin inhibits phosphorylation of zidovudine	Avoid

[a]PI: Protease inhibitors: amprenavir, indinavir, lopinavir, nelfinavir, ritonavir, saquinavir
[b]Also note additional drug interactions above.
SDC: serum drug concentration
(This list is meant to include major interactions and is not exhaustive. Individual package inserts along with the primary literature should be consulted as new interactions continue to be studied and reported. Avoid combinations of drugs with overlapping toxicities whenever possible.)

setting for upper respiratory tract infections (e.g., pharyngitis, bronchitis, sinusitis, and otitis media), lower respiratory tract infections, skin and soft-tissue infections, uncomplicated urinary tract infections, and selected sexually transmitted diseases may receive oral therapy.

DRUG TOXICITY

It is incumbent on health professionals to avoid toxic drugs whenever possible. Antibiotics associated with CNS toxicities, usually when not dose adjusted for renal function, include penicillins, cephalosporins, quinolones, and imipenem. Hematologic toxicities are generally manifested with prolonged use of nafcillin (neutropenia), piperacillin (platelet dysfunction), cefotetan (hypoprothrombinemia), chloramphenicol (bone marrow suppression, both idiosyncratic and dose-related toxicity), and trimethoprim (megaloblastic anemia). Reversible nephrotoxicity is classically associated with aminoglycosides and vancomycin. Reversible ototoxicity can occur with aminoglycosides or erythromycin. In the outpatient setting, patients must be cautioned regarding photosensitivity with azithromycin, quinolones, tetracyclines, pyrazinamide, sulfamethoxazole, and trimethoprim. Lastly, all antibiotics have been implicated in causing diarrhea and colitis secondary to *Clostridium difficile* (see Chap. 111).[34]

Aside from consideration of drug toxicity, some antimicrobial use requires more intensive risk-benefit analysis. An example of this is the decision to use isoniazid prophylactically to prevent tuberculosis. Because the hepatotoxicity of isoniazid increases in frequency with age, older persons who are candidates for isoniazid prophylaxis (positive skin test) must have additional risk factors for tuberculosis to balance the potential toxic effects. These include evidence of recent skin test conversion, immunosuppression, or previous gastrectomy. Older patients without additional risk factors are more likely to suffer toxicity from isoniazid than derive benefit from its use.[35]

COST

The costs of drug therapy are increasing dramatically, especially as new products, derived from biotechnology, are introduced. Greater attention is being paid to the pharmacoeconomics of drug therapy, where patient outcomes are valued and the costs to arrive at those outcomes are estimated. With increasing numbers of patients enrolled in managed care organizations, understanding the true cost of antimicrobial therapy is more important than ever. The total cost of antimicrobial therapy includes much more than just the acquisition cost of the drugs.[36]

Many ancillary costs and factors affect the true cost of therapy. These include factors such as storage, preparation, distribution, and administration, as well as all of the costs incurred from monitoring for adverse effects and factors such as length of hospitalization, readmissions, and all directly provided health care goods and services. More difficult to value, but equally as important, are indirect costs, such as patient quality-of-life issues. Pharmacoeconomic and outcomes analysis are becoming more widely applied and used, in order to derive values such as cost-benefit ratios and the cost effectiveness of various products as compared to each other. A detailed review of pharmacoeconomic analyses is beyond the scope of this chapter, but excellent reviews of the subject are available.[37] A great deal more research in this area is needed, and multidisciplinary, collaborative efforts with the involvement of pharmacy, medicine, nursing, and microbiology are essential.[38]

Many new oral antimicrobials have been approved, including cephalosporins, β-lactam β-lactamase inhibitors, macrolides, and fluoroquinolones, that can be used in place of more expensive parenteral therapy. These agents offer extended spectrum killing activity, increased tissue penetration, and excellent safety and pharmacokinetic profiles. Many older, less expensive oral agents also remain appropriate choices. When oral therapy is being considered, the choice between convenient once-a-day expensive agents versus multiple-dose inexpensive agents arises. It is easy to calculate the difference in acquisition cost; however, the overall cost between agents is more difficult to determine. Factors to weigh include safety, effectiveness, tolerability, patient compliance, and potential drug-drug interactions. In some instances, more expensive agents may be warranted to avoid adverse outcomes.[39]

COMBINATION ANTIMICROBIAL THERAPY

In selecting a drug regimen for a given patient, consideration must be given to the necessity of using more than one drug. Combinations of antimicrobials are generally used to broaden the spectrum of coverage for empiric therapy, achieve synergistic activity against the infecting organism, and prevent the emergence of resistance.[40]

BROADENING THE SPECTRUM OF COVERAGE

Increasing the coverage of antimicrobial therapy is generally necessary in mixed infections where multiple organisms are likely to be present. This is the case in intra-abdominal and female pelvic infections in which a variety of aerobic and anaerobic bacteria may produce disease.[41] Traditionally, a combination of a drug active against aerobic gram-negative bacilli, such as an aminoglycoside, and a drug active against anaerobic bacteria, such as metronidazole or clindamycin, is selected. Newer β-lactam compounds, which possess good activity against both of these types of organisms, such as the cephamycins, imipenem, or the β-lactam and β-lactamase inhibitor combinations may be adequate to replace the combination and, thereby, reduce the cost of therapy. The other clinical situation in which an increased spectrum of activity is desirable is with nosocomial infections.[32]

SYNERGISM

Laboratory tests to identify synergy between antibiotic combinations are described in Chap. 103. The achievement of synergistic antimicrobial activity is advantageous for infections caused by enteric gram-negative bacilli in immunosuppressed patients. Traditionally, combinations of aminoglycosides and β-lactams have been used because these drugs together generally act synergistically against a wide variety of bacteria. The data supporting superior efficacy of synergistic over non-synergistic combinations is weak, however. At best, it would appear that synergistic combinations produce better results in infections caused by *P. aeruginosa*, in certain infections caused by *Enterococcus spp.*, and, perhaps, in patients with profound, persistent neutropenia.[42,43]

The most obvious example of the use of synergy is the treatment of enterococcal endocarditis. The causative organism is usually only inhibited by penicillins, but it is rapidly killed by the addition of streptomycin or gentamicin to a penicillin.[42] The necessity for bactericidal activity in the treatment of endocarditis underscores the need for these synergistic combinations.

PREVENTING RESISTANCE

The use of combinations to prevent the emergence of resistance is widely applied but not often realized. The only circumstance where this has been clearly effective is in the treatment of tuberculosis. The prevalence of resistance to a first-line drug, such as isoniazid or rifampin, in a population of organisms may be as high as 1 in 10^6 to 10^8. Because the bacterial load in a patient with active tuberculosis often exceeds this, two drugs are given to reduce the likelihood of encountering resistance to less than 1 in 10.[35] There is ample evidence from *in vitro* data and experimental bacterial infections that combinations of drugs with different mechanisms are effective in the prevention of the emergence of resistance. Data from clinical trials, however, are either conflicting or do not convincingly support this concept.[44]

DISADVANTAGES OF COMBINATION THERAPY

Although there are potentially beneficial effects from combining drugs, there also are potential disadvantages. Examples include additive nephrotoxicity from drugs, such as aminoglycosides, amphotericin, and, possibly, vancomycin.[45] Inactivation of aminoglycosides by penicillins may be clinically significant when excessive doses of penicillin are given to a patient in renal failure.[46]

The combination of two or more antibiotics may result in antagonistic effects (see Chap. 103). Clinically, the effect of antagonism may be evident when one drug induces β-lactamase production and another drug is β-lactamase unstable.[47] Cefoxitin and imipenem are examples of drugs capable of inducing β-lactamases and may result in more rapid inactivation of penicillins when used together.

MONITORING THERAPEUTIC RESPONSE

After antimicrobial therapy has been instituted, the patient must be monitored carefully for a therapeutic response. Culture and sensitivity reports from specimens sent to the microbiology laboratory must be reviewed, and the therapy changed accordingly. Use of agents with the narrowest spectrum of activity against identified pathogens is recommended. If anaerobes are suspected, even if they are not identified, anaerobic therapy should be continued.

Patient monitoring should include many of the same parameters used to diagnose the infection. The WBC count and temperature should start to normalize. Physical complaints from the patient should also diminish (i.e., decreased pain, shortness of breath, cough, or sputum production). Appetite should improve. Radiologic improvement may lag behind clinical improvement. Determinations of serum (or other fluid) levels of antimicrobials may be useful in assuring outcome, preventing toxicity, or both. There are only a few antimicrobials that require serum concentration monitoring, and then only in selected situations. These include the aminoglycosides, flucytosine, and chloramphenicol. Achievement of adequate aminoglycoside concentrations within the first few days of therapy of gram-negative infection has been correlated with better therapeutic outcome.[48] In addition, assuring that excessive concentrations of flucytosine or chloramphenicol (in neonates) are avoided will prevent toxicity.

Changes in the distribution volume may have significant impact on the efficacy, safety, or both of therapy. An unexpectedly low volume of distribution (such as in the dehydrated patient) will result in higher, potentially toxic drug concentrations, whereas a larger-than-expected volume (such as in patients with edema or ascites) will result in low, potentially subtherapeutic concentrations. The most effective methods use measured serum concentrations of the drugs rather than estimations from renal function tests to assess true drug clearance from the body.

As patients improve clinically, the route of administration should be reevaluated. Streamlining therapy from parenteral to oral (switch therapy) has become an accepted practice for many infections outside the bloodstream and CNS.[33,49] Criteria that should be present to justify switch to oral therapy include (a) overall clinical improvement; (b) afebrile for 24 to 48 hours; (c) decreased WBC count; and (d) functioning GI tract. Drugs that exhibit excellent oral bioavailability when compared to intravenous formulations include amoxicillin, azithromycin, ciprofloxacin, clindamycin, doxycycline, gatifloxacin, levofloxacin, metronidazole, moxifloxacin, sparfloxacin, linezolid, and trimethoprim-sulfamethoxazole.

FAILURE OF ANTIMICROBIAL THERAPY

A variety of factors may be responsible for an apparent lack of response to therapy.[50] Patients who fail to respond over 2 to 3 days require a thorough reevaluation. It is possible that the disease is not infectious, is nonbacterial in origin, or there is an undetected pathogen in a polymicrobial infection. Other factors include those directly related to drug selection, the host, or the pathogen. Laboratory error in identification, susceptibility testing, or both (presence of inoculum effect or resistant subpopulations) are rare causes of antimicrobial failure.

FAILURES CAUSED BY DRUG SELECTION

Factors directly related to the drug selection include an inappropriate drug selection or dosage or route of administration. Malabsorption of a drug product because of GI disease, such as a short-bowel syndrome, or a drug interaction, such as complexation of fluoroquinolones with multivalent cations resulting in reduced absorption, may lead to potentially subtherapeutic serum concentrations. Accelerated drug elimination is also possible. This may occur in patients with cystic fibrosis or during pregnancy, when more rapid clearance or larger volumes of distribution may result in low serum concentrations, particularly for aminoglycosides. A common cause of failure of therapy is poor penetration into the site of infection. This is especially true for sites such as the CNS, eye, and prostate gland. Drug failure can also result from drugs that are highly protein bound or that are chemically inactivated at the site of infection.

FAILURES CAUSED BY HOST FACTORS

Host defenses must be considered when evaluating a patient who is not responding to antimicrobial therapy. Patients who are immunosuppressed (e.g., granulocytopenia from chemotherapy, or AIDS) may respond poorly to therapy because their defenses are inadequate to eradicate the infection despite seemingly adequate drug regimens. A good example is the poor response of infection in granulocytopenic patients that is seen when their WBC counts remain low during therapy. This contrasts to a much better response when granulocyte counts rise during therapy.[51]

Other host factors are related to the necessity for surgical drainage of abscesses or removal of foreign bodies, necrotic tissue, or both. If these situations are not corrected, they result in persistent infection and, occasionally, bacteremia, despite adequate antimicrobial therapy.

FAILURES CAUSED BY MICROORGANISMS

Factors related to the pathogen include the development of drug resistance during therapy.[52] Primary resistance refers to the intrinsic resistance of the pathogens producing the infection. Several infections are more likely to result in drug resistance because of drug inaccessibility (e.g., pneumonia, endocarditis, abdominal and deep-seated skin and soft tissue infections). It has become increasingly obvious that, despite the development and introduction of numerous new antimicrobial agents, bacterial resistance has continued to increase, both within and across different bacterial genera.

Most of the newer antibacterial agents developed and licensed in the past 10 years are targeted toward improved activity against gram-negative bacteria. This list includes parenteral and oral fluoroquinolones, carbapenems, β-lactam β-lactamase inhibitor combinations, and newer cephalosporins. Organisms in which resistance has increased most dramatically include enterococci, pneumococci, and *Mycobacterium tuberculosis*. Enterococci have been isolated with multiple resistance patterns. They may be resistant to β-lactams (by virtue of β-lactamase production, altered penicillin-binding proteins [PBP], or both), vancomycin (via alterations in peptidoglycan synthesis), and high levels of aminoglycosides (via enzymatic degradation).

Pneumococci resistant to penicillins, certain cephalosporins, and macrolides are increasingly common. These organisms are generally susceptible to vancomycin and cefotaxime or ceftriaxone. *M. tuberculosis* resistant to one or more first-line antitubercular agents (isoniazid [INH], rifampin, ethambutol, streptomycin, and pyrazinamide) have increased in frequency as well. This has been observed principally in populations of prison inmates and patients with AIDS.

The increase in resistance among these organisms is believed to be a result of continued overuse of antimicrobials in the community, as well as in hospitals, and the increasing prevalence of immunosuppressed patients receiving long-term suppressive antimicrobials for the prevention of infections. These resistance patterns are regionally variable, and susceptibility patterns in the community (or hospital) should be monitored closely to promote rational antimicrobial selection.[53]

The most recently approved antimicrobial agents such as quinupristin/dalfopristin and linezolid have been targeted at resistant gram-positive bacteria. Numerous other drugs currently in development also have enhanced activity against these bacteria.

The emergence of resistance during antimicrobial therapy is reported most frequently in pulmonary or other deep-seated infections caused by *P. aeruginosa.* This occurs in 20% to 30% of cases and with all the available antibacterial agents, including imipenem. This organism and a group of enteric gram-negative bacilli (*Enterobacter aerogenes, Enterobacter cloacae, Citrobacter freundii, Serratia marcescens,* and a few others) can produce a β-lactamase that is capable of hydrolyzing broad-spectrum cephalosporins and, to a lesser extent, penicillins.[53] These enzymes are categorized as Richmond-Sykes type I, and their genetic code is found on the chromosome. Resistant mutants of these aforementioned organisms that produce large quantities of these enzymes may be present within an infection and may be responsible for the emergence of resistance during therapy. The mutants occur at a frequency of 1 in 10^6 to 1 in 10^8 bacteria, the numbers of bacteria commonly encountered in clinical infections.[53] Because only 10^4 to 10^5 bacteria are tested for susceptibility in the microbiology laboratory, however, this potential resistance may not be detected.

Treatment of an infection caused by *Enterobacter, Citrobacter, Serratia,* or *P. aeruginosa* with a third-generation cephalosporin or aztreonam may produce an initial clinical response by eradicating all of the susceptible bacteria in the population. Within a few days, however, the highly resistant subpopulations have a selective advantage and may overgrow the infection site to produce a relapse.[53] These bacteria usually retain susceptibility to aminoglycosides, imipenem, and fluoroquinolones but are resistant to all other β-lactams. It should be obvious that host defenses are extremely important in this scenario. Debilitated patients with pulmonary infections, abscesses, or osteomyelitis are at high risk for drug failure. In these situations, a combination regimen to prevent the emergence of resistance or the use of imipenem or a fluoroquinolone may be warranted for empiric therapy.

ANTIMICROBIAL USE MANAGEMENT

ANTIBIOTIC FORMULARY

Institutions must make decisions regarding which antibiotics to include on their formularies. The actual decision to have a formulary remains controversial; however, restricting choices does encourage familiarity with a core of antibiotics for residents and attending physicians. Open formularies allow the empiric use of any commercially available antibiotics with recommended guidelines for changes when culture and sensitivity results are finalized. Many institutions have organized an antibiotic subcommittee to the Pharmacy and Therapeutics Committee, which meets to discuss trends in resistance and review new agents. The subcommittee is generally a multidisciplinary group, including representation from microbiology, infection control, pharmacy, and physicians from several disciplines, including infectious disease. The actual implementation of the guidelines and restrictions recommended by such groups requires the cooperation of the entire medical staff. Education plays a major role in the success of the antibiotic formulary.[54]

ANTIMICROBIAL SWITCHING

An interesting topic in formulary management that continues to gain interest despite little scientific research is *antimicrobial switching*. Antimicrobial switching is a predetermined change in an antimicrobial recommendation for empiric therapy of a specific infection at a predetermined time.[55] It has also been called "cycling" or "rotation" of antimicrobials. Importantly, this strategy should not be confused with *antimicrobial switch therapy* that involves change in route of administration of antimicrobial therapy (i.e., intravenous to oral).

Antimicrobial switching is employed as a mechanism to reduce or prevent antimicrobial resistance. *Proactive switching* is a planned switch to preempt resistance at a predetermined point or series of points with a predetermined schedule. *Reactive switching* is a response to high or unacceptable resistance and is often a one-time switch. Most programs incorporate aspects of both types of switching. Cycling implies returning to the original drug after other choices have been used. Rotation implies several planned changes.

Antimicrobial switching is based on the assumptions that the resistance problem being dealt with is (a) caused by the overuse of a particular agent or class of agents and (b) that discontinuation of the particular agent or class of agents will restore susceptibility. These assumptions correlate best with nosocomial gram-negative organisms that can rapidly develop resistance. Theoretically, antimicrobial agents should be sequenced in such an order that mechanisms of resistance do not overlap (i.e., changing drug classes).[55] Experts have expressed the need for further well-controlled, long-term studies. The Centers for Disease Control is currently accepting applications for funding of antimicrobial switch programs.

KEEPING CURRENT

Attention must be paid to the literature on antimicrobials to assist in the selection of therapy. The results from prospective, controlled, randomized clinical trials should be evaluated whenever possible when considering appropriate antimicrobial therapy. Results from prelicensing open trials offer only limited information that may be useful in this regard, because patients in these trials are generally not seriously ill, are not infected with multiply resistant bacteria, and other confounding factors found in most clinical situations are excluded by virtue of the study design. Therefore, comparative data in more seriously ill patients is essential for the appropriate application of new agents.[56]

Postmarketing trials are also important as results may demonstrate superiority of one regimen over another, either in efficacy, safety, or cost effectiveness. Appropriate antimicrobial therapy may change as new organisms are discovered, susceptibility patterns change, new drugs become available, and new clinical trial results are published. Classical thinking in the treatment of infectious diseases will continue to change and evolve to maintain antimicrobial efficacy. Optimal use of modern antimicrobials is just beginning to be defined.[57]

▶ PRINCIPLES OF PHARMACOTHERAPY

- Every attempt should be made to obtain specimens for culture and sensitivity testing prior to initiating antibiotics.
- Empiric antibiotic therapy should be based on knowledge of likely pathogens for the site of infection, information from patient history (recent hospitalizations, work-related exposure, travel, pets), and local susceptibility.
- Patients with delayed reactions to penicillin (skin rash) can generally receive cephalosporins. Patients with type I hypersensitivity reactions to penicillins (anaphylaxis) should not receive cephalosporins (alternatives include aztreonam, quinolones, sulfa drugs, or vancomycin based on type of coverage indicated).
- Estimated renal function should be calculated for every patient who is to receive antibiotics and the dose interval adjusted accordingly. Hepatic function should be considered for drugs eliminated through the hepatobiliary system, such as clindamycin, erythromycin, and metronidazole.
- All concomitant drugs and nutrient supplements should be reviewed when an antibiotic is added to a patient's therapy.
- Combination antibiotic therapy may be indicated for polymicrobial infections (abdominal, gynecologic infections) to produce synergistic killing (β-lactam plus aminoglycoside versus *P. aeruginosa*) or to prevent the emergence of resistance.
- Positive cultures must be interpreted with caution to distinguish true infection from colonization or contamination.
- Treatment for the specific organisms identified should include an agent(s) with the narrowest spectrum of activity. Improvement on broad-spectrum regimen is not enough reason not to streamline therapy. Antibiotic route of administration should be evaluated daily and streamlining from intravenous to oral should be attempted as signs of infection improve for patients with functioning GI tracts (general exceptions are bloodstream and CNS infections).
- All patients receiving antibiotics should be monitored for efficacy (e.g., decreasing temperature and WBC count, diminishing signs and symptoms of infection), toxicity (hypersensitivity: β-lactams, cephalosporins; nephrotoxicity: aminoglycosides, amphotericin; diarrhea: all), and development of superinfection (fungal infection).
- Patients not responding to an appropriate treatment in 2 to 3 days should be reevaluated to ensure (a) that infection is the correct diagnosis; (b) therapeutic drug concentrations are being achieved; (c) patient is not immunosuppressed; (d) patient does not have isolated infection (abscess, foreign body); or (e) resistance has not developed.

REFERENCES

1. Hessen TM, Kaye D. Principles of selection and use of antibacterial agents: in vitro activity and pharmacology. Infect Dis Clin North Am 2000;14:265–279.
2. Dinarello CA, Cannon JG, Wolff SM. New concepts on the pathogenesis of fever. Rev Infect Dis 1988;10:168–189.
3. Mackowiak PA, Durach DT. Fever of unknown origin. In: Mandell GL, Bennett JE, Dolin R, eds. Mandell, Douglas and Bennett's Principles and Practice of Infectious Diseases, 5th ed. Philadelphia, Churchill Livingstone, 2000:622–633.
4. Johnson DH, Cunha BA. Drug fever. Infect Dis Clin North Am 1996;10: 85–91.
5. Niederman MS, Bass JB, Campbell GD, et al. Official ATS statement: Guidelines for the initial management of adults with community-acquired pneumonia—Diagnosis, assessment of severity, and initial antimicrobial therapy. Am Rev Resp Dis 1993;148:1418–1426.
6. Andes DR, Craig WA. Pharmacokinetics and pharmacodynamics of antibiotics in meningitis. Infect Dis Clin North Am 1999;13:595–618.
7. Washington JA. The microbiological diagnosis of infective endocarditis. J Antimicrob Chemother 1987;20(suppl A):29–36.
8. Wilson ML. General principles of specimen collection and transport. Clin Infect Dis 1996;22:766–777.
9. Weiss ME. Drug allergy. Med Clin North Am 1992;76:857–882.
10. Saxon A. Immediate hypersensitivity reactions to beta-lactam antibiotics. Rev Infect Dis 1983;5(suppl 2):S368–S378.
11. Saxon A, Swabb EA, Adkinson NF. Investigation into the immunologic cross-reactivity of aztreonam with other beta-lactam antibiotics. Am J Med 1985;78(suppl 2A):19–26.
12. Saez-Llorens X, McCraken GH. Bacterial meningitis in neonates and children. Infect Dis Clin North Am 1990;4:623–644.
13. Powell DA, Nahata MC. Chloramphenicol: New perspectives on an old drug. Drug Intell Clin Pharm 1982;16:295–300.
14. Kantor HI, Sutherland DA, Leonard JT, et al. Effect of bilirubin metabolism in the newborn of sulfisoxazole administered to the mother. Obstet Gynecol 1961;17:494–500.
15. San Joaquin VH, Stull TL. Antibacterial agents in pediatrics. Infect Dis Clin North Am 2000;14:341–355.
16. Pichichero ME. Empiric antibiotic selection criteria for respiratory infections in pediatric practice. Pediatr Infect Dis J 1997;16:S60–S64.
17. Stalam M, Kaye D. Antibiotic agents in the elderly. Infect Dis Clin North Am 2000;14:357–369.
18. Duff P. Antibiotic selection in obstetric patients. Infect Dis Clin North Am 1997;11:1–12.
19. Relling MV. Polymorphic drug metabolism. Clin Pharm 1989;8:852–863.
20. Tabbara IA. Hemolytic anemias: Diagnosis and management. Med Clin North Am 1992;76:649–668.
21. Livornese LL, Slavin D, Benz RL, et al. Use of antibacterial agents in renal failure. Infect Dis Clin North Am 2000;14:371–389.
22. Tschida SJ, Vance-Bryan K, Zaske DE. Anti-infective agents in hepatic disease. Med Clin North Am 1995;79:895–917.
23. Hughes WT, Armstrong D, Bodey GP, et al. 1997 Guidelines for the use of antimicrobial agents in neutropenic patients with unexplained fever:

Guidelines from the Infectious Diseases Society of America. Clin Infect Dis 1997;25:551–573.

24. USPHS/IDSA guidelines for the prevention of opportunistic infections in persons infected with human immunodeficiency virus: A summary. MMWR Morb Mortal Wkly Rep 1999;48(RR-10):1–59.
25. Levison ME. Pharmacodynamics of antibacterial agents. Infect Dis Clin North Am 2000;14:281–291.
26. Spivey JM. The post-antibiotic effect. Clin Pharm 1992;11:865–875.
27. Forest A, Nix DE, Ballow CH, et al. Pharmacodynamics of intravenous ciprofloxacin in seriously ill patients. Antimicrob Agents Chemother 1993;37:1073–1081.
28. Thomas JK, Forest A, Bhavnani SM, et al. Pharmacodynamic evaluation of factors associated with the development of bacterial resistance in acutely ill patients during therapy. Antimicrob Agents Chemother 1998;42:521–527.
29. Craig WA, Ebert SC. Continuous infusion of beta-lactam antibiotics. Antimicrob Agents Chemother 1992;36:2577–2583.
30. Nix DE, Goodwin SD, Peloquin CA, et al. Antibiotic tissue penetration and its relevance: Impact of tissue penetration on infection response. Antimicrob Agents Chemother 1991;35:1953–1959.
31. Quagliarello VJ, Scheld WM. Treatment of bacterial meningitis. N Engl J Med 1997;336:708–716.
32. Campbell GD, Niederman MS, Broughton WA, et al. Official ATS statement: Hospital-acquired pneumonia in adults: Diagnosis, assessment of severity, initial antimicrobial therapy and preventative strategies. Am J Respir Crit Care Med 1995;153:1711–1725.
33. Ramierez JA. Switch therapy in community-acquired pneumonia. Diagn Microbiol Infect Dis 1995;22(1–2):219–223.
34. Johnson S, Gerding DN. *Clostridium difficile*-associated diarrhea. Clin Infect Dis 1998;26:1027–1034.
35. American Thoracic Society. Treatment of tuberculosis and tuberculosis infection in adults and children. Am J Respir Crit Care Med 1994;149:1359–1374.
36. Guglielmo BJ, Brooks GF. Antimicrobial therapy—Cost-benefit considerations. Drugs 1989;38:473–480.
37. McGhan WF. Pharmacoeconomics and the evaluation of drugs and services. Hosp Formul 1993;28:365–378.
38. Marr JJ, Moffet HL, Kunin CM. Guidelines for improving the use of antimicrobial agents in hospitals: A statement by the Infectious Diseases Society of America. J Infect Dis 1988;157:869–876.
39. Nightingale CH, Quintiliani R. Cost of oral antibiotic therapy. Pharmacother 1997;17:302–307.
40. Rybak MJ, McGrath BJ. Combination antibacterial therapy for bacterial infections: Guidelines for the clinician. Drugs 1996;52:390–405.
41. Landers DV, Wolner-Hanssen P, Paavonen J, et al. Combination antimicrobial therapy in the treatment of acute pelvic inflammatory disease. Am J Obstet Gynecol 1991;164:849–858.
42. Eliopoulos GM. The ten most commonly asked questions about resistant enterococcal infections. Infect Dis Clin Pract 1994;3:125–129.
43. Hilf M, Yu VL, Sharp J, et al. Antibiotic therapy for *Pseudomonas aeruginosa* bacteremia: Outcome correlations in a prospective study of 200 patients. Am J Med 1989;87:540–546.
44. Barriere SL. Bacterial resistance to beta-lactams and its prevention with combination antimicrobial therapy. Pharmacotherapy 1992;12:391–396.
45. Rybak MJ, Albrecht LM, Boike SC, et al. Nephrotoxicity of vancomycin, alone and with aminoglycoside. J Antimicrob Chemother 1990;25:679–687.
46. Manian FA, Stone WJ, Alford RH. Adverse antibiotic effects associated with renal insufficiency. Rev Infect Dis 1989;10:43–55.
47. Sanders CC, Sanders E Jr. Microbial resistance to newer generation β-lactam antibiotics: Clinical and laboratory implications. J Infect Dis 1985;151:399–406.
48. Moore RD, Smith CR, Lietman PS. Association of aminoglycoside plasma levels with therapeutic outcome in gram-negative pneumonia. Am J Med 1984;77:657–662.
49. Cunha BA. Intravenous-to-oral antibiotic switch therapy. Postgrad Med 1997;101:111–128.
50. Cunha BA, Ortega AM. Antibiotic failure. Med Clin North Am 1995;79:663–672.
51. Pizzo PA. Management of fever in patients with cancer and treatment-induced neutropenia. N Engl J Med 1993;328:1323–1332.
52. Kaye KS, Fraimiw HS, Abrutyn E. Pathogens resistant to antimicrobial agents: Epidemiology, molecular mechanisms, and clinical management. Infect Dis Clin North Am 2000;14:293–319.
53. Murray BE. The problems and dilemma of antimicrobial resistance. Pharmacotherapy 1992;12(6 part 2):86s–93s.
54. Quintiliani R, Nightingale CH, Crowe HM, et al. Strategic antibiotic decision-making at the formulary level. Rev Infect Dis 1991;13 (suppl 9):S770–S777.
55. McGowan JE Jr. Strategies for study of the role of cycling on antimicrobial use and resistance. Infect Control Hosp Epidemiol 2000;21:S36–S43.
56. Gilbert DN. Guidelines for evaluating new antimicrobial agents. J Infect Dis 1987;156:934–941.
57. Polk R. Optimal use of modern antibiotics: Emerging trends. Clin Infect Dis 1999;29:264–274.

APPENDIX 104–1A
Drugs of Choice, First Choice, *Alternative(s)*

GRAM-POSITIVE COCCI

Enterococcus faecalis **(generally not as resistant to antibiotics as *Enterococcus faecium*)**
- Serious infection (endocarditis, meningitis, pyelonephritis with bacteremia)
- Ampicillin (or penicillin G) + (gentamicin or streptomycin)
- *Vancomycin + (gentamicin or streptomycin)*
- Urinary tract infection (UTI)
- Ampicillin, amoxicillin
- *Doxycycline,[a] ciprofloxacin,[b] levofloxacin,[b] or fosfomycin*

Enterococcus faecium **(generally more resistant to antibiotics than *Enterococcus faecalis*)**
- Recommend consultation with infectious disease specialist.

Staphylococcus aureus/Staphylococcus epidermidis
- Methicillin (oxacillin)-sensitive
- PRP[c]
- *FGC,[d,e] trimethoprim-sulfamethoxazole, clindamycin,[f] or BLIC[g]*
- Methicillin (oxacillin)-resistant
- Vancomycin ± (gentamicin or rifampin)
- *Per sensitivities: Trimethoprim-sulfamethoxazole, doxycycline,[a] either ± rifampin*

Streptococcus **(groups A, B, C, G, and *S. bovis*)**
- Penicillin G[h] or V[i] or ampicillin
- *FGC,[d,e] erythromycin, azithromycin, clarithromycin,[j] or vancomycin*

Streptococcus pneumoniae
- Penicillin-sensitive (MIC <0.1 μg/mL)
- Penicillin G or V or ampicillin
- *Erythromycin, FGC,[d,e] azithromycin, or clarithromycin[j]*
- Penicillin intermediate (MIC 0.1–1.0 μg/mL)
- High-dose penicillin (12 million units/day for adults) or ceftriaxone[e] or cefotaxime[e]
- *Levofloxacin[b] or vancomycin*
- Penicillin-resistant (MIC ≥2.0 μg/mL)
- Recommend consultation with infectious disease specialist.
- Vancomycin ± rifampin
- *Per sensitivities: TGC,[e,k] imipenem, meropenem, levofloxacin,[b] sparfloxacin,[b] gatifloxacin,[b] or moxifloxacin[b]*

***Streptococcus*, viridans group**
- Penicillin G ± gentamicin[l]
- *FGC,[d,e] erythromycin, azithromyxcin, clarithromycin,[j] or vancomycin ± gentamicin*

GRAM-NEGATIVE COCCI

Moraxella (Branhamella) catarrhalis
- BLIC[g]
- *Trimethoprim-sulfamethoxazole, erythromycin, azithromycin, clarithromycin,[j] doxycycline,[a] SGC,[e,m] TGC,[e,k] or TGCpo[e,n]*

Neisseria gonorrhoeae (also give concomitant treatment for ***Chlamydia trachomatis***)
- Disseminated gonococcal infection
- Ceftriaxone[e] or cefotaxime[e]
- *Oral followup: Cefixime,[e] cefpodoxime,[e] ciprofloxacin,[b] or ofloxacin[b]*
- Uncomplicated infection
- Ceftriaxone[e] or cefotaxime,[e] cefixime,[e] or cefpodoxime[e]
- *Ciprofloxacin[b] or ofloxacin[b]*

Neisseria meningitidis
- Penicillin G
- *TGC[e,k]*

GRAM-POSITIVE BACILLI

Clostridium perfringens
- Penicillin G ± clindamycin
- *Metronidazole, clindamycin, doxycycline,[a] cefazolin,[e] or imipenem[o]*

Clostridium difficile
- Oral metronidazole
- *Oral vancomycin*

GRAM-NEGATIVE BACILLI

Acinetobacter spp.
- Imipenem or meropenem either ± aminoglycoside[p] (amikacin usually most effective)
- *Ciprofloxacin,[b] trimethoprim-sulfamethoxazole, or ampicillin/sulbactam*

Bacteroides fragilis **(and others)**
- Metronidazole
- *BLIC,[g] clindamycin, cephamycin,[e,q] or imipenem[o]*

Enterobacter spp.
- Imipenem, meropenem, or cefepime any plus aminoglycoside[p]
- *Ciprofloxacin,[b] trimethoprim-sulfamethoxazole, TGC,[e,k] or TGCpo[e,n]*

Escherichia coli
- Meningitis
- TGC[e,k] or meropenem
- Systemic infection
- TGC,[e,k]
- *Ampicillin/sulbactam, FGC,[d,e] trimethoprim-sulfamethoxazole, SGC,[e,m] fluoroquinolone,[b,o,r] imipenem,[o] or meropenem[o]*
- Urinary tract infection
- Most oral agents: check sensitivities.
- Ampicillin, amoxicillin/clavulanate, trimethoprim-sulfamethoxazole, or cephalexin[e]
- *Aminoglycoside, FGC[d,e] or fluoroquinolone[b,o,r]*

Gardnerella vaginalis
- Metronidazole
- *Clindamycin*

Haemophilus influenzae
- Meningitis
- Cefotaxime[e] or ceftriaxone[e]
- *Meropenem[o] or chloramphenicol[r]*
- Other infections
- BLIC,[g] or if β-lactamase negative, ampicillin or amoxicillin

Trimethoprim-sulfamethoxazole, cefuroxime,[e] erythromycin, azithromycin, clarithromycin,[j] or fluoroquinolone[b,o,r]

Klebsiella pneumoniae

TGC[e,k] (if UTI only: aminoglycoside[p])

Trimethoprim-sulfamethoxazole, cefuroxime,[e] fluoroquinolone,[b,r] BLIC,[g] imipenem,[o] or meropenem[o]

Legionella spp.

Erythromycin $\pm$ rifampin or fluoroquinolone[b,r]

Trimethoprim-sulfamethoxazole, fluoroquinolone,[b,r] clarithromycin,[j] azithromycin, or doxycycline[a]

Pasteurella multocida

Penicillin G

Doxycycline,[a] BLIC,[g] trimethoprim-sulfamethoxazole or ceftriaxone[e,k]

Proteus mirabilis

Ampicillin

Trimethoprim-sulfamethoxazole, most antibiotics except PRP[c]

***Proteus* (indole-positive) (including *Providencia rettgeri, Morganella morganii, Proteus vulgaris*)**

TGC[e,k] or fluoroquinolone[b,r]

Trimethoprim-sulfamethoxazole, BLIC,[g] aztreonam,[t] imipenem,[o] or TGCpo[e,n]

Providencia stuartii

TGC[e,k] or fluoroquinolone[b,r]

Trimethoprim-sulfamethoxazole, aztreonam,[t] imipenem,[o] or meropenem[o]

Pseudomonas aeruginosa

Piperacillin or ceftazidime plus aminoglycoside[p]

Cefepime,[e] ciprofloxacin,[b] aztreonam,[t] imipenem,[o] or meropenem[o]

UTI only: Aminoglycoside[p]

Ciprofloxacin[b]

Salmonella typhi

Ciprofloxacin,[b] ceftriaxone,[e] or cefotaxime[e]

Trimethoprim-sulfamethoxazole

Serratia marcescens

TGC[e,k] $\pm$ gentamicin

Trimethoprim-sulfamethoxazole, ciprofloxacin,[b] aztreonam,[t] imipenem,[o] or meropenem[o]

Stenotrophomonas (Xanthomonas) maltophilia

Trimethoprim-sulfamethoxazole

Generally very resistant to all antimicrobials; check sensitivities to ceftazidime,[e] ticarcillin/clavulanate, doxycycline,[a] and minocycline[a]

MISCELLANEOUS MICROORGANISMS

Chlamydia pneumoniae

Doxycycline[a]

Erythromycin, azithromycin, clarithromycin,[j] or fluoroquinolone[b,r]

Chlamydia trachomatis

Doxycycline[a] or azithromycin

Levofloxacin[b] or ofloxacin[b]

Mycoplasma pneumoniae

Erythromycin, azithromycin, clarithromycin[j]

Doxycycline[a] or fluoroquinolone[b,r]

SPIROCHETES

Treponema pallidum

Neurosyphilis

Penicillin G

Ceftriaxone[e]

Primary or secondary

Benzathine penicillin G

Doxycycline[a] or ceftriaxone[e]

***Borrelia burgdorferi* (choice depends on stage of disease)**

Ceftriaxone,[e] or cefuroxime axetil,[e] doxycycline,[a] amoxicillin

High-dose penicillin, cefotaxime,[e] azithromycin, or clarithromycin[j]

[a] *Not for use in pregnant patients or children younger than 8 years old.*

[b] *Not for use in pregnant patients or children younger than 18 years old.*

[c] *Penicillinase-resistant penicillin: nafcillin or oxacillin.*

[d] *First-generation cephalosporins. IV: cefazolin; PO: cephalexin, cephradine, or cefadroxil.*

[e] *Some penicillin-allergic patients may react to cephalosporins.*

[f] *Not reliably bactericidal, should not be used for endocarditis.*

[g] *β-Lactamase inhibitor combination. IV: ampicillin/sulbactam; PO: amoxicillin/clavulanate.*

[h] *Either aqueous penicillin G or benzathine penicillin G (pharyngitis only).*

[i] *Only for soft-tissue infections or upper respiratory infections (pharyngitis, otitis media).*

[j] *Do not use in pregnant patients.*

[k] *Third-generation cephalosporins. IV: cefotaxime, ceftriaxone.*

[l] *Gentamicin should be added if tolerance or moderately susceptible (MIC >0.1 g/mL) organisms are encountered; streptomycin is used but may be more toxic.*

[m] *Second-generation cephalosporins. IV: cefuroxime; PO: cefuroxime axetil, cefaclor, cefprozil.*

[n] *Third-generation cephalosporins. PO: cefixime, cefetamet, cefpodoxime, ceftibuten.*

[o] *Reserve for serious infection.*

[p] *Aminoglycosides: gentamicin, tobramycin, amikacin—use per sensitivities.*

[q] *Cefoxitin, cefotetan, cefmetazole.*

[r] *IV/PO: ciprofloxacin, ofloxacin, levofloxacin, gatifloxacin, PO: moxifloxacin, sparfloxacin.*

[s] *Reserve for serious infection when less toxic drugs are not effective.*

[t] *Generally reserved for patients with hypersensitivity reactions to penicillin.*

105

CENTRAL NERVOUS SYSTEM INFECTIONS

Gigi H. Ross, Brent W. Gunderson, Khalid H. Ibrahim, Christopher J. Sullivan, and John C. Rotschafer

Central nervous system (CNS) infections are caused by various pathogens, including bacteria, viruses, fungi, and parasites. Infections are the result of hematogenous spread from a primary infection site, seeding from a parameningeal focus, reactivation from a latent site, trauma, or congenital defects in the CNS. Newer diagnostic techniques enable more rapid and definitive diagnoses, thus diminishing the number of unknown "aseptic meningitis" diagnoses and improving targeted therapy. Bacteria resistant to multiple antibiotics present new challenges in the management of meningitis. This chapter presents the etiologies, pathophysiology, therapy, and prophylaxis of these infections, but concentrates predominately on bacterial meningitis.

EPIDEMIOLOGY

The incidence of acute bacterial meningitis in the United States is approximately 3 cases per 100,000 persons per year.[1] Overall mortality rates for patients with meningitis range from 3% to 33%.[2–5] Neurologic sequelae frequently associated with meningitis include seizures, sensorineural hearing loss, and hydrocephalus. Risk for the development of neurologic sequelae is dependent on the infecting organism. Generally, 10% of patients who survive meningitis may develop neurologic disabilities. Patients surviving gram-negative bacillary meningitis, however, have a 60% chance of developing complications from their infection.[2–5] Despite the availability of antimicrobial therapy against the most common CNS pathogens, CNS infections continue to have significant morbidity and mortality.

ETIOLOGY

Central nervous system infections are caused by a variety of microorganisms. Historically, CNS infections were primarily community acquired; however, an increasing number are now nosocomial.[5] Surveillance studies of bacterial meningitis in the United States were conducted in 1986 and, in a smaller study, again in 1995.[6,7] In 1986, *Haemophilus influenzae* was the most commonly identified cause of bacterial meningitis (45%), followed by *Streptococcus pneumoniae* (18%) and *Neisseria meningitidis* (14%). In 1995, approximately 5 years after the introduction of the *H. influenzae* type b vaccine (HIB), *S. pneumoniae* was the most commonly identified cause of bacterial meningitis (47%) followed by *N. meningitidis* (25%), *Listeria monocytogenes* (8%), and *H. influenzae* (7%).

The CDC reported an 82% decrease in the incidence of *H. influenzae* type b infections between 1985 and 1991 for children younger than 5 years old, which coincides with the increased distribution of the HIB vaccine in this age group.[3,8] A similar phenomenon will likely be observed with the introduction of the new pediatric pneumococcal vaccine. Mass immunization with the HIB vaccine has also resulted in alterations in the age distribution of bacterial meningitis. While the median age was 15 months in 1986, by 1995, that age increased to 25 years. Accordingly, the proportion of cases in those 18 years of age and older increased from 20.8% to 51.5%.[7]

ANATOMY AND PHYSIOLOGY OF THE CENTRAL NERVOUS SYSTEM

MENINGES

The skull and vertebrae protect the CNS from blunt or penetrating trauma (Fig. 105–1). The brain is suspended in these structures by cerebrospinal fluid (CSF) and is surrounded by the meninges. The meninges are made up of three separate membranes: dura mater, arachnoid, and pia mater.[9,10] Dura mater, or pachymeninges, lies directly beneath and is adherent to the skull. The other two membranes are referred to collectively as leptomeninges. Pia mater lies directly over brain tissue. Arachnoid, the middle layer, lies between the dura mater and the pia mater. The subarachnoid space, located between the arachnoid and pia mater, is the conduit for CSF. By definition, meningitis refers to inflammation of the subarachnoid space or spinal fluid, whereas encephalitis is an inflammation of the brain itself. Because infectious microorganisms are frequently an underlying cause of these inflammatory processes, the terms meningitis and encephalitis are frequently used to denote an infectious process. The decision regarding the diagnosis of meningoencephalitis depends on radiographic, laboratory, and clinical information, but would refer to inflammation of both tissue and fluid.

CEREBROSPINAL FLUID

Approximately 85% of the CSF is produced within the fourth and lateral ventricles by the choroid plexus (Fig. 105–1). Cerebrospinal fluid volume in the CNS is related to patient age: infants have approximately 40–60 mL of CSF, children have 60–100 mL, and adults have 110–160 mL. Normally, CSF is produced at the rate of approximately 500 mL/d and flows unidirectionally downward through the spinal cord. The CSF is removed by the arachnoid villi and vertebral venous plexus located in the spinal cord and does not recommunicate with the point of production.[9]

The CSF is normally clear with a protein content of <50 mg/dL, a glucose concentration of approximately 50% to 66% of the simultaneous peripheral serum glucose concentration, a pH of approximately 7.4, and typically contains fewer than five white blood cells (WBCs) per mm^3, all of which should be lymphocytes (Table 105–1).

BLOOD-BRAIN BARRIER/BLOOD-CEREBROSPINAL FLUID BARRIER

Natural barriers to the exchange of drugs and endogenous compounds among the blood, brain, and CSF are the blood-brain barrier (BBB) and blood-CSF barrier (BCSFB) (Fig. 105–2). The BBB consists of

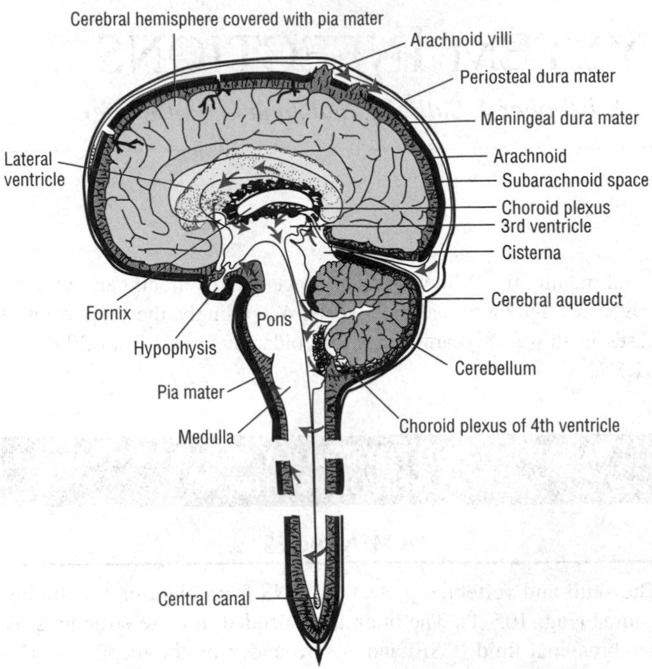

FIGURE 105–1. The central nervous system.

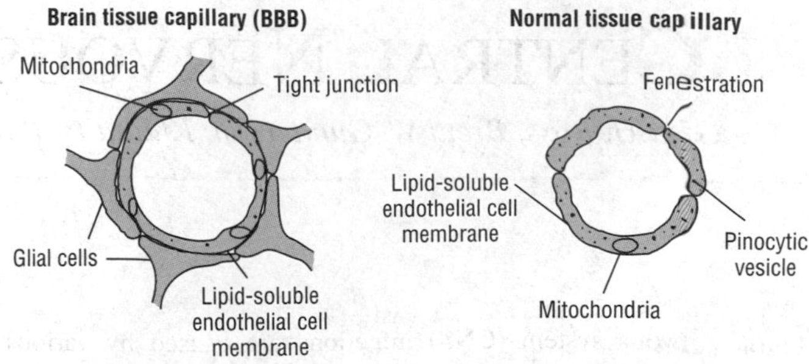

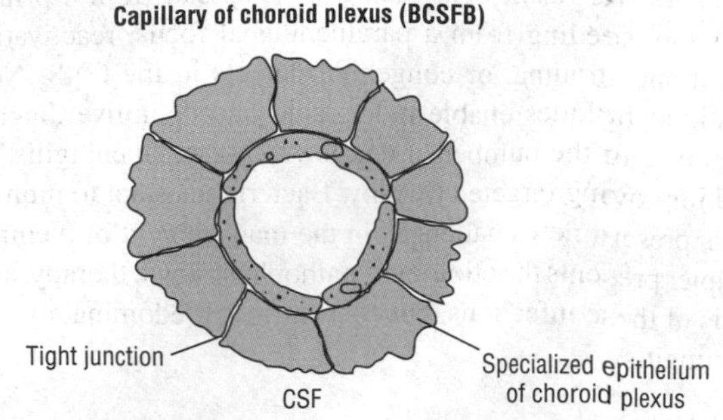

FIGURE 105–2. Representation of a brain tissue capillary, normal tissue capillary, and blood-cerebrospinal fluid barrier capillary. *(From Zabinski RA, Vance-Bryan K, Rotschafer JC. The management of central nervous system infection. J Pharm Pract 1991;4(3):170–191, with permission.)*

tightly joined capillary endothelial cells. Drug entry into brain tissue is accomplished by direct passage through the capillary endothelial cells and further penetration of the glial cells that envelop the capillary structure.[9]

Passage of drugs into the CSF is controlled by the BCSFB. Ependymal cells of the choroid plexus, which function as an active transport system similar to the renal tubular epithelial cells, create this barrier. The inflammatory process associated with meningitis inhibits the active transport system of the choroid plexus.[11] Like the active transport system in the kidney, the secretion of substances out of the choroid plexus can also be inhibited by the administration of probenecid.[12]

PATHOPHYSIOLOGY OF THE CENTRAL NERVOUS SYSTEM INFECTION

The critical first step in the acquisition of acute bacterial meningitis is nasopharyngeal colonization of the host. Bacterial pathogens attach themselves to nasopharyngeal epithelial cells via surface structures called lectins and are phagocytized across nonciliated columnar nasopharyngeal cells into the host's bloodstream.[2] Immunoglobulins (Ig) such as secretory IgA are found in high concentrations within nasopharyngeal secretions and work to inhibit bacterial colonization.[2]

After accessing the patient's bloodstream, bacteria must overcome the host's defense mechanisms. Commonly, CNS bacterial pathogens will produce an extensive polysaccharide capsule resistant to neutrophil phagocytosis and complement opsonization. Studies with *H. influenzae, Escherichia coli,* and *N. meningitidis* found that strains lacking polysaccharide capsules are unable to cause meningitis. Capsular polysaccharides activate the alternate complement pathway, which promotes phagocytosis and clearance of infecting pathogens. Patients unable to activate the alternative complement pathway, such as asplenic and sickle cell patients, are predisposed to bacterial infections caused by encapsulated microorganisms and are, therefore, at risk for meningitis.

Although the exact site and mechanism of bacterial invasion into the CNS is unknown, studies suggest invasion into the subarachnoid space occurs by continuous exposure of the CNS to large bacterial inocula. Bacteremia with inoculum densities of at least 10^3 colony forming units/mL appears to be essential for subarachnoid space invasion.[2] Although several sites of bacterial invasion have been theorized, the

TABLE 105–1. Mean Values of the Components of Normal and Abnormal Cerebrospinal Fluid[18]

Type	Normal	Bacterial Infection	Viral Infection	Fungal Infection	Tuberculosis
WBC (mm^3)	<5	400–100,000	5–500	40–400	100–1,000
Differential	>90%[a]	>90 PMN	50[b,c]	>50[b]	>80[b,c]
Protein (mg/dL)	<50	80–500	30–150	40–150	≤40–150
Glucose (mg/dL)	2/3 serum	<1/2 serum	<30–70	<30–70	<30–70

[a]Monocytes
[b]Lymphocytes
[c]Initial cerebrospinal fluid (CSF) white blood cell (WBC) may reveal a predominance of polymorphonuclear neutrophils (PMNs).

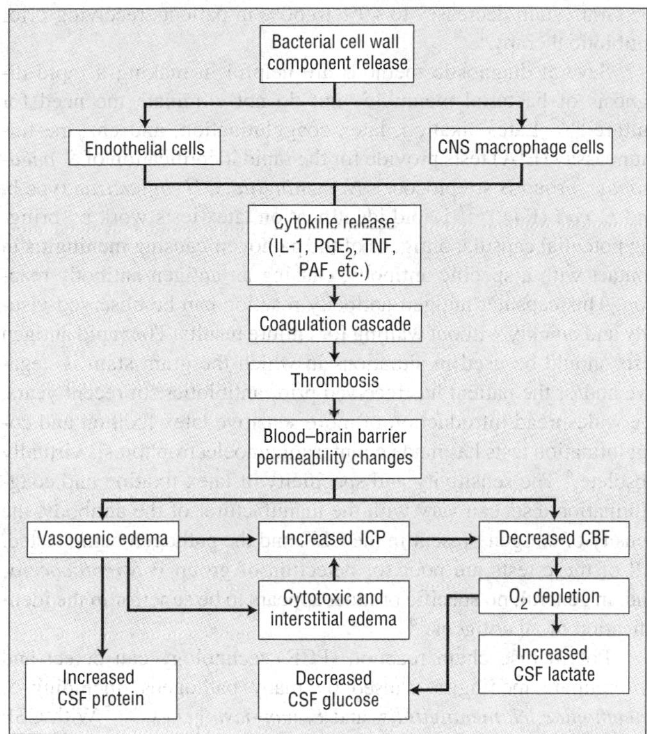

FIGURE 105–3. Hypothetical schema of pathophysiology events that occur during bacterial meningitis. CBF, cerebral blood flow; CSF, cerebrospinal fluid; ICP, intracranial pressure; IL-1, interleukin-1; PAF, platelet-activating factor; PGE_2, prostaglandin E_2; TNF, tumor necrosis factor.

most plausible sites are those highly perfused, such as the choroid plexus (with blood flow rates approximately 200 mL/g/min). Additionally, cells of the choroid plexus possess receptors that facilitate bacterial adherence and allow bacterial transport into the subarachnoid space.[2] Host defense mechanisms within the subarachnoid space are inadequate to combat bacterial pathogens; bacteria, therefore, replicate freely within the CSF until either overgrowth occurs or an effective antibiotic regimen is administered that terminates the process.

Bacterial cell death can cause the release of cell wall components, such as lipopolysaccharide (LPS), lipid A (endotoxin), lipoteichoic acid, teichoic acid, and peptidoglycan, depending on whether the pathogen is gram-positive or gram-negative (Fig. 105–3). These cell wall components cause capillary endothelial cells and CNS macrophages to release cytokines (interleukin-1 [IL-1] and tumor necrosis factor [TNF]). Cytokines interact with capillary endothelial cells and CNS leukocytes to release products of the cyclooxygenase-arachidonic acid pathway (prostaglandins and thromboxanes) and platelet-activating factor (PAF). The PAF activates the coagulation cascade, and arachidonic acid metabolites stimulate vasodilation. These events propagate other sequential events and cytokines, which lead to cerebral edema, elevated intracranial pressure, CSF pleocytosis, disseminated intravascular coagulation (DIC), syndrome of inappropriate antidiuretic hormone (SIADH) secretion, decreased cerebral blood flow, cerebral ischemia, and death.[2,13]

CLINICAL PRESENTATION AND DIAGNOSIS

The clinical signs and symptoms of meningitis are variable and dependent on the age of the patient. Adult patients with bacterial meningitis often present with the classic signs and symptoms of meningitis, such as headache, fever, stiffness of the neck, back, or both, nuchal rigidity,

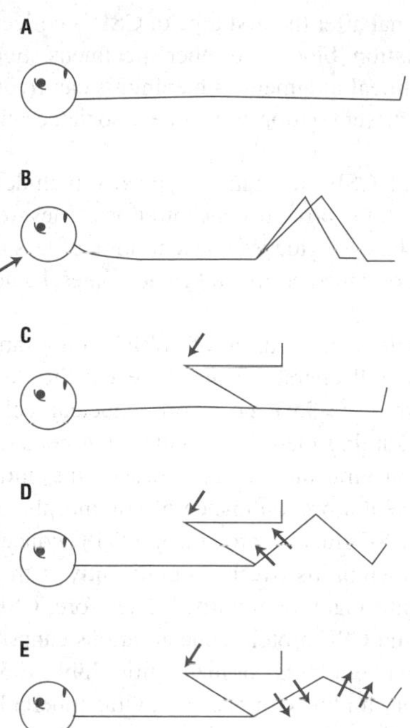

FIGURE 105–4. **A** and **B**, Brudzinski's neck sign. Flexion of the neck by the examiner produces hip and knee flexion (**B**). **C–E**, Brudzinksi's leg signs. **C**, Examiner passively flexes patient's leg (*arrow*). **D**, The identical contralateral sign: contralateral leg begins to flex (*arrows*). **E**, The reciprocal contralateral sign: the same leg that extended the active flexion begins to extend spontaneously, a reflex resembling a little kick (*double arrows*). *(From Verghese A, Gallemore G. Kernig's and Brudzinski's signs revisited. Rev Infect Dis 1987;9:1187–1192, with permission.)*

Brudzinski's sign (Fig. 105–4), Kernig's sign (Fig. 105–5), or both, and photophobia.[14] Later in the course of the disease, the patient may experience obtundation, seizures, focal neurologic deficits, and hydrocephalus. Conversely, young infants with bacterial meningitis may have nonspecific symptoms, such as irritability, altered sleep patterns, vomiting, high-pitched crying, decreased oral intake, or seizures.[15] As a child ages, a more CNS-specific clinical picture becomes prevalent; changes in activity level, somnolence, confusion, or lethargy are frequently reported.[15] Up to 50% of patients diagnosed with meningitis have received prior antibiotic therapy.[4] These patients may present less frequently with fever or mental status changes and may have a longer duration of symptoms.[16]

A presumptive diagnosis of bacterial meningitis is based on the initial results of the CSF collected. Typically, four tubes of CSF are collected via lumbar puncture for chemistry, microbiology, and hematology tests.[16] Any contamination with skin flora and disinfectant

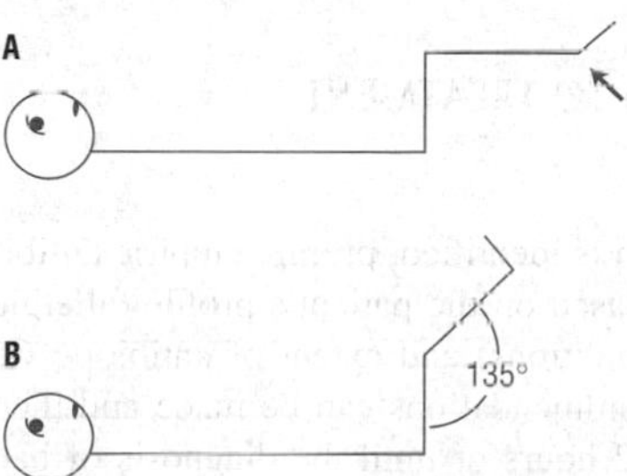

FIGURE 105–5. Kernig's sign. **A**, Examiner flexes hip 90 degrees to the trunk and attempts to extend the knees. **B**, "Contracture" or extensor spasm at the knee 135 degrees. *(From Verghese A, Gallemore G. Kernig's and Brudzinski's signs revisited. Rev Infect Dis 1987;9:1187–1192, with permission.)*

should be minimal after the first tube of CSF is collected. In addition to CSF examination, blood and other specimens should be cultured according to clinical judgment as meningitis can frequently arise via hematogenous dissemination or can be associated with infections at other sites.

Analysis of CSF chemistries typically includes measurement of glucose and total protein concentrations. Elevated CSF protein ≥50 mg/dL and a CSF glucose concentration of less than 50% of the simultaneously obtained peripheral value suggest bacterial meningitis (Table 105–1).

Hematologic examination of WBC count and accompanying differential will characteristically reveal the presence of 200–10,000 WBC/mm^3 (>95% polymorphonuclear cells) in bacterial meningitis, presuming there is no underlying hematologic disorder. In some cases of viral meningitis, however, the initial examination of CSF may reveal a predominance of polymorphonuclear cells.[9,17] The values for CSF glucose, protein, and WBC concentrations found with bacterial meningitis overlap significantly with those for viral, tuberculous, and fungal meningitis.[18] Therefore, CSF WBC counts, CSF glucose, and CSF protein concentrations cannot always distinguish the different etiologies of meningitis. Table 105–1 summarizes typical laboratory findings for bacterial, viral, tuberculous, and fungal CNS infections.[18]

Gram stain and culture of the CSF are the most important laboratory tests performed for bacterial meningitis. Recovery of bacterial pathogens from both culture and Gram stain can be greatly influenced by the quantity of CSF available for culture and prior use of antimicrobial therapy.[4] When performed before antibiotic therapy is initiated, Gram stain is both rapid and sensitive and can confirm the diagnosis of bacterial meningitis in 60% to 90% of cases.[10,17] The sensitivity of the Gram stain decreases to 40% to 60% in patients receiving prior antibiotic therapy.[4]

Several diagnostic methods are helpful in making a rapid diagnosis of bacterial meningitis but do not eliminate the need for culture.[10,17] Latex fixation, latex coagglutination, and enzyme immunoassay (EIA) tests provide for the rapid identification of *S. pneumoniae*, group B streptococci, *N. meningitidis*, *H. influenzae* type b, and *E. coli* (K1).[10,17] Rapid identification latex tests work by bringing potential capsular antigens of the pathogen-causing meningitis in contact with a specific antibody, causing an antigen-antibody reaction. This capsular antigen-antibody reaction can be observed visually and quickly without waiting for culture results. The rapid antigen tests should be used in situations in which the gram stain is negative and/or the patient has received prior antibiotics. In recent years, the widespread introduction of more sensitive latex fixation and coagglutination tests has made counterimmunoelectrophoresis virtually obsolete.[4] The sensitivity and specificity of latex fixation and coagglutination tests can vary with the manufacturer of the antibody, the density of antigen present in the CSF, and the pathogen being tested. All of these tests are poor for detection of group B *Streptococcus*, and, in general, no specific product appears to be superior in the identification of all antigens.[10,17]

Polymerase chain reaction (PCR) technology can detect and differentiate meningitis caused by many pathogens, including *S. pneumoniae*, *N. meningitidis*, and *L. monocytogenes*.[19,20] With CSF samples, the sensitivity and specificity of these methods approach 90% and 100%, respectively.[19] Unfortunately, PCR testing can be time-consuming and expensive, both of which have hindered the widespread use of the technology. PCR testing is also useful in documenting CNS infections caused by viruses, mycobacteria, or fungi.

▶ TREATMENT: Central Nervous System Infections

DESIRED OUTCOME

The importance of supportive care, particularly early in the course of treatment, cannot be emphasized enough. Administration of fluids, electrolytes, antipyretics, analgesia, and other supportive measures are indicated for patients presenting with acute bacterial meningitis. Although supportive care is initially important, appropriate antibiotic therapy (empiric or definitive) should be started as soon as possible. Understanding antibiotic selection and the issues surrounding their penetration will assist in meeting the goals of treatment, which include eradication of infection with amelioration of signs and symptoms, and prevention of neurologic sequelae, such as seizures, deafness, coma, and death.

APPROACH TO TREATMENT

Until a pathogen is identified, prompt empiric antibiotic coverage is often needed. Based on the patient's profile (allergies, age, concurrent medical conditions) and extent of antibiotic CNS penetration, appropriate recommendations can be made and therapy should last at least 48 to 72 hours or until the diagnosis of bacterial meningitis can be ruled out (Tables 105–2 and 105–3). Continued therapy should be based on the assessment of clinical improvement, cultures, and sensitivity testing results. After a pathogen is identified, antibiotic therapy should be tailored toward the specific pathogen (Tables 105–4 and 105–5). Throughout the course of treatment, various efficacy parameters, such as signs and symptoms, microbiologic findings, and CSF examination should be followed to evaluate the success of meeting the desired outcomes. The following section discusses issues surrounding the approach to treatment, such as antibiotic penetration within the CNS, the duration of antibiotic therapy, and the use of adjunctive steroids.

Several factors influence the transfer of antibiotic from capillary blood into the CNS, including inflammation of the meninges, which increases antibiotic penetration through damage to tight junctions between capillary endothelial cells and decreases the activity of an energy-dependent efflux pump in the choroid plexus responsible for movement of penicillins, and, to a much lesser extent, fluoroquinolones and aminoglycosides (Table 105–3). Antibiotics having low molecular weight are more easily passed through biologic barriers than are compounds of higher molecular weight. Only antibiotics that are nonionized at physiologic or pathologic pH are capable of diffusion. Highly lipid-soluble compounds penetrate more readily than water-soluble compounds. Antibiotics that are not extensively protein bound in the serum provide a larger free fraction of drug capable of passing into the CSF. Passage of large, polar antibiotics into the CSF may be assisted, however, by a carrier transport system.

Problems of CSF penetration may be overcome by direct instillation of antibiotics intrathecally, intracisternally, or intraventricularly (Table 105–6).[21–26] Advantages of direct instillation, however, must be weighed against the risks of invasive CNS procedures. Intrathecal administration of antibiotics is unlikely to produce therapeutic

TABLE 105–2. Bacterial Meningitis: Most Likely Organisms and Empiric Therapy by Age Group

Age Commonly Affected	Most Likely Organisms	Empiric Therapy	Risk Factors for All Age Groups
Newborn–1 month	Gram-negative enterics* Group B streptococcus *Listeria monocytogenes*	Ampicillin + CTX or CTR or AG	Respiratory tract infection Otitis media Mastoiditis
1 month–4 years	*H. influenzae* *N. meningitidis* *S. pneumoniae*	CTX or CTR and VM	Head Trauma Alcoholism High-dose steroids
5–29 years	*N. meningitidis* *S. pneumoniae* *H. influenzae*	CTX or CTR and VM	Splenectomy Sickle cell disease Immunoglobulin deficiency
30–60 years	*S. pneumoniae* *N. meningitidis*	CTX or CTR and VM	Immunosuppression
> 60 years	*S. pneumoniae* Gram-negative enterics *L. monocytogenes*	Ampicillin + CTR or CTR or AG and VM	

**Escherichia coli, Klebsiella spp., Enterobacter spp.* common. AG, aminoglycoside; CTX, cefotaxime; CTR, ceftriaxone; VM, vancomycin. (Use should be based on local incidence of penicillin-resistant *S. pneumoniae* and until CTX or CTR minimal inhibitory concentration results are available.)

concentrations in the ventricles because of the unidirectional flow of CSF.[22] Although intraventricular administration may be preferred over intrathecal administration from a therapeutic standpoint, the former requires neurosurgical placement of an Ommaya or a Rickham reservoir.[23] Intraventricular delivery may be necessary when bacteria such as *L. monocytogenes, Pseudomonas aeruginosa,* or enterococci that may require treatment with aminoglycosides are isolated. In a review of antibiotic-induced endotoxin release, children receiving both parenteral antibiotics and intrathecal gentamicin had higher CSF endotoxin levels, higher CSF IL-1 β levels, and higher mortality than did children receiving only parenteral antibiotics.[27] Interestingly, the differences were attributed to direct CSF administration of gentamicin, which is generally thought to blunt the endotoxin release caused by β-lactam antibiotics.[27]

TABLE 105–3. Penetration of Antimicrobial Agents into the Cerebrospinal Fluid

Therapeutic Levels in CSF With or Without Inflammation	
Sulfonamides	Trimethoprim
Choramphenicol	Isoniazid
Rifampin	Pyrazinamide
Ethionamide	Cycloserine
Metronidazole	
Therapeutic Levels in CSF With Inflammation of Meninges	
Penicillin G	Ampicillin ± sulbactam
Carbenicillin	Ticarcillin ± clavulanic acid
Nafcillin	Mezlocillin
Piperacillin	Cefuroxime
Cefotaxime	Ceftizoxime
Ceftriaxone	Ceftazidime
Imipenem	Aztreonam
Meropenem	Ofloxacin
Vancomycin	Ciprofloxacin
Vidarabine	Ethambutol
Flucytosine	Fluconazole
Pyrimethamine	Ganciclovir
Acyclovir	Foscarnet
Nontherapeutic Levels in CSF With or Without Inflammation	
Aminoglycosides	First generation cephalosporins
Cefoperazone	Second-generation cephalosporins[a]
Clindamycin[b]	Ketoconazole
Amphotericin B	Itraconazole[c]

[a]Cefuroxime is an exception.
[b]Achieves therapeutic brain tissue concentrations.
[c]Achieves therapeutic concentrations for *Cryptococcus neoformans* therapy.
CSF, cerebrospinal fluid.

Although the length of treatment for bacterial meningitis is generally based on causative organism, there is no universally accepted standard. Meningitis caused by *S. pneumoniae, N. meningitidis,* and *H. influenzae* is successfully treated with 7 to 14 days of antibiotic therapy. In contrast, a longer duration of 14 to 21 days is recommended for patients infected with *L. monocytogenes,* group B streptococci, and enteric gram-negative bacilli because of a high probability of relapse. Therapy should be individualized, and some patients may require longer courses.[1,28,29]

CAUSATIVE AGENTS

NEISSERIA MENINGITIDIS (MENINGOCOCCUS)

N. meningitidis is most commonly found in children and young adults. The source of infection is usually an asymptomatic carrier. Most cases occur in the winter or spring at a time when viral meningitis is relatively uncommon. Five serogroups of *N. meningitidis* (A, B, C, Y, and W-135) are primarily responsible. Clusters of meningococcal disease, defined as two or more cases of the same serogroup that are closer in time and space than expected for the population or group under observation are generally associated with schools.[30,31] Although some of these clusters have been caused by serogroup B, the majority have been caused by serogroup C. Serogroup A, although associated with meningococcal outbreaks in Africa and Asia, is a rare cause of disease in the United States.[32] Serogroup Y, although frequently associated with pneumonia, is emerging as an important cause of invasive meningococcal disease in select areas.[33] Overall, *N. meningitidis* accounts for 25% of all meningitis cases, 60% of cases in persons ages 2 to 18 years, and carries a case fatality rate of approximately 3%.[7]

Initially, patients are colonized and, at some point, develop a bacteremia, which most likely occurs prior to hospital admission. Metastatic seeding to the meninges, the most common site, occurs as a result of the bacteremia.[13,34] After the acute phase of meningitis has

TABLE 105–4. Antimicrobial Agents of First Choice and Alternative Choice in Treatment of Meningitis Caused by Gram-positive Microorganisms

Organism	Antibiotic of First Choice[a]	Alternative Antibiotics[a]
Streptococcus pneumoniae		
Penicillin susceptible	Penicillin G 200,000–300,000 U/kg/day in 6 divided doses IV max: 4 million U q4h IV	Cefotaxime 200 mg/kg/day in 6 divided doses max 2 g q4h Ceftriaxone 100 mg/kg/day in one dose IV[b] max: adults 2 g q12 h Chloramphenicol 100 mg/kg/day in 4 divided doses max 1.5 g q6h
Penicillin resistant[c]	Cefotaxime or ceftriaxone and vancomycin 30–40 mg/kg/day IV	Cefepime 50 mg/kg/dose q12h[b] max: adult 2g q8h IV *or* Meropenem 40 mg/kg q8h IV[b] max: adults 1 g q8h IV with vancomycin
Group B streptococcus	Penicillin ± gentamicin	Ampicillin Cefotaxime Ceftriaxone Chloramphenicol
Staphylococcus aureus		
Penicillin resistant	Nafcillin 200 mg/kg/day in 6 divided doses IV max: 2 g q4h IV	Vancomycin
Methicillin resistant	Vancomycin	—
Staphylococcus epidermidis		
Penicillin resistant	Nafcillin	Vancomycin
Methicillin resistant	Vancomycin	
Listeria monocytogenes	Ampicillin 220–400 mg/kg/day in 4 divided doses IV or penicillin G max: 2 g q4h IV plus gentamicin	Trimethoprim 10 mg/kg/day and sulfamethoxazole 50 mg/kg/day in 4 divided doses Vancomycin + gentamicin

[a]Recommended doses for adults and pediatric patients with normal renal and/or hepatic function.
[b]Pediatrics.
[c]Incidence of resistance is 30% to 40%.

TABLE 105–5. Antimicrobial Agents of First Choice and Alternative Choice in Treatment of Meningitis Caused by Gram-negative Microorganisms

Organism	Antibiotic of First Choice[a]	Alternative Antibiotics[a]
Neisseria meningitidis (meningococcal)	Penicillin G 200,000–300,000 U/kg/day	Cefotaxime 200 mg/kg/day in 6 divided doses max: 2 g IV q4h Ceftriaxone 100 mg/kg/day in one dose[b] max: adults 2 g IV q12h Chloramphenicol 100 mg/kg/day in 4 divided doses max: 1.5 g IV q6h
Escherichia coli	Cefotaxime or ceftriaxone	Cefepime 50 mg/kg/dose q12h[b] max: adult 2 g q8h IV Meropenem 40 mg/kg q8h IV[b] max: adults 1 g q8h IV
Haemophilus influenzae		
β-Lactamase positive	Cefotaxime	Ceftriaxone
β-Lactamase negative	Ampicillin 200–400 mg/kg/day in 4 divided doses IV max: 2 g q4h IV	Cefotaxime Ceftriaxone
Pseudomonas aeruginosa	Ceftazidime 85 mg/kg/day max 2 g IV q6h plus tobramycin 5–7.5 mg/kg/day IV[c]	Meropenem Piperacillin 200–300 mg/kg/day max: 3 g q4h IV plus tobramicin
Enterobacteriaceae	Cefotaxime	Ceftriaxone Piperacillin plus aminoglycoside Meropenem

[a]Recommended doses for adults and pediatric patients with normal renal and/or hepatic function.
[b]Pediatrics.
[c]Direct central nervous system administration may be added; see Table 105–6 for dosage.

TABLE 105–6. Intraventricular and Intrathecal Antibiotic Dosage Recommendation

Antibiotic	Dose (mg)	Expected CSF Concentration* (mg/L)	Reference
Ampicillin	10–50	60–300	114–116
Methicillin	25–100	160–600	114–116
Nafcillin	75	500	115
Cephalothin	25–100	160–600	114–116
Chloramphenicol	25–100	160–600	114,116,117
Gentamicin	1–10	6–60	22,114–117
Tobramycin	1–10	6–60	22
Vancomycin	5	30	51,118,119
Amphotericin B	0.05–0.25 mg/d to 0.05–1 mg 1 to 3 times weekly	—	24

*Assumes adult CSF volume = 150 mL.
CSF, cerebrospinal fluid.

resolved, there is a unique immune reaction that distinguishes meningococcal meningitis from other bacterial causes. The patient develops a characteristic immunologic reaction of fever, arthritis (usually involving large joints), and pericarditis approximately 10 to 14 days after the onset of disease and despite successful treatment.[35] At this time, examination of the synovial fluid reveals a large number of polymorphonuclear cells, elevated protein concentrations, normal glucose concentrations, and sterile cultures. The reaction may last a week or longer, and no additional antibiotic therapy is required. Patients, however, may benefit from nonsteroidal anti-inflammatory agents and supportive care.[35]

Seizures and coma are uncommon with meningococcal meningitis. Patients may behave aggressively, however, and are often maniacal. Patients may develop deafness and transiently impaired ocular movements. Deafness unilaterally, or more commonly bilaterally, may develop early or late in the disease course.[35] Hearing loss secondary to sensory nerve damage (sensorineural hearing) is usually permanent, whereas conductive hearing impairment, such as damage to the tympanic membrane, is often reversible. Incidence of sensorineural hearing loss varies with the etiologic organism (*S. pneumoniae,* 31%; *N. meningitidis,* 10.5%; and *H. influenzae,* 6%).[36] Many of the neurologic deficits are transient and resolve within 1 year following meningitis.[37]

Presence of petechiae may be the primary clue that the underlying pathogen is *N. meningitidis.* Approximately 50% of patients with meningococcal meningitis have purpuric lesions, petechiae, or both. Patients may have an obvious or subclinical picture of DIC, which may progress to infarction of the adrenal glands and renal cortex and cause widespread thrombosis.

Aggressive, early intervention with high-dose IV crystalline penicillin G, 50,000 U/kg every 4 hours, is usually recommended for the treatment of *N. meningitidis* meningitis. Chloramphenicol is bactericidal for *N. meningitidis* and may be used in place of penicillin G. Several third-generation cephalosporins (cefotaxime, ceftazidime, ceftizoxime, ceftriaxone, and cefuroxime) have indications for the treatment of meningitis and are acceptable alternatives to penicillin G (Table 105–5).

Cases of meningitis caused by relatively and completely penicillin-resistant meningococci have been reported.[38] Prevalence varies geographically, ranging from 0.4% to 42.6%.[39] The clinical significance of this resistance is unknown because resistance has not been correlated with any treatment failures. Completely resistant strains produce β-lactamase, whereas relatively resistant strains altered penicillin-binding proteins. In 1991, strains with altered penicillin-binding proteins represented approximately 4% of meningococcal isolates.[32] These resistance patterns may necessitate a future change away from penicillin as the antibiotic treatment of choice for meningococcal meningitis.

Close contacts of patients contracting *N. meningitidis* meningitis are at an increased risk of developing meningitis. Secondary cases of meningitis usually develop within the first week following exposure, but they may take up to 60 days after contact with the index case.[40] Risk factors in these contacts have been estimated at 200 to 1,000 times that of the general population.[41,42] Young children are at the greatest risk of contracting *N. meningitidis;* however, persons of all ages are at risk, especially close contacts who are exposed via household, day care, or military contact.

Prophylaxis of close contacts should be started only after consultation with the local health department. In general, rifampin is given as prophylaxis for 2 days.[32] The adult dose is 600 mg every 12 hours, while infants and children aged 1 month and older should receive 10 mg/kg and infants younger than 1 month should receive 5 mg/kg. Further discussion of who should receive prophylaxis is beyond the scope of this text; interested readers can refer to the recommendations of the United States Centers for Disease Control and Prevention for that information.[43]

STREPTOCOCCUS PNEUMONIAE (PNEUMOCOCCUS OR DIPLOCOCCUS)

S. pneumoniae is the most common cause of meningitis in persons less than 19 years of age, and also is frequently implicated in those between 1 month and 18 years of age. Overall, the case fatality rate is approximately 20%.[7] Approximately 50% of cases are secondary infections resulting from primary infections of parameningeal foci such as the ear or paranasal sinuses. Pneumonia, endocarditis, CSF leak secondary to head trauma, splenectomy, alcoholism, sickle cell disease, and bone marrow transplantation may predispose the patient to the development of pneumococcal meningitis.

Neurologic complications, such as coma and seizures, are common with pneumococcal meningitis; however, bacteremia tends to be less common than with *N. meningitidis.*[35] Risk factors for recurrent pneumococcal meningitis include traumatic tears of the dura, fracture of the cribriform plate or paranasal sinuses, nasal meningoceles, repeated episodes of otitis media, basilar skull fractures and cerebrospinal fluid leaks.

Treatment with IV crystalline penicillin G (50,000 U/kg every 4 hours) in adult patients with a drug-susceptible isolate and normal renal function usually results in a favorable outcome. As approximately 35% of *S. pneumoniae* strains are either intermediately penicillin-resistant (MIC 0.1–1.0 mg/L) or highly penicillin-resistant (MIC > 1.0 mg/L),[44–47] meticulous testing of all CSF isolates for penicillin resistance is recommended. Ceftriaxone and cefotaxime have served as alternatives to penicillin in the treatment of penicillin intermediate- and highly resistant pneumococci. Treatment failures with third-generation cephalosporins in the management of penicillin-resistant pneumococci have been reported.[48,49] Therapeutic approaches to cephalosporin-resistant pneumococcus include vancomycin and rifampin, which have demonstrated synergistic activity with ceftriaxone. However, no data from controlled clinical trials supporting the use of rifampin are available. Therefore, the combination of vancomycin and ceftriaxone has been suggested as empiric treatment until the results of antimicrobial susceptibility testing are available.[50]

Ceftriaxone and vancomycin are the agents of choice to empirically treat presumed pneumococcal meningitis until the susceptibility is known. Penicillin may be used for drug-susceptible isolates with MICs ≤ 0.06 mg/L, but for intermediate isolates, ceftriaxone is used, and for highly drug-resistant isolates, a combination of ceftriaxone and vancomycin should be used. In especially severe cases, therapeutic drug monitoring of the CSF, and possibly even direct antibiotic instillation, may be necessary.

Outcomes in pneumococcal meningitis depend on the serotype of the microorganism (especially type 3), whether the infection is primary or secondary, and the number of WBCs in the CSF.[35] Cefotaxime, ceftriaxone, meropenem, and vancomycin are potentially useful for penicillin-sensitive (MIC ≤ 0.06 mg/L) and resistant strains of pneumococcus. Some concern is warranted with the use of imipenem for CNS infections because of the possibility of drug-induced seizures, especially if the dose is not adjusted for renal function. The newer fluoroquinolones represent another therapeutic option because of favorable activity against multidrug-resistant pneumococci and good penetration into the CSF. However, clinical data to date regarding fluoroquinolone treatment of pneumococcal meningitis is mainly limited to animal models. Comparative, controlled, clinical efficacy trials in patients with meningitis are necessary before routine use of the fluoroquinolones is viable. Quinupristin/dalfopristin and linezolid have emerged as therapeutic options for treating multidrug-resistant gram-positive infections. However, because no data is yet available, these agents cannot be recommended. Vancomycin in combination with ceftriaxone is probably the most effective option at the present time.[44,45,50]

As the guidelines in this chapter demonstrate, patients with proven or suspected *S. pneumoniae* meningitis, as well as those with penicillin allergies, require treatment with vancomycin. Although vancomycin appears to distribute well into most tissues of the body, distribution into the CSF is limited, especially when the meninges are not inflamed. Some authors suggest consideration of intraventricular administration for bacterial meningitis, but only if the patient does not respond clinically to intravenous administration. Congeni and coworkers suggested a daily 5-mg intraventricular dose in addition to continued intravenous administration in this situation.[51] Other investigators support this recommendation.[52]

Clinicians should appreciate that the pharmacokinetics of vancomycin are different inside and outside the CNS, and that the dose and frequency of administration may need to be altered. Considering that vancomycin kills in a concentration-independent manner, the critical factor is the relationship between the concentration of vancomycin present in the CNS and susceptibility of the infecting bacterial pathogen, not the concentration in the serum. Concentrations of vancomycin in the CNS need to be maintained above the minimal inhibitory concentration for 90% of the likely bacterial pathogens to assure a satisfactory clinical outcome. Although data from animal models indicate vancomycin penetration into the CNS is decreased when dexamethasone is given concomitantly, this may not represent an issue in the clinical setting.[53–55] Furthermore, higher doses of vancomycin may provide the driving force needed to achieve therapeutic CNS concentrations even when dexamethasone is given.[56] Because of the lack of clinical data in adults, concomitant use of steroids with vancomycin should probably be reserved for special cases.

Pneumococcal vaccines now available may help in reducing the risk of invasive pneumococcal disease. Virtually all serotypes of *S. pneumoniae* exhibiting intermediate or complete resistance to penicillin are found in the 23-serotype pneumococcal vaccine. All patients for whom the vaccine is indicated, persons 65 years old and older, and asplenic or immunocompromised patients, should be immunized.[45,47] Unfortunately, because of variability in the host's inability to mount an immune response to the vaccine, the efficacy of this product in children younger than 2 years of age and immunocompromised adults limits the usefulness of the vaccine as a solution to the problem of penicillin-resistant pneumococci. A new heptavalent pneumococcal conjugate vaccine (Prevnar) was recently approved for use in infants and children between 2 months and 9 years of age and appears to be highly effective in preventing invasive disease.[57] Widespread vaccination may have a significant impact on the prevalence of pneumococcal meningitis, including infection caused by antibiotic-resistant strains. A recent cohort study of 3.8 million healthy infants projected that vaccination would prevent more than 12,000 cases of invasive disease for each US birth cohort, resulting in substantial decreases in morbidity and mortality, as well possible dollar savings.[58] Current recommendations are for all healthy infants and children younger than 2 years of age to be immunized with the heptavalent vaccine at 2, 4, 6, and 12 to 15 months. The recommendations are extended to include Alaskan Native, Native American, and African American children between the ages of 2 years and 5 years.

Chemoprophylaxis with oral penicillin and vaccination for close contacts of an index case with *S. pneumoniae* meningitis are generally not recommended because the risk of acquiring pneumococcal disease is similar to the infection rate in the general population.[41,42] Vaccination and chemoprophylaxis, however, reduces the incidence of pneumococcal septicemia and meningitis in young patients with sickle cell disease.[41]

HAEMOPHILUS INFLUENZAE

In the past, *H. influenzae* was the most common cause of meningitis in infants and children 6 months to 3 years of age. Since the introduction of effective vaccines, however, the incidence of *H. influenzae* type b disease in the United States has declined dramatically.[8] Now, *H. influenzae* is implicated in only 7% of all meningitis cases with an incidence of 0.2 per 100,000 persons per year.[7] The case fatality rate is approximately 6%.[7] In children older than 3 years of age and in adults, meningitis caused by *H. influenzae* may indicate a parameningeal focus of infection such as middle-ear infection, paranasal sinus infection, or CSF leakage. Spread of the organism occurs either through draining of these areas via the veins or from bacteremia originating from the local focus of infection.[13,34]

In the past, ampicillin and chloramphenicol were the drugs of choice to treat pediatric meningitis. However, because approximately 30% to 40% of *H. influenzae* are now ampicillin resistant, many clinicians use a third-generation cephalosporin or chloramphenicol and ampicillin for initial antimicrobial therapy. If the organism is shown to be sensitive to ampicillin, the patient can then be switched from the third-generation cephalosporin to ampicillin and chloramphenicol, if used initially, can be discontinued. Most clinicians consider third-generation cephalosporins as the drugs of choice for meningitis caused by *H. influenzae*. Third-generation cephalosporins (cefotaxime and ceftriaxone) are very active against β-lactamase-producing and non-β-lactamase-producing strains of *H. influenzae,* are relatively free of toxicity, and do not require serum concentration monitoring. Serum concentration monitoring is required for chloramphenicol to avoid toxicity and subtherapeutic levels.

Secondary cases resulting from close contact with an index case occur within 30 days of the onset of disease. As with meningococcal meningitis, close contacts may be at 200 to 1,000 times the risk of the general population for acquiring *H. influenzae* meningitis.[41] Close contacts are usually defined as household members, individuals sharing sleeping quarters, day care attendees, nursing home residents, and crowded confined populations.[41] The risk of acquiring *H. influenzae* meningitis is low without intimate contact with the index patient's respiratory secretions.[41]

Prophylaxis is to protect close contacts from the index case by eliminating nasopharyngeal and oropharyngeal carriage of *H. influenzae*. Invasive disease should be reported to the local public health department and the United States Centers for Disease Control and Prevention. Prophylaxis of close contacts should be started only after consultation with the local health department. In general, children should receive rifampin 20 mg/kg (maximum 600 mg), and adults 600 mg daily in one dose for 4 days.[32] Individuals fully vaccinated should not receive prophylaxis.[32] Further discussion of who should receive prophylaxis is beyond the scope of this text; interested readers can refer to the recommendations of the American Academy of Pediatrics for that information.[59]

There are several HIB conjugate vaccines available in the United States (HbOC [HibTITER, TETRAMUNE], PRP-OMP [Pedvax-HIB], PRP-T [ActHIB, OmniHIB] and PRP-D [ProHIBIT—for use only in children 12 months of age or older]).[60] Vaccination includes a series of doses and is usually begun in infants at 2 months of age. In addition to pediatric immunization, the vaccine should also be considered in patients older than 5 years of age with these underlying conditions: sickle cell disease, asplenia, and immunocompromising diseases. Refer to Chap. 122 for further information on dosing and administration.

GRAM-NEGATIVE MENINGITIS

During the last 20 years, the incidence of gram-negative bacillary meningitis, excluding *H. influenzae,* has been increasing. Enteric gram-negative organisms are the fourth leading cause of meningitis, with only *S. pneumoniae, H. influenzae,* and *N. meningitidis* having a higher incidence.

Several factors predispose patients to the development of gram-negative meningitis: congenital defects involving the CNS; accidental cranial trauma; neurosurgery; the use of antimicrobial agents with exclusive gram-positive activity preoperatively in neurosurgery; any form of communication between the skin and subarachnoid space, such as a dermal sinus; diabetes; malignancy; urinary tract infection in neonates; cirrhosis; parameningeal infection; spinal anesthesia; and hospitalization in general.

Elderly debilitated patients are at an increased risk of gram-negative meningitis but typically lack the classic signs and symptoms of the disease. Nuchal rigidity may be difficult to detect secondary to cervical arthritis. Presence of a low-grade fever and changes in mental status, without other obvious cause, should prompt consideration of meningitis and a lumbar puncture. Neonates are also at risk for gram-negative meningitis with *E. coli* and *Klebsiella pneumoniae,* which are responsible for 60% to 70% of cases.

Optimal antimicrobial therapies for gram-negative bacillary meningitis have not been fully defined. The therapy of gram-negative meningitis is complex because of the variety of organisms that can infect the CNS. The treatment of meningitis caused by *P. aeruginosa* remains a special problem because antibiotics showing good antibacterial activity against *P. aeruginosa,* such as antipseudomonal penicillins and aminoglycosides, penetrate the CSF poorly. Initially, cases of *P. aeruginosa* meningitis should be treated with an extended spectrum β-lactam such as ceftazidime, piperacillin, cefepime or meropenem plus an aminoglycoside, usually tobramycin.[61,62] Because aminoglycosides penetrate the CSF poorly, their inclusion is predominantly to aid in the treatment of extracerebral infections. If multidrug-resistant pseudomonas is initially suspected, intraventricular administration of aminoglycoside should be considered along with IV administration. Preservative-free forms of gentamicin and tobramycin are available and should be used for direct administration into the CSF. Intraventricular aminoglycoside dosages should be adjusted to the estimated CSF volume (0.03 mg of tobramycin or gentamicin/mL of CSF and 0.1 mg of amikacin/mL of CSF every 24 hours). The CSF flows unidirectionally with gravity, and most data suggest intraventricular aminoglycoside administration is more likely to produce therapeutic concentrations throughout the CSF than intrathecal administration.[22,62] Ventricular levels of aminoglycoside should be monitored every 2 or 3 days, just prior to the next intraventricular dose, and should approximate 2–10 mg/L. Interpretation of drug levels may be difficult to assess because determinations are often contaminated with residual aminoglycoside from the previous dose.

Other gram-negative organisms causing meningitis, excluding *P. aeruginosa,* can most likely be treated with a third-generation cephalosporin, such as cefotaxime, ceftriaxone, or ceftazidime. Ceftazidime, however, may not be the best choice of empiric antibiotic for situations where the offending organism is not initially known because CSF antibiotic concentrations greater than 10 times the minimal bactericidal concentration (MBC) may not be reliably produced for gram-positive organisms. In adults, daily doses of 8–12 g/day of third-generation cephalosporins (2 g twice a day of ceftriaxone) should produce CSF concentrations of 5–20 mg/L.

Trimethoprim-sulfamethoxazole (TMP/SMX) is useful in the management of the Enterobacteriaceae family, and may also be useful in the management of *Acinetobacter spp.* and *L. monocytogenes*.[63] One advantage of TMP/SMX is that its penetration into the CSF is not dependent on meningeal inflammation. TMP/SMX is not, however, bactericidal. TMP/SMX produces CSF levels of 1.9–5.7 mg/L for the former and 20–63 mg/L for the latter when given parenterally in doses of 10 mg/kg/day (trimethoprim) and 50 mg/kg/day (sulfamethoxazole).

Fluoroquinolones are not approved for the treatment of gram-negative bacterial meningitis, and clinical experience is minimal. Fluoroquinolones should only be considered when multidrug-resistant gram-negative rods are suspected.[64]

Cerebrospinal fluid cultures may remain positive for 10 days or more with a regimen that will eventually be curative. Therapeutic efficacy can be monitored through bacterial colony counts every 2 or 3 days, which should progressively decrease over the period of therapy. Therapy for gram-negative meningitis should be continued for a minimum of 21 days from the start of treatment.[65]

LISTERIA MONOCYTOGENES

L. monocytogenes is a gram-positive diphtheroid-like organism responsible for 8% of all reported cases of meningitis.[7] This disease primarily affects neonates, alcoholics, immunocompromised patients, and the elderly. *L. monocytogenes* is implicated in 20% of meningitis cases in persons >60 years old, and carries a case fatality rate of approximately 15%.[7]

Transmission usually involves colonization of the patient's GI tract with the organisms, which then penetrate the gut lumen. Coleslaw, pasteurized milk, Mexican-style soft cheese, ready-to-eat foods, and raw beef and poultry have all been identified as sources of this food-borne pathogen.[32] If a sufficient cell-mediated immune response (T lymphocyte, macrophages) is not produced, bacteremia, meningitis, meningoencephalitis, or cerebritis may develop.[66] Infection of the CNS may be diffuse or localized, possibly involving the cerebral hemispheres, thalamus, and brainstem. In immunocompromised hosts, approximately 75% of *L. monocytogenes* infections result in transmission into the CNS.[66]

The incidence of *L. monocytogenes* meningitis tends to peak in the summer and early fall. As with gram-negative meningitis, presentation may be subtle and insidious and clinical suspicion should prompt lumbar puncture. *L. monocytogenes* produces primarily a mononuclear CSF response.[66] One common laboratory error seen with *L. monocytogenes* is a tendency to misidentify the organism on Gram stain as a diphtheroid, streptococcus, or a poorly staining gram-negative rod.

Treatment of *L. monocytogenes* meningitis with penicillin G or ampicillin may result in only a bacteriostatic effect and possible persistence of infection. Usually the combination of penicillin G or ampicillin with an aminoglycoside results in a bactericidal effect. Patients should be treated for 2 to 3 weeks after defervescence to prevent the possibility of relapse.[66] Combination therapy is usually employed for at least 10 days with the remaining course of therapy completed with penicillin G or ampicillin alone. Trimethoprim-sulfamethoxazole may be an effective alternative as adequate CSF penetration is achieved. Vancomycin may be also used, although *in vivo* failures have been reported.[65] Chloramphenicol, which is bactericidal against *H. influenzae, N. meningitidis,* and *S. pneumoniae,* is bacteriostatic against *L. monocytogenes.* None of the third-generation cephalosporins are effective for *L. monocytogenes.*

Dexamethasone as an Adjunctive Treatment for Meningitis

In addition to antibiotics, dexamethasone has become a commonly used therapy for the treatment of pediatric meningitis.[67] Corticosteroids inhibit the production of both TNF and IL-1. A series of clinical studies assessing the efficacy of corticosteroid therapy for the initial treatment of bacterial meningitis have reported conflicting results.[68–72] The majority of trials were conducted on small sample populations, each with different pathogenic bacterial causes and treatment modalities. Several meta-analyses have shown significant improvement in markers of active infection, such as CSF glucose concentrations, as well as CSF protein and lactate concentrations after corticosteroid administration as adjunctive treatment.[73]

Consistently, a significantly lower incidence of neurologic sequelae commonly associated with bacterial meningitis was detected with corticosteroid use. In trials that measured inflammatory mediators, lower levels of TNF, PAF, or IL-1 were detected in patients treated with dexamethasone.[68,69,72] No study, however, has detected a significant difference in time to bacterial eradication. Only one study detected a significant difference in mortality between patients treated with dexamethasone plus antibiotics and antibiotic therapy alone, favoring the use of the corticosteroid.[70] Based on these investigations, some authors advocate all infants (>2 months) and children with suspected bacterial meningitis receive dexamethasone.[3,68,69,71,72]

Routine use of dexamethasone in meningitis is not without controversy, and several authors have outlined shortcomings regarding the clinical evidence supporting the use of dexamethasone in pediatric bacterial meningitis.[3,74] A potential concern is that adjunctive dexamethasone therapy might reduce the penetration of antibiotics into the CSF by inhibiting meningeal inflammation. In experimental models of meningitis, steroids decreased the CSF concentrations of ampicillin, rifampin, vancomycin, and gentamicin[54,72] and ceftriaxone penetration into CSF was unaffected by concurrent dexamethasone administration in pediatric patients.[75]

A fundamental problem with corticosteroid investigations to date is that the majority of patients in the trials had *H. influenzae* meningitis. Although *H. influenzae* was the most commonly identified causative pathogen responsible for bacterial meningitis in the United States in 1986, the incidence of *H. influenzae* meningitis has decreased dramatically because of the introduction of polysaccharide conjugate vaccines.[3,8] Whether or not steroids are beneficial in meningitis caused by *S. pneumoniae, N. meningitidis,* and group B streptococci is unclear. A retrospective analysis of pediatric patients with pneumococcal meningitis and one unblinded, noncontrolled trial suggested that adjunctive steroids may decrease the neurologic sequelae and mortality associated with *S. pneumoniae* meningitis.[68,76] A recent meta-analysis suggests that, with the possible exception of hearing loss, dexamethasone does not protect against neurologic sequelae.[77] The protective effect of dexamethasone was observed to be strongest in those with meningitis caused by *H. influenzae.*

The American Academy of Pediatrics suggests dexamethasone be considered for infants and children 2 months of age or older with pneumococcal meningitis and that it be given to those with *H. influenzae* meningitis.[59,78] The commonly used intravenous dose is 0.15 mg/kg every 6 hours for 4 days. Alternatively, prospective, randomized, double-blind studies have found dexamethasone 0.15 mg/kg every 6 hours for 2 days or dexamethasone 0.4 mg/kg every 12 hours for 2 days to be equally effective and potentially less toxic.[72,79] Dexamethasone should be administered prior to the first antibiotic dose and serum hemoglobin and stool guaiac should be monitored for evidence of GI bleeding.[69,71,74,76,79]

MYCOBACTERIUM TUBERCULOSIS

Mycobacterium tuberculosis is the primary cause of tuberculous meningitis. Tuberculous meningitis is associated with significant morbidity and mortality and is difficult to diagnose in a timely manner.[80] The epidemiology of tuberculous meningitis as a cause of extrapulmonary tuberculosis has changed. Between the years 1990 and 1997, an average of 193 cases of tuberculosis meningitis were reported to the CDC, representing 4.7% of extrapulmonary cases.[81] The number of cases reported in 1990 was 284, or 6.2% of extrapulmonary cases.[81] This change is most likely secondary to HIV/AIDS and rising rates among minority adults leading to increased tuberculosis in their children.[81]

The most useful clue to tubercular meningitis is the presence of inflammation of the CSF in an individual who is at epidemiologic risk for tuberculosis. Although as many as 40% of patients may present with evidence of pulmonary involvement with hilar adenopathy, tuberculous meningitis may still exist in the absence of disease in the lung or extrapulmonary sites. The tuberculin skin test (purified protein derivative [PPD]) is also negative in 5% to 50% of cases.[80]

Upon initial examination, CSF usually contains from 100–1,000 WBC/mm^3, which may be 75% to 80% polymorphonuclear cells.[80,82] Over time, the pattern of WBC in the CSF will shift to lymphocytes and monocytes (Table 105–1). Cerebrospinal fluid glucose may initially be normal, but gradually decreases as the disease progresses.[80,82] Protein concentration within the CSF may be normal or elevated, with high protein levels shown to correlate with advanced disease.[80,82,83]

One potentially useful diagnostic sign unique to tuberculous meningitis is paralysis of the VI cranial nerve, which initially is unilateral and then progresses to bilateral.[35] Initial acid-fast bacilli (AFB) smears are approximately 37% sensitive and as much as 87% sensitive following subsequent smears. Sensitivity of the AFB smear is enhanced by the examination of multiple CSF specimens collected on consecutive days. Cultures of CSF are positive in 45% to 90% of cases depending on the quantity of CSF used in the culture, pathogen density, and experience of the laboratory in culturing *M. tuberculosis*. Some clinicians will obtain fluid from the base of the brain or the ventricles in an attempt to increase the yield. Positive culture results may take up to 8 weeks, providing little help with initial diagnosis.[80,82] The Bactec system, a newer broth-based media with radioactive isotope detectors, has considerably shortened the time to detection and is capable of detecting organisms in an average of 9 days, and of determining identification in 5 days.[84] Other methods to shorten the time to detection and increase sensitivity are being developed and include genetic probes and immunoassays (radioimmunoassay ([RIA], enzyme-linked immunosorbent assay [ELISA]).[84]

Unfortunately, the incidence of multidrug-resistant strains of *M. tuberculosis* has increased, necessitating the use of at least four or five antitubercular agents to treat active pulmonary disease.[85,86] As of 1993, the CDC recommends a regimen of four drugs for empiric treatment of *M. tuberculosis,* unless resistance to isoniazid in the area is less than 4%.[86] This regimen consists of isoniazid, rifampin, pyrazinamide, and ethambutol 15–25 mg/kg/day (maximum 2.5 g/day) or streptomycin 15–30 mg/kg/day (maximum 1 g/day) for the first 2 months, generally followed by isoniazid plus rifampin for the duration of therapy. Of relevance in meningitis is that streptomycin does not readily penetrate into the CNS. The recommended therapy for HIV-positive individuals is the same as for immunocompetent patients, although rifabutin may be considered in place of other rifamycins in an effort to minimize drug interactions with protease inhibitors and nonnucleoside reverse transcriptase inhibitors. Therapy in HIV-negative and -positive patients should be individualized based on susceptibility patterns and guidelines from the Centers for Disease Control and Prevention and The American Thoracic Society which are frequently updated and available on the Internet [http://www.cdc.gov/nchstp/tb/pubs/mmwrhtml/maj_guide.htm]. Patients with *M. tuberculosis* meningitis should be treated for 9 months or longer with multiple-drug therapy and patients with rifampin-resistant strains should receive 18 to 24 months of therapy.

Isoniazid, the mainstay in virtually any regimen to treat *M. tuberculosis,* penetrates the CSF with or without meningeal inflammation and achieves concentrations of more than 30 times the MIC of *M. tuberculosis* (MICs of 0.05–0.2 mg/L).[66,80,82] Rifampin's penetration of CSF approximates only 20% of serum concentrations in the presence of meningeal inflammation. *M. tuberculosis* is so exquisitely sensitive to rifampin, however, that its low penetration ratio is of little clinical significance.[80,82,87] The incidence of *M. tuberculosis* resistance to rifampin has also increased, necessitating empiric multiple antibiotic regimens.

Pyrazinamide is a small molecule that penetrates the CSF well in the presence or absence of meningeal inflammation. Streptomycin, an aminoglycoside, penetrates CSF poorly, even in the presence of meningeal inflammation. Ethambutol is a weak antitubercular agent and reaches the CSF in moderate concentrations. Ethambutol's use is also limited by a high incidence of dose-related optic neuritis. Ethionamide and cycloserine are two other agents that are sometimes used to treat tuberculous meningitis. These agents both penetrate the CSF well in the absence of meningeal inflammation.[80,82]

The usual dose of isoniazid in children is 10–20 mg/kg/day (maximum 300 mg/day), and adults usually receive 5–10 mg/kg/day or a daily dose of 300 mg. Supplemental doses of pyridoxine hydrochloride (vitamin B_6) 50 mg/day are recommended to prevent the peripheral neuropathy associated with isoniazid administration.[80,82] Concurrent administration of rifampin is recommended at doses of 10–20 mg/kg/day (maximum 600 mg/day) for children and 600 mg/day for adults.[80,82] The addition of pyrazinamide (children and adults 15–30 mg/kg/day; maximum in both 2 g/day) to the regimen of isoniazid and rifampin is recommended.[80,86] Duration of concomitant pyrazinamide therapy generally should be limited to 2 months in order to avoid hepatotoxicity.

The role of steroids in the management of tuberculous meningitis remains controversial. In some cases, administration of oral prednisone 40–60 mg/day or 0.2 mg/kg/day of IV dexamethasone has resulted in a dramatic clearing of sensorium, remission of CSF abnormalities, reduction in fever, and elimination of headaches.[80,82] Concerns regarding the use of steroids include a possible interference with CSF chemistry studies and decreased penetration of antitubercular agents because of a decrease in inflammation. In addition, a small study of 23 patients, in 1969, found that while dexamethasone improved CSF leukocytosis as well as CSF protein and glucose concentrations, only a reduction in cerebral edema/intracranial hypertension correlated with improved mortality.[88] Despite the controversy, the trend toward an improved outcome generally supports their use for tuberculous meningitis.[89]

Tuberculous meningitis has a mortality rate of 10% to 50%, despite early diagnosis and treatment.[80,82,89] The level of patient consciousness at the start of therapy is the most useful prognostic indicator. Patients who are comatose at the beginning of therapy have a mortality rate of approximately 75%.[82] Other negative prognostic factors include old age, poor nutrition, evidence of miliary disease, high initial CSF protein concentrations, presence of hydrocephalus, and evidence of elevated intracranial pressure.[82] Ten percent to 30% of patients surviving the disease have physical or mental sequelae, including deafness, vertigo, and short-term memory loss.[80,82]

CRYPTOCOCCUS NEOFORMANS

Cryptococcal meningitis is the most common form of fungal CNS infection in the United States and is a major cause of morbidity and mortality in immunosuppressed patients. Patients with HIV have a 5% to 10% risk of developing cryptococcus during their lifetime.[90] *Cryptococcus neoformans* is a soil fungus acquired by inhalation of spores from the environment leading to a pneumonia which may not be clinically manifest. Secondary fungemia leads to dissemination, especially in immunocompromised hosts, and infection of the central nervous system and other sites such as the skin, prostate, bone, kidneys, eyes, liver, spleen, adrenal glands, and lymph nodes.[91] The incubation period in AIDS patients may be very short, as opposed to a relatively normal host in whom it may be very long.

Symptoms of cryptococcus meningitis are insidious and may be present for varying periods depending on the host involved before the definitive diagnosis is made. Fever and a history of headaches are the most common symptoms, although altered mentation and evidence of focal neurologic deficits may be present. Examination of the CSF usually reveals small numbers of WBCs (<150/mm^3), which are primarily lymphocytes (Table 105–1). Diagnosis is based on the presence of a positive CSF, blood, sputum, or urine culture for *C. neoformans*. The CSF cultures are positive in more than 90% of cases. Organisms may be seen microscopically when stained with India ink and are more likely to be seen in AIDS patients than in other hosts. An additional rapid test helpful in diagnosis is latex agglutination, which detects the presence of cryptococcal antigens.[91] Latex agglutination is positive in more than 90% of culture-positive cases. A cryptococcal antigen test can be used to follow the prognosis of non-AIDS patients, but cryptococcal antigen titers do not correlate well with treatment efficacy in AIDS patients.[92] A cryptococcal antigen detection test needs to be considered in any patient initially presenting with meningitis. Risk factors predictive of a poor outcome include lethargy at presentation, high CSF cryptococcal antigen titer, and low CSF WBC count.[93]

Despite poor penetration into the CSF, amphotericin B has long been the drug of choice for the treatment of acute *C. neoformans* meningitis. Amphotericin B 0.5–1 mg/kg/day combined with flucytosine 100 mg/kg/day is more effective than amphotericin alone, with successful outcomes in 75% of non-AIDS patients and in 50% of AIDS patients.[94] Unfortunately, in the AIDS population, flucytosine is often poorly tolerated, causing bone marrow suppression and GI distress. Amphotericin B alone, although less effective, has been used in AIDS patients with preexisting granulocytopenia.[94,95] Intraventricular amphotericin B with intravenous amphotericin B plus flucytosine has been suggested as initial therapy. Intraventricular amphotericin B, however, is generally reserved for those patients who fail to respond to systemic therapy.[91] Because of the high acute mortality rate of up to 40% and a relapse rate of 50% in AIDS patients receiving therapy, many new agents and regimens are being investigated in this population.[93] A small, noncomparative open study evaluating the safety and efficacy of liposomal amphotericin B (AmBisome) found the product to be well tolerated and moderately effective.[96] A second study found high-dose liposomal amphotericin B (4 mg/kg) to more rapidly clear CSF cultures as compared to standard amphotericin B, although clinical efficacy was not significantly different.[97]

Azole therapy is the most studied alternative regimen for the treatment of *C. neoformans* meningitis in AIDS patients. Fluconazole at doses of 200 mg/day was compared to amphotericin B alone (0.4 mg/kg/day) with no significant difference in overall mortality between groups.[98] Patients receiving fluconazole had a higher 2-week mortality rate and time to CSF conversion.[98] High-dose fluconazole therapy (800 mg/day) was tried as salvage therapy in eight AIDS patients who failed previous antifungal therapy, but success was limited.[99] Itraconazole 200 mg orally twice daily was less effective than amphotericin B plus flucytosine in a small nonblinded study.[100]

Patients with AIDS often require lifelong maintenance or suppressive therapy because of high relapse rates following acute therapy for *C. neoformans*. A large, multicenter, controlled trial compared fluconazole (200 mg/day) and amphotericin B (1 mg/kg/wk) in the prevention of relapse.[101] Two percent of patients receiving fluconazole versus 18% of patients on amphotericin B relapsed. In addition, the amphotericin B group had significantly more frequent bacterial infections, bacteremias, and drug-related toxicity.[101] One study suggested itraconazole (200 mg twice daily) might be a suitable alternative in those patients who are unable to receive fluconazole (400 mg daily) for consolidation therapy (8 weeks of therapy that follows an initial 2 weeks of therapy, which includes amphotericin B plus flucytosine).[102] Therefore, patients with AIDS-associated cryptococcal meningitis should receive primary therapy, generally using amphotericin B with or without flucytosine or fluconazole alone, followed by maintenance therapy with fluconazole or itraconazole, for the life of the patient.[90] However, treatment recommendations are controversial and treatment needs to be individualized.

VIRAL ENCEPHALITIS

The epidemiology of viral encephalitis in the United States has changed dramatically since the mid-1960s because of the introduction of large-scale polio and mumps immunization programs. In the United States, the incidence of mumps has decreased 98% between 1967 and 1985. Worldwide, mumps remains a causative agent of viral encephalitis in countries with low vaccination rates. Poliomyelitis, once a significant cause of encephalitis, is now confined to only a few less-developed countries and will likely soon be eradicated as an infectious agent.

Nonpolio enteroviruses such as coxsackieviruses A and B, echoviruses, and enteroviruses 70 and 71 cause approximately 85% of all viral encephalitis cases.[18,103] The remaining 15% of viral encephalitis cases are caused by a variety of pathogens, such as arboviruses, adenoviruses, influenzae virus A and B, rotavirus, coronavirus, cytomegalovirus, varicella-zoster, herpes simplex, Epstein-Barr virus, and lymphocytic choriomeningitis.[18,104,105] The St. Louis and LaCrosse viruses are the most common cause of arbovirus encephalitis and are associated with infections in the late summer and fall.[103]

Viral encephalitis is acquired primarily by hematogenous spread or alternatively by neuronal spread of the causative pathogen.[106] After entry into the host, viral replication occurs, resulting in dissemination through the reticuloendothelial system or vasculature. Infection of the capillary endothelial cells and choroid plexus may provide a conduit for CNS infections.[106] Viruses, such as polio, herpes, and varicella-zoster, may also gain access to the CNS by axonal retrograde transmission from peripheral nerve endings.[106] After a particular virus gains access to the CNS, the course of infection is dependent on the virulence of the particular virus and host immune response. Host response to aseptic CNS infections is mediated by a complex cascade of inflammatory cytokines in a manner similar to purulent meningitis. In contrast to purulent meningitis, host response to viral encephalitis is primarily mediated through cytotoxic T-lymphocytes. Although TNF is a prominent mediator in purulent bacterial meningitis, TNF concentrations are not increased in viral encephalitis, whereas increases in concentrations of IL-1 and interferon (INF) α and γ occur.[107] Tumor necrosis factor concentrations have been suggested as a diagnostic tool for differentiating between bacterial meningitis and viral encephalitis.[107] While cytokine assays are available for investigational use, they are not routinely used in the clinical diagnosis of viral encephalitis.

The clinical syndrome associated with viral encephalitis is generally independent of viral etiology and may vary depending on the patient's age. Common signs in adults include headache, mild fever (<40°C/104°F), nuchal rigidity, malaise, drowsiness, nausea, vomiting, and photophobia. Only fever and irritability may be evident in the infant, and meningitis must be ruled out as a cause of fever when no other localized findings are observed in a child. Duration of symptoms generally last 1 to 2 weeks, and specific manifestations outside of the meninges can also occur depending on viral etiology.

Laboratory examination of the CSF usually reveals a pleocytosis with 10–1,000 WBCs/mm^3, which are primarily lymphocytic; however, 20% to 75% of patients with viral encephalitis may have a predominance of polymorphonuclear cells on initial examination of the CSF, especially in enteroviral meningitis.[18] Upon repeat lumbar puncture, 90% of patients initially presenting with a predominance of neutrophils experience a shift to a predominance of mononuclear cells. Other laboratory findings include normal to mildly elevated protein concentrations and normal or mildly reduced glucose concentrations[18] (Table 105–1).

Historically, pathogens responsible for viral encephalitis were not identified.[108] Poor laboratory recovery of viral pathogens and limited treatment options for viral encephalitis made the need for specific identification of pathogens of questionable value. Advances in diagnostic laboratory techniques and the potential for decreased costs associated with longer duration of hospitalization for patients with unconfirmed viral encephalitis have led to a reevaluation of the need for confirmatory pathogen diagnosis.[105] When clinical signs warrant pathogen identification, appropriate laboratory diagnostic techniques, including PCR, should be undertaken.

Although there are numerous pathogenic causes of viral encephalitis, much of the clinical presentation, diagnosis, and treatment is similar. The most commonly isolated viral etiologies are described next.

Nonpolio enteroviruses are unenveloped single-strand RNA viruses. Commonly, the incidence of enteroviral encephalitis peaks in late summer and continues into early fall. Enteroviruses are transmitted in the host via the fecal-oral route. Clinical presentation of enteroviral infection is frequently nonspecific and characterized by fever, nausea, vomiting, and malaise; however, GI symptoms may not be present. Following a prodrome of 1 to 2 days, headache, photophobia, and neck stiffness develop. Diagnosis can be confirmed by cell culture from the CSF where the incidence of successful isolation has ranged from 40% to 80%.[107] In addition, enterovirus can be isolated from throat swabs (60%) and stool cultures (80%), but they are not necessarily diagnostic because the virus is shed in the stool for 1 to 2 weeks following infection.[108] Conversely, an enterovirus-specific reverse transcriptase polymerase chain reaction (EV-PCR) test can provide prompt results within 24 hours with a sensitivity and a specificity of 100%.[109] Treatment for enteroviral encephalitis consists of supportive care, fluids, antipyretics, and analgesics. Generally, disease progression is self-limiting, and the patient recovers fully without long-term neurologic complications.

Both herpes simplex virus types 1 and 2 have been associated with infections of the CNS.[110] Herpes simplex type 1 (HSV-1) is associated with encephalitis in adults, whereas herpes simplex type 2 (HSV-2) is associated predominantly with encephalitis in newborns.[103] An HSV infection of the central nervous system is most likely spread via retrograde movement from the dorsal root ganglion. Sexually active adults acquire herpes simplex meningitis during or after an attack of genital or rectal herpes. Although HSV-2 can frequently be cultured from CSF, HSV-1 cannot. As such, PCR may be more useful than culture in detecting infection with HSV; diagnosis is usually made by PCR, culture or by a fourfold rise in complement-fixing antibody to the virus. Establishing the correct diagnosis as early as possible is paramount because mortality rates are between 50% and 85% without treatment, and unlike other viral encephalitides, specific and effective therapy is available. As a result, empiric therapy of suspected HSV encephalitis while laboratory results are pending is necessary. Additionally, a clinical decision to treat may need to be made regardless of test results. Although herpes simplex may be strongly suspected on the basis of local findings after clinical evaluation, only half of these patients will have a diagnosis confirmed by brain biopsy.[110]

Acyclovir is the drug of choice for herpes simplex encephalitis. In patients with normal renal function, acyclovir is usually administered as 10 mg/kg IV every 8 hours for 2 to 3 weeks.[103] Herpes virus resistance to acyclovir has been reported with increasing incidence, particularly from immunocompromised patients with prior or chronic exposures to acyclovir.[111] The alternative treatment for acyclovir-resistant herpes simplex virus is foscarnet.[103] The major toxicity of foscarnet is renal impairment, and doses must be individualized for renal function.[112] The dose for patients with normal renal function is 40 mg/kg infused over 1 hour every 8 to 12 hours for 2 to 3 weeks. Ensuring adequate hydration is imperative. In addition, patients receiving foscarnet should be monitored for seizures related to alterations in plasma electrolyte levels.

Although arboviruses cause up to 10% of viral encephalitis cases, these viruses are most commonly associated with encephalitis.[106] The four most common pathogens are the St. Louis virus, the California virus, and the eastern and western equine viruses. Transmission of these viruses occurs through the bites of mosquitoes. Typically, an incubation period of 2 to 14 days precedes the onset of clinical symptoms. Infection of the brain tissue results in fever, headache, paralysis, and coma. While many patients have a benign presentation, symptomatic cases are associated with a higher degree of mortality. Mortality rates of 50% to 75% have been reported for eastern equine virus, whereas mortality rates for western equine and St. Louis viruses are 3% to 4% and 10% to 20%, respectively.[103,106] Treatment is supportive, including treatment for seizures and increased intracranial pressure, and in the majority of cases, the disease is self-limiting.[106]

HIV encephalitis is the most common CNS complication associated with AIDS. Frequently, patients may complain of headache, photophobia, or stiff neck at the time of presumed seroconversion. As the disease progresses, however, neurologic symptoms are frequently reported secondary to other opportunistic infections. Diagnosis of viral encephalitis is difficult because mental status and neurologic exams are not sensitive enough to detect early changes. Direct evidence of HIV encephalitis can be obtained through CSF culture, p24 antigen testing, or qualitative or quantitative PCR for HIV-RNA. Diagnostic workup of other potential copathogens, such as HSV, *Toxoplasma gondii, M. tuberculosis, Aspergillus spp.*, and cryptococcus should also be performed. Refer to Chap. 123 for a complete discussion of infectious complications in HIV-positive individuals.

EVALUATION OF THERAPEUTIC OUTCOMES

SIGNS AND SYMPTOMS

Because of the potential for rapid deterioration associated with meningitis, signs and symptoms of fever, headache, meningismus (nuchal rigidity, Brudzinski's sign, or Kernig's sign), vital signs, and signs of cerebral dysfunction should be evaluated every 4 hours for the initial 3 days and then daily thereafter. The Glasgow Coma Scale should be used in severely ill patients. Trends in improvement and resolution rather than single evaluations in time are more important in monitoring the signs and symptoms of meningitis.

MICROBIOLOGIC FINDINGS

Cerebrospinal fluid and blood samples (two sets) for Gram stain, cultures, and sensitivity testing should be taken prior to starting antibiotic therapy. If lumbar puncture is delayed, however, antibiotics should be started. Studies show that even 24 hours after initiating antibiotics, up to 38% of CSF cultures were positive.[113] Gram stain results can be obtained immediately and can guide empiric antibiotic treatment. Identification of the organism can be made within 24 to 36 hours, and sensitivities should be available within 48 to 60 hours. Repeat cultures should be performed to help determine if sterilization is achieved. A second tube of blood should be taken to allow for latex agglutination tests of antigens to common meningeal pathogens (*H. influenzae, S. pneumoniae, N. meningitidis, E. coli,* and group B streptococcus) if the Gram stain has not been helpful.

CEREBROSPINAL FLUID EXAMINATION

In bacterial meningitis, the CSF WBC count is usually greater than 1,000/mm^3, the CSF protein is elevated, and the CSF glucose (hypoglycorrhachia) is often low (<50 μg/dL or 50% to 60% of a simultaneous blood glucose value). Viral encephalitis, in contrast, results in relatively normal CSF protein and glucose levels and typically does not result in greater than 90% PMNs in the CSF (Table 105–1).

▶ PRINCIPLES OF PHARMACOTHERAPY

In cases of meningitis, initial findings can include:

- *Presenting signs and symptoms:* fever, headache, nuchal rigidity, Brudzinski's or Kernig's sign, and altered mental status.
- *Abnormal CSF chemistries:* elevated WBC (>100/mm^3), elevated protein (>50 mg/dL), and decreased glucose levels (<40 mg/dL).
- The three most likely pathogens of bacterial meningitis are *S. pneumoniae, N. meningitidis,* and *H. influenzae.*

Three main microbiologic tests that should be obtained include:

- *Gram stain of the CSF:* identifies the organism in 50% to 90% of cases.
- *CSF cultures:* are positive in 80% of patients.
- *Blood cultures.*

Three primary goals of treatment in meningitis include:

- *Amelioration* of signs and symptoms.
- *Eradication* of infection.
- *Prevention* of the development of neurologic sequelae, such as seizures, deafness, coma, and death.

- Empiric coverage with an appropriate antibiotic should be started as soon as possible when clinical suspicion of meningitis exists. If there is a delay in doing a lumbar puncture (even a delay of 30 to 60 minutes), the first dose of an antibiotic *should not* be withheld. Changes in the CSF after initiation of antibiotics usually take 12 to 24 hours.
- When selecting antibiotics, the clinician must consider the antibiotic's ability to concentrate at the site of infection, as well as the spectrum of antibacterial activity. Empiric choices should be based on age and predisposing conditions.
- *Ceftriaxone* or *cefotaxime* and *vancomycin* are reasonable initial choices for empiric coverage of community-acquired meningitis in adult patients.
- *Listeria monocytogenes* is a common pathogen in infants and in the elderly. Therefore, *ampicillin* should be empirically added to antimicrobial coverage.
- In contrast to the treatment of other infectious diseases, antibiotic dosages in the treatment of meningitis should be maximized to optimize CNS penetration.
- The duration of antibiotic treatment for meningitis has not been standardized; however, the duration of antibiotic therapy is generally based on the causative organism and the individual case, and may range from 7 to 21 days.
- Steroid treatment includes dexamethasone 0.15 mg/kg/dose to be given four times daily for 4 days in infants and children older than 2 months of age with proven or strongly suspected bacterial meningitis, and in adults with a high concentration of bacteria in CSF and evidence of increased intracranial pressure. Steroids should be given prior to antibiotics.
- Close contacts and relatives of the index case should be assessed for appropriate prophylaxis, particularly with *N. meningitidis* and *H. influenzae* meningitis.

REFERENCES

1. Segreti J, Harris AA. Acute bacterial meningitis. Infect Dis Clin North Am 1996;10(4):797–809.
2. Tunkel AR, Wispelwey B, Scheld WM. Pathogenesis and pathophysiology of meningitis. Infect Dis Clin North Am 1990;4(4):555–581.
3. Quagliarello VJ, Scheld WM. New perspectives on bacterial meningitis. Clin Infect Dis 1993;17(4):603–608; quiz 609–610.
4. Gray LD, Fedorko DP. Laboratory diagnosis of bacterial meningitis. Clin Microbiol Rev 1992;5(2):130–145.
5. Durand ML, Calderwood SB, Weber DJ, et al. Acute bacterial meningitis in adults. A review of 493 episodes [see comments]. N Engl J Med 1993;328(1):21–28.
6. Wenger JD, Hightower AW, Facklam RR, Gaventa S, Broome CV. Bacterial meningitis in the United States, 1986: Report of a multistate surveillance study. The Bacterial Meningitis Study Group. J Infect Dis 1990;162(6):1316–1323.
7. Schuchat A, Robinson K, Wenger JD, et al. Bacterial meningitis in the United States in 1995. Active Surveillance Team. N Engl J Med 1997;337(14):970–976.
8. Adams WG, Deaver KA, Cochi SL, et al. Decline of childhood Haemophilus influenzae type b (HIB) disease in the HIB vaccine era [see comments]. JAMA 1993;269(2):221–226.
9. Greenlee J. Anatomic considerations in central nervous system infections. In: Mandell G, Douglas R, Bennett J, eds. Principles and Practice of Infectious Diseases. New York, Churchill Livingstone, 1990:732–741.
10. Greenlee JE. Approach to diagnosis of meningitis. Cerebrospinal fluid evaluation. Infect Dis Clin North Am 1990;4(4):583–598.

11. Spector R, Lorenzo AV. Inhibition of penicillin transport from the cerebrospinal fluid after intracisternal inoculation of bacteria. J Clin Invest 1974;54(2):316–325.
12. Dacey RG, Sande MA. Effect of probenecid on cerebrospinal fluid concentrations of penicillin and cephalosporin derivatives. Antimicrob Agents Chemother 1974;6(4):437–441.
13. Saez-Llorens X, Ramilo O, Mustafa MM, Mertsola J, McCracken GH Jr. Molecular pathophysiology of bacterial meningitis: Current concepts and therapeutic implications. J Pediatr 1990;116(5):671–684.
14. Verghese A, Gallemore G. Kernig's and Brudzinski's signs revisited. Rev Infect Dis 1987;9(6):1187–1192.
15. Lipton JD, Schafermeyer RW. Evolving concepts in pediatric bacterial meningitis—Part I: Pathophysiology and diagnosis [see comments]. Ann Emerg Med 1993;22(10):1602–1615.
16. Rothrock SG, Green SM, Wren J, Letai D, Daniel-Underwood L, Pillar E. Pediatric bacterial meningitis: Is prior antibiotic therapy associated with an altered clinical presentation? Ann Emerg Med 1992;21(2):146–152.
17. Robinson RO, Roberts H. Acute bacterial meningitis. I: Diagnosis. Dev Med Child Neurol 1990;32(1):83–86.
18. Maxson S, Jacobs RF. Viral meningitis. Tips to rapidly diagnose treatable causes. Postgrad Med 1993;93(8):153–156, 159–160, 163–166.
19. Kaplan SL. Clinical presentations, diagnosis, and prognostic factors of bacterial meningitis. Infect Dis Clin North Am 1999;13(3):vi–vii, 579–594.
20. Backman A, Lantz P, Radstrom P, Olcen P. Evaluation of an extended diagnostic PCR assay for detection and verification of the common causes of bacterial meningitis in CSF and other biological samples. Mol Cell Probes 1999;13(1):49–60.
21. Klein O, Neu HC. Use of antimicrobial agents to treat central nervous system infection. Neurosurg Clin N Am 1992;3(2):323–342.
22. Kaiser AB, McGee ZA. Aminoglycoside therapy of gram-negative bacillary meningitis. N Engl J Med 1975;293(24):1215–1220.
23. Ratcheson RA, Ommaya AK. Experience with the subcutaneous cerebrospinal-fluid reservoir. Preliminary report of 60 cases. N Engl J Med 1968;279(19):1025–1031.
24. Wen DY, Bottini AG, Hall WA, Haines SJ. Infections in neurologic surgery. The intraventricular use of antibiotics. Neurosurg Clin N Am 1992;3(2):343–354.
25. Wright PF, Kaiser AB, Bowman CM, McKee KT Jr, Trujillo H, McGee ZA. The pharmacokinetics and efficacy of an aminoglycoside administered into the cerebral ventricles in neonates: Implications for further evaluation of this route of therapy in meningitis. J Infect Dis 1981;143(2):141–147.
26. Thea D, Barza M. Use of antibacterial agents in infections of the central nervous system. Infect Dis Clin North Am 1989;3(3):553–570.
27. Prins JM, van Deventer SJ, Kuijper EJ, Speelman P. Clinical relevance of antibiotic-induced endotoxin release. Antimicrob Agents Chemother 1994;38(6):1211–1218.
28. Rockowitz J, Tunkel AR. Bacterial meningitis. Practical guidelines for management. Drugs 1995;50(5):838–853.
29. Quagliarello VJ, Scheld WM. Treatment of bacterial meningitis [see comments]. N Engl J Med 1997;336(10):708–716.
30. Gold R. Epidemiology of bacterial meningitis. Infect Dis Clin North Am 1999;13(3):v, 515–525.
31. Anonymous. Meningococcal disease prevention and control strategies for practice-based physicians. Committee on Infectious Diseases, American Academy of Pediatrics. Infectious Diseases and Immunization Committee, Canadian Paediatric Society. Pediatrics 1996;97(3):404–412.
32. Spach DH, Jackson LA. Bacterial meningitis. Neurol Clin 1999;17(4):711–735.
33. Racoosin JA, Whitney CG, Conover CS, Diaz PS. Serogroup Y meningococcal disease in Chicago, 1991–1997. JAMA 1998;280(24):2094–2098.
34. Tunkel AR, Scheld WM. Pathogenesis and pathophysiology of bacterial meningitis. Clin Microbiol Rev 1993;6(2):118–136.
35. Weinstein L. Bacterial meningitis. Specific etiologic diagnosis on the basis of distinctive epidemiologic, pathogenetic, and clinical features. Med Clin North Am 1985;69(2):219–229.
36. Dodge PR, Davis H, Feigin RD, et al. Prospective evaluation of hearing impairment as a sequela of acute bacterial meningitis. N Engl J Med 1984;311(14):869–874.
37. Pomeroy SL, Holmes SJ, Dodge PR, Feigin RD. Seizures and other neurologic sequelae of bacterial meningitis in children. N Engl J Med 1990;323(24):1651–1657.
38. Van Esso D, Fontanals D, Uriz S, et al. *Neisseria meningitidis* strains with decreased susceptibility to penicillin. Pediatr Infect Dis J 1987;6(5):438–439.
39. Klugman KP, Madhi SA. Emergence of drug resistance. Impact on bacterial meningitis. Infect Dis Clin North Am 1999;13(3):vii, 637–646.
40. Schwartz B. Chemoprophylaxis for bacterial infections: Principles of and application to meningococcal infections. Rev Infect Dis 1991;13(suppl 2):S170–S173.
41. Lieberman JM, Greenberg DP, Ward JI. Prevention of bacterial meningitis. Vaccines and chemoprophylaxis. Infect Dis Clin North Am 1990;4(4):703–729.
42. Cuevas LE, Hart CA. Chemoprophylaxis of bacterial meningitis. J Antimicrob Chemother 1993;31(suppl B):79–91.
43. Anonymous. Prevention and control of meningococcal disease. Recommendations of the Advisory Committee on Immunization Practices (ACIP). MMWR Morb Mortal Wkly Rep 2000;49(RR-7):1–10.
44. Appelbaum PC. Antimicrobial resistance in Streptococcus pneumoniae: An overview. Clin Infect Dis 1992;15(1):77–83.
45. Caputo GM, Appelbaum PC, Liu HH. Infections due to penicillin-resistant pneumococci. Clinical, epidemiologic, and microbiologic features [see comments]. Arch Intern Med 1993;153(11):1301–1310.
46. Anonymous. Prevalence of penicillin-resistant *Streptococcus pneumoniae*—Connecticut, United States, 1992–1993. Can Commun Dis Rep 1994;20(9):71–73.
47. Jacobs MR. Treatment and diagnosis of infections caused by drug-resistant *Streptococcus pneumoniae*. Clin Infect Dis 1992;15(1):119–127.
48. John CC. Treatment failure with use of a third-generation cephalosporin for penicillin-resistant pneumococcal meningitis: Case report and review. Clin Infect Dis 1994;18(2):188–193.
49. Catalan MJ, Fernandez JM, Vazquez A, Varela de Seijas E, Suarez A, Bernaldo de Quiros JC. Failure of cefotaxime in the treatment of meningitis due to relatively resistant *Streptococcus pneumoniae*. Clin Infect Dis 1994;18(5):766–769.
50. Friedland IR, Paris M, Ehrett S, Hickey S, Olsen K, McCracken GH Jr. Evaluation of antimicrobial regimens for treatment of experimental penicillin- and cephalosporin-resistant pneumococcal meningitis. Antimicrob Agents Chemother 1993;37(8):1630–1636.
51. Congeni B, Tan J, Salstrom S. Kinetics of vancomycin after intraventricular and intravenous administration. Pediatr Res 1979;13:459–463.
52. Luer MS, Hatton J. Vancomycin administration into the cerebrospinal fluid: a review. Ann Pharmacother 1993;27(7–8):912–921.
53. Cabellos C, Martinez-Lacasa J, Martos A, et al. Influence of dexamethasone on efficacy of ceftriaxone and vancomycin therapy in experimental pneumococcal meningitis. Antimicrob Agents Chemother 1995;39(9):2158–2160.
54. Paris MM, Hickey SM, Uscher MI, Shelton S, Olsen KD, McCracken GH Jr. Effect of dexamethasone on therapy of experimental penicillin- and cephalosporin-resistant pneumococcal meningitis. Antimicrob Agents Chemother 1994;38(6):1320–1324.
55. Paris MM, Ramilo O, McCracken GH Jr. Management of meningitis caused by penicillin-resistant *Streptococcus pneumoniae*. Antimicrob Agents Chemother 1995;39(10):2171–2175.
56. Ahmed A, Jafri H, Lutsar I, et al. Pharmacodynamics of vancomycin for the treatment of experimental penicillin- and cephalosporin-resistant pneumococcal meningitis. Antimicrob Agents Chemother 1999;43(4):876–881.
57. Black S, Shinefield H, Fireman B, et al. Efficacy, safety and immunogenicity of heptavalent pneumococcal conjugate vaccine in children. Northern California Kaiser Permanente Vaccine Study Center Group [see comments]. Pediatr Infect Dis J 2000;19(3):187–195.

58. Lieu TA, Ray GT, Black SB, et al. Projected cost-effectiveness of pneumococcal conjugate vaccination of healthy infants and young children. JAMA 2000;283(11):1460–1468.
59. American Academy of Pediatrics. Haemophilus influenzae infections. In: Pickering LK, ed. 2000 Red Book: Report of the Committee on Infectious Diseases, 25th ed. Elk Grove Village, IL: American Academy of Pediatrics, 2000:262–272.
60. Anonymous. Recommendations for use of Haemophilus b conjugate vaccines and a combined diphtheria, tetanus, pertussis, and Haemophilus b vaccine. Recommendations of the advisory Committee on Immunization Practices (ACIP). MMWR Morb Mortal Wkly Rep 1993;42(RR-13): 1–15.
61. Korvick JA, Yu VL. Antimicrobial agent therapy for *Pseudomonas aeruginosa*. Antimicrob Agents Chemother 1991;35(11):2167–2172.
62. Rodriguez WJ, Khan WN, Cocchetto DM, Feris J, Puig JR, Akram S. Treatment of *Pseudomonas meningitis* with ceftazidime with or without concurrent therapy. Pediatr Infect Dis J 1990;9(2):83–87.
63. Wolff MA, Young CL, Ramphal R. Antibiotic therapy for Enterobacter meningitis: A retrospective review of 13 episodes and review of the literature. Clin Infect Dis 1993;16(6):772–777.
64. Wolff M, Boutron L, Singlas E, Clair B, Decazes JM, Regnier B. Penetration of ciprofloxacin into cerebrospinal fluid of patients with bacterial meningitis. Antimicrob Agents Chemother 1987;31(6):899–902.
65. Saez-Llorens X, McCracken GH Jr. Antimicrobial and anti-inflammatory treatment of bacterial meningitis. Infect Dis Clin North Am 1999;13 (3):vii, 619–636.
66. Rubin RH, Hooper DC. Central nervous system infection in the compromised host. Med Clin North Am 1985;69(2):281–296.
67. Lebel MH. Dexamethasone therapy of bacterial meningitis. Antibiot Chemother 1992;45:169–183.
68. Girgis NI, Farid Z, Mikhail IA, Farrag I, Sultan Y, Kilpatrick ME. Dexamethasone treatment for bacterial meningitis in children and adults. Pediatr Infect Dis J 1989;8(12):848–851.
69. Lebel MH, Freij BJ, Syrogiannopoulos GA, et al. Dexamethasone therapy for bacterial meningitis. Results of two double-blind, placebo-controlled trials. N Engl J Med 1988;319(15):964–971.
70. Lebel MH, Hoyt MJ, Waagner DC, Rollins NK, Finitzo T, McCracken GH Jr. Magnetic resonance imaging and dexamethasone therapy for bacterial meningitis. Am J Dis Child 1989;143(3):301–306.
71. Odio CM, Faingezicht I, Paris M, et al. The beneficial effects of early dexamethasone administration in infants and children with bacterial meningitis [see comments]. N Engl J Med 1991;324(22):1525–1531.
72. Schaad UB, Lips U, Gnehm HE, Blumberg A, Heinzer I, Wedgwood J. Dexamethasone therapy for bacterial meningitis in children. Swiss Meningitis Study Group. Lancet 1993;342(8869):457–461.
73. Havens PL, Wendelberger KJ, Hoffman GM, Lee MB, Chusid MJ. Corticosteroids as adjunctive therapy in bacterial meningitis. A meta-analysis of clinical trials. Am J Dis Child 1989;143(9):1051–1055.
74. Anonymous. Should we use dexamethasone in meningitis? The Meningitis Working Party of the British Paediatric Immunology and Infectious Diseases Group. Arch Dis Child 1992;67(11):1398–1401.
75. Gaillard JL, Abadie V, Cheron G, et al. Concentrations of ceftriaxone in cerebrospinal fluid of children with meningitis receiving dexamethasone therapy. Antimicrob Agents Chemother 1994;38(5):1209–1210.
76. Kennedy WA, Hoyt MJ, McCracken GH Jr. The role of corticosteroid therapy in children with pneumococcal meningitis. Am J Dis Child 1991;145(12):1374–1378.
77. McIntyre PB, Berkey CS, King SM, et al. Dexamethasone as adjunctive therapy in bacterial meningitis. A meta-analysis of randomized clinical trials since 1988. JAMA 1997;278(11):925–931.
78. American Academy of Pediatrics. Pneumococcal infections. In: Pickering LK, ed. 2000 Red Book: Report of the Committee on Infectious Diseases, 25th ed. Elk Grove Village, IL: American Academy of Pediatrics, 2000:452–460.
79. Syrogiannopoulos GA, Lourida AN, Theodoridou MC, et al. Dexamethasone therapy for bacterial meningitis in children: 2- versus 4-day regimen. J Infect Dis 1994;169(4):853–88.
80. Leonard JM, Des Prez RM. Tuberculous meningitis. Infect Dis Clin North Am 1990;4(4):769–787.
81. Iseman MD. Extrapulmonary Tuberculosis in Adults. A Clinician's Guide to Tuberculosis. Philadelphia, Lippincott Williams & Wilkins, 2000:145–197.
82. Holdiness MR. Management of tuberculosis meningitis. Drugs 1990;39(2):224–233.
83. Kent SJ, Crowe SM, Yung A, Lucas CR, Mijch AM. Tuberculous meningitis: A 30-year review [see comments]. Clin Infect Dis 1993;17(6):987–994.
84. Daniel TM. The rapid diagnosis of tuberculosis: A selective review. J Lab Clin Med 1990;116(3):277–282.
85. Bloch AB, Cauthen GM, Onorato IM, et al. Nationwide survey of drug-resistant tuberculosis in the United States [see comments]. JAMA 1994;271(9):665–671.
86. Anonymous. Initial therapy for tuberculosis in the era of multidrug resistance. Recommendations of the Advisory Council for the Elimination of Tuberculosis [published erratum appears at MMWR Morb Mortal Wkly Rep 1993;42(27):536]. MMWR Morb Mortal Wkly Rep 1993;42 (RR-7):1–8.
87. Ellard GA, Humphries MJ, Allen BW. Cerebrospinal fluid drug concentrations and the treatment of tuberculous meningitis. Am Rev Resp Dis 1993;148(3):650–655.
88. O'Toole RD, Thornton GF, Mukherjee MK, Nath RL. Dexamethasone in tuberculous meningitis. Relationship of cerebrospinal fluid effects to therapeutic efficacy. Ann Intern Med 1969;70(1):39–48.
89. Alzeer AH, FitzGerald JM. Corticosteroids and tuberculosis: Risks and use as adjunct therapy [see comments]. Tuber Lung Dis 1993;74(1):6–11.
90. Dismukes WE. Management of cryptococcosis [see comments]. Clin Infect Dis 1993;17(suppl 2):S507–S512.
91. Sugar AM, Stern JJ, Dupont B. Overview: Treatment of cryptococcal meningitis. Rev Infect Dis 1990;12(suppl 3):S338–S348.
92. Powderly WG, Cloud GA, Dismukes WE, Saag MS. Measurement of cryptococcal antigen in serum and cerebrospinal fluid: Value in the management of AIDS-associated cryptococcal meningitis. Clin Infect Dis 1994;18(5):789–792.
93. Powderly WG. Therapy for cryptococcal meningitis in patients with AIDS. Clin Infect Dis 1992;14(suppl 1):S54–S59.
94. Bennett JE, Dismukes WE, Duma RJ, et al. A comparison of amphotericin B alone and combined with flucytosine in the treatment of cryptococcal meningitis. N Engl J Med 1979;301(3):126–131.
95. Chuck SL, Sande MA. Infections with *Cryptococcus neoformans* in the acquired immunodeficiency syndrome [see comments]. N Engl J Med 1989;321(12):794–799.
96. Coker RJ, Viviani M, Gazzard BG, et al. Treatment of cryptococcosis with liposomal amphotericin B (AmBisome) in 23 patients with AIDS. AIDS 1993;7(6):829–835.
97. Leenders AC, Reiss P, Portegies P, et al. Liposomal amphotericin B (AmBisome) compared with amphotericin B both followed by oral fluconazole in the treatment of AIDS-associated cryptococcal meningitis. AIDS 1997;11(12):1463–1471.
98. Saag MS, Powderly WG, Cloud GA, et al. Comparison of amphotericin B with fluconazole in the treatment of acute AIDS-associated cryptococcal meningitis. The NIAID Mycoses Study Group and the AIDS Clinical Trials Group [see comments]. N Engl J Med 1992;326(2):83–89.
99. Berry AJ, Rinaldi MG, Graybill JR. Use of high-dose fluconazole as salvage therapy for cryptococcal meningitis in patients with AIDS. Antimicrob Agents Chemother 1992;36(3):690–692.
100. de Gans J, Portegies P, Tiessens G, et al. Itraconazole compared with amphotericin B plus flucytosine in AIDS patients with cryptococcal meningitis. AIDS 1992;6(2):185–190.
101. Powderly WG, Saag MS, Cloud GA, et al. A controlled trial of fluconazole or amphotericin B to prevent relapse of cryptococcal meningitis in patients with the acquired immunodeficiency syndrome. The NIAID AIDS Clinical Trials Group and Mycoses Study Group [see comments]. N Engl J Med 1992;326(12):793–798.
102. van der Horst CM, Saag MS, Cloud GA, et al. Treatment of cryptococcal meningitis associated with the acquired immunodeficiency syndrome.

National Institute of Allergy and Infectious Diseases Mycoses Study Group and AIDS Clinical Trials Group [see comments]. N Engl J Med 1997;337(1):15–21.

103. Roos KL. Encephalitis. Neurol Clin 1999;17(4):813–833.
104. Nelsen S, Sealy DP, Schneider EF. The aseptic meningitis syndrome. Am Fam Physician 1993;48(5):809–815.
105. Dalton M, Newton RW. Aseptic meningitis. Dev Med Child Neurol 1991;33(5):446–451.
106. Rubeiz H, Roos RP. Viral meningitis and encephalitis. Semin Neurol 1992;12(3):165–177.
107. Glimaker M. Enteroviral meningitis. Diagnostic methods and aspects on the distinction from bacterial meningitis. Scand J Infect Dis Suppl 1992;85:1–64.
108. Overall JC Jr. Is it bacterial or viral? Laboratory differentiation. Pediatr Rev 1993;14(7):251–261.
109. Sawyer MH, Holland D, Aintablian N, Connor JD, Keyser EF, Waecker NJ Jr. Diagnosis of enteroviral central nervous system infection by polymerase chain reaction during a large community outbreak. Pediatr Infect Dis J 1994;13(3):177–182.
110. Connolly KJ, Hammer SM. The acute aseptic meningitis syndrome. Infect Dis Clin North Am 1990;4(4):599–622.
111. Gateley A, Gander RM, Johnson PC, Kit S, Otsuka H, Kohl S. Herpes simplex virus type 2 meningoencephalitis resistant to acyclovir in a patient with AIDS. J Infect Dis 1990;161(4):711–715.
112. Foscavir injection: Package insert. Astra USA, Inc., 1999.
113. Talan DA, Hoffman JR, Yoshikawa TT, Overturf GD. Role of empiric parenteral antibiotics prior to lumbar puncture in suspected bacterial meningitis: State of the art [see comments]. Rev Infect Dis 1988;10(2): 365–376.
114. Salmon JH. Ventriculitis complicating meningitis. Am J Dis Child 1972;124(1):35–40.
115. Wald SL, McLaurin RL. Cerebrospinal fluid antibiotic levels during treatment of shunt infections. J Neurosurg 1980;52(1):41–46.
116. McLaurin RL. Infected cerebrospinal fluid shunts. Surg Neurol 1973; 1(4):191–195.
117. Sells CJ, Shurtleff DB, Loeser JD. Gram-negative cerebrospinal fluid shunt-associated infections. Pediatrics 1977;59(4):614–618.
118. Pau AK, Smego RA Jr, Fisher MA. Intraventricular vancomycin: Observations of tolerance and pharmacokinetics in two infants with ventricular shunt infections. Pediatr Infect Dis J 1986;5(1):93–96.
119. Visconti EB, Peter G. Vancomycin treatment of cerebrospinal fluid shunt infections. Report of two cases. J Neurosurg 1979;51(2):245–246.

106

Lower Respiratory Tract Infections

Mark L. Glover and Michael D. Reed

Respiratory infections remain the major cause of morbidity from acute illness in the United States, and most likely represent the single most common reason patients seek medical attention. This chapter focuses on bacterial and viral infections involving the lower respiratory tract, which includes the tracheobronchial tree and lung parenchyma.

The respiratory tract has an elaborate system of host defenses, including humoral immunity, cellular immunity, and anatomic mechanisms.[1–4] When functioning properly, the host defenses of the respiratory tract are markedly effective in protecting against pathogen invasion and removing potentially infectious agents from the lungs.[2–4] For the most part, infections in the lower respiratory tract occur only when these defense mechanisms are impaired, such as with dysgammaglobulinemia or compromised ciliary function caused by the chronic inflammation that accompanies cigarette smoking. In addition, local defenses may be overwhelmed when a particularly virulent microorganism or excessive inoculum invades lung parenchyma. The majority of pulmonary infections follow colonization of the upper respiratory tract with potential pathogens, which, after achieving sufficiently high concentrations, gain access to the lung via aspiration of oropharyngeal secretions. Less commonly, microbes enter the lung via the blood from an extrapulmonary source or by the inhalation of infected aerosolized particles. The specific type of pulmonary infection caused by an invading microorganism is determined by a variety of host factors, including age, anatomic features of the airway, and specific characteristics of the infecting agent.

The most common infections involving the lower respiratory tract include bronchitis, bronchiolitis, and pneumonia. Lower respiratory tract infections in children and adults are most commonly a result of either viral or bacterial invasion of lung parenchyma. The diagnosis of viral infections rests primarily on the recognition of a characteristic constellation of clinical signs and symptoms. Because treatment is largely supportive, only occasionally does the diagnosis require laboratory confirmation; this is achieved through serologic tests or the identification of the organism by culture or antigen detection in respiratory secretions. New laboratory techniques employing polymerase chain reaction (PCR) technology are emerging as a means to identify specific pathogens rapidly and accurately.

In contrast, because bacterial pneumonia usually necessitates expedient, effective, and specific antibiotic therapy, its management depends, in large part, on isolation of the etiologic agent by culture from lung tissue or secretions. The pharynx is colonized with many organisms that can potentially cause pneumonia; therefore, culture of expectorated sputum can be misleading unless the specimen is examined to ensure that it has originated from the lower respiratory tract.[5] The Gram stain provides the easiest method to distinguish lower from upper respiratory tract secretions; moreover, through determination of the shape and color of the bacteria, the Gram stain frequently narrows the microbiologic differential diagnosis sufficiently to allow accurate initial therapy. Scanned under low-power microscopy, Gram-stained expectorated upper respiratory tract secretions contain many irregularly shaped epithelial cells with little evidence of inflammation. Microorganisms of a variety of morphologies are present (Fig. 106–1). In contrast, a lower-tract specimen from a patient with bacterial pneumonia usually contains multiple neutrophils per high-powered field and a single or predominant bacterial species. Culture of specimens confirmed to originate from the lower tract by Gram stain provides valuable diagnostic information in the majority of patients with bacterial pneumonia.[6,7]

An appropriate treatment regimen for the patient with an uncomplicated lower respiratory tract infection can usually be established by the history, physical examination, chest radiograph, and properly collected sputum cultures interpreted in light of the most common lung pathogens and their antibiotic susceptibility patterns within one's community. More sophisticated or invasive diagnostic methods (such as computerized tomography, bronchoscopy, or lung biopsy)[8–11] should be reserved for very ill patients who are unable to expectorate sputum or who are not responding to empiric therapy, or for pulmonary infections occurring in the immunocompromised patient.

BRONCHITIS

Bronchitis and bronchiolitis are inflammatory conditions of the large and small elements, respectively, of the tracheobronchial tree. The inflammatory process does not extend to the alveoli. Bronchitis is frequently classified as acute or chronic. Acute bronchitis occurs in all ages, and chronic bronchitis primarily affects adults. Bronchiolitis is a disease of infancy.

ACUTE BRONCHITIS

EPIDEMIOLOGY AND ETIOLOGY

Acute bronchitis most commonly occurs during the winter months, following a pattern similar to those of other acute respiratory tract infections. Cold, damp climates, the presence of high concentrations of irritating substances, such as air pollution or cigarette smoke, or both, may precipitate attacks.[12,13]

Respiratory viruses are by far the most common infectious agents associated with acute bronchitis. The common cold viruses, rhinovirus and coronavirus, and lower respiratory tract pathogens, including influenza virus, adenovirus, and respiratory syncytial virus, account for the majority of cases. In children, similar pathogens are observed with the addition of the parainfluenza viruses. While the true incidence remains to be defined, *Mycoplasma pneumonia* also appears to be a frequent cause of acute bronchitis. Additionally, *Chlamydia pneumoniae*[14] and *Bordetella pertussis* (the agent responsible for whooping cough) have been associated with acute respiratory tract infections. Although a variety of bacteria, including *Streptococcus pneumoniae, Streptococcus spp., Staphylococcus spp.,* and *Haemophilus spp.* may be isolated from throat or sputum culture, it is probable that these organisms represent contamination by normal flora of the upper respiratory tract rather than true pathogens.

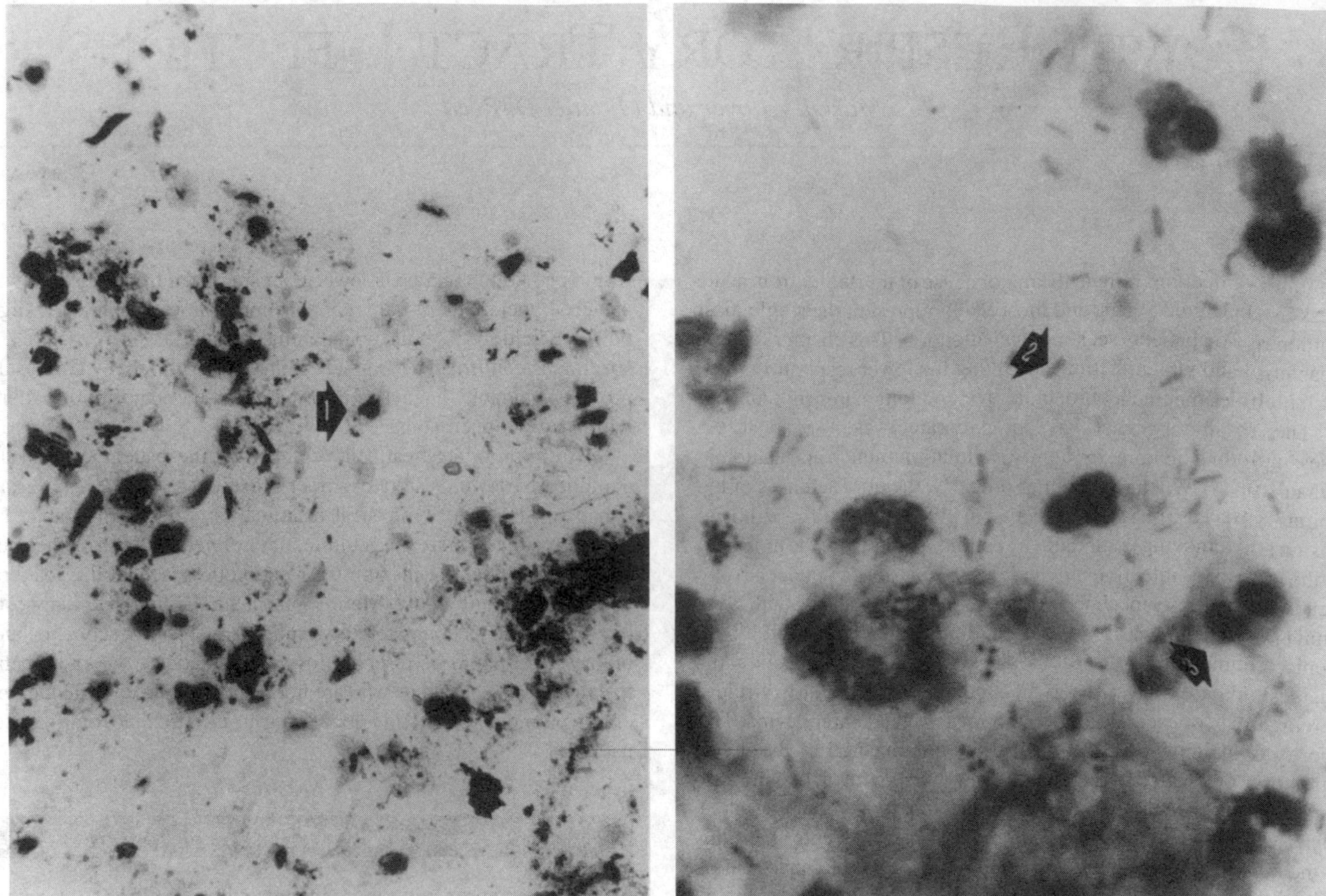

FIGURE 106–1. Gram stain of sputum. *Left panel.* Scanned under low power (10x), this sample contains many irregularly shaped epithelial cells (*arrow 1*) and no inflammatory cells, indicating that the specimen was derived from the upper respiratory tract. *Right panel.* Under oil immersion (100x), this specimen contains a predominance of gram-negative rods (*arrow 2*) and many polymorphonuclear cells (*arrow 3*) per high-power field, confirming that this specimen was derived from the lower respiratory tract. The sample grew *Klebsiella pneumoniae.*

Although a primary bacterial etiology for acute bronchitis appears rare, secondary bacterial infection may be involved.

PATHOGENESIS

Because acute bronchitis is primarily a self-limiting illness and rarely a cause of death, few data are available to describe the pathology. In general, infection of the trachea and bronchi yields hyperemic and edematous mucous membranes with an increase in bronchial secretions. Destruction of respiratory epithelium can range from mild to extensive and may affect bronchial mucociliary function. In addition, the increase in bronchial secretions, which can become thick and tenacious, further impairs mucociliary activity. The probability of permanent damage to the airways as a result of acute bronchitis remains unclear; however, epidemiologic evaluations support the belief that recurrent acute respiratory infections may be associated with increased airway hyperreactivity and possibly the pathogenesis of asthma or chronic obstructive lung disease.[13,15]

CLINICAL PRESENTATION

Acute bronchitis usually begins as an upper respiratory infection. Nonspecific complaints, including malaise and headache, frequently accompany coryza and sore throat. Cough is the hallmark of acute bronchitis and occurs early. The onset of cough may be insidious or abrupt, and the symptoms persist despite the resolution of nasal or nasopharyngeal complaints. Frequently, the cough is initially nonproductive but progresses, yielding mucopurulent sputum. In older children and adults, the sputum is raised and expectorated; in the young child, sputum is often swallowed and can result in gagging and vomiting. Substantial discomfort may result from the coughing. Dyspnea, cyanosis, or signs of airway obstruction are rarely observed unless the patient has underlying pulmonary disease, such as emphysema or chronic obstructive pulmonary disease. Fever, when present, rarely exceeds 39°C (102.2°F) and appears most commonly with adenovirus, influenza virus, and *M. pneumonia* infections.

The chest examination in acute bronchitis may reveal rhonchi and coarse, moist, bilateral rales. Chest radiographs are usually normal. The diagnosis is typically made on the basis of a characteristic history and physical examination. Bacterial cultures of expectorated sputum are generally of limited use because of the inability to avoid normal nasopharyngeal flora by the sampling technique. In routine cases, viral cultures are unnecessary and frequently unavailable. Viral antigen detection tests, developed to identify respiratory viral antigens from nasal secretions rapidly, can be obtained in many hospital laboratories and in some practice settings when a specific diagnosis is necessary for clinical or epidemiologic reasons.[16] Cultures or serologic diagnosis of *M. pneumonia* and culture or direct fluorescent antibody detection for *B. pertussis* should be obtained in prolonged or severe cases when epidemiologic considerations would suggest their involvement.[17]

▶ TREATMENT: Acute Bronchitis

DESIRED OUTCOME

In the absence of a complicating bacterial superinfection, acute bronchitis is almost always self-limiting. The goals of therapy, therefore, are to provide comfort to the patient, and, in the unusually severe case, to treat associated dehydration and respiratory compromise.

GENERAL APPROACH TO TREATMENT

The treatment of acute bronchitis is symptomatic and supportive in nature. Reassurance and antipyretics frequently are all that are needed.

NONPHARMACOLOGIC THERAPY

Bed rest for comfort may be instituted as desired. Patients should be encouraged to drink fluids to prevent dehydration and to possibly decrease the viscosity of respiratory secretions. Mist therapy, the use of a vaporizer, or both may further promote the thinning and loosening of respiratory secretions.

PHARMACOLOGIC THERAPY

Mild analgesic-antipyretic therapy is often helpful in relieving the associated lethargy, malaise, and fever. Aspirin or acetaminophen (650 mg in adults or 10–15 mg/kg/dose in children; maximum daily pediatric dose 60 mg/kg; maximum daily adult dose 4 g) or ibuprofen (200–400 mg in adults or 10 mg/kg/dose in children; maximum daily pediatric dose 40 mg/kg; maximum daily adult dose 3.2 g) should be administered every 4 to 6 hours. In children, aspirin should be avoided and acetaminophen used as the preferred agent because of the possible association between aspirin use and the development of Reye's syndrome.[18]

The use of ibuprofen as an antipyretic has increased. The drug's antipyretic efficacy appears identical to that of aspirin or acetaminophen, although its duration of antipyretic effect may be slightly longer (e.g., 3 to 4 hours for aspirin and acetaminophen vs 5 to 6 hours for ibuprofen). Caution should be exercised in the administration of ibuprofen in those less than 3 months of age and elderly patients and individuals with poor renal function. Aspirin and ibuprofen inhibit prostaglandin synthesis and may adversely influence renal function in these predisposed patient populations.

Patients suffering from acute bronchitis frequently medicate themselves with over-the-counter cough and cold remedies containing various combinations of antihistamines, sympathomimetics, and antitussives despite the lack of definitive evidence supporting their effectiveness.[19] In fact, the tendency of these agents to dehydrate bronchial secretions could potentially aggravate and prolong the recovery process. Persistent, mild cough, which may be bothersome, can be treated with dextromethorphan; more severe coughs may require intermittent codeine or other similar agents. In severe cases, cough may be persistent enough to disrupt sleep, and the use of a mild sedative-hypnotic, concomitantly with a cough suppressant, may be desirable; however, antitussives should be used cautiously when the cough is productive. The primary or supplemental use of expectorants is questionable because their clinical effectiveness has not been well established.

Routine use of antibiotics in the treatment of acute bronchitis should be discouraged;[20,21] however, in patients who exhibit persistent fever or respiratory symptoms for more than 4 to 6 days, the possibility of a concurrent bacterial infection should be suspected. When possible, antibiotic therapy should be directed toward anticipated respiratory pathogen(s) (*S. pneumoniae, Haemophilus influenzae*). *Mycoplasma pneumoniae,* if suspected by history or positive cold agglutinins (titers > 1:32), or if confirmed by culture or serology, may be treated with erythromycin or its analogs (clarithromycin, azithromycin). Alternatively and empirically, a fluoroquinolone with activity against these pathogens (e.g., gatifloxacin, increased dose levofloxacin) may be used. During known epidemics involving the influenza A virus, amantadine or rimantadine may be effective in minimizing associated symptoms if administered early in the course of the disease.[22] The recently marketed neuraminidase inhibitors, zanamivir and oseltamivir, are active against both influenza A and B viral infections and may reduce the severity and duration of the influenza episode if administered promptly during the onset of the viral infection.[23,24]

CHRONIC BRONCHITIS

EPIDEMIOLOGY AND ETIOLOGY

Chronic bronchitis is a nonspecific disease that primarily affects adults. Between 10% and 25% of the adult population 40 years of age or older suffer from chronic bronchitis, resulting in substantial health care dollar expenditures and lost wages.[25–27] This disease is so common that acute bronchitis and acute exacerbations of chronic bronchitis result in approximately 14 million physician visits per year in the United States. Similar to acute bronchitis, cold, damp climates and the presence of elevated airborne concentrations of irritating substances may favor this disease.[25–27] Chronic bronchitis occurs more commonly in men than in women.

Chronic bronchitis is a result of several contributing factors, the most prominent of these include cigarette smoking, exposure to occupational dusts, fumes, environmental pollution, and bacterial (and possibly viral) infection. The influence that each of these factors and others, either alone or in combination, contributes to chronic bronchitis is unknown. Cigarette smoke is a well-known airway irritant and is believed by many to be the predominant factor in the etiology of chronic bronchitis. Studies of lungs from smoking and nonsmoking individuals have clearly demonstrated a substantial increase in the number of alveolar macrophages, as well as the presence of bronchial inflammation, in individuals who smoke cigarettes. Although the majority of patients who suffer from chronic bronchitis have a positive smoking history, no history of smoking can be identified in as many as 10% of cases. These findings suggest that additional airway irritants, either alone or more probably in combination, are responsible for the pathogenesis of chronic bronchitis. The only known genetic abnormality leading to chronic obstructive pulmonary disease (COPD) is α_1-antitrypsin deficiency occurring in less than 1% of COPD in the United States.

In addition, the influence of recurrent respiratory tract infections during childhood or young adult life on the later development of chronic bronchitis remains obscure. Recurrent respiratory infections at a young age may predispose individuals to the development of chronic bronchitis;[15,28] however, it is unclear whether these recurrent respiratory tract infections are a result of unrecognized anatomic abnormalities of the airways or impaired pulmonary defense mechanisms.

PATHOGENESIS

The chronic inhalation of an irritating noxious substance compromises the normal secretory and mucociliary function of bronchial mucosa. In chronic bronchitis, the bronchial wall is thickened and the number of mucus-secreting goblet cells in the surface epithelium of both larger and smaller bronchi is markedly increased.[29] In contrast, goblet cells are generally absent from the smaller bronchi of normal individuals. In addition to the increased number of goblet cells, hypertrophy of the mucous glands and dilation of the mucous gland ducts are also observed. As a result of these changes, chronic bronchitics have substantially more mucus in their peripheral airways, further impairing normal lung defenses. This increased quantity of tenacious secretions within the bronchial tree frequently causes mucous plugging of the smaller airways. Accompanying these changes are squamous cell metaplasia of the surface epithelium, edema and increased vascularity of the basement membrane of larger airways, and variable chronic inflammatory cell infiltration. Continued progression of this pathology can result in residual scarring of small bronchi, augmenting airway obstruction and weakening of bronchial walls.

CLINICAL PRESENTATION

The hallmark of chronic bronchitis is a cough that may range from a mild "smoker's" cough to severe incessant coughing productive of purulent sputum. Coughing may be precipitated by multiple stimuli, including simple, normal conversation. Expectoration of the largest quantity of sputum usually occurs upon arising in the morning, although many patients expectorate sputum throughout the day. The expectorated sputum is usually tenacious and can vary in color from white to yellow-green. As a result, many patients complain of a frequent bad taste in their mouth and of halitosis.

The diagnosis of chronic bronchitis is based primarily on clinical assessment and history. Any patient who reports the coughing up of sputum on most days for at least 3 consecutive months each year for 2 consecutive years presumptively has chronic bronchitis.[26,27] The diagnosis of chronic bronchitis is made only when the possibilities of bronchiectasis, cardiac failure, cystic fibrosis, and lung carcinoma have been effectively excluded. In an attempt to be more specific in the diagnosis, some investigators have added lost wages for 3 or more weeks to the criteria. In addition, many clinicians attempt to subdivide their patients into one of three subgroups: (a) those patients with simple chronic bronchitis; (b) those with chronic or recurrent mucopurulent bronchitis (based on the presence of mucopurulent sputum confirmed by microscopic analysis); and (c) those with chronic obstructive bronchitis (based on the clinical history and presence of airway obstruction documented by pulmonary function testing). More recently, an ad hoc international committee comprised of pulmonary and infectious disease physicians developed a classification system that can serve as a practical guide for initial patient assessment and management (Table 106–1) for patients with chronic bronchitis.[27]

TABLE 106–1. Useful Classification System for Patients With Chronic Bronchitis and Initial Treatment Options[27]

Baseline Status	Criteria or Risk Factors	Usual Pathogens		Initial Treatment Options
Class I				
Acute tracheobronchitis	No underlying structural disease	Usually a virus	1st	None unless symptoms persist
			2nd	Amoxicillin; amoxicillin-clavulanate; or a macrolide/azithromycin
Class II				
Chronic bronchitis	FEV_1 >50% predicted value, increased sputum volume and purulence	*Haemophilus influenzae, Haemophilus spp., Moraxella catarrhalis, Streptococcus pneumoniae* (β-lactam resistance possible)	1st	Amoxicillin, or quinolone if prevalence of *H. influenzae* resistance to amoxicillin is >20%
			2nd	Quinolone, amoxicillin-clavulanate, azithromycin, tetracycline, or trimethoprim-sulfamethoxazole
Class III				
Chronic bronchitis with complications	FEV_1 <50% predicted value, increased sputum volume and purulence, advanced age, at least four flares/year, or significant comorbidity	Same as class II; also *Klebsiella pneumoniae, Pseudomonas aeruginosa, K. pneumoniae,* and other gram-negative organisms (β-lactam resistance common)	1st	Quinolone
			2nd	Expanded spectrum cephalosporin, amoxicillin-clavulanate, or azithromycin
Class IV				
Chronic bronchial infection	Same as for class III plus yearlong production of purulent sputum	Same as class III	1st	Oral or parenteral quinolone, carbapenem or expanded spectrum cephalosporin followed by high-dose oral ciprofloxacin or routine dose trovafloxacin

1st, first choices; 2nd, alternate treatment options.
Quinolone: ciprofloxacin, gatifloxacin, levofloxacin.
Tetracycline: tetracycline HCl, doxycycline.
Carbapenem: imipenem/cilastatin, meropenem.
Expanded spectrum cephalosporin: ceftazidime, cefepime.

Chest auscultation usually reveals inspiratory and expiratory rales, rhonchi, and mild wheezing with an expiratory phase that is frequently prolonged. Normal vesicular breathing sounds are diminished. Depending on the severity of the disease, an increase in the anteroposterior diameter of the thoracic cage (observed as a barrel chest), hyperresonance on percussion with obliteration of the area of cardiac dullness, and depressed diaphragms with limited mobility are often observed. In more advanced stages, cyanosis is common and may be accompanied by a compensatory erythrocytosis. Clubbing of the digits is infrequent, but when observed is usually reflective of advanced disease. In more progressed stages of chronic bronchitis, physical findings associated with cor pulmonale, including cardiac enlargement, hepatomegaly, and edema of the lower extremities, are observed. In general, chronic bronchitics tend to maintain at least normal body weight and are commonly obese. Radiographic studies are of limited value either in the diagnosis or as a means of sequentially following a patient. A decrease in vital capacity and a prolongation of expiratory flow are usually found from pulmonary function studies.

The microscopic and laboratory assessment of sputum is considered an important component in the overall evaluation of patients with chronic bronchitis. A fresh sputum specimen obtained as an early morning sample is preferred. Comparison of the cellular constituents of chronic bronchitic sputum with those of normal sputum can provide insight into the degree of activity of the disease processes.[25] An increased number of polymorphonuclear granulocytes often suggests continual bronchial irritation, whereas an increased number of eosinophils suggests an allergic component that should be further investigated. Gram staining of the sputum often reveals a mixture of both gram-positive and gram-negative bacteria, reflecting normal oropharyngeal flora and tracheal colonization by *S. pneumoniae, H. influenzae,* and *Moraxella catarrhalis.* Table 106–2 outlines the most common bacterial isolates identified from sputum culture in patients experiencing an acute exacerbation of chronic bronchitis.

TABLE 106–2. Common Bacterial Pathogens Isolated From the Sputum of Patients With an Acute Exacerbation of Chronic Bronchitis

Pathogen	Estimated Incidence[a]
Haemophilus influenzae[b]	24–26
Haemophilus parainfluenzae	20
Streptococcus pneumoniae[c]	15
Moraxella catarrhalis[b]	15
Klebsiella pneumoniae	4
Serratia marcescens	2
Neisseria meningitidis[b]	2
Pseudomonas aeruginosa	2

[a]Expressed as percent of cultures.
[b]Often β-lactamase positive.
[c]As many as 25% of strains may be intermediate or highly resistant to penicillin.

▶ TREATMENT: Chronic Bronchitis

DESIRED OUTCOME

The goals of therapy for chronic bronchitis are twofold: first, to reduce the severity of the chronic symptoms and second, to ameliorate acute exacerbations and to achieve prolonged infection-free intervals.

GENERAL APPROACH TO TREATMENT

The approach to the treatment of chronic bronchitis is multifactorial. First and foremost, attempts must be made to reduce the patient's exposure to known bronchial irritants (e.g., smoking). Additionally, measures to provide pulmonary toilet can be instituted. Finally, in the face of an acute exacerbation, a trial of antibiotics directed against the most likely underlying pathogens can be initiated.

NONPHARMACOLOGIC THERAPY

A complete occupational and environmental history for the determination of exposure to noxious, irritating gases, as well as preference toward cigarette smoking must be assessed. Often easier discussed than accomplished, honest, yet reasonable, attempts should be made with the patient to reduce or eliminate completely the number of cigarettes smoked daily and to reduce his or her exposure to second hand smoke. In an organized, coordinated cessation program, which includes counseling and hypnotherapy, the adjunctive use of nicotine substitutes, such as a nicotine gum or patch, may promote the reduction or complete withdrawal from cigarette smoking. Often just as difficult is the modification of exposure to irritating substances within the home and workplace.

During acute pulmonary exacerbations of the disease, a patient's ability to mobilize and expectorate sputum may be dramatically reduced. In these instances, attempts at postural drainage techniques, with instruction, active participation, or both from a respiratory therapist, may assist in promoting clearance of pulmonary secretions. In addition, humidification of inspired air may promote the hydration (liquefaction) of tenacious secretions allowing for more productive removal. The use of mucolytic aerosols, such as *N*-acetylcysteine and DNAse, is of questionable therapeutic value, particularly considering their propensity to induce bronchospasm (*N*-acetylcysteine) and their excessive cost. Oral or aerosolized bronchodilators may benefit some patients during acute pulmonary exacerbations.

PHARMACOLOGIC THERAPY

For those patients who consistently demonstrate clinical limitation in airflow, a therapeutic challenge of bronchodilators (such as albuterol aerosol) should be considered. Pulmonary function tests can be performed pre- and post-β_2-agonist aerosol to more objectively determine a patient's propensity to benefit from supplemental aerosol therapy. However, this laboratory assessment, often performed at times of better health, may not accurately predict a patient's potential benefit from β_2 aerosols during an acute exacerbation of their chronic bronchitis. Although chronic theophylline administration has been extensively used in the past, this therapy is being employed with decreasing frequency in favor of aerosolized β_2-receptor agonists. Albuterol is most commonly used, one to two puffs of the metered dose inhaler three to four times daily.[26] The role of aerosolized surfactant has also been assessed in patients with stable chronic bronchitis.[30] This preliminary study reveals very encouraging results with surfactant demonstrating improvement in pulmonary function and sputum transport by cilia (i.e., clearance). The role of surfactant as a carrier vehicle for other aerosol medications also appears promising and will most likely be evaluated over the next several years.

Numerous comparative evaluations, including placebo-controlled studies of antibiotic administration with acute and chronic treatment of chronic bronchitics, have suggested definite clinical benefit, whereas other similar studies have not.[26,27,31–33] The antibiotics most frequently selected (ampicillin, tetracycline [or doxycycline], chloramphenicol, trimethoprim-sulfamethoxazole) possess variable *in vitro* activity against the common sputum isolates *H. influenzae, S. pneumoniae, M. catarrhalis,* and *M. pneumoniae.*

In general, these conflicting results appear independent of which antibiotic was used or regimen compared. The wide disparity that exists in the results from these studies, combined with the difficulties in recognition and lack of standardized diagnostic criteria for acute exacerbation of chronic bronchitis[31] serves as the basis for the enormous controversy surrounding the use of antibiotics in this condition.[34,35]

Further complicating antibiotic selection is the increasing resistance of the common bacterial pathogens to first-line agents. As many as 30% to 40% of *H. influenzae* and 95% of *M. catarrhalis* produce β-lactamase. Moreover, up to as many as 30% of *S. pneumoniae* isolates demonstrate resistance to penicillin (MIC $\geq$ 0.1 mg/L) with approximately 14% of isolates being highly resistant (MIC $>$ 2 mg/L).[36,37] In addition, *S. pneumoniae* resistance is becoming more concerning as the incidence of macrolide resistance is approximately 20%.[33,38] Despite these changes in bacterial susceptibility, it is recommended to initiate therapy with first-line agents in less severely affected patients. The scheme outlined in Table 106–1 can be used as an initial guide to the selection of antibiotics based on disease severity (class I through class IV). Regardless of which antibiotic is selected, careful attention to predetermined outcome measures should be closely monitored in each patient to determine the success or failure of the therapeutic intervention.[35] Thus, oral antibiotics with broader antibacterial spectrums (cefixime, amoxicillin-clavulanate, quinolones, or azilides), that possess more potent *in vitro* activity against sputum isolates are generally not needed as initial therapy because clinical response often appears independent of the pathogens' *in vitro* susceptibility for many patients.[26,27,32,33]

An important clinical outcome variable directing drug selection and criteria for beginning antibiotics in individual patients is the infection-free period when chronic bronchitics are off antibiotics. The actual length of the infection-free time period, as well as the change in the number of physician office visits and hospital admissions with a particular antibiotic regimen, is extremely important to identify, whenever possible, for each patient. The longest infection-free period defines that antibiotic regimen as the "regimen of choice" for the specific patient for future acute exacerbations of their disease. However, the impact this preferred therapy may have on the disease or its progression, if incorporated as an aggressive targeted strategy over time, is less-well characterized.

Antibiotics should be selected that are effective against responsible pathogens, that demonstrate the least risk of drug interactions, and can be administered in a manner that promotes compliance. Antibiotics commonly used in the treatment of these patients and their respective adult starting doses are outlined in Table 106–3. It is important to note that doses of antibiotics should be adjusted as needed to the desired clinical effect and the lowest incidence of acceptable side effects. A frequent, successful clinical strategy to enhance the duration of symptom-free periods incorporates higher dose antibiotic regimens using the upper limit of the recommended daily antibiotic dose for a period of 10 to 14 days.[33]

TABLE 106–3. Oral Antibiotics Commonly Used for the Treatment of Acute Respiratory Exacerbations in Chronic Bronchitis

Antibiotic	Usual Adult Dose (g)	Dose Schedule (doses/day)
Preferred Drugs		
Ampicillin	0.5–1	4
Amoxicillin	0.5–1	3
Cefprozil	0.5	2
Cefuroxime	0.5	2
Ciprofloxacin	0.5–0.75	2
Gatifloxacin	0.4	1
Levofloxacin	0.5–0.75	1
Doxycycline	0.1	2
Minocycline	0.1	2
Tetracycline HCl	0.5	4
Amoxicillin-clavulanate	0.5	3
Trimethoprim-sulfamethoxazole	1 DS*	2
Supplemental Drugs		
Azithromycin	0.25–0.5	1
Erythomycin	0.5	4
Clarithromycin	0.25–0.5	2
Cefixime	0.4	1
Cephalexin	0.5	4
Cefaclor	0.25–0.5	3

*DS, double-strength tablet (160 mg trimethoprim/800 mg sulfamethoxazole).

Ampicillin is often considered the drug of choice for the treatment of acute exacerbations of chronic bronchitis. Unfortunately, the need for multiple repeat daily doses (four times daily), increased incidence of gastrointestinal side effects, and the increasing incidence of penicillin-resistant β-lactamase-producing strains of bacteria (Tables 106–1 and 106–2) have limited the usefulness of this safe and very cost-effective antibiotic. As stated earlier, the proposed classification system outlined in Table 106–1 offers first- and second-line treatment options for acute exacerbations of chronic bronchitis, which is directed by the baseline clinical status of the patient. These treatment recommendations can be used to initiate therapy in patients with class I through class IV disease.

The value of the erythromycins when mycoplasma is involved is unquestionable, whereas the value, if any, of the newer erythromycin analogs, azithromycin or clarithromycin, as first-line agents in the treatment of these patients is unknown. Azithromycin should be considered as the macrolide/azilide of choice when considering the drug's *in vitro* antibacterial spectrum of activity, tissue distribution characteristics, and lack of metabolic based drug-drug interactions.[39] In contrast, the fluoroquinolones have emerged as effective alternative agents, particularly when gram-negative pathogens are involved or in more clinically or severely ill patients (Table 106–1). The increasing resistance of selected pathogens to ciprofloxacin may necessitate the use of newer analogs with greater *in vitro* antibacterial activity, including penicillin tolerant or resistant *S. pneumoniae* (e.g., gatifloxacin). The increased cost of fluoroquinolones must be carefully weighed against the possible superiority of quinolones in their apparent initial success rate and more prolonged infection-free time period.[26,27]

In the patient whose history suggests recurrent exacerbations of disease that might be attributable to specific events (that is, it is seasonal or related to the winter months), a trial of prophylactic antibiotics might be beneficial. If no clinical improvement is noted over an appropriate time period (2 to 3 months per year for 2 to 3 years), one might elect to discontinue further attempts at prophylactic therapy. Similarly, such patient-specific trials could be performed in individuals experiencing acute exacerbations, focusing on defining the infection-free period. Although less than desirable, this method of clinical assessment might distinguish those patients who will benefit from prophylactic antibiotic therapy from those patients who will not benefit.

BRONCHIOLITIS

EPIDEMIOLOGY AND ETIOLOGY

Bronchiolitis is an acute viral infection of the lower respiratory tract most commonly affecting infants during the first year of life with peak attack rates occurring in infants between the ages of 2 and 10 months. Infectious bronchiolitis is unusual in children older than 2 years of age. The occurrence of bronchiolitis peaks during the winter months and persists through early spring. Bronchiolitis remains a major reason why infants under 6 months of age require hospitalization. The hospitalization rate for infants younger than 6 months of age for bronchiolitis approximates 6 per 1,000 children per year. The incidence of bronchiolitis appears to be more common in males than in females.[12,13,40]

Respiratory syncytial virus is the most common cause of bronchiolitis, accounting for 45% to 60% of all cases. During epidemic periods, the incidence of respiratory syncytial virus-induced bronchiolitis can exceed 80% of cases. Parainfluenza viruses type 3 (10% to 15%), type 1 (5% to 10%), and type 2 (1% to 5%) are the second most common pathogens, constituting as a group nearly 25% of cases. Bacteria serve as secondary pathogens in only a small minority of cases.

CLINICAL PRESENTATION

A prodrome suggesting an upper respiratory tract infection, usually lasting from 2 to 7 days, precedes the onset of clinical symptoms. During this prodromal period, infants may be irritable and restless and have a mild fever. The most common clinical signs of bronchiolitis are cough and coryza. As symptoms progress, infants may experience vomiting, diarrhea, noisy breathing, and an increase in respiratory rate. For those infants presenting to a hospital, examination reveals a rapid pulse and a respiratory rate between 40 and 80 breaths per minute. Breathing is labored with retractions of the chest wall, nasal flaring, and grunting. Chest auscultation reveals wheezing and inspiratory rales. Mild conjunctivitis may be observed in up to one-third of infants, whereas 5% to 10% may have a concurrent otitis media.

As a result of limited oral intake because of coughing combined with fever, vomiting, and diarrhea, infants are frequently dehydrated. The increased work of breathing and tachypnea most likely further increases fluid loss. In most cases, this clinical picture persists between 3 and 7 days. Although the hospital course of bronchiolitic children is often variable, substantial clinical improvement is usually observed within the first 2 days, with gradual improvement and resolution over the next 7 to 21 days.

The diagnosis of bronchiolitis is based primarily on history and clinical findings. It is important for the clinician to attempt to differentiate between bronchiolitis and a host of other clinical entities affecting infants, which may produce a similar picture of dyspnea and wheezing. Asthma, congestive heart failure, anatomic airway abnormalities, cystic fibrosis, foreign bodies, and gastroesophageal reflux are the primary disease entities that may present with wheezing on physical examination in children. The isolation of a viral pathogen in the respiratory secretions of a wheezing child establishes a presumptive diagnosis of infectious bronchiolitis. The ability to identify specific viral pathogens is, however, often hindered by the limited availability of special virology laboratories. The proliferation of commercial enzyme-linked immunosorbent assays (ELISA) and fluorescent antibody staining techniques of nasopharyngeal secretions has increased the ability to identify viral antigens within several hours.[16] Identification of respiratory syncytial virus (RSV) by PCR should be routinely available from most clinical laboratories but its relevance to the clinical management of bronchiolitis remains obscure.

Multiple clinical laboratory determinations have been used to assist in the management of cases of bronchiolitis. Roentgenographic evaluation of the chest in children with bronchiolitis yields variable findings but may help to distinguish this illness from other entities characterized by wheezing.[28] The peripheral white blood cell (WBC) count is usually normal or only slightly elevated. In those children requiring hospitalization, abnormalities in blood gas tensions are frequent and appear to relate to disease severity. Hypoxemia is common and increases the respiratory drive, whereas hypercarbia is seen only in the most severe cases. Despite the presence of moderate degrees of hypoxemia, clinical cyanosis is unusual.

▶ TREATMENT: Bronchiolitis

DESIRED OUTCOME

In the well infant, bronchiolitis is usually a self-limiting illness, and reassurance and antipyretics are usually all that are necessary while waiting for resolution of the underlying viral infection. In-hospital support is necessary for the child suffering from respiratory failure or dehydration; underlying cardiac and pulmonary disease potentiate these conditions.

GENERAL APPROACH TO TREATMENT

Almost all otherwise healthy babies with bronchiolitis can be followed as outpatients. Such infants are treated for fever, provided generous amounts of oral fluids, and closely observed for evidence of respiratory deterioration. In severely affected children, the mainstays of therapy for bronchiolitis are oxygen therapy and intravenous fluids. In a subset of patients, aerosolized bronchodilators may have a role. In selected infants, particularly those with underlying pulmonary or cardiac disease or both, with severe acute infection, therapy with the antiviral agent ribavirin may be considered.

PHARMACOLOGIC THERAPY

Aerosolized β_2-adrenergic therapy appears to offer little benefit for the majority of patients and may even be detrimental.[13,40,41] However, this therapy may offer some benefit to the child with a predisposition toward bronchospasm. In hospitalized patients, bronchodilator therapy may be offered initially but should not be pursued in the absence of a clear-cut clinical benefit. Similarly, controlled trials of corticosteroids have failed to reveal any therapeutic benefit (or harmful effect) when administered to bronchiolitic infants.[40,41] As a result, the routine use of systemically administered corticosteroids is discouraged. Although it has been common practice to place children with bronchiolitis in mist tents, there are no data to document the effectiveness of this practice. Because bacteria do not represent primary pathogens in the etiology of bronchiolitis, antibiotics should not be routinely administered. Despite this, many clinicians frequently administer antibiotics initially while awaiting culture results, because the clinical and radiographic findings in bronchiolitis are often suggestive of a possible bacterial pneumonia.[42]

Ribavirin may offer benefit to a subset of infants with bronchiolitis. Although ribavirin, a synthetic nucleoside, possesses *in vitro* antiviral properties against a variety of RNA and DNA viruses, including influenza A, influenza B, parainfluenza, and adenovirus,[43] it is approved only in aerosolized form against RSV.[44] Use of the drug requires special equipment (small-particle aerosol generator) and specially trained personnel for administration via oxygen hood or mist tent.[13] Special care must be taken to avoid drug particle deposition and the resultant clogging of respiratory tubing and valves in mechanical ventilators.[45]

Among hospital admissions for RSV, ribavirin therapy failed to decrease length of hospital stay, number of days in the intensive care unit, or the number of days receiving mechanical ventilation.[46] Consequently, the American Academy of Pediatrics has modified its recommendation for the use of ribavirin from "should be used" to "may be considered."[47] In light of this and because of the requirement for special aerosolization equipment and the cost of the drug itself, most experts recommend reserving use of ribavirin for severely ill patients, especially those with chronic lung disease (particularly bronchopulmonary dysplasia), congenital heart disease, prematurity, and immunodeficiency (especially severe combined immunodeficiency and human immunodeficiency virus [HIV] infection).[48,49] Ribavirin also may be considered in otherwise healthy patients with severe distress because of RSV.

In a select group of infants, prophylaxis against RSV may be warranted. When administered monthly during the RSV season, both respiratory syncytial virus immune globulin (RSVIG)[50] and palivizumab[51] (a monoclonal antibody for RSV) may decrease the number of RSV episodes and the need for hospitalization. Among the two, palivizumab appears to be preferred, given its ease of administration, lack of administration-related adverse effects, and noninterference with select immunizations.

PNEUMONIA

EPIDEMIOLOGY

Pneumonia is the most common infectious cause of death in the United States, where approximately 4 million cases are diagnosed annually at a cost of $23 billion dollars to the health care system. Pneumonia occurs throughout the year, with the relative prevalence of disease resulting from different etiologic agents varying with the seasons. It occurs in persons of all ages, although the clinical manifestations are most severe in the very young, the elderly, and the chronically ill.

PATHOGENESIS

Microorganisms gain access to the lower respiratory tract by three routes. They may be inhaled as aerosolized particles, or they may enter the lung via the bloodstream from an extrapulmonary site of infection; however, aspiration of oropharyngeal contents, a common occurrence in both healthy and ill persons during sleep, is the major mechanism by which pulmonary pathogens gain access to the normally sterile lower airways and alveoli. When pulmonary defense mechanisms are functioning optimally, aspirated microorganisms are cleared from the region before infection can become established;[1–4] however, aspiration of potential pathogens from the oropharynx can result in pneumonia if lung defenses are impaired. Factors that promote aspiration, such as altered sensorium and neuromuscular disease, may result in an increase in the size of the inoculum delivered to the lower respiratory tract, thereby overwhelming local defense mechanisms. Lung infections with viruses suppress the antibacterial activity of the lung by impairing alveolar macrophage function and mucociliary clearance, thus setting the stage for secondary bacterial pneumonia. Mucociliary transport is also depressed by ethanol and narcotics, and by obstruction of a bronchus by mucus, tumor, or extrinsic compression. All of these factors can severely impair the pulmonary clearance of aspirated bacteria.[1–4]

The most prominent pathogens causing community-acquired pneumonia in otherwise healthy adults are *S. pneumoniae* (pneumococcus) and *M. pneumoniae.* Pneumococcus is the most common cause of bacterial pneumonia in all age groups and accounts for up to 70% of all acute bacterial pneumonias in the United States. *Mycoplasma pneumoniae* is believed to account for 10% to 20% of cases. Legionella, *C. pneumoniae,* and a variety of viruses, also cause pneumonia among otherwise healthy persons.[52] Community-acquired pneumonias caused by *Staphylococcus aureus* and gram-negative rods are observed primarily in the elderly, especially those residing in nursing homes, and in association with alcoholism and other debilitating conditions.[53] The term "atypical" may be applied to pneumonia to indicate that the pneumonia may be caused by an atypical pathogen. Although this is older terminology which is slowly fading to the history books, a reference to atypical pneumonia or atypical pathogens refers to pneumonia (i.e., bilateral lobar pneumonia with a negative Gram stain) caused by *Mycoplasma pneumoniae, Chlamydia pneumoniae*, or Legionella.

Gram-negative aerobic bacilli and *S. aureus* are also the leading causative agents in hospital-acquired pneumonia.[54] Anaerobic bacteria are the most common etiologic agents in pneumonia that follows the gross aspiration of gastric or oropharyngeal contents.

Pneumonia in infants and children is caused by a wider range of microorganisms and, unlike adults, nonbacterial pathogens predominate. Most pneumonias in the pediatric age group are caused by viruses, especially RSV, parainfluenza, and adenovirus. *Mycoplasma pneumoniae* is an important pathogen in older children. Beyond the neonatal period, the pneumococcus is the major bacterial pathogen in childhood pneumonia followed by group A streptococcus and *S. aureus. Haemophilus influenzae* type b, once a major childhood pathogen, has become an infrequent cause of pneumonia since the introduction of active vaccination against this organism in the late 1980s.

CLINICAL PRESENTATION

BACTERIAL PNEUMONIA

Bacterial pneumonia is most commonly caused by the gram-positive streptococci and staphylococci and by gram-negative organisms that normally inhabit the gastrointestinal tract (enterics) and soil and water (nonenterics). In addition, *Legionella pneumophila,* itself a weakly staining gram-negative nonenteric organism, accounts for a small percentage of community- and hospital-acquired bacterial pneumonia. Finally, *Mycobacterium tuberculosis,* an acid-fast staining bacillus, has reemerged as an important cause of pneumonia in urban centers throughout the United States.

Although a wide array of gram-positive and gram-negative organisms can cause pneumonia, they usually present a similar clinical appearance. Typically, the onset of illness is abrupt or subacute, with fever, chills, dyspnea, and productive cough predominating. Pneumococcus, staphylococcus, the enteric gram-negative rods, and occasionally other organisms may produce local irritation or destruction of blood vessels leading to rust-colored sputum or hemoptysis. On physical examination the patient is tachypneic and tachycardic, frequently with chest wall retractions and grunting respirations. Consolidation of the underlying lung is reflected in diminished breath sounds on auscultation over the affected area accompanied by inspiratory crackles as pus-filled alveoli open during lung expansion. Other signs of localized lung consolidation include dullness to percussion, increased tactile fremitus, whisper pectoriloquy, and egophony. Pleural effusions, both sterile and empyematous, may be associated with many of these entities, evidenced by distant breath sounds and a wide area of dulled percussion.

The chest radiograph and sputum examination and culture are the most useful diagnostic tests in gram-positive and gram-negative bacterial pneumonia. Typically, the chest radiograph reveals a dense lobar or segmental infiltrate. Patchy consolidation occasionally may be seen, however, with virtually all these pathogens. Occasionally, pneumonia resulting from hematogenous spread of the organisms results in a diffuse, alveolar pattern on chest radiograph. Gram stain of the expectorated sputum demonstrates many polymorphonuclear cells per high-powered field in the presence of a predominant organism (see Fig. 106–1), which is reflected in heavy growth of a single species on culture. Other laboratory tests are less sensitive or specific. Blood cultures may be helpful in identifying the offending organism but are positive in only a minority of cases. The complete blood count usually reflects a leukocytosis with a predominance of polymorphonuclear cells; in some instances, particularly pneumococcus, the elevation of the WBC count may be pronounced. Normal or mildly elevated WBC counts, however, do not exclude bacterial pneumonic disease. The patient may also be hypoxic as reflected by low oxygen saturation on arterial blood gas or pulse oximetry.

Although the clinical appearance of the gram-positive and gram-negative pneumonias are similar, there are epidemiologic and clinical clues that render one more likely than the others.

Gram-Positive Bacteria

Pneumococcus is the most common community-acquired bacterial pneumonia, accounting for 25% to 70% of cases. It is particularly prevalent and severe in patients with splenic dysfunction, diabetes mellitus, chronic cardiopulmonary or renal disease, or HIV infection. *S. aureus* pneumonia occurs in both the community and hospital setting.[54] Community-acquired disease with *S. aureus* is identified most frequently in young infants, patients with early cystic fibrosis, and those recovering from an antecedent respiratory viral infection. *S. aureus* is a prominent cause of nosocomial pneumonia and may result from hematogenous spread from a distant source. In both settings, it is characteristically severe and accompanied by the formation of pneumatoceles (air-containing cavities within the lung). Group B streptococcus, although rare in adults, is the most common cause of bacterial pneumonia among neonates, where it typically causes a clinical and radiographic picture nearly indistinguishable from hyaline membrane disease.[55] Group A streptococcus is an uncommon cause of community-acquired pneumonia and frequently occurs after a viral respiratory tract infection. Only occasionally is it associated with streptococcal pharyngitis. The organism is pyogenic, and the presentation can be severe.

Enteric Gram-Negative Bacteria

Community-acquired enteric gram-negative pneumonia is identified most frequently among patients with chronic illness, especially alcoholism and diabetes mellitus. The enteric gram-negative bacteria are also leading causes of nosocomial pneumonia, because the upper respiratory tract becomes rapidly colonized with gram-negative organisms after hospitalization, particularly among critically ill patients and those receiving antibiotics. Outbreaks of nosocomial disease occasionally may be caused by contaminated respiratory therapy equipment. *Klebsiella pneumoniae* is the most frequently encountered pathogen among the gram-negative enteric bacteria, although the relative prominence of these organisms varies from hospital to hospital. The gram-negative bacilli are associated with high mortality, sometimes exceeding 50%; their potential to produce significant morbidity and mortality has also been enhanced by the emergence of highly antibiotic-resistant organisms in some hospital settings.[56]

Nonenteric Gram-Negative Bacteria

The most prominent nonenteric gram-negative rods associated with pneumonia include *Pseudomonas, Haemophilus,* and *Moraxella.* Like the enteric gram-negative organisms, *Pseudomonas aeruginosa* is a frequent cause of hospital-acquired pneumonia and is particularly prominent among neutropenic and burn patients.[56] In addition, cystic fibrosis patients suffer from chronic, multilobar infections with *P. aeruginosa,* as well as other pseudomonas species; these infections are punctuated with acute exacerbations.[57] *H. influenzae* type b historically has been a prominent pathogen in childhood pneumonia. Since the introduction of the conjugated haemophilus vaccines in the late 1980s, however, there has been a dramatic drop in the incidence of all invasive disease because of this organism in the pediatric age group Two different clinical presentations of *H. influenzae* pneumonia are still seen in adults, however. The most common by far is the bronchopneumonia form, which develops most frequently in patients with underlying chronic lung disease and is believed to represent, in most patients, an exacerbation of chronic bronchitis. In the second form of *H. influenzae* pneumonia, segmental or lobar involvement predominates. The course of this illness is more acute, with sudden onset of cough, fever, and pleuritic chest pain. Finally, *M. catarrhalis,* an important cause of otitis media and sinusitis, has been found to be an increasingly important cause of lower respiratory tract infections in immunoincompetent and hospitalized patients.

Legionella pneumophila

Of the several *Legionella* species known to cause pneumonia in humans, *L. pneumophila* is by far the most important and accounts for 2% to 15% of all community-acquired pneumonias in North America and Europe.[58] *Legionella* is a water and soil organism and is most probably transmitted by the inhalation of aerosols containing the organism or by microaspiration of contaminated water. Outbreaks of illness caused by *L. pneumophila* have been linked to excavation sites and to contaminated water from air conditioners and showers. Person-to-person transmission has not been demonstrated. In addition to epidemics, *L. pneumophila* causes sporadic illness that peaks in summer and fall. Individuals who are male, middle age or older, immunocompromised, chronic bronchitics, or cigarette smokers are at increased risk.

Infection with *L. pneumophila* is characterized by multisystem involvement, including rapidly progressive pneumonia. It has a gradual onset, with prominent constitutional symptoms, such as malaise, lethargy, weakness, and anorexia, occurring early in the course of the illness. A dry, nonproductive cough is initially present, which becomes productive of mucoid or purulent sputum over several days. Fevers exceeding 40°C (104°F) develop in more than half of patients and are typically unremitting and associated with a relative bradycardia. Pleuritic chest pain and progressive dyspnea may be seen. Extrapulmonary symptoms remain evident throughout the course of the illness, particularly diarrhea, nausea, and vomiting. Myalgias and arthralgias also occur. Substantial changes in a patient's mental status, often out of proportion to the degree of fever, are seen in approximately one-fourth of patients. Obtundation, hallucinations, grand mal seizures, and focal neurologic findings are also associated with this illness. Chest roentgenograms initially reveal patchy alveolar infiltrates that may be bilateral. Progression to lobar or multilobar consolidation is frequent, as are small pleural effusions.

Laboratory findings include leukocytosis with a predominance of mature and immature granulocytes in 50% to 75% of patients. Urinalysis may reveal proteinuria, hematuria, and casts; liver function tests may be abnormal. Hyponatremia and hypophosphatemia have also been frequently reported. Because *L. pneumophila* stains poorly with commonly used stains, routine microscopic examination of sputum is of little diagnostic value. While it exhibits slow growth and has highly selective growth requirements, *L. pneumophila* has been successfully isolated from tissue using a specialized medium. Direct fluorescent antibody examination of respiratory tract secretions, lung tissue, or pleural fluid is the most rapid means of establishing the diagnosis. The sensitivity of this method approaches 70% for sputum and 90% for lung tissue, and diagnostic specificity is high for both.[58] Commercially available urine antigen tests have been developed for *L. pneumophila;* these tests are 70% sensitive and remain positive for weeks, even after effective antibiotics have been started. Because these diagnostic tests are unavailable in many clinical laboratories, the diagnosis of Legionnaire's disease often is presumptive and based on a suggestive clinical presentation.

Anaerobic Pneumonia

Anaerobic pneumonitis is most likely to occur in individuals predisposed to aspiration by impaired consciousness and may be more prevalent in those with periodontal disease or dysphagia. In addition, bronchogenic carcinoma is an associated underlying condition. A variety of gram-positive and gram-negative anaerobic bacteria indigenous to the upper airway may cause pneumonitis when large quantities of oropharyngeal secretions are aspirated into the lower airways. The organisms most frequently implicated are *Peptostreptococcus spp., Fusobacteria, Bacteroides melaninogenicus, Bacteroides fragilis,* and *Peptococcus spp.;* polymicrobial infections with anaerobes and aerobes, such as *S. aureus, S. pneumoniae,* and gram-negative bacilli, are common.[59]

The course of illness is typically indolent with cough, low-grade fever, and weight loss, although an acute presentation may occur. Rigors are notably absent, and bacteremia is rare. Putrid sputum, when present, is highly suggestive of the diagnosis. Chest radiographs reveal infiltrates typically located in dependent lung segments, and lung abscesses develop in 20% of patients 1 to 2 weeks into the course of the illness.[59]

Tuberculosis

The acid-fast bacillus *M. tuberculosis* causes tuberculosis. After years of steady decline, the number of cases of pneumonia caused by *M. tuberculosis* in the United States began to increase in the mid- to late 1980s. The new epidemic was a consequence of an increased incidence in prison inmates, intravenous drug abusers, immigrants, and, most prominently, HIV-infected patients,[60] and is most prominent in urban neighborhoods afflicted with crowded conditions and poor access to health care. Unlike previous eras in which tuberculosis was most frequently seen in elderly men, infection currently is identified in increasing numbers of young minority adults.[61] The reason for the resurgence of tuberculosis is at least partially related to coinfection with HIV; HIV-infected patients are more likely to develop symptomatic disease with its associated fits of coughing than their immunocompetent counterparts, and this enables further spread of infection.[62] Other groups prone to tuberculosis include the homeless and patients in chronic care facilities and homes for the elderly. Fortunately, since 1992 the incidence of tuberculosis in the United States has declined, reaching a record low. However, worldwide, the incidence continues to increase. Both this sustained worldwide increase of tuberculosis and the past reemergence of tuberculosis in the United States are important reasons for the development of multiple-drug resistance, that is, of mycobacteria that are resistant to two or more of the first-line antituberculosis drugs. Infection caused by these organisms is poorly responsive to alternative therapy and is associated with mortality rates exceeding 50% (see Chap. 110).

Tuberculosis is spread person-to-person through the inhalation of droplet nuclei generated by vigorous coughing. The majority of patients who become infected with *M. tuberculosis* remain asymptomatic despite life-long infection and have a normal chest radiograph. Infection in these patients is detected only through routine skin testing. Less frequently, particularly in those with poor immunity, the infection cannot be contained by local macrophages, and the tuberculous burden grows sufficiently to cause clinical manifestations.

Adult disease (from adolescence onward) begins with constitutional complaints followed by a prominent chronic, troublesome cough productive of mucopurulent material. The infection initially appears in the lung apices with little or no hilar adenopathy and, in advanced disease, results in lung necrosis, producing a cavity containing enormous numbers of organisms. With sufficient cough, the cavitary contents are mobilized and aspirated into other areas of the lung, where additional cavities may be formed.

In contrast, pediatric tuberculosis commonly is associated with little cough even in the presence of extensive pulmonary infection. Instead, the child presents with a subacute course of poor appetite, weight loss, lethargy, fever, and sweats. The chest radiograph reveals a widened mediastinum representing enlarged hilar lymph nodes reacting to the tuberculin inoculum. In progressive cases, the nodes impinge upon or erode through a large bronchus, resulting in a dense consolidation of the segment distal to the lesion. Cavitary disease is uncommon.

Nonbacterial Pneumonia

Viruses, mycoplasma species, chlamydial species, and fungi are recognized causes of pneumonia syndromes in all age groups. The designation atypical pneumonia, distinct from the typical bacterial pneumonia most commonly seen in adults, has been used to describe the illness caused by many of these agents.[63]

Mycoplasma Pneumonia

Taxonomically, the mycoplasmas are included in their own class labeled Mollicutes. Although their small size and filterability are similar to viruses, the structure of their ribosomal RNA indicates that they have evolved from bacteria, and, unlike any virus, they contain cytoplasm and can replicate in an extracellular environment. They are distinguished from eubacteria by their low genetic content; in addition, the mycoplasmas lack a cell wall and are surrounded instead by a lipid membrane.[63]

Mycoplasma pneumonia causes human disease throughout the year, with a slightly increased incidence in fall and early winter. During the summer months when other causes of pneumonia are less common, *M. pneumoniae* is responsible for a greater proportion of cases. Both infection and disease from *M. pneumoniae* are common, with two-thirds of children ages 2 to 5 years and 97% of persons older than 17 years of age having detectable serum antibody to the organism. Overall, *M. pneumoniae* is responsible for approximately 20% of pneumonia cases, although in enclosed populations, such as military recruits and college dormitory residents, it may cause more than 50%. Infection is spread by close person-to-person contact, and the incubation period is 2 to 3 weeks. *Mycoplasma pneumoniae* infections are unusual in children under 5 years of age and show a peak incidence in older children and young adults. Only 3% to 10% of persons infected with *M. pneumoniae* develop pneumonia, with the majority of respiratory tract involvement being manifested as pharyngitis and tracheobronchitis. Asymptomatic infection is apparently common.

Mycoplasma pneumoniae presents with a gradual onset of fever, headache, and malaise, with the appearance 3 to 5 days after the onset of illness of a persistent, hacking cough that initially is nonproductive. Sore throat, ear pain, and rhinorrhea are often present. Chills are only occasionally seen, and pleuritic pain is uncommon. Lung findings are generally limited to rales and rhonchi; findings of consolidation are rarely present. Nonpulmonary manifestations are extremely common and include nausea, vomiting, diarrhea, myalgias, arthralgias, polyarticular arthritis, skin rashes, myocarditis and pericarditis, hemolytic anemia, meningoencephalitis, cranial neuropathies, and Guillain-Barré syndrome. Systemic symptoms generally clear in 1 to 2 weeks, while respiratory symptoms may persist for up to 4 weeks. Although the course of mycoplasmal pneumonia is usually benign and self-limited, severe respiratory disease may develop in patients with sickle cell disease, agammaglobulinemia, and chronic obstructive lung disease.[63]

Radiographic findings are generally more impressive than the patient's physical findings and include patchy or interstitial infiltrates, which are most commonly seen in the lower lobes. Small unilateral, transient pleural effusions are common, but large effusions and empyema are rare. Roentgenographic abnormalities resolve slowly, and 4 to 6 weeks may be required for complete resolution.

Sputum Gram stain may reveal mononuclear or polymorphonuclear leukocytes, with no predominant organism. Although *M. pneumoniae* can be cultured from respiratory secretions using specialized medium, its growth is slow and 2 to 3 weeks may be necessary for culture identification. Indirect evidence of infection by *M. pneumoniae* is the presence of elevated levels of serum cold hemagglutinins. These immunoglobulin M (IgM) antibodies develop in approximately half of patients with mycoplasmal pneumonia and can be elevated in other illnesses, especially viral infection. A definitive diagnosis can also be made by demonstrating a fourfold or greater rise in serum antibodies to *M. pneumoniae;* however, because this test also requires 2 to 4 weeks for results, the diagnosis of mycoplasmal pneumonia during the acute phase of the illness must be based on the characteristic history, appropriate clinical setting, and typical physical findings.

Chlamydial Pneumonia

Chlamydia pneumoniae, formally designated the "TWAR agent," after the laboratory designations for the first two isolates, is a relatively recently identified pathogen antigenically similar to *Chlamydia psitttaci. Chlamydia pneumoniae* infection is ubiquitous worldwide, but only a small percentage of infections results in clinically apparent pneumonia.[64] Conversely, approximately 5% to 15% of pneumonia is associated with this pathogen. Primary-infection chlamydia pneumonia typically occurs in young adults and is characterized by mild respiratory symptoms with a gradual onset. Constitutional manifestations, particularly fever and headache, are common. The radiographic findings are nonspecific and usually consist of multilobular interstitial infiltrates. Immunity is incomplete, and reinfection with *C. pneumoniae* is common, particularly among the elderly. The definitive diagnosis of *C. pneumoniae*-associated pneumonia depends on identification of the organism in sputum. Culture of this organism is difficult, however, and antigen detection systems, though commercially available, are insensitive.

Viral Pneumonia

Viruses are an uncommon cause of pneumonia in adults except in the immunosuppressed. Influenza virus, usually type A, is the most common cause of pneumonia in the adult civilian population, whereas adenoviruses cause most cases in military trainees. In contrast, viruses are by far the most common agents producing pneumonia in infants and young children, with RSV, parainfluenza, and adenovirus producing most cases.

All viral respiratory tract infections occur more commonly in the winter, and rapid person-to-person spread through susceptible populations is typical. Underlying cardiac or pulmonary disease predisposes to an increased incidence and severity of viral lower respiratory tract infection, especially with influenza virus in adults and RSV in children. Radiographic findings are nonspecific and include bronchial wall thickening and perihilar and diffuse interstitial infiltrates. Pleural effusions may be seen, especially in adenovirus and parainfluenza pneumonia.

The clinical pictures produced by respiratory viruses are sufficiently variable and overlap to such a degree that an etiologic diagnosis cannot confidently be made on clinical grounds alone. Although virus isolation in tissue culture is possible, 7 or more days is often required for virus identification; thus, this method usually cannot be relied on for definitive diagnosis during the acute phase of illness. Serologic tests for virus-specific antibodies are often used in the diagnosis of viral infections. The diagnostic fourfold rise in titer between acute and convalescent phase sera may require 2 to 3 weeks to develop. Same-day diagnosis of viral infections is now possible through the use of indirect immunofluorescence tests on exfoliated cells from the respiratory tract. The immunofluorescence technique frequently employs a battery of monoclonal antibodies, including those against influenza A and B, RSV, parainfluenza, and adenovirus to provide rapid diagnosis of a range of viral infections.[16]

TABLE 106–4. Pulmonary Complications of Human Immunodeficiency Virus Infection[66]

Infections
- Viruses
  - Cytomegalovirus
  - Herpes simplex virus
  - Varicella-zoster virus
  - Respiratory syncytial virus and other common respiratory pathogens (parainfluenza virus, adenovirus)
  - Measles virus
- Bacteria
  - Pyogenic organisms (especially *Streptococcus pneumoniae, Haemophilus influenzae*; in late disease, *S. aureus* and gram-negatives)
  - *Mycobacterium tuberculosis*
  - *Mycobacterium avium* complex and other nontuberculous mycobacteria
- Fungi
  - *Histoplasma capsulatum*
  - *Coccidioides immitis*
  - *Cryptococcus neoformans*
  - *Candida spp.*
  - *Aspergillus spp.*
- Parasites
  - *Pneumocystis carinii*
  - *Toxoplasma gondii*
  - Cryptosporidia
  - *Strongyloides stercoralis*
- Malignancies
  - Kaposi's sarcoma
  - Non-Hodgkin's lymphoma
  - Smooth-muscle tumors
- Lymphocytic interstitial pneumonitis
- Nonspecific interstitial pneumonitis
- Drug-induced pneumonitis

PNEUMONIA IN SPECIAL CLINICAL CIRCUMSTANCES

Pneumonia in the Human Immunodeficiency Virus-Infected Patient

Human immunodeficiency virus infects and destroys helper T lymphocytes bearing the CD4 surface molecule; these cells are critical for orchestrating a wide variety of immunologic responses. Their depletion consequently results in the dysfunction of both cell-mediated and humoral immunity. As a result, a broad range of pathogens can cause pneumonia in HIV infection (Table 106–4).[65–67] The HIV-infected patient may be afflicted with pneumonia multiple times in his or her lifetime, particularly in the advanced stages of the disease, and a given episode may be caused by more than one species.

The clinical presentation of pneumonia in HIV-infected persons is frequently not helpful in distinguishing one pathogen from another. The pneumonia usually is subacute in onset and consists of fever, nonproductive cough, and dyspnea. Radiographically, most of these entities produce a multilobular or diffuse pattern. Some practitioners initially treat the HIV-infected patient with pneumonia empirically, covering the most common entities (bacteria and *P. carinii*). More frequently, however, given the wide array of possible pathogens, a specific microbiologic diagnosis is aggressively pursued early in the patient's course through sputum induction or bronchoalveolar lavage to allow a rational choice of an antimicrobial regimen.[65–67] The diagnosis and treatment of HIV-infected patients with pulmonary disease is discussed in detail in Chap. 123.

Pneumonia in the Neutropenic Host

Neutropenia in the cancer patient is a common complication of aggressive chemotherapy but occasionally can result from the cancer itself. The risk of infection in the cytopenic patient is significantly increased when the absolute neutrophil count falls below 500 cells/mm^3 and the neutropenia persists for longer than 7 days.[68–70] In many patients, the duration of chemotherapy-induced cytopenia can be reduced by the judicious application of colony-stimulating factors.[71]

The organisms that cause pneumonia in the cytopenic cancer patient include a broad range of bacteria and fungi. Prominent among these are enteric and nonenteric (particularly pseudomonas) gram-negative rods, streptococci, and staphylococci, as well as the fungi candida, aspergillus, and mucor.[68–70] The chest radiograph may reveal the lobar pattern typical of bacterial infection in the normal host, or it may exhibit a diffuse pattern; sometimes the pneumonia remains invisible by chest radiograph until the neutropenia resolves. Noninfectious entities may also cause pulmonary symptoms; these include toxicity from radiation or chemotherapy or infiltration of the lung parenchyma by the tumor itself.

Nosocomial Pneumonia

After the urinary tract and the bloodstream, the lungs are the most frequent site of infection acquired in the hospital.[56,72] Nosocomial pneumonia is seen most commonly in critically ill patients. Several factors that predispose to the development of nosocomial pneumonia include the severity of illness, duration of hospitalization, and prior antibiotic exposure. The strongest predisposing factor, however, is mechanical ventilation (intubation), which bypasses the natural airway defenses against the migration of upper respiratory tract organisms into the lower tract. This situation is exacerbated by the wide use of H_2-receptor blocking agents in the intensive care unit.[56,73] Such use increases the pH of gastric secretions and may promote the proliferation of microorganisms in the upper gastrointestinal tract. Subclinical microaspirations are events that occur routinely in intubated patients resulting in the inoculation of bacteria-contaminated gastric contents into the lung and a higher incidence of nosocomial pneumonia. Ventilator-associated pneumonia can be accurately diagnosed by any one of multiple standard criteria including histopathologic examination of lung tissue obtained by open-lung biopsy; rapid cavitation of a pulmonary infiltrate in the absence of cancer or tuberculosis; positive pleural fluid culture; and same species with an identical antibiogram for a pathogen(s) isolated from blood and respiratory secretions without another identifiable source of bacteremia.[74]

The organisms most commonly associated with nosocomial pneumonia are *S. aureus* and enteric (e.g., *Klebsiella* or *E. coli*) and nonenteric (e.g., *Pseudomonas*) gram-negative bacilli, the organisms that colonize the pharynx of the hospitalized, critically ill patient. The diagnosis of nosocomial pneumonia is usually established by the presence of a new infiltrate on chest radiograph, fever, worsening respiratory status, and the appearance of thick, neutrophil-laden respiratory secretions. In actuality, the diagnosis is often difficult to make in the intensively ill patient with underlying lung pathology that can itself be associated with an abnormal, changing radiograph, such as congestive heart failure or chronic lung disease. Broad-spectrum antibiotics frequently are empirically started even in equivocal circumstances, with bronchoscopy reserved for poorly responsive cases.[73,75]

▶ TREATMENT: Pneumonia

DESIRED OUTCOME

Eradication of the offending organism through the selection of the appropriate antibiotic and complete clinical cure are the goals of therapy for bacterial pneumonia. Therapy should minimize associated morbidity, including either one or both of these: reversible or irreversible disease and drug-induced organ toxicity (e.g., renal, lung, or hepatic dysfunction). Most cases of viral pneumonia are self-limiting, although therapy of influenza pneumonia with specific antiviral agents (amantidine or rimantidine) may hasten recovery. All efforts should focus on the design of the most cost-effective approach to therapy. Whenever possible, the oral (versus parenteral) route for drug administration should be selected, encouraging outpatient management rather than hospitalization.

GENERAL APPROACH TO TREATMENT

The first priority in assessing the patient with pneumonia is to evaluate the adequacy of respiratory function and to determine whether there are signs of systemic illness, specifically dehydration or sepsis with resulting circulatory collapse. Oxygen or, in severe cases, mechanical ventilation and fluid resuscitation should be provided as necessary. The second priority is to obtain appropriate sputum samples to determine the microbiologic etiology. In many cases of community-acquired pneumonia, an antibiotic can be appropriately selected without sputum sampling, but in complicated cases (for example, the immunocompromised host) samples may have to be obtained through invasive means. Rehydration should be provided to replace losses that may have occurred because of fever, poor intake, associated vomiting, or all of these. Finally, selection of an appropriate antimicrobial must be made based on the patient's probable or documented microbiology, distribution in the respiratory tract, side effects, and cost.

NONPHARMACOLOGIC THERAPY

The supportive care of the patient with pneumonia includes humidified oxygen for hypoxemia, administration of bronchodilators (albuterol) when bronchospasm is present, and chest physiotherapy with postural drainage if there is evidence of retained secretions. Additional therapeutic adjuncts include adequate hydration (intravenously if necessary), optimal nutritional support, and control of fever.

PHARMACOLOGIC THERAPY

ANTIBIOTIC CONCENTRATIONS

Antibiotic concentrations in respiratory secretions in excess of the pathogen minimal inhibitory concentration (MIC) are necessary for successful treatment of pulmonary infections.[76,77] The concept of a blood-bronchus barrier, analogous but dissimilar to the blood-brain barrier, has been used to assess the characteristics of drug penetration into pulmonary secretions. The ability of a drug to penetrate respiratory secretions depends on multiple physicochemical factors, including molecular size, lipid solubility, and degree of ionization at serum and biologic fluid pH and extent of protein binding. Studies performed in animals and cystic fibrosis patients suggest that larger molecular size favors the accumulation of drugs in bronchial secretions. This finding contrasts with data on drug penetration of other physiologic compartments, such as the cerebrospinal fluid, and may be a result of the trapping of lower-molecular-weight compounds in mucin pores. Nevertheless, the rate at which a drug may accumulate in certain respiratory secretions would appear to remain an important factor relative to the drug's clinical efficacy in treating pulmonary infections. The un-ionized form of a drug and lipid solubility also appear to favor drug penetration. It should be noted that the pH of the infected bronchi is often more acidic than that of normal tissue and blood.[77–79]

Fewer data are available for assessing the influence of drug protein binding on the rate and amount of respiratory secretion penetration. Clearly, it is the free antibiotic fraction reaching the infected site capable of binding to the bacterial cell target that is responsible for antibacterial activity. As the degree of protein binding influences a drug's ability to traverse membranes, a similar relationship would be expected within the lung. However, focusing on the absolute amount for which an antibiotic is bound to plasma/tissue proteins without accounting for the drug's overall antibacterial potency is errant. To completely assess an antibiotic's therapeutic potential in the treatment of pneumonia, or any infectious process, it is prudent to assess the antibiotic's integrated pharmacokinetic-pharmacodynamic characteristics (i.e., bacterial killing may be concentration-dependent or time-dependent) that accounts for the drug's degree of binding to serum proteins, tissue distribution, and *in vitro* potency. Thus, simply focusing on a drug's degree of protein binding is an errant, oversimplistic approach that does not account for the drug's inherent antibacterial activity or distribution characteristics.

The concepts relating to antibiotic activity and overall drug penetration of respiratory secretions outlined above have supported the clinical practice of administering certain antibiotics (aminoglycosides) to achieve high peak serum concentrations on the assumption that higher (and possibly more effective) biologic fluid concentrations of the drug will be achieved. The aminoglycosides are large, polar molecules which diffuse poorly into tissue and respiratory secretions; however, with increasing concentrations as obtained with once daily dosing, increased target tissue concentrations would be expected with increasing individual doses. Substantial clinical experience supports this practice for treating pulmonary infections with certain antibiotics (i.e., concentration-dependent antimicrobials), although more data are needed to describe the relationships between these variables and clinical response (see Chap. 104).

Prior to the availability of newer β-lactam and quinolone antibiotics possessing consistently potent activity against multiple gram-negative pathogens, the administration of antibiotics by direct endotracheal instillation was promoted by some investigators.[77,79] This method of drug administration is an attempt to provide increased topical concentrations of antibiotics that do not appear to penetrate respiratory secretions effectively while reducing the likelihood of systemic toxicity. In addition, greater local concentrations of antibiotics, particularly for the polymyxins and aminoglycosides, are believed to overcome partially the substantial decrease in antibiotic bioactivity observed when these agents interact with the purulent material present in infectious foci.[77–79] Despite these potential theoretical advantages, the role of antibiotic aerosols or direct endotracheal instillation in clinical practice remains controversial.

Sputum is frequently assessed as possibly representing the pharmacodynamic interface for pulmonary infections. However, sputum represents only one of many pulmonary fluids and secretions, although sputum may serve as a reservoir for pathogen growth. These beliefs have led many investigators to assess antibiotic concentrations in sputum, frequently describing sputum drug concentrations as a ratio of serum to sputum drug concentration. Although sputum drug concentrations provide us with some insight into the characteristics of drug penetration of respiratory secretions, caution should be exercised in the interpretation of these data. Data describing sputum drug concentrations are often difficult to interpret because of differences in analytic techniques, method of sputum sampling, and random nature of sampling times relative to drug dose. Moreover, representation of sputum drug concentrations as a ratio of serum drug concentration can be misleading and most probably should be described relative to absolute drug concentration or apparent area under the drug-concentration curve in sputum. To more accurately describe the distribution characteristics of antimicrobial agents in sputum, research studies should be designed to allow sequential repeated sputum sampling over a dosage interval under both first-dose and steady-state conditions. Thus, until greater sophistication is realized in our understanding of the relationships between antibiotic concentrations in specific anatomic sites, plasma (blood)-based integrated pharmacokinetic-pharmacodynamic correlates should be used for antibiotic and dose selection.

SELECTION OF ANTIMICROBIAL AGENTS

The treatment of bacterial pneumonia, like the treatment of most infectious diseases, initially involves the empiric institution of a relatively broad-spectrum antibiotic that is effective against probable pathogens after appropriate cultures and specimens for laboratory evaluation have been obtained.[80] Therapy should be narrowed to cover specific pathogens after the results of cultures are known. Multiple factors that help define the potential pathogens involved include patient age, previous and current medication history, underlying disease(s), major organ function, and present clinical status. These factors must be evaluated to select properly an effective empiric antibiotic regimen, as well as the most appropriate route for drug administration (oral, parenteral). For a more detailed discussion on the principles of antibiotic selection, see Chap. 104.

Numerous antibiotics are available, and the majority are effective in the treatment of bacterial pneumonia. Superiority of one compound over another when both demonstrate similar *in vitro* activity and tissue distribution characteristics is difficult to define. Our opinions on appropriate empiric choices for the treatment of bacterial pneumonias relative to a patient's underlying disease are shown in Table 106–5 for adults and Table 106–6 for children. A complete listing of antimicrobial agents for specific pathogens is beyond the scope of this chapter and is presented in Chap. 104. Table 106–7 lists dosages for the treatment of bacterial pneumonia.

The list of commercially available antimicrobial agents with documented bacterial and clinical effectiveness in the treatment of pneumonia appears endless. The large number of expensive drugs mandates critical evaluation for formulary selection and clinical use. Similarities of *in vitro* activity, resistance to bacterial-inactivating enzymes, and overall effectiveness often make rational therapeutic decisions difficult and even appear random. Some general principles, however, may be applied to guide rational antibiotic choice including direct comparison of the antibiotic's likely attainment of

TABLE 106–5. Empiric Antimicrobial Therapy for Pneumonia in Adults[a]

Clinical Setting	Usual Pathogen(s)	Presumptive Therapy
Previously healthy, ambulatory patient	Pneumococcus, *Mycoplasma pneumoniae*	Macrolide/azilide,[b] tetracycline[c]
Elderly	Pneumococcus, gram-negative bacilli (such as *Klebsiella pneumoniae*); *Staphylococcus aureus, Haemophilus influenzae*	Piperacillin/tazobactam, cephalosporin[d]; carbapenem[e]
Chronic bronchitis	Pneumococcus, *H. influenzae, M. catarrhalis*	Amoxicillin, tetracycline,[c] TMP/SMZ,[f] cefuroxime, amoxicillin/clavulanate, macrolide/azilide,[b] quinolone
Alcoholism	Pneumococcus, *K. pneumoniae, S. aureus, H. influenzae,* possibly mouth anaerobes	Ticarcillin/clavulanate, piperacillin/tazobactam, plus aminoglycoside; carbapenem,[e] quinolone[g]
Aspiration		
Community	Mouth anaerobes	Penicillin or clindamycin
Hospital/residential care	Mouth anaerobes, *S. aureus,* gram-negative enterics	Clindamycin, ticarcillin/clavulanate, piperacillin/tazobactam, plus aminoglycoside
Nosocomial pneumonia	Gram-negative bacilli (such as *K. pneumoniae, Enterobacter spp., Pseudomonas aeruginosa*), *S. aureus*	Piperacillin/tazobactam, carbapenem[e] or expanded spectrum cephalosporin[h] plus aminoglycoside, quinolone[g]

[a]See section on treatment of bacterial pneumonia.
[b]Macrolide/azilide: erythromycin, clarithromycin/azithromycin.
[c]Tetracycline: tetracycline HCl, doxycycline.
[d]Cephalosporin: cefuroxime, ceftriaxone, cefotaxime.
[e]Carbapenem: imipenem/cilastatin, meropenem.
[f]TMP/SMZ, trimethoprim-sulfamethoxazole.
[g]Quinolone: ciprofloxacin, gatifloxacin, levofloxacin.
[h]Expanded spectrum cephalosporin: ceftazidime, cefepime.

TABLE 106–6. Empiric Antimicrobial Therapy for Pneumonia in Pediatric Patients[a]

Age	Usual Pathogen(s)	Presumptive Therapy
1 month	Group B streptococcus, *Haemophilus influenzae* (nontypable), *Escherichia coli*, *Staphylococcus aureus*, *Listeria*	Ampicillin/sulbactam, cephalosporin[b] carbapenem[c]
	CMV, RSV, adenovirus	Ribavirin for RSV
1–3 months	*Chlamydia*, possibly *Ureaplasma*, CMV, *Pneumocystis carinii* (afebrile pneumonia syndrome)	Macrolide/azilide,[d] TMP/SMZ
	RSV	Ribavirin
	Pneumococcus, *S. aureus*	Semisynthetic penicillin[e] or cephalosporin[f]
3 months–6 years	Pneumococcus, *H. influenzae*, RSV, adenovirus, parainfluenza	Amoxicillin or cephalosporin[f] Ampicillin/sulbactam, amoxicillin/clavulanate Ribavirin for RSV
>6 years	Pneumococcus, *Mycoplasma pneumoniae*, adenovirus	Macrolide/azilide[d] Cephalosporin,[f] amoxicillin/clavulanate

CMV, cytomegalovirus; RSV, respiratory syncytial virus; TMP/SMZ, trimethoprim-sulfamethoxazole.
[a]See section on treatment of bacterial pneumonia.
[b]Third-generation cephalosporin: ceftriaxone, cefotaxime, cefepime. Note that cephalosporins are not active against *Listeria*.
[c]Carbapenem: imipenem/cilastatin, meropenem.
[d]Macrolide/azilide: erythromycin, clarithromycin, azithromycin.
[e]Semisynthetic penicillin: nafcillin, oxacillin.
[f]Second-generation cephalosporin: cefuroxime, cefprozil.
See text for details regarding ribavirin treatment for RSV infection.

the defined pharmacokinetic-pharmacodynamic target correlate for specific bacterial species within the infected site. For the treatment of bacterial pneumonia, it is projected that for concentration-independent antimicrobials (e.g., β-lactams, carbapenems) that the plasma drug concentration exceed the pathogen MIC for >50% of the dosing interval; for concentration-dependent antimicrobials (i.e., aminioglycosides, fluoroquinolones) the peak drug concentration to pathogen MIC ratio >8–10 or the ratio of the pathogen MIC/antibiotic area under the curve (AUC) >25–40 for gram-positive pathogens and >100 for gram-negative pathogens correlates with bacteriologic cure. An understanding and application of these inherent drug characteristics would appear to be of the utmost importance for the selection of an optimal therapeutic regimen. Thus, whenever possible, identification of the causative pathogen and expected/defined antibiotic activity (i.e., MIC) is of paramount importance to the selection/design of the optimal antibiotic regimen.

COMMUNITY-ACQUIRED PNEUMONIA

For community-acquired pneumonia, the bacterial causes are relatively constant, even across geographic areas and patient populations.

TABLE 106–7. Antibiotic Doses for the Treatment of Bacterial Pneumonia

Antibiotic class		Daily Antibiotic dose Pediatric (mg/kg/day)	Adult (total dose/day)
Macrolide	Clarithromycin	15	0.5–1 g
	Erythromycin	30–50	1–2 g
Azilide	Azithromycin	10 mg/kg × 1 day, then 5 mg/kg/day × 4 days	500 mg/day 1, then 250 mg/day × 4 days
Tetracycline[a]	Tetracycline HCl	25–50	1–2 g
	Oxytetracycline	2–4	0.1–0.2 g
Penicillin (combinations)	Ampicillin/amoxicillin	100–200	2–6 g
	Amoxicillin/clavulanate[b]	40–90	0.75–1 g
	Piperacillin/tazobactam	200–300	12 g
	Ampicillin/sulbactam	100–200	4–8 g
Extended-spectrum cephalosporins	Ceftriaxone	50–75	1–2 g
	Ceftazidime	150	2–6 g
	Cefepime	100–150	2–4 g
Quinolones	Gatifloxicin[c]	10–20	0.4 g
	Levofloxacin	10–15	0.5–0.75 g
	Ciprofloxacin	20–30	0.5–1.5 g
Aminoglycosides	Gentamicin	7.5	4–6 mg/kg/day
	Tobramycin	7.5	4–6 mg/kg/day

Doses may be increased for more severe disease and may require modification in patients with organ dysfunction.
[a]Tetracyclines are rarely used in pediatric patients, particularly in those younger than 8 years of age because of tetracycline-induced permanent tooth discoloration.
[b]Higher dose amoxicillin, amoxicillin-clavulanate (e.g., 90 mg/kg/day is used for penicillin-resistant *S. pneumoniae*)
[c]Quinolones are avoided in pediatric patients because of the potential for cartilage damage; however, their use in pediatrics is emerging. Doses shown are extrapolated from adults and will require further study.

Unfortunately, pathogen resistance to standard antimicrobials is increasing (e.g., penicillin-resistant pneumococci) necessitating careful attention by the clinician to local and regional bacterial susceptibility patterns.[81] Thus, whenever possible, based on presumed antibacterial susceptibility, initial therapy should consist of older, less-expensive agents, with newer antibiotics (e.g., latest fluoroquinolone or newest antimicrobial released) reserved for unresponsive illness or special circumstances. The indiscriminate use of recently introduced agents increases health care costs and, in some instances (such as with the widespread use of quinolones), induces resistance among a significant percentage of community-acquired organisms.[82,83] It must be emphasized, however, that the rapidly evolving epidemiology of bacterial resistance, including the increasing emergence of penicillin-resistant pneumococcus in many areas of the United States and Europe,[84] forces the clinician to be vigilant and knowledgeable about antibiotic sensitivity patterns in each community. The indiscriminate use of antimicrobials for the treatment of pneumonia has contributed to the problem of antimicrobial resistance underscoring the need for defining the optimal antibiotic regimen for each patient.[80,81]

NOSOCOMIAL PNEUMONIA

Antibiotic selection within the hospital environment demands greater care because of constant changes in antibiotic resistance patterns *in vitro* and *in vivo*. Ironically, some β-lactam antibiotics, which were developed to treat multiple antibiotic-resistant hospital-acquired organisms, can themselves induce broad-spectrum bacterial β-lactamases and thereby lead to even greater problems with resistance.[84] These facts underscore the importance of regularly documenting the epidemiology of pathogens and infectious diseases within a specific practice or institution. As a result, an antimicrobial agent for a specific infectious disease favored in one practice site may not be the most desirable selection in another, despite similarities in size and patient profile. Strict and careful control and, possibly, rotation of empiric antibiotics in the hospital environment may help to limit the emergence of resistant organisms. Newer antibiotics developed to treat resistant, hospital-acquired pathogens are, however, costly; therefore, their use must be moderated to some extent in an era where capitated hospital costs and mandated budget cuts will not tolerate careless antibiotic use.

FLUOROQUINOLONE ANTIBIOTICS

The *in vitro* spectrum of antibacterial activity of systemically absorbed fluoroquinolone antibiotics, such as ciprofloxacin, levofloxacin, moxifloxacin, and gatifloxacin, suggests that these drugs have an important role in the treatment of bacterial infections of the lower respiratory tract. Numerous clinical studies describe the efficacy of these drugs for the treatment of purulent bronchitis, acute exacerbations of chronic bronchitis, pneumonia, and cystic fibrosis.[85] The widespread use of earlier analogs (ciprofloxacin) by primary care physicians has led, however, to pathogen resistance and treatment failures, including, perhaps most important, isolates of *S. pneumonia.* Although newer quinolones are more active against common respiratory tract pathogens than older agents, this experience renders it difficult to recommend their indiscriminate use for routine community-acquired pneumonia. Nevertheless, these drugs may be effective alternative agents for the treatment of community-acquired pneumonia or in the initial treatment of nosocomial pneumonia for hospitalized patients and patients residing in extended-care facilities. The availability of newer analogs with broad spectra of antibacterial activity, including *S. pneumoniae* (e.g., gatifloxacin) further enhances the desirability of a quinolone as a first-line agent, expanding the therapeutic armamentarium for both community-acquired and nosocomially acquired pneumonia. At present, quinolone use in pediatrics remains restricted and limited because of possible fluoroquinolone-induced destructive lesions of growing cartilage primarily of the weight-bearing joints. These quinolone-associated arthritic lesions were determined in animals following large doses but have not been reflected in the human experience. The need for quinolones for the treatment of selected infections arising in pediatric patients continues, and their continued safety in these patients has served as the foundation for ongoing controlled, clinical efficacy and safety trials in pediatric patients. United States Food and Drug Administration approval for use of a quinolone antibiotic in children is anticipated within the next few years.

MACROLIDE/AZOLIDE ANTIBIOTICS

Among the more recently introduced classes of oral antibiotics, the newer macrolides possess excellent activity against most *S. pneumoniae* and mycoplasma. Azithromycin and clarithromycin appear to offer viable alternative agents to erythromycin, particularly in those patients who are intolerant to erythromycin analogs (e.g., gastrointestinal upset) and, for azithromycin, in those patients who are taking medications that may result in a clinically significant drug-drug interaction (e.g., erythromycin with carbamazepine or theophylline).[39] Azithromycin offers the added advantage of once-daily dosing and short-course therapy because of the drug's extensive tissue distribution characteristics and prolonged elimination half-life.[39]

PREVENTION

Prevention of some cases of pneumonia is possible through the use of vaccines and medications against selected infectious agents. Polyvalent polysaccharide vaccines are available for two of the leading causes of bacterial pneumonia, pneumococcus and *H. influenzae* type b. Inactivated influenza virus vaccines formulated annually to contain antigens representative of expected prevalent strains are widely available and generally well tolerated. Immunization is recommended for individuals likely to experience serious complications from influenza infection, such as patients with underlying heart or lung disease, chronic renal disease, and the elderly. For a detailed description of the use of these vaccines, see Chap. 122. Although it should not replace active immunization, amantadine may be administered for prevention of influenza A infection, beginning as soon as possible after exposure and continuing for at least 10 days. The recommended dose is 5 mg/kg/day in two to three divided doses not to exceed 150 mg/day in children 1 to 9 years of age and 200 mg/day in two divided doses in patients 9 years of age or older. More recently, the discovery of the importance of neuraminidase to the viability of the influenza A and B virus has led to the development of the most effective drugs available for the prevention and treatment of influenza disease. Oseltamivir and zanamivir are the first of a new class of neuraminidase inhibitors. The influenza virus contains two surface glycoproteins, hemagglutinin and neuraminidase, which interact with viral receptors containing neuraminic acid. Neuraminidase is a tetramer where the highly active site has been conserved among all influenza A and B strains. Under normal conditions, neuraminidase destroys receptors recognized by hemagglutinin, which allows the virus to penetrate secretions, viral replication, and viral release from the cell surface, all of which are necessary for viral propagation and virulence. Thus, inhibition of the activity of neuraminidase by these drugs prevents influenza infection by inhibiting the release of newly formed virus from the surface of infected cells combined with the prevention of viral spreading across the respiratory tract epithelium. Zanamivir is available for aerosol administration, leading to some concern over aerosolization in patients with disease-induced hyperactive airways, whereas oseltamivir is available for oral administration. Both agents are effective in preventing disease, particularly if therapy is begun within 30 hours of symptom onset or exposure (e.g., epidemics) and for treatment in febrile individuals.[86,87]

EVALUATION OF THERAPEUTIC OUTCOMES

After therapy has been instituted, appropriate clinical parameters should be monitored to ensure efficacy and safety of the therapeutic regimen. In patients with bacterial infections of the upper or lower respiratory tract, the time to resolution of initial presenting symptoms and the lack of appearance of new associated symptomatology is important to determine. In patients with community-acquired pneumonia or pneumonia from any source of mild to moderate clinical severity, the time to resolution of cough, decreasing sputum production, and fever, as well as other constitutional symptoms of malaise, nausea, vomiting, and lethargy should be noted. If the patient requires supplemental oxygen therapy, the amount and need should also be regularly assessed. A gradual and persistent improvement in the resolution of these symptoms and therapies should be observed. Initial resolution should be observed within the first 2 days, progressing to complete resolution within 5 to 7 days, but usually in no more than 10 days. In patients with nosocomial pneumonia or substantial underlying diseases, or both, additional parameters can be followed including the magnitude and character of the peripheral blood WBC count, chest radiograph, and blood gas determinations. Similar to patients with less-severe disease, some resolution of symptoms should be observed within 2 days of instituting antibiotic therapy. If within 2 days of starting seemingly appropriate antibiotic therapy, no resolution of symptoms are observed, or if the patient's clinical status is deteriorating, the appropriateness of initial antibiotic therapy should be critically reassessed. The patient should be carefully evaluated for deterioration in their underlying concurrent disease(s). Additionally, the caregiver should consider the possibility of changing the initial antibiotic therapy to expand antimicrobial coverage not included in the original regimen (e.g., mycoplasma, legionella, and anaerobes). Furthermore, the possible need for antifungal therapy (amphotericin B) should be considered. Some resolution of symptoms should be observed within 2 days of starting proper antibiotic therapy, with complete resolution expected within 10 to 14 days.

▶ PRINCIPLES OF PHARMACOTHERAPY

- In the United States, respiratory infections remain the major cause of morbidity from acute illness and most likely represent the most common reasons why patients seek medical attention.
- The majority of pulmonary infections follow colonization of the upper respiratory tract with potential pathogens, whereas less commonly, microbes gain access to the lung via the blood from an extrapulmonary source or by inhalation of infected aerosol particles. The competency of a patient's immune status is an important factor influencing the susceptibility to infection, etiologic cause, and disease severity.
- An appropriate treatment regimen for the patient with uncomplicated lower respiratory tract infection can usually be established by patient history, physical examination, chest radiograph, and properly collected sputum for culture interpreted in light of current knowledge of the most common lung pathogens and their antibiotic susceptibility patterns within one's community.
- Acute bronchitis is most commonly caused by respiratory viruses and almost always is self-limiting with therapy targeting associated symptoms, such as lethargy, malaise, or fever (ibuprofen or acetaminophen); fluids for rehydration; and in some patients, cough suppressants. The routine use of antibiotics should be avoided.
- Chronic bronchitis is a result of several contributing factors; the most prominent of these are cigarette smoking, exposure to occupational dusts, fumes, environmental pollution, and bacterial (and possibly viral) infection. The hallmark of this disease is chronic cough productive of purulent sputum and the persistent presence of microorganisms in the patient's sputum.
- The treatment of acute exacerbations of chronic bronchitis include attempts to mobilize and enhance sputum expectoration (chest physiotherapy, humidification of inspired air), oxygen if needed, aerosolized bronchodilators (albuterol) in select patients with demonstrated benefit and antibiotics.
- Antibiotic selection for the treatment of acute exacerbations of chronic bronchitis is dependent on the drug's inherent activity against presumed and identified pathogens, the patient's severity of disease (see Table 106–1), least propensity for drug-drug interactions, and cost.
- Respiratory syncytial virus is the most common cause of acute bronchiolitis, an infection that mostly affects infants during their first year of life. In the well infant, bronchiolitis is usually a self-limiting viral illness, whereas in the child with underlying respiratory or cardiac disease, or both, the child may develop severe respiratory compromise (failure) necessitating in-hospital treatment (such as rehydration, oxygen, and, in select patients, bronchodilator, ribavirin aerosol, or both).
- The most prominent pathogens causing community-acquired pneumonia in otherwise healthy adults are *S. pneumoniae* (70%) and *M. pneumoniae* (10% to 20%), whereas the most common pathogens causing hospital-acquired pneumonia (including nursing home residents) are *S. aureus* and gram-negative aerobic bacilli. Anaerobic bacteria are the most common etiologic agents in pneumonia that follows aspiration of gastric or oropharyngeal contents.
- Uncomplicated community-acquired pneumonia can usually be effectively treated with oral antibiotics. Humidified oxygen for hypoxemia, bronchodilators (albuterol) when bronchospasm is present, rehydration fluids, and chest physiotherapy for marked accumulation of retained respiratory secretions may be needed. Antibiotic regimens should be selected based on presumed causative pathogens (see Tables 106–5 and 106–6) and pulmonary distribution characteristics, and they should be adjusted to provide optimal activity against pathogens identified by culture (sputum or blood).

- The treatment of nosocomial pneumonia requires aggressive therapy with careful consideration to the dominance and susceptibility patterns of the pathogens present within the institution. The epidemiology of these common pathogens should be evaluated on a regular basis to identify changing resistance patterns and subsequent alternation of treatment guidelines.

REFERENCES

1. DeLong PA, Kotloff RM. An overview of pulmonary host defenses. Semin Roentgenol 2000;35:118–123.
2. Ward PA. Role of complement, chemokines and regulatory cytokines in acute lung injury. Ann N Y Acad Sci 1996;796:104–112.
3. Brandtzaeg P. The role of humoral mucosal immunity in the induction and maintenance of chronic airway infections. Am J Respir Crit Care Med 1995;151:2081–2087.
4. Standiford TJ. Cytokines and pulmonary defenses. Curr Opin Pulm Med 1997;3:81–88.
5. Yungbluth M. The laboratory diagnosis of pneumonia: The role of the community hospital pathologist. Clin Lab Med 1995;15:209–234.
6. Griffen JJ, Meduri GU. New approaches in the diagnosis of nosocomial pneumonia. Med Clin North Am 1994;78:1091–1122.
7. Cook DJ, Brun-Buisson C, Guyatt GH, et al. Evaluation of new diagnostic technologies: Bronchoalveolar lavage and the diagnosis of ventilator associated pneumonia. Crit Care Med 1994;22:1314–1322.
8. Galvin JR, Gingrich RD, Hoffman E, et al. Ultrafast computed tomography of the chest. Radiol Clin North Am 1994;32:775–793.
9. Marik PE, Brown WJ. A comparison of bronchoscopic vs. blind protected specimen brush sampling in patients with suspected ventilator-associated pneumonia. Chest 1995;108:203–207.
10. Kirtland SH, Corley DE, Winterbauer RH, et al. The diagnosis of ventilator-associated pneumonia: A comparison of histologic, microbiologic, and clinical criteria. Chest 1997;112:445–457.
11. Jimenez P, Saldias F, Meneses M, et al. Diagnostic bronchoscopy in patients with community-acquired pneumonia: Comparison between bronchoalveolar lavage and telescoping plugged catheter cultures. Chest 1993;103:1023–1027.
12. Stark JM. Lung infections in children. Curr Opin Pediatr 1993;5: 273–280.
13. Everard ML. Bronchiolitis: Origins and optimal management. Drugs 1995;49:885–896.
14. Falck G, Gnarpe J, Gnarpe H. Prevalence of *Chlamydia pneumoniae* in healthy children and in children with respiratory tract infections. Pediatr Infect Dis J 1997;16:549–554.
15. Rodriguez WJ. Management strategies for respiratory syncytial virus infections in infants. J Pediatr 1999;135(suppl 2):S45–S50.
16. Adcock PM, Stout GG, Hauck MA, Marshall GS. Effect of rapid viral diagnosis on the management of children hospitalized with lower respiratory tract infection. Pediatr Infect Dis J 1997;16: 842–846.
17. Black S. Epidemiology of pertussis. Pediatr Infect Dis J 1997;16 (suppl 4):S85–S89.
18. Visentin M, Salmona M, Tacconi MT. Reye's and Reye-like syndromes: Drug-related diseases? Drug Metab Rev 1995;27:517–539.
19. Katcher ML. Cold, cough, and allergy medications: Uses and abuses. Pediatr Rev 1996;17:12–17.
20. MacKay DN. Treatment of acute bronchitis in adults without underlying lung disease. J Gen Intern Med 1996;11:557–562.
21. O'Brien KL, Dowell SF, Schwartz B, et al. Cough illness/bronchitis—Principles of judicious use of antimicrobial agents. Pediatrics 1998;101: 178–181.
22. Nicholson KG. Use of antivirals in influenza in the elderly: Prophylaxis and therapy. Gerontology 1996;42:280–289.
23. Treanor JJ, Hayden FG, Vrooman PS, et al. Efficacy and safety of the oral neuraminidase inhibitor oseltamivir in treating acute influenza: A randomized controlled trial. JAMA 2000;283(8):1016–1024.
24. Monto AS, Webster A, Keene O. Randomized, placebo-controlled studies of inhaled zanamivir in the treatment of influenza A and B: Pooled efficacy analysis. J Antimicrob Chemother 1999;44(suppl B):23–29.
25. Adams SG, Anzueto A. Antibiotic therapy in acute exacerbations of chronic bronchitis. Semin Respir Infect 2000;15:234–247.
26. American Thoracic Society. Standards for the diagnosis and care of patients with chronic bronchitis. Am J Respir Crit Care Med 1995;152 (suppl):S78–S122.
27. Grossman RF. Acute exacerbations of chronic bronchitis. Hosp Pract 1997;132:85–94.
28. Godfrey S. Bronchioloitis and asthma in infancy and early childhood. Thorax 1996;51(suppl 2):S60–S64.
29. Wilson R, Wilson CB. Defining subsets of patients with chronic bronchitis. Chest 1997;112:303S–309S.
30. Anzueto A, Jubran M, Ohan JA, et al. Effects of aerosolized surfactant in patients with stable bronchitis: A prospective randomized controlled trial. JAMA 1997;278:957–960.
31. Wilson R, Tillotson G, Ball P. Clinical studies in chronic bronchitis: A need for better definition and classification of severity. J Antimicrob Chemother 1996;37:205–208.
32. Saint S, Bent S, Vittinghoff E, Grady D. Antibiotics in chronic obstructive pulmonary disease exacerbations: A meta analysis. JAMA 1995;273:957–960.
33. Russo RL, D'Aprile MD. Role of antimicrobial therapy in acute exacerbations of chronic obstructive pulmonary disease. Ann Pharmacother 2001;35:576–581.
34. Ball P. Epidemiology and treatment of chronic bronchitis and its exacerbations. Chest 1995;108:43S–52S.
35. Wilson R. Outcome predictors in bronchitis. Chest 1995;108(suppl): 53S–57S.
36. Lund BC, Ernst EJ, Klepser ME. Strategies in the treatment of penicillin-resistant *Streptococcus pneumoniae*. Am J Health Syst Pharm 1998;55:1987–1994.
37. Harwell JI, Brown RB. The drug-resistant pneumococcus: Clinical relevance, therapy, and prevention. Chest 2000;117:530–541.
38. Campbell GD, Silberman R. Drug-resistant *Streptococcus pneumoniae*. Clin Infect Dis 1998;26:1188–1195.
39. Reed MD, Blumer JL. Azithromycin: A critical review of the first azilde antibiotic and its role in pediatric practice. Pediatr Infect Dis J 1997;16:1069–1083.
40. Klassen TP. Recent advances in the treatment of bronchiolitis and laryngitis. Pediatr Clin North Am 1997;44:249–261.
41. Klassen TP, Sutcliff T, Watters LK, et al. Dexamethasone in salbutamol-treated inpatients with acute bronchiolitis: A randomized controlled study. J Pediatr 1997;130:191–196.
42. Muller NL, Miller RR. Diseases of the bronchioles: CT and histopathologic findings. Radiology 1995;196:3–12.
43. Ottolini MG, Hemming VG. Prevention and treatment recommendations for respiratory syncytial virus infection. Drugs 1997;54:867–884.
44. McCarthy CA, Hall CB. Recent approaches to the management and prevention of respiratory syncytial virus infection. Curr Clin Top Infect Dis 1998;18:1–18.
45. Englund JA, Piedra PA, Ahn YM, et al. High-dose, short-duration ribavirin aerosol therapy compared with standard ribavirin therapy in children with suspected respiratory syncytial virus infection. J Pediatr 1994;125:635–641.
46. Darville T, Yamauchi T. Respiratory syncytial virus. Pediatr Rev 1998;19:55–61.
47. Committee on Infectious Diseases. Reassessment of the indications for ribavirin therapy in respiratory syncytial virus infections. Pediatrics 1996;97:137–140.
48. Committee on Infectious Diseases. 1997 Redbook: Report of the Committee on Infectious Diseases, 24th ed. Elk Grove Village, IL, American Academy of Pediatrics, 1997:445.
49. Meert KL, Sarnaik AP, Gelmini MJ, et al. Aerosolized ribavirin in mechanically ventilated children with respiratory syncytial virus lower respiratory tract disease: A prospective, double-blind, randomized trial. Crit Care Med 1994;22:566–572.

50. The Prevent Study Group. Reduction of respiratory syncytial virus hospitalizations among premature infants and infants with bronchopulmonary dysplasia using respiratory syncytial virus immune globulin prophylaxis. Pediatrics 1997;99:93–99.
51. The Impact-RSV Study Group. Palivizumab, a humanized respiratory syncytial virus monoclonal antibody, reduces hospitalization from respiratory syncytial virus infection in high-risk infants. Pediatrics 1998;102:531–537.
52. Cunha BA. Community-acquired pneumonia. Diagnostic and therapeutic approach. Med Clin North Am 2001;85:43–77.
53. Mandell LA. Community-acquired pneumonia: Etiology, epidemiology and treatment. Chest 1995;108(suppl):35S–42S.
54. Cunha BA. Nosocomial pneumonia: Diagnostic and therapeutic considerations. Med Clin North Am 2001;85:79–114.
55. Baker CJ, Edwards MS. Group B streptococcal infections. In: Remington JS, Klein JO, eds. Infectious Diseases of the Fetus and Newborn Infant, 4th ed. Philadelphia, Saunders, 1995:980–1054.
56. American Thoracic Society. Hospital-acquired pneumonia in adults: Diagnosis, assessment of severity, initial antimicrobial therapy, and preventative strategies. Am J Respir Crit Care Med 1996;153:1711– 1725.
57. Beringer PM. New approaches to optimizing antimicrobial therapy in patients with cystic fibrosis. Curr Opin Pulm Med 1999;5:371–377.
58. Stout JE, Yu VL. Legionellosis. N Engl J Med 1997;337:682–687.
59. Bartlett JG. Anaerobic bacterial infections of the lung and pleural space. Clin Infect Dis 1993;16(suppl 4):S248–S255.
60. Martin G, Lazarus A. Epidemiology and diagnosis of tuberculosis. Postgrad Med 2000;108:42–54.
61. McCray E, Weinbaum CM, Braden CR, et al. The epidemiology of tuberculosis in the United States. Clin Chest Med 1997;18:99–113.
62. Telzak EE. Tuberculosis and human immunodeficiency virus infection. Med Clin North Am 1997;81:345–360.
63. Plouffe J. Importance of typical pathogens of community acquired pneumonia. Clin Infect Dis 2000;31(suppl 2):S35–S39.
64. File TM, Tan JS, Plouffe JF. The role of atypical pathogens: *Mycoplasma pneumoniae, Chlamydia pneumoniae* and *Legionella pneumophila* in respiratory infection. Infect Dis Clin North Am 1998;12:569–592.
65. Ashley EA, Johnson MA, Lipman MC. Human immunodeficiency virus and respiratory infection. Curr Opin Pulm Med 2000;6:240–245.
66. Schneider RF, Rosen MJ. Pulmonary complications of HIV infection. Curr Opin Pulm Med 1997;3:151–158.
67. Noskin GA, Glassroth J. Bacterial pneumonia associated with HIV-1 infection. Clin Chest Med 1996;17:713–723.
68. Pizzo PA. Management of fever in patients with cancer and treatment-induced neutropenia. N Engl J Med 1993;328:1323–1332.
69. Hughes WT, Armstrong D, Bodey GP, et al. 1997 guidelines for the use of antimicrobial agents in neutropenic patients with unexplained fever. Clin Infect Dis 1997;25:551–573.
70. Whimbey E, Goodrich J, Bodey GP. Pneumonia in cancer patients. Cancer Treat Rep 1995;79:185–210.
71. Mayhall CG. Ventilator-associated pneumonia or not? Contemporary diagnosis. Emerg Infect Dis 2001;7:200–204.
72. ASCO Ad Hoc Colony-Stimulating Factor Guidelines Expert Panel. Update of recommendations for the use of hematopoietic colony-stimulating factors: Evidence-based clinical practice guidelines. J Clin Oncol 1996;14:1957–1960.
73. Gallego M, Valles J, Rello J. New perspectives in the diagnosis of nosocomial pneumonia. Curr Opin Pulm Med 1997;3:116–119.
74. Young PJ, Ridley SA. Ventilator-associated pneumonia: Diagnosis and prevention. Anaesthesia 1999;54:1183–1197.
75. Estes RJ, Meduri GU. The pathogenesis of ventilator-associated pneumonia: I. Mechanisms of bacterial transcolonization and airway inoculation. Intensive Care Med 1995;21:365–383.
76. Amsden GW, Duran JM. Interpretation of antibacterial susceptibility reports: *In vitro* clinical breakpoints. Drugs 2001;61:163–166.
77. Honeybourne D. Antibiotic penetration in the respiratory tract and implications. Curr Opin Pulm Med 1997;3:170–174.
78. Bodem CR, Lampton LM, Miller DP, et al. Endobronchial pH: Relevance to aminoglycoside activity in gram-negative bacillary pneumonia. Am Rev Resp Dis 1983;127:39–41.
79. Smaldone GC, Palmer LB. Aerosolized antibiotics: Current and future. Respir Care 2000;45:667–675.
80. Barlett JG, Dowell SF, Mandell LA, et al. Practice guidelines for the management of community-acquired pneumonia in adults. Clin Infect Dis 2000;31:347–382.
81. Heffelfinger JD, Dowell SF, Jorgensen JH. Management of community-acquired pneumonia in the era of pneumococcal resistance. A report from the Drug-Resistant *Streptococcus pneumoniae* Therapeutic Working Group. Arch Intern Med 2000;160:1399–1408.
82. Jacoby GA. Prevalence and resistance mechanisms of common bacterial respiratory pathogens. Clin Infect Dis 1994;18:951–957.
83. Collignon P, Turnidge JD. Antibiotic resistance in *Streptococcus pneumoniae*. Med J Aust 2000;173(suppl):S58–S64.
84. Shlaes DM, Gerding DN, John JF, et al. Society for Healthcare Epidemiology of America and Infectious Diseases Society of America Joint Committee on the Prevention of Antimicrobial Resistance: Guidelines for the prevention of antimicrobial resistance in hospitals. Clin Infect Dis 1997;25:584–599.
85. Aminimanizani A, Beringer P, Jelliffe R. Comparative pharmacokinetics and pharmacodynamics of the newer fluoroquinolone antibacterials. Clin Pharmacokinet 2001;40:169–187.
86. Gubareva LV, Kaiser L, Hayden FG. Influenza virus neuraminidase inhibitors. Lancet 2000;355:827–835.
87. McNicholl IR, McNicholl JJ. Neuraminidase inhibitors: Zanamivir and oseltamivir. Ann Pharmacother 2001;35:57–70.

107

UPPER RESPIRATORY TRACT INFECTIONS

Monique Richer and Michel Deschênes

Otitis media, pharyngitis, croup, and sinusitis are the most common acute upper respiratory tract infections of early childhood. Epiglottitis, otitis media, pharyngitis, and sinusitis also occur in adults. This group of diseases represents one of the most frequent reasons for medical care in North America. Approximately 75% of all outpatient prescriptions for antimicrobial medications are issued for these conditions.[1] Understanding the underlying microbiology, pathophysiology, and predisposing factors, as well as the advent of an armamentarium of new antimicrobial agents, significantly improves their management and outcome, as well as the quality of life of those who suffer from these infections.

OTITIS MEDIA

Otitis media is a nonspecific term describing an inflammation of the middle ear, and it is classified according to clinical presentation.[2] Acute otitis media (AOM) involves the rapid onset of signs and symptoms of infection in the middle ear.

Otitis media with effusion (accumulation of liquid in the middle ear cavity) differs from acute otitis media in that signs and symptoms of an acute infection are absent. The opacity of the tympanic membrane makes the type of effusion (serous, mucous, purulent) difficult to determine.

Chronic purulent otitis media, characterized by a chronic inflammation of the middle ear and otitis media without effusion are rare conditions and are not discussed at length in this chapter.

EPIDEMIOLOGY

Acute otitis media is the most frequent diagnosis in infants and children who visit physicians because of illness.[1] Acute episodes are more frequent during the first 3 years of life: by the age of 1 year, 50% of children will have had one episode of otitis media, and by the age of 3 years, 60% will have had one episode and 30% will have had at least three episodes.[2,3] It is the most common reason for outpatient treatment in the United States.[4] Data from the US National Health Interview Survey (NHIS) indicate that the prevalence rate of recurrent AOM increased from 18.7% in 1981 to 26.9% in 1988. The greatest increase occurred in infants younger than 12 months of age.[5] Acute otitis media also presents in adults, albeit less frequently.[2]

ETIOLOGY

Several risk factors contribute to the higher incidence and increased frequency of otitis media.

SEASON

The frequency of otitis media is greater in winter months and appears to parallel the outbreaks of viral infections of the respiratory tract.[6] A child born in the fall has a higher risk of recurrent otitis media possibly because these children are exposed to winter respiratory pathogens while being vulnerable.[7]

MALFORMATIONS

Infants with anatomic problems, such as cleft palate, adenoid hypertrophy, and Down's syndrome, are particularly at risk for the development of acute otitis media and recurrences.

ENVIRONMENTAL FACTORS

A history of recurrent acute otitis media or respiratory tract infections in a sibling doubles the risk of developing acute otitis media. A prospective, longitudinal study of twins and triplets shows a strong genetic component in the amount of time with middle ear effusion, episodes with middle ear effusion, and AOM.[8] Attending day care centers and parental smoking increases the risk, and breast feeding appears as a significant protective factor.[5–7,9,10]

RACE

The incidence of acute otitis media is more predominant in whites than in the American black population.[5] Native Americans and the Inuit represent a population particularly at risk.[11] The differences observed among races are attributed to factors such as anatomic differences of the eustachian tube, living conditions, availability of medical care, and the small sample sizes of the groups studied.

AGE AT FIRST EPISODE

The earlier children experience their first episode of otitis media, the greater the risk of developing more severe, persistent, and recurrent episodes. Infants with a first episode before the age of 6 months have a relative risk of 1.5 of AOM within the next 24 months as compared to infants and children who have a first episode at an age older than 6 months.[5,6]

ANATOMY AND PATHOPHYSIOLOGY

The middle ear is best described as an air-filled cavity that begins at the tympanic membrane and extends to the nasopharynx via the eustachian tube (Fig. 107–1). It is contiguous with air-filled cells of

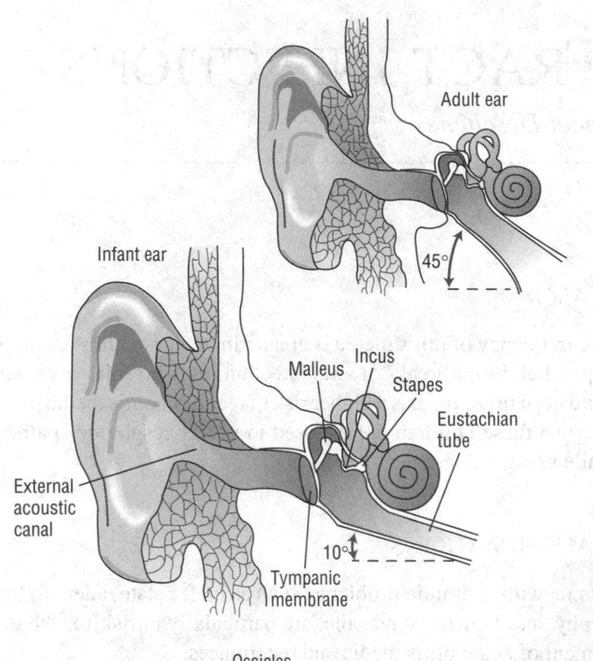

FIGURE 107–1. Anatomic differences between the angle of the eustachian tube of the infant and the adult.

the mastoid, but it also shares the same respiratory mucosa as the nose, nasopharynx, and eustachian tubes.

The eustachian tube lies at a 45-degree angle to the horizontal plane in adults and at a 10-degree angle in infants (Fig. 107–1). Its primary functions with respect to the middle ear are (a) regulation of atmospheric pressure between both sides of the tympanic membrane, (b) protection from nasopharyngeal secretions, and (c) draining secretions from the middle ear into the nasopharynx. In infants, this difference in angulation may cause improper drainage of the middle ear as a result of decreased gravitational effects on the eustachian tube. In addition, the muscle responsible for eustachian tube opening, the tensor veli palatini, is less efficient. Thus, abnormal function of the eustachian tubes seems to be the pathogenic basis of middle ear disease, causing reflux transudation of liquid in the middle ear, and finally proliferation of bacteria in these secretions, resulting in acute otitis media.

MICROBIOLOGY

Streptococcus pneumoniae is the predominant bacterial pathogen associated with recurrent AOM.[12] *S. pneumoniae* causes approximately 7 million cases of otitis media annually in the United States.[13] The second and third most frequently cultured pathogens are *Haemophilus influenzae* and *Moraxella catarrhalis*, respectively.[14] To a lesser extent, *Staphylococcus aureus, Streptococcus pyogenes, Escherichia coli,* and a few other strains (*Pseudomonas aeruginosa* and group B streptococci) have been isolated. The bacteriology of middle ear effusion has changed from the 1980s when β-lactam resistance in non-type b strains of *H. influenzae* (15% to 30%) and *M. catarrhalis* (75%) was of primary concern.[15] In the 1990s, the percentage of *S. pneumoniae* strains found to demonstrate a reduced susceptibility to amoxicillin ranges from 30% to 60% in the United States.[16] This change has caused health authorities to reassess the treatment of acute otitis media. In addition, the proportion of β-lactamase producing *H. influenzae* and *M. catarrhalis* strains in acute otitis media has nearly tripled in the last decade. Resistance has gone from 15% to 55% for *H. influenzae* to nearly 100% for *M. catarrhalis*.[12,14] Anaerobic bacteria, such as *Chlamydia trachomatis,* as well as viruses and *Mycoplasma* are suspected of playing a role in otitis media[17,18] Their contribution to the disease process is obscured by the difficulty in isolating these pathogens.

CLINICAL PRESENTATION

Acute otitis media involves the rapid onset of signs and symptoms of inflammation in the middle ear that manifests clinically as one or more of the following: otalgia (denoted by pulling of the ear in some infants), hearing loss (secondary to effusion), and fever. Clinical presentation may include nonspecific symptoms, particularly in young children, such as irritability, lethargy, anorexia, or vomiting. This usually occurs in a child who has had an upper respiratory tract infection for several days. Otitis media may be present, however, without the aforementioned characteristics, which reinforces the need for regular otoscopic examination in the presence of fever.[2,11]

The diagnosis of otitis media is confirmed by the examination of the tympanic membrane. Redness or opacity of the tympanic membrane, the absence of light reflection, bulging, and immobility of the tympanic membrane to pneumatic otoscopy are all indicative of a middle ear effusion and suggestive of otitis media. Redness of the tympanic membrane, however, can also result from crying, sneezing, coughing, or fever. Otorrhea (purulent discharge) through perforation of the tympanic membrane or through tympanostomy tubes is also indicative of otitis media. Evaluation of the mobility of the tympanic membrane by insufflation with a pneumatic otoscope or determined by a tympanometer is considered essential for the proper diagnosis of acute otitis media.[11] The tympanometer uses the reflection of sounds by the eardrum to detect the presence of liquid by the middle ear cavity, which is recognized by a flat tympanogram instead of the normal bell-shaped diagram. In difficult cases, the use of tympanocentesis provides a definitive diagnosis of otitis media and yields identification and susceptibility patterns of the pathogens.

Acute otitis media resolves spontaneously in the majority of children regardless of whether the tympanic membrane ruptures, a myringotomy is performed or antibiotics are prescribed.[19] In as many as one-third of ears, there will still be sufficient fluid in the middle ear 4 weeks later to cause a slight hearing loss. By 11 weeks, there will be no otoscopic or tympanometric evidence of middle ear fluid in 95% of children.[19] The incidence of acute mastoiditis is low. The intracaranial complications, meningitis, mastoiditis, and brain abcess are infrequent.[19] However, children younger than 12 months of age are particularly at risk for complications and otitis media should be treated in this age group.[19]

The difference between acute otitis media and otitis media with effusion is that the child is asymptomatic with the latter. Because of unsuccessful attempts to culture bacteria, it was once thought that the effusion was sterile. Studies have demonstrated the presence of bacteria in approximately 50% of the cases of otitis media with effusion. The bacteria are similar to those isolated in acute otitis media but with a slightly different distribution: *H. influenzae,* 12% to 50%; *S. pneumoniae,* 3% to 40%; and *Staphylococcus epidermidis,* 19% to 37%. *S. aureus* and *M. catarrhalis* are encountered less frequently.[2,20]

▶ TREATMENT: Otitis Media

DESIRED OUTCOME

The goals of treatment of otitis media include the control of pain, the eradication of infection, the prevention of complications, the avoidance of unnecessary antibiotics, and the minimization of adverse effects of treatment (Table 107–1).

GENERAL APPROACH TO TREATMENT

Although a significant percentage of children will have cured their acute episode of otitis media with symptomatologic treatment only, oral antibiotic therapy remains the mainstay of therapy. However, the inaccurate dignosis of acute otitis media can result in the overprescribing of antibiotics, thus contributing to antibiotic resistance. Unfortunately, clinical criteria that can distinguish patients who will require antibiotic therapy are not always used. It is strongly suggested that the diagnostic accuracy of acute otitis media be improved with the use of pneumatic otoscopy and when required, tympanocentesis.[21]

TABLE 107–1. Recommendations for Providing Pharmaceutical Care to URTI Patients Receiving Antibiotic Therapy

1. Recommend drug treatment as presented in the chapter text and in the Principles of Pharmacotherapy.
2. Counsel patient or parent of patient with recurrent otitis media on the possible benefits of decreasing exposure to tobacco smoke and of the contribution of factors such as exposure to respiratory pathogens (day care, siblings, winter months) to the incidence of URTI.
3. Assess the likelihood of patient or parent and child compliance to the antibiotic regimen. Advocate the most effective, the most palatable, but the simplest drug regimen.
4. Assess the patient's allergy status to penicillin or other antibiotics.
5. Provide appropriate tools (graduated syringes or spoons) in order to ensure adequate dispensing of the medication by the caregiver.
6. Assess and monitor patients for potential side effects such as diarrhea, abdominal cramps, and rash.
7. Assess and monitor patients for possible drug interactions, especially those receiving erythromycin, clarithromycin, or azithromycin, or women taking birth-control medication.
8. Assess noncompliance and the possibility of antibiotic resistance, especially with standard dose amoxicillin.
9. Provide patient education to patients or parents of children with URTI. Information should include:
   Cause: URTI can be caused by bacteria or viruses.
   Treatment: Treatment includes symptom and fever relief with acetaminophen or ibuprofen. When a bacterial cause is suspected, the treatment consists of the former and antibiotics.
   Administration: Instruct the patient or the parent on when, how, and how long to take the medication.
   Adverse effects: Counsel the patient or the parent to report intolerable effects
   Complete treatment: Advise the patient or the parent to complete the treatment even if the child or the patient is feeling better.
   Compliance: Explain the importance of compliance to the drug regimen and the contribution of noncompliance to the development of bacterial resistance.
   Alarm symptoms: Instruct the patient or the parent to report lack of improvement of symptoms, persistent diarrhea, poor feeding, persistent fever or rash.

NONPHARMACOLOGIC THERAPY

Supportive therapy with analgesics, antipyretics, and local heat is beneficial in the comfort of the child.[21] Although antihistamines and decongestants have been used for the symptomatic relief of acute otitis media, they are not efficacious in the resolution of effusion or the relief of symptoms.[11]

A frequent nonpharmacologic approach to the treatment of recurrent episodes of otitis media is myringotomy and insertion of tympanostomy tubes. An incision of the tympanic membrane is made under anesthesia, the middle ear effusion is aspirated, and a short biflanged tympanostomy tube is inserted. The insertion of tympanostomy tubes reduces recurrent episodes of otitis media by 50% with an infection-free period of 3 months for most patients.[22] The insertion of tympanostomy tubes interrupts the cycle of recurrent infections, rapidly restores essential hearing for a short period, and relieves the discomfort that causes irritability in children. The advantages associated with tube placement are not reached without potential risks, primarily, exposure to general anesthesia and permanent scarring of the tympanic membrane.

PHARMACOLOGIC THERAPY

ANTIBIOTIC THERAPY

Uncomplicated acute otitis media has a favorable natural history, regardless of antibiotic therapy. A meta-analysis of studies conducted from 1966 to 1992 concluded that the overall rate of spontaneous resolution of acute otitis media was 81%.[23] The data revealed that the benefit of antibiotics in acute otitis media was 13.7% over placebo. In another study, antibiotics were assessed to resolve pain approximately two days sooner than when no antibiotic therapy was given or when analgesics alone were given.[24] In a study performed in the Netherlands, the authors concluded that early symptom resolution was more common with amoxicillin therapy (40 mg/kg/day) but that seven to eight children require treatment for one child to have improved symptoms at day 4.[25] Although the policy of nonantibiotic treatment of acute otitis media has been recommended in the Netherlands, Iceland, and the United Kingdom, it has not gained wide acceptance in North America.

If the decision has been made to treat with an antibiotic, selection of the appropriate antibiotic is based on antimicrobial susceptibility, penetration into the middle ear fluid, clinical efficacy, compliance factors, adverse effects profile, and cost. Table 107–2 summarizes the recommended doses and dosing schedules of the most frequently used antibiotics for treatment of otitis media.

Amoxicillin is still considered as the first line of treatment. With its excellent *in vitro* activity against *S. pneumoniae* and most *H. influenzae* isolates from the middle ear, amoxicillin remains the antibiotic of choice according to the CDC.[26] Higher dosages of amoxicillin are recommended to address the issue of penicillin-resistant pneumocci by producing higher levels of amoxicillin in

TABLE 107–2. Dosing Regimen and Cost of Antibiotic Use in Upper Respiratory Tract Infections[14,17,46,47,49,60]

Antibiotic(s)	Daily Pediatric Dose	Likelihood of Clinical Success in OM and Sinusitis[c] β-Lactamase + *H. influenzae*	Resistant *S. pneumoniae*	Adult Dosage	Regimen	Cost ($)
Amoxicillin	40 mg/kg	3	1	250–500 mg	every 8 hours	$
	80–90 mg/kg[a]	4	1			
Pivampicillin	40–60 mg/kg	3	1	500 mg	every 12 hours	$$
Amoxicillin-clavulanate	40–45 mg/kg as amoxicillin	3	5	250–500 mg	every 8 hours	$$$
	80–90 mg/kg as amoxicillin; 6.4 mg/kg of clavulanate[ab]	4	5			
Trimethoprim-sulfamethoxazole	8–10 mg/kg trimethoprim	2	3	160/800 mg	every 12 hours	$
Cefaclor	20–40 mg/kg	2	3	250–500 mg	every 8 or 12 hours	$$$
Cefprozil	7.5–15 mg/kg	3	4	250–500 mg	every 12 or 24 hours	$$$
Cefuroxime axetil	30–40 mg/kg	3	4	250–500 mg	every 12 hours	$$$
Loracarbef	7.5–15 mg/kg	2	3	200–400 mg	every 12 hours	$$$
Cefixime	8–9 mg/kg	1	5	400 mg	every 12 or 24 hours	$$$
Cefpodoxime proxetil	10 mg/kg	3	5	100–200 mg	every 12 or 24 hours	$$$
Ceftibuten	9 mg/kg	1	5	400 mg	every 24 hours	$$$
Cefdinir	14 mg/kg	1	5	300–600 mg	every 12 or 24 hours	$$$
Ceftriaxone[d]	50 mg/kg I.M.	4	5	1 g	every 24 hours	
Erythromycin-sulfisoxazole	40 mg/kg of erythromycin	1	3	—	every 8 or 12 hours	$$
Clarithromycin	7.5–15 mg/kg	2	3	250–500 mg	every 12 hours	$$$
Azithromycin	10 mg/kg day 1, 5 mg/kg days 2–5 (OM) 12 mg/kg × 5 days (SP)	2	3	500 mg day 1, 250 mg days 2–5	every 24 hours	$$$
Ciprofloxacin	—	5	1	500–700 mg	every 12 hours	$$$
Levofloxacin	—	1	1	500 mg	every 24 hours	$$$
Gatifloxacin	—	1	1	400 mg	every 24 hours	$$$
Moxifloxacin	—	1	1	400 mg	every 24 hours	$$$

OM, otitis media; SP, streptococcal pharyngitis.
$, <$10 $$, $10–20 $$$, >$20
[a]CDC Working group treatment recommendations for acute otitis media.
[b]The amoxicillin-clavulanate regimen would require two prescriptions: one for amoxicillin (40–50 mg/kg/d) and one for amoxicillin clavulanate (40 mg/kg/d as amoxicillin).
[c]Adapted from reference 14. Ordinal scale 1 (least likely to be effective) to 5 (most likely to be effective).
[d]Ceftriaxone efficacy against intermediately resistant and resistant *S. pneumoniae* has been optimal when administered as three injections on three consecutive days.

the middle ear fluid. The CDC Working group recommends that when no antibiotics were given in the prior month, standard-dose amoxicillin (40 mg/kg/day) or high-dose amoxicillin (80–90 mg/kg/day) be administered. In the event of clinically defined treatment failure on day 3, amoxicillin should be discontinued and high-dose amoxicillin-clavulanate (90 mg/kg/day of amoxicillin and 6.4 mg/kg/day of clavulanate—formulation not available in North America), cefuroxime axetil, or intramuscular ceftriaxone be administered. In the presence of recurrent acute otitis media, high-dose amoxicillin, high-dose amoxicillin-clavulanate, or cefuroxime axetil should be considered. In the event of treatment failure, a 3-day course of intramuscular ceftriaxone, clindamycin (*S. pneumoniae* determined by tympanocentesis), or tympanocentesis should be considered.[26] In the case of uncomplicated acute otitis media, a single injection of ceftriaxone is acceptable.[17] Other cephalosporins (cefprozil, cefpodoxime, cefdinir) or macrolides are also good alternatives.[17]

Regardless of the dosage, amoxicillin will not eradicate β-lactamase-producing *H. influenzae* or *M. catarrhalis.* When there is documentation of regional resistance to β-lactam agents, β-lactamase-resistant antibiotics should be used. Appropriate choices include trimethoprim-sulfamethoxazole (TMP/SMX), cefixime, cefuroxime axetil, cefaclor, ceftibuten, cefprozil, cefpodoxime proxetil, loracarbef, azithromycin, clarithromycin, and erythromycin-sulfisoxazole.[27–32] TMP/SMX offers good activity against *H. influenzae*, but its activity against group A *Streptococcus* is poor, and pneumococcal resistance is increasing. Pneumococcus, as well as *S. pyogenes,* are showing increasing resistance to both TMP/SMX and the macrolides. The combination of sulfisoxazole with erythromycin also provides coverage for the primary pathogens. In addition, it is a useful alternative for patients who are allergic to penicillins and cephalosporins. Cefaclor has demonstrated good activity against most pathogens. The isolation of resistant strains of *H. influenzae* and *M. catarrhalis* is, however, increasing.[27] The *in vitro* spectrum of activity of azithromycin and clarithromycin includes most pathogens that cause otitis media. Streptococci that are resistant to erythromycin can exhibit cross-resistance to azithromycin.[33] The combination of clarithromycin and its active metabolite has synergistic or additive activity against *H. influenzae.*[33] A 10-day course of antimicrobial therapy is recommended. However, patients prefer a shorter course of therapy (5 days or less). Reviews of comparative trials of shorter and longer courses of antibiotics show that shortened courses of antibiotics are likely to be successful in most patients older than 2 years of age.[34,35]

Chronic otitis media with effusion is described as an effusion lasting more than 3 months. A short course of antibiotics appears to be effective in the short-term clearance of the effusion.[36,37] The effect is limited, however, and is of relatively short duration.[36] Improvement of effusion is best seen with insertion of tympanostomy tubes. Tympanostomy should be considered in the following instances: (a) occurrence in infants <12 months of age because of their inability to communicate symptoms; (b) concurrence of an acute purulent upper respiratory tract infection; (c) the presence of permanent conductive-sensorineural hearing loss; (d) vertigo or tinnitus; (e) the presence of severe atelectasis; (f) changes of the middle ear, such as adhesive otitis or ossicular involvement; (g) presence of effusion for 2 to 3 months or longer; or (h) frequent episodes of effusion, resulting in the accumulation of time of effusion during a period of 6 of 12 months.[11]

Chemoprophylaxis

Several studies have demonstrated the effectiveness of chemoprophylaxis, but the indications, duration, and selection of the most effective agent are still controversial.[36] The following regimens have been advocated: (a) amoxicillin (20–30 mg/kg/day) in one dose at bedtime or in two divided doses every 12 hours; (b) sulfisoxazole (80–100 mg/kg/day) every 24 hours; and (c) TMP/SMX (equivalent of 4 mg/kg/day of TMP) every 24 hours. The Food and Drug Administration has not approved TMP/SMX for this indication. Prophylactic therapy appears to have a beneficial but limited effect on recurrent otitis media. It should be initiated during the winter and early spring when recurrences are highest and continued for 3 months or until there is a failure of therapy.[20] The appropriate course of treatment in patients who develop acute otitis media while on prophylaxis is to treat the acute episode with the usual 10 days of antibiotic therapy, using an alternative agent if amoxicillin was used for prophylaxis.

The antipneumococcal vaccines Pnu-Imune and Pneumovax contain frequently encountered pneumococcal antigens associated with otitis media. In children older than 2 years of age, this vaccine has been responsible for an approximately 10% to 20% reduction of acute otitis media (33% in day care centers).[37] Unfortunately, children younger than 2 years of age respond poorly to most polysaccharide vaccines. The *H. influenzae* type b (HIB) polysaccharide vaccine is not useful in the prevention of acute otitis media because nontypeable strains of *H. influenzae* are most frequently implicated.

Clinical Efficacy

Evaluating the efficacies of the antibiotics used in the treatment of otitis media is not straightforward. The majority of clinical trials of antibiotic therapy are comparative and often determine both clinical and bacteriologic outcomes.[29–32] A greater than 90% clinical success rate, generally defined as an absence of all presenting signs and symptoms of acute otitis media, can be achieved in the presence of bacteriologic cure (sterile middle ear fluid culture) and a 62% clinical cure can be observed with bacteriologic failure.[38] An 80% clinical success rate was demonstrated in nonbacterial otitis media. It is also important to consider that symptomatic improvement can be observed without antibacterial therapy. A meta-analysis evaluating the complete clinical resolution of otitis media (exclusive of middle ear effusion) reported that the spontaneous rate of resolution without antibiotics or tympanocentesis was 81%.[23] The use of antibiotics increased resolution by 13.7%. Albeit modest, the impact of antibiotic use on clinical resolution was significant. Conversely, symptoms can persist despite effective antibacterial therapy, especially in the presence of viral infections.

Compliance Factors

Most children with otitis media become asymptomatic within 24 to 72 hours of the initiation of therapy. It is, therefore, not surprising that less than 50% of the children treated for otitis media complete the full course of antimicrobials.[39] The number of daily doses to be administered has an impact on the compliance to a therapeutic regimen, making duration of therapy and cost important issues in the choice of therapy. Short dosing intervals and the recommended 10-day course of antimicrobial therapy for acute otitis media certainly represent contributory factors to noncompliance, and antibiotics that offer longer dosing intervals are advantageous. In some instances, a shorter course of oral therapy is effective.[40] In this study, tympanocentesis was performed in every patient and may have had an impact on outcome. In a randomized, double-blind clinical trial, rates of improvement, failure, relapse, and reinfection with a single dose of ceftriaxone (50 mg/kg IM) were comparable to a 10-day course of oral amoxicillin (40 mg/kg/day) in children with acute otitis media.[41,42]

Although liquid formulations of antimicrobials offer flexibility in dosage adjustment for children, palatability of these preparations impacts on compliance.[43] Fortunately, the majority of the antimicrobial suspensions on the market for children are flavored.

Adverse Effects

There is little to distinguish one antibiotic from another in terms of safety profile. All of the antibiotics used in the treatment of otitis media are quite safe. The most frequent adverse reactions associated with the use of antimicrobials in the treatment of acute otitis media are gastrointestinal and cutaneous. The incidence of diarrhea is highest with amoxicillin (>20%) and may be increased when higher doses (80–90 mg/kg/day) are used. The addition of clavulanic acid to amoxicillin increases, in a dose-related manner, the incidence of diarrhea, nausea, and vomiting when compared to amoxicillin alone. Cefixime is reported to cause diarrhea more often than cefaclor (11% to 20%). The incidences of rashes and diarrhea with the newer cephalosporins (cefpodoxime, proxetil, cefprozil, and loracarbef) range from 1% to 3% and are similar to that of other cephalosporins and penicillins. Erythromycin-sulfisoxazole has been associated with abdominal cramping, as well as diarrhea, when the erythromycin component exceeded 40 mg/kg/day. Gastrointestinal disturbances were reported less frequently with azithromycin and clarithromycin than with erythromycin.

The potential for hypersensitivity reactions with β-lactams and sulfonamide-containing antimicrobials is well recognized. The nonallergic rash, well described with aminopenicillins, is reported in approximately 10% of treated patients. Agents containing sulfonamides (TMP/SMX, erythromycin-sulfisoxazole) are known to cause rare hematologic effects and cutaneous reactions that could be as severe as exfoliative dermatitis or Stevens-Johnson syndrome. Cefaclor has been linked to the development of a serum sickness-like illness associated with erythema multiforme (1.1%), which is reversible with discontinuation of treatment.

PHARMACOECONOMIC CONSIDERATIONS

The total cost of treating otitis media in the United States is estimated at more than 3.5 billion dollars annually.[44] Since the efficacy, antimicrobial activity, and adverse-effect profiles of many of the treatment regimens are comparable, cost of treatment becomes the issue. Table 107–2 lists the average wholesale price for different antimicrobial agents for the 10-day regimen for a 20-kg child as well as for adults. Amoxicillin-clavulanate and the newer molecules offer broader bacterial coverage but are by far more expensive.

EVALUATION OF THERAPEUTIC OUTCOMES

With proper treatment, symptoms of acute otitis media in most children will abate within 24 to 72 hours. It is useful, however, to reexamine the patient at the end of therapy. Even with efficacious antibiotic treatment, effusion of the middle ear may be present and persist in 10% of cases. Otitis media with effusion is classified according to the duration of the effusion: subacute—3 weeks to 3 months, and chronic—longer than 3 months. Middle-ear effusion declines exponentially over a period of weeks to months. Thirty-six percent to 77% of episodes will resolve within 1 month and 9% to 32% of children will have had an episode lasting more than 3 months.[2] The following treatment options could be offered to patients beyond this time: (a) amoxicillin (20 mg/kg/day) or TMP/SMX (4/20 mg/kg/day) continuously while the effusion persists; (b) appropriate antimicrobial therapy of each episode of acute otitis media; or (c) myringotomy and tympanostomy tube placement. If acute otitis media occurs while the patient has tympanostomy tubes, *P. aeruginosa* infection should be considered and appropriate antimicrobial treatment should be initiated. If the effusion persists beyond 2 to 3 months, it is termed otitis media with effusion and should be treated as a chronic otitis media.

If the signs and symptoms of acute otitis media occur within 1 month of the initial episode, it is assumed that the same microorganism caused the infection. Emergence of resistance to *S. pneumoniae* or a β-lactamase-producing organism may be suspected. This new episode should be treated with high-dose amoxicillin or an antibiotic that is stable to β-lactamase. If the new episode occurs over 1 month after the initial infection in a child who was completely free of signs and symptoms between episodes, the management of the recurrent episode is the same as the first episode. If a child exhibits more than four episodes in a 6-month period, or six episodes in a 12-month period, this patient can be managed by chemoprophylaxis with antimicrobials, myringotomy and insertion of tympanostomy tubes, or both.

PHARYNGITIS

The evaluation, diagnosis, and treatment of patients with pharyngitis is a common problem for all providers of primary health care. In the United States, approximately 15 million patients annually seek care for the relief of sore throat symptoms. Upper respiratory tract infections account for about 12% of visits to family physicians in Ontario, Canada.[45] Decisions about management often relate to whether or not there is a possibility of group A β-hemolytic streptococcus (GAS) because of the risk of rheumatic heart disease and because streptococcal pharyngitis is the only common form of the disease for which antimicrobial therapy is indicated.[46,47]

Pharyngitis is an inflammation of the pharynx and surrounding lymphoid tissue that may be of viral or bacterial origin. Viruses appear to be the cause of the majority of episodes, often as constituents of the common cold. A significant number are of bacterial origin, however, with group A β-hemolytic streptococci *(S. pyogenes)* being the most prevalent microorganism. It is important to differentiate viral from streptococcal tonsillopharyngitis because of the sequelae of group A β-hemolytic *Streptococcus* pharyngitis and its favorable response to antibiotic treatment.

ETIOLOGY AND PATHOPHYSIOLOGY

Microbiologic etiology of acute pharyngitis varies depending on the age of the patients. In children younger than 4 years of age, the etiology is usually viral. The peak incidence of GAS is between 4 and 14 years of age.[48] The rarity of this disease in children younger than 4 years of age has been attributed to the low adherence of GAS to the buccal epithelial cells. Viral sore throats attributed to rhinoviruses and coronaviruses are associated with mild episodes, whereas adenoviruses and herpes simplex viruses, although less prevalent, are attributed to the more severe episodes of pharyngitis. Epstein-Barr (infectious mononucleosis), influenza, measles, and varicella viruses are capable of producing symptoms of pharyngitis as part of their viradrome. Mononucleosis is a disease transmitted by blood and saliva and is diagnosed mainly in adolescents and young adults.

Bacterial pathogens constitute 10% to 30% of all pharyngitis, and the symptomatology generally overlaps that of viral pharyngitis. The normal pharynx is host to gram-positive and gram-negative cocci and rods, both aerobic and anaerobic in nature. Normal flora is constituted by various bacteria of low pathogenicity. The pathogenic pneumococci (group A, C, G streptococci), *Corynebacterium diphtheriae, Chlamydia pneumoniae, Mycoplasma pneumoniae,* and *H. influenzae* are present in accountable numbers as well. GAS, the most prevalent bacterial pathogen in symptomatic pharyngitis, is responsible for 10% of pharyngitis in adults and 30% in children.[46,47] Complications of GAS pharyngitis can be infectious (peritonsillar or retropharyngeal abscess) or noninfectious (rheumatic fever or glomerulonephritis). The prompt diagnosis and treatment of GAS pharyngitis has decreased the incidence of rheumatic fever but has no effect on the incidence of acute poststreptococcal glomerulonephritis. The endemic incidence of rheumatic fever is 0.3% and can increase to 3% following a streptococcal pharyngitis epidemic.[49] Other groups of streptococci (B, C, and G) have been associated with acute episodes of pharyngitis but are not associated with the development of rheumatic fever or poststreptococcal glomerulonephritis.

Finally, toxigenic strains of *C. diphtheriae* can cause pharyngitis and lead to diphtheria. Like GAS, diphtheria is spread through respiratory secretions and has an incubation period of 2 to 5 days. Fortunately, as a result of immunization programs, diphtheria is rare in North America, but the complications associated with this pathogen warrant accurate diagnosis and immediate treatment. The clinical characteristics of diphtheria are a grayish membrane overlaying the tonsils, cervical adenopathy with edema, and a toxic appearance.

When there is a difficulty in establishing a diagnosis, noninfectious causes of pharyngitis should be considered. Allergies, sinusitis, postnasal drip, and certain malignancies affect the upper respiratory tract or pharynx directly and should be evaluated before initiation of antibiotic therapy. The exposure to irritating substances (e.g., cigarette smoke, environmental pollutants, ingestion of caustic substances, and ingestion of hot foods or liquids) or direct trauma to the pharynx may cause pharyngitis and should be excluded as primary causes.

CLINICAL PRESENTATION

The diagnosis of acute GAS pharyngitis should be suspected on clinical and epidemiologic grounds and then supported by the results of a laboratory test. Symptoms of pharyngitis include a sore throat that is associated with dysphagia and fever. In the presence of a bacterial infection, symptoms appear 1 to 5 days following contact with the microorganism. On physical examination, hyperemia of the pharynx and hypertrophied tonsils can be observed. Occasionally, tonsillar exudates, as well as vesicles, are noted. Examination can further reveal the presence of cervical lymph nodes, as well as a scarlitinous rash. In the majority of cases of acute pharyngitis, however, it is not possible to differentiate, on a clinical basis, between viral and bacterial etiology.[48] In fact, throat findings are similar among those with and without GAS pharyngitis. Consequently, sole reliance on the presence of a red throat would result in up to 80% of those with a negative sore throat culture to be incorrectly diagnosed as having GAS pharyngitis. Pharyngeal or tonsillar exudate has a higher specificity but will miss 75% of GAS cases.

For any symptom or sign, there is a considerable overlap between those with and without GAS pharyngitis. This observation led investigators to develop scoring systems and clinical rules based on a combination of findings to optimize diagnostic accuracy. A sore throat score developed by Centor and associates[50] was derived from a study of 286 consecutive patients older than 15 years of age who presented complaining of a sore throat. Four findings independently predicted a positive throat culture for GAS: the presence of a tonsillar exudate, swollen and tender cervical nodes, lack of cough, and a history of fever greater than 38°C (101°F).[50,51]

The sore throat score has proven to have a higher sensitivity than clinical judgment, but its specificity is unsatisfactory for making treatment decisions.[52] This can be corrected by linking the score with explicit decisions about throat culture use (Fig. 107–2).

For patients with none or only one of the clinical findings, the probability of GAS is less than 10%. No throat culture should be taken and no antibiotic should be prescribed to this group. In those with two or three findings, a throat culture should be taken and the treatment decision postponed until culture results are available; more than 70% of the throat cultures in this group will be negative. The third group represents about 10% to 15% of individuals who present with all four characteristics. These individuals have the highest probability of GAS pharyngitis, are likely to be sicker, and sometimes gain the most benefit from relief of symptoms. For these patients, a throat culture should be taken and the decision to initiate antibiotic treatment should be based on clinical grounds.[51] Epidemiologic factors, such as family history, history of contact with patients having a cold or influenza, and time of the year, can provide further information to establish the appropriate diagnosis. In a followup study, McIsaac evaluated the performance of the score approach in a population of family medicine patients (621 patients, 3 years of age and older) undergoing routine clinical care from their family physicians in 49 Ontario communities.[53] In this study, the prevalence of GAS was 17% (10% to 20% in general practice setting) and the prevalence was higher among children than among adults. The sensitivity of the score approach was 76.5% and the specificity was 92.1%. Physicians prescribed antibiotics to 28% of the patients. Of these prescriptions, 63% were given to patients whose culture results were negative for GAS. As compared to usual physician care, management according to the sore throat score would have resulted in a 52.3% reduction in antibiotic prescriptions, a 63.7% reduction in unnecessary antibiotic prescriptions, and a 35.8% reduction in the culture of throat samples ($p < 0.01$).

Does the patient meet the following criteria?

- Absence of cough
- History of fever > 38°C (101°F)
- Tonsillar exudate
- Swollen, tender anterior cervical nodes

Number of criteria met*	Percent chance of streptococcal infection**	Suggested action
0 1	2–3 3–7	No culture or antibiotic required
2 3	8–16 19–34	Culture all; treat only if culture is positive
4	41–61	Culture all; treat with penicillin on clinical grounds***

FIGURE 107–2. Determination of the sore throat score. *This score should not be applied to those younger than 15 years of age or in a community in which an outbreak of GAS is occurring. **In a community with the usual levels of infection. ***If patient has a higher fever or is clinically unwell, and presents early in disease course. *(Adapted from reference 43.)*

The primary purpose of obtaining a throat culture in a patient who presents with signs and symptoms of pharyngitis is to identify the GAS, initiate treatment, and avoid sequelae. Table 107–3 lists the criteria for the identification of individuals with pharyngitis in whom a culture is recommended.

A throat culture obtained from the surface of the tonsils and the posterior pharyngeal wall is the most commonly used test for the identification of GAS. Because the time necessary to obtain results is approximately 24 to 48 hours, rapid streptococcal tests were developed for the identification of GAS. These tests detect the GAS antigen directly from a throat swab with a specificity greater than 90% in the 10 minutes to 70 minutes required for completion (depending on the test).[47] This enables patients to be treated earlier, lowering the risk of transmission of GAS. Even though these rapid test kits provide a faster diagnosis than the aerobic culture, they are less sensitive. The recommendation is to perform a throat culture if a negative result is obtained with the rapid test kits. It is important to note that a rapid diagnosis for the prevention of acute rheumatic fever is not essential, because antibiotic therapy can be initiated as late as 9 days after the onset of streptococcal pharyngitis and still be effective.[47]

Tests for antibodies, such as antistreptolysin O (ASO) and antideoxyribonuclease B (ADNase B), are useful in confirming a recent GAS infection.[49] These tests can aid in the diagnosis of patients with acute rheumatic fever or acute glomerulonephritis. They are of no immediate value, however, in the diagnosis and management of acute streptococcal infection.

TABLE 107–3. Conditions in Which a Throat Culture Is Recommended in Pharyngitis

Children aged 4–15 years with an elevated temperature and sore throat as the primary complaint
Close contact with a person with streptococcal pharyngitis
Individuals with a history of rheumatic fever or heart disease
Epidemic of group A β-hemolytic streptococcus or *Corynebacterium diphtheria*
Adults presenting with pharyngitis and two or more of the following signs and symptoms:
- Fever over 38°C (101°F)
- Tonsillar exudate
- Absence of cough
- Swollen, tender, anterior cervical lymph nodes

With mononucleosis, a 3- to 5-day prodrome consisting of a sore throat, fever, and asthenia is observed after a 30- to 50-day incubation period. Physical examination usually reveals pharyngitis with tonsillar exudates, palatal petechiae, and posterior cervical adenopathies. In 50% to 75% of cases, splenomegaly can be palpated after 2 weeks of active disease. A macular erythematous rash is present in 10% of cases but increases to 50% in cases in which ampicillin has been prescribed. Finally, jaundice can be documented in 5% of patients, whereas elevated liver transaminases (aspartate transaminase [AST], alanine transaminase [ALT]) are reported in 40% of cases.

Diagnosis of mononucleosis is confirmed by blood analysis, which should reveal lymphocytosis and the presence of atypical lymphocytes. A positive Monospot screen (Paul-Bunnell test) for the presence of heterophil (IgM) antibodies confirms the diagnosis of mononucleosis. However, these antibodies are only present in sufficient quantities after 2 weeks of active disease. Possible complications of tonsillar hypertrophy, albeit rare, include upper respiratory airway obstruction, thrombocytopenia, and traumatic or spontaneous splenic rupture.

▶ TREATMENT: Pharyngitis

DESIRED OUTCOME

The goals of treatment of pharyngitis are to resolve symptoms as quickly as possible, limit spread of infection, and prevent complications such as rheumatic heart disease. Treatment of pharyngitis varies depending on etiology. The treatment of viral pharyngitis is symptomatic. With a negative throat culture, antibiotics can safely be withheld, as GAS is almost always found on culture in individuals with active infections. When required, antibiotic therapy for GAS infection shortens the clinical course of the disease, prevents acute rheumatic fever, reduces the period of contagion to 24 hours, limits the spread of infection, and reduces the incidence of suppurative complications.[47]

PHARMACOLOGIC THERAPY

Penicillin has long been the drug of choice for pharyngitis caused by GAS.[46–49,54] Despite the development of antimicrobial resistance among most common pediatric pathogens, group A streptococci remains uniformly susceptible to penicillin. Therefore, penicillin remains the drug of choice and is recommended by the Academy of Pediatrics and the American Heart Association. Children younger than 12 years old with GAS pharyngitis should receive penicillin V 250 mg twice daily given orally for 10 days or benzathine penicillin (600,000 units if $\leq$27 kg; 1,200,000 units if >27 kg) intramuscularly as a single dose.[46,47] A recent meta-analysis concluded that twice-daily dosing of 10-day penicillin is as efficacious as more frequent dosing regimens in the treatment of GAS pharyngitis. Decreased efficacy was noted with a daily dose of the regimen. In contrast, this decreased efficacy was not found with daily dosing of amoxicillin and warrants further investigation.[55] The use of the injectable form of penicillin favors compliance but is painful and increases the risk of allergic reactions. For adolescents and adults, penicillin V 500 mg twice daily orally for 10 days should be given.

For the penicillin-allergic patient, erythromycin estolate 20–40 mg/kg/day in two to four divided doses or erythromycin ethylsuccinate 40–50 mg/kg/day in two to four divided doses for 10 days are suitable alternatives.[47] Resistance of GAS to erythromycin has, however, been observed in the United States in approximately 5% of the strains isolated. An oral cephalosporin is also a reasonable alternative to penicillin. Treatment with a number of antimicrobial agents (Table 107–2) has resulted in rates of eradication at 5 days that are comparable to those rates of eradication achieved after 10 days of penicillin.[47,56] Reports suggest changes to the recommended regimen of 10 days of oral penicillin, such as the use of an alternative agent with a broader antimicrobial spectrum, particularly against penicillinase-producing strains of oral bacteria and a decrease in the duration of therapy. However, costs and effect on patterns of antimicrobial resistance must be considered.

Approximately 25% of individuals within the household of an index patient may also harbor GAS in their upper respiratory tract. It is usually unnecessary to perform throat cultures or to treat them if they are asymptomatic.[47] When a larger group (e.g., schools, day care center) is involved in a documented outbreak of GAS, throat cultures should be performed for all involved. However, only those with positive throat cultures should be treated with antimicrobials.[47]

EVALUATION OF THERAPEUTIC OUTCOMES

Approximately 10% to 20% of children and adults with GAS pharyngitis who are treated adequately will relapse. Patients who fail to respond to penicillin may harbor a greater number of penicillin-resistant, β-lactamase-producing microorganisms. Other causes besides copathogenicity include lack of compliance and recurrent exposure. A recurrent episode of pharyngitis should be classified as either a relapse (because of the same bacterial strain), as a reinfection (caused by a new strain), or as persistence of the carrier state. Streptococcal carriers do not ordinarily require further antimicrobial therapy. For a relapse, it is appropriate to change the antimicrobial agent. Antibiotics listed in Table 107–2 are good alternatives. If a new strain is present, the initial antimicrobial can be reinstated. With persistent recurrent episodes, clindamycin, amoxicillin/clavulanate, or a single dose of benzathine penicillin with rifampin 10 mg/kg twice daily for 4 days are appropriate alternatives.[47,57]

Tonsillectomy and adenoidectomy in children with recurrent pharyngitis do not significantly decrease the number of GAS infections when compared with controls who did not undergo surgery. The recommended approach in children with severe and recurrent pharyngitis is to delay the surgery hoping for an eventual improvement. If no improvement is seen, tonsillectomy can be considered.

SINUSITIS

Acute sinusitis is a common condition affecting children and adults and is associated with both bacterial and viral infections of the upper

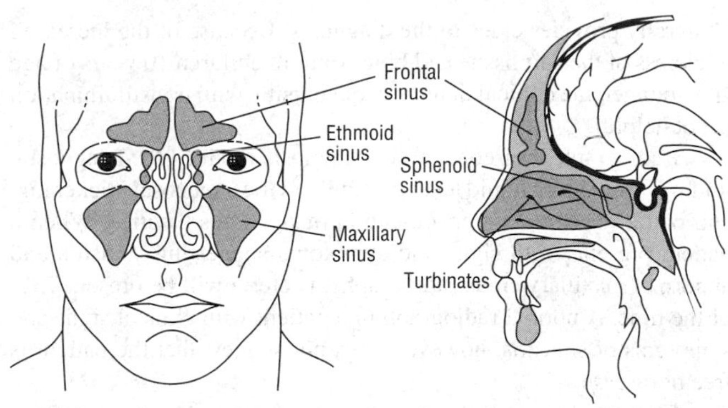

FIGURE 107–3. Anatomy of the sinus cavities.

respiratory tract. Children have between six and eight common colds per year, depending on age, number of siblings, and type of day care services. Adults experience approximately two to three common colds per year, and incidence may increase while parenting or working with young children. Of these upper respiratory infections, 0.5% are complicated by acute sinusitis. Acute sinusitis accounts for 5% of physician visits by young adults.[58]

The sinuses are four paired, air-filled cavities that are situated around the nasal cavity and adjoin the orbits and anterior cranial fossa (Fig. 107–3). The maxillary and ethmoid sinuses are well developed at birth. The sphenoid sinus originates from the ethmoid sinuses and develops when the child is between 3 and 7 years of age. The frontal sinuses develop by the time that the child is 12 years of age. The sinuses are contiguous with mucosa of the upper respiratory tract and are lined with ciliated pseudocolumnar epithelium. Small tubular openings called the sinus ostia connect the sinus cavities and facilitate drainage of the sinuses into the nasal cavity through the activity of the ciliated cells.[58]

Sinusitis is classified as acute or chronic primarily on the basis of pathologic findings and duration of infection. Acute sinusitis is defined as any infection process in the sinus that lasts up to 4 weeks.[59] If the disease persists for 12 weeks, it is classified as chronic. As well, individuals who experience more than three or four episodes annually or who repeatedly fail to respond to medical therapy may be considered to have chronic disease.[59]

ETIOLOGY AND PATHOGENESIS

The causative organisms of acute bacterial sinusitis are similar to those of acute otitis media. Studies in which culture specimens were obtained by sinus puncture reveal that the dominant organisms are *S. pneumoniae* (30% to 40%), nontypeable *H. influenzae* (20% to 30%) and *M. catarrhalis* (12% to 20%). The prevalence of sinusitis is greater among children than among adults (26% vs 2%).[60] Infrequently encountered bacteria include *S. pyogenes*, which may be a concurrent infection in 15% to 20% of children, *S. aureus*, and anaerobic bacteria. Viruses, such as rhinovirus, influenza virus, adenovirus, and the parainfluenza virus, are isolated in 15% of aspirates and are generally remnants of upper respiratory tract viral infections.[59,61] As with otitis media, bacterial resistance is increasing with similar resistance patterns. The overuse of antibiotics, inappropriate dosing and the use of broad-spectrum antibiotics as first-line treatment have contributed to the rising incidence of drug-resistant strains of bacteria.[59]

Conditions that affect the patency of the sinus ostia, normal function of the mucociliary sinus epithelium, normal immune defenses of the upper respiratory tract, or events that introduce microorganisms into the sinuses predispose to sinus infections. Bacterial and viral infections of the respiratory tract and allergic inflammation are conditions that cause sinus ostia obstruction and lead to the retention of secretions. Preceding viral infection or epithelial damage weakens mucosal defenses and facilitates penetration of bacteria into the sinus mucosa. Although nasal allergies contribute to edema and swelling of the nasal mucosa, little information is available concerning their role in acute sinusitis.

CLINICAL PRESENTATION

The clinical presentation of sinusitis is dependent on the acuteness or chronicity of the infection, as well as the patient's age. Many symptoms of acute sinusitis are nonspecific and may be difficult to differentiate from symptoms of upper respiratory tract infection or allergic rhinitis. The most commonly encountered symptoms include mucopurulent nasal discharge, nasal congestion, facial pain (particularly unilateral), maxillary toothache, and fever.[58]

The persistence of nasal discharge and a cough for more than 10 days following a viral infection of the upper respiratory tract is indicative of sinusitis. The previously clear, thin nasal discharge associated with viral infections may become mucoid or purulent with an increase in both viscosity and quantity. A poor response to decongestants also increases the likelihood of sinusitis.[58] Progression of the cough is the symptom for which parents seek medical attention, even though the child may not appear ill despite a low-grade fever. In children, the presence of malodorous breath (halitosis) in the absence of pharyngitis and poor dental hygiene, or morning periorbital swelling with or without pain, may be signs of a sinus infection. Headaches caused by sinusitis respond poorly to analgesics. The pain corresponds to the sinuses affected and is described as a feeling of fullness or a dull ache. The incidence of this type of headache in children younger than 5 years of age is rare because the frontal sinuses are not fully developed.

No single clinical finding is predictive of acute sinusitis. Three symptoms (maxillary toothache, poor response to decongestants, and colored nasal discharge) and two signs (purulent nasal secretions and abnormal transillumination) are the best clinical predictors of acute sinusitis. When four or more of the signs and symptoms are present, the likelihood of sinusitis is high; when fewer than two of the above signs or symptoms are present, acute sinusitis can be ruled out.[62] In another report, the presence of one major diagnostic factor (facial pain or pressure [requires another major factor]; facial congestion or fullness; nasal obstruction; nasal purulence; hyposmia; fever) and two minor factors (headache; halitosis; fatigue; dental pain; cough; ear pain or fullness; or fever in nonacute sinusitis) were predictive of sinusitis.[63] In between these values, the diagnosis is unclear and sinus radiography may be helpful.

Symptoms in children are different and more nonspecific than those in adults and are more difficult to distinguish from the common cold and vasomotor rhinitis. The most common complaints are cough and nasal discharge.[59]

In addition to history and physical examination, the diagnosis of sinusitis may require transillumination of maxillary sinuses, radiography of the sinuses for adults and children older than 1 year of age, and, occasionally, computed tomography or magnetic resonance imaging. Sinus puncture with aspiration and culture of sinus secretions remains the gold standard for diagnosis; unfortunately, this technique is invasive and impractical.

A useful laboratory tool is the cytologic examination of fresh nasal secretions. On microscopic examination, a high concentration of polymorphonuclear cells with intracellular bacteria is often observed. Polymorphonucleocytes generally predominate during viral infections, but when present in high numbers in a chronic and profuse rhinorrhea, they are suggestive of sinusitis. A differentiation between chronic sinusitis and allergic rhinitis can be made when eosinophils predominate. If the smear is devoid of eosinophils, chronic sinusitis can be suspected. However, this test is rarely performed in clinical practice.

Transillumination is helpful in the diagnosis of maxillary and frontal sinusitis. Both the patient and examiner must be in a darkened room. Interpretation of the transillumination of the frontal sinuses is difficult because they are naturally asymmetric. Hence, only maxillary sinuses can be adequately evaluated.[58] The maxillary sinuses are transilluminated when a high-intensity light source, shielded from the examiner, is placed over the midpoint of the inferior orbital rim. Light transmission through the hard palate is assessed by the examiner with the patient's mouth open. Assessment of the symmetry of the blush bilaterally provides clues to the diagnosis. Because of the increased thickness of the soft tissue and bony vault in children 10 years of age and younger, the clinical diagnosis of sinusitis with transillumination is not helpful.

Radiography can confirm the diagnosis of sinusitis. Diagnostic findings include air-liquid levels in sinus cavities, mucosal thickening, and partial or complete opacification of the sinus cavities. When a patient presents with signs and symptoms suggesting sinusitis and abnormal maxillary sinus radiography, bacteria will be present 75% of the time. A normal radiograph in a patient with clinical signs and symptoms of sinusitis, however, does not suggest that the patient is free of disease.

Computed tomography and magnetic resonance imagery are useful in cases of sinusitis that are complicated by intracranial or intraorbital suppuration. They are not otherwise cost-effective and should not be used routinely to diagnose acute sinusitis.

▶ TREATMENT: Sinusitis

DESIRED OUTCOME

Many symptoms of sinusitis will resolve without medical therapy within 48 hours. When they persist, the goals of treatment include symptomatic relief, restoring and improving sinus function, preventing intracranial complications (periorbital cellulitis, meningitis, facial osteomyelitis), preventing the progression to chronic sinusitis and eradicating the causative pathogen.

PHARMACOLOGIC THERAPY

Although 40% of sinusitis patients will recover spontaneously, antibiotics are the mainstay of therapy in toxic-appearing patients, those who fail initial therapy with topical decongestants, and patients with co-morbid conditions.[60] Selection of the appropriate agent is directed against the most likely pathogens (Table 107–2). Amoxicillin or TMP/SMX are still considered to be a first-line treatment of acute bacterial sinusitis.[58,59] It is recommended that the amoxicillin dose be doubled as in the treatment of otitis media, especially in areas in which resistance to *S. pneumoniae* is high.[59] However, the clinical benefits of using higher doses of amoxicillin in the treatment of sinusitis remains to be evaluated. In adults, TMP/SMX is efficacious but may be ineffective in group A streptococcal infections. It can be considered for first-line therapy in patients allergic to penicillin. Bacteriologic cure rates for amoxicillin-clavulanate, loracarbef, azithromycin, clarithromycin, cefuroxime axetil, cefixime, cefaclor, and erythromycin-sulfisoxazole were comparable.[58] β-Lactams are considered second-line choices for the treatment of sinusitis. The first-generation agents have poor *H. influenzae* coverage. Several second- and third-generation cephalosporins have excellent activity against all major pathogens except resistant *S. pneumoniae*. Fluoroquinolones (levofloxacin, gatifloxacin, moxifloxacin) offer excellent coverage against all major pathogens, resistant or not, as well as excellent penetration into the sinuses. Table 107–2 decribes dosages and costs.

Acute sinusitis is treated for 10 to 14 days, but duration can be extended to 30 days in protracted cases.[64] Adverse effects and pharmacoeconomic factors are similar to those described in the section on otitis media.

ADJUNCT THERAPY

In the immunocompromised host, initial treatment should consist of topical decongestants and steam inhalations every four hours. If the maxillary sinuses are involved, patients should be advised to sleep in a semi-upright position to facilitate drainage. Adjunctive treatments are designed to promote ciliary function and to decrease edema.[59] Although there are no published placebo-controlled studies of decongestants, these medications are often included in the treatment of uncomplicated acute sinusitis. Nasal spray decongestants, such as phenylephrine hydrochloride (0.5%) or oxymetazoline hydrochloride (0.05%) may facilitate drainage.[59] The use of such agents should not exceed more than 72 hours because of a tolerance effect and possible rebound congestion. Purulent secretions present in the nose should be removed before administration.

Oral decongestants (pseudoephedrine) reduce nasal blood flow through their α-adrenergic activity. Their use improves nasal patency by increasing the functional diameter of the maxillary ostium.[58] Systemic decongestants are not recommended in the pediatric population because of the potential for cardiac stimulation, hypertension, or neurologic complications.[65]

Antihistamines are ineffective in the management of acute sinusitis, and they may interfere with the clearance of purulent mucous secretions because of their potential to cause dryness of mucosal membranes (anticholinergic effect). The use of an intranasal corticosteroid can increase ostium patency; however, this effect is inconsistent. Because corticosteroids take a long time to act, an episode of acute sinusitis may resolve before their beneficial effects are noticed. Irrigation of the nasal cavity using a saline solution in a squeeze spray bottle may provide symptomatic relief.

EVALUATION OF THERAPEUTIC OUTCOMES

With proper treatment, symptoms of acute sinusitis will abate in 2 to 5 days. It is necessary to stress the importance of continuing antibiotic therapy for 10 days. Appropriate followup should be initiated in order to promote compliance. If treatment failure occurs and the patient has not responded to first-line therapy, additional evaluations are necessary and second-line therapy can be used. Patients with recurrent episodes of acute sinusitis who do not have anatomic anomalies may benefit from second-line therapy. Complications of sinusitis include periorbital cellulitis, particularly in children, as well as meningitis. Finally, unrecognized sinusitis is a rather frequent cause of poorly controlled asthma. Occult sinusitis should be sought in patients with uncontrolled asthma not responding to bronchodilators and corticosteroids.

EPIGLOTTITIS AND LARYNGITIS (CROUP)

Laryngeal dyspnea is frequently encountered in children. The most frequent cause is the infection affecting supra- or subglottic structures. Supraglottic infections include epiglottitis, retropharyngeal abscess, peritonsillar abscess, Ludwig's angina, and acute tonsillitis. Subglottic manifestations (croup) can result in spasmodic laryngitis, as well as viral or bacterial laryngotracheitis. Other etiologies include foreign body aspiration, trauma to the larynx, angioneurotic edema (allergic), and congenital abnormalities.

To better understand the manifestations of epiglottitis and croup, it is important to review the anatomic particularities of the upper respiratory tract in children. The epiglottis is one of the main cartilages of the larynx that blocks entry to the glottis during swallowing. In children, the larynx is located higher (the glottis is at the C2-C3 level) and in a position anterior to that in the adult. Unlike adults, the narrowest area of the upper respiratory airway in children is the cricoid ring. Finally, the glottis is of a small caliber (4 × 7 mm). A 1-mm edema of the wall will result in a 35% reduction of the aperture, thereby increasing airway resistance by a factor of 16.

EPIGLOTTITIS

Epiglottitis is a true airway emergency in which acute airway obstruction can occur. It is caused primarily by HIB. Epiglottitis is more prevalent in children ages 2 to 6 years, but its incidence has decreased significantly since the advent of the HIB vaccine.[66] The onset of the disease is rapid, and the evolution is often brisk. Respiratory distress, drooling, dysphagia, and dysphonia are the typical signs of the disease (the "four Ds"). Fever is usually high and often manifests as the first symptom. The airway obstruction evolves rapidly and manifests by respiratory distress, an inspiratory stridor, loss of voice, and the presence of intercostal drawing. The typical posture of the child (tripod) with arms at the side, upper body set forward, neck extended with the chin thrust forward, and mouth wide open maximizes the size of the supraglottic airway. One can observe over a period of 2 to 4 hours the signs of upper respiratory airway obstruction, and in half of the cases and sometimes late in the course of the disease, hypersalivation (drooling). Once epiglottitis is suspected, the diagnosis should be confirmed by a person who is prepared for immediate airway intervention. When there is doubt as to the diagnosis, if the condition of the patient permits and the physician is present at bedside, a lateral neck radiograph obtained in a sitting position will show an edematous epiglottis in 95% of cases (thumb sign). When the airway has been stabilized, blood gases, as well as blood and epiglottal cultures, can be obtained.

It is important to note that epiglottitis can also manifest itself in adults and usually presents as intense dysphagia progressing over a period of a few days.[67] When compared to children, dyspnea appears later in the course of the disease, thus delaying diagnosis.

▶ TREATMENT: Epiglottitis

NONPHARMACOLOGIC THERAPY

The primary concern in the management of epiglottitis is establishing and maintaining the airway. It is important to maintain the patient in a sitting position, to avoid manipulations (e.g., blood drawing), and to not attempt a throat exam. If the child presents with imminent respiratory insufficiency, humidified oxygen (Fio_2 of 1.0) in a way best tolerated, with or without manual insufflations, should be administered while preparing for intubation. The optimal treatment consists of transporting the child to the operating room and performing a direct laryngoscopy followed by intubation if epiglottitis is confirmed.

PHARMACOLOGIC THERAPY

After the airway has been established, antibiotic therapy should be instituted and empirically directed against HIB. The second- or third-generation cephalosporins cefuroxime (150 mg/kg/day given every 8 hours), cefotaxime (150–225 mg/kg/day given every 6 hours), or ceftriaxone (80–100 mg/kg/day given every 12 hours) are appropriate. Once the condition improves, the patient is extubated, and oral antibiotic therapy is recommended and continued for a total of 10 days. Corticosteroids (dexamethasone) can be used to decrease laryngeal edema.

Isolation of the hospitalized patient is indicated until 24 hours after initiation of effective therapy. Household contacts, defined as individuals residing in the home of the index patient or nonresidents who spent 4 or more hours with the index patient for at least 5 of the 7 days preceding the day of hospitalization, should receive chemoprophylaxis with rifampin (20 mg/kg/day for 4 days given once a day, maximum 600 mg/day). Management of day care and nursery school contact groups should be individualized.

TABLE 107–4. Differentiating Clinical Features of Epiglottitis, Viral Croup, and Laryngotracheitis

Feature	Epiglottitis	Viral Croup	Bacterial Croup
Pathogens	HIB	Parainfluenzae virus RSV	*S. aureus*
Age	2–6 years	6 months to 3 years	1 month – 6 years
Season	All seasons	Fall-winter	All seasons
Time of day	Anytime	Beginning of night	Anytime
Signs and symptoms			
Clinical presentation	Toxic, typical posture	Nontoxic, supine	Toxic supine
Progression	Rapid (2–4 hours)	Rapid	Slow
Fever	High	Absent or low	Moderate
Stridor	Muffled	Loud	Loud
Barking cough	No	Yes	Yes
Sore throat (dysphagia)	Yes	No	No
Drooling	Yes (50% of cases)	No	No
Laboratory evaluation			
Leukocytosis	Elevated	Normal	Elevated
Blood culture	Positive (70% to 90% of cases)	Negative	Positive in some cases

HIB, *a Haemophilus influenzae* type b; RSV, respiratory syncytial virus.

LARYNGITIS (CROUP)

Laryngitis (croup) is the most frequent cause of laryngeal dyspnea in children. It is characterized by the presence of stridor and presents most often in the early hours of the night in children younger than 3 years of age. In contrast to epiglottitis, a barking cough and an absence of drooling is observed (Table 107–4). Laryngitis can be divided into three groups.

SPASMODIC LARYNGITIS

The etiology is not well defined and could be of viral or allergic origin. The onset is rapid, without a prodrome or fever, and the manifestations resolve rapidly.

VIRAL LARYNGOTRACHEITIS

It is caused primarily by parainfluenza (types 1 and 2).[66] It is preceded by an upper respiratory tract infection and fever (1 to 3 days), and occasionally it progresses toward respiratory distress. This syndrome generally resolves, however, without any specific treatment within 4 days, during which time the symptoms become intermittent with nocturnal exacerbations.

BACTERIAL LARYNGOTRACHEITIS (*PSEUDOMEMBRANOUS LARYNGITIS*)

This is another form of croup that is rare but life-threatening. Most cases are caused by a secondary infection following a viral laryngitis, the only primary laryngotracheitis being caused by diphtheria. The clinical presentation includes copious purulent secretions and, occasionally, the presence of a membranous film in the trachea. Bacteria involved include *S. aureus,* group A β-hemolytic streptococcus, HIB, *M. catarrhalis,* and pneumococcus. Progressive symptoms of stridor, fever, and frequent hoarse cough are usually observed. Contrary to viral laryngitis, this disease evolves toward respiratory distress. A radiograph of the soft tissues of the neck and lungs may reveal an irregularity of the tracheal mucosa (in 10% of cases) or pulmonary infiltrates.

Whatever the cause of laryngitis, it is important to evaluate the severity of the respiratory distress because this will guide the choice of treatment. Severity is determined on physical exam by the presence of stridor, intercostal drawing, vesicular murmur upon pulmonary auscultation, skin coloration, and level of consciousness. The presence of cyanosis and a decrease in the level of consciousness are indicative of severity. The anterior-posterior view of the soft tissues of the neck on radiography can reveal a narrowing of the air column as a result of subglottic edema. This, however, is not pathognomonic of laryngitis, and the severity of the disease is not well-correlated with the amount of subglottic edema.

▶ TREATMENT: Laryngitis

Treatment varies according to the severity (mild, moderate, severe) of the laryngitis. Most cases can be treated as outpatients. Therapeutic options include humidified oxygen, racemic epinephrine, and corticosteroids.

NONPHARMACOLOGIC THERAPY

Humidified oxygen should be administered in the presence of suspected or documented hypoxia ($SAO_2 < 90\%$). Cold humidity can relieve symptoms of laryngitis, although its efficacy has not been proven scientifically. It is believed to act by liquefying secretions and soothing the irritated laryngeal mucosa. If the child is in mild respiratory distress, parents can take the child outdoors for a period of approximately 15 minutes, weather permitting. This is efficacious in relieving less severe symptoms but does not allow for close monitoring of the child. Alternatively, a humidified oxygen tent allows the child to be exposed to cold humidity in a 40% oxygen environment. If the child is cooperative, application of a face mask and nebulizer is an option. This also ensures the delivery of cold humidified air (ice and physiologic saline) while allowing for higher oxygen concentrations (35% to 60% with a flow of 6–10 L/min). Whatever the method used, it is important to keep the child calm and ensure the parents' cooperation.

PHARMACOLOGIC THERAPY

Racemic epinephrine, an α- and β-adrenergic agonist, can be used in moderate to severe laryngitis. Its benefits are derived from its α-receptor activity, which results in vasoconstriction and a decrease in subglottic edema. In addition, its β-receptor effects cause bronchodilation and relieve airway obstruction.[68]

A 0.5-mL dose of 2.25% racemic epinephrine (Vaponetrin) diluted in 2.5–3.5 mL of physiologic saline is recommended.[69] Administration by nebulization with a face mask is preferred. A single dose is usually sufficient to relieve the symptoms of obstruction, but additional doses can be administered every 30 minutes if stridor persists while the child is at rest. The time to peak effect is 10 to 30 minutes, and the duration of action is 2 to 3 hours. Contrary to general belief, there is no rebound effect; however, obstructive symptoms can return upon cessation of treatment. A period of observation of a minimum of 3 hours is recommended, with subsequent reevaluation of the respiratory status.

Corticosteroids are used in moderate to severe laryngitis. Several studies, as well as a meta-analysis, confirm the benefits of corticosteroids in laryngitis.[70–72] Their use in hospitalized patients significantly improved the patients' respiratory status in 12 to 24 hours following administration, thereby decreasing the need for intubation and allowing for earlier discharge. Dexamethasone is preferred because of its rapid onset of action (<2 hours), its peak of action (6 to 8 hours), and its long half-life (36 to 72 hours). A dose-effect relationship has been noted, the optimal dose of dexamethasone being 0.6 mg/kg given orally or intramuscularly (maximum dose of 8 mg).[73] One study showed, however, that, when compared to doses of 0.3 and 0.6 mg/kg, no significant difference was noted when a dose of 0.15 mg/kg of dexamethasone was used.[74] Its pharmacokinetics allow for single-dose administration, although a second identical dose can be administered after 24 hours if respiratory distress persists. At this point, it is recommended that any child requiring the administration of racemic epinephrine be given 0.6 mg/kg of dexamethasone.

Studies show the benefit of inhaled steroids. Two milligrams of nebulized budesonide provides short-term clinical effects similar to racemic epinephrine when used in mild to moderate laryngitis. It has an onset of action of 30 minutes and a duration of action of 2 hours.[75–78] The proposed mechanism of action is a topical vasoconstrictive effect on the edematous laryngeal mucosa, thereby reducing capillary permeability. Budesonide offers an interesting alternative in the treatment of laryngitis. When compared to 0.6 mg/kg of dexamethasone and placebo, 4 mg of nebulized budesonide showed greater improvement in croup scores than placebo and a lower hospitalization rate.[79]

The meta-analysis performed by the Cochrane library reveals that children presenting with croup require fewer adrenaline treatments when receiving dexamethasone (decrease of 12%) or budesonide (decrease of 9%).[72] There is also a decrease in the length of time spent in the emergency department. Both dexamethasone and budesonide are effective in relieving the symptoms of croup as early as 6 hours after treatment.

Antibiotics should only be used when the diagnosis of bacterial laryngotracheitis is made, in which case, antibiotics targeting *S. aureus,* streptococcus, and HIB should be used. Cefuroxime is a good first choice, followed by a combination of cloxacillin and cefotaxime, and finally the combination of vancomycin in association with an aminoglycoside. The combined therapy is preferred when laryngitis was contracted in the hospital. Enterobacteria are often implicated if the patient is immunosuppressed. Adjunct therapy includes intubation, which provides adequate humidity and aspirates airway secretions. Bacterial laryngotracheitis is fatal if not recognized early.

▶ PRINCIPLES OF PHARMACOTHERAPY

- Practitioners should be aware of resistance patterns for upper respiratory tract infections in their specific communities.
- The diagnosis of otitis media is confirmed by the examination of the tympanic membrane. Redness or opacity of the tympanic membrane, the absence of light reflection, bulging, and immobility of the tympanic membrane to pneumatic otoscopy are all indicative of a middle ear effusion and are suggestive of otitis media.
- Otitis media can be caused by *Streptococcus pneumoniae*, nontypeable strains of *Haemophilus influenzae*, and *Moraxella catarrhalis.*
- The percentage of *S. pneumoniae* strains found to demonstrate a reduced susceptibility to amoxicillin has significantly increased. The proportion of β-lactamase producing *H. influenzae* and *M. catarrhalis* strains in acute otitis media has nearly tripled in the last decade.
- Oral antibiotics remain the mainstay of therapy for acute otitis media, and amoxicillin for 10 days is still the drug of choice. In addition to antimicrobial therapy, supportive therapy with analgesics, antipyretics, and local heat are beneficial.
- When resistant *S. pneumoniae* are suspected, high-dose amoxicillin or the use amoxicillin/clavulanate should be considered.

- Viruses appear to be the cause of the majority of episodes of pharyngitis, often as constituents of the common cold. A significant number of sore throats are of bacterial origin, with group A β-hemolytic streptococci being the most prevalent microorganism.
- A throat culture obtained from the surface of the tonsils and the posterior pharyngeal wall is the most commonly used test for the identification of GAS.
- Penicillin is the drug of choice for pharyngitis caused by GAS. The recommended duration of therapy is 10 days.
- The predominant organisms that cause sinusitis are *S. pneumoniae* and nontypeable *H. influenzae*. As in otitis media, resistance is increasing.
- Three symptoms (maxillary toothache, poor response to decongestants, and history of colored nasal discharge) and two signs (purulent nasal secretions and abnormal transillumination) are the best clinical predictors of acute sinusitis.
- Oral antibiotics remain the mainstay of therapy for acute sinusitis, and amoxicillin (for 10 days) is still the drug of choice. Nasal spray decongestants, such as phenylephrine hydrochloride (0.5%) or oxymetazoline hydrochloride (0.05%), may facilitate drainage in uncomplicated cases.
- Epiglottitis is a true airway emergency in which acute airway obstruction can occur. It is caused primarily by HIB and should be treated with humidified oxygen and an intravenous second- or third-generation cephalosporin.
- Racemic epinephrine, administered by nebulization, can be used in moderate to severe laryngitis.
- Children presenting with croup require fewer adrenaline treatments when receiving glucocorticoids. Both dexamethasone and budesonide are effective in relieving the symptoms of croup as early as 6 hours after treatment, which results in less time spent in the emergency department.

REFERENCES

1. McCaig LF, Hughes JM. Trends in antimicrobial prescribing among office-based physicians in the United States [published erratum in JAMA 1998;11:279]. JAMA 1995;273:241–249.
2. Bluestone CD, Klein JO. Otitis media, atelectasis, and eustachian tube dysfunction. In: Bluestone CD, Stool SE, Scheetz MD, eds. Pediatric Otolaryngology. Philadelphia, Saunders, 1990:322–334.
3. Rosenfeld RM. An evidence-based approach to treating otitis media. Pediatr Clin North Am 1996;43:1165–1181.
4. Froom J, Culpepper L, Jacob M, et al. Antimicrobials for acute otitis media? A review from the International Primary Care Network. BMJ 1997;315:98–102.
5. Lanphear BP, Byrd RS, Auinger P, et al. Increasing prevalence of recurrent otitis media among children in the United States. Pediatrics 1997;99: 1–7.
6. Pelton SI. New concepts in the pathophysiology and management of middle ear disease in childhood. Drugs 1996;52(suppl 2):62–66.
7. Daly KA, Brown JE, Lindgren BR, et al. Epidemiology of otitis media onset by six months of age. Pediatrics 1999;103:1158–1166.
8. Casselbrant ML, Mandel EM, Fall PA, et al. The heritability of otitis media. A twin and triplet study. JAMA 1999;282:2125–2130.
9. Uhari M, Mäntysaari K, Niemelä M;. A meta-analytic review of the risk factors for acute otitis media. Clin Infect Dis 1996;22:1079–1083.
10. Duncan B, Ey J, Holberg CJ, et al. Exclusive breast-feeding for at least 4 months protects against otitis media. Pediatrics 1993;91:867–872.
11. Swanson JA, Hoecker JL. Otitis media in young children. Mayo Clin Proc 1996;71:179–183.
12. Block WSl. Causative pathogen, antibiotic resistance and therapeutic considerations in acute otitis media. Pediatr Infect Dis 1997;16:449–456.
13. Centers for Disease Control and Prevention. Defining the public health impact of drug-resistant *Streptococcus pneumoniae*: Report of a working group. MMWR Morb Mortal Wkly Rep 1996;45(RR-1 suppl):1–20.
14. Pichichero M, Reiner SA, Brook I, et al. Controversies in the medical management of persistent and recurrent acute otitis media. Recommendations of a clinical advisory committee. Ann Otol Laryngol 2000;109:2–12.
15. Carlin SA, Marchant CD, Shurin PA, et al. Host factors and early therapeutic response in acute otitis media. J Pediatr 1991;118:178–183.
16. Jacobs MR, Dagan R, Applebaum DJ, et al. Prevalence of antimicrobial resistant-pathogens in middle ear fluid: Multinational study of 917 children with acute otitis media. Antimicrob Agents Chemother 1998;42:589–595.
17. Pichichero ME. Acute otitis media: Part II. Treatment in an era of increasing antibiotic resistance. Am Fam Physician 2000;61(8):2410–2418.
18. Heikkinen T, Thint M, Chonmaintree T. Prevalence of various respiratory viruses in the middle ear during acute otitis media. N Engl J Med 1999;340:260–264.
19. Walsh RM, Bath AP, Hawke M, et al. Acute otitis media: Four out of five kids. Can J Diagn 1999;16:106–121.
20. Berman S. Management of acute and chronic otitis media in pediatric practice. Curr Opin Pediatr 1995;7:513–522.
21. Pichichero ME. Changing the treatment paradigm for acute otitis media in children. JAMA 1998;279:1748–1750.
22. Bluestone CD, Klein JO, Gates GA. "Appropriateness" of tympanostomy tubes: Setting the record straight. Arch Otolaryngol Head Neck Surg 1994;120:1051–1053.
23. Rosenfeld RM, Vertrees JE, Carr J, et al. Clinical efficacy of antimicrobial drugs for acute otitis media: Meta-analysis of 5400 children from 33 randomized trials. J Pediatr 1994;124:355–367.
24. Del Mar C, Galsziou P, Hayem M. Are antibiotics indicated as initial treatment for children with acute otitis media? A meta-analysis. BMJ 1997;314:1526–1529.
25. Damoiseaux RAM, van Balen AM, Hoes AW, et al. Primary care based randomized, double-blind trial of amoxicillin versus placebo for acute otitis media in children under 2 years. BMJ 2000;320:350–353.
26. Dowell SF, Butler JC, Giebink GS, et al. Acute otitis media: Management and surveillance in an era of pneumococcal resistance—A report from the Drug-Resistant *Streptococcus pneumoniae* Therapeutic Working Group. Pediatr Infect Dis 1999;18:1–9.
27. Force RW, Nahata MC. Loracarbef: A new orally administered carbacephem antibiotic. Ann Pharmacother 1993;27:321–329.
28. Chocas EC, Paap CM, Godley PJ. Cefpodoxime proxetil: A new, broad-spectrum, oral cephalosporin. Ann Pharmacother 1993;27:1369–1377.
29. Blumer JL, Forti WP, Summerhouse TL. Comparison of the efficacy and tolerability of once-daily ceftibuten and twice daily cefprozil in the treatment of children with acute otitis media. Clin Ther 1996;18:811–820.
30. Khurana CM. A multicenter, randomized, open label comparison of azithromycin and amoxicillin/clavulanate in acute otitis media among children attending day care or school. Pediatr Infect Dis J 1996;15 (9 suppl):S24–S29.
31. Gehanno P, Berche P, Boucot I, et al. Comparative efficacy and safety of cefprozil and amoxicillin/clavulanate in the treatment of acute otitis media in children. J Antimicrob Chemother 1994;33:1209–1218.
32. Aspin MM, Hoberman A, McCarty J, et al. Comparative study of the safety and efficacy of clarithromycin and amoxicillin/clavulanate in the treatment of acute otitis media in children. J Pediatr 1994;125:136–141.
33. Piscitelli SC, Danziger LH, Rodvold KA. Clarithromycin and azithromycin: New macrolide antibiotics. Clin Pharm 1992;11:137–152.
34. Pichichero ME, Cohen R. Shortened course of antibiotic therapy for acute otitis media, sinusitis and tonsillopharyngitis. Pediatr Infect Dis J 1997;16:680–695.
35. Kozyrskyj AL, Hildes-Ripstein GE, Longstaffe SE, et al. Treatment of acute otitis media with a shortened course of antibiotics: A meta-analysis. JAMA 1998;279:1736–1742.

36. Williams RL, Chalmers TC, Stange KC, et al. Use of antibiotics in preventing recurrent acute otitis media and in treating otitis media with effusion: A meta-analytic attempt to resolve the brouhaha. JAMA 1993;270:1344–1351.
37. American Academy of Pediatrics. Report of the Committee on Infectious Diseases. Evanston, IL, American Academy of Pediatrics, 1994.
38. Marchant CD, Carlin SA, Johnson CE, Shurin PA. Measuring the comparative efficacy of antibacterial agents for acute otitis media: The "Pollyanna phenomenon." J Pediatr 1992;120:120–127.
39. Mattar ME, Markello J, Yaffe SJ. Pharmaceutical factors affecting pediatric compliance. Pediatrics 1975;55:101–108.
40. McLinn S. Double-blind and open label studies of azithromycin in the management of acute otitis media in children: A review. Pediatr Infect Dis J 1995;14(suppl):S62–S66.
41. Green SM, Rothrock SG. Single-dose intramuscular ceftriaxone for acute otitis media in children. Pediatrics 1993;91:23–30.
42. Cohen R, Navel M, Grunberg J, et al. One dose-ceftriaxone vs. ten days of amoxicillin-clavulanate therapy for acute otitis media: Clinical efficacy and change in nasopharyngeal flora. Pediatr Infect Dis J 1999;18:403–409.
43. Dagan R, Shvartzman P, Liss Z. Variation in acceptance of common oral antibiotic suspensions. Pediatr Infect Dis J 1994;13:686–690.
44. Wandstrat TL, Kaplan B. Pharmacoeconomic impact of factors affecting compliance with antibiotic regimens in the treatment of acute otitis media. Pediatr Infect Dis J 1997;16(2 suppl):S27–S29.
45. McIsaac WJ, Goel V, Slaughter PM, et al. Reconsidering sore throats: 1. Can Fam Physician 1997;43:485–493.
46. Bisno AL. Acute pharyngitis. N Engl J Med 2001;344(3):205–211.
47. Bisno AL, Gerber MA, Gwaltney JM, et al. Diagnosis and management of group A streptococcal pharyngitis: A practice guideline. Clin Infect Dis 1997;25:574–583.
48. Pichichero ME. Controversies in the treatment of streptococcal pharyngitis. Am Fam Physician 1990;42:1567 1576.
49. Dajani A, Taubert K, Ferrieri P, et al. Treatment of acute streptococcal pharyngitis and prevention of rheumatic fever: A statement for health professionals. Pediatrics 1995;96;758–764.
50. Centor RM, Witherspoon JM, Dalton HP, et al. The diagnosis of strep throat in adults in the emergency room. Med Decis Making 1981;1:239–246.
51. McIsaac WJ, Goel V, Slaughter PM, et al. Reconsidering sore throats: 2. Can Fam Physician 1997;43:495–500.
52. Ebell MH, Smith MA, Barry HC, et al. Does this patient have strep throat? JAMA 2000;284:2912–2918.
53. McIsaac WJ, Goel V, To T, et al. The validity of a throat score in family practice. CMAJ 2000,163(7):811–815.
54. Treatment of group A streptococcal pharyngitis. Pediatr Child Health 1997;2(2):97–98.
55. Lan AJ, Colford JM. The impact of dosing frequency on the efficacy of 10-day penicillin or amoxicillin therapy for streptococcal tonsillopharyngitis: A meta-analysis. Pediatrics 2000;105(2):423–410.
56. Adam D, Acholtz H, Helmerking M. Short-course antibiotic treatment of 4782 culture-proven cases of group A streptococcal tonsillopharyngitis and incidence of poststreptococcal sequelae. J Infect Dis 2000;182:509–516
57. Tanz RR, Shulman ST, Barthel MJ, et al. Penicillin plus rifampin eradicates pharyngeal carriage of group A streptococci. J Pediatr 1985;106:876–880.
58. Low DE, Desrosiers M, McSherry J, et al. A practical guide for the diagnosis and treatment of acute sinusitis. CMAJ 1997;156(6 suppl):S1–S14.
59. Brook I, Gooch WM, Jenjins SG, et al. Medical management of acute bacterial sinusitis. Recommendations of a clinical advisory committee on pediatric and adult sinusitis. Ann Otol Rhinol Laryngol 2000;109:2–20.
60. Ahuja GS, Thompson J. What role for antibiotics in otitis media and sinusitis? Postgrad Med 1998;104:93–99, 103–104.
61. Wald ER. Expanded role of group A streptococci in children with upper respiratory infections. Pediatr Infect Dis J 1999;18:663–665.
62. Williams JW, Simel DL, Roberts L, et al. Clinical evaluation for sinusitis: Making the diagnosis by history and physical examination. Ann Intern Med 1992;117:705–710.
63. Lanza DC, Kennedy DW. Adult rhinosinusitis defined. In: Anon JB, ed. Report of the Rhinosinusitis Task Force Committee meeting. Otolaryngol Head Neck Surg 1997;117(suppl):S1–S7.
64. Williams JW, Holleman DR, Samsa GP, et al. Randomized controlled trial of 3 vs 10 days of trimethoprim/sulfamethoxazole for acute maxillary sinusitis. JAMA 1995;273:1015–1021.
65. Katcher ML. Cold, cough, and allergy medications: Uses and abuses. Pediatr Rev 1996;17:12–17.
66. Cressman WR, Myer CW. Diagnosis and management of croup and epiglottitis. Pediatr Clin North Am 1994;41:265–276.
67. Strausbaugh LJ. *Haemophilus influenzae* infections in adults: A pathogen in search of respect. Postgrad Med 1997;101:191–192.
68. Hoffman BB, Lefkowitz RJ. Catecholamines, sympathomimetic drugs and adrenergic receptor antagonists. In: Hardman JG, Limberg LE, eds. Goodman and Gilman's The Pharmacological Basis of Therapeutics, 9th ed. New York, McGraw-Hill, 1996:199–248.
69. Folland DS. Treatment of croup: Sending home an improved child and relieved parents. Postgrad Med 1997;101:271–273.
70. Cruz MN, Stewart G, Rosenberg N. Use of dexamethasone in the outpatient management of acute laryngotracheitis. Pediatrics 1995;96 (2 part 1):220–223.
71. Geelhoed GC, Macdonald WB. Oral and inhaled steroids in croup: A randomized, placebo-controlled trial. Pediatr Pulmonol 1995;20:355–361.
72. Ausejo M, Saenz A, Pham B, et al. Glucocorticoids for croup (Cochrane review). Cochrane Database Syst Rev 2001;1.
73. Rittichier KK, Ledwith CA. Outpatient treatment of moderate croup with dexamethasone: Intramuscular versus oral dosing. Pediatrics 2000;106:1344–1348.
74. Geelhoed GC, Macdonald WB. Oral dexamethasone in the treatment of croup: 0.15 mg/kg versus 0.3 mg/kg versus 0.6 mg/kg. Pediatr Pulmunol 1995;20:362–368.
75. Godden CW, Campbell MJ, Hussey M, et al. Double-blind placebo-controlled trial of nebulized budesonide for croup. Arch Dis Child 1997; 76:155–158.
76. Fitzgerald D, Mellis C, Johnson M, et al. Nebulized budesonide is as effective as nebulized adrenaline in moderately severe croup. Pediatrics 1996;97:722–725.
77. Klassen TP, Feldman ME, Watters LK, et al. Nebulized budesonide for children with mild-to-moderate croup. N Engl J Med 1994;331:285–289.
78. Johnson DW, Schuh S, Koren G, et al. Outpatient treatment of croup with nebulized dexamethasone. Arch Pediatr Adolesc Med 1996;150:349–355
79. Johnson DW, Jacobson S, Edney PC, et al. A comparison of nebulized budesonide, intramuscular dexamethasone, and placebo for moderately severe croup. N Engl J Med 1998;339:498–503.

108

SKIN AND SOFT TISSUE INFECTIONS

Larry H. Danziger, Douglas N. Fish, and Susan L. Pendland

Infections of the skin and soft tissues are among the most common infections seen in both community and hospital settings. These infections may involve any or all layers of the skin, fascia, and muscle. They may also spread far from the initial site of infection and lead to more severe complications, such as endocarditis, gram-negative sepsis, or streptococcal glomerulonephritis. The treatment of skin and soft tissue infections may at times necessitate both medical and surgical management. This chapter presents details of the pathogenesis and management of some of the most common infections involving the skin and soft tissues. The first part of this chapter discusses a variety of skin and soft tissue infections that range in severity from superficial to life threatening. The remainder of the chapter discusses diabetic foot infections, pressure sores, and human and animal bites.

PATHOPHYSIOLOGY

The skin serves as a barrier between humans and their environment and therefore functions as a primary defense mechanism against infections. The skin consists of the epidermis, the dermis, and subcutaneous fat. The epidermis is the outermost, nonvascular layer of the skin. It varies in thickness, from approximately 0.1 mm on most areas of the body to a maximum of 1.5 mm on the soles of the feet. Although extremely thin, the epidermis is composed of several layers. The innermost layer consists of continuously dividing cells. The outer layers are renewed as cells are gradually pushed outward. As the cells approach the surface, they become flattened, lose their nuclei, and are filled with keratin. The outermost layer, the stratum corneum, is composed of flattened, cornified, nonnucleated cells. The dermis is the layer of skin directly beneath the epidermis. It consists of connective tissue and contains blood vessels and lymphatics, sensory nerve endings, sweat and sebaceous glands, hair follicles, and smooth-muscle fibers. Beneath the dermis is a layer of loose connective tissue containing primarily fat cells. This subcutaneous fat layer is of variable thickness over the body. Beneath the subcutaneous fat lies the fascia, which separates the skin from underlying muscle. It is generally divided into superficial fascia, which is located immediately beneath the skin, and deep fascia, which forms sheaths for muscles.

The skin and subcutaneous tissues are normally extremely resistant to infection. Even when high concentrations of bacteria are applied topically or injected into the soft tissue, resultant infections are rare.[1] Several host factors act together to confer protection against skin infections. The surface of the skin is relatively dry and is not conducive to bacterial growth. Also, continuous renewal of the epidermal layer results in the shedding of keratocytes, as well as skin bacteria. In addition, sebaceous secretions are hydrolyzed to form free fatty acids that strongly inhibit the growth of many bacteria and fungi.[1] The conditions that may predispose a patient to the development of skin infections include (a) a high concentration of bacteria ($>10^5$ microorganisms); (b) excessive moisture of the skin; (c) inadequate blood supply; (d) availability of bacterial nutrients; and (e) damage to the corneal layer allowing for bacterial penetration.[1,2]

The majority of skin and soft tissue infections result from the disruption of normal host defenses by processes such as skin puncture, abrasion, or underlying diseases (e.g., diabetes). The nature and severity of the infection depends on both the type of microorganism present and the site of inoculation. A large percentage of these infections are caused by normal skin flora (Table 108–1). Exposed areas of the body (face, neck) generally have the highest bacterial density and *Staphylococcus epidermidis* is the most common microorganism, whereas moister areas (axilla and groin) are most frequently colonized with gram-negative bacilli.[2]

Common bacterial infections of the skin can be classified as primary or secondary (Table 108–2). Primary bacterial infections usually involve areas of previously healthy skin and are typically caused by a single pathogen. In contrast, secondary infections occur in areas of previously damaged skin and are frequently polymicrobic.

FOLLICULITIS, FURUNCLES, AND CARBUNCLES

Folliculitis is a superficial infection surrounding the hair follicles. This condition is commonly referred to as a stye when it occurs at the base of the eyelid. Most cases of folliculitis are caused by *Staphylococcus aureus*. Inadequate chlorine levels in whirlpools, hot tubs, and swimming pools have been responsible for outbreaks of folliculitis caused by *Pseudomonas aeruginosa*.[3] Pruritic, erythematous papules appear 48 hours after exposure to large numbers of organisms. The papules evolve into pustules that generally heal in several days.

Furuncles, more commonly referred to as boils, are an extension of folliculitis, in which inflammation extends from around the hair shaft to involve the dermis. Furuncles can occur anywhere on hairy skin, but generally develop in areas subject to friction and perspiration. The lesion starts as a firm, tender, red nodule that becomes painful and fluctuant.[4] Surgical incision is occasionally used; however, the lesions often drain spontaneously. Furuncles are discrete lesions, whether occurring as singular or multiple nodules. They are called carbuncles when the lesions coalesce and extend to the subcutaneous tissue. Unlike infections with folliculitis and furuncles, carbuncles are commonly associated with fever, chills, and malaise. Bacteremia with secondary spread to other tissues is common.

▶ TREATMENT: Folliculitis, Furuncles, and Carbuncles

Treatment of folliculitis generally requires only local measures, such as warm saline compresses or topical antibacterials (clindamycin, erythromycin, mupirocin). Small furuncles can generally be treated with moist heat, which promotes localization and drainage of pus.[4] Large and/or multiple furuncles and carbuncles are generally treated with a penicillinase-resistant penicillin (dicloxacillin 250 mg po every 6 hours for 7 to 10 days). Alternative agents for penicillin allergic patients include clindamycin (150–300 mg po every 6 hours) and

TABLE 108–1. Predominant Microorganisms of Normal Skin

Bacteria
Gram positives
Staphylococcus epidermidis
Staphylococcus aureus
Diphtheroids
Corynebacterium spp.
Propionibacterium spp.
Streptococcus spp.
Peptostreptococcus spp.
Bacillus spp.
Micrococcus spp.
Gram negatives
Enterobacteriaceae
Yeast
Pityrosporum ovale
Candida

erythromycin (250–500 mg po every 6 hours). Surgical incision is indicated for large and fluctuant lesions that do not spontaneously drain.[4]

ERYSIPELAS

Erysipelas (Saint Anthony's fire) is a distinct type of superficial cellulitis with extensive lymphatic involvement.[4] This infection is almost always caused by group A streptococci (*Streptococcus pyogenes*). The organism most likely gains access via some small break in the skin. Other streptococci (group B in the newborn) and *S. aureus* are rare causes of erysipelas.

Erysipelas most commonly occurs in infants, young children, the elderly, and patients with nephrotic syndrome. This infection also occurs in areas of preexisting lymphatic obstruction or edema. The lower extremities are the most common sites for erysipelas. The lesion is bright red, edematous, indurated, and painful. Fever and leukocytosis are common. The clinical presentation of erysipelas differs from cellulitis in that the lesion is sharply circumscribed by an elevated border. The causative organism usually cannot be cultured from the surface skin lesion but may sometimes be aspirated from the edge of the advancing lesion.[5,6] Diagnosis is made on the basis of the characteristic appearance of the lesion.

▶ TREATMENT: Erysipelas

The goal of treatment of erysipelas is rapid eradication of the infection. Mild to moderate cases of erysipelas are treated with procaine penicillin G 600,000 units IM twice daily or penicillin VK 250–500 mg po four times daily (in children 1–18 years of age, 25,000–90,000 U/kg/day divided into four doses) for 7 to 10 days.[4,7,8] Penicillin-allergic patients can be treated with erythromycin, although caution is warranted as some strains may be resistant.[4,7,8] For more serious infections, the patient should be hospitalized and aqueous penicillin G 2–8 million units daily should be administered intravenously.[4,5] The infection may appear to worsen shortly after treatment, as dying organisms release toxins responsible for many of the clinical features.

IMPETIGO

Impetigo is another distinct type of superficial cellulitis that is caused by *S. aureus* and/or group A streptococci (*S. pyogenes*). In the past, most cases were caused by group A streptococci. In recent years, *S. aureus*, either alone or in combination with group A streptococci, has emerged as the principal cause of impetigo. This superficial skin infection is most common during hot, humid weather, which facilitates microbial colonization of the skin. Minor trauma, such as scratches or insect bites, then allows entry of organisms into the superficial layers of skin, and infection ensues. Impetigo occurs most commonly in children. It is also highly communicable and readily spread through close contact, especially among siblings, day care centers, and schools.[4,5]

Impetigo manifests initially as small, fluid-filled vesicles. These lesions then rapidly develop into pus-filled blisters that readily rupture. The purulent discharges of these lesions dry to form golden-yellow crusts that are characteristic of impetigo. Pruritus is common, and scratching of the lesions may further spread infection through excoriation of the skin. Other systemic signs of infection are minimal.

The bullous form of impetigo is seen in newborns and young children and accounts for approximately 10% of all cases of impetigo. The bullous form is caused by strains of *S. aureus* capable of producing exfoliative toxins. The lesions begin as vesicles and turn into bullae containing clear yellow fluid. The bullae soon rupture, forming thin, light brown crusts.

TABLE 108–2. Bacterial Classification of Important Skin and Soft Tissue Infections

Primary Infections	
Erysipelas	Group A streptococci
Impetigo	*Staphylococcus aureus*, group A streptococci
Lymphangitis	Group A streptococci; occasionally *S. aureus*
Cellulitis	Group A streptococci, *S. aureus;* occasionally other gram-positive cocci, gram-negative bacilli, and/or anaerobes
Necrotizing fasciitis	
Type I	Anaerobes (*Bacteroides spp., Peptostreptococcus spp.*) and facultative bacteria (streptococci, Enterobacteriaceae)
Type II	Group A streptococci
Secondary Infections	
Diabetic foot infections	*S. aureus*, streptococci, Enterobacteriaceae, *Bacteroides spp., Peptostreptococcus spp., Pseudomonas aeruginosa*
Pressure sores	*S. aureus*, streptococci, Enterobacteriaceae, *Bacteroides spp., Peptostreptococcus spp., Pseudomonas aeruginosa*
Bite wounds	
Animal	*Pasteurella multocida, S. aureus*, streptococci, *Bacteroides spp.*
Human	*Eikenella corrodens, S. aureus*, streptococci, *Corynebacterium spp., Bacteroides spp., Peptostreptococcus spp.*
Burn wounds	*Pseudomonas aeruginosa*, Enterobacteriaceae, *S. aureus*, streptococci

▶ TREATMENT: Impetigo

Although impetigo may resolve spontaneously, treatment is indicated to relieve symptoms, prevent formation of new lesions, and prevent complications, such as cellulitis. Penicillinase-resistant penicillins (dicloxacillin 12.5 mg/kg po daily in four divided doses for children) are preferred for treatment because of the increased incidence of infections caused by *S. aureus*. First-generation cephalosporins are also effective, although they are generally more expensive. Cephalexin (25–50 mg/kg po daily in two divided doses for children) and cefadroxil (30 mg/kg po daily in two divided doses for children) are commonly used. Penicillin, administered as either a single IM dose of benzathine penicillin G (300,000–600,000 units in children, 1.2 million units in adults) or as oral penicillin VK, is effective for infections caused by group A streptococci. Penicillin-allergic patients can be treated with oral erythromycin (30–50 mg/kg/day in four divided doses for children; 250–500 mg po every 6 hours for adults). The duration of therapy is 7 to 10 days. Topical antibiotics, such as mupirocin and bacitracin have been used to treat nonbullous impetigo. Mupirocin ointment (applied 3 times daily for 7 days) is as effective as erythromycin.[9] With proper treatment, healing of skin lesions is generally rapid and occurs without residual scarring. Removal of crusts by soaking in soap and warm water may also be helpful in providing symptomatic relief.[4,7]

LYMPHANGITIS

Acute lymphangitis refers to an inflammation involving subcutaneous lymphatic channels. Most infections are caused by group A streptococci.[7,10] Lymphangitis usually occurs secondary to puncture wounds, infected blisters, or other skin lesions. Systemic manifestations of infection (fever, chills, malaise, headache, and leukocytosis) often develop rapidly before any sign of infection is evident at the initial site of inoculation or even after the initial lesion has subsided. The systemic symptoms are often more profound than would be expected from examination of the cutaneous lesion. Acute lymphangitis is characterized by the rapid development of fine red linear streaks extending proximally from the initial site of infection toward the regional lymph nodes, which are usually enlarged and tender. Pain and peripheral edema of the involved extremity may often be present.[7,10] Lymphadenitis (acute or chronic inflammation of the lymph nodes) may also occur when microorganisms reach the lymph nodes and elicit an inflammatory response.

Identification of a peripheral lesion associated with proximal red linear streaks directed toward the regional lymph nodes is diagnostic of acute lymphangitis. At times, thrombophlebitis and acute lymphangitis in the lower extremities may be confused, because both are associated with red linear streaking and tender areas; however, in thrombophlebitis, no portal of entry is identifiable. Cultures of the affected lesions often yield negative results, as the infection resides within the lymphatic channels; however, the offending pathogen can often be identified by Gram stain of the initial lesion if done early in the course of the disease.

▶ TREATMENT: Lymphangitis

The goal of therapy for lymphangitis is rapid eradication of infection and prevention of further systemic complications. Penicillin is the antibiotic of choice. Because this infection is potentially serious and rapidly progressive, initial treatment should be with IV penicillin G. Lymphangitis usually responds rapidly to appropriate therapy; signs and symptoms often are markedly decreased or absent within 24 hours of starting antibiotics. Parenteral treatment should be continued for 48 to 72 hours, followed by oral penicillin VK for a total of 10 days.[10,11] Nondrug therapy includes immobilization and elevation of the affected extremity and warm-water soaks every 2 to 4 hours.[7] For penicillin-allergic patients, erythromycin or clindamycin may be used.

CELLULITIS

Cellulitis is an acute, infectious process that initially affects the epidermis and dermis and may subsequently spread within the superficial fascia. Cellulitis is characterized by erythema and edema of the skin. Inflammation is generally present with little or no necrosis or suppuration of soft tissue. The lesion, which may be extensive, is hot, painful, nonelevated, and has poorly defined margins. Tender lymphadenopathy associated with lymphatic involvement is common. Malaise, fever, chills, and leukocytosis are also commonly present. There is usually a history of an antecedent wound from a minor trauma, abrasion, ulcer, or surgery.

Cellulitis is considered a serious disease because of the propensity of the infection to spread through lymphatic tissue and to the bloodstream. Bacteremia may be present in as much as 30% of cases of cellulitis. In older patients, cellulitis of the lower extremities may also be complicated by thrombophlebitis. Other complications of cellulitis include local abscess, osteomyelitis, and septic arthritis.[7,8]

Group A streptococci (*S. pyogenes*) or *S. aureus* are the most frequent etiologic agents. However, a variety of bacteria have been implicated in various types of cellulitis (Table 108–2). A Gram stain of fluid obtained by injection and aspiration of 0.5 mL of saline (using a small 22-gauge needle) into the advancing edge of the lesion may aid the microbiologic diagnosis, but often yields negative results.[6] Diagnosis is usually made on clinical grounds, that is, the appearance of the lesion.

Injection drug users are predisposed to a number of infectious complications, including abscess formation and cellulitis at the site of injection.[12] These skin and soft tissue infections are most frequently located on the upper extremities and are often polymicrobic in nature.[13] *S. aureus* or streptococci are the most common pathogenic organisms isolated from these infections (37% to 61% of patients). Anaerobic bacteria are also commonly found (6% to 67% of patients), although the role of these bacteria in the pathogenesis of infection is unclear.[13] Fungal infections (primarily *Candida*) have also been noted to be a cause of skin and soft tissue infections in injection drug users.[14] These various organisms are believed to originate as normal flora of the skin, as well as from the mouth and contaminated needles, syringes, and diluents.[13]

Acute cellulitis with mixed aerobic and anaerobic flora generally occurs in diabetics, where the skin is adjacent to some site of trauma, at sites of surgical incisions to the abdomen or perineum, or where host defenses have been otherwise compromised (vascular insufficiency). As with other types of cellulitis, warmth, redness, and induration are observed; there may also be gas formation (crepitus). If the cellulitis progresses, it can lead to areas of gangrene. Because these infections often occur in patients with alterations in host defense mechanisms, poor nutrition, or both, systemic findings such as hypotension, dehydration, and altered mental status, are common. Needle aspiration of the leading edge of the lesion and subsequent Gram staining and culture may be helpful in isolating the potential pathogens.

▶ TREATMENT: Cellulitis

The goal of therapy of acute bacterial cellulitis is rapid eradication of the infection and prevention of further complications. Antimicrobial therapy of bacterial cellulitis is directed against the type of bacteria either documented, or suspected to be present based on the clinical presentation. Local care of cellulitis includes elevation and immobilization of the involved area to decrease swelling. Cool sterile saline dressings can decrease pain and can be followed later with moist heat to aid in localization of the cellulitis. Surgical intervention (incision and drainage) as a mode of therapy is rarely indicated in the treatment of cellulitis.

As staphylococcal and streptococcal cellulitis are clinically indistinguishable,[5] administration of a semisynthetic penicillin (nafcillin or oxacillin) is recommended until a definitive diagnosis, by skin or blood cultures, can be made (Table 108–3).[4,7,8] Mild to moderate infections not associated with systemic symptoms may be

TABLE 108–3. Initial Treatment Regimens for Cellulitis Caused by Various Pathogens

Antibiotic	Adult Dose and Route	Pediatric Dose and Route
Staphylococcal or Unknown Gram-Positive Infection		
Mild infection	Dicloxacillin 0.25–0.5 g PO every 6 h[a,b]	Dicloxacillin 25–50 mg/kg/day PO in four divided doses[a,b]
Moderate–severe infection	Nafcillin or oxacillin 1–2 g IV every 4–6 h[a,b]	Nafcillin or oxacillin 150–200 mg/kg/day (not to exceed 12 g/24 h) IV in four to six equally divided doses[a,b]
Streptococcal (Documented)		
Mild infection	Penicillin VK 0.5 g PO every 6 h[a] or procaine penicillin G 600,000 units IM every 8–12 h[a]	Penicillin VK 125–250 mg PO every 6–8 h, or procaine penicillin G 25,000–50,000 units/kg (not to exceed 600,000 units) IM every 8–12 h[a]
Moderate–severe infection	Aqueous penicillin G 1–2 million units IV every 4–6 h[a,c]	Aqueous penicillin G 100,000–200,000 units/kg/day IV in four divided doses[a]
Gram-Negative Bacilli		
Mild infection	Cefaclor 0.5 g PO every 8 h[d] or cefuroxime axetil 0.5 g PO every 12 h[d]	Cefaclor 20–40 mg/kg/day (not to exceed 1 g) PO in three divided doses or cefuroxime axetil 0.125–0.25 g (tablets) PO every 12 h
Moderate–severe to infection	Aminoglycoside[e] or IV cephalosporin (first- or second-generation depending on severity of infection or susceptibility pattern)[d]	Aminoglycoside[e] or intravenous cephalosporin (first- or second-generation depending on severity of infection or susceptibility pattern)
Polymicrobic Infection Without Anaerobes	Aminoglycoside[e] + penicillin G 1–2 million units every 4–6 h or a semisynthetic penicillin (nafcillin 1–2 g every 4–6 h) depending on isolation of staphylococci or streptococci[b]	Aminoglycoside[e] + penicillin G 100,000 to 200,000 units/kg/day IV in four divided doses or a semisynthetic penicillin (nafcillin 150–200 mg/kg/day [not to exceed 12 g/24 h] IV in four to six equally divided doses) depending on isolation of staphylococci or streptococci[b]
Polymicrobic Infection With Anaerobes		
Mild infection	Amoxicillin/clavulanate 0.875 g PO every 12 h *or* A fluoroquinolone (ciprofloxacin 0.4 g PO every 12 h or levofloxacin 0.5–0.75 g PO every 24 h) plus clindamycin 0.3–0.6 g PO every 8 h or metronidazole 0.5 g PO every 8 h	Amoxicillin/clavulanic acid 20 mg/kg/day PO in three divided doses
Moderate–severe infection	Aminoglycoside[e,f] + clindamycin 0.6–0.9 g IV every 8 h or metronidazole 0.5 g IV every 8 h *or* Monotherapy with second- or third-generation cephalosporin (cefoxitin 1–2 g IV every 6 h or ceftizoxime 1–2 g IV every 8 h) *or* Monotherapy with imipenem 0.5 g IV every 6–8 h, meropenem 1 g IV every 8 h, or extended-spectrum penicillins with a β-lactamase inhibitor (piperacillin/tazobactam 4.5 g IV every 6 h)	Aminoglycoside[e] plus clindamycin 15 mg/kg/day IV in three divided doses or metronidazole 30–50 mg/kg/day IV in three divided doses

[a]For penicillin-allergic patients, use erythromycin 0.5–1.0 g every 6 h (pediatric dosing 30–40 mg/kg/day in divided doses).
[b]For methicillin-resistant staphylococci, use vancomycin 0.5–1 g every 6–12 h (pediatric dosing 40 mg/kg/day in divided doses) with dosage adjustments made for renal dysfunction.
[c]For type II necrotizing fasciitis, use clindamycin 0.6–0.9 g IV every 8 h (in children, clindamycin 15 mg/kg/day IV in 3 divided doses) should be added.
[d]For penicillin-allergic adults, use a fluoroquinolone (ciprofloxacin 0.5–0.75 g PO every 12 h or 0.4 g IV every 12 h; levofloxacin 0.5–0.75 g PO or IV every 24 h; gatifloxacin 0.4 g PO or IV every 24 h; or moxifloxacin 0.4 g PO or IV every 24 h).
[e]Gentamicin or tobramycin, 2 mg/kg loading dose, then maintenance dose determined by serum concentrations.
[f]A fluoroquinolone or aztreonam 1 g IV every 6 h may be used in place of the aminoglycoside in patients with severe renal dysfunction or other relative contraindications to aminoglycoside use.

treated orally with dicloxacillin. If documented to be a mild cellulitis secondary to streptococci, oral penicillin VK or intramuscular (IM) procaine penicillin may be administered. More severe infections, either staphylococcal or streptococcal, should be initially treated with intravenous (IV) antibiotic regimens.[6] Ceftriaxone 50–100 mg/kg as a single daily dose is efficacious in the treatment of cellulitis in pediatric patients.[15] The usual duration of therapy for cellulitis is 7 to 10 days.[4,7,8] If treated promptly with appropriate antibiotics, the majority of patients with cellulitis are rapidly cured. Failure to respond to therapy may be indicative of an underlying local or systemic problem or a misdiagnosis.

In penicillin-allergic patients, oral or parenteral erythromycin may be used.[4,7] Alternatively, a first-generation cephalosporin, such as cefazolin (1–2 g IV every 8 hours), may be used cautiously for patients who have not experienced immediate or anaphylactic penicillin reactions and are negative for a penicillin skin test. In mild cases in which an oral cephalosporin can be used, cefadroxil 500 mg twice daily or cephalexin 250–500 mg four times daily is recommended. Other oral cephalosporins, such as cefaclor, cefprozil, and cefpodoxime proxetil, are also effective in the treatment of cellulitis but are considerably more expensive.[7] Clarithromycin, azithromycin, and clindamycin may also be effective alternatives for the treatment of cellulitis caused by gram-positive organisms, but they appear to offer no therapeutic advantages and are also relatively expensive. In severe cases in which erythromycin or cephalosporins cannot be used because of documented methicillin-resistant staphylococci or severe allergic reactions to β-lactam antibiotics, vancomycin should be administered.

The carbapenems (imipenem and meropenem) and the β-lactamase inhibitor combination antibiotics (ampicillin/sulbactam, ticarcillin/clavulanic acid, and piperacillin/tazobactam) also appear to be equivalent to standard therapies in adults.[16–18] The cost of these newer agents without increased efficacy compared to other reliable regimens, however, makes them less desirable. Oral fluoroquinolones have demonstrated efficacy similar to parenteral cephalosporins in the treatment of soft tissue infections caused by gram-positive organisms.[19–22] The use of fluoroquinolones is of concern, however, because of increasing reports of resistance among gram-positive bacteria, particularly staphylococci. Sensitivity testing is recommended when a fluoroquinolone is to be used. Also, fluoroquinolones are not approved for use in children because of toxicity concerns.

Two newer agents, linezolid and the combination product quinupristin/dalfopristin, are also indicated for the treatment of severe skin and soft tissue infections caused by staphylococci and streptococci. These agents are clearly effective for therapy of these infections and appear to be equivalent to standard therapies.[23,24] However, the excellent activity of these drugs against resistant gram-positive pathogens such as methicillin-resistant staphylococci and significantly higher cost make them most appropriate for treatment of complicated or refractory infections, or those caused by multi-drug-resistant pathogens.

For cellulitis caused by gram-negative bacilli or a mixture of microorganisms, immediate antimicrobial chemotherapy, as determined by Gram stain, is essential (Table 108–3). Surgical excision of necrotic tissue and drainage may also be appropriate. Gram negative cellulitis may be appropriately treated with an aminoglycoside or first- or second-generation cephalosporin. If gram-positive aerobic bacteria are also present, penicillin G or a semisynthetic penicillin should be added to the regimen. Ceftazidime and the fluoroquinolones are effective in the treatment of cellulitis caused by both gram-negative and gram-positive bacteria.[19–22,25]

If there is no obvious focus of infection, some internal source should be sought, such as a perforated viscus or a rectal tear, and repaired if possible. As these types of infections are often polymicrobic in nature, antibiotic regimens should be broadened to include agents with good activity against not only gram-negative enteric bacilli, but also anaerobic bacteria. Many different treatment regimens are possible, depending on the bacteriology of the lesion (Table 108–3). Usually an aminoglycoside combined with an antianaerobic cephalosporin, extended spectrum penicillin, or clindamycin is used. Second- or third-generation cephalosporins have been suggested as single-agent therapy in certain instances.[26,27] Monotherapy with a β-lactam plus β-lactamase inhibitor combination antibiotic or a carbapenem may also be appropriate in seriously ill patients. Therapy should be 10 to 14 days in duration.

Because gram-negative and mixed aerobic-anaerobic cellulitis can progress quickly to serious tissue invasion, therapeutic intervention should be immediate. If treated early, a quick response can be seen. Unfortunately, because this infection often occurs in patients with compromised immune defenses, the infection may still progress, even with therapeutic intervention. If the infectious process is secondary to a systemic cause (e.g., diabetes), the treatment course can be prolonged and may be associated with high morbidity and mortality.

Infections in injection drug users are generally treated similarly to those in other types of patients. It is important that blood cultures be obtained, as 25% to 35% of patients may be bacteremic.[13,28] Also, patients should be assessed for the presence of abscesses; incision, drainage, and culture of these lesions are of extreme importance, when indicated. Seriously ill-appearing patients, or patients with extensive cellulitis or deep-seated infections should receive a parenteral antistaphylococcal penicillin plus an aminoglycoside because of the risk of polymicrobial infections.[4,13,14] In addition, if the patient presents with an infection associated with systemic toxicity and watery, foul-smelling exudate, the suspicion should be high that anaerobes are present, and appropriate therapy instituted. Treatment with either amphotericin B or an azole antifungal agent (fluconazole, itraconazole) is warranted if *Candida albicans* is identified.[14]

NECROTIZING SOFT TISSUE INFECTIONS

Necrotizing soft tissue infections consist of a group of highly lethal infections that require early and aggressive surgical débridement, in addition to appropriate antibiotics and intensive supportive care.[29] A variety of different descriptive terms have been used to classify necrotizing infections. These have been based upon factors such as predisposing conditions, onset of symptoms, pain, skin appearance, etiologic agent, gas production, muscle involvement, and systemic toxicity. While many of the necrotizing soft tissue infections have been designated as unique infectious processes, they all share similar pathophysiologies, clinical features, and treatment approaches.[29] The major clinical entities of necrotizing infections are necrotizing fasciitis and clostridial myonecrosis (gas gangrene).[29] These infections may occur in almost any anatomic location, but most frequently involve the abdomen, the perineum, and the lower extremities.[29] Patients often have predisposing factors such as diabetes mellitus, local trauma or infection, or recent surgery.

Necrotizing fasciitis is a rare, but very severe infection of the subcutaneous tissue that results in progressive destruction of the superficial fascia and subcutaneous fat. It is generally characterized as two different types based on bacterial etiology. Type I necrotizing fasciitis generally occurs after trauma and surgery and involves a mixture of anaerobes (*Bacteroides*, *Peptostreptococcus*) and facultative bacteria (streptococci and members of the Enterobacteriaceae), which act synergistically to cause destruction of fat and fascia. Necrotizing fasciitis affecting the male genitalia has been termed Fournier's gangrene. Type II necrotizing fasciitis is caused by virulent strains of group A streptococci (*S. pyogenes*), and is more commonly referred to as streptococcal gangrene. This type of infection has received considerable attention in recent years because of reports of "flesh-eating bacteria" by the lay press. Unlike previous reports of streptococcal gangrene that affected older individuals with underlying diseases, recent reports have occurred primarily in young, previously healthy adults following some type of minor trauma. It differs from the polymicrobial type I infections in its clinical presentation. In type I infections, the skin may be spared and the speed at which the infection spreads is somewhat slower. Type II infections have rapidly extending necrosis of subcutaneous tissues and skin, gangrene, severe local pain, and systemic toxicity.[5] These infections are also highly associated with an early onset of shock and organ failure, and are present in approximately half of the cases of streptococcal toxic shock-like syndrome.[5]

At the beginning of an infection, it may be difficult to differentiate between necrotizing fasciitis and cellulitis. Like cellulitis, the affected area is initially hot, swollen, and erythematous without sharp margins. The area is shiny, exquisitely tender, and painful. Diffuse swelling of the area is followed by the appearance of bullae filled with clear fluid. The infectious process progresses rapidly, with the skin taking on a maroon or violaceous color after several days.[5] Without appropriate intervention, the infection will rapidly evolve into a frank cutaneous gangrene, sometimes with myonecrosis (involvement of skin and muscle).[5] There are generally marked systemic symptoms (fever, chills, leukocytosis), which may include shock and organ failure, especially in patients with type II infections. Because of the aggressive nature and high mortality (20% to 50%) associated with these infections,[4] a rapid diagnosis is critical. In general, pain in the affected area and systemic toxicity are more pronounced than would be expected with cellulitis.[29] Although computerized tomography and magnetic resonance imaging studies can distinguish these infections, the best and most rapid diagnosis is obtained via surgical exploration.[29]

Clostridial myonecrosis is a necrotizing infection that involves the skeletal muscle. Gas production and muscle necrosis are prominent features of this infection, which readily explains why this infection is commonly referred to as "gas gangrene."[29] Most infections occur after surgery or trauma, with *Clostridium perfringens* identified as the most common etiologic agent. Unlike necrotizing fasciitis, clostridial myonecrosis shows little inflammation on histologic exam.[29] The infection advances rapidly, often over a matter of a few hours.[29]

▶ TREATMENT: Necrotizing Soft Tissue Infections

After the diagnosis is made, immediate and aggressive surgical débridement of all necrotic tissue is essential.[29] Broad-spectrum antibiotics should be administered, with coverage against streptococci, Enterobacteriaceae, and anaerobes. A variety of antibiotic regimens have been successfully used to treat necrotizing soft tissue infections; these are generally similar to those used for severe polymicrobic cellulitis involving anaerobes (Table 108–3). Other combination antibiotic regimens that may be used prior to obtaining bacteriologic data include ampicillin, gentamicin, and clindamycin (or metronidazole); ampicillin-sulbactam and gentamicin; or imipenem and metronidazole.[4] Antibiotic therapy can be modified after Gram stain and culture reports are available. If a diagnosis of type II necrotizing fasciitis is established, the broad-spectrum empiric therapy should be replaced with the combination of penicillin and clindamycin.[5] While *S. pyogenes* remains susceptible to penicillin, clindamycin has been experimentally shown to be more effective.[5] A variety of factors have been postulated to explain the higher efficacy of clindamycin. These include the mechanism of action (inhibition of protein synthesis), which is not affected by the size of the inoculum or the stage of bacterial growth.[5] In addition, clindamycin has immunomodulatory properties that may account for the higher efficacy.[5] The combination of penicillin and clindamycin is also recommended for treatment of clostridial myonecrosis.[29] In addition, hyperbaric oxygen has been reported to be of some benefit for clostridial myonecrosis.[29]

DIABETIC FOOT INFECTIONS

Disorders of the foot are among the most common complications of diabetes, accounting for as much as 20% of all hospitalizations in diabetic patients at an annual cost of 200 million to 350 million dollars.[30,31] It is estimated that 25% of diabetic patients experience significant soft tissue infection at some time during the course of their lifetime. Approximately 55,000 lower extremity amputations, often sequelae of uncontrolled infection, are performed each year on diabetic patients; this represents 50% of all nontraumatic amputations in the United States.[31] Studies show that 10% to 20% of diabetics will undergo additional surgery or amputation of a second limb within 12 months of the initial amputation.[32] By 5 years this increases to 25% to 50%, with death reported in as much as two-thirds of cases.[32]

PATHOPHYSIOLOGY

Three key factors are involved in the development of diabetic foot problems: (a) neuropathy; (b) angiopathy and ischemia; and (c) immunologic defects. Any of these disorders can occur in isolation; however, they frequently occur together.

Neuropathic changes to the autonomic nervous system as a consequence of diabetes may affect the motor nerve supply of small intrinsic muscles of the foot, resulting in muscular imbalance, abnormal stresses on tissues and bone, and repetitive injuries.[33] Diminished sensory perception causes an absence of pain and unawareness of minor injuries and ulceration. Also, the sympathetic nerve supply may be damaged and can result in an absence of sweating; this leads to dry cracked skin, which can become secondarily infected.[30]

Atherosclerosis is more common, appears at a younger age, and progresses more rapidly in the diabetic than in the nondiabetic. Diabetics may have problems with both small vessels (microangiopathy) and large vessels (macroangiopathy) that can result in varying degrees of ischemia, ultimately leading to skin breakdown and infection.

Diabetic patients typically have normal humoral immunity, normal levels of immunoglobulins, and normal antibody responses. Patients with diabetes, however, have impaired phagocytosis and intracellular microbicidal function as compared to nondiabetics; this may

TABLE 108–4. Bacterial Isolates from Foot Infections in Diabetic Patients

Organisms	Percentage of Isolates
Aerobes	69%
Gram-positive	45%
Staphylococcus aureus	13%
Streptococcus spp.	11%
Enterococcus spp.	8%
Coagulase-negative staphylococci	7%
Gram-negative	24%
Proteus spp.	5%
Enterobacter spp.	3%
Escherichia coli	3%
Klebsiella spp.	2%
Pseudomonas aeruginosa	2%
Other gram-negative bacilli	7%
Anaerobes	31%
Peptostreptococcus spp.	13%
Bacteroides fragilis group	5%
Other *Bacteroides spp.*	4%
Clostridium spp.	2%
Other anaerobes	7%

From Ref. 34 with permission.

be related to angiopathy and low tissue-levels of oxygen.[30] These defects in cell-mediated immunity make patients with diabetes more susceptible to certain types of infection and impair the patients' ability to heal wounds adequately.[33]

ETIOLOGY AND CLINICAL PRESENTATION

Diabetic foot infections are polymicrobic in nature with an average of 4.1 to 5.8 isolates per culture (Table 108–4).[34] Staphylococci (especially *S. aureus*) and streptococci are the most common pathogens, although gram-negative bacilli and/or anaerobes occur in approximately 50% of cases.[35] Common gram-negative bacilli isolated includes *E. coli*, *Klebsiella* species, *Proteus* species, and *P. aeruginosa*. *Bacteroides fragilis* and *Peptostreptococcus* species are among the most common anaerobes isolated.

The optimum technique for obtaining culture material from ulcerated lesions is still debated.[36] Routine swab cultures of ulcerative lesions are difficult to interpret because of organisms that colonize the surface of the wounds. Cultures of material from sinus tracts are also unreliable. The correlation between these superficial cultures and true deep cultures (via biopsy or needle aspiration of drainage or abscess fluid) is poor.[34,35,37] Therefore, cultures and sensitivity tests should be done with specimens obtained from a deep culture whenever possible. Before the wound is cultured, it should be vigorously scrubbed with saline-moistened sterile gauze to remove any overlying necrotic debris.[38] Cultures then can be obtained from the wound base, preferably from expressed pus.[38] Specimens obtained from curettage of the base of the ulcer correlate best with results from deep-tissue or bone biopsies.[38] Because of the complex microbiology of these infections, wounds must be cultured for both aerobic and anaerobic specimens.[34,35,37]

Clinical signs and symptoms of infection in the diabetic foot may not be present secondary to the angiopathy and neuropathy. Infections are often much more extensive than they initially appear. Diabetic foot infections begin with local bacterial invasion.[32] Patients with peripheral neuropathy often do not experience pain, but seek medical care for swelling or erythema in the foot.[32] There are three major types of foot infections seen in diabetic patients: deep abscesses, cellulitis of the dorsum, and mal perforans ulcers.[36] The majority of deep abscesses involve the central plantar space (arch), and are caused by minor penetrating trauma or by an extension of infection of a nail or web space of the toes. Skin infections of the dorsal area generally arise from infections in the toes that are related to routine care of the nails, nailbeds, and calluses of the toes. Mal perforans ulcer is a chronic ulcer of the sole of the foot. The ulcer develops on thickened, hardened calluses over the first or fifth metatarsal. Mal perforans ulcers are associated with neuropathy, which is responsible for the misalignment of the weight-bearing bones of the foot.[36] Osteomyelitis is one of the most serious complications of foot problems in diabetic patients and may occur in 30% to 40% of infections.[30,37,39]

▶ TREATMENT: Diabetic Foot Infections

The goal of therapy of diabetic foot infections is preservation of as much normal limb function as possible while preventing additional infectious complications. Up to 90% of these infections can be successfully treated with a comprehensive treatment approach that includes both wound care and antimicrobial therapy.[37] After carefully assessing the extent of the lesion and obtaining necessary cultures, necrotic tissue must be thoroughly débrided with wound drainage and amputation as required. Wounds are kept clean, and dressings changed frequently (two to three times daily). The presence of osteomyelitis must also be assessed via radiograph, bone scan, or both, as appropriate. Because of the relationship between hyperglycemia and immune system defects, glycemic control must be maximized to ensure optimal wound healing. In addition, the patient's activities should initially be restricted to bedrest for leg elevation and control of edema, if present. Finally, appropriate antimicrobials must be initiated.[30,31,37,39] However, the optimal antimicrobial therapy for diabetic foot infections has yet to be defined.

The majority of mild, uncomplicated infections can be successfully managed on an outpatient basis with oral antimicrobials and good wound care. Many different agents have been studied, including cefaclor, cephalexin, fluoroquinolones, clindamycin, and amoxicillin/clavulanic acid; these agents provide clinical cure rates of 60% to 85% in published studies.[33,35,39,40] However, significant failure rates and/or relapse rates have been reported with the use of oral agents. In addition, the development of resistance was problematic in some infections involving *P. aeruginosa* and staphylococci.[41] Many clinicians consider amoxicillin/clavulanic acid to be the most favorable agent because of its broad spectrum of activity, which includes staphylococci, streptococci, enterococci, and many Enterobacteriaceae and anaerobes.[35] However, this agent does not have activity against *P. aeruginosa*. Fluoroquinolones, which provide coverage against *P. aeruginosa*, have been extensively studied as monotherapy, but they are perhaps most appropriately used in combination with metronidazole or clindamycin to provide anaerobic activity.[33,35,42] Oral antimicrobials should be used cautiously in serious infections, especially those complicated by osteomyelitis, extensive ulceration, areas of necrosis, or a combination of these. Therapy should be carefully reevaluated after 48 to 72 hours to assess favorable response.

Intravenous therapy should be considered if clinical improvement is not observed at this time.

Initial therapy for patients requiring hospitalization for moderate to severe infections is similar to that for polymicrobic cellulitis with anaerobes (Table 108–3). Monotherapy with broad-spectrum parenteral antimicrobials along with appropriate medical or surgical management, or both, is often effective in treating these infections, including those in which osteomyelitis is present.[43,44] Monotherapy is particularly attractive because of the potential advantages of convenience, cost, and avoidance of toxicities. Microbiologic and clinical cure rates ranging from 60% to 90% may be expected from any of these agents; selection of a specific regimen is primarily determined by cost. In penicillin-allergic patients, metronidazole or clindamycin plus either a fluoroquinolone, aztreonam, or possibly a third-generation cephalosporin are appropriate choices.[33,35,39] Vancomycin is also frequently used in severe infections because of its excellent activity against gram-positive pathogens. Because these patients may already have some degree of diabetic nephropathy that may place them at higher risk of nephrotoxicity, recommendations have strongly advocated the avoidance of aminoglycoside antibiotics unless no alternative agents are available.[30] When an aminoglycoside is used, care must be taken to avoid further compromising renal function. All antibiotic regimes should be adjusted as necessary for renal dysfunction.

Empiric therapy that is totally comprehensive in its coverage of all possible pathogens may not be necessary unless the infection is life-threatening.[35,43,44] No differences were reported in the efficacy of ampicillin/sulbactam versus imipenem/cilastatin for treatment of limb-threatening diabetic foot infections, despite the higher incidence of potential pathogens resistant to the ampicillin/sulbactam regimen.[43] For optimal results, drug therapy should be appropriately modified according to information from deep tissue culture and the clinical condition of the patient. Infections in diabetic patients often require extended courses of therapy because of impaired host immunity and poor wound healing. Mild infections can be treated with oral agents and should generally be treated for at least 10 to 14 days, while more severe infections dictate initial parenteral therapy and often require up to 21 days or more of antibiotic therapy. In cases of underlying osteomyelitis, treatment should continue for 6 to 12 weeks.[30,33,35,39] After healing of the infection has occurred, a well-designed program for prevention of further infections should be instituted.

PRESSURE SORES

The terms decubitus ulcer, bed sore, and pressure sore are used interchangeably. The decubitus ulcer and the bed sore are types of pressure sores. The term decubitus ulcer is derived from the Latin word *decumbere,* meaning "lying down." Pressure sores, however, can develop regardless of a patient's position. Pressure sores are most frequently seen in chronically debilitated persons, the elderly, and persons with serious spinal cord injury. Generally, those patients who are at risk for pressure sores are elderly or chronically ill young patients who are immobilized either in bed or to a wheelchair and who may have altered mental status and/or incontinence.

PATHOPHYSIOLOGY

Many factors are thought to predispose patients to the formation of pressure sores: paralysis, paresis, immobilization, malnutrition, anemia, infection, and advanced age. Four factors thought to be most critical to their formation are pressure, shearing forces, friction, and moisture; however, there is still debate as to the exact pathophysiology of pressure sore formation.

Pressure is the essential element in the formation of pressure sores. The areas of highest pressure are most often generated over the bony prominences. Studies show that when the pressure is relieved intermittently within a 2-hour period, only minimal changes occur in soft tissue and skin structures.[45] Therefore, both the degree of pressure and the length of time that the pressure is applied are important.

Shearing forces are caused by the sliding of adjacent parallel surfaces of soft tissues in an unequal fashion. This situation can occur when the head of a bed is raised, causing the upper torso to slide downward, transmitting pressure to the sacrum and other areas. This effect results in occlusion or distortion of vessels, leading to compromise of the dermis. At the same time, sitting and gravity create shearing forces; the posterior sacral skin area can become fixed secondary to friction with the bed. The effects of friction and shearing forces combine, resulting in transmission of force to the deep portion of the superficial fascia and leading to further damage of soft tissue structures.

Compounding the problems of shearing and friction forces are the macerating effects of excessive moisture in the local environment, resulting from incontinence and perspiration. This factor is of critical importance because when combined with the other forces, it increases the risk of pressure sore formation fivefold.[46]

CLINICAL PRESENTATION

The persistence of pressure, shearing forces, friction, and moisture often results in pressure sore formation. Without treatment an initial small, localized area of ulceration can rapidly progress to 5–6 cm within days. The visible ulcer is just a small portion of the actual wound; up to 70% of the total wound is below the skin. A pressure gradient phenomenon is created by which the wound takes on a conical nature; the smallest point is at the skin surface and the largest portion of the defect is at the base of the ulcer (Fig. 108–1).

Numerous systems for classification of pressure sores have been described. The two most frequently used systems are those of Shea[47] and the 1989 National Pressure Ulcer Advisory Panel.[48] These

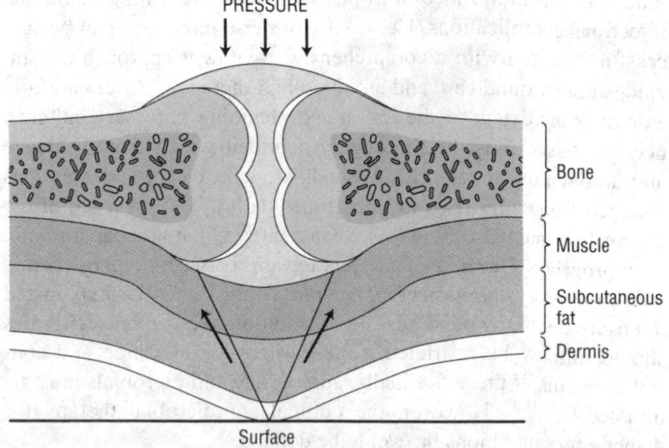

FIGURE 108–1. Distribution of forces involved with sore formation in a conical fashion.

TABLE 108–5. **Pressure Sore Classification**[48]

Stage 1	Pressure sore is generally reversible, is limited to the epidermis, and resembles an abrasion. It is best described as an irregularly shaped area of soft tissue swelling with induration and heat.
Stage 2	A stage 2 sore may also be reversible; it extends through the dermis to the subcutaneous fat along with extensive undermining.
Stage 3*	In this instance, the sore or ulcer extends further into subcutaneous fat along with extensive undermining.
Stage 4*	The sore or ulcer is characterized by penetration into deep fascia involving both muscle and bone.

*Stage 3 and 4 lesions are unlikely to resolve on their own and often require surgical intervention.

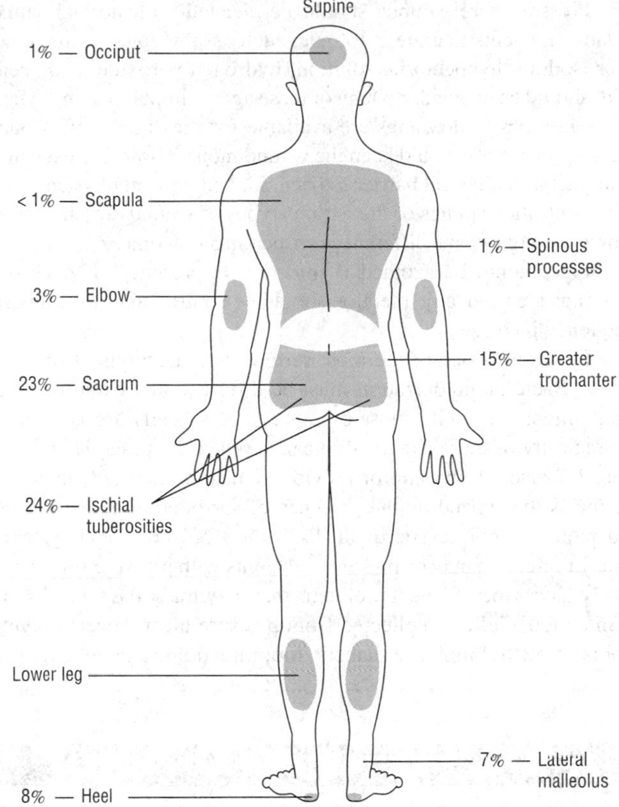

FIGURE 108–2. Supine view of areas where pressure sore formation tends to occur.

classification systems define the various stages of progression through which a pressure sore may pass (Table 108–5).

Pressure sores can occur anywhere on the body. More than 95% of all pressure sores are located on the lower part of the body (65% in the region of the pelvis and 3.4% on the lower extremities) (Fig. 108–2). The most common sites on the lower portion of the body are the sacral and coccygeal areas, ischial tuberosities, and greater trochanter.

Complications of pressure sores are not uncommon and may be life-threatening. The most frequently encountered complications are infectious in nature. Pressure sores are routinely colonized by a wide variety of microorganisms; gram-negative aerobes and anaerobes are most often associated with pressure sore infections.[49] Systemic infections are not infrequent. Extension to the bone can occur and can lead to osteomyelitis.

▶ TREATMENT: Pressure Sores

Prevention is the single most important aspect in the management of pressure sores. Prevention is far easier and less costly than the intensive care necessary for the healing and eventual closure of pressure sores. Of primary importance, then, is the ability to identify those patients who are at high risk so that preventive measures may be instituted.

The medical approach to the treatment of pressure sores depends on the stage of the disease. Medical management is generally indicated for lesions that are of moderate size and relatively shallow depth (stage 1 or 2 lesions) and are not located over a bony prominence. Depending on their location and severity, from 30% to 80% of these ulcers will heal without an operation. Surgical intervention is almost always necessary for ulcers that extend through superficial fascia or into bone (stage 3 and 4 lesions).

The goal of therapy is to clean and decontaminate the ulcer to promote wound healing by permitting the formation of healthy granulation tissue, or to prepare the wound for an operative procedure. The main factors to be considered for successful topical therapy (local care) are (a) relief of pressure, (b) débridement of necrotic tissue as needed, (c) wound cleansing, (d) dressing selection, and (e) prevention, diagnosis, and treatment of infection.[50]

Friction and shearing forces can be minimized with proper positioning. Skin care and prevention of soilage are important, with the intent being to keep the surface relatively free of moisture. Patients with problems of incontinence should be frequently cleaned, and efforts should be made to keep the involved areas dry. Natural sheepskin is believed to be useful in minimizing the effects of moisture, shearing forces, and friction. Relief of pressure is probably the single most important factor in preventing pressure sore formation. Relief for a period of only 5 minutes once every 2 hours is believed to give protection against pressure sore formation.[45]

The goals of débridement and cleansing measures are removal of devitalized tissue and reduction of bacterial contamination, which can slow granulation time and, therefore, impede healing. Débridement can be accomplished by surgical, mechanical, or chemical means. Surgical débridement rapidly removes necrotic material from the wound and is recommended for urgent situations (e.g., cellulitis and sepsis).[50] Mechanical débridement generally involves wet-to-dry dressing changes. Saline-soaked gauze is applied to the wound; after drying, the gauze is removed and with it any adherent necrotic tissue. Other effective mechanical therapies include hydrotherapy (use of the whirlpool [Hubbard tank] to remove necrotic tissue and debris), wound irrigation, and dextranomers (beads placed in the wound to absorb exudate and bacteria). Chemical débridement includes enzymatic and autolytic agents. Enzymatic débridement involves application of topical debriding agents to remove devitalized tissue. This method is recommended for patients who cannot tolerate surgery or are in a long-term care or home setting. Autolytic débridement involves the use of synthetic dressings that allow devitalized tissue to self-digest via enzymes present in wound fluids. Autolytic débridement is contraindicated in the treatment of infected pressure sores.

Pressure sore wounds should be cleaned with normal saline. Cleansing agents that are cytotoxic, such as povidone iodine, iodophor, sodium hypochlorite solution, hydrogen peroxide, and acetic acid, should be avoided.[50] Many of these agents impair healing. Many different types of dressings are available for pressure sores. Wound dressing materials should keep the wound moist, allow free exchange of air, act as a physical barrier to bacteria, and prevent physical damage. Controlled studies of the various types of wound dressings have shown no significant differences in healing outcomes.[50] Occlusive dressings should be avoided if infection is present.[51] If occlusive dressings are used, any infection should be controlled or the dressing frequency increased.

Infection is one of the most serious complications of pressure ulcers. Bacterial colonization must be differentiated from true bacterial infection. While most pressure sore wounds are colonized, the majority of these eventually heal.[52] When the tissue is infected, there is bacterial invasion of previously healthy tissue. Clinical infection is recognized by the presence of surrounding redness, heat, and pain. In addition, purulent discharge, foul odor, and systemic signs of infection may be present.[52] Patients with pressure sores commonly have other medical problems that may mask the typical signs of infection. Cultures collected from pressure ulcers reveal polymicrobial growth. Similar to diabetic foot infections, a large variety of aerobic gram-positive and gram-negative organisms, as well as anaerobes, are frequently isolated from wound cultures. A culture collected by swab is likely to identify surface bacteria colonizing the wound rather than to diagnose the infection.[51] Cultures should be collected from either a biopsy or from fluid obtained by needle aspiration.[51] Clinicians must also be aware of the possibility of underlying osteomyelitis.

Systemic treatment of an infected pressure ulcer should be guided by results from appropriately collected cultures. Curettage of the ulcer base after débridement provides more reliable culture information than does needle aspiration.[52] Biopsy specimens give the most reliable data, but may not be practical to obtain. Deep-tissue cultures from different sites may give different results. Systemic antibiotics are generally reserved for treatment of bacteremia, sepsis, cellulitis, or osteomyelitis.[51] However, a short 2-week trial of topical antibiotics (silver sulfadiazine or triple antibiotic) is recommended for a clean ulcer that is not healing or is producing a moderate amount of exudate despite appropriate care.[51]

Other nonpharmacologic approaches to shortening the healing time have included the use of hyperbaric oxygenation, hydrotherapy, high-frequency/high-intensity sound waves, and electrotherapy.[52,53] Electrical stimulation is the only adjunctive therapy that has been shown to be effective.[52,53]

INFECTED BITE WOUNDS

It has been estimated that half of the population in the United States will be bitten by either an animal or another human sometime during their lifetimes.[54] Bite wounds have a substantial potential for infectious complications. If left untreated, complications such as soft tissue infection or osteomyelitis may occur, possibly requiring extensive débridement or amputation. Most of the therapeutic decisions surrounding bite wounds are controversial, because most of the available data are derived from anecdotal case reports.

DOG BITES

Dog bites account for approximately 80% of all animal bite wounds requiring medical attention. A survey of US emergency departments reported an annual adjusted total of 333,687 visits from 1992 to 1994 for new dog bite-related injuries.[55] Based on the data gathered in this study, approximately 914 new dog bite injuries are seen in emergency departments every day. Dog bites commonly occur in individuals younger than 20 years of age (52.2% of reported cases) who are most often male (57.8%). More than 70% of bites are to the extremities.[54] Occasionally, facial bites may occur, and these are seen most often in children younger than 15 years of age and can be a lethal event via exsanguination. From 1979 through 1994, 279 deaths were the result of attacks by dogs.[56]

Health care providers see two distinct groups of patients seeking medical attention for dog bites.[57] The first group of patients presents 8 to 12 hours after the injury. These patients require general wound care, repair of tear wounds, or rabies and/or tetanus treatment. The second group of patients presents more than 12 hours after the injury has occurred. These patients usually have clinical signs of infection and seek medical attention for infection-related complaints (i.e., pain, purulent discharge, swelling). Those patients at greatest risk of acquiring an infection after a bite have had a puncture wound (usually the hand), have not sought medical attention within 12 hours of the injury, and are older than 50 years of age.[58,59]

Infected dog bites generally present as a localized cellulitis with pain at the site of injury. The cellulitis usually spreads proximally from the initial site of injury and a gray malodorous discharge may be encountered. If *Pasteurella multocida* is present, a rapidly progressing cellulitis is observed with pain and swelling developing within 24 (70%) to 48 (90%) hours of initial injury.[60] Fewer than 20% of patients have a concomitant adenopathy or lymphangitis. Fever is uncommon. Wounds close to bones or joints may lead to infections of these structures.

Infections from dog bite wounds are caused predominantly by organisms documented to be from the dog's oral flora.[59] Most infections are polymicrobial, with approximately five bacterial isolates per culture.[61] *Pasteurella* species are the most frequent isolates. Other common aerobes include streptococci, staphylococci, *Moraxella,* and *Neisseria.* The most common anaerobes are *Fusobacterium, Bacteroides, Porphyromonas,* and *Prevotella.*[61] Wound-site cultures in both infected and noninfected patients have similar bacteria present, with aerobic organisms isolated from 74% to 90% and anaerobic organisms isolated from 41% to 49%.[61–63] Unfortunately, cultures obtained from early, noninfected bite wounds are not of value in predicting the subsequent development of infection. Documentation of the mechanism of injury is important; if possible, an immunization history of the animal should be obtained. It is also important for the patient's tetanus immune status to be determined.

Wounds should be thoroughly irrigated with a copious volume (>150 mL) of sterile normal saline. Proper irrigation will reduce the bacterial count in the wound. Antibiotic or iodine solutions do not offer any advantage over saline and may actually increase tissue irritation. Several management techniques used in the treatment of bite wounds remain controversial; these include the extent and type of débridement,[57] the use of primary closure within 24 hours of the injury,[63] and indications for the use of antibiotics.

The role of prophylactic antimicrobial therapy for the early, noninfected bite wound remains controversial.[54,64] Unfortunately, suggestions concerning the use of prophylactic antibiotics are based on minimal data because few clinical trials have been performed.

Most reports are of retrospective studies or observations of complicated cases. A meta-analysis of eight randomized trials of dog-bite wounds evaluated the use of antibiotics for prophylaxis for the prevention of infectious complications.[65] The overall occurrence of infectious complications ranged from 3.2% to 45.8%. All studies used oral antibiotics with six of the eight using either penicillin or a penicillinase-resistant penicillin. Five of the eight studies documented a reduced risk for infection in those patients receiving antimicrobial prophylaxis.

Controlled studies have not definitively shown benefits with prophylactic antibiotics for noninfected bites. Because up to 20% of bite wounds may become infected, a 3- to 5-day course of antimicrobial therapy is generally recommended.[54] This is especially important for those patients at greater risk for infection (patients older than 50 years of age, puncture wounds, wounds to the hands, and wounds in immunocompromised hosts).[66,67] Treatment should be directed at the typical aerobic and anaerobic oral flora of dogs, as well as at potential pathogens from the skin flora of the bite victim. To date, there is no single, universally agreed upon treatment regimen for bite wounds. Penicillin provides excellent coverage for *P. multocida*, but not for *S. aureus* and most of the other staphylococci that are commonly isolated from bite wounds. Although penicillinase-resistant penicillins, first-generation cephalosporins, erythromycin, and clindamycin have excellent activity against staphylococci, these agents are not active against most strains of *P. multocida*.

Antibiotic regimens suggested for empiric therapy of dog bite wounds include (a) a combination of a β-lactam antibiotic and a β-lactamase inhibitor; (b) a second-generation cephalosporin with anaerobic activity; or (c) penicillin in combination with a first-generation cephalosporin or clindamycin. Tetracyclines (e.g., doxycycline) and trimethoprim-sulfamethoxazole have activity against *P. multocida* and are often recommended as an alternative form of therapy for those patients allergic to penicillins. However, tetracyclines should not be used in children and/or pregnant women; trimethoprim-sulfamethoxazole should also be avoided during pregnancy. Erythromycin may be considered an alternative in growing children or pregnant women. If erythromycin is selected, bacterial sensitivities should be obtained and clinical response carefully monitored, as most strains of *P. multocida* are resistant.

In addition to irrigation and antibiotics, when indicated, the injured area should be immobilized and elevated. Clinical failures due to edema have occurred despite appropriate antibiotic therapy.[54] Therefore it is important to stress to patients that the affected area should be elevated for several days or until edema has resolved.

Infections developing within the first 24 hours of a bite are most often caused by *P. multocida* and should be treated with penicillin VK 500 mg po four times daily (in children, 80,000–90,000 U/kg/day po divided into four doses) or amoxicillin 500 mg po three times daily (in children, 40 mg/kg/day po divided into three doses). Tetracycline is an alternative for penicillin-allergic children and nonpregnant adults (500 mg po four times daily; in children, 50 mg/kg/day po divided into four doses).[66] For severe infections, IV penicillin (1.2 million units every 4 to 6 hours) therapy should be started and followed by oral therapy when the signs of cellulitis have subsided. Treatment should be given for 10 to 14 days.

For those infections developing more than 36 to 48 hours after the bite, the risk of *P. multocida* being involved dramatically decreases. In these patients, staphylococci or streptococci are the most likely causative pathogens. Therapy, in this instance, includes a penicillinase-resistant penicillin (dicloxacillin 250–500 mg po four times daily; in children, 25–50 mg/kg/day po divided into four doses) or a cephalosporin (cefuroxime axetil 500 mg po twice daily; or children 20–30 mg/kg/day po divided into two doses) and should be given for a full 10 to 14 days.[66] Results of a Gram stain should be used to confirm the appropriateness of therapy.

The fluoroquinolones are highly active *in vitro* against *Pasteurella* and other common aerobic isolates found in these bite wounds; however, they have very little activity against the anaerobes isolated in these infections. The role of fluoroquinolones in the therapy of bite wounds has yet to be defined.

Tetanus does not commonly occur after dog bites; however, it is a theoretical possibility. If the immunization history of a patient with anything other than a clean, minor wound is unknown, tetanus-diphtheria (TD) toxoids and tetanus immune globulin (TIg) should be administered.[68] Patients with wounds that do not require immunization with TD toxoids are those who have had three or more immunization doses of TIg within the past 5 years. Patients who have received three or more doses of TIg within the last 10 years or patients who received two doses of TIg within the first 24 hours of injury do not require additional TIg therapy.[68]

Because the rabies virus can be transmitted via saliva, rabies may be a potential complication of a bite. When the symptoms of rabies develop after a bite, the prognosis for survival is poor. Roughly 3% of rabies cases documented in animals were in dogs (the most frequent vectors are skunks, raccoons, and bats).

After a patient has been exposed to rabies, the treatment objectives consist of thorough irrigation of the wound, tetanus prophylaxis, antibiotic prophylaxis, if indicated, and immunization. Prompt, thorough irrigation of the wound with soap or iodine solution may reduce the development of rabies.[60] Postexposure prophylaxis immunization consists of the administration of both passive antibody and vaccine. The only exceptions to antibody administration are patients who have been previously immunized and have the appropriate degree of documented rabies antibody titers.

CAT BITES

Cat bites, with an estimated incidence of 5% to 15% of all animal bites, are the second most common cause of animal bite wounds in the United States.[60] Bites and scratches most commonly occur on the upper extremities, with most injuries reported in women.[54] Infection rates, estimated at 30% to 50%, are more than double those seen with dog bites.[54,60] These infections are frequently (75%) caused by *P. multocida,* which has been isolated in the oropharynx of 50% to 70% of healthy cats.[58] Mixed aerobic and anaerobic infections have been reported in 63% of cat bite wounds, while approximately one-third of cultures grow aerobes only.[61] Both tularemia (*Pasteurella tularensis*) and rabies have also been transmitted by cat bites.[58]

The management of cat bites is similar to that discussed for dog bites. Cat scratches typically involve the same organisms as bites and should be treated accordingly. Antibiotic therapy with penicillin is the mainstay, and therapy is as described for dog bites.

HUMAN BITES

Human bites are the third most frequent type of bite. Infected human bites can occur as bites from the teeth or from blows to the mouth (clenched-fist injuries). Human bites are generally more serious than animal bites and carry a higher likelihood of infection than do most animal bites. Infectious complications occur in 10% to 50% of patients with human bites.[60,69,70]

Self-inflicted bites most commonly occur on the lips or around the fingernails (from sucking or biting the nails). Bites by others can occur to any part of the body, but most often involve the hands. Bites to the hand are most serious and more frequently become infected. The clenched-fist injury is a traumatic laceration caused by one person hitting another in the mouth and is a very serious bite wound. The areas most commonly affected by this injury are the third and fourth metacarpophalangeal joints.

Patients with infected bites to the hand may develop a painful, throbbing, swollen extremity. The wound often has a purulent discharge, and the patient complains of a decreased range of motion. In addition to a cellulitis, other complications, such as osteomyelitis, septic arthritis, and tenosynovitis, can occur. Loss of a digit or hand has been reported.

Infections caused by these injuries are similar, and most often are caused by the normal oral flora, which include both aerobic and anaerobic microorganisms. *S. aureus* is the most common aerobic isolate followed by *Streptococcus* species, *Corynebacterium* species, and *Eikenella corrodens*. *E. corrodens* is isolated from human bite wounds approximately 30% of the time. It is usually susceptible to penicillin but is resistant to penicillinase-resistant penicillins and to first-generation cephalosporins. Anaerobic microorganisms have been isolated in approximately 40% of human bites and 55% of clenched-fist injuries. The anaerobes most frequently recovered from human bite infections are similar to those seen in animal bite wounds and include *Bacteroides fragilis* and *Peptostreptococcus* species.[60]

Management of bite wounds consists of aggressive irrigation, surgical débridement, and immobilization of the affected area. Primary closure for human bites is not generally recommended. If damage to a bone or joint is suspected, radiographic evaluation should be undertaken. Tetanus toxoid and antitoxin may be indicated. Transmission of viruses has been documented through human bites, therefore information about the biter is important. Although the possibility of acquiring the human immunodeficiency virus (HIV) through bites is believed to be unlikely, the presence of the virus in the saliva makes disease transmission possible. If the biter is HIV-positive, the victim should have a baseline blood specimen drawn to determine preexposure HIV status and then be retested in 3 months and 6 months.[70] The bite wound should be thoroughly and vigorously irrigated with a virucidal agent such as povidone-iodine.[60] Bite victims exposed to blood-tainted saliva should be offered antiretroviral chemoprophylaxis.

Patients with noninfected hand bite injuries should be given prophylactic antibiotic therapy. Initial therapy should consist of a penicillinase-resistant penicillin (dicloxacillin 250–500 mg po four times daily; in children, 25–50 mg/kg/day po divided into four doses) in combination with penicillin VK 250–500 mg po four times daily (in children, 40,000–90,000 U/kg/day po divided into four doses). Prophylactic therapy should be given for 3 to 5 days as for dog bites.[71] A first-generation cephalosporin or macrolide is not recommended, as the sensitivity of these agents to *E. corrodens* is variable.[72]

For infected bite wounds, penicillin and a penicillinase-resistant penicillin or amoxicillin/clavulanic acid 875 mg/125 mg po twice daily (40 mg/kg/day po of the amoxicillin component divided into two doses) should be empirically started pending the culture results. Tetracyclines or a combination of clindamycin plus a fluoroquinolone or trimethoprim-sulfamethoxazole may be used as an alternative therapy for the penicillin-allergic patient. Hospitalization for minor wounds is not necessary if surgical repair of vital structures has not been performed. Those patients suffering serious injuries or clenched-fist injuries should be started on IV antibiotics. Duration of therapy for infected bite injuries should be 7 to 14 days.

Antibiotic therapy should always be used in clenched-fist injuries. Therapy should include penicillin (or ampicillin) plus a penicillinase-resistant penicillin until the final cultures are available. Therapeutic failures have been documented when either first-generation cephalosporins or penicillinase-resistant penicillins have been used alone, most likely because of their poor and variable activity against *E. corrodens*.[73,74] Therapy should be continued from 7 to 14 days.[71]

Guidelines for therapy of infections associated with bites are:

1. Determine the time frame of injury to presentation.
2. Determine rabies, tetanus, and HIV status, and administer prophylaxis when necessary.
3. All wounds should be thoroughly cleaned.
4. If the wound looks benign, without infection, or indication of other than local involvement, the patient can be sent home on oral antimicrobial agents (3 to 5 days) based on the type of bite injury.
5. Wounds that are swollen, tender, erythematous, and with lymphadenopathy require hospitalization for observation. In this instance, parenteral antimicrobials along with elevation and splinting of the injured area are the mainstays of therapy (total duration of therapy 7 to 14 days).
6. If improvement is not seen within 24 hours, then aggressive operative débridement is indicated.

► PRINCIPLES OF PHARMACOTHERAPY

- Folliculitis is a superficial infection surrounding hair follicles. Most infections are caused by *S. aureus*. Treatment generally consists of local measures such as warm moist compresses or topical antibiotics.
- Furuncles (boils) and carbuncles are infections that are around hair follicles, but which also invade the surrounding dermis. Lesions characteristically begin as firm, tender, red nodules that become painful and fluctuant. Most drain spontaneously; if not, surgical incision is indicated for large and fluctuant lesions. Small furuncles are generally treated with warm moist heat, whereas large furuncles and carbuncles are most often treated with dicloxacillin.
- Erysipelas is a type of superficial cellulitis with extensive lymphatic involvement. It differs from cellulitis in that the lesion is sharply demarcated by an elevated border. Erysipelas is caused by group A streptococci and is treated with penicillin. Serious infections should be treated with intravenous antibiotics.
- Impetigo is a type of superficial cellulitis caused by *S. aureus* and/or group A streptococci. It occurs most commonly in children. Lesions start as small, fluid-filled vesicles that rapidly develop into pus-filled blisters. The blisters rupture and dry to form golden-yellow crusts, which are the characteristic feature of this infection. Dicloxacillin is commonly used for treatment, although topical antibiotics such as mupirocin are also effective.
- Lymphangitis is an infection of the subcutaneous lymphatic channels. It is generally caused by group A streptococci. Acute lymphangitis is characterized by the rapid development of fine red linear streaks extending from the initial infection site toward the regional lymph nodes, which are usually enlarged and tender. Penicillin is the drug of choice.
- Cellulitis is an infection of the epidermis, dermis, and superficial fascia. Lesions are generally hot, painful, and erythematous, with

nonelevated, poorly defined margins. The most common causes of cellulitis are group A streptococci and *S. aureus*. Treatment generally consists of a penicillinase-resistant penicillin for 7 to 10 days, although other agents may be needed if gram-negative bacilli or anaerobes are suspected.

- Necrotizing fasciitis is a rare, but life-threatening infection of subcutaneous tissue that results in progressive destruction of superficial fascia and subcutaneous fat. Type I infections are caused by a mixture of anaerobes and facultative bacteria (streptococci, Enterobacteriaceae) and are treated with broad-spectrum antibiotics. Type II infections are caused by group A streptococci and are treated with the combination of penicillin and clindamycin. Early and aggressive surgical débridement is an essential part of therapy for both types of necrotizing fasciitis.
- The majority of diabetic foot infections may be successfully managed with a comprehensive treatment approach that includes both proper wound care and antimicrobial therapy. Antimicrobial regimens for diabetic foot infections should include broad-spectrum coverage of staphylococci, streptococci, enteric gram-negative bacilli, and anaerobes. Outpatient therapy with oral antimicrobials should be utilized whenever possible.
- Prevention is the single most important aspect in the management of pressure sores. After a sore develops, successful local care includes a comprehensive approach consisting of relief of pressure, proper cleaning (débridement), disinfection, and appropriate antimicrobial therapy if an infection is present. Good wound care is crucial to successful management.
- All bite wounds (either animal or human) should be thoroughly irrigated with large volumes of sterile normal saline, and the injured area should be immobilized and elevated. Antimicrobial prophylaxis of dog or cat bites is not routinely recommended, although the need for tetanus-diphtheria toxoids and tetanus immune globulin should be considered for more severe wounds.
- Infections developing within the first 24 hours of a dog or cat bite are caused most often by *Pasteurella multocida* and should be treated with penicillin or amoxicillin for 10 to 14 days. Infections developing more than 36 to 48 hours after a bite are most likely caused by staphylococci or streptococci and should be treated with an antistaphylococcal penicillin or cephalosporin.
- Patients with noninfected human bite injuries of the hand should be given prophylactic antimicrobial therapy with penicillin plus dicloxacillin for 3 to 5 days. Infected wounds of the hand, particularly clenched-fist injuries, should be treated with penicillin plus dicloxacillin or amoxicillin/clavulanate for 7 to 14 days.

REFERENCES

1. Yagupski P. Bacteriologic aspects of skin and soft tissue infections. Pediatr Ann 1993;22:217–224.
2. Ducan WC, McBride ME, Knox JM. Experimental production of infection in humans. J Invest Dermatol 1970;54:319–323.
3. Gustafson LT, Band JD, Hutchinson RH, et al. *Pseudomonas* folliculitis: An outbreak and review. Rev Infect Dis 1983;5:1–8.
4. Swartz MN. Cellulitis and subcutaneous tissue infections. In: Mandell GL, Bennett JE, Dolin R, eds. Principles and Practice of Infectious Diseases, 5th ed. Philadelphia, Churchill Livingstone, 2000:1037–1057.
5. Bisno AL, Stevens DL. Streptococcal infections of skin and soft tissues. N Engl J Med 1996;334:240–245.
6. Hook EW, Hooton TM, Horton C, et al. Microbiologic evaluation of cutaneous cellulitis in adults. Arch Intern Med 1986;146:295–297.
7. Sadick NS. Current aspects of bacterial infections of the skin. Dermatol Clin 1997;15:341–349.
8. Ben-Amitai D, Ashkenazi S. Common bacterial skin infections in childhood. Pediatr Ann 1993;22:225–233.
9. Britton JW, Fajardo JE, Krafte-Jacobs B. Comparison of mupirocin and erythromycin in the treatment of impetigo. J Pediatr 1990;117:827–829.
10. Swartz MN. Lymphadenitis and lymphangitis. In: Mandell GL, Bennett JE, Dolin R, eds. Principles and Practice of Infectious Diseases, 5th ed. Philadelphia, Churchill Livingstone, 2000:1066–1075.
11. Bass JW. Treatment of skin and skin structure infections. Pediatr Infect Dis J 1992;11:152–155.
12. Binswanger IA, Kral AH, Bluthenthal RN, Rybold DJ, Edlin BR. High prevalence of abscesses and cellulitis among community-recruited injection drug users in San Francisco. Clin Infect Dis 2000;30:579–581.
13. Orangio GR, Pitlick SD, Latta PD, et al. Soft tissue infections in parenteral drug abusers. Ann Surg 1984;199:97–100.
14. Bisbe J, Miro J, Latorre, et al. Disseminated candidiasis in addicts who use brown heroin: Report of 83 cases and review. Clin Infect Dis 1992;15:910–923.
15. Dagan R, Moshe P, Watemberg N, et al. Outpatient treatment of serious community-acquired pediatric infections using once daily intramuscular ceftriaxone. Pediatr Infect Dis J 1987;6:1080–1084.
16. Gould IM, Hudson M, Morris J, et al. Imipenem versus standard therapy in the treatment of serious soft tissue infection. Drugs Exp Clin Res 1988;14(8):555–558.
17. Kulhanjian J, Dunphy M, Hamstra S, et al. Randomized comparative study of ampicillin/sulbactam vs. ceftriaxone for treatment of soft tissue and skeletal infections in children. Pediatr Infect Dis J 1989;8:605–610.
18. Tan JS, Wishnow RM, Talan DA, et al. Treatment of hospitalized patients with complicated skin and skin structure infections: Double-blind, randomized, multicenter study of piperacillin-tazobactam versus ticarcillin-clavulanate. Antimicrob Agents Chemother 1993;37:1580–1586.
19. Gentry LO, Ramirez-Ronda CH, Rodriquez-Noriega E, et al. Oral ciprofloxacin vs. parenteral cefotaxime in the treatment of difficult skin and skin structure infections. Arch Intern Med 1989;148:2579–2583.
20. Gentry LO. Therapy with newer oral β-lactam and quinolone agents for infections of the skin and skin structures: A review. Clin Infect Dis 1992;14:285–297.
21. Gentry LO, Rodriguez-Gomez G, Zeluff BJ, et al. A comparative evaluation of oral ofloxacin versus intravenous cefotaxime therapy for serious skin and skin structure infections. Am J Med 1989;87(suppl 6C):57S–S60.
22. Thadepalli H, Mathai D, Chuah SK, et al. Ciprofloxacin versus ceftazidime in skin and soft tissue infections. J Chemother 1989;1(1):30–34.
23. Stevens DL, Smith LG, Bruss JB, et al. Randomized comparison of linezolid (PNU-100766) versus oxacillin-dicloxacillin for treatment of complicated skin and soft tissue infections. Antimicrob Agents Chemother 2000;44:3408–3413.
24. Nichols RL, Graham DR, Barriere SL, et al. Treatment of hospitalized patients with complicated gram-positive skin and skin structure infections: Two randomized, multicentre studies of quinupristin/dalfopristin versus cefazolin, oxacillin or vancomycin. Synercid Skin and Skin Structure Infection Group. J Antimicrob Chemother 1999;44:263–273.
25. Dominquez J, Palma F, Vega ME, et al. Brief report: Prospective, controlled, randomized non-blind comparison of intravenous/oral ciprofloxacin with intravenous ceftazidime in the treatment of skin or soft tissue infections. Am J Med 1989;87(suppl 5A)13:136S–137S.
26. LeFrock J, Blais F, Schell, et al. Cefoxitin in the treatment of diabetic patients with lower extremity infections. Infect Surg 1983;2:361–374.
27. Hughes C, Johnson C, Bamberger D, et al. Treatment and long-term follow-up of foot infections in patients with diabetes or ischemia: A randomized, prospective, double blind comparison of cefoxitin and ceftizoxime. Clin Ther 1987;10(suppl A):36–49.
28. Crane L, Levine D, Acrvos M, et al. Bacteremia in narcotic addicts at Detroit Medical Center: Microbiology, epidemiology, risk factors, and empiric therapy. Rev Infect Dis 1986;8:364–373.
29. Urschel JD. Necrotizing soft tissue infections. Postgrad Med J 1999;75:645–649.

30. Lipsky BA, Pecoraro RE, Wheat LJ. The diabetic foot: Soft tissue and bone infection. Infect Dis Clin North Am 1990;4:409–432.
31. Levin ME. Foot lesions in patients with diabetes mellitus. Endocrinol Metab Clin North Am 1996;25:447–462.
32. Slovenkai MP. Foot problems in diabetes. Med Clin North Am 1998; 82:949–971.
33. West NJ. Systemic antimicrobial treatment of foot infections in diabetic patients. Am J Health Syst Pharm 1995;52:1199–207.
34. Gerding DN. Foot infections in diabetic patients: The role of anaerobes. Clin Infect Dis 1995;20(suppl 2):S283–S288.
35. Grayson ML. Diabetic foot infections: Antimicrobial therapy. Infect Dis Clin North Am 1995;9:143–161.
36. Gentry LO. Diagnosis and management of the diabetic foot ulcer. J Antimicrob Chemother 1993;32(suppl A):77–89.
37. Caputo GM, Cavanagh PR, Ulbrecht JS, et al. Assessment and management of foot disease in patients with diabetes. N Engl J Med 1994;331:854–860.
38. Shea KW. Antimicrobial therapy for diabetic foot infections. Postgrad Med 1999;106:85–94.
39. Smith AJ, Daniels T, Bohnen JMA. Soft tissue infections and the diabetic foot. Am J Surg 1996;172(suppl 6A):7S–12S.
40. Parish LC, Aten EM. Treatment of skin and skin structure infections: A comparative study of Augmentin and cefaclor. Cutis 1984;34:567–570.
41. Eron LJ, Harvey L, Hixon DL, et al. Ciprofloxacin therapy of infections caused by *Pseudomonas aeruginosa* and other resistant bacteria. Antimicrob Agents Chemother 1985;28:308–310.
42. Sesin PG, Paszko A, O'Keefe E. Oral clindamycin and ciprofloxacin therapy for diabetic foot infections. Pharmacotherapy 1990;10:154–156.
43. Grayson ML, Gibbons GW, Habershaw GM, et al. Use of ampicillin/sulbactam versus imipenem/cilastatin in the treatment of limb-threatening foot infections in diabetic patients. Clin Infect Dis 1994;18:683–693.
44. Lipsky BA, Baker PD, Landon GC, et al. Antibiotic therapy for diabetic foot infections: Comparison of two parenteral-to-oral regimens. Clin Infect Dis 1997;24:643–648.
45. Goode PS, Allman RM. The prevention and management of pressure sores. Med Clin North Am 1989;73:1511–1524.
46. Reuler JB, Cooney TG. The pressure sore: Pathophysiology and principles of management. Ann Intern Med 1981;94:661–666.
47. Shea JD. Pressure sores—Classification and management. Clin Orthop 1975;112:89–100.
48. National Pressure Ulcer Advisory Panel. Pressure ulcers: Incidence, economics, risk. Consensus Development Conference statement. Decubitus 1989;2:24–29.
49. Gradon J, Adamsom C. Infections of pressure ulcers: Management and controversies. Infect Dis Clin Pract 1995;1:11–16.
50. Cervo FA, Cruz AC, Posillico JA. Pressure ulcers. Analysis of guidelines for treatment and management. Geriatrics 2000;55:55–60.
51. Findlay D. Practical management of pressure ulcers. Am Fam Physician 1996;54:1519–1528.
52. Kanj LF, Wilking SVB, Phillips TJ. Pressure ulcers. J Am Acad Derm 1998;38:517–536.
53. Cuddigan J, Frantz RA. Pressure ulcer research: Pressure ulcer treatment. A monograph from the National Pressure Ulcer Advisory Panel. Adv Wound Care 1998;2:294–300.
54. Goldstein E. Bite wounds and infection. Clin Infect Dis 1992;14:633–640.
55. Weiss HB, Friedman DI, Coben JH. Incidence of dog bite injuries treated in emergency departments. JAMA 1998;279:51–53.
56. Anonymous. Dog bite related fatalities—United States, 1995–1996. MMWR Morb Mortal Wkly Rep 1997;46:463–467.
57. Callaham ML. Treatment of common dog bites: Infection risk factors. J Am Coll Emerg Phys 1978;7:83–87.
58. Rest JG, Goldstein EJC. Management of human and animal bite wounds. Emerg Med Clin North Am 1985;3:117–126.
59. Goldstein EJC, Citron DM, Finegold SM. Role of anaerobic bacteria in bite wound infections. Rev Infect Dis 1984;6(suppl 1):S177–S183.
60. Griego RD, Rosen T, Orengo IF, et al. Dog, cat, and human bites: A review. J Am Acad Dermatol 1995;33:1019–1029.
61. Talan DA, Citron DM, Abrahamian FM, et al. Bacteriologic analysis of infected dog and cat bites. N Engl J Med 1999;340:85–92.
62. Wiggins ME, Akelamn E, Weiss AP. The management of dog bites and dog bite infections to the hand. Orthopedics 1994;17:617–623.
63. Goldstein EJC, Citron DM, Finegold SM. Dog bite wounds and infection: A prospective clinical study. Ann Emerg Med 1980;9:508–512.
64. Elenbass RM, McNaoney WK, Robinson WA. Prophylactic oxacillin in dog bite wounds. Ann Emerg Med 1982;11:248–251.
65. Cummings P. Antibiotics to prevent infections in patients with dog bite wounds: A meta-analysis of randomized trials. Ann Emerg Med 1994;23:535–540.
66. Elliot DL, Tolle SW, Goldberg L, et al. Pet-associated illness. N Engl J Med 1985;313:985–995.
67. Goldstein E, Citron DM, Richwals GA. Lack of *in vitro* efficacy of oral forms of certain cephalosporins, erythromycin, and oxacillin against *Pasteurella multocida*. Antimicrob Agents Chemother 1988;32(2):213–215.
68. Goldstein EJ, Reinhardt JF, Murray PM, et al. Outpatient therapy of bite wounds: Demographic data, bacteriology, and a prospective, randomized trial of amoxicillin/clavulanic acid versus penicillin (dicloxacillin). Int J Derm 1987;26(2):123–127.
69. Mann RJ, Hoffield TA, Farmer CB. Human bites of the hand: Twenty years of experience. J Hand Surg 1977;2:97–99.
70. Bunzli WF, Wright DH, Hoang AD, et al. Current management of human bites. Pharmacotherapy 1998;18:227–234.
71. Talan D. Infectious disease issues in the emergency department. Clin Infect Dis 1996;23:1–14.
72. Goldstein E, Gombert M, Agyare E. Susceptibility of *Eikenella corrodens* to newer beta-lactam antibiotics. Antimicrob Agents Chemother 1980;18:832–833.
73. Goldstein E, Miller T, Citron D, et al. Infections following clenched-fist injury: A new perspective. J Hand Surg 1978;3:455–459.
74. Goldstein E, Barene M, Miller TA. *Eikenella corrodens* in hand infections. J Hand Surg 1983;8:563–566.

109
INFECTIVE ENDOCARDITIS

Michael A. Crouch

Endocarditis is an inflammation of the endocardium, the membrane lining the chambers of the heart and covering the cusps of the heart valves.[1,2] More commonly, endocarditis refers to infection of the heart valves by various microorganisms. Although bacteria primarily cause endocarditis, fungi and other atypical microorganisms can lead to the disease; thus, the more encompassing term *infective endocarditis* (IE) is preferred.

Endocarditis is often referred to as acute or subacute, depending on the clinical presentation. The acute, fulminating form is associated with high fevers and systemic toxicity. Virulent bacteria, such as *Staphylococcus aureus*, frequently cause this syndrome and if untreated, death occurs within a few days to weeks. On the other hand, subacute IE is more indolent and is caused by less-invasive organisms, such as viridans streptococci, usually occurring in preexisting valvular heart disease. IE is best classified based on the etiologic organism, the anatomic site of infection, and pathogenic risk factors.[2] Infection may also follow surgical insertion of a prosthetic heart valve, resulting in prosthetic valve endocarditis (PVE).[3]

EPIDEMIOLOGY AND ETIOLOGY

Infective endocarditis is an uncommon infection, accounting for approximately 1 of every 1,000 hospital admissions.[1] Yet, the incidence of IE may be increasing and it is now the fourth leading cause of infectious disease syndromes that are life-threatening, after urosepsis, pneumonia, and intra-abdominal sepsis.[4] The male-to-female ratio is 1.7:1. Overall, a majority of cases occur in individuals older than 50 years of age and it is uncommon in children.[1,2] As the population ages and as valve replacement surgery becomes more common, the mean age of patients with IE increases. However, intravenous (IV) drug abusers, who tend to be younger males, are also at high risk of IE. Other conditions associated with a higher incidence of IE include diabetes, long-term hemodialysis, and poor dental hygeine.

Most persons with IE have risk factors, such as preexisting cardiac valvular abnormalities. Many types of structural heart disease result in turbulence of blood flow that increases the risk for IE. A predisposing factor, however, may be absent in up to 25% of cases. Some of the more important risk factors include:[5]

- Presence of a prosthetic valve (400-fold increased risk)
- Previous endocarditis (400-fold increased risk)
- Complex cyanotic congenital heart disease (e.g., single ventricle states)
- Surgically constructed systemic pulmonary shunts or conduits
- Acquired valvular dysfunction (e.g., rheumatic heart disease)
- Hypertrophic cardiomyopathy
- Mitral valve prolapse with regurgitation
- IV drug abuse

In the past, rheumatic heart disease was a prevalent risk factor for IE, although the incidence of this disease continues to decline. The risk of IE in persons with mitral valve prolapse and regurgitation is small, but because the condition is prevalent, it is an important contributor to the overall number of IE cases.[5] Prosthetic valve endocarditis occurs in 1% to 4% of patients undergoing valve replacement surgery.[3]

Nearly every organism causing human disease has been reported to cause IE (Table 109–1). Three groups of organisms, however, cause a majority of cases: streptococci (55% to 62%), staphylococci (30% to 40%), and enterococci (5% to 18%).[1,7] Recently, the incidence of staphylococci, particularly *S. aureus*, has increased.[5] In general, streptococci cause IE in patients with underlying cardiac abnormalities, such as mitral valve prolapse or rheumatic heart disease. Staphylococci (*S. aureus* and coagulase-negative staphylococci) are the most common cause of PVE within the first year after valve surgery, and *S. aureus* is common in the IV drug abuser. Enterococcal endocarditis tends to follow genitourinary manipulations (older men) or obstetric procedures (younger women). There are many exceptions to the preceding generalizations; thus, isolation of the causative pathogen and determination of its antimicrobial susceptibilities offer the best chance for successful therapy.

The mitral and aortic valves are most commonly affected in cases involving a single valve. Subacute endocarditis tends to involve the mitral valve whereas acute disease involves the aortic valve. Up to 35% of cases involve concomitant infections of both the aortic and the mitral valves. Infection of the tricuspid valve is less common, with a majority of these cases occurring in patients with IV drug abuse. It is rare for pulmonary valves to be infected.[1,2]

PATHOGENESIS AND PATHOPHYSIOLOGY

The development of IE via hematogenous spread, the most common route, requires the sequential occurrence of several factors. These components are complex and not fully elucidated:[1,2]

- *The endothelial surface of the heart is damaged.* This injury occurs with turbulent blood flow associated with the valvular lesions previously described.
- *Platelet and fibrin deposition occurs on the abnormal epithelial surface.* These platelet-fibrin deposits are referred to as nonbacterial thrombotic endocarditis (NBTE).
- *Bacteremia gives organisms access to and results in colonization of the endocardial surface.* Bacteremia is the result of trauma to a mucosal surface with a high concentration of resident bacteria, such as the oral cavity and gastrointestinal tract. Transient bacteremia commonly follows certain dental, gastrointestinal, urologic, and gynecologic procedures. Staphylococci, viridans streptococci, and enterococci are most likely to adhere to NBTE, probably because of production of specific adherence factors, such as dextran by some oral streptococci and glycocalyx for staphylococci.[2,8] Gram-negative bacteria rarely adhere to heart valves and are uncommon causes of IE.

TABLE 109–1. Etiologic Agents in Infective Endocarditis

Agent	Percentage of Cases
Streptococci	55–62
Viridans streptococci	30–40
Other streptococci	15–25
Staphylococci	20–35
Coagulase-positive	10–27
Coagulase-negative	1–3
Enterococci	5–18
Gram-negative aerobic bacilli	1.5–13
Fungi	2–4
Miscellaneous bacteria	< 5
Mixed Infections	1–2
"Culture negative"	< 5–24

(Adapted from Ref. 1.)

- *After colonization of the endothelial surface, a "vegetation" of fibrin, platelets, and bacteria forms.* The protective cover of fibrin and platelets allows unimpeded bacterial growth to concentrations as high as 10^9 to 10^{10} organisms per gram of tissue.

The pathogenesis of early PVE differs from the IE acquired by the hematogenous route in that surgery may directly inoculate the valve with bacteria from the patient's skin or operating room personnel. The recently placed, nonendothelialized valve is more susceptible to bacterial colonization than native valves. Bacteria may also colonize the new valve from contaminated bypass pumps, cannulas, and pacemakers, or from a nosocomial bacteremia subsequent to an intravascular catheter.[3,9,10] The mechanism of bacterial colonization and pathogenesis in late PVE is similar to native valve endocarditis.[3]

The vegetations seen in IE may be single or multiple, and vary in size from a few millimeters to centimeters. Bacteria within the vegetation grow slowly and are protected from antibiotics and host defenses. The adverse effects of IE and the resulting lesions can be far reaching and include (a) local perivalvular damage, (b) embolization of septic fragments with potential hematogenous seeding of remote sites, and (c) formation of antibody complexes.

Formation of vegetations may destroy valvular tissue, and continued destruction can lead to acute heart failure via perforation of the valve leaflet, rupture of the chordae tendineae or papillary muscle, or, in the patient with PVE, valve dehiscence. Occasionally, valvular stenosis may occur. Abscesses can develop in the valve ring or in myocardial tissue itself. Even with the resolution of the process, fibrosis of tissue with some residual dysfunction is possible.

Vegetations may be friable, and fragments released downstream. These infected particles, termed septic emboli, can result in an organ abscess or infarction. Septic emboli from right-sided endocarditis commonly lodge in the lung, causing pulmonary abscesses. Emboli from left-sided vegetations commonly affect organs with high blood flow, such as the kidneys, spleen, and brain. Metastatic abscesses are often small and miliary.[2]

Circulating immune complexes consisting of antigen, antibody, and complement may deposit in organs, producing local inflammation and damage (glomerulonephritis in the kidneys). Other potential pathologic changes that result from immune complex deposition or septic emboli include the development of "mycotic" aneurysms (although the aneurysm is usually bacterial in origin, not fungal), cerebral infarction, splenic infarction and abscess, and skin manifestations, such as petechiae, Osler nodes, and Janeway lesions.

TABLE 109–2. Clinical Manifestations of Infective Endocarditis

Symptoms	Percentage	Signs	Percentage
Fever	80	Fever	90
Chills	40	Heart murmur	85
Weakness	40	Changing murmur	5–10
Dyspnea	40	New murmur	3–5
Sweats	25	Embolic phenomena	>50
Anorexia	25	Skin manifestations	18–50
Weight loss	25	Osler nodes	10–23
Malaise	25	Splinter hemorrhages	15
Cough	25	Petechiae	20–40
Skin lesions	20	Janeway lesion	<10
Stroke	20	Splenomegaly	20–57
Nausea/vomiting	20	Septic complications (e.g., pneumonia, meningitis)	20
Headache	20		
Myalgia/arthralgia	15		
Edema	15	Mycotic aneurysms	20
Chest pain	15	Clubbing	12–52
Abdominal pain	15	Retinal lesion	2–10
Delirium/coma	10–15	Signs of renal failure	10–15
Hemoptysis	10		
Back pain	10		

(Adapted from Ref. 1.)

CLINICAL PRESENTATION

The clinical presentation of IE is highly variable (Table 109–2). Fever is a common finding and is often accompanied by other nonspecific symptoms. The fever may be relatively low grade, particularly in subacute cases. Heart murmurs are found in 85% of patients, with a much lower percentage documented as new or changing murmurs. In patients with subacute disease, evidence of long-standing infection may include embolic phenomena, such as splenic or renal infarction and skin lesions. Infective endocarditis usually begins insidiously and gradually worsens. Patients may present with nonspecific findings, such as fatigue, weakness, low-grade fever, anorexia, and weight loss. Arthralgias and myalgias are also common. In contrast, patients with acute disease, such as the IV drug abuser with *S. aureus* IE, may appear with classic signs of sepsis.

Other important clinical signs, especially prevalent in subacute illness, may include the following peripheral manifestations ("stigmata") of endocarditis:[1,2]

- *Osler nodes:* Purplish or erythematous subcutaneous papules or nodules on the pads of the fingers and toes. These lesions are 2–15 mm in size and are painful and tender. These nodes are not specific for IE and may be the result of embolism, immunologic phenomena, or both.
- *Janeway lesions:* Hemorrhagic, painless plaques on the palms of the hands or soles of the feet. These lesions are believed to be embolic in origin.
- *Splinter hemorrhages:* Thin, linear hemorrhages found under the nailbeds of the fingers or toes. These lesions are not specific for IE and are more commonly the result of traumatic injuries. Distal lesions are more likely the result of trauma, whereas proximal lesions tend to be associated with IE.
- *Petechiae:* Small (usually 1–2 mm in diameter), erythematous, painless, hemorrhagic lesions. These lesions appear anywhere on the skin but more frequently on the anterior trunk, buccal mucosa and palate, and conjunctivae. Petechiae are nonblanching and resolve after a few days.

- *Clubbing of the fingers:* Proliferative change in the soft tissues about the terminal phalanges, observed in long-standing bacterial endocarditis.
- *Roth spots:* Retinal infarct with central pallor and surrounding hemorrhage.
- *Emboli:* Embolic phenomena occur in up to one-third of cases and may result in significant complications. Left-sided endocarditis can result in renal artery emboli causing flank pain with hematuria, splenic artery emboli causing abdominal pain, and cerebral emboli, which may result in hemiplegia or alteration in mental status. Right-sided endocarditis may result in pulmonary emboli, causing pleuritic pain with hemoptysis and pneumonia. Splenomegaly is also a frequent finding in patients with prolonged endocarditis.

LABORATORY FINDINGS

Patients with IE typically have laboratory abnormalities; however, none of these changes are specific for the disease.[11] A normocytic, normochromic anemia with a low serum iron and low iron-binding capacity is seen in 70% to 90% of patients, typically in those with subacute disease. Patients may also present with thrombocytopenia, although this is less common than anemia. In addition, the white blood cell (WBC) count is normal or slightly elevated, sometimes with a mild left shift. Acute endocarditis, however, may present with an elevated WBC count, consistent with a fulminant infection. The erythrocyte sedimentation rate is elevated in 90% to 100% of patients, and the level of C-reactive protein may also be elevated.[1] The urinary analysis is often abnormal with proteinuria and microscopic hematuria occurring in approximately 50% of individuals.

BLOOD CULTURES

The hallmark of IE is a continuous bacteremia caused by bacteria shedding from the vegetation into the bloodstream; more than 95% of patients with IE have positive blood cultures.[1,2,11] Three sets of blood cultures, each from separate venipuncture sites, should be collected over 24 hours, and antibiotics should be withheld until adequate blood cultures are obtained. On the other hand, if a patient has a toxic appearance several blood cultures should be collected promptly, followed by immediate, empiric antimicrobial treatment. In those patients with blood cultures initially showing no growth, the laboratory should be advised and cultures held for up to a month to detect growth of fastidious organisms. The blood cultures in patients who have received previous antibiotics should also be monitored more closely because pathogen growth may be suppressed. In contrast to bacterial valvular infections, only about one-half of fungal endocarditis infections have positive blood cultures. "Culture-negative" endocarditis describes a patient in whom a clinical diagnosis of IE is likely, but blood cultures do not yield a pathogen.[11] This condition is often the consequence of previous antibiotic therapy, slow-growing fastidious organisms, nonbacterial etiologies (e.g., fungi), and improperly collected blood cultures.[4]

OTHER DIAGNOSTIC TESTS

An electrocardiogram, chest radiograph, and echocardiogram are commonly performed in those suspected of endocarditis. The electrocardiogram rarely shows important diagnostic findings, but may reveal heart block suggesting extension of the infection. The chest radiograph may provide more diagnostic information, especially in a patient with right-sided endocarditis. Septic pulmonary emboli may occur leading to multiple lung foci. The echocardiogram is the most important test, and should be performed in all patients suspected of this infection.

Echocardiography using the transthoracic (TTE) or transesophageal (TEE) technique plays an important role in the diagnosis and management of IE.[4] The TEE technique is far more sensitive for detecting vegetations (90% to 100%) as compared to TTE (58% to 63%),[2] and TEE maintains good specificity (85% to 95%). Consequently, TEE is preferred in high risk patients such as those with a prosthetic heart valve, congenital heart disease, previous endocarditis, a new murmur, or stigmata of endocarditis.[4] The lack of vegetation on echocardiogram does not exclude infection even if the transesophageal approach is used. Conversely, the test may reveal an unsuspected large vegetation, extension of the disease into surrounding tissue, valvular defects, abscess formation, cordial rupture, or an intracardiac fistula. Thus, in addition to helping in the diagnosis of IE, the echocardiogram allows the physician to evaluate hemodynamic stability and the need for urgent surgical intervention; it also provides a rough estimate of the likelihood of embolism.[12,13]

DIAGNOSIS

The signs and symptoms of IE are not specific, and the diagnosis is often unclear.[1,2,4] The diagnosis of IE requires the integration of clinical, laboratory, and echocardiographic findings. The most recent diagnostic criteria (the Duke criteria) include major variables (persistent bacteremia and echocardiographic findings) and minor variables (predisposition, fever, vascular phenomena, and microbiologic and echocardiographic findings not meeting major criteria).[14] Based on the number of major and minor criteria that are positive, patients suspected of IE are divided into three separate categories: "definite IE," "possible IE," or "IE rejected." Although a modified version of these criteria has been proposed, these criteria remain the standard method of diagnosis and have increased the number of patients diagnosed with definite IE.[4,14]

PROGNOSIS

The outcome for endocarditis is improved with rapid diagnosis, appropriate treatment (antimicrobial therapy, surgery, or both), and prompt recognition of complications, should they arise. Factors associated with increased mortality include (a) heart failure; (b) culture-negative endocarditis; (c) endocarditis caused by resistant organisms, such as fungi or gram-negative bacteria; (d) left-sided endocarditis caused by *S. aureus;* and (e) prosthetic valve endocarditis.[1,15] The presence of heart failure has the greatest negative impact on the short-term prognosis.[4] For native valve IE, mortality rates range from 16% to 27%; lower rates occur with viridans streptococci (4% to 9%) and higher rates occur with left-sided IE caused by enterococci (15% to 20%) and staphylococci (25% to 47%). Even higher rates of mortality are seen with unusually encountered organisms (e.g., gram-negative bacilli). After appropriate treatment and recovery, the risk of morbidity and mortality following IE persist for years, although it gradually declines annually. Morbidity remains elevated because of a greater likelihood of recurrent IE, heart failure, and embolism, or if a valve is replaced, the risk of anticoagulation, valve thrombosis, or additional valve surgery.[16]

▶ TREATMENT: Infective Endocarditis

DESIRED OUTCOMES

The desired outcomes for treatment and prophylaxis of IE are to:

- Relieve the signs and symptoms of the disease.
- Decrease morbidity and mortality associated with the infection.
- Eradicate the causative organism with minimal drug exposure.
- Provide cost-effective antimicrobial therapy, determined by the likely or identified pathogen, drug susceptibilities, hepatic and renal function, drug allergies, and anticipated drug toxicities.
- Prevent IE from occurring or recurring in high-risk patients with appropriate prophylactic antimicrobials.

GENERAL APPROACH TO TREATMENT

The most important approach in the treatment of IE is isolation of the infecting pathogen followed by high-dose, parenteral, bactericidal antibiotics for an extended period.[1,2,17] Large doses of parenteral antimicrobials are usually necessary to achieve bactericidal concentrations within vegetations. An extended duration of therapy is required, even for susceptible pathogens, because microorganisms are enclosed within valvular vegetations and fibrin deposits. These barriers impair host defenses and protect microbes from phagocytic cells. In addition, the high bacterial concentrations within vegetations may result in an inoculum effect that further resists killing. Many bacteria are not actively dividing, further limiting the rate of bacterial death. For most patients, 4 to 6 weeks of therapy is required.

For some pathogens, such as enterococci, the use of synergistic antimicrobial combinations is essential to obtain a bactericidal effect. Combination antibiotics may also decrease the emergence of resistant organisms during treatment (e.g., PVE caused by coagulase-negative staphylococci), and hasten the pace of clinical and microbiologic response (e.g., some streptococcal and staphylococcal infections). Occasionally, the combination treatment will result in a shorter treatment course.

Pharmacodynamic investigations in the IE animal model allow quantitation of bacterial densities within vegetations over time as a function of antibiotic concentration. These models empirically confirm many of the observed IE treatment principles.[18,19] The effective antibiotic concentration in serum may be many times the minimal bactericidal concentration (MBC) of the infecting pathogen, depending on additional characteristics. The most effective antibiotics have a rapid and homogeneous distribution into the vegetation, kill bacteria rapidly, and are least susceptible to a large inoculum. Aminoglycosides have the most favorable characteristics, followed by β-lactams, and then glycopeptides.[19]

NONPHARMACOLOGIC THERAPY

Surgery is an important adjunct in the management of endocarditis. In most surgical cases, valvectomy and valve replacement are performed to remove infected tissue and to restore hemodynamic function. Echocardiographic features that suggest the need for surgery include persistent vegetation or an increase in vegetation size after prolonged treatment, valve dysfunction, or perivalvular extension (e.g., abscess).[4] Surgery may also be considered in cases of PVE, endocarditis caused by resistant organisms (e.g., fungi or gram-negative bacteria), or if there is persistent bacteremia or other evidence of failure despite appropriate antimicrobial therapy.[3,20,21] The major indications for surgical intervention in the past have been heart failure in left-side IE and persistent infection in right-sided IE.[1]

PHARMACOLOGIC THERAPY

Specific treatment recommendations from the American Heart Association (AHA) provide guidance for the management of the more common causes of IE.[22] These recommendations are summarized in Tables 109–3 through 109–8 and are discussed in more detail in the following sections. Because these guidelines address only common causes of endocarditis, readers are referred to other references for more in-depth discussion of unusually encountered organisms.[4] Subsequent to the most recent publication of the AHA guidelines (1995), the British Society for Antimicrobial Chemotherapy (BSAC) published treatment recommendations.[23] Although derived separately, these recommendations are quite similar to those of the AHA in regards to organism specific treatment. The only major difference in these two guidelines pertains to empiric treatment of endocarditis. After appropriate blood cultures are obtained, the BSAC guidelines suggest empiric therapy with penicillin plus gentamicin for most patients, but when staphylococcal infection is suspected, they recommend vancomycin plus gentamicin. Although community-acquired staphylococcal infections rarely are methicillin-resistant, the BSAC guidelines recommend vancomycin for all suspected staphylococcal infections as an attempt to simplify recommendations, at least during the initial phase of treatment. While not specifically mentioned in the BSAC guidelines, a penicillinase-resistant penicillin (e.g., nafcillin) is a reasonable alternative to vancomycin during the short-term empiric treatment of community-acquired infection suspected to be staphylococci while identification and susceptibilities are obtained.

STREPTOCOCCAL ENDOCARDITIS

Streptococci cause a majority of IE cases with most isolates being viridans streptococci. Viridans streptococci refer to a large number of different species, such as *Streptococcus mutans, Streptococcus sanguis,* and *Streptococcus mitis.* These bacteria are common inhabitants of the human mouth and gingiva and they are especially common causes of endocarditis involving native valves.[1,24] During dental surgery and even when brushing the teeth, these organisms can cause a transient bacteremia that can result in IE in the susceptible individual. Streptococcal endocarditis is usually subacute, and the response to medical treatment is good. *Streptococcus bovis* is not a viridans streptococcus, but it is included in this group because it is penicillin sensitive and requires the same treatment as viridans streptococci. *Streptococcus bovis* is a group D streptococcus that resides in the gastrointestinal (GI) tract. IE caused by this organism is often associated with a GI pathology, especially colon carcinoma. Endocarditis caused by *Streptococcus pneumoniae, Streptococcus pyogenes*, and Groups B, C, and G streptococci are relatively uncommon and their treatment is not well defined.[1]

TABLE 109–3. Suggested Regimens for Therapy of Native Valve Endocarditis Caused by Penicillin-Susceptible Viridans Streptococci and *Streptococcus bovis* (Minimal Inhibitory Concentration ≤0.1 μg/mL)*

Antibiotic	Dosage and Route	Duration, wk	Comments
Aqueous crystalline penicillin G sodium	12–18 million U/24 h IV either continuously or in six equally divided doses	4	Preferred in most patients older than 65 y and in those with impairment of the eighth nerve or renal function
or			
Ceftriaxone sodium	2 g once daily IV or IM†	4	
Aqueous crystalline penicillin G sodium	12–18 million U/24 h IV either continuously or in six equally divided doses	2	
With gentamicin sulfate‡	1 mg/kg IM or IV every 8 h	2	When obtained 1 h after a 20- to 30-min IV infusion or IM injection, serum concentration of gentamicin of approximately 3 μg/mL is desirable; trough concentration should be <1 μg/mL.
Vancomycin hydrochloride§	30 mg/kg per 24 h IV in two equally divided doses, not to exceed 2 g/24 h unless serum levels are monitored	4	Vancomycin therapy is recommended for patients allergic to β-lactams; peak serum concentrations of vancomycin should be obtained 1 h after completion of the infusion and should be in the range of 30–45 μg/mL for twice-daily dosing

*Dosages recommended are for patients with normal renal function. For nutritionally variant streptococci, see Table 109–7. IV, intravenous; IM, intramuscular.

†Patients should be informed that IM injection of ceftriaxone is painful.

‡Dosing of gentamicin on a mg/kg basis will produce higher serum concentrations in obese patients than in lean patients. Therefore, in obese patients, dosing should be based on ideal body weight. (Ideal body weight for men is 50 kg + 2.3 kg per inch over 5 feet in height, and ideal body weight for women is 45.5 kg + 2.3 kg per inch over 5 feet in height.) Relative contraindications to the use of gentamicin are age >65 y, renal impairment, or impairment of the eighth nerve. Other potentially nephrotoxic agents (e.g., nonsteroidal anti-inflammatory drugs) should be used cautiously in patients receiving gentamicin.

§Vancomycin dosage should be reduced in patients with impaired renal function. Vancomycin given on a mg/kg basis will produce higher serum concentrations in obese patients than in lean patients. Therefore, in obese patients, dosing should be based on ideal body weight. Each dose of vancomycin should be infused over at least 1 h to reduce the risk of the histamine-release ("red man" syndrome).

(From Wilson WR, Karchmer AW, Dajani AS, et al. Antibiotic treatment of adults with infective endocarditis due to streptococci, enterococci, and staphylococci, and HACEK microorganisms. JAMA 1995;274:1706–1713, with permission.)

Antimicrobial regimens for viridans streptococci are well studied and, in uncomplicated cases, response rates as high as 98% can be expected. Viridans streptococci are penicillin susceptible, although some are more susceptible than others. Most are exquisitely sensitive to penicillin G and have minimal inhibitory concentrations (MICs) ≤ 0.1 μg/mL.[22,24] Approximately 10% to 20% are moderately susceptible (MIC 0.1–0.5 μg/mL). This difference in *in vitro* susceptibility led to recommendations that the MIC be determined for all viridans streptococci, and that the results be used to guide therapy. Some streptococci are deemed tolerant to the killing effects of penicillin, where the MBC exceeds the MIC by 32 times. A tolerant organism is inhibited, but not killed by an antibiotic normally considered bactericidal.[25] Bactericidal activity is required for successful treatment of IE; therefore, infections with a tolerant organism may relapse after treatment. Despite some animal studies of endocarditis suggesting that tolerant strains do not respond as readily to β-lactam therapy as nontolerant ones, this phenomenon is primarily a laboratory finding with little clinical significance.[17,26] Treatment for tolerant strains is identical to nontolerant organisms and measurement of the MBC is not recommended.[22,23]

An assortment of regimens can be used to treat uncomplicated endocarditis caused by fully susceptible viridans streptococci (Table 109–3). Two single-drug regimens consist of either high-dose parenteral penicillin G or ceftriaxone for 4 weeks. If a shorter course of therapy is desired, the guidelines suggest high-dose parenteral penicillin G plus an aminoglycoside.[22,24] When used in select patients, this combination is equally effective to 4 weeks of penicillin alone. Although streptomycin was listed in previous guidelines, gentamicin is the preferred aminoglycoside because serum drug concentrations are easily obtained, clinicians are more familiar with its use, and the

TABLE 109–4. Therapy for Native Valve Endocarditis Caused by Strains of Viridans Streptococci and *Streptococcus bovis* Relatively Resistant to Penicillin G (Minimal Inhibitory Concentration >0.1 μg/mL and <0.5 μg/mL)*

Antibiotic	Dosage and Route	Duration, wk	Comments
Aqueous crystalline penicillin G sodium	18 million U/24 h IV either continuously or in six equally divided doses	4	Cefazolin or other first-generation cephalosporins may be substituted for penicillin in patients whose penicillin hypersensitivity is not of the immediate type
With gentamicin sulfate†	1 mg/kg IM or IV every 8 h	2	
Vancomycin hydrochloride‡	30 mg/kg per 24 h IV in two equally divided doses, not to exceed 2 g/24 h unless serum levels are monitored	4	Vancomycin therapy is recommended for patients allergic to β-lactams

*Dosages recommended are for patients with normal renal function. IV, intravenous; IM, intramuscular.
†For specific dosing adjustment and issues concerning gentamicin (obese patients, relative contraindications), see Table 109–3 footnotes.
‡For specific dosing adjustment and issues concerning vancomycin (obese patients, length of infusion), see Table 109–3 footnotes.
(From Wilson WR, Karchmer AW, Dajani AS, et al. Antibiotic treatment of adults with infective endocarditis due to streptococci, enterococci, and staphylococci, and HACEK microorganisms. JAMA 1995;274:1706–1713, with permission.)

few strains of streptococci resistant to the effects of streptomycin-penicillin remain susceptible to gentamicin-penicillin. Other aminoglycosides are not recommended.

The decision of which regimen to use depends on the perceived risk versus benefit. For example, a 2-week course of gentamicin in an elderly patient with renal impairment may be associated with ototoxicity, worsening renal function, or both. Furthermore, the 2-week regimen is not recommended for patients with complications such as extracardiac foci. On the other hand, a 4-week course of penicillin alone generally entails greater expense, especially if the patient remains in the hospital. Monotherapy with once-daily ceftriaxone offers ease of administration, facilitates home health care treatment, and may be cost-effective.[27]

The BSAC guidelines suggest that all of the following conditions be present to consider a 2-week treatment regimen for penicillin-sensitive streptococcal endocarditis:[23,28]

- Penicillin-sensitive viridans streptococcus or *S. bovis* (penicillin MIC < 0.1 μg/mL).
- No cardiovascular risk factors such as heart failure, aortic insufficiency, or conduction abnormalities.
- No evidence of thromboembolic disease.
- Native valve infection.
- No vegetation of >5 mm diameter on echocardiogram.
- Clinical response within 7 days. The temperature should return to normal, the patient should feel well, and the patient's appetite should return to normal.

When a patient has a history of an immediate-type hypersensitivity to penicillin, vancomycin is the drug of choice for IE caused by viridans streptococci. When vancomycin is chosen, the addition of gentamicin is not recommended.[22] First-generation and some third-generation cephalosporins (ceftriaxone) are alternatives in patients with a history of delayed penicillin reactions. Most patients who report a penicillin allergy have a negative penicillin skin test and are consequently at low risk of anaphylaxis.[29] The published experience with penicillin is more extensive than with alternative regimens; therefore, a thorough allergy history must be obtained before a second-line therapy is administered.

In patients with complicated infections (e.g., extracardiac foci) or when the streptococcus has an MIC of 0.1–0.5 μg/mL, combination therapy with an aminoglycoside and penicillin (higher dose preferred) for the first 2 weeks, followed by penicillin alone for an additional 2 weeks is recommended (Table 109–4).[22,24] Some viridans streptococci have biologic characteristics that complicate diagnosis and treatment. For example, some bacteria have nutritional deficiencies that hinder growth in routine culture media.[2] These organisms require special broth supplemented with pyridoxal hydrochloride or cysteine. For patients infected with nutritionally variant streptococci or when the streptococcus has an MIC ≥ 0.5 μg/mL, treatment should follow the enterococcal endocarditis treatment guidelines.[22]

The rationale for combination therapy of penicillin-susceptible viridans streptococci is that enhanced activity against these organisms is usually observed when cell wall active agents are combined with aminoglycosides *in vitro*.[17,22,24] Combined treatment results in quicker sterilization of vegetations in animal models of endocarditis and probably explains the high response rates observed in patients treated for a total of 2 weeks.[22] The combined treatment, however, is not superior to penicillin alone. For IE caused by streptococci relatively resistant to penicillin (MIC of 0.1–0.5 mg/mL), combination therapy for 2 weeks is recommended, followed by penicillin alone for 2 additional weeks.[22,24] Some authors question the need for combination therapy for such relatively resistant streptococci, emphasizing that few human data suggest that patients with endocarditis caused by these organisms respond less well to penicillin alone.[30]

Whether or not extended interval aminoglycoside dosing has a role in IE is controversial. This dosing approach, as compared to thrice daily dosing, appears to have an equal and possibly greater efficacy in streptococcal endocarditis.[31–34] One recent study specifically evaluated the combination of ceftriaxone (2 g daily) with gentamicin (3 mg/kg daily) for 2 weeks compared to ceftriaxone (2 g daily) alone for 4 weeks for penicillin-sensitive streptococci. Both regimens were safe and effective with similar clinical cure rates at 3 months following treatment.[35]

STAPHYLOCOCCAL ENDOCARDITIS

Endocarditis caused by staphylococci is becoming more prevalent, mainly because of increased IV drug abuse, more frequent use of peripheral and central venous catheters, and increased frequency of valve replacement surgery.[8,36,37] *Staphylococcus aureus* is the most common organism causing IE among IV drug abusers and persons with venous catheters. Coagulase-negative staphylococci (usually *Staphylococcus epidermidis*) are prominent causes of PVE.

Staphylococcal endocarditis is not a homogeneous disease; appropriate management requires consideration of several questions, such as: Is the organism methicillin resistant? Should combination therapy be used? Is the infection on a native or prosthetic valve? Is the patient an IV drug abuser? Is the infection on the left or right side of the heart? Another consideration in staphylococcal endocarditis is that some organisms may exhibit tolerance to antibiotics. However, similar to streptococci the concern for tolerance among staphylococci should not affect antibiotic selection.[22]

Any patient who develops staphylococcal bacteremia is at risk for endocarditis. Many investigators have attempted to develop criteria that identify the bacteremic patient likely to have IE.[37] In hospitalized patients with *S. aureus* bacteremia and an identified focus of infection, such as a vascular catheter, the risk of concomitant IE is low and treatment of the bacteremia can be reduced to 2 weeks. This approach applies only if the patient does not have a prosthetic valve or additional clinical evidence for endocarditis.[36,37] On the other hand, the following parameters predict higher risk of IE in patients with *S. aureus* bacteremia: (a) the absence of a primary site of infection; (b) community acquisition of infection; (c) metastatic signs of infection; and (d) valvular vegetations detected by echocardiography.[1,4]

The recommended therapy for patients with left-sided IE caused by methicillin-sensitive *S. aureus* (MSSA) is 4 to 6 weeks of nafcillin or oxacillin, often combined with a short course of gentamicin (Table 109–5). From *in vitro* studies, the combination of an aminoglycoside and penicillinase-resistant penicillin or vancomycin enhances the activity of these drugs towards MSSA. In animal models of endocarditis combinations of penicillin with an aminoglycoside eradicate organisms from vegetations more rapidly than penicillins alone.[36] In human studies, the addition of an aminoglycoside to nafcillin for the first week of therapy hastens the resolution of fever and bacteremia, but it does not affect survival or relapse rates.[38]

If a patient has a mild, delayed allergy to penicillin, first-generation cephalosporins are effective alternatives, but they should be avoided in patients with a history of immediate-type hypersensitivity reactions (Table 109–5). The potential for a true immediate-type allergy should be carefully assessed and a penicillin skin test used before receiving antibiotic treatment to evaluate the patient claiming an allergy.[39] In patients with a positive skin test or a history of immediate hypersensitivity to penicillin, vancomycin is the agent of choice. Vancomycin, however, kills *S. aureus* slowly and is regarded as inferior to penicillinase-resistant penicillins for MSSA. Rifampin as an adjunctive therapy is controversial; however, this agent, added to vancomycin in refractory or complicated infections in patients with left-sided IE, may result in dramatic patient improvement.[36,37] Generally, antibiotic therapy should be continued for 4 to 6 weeks. Unfortunately, left-sided IE caused by *S. aureus* continues to have a poor prognosis with a mortality rate of 25% to 47%.[15,22] For reasons discussed in the following section, IV drug abusers have a more favorable response to therapy.

During the past decade, greater numbers of staphylococci became resistant to penicillinase-resistant penicillins (e.g., methicillin). Vancomycin is the drug of choice for these organisms because most methicillin-resistant *S. aureus* (MRSA) and coagulase-negative staphylococci are susceptible to it (Table 109–5). The presence or lack of a prosthetic heart valve in patients with a methicillin-resistant organism guides therapy and determines whether vancomycin should be used alone or, if a prosthetic valve is present, whether combination therapy is necessary (Table 109–6).[3,22]

Staphylococcus Endocarditis: Intravenous Drug Abuser

Infective endocarditis in the IV drug abuser is frequently (60% to 80%) caused by *S. aureus,* although other organisms may be common in certain geographic locations.[40] In this setting, the tricuspid valve is frequently infected, resulting in right-sided IE. Most patients have no history of valve abnormalities, are usually otherwise healthy, and

TABLE 109–5. Therapy for Endocarditis Caused by *Staphylococcus* in the Absence of Prosthetic Material*

Antibiotic	Dosage and Route	Duration	Comments
Methicillin-Susceptible Staphylococci			
Regimens for non–β-lactam-allergic patients			
Nafcillin sodium or oxacillin sodium	2 g IV every 4 h	4–6 wk	Benefit of additional aminoglycosides has not been established
With optional addition of gentamicin sulfate†	1 mg/kg IM or IV every 8 h	3–5 days	
Regimens for β-lactam-allergic patients			
Cefazolin (or other first-generation cephalosporins in equivalent dosages)	2 g IV every 8 h	4–6 wk	Cephalosporins should be avoided in patients with immediate-type hypersensitivity to penicillin
With optional addition of gentamicin†	1 mg/kg IM or IV every 8 h	3–5 days	
Vancomycin hydrochloride‡	30 mg/kg per 24 h IV in two equally divided doses, not to exceed 2 g/24 h unless serum levels are monitored	4–6 wk	Recommended for patients allergic to penicillin
Methicillin-Resistant Staphylococci			
Vancomycin hydrochloride‡	30 mg/kg per 24 h IV in two equally divided doses, not to exceed 2 g/24 h unless serum levels are monitored	4–6 wk	

*For treatment of endocarditis caused by penicillin-susceptible staphylococci (minimal inhibitory concentration ≤0.1 μg/mL), aqueous crystalline penicillin G sodium (Table 109–3, first regimen) can be used for 4 to 6 wk instead of nafcillin or oxacillin. Shorter antibiotic courses have been effective in some drug addicts with right-sided endocarditis caused by *Staphylococcus aureus* (see text). See text for comments on use of rifampin. IV, intravenous; IM, intramuscular.

†For specific dosing adjustment and issues concerning gentamicin (obese patients, relative contraindications), see Table 109–3 footnotes.

‡For specific dosing adjustment and issues concerning vancomycin (obese patients, length of infusion), see Table 109–3 footnotes.

(From Wilson WR, Karchmer AW, Dajani AS, et al. Antibiotic treatment of adults with infective endocarditis due to streptococci, enterococci, and staphylococci, and HACEK microorganisms. JAMA 1995;274:1706–1713, with permission.)

TABLE 109–6. Treatment of Staphylococcal Endocarditis in the Presence of a Prosthetic Valve or Other Prosthetic Material*

Antibiotic	Dosage and Route	Duration, wk	Comments
Regimen for Methicillin-Resistant Staphylococci			
Vancomycin hydrochloride[†]	30 mg/kg per 24 h IV in 2 or 4 equally divided doses, not to exceed 2 g/24 h unless serum levels are monitored	≥ 6	
With rifampin[‡]	300 mg orally every 8 h	≥ 6	Rifampin increases the amount of warfarin sodium required for antithrombotic therapy.
And with gentamicin sulfate[§]	1 mg/kg IM or IV every 8 h	2	
Regimen for Methicillin-Susceptible Staphylococci			
Nafcillin sodium or oxacillin sodium	2 g IV every 4 h	≥ 6	First-generation cephalosporins or vancomycin should be used in patients allergic to β-lactam. Cephalosporins should be avoided in patients with immediate-type hypersensitivity to penicillin or with methicillin-resistant staphylococci.
With rifampin[‡]	300 mg orally every 8 h	≥ 6	
And with gentamicin sulfate[§††]	1 mg/kg IM or IV every 8 h	2	

*Dosages recommended are for patients with normal renal function. IV, intravenous; IM, intramuscular.
†For specific dosing adjustment and issues concerning vancomycin (obese patients, length of infusion), see Table 109–3 footnotes.
‡Rifampin plays a unique role in the eradication of staphylococcal infection involving prosthetic material (see text); combination therapy is essential to prevent emergence of rifampin resistance.
§For specific dosing adjustment and issues concerning gentamicin (obese patients, relative contraindications), see Table 109–3 footnotes.
††Use during initial 2 wk.
(From Wilson WR, Karchmer AW, Dajani AS, et al. Antibiotic treatment of adults with infective endocarditis due to streptococci, enterococci, and staphylococci, and HACEK microorganisms. JAMA 1995;274:1706–1713, with permission.)

have a good response to medical treatment. Nonetheless, surgery may be required in up to 25% of cases.

Standard treatment for MSSA endocarditis is 4 weeks of monotherapy with a penicillinase-resistant penicillin (Table 109–5). In the IV drug abuser, however, the clinical response with right-sided MSSA endocarditis is usually excellent. Emerging data suggest that these patients may be effectively treated (clinical and microbiologic cure exceeding 90%) with a 2-week course of nafcillin or oxacillin plus an aminoglycoside.[41–46] Short-course vancomycin, in place of nafcillin or oxacillin, appears to be ineffective.[44] A more recent trial suggested that a 2-week regimen of a penicillinase-resistant penicillin alone, without the addition of an aminoglycoside, is as effective as combined therapy in MSSA tricuspid valve endocarditis.[47] Although these data suggest an aminoglycoside is unnecessary for short-course treatment in the IV drug abuser with right-sided IE, most clinicians are uncomfortable with monotherapy and choose combination treatment in this situation. Short-course therapy should not be used in metastatic or left-sided endocarditis and is inappropriate in patients with underlying acquired immunodeficiency syndrome (AIDS) or substantial pulmonary complications, such as lung abscess from right-sided IE.[22]

Vancomycin historically has been regarded as therapeutically equivalent to penicillins for MSSA infections. A small investigation, however, demonstrated that approximately one-third of IV drug abusers with MSSA IE responded unsatisfactorily to vancomycin, a poorer response rate than penicillinase-resistant penicillins.[48] This decreased response rate may be related to a slower rate of *in vitro* killing of *S. aureus* by vancomycin as compared to nafcillin. This finding is consistent with a prospective study in 42 patients with MRSA IE.[49] Patients treated with vancomycin remained bacteremic for a median duration of 7 days, which is substantially longer than studies with β-lactam therapy. A second proposed reason why penicillin should be used before vancomycin is the increasing prevalence of vancomycin-resistant enterococci (VRE). It has been suggested that frequent, inappropriate use of vancomycin for the treatment of MSSA is associated with the selection of VRE.[50,51] This association, however, has been questioned by a meta-analysis.[52] Irrespective of whether this association exists, the concerns of efficacy emphasize the importance of documenting a patient's penicillin allergy before initiating vancomycin. If vancomycin is selected, a full 4 weeks of therapy is recommended.

An intriguing therapeutic approach for staphylococcal endocarditis in the IV drug abuser is oral treatment. Preliminary data have suggested short-course intravenous treatment (primarily nafcillin; mean 16.4 days) followed by oral treatment (dicloxacillin or oxacillin; mean 26 days) might be effective for tricuspid valve MSSA endocarditis.[53] The positive results of this trial can be explained by the duration of IV antibiotics (greater than 2 weeks), which may be a sufficient treatment course in this patient population. Yet, two other studies, which used predominately oral therapy (ciprofloxacin and rifampin), found this regimen to be effective (cure rates exceeding 90%) in addicts with uncomplicated right-sided endocarditis caused by MSSA.[54,55] At this time, concerns with resistance (e.g., ciprofloxacin) and limited published data preclude routine use of oral antibacterial regimens for the treatment of IE in the IV drug abuser.

Staphylococcal Endocarditis: Prosthetic Valves

PVE accounts for approximately 15% of all IE cases.[56] An episode of PVE occurring within 2 months of surgery strongly suggests the cause is staphylococci implanted during the procedure.[3] Yet, the risk of staphylococcal endocarditis remains elevated for up to 12 months after valve replacement. Because this type of IE is typically a nosocomial infection, methicillin-resistant organisms are common and vancomycin is the cornerstone of therapy. Combination antimicrobials are recommended because of the high morbidity and mortality associated with PVE and its refractoriness to therapy.[3,22] Although the addition of rifampin to a penicillinase-resistant penicillin or vancomycin does not result in predictable bacterial synergism, rifampin may have unique activity against staphylococcal infection that involves prosthetic material where its addition results in a higher microbiologic cure rate.[2] Combination therapy also decreases the emergence of resistance to rifampin, which frequently occurs when used alone. For methicillin-resistant staphylococci (both MRSA and coagulase-negative staphylococci), vancomycin is recommended with rifampin for ≥6 weeks (Table 109–6). An aminoglycoside is added for the first 2 weeks, if the organism is aminoglycoside-susceptible. For MSSA, a penicillinase-resistant penicillin is administered in place of vancomycin. PVE responds poorly to medical treatment and has a higher mortality compared to native valve endocarditis. Valve dehiscence and incompetence can result in acute heart failure, and surgery is often an essential component of treatment.[3]

After 12 months, the likely organism for PVE parallels that of native valve endocarditis. As with native valve endocarditis, antimicrobial therapy should be based on the identified organism and *in vitro* susceptibility. If an organism is identified other than staphylococci, the treatment regimen should be guided by susceptibilities and at least 6 weeks in duration.[3,23] Additionally, a concomitant aminoglycoside is recommended if streptococci or enterococci are identified. Once-daily aminoglycoside regimens have not been evaluated in PVE and are not recommended.[3]

The use of anticoagulation is controversial in PVE. However, patients with an infected mechanical valve still receive benefit of anticoagulation; thus, those who require anticoagulation for prosthetic valves should cautiously continue the anticoagulant during endocarditis therapy, unless a contraindication to therapy exists.

ENTEROCOCCAL ENDOCARDITIS

Enterococci are normal inhabitants of the human GI tract and, occasionally, of the anterior urethra. These organisms are usually of low virulence but can become a pathogen in predisposed patients following genitourinary manipulations (older men) or obstetric procedures (younger women).[2] Historically, enterococci were considered group D streptococci, but they have been reclassified into the genus *Enterococcus (E. faecalis* and *E. faecium). E. faecalis* is the most common clinical isolate (approximately 90%) of the two species. Enterococci cause 5% to 18% of endocarditis cases, but it is more resistant to therapy as compared to staphylococci and streptococci. This organism is noteworthy for these reasons: (a) no single antibiotic is bactericidal; (b) MICs to penicillin are relatively high (1–25 mg/mL); (c) intrinsic resistance occurs to all cephalosporins and relative resistance occurs to aminoglycosides (e.g., "low-level" aminoglycoside resistance); (d) combinations of a cell wall active agent, such as a penicillin or vancomycin, plus an aminoglycoside are necessary for killing; and (e) resistance to all available drugs is increasing.[1,22,57]

Monotherapy with penicillin for IE caused by enterococci results in relapse rates of 50% to 80%. When used alone, penicillins are only bacteriostatic against enterococci and combination therapy is always recommended for susceptible strains.[57] The relapse rate following penicillin-gentamicin therapy for susceptible strains is less than 15%.[13] The killing of enterococci by the bactericidal combination of an aminoglycoside and a penicillin is the best clinical example of antibiotic synergy. Because the aminoglycoside cannot penetrate the bacterial cell in the absence of the penicillin, enterococci will usually appear to be resistant to aminoglycosides by routine susceptibility testing (low-level resistance). However, in the presence of an agent that disrupts the cell wall such as penicillin or vancomycin, the aminoglycoside can gain entry, attach to bacterial ribosomes, and cause rapid cell death. An aminoglycoside-vancomycin combination is also synergistic against enterococci and is appropriate therapy for the penicillin-allergic patient.[58]

Enterococcal endocarditis ordinarily requires 4 to 6 weeks of high-dose penicillin G or ampicillin, plus an aminoglycoside for cure (Table 109–7). Ampicillin has greater *in vitro* activity as compared to penicillin G, although there are no clinical data to document differences in efficacy. A 6-week course is recommended for patients with symptoms lasting longer than 3 months, recurrent cases, and mitral valve involvement. Streptomycin has been the most extensively studied aminoglycoside, but gentamicin is presently favored. Other aminoglycosides cannot be routinely substituted. In the treatment of enterococcal endocarditis, relatively low serum

TABLE 109–7. Standard Therapy for Endocarditis Caused by Enterococci*

Antibiotic	Dosage and Route	Duration, wk	Comments
Aqueous crystalline penicillin G sodium	18–30 million U/24 h IV either continuously or in six equally divided doses	4–6	4-wk therapy recommended for patients with symptoms <3 mo in duration; 6-wk therapy recommended for patients with symptoms >3 mo in duration
With gentamicin sulfate†	1 mg/kg IM or IV every 8 h	4–6	
Ampicillin sodium	12 g/24 h IV either continuously or in six equally divided doses	4–6	
With gentamicin sulfate†	1 mg/kg IM or IV every 8 h	4–6	
Vancomycin hydrochloride†‡	30 mg/kg per 24 h IV in two equally divided doses, not to exceed 2 g/24 h unless serum levels are monitored	4–6	Vancomycin therapy is recommended for patients allergic to β-lactams; cephalosporins are not acceptable alternatives for patients allergic to penicillin
With gentamicin sulfate†	1 mg/kg IM or IV every 8 h	4–6	

*All enterococci causing endocarditis must be tested for antimicrobial susceptibility in order to select optimal therapy (see text). This table is for endocarditis caused by gentamicin- or vancomycin-susceptible enterococci, viridans streptococci with a minimal inhibitory concentration of >0.5 μg/mL, nutritionally variant viridans streptococci, or prosthetic valve endocarditis caused by viridans streptococci or *Streptococcus bovis*. Antibiotic dosages are for patients with normal renal function. IV, intravenous; IM, intramuscular.

†For specific dosing adjustment and issues concerning gentamicin (obese patients, relative contraindications), see Table 109–3 footnotes.

‡For specific dosing adjustment and issues concerning vancomycin (obese patients, length of infusion), see Table 109–3 footnotes.

(From Wilson WR, Karchmer AW, Dajani AS, et al. Antibiotic treatment of adults with infective endocarditis due to streptococci, enterococci, and staphylococci, and HACEK microorganisms. JAMA 1995;274:1706–1713, with permission.)

concentrations of aminoglycosides appear adequate for successful therapy, such as a gentamicin peak concentration of approximately 3 μg/mL.[59] Even though this dosing approach remains to be advocated in the most recent treatment guidelines, this low-level peak gentamicin recommendation is debatable because it has not been well documented to be equally or more efficacious than higher serum concentrations.[60] Treatment of enterococcal endocarditis does not have the high success rate seen with IE caused by viridans streptococci, presumably because the organism is more resistant to killing.

Although some data support the use of extended interval aminoglycoside dosing for other types of endocarditis (i.e., streptococci), the data are more vague regarding this strategy in enterococcal IE.[61] While some data suggest drug efficacy in enterococcal endocarditis is not affected by this dosing regimen[62–64] discordant studies have been published that imply large aminoglycoside doses at infrequent intervals may not be optimal.[65,66] Despite a case report successfully using once-daily gentamicin in a patient with right-sided enterococcal endocarditis,[67] the paucity of human data precludes routine use of this dosing strategy at this time.

Resistance among enterococci to penicillins and aminoglycosides is increasing.[57] Enterococci that exhibit high-level resistance to streptomycin (MIC > 2,000 μg/mL) are not synergistically killed by penicillin and streptomycin because the aminoglycoside either no longer binds to the ribosome or is inactivated by an aminoglycoside-modifying enzyme, streptomycin adenylase. Because enterococci will appear resistant to aminoglycosides on routine susceptibility testing, the only way to distinguish high-level from low-level resistance is by performing special susceptibility tests using 500–2,000 μg/mL of the aminoglycoside. High-level streptomycin-resistant enterococci occur with a frequency of 40% to 50%, and high-level resistance to gentamicin is now found in 10% to 50% of isolates. Although most gentamicin-resistant enterococci are resistant to all aminoglycosides (including amikacin), 30% to 50% remain susceptible to streptomycin.[57] High-level gentamicin resistance is mediated by a bifunctional aminoglycoside-modifying enzyme, 6′-acetyltransferase/2′-phosphotransferase, and most strains also possess streptomycin adenylase. These organisms do not commonly cause IE; data on appropriate therapy are sparse, and therapeutic options are few. Case reports indicate that some patients will respond to very high doses of ampicillin, as observed in the early trials of penicillin monotherapy.[68]

In addition to isolates with high-level aminoglycoside resistance, β-lactamase-producing enterococci (especially *E. faecium*) have been reported.[69] If these organisms are discovered, vancomycin or ampicillin-sulbactam should be considered. VRE are increasingly reported, primarily with *E. faecium.* Vancomycin resistance occurs when the bacterium replaces the normal vancomycin target, d-alanine, d-alanine, with a peptidoglycan precursor that does not bind vancomycin, d-alanine, d-lactate.[70] Combination therapies including teicoplanin, quinupristin/dalfopristin, or linezolid appear to be the most promising treatments.

LESS COMMON TYPES OF INFECTIVE ENDOCARDITIS

HACEK Group

Gram-negative bacteria from the HACEK group *(Haemophilus parainfluenzae, Haemophilus aphrophilus, Actinobacillus actinomycetemcomitans, Cardiobacterum hominis, Eikenella corrodens,* and *Kingella kingae)* are unusual causes of IE. Frequently, this type of IE presents as a subacute illness with large vegetations and emboli.[71] These oropharyngeal organisms are typically slow growing and should be considered as possible causes of "culture-negative" endocarditis. Ceftriaxone or high doses of ampicillin with gentamicin for 4 weeks is the recommended therapy, although ceftriaxone may be preferred (Table 109–8).[22] Valve replacement is occasionally required.

Culture-Negative Endocarditis

Sterile blood cultures are reported in up to 5% of patients with IE, if strict diagnostic criteria are used.[1,5,72] This type of IE may occur as a result of unidentified subacute right-sided IE, previous antibiotic therapy, slow-growing fastidious organisms, nonbacterial etiologies (e.g., fungi), and improperly collected blood cultures. In patients that do not abuse IV drugs, culture-negative IE treatment will usually

TABLE 109–8. Therapy for Endocarditis Caused by HACEK Microorganisms (*Haemophilus parainfluenzae, Haemophilus aphrophilus, Actinobacillus actinomycetemcomitans, Cardiobacterium hominis, Eikenella corrodens,* and *Kingella kingae*)*

Antibiotic	Dosage and Route	Duration, wk	Comments
Ceftriaxone sodium†	2 g once daily IV or IM†	4	Cefotaxime sodium or other third-generation cephalosporins may be substituted
Ampicillin sodium‡	12 g/24 h IV either continuously or in six equally divided doses	4	
	1 mg/kg IM or IV every 8 h		
With gentamicin sulfate§		4	

*Antibiotic dosages are for patients with normal renal function. IV, intravenous; IM, intramuscular.
†Patients should be informed that IM injection of ceftriaxone is painful.
‡Ampicillin should not be used if laboratory tests show β-lactamase production.
§For specific dosing adjustment and issues concerning gentamicin (obese patients, relative contraindications), see Table 109–3 footnotes.
(From Wilson WR, Karchmer AW, Dajani AS, et al. Antibiotic treatment of adults with infective endocarditis due to streptococci, enterococci, and staphylococci, and HACEK microorganisms. JAMA 1995;274:1706–1713, with permission.)

follow an approach that encompasses treatment for enterococci, the HACEK group, and nutritionally variant streptococci.

Although controversial, therapy of culture-negative endocarditis consists of penicillin or ampicillin, an aminoglycoside (e.g., gentamicin), and ceftriaxone. In the IV drug abuser, where staphylococci is suspected, a penicillinase-resistant penicillin or a cephalosporin with activity against staphylococci could be added to the above regimen. Extended antimicrobial treatment is required (e.g., 6 weeks), although the aminoglycoside may be removed after a 2 weeks, if clinical improvement is observed.[1] This empiric approach highlights the need for proper collection of blood cultures and an extensive medication history. Continued observation for the pathogen is essential and blood culture initially showing no growth should be held for as long as 4 weeks to identify slow-growing organisms.

Gram-Negative Bacilli

Endocarditis caused by gram-negative bacilli is relatively uncommon, despite an increasing rate of gram-negative bacteremia. Patients at higher risk include IV drug abusers and those with prosthetic heart valves. Numerous cases of *Pseudomonas*-induced endocarditis have been reported, with a majority occurring in IV drug abusers. Other gram-negative bacilli that have been implicated in IE include *Salmonella spp., E. coli, Citrobacter spp., Klebsiella-Enterobacter spp., S. marcescens, Proteus spp.*, and *Providencia spp.*[1] Generally, these infections have a poor prognosis, with mortality rates as high as 60% to 80%.[15]

Overall, there is little clinical information on which to base solid treatment recommendations for this category of IE. For many cases, identification of the organisms and determination of *in vitro* susceptibility will guide therapy. Often, early valve replacement is necessary, especially if *Pseudomonas* is identified. Many cases of gram-negative IE require the combination of a β-lactam antibiotic and an aminoglycoside for an extended period (e.g., 6 weeks).[1] The choice of β-lactam depends on the organism. Ampicillin or ceftriaxone are reasonable options if *E. coli* is identified, whereas ceftazidime or an extended-spectrum penicillin (e.g., piperacillin) would be chosen for *Pseudomonas*. Higher doses of the amionoglycoside (e.g., 8 mg/kg/d) may improve the survival rates of *Pseudomonas* IE, especially when combined with surgery.[71,73]

Fungal Endocarditis

Fungi cause between 2% and 4% of endocarditis cases; most patients with fungal endocarditis have undergone recent cardiovascular surgery, are IV drug abusers, have received prolonged treatment with IV catheters or antibiotics, or are immunocompromised.[1,2,7,74] *Candida spp.* and *Aspergillus spp.* are the most commonly involved, and the mortality rate is high for these reasons: (a) large, bulky vegetations that often form; (b) systemic septic embolization that may occur; (c) the tendency for fungi to invade the myocardium; (d) poor penetration of vegetations by antifungals; (e) the low toxic:therapeutic ratio of agents, such as amphotericin B; and (f) the lack of consistent fungicidal activity of available antifungal agents.[1]

When fungal IE is identified, the combined medical-surgical approach is recommended. Because these infections occur infrequently, scant clinical data are available to make solid treatment recommendations; however, the use of antifungal agents alone has been globally unsuccessful. Amphotericin B is the mainstay pharmacologic approach with the possible addition of flucytosine. The usefulness of fluconazole and itraconazole remain unknown at this time, although high-dose itraconazole may be of worth in *Aspergillus* endocarditis and fluconazole has had limited success in *Candida* IE. Surgical therapy, in combination with an antifungal, may improve the patient's prognosis.[74]

EVALUATION OF THERAPEUTIC OUTCOMES

The evaluation of patients treated for IE includes assessment of disease signs and symptoms, blood cultures, microbiologic tests, serum drug concentrations, and other tests that evaluate organ function.

PHARMACOECONOMIC CONSIDERATIONS

Infective endocarditis remains an uncommon disease, but the cost of treatment can be substantial. In the past, the long duration of hospitalization required to administer IV antimicrobials was the major expense. In selected cases, abbreviated, outpatient, and possibly in the future oral antimicrobial therapy may appreciably reduce the cost of care.

Shorter-course antimicrobial regimens are advocated when possible. For instance, in exquisitely sensitive streptococcal endocarditis (MICs $\leq 0.1\ \mu$g/mL), a 2-week regimen of high-dose parenteral penicillin G in combination with an aminoglycoside is as effective as 4 weeks of penicillin alone.[22,24] Uncomplicated, right-sided MSSA endocarditis in the IV drug abuser may also be treated with a 2-week course. Treatment with nafcillin or oxacillin, in combination with an aminoglycoside, appears to be cost-effective.

The initiation of outpatient parenteral antibiotics should be considered early in treatment of IE, after the patient is clinically stable and responds favorably to initial antibiotics. Outpatient treatment has been demonstrated to be safe and effective in select situations.[75] Patients considered for home therapy must be hemodynamically stable, compliant with therapy, have careful medical monitoring, understand the potential complications of the disease, and have immediate access to medical care. Advances in technology allow for the outpatient administration of complex antibiotic regimens that significantly reduce the cost of therapy. Simple regimens, such as single daily doses of ceftriaxone for streptococcal IE, are particularly attractive. Although endocarditis is common in the IV drug abuser, and home health care would substantially reduce the cost of treatment, many clinicians are uncomfortable with outpatient IV therapy because central venous access is required. Sudden cardiac decompensation in an outpatient setting is also of concern.

SIGNS AND SYMPTOMS

Fever usually subsides within 1 week of initiating therapy.[1,2] Persistence of fever may indicate ineffective antimicrobial therapy, emboli, infections of intravascular catheters, or drug reactions. In some patients, low-grade fever may persist even with appropriate antimicrobial therapy. With defervescence, the patient should begin to feel better and other symptoms, such as lethargy or weakness, should subside.

BLOOD CULTURES

Blood cultures should be negative within a few days, although microbiologic response to vancomycin may be slower.[1,2] If bacteria continue to be isolated from blood beyond the first few days of therapy, it may indicate that the antimicrobials are inactive against the pathogen or that the doses are not producing adequate concentrations at the site of infection. After the initiation of therapy, blood cultures should be rechecked until negative. During the remainder of therapy, frequent blood culturing is not necessary. Additional blood cultures should be rechecked after successful treatment (e.g., once or twice within the 8 weeks after treatment) to ensure cure.

MICROBIOLOGIC TESTS

For all isolates from blood cultures MICs should be determined; MBCs are no longer recommended.[22,23] The agent currently being used should be tested as well as alternatives that may be required if intolerance, allergy, or resistance occurs. Occasionally, it is useful to determine whether synergy exists for antimicrobial combinations, although synergistic regimens can usually be predicted from the literature. Methods for *in vitro* determinations of synergy are summarized in Chap. 103.

Serum bactericidal titers (SBTs; also called Schlicter tests) have been used for many years and in association with a number of infectious diseases.[76,77] The SBT is the greatest dilution of a patient's serum sample, which is obtained while receiving antimicrobial treatment that kills greater than 99.9% of an inoculum of the infecting pathogen *in vitro* over 18 to 24 hours. In animal models of endocarditis, studies suggest that an SBT of 1:8 is predictive of response.[18] In humans with endocarditis, however, the correlation with SBTs and outcome is less clear. One investigation found peak and trough SBT ratio of 1:64 or greater and 1:32 predicted cure, although a lower titer did not predict failure.[78] Serum bactericidal titers $\geq$1:32 are easily achieved for most streptococci causing endocarditis because the MBC is low relative to achievable concentrations of penicillin; however, for enterococci, methicillin-resistant staphylococci, and gram-negative bacilli, high SBTs may be difficult to achieve.

At present, SBTs have little value in monitoring treatment of common types of IE and should not be routinely recommended.[22,23] This test may be useful when the causative organisms are only moderately susceptible to antimicrobials, when less well-established regimens are used, or when response to therapy is suboptimal and dosage escalation is considered.

SERUM DRUG CONCENTRATIONS

Of the agents commonly used for IE, measurement of serum drug concentrations is routinely available for aminoglycosides (except streptomycin) and vancomycin. Few data, however, support attaining any specific serum concentrations in patients with IE. In general, serum concentrations of the antimicrobial should exceed the MBC of the organisms, but in practice, this principle is usually not helpful in monitoring patients with endocarditis. Aminoglycoside concentrations rarely exceed the MBC for certain organisms, such as streptococci and enterococci, and concentrations have not been correlated with response, such as aminoglycosides and vancomycin for staphylococci.[78,79]

When aminoglycosides are administered for IE caused by gram-positive cocci with a traditional thrice-daily regimen, peak serum concentrations are recommended to be on the low side of the traditional ranges (3 μg/mL for gentamicin). If extended interval dosing is used, the most appropriate method of monitoring has not been determined. When vancomycin is administered, the most recent treatment guidelines (1995) recommend serum drug monitoring.[22]

PREVENTION

Antimicrobial prophylaxis is used to prevent IE in patients at high risk.[80,81] The use of antimicrobials for this purpose requires consideration of (a) cardiac conditions associated with endocarditis; (b) procedures causing bacteremia; (c) organisms likely to cause endocarditis; and (d) pharmacokinetics, spectrum, cost, adverse effects, and ease of administration of available antimicrombial agents. The objective of prophylaxis is to diminish the likelihood of IE in high-risk individuals (Table 109–9) who are undergoing procedures that cause transient bacteremia (Tables 109–10 and 109–11). Although there are no prospective, controlled human trials demonstrating that prophylaxis in high-risk individuals protects against the development of endocarditis during bacteremia-induced procedures, animal studies suggest possible benefit.[82] Most causes of IE, however, appear not to be secondary to an invasive procedure. Bacteremia as a consequence of daily activities may in fact be the major culprit and the value of antibiotic prophylaxis before bacteremia-causing procedures has been questioned.[83] Yet, retrospective human studies support that a reduction of endocarditis occurs in selected cases following dental surgery where prophylaxis is employed.[84] The mechanism of a beneficial effect in humans is unclear, but antibiotics may decrease the number of bacteria at the surgical site, kill bacteria after they are introduced into the blood, and prevent adhesion of bacteria to the valve. Studies have found that prophylaxis does not reduce the frequency of bacteremia immediately following tooth extraction as

TABLE 109–9. Cardiac Conditions Associated With Endocarditis

Endocarditis Prophylaxis Recommended

High-risk category
- Prosthetic cardiac valves, including bioprosthetic and homograft valves
- Previous bacterial endocarditis
- Complex cyanotic congenital heart disease (e.g., single ventricle states, transposition of the great arteries, tetralogy of Fallot)
- Surgically constructed systemic pulmonary shunts or conduits

Moderate-risk category
- Most other congenital cardiac malformations (other than above and below)
- Acquired valvular dysfunction (e.g., rheumatic heart disease)
- Hypertrophic cardiomyopathy
- Mitral valve prolapse with valvular regurgitation and/or thickened leaflets

Endocarditis Prophylaxis Not Recommended

Negligible-risk category (no greater risk than the general population)
- Isolated secundum atrial septal defect
- Surgical repair of atrial septal defect, ventricular septal defect, or patent ductus arteriosus (without residua beyond 6 mo)
- Previous coronary artery bypass graft surgery
- Mitral valve prolapse without valvular regurgitation
- Physiologic, functional, or innocent heart murmurs
- Previous Kawasaki disease without valvular dysfunction
- Previous rheumatic fever without valvular dysfunction
- Cardiac pacemakers (intravascular and epicardial) and implanted defibrillators

(From Dajani AS, Taubert KA, Wilson W, et al. Prevention of bacterial endocarditis: Recommendations by the American Heart Association. JAMA 1997;277:1794–1801, with permission.)

TABLE 109–10. Dental Procedures and Endocarditis Prophylaxis

Endocarditis Prophylaxis Recommended*
- Dental extractions
- Periodontal procedures including surgery, scaling and root planing, probing, and recall maintenance
- Dental implant placement and reimplantation of avulsed teeth
- Endodontic (root canal) instrumentation or surgery only beyond the apex
- Subgingival placement of antibiotic fibers or strips
- Initial placement of orthodontic bands but not brackets
- Intraligamentary local anesthetic injections
- Prophylactic cleaning of teeth or implants where bleeding is anticipated

Endocarditis Prophylaxis Not Recommended
- Restorative dentistry† (operative and prosthodontic) with or without retraction cord‡
- Local anesthetic injections (nonintraligamentary)
- Intracanal endodontic treatment; postplacement and buildup
- Placement of rubber dams
- Postoperative suture removal
- Placement of removable prosthodontic or orthodontic appliances
- Taking of oral impressions
- Fluoride treatments
- Taking of oral radiographs
- Orthodontic appliance adjustment
- Shedding of primary teeth

*Prophylaxis is recommended for patients with high- and moderate-risk cardiac conditions.
†This includes restoration of decayed teeth (filling cavities) and replacement of missing teeth.
‡Clinical judgment may indicate antibiotic use in selected circumstances that may create significant bleeding.
(From Dajani AS, Taubert KA, Wilson W, et al. Prevention of bacterial endocarditis: Recommendations by the American Heart Association. JAMA 1997;277:1794–1801, with permission.)

TABLE 109–11. Other Procedures and Endocarditis Prophylaxis

Endocarditis Prophylaxis Recommended
- Respiratory tract
  - Tonsillectomy and/or adenoidectomy
  - Surgical operations that involve respiratory mucosa
  - Bronchosopy with a rigid bronchoscope
- Gastrointestinal tract*
  - Sclerotherapy for esophageal varices
  - Esophageal stricture dilation
  - Endoscopic retrograde cholangiography with biliary obstruction
  - Biliary tract surgery
  - Surgical operations that involve intestinal mucosa
- Genitourinary tract
  - Prostatic surgery
  - Cystoscopy
  - Urethral dilation

Endocarditis Prophylaxis Not Recommended
- Respiratory tract
  - Endotracheal intubation
  - Bronchoscopy with a flexible bronchoscope, with or without biopsy†
  - Tympanostomy tube insertion
- Gastrointestinal tract
  - Transesophageal echocardiography†
  - Endoscopy with or without gastrointestinal biopsy†
- Genitourinary tract
  - Vaginal hysterectomy†
  - Vaginal delivery†
  - Caesarean section
  - In uninfected tissue:
    - Urethral catheterization
    - Uterine dilation and curettage
    - Therapeutic abortion
    - Sterilization procedures
    - Insertion or removal of intrauterine devices
- Other
  - Cardiac catheterization, including balloon angioplasty
  - Implanted cardiac pacemakers, implanted defibrillators, and coronary stents
  - Incision or biopsy of surgically scrubbed skin
  - Circumcision

*Prophylaxis is recommended for high-risk patients; optional for medium-risk patients.
†Prophylaxis is optional for high-risk patients.
(From Dajani AS, Taubert KA, Wilson W, et al. Prevention of bacterial endocarditis. Recommendations by the American Heart Association. JAMA 1997;277:1794–1801, with permission.)

compared to a control group, suggesting that a reduction in adhesion or effects after the bacteria adhere to the endocardium are more likely mechanisms.[85,86]

PATIENTS AT RISK

Patients with certain cardiac lesions, particularly those with prosthetic heart valves or a history of bacterial endocarditis, are at high risk for developing IE (Table 109–9). Nevertheless, only 15% to 25% of patients who develop IE are in a definable high-risk category.[80] Few cases of IE are preventable with antibiotic prophylaxis, even with 100% effectiveness.[87] Despite the low probability that IE will develop, prophylaxis is recommended for some dental, respiratory, GI, and genitourinary procedures (Tables 109–10 and 109–11) because of the significant morbidity associated with the disease. Patients undergoing valve implant surgery are at a much greater risk for IE than are those patients undergoing dental surgery.

PROCEDURES CAUSING BACTEREMIA

Bacteremia accompanies many everyday events, such as brushing the teeth and chewing, although certain medical and surgical procedures are more likely to cause a transient bacteremia (Tables 109–10 and 109–11). Antibiotic prophylaxis is recommended in patients at risk undergoing a bacteremia-causing procedure. For dental procedures of the gums and oral structures that cause bleeding, viridans streptococci frequently cause bacteremia, whereas instrumentation and surgery of the GI and genitourinary tracts more often result in enterococcal bacteremia.[1]

ANTIBIOTIC REGIMENS

The American Heart Association routinely publishes guidelines regarding the prevention of IE, with the most recent revision occurring in 1997.[82] A single 2-g dose of amoxicillin is recommended for adult patients at risk, given 1 hour before undergoing procedures associated with bacteremia (Table 109–12). Because the duration of antimicrobial prophylaxis appears to be relatively short, these guidelines do not advocate a second oral dose of amoxicillin, which was recommended previously. Alternative prophylaxis regimens for patients allergic to penicillins, those unable to take oral medications, and regimens for genitourinary and GI procedures are provided (Tables 109–12 and 109–13). A recent report highlights the need to educate physicians and patients regarding these guidelines, as overuse of IE prophylaxis occurs in low-risk patients, and underusage is common in moderate-risk patients.[88]

TABLE 109–12. Prophylactic Regimens for Dental, Oral, Respiratory Tract, or Esophageal Procedures

Situation	Agent	Regimen*
Standard general prophylaxis	Amoxicillin	Adults: 2 g; children: 50 mg/kg orally 1 h before procedure
Unable to take oral medications	Ampicillin	Adults: 2 g intramuscularly (IM) or intravenously (IV); children: 50 mg/kg IM or IV within 30 min before procedure
Allergic to penicillin	Clindamycin or	Adults: 600 mg; children: 20 mg/kg orally 1 h before procedure
	Cephalexin† or cefadroxil† or	Adults: 2 g; children: 50 mg/kg orally 1 h before procedure
	Azithromycin or clarithromycin	Adults: 500 mg; children: 15 mg/kg orally 1 h before procedure
Allergic to penicillin and unable to take oral medications	Clindamycin or	Adults: 600 mg; children: 20 mg/kg IV within 30 min before procedure
	Cefazolin†	Adults 1 g; children: 25 mg/kg IM or IV within 30 min before procedure

*Total children's dose should not exceed adult dose.
†Cephalosporins should not be used in individuals with immediate-type hypersensitivity reaction (urticaria, angioedema, or anaphylaxis) to penicillins.
(From Dajani AS, Taubert KA, Wilson W, et al. Prevention of bacterial endocarditis: Recommendations by the American Heart Association. JAMA 1997;277:1794–1801, with permission.)

TABLE 109–13. Prophylactic Regimens for Genitourinary and Gastrointestinal (Excluding Esophageal) Procedures

Situation	Agent*	Regimen†
High-risk patients	Ampicillin plus Gentamicin	Adults: ampicillin 2 g intramuscularly (IM) or intravenously (IV) plus gentamicin 1.5 mg/kg (not to exceed 120 mg) within 30 min of starting the procedure; 6 h later, ampicillin 1 g IM/IV or amoxicillin 1 g orally. Children: ampicillin 50 mg/kg IM or IV (not to exceed 2 g) plus gentamicin 1.5 mg/kg within 30 min of starting the procedure; 6 h later, ampicillin 25 mg/kg IM/IV or amoxicillin 25 mg/kg orally.
High-risk patients allergic to ampicillin/amoxicillin	Vancomycin plus Gentamicin	Adults: vancomycin 1 g IV over 1–2 h plus gentamicin 1.5 mg/kg IV/IM (not to exceed 120 mg); complete injection/infusion within 30 min of starting the procedure. Children: vancomycin 20 mg/kg IV over 1–2 h plus gentamicin 1.5 mg/kg IV/IM; complete injection/infusion within 30 min of starting the procedure.
Moderate-risk patients	Amoxicillin or Ampicillin	Adults: amoxicillin 2 g orally 1 h before procedure, or ampicillin 2 g IM/IV within 30 min of starting the procedure. Children: amoxicillin 50 mg/kg orally 1 h before procedure, or ampicllin 50 mg/kg IM/IV within 30 min of starting the procedure.
Moderate-risk patients allergic to ampicillin/amoxicillin	Vancomycin	Adults: vancomycin 1 g IV over 1–2 h; complete infusion within 30 min of starting the procedure. Children: vancomycin 20 mg/kg IV over 1–2 h; complete infusion within 30 min of starting the procedure.

*Total children's dose should not exceed adult dose.
†No second dose of vancomycin or gentamicin is recommended.
(From Dajani AS, Taubert KA, Wilson W, et al. Prevention of bacterial endocarditis: Recommendations by the American Heart Association. JAMA 1997;277:1794–1801, with permission.)

▶ PRINCIPLES OF PHARMACOTHERAPY

- Infective endocarditis is an uncommon infection usually occurring in persons with preexisting cardiac valvular abnormalities (prosthetic heart valves) or with other specific risk factors (IV drug abuse).
- Three groups of organisms generally cause IE: streptococci (50% to 62%), staphylococci (30% to 40%), and enterococci (5% to 18%).
- The clinical presentation of IE is highly variable and nonspecific, although a fever and murmur are usually present. Classical, peripheral manifestations (Osler nodes) may or may not occur.
- The diagnosis of IE is often unclear. Nonspecific signs, symptoms, and laboratory findings are important but do not reliably determine infection. The two major diagnostic criteria are blood cultures, to identify the infecting pathogen, and an echocardiogram, to determine the presence of a valvular vegetation.
- Isolation of the infecting pathogen and determination of antimicrobial susceptibilities are the most important approach in the treatment of IE. High-dose, parenteral, bactericidal anti-infectives are necessary for an extended period (usually 4 to 6 weeks).
- Surgical replacement of the infected heart valve is an important adjunct to endocarditis treatment in certain situations (e.g., patients with acute heart failure).
- β-Lactam antibiotics, such as penicillin G, nafcillin, and ampicillin, remain the drugs of choice for streptococcal, staphylococcal, and enterococcal endocarditis, respectively.
- Aminoglycosides are essential to obtain a synergistic bactericidal effect in the treatment of enterococcal endocarditis. Adjunctive aminoglycosides may also hasten the pace of clinical or microbiologic cure (such as in case of streptococcal and staphylococcal endocarditis) and prevent the emergence of resistant organisms (PVE caused by coagulase-negative staphylococci).
- Vancomycin is reserved for the treatment of resistant organisms and patients with immediate β-lactam allergies.
- Patients at high risk of IE, such as persons with prosthetic heart valves, should receive antimicrobial agents before a bacteremia-causing procedure (dental extraction). The agent is determined by the likely organism(s) leading to bacteremia and drug-specific parameters.

REFERENCES

1. Bayer AS, Scheld WM. Endocarditis and intravascular infections. In: Mandell GL, Bennett JE, Dolin R, eds. Principles and Practice of Infectious Diseases, 5th ed. Philadelphia, Churchill Livingstone, 2000:857–902.
2. Karchmer AW. Infective endocarditis. In: Braunwald E, ed. Heart Disease: A Textbook of Cardiovascular Medicine, 5th ed. Philadelphia, Saunders, 1997:1077–1104.
3. Karchmer AW. Infections of prosthetic valves and intravascular devices. In: Mandell GL, Bennett JE, Dolin R, eds. Principles and Practice of Infectious Diseases, 5th ed. Philadelphia, Churchill Livingstone, 2000:903–917.
4. Bayer AS, Bolger AF, Taubert KA, et al. Diagnosis and management of infective endocarditis and its complications. Circulation 1998;98:2936–2948.
5. Mylonakis E, Calderwood SB. Infective endocarditis in adults. N Engl J Med 2001;345:1318–1320.
6. Steckelberg JM, Wilson WR. Risk factors for infective endocarditis. Infect Dis Clin North Am 1993;7:9–19.
7. Tunkel AR. Infecting microorganisms. In: Kaye D, ed. Infective Endocarditis, 2nd ed. New York, Raven Press, 1992:85–97.
8. Johnson CM. Adherence events in the pathogenesis of infective endocarditis. Infect Dis Clin North Am 1993;7:21–36.
9. Fang G, Keys TF, Gentry LO, et al. Prosthetic valve endocarditis resulting from nosocomial bacteremia: A prospective, multicenter study. Ann Intern Med 1993;119:560–567.
10. Whitener C, Caputo GM, Weitekamp MR, Karchmer AW. Endocarditis due to coagulase-negative staphylococci: Microbiologic, epidemiologic, and clinical considerations. Infect Dis Clin North Am 1993;7:81–96.
11. Kaye KM, Kaye D. Laboratory findings including blood cultures. In: Kaye D, ed. Infectious Endocarditis, 2nd ed. New York, Raven Press, 1992: 117–124.
12. Mugge A. Echocardiographic detection of cardiac valve vegetations and prognostic implications. Infect Dis Clin North Am 1993;7:877–898.
13. Flachskampf FA, Daniel WG. Role of transoesophageal echocardiography in infective endocarditis. Heart 2000;84:3–4.
14. Durack DT, Lukes AS, Bright DK. New criteria for diagnosis of infective endocarditis: Utilization of specific echocardiographic findings. Am J Med 1994;96:200–209.
15. Gold MJ. Cure rates and long-term prognosis. In: Kaye D, ed. Infective Endocarditis, 2nd ed. New York, Raven Press, 1992:455–464.
16. Pokorski RJ. Long-term survival of patients with infective endocarditis. J Insur Med 1998;30:76–87.
17. Baldassarre JS, Kaye D. Principles and overview of antibiotic therapy. In: Kaye D, ed. Infectious Endocarditis, 2nd ed. New York, Raven Press, 1992:169–190.
18. Tunkel AR, Scheld WM. Experimental models of endocarditis. In: Kaye D, ed. Infectious Endocarditis, 2nd ed. New York, Raven Press, 1992:37–56.
19. Carbon C, Cremieux A-C, Fantin B. Pharmacokinetics and pharmacodynamic aspects of therapy of experimental endocarditis. Infect Dis Clin North Am 1993;7:37–51.
20. Douglas JL, Dismukes WE. Surgical therapy of infective endocarditis on natural valves. In: Kaye D, ed. Infectious Endocarditis, 2nd ed. New York, Raven Press, 1992:397–411.
21. Ferguson E, Reardon MJ, Letsou GV. The surgical management of bacterial valvular endocarditis. Curr Opin Cardiol 2000;15:82–85.
22. Wilson WR, Karchmer AW, Dajani AS, et al. Antibiotic treatment of adults with infective endocarditis due to streptococci, enterococci, staphylococci, and HACEK microorganisms. JAMA 1995;274:1706–1713.
23. Simmons NA, Ball AP, Eykyn SJ, et al. Antibiotic treatment of streptococcal, enterococcal, and staphylococcal endocarditis. Heart 1998;79:207–210.
24. Roberts RB. Streptococcal endocarditis: The viridans and beta-hemolytic streptococci. In: Kaye D, ed. Infectious Endocarditis, 2nd ed. New York, Raven Press, 1992:191–208.
25. Levison ME. *In vitro* assays. In: Kaye D, ed. Infectious Endocarditis, 2nd ed. New York, Raven Press, 1992:151–167.
26. Sherris J. Problems in *in vitro* determination of antibiotic tolerance in clinical isolates. Antimicrob Agents Chemother 1986;30:633–637.
27. Francioli PB. Ceftriaxone and outpatient treatment of infective endocarditis. Infect Dis Clin North Am 1993;7:97–116.
28. Shanson DC. New guidelines for the antibiotic treatment of streptococcal, enterococcal and staphylococcal endocarditis. J Antimicrob Chemother 1998;42:292–296.
29. Weiss ME, Adkinson NF. Beta lactam allergy. In: Mandell GL, Bennett JE, Dolin R, eds. Principles and Practice of Infectious Diseases, 5th ed. Philadelphia, Churchill Livingstone, 2000:299–305.
30. DiNubile MJ. Treatment of endocarditis caused by relatively resistant nonenterococcal streptococci: Is penicillin enough? Rev Infect Dis 1990;12:112–115.
31. Blatter M, Fluckiger U, Entenza J, et al. Simulated human serum profiles of one daily dose of ceftriaxone plus netilmicin in treatment of

experimental streptococcal endocarditis. Antimicrob Agents Chemother 1993;37:1971–1976.

32. Francioli PB, Glauser MP. Synergistic activity of ceftriaxone combined with netilmicin administered once daily for treatment of experimental streptococcal endocarditis. Antimicrob Agents Chemother 1993;37:207–212.
33. Gavalda J, Pahissa A, Almirante B, et al. Effect of gentamicin dosing interval on therapy of viridans streptococcal experimental endocarditis with gentamicin plus penicillin. Antimicrob Agents Chemother 1995;39:2098–2103.
34. Francioli P, Ruch W, Stamboulian D, et al. Treatment of streptococcal endocarditis with a single daily dose of ceftriaxone and netilmicin for 14 days: A prospective multicenter study. Clin Infect Dis 1995;21:1406–1410.
35. Sexton DJ, Tenenbaum MJ, Wilson WR, et al. Ceftriaxone once daily for 4 weeks compared to ceftriaxone plus gentamicin once daily for 2 weeks for treatment of penicillin-susceptible streptococcal endocarditis. Clin Infect Dis 1998;27:1470–1474.
36. Karchmer A. Staphylococcal endocarditis. In: Kaye D, ed. Infectious Endocarditis, 2nd ed. New York, Raven Press, 1992:225–249.
37. Mortara LA, Bayer AS. *Staphylococcus aureus* bacteremia and endocarditis: New diagnostic and therapeutic concepts. Infect Dis Clin North Am 1993;7:53–68.
38. Korzeniowski O, Sande MA. The National Collaborative Endocarditis Study Group: Combination antimicrobial therapy for *Staphylococcus aureus* endocarditis in patients addicted to parenteral drugs and in nonaddicts. Ann Intern Med 1982;97:496–503.
39. Dodek P, Phillip P. Questionable history of immediate-type hypersensitivity to penicillin in staphylococcal endocarditis: treatment based on skin test results versus empirical alternative treatment—A decision analysis. Clin Infect Dis 1999;29:1251–1256.
40. Sande MA, Lee B, Mills J, Chambers HF. Endocarditis in intravenous drug abusers. In: Kaye D, ed. Infectious Endocarditis, 2nd ed. New York, Raven Press, 1992:345–357.
41. Chambers HF. Short-course combination and oral therapies of *Staphylococcus aureus* endocarditis. Med Clin North Am 1993;7:69–80.
42. DiNubile MJ. Abbreviated therapy for right-sided *Staphylococcus aureus* endocarditis in injection drug users: The time has come? Eur J Clin Microbiol Infect Dis 1994;13:533–534.
43. DiNubile MJ. Short-course antibiotic therapy for right-sided *Staphylococcus aureus* endocarditis in injection drug users. Ann Intern Med 1994;121:873–876.
44. Chambers HF, Miller T, Newman MD. Right-sided endocarditis in intravenous drug abusers: Two-week combination therapy. Ann Intern Med 1988;109:619–624.
45. Espinosa FJ, Valdes M, Martin-Luengo M, et al. Right sided endocarditis caused by *Staphylococcus aureus* in parenteral drug addicts: Evaluation of a combined therapeutic scheme for 2 weeks versus conventional treatment. Enferm Infecc Microbiol Clin 1993;11:235–240.
46. Torres-Tortosa M, de Cueto M, Vergara A, et al. Prospective evaluation of a two-week course of intravenous antibiotics in intravenous drug addicts with infective endocarditis. Eur J Clin Microbiol Infect Dis 1994;13:559–564.
47. Ribera E, Gomez-Jimenez J, Cortes E, et al. Effectiveness of cloxacillin with and without gentamicin in short-term therapy for right-sided *Staphylococcus aureus* endocarditis: A randomized, controlled trial. Ann Intern Med 1996;125:969–974.
48. Small PM, Chambers HF. Vancomycin for *Staphylococcus aureus* endocarditis in intravenous drug users. Antimicrob Agents Chemother 1990;34:1227–1231.
49. Levine DP, Fromm BS, Reddy BR. Slow response to vancomycin or vancomycin plus rifampin in methicillin-resistant *Staphylococcus aureus* endocarditis. Ann Intern Med 1991;115:674–680.
50. Ena J, Dick R, Jones R, et al. The epidemiology of intravenous vancomycin usage in a university hospital. JAMA 1993;269:598–602.
51. Hospital Infection Control Practices Advisory Committee (HICPAC). Recommendations for preventing the spread of vancomycin resistance. Infect Control Hosp Epidemiol 1995;16:105–113.
52. Carmeli Y, Samore MH, Huskins C. The association between antecedent vancomycin treatment and hospital-acquired vancomycin-resistant enterococci: A meta-analysis. Arch Intern Med 1999;159:2641–2648.
53. Parker RH, Fossieck BE. Intravenous followed by oral antimicrobial therapy for staphylococcal endocarditis. Ann Intern Med 1980;93:832–834.
54. Dworkin RJ, Lee BL, Sande MA, Chambers HF. Treatment of right-sided *Staphylococcus aureus* endocarditis in intravenous drug abusers with ciprofloxacin and rifampin. Lancet 1989;2:1071–1073.
55. Heldman AW, Hartert TV, Ray SC, et al. Oral antibiotic treatment of right-sided staphylococcal endocarditis in injection drug users: Prospective randomized comparison with parenteral therapy. Am J Med 1996;101:68–76.
56. Berlin JA, Abrutyn E, Strom BL, et al. Incidence of infective endocarditis in the Delaware Valley, 1988–1990. Am J Cardiol 1995;76:933–936.
57. Eliopolis GM. Enterococcal endocarditis. In: Kaye D, ed. Infective Endocarditis, 2nd ed. New York, Raven Press, 1992:209–223.
58. Murray BE. The life and times of the enterococcus. Clin Microbiol Rev 1990;3:46–65.
59. Wilson WR, Wilkowske CJ, Wright AJ, et al. Treatment of streptomycin-susceptible and streptomycin resistant enterococcal endocarditis. Ann Intern Med 1984;100:816–823.
60. Eliopolis GM. Aminoglycoside resistant enterococcal endocarditis. Infect Dis Clin North Am 1993;7:117–133.
61. Tam VH, Preston SL, Briceland LL. Once-daily aminoglycosides in the treatment of gram-positive endocarditis. Ann Pharmacother 1999;33:600–606.
62. Houlihan HH, Stokes DP, Rybak MJ. Pharmacodynamics of vancomycin and ampicillin alone and in combination with gentamicin once daily or thrice daily against *Enterococcus faecalis* in an *in vitro* infection model. J Antimicrob Chemother 2000;46:79–86.
63. Gavalda J, Cardona PJ, Almirante B, et al. Treatment of experimental endocarditis due to *Enterococcus faecalis* using profiles of ampicillin in human serum. Antimicrob Agents Chemother 1996;40:173–178.
64. Schwank S, Blaser J. Once versus thrice-daily netilmicin combined with amoxicillin, penicillin, or vancomycin against *Enterococcus faecalis* in a pharmacodynamic *in vitro* model. Antimicrob Agents Chemother 1996;40:2258–2261.
65. Fantin B, Carbon C. Importance of the aminoglycoside dosing regimen in the penicillin-netilmicin combination for treatment of *Enterococcus faecalis*-induced experimental endocarditis. Antimicrob Agents Chemother 1990;34:2387–2391.
66. Marangos MN, Nicolau DP, Quintiliani R, Nightingale CH. Influence of gentamicin dosing interval on the efficacy of penicillin-containing regimens in experimental *Enterococcus faecalis* endocarditis. J Antimicrob Chemother 1997;39:519–522.
67. Tam VH, McKinnon PS, Levine DP, Brandel SM, Rybak MJ. Once-daily aminoglycoside in the treatment of *Enterococcus faecalis* endocarditis: Case report and review. Pharmacotherapy 2000;20:1116–1119.
68. Lipman ML, Silva J. Endocarditis due to *Streptococcus faecalis* with high-level resistance to gentamicin. Rev Infect Dis 1989;11:325–328.
69. Wells VD, Wong ES, Murray BE, et al. Infections due to beta-lactamase-producing, high-level gentamicin-resistant *Enterococcus faecalis*. Ann Intern Med 1992;116:285–292.
70. Tailor SA, Bailey EM, Rybak MJ. *Enterococcus*: An emerging pathogen. Ann Pharmacother 1993;27:1231–1242.
71. Hessen MT, Abrutyn E. Gram-negative bacterial endocarditis. In: Kaye D, ed. Infective Endocarditis, 2nd ed. New York, Raven Press, 1992:251–264.
72. Tunkel AR, Kaye D. Endocarditis with negative blood cultures. N Engl J Med 1992;326:1215–1217.
73. Reyes MP, Lerner AM. Current problems in the treatment of infective endocarditis due to *Pseudomonas aeruginosa*. Rev Infect Dis 1983;5:314–321.
74. Moyer DV, Edwards JE. Fungal endocarditis. In: Kaye D, ed. Infective Endocarditis, 2nd ed. New York, Raven Press, 1992:299–312.
75. Rehm SJ. Outpatient intravenous antibiotic therapy for endocarditis. Infect Dis Clin North Am 1998;12:879–901.
76. Santoro J, Ingerman M. Response to therapy: Relapse and reinfections. In: Kaye D, ed. Infective Endocarditis, 2nd ed. New York, Raven Press, 1992:423–433.

77. Levinson ME. *In vitro* assays. In: Kaye D, ed. Infective Endocarditis, 2nd ed. New York, Raven Press, 1992:151–167.
78. Weinstein MP, Stratton CW, Ackley A, et al. Multicenter collaborative evaluation of a standardized serum bactericidal test as a prognostic indicator in infective endocarditis. Am J Med 1985;78:262–269.
79. McCormack JP, Jewesson PJ. A critical reevaluation of the "therapeutic range" of aminoglycosides. Clin Infect Dis 1992;14:320–339.
80. Durack DT. Prophylaxis of infective endocarditis. In: Mandell GL, Bennett JE, Dolin R, eds. Principles and Practice of Infectious Diseases, 5th ed. Philadelphia, Churchill Livingstone, 2000:917–925.
81. Durack DT. Prevention of infective endocarditis. N Engl J Med 1995;332:38–44.
82. Dajani AS, Taubert KA, Wilson W, et al. Prevention of bacterial endocarditis: Recommendations by the American Heart Association. JAMA 1997;277:1794–1801.
83. Roberts GJ. Dentist are innocent! "Everyday" bacteremia is real culprit: A review and assessment of the evidence that dental surgical procedures are a principal cause of bacterial endocarditis. Pediatr Cardiol 1999;20:317–325.
84. Greenman RL, Bisno AL. Prevention of bacterial endocarditis. In: Kaye D, ed. Infective Endocarditis, 2nd ed. New York, Raven Press, 1992:465–481.
85. Hall G, Hedstrom SA, Heimdahl A, Nord CE. Prophylactic administration of penicillins for endocarditis does not reduce the incidence of postextraction bacteremia. Clin Infect Dis 1993;17:188–194.
86. Van der Meer JT, Van Wijk W, Thompson J, et al. Efficacy of antibiotic prophylaxis for prevention of native-valve endocarditis. Lancet 1992;339:135–139.
87. Strom BL, Abrutyne E, Berlin JA, et al. Dental and cardiac risk factors for infective endocarditis: A population-based, case-control study. Ann Intern Med 1998;129:761–769.
88. Seto TB, Kwiat D, Taira DA, Douglas PS, Manning WJ. Physicians' recommendations to patients for use of antibiotic prophylaxis to prevent endocarditis. JAMA 2000;284:68–71.

110

TUBERCULOSIS

Charles A. Peloquin

Tuberculosis (TB) is the leading infectious killer on earth. TB is caused by *Mycobacterium tuberculosis,* which can produce a silent, latent infection, or active disease.[1] Although TB in the United States is at an all-time low, it remains largely out of control in many countries. TB currently infects roughly one-third of the world's population.[1] Given the increase in drug resistance, it is critical that a major effort be made to control TB before it is too late.

EPIDEMIOLOGY

TB is a very old disease, with ancient human remains showing evidence consistent with TB.[1–3] TB was originally termed "phthisis" because of the emaciated features of patients with the disease, and later became known as "consumption."[1] TB rates tend to increase with increasing urbanization, especially when overcrowding occurs.[3]

It appears likely that *M. tuberculosis* is a variant of *M. bovis,* which causes a tuberculosis-like disease in livestock. TB probably emerged as a significant pathogen in Europe during the Middle Ages, and expanded its grip during the Industrial Revolution.[3] During the eighteenth and nineteenth centuries, as many as 25% of recorded adult deaths in Europe and the United States could be attributed to TB.[1–3] Many advances in the prevention of infection, such as pasteurization of milk and isolation of infected persons, are the result of the threat of TB.

Globally, 2 to 3 million people die from TB each year.[1,2,4] In the United States, approximately 13 million people are latently infected with *M. tuberculosis.* There were 18,361 cases of active disease in 1998, and 17,531 cases in 1999, and roughly 10% of these patients died before completing TB treatment.[5] (For detailed data analysis visit the Centers for Disease Control and Prevention [CDC] Web site at http://www.cdc.gov/nchstp/tb.) From the 1950s to the early 1980s, the annual incidence of TB in the United States declined steadily by nearly 5% per year (Fig. 110–1). In 1984, however, this decline slowed, and the incidence of TB in the United States actually increased during 1988 to 1992, from 9.3 to 10.5 cases/100,000 general population. Since then, implementation of more stringent screening criteria, infection control practices, and treatment protocols have resulted in case rates of <7 cases/100,000. Although this represents significant improvement, the eradication of TB in the United States remains a distant goal.[4]

RISK FACTORS FOR INFECTION

LOCATION AND PLACE OF BIRTH

Entry points to the United States have the highest number of TB cases. California, New York, Texas, and Florida each had more than 1000 new TB cases in 1999 (CDC data).[5] Nationally, the percentage of foreign born TB patients has increased yearly since 1986 (41% in 1998; 43% in 1999). Nearly two-thirds of these patients come from seven countries: Mexico (23%), the Philippines (13%), Vietnam (10%), India (7%), China (5%), Haiti (4%), and South Korea (3%).

Within the United States, TB is most prevalent in large urban areas.[4] Five cities—New York, Los Angeles, Chicago, Houston, and San Francisco—accounted for 3078 cases in 1999 (17.5% of all U.S. cases), with 15 cities accounting for 25% of all new cases (CDC data).[5] Close contacts of patients with pulmonary TB (>40 h/wk) have infection rates of 25% to 30%.[5,6] TB patients frequently have limited access to health care, live in crowded conditions, or are immunocompromised.[2,4] In 1999, 58% of all TB patients were unemployed for >2 years at the time of diagnosis, and 6% were homeless. Approximately 16% had a history of alcohol abuse, 8% were noninjecting drug users, and 3% were injecting drug users. These concurrent social problems make treating these patients particularly difficult.

RACE AND ETHNICITY

TB disproportionately affects ethnic minorities in the United States. From 1985 to 1992, TB rates in the United States increased by 12.9%, from 9.3 to 10.5 cases/100,000 population. During this period, the incidence of TB in whites decreased by 11%, but it increased in Hispanic Americans by 5%, in Asian-Pacific Islanders by 12%, and in non-Hispanic blacks by 38%. Some of these increases were a result of immigration from high-incidence countries.[4] Fortunately, from 1993 to 1998, there was a 19% decrease in TB among Hispanics, and a 22% decrease in non-Hispanic blacks. The modest 1.5% decrease among Asian-Pacific Islanders probably reflects ongoing activation of latent infection among recent immigrants to the United States.

AGE, GENDER, AND OCCUPATION

By the mid-1980s, the highest prevalence of TB in the United States was found in the elderly.[3,4] In 1987, the elderly accounted for 12% of the total population, but 27% of TB cases, with a case rate of 20.6/100,000.[7] Many of these patients were infected in the early 1900s, when TB was much more common. However, others were recently infected in settings such as nursing homes, where TB rates are twice that for other elderly populations.[7]

TB rates among 25- to 44-year-olds shot up in the late 1980s, especially in minority populations (Fig. 110–2).[4] This led to a concurrent increase of TB in children. Nearly 80% of all pediatric TB cases occurred in ethnic minorities.[4] Men were twice as likely as women to have TB, and workers in hospitals, long-term care facilities, and correctional facilities also were at greater risk of TB than the general population. This risk led to substantial efforts to control the spread of TB in these facilities.[4,8,9]

COINFECTION WITH HUMAN IMMUNODEFICIENCY VIRUS (HIV)

TB and HIV make a bad combination. Each infection appears to facilitate the growth of the other. In 1998, an estimated 10% of TB

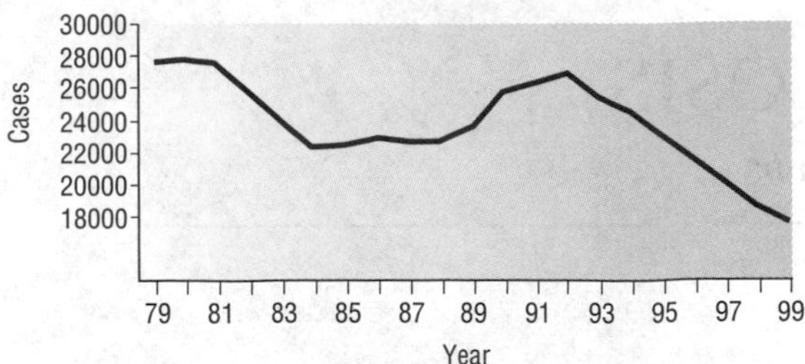

FIGURE 110–1. Reported TB cases in the United States, 1979–1999.

patients in the United States were coinfected with HIV, and roughly 20% of TB patients ages 25 to 44 years were coinfected.[4,5,10] HIV coinfection may not increase the risk of tuberculous infection, but it does increase the likelihood of infection progressing to active disease. TB and HIV patients share a number of behavioral risk factors which contribute to the high coinfection rates.[2,11,12]

RISK FACTORS FOR DISEASE

After infection, the lifetime risk of developing active TB disease is roughly 1 in 10, with the greatest risk during the first 2 years after infection. Children younger than 2 years of age and the elderly are considered to have a two to five times greater risk for developing active disease, as compared to other groups. Patients with underlying immune suppression (renal failure, cancer, and immunosuppressive drug treatment) have an estimated risk 4- to 16-fold higher than other patients. Finally, the CDC estimates that HIV-infected patients with tuberculous infection are 100 times more likely to develop active TB.[4,13] Unlike normal hosts, their *annual* risk of disease reactivation is about 1 in 10. Therefore, all patients with HIV infection should be screened for tuberculous infection, and vice versa.

ETIOLOGY

M. tuberculosis is a slender, straight, or slightly curved bacillus, ranging from 1 to 4 μm in length.[1,14,15] Because of its waxy outer layer, *M. tuberculosis* does not stain well with Gram's stain.[1] The Ziehl-Neelsen or the fluorochrome stains must be used instead.[1] After staining the organisms with carbol-fuchsin, mycobacteria retain the red color despite acid-alcohol washes, hence they are called acid-fast bacilli (AFB).[14] Microscopic examination can detect about 10,000 organisms/mL of specimen, but it cannot differentiate species or viability.[1,14,15] Most strains of mycobacteria are slow growing, with doubling times approaching 24 hours, as compared to every 20 to 40 minutes for bacteria.

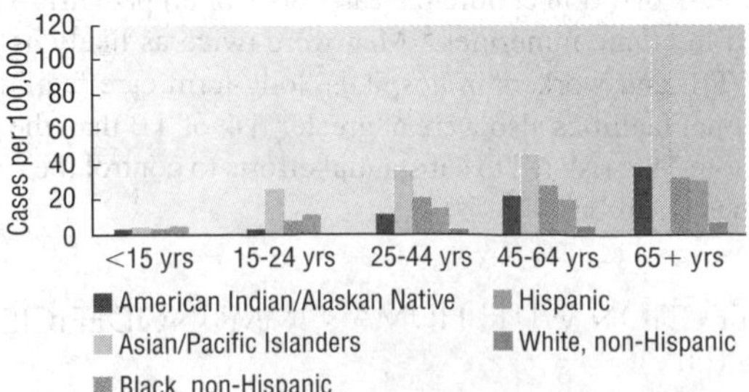

FIGURE 110–2. TB case rates by age group and race/ethnicity in the United States, 1999.

Among the mycobacteria, only *M. tuberculosis* is a frequent human pathogen. Some nontuberculous mycobacteria, such as *M. kansasii, M. fortuitum,* and *M. avium* complex (MAC) cause infections in patients with underlying diseases, most notably those with acquired immunodeficiency syndrome (AIDS). Treatment of these pathogens is discussed in Chap. 123.

CULTURE AND SUSCEPTIBILITY TESTING

Specialized media are needed to grow mycobacteria.[1,14,15] Direct susceptibility testing involves inoculating the test media with organisms taken directly from a concentrated, smear-positive specimen. This approach produces susceptibility results in 2 to 3 weeks. Indirect susceptibility testing involves inoculating the test media with organisms obtained from a pure culture of the organisms, which can take several weeks longer. The most common agar method, known as the proportion method, uses the ratio of colony counts on drug-containing agar to that on drug-free agar.[1,15] In the United States, the critical proportion for resistance is 1%. The proportion method's limitations include several weeks to obtain results, drug degradation during the incubation, and a qualitative result (susceptible or resistant). The BACTEC system (Becton-Dickinson, Sparks, MD) uses liquid media (7H12 broth) and detects live mycobacteria based on the release radiolabeled CO_2.[14] Advantages of the BACTEC system include reduced incubation time, reduced drug loss in the media, and, when multiple concentrations are tested, a truly quantitative end point.[1,14,15] Newer, nonradiometric rapid methods are now being marketed.

Several new rapid-identification tests are available. Nucleic acid probes such as the AccuProbe (Gen-Probe, San Diego, CA), use DNA probes to identify the presence of complementary rRNA for several mycobacterial species.[14,16] DNA fingerprinting using restriction fragment length polymorphism (RFLP) analysis has been used to identify clusters of cases.[1,14,16] Amplification of the genetic material can be achieved through polymerase chain reaction (PCR; Roche Molecular Systems, Branchburg, NJ), amplified *M. tuberculosis* direct test (MTD; Gen-Probe, San Diego, CA), and strand displacement amplification (SDA; Becton-Dickinson, Sparks, MD).[14,17] Thin layer chromatography (TLC), high-performance liquid chromatography (HPLC) for mycolic acid identification, and gas chromatography (GC) for short-chain fatty acids (methyl esters) have been used to speciate mycobacterial isolates.[1,14,16]

TRANSMISSION

M. tuberculosis is transmitted from person-to-person by coughing or sneezing. This produces droplet nuclei that are dispersed in the air.[5] Each droplet nuclei contains one to three organisms. Riley and colleagues showed that air circulated from a hospital TB ward could cause disease in guinea pigs.[18] When this air was filtered or treated with ultraviolet radiation, the animals were not infected.[18] About 30% of individuals who experience prolonged contact with an infectious TB patient will become infected.

A person with cavitary, pulmonary TB and a cough may infect roughly one person per month until they are effectively treated, although this number can vary significantly. A person with the uncommon laryngeal form of TB can spread organisms even when talking, so the transmission rates can be very high. While immunocompromised conditions, such as AIDS, may not change the acquisition of the organisms, the weakened immune function of these patients puts them at higher risk for active disease.[2]

PATHOPHYSIOLOGY

IMMUNE RESPONSE

The macrophages and T lymphocytes are primarily responsible for fighting mycobacteria. T lymphocytes with an $\alpha\beta$ T cell receptor (TCR) compose 95% of T lymphocytes, and are capable of recognizing both cellular and soluble antigens. The $\alpha\beta$ T lymphocytes are further divided into CD4 (helper) and CD8 (cytotoxic/suppressor) lymphocytes. One subset of these CD4 lymphocytes appears to act against mycobacteria (Th-1 cells). These differ from the Th-2 subpopulation of CD4 cells that activate B cells. Th-1 cells recognize the antigen presented by macrophages, are activated by interleukin-12 (IL-12), and are suppressed by IL-4 and IL-10. These lymphocytes secrete interferon (IFN)-γ, which activates macrophages to destroy mycobacteria. Later, cytolytic T lymphocytes join in, destroying cells harboring mycobacteria.[19] A third group of T lymphocytes possesses a $\gamma\delta$ TCR. These cells appear to recognize ligands different from those of $\alpha\beta$ T cells.[19] Having an immunoregulatory role, they appear to contribute to host resistance to infection. Because the CD4 T cells are depleted by HIV infection, one can see how AIDS patients would have difficulty controlling an *M. tuberculosis* infection.

PRIMARY INFECTION

As described above, primary infection results from inhaling organisms contained in droplet nuclei. These particles are small enough (1–5 mm) to reach the alveolar surface. The progression to clinical disease depends on the inoculum size and the host's cell-mediated immune system.[5,20,21] Once implanted, the organisms multiply, and are ingested by pulmonary macrophages, where they continue to multiply more slowly. Intracellular organisms then spread to the regional lymph nodes in the hilar, mediastinal, and retroperitoneal areas. At this point (days 5 to 15), $\alpha\beta$ CD4 lymphocytes are presented with antigen, activate, and secrete IFN-γ, which stimulates macrophages to become bactericidal. Depending on the inflammatory response, tissue necrosis and calcification of the infection site plus the regional lymph nodes may occur. Most signs of the infection disappear, although some patients are left with a radiodense area on chest x-ray called a Ghon complex.

During lymph node involvement, the organisms may be held in check. More frequently, they may spread throughout the body through the bloodstream. They may infect any organ system, and most commonly infect the posterior apical region of the lungs. Nodular infiltrates, called Simon foci, may be seen in the apices of the lungs. By this time (days 15 to 25), macrophages have begun to form granulomas to contain the organisms. In addition, $\gamma\delta$ T lymphocytes may begin to destroy AFB-containing macrophages. This acts to reduce the number of bacteria, but also probably prevents "overstimulation" of the immune system, which otherwise might result in autoimmunity.[19]

At the same time, delayed hypersensitivity develops through activation and multiplication of CD4 lymphocytes. Over 1 to 3 months, activated lymphocytes reach an adequate number, and tissue hypersensitivity results. This is shown by a positive tuberculin skin test. Note that the immune mediated containment of TB (Th-1 response) and the development of cutaneous hypersensitivity are two separate events. By days 20 to 40, cytolytic T cells begin to destroy macrophages containing AFB. Dissemination is halted, and the remaining mycobacteria reside within granulomas or macrophages that have avoided detection and lysis.[19]

There are two types of granulomas. Proliferative granulomas are stable and can effectively limit the spread of the organism. Caseating granulomas, so named for their cheese-like appearance, have a necrotic center and are relatively unstable. They permit the limited growth of *M. tuberculosis* within them.[5,20,21]

Approximately 90% of infected patients have no further clinical manifestations. Most only show a positive skin test (70%), while some also have radiographic evidence of stable granulomas (15% to 20%). Approximately 3% to 5% of patients (usually children, the elderly, or the immunocompromised) experience "progressive primary" disease, which occurs before skin test conversion.[22,23] This presents as progressive pneumonia, usually in the lower lobes. Disease frequently spreads, leading to meningitis and other severe forms of TB.[22,23]

REACTIVATION DISEASE

About 7% to 10% of infected patients develop reactivation disease. Nearly one-half of these cases occur within 2 years of infection.[20] In the United States, most cases of TB result from reactivation. Reinfection is uncommon in the United States because of the low rate of exposure, and because previously sensitized individuals possess some degree of immunity to reinfection. Exceptions include patients coinfected with HIV who live in areas of higher exposure to *M. tuberculosis.*

The apical areas of the lungs are the most common sites for reactivation (85% of cases). For reasons that are not entirely known (waning cellular immunity, loss of specific T-cell clones, blocking antibody), organisms within granulomas emerge and begin multiplying extracellularly.[24] The inflammatory response produces caseating granulomas, which will eventually liquefy and cavitate. The immune response contributes to the severity of the damage. Pulmonary cavities are caused by invasion of neutrophils into lung parenchyma. This aerobic environment enhances growth of the organism, producing bacterial counts in the cavity which may be as high as 10^8 per milliliter of sputum. Fluid in the cavity is aerosolized by coughing, spreading the organisms within the lungs, and externally to other hosts. Partial healing may result from fibrosis, but these areas may reactivate.[5,20] If left untreated, pulmonary TB spreads to involve the entire respiratory tract, resulting in hypoxia, respiratory acidosis, and death.

EXTRAPULMONARY AND MILIARY TUBERCULOSIS

Caseating granuloma at extrapulmonary sites can undergo liquefaction, releasing tubercle bacilli and causing symptomatic disease. Extrapulmonary TB is uncommon in normal hosts, but more common in HIV-infected patients (Table 110–1). Because of the unusual presentation, diagnosis is difficult and often delayed. Lymphatic and pleural disease are most common, followed by bone, joint, genitourinary, meningeal, and other forms of disease.[20] Left untreated, these forms also may result in death.

Occasionally, a massive inoculum of organisms enters the bloodstream, causing widely disseminated disease known as miliary TB. It is named for the millet seed appearance of the small granulomas seen on chest radiograph, and it can be rapidly fatal.[20]

INFLUENCE OF HIV INFECTION ON PATHOGENESIS

As CD4 lymphocytes multiply in response to the mycobacterial infection, HIV multiplies within these cells, and selectively destroys them. In turn, the TB-fighting lymphocytes are depleted.[19] This vicious cycle puts HIV-infected patients at 100 times the risk of active TB disease.[25] In addition, the combination of HIV infection and

TABLE 110–1. Likelihood of Various Clinical Presentations of Tuberculous Infection in Different Patient Groups

Status at Exposure	Asymptomatic Infection	Progressive Primary Infection	Reactivation Pulmonary	Extrapulmonary Disease	Miliary Tuberculosis
<1 yr old	++	+++	+/−	++	+
1–5 yr	++	++	+/−	++	+
6–10 yr	++	+	+	+	+
11–17 yr	+++	+/−	+	+	+/−
HIV (−) adult	+++	+/−	+	+	+/−
HIV (+) adult	+	++	+	++	+

+++, predominant feature; ++, common; +, occasional; +/−, rare.

certain social behaviors increase the risk of newly acquired TB. Recent studies also show that, in selected areas of the United States, 40% to 50% of new TB cases are the result of recent infection, particularly among HIV-infected individuals.[26–28]

While mycobacteria are spreading in the body, HIV replication accelerates in lymphocytes and macrophages. This leads to progression of HIV disease.[29] HIV-infected patients infected with TB deteriorate more rapidly unless they receive antimycobacterial chemotherapy for latent TB infection.[25,30] This has prompted widespread screening for tuberculous infection in HIV-infected patients, and empiric chemoprophylaxis for those in whom infection cannot be ruled out.

CLINICAL PRESENTATION

TB can present with generalized symptoms of weight loss, malaise, fever, and night sweats.[1,5,21] Typically, the patient develops a persistent cough, productive of sputum. Often, the onset of TB is insidious, and the diagnosis may not be considered until a chest radiograph is performed. Typical radiographic findings include patchy or nodular infiltrates in the apical areas of the upper lobes or the superior segment of the lower lobes. As the infection progresses, cavitation is often seen, with or without air-fluid levels. Unfortunately, many patients do not seek medical attention until more dramatic symptoms, such as hemoptysis, occur. At this point, patients typically have large cavitary lung lesions with high mycobacterial burdens. Expectoration or swallowing of sputum containing large numbers of organisms may result in extension of disease to other areas. Ulceration of the pharynx, larynx, tongue, and oral mucosa, as well as otitis media, gastric ulceration, and perirectal abscess may occur.[1,5,21] Physical exam is nonspecific, but suggestive of progressive pulmonary disease. Dullness to chest percussion suggests consolidation in the involved areas of the lung. Rales and increased vocal fremitus are frequently observed on auscultation. Respiratory insufficiency may lead to cyanosis and clubbing of the digits. Abnormal laboratory data usually are limited to moderate elevations in the white blood cell (WBC) count with a lymphocyte predominance.

The presentation of TB in patients coinfected with HIV varies, depending on the stage of HIV infection (Table 110–2). TB often occurs early in the course of immunosuppression.[1,31–33] As their CD4 counts decline, AIDS patients are less likely to have cavitary pulmonary TB, a positive skin test, or fever. Pulmonary radiographic findings may be minimal or absent. Patients infected with HIV have a higher incidence of extrapulmonary TB, and are much more likely to present with progressive primary disease. Because their symptoms are not specific to TB, the diagnosis is often delayed. Postmortem diagnoses of TB account for roughly 5% of all reported cases.[34]

Extrapulmonary TB typically presents as a slowly progressive decline in organ function. Patients may have low-grade fever and other constitutional symptoms. Patients with genitourinary TB may present with sterile pyuria and hematuria. Lymphadenitis often involves the cervical and supraclavicular nodes, and may appear as a neck mass with spontaneous drainage. Tuberculous arthritis and osteomyelitis most commonly occur in the elderly, and usually affect the lower spine and weight-bearing joints. Abnormal behavior, headaches, or convulsions suggest tuberculous meningitis. Involvement of the peritoneum, pericardium, larynx, and adrenal glands also occurs.[21]

THE ELDERLY

TB in the elderly is easily confused with other respiratory diseases. Many clinical findings are muted or absent altogether. As compared to younger patients, TB in the elderly is far less likely to present with positive skin tests, fevers, night sweats, sputum production, or hemoptysis.[35,36] Weight loss may occur, but is nonspecific. In contrast, mental status changes are twice as common in the elderly, and mortality is six times higher.[35] TB is a preventable cause of death in the elderly that should not be overlooked.

CHILDREN

TB in children may present as a typical bacterial pneumonia, called progressive primary TB.[22,23] Clinical disease often begins 1 to

TABLE 110–2. Clinical Features of Tuberculosis in HIV-Positive versus HIV-Negative Patients

	HIV-negative (Immunocompetent)	HIV-positive (AIDS)
Onset	Gradual	More abrupt as CD4 count drops
Presentation	Reactivation	More progressive; primary abrupt as CD4 count drops
PPD result	Usually positive	Often negative
Chest radiograph	Apical infiltrate	More diffuse as CD4 count drops; may involve lower lobes
Extrapulmonary forms	Occasional	Common
Other pathogens present	Occasional	Common
AFB-positive sputum	Usually	Usually
Response to therapy	Excellent	Good

PPD, purified protein derivative.

2 months after exposure, and precedes cutaneous hypersensitivity. Unlike adults, pulmonary TB in children often involves the lower and middle lobes.[22,23,37] Dissemination to the lymph nodes, GI and genitourinary tracts, bone marrow, and meninges is fairly common. Because of delays in recruitment of cellular immunity, cavitary disease is infrequent, and the number of organisms present is typically smaller than in an adult. Because cavitary lesions are uncommon, children do not spread the disease readily. Pediatric TB, however, can be rapidly fatal, and it requires the prompt introduction of effective chemotherapy.

DIAGNOSIS

SKIN TESTING

The key to stopping the spread of TB is early identification of infected individuals.[1,21,25,38] This is done with the tuberculin purified protein derivative (PPD) skin test. Table 110–3 lists those populations that might benefit most from skin testing. Members of these high-risk groups should be tested for TB infection, and they also should be educated about TB in an effort to reduce transmission.

Because it is quantitative, the Mantoux test is preferred to the Heaf or tine test. The standard 5 tuberculin unit (5 TU) PPD dose is placed intracutaneously on the volar aspect of the forearm with a 26- or 27-gauge needle.[6,25] This injection should produce a small, raised, blanched wheal. It is important that the injection not be placed too deeply, or it may be read falsely as negative. An experienced professional should read the test in 48 to 72 hours, although the test may remain positive as long as 5 days. The area of induration (not erythema) is the important end point. For most immunocompetent patients with some risk of exposure, an area of ≥10 mm is considered positive, and for HIV-infected individuals and recent contacts of TB patients, ≥5 mm is considered positive.[21,25,38,39] For young children or AIDS patients recently exposed to TB, any induration might be read as positive.

A control skin test panel of *Candida,* trichophytin, and mumps antigens may used in HIV-infected individuals to rule out anergy.[25,40] Anergy panels are imperfect tools, but they can provide additional information regarding a specific patient's immune response. However, the CDC does not recommend the routine use of anergy panels.[25,40] Patients known to be HIV positive should be tested for TB, and patients with positive TB skin tests should be considered for HIV testing. A further diagnostic workup in HIV patients is recommended to diagnose or to rule out TB adequately.[21,38,39]

Although three test strengths of purified protein derivative-standard (PPD-S) are available, the intermediate-strength form (5-TU) is almost always used. Few data exist with which to interpret the tests performed with the other strengths.[41] Two 5-TU products, Aplisol and Tubersol, are commercially available, but because of more predictable results, Tubersol appears to be the preferred product.

Although the tuberculin skin test alone cannot induce cutaneous hypersensitivity *de novo,* it may enhance low-level reactivity in some patients, converting a negative test to a positive after a second test. This "booster effect" usually occurs in patients with past tuberculous infection, immunization with bacillus Calmette-Guérin (BCG) vaccine, or from infection with nontuberculous mycobacteria.[21] In individuals who will be skin tested periodically (such as in health care workers), the two-stage method is recommended for the first test to detect boosters (i.e., PPD tests are placed twice within a 1- to 2-week period).[42] All individuals who initially boost should be further examined for evidence of active TB. Clinicians also should consider other factors (history of exposure, signs, and symptoms) in making decisions to treat. Nonboosters are considered to be without infection, and any subsequent positive skin test should be viewed as evidence of recent infection requiring treatment.[21,25]

False-negative results have many causes. These include faulty test material, poor administration technique, observer error, and a weak host immune system. In addition, up to 20% of patients with active TB disease are PPD negative, presumably because the immune system is preoccupied by the lesions.[38] False-positive results are more

TABLE 110–3. Criteria for Tuberculin Positivity, by Risk Group

Reaction ≥ 5 mm of Induration	Reaction ≥ 10 mm of Induration	Reaction ≥ 15 mm of Induration
Human immunodeficiency virus (HIV)-positive persons	Recent immigrants (i.e., within the last 5 yr) from high prevalence countries	Persons with no risk factors for TB
Recent contacts of tuberculosis (TB) case patients	Injection drug users	
Fibrotic changes on chest radiograph consistent with prior TB	Residents and employees† of the following high-risk congregate settings: prisons and jails, nursing homes and other long-term facilities for the elderly, hospitals and other health care facilities, residential facilities for patients with acquired immunodeficiency syndrome (AIDS), and homeless shelters	
Patients with organ transplants and other immunosuppressed patients (receiving the equivalent of ≥ 15 mg/d of prednisone for 1 mo or more)*	Mycobacteriology laboratory personnel	
	Persons with the following clinical conditions that place them at high risk: silicosis, diabetes mellitus, chronic renal failure, some hematologic disorders (e.g., leukemias and lymphomas), other specific malignancies (e.g., carcinoma of the head or neck and lung), weight loss of ≥ 10% of ideal body weight, gastrectomy, and jejunoileal bypass	
	Children younger than 4 yr of age or infants, children, and adolescents exposed to adults at high risk	

*Risk of TB in patients treated with corticosteroids increases with higher dose and longer duration.
†For persons who are otherwise at low risk and are tested at the start of employment, a reaction of ≥ 15 mm induration is considered positive.
Source: Adapted from Centers for Disease Control and Prevention. Screening for tuberculosis and tuberculosis infection in high risk populations: recommendations of the Advisory Council for the Elimination of Tuberculosis. MMWR 1995;44(No. RR-11):19–34.

common in low-risk patients, and in those patients recently vaccinated with BCG. A BCG vaccination, however, should not lead one to ignore a positive PPD result. Such patients require careful evaluation for active disease, and preventive therapy may be considered.

ADDITIONAL TESTS

Patients with proven or suspected tuberculous infection should undergo testing to rule out active disease. The diagnosis of active TB can be made with physical examination, radiographs, and microbiologic examination of sputum or other infected material.[21,43] Attempts should be made to isolate *M. tuberculosis* from the site of infection. Sputum collected in the morning usually has the highest number of organisms per volume and, hence, the highest yield.[14,15] Daily sputum collections over three consecutive days are recommended.

For patients unable to expectorate, sputum induction with aerosolized hypertonic saline may produce a diagnostic sample. Bronchoscopy, or aspiration of gastric fluid via a nasogastric tube, may be attempted in selected patients.[21] For patients with suspected extrapulmonary TB, samples of draining fluid, biopsies of the infected site, or both may be attempted. Blood cultures are positive occasionally, more commonly in AIDS patients.[44]

▶ TREATMENT: Tuberculosis

DESIRED OUTCOME

The desired outcomes in the treatment of tuberculosis are:

1. Rapid identification of a new TB case.
2. Isolation of the patient with active disease to prevent the spread of the disease.
3. Collection of appropriate samples for smears and cultures.
4. Initiation of specific antituberculosis treatment.
5. Prompt resolution of the signs and symptoms of disease.
6. Achievement of a noninfectious state in the patient, thus ending isolation.
7. Adherence to the treatment regimen by the patient.
8. Cure of the patient as quickly as possible (generally at least 6 months of treatment).

Secondary goals are the identification of the index case that infected the patient, the identification of all persons infected by both the index case and the new case of TB, and the completion of appropriate treatments for those individuals.

GENERAL APPROACHES TO TREATMENT

Drug treatment is the cornerstone of TB management. Monotherapy can be used only for infected patients who do not have active TB (latent infection as shown by positive skin test). Once active disease is present, a minimum of two drugs, and generally three or more drugs must be used simultaneously. The duration of treatment depends on the condition of the host, extent of disease, presence of drug resistance, and tolerance of medical interventions. The shortest duration of treatment is generally 6 months, and 2 to 3 years of treatment may be necessary in extreme cases of multidrug-resistant TB (MDR-TB). Because the duration of therapy is so long, and because patients may feel relatively well after a few weeks of treatment, careful followup is required. It increasingly has been shown that directly observed therapy by a health care worker is a cost-effective way to ensure the completion of treatment.[45,46]

PRINCIPLES FOR TREATING INFECTION AND TREATING DISEASE

Asymptomatic patients with tuberculous infection have a bacillary load of approximately 10^3 organisms, as compared to 10^{11} organisms in a patient with cavitary pulmonary TB.[6,37,47] As the number of organisms increases, the likelihood of finding naturally occurring, drug-resistant mutants also increases. Naturally occurring mutants are found at rates of 1 in 10^6 to 1 in 10^8 organisms for the antituberculosis drugs. When treating asymptomatic latent infection with isoniazid (INH) monotherapy, the risk of selecting out INH-resistant organisms is low. The INH mutation rate is about 1 in 10^6, but only about 10^3 organisms are present in the body. In contrast, the risk of selecting out INH-resistant organisms would be unacceptably high in patients with cavitary TB. One can guard against selecting out these INH-resistant mutants by adding another drug, such as rifampin (RIF). The rates for multiple-drug mutations occur as an additive function of the individual rates; only 1 in 10^{13} (INH rate of 10^6 plus RIF rate of 10^7) organisms would be resistant to both drugs by natural mutation. Because this number is larger than the number of organisms typically found in a cavitary lesion, it is unlikely that many such organisms are present. Therefore, combination chemotherapy is required for treating active TB disease; and the patient should be on at least two drugs to which the isolate is susceptible. RIF and INH are the antimycobacterial agents most capable of preventing resistance, followed by ethambutol (EMB), streptomycin (SM), and pyrazinamide (PZA).[37,47]

Three subpopulations of mycobacteria are proposed to exist within the body, each of which appears to be most susceptible to certain drugs.[15,37,47] Most numerous (possibly 10^7 to 10^9 organisms) are the extracellular, rapidly dividing bacteria, often found within cavities. These are inhibited or killed most readily by INH, followed by RIF, SM, and the other antimycobacterial drugs. A second group (possibly 10^5 to 10^7 organisms) is comprised of organisms residing within caseating granulomas; these organisms are usually in a semi-dormant metabolic state, but on occasion will increase their activity for short periods of time. It is believed that PZA, through its conversion to pyrazinoic acid is active against such organisms. RIF and INH are also likely to be active against this subpopulation. The final subset is the intracellular mycobacteria, present within macrophages (10^4 to 10^6). Debate continues regarding the percentage of such cells that produce an acidic environment, because *M. tuberculosis* appears to block the normal fusion and acidification of the phagosomes with the lysosomes. RIF, INH, and the quinolones appear to be most active against intracellular *M. tuberculosis*. Although these theories appear to explain what happens during the treatment of TB, there is no practical way to quantitate these populations within a given patient.

NONPHARMACOLOGIC THERAPY

These interventions aim to (a) prevent the spread of TB, (b) find where TB has already spread through contact investigation, and (c) replenish the weakened (consumptive) patient to a state of normal weight and well being. The first two are the purview of the public health department. Pharmacists involved in the treatment of TB should verify that the local health department has been notified of a new case of TB. While it is often assumed that the physician or laboratory has already done this, studies repeatedly show that as many as 37% of cases are not properly reported.[4] Workers in hospitals and other institutions must be very conscious of the potential for spreading TB within their facilities, and appropriate steps need to be taken to prevent this.[8,9] Pharmacists caring for TB patients should learn and follow the institution's infection control guidelines. Debilitated TB patients may require therapy for multiple medical problems, including substance abuse and HIV infection, and some may desperately need nutritional reconstitution. Therefore, pharmacists involved in substance abuse rehabilitation and nutritional support services should be familiar with the particular needs of TB patients.

Other nonpharmacologic interventions include surgery for advanced cases of pulmonary disease, tuberculomas, and certain extrapulmonary lesions. Vaccines against TB include BCG (discussed later) and *M. vaccae*. The latter is an experimental treatment designed to shift the immune response toward the more effective and less destructive Th-1 response. There is no vaccine, however, that can prevent infection by *M. tuberculosis*, which is what is truly needed.

PHARMACOLOGIC THERAPY

Most importantly, the treatment of active TB involves multiple drugs. There are two primary antituberculosis drugs—INH and RIF—with the rest of the drugs playing specific roles. Isoniazid and RIF should be used together whenever possible. Tables 110–4 and 110–5 list these and other drugs by their primary targets: drugs that work primarily against the mycobacterial cell wall and those that work primarily against intracellular targets.[2] It is clear from these data that INH and RIF are much more potent than the other drugs against *M. tuberculosis*. Depending on the dosing strategy, the aminoglycosides (as shown by streptomycin, but including kanamycin and amikacin) can display considerable activity versus *M. tuberculosis*. The remaining drugs are considerably weaker, and without INH and RIF, their use requires much longer durations of treatment. These parameter estimates are based on published minimal inhibitory concentrations (MICs) and pharmacokinetic data. Using the midpoint of the proposed normal ranges for the maximum serum concentration

TABLE 110–4. Potency of Antimycobacterial Drugs That Act Primarily Against the Cell Wall

Drug	Cmax:MIC	T > MIC	AUC > MIC
Cycloserine	3.8	22.5	195.5
Ethambutol 25 mg/kg	10.0	13.0	23.4
Ethionamide	1.6	1.5	1.0
Isoniazid			
(f)	40.0	9.0	11.6
(s)	40.0	18.0	19.2
Thiacetazone	1.3	5.5	1.2

AUC, area under the serum concentration time curve; Cmax, maximum serum concentration; f, fast acetylator, MIC, minimal inhibitory concentration; s, slow acetylator; T > MIC, time serum concentrations remain above the MIC (hours).
(From Ref. 1, with permission.)

TABLE 110–5. Potency of Antimycobacterial Drugs That Act Primarily Against Intracellular Targets

Drug	Cmax:MIC	T > MIC	AUC > MIC
Rifampin	24.0	9.0	39.9
Streptomycin			
(h)	18.8	11.0	274.6
(c)	10.0	8.0	124.5
Aminosalicylate[a]	75.0	4.0	153.7
Ciprofloxacin	5.0	10.5	16.9
Ofloxacin	5.0	15.5	47.4

AUC, area under the serum concentration time curve; c, 12–15 mg/kg IV five times per week; Cmax, maximum serum concentration; h, 22–25 mg/kg three times per week; MIC, minimal inhibitory concentration; T > MIC, time serum concentrations remain above the MIC (hours).
[a]Despite the high Cmax:MIC ratio, aminosalicylate is known to be a relatively weak agent versus TB. Its mechanism of action is poorly understood but is primarily bacteriostatic. Aminosalicylate may be misclassified as an intracellular agent.
(From Ref. 1, with permission.)

(Cmax) and typical first-order elimination half-lives, the pharmacodynamic parameters Cmax:MIC ratio, area under the curve (AUC) > MIC, and time > MIC were derived.[2] The use of higher doses of the TB drugs to treat moderately resistant organisms has not been systematically studied. Typically, *M. tuberculosis* is either very susceptible or very resistant to a given drug. This contrasts with *M. avium*, where moderately resistant organisms are a frequent occurrence. Theoretically, MIC results could be used to guide dosing in the treatment of moderately resistant *M. tuberculosis*, but this remains to be prospectively studied.[2]

DRUG TREATMENTS OF FIRST CHOICE AND ALTERNATIVE TREATMENTS

Treating Latent Infection

The treatment of latent infection can reduce the risk that a patient will progress to active disease. This is good not only for the patient in question, but it also prevents additional cases of TB that might have occurred had the patient developed active disease. This early intervention is called prophylaxis, chemoprophylaxis, or preventive treatment, although referring to it as treatment of latent TB infection is most accurate. Table 110–6 lists treatment regimens for latent TB infection. In particular, children younger than 5 years old, or HIV-positive patients with recent exposures to infectious cases of TB, should be evaluated for active disease. Once this is ruled out, they should be given preventive treatment.[2,22,23,39] In children, therapy should be continued for 3 months after contact with the source case is ended.[23] If the repeat skin test is negative at that time, treatment can be stopped. Otherwise, children should be treated for a total of 9 months.[23] Preventive treatment for HIV-positive patients is generally as long as for HIV negative patients.[25,48]

Isoniazid-preventive therapy (typically given as 300 mg daily to an adult) is the primary treatment for latent TB infection in the United States.[2] It is effective in about 69% of patients, but it approaches 93% efficacy when patients adhere to a 52-week regimen.[2,39,49–51] The keys to success are (a) infection caused by an INH-susceptible isolate, (b) adherence to the INH regimen for 6 to 12 months, and (c) a low risk of exogenous reinfection.[2] The 52-week regimens are somewhat more effective than the 24-week regimens, with the greatest benefit

TABLE 110–6. Recommended Drug Regimens for Treatment of Latent Tuberculosis (TB) Infection in Adults

Drug	Interval and Duration	Comments	Rating* (Evidence)† HIV−	HIV+
Isoniazid	Daily for 9 mo‡,§	In human immunodeficiency virus (HIV)-infected patients, isoniazid may be administered concurrently with nucleoside reverse transcriptase inhibitors (NRTIs), protease inhibitors, or non-nucleoside reverse transcriptase inhibitors (NNRTIs)	A (II)	A (II)
	Twice weekly for 9 mo‡,§	Directly observed therapy (DOT) must be used with twice-weekly dosing	B (II)	B (II)
Isoniazid	Daily for 6 mo§	Not indicated for HIV-infected persons, those with fibrotic lesions on chest radiographs, or children	B (I)	C (I)
	Twice weekly for 6 mo§	DOT must be used with twice-weekly dosing	B (II)	C (I)
Rifampin plus pyrazinamide	Daily for 2 mo	May also be offered to persons who are contacts of patients with isoniazid-resistant, rifampin-susceptible TB In HIV-infected patients, protease inhibitors or NNRTIs should generally not be administered concurrently with rifampin; rifabutin can be used as an alternative for patients treated with indinavir, nelfinavir, amprenivir, ritonavir, or efavirenz, and possibly with nevirapine or soft-gel saquinavir¶	B (II)	A (I)
	Twice weekly for 2–3 mo	DOT must be used with twice-weekly dosing	C (II)	C (I)
Rifampin	Daily for 4 mo	For persons who cannot tolerate pyrazinamide For persons who are contacts of patients with isoniazid-resistant, rifampin-susceptible TB who cannot tolerate pyrazinamide	B (II)	B (III)

*Strength of recommendation: A = preferred; B = acceptable alternative; C = offer when A and B cannot be given.
†Quality of evidence: I = randomized clinical trial data; II = data from clinical trials that are not randomized or were conducted in other populations; III = expert opinion.
‡Recommended regimen for children younger than 18 yr of age.
§Recommended regimens for pregnant women. Some experts would use rifampin and pyrazinamide for 2 mo as an alternative regimen in HIV-infected pregnant women, although pyrazinamide should be avoided during the first trimester.
¶Rifabutin should not be used with ritonavir, hard-gel saquinavir, or delavirdine. When used with other protease inhibitors or NNRTIs, dose adjustment of rifabutin may be required.

appearing by 9 months of treatment.[2,49] Isoniazid doses of 5–10 mg/kg of body weight, up to 300 mg per day, are used in adults (Table 110–7).[52] Doses lower than this are less effective.[2,49] Whenever possible, INH should be given on an empty stomach, and antacids should be avoided within 2 hours of dosing. When adherence is an issue, twice-weekly INH (900 mg in an adult) can be given using directly observed therapy. Nine months is preferred, but if that is not possible, 6 months still provides considerable benefit.

When the isolate from the presumed source case is resistant to INH alone, RIF has been the primary alternative drug.[2,25,48,49] RIF 600 mg (or rifabutin [RBN] 300 mg) is given daily for 4 months. Twice-weekly treatment is not recommended. Concern has been expressed over the possibility of selecting for RIF resistance in previously INH-resistant organisms. This seems unlikely, and has not been proven to occur in humans. A more conservative approach is to add another drug, such as PZA to the regimen. Short-course chemoprophylaxis is now recommended as an alternative to INH: 2 months of RIF 600 mg and PZA 15–20 mg/kg (or RBN 300 mg and PZA 15–20 mg/kg).[25] Twice-weekly directly observed therapy is also possible for this two-drug regimen. The rifampin doses are not changed, but the PZA dose is increased to 50 mg/kg.

When the isolate from the presumed source case is resistant to INH and RIF (MDR-TB), there is no alternative regimen proven to be effective.[2] Based on the known or likely susceptibility pattern of the infecting organism, regimens of PZA plus EMB or EMB plus a fluoroquinolone (ofloxacin [OFLOX] or levofloxacin [LEVO]), have been proposed.[2,25,39] Because none of these agents are as potent as INH or RIF, it is not known how effective such regimens may be. The current recommended duration is 6 to 12 months.

Some physicians are hesitant to treat asymptomatic patients with positive skin tests for fear of INH hepatotoxicity. It has been documented repeatedly that the risk of infection outweighs the risk for drug toxicity in patients eligible for treatment. In fact, reports suggest that elderly patients and patients at lower risk for developing TB still benefit.[53] Patients treated with INH may receive pyridoxine (vitamin B_6) 10–50 mg daily to reduce the incidence of central nervous system (CNS) effects or peripheral neuropathies. Pregnant women, alcoholics, and others with poor diets definitely should receive vitamin B_6. All patients who receive chemoprophylaxis should be monitored monthly for improvement or worsening of symptoms. Any worsening of the clinical condition should prompt a chest radiograph and sputum analysis for AFB.

Treating Active Disease

Drug susceptibility data from the index case isolate should guide the initial drug selection.[2] If this data is not available, the drug resistance pattern in the area where the patient likely acquired TB must be taken into account.[2] If the patient is being evaluated for the retreatment of TB, it is imperative to know what drugs were used previously and for how long.[2] At the National Jewish Medical and Research Center, the patient's drug history calendar is known as a Drug-O-Gram, which shows the start and stop dates of all antimycobacterial drugs on a horizontal bar graph.[2,54] The failure to reconstruct the drug history carefully can seriously compromise any effort at retreatment. Finally, appropriate samples should be sent for culture and susceptibility testing prior to initiating therapy.[2]

TABLE 110–7. Dosing Information

Drug	Route and Frequency	Adult Daily	Adult 2 × Weekly	Pediatric Daily	Pediatric 2 × Weekly	Dose: Renal Failure	CSF Penetration
Amikacin (AK)	IM, IV qd	12–15 mg/kg	25–30 mg/kg[a]	12–15 mg/kg 15–30 mg/kg[a]	(Presumably as adults)	12–15 mg/kg 3 × weekly	20%–40% est.
Aminosalicylic acid (PAS)	Oral [IV[b]] bid or tid	4 g/dose 8–12 g total 150 mg/kg[a]	Not known divided tid	150 mg/kg[a]	Not known	Unknown; avoid if possible	10%–50%
Capreomycin (CM)	IM, IV qd	12–15 mg/kg	Not known	12–15 mg/kg 15–30 mg/kg[a]	Not known	12–15 mg/kg 3 × weekly	20%–40% est.
Ciprofloxacin (CIPRO)	Oral qd	750–1000 mg	Not known	Not known 8–10 mg/kg?	Not known	Unchanged unless severe	4%–10%
Clofazimine[d] (CFZ)	Oral qd	100–200 mg	Not known	Not known 2–3 mg/kg?	Not known	Unchanged	Not known, est. poor
Cycloserine[e] (CSN)	Oral qd or bid	250–500 mg/dose 750–1000 mg total	Not known	15–20 mg/kg[a]	Not known	250–500 mg 3 × weekly	50%–80%
Ethambutol (EMB)	Oral, [IV[b]] qd	25 mg/kg (2 mo) then 15 mg/kg	50 mg/kg	25 mg/kg (2 mo) then 15 mg/kg	50 mg/kg	15–25 mg/kg 3 × weekly	5%–65% est; variable inflammation
Ethionamide[e] (ETA)	Oral qd or bid	250–500 mg/dose 750–1000 mg total	Not known	15–20 mg/kg	Not known	Unchanged	20%–100% est.
Isoniazid (INH)	Oral, IM, IV[c] qd	300 mg (5 mg/kg)	15 mg/kg 900 mg max[a]	10–20 mg/kg 300 mg max[a]	20–40 mg/kg 900 mg max[a]	Unchanged or reduced to qod	20%–100%
Kanamycin (KM)	IM, IV qd	12–15 mg/kg	25–30 mg/kg[a]	12–15 mg/kg 15–30 mg/kg[a]	(Presumably as adults)	12–15 mg/kg 3 × weekly	20%–40% est.
Levofloxacin (LEVO)	Oral qd	750–1000 mg	Not known	Not known, 8–10 mg/kg	Not known	~800 mg 3 × weekly	30%–90%
Pyrazinamide (PZA)	Oral qd or bid	15–30 mg/kg 2 g max[a]	35–70 mg/kg 4 g max[a]	15–30 mg/kg 2 g max[a]	35–70 mg/kg 4 g max[a]	15–30 mg/kg 3 × weekly	50%–100%
Rifabutin (RBN)	Oral qd	300–450 mg	300–450 mg proposed	5–10 mg/kg proposed	Not known	Unchanged in most patients	30%–70%
Rifampin (RIF)	Oral, IV qd	450–600 mg (10 mg/kg)	450–600 mg (10 mg/kg)	10–20 mg/kg 600 mg max[a]	10–20 mg/kg 600 mg max[a]	Unchanged in most patients	5%–20% est.; variable, inflammation
Streptomycin (SM)	IM, IV[c] qd	12–15 mg/kg	25–30 mg/kg[a]	12–15 mg/kg 20–40 mg/kg[a]	25–30 mg/kg[a]	12–15 mg/kg 3 × weekly	20%–40% est.
Thiacetazone (TB-1)	[Oral[b]] qd	150 mg	Not known	2–5 mg/kg proposed	Not known	Not known; avoid if possible	Not known

[a]ATS/CDC 1994 guidelines, which may differ from practice at National Jewish Center.
[b]Available outside of United States; may be imported under IND, an investigational new drug application.
[c]IV route of administration not FDA approved.
[d]Various intermittent clofazimine regimens have been proposed for leprosy, but not MTB or MAC.
[e]Introduce gradually over several days.
CSF, cerebrospinal fluid; est., estimated; FDA, Food and Drug Administration; MTB, *Mycobacterium tuberculosis;* MAC, *Mycobacterium avium* complex; ATS, American Thoracic Society; CDC, Centers for Disease Control and Prevention.

TABLE 110–8. Regimen Options for the Initial Treatment of Active Tuberculosis Among Children and Adults

TB Without HIV Infection		
Option 1	*Option 2*	*Option 3*
Administer daily INH, RIF, and pyrazinamide for 8 wk followed by 16 wk of INH and RIF daily or two to three times/wk[a] in areas where the INH resistance rate is not documented to be <4%. Ethambutol or streptomycin should be added to the initial regimen until susceptibility to INH and RIF is demonstrated. Continue treatment for at least 6 mo and 3 mo beyond culture conversion. Consult a TB medical expert if the patient is symptomatic or smear or culture positive after 3 mo.	Administer daily INH, RIF, pyrazinamide, and streptomycin or ethambutol for 2 wk followed by two times/wk[a] administration of the same drugs for 6 wk (by DOT), and subsequently, with two times/wk administration of INH and RIF for 16 wk (by DOT). Consult a TB medical expert if the patient is symptomatic or smear or culture positive after 3 mo.	Treat by DOT three times/wk[a] with INH, RIF, pyrazinamide and ethambutol or streptomycin for 6 mo. Consult a TB medical expert if the patient is symptomatic or smear or culture positive after 3 mo.

DOT = directly observed therapy; HIV = human immunodeficiency virus; INH = isoniazid; RIF = rifampin; TB = tuberculosis.
[a]All regimens administered two times/wk or three times/wk should be monitored by DOT for the duration of therapy.
[b]The strongest evidence from clinical trials is the effectiveness of all four drugs administered for the full 6 mo. There is weaker evidence that streptomycin can be discontinued after 4 mo if the isolate is susceptible to all drugs. The evidence for stopping pyrazinamide before the end of 6 mo is equivocal for the three times/wk regimen, and there is no evidence on the effectiveness of this regimen with ethambutol for less than the full 6 mo.
From Ref. 2, with permission.

It is possible to cure most cases of drug-susceptible TB with just 9 months of INH and RIF treatment. The addition of 2 months of PZA shortens the duration of treatment to 6 months for such patients. The recommended treatment regimens for drug-susceptible disease in HIV negative and positive patients are shown in Tables 110–8 and 110–9, respectively. Section 3, 6-month RIF-based therapy, is the standard treatment for HIV negative patients of all ages. EMB is used cautiously in children. Note that for drug-susceptible TB, treatment can be given daily or intermittently. When intermittent therapy is used, directly observed therapy is essential. Missed doses during an intermittent regimen can seriously compromise the efficacy of the treatment and increase the relapse rate.

Different end points may be reached during the treatment of TB. First, the patient may convert to a negative sputum smear. When this occurs, the patient has less than 10,000 organisms/mL of sputum and is at reduced risk of spreading TB. Such patients can be removed from respiratory isolation, provided that they are careful not to cough on others. It is still advisable that they meet with others only in well-ventilated places, particularly outdoors. The combination of air movement and ultraviolet radiation from the sun eliminates the risk of spreading TB.

Patients can be smear negative but culture positive. These patients must continue treatment because they still harbor many live organisms. Once the patients are smear and culture negative consistently, they are on their way to cure. Occasionally, patients will have isolated positive smears or cultures. TB patients with positive smears and negative cultures typically have dead organisms in their samples, indicating effective chemotherapy. They may be releasing organisms that were contained in a previously closed cavity. Provided that subsequent smears and cultures remain negative, such patients can complete standard or slightly prolonged treatment courses.

With rare exceptions, patients must complete 6 months or more of treatment. It has been argued that HIV-positive patients should be treated for an additional 3 months and for at least 6 months from the time that they convert to smear and culture negativity.[2,6] When INH and RIF cannot be used, treatment durations become 2 years or more, regardless of immune status.

EMB or SM are typically added to INH, RIF, and PZA at the start of treatment until susceptibility data are available.[2,6,39,55] This provides a good regimen in the event of INH resistance, and avoids monotherapy in the event of initial two-drug resistance. Adjustments to the regimen should be made once the susceptibility data are available.[2,55] If the organism is drug-susceptible, a regimen of INH and RIF for 6 months, supplemented in the first 2 months by PZA, can be used. If the organism is drug-resistant, careful consideration of the remaining therapeutic options must be made. Two or more drugs with *in vitro* activity against the patient's isolate, and that the patient has not received previously, should be added to the regimen, as needed. TB specialists should be consulted regarding cases of drug-resistant TB.[2,55]

There is no standard regimen for MDR-TB.[2,55] Each patient's exposure history (known source case or location where infection likely occurred), previous treatment history (including toxicity and adherence issues), and current susceptibility data must be considered simultaneously. In addition to avoiding monotherapy, it is critical to avoid adding only a single drug to a failing regimen.[2,54,55] This leads to the sequential selection of drug resistance, and eventually there are no drugs left. TB specialists should manage the treatment of MDR-TB. It is important to realize that it may take several months for a patient with MDR-TB to become culture negative, because the drugs used lack the potency of INH and RIF.[2] Therefore, prolonged respiratory isolation may be required.

Drug resistance should be suspected in these situations:

- Patients who have received prior therapy for TB.
- Patients from areas with a high prevalence of resistance (New York City, Mexico, Southeast Asia, and the former Soviet states).
- Patients who are homeless, institutionalized, IV drug abusers, or infected with HIV.
- Patients who still have AFB-positive sputum smears after 2 months of therapy.
- Patients who still have positive cultures after 3 to 4 months of therapy.
- Patients who require retreatment.

These patients, those in whom therapy is failing, and those with documented exposure to drug-resistant organisms, should be considered to be infected with resistant organisms until proven otherwise. In patients with prior treatment, therapy should be modified to include two

TABLE 110–9. Treatment Regimens for Human Immunodeficiency Virus (HIV)-Related Tuberculosis (TB)

	Induction Phase		Continuation Phase			
Rating	Drugs	Interval and Duration	Drugs	Interval and Duration	Considerations for HIV Therapy	Comments
Six-month RFB-based therapy (may be prolonged* to 9 months)						
A.II	•INH •RFB •PZA† •EMB†	Daily for 2 months (8 weeks)	•INH •RFB	Daily or 2 times/week for 4 months (18 weeks)	RFB should not be used concurrently with ritonavir, hard-gel saquinavir (Invirase), or delavirdine.	If the patient also is taking indinavir, nelfinavir, or amprenavir, the daily dose of RFB is decreased from 300 mg to 150 mg. The twice-weekly dose of RFB (300 mg) remains unchanged if the patient is also taking these protease inhibitors.
		or		or	A 20%–25% increase in the dose of protease inhibitors or NNRTIs might be necessary.	
	•INH •RFB •PZA† •EMB†	Daily for 2 weeks and then 2 times/week for 6 weeks	•INH •RFB	2 times/week for 4 months (18 weeks)	The patient should be monitored carefully for RFB drug toxicity (arthralgia, uveitis, leukopenia) if RFB is used concurrently with protease inhibitors or NNRTIs.	If the patient also is taking efavirenz, the daily or twice weekly dose of RFB is increased from 300 mg to 450 mg.
					Evidence of decreased antiretroviral drug activity should be assessed periodically with HIV RNA levels.	Three-times-a-week administration of RFB used in combination with antiretroviral therapy has not been studied.
					No contraindication exists for the use of RFB with NRTIs.	
Nine-month SM-based therapy (may be prolonged* to 12 months)						
B.II	•INH •SM •PZA •EMB	Daily for 2 months (8 weeks)	•INH •SM •PZA	2–3 times/week for 7 months (30 weeks)	Can be used concurrently with antiretroviral regimens that include protease inhibitors, NRTIs, and NNRTIs.	SM is contraindicated for pregnant women.
		or		or		Every effort should be made to continue administering SM for the total duration of treatment. When SM is not used for the recommended 9 months, EMB should be added to the regimen and the treatment duration should be prolonged from 9 months (38 weeks) to 12 months (52 weeks).
	•INH •SM •PZA •EMB	Daily for 2 weeks and then 2–3 times/week for 6 weeks	•INH •SM •PZA	2–3 times/week for 7 months (30 weeks)		

TABLE 110–9. (Continued)

Rating	Induction Phase: Drugs	Induction Phase: Interval and Duration	Continuation Phase: Drugs	Continuation Phase: Interval and Duration	Considerations for HIV Therapy	Comments
Six-month RIF-based therapy (may be prolonged* to 9 months)						
A.I	• INH • RIF • PZA[§] • EMB[§] (or SM)	Daily for 2 months (8 weeks) or	• INH • RIF	Daily or 2–3 times/week for 4 months (18 weeks) or	Protease inhibitors or NNRTIs should not be administered concurrently with RIF. NRTIs can be administered concurrently with RIF. If appropriate, patients should be assessed every 3 months to evaluate the decision to initiate antiretroviral therapy. A 2-week "P-450 induction washout" period may be necessary between the last dose of RIF and the first dose of protease inhibitors or NNRTIs.	SM is contraindicated for pregnant women.
	• INH • RIF • PZA[§] • EMB[§] (or SM)	Daily for 2 weeks and then 2–3 times/week for 6 weeks or	• INH • RIF	2–3 times/week for 4 months (18 weeks) or		
	• INH • RIF • PZA • EMB (or SM)	3 times/week for 2 months (8 weeks)	• INH • RIF • PZA • EMB (or SM)	3 times/week for 4 months (18 weeks)		

EMB = ethambutol; INH = isoniazid; PZA = pyrazinamide; RFB = rifabutin; RIF = rifampin SM = streptomycin.
NNRTI = nonnucleoside reverse transcriptase inhibitor; NRTI = nucleoside reverse transcriptase inhibitor.
*Duration of therapy should be prolonged for patients with delayed response to therapy. Criteria for delayed response should be assessed at the end of the 2-month induction phase and include a) lack of conversion of the *Mycobacterium tuberculosis* culture from positive to negative or b) lack of resolution or progression of signs or symptoms of TB.
[†]Continue PZA and EMB for the total duration of the induction phase (8 weeks).
[§]Continue PZA for the total duration of the induction phase (8 weeks). EMB can be stopped after susceptibility test results indicate *Mycobacterium tuberculosis* susceptibility to INH and RIF.

additional drugs that have not been used previously. For empiric therapy of suspected drug-resistant TB, at least four drugs should be used (INH, RIF, PZA, EMB, or SM). These regimens may be altered when the susceptibility pattern becomes known. If the index case is known, then the same effective regimen should be employed for the new case. Again, MDR-TB cases should be referred to specialists.

SPECIAL POPULATIONS

Tuberculous Meningitis and Extrapulmonary Disease

In general, INH, PZA, ethionamide (ETA), and cycloserine (CS) penetrate the cerebrospinal fluid (CSF) readily, but RIF, EMB, and SM have variable CNS penetration.[56] Of the quinolones, levofloxacin (LEVO) may be preferred. Patients with CNS tuberculosis are often treated for longer periods (9 to 12 months).[22] Extrapulmonary TB of the soft tissues can be treated with conventional regimens. TB of the bone is typically treated for 9 to 12 months, occasionally with surgical débridement.[2,6,57]

Children

TB in children may be treated with regimens similar to those used in adults, although some physicians still prefer to extend treatment to 9 months.[22,23,37,57] Pediatric doses of INH and RIF on a milligram per kilogram basis are higher than those used in adults (see Table 110–7).[52]

Pregnancy

Women with TB should be cautioned against becoming pregnant, as the disease poses a risk to the fetus as well as to the mother. Studies that have examined the incidence of birth defects resulting from various antituberculosis drugs concluded that the risk to infants born to mothers treated with INH or EMB was equal to that in normal populations.[56–59] It appears that INH is relatively safe when used during pregnancy, despite its ability to cross the placenta. Supplementation with B vitamins is particularly important during pregnancy. RIF is not frequently associated with birth defects, but those seen are occasionally severe, including limb reduction and CNS lesions.[56] Some have proposed that RIF be reserved for cases in which the mother has more advanced disease requiring more aggressive therapy. PZA has not been studied in pregnant women. Given the fact that it is similar to INH and ETA in size and general structure, it probably crosses the placenta readily. Data on its potential teratogenicity are not available. Reports on the use of EMB during pregnancy indicate that it is relatively safe.[56–59]

SM has been associated with varying degrees of hearing impairment in the newborn, including complete deafness, so the use of this agent must be reserved for situations in which it is an essential component of the therapy in the mother.[56] Fortunately, it appears that the majority of infants exposed to SM *in utero* have no ill effects from the drug, so there is hope for a favorable outcome in those situations in which it must be used. The other aminoglycosides have also been shown to cross the placenta, presenting similar risks. Although capreomycin (CM) has not been studied, it probably acts like SM.

ETA may be associated with premature delivery and congenital deformities when used during pregnancy.[56] Mongolism has also been reported in the offspring of mothers who took ETA during pregnancy. Despite occasional reports of ETA's safe use during pregnancy, ETA cannot be recommended in this setting. Para-aminosalicylic acid (PAS) has been used in pregnancy, apparently without ill effect. CS is known to cross the placenta. The effect that CS may have on the developing fetus, however, is unknown. Therefore, CS generally cannot be recommended during pregnancy, although it may have some future role in selected cases.[56]

Ciprofloxacin (CIPRO), OFLOX, LEVO, and the other quinolones, although not shown to be teratogens, have been associated with permanent damage to cartilage in the weight-bearing joints of immature animals, especially dogs and rabbits.[56] Although these drugs frequently do not cause joint problems in humans, other antituberculosis agents should be used during pregnancy.

Pregnant women with active TB should receive INH and RIF for a period of 9 months. If a third drug is necessary, EMB may be added. Therapy with INH for asymptomatic tuberculous infection may be delayed until after pregnancy or, if recent skin test conversion has occurred, started during the second trimester of pregnancy.[56–59] Although most antituberculosis drugs are excreted in breast milk, the amount of drug received by the infant through nursing is insufficient to cause toxicity. Quinolones should be avoided in nursing mothers if possible.

Human Immunodeficiency Virus

Patients with AIDS and other immunocompromised hosts may be managed with chemotherapeutic regimens similar to those used in immunocompetent individuals, although treatment is often extended (9 to 12 months).[2,5,33,57] Prognosis has been particularly poor for HIV-infected patients infected with MDR-TB. Differentiation must be made between infection with *M. tuberculosis* and nontuberculous mycobacteria, such as *M. avium* complex, because the drugs used are different. While awaiting laboratory results, the patient can be empirically treated for TB if there is any doubt about the causative organism. Some patients with AIDS malabsorb their oral medications; this is discussed later under therapeutic drug monitoring.[2] The major issue of drug interactions is discussed further below, under rifampin.

Renal Failure

Table 110–7 provides details regarding the excretion of the antimycobacterial drugs.[52,60,61] Antituberculosis drugs that rely on renal clearance for most of their elimination include the aminoglycosides (amikacin [AK], kanamycin [KM], and SM), the polypeptide CM (and viomycin [VM]), EMB, CS, OFLOX, and LEVO. CIPRO is about 50% cleared by the kidneys.[56] In addition, some of the metabolites of the antituberculosis drugs, particularly those of INH, PZA, and PAS, are cleared primarily by the kidneys. The precise role of these metabolites in the toxicity profiles of their parent compounds is largely unknown, so the danger of their accumulation in renal failure has not been determined.

INH is primarily excreted through metabolism in the liver.[56,60] It has been recommended that most patients receive standard doses (300 mg daily) of INH, preferably after hemodialysis. RIF can be given in normal daily doses to patients in renal failure after dialysis.[60] Pyrazinamide is converted primarily to pyrazinoic acid and 5-hydroxypyrazinoic acid, which are renally eliminated. Normal doses of PZA (20–35 mg/kg) can be administered approximately three times per week following each dialysis session.[60] Patients with decreased renal function may accumulate EMB, as renal elimination accounts for about 80% of the dose.[60] A dose of 15 mg/kg three times per week after dialysis appears reasonable. It is essential that such patients have frequent examinations for visual acuity and red-green color discrimination.

Aminoglycosides and CM (and VM) should also be avoided in patients with end-stage renal disease whenever possible. Otherwise, two to three doses per week should be the maximum. ETA and its sulfoxide metabolite are not found in significant quantities in the urine, so dosing is generally unchanged.[61] PAS is converted largely to metabolites prior to renal elimination; these metabolites may accumulate in renal failure.[61] CS is dependent on renal clearance for elimination and will accumulate in renal failure.[61] Serum concentration monitoring must be performed to avoid dose-related toxicities in renal failure patients.[56,60–62] CIPRO is only partially dependent on renal clearance, so it may be the preferred quinolone in this setting.

Hepatic Failure

Antituberculosis drugs that rely on hepatic clearance for most of their elimination from the body include INH, ETA, RIF, PZA, and PAS.[56] CIPRO is about 50% cleared by the liver. Reports have indicated a decreased clearance of INH and RIF in liver disease, with moderate increases in the half-life of each agent (30% to 100%). Specific information regarding the effects of hepatic dysfunction on the clearance of ETA are not available. One paper was published that showed significant accumulation of PZA in icteric TB patients, with concentrations in some patients reaching 300 μg/mL. In another study, PAS pharmacokinetics were not substantially altered in patients with a variety of liver diseases. CIPRO concentrations are not substantially altered in hepatic disease. Unfortunately, elevations of serum transaminase concentrations may indicate damage to the liver, but transaminase concentrations generally are not correlated with the residual capacity of the liver to metabolize drugs. Additional consideration should be given to avoiding drugs known to produce hepatotoxicity, such as INH, RIF, and PZA, and to a lesser degree, ETA, PAS, and rarely, EMB, if the risk of further liver damage outweighs the benefits of the drugs in controlling the mycobacterial infection.[56] Serum concentration monitoring may be considered for such patients.

Morbid Obesity

Only limited information on the volume of distribution of most of the antituberculosis drugs is available, so the proper doses of these drugs in morbid obesity is still unclear.[56] Hydrophilic drugs (INH, PZA, the aminoglycosides, CM, EMB, PAS, CS), or those that typically display relatively small volumes (INH, RIF, the aminoglycosides, CM, EMB) should initially be used in doses based on ideal body weight (IBW). These drugs can be expected to remain largely in the vascular space and the extracellular fluid and not attain high concentrations in adipose tissue. Elevated serum concentrations can be avoided by initially prescribing doses of these drugs based on IBW, followed by serum concentration monitoring to confirm that effective concentrations can be maintained in the serum.

DRUG CLASS INFORMATION

This section summarizes information regarding the antimycobacterial drugs. The interested reader also is referred to several other publications that provide additional detail regarding these drugs.[2,5,15,22,37,47,49,56,57,61–73] Credit is given to those authors for providing the information that is summarized here. Please refer to Tables 110–7, 110–8, and 110–9 for specific dosing information.

Primary Antituberculosis Drugs

Isoniazid.

INH is highly specific for mycobacteria, with an MIC against *M. tuberculosis* of 0.01–0.25 μg/mL. Most nontuberculous mycobacteria are resistant to INH, although *M. kansasii* and *M. xenopi* are susceptible. The most common mechanism of resistance results from mutations in the katG gene, leading to the loss of catalase-peroxidase activity and the failure to produce the toxic INH derivatives.

INH is readily absorbed from the GI tract and from IM injection sites. It can also be given as a short IV infusion over 5 minutes if diluted in about 20 mL of normal saline.[74] Food and possibly antacids may reduce isoniazid's absorption; INH should be given on an empty stomach whenever possible.[75,76] Hepatic and possibly intestinal *N*-acetyltransferase form the principle metabolite, acetylisoniazid, which lacks antimycobacterial activity. The rate at which humans acetylate isoniazid is genetically determined; slow acetylation is an autosomal recessive trait and is a result of a relative *N*-acetyltransferase deficiency. Fast acetylators (INH half-life less than 2 hours) are heterozygous or homozygous dominants, with approximately 50% of whites and blacks and 80% to 90% of Asians and Eskimos being rapid acetylators. Slow acetylators (INH half-life typically 3 to 4 hours) may be at an increased risk of hepatotoxicity. The association of acetylator status and risk of hepatotoxicity from clinical trials, however, appears to be weak.

Transient elevations of the serum transaminases occur in 12% to 15% of patients receiving INH, and usually occur within the first 8 to 12 weeks of therapy. Overt hepatotoxicity, however, occurs in only 1% of cases. Risk factors for hepatotoxicity include patient age (Table 110–10), preexisting liver disease, pregnancy, and the postpartum state. Moderate consumption of alcohol is probably not a risk factor if it has not resulted in preexisting liver disease.

INH also may result in neurotoxicity, most frequently presenting as peripheral neuropathy or, in overdose, seizures and coma. Central nervous system effects, such as ataxia, mental status changes, or exacerbation of preexisting convulsive disorders, are also occasionally observed. INH appears to exert its neurotoxic effect through enhanced elimination of pyridoxine, competitive inhibition with pyridoxine in its action as a cofactor in the synthesis of synaptic neurotransmitters, or both. Patients with pyridoxine deficiency, such as alcoholics, children, and the malnourished, are at increased risk, as are patients who are slow acetylators of INH and those predisposed to neuropathy, such as diabetics. Coadministration of as little as 6 mg of pyridoxine daily will reduce the incidence of these neurotoxic effects from 20% to less than 1%. Isoniazid reportedly inhibits the

TABLE 110–10. Effect of Age on Incidence of Hepatitis From Isoniazid

Age (years)	Frequency (%)
0–19	0.3–0.6
20–34	0.3–2.2
35–49	1.2–3.2
50–64	2.3–3.4
>65	2.3–4.2

metabolism of phenytoin, carbamazepine, primidone, and warfarin. Patients who are being treated with these agents should be monitored closely, and appropriate dose adjustments should be made when necessary.

Rifampin. The introduction of RIF into routine use during the 1970s allowed for true short-course treatment of TB (6 to 9 months). Without RIF, treatment is generally 18 months or longer. Drug resistance to RIF is one of the most ominous prognostic factors influencing the outcome of therapy, because it is frequently associated with INH resistance and leaves the patient with few good therapeutic options.

RIF shows bactericidal activity against *M. tuberculosis* and several other mycobacterial species, including *M. bovis and M. kansasii.* Other nontuberculous mycobacteria, including *M. avium* complex, show variable susceptibility to RIF. RIF also is active against a broad array of other bacteria. Alteration of the target site on RNA polymerase, primarily through changes in the rpoB gene, leads to most forms of RIF resistance.

RIF is usually given orally, but it can also be given as a 30-minute IV infusion.[65,75,77] Patients with AIDS, diabetes, and other GI problems appear to have difficulty absorbing RIF after oral doses, which is associated with therapeutic failures in some cases. RIF is metabolized to 25-desacetylrifampin, which retains most of RIF's activity; most of RIF and its metabolite are cleared in the bile.

Elevations in hepatic enzymes have been attributed to RIF in 10% to 15% of patients, with overt hepatotoxicity occurring in less than 1%. More frequent adverse effects of RIF include rash, fever, and GI distress. Allergic reactions to RIF have been reported and occur more frequently with intermittent RIF doses $\geq$900 mg twice weekly. These reactions may take the form of a flu-like syndrome, with development of fever, chills, headache, arthralgias, and, rarely, hypotension and shock. Alternatively, hemolytic anemia or acute renal failure may occur, requiring permanent discontinuation.

RIF's potent induction of hepatic enzymes, especially CYP 3A4, may enhance the elimination of many other drugs, most notably the protease inhibitors used to treat HIV. This has lead to a rethinking of the regimens recommended for HIV-positive patients (Table 110–9).[78–80] Also, women who use oral contraceptives must use another form of contraception during therapy, because increased clearance of the hormones may lead to unexpected pregnancies. Patient records should be reviewed for potential drug interactions before dispensing RIF.[65] RIF may turn urine and other secretions orange-red and may permanently stain some types of contact lenses.

Other Rifamycins. Rifabutin (RBN), used primarily for disseminated *M. avium* infection in AIDS patients, also is quite active against *M. tuberculosis.* A very limited number of RIF-resistant organisms are susceptible to RBN, although most are resistant to all rifamycins. Because RBN is a less-potent enzyme inducer than RIF, it may be considered for patients receiving protease inhibitors.[78–80] Regimens that use mostly intermittent RBN (twice weekly) for TB are being investigated. Rifapentine is a long acting rifamycin also being studied for TB. It is approved for use in HIV-negative TB patients. It is about 85% as potent an enzyme inducer as RIF, so similar drug-interaction precautions must be taken.

Other First-Line Antituberculosis Drugs

After INH and RIF, all TB drugs are much weaker and, without INH and RIF, cannot effect a cure in less than 2 years. Judicious use of these drugs can, however, shorten the duration of treatment and prevent the development of drug resistance.

Pyrazinamide. Adding PZA to the first 2 months of treatment with INH and RIF shortens the duration to as little as 6 months. The drug can be used daily or intermittently, and it is used exclusively for TB. PZA is well absorbed after oral doses and is largely converted to pyrazinoic acid (active metabolite) and 5-hydroxypyrazinoic acid, which are subsequently excreted renally.[75,81] The most common toxicities of PZA are GI distress, arthralgias, and elevations in the serum uric acid concentrations. Most patients are free from gouty symptoms and do not require therapy for this laboratory "toxicity". Hepatotoxicity is the major limiting adverse effect, but it is far less common with current dosing regimens.

A fixed combination product (Rifater, Aventis) of RIF 120 mg, INH 50 mg, and PZA 300 mg is now available in the United States. It is designed to prevent drug resistance by keeping the self-medicating patient from using only one drug at a time. If the patient is receiving directly observed therapy, there is no particular advantage to this product. The typical daily dose of Rifater will be five to six tablets daily. When PZA is discontinued after 2 months of treatment, the combination product Rifamate (INH 150 mg and RIF 300 mg) can be substituted.

Ethambutol. EMB replaced PAS as a first-line agent in the 1960s because it was better tolerated by patients. EMB is used as a fourth drug for TB while awaiting susceptibility data. If the organism is susceptible to INH, RIF, and PZA, EMB can be stopped. EMB is active against most mycobacteria, including *M. tuberculosis* and *M. avium,* but it is generally bacteriostatic.

EMB displays adequate absorption after oral doses, but like RIF, appears to have variable absorption in patients with AIDS, diabetes, cystic fibrosis, and others with GI problems.[62,82] An IV form is available in Europe and can be obtained from the U.S. manufacturer under an investigational new drug application. The EMB dose should be reduced to three times per week in patients with renal failure.[60,83]

Retrobulbar neuritis is the major adverse effect noted in patients treated with EMB. Incidence is dose related, with occurrence rates of 5% or more in patients receiving daily doses of >30 mg/kg/d. Patients usually complain of a change in visual acuity, the inability to see the color green, or both. They should be monitored monthly while on the drug using Snellen wall charts for visual acuity and Ishihara red-green color discrimination cards. EMB is sometimes avoided in children because of the difficulty in monitoring visual acuity in this group; however, the drug appears to be safe even in this group.[37,84] Other adverse effects that may be observed include rash, fever, arthralgias, and GI irritation.

Streptomycin. SM is one of three aminoglycoside antibiotics (along with AK and KM) that are active against mycobacteria. SM is quite active against MAC and several other mycobacteria, *Enterococci, Brucella, Yersinia,* and various other bacteria. Like EMB, SM is used as a fourth drug for TB while awaiting susceptibility data or in cases of MDR-TB.

Although labeled only for IM dosing, SM (and CM) can be given safely as IV infusions (100 mL of dextrose 5% water or normal saline) over 30 minutes, similar to the other aminoglycosides.[85] SM, like other aminoglycosides, is renally cleared by glomerular filtration and must be given less often in patients with renal dysfunction.

SM occasionally causes nephrotoxicity, although it tends to be mild and reversible. It also is capable of causing ototoxicity (vestibular and cochlear), which may become permanent with continued use. SM is said to have more ototoxicity and less nephrotoxicity than other aminoglycosides, but this largely reflects different patterns of use. SM is given daily (12–15 mg/kg) or twice weekly (22–27 mg/kg) for several months, while other aminoglycosides are typically given in smaller doses every 8 to 24 hours for only 1 to 2 weeks. Toxicity profiles cannot be accurately compared from such divergent practices. Neuromuscular blockade has been reported to occur rarely with SM.

AK, KM, CM and VM share many features with SM, and the previous discussion also pertains to them. Resistance to amikacin and kanamycin are highly linked, but they are independent of resistance to SM, which is also independent of resistance to CM and VM. Therefore, susceptibility tests should guide the selection of these injectable drugs. Aminosidine (paromomycin) is also being studied for use against TB through an investigational new drug designed by the University of Illinois in Chicago.

Second-line Antituberculosis Drugs

Para-aminosalicylic Acid. PAS is a synthetic structural analog of aminobenzoic acid. In the United States, only the enteric-coated, sustained-release granule form (Paser) is available.[86–88] An IV form is available in Europe; if imported under an investigational new drug application, it is essential to test for the toxic breakdown product *m*-aminophenol before administering it to the patient. Both PAS and the *N*-acetyl metabolite are renally excreted. Traditionally, this drug was avoided in renal failure, although the basis for this is weak. PAS does not affect clotting time and generally should not alter symptoms of uremia. Therefore, PAS can be given cautiously to patients with renal failure.[61]

Gastrointestinal disturbances are the most common adverse effects from PAS. With the older dosage forms, nausea, vomiting, abdominal pain, and diarrhea were very common. The new Paser granules have offered significant relief from the nausea, vomiting, and abdominal pain; however, diarrhea remains a significant problem.[86] This diarrhea is usually self-limited, with symptoms improving after the first 1 to 2 weeks of therapy. Occasionally, a few doses of an opioid will resolve the problem. It is also important to tell the patient that the empty granules will appear in the stool. Although FDA approved for three daily doses, pharmacokinetic data support twice-daily dosing.[87]

Various types of malabsorption, including steatorrhea, were reported with previous dosage forms of PAS. Hypersensitivity may occur, and rarely, severe hepatitis. Mortality associated with PAS-induced hepatitis may be as high as 21%. PAS may cause a positive direct Coombs' test, which may lead to hemolytic anemia in patients with glucose-6-phosphate dehydrogenase deficiency. PAS is known to produce goiter, with or without myxedema, that seems to occur more frequently with concomitant therapy with ETA.

Cycloserine. CS has moderate activity versus *M. tuberculosis* and selected nontuberculous mycobacteria. It possesses marginal activity against other organisms, such as *Staphylococcus aureus* and some gram-negative bacilli, such as *Escherichia coli*. CS is well-absorbed orally and is best taken on an empty stomach.[88] It is cleared primarily through the kidneys by glomerular filtration, and requires dosage reduction in renal failure. CS can produce dose-related CNS toxicity, including lethargy, confusion, or unusual behavior. Seizures, although reported, are exceedingly rare. Therapy is vastly improved by maintaining 2-hour postdose serum concentrations between 20 and 35 μg/mL.[62] Most patients reach a maximum dose of 750 mg daily, divided unevenly into two doses. This can be achieved by starting CS 250 mg daily for 2 days, followed by 250-mg increments over 2-day intervals. This dose can be maintained if the patient complains of only occasional, mild CNS effects, such as difficulty concentrating. Serum concentrations can be checked 1 to 2 weeks into therapy. The addition of pyridoxine 50 mg daily may improve patient tolerance of cycloserine.

Ethionamide. ETA shares structural features with two other antimycobacterial agents—INH and, more distantly, thiacetazone. Prothionamide, the *n*-propyl derivative of ethionamide, is used in Europe. ETA is only active against organisms of the genus *Mycobacterium*, and it should be considered primarily bacteriostatic, as it is difficult to achieve serum concentrations that would be bactericidal.

Gastrointestinal toxicity is the dose-limiting adverse effect. The drug should be introduced gradually in 250-mg increments, as described earlier for CS. Rarely will a patient tolerate more than 1000 mg daily in divided oral doses. ETA may be administered with a light snack or prior to bedtime to minimize GI intolerance. Food does not affect the absorption of ETA significantly.[89] ETA suppositories, while better tolerated, produce serum concentrations that are approximately 50% of those achieved with oral doses. Little ETA is recovered in the urine, so doses remain the same in renal failure.

ETA is associated with hepatocellular injury and, rarely, with various CNS effects, such as headache, drowsiness, giddiness, depression, psychosis, peripheral neuritis, and visual disturbances. Other adverse effects include goiter, with or without hypothyroidism (especially when given with PAS), gynecomastia, alopecia, impotence, menorrhagia, photodermatitis, and acne. The management of diabetes may also be more difficult in patients receiving ETA.

Clofazimine. Clofazimine is a drug with good activity against *M. leprae* and weak activity against *M. tuberculosis* and *M. avium*. It is used in doses of 100–200 mg daily in advanced cases of MDR-TB or MAC, especially when therapeutic options are limited.[89,90] The drug has a terminal elimination half-life weeks long. Gastrointestinal distress and skin discoloration are the most important adverse reactions. Although uncommon, severe GI pain may occur because of deposition of clofazimine crystals within the intestines; this may require surgical correction.

Thiacetazone. Thiacetazone is a weak agent still used in parts of the developing world because of its low cost. Skin reactions, including rash and Stevens-Johnson syndrome, may occur; thiacetazone must be permanently discontinued as soon as a rash appears. Similar to trimethoprim-sulfamethoxazole, the incidence of skin reactions is much higher in AIDS patients.[91]

Quinolones. OFLOX, LEVO, CIPRO, and sparfloxacin have been used in the treatment of TB. They are bactericidal against extracellular *M. tuberculosis* and achieve good intracellular concentrations. These agents are also useful because most are available in both oral and IV dosage forms. OFLOX, and now LEVO, are generally favored over CIPRO because of higher serum concentrations in relationship to *in vitro* activity.[92,93] LEVO is twice as active as ofloxacin, and it may emerge as the preferred quinolone for MDR-TB. New quinolones, including moxifloxacin and gatifloxacin, have good activity against

M. tuberculosis and may evolve into acceptable TB drugs as experience is gained with them.

LEVO is renally cleared, and may be given three times weekly to patients on hemodialysis. CIPRO is both hepatically and renally cleared, and may be preferred in that situation. Adverse effects, including headache, dizziness, confusion, and caffeine-like effects, including insomnia, joint pain, GI distress, and dysuria. Limited experience suggests that these drugs may be used safely in children with MDR-TB. Sparfloxacin, while most active among quinolones in animal models, has dose-limiting adverse effects, including photosensitization and prolongation of the QTc interval. These toxicities make this agent less attractive compared to LEVO or CIPRO. The combination of OFLOX and PZA has been reported to have a higher than expected incidence of toxicity when used as chemoprophylaxis in patients exposed to MDR-TB. This may be idiosyncratic, or it may represent an interaction, such as competition for renal secretion between OFLOX and the PZA metabolites. LEVO would be expected to produce the same effects.

β-Lactam and β-Lactamase Inhibitor Combinations. The β-lactams have limited activity against mycobacteria because these organisms produce β-lactamases and because β-lactams fail to enter macrophages.[94] Cefoxitin, a β-lactamase-stable cephalosporin, has useful activity against rapidly growing mycobacteria, such as *M. fortuitum* and *M. chelonae*. Combinations of β-lactams with β-lactamase inhibitors have been used in salvage regimens for patients with no other options.

Macrolides/Azalides. The macrolide, clarithromycin, and azalide, azithromycin, represent substantial advances in the treatment of *M. avium* complex, but demonstrate limited activity against *M. tuberculosis,* and are infrequently used for TB.

New Drugs and Delivery Systems. The 5-nitroimidazoles, including the new compound PA 824, are chemically related to metronidazole and tinidazole.[95] This class, along with the oxazolidinones may produce useful agents for TB. Linezolid has been used in a few patients with TB.[96] Long-term use of linezolid requires careful monitoring of hematologic indices. Chemical modification of existing compounds, such as PZA, may produce new TB drugs. Finally, continuing research on the construction of the mycobacterial cell wall and intracellular pathways may lead to agents with unique activity against this genus.

Liposomes have been investigated as delivery systems for various agents against mycobacteria, including INH, RIF, and the aminoglycosides. Liposomes could also be used to deliver β lactams or other agents that are generally excluded from macrophages. By changing the pharmacokinetic profile of such agents, their use in the treatment of mycobacterial infections could be greatly enhanced.

Corticosteroids. Adjunctive therapy with corticosteroids may be of benefit in some patients with tuberculous meningitis or pericarditis to relieve inflammation and pressure.[97] They should be avoided in most other circumstances, as they detract from the immune response to TB.

Bacille Calmette-Guérin Vaccine. The BCG vaccine is an attenuated, hybridized strain of *M. bovis*. It was originally developed in 1921 and is used as a prophylactic vaccine against TB. Administration of BCG vaccine is compulsory in many developing countries and is officially recommended in many others. Vaccination with BCG produces a subclinical infection resulting in sensitization of T lymphocytes and cross-immunity to *M. tuberculosis,* as well as cutaneous hypersensitivity and, in many cases, a positive tuberculin skin test.

In the published clinical trials, several different BCG preparations were used, and the efficacy of these vaccinations ranged from negative 56% (some patients did worse with the vaccine) to positive 80%.[2] Trials within the United States and Puerto Rico show efficacy rates of 6% to 29%. The primary benefit of BCG vaccination appears to be the prevention of severe forms of TB in children. Data from the BCG trials show that the incidence of tuberculous meningitis and miliary TB is 52% to 100% lower and that the incidence of pulmonary TB is 2% to 80% lower in vaccinated children younger than 15 years of age than it was in unvaccinated controls.

Unfortunately, BCG does not appear to be very reliable in preventing disease by *M. tuberculosis* in other segments of the population. Side effects occur in 1% to 10% of vaccinated persons and usually include severe or prolonged ulceration at the vaccination site, lymphadenitis, and lupus vulgaris. It is recommended that pregnant women and patients with impaired immune systems, including those with HIV infection, avoid vaccination. The World Health Organization (WHO) recommends, however, that in populations where the risk of TB is high, HIV-infected infants who are asymptomatic should receive BCG vaccine at birth or as soon as possible thereafter. Because BCG infection has occurred in AIDS patients given the vaccine, individuals with symptomatic HIV infection should not be vaccinated.[2]

In the United States, BCG vaccination is recommended only for uninfected children who are at unavoidable risk of exposure to TB and for whom other methods of prevention and control have failed or are not feasible.[2] Its use is very limited.

PHARMACOECONOMIC CONSIDERATIONS

The WHO and the World Bank agree that the control of TB is one of the most cost-effective health interventions that any nation can pursue. Early identification of TB cases and the effective use of INH, RIF, PZA (plus EMB or SM) while the isolate is still drug-susceptible should always be the primary goals of public health departments. Contact investigation and treatment of those infected but without disease are important secondary goals to reduce the number of future cases.

Patients who complete all of their treatment for drug-susceptible TB have cure rates approaching 100%. Noncompliance (nonadherence), drug resistance, extrapulmonary disease, and concomitant disease states reduce the overall effectiveness of chemotherapy of TB to about 75%.

The treatment of TB is not particularly expensive, especially if hospitalization is not required.[98] Furthermore, TB is quite curable. Because the various TB drugs each have a role to play in the treatment of TB or MDR-TB, all of the FDA-approved antituberculosis drugs should be on institutional formularies. Centers that see little MDR-TB need not keep stocks of the second-line drugs, provided that they are readily available should the need arise. Because the treatment of MDR-TB is difficult, and because missteps are potentially disastrous, such patients should be referred to centers experienced in the management of MDR-TB.[99,100]

EVALUATION OF THERAPEUTIC OUTCOMES

MONITORING OF THE PHARMACEUTICAL CARE PLAN

The most serious problem with TB therapy is patient nonadherence to the prescribed regimens.[101–104] Unfortunately, there is no reliable way to identify such patients a priori. In the study by Brudney and Dobkin, 89% of the patients were noncompliant with therapy.[103] It is critical to the control of TB that adherence rates be dramatically improved. The most effective way to achieve this end is with directly observed therapy.[45,46,57] Despite criticisms that it will cost more money, it is far cheaper in the long run to prevent the further spread of disease with directly observed therapy than it is to continuously track down and treat additional cases of TB.

It is assumed that the homeless and other underprivileged individuals constitute the group of patients considered "unreliable" and that directly observed therapy should be reserved for them; it is also assumed that "responsible" patients cared for by private physicians may be treated with daily, unsupervised therapy. A study conducted in Baltimore, MD, however, compared outcomes (sputum culture conversion to negative at 3 months) in patients with pulmonary TB who were treated by private physicians with outcomes in patients treated via directly observed therapy in a city-run clinic. Surprisingly, 3-month culture conversion occurred in only 40% of the private-care patients, as compared to 90% in the city-clinic-care patients.[105] Clearly, expansion of the use of directly observed therapy to nearly all patients with TB may be beneficial.

Patients should have sputum samples sent for AFB stains every few days until smears are negative. This may take 10 to 14 days. After the patient is consistently smear negative, the patient may be removed from isolation and, if symptomatically improved, discharged from the hospital. Once on maintenance therapy, sputum cultures can be performed monthly until negative, which generally occurs within 2 months. If sputum cultures continue to be positive after 2 months, drug susceptibility testing should be repeated, and serum concentrations of the drugs should be checked.

Serum chemistries, including blood urea nitrogen (BUN), creatinine, aspartate transaminase (AST), and alanine transaminase (ALT), and a complete blood count with platelets may be performed at baseline and periodically thereafter, depending on the presence of other factors that may increase the likelihood of toxicity (advanced age, alcohol abuse, pregnancy). Hepatotoxicity should be suspected in patients whose transaminases exceed five times the upper limit of normal or whose total bilirubin exceeds 3 mg/dL. At this point, the offending agent(s) should be discontinued. Sequential reintroduction of the drugs with frequent testing of liver enzymes is often successful in identifying the offending agent; other agents may be continued. Alternative agents should be selected as needed. Audiometric testing should be performed at baseline and monthly in patients who must receive SM for more than 1 to 2 months. Vision testing should be performed on all patients who receive EMB. All patients diagnosed with TB should be tested for HIV infection.

THERAPEUTIC DRUG MONITORING

Therapeutic drug monitoring, or applied pharmacokinetics, is the use of serum drug concentrations to optimize therapy.[2,62,69] Non-AIDS patients with drug-susceptible TB generally do well, and therapeutic drug monitoring should only be used if these patients are failing appropriate directly observed therapy (no clinical improvement after 2 to 4 weeks or smear positive after 4 to 6 weeks). On the other hand, patients with AIDS, diabetes, cystic fibrosis, and various GI disorders often fail to absorb these drugs properly and are candidates for therapeutic drug monitoring. Also, patients with hepatic or renal disease should be monitored, given their potential for overdoses.

In the treatment of MDR-TB, the differences between the Cmax and MIC for the second-line agents are much smaller that with INH and RIF. Therefore, alterations in the absorption of these drugs can have significant impact on the outcome of therapy.[62] Although the optimal serum concentrations for TB are not known, target serum peak concentrations have been proposed.[62] Blood collected at 2 and 6 hours postdose have been used with some success, although they may not be the optimal sampling times for all of the drugs. Long half-life drugs (PZA, CS, LEVO) can be sampled at 2 and 10 hours if an estimate of the half-life is desired.[60] Finally, therapeutic drug monitoring of the TB and HIV drugs is perhaps the most logical way to untangle the complex drug interactions that take place (Tables 110–11 and 110–12).[106]

CONCLUSIONS

Good patient compliance is the cornerstone to effective antimycobacterial chemotherapy. Pharmacists should monitor TB therapy with particular interest in drug-drug interactions, drug malabsorption, and avoiding the error of adding a single drug to a failing regimen. They should educate patients on the importance of continuing their chemotherapy, despite symptomatic improvement. Pharmacists should become part of a multidisciplinary team (with nurses, physicians, social workers) devoted to successful chemotherapy of TB patients and their families.

TABLE 110–11. Effects of Coadministration of Rifamycins (Rifabutin, Rifampin) and HIV-1 Protease Inhibitors (PI) on the Systemic Exposure (AUC) of Each Drug, Expressed as a Percentage Change in AUC of the Concomitant Treatment Relative to That of the Drug-Alone Treatment

	Rifabutin		Rifampin	
Protease Inhibitor (PI)	Effect of Rifabutin on PI	Effect of PI on Rifabutin	Effect of Rifampin on PI	Effect of PI on Rifampin
Saquinavir	↓ 45%	NR	↓ 80%	NR
Ritonavir[a]	NR	↑ 293%	↓ 35%	Unchanged
Indinavir	↓ 34%	↑ 173%	↓ 92%	NR
Nelfinavir	↓ 32%	↑ 207%	↓ 82%	NR
Amprenavir	↓ 14%	↑ 200%	↓ 81%	NR

[a]Data from only two subjects. NR = Not reported.

Adapted from Burman WJ, Gallicano K, Peloquin C. Clin Infect Dis 1999;28:419–430. With permission.

TABLE 110–12. Effects of Coadministration of Rifamycins (Rifabutin, Rifampin) and Currently Approved Nonnucleoside Reverse Transcriptase Inhibitors (NNRTIs) on the (AUC) of Each Drug

	Rifabutin		Rifampin	
NNRTI	Effect of Rifabutin on NNRTI	Effect of NNRTI on Rifabutin (predicted)[a]	Effect of Rifampin on NNRTI	Effect of NNRTI on Rifampin (predicted)[a]
Nevirapine	↓ 16%	NR (↓)	↓ 37%	NR(unchanged)
Delavirdine	↓ 80%	↑ 342%	↓ 96%	Unchanged
Efavirenz	↓ 10%	↓ 38%	↓ 13%	Unchanged

[a]Predicted using existing knowledge regarding metabolic pathways for the two drugs.
NR = Not reported.
Adapted from Burman WJ, Gallicano K, Peloquin C. Clin Infect Dis 1999;28:419–430. With permission.

▶ PRINCIPLES OF PHARMACOTHERAPY

- TB is the most prevalent communicable infectious disease on earth.
- In the United States, TB disproportionately affects ethnic minorities as compared to whites.
- Coinfection with HIV and TB accelerates the progression of both diseases, thus requiring rapid diagnosis and treatment of both diseases.
- Mycobacteria are slow-growing organisms; in the laboratory, they require special stains, special growth media, and long periods of incubation.
- TB can produce atypical signs and symptoms in infants and immunocompromised hosts, and it can progress rapidly in these patients.
- Latent TB infection can lead to reactivation disease years after the primary infection occurred.
- Patients suspected of having active TB disease must be isolated until the diagnosis is confirmed and they are no longer contagious.
- Isoniazid and rifampin are the two most important TB drugs; organisms resistant to both of these drugs (MDR-TB) are much more difficult to treat.
- Never add a single drug to a failing regimen.
- Directly observed treatment should be used whenever possible to reduce treatment failures and the selection of drug-resistant isolates.

ACKNOWLEDGMENT

This chapter is based on earlier editions written by Steve C. Ebert, Pharm.D.

REFERENCES

1. WHO Report on the Global Tuberculosis Epidemic 1998.
2. Peloquin CA, Berning SE. Infections due to *Mycobacterium tuberculosis*. Ann Pharmacother 1994;28:72–84.
3. Stead WW. The origin and erratic global spread of tuberculosis. Clin Chest Med 1997;18:65–77.
4. McCray E, Weinbaum CM, Braden CR, Onorato IM. The epidemiology of tuberculosis in the United States. Clin Chest Med 1997;18:99–113.
5. Centers for Disease Control and Prevention. Reported Tuberculosis in the United States, 1999. August, 2000:1–57.
6. Haas DW, Des Prez RM. Mycobacterium tuberculosis. In: Mandell GL, Bennett JE, Dolin R, eds. Principles and Practice of Infectious Diseases, 4th ed. New York, John Wiley, 1995:2213–2243.
7. Bentley DW. Tuberculosis in long-term care facilities. Infect Control Hosp Epidemiol 1990;11:42–46.
8. Fennelly KP. Personal respiratory protection against *Mycobacterium tuberculosis*. Clin Chest Med 1997;18:1–17.
9. Davis YM, McCray E, Simone PM. Personal respiratory protection against *Mycobacterium tuberculosis*. Clin Chest Med 1997;18:19–33.
10. Rosenblum LS, Castro KG, Dooley S, Morgan M. Effect of HIV infection and tuberculosis on hospitalizations and cost of care for young adults in the United States, 1985 to 1990. Ann Intern Med 1994;121:786–792.
11. Small PM, Shafer RW, Hopewell PC, et al. Exogenous reinfection with multidrug-resistant Mycobacterium tuberculosis in patients with advanced HIV infection. N Engl J Med 1993;328:1137–1144.
12. Beck-Sague C, Dooley SW, Hutton MD, et al. Hospital outbreak of multidrug-resistant *Mycobacterium tuberculosis* infections: Factors in transmission to staff and HIV-infected patients. JAMA 1992;268:1280–1286.
13. Centers for Disease Control and Prevention. Meeting the challenge of multidrug-resistant tuberculosis: Summary of a conference. MMWR Morb Mortal Wkly Rep 1992;41(R-11):51–71.
14. Heifets L. Mycobacteriology laboratory. Clin Chest Med 1997;18:35–53.
15. Heifets LB. Drug susceptibility tests in the management of chemotherapy of tuberculosis. In: Heifets LB, ed. Drug Susceptibility in the Chemotherapy of Mycobacterial Infections. Boca Raton, FL, CRC Press, 1991:89–122.
16. Roberts GD, Böttger EC, Stockman L. Methods for the rapid identification of mycobacterial species. Clin Lab Med 1996;16:603–615.
17. Sandin RL. Polymerase chain reaction and other amplification techniques in mycobacteriology. Clin Lab Med 1996;16:617–39.
18. Riley RL, Mills CC, Nyka W, et al. Aerial dissemination of pulmonary tuberculosis: A two-year study of contagion in a tuberculosis ward. Am J Hygiene 1959;70:185–196.
19. Orme IM, Andersen P, Boom WH. T cell response to Mycobacterium tuberculosis. J Infect Dis 1993;167:1481–1497.
20. Haque AK. The pathology and pathophysiology of mycobacterial infections. J Thorac Imag 1990;5:8–16.
21. American Thoracic Society. Diagnostic standards and classification of tuberculosis in adults and children. Am J Respir Crit Care Med 2000;161:1376–1395.
22. Peloquin CA, Berning SE. Tuberculosis and multi-drug resistant tuberculosis in children. Pediatr Nurs 1995;21:566–572.
23. Correa AG. Unique aspects of tuberculosis in the pediatric population. Clin Chest Med 1997;18:89–98.
24. Kleinhenz ME, Ellner JJ. Antigen responsiveness during tuberculosis: Regulatory interactions of T cell subpopulations and adherent cells. J Lab Clin Med 1987;110:31–40.

25. American Thoracic Society. Targeted tuberculin skin testing and treatment of latent tuberculosis infection. Am J Respir Crit Care Med 2000;161:S221–S247.
26. Alland D, Kalkut GE, Moss AR, et al. Transmission of tuberculosis in New York City: An analysis of DNA fingerprinting and conventional epidemiologic methods. N Engl J Med 1994;330:1710–1716.
27. Small PM, Hopewell PC, Singh SP, et al. The epidemiology of tuberculosis in San Francisco: A population-based study using conventional and molecular methods. N Engl J Med 1994;330:1703–1709.
28. Daley CL, Small PM, Schecter GF, et al. An outbreak of tuberculosis with accelerated progression among persons infected with the human immunodeficiency virus: An analysis using restricted-fragment-length polymorphisms. N Engl J Med 1992;326:231–235.
29. Wallis RS, Vjecha M, Amir-Tahmasseb M, et al. Influence of tuberculosis on human immunodeficiency virus (HIV-1): Enhanced cytokine expression and elevated beta-2-microglobulin in HIV-1-associated tuberculosis. J Infect Dis 1993;167:43–48.
30. Pape JW, Jean SS, Ho JL, et al. Effect of isoniazid prophylaxis on incidence of active tuberculosis and progression of HIV infection. Lancet 1993;342:268–272.
31. Barnes PF, Bloch AB, Davidson PT, Snider DE. Tuberculosis in patients with human immunodeficiency virus infection. N Engl J Med 1991;324:1644–1650.
32. American Thoracic Society/Centers for Disease Control and Prevention. Joint statement: Mycobacterioses and the acquired immunodeficiency syndrome. Am Rev Respir Dis 1987;136:492–496.
33. Cohn DL, Dobkin JF. Treatment and prevention of tuberculosis in HIV infection. AIDS 1993;7(suppl 1):S195–S202.
34. Snider DE. Recognition and elimination of tuberculosis. Adv Intern Med 1993;38:169–187.
35. Alvarez S, Shell C, Berk SL. Pulmonary tuberculosis in elderly men. Am J Med 1987;82:602–606.
36. Umeki S. Comparison of younger and elderly patients with pulmonary tuberculosis. Respiration 1989;55:75–83.
37. Starke JR. Multidrug therapy for tuberculosis in children. Pediatr Infect Dis J 1990;9:785–793.
38. American Thoracic Society/Centers for Disease Control and Prevention. Joint statement: Control of tuberculosis in the United States. Am Rev Respir Dis 1992;146:1623–1633.
39. Centers for Disease Control and Prevention. Management of persons exposed to multidrug-resistant tuberculosis. MMWR Morb Mortal Wkly Rep 1992;41:61–71.
40. Centers for Disease Control and Prevention. Anergy skin testing and preventive therapy for HIV-infected persons: Revised recommendations. MMWR Morb Mortal Wkly Rep 1997;46(RR-15):1–10.
41. Sbarbaro JA. Skin testing in the diagnosis of tuberculosis. Semin Respir Infect 1986;1:234–238.
42. Rosenberg T, Manfreda J, Hershfield ES. Two-step tuberculin testing in staff and residents of a nursing home. Am Rev Resp Dis 1993;148:1537–1540.
43. Barnes PE, Steele MA, Young SMM, Vachon LA. Tuberculosis in patients with human immunodeficiency virus infection: How often does it mimic *Pneumocystis carinii* pneumonia? Chest 1992;102:428–432.
44. Bouza E, Diaz-Lopez MD, Moreno S, et al. Mycobacterium tuberculosis bacteremia in patients with and without human immunodeficiency virus infection. Arch Intern Med 1993;153:496–500.
45. Fujiwara PI, Larkin C, Frieden TR. Directly observed therapy in New York City. Clin Chest Med 1997;18:135–148.
46. Weis SE. Universal directly observed therapy. Clin Chest Med 1997; 18:155–163.
47. Mitchison DA. Basic mechanisms of chemotherapy. Chest 1979;76 (suppl):771–781.
48. Bishai WR, Chaisson RE. Short-course chemoprophylaxis for tuberculosis. Clin Chest Med 1997;18:115–122.
49. Comstock GW, Woolpert SH. Prophylaxis. In: Schlossberg D, ed. Tuberculosis, 2nd ed. New York, Springer-Verlag, 1986:55–59.
50. Comstock GW. Evaluating isoniazid preventive therapy: The need for more data. Ann Intern Med 1981;94:817–819.
51. Snider DE. Decision analysis for isoniazid preventive therapy: Take it or leave it? Am Rev Respir Dis 1988;137:2–4.
52. Peloquin CA, Iseman MD. Antimycobacterial agents. In: Root RK, ed. Clinical Infectious Diseases: A Practical Approach. New York, Oxford University Press, 1999; p327–35.
53. Stead WW, To T, Harrison RW, et al. Benefit-risk considerations in preventive treatment for tuberculosis in elderly persons. Ann Intern Med 1987;107:843–845.
54. Goble M. Drug-resistant tuberculosis. Semin Respir Infect 1986;1:220–229.
55. Centers for Disease Control and Prevention. Initial therapy for tuberculosis in the era of multidrug resistance. MMWR Morb Mortal Wkly Rep 1993;42(RR-7):1–8.
56. Peloquin CA. Antituberculosis drugs: Pharmacokinetics. In: Heifets LB, ed. Drug Susceptibility in the Chemotherapy of Mycobacterial Infections. Boca Raton, FL, CRC Press, 1991:59–88.
57. American Thoracic Society. Treatment of tuberculosis and tuberculosis infection in adults and children. Am J Respir Crit Care Med 1994; 149:1359–1374.
58. Hamadeh MA, Glassroth J. Tuberculosis and pregnancy. Chest 1992;101:1114–1120.
59. Vallejo JG, Starke JR. Tuberculosis and pregnancy. Clin Chest Med 1992;13:693–707.
60. Malone RS, Fish DN, Spiegel DM, Childs JM, Peloquin CA. The effect of hemodialysis on isoniazid, rifampin, pyrazinamide, and ethambutol. Am J Respir Crit Care Med 1999;159:1580–1584.
61. Malone RS, Fish DN, Spiegel DM, Childs JM, Peloquin CA. The effect of hemodialysis on cycloserine, ethionamide, para-aminosalicylate, and clofazimine. Chest 1999;116:984–990.
62. Peloquin CA. Using therapeutic drug monitoring to dose the antimycobacterial drugs. Clin Chest Med 1997;18:79–87.
63. Offe HA. Historical introduction and chemical characteristics of antituberculosis drugs. In: Bartmann K, ed. Antituberculosis Drugs. Berlin, Springer-Verlag, 1988:1–30.
64. Kucers A, Bennett N McK, eds. The Use of Antibiotics, 4th ed. Philadelphia, Lippincott, 1988.
65. McEvoy GK, ed. AHFS Drug Information. American Soc Health-Systems Pharmacists, Bethesda, MD, 2000.
66. Yu VL, Merigan TC, Barriere S, White NJ, eds. Antimicrobial Chemotherapy. Baltimore, MD, Williams and Wilkins, 1998.
67. Girling DJ. Adverse effects of antituberculous drugs. Drugs 1982;23: 56–74.
68. Holdiness MR. Clinical pharmacokinetics of the antituberculosis drugs. Clin Pharmacokinet 1984;9:511–544.
69. Peloquin CA. Pharmacology of the antimycobacterial drugs. Med Clin North Am 1993;77:1253–1262.
70. Blanchard JS. Molecular mechanisms of drug resistance in *Mycobacterium tuberculosis*. Ann Rev Biochem 1996;65:215–239.
71. Verbist L. Mode of action of antituberculous drugs: I. Medicon Intl 1974;3:11–23.
72. Verbist L. Mode of action of antituberculous drugs: II. Medicon Intl 1979;3:3–17.
73. Winder FG. Mode of action of the antimycobacterial agents and associated aspects of the molecular biology of the mycobacteria. In: Ratledge C, Stanford J, eds. The Biology of Mycobacteria: Vol 1. Physiology, Identification, and Classification. London, Academic Press, 1982: 353–438.
74. Crabbe SJ. Drug infosearch—Intravenous isoniazid. P&T 1990;15: 1483–1484.
75. Peloquin CA, Jaresko GS, Yong CL, Keung ACF, Bulpitt AE, Jelliffe RW. Population pharmacokinetic modeling of isoniazid, rifampin, and pyrazinamide. Antimicrob Agents Chemother 1997;41:2670–2679.
76. Peloquin CA, Namdar R, Dodge AA, Nix DE. Pharmacokinetics of isoniazid under fasting conditions, with food, and with antacids. Int J Tuberc Lung Dis 1999;3:703–710.
77. Peloquin CA, Namdar R, Singleton MD, Nix DE. Pharmacokinetics of rifampin under fasting conditions, with food, and with antacids. Chest 1999;115:12–18.

78. Centers for Disease Control and Prevention. Prevention and treatment of tuberculosis among patients infected with human immunodeficiency virus: Principles of therapy and revised recommendations. MMWR Morb Mortal Wkly Rep 1998;47(No. RR-20):1–58.
79. Centers for Disease Control and Prevention. Updated guidelines for the use of rifabutin or rifampin for the treatment and prevention of tuberculosis among HIV-infected patients taking protease inhibitors on nonnucleoside reverse transcriptase inhibitors. MMWR Morb Mortal Wkly Rep 2000;49:185–189.
80. Burman WJ, Gallicano K, Peloquin CA. Therapeutic implications of drug interactions in the treatment of HIV-related tuberculosis. Clin Infect Dis 1999;28:419–430.
81. Peloquin CA, Bulpitt AE, Jaresko GS, Jelliffe RW, James GT, Nix DE. Pharmacokinetics of pyrazinamide under fasting conditions, with food, and with antacids. Pharmacotherapy 1998;18:1205–1211.
82. Peloquin CA, Bulpitt AE, Jaresko GS, Jelliffe RW, Childs JM, Nix DE. Pharmacokinetics of ethambutol under fasting conditions, with food, and with antacids. Antimicrob Agents Chemother 1999;43:568–572.
83. Summers KK, Hardin TC. Treatment of tuberculosis in hemodialysis patients. J Infect Dis Pharmacother 1996;2:37–55.
84. Trébucq A. Should ethambutol be recommended for routine treatment of tuberculosis in children? A review of the literature. Int J Tuberc Lung Dis 1997;1:12–15.
85. Peloquin CA, Berning SE. Comment: Intravenous streptomycin. Ann Pharmacother 1993;27:1546–1547. Letter.
86. Peloquin CA, Henshaw TL, Huitt GA, Berning, SE, Nitta AT, James GT. Pharmacokinetic evaluation of *p*-aminosalicylic acid granules [correction: Pharmacotherapy 1994;14(4):2]. Pharmacotherapy 1994;14: 40–46.
87. Peloquin CA, Berning SE, Huitt GA, Childs JM, Singleton MD, James GT. Once-daily and twice-daily dosing of *p*-aminosalicylic acid (PAS) granules. Am J Respir Crit Care Med 1999;159:932–934.
88. Peloquin CA, Zhu M, Nix DE. Effect of food and antacids on cycloserine and *p*-aminosalicylic acid pharmacokinetics. Abstract, 40 Interscience Conference on Antimicrobial Agents and Chemotherapy, Toronto, CA, September 17–20, 2000.
89. Peloquin CA, Auclair B, Nix DE. Effect of food and antacids on ethionamide (ETA) and clofazimine (CF) pharmacokinetics (PK). Abstract, 39th Interscience Conference on Antimicrobial Agents and Chemotherapy, San Francisco, CA, September 26–29, 1999, and National Jewish Medical and Research Center Centennial Festschrift Celebration, Denver, CO, October 1, 1999.
90. Garrelts J. Clofazimine: A review of its use in leprosy and Mycobacterium avium complex infection. Ann Pharmacother 1991;25:525–531.
91. Elliott AM, Foster SD. Thiacetazone: Time to call a halt? Tuber Lung Dis 1996;77:27–29.
92. Berning SE, Madsen L, Iseman MD, Peloquin CA. Long-term safety of ofloxacin and ciprofloxacin in the treatment of mycobacterial infections. Am J Respir Crit Care Med 1995;151:2006–2009.
93. Peloquin CA, Berning SE, Madsen L, Iseman MD. Ofloxacin and ciprofloxacin in the treatment of mycobacterial infections: Development of resistance and drug interactions. J Infect Dis Pharmacother 1995;1:45–65.
94. Zhang Y, Steingrube VA, Wallace RJ. Beta-lactamase inhibitors and the inducibility of the beta-lactamase of *Mycobacterium tuberculosis*. Am Rev Resp Dis 1992;145:657–660.
95. Stover CK, Warrener P, VanDevanter DR, et al. A small-molecule nitroimidazopyran drug candidate for the treatment of tuberculosis. Nature 2000;405:962–966.
96. Clemett D, Markham A. Linezolid. Drugs 2000;59:815–827.
97. Kaojarern S, Supmonchai K, Phuapradit P, et al. Effect of steroids on cerebrospinal fluid penetration of antituberculous agents in tuberculous meningitis. Clin Pharmacol Ther 1991;49:6–12.
98. Reves R, Burman W, Dalton C, et al. A cost-effectiveness analysis of directly observed therapy versus self-administered therapy for treatment of tuberculosis. Am J Resp Crit Care Med 1997;155(suppl):A33. Abstract.
99. Goble M, Iseman MD, Madsen LA, et al. Treatment of 171 patients with pulmonary tuberculosis resistant to isoniazid and rifampin. N Engl J Med 1993;328:527–532.
100. Iseman MD. Treatment of multidrug-resistant tuberculosis. N Engl J Med 1993;329:784–791.
101. Bloch AB, Cauthen GM, Onorato IM, et al. Nationwide survey of drug-resistant tuberculosis in the United States. JAMA 1994;271:665–671.
102. Frieden TR, Sterling T, Pablos-Mendez A, et al. The emergence of drug-resistant tuberculosis in New York City. N Engl J Med 1993;328:521–526.
103. Brudney K, Dobkin J. Resurgent tuberculosis in New York City: Human immunodeficiency virus, homelessness, and the decline of tuberculosis control programs. Am Rev Resp Dis 1991;144:745–749.
104. Mahmoudi A, Iseman MD. Pitfalls in the care of patients with tuberculosis: Common errors and their association with the acquisition of drug resistance. JAMA 1993;270:65–68.
105. Chaulk CP, Bartlett JG, Chaisson RE. 15 years of directly observed therapy for TB. Program and Abstracts, 32nd Annual Meeting, Infectious Diseases Society of America, Orlando, FL, October 7–9, 1994. Abstract 181.
106. Peloquin CA. Agents for tuberculosis. In: Piscitelli SC, Rodvold KA, eds. Drug Interactions in Infectious Diseases. Totowa, NJ, Humana Press, 2001:109–120.

111

Gastrointestinal Infections and Enterotoxigenic Poisonings

J.D. Anderson, Todd D. Lemke, Laura J. Odell, and Tom A. Larson

Collectively, gastrointestinal (GI) infections are among the more common causes of morbidity and mortality around the world. In underdeveloped and developing countries, dehydrating diarrhea is the leading cause of death in infants and children under 5 years of age. The prevalence of diarrhea is estimated to be 3 to 5 billion cases per year and results in as many as 10 million deaths per year.[1] Developed countries, including the United States, are not isolated from diarrheal illness. Diarrhea is responsible for approximately 10% of hospitalizations in children younger than 5 years of age, or approximately 220,000 admissions per year. Between 300 and 500 children in the United States die each year from dehydration caused by diarrhea.[2–4] These figures underscore the severity of diarrhea in children and the urgency for timely reversal of progressive dehydration.

Children are at increased risk of dying from diarrheal illness because of the high turnover of body fluid proportional to body weight, but other groups are at risk as well. These groups include travelers and campers, immunocompromised patients, such as those with AIDS, patients in chronic care facilities, and military personnel assigned overseas. The elderly are also at increased risk because of decreased immune function, achlorhydria, and colonic dysmotility.

Because of the self-limited nature of infectious diarrhea after appropriate rehydration and the economic burden of identification, the infectious agents often go unidentified. Bacteria, viruses, and protozoans account for the vast majority of infectious diarrhea. This chapter focuses on the bacterial and viral etiologies of GI infections and their treatment.

REHYDRATION THERAPY

Fluid replacement is the cornerstone of therapy for diarrhea regardless of etiology. Infection may require specific antimicrobial therapy in certain cases (Table 111–1). Initial assessment of fluid loss is essential for rehydration; however, an accurate baseline weight may not be available. Weight loss is the most reliable means of determining the extent of water loss. Clinical signs can be helpful in determining approximate deficits[5] (Table 111–2). Electrolyte levels should be measured. Physical assessment is generally more reliable in young children and infants than in adults.

Glucose-based oral rehydration therapy (ORT) is able to reverse dehydration in nearly all cases of mild-to-moderate diarrhea.[6] Treatment failure is infrequent (3% to 6%).[7] Oral rehydration therapy offers the advantages of being inexpensive, noninvasive, and does not require hospitalization to administer. Glucose-based ORT generally does not decrease the duration of diarrhea or stool volume, but it does prevent dehydration, which is responsible for most diarrheal deaths.[8,9] Fluid loss greater than 10% of body water is considered severe and requires intravenous (IV) fluid replacement with Ringer lactate or normal saline. IV therapy is also indicated in patients with uncontrolled vomiting, presence of a paralytic ileus, stool output greater than 10 mL/kg/h, shock, or loss of consciousness.[7] Rapid IV rehydration is preferred over more prolonged deficit replacement regimens for restoring extracellular fluids and electrolytes, as it more effectively reestablishes gastrointestinal and renal perfusion.[10] Table 111–2 summarizes fluid replacement guidelines for each dehydration category.

The necessary components of ORT solutions include glucose, sodium, potassium, chloride, and water (Table 111–3). Oral rehydration therapy takes advantage of glucose-coupled sodium transport in the small bowel. Glucose enhances sodium, and subsequently, water transport across intestinal walls. Glucose concentrations greater than 5% may produce an osmotic diarrhea. Low osmolarity ORT solutions (rice- or cereal-based) reduce the diarrhea stool number, volume, and frequency, as well as the duration of diarrhea and the ORT solution volume requirements when compared with isotonic high-glucose ORT solutions similar to the World Health Organization (WHO) formulation.[9,11–13] The efficacy of rice-based ORT solutions may be in part a result of their hypotonicity, which promotes intestinal water absorption.[12,14] Also, slow rice hydrolysis allows some rice (glucose) absorption to take place before hydrolysis occurs. Starch and simple proteins provide more cotransport molecules with little osmotic penalty, thus increasing fluid and electrolyte uptake by enterocytes and reducing stool losses.[15] Therefore, a larger carbohydrate load can be given with rice solutions, resulting in a greater nutritional advantage.[11,14] Amylase-resistant starch added to standard ORT shortened the duration of diarrhea in cholera patients as compared to standard ORT and rice-based ORT.[16] Human breast milk, cow's milk, glycine, soy fiber formulas, and cereal preparations have been used successfully as rehydration substrates.[17–19]

Sodium content for oral replacement solutions should be between 50 and 90 mEq/L for initial rehydration. The American Academy of Pediatrics (AAP) recommends rehydration with a more electrolyte-concentrated rehydration phase and a subsequent maintenance phase using the more dilute solutions and larger volume (Table 111–2).[15] In children with vomiting and diarrhea, ORT may be given as 5 mL every 2 to 3 minutes in a teaspoon or oral syringe. Nasogastric administration of ORT is an alternative method of administration in a child with persistent vomiting.[12] Maintenance rehydration requires sodium concentrations between 40 and 60 mEq/L. Oral rehydration therapy solutions with high sodium content may be alternated with water if a low sodium fluid is not available. The maintenance phase should provide 100–150 mL/kg/d plus additional replacement for stool losses. Traditional clear fluids, such as soda, apple juice, broth, and Gatorade are hyperosmolar solutions that may draw free water into the gut lumen and cause hypernatremia. Use of these solutions should be avoided.

Early refeeding as tolerated is recommended.[3,5,20,21] The AAP guidelines recommend age-appropriate diet resumption as soon as dehydration is corrected.[15] Breast milk, lactose-free soy formula, and cow's milk-based formulas can often be continued.[20] Early initiation of feeding has shortened the course of diarrhea. In a study of severely malnourished children under 5 years of age with diarrhea,

TABLE 111–1. Antibiotic Selection

Organism	First Choice	Alternatives
Campylobacter	Macrolides, fluoroquinolones	Tetracyclines, chloramphenicol, clindamycin, aminoglycosides
C. difficile	Metronidazole	Vancomycin, bacitracin
E. coli	TMP/SMX[a,b], fluoroquinolones	Aminoglycosides, chloramphenicol, cephalosporins
Salmonella	Fluoroquinolones, TMP/SMX	Third-generation cephalosporins, ampicillin, chloramphenicol, azithromycin
Shigella (in US)	TMP/SMX	Fluoroquinolones, azithromycin
Shigella (outside US)	Fluoroquinolones	Azithromycin
V. cholera	Fluoroquinolones, tetracycline	Doxycycline, TMP/SMX[c]
Y. enterocolitica	Fluoroquinolones	Doxycycline, TMP/SMX, aminoglycosides, ceftriaxone, chloramphenicol
Traveler's (empiric)	Fluoroquinolones, TMP/SMX[b]	
	General Dosing Guidelines	
Drug	***Children***	***Adult***
Amikacin (IV)	10 mg/kg every 8 h	7.5 mg/kg every 12 h
Ampicillin (IV)	50 mg/kg every 6 h	150–200 mg/kg/day divided every 6 h
Ampicillin (po)	50–100 mg/kg/day divided every 6 h	250–500 mg every 6 h
Azithromycin (po)	10–12 mg/kg on day 1, 5 mg/kg/day for 4 days	500 mg day 1, then 250 mg for 4 days
Bacitracin (po)	800–1,200 U/kg/day divided every 8 h	25,000 U every 6 h
Cefotaxime (IV)	50 mg/kg every 6 h	1–2 g every 4–12 h
Ceftriaxone (IV)	50–100 mg/kg every 24 h	1–2 g/day divided every 12–24 h
Chloramphenicol (IV)	12.5–25 mg/kg every 6 h	50 mg/kg every 6 h
Ciprofloxacin (IV)	NR	200–400 mg every 12 h
Ciprofloxacin (po)	NR	500–750 mg every 12 h
Clindamycin (po)	5–6 mg/kg every 8 h	150–450 mg every 6 h
Clindamycin (IV)	7.5 mg/kg every 6 h	600–900 mg every 8 h
Doxycycline (po)	(age 8 or older) 2–4 mg/kg/day divided q 12 h	100 mg every 12 h
Erythromycin (po)	10 mg/kg every 6 h	250–500 mg every 6 h
Gentamicin (IV)	2.5 mg/kg every 8 h	3–5 mg/kg/day divided every 8 h
Metronidazole (po)	7.5 mg/kg every 6 h	250–500 mg every 6–8 h
Norfloxacin (po)	NR	400 mg every 12 h
Ofloxacin (po)	NR	200–400 mg every 12 h
Tetracycline (po)	(age 8 or older) 25–50 mg/kg/day divided q 6 h	250–500 mg every 6 h
TMP/SMX (po)	8–12 mg/kg/day divided every 12 h	160 mg every 12 h
Tobramycin (IV)	2.5 mg/kg every 8 h	3–5 mg/kg/day divided every 8 h
Vancomycin (po)	10–50 mg/kg/day divided every 6 h, max 125 mg per dose	125 mg every 6 h

[a]TMP/SMX, trimethoprim-sulfamethoxazole
[b]With ETEC and traveler's, TMP/SMX useful in Mexico; however, resistance is seen in Asia, Africa, and South America
[c]Strain 0139 is resistant to TMP/SMX
(Adapted from Refs. 29 and 31.)
NR, not recommended.

using a standardized protocol of slower oral rehydration, immediate feeding, and intensive management of complications resulted in a significant reduction of mortality as compared to standard therapy.[22] Initially, easily digested foods, such as bananas, applesauce, and cereal, may be added. Foods high in fiber, sodium, and sugar should be avoided. Lactase deficiency may be exacerbated among known lactase-deficient patients and may persist up to 10 days.

After starting rehydration therapy, parents should be instructed to observe the child for a reversal of the signs of dehydration, increased stool consistency, and decreased stool frequency. If ORT is not improving the fluid status and the patient continues to produce frequent large volume watery stools, close supervision with medical support is justified.[23,24]

A variety of pathogens can be responsible for acute infectious diarrhea. Viruses are the most common cause of gastroenteritis in children. Bacterial species that are commonly associated with infectious diarrhea in the United States are *Shigella* spp., *Salmonella* spp., *Campylobacter* spp., *Yersinia* spp., *Escherichia* spp., *Clostridium* spp., and *Staphylococcus* spp. Although not a major cause in North America, *Vibrio* spp. is a leading cause of bacterial gastroenteritis on a global scale. The diarrhea is generally referred to as either watery (enterotoxigenic) or dysentery (invasive). Clinical signs and symptoms may point to the etiology (Table 111–4). A simple generalization implies that dysentery diarrhea requires antimicrobial therapy, laboratory monitoring, and intensive follow-up, whereas watery diarrhea is self-limiting.

TABLE 111–2. Clinical Assessment of Degree of Dehydration in Children Based on Percentage of Body Weight Loss*

Variable	Mild, 3%–5%	Moderate, 6%–9%	Severe, ≥10%
Blood pressure	Normal	Normal	Normal to reduced
Quality of pulses	Normal	Normal or slightly decreased	Moderately decreased
Heart rate	Normal	Increased	Increased (bradycardia in severe cases)
Skin turgor	Normal	Decreased	Decreased
Fontanelle	Normal	Sunken	Sunken
Mucous membranes	Slightly dry	Dry	Dry
Eyes	Normal	Sunken orbits/decreased tears	Deeply sunken orbits/decreased tears
Extremities	Warm, normal capillary refill	Delayed capillary refill	Cool, mottled
Mental status	Normal	Normal to listless	Normal to lethargic or comatose
Urine output	Slightly decreased	<1 mL/kg/h	<1 mL/kg/h
Thirst	Slightly increased	Moderately increased	Very thirsty or too lethargic to indicate
Fluid replacement	ORT 50 mL/kg over 2–4 hrs	ORT 100 mL/kg over 2–4 h	Ringer lactate 40 mL/kg in 15–30 min, then 20–40 mL/kg if skin turgor, alertness, and pulse have not returned to normal *or* Ringer lactate or NS 20 mL/kg, repeat if necessary, and then replace water and electrolyte deficits over 1–2 days
	Replace ongoing losses with low-sodium ORT (40–60 mEq/L Na^+) at 10 mL/kg per stool or emesis	Replace ongoing losses with low-sodium ORT (40–60 mEq/L Na^+) at 10 mL/kg per stool or emesis	Followed by ORT 100 mL/kg over 4 hours. Replace ongoing losses with low-sodium ORT (40–60 mEq/L Na^+) at 10 mL/kg per stool or emesis

*Percentages vary among authors for each dehydration category; hemodynamic and perfusion status is most important; when unsure of category, therapy for more severe category is recommended.
ORT, oval rehydration therapy.
(Adapted from Refs. 10 and 15.)

BACTERIAL INFECTIONS

ENTEROTOXIGENIC (CHOLERA-LIKE) DIARRHEA

CHOLERA (*VIBRIO CHOLERAE*)

Epidemiology and Etiology

Cholera has been endemic in the Ganges delta, West Bengal, Bangladesh, and southern Asia (including Southeast Asia) since at least 1817. A 1994 outbreak of a multidrug-resistant strain of cholera among Rwandan refugees resulted in more than 20,000 deaths.[25] Cholera epidemics in 1991 and 1998 caused more than 1 million deaths in Latin America. As international travel increases, the occurrence of cholera in the United States also increases. Cholera has been reported in all major regions of the United States. However, the incidence, 1 case per 1 million persons, makes it extremely rare.[26,27]

Vibrio cholerae O1 is the most common serotype associated with epidemics and pandemics. Other serotypes have also been associated with epidemics—*V. cholerae* O139 Bengal appeared in India in 1992 and spread rapidly through Southeast Asia. *V. cholerae* O139 has also been isolated from food-production animals in the Netherlands.[28] Four mechanisms for transmission have been proposed, including animal reservoirs, chronic carriers, asymptomatic or mild disease victims, or water reservoirs. A relatively large inoculum is required to produce clinical disease. The majority of people infected with *V. cholerae* O1 have no symptoms, and only 2% to 5% will develop severe diarrhea, which may cause death within 24 hours. An estimated 25% to 50% of cases are fatal if left untreated.

TABLE 111–3. Comparison of Common Solutions Used in Oral Rehydration and Maintenance

Product	Na (mEq/L)	K (mEq/L)	Base (mEq/L)	Carbohydrate (mmol/L)	Osmolality (mOsm/L)
Naturalyte (unlimited beverage)	45	20	48	140	265
Pediatric electrolyte (NutraMax)	45	20	30	140	250
Pedialyte (Ross)	45	20	30	140	250
Infalyte (formerly Ricelyte; Mead Johnson)	50	25	30	70	200
Rehydralyte (Ross)	75	20	30	140	310
WHO/UNICEF oral rehydration salts	90	20	30	111	310
Cola	2	0	13	700	750
Apple juice	5	32	0	690	730
Chicken broth	250	8	0	0	500
Sports beverage	20	3	3	255	330

(Adapted from Ref. 15.)

TABLE 111–4. Acute Infectious Diarrhea Clinical Syndromes: Watery vs. Dysenteric

	Watery	Dysenteric
Percentage of Patients	90	5–10
Stools		
Appearance	Watery	Bloody
Volume	Increased: ++/+++	Increased: +/++
Number per day	<10	>10
Reducing substances	0 to +++	0
pH	5.0–7.5	6.0–7.5
Occult blood	Negative	Positive
Fecal PMN cells	Absent or few	Many
Mechanisms	Toxins Reduced absorption	Mucosal invasion
Complications		
Dehydration	Could be severe	Mild
Others	Acidosis, shock, electrolyte imbalance	Tenesmus, rectal prolapse, seizures
Etiology	Rotaviruses Enterotoxigenic *E. coli* *V. cholerae*	*Shigella* spp. *Campylobacter* spp. *S. enteritidis*

(Adapted from Ref. 7.)

Pathophysiology

Most pathology of cholera is thought to result from an enterotoxin (cholera toxin) produced by the bacteria.[1] Cholera toxin stimulates adenylate cyclase, which increases intracellular cAMP and results in increased secretion of fluids and electrolytes. The toxin likely acts along the entire intestinal tract; however, most fluid loss occurs in the duodenum. The net effect of cholera toxin is isotonic secretion (primarily in the small intestine), which exceeds the absorptive capacity of the intestinal tract (primarily the colon).

Clinical Presentation

The average incubation period of *V. cholerae* is 1 to 3 days. The clinical presentation can vary from asymptomatic to the most severe typical cholera syndrome. In the most severe state, this disease can progress to death in 2 to 4 hours if not treated. Initial stools generally do not have the "rice water" appearance that is classically seen with cholera.

Most signs and symptoms are a direct result of fluid and electrolyte loss, and generally correlate well with the severity of fluid loss (Table 111–2). Fluid collection within the intestines may cause further intravascular depletion without diarrhea. Patients may lose up to a liter of isotonic fluid every hour.

Hypokalemia is often seen in children, perhaps as a reflection of a greater potassium loss with diarrhea than seen with adults. Altered consciousness, hypoglycemia, muscle weakness and cramping, cardiac arrhythmias, and ileus may be manifestations of electrolyte losses. Other complications include acidosis, renal failure secondary to volume depletion, iatrogenic water intoxication from overrehydration, and aspiration pneumonia.

▶ TREATMENT: Enterotoxigenic Diarrhea

FLUID AND ELECTROLYTE REPLACEMENT

- Rice- or cereal-based formula is preferred.[16,30]
- Intravenous fluids, preferably Ringer lactate, should be used in severe dehydration or when intractable vomiting prevents sufficient fluid replacement with ORT.[29]

ANTIBIOTICS

- Antibiotics are always indicated and shorten duration of diarrhea, decrease fluid loss, and shorten duration of carrier state.[29]
- Table 111–1 provides recommendations on antibiotic selection. Recommended regimens include:
  - Tetracycline 500 mg orally 4 times a day × 3 days; doxycycline 300 mg orally, single dose (as efficacious as tetracycline but associated with prolonged fecal excretion of bacteria)
  - Norfloxacin 400 mg orally 2 times a day × 3 days, ciprofloxacin 500 mg orally 2 times a day × 3 days or 1,000 mg orally × 1 (preferred where tetracycline resistance is common[25]). Quinolones are the drugs of choice for known *V. cholerae* O139 infections.[32]
  - TMP/SMX DS tablet orally 2 times a day × 3 days. TMP/SMX is preferred in pregnancy and in children. However strain O139 may be resistant to TMP/SMX.
  - Chloramphenicol, erythromycin, and furazolidone have been effective.

VACCINE

The manufacture and sale of the only licensed cholera vaccine in the United States has been discontinued. Two vaccines are available in other countries.[33] These vaccines are given as two doses (2 weeks apart) with booster after 1 year.

The vaccines are not recommended for travelers because of transient immunity. The World Health Organization does not require vaccination for international travel to or from endemic areas because the series of two injections is effective in only 50% of people and immunity wanes in 6 months or less.

ESCHERICHIA COLI

EPIDEMIOLOGY AND ETIOLOGY

Escherichia coli is a gram-negative bacillus commonly found in the human GI tract.[34] It is divided into five groups based on mechanisms of diarrheal disease and toxin production: enterotoxigenic *E. coli* (ETEC), enteroinvasive *E. coli* (EIEC), enteropathogenic *E. coli* (EPEC), enteroadhesive *E. coli* (EAEC), and enterohemorrhagic *E. coli* (EHEC).

The most common group is ETEC; it accounts for about half of all cases of *E. coli* diarrhea and for more than 79,000 cases in the United States each year.[35,36] Enterotoxigenic *E. coli* is incriminated as being the most common cause of traveler's diarrhea and a common cause of food- and water-associated outbreaks.[1,30] Recognized as a common and potentially deadly cause of infectious diarrhea, EHEC is believed to be the major etiological factor responsible for the development of hemolytic uremic syndrome (HUS), which is potentially fatal. The first human cases of EHEC were reported in 1982 and were caused by contaminated hamburgers. There were 38 infectious outbreaks caused by the EHEC serotype 0157:H7 reported to the Center for Disease Control and Prevention in 1999. The transmission usually occurs via food and water, and outbreaks have been associated with undercooked ground beef.[37] Reports of EHEC enteritis continue to increase. Antibiotic treatment of this serotype in children may increase the risk of developing HUS by lysing bacteria and increasing toxin release.[38]

PATHOPHYSIOLOGY

Enterotoxigenic *E. coli* are capable of producing two plasmid-mediated enterotoxins: heat-labile toxin (HLT) and heat-stable toxin (HST). A cholera-like toxin, HLT has two subunits (A and B) that have similar antigenic properties and action on the gut mucosa. The net effect of this toxin on the mucosa is production of a cholera-like secretory diarrhea. With a rapid onset of action, HST is nonantigenic, has a low molecular weight, and probably acts only on the small intestine.[39] The pathogenicity of EHEC is related to the production of cytotoxins, commonly called shiga-like toxins because of their resemblance to the shiga toxin of *Shigella dysenteriae*.[40]

CLINICAL PRESENTATION

Nausea and watery stools, with or without abdominal cramping, characterize the disease caused by ETEC. Usually, there is no blood or pus in the stool. Signs and symptoms are directly dependent on the extent of fluid loss, which in most cases is subclinical. Most ETEC diarrhea resolves within 24 to 48 hours without complication.

Symptoms from EHEC infection can be severe, with as many as 11 to 12 bloody stools per day.[40,41] Cramping and severe abdominal pain are common, nausea occurs in about two-thirds of patients, and vomiting occurs in less than one-third. Symptoms usually last 1 week. The white blood cell (WBC) count is elevated and accompanied by a left shift, but patients often remain afebrile. Stool cultures should be performed when EHEC is suspected.[37] Death may rarely occur, usually as a result of HUS and postdiarrheal thrombocytopenic purpura (TTP).[37]

▶ TREATMENT: Enterohemorrhagic *Escherichia coli* Diarrhea

Fluid and electrolyte replacement (95% of cases resolve).[31]

Antibiotic use is controversial, as it may increase the risk of HUS.[29,31,38]

Antimotility agents are contraindicated (increase duration of bloody diarrhea caused by toxin retention in the colon).[29,35]

Oral vaccines that target colonization factor antigens are under development.[42]

TRAVELER'S DIARRHEA[43,44]

Traveler's diarrhea is the passage of unformed or liquid stools by persons traveling outside their home region or by persons who have returned home from such travel 10 or fewer days before the onset of symptoms.[43] The severity of the syndrome can be determined by the number of stools per day and the presence or absence of cramping, nausea, and vomiting.[43] An estimated 20% to 50% of people traveling to high-risk areas will develop the illness. It is rarely life-threatening, and is caused by fecally contaminated food or water. Especially risky foods include raw or undercooked meat and seafood, and raw fruits and vegetables. Tap water, ice, and unpasteurized milk and dairy products may be associated with increased risk.

Onset usually occurs during the first week, but can occur any time during the visit or shortly after returning home. The median duration is 3 to 4 days, with only 10% of cases lasting more than 1 week. High-risk areas include Central America, Africa, Asia, India, and the Middle East. Southern Europe and the Caribbean islands are considered intermediate risk regions.

The most common pathogens include ETEC (20% to 72%), *Shigella* (3% to 25%), *Campylobacter* (3% to 17%), *Salmonella* (3% to 7%), and viruses (0% to 30%).

High-risk populations include the immunocompromised, those who have achlorhydria or inflammatory bowel disease, and people taking diuretics, digoxin, lithium or insulin (because of the need for appropriate hydration).

PROPHYLAXIS

Patient education promoting food and beverage consumption:

- "Peel it, boil it, cook it, or forget it"
- Use water purification or reliable bottled beverages
- Bring a travel kit including a thermometer, loperamide, 3 days of antibiotics (see below), oral rehydration solution salts, and a water purification method

Nonantibiotic regimens[29]

- Bismuth subsalicylate, 525 mg orally once to four times daily for up to 3 weeks
- Diphenoxylate and loperamide are ineffective

Antibiotics (see Table 111–1)[29] are used in high-risk individuals and in situations in which short-term illness could ruin the purpose of the trip. The CDC does not recommend this use of antibiotics because of ETEC-resistant strains,[30] side effects, and an imposed false sense of security.

- TMP/SMX DS tablet orally once daily (in Mexico)
- Norfloxacin 400 mg or ciprofloxacin 500 mg orally once daily (in Asia, Africa, and South America)
- Doxycycline is no longer used because of widespread resistance.[29]

No vaccines are currently marketed in United States, and those that are available and in development are ineffective.

► TREATMENT: Traveler's Diarrhea

Fluid and electrolyte replacement should be initiated at the onset of diarrhea. (ORT is generally not required in healthy individuals; flavored mineral water offers a good source of sodium and glucose).

Agents used to treat symptoms include:

- Loperamide (preferred because of its quicker onset and longer duration of relief relative to bismuth): initially 4 mg orally, then 2 mg with each subsequent loose stool to a maximum of 16 mg/d in patients without bloody diarrhea; discontinue if symptoms persist for over 48 hours.
- Bismuth subsalicylate 525 mg every 30 minutes up to 8 doses

The following antibiotics (see Table 111–1) are recommended in addition to loperamide in moderate or severe diarrhea with systemic symptoms:

- Norfloxacin 400 mg or ciprofloxacin 500 mg orally twice daily × 3 days
- TMP/SMX DS tablet orally twice daily × 3 days (drug of choice in Mexico only, as resistance common in tropics)
- Azithromycin 500 mg orally once daily × 3 days (only in areas of high prevalence of *Campylobacter* species resistant to quinolones, such as Thailand)[29]

PSEUDOMEMBRANOUS COLITIS (*CLOSTRIDIUM DIFFICILE*)

Pseudomembranous colitis (PMC) was first reported in 1893, and was associated with antibiotic therapy in 1955. Although described in the preantibiotic era, the incidence has increasingly been associated with antibiotic administration. *Clostridium difficile* colitis is the *most common* nosocomial infection, infecting *16% to 20% of inpatients,* one-third of whom are symptomatic.[29]

EPIDEMIOLOGY AND ETIOLOGY

Clostridium difficile is a gram-positive spore-forming anaerobic bacillus. The incidence of intestinal colonization is variable, ranging from 30% to 70% in infants to 3% to 5% in healthy adults.[45,46] The relationship between the colonized state and active disease is poorly understood. Many people are colonized with the bacteria yet do not go on to develop PMC.

The exact incidence of PMC within the United States is unknown. It occurs most often in high-risk groups, such as the elderly, debilitated patients, cancer patients, surgical patients, any patient receiving antibiotics, patients with nasogastric tubes, and patients who frequently use laxatives.[47] Pseudomembranous colitis has been associated with use of broad-spectrum antimicrobials, including clindamycin, ampicillin, or third-generation cephalosporins.[48] Other agents that have been implicated, albeit at a lower incidence rate, include aminoglycosides, erythromycin, fluoroquinolones, TMP/SMX, and, surprisingly, vancomycin and metronidazole, two of the most commonly used antimicrobials for treatment of *C. difficile*.[48,49]

PATHOPHYSIOLOGY

Clostridium difficile colitis is a toxin-mediated disease. Two toxins (A and B) have been described. Toxin A is the major pathogenic factor and has been characterized as an enterotoxin that causes disease through actin disaggregation, intracellular calcium release, and damaging neurons.[45] Toxin B is a nonenterotoxic cytotoxin that causes depolymerization of filamentous actin. The toxins appear to act on mucosal membranes, causing necrosis, inflammation, increased peristalsis, and loss of fluid and electrolytes.

CLINICAL PRESENTATION

Pseudomembranous colitis is characterized by vomiting, fever, cramping, abdominal pain and tenderness, and profuse greenish diarrhea either during or after antibiotic therapy. Fevers and marked leukocytosis can also occur. Symptoms can start a few days after the start of antibiotic therapy or several weeks after antibiotics have been discontinued. The onset of illness is often abrupt.

The American College of Gastroenterology published guidelines for diagnosis and treatment of *C. difficile*-associated diarrhea.[50] The diagnosis of PMC should be suspected in patients with diarrhea who have received antibiotics within the previous 2 months or whose diarrhea began 72 hours or more after hospitalization. Diagnosis can be made by demonstration in stool samples of toxin A or B, stool culture for *C. difficile,* or endoscopy. If the stool sample is negative, a second is recommended, as the testing sensitivity may be increased with the second analysis and *C. difficile* enterocolitis in hospitals often goes unrecognized.[49] Endoscopy should be reserved for situations when rapid diagnosis is needed, ileus is present, and a stool is not available, or when other colonic diseases are in the differential.

► TREATMENT: Pseudomembranous Colitis

- Discontinue or switch to an alternative antibiotic (15% to 23% of patients will self-resolve).[48]
- Fluid and electrolyte replacement as necessary.

Metronidazole 250 mg orally 4 times a day or 500 mg orally 3 times a day × 10 days is the first drug of choice. It is similar to vancomycin in duration of diarrhea, incidence of side effects, and relapse. However, it is less expensive than vancomycin.

Concern for vancomycin resistance promotes metronidazole use.

Oral vancomycin 125 mg 4 times a day × 10 days is the second-line treatment. It is used when the patient has not responded to oral metronidazole; the organism is resistant to metronidazole; the patient is allergic to metronidazole, is unable to tolerate it, or is being treated with ethanol containing solutions; the patient is either pregnant or is younger than 10 years of age; the patient is critically ill because of *C. difficile* diarrhea or colitis (the duration of diarrhea is reduced to 3 days vs 4.6 days with metronidazole);[29] there is evidence suggesting that the diarrhea is caused by *Staphylococcus aureus;* or when IV vancomycin does not achieve gut lumen concentrations high enough for effective bacterial elimination.

Bacitracin is the third-line treatment. In resolving symptoms, 80,000 units of bacitracin orally daily is as effective as vancomycin, but is not as effective in irradicating the organism. Bacitracin's poor taste, which increases patients' resistance, limits its use.[50,51] Teicoplanin and fusidic acid have been effective in resolving symptoms and irradicating the organism.[48]

Relapse after antibiotic treatment occurs in about 10% to 25% of patients and does not appear to be influenced by whether metronidazole or vancomycin was used for treatment or by the dose or duration of treatment of the initial episode.[29] Recurrences occur because of the persistence of the spore forms of *C. difficile* that are not killed by antibiotic therapy or reinfection by a new strain. Recurrences usually occur 2 to 10 days after antibiotics are stopped. Retreatment with metronidazole or vancomycin with the previous dose for 10 to 14 days is generally successful. The addition of rifampin to vancomycin has been effective.[48]

Some investigators have found prophylaxis with competing, nonpathogenic organisms, such as *Lactobacillus* spp. or *Saccharomyces* spp., to be helpful in preventing relapse in small numbers of patients.[52,53] It is thought that these organisms help to restore the natural flora in the gut and make patients more resistant to colonization by *C. difficile*.

Vancomycin has been used in combination with anion exchange resins, dosed to avoid drug-resin binding, and this has been successfully used in a small number of cases.[29] Cholestyramine 4 g three to four times daily or colestipol 5 g twice daily have been used as alternatives to antibiotics in mild cases.

Drugs that inhibit peristalsis, such as diphenoxylate, are contraindicated in PMC. Slowing of fecal transit time is thought to result in extended toxin-associated damage.

INVASIVE (DYSENTERY-LIKE) DIARRHEA

BACILLARY DYSENTERY (SHIGELLOSIS)

Epidemiology and Etiology

The shigellae are gram-negative bacilli belonging to the family Enterobacteriaceae. Four species most often associated with disease are *Shigella dysenteriae* type I, *S. flexneri, S. boydii,* and *S. sonnei.* The shigellae have worldwide distribution, with regional differences in prevalence of subgroups responsible for disease. For example, in the United States, the common causes of shigellosis are *S. sonnei* and *S. flexneri.* Cases caused by other shigellae are most often acquired during travel to developing countries. Because of overuse of antibiotics in human and animal feed, Southeast Asia and India have higher levels of resistance. Poor sanitation, poor personal hygiene, inadequate water supply, malnutrition, and increased population density are associated with an increased risk of shigella gastroenteritis epidemics, even in developed countries.

The majority of cases result from fecal–oral transmission. A few well-documented food- and water-associated outbreaks have been reported. Peak incidence in the United States is in late summer. Estimates indicate 450,000 cases of shigellosis occur in the United States and 165 million cases occur in the world annually, resulting in over 1 million deaths worldwide each year.[54]

Shigellosis is primarily a disease of children, with the highest incidence between ages 6 months and 5 years. Infection among infants is uncommon, and only one-third of all cases occur in adults.

Pathogenesis

Ingestion of as few as 10 to 200 viable organisms of the shigella species causes disease in healthy adults, explaining the ease with which the disease is transmitted from person to person.[55] The bacteria multiply and spread within the submucosa, but they rarely extend beyond the mucosa. Penetration of the mucosa is genetically conferred by large "invasion plasmids" and results in distortion of the crypts, death to intestinal epithelium causing focal ulceration, sloughing of mucosal cells, bloody mucoid exudate into the gut lumen, and submucosal accumulation of inflammatory cells with microabscess formation. Microabscesses may eventually coalesce, forming larger abscesses. Infection frequently involves the entire colon. Some *Shigella* spp. produce a cytotoxin, or shiga-toxin, the pathogenic role of which is unclear, although it is thought to damage endothelial cells of the lamina propria, resulting in microangiopathic changes that can progress to HUS. Watery diarrhea commonly precedes the dysentery and may be a result of these toxins.

Clinical Presentation

Signs and symptoms are initially nonspecific. Frequent watery stools appear within 48 hours and are followed by bloody diarrhea and other signs of dysentery within a few days (Table 111–4). Stools are often greenish in color and contain leukocytes.

Fluid and electrolyte loss may be significant, particularly in infants and elderly patients. Stool culture will establish *Shigella* spp. as the causative agent. A rapid diagnostic test kit, which uses DNA amplification by the polymerase chain reaction, is available.

If untreated, bacillary dysentery usually lasts about 1 week (range, 1 to 30 days). Complications are unusual but may include severe dehydration, generalized seizures, septicemia, toxic megacolon, perforated colon, arthritis, protein-losing enteropathy, and HUS. Mortality is rare, but it may be more likely with *S. dysenteriae* type I. Less than 3% of persons who are infected with *Shigella flexneri* will later develop Reiter's syndrome, characterized by pains in the joints, irritation of the eyes, and painful urination. This can lead to chronic arthritis.

▶ TREATMENT: Shigellosis

Shigelloisis is usually a self-limiting disease. Most patients recover in 4 to 7 days, although 10% may experience a recurrence. Oral fluid and electrolyte replacement is the foundation of treatment (dysentery is not generally associated with significant fluid loss).

Antibiotic treatment is indicated in the infirm, those who are immunocompromised, children in day care centers, elderly, malnourished children, and health care workers (shortens period of fecal shedding and attenuates the clinical illness).

The choice of agent depends upon location (see Table 111–1).[29,31] For infections acquired in the United States, the agents of choice are TMP/SMX DS tablet orally twice daily × 5 days (only 4% resistance)[29] or ciprofloxacin, norfloxacin, or azithromycin, as dosed below. For infections acquired outside the United States, the agents of choice are ciprofloxacin 500 mg or norfloxacin 400 mg orally twice daily × 5 days or azithromycin 500 mg orally, then 250 mg orally once daily × 4 days.[56]

Quinolones have been used for shigellosis in children[31] and shorter therapies have been used successfully for mild disease.[29] *Shigella* resistance has reduced the effectiveness of tetracyclines, ampicillin, and TMP/SMX, all former first-line agents.[57,58] Antimotility agents are contraindicated as they prolong fever and diarrhea. Oral vaccines currently in development contain attenuated strains of *Shigella* and provide protection against shigellosis in human challenges.[59,60] Commercial production of such vaccines is not yet available.

SALMONELLOSIS

Epidemiology and Etiology

Salmonella spp. are gram-negative bacilli belonging to the family Enterobacteriaceae. The genus *Salmonella* has three species *(S. typhi, S. enteritidis,* and *S. choleraesuis).* Human disease caused by salmonella generally falls into four categories: acute gastroenteritis (enterocolitis), bacteremia, extraintestinal localized infection, and enteric fever (typhoid and paratyphoid fever). Salmonellosis is a disease primarily of infants, children, and adolescents. Children younger than 5 years of age account for about 25% of all diagnosed cases.[61] Approximately 1 to 2 million cases of salmonellosis occur in the United States annually.[2] More than 500 cases per year are fatal.[62] Contaminated food or water has been implicated in the majority of cases. Direct fecal–oral transmission occurs less frequently but is particularly important in children. Foods most often implicated in human salmonellosis are poultry, poultry products, beef, pork, and dairy products. An outbreak of *S. enteritidis* in the Midwest, in 1994, affecting more than 2,000 people was traced to ice cream produced in a single location.[63] Pets, particularly reptiles, have been shown to be a common source of infection.[55,61]

Most reports of outbreaks occur sporadically within households and institutions. It is quite common for family contacts to acquire infection. While the incidence of salmonella infection overall has increased over the past decade, that attributed to *S. typhi* has declined. Conditions that may predispose to infection include those that decrease gastric acidity, antibiotic use, malnutrition, and immunodeficient states.[55]

Pathophysiology

Salmonellae enterocolitis appears to occur secondary to mucosal invasion of microorganisms.[2] *S. enteritidis,* the most common serotype in North America and Europe, causes enterocolitis.[29] The different serotypes have a broad range of invasive potential. Some salmonellae, such as *S. choleraesuis,* which is the most invasive, are frequently associated with bacteremia and metastatic localization, whereas others seldom cause disease. There is evidence that an enterotoxin may be produced, perhaps within the enterocyte.[64] Other as yet unclear mechanisms may also play a role.

Clinical Presentation

Enterocolitis. Most patients experience symptoms within 72 hours of ingestion of the bacteria. Patients often complain of nausea and vomiting followed by abdominal cramps, headache, fever, and diarrhea, although the actual presentation is quite variable. Some patients do not have increased stool frequency, whereas others have more than one stool per hour. Stools are generally loose and may be mucoid or bloody (dysentery-like), or both. Temperatures usually range between 100°F (37.7°C) and 102°F (38.8°C), but may be higher. Some evidence suggests that higher fever, greater than or equal to 104°F (40°C), is associated with shorter bacterial excretion.[65] Diarrhea and fever usually spontaneously resolve within 1 to 5 days, but may last 2 weeks.

Stool cultures inevitably yield the causative organism if obtained early (i.e., in patients hospitalized ≤3 days).[49] Recovery of organisms continues to decrease with time, however, so that by 3 to 4 weeks, only 5% to 15% of adult patients are passing salmonella. Infants and children tend to pass bacteria for longer periods than adults. Some patients may continue to shed salmonella for a year or longer. These "chronic carrier" states are rare for serotypes other than *S. typhi.*

Bacteremia. Salmonellae can produce bacteremia without classic enterocolitis or enteric fever. Bacteremia rarely occurs in older adults, but it can occur in up to 40% of infants.[55] The clinical syndrome is characterized by persistent bacteremia and prolonged intermittent fever with chills. Stool cultures are frequently negative. This is most frequent, and highly likely, with serotype *S. choleraesuis* infections (50%). Leukocyte counts are often within the normal range.

Localized Infections. Extraluminal infection or abscess formation or both can occur at any site. They may follow any of the other syndromes, or they may be the primary presentation. Metastatic infections have been reported to involve bone, cysts, heart, kidney, liver, lungs, pericardium, spleen, and tumors. The clinical presentation is usually determined by the organ systems involved. Polymorphonuclear leukocyte counts are often elevated.

Enteric Fever (Typhoid and Paratyphoid). Enteric fever caused by *S. typhi* is called typhoid fever. If caused by any other serotype, it is referred to as paratyphoid fever. The clinical presentations of typhoid fever and paratyphoid fever are generally indistinguishable, although in retrospect, paratyphoid fever tends to be less severe than typhoid fever. Incubation time can range from 10 to 14 days. The onset of symptoms is gradual. Nonspecific symptoms of fever, dull headache, malaise, anorexia, and myalgias are most common. Initially, fever tends to be remittent, but gradually progresses over the first week to temperatures that are often sustained over 104°F (40°C). Other frequently encountered symptoms include chills, nausea, vomiting, cough, weakness, and sore throat. Symptoms slowly subside within 4 weeks.

Physical examination generally reveals an acutely ill patient. An erythematous maculopapular rash, known as rose spots, appears primarily on the abdomen in 15% to 50% of patients. The abdomen may also be tender, particularly in the lower quadrants. Hepatomegaly, splenomegaly, or both may also be present in 50% of the cases, and cervical lymph nodes may be enlarged.

A normochromic anemia may develop rapidly without evidence of GI blood loss, although intestinal bleeding may be contributory. Leukopenia may be reflective of a relative decrease in polymorphonuclear leukocytes. White cell counts may range from 1,200 to 20,000 cells/mm^3. As many as one-third of the patients have elevated levels of the liver enzymes glutamic-oxaloacetic transaminase and alkaline phosphatase in serum. About 80% of patients have positive blood cultures. Bacteremia persists in about one-third of cases for several weeks if not treated. Intestinal perforation, thrombophlebitis, toxemia with circulatory collapse, intestinal hemorrhage, and pneumonia all contribute to a fatality rate of 1% to 2%. Without treatment, mortality may be 10%.

▶ TREATMENT: Salmonellosis

ENTEROCOLITIS

Fluid and electrolyte replacement is the primary mode of treatment. Most patients respond well to ORT (self-limited illness).

Antidiarrheal drugs should be avoided as they increase the risk of mucosal invasion and complications. Antibiotic therapy is *not* indicated in healthy adults (it has no effect on duration of fever or diarrhea, and frequent use increases resistance and duration of fecal shedding).[29]

Antibiotics should be used in: (a) neonates or infants younger than 6 months of age because young children have an increased risk of complicated infection; (b) patients with primary or secondary immunodeficiency, such as AIDS or chemotherapy patients; (c) severely symptomatic patients with fever and bloody diarrhea; and (d) patients after splenectomy.[2,29] Susceptibility testing is recommended because many drug-resistant strains of salmonella have emerged.[34]

Recommended antibiotics include:

- Ciprofloxacin 500 mg or norfloxacin 400 mg orally twice daily × 3 to 7 days (resistance to these drugs is increasing; although not approved for children, these drugs have been safely used in this group.
- Azithromycin 1,000 mg orally × 1 day, followed by 500 mg orally once daily × 6 days
- Third-generation cephalosporins (ceftriaxone 2 g IV once daily or cefotaxime 2 g IV three times daily × 5 days)

BACTEREMIA AND LOCALIZED INFECTIONS

Chloramphenicol or ampicillin is the most frequently used drug for treatment. TMP/SMX, which is effective in treatment of localized salmonella infections, should be considered when the organism is resistant to the first-line agents. Ampicillin is the preferred agent when bactericidal activity is desired, as with endocarditis or other intravascular infections, although fluoroquinolones and third-generation cephalosporins have also been used. The duration of antibiotic therapy is dictated by the site of infection; for example, osteomyelitis should be treated for 4 to 6 weeks or longer.

ENTERIC FEVER (TYPHOID AND PARATYPHOID)

Antibiotic choice is dictated by susceptibility testing.[29,31] Ciprofloxacin 500 mg orally twice daily × 10 days is the drug of choice for adults in areas where multidrug resistance (MDR) is common.[66,67] However, quinolone-resistant strains are emerging. One study showed decreased sensitivity to ciprofloxacin in 21% of *S. typhi* infections.[29,68] Although quinolones are not recommended in children, use of ciprofloxacin in areas where multidrug-resistant *S. typhi* occurs is acceptable. Ceftriaxone 2 g IV once daily × 5 days is an alternative drug choice. One study showed it to be inferior to ofloxacin in patients with MDR strains.[29,31,61]

Other drugs of choice include azithromycin 1,000 mg orally × 1 day followed by 500 mg once daily × 5 days, as well as cefixime, cefotaxime, and cefuroxime, which are effective in treating enteric fever caused by MDR strains.[29,68] Chloramphenicol 500 mg 4 times daily orally or IV × 14 days was once the drug of choice, but now has a high level of resistance. In 1994–1995, 35% of isolates in Great Britain were resistant.[69] However, with the declining use of chloramphenicol in the past decades, sensitive strains to this agent may be reemerging.[29]

Outbreaks of multidrug-resistant *S. typhi* have been reported in many developing countries, including Pakistan, India, Southeast Asia, and North and South Africa.[57] Resistance is often transferred via plasmids to sulfonamides, tetracycline, and streptomycin. Ampicillin, amoxicillin, and TMP/SMX are sometimes effective, although resistance has been reported with these agents as well.

Therapy should be continued for 10 to 14 days. Clinical response to antibiotics is often seen within 2 days; however, temperatures slowly normalize within 3 to 5 days.

Dexamethasone 1 mg/kg every 6 hours for 24 to 48 hours has been used with some success in the severely ill.[31,61] Vaccines are recommended for high-risk groups, including household contacts of *S. typhi* carriers, laboratory technicians with repeated exposure, sanitation workers in endemic areas, and travelers to developing countries.

Three vaccines against *S. typhi* are licensed in the United States: a heat-phenol-inactivated parenteral vaccine (Typhoid Vaccine, USP), an orally administered vaccine (Ty21a, Vivotif Berna), and a parenteral polysaccharide vaccine (ViCPS, Typhim Vi).[70–72] Efficacy of vaccines ranges from 42% to 77% and immunity persists for 3 to 5 years. The parenteral inactivated vaccine causes substantially more adverse reactions than the other two, but provides more prolonged protection.[73] The oral typhoid vaccine should not be administered to immunocompromised persons, patients taking antibiotics, or patients with gastroenteritis. An oral vaccine in Phase 2 trials provides protection with fewer doses than Ty21a and may be the better choice in people who are immunocompromised.[74]

"CHRONIC-CARRIERS" OF SALMONELLA

"Chronic-carriers" of salmonella usually have negative stool cultures at 12 weeks after the onset of illness, but some may have continued positive stool cultures at 6 to 12 months. Chronic fecal shedding of salmonella has been associated with chronic biliary infection and cholelithiasis. The drug of choice is norfloxacin 400 mg orally twice daily × 28 days. It is effective in eradicating the bacteria.[29] These patients should take preventative measures (i.e., antibiotics and hygiene) so that they do not serve as reservoirs of infection to the community.

CAMPYLOBACTERIOSIS

EPIDEMIOLOGY AND ETIOLOGY

The *Campylobacter* spp. are flagellated, curved, gram negative rods. *Campylobacter jejuni* is the species responsible for more than 99% of *Campylobacter*-associated gastroenteritis.[75] The true incidence is difficult to estimate because *Campylobacter* is difficult to culture and is not included in routine stool cultures, but an estimated 2.4 million persons are affected each year. *Campylobacter* spp. are thought to be a major cause of diarrhea in children, with an incidence greater than *Salmonella* or *Shigella*.[76] The peak incidence is in young children and young adults. Patients with AIDS are particularly susceptible; the incidence in AIDS patients is 40 times that of the general population.[75] The incidence is also higher in males than females, although the reason for this is unknown. Most reported cases occur during the summer months.

Transmission of infection appears to be by ingestion of contaminated food or water. Mammals, such as livestock, puppies, cats, and birds, including poultry, are believed to be the primary reservoir of *Campylobacter*. Epidemiologic studies suggest that previous exposure confers immunity to the infecting strain.

PATHOPHYSIOLOGY

Campylobacter spp. is susceptible to acid, much like *Salmonella*. Therefore, an inoculum of approximately 800 organisms is required to initiate infection. Conditions in the upper small intestine are favorable for multiplication. Flagella-mediated adherence and tissue invasion by bacteria have been demonstrated in the jejunum, ileum, and colon. Infection results in an acute, inflammatory enteritis. *Campylobacter jejuni* can produce an enterotoxin or cytotoxin.[77] Both cytotoxins and enterotoxins may be produced in many strains.

CLINICAL PRESENTATION

The average incubation period of *Campylobacter* is 2 to 4 days. The most common presenting symptoms include diarrhea of varying consistency and severity, abdominal pain, and fever. Nausea, vomiting, headache, myalgias, and malaise may also occur. Bowel movements may be numerous, bloody (dysentery-like), foul smelling, and range from loose to watery. Cramping and abdominal pain are usually relieved by defecation.

The disease is usually self-limited to about 1 week, but it may persist longer in 10% to 20% of patients. A reactive arthritis may be seen in as many as 5% of cases. Complications, including pseudoappendicitis, thrombophlebitis, abscess, septicemia, peritonitis, empyema, urinary tract infection, and cholecystitis are uncommon but occur more frequently in those who are immunocompromised. *Campylobacter jejuni* has been associated with Guillain-Barré syndrome, but the relationship is not well understood.[75,76,78] Diagnosis is made by stool culture, but the bacteria are sometimes identifiable with Gram stain or carbol-fuchsin stain.

▶ TREATMENT: Campylobacteriosis

The primary treatment of campylobacteriosis is oral fluid and electrolyte replacement. Most people recover from this self-limiting disease in 4 to 7 days. Antibiotics are *not* useful unless started within 4 days of the start of the illness, as they do not shorten the duration or severity of diarrhea, but only shorten the duration of bacterial excretion. However, antibiotics are warranted in the very young, the very old, the immunocompromised, and in those with severe bloody diarrhea[29,31] (Table 111–1).

Ciprofloxacin 500 mg or norfloxacin 400 mg orally twice daily × 5 days are agents of choice. Quinolone resistance has increased to 10% to 13% in the United States (41% to 88% in Europe and Asia) in recent years, and may be partially a result of their use in poultry feed and their frequent use overseas in treating enteric infections.[29,79]

Other treatment agents include azithromycin 500 mg orally once daily × 3 days, and erythromycin stearate 500 mg once daily × 5 days. Tetracycline, chloramphenicol, clindamycin, and aminoglycosides may be effective.[75]

Antimotility agents (such as loperamide) are contraindicated, because slowing fecal transit time may extend the duration of infection and increase toxin mucosal invasion.

YERSINIOSIS

Yersinia is an anaerobic gram-negative coccobacillus that is widely distributed in nature. The genus *Yersinia* includes six species known to cause disease in humans. Of these, *Y. enterocolitica* is most likely to be associated with intestinal infection, and most likely in young children. More than 50 serotypes exist; of these, serotypes 0:3, 0:8, and 0:9 are most frequently associated with enterocolitis. Peak incidence occurs during the winter months.

The organisms have been isolated from a variety of food sources, including pigs and raw goat and cow milk. Refrigeration does not deter the development of adherence and invasive virulence factors. *Yersinia pestis* is the causative agent of plague and is usually spread by bites from infected animals, such as fleas, rodents, or cats.[80,81] Plague is rare in the United States. Only 10 confirmed cases were reported to the Centers for Disease Control and Prevention (CDC) in 1993.[82]

Yersinia enterocolitica invade the intestinal epithelium and penetrate the intestinal mucosa.[83] Most strains produce an enterotoxin, but the role of toxin production in causing diarrhea is not well established.

These bacteria cause a wide spectrum of clinical syndromes. The majority of cases present with enterocolitis that is mild and self-limiting. Symptoms include vomiting, abdominal pain, diarrhea, and fever; up to 60% of patients will have blood-streaked stools. Diarrhea resolves after 1 to 4 weeks, but the bacteria excretion may continue for up to 3 months after diarrhea subsides. In older children who can report symptoms, pain symptoms may closely mimic appendicitis. Infants younger than 3 months are at greatest risk of developing bacteremia. Other patients associated with high risk of bacteremia include those with cirrhosis and iron-overloaded patients.[29] Other complications that may occur include peritonitis, cholangitis, intestinal perforation, ileocolic intussusception, and toxic megacolon. Many patients develop a reactive arthritis 1 to 2 weeks after recovery from enteritis. The arthritis usually resolves in 1 to 4 months but may persist in about 10% of cases.[84] Other postinfection complications include erythema nodosum and exudative pharyngitis.

▶ TREATMENT: Yersiniosis

Oral fluid and electrolyte replacement (self-limiting disease) are an important initial approach. Antibiotics may not alter the time to resolution of the diarrhea or the rate of bacteriologic cure. Antibiotics should be used in high-risk patients who may develop bacteremia (i.e., infants younger than 3 months of age, and patients with cirrhosis or iron overload) or in those patients with bone and joint infections.[29,31]

Fluoroquinolones alone or in combination with third-generation cephalosporins or aminoglycosides may be effective for *Yersinia* bacteremia, or in those with bone and joint infections.[29] Other antibiotics effective *in vitro* are chloramphenicol, tetracyclines, and TMP/SMX. Agents frequently resistant to *Yersinia* are penicillin G, ampicillin, and first-generation cephalosporins. Plague is generally treated with streptomycin. Tetracyclines, gentamicin, and chloramphenicol may also be used.[81]

A formalin-inactivated plague vaccine is effective in preventing flea-borne transmission. The vaccine is recommended for laboratory personnel frequently exposed to *Y. pestis* and for people with regular contact with wild rodents or their fleas in endemic areas.[80]

ACUTE VIRAL GASTROENTERITIS

Acute viral gastroenteritis was unknown until the 1970s. Viruses are now recognized as the leading cause of diarrhea in the world, although in many cases an exact pathogen cannot be determined. Viruses that have been recovered from the stools of patients with gastroenteritis include rotavirus, enteric adenovirus, Norwalk virus, calicivirus, astrovirus, and coronavirus.

ROTAVIRUSES

EPIDEMIOLOGY AND ETIOLOGY

Rotavirus is the major cause of severe diarrhea worldwide and accounts for approximately 70,000 hospitalizations and 100 deaths in the United States per year. One million people worldwide die annually from rotavirus infection. The fecal–oral route is thought to be the most common mode of transmission.[85] Although infection is most often seen in children ages 3 to 24 months, adults can be infected and may act as a reservoir for transmission. Serologic surveys show that nearly all children are infected by age 4 years. Rotavirus infection rates peak from November to May each year. In the first 5 years of life, four of five children in the United States will develop diarrhea from a rotavirus infection.

Rotaviruses are double-stranded wheel-shaped RNA viruses. Rotaviruses cause diarrhea by infecting the small intestinal villi. Changes to villi include shortening of villi, crypt hyperplasia, and mononuclear cell infiltration of the lamina propria. Diarrhea results from decreased absorption across intestinal mucosal surface.[85]

CLINICAL PRESENTATION

The rotavirus incubation period is less than 48 hours. Clinical manifestations of rotavirus infections vary from asymptomatic (which is common in adults) to severe nausea, vomiting, and diarrhea with dehydration. The first infection tends to be the most severe. Symptoms are characterized initially by nausea and vomiting (67% to 90%). Fever occurs in about two-thirds of children. Diarrhea occurs in most patients and lasts from 1 to 9 days. Other signs and symptoms include respiratory symptoms, irritability, lethargy, pharyngeal erythema, rhinitis, red tympanic membranes, and palpable cervical lymph nodes. Dehydration and electrolyte disturbances occur more frequently in children.

Laboratory findings reflect the degree of vomiting, diarrhea, or both. Transient rises in liver enzymes may be seen in 60% of children hospitalized for rotavirus diarrhea. The WBC count is usually normal. Stools rarely contain blood or leukocytes. Rotavirus detection in stool samples is possible with an enzyme immunoassay and a latex agglutination assay, both of which are commercially available.

Vaccines to prevent rotavirus infection showed early promise, and the first was licensed for use in the United States in 1998. One vaccine approved for use by the FDA, RotaShield, was withdrawn from the market after 1.5 million doses were administered. Although efficacious, infants receiving the vaccine showed an increased rate of idiopathic intussusception.[86] The future of rotavirus vaccine development includes the creation of virus-like particles and DNA vaccines.

► TREATMENT: Rotavirus Infection

Oral fluid and electrolyte replacement is the cornerstone of treatment.[87]

Oral *Lactobacillus* therapy may reduce the duration of diarrhea and of rotavirus excretion.[88]

Bismuth subsalicylate, although shown to decrease duration of diarrhea and stool output, is not recommended for routine use because of the self-limiting nature of the disease and the risk of bismuth subsalicylate overdose. Antimotility agents are not recommended, as they have not been shown to decrease the duration or volume of diarrhea.

A live attenuated oral human rotavirus vaccine was recently studied in infants in the United States in a randomized, double-blind, placebo-controlled trial. It was found to be effective, with subsequent rotaviral disease occurring in 18 of 107 placebo recipients versus 2 of 108 active vaccine recipients, an efficacy of 89%. No significant adverse events other than mild fever were reported.[89]

NORWALK AND NORWALK-LIKE AGENTS

EPIDEMIOLOGY

Parvovirus-like agents constitute a group of viruses that can cause acute gastroenteritis. The Norwalk virus was the first of these agents to be described in 1972. Agents of this group are named according to the location of the outbreak of illness or contaminated source, such as Norwalk, Hawaii, Montgomery County, Ditchling, Cockle, Paramatta, Snow Mountain, and Marin County.[90]

As with most viruses, the epidemiology of the Norwalk-like agents is not well understood. The disease commonly affects children and adults, but it is not often associated with disease in neonates and preschool children.[91] Outbreaks have been documented in families, health care systems, cruise ships, and college dormitories.[92]

to weeks. Other symptoms can include blurred vision, photophobia (90%), dysphagia (76%), generalized weakness (58%), nausea and vomiting (56%), and dysphonia (55%).

Diagnosis is made by culturing *C. botulinum* from the stool. Treatment consists primarily of respiratory support and use of botulinum antitoxin. Respiratory failure may occur prior to involvement of other upper muscle groups. If evaluation is performed within several hours of ingestion, gastric lavage or induction of vomiting is suggested. Cathartics and enemas can also be used to remove residual toxin from the bowel, but they are contraindicated in cases of ileus.

Although the effectiveness of antitoxins is unknown, patients diagnosed with botulism should receive botulinum antitoxin. Botulinum antitoxin is a concentrated preparation of equine globulins obtained from horses immunized with toxins A, B, and E. Because trivalent antitoxin is equine in origin, patients should be tested for hypersensitivity before receiving the product intravenously.

Other agents used experimentally as adjunctive therapy are guanidine, which antagonizes the effect of botulinum toxin at the neuromuscular junction, and 4-aminopyridine, which increases acetylcholine release.[101] Newer and more effective methods of treatment and prevention are under development, including a botulinum toxin vaccine consisting of nontoxic botulinum fragments.

Prevention should always be stressed. Botulinum toxins are heat labile and readily destroyed by 10 minutes of boiling. All home-canned foods should be processed according to directions and boiled, not just warmed, prior to consumption.

EVALUATION OF THERAPEUTIC OUTCOMES

Appropriate follow-up care of patients with acute diarrhea is based on assessing for successful restoration of fluid losses. The clinical signs and symptoms (Table 111–2) that led to diagnosis can also indicate rehydration success and should be assessed frequently. Because oral rehydration therapy is now preferred, routine laboratory testing is often unnecessary. Electrolytes should be measured in those receiving parenteral fluids, when oral replacement fails, or when signs of hypernatremia or hypokalemia are present.[102] Follow-up stool samples to ensure complete evacuation of the infecting pathogen may only be necessary in patients at high risk to initiate or contribute to a community outbreak. All patients should be monitored for complications associated with the infecting pathogen, resolution of the diarrhea, and adverse reactions to the pharmacologic agents used. One panel suggests prompt discharge of hospitalized children should occur when rehydration is achieved, IV fluids have not been required, oral intake equals or exceeds losses, and adequate family education and medical follow-up is assured.[103] For most patients, discharge can occur in 16 to 24 hours.

PHARMACOECONOMIC CONSIDERATIONS OF GASTROINTESTINAL INFECTIONS

Although infectious diarrhea in the United States is often self-limited, the economic impact of GI infections is enormous. Traveler's diarrhea interferes with planned activities or work in 30% of those affected, accounting for unknown but substantial direct and indirect lost dollars because of decreased productivity.[43]

Diarrheal illness accounts for 2 to 3.7 million doctor visits and 200,000 hospitalizations per year in children younger than 5 years of age in the United States. Avendano and associates evaluated the costs of diarrhea episodes resulting in a physician visit in children younger than 5 years of age.[102] They estimated the total cost per episode to be approximately $290. This extrapolates to a cost of over $2 billion per year for children younger than 5 years of age.[15] In 50% of cases, diarrheal illness leads to at least 1 full day of lost activity by the patient or parents of patients. This results in a total projected cost of $23 billion per year in the United States based on estimated medical costs and lost productivity.[1]

▶ PRINCIPLES OF PHARMACOTHERAPY

- Etiologies of infectious diarrhea include bacteria, viruses, and protozoans. Viral infections are the leading cause of diarrhea in the world.
- Fluid and electrolyte replacement is the cornerstone of therapy. Most cases of mild and moderate diarrhea can be treated with oral rehydration therapy.
- The necessary components of oral replacement therapy are glucose, sodium, potassium, chloride, and water.
- Metronidazole is the treatment of choice for *C. difficile* colitis. Vancomycin is an alternative.
- Antimicrobial therapy is often not indicated for enteritis as many cases are mild and self-limited or are viral in nature.
- When antimicrobials are used for enteritis they should be active against the most likely pathogen based on clinical symptoms, epidemiologic patterns, and resistance patterns in the area.
- Food poisoning may be responsible for over 76 million cases of diarrhea per year. Common pathogens include *Staphylococcus, Salmonella, Shigella,* and *Clostridium.*
- Patient education and prevention strategies are important in preventing and treating traveler's diarrhea. Prophylaxis with antibiotics is appropriate in certain situations.

REFERENCES

1. Cheney CP, Wong RKH. Acute infectious diarrhea. Med Clin North Am 1993;77:1169–1196.
2. Laney DW, Cohen MB. Approach to the pediatric patient with diarrhea. Gastroenterol Clin North Am 1993;22:499–515.
3. Brown KH. Dietary management of acute diarrheal disease: Contemporary scientific issues. Am Inst Nutr 1994;124:1455S–1460S.
4. Glass RI, Lew JF, Gangarosa RE, et al. Estimates of morbidity and mortality rates for diarrheal disease in American children. J Pediatr 1991;118:S27–S33.
5. Meyers A. Modern management of acute diarrhea and dehydration in children. Am Fam Phys 1995;51:1103–1115.
6. Gavin N, Merrick N, Davidson B. Efficacy of glucose-based oral rehydration therapy. Pediatrics 1996;98:45–51.
7. Gastañaduy AS, Begue RE. Acute gastroenteritis. Clin Pediatr 1999;38:1–12.
8. Lebenthal E, Khin-Maung-U, Rolston DDK, et al. Thermophilic amylase-digested rice-electrolyte solution in the treatment of acute diarrhea in children. Pediatrics 1995;95:198–202.
9. Islam A, Molla AM, Ahmed MA, et al. Is rice based oral replacement therapy effective in young infants? Arch Dis Child 1994;71:19–23.
10. Holliday MA, Friedman AL, Wassner SJ. Extracellular fluid restoration in dehydration: A critique of rapid versus slow. Pediatr Nephrol 1999;13:292–297.
11. Molina S, Vettorazzi C, Peerson JM. Clinical trial of glucose-oral rehydration solution (ORS), rice dextrin-ORS, and rice flour-ORS for the management of children with acute diarrhea and mild or moderate dehydration. Pediatrics 1995;95:191–197.

12. Liebelt EL. Clinical and laboratory evaluation and management of children with vomiting, diarrhea, and dehydration. Curr Opin Pediatr 1998;10:461–469.
13. Valentiner-Branth P, Steinsland H, Gjessing HK, et al. Community-based randomized controlled trial of reduced osmolarity oral rehydration solution in acute childhood diarrhea. Pediatr Infect Dis J 1999;18:789–795.
14. Thillainayagam AV, Hunt JB, Farthing MJG. Enhancing clinical efficacy of oral rehydration therapy: Is low osmolality the key? Gastroenterology 1998;114:197–210.
15. American Academy of Pediatrics. Practice parameter: The management of acute gastroenteritis in young children. Pediatrics 1996;97:424–435.
16. Ramakrishna BS, Venkataraman S, Srinivasan P, et al. Amylase-resistant starch plus oral rehydration solution for cholera. N Engl J Med 2000; 342:308–313.
17. Vanderhoof JA, Murray ND, Paule CL, Ostrom KM. Use of soy fiber in acute diarrhea in infants and toddlers. Clin Pediatr 1997;36:135–139.
18. Goepp JG, Katz SA. Oral rehydration therapy. Am Fam Phys 1993; 47:843–848.
19. Gore SM, Fontaine O, Pierce MF. Impact of rice-based oral rehydration solution on stool output and duration of diarrhoea: Meta-analysis of 13 clinical trials. BMJ 1992;304:287–291.
20. Fayed IM, Hashem M, Hussein A, et al. Comparison of soy-based formulas with lactose and with sucrose in the treatment of acute diarrhea in infants. Arch Pediatr Adolesc Med 1999;153:675–680.
21. Sullivan PB. Nutritional management of acute diarrhea. Nutrition 1998; 14:758–762.
22. Ahmed T, Ali M, Ullah MM, et al. Mortality in severely malnourished children with diarrhoea and use of a standardised management protocol. Lancet 1999;353:1919–1922.
23. Alam NH, Ahmed T, Khatun M, Molla AM. Effects of food with two oral rehydration therapies: A randomized, controlled clinical trial. Gut 1992;33:560–562.
24. Faruque ASG, Mahalanabis D, Islam A, et al. Breast feeding and oral rehydration at home during diarrhoea to prevent dehydration. Arch Dis Child 1992;67:1027–1029.
25. Khan WA, Bennish ML, Seas C, et al. Randomised controlled comparison of single-dose ciprofloxacin and doxycycline for cholera caused by *Vibrio cholerae* 01 or 0139. Lancet 1996;348:296–300.
26. Mahon BE, Mintz ED, Greene KD, et al. Reported cholera in the United States, 1992–1994. JAMA 1996;276:307–312.
27. Anonymous. Update: *Vibrio cholerae* O1—Western Hemisphere, 1991–1994, and *V. cholerae* O139—Asia, 1994. MMWR Morb Mortal Wkly Rep 1995;44(11):215–219.
28. Cheasty T, Said B, Threlfall EJ. *V. cholerae* non-O1: Implications for man? Lancet 1999;354:89–90.
29. Banerjee S, LaMont JT. Treatment of gastrointestinal infections. Gastroenterology 2000;118(2 suppl 1):S48–67.
30. Afghani B, Stutman HR. Toxin-related diarrheas. Pediatr Ann 1994;23: 549–555.
31. Gilbert DN, Moellering RC, Sande MA. The Sanford Guide to Antimicrobial Therapy, 30th ed. Hyde Park, VT: Antimicrobial Therapy, 2000:12–13.
32. Dutta D, Bhattacharya SK, Bhattacharya MK, et al. Efficacy of norfloxacin and doxycyline for treatment of *Vibrio cholerae* 0139 infection. J Antimicrob Chemother 1996;37;575–581.
33. Taylor DN, Cardenas V, Sanchez JL, et al. Two-year study of the protective efficacy of the oral whole cell plus recombinant B subunit cholera vaccine in Peru. J Infect Dis 2000;181:1667–1673.
34. Isada CM, Kasten BL, Goldman CM, et al. Infectious Disease Handbook 1997–1998, 2nd ed. Hudson, OH, Lexi-Comp, 1996:136–138.
35. Cantey JR. *Escherichia coli* diarrhea. Gastroenterol Clin North Am 1993;22:609–622.
36. Anonymous. Diarrheagenic *Escherichia coli* (non-Shiga toxin-producing *E. coli*). CDC Web site, URL: http://www.cdc.gov/ncidod/dbmd/diseaseinfo/diarrecoli_t.htm, Updated April 2000.
37. Anonymous. *Escherichia coli* O157: H7. CDC Web site, URL: http://www.cdc.gov/ncidod/dbmd/diseaseinfo/escherichiacoli_t.htm Updated May 2000.
38. Wong CS, Jelacic S, Habeeb RL, et al. The risk of the hemolytic-uremic syndrome after antibiotic treatment of *Escherichia coli* O157:H7 infections. N Engl J Med 2000;342:1930–1936.
39. Brook MG, Bannister BA. Diarrhoea-causing *Escherichia coli*. Dig Dis 1993;11:288–297.
40. Slutsker L, Ries AA, Greene KD, et al. *Escherichia coli* O157:H7 diarrhea in the United States: Clinical and epidemiologic features. Ann Intern Med 1997;126:505–513.
41. Mead PS, Griffin PM. *Escherichia coli* O157:H7. Lancet 1998;352: 1207–1212.
42. Ahren C, Jertborn M, Svennerholm A. Intestinal immune responses to an inactivated oral enterotoxigenic *Escherichia coli* vaccine and associated immunoglobulin A responses in blood. Infect Immunol 1998;66(7): 3311–3316.
43. Passaro DJ, Parsonnet J. Advances in the prevention and management of traveler's diarrhea. Curr Clin Top Infect Dis 1998;18:217–236.
44. Centers for Disease Control and Prevention. Health Information for International Travel 1999–2000. Atlanta, GA: Department of Health and Human Services [also URL: http://www.cdc.gov/travel/diarrhea.htm].
45. Reinke CM, Messick CR. Update on *Clostridium difficile*-induced colitis: 1. Am J Hosp Pharm 1994;51:1771–1781.
46. Caputo GM, Weitekamp MR, Bacon AE, Whitener C. *Clostridium difficile* infection: A common clinical problem for the general internist. J Gen Intern Med 1994;9:528–533.
47. Taylor ME, Oppenheim BA. Hospital-acquired infection in elderly patients. J Hosp Infect 1998;38:245–260.
48. Johnson S, Gerding DN. *Clostridium difficile*-associated diarrhea. Clin Infect Dis 1998;26:1027–1036.
49. Rohner P, Pittet D, Pepey B, et al. Etiological agents of infectious diarrhea: Implications for requests for microbial culture. J Clin Microbiol 1997;35:1427–1432.
50. Feteky R. Guidelines for the diagnosis and management of *Clostridium difficile*-associated diarrhea and colitis. Am J Gastroenterol 1997;92: 739–750.
51. Reinke CM, Messick CR. Update on *Clostridium difficile*-induced colitis: 2. Am J Hosp Pharm 1994;51:1892–1901.
52. Elmer GW, Surawicz CM, McFarland LV. Biotherapeutic agents: A neglected modality for the treatment and prevention of selected intestinal and vaginal infections. JAMA 1996;275:870–876.
53. Vanderhoof JA, Young RJ. Use of probiotics in childhood gastrointestinal disorders. J Pediatr Gastroenterol Nutr 1998;27:323–331.
54. Kotloff KL, Winickoff B, Ivanoff JD, et al. Global burden of Shigella infections: Implications for vaccine development and implementation. Bull WHO 1999;77:651–656.
55. Stutman HR. Salmonella, Shigella, and Campylobacter: Common bacterial causes of infectious diarrhea. Pediatr Ann 1994;23:538–543.
56. Khan WA, Seas C, Dhar U, et al. Treatment of shigellosis: V. Comparison of azithromycin and ciprofloxacin. Ann Intern Med 1997;126:697–703.
57. Sack RB, Rahman M, Yunus M, Khan EH. Antimicrobial resistance in organisms causing diarrheal disease. Clin Infect Dis 1997;24(suppl 1): S102–S105.
58. Patwari AK. Multidrug resistant Shigella infections in children. J Diarrhoeal Dis Res 1994;12:182–186.
59. Coster TS, Hoge CW, VanDeVerg LL, et al. Vaccination against shigellosis with attenuated *Shigella flexneri* 2a strain SC602. Infect Immunol 1999;67(7):3437–3443.
60. Kotloff KL, Noriega FR, Samandari T, et al. *Shigella flexneri* 2a strain CVD 1207, with specific deletions in virG, sen, set, and guaBA, is highly attenuated in humans. Infect Immun 2000;68(3):1034–1039.
61. Hogan DE. The emergency department approach to diarrhea. Emerg Med Clin North Am 1996;14:673–694.
62. Anonymous. Salmonellosis. CDC Web site, URL: http://www.cdc.gov/ncidod/dbmd/diseaseinfo/salmonellosis_t.htm Updated March 2000.
63. Anonymous. Outbreak of *Salmonella enteritidis* associated with nationally distributed ice cream products—Minnesota, South Dakota, and Wisconsin, 1994. MMWR Morb Mortal Wkly Rep 1994;43:740–741.
64. Anonymous. U.S. Food & Drug Administration Center for Food Safety and Applied Nutrition Foodborne Pathogenic Microorganisms and

Natural Toxins, 1992, Washington, DC, Dept. Health and Human Services. Also: www.cfsan.fda.gov/~mow/intro.html.
65. El-Radhi AS, Rostila T, Vesikari T. Association of high fever and short bacterial excretion after salmonellosis. Arch Dis Child 1992;67:531–532.
66. Alam MN, Haq SA, Das KK, et al. Efficacy of ciprofloxacin in enteric fever: Comparison of treatment duration in sensitive and multidrug-resistant Salmonella. Am J Trop Med Hyg 1995;53:306–311.
67. Hosek G, Leschinsky D, Irons S, Safranek TJ. Multidrug-resistant Salmonella serotype typhimurium—United States, 1996. JAMA 1997; 277:1513.
68. Threlfall EJ, Ward LR, Skinner JA, et al. Ciprofloxacin-resistant *Salmonella typhi* and treatment failure. Lancet 1999;353:1590–1591.
69. Rowe B, Ward L, Threlfall EJ. Multidrug-resistant *Salmonella typhi*: A worldwide epidemic. Clin Infect Dis 1997;24(suppl 1):S106–S109.
70. Conrad DA, Jenson HB. New and improved vaccines: Promising weapons against varicella, hepatitis A, and typhoid fever. Postgrad Med 1996;100:113–126.
71. Plotkin SA, Bouveret-LeCam N. A new typhoid vaccine composed of the Vi capsular polysaccharide. Arch Intern Med 1995;155:2293–2299.
72. Anonymous. Typhoid immunization recommendations of the Advisory Committee on Immunization Practices (ACIP). MMWR Morb Mortal Wkly Rep 1994;43(RR-14):1–7.
73. Engels EA, Lau J. Vaccines for preventing typhoid fever. Cochrane Database Syst Rev 2000;3(2):CD $\phi\phi$ 1261.
74. Tacket CO, Szetein MB, Wasserman SS, et al. Phase 2 clinical trial of attenuated *Salmonella enterica* serovar *typhi* oral live vector vaccine CVD 908-htrA in U.S. volunteers. Infect Immunol 2000;68(3):1196–1201.
75. Allos BM, Blaser MJ. *Campylobacter jejuni* and the expanding spectrum of related infections. Clin Infect Dis 1995;20:1092–1101.
76. Peterson MC. Clinical aspects of *Campylobacter jejuni* infections in adults. West J Med 1994;161:148–152.
77. Wallis MR. The pathogenesis of *Campylobacter jejuni*. Br J Biomed Sci 1994;51:57–64.
78. Ketley JM. Pathogenesis of enteric infection by *Campylobacter*. Microbiology 1997;143:5–21.
79. Sjögren E, Lindblom GB, Kaijser B. Norfloxacin resistance in *Campylobacter jejuni* and *Campylobacter coli* isolates from Swedish patients. J Antimicrob Chemother 1997;40:257–261.
80. Gage KL, Dennis DT, Tsai TF. Prevention of plague: Recommendations of the advisory committee on immunization practices (ACIP). MMWR Morb Mortal Wkly Rep 1996;45(RR14):1–15.
81. Perry RD, Fetherston JD. *Yersinia pestis*—Etiologic agent of plague. Clin Microbiol Rev 1997;10:35–66.
82. Werner SB, Murray R, Reilly K, et al. Human plague—United States, 1993–1994. JAMA 1994;271:1312.
83. San Joaquin VH. Aeromonas, Yersinia, and miscellaneous bacterial enteropathogens. Pediatr Ann 1994;23:544–548.
84. Baert F, Peetermans W, Knockaert D. Yersinosis: The clinical spectrum. Acta Clinica Belgica 1994;49:76–85.
85. Lieberman JM. Rotavirus and other viral cases of gastroenteritis. Pediatr Ann 1994;23:529–535.
86. Anonymous. Withdrawal of rotavirus vaccine recommendation. MMWR Morb Mortal Wkly Rep 1999;48(43):1007.
87. Nappert G, Barrios JM, Zello GA, Naylor JM. Oral rehydration solution therapy in the management of children with rotavirus diarrhea. Nutr Rev 2000;58:80–87.
88. Guarino A, Canani RB, Spagnuolo MI, et al. Oral bacterial therapy reduces the duration of symptoms and of viral excretion in children with mild diarrhea. J Pediatr Gastroenterol Nutr 1997;25:516–519.
89. Bernstein DI, Sack DA, Rothstein E, et al. Efficacy of live, attenuated, human rotavirus vaccine 89–12 in infants: A randomized placebo-controlled trial. Lancet 1999;354:287–290.
90. Caul EO. Viral gastroenteritis: Small round structured viruses, caliciviruses, and astroviruses: I. The clinical and diagnostic perspective. J Clin Pathol 1996;49:874–880.
91. Taterka JA, Cuff CF, Rubin DH. Viral gastrointestinal infections. Gastroenterol Clin North Am 1992;21:303–329.
92. Caul EO. Viral gastroenteritis: Small round structured viruses, caliciviruses, and astroviruses: II. The epidemiological perspective. J Clin Pathol 1996;49:959–964.
93. Aristeguieta C, Koenders I, Windham D, et al. Multistate outbreak of viral gastroenteritis associated with consumption of oysters—Apalachicola Bay, Florida, December 1994–January 1995. JAMA 1995;273:452.
94. Cirino J, Cumberland D, Pollack L, et al. Multistate outbreak of viral gastroenteritis related to consumption of oysters—1993. JAMA 1994; 271:183–184.
95. Ball JM, Graham DY, Opekun AR, et al. Recombinant Norwalk virus-like particles given orally to volunteers: Phase I study. Gastroenterology 1999;117:40–48.
96. Grohmann GS, Glass RI, Pereira HG, et al. Enteric viruses and diarrhea in HIV-infected patients. N Engl J Med 1993;329:14–20.
97. Smith PD. Infectious diarrheas in patients with AIDS. Gastroenterol Clin North Am 1993;22:535–548.
98. Anonymous. Preliminary FoodNet Data on the Incidence of Foodborne Illnesses—Selected Sites, United States, 1999. MMWR Morb Mortal Wkly Rep 2000;49(10):201–205.
99. Hatheway CL. Toxigenic Clostridia. Clin Microbiol Rev 1990;3:66–98.
100. Roblot P, Roblot F, Fauchere JL, et al. Retrospective study of 108 cases of botulism in Poitiers, France. J Med Microbiol 1994;40:379–384.
101. Middlebrook JL. Protection strategies against botulinum toxin. Adv Exper Med Biol 1995;383:93–98.
102. Avendano P, Matson DO, Long J, et al. Costs associated with office visits for diarrhea in infants and toddlers. Pediatr Infect Dis J 1993;12:897–902.

112

INTRA-ABDOMINAL INFECTIONS

Joseph T. DiPiro and Thomas R. Howdieshell

Intra-abdominal infections are those contained within the peritoneum or retroperitoneal space. The peritoneal cavity extends from the undersurface of the diaphragm to the floor of the pelvis and contains the stomach, small bowel, large bowel, liver, gallbladder, and spleen. The duodenum, pancreas, kidneys, adrenal glands, great vessels (aorta and vena cava), and most mesenteric vascular structures reside in the retroperitoneum. Intra-abdominal infections may be generalized or localized. They may be contained within visceral structures, such as the liver, gall bladder, spleen, pancreas, kidney, or female reproductive organs. Two general types of intra-abdominal infection are discussed throughout this chapter: peritonitis and abscess. Peritonitis is defined as the acute, inflammatory response of the peritoneal lining to microorganisms, chemicals, irradiation, or foreign body injury. This chapter deals only with peritonitis of infectious origin.

An abscess is a purulent collection of fluid separated from surrounding tissue by a wall comprised of inflammatory cells and adjacent organs. It usually contains necrotic debris, bacteria, and inflammatory cells. These processes differ considerably in presentation and approach to treatment.

EPIDEMIOLOGY

Peritonitis may be classified as either primary or secondary. Primary peritonitis, also called "spontaneous bacterial peritonitis," is best defined as infection of the peritoneal cavity without an evident source in the abdomen.[1] Bacteria may be transported from the bloodstream to the peritoneal cavity where the inflammatory process begins. In secondary peritonitis, a focal disease process is evident within the abdomen. Secondary peritonitis may involve perforation of the gastrointestinal (GI) tract (possibly because of ulceration, ischemia, or obstruction), postoperative peritonitis, or post-traumatic peritonitis (blunt or penetrating trauma). Primary peritonitis is relatively uncommon in adults and normal infants and children. Primary peritonitis develops in up to 25% of patients with alcoholic cirrhosis.[2] Approximately 60% of all patients on chronic ambulatory peritoneal dialysis (CAPD) will have at least one episode of peritonitis during the first year.[3] The average incidence of peritonitis in patients undergoing continuous ambulatory peritoneal dialysis is from 1.3 episodes per year to 1 episode every 19 months.[2,4] Epidemiologic data for secondary intra-abdominal infections is limited. Any of numerous intra-abdominal processes may give rise to secondary peritonitis including perforation of a peptic ulcer; traumatic perforation of the stomach, small or large bowel, uterus, or urinary bladder; appendicitis; pancreatitis; diverticulitis; bowel infarction; cholecystitis; operative contamination of the peritoneum; and diseases of the female genital tract such as septic abortion, postoperative uterine infection, endometritis, or salpingitis. Appendicitis is one of the most common causes of intra-abdominal infection. In 1998, 278,000 appendectomies were performed in the United States for suspected appendicitis.[5]

ETIOLOGY

Primary peritonitis in adults most commonly occurs in association with alcoholic cirrhosis, especially in its end stage. It has also been reported with ascites caused by post-necrotic cirrhosis, chronic active hepatitis, acute viral hepatitis, congestive heart failure, malignancy, systemic lupus erythematosus, and nephritic syndrome. It may also result from the use of a peritoneal catheter for dialysis or central nervous system ventriculoperitoneal shunting. Rarely, primary peritonitis occurs with no apparent underlying disease.

Table 112–1 summarizes many of the potential causes of bacterial peritonitis. These include inflammatory processes of the GI tract or abdominal organs, bowel obstruction, vascular occlusions that may lead to gangrene of the intestines, and neoplasia that may cause intestinal perforation or obstruction. Other possible causes include those resulting from traumatic injuries or postoperative infections.

Abscesses are the result of chronic inflammation and may occur without preceding generalized peritonitis. They may be located within one of the spaces of the peritoneal cavity or within one of the visceral organs and may range from a few milliliters to a liter or more in volume. These collections often have a fibrinous capsule and may take from a few months to years to form.

The causes of intra-abdominal abscess overlap those of peritonitis and, in fact, may occur sequentially or simultaneously. Appendicitis is the most frequent cause of abscess. Other potential causes of intra-abdominal abscess include pancreatitis, diverticulitis, lesions of the biliary tract, genitourinary tract infections, perforating tumors in the abdomen, trauma, and leaking intestinal anastomosis. In addition, pelvic inflammatory disease in women may lead to tuboovarian abscess. For certain diseases, such as appendicitis and diverticulitis, abscesses occur more frequently than generalized peritonitis.

MICROFLORA OF THE GASTROINTESTINAL TRACT AND FEMALE GENITAL TRACT

A full appreciation of intra-abdominal infection requires an understanding of the normal microflora within the GI tract. There are striking differences in bacterial species and concentrations of flora within the various segments of the GI tract (Table 112–2), and this bacterial environment usually determines the severity of infectious processes in the abdomen. Generally, the low gastric pH eradicates bacteria that enter the stomach. With achlorhydria, bacterial counts may rise to 10^5 to 10^7 organisms/mL. The normally low bacterial count may increase by 1,000- or 10,000-fold with gastric outlet obstruction, gastric cancer, and in patients receiving histamine-2 (H_2) receptor antagonists, proton pump inhibitors, or antacids, and in the presence of blood.

The biliary tract (gallbladder and bile ducts) is sterile in most healthy individuals but in certain groups (patients older than 70 years with acute cholecystitis, jaundice, or common bile duct stones), it is likely to be colonized by aerobic gram-negative bacilli (particularly *Escherichia coli* and *Klebsiella* spp.) and enterococci.[6] Patients

TABLE 112–1. Causes of Bacterial Peritonitis

Primary Bacterial Peritonitis
- Peritoneal dialysis
- Cirrhosis with ascites
- Nephrotic syndrome

Secondary Bacterial Peritonitis
- Miscellaneous causes
  - Diverticulitis
  - Appendicitis
  - Inflammatory bowel diseases
  - Salpingitis
  - Biliary tract infections
  - Necrotizing pancreatitis
- Neoplasms
  - Intestinal obstruction
  - Perforation
- Mechanical gastrointestinal problems
  - Any cause of small bowel obstruction (adhesions, hernia)
- Vascular causes
  - Mesenteric arterial or venous occlusion (atrial fibrillation)
  - Mesenteric ischemia without occlusion
- Trauma
  - Blunt abdominal trauma with rupture of intestine
  - Penetrating abdominal trauma
- Iatrogenic intestinal perforation (endoscopy)
- Intraoperative events
- Peritoneal contamination during abdominal operation
- Leakage from gastrointestinal anastomosis

with biliary tract bacterial colonization are at greater risk of intra-abdominal infection.

In the distal ileum, bacterial counts of aerobes and anaerobes are quite high. In the colon, there may be 400 to 500 different types of bacteria with concentrations often reaching 10^{11} organisms/mL, and anaerobic bacteria outnumbering aerobic bacteria by more than 1,000 to 1. In fact, up to 50% of the dry mass of stool is bacteria. Fortunately, most colonic bacteria are not pathogens because they cannot survive in environments outside the colon. Perforation of the colon results in the release of very large numbers of anaerobic and aerobic bacteria into the peritoneum. The colonic flora is generally consistent unless broad-spectrum antimicrobials have been used, in which case there are increases in *Candida* or gram-negative bacteria.

The lower female genital tract is generally colonized by a large number of aerobic and anaerobic bacteria. Anaerobes may number 10^9 organisms/mL and often include lactobacilli, eubacteria, clostridia, anaerobic streptococci, and, less frequently, *Bacteroides fragilis.* Aerobic bacteria are most often streptococci and *Staphylococcus epidermidis,* and these may number 10^8 organisms/mL.

PATHOPHYSIOLOGY

Intra-abdominal infection results from bacterial entry into the peritoneal or retroperitoneal spaces or from bacterial collections within intra-abdominal organs. In primary peritonitis, bacteria may enter the abdomen via the bloodstream or the lymphatic system by transmigration through the bowel wall, or via the fallopian tubes in females. Hematogenous bacterial spread (through the bloodstream) occurs more frequently with tuberculosis peritonitis or peritonitis associated with cirrhotic ascites. When peritonitis results from peritoneal dialysis, skin surface flora are introduced via the peritoneal catheter.[7] In secondary peritonitis, bacteria most often enter the peritoneum or retroperitoneum as a result of perforation of the GI or female genital tracts caused by diseases or traumatic injuries. Also, peritonitis or abscess may result from contamination of the peritoneum during a surgical procedure or following anastomotic leak.

The physiologic characteristics of the peritoneal cavity determine the nature of the response to infection or inflammation within it. The peritoneum is lined by a highly permeable, serous membrane with a surface area approximately that of skin. The peritoneal cavity is lubricated with 20–50 mL of sterile, clear yellow fluid, normally with fewer than 300 cells/mm^3, a specific gravity below 1.016, and protein below 3 g/dL. These conditions change drastically with peritoneal infection or inflammation, as is described later.

After bacteria are introduced into the peritoneal cavity, there is an immediate response to contain the insult. Humoral and cellular defenses respond first; then the omentum migrates to the affected area. A

TABLE 112–2. Usual Microflora of the Gastrointestinal Tract

		Approximate Concentration (Log No. Organisms/mL)	
Site	**Commonly Found Bacteria**	**Aerobes**	**Anaerobes**
Stomach[a]	Streptococcus, Lactobacillus	10–100	Rare
Biliary tract	Normally sterile (*Escherichia coli,* Klebsiella, or enterococci in some patients)	0	0
Proximal small bowel	Streptococcus (including enterococci), *E. coli,* Klebsiella, Lactobacillus, diphtheroids	100	Few
Distal ileum	*E. coli,* Klebsiella, Enterobacter, enterococci, *Bacteroides fragilis,* Clostridium, peptostreptococci	10^4–10^6	10^5–10^7
Colon	*Bacteroides* spp., peptostreptococci, Clostridium, *E. coli,* Klebsiella, enterococci, Enterobacter, and many others	10^5–10^8	10^9–10^{11}

[a]With achlorhydria, H_2-antagonist therapy, gastric cancer, or gastric outlet obstruction, bacterial counts may rise to 10^5/mL.

limited bacterial inoculum is rapidly handled by defense mechanisms including complement activation. Under certain conditions the bacterial insult is not contained, and bacteria disseminate throughout the peritoneal cavity, resulting in peritonitis. This is more likely to occur in the presence of a foreign body, hematoma, dead tissue, or where there is a large bacterial inoculum, continuing bacterial contamination, and contamination involving a mixture of synergistic organisms. Protein-calorie malnutrition, antecedent steroid therapy, and diabetes mellitus may also contribute to the formation of an intra-abdominal abscess.

When bacteria become dispersed throughout the peritoneum, the inflammatory process involves the majority of the peritoneal lining. There is an outpouring into the peritoneum of fluid containing leukocytes, fibrin, and other proteins that form exudates on the inflamed peritoneal surfaces and begin to form adhesions between peritoneal structures. This process, combined with a paralysis of the intestines (ileus), may result in confinement of the contamination to one or more locations within the peritoneum. Fluid also begins to collect in the bowel lumen and wall, and distention may result.

The fluid and protein shift into the abdomen (third-spacing) may be so dramatic that circulating blood volume is decreased, which causes decreased cardiac output and shock. Accompanying fever, vomiting, or diarrhea may worsen the fluid imbalance. A reflex sympathetic response, manifested by sweating, tachycardia, and vasoconstriction, may be evident. With an inflamed peritoneum, bacteria and endotoxins are easily absorbed into the bloodstream (translocation), and this may result in septic shock. Other foreign substances present in the peritoneal cavity potentiate peritonitis. These adjuvants, notably feces, dead tissues, barium, mucus, bile, and blood, have detrimental effects on host defense mechanisms, particularly on bacterial phagocytosis.

Many of the manifestations of intra-abdominal infections, particularly peritonitis, result from cytokine activity. Inflammatory cytokines, such as tumor necrosis factor (TNF)-α, interleukin-1 (IL-1), IL-6, IL-8, and interferon (INF)-γ, are produced by macrophages and neutrophils in response to bacteria and bacterial products, or to tissue injury resulting from the surgical incision.[8] These cytokines produce wide-ranging effects on the endothelium of organs, particularly the liver, lungs, kidneys, and heart. With uncontrolled activation of these mediators, sepsis may result (see Chap. 117).

Peritonitis may result in mortality because of the effects on major organ systems. As mentioned earlier, fluid shifts and endotoxin may cause hypotension and shock. Fluid loss from the vasculature with generalized peritonitis is similar to that which occurs after a 50% second-degree burn. Hypoalbuminemia may result from protein loss into the peritoneum. Pulmonary function may be compromised because the inflamed peritoneum causes splinting (muscle rigidity caused by pain) that inhibits proper diaphragmatic movement. Atelectasis and pulmonary shunting of blood may result in the onset of the adult respiratory distress syndrome and associated hypoxemia. With fluid loss, and hypotension, or endotoxemia, renal perfusion may be compromised, and acute renal failure is a potential threat. In addition, endotoxin is also hepatotoxic, and exposure during sepsis may lead to hepatic dysfunction.

If the body is successful in localizing peritoneal contamination but fails to eliminate bacteria completely, an abscess results. This collection of necrotic tissue, bacteria, and white blood cells (WBCs) may be at single or multiple sites, and may be within one of the spaces of the peritoneal cavity, or in one of the visceral organs. The location of the abscess is often related to the site of primary disease. For example, abscesses resulting from appendicitis tend to appear in the right lower quadrant or the pelvis; those resulting from diverticulitis tend to appear in the left lower quadrant or pelvis.

An abscess begins by the combined action of inflammatory cells (such as neutrophils), bacteria, fibrin, and other inflammatory components. Bacteria may release heparinases that cause local thrombosis and tissue necrosis, or fibrinolysins, collagenases, or other enzymes that allow extension of the process into surrounding tissues. Neutrophils gathered in the abscess cavity die in 3 to 5 days, releasing lysosomal enzymes that liquefy the core of the abscess. A mature abscess may have a fibrinous capsule that isolates bacteria and the liquid core from antimicrobials and immunologic defenses.

Within the abscess, the oxygen tension is low, anaerobic bacteria thrive, and the size of the abscess may increase because it is hypertonic, resulting in an additional influx of fluid. Hypertonicity promotes the formation of bacterial L forms, which are resistant to antimicrobial agents that disrupt cell walls. Abscess formation may continue and stabilize for long periods of time, and may not be readily evident to patient or physician. In some instances, the abscess may resolve spontaneously, and, infrequently, it may erode into adjacent organs, or rupture and cause diffuse peritonitis. If the abscess erodes through the skin, it may result in a fistula, connecting bowel to skin, or in a noncommunicating sinus tract.

MICROBIOLOGY OF INTRA-ABDOMINAL INFECTION

Primary bacterial peritonitis is often caused by a single organism. In children, the pathogen is usually *Streptococcus pneumoniae* or a group A Streptococcus.[8] When peritonitis occurs in association with cirrhotic ascites, enteric organisms are usually responsible.[9,10] *Escherichia coli* is isolated most frequently, followed by *Streptococcal* spp. (including pneumococcus), *Klebsiella, Bacteroides* spp., *Pseudomonas aeruginosa,* and numerous other organisms. Occasionally, primary peritonitis may be caused by *Mycobacterium tuberculosis*. Peritonitis in patients undergoing peritoneal dialysis is most often caused by common skin organisms, such as *S. epidermidis, Staphylococcus aureus,* Streptococci, and Diphtheroids.[9] Occasionally, aerobic gram-negative bacilli may cause infections, particularly in patients undergoing dialysis during hospitalization. Mortality from primary peritonitis caused by gram-negative bacteria is much greater than for gram-positive bacteria.[11]

Because of the diverse bacteria present in the GI tract, secondary intra-abdominal infections are often polymicrobial.[12] The mean number of different bacterial species isolated from infected intra-abdominal sites ranged from 2.9 to 3.7, including an average of 1.3 to 1.6 aerobes and 1.7 to 2.1 anaerobes.[13,14] With proper anaerobic specimen collection, anaerobic organisms are isolated in most patients. In one report of patients with gangrenous and perforated appendicitis, an average of 10.2 different organisms was isolated from each patient, including 2.7 aerobes and 7.5 anaerobes.[15] Purely aerobic or anaerobic infections are uncommon, as are infections caused by fungi. The frequencies with which specific bacteria were isolated in intra-abdominal infections are given in Table 112–3.[16] *Escherichia coli, Streptococcus* spp., and *Bacteroides* spp. were most often isolated from the infection site, as well as from blood cultures. In patients diagnosed with severe infections, the pattern of bacterial isolates may change and commonly includes *Candida, Enterococci, Enterobacter,* and S. *epidermidis*.[16]

Visceral abscesses differ in character from the typical intra-abdominal abscess. Hepatic abscesses may be polymicrobial (involving *E. coli* and anaerobes) or occasionally may be caused by amoeba. Pancreatic abscesses are often polymicrobial, involving enteric bacteria that ascend through the biliary system. Splenic abscesses usually result from hematogenous dissemination of bacteria, such as *S. aureus,* Streptococci, and, occasionally, *salmonella* or anaerobic organisms. Pelvic inflammatory disease is initially associated with

TABLE 112–3. Pathogens Isolated from 255 Patients With Intra-Abdominal Infections[1]

Aerobic Bacteria	Number of Isolates	Anaerobic Bacteria	Number of Isolates
E. coli	140	*Bacteroides* spp.	305
Klebsiella spp.	33	Peptostreptococcus	78
Enterobacter spp.	19	Fusobacteria	48
Proteus spp.	15	Clostridium	35
Pseudomonas spp.	33	Prevotella	27
Streptococcus	184	Gemella	26
Enterococcus	35	Porphyromonas	18
Staphylococcus	34		
Others	24		

(Adapted from Ref 1.)

Neisseria gonorrhoeae or *Chlamydia trachomatis*. However, tuboovarian abscesses are usually polymicrobial having a mix of gram-positive and gram-negative aerobes and anaerobes.

BACTERIAL SYNERGISM

The size of the bacterial inoculum and the number and types of bacterial species present in intra-abdominal infections influence patient outcome. The combination of aerobic and anaerobic organisms appears to increase the severity of infection greatly. In animal studies, combinations of aerobic and anaerobic bacteria were much more lethal than infections caused by aerobes or anaerobes alone.

Facultative bacteria may provide an environment conducive to the growth of anaerobic bacteria.[12] Although many bacteria isolated in mixed infections are nonpathogenic by themselves, their presence may be essential for the pathogenicity of the bacterial mixture.[2] The role of facultative bacteria in mixed infections can include (a) promotion of an appropriate environment for anaerobic growth through oxygen consumption; (b) production of nutrients necessary for anaerobes; or (c) production of extracellular enzymes that promote tissue invasion by anaerobes.

Rat models of intra-abdominal infection demonstrate that uncontrolled infection with a mix of aerobes and anaerobes leads to a two-stage infectious process. During the first 5 days after intra-abdominal implantation of gelatin capsules containing a mixture of 22 aerobic and anaerobic bacteria, acute generalized peritonitis was observed, and the mortality rate was about 40%. After 5 days, mortality from intra-abdominal infection was not observed; however, almost all surviving animals had intra-abdominal abscesses when sacrificed at 2 weeks. During the peritonitis stages, *E. coli* was noted in the bloodstream of most animals, and *E. coli, B. fragilis,* and Enterococci were isolated from peritoneal exudates. Bacteremia could not be demonstrated during the abscess stage, but abscesses were found to contain predominantly anaerobic bacteria *(B. fragilis* and *Fusobacterium varium). E. coli* and Enterococcus were also isolated from the abscess cavity. These experiments and others support the concept that aerobic enteric organisms and anaerobes are pathogens in intra-abdominal infection. Aerobic bacteria, particularly *E. coli,* appear responsible for the early mortality from peritonitis, whereas anaerobic bacteria are major pathogens in abscesses, with *B. fragilis* predominating. *B. fragilis* has a capsular polysaccharide complex that promotes the formation of intra-abdominal abscesses.[17]

Enterococcus can be isolated from many intra-abdominal infections in humans, but its role as a pathogen is not clear.[18] Antimicrobial regimens that are ineffective against enterococcus *in vitro* have been successful in treating intra-abdominal infections. Enterococcal infection occurs in the presence of specific risk factors, indicating failure of the host's defenses (immunocompromised patients). One report suggested that isolation of enterococcus from an intra-abdominal focus was a predictor of treatment failure in complicated intra-abdominal infections.[19]

CLINICAL PRESENTATION

Intra-abdominal infections have a wide spectrum of clinical features, often depending on the specific disease process, the location and magnitude of bacterial contamination, and concurrent host factors. Peritonitis is usually easily recognized but intra-abdominal abscess may often continue for considerable periods of time, either going unrecognized or attributed to an unrelated disease process.

Generalized bacterial peritonitis usually commands the immediate attention of the physician, because the patient most often presents in acute distress. The patient lies still, usually on his or her back, possibly with hips slightly flexed. Any movement of the patient, including rocking the bed or breathing worsens the generalized abdominal pain. The patient exhibits voluntary guarding of the abdominal musculature and respirations are shallow and frequent. There is generalized abdominal tenderness on examination, and after a short period of time the abdominal muscles become rigid, a product of involuntary guarding; this is called a "board-like abdomen." Bowel sounds are at first faint, then become absent as peristalsis ceases and abdominal distention ensues. Frequently, the patient has nausea often accompanied by vomiting. The secretion of fluid into the peritoneal cavity causes the vascular volume to contract. This, as well as the physiologic response to stress, causes a reflex tachycardia. Initially, the patient's temperature is normal, but increases to 100°F to 102°F (37.7°C to 38.8°C) within the first few hours, and may continue to rise for the next several hours. Because of the fluid loss into the peritoneum as well as vomiting, the patient may appear dehydrated, and a decreased urine output is noted.

If peritonitis continues untreated, the patient may experience hypovolemic shock from third-space fluid loss into the peritoneum, bowel wall, and lumen. This may be accompanied by sepsis because the inflamed peritoneum absorbs bacteria and toxins from the suppurative process into mesenteric blood vessels and lymph nodes, initiating production of inflammatory cytokines. Hypovolemic shock is the major factor contributing to mortality in the early stage of peritonitis.

Laboratory evaluations usually demonstrate leukocytosis (15,000 to 20,000 WBC/mm^3), with neutrophils predominating and an elevated percentage of immature neutrophils (bands). The hematocrit and the blood urea nitrogen may be elevated because of the dehydration. Early after the insult, the patient is usually alkalotic because of hyperventilation and vomiting. As the process progresses, the patient may become acidotic from hypovolemia or presence of devitalized tissue, leading to anaerobic metabolism. At this stage, serum lactic acid will be elevated. Abdominal radiographs may be useful, as free air in the abdomen (indicating intestinal perforation) or distention of the small or large bowel is often evident.

The presentation of primary peritonitis can be quite different from that of secondary peritonitis. Primary peritonitis can develop over a period of days to weeks and is evident as an acute febrile illness. Usually the patient has nausea, vomiting (sometimes with diarrhea), abdominal tenderness, and hypoactive bowel sounds, although the abdominal signs are variable. The patient's temperature or WBC count may be only mildly elevated. The cirrhotic patient may have worsening encephalopathy.

Patients with peritonitis related to chronic peritoneal dialysis usually have abdominal pain and tenderness, possibly with nausea and vomiting, but fever is not a consistent finding. In these patients, a cloudy dialysate effluent is often noted as a first sign of peritonitis, indicating the presence of bacteria and inflammatory cells.

With primary peritonitis, routine evaluative procedures should be performed (serum chemistries, complete blood count, abdominal radiographs, blood cultures), and, if possible, the ascitic fluid, collected by paracentesis or drainage of peritoneal dialysate, should be examined. In the presence of peritonitis, ascitic fluid usually contains greater than 300 leukocytes/mm^3 and bacteria may be evident on Gram stain of a centrifuged specimen; however, in 60% to 80% of patients with cirrhotic ascites the Gram stain is negative.

Intra-abdominal abscess may pose a difficult diagnostic challenge because the symptoms are often neither specific nor dramatic. The patient may complain of abdominal pain or discomfort, but these symptoms are not reliable. Fever is usually present; often it is low grade, but it may be high, with a spiking pattern. The patient may have a paralytic ileus and abdominal distention. The abdominal examination is unreliable; tenderness and pain may be present, and a mass may be palpated.

Peritonitis may result from an abscess that ruptures, spreading bacteria and toxins throughout the peritoneum. In other patients, the entry of bacterial toxins into the systemic circulation from the abscess may lead to sepsis and progressive multisystem organ failure (renal, hepatic, pulmonary, or cardiac).

Laboratory studies are generally not helpful in the diagnosis of intra-abdominal abscess, although most patients will have leukocytosis. Some patients may have positive blood cultures, whereas others, particularly diabetics, may have hyperglycemia. The finding of *Bacteroides* or any two enteric bacteria in the bloodstream is often indicative of an intra-abdominal infectious process.

Radiographic methods are used to make the diagnosis of an intra-abdominal abscess. Plain radiographs may show air-fluid levels or shift of normal intra-abdominal contents by the abscess mass. Gastrointestinal contrast studies may also demonstrate this displacement of abdominal structures. Both of these modalities provide indirect evidence of abscess presence, but are not generally helpful in precisely locating the abscess.

Ultrasound is frequently the first diagnostic method used when an intra-abdominal abscess is suspected. The procedure may be done at the bedside, which is particularly helpful in the patient in the intensive care unit. The other advantage of this procedure is that it involves no radiation exposure. Limitations of ultrasound include difficulty in distinguishing between an early abscess and loops of intestine. In some patients, particularly the obese, it is technically difficult to perform the exam.[20]

Computed tomography (CT) scan is frequently used to evaluate the abdomen for the presence of an abscess and is the imaging modality of greatest value. Oral radiocontrast agents may be given to allow differentiation of the abscess from the bowel. Intravenous radiocontrast agents will be taken up preferentially in the wall of the abscess, creating a unique radiographic appearance.

Magnetic resonance imaging might be used to locate an intra-abdominal abscess, particularly in the retroperitoneum, but this modality offers no significant advantage when compared to CT scan, and is infrequently used.

The final diagnostic imaging modality is radioactive isotope imaging. Specific techniques include the use of ^{67}Ga citrate-, ^{99m}Tc-, and ^{111}In-labeled leukocytes.[21] These studies require a long period of imaging and are not routinely employed unless CT scanning fails to demonstrate a suspected abscess.

Intra-abdominal infection caused by disease processes at specific sites often produces characteristic manifestations that are helpful in diagnosis. For example, a patient with diverticulitis may exhibit stabbing left-lower-quadrant abdominal pain and constipation. Fever and leukocytosis are often present, and a tender mass is sometimes palpable. With appendicitis, the findings may be inconsistent, but many patients have a sudden onset of periumbilical or epigastric pain, which is usually colicky and shifts to the right lower quadrant. The location of pain may vary, as the appendix can be in many locations in the abdomen. A mass may be palpable on abdominal or rectal examination. The patient's temperature is generally mildly elevated early and then increases. If perforation and peritonitis occur, findings would include diffuse abdominal pain, rigidity, and sustained fever. More frequently, however, appendiceal perforation results in a local abscess.

Abscesses in specific locations may produce clues to their existence. Pelvic abscesses may be palpable by pelvic or rectal examination. A subdiaphragmatic abscess may result in pleural effusion noted on chest X-ray. Retroperitoneal abscesses may cause lumbar or psoas muscle spasm resulting in lower back pain and hip flexion.

The presentation and outcome of any intra-abdominal infection may be influenced by patient-specific factors. Those who are malnourished, who have sustained multiple traumatic injuries, or who are at the extremes of age are more likely to succumb to intra-abdominal infection or to require an extended period for recovery. In addition to these factors, those with associated diseases, such as diabetes mellitus, malignancy, renal failure, or cirrhosis, and who are recognized to be immunocompromised, are at greater risk for most infectious processes, including intra-abdominal infection. Other risk factors often related to intra-abdominal infection include the use of corticosteroids, particularly in patients with Crohn's disease, and radiation therapy for tumors. Also, concurrent use of antimicrobial agents may prevent the prompt diagnosis of abscesses. In some instances, acute intra-abdominal infectious processes may become chronic with the initiation of antimicrobial agents. Geriatric patients with intra-abdominal infection frequently present without the typical signs and symptoms of abdominal pain, nausea, vomiting, diarrhea, and fever.[22]

▶ TREATMENT: Intra-Abdominal Infections

DESIRED OUTCOME

The goals of treatment are the correction of intra-abdominal disease processes or injuries that have caused infection and the drainage of collections of purulent material (abscess). A secondary objective is to achieve a resolution of infection without major organ system complications (obstruction, fistula, or renal failure) or adverse drug effects. Ideally, the patient should be discharged from the hospital with full function for self-care and routine daily activities.

GENERAL APPROACH TO TREATMENT

The treatment of intra-abdominal infection most often requires the coordinated use of three major modalities: (a) prompt drainage, (b) support of vital functions, and (c) appropriate antimicrobial therapy to treat infection not removed by surgery.

Antimicrobials are an important adjunct to drainage procedures in the treatment of intra-abdominal infections; however, the use of antimicrobial agents without surgical intervention is usually inadequate. For specific situations (e.g., most cases of primary peritonitis), drainage procedures may not be required, and antimicrobial agents become the mainstay of therapy.

In the early phase of serious intra-abdominal infections, attention should be given to the maintenance of organ system functions. With generalized peritonitis, large volumes of intravenous (IV) fluids are required to restore vascular volume, to improve cardiovascular function, and to maintain adequate tissue perfusion and oxygenation. Adequate urine output should be maintained to ensure proper renal function. Correcting hypovolemia and restoring cardiac output does this. Respiratory function can be assisted by a variety of methods, including ventilatory support in severely ill patients. Often, the critically ill patient with intra-abdominal infection will require intensive care monitoring, particularly if there is cardiovascular or respiratory instability. Also, isolation procedures may be required if the infectious process poses a threat to other hospitalized patients.

An additional important component of therapy is nutrition. Intra-abdominal infections often directly involve the GI tract or disrupt its function (paralytic ileus). The return of GI motility may take days, weeks, and occasionally months. In the interim, enteral or parenteral nutrition as indicated allows improved immune function and wound to ensure recovery.

NONPHARMACOLOGIC TREATMENT

DRAINAGE PROCEDURES

Primary peritonitis is treated with antimicrobials and rarely requires drainage. Secondary peritonitis requires surgical correction of the underlying pathology. The drainage of the purulent material is the critical element in the management of an intra-abdominal abscess. Without adequate drainage of the abscess, antimicrobial therapy and fluid resuscitation can be expected to fail.

Secondary peritonitis is treated surgically. At the time of laparotomy, attempts are made to correct the cause of the peritonitis. This may include patching a perforated ulcer with omentum, resection of a segment of perforated colon, or resection of a portion of gangrenous small intestine. The goal of all of these procedures is to remove the inflamed or gangrenous viscus and to prevent further bacterial contamination. The presence of active inflammation increases the difficulty of the surgical procedure. This results in a higher morbidity and mortality rate than if the same procedures were performed in an elective setting without inflammation.

The presence of active inflammation may make it technically impossible to perform the ultimate surgical procedure. In this situation, attempts are made to provide drainage of the infected or gangrenous structures. An example of this situation is empyema of the gallbladder. If it is unsafe or impossible to perform the cholecystectomy, then a tube is placed into the gallbladder. This procedure—cholecystostomy—provides for drainage of the purulent material present in the gallbladder. The gallbladder would then be removed at a subsequent operation following resolution of the inflammation.

If an intra-abdominal abscess, separate from any intra-abdominal organ, is discovered during an exploratory laparotomy, then it may be dèbrided, excised, or drained. If the intra-abdominal abscess involves an abdominal structure, then a resection of part or all of that organ may be required. An example of this situation is an abscess associated with diverticular disease of the colon. Management may include drainage of the abscess and resection of the involved colon. All foreign material, necrotic tissue, feces, blood, or pus should be removed from the operative field, and the peritoneum should be copiously irrigated with 0.9% sodium chloride to decrease the concentrations of bacteria or other noxious substances.

After an abscess is located, it must be drained. This may be performed surgically or using percutaneous, image-guided techniques.[23,24] Typically, image-guided techniques are done using ultrasound or CT. The management of intra-abdominal abscess with percutaneous catheter drainage may represent the ultimate procedure. The patient may require a subsequent procedure to treat the underlying conditions. In this latter circumstance, a significant advantage is obtained by first draining the abscess percutaneously. This allows the surgical procedure to be performed on a patient who is no longer suffering the systemic manifestations of uncontrolled infection.

A number of drainage techniques have been described using endoscopy and laparoscopy.[25,26] These minimal access techniques may offer advantages when compared to traditional surgery, but will probably be used less often than radiologically assisted percutaneous drainage techniques.

The most valuable microbiologic information may be obtained at the time of operation or percutaneous abscess drainage. If pus or fluids is found that is believed to be infected, it is best to aspirate 2–3 mL into a syringe, remove any air, and tightly cap the syringe. The specimen should be taken promptly to the microbiology laboratory where a Gram stain should be performed immediately and cultures prepared for identification of aerobic and anaerobic bacteria. If there is no fluid available for collection, culture swab devices may be applied to the infected area. Swabs transported under aerobic and anaerobic conditions are required, and should be analyzed as just described.

FLUID THERAPY

Aggressive fluid repletion and management are required for successful treatment of intra-abdominal infections. Fluid therapy is instituted for the purposes of achieving or maintaining proper intravascular volume to ensure adequate urine output and correction of acidosis. Intravascular volume is often decreased in patients with severe intra-abdominal infection because fluid accumulates in the abdomen; collecting in a third space at the expense of the plasma volume. Loss of fluid through vomiting, diarrhea, or a nasogastric suction tube contributes to dehydration. Intravascular volume can be assessed by blood pressure and heart rate, but more accurately by measurement of central venous pressure or pulmonary capillary wedge pressure. When a contracted vascular volume is accompanied by hemorrhage, the hematocrit initially is about normal, but if there is no associated hemorrhage, the hematocrit is usually elevated as an indication of hemoconcentration. Urine output should be continuously monitored in severely ill patients by use of a transurethral bladder catheter, quantitated hourly, and it should equal or exceed 0.5 mL/kg body weight/h.

In patients with peritonitis, hypovolemia is often accompanied by acidosis, so a reasonable IV fluid would be lactated Ringer, which contains the bicarbonate precursor, lactate, as well as sodium, chloride,

TABLE 112–4. Likely Intra-Abdominal Pathogens

Type of Infection	Aerobes	Anaerobes
Primary Bacterial Peritonitis		
Children (spontaneous)	Pneumococci, group A *Streptococcus*	—
Cirrhosis	*E. coli, Klebsiella,* pneumococci (many others)	—
Peritoneal dialysis	*Staphylococcus, Streptococcus*	—
Secondary Bacterial Peritonitis		
Gastroduodenal	*Streptococcus, E. coli*	—
Biliary tract	*E. coli, Klebsiella,* enterococci	Clostridium or Bacteroides (infrequent)
Small or large bowel	*E. coli, Klebsiella* spp., *Proteus* spp.	*Bacteroides fragilis* and other *Bacteroides, Clostridium*
Appendicitis	*E. coli, Pseudomonas*	*Bacteroides* spp.
Abscesses	*E. coli, Klebsiella,* enterococci	*B. fragilis* and other *Bacteroides, Clostridium,* anaerobic cocci
Liver	*E. coli, Klebsiella,* enterococci staphylococci, amoeba	*Bacteroides* (infrequent)
Spleen	*Staphylococcus, Streptococcus*	

potassium, and calcium. In the initial hour of treatment, large volumes of solution may need to be administered to restore intravascular volume. For a few hours thereafter, fluids may be required at a rate of 1 L/h. Maintenance fluids should be instituted (after intravascular volume is restored) with 0.9% sodium chloride and potassium chloride (20 mEq/L) or 5% dextrose and 0.45% sodium chloride with potassium chloride (20 mEq/L). The administration rate should be based on estimated daily fluid loss through urine and nasogastric suction, including 0.5–1.0 L for insensible fluid loss. Potassium would not routinely be included if the patient is hyperkalemic or has renal failure.

In patients with significant blood loss, blood transfusion may be indicated. This is generally in the form of packed red blood cells. The criteria for blood transfusion are controversial, but a hematocrit of 25% is generally accepted. In the individual patient, the decision is often determined by the overall clinical status and the ability of the patient to compensate for the reduction in oxygen-carrying capacity associated with an acute anemia. Additional blood-component therapy with fresh-frozen plasma or platelets is also based on the needs of the individual patient. Aggressive fluid therapy must often be continued in the postoperative period, as fluid will continue to sequester in the peritoneal cavity, bowel wall, and lumen.

PHARMACOLOGIC TREATMENT

ANTIMICROBIAL THERAPY

The goals of antimicrobial therapy are (a) to control bacteremia and prevent the establishment of metastatic foci of infection, (b) to reduce suppurative complications after bacterial contamination, and (c) to prevent local spread of existing infection. After suppuration has occurred (e.g., an abscess has formed), a cure by antibiotic therapy alone is very difficult to achieve; antimicrobials may serve to improve the results with surgery alone.

An empiric antimicrobial regimen should be started as soon as the presence of intra-abdominal infection is suspected. Therefore, antibiotics are usually initiated before identification of the infecting organisms is complete. Therapy must be initiated based on the likely pathogens. Predominant pathogens, as discussed in the previous section, vary depending on the site of intra-abdominal infection and the underlying disease process. Table 112–4 lists the likely pathogens against which antimicrobial agents should be directed.

Antimicrobial Experience

Many studies have been conducted evaluating or comparing the effectiveness of antimicrobials for treatment of intra-abdominal infections. Substantial differences in patient outcomes from treatment with a variety of agents have generally not been demonstrated. One investigator found that there was no difference in clinical outcomes between two regimens with quite different activity against intra-abdominal isolates (cefoxitin and imipenem/cilastatin).[27] Ninety-eight percent of isolates were susceptible to imipenem/cilastatin and 72% to cefoxitin.

Important findings from the last 20 years of clinical trials regarding selection of antimicrobials for intra-abdominal infections are:

- Antimicrobial regimens should cover a broad spectrum of aerobic and anaerobic bacteria from the gastrointestinal tract.
- Single-agent regimens (such as second-generation cephalosporins, extended-spectrum penicillins, or carbapenems) have been as effective as combinations of aminoglycosides with antianaerobic agents. This is also true for antimicrobial treatment of acute bacterial contamination from penetrating abdominal trauma.[28,29]
- Clindamycin and metronidazole appear to be equivalent in efficacy when combined with agents effective against aerobic, gram-negative bacilli (gentamicin or aztreonam).

A number of studies have been conducted in patients with established intra-abdominal infections. Table 112–5 is a compilation of notable studies. Generally, published studies do not demonstrate clinical differences between agents, although it is doubtful that many of the studies would have detected clinically significant differences in patient outcome because the numbers of patients studied were often too few.

Intra-abdominal infection presents in many different ways and with a wide spectrum of severity. The regimen employed and duration of treatment depend on the specific clinical circumstances (i.e., the nature of the underlying disease process and the condition of the patient). Compromised patients require more aggressive therapies

TABLE 112–5. Some Comparative Studies of Intra-Abdominal Infection

Investigators	Agent(s) Tested	Number of Patients Studied	Percent of Patients with Satisfactory Outcome
Solomkin et al., 1990[29]	Imipenem/cilastatin	81	83
	Tobramycin/clindamycin	81	70
Brismar et al., 1992[30]	Imipenem/cilastatin	58	69
	Piperacillin/tazobactam	55	93
Wilson, 1997[31]	Meropenem	97	92
	Tobramycin/clindamycin	94	86
Cohn, et al., 2000[32]	Ciprofloxacin plus metronidazole	151	74
	Piperacillin/tazobactam	131	63 $p = 0.047$
Barrie, et al., 1997[33]	Cefepime plus metronidazole	95	88
	Imipenem/cilastatin	122	76 $p = 0.02$

than do otherwise healthy patients who experience the same intra-abdominal infection.

Recommendations

For most intra-abdominal infections, the antimicrobial regimen should be effective against both aerobic and anaerobic bacteria.[34] Although it is impossible to provide antimicrobial activity against every possible pathogen, agents with activity against enteric gram-negative bacilli, such as *E. coli* and *Klebsiella,* and anaerobes such as *B. fragilis* and *Clostridia* spp., should be administered. If most of the organisms can be eliminated through drainage or antimicrobials, the synergistic effect may be removed and the patient's defenses may be able to eradicate the remaining infection.

Table 112–6 presents recommended and alternative regimens for selected situations. These are general guidelines, not rules, because there are many factors that cannot be incorporated into such a table.

Most patients with severe intra-abdominal infections, when there is generalized peritonitis or sepsis, should be placed on a carbapenem such as imipenem or meropenem or a penicillin/β-lactamase inhibitor combination. Combinations of an aminoglycoside with an antianaerobic agent, such as clindamycin or metronidazole, may be used, but some authors consider such combinations to be obsolete.[1] Gentamicin is the aminoglycoside of choice based on its lower cost. Other aminoglycosides, such as tobramycin, amikacin, and netilmicin, have no advantages in intra-abdominal infections and are generally not drugs of first choice. Aztreonam may be used as an alternative to aminoglycoside to avoid potential nephrotoxicity. Additionally, ciprofloxacin with metronidazole may be used.

The dosage for aminoglycosides should initially be determined based on the patient's weight and renal function. Dosage adjustment should be performed by applying pharmacokinetic principles and by using peak and trough serum drug levels. Because the enteric gram-negative bacilli are usually very susceptible to aminoglycosides, and because the aminoglycosides are well distributed into peritoneal fluid,[35,36] high serum aminoglycoside concentrations are generally not required. Unless relatively resistant bacteria are suspected, a gentamicin or tobramycin peak concentration of 5–6 μg/mL is usually effective. To achieve these serum concentrations, gentamicin or tobramycin dosage may range from 1 to 3 mg/kg per dose given as often as every 6 hours or as infrequently as every 48 hours if the patient has renal failure. Because aminoglycosides have concentration-dependent killing and a relatively long postantibiotic effect for aerobic gram-negative bacilli, once-daily administration (5–7 mg/kg) is a reasonable alternative and appears to be equivalent to multiple daily dosing.

When used for intra-abdominal infection, aminoglycosides should be combined with agents that are effective against the majority of *B. fragilis.* Clindamycin or metronidazole is the agent of first choice, but others, such as antianaerobic cephalosporins (cefoxitin, cefotetan, or ceftizoxime), piperacillin, mezlocillin, and combinations of extended-spectrum penicillins with β-lactamase inhibitors, would be suitable alternatives. Clindamycin should be administered intravenously in a dosage of 600 or 900 mg every 8 hours. Patients receiving multiple, broad-spectrum antimicrobial agents who are immunocompromised should receive an oral antifungal agent for prevention of fungal overgrowth in the mouth and GI tract. The benefits of systemic antifungal prophylaxis (with fluconazole) have not been established for intra-abdominal infection and should not routinely be used.

With intra-abdominal contamination from the upper GI tract (perforation of a peptic ulcer or biliary tract disease), *B. fragilis* is an uncommon pathogen and other agents may, therefore, be substituted for clindamycin or metronidazole. Alternatives include ampicillin, penicillin, or first-generation cephalosporins.

Ampicillin may be added to combinations of aminoglycosides and clindamycin or metronidazole to assure antimicrobial coverage for enterococci, although this is controversial.[37] Regimens without activity against enterococci (gentamicin with clindamycin or cephalosporins) are generally effective in treating these infections; however, there are numerous reports of enterococcal superinfection in immunocompromised patients, particularly after cephalosporin use.

The failure of host defenses may be a critical factor in the pathogenicity of enterococci. In immunocompromised patients or patients with valvular heart disease or a prosthetic heart valve,[38] there is justification to provide specific antimicrobial activity against enterococci. Ampicillin or other penicillins that are active against enterococci (penicillin, piperacillin, mezlocillin) should be used in patients at high risk, patients with persistent or recurrent intra-abdominal infection, patients in shock, or patients who are immunosuppressed, such as after organ transplantation. Ampicillin remains the drug of choice for this purpose because it is most active *in vitro* against enterococci and is relatively inexpensive. Vancomycin is active against most enterococci; however, resistance is increasing, and this agent should be reserved for established infections when first-line therapies cannot be used.

With peritonitis that occurs from CAPD, the antimicrobial regimen used should be tailored to the isolated organism. The selection of a specific agent or combination should be based on culture and susceptibility data. If microbiologic data are unavailable, empiric therapy with a first-generation cephalosporin plus an aminoglycoside is recommended. In less-severe infections, a first-generation

TABLE 112–6. Recommendations for Initial Antimicrobial Agents for Intra-Abdominal Infections

	Primary Agents	Alternatives
Primary Bacterial Peritonitis		
Cirrhosis	Cefotaxime	1. Add clindamycin or metronidazole if anaerobes are suspected 2. Other third-generation cephalosporins, extended-spectrum penicillins, aztreonam, and imipenem as alternatives 3. Aminoglycoside with antipseudomonal penicillin
Peritoneal dialysis	Regimen based on organism isolated 1. Staphylococcus: penicillinase-resistant penicillin or first-generation cephalosporin 2. *Streptococcus:* penicillin G 3. Aerobic gram-negative bacilli: cefotaxime, ceftazidime, or aminoglycoside plus an antipseudomonal penicillin 4. *Pseudomonas aeruginosa*: aminoglycoside plus antipseudomonal penicillin or ceftazidime	1. Alternative for resistant staphylococci is vancomycin 2. Alternative for Streptococcus is a first-generation cephalosporin 3. Alternatives for gram-negative bacilli are other third-generation cephalosporins, aztreonam, and extended-spectrum penicillins with β-lactamase inhibitors
Secondary Bacterial Peritonitis		
Perforated peptic ulcer	First-generation cephalosporins	1. Antianaerobic cephalosporins[a] 2. Possibly add aminoglycoside if patient condition is poor
Other	Imipenem/cilistatin, meropenem, or extended-spectrum penicillins with β-lactamase inhibitor	1. Aminoglycoside with clindamycin or metronidazole; add ampicillin if patient is immunocompromised or if biliary tract origin of infection 2. Aztreonam with clindamycin 3. Antianaerobic cephalosporins[a] 4. Ciprofloxacin with metronidazole
Abscess		
General	Imipenem/cilastatin, meropenem or extended-spectrum penicillins with β-lactamase Inhibitor	1. Aztreonam with clindamycin 2. Aminoglycoside with clindamycin or metronidazole; add ampicillin 3. Ciprofloxacin with metronidazole
Liver	As above but add a first-generation cephalosporin	Use metronidazole if amoebic liver abscess is suspected
Spleen	Aminoglycoside plus penicillinase-resistant penicillin	Alternatives for penicillinase-resistant penicillin are first-generation cephalosporins or vancomycin
Appendicitis		
Normal or inflamed	Antianaerobic cephalosporins[a] (discontinued immediately postoperation)	1. Aminoglycoside with clindamycin or metronidazole
Gangrenous or perforated	Imipenem/cilastatin, meropenem, antianaerobic cephalosporins* or extended-spectrum penicillins with β-lactamase inhibitor	1. Aztreonam with clindamycin 2. Aminoglycoside with clindamycin or metronidazole 3. Ciprofloxacin with metronidazole
Acute Cholecystitis	First-generation cephalosporin	Aminoglycoside plus ampicillin if severe infection
Cholangitis	Aminoglycoside with ampicillin with or without clindamycin or metronidazole	Use vancomycin instead of ampicillin if patient is allergic to penicillin
Acute Contamination from Abdominal Trauma	Antianaerobic cephalosporins[a] or extended-spectrum penicillins	Aminoglycoside with one of the following: clindamycin, metronidazole, or antianaerobic cephalosporins*
Pelvic Inflammatory Disease	Cefotetan or cefoxitin with doxycycline	1. Clindamycin with gentamicin 2. Ofloxacin with metronidazole 3. Ampicillin/sulbactam with doxycycline 4. Ciprofloxacin with doxycycline and metronidazole

[a]Cefoxitin, cefotetan, and ceftizoxime.

cephalosporin alone given intraperitoneally may suffice. Infection with staphylococci may be treated with a penicillinase-resistant penicillin (methicillin, nafcillin, oxacillin), first-generation cephalosporins, or vancomycin if the patient is allergic to penicillin or the isolate is resistant to methicillin. For streptococcal infections, penicillin or ampicillin would be preferable to penicillinase-resistant penicillins. Most aerobic gram-negative bacilli may be effectively treated with an aminoglycoside. For infections caused by *P. aeruginosa,* an antipseudomonal penicillin (ticarcillin, piperacillin, mezlocillin, or azlocillin) or ceftazidime may be added.

Patients with peritonitis who are undergoing CAPD may receive parenteral, as well as intraperitoneal, antimicrobial agents. Intraperitoneal antimicrobial agents alone are often sufficient, unless severe infection is present. A number of agents may be instilled through peritoneal catheters. Recommended concentrations of antimicrobial agents for intraperitoneal irrigation solutions are 8 mg/L for gentamicin and tobramycin; 1–3 mg/L for clindamycin; 50,000 U/L for penicillin G; 125 mg/L for cephalosporins; 100–150 mg/L for ticarcillin or carbenicillin; 50 mg/L for ampicillin; 100 mg/L for methicillin; 30 mg/L for vancomycin; and 3 mg/L for amphotericin B.[39]

The usual duration of therapy for peritonitis associated with CAPD is 10 to 14 days, but up to 3 weeks of therapy may be required. Antimicrobial therapy should be continued until dialysate fluid is clear, cultures are negative for 2 to 3 days, and the patient is asymptomatic. When parenteral agents are administered, the initial dose would be the same as that for patients with normal renal function, while subsequent doses should be much less or given less frequently for renally excreted agents, and should account for possible loss through peritoneal dialysis. Serum concentrations should be performed for aminoglycosides and vancomycin. Some studies have demonstrated that for patients with spontaneous bacterial peritonitis associated with cirrhotic ascites, treatment duration may be a short as 5 days when ascitic fluid polymorphonuclear cell counts are used to guide treatment.[40,41]

After acute bacterial contamination, such as with abdominal trauma where GI contents spill into the peritoneum, combination antimicrobial regimens are not required. If the patient is seen soon after injury (within 2 hours) and surgical measures are instituted promptly, single-agent regimens, such as antianaerobic cephalosporins (such as cefoxitin or cefotetan) or extended-spectrum penicillins, are effective in preventing most infectious complications. Antimicrobials should be administered as soon as possible after injury.

For appendicitis, the antimicrobial regimen used should depend on the appearance of the appendix at the time of operation, which may be normal, inflamed, gangrenous, or perforated. Because the condition of the appendix is unknown preoperatively, it is advisable to begin antimicrobial agents before the appendectomy is performed. Reasonable regimens would be antianaerobic cephalosporins or, if the patient is seriously ill, a combination of aminoglycoside with clindamycin or metronidazole. If, at operation, the appendix is found to be normal or inflamed, postoperative antimicrobials would not be required. If the appendix is gangrenous or perforated, a treatment course of 7 to 10 days with the agents listed in Table 112–6 is appropriate.

The necessary duration of treatment for intra-abdominal infections is not clearly defined. Acute intra-abdominal contamination, such as after a traumatic injury, may be treated with a very short course (24 hours).[42] For established infections (peritonitis or intra-abdominal abscess), an antimicrobial course of 5–7 days is justified. This allows eradication of bacteria remaining in the peritoneum after a surgical procedure or bacteria that may enter the peritoneum through healing suture lines. Comparative studies examining shorter courses of therapy (2 or 3 days) have not been conducted to verify that longer courses are essential. Under certain conditions, therapy for longer than 7 days would be justified; for example, if the patient remains febrile or is in poor general condition, when relatively resistant bacteria are isolated, or when a focus of infection in the abdomen may still be present. For some abscesses, such as pyogenic liver abscess, antimicrobials may be required for a month or longer.

Intraperitoneal irrigation of antimicrobial agents for treatment of intra-abdominal infection has often been studied with conflicting results.[43] Intraoperative antimicrobial irrigation has not been shown to improve patient outcomes in comparison with copious intraoperative irrigation with normal saline. Possibly the most important aspect of peritoneal irrigation is the dilutional effect on bacteria and adjuvants that promote infection (intestinal contents and hemoglobin). As discussed before, investigators have shown that most systemically administered antimicrobials easily cross the peritoneal membrane so that peritoneal fluid concentrations are similar to serum.[35,44] Confined areas, such as an abscess, can be expected to attain much lower antimicrobial concentrations.

EVALUATION OF THERAPEUTIC OUTCOMES

Whichever antimicrobial regimen is chosen, the patient should be continually reassessed to determine the success or failure of therapies. The clinician should recognize that there are many reasons for poor outcome of patients with intra-abdominal infection; improper antimicrobial administration is only one. The patient may be immunocompromised, which decreases the likelihood of successful outcome with any regimen. It is impossible for antimicrobials to compensate totally for a nonfunctioning immune system. There may be surgical reasons for poor patient outcome. Failure to identify all intra-abdominal foci of infection or leaks from a GI anastomosis may cause continued intra-abdominal infection. Even when intra-abdominal infection is controlled, accompanying organ system failure, most often renal or respiratory, but possibly hepatic or cardiac, may lead to patient demise.

The outcome from intra-abdominal infection is not determined solely by what transpires in the abdomen. Unsatisfactory outcomes in patients with intra-abdominal infections may result from complications that arise in other organ systems. A complication commonly associated with mortality after intra-abdominal infection is pneumonia.[45,46] In fact, one investigator found that the cause of death in patients with intra-abdominal infection was more likely related to the lower respiratory tract than the abdomen.[45] A high APACHE (acute physiology and chronic health evaluation) II score, low serum albumin, and high New York Heart Association cardiac function status were significantly and independently associated with increased mortality from intra-abdominal infection.[47]

Once antimicrobials are initiated, and the other important therapies described earlier are used, most patients should show improvement within 2 to 3 days. Usually, temperature will return to near normal, vital signs should stabilize, and the patient should not appear in distress, with the exception of recognized discomfort and pain from incisions, drains, and nasogastric tube. At 24 to 48 hours, aerobic bacterial culture results should return. If a suspected pathogen is not sensitive to the antimicrobial agents being given, the regimen should be changed if the patient has not shown sufficient improvement. If the isolated pathogen is extremely sensitive to one antimicrobial and the patient is progressing well, concurrent antimicrobial therapy may often be discontinued. Although some investigators suggest that routine culturing of patients with community-acquired intra-abdominal infections contributes little to their management,[48] other investigators suggest that antimicrobial therapy should be based on susceptibility of the flora collected from the operative site because this has been shown to correlate with clinical outcome.[49]

With present anaerobic culturing techniques and the slow growth of these organisms, anaerobes are often not identified until 4 to 7 days after culture, and sensitivity information is difficult to obtain. For this reason, there are usually few data with which to alter the antianaerobic component of the antimicrobial regimen. A report indicating that anaerobes were not isolated should not be the sole justification for discontinuing antianaerobic drugs because anaerobic bacteria that were present in the infectious process may not have been properly transported to the microbiology laboratory, or other problems may have led to cell death *in vitro*.

Reasons for antimicrobial failure may not always be apparent. Even when antimicrobial susceptibility tests indicate that an organism is susceptible to the antimicrobial *in vitro,* therapeutic failures may occur. Possibly there is poor penetration of the antimicrobial into the focus of infection, or bacterial resistance may develop after initiation of antimicrobial therapy. Also, it is possible that an antimicrobial regimen may encourage the development of infection by organisms not susceptible to the regimen being used. Superinfection in patients being treated for intra-abdominal infection can be caused by *Candida;* however, enterococci or opportunistic gram-negative bacilli such as *Pseudomonas* or *Serratia* may be involved.

Treatment regimens for intra-abdominal infection can be judged as successful if the patient recovers from the infection without recurrent peritonitis or intra-abdominal abscess, and without the need for additional antimicrobials. A regimen can be considered unsuccessful if a significant adverse drug reaction occurs, reoperation is necessary, or patient improvement is delayed beyond 1 or 2 weeks.

▶ PRINCIPLES OF PHARMACOTHERAPY

- Most secondary intra-abdominal infections are caused by a defect in the gastrointestinal tract that must be treated by surgical drainage and repair.
- Secondary intra-abdominal infections are usually caused by a mixture of enteric gram-negative bacilli and anaerobes.
- For peritonitis, early and aggressive intravenous fluid and electrolyte therapy is essential.
- Antimicrobial regimens for secondary intra-abdominal infections should include coverage for enteric gram-negative bacilli and anaerobes. Regimens that may be used for treatment of secondary intra-abdominal infections include (a) an aminoglycoside plus clindamycin (or metronidazole); (b) aztreonam plus clindamycin; (c) imipenem/cilastatin or meropenem; (d) extended-spectrum penicillins with β-lactamase inhibitors; (e) ciprofloxacin with metronidazole; and (e) antianaerobic cephalosporins.
- Cultures of secondary intra-abdominal infection sites are generally not useful for directing antimicrobial therapy.
- Antimicrobial regimens should be adjusted to provide excellent activity against any pathogens isolated from blood specimens.
- The duration of antimicrobial treatment has not been well established but should be a total of 5–7 days for most intra-abdominal infections.
- Primary peritonitis is generally caused by a single organism (*S. aureus* in patients undergoing CAPD, or *E. coli* in patients with cirrhosis).
- Treatment of primary peritonitis for CAPD patients should include an antistaphylococcal antimicrobial, such as a first-generation cephalosporin or vancomycin (usually given by the intraperitoneal route).
- Patients treated for intra-abdominal infections should be assessed for the occurrence of drug-related adverse effects, particularly hypersensitivity reactions (β-lactam antimicrobials), diarrhea (most agents), fungal infections (most agents), and nephrotoxicity (aminoglycosides).

REFERENCES

1. Whittmann DH, Schein M, Condon RE. Management of secondary peritonitis. Ann Surg 1996;224:10–18.
2. Johnson CC, Baldessarre J, Levinson ME. Peritonitis: Update on pathophysiology, clinical manifestations, and management. Clin Infect Dis 1997;24:1035–1047.
3. Saklayen MG. CAPD peritonitis. Incidence: pathogens, diagnosis, and management. Med Clin North Am 1990;74:997–1010.
4. Suh H, Wadhwa NK, Cabralda T, Sorrento J. Endogenous peritonitis and related outcome in peritoneal dialysis patients. Adv Perit Dial 1996;12:192–195.
5. Hall MJ, Popovic JR. 1998 Summary: National Hospital Discharge Survey, #316. National Center for Health Statistics, 2000.
6. Toloza EM, Wilson SE. Cholecystitis and cholangitis. In: Fry DE, ed. Surgical Infections. Boston, Little, Brown, 1995:254–263.
7. Keene WF, Alexander SR, Bailie GR, et al. Peritoneal dialysis—Related peritonitis treatment recommendations: 1996 update. Perit Dial Int 1996; 16:557–573.
8. Schein M, Wittman DH, Holzheimer R, et al. Hypothesis: Compartmentalization of cytokines in intraabdominal infection. Surgery 1996;119: 694–700.
9. Bhuva M, Ganger D, Jensen D. Spontaneous bacterial peritonitis: An update on evaluation, management, and prevention. Am J Med 1994;97: 169–175.
10. Gilbert J, Kamath PS. Spontaneous bacterial peritonitis: An update. Mayo Clin Proc 1995;70:365–370.
11. Troidle L, Gordon-Brennan N, Kliger A, Finkelstein F. Differing outcomes of gram-positive and gram-negative peritonitis. Am J Kidney Dis 1998;32:623–628.
12. McClean KL, Shhehan GJ, Harding GKM. Intraabdominal infection: A review. Clin Infect Dis 1994;19:100–116.
13. Brook I, Frazier EH. Microbiology subphrenic abscesses. A 14 year experience. Am Surg 1999;65:1049–1053.
14. Brook I, Frazier EH. Aerobic and anaerobic microbiology of retroperitoneal abscesses. Clin Infect Dis 1998;26:938–941.
15. Bennion RS, Baron EJ, Thompson JE, et al. The bacteriology of gangrenous and perforated appendicitis—Revisited. Ann Surg 1990;211:165–171.
16. Sawyer RG, Rosenlof LK, Adams RB, et al. Peritonitis into the 1990s: Changing pathogens and changing strategies in the critically ill. Am Surg 1992;58:82–87.
17. Tzianabos AO, Kasper DL, Onderdonk AB. Structure and function of *Bacteroides fragilis* capsular polysaccharides: Relationship to induction and prevention of abscesses. Clin Infect Dis 1995;20(suppl 2):S132–S140.
18. Montravers P, Andremont A, Massias L, Carbon C. Investigation of the potential role of *Enterococcus faecalis* in the pathophysiology of experimental peritonitis. J Infect Dis 1994;169:821–830.
19. Burnett RJ, Haverstock DC, Dellinger EP, et al. Definition of the role of enterococcus in intra-abdominal infection: Analysis of a prospective randomized trial. Surgery 1995;118:721–723.
20. Gazelle GS, Mueller PR. Abdominal abscess: Imaging and intervention. Radiol Clin North Am 1994;32:913–932.

21. Datz FL. Abdominal abscess detection: Gallium-, ^{111}In-, and ^{99m}Tc-labeled leukocytes, and polyclonal and monoclonal antibodies. Semin Nucl Med 1996;26:51–64.
22. Cooper GS, Shlaes DM, Salata RA. Intra-abdominal infection: Differences in presentation and outcome between younger patients and the elderly. Clin Infect Dis 1994;19:146–148.
23. Montgomery RS, Wilson SE. Intraabdominal abscesses: Image-guided diagnosis and therapy. Clin Infect Dis 1996;23:28–36.
24. Shuler FW, Newman CN, Angood PB, et al. Nonoperative management for intra-abdominal abscesses. Am Surg 1996;62:218–222.
25. Robles PJ, Lancaster B. Laparoscopic drainage of right subphrenic abscess: Report of one case. J Laparoendosc Surg 1996;6:55–60.
26. Kim HB, Gregor MB, Boley SJ, Kleinhaus S. Digitally assisted laparoscopic drainage of multiple intra-abdominal abscesses. J Laparoendosc Surg 1993;3:477–479.
27. Christou NV, Turgeon P, Wassef R, et al. Management of intra-abdominal infections: The case for intraoperative cultures and comprehensive broad spectrum antibiotic coverage. Arch Surg 1996;131:1193–1201.
28. Hooker KD, DiPiro JT, Wynn JJ. Aminoglycoside combinations versus single β-lactams for penetrating abdominal trauma: A meta analysis. J Trauma 1991;31:1155–1160.
29. Solomkin JS, Dellinger EP, Christou NV, et al. Results of a multicenter trial comparing imipenem/cilastatin to tobramycin/clindamycin for intra-abdominal infections. Ann Surg 1990;212:581–591.
30. Brismar B, Malmborg AS, Tunevall G, et al. Piperacillin-tazobactam versus imipenem-cilastatin for treatment of intra-abdominal infections. Antimicrob Agents Chemother 1992;36:2766–2773.
31. Wilson SE. Results of a randomized, multicenter trial of meropenem versus clindamycin/tobramycin for the treatment of intra-abdominal infections. Clin Infect Dis 1997;24(suppl 2):S197–206.
32. Cohn SM, Lipsett PA, Buchman TG, et al. Comparison of intravenous/oral ciprofloxacin plus metronidazole versus piperacillin/tazobactam in the treatment of complicated intra-abdominal infections. Ann Surg 2000; 232:254–262.
33. Barie PS, Vogel SB, Dellinger EP, et al. A randomized, double-blind clinical trial comparing cefepime plus metronidazole with imipenem-cilastatin in the treatment of complicated intra-abdominal infections. Arch Surg 1997;132:1294–1302.
34. Bohnen JMA, Solomkin JS, Dellinger EP, et al. Guidelines for clinical care: Anti-infective agents for intra-abdominal infection. Arch Surg 1992;127:83–89.
35. Serour F, Dan M, Gorea A, et al. Penetration of aminoglycosides into human peritoneal tissue. Chemotherapy 1990;36:251–253.
36. Hodgman T, Dasta JK, Armstrong DK, et al. Tobramycin disposition into ascitic fluid. Clin Pharm 1984;3:203–205.
37. Dougherty SH. Role of enterococcus in intraabdominal sepsis. Am J Surg 1984;148:308–312.
38. Barrie PS, Christou NV, Dellinger EP, et al. Pathogenicity of the enterococcus in surgical infections. Ann Surg 1990;212:155–159.
39. Levison ME, Pontzer RE. Peritonitis and other intra-abdominal infections. In: Mardell GL, Douglas RG, Bennett JE, eds. Principles and Practice of Infectious Diseases. New York, John Wiley, 1985:488.
40. Fong T, Akriviadis ES, Runyon BA, et al. Polymorphonuclear cell count response and duration of antibiotic therapy in spontaneous bacterial peritonitis. Hepatology 1989;9:423–426.
41. Runyon BA, McHutchison JG, Antillon MR, et al. Short-course versus long-course antibiotic treatment of spontaneous bacterial peritonitis. Gastroenterol 1991;100:1737–1742.
42. Bozorgzadeh A, Pizzi WF, Barie PS, et al. The duration of antibiotic administration in predicting abdominal trauma. Am J Surg 1999;172: 125–135.
43. Schein M, Gecelter G, Freinkel W, et al. Peritoneal lavage in abdominal sepsis: A controlled clinical study. Arch Surg 1990;125:1132–1135.
44. Wittman DH, Schassan HH. Penetration of eight β-lactam antibiotics into peritoneal fluid. Arch Surg 1983;118:205–213.
45. Mustard RA, Bohnen JMA, Rosati C, Schouten D. Pneumonia complicating abdominal sepsis. Arch Surg 1991;126:170–175.
46. Richardson JD, DeCamp MM, Garrison RN, Fry DE. Pulmonary infection complicating intra-abdominal sepsis. Ann Surg 1982;195:732–737.
47. Christou NV, Barie PS, Dellinger EP, et al. Surgical infection society intra-abdominal infection study. Arch Surg 1993;128:193–199.
48. Dougherty SH. Antimicrobial culture and susceptibility testing has little value for routine management of secondary bacterial peritonitis. Clin Infect Dis 1997;25(suppl 2):S258–S261.
49. Wilson SE, Hopkins JA. Clinical correlates of anaerobic bacteriology in peritonitis. Clin Infect Dis 1995;20(suppl 2):S251–S256.

113
PARASITIC DISEASES

J.V. Anandan

Parasitic diseases are receiving increasing attention from clinicians in the United States because of the high frequency of travel, deployment of personnel for humanitarian and military missions (e.g., Peace Corps volunteers), inflow of immigrants from a wider geographic distribution, and the presence of immunosuppressed populations (AIDS, transplant patients). Migrant farm workers who work and live in substandard hygienic conditions, the large and growing Central and South American immigrant population, and other poorly screened immigrants from Asia, represent significant sources of parasitic infections in the United States.[1–9] Clinicians need to have a heightened awareness for parasitic diseases and how to treat them. Clinical signs and symptoms, together with patient's travel history, should be used with other diagnostic aids in the identification of parasitic diseases. Parasitic infections caused by pathogenic protozoa or helminths affect more than 3 billion people worldwide and impose tremendous health and economic burdens on developing countries.[9]

This chapter discusses the major parasitic diseases, including protozoan diseases (amebiasis, malaria), helminthic infections (ascariasis, enterobiasis), and ectoparasitic infestations (head and body lice). Emphasis is placed on diseases more frequently seen in the United States. World distribution of parasites is dependent on the presence of suitable hosts, habitats, and environmental conditions.[9] A human parasite that does not use an intermediate host is likely to be found in any inhabited region of the world, as long as the environmental conditions are suitable. Ascaris (round worm) and Trichuris (whip worm) require carelessness of habits for transfer and require time outside the body, where they are exposed to heat and dryness, to reach the infective stage. The distribution of the hookworm is more limited, because the free-living forms are unprotected by resistant shells or cysts. African trypanosomiasis never occurs outside the range of the tsetse fly, malaria never occurs beyond the range of the infective *Anopheles* mosquito, and schistosomiasis never occurs in the absence of a specific water snail. The prevalence of clonorchiasis (Chinese liver fluke) is an example of the impact of both environmental and geographic factors. Clonorchiasis not only requires simultaneous presence of humans, specific snail species, and certain fish, but also unsanitary conditions that make the eggs accessible to the snails, an association of the snail and fish, and the established local habit of eating raw fish. The ability of some parasites to infect hosts other than humans may perpetuate an infection, even when human habits preclude the possibility of more than occasional access to the human body. In North America, the broad tapeworm (*Diphyllobothrium latus*) would perish if it were not that dogs and other carnivores, such as the brown bear, serve as reservoir hosts.

HOST–PARASITE RELATIONSHIP

Symbiosis is the association of two species for the purpose of obtaining food for either one or the other. Parasitism is a symbiotic relationship in which one species, the host, is injured through the activities of the other. Through evolution, parasites have made specific morphologic adaptations. Adaptation to the host has taken a number of forms: loss of locomotor organelles in the protozoan *Sporozoa;* partial and complete lack of digestive systems in the trematodes and cestodes, respectively; elaboration of proteolytic enzymes to penetrate the host intestinal mucosa by *Entamoeba histolytica,* the cercariae of the blood fluke that penetrate the skin of the host by elaborate enzymes; and, finally, the ability to infect an intermediate host to increase reproductive capacity as seen among the cestodes and trematodes.[9] Parasites normally inflict some degree of injury to the host, the extent of which is dependent on such factors as parasite load, nutritional status, and immunologic competence of the host. *Entamoeba coli* is considered commensal because it subsists on the bacterial flora of the gut and does not cause any harm to the host. Unlike *Entamoeba coli, Fasciolopsis buski,* the giant intestinal fluke, and *Entamoeba histolytica* can produce severe local damage to the intestinal wall. *Ascaris,* the roundworm, can perforate the bowel wall, cause intestinal obstruction, and invade the appendix and bile duct. Malarial parasites destroy red cells by multiplying inside them. *Diphyllobothrium latum,* or the broad fish tapeworm, removes vitamin B_{12} from the gastrointestinal tract (GI) tract, resulting in megaloblastic anemia.[9]

PROTOZOAN DISEASES

MALARIA

Malaria represents the most devastating disease in terms of human suffering and economics. It affects the largest number of people (between 300 and 500 million new infections are reported annually) in the world, with more than 2 million deaths worldwide.[10,11]

EPIDEMIOLOGY

The exact geographic distribution of the various species is not well documented; however, it is reported that *P. vivax* is more prevalent in India, Pakistan, Bangladesh, Sri Lanka, and Central America, while *P. falciparum* is predominantly in Africa, Haiti, Dominican Republic, Amazon region of South America, and New Guinea. Both *P. falciparum* and *P. vivax* are prevalent in all of Southeast Asia, South America, Middle East, North Africa, Ethiopia, Somalia, and Sudan.[12,13] Most of the infections with *P. ovale* occur in Africa and the distribution of *Plasmodium malariae* is considered worldwide.

In the United States, most cases of malaria are reported in immigrants from endemic areas and in American travelers. Blood transfusion has also been cited as a cause of malarial infection.[14] The transmission of malaria from recent immigrants from endemic areas is a real threat because of the presence of two mosquito vectors—*Anopheles albimanus* and *A. freeborni*—in the United States.[12]

ETIOLOGY

Malaria is transmitted by the bite of an infected *Anopheles* mosquito which introduces the sporozoites (tissue parasites) of the plasmodia

(*Plasmodium falciparum, P. vivax, P. malariae,* and *P. ovale*) into the bloodstream. The asexual reproduction stage develops in humans, whereas the sexual stage occurs in the mosquito.[9,12] The sporozoites invade parenchymal hepatocytes, multiply in stages referred to as exo-erythrocytic stages, and become hepatic vegetative forms or schizonts. Schizonts rupture to release daughter cells, or merozoites, which then infect erythrocytes.

P. falciparum and *P. malariae* remain in the primary exoerythrocytic stage in the liver for about 4 weeks before invading erythrocytes, whereas *P. vivax* and *P. ovale* can exist in the liver in the latent exoerythrocytic form for extended periods, and therefore infected subjects can experience relapses. The merozoites that invade the erythrocytes develop sequentially into ring forms, trophozoites, schizonts, and, finally, into merozoites, which can invade other erythrocytes, or can develop into gametocytes, which undergo the sexual stage in the *Anopheles* vector. Erythrocytic forms never reinvade the liver without developing into sporozoites in the vector and therefore malaria infections from transfusion never result in the exoerythrocytic or "liver" form.[9,12] *P. falciparum* can result in high levels of parasitemia because of its ability to invade erythrocytes of all ages, unlike *P. vivax* and *P. ovale,* which only invade young cells.[12]

PATHOLOGY

Patients with malaria usually present with nonspecific fever, headache, malaise, and vomiting.[11] The malarial paroxysm characterized by fever, chills, and rigor can cause vasodilation and orthostatic hypotension. The high fever, marked diaphoresis, and vomiting can lead to serious fluid and electrolyte abnormalities. The erythrocytic phase causes extensive hemolysis, which results in anemia and splenomegaly. The most serious complications are usually associated with *P. falciparum* infections, and include hypoglycemia; acute renal failure; pulmonary edema; severe anemia; thrombocytopenia; high-output heart failure; cerebral congestion; seizures and coma; and adult respiratory syndrome.[15–21] Infants and children younger than 5 years of age, and nonimmune women who are pregnant, are at high risk for severe complications from falciparum malaria.[15,17] The complications associated with falciparum malaria are primarily a result of the high parasitemia and the ability of the parasites to sequester in capillaries and postcapillary vessels of organs such as the brain and the kidney. It has been postulated that tissue hypoxia from anemia, together with *P. falciparum*-parasitized red cell adherence to endothelial cells in capillaries, contributes to extensive vascular disease and severe metabolic effects.[12,15] *P. malariae* is implicated in immune-mediated glomerulonephritis and nephrotic syndrome.[12]

CLINICAL PRESENTATION

The erythrocytic phase of malaria is preceded by a prodrome that includes headache, anorexia, malaise, fatigue, and myalgias. Patients may also have nonspecific complaints such as abdominal pain, diarrhea, chest pain, and arthralgias. The prodromal period is followed by the paroxysm, manifested as high fever, chills, and rigor.[11] The typical malarial paroxysm is usually followed by a "cold phase," severe pallor, cyanosis of the lips and nail bed, and cutis anserina ("goose flesh").[11,12] These symptoms are replaced by a "hot phase" in which the patient's fever may be between 40.5°C (104.9°F) and 41°C (105.8°F). The "hot" phase is followed in 2 to 6 hours by a "sweating" phase in which the fever resolves and the patient shows marked fatigue and drowsiness. Other symptoms during this phase include warm, dry skin; tachycardia; cough; severe headache; nausea; vomiting; abdominal pain; diarrhea; and delirium. Lactic acidosis and hypoglycemia have been reported as a complication of falciparum malaria.[12,15] Patients are usually asymptomatic between the malarial paroxysms.

To ensure a positive diagnosis, blood smears should be obtained every 12 to 24 hours for 3 consecutive days.[9,12,15] The presence of parasites in the blood 3 to 5 days after initiation of therapy suggests drug resistance. Recent advances for detecting malaria parasite have included DNA or RNA probes by polymerase chain reaction and a rapid dipstick test (PARASIGHT F, Becton-Dickinson, Cockeysville, MD).[9,12,22] The dipstick is reported to have a sensitivity of 88% and specificity of 97%, which is comparable to microscopy.[22]

▶ TREATMENT: Malaria

DESIRED OUTCOME

The primary goal in the management of malaria is the rapid diagnosis of the *Plasmodia* spp. by blood smears (repeated every 12 hours for 3 days), so as to initiate timely antimalarial therapy to eradicate the infection within 48 to 72 hours and to avoid complications such as hypoglycemia, pulmonary edema, and renal failure that are responsible for increased mortality in malaria.

PHARMACOLOGIC THERAPY

In adults, the chemoprophylaxis for all species of *Plasmodia* is chloroquine phosphate 300 mg (base) once weekly, beginning 1 week prior to departure and continued for 4 weeks after leaving an endemic area.[10,11,12,23,24] The pediatric dose of chloroquine phosphate is 5 mg (base)/kg (maximum 300 mg). When visiting or leaving an area endemic for *P. vivax* or *P. ovale,* primaquine phosphate (Primaquine) 15 mg (base) daily for 14 days beginning the last 2 weeks of chloroquine prophylaxis should be added to the regimen. The pediatric dose of primaquine is 0.3 mg (base)/kg/day for 14 days. The pediatric doses of chloroquine can be calculated based on body weight, and the tablets can be pulverized and placed in gelatin capsules. Parents can be instructed to suspend the dose in food, simple syrup, chocolate milk, or drink.[15]

In areas where chloroquine-resistant *P. falciparum* strains exist, travelers should receive mefloquine (Lariam) for prophylaxis. The adult dose of mefloquine is 250 mg once weekly, beginning 1 week prior to departure and continuing for the full period of exposure, followed by 250 mg for 4 weeks after last exposure.[23–27] The pediatric dose of mefloquine for prophylaxis is:

Body weight (kg)	Dose
15–19	1/4 tablet
20–30	1/2 tablet
31–45	3/4 tablet
>45	1 tablet

In travelers who are at immediate risk to drug-resistant falciparum malaria, a loading dose of mefloquine may be considered. Mefloquine is administered at 250 mg daily for 3 days before travel, followed by 250 mg once weekly while in the endemic area, and continued for 4 weeks after last exposure.[11,25,26] Some patients may experience neuropsychiatric reactions from this regimen and may need to be monitored closely.[11]

An alternative regimen for prophylaxis in chloroquine-resistant areas for those who cannot tolerate mefloquine, is to take doxycycline 100 mg daily starting 1 to 2 days prior to departure, during the exposure period, and continuing for 4 weeks after leaving the endemic area.[12,24] Children older than 8 years of age should receive 2 mg/kg/day (up to 100 mg) of doxycycline. Doxycycline is contraindicated in children under 8 years of age, in pregnant women, and during breast-feeding.[11,23,24,28]

A study comparing azithromycin (Zithromax) 250 mg daily and doxycycline 100 mg daily for prophylaxis for malaria, demonstrated that azithromycin may be an alternative to doxycycline.[29] Daily Primaquine 15 mg (base) has also been recommended for prophylaxis for both *P. vivax* and *P. falciparum* malaria.[30]

In an uncomplicated attack of malaria (for all plasmodia except chloroquine-resistant *P. falciparum*), the recommended regimen is chloroquine 600 mg (base) initially, followed by 300 mg (base) 6 hours later, and then 300 mg (base) daily for 2 days. In severe illness, or when oral therapy is not tolerated, quinidine gluconate 10 mg/kg as a loading dose (maximum 600 mg) in 250 mL normal saline should be administered slowly over 1 to 2 hours followed by continuous infusion of 0.02 mg/kg/min until oral therapy can be started.[23,24] In patients who have either received quinine or mefloquine, the loading dose of quinidine should be omitted. Oral quinine (300 mg every 8 hours) should follow the intravenous dose of quinidine to complete 3 days for all infections, except for *P. falcipraum* acquired in Thailand, in which case, a full 7-day course should be given.[23,24] The pediatric dose of intravenous quinidine gluconate is the same as the dose for adults.[24] The pediatric dose of quinine is 25 mg/kg/d in three divided doses for 3 or 7 days.[24]

In *P. falciparum* (chloroquine-resistant) infections, a single dose of mefloquine 1,250 mg should be used. The pediatric dose of mefloquine is 25 mg/kg (<45 kg) as a single dose.[12,24] Intravenous quinidine gluconate followed by oral quinine should be administered for severe illness, as already indicated.[11,12,24] A second drug needs to be administered in chloroquine-resistant *P. falciparum*, and this second drug should follow the oral quinidine regimen: either a single dose of three tablets of pyrimethamine/sulfadoxine (Fansidar)on the last day of intravenous quinidine, or clindamycin 900 mg three times daily for 3 to 5 days.[23,24] An alternative oral treatment for chloroquine-resistant *P. falciparum* infection is the combination of atovaquone 250 mg and proguanil 100 mg (Malarone) (dose: 4 tablets daily × 3 days).[24] The intravenous quinidine regimen requires close monitoring of the electrocardiogram and other vital signs (e.g., hypotension, hypoglycemia).[15,23,24] Because falciparum malaria is associated with serious complications including pulmonary edema, hypoglycemia, jaundice, renal failure, confusion, delirium, seizures, coma, and death, careful monitoring of fluid status and hemodynamic parameters is mandatory.[15,23,24] Exchange transfusion may be required in patients with *P. falciparum* malaria where parasitemia is 5% to 15%; this may manifest as mental status changes, pulmonary edema, or renal failure.[15,23] Either peritoneal or hemodialysis may be indicated in renal failure.

Malarial infection does not produce immunity in patients and active research has been initiated to develop a malaria vaccine.[12,31–34] A vaccine that blocks the entry of sporozoites into the liver cells will prevent malaria at this stage. However, immunity to sporozoites does not protect the host against parasites in the erythrocytic cycle.[32] Infective sporozoites of *P. falciparum* are covered by a polypeptide, circumsporozoite protein.[31] Isolation and identification of the gene encoding for this circumsporozoite protein has led to the development of a monoclonal antibody by recombinant DNA technology; *P. falciparum* sporozoite vaccine is now under investigation.[31,33]

EVALUATION OF THERAPEUTIC OUTCOMES

When advising potential travelers on prophylaxis for malaria, be aware of the incidence of chloroquine-resistant *P. falciparum* malaria and the countries where this is prevalent.[11,15,24,27] Detailed recommendations for prevention of malaria may be obtained by checking the World Wide Web (e.g., http://www.cdc.gov/travel/; http://www2.cdc.gov/mmwr/;),[34] or by calling the Centers for Disease Control and Prevention (CDC) (see Appendix 113–1). A number of newer drugs are under active study and include the water-soluble artesunate and the oil-soluble artemether, Lumefantrine (also known as benflumetol) and combinations of this with other agents, and the recent approval in the United States of the combination atovaquone and proguanil (Malarone).[10,36–40] Halofantrine (Halfan), approved in 1992, is indicated for multidrug-resistant *P. falciparum* but has poor bioavailability, prolongs QTc interval at the recommended doses, and has been reported with therapeutic failures.[24]

Acute *P. falciparum* malaria resistant to chloroquine should be treated with intravenous quinidine. These patients should have a central venous catheter to follow fluid status and the electrocardiogram should be closely monitored. Hypoglycemia that is associated with *P. falciparum* should be checked and corrected with dextrose infusions.[15] Quinidine infusion should be temporarily slowed or stopped if a QT interval >0.6 seconds, an increase in QRS complex >50%, or hypotension unresponsive to fluid challenge results. The suggested quinidine levels should be maintained at 3–7 mg/L.[15,23] Blood smears should be checked every 12 hours until parasitemia is <1%. Resolution of fever should take place between 36 and 48 hours after initiation of the IV quinidine therapy, and the blood should be clear of parasites in 5 days.[15,23] If parenteral therapy is required for more than 48 hours it is suggested that the dose of quinidine be lowered by half.[24]

Travelers to endemic areas for malaria should be advised to remain in well-screened areas, to wear clothes that cover most of the body, and to sleep in mosquito nets.[41] It is prudent to carry the insect repellent DEET (*N,N*-diethylmetatoluamide) or other insect sprays containing DEET for use in mosquito-infested areas. Readers are urged to check publications from the CDC for the list of countries where chloroquine-resistant *P. falciparum* exist.[24,34]

AMEBIASIS

EPIDEMIOLOGY AND ETIOLOGY

Because of its worldwide distribution and serious gastrointestinal manifestations, amebiasis is one of the most important parasitic diseases of humans.[9,42–45] The major causative organism in amebiasis is *Entamoeba histolytica*, which inhabits the colon, and must be differentiated from the *E. dispar*, which is associated with an asymptomatic carrier state and is considered nonpathogenic. Although *E. histolytica* and *E. dispar* are indistinguishable morphologically, recent research using monoclonal antibodies have been able to separate the two.[44,45] Invasive amebiasis is almost exclusively the result of *E. histolytica* infection. It is estimated that 50 million cases of invasive disease result each year worldwide, leading to an excess of 100,000 deaths.[44] In the United States, the incidence of amebiasis is estimated at about 4% in the general population.[45] The highest incidence is found in institutionalized mentally retarded patients, sexually active homosexuals, patients with acquired immune deficiency syndrome (AIDS), the Native American population, and new immigrants from endemic areas (e.g., Mexico, India, West and South Africa and portions of Central and South America).[44–50]

PATHOLOGY

E. histolytica invades mucosal cells of colonic epithelium producing the classic flask-shaped ulcer in the submucosa.[42,44,45] The trophozoite has a cytolethal effect on cells through a toxin. If the trophozoite gets into the portal circulation, it will be carried to the liver where it produces abscess and periportal fibrosis. Amebic ulcerations can affect the perineum and genitalia, and abscesses may occur in the lung and brain.[46–54]

CLINICAL PRESENTATION

The most frequent clinical manifestations of the disease are gastrointestinal, with vague complaints of abdominal discomfort and malaise to severe abdominal cramps, flatulence, and bloody diarrhea with mucus (heme-positive in 100% of cases).[42,45]

Right upper quadrant pain, hepatomegaly, and liver tenderness, with referred pain to the left or right shoulder, usually suggest an amebic liver abscess. Liver abscesses that are located in the right lobe can spread to the lungs and pleura.[42–45] Pericardial infection, although rare, may be associated with extension of the amebic abscess from the left lobe of the liver. Erosion of liver abscesses also present as peritonitis.[42,47,51,52]

Eosinophilia is usually absent, although mild leukocytosis is not unusual in intestinal amebiasis.[42] A patient with liver abscess, however, will usually present with high fever, significant leukocytosis with left shift, elevated alkaline phosphatase, and liver tenderness on palpation.[42,44,45]

Review of the patient's history and recent travel, cannot be overemphasized. Intestinal amebiasis is diagnosed by demonstrating *E. histolytica* cysts or trophozoites (may contain ingested erythrocytes) in fresh stool or from a specimen obtained by sigmoidoscopy. Three stool samples obtained 24 hours apart will produce a 60% to 90% yield for *E. histolytica*. Microscopy may not differentiate between the pathogenic *E. histolytica* and the nonpathogenic *E. dispar* in stools. Monoclonal antibodies are used in antigen capture enzyme-linked immunosorbent assays (ELISA).[42,44,45] Endoscopy with scraping or biopsy may provide more definitive diagnosis where stool examinations do not provide adequate evidence.[44]

When amebic liver abscess is suspected from initial physical examination and history, confirmatory diagnostic procedures will include serology and liver scans (using isotopes by ultrasound or computerized tomography) or magnetic resonance imaging.[42,44,55] Leukocytosis (>10,000/mm^3) and elevated alkaline phosphatase (>75%) are common findings. In rare instances, needle aspiration of the hepatic abscess may be attempted using ultrasound guidance.[52]

▶ TREATMENT: Amebiasis

DESIRED OUTCOME

In amebiasis, the goals of therapy are initially to eradicate the parasite by use of specific amebicides and then to render supportive therapy.

TREATMENT REGIMENS

A number of different regimens have been suggested, depending on the category of amebiasis: asymptomatic cyst-passers, intestinal amebiasis, and amebic liver abscess.[42–45] Electrolyte replacement and nutritional support are essential adjunctive treatment modalities. Large hepatic abscess or amebic pericarditis may require needle aspiration, percutaneous catheter drainage, or, rarely, surgery before drug therapy.[42,43,45] Most regimens require a combination of drugs administered concurrently or sequentially.[24]

HISTORY

Careful history should be taken when one of the differential diagnoses is ulcerative colitis, because corticosteroid administration has the potential to unmask amebiasis and produce toxic megacolon.[45] All patients diagnosed as having inflammatory bowel disease should have their stools carefully examined and serologic testing done for amebiasis, to avoid the serious consequence that results from administration of corticosteroids.

PHARMACOLOGIC THERAPY

Metronidazole (Flagyl), tetracycline, dehydroemetine, and chloroquine (Aralen) are tissue-acting agents, whereas iodoquinol (Yodoxin), diloxanide furoate (Furamide), and paromomycin (Humatin) are luminal amebicides. A systemic agent may be so well absorbed that only small amounts of the drug stays in the bowel, which might prove ineffective as a luminal agent.[24,42,45,56,57] A luminal-acting agent, on the other hand, may be too poorly absorbed to be effective in the tissue. In the asymptomatic cyst-passer, it is necessary to eradicate the causative agent from lumen to prevent intestinal amebiasis or the development of amebic liver abscess. Drug effectiveness must be monitored by stool examination; that is, from one to three negative specimens from 1 to 3 months after treatment.

Asymptomatic cyst passers and patients with mild intestinal amebiasis should receive one of the following luminal agents: paromomycin 25–30 mg/kg/day three times daily for 7 days, or iodoquinol 650 mg three times daily for 20 days, or diloxanide furoate 500 mg three times daily for 10 days. These regimens have cure rates between 85% and 94%.[45] Diloxanide furoate is only available from the CDC.[24] The pediatric dose for paromomycin is the same as in adults, whereas the dose of iodoquinol is 30–40 mg/kg/day in 3 doses for 20 days, and the dose of diloxanide furoate is 20 mg/kg/day in 3 doses for 10 days.[24] Paromomycin is the preferred luminal agent in pregnant patients.[24,43]

Patients with severe intestinal disease or liver abscess should receive metronidazole 750 mg three times daily for 10 days, followed by a course of one of the luminal agents indicated above.[24,42–45] An alternative regimen of metronidazole 2.4 g/day for 2 days has been suggested to treat intestinal amebiasis.[45] In the pediatric patient, the dose of oral metronidazole is 50 mg/kg/day in divided doses to be followed by a luminal agent.[24] Patients who are too ill to take oral metronidazole should receive the drug in equivalent doses by the IV route.[42,45]

EVALUATION OF THERAPEUTIC OUTCOMES

Followup in patients with amebiasis should include repeat stool examination, serology, colonoscopy (in colitis) or computed tomography (CT; in liver abscess) between days 5 and 7, at the end of the course of therapy, and a month after the end of therapy.[42] Most patients with either intestinal amebiasis or colitis will respond in 3 to 5 days with amelioration of symptoms. Patients with liver abscesses may take from 7 to 10 days to respond; patients not responding during this period may require aspiration of abscesses or exploratory laparotomy. Serial liver scans have demonstrated healing of liver abscesses over 4 to 8 months after adequate therapy.[42]

SANITATION AND PREVENTIVE MEASURES

Travelers and tourists visiting an epidemic area should avoid local tap water, ice, salad, and unpeeled fruits. Water can be disinfected by use of iodine (tincture of iodine or commercial sources: Potable Aqua tablet, Wisconsin Pharmacal, or Globaline, Wallace & Trernain) or strong chlorine (laundry bleach) solution, but boiled water is probably the safest. An alternative or additional measure may be to carry a portable water purifier (Safewater, Durango, CO). Because food handlers in Asia and Latin America may be a source of amebiasis, travelers should avoid eating at food stalls and open markets.

GIARDIASIS

EPIDEMIOLOGY AND ETIOLOGY

Giardia lamblia (also known as *G. intestinalis* or *G. duodenalis*), an enteric protozoan, is the most common intestinal parasite responsible for diarrheal syndromes throughout the world.[58–62] *Giardia* is the most frequently identified intestinal parasite in the United States with a prevalence rate of 16% in some areas. *G. lamblia* has been identified as the first enteric pathogen seen in children in developing countries with prevalence rates between 15% and 30%.[59,60]

There are two stages in the life cycle of *G. lamblia:* the trophozoite and the cyst. *G. lamblia,* which is found in the small intestine, the gallbladder, and in the biliary drainage, is a pear-shaped trophozoite with four pairs of flagella. Two nuclei lie in the area of the sucking disk, giving the protozoan a characteristic face-like image.

The distribution of giardiasis is worldwide. Children seem to be more frequently affected than adults. Children in day care centers may infect parents and other family members.[60] In less-developed countries, fecal contamination of the environment, lack of potable water, education, and housing continue to be risk factors for giardiasis among children.

PATHOLOGY

Giardiasis results from ingestion of *G. lamblia* cysts in fecally contaminated water or food. The protozoan excysts under the stimulus of low gastric pH to release the trophozoite.[59] Colonization and multiplication of the trophozoite leads to mucosal invasion, localized edema, and flattening of the villi resulting in malabsorption states in the host.[59–62]

Lactose intolerance precipitated by giardiasis can persist even after eradication of the protozoan. Achlorhydria, hypogammaglobulinemia, or deficiency in secretory immunoglobulin A (IgA) are predispositions for giardiasis.[58–60]

CLINICAL PRESENTATION

Following an incubation period of 1 to 2 weeks after ingestion of the *G. lamblia* cysts, symptomatic giardiasis is marked by acute onset of diarrhea, cramplike abdominal pains, bloating, and flatulence.[58–61] Complaints from patients include malaise, nausea, anorexia, and belching. Signs and symptoms may be confused for other gastrointestinal conditions.[63,64] Chronic diarrhea may continue with foul smelling, copious, light-colored fatty stools and weight loss. Periods of diarrhea may alternate with constipation. Patients will complain of malaise, headache, and abdominal and epigastric discomfort frequently exacerbated by eating. Giardiasis can cause steatorrhea and vitamin B_{12} and fat-soluble vitamin deficiencies if left untreated.[63,65–67]

Diagnosis of giardiasis is made by examination of fresh stool or a preserved specimen during the acute diarrheal phase. Fresh stool specimens may show the trophozoites, whereas preserved specimens usually yield the cysts. The alternative method is to use the string or Entero-Test (Hedeco, Palo Alto, CA). The Entero-Test consists of a weighted gelatin capsule secured to a nylon string, the free end of which is secured at the mouth while the capsule is swallowed. The string is removed in 4 to 6 hours and the end, which is normally located in the jejunum, is checked for trophozoites under a microscope.[60,61] If both the stool exam and string test prove unsuccessful, it may be necessary to attempt duodenal aspiration and biopsy to confirm the diagnosis; this may be more important in AIDS patients or in patients with hypogammaglobulinemia.[61] Most clinicians would advocate a clinical trial of the standard therapy before undertaking invasive diagnostic tests.[60,61] An indirect fluorescent antibody (IFA) that uses a monoclonal antibody to a protein in *Giardia* cyst is commercially available for detection of the *Giardia* antigen (Meridan Diagnostics, Cincinnati, OH).[60,61,63]

▶ TREATMENT: Giardiasis

DESIRED OUTCOME

To reduce morbidity and to avoid complications in patients identified with prolonged diarrhea and malabsorption, and who have a recent history of travel to an endemic area, rapid identification by ova and parasite (O&P) examination or by antigen detection test, should be used to institute appropriate therapy.

PHARMACOLOGIC THERAPY

All symptomatic adults and children older than 8 years of age should be treated with metronidazole 250 mg three times daily for 7 days. The alternative drugs include furazolidone 100 mg four times or paromomycin 25–30 mg/kg/day in divided doses daily for 1 week.[24,58–61] Paromomycin or bacitracin or bacitracin zinc may be safe agents in pregnancy.[24] The pediatric dose for metronidazole is 15 mg/kg/day three times daily for 5–7 days.[24] Furazolidone suspension (50 mg per 15 mL) is an alternative drug for pediatrics. Quinacrine, which was the drug of choice in giardiasis, has been discontinued by the manufacturer in the United States. A recent study indicated that albendazole 400 mg daily for 5 days had cure rates of 97% and was equivalent to metronidazole in children.[9,60,61]

EVALUATION OF THERAPEUTIC OUTCOMES

Patients with symptomatic giardiasis, positive stool samples, or detection of *Giardia* antigen by IFA or ELISA, should be treated with metronidazole for 7 days. Metronidazole produces cure rates between 85% and 95%.[59–61] Diarrhea will stop within a few days, although in some patients, it may take 1 to 2 weeks. Cyst excretion will cease within days; however, intestinal dysfunction (manifested as increased transit time) and radiologic changes (irregular thickening of the folds in the upper small intestine) may take a few months to resolve.[68] Patients who fail initial therapy with metronidazole should receive a second course of therapy. Pregnant patients can receive paromomycin 25–30 mg/kg/day in divided doses for 7 days. Metronidazole has been used in the second and third trimester of pregnancy.[60]

Giardiasis can be prevented by good personal hygiene and by caution in food and drink consumption. Preventive measures are similar to those discussed in amebiasis (see "Sanitation and Preventive Measures").

LEISHMANIASIS

EPIDEMIOLOGY AND ETIOLOGY

This disease is caused by a protozoan belonging to the genus *Leishmania*. The three variations of the disease are visceral leishmaniasis (*kala-azar,* "black fever," or Assam fever), cutaneous leishmaniasis, and mucocutaneous leishmaniasis.[69–73] The visceral form is predominantly caused by *Leishmania donovani,* while the other two forms are caused by other species. Leishmaniasis is a complex disease, but space constraints do not justify an extended discussion here; interested readers are urged to consult other sources.[69,73,74]

Leishmania exists in two forms: as a flagellated extracellular parasite in the sandfly vector (*Phlebotomus* in the Indian subcontinent and *Lutzomyia* and *Psychodopygus* in North and South America, Africa, or the Middle East) and an aflagellar amastigote (intracellular form) in the host.[73,74] The major reservoirs for *Leishmania,* depending on geographic location, are dogs, foxes, squirrels, and rodents. In the United States, a rodent reservoir (*Neotoma micropus*) has been traced to 27 cutaneous leishmaniasis cases in Texas.[75] The sandflies ingest the parasite when they feed on the reservoir animals. After metamorphosis in the gut of the sandfly, the parasite is transferred to the human host when the infected sandfly takes a blood meal. Cutaneous leishmaniasis seen most frequently in the United States is caused by either *Leishmania braziliensis* or *L. mexicana,* which are endemic to south Mexico and Central America.[73,74]

The disease can range from cutaneous ulcers to the mucocutaneous form affecting the nose, oral cavity, and pharynx. The highest incidence is usually seen in the summer months, especially in subjects working near forested areas. Visceral leishmaniasis may be acquired from transfusion of contaminated blood and accidental needle stick injuries.[69,73] Patients with advanced stage acquired immunodeficiency syndrome (AIDS) are reported to be highly susceptible to leishmaniasis.[73]

CLINICAL PRESENTATION

Visceral leishmaniasis usually begins as a papule, which may or may not ulcerate. Subsequently, the amastigote disseminates throughout the reticuloendothelial system to include the spleen, liver, bone marrow, and lymphatic nodes. Hypertrophy of the spleen and liver can take place. Visceral ("viscerotropic") leishmaniasis usually develop between 3 and 8 months (range, 10 days to 2 years) after exposure.[71,73] Patients may present with fever, chills, malaise, weight loss, abdominal distention and hepatosplenomegaly.[71,73]

In the cutaneous disease, the initial lesion appears between 2 and 8 weeks following the bite of the infected sandfly and progresses to a raised ulcer that may persist for months and years.[72] The mucocutaneous form, which is usually caused by *L. braziliensis,* will result in mutilating mucosal infections affecting the nose, soft palate, and the trachea. Demonstration of amastigote in tissue or bone marrow confirms the diagnosis of leishmaniasis.[69–73]

▶ TREATMENT: Leishmaniasis

DESIRED OUTCOME

The major goal is to eradicate the amastigote in the tissue and to minimize the ensuing complications of leishmaniasis.

PHARMACOLOGIC THERAPY

All three forms of leishmaniasis are treated with stibogluconate sodium (antimony sodium gluconate-pentavalent antimony-Pentostam) which is obtained from the CDC. In the adult, both the cutaneous and mucocutaneous forms (*L. braziliensis* and *L. mexicana*) are treated with stibogluconate 20 mg SB/kg/day for 20 to 28 days.[24] The drug may be administered by either the IV or intramuscular (IM) route. Therapy for all forms of leishmaniasis may be repeated.[24] The alternative drug for the visceral form is amphotericin B (Fungizone) or liposomal amphotericin B (AmBisome) while pentamidine isethionate (Pentam 300) is recommended for mucocutaneous and cutaneous forms.[24,76–79] Pediatric patients receive the same dose as adults (see Appendix 113–1 for side effects of drugs). Pentavalent antimony therapy combined with γ-interferon or liposomal amphotericin may be alternatives in refractory leishmaniasis.[24] Other combination therapies and alternative agents for the various forms of leishmaniasis are discussed in details by a number of authors.[69,70,78,79]

EVALUATION OF THERAPEUTIC OUTCOMES

The presence of dead amastigotes in tissue and bone marrow, resolution of anemia and leukopenia, and disappearance of splenomegaly and hepatomegaly may be used as monitoring parameters for the disease. Travelers to endemic areas should use insect repellents and sleep in fine-mesh netting to avoid exposure to the sandfly.[73] No effective chemoprophylaxis against leishmaniasis is available.

AMERICAN TRYPANOSOMIASIS

ETIOLOGY

Two distinct forms of the genus *Trypanosoma* occur in humans. One is associated with African trypanosomiasis (sleeping sickness) and the other with American trypanosomiasis (Chagas disease).[80–82] *Trypanosoma brucei gambiense* and *Trypanosoma brucei rhodesiense* are the causative organisms for African trypanosomiasis. In Chagas disease, the trypomastigote is found in the bloodstream and an ovoid, unflagellated, intracellular form is found in cardiac and other tissues.[80,81]

Trypanosoma cruzi is the agent that causes American trypanosomiasis. American trypanosomiasis is transmitted by a number of species of a reduviid bug (*Triatoma infestans, Rhodrium prolixus*) which live in wall cracks of houses in rural areas of North, Central, and South America. The reduviid bug is infected by sucking blood from animals (opossums, dogs, and cats) or humans infected with circulating trypomastigotes.

CLINICAL PRESENTATION

Acute infection is frequently seen in children, although Chagas disease in adults can also be present with the acute phase. Unilateral orbital edema (Romana's sign) because of local inflammation produced by the multiplying parasite may be seen. A local inoculation granuloma or chagoma appearing as a dusty erythematous lesion may be present, indicating the site of entry of the parasite. Fever, hepatosplenomegaly, and lymphadenopathy may also be present.

In chronic disease, patients present with cardiomyopathy and congestive heart failure. Electrocardiograms are usually abnormal, demonstrating extrasystoles, first-degree heart block, right-bundle-branch block, and other serious conduction disturbances.[81,82] Degeneration of the autonomic ganglia in the smooth muscle of the esophagus and colon lead to uncoordinated peristalsis. The end result has been reported to be "mega syndromes" of affected organs.[83,84] Penetration of central nervous system results in meningoencephalitis, seizures, and focal paralysis.[85–87]

A history to verify the possible exposure to *T. cruzi* should be an important initial diagnostic workup. Recovery of *T. cruzi* is definitive; however, this is not always possible, especially in chronic disease. Positive serologic tests using indirect hemagglutination test, ELISA (Chagas EIA, Abbott Labs), and a complement fixation (CF) test are used.[80] The CDC has used polymerase chain reaction (PCR) to diagnosis *T. cruzi*.[88] Specimens may be sent to the CDC for testing. False-positive reactions are seen especially in those exposed to leishmaniasis, syphilis, or malaria.[80]

▶ TREATMENT: American Trypanosomiasis

DESIRED OUTCOME

The primary goal of drug therapy in trypanosomiasis is to reduce the duration and severity of the illness, and possibly to decrease mortality.

PHARMACOLOGIC THERAPY

The drugs that have been used to treat *T. cruzi* infections: nifurtimox (Lampit, Bayer 2502) and benznidazole (Rochagan).[24,89,90] Oral nifurtimox is available from the CDC, while benznidazole is only available in Brazil. The adult dose of nifurtimox is 8–10 mg/kg/day in divided doses for 120 days. Because pediatric patients tolerate the drug better than adults, the dose for children ages 1 to 10 years is 15–20 mg/kg/day, and for children ages 11 to 16 years it is 12.5–15 mg/kg/day in divided doses.[24] Symptomatic treatment for heart failure include digitalis and diuretics; the gastrointestinal complications, however, may require surgical revisions and reconstruction.[81]

EVALUATION OF THERAPEUTIC OUTCOMES

American trypanosomiasis (Chagas disease) which is endemic in all Latin American countries can be transmitted congenitally, by blood transfusion, and by organ transplantation.[80–82] Treatment with nifurtimox of the acute phase (fever, malaise, edema of face, generalized lymphadenopathy, and hepatosplenomegaly) produces between 50% and 75% cure rates.[80,82] Treatment of chronic infection with nifurtimox is not recommended. It is essential to identify *T. cruzi*-infected patients by serology and to monitor the cardiovascular status of these patients by electrocardiogram periodically. The congestive failure of cardiomyopathic Chagas disease is treated the same way as cardiomyopathies from other causes.[81]

HELMINTHIC DISEASES

The majority of intestinal helminthic infections may not be associated with clearly defined manifestation of disease, but they can cause significant pathology.[91–102] One factor that determines the pathogenicity of helminths is their population density. Light infections may be fairly well tolerated, whereas high populations of intestinal helminths can result in predictable disease presentations. In the United States, these infections are most frequently seen in recent immigrants from Southeast Asia, the Caribbean, Mexico, and Central America.[1,3,9,100] There is a higher incidence of helminthic infections in the southern states. Other populations that have a high risk of infestation include institutionalized patients (both young and elderly), preschool children in day care centers, residents of Indian reservations, and homosexual individuals. Certain conditions and drugs (fever, corticosteroids, and anesthesia) can cause atypical localization of worms.[9,101,102] Immunocompromised hosts can be overwhelmed by some helminthic infections, such as strongyloidiasis.[102]

NEMATODES

HOOKWORM DISEASE

This is an infection of the small intestine caused by either *Ancylostoma duodenale* or *Necator americanus*. *N. americanus* is found in the southeastern United States, where the temperature and humidity provide the proper environment. *Ancylostoma* is rarely seen in the United States.

The life cycles of both species of hookworm are similar. The adult worms live in the small intestine attached to the mucosa. The females liberate eggs, which are eliminated in the feces and develop into larvae. Infective larva enter the host in contaminated food or water, or penetrate the skin, where a papular eruption with localized edema and erythema can result.

In the small intestine, where the adult worm lives attached to the mucosa, injury is usually caused by mechanical and lytic destruction of tissue. The loss of blood can lead to anemia and hypoproteinemia.[9,95–98]

Stool should be examined for eggs and the rhabditiform larvae. Eosinophilia (30% to 60%) is present in patients with chronic infection.

▶ TREATMENT: Hookworm Disease

Mebendazole (Vermox), an oral synthetic benzimidazole, is the agent of first choice. It is also effective against ascariasis, enterobiasis, and trichuriasis.[24,25,103–106] The adult dose for treatment of hookworm infestation is 100 mg twice daily for 3 days. Pediatric patients older than 2 years of age should receive the same dose as adults.[24]

ASCARIASIS

Ascariasis is caused by the giant roundworm *Ascaris lumbricoides*. Female worms range from 20–35 cm in length. The worm is found worldwide, but more commonly in areas where sanitation is poor. In the United States, endemic areas include southeastern parts of the Appalachian range and the Gulf Coast states.[9] It is estimated that about 4 million people in the United States have ascariasis.

Clinical Manifestations

During the migration of the larvae through the lungs, patients can present with pneumonitis, fever, cough, eosinophilia, and pulmonary infiltrates.[9,91,101] Other symptoms of ascariasis include abdominal discomfort, abdominal obstruction, vomiting, and appendicitis.[92–94,101] Diagnosis is made by demonstrating the characteristic egg in the stool.

▶ TREATMENT: Ascariasis

In both adults and pediatric patients older than 2 years of age, the treatment for ascariasis is mebendazole (Vermox) 100 mg twice daily for 3 days. An alternative drug for ascariasis is pyrantel pamoate (Antiminth).[24,106]

ENTEROBIASIS

Enterobiasis or pinworm infection is caused by *Enterobius vermicularis*. The pinworm is a small thread-like spindle-shaped worm about 1 cm in length. It is the most widely distributed helminthic infection in the world. There are estimated to be 42 million cases in the United States.[91,107] The majority of those infected are children.

There are no significant pathologic changes with the infection. The most common problem is cutaneous irritation in the perianal region, made by the migrating females or presence of eggs. The intense pruritus and scratching can cause dermatitis and secondary bacterial infections. In children, the itching can cause loss of sleep and restlessness.

The most effective method of diagnosing pinworm infections is by the use of perianal swab using Scotch tape. The Scotch tape, which is applied to the perianal region with a tongue depressor, is microscopically examined for eggs.[9,91,107]

▶ TREATMENT: Enterobiasis

Helminthic drugs are used to eradicate or reduce the parasitic load in patients. The common agents for treatment include pyrantel pamoate, mebendazole, or albendazole (Zentel). The dose of pyrantel pamoate is 11 mg/kg (maximum 1 g) as a single dose that can be repeated in 2 weeks. The dose of mebendazole for adults and children older than 2 years of age is 100 mg as a single dose; this may be repeated in 2 weeks.[24,25] Following treatment, all bedding and underclothes should be sterilized by steaming or washing in the hot water cycle of a regular washing machine; this will eradicate the eggs. Bathroom rugs and toilet accessories should also be cleaned in a similar way.

EVALUATION OF THERAPEUTIC OUTCOME: NEMATODES

Morbidity and disease with intestinal nematodes is related to the intensity of infection or worm burden; subjects with transient exposure have less-severe disease. The major adverse effects of intestinal nematodes are malnutrition, fatigue, and diminished work capacity. Treatment with antihelmintic agents results in complete eradication and significant change in well being of subjects. Unlike other nematodes, strongyloidiasis can perpetuate itself by autoinfection, and under immunosuppression, the filariform can invade various organs (lungs, central nervous system, and the like) to produce disseminated infection that can be fatal.[9,91,102]

ECTOPARASITES

A parasite that lives on the outside of the body of the host is called an ectoparasite. It is estimated that 6 to 12 million people become infested with pediculosis yearly in the United States.[108] Pediculosis is usually associated with poor personal hygiene, and infections are passed from person-to-person through social and sexual contact. The three types of human lice belong to two genera: *Pediculus,* including the head and body lice, and *Phthirus,* with only one species, the crab louse.[9,108–113] The human louse is detectable to the human naked eye and measures approximately 2–3 mm in length.

LICE

The two species that belong to this group include *Pediculus humanus capitis* (head louse) and *P. humanus corporis* (body louse). Female lice deposit eggs on the hair. The eggs (or nits) remain firmly attached to the hair and in about 10 days the lice hatch to form nymphs, which mature in 2 weeks. Using both their piercing mouth parts and a pumping device, the larvae and adults feed on the blood of the host. The body louse and head louse are essentially identical, although they live on different parts of the body. Unlike the head louse, which lives on the hair, the body louse is more frequently found on clothing of the infected host.

The pubic or crab louse is found on the hairs around the genitals, although they can occur in other areas of the body (e.g., eyelashes, beards, axillae).

Patients usually complain of severe pruritus from papular lesions produced by the bite of the louse. Hypersensitivity to foreign material injected by the lice can produce macular swellings and can occasionally lead to secondary bacterial infections. As a result of long-standing pediculosis and secondary infections, hyperpigmentation and thickening of the skin can take place, a condition referred to as "vagabond's" disease.[109]

► TREATMENT: Lice

The goal of therapy is to eradicate the causative organisms and provide symptomatic relief to patients. The agent of choice for all the three infections (body, head, and crab lice) is 1% permethrin (Nix).[108–115] Permethrin is a derivative of the flowers of the plant *Chrysanthemum cinerariifolium.* The term "pyrethrin" is usually applied to several esters of chrysanthemic acid and pyrethric acid. Permethrin has both pediculicidal and ovicidal activity against *Pediculus humanus var capitis*. The cure rate is reported to be in the range of 97% to 99%.[116–118] Individuals who have a history of ragweed or chrysanthemum allergy should use this compound with caution. The side effects reported with permethrin products include itching, burning, stinging, and tingling.[116,117] Permethrin 1% is applied to the scalp after the hair has been dried following a shampooing. The scalp should be saturated with permethrin liquid and a towel should be wrapped around the scalp to allow the application to stay on for 10 minutes. The hair should then be rinsed off. A cream rinse of permethrin 1% (Nix-Creme Rinse) is also available and is as effective as lindane.[113] Either of these two preparations may also be used for *Phthirus pubis* and *Pediculus humanus* infestations.[24] Other members of the family or sexual partners should also be treated. All bedding and clothes should be sterilized by boiling or washing in the hot water cycle of the washing machine to avoid reinfections. Seams of clothes should be examined to verify that all organisms are eradicated. An ocular lubricant (e.g., Lacri-Lube S.O.P.), applied twice daily, may be used to remove crab louse infection of the eyelids.

Another alternative for pediculosis is pyrethrin 0.3% combined with 3% piperonyl butoxide and 1.2% petroleum distillate (R&C, RID).[109,113,115] The same directions for permethrin should be followed when applying this preparation. For the relief of pruritus, a soothing lotion of calamine liniment or lotion with 0.1% menthol may be used.

SCABIES

Scabies is caused by the itch mite *Sarcoptes scabei,* which affects both humans and animals. Mange in domestic animals is caused by the same organism. Infection usually affects the interdigital and popliteal folds, axillary folds, the umbilicus, and scrotum.[108,110]

CLINICAL PRESENTATION

Patients will complain of severe itching and an inability to sleep, and may have excoriations in the interdigital web spaces, wrists, elbows, buttocks, groin, and scalp. Excoriations may lead to secondary bacterial infections. The diagnosis is made by looking for burrows formed by the mite and taking skin scrapings, which will demonstrate the mite on a wet mount.

► TREATMENT: Scabies

Because these infections cause a great deal of discomfort and distress to patients and families, the goals of therapy are to eradicate the infestations rapidly, to institute symptomatic treatment, and to provide counseling and reassurance. The treatment of choice is permethrin 5% (Elimite) cream.[24,110,113,118,119] To initiate the treatment, the skin should be scrubbed thoroughly in a warm soapy bath, using a soft brush to remove all scabs. The lotion is then applied to the whole body, avoiding the face, mucous membranes, and eyes. The application should be left on for 8 to 14 hours before bathing.[24] A single application eradicates 91% of scabies in subjects.[113,119] All close contacts should be checked and treated appropriately.

Other agents used to treat scabies are γ-benzene hexachloride 1% lotion (Kwell, Lindane) and Crotamiton 10% (Eurax). These should be used in patients who have hypersensitivity to permethrin preparations. Topical corticosteroids and antihistamines may be used to decrease pruritus.

Permethrin (1% to 5%) for pediculosis and scabies is the preferred agent and remains the safest agent especially in infants and children.[113,118] One application of permethrin is consistently effective in eradicating more than 90% of all infections. However, pruritus may persist for 2 to 4 weeks because of the remnants of mite parts in the skin.

▶ PRINCIPLES OF PHARMACOTHERAPY

- All deaths for malaria are preventable. The primary reasons for deaths are failure to take chemoprophylaxis, delay in seeking medical care, and misdiagnosis.
- Falciparum malaria, primarily affecting travelers to Africa, which may be resistant to chloroquine, should be treated with quinidine. The estimated median cost of treating one case of severe *P. falciparum* infection is $12,516 as compared to $56 for a 23-day full-prophylactic course of mefloquine.
- Either chloroquine or quinidine may be used for malaria during pregnancy.
- Patients with severe intestinal disease or liver abscess caused by amebiasis should receive metronidazole 750 mg tid × 10 days followed by a full course of a luminal agent (either iodoquinol or paromomycin).
- Paromomycin 25–30 mg/kg tid × 7 days is the preferred luminal agent for amebiasis in pregnant patients.
- If three stools for ova and parasites are negative for giardiasis, consider treating empirically with metronidazole 250 mg tid × 5 days. Alternatives: small bowel sampling (Entero test) and endoscopy for biopsy; if these are negative, consider another diagnosis.
- The treatment of choice for leishmaniasis is sodium stibogluconate: 20 mg SB/kg/day × 20 to 28 days. An alternative therapy is amphotericin-B lipid complex 1–3 mg/kg/day for 5 days.
- Patient history, including blood transfusions and serology, should be reviewed to establish diagnosis of trypanosomiasis (Chagas disease).
- All cardiac manifestations, which are chronic symptoms of Chagas disease, are treated with standard regimens for cardiomyopathies: diuretics, digoxin, and antiarrhythmic drugs.
- Either mebendazole 100 mg bid × 3 days or albendazole 400 mg daily (approved in the United States for neurocysticercosis) are appropriate therapy for all helminthic infestations (except for pinworms where a single dose repeated after 2 weeks is the therapy).
- The drug of choice for both pediculosis and scabies is permethrin (Nix, and Elimite, respectively). An alternate therapy for pediculosis is ivermectin (Mectizan) 200 mg/kg as a single oral dose.

REFERENCES

1. Freedman DO, Woodall J. Emerging infectious diseases and the risk to the traveler. Med Clin North Am 1999;83:865–883.
2. Bechtel GA. Parasitic infections among migrant farm families. J Community Health Nurs 1998;15:1–7.
3. Walker PF, Jaranson J. Refuge and immigrant health care. Med Clin North Am 1999;83:1103–1120.
4. Kitchen LW. Case studies in international medicine. Am Fam Physician 1999;59:3040–3044.
5. Viani RM, Bromberg K. Pediatric imported malaria in New York: Delayed diagnosis. Clin Pediatr 1999;38:333–337.
6. Beigel Y, Greenberg Z, Ostfeld I. Letting the patient off the hook. N Engl J Med 2000;342:1658–1661.
7. Parkas V, Godwin J, Murray HW. Kala-Azar comes to New York. Arch Intern Med 1997;157:921–923.
8. Sinha A, Grace C, Alston WK, et al. African trypanosomiasis in two travelers from the United States. Clin Infect Dis 1999;29:840–844.
9. Markell EK, John DT, Krotoski WA. Markell and Voge's Medical Parasitology, 8th ed. Philadelphia, Saunders, 1999.
10. Baird JK, Hoffman SL. Prevention of malaria in travelers. Med Clin North Am 1999;83:923–944.
11. Kain KC, Keystone JS. Malaria in travelers: Epidemiology, disease and prevention. Infect Dis Clin North Am 1998;12:267–284.
12. Krogstad DJ. Plasmodium species (Malaria). In: Mandell GL, Dolin R, Bennett JE, eds. Principles and Practice of Infectious Diseases, 5th ed. New York, Churchill Livingstone, 2000:2817–2831.
13. Lobel HO, Kozarsky PE. Update on prevention of malaria for travelers. JAMA 1997;278:1767–1771.
14. Herwaldt BL, Juranek DD. Laboratory-acquired malaria, leishmaniasis, trypanosomiasis, and toxoplasmosis. Am J Trop Med Hyg 1993;48:313–323.
15. Murphy GS, Oldfield EC III. Falciparum malaria. Infect Dis Clin North Am 1996;10:747–775.
16. Mhlanga JDM, Bentivoglio M, Kristensson K. Neurobiology of cerebral malaria and African sleeping sickness. Brain Res Bull 1997;44:579–589.
17. Luxenburger C, Ricci F, White NJ, et al. The epidemiology of severe malaria in an area of low transmission in Thailand. Trans R Soc Trop Med Hyg 1997;91:256–262.
18. Zinna S, Vathsala A, Woo KT. A case series of Falciparum malaria-induced acute renal failure. Ann Acad Med Singapore 1999;28:578–582.
19. Schellenberg D, Menendez C, Kahigwa E, et al. African children with malaria in an area of intensive *Plasmodium falciparum* transmission: Features on admission to the hospital and risk factors for death. Am J Trop Med Hyg 1999;61:431–438.
20. Mordmullaer B, Kremsner PG. Hyperparasitemia and blood exchange transfusion for treatment of children with Falciparum malaria. Clin Infect Dis 1998;26:850–852.
21. Kemper CA. Pulmonary disease in selected protozoal infections. Semin Respir Infect 1997;12:113–121.
22. Humar A, Ohrt C, Kain KC, et al. PARASIGHT F test compared with the polymerase chain reaction and microscopy for the diagnosis of *Plasmodium falciparum* malaria in travelers. Am J Trop Med Hyg 1997;56:44–48.
23. White NJ. The treatment of malaria. N Engl J Med 1996;335:800–806.
24. Anonymous. Drugs for parasitic infections. Med Lett 1998;40:1–12.
25. Rosenblatt JE. Parasitic agents. Mayo Clin Proc 1999;74:1161–1175.
26. Schlagenhauf P. Mefloquine for malaria chemoprophylaxis 1992–1998: A review. J Travel Med 1999;6:122–133.
27. Taylor TE, Strickland GT. Infections of the blood and reticuloendothelial system: Malaria. In: Strickland GT, ed. Hunter's Tropical Medicine and Emerging Infectious Diseases, 8th ed. Philadelphia, Saunders, 2000:614–643.
28. Silver HM. Malarial infection during pregnancy. Infect Dis Clin North Am 1997;11:99–107.
29. Anderson SL, Oloo AJ, Gordon DM, et al. Successful double-blind, randomized, placebo-controlled field trial of azithromycin and doxycycline as prophylaxis for malaria in Western Kenya. Clin Infect Dis 1998;26:146–150.

30. Schwartz E, Regev-Yochay G. Primaquine as prophylaxis for malaria for nonimmune travelers: A comparison with mefloquine and doxycycline. Clin Infect Dis 1999;29:1502–1506.
31. Stoute JA, Slaoui M, Cohen JD, et al. A preliminary evaluation of a recombinant circumsporozoite protein vaccine against *Plasmodium falciparum* malaria. N Engl J Med 1997;336:86–91.
32. Nussenzweig RS, Zavala F. A malaria vaccine based on a sporozoite antigen. N Engl J Med 1997;336:128–130.
33. Thompson RF, Baas DM, Hoffman SL. Travel vaccines. Infect Dis Clin North Am 1999;13:149–167.
34. Freedman DO. Keeping current. Travel medicine resources available on the Internet. Infect Dis Clin North Am 1998;12:543–547.
35. Gardner MJ. The genome of the malaria parasite. Curr Opin Genet Dev 1999;9:704–708.
36. Newton P, Suputtamongkol Y, White NJ, et al. Antimalarial bioavailability and disposition of artesunate in acute falciparum malaria. Antimicrob Agents Chemother 2000;44:972–977.
37. Ezzet F, van Vugt M, Nosten F, Looareesuwan S, White NJ. Pharmacokinetics and pharmacodynamics of lumefantrine (Benflumetol) in acute falciparum malaria. Antimicrob Agents Chemother 2000:44: 697–704.
38. Looareesuwan S, Wilairatana P, Royce C at al. A randomized, double-blind, comparative trial of a new oral combination of artemether and benflumetol (CGP 56697) with mefloquine in the treatment of acute *Plasmodium falciparum* malaria in Thailand. Am J Trop Med Hyg 1999;60:238–243.
39. Looareesuwan S, Chulay JD, Canfield CJ, Hutchinson DBA for Malarone clinical trials study group. Malarone (atovaquone and proguanil hydrochloride): Review of its clinical development for treatment of malaria. Am J Trop Med Hyg 1999;60:533–541.
40. Looareesuwan S, Wilairatana P, Hutchinson DBA, et al. Efficacy and safety of atovaquone/proguanil compared with mefloquine for treatment of acute *Plasmodium falciparum* malaria in Thailand. Am J Trop Med Hyg 1999;60:526–532.
41. Fradin MS. Mosquitoes and mosquito repellents: A clinician's guide. Ann Intern Med 1998;128:931–940.
42. Jackson TFHG, Gathiram V. Intestinal and genital infections. Amebiasis. In: Strickland GT, ed. Tropical Medicine and Emerging Infections, 8th ed. Philadelphia, Saunders, 2000:577–588.
43. Li E, Stanley SL Jr. Protozoa. Amebiasis. Gastroenterol Clin North Am 1996;25:471–492.
44. Petr WA, Singh U. Diagnosis and management of amebiasis. Clin Infect Dis 1999;29:1117–1125.
45. Ravdin J. *Entamoeba histolytica* (amebiasis). In: Mandell GL, Dolin R, Bennett JA, eds. Principles and Practice of Infectious Diseases, 5th ed. New York, Churchill Livingstone, 2000:2798–2810.
46. Shandera WX, Bollam P, White C Jr, et al. Hepatic amebiasis among patients in a public hospital. South Med J 1998;91:829–837.
47. Hoffner R, Kilaghbian T, Esekogwa VI, Henderson SO. Common presentations of amebic liver abscess. Ann Emerg Med 1999;34:351–355.
48. Antony S, Lopez-Po P. Genital amebiasis: Historical perspective of an unusual disease presentation. Urology 1999;54:952–955.
49. Yoshikawa I, Murata I, Yano K, Kume K, Otsuki M. Asymptomatic amebic colitis in a homosexual man. Am J Gastroenterol 1999;94:2306–2308.
50. Palau LA, Kemmerly SA. First report of invasive amebiasis in an organ transplant recipient. Transplantation 1997;64:936–937.
51. Sachdev GK, Dhol P. Colonic involvement in patients with amebic liver abscess: Endoscopic findings. Gastrointest Endosc 1997;46:37–39.
52. Akgun Y, Tacyildiz I, Celik Y. Amebic liver abscess: Changing trends over 20 years. World J Surg 1999;23:102–106.
53. Hejase MJ, Bihrle R, Castillo G, Coogan CL. Amebiasis of the penis. Urology 1996;48:151–154.
54. Lyche KD, Jensen WA. Pleuropulmonary amebiasis. Semin Respir Infect 1997;12:106–112.
55. Kimura K, Stoopen M, Reeder MM, Moncado R. Amebiasis: Modern diagnostic imaging with pathological and clinical correlation. Semin Roentgenol 1997;32:250–275.
56. Tracy JW, Webster LT Jr. Drugs used in the chemotherapy of protozoal infections. In: Hardman JG, Limbird LE, Molinoff PB, Ruddon RW, Gilman AG, eds. The Pharmacological Basis of Therapeutics, 9th ed. New York, Pergamon Press, 1996:987–1008.
57. Goldsmith R. Antiprotozoal drugs. In: Katzung BG, ed. Basic and Clinical Pharmacology, 7th ed. Stamford, CT, Appleton & Lange, 1998:838–861.
58. Wright SG. Giardiasis. In: Strickland GT, ed. Tropical Medicine and Emerging Infectious Diseases, 8th ed. Philadelphia, Saunders, 2000: 589–593.
59. Farthing MJ. Giardiasis. Gastroenterol Clin North Am 1996;25:493–515.
60. Hill DR. *Giardia lamblia*. In: Mandell GL, Dolin R, Bennett JE, eds. Principles and Practice of Infectious Diseases, 5th ed. Philadelphia, Churchill Livingstone, 2000:2888–2894.
61. Ortega YR, Adam RD. Giardia: Overview and update. Clin Infect Dis 1997;25:545–550.
62. Heregi G, Cleary TG. Giardia. Pediatr Rev 1997;18:243–247.
63. Thielman NM, Guerrant RL. Persistent diarrhea in the returned traveler. Infect Dis Clin North Am 1998;12:489–501.
64. Oberhuber G, Stolte M. Symptoms in patients with giardiasis undergoing upper gastrointestinal endoscopy. Endoscopy 1997;29:716–720.
65. Bai JC. Malabsorption syndromes. Digestion 1998;59:530–546.
66. Carroccio A, Montalto G, Notarbartolo A, et al. Secondary impairment of pancreatic function as a cause of severe malabsorption in intestinal giardiasis: A case report. Am J Trop Med Hyg 1997;56:599–602.
67. Springer SC, Key JD. Vitamin B_{12} deficiency and subclinical infection with *Giardia lamblia* in an adolescent with agammaglobulinemia of Bruton. J Adolesc Health 1997;20:58–61.
68. Reeder MM. Radiological diagnosis of giardiasis. Semin Roentgenol 1997;32:291–300.
69. Herwaldt B. Leishmaniasis. Lancet 1999;354:1191–1199.
70. Berman JD. Human leishmaniasis: Clinical, diagnostic, and chemotherapeutic development in the last 10 years. Clin Infect Dis 1997;24:684–703.
71. Davidson RN. Visceral leishmaniasis in clinical practice. J Infect 1999;39:112–116.
72. Salman SM, Rubeiz NG, Kibbi A. Cutaneous leishmaniasis: Clinical features and diagnosis. Clin Dermatol 1999;17:291–296.
73. Pearson RD, De Queiroz Souza A, Jeronimo SMB. Leishmania species: Visceral (KALA-AZAR), cutaneous, and mucosal leishmaniasis. In: Mandell GL, Bennett JE, Dolin R, eds. Principles and Practice of Infectious Diseases, 5th ed. Philadelphia, Churchill Livingstone, 2000:2831–2845.
74. Magill AJ. Leishmaniasis. In: Strickland GT, ed. Hunter's Tropical Medicine and Emerging Infectious Diseases, 8th ed. Philadelphia, Saunders, 2000:665–687.
75. McHugh CP, Melby PC, LaFon G. Leishmaniasis in Texas: Epidemiology and clinical aspects of human cases. Am J Trop Med Hyg 1996;55:547–555.
76. Sundar S, Agrawal NK, Murray HW, et al. Short-course, low-dose amphotericin-B lipid complex therapy for visceral leishmaniasis unresponsive to antimony. Ann Intern Med 1997;127:133–137.
77. Meyerhoff A. U.S. Food and Drug Administration approval of AmBisome (liposomal amphotericin B) for treatment of visceral leishmaniasis. Clin Infect Dis 1999;28:42–48.
78. Davidson RN. Practical guide for the treatment of leishmaniasis. Drugs 1998;56:1009–1018.
79. Moskowitz PF, Kurban AK. Treatment of cutaneous leishmaniasis: Retrospectives and advances for the 21st century. Clin Dermatol 1999;17:305–315.
80. Magill AJ, Reed SG. American trypanosomiasis. In: Strickland GT, ed. Hunter's Tropical Medicine and Emerging Infectious Diseases, 8th ed. Philadelphia, Saunders, 2000:653–664.
81. Prata A. Chagas' disease. Infect Dis Clin North Am 1994;8:61–76.
82. Kirchhoff LV. Trypanosoma species (American trypanosomiasis, Chagas' disease): Biology of trypanosomes. In: Mandell GL, Bennett JE, Dolin R, eds. Principles and Practice of Infectious Diseases, 5th ed. Philadelphia, Churchill Livingstone, 2000:2845–2853.

83. de Oliveira RB, Troncon LEA, Dantas RO, Meneghelli UG. Gastrointestinal manifestations of Chagas' disease. Am J Gastroenterol 1998;93:884–889.
84. Mattoso LF, Reeder MM. Radiological diagnosis of Chagas' disease (American trypanosomiasis). Semin Roentgenol 1998;33:26–46.
85. Chemelli L, Scaravilli F. Trypanosomiasis. Brain Pathol 1997;7:599–611.
86. Silva N, O'Bryan L, Masur H, et al. *Trypanosoma cruzi* meningoencephalitis in HIV-infected patients. J Acquir Immune Defic Syndr 1999;20:342–349.
87. Ferreira MS, Nishioka SA, Rocha A, et al. Reactivation of Chagas' disease in patients with AIDs: Report of three cases and review of the literature. Clin Infect Dis 1997;25:1397–1400.
88. Herwaldt BL, Grijalva MJ, Newsome AL, et al. Use of polymerase chain reaction to diagnose the fifth reported US case of autochthonous transmission of *Trypanosoma cruzi,* in Tennessee, 1998. J Infect Dis 2000;181:395–399.
89. Estani SS, Segura EL, Ruiz AM, et al. Efficacy of chemotherapy with benznidazole in children in the indeterminate phase of Chagas' disease. Am J Trop Med Hyg 1998;39:526–529.
90. de Andrade ALSS, Zicker F, de Oliveira RM, et al. Randomized trial of efficacy of benznidazole in treatment of early *Trypanosoma cruzi* infection. Lancet 1996;348:1407–1413.
91. Mahmoud AA. Intestinal nematodes (roundworms). In: Mandell GL, Bennett JE, Dolin R, eds. Principles and Practice of Infectious Diseases, 5th ed. Philadelphia, Churchill Livingstone, 2000:2938–2943.
92. Ferreyra NP, Cerri GG. Ascariasis of the alimentary tract, liver, pancreas and biliary system: Its diagnosis by ultrasonography. Heptogastroenterology 1998;45:932–937.
93. Goenka MK, Chowdhury A, Das K. Appendicular ascariasis: colonoscopic management. Gastrointest Endosc 1999;50:435–436.
94. Javid G, Wani N, Gulzar Gm, et al. Gallbladder ascariasis: Presentation and management. Br J Surg 1999;86:1526–1527.
95. Brooker S, Peshu N, Warn PA, et al. The epidemiology of hookworm infection and its contribution to anaemia among pre-school children in the Kenya Coast. Trans R Soc Trop Med Hyg 1999;93:240–246.
96. Olsen A, Magnussen P, Ouma JH, Andreassen J, Friis H. The contribution of hookworm and other parasitic infections to haemoglobin and iron status among children and adults in Western Kenya. Trans R Soc Trop Med Hyg 1998;92:643–649.
97. Stoltzfus RJ, Chwaya HM, Tielsch JM, et al. Epidemiology of iron deficiency anemia in Zanzibari school children: The importance of hookworms. Am J Clin Nutri 1997;65:153–159.
98. Hotez PJ, Ghosh K, Hawdon J, et al. Vaccines for hookworm infection. Pediat Infect Dis J 1997;16:935–940.
99. De Silva NR, Guyatt HL, Bundy DA. Morbidity and mortality due to ascaris-induced intestinal obstruction. Trans R Soc Trop Med Hyg 1997;91:31–36.
100. Kappas KD, Lundgren RG, Juranek DD. Intestinal parasitism in the United States: Update on a continuing problem. Am J Trop Med Hyg 1994;50:705–713.
101. Bundy DAP, De Silva N. Intestinal Nematodes that migrate through lungs (ascariasis). In: Strickland GT, ed. Hunter's Tropical Medicine and Emerging Infectious Diseases, 8th ed. Philadelphia, Saunders, 2000:726–730.
102. Gilman RH. Intestinal nematodes that migrate through skin and lung. Strongyloides infections. In: Strickland GT, ed. Hunter's Tropical Medicine and Emerging Infectious Diseases, 8th ed. Philadelphia, Saunders, 2000:736–740.
103. Albonico M, Stoltzfus RJ, Savioli L, Chwaya HM, d'Harcourt E. Controlled evaluation of two school-based anthelminthic chemotherapy regimens on the intensity of intestinal helminth infections. Int J Epidemiol 1999;28:591–596.
104. Bennett A, Guyatt H. Reducing intestinal nematode infection: Efficacy of albendazole and mebendazole. Parasitol Today 2000;16:71–74.
105. de Silva NR, Sirisena JLGJ, Gunasekera DPS, Ismail MM, de Silva HJ. Effect of mebendazole therapy during pregnancy on birth outcome. Lancet 1999;353:1145–1149.
106. Goldsmith RS. Clinical pharmacology of the anthelmintic drugs. In: Katzung BG, ed. Basic and Clinical Pharmacology, 8th ed. Stamford, CT, Appleton & Lange, 1998:862–880.
107. Bundy DA, Cooper E. Nematodes limited to the intestinal tract (*Enterobius vermicularis*, *Trichuris trichiura* and *Capillaria philippinensis*). In: Strickland GT, ed. Hunter's Tropical Medicine and Emerging Infectious Diseases, 8th ed. Philadelphia, Saunders, 2000:719–726.
108. Chosidow O. Scabies and pediculosis. Lancet 2000;355:819–826.
109. Mathieu ME, Wilson BB. Lice (pediculosis). In: Mandell GL, Bennett JR, Dolin R,eds. Principles and Practice of Infectious Diseases, 5th ed. Philadelphia, Churchill Livingstone, 2000:2972–2974.
110. Parish LC, Witkowski JA. The saga of ectoparasitosis: Scabies and pediculosis. Int J Dermatol 1999;38:432–433.
111. Meinking TL, Taplin D. Infestations: Pediculosis. Curr Probl Dermatol 1996;24:157–163.
112. Ibarra J, Hall DMB. Head lice in schoolchildren. Arch Dis Childhood 1996;75:471–473.
113. Brown S, Becher J, Brady W. Treatment of ectoparasitic infections: Review of the English-language literature, 1982–1992. Clin Infect Dis 1995;20(suppl 1):S104–S109.
114. Taplin D, Meinking TL. Permethrin. Curr Probl Dermatol 1996;24:255–260.
115. Burhart CG, Burhart CN, Burhart KM. An assessment of topical and oral prescription and over-the-counter treatments for head lice. J Am Acad Dermatol 1998;38:979–982.
116. Stichele RHV, Dezeure EM, Bogaert MG. Systematic review of the clinical efficacy of topical treatments for head lice. BMJ 1995;311:604–608.
117. Anonymous. Drugs for head lice. Med Lett 1997;39:6–7.
118. Taplin D, Meinking TL. Safety of permethrin vs lindane for treatment of scabies. Arch Dermatol 1996;132:959–962.
119. Elgart ML. A risk-benefit assessment of agents used in the treatment of scabies. Drug Saf 1996;14:386–393.

A

Appendix 113–1 Antiparasitic drugs

Drug	Indications	Side Effects	Comments	References
Albendazole 200-mg tablet (Zentel)	Giardiasis Ascariasis Neurocysticercosis	GI: Abdominal pain, nausea, diarrhea, increase in liver function enzymes	Not recommended in children <2 years old	9, 24, 104, 106
Atovaquone 250 mg *plus* Proguanil 100 mg (Malarone)[a]	Prevention and treatment of *P. falciparum* malaria	Abdominal pain, nausea, vomiting, and headache		9, 24, 27, 39–40
Chloroquine phosphate (Aralen, Nivaquine) 250- and 500-mg tablets; 50 mg/mL (as HCl); 5 mL ampule	Malaria	GI: Nausea, vomiting, diarrhea CNS: Dizziness, headache, blurring of vision, confusion, fatigue Derm: Pruritus	Administer oral dose after meals IV route: Recommend EKG monitoring *Contraindication*: Patients with psoriasis or porphyria	9–13, 23, 24, 27, 28
Dehydroemetine Dihydrochloride[b] 30 mg/mL; 2 mL ampule	Amebiasis	GI: Nausea, vomiting, diarrhea Card: Hypotension, arrhythmias, cardiac failure Other: Muscular pains, paralysis, death Cumulative toxicity: Doses > 650 mg	Prolongation: QT, PR, QRS, ST segment on EKG (may be indication to stop therapy) *Contraindication*: Cardiac and renal disease	9, 24, 43, 45, 56, 57
Diloxanide furoate[b] (Furamide) 500 mg tablet	Amebiasis	GI: Nausea, flatulence Derm: Pruritus		9, 24, 44, 56, 57
Furazolidone (Furoxone) 100-mg tablet Suspension: 50 mg/ 5 mL	Giardiasis Alternative to metronidazole	GI: Nausea, vomiting Hypersensitivity: Hypotension, fever, arthralgia, urticaria Other: Headache	Disulfiram-like reaction with alcohol; avoid in G6PD[b] deficiency; may cause hemolysis; changes color of urine to brown	24, 59, 60–62
Halofantrine (Halfan) 250-mg tablet	*P. falciparum* malaria	GI: abdominal pain, diarrhea Card: Prolongation of QT interval	Should not be taken with fatty meals *Contraindication*: Preexisting conduction defects	12, 23, 24
Iodoquinol (Yodoxin) 210-mg tablet	Amebiasis	GI: Abdominal pain, diarrhea Derm: Rash	May interfere with thyroid function test *Contraindication*: Patients with iodine intolerance	24, 42–45, 56, 57
Ivermectin (Stromectol) 6-mg tablet	Strongyloidiasis Pediculosis	Dizziness, somnolence, tremor, vertigo, pruritus, abdominal pain	Should be taken with a full glass of water	24, 57
Mebendazole (Vermox) 100-mg chewable tablet	Ascariasis, trichuriasis, hookworm, pinworm	GI: Abdominal pain, diarrhea CNS: Headache, dizziness Other: Pyrexia, neutropenia	Drug should be taken with meals *Contraindication*: Pregnancy *Drug interaction*: Can increase serum levels of theophylline	24, 91, 104, 105–107
Mefloquine (Lariam) 250-mg tablet	*P. falciparum* malaria	Incidence 17% GI: Nausea, vomiting, abdominal pain, diarrhea Card: Sinus bradycardia CNS: vertigo, dizziness, confusion, hallucinations, psychosis, convulsions Derm: Itching, skin rash	Patients given doses in excess of 12 mg/kg should be carefully monitored as the side effects are dose related	10–13, 15, 23, 24–26

Drug	Indications	Side Effects	Comments	References
Metronidazole (Flagyl) Oral: 250-mg, 500-mg tablets	Amebiasis giardiasis	GI: Nausea, anorexia, vomiting, diarrhea, abdominal cramping, glossitis, metallic taste CNS: Dizziness, vertigo, headache, paresthesias	Avoid alcohol; alcohol ingestion will cause the disulfiram reaction: abdominal distress, vomiting, hypotension *Contraindication*: First trimester of pregnancy	24, 42–45, 56–62
Nifurtimox[b] (Lampit, Bayer 2502)	South American trypanosomiasis	GI: Anorexia, nausea CNS: Peripheral neuritis, psychosis Hemat: Hemolysis in G6PD[c] deficient patients	Monitor pulmonary function and hematologic parameters	24, 56, 80–82
Primaquine phosphate 26.3-mg tablet	Malaria (*P. vivax*) (*P. ovale*)	GI: Nausea, abdominal pain CNS: Mental depression	In G6PD[c] deficiency can cause hemolysis	9, 10–12, 23, 24, 30
Pyrantel pamoate (Antiminth) 50-mg/mL suspension	Pinworm Hookworm	GI: Anorexia, nausea, abdominal cramps, diarrhea CNS: Headache, dizziness		24, 91, 106, 107
Pyrimethamine (Daraprim) 25-mg tablet	Malaria (see pyrimethamine-sulfadoxime)	GI: Abdominal pain, vomiting, glossitis Hemat: Megaloblastic anemia, hemolytic anemia	Recommended that folinic acid 1–5 mg/day be concurrently administered; can cause hemolysis in patients with G6PD[c] deficiency	24, 27, 56
Pyrimethamine 25 mg *plus* sulfadoxine 500 mg (Fansidar)	*P. falciparium* resistant malaria	For pyrimethamine see above GI: Nausea, abdominal pain, stomatitis Hemat: Agranulocytosis, aplastic anemia, leukopenia	Combination has recently been reported to cause the Stevens-Johnson syndrome; patients should be advised to call their physician/pharmacist if a skin rash or other reactions are seen	9, 10–12, 23, 24, 27
Quinidine gluconate 500 mg base/mL; 10 mL	Acute malaria	GI: Nausea, vomiting, diarrhea Card: Hypotension, widening of QRS and QT on EKG, heart block	Administration of IV quinidine requires close monitoring; should normally monitor EKG and all vital signs	9, 12, 15, 23, 24
Quinine sulfate 325-mg and 650-mg tablets	Acute malaria	Cinchonism: Flushing, dizziness, nausea, vomiting, diarrhea (levels over 10 μg/mL) Card: Hypotension, widening of QRS complex Hemat: Hemolysis, leukopenia, thrombocytopenia	When drug is administered IV it should be administered by slow infusion (600 mg over 8 h); close monitoring of vitals and EKG *Avoid use:* IM administration	9, 18, 23–25, 57
Sodium stibogluconate (Pentostam)[b]	Leishmaniasis	GI: Nausea, vomiting, abdominal pain, pancreatitis, increase LFTs Musculoskel: Myalgia, fatigue Card: T-wave inversion, bradycardia Hemat: Leukopenia, thrombocytopenia pancreatitis	Highly toxic, requires careful monitoring—vitals and EKG; caution in patients with liver or cardiac problems	69–71, 73, 74, 78

[a]Atovaquone 62.5 mg/proguanil 25 mg (Malarone)—pediatric dosage strength

[b]Investigational drugs obtained from The Centers for Disease Control and Prevention Parasitic Disease Drug Service, Atlanta, GA 30333. (707) 488-7760 (business hours: 8:00 AM to 4:30 PM EST), (404) 639-2888 (night, weekend, or holiday—for emergency calls only). Readers may also call local state health offices for specific information on travel information and parasitic diseases. Internet: CDC International Travel Information: http://www.cdc.gov/travel/travel.htm.[34]

[c]G6PD, glucose-6-phosphate dehydrogenase.

114

URINARY TRACT INFECTIONS AND PROSTATITIS

Elizabeth A. Coyle and Randall A. Prince

Infections of the urinary tract represent a wide variety of syndromes, including urethritis, cystitis, prostatitis, and pyelonephritis. Urinary tract infections (UTIs) are one of the most commonly occurring bacterial infections and account for 8 million patient visits annually.[1,2] It is estimated that 20% of all women will suffer a symptomatic UTI at some point in their lives, with many women having multiple recurrences.[3] Infections in men occur much less frequently until the age of 65, at which point the incidence rates in men and women are similar.

A UTI is defined as the presence of microorganisms in the urinary tract that cannot be accounted for by contamination. The organisms present have the potential to invade the tissues of the urinary tract and adjacent structures. Infection may be limited to the growth of bacteria in the urine, which frequently may not produce symptoms. A UTI can present as several syndromes associated with an inflammatory response to microbial invasion and can range from asymptomatic bacteriuria to pyelonephritis with bacteremia or sepsis.

Generally speaking, UTIs are be classified by several methods. Typically, they have been described by anatomic site of involvement. Lower tract infections include cystitis (bladder), urethritis (urethra), prostatitis (prostrate gland), and epididymitis. Pyelonephritis is an infection involving the kidneys and represents upper tract infection.

Also, UTIs are designated as uncomplicated or complicated. Uncomplicated infections occur in individuals who lack structural or functional abnormalities of the urinary tract that interfere with the normal flow of urine or voiding mechanism. These infections occur in females of childbearing age (15–45 years) who are otherwise normal, healthy individuals. Infections in males are generally not classified as uncomplicated because these infections are rare, and most often represent a structural or neurologic abnormality.

Complicated UTIs are the result of a predisposing lesion of the urinary tract, such as a congenital abnormality or distortion of the urinary tract, a stone, indwelling catheter, prostatic hypertrophy, obstruction, or neurologic deficit that interferes with the normal flow of urine and urinary tract defenses. Complicated infections occur in both genders and frequently involve the upper and lower urinary tract.

Recurrent UTIs are characterized by multiple symptomatic infections with asymptomatic periods occurring between each episode. Either reinfection or relapse causes these infections. Reinfections are caused by a different organism than originally isolated and account for the majority of recurrent UTIs. Relapse is the development of repeated infections with the same initial organism and usually indicates a persistent infectious source.

Asymptomatic bacteriuria is a common finding, particularly among those $\geq$65 years of age, when there is significant bacteriuria ($>10^5$ bacteria/mL of urine) in the absence of symptoms. Symptomatic abacteriuria or acute urethral syndrome consists of symptoms of frequency and dysuria in the absence of significant bacteriuria. This syndrome is commonly associated with chlamydia infections.

Significant bacteriuria is a term used to distinguish the presence of microorganisms that represent true infection versus contamination of the urine as it passes through the distal urethra prior to collection. Historically, bacterial counts equal to or greater than 100,000 organisms/mL of urine in a clean catch specimen were judged to indicate true infection.[4]

Counts less than 100,000, however, may represent true infection in certain situations; for example, with concurrent antibacterial drug administration, rapid urine flow, low urinary pH, or upper tract obstruction.[5] Table 114–1 lists the clinical definitions of significant bacteriuria that are dependent on the clinical setting and the method of specimen collection.[4] These criteria allow for more appropriate specificity and sensitivity in documenting infection under differing clinical circumstances.

EPIDEMIOLOGY

The prevalence of UTIs varies with age and gender. In newborns and infants up to 6 months of age, the prevalence of bacteriuria is about 1% and is more common in boys. Most of these infections are associated with structural or functional abnormalities of the urinary tract, and have been correlated to the lack of circumcision.[6] Between the ages of 1 and 5 years, UTIs occur more frequently in females. The prevalence of bacteriuria in females and males of this age group is 4.5% and 0.5%, respectively.[7] Infections occurring in preschool boys usually are associated with congenital abnormalities of the urinary tract. These infections are difficult to recognize because of the age of the patient, but they often are symptomatic. In addition, it is believed that the majority of renal damage associated with UTI develops at this age.[7]

Through grade school and before puberty, the prevalence of UTI is about 1%, with 5% of females reported to have significant bacteriuria prior to leaving high school. This percentage increases dramatically to 1% to 4% after puberty in nonpregnant females, primarily as a result of sexual activity. It is estimated that one in five women will suffer a symptomatic UTI at some point in their lives. Many women have recurrent infections, with a significant proportion of these women having a history of childhood infections. In contrast, the prevalence of bacteriuria in adult men is very low ($<0.1\%$).[8]

In the elderly, the ratio of bacteriuria in women and men is altered dramatically and is approximately equal in persons over the age of 65.[9] The overall incidence of UTI increases substantially in this population with the majority of infections being asymptomatic. The rate of infection increases further for those elderly persons who are residing in nursing homes, particularly those persons who are frequently hospitalized. The increase is probably the result of a number of factors, including obstruction from prostatic hypertrophy in males; poor bladder emptying as a result of prolapse in females; fecal incontinence in demented patients; neuromuscular disease, including strokes; and increased urinary instrumentation (catheterization).

ETIOLOGY

The bacteria causing UTIs usually originate from bowel flora of the host. Although virtually every organism is associated with UTIs,

TABLE 114–1. Diagnostic Criteria for Significant Bacteriuria

$\geq 10^2$ CFU coliforms/mL or $\geq 10^5$ CFU noncoliforms/mL in a symptomatic female
$\geq 10^3$ CFU bacteria/mL in a symptomatic male
$\geq 10^5$ CFU bacteria/mL in a symptomatic individuals on two consecutive specimens
Any growth of bacteria on suprapubic catheterization in a symptomatic patient
$\geq 10^2$ CFU bacteria/mL in a catheterized patient

CFU, Colony-forming unit.

certain organisms predominate as a result of specific virulence factors. The most common cause of uncomplicated UTIs is *Escherichia coli,* which accounts for 85% of community-acquired infections. Additional causative organisms in uncomplicated infections include *Staphylococcus saprophyticus* (5% to 15%), *Klebsiella pneumoniae, Proteus* spp., *Pseudomonas aeruginosa,* and *Enterococcus* spp. (5% to 10%).

Because *S. epidermidis* is frequently isolated from the urinary tract, it should be considered a contaminant initially. Repeat cultures should be performed to help confirm the organism as a real pathogen.

Organisms isolated from individuals with complicated infections are more varied and are generally more resistant than those found in uncomplicated infections. *E. coli* is a frequently isolated pathogen, but it accounts for less than 50% of infections. Other frequently isolated organisms include *Proteus* spp., *K. pneumoniae, Enterobacter* spp., *P. aeruginosa,* staphylococci, and enterococci. *Enterococcus faecalis* represents the second most frequently isolated organism in hospitalized patients.[10] In part, this finding may be related to the extensive use of third-generation cephalosporin antibiotics, which are not active against the enterococci. *E. faecalis* resistance to vancomycin has become more widespread and is a major therapeutic, as well as infection control, issue.[11]

S. aureus infections may arise from the urinary tract, but they are more commonly a result of bacteremia producing metastatic abscesses in the kidney. *Candida* spp. are common causes of UTI in the critically ill and chronically catheterized patient.

The majority of UTIs are caused by a single organism; however, in patients with stones, indwelling urinary catheters, or chronic renal abscesses, multiple organisms may be isolated. Depending on the clinical situation, the recovery of multiple organisms may represent contamination and a repeat evaluation should be done.

PATHOPHYSIOLOGY

ROUTE OF INFECTION

In general, organisms gain entry into the urinary tract via three possible routes: the ascending, hematogenous (descending), and lymphatic pathways. The female urethra is usually colonized with bacteria believed to originate from the fecal flora. The short length of the female urethra and its proximity to the perirectal area make colonization of the urethra likely. Other factors that promote urethral colonization include the use of spermicides and diaphragms as methods of contraception.[2] Although there is evidence in females that bladder infections follow the colonization of the urethra, the mode of ascent of the microorganisms is not completely understood. Massage of the female urethra and sexual intercourse allow bacteria to reach the bladder.[12] Once bacteria have reached the bladder, the organisms quickly multiply and can ascend the ureters to the kidneys. This sequence of events is more likely to occur if vesicoureteral reflux (reflux of urine into the ureters and kidneys while voiding) is present. The fact that UTIs are more common in females than males because of the anatomic differences in location and length of the urethra tends to support the ascending route of infections as the primary acquisition route.

Infection of the kidney by hematogenous spread of microorganisms usually occurs as the result of dissemination of organisms from a distant primary infection in the body. Infections via the descending route are uncommon and involve a relatively small number of invasive pathogens. Bacteremia caused by *S. aureus* may produce renal abscesses. Additional organisms include *Candida* spp., *Mycobacterium tuberculosis, Salmonella* spp., and *Enterococcus* spp. Of particular interest, it is difficult to produce experimental pyelonephritis by intravenously administering common gram-negative organisms, such as *E. coli* and *P. aeruginosa.* Overall, less than 5% of documented UTIs result from hematogenous spread of microorganisms.

There appears to be little evidence supporting a significant role for renal lymphatics in the pathogenesis of UTIs. There are lymphatic communications between the bowel and kidney, as well as the bladder and kidney. There is no evidence, however, that microorganisms are transferred to the kidney via this route.

After bacteria reach the urinary tract, three factors determine the development of infection: the size of the inoculum, the virulence of the microorganism, and the competency of the natural host defense mechanisms. The majority of UTIs reflect a failure in host defense mechanisms.

HOST DEFENSE MECHANISMS

The normal urinary tract is generally resistant to invasion by bacteria and is very efficient in rapidly eliminating microorganisms that reach the bladder. The urine under normal circumstances is capable of inhibiting and killing microorganisms. The factors thought to be responsible include a low pH, extremes in osmolality, high urea concentration, and high organic acid concentration. Bacterial growth is further inhibited in males by the addition of prostatic secretions.[13,14]

The introduction of bacteria into the bladder stimulates micturition with increased diuresis and efficient emptying of the bladder. These factors are critical in preventing the initiation and maintenance of bladder infections. Patients who are unable to void urine completely are at greater risk of developing UTIs and frequently have recurrent infections. Also, patients with even small residual amounts of urine in their bladder respond less favorably to treatment than patients who are able to empty their bladders completely.[15]

An important virulence factor of bacteria is their ability to adhere to urinary epithelial cells, resulting in colonization of the urinary tract, bladder infections, and pyelonephritis. Various factors that act as antiadherence mechanisms are present in the bladder, preventing bacterial colonization and infection. The epithelial cells of the bladder are coated with a urinary mucus or slime called glycosaminoglycan. This thin layer of surface mucopolysaccharide is hydrophilic and strongly negatively charged. When bound to the uroepithelium, it attracts water molecules and forms a layer between the bladder and urine. The antiadherence characteristics of the glycosaminoglycan layer are nonspecific and, when removed by dilute acid solutions, result in rapid bacterial adherence.[16]

In addition, the Tamm-Horsfall protein is a glycoprotein produced by the ascending limb of Henle and distal tubule, which is secreted into the urine and contains mannose residues. These mannose residues bind *E. coli* that contain small surface projecting organellae on its surface called pili or fimbriae. Type 1 fimbriae are mannose sensitive, and this interaction prevents the bacteria from binding to similar receptors present on the mucosal surface of the bladder. Other factors that possibly prevent adherence of bacteria include immunoglobulins (Ig) G and A. Investigators have documented both systemic and local kidney Ig synthesis in upper tract infections. The role of Igs in preventing bladder infection is less clear. Patients with reduced urinary levels of secretory IgA are, however, at increased risk of infections of the urinary tract.[13]

After bacteria have actually invaded the bladder mucosa, an inflammatory response is stimulated with the mobilization of polymorphonuclear leukocytes (PMNs) and resulting phagocytosis. PMNs are primarily responsible for limiting the tissue invasion and controlling the spread of infection in the bladder and kidney. They do not play a role in preventing bladder colonization or infections, and actually contribute to renal tissue damage.

Other host factors that may play a role in the prevention of UTIs are the presence of lactobacillus in the vaginal flora and circulating estrogen levels. In premenopausal women, circulating estrogen supports the vaginal tract growth of lactobacilli, which produce lactic acid to help maintain a low vaginal pH, thereby preventing *E. coli* vaginal colonization. Spermicide use, β-lactam antimicrobials use, lower estrogen levels, intercourse with a new partner, and douching can lead to decreases in lactobacilli colonization.[17,18]

BACTERIAL VIRULENCE FACTORS

Pathogenic organisms have differing degrees of pathogenicity (virulence), which play a role in the development and severity of infection. Bacteria that adhere to the epithelium of the urinary tract are associated with colonization and infection. The mechanism of adhesion of gram-negative bacteria, particularly *E. coli,* is related to bacterial fimbriae that are rigid hair-like appendages of the cell wall.[19] These fimbriae adhere to specific glycolipid components on epithelial cells. The most common type of fimbriae is type 1, which binds to mannose residues present in glycoproteins. Glycosaminoglycan and Tamm-Horsfall protein are rich in mannose residues that readily trap those organisms that contain type 1 fimbriae, which are then washed out of the bladder.[20] Other fimbriae are mannose resistant and are more frequently associated with pyelonephritis, such as P fimbriae, which bind avidly to specific glycolipid receptors on uroepithelial cells. These bacteria are resistant to washout or removal by glycosaminoglycan and are able to multiply and invade tissue, especially the kidney. In addition, PMNs, as well as secretory IgA antibodies, contain receptors for type 1 fimbriae, which facilitates phagocytosis, but they lack receptors for P fimbriae.

Other virulence factors include the production of hemolysin and aerobactin.[19] Hemolysin is a cytotoxic protein produced by bacteria that lyse a wide range of cells, including erythrocytes, PMNs, and monocytes. *E. coli* and other gram-negative bacteria require iron for aerobic metabolism and multiplication. Aerobactin facilitates the binding and uptake of iron by *E. coli;* however, the significance of this property in the pathogenesis of UTIs remains unknown.

PREDISPOSING FACTORS TO INFECTION

The normal urinary tract is typically resistant to infection and colonization by pathogenic bacteria. In patients with underlying structural abnormalities of the urinary tract, the typical host defenses previously discussed are usually lacking. There are several known abnormalities of the urinary tract system that interfere with its natural defense mechanisms, the most important of which is obstruction. Obstruction can inhibit the normal flow of urine, disrupting the natural flushing and voiding effect in removing bacteria from the bladder and resulting in incomplete emptying. Common conditions that result in residual urine volumes include prostatic hypertrophy, urethral strictures, calculi, tumors, bladder diverticula, and drugs, such as anticholinergic agents. Additional causes of incomplete bladder emptying include neurologic malfunctions associated with stroke, diabetes, spinal cord injuries, tabes dorsalis, and other neuropathies.

Vesicoureteral reflux represents a condition in which urine is forced up the ureters to the kidneys. Urinary reflux is not only associated with an increased incidence of UTIs and pyelonephritis, but it is also associated with renal damage.[21] Reflux may be the result of a congenital abnormality or more commonly the result of bladder overdistention from obstruction.

Other risk factors include urinary catheterization, mechanical instrumentation, pregnancy, and the use of spermicides and diaphragms.

CLINICAL PRESENTATION

CLINICAL FINDINGS

The presenting signs and symptoms of UTIs in adults are easily recognized. The typical manifestations of lower tract infections include dysuria, urgency, frequency, nocturia, and suprapubic heaviness. Women will frequently report gross hematuria. Systemic symptoms, including fever, are typically absent in this setting. Unfortunately, large portions of patients with significant bacteriuria are asymptomatic. These patients may be normal healthy patients, elderly patients, children, pregnant patients, and patients with indwelling catheters.

The manifestations of upper tract infections classically involve systemic symptoms, including flank pain, costovertebral tenderness, abdominal pain, fever, nausea, vomiting, and malaise. Lower tract symptoms may or may not precede upper tract infections but often occur 1 to 2 days prior to systemic symptoms. It is important to note that attempts at differentiating upper tract from lower tract infections on the basis of symptoms alone are not reliable.

Elderly patients frequently do not experience specific urinary symptoms, but they will present with altered mental status, change in eating habits, or gastrointestinal symptoms. In addition, patients with indwelling catheters or neurologic disorders will commonly not have lower tract symptoms, while flank pain and fever may be recognized. Many of the aforementioned patients will, however, frequently develop upper tract infections with bacteremia with no or minimal urinary tract symptoms.

Acute bacterial prostatitis (ABP) presents as other acute infections. Common symptoms include perineal, sacral, or suprapubic pain; fever; urinary retention; and other urinary tract symptoms (frequency, dysuria, nocturia). Digital palpation of the prostate via the rectum typically reveals a swollen, tender, warm, and indurated prostate.

In contrast to acute bacterial prostatitis, manifestations of chronic bacterial prostatitis (CBP) are more variable. Presenting symptoms include the vague description of voiding difficulties, such as frequency, dysuria, and urgency, along with low back pain and perineal and suprapubic discomfort. Many patients are asymptomatic, but most have varying degrees of voiding discomfort. Although the physical examination is frequently unremarkable, the prostate gland may feel boggy, indurated, or normal.

LABORATORY FINDINGS

Symptoms alone are unreliable for the diagnosis of bacterial UTIs. The key to the diagnosis of UTI is the ability to demonstrate significant numbers of microorganisms in an appropriate urine specimen to distinguish contamination from infection. The type and extent of laboratory examination required depends on the clinical situation.

URINE COLLECTION

Examination of the urine is the cornerstone of laboratory evaluation for UTIs. There are three acceptable methods of urine collection. The first is the midstream clean-catch method. After cleaning the urethral opening area in both men and women, 20–30 mL of urine is voided and discarded. The next part of the urine flow is collected and should be processed immediately (refrigerated as soon as possible). Specimens that are allowed to sit at room temperature for several hours may result in falsely elevated bacterial counts. The midstream clean catch is the preferred method for the routine collection of urine for culture. When a routine urine specimen cannot be collected or contamination occurs, alternative collection techniques must be used.

The two acceptable alternative methods include catheterization and suprapubic bladder aspiration. Catheterization may be necessary for patients who are uncooperative or who are unable to void urine. If catheterization is performed carefully with aseptic technique, the method yields reliable results. Note, however, that introduction of bacteria into the bladder may result, and the procedure is associated with infection in 1% to 2% of patients. Suprapubic bladder aspiration involves inserting a needle directly into the bladder and aspirating the urine. This procedure bypasses the contaminating organisms present in the urethra, and any bacteria found using this technique are generally considered to represent significant bacteriuria. Suprapubic aspiration is a safe and painless procedure that is most useful in newborns, infants, paraplegics, seriously ill patients, and others when infection is suspected and routine procedures have provided confusing or equivocal results.

BACTERIAL COUNT

The diagnosis of UTI is based on the isolation of significant numbers of bacteria from a urine specimen. Microscopic examination of a urine sample is an easy to perform and reliable method for the presumptive diagnosis of bacteriuria. The examination may be performed by preparing a Gram stain of unspun or centrifuged urine. The presence of at least one organism per oil-immersion field in a properly collected uncentrifuged specimen correlates well with >100,000 bacteria/mL of urine. For detecting smaller numbers of organisms, a centrifuged specimen is more sensitive. Such examinations detect $>10^5$ bacteria/mL with a sensitivity >90% and a specificity >70%.[22] Counts of less than 30,000, however, are usually not reliably recognized by these methods.[23]

PYURIA, HEMATURIA, AND PROTEINURIA

Microscopic examination of the urine for leukocytes is also used to determine the presence of pyuria. The presence of pyuria in a symptomatic patient correlates with significant bacteriuria.[24] Pyuria is defined as a white blood cell (WBC) count of greater than 10 WBC/mm^3 of urine. A count of 5–10 WBC/mm^3 is accepted as the upper limit of normal. It should be emphasized that pyuria is nonspecific and signifies only the presence of inflammation and not necessarily infection. Thus, patients with pyuria may or may not have infection. Sterile pyuria has long been associated with urinary tuberculosis, as well as chlamydial and fungal urinary infections.

Hematuria, microscopic or gross, is frequently present in patients with UTI, but is nonspecific. Hematuria may indicate the presence of other disorders, such as renal calculi, tumors, or glomerulonephritis. Proteinuria is commonly found in the presence of infection.

CHEMISTRY

Several biochemical tests have been developed for screening urine for the presence of bacteria. A common dipstick test detects the presence of nitrite in the urine, which is formed by bacteria that reduce nitrate normally present in the urine. False-positive tests are uncommon. False-negative tests are more common and are frequently caused by the presence of gram-positive organisms or *P. aeruginosa* that do not reduce nitrate.[25] Other causes of false tests include low urinary pH, frequent voiding, and dilute urine.

The leukocyte esterase (LE) dipstick test is a rapid screening test for detecting the presence of pyuria. Leukocytes esterase is found in primary neutrophil granules and indicates the presence of WBCs. The LE test is a sensitive and highly specific test for detecting more than 10 WBC/mm^3 of urine. When the LE test is used with the nitrite test, the range of reported sensitivity and specificity is 45.5% to 100% and 60% to 98%, respectively, for the detection of bacteriuria.[26,27] These tests can be useful in the outpatient evaluation of uncomplicated UTIs. However, urine culture is still the "gold standard" test in determining the presence of UTIs.

CULTURE

The most reliable method of diagnosing UTI is by quantitative urine culture. Urine in the bladder is normally sterile, making it statistically possible to differentiate contamination of the urine from infection by quantifying the number of bacteria present in a urine sample. This criterion is based on a properly collected midstream clean-catch urine specimen. Patients with infection usually have greater than 10^5 bacteria/mL of urine. It should be emphasized that as many as one-third of women with symptomatic infection have less than 10^5 bacteria/mL. A significant portion of patients with UTIs, either symptomatic or asymptomatic, also have less than 10^5 bacteria/mL of urine.

Several laboratory methods are used to quantify bacteria present in the urine. The most accurate method is the pour-plate technique. This method is unsuitable for a high-volume laboratory because it is expensive and time consuming. The streak-plate method is an alternative that involves using a calibrated loop technique to streak a fixed amount of urine on an agar plate. This method is used most commonly in diagnostic laboratories because it is simple to perform and less costly.

After identification and quantification are complete, the next step is to determine the susceptibility of the organism. There are several methods by which bacterial susceptibility testing may be performed. Knowledge of bacterial susceptibility and achievable urine concentration of the antibiotics puts the clinician in a better position to select an appropriate agent for treatment.

Infection Site

Several methods have been evaluated to determine the location of infection within the urinary system and differentiate upper tract involvement from lower tract. The most direct method is a ureteral catheterization procedure as described by Stamey and colleagues.[28] The method involves the passage of a catheter into the bladder and then into each ureter where quantitative cultures are obtained. History and physical examination were of little value in predicting the site of infection. Although this method provides direct quantitative evidence for UTI, it is invasive, technically difficult, and expensive. The Fairley bladder washout technique is a modification of the Stamey procedure, which involves Foley catheterization only.[29] After the catheter is passed, bladder samples are obtained and the bladder is washed out with culture samples taken at 10, 20, and 30 minutes. The procedure shows that up to 50% of patients have renal involvement, regardless of signs and symptoms. Other investigators found 10% to 20% of tests to be equivocal.[30]

Noninvasive methods of localization may be more acceptable for routine use; however, they have limited clinical value. Patients with pyelonephritis can have abnormalities in urinary concentrating ability. The use of concentrating ability for localization of UTIs is, however, associated with a high false-positive and false-negative response, and is not useful clinically.[25] The antibody coated bacteria (ACB) test is an immunofluorescent method that detects bacteria coated with Ig in freshly voided urine. The sensitivity and specificity of this test to localize the site of infection is reported to average 88% and 76%, respectively.[30] Because of the high incidence of false-positive and false-negative results, ACB testing is not routinely used in the management of UTIs.

Virtually all patients with uncomplicated lower tract infections can be cured with a short course of antibiotic therapy, and this assumption can sometimes be used to distinguish patients with lower and upper tract infections. Those patients who do not respond or who relapse do so because of upper tract involvement. It is rarely necessary to localize the site of infection to direct the clinical management of the patient.

▶ TREATMENT: Urinary Tract Infections

DESIRED OUTCOME

The goals of UTI treatments are: (a) to prevent or to treat systemic consequences of infection; (b) to eradicate the invading organism; (c) to prevent the reoccurrence of infection; and (d) to prevent any adverse effects of therapy.

MANAGEMENT

The management of a patient with a UTI includes initial evaluation, selection of an antibacterial agent and duration of therapy, and follow-up evaluation. The initial selection of an antimicrobial agent for the treatment of UTI is primarily based on the severity of the presenting signs and symptoms, the site of infection, and whether the infection is determined to be uncomplicated or complicated. Other considerations include antibiotic susceptibility, side-effect potential, cost, and the comparative inconvenience of different therapies.

Various pharmacologic factors may affect the action of antibacterial agents. Certainly the ability of the agent to achieve appropriate concentrations in the urine is of utmost importance. Factors that affect the rate and extent of excretion through the kidney include the patient's glomerular filtration rate and whether or not the agent is actively secreted. Filtration depends on the molecular size and degree of protein binding of the agent. Agents, such as sulfonamides, tetracyclines, and aminoglycosides, enter the urine via filtration. As the glomerular filtration rate is reduced, the amount of drug that enters the urine is reduced. Most β-lactam agents and quinolones are filtered and are actively secreted into the urine. For this reason, these agents achieve high urinary concentrations, despite unfavorable protein-binding characteristics or the presence of renal dysfunction.

The ability to eradicate bacteria from the urine is directly related to the sensitivity of the microorganism and the achievable concentrations of the antimicrobial agent in the urine. Unfortunately, most susceptibility testing is directed at achievable concentrations in the blood. There is a poor correlation between achievable blood levels of antimicrobial agents and the eradication of bacteria from the urine.[31] In the treatment of lower tract infections, plasma concentrations of antibacterial agents may not be important; however, achieving appropriate plasma concentrations appears critical in patients with bacteremia and renal abscesses.

There are a number of nonspecific therapies that have been advocated in the treatment and prevention of UTIs. Fluid hydration has been used to produce rapid dilution of bacteria and removal of infected urine by increased voiding. A critical factor appears to be the amount of residual volume remaining after voiding. As little as 10 mL of residual urine can significantly alter the eradication of infection.[15] Paradoxically, increased diuresis also may promote susceptibility to infection by diluting the normal antibacterial properties of the urine. Often in clinical practice, the concentrations of antimicrobial agents in the urine are so high that dilution has little effect on efficacy.

The antibacterial activity of the urine is related to the low pH, which is the result of high concentrations of various organic acids. Large volumes of cranberry juice increase the antibacterial activity of the urine and prevent the development of UTIs.[32] Apparently, the cranberry juice content of fructose and other unknown substances acts to interfere with adherence mechanisms of some pathogens, thereby preventing infection. Acidification of the urine by cranberry juice does not appear to play a significant role. The use of other agents (ascorbic acid) to acidify the urine to hinder bacterial growth does not achieve significant acidification. Therefore, attempts to acidify urine with systemic agents are not recommended. Lactobacillus probiotics also may aid in the prevention of female UTIs by increasing the vaginal pH, thereby decreasing *E. coli* colonization.[18] In postmenopausal women, estrogen replacement may be help in the prevention of recurrent UTIs. After 1 month of topical estrogen replacement, increases in vaginal Lactobacillus and pH, as well as decreases in *E. coli* colonization, have been found.[17]

Urinary analgesics, such as phenazopyridine hydrochloride (Pyridium), are frequently used by many clinicians. If the pain or dysuria present in an UTI is a consequence of infection, then urinary analgesics have little clinical role as most patients' symptoms respond quite rapidly to appropriate antibacterial therapy. Urinary analgesics also may mask signs and symptoms of UTIs not responding to antimicrobial therapy.

PHARMACOLOGIC THERAPY

Ideally, the antimicrobial agent chosen should be well tolerated, well absorbed, achieve high urinary concentrations, and have a spectrum of activity limited to the known or suspected pathogen(s). Table 114–2 lists the most common agents used in the treatment of UTIs along with comments concerning their general use. Table 114–3 presents an overview of various therapeutic options for outpatient therapy of UTI. Table 114–4 describes empiric treatment regimens for selected clinical situations.

TABLE 114–2. Commonly Used Antimicrobial Agents in the Treatment of Urinary Tract Infections

Oral Therapy	Comments
Sulfonamides	These agents have generally been replaced by more agents because of resistance.
Trimethoprim-sulfamethoxazole	This combination is highly effective against most aerobic enteric bacteria except *P. aeruginosa*. High urinary tract tissue levels and urine levels are achieved, which may be important in complicated infection treatment. Also effective as prophylaxis for recurrent infections.
Penicillins Ampicillin Amoxicillin Amoxicillin/clavulanic acid Carbenicillin indanyl	Ampicillin is the standard penicillin that has broad-spectrum activity. Increasing *E. coli* resistance has limited its use in acute cystitis. Drug of choice for enterococci sensitive to penicillin. Amoxicillin-clavulanate is preferred for resistance problems. Carbenicillin indanyl is only indicated for the treatment of urinary tract infections.
Cephalosporins Cephalexin Cephradine Cefaclor Cefadroxil Cefuroxime Cefixime Cefzil Cefpodoxime	There are no major advantages of these agents over other agents in the treatment of urinary tract infections and they are more expensive. They may be useful in cases of resistance to amoxicillin and trimethoprim-sulfamethoxazole. These agents are not active against enterococci.
Tetracyclines Tetracycline Doxycycline Minocycline	These agents have been effective for initial episodes of urinary tract infections, however, resistance develops rapidly and their use is limited. These agents also lead to candidal overgrowth. They are primarily useful for chlamydial infections.
Quinolones Ciprofloxacin Norfloxacin Levofloxacin Gatifloxacin Moxifloxacin	The newer quinolones have a greater spectrum of activity including *P. aeruginosa*. These agents are effective for pyelonephritis and prostatitis. Avoid use in pregnant women and children.
Nitrofurantoin	This agent is effective as both a therapeutic and prophylactic agent in patients with recurrent UTIs. Main advantage is the lack of resistance even after long courses of therapy. Adverse effects may limit use (GI intolerance, neuropathies, pulmonary reactions).
Azithromycin	Single-dose therapy for chlamydial infections.
Methanamine hippurate/mandalate	These agents are reserved for prophylactic therapy or suppressive use between episodes of infection.
Fosfomycin	Single-dose therapy for uncomplicated infections.
Parenteral Therapy	
Aminoglycosides Gentamicin Tobramycin Amikacin Netilmicin	Gentamicin and tobramycin are equally effective; gentamicin is less expensive. Tobramycin has better pseudomonal activity, which may be important in serious systemic infections. Amikacin is generally reserved for multiresistant bacteria.
Penicillins Ampicillin Ampicillin/sulbactam Ticarcillin/clavulanate Piperacillin Piperacillin/tazobactam	These agents are generally equally effective for susceptible bacteria. The extended-spectrum penicillins are more active against *P. aeruginosa* and enterococci and often are preferred over cephalosporins. They are very useful in renally impaired patients or when an aminoglycoside is to be avoided.
Cephalosporins—first, second, and third generation	Second- and third-generation cephalosporins have a broad spectrum of activity against gram-negative bacteria, but are not active against enterococci and have limited activity against *P. aeruginosa*. Ceftazidime and cefepime are active against *P. aeruginosa*. They are useful for nosocomial infections and urosepsis caused by susceptible pathogens.
Imipenem/cilastin Meropenem	These agent have broad spectrum of activity including gram-positive, gram-negative, and anaerobic bacteria. They are active against *P. aeruginosa* and enterococci, but may be associated with candidal superinfections.
Aztreonam	A monobactam that is only active against gram-negative bacteria, including some strains of *P. aeruginosa*. Generally useful for nosocomial infections when aminoglycosides are to be avoided and in penicillin-sensitive patients.
Quinolones Ciprofloxacin Levofloxacin Gatifloxacin	These agents have broad spectrum activity against both gram-negative and gram-positive bacteria. They provide urine and high tissue concentrations and are actively secreted in reduced renal function.

TABLE 114–3. Overview of Outpatient Antimicrobial Therapy for Lower Tract Infections in Adults

Indications	Antibiotic	Dose*	Interval	Duration
Lower tract Infections		2 DS tablets	Single dose	1 day
Uncomplicated	Trimethoprim-sulfamethoxazole	1 DS tablet	bid	3 days
	Ciprofloxacin	250 mg	bid	3 days
	Norfloxacin	400 mg	bid	3 days
	Gatifloxacin	200–400 mg	qd	3 days
	Levofloxacin	250 mg	qd	3 days
	Moxifloxacin (po only)	400 mg	qd	3 days
	Lomefloxacin	400 mg	qd	3 days
	Enoxacin	200 mg	bid	3 days
	Amoxicillin	6 × 500 mg	Single dose	1 day
		500 mg	bid	3 days
	Amoxicillin/clavulanate	500 mg	tid	3 days
	Trimethoprim	100 mg	bid	3 days
	Nitrofurantoin	100 mg	qid	3 days
	Fosfomycin	3 g	Single dose	1 day
Complicated	Trimethoprim-sulfamethoxazole	1 DS tablet	bid	7–10 days
	Trimethoprim	100 mg	bid	7–10 days
	Norfloxacin	400 mg	bid	7–10 days
	Ciprofloxacin	250–500 mg	bid	7–10 days
	Gatifloxacin	400 mg	qd	7–10 days
	Moxifloxacin (po only)	400 mg	qd	7–10 days
	Lomefloxacin	400 mg	qd	7–10 days
	Levofloxacin	250 mg	qd	7–10 days
	Amoxicillin/clavulanate	500 mg	tid	7–10 days
Recurrent Infections	Nitrofurantion	50 mg	qd	6 months
	Trimethoprim	100 mg	qd	6 months
	Trimethoprim-sulfamethoxazole	1/2 SS tablet	qd	6 months
Acute Urethral Syndrome	Trimethoprim-sulfamethoxazole	1 DS	bid	3 days
Failure of TMP/SMX	Azithromycin	1 g	Single dose	
	Doxycycline	100 mg	bid	7 days
Acute Pyelonephritis	Trimethoprim-sulfamethoxazole	1 DS tablet	bid	14 days
	Ciprofloxacin	500 mg	bid	14 days
	Gatifloxacin	400 mg	qd	14 days
	Norfloxacin	400 mg	bid	14 days
	Levofloxacin	250 mg	qd	14 days
	Moxifloxacin (po only)	400 mg	qd	14 days
	Lomefloxacin	400 mg	qd	14 days
	Enoxacin	400 mg	bid	14 days
	Amoxicillin/clavulanate	500 mg	tid	14 days

*Dosing intervals for normal renal function.
DS = double strength; SS = single strength.

TABLE 114–4. Empiric Treatment of Urinary Tract Infections and Prostatitis

Diagnosis	Pathogens	Treatment	Comments
Acute uncomplicated cystitis	*E. coli* *S. saprophyticus*	1. TMP/SMX × 3 days 2. Quinolone × 3 days	Short-course therapy more effective than single dose
Pregnancy	As above	1. Amox/clav × 7 days 2. Cephalosporin × 7 days 3. TMP/SMX × 7 days	Avoid TMP/SMX during third trimester
Acute pyelonephritis			
Uncomplicated	*E. coli*	1. TMP/SMX × 14 days 2. Quinolone × 14 days	Can be managed as outpatient
Complicated	*E. coli, P. mirabilis, K. pneumoniae, P. aeruginosa, E. faecalis*	1. Quinolone × 14 days 2. Extended spectrum penicillin plus aminoglycoside	Severity of illness will determine duration of IV therapy. Culture results should direct therapy. Oral therapy may complete 14 days of therapy
Prostatitis	*E. coli, K. pneumoniae, Proteus* spp., *P. aeruginosa*	1. TMP/SMX × 4–6 weeks 2. Quinolone × 4–6 weeks	Acute prostatitis may require IV therapy initially Chronic prostatitis may require longer treatment periods or surgery

The therapeutic management of UTIs is best accomplished by first categorizing the type of infection: acute uncomplicated cystitis, symptomatic bacteriuria, asymptomatic bacteriuria, complicated UTIs, recurrent infections, or prostatitis.

In choosing the appropriate antibiotic therapy, it is important to be aware of the increasing resistance of *E. coli* and other pathogens to many antimicrobials. Resistance to *E. coli* is as high as 30% for amoxicillin and cephalosporins.[33,34] Overall trimethoprim-sulfamethoxazole remains susceptible, although resistance as high as 15% has been reported in various places.[34,35] Prior antibiotic exposure is the most significant risk factor associated with the resistance.[35,36] Antibiotic therapy should be determined based on the geographic resistance patterns of the prescriber, as well as the patient's recent history of antibiotic exposure.

ACUTE UNCOMPLICATED CYSTITIS

Acute uncomplicated cystitis is the most common form of UTI. These infections typically occur in women of childbearing age and are often related to sexual activity. Although the presence of dysuria, frequency, urgency, and suprapubic discomfort are frequently associated with lower tract infection, a significant number of patients have upper tract involvement as well.[37] Because these infections are predominantly caused by *E. coli,* antimicrobial therapy should initially be directed against this organism. Other common causes include *S. saprophyticus* and, occasionally, *K. pneumoniae* and *Proteus mirabilis.* Because the causative organisms and their susceptibility are generally known, many clinicians advocate a cost-effective approach to management. This approach includes a urinalysis and initiation of empiric therapy without a urine culture[37] (Fig. 114–1).

The goal of treatment for uncomplicated cystitis is to eradicate the causative organism and to reduce the incidence of recurrence caused by relapse or reinfection. The ability to reduce the chance of recurrence is dependent on the agent's efficacy in eradicating the uropathogenic bacteria from the vaginal and gastrointestinal reservoir. In the past, conventional therapy consisted of an effective oral antibiotic administered for 7 to 14 days. It is now apparent, however, that acute cystitis is a superficial mucosal infection that can be eradicated with much shorter courses of therapy. Advantages of

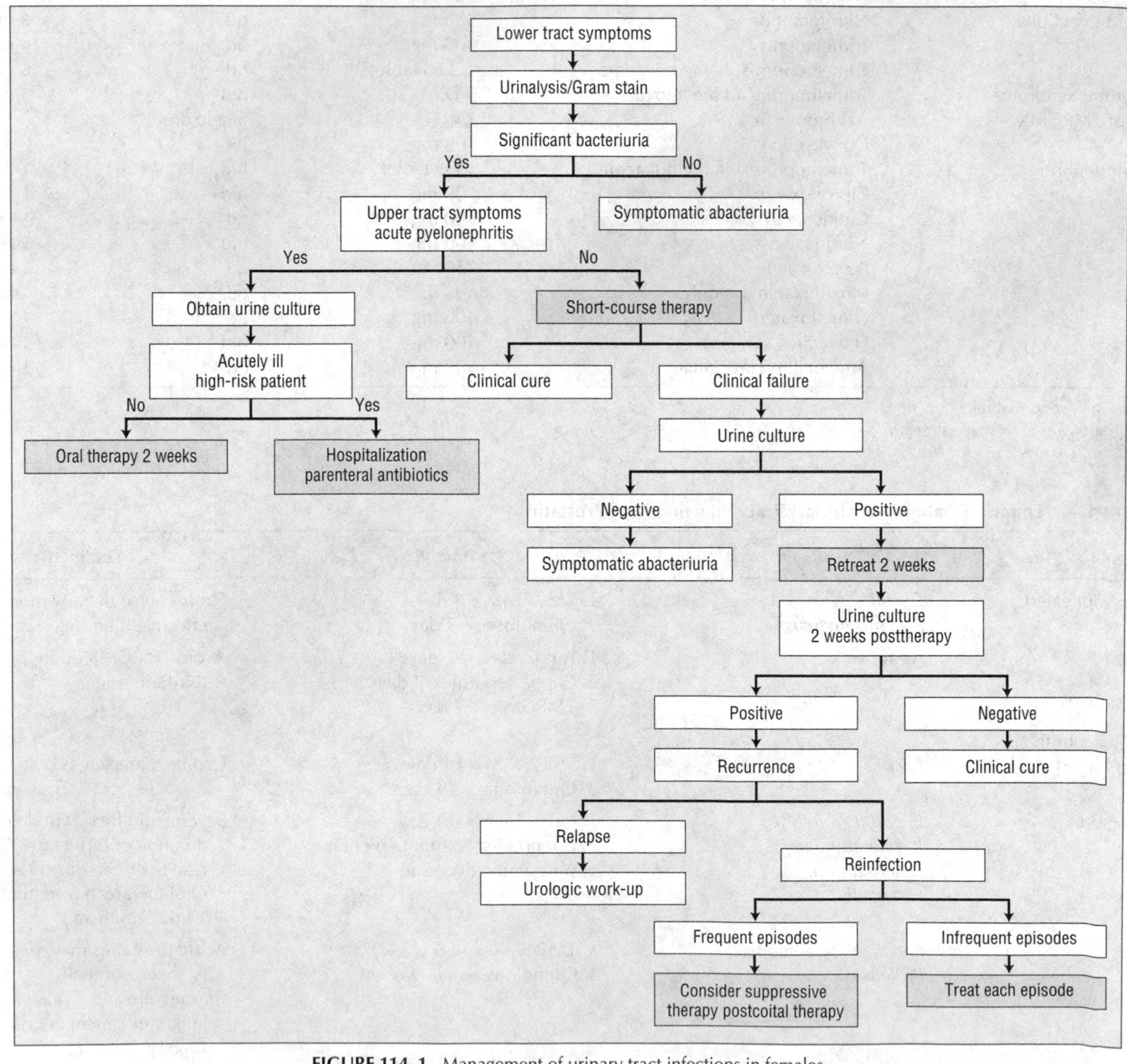

FIGURE 114–1. Management of urinary tract infections in females.

short-course therapy include increased compliance, fewer side effects, decreased cost, and less potential for the development of resistance. Single-dose therapy is frequently used although it can be associated with lower cure rates and increased reoccurrence compared to longer therapies.[1,31,39] Clinicians should not assume that all antimicrobial agents are effective as single-dose therapies. Data suggest that trimethoprim-sulfamethoxazole or the fluoroquinolones are most efficacious as single-dose therapies. Fosfomycin once daily has also been used, although other therapies appear superior.[1,40] The efficacy of these agents is probably related to observations that *E. coli* causing community-acquired UTIs are increasingly resistant to ampicillin, amoxicillin, and sulfonamides. In addition, oral β-lactam antibiotics are eliminated more rapidly and do not achieve high renal tissue concentrations as compared to trimethoprim-sulfamethoxazole and are less successful in eradicating uropathogens from the vaginal and gastrointestinal reservoirs.

Three-day courses of trimethoprim-sulfamethoxazole or a fluoroquinolone are superior to single-dose therapies.[38] The use of amoxicillin, sulfonamides, and nitrofurantoin is not recommended because of the high incidence of resistant *E. coli*. For most adult females, short-course therapy is the treatment of choice for uncomplicated lower UTIs. Short-course therapy is inappropriate for those patients who have had previous infections caused by resistant bacteria, for male patients, and for patients with complicated UTIs. If symptoms do not respond or recur, a urine culture should be obtained and conventional therapy with a suitable agent instituted.[1,41–43]

SYMPTOMATIC ABACTERIURIA

Symptomatic abacteriuria or acute urethral syndrome represents a clinical syndrome in which females present with dysuria and pyuria, but the urine culture reveals less than 10^5 bacteria/mL of urine. Acute urethral syndrome is estimated to account for more than half of the complaints of dysuria seen in the community today. These women are most likely to be infected with small numbers of coliform bacteria including *E. coli, Staphylococcus* spp., or *Chlamydia trachomatis*. Additional causes include *Neisseria gonorrhoeae, Gardnerella vaginalis,* and *Ureaplasma urealyticum.*

Most patients presenting with pyuria will, in fact, have infection that requires treatment. Single-dose or short-course therapy with trimethoprim-sulfamethoxazole has been used effectively, and prolonged courses of therapy are not necessary for the majority of patients. If single-dose or short-course therapy is ineffective, a culture should be obtained. If the patient reports recent sexual activity, therapy for *C. trachomatis* should be considered. Chlamydial treatment should consist of a 1-g dose of azithromycin or doxycycline 100 mg bid for 7 days. Often, concomitant treatment of all sexual partners is required to cure chlamydial infections and prevent reacquisition (see Chap. 115).

ASYMPTOMATIC BACTERIURIA

Asymptomatic bacteriuria represents those patients who, in the absence of urinary symptoms, are found to have two consecutive urine cultures with $>10^5$ of the same organism. The majority of patients with asymptomatic bacteriuria are elderly and female. Pregnant women are another group of patients that frequently present with asymptomatic bacteriuria. Although this group of patients typically responds to treatment, relapse and reinfection are very common and chronic asymptomatic bacteriuria is difficult to eradicate.

The management of asymptomatic bacteriuria is dependent on the age of the patient and whether or not they are pregnant. In children, because of a greater risk of developing renal scarring and long-standing renal damage, treatment should consist of conventional courses of therapy as that for symptomatic infection. The greatest risk of renal damage occurs during the first 5 years of life.[44] In the nonpregnant female, therapy is controversial; however, treatment has little effect on the natural course of infections.

Two groups characterize asymptomatic bacteriuria in the elderly: those with persistent bacteriuria and those with intermittent bacteriuria. Most clinicians feel that asymptomatic bacteriuria in the elderly is a benign disease and does not warrant treatment. Most data indicate that the patient without urinary tract obstruction is not destined to develop progressive renal damage. Investigators who have demonstrated an association between bacteriuria and decreased survival, however, have questioned this approach. In this setting, there is no apparent urgency in initiating therapy, so two cultures should be obtained to confirm the presence of bacteriuria. Treating ambulatory, nonhospitalized elderly women is effective in eliminating bacteria for at least 6 months and may protect against the development of symptomatic bacteriuria; however, only 50% of patients remained free of bacteria after 1 year.[45]

Several studies in hospitalized elderly subjects, however, have not found antimicrobial therapy to be efficacious.[46,47] A number of questions remain unanswered; for example, the effect of eradication of bacteriuria on life expectancy, the cost-effectiveness and risk:benefit ratio of therapy, and the effect on morbidity. Certainly, with the information available and the high adverse reaction rate in the elderly, vigorous treatment and screening programs cannot be advocated.

COMPLICATED URINARY TRACT INFECTIONS

Acute Pyelonephritis

The presentation of high-grade fever (>38.3°C/100.9°F) and severe flank pain should be treated as acute pyelonephritis, warranting aggressive management. Severely ill patients with pyelonephritis should be hospitalized and intravenous antimicrobials administered initially. However, milder cases may be managed with orally administered antibiotics in an outpatient setting. Symptoms of nausea, vomiting, and dehydration may require hospitalization.

At the time of presentation, a Gram stain of the urine should be performed along with a urinalysis, culture, and sensitivity tests. The Gram stain should indicate the morphology of the infecting organism(s) and help direct the selection of an appropriate antibiotic. However, the precise identity and susceptibility of the infecting organism(s) will be unknown initially, warranting empiric therapy.

The goals of treatment include the achievement of therapeutic concentrations of an antimicrobial agent in the bloodstream and urinary tract to which the invading organism is susceptible and sufficient therapy to eradicate residual infection in the tissues of the urinary tract.

In the mild-to-moderate symptomatic patient in which oral therapy is considered, an effective agent should be administered for at least a 2-week period, although use of highly active agents for 7 to 10 days may be sufficient.[1,48] Oral antibiotics that are highly active against the probable pathogens and are sufficiently bioavailable are preferred. Although the sulfonamides and ampicillin or amoxicillin have been the primary choices for the treatment of gram-negative bacillary infections, they are no longer considered reliable agents for UTIs.[31] Reports of increasing resistance to *E. coli* have tempered their use. In addition, treatment with trimethoprim-sulfamethoxazole (one double-strength tablet twice daily) for 2 weeks was superior to ampicillin, despite the organism being susceptible to both agents.[49] Agents such as trimethoprim-sulfamethoxazole and the fluoroquinolones are the agents of choice. If a Gram stain reveals gram-positive cocci, *E. faecalis* should be considered and treatment directed against this potential pathogen (ampicillin). Close follow-up of outpatient treatment is mandatory to assure success.

In the seriously ill patient, parenteral therapy should be administered initially. Therapy should provide a broad spectrum of coverage and should be directed toward bacteremia or sepsis, if present. A number of antibiotic regimens have been used as empiric therapy, including an intravenous fluoroquinolone, an aminoglycoside with or without ampicillin, extended spectrum cephalosporins with or without an aminoglycoside.[1] Other options include aztreonam, the β-lactamase inhibitor combinations (ampicillin/sulbactam, ticarcillin/clavulanate, and piperacillin/tazobactam), imipenem or IV trimethoprim-sulfamethoxazole. If the patient has been hospitalized within the past 6 months, has a urinary catheter, or is a nursing home resident, the possibility of *P. aeruginosa* and enterococci, as well as multiply resistant organisms, should be considered. In this setting, ceftazidime, ticarcillin/clavulanate, piperacillin, aztreonam, or imipenem in combination with an aminoglycoside is recommended. The rationale for combination therapy is that in experimental animals, 3 days of aminoglycoside combination therapy followed by nonaminoglycoside single-agent therapy for 7 days resulted in a 100% cure rate.[50] If the patient responds to initial combination therapy, the aminoglycoside may be discontinued after 3 days. Although the aminoglycoside therapy is stopped, renal tissue concentrations of the aminoglycoside will persist for days. Based on sensitivity data, the patient can then be maintained or switched to a less-expensive single agent and, ultimately, an appropriate oral agent may be used.

Effective therapy should stabilize the patient within 12 to 24 hours. A significant reduction in urine bacterial concentrations should occur in 48 hours. If bacteriologic response has not occurred, an alternative agent should be considered based on susceptibility testing. If the patient fails to respond clinically within 3 to 4 days or has persistently positive blood or urine cultures, further investigation is needed to exclude bacterial resistance, possible obstruction, papillary necrosis, intrarenal or perinephric abscess, or some other disease process. Usually by the third day of therapy, the patient is afebrile and significantly less symptomatic. In general, after the patient has been afebrile for 24 hours, parenteral therapy may be discontinued, and oral therapy instituted to complete a 2-week course. Follow-up urine cultures should be obtained 2 weeks after completion of therapy to ensure a satisfactory response and detect possible relapse.

Urinary Tract Infections in Males

The management of UTIs in males is distinctly different and often more difficult than in females. Infections in male patients are considered to be complicated because endogenous bacteria in the presence of functional or structural abnormalities that disrupt the normal defense mechanisms of the urinary tract cause them. The incidence of infections in males younger than 60 years of age is much less than the incidence in females. During the adult years, the occurrence of infection can be directly related to some manipulation of the urinary tract. The most common causes are instrumentation of the urinary tract, catheterization, and renal and urinary stones. Uncomplicated infections are rare, but they may occur in young males as a result of homosexual activity, lack of circumcision, and having sex with partners who are colonized with uropathogenic bacteria. As the patient ages, the most common cause of infection is related to bladder outlet obstruction because of prostatic hypertrophy. In addition, the prostate gland may become infected and provide a nidus for recurrent infection in males.

The conventional view is that therapy in males requires prolonged treatment (Fig. 114–2). A urine culture should be obtained before treatment because the cause of infection in men is not as predictable as in women. Single-dose or short-course therapy is not recommended in this setting. Considerably fewer data are available comparing various antimicrobial agents in males as compared to females. If gram-negative bacteria are presumed, trimethoprim-sulfamethoxazole or the quinolone antimicrobials should be considered because these agents achieve high renal tissue, urine, and prostatic concentrations.[14]

Initial therapy should be for 10 to 14 days. Factors associated with treatment success are isolation of a single organism, the absence of significant obstruction or anatomic abnormalities, a normal functioning urinary tract, and the absence of prostatic involvement. Parenteral therapy may be required in certain situations, such as in severely ill patients, the presence of acute prostatitis, or epididymitis, and in patients who cannot tolerate oral medications. A comparison of 2-week versus 6-week therapy in males with recurrent infections who were given trimethoprim-sulfamethoxazole had cure rates of 29% and 62%, respectively.[51] Other investigators advocate longer treatment periods in males as well.[52] Follow-up cultures at 4 to 6 weeks after treatment are important in males to ensure bacteriologic cure. Many patients require longer periods of treatment and possible alterations in antibiotics, depending on culture and sensitivity results and clinical response.

Recurrent Infections

Recurrent episodes of UTI account for a significant portion of all UTIs. Of those patients suffering from recurrent infections, 80% can be considered reinfections; that is, the recurrence of infection by an organism different than the organism isolated from the preceding infection. These patients are most commonly female and recurrence develops in about 20% of them with cystitis. Reinfections can be divided into two groups: those with less than two or three episodes per year and those who develop more frequent infections.

Management strategies depend on predisposing factors, number of episodes per year, and patient's preference. Factors that have commonly been associated with recurrent infections include sexual intercourse and diaphragm or spermicide use for birth control. Therapeutic options include self-administered therapy, postcoital therapy, and continuous low-dose prophylaxis. In those patients with infrequent infections (less than three infections per year), each episode should be treated as a separately occurring infection. Short-course therapy is appropriate in this setting. Many women have been successfully treated with self-administered short-course therapy at the onset of symptoms.[53]

In those patients with more frequent symptomatic infections and no apparent precipitating event, long-term prophylactic antimicrobial therapy may be instituted. Prophylactic therapy has been found to reduce the frequency of symptomatic infections in elderly men, women, and children. In women, most studies show a reinfection rate of two to three per patient year reduced to 0.1 to 0.2 per patient year with treatment.[54] Before prophylaxis is initiated, patients should be treated conventionally with an appropriate agent. Trimethoprim-sulfamethoxazole (one-half of a single-strength tablet), trimethoprim (100 mg daily), a fluoroquinolone (one tablet), or nitrofurantoin (50 or 100 mg daily) all reduce the rate of reinfection as single-agent

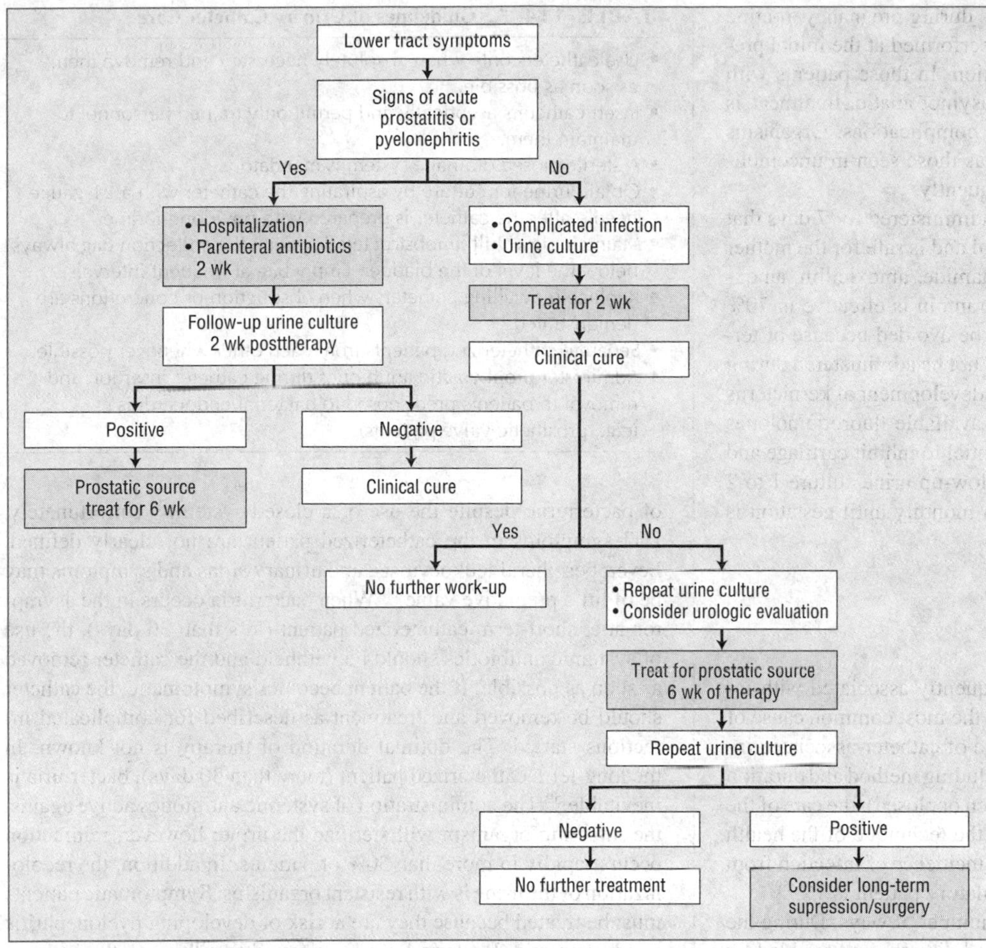

FIGURE 114–2. Management of urinary tract infections in males.

therapy.[12] Full-dose therapy with these agents is unnecessary, and single daily doses can be used. Therapy is generally prescribed for a period of 6 months, during which time urine cultures are followed monthly. If symptomatic episodes develop, the patient should receive a full course of therapy with an effective agent and should be restarted on prophylactic therapy.

In those women who experience symptomatic reinfections in association with sexual activity, voiding after intercourse may help prevent infection. Also, single-dose prophylactic therapy with trimethoprim-sulfamethoxazole taken after intercourse has been found to reduce the incidence of recurrent infection significantly.[55]

In postmenopausal women with recurrent infections, the lack of estrogen results in changes of the bacterial flora of the vagina, resulting in increased colonization with uropathogenic *E. coli*. Topically administered estrogen cream is reported to reduce the incidence of infections in this population.[42]

The remaining 20% of recurrent UTIs are relapses. That is, persistence of infection with the same organism after therapy for an isolated UTI. The recurrence of symptomatic or asymptomatic bacteriuria after therapy usually indicates that the patient has renal involvement, a structural abnormality of the urinary tract, or chronic bacterial prostatitis. In the absence of structural abnormalities, relapse is often related to renal infection and requires a long duration of treatment. Women who relapse after short course therapy should receive a 2-week course of therapy. In patients who relapse after 2 weeks of therapy, therapy should be continued for another 2 to 4 weeks. If relapse occurs after 6 weeks of therapy, urologic evaluation should be performed and any obstructive lesion should be corrected. If this is not possible, therapy for 6 months or longer may be considered. Asymptomatic adults who have no evidence of urinary obstruction should not receive long-term therapy.

In males, relapse usually indicates bacterial prostatitis, the most common cause of persistent bacteriuria. Many agents have been used for long-term therapy of relapses; however, trimethoprim-sulfameth oxazole and the fluoroquinolones appear to be highly effective.

SPECIAL CONDITIONS

Urinary Tract Infections in Pregnancy

During pregnancy, significant physiologic changes occur to the entire urinary tract that dramatically alter the prevalence of UTIs and pyelonephritis. Severe dilation of the renal pelvis and ureters, decreased ureteral peristalsis, and reduced bladder tone occur during pregnancy.[56,57] These changes result in urinary stasis and reduced defenses against reflux of bacteria to the kidneys. In addition, increased urine content of amino acids, vitamins, and nutrients encourage bacterial growth. All these factors increase the incidence of bacteriuria resulting in symptomatic infections, especially during the third trimester.

Asymptomatic bacteriuria occurs in 4% to 7% of pregnant patients. Of these, 20% to 40% will develop acute symptomatic pyelonephritis during pregnancy. If untreated, asymptomatic bacteriuria has the potential to cause significant adverse effects, including prematurity, low birth weight, and stillbirth.[58] As pyelonephritis is associated with significant adverse events during pregnancy, routine screening tests for bacteriuria should be performed at the initial prenatal visit and again at 28 weeks' gestation. In those patients with significant bacteriuria, symptomatic or asymptomatic, treatment is recommended in order to avoid possible complications. Organisms associated with bacteriuria are the same as those seen in uncomplicated UTIs with *E. coli* isolated most frequently.

Therapy should consist of an agent administered for 7 days that has a relatively low adverse effect potential and is safe for the mother and baby. The administration of a sulfonamide, amoxicillin, amoxicillin/clavulanate, cephalexin, or nitrofurantoin is effective in 70% to 80% of patients. Tetracyclines should be avoided because of teratogenic effects, and sulfonamides should not be administered during the third trimester because of the possible development of kernicterus and hyperbilirubinemia. In addition, the available fluoroquinolones should not be given because of their potential to inhibit cartilage and bone development in the newborn. A follow-up urine culture 1 to 2 weeks after completing therapy and then monthly until gestation is complete is recommended.

Catheterized Patients

The use of an indwelling catheter is frequently associated with infection of the urinary tract and represents the most common cause of hospital-acquired infection. The incidence of catheter-associated infection is related to a variety of factors, including method and duration of catheterization, the catheter system (open or closed), the care of the system, susceptibility of the patient, and the technique of the health care personnel inserting the catheter. The incidence of infection from a single catheterization in a healthy ambulatory patient is 1%.[59]

Bacteria may enter the bladder in a number of ways. During the catheterization, bacteria may be introduced directly into the bladder from the urethra. Once the catheter is in place, bacteria may pass up the lumen of the catheter via the movement of air bubbles, by motility of the bacteria, or by capillary action. In addition, bacteria may reach the bladder from around the exudative sheath that surrounds the catheter in the urethra. Cleaning the periurethral area thoroughly and applying an antiseptic (povidone-iodine) can minimize infection occurring during the insertion of the catheter. The use of closed drainage systems has significantly reduced the ability of bacteria to pass up the lumen of the catheter and cause infection. A bacterium passing around the catheter sheath in the urethra is probably the most important pathway for infection. Avoiding manipulation of the catheter and trauma to the urethra and urethral meatus can minimize this path of acquisition.

Patients with indwelling catheters acquire UTIs at a rate of 5% per day.[59] The closed systems are capable of preventing bacteriuria in most patients for up to 10 days with appropriate care. After 30 days of catheterization, however, there is a 78% to 95% incidence of bacteriuria, despite the use of a closed system.[59] Unfortunately, UTI symptoms in the catheterized patient are not clearly defined. Fever, peripheral leukocytosis, and urinary signs and symptoms may be of little predictive value.[60] When bacteriuria occurs in the asymptomatic, short-term catheterized patient (less than 30 days), the use of systemic antibiotics should be withheld and the catheter removed as soon as possible. If the patient becomes symptomatic, the catheter should be removed and treatment as described for complicated infections started. The optimal duration of therapy is not known. In the long-term catheterized patient (more than 30 days), bacteriuria is inevitable.[59] The administration of systemic antibiotics active against the infecting organism will sterilize the urine; however, reinfection occurs rapidly in more than 50% of patients. In addition, the recolonization of the urine is with resistant organisms. Symptomatic patients must be treated because they are at risk of developing pyelonephritis and bacteremia. Bacteria have been found to adhere to the catheter and to produce a biofilm consisting of bacterial glycocalyces, Tamm-Horsfall protein, and apatite and struvite salts, which act to protect the bacteria from antibiotics.[61] Recatheterization with a new, sterile unit should be performed in those symptomatic patients, if the existing catheter has been in place for more than 2 weeks.

TABLE 114–5. Guidelines of Urinary Catheter Care

- Use catheters only when absolutely necessary and remove them as soon as possible.
- Insert catheters aseptically and permit only trained personnel to maintain them.
- A sterile closed drainage system is mandatory.
- Obtain urine for culture by aspirating the catheter with a 21-gauge needle after the catheter is prepared with povidone-iodine.
- Maintain downhill, unobstructed flow with the collection bag always below the level of the bladder. Empty bag at frequent intervals.
- Replace indwelling catheters when obstruction or concretions are demonstrated.
- Separate catheterized patients from each other whenever possible.
- Administer prophylactic antibiotics during catheter insertion and removal to patients predisposed to bacterial endocarditis (e.g., prosthetic valve patients).

Various methods have been proposed to prevent the development of bacteriuria and infection in the patient with an indwelling catheter (Table 114–5). The success of these methods depends on the type of catheter and the length of time it is in place. The use of constant bladder irrigation with antiseptic or antibacterial solutions has been investigated and found to reduce the incidence of infection in those with open drainage systems, but they have no advantage in those with closed systems. The use of prophylactic systemic antibiotics in patients with short-term catheterization reduces the incidence of infection over the first 4 to 7 days.[62] In long-term catheterized patients, however, antibiotics only postpone the development of bacteriuria and lead to the emergence of resistant organisms.

PROSTATITIS

Bacterial prostatitis is an inflammation of the prostate gland and surrounding tissue as a result of infection. It is classified as either acute or chronic. By definition, pathogenic bacteria and significant inflammatory cells must be present in prostatic secretions and urine to make the diagnosis of bacterial prostatitis. Prostatitis rarely occurs in young males, but it is commonly associated with recurrent infections in persons older than 30 years. As many as 50% of all males develop some form of prostatitis at some period in their life.[63] The acute form is typically an acute infectious disease characterized by a sudden onset of fever, tenderness, and urinary and constitutional symptoms. Chronic prostatitis presents with few symptoms related to the prostate, but rather symptoms of urinating difficulty, low back pain, perineal pressure, or a combination of these. It represents a recurring infection, with the same organism that results from incomplete eradication of bacteria from the prostate gland.

PATHOGENESIS AND ETIOLOGY

The exact mechanism of bacterial infection of the prostate is not well understood. The possible routes of infection are the same as those for UTIs. Reflux of infected urine into the prostate gland is thought to play an important role in causing infection. Studies suggest that intraprostatic reflux of urine occurs commonly and results in direct inoculation of infected urine into the prostate.[64] In addition, intraprostatic reflux of sterile urine can result in a chemical prostatitis and may be the cause of nonbacterial prostatitis. Sexual intercourse may contribute to infection of the prostate gland, because prostatic secretions from men with chronic prostatitis and vaginal cultures from their sexual partners grew identical organisms.[65] Other known causes of bacterial prostatitis include indwelling urethral and condom catheterization, urethral instrumentation, and transurethral prostatectomy in patients with infected urine.

A number of physiologic factors are believed to contribute to the development of prostatitis. Functional abnormalities found in bacterial prostatitis include altered prostate secretory functions. Prostatic fluid obtained from normal males contains prostatic antibacterial factor (PAF). This heat-stable, low-molecular-weight cation is a zinc-complexed polypeptide that is bactericidal to most urinary tract pathogens.[66] The antibacterial activity of PAF is directly related to the zinc content of prostatic fluid. Prostate fluid zinc levels and PAF activity also appear diminished in patients with prostatitis, as well as in the elderly.[64] Whether these changes are a cause or effect of prostatitis remains to be determined.

The pH of prostatic secretions in patients with prostatitis has also been reported to be altered.[67] Normal prostatic secretions have a pH in the range of 6.6 to 7.6. With increasing age, the pH tends to become more alkaline. In patients with inflammation of the prostate, prostatic secretions may have an alkaline pH in the range of 7 to 9. These changes suggest a generalized secretory dysfunction of the prostate, which can not only affect the pathogenesis of prostatitis, but can also influence the mode of therapy.

Gram-negative, enteric organisms are the most frequent pathogens in acute bacterial prostatitis.[64] *E. coli* is the predominant organism, occurring in 75% of cases. Other gram-negative organisms frequently isolated include *K. pneumoniae, P. mirabilis,* and, less frequently, *P. aeruginosa, Enterobacter* spp., and *Serratia* spp. Occasionally, cases of gonococcal and staphylococcal prostatitis occur, but they are infrequent.

E. coli most commonly causes chronic bacterial prostatitis with other gram-negative organisms isolated less frequently. The importance of gram-positive organisms in chronic bacterial prostatitis remains controversial. *S. epidermidis, S. aureus,* and diphtheroids have been isolated in some studies.

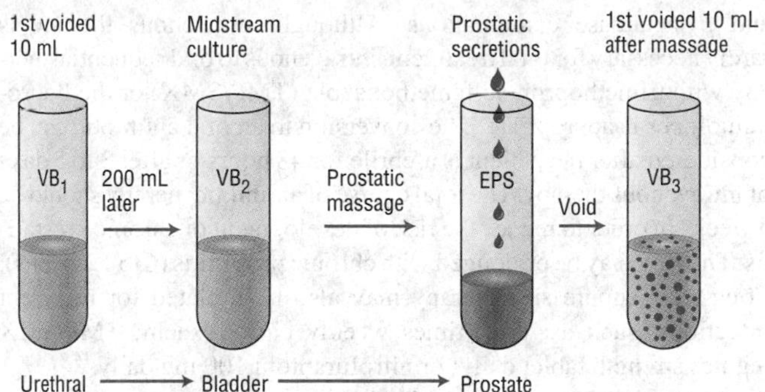

FIGURE 114–3. Segmented cultures of the lower urinary tract in men.

CLINICAL PRESENTATION

Acute bacterial prostatitis presents as other acute infections. Common symptoms include high fever, chills, malaise, myalgia, localized pain (perineal, rectal, sacrococcygeal), and other urinary symptoms (frequency, urgency, dysuria, nocturia, retention). Digital palpation of the prostate via the rectum may reveal a swollen, tender, warm, tense, or indurated gland. Massage of the prostate will express a purulent discharge, which will readily grow the pathogenic organism. Prostatic massage is contraindicated in ABP, however, because of the risk of inducing bacteremia and associated local pain. The diagnosis of ABP can be made from the patient's clinical presentation and the presence of significant bacteriuria. As with other UTIs, the infecting organism can be isolated from a midstream specimen.

In contrast, CBP is more difficult to diagnose and treat. Chronic bacterial prostatitis is typically characterized by recurrent UTIs with the same pathogen and is the most common cause of recurrent UTI in males. Although examination of the prostate gland often reveals a normal gland, most will have prostatic enlargement. The patient's clinical presentation can vary widely. Presenting symptoms include the vague description of voiding difficulties, such as frequency, urgency, and dysuria. In addition, symptoms of low back pain and perineal and suprapubic discomfort are present. Many adults, however, are asymptomatic.

Because physical examination of the prostate is often normal, urinary tract localization studies are critical to the diagnosis of CBP. The method of quantitative localization culture, as described by Meares and Stamey, remains the diagnostic standard[68] (Fig. 114–3). The method compares the bacterial growth in sequential urine and prostatic fluid cultures obtained during micturition. The first 10 mL of voided urine is collected (voiding bladder 1 or VB1) and constitutes urethral urine. After approximately 200 mL of urine has been voided, a 10-mL midstream sample is collected (VB2). This specimen represents bladder urine. After the patient voids, the prostate is massaged and expressed prostatic secretions (EPS) are collected. After prostatic massage, the patient voids again and 10 mL of urine is collected (VB3).

The diagnosis of bacterial prostatitis is made when the number of bacteria in EPS is 10 times that of the urethral sample (VB1) and midstream sample (VB2). If no EPS is available, the urine sample following massage (VB3) should contain a bacterial count 10-fold greater than that of VB1 or VB2. If significant bacteriuria is present, ampicillin, cephalexin, or nitrofurantoin should be given for 2 to 3 days to sterilize the urine prior to performing the localization study.

▶ TREATMENT: Prostatitis

The goals in the management of bacterial prostatitis are, in general, the same as those for UTIs. Acute bacterial prostatitis responds well to appropriate antimicrobial therapy that is directed at the most commonly isolated organisms. Prostatic penetration of antimicrobials occurs because the acute inflammatory reaction alters the cellular membrane barrier between the bloodstream and the prostate. The majority of patients can be managed with oral antimicrobial agents, such as trimethoprim-sulfamethoxazole and the fluoroquinolones (ciprofloxacin, levofloxacin, gatifloxacin, moxifloxacin). Other effective agents in this setting include cephalosporins and β-lactam and β-lactamase combinations. Although intravenous therapy is rarely necessary for total treatment, intravenous to oral sequential therapy with trimethoprim-sulfamethoxazole (TMP/SMX) or the fluoroquinolones is appropriate. The conversion to an oral antibiotic can be considered after the patient is afebrile for 48 hours or after 3 to 5 days of intravenous therapy. The total course of antibiotic therapy should be 4 weeks in order to reduce the risk of development of chronic prostatitis. Therapy may be prolonged with chronic prostatitis (6 to 12 weeks). Long-term suppressive therapy may also be initiated for recurrent infections, such as: three-times weekly ciprofloxacin; TMP/SMX regular strength tablet daily; or nitrofurantoin 100 mg daily.[14]

Chronic bacterial prostatitis often presents a more vexing situation because cures are rarely obtained. In the past, it was recognized that despite high serum concentrations of antibacterial drugs in excess of the minimal inhibitory concentrations of the infecting organisms, bacteria persisted in prostatic fluid. Most likely, the failure to eradicate sensitive bacteria was owing to the inability of antibiotics to reach sufficient concentrations in the prostatic fluid and cross the prostatic epithelium.

Several factors that determine antibiotic diffusion into prostatic secretions were delineated from the canine model. Lipid solubility is a major determinant in the ability of drugs to diffuse from plasma across epithelial membranes. The degree of ionization in plasma also affects the diffusion of drugs. Only un-ionized molecules can cross the lipid barrier of prostatic cells and the drug's pK_a directly determines the fraction of unchanged drug.

The pH gradient across the membrane has an influence on tissue penetration as well. A pH gradient of at least one pH unit between separate compartments allows for ion trapping. As the un-ionized drug crosses the epithelial barrier into prostatic fluid, it becomes ionized, allowing less drug to diffuse back across the lipid barrier. In early studies with the canine model, the prostatic pH was reported to be acidic (6.4).[64] More recent studies in man, however, have reported that the pH of prostatic secretions from an inflamed prostate is actually basic (8.1 to 8.3).[64]

The choice of antibiotics in CBP should include those agents that are capable of reaching therapeutic concentrations in the prostatic fluid and that possess the spectrum of activity to be effective. Agents that achieve therapeutic prostatic concentrations include trimethoprim and the fluoroquinolones. Sulfamethoxazole penetrates poorly and probably contributes very little to trimethoprim. The fluoroquinolones appear to provide the best therapeutic options in the management of CBP. Trimethoprim-sulfamethoxazole is also effective. Therapy should be continued for 4 to 6 weeks initially. Longer treatment periods may be necessary in some cases. If therapy fails with these regimens, chronic suppressive therapy may be used or surgery considered.

PHARMACOECONOMIC CONSIDERATIONS

The cost-effective management of UTIs requires knowledge of its pathogenesis and causative organisms associated with the various clinical syndromes described in this chapter. The costs associated with managing a UTI include direct costs, such a laboratory tests, medication, and health care visits. The indirect costs include lost work time and general quality of life issues, such as disease or therapy adverse effects.

Direct costs are those associated with diagnosis, treatment, and follow-up. Reported percentages for these costs in cystitis are physician consultation 23%, laboratory costs 64%, and pharmaceuticals 13%.[69] The cost of pharmaceuticals varies according to the agents used and the duration of therapy. When trimethoprim-sulfamethoxazole and amoxicillin have been compared, trimethoprim-sulfamethoxazole results in a higher cure rate, lower relapse, fewer symptoms, and lower costs.[70] The fluoroquinolones have also been found to be highly effective agents but are generally more expensive. The outcome and total cost are dependent on whether therapy is empiric or definitive (based on a culture diagnosis for acute infection).

▶ PRINCIPLES OF PHARMACOTHERAPY

- Urinary tract infections are classified as uncomplicated and complicated. Uncomplicated refers to an otherwise healthy female who lacks structural or functional abnormalities of the urinary tract. Most often, complicated infections are associated with a predisposing lesion of the urinary tract; however, the term may be used to refer to all other infections, except for those in the otherwise healthy adult female.
- Significant bacteriuria has traditionally been defined as bacterial counts of greater than 100,000 (10^5)/mL of urine. Many clinicians, however, have challenged this as a too general statement. Indeed, significant bacteriuria in patients with symptoms of a urinary tract infection may be defined as greater than 10^2 organisms/mL.
- The most frequent mechanism of infections is via the ascending route with organisms that originate from the fecal flora.
- Eighty-five percent of uncomplicated urinary tract infections are caused by *E. coli* and the remainder primarily by *S. saprophyticus, Proteus* spp., and *Klebsiella* spp. Complicated infections are more frequently associated with gram-negative organisms and *E. faecalis*.
- The key to the diagnosis of urinary tract infections is the ability to demonstrate significant numbers of microorganisms in an appropriate urine specimen. The extent of laboratory examination depends on the clinical situation.
- The goals of treatment of urinary tract infections are to prevent or treat systemic consequences of infections, eradicate the invading organism, and prevent the reoccurrence of infection.
- Uncomplicated urinary tract infections can be most effectively managed with short-course (3 to 5 days) therapy with either trime-thoprim-sulfamethoxazole or a fluoroquinolone. Complicated infections require longer treatment periods (2 weeks) with one of these agents.
- Acute bacterial prostatitis can be managed with many agents that have activity against the causative organism. Chronic prostatitis requires an agent that is not only active against the causative organism, but also concentrates in the prostatic secretions. Therapy with trimethoprim-sulfamethoxazole or a fluoroquinolone are preferred for 4 to 6 weeks.

REFERENCES

1. Warren JW, Abrutyn E, Hebel JR, Johnson JR, Schaeffer AJ, Stamm WE. Guidelines for antimicrobial treatment of uncomplicated acute bacterial cystitis and acute pyelonephritis. Clin Infect Dis 1999;29:745–758.
2. Bacheller CD, Bernstein JM. Urinary tract infections. Med Clin North Am 1997;81:719–729.

3. Plumridge RJ, Golledge CL. Treatment of urinary tract infection: Clinical and economic considerations. Pharmacoeconomics 1996;9:295–306.
4. Johnson CC. Definitions, classification, and clinical presentation of urinary tract infections. Med Clin North Am 1991;75:241–252.
5. Platt R. Quantitative definition of bacteriuria. Am J Med 1983;75:44–52.
6. Stull TL, LiPuma JJ. Epidemiology and natural history of urinary tract infections in children. Med Clin North Am 1991;75:287–298.
7. Smellie JM. Reflections of thirty years of treating children with urinary tract infections. J Urol 1991;146:665–668.
8. Sobel JD, Kaye D. Urinary tract infections. In: Mandell GL, Bennett JE, Dolin R, eds. Principles and Practice of Infectious Diseases, 4th ed. New York, Churchill Livingstone, 1995:662–690.
9. Baldassarre JS, Kaye D. Special problems in urinary tract infections in the elderly. Med Clin North Am 1991,75:375–390.
10. Turck M, Stamm WE. Nosocomial infection of the urinary tract. Am J Med 1981;70:651–654.
11. Boyce JM. Vancomycin-resistant Enterococcus: Detection, epidemiology, and control measures. Infect Dis Clin North Am 1997;11:367–384.
12. Nicolle LE, Harding GKM, Preiksaitis J, et al. The association of urinary tract infection with sexual intercourse. J Infect Dis 1982;146:579–583.
13. Stamey TA, Fair WR, Timothy MM, et al. Antibacterial nature of prostatic fluid. Nature 1968;218:444–447.
14. Lipsky BA. Prostatitis and urinary tract infection in men: What's new; what's true? Am J Med 1999;106:327–334.
15. Shand DG, Nimmon CC, O'Grady F, et al. Relation between residual urine volume and response to treatment of urinary infection. Lancet 1970;1:1305–1306.
16. Parsons CL, Schrom SH, Hanno P, et al. Bladder surface mucin: Examination of possible mechanisms for its antibacterial effect. Invest Urol 1978;6:196–200.
17. Raz R, Stamm WE. A controlled trial of intravaginal estriol in postmenopausal women with recurrent urinary tract infections. N Engl J Med 1993;329(11):753–756.
18. Gupta K, Stapleton AE, Hooton TM, Roberts PL, Fennell CL, Stamm WE. Inverse association of H_2O_2-producing lactobacilli and vaginal *Escherichia coli* colonization in women with recurrent urinary tract infections. J Infect Dis 1998;178:446–450.
19. Sobel JD. Bacterial etiologic agents in the pathogenesis of urinary tract infections. Med Clin North Am 1991;75:253–273.
20. Orskov I, Ferencz A, Orskov F. Tamm-Horsfall protein or uromucoid is the normal urinary slime that traps type-1 fimbriated *Escherichia coli.* Lancet 1980;1:887.
21. Measley RE, Levison ME. Host defense mechanisms in the pathogenesis of urinary tract infection. Med Clin North Am 1991;75:275–286.
22. Jenkins RD, Fenn JP, Matsen JM. Review of urine microscopy for bacteriuria. JAMA 1986;255:3397–3403.
23. Pezzlo M. Detection of urinary tract infections by rapid methods. Clin Microbiol Rev 1988;2:268–280.
24. Stamm WE. Measurement of pyuria and its relation to bacteriuria. Am J Med 1983;75(suppl 1):53–58.
25. Pappas PG. Laboratory in the diagnosis and management of urinary tract infections. Med Clin North Am 1991;75:313–325.
26. Pels RJ, Bor DH, Woolhandler S, et al. Dipstick urinalysis screening of asymptomatic adults for urinary tract disorders. JAMA 1989;262:1221–1224.
27. VanNostrand JD, Junkins AD, Bartholdi RK. Poor predictive ability of urinalysis and microscopic examination to detect urinary tract infection. Am J Clin Pathol 2000;113:709–713.
28. Stamey TA, Govan DE, Palmer JM. The localization and treatment of urinary tract infections: The role of bactericidal urine levels as opposed to serum levels. Medicine 1965;44:1–36.
29. Fairley KF, Bond AG, Brown RB, et al. Simple test to determine the site of urinary tract infection. Lancet 1967;2:427–428.
30. Thomas VC, Forland M. Antibody coated bacteria in urinary tract infection. Kidney Int 1982;21:1–7.
31. Stamey TA, Fair WR, Timothy MM, et al. Serum versus urinary antimicrobial concentrations in cure of urinary tract infections. N Engl J Med 1974;291:1159–1163.
32. Avorn J, Monane M, Gurwitz JH, et al. Reduction of bacteriuria and pyuria after ingestion of cranberry juice. JAMA 1994;271:751–754.
33. Barrett SP, Savage MA, Rebec MP, Guyot A, Andrews N, Shrimpton SB. Antibiotic sensitivity of bacteria associated with community acquired UTI in Britain. J Antimicrob Chemother 1999;44:359–365.
34. Kahlmeter G. The ECO-SENS Project: A prospective, multinational, multicentre, epidemiological survey of the prevalence and antimicrobial susceptibility of urinary tract pathogens-interim report. J Antimicrob Chemother 2000;46(suppl S1):15–22.
35. Steinke DT, Seaton RA, Phillips G, MacDonald TM, Davey PG. Factors associated with trimethoprim-resistant bacteria isolated from urine samples. J Antimicrob Chemother 1999;43:841–843.
36. Goettsch W, VanPelt W, Naglekerke N, et al. Increasing resistance to fluoroquinolones in *Escherichia coli* from urinary tract infections in the Netherlands. J Antimicrob Chemother 2000;46:223–228.
37. Johnson JR, Stamm WE. Urinary tract infection in women: Diagnosis and treatment. Ann Intern Med 1989;11:906–917.
38. Stamm WE, Hooton TM. Management of urinary tract infections in adults. N Engl J Med 1993;329:1328–1334.
39. Naber KG. Treatment options for acute uncomplicated cystitis in adults. J Antimicrob Chemother 2000;46(suppl S1):23–27.
40. Stein GE. Comparison of Single-dose fosfomycin and a 7-day course of nitrofurantoin in female patients with uncomplicated urinary tract infections. Clin Ther 1999;21(11):1864–1872.
41. Irvani A, Klimberg I, Briefer C, Munera C, Kowalsky SF, Echols RM. A trial comparing low-dose, short-course ciprofloxacin and standard 7-day therapy with co-trimoxazole or nitrofurantoin in the treatment of uncomplicated urinary tract infections. J Antimicrob Chemother 1999;43(suppl A):67–75.
42. McCarty JM, Richard G, Huck W, et al. A randomized trial of short-course ciprofloxacin, ofloxacin, or trimethoprim-sulfamethoxazole for treatment of acute urinary tract infections in women. Am J Med 1999;106:292–299.
43. Tice AD. Short course therapy of acute cystitis: A brief review of therapeutic strategies. J Antimicrob Chemother 1999;43(suppl A):85–93.
44. Sherbotie JR, Cornfield D. Management of urinary tract infections in children. Med Clin North Am 1991;75:327–338.
45. Boscia JA, Kobasa WD, Knight RA, et al. Therapy versus no therapy for bacteriuria in elderly ambulatory non-hospitalized women. JAMA 1987;257:1067–1071.
46. Nicolle LE, Mayhew WJ, Bryan L. Prospective, randomized comparison of therapy and no therapy for asymptomatic bacteriuria in institutionalized women. Am J Med 1987;83:27–33.
47. Nicolle LE, Bjornson J, Harding GKM, et al. Bacteriuria in elderly institutionalized men. N Engl J Med 1983;309:1420–1425.
48. Melekos MD, Naber KG. Complicated urinary tract infections. Int J Antimicrob Agents 2000;15:247–256.
49. Norrby SR. Short-term treatment of uncomplicated lower urinary tract infections in women. Rev Infect Dis 1990;12:458–467.
50. Bergeron MG, Beauchamp D, Poirier A, et al. Continuous vs. intermittent administration of antimicrobial agents: Tissue penetration and efficacy *in vivo*. Rev Infect Dis 1985;3:84–97.
51. Gleckman R, Crowley M, Natsios GA. Therapy of recurrent invasive urinary tract infection in men. N Engl J Med 1979;301:878–880.
52. Lipsky GA. Urinary tract infections in men: Epidemiology, pathophysiology, diagnosis, and treatment. Ann Intern Med 1989;110:138–150.
53. Wong ES, McKevitt M, Running K, et al. Management of recurrent urinary tract infections with patient-administered single-dose therapy. Ann Intern Med 1985;102:302–307.
54. Nicolle LE, Ronald AR. Recurrent urinary tract infection in adult women: Diagnosis and treatment. Infect Dis Clin North Am 1987;1:793–806.
55. Stapleton A, Latham RH, Johnson C, et al. Post-coital antimicrobial prophylaxis for recurrent urinary tract infection. JAMA 1990;264:703–706.
56. Andriole VT, Patterson TF. Epidemiology, natural history, and management of urinary tract infection in pregnancy. Med Clin North Am 1991;75:359–373.
57. Christensen B. Which antibiotics are appropriate for treating bacteriuria in pregnancy. J Antimicrob Chemother 2000;46(suppl S1):29–34.

58. McGrady GA, Daling JR, Peterson DR. Maternal urinary tract infection and adverse fetal outcomes. Am J Epidemiol 1985;121:377–381.
59. Warren JW. The catheter and urinary tract infection. Med Clin North Am 1991;75:481–493.
60. Tambyah PA, Maki DG. Catheter-associated urinary tract infection is rarely symptomatic. Arch Intern Med 2000;160:678–682.
61. Ohkawa M, Sugata T, Sawaki M, et al. Bacterial and crystal adherence to the surfaces of indwelling urethral catheters. J Urol 1990;143:717–721.
62. Stamm WE. Catheter-associated urinary tract infection: Epidemiology, pathogenesis, and prevention. Am J Med 1991;91(suppl 3):65s–71s.
63. Schaefer AJ. Urinary tract infection in men: State of the art. Infection 1994;22(suppl 1):S19–S21.
64. Meares EM. Prostatitis. Med Clin North Am 1991;75:405–424.
65. Stamey TA. Urinary infections in males. In: Pathogenesis and Treatment of Urinary Tract Infections. Baltimore, Williams & Wilkins, 1980:342–429.
66. Fair WR, Couch J, Wehner M. Prostatic antibacterial factor: Identity and significance. Urology 1976;7:169–177.
67. Pfau A, Perlberg S, Shapiro A. The pH of prostatic fluid in health and disease: Implications of treatment in chronic bacterial prostatitis. J Urol 1978;119:384–387.
68. Meares EM, Stamey TA. Bacteriologic localization patterns in bacterial prostatitis and urethritis. Invest Urol 1968;5:492–518.
69. Patton JP, Nash DB, Abrutyn E. Urinary tract infection: Economic considerations. Med Clin North Am 1991;75:495–513.
70. MacDonald TM, Collins D, McGilchrist MM, et al. The utilization and economic evaluation of antibiotics prescribed in primary care. J Antimicrob Chemother 1995;35:191–204.

115

SEXUALLY TRANSMITTED DISEASES

Leroy C. Knodel

Over the years, the spectrum of sexually transmitted diseases (STDs) has broadened from the classic venereal diseases—gonorrhea, syphilis, chancroid, lymphogranuloma venereum, and granuloma inguinale—to include a variety of pathogens known to be spread by sexual contact (Table 115–1).[1–3] Because of the large number of infected individuals, the diversity of clinical manifestations, the changing drug susceptibility patterns of some pathogens, and the high frequency of multiple STDs occurring simultaneously in infected individuals, the diagnosis and management of patients with STDs are much more complex today than they were even a decade ago.

Despite a higher reported incidence of all major STDs in men, the complications of STDs generally are more frequent and severe in women. In particular, serious effects on maternal and infant health during pregnancy are well documented. Damage to reproductive organs, increased risk of cancer, complications associated with pregnancy, and transmission of disease to the fetus or newborn are associated with several STDs. As a result of the physiologic, psychosocial, and economic consequences of STDs and because of the increasing prevalence of some viral STDs, such as human immunodeficiency virus (HIV) and genital herpes, for which curative therapy is not available, there has been a resurgence of interest in STD research and the primary prevention of these diseases.[1–3]

With the exception of human immunodeficiency virus infection, which is reviewed in detail in Chap. 123, the most frequently occurring STDs in the United States are discussed in this chapter. For other less-common STDs, only recommended treatment regimens are presented. The most current information on the epidemiology, diagnosis, and treatment of STDs provided by the Centers for Disease Control and Prevention (CDC) can be obtained at their Website on the Internet (http://www.cdc.gov/).

Numerous interrelated factors contribute to the epidemic nature of sexually transmitted diseases. Sociocultural, demographic, and economic factors together with patterns of sexual behavior, host susceptibility to infection, changing properties of the causative pathogens, disease transmission by asymptomatic individuals, and environmental factors are important determinants of the frequency and distribution of STDs in the United States and worldwide.[2,3]

Age is one of the most important demographic determinants of STD incidence. Overall, two-thirds of STD cases each year occur in persons in their teens and twenties, the peak years of sexual activity. With increasing age, the incidence of most STDs decreases exponentially. In sexually active teenagers, STD rates are highest in the youngest, suggesting that physiologic differences may contribute to increased susceptibility.[2–5]

Age-specific rates of STDs are higher in men than in women; however, reported rates may not represent true gender differences, but rather may reflect greater ease of detection in men. In recent years, the ratio of male-to-female cases for most STDs has declined, possibly reflecting improvements in the diagnosis of STDs in asymptomatic women or changes in female sexual behavior following the availability of improved methods of contraception. Although some racial disparity exists for rates of STD infection, it is possible that this is a reflection of socioeconomic differences.[2–5]

Epidemiologic data have shown that the single greatest risk factor for contracting STDs is the number of sexual partners. As the number of sexual partners increases, the risk of being exposed to someone infected with an STD increases. Sexual preference also plays a major role in the transmission of STDs. For all major STDs, rates are disproportionately greater in men who have sex with men (MSM) than in heterosexuals. Also, a number of less common STDs, including several caused by enteric protozoans and bacterial pathogens, occur primarily in MSM. The major risk factors for MSM appear to be related to the greater number of sexual partners and the practice of unprotected anal-genital, oral-genital, and oral-anal intercourse. In addition, prostitution and illicit drug use continue to be associated with a higher incidence of most STDs.[2,4,5]

Some of the most serious sequelae of STDs are associated with congenital or perinatal infections. The majority of neonatal infections are acquired at birth, after infant passage through an infected cervix or vagina. Neonatal *Chlamydia trachomatis, Neisseria gonorrhoeae,* and herpes simplex virus (HSV) infections are associated with this type of spread. For pregnant women with syphilis, infection is usually transmitted transplacentally, producing a congenital infection. Depending on the organism, neonatal infections can manifest in a variety of ways. Ophthalmia neonatorum can result from chlamydial or gonorrheal infections, while syphilis and herpes infections can produce more severe complications, including neurologic impairment. Neonatal herpes infections also are associated with a high mortality.[1–3]

Other than complete abstinence, the most effective way to prevent STD transmission is by maintaining a mutually monogamous sexual relationship between uninfected partners. Short of this, use of barrier contraceptive methods, such as the male and female condoms, diaphragm, cervical cap, vaginal sponges, and vaginal spermicides alone or in combination, provide varying degrees of protection from a number of STDs. When used correctly and consistently, male latex condoms with or without spermicide are more effective than natural skin condoms in protecting against STD transmission, including HIV, gonorrhea, chlamydia, HSV, and hepatitis B.[5–8] When lubrication is desired with latex condoms, water-based products, such as K-Y Jelly, are recommended because oil-based agents (e.g., petroleum jelly) can weaken latex condoms and reduce their effectiveness. The female condom is a lubricated polyurethane sheath with a diaphragm-like ring on each end that can be used as a protective device for women with male sexual partners who do not desire to use a condom. When inserted into the vagina, it may act as a mechanical barrier to disease transmission. Limited data suggest that the female condom blocks penetration of viruses, including HIV; for nonviral STDs, it is believed that the female condom provides STD protection similar to the male condom. Use of nonoxynol-9, a vaginal spermicide with cytolytic activity, reduces the risk for acquiring cervical gonorrhea and chlamydia when used alone. Although *in vitro* data suggest that nonoxynol-9 possesses some activity against HIV, there is no evidence that it prevents transmission of the virus or provides any additional benefit in preventing

TABLE 115–1. Sexually Transmitted Diseases

Disease	Associated Pathogens
Bacterial	
Gonorrhea	*Neisseria gonorrhoeae*
Syphilis	*Treponema pallidum*
Chancroid	*Haemophilus ducreyi*
Granuloma inguinale	*Calymmatobacterium granulomatis*
Enteric disease	*Salmonella* spp., *Shigella* spp., *Campylobacter fetus*
Campylobacter infection	*Campylobacter jejuni*
Bacterial vaginosis	*Gardnerella vaginalis, Mycoplasma hominis, Bacteroides* spp., *Mobiluncus* spp.
Group B streptococcal infections	Group B streptococcus
Chlamydial	
Nongonococcal urethritis	*Chlamydia trachomatis*
Lymphogranuloma venereum	*Chlamydia trachomatis,* type L
Viral	
Acquired Immunodeficiency Syndrome (AIDS)	Human immunodeficiency virus
Herpes genitalis	Herpes simplex virus, type I and II
Viral Hepatitis	Hepatitis A, B, C, D viruses
Condylomata acuminata	Human papillomavirus
Molluscum contagiosum	Poxvirus
Cytomegalovirus infection	Cytomegalovirus
Mycoplasmal	
Nongonococcal urethritis	*Ureaplasma urealyticum*
Protozoal	
Trichomoniasis	*Trichomonas vaginalis*
Amebiasis	*Entamoeba histolytica*
Giardiasis	*Giardia lamblia*
Fungal	
Vaginal Candidiasis	*Candida albicans*
Parasitic	
Scabies	*Sarcoptes scabiei*
Pediculosis pubis	*Phthirus pubis*
Enterobiasis	*Enterobius vermicularis*

HIV transmission when used in conjunction with latex condoms. Some evidence exists that diaphragms may protect against cervical gonorrheal, chlamydial, and trichomonal infections. Although vaginal spermicides and diaphragms may confer some protection to women, their effect on preventing disease transmission to men has not been evaluated.[6–8] The varied spectrum of clinical syndromes produced by common STDs is determined not only by the etiologic pathogen(s), but also by differences in male and female anatomy and reproductive physiology. For a number of STDs, the signs and symptoms overlap sufficiently to prevent accurate diagnosis without microbiologic confirmation. Frequently, symptoms are minimal or absent despite the presence of infection. Table 115–2 lists common clinical syndromes associated with STDs.[1,2,5]

GONORRHEA

EPIDEMIOLOGY AND ETIOLOGY

Neisseria gonorrhoeae is a gram-negative diplococcus estimated to cause up to 1 million infections per year in the United States. Although the number of reported cases of gonorrhea in the United States declined substantially from 1981 to 1996, the CDC notes an increase in reported cases between 1997 and 1999. Of even greater concern, a substantial number of infections remain unreported.[1,9,10] Humans are the only known natural host of this intracellular parasite. Because of its rapid incubation period and the large number of infected individuals with asymptomatic disease, gonorrhea is difficult to control.[1,10]

The risk of a female acquiring a cervical infection after a single episode of vaginal intercourse with an infected male is approximately 50% to 60%, and the risk increases with multiple exposure.[10] While the risk of disease transmission from an infected female to an uninfected male is less, it still is as high as 20% to 30% following a single act of coitus. No data are available on the risk of transmission after other types of sexual contact.[10,11]

PATHOPHYSIOLOGY

On contact with a mucosal surface lined by columnar, cuboidal, or noncornified squamous epithelial cells, the gonococci attach to cell membranes by means of surface pili and are then pinocytosed. The virulence of the organism is mediated primarily by the presence of pili and other outer membrane proteins. After mucosal damage is established, polymorphonuclear leukocytes invade the tissue, submucosal abscesses form, and purulent exudates are secreted.[10]

CLINICAL PRESENTATION

Infected individuals may be symptomatic or asymptomatic, may have complicated or uncomplicated infections, and may have infections involving several anatomic sites. Urethritis is the most common presenting manifestation in males, and it usually develops within 2 to 8 days of exposure. Dysuria and urinary frequency are seen initially, followed in 1 to 2 days by a profuse, purulent urethral discharge. In approximately 25% of cases, the discharge is scant and only minimally purulent, making it almost indistinguishable from nongonococcal urethritis (NGU). Because most men seek treatment from discomforting symptoms, complications resulting from extension of the infection in males, such as epididymitis, prostatitis, inguinal lymphadenopathy, and urethral stricture, are rarely seen today. The majority of symptomatic patients who are not treated become asymptomatic within 6 months, with only a few becoming asymptomatic carriers of the disease.[10–12]

The most common site of gonococcal infection in women is the endocervical canal. Anterior spread of infected vaginal secretions produces urethritis. The incubation period is more variable in females, but symptoms typically appear within 10 days following exposure. Symptoms are relatively nonspecific and include dysuria, urinary frequency, abnormal vaginal discharge, and abnormal uterine bleeding. Diagnosis based on symptoms alone is confounded because infection with other organisms may produce similar manifestations. The majority of gonococcal urethral or cervical infections in females are either asymptomatic or produce minimal symptoms.[10–12]

Other sites of gonococcal infection include the rectum, oropharynx, and eye. Anorectal gonococcal infections are common in females and MSM. In MSM, rectal intercourse is the primary cause, whereas most infections in women are caused by perineal contamination with vaginal discharge. Many patients with anorectal gonorrhea have minimal, if any, symptoms. When present, symptoms range from mild pruritus to severe rectal pain, tenesmus, and a mucopurulent rectal discharge.[11,12]

Like rectal infections, pharyngeal infections are more common in females and MSM. Symptoms can mimic pharyngitis or tonsillitis, although patients are typically asymptomatic. Gonococcal conjunctivitis is rare and usually results from autoinoculation via the fingers from an anogenital infection.[11,12] As a result of the nonspecific signs and symptoms, many women do not seek treatment until after the

TABLE 115–2. Selected Syndromes Associated with Common Sexually Transmitted Pathogens

Syndrome	Commonly Implicated Pathogens	Common Clinical Manifestations[a]
Urethritis	*Chlamydia trachomatis,* herpes simplex virus, *Neisseria gonorrhoeae, Trichomonas vaginalis, Ureaplasma urealyticum*	Urethral discharge, dysuria
Epididymitis	*C. trachomatis, N. gonorrhoeae*	Scrotal pain, inguinal pain, flank pain, urethral discharge
Cervicitis/Vulvovaginitis	*C. trachomatis, Gardnerella vaginalis,* herpes simplex virus, human papillomavirus, *N. gonorrhoeae, T. vaginalis*	Abnormal vaginal discharge, vulvar itching/irritation, dysuria, dyspareunia
Genital Ulcers (painful)	*Haemophilus ducreyi,* herpes simplex virus	Usually multiple vesicular/pustular (herpes) or papular/pustular (*H. ducreyi*) lesions that may coalesce; painful, tender lymphadenopathy[b]
Genital Ulcers (painless)	Treponema pallidum	Usually single papular lesion
Genital/Anal Warts	Human papillomavirus	Multiple lesions ranging in size from small papular warts to large exophytic condylomas
Pharyngitis	*C. trachomatis* (?), herpes simplex virus, *N. gonorrhoeae*	Symptoms of acute pharyngitis, cervical lymphadenopathy, fever[c]
Proctitis	*C. trachomatis,* herpes simplex virus *N. gonorrhoeae, T. pallidum*	Constipation, anorectal discomfort, tenesmus, mucopurulent rectal discharge
Salpingitis	*C. trachomatis, N. gonorrhoeae*	Lower abdominal pain, purulent cervical or vaginal discharge, adnexal swelling, fever[d]

[a]For some syndromes, clinical manifestations may be minimal or absent.
[b]Recurrent herpes infection may manifest as a single lesion.
[c]Most cases of pharyngeal gonococcal infection are asymptomatic.
[d]Salpingitis increases the risk of subsequent ectopic pregnancy and infertility.

development of serious complications, such as pelvic inflammatory disease (PID). Approximately 15% of women with gonorrhea develop PID. Left untreated, PID can be an indirect cause of infertility and ectopic pregnancies. In 0.5% to 3.0% of patients with gonorrhea, the gonococci invade the bloodstream and produce disseminated disease. Disseminated gonorrhea infection (DGI) is three times more common in women than in men. The usual clinical manifestations of DGI are tender necrotic skin lesions, tenosynovitis, and monarticular arthritis. Occasionally, mild hepatitis, myocarditis, and endocarditis occur; very rarely, gonococcal meningitis is reported.[1,10–13]

DIAGNOSIS

Diagnosis of gonococcal infections can be made by Gram-stained smears, culture, or newer methods based on the detection of cellular components of the gonococcus (enzymes, antigens, DNA, or lipopolysaccharide) in clinical specimens. Various stains have been used to identify gonococci microscopically, with the Gram stain the most widely used in clinical practice. Gram-stained smears are positive for gonococci when gram-negative diplococci of typical kidney bean morphology are identified within polymorphonuclear leukocytes.[11] In the presence of equivocal smears (extracellular gonococcal forms that can be nonpathogenic, commensal *Neisseria,* or gram-negative diplococci of atypical morphology), culture is mandatory. In urethral smears from men with symptomatic urethritis, the smear is highly sensitive and specific, and culture is considered optional. Gram-stained smears are specific but insensitive for endocervical, rectal, cutaneous, and asymptomatic male urethral infections. In these situations, culture is the most reliable means of diagnosis.[10,13,14] Because of the presence of nonpathogenic *Neisseria* in the pharynx of most people, the Gram stain is not useful in the diagnosis of pharyngeal infection.[12]

Culture is considered the most reliable means of diagnosing gonococcal infections. Anatomic sites to be cultured depend on the individual's sexual preferences and body areas exposed. In women, because the urethra and other sites are rarely the sole locus of infection, cervical cultures produce the highest yield and are frequently performed in conjunction with rectal cultures. Urethral cultures are recommended in women who have had hysterectomies and heterosexual men. In MSM, anorectal cultures generally produce the highest yields, and pharyngeal and urethral cultures are considered optional.[10,13,14]

Because technical constraints and cost preclude the use of culture techniques in most office settings and clinics, alternative methods of diagnosis have been developed, including enzyme immunoassay, DNA probe techniques and nucleic acid amplification techniques employing polymerase chain reaction (PCR) and ligase chain reaction (LCR). With the exception of Gram stain for symptomatic gonococcal urethritis, these tests offer increased sensitivity and/or specificity over both Gram stain and culture.[10] Additionally, many of these tests can provide a more rapid means of diagnosis than culture. Of particular clinical importance is the high sensitivity of DNA probe and PCR methods for detecting *N. gonorrhoeae* in first-void urine samples of infected individuals and the extension of this technology to concurrently test for *C. trachomatis* in a single specimen.[11,13–16]

► TREATMENT: Gonorrhea

Neisseria gonorrhoeae are susceptible to a variety of antibiotics. The development of chromosomally mediated and plasmid-mediated resistance has resulted, however, in an increasing number of isolates resistant to former first-line antibiotics, such as penicillin, ampicillin, amoxicillin, and tetracycline.[10,16–19]

All gonorrhea treatment regimens recommended by the CDC consist of various oral or parenteral cephalosporins and fluoroquinolones given as a single dose (Table 115–3).[1] These regimens have documented efficacy in the treatment of urethral, cervical, rectal, and pharyngeal infections. Coexisting chlamydial infection, which is documented in as many as 60% of women and in as many as 25% of men with gonorrhea, constitutes the major cause of postgonococcal urethritis, cervicitis, and salpingitis in patients treated for gonorrhea.[10,13,16] As a result, concomitant treatment with doxycycline or azithromycin is recommended in all patients treated for gonorrhea. While none of the single-dose regimens recommended for gonorrhea in the CDC guidelines is effective against chlamydia, azithromycin (2 g) as a single dose is highly effective in eradicating both gonorrhea and chlamydia. Concerns over gastrointestinal (GI) adverse effects, as well as cost, preclude azithromycin's routine use at this time.[10,16,17] Ceftriaxone, the only parenteral agent included in CDC recommended first-line agents for the treatment of gonorrhea, is administered intramuscularly (IM) as a single 125-mg dose. Unfortunately, vials containing less than 250 mg are unavailable, and ceftriaxone remains an expensive alternative to recommended oral antibiotics.[1,17]

Although oral therapy offers a promising alternative to the expense and pain associated with parenteral therapy, it may not be preferred for all cases of gonorrhea. Of the regimens of choice, only ceftriaxone is effective in eradicating both gonorrhea and incubating syphilis. Because the overall incidence of concomitant infection with both gonorrhea and syphilis appears low in most areas, selection of ceftriaxone based on this criterion should be considered only in areas in which the incidence of syphilis infection is high.[17] Resistance to the broad-spectrum cephalosporins recommended for the treatment of gonorrhea has not been reported. However, the development of high-level resistance to fluoroquinolones has resulted in a high prevalence of treatment failures in some parts of the world.[10,16] This appears to be a particular problem in Asia and Western Pacific nations, where more than 50% of isolates exhibit intermediate-level resistance.[11] Despite reports of low-level resistance to fluoroquinolones in some US cities, widespread, clinically significant resistance is not a problem in the United States at present.

Ofloxacin is useful in eradicating both *N. gonorrhoeae* and *C. trachomatis;* however, different dosage regimens are required for each pathogen, and it is unknown whether the lower, multiple-dose daily regimen used in chlamydial infections is effective in eradicating gonorrheal infections.[1,17,18] Spectinomycin is still the preferred alternative for patients unable to tolerate the recommended cephalosporin or fluoroquinolone regimens. Although some resistance to spectinomycin is reported, its limited use appears to have prevented widespread resistance from developing. Unlike ceftriaxone and the fluoroquinolones, spectinomycin has only limited efficacy in treating pharyngeal infections.[1,10]

Pregnant women infected with *N. gonorrhoeae* should be treated with either a cephalosporin or spectinomycin because fluoroquinolones are contraindicated.[1,18] For the treatment of presumed or diagnosed concurrent *C. trachomatis* infection, erythromycin or amoxicillin are the preferred treatments.[1,10,17,18]

Ceftriaxone is the recommended therapy for DGI, gonococcal meningitis, endocarditis, and any type of gonococcal infection in children. Parenteral therapy is suggested for children less than 12 years of age primarily because oral regimens have not been adequately studied. In cases of DGI, patients should be hospitalized and treated initially with ceftriaxone, or ceftizoxime, or cefotaxime. Although marked improvement is usually noted within 48 hours of initiating therapy, treatment should be continued as an outpatient with cefixime, or ciprofloxacin, or ofloxacin to complete a total of 7 days of antibiotic therapy.[1] Children and pregnant or lactating women should not receive ciprofloxacin or ofloxacin because of the concern for bone and joint disorders. In MSM with DGI, ceftriaxone is preferred because of its efficacy in treating coexisting rectal, pharyngeal, and urethral infections.[1,10,18]

Gonococcal ophthalmia is highly contagious in adults and neonates and requires IM ceftriaxone therapy. Single-dose therapy is adequate for gonococcal conjunctivitis, although some physicians recommend continuing therapy until cultures are negative at 48 to 72 hours. Topical antibiotics are not sufficiently effective when used alone for ocular infections and are not necessary with appropriate systemic therapy. Infants with either type of ophthalmologic infection should be evaluated for signs of DGI.[1,10,16,18]

Treatment of gonorrhea during pregnancy is essential to prevent ophthalmia neonatorum. Gonococcal infection in newborns results primarily from passage through an infected birth canal, but it also can be transmitted *in utero*. Ophthalmia neonatorum is the most common ophthalmic infection in newborns (1.6% to 12%), although membranes of the vagina, pharynx, or rectum also can become colonized. Conjunctival involvement usually develops within 7 days of delivery and is characterized by intense, bilateral conjunctival inflammation with chemosis. If not promptly treated, corneal ulceration and blindness can develop. Because the law in most states requires neonatal prophylaxis with topical ocular antimicrobials, gonococcal ophthalmia neonatorum is rare in the United States. The American Academy of Pediatrics recommends that either silver nitrate (1%), tetracycline (1%), or erythromycin (0.5%) be instilled in each conjunctival sac immediately postpartum. Of these agents, silver nitrate is the only one with documented efficacy in preventing ophthalmia caused by penicillinase-producing *N. gonorrhoeae*. Approximately 2% of infants at risk of infection fail prophylaxis with recommended ophthalmic antibiotics. As a result, infants born to infected mothers should also receive an IM or intravenous (IV) injection of ceftriaxone 50 mg/kg for 7 days.[1,16,18,20–22]

EVALUATION OF THERAPEUTIC OUTCOMES

Although some clinicians recommend obtaining followup cultures at least 3 days after treatment, combination gonorrhea and chlamydial therapy rarely results in treatment failures, and routine followup of patients treated with a regimen included in the CDC guidelines is not recommended. Persistence of symptoms following any treatment requires culture of the site(s) of gonorrheal infection, as well as susceptibility testing if gonococci are isolated. In most cases, the presence of gonococci indicates reinfection rather than treatment failure and reflects the need for improved patient education and sex-partner referral. Persistence of symptoms can also be caused by other infectious causes, such as *C. trachomatis.*[1]

TABLE 115–3. Treatment of Gonorrhea

Type of Infection	Recommended Regimens[a]	Alternative Regimens[b]
Uncomplicated infections of the cervix, urethra, and rectum in adults[c,d]	Ceftriaxone 125 mg IM once;[e] or Ciprofloxacin 500 mg po once;[e] or Cefixime 400 mg po once; or Ofloxacin 400 mg po once[e] *plus* A treatment regimen for presumptive *C. trachomatis* coinfection (see Table 115–5)	Spectinomycin 2 g IM once; or Ceftizoxime 500 mg IM once; or Cefotaxime 500 mg IM once; or Cefotetan 1 g IM once; or Cefoxitin 2 g IM once with probenecid 1 g po once; or Lomefloxacin 400 mg po once; or Enoxacin 400 mg po once; or Norfloxacin 800 mg po once *plus* A treatment regimen for presumptive *C. trachomatis* coinfection (see Table 115–5)
Gonococcal infections in pregnancy	Ceftriaxone 125 mg IM once[f,g] *plus* A recommended treatment regimen for presumptive *C. trachomatis* infection during pregnancy[g] (see Table 115–5)	Spectinomycin 2.0 g IM once *plus* A recommended treatment regimen for presumptive *C. trachomatis* infection during pregnancy[g] (see Table 115–5)
Disseminated gonococcal infection in adults (>45 kg)[g,h,i,j]	Ceftriaxone 1 g IM or IV every 24 hours[k]	Ceftizoxime 1 g IV every 8 hours[k] *or* Cefotaxime 1 g IV every 8 hours[k]
Uncomplicated infections of the cervix, urethra, and rectum in children (<45 kg)	Ceftriaxone 125 mg IM once[l]	Spectinomycin 40 mg/kg IM once (not to exceed 2 g)
Gonococcal conjunctivitis in adults	Ceftriaxone 1 g IM once[m]	
Ophthalmia neonatorum	Ceftriaxone 25–50 mg/kg IV or IM once (not to exceed 125 mg)	
Infants born to mothers with gonococcal infection (prophylaxis)	Ceftriaxone 25–50 mg/kg IV or IM once (not to exceed 125 mg)	

[a]Recommendations are those of the CDC.
[b]A number of other antimicrobials have demonstrated efficacy in treating uncomplicated gonorrhea but are not included in the CDC guidelines.
[c]Treatment failures are usually a result of reinfection and necessitate patient education and sex-partner referral; additional treatment regimens for gonorrhea and chlamydia infections should be administered. Epididymitis should be treated for 10 days (see Table 115–5).
[d]Patients allergic to β-lactams should receive a quinolone. Persons unable to tolerate a β-lactam (penicillin or cephalosporin) or a quinolone should receive spectinomycin.
[e]Also recommended for the treatment of uncomplicated infections of the pharynx in combination with a treatment regimen for presumptive *C. trachomatis* infection.
[f]Another recommended IM or po cephalosporin also may be used.
[g]The fluoroquinolones, doxycycline, and erythromycin ethylsuccinate are contraindicated during pregnancy.
[h]Patients treated with one of the recommended regimens should be treated with doxycycline or azithromycin for possible coexistent chlamydial infection.
[i]Patients with gonococcal meningitis should be treated for 10 to 14 days and those with endocarditis should be treated for at least 4 weeks with ceftriaxone 1–2 g IV every 12 hours.
[j]All treatment regimens should be continued for 24 to 48 hours after improvement begins; at this time therapy can be switched to one of the following oral regimens to complete a 7-day course of treatment: cefixime 400 mg po twice daily, or ciprofloxacin 500 mg po two times daily, or ofloxacin 400 mg po twice daily.
[k]All regimens should be continued for 24 to 48 hours after improvement begins; at this time therapy can be switched to one of the following oral regimens to complete a 7-day course of treatment: cefixime 400 mg po twice daily, or ciprofloxacin 500 mg twice daily, or ofloxacin 400 mg po twice daily.
[l]Patients with bacteremia or arthritis should receive ceftriaxone 50 mg/kg (maximum 1 g) IM or IV once daily for 7 days.
[m]The eye should be lavaged one time with saline solution.

SYPHILIS

EPIDEMIOLOGY AND ETIOLOGY

Although syphilis was the sixth most frequently reported communicable disease in the United States in 1998, the incidence of this disease has declined by more than 80% since 1990.[9,23] In addition to being highly contagious, syphilis is of major concern because, if left untreated, it can progress to a chronic systemic disease that can be fatal or seriously disabling.[24–27]

Syphilis is usually acquired by sexual contact with infected mucous membranes or cutaneous lesions, although on rare occasions it can be acquired by nonsexual personal contact, accidental inoculation, or blood transfusion. The causative organism of syphilis is *Treponema pallidum,* a spirochete. The risk of acquiring syphilis from an infected individual after a single sexual encounter is approximately 50% to 60%. After sexual contact, the organism penetrates the intact mucous membrane or a break in the cornified epithelium and spirochetemia occurs.[23–27]

Evidence of a strong association between syphilis and HIV infection has been noted. Although complex and incompletely understood, it appears that syphilis, similar to other sexually transmitted genital ulcer diseases, can increase the risk of acquiring HIV in exposed individuals. Also, immunologic defects in HIV-infected individuals can modify the serologic response to syphilis. In particular, the possibility of delayed seroreactivity, markedly elevated serologic titers, and increased false-positive results could complicate the diagnosis, as well as assessment of treatment efficacy, in HIV-positive individuals infected with syphilis. Furthermore, anecdotal evidence suggests compromised immune function may result in an accelerated progression of syphilis, particularly to neurosyphilis, requiring more aggressive antibiotic therapy in comparison to an immunocompetent host.[12,23–25,27,28] As a result of this association, the CDC recommends that all patients diagnosed with syphilis be tested for HIV infection.[1]

CLINICAL PRESENTATION

PRIMARY SYPHILIS

After exposure and an incubation period of 10 to 90 days (average, 21 days), a painless lesion or chancre appears at the site of inoculation. Classically, the chancre is single, but multiple lesions are reported in up to 30% of infections.[24] The chancre usually begins as a dull red macule that subsequently develops into a papule that erodes and ulcerates. Although chancres vary markedly in appearance, most are rounded or oval in shape, indurated, and well marginated with a clear base. Oral and anorectal chancres are common in MSM and frequently have an atypical appearance. All chancres are highly infectious, although they are generally painless lesions unless secondarily infected or located at extragenital sites. Even without treatment, chancres persist only for 1 to 8 weeks before spontaneously healing. During this stage, painless, nonsuppurative inguinal lymphadenopathy is not uncommon. Because syphilitic chancres can be confused with other infectious etiologies, appropriate diagnostic testing is important.[11,23–26]

SECONDARY SYPHILIS

The secondary stage of syphilis develops 2 to 8 weeks after the onset of the primary stage in untreated or inadequately treated patients. This stage is characterized by a variety of mucocutaneous eruptions, resulting from widespread hematogenous and lymphatic spread of *T. pallidum.* Skin lesions can either be generalized or localized to a small portion of the body and, with the exception of follicular lesions, are nonpruritic. Lesions often appear on the palms of the hands and the soles of the feet. Because palm and sole manifestations characterize few dermatologic conditions, involvement of these areas is highly suggestive of syphilis. In addition to the skin lesions, mild and transitory malaise, fever, pharyngitis, headache, anorexia, and arthralgia are common. Generalized lymphadenopathy also is seen in the majority of patients. In untreated individuals, signs and symptoms of secondary syphilis disappear in 4 to 10 weeks; however, lesions may recur at any time within 4 years if the patient remains untreated.[11,23–26]

LATENT SYPHILIS

By definition, persons with a positive serologic test for syphilis but with no other evidence of disease have latent syphilis. Latent syphilis is further divided into early and late latency. During early latency the patient is considered potentially infectious because of the 25% risk of spontaneous mucocutaneous relapse. The US Public Health Service defines early latency as 1 year from the onset of infection, although other investigators propose a longer interval, such as 2 to 4 years. With the exception of pregnancy in which the mother may pass the disease to the fetus, late latency is considered noninfectious, although the patient remains a host.[1,11,23,27]

Most untreated patients with late latent syphilis have no further sequelae; however, approximately 25% to 30% progress either to neurosyphilis or to late syphilis with clinical manifestations other than neurosyphilis. Treatment of all patients with latent syphilis is essential because there is no way to predict which patients will have progression of their disease.[23,24]

TERTIARY SYPHILIS AND NEUROSYPHILIS

If left untreated, syphilis can slowly produce an inflammatory reaction in virtually any organ in the body. Manifestations of this disease progression were previously referred to as tertiary syphilis.[24] These clinical manifestations now are differentiated into two subgroups based on the presence or absence of central nervous system (CNS) involvement: neurosyphilis or tertiary syphilis (i.e., gumma and cardiovascular syphilis). Most typically, evidence of disease progression is not apparent until 10 to 30 years following the initial infection.[23–27]

Classically, neurosyphilis was used to describe the approximately 20% of patients experiencing disease progression from the latent stage and manifesting with signs of general paresis, eighth cranial nerve deafness, optic atrophy and blindness, progressive dementia, meningovascular complications, or tabes dorsalis. Currently, the term encompasses any patient with cerebrospinal fluid (CSF) abnormalities consistent with central nervous system infection.[23–27] It is estimated that approximately 40% of patients with primary or secondary syphilis exhibit such abnormalities, although most remain asymptomatic. Persistence of CSF abnormalities into late latency is associated with a greater risk of progression to symptomatic neurosyphilis. Because of the availability of effective antibiotic therapy, the manifestations of severe late syphilis are rare, particularly for patients with intact immune systems. Although data are conflicting, some investigators suggest that HIV-infected patients are at greater risk of developing symptomatic neurosyphilis.[24–27,29]

Rarely seen, the most common manifestations of disease progression from late latency are benign gumma formation and cardiovascular syphilis. The gumma, a nonspecific granulomatous lesion, is the classic lesion of late syphilis and develops in 50% of patients with disease progression. These chronic, destructive lesions characteristically infiltrate the skin, bone, soft tissue, and liver, but can be found in any organ or tissue. Gummas of critical organs, such as the heart or brain, can be fatal. Aortitis and aortic insufficiency characterize cardiovascular syphilis. Syphilitic aortic aneurysms also are common.[23,25,26,28,29]

CONGENITAL SYPHILIS

In pregnant women with syphilis, *T. pallidum* can cross the placenta at any time during pregnancy. The risk of fetal infection is greatest in pregnant women with primary and secondary syphilis, and declines in pregnant women with late disease.[23] Transmission of syphilis during pregnancy primarily occurs transplacentally and can result in fetal death, prematurity, or congenital syphilis. Symptoms can be seen during the first months of life (early congenital syphilis) or later in childhood or adolescence (late congenital syphilis). Manifestations of early congenital syphilis resemble those of secondary syphilis, although those of late congenital syphilis correspond to the tertiary stage in adults.[12,22,23]

DIAGNOSIS

Because *T. pallidum* is difficult to culture *in vitro*, diagnosis is based primarily on microscopic examination of serous material from a suspected syphilitic lesion or on results from serologic testing. In primary syphilis, diagnosis is established by the presence of *T. pallidum* on dark-field microscopic examination of material from cutaneous lesions and enlarged lymph nodes in patients with secondary syphilis. In incubating syphilis, confirmation is frequently by dark-field microscopic examination, because serologic tests can be unreactive early in the disease.[29–32] Another method of direct microscopic examination, the direct fluorescent antibody test (DFA-TP), which uses monoclonal or polyclonal antibodies specific for *T. pallidum,* has greater specificity and sensitivity than does dark-field examination and does not require the immediate examination of fresh specimens.[11,23,30–32]

Serologic tests are the mainstay in the diagnosis of syphilis and are traditionally categorized as nontreponemal or treponemal. Common nontreponemal tests include the Venereal Disease Research Laboratory (VDRL) slide test and the more frequently used rapid plasma reagin (RPR) card test.[23,28] Nontreponemal tests, which are inexpensive and easily performed, rely on the detection of reagin, a heterogeneous group of antibodies. A positive nontreponemal test can indicate the presence of any stage of syphilis or congenital syphilis, although incubating syphilis and very early primary syphilis produce a negative reaction; however, because they are nonspecific tests, false-positive reactions occur, making them inappropriate to confirm the diagnosis alone. Transiently false-positive results can be seen in patients with acute febrile illnesses, after immunizations, and during pregnancy. Chronic false-positive results are commonly associated with heroin addiction, aging, chronic infections, autoimmune diseases, and malignant disease. In some cases, false-positive reactions are familial and are related to abnormal serum globulin levels.[11,12,23,29,31,32]

Nontreponemal tests are used primarily as screening tests; however, because reaginic antibody titers also can be quantitated by testing serial dilutions of the patient's serum for reactivity, they are useful in following the progression of the disease, recovery after therapy, and possible reinfection. Because antibody titers vary to some extent between tests, it is important that sequential serologic testing be performed using the same method each time. In patients successfully treated for primary and secondary syphilis, nontreponemal tests will almost always return to seronegativity. If these tests are going to return to negative in patients with early latent syphilis, they will do so within the first 4 years after adequate therapy; patients with disease of longer duration usually remain seropositive for life. In addition to its use in serologic testing, the VDRL is often used on CSF to diagnose neurosyphilis.[12,28,30–32]

In some patients with secondary syphilis, a prozone phenomenon occurs that produces a negative VDRL despite the presence of high reaginic antibody titers.[28] This is corrected by diluting the patient's serum prior to testing.[12,32] For HIV-positive individuals with syphilis, the reactivity of nontreponemal tests can vary depending on the stage of the HIV infection. In the early stages, reaginic titers higher than in non-HIV-infected patients have been seen, resulting in the prozone phenomenon. During the later stages of HIV infection, however, when immune function deteriorates to a greater extent, serologic responses can be reduced or delayed. As a result, the diagnosis of syphilis in HIV-infected individuals can be more difficult.[24,28,30–32]

In diagnosing all stages of syphilis, treponemal tests are more sensitive than nontreponemal tests. Because these tests are technically more demanding and are more expensive, they are used primarily as confirmatory rather than as screening tests. The fluorescent treponemal antibody absorption (FTA-ABS) test is the most frequently used treponemal test. The FTA-ABS test uses the *T. pallidum* antigen to detect specific antibodies to treponemal organisms. The FTA-ABS test becomes positive earlier than nontreponemal tests in primary syphilis. After adequate antibiotic therapy for any stage of syphilis, the FTA-ABS test usually remains reactive for life, and, therefore, is not useful in assessing serologic response to therapy, relapse, or reinfection. In suspected neurosyphilis when the VDRL for CSF is negative, testing of CSF with the FTA-ABS is sometimes recommended. While less specific than the VDRL for CSF involvement, the FTA-ABS appears highly sensitive.[27] Other serologic tests that are specific for the treponemal antibody are the *T. pallidum* hemagglutination assay (TPHA) and the microhemagglutination assay for antibodies to *T. pallidum* (MHATP).[32] PCR-based tests also are being investigated, particularly in situations in which serologic testing has poor sensitivity and specificity (congenital syphilis, early primary syphilis, neurosyphilis).[13,23,30,32] Additionally, multiplex PCR tests that can identify the presence of *T. pallidum*, HSV 1 and 2, and *Haemophilus ducreyi* from genital ulcer specimens are under study.[30]

▶ TREATMENT: Syphilis

Table 115–4 presents the CDC's treatment recommendations.[1] Parenteral penicillin G is the treatment of choice for all stages of syphilis. Because *T. pallidum* multiplies slowly, single doses of short- or intermediate-acting penicillins do not provide the prolonged, low-level exposure to penicillin required for eradication of the treponeme. As a result, benzathine penicillin G is the only penicillin effective for single-dose therapy.[1,11–13,24–27]

The recommended treatment for syphilis of less than 1 year's duration is benzathine penicillin G 2.4 million units as a single dose. Although the relapse rate for this regimen is less than 3%, some investigators advocate that 2.4 million units be administered once a week for 2 consecutive weeks. In patients with syphilis of greater than 1 year's duration and normal CSF examination, benzathine penicillin G is administered weekly for three successive doses. Although not specifically recommended by the CDC, this three-dose regimen is used by some experts to treat HIV-infected patients with syphilis of less than 1 year's duration based on data suggesting a greater risk of treatment failure with single-dose therapy.[26] Some experts even prefer to treat all patients with syphilis of less than 1 year's duration with the three-dose regimen since single-dose therapy is not consistently effective in eradicating treponemes from the CSF; this is of primary concern in patients with undiagnosed CSF involvement, such as HIV-infected individuals.[28]

Patients with abnormal CSF findings should be treated as having neurosyphilis. Preferred regimens for neurosyphilis provide treatment over 10 to 14 days with parenteral penicillin G administered every 4 hours. Benzathine penicillin G alone in standard weekly doses or procaine penicillin G in doses under 2.4 million units do not consistently

TABLE 115–4. Drug Therapy and Followup of Syphilis

Stage/Type of Syphilis	Recommended Regimens[a]	Followup Serology
Primary, secondary, or latent syphilis of less than 1 year's duration (early latent syphilis)	Benzathine penicillin G 2.4 million units IM in a single dose[b]	Quantitative nontreponemal tests at 3 months for primary and secondary syphilis; at 6 and 12 months for early latent syphilis[c]
Latent syphilis of more than 1 year's duration (late latent syphilis) or syphilis of unknown duration	Benzathine penicillin G 2.4 million units IM once a week for 3 successive weeks (7.2 million units total)	Quantitative nontreponemal tests at 6, 12, and 24 months[d]
Neurosyphilis	Aqueous crystalline penicillin G 18–24 million units IV (3–4 million units every 4 hours) for 10 to 14 days,[e] *or* Aqueous procaine penicillin G 2.4 million units IM daily plus probenecid 500 mg po four times daily, both for 10 to 14 days[e]	CSF[f] examination every 6 months until the cell count is normal; if it has not decreased at 6 months or is not normal by 2 years, retreatment should be considered
Congenital syphilis	Aqueous crystalline penicillin G 50,000 U/kg IV every 12 hours during the first 7 days of life and every 8 hours thereafter for a total of 10 days *or* Procaine penicillin G 50,000 U/kg IM daily for 10 days	Quantitative nontreponemal tests every 2 to 3 months until nonreactive or titers have decreased fourfold
Penicillin-allergic patients[g] Primary, secondary, or early latent syphilis	Doxycycline 100 mg po twice daily for 2 weeks[h,i] *or* Tetracycline 500 mg po four times daily for 2 weeks[h,i]	Same as for nonpenicillin-allergic patients
Latent syphilis of more than 1 year's duration (late latent syphilis) or syphilis of unknown duration	Doxycycline 100 mg po twice daily for 4 weeks[i] *or* Tetracycline 500 mg po four times daily for 4 weeks[i]	Same as for nonpenicillin-allergic patients

[a]Recommendations are those of the CDC.
[b]Some experts recommend multiple doses of benzathine penicillin G or other supplemental antibiotics in addition to benzathine penicillin G in HIV-infected patients with primary or secondary syphilis; HIV-infected patients with early latent syphilis should be treated with the recommended regimen for latent syphilis of more than 1 year's duration.
[c]More frequent followup (i.e., at 3, 6, 9, 12, and 24 months) recommended for HIV-infected patients.
[d]More frequent followup (i.e., at 6, 12, 18, and 24 months) recommended for HIV-infected patients.
[e]Some experts administer benzathine penicillin G 2.4 million units IM after completion of the neurosyphilis regimens to provide a total duration of therapy comparable to that used for late syphilis in the absence of neurosyphilis.
[f]CSF, cerebral spinal fluid.
[g]For nonpregnant patients; pregnant patients should be treated with penicillin after desensitization.
[h]Although less effective than either the doxycycline or tetracycline regimen, erythromycin 500 mg po four times daily can be considered as an alternative regimen for nonpregnant patients.
[i]Pregnant patients allergic to penicillin should be desensitized and treated with penicillin.

provide treponemicidal levels in the CSF and have resulted in treatment failures.[1,24–27]

Because *T. pallidum* resistance to penicillin has not emerged, the primary need for alternative drugs in treating syphilis is for penicillin-allergic patients. Alternative regimens recommended for penicillin-allergic patients are doxycycline 100 mg orally twice daily or tetracycline 500 mg orally four times daily for 2 to 4 weeks, depending on the duration of syphilis infection. Although erythromycin 500 mg orally four times daily was recommended in the past as an alternative regimen in nonpregnant, penicillin-allergic patients, evidence suggests that it is not as effective as other recommended regimens.[1,29]

Alternative treatment regimens should be used only in cases of documented penicillin allergy and, given concerns regarding patient compliance with these regimens, followup serologic testing is of particular importance.[12,13,24–27]

Other antibiotics used successfully in treating syphilis include various β-lactam antibiotics; however, none offer significant advantages over benzathine penicillin G. Even though ceftriaxone is considered effective in eradicating incubating syphilis when given as a single 125-mg dose, higher doses and more frequent administration (e.g., 250–1,000 mg daily for 8 to 10 days) appear necessary for more advanced syphilis, and treatment failures are reported in HIV-infected patients.[1,25,26] Preliminary data indicate that azithromycin 500 mg once daily for 10 days produces good results in patients with early syphilis.[28]

For pregnant patients, penicillin is the treatment of choice at the dosage recommended for that particular stage of syphilis. To assure treatment success and prevent transmission to the fetus, some experts advocate an additional IM dose of benzathine penicillin G 2.4 million units 1 week after completion of the recommended regimen. This may be particularly beneficial in women diagnosed and treated during the third trimester or those with secondary syphilis. In women allergic to penicillin, safe and effective alternatives are not available; therefore, skin testing should be performed to confirm a penicillin allergy. It is recommended that women with positive skin tests undergo penicillin desensitization and receive the appropriate treatment regimen for their stage of disease.[1,11,28]

The majority of patients treated for primary and secondary syphilis experience the Jarisch-Herxheimer reaction after treatment. This benign, self-limiting reaction is characterized by flu-like symptoms, such as transient headache, fever, chills, malaise, arthralgia, myalgia, tachypnea, peripheral vasodilation, and aggravation of syphilitic lesions. The exact mechanism of the reaction is unknown, although proposed etiologies, including immunologic mechanisms and release of endotoxin or other toxic treponemal products, are not substantiated.[19,20,28] The Jarisch-Herxheimer reaction is independent of the drug and dose used and should not be confused with penicillin allergy. It usually begins within 2 to 4 hours of initiating therapy, peaks at 8 hours, and is complete within 12 to 24 hours. Most reactions can be managed symptomatically with analgesics, antipyretics, and rest. Steroids and antihistamines have been administered prior to initiation of syphilitic therapy but are of limited value.[1,11,12,27–29]

EVALUATION OF THERAPEUTIC OUTCOMES

Table 115–4 lists the CDC recommendations for serologic followup of patients treated for syphilis.[1] Quantitative nontreponemal tests should be performed at 6 and 12 months in all patients treated for primary and secondary syphilis and at 6, 12, and 24 months for early and late latent disease. The CDC recommends more frequent monitoring of HIV-infected individuals. In general, the time to reach seronegativity is proportional to the duration of the disease. Table 115–4 also includes specific testing recommendations for other stages of syphilis. Despite adequate therapy, some patients may remain seropositive based on nontreponemal test results. In these cases, stabilization of low reaginic titers is indicative of adequate therapy.[1,28,30,31] For women treated during pregnancy, monthly quantitative nontreponemal tests are recommended until the adequacy of therapy is established. Women who do not demonstrate a fourfold decrease in titer over a 3-month period, or who show a fourfold increase in titer between tests, should be retreated.[1,11,23,27,29,31]

CHLAMYDIA TRACHOMATIS

EPIDEMIOLOGY AND ETIOLOGY

Based on reporting to the CDC it is estimated that 3 to 4 million new cases of chlamydia are treated annually in the United States, ranking it as the most frequently reported infectious disease in this country. Similar to other STDs, gross underreporting is believed to exist, partly because of the large number of individuals who are treated presumptively without confirmatory microbiologic testing, and partly because of the large number of individuals with asymptomatic infections. Chlamydial infections represent the most common cause of NGU, accounting for as much as 50% of such infections.[9,32,33]

PATHOPHYSIOLOGY

Chlamydia trachomatis is an obligate intracellular parasite that shares properties of both viruses and bacteria. Like viruses, chlamydiae require cellular material from host cells for replication; however, unlike viruses, chlamydiae maintain their cellular identity throughout development. Although *C. trachomatis* lacks a cell wall peptidoglycan, its major outer membrane is similar to gram-negative bacteria. At least 18 serovars (subspecies) of *C. trachomatis* exist, of which only the lymphogranuloma venereum strains produce potentially invasive infections. The remaining serovars are involved primarily with superficial infection of epithelial cells.[33–37]

The risk of transmissibility of chlamydia after exposure is unknown, but is believed to be substantially less than that following exposure to *N. gonorrhoeae*.[33] It is estimated that coinfection with chlamydia occurs in up to 60% of individuals with gonorrhea.[10,11,13] All individuals diagnosed with *N. gonorrhoeae* should be assumed also to have *C. trachomatis* present.[16] Of major concern are recent data indicating that chlamydial cervicitis can increase the risk of acquisition of HIV.[33] In addition to genital infections, ocular and pharyngeal infections are reported and usually occur secondary to vaginal delivery through an infected birth canal and from orogenital contact, respectively.[35]

CLINICAL PRESENTATION

In males, the most common symptoms of chlamydial genital tract infections are dysuria, urinary frequency, and a mucoid urethral discharge occurring 7 to 21 days after exposure. The discharge is usually less profuse and more mucoid or watery than the urethral discharge associated with gonorrhea. Typically, it is more obvious in the morning. In many cases, the discharge is not noticeable, and crusting of the meatus or staining of undergarments may be the only sign. In as many as 50% of infected heterosexual males, no signs or symptoms are present. *C. trachomatis* is responsible for approximately 50% of all cases of acute epididymitis reported in the United States annually.[1,33,34,36] Rectal infections occur in men practicing receptive anal intercourse, and while these infections are usually asymptomatic, they can produce complications, such as proctitis or proctocolitis.[33,34]

The majority of women with chlamydial infections are asymptomatic. In women with urethral infections, dysuria and frequency are uncommon. When symptomatic, the most common manifestation of infection is endocervicitis with a mucopurulent discharge. On exam, the cervix tends to be friable and ectopic. Chlamydia has been recognized as a major cause of PID and its associated complications, such as infertility and ectopic pregnancy.[33–35]

Similar to gonorrhea, chlamydia may be transmitted to an infant during contact with infected cervicovaginal secretions. Nearly two-thirds of infants acquire chlamydial infection after endocervical exposure, with the primary morbidity associated with seeding of the infant's eyes, nasopharynx, rectum, or vagina. In exposed infants, neonatal conjunctivitis develops in as many as 50% and pneumonia develops in up to 16%. Inclusion conjunctivitis in newborns is usually self-limited, but it can result in scarring and micropannus of the cornea. Interstitial pneumonitis occurring secondary to carriage in the nasopharynx is typically mild, but it can be severe and require hospitalization.[16,33–35]

DIAGNOSIS

Because of the high rate of asymptomatic disease and the disease's high prevalence in sexually active adolescent females, the CDC recommends that these individuals undergo screening during routine annual pelvic examinations.[1,32] Laboratory confirmation of chlamydial infection is important because of the relative lack of specificity of symptoms when present. Cell culture is the reference standard against which all other diagnostic tests are measured. Because chlamydiae are obligate intracellular parasites, specimens for culture must be obtained from endocervical (women) or urethral (men) epithelial cell scrapings rather than from urine or urethral discharges. Although tissue culture techniques have close to a 100% specificity, their sensitivity is reported to be as low as 70%, in part because of problems of improper specimen collection, transport, or processing. Because of the technical demands, expense, and length of time until results are available (3 to 7 days), culture is not as widely used for diagnostic purposes today. However, culture remains the diagnostic standard in medicolegal cases such as sexual assault and child abuse because of its high specificity and ability to detect only viable organisms. Serologic tests are of limited value in diagnosing genital chlamydial infections and are used primarily as a research tool.[32,34,37–39]

Tests that detect chlamydial antigens and nucleic acid provide more rapid results, are technically less demanding to perform, are less costly, and, in some situations, have greater sensitivity than culture. The most commonly used nonculture tests for detection of *C. trachomatis* are the enzyme immunoassay (EIA), DNA hybridization probe, and the direct fluorescent monoclonal antibody (DFA) test. In comparison to culture, these tests have reduced sensitivities and slightly reduced specificities overall. Although the DFA test can be conducted in a short period of time, its sensitivity is highly dependent on skilled personnel in preparing the specimen for viewing under a fluorescent microscope and in interpreting the results. This test is frequently used as a confirmatory test for positive results seen with other nonculture tests. Most commercially available tests used to detect *C. trachomatis* use EIA techniques that detect chlamydial lipopolysaccharide (LPS) antigen. Some EIA methods, however, are not specific for *C. trachomatis,* and false-positive results are reported with other chlamydia species, as well as with some gram-negative bacteria. The sensitivity and specificity of the test are generally lower when urine specimens are used.[34,36–41]

Rapid office tests that employ EIA technology for diagnosing chlamydial infections are widely available, and most provide results in 30 minutes. These tests are generally much less sensitive and specific than laboratory-performed EIA, and they are subject to a high false-positive rate because of the cross-reactivity of LPS from other microorganisms. As a result, a positive rapid office test should only be considered presumptive, and test results should be confirmed by a laboratory-based method.[34,36,37] The greatest advances in the detection of chlamydial infection involved the development of various nucleic acid detection methods. Similar to EIA, the DNA hybridization probe test is easy to perform and a large number of samples can be processed at the same time. Overall, the sensitivity and specificity of the DNA probe tests are greater than with EIA.[33,37,39,40,41]

Of all the advances in the diagnosis of *C. trachomatis* infections, the development of DNA amplification tests (PCR or LCR) that can detect small amounts of chlamydial DNA has been the most important. These tests are highly sensitive and specific for detecting infection in both urogenital specimens and urine. Use of self-collected vaginal swabs or first-void urine samples offer greater patient acceptability, particularly when used to screen asymptomatic individuals. However, because of their ability to detect as little as a single gene copy in a specimen, nucleic acid residues that persist following successful antibiotic therapy of a chlamydial infection can result in a false-positive test for several weeks following eradication of the organism.[32–34,37,38,39–41]

▶ TREATMENT: Chlamydia

A number of antimicrobials, including tetracyclines, macrolides, and some fluoroquinolones, particularly ofloxacin, display good *in vitro* and *in vivo* activity against *C. trachomatis.*[16] In most clinical trials, cure rates exceeding 90% are reported for these agents. All of these antimicrobials also appear to have good efficacy against *Ureaplasma urealyticum,* the second most common cause of NGU.[21,35–38,42,43]

Azithromycin 1 g orally as a single dose or doxycycline 100 mg orally twice daily are the regimens of choice for the treatment of chlamydial infections (Table 115–5).[1] Because of its prolonged serum and tissue half-life, azithromycin is the only single-dose therapy that is effective in treating *C. trachomatis.*[1,42] Despite a higher acquisition cost than generic doxycycline, azithromycin may be a more cost-effective alternative in patient populations in which compliance is a problem.[43,44] Unlike the capsule dosage form that should be taken on an empty stomach, the single 1 g azithromycin dose packet for oral suspension can be taken without regard to meals.

Ofloxacin is the only fluoroquinolone with well-documented efficacy in *C. trachomatis* infections and is considered an alternative to both doxycycline and azithromycin. Ofloxacin is dosed twice daily for 7 days like doxycycline, but it is more expensive. Although ciprofloxacin has activity against *C. trachomatis* and *U. urealyticum,* dosages as high as 2 g per day have not consistently eradicated chlamydial infections.[33,35,36,42,44]

For pregnant women with chlamydial urogenital infections, treatment can significantly reduce the risk of pregnancy complications and transmission to the newborn. Because the use of doxycycline and ofloxacin are contraindicated during pregnancy, erythromycin base or amoxicillin are the recommended drug treatments (Table 115–5).[1,35,44] Some clinicians prefer amoxicillin over erythromycin because of better patient tolerability and, as a result, improved patient compliance.[33] Patients intolerant of the recommended erythromycin dosage can be treated with half of the daily dose for 2 weeks instead of 1 week. Recommended alternatives to erythromycin base are erythromycin ethylsuccinate and azithromycin. Although not recommended as first-line therapy because data on its use in pregnancy are limited, azithromycin is the only agent with documented efficacy in a single dose. Like erythromycin, azithromycin is in pregnancy category B and is probably an acceptable agent for use during pregnancy. It is recommended that posttreatment cultures be obtained for pregnant patients treated for chlamydial infections to ensure eradication of the infection.[1,35]

C. trachomatis transmission during perinatal exposure can result in infections of the eye, oropharynx, lungs, urogenital tract, and rectum of the neonate or infant. Despite their efficacy in preventing gonococcal ophthalmia, topical erythromycin ointment (0.5%), tetracycline ointment (1%), and silver nitrate solution (1%) appear less

TABLE 115–5. Treatment of Chlamydial Infections

Infection	Recommended Regimens[a]	Alternative Regimen
Uncomplicated urethral, endocervical, or rectal infection in adults	Azithromycin 1 g po once *or* Doxycycline 100 mg po twice daily for 7 days	Ofloxacin 300 mg po twice daily for 7 days *or* Erythromycin base 500 mg po four times daily for 7 days *or* Erythromycin ethyl succinate 800 mg po four times daily for 7 days
Urogenital infections during pregnancy	Erythromycin base 500 mg po four times daily for 7 days *or* Amoxicillin 500 mg po three times daily for 7 days	Erythromycin base 250 mg po four times daily for 14 days *or* Erythromycin ethyl succinate 800 mg po four times daily for 7 days (or 400 mg po four times daily for 14 days) *or* Azithromycin 1 g po as a single dose[b]
Conjunctivitis of the newborn or pneumonia in infants	Erythromycin base 50 mg/kg/day po in four divided doses for 10 to 14 days[c]	
Epididymitis	Ceftriaxone 250 mg IM *plus* Doxycycline 100 mg po twice daily for 10 days	

[a]Recommendations are those of the CDC.
[b]Data are insufficient to recommend routine use of azithromycin in pregnant women at this time.
[c]Topical therapy alone is inadequate and is unnecessary when systemic therapy is administered.

effective in preventing chlamydial ophthalmia.[1] Additionally, topical therapy has no effect on nasal carriage or colonization of other parts of the infant's body, so the potential for other infections, including pneumonia, still remains.[22,35,44] Because of the high percentage of treatment failures, topical therapy should not be used to treat ophthalmia caused by *C. trachomatis.* Instead, oral erythromycin 50 mg/kg/d in four divided doses for 10 to 14 days is recommended.[1,44]

EVALUATION OF THERAPEUTIC OUTCOMES

Treatment of chlamydial infections with the recommended regimens is highly effective, therefore, posttreatment laboratory testing is not routinely recommended unless symptoms persist or there are other specific concerns (e.g., pregnancy). Posttreatment tests should not be performed for at least 3 weeks following completion of therapy.[1] When posttreatment tests are positive, they usually represent noncompliance, failure to treat sexual partners, or laboratory error, rather than inadequate therapy or resistance to therapy. Infants with pneumonitis should receive followup testing because erythromycin is only 80% effective and a second course of therapy may be necessary.[1,34,40,41]

GENITAL HERPES

EPIDEMIOLOGY AND ETIOLOGY

Genital herpes infections represent the most common cause of genital ulceration seen in the United States. It is estimated that more than 45 million Americans have genital herpes and that this number is increasing by approximately 500,000 each year.[15–18] Because of its morbidity, recurrent nature, and potential for complications, as well as its ability to be transmitted asymptomatically, genital herpes is receiving increased attention.[13,45–54] Similar to syphilis and other STDs, the presence of genital herpes lesions is associated with an increased risk of acquiring HIV following exposure.[47,54]

PATHOPHYSIOLOGY

Herpes comes from the Greek word meaning "to creep" and is used to describe two distinct but antigenically related serotypes of herpes simplex virus. Herpes simplex virus type 1 (HSV-1) is most commonly associated with oropharyngeal disease, and herpes simplex virus type 2 (HSV-2) is most closely associated with genital disease; however, each virus is capable of causing infections clinically indistinguishable in both anatomic areas.[46,47,50,54,55]

Humans are the sole known reservoir for HSV. Infection is transmitted via inoculation of virus from infected secretions onto mucosal surfaces (e.g., urethra, oropharynx, cervix, conjunctivae) or through abraded skin. Evidence that the virus survives for a limited time on environmental surfaces suggests the possibility of fomitic transfer as a nonvenereal route of transmission.[46,50,56]

The cycle of HSV infection occurs in five stages: primary mucocutaneous infection, infection of the ganglia, establishment of latency, reactivation, and recurrent infection. After viral inoculation, HSV infection is associated with cytoplasmic granulation, ballooning degeneration of cells, and production of mononucleated giant cells. Initially, the cellular response is predominantly polymorphonuclear, followed by a lymphocytic response. Replication occurs with viral spread to contiguous cells and peripheral sensory nerves. Latency then is established in sensory or autonomic nerve root ganglia. Latency appears to be lifelong, interrupted only by reactivation of the viral infection. It is unclear what factors are important in maintaining latency, but immune responses and emotional and physical stresses appear important in reactivating latent virus.[46,48]

CLINICAL PRESENTATION

The clinical manifestations of first episodes of genital herpes usually appear within 2 to 14 days after exposure. The signs and symptoms are influenced by many factors, including previous exposure to HSV, viral type, and host factors, such as age and site of infection. On the basis of retrospective studies, it is estimated that up to 50% of genital HSV infections are asymptomatic, and these infections may represent the most common source of transmission of genital and neonatal herpes infections.[32,46,47,54] As a result, identification of individuals with asymptomatic disease may prove beneficial in the control of genital herpes transmission.[13,46,53,55] In terms of the natural history of genital herpes infection and its treatment, it is important to distinguish between first-episode primary, first-episode nonprimary, and recurrent infections.

FIRST-EPISODE INFECTIONS

First-episode primary infections are classified as infections occurring in persons lacking antibody to either type of HSV. These infections are characterized by a prolonged duration of systemic and local symptoms, sometimes requiring hospitalization. More than 50% of patients with primary infections experience flu-like symptoms of fever, headache, malaise, and myalgias. These symptoms gradually resolve over the course of a week. Local symptoms include development of pustular or ulcerative lesions on the external genitalia. Lesions usually begin as papules or vesicles that rapidly spread over the genitalia. Clusters of the lesions coalesce into large areas of ulceration, which, over 2 to 3 weeks, crust, reepithelialize, or both. Genital lesions are described as painful by more than 90% of infected men and women. Development of new lesions is fairly common during the first 10 days of a primary infection. Other local symptoms can include itching, dysuria, vaginal or urethral discharge, and tender inguinal adenopathy; the latter is usually the last symptom to resolve. Viral shedding lasts approximately 11 to 12 days.[13,47,48,53,56]

First-episode nonprimary genital herpes is defined as an infection in individuals who have clinical or serologic evidence of prior HSV (usually HSV-1) infection at another body site. These infections tend to be milder than true primary infections, with a lower incidence of constitutional symptoms and a shorter duration of local symptoms. Viral shedding usually lasts about 7 days.[13,50,51,53] Some data suggest that immunity produced by a prior HSV-1 infection may reduce the risk of acquiring a genital HSV-2 infection.[47,48,54,56]

RECURRENT INFECTIONS

In contrast to first-episode primary and first-episode nonprimary infections, recurrent infections are infrequently associated with systemic manifestations. Recurrent infection is localized to the genital area and is milder and of a shorter duration (8 to 12 days). Viral shedding lasts approximately 4 days. Approximately 50% of patients with genital herpes experience a prodrome prior to the appearance of recurrent lesions. This typically consists of a mild tingling or itching sensation hours to a few days prior to the appearance of vesicles. In a few patients, symptoms of sacral neuralgia are seen.[13,47,48,51,53,54]

As with a first-episode infection, symptoms of recurrent infection tend to be more severe in women, primarily as a result of the greater genital surface area involved. Also, recurrent genital infections caused by HSV-2 tend to be more severe than those associated with HSV-1 infection. Approximately 80% to 90% of patients with a first-episode HSV-2 genital infection experience a recurrence within 12 months compared with approximately 50% to 60% infected with HSV-1.[50,51] The median number of recurrences is estimated at four per year when infection is caused by HSV-2, versus only one per year for HSV-1 infections.[46–48,54] Symptoms of first-episode and recurrent infections tend to be more severe and prolonged in immunocompromised patients than in immunocompetent patients. In addition, immunocompromised patients are more susceptible to initial genital infection and subsequent recurrences, as well as generalized systemic infection.[47,48,51,53,54]

COMPLICATIONS

Complications from genital herpes infections result from both genital spread and autoinoculation of the virus, and occur most commonly with primary first episodes. Lesions at extragenital sites, such as the eye, rectum, pharynx, and fingers, are not uncommon. Central nervous system involvement is occasionally seen and may take several forms, including an aseptic meningitis, transverse myelitis, or sacral radiculopathy syndrome.[47,50,51,54]

A major concern is the effect of genital herpes on neonates exposed during pregnancy. Neonatal herpes is associated with a high mortality and significant morbidity. It is transmitted to the newborn primarily through exposure to HSV in the birth canal but, in rare cases, also is transmitted transplacentally. The risk of transmission during birth appears much greater for first-episode primary infections than for recurrent infections. Neonatal herpes infection has a case-fatality rate of approximately 50%, with a large proportion of surviving infants experiencing significant morbidity, including permanent neurologic damage.[13,50,55]

DIAGNOSIS

Confirmation of a genital herpes infection can be made only with laboratory testing. Tissue culture is the most specific (100%) and sensitive method (80% to 90%) of confirming the diagnosis of first-episode genital herpes; however, culture is relatively insensitive in detecting HSV in ulcers in the latter stages of healing and in recurrent infections, as a result, in part, of reduced viral load. Viral culture is expensive and time-consuming, and improper collection or transport of specimens can result in false-negative results. In most situations, HSV isolation on tissue culture takes 48 to 96 hours. Following isolation, it is recommended that typing of the virus be performed because of prognostic implications (HSV-1 is associated with a lower rate of asymptomatic and symptomatic recurrence).[54] In instances in which rapid detection is necessary, such as an impending birth, other detection methods may be more useful. Amplified culture techniques that combine cell culture for 24 hours and subsequent staining for HSV antigen have sensitivities and specificities only slightly less than those of culture.[46,47,49,50,52,53] The Tzanck test is a rapid detection method in which cells from suspected lesions are stained and examined for the presence of characteristic multinucleated giant cells. While easy to perform and inexpensive, the specificity and sensitivity are low. Antigen detection methods, such as direct immunofluorescence, immunoperoxidase staining, and EIA, provide more rapid results than culture and are less expensive.[14,48,53,54,57]

The majority of patients infected with either HSV-1 or HSV-2 develop circulating antibodies to HSV antigens; however, commercially available serologic assays for detection of HSV antibodies are often overused and have only limited use in the diagnosis of genital herpes. The cross-reactivity of antibodies to HSV-1 and HSV-2 in most of these assays, coupled with the high prevalence of HSV-1 antibody in the adult population, makes it difficult to interpret the results. Type-specific antibody tests that can identify carriers of HSV-2 have been developed and may soon replace other nonspecific tests in diagnosing HSV infections.[46,54]

While the diagnosis of genital herpes can be confirmed only by laboratory tests, less stringent diagnostic criteria (e.g., characteristic physical findings or clinical history) frequently are used in clinical practice. A presumptive diagnosis of genital herpes commonly is made based on the presence of dark-field-negative, vesicular, or ulcerative genital lesions. A prior history of similar lesions or recent sexual contact with an individual with similar lesions also is useful in making the diagnosis. Other STDs, including chancroid, lymphogranuloma venereum, and granuloma inguinale, and causes, such as trauma, allergic reactions, and bacterial or fungal infections, are considered in the differential diagnosis.

▶ TREATMENT: Genital Herpes

The most achievable goals in the management of genital herpes are to relieve symptoms and to shorten the clinical course, to prevent complications and recurrences, and to decrease disease transmission. Although research has focused primarily on the treatment of active infection and suppression of recurrences, increasing emphasis is being placed on various approaches, including immunotherapy that might provide protection from disease transmission or possibly eliminate established latency.[47,51,55]

Palliative and supportive measures are the cornerstone of therapy for patients with genital herpes. Pain and discomfort usually respond to warm saline baths or the use of analgesics, antipyretics, or antipruritics; good genital hygiene can prevent the development of bacterial superinfection. Specific chemotherapeutic approaches to treating genital herpes include antiviral compounds, topical surfactants, photodynamic dyes, immune modulators, vaccines, and interferons. Few of these have undergone extensive evaluation, however, and only the antiviral agents have demonstrated any consistent clinical efficacy.[49–53,57,58] The most recent CDC recommendations for the treatment of genital herpes include the antiviral agents acyclovir, valacyclovir, and famciclovir (Table 115–6).[1] Valacyclovir, a prodrug of acyclovir, and famciclovir, a prodrug of penciclovir, possess improved pharmacokinetic profiles over acyclovir, allowing them to be dosed less frequently. Their overall efficacy in treating genital HSV infection, however, appears comparable to acyclovir.[44,47,50,55,56]

FIRST-EPISODE INFECTIONS

Oral formulations of acyclovir, famciclovir, and valacyclovir have demonstrated efficacy in reducing viral shedding, duration of symptoms, and time to healing of first-episode genital herpes infections, with maximal benefits seen when therapy is initiated at the earliest stages of infection.[55] In contrast, topical acyclovir or penciclovir therapy, when used alone or in combination with oral therapy, is considered of little or no benefit in most patients. Table 115–6 lists the recommended acyclovir, famciclovir, and valacyclovir oral regimens for first-episode infections. Although the valacyclovir and famciclovir dosage regimens are more convenient than the five times daily acyclovir regimen and offer the potential for greater patient compliance, no therapeutic advantages over acyclovir are apparent at this time.[32,47,48,50] In immunocompromised patients or those with severe symptoms or complications necessitating hospitalization, parenteral acyclovir may be beneficial; however, the IV regimen has been associated with renal, GI, bone marrow, and central nervous system toxicity, particularly in patients with renal dysfunction receiving high doses. No antiviral regimen is known to prevent latency or alter the subsequent frequency and severity of recurrences in humans.[32,47,50,51,55]

RECURRENT INFECTIONS

The role of antiviral agents in the treatment of most recurrent genital herpes episodes is controversial. Because signs and symptoms of recurrent infections are generally milder and of shorter duration than those of first-episode infections in immunocompetent hosts, demonstration of clinically important therapeutic benefits is difficult. There are two approaches to management of recurrent episodes: episodic or chronic suppressive therapy.[32,47,50,51,55,56]

Episodic therapy is initiated early during the course of the recurrence, preferably at the onset of prodromal symptoms, but no more than 48 hours after symptom onset. In most patients, appreciable effects on symptomatology are not seen. Patients with prolonged episodes of recurrent infection or severe symptomatology are most likely to benefit from episodic therapy. Table 115–6 lists the recommended acyclovir, famciclovir, and valacyclovir suppressive regimens. Because of the relative mildness and brevity of recurrent infections, parenteral administration of acyclovir is not justifiable.[32,47,51,55,56]

Cost and the potential for adverse effects preclude available antiviral agents from being recommended for routine use as suppressive therapy in all patients with recurrent genital herpes. Patients with frequent (greater than six per year) and physically or psychologically distressing recurrences, however, are candidates for suppressive therapy.[32,55,56] Continuous therapy with recommended antivirals has been shown to reduce the frequency and severity of recurrences in 70% to 90% of patients experiencing frequent recurrences. Asymptomatic viral shedding is reduced by 95% in patients receiving suppressive therapy; however, a significant decrease in disease transmission to sexual partners has not been documented. This is likely a result of low-level shedding that still occurs during suppressive therapy.[32,54,55] Resistant HSV isolates have been identified in some patients experiencing breakthrough recurrences while taking acyclovir. Although there is concern about the development of resistant strains with suppressive therapy, clinical trials have found no evidence of cumulative toxicity or significant resistance in patients treated continuously with the recommended antivirals.[44,46,47,50,56]

SELECTED POPULATIONS

Immunocompromised patients are at greatest risk for severe and recurrent HSV infections but do benefit from therapy with all oral, intravenous, and topical antivirals. As with the immunocompetent host, effects are more pronounced with systemic administration. Acyclovir, valacyclovir, and famciclovir have been used to prevent

TABLE 115–6. Treatment of Genital Herpes

Type of Infection	Recommended Regimens[a,b]	Alternative Regimen
First clinical episode of genital herpes[c]	Acyclovir 400 mg po three times daily for 7 to 10 days *or* Acyclovir 200 mg po five times daily for 7 to 10 days *or* Famciclovir 250 mg po three times daily for 7 to 10 days *or* Valacyclovir 1 g po twice daily for 7 to 10 days	Acyclovir 5–10 mg/kg IV every 8 hours for 5 to 7 days or until clinical resolution occurs[d]
First clinical episode of herpes proctitis or oral infection including stomatitis or pharyngitis	Acyclovir 400 mg po five times daily for 7 to 10 days[e]	Acyclovir 5–10 mg/kg IV every 8 hours for 5 to 7 days or until clinical resolution occurs[d]
Recurrent infection Treatment	Acyclovir 200 mg po five times daily, or 400 mg po three times daily, or 800 mg po two times daily for 5 days[f] *or* Famciclovir 125 mg po twice daily for 5 days[f] *or* Valacyclovir 500 mg po twice daily for 5 days[f]	
Suppression	Acyclovir 400 mg po twice daily[g] *or* Famciclovir 250 mg po twice daily *or* Valacyclovir 500 mg *or* 1,000 mg po once daily[h]	

[a]Recommendations are those of the CDC.
[b]HIV-infected patients may require more aggressive therapy.
[c]Primary or nonprimary first episode.
[d]Only for patients with severe symptoms or complications that necessitate hospitalization.
[e]Recommendations based on studies using this dosage regimen rather than the lower dosage regimens recommended for first clinical episodes of genital herpes. It is not clear whether lower dosage regimens would have comparable efficacy. Famciclovir and valacyclovir are probably also effective for proctitis and oral infection, but clinical experience is limited.
[f]Treatment should be limited to patients with severe symptoms. Treatment is most beneficial when instituted at the earliest sign of recurrence (i.e., prodrome); therapy initiated 48 hours or more after the onset of symptoms has no effect.
[g]Indicated only for patients with frequent and/or severe recurrences; although safety and efficacy are documented in patients receiving acyclovir daily therapy for as long as 6 years and valacyclovir and famciclovir therapy for 1 year, it is recommended that therapy be discontinued after 1 year of continuous suppressive therapy to assess the patient's rate of recurrent episodes.
[h]Valacyclovir 500 mg appears less effective than valacyclovir 1,000 mg in patients with ≥10 recurrences per year.

reactivation of infection in patients seropositive for HSV who undergo transplantation procedures or induction chemotherapy for acute leukemia. Immunocompromised individuals, such as patients with AIDS, who fail treatment or prophylaxis with recommended antiviral doses, frequently demonstrate improved response with higher doses. If resistance is suspected or confirmed with recommended first-line antivirals, alternative agents, such as foscarnet or vidarabine, are usually effective. Their use is associated, however, with a greater risk of serious adverse effects.[45,51,52,56]

The safety of acyclovir, famciclovir, and valacyclovir during pregnancy is not established, although considerable experience with acyclovir in pregnant patients has produced no evidence of teratogenic effects. Because of the high maternal and infant morbidity associated with first-episode primary genital infections at or near term, many clinicians advocate the use of systemic acyclovir as the standard of care in such cases; however, the effectiveness of such therapy is unknown. The use of acyclovir to treat or suppress recurrent episodes near-term is more controversial, primarily because of the lack of data demonstrating significant benefits in this situation.[32,50,55,56,59–61]

With the increasing prevalence of genital herpes worldwide, the potential exists for widespread use and misuse of acyclovir, valacyclovir, and famciclovir, resulting in development of resistant HSV isolates. *In vitro* resistance to these three agents is usually mediated by alterations in viral thymidine kinase; most resistant isolates are either thymidine kinase deficient or have altered thymidine kinase. The incidence and clinical implications of HSV resistance require further study, particularly with respect to immunocompromised hosts in whom resistance may develop with greater frequency and be of greater clinical importance. Unlike acyclovir, valacyclovir, and famciclovir, foscarnet does not require the presence of thymidine kinase to be effective.[47,50,52,55,56]

Numerous agents for the prophylaxis and treatment of genital herpes infections are being studied. Neither topical nor systemic interferons have demonstrated consistent beneficial effects in genital HSV infections; however, a reduction in pain and time of healing of lesions has been reported with an interferon preparation incorporated into a gel containing nonoxynol-9. Other treatments under investigation include cidofovir and immune modulators, such as imiquimod.[47,53,56] Agents that can eliminate ganglionic latency and prevent recurrent HSV infections are not expected to be available in the near future. Much more promising for the near future are vaccines under development. Unfortunately, safety concerns with live attenuated virus vaccines resulted in research focused primarily on recombinant protein vaccines that have exhibited relatively poor immunogenicity. In recent years investigations using replication-defective HSV mutants that are not pathogenic, as well as DNA vaccines that foster host cell uptake of foreign DNA that encodes for an antigenic viral protein, have shown that they induce long-standing immunity in animal models. Studies in humans are currently underway. Use of heterologous vaccines (bacillus Calmette-Guérin and influenza vaccines) to stimulate the immune system in patients with recurrent genital herpes have proven of no significant benefit.[47,55,62–64]

EVALUATION OF THERAPEUTIC OUTCOMES

Available antiviral compounds are of greatest benefit in patients experiencing first-episode primary infections, immunocompromised patients, and patients with frequent or severe recurrent infections. Antivirals, however, are palliative and not curative, and patients receiving these agents should be monitored closely for adverse drug effects. CDC guidelines suggest that discontinuation of suppressive therapy after 1 year be considered to assess for possible changes in the patient's intrinsic pattern of recurrence. In many patients, decreases in recurrence rates and the severity of symptoms occur over time. However, some clinicians prefer to continue suppressive therapy indefinitely because it significantly reduces asymptomatic viral shedding, a potential benefit in reducing the risk of disease transmission to uninfected sexual partners.[1,65,66]

TRICHOMONIASIS

EPIDEMIOLOGY AND ETIOLOGY

Trichomonas vaginalis, a flagellated, motile protozoan is responsible for an estimated 2.5 to 3 million cases of trichomoniasis annually in the United States. Humans are host to two other *Trichomonas* species, *T. tenax* and *T. hominis,* but *T. vaginalis* is the only species thought to be pathogenic.[67–72] Although infection by nonsexual contact is reported, it is uncommon. Contamination of inanimate objects and spread of infection via communal bathing or contact with infected bath or toilet articles is possible because *T. vaginalis* can survive for several hours on moist surfaces.[71,72] Neonatal infections also represent another possible nonvenereal route of disease transmission.[67–71,73,74]

Coinfection with other STDs is not unusual in patients diagnosed with trichomoniasis. Women infected with *T. vaginalis* are three times more likely to have gonorrhea than those who do not have trichomoniasis; approximately 20% of men with gonococcal urethritis also have trichomoniasis.[69] In patients treated appropriately for genital *C. trachomatis* or *U. urealyticum* infection, persistent urethritis can result from coexisting trichomonal infection.[13,67,68,70] Although not well documented, it is proposed that the inflammatory response produced by trichomoniasis may increased the risk of acquiring HIV.[71,74]

PATHOPHYSIOLOGY

Trichomonads are isolated from the vagina, urethra, and Skene glands in 90% to 95% of infected women. Infrequently, they are recovered from the endocervix. Extragenital sites are epidemiologically important, because infection can persist and result in reinfection of the vagina if local therapy alone is used.[71,72] This may account for the higher relapse rates reported for local versus systemic therapy.[71,72,75] After attachment to the vaginal or urethral mucosa, trichomonads usually elicit an inflammatory response that manifests as a discharge containing large numbers of polymorphonuclear leukocytes.[68–72]

CLINICAL PRESENTATION

Trichomonal infections are much more common in women than in men. This may in part be because of the reported greater transmissibility of the organism from men to women. The incubation period of trichomoniasis is 3 to 28 days, with as many as 50% of infected women remaining asymptomatic.[68,72] When symptomatic, females can present with mild-to-severe vaginal discharge, vulvar pruritus, dyspareunia, and dysuria. Symptoms frequently worsen during menstruation when the pH of the vagina is optimal for growth of trichomonads. Vaginal discharge is noted in approximately 50% to 75% of infected women and classically has been described as malodorous, foamy, and yellow-green in color; however, more typically the discharge is grayish and only mildly odoriferous. Severe pruritus is noted in as many as 50% of women.[68,70,73,76]

On examination of symptomatic women, the vulva and surrounding areas may be diffusely erythematous and excoriated as a result of scratching. Secondary infection of excoriated areas is not uncommon. The vagina is often erythematous, and surface erosions of the cervix ("strawberry" vagina and cervix) may be seen. Tender inguinal lymphadenopathy and lower abdominal pain occur infrequently. In a small percentage of patients, there may be no abnormal findings on vaginal examination. There is no evidence that trichomonads spread beyond the cervix to cause PID or disseminated disease; however, it is suggested that cervical erosion secondary to trichomoniasis may contribute to malignant transformation.[68–70,72,74]

Trichomoniasis may be responsible for causing premature rupture of the membranes and preterm delivery.[13,29] It also can be transmitted to neonates after passage through an infected birth canal. Although the risk is low (5%) and most cases of neonatal infections are self-limited, persistent vaginal or urethral infections during pregnancy should be treated.[1,68,71,75]

The majority of trichomonal infections in men are asymptomatic, largely because of the smaller number of organisms usually present.[13,72] It is likely that differences in pathogenicity of trichomonads in men and women reflect differences in the microenvironment of the vagina and urethra. The most common site of infection in men is the urethra, and when symptoms are present, urethral discharge is seen most commonly, followed by pruritus and dysuria. The discharge can range from mucoid to purulent. For most men, trichomonal urethritis is associated with a high spontaneous cure rate. Complications of infection in men are uncommon, although some cases of prostatitis and epididymitis have been attributed to *T. vaginalis.*[67,70–72]

DIAGNOSIS

Trichomonas vaginalis produces nonspecific symptoms also consistent with bacterial vaginosis; as a result, laboratory diagnosis is required. Because *T. vaginalis* requires a pH range of 4.9 to 7.5 for survival, a vaginal discharge pH of greater than 5.0 usually indicates the presence of either *T. vaginalis* or *Gardnerella vaginalis,* a common cause of bacterial vaginosis. The simplest and most reliable means of diagnosis is a wet-mount examination of the vaginal discharge.[67,70–72] Trichomoniasis is confirmed if characteristic pear-shaped, flagellating organisms are observed. The wet mount is only about 75% to 80% sensitive in detecting the presence of trichomonads, with lower sensitivities reported in men and in women with low-grade, subacute, or chronic infections.[68–70,72,76]

Although the presence of trichomonads may be reported on a Papanicolaou (Pap) smear, the sensitivity of this cytologic technique is less than for wet mount and also is associated with a number of false-positive results. Stained smears of cervical specimens have been used in diagnosis, but they are less sensitive and more time-consuming than the wet mount and, therefore, are not recommended.[72] Culture techniques for trichomonads are highly specific and more sensitive than the wet mount, but they are not useful in rapid diagnosis because up to 48 hours or longer is necessary for growth. Cultures may be necessary, however, to confirm the diagnosis in the absence of a positive wet mount, or to determine antimicrobial susceptibility in intractable cases.[13,67–72,76] Recently, several rapid diagnostic tests that use monoclonal antibody or DNA probe techniques have been shown to have high sensitivities and specificities in the diagnosis of trichomoniasis. Such tests could replace more traditional diagnostic tests in the near future.[71,72]

In males, demonstration of trichomonads in urethral specimens or urine sediment by wet mount is difficult, and diagnosis depends largely on culture. Specimens from males should be taken prior to first voiding, as the small number of trichomonads in males may be reduced by micturition.[13,70–72]

▶ TREATMENT: Trichomoniasis

Metronidazole is the only antimicrobial agent available in the United States that is consistently effective in *T. vaginalis* infections. In only a few cases have *T. vaginalis* isolates been resistant to standard metronidazole doses. In these instances, longer courses of therapy or doses higher than those routinely recommended as initial therapy usually produces a cure.[1,67,68,70–75,77]

Table 115–7 provides treatment recommendations for *Trichomonas* infections.[1] The standard therapy for trichomoniasis is metronidazole 2 g orally as a single dose; cure rates are comparable to the recommended alternative regimen of 500 mg twice daily for 7 days. When sexual partners are treated simultaneously, cure rates greater than 95% are reported.[13,68] If sexual partners are not treated concurrently, cure rates are in the range of 80% to 90%.[68–70,78] In limited clinical testing, single metronidazole doses of less than 1.5 g are associated with high failure rates.[71]

Advantages of single-dose therapy over the multidose alternative regimen include better patient compliance, lower total dose, lower cost, and shorter exposure of the patient's GI and urogenital anaerobic bacterial flora to the drug. As a result of the latter, the likelihood of developing pseudomembranous colitis or symptomatic candidal vulvovaginitis is decreased.[68,69,71,76,77] Because high doses of metronidazole have mutagenic effects in bacteria and oncogenic effects in mice, a reduced time of exposure in humans may be beneficial. There is no conclusive evidence for either of these effects in humans after short-term therapy with recommended doses.[69,71,75,76] Gastrointestinal complaints (e.g., anorexia, nausea, vomiting, diarrhea) are more common with the single 2-g dose, occurring in 5% to 10% of treated patients. Some patients also complain of a bitter metallic taste in the mouth. Patients intolerant of the single 2-g dose because of GI adverse effects usually tolerate the multidose regimen.[68–72,74,79]

To achieve maximal cure rates and prevent relapse with the single 2-g dose of metronidazole, simultaneous treatment of infected sexual partners is necessary. In women treated with the alternative 7-day course, however, relapse rates are not appreciably different regardless of whether or not sexual partners are treated. It is speculated that in men spontaneous resolution of trichomonal infection or a reduction in the number of trichomonads below the inoculum necessary to transmit disease may occur during the 7 days of a female's therapy.[68,70–72]

Patients who fail to respond to an initial course of metronidazole therapy usually respond to a second course. In these cases, sexual partners also should be retreated. For some *T. vaginalis* strains, higher dosages (2–7.5 g daily for 3 to 14 days) are effective. Good response

TABLE 115–7. Treatment of Trichomoniasis

Type	Recommended Regimen[a]	Alternative Regimen
Symptomatic and asymptomatic infections	Metronidazole 2 g po in a single dose[b]	Metronidazole 500 mg po twice daily for 7 days[c]
Treatment in pregnancy	Metronidazole 2 g po in a single dose[d]	
Neonatal infections[e]	Metronidazole 10–30 mg/kg daily for 5 to 8 days	

[a]Recommendations are those of the CDC.
[b]Treatment failures should be treated with metronidazole 500 mg po twice daily for 7 days. Persistent failures should be managed in consultation with an expert. Metronidazole 2 g po daily for 3 to 5 days is effective in patients infected with *T. vaginalis* strains that are mildly resistant to metronidazole, but experience is limited; higher doses also have been used.
[c]Metronidazole labeling approved by the FDA does not include this regimen. Dosage regimens for treatment of trichomoniasis included in the product labeling are the single 2-g dose; 250 mg three times daily for 7 days; and 375 mg twice daily for 7 days. The 250-mg and 375-mg dosage regimens are currently not included in the CDC recommendations.
[d]Metronidazole is contraindicated in the first trimester of pregnancy. While the CDC recommends a single 2-g dose for treatment during pregnancy, a 7-day regimen is preferred by some experts because it produces lower peak serum drug concentrations.
[e]Only infants with symptomatic trichomoniasis or with urogenital trichomonal colonization that persists beyond the fourth week of life.

rates also are reported for metronidazole 2–3 g orally plus either a single 500-mg tablet administered intravaginally or intravaginal metronidazole gel (0.75%) for 7 to 14 days.[71,80] One report described the successful use of intravaginal nonoxynol-9 in treating a trichomonal infection resistant to metronidazole. Use of IV metronidazole may be warranted for rare cases of intolerance to oral medication or infections resistant to high-dose oral metronidazole.[68,70,72,74,76,77,79]

Patients taking metronidazole should be instructed to avoid alcohol ingestion during therapy and for 1 to 2 days after completion of therapy because of a possible disulfiram-like effect. Metronidazole can potentiate the hypoprothrombinemic effects of warfarin, but a clinically significant effect is unlikely with single-dose regimens. Because metronidazole is secreted in breast milk, it is recommended that breast feeding be interrupted for at least 24 hours after maternal ingestion of a single 2-g dose.[1,70,75–77,79]

No consensus exists on treating *Trichomonas* infections in pregnant women. Although metronidazole is contraindicated during the first trimester of pregnancy (based on FDA-approved labeling) and some experts recommend avoiding its use throughout pregnancy, other experts advocate its use during any stage of pregnancy because of the potential adverse pregnancy outcomes associated with trichomoniasis (e.g., premature rupture of membranes, neonatal respiratory tract infection, low-birth-weight infants).[1,71,74,75] Metronidazole easily crosses the placenta, and fetal blood levels are comparable to maternal levels. However, a clear association between teratogenic effects and maternal ingestion during pregnancy has not been shown.[1,68–70,75,76,79]

Various local therapies for trichomoniasis have been proposed, particularly for pregnant patients. Clotrimazole vaginal suppositories, 100 mg at bedtime for 1 to 2 weeks, relieve symptoms in many women and produce cure rates of 50% or greater.[68,72–74,76] An alternative therapy is gentle douching with either a diluted solution of vinegar or a 1% zinc sulfate solution until symptoms improve, then less frequently thereafter. This therapy generally provides some symptomatic improvement but few cures. Although once recommended, povidone-iodine douches should be avoided during pregnancy because of the risk of fetal thyroid suppression.[70,71,74,75]

Several 5-nitroimidazole antibiotics related to metronidazole (tinidazole, nimorazole, ornidazole, carnidazole) are being investigated worldwide for the treatment of trichomoniasis. Unfortunately, none of these agents differs significantly from metronidazole in terms of efficacy or toxicity against metronidazole-susceptible strains of *T. vaginalis*. Tinidazole is reported to have produced cures in a small percentage of metronidazole-resistant infections, but overall, cross-resistance between metronidazole and other 5-nitroimidazoles is high.[69–71,74,77,79]

EVALUATION OF THERAPEUTIC OUTCOMES

Followup is considered unnecessary in patients who become asymptomatic after treatment with metronidazole. When patients remain symptomatic, it is important to determine if reinfection has occurred. In these cases, a repeat course of therapy, as well as identification and treatment or retreatment of infected sexual partners, is recommended. In situations in which reinfection can be excluded, a relative resistance to metronidazole should be assumed and an alternative, multidose metronidazole regimen should be prescribed. Culture and sensitivity are warranted for infections unresponsive to alternative metronidazole regimens.

HUMAN PAPILLOMAVIRUS AND OTHER SEXUALLY TRANSMITTED DISEASES

Several STDs other than those previously discussed occur with varying frequency in the United States and throughout the world. While an in-depth discussion of these diseases is beyond the scope of this chapter, Table 115–8 lists recommended treatment regimens.[1] Of notable importance among these other STDs, however, is genital human papillomavirus (HPV) infection, the most common viral STD in the United States. More than 83 HPV types have been characterized by genomic makeup, with more than 25 types associated with genital tract lesions. Of these, types 6 and 11 are most commonly associated with the development of low-grade dysplasia manifested as exophytic genital warts. In most individuals, genital infection with HPV is subclinical and patients with visible acuminate warts represent less than 1% of all infected individuals. When present, genital warts can be large and multifocal, producing variable degrees of discomfort. Based on HPV DNA detection methods, the majority of warts will regress spontaneously within 1 to 2 years of their initial appearance. However, reinfection is common in young, sexually active populations.[1,80–82]

Infection with several HPV types (i.e., types 16, 18, 45, and 56) is considered the major risk factor for the development of cervical neoplasia, the second most common cancer in women worldwide. While epidemiologic, virologic, and clinical data strongly support this association, HPV infection alone is insufficient to cause cervical cancer development because only a small percentage of infected women develop the disease. It appears that the interplay of host immune defenses, genetic factors, and infection with HPV types containing a more aggressive variant all contribute to the risk of developing cervical neoplasia.[1,80–82]

The Pap smear is the most cost-effective and frequently used diagnostic test for HPV. It can detect abnormal cytology in patients with clinical manifestations and those with subclinical disease (i.e., no overt condylomata). Unfortunately, the Pap smear is unable to detect latent HPV infection. No consensus exists on the best approach to treating patients with genital HPV infection, particularly because most cases appear to be transient with spontaneous regression of lesions. A variety of treatments are recommended (Table 115–8), but none is clearly superior to the others. Treatment generally is directed toward patients with manifestations of genital warts, with the goal of removing or destroying these lesions and grossly infected surrounding tissue. Because such treatment neither stops viral expression in surrounding tissue nor eliminates viral latency, recurrence of lesions is not uncommon. The development of a vaccine against HPV is a major focus of research related to genital HPV infections. An important consideration in vaccine development is the need to incorporate viral particles from multiple HPV types because there is limited cross-protection between the different HPV types known to cause genital infections. Current research emphasis is on the development of polyvalent vaccines that would offer protection against the most common types of HPV as well as those types known to be associated with cervical cancer. Additionally, therapeutic vaccines aimed at either suppressing replicating virus or reversing neoplastic transformation in infected individuals are being evaluated.[1,80–82]

CONCLUSIONS

More than 20 different diseases have been identified for which sexual transmission is epidemiologically important. For most STDs, curative

TABLE 115–8. Treatment Regimens for Miscellaneous Sexually Transmitted Diseases

Infection	Recommended Regimen[a]	Alternative Regimen
Chancroid (*Haemophilus ducreyi*)	Azithromycin 1 g po in a single dose *or* Ceftriaxone 250 mg IM in a single dose *or* Ciprofloxacin 500 mg po twice daily for 3 days[b] *or* Erythromycin base 500 mg po four times daily for 7 days	
Lymphogranuloma venereum	Doxycycline 100 mg po twice daily for 21 days	Erythromycin base 500 mg po four times daily for 21 days
Human papillomavirus (HPV) infection	*Provider-Administered Therapies*	
External genital warts	Cryotherapy (e.g., liquid nitrogen or cryoprobe) *or* Podophyllin 10% to 25% in compound tincture of benzoin applied to lesions; repeat weekly if necessary[c,d] *or* Trichloroacetic acid (TCA) 80% to 90% or bichloroacetic acid (BCA) 80% to 90% applied to warts; repeat weekly if necessary *or* Surgical removal (tangential scissor excision, tangential shave excision, curettage, or electrosurgery)	Intralesional interferon or laser surgery
	Patient-Applied Therapies	
	Podofilox 0.5% solution or gel applied twice daily for 3 days, followed by 4 days of no therapy; cycle is repeated as necessary for a total of four cycles[c,d,e] *or* Imiquimod 5% cream applied at bedtime three times weekly for up to 16 weeks[c]	
Vaginal and anal warts	Cryotherapy with liquid nitrogen *or* TCA or BCA 80% to 90% as for external HPV warts *or* Podophyllin 10% to 25% in compound tincture of benzoin applied at weekly intervals (*not* for anal warts)[c,d,f] *or* Surgical removal (*not* for vaginal warts)	

[a]Recommendations are those of the CDC.
[b]Ciprofloxacin is contraindicated for pregnant and lactating women and for persons aged younger than 18 years of age.
[c]Safety during pregnancy is not established.
[d]Some experts recommend washing podophyllin off after 1 to 4 hours to minimize local irritation.
[e]Genital warts only.
[f]Some experts caution against vaginal use because of potential systemic absorption; care must be taken to ensure that the treated area is dry before removing the speculum.

drug therapies are available; however, therapeutic approaches to viral STDs, such as genital herpes, provide only palliation and suppression of symptoms. Technologic advances in laboratory medicine have resulted in improved and more rapid diagnostic capabilities for many STDs. These advances are of particular importance for individuals with undiagnosed, asymptomatic disease who comprise a vast reservoir for continued disease transmission. Sexually active persons can reduce their risk of transmitting or acquiring an STD by avoidance of unsafe sexual practices, maintaining a mutually monogamous sexual relationship, or proper use of physical and chemical barriers during intercourse. In the future, vaccines providing protection from common STDs may have a significant effect on reducing the incidence of these infections.

▶ PRINCIPLES OF PHARMACOTHERAPY

- STDs are the most common infectious diseases in the United States, with nearly two-thirds of all cases occurring in individuals younger than 25 years of age.

- Individuals diagnosed with one STD are at a high risk of having a second or third coincident STD.
- For hormonal and anatomic reasons, STDs generally are more easily transmitted to and more difficult to diagnose in women. Similarly, serious or life-threatening complications of undiagnosed or inadequately treated STDs are much more likely to occur in women, including pelvic inflammatory disease, infertility, ectopic pregnancy, and cervical cancer.
- A high percentage of cases of many STDs are asymptomatic or minimally symptomatic, which adds to the difficulty in controlling their transmission.
- With the exception of viral STDs, such as genital herpes, HPV, or HIV, most STDs are easily cured with available antibiotics.
- The CDC guidelines for treatment of STDs should be followed (available on the Internet at www.cdc.gov).
- Single-dose therapies are preferred for the treatment of STDs to improve patient compliance, but they may not be economically feasible in some settings.
- Treatment failures for most STDs are generally a result of reinfection or noncompliance with multidose antibiotic regimens rather than a lack of efficacy of recommended regimens.
- Infection with many common STDs appears to facilitate the transmission of HIV.
- Other than abstinence or a monogamous sexual relationship between two uninfected individuals, barrier methods of contraception, such as latex condoms, diaphragms, and spermicides, offer the only available methods for providing some degree of protection from transmission of some STDs.

REFERENCES

1. Anonymous. 1998 Guidelines for treatment of sexually transmitted diseases. MMWR Morb Mortal Wkly Rep 1998;47(RR-1):1–116.
2. Holmes KK, Handsfield HH. Sexually transmitted diseases: Overview and clinical approach. In: Fauci AS, Braunwald E, Isselbacher KJ, et al., eds. Harrison's Principles of Internal Medicine, 14th ed. New York, McGraw-Hill, 1998:801–812.
3. Braverman PK. Sexually transmitted diseases in adolescents. Med Clin North Am 2000;84:869–889.
4. Handsfield HH. Sex, science, and society: A look at sexually transmitted diseases. Postgrad Med 1997;101:268–273, 277–278.
5. Adimora AA, Hamilton H, Holmes KK, Sparling PF. Sexually Transmitted Diseases, 2nd ed., Companion Handbook. New York, McGraw-Hill, 1994:1–9.
6. McCree DH. The use of condoms and spermicides in preventing STDs. Pharm Times 1996;62(5):85, 88, 92–94, 97, 99.
7. Gilliam ML, Derman RJ. Barrier methods of contraception. Obstet Gynecol Clin North Am 2000;27:841–858.
8. Kelaghan J. Physical barrier methods: Acceptance, use and effectiveness. In: Stanberry LR, Bernstein DI, eds. Sexually Transmitted Diseases: Vaccines, Prevention and Control. New York, Academic Press, 2000:139–148.
9. Anonymous. Summary of notifiable diseases, United States, 1998. MMWR Morb Mortal Wkly Rep 1999;47(53):1–94.
10. Sparling PF, Handsfield HH. *Neisseria gonorrhoeae*. In: Mandell GL, Bennett JE, Dolin R, eds. Principles and Practice of Infectious Diseases, 5th ed. Philadelphia, Churchill Livingstone, 2000:2242–2257.
11. Emmert DH, Kirchner JT. Sexually transmitted diseases in women: Gonorrhea and syphilis. Postgrad Med 2000;107:181–197.
12. Siegel MA. Syphilis and gonorrhea. Dent Clin North Am 1996;40: 369–383.
13. Anderson JR. Genital tract infections in women. Med Clin North Am 1995;79:1271–1298.
14. Woods GL. Update on laboratory diagnosis of sexually transmitted diseases. Clin Lab Med 1995;15:665–684.
15. Koumans EH, Johnson RE, Knapp JS, St. Louis ME. Laboratory testing for *Neisseria gonorrhoeae* by recently introduced nonculture tests: A performance review with clinical and public health considerations. Clin Infect Dis 1998:27:1171–1180.
16. Mahony JB. Multiplex polymerase chain reaction for the diagnosis of sexually transmitted diseases. Clin Lab Med 1996;16:61–71.
17. Moran JS, Levine WC. Drugs of choice for the treatment of uncomplicated gonococcal infections. Clin Infect Dis 1995;20(suppl 1):S47–S65.
18. Bignell C. Antibiotic treatment of gonorrhoea—Clinical evidence for choice. Genitourin Med 1996;72:315–320.
19. Fox KK, Knapp JS, Holmes KK, et al. Antimicrobial resistance in *Neisseria gonorrhoeae* in the United States, 1988–1994: The emergence of decreased susceptibility to the fluoroquinolones. J Infect Dis 1997;175:1396–1403.
20. Hammerschlag MR. Neonatal conjunctivitis. Pediatr Ann 1993;22: 346–351.
21. O'Hara MA. Ophthalmia neonatorum. Pediatr Clin North Am 1993;40: 715–725.
22. Smith J, Finn A. Antimicrobial prophylaxis. Arch Dis Child 1999;80: 388–392.
23. Singh AE, Romanowski B. Syphilis: Review with emphasis on clinical, epidemiologic, and some biologic features. Clin Microbiol Rev 1999; 12:187–209.
24. Tramont EC. Syphilis in adults: From Christopher Columbus to Sir Alexander Fleming to AIDS. Clin Infect Dis 1995;21:1361–1371.
25. Goens JL, Janniger CK, de Wolf K. Dermatologic and systemic manifestations of syphilis. Am Fam Physician 1994;50:1013–1020.
26. Flores JL. Syphilis—A tale of twisted treponemes. West J Med 1995;163: 552–559.
27. Anonymous. Syphilis. USP DI Update (Vols I, II). Rockville, MD, The United States Pharmacopeial Convention, 1997:434–444.
28. van Voorst Vader PC. Syphilis management and treatment. Dermatol Clin 1998;16:699–711.
29. Birnbaum NR, Goldschmidt RH, Buffett WO. Resolving the common clinical dilemmas of syphilis. Am Fam Physician 1999;59:2233–2240.
30. Wicher K, Horowitz HW, Wicher V. Laboratory methods of diagnosis of syphilis for the beginning of the third millennium. Microbes Infect 1999;1:1035–1049.
31. Clyne B, Jerrard DA. Syphilis testing. J Emerg Med 2000;18:361–367.
32. Kirchner JT, Emmert DH. Sexually transmitted diseases in women: *Chlamydia trachomatis* and herpes simplex infections. Postgrad Med 2000:107:55–58, 61–65.
33. Jones RB, Batteiger BE. *Chlamydia trachomatis* (trachoma, perinatal infections, lymphogranuloma venereum, and other genital infections). In: Mandell GL, Bennett JE, Dolin R, eds. Principles and Practice of Infectious Diseases, 5th ed. Philadelphia, Churchill Livingstone, 2000:1989–2004.
34. Black CM. Current methods of laboratory diagnosis of *Chlamydia trachomatis* infections. Clin Microbiol Rev 1997;10:160–184.
35. Weinstock H, Dean D, Bolan G. *Chlamydia trachomatis* infections. Infect Dis Clin North Am 1994;8:797–819.
36. Heath CB, Heath JM. Chlamydia trachomatis infection update. Am Fam Physician 1995;52:1455–1461.
37. Morton RS, Kinghorn GR. Genitourinary chlamydial infection: A reappraisal and hypothesis. Int J STD AIDS 1999;10:765–775.
38. Anonymous. National guideline for the management of *Chlamydia trachomatis* genital tract infection. Sex Transm Infect 1999;75(suppl 1): 4S–8S.
39. Schubiner H, LeBar W. *Chlamydia trachomatis* infections in women. Curr Probl Dermatol 1996;24:25–33.
40. LeBar WD. Keeping up with the new technology: New approaches to diagnosis of *Chlamydia* infection. Clin Chem 1996;42:809–812.
41. Skolnik NS. Screening for *Chlamydia trachomatis* infection. Am Fam Physician 1995;51:821–826.
42. Nickel P, Naher H. Nongonococcal urethritis. Curr Probl Dermatol 1996;24:97–104.

43. Nuovo J, Melnikow J, Paliescheskey M, et al. Cost-effectiveness analysis of five different antibiotic regimens for the treatment of uncomplicated *Chlamydia trachomatis* cervicitis. J Am Board Fam Pract 1995;8:7–16.
44. Anonymous. Drugs for sexually transmitted infections. Med Lett Drugs Ther 1999;41:85–90.
45. Conant MA, Berger TG, Coates TJ, et al. Genital herpes: An integrated approach to management. J Am Acad Dermatol 1996;35:601–605.
46. Corey L. Herpes simplex virus. In: Mandell GL, Bennett JE, Dolin R, eds. Principles and Practice of Infectious Diseases, 5th ed. Philadelphia, Churchill Livingstone, 2000:1564–1580.
47. Marques AR, Straus SE. Herpes simplex Type 2 infections—An update. Dis Mon 2000;46:327–359.
48. Sacks SL. Improving the management of genital herpes. Hosp Pract (Off Ed) 1999;34(2):41–49.
49. Mertz GJ. Epidemiology of genital herpes infections. Infect Dis Clin North Am 1993;7:825–839.
50. White C, Wardropper AG. Genital herpes simplex infection in women. Clin Dermatol 1997;15:81–91.
51. Clark JL, Tatum NO, Noble SL. Management of genital herpes. Am Fam Physician 1995;51:175–182.
52. Mertz GJ. Management of genital herpes. Adv Exp Med Biol 1996;394: 1–10.
53. McDonald LL, Stites PC, Buntin DM. Sexually transmitted diseases update. Dermatol Clin 1997;15:221–232.
54. Ashley RL, Wald A. Genital herpes: Review of the epidemiologic and potential use of type-specific serology. Clin Microbiol Rev 1999;12:1–8.
55. Leung DT, Sacks SL. Current recommendations for the treatment of genital herpes. Drugs 2000;60:1329–1352.
56. Geers TA, Isada CM. Update on antiviral therapy for genital herpes infection. Cleve Clin J Med 2000;67:567–573.
57. Hoffman IF, Schmitz JL. Genital ulcer disease: Management in the HIV era. Postgrad Med 1995;98(3):67–70, 73–76, 79–82.
58. Thin RN. Diagnosis of genital herpes simplex infections. Curr Probl Dermatol 1996;24:50–56.
59. Blanchier H, Huraux J-M, Huraux-Rendu C, Sainte-Croix le Baleur A. Genital herpes and pregnancy—Preventive measures. Eur J Obstet Gynecol Reprod Biol 1994;53:33–38.
60. Whitley RJ. Neonatal herpes simplex virus infections. J Med Virol 1993;(suppl 1):13–21.
61. Scott LL. Prevention of perinatal herpes: Prophylactic antiviral therapy? Clin Obstet Gynecol 1999;42:134–148.
62. McKenzie R, Straus SE. Therapeutic immunization for recurrent herpes simplex virus infections. Adv Exp Med Biol 1996;394:67–83.
63. Adimora A, Sparling PF, Cohen MS. Vaccines for classic sexually transmitted diseases. Infect Dis Clin North Am 1994;8:859–876.
64. Krause PR, Straus SE. Herpesvirus vaccines: Development, controversies, and applications. Infect Dis Clin North Am 1999;13:61–81.
65. Beutner KR. Genital herpes. Curr Probl Dermatol 1996;24:132–139.
66. Wald A, Corey L, Cone R, et al. Frequent genital herpes simplex virus 2 shedding in immunocompetent women: Effect of acyclovir treatment. J Clin Invest 1997;99:1092–1097.
67. Krieger JN. Trichomoniasis in men: Old issues and new data. Sex Transm Dis 1995;22:83–96.
68. Heine P, McGregor JA. *Trichomonas vaginalis:* A reemerging pathogen. Clin Obstet Gynecol 1993;36:137–144.
69. Moldwin RM. Sexually transmitted protozoal infections. Urol Clin North Am 1992;19:93–101.
70. Adimora AA, Hamilton H, Holmes KK, Sparling PF. Sexually Transmitted Diseases, 2nd ed, Companion Handbook. New York, McGraw-Hill, 1994:212–222.
71. Rein MF. *Trichomonas vaginalis*. In: Mandell GL, Bennett JE, Dolin R, eds. Principles and Practice of Infectious Diseases, 5th ed. Philadelphia, Churchill Livingstone, 2000:2894–2898.
72. Petrin D, Delgaty K, Bhattt R, Garber G. Clinical and microbiological aspects of *Trichomonas vaginalis*. Clin Microbiol Rev 1998;11:300–317.
73. Goode MA, Grauer K, Gums JG. Infectious vaginitis: Selecting therapy and preventing recurrence. Postgrad Med 1994;96(6):85–88, 91, 93–96, 98.
74. Carr PL, Felsenstein D, Friedman RH. Evaluation and management of vaginitis. J Gen Intern Med 1998;13:335–346.
75. Murphy PA, Jones E. Use of oral metronidazole in pregnancy: Risks, benefits, and practice guidelines. J Nurse Midwif 1994;39:214–220.
76. Sweet RL, Gibbs RS. Infectious Diseases of the Female Genital Tract, 3rd ed. Baltimore, William & Wilkins, 1995:343–347.
77. Sobel JD. Vaginitis. N Engl J Med 1997;337:1896–1903.
78. Spence MR, Harwell TS, Davies MC, Smith JL. The minimum single oral metronidazole dose for treating trichomoniasis: A randomized, blinded study. Obstet Gynecol 1997;89:699–703.
79. Schwebke JR. Metronidazole: Utilization in the obstetric and gynecologic patient. Sex Transm Dis 1995;22:370–376.
80. Carr J, Gyorfi T. Human papillomavirus: Epidemiology, transmission, and pathogenesis. Clin Lab Med 2000;20:235–255.
81. Sedlacek TV. Advances in the diagnosis and treatment of human papillomavirus infections. Clin Obstet Gynecol 1999;42:206–220.
82. Kaufman RH, Adam E, Vonka V. Human papillomavirus infection and cervical carcinoma. Clin Obstet Gynecol 2000;43:363–380.

116

BONE AND JOINT INFECTIONS

Edward P. Armstrong

Bone and joint infections are comprised of two disease processes known respectively as osteomyelitis and septic, or infectious, arthritis. As such, they are unique and separate infectious entities, with different signs and symptoms and infecting organisms. Introduction of oral antibiotic therapy has dramatically impacted antibiotic regimens used to treat these diseases. In spite of advances in therapy, however, these infections continue to cause significant morbidity from residual damage and chronic recurring infections. Emphasis on initiating antibiotic therapy as soon as possible is important in reducing long-term complications.

EPIDEMIOLOGY

Osteomyelitis is generally an uncommon disease. One classic publication reported that 247 patients had osteomyelitis in a prominent American teaching hospital during a 4-year period.[1] Acute osteomyelitis has an estimated annual incidence of 0.1 per 1,000 children.[2] Osteomyelitis caused by contiguous spread, including postoperative, direct puncture, and that associated with adjacent soft-tissue infections, comprises 47% of infections. Hematogenous osteomyelitis comprises 19% of infections, and osteomyelitis occurring in patients with significant peripheral vascular disease comprises 34% of infections. A review of osteomyelitis cases based on duration of disease shows that acute disease constitutes 56% of patients and that chronic osteomyelitis, defined as having a previous hospitalization for the same infection, constitutes 44% of patients.

Infectious or septic arthritis is an inflammatory reaction within the joint space. Distinct from osteomyelitis, septic arthritis is a more common disease and is known to be one of the most common causes of new cases of arthritis. One study identified 1,158 cases of septic arthritis in a 4-year period.[3] Another hospital study reported 64 children with septic arthritis during a 6-year time frame.[4]

ETIOLOGY

OSTEOMYELITIS

The most common method of classifying osteomyelitis is based on the route in which the infecting organism reaches the bone. Infection that results from spread through the bloodstream is termed *hematogenous osteomyelitis.* When the organism reaches the bone from an adjoining soft-tissue infection, it is termed *contiguous osteomyelitis.* Osteomyelitis that results from direct inoculation, such as from trauma, puncture wounds, or surgery, generally is also classified under the contiguous osteomyelitis category. Patients with peripheral vascular disease are at risk for development of osteomyelitis, and these patients are often separated into a third distinct category because of their unique management features.

Osteomyelitis may also be classified based on the duration of the disease. Acute osteomyelitis describes infections of recent onset, usually several days to 1 week, while chronic infections are those of a longer duration. Some authors describe chronic infections as those with symptoms for more than 1 month before therapy, while other authors define chronic infections as relapse of an initial infection. Yet a third system sometimes used to classify osteomyelitis has been developed.[5,6] It is a staging system based on the anatomic location of the infection (medullary or superficial) and the physiologic status of the patient (otherwise healthy, systemic immunologic compromise, local immunologic compromise). This classification system may be useful when comparing patients between different studies and attempting to categorize the severity of infection.

INFECTIOUS ARTHRITIS

Infectious arthritis may occur from many different types of microorganisms. Most infecting organisms are known to produce an infection in a single joint, termed *monarticular infections;* however, infections also may involve two or more joints.[7] As with osteomyelitis, joint infections also may be classified according to the mechanisms by which the infecting organism reaches the joint. Infectious arthritis may result from the spread of an adjacent bone infection, direct contamination of the joint space, or hematogenous dissemination. Hematogenous spread of the disease comprises the majority of infections; spread from osteomyelitis and direct inoculation are much less frequent.[8] Infectious arthritis most commonly occurs in patients older than age 16; 24% of cases occur in children 15 years of age or younger.[9]

PATHOPHYSIOLOGY

HEMATOGENOUS OSTEOMYELITIS

Hematogenous osteomyelitis is classically described as a disease of children because most cases occur in patients younger than 16 years of age.[6] Table 116–1 summarizes the primary characteristics of osteomyelitis. Less commonly, these infections occur in adults. One exception, vertebral osteomyelitis, involves the vertebrae and occurs most frequently in patients older than 50 years of age.

Unique features of the anatomy and physiology of some bones appears to predispose them to become infected.[10] The vascular structure within the long bones appears to predispose the bone for hematogenous infections to begin within the metaphyses (Fig. 116–1). The nutrient arteries of the long bones divide within the medullary canal of the bone into small arterioles.[11] These end in hairpin turns near the growth plate and flow into veins, of much wider diameter, that drain the medullary cavity. An infection in hematogenous disease is initiated within the bend of the arterioles. There is considerable slowing of blood flow passing through the hairpin turns within the arterioles and then into the wider venous structures. This sludging of blood flow allows bacteria present within the bloodstream to settle and initiate an inflammatory response. In addition to these structural features, there also appears to be less active phagocytosis within the metaphysis. After the bacteria settle in the bone, avascular

TABLE 116–1. Types of Osteomyelitis, Age Distribution, Common Sites, and Risk Factors

Type of Osteomyelitis	Typical Age (y)	Site(s) Involved	Risk Factors
Hematogenous	Younger than 1	Long bones and joints	Prematurity, umbilical catheter or venous cutdown, respiratory distress syndrome, perinatal asphyxia
	1–20	Long bones (femur, tibia, humerus)	Infection (pharyngitis, cellulitis, respiratory infections), sickle cell disease, puncture wounds to feet
	Older than 50	Vertebrae	Diabetes mellitus, blunt trauma to spine, urinary tract infection
Contiguous	Older than 50	Femur, tibia, mandible	Hip fractures, open fractures
Vascular insufficiency	Older than 50	Feet, toes	Diabetes mellitus, peripheral vascular disease, pressure sores

necrosis may occur from occlusion of the nutrient vessels and release of bacterial enzymes.

In addition to these anatomic and functional features, there is some evidence that trauma is associated with developing an infection in specific bones. Children who develop hematogenous osteomyelitis may report some type of trauma as an etiologic event. Animal data also indicate that traumatized bone is more likely to become infected than normal bone.

Once the infection is initiated, exudate begins to form within the bone, which produces increased pressure. The age of the patient largely determines the next stage in the pathophysiology. In children older than 12 to 18 months, the infection that started in the metaphysis of a long bone is prevented from spreading into the joint because of the growth plate; however, the exudate often expands laterally through the thin outer cortex of the bone and raises the loose periosteum. The periosteum is thick and not easily broken, and the resulting pus usually remains subperiosteal. If there is significant periosteal damage, a soft-tissue abscess may develop. Impairment of blood flow to the outer portion of the cortical bone may occur, producing dead bone that separates from healthy bone, termed *sequestra.* The elevated periosteum remains viable because its blood supply, derived from the overlying muscle, is unaffected. The raised periosteum will continue to produce bone; however, this new bone is now separated from the cortex because the periosteum has been raised from the infection. This new bone is termed *involucrum.*

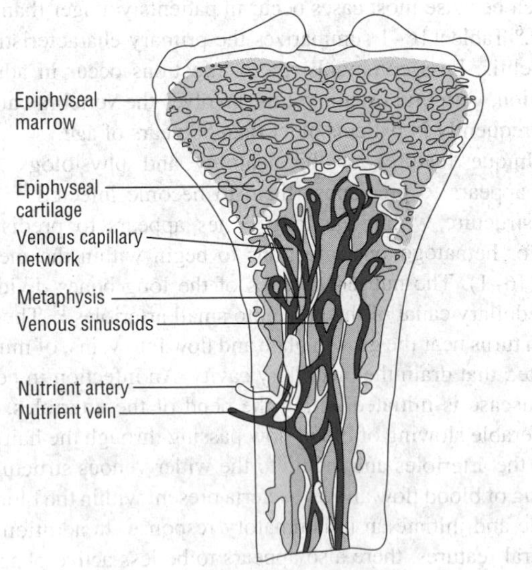

FIGURE 116–1. Cross-section of normal bone.

In adults, the periosteum is tightly bound, and the cortex is thick. These anatomic features generally cause the infections to remain intramedullary. As expected, subperiosteal abscess formations are less common in this population. The infection may spread to adjacent bone structures through the Haversian and Volkmann canals. Chronic osteomyelitis is more likely to occur if large segments of bone become avascular and necrotic.

Neonatal patients also have unique characteristics. In these patients, there are blood vessels that spread through the cortex of the metaphyses and up into the epiphyses. This enables an infection that started within the metaphyseal area to spread easily to involve the epiphyses and then into the joint. Therefore, in infants, not only can the infection spread to involve the periosteum and the shaft as in children, but the infection can also spread to involve the joint.

Hematogenous osteomyelitis also is known to have a predilection for certain bones. The specific bones most likely to be involved also depend on the age of the patient. Children most commonly develop infections within the femur, tibia, humerus, and fibula. Vertebral infections are more common in patients older than 50 years of age. Neonatal infections commonly involve multiple bones.

The bacteriology of hematogenous osteomyelitis is unique compared with osteomyelitis caused by other routes of infection. A single organism is responsible for the vast majority of hematogenous infections. *Staphylococcus aureus* is isolated from 60% to 90% of the hematogenous infections in children. In one report of children with acute osteomyelitis during a 30-year period, *S. aureus* was responsible in 76% and *Haemophilus influenzae* type b was responsible in 13% of the 46 cases for which organisms were identified.[2] Neonatal osteomyelitis has a wider spectrum in infecting organisms.[12] The three most common etiologic agents are *S. aureus,* group B streptococcus, and *Escherichia coli.* The infections from *S. aureus* and *E. coli* have been linked to complications occurring during pregnancy or delivery, and they are most frequently involved in multiple bone infections.

Vertebral osteomyelitis has several unique features. Vertebral osteomyelitis most commonly occurs in adults. The highest incidence is noted in patients in their fifties and sixties. The lumbar and thoracic regions are the locations of the majority of infections. Hematogenous infections are most likely to develop in the vascular areas near the subchondral plate region of the vertebral body. Staphylococci cause approximately 60% of these infections; however, gram-negative organisms now play a significant role. It is presumed that these gram-negative organisms, particularly *E. coli,* most likely originate within the urinary tract. *E. coli* vertebral infections have been associated with urinary tract infections, positive urine cultures, and bacteremias. *Mycobacterium tuberculosis* also is known to cause infections in the spine.[11] Skin and respiratory tract infections are other foci of infections known to lead to vertebral infections.

A unique category of osteomyelitis patients are those individuals with a history of intravenous (IV) drug abuse. More than 50% of the osteomyelitis infections in this group of patients are found in the vertebral column. Less than 20% of infections are located in either the sternoarticular or pelvic girdle. Infections are much less frequent within the extremities. A very unusual feature of osteomyelitis in the IV drug-abusing population is the spectrum of organisms. Gram-negative organisms are responsible for 88% of infections. *Pseudomonas aeruginosa,* either singly or in combination with other organisms, is cultured in 78% of all infections. *Klebsiella, Enterobacter,* and *Serratia* also may be found, but less commonly. In addition, staphylococcal and streptococcal organisms may be cultured.

Patients with sickle cell anemia and related hemoglobinopathies have a much higher rate of infection with *Salmonella* as compared to other populations.[13] *Salmonella* species are responsible for two-thirds of the infections in these patients. It is believed that bowel infarctions from the sickle cell disease may facilitate salmonellae entry into the bloodstream from the colon and spread hematogenously to the bone. Osteomyelitis in patients with sickle cell disease may occur in any bone, but it is observed to be most common in the medullary cavity of long or tubular bones. Because of the difficulty in separating bone pain during a sickle cell crisis from that of an infection, osteomyelitis may be relatively advanced in these patients when the diagnosis is made. Although salmonellae are cultured most frequently, staphylococci and other gram-negative organisms also may be isolated.

CONTIGUOUS-SPREAD OSTEOMYELITIS

This category of osteomyelitis includes those infections caused by direct entrance of organisms from a source outside of the body or progressive spread of an infection from tissue adjacent to the bone.[13] Penetrating wounds (e.g., trauma), open fractures, or various invasive orthopedic procedures may result in direct inoculation of organisms into the bone. More than 80% of cases of postoperative osteomyelitis are known to occur following open reductions of fractures. Specifically, these infections occur most commonly after internal fixation of a hip fracture or femoral or tibial shaft fracture.

Osteomyelitis secondary to an adjoining soft-tissue infection comprises another very important group of contiguous infections, and most often involves the fingers and toes. Less commonly, infections may spread from infected teeth to involve the mandible or occur secondary to sinus infections by spreading through the mucosal lining of the sinuses into the vascular system surrounding the bone.

In contrast to hematogenous osteomyelitis, which most commonly occurs in children, contiguous-spread osteomyelitis most commonly occurs in patients older than age 50. Most likely this is because of the fact that important predisposing factors, such as hip fractures, are more common in this age group.

Contiguous-spread disease has several important differences compared with hematogenous osteomyelitis. Although *S. aureus* is still the most common organism isolated, infections with multiple organisms, including gram-negative bacilli, frequently occur. *P. aeruginosa, Proteus, Streptococcus, E. coli, S. epidermidis,* and anaerobes all may be isolated. One important exception to this wide range of organisms is puncture wounds of the feet. There is a strong correlation between puncture wounds of the feet and gram-negative osteomyelitis, especially infections caused by *P. aeruginosa.*[13,14]

Patients with osteomyelitis in association with severe vascular insufficiency are extremely difficult to manage.[15] As anticipated, most of these patients have diabetes mellitus or severe atherosclerosis, and they develop their infections from contiguous-spread mechanisms. Generally, these patients are between the ages of 50 and 70 years when they develop osteomyelitis. Frequently, patients with vascular disease develop osteomyelitis in their toes and fingers, and there is usually an adjacent area of infection, such as cellulitis or dermal ulcers.

Another important characteristic of osteomyelitis in association with vascular insufficiency is the spectrum of infecting organisms. Infections in these patients almost always include multiple organisms. The mixed floral infections often include *Staphylococcus* and *Streptococcus* or the combination of *Staphylococcus, Streptococcus,* and Enterobacteriaceae. *Enterococcus* and anaerobic organisms also may be seen.

Anaerobic organisms also play a role in osteomyelitis. When anaerobes are grown from cultures, they usually are found in association with other organisms, including aerobic bacteria. The two most common predisposing factors in patients who have anaerobic osteomyelitis are previous fractures and diabetes mellitus. The anaerobic infections in association with diabetes mellitus occur almost always within the feet. *Bacteroides fragilis* and *B. melaninogenicus* comprise the majority of anaerobic isolates.

INFECTIOUS ARTHRITIS

Distinct from osteomyelitis, infectious arthritis is usually acquired by hematogenous spread.[16] The synovial tissue is very vascular and does not have a basement membrane, so organisms in the blood can easily reach the synovial fluid. Table 116–2 summarizes the characteristics of acute infectious arthritis. Some organisms, such as *Neisseria gonorrhoeae,* are especially likely to infect a joint during bacteremia. In addition, organisms also may gain access to the joint from a deep-penetrating wound, an intra-articular steroid injection, arthroscopy, prosthetic joint surgery, and contiguous osteomyelitis expansion into the joint.[3]

The risk factors associated with adult infectious arthritis (more than one factor may be present) are:

- Systemic corticosteroid use
- Preexisting arthritis
- Arthrocentesis
- Distant infection
- Diabetes mellitus
- Trauma
- Other diseases

Trauma also appears to be a risk factor in facilitating microorganism entry into the synovial space. One study found that 35% of patients with infectious arthritis had preexisting joint disease.[9] Unlike children, adults often have significant systemic diseases that predispose them to infectious arthritis, such as diabetes mellitus, immunosuppressive states (cancer, liver disease), or preexisting arthritis. Intravenous drug abusers also are prone to develop septic arthritis. Arthritis, joint trauma, and surgery are other important risk factors, because chronic inflammation or trauma makes the joint more susceptible to infection.[17] In addition, rheumatoid arthritis patients may be prone to bacterial infection because of an inherent phagocytic defect, as well as concomitant corticosteroid therapy. Hormonal factors appear to play a role in *N. gonorrhoeae* infectious arthritis. Women are more prone to develop disseminated gonococcal infections than men. The second and third trimesters of pregnancy and during menstruation appear to be the times of greatest risk for developing gonococcal bacteremia.

TABLE 116–2. Characteristics of Acute Infectious Arthritis

Feature	Finding
Peak incidence	Children younger than 16 years of age Adults older than 50 years of age
Clinical findings	Fever of 38°C–40°C (100.4°F–104°F) in children; painful swollen joint in the absence of trauma Physical exam: effusion, restriction of joint motion, tenderness and warmth of joint
Most commonly affected joints	Knee, hip, ankle, elbow, wrist, and shoulder
Laboratory findings	
Erythrocyte sedimentation rate	Elevated in 90% of cases
White blood cell count	Elevated in 30% to 60% of cases
Left shift	Seen in two-thirds of patients
Blood culture	Positive in 40% of cases
Needle aspiration of joint	Gram-stain diagnostic in 30% to 50% of cases. Synovial fluid cultures are positive in 60% to 80% of cases. Synovial fluid differential reveals 90% polymorphonuclear leukocytes. Synovial fluid glucose decreased relative to serum glucose. Lactic acid levels elevated in nongonococcal infectious arthritis, but not in gonococcal infectious arthritis

After bacteria gain access to the joint, the organisms begin to multiply and produce a persistent purulent effusion within the joint. If this joint effusion is present beyond 7 days, chronic, and sometimes irreversible, damage may occur. Purulent effusions may promote cartilage destruction by increasing leukocyte enzyme activity. In conjunction with the development of the effusion, almost all patients will develop a hot, swollen, painful joint. The proteolytic enzymes within the effusion and pressure necrosis may lead to cartilage and bone damage.

S. aureus is the single most common infecting organism; it is found in 48% of cases of nongonococcal bacterial arthritis. Streptococcal infections account for 18% of cases and gram-negative organisms are less common.[9] Overall, *E. coli* is the most common of the gram-negative organisms; however, *P. aeruginosa* is the most frequent organism in IV drug abusers.

Neonates may have infectious arthritis because of a broad range of organisms, with *S. aureus, Streptococcus,* and gram-negative organisms being most common. *S. aureus, H. influenzae* type b, and *Streptococcus* are the most common pathogens in children younger than 5 years of age. Other countries, however, may observe a lower frequency of *S. aureus* infection.[18] Within the adult population, *S. aureus* is responsible for the vast majority of nongonococcal infections. The most common cause of bacterial arthritis in adults 18–30 years of age is *N. gonorrhoeae,* which are the most common infections in women. Although less common, nonbacterial causes of osteomyelitis and septic arthritis include fungi and viruses.[19]

CLINICAL PRESENTATION

OSTEOMYELITIS

The specific signs and symptoms seen in osteomyelitis vary depending on the route by which the organism reached the bone and the age of the patient. Most patients with hematogenous osteomyelitis complain of significant tenderness of the infected area, pain, swelling, fever, chills, decreased motion, and malaise. Although this presentation is classic, some patients with hematogenous disease may only have mild tenderness and a low-grade fever. Although hematogenous neonatal osteomyelitis infections may rapidly spread to involve the joint, often there are few systemic symptoms present. A joint effusion, present in 60% to 70% of neonatal infections, decreased limb motion, and edema over the affected area may be the only signs from which to make a diagnosis.

A commonly described diagnostic dilemma is pyogenic vertebral osteomyelitis. Many patients complain of nonspecific symptoms, such as severe back pain, fever or night sweats, and weight loss. Other patients may note a gradual onset in symptoms with a possible low-grade fever and complaints of continuous back pain. The pain is typically described as being present at rest and increasing in severity with movement. Of great concern is that if the infection extends and compresses the spinal cord, neurologic symptoms may develop.[20]

Signs and symptoms of osteomyelitis caused by spread of infection from a contiguous focus depend on the precipitating cause. If the infection follows surgery or bone trauma, the symptoms of the infection are usually noted within 1 month. The most frequent symptom is simply pain in the area of infection. Less commonly, patients also may develop a fever and elevated white blood cell (WBC) count. On physical examination, a patient with contiguous-spread osteomyelitis may have an area of localized tenderness, warmth, edema, and erythema over the infected site. Patients with significant vascular insufficiency usually have local symptoms, such as pain, swelling, and redness. Less commonly, patients with vascular disease also may have a fever and elevated WBC count.

INFECTIOUS ARTHRITIS

Because the differences in the clinical presentation and microbiologic characteristics of infectious arthritis are major, it is useful to separate this disease into nongonococcal and gonococcal bacterial arthritis. Patients with nongonococcal bacterial arthritis almost always present with a fever, and 50% of patients have an elevated WBC count. The average initial synovial WBC count is 100,000 cells/mm^3 or greater in nongonococcal bacterial disease.

Nongonococcal bacterial arthritis almost always involves only a single joint.[7] The knee is the most commonly involved joint, but infections also may occur in the shoulder, wrist, hip, ankle, interphalangeal, and elbow joints. Usually, the initial focus of infection that acted as the source for bacterial or microbial entrance can be identified. Common routes for bacterial entrance include infections of the respiratory tract, skin, and urinary tract. Blood cultures are important in these patients because they may be positive in 50% of patients.

In contrast to the other forms of infectious arthritis, the most frequent initial sign of disseminated gonococcal infections is a migratory polyarthralgia.[21] In addition, two-thirds of patients also complain of fever, dermatitis, and tenosynovitis (inflammation of the tendon sheath). Unique to gonococcal disease, 50% of these patients have polyarthritis. Small papules on the trunk or extremities are the most frequent skin lesions seen in these infections, but only 30% to 40% of patients with disseminated gonococcal infection present with the classic hot, swollen, purulent joint. The mean synovial WBC count in gonococcal arthritis is usually 50,000 cells/mm^3 or more.

Another type of infectious arthritis occurs following prosthetic joint surgery. Because joint operations are being performed more frequently, more cases are now occurring. Fortunately, the risk of developing a joint infection following surgery is low. Because these are clean operations, the risk of developing a postoperative infection is estimated to be less than 5%. Infections are observed, however, more commonly after surgical revision of prosthetic joints. As anticipated, the candidates for this surgical procedure are usually elderly and have a history of either osteoarthritis or rheumatoid arthritis. When patients develop infectious arthritis following joint surgery, they often state that they have experienced some pain in the area. With an infection present, their erythrocyte sedimentation rate is usually elevated, although a leukocytosis often is absent. Infections that result from postoperative contamination usually become apparent within 1 year of surgery. If an infection occurs after this period, it is usually the result of hematogenous spread rather than from the surgery itself. Staphylococci continue to comprise the most common infecting organisms. *S. epidermidis* is responsible for 40% of prosthetic joint infections, and *S. aureus* is responsible for 20% of infections. Multiple organisms and anaerobic bacteria, however, also may be seen in some infections.

RADIOLOGIC AND LABORATORY TESTS

The evaluation of a patient who may potentially have osteomyelitis has several unusual aspects. Radiographs of the involved area should be obtained; however, bone changes characteristic of osteomyelitis are not seen for at least 10 to 14 days after the onset of the infection.[22] Radiologists may note soft-tissue swelling before any bone changes become obvious. Bone lesions do not appear on roentgenogram films until 10 days after infection because more than 50% of the bone matrix must be removed before the lesions can be detected. As an aide to improve the diagnosis, bone scanning is commonly used.[23] Technetium and gallium scanning may be positive as early as 1 day after the onset of symptoms, well before any radiographic changes may be seen.

Despite the seriousness of osteomyelitis, often there are few laboratory abnormalities. Often, the erythrocyte sedimentation rate and the WBC count are the only laboratory abnormalities. The degree of abnormality of these two laboratory findings does not correlate with the disease outcome; however, they are useful for monitoring therapy.

When a clinical assessment of osteomyelitis is suspected, it is important to establish a bacteriologic diagnosis by culture of the infected bone. Accurate culture information is especially important as a guide for treatment of osteomyelitis. Bone aspiration is valuable in determining an accurate bacteriologic diagnosis. In addition, performing a bone aspiration determines whether or not there is an abscess present. If an abscess is located, the pus is cultured and a Gram stain is performed. If an abscess is found, the fluid needs to be drained and cultured. Aspirates of subperiosteal pus or metaphyseal fluid yield a pathogen in 70% of cases. Cultures should be done for both aerobic and anaerobic bacteria. A Gram stain of the aspirate may be useful in initiating empiric antibiotic therapy. This allows a more appropriate choice of antibiotics from the first day of therapy, rather than waiting several days while culture results are pending.

If a specimen is obtained from a previously undrained or unopened wound abscess, the pathogen usually can be identified. In chronic osteomyelitis, however, identification may be more difficult. Open wounds and draining sinuses frequently are contaminated with other organisms and, thus, provide inaccurate culture information. Therefore, because of the inaccuracies with sinus tract cultures, they cannot be relied on to reflect the pathogen. Cultures of loculated pus aspirates in the area of orthopedic devices removed from infected bone can be trusted, however, to identify the infecting organism. The preferable time to obtain culture material in a patient with chronic draining sinus is at the time of open surgical débridement.

In addition to performing cultures from the involved bone, it also is important to obtain cultures from any site believed to be the source of a bacteremia. It also is important to obtain blood cultures. Approximately 50% of patients with hematogenous osteomyelitis will have positive blood cultures.

When evaluating the possibility of a patient having infectious arthritis, immediate joint aspiration with subsequent analysis of the synovial fluid is extremely important. The presence of purulent fluid usually indicates the presence of a septic joint. The synovial fluid WBC count is usually 50,000–200,000 cells/mm^3 when an infection is present. Approximately half of the patients with an infected joint have a low synovial glucose level, usually less than 40 mg/dL.

Gram stains of joint fluid demonstrate bacteria in 50% of patients with septic arthritis; however, such stains may be positive in only 25% of patients with gonococcal arthritis infections. Synovial fluid cultures usually are positive in patients with nongonococcal infections. Both blood and joint fluid should be cultured aerobically and anaerobically in a patient suspected of having an infected joint. Blood cultures are positive in one-half of patients with nongonococcal infections, but in only 20% of those with gonococcal infections. Pharyngeal, rectal, cervical, or urethral smears and cultures should be performed if a disseminated gonococcal infection is considered. As with osteomyelitis, most patients will have an elevated erythrocyte sedimentation rate.

Radiographs of infected joints often reveal distention of the joint capsule with soft-tissue swelling in the adjacent space. Magnetic resonance imaging may be helpful in identifying an infected hip. In patients who have developed an infected prosthetic joint, loosening of the prosthesis may be seen radiographically.

▶ TREATMENT: Bone and Joint Infections

DESIRED OUTCOME

The goals of treatment are resolution of the infection and prevention of long-term sequelae. The ultimate outcome of osteomyelitis depends on the acute or chronic nature of the disease and how rapidly appropriate therapy is initiated. Patients with acute osteomyelitis have the best prognosis. Cure rates exceeding 80% may be expected for patients with acute osteomyelitis who have surgery as indicated and received injectable antibiotics for 4 to 6 weeks.

In contrast, patients with chronic osteomyelitis have a much poorer prognosis.[24] Dead bone and other necrotic material from the infection act as a bacterial reservoir and make the infection very difficult to eliminate. Adequate surgical débridement to remove all the dead bone and necrotic material combined with prolonged administration of antibiotics provide the best chance to obtain a cure. The inability to remove all the dead bone may allow residual infection and require suppressive antibiotics to control the infection.

In comparison, many patients who develop infectious arthritis recover with no long-term sequelae. Gonococcal arthritis usually resolves rapidly with antibiotics; however, patients with staphylococcal arthritis have a higher incidence of joint damage. Individuals at greatest risk for long-term sequelae are those patients who have symptoms present for more than 7 days before starting therapy, infections occurring within the hip joint, and infections caused by gram-negative organisms. Common, long-term residual effects following infectious arthritis are limited joint motion and persistent pain. Shortening of the affected extremity is another well-known complication. More than half the children who subsequently developed residual joint damage were believed normal at the time of hospital discharge.

GENERAL APPROACH TO TREATMENT

Following completion of the steps needed to determine the infecting organism, the most important treatment modality of acute osteomyelitis is the administration of appropriate antibiotics in adequate doses for a sufficient length of time. It is important to stress that early antibiotic therapy may avoid the need for surgery.[25] A delay in treatment may allow bone necrosis to occur and make eradication of the infection much more difficult. In these patients, recurrent exacerbations of the infection may result if all necrotic tissue is not removed surgically and all microorganisms eliminated.

If a patient with hematogenous osteomyelitis does not respond by having a decrease in fever, local swelling, redness, and pain following the initiation of adequate antibiotic therapy, the patient should undergo surgical débridement of the infected area. It is important to emphasize the priority of starting antibiotics immediately after the cultures have been obtained. No treatment failures have been reported if injectable antibiotics were started within 48 hours from the onset of symptoms in children with osteomyelitis.

PHARMACOLOGIC THERAPY

ANTIBIOTIC BONE CONCENTRATION

Antibiotics used in the management of acute osteomyelitis are generally given in high doses (adjusted for weight, renal function, hepatic function, or both) so that adequate antimicrobial concentrations are reached within the infected bone. Eight to 12 g/d of a penicillinase-resistant penicillin (nafcillin or oxacillin), ampicillin, or cephalosporin, or a similar large dose of another parenteral antibiotic is used in the initial management of adults with osteomyelitis. These dosing recommendations are, however, empiric; the relationship between a specific dose of a given antibiotic and its resultant concentration within the infected bone is largely unknown.[26] Semisynthetic penicillins, cephalosporins, clindamycin, and the aminoglycosides can be detected in bone homogenates soon after their administration.

DURATION OF ANTIBIOTIC THERAPY

The specific duration of antibiotic therapy needed in the management of osteomyelitis is usually 4 to 6 weeks.[27] Failures approaching 20% have been observed in children treated with injectable antibiotics for 3 weeks or less. Thus, with the data indicating a minimum of 3 weeks of antibiotic therapy, the standard treatment for osteomyelitis has been parenteral antibiotics for 4 to 6 weeks. Although these data were determined in children, this duration of therapy recommendation is also used in adults. A recent trial assessing ceftriaxone 2g IV once daily for at least 6 weeks for *S. aureus* osteomyelitis found a cure rate of 77%.[28] The failures in this study were in patients with infected necrotic bone or infected hardware (wires, plates, screws, and rods) that could not be removed.

A modification of this recommendation has been used in some patients. Children receiving an appropriate oral antibiotic regimen and adults receiving an oral fluoroquinolone antibiotic, such as ciprofloxacin, for a duration of 6 weeks have been treated successfully. Monitoring the patient's clinical signs and symptoms and their erythrocyte sedimentation rate are important parameters in order to assess therapy. If signs or symptoms are still present at 6 weeks, therapy should be extended.

ORAL ANTIBIOTIC THERAPY

One of the most significant changes in the management of osteomyelitis is the use of oral antibiotics to complete therapy.[29] Criteria for the use of oral outpatient antibiotic therapy for osteomyelitis are:

- Confirmed osteomyelitis
- Organism identified
- Antibiotic sensitivity determined
- Suitable oral agent available
- Compliance assured

Suitable candidates are children with good clinical response to IV therapy and adults without diabetes mellitus or peripheral vascular disease.

Two primary populations have benefited from oral treatment. Children responding to initial parenteral therapy may be excellent candidates to receive followup oral therapy with an agent such as dicloxacillin, cephalexin, or ampicillin, depending on their culture and sensitivity results.[30,31] Although more controversial, the other population to benefit from oral therapy is adults with an infecting organism sensitive to a fluoroquinolone.[32] These two populations now no longer routinely require expensive and complicated courses of long-term parenteral antibiotics.

The use of oral antibiotics is well studied in children. Several studies documenting the effectiveness of oral therapy used injectable antibiotics initially and then switched to oral antibiotics when there was a decrease in the signs of inflammation and the erythrocyte sedimentation rate, or when the patient was afebrile for 3 days.[31] If pus was obtained on the initial needle aspirate or if a reduction in fever, local swelling, and tenderness did not occur despite adequate rest, immobilization, and intensive antibiotic therapy, the patients underwent surgical drainage.

The patients enrolled in oral antibiotic trials generally had disease of recent onset, identification of a specific infecting organism, enforced compliance, and surgery as indicated. In patients who meet these criteria, oral antibiotics appear to offer a great advantage in the treatment of osteomyelitis. Patients not meeting these criteria are more likely to develop chronic osteomyelitis with resultant recurrent exacerbations of the infection if oral therapy is attempted. One recent trial found no treatment failures in children with acute *S. aureus* osteomyelitis who were treated with either 150 mg/kg/d of cephradine or 40 mg/kg/d of clindamycin that was started initially IV and converted to oral therapy within 4 days.[33]

Ciprofloxacin is effective in the treatment of osteomyelitis caused by gram-negative strains, such as *Enterobacter cloacae* and *Serratia marcescens*.[34] Many strains of streptococci are relatively resistant. Its activity against gram-negative bacilli allows patients to be treated orally and avoids the potential toxic complications of 4 to 6 weeks of aminoglycoside therapy. Ciprofloxacin and other fluoroquinolones have also demonstrated effectiveness in the treatment of chronic osteomyelitis along with adequate surgical débridement.[35,36] Another benefit with this agent is that it may be administered on an every-12-hour schedule. An important limitation of the drug, however, is that it should not be used in children younger than 16 to 18 years of age or in pregnant women because of its potential to cause cartilage damage. Other limitations of ciprofloxacin are that it has poor coverage against anaerobic organisms and staphylococci and that *P. aeruginosa* may develop resistance.[37]

Concern has been raised with staphylococci resistance to fluoroquinolones. Methicillin-resistant *S. aureus* infections do not respond well to ciprofloxacin; however, resistance may also be troublesome for methicillin-sensitive strains. It is now recommended that when ciprofloxacin is to be used to treat osteomyelitis with mixed etiologies that include *S. aureus,* ciprofloxacin should be combined with an antistaphylococcal drug.[37]

ANTIBIOTIC SELECTION

A critical component in the management of osteomyelitis is the selection of appropriate antibiotics. Empiric therapy must be selected on the basis of the most likely infecting organism while the results of culture and sensitivity data are pending. Table 116–3 summarizes empiric therapy recommendations. Dosages expressed in terms of milligrams per kilograms per day are generally given in divided doses every 6 to 8 hours (three to four times a day).

Because *S. aureus,* streptococci, and *E. coli* are the most common infecting organisms in newborns, an IV dosage of 40 mg/kg/d (given in two divided doses) of cefazolin is appropriate. For children 5 years of age or younger, *S. aureus, H. influenzae* type b, and streptococci are the most common infecting organisms. Appropriate therapy in this age group is cefuroxime IV 100 mg/kg/d. For children older than 5 years, *S. aureus* is the most likely infecting organism, and either nafcillin 100 mg/kg/d IV or cefazolin 100 mg/kg/d IV are recommended. If patients are allergic to penicillins or cephalosporins, vancomycin or clindamycin may be used for *S. aureus* coverage. Children with osteomyelitis usually can be successfully treated with 4 weeks of parenteral therapy.

An oral regimen may be an alternative to the previous recommendation in many cases of osteomyelitis in children. Children in whom the infecting organism is identified, who have undergone surgery if needed, and have had a good clinical response to IV therapy may be candidates for the alternate oral antibiotic regimen. It is recommended that parenteral antibiotic therapy be initiated and continued until there has been a resolution in the erythema, swelling, and tenderness, and until the patient is afebrile. Dicloxacillin, cloxacillin, and cephalexin (100 mg/kg/d) are effective oral agents. Patients should be monitored with periodic WBC counts, erythrocyte sedimentation rates, and radiographic findings. When oral antibiotics are used, the total duration of oral and injectable therapy is usually at least 4 to 6 weeks. As previously stated, because of the risk of cartilage damage, fluoroquinolones should not be used in children.

Hematogenous osteomyelitis in adults is most frequently caused by *S. aureus* and, thus, is appropriately treated with 8–12 g/day of a penicillinase-resistant penicillin, such as nafcillin. A similar dose of a first-generation cephalosporin (e.g., cefazolin), clindamycin 2.4 g/day or vancomycin 2 g/day (with normal renal function), may be used in those individuals allergic to penicillin; however, if the infection is located within the vertebrae, *E. coli* must be considered, and, thus, depending on the culture and sensitivity data, a switch to a cephalosporin may be needed.[38] After institution of appropriate antibiotic therapy, the antimicrobial agent should be continued for at least 4 to 6 weeks total (parenteral plus oral).

Special Populations

Osteomyelitis in a patient with a hemoglobinopathy, such as sickle cell anemia, is commonly caused by either *Salmonella* or *S. aureus*. Thus,

TABLE 116–3. Empiric Treatment of Osteomyelitis

Patient Subtype	Likely Infecting Organism	Antibiotic[a]
Newborn	*S. aureus,* streptococci, *E. coli*	Cefazolin 100 mg/kg/day IV
Children 5 years of age or younger	*S. aureus, H. influenzae* type b, streptococci	Cefuroxime 100 mg/kg/day IV
Children older than 5 years of age	*S. aureus*	Nafcillin 40 mg/kg/day IV *or* cefazolin 100 mg/kg/day IV
Adults	*S. aureus*	Nafcillin 2 g IV every 4 hours *or* cefazolin 2 g IV every 8 hours
Intravenous drug abusers	Pseudomonas	Ciprofloxacin 750 mg po twice daily *or* ceftazidime 2 g IV every 8 hours plus tobramycin 5 mg/kg/day IV
Postoperative or posttrauma patients	Gram-positive and gram-negative organisms	Nafcillin 2 g IV every 4 hours plus ceftazidime 2 g IV every 8 hours *or* ticarcillin–clavulanate 3.1 g IV every 4 hours
Patients with vascular insufficiency	Gram-positive and gram-negative organisms	Nafcillin 2 g IV every 4 hours *or* cefazolin 2 g IV every 8 hours plus ceftazidime 2 g IV every 8 hours
	If anaerobes suspected	Cefotetan 2 g IV every 12 hours *or* clindamycin 900 mg IV every 8 hours plus ceftazidime 2 g IV every 8 hours

[a]Dosage should be adjusted for some agents in patients with renal and/or hepatic dysfunction.

empiric antibiotics of first choice are a penicillinase-resistant penicillin plus ampicillin. Alternatives to ampicillin are a third-generation cephalosporin, chloramphenicol, or ciprofloxacin (in adults).

Bone infections in patients with a history of IV drug abuse require coverage for gram-negative organisms; therefore, empiric treatment with ceftazidime 2 g IV every 8 hours plus an aminoglycoside is indicated. If compliance can be assured, these patients are excellent candidates to receive oral ciprofloxacin 750 mg twice daily. Antibiotic therapy in these patients should be continued for at least 4 to 6 weeks.

As previously discussed, several microorganisms can cause bone infections that occur after surgery or from contiguous spread of an adjacent soft-tissue infection. *S. aureus* is the single most common organism, but multiple organisms may be involved. To provide the required broad-spectrum coverage, nafcillin 2 g IV every 4 hours plus ceftazidime 2 g IV every 8 hours should be used as initial therapy. An alternative single agent is ticarcillin/clavulanate potassium 3.1 g IV every 4 hours; however, there is less experience with this agent. The antibiotic regimen may require modification after culture and sensitivity information is evaluated. Based on the culture and sensitivity data, ciprofloxacin may be an appropriate oral alternative for these patients. Frequently, the antibiotics must be continued for 6 weeks to obtain a cure, and surgery often is required to remove any infected or devitalized tissue.

Patients with established vascular insufficiency who subsequently develop osteomyelitis are extremely difficult to manage.[39,40] Impaired blood flow to the extremities impedes the healing process possibly requiring vascular bypass surgery.[41] Infections in these patients include a wide range of organisms, including *S. aureus, Streptococcus,* anaerobes, and gram-negative organisms. Broad-spectrum therapy with a penicillinase-resistant penicillin in combination with ceftazidime is the preferred initial therapy. If anaerobes are suspected, an antianaerobic cephalosporin (e.g., cefoxitin) or clindamycin plus ceftazidime may be substituted. Ampicillin may need to be added to the regimen to provide coverage against *Enterococcus*. In spite of aggressive antibiotic therapy along with surgical débridement, these patients continue to have very low cure rates. Amputation of the involved area may be required to obtain a cure of the infection.[42]

Home Antibiotic Therapy

Because the management of bone and joint infections frequently requires prolonged parenteral antibiotics, newer antibiotic regimens are being evaluated. Administration of antibiotics in the home environment and the use of antibiotics with extended elimination half-lives are being studied.[43] Although acute osteomyelitis is one of the more common infectious diseases that may be treated with home IV antibiotics, not all patients are acceptable candidates for home administration.[44] Patients must be screened to include only those patients who are receiving a stable treatment program, those patients who are interested and are motivated in participating, and those patients who have good venous access, as well as those patients who have support from family members or neighbors and have home facilities for storage and refrigeration. Patients with adequate vascular access may be able to use a peripheral IV catheter; however, a central IV catheter may be required if venous access difficulties occur. Certain exclusion criteria also must be considered. Complications of other preexisting diseases, such as diabetic retinopathy, intention tremor, disabling inflammation or degenerative joint disease, coagulopathies, or various neurologic disorders may prevent individuals from receiving home antibiotics. Histories of alcoholism and IV drug abuse also are important exclusion criteria. Patients who are fluent in only a foreign language and patients who are illiterate or hard of hearing may have to be excluded if a qualified guardian is unavailable. In addition to meeting these initial screening criteria, patients must successfully complete a thorough training program before hospital discharge. Aseptic technique, proper catheter care, and correct administration techniques must be documented. Once a patient is receiving therapy in the home environment, continued monitoring of their antimicrobial therapy is important. It is vital to ensure compliance with the antimicrobial regimen.

In addition, the specific antibiotic regimen characteristics must be considered when evaluating a patient for home antibiotics.[45] Some important features are microbiologic culture and sensitivity data, the number of required daily antimicrobial doses, antibiotic stability data, and requirements for unique monitoring for the specific antimicrobial regimen, such as serum creatinine and peak and trough concentration measurements with aminoglycosides. Although an organism may be sensitive to several antimicrobial agents, one antibiotic may provide practical benefits over other agents. Patients who have an infecting organism sensitive to one of the longer acting (less frequently dosed) cephalosporins and who are resistant to less-expensive agents (cefazolin) may benefit from the newer antibiotics. It is important, however, to monitor for the development of resistant strains and superinfections.

Infectious Arthritis

The three most important therapeutic maneuvers in the management of infectious arthritis are appropriate antibiotics, joint drainage, and joint rest.[46] Initial smears of the synovial fluid may be useful in initially selecting appropriate antibiotic therapy. If bacteria are not observed on the Gram stain in a patient who has a purulent joint effusion, antibiotics should still be initiated because of the high risk of an infection being present.[47] A delay in initiating antibiotics significantly increases the likelihood for long-term complications.

The specific antibiotic selected depends on the most likely infecting organism. In infants less than 1 month old, the infecting organisms vary widely and empiric therapy must, thus, provide broad-spectrum coverage. A penicillinase-resistant penicillin, such as nafcillin or oxacillin (50 mg/kg/day), plus an aminoglycoside is appropriate. Children younger than 5 years of age may be infected with *H. influenzae,* for which ampicillin therapy is indicated. The substitution of cefuroxime may be required if the patient is located in a geographic area with a high level of ampicillin resistance.[48]

In children older than 5 years of age and in adults, initial therapy with a penicillinase-resistant penicillin is appropriate to provide the necessary coverage against *S. aureus*. Therapy should be changed to vancomycin if the *S. aureus* is resistant to methicillin. Preliminary data indicate children with infectious arthritis may be converted to oral therapy after initial IV therapy.[49,50] As with osteomyelitis, IV drug abusers require coverage for *P. aeruginosa* and, therefore, combination therapy with an aminoglycoside is needed. The antibiotics selected are usually administered parenterally. Antibiotics administered by this route achieve sufficient concentrations within the synovial fluid, and, thus, intra-articular antibiotic injections are unnecessary. Although studies to define clearly the appropriate length of therapy have not been conducted, 2 to 3 weeks of antibiotic therapy is generally adequate in nongonococcal infections. Joint fluid cultures are usually no longer positive after 7 days of antibiotics.

Disseminated gonococcal infections often respond quickly to antibiotics.[51] Ceftriaxone 1 g/day for 7 to 10 days is the treatment of choice. After culture and sensitivity results are available, and the organism is sensitive, therapy can be switched on the fourth day to oral amoxicillin, or to doxycycline, or to tetracycline to complete the 7- to 10-day course of antibiotic therapy. Clinical resolution of signs and symptoms is usually rapid.

Closed-needle aspiration is recommended for all infected joints except the hip. Joint drainage may be repeated daily for 5 to 7 days until effusions no longer reaccumulate. Open drainage is required in hip infections because closed-needle aspiration is difficult. During the initial phase of the infection, weight bearing, such as walking, on the joint should be avoided. Passive range-of-motion exercises should be initiated when the pain begins to subside in order to maintain joint mobility.[52] Approximately one-third of patients with bacterial arthritis have a bad joint outcome such as severe functional deterioration.[53] Poor joint outcomes are associated with older patients, those with preexisting joint disease, and patients with an infected joint containing synthetic material.

PHARMACOECONOMIC CONSIDERATIONS

Cost and outcome issues are important in osteomyelitis and infectious arthritis. If long-term sequelae develop, such as impaired joint motion or draining sinus tracts, or if amputation is required, patient quality of life may be significantly diminished. Cost and quality of life issues have clearly played a major role in evaluating other treatment alternatives (oral therapy or home antibiotic treatment) rather than requiring patients to remain hospitalized to receive 4 to 6 weeks of parenteral antibiotics.[45] More recently, a Markov model compared different treatments in non-insulin-dependent diabetes mellitus patients who had foot infections and suspected osteomyelitis.[15] This study found that a 10-week course of culture-guided oral antibiotics after surgical débridement may be as effective and less costly than other treatment approaches, such as immediate amputation.

EVALUATION OF THERAPEUTIC OUTCOMES

Patients with bone and joint infections must be monitored closely. Table 116–4 summarizes a pharmaceutical care monitoring protocol. An assessment of a therapy's success or failure is based on the patient's clinical findings and laboratory values. The clinical signs of inflammation, such as swelling, tenderness, pain, redness, and fever, should resolve with appropriate therapy. Initially, the clinical signs are assessed daily until improvement, then periodically thereafter. Elevations in WBC count also should gradually decline. The WBC count is usually obtained once or twice per week until it returns to the normal range. The erythrocyte sedimentation rate is usually determined weekly. Elevations in the erythrocyte sedimentation rate may not return to normal for several weeks of therapy. If, by the end of the 4- to 6-week antibiotic course, the clinical findings of osteomyelitis are no longer present and the erythrocyte sedimentation rate is within normal limits, the patient may be considered a clinical cure. Patients may relapse, however, after initially appearing to be cured. No relapse for 1 year is generally considered a complete cure.

If a patient fails to resolve the clinical signs and symptoms of inflammation after appropriate empiric antibiotics, surgical débridement may be needed. In addition, the patient may have a resistant infecting organism that may require a modification of the antibiotic therapy. It is especially important to note the infecting organism and its sensitivity pattern. Followup cultures at subsequent débridements may be useful to assess the antibiotic therapy.

Despite apparently adequate surgery and antibiotics, some patients may fail therapy and have recurrent relapses in their infection. This scenario is more common in the population with chronic osteomyelitis. These patients may require long-term oral antibiotics in order to keep the infection under control.

▶ PRINCIPLES OF PHARMACOTHERAPY

- The most common cause of osteomyelitis (particularly that acquired by hematogenous spread) and infectious arthritis is *S. aureus*.
- Culture and susceptibility information are essential as a guide for antimicrobial treatment of osteomyelitis and infectious arthritis.
- Joint aspiration and examination of synovial fluid are extremely important to evaluate the possibility of infectious arthritis.
- The most important treatment modality of acute osteomyelitis is the administration of appropriate antibiotics in adequate doses for a sufficient length of time.
- Antibiotics are generally given in high doses so that adequate antimicrobial concentrations are reached within infected bone and joints.

TABLE 116–4. Monitoring Protocol

Parameter	Frequency	Notes
Culture and sensitivity	At initiation of treatment	
White blood cell count	1–2 times/wk until within normal range	
Erythrocyte sedimentation rate	Weekly	May not decrease to normal range until several weeks of therapy
Clinical signs of inflammation (redness, pain, swelling, tenderness, fever)	Daily during initiation of therapy	
Compliance of outpatient therapy	Reinforce before starting oral therapy and with each health care visit	Compliance is critical if treatment is to be successful

- The standard duration of antimicrobial treatment for osteomyelitis is 4 to 6 weeks.
- Oral antimicrobial therapy may be used for osteomyelitis to complete a parenteral regimen in children who have had a good clinical response to IV antibiotics or in adults without diabetes mellitus or peripheral vascular disease, when the organism is susceptible to the oral antimicrobial, a suitable oral agent is available, and compliance is assured.
- The three most important therapeutic maneuvers in the management of infectious arthritis are appropriate antibiotics, joint drainage, and joint rest.

REFERENCES

1. Waldvogel FA, Medoff G, Swartz MN. Osteomyelitis: A review of clinical features, therapeutic considerations and unusual aspects. N Engl J Med 1970;282:198–206, 260–266, 316–322.
2. Dahl LB, Hoyland AL, Dramsdahl H, Kaaresen PI. Acute osteomyelitis in children: A population-based retrospective study 1965 to 1994. Scand J Infect Dis 1998;30:573–577.
3. Atkins BL, Bowler CJW. The diagnosis of large joint sepsis. J Hosp Infect 1998;40:263–274.
4. Luhmann JD, Luhmann SJ. Etiology of septic arthritis in children: An update for the 1990s. Pediatr Emerg Care 1999;15:40–42.
5. Mader JT, Ortiz M, Calhoun JH. Update on the diagnosis and management of osteomyelitis. Clin Podiatr Med Surg 1996;13:701–724.
6. Mader JT, Shirtliff M, Calhoun JH. Staging and staging application in osteomyelitis. Clin Infect Dis 1997;25:1303–1309.
7. Smith JW, Piercy EA. Infectious arthritis. Clin Infect Dis 1995;20: 225–231.
8. Stimmler MM. Infectious arthritis: Tailoring initial treatment to clinical findings. Postgrad Med 1996;99:127–139.
9. Weston VC, Jones AC, Bradbury N, Fawthrop F, Doherty M. Clinical features and outcomes of septic arthritis in a single UK Health District 1982–1991. Ann Rheum Dis 1999;58:214–219.
10. Lew DP, Waldvogel FA. Osteomyelitis. N Engl J Med 1997;336: 999–1007.
11. Sonnen GM, Henry NK. Pediatric bone and joint infections. Pediatr Clin North Am 1996;43:933–947.
12. Barton LL, Villar RG, Rice SA. Neonatal group B streptococcal vertebral osteomyelitis. Pediatrics 1996;98(3 Pt 1):459–461.
13. Haas DW, McAndrew MP. Bacterial osteomyelitis in adults: Evolving considerations in diagnosis and treatment. Am J Med 1996;101: 550–561.
14. Puffingarger WR, Gruel CR, Herndon WA, Sullivan JA. Osteomyelitis of the calcaneus in children. J Pediatr Orthop 1996;16:224–230.
15. Eckman MH, Greenfield S, Mackey WC, et al. Foot infections in diabetic patients: Decision and cost-effectiveness. JAMA 1995;273:712–720.
16. Norman DC, Yoshikawa TT. Infections of the bone, joint, and bursa. Clin Geriatr Med 1994;10:703–718.
17. Kaandorp CJE, van Schaardenburg D, Krijnen P, et al. Risk factors for septic arthritis in patients with joint disease. Arthritis Rheum 1995;38: 1819–1825.
18. Yagupsky P, Bar-Ziv Y, Howard CB, Dagan R. Epidemiology, etiology, and clinical features of septic arthritis in children younger than 24 months. Arch Pediatr Adolesc Med 1995;149:537–540.
19. Perez-Gomez A, Prieto A, Torresano M, et al. Role of the new azoles in the treatment of fungal osteoarticular infections. Semin Arthritis Rheum 1998;27:226–244.
20. Ozuna RM, Delamarter RB. Pyogenic vertebral osteomyelitis and postsurgical disc space infections. Orthop Clin North Am 1996;27: 87–94.
21. Cucurull E, Expinoza LR. Gonococcal arthritis. Rheum Dis Clin North Am 1998;24:305–322.
22. Roy DR. Osteomyelitis. Pediatr Rev 1995;16:380–385.
23. Sutter CW, Shelton DK. Three-phase bone scan in osteomyelitis and other musculoskeletal disorders. Am Fam Physician 1996;54:1639–1647.
24. Eckardt JJ, Wirganowicz PZ, Mar T. An aggressive surgical approach to the management of chronic osteomyelitis. Clin Orthop 1994;298: 229–239.
25. Hamdy RC, Lawton L, Carey T, et al. Subacute hematogenous osteomyelitis: Are biopsy and surgery always indicated? J Pediatr Orthop 1996;16:220–223.
26. Xue IB, Davey PG, Phillips G. Variation in postantibiotic effect of clindamycin against clinical isolates of *Staphylococcus aureus* and implications for dosing of patients with osteomyelitis. Antimicrob Agents Chemother 1996;40:1403–1407.
27. Mader JT, Shirtliff ME, Bergquist SC, Calhoun J. Antimicrobial treatment of chronic osteomyelitis. Clin Orthop Res 1999;360:47–65.
28. Guglielmo BJ, Luber AD, Paletta D, Jacobs RA. Ceftriaxone therapy for staphylococcal osteomyelitis: A review. Clin Infect Dis 2000;30:205–207.
29. Karwowska A, Davies HD, Jadavji T. Epidemiology and outcome of osteomyelitis in the era of sequential intravenous-oral therapy. Pediatr Infect Dis J 1998;17:1021–1026.
30. Lane-O'Kelly A, Moloney AC. Acute haematogenous osteomyelitis—Evaluation of management in the 1990s. Ir J Med Sci 1995;164:285–288.
31. Peltola H, Unkila-Kallio L, Kallio MJT. Simplified treatment of acute staphylococcal osteomyelitis of childhood. Pediatrics 1997;99:846–850.
32. Greenberg RN, Newman MT, Shariaty S, Pectol RW. Ciprofloxacin, lomefloxacin, or levofloxacin as treatment for chronic osteomyelitis. Antimicrob Agents Chemother 2000;44:164–166.
33. Peltola H, Unkila-Kallio L, Kallio MJT, Finnish Study Group. Simplified treatment of acute staphylococcal osteomyelitis of childhood. Pediatrics 1997;99:846–850.
34. Lew DP, Waldvogel FA. Use of quinolones in osteomyelitis and infected orthopaedic prosthesis. Drugs 1999;58 (suppl 2):85–91.
35. Rissing JP. Antimicrobial therapy for chronic osteomyelitis in adults: role of the quinolones. Clin Infect Dis 1997;25:1327–1333.
36. Galanakis N, Giamarellou H, Moussas T, Dounis E. Chronic osteomyelitis caused by multi-resistant gram-negative bacteria: Evaluation of treatment with newer quinolones after prolonged follow-up. J Antimicrob Chemother 1997;39:241–246.
37. Lew DP, Waldvogel FA. Quinolones and osteomyelitis: State-of-the-art. Drugs 1995;49(suppl 2):100–111.
38. Sapico FL. Microbiology and antimicrobial therapy of spinal infections. Orthop Clin North Am 1996;27:9–13.
39. LeFrock JL, Joseph WS. Bone and soft-tissue infections of the lower extremity in diabetics. Clin Podiatr Med Surg 1995;12:87–103.
40. HaVan G, Siney H, Danan JP, et al. Treatment of osteomyelitis in the diabetic foot: Contribution of conservative surgery. Diabetes Care 1996;19:1257–1260.
41. Hill SL, Holtzman GI, Buse R. The effects of peripheral vascular disease with osteomyelitis in the diabetic foot. Am J Surg 1999;177:282–286.
42. Eneroth M, Larsson J, Apelqvist J. Deep foot infections in patients with diabetes and foot ulcer: An entity with different characteristics, treatments, and prognosis. J Diabetes Complications 1999;13:254–263.
43. Williams DN, Rehm SJ, Tice AD, Bradley JS, Kind AC, Craig WA. Practice guidelines for community-based parenteral anti-infective therapy. Clin Infect Dis 1997;25:787–801.
44. Tice AD. Outpatient antimicrobial therapy for osteomyelitis. Infect Dis Clin North Am 1998;12:903–919.
45. Mauceri AA. Treatment of bone and joint infections utilizing a third-generation cephalosporin with an outpatient drug delivery device. Am J Med 1994;97(suppl 2A):14–22.
46. Cimmino MA. Recognition and management of bacterial arthritis. Drugs 1997;54:50–60.
47. Lyon RM, Evanich JD. Culture-negative septic arthritis in children. J Pediatr Orthop 1999;19:655–659.

48. Mader JT, Mohan D, Calhoun J. A practical guide to the diagnosis and management of bone and joint infections. Drugs 1997;54:253–264.
49. Newton PO, Ballock RT, Bradley JS. Oral antibiotic therapy of bacterial arthritis. Pediatr Infect J 1999;18:1102–1103.
50. Kim HKW, Alman B, Cole WG. A shortened course of parenteral antibiotic therapy in the management of acute septic arthritis of the hip. J Pediatr Orthop 2000;20:44–47.
51. Angulo JM, Espinoza LR. Gonococcal arthritis. Comp Ther 1999;25: 155–162.
52. Boustred AM, Singer M, Hudson DA, Bolitho GE. Septic arthritis of the metacarpophalangeal and interphalangeal joints of the hand. Ann Plast Surg 1999;42:623–629.
53. Kaandorp CJE, Krijnen P, Bernelot Moens HJ, Habbema JDF, van Schaardenburg D. The outcome of bacterial arthritis. Arthritis Rheum 1997;40:884–892.

117

SEPSIS AND SEPTIC SHOCK

S. Lena Kang-Birken and Joseph T. DiPiro

Sepsis and septic shock are increasing problems for the national health care system. In 1998, septicemia discharges totaled 347,000, and it was also responsible for the third longest average length of hospital stay (7.6 days), following malignant neoplasms and psychoses.[1] From 1979 to 1997, death caused by septicemia increased by 82.6%. Of the 15 leading causes of death, septicemia was the 12th leading cause in 1997.[2] Sepsis and associated sequelae continue to be the leading causes of death in intensive care units. Sepsis may occur in 25% of intensive care unit (ICU) patients in comparison to 2% to 3% of non-ICU patients.[3] More than half of these patients further develop severe sepsis and 25% of patients with severe sepsis have shock. The prognosis of patients with sepsis is related to underlying diseases and the initial presentation with shock and organ failures. While the emphasis within the health care system is shifting toward disease prevention and the outpatient management of chronic diseases, there remains a vital need for clinicians to comprehend the pathophysiology and to appreciate the management options available for acutely ill patients with sepsis or septic shock.

DEFINITIONS

Differentiation of the terms associated with sepsis and septic shock are important to the understanding of the events that occur when microorganisms invade the bloodstream. *Septicemia* is an imprecise term classically associated with severe clinical signs and symptoms characteristic of systemic toxicity secondary to bloodstream invasion by microorganisms or associated toxins. *Sepsis* describes the physiologic manifestations in response to an infection. In 1992, a joint committee of the American College of Chest Physicians and the Society of Critical Care Medicine standardized the terminology related to sepsis for several reasons: (a) widespread confusion with the use of these terms; (b) the need to provide a flexible classification scheme for patient identification; (c) identification of an earlier therapeutic intervention; (d) standardization of research protocols (Table 117–1).[4]

The criteria for the new terms provide specific physiologic variables that can be used to categorize a patient as having bacteremia, systemic inflammatory response syndrome (SIRS), sepsis, severe sepsis (consistent with the older term *sepsis syndrome*), septic shock, or multiple organ dysfunction syndrome (MODS), suggesting an important continuum of progressive physiologic decline. Introduction of the term SIRS reflects the knowledge that a physiologically similar systemic inflammatory response can be seen even in the absence of identifiable infection (Fig. 117–1).[5,6] It is important to note that progression from sepsis to MODS can occur in the absence of an intervening period of septic shock. The concept of a compensatory anti-inflammatory response syndrome (CARS) describes physiological response to systemic inflammatory syndrome in cases of infection or injury.[7] Although the consensus committee has achieved its original aim of standardization of terminology, a continuing evolution in our understanding of the pathogenesis of sepsis suggests a need for refinement of definitions.[8,9]

ETIOLOGY

While almost any microorganism can be associated with the clinical development of sepsis and septic shock, the most common etiologic pathogens are gram-negative bacteria, gram-positive bacteria, and fungi. Certain viruses and rickettsiae may produce a similar syndrome.

GRAM-NEGATIVE BACTERIAL SEPSIS

The incidence of gram-negative bacterial infection has increased greatly in the last 20 years. A greater proportion of patients with gram-negative bacteremia develop clinical sepsis, and gram-negative bacteria are also more likely to produce septic shock in comparison to gram-positive organisms, 50% versus 25%, respectively.[10]

Summaries of gram-negative sepsis show that *Escherichia coli* is the most commonly isolated pathogen in sepsis.[11] Other common gram-negative pathogens include *Klebsiella* spp., *Serratia* spp., *Enterobacter* spp., and *Proteus* spp. *Pseudomonas aeruginosa,* although not considered a predominant endogenous flora, is found widely in the environment and is the most frequent cause of sepsis fatality. These commensal organisms are generally not aggressive pathogens because normal host flora inhibit the overgrowth of potentially pathogenic organisms. However, when the body's immunity breaks down, these organisms extend beyond normal sites and often progress from colonization to illness. With the administration of antimicrobial agents having broad spectra of activity, the protective flora are presumably removed, thus allowing overgrowth of more virulent species. Additionally, the integrity of the gastrointestinal mucosa as a mechanical barrier is critical. The infectious implications of trauma, penetrating wounds, small surface ulcerations, mechanical obstructions, and ischemic necrosis of the bowel carry a high risk of subsequent gram-negative infection that often progresses to sepsis.

Gram-negative sepsis results in a higher mortality rate compared with sepsis from any other groups of organisms.[10,11] The major factor associated with the outcome of gram-negative sepsis appears to be the severity of any underlying condition. Patients with rapidly fatal conditions, such as acute leukemia, aplastic anemia, and $>$ 70% of the body's surface burn injury, have a significantly worse prognosis than do those patients with nonfatal underlying conditions, such as diabetes mellitus or chronic renal insufficiency.[11] Age does not appear to be an independent determinant of mortality with gram-negative sepsis.

GRAM-POSITIVE BACTERIAL SEPSIS

Gram-positive organisms are becoming more frequent pathogens in sepsis and septic shock, accounting for approximately 50% of bacteremic events. They are commonly caused by *Staphylococcus aureus*, *Staphylococcus epidermidis*, *Streptococcus pneumoniae*, and *Enterococcus faecalis*. *Streptococcus pyogenes*, viridans streptococci, and *Clostridium perfringens* are less commonly involved.[11,12]

TABLE 117–1. Definitions Related to Sepsis

Condition	Definition
Bacteremia (fungemia)	Presence of viable bacteria (fungi) in the bloodstream.
Infection	Inflammatory response to invasion of normally sterile host tissue by the microorganisms.
Systemic inflammatory response syndrome (SIRS)	Systemic inflammatory response to a variety of clinical insults which can be infection, but can be noninfectious etiology. The response is manifested by two or more of the following conditions: T > 38°C (100.4°F) or < 36°C (96.8°F); HR > 90 beats/min; RR > 20 breaths/min or $Paco_2$ < 32 torr; WBC > 12,000 cells/mm^3, < 4,000 cells/mm^3, or > 10% immature (band) forms.
Sepsis	The SIRS secondary to infection.
Severe sepsis	Sepsis associated with organ dysfunction, hypoperfusion, or hypotension. Hypoperfusion and perfusion abnormalities may include, but are not limited to, lactic acidosis, oliguria, or acute alteration in mental status.
Septic shock	Sepsis with hypotension, despite fluid resuscitation, along with the presence of perfusion abnormalities. Patients who are on inotropic or vasopressor agents may not be hypotensive at the time perfusion abnormalities are measured.
Multiple organ dysfunction syndrome (MODS)	Presence of altered organ function requiring intervention to maintain homeostasis.
Compensatory anti-inflammatory response syndrome (CARS)	Compensatory physiologic response to systemic inflammatory response syndrome that is considered secondary to the actions of anti-inflammatory cytokine mediators.

HR, heart rate; RR, respiratory rate; T, temperature
(From Ref. 5.)

S. epidermidis is most often related to infected intravascular devices, such as artificial heart valves and stents and the use of intravenous and intra-arterial catheters. Although the report of a single blood or tissue culture being positive for coagulase-negative staphylococci is often considered a contaminant and clinically innocuous, severe life-threatening sepsis secondary to *S. epidermidis* has been described. *S. pneumoniae* is associated with an overall mortality rate of over 25%. Factors related to a higher mortality include shock, respiratory insufficiency, preexisting renal failure, and the presence of a rapidly fatal underlying disease. The rates of nosocomial enterococcal bacteremia and associated sepsis are also increasing. Enterococci are isolated most commonly in blood cultures following a prolonged hospitalization and treatment with broad-spectrum cephalosporins.

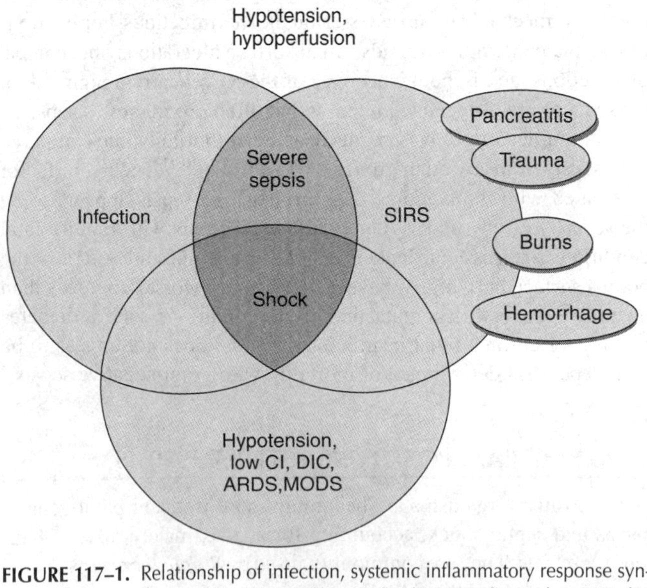

FIGURE 117–1. Relationship of infection, systemic inflammatory response syndrome (SIRS), sepsis, severe sepsis, and septic shock. CI, cardiac index; DIC, disseminated intravascular coagulation; ARDS, acute respiratory distress syndrome; MODS, multiple organ dysfunction syndrome.

ANAEROBIC AND MISCELLANEOUS BACTERIAL SEPSIS

Anaerobes are usually considered low-risk organisms for the development of sepsis. If present, anaerobes are often found together with other pathogenic bacteria that are commonly found in sepsis. Mortality rates are similar to sepsis caused by a single organism. Although some clinicians believe the particular combination of organisms present in polymicrobial sepsis may provide clues to the source of infection, no clear source for the infection can be identified in up to 25% of cases. Other less common pathogens include meningococcus, gonococcus, rickettsia, chlamydia, and spirochetes.[11]

FUNGAL SEPSIS

Candida spp. (especially *C. albicans, C. krusii, C. parapsilosis,* and *C. glabrata*), are common causes of fungal sepsis in hospitalized patients. Other fungi identified as causes of sepsis include *Cryptococcus, Coccidioides, Fusarium,* and *Aspergillus*. Risk factors include abdominal surgery; poorly controlled diabetes mellitus; prolonged granulocytopenia; broad-spectrum antibiotic treatment;

corticosteroid treatment; prolonged hospitalization; central venous catheter; total parenteral nutrition; hematologic malignancy; and chronic, indwelling bladder (Foley) catheter. The rates of nosocomial candidemia have been increasing, possibly because of the use of broad-spectrum antibiotics and the advancements in critical care, allowing for longer survival of critically ill patients. Mortality ranges from 41% to 71% in patients with fungemia.[13] Hematologic diseases, neutropenia, and a higher number of positive blood cultures were associated with poor outcome irrespective of patient's gender, age, or days of antifungal drug treatment.

VIRAL SEPSIS

Viremia is common to many viral illnesses, but it does not usually lead to the development of clinical sepsis. Development of hypotension and disseminated intravascular coagulation (DIC) may occur with unusual viruses, such as Ebola virus and Lassa fever virus, and may be seen occasionally with influenza A, arbovirus, and possibly severe measles.[11]

PATHOPHYSIOLOGY

The pathophysiologic sequelae resulting from the interaction between the invading pathogen and the human host are diverse, complex, and incompletely understood.[14] Definitive relationships between infection and progression to septic shock have been difficult to demonstrate. Furthermore, clinical and histopathologic changes attributed to infection may be similar to those of coexisting conditions. Finally, observations from work with animal models of sepsis are difficult to apply to humans because of potential marked differences in responses.

CELLULAR COMPONENTS FOR INITIATING THE INFLAMMATORY PROCESS

The pathophysiologic focus of gram-negative sepsis has been on the lipopolysaccharide component of the bacterial cell wall. Commonly referred to as endotoxin, this substance is unique to the outer membrane of the gram-negative cell wall, and is generally released with bacterial lysis. The lipopolysaccharide molecule consists of three distinct regions. The outermost component, referred to as *O-antigen,* has diverse antigenicity, depending on bacterial species. The middle region, the *core,* has less antigenic diversity. Lipid A is the innermost region, found in both aerobic and anaerobic gram-negative bacilli. Lipid A is highly immunoreactive, and is considered responsible for most of the toxic effects observed with gram-negative sepsis. Although lipid A may affect tissues directly, its predominant effect is to activate macrophages and trigger inflammatory cascades critical in the progression to sepsis and septic shock.[14,15] After being released from gram-negative bacteria, the endotoxin associates with a protein called a lipopolysaccharide-binding protein. This complex then engages the specific CD14 receptor on the surface of the macrophage, leading to activation and release of cytokine mediators.

In gram-positive sepsis, peptidoglycan appears to exhibit proinflammatory activity. Unlike gram-negative organisms, peptidoglycan comprises up to 40% of gram-positive cell mass, and is exposed on the bacterial cell wall surface. Although it competes with lipid A for similar binding sites on CD14, the potency of peptidoglycan is less than that of endotoxin.[12]

PRO- AND ANTI-INFLAMMATORY MEDIATORS

Sepsis involves activation of inflammatory pathways, and a complex interaction between proinflammatory and anti-inflammatory mediators play a major role in the pathogenesis of sepsis. Proinflammatory cytokines facilitate a wide range of inflammatory processes.[16] The key proinflammatory mediators include tumor necrosis factor-α (TNF-α), interleukin-1β (IL-1β), and interleukin-6 (IL-6), which are released by activated macrophages. Other cytokines that may be important for the pathogenesis of sepsis include interleukin-8 (IL-8), platelet activating factor (PAF), leukotrienes, and thromboxane A_2.[14,16,17] The significant anti-inflammatory mediators include interleukin-1 receptor antagonist (IL-1ra), IL-4, and IL-10.[15,17,18] These anti-inflammatory cytokines interfere with the inflammatory processes by inhibiting the production of the proinflammatory cytokines and down-regulating some inflammatory cells.

The TNF-α is considered the primary mediator of sepsis.[14–17] In healthy humans who were injected with endotoxin, free TNF-α was detected in plasma, and these volunteers developed many symptoms associated with gram-negative infection. Coincidentally, the TNF-α level is highly elevated, although for a short period of time, in most patients with sepsis. In meningococcemia, increased morbidity and mortality are associated with high plasma concentrations of TNF-α. Anti-TNF-α monoclonal antibodies injected into animals have a protective effect, particularly when the antibody was administered prior to the endotoxin challenge. The TNF-α release leads to activation of other cytokines (IL-1β and IL-6) associated with cellular damage. In addition, TNF-α stimulates the release of cyclooxygenase-derived arachidonic acid metabolites (thromboxane A_2 and prostaglandins) that contribute to vascular endothelial damage. TNF-α also causes endothelial cells to express adhesion molecules, facilitating influx of granulocytes.

The net effect of a given mediator can vary depending on the state of activation of the target cell, the presence of other mediators near the target cell, and the ability of the target cell to release mediators that can augment or inhibit the primary mediator. When the balance in the localized response is lost, the patient becomes systemically ill. As Figure 117–2 illustrates, when there is a systemic spillover of excessive proinflammatory mediators, the patient presents with SIRS and possibly MODS. Shortly after this initial phase, counterregulatory pathways become activated, and there is a systemic spillover of excessive anti-inflammatory mediators (CARS). The balance between pro- and anti-inflammatory mechanisms determines the degree of inflammation, ranging from local antibacterial activity to systemic tissue toxicity or organ failure[7,14,17]

CASCADE OF SEPSIS

The cascade leading to development of sepsis is complex and multifactorial, involving various mediators and cell lines (Fig. 117–3).[16,17,19] Through the actions of the mediators, a variety of cells become activated, initiating detrimental cascades. Initially, macrophages become activated and produce inflammatory cytokines. These cytokines then influence a wide range of cells, including endothelial cells, lymphocytes, hepatocytes, neutrophils, and platelets. Endothelial cells that respond to and produce a variety of cytokines mediate a primary mechanism of injury with sepsis. When injured, endothelial cells allow circulating cells (granulocytes) and plasma constituents to enter inflamed tissues, which may result in organ damage. The microcirculation is affected by sepsis-induced inflammation.[20] The arterioles become less responsive to either vasoconstrictors or vasodilators. The capillaries are less perfused, and there is neutrophil infiltration and protein leakage into the venules. Pulmonary dysfunction may result

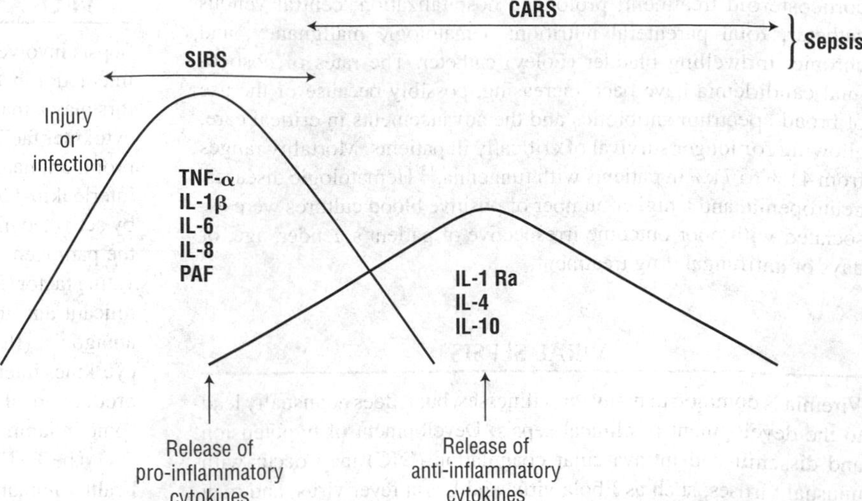

FIGURE 117–2. Pro- and anti-inflammatory events during sepsis.[14]

from the destructive mechanisms (proteolytic enzymes and reactive oxygen species) of neutrophils that are attracted to lung tissue through the action of IL-8 (and other chemoattractants).

Activation of complement in sepsis leads to pathophysiologic consequences including generation of anaphylatoxins and other substances that augment or exaggerate the inflammatory response. Stimulation of leukocyte chemotaxis, phagocytosis with lysosomal enzyme release, increased aggregation and adhesion of platelets and neutrophils, and the production of toxic superoxide radicals are attributed, in part, to complement activation. Among these responses is the release of histamine from mast cells and the resultant increase in capillary permeability and the "third-spacing" of fluid in interstitial spaces.

The inflammatory process in sepsis is directly linked to the coagulation system. Proinflammatory mechanisms that promote sepsis are also procoagulant and antifibrinolytic, whereas fibrinolytic mechanisms may be anti-inflammatory. A key endogenous substance involved in inflammation of sepsis is activated protein C, which enhances fibrinolysis and inhibits inflammation. Levels of protein C are reduced in patients with sepsis.[21]

MARKERS PREDICTING THE SEVERITY

Measurement of endotoxin and cytokine levels in plasma has been proposed as a method to detect sepsis in its early stages or to quantify

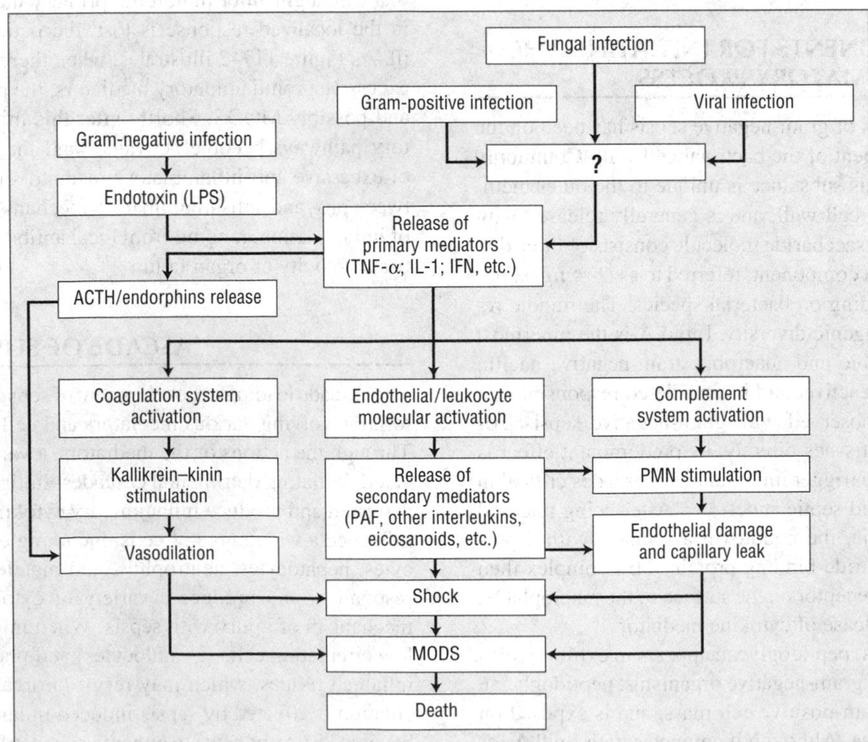

FIGURE 117–3. Cascades of sepsis. ACTH, advenocorticotropic hormone.

the severity of sepsis.[22–27] The TNF-α level is transiently elevated in the plasma of most patients with sepsis. However, the TNF-α levels may also be increased in patients with a variety of diseases and in many healthy people.[15] There is a correlation of TNF-α levels with the severity of sepsis, and high TNF-α levels are found in patients with septic shock. In contrast, IL-1 levels have been inconsistently associated with sepsis. IL-6 may be a more consistent predictor of sepsis, because it remains elevated for a longer period of time than does TNF-α, and it appears to be related to sepsis severity and mortality.[23–26] Circulating concentrations of IL-8 have also been related to severity of sepsis and mortality.[27] Although the plasma endotoxin concentration does not correlate to the development of gram-negative sepsis or outcome from infection, decreased antiendotoxin core immunoglobulin G concentrations are associated with increased mortality in patients with sepsis syndrome.[28,29]

COMPLICATIONS

Shock is the most ominous complication associated with sepsis, and mortality occurs in approximately half of the patients with septic shock. Severe hypotension associated with sepsis appears to be caused, in part, by the release of vasoactive peptides, such as bradykinin and serotonin, and by endothelial cell damage leading to the extravasation of fluids into interstitial spaces. Septic shock is associated with several complications including disseminated intravascular coagulation, acute respiratory distress syndrome, and multiple organ failure.

DISSEMINATED INTRAVASCULAR COAGULATION

DIC is a frequent complication of gram-negative sepsis. Nearly every case of severe shock caused by trauma, or sepsis, or both results in DIC.[19] It is primarily attributed to the activation of factor XII (Hageman factor) by endotoxin. The subsequent activation and consumption of coagulation factors II, V, VIII, and platelets far exceed the rate of synthesis, resulting in an inability to maintain hemostasis. Paradoxic bleeding may occur because of the consumption of clotting factors and the rapid lysis of clots resulting from the simultaneously activated plasminogen (fibrinolytic system). Fibrin breakdown results in circulating soluble peptides called fibrin degradation products. Complications of DIC vary and depend on the target organ affected and severity of the coagulopathy. DIC may produce acute renal failure, hemorrhagic necrosis of the gastrointestinal mucosa, liver failure, acute pancreatitis, acute respiratory distress syndrome, and pulmonary failure.

ACUTE RESPIRATORY DISTRESS SYNDROME

Acute respiratory distress syndrome (ARDS), a pulmonary manifestation of multiple organ dysfunction syndrome, occurs in approximately 25% of SIRS patients, and in many patients with gram-negative sepsis.[30] It is a functional lung injury, characterized by diffuse alveolar damage, that leads to noncardiogenic pulmonary edema through increased vascular permeability.[30,31] Consequently, air spaces fill with fluid, and there is deterioration of gas exchange of the lung, impaired compliance, and refractory hypoxemia. This has been defined as acute lung injury with detection of bilateral pulmonary infiltrates on the frontal chest radiograph, a pulmonary artery wedge occlusion pressure (PAWP) of $\leq$ 18 mm Hg (or no clinical evidence of elevated left atrial pressure on the basis on chest radiograph and other clinical data), and a ratio of Pao_2 to $Fio_2 < 200$ (regardless of the level of positive end-expiratory pressure).[32] It is associated with mortality rate of 60% to 90%.[33]

In sepsis caused by *S. aureus,* pulmonary involvement was reported in 82% of the patients.[34] The pulmonary findings including bronchopneumonic infiltration, lobar consolidation, and pleurisy resulted in a mortality rate of approximately 19%.

HEMODYNAMIC EFFECTS

The hallmark of the hemodynamic effect of sepsis is the hyperdynamic state characterized by high cardiac output and an abnormally low systemic vascular resistance (SVR).[35] A low cardiac output appears to reflect inadequate maintenance of the circulating volume. Evidence suggests that myocardial function is impaired. In one dramatic study, small doses of endotoxin from *E. coli* were injected into normal volunteers to study the cardiovascular effects in comparison to controls who received saline.[36] In subjects who received endotoxin, the cardiac index before volume loading increased by 53%, the heart rate increased by 36%, and the SVR decreased by 46%. After volume loading, the ejection fraction decreased by 1% from the baseline value in subjects who received endotoxin, but increased by 14% in controls. Left ventricular end-diastolic and end-systolic indices increased by 14% and 24%, respectively. Finally, left ventricular performance as measured by the ratio of the peak systolic pressure to the end-systolic volume index was depressed in subjects who received endotoxin and increased in the control group. These data suggest that endotoxin depresses left ventricular function independent of changes in left ventricular volume or vascular resistance. These findings are consistent with those seen in septic shock and suggest that endotoxin or secondary mediators such as TNF-α directly depress cardiovascular function.

Sepsis-associated hypotension raises concern for the balance of oxygen delivery to the tissues (Do_2) and oxygen consumption by the tissues (Vo_2).[37] Sepsis results in a distributive shock characterized by inappropriately increased blood flow to selected tissues at the expense of other tissues, which is independent of specific tissue oxygen needs. This perfusion defect is accentuated by an increased precapillary atrioventricular (AV) shunt. If perfusion decreases, oxygen extraction increases and the arteriovenous oxygen gradient widens. Cellular Do_2 is decreased, but Vo_2 remains unaffected. When increased oxygen demand occurs without increased blood flow, the increased Vo_2 is compensated by increased oxygen extraction. If perfusion decreases sufficiently in the face of high metabolic demands, then the reserve Do_2 can be exceeded and tissue ischemia results. Significant tissue ischemia leads to organ dysfunction and failure, and ultimately to death, if not reversed.

CLINICAL PRESENTATION

Table 117–2 lists some of the common clinical features of sepsis, although a number of these findings are not limited to infectious processes. The initial clinical presentation can be referred to as signs and symptoms of early sepsis, and they typically include fever, chills, and change in mental status. Hypothermia may occur with a systemic infection, and this is often associated with a poor prognosis.[11] In patients with sepsis caused by gram-negative bacilli, hyperventilation may occur even before fever and chills, and it may lead to respiratory alkalosis as the earliest metabolic change.

TABLE 117–2. Signs and Symptoms Associated with Sepsis

Early Sepsis	Late Sepsis
Fever or hypothermia	Lactic acidosis
Rigors, chills	Oliguria
Tachycardia	Leukopenia
Tachypnea	DIC
Nausea, vomiting	Myocardial depression
Hyperglycemia	Pulmonary edema
Myalgias	Hypotension (shock)
Lethargy, malaise	Hypoglycemia
Proteinuria	Azotemia
Hypoxia	Thrombocytopenia
Leukocytosis	ARDS
Hyperbilirubinemia	Gastrointestinal hemorrhage
	Coma

Progression of uncontrolled sepsis leads to clinical evidence of organ system dysfunction as represented by the signs and symptoms attributed to late sepsis. With the exception of rapidly progressing cases as in meningococcemia, *P. aeruginosa,* or *Aeromonas* infection, the onset of shock is slow and usually follows a period of several hours of hemodynamic instability. Oliguria often follows hypotension. Increased glycolysis with impaired clearance of the resulting lactate by the liver and kidneys and tissue hypoxia because of hypoperfusion result in elevated lactate levels, contributing to metabolic acidosis. Altered glucose metabolism, including impaired gluconeogenesis and excessive insulin release, is evidenced by either hyperglycemia or hypoglycemia. The distinction between early and late sepsis is arbitrary, and it is recognized that sepsis represents a spectrum of clinical findings.[37]

▶ TREATMENT: Sepsis and Septic Shock

The treatment of sepsis should be targeted toward medical and surgical treatment of the infection site and toward support of organ function. Therapy can be divided into immediate stabilization, followed by more definitive therapeutic interventions. In addition to immediate, aggressive antimicrobial therapy, priorities in the management of sepsis include rapid reversal of hypotension and hypoperfusion. Other supportive care such as stress ulcer prophylaxis and nutritional support is important to prevent complications during the stay in the intensive care unit.

The primary goals of therapy for patients with sepsis include (a) timely diagnosis and identification of pathogen; (b) rapid elimination of the source of infection; (c) early initiation of aggressive antimicrobial therapy; (d) interruption of pathogenic sequence leading to septic shock; (e) avoidance of organ failure.

DIAGNOSIS AND IDENTIFICATION OF PATHOGEN

The presence of clinical features suggesting sepsis should prompt further evaluation of the patient. In addition to obtaining a careful history of any underlying conditions and recent travel, injury, animal exposure, infection or use of antibiotics, a complete physical examination should be performed to determine the cause of the infection. A collection of specimens should be sent for culture prior to initiating any antimicrobial therapy. Generally, at least two sets of blood samples should be sent for aerobic and anaerobic culture, and samples of urine and sputum should also be sent for culture. If the patient is confused, complains of severe headache, or experiences a seizure, then a lumbar puncture is indicated, assuming intracranial pressure is not increased and there are no focal cranial lesions identified by computed tomography scan. Further tests may be indicated to assess any systemic organ dysfunction due to severe sepsis. The laboratory tests should include hemoglobin, white blood cell count with differential, platelet count, complete chemistry profile, coagulation parameters, serum lactate, and arterial blood gases.[39]

ELIMINATION OF SOURCE OF INFECTION

After the source of infection is identified, prompt efforts to remove or to eliminate the source should be initiated. Often gram-positive bacterial and fungal bloodstream infections are associated with infected intravascular catheters, and if suspected, these catheters should be removed and cultured. Urinary tract catheters may be associated with gram-negative bacterial and fungal infections of the genitourinary tract, and these should be removed in situations in which association with sepsis is suspected. Suspicion of soft tissue (cellulitis or wound infection) or bone involvement should lead to aggressive débridement of the affected area. Evidence of an abscess or sepsis associated with any intra-abdominal pathology should prompt surgical intervention.

ANTIMICROBIAL THERAPY

Aggressive, early antimicrobial therapy is critical in the management of septic patients because of high incidence of complications and mortality. Because of the inherent problems associated with the timely identification of the infecting organism or organisms, empiric antimicrobial regimens are usually started initially. Selection of empiric regimen should be based on the suspected site of infection, most likely pathogens, acquisition of the organism from the community or hospital, the patient's immune status, and the antibiotic susceptibility and resistance profile for the institution. All patients should be treated initially with parenteral antibiotics for optimal drug concentrations. Empiric therapy for an immunocompromised patient should consist of antimicrobial combinations likely to be synergistic. After the pathogen is identified, a change to more specific antimicrobial therapy should be made.

SELECTION OF ANTIMICROBIAL AGENTS

The development of new antibiotics with an expanded spectrum of activity and enhanced *in vitro* activities provide the clinician with a wide range of potential choices. However, few controlled trials have evaluated comparative antibiotic regimens in the treatment of sepsis, and the optimal choice of antimicrobial therapy for sepsis is not often clear.[40] Nevertheless, some general guidelines exist for selecting the empiric antimicrobial regimen.

When serious gram-negative sepsis is suspected, aggressive therapy with activity against *P. aeruginosa* and *Enterobacter* spp. should be instituted. A combination regimen is generally recommended in order to provide additive or synergistic effects, to expand the spectrum of coverage, and to reduce the emergence of resistant bacterial subpopulations. For instance, either an antipseudomonal cephalosporin or antipseudomonal penicillin can be combined with an aminoglycoside.[41] When an aminoglycoside is undesirable, a fluoroquinolone can be used instead. However, synergistic activity with this particular combination is not uniformly observed.

A few studies compared monotherapy with standard combination regimens in selected clinical situations and demonstrated equal efficacy. For example, ceftazidime alone appears equivalent to an antipseudomonal penicillin plus aminoglycoside combination in febrile neutropenic patients. It is critical, however, to pay particular attention to local resistance patterns when considering monotherapy. If anaerobes are a possible cause, metronidazole should be added.

Recently, gram-positive pathogens have become more predominant in nosocomial infections including sepsis. If methicillin-resistant *S. aureus* or coagulase-negative staphylococci are suspected in cases of catheter- or medical device-related infections, vancomycin should be added. However, worldwide emergence of glycopeptide intermediately resistant *S. aureus* and vancomycin-resistant enterococci has lead to development of alternative antimicrobial agents such as teicoplanin, quinupristin/dalfopristin and linezolid.[42–44]

Table 117–3 lists antimicrobial regimens that can be used empirically based on the possible source of infection. In the nonneutropenic patient with an urinary tract infection, a third-generation cephalosporin, fluoroquinolone, or extended-spectrum penicillin, each with or without an aminoglycoside, should be considered.[40,41] *S. pneumoniae* is the most common cause of community-acquired pneumonia, and it accounts for approximately 60% of all deaths. The rising incidence of penicillin-resistant *S. pneumoniae* requires empiric use of third-generation cephalosporin. Macrolides are very effective against atypical pathogens including *Legionella pneumophila, Mycoplasma pneumoniae,* and *Chlamydia pneumoniae*. However, newer macrolides, such as clarithromycin and azithromycin, are better tolerated than erythromycin. A newer fluoroquinolone, such as levofloxacin, can be used as monotherapy, because unlike ciprofloxacin, newer fluoroquinolones generally offer excellent coverage against penicillin-resistant pneumococci and aerobic gram-negative bacteria, as well as atypical pathogens.[45,46] In nosocomial pneumonia, enteric gram-negative bacteria such as *Enterobacter* and *Klebsiella* spp., *P. aeruginosa,* and *S. aureus* are the major pathogens. If *P. aeruginosa* infection is suspected, a dual regimen of antipseudomonal penicillin or third- or fourth-generation cephalosporin and an aminoglycoside is recommended because of the high mortality rate associated with *Pseudomonas* infection.

Secondary peritonitis as a consequence of perforation of the gastrointestinal tract is usually polymicrobial involving enteric aerobes and anaerobes, and as many as five organisms are isolated per patient. In addition to surgical intervention, broad-spectrum antibiotics such as β-lactamase inhibitor combination agents (piperacillin/tazobactam or ticarcillin/clavulanate) are appropriate in intra-abdominal infections.

TABLE 117–3. Empiric Antimicrobial Regimens in Sepsis

Infection (Site or Type)	Antimicrobial Regimen: *Community Acquired*	Antimicrobial Regimen: *Hospital Acquired*
Urinary tract	Fluoroquinolone[a]	Extended-spectrum penicillin[b] or 3rd-generation cephalosporin[c] ± AMG[g] or Fluoroquinolone
Respiratory tract	Newer fluoroquinolone[d] or Ceftriaxone plus Clarithromycin/Azithromycin	3rd-generation cephalosporin or 4th-generation cephalosporin[e] + AMG[g] or Newer fluoroquinolone[d]
Intra-abdominal	β-Lactamase inhibitor combo[f] or Ampicillin plus Metronidazole + AMG[g]	Meropenem or β-Lactamase inhibitor combo[f] plus AMG[g]
Skin/soft tissue	Nafcillin or Cefazolin	3rd-generation cephalosporin[c] +/− Vancomycin
Catheter-related		Vancomycin
Unknown		Extended-spectrum penicillin[b] or Ceftazidime/Cefipime + AMG[g] ± Vancomycin or Meropenem

[a]Ciprofloxacin.
[b]Piperacillin.
[c]Cefetazidime, ceftriaxone.
[d]Levofloxacin, gatifloxacin.
[e]Cefipime.
[f]Ampicillin/sulbactam, piperacillin/tazobactam.
[g]AMG, Aminoglycoside (gentamicin, tobramycin).

Imipenem or meropenem may be indicated if resistance patterns prohibit use of other, less-expensive therapies.[47,48] Currently, most clinicians prefer meropenem to imipenem because it offers similar activity as imipenem with less propensity to cause seizure. In a multicenter study, meropenem has been shown efficacious and safe for the treatment of sepsis syndrome in patients who are 65 years of age or older when compared to a combination regimen of cefuroxime and gentamicin.[47] Trovafloxacin is the first fluoroquinolone with expanded spectrum of activity including anaerobes.[49] However, since the introduction of trovafloxacin in late 1997, 152 cases of serious hepatic events most likely related to trovafloxacin have been reported to the US Food and Drug Administration and to the European Agency for the Evaluation of Medical Products.[50] Subsequently, the manufacturer withdrew trovafloxacin from European markets in 1999, and although the drug remains available in the United States, it is limited to complicated infections that do not respond to other therapy.[51] Against anaerobes, metronidazole is preferred over clindamycin because approximately 20% of *Bacteroides* spp. are resistant to clindamycin.[52]

In soft-tissue infection caused by group A streptococcus, streptococcal toxic shock syndrome may occur. Although penicillin and cefazolin are efficacious, experimental models of group A streptococcal infection show clindamycin to be more effective than penicillin.[41]

THERAPEUTIC CONSIDERATIONS WITH AMINOGLYCOSIDES

In vitro, tobramycin appears somewhat more active (based on concentrations achievable in serum relative to usual minimum inhibitory concentration) than gentamicin against *P. aeruginosa.* Gentamicin, however, appears more active than tobramycin against *Serratia* spp. Overall, amikacin exhibits most *in vitro* activity against the *Klebsiella-Enterobacter-Serratia* group. Among aminoglycosides, amikacin is less susceptible than gentamicin and tobramycin to plasmid-mediated enzyme inactivation, and it should be reserved as an alternative in situations of suspected or established resistance to gentamicin and tobramycin.

Although aminoglycosides have been traditionally administered in divided doses, there has been widespread acceptance of administering aminoglycosides in a single daily dose of 4–7 mg/kg for gentamicin and tobramycin and 10–15 mg/kg for amikacin.[53–56] The practice of single daily dose optimizes the pharmacodynamic parameters of aminoglycosides. Even before the practice of single daily dose of aminoglycoside was introduced, early (within the first 24 hours of therapy) attainment of high peak concentration was reported to be associated with improved outcome and reduced mortality for serious gram-negative infections.[57] A high peak concentration is achieved with single daily dose administration, and single daily dose maximizes the well-defined, concentration-dependent killing activity of aminoglycosides, as well as the prolonged postantibiotic effect against gram-negative bacterial pathogens. Furthermore, nephrotoxicity is significantly reduced. With single daily dose, there is a prolonged drug-free period during which the reported saturable, or rate-limited, uptake of aminoglycosides into proximal renal tubular cells can be completed.[58] Despite some controversies, growing literature supports the single daily dose administration of aminoglycosides in most patients.[59,60] A recent survey of acute care hospitals in the United States indicated that approximately 75% of the hospitals have adopted the extended interval dosing of aminoglycoside.[56] Because of insufficient clinical data, single daily dose administration should not be used in pediatric patients, burn victims, pregnant patients, patients with preexisting or progressive renal dysfunction, or patients requiring aminoglycosides for synergy against gram-positive pathogens.

THERAPEUTIC MONITORING OF AMINOGLYCOSIDE SERUM CONCENTRATIONS

There is marked variability in aminoglycoside pharmacokinetic parameters between individual patients, which leads to variable serum concentrations relative to the dose administered.[61] Furthermore, nephrotoxicity and ototoxicity from aminoglycosides is considered secondary to accumulation of the drug within the body. Hence, appropriate monitoring of aminoglycoside serum concentrations becomes imperative. With traditional dosing, peak concentrations in the range of 6–10 μg/mL and 20–40 μg/mL are desirable with gentamicin (and tobramycin) and amikacin, respectively.[62] Target trough concentrations should be less than 2 μg/mL for gentamicin and tobramycin, and less than 7 μg/mL for amikacin.

When single daily dosing of aminoglycosides is employed, recommendations for serum concentration monitoring vary.[53,58] Although there are several published nomograms and monitoring schemes, an aminoglycoside trough concentration that is undetectable is consistently desired.[53,63] The trouble with only monitoring a trough in many patients is that if an undetectable value is obtained, it is not known how long the concentration has been undetectable, and the dosing regimen cannot be satisfactorily assessed. For most institutions that have adopted the single daily dose, monitoring of serum concentrations has shifted from peak and trough levels to obtaining a single level at 6–18 hours following infusion. Less than one-third of these hospitals reported measuring only the trough concentration.[56] Most institutions relied on the clinical judgment for the frequency of monitoring concentrations.

ANTIFUNGAL THERAPY

Candida species are most frequently associated with fungal infections.[64] Candidemia is frequently associated with sepsis syndrome and a high mortality rate.[65] Both amphotericin B and the azoles are similarly effective in treating mycotic infections. Azoles are less toxic and easier to administer. However, suspected systemic mycotic infection leading to sepsis should be empirically treated with parenteral amphotericin B because of its greater activity against Candida species, including against nonalbicans species.[65]

Amphotericin B should be infused daily over a period of 2–4 hours based on patient tolerance. If the patient suffers from infusion-related fever, chills, rigors, headache, nausea, and vomiting, pretreatment with acetaminophen and diphenhydramine may be useful. Parenteral meperidine can be used to stop rigors, but it is not recommended as a pretreatment.[66] Three new lipid formulations of amphotericin (amphotericin B lipid complex, amphotericin B cholesteryl sulfate, and liposomal amphotericin B) offer several advantages over amphotericin B deoxycholate.[67,68] They are less nephrotoxic, allow increased daily dose, have high tissue concentrations in the reticuloendothelial organs such as lungs, liver, and spleen, and have decreased infusion-associated side effects. However, they are costly and a recent pharmacoeconomic study suggested that the overall benefit of using a lipid formulation did not significantly offset the cost of the product.[69] Furthermore, superior clinical efficacy over the conventional amphotericin B or between the lipid formulations has not clearly established in comparative clinical trials. Consequently, conventional amphotericin B remains the standard therapy for invasive or life-threatening mycotic infections. However, in cases of intolerance or clinical failure, a change to a lipid formulation should be considered.

ANTIVIRAL THERAPY

When sepsis is caused by a systemic viral infection, the choice of therapy is dependent on the suspected or documented viral pathogen. Parenteral antivirals that may be employed include acyclovir, ganciclovir, foscarnet, and ribavirin. Aerosol administration of ribavirin may be indicated in serious illness secondary to respiratory syncytial virus.

DURATION OF THERAPY

The average duration of antimicrobial therapy in the normal host with sepsis is 10–14 days.[11] However, the duration may vary depending on the site of the infection, as well as the overall response to therapy. After the patient is hemodynamically stable, has been afebrile for 48–72 hours, has a normalizing white blood cell (WBC) count, and is able to take oral medications, then a "step-down" from parenteral to oral antibiotics can be considered for the duration of therapy. Treatment may continue considerably longer if the infection is persistent. In a neutropenic patient, therapy is usually continued until the patient is no longer neutropenic and has been afebrile for at least 72 hours.

HEMODYNAMIC SUPPORT

A high cardiac output and a low systemic vascular resistance characterize septic shock. Patients may have hypotension as a result of low systemic vascular resistance and abnormal distribution of blood flow in the microcirculation, resulting in compromised tissue perfusion. Because approximately half of patients with septic shock die of multiple organ system failure, they should be monitored carefully and aggressive hemodynamic support should be initiated. Patients with septic shock should be monitored with a right-sided heart catheter for hemodynamic assessment in an intensive care unit.[70] Hemodynamics change rapidly in sepsis and noninvasive evaluation may give inaccurate assessment of filling pressures and cardiac output. Hemodynamic support can be divided into three main categories: fluid therapy, vasopressor therapy, and inotropic therapy.

FLUID THERAPY

Septic patients have enormous fluid requirements as a result of peripheral vasodilation and capillary leakage.[40,71] Rapid fluid resuscitation is the best initial therapeutic intervention for treatment of hypotension in sepsis. The goal of fluid therapy is to maximize cardiac output by increasing the left ventricular preload, which will ultimately restore tissue perfusion.[70] Fluid administration should be titrated to clinical endpoints such as heart rate, urine output, and blood pressure. An increased serum lactate, a by-product of cellular anaerobic metabolism, should normalize as the tissue perfusion improves.

Isotonic crystalloids, such as 0.9% NaCl (normal saline) or lactated Ringer solution are commonly used for fluid resuscitation. A patient in septic shock typically requires up to 10 L of crystalloid solution during the first 24-hour period. These solutions distribute into the extracellular compartment. Approximately 25% of the infused volume of crystalloid remains in the intravascular space, while the balance distributes to extravascular spaces. Although this could impair diffusion of oxygen to tissues, clinical impact is unproven.

Most commonly used colloids are 5% albumin, naturally occurring plasma protein and 6% hetastarch, a synthetic colloid formulation. These solutions offer more rapid restoration of intravascular volume because they produce greater intravascular volume expansion per quantity of volume infused. Colloids produce less peripheral edema than crystalloid, but there is no significant clinical impact. The use of colloid solutions and blood products may be particularly important if there is significant blood loss associated with sepsis or if the patient had severe preexisting anemia.[71]

The major complications with fluid resuscitation are pulmonary and systemic edema. Aggressive volume expansion may cause increase in pulmonary capillary pressure leading to an increase in lung water and associated hypoxemia. Currently available studies and reports suggest that there is no significant difference in the incidence of pulmonary edema between the crystalloid and colloid solutions.

Septic shock can be managed successfully with either crystalloid or colloids.[72] Although crystalloid solutions require 2–4 times more volume than colloids, they are the usual choice for fluid resuscitation because the cost is significantly less than colloids. However, colloids may be preferred especially when the serum albumin is less than 2.0 g/dL. In summary, there is controversy in the use of colloids or crystalloids. Until future information proves otherwise, crystalloids are recommended for routine volume expansion.

INOTROPE AND VASOPRESSOR THERAPY

When fluid resuscitation alone provides inadequate arterial pressure and organ perfusion, vasopressors and inotropic agents should be initiated. Inotropic agents such as dopamine and dobutamine have been effective in improving cardiac output. Vasopressors should be considered when mean arterial pressure (MAP) is initially very low or when MAP is persistently low ($<$ 60–65 mm Hg) after adequate left ventricular preload and inotrope therapy. Although inotropes and vasopressors are effective in life-threatening hypotension and in improving cardiac index, there are significant complications such as tachycardia and myocardial ischemia and infarction as a result of change in myocardial oxygen consumption in patients with coexisting coronary disease. Thus, a catecholamine infusion should be titrated gradually to restore MAP without impairing stroke volume.

Agents commonly considered for vasopressor or inotropic support include dopamine, dobutamine, norepinephrine, phenylephrine, and epinephrine (Table 117–4).[40,73,74] Dopamine, an α- and β-adrenergic agent with dopaminergic activity, appears to increase MAP effectively in patients who remain hypotensive with reduced cardiac function after aggressive fluid resuscitation. Thus, it is often the initial choice in sepsis because of combined vasopressor and inotropic effects. While low-dose dopamine (1–5 μg/kg/min) is effective in maintaining renal perfusion, higher doses (>5 μg/kg/min) exhibit α and β activity and are frequently used to support blood pressure and to improve cardiac function such as increase in cardiac index (CI).

Dobutamine is a β-adrenergic inotropic agent that many clinicians consider to be the preferred drug for improvement of cardiac output and oxygen delivery, particularly in early sepsis before significant peripheral vasodilation has occurred. Doses of 2–20 μg/kg/min increased the CI, ranging from 20% to 66%. However, heart rate often increased significantly.[70] Dobutamine should be considered in

TABLE 117–4. Receptor Activity of Cardiovascular Agents Commonly Used in Septic Shock

Agent	α_1	α_2	β_1	β_2	Dopaminergic
Dopamine	++/+++	?	++++	++	++++
Dobutamine	+	+	++++	++	0
Epinephrine	++++	++++	++++	+++	0
Norepinephrine	+++	+++	+++	+/++	0
Phenylephrine	++/+++	+	?	0	0

α_1, α_1-adrenergic receptor; α_2, α_2-adrenergic receptor; β_1, β_1-adrenergic receptor; β_2, β_2-adrenergic receptor; 0, no activity; ++++; maximal activity; ?, unknown activity.
(From Ref. 55.)

severely septic patients with adequate filling pressures and blood pressure but low CI.

Norepinephrine is a potent α-adrenergic agent with less pronounced β-adrenergic activity, and it can be useful in septic shock when the clinician desires potent vasoconstriction of peripheral vascular beds. Doses of 0.01–3 μg/kg/min can reliably increase blood pressure with little changes in heart rate or cardiac index. Early human and animal studies suggest that norepinephrine decreases renal blood flow. In comparison to norepinephrine alone, a combination of low-dose dopamine and norepinephrine improves renal function in animals and healthy volunteers while successfully increasing the blood pressure.[75]

Phenylephrine, a selective α_1-agonist, has a rapid onset, short duration, and primary vascular effects, making it an attractive agent in the management of hypotension associated with septic shock. The limited available information suggests that it can increase blood pressure in fluid-resuscitated patients, and it does not appear to impair cardiac or renal function. Phenylephrine appears useful when tachycardia limits the usage of other vasopressors.

Epinephrine, a nonspecific α- and β-adrenergic agonist, is capable of increasing CI and producing significant peripheral vasoconstriction in doses of 0.1–0.5 μg/kg/min. However, because of its undesirable effects, including a propensity to increase lactate level and to impair blood flow to the splanchnic system, it should be reserved for patients who fail to respond to traditional therapies for increasing or maintaining blood pressure.

In summary, for the septic patient with clinical signs of shock and significant hypotension unresponsive to aggressive fluid therapy, dopamine is the preferred agent for increasing the blood pressure. If dopamine does not produce the desired hemodynamic response, norepinephrine can be used with low-dose dopamine to increase renal blood flow. Epinephrine should be considered for refractory hypotension. In a septic patient with low cardiac index after adequate fluid therapy and an adequate MAP, dobutamine is the first-line agent. This strategy often is successful in increasing cardiac output and improving organ perfusion. Alternatively, dopamine in moderate doses (5–10 μg/kg/min) can also be used as an initial agent because of its selective effect on increasing cardiac output with its minimal effect on the systemic vascular resistance.

ADJUNCTIVE THERAPIES

ARDS and hypoxia are common in septic patients, even in septic patients without pulmonary infection. Oxygen therapy is indicated to maintain oxygen saturation greater than 90%, and with progressive pulmonary insufficiency, the patient may require assisted ventilation. The management of patients with ARDS is primarily supportive. Uncontrolled reports suggest that IV methylprednisolone, in doses of 75–250 mg every 6 hours, may improve survival in severely ill patients with refractory late ARDS.[76,77] Other agents have been evaluated as interventions in ARDS, including exogenous surfactant, acetylcysteine, and cyclooxygenase inhibitors, but none consistently improves outcome.[40,73]

Ketoconazole reduced the progression to ARDS and increased survival in a small study of septic surgical patients, possibly as a result of its inhibitory effects on alveolar macrophage production of leukotriene B_4 and thromboxane A_2.[78] Early work with inhaled administration of nitric oxide (NO), a potent endogenous vasodilator, in patients with ARDS suggests improved arterial oxygenation and reduced pulmonary artery pressures.[79] NO is believed to protect endothelial cells from injury induced by free radicals released from activated neutrophils.[80,81] Additional work is needed to define any role for NO in the management of sepsis because NO is also associated with the initiation and maintenance of hypotension in sepsis, as well as being an important mediator of sepsis-induced refractoriness to the vasopressor effects of catecholamines.[70]

The corticosteroids have been the subject of much controversy in the management of septic patients.[82,83] Corticosteroids suppress the activation of polymorphonuclear leukocytes, complement activation, release of TNF, and the activation of the coagulation system involved in the cascades of sepsis. However, well-designed prospective studies showed no benefit from empiric high-dose steroid treatment initiated early in septic shock. While a recent study demonstrated improved outcome with lower doses of steroids in patients with persistent vasopressor requirements, routine use of corticosteroids in patients with sepsis or septic shock is not supported.[39,84]

Heparin therapy for DIC is discouraged by most clinicians as there is no evidence that heparin prolongs the survival of patients despite its effect on hypercoagulable condition found in DIC.[85] Hemorrhage is best managed by the replacement of clotting factors, platelets, and packed red blood cells.

Patients with severe sepsis are susceptible to progressive malnutrition secondary to the hypermetabolism associated with severe illness and injury.[86] Hence, early enteral nutrition is recommended in patients with severe sepsis and septic shock. Nonprotein caloric requirement range from 25 to 40 kcal/kg/day, and overfeeding of carbohydrates should be avoided to reduce the ventilatory requirements of the patient. Hyperglycemia associated with insulin-resistance is common, and management of elevated serum glucose may not be satisfactory with insulin therapy alone. The use of increased amounts of lipid to meet nonprotein caloric needs while reducing carbohydrate administration may be useful in this setting. Protein requirements are increased to 1.5–2.5 g/kg/day, and increased amounts of branched-chain amino acids may be beneficial in septic patients.[87]

IMMUNOTHERAPY

A variety of strategies have been used to reverse or control the inflammatory process initiated during sepsis (Table 117–5).[88,89] Recognizing the major role that endotoxin plays in the inflammatory progression of gram-negative sepsis and the similarity of lipid A among gram-negative bacteria, monoclonal antibodies against endotoxin were first to be tested. Studies conducted with monoclonal antibodies (E5, HA-1A) that bind to the lipid A portion of the endotoxin molecule have failed to demonstrate beneficial effects when administered to patients with clinical evidence of sepsis. Timing of the treatment was thought to be critical in reducing the initiation of the sepsis cascades.[90–92]

Additional approaches include inhibition of inflammatory cytokines by antibodies that bind the cytokines, competitive inhibitors of cytokine receptor binding, or soluble receptors that interact with the cytokine but do not lead to activation of target cells. Administration of anti-inflammatory cytokines (e.g., IL-4 and IL-10) and proinflammatory cytokines (e.g., interferon-γ), and use of pentoxifylline, which is known to reduce cytokine production and to release from leukocytes, are under investigation.[93–101] Despite the initial enthusiasm in immunotherapeutic interventions for sepsis, overall results have been generally disappointing. A recent approach has been the administration of activated protein C (drotrecogin) to promote fibrinolysis and associated anti-inflammatory mechanisms.[21]

TABLE 117–5. Summary of Selected Recently Completed Clinical Trials for Sepsis

Experimental Agent	Comments
HA-1A (anti-lipid A MAb)[75,76]	No overall benefit; favorable trend in meningococcemia (preliminary report)
E5 (antilipid A MAb)[71]	No overall benefit; improved organ dysfunction in some subgroups
Interleukin-1-receptor antagonist[77]	No overall benefit
Platelet-activating factor inhibitors[78]	No overall benefit; favorable trend in gram-negative sepsis
Bradykinin antagonists[79]	No overall benefit; favorable trend in gram-negative sepsis
Immunoglobulins[70]	No overall benefit
Anti-TNF Mab[80,81]	No overall benefit; some evidence of improvement in subgroups of shock patients
TNF receptor: immunoglobulin constructs[82,83]	Phase II—p75 receptor—worsened outcome ($P < 0.01$); p55 receptor—no overall benefit in phase III despite favorable trends in phase II
L-N-Mono methyl arginine[84]	No overall benefit (preliminary report)
Drotrecogin[21] (activated protein C)	Significant reduction in mortality with severe sepsis

(From Ref. 74.)

▶ PRINCIPLES OF PHARMACOTHERAPY

- The etiologies of sepsis and septic shock include gram-negative bacterial pathogens; but also increasingly common are gram-positive bacterial and fungal pathogens.
- Sepsis represents a complex pathophysiology, resulting from important interactions between the pathogen and host, progressing to a systemic inflammatory state mediated by dysregulation of proinflammatory and anti-inflammatory mediators.
- Timely diagnosis and identification of the pathogen are critical to successful management of the septic patient.
- Prompt, aggressive initiation of broad-spectrum, parenteral antibiotic therapy is required. Antibiotic selection should be based on clinical presentation, site of infection, and suspected pathogens.
- Significant fluid leaks from the vasculature occur with sepsis, and administration of large volumes of fluid is required. Crystalloid solutions, such as normal saline, are generally recommended.
- Hemodynamic support using inotropic agents and vasopressors should be initiated in patients who cannot maintain acceptable cardiac output or blood pressure with aggressive fluid therapy alone.
- Supplemental oxygen and assisted ventilatory support may be required in many patients with progressive sepsis and acute respiratory distress syndrome.
- Early enteral nutrition is recommended in patients with severe sepsis who are susceptible to malnutrition secondary to the hypermetabolism associated with severe illness.
- The role of immunotherapy in sepsis is not defined, and such interventions remain investigational.

REFERENCES

1. National Center for Health Statistics. National hospital discharge survey: Annual summary, 1998. Vital Health Stat 13 2000;148.
2. Centers for Disease Control and Prevention, National Center for Health Statistics. Mortality patterns—United States, 1997. MMWR Morb Mortal Wkly Rep 1999;48:644–680.
3. Brun-Buisson C. The epidemiology of the SIRS. Intensive Care Med 2000;26(suppl 1):S64–S74.
4. American College of Chest Physicians/Society of Critical Care Medicine Consensus Conference. Definitions for sepsis and organ failure and guidelines for the use of innovative therapies in sepsis. Crit Care Med 1992;20:864–874.
5. Fry DE. Sepsis syndrome. Am Surg 2000;66:126–132.
6. Nystrom PO. The systemic inflammatory response syndrome: Definitions and aetiology. J Antimicrob Chemother 1998;41(suppl A): 1–7.
7. Bone RC. Sir Isaac Newton, sepsis, SIRS, and CARS. Crit Care Med 1996;24:1125–1128.
8. Muckart DJJ, Bhagwanjee B. American College of Chest Physicians/Society of Critical Care Medicine Conference definitions of the systemic inflammatory response syndrome and allied disorders in relation to critically injured patients. Crit Care Med 1997;25:1789–1795.
9. Abraham E, Matthay MJ, Dinarello CA, et al. Consensus conference definitions for sepsis, septic shock, acute lung injury, and acute respiratory distress syndrome: Time for a reevaluation. Crit Care Med 2000;28:232–235.
10. Lazaron V. Gram-negative sepsis and the sepsis syndrome. Urol Clin North Am 1999;26:687–699.

11. Young LS. Sepsis syndrome. In: Mandell GL, Bennett JE, Dolin R, eds. Principles and Practice of Infectious Diseases, 5th ed. New York, Churchill Livingstone, 2000;806–819.
12. Sriskandan S, Cohen J. Gram-positive sepsis. Infect Dis Clin North Am 1999;13:397–412.
13. Costa SF, Marinho I, Araujo EA, et al. Nosocomial fungaemia: A 2-year prospective study. J Hosp Infect 2000;45:69–72.
14. Bone RC, Grodzin CJ, Balk RJ. Sepsis: A new hypothesis for the pathogenesis of the diseases process. Chest 1997;112:235–243.
15. Marie C, Muret J, Fitting C, et al. Interleukin-1 receptor antagonist production during infectious and noninfectious systemic inflammatory response syndrome. Crit Care Med 2000;28:2277–2282.
16. Kim PK, Deutschman CS. Inflammatory responses and mediators. Surg Clin North Am 2000;80:885–894.
17. Van der Poll T, van Deventer SJH. Cytokines and anticytokines in the pathogenesis of sepsis. Infect Dis Clinic North Am 1999;13:413–426.
18. Van der Poll T, Malefyt RW, Coyle SM, Lowry SF. Antiinflammatory cytokine responses during clinical sepsis and experimental endotoxemia: Sequential measurements of plasma soluble interleukin (IL)-1 receptor type II, IL-10, IL-13. J Infect Dis 1997;175:118–122.
19. Hardaway RM. A review of septic shock. Am Surg 2000;66:22–29.
20. Lush CW, Kvietys PR. Microvascular dysfunction in sepsis. Microcirculation 2000;7:83–101.
21. Bernard GR, Vincent JL, Laterre PF, et al. Efficacy and safety of recombinant human activated protein C for severe sepsis. N Engl J Med 2001;344:699–709.
22. Damas P, Canivet J, De Groote D, et al. Sepsis and serum cytokine concentrations. Crit Care Med 1997;25:405–412.
23. Damas P, Ledoux D, Nys M, et al. Cytokine serum level during sepsis in human IL-6 as a marker of severity. Ann Surg 1992;215:356–362.
24. Damas P, Reuter A, Gysen P, et al. Tumor necrosis factor and interleukin-1 serum levels during severe sepsis in humans. Crit Care Med 1989;17:975–978.
25. Casey LC, Balk RA, Bone RC. Plasma cytokine and endotoxin levels correlate with survival in patients with sepsis syndrome. Ann Intern Med 1993;119:771–778.
26. Steinmetz HT, Herbertz A, Bertram M, Diehl V. Increase in interleukin-6 serum level preceding fever in granulocytopenia and correlation with death from sepsis. J Infect Dis 1995;171:225–228.
27. Marty C, Misset B, Tamion F, et al. Circulating interleukin-8 concentrations in patients with multiple organ failure of septic and nonseptic origin. Crit Care Med 1994;22:673–679.
28. Guidet B, Barakett V, Vassal T, et al. Endotoxemia and bacteremia in patients with sepsis syndrome in the intensive care unit. Chest 1994;106:1194–1201.
29. Strutz F, Heller G, Krasemann K, et al. Relationship of antibodies to endotoxin core to mortality in medical patients with sepsis syndrome. Intensive Care Med 1999;25:435–444.
30. Kollef MH, Schuster DP. The acute respiratory distress syndrome. N Engl J Med 1995;332:27–37.
31. Sessler CN, Bloomfield GL, Fowler AA. Current concepts of sepsis and acute lung injury. Clin Chest Med 1996;17:213–235.
32. Bernard GR, Artgas A, Brigham KL, et al. The American-European Consensus Conference on ARDS: Definitions, mechanisms, relevant outcomes and clinical coordination. Am J Resp Crit Care Med 1994; 149:818–824.
33. Martin MA, Silverman HJ. Gram-negative sepsis and the adult respiratory distress syndrome. Clin Infect Dis 1992;14:1213–1228.
34. Caksen H, Ozturk MK, Uzum K, et al. Pulmonary complications in patients with staphylococcal sepsis. Pediatr Int 2000;42:268–271.
35. Bunnell E, Parrillo JE. Cardiac dysfunction during septic shock. Clin Chest Med 1996;17:237–248.
36. Suffredini AF, Fromm RE, Parker MM, et al. The cardiovascular response of normal humans to the administration of endotoxin. N Engl J Med 1990;321:280–287.
37. Chittock DR, Russell JA. Oxygen delivery and consumption during sepsis. Clin Chest Med 1996;17:263–278.
38. Conboy K, Welage LS, Walawander MA, et al. Sepsis syndrome associated sequelae in patients at high risk for gram-negative sepsis. Pharmacotherapy 1995;15:66–77.
39. Dellinger RP. Current therapy for sepsis. Infect Dis Clin North Am 1999;13:495–509.
40. Wiessner WH, Casey LC, Zbilut JP. Treatment of sepsis and septic shock: A review. Heart Lung 1995;24:380–392.
41. Simon D, Trenholme G. Antibiotic selection for patients with septic shock. Crit Care Clin 2000;16:215–231.
42. Wood MJ. Chemotherapy for gram-positive nosocomial sepsis. J Chemother 1999;11:446–452.
43. Harding I, MacGowan AP, White LO, et al. Teicoplanin therapy for *Staphylococcus aureus* septicaemia: Relationship between predose serum concentrations and outcome. J Antimicrob Chemother 2000;45; 835–841.
44. Chien JW, Kucia ML, Salata RA. Use of linezolid, an oxazolidinone, in the treatment of multidrug-resistant gram-positive bacterial infections. Clin Infect Dis 2000;30:146–151.
45. Kays MB, Conklin M. Comparative in vitro activity and pharmacodynamics of five fluoroquinolones against clinical isolates of *Streptococcus pnueumoniae*. Pharmacotherapy 2000;20:1310–1317.
46. Blondeau JM. A review of the comparative in-vitro activities of 12 antimicrobial agents, with a focus on five new "respiratory quinolones." J Antimicrob Chermother 1999;43(suppl B):1–11.
47. Jaspers CA, Kieft H, Speelberg B, et al. Meropenem versus cefuroxime plus gentamicin for treatment of serious infections in elderly patients. Antimicrob Agents Chemother 1998;42;1233–1238.
48. Bradley JS, Garau J, Lode H, et al. Carbapenems in clinical practice: A guide to their use in serious infection. Int J Antimicrob Agents 1999;11:93–100.
49. Thadepalli H, Reddy U, Chuah SK, et al. *In vivo* efficacy of trovafloxacin (CP-99,217), a new quinolone, in experimental intra-abdominal abscesses caused by *Bacteroides fragilis* and *Escherichia coli*. Antimicrob Agents Chemother 1997;41:583–586.
50. Lucena MI, Andrade RJ, Rodrigo L, et al. Trovafloxacin-induced acute hepatitis. Clin Infect Dis 2000;30:400–401.
51. European Agency for the Evaluation of Medicinal Products. Public statement on trovafloxacin/alatrofloxacin: Recommendation to suspend the marketing authorisation in the European Union. London, 15 June 1999. Available at: www.emea.eu.int/pdfs/human/press/pus/1804699EN.pdf (Accessed December 10, 2001).
52. Dalmau D, Cayouette M, Lamothe F, et al. Clindamycin resistance in *Bacteroides fragilis* group: Association with hospital-acquired infection. Clin Infect Dis 1997:24:874–877.
53. Nicolau DP, Freeman CD, Belliveau PP, et al. Experience with a once-daily aminoglycoside program administered to 2,184 adult patients. Antimicrob Agents Chemother 1995;39:650–655.
54. Hatala R, Dinh T, Cook DJ. Once-daily aminoglycoside dosing in immunocompetent adults: A meta-analysis. Ann Intern Med 1996;124: 717–725.
55. Hatala R, Dinh T, Cook DJ. Single daily dosing of aminoglycosides in immunocompromised adults: A systemic review. Clin Infect Dis 1997; 24:810–815.
56. Chuck SK, Raber SR, Rodvold KA, Areff D. National survey of extended-interval aminoglycoside dosing. Clin Infect Dis 2000;30:433–439.
57. Moore RD, Lietman PS, Smith CR. The association of aminoglycoside plasma levels with mortality in patients with gram-negative bacteremia. J Infect Dis 1984;149:443–448.
58. Gilbert DN. Once daily dosing of aminoglycoside therapy. Antimicrob Agents Chemother 1991;35:339–405.
59. Bertino JS, Rotschafer JC. Single daily dosing of aminoglycosides—A concept whose time has not yet come. Clin Infect Dis 1997;24:820–823. Editorial response.
60. Brown GH, Bertino JS, Rotschafer J. Single daily dosing of aminoglycosides—A community standard? Clin Infect Dis 2000;30: 440–441. Editorial response.

61. Fry DE. The importance of antibiotic pharmacokinetics in critical illness. Am J Surg 1996;172(suppl 6A):20S–25S.
62. Moore RD, Lietman PS, Smith CR. Clinical response to aminoglycoside therapy: Importance of the ratio of peak concentration to minimum inhibitory concentration. J Infect Dis 1987;155:93–97.
63. Bailey TC, Little JR, Littenberg B, et al. A meta-analysis of extended-interval dosing versus multiple daily dosing of aminoglycosides. Clin Infect Dis 1997;24:786–795.
64. Berrouane YF, Herwaldt LA, Pfaller MA. Trends in antifungal use and epidemiology of nosocomial yeast infections in a university hospital. J Clin Microbiol 1999;37:531–537.
65. Rex JH, Walsh TJ, Sobel JD, et al. Practice guidelines for the treatment of candidiasis. Infectious Diseases Society of America. Clin Infect Dis 2000;30:662–678.
66. Goodwin SD, Cleary JD, Walawander CA, et al. Pretreatment regimens for adverse events related to infusion of amphotericin B. Clin Infect Dis 1995;20:755–761.
67. Robinson RF, Nahata MC. A comparative review of conventional and lipid formulations of amphotericin B. J Clin Pharm Ther 1999;24:249–257.
68. Dismukes WE. Introduction to antifungal drugs. Clin Infect Dis 2000;30:653–657.
69. Cagnoni PJ, Walsh TJ, Prendergast MM, et al. Pharmacoeconomic analysis of liposomal amphotericin B versus conventional amphotericin B in the empirical treatment of persistently febrile neutropenic patients. J Clin Oncol 2000;18:2476–2483.
70. Practice parameters for hemodynamic support of sepsis in adult patients in sepsis. Task force of the American College of Critical Care Medicine, Society of Critical Care Medicine. Crit Care Med 1999;27:639–660.
71. Ognibene FP. Hemodynamic support during sepsis. Clin Chest Med 1996;17:279–287.
72. Boldt J, Muller M, Mentges D, et al. Volume therapy in the critically ill: Is there a difference? Intensive Care Med 1998;24:28–36.
73. Weikert LF, Bernard GR. Pharmacotherapy of sepsis. Clin Chest Med 1996;17:289–305.
74. Rudis MI, Basha MA, Zarowitz BJ. Is it time to reposition vasopressors and inotropes in sepsis? Crit Care Med 1996;24:525–537.
75. Schaer GL, Fink MP, Parilto JE. Norepinephrine alone versus norepinephrine plus low-dose dopamine: Enhanced renal blood flow with combination pressor therapy. Crit Care Med 1985;13:492–496.
76. Hooper RG, Kearl RA. Established adult respiratory distress syndrome successfully treated with corticosteroids. South Med J 1996;89:449–451.
77. Biffl WL, Moore FA, Moore EE, et al. Are corticosteroids salvage therapy for refractory acute respiratory distress syndrome? Am J Surg 1995;170:591–596.
78. Yu M, Tomasa G. A double-blind, prospective, randomized trial for ketoconazole, a thromboxane synthetase inhibitor, in the prophylaxis of the adult respiratory distress syndrome. Crit Care Med 1993;21:1635–1642.
79. Rossaint R, Falke KJ, Lopez F, et al. Inhaled nitric oxide for the adult respiratory distress syndrome. N Engl J Med 1993;328:339–405.
80. Payen D, Bernard C, Beloucif S. Nitric oxide in sepsis. Clin Chest Med 1996;17:333–350.
81. Fink MP, Payen D. The role of nitric oxide in sepsis and ARDS: Synopsis of a roundtable conference held in Brussels on 18–20 March 1995. Intensive Care Med 1996;22:158–165.
82. Cronin L, Cook DJ, Carlet J, et al. Corticosteroid treatment for sepsis: A critical appraisal and meta-analysis of the literature. Crit Care Med 1995;23:1430 1439.
83. Lefering R, Neugebauer AEM. Steroid controversy in sepsis and septic shock: A meta-analysis. Crit Care Med 1995;23:1294–1303.
84. Bollaert PE, Charpentier C, Levy B, et al. Reversal of late septic shock with supraphysiological doses of hydrocortisone. Crit Care Med 1998;26:645–650.
85. Staudinger T, Locker GJ, Frass M. Management of acquired coagulation disorders in emergency and intensive-care medicine. Semin Thromb Hemostasis 1996;22:93–104.
86. DeWitt RC, Kudsk KA. The gut's role in metabolism, mucosal barrier function, and gut immunology. Infect Dis Clin North Am 1999;13:465–481.
87. Garcia-de-Lorenzo A, Ortiz-Leyba C, Planas M, et al. Parenteral administration of different amounts of branch-chain amino acids in septic patients: Clinical and metabolic aspects. Crit Care Med 1997;25:418–424.
88. Ralston DR, St. John RC. Immunotherapy for sepsis. Clin Chest Med 1996;17:307–317.
89. Opal SM, Cross AS. Clinical trials for severe sepsis: past failures and future hopes. Infect Dis Clin North Am 1999;13:285–297.
90. Bone RC, Balk RA, Fein AM, et al. A second large controlled clinical study of E5, a monoclonal antibody to endotoxin: Results of a prospective, multicenter, randomized, controlled trial. Crit Care Med 1995;23:994–1006.
91. Ziegler EJ, Fisher CJ Jr, Sprung CL, et al. Treatment of gram-negative bacteremia and septic shock with HA1A human monoclonal antibody against endotoxin. N Engl J Med 1991;324:429–436.
92. McCloskey RV, Straube RC, Sanders C, et al, for the CHESS Trial Study Group. Treatment of septic shock with human monoclonal antibody HA1A: Randomized, double-blind, placebo-controlled trial. Ann Intern Med 1994;120:1–5.
93. Doche WD, Randow F, Syrbe U, et al. Monocyte deactivation in septic patients: Restoration by IFN-γ treatment. Nat Med 1997;3:678–681.
94. Opal SM, Fisher CJ, Pribble JP, et al. The confirmatory interleukin-1 receptor antagonist trial in sepsis: A phase III randomized, double-blind, placebo-controlled, multicenter trial. Crit Care Med 1997;25:1115–1124.
95. Dhainaut JF, Tenaillon A, LeTulzo J, et al. Platelet activity factor antagonist BN52021 in the treatment of severe sepsis: A randomized, double-blind, placebo-controlled multicenter trial. Crit Care Med 1994;22:1720–1728.
96. Fein AM, Bernard GR, Criner GJ, et al. Treatment of severe systemic inflammatory response syndrome and sepsis with a novel bradykinin antagonist, Deltibant (CP-0127). JAMA 1997;277;482–487.
97. Abraham E, Anzueto A, Gutierrez G, et al. Double-blind, randomized, controlled trial of monoclonal antibody to human tumor necrosis factor in treatment of septic shock. Lancet 1998;351:929–933.
98. Cohen J, Carlet J. INTERSEPT: An international, multicenter, placebo-controlled trial of monoclonal antibody to human tumor necrosis factor-α in patients with sepsis. Crit Care Med 1996;24:1431–1440.
99. Abraham E, Glauser MP, Butler T, et al. p55 tumor necrosis factor receptor fusion protein in the treatment of patients with severe sepsis and septic shock. JAMA 1997;277;1531–1534.
100. Fisher CJ, Agosti JM, Pal SM, et al. Treatment of septic with the tumor necrosis factor receptor: Fc fusion protein. N Engl J Med 1996;334:1697–1702.
101. Grover R, Zaccardelli D, Colice G, et al. An open-label dose escalation study of the nitric oxide synthase inhibitor, N^6-methyl-L-arginine hydrochloride (546C88), in patients with septic shock. Crit Care Med 1999;27:913–922.

118
Superficial Fungal Infections

Thomas E. R. Brown and Thomas W. F. Chin

Superficial mycoses are among the most common infections in the world and fungal infections are the second most common vaginal infection in North America. Oral fungal infections in humans were reported as far back as 1839. Over the last 15 to 20 years, the occurrence rates of some fungal infections have increased dramatically. The prevalence of fungal skin infections varies throughout different parts of the world from the most common causes of skin infections in the tropics to relatively rare disorders in the United States. This chapter reviews the pharmacotherapy of vulvovaginal candidiasis, oropharyngeal and esophageal candidiasis, and common dermatophyte infections.

VULVOVAGINAL CANDIDIASIS

Vulvovaginal candidiasis (VVC) refers to infections in individuals with or without symptoms who have positive vaginal cultures for candida. Depending on episodic frequency VVC can be classified as either sporadic or recurrent.[1] This classification is essential to understanding the pathophysiology, as well as the pharmacotherapy, in the treatment of VVC. Furthermore, VVC may be defined as uncomplicated, which refers to sporadic infections that are susceptible to all forms of antifungal therapy regardless of the duration of treatment, or as complicated infections in which consideration of factors affecting the host, microorganism and pharmacotherapy all have an essential role in successful treatment.[1] Complicated VVC includes recurrent VVC, severe disease, non-*albicans* candidiasis, and abnormal host factors, including diabetes mellitus, immunosuppression, and pregnancy.[1]

EPIDEMIOLOGY

Minimal information on the incidence and prevalence of VVC exists. It is a nonnotifiable disease therefore estimates are derived from self-reported histories. Further limiting reliable estimates is the fact that VVC is usually diagnosed without microscopy and or cultures and antifungal preparations are available over-the-counter for self-treatment.[1] By 25 years of age, approximately 50% of college students will have had at least 1 episode of VVC.[1] It is rare before menarche and increases dramatically around 20 years of age, with the peak incidence between 30 and 40 years of age. It is associated with the initial act of sexual intercourse. As many as 75% of women experience one bout of symptomatic VVC in their lifetime. Forty percent to 50% of women who experience one episode of VVC experience a second episode, and 5% experience recurrent VVC.[2,3] Black women appear to be at higher risk of developing VVC as compared to whites (62.8% vs 55%, respectively).[4] The incidence after menopause remains unknown.

PATHOPHYSIOLOGY

Candida albicans is the major pathogen responsible, accounting for 80% to 92% of symptomatic episodes of VVC. The remainder are caused by non-*albicans* species with *C. glabrata* dominating.[5] The number of cases of non-*albicans* candidiasis appears to be increasing, possibly related to the use of over-the-counter vaginal antifungal preparations, short-course therapy, and/or the increased use of long-term maintenance therapy in preventing recurrent infections.[1]

Candidal species can act as commensal members of the vaginal flora. Asymptomatic colonization with candida has been found in 10% to 20% of reproductive aged women.[5,6] Candidal organisms are dimorphic, blastospores are believed to be responsible for colonization (transmission and spread), while germinated candida forms are associated with tissue invasion and symptomatic infections.[7] To colonize the vagina, candida must be able to attach to the mucosa. The attachment process is complex. Not only are candidal surface structures important for attachment, but appropriate receptors for attachment must be present in the epithelial tissue. Not all women have the same range of receptors, which may explain variation in colonization.[6] Changes in the host's vaginal environment or response are necessary to induce a symptomatic infection. Unfortunately, in most cases of symptomatic VVC, no precipitating factor can be identified.[7]

RISK FACTORS

Several factors are considered as predisposing a woman to VVC. Vulvovaginal candidiasis is not considered to be a sexually transmitted disease, although sexual factors may be important. There is a dramatic increase in the frequency of VVC when women become sexually active. In addition, oral genital contact may increase the risk.[1] However, current guidelines do not recommend the treatment of asymptomatic partners.[5] Contraceptive agents including the diaphragm with spermicide, contraceptive sponge, and the intrauterine device increase the risk of VVC. Oral contraceptive users demonstrated increase risk of candidiasis; however, these reports were with the higher-dose oral contraceptive pills and the risk may not be as great with the lower-estrogen-dose-containing oral contraceptives.[8]

Antibiotic use may increase the risk of VVC, however it is only significant in a small number of women. The mechanism by which antibiotics can increase the risk of VVC is unknown; colonization, however, is a prerequisite.[1] Diet (excess refined carbohydrate), douching, and tight fitting clothing are often listed as important risk factors; however, no association has been established between these factors and increased risk of VVC.[1]

CLINICAL PRESENTATION

The symptoms of vulvovaginal candidiasis include intense vulvar itching, soreness, irritation, burning on micturition, and dyspareunia. Signs of VVC may include erythema, fissuring, curdy "cheese-like" (nonoffensive) discharge, satellite lesions, and edema.[1,5] These signs and symptoms are not pathognomonic, and a reliable diagnosis can not be made without laboratory tests. Self-diagnosis has a sensitivity of 35% and specificity of 89% with a positive predictive value of 62%.[4] One study showed that more than 50% of women who had self-diagnosed VVC did not have yeast as the causative agent.[9] Diagnosis should be based on both clinical presentation and investigations, including vaginal pH, saline microscopy, and 10% potassium hydroxide microscopy. The vaginal pH remains normal in VVC and microscopic investigations should detect blastospores or pseudohyphae. Candidal cultures are usually not required in the diagnosis of uncomplicated VVC; however, they are recommended when an individual presents with classic signs/symptoms of VVC and has a normal vaginal pH, but microscopy is inconclusive or recurrence is suspected.[5]

▶ TREATMENT: Vulvovaginal Candidiasis

GOALS OF THERAPY

The goal of therapy is to treat symptomatic VVC for complete resolution of symptoms. Test of cure is not necessary if symptoms resolve.[5] Antimycotic agents used in the treatment of VVC do not meet the definition of being a fungicidal agent because of their slower killing rate. At the end of therapy, the number of viable organisms drops below the detectable range. However, by 6 weeks, after a course of therapy, 25% to 40% of women will have positive yeast cultures and remain asymptomatic.[1] Asymptomatic colonization with candida does not require therapy.

GENERAL APPROACHES TO TREATMENT

The approach to therapy is to remove or improve any predisposing factors if they can be identified. A pharmacologic agent should have limited local and systemic side effects, a high cure rate, and easy administration. Additionally, it would be advantageous to use a therapy that was able to resolve symptoms within 24 hours, that had broad antimycotic activity (to cover increasing rates on non-*albicans Candida*), that prevented recurrence, and that could be used over a shortened period of time 1 to 3 days.

NONPHARMACOLOGIC TREATMENTS

Avoid harsh soaps and perfumes to reduce vulvar irritation. Keep the genital area clean and dry by avoiding constrictive clothing and frequent or prolonged exposure to the use of hot tubs.[3] Cool baths may be used to soothe the skin.[3] Daily ingestion of 240 mL of yogurt containing *Lactobacillus acidophilus* decreased colonization and symptomatic infections of VVC in women with recurrent infections.[10]

PHARMACOLOGIC TREATMENTS

UNCOMPLICATED VULVOVAGINAL CANDIDIASIS

Cure rates for uncomplicated VVC are between 80% and 95% with topical or oral azoles and between 70% and 90% with nystatin preparations. Table 118–1 lists available topical and oral preparations for the treatment of uncomplicated VVC. There are many topical over-the-counter preparations for the treatment of VVC. No significant differences in *in vitro* activity, or clinical efficacy exist between the topical azole agents.[1,3,5] The selection of a topical azole should be based primarily on an individual patient's preference as to product formulation. Some topical products may cause vaginal burning, stinging, or irritation; on the other hand the vehicle used in topical creams or gels can provide initial symptomatic relief.[1] Most topical preparations can decrease the efficacy of latex condoms or diaphragms.

Oral azoles have been used in the treatment of VVC. One study demonstrated patients' preference to oral therapy because of its convenience.[11] There is therapeutic equivalence between oral and topical therapy.[1] In the treatment of uncomplicated VVC, the duration of therapy is not critical. Cure rates with different lengths of treatment have not demonstrated that one therapy is significantly better.[12,13] Shorter duration therapies (i.e., clotrimazole 1-day therapy) consist of higher concentrations of azoles that maintain the local therapeutic effect for up to 72 hours and allow for resolution of signs and symptoms.[14] A review of 14 trials that examined 1-day treatments showed less than 7% difference in short-term cure rates or improvement between any two treatments in any two studies and no significant differences in short- or long-term clinical cure rates between 1-day regimens.[12]

If the vulva is significantly irritated, topical application of a low potency corticosteroid may be beneficial.[1,3,5] Anecdotal evidence suggests that high potency corticosteroids may initially exacerbate the burning sensation.[1] Table 118–1 lists the therapeutic options for the treatment of uncomplicated VVC.

TABLE 118–1. Treatment for Uncomplicated Vulvovaginal Candidiasis

Active Ingredient	Preparation	Regimen
Over the Counter	**Vaginal Products**	
Butoconazole	2% cream	1 applicator × 3 days
Clotrimazole	1% cream	1 applicator or
	100 mg tablet	1 100 mg tablet × 7 days
	2% cream	1 applicator or
	200 mg tablet	1 200 mg tablet × 3 days
	10% cream	1 applicator or
	500 mg tablet	1 500 mg tablet × 1 day
Miconazole[a]	2% cream	1 applicator or
	100 mg suppository	1 suppository × 7 days
	200 mg suppository	1 suppository × 3 days
	1200 mg ovule	1 ovule × 1 day
Ticonazole	6.5% ointment	1 applicator or
	300 mg ovule	1 ovule × 1 day
Prescription		
Econazole	150 mg tablet	1 tablet × 3 days
Fenticonazole	2% cream	1 applicator × 7 days
Nystatin	100,000 unit tablet	1 tablet × 14 days
Terconazole	0.4% cream	1 applicator × 7 days
	0.8% cream	1 applicator or
	80 mg suppository	1 suppository × 3 days
Oral Products		
Ketoconazole	200 mg	1 tablet bid × 5 days
Itraconazole	200 mg	1 tablet bid × 1 day
Fluconazole	150 mg	1 tablet × 1 day

[a]The US Food and Drug Administration warns of possible increase in anticoagulant effects of warfarin with concomitant use.

COMPLICATED VULVOVAGINAL CANDIDIASIS

Complicated VVC occurs in patients who are immunocompromised or have uncontrolled diabetes mellitus.[1] The main approach to the treatment of these individuals is to increase the length of therapy. Current recommendations are to lengthen therapy to 10 to 14 days regardless of the route of administration.[16] Therapeutic options would include those listed in Table 118–1; however, regimens should be continued for 10 to 14 days. In a study of patients experiencing severe infections, better outcomes were achieved with 7-day topical azole therapy as compared to single-dose fluconazole.[16] Length of therapy should also be extended in infections caused by non-*albicans* species. Most of these organisms have higher minimum inhibitory concentrations to the azoles as compared to *C. albicans*. They are still susceptible to the azoles, but require a longer duration of treatment.[1]

VVC during pregnancy may also be considered complicated because consideration of host factors such as hormonal changes that can affect normal flora are essential in selecting therapeutic regimens. Topical agents are considered to be safe throughout pregnancy. Nystatin topical cream used for treating VVC was considered to be the regimen of choice in the first trimester, but recent guidelines recommend the use of topical azoles and that 10 to 14 days of treatment may be necessary.[5] Oral agents are contraindicated in pregnancy because of the concern of fetal complications. However, a prospective assessment of pregnancy outcomes in 226 women exposed to fluconazole in the first trimester did not indicate increased risk of congenital abnormalities or other adverse outcomes.[17] The median dose of fluconazole was 200 mg with 46.5% of the cohort receiving a single dose of fluconazole 150 mg.

RECURRENT VULVOVAGINAL CANDIDIASIS

Recurrent vulvovaginal candidiasis (RVVC) is defined as having more than four episodes of VVC within a 12-month period.[1,5] Fewer than 5% of women develop RVVC and its pathogenesis is poorly understood. A proper diagnosis should be obtained to rule out other infections or nonmycotic contact dermatitis. Most of the therapies are empirical and not based on proper randomized controlled trials.[5] Treatments include induction therapy, which should be administered for a minimum of 14 days or until clinical remission, and negative cultures have been obtained.[1] Table 118–1 lists the medications used for induction therapy. Induction therapy should be followed by a maintenance regimen that is used for 6 months. The following are recommended maintenance regimens.

Clotrimazole 500 mg vaginally once weekly × 6 months
Fluconazole 100 mg once weekly × 6 months
Ketoconazole 100 mg daily × 6 months
Itraconazole 400 mg once monthly × 6 months

Fifty percent of women may experience a relapse after maintenance therapy is discontinued.[5] A relapse may be treated as an individual episode if relapses are infrequent. However, if the relapses establish a repetitive pattern, then induction and maintenance regimens are indicated.[1]

ANTIFUNGAL RESISTANT VULVOVAGINAL CANDIDIASIS

Resistance to azole antifungals should be considered in individuals who have persistently positive yeast cultures and fail to respond to therapy despite adherence to prescribed regimens.[1] These infections can be treated with boric acid or 5-flucytosine.[18,19] Boric acid is administered as a 600-mg intravaginal capsule daily for 14 days of induction therapy, followed by a maintenance regimen of one capsule intravaginally twice weekly. Boric acid is toxic if administered orally. 5-Flucytosine cream is administered vaginally; 1,000 mg inserted nightly for 7 days.

PHARMACOECONOMIC CONSIDERATIONS

There is little information on the pharmacoeconomics associated with VVC. One study examined the direct costs including medical expenses (medications, clinic charges) and nonmedical expenses (costs of travel and time required in obtaining treatment) of VVC. Indirect costs (output loss through disability and premature death) were excluded from their estimates. The estimated total cost for all episodes of VVC in the United States in 1995 was $1.8 billion. The costs were higher in black women compared to white women ($34 versus $16 per capita cost, respectively). This difference is largely a result of the higher incidence of VVC among black women and because black women tend to seek medical advice, rather than relying on self-diagnosis and treatment.[4]

EVALUATION OF THERAPEUTIC OUTCOME

Treatment of VVC will be considered to have positive outcomes if the symptoms of VVC are resolved within 24–48 hours and no adverse medication events are experienced. Self assessment of symptom relief is appropriate for most cases of VVC. If symptoms remain unresolved or recur, then further testing and treatment may be required.

OROPHARYNGEAL AND ESOPHAGEAL CANDIDIASIS

Candida is the predominant fungi responsible for the majority of oral fungal infections, and *Candida albicans* is the principal species causing the infection, commonly referred to as candidiasis (the proper but less commonly used term being candidosis).

EPIDEMIOLOGY AND MICROBIOLOGY

Candida species are present as a part of the natural microflora of the oral cavity, as well as the intestinal tract and vagina. *Candida* can be isolated from the oral cavity in 30% to 60% of healthy adults with no evidence of infection.[20,21] Colonization rates increase with severity of illness and duration of hospitalization, as well as with age. In adults over age 60 years, colonization rate was reported to be 59% as compared to 21% in persons ages 5 to 7 years.[22] In hospitalized patients, without human immunodeficiency virus (HIV) disease, *C. albicans* was detected in 70% to 80% of oral isolates, while non-*albicans Candida* species accounted for less than 10% of the isolates.[21]

The incidence of oropharyngeal candidiasis (OPC) has increased significantly over the past 15 to 20 years, with the rates of OPC increasing almost fivefold from 1980 to 1989.[20,23] Oropharyngeal candidiasis is the most common opportunistic infection in patients with HIV disease, and it may be the first clinical manifestation of the HIV infection in up to 70% of patients.[24,25] Eighty percent to 90% of HIV-infected patients will develop at least one episode of OPC at some stage during a progressive course of their disease.[21,23,25] The incidence of OPC in HIV-infected patients without acquired immune deficiency syndrome (AIDS) range from 7% to 48%.[21,25] The incidence increases as the CD4 lymphocyte cell count decreases, and OPC will occur in approximately 60% of those with a CD4 cell count $<$100–200 cells/mm^3, more than half of whom will experience a recurrence. In non-HIV diseases, such as leukemia, OPC is reported in up to one-third of leukemic patients.[26]

The prevalence of esophageal candidiasis has increased mainly because of its frequency in AIDS. Esophageal candidiasis is the first opportunistic infection in 3% to 10% of HIV-infected patients, and is the second most common AIDS-defining disease after *Pneumocystis carinii* pneumonia.[23] The mean incidence of esophageal candidiasis among HIV-infected patients ranges from 10% to 20%.[21,23]

Although oral candidiasis is usually synonymously linked with *C. albicans* infection, a number of other *Candida* species can also be pathogenic. These include *C. glabrata* (formerly *Torulopsis*), *C. tropicalis, C. krusei, C. guilliermondi, C. parapsilosis,* and others.[20,21,23] There has been a noteworthy increase in the frequency of infections caused by these non-*albicans Candida* species, with the rate increased by about fivefold to 17% of candidal infections in the early 1990s.[21,23] However, in patients with cancer, almost half (46%) of all *Candida* infections are caused by non-*albicans Candida* species.[23]

C. albicans is also the most common cause of esophageal candidiasis, accounting for approximately 80% of cases. Nonalbicans species responsible include *C. glabrata, C. tropicalis, C. krusei,* and *C. parapsilosis*.[23]

The epidemiology of mucosa candidiasis has been impacted by two factors. The widespread use of the azoles has led to a decline in the prevalence of mucosa candidiasis while leading to the emergence of refractory infections that have become difficult to treat. The introduction of highly active antiretroviral therapy (HAART) appears to have resulted in a significant decline in the prevalence of OPC and esophageal candidiasis by 50% to 60%.[25]

PATHOPHYSIOLOGY

Significant differences exist in the virulence among *Candida* species. Although the virulence factors of *Candida* are not well characterized, the main factors are surface molecules that permit adherence of the organisms to other structures (cells, extracellular matrix, and hardware), hydrolytic enzymes, and the ability to convert to a hyphal form.

The presence of *Candida* usually stimulates antibody formation and cell-mediated immunity in most healthy adults without causing any signs or symptoms of infection. Effective antifungal host-defense mechanisms in the oral cavity play an important role in maintaining the colonizing organisms in low numbers for years in the absence of inflammation. The changeover of the role of *Candida* from commensal to pathogenic in the human host usually occurs when host defenses are impaired, such as the T-lymphocyte-mediated immune system and neutrophils. Hence, in HIV infection, oral carriage of yeasts and risk of mucosal invasion increase with progressive decline in CD4 cells. Cytokines, especially γ-interferon, inhibit transformation of *Candida* blastoconidia to the more invasive hyphal phase.[21] Neutropenic patients are at highest risk of developing candidiasis, which underscores the importance of neutrophils in host defense against *Candida*.

Inherited or acquired immune impairment will usually result in an overgrowth of the oral fungal flora with subsequent development of OPC. Several factors contribute to the ability of *Candida* to cause infection. Structural host defects associated with *Candida* infection include breaks in the integrity of skin or mucous membranes caused by burns, trauma, or occlusion and maceration. Exogenous causes include the use of broad-spectrum antimicrobials that alter the colonizing flora, and use of corticosteroids and immunosuppressive drugs for prolonged periods. Alteration of the oral environment can be caused by dentures, nonpolished inner surface of which provides a milieu conducive to survival of *Candida* and other microorganisms.

Oropharyngeal candidiasis is considered one of the earliest indicators of HIV infection, and is a relatively reliable indirect marker of disease progression.[25] Although OPC is usually not a life-threatening infection, it may predispose patients to develop more invasive disease, including esophageal candidiasis.[23] The combination of OPC and esophageal symptoms is both specific and sensitive in predicting esophageal disease. The presence of OPC or esophageal candidiasis usually suggest a reduced CD4 cell count and/or elevated HIV load, and may be predictive of the progression and prognosis of HIV infection. The incidence of OPC increases, especially when the CD4 cells falls to between 500 and 200 cells/mm^3.[27] Esophageal candidiasis can be as common or even more common than OPC in patients with more advanced HIV infection. It occurs more commonly later in the natural history of AIDS, and almost invariably at a lower CD4 count (range, 10–105 cells/mm^3).[21] In more than half of HIV-infected patients, HIV infection evolves into AIDS as early as 1 to 3 years after the appearance of oral candida lesions, if the HIV infection remains inadequately controlled. Thus OPC has become one of the criteria frequently used in staging systems for HIV infection. For example, the Centers for Disease Control and Prevention classifies OPC as indicative of symptomatic HIV infection, but does not similarly classify it as AIDS.[23,24] Several studies show, that OPC, regardless of CD4 cell count, predicts the development of AIDS-related illnesses.[24]

RISK FACTORS

Local and systemic factors, as well as characteristics of the organism itself can increase the susceptibility of an individual to *Candida* infections. Table 118–2 summarizes the local and systemic factors that predispose to development of oropharyngeal candidiasis.[20,26] Other endocrine disorders besides diabetes mellitus, such as hypothyroidism, hypoparathyroidism, and hypoadrenalism, can also predispose patients to *Candida* overgrowth.[20] Patients with primary immune deficiencies such as lymphocytic abnormalities, phagocytic dysfunction, IgA deficiency, viral-induced immune paralysis, and severe congenital immunodeficiencies are also at risk for oropharyngeal candidiasis as well as disseminated candidiasis. Oral mucosal disease, such as lichen planus, can be preexistent causes of candidiasis. Smoking has been suggested as a predisposing risk factor. In many cases, multiple concurrent predisposing factors to candidiasis may exist; e.g., xerostomia with mucositis and break in epithelial surface or immunosuppression as might occur in a leukemic patient receiving radiation and chemotherapy. The severity and extent of *Candida* infections increase with the number and severity of predisposing risk factors.

CLINICAL PRESENTATION AND DIAGNOSIS

The clinical features of OPC can be quite diverse. Depending on the nature of the involvement, symptoms may range from none to sore, painful mouth, burning tongue, metallic taste, difficulty in speaking, and dysphagia. Similarly, clinical signs are variable, and lesions may occur on surfaces of the buccal mucosa, throat, tongue, or gums. Table 118–3 summarizes the five major forms of OPC. Pseudomembranous

TABLE 118–2. Risk Factors for Developement of Oropharyngeal Candidiasis

Local Factors	Potential Mechanisms
Use of steroids and antibiotics	Suppression of cellular immunity and inhibition of phagocytosis by steroids including chronic use of inhaled and topical steroids. Alteration of endogenous oral flora by broad-spectrum antibiotics, especially when used with steroids, creates a milieu for proliferation of *Candida* because of reduced environmental and nutritional competition.
Dentures	Enhanced adherence of *Candida* to acrylic material of dentures, reduced saliva flow under surfaces of denture fittings, improperly fitted dentures, or poor oral hygiene.
Xerostomia caused by drugs (e.g., tricyclic antidepressants, phenothiazine) and chemotherapy, radiotherapy to head-neck and various diseases (e.g., Sjögren's syndrome, HIV, cancer of head-neck, bone marrow transplant recipients)	Reduced dilutional and cleansing effect because of low secretion rate and low pH in saliva. Saliva and mucosa secretions have defense factors, such as lactoferrin, sialoperoxidase, lysozyme, histidine-rich polypeptide, secretory IgA antibodies, and specific anti-*Candida* antibodies, which help to prevent adhesion and overgrowth of *Candida*.
Disruption of oral mucosa due to chemotherapy and radiotherapy, ulcers, endotracheal intubation trauma, burns, and smoking	Oral mucositis induced by radiation and breaks in physical barrier of oral epithelium, which is protective against invasion by microorganisms; altered rate of mucosa regeneration by cancer chemotherapy, which increases vulnerability to infection.
Systemic Factors	**Potential Mechanisms**
Drugs (cytotoxic agents, corticosteroids, immunosuppressants postorgan transplant), environmental chemicals (benzene, pesticides)	Reduced immunity as a result of drug-induced neutropenia or cell-mediated immunity.
Neonates or advanced age	Immature immune system of neonates who usually acquire infection during birth to a mother with vaginal candidiasis, or from exposure to infected bottle nipples or to skin of adult care giver.
HIV infection/AIDS	Depletion of CD4 T lymphocytes, especially below 200–300 cells/mm^3; anti-*Candida* protective mechanism of T lymphocytes at a mucosal level is unclear but may be a result of altered cytokines, especially γ-interferon, which inhibit transformation of *Candida* blastocondia to the more invasive hyphal phase.
Diabetes	Higher than normal numbers of *C. albicans* cultured from saliva of daibetic patients. May be related to the elevated glucose levels and reduced chemotactic factor in saliva, altered neutrophil function, and reduced saliva volume and flow.
Malignancies (e.g., leukemia, head-neck cancer)	Use of intensive radiotherapy and chemotherapy can disrupt oral mucosa and can also cause xerostomia; also, prolonged use of broad-spectrum antibiotics in neutropenic patients can alter the normal oral flora. Because of the prolonged neutropenia, the principal immune defect, which is especially seen in leukemic patients, the initial oropharyngeal candidiasis can become systemic or invasive.
Nutritional deficiencies (e.g., iron, folate, vitamins B_1, B_2, B_6, B_{12}, C)	May be related to dietary restriction or GI absorption problems. Deficiencies may serve to enhance the pathogenic potential of the *Candida* inhabitants, alter host defense mechanisms, or cause a change in epithelial barrier integrity.

TABLE 118–3. Clinical Classification of Oropharyngeal Candidiasis

Types	Population at Risk	Clinical Signs and Appearance
Pseudomembranous (thrush)	Neonates; patients with HIV or cancer; debilitated elderly; patients on broad-spectrum antibiotics, steroid inhalers; patients with dry mouth from various causes; smokers	Yellowish white, soft plaques (or milk curds) overlying areas of erythema on the buccal mucosa, tongue, gums, and throat; plaques are easily removed by vigorous rubbing but may leave red or bleeding sites when removed; lesions on the tongue dorsum gives it a bald depapillated appearance.
Erythematous	Patients with HIV; patients on broad-spectrum antibiotics, steroid inhalers	Sensitive and painful erythematous mucosa with few, If any, white plaques; lesions are generally on dorsal surface of tongue or hard palate, occasionally on soft palate, but any part of mucosa can be involved; appear as flat red patches on the palate or atrophic patches on tongue dorsum with loss of papillae.
Hyperplastic (leukoplakic)	Smokers; uncommon in patients with HIV	Thick white and adherent keratotic plaques on the buccal mucosa, tongue, lips and bottom of mouth; plaques cannot be easily scraped off or only partially removed.
Angular cheilitis	Patients with HIV; denture wearers	Painful red, ulcerative, cracking or fissuring lesion at one or both corners of the mouth as a result of inflammatory reaction; lesions are usually small and rather punctate, but occasionally may extend in a linear fashion from the angles onto the facial skin.
Denture stomatitis	Denture wearers who tend to be the elderly and have poor oral hygiene	Red, flat lesions on mucosa beneath the denture that extend right up to the denture border; more commonly located beneath a maxillary denture although can be encountered beneath a mandibular denture.

candidiasis, commonly known as oral thrush, is the most common type, while in HIV infection pseudomembranous candidiasis, erythematous candidiasis, and angular cheilitis constitute the three most common forms. Patients with OPC may be asymptomatic even with large areas of affected mucosa. Symptomatic patients may report taste disturbances, a burning sensation, change in sense of smell, or a dry mouth, occasionally resulting in a decreased appetite and oral intake. Recurrences may have the initial type of presentation or as a different form. Dysphagia and odynophagia may occur in those with involvement of the oropharynx. It is important to note that OPC may appear with more than one group of symptoms simultaneously, or in conjunction with concurrent mucositis of other etiologies.[20]

The diagnosis of oropharyngeal candidiasis is primarily a clinical one, made by identification of the characteristic appearance in the oral mucosa.[24] For a more definitive diagnosis, cytology, culture, and biopsy procedures are needed to corroborate the clinical diagnosis. However, a positive cytology or isolation of *Candida* does not necessarily confirm infection by itself because *Candida* is a common commensal in the oral flora. In clinical practice, the more common approach is to treat the patient with a full therapeutic course of an antifungal. Restoration of an asymptomatic, healthy, pink oral mucosa would confirm the diagnosis of candidiasis. This approach has the advantages of being simple, painless, and inexpensive. However, hyperplastic candidiasis can be resistant to antifungal therapy and may be difficult to confirm with this method. Use of smears or cultures from swabs, whole saliva samples, or saline rinses may be used in cases of recalcitrant candidiasis to determine the infecting species and to predict likely drug resistance.

Esophageal candidiasis usually occurs as an extension of OPC. However, in many published reports, the esophagus was the only site involved, with the distal two-thirds, rather than the proximal one-third, as the most common site.[21] Esophageal candidiasis commonly causes odynophagia, dysphagia, or retrosternal pain. These symptoms may be severe enough to result in significant weight loss. Some patients with esophageal candidiasis may be completely asymptomatic despite objective esophageal involvement.[21] The diagnosis of esophageal candidiasis may be suggested by the characteristic findings of multiple plaque-like lesions on a barium esophagogram.[24] A definitive diagnosis requires endoscopy with brushing of the lesions or mucosal biopsy. Diagnostic testing may be done if the symptoms fail to resolve after adequate therapeutic trial. However, as with OPC, a therapeutic course with antifungal agent is usually employed before carrying out the invasive diagnostic procedures. The presence of OPC also serves as a moderately useful diagnostic marker for esophageal candidiasis.

▶ TREATMENT: Oropharyngeal Candidiasis

DESIRED OUTCOMES

The primary desired outcome in the management of OPC is the elimination of the associated clinical signs and symptoms. In the most severe cases, the patient's quality of life may be impaired, and may result in decreased fluid and food intake. If untreated or inappropriately treated, oropharyngeal candidiasis may lead to more extensive oral disease, especially in patients who are immunocompromised. The most serious complication of untreated OPC is extension of the infection to esophageal candidiasis. Because esophageal candidiasis is more debilitating, the patient's quality of life is more affected. It is important to initiate appropriate antifungal therapy for both oropharyngeal and esophageal candidiasis. Preventing or minimizing the number of future relapses of both types of candidiasis is an equally important outcome. The approach depends largely on the underlying predisposing conditions.

Minimizing toxicities of systemic antifungal agents, as well as ensuring that the patient takes the medication appropriately, are important secondary outcomes of therapy. Factors to consider include potential drug interactions and liver toxicity of the azoles, and renal toxicity of amphotericin B. Patients need to know how to best use topical agents for maximum effectiveness, as well as be aware if an agent should be taken with or without food.

GENERAL APPROACH TO TREATMENT

The management of *Candida* infections should be individualized for each patient, taking into consideration the underlying immune status, other concurrent mucosal and medical diseases, concomitant medications, and exogenous infectious sources. If possible, it is desirable to minimize all predisposing factors, such as administration of corticosteroids, chemotherapeutic agents and antimicrobials, as well as institution of proper oral hygiene, and resolving concurrent conditions such as denture stomatitis. Selection of an appropriate antifungal agent for treatment of candidiasis requires consideration of several factors, including patient's drug adherence; adequate saliva for dissolution of solid topical medications; risk of caries from sucrose or dextrose-containing preparations; potential drug interactions; coexisting medication conditions (e.g., liver disease may affect certain systemic drugs); location and severity of the infection; and the need for long-term maintenance therapy.[28] Another factor, which could impact drug selection, is the emergence of fluconazole-resistant species of *C. albicans,* and in some cases to all azoles, and other intrinsically more resistant species such as *C. krusei, C. glabrata,* and *C. tropicalis*. In patients with HIV disease, it is equally important for patients to be receiving optimal antiretroviral therapy to minimize future relapses.

Topical therapies should be the first choice for local and regional infections. The efficacy of antifungal agents for OPC varies in different patient populations. Until the polyene antifungal agents became available in the 1950s, gentian violet, an aniline dye, was commonly used to treat oropharyngeal candidiasis.[26] Problems with gentian violet include fungal resistance, skin irritation, and especially the unaesthetic staining of the oral mucosa. Current topical agents, such as nystatin and clotrimazole, have been the standard of treatment for uncomplicated oropharyngeal candidiasis, and are generally effective for treatment in otherwise healthy adults and infants. Topical agents are available in an assortment of formulations, including oral rinses (suspension), troches, powder, vaginal tablets, and creams. The two most common types of formulations currently used are the suspension and troches. Tables 118–4 and 118–5 summarize considerations for selection of a topical agent and the dosing regimen.

Systemic therapy is necessary in patients with OPC that is refractory to topical treatment, those who cannot tolerate topical agents, and those at high risk for disseminated systemic or invasive candidiasis. Effective treatment of esophageal candidiasis generally requires the use of systemic antifungal agents. However, these agents have the disadvantage of producing more side effects and drug-drug interactions (Tables 118–4 and 118–5). Limiting the use of systemic azole agents assists in preventing unnecessary drug exposure, and minimizes the

TABLE 118–4. Therapeutic Options for Mucosal Candidiasis

Antifungal	Preparation	Use	Treatment Dosage/Duration	Long-Term Suppressive Dosage
Clotrimazole	10 mg troche	OC	10 mg held in mouth for 15 to 20 minutes for slow dissolution, four to five times daily for 7 to 14 days	OC: same dose
Nystatin	100,000 U/mL suspension	OC	5 mL swish and swallow qid for 7 to 14 days	OC: same dose
	200,000 units troche	OC	1–2 troches qid for 7 to 14 days	
Amphotericin B	100 mg/mL suspension injection	OC	1 mL swish and swallow four to five times daily for 7 to 14 days	
		EC	Moderate disease: 0.15–0.3 mg/kg/day or 10–20 mg IV infusion for 10 days Severe disease: 0.3–0.6 mg/kg/day IV infusion for 10–14 days	
Ketoconazole	200 mg tablets	OC	200 mg daily for 7 to 14 days	200 mg daily
		EC	400 mg daily for 14 to 21 days	
Fluconazole	100 mg tablets	OC	100–200 mg daily for 7 to 14 days	OC: 100–200 mg daily
		EC	200–400 mg daily for 14 to 21 days	EC: 100–200 mg daily
Itraconazole	10 mg/mL solution	OC	100–200 mg (solution) or 200 mg (tablets) daily for 7 to 14 days	OC/EC: same dose
	100 mg tablet	EC	Same dose but for 14 to 21 days	

OC, oropharyngeal candidiasis; EC, esophageal candidiasis.

potential of drug-resistant candidiasis, particularly fluconazole resistance.

Antifungals are generally less efficacious in patients with HIV infection than in patients with cancer, and the time to response is also more prolonged.[21] In addition, treatment in HIV-infected patients usually produces a transient clinical response by lowering the quantity of organisms in the affected area without completely eradicating the yeast. The relapse rates are also higher in the HIV-infected patients than in other patient populations. As HIV infection progresses and antiretroviral treatment is suboptimal, patients usually experience more frequent recurrences of oropharyngeal, as well as esophageal candidiasis. This leads to more exposure to antifungals, to increased risk of antifungal resistance, and to more severe morbidity. The potential for antifungal cross-resistance creates an additional real concern. It is important to ensure that patients with oropharyngeal and/or esophageal candidiasis are also receiving optimal antiretroviral therapy that will help in the immune reconstitution.

OROPHARYNGEAL CANDIDIASIS—HIV-INFECTED PATIENTS

Any HIV-infected patient who presents with oropharyngeal and/or esophageal candidiasis should be assessed for adequacy and effectiveness of antiretroviral therapy and immunodeficiency status because the development of oropharyngeal/esophageal candidiasis reflects immunologic impairment or deterioration. Ensuring that the patient is receiving appropriate antiretroviral therapy will, in the long run, improve success in the management of the infection. It is appropriate to initiate therapy with topical agents for initial or recurrent episodes of OPC, provided that clinical symptoms are not severe and there is minimal risk of esophageal involvement.[25] Clinical responses with the resolution of signs and symptoms generally occur within 5 to 7 days of starting treatment.[21,25] Clotrimazole appears to be the most effective topical agent and demonstrates comparable clinical response rates with both fluconazole and itraconazole.[23,25] However, the mycologic cure rates are generally significantly lower and the 4 week relapse rates tend to be higher for clotrimazole as compared with the systemic triazoles.[23] This may be of limited clinical significance in patients receiving effective antiretroviral therapy owing to their decreased susceptibility to opportunistic infection. Nystatin suspension, although still frequently used, appears to be the least-effective agent, and is associated with frequent treatment failures and early relapses, especially in patients with advanced HIV disease or neutropenia.[23,26]

Systemic oral azoles could be reserved for use in the more severe episodes of OPC unresponsive to topical agents, or with concurrent esophageal involvement.[21,23,25] Ketoconazole was the first oral systemic azole agent to be used successfully in patients with malignancy and AIDS.[21] However, in several comparative trials the clinical efficacy was greater with the newer triazoles such as fluconazole and itraconazole (greater than 85%) than with ketoconazole (62% to 83%). Mycologic cure rates and relapse-free periods, as well as safety profiles, are also generally better with fluconazole and itraconazole.[21,23] Although clinical response in more than 80% of patients can be obtained with 50–100 mg daily doses of fluconazole, complete mycologic cure is more difficult to attain with the lower dose, especially in more advanced disease.[21] There is also concern raised about the potential of the lower dose contributing to selection of resistance. Itraconazole oral solution with an improved absorption profile compared with the capsule formulation, is comparable to fluconazole with respect to clinical and mycologic response, and relapse rates.[21,29] A 14-day treatment course of itraconazole seems to be more effective than a 7-day course—the shorter course is associated with lower rates of mycologic cure and higher relapse rates.[29] Itraconazole solution can be used as first-line therapy for OPC and it may be effective for cases refractory to fluconazole.[23,25]

OROPHARYNGEAL CANDIDIASIS—NON–HIV-INFECTED PATIENTS

This patient population includes those patients with hematologic malignancy (e.g., leukemia) or bone marrow transplant who are receiving cytotoxic chemotherapy; those patients with solid tumors; those patients with solid organ transplants who are receiving immunosuppressive therapy; and those patients with diabetes mellitus; as well as patients on prolonged courses of antibiotics or corticosteroids, and the debilitated elderly.[30] Factors to consider in deciding whether to use

TABLE 118–5. Antifungal Pharmacotherapy

Antifungal	Pharmaceutical Considerations	Common/Significant Side Effects	Drug Interactions
Topical Agents	• Not absorbed systemically—do not cause significant systemic adverse effects and drug interactions. • Requires frequent applications because of short contact time; ideal contact time between the drug and oral mucosa is 20 to 30 minutes • Requires sufficient saliva to dissolve troches; too much saliva can produce a dilutional effect especially for suspensions **Clotrimazole troche** • Has a pleasant taste; an alternative for patients who do not like the taste of nystatin • May be poorly soluble in presence of xerostomia, and the rough surface of tablet may become irritating to the oral soft tissue • Contains dextrose, which has cariogenic potential **Clotrimazole, Ketoconazole, Miconazole, or Nystatin cream** • Easier to apply to corners of mouth in angular cheilitis, three times daily **Nystatin suspension** • Has unpleasant taste • Has high sucrose content—cariogenic potential particularly in dentate patients, and caution when used in diabetics; sucrose-free formulation available in UK • A better choice for patients with xerostomia • Nausea/vomiting may be a problem in cancer patients already nauseated from chemotherapy **Nystatin troche** • Also contains sucrose • Has bitter taste and licorice flavor may be unpalatable to some patients • Problematic for patients with xerostomia • Vaginal tablets used as a troche have advantage of not containing sucrose, but unpalatable psychologically **Amphotericin B oral suspension** • Must be given four times daily • Has a pleasant taste	**Clotrimazole** • Altered taste • Mild gastrointestinal upset **Nystatin** • Usually mild—nausea, vomiting, diarrhea **Amphotericin B** • Nausea, vomiting, diarrhea with higher doses	**Clotrimazole** • None **Nystatin** • None
Systemic Azoles	• Convenient to take, usually dosed once to twice daily • Contraindicated during pregnancy, especially during the first trimester, except in severe disseminated cases **Ketoconazole** • Requires gastric acidity for absorption, which may be problematic in AIDS patients with achlorhydric; may be overcome by administering with acidic beverages such as Coca Cola **Fluconazole** • Better tolerated than ketoconazole • More completely absorbed than ketoconazole and itraconazole, with oral bioavailability of 90%, and is unaffected by food or gastric pH	**Ketoconazole** • Most common are nausea, vomiting, abdominal pain, itching, and headache[26] • Hepatotoxicity usually associated with long-term use; manifest more commonly as asymptomatic elevations in serum transaminases, reported in 2% to 10% of patients, and less commonly, hepatitis with jaundice, and rarely, hepatic failure; incidence of serious hepatotoxicity is reported to be in the range of 1:10,000 to 1:2,000[26] • Endocrine effects • Lichenoid mucosa reactions have been associated with long-term use[20] **Fluconazole** • Gastrointestinal upset	**Ketoconazole** Efficacy ↓ by • Antacids, H_2-blockers, proton-pump inhibitors • Carbamazepine, phenobarbital, phenytoin • Didansosine • Isoniazid, Rifampin ↑ Toxicity of • Atovaquone • Cisapride • Contraceptives, prednisone • Cyclosporin • Macrolides • Midazolam • Oral hypoglycemics • Rifabutin

TABLE 118–5. (Continued)

Antifungal	Pharmaceutical Considerations	Common/Significant Side Effects	Drug Interactions
	• Oral solution is now available **Itraconazole** • Capsule is more variably absorbed and is reduced by hypoacidity, and should be taken with food for optimum absorption; however, its greater potency than ketoconazole may enable effective plasma concentrations to be achieved even with incomplete absorption • Bioavailability of aqueous solution (in hydroxypropyl cyclodextrin) is improved by 30% as compared to the capsule • Absorption of solution is greater in fasting state than in the postprandial state • Solution also provides the benefits of both topical effects to the oral mucosa and systemic availability of the drug following absorption • Beneficial to patients with swallowing problems, mucositis, hypoacidity, or reduced gastric function.	• Hepatitis **Itraconazole** • Gastrointestinal upset • Hepatotoxicity[a] • CHF, pulmonary edema	• Theophylline • Warfarin **Fluconazole** Efficacy ↓ by • Rifampin ↑ Toxicity of • Cyclosporin • Contraceptives, prednisone • Sulfonylureas • Theophylline • Warfarin **Itraconazole** • Digoxin levels increased • Same drugs as ketoconazole
Intravenous	**Amphotericin B** • Requires sterile preparation	**Amphotericin B** • Fever, chills, sweat • Nephrotoxicity, electrolyte disturbance • Bone marrow	**Amphotericin B** Toxicity enhanced by • Aminoglycosides • Antineoplastics • Cyclosporin • Digoxin • Pentamidine

[a]See discussion under onychomycosis.

topical or systemic antifungal therapy include the severity and extent of mucosal involvement (oropharyngeal vs esophageal), predisposing risk factors, and risk for dissemination. Patients who develop neutropenia (e.g., leukemic and bone marrow transplant patients) are usually at higher risk for disseminated candidiasis, and treatment is more aggressive. Patients with cell-mediated immune deficits but who have normal or near-normal granulocyte function and number (e.g., solid tumors, solid organ transplants, or diabetic patients) are at low risk for dissemination of infection.

In immunocompromised patients, specific antifungal therapy may be unnecessary for the asymptomatic patients at relatively low risk for disseminated candidiasis, such as those who are not granulocytopenic or who are expected to have a short duration of granulocytopenia.[31] Many of these infections will clear spontaneously after recovery of the granulocytes, or discontinuation of antibiotic and/or immunosuppressive therapy. However, antifungal therapy is usually required for patients who have persistent infection, or who have significant symptoms, usually pain, or who are granulocytopenic with relatively high risk of fungal dissemination.[31] Topical agents may be first given a therapeutic trial depending on severity of infection and degree of immunosuppression. Although both nystatin and clotrimazole can be effective in treating OPC, nystatin suspension does not effectively reduce the incidence of either oropharyngeal or systemic candida infections in the immunocompromised patients receiving chemotherapy or radiation; its use is often associated with frequent treatment failures and early relapses.[26,31,32] Clotrimazole appears to more effective in reducing colonization and treating acute episodes in cancer patients who are immunocompromised. The recent availability of oral amphotericin B solution seems to be a reasonable alternative for patients not responding to clotrimazole; however, clinical trials are needed to evaluate its efficacy.

Use of systemic azole agents (ketoconazole, fluconazole, and itraconazole) should be considered for treating OPC in patients who have failed or who are unable to take topical therapy.[26,31] Fluconazole 100–200 mg daily tends to be more commonly used because of more extensive experience with its use, and it has a more favorable absorption and side effect profile as compared to ketoconazole. Ketoconazole is felt to be of no or limited benefit in treatment of *Candida* infections in neutropenic patients at high risk of dissemination.[30] If the oral route is not feasible for reasons, such as severe chemotherapy-induced mucositis, fluconazole may be administered intravenously. There is less experience with itraconazole, although the solution would seem a better choice because of enhanced oral absorption than the tablet formulation. In cases unresponsive to azoles, intravenous amphotericin B in relatively low doses of 0.1–0.3 mg/kg/day may be tried.[30,31] Because of the higher risk for dissemination in patients who are severely neutropenic ($<0.1 \times 10^9$ neutrophils/L) or clinically unstable (hypotensive, febrile), some clinicians may prefer to initiate therapy with intravenous amphotericin B at 0.6 mg/kg/day, with therapy continued until the neutropenia has resolved.[30,31]

Topical therapy with clotrimazole or nystatin for 7 days is usually adequate for treating mucocutaneous candidiasis in the majority of solid organ transplant patients.[33] Use of topical therapy will reduce the number of systemic drugs that these patients receive, and hence minimize the risk of drug-drug interactions. Failure to respond to topical agents warrants the use of fluconazole 200–400 mg daily. Low-dose amphotericin B, 5–10 mg daily for 7 to 10 days, is reserved for the unusual cases of treatment failure.

Patients who develop OPC because of prolonged antibiotic use or aerosolized corticosteroids use, can usually be managed successfully by discontinuation of the offending agent, and the infection will usually resolve. If there is strong desire to treat because of discomfort or need to hasten symptom resolution, or inability to stop the offending agent, therapy with a topical agent, either clotrimazole or nystatin, is effective in most cases. The advantage of systemic azoles is the convenience of less frequent dosing. Symptoms usually improve in 3 to 4 days. Amphotericin B oral suspension offers another option. Infants should be given smaller amounts more frequently (e.g., nystatin 100,000 units every 2 to 3 hours) to ensure better contact time. If the underlying cause for the infection is dentures, the patient should be instructed on proper disinfection by removing the dentures every night and soaking in antiseptic solution. Appropriate antiseptics for disinfection include chlorhexidine gluconate 0.12%, or a quaternary ammonium compound (1:750 benzalkonium chloride), or sodium hypochlorite as a 1:50 dilution of household bleach in tap water.[20]

ESOPHAGEAL CANDIDIASIS—HIV-INFECTED PATIENTS

Treatment of esophageal candidiasis requires systemic antifungal agents. Topical antifungal therapy with clotrimazole or nystatin is usually of limited value, except in the very mild forms of esophageal candidiasis in non–HIV-infected patients.[21] Fluconazole is more effective than ketoconazole, with respect to endoscopic cure and clinical response, and usually produces a more rapid onset of action and resolution of symptoms.[23] Fluconazole is also more effective than oral itraconazole capsules with respect to short-term (2 or 3 weeks) endoscopic and/or clinical cure, but equivalent with respect to long-term (12 months) cure.[23] However, itraconazole solution is as effective as fluconazole.[21,23] The use of fluconazole solution is an effective alternative, although there have been no comparative trials conducted.

In the more advanced esophageal disease, oral azole treatment may be ineffective. Systemic amphotericin B is reserved primarily for patients with endoscopically proven disease who are refractory to fluconazole therapy.[21]

ESOPHAGEAL CANDIDIASIS—NON–HIV-INFECTED PATIENTS

As in the case of HIV-infected patients, topical agents like nystatin and clotrimazole are not as effective as fluconazole for treatment of esophageal candidiasis. Most nongranulocytopenic patients respond favorably to fluconazole 200–400 mg daily given for 1 to 2 weeks.[31] However, in the severely symptomatic patients who are clinically stable (afebrile, nonhypotensive), intravenous fluconazole may be considered. Failure to respond because of potential resistant organisms to fluconazole warrants use of intravenous amphotericin B 0.6 mg/kg/day.

Granulocytopenic patients with mild to moderate symptoms who are clinically stable may be initiated on a trial of fluconazole 400 mg daily. If the symptoms worsen or fail to respond, intravenous amphotericin B may be used. Intravenous amphotericin B may be considered for initial therapy in granulocytopenic patients who present initially with severe symptoms, or who are at high risk for dissemination of *Candida,* such as those receiving other aggressive immunosuppressive therapy (e.g., corticosteroids, total body irradiation, antithymocyte globulin), and who have documented evidence of esophageal candidiasis, or who have failed an initial empirical trial of oral nonabsorbable agents or fluconazole.[31] Amphotericin B should be continued until at least the neutropenia resolves. For patients whose symptoms have resolved, and who are afebrile and clinically stable, amphotericin B should be discontinued and monitored closely for recurrence. In high-risk patients, particularly those with persistent fever and granulocytopenia, the potential presence of clinically occult, diffuse GI, or disseminated candidiasis should be considered.

ANTIFUNGAL PROPHYLAXIS IN HIV-INFECTED PATIENTS

Most antifungal agents (e.g., the azoles) currently employed to treat acute candidiasis infections are fungistatic rather than fungicidal. Thus, they primarily reduce the quantity of organisms and do not effectively eradicate the fungi permanently from the mucosal surfaces and skin which are home to these ubiquitous organisms. Initial therapeutic success of treatment may be followed by clinical relapses, especially in patients with predisposing immunodeficiency or other concurrent mucosal diseases. The risk for relapse appears to depend on duration of therapy and degree of immunosuppression, and may occur sooner after topical therapy and ketoconazole than after itraconazole or fluconazole therapy.[21]

Fluconazole is effective in reducing the risk for mucosal (oropharyngeal, esophageal, and vaginal) candidiasis in patients with advanced HIV disease, although it does not provide complete protection and breakthrough infections may still occur.[21] However, recent guidelines from the USPHS/IDSA do not recommend routine primary prophylaxis for mucosal candidiasis.[34] The rationale includes effectiveness of therapy for acute episodes; low incidence of serious invasive fungal disease; low mortality associated with mucosal candidiasis; the potential development of resistant candidiasis; the possibility of drug interactions; and the prohibitive long-term cost of prophylaxis. For the same reasons, chronic suppressive therapy (i.e., secondary prophylaxis of recurrent OPC) is also not recommended.[34] Clinicians should treat each acute episode of OPC as it occurs. However, in some HIV-infected patients with multiple recurrent episodes of symptomatic OPC, or when the disease is sufficiently severe, or who are at risk of developing esophageal candidiasis, chronic suppressive therapy (i.e., secondary prophylaxis) may be considered with fluconazole or itraconazole solution; ketoconazole is a less-desirable alternative.[21,34] On the other hand, patients with a history of documented esophageal candidiasis, particularly multiple episodes, are candidates to be considered for chronic suppressive therapy preferably with fluconazole or itraconazole solution.[34] It is important that HIV-infected patients receive concurrent effective antiretroviral therapy that appears to contribute to reduction in recurrence of mucosal candidiasis, likely via immune reconstitution.

ANTIFUNGAL PROPHYLAXIS IN NON–HIV-INFECTED PATIENTS

The use of antifungal prophylaxis in patients with cancer is a complex and controversial issue. Superficial fungal infections are unlikely to be fatal. However, neutropenic patients are at increased risk of systemic infection as a complication of superficial infection, especially if they are also taking antibiotics. The use of antifungal prophylaxis needs to be considered in the broader context of not only reducing colonization and risk of superficial candidiasis, but more importantly, in reducing the risk for disseminated or invasive candidiasis, and in improving mortality in the neutropenic patients. Ketoconazole, fluconazole, itraconazole, and clotrimazole all appear to have efficacy as antifungal prophylaxis.[35] However, comparative trials of the efficacy of these agents are lacking. The most data and experience relate to the use of fluconazole. Ketoconazole can reduce colonization rates with *Candida* species in susceptible populations, but it is not considered effective in preventing disseminated candidiasis. Prophylactic use of itraconazole seems effective, but prospective comparative trials are needed to better define its role. Nystatin is relatively ineffective in reducing the incidence of either oropharyngeal or systemic candidiasis in immunocompromised patients receiving chemotherapy or radiation.[32,36] Two meta-analyses indicate that there is beneficial effect of antifungal prophylaxis for OPC in cancer patients.[36,37] The partially absorbed agents (e.g., clotrimazole) seem to be more effective than the systemic azoles; the nonabsorbable agents (nystatin, amphotericin B) do not seem to be effective.[36] Despite the clinical data supporting the relative efficacy of antifungal prophylaxis for mucocutaneous candidiasis, they are largely ineffective in the prevention of disseminated candidiasis or improvement of survival in neutropenic leukemic patients.[33] The problems associated with the use of prophylaxis include development of fluconazole-resistant *C. albicans* strains and the shift in the incidence to more non-*albicans* species, as well as emergence of *Candida* isolates resistant to both amphotericin B and the newer azoles. Thus, there is concern regarding the widespread use of prophylaxis in the neutropenic leukemic patients considering the lack of solid data supporting their prophylactic efficacy coupled with the problems of drug resistance.

There is consensus regarding the value of fluconazole prophylaxis in patients undergoing allogeneic and high-risk autologous bone marrow transplantation (BMT). Fluconazole is effective in preventing superficial and disseminated candidiasis, and is associated with a lower overall mortality.[33] The current recommended dose of fluconazole is 400 mg daily orally or intravenously, although based on a retrospective study, 100–200 mg daily may be effective.[33] More recent data suggest that prolonged administration of fluconazole 400 mg daily for 75 days after allogeneic BMT is associated with an overall improved survival benefit because of decreased graft-versus-host disease, a persistent protection against disseminated candidal infections, and candidiasis-related death.[38] In a prospective trial in a mixed population of patients with leukemia or who were undergoing autologous BMT, itraconazole 400 mg daily as oral solution reduced the risk of invasive candidiasis from 4% to 0.5%.[39] When given prophylactically in low doses to neutropenic autologous bone marrow transplant recipients, amphotericin B may be beneficial in certain high-risk patients.[26] It may also be used prophylactically in solid organ transplant recipients.[26]

ANTIFUNGAL-REFRACTORY MUCOSAL CANDIDIASIS

Resistant and refractory candidiasis are often used interchangeably to describe difficult-to-treat cases of OPC. Resistant candidiasis more appropriately indicates a lack of *in vitro* susceptibility, whereas the refractory disease, as well as clinical failures and clinically unresponsive disease, indicate failure of episodes of OPC to respond to appropriate antifungal regimens.[25] Development of drug-resistant *Candida* is one factor associated with occurrence of refractory disease. In particular, the emergence of fluconazole-resistant *C. albicans* has become a significant therapeutic problem. In addition there is selection of other, inherently more resistant *Candida* species, such as *C. krusei, C. glabrata,* and, more recently, *C. dubliniensis*.[25] Other potential risk factors associated with the development of refractory disease and resistant candidiasis are similar and include frequent episodes, advanced AIDS with low CD4 cell count (<50 cells/μL), repeated courses and prolonged duration of various antifungal therapy, and prolonged systemic azole use.[21,23,25] Clinical failures of OPC may be a result of poor drug adherence, reduced drug absorption associated with hypochlorhydria, drug-drug interactions, or advanced immunosuppression, and should be distinguished from true refractory and drug-resistant disease.[21,25]

Treatment of refractory disease is frequently unsatisfactory, and clinical response is usually short-lived, with rapid and periodic recurrences. Improving immune function with effective potent antiretroviral therapy if available is often beneficial.[25,40] Doubling of the fluconazole dosage, to 400 mg or 800 mg daily, may be effective in some patients with infection caused by *Candida* of intermediate resistance, although the response may be just transient.[21] The increased dosage is usually ineffective for truly resistant strains unless drug interaction or poor patient adherence is causing the reduced serum drug concentrations. Fluconazole oral suspension may be beneficial in some patients because of increased salivary concentrations obtained when the suspension is taken with the swish-and-swallow technique.[21] Itraconazole oral suspension is effective in 55% to 70% of patients; however, the benefit is short-lived if chronic suppressive therapy is not maintained, and there is a high likelihood of the development of itraconazole resistance.[21] Amphotericin B oral suspension provides another option, although results from several small studies yielded mixed results, with clinical efficacy of 50% to 75%, and a high relapse rate.[21,25] Patients with severe disease unresponsive to other agents, require intravenous amphotericin B 0.4–0.6 mg/kg/day for 7 to 10 days to achieve clinical response.[21] After response, suppressive therapy with amphotericin B is required to increase disease-free intervals. Patients who fail to respond to amphotericin B and require >1 mg/kg/day may be candidates for liposomal amphotericin B preparations because of renal and/or bone marrow toxicities, although at a markedly higher cost. Flucytosine is usually not used as monotherapy because of rapid development of resistance, but may be used in combination with an azole or amphotericin B.

EVALUATION OF THERAPEUTIC OUTCOMES

Efficacy end points for oropharyngeal and esophageal candidiasis include rapid relief of symptoms, prevention of complications without early relapse after completion of course of therapy. Sterilization of the oral cavity is not a feasible end point as mycologic eradication is rarely achievable, especially in HIV-positive patients. Symptomatic relief of presenting signs and symptoms generally occur within 2 to 3 days of starting therapy, with complete resolution by 7 to 10 days. Patients should be advised about the time course and to return for reassessment when signs and symptoms recur. It is usually unnecessary for the patient to be reassessed soon after finishing the treatment course. However, HIV patients should be questioned and examined for occurrence of mucosa candidiasis as part of their regular follow-up. The frequency of monitoring may be more frequent in neutropenic patient because of concern for dissemination of candidiasis. During the period of neutropenia, temperature should be monitored daily, as well as signs of dissemination (see Chap. 119). Hospitalized patients who are receiving intravenous amphotericin B also require daily monitoring by the pharmacist.

Efficacy of the antifungal agent is partly influenced by patient adherence to the medication regimen. Patients must be counseled on proper administration and dosing, in particular for topical agents. Table 118–6 lists counseling tips.

The likelihood of drug-related problems pertaining to drug toxicity and drug interactions depends on which antifungal agent is used.

TABLE 118–6. Patient Counseling Tips for Oropharyngeal Candidiasis[30]

1. Clean the oral cavity prior to administering the topical antifungal agent. Daily fluoride rinses may help reduce the risk of caries when using an agent containing sucrose or dextrose.
2. Use the topical antifungal agent after meals because saliva flow and mouth movements can reduce the contact time.
3. Troches should be slowly dissolved in mouth, not chewed or swallowed whole, over 15 to 30 minutes and the saliva swallowed.
4. Suspension should be swished around the mouth in the oral cavity to cover all areas for as long as possible, ideally at least 1 minute, and then gargled and swallowed.
5. Remove dentures while medication is being applied to the oral tissues.
6. Dentures should be removed and disinfected overnight using an antiseptic solution such as benzalkonium chloride 1:750, chlorhexidine 0.12–0.2%, or sodium hypochlorite 1–2%. Disinfect oral tissues in addition to dental prosthesis.
7. Use a suspension instead of a troche if xerostomia is present; if a troche is preferred, the patient should rinse or drink water prior to dosing. For xerostomia, suggest nonpharmacologic measures for symptomatic relief, such as ice chips, sugarless gum or hard candy, and citrus beverages.
8. Complete treatment course even though symptomatic improvement may occur in 48 to 72 hours.

Safety end points include monitoring for occurrence of the relevant drug side effects and drug interactions.

MYCOTIC INFECTIONS OF THE SKIN, HAIR, AND NAILS

Superficial mycotic infections of the skin are referred to as dermatophytoses. They are common infections, which are usually caused by dermatophytes classified by genera: Trichophyton, Epidermophyton, or Microsporum.[42] Dermatophytes have the ability to penetrate keratinous structures of the body. These infections affect both male and female genders and all races. Reservoirs of mycotic infections include humans, animals, or soil.[42] Individuals may develop an infection if they come in contact with a reservoir in addition to having a conducive environment for mycotic growth (i.e., moist conditions).[43] Risk factors for the development of an infection include prolonged exposure to sweaty clothes, failure to bathe regularly, many skin folds, sedentariness, and confinement to bed.[43]

Mycotic infections of the skin have a classic appearance which consists of a central clearing surrounded by an advancing red, scaly, elevated border.[43] Infections of the nail can appear chalky and dull, yellow or white, and become brittle and crumbly.

Diagnosis is usually based on the patient history as well as the physical examination.[44] Diagnostic tests include direct microscopic examination of a specimen after the addition of potassium chloride (KOH) or fungal cultures. The KOH test is quick, inexpensive, and easy to perform, whereas cultures are more expensive and take longer to obtain results. Diagnostic tests are recommended when systemic therapy is likely to be prescribed.[44]

Superficial mycotic infections are categorized by the pattern and site of infection.[42] The most commonly occurring infections in North America are detailed below. A general approach to treatment includes keeping the infected area dry and clean and limiting exposure to the infected reservoir. Table 118–7 lists specific treatments for each mycotic infection.

TINEA PEDIS

Tinea pedis is the most common dermatophytoses (affecting approximately 70% of adults). It is better known as "athletes foot" and occurs in hot weather, exposure to surface reservoirs (locker room floors) and with the use of occlusive footwear.[43] Treatment with topical therapy for 2 to 4 weeks is often adequate for mild infections; however, severe infections or involvement of the nails requires oral therapy (Table 118–7).[43] Recurrence of infection occurs in up to 70% of individuals. Prolonged treatment with either topical or systemic therapy may be required.[44]

TINEA MANUUM

Tinea manuum usually involves the palmar surface of the hands, is unilateral, and may involve the feet. Treatment of this infection is similar to T. pedis (Table 118–7). Emollients that contain lactic acid may also be useful.[43]

TINEA CRURIS

Tinea cruris is an infection of the proximal thighs and buttocks.[44] It is referred to as "jock itch" and is more common in males. The scrotum and penis are often spared from infection. Treatment with topical therapy is recommended and should continue for 1 to 2 weeks after symptom resolution. Severe infections may require oral therapy (Table 118–7). Relief of pruritus and burning may be facilitated by the use of short-term (2 to 3 days) topical steroids (2.5% hydrocortisone).[43]

TINEA CORPORIS

Tinea corporis is an infection the glabrous skin of the trunk and extremities. Therapy is similar to T. pedis, T. manuum, and T. cruris (Table 118–7).

TINEA CAPITIS

Tinea capitis is a mycotic infection involving the scalp, hair follicles, and adjacent skin,[45] that primarily affects children. Treatment should consist of oral therapy as well as the cleaning of combs and brushes, which may be contaminated (Table 118–7).[2] Daily shampooing is recommended for removal of scales. Some children and adults may be asymptomatic carriers, thereby facilitating spread of the infection.[45] Family members who culture positive for T. tonsurans should be treated with a antifungal shampoo (ketoconazole, selenium sulfide, or povidone-iodine).[45]

TINEA BARBAE

Tine barbae affects the hairs and follicles of beards and mustaches.[45] Treatment is similar to T. capitis (Table 118–7). Removal of the beard or mustache is recommended.[43]

PITYRIASIS VERSICOLOR

Hyperpigmented and hypopigmented scaly patches characterize pityriasis versicolor. These patches are found on the trunk and extremities.[46] It is more common in adults and in areas with tropical ambient temperatures. Topical treatment is usually adequate unless there is extensive involvement, recurrent infections, or failure of topical therapy (Table 118–7).[46]

TABLE 118–7. Treatment of Mycoses of the Skin, Hair, and Nails

	Topical*+	Oral+#
T. pedis T. manuum T. cruris T. corporis	Butenafine qd Ciclopirox bid Clotrimazole bid Econazole qd Haloprogen bid Ketoconazole cream qd Miconazole bid Naftifine cream qd, gel bid Oxiconazole bid Sulconazole bid Terbinafine bid Tolnaftate bid Triacetin cream, solution tid Undecylenic acid—various preparations apply as directed	Fluconazole 150 mg once weekly for 1 to 4 weeks Ketoconazole 200 mg qd × 4 wk Itraconazole 200–400 mg per day × 1 wk Terbinafine 250 mg per day × 2 wk Griseofulvin 500 mg per day × 2–4 weeks (T. corporis), × 4–8 weeks (T. pedis)
T. capitis T. barbae	Shampoo only in conjunction with oral therapy or for treatment of asymptomatic carriers Ketaconazole twice weekly for 4 weeks Selenium sulfide daily for 2 weeks	Terbinafine 250 mg per day 4–8 wk Ketoconazole 200 mg qd × 4 wk Itraconazole 100–200 mg per day × 4–6 wk Griseofulvin 500 mg per day × 4–6 wk
Pityriasis versicolor	Clotrimazole bid Econazole qd Halprogin bid Ketoconazole qd Miconazole bid Oxiconazole cream only bid Sulconazole bid Terbinafine bid Tolnaftate tid	Ketoconazole 400 mg once Fluconazole 400 mg once Itraconazole 200 mg qd × 3–7 days
Onychomycosis (Fingernail, Toenail)	Ciclopirax nail lacquer—apply solution qhs for up to 48 weeks	Terbinafine 250 mg per day × 6 wk (finger), 12 wk (toe) Itraconazole 200 mg bid × 1 wk/mo × 2 mo (finger) × 3–4 mo (toe) *or* 200 mg per day × 2 mo (finger), × 3 mo (toe) Fluconazole 150–300 mg × 1/wk × 3–6 mo (finger), × 6–12 mo (toe)

*Other products are available including combination products.
+Length of therapy depends on mycotic sensitivity and severity of infection.
#See discussion under onychomycosis regarding potential toxicity of terbinafine and itraconazole.

ONYCHOMYCOSIS (TINEA UNGUIUM)

Onychomycosis is a fungal infection of the nails. It is more common in the toenails than in the fingernails. Topical therapy alone may not be successful. The US Food and Drug Administration recently approved a topical nail lacquer—ciclopirox 8% (Penlac)—for treatment of mild-to-moderate onychomycosis caused by T. rubrum, that does not involve the lunula.[47] Ciclopirox, a hydroxypyridine, has a broad spectrum of antifungal activity, although its mechanism of action is unknown. Initial improvement may take as long as 6 months to occur. However, complete cure is reported in less than 10% of treated patients, with only about 60% of responders still remaining disease-free at 12 weeks after stopping treatment. Griseofulvin was the first effective systemic antifungal agent for treatment of dermal mycoses, including onychomycoses. It has a narrow spectrum of activity, limited primarily to dermatophytes. Long-term success rates for toenail onychomycosis is less than 40%, and relapse rates are high despite therapy of a year or longer.[48,49] It is rarely used today with the advent of the azoles and terbinafine. Because of the potentially serious toxicity associated with long term use (12 to 18 months) of ketoconazole, and because of cure rates not much higher than those seen with griseofulvin, ketoconazole's use has been replaced by the newer triazole agents itraconazole and fluconazole.

Terbinafine, an allylamine, has the greatest *in vitro* activity against dermatophytes as compared to itraconazole and griseofulvin.[48] It is also active against molds, but is less active against yeasts. In contrast to the azoles, terbinafine is fungicidal and has lower affinity for the cytochrome P450 3A4 enzymes, and thus less propensity for drug interactions. However, terbinafine inhibits CYP2D6 enzymes, which are responsible for metabolism of tricyclic antidepressants and other psychotropic drugs.[50] Case reports document nortriptyline toxicity when given concomitantly with terbinafine. Clearance of terbinafine is reduced by cimetidine and enhanced by enzyme inducers such as, rifampin, rifabutin, and phenobarbital.[49,50] Terbinafine achieves maximum effective concentrations in the nail after 18 weeks with a 6-week treatment, and it has an average plasma half-life of about 3 weeks. Treatment of toenail onychomycosis requires a 12-week course, while a 6-week course is generally adequate for fingernail onychomycosis (Table 118–7).[48,50] Terbinafine achieves cure rates of up to 90% for fingernail infection and 60% to 80% for toenail infection, with 12-month relapse rates of 6% and 12%, respectively.[48–51]

Terbinafine pulse therapy may also be effective, although data are insufficient to recommend this method of administration.[52] The more common adverse effects reported with terbinafine are gastrointestinal (diarrhea, dyspepsia, nausea, abdominal path), dermatologic (rash, urticaria, pruritus), and headache; less common adverse effects include taste disturbances, fatigue, inability to concentrate, and asymptomatic liver enzyme abnormalities.[48,49,50] Although uncommon, severe adverse effects have been reported with terbinafine, including erythema multiforme, Stevens-Johnson syndrome, neutropenia, and hepatotoxicity. In May 2001, the Food and Drug Administration (FDA) issued a Public Health Advisory on the association of terbinafine tablets with serious hepatotoxicity, including liver failure, transplantation, and death.[53] Terbinafine is not recommended for patients with chronic or active liver disease, although hepatotoxicity may occur in patients with no preexisting liver disease or serious underlying medical condition. Prior to initiating terbinafine treatment, it is recommended to obtain appropriate nail specimens for laboratory testing to confirm the diagnosis of onychomycosis. Liver function parameters (serum transaminases) should be assessed prior to and periodically during treatment with terbinafine.

The clinical efficacy rates of itraconazole for onychomycosis range from 40% to 80%.[48,49] Compared to terbinafine, itraconazole seems to be slightly less superior.[48] Itraconazole may be administered as continuous or pulse therapy (Table 118–7). Pharmacokinetic features of itraconazole that favor its use for onychomycosis include strong affinity for keratinized tissue, high tissue binding, and slow elimination from tissues. Pulse therapy is possible with itraconazole because effective drug concentrations in the nail matrix and bed are achievable within a week of starting treatment, and effective concentrations remain present in the nail for six to nine months after drug discontinuation. Adverse drug effects are minimized with pulse therapy and patient compliance is enhanced. The common adverse effects of itraconazole are similar to terbinafine, such as gastrointestinal, dermatologic, and headache; less common adverse effects include dizziness, fatigue, fever, decreased libido, and asymptomatic liver enzyme abnormalities.[48–50] However, serious cases of liver failure, transplantation, and death have been reported with the use of itraconazole, resulting in a recent FDA Health Advisory warning.[53] Itraconazole is best avoided in patients with chronic or active liver disease. In addition, there is an FDA warning on the risk of developing congestive heart failure (CHF) associated with the use of itraconazole, possibly related to its potential negative inotropic effect.[53] Therefore, itraconazole should not be used in patients with evidence of history of ventricular dysfunction such as CHF. Prior to initiating itraconazole treatment, it is recommended to obtain appropriate nail specimens for laboratory testing to confirm the diagnosis of onychomycosis. Liver function parameters (serum transaminases) should be assessed prior to and periodically during treatment with itraconazole. Symptomatic assessment for development of CHF also should be included as part of therapy monitoring.

Fluconazole has only been recently evaluated in therapy of onychomycosis, and comparative data with other antifungal agents are lacking. Fluconazole may be given as continuous or pulse therapy. Clinical success rates greater than 75% are associated with use of fluconazole.[49] However, the range of dosages studied is wider than for itraconazole (Table 118–7).

Factors associated with poor response to systemic therapy include compromised immune system (AIDS); reduced blood flow (diabetes, peripheral vascular disease, vasculitis, connective tissue disease, congestive heart failure); coexistent nail disease (psoriasis); nail factors (slow growth, thick nails, severe disease); drug-resistant organisms because of extensive prior drug exposure; and reduced bioavailability (absorption problems, poor compliance, drug interactions).[54] A new nail may require 3 to 12 months to grow out. Thus, after completion of a treatment course, the nail may not appear clinically cured. Patients should be counseled that infection of fingernails requires 4 to 6 months, or even longer for toenails, to resolve.

▶ PRINCIPLES OF PHARMACOTHERAPY

- Self-diagnosis of VVC has a positive predictive value of 62%, therefore diagnosis should be based on clinical symptoms as well as vaginal pH and microscopy.
- Asymptomatic colonization of *Candida* in the vagina does not require therapy.
- Short courses of antimycotic agents are useful in the treatment of uncomplicated VVC. Therapy should be increased to 10 to 14 days in length when treating those with complicated VVC (i.e., immunosuppression, uncontrolled diabetes, severe infections, or pregnancy).
- Recurrent VVC defined as more than four episodes within 1 year should be treated with induction therapy (of at least 14 days or until clinical remission with negative cultures). Maintenance therapy for 6 months should follow induction therapy.
- The predominant pathogen in initial and recurrent episodes of OPC is *C. albicans*. The major factor that leads to the development of OPC is impairment of the host defense mechanisms, such as T-lymphocyte–mediated immune system and neutrophils. OPC is the most common opportunistic infection seen in patients with HIV infection, and the incidence and severity of OPC increase with disease progression. OPC may predispose patients to develop more invasive disease such as esophageal disease.
- Antifungal therapy is generally less efficacious in treatment of mucosal candidiasis in the HIV- infected patients than patients with cancer, and relapse rates are also higher in HIV-infected patients. It is important that these patients also be receiving optimal antiretroviral therapy.
- Selection of specific antifungal agents should consider factors, such as formulation characteristics; drug pharmacokinetics and interactions; side effects; patient adherence factors (convenience, taste, cost); severity and nature of the infection; underlying immune status; and emergence of drug resistance.
- Topical antifungal therapy should be considered first-line for treatment of initial or recurrent cases of uncomplicated OPC to minimize the risk of drug resistance. Systemic azole therapy should be reserved for cases unresponsive to topical therapies or for more severe OPC with esophageal involvement or profound neutropenia. Topical therapy is usually ineffective in treatment of esophageal candidiasis, which requires initiation of systemic azole agents.
- Neither primary nor secondary antifungal prophylaxis is routinely recommended for mucosal candidiasis in HIV-infected patients, except for patients with multiple recurrent episodes of symptomatic OPC or esophageal candidiasis, where secondary prophylaxis may be considered. In neutropenic leukemic patients, there is concern regarding use of antifungal prophylaxis because there are no solid data to support its efficacy coupled with potential for development of drug resistance. There is consensus regarding the value of antifungal prophylaxis in patients undergoing allogeneic and high-risk autologous BMT.

- Topical therapy is the route of choice in mild to moderate infections of T. pedis, T. manuum, T. cruris, T. corporis, and Pityriasis versicolor. Oral therapy is the route of choice for T. capitis, T. barbae, and onychomycosis.

REFERENCES

1. Sobel JD, Faro S, Force R, et al. Vulvovaginal candidiasis: Epidemiologic, diagnostic and therapeutic considerations. Am J Obstet Gynecol 1998; 178:203–211.
2. Hurley R. Recurrent *Candida* infection. Clin Obstet Gynecol 1981;8:209–213.
3. Haefner HK. Current evaluation and management of vulvovaginitis. Clin Obstet Gynecol 1999;42:184–195.
4. Foxman B, Barlow R, D'arcy H, Gillespie B, Sobel JD. *Candida* vaginitis self-reported incidence and associated costs. Sex Transm Dis 2000; 27:230–235.
5. Clinical Effectiveness Group. National guideline for the management of vulvovaginal candidiasis. Sex Transm Infect 1999;75(suppl 1):S19–S20.
6. Larsen B. Vaginal flora in health and disease. Clin Obstet Gynecol 1993; 36:107–121.
7. Sobel JD. Clinical vulvovaginitis. Clin Obstet Gynecol 1993;36:153–165.
8. Barbone F, Austin H, Louv WC, Alexander WJ. A follow-up study of the methods of contraception, sexual activity, and rates of trichomoniasis, candidiasis, and bacterial vaginosis. Am J Obstet Gynecol 1990;163:510–514.
9. Ferris DG, Dekle C, Litaker MS. Women's use of over-the-counter antifungal pharmaceutical products for gynecologic symptoms. J Fam Pract 1996;42:595–600.
10. Hilton E, Isenberg HD, Alperstein P, France K, Borenstein MT. Ingestion of yogurt containing *Lactobacillus acidophilus* as prophylaxis for candidal vaginitis. Ann Intern Med 1992;116:353–357.
11. Tooley PJ. Patient and doctor preferences in the treatment of vaginal candidiasis. Practitioner 1985;229:655–662.
12. Edelman DA, Grant S. One-day therapy for vaginal candidiasis a review. J Reprod Med 1999;44:543–547.
13. Perry CM, Whittington R, McTavish D. Fluconazole: An update of its antimicrobial activity, pharmacokinetic properties, and therapeutic use in vaginal candidiasis. Drugs 1995;49:984–1006.
14. Mendling W, Plempel M. Vaginal secretion levels after 6 days, 3 days and 1 day of treatment with 100-, 200-, 500-mg vaginal tablets of clotrimazole and their therapeutic efficacy. Chemotherapy 1982;28(suppl 1):43–47.
15. Kaplan B, Royburt M, Rabinerson D, Neri A. Once-daily fluocinonide-bifonazole combination for the treatment of vulvar itching and vulvovaginal candidiasis. Preliminary study. Clin Exp Obstet Gynecol 1996;23:173–176.
16. Sobel JD, Brooker JD, Stein GE, et al. Single oral dose of fluconazole compared with conventional clotrimazole topical therapy of candida vaginitis. Am J Obstet Gynecol 1995;172:1263–1268.
17. Mastroiacovo P, Mazzone T, Botto L, et al. Prospective assessment of pregnancy outcomes after first-trimester exposure to fluconazole. Am J Obstet Gynecol 1996;175:1645–1650.
18. Horowitz BJ. Topical flucytosine therapy for chronic recurrent candida tropicalis infections. J Reprod Med 1986;31:821–824.
19. Sobel JD, Chaim W. Treatment of *Torulopsis glabrata* vaginitis: Retrospective review of boric acid therapy. Clin Infect Dis 1996;22:336–340.
20. Fotos PG, Lilly JP. Clinical management of oral and perioral candidosis. Dermatol Clin 1996;14(2):273–280.
21. Vazquez JA. Options for the management of mucosal candidiasis in patients with AIDS and HIV infection. Pharmacotherapy 1999;19(1):76–87.
22. Kleinegger CL, Lockhart SR, Vargas K, Soll DR. Frequency, intensity, species and strains of oral candida vary as a function of host age. J Clin Microbiol 1996;34:2246–2254.
23. Darouiche RO. Oropharyngeal and esophageal candidiasis in immunocompromised patients: Treatment issues. Clin Infect Dis 1998;26:259–274.
24. Minamoto GY, Rosenberg AS. Fungal infections in patients with acquired immunodeficiency syndrome. Med Clin North Am 1997;81(2):381–409.
25. Powderly WG, Mayer KH, Perfect JR. Diagnosis and treatment of oropharyngeal candiasis in patients infected with HIV: A critical reassessment. AIDS Res Hum Retroviruses 1999;15:1405–1412.
26. Epstein JB, Polsky B. Oropharyngeal candidiasis: A review of its clinical spectrum and current therapies. Clin Ther 1998;20(1):40–57.
27. Powderly WG, Gallant JE, Ghannoum MA, Mayer KH, et al. Oropharyngeal candidiasis in patients with HIV: Suggested guidelines for therapy. AIDS Res Hum Retroviruses 1999;15:1619–1623.
28. Greespan D, Shirlaw PS. Management of the oral mucosal lesions seen in association with HIV infection. Oral Dis 1997;3(suppl 1):S228–S234.
29. Graybill JR, Vazquez J, Darouiche RO, et al. Itraconazole oral solution: A novel and effective treatment for oropharyngeal candidiasis in HIV/AIDS patients. Am J Med 1998;104:33–39.
30. Bombassaro AM. Oral candidiasis—a review of signs, symptoms and management. Pharm Pract 1995;11(4):54–60.
31. Freifeld AG, Walsh TJ, Pizzo PA. Clinical approaches to infections in the compromised host. In: Hoffman R, Benz EJ Jr, Shattil SJ, et al., eds. Hematology: Basic Principles and Practice, 3rd ed. Philadelphia, Churchill Livingstone, 2000.
32. Gotzsche PC, Johansen HK. Nystatin prophylaxis and treatment in severely immunodepressed patients. Cochrane Database Syst Rev 2000;3.
33. Anonymous. International conference for the development of a consensus on the management and prevention of severe candidal infections. Clin Infect Dis 1997;25:43–59.
34. USPHS/IDSA Prevention of Opportunistic Infections Working Group. 1999 USPHS/IDSA guidelines for the prevention of opportunistic infections in persons infected with human immunodeficiency virus. Clin Infect Dis 2000;30:S29–S65.
35. Preston SL, Briceland LL. Fluconazole for antifungal prophylaxis in chemotherapy-induced neutropenia. Am J Health Syst Pharm 1995;52: 164–173.
36. Clarkson JE, Worthington HV, Eden OB. Prevention of oral mucositis or oral candidiasis for patients with cancer receiving chemotherapy (excluding head and neck cancer. Cochrane Database Syst Rev 2000;2.
37. Meunier F, Paesmans M, Autier P. Value of antifungal prophylaxis with antifungal drugs against oropharyngeal candidiasis in cancer patients. Oral Oncol–Europ J Cancer 1994;30(3):196–199.
38. Kieren A, Seidel K, Slavin MA, Bowden RA, et al. Prolonged fluconazole prophylaxis is associated with persistent protection against candidiasis-related death in allogeneic marrow transplant recipients: Long-term follow-up of a randomized placebo-controlled trial. Blood 2000;96:2055–2061.
39. Menichetti F, Del Favero A, Martino P, et al. Itraconazole oral solution as prophylaxis for fungal infections in neutropenic patients with hematologic malignancies: A randomized, placebo-controlled, double-blind, multicenter trial. Clin Infect Dis 1999;28:250–255.
40. Valdez H, Gripshover BM, Salata RA, Lederman MM. Resolution of azole-resistant oropharyngeal candidiasis after initiation of potent combination antiretroviral therapy. AIDS 1998;12:538.
41. Piscitelli SG, Flexner C, Minor JR, et al. Drug interactions in patients infected with human immunodeficiency virus. Clin Infect Dis 1996;23:685–693.
42. Nowak MA, Brodell RT. Rapid diagnosis of superficial fungal infections. Postgrad Med 1999;2:179–180.
43. Goldstein AO, Smith KM, Ives TJ, Goldstein B. Mycotic infections effective management of conditions involving the skin, hair, and nails. Geriatrics 2000;55:40–52.
44. Drake LA, Dinehart SM, Farmer ER, et al. Guidelines of care for superficial mycotic infections of the skin: Tinea corporis, tinea cruris, tinea faciei, tinea manuum, and tinea pedis. J Am Acad Dermatol 1996;34:282–286.
45. Drake LA, Dinehart SM, Farmer ER, et al. Guidelines of care for superficial mycotic infections of the skin: Tinea capitis and tinea barbae. J Am Acad Dermatol 1996;34:290–294.
46. Drake LA, Dinehart SM, Farmer ER, et al. Guidelines of care for superficial mycotic infections of the skin: Pityriasis (tinea) versicolor. J Am Acad Dermatol 1996;34:287–289.

47. Ciclopirox (Penlac) nail lacquer for onychomycosis. Med Lett 2000;42: 51–52.
48. Niewerth M, Korting HC. Management of onychomycosis. Drugs 1999; 58:283–296.
49. Scher RK. Onychomycosis: Therapeutic update. J Am Acad Dermatol 1999;40:S21–S26.
50. Smith EB. The treatment of dermatophytosis: Safety considerations. J Am Acad Dermatol 2000;43(suppl 5):S113–S119.
51. Goldstein AO, Smith KM, Ives IJ, Goldstein B. Effective management of conditions involving the skin, hair and nails. Geriatrics 2000;55:40–52.
52. Noble SL, Forbes RC, Stamm PL. Diagnosis and management of common tinea infections. Am Fam Phys 1998;58:163–174.
53. Anon. FDA issues health advisory regarding the safety of Sporanox products and Lamisil tablets to treat fingernail infections. www.fda.gov/cder/drug/advisory/sporanox-lamisil/advisory.htm.
54. Mayeaux EJ Jr. Nail disorders. Prim Care 2000;27:333–354.

119
INVASIVE FUNGAL INFECTIONS

Peggy L. Carver

For many years, fungal infections were classified as either superficial "nuisance diseases," such as athlete's foot or vulvovaginal candidiasis, or as relatively rare infections confined primarily to endemic areas of the country. When invasive fungal infections were encountered, amphotericin B was the only consistently effective, systemically active agent available for the treatment of systemic mycoses. Advances in medical technology, including organ and bone marrow transplantation, cytotoxic chemotherapy, the widespread use of indwelling intravenous (IV) catheters, and the increased use of potent, broad-spectrum antimicrobial agents have all contributed to the dramatic increase in the incidence of fungal infections worldwide. Fungal infections have emerged as a major cause of death among cancer patients and transplant recipients.[1–4] In addition, patients with acquired immunodeficiency syndrome (AIDS) experience substantially more frequent and severe forms of cryptococcosis, histoplasmosis, coccidioidomycosis, and mucocutaneous (esophageal, oral, and vulvovaginal) candidiasis.

Problems remain in the diagnosis, prevention, and treatment of fungal infections. Unlike the available diagnostic techniques for most bacterial pathogens, there remains a host of unresolved issues regarding standardization of susceptibility testing methods, *in vitro* and *in vivo* models of infection, the utility of monitoring antifungal plasma concentrations, and the development and identification of resistant pathogens.[1,5,6,7] Recently, the Infectious Diseases Society of America published guidelines for the treatment of many commonly encountered fungal infections. These guidelines provide summaries of the literature and a consensus of expert opinions regarding the treatment of these difficult infections.[7]

MYCOLOGY

Fungi are eucaryotic organisms with a defined nucleus enclosed by a nuclear membrane; a cytoplasmic membrane containing lipids, glycoproteins and sterols, mitochondria, Golgi apparatus, ribosomes bound to endoplasmic reticulum; and a cytoskeleton with microtubules, microfilaments, and intermediate filaments. Fungi have rigid cell walls composed of chitin, cellulose, or both, that stain with Gomori methenamine silver or periodic acid-Schiff reagent. Most fungi, except *Candida*, are too weakly gram-positive to be seen well on Gram's stain. *Cryptococcus neoformans* has a polysaccharide capsule surrounding the cell wall.[7]

Morphologically, pathogenic fungi can be grouped as either filamentous molds or unicellular yeasts. *Molds* grow as multicellular branching, thread-like filaments (hyphae) that are either septate (divided by transverse walls) or coenocytic (multinucleate without cross walls) (Fig. 119–1). On agar media, molds grow outward from the point of inoculation by extension of the tips of filaments, and then branch repeatedly, interweaving to form fuzzy, matted growths called *mycelium*. Yeasts are oval or spherically shaped unicellular forms that generally produce pasty or mucoid colonies on agar media, similar to those observed with bacterial cultures. Yeasts have rigid cell walls that reproduce by budding, a process in which daughter cells arise from pinching off a portion of the parent cell.

Fungi reproduce by forming spores asexually via mitosis to produce motile sporangiospores or nonmotile conidia (singular, conidium), or they reproduce sexually through meiosis to produce ascospores, basidiospores, oospores, or zygospores. Although terms such as *spore* and *conidia* should no longer be used interchangeably, some newer literature and much of the older medical literature continue to confuse these terms.

In the past, clinical identification and naming of fungi was based on observations of the fruiting structures (often the asexual form) associated with the development of conidia. In more recent years, complete life cycles of many clinically relevant fungi have been elucidated, and additional names have been added to describe their sexual forms. Many microbiology laboratories and clinicians, however, continue to use the older names assigned to the asexual forms because most fungi isolated in the clinical laboratory are found in the asexual form, and the human diseases resulting from the pathogen are often based on this name. For example, *Blastomyces dermatitidis,* the etiologic agent of human blastomycosis, was named in 1898, based on its asexual (conidial) characteristics. In 1968, the life cycle of the fungus was found to include a meiotic stage that produces ascospores. A new name, *Ajellomyces dermatitidis,* was chosen to describe the sexual (ascomycetous) form; however, because the form isolated in clinical microbiology laboratories is *B. dermatitidis,* this name is retained for clinical use.

Many pathogenic fungi, termed *dimorphic fungi,* exist as either a yeast or a mold, depending on pathogen, site of growth (in the host or in the laboratory setting), and temperature. Usually, yeasts are the parasitic form that invade human or animal host tissue, while molds are the free-living form found in the environment. For example, *Histoplasma capsulatum* exists as a yeast in humans and as a mold in the laboratory.[1,8]

SUSCEPTIBILITY TESTING OF ANTIFUNGAL AGENTS

Most laboratories do not routinely perform susceptibility tests on fungal isolates, but standardized methods for performing these tests are being developed.[5] Standardized testing methods are now available for testing selected yeasts, including most *Candida* species; however, testing methods for *Aspergillus* and other filamentous fungi are still under development. Interpretive breakpoints are available for testing the susceptibility of *Candida* species to fluconazole, itraconazole, and flucytosine (Table 119–1). It is important that the breakpoints be used following testing with the standardized, reproducible laboratory methodology (NCCLS 27-A) used to develop the test, and that they be interpreted in the context of the delivered dose of the antifungal agent. For further detail, refer to the section outlining treatment of *Candida* infections. Reliable and convincing interpretive breakpoints are not yet available for amphotericin B. The NCCLS M27-A methodology does not reliably identify amphotericin-B resistant isolates; variations of the methodology using different media appear to enhance detection of resistant isolates.[5,9]

Because *in vitro* correlations with *in vivo* outcomes in patients are not yet known, the role of routine susceptibility testing is unknown at

(absolute neutrophil count <1,000/L). The potential benefits of prophylactic therapy must be weighed against the potential risks inherent in each regimen. Perfect[15] suggested that each clinician consider at least six criteria before justifying antifungal prophylaxis: (a) safety; (b) efficacy; (c) cost; (d) consequence; (e) prevalence; and (f) resistance.

Early empirical therapy is the administration of systemic antifungal agents at the onset of fever and neutropenia.

Empirical therapy with systemic antifungal agents is administered to granulocytopenic patients with persistent or recurrent fever despite the administration of appropriate antimicrobial therapy.

Secondary prophylaxis (or suppressive therapy) refers to administration of systemic antifungal agents (generally prior to and throughout the period of granulocytopenia) to prevent relapse of a documented invasive fungal infection that was treated during a previous episode of granulocytopenia.

Although these treatment classifications have also been applied to the treatment of fungal infections in AIDS, patients with AIDS rarely acquire systemic infections caused by *Candida* or *Aspergillus* spp. unless they become granulocytopenic because of disease or drugs. The use of antifungal prophylaxis is much less widely studied in this population, although studies suggest that early antifungal prophylaxis decreases the incidence of invasive cryptococcal disease.[16] Suppressive therapy is generally necessary following acute therapy for histoplasmosis, coccidioidomycosis, and cryptococcosis because of the high rates of relapse when antifungal therapy is discontinued.

PROPHYLAXIS OF HUMAN IMMUNODEFICIENCY VIRUS-INFECTED PATIENT

Fluconazole prevented cryptococcosis and local *Candida* infections, including esophagitis, but overall mortality was not improved.[10] Because of the high costs of long-term prophylaxis, improved therapeutic regimens available for treating cryptococcal meningitis, and increasing reports of fluconazole resistance among *Candida* isolates from AIDS patients, many clinicians prefer not to use fluconazole prophylaxis in AIDS patients. For some patients with very low CD4 counts, however, some clinicians feel it is cost-effective to use fluconazole prophylaxis to prevent cryptococcosis.[10]

HISTOPLASMOSIS

In humans, histoplasmosis is caused by inhalation of dust-borne microconidia of the dimorphic fungus *Histoplasma capsulatum*. Although there exist two dimorphic varieties of *H. capsulatum,* the small-celled (2–5 μm) form (var. *capsulatum*) occurs globally, while the large-celled (8–15 μm) form (var. *duboisii*) is confined to the African continent and Madagascar. *H. capsulatum* was originally named on the basis of intrahistiocytic plasmodia-like organisms recovered from tissues; however, the pseudoencapsulated appearance proved to be an artifact caused by cytoplasmic shrinkage from the rigid cell wall during tissue fixation. In tissues stained by conventional techniques, *H. capsulatum* appears as an oval or round, narrow-pore, budding, unencapsulated yeast.[17]

EPIDEMIOLOGY

Although histoplasmosis is found worldwide, certain areas of North and Latin America are recognized as endemic areas; in the United States, most disease is localized along the Ohio and Mississippi river valleys, where >90% of residents may be affected. Precise reasons for this endemic distribution pattern are unknown but are thought to include moderate climate, humidity, and soil characteristics. *H. capsulatum* is found in nitrogen-enriched soils, particularly those heavily contaminated by avian or bat guano, that accelerate sporulation. Blackbird or pigeon roosts, chicken coops, and sites frequented by bats, such as caves, attics, or old buildings, serve as "microfoci" of infections. Although birds are not infected because of their high body temperature, bats (mammals) may be infected and can pass yeast forms in their feces, allowing the spread of *H. capsulatum* to new habitats. Air currents carry the spores for great distances, exposing individuals who were unaware of contact with the contaminated site.[17–19]

PATHOPHYSIOLOGY

At ambient temperatures, *H. capsulatum* grows as a mold. The mycelial phase consists of septate branching hyphae with terminal micro and macroconidia that range in size from 2 to 14 μm in diameter. When soil is disturbed, these conidia become aerosolized and reach the bronchioles or alveoli.[17]

Animal studies demonstrate that within 2 to 3 days after reaching lung tissue, the conidia germinate, releasing yeast forms that begin multiplying by binary fission. During the next 9 to 15 days, organisms are ingested but not destroyed by large numbers of macrophages that are recruited to the infected site, resulting in small infiltrates. Infected macrophages migrate to the mediastinal lymph nodes and other sites within the mononuclear phagocyte system, particularly the spleen and liver. At this time, the onset of specific T-cell immunity in the nonimmune host activates the macrophages, rendering them capable of fungicidal activity. Tissue granulomas form, many of which develop central caseation and necrosis over the next 2 to 4 months. Over a period of several years, these foci become encapsulated and calcified, often with viable yeast trapped within the necrotic tissue.[17,20]

Cellular immunity, as measured by histoplasmin skin test reactivity, wanes in the absence of occasional reexposure. Although exposure to heavy inocula may overcome these immune mechanisms, resulting in severe disease, reinfection occurs frequently in endemic areas. In the immune individual, the reactions of acquired immunity begin 24 to 48 hours after the appearance of yeast forms, resulting in milder forms of illness and little proliferation of organisms. Although viable organisms may be found within granulomas years after initial infection, the organisms appear to have little ability to proliferate within the fibrous capsules, except in immunocompromised patients.[17,20]

CLINICAL PRESENTATION

The outcome of infection with *H. capsulatum* depends on a complex interplay of host, pathogen, and environmental factors. Host factors include the degree of immunosuppression and the presence of immunity (from prior infection). Environmental factors include inoculum size, exposure within an enclosed area, and duration of exposure. Hematogenous dissemination from the lungs to other tissues probably occurs in all infected individuals during the first 2 weeks of infection before specific immunity has developed, but is nonprogressive in the majority of cases, which leads to the development of calcified granulomas of the liver and/or spleen. Progressive pulmonary infection is common in patients with underlying centrilobular emphysema. A variety of acute and chronic manifestations of histoplasmosis appear to result from unusual inflammatory or fibrotic responses to the pathogen, including pericarditis and rheumatologic syndromes during the first year after exposure, with chronic mediastinal inflammation or fibrosis, broncholithiasis, and enlarging parenchymal granulomas later in the course of disease.[17,20]

ACUTE PULMONARY HISTOPLASMOSIS

In the vast majority of patients, low-inoculum exposure to *H. capsulatum* results in *mild* or *asymptomatic* pulmonary histoplasmosis. The course of disease is generally benign, and symptoms usually abate within a few weeks of onset. Therapy may be helpful in symptomatic patients whose conditions have not improved during the first month of infection. Fever persisting >3 weeks may indicate that the patient is developing progressive disseminated disease, which may be aborted by antifungal therapy. Whether antifungal therapy hastens recovery or prevents complications is unknown, because it has never been studied in prospective trials.

Patients exposed to a higher inoculum during an acute primary infection or reinfection may experience an acute, self-limited illness with flu-like pulmonary symptoms, including fever, chills, headache, myalgia, and a nonproductive cough. Patients with *diffuse pulmonary histoplasmosis* may have diffuse radiographic involvement, become hypoxic, and require ventilatory support. A small percentage of patients present with arthritis, erythema nodosum, pericarditis, or mediastinal granuloma, which may require the addition of anti-inflammatory agents to their therapy.[17]

CHRONIC PULMONARY HISTOPLASMOSIS

Chronic pulmonary histoplasmosis generally presents as an opportunistic infection imposed on a preexisting structural abnormality, such as lesions resulting from emphysema. Patients demonstrate chronic pulmonary symptoms and apical lung lesions that progress with inflammation, calcified granulomas, and fibrosis. Patients with early, noncavitary disease often recover without treatment. Progression of disease over a period of years, seen in 25% to 30% of patients, is associated with cavitation, bronchopleural fistulas, extension to the other lung, pulmonary insufficiency, and often death.[19]

DISSEMINATED HISTOPLASMOSIS

In patients exposed to a large inoculum and in immunocompromised hosts, successful containment of the organism within macrophages may not occur, resulting in a progressive illness characterized by yeast-filled phagocytic cells and an inability to produce granulomas. This disease, termed *disseminated histoplasmosis,* is characterized by persistent parasitization of macrophages. The clinical severity of the diverse forms of disseminated histoplasmosis (Table 119–2) generally parallels the degree of macrophage parasitization observed.[17]

Acute (infantile) disseminated histoplasmosis is characterized by massive involvement of the mononuclear phagocyte system by yeast-engorged macrophages. Classically, this severe type of infection is seen in infants and young children and (rarely) in adults with Hodgkin's disease or other lymphoproliferative disorders. In infants or children, acute disseminated histoplasmosis is characterized by unrelenting fever, anemia, leukopenia or thrombocytopenia, enlargement of the liver, spleen, and visceral lymph nodes, and GI symptoms, particularly nausea, vomiting, and diarrhea. The chest roentgenogram often demonstrates remnants of the initiating acute pulmonary lesion. Untreated disease is uniformly fatal in 1 to 2 months. A less severe "subacute" form of the disease, which occurs in both infants and immunocompetent adults, is characterized by focal destructive lesions in various organs, weight loss, weakness, fever, and malaise. Untreated disease is generally fatal in approximately 10 months.[17,19]

Most adults with disseminated histoplasmosis demonstrate a mild, chronic form of the disease. Untreated patients are often ill for 10 to 20 years, demonstrating long asymptomatic periods interrupted by relapses of clinical illness, characterized primarily by weight loss, weakness, and fatigue. Chronic disseminated histoplasmosis can be seen in patients with lymphoreticular neoplasms (Hodgkin's disease) and patients undergoing immunosuppressant chemotherapy for organ transplantation or for rheumatic diseases. Although central nervous system (CNS) involvement occurs in 10% to 20% of patients with severe underlying immunosuppressive conditions, focal organ involvement is uncommon. The disease is characterized by the development of focal granulomatous lesions, often with bone marrow involvement resulting in thrombocytopenia, anemia, and leukemia. Fever, hepatosplenomegaly, and GI ulceration are common.[17,19]

HISTOPLASMOSIS IN HIV-INFECTED PATIENTS

Adult patients with AIDS demonstrate an acute form of disseminated disease that resembles the syndrome seen in infants and children. Progressive disseminated histoplasmosis (PDH) can occur as the direct result of initial infection or because of the reactivation of dormant foci. In endemic areas, 50% of AIDS patients demonstrate PDH as the first manifestation of their disease. Progressive disseminated histoplasmosis is characterized by fever (75% of patients), weight loss, chills, night sweats, enlargement of the spleen, liver, or lymph nodes, and anemia. Pulmonary symptoms occur in only one-third of patients and do not always correlate with the presence of infiltrates on chest roentgenogram. A clinical syndrome resembling septicemia is seen in approximately 25% to 50% of patients.[17,19]

DIAGNOSIS

Detection of single, yeast-like cells 2–5 μm in diameter with narrow-based budding in direct exam or histologic study of blood smears or tissues should raise strong suspicion of infection with *H. capsulatum,* because colonization does not occur as with *Aspergillus* or *Candida* infection. Identification of mycelial isolates from clinical cultures can be made by conversion of the mycelium to the yeast form (requires 3 to 6 weeks) or via a rapid (2-hour) and 100% sensitive DNA probe that recognizes ribosomal DNA. In patients with suspected disseminated or chronic cavitary histoplasmosis, two to three blood, sputum, and bone marrow cultures and stains should be obtained using the lysis centrifugation technique, and the cultures held for 14 to 21 days for optimal yield of *H. capsulatum.* In patients with acute self-limited histoplasmosis, extensive testing to verify the diagnosis may not be necessary.[14,17,20]

In most patients, serologic evidence remains the primary method in the diagnosis of histoplasmosis. Results obtained from commercially available complement fixation (CF), immunodiffusion (ID), and latex agglutination (LA) antibody tests are used alone or in combination. In general, the use of histoplasmin skin tests is of little value except in epidemiologic studies, because histoplasmin reactivity waxes in the absence of occasional reexposure. In addition, histoplasmin skin testing may result in a false increase in the CF titer for mycelial antigen (CF-M) to *H. capsulatum.* A fourfold rise in the CF titer is

TABLE 119–2. Clinical Manifestations and Therapy of Histoplasmosis

Type of Disease and Common Clinical Manifestations	Approximate Frequency (%)[a]	Therapy/Comments
Nonimmunosuppressed host		
Acute pulmonary histoplasmosis		
Asymptomatic or mild disease	50–99	*Asymptomatic, mild, or symptoms <4 weeks*: No therapy generally required. *Symptoms >4 weeks*: Itraconazole 200 mg once daily × 6–12 weeks
Self-limited disease	1–50	*Self-limited disease*: AmB[b] 0.3–0.5 mg/kg/day × 2–4 weeks (total dose 500 mg) or ketoconazole 400 mg orally daily × 3–6 months may be beneficial in patients with severe hypoxia following inhalation of large inocula. Antifungal therapy generally not useful for arthritis or pericarditis. NSAIDs[c] or corticosteroids may be useful in some cases. *Mediastinal granulomas*: Most lesions resolve spontaneously. Surgery or antifungal therapy with AmB 40–50 mg/day × 2–3 weeks or ketoconazole 400 mg/day orally × >30 months may be beneficial in some cases.
Severe diffuse pulmonary disease		AmB 0.7 mg/kg/day, for a total dose of ≤35 mg/kg (or 3 mg/kg/day of one of the lipid preparations) + prednisone 60 mg daily × 2 weeks;[d] followed by itraconazole 200 mg once or twice daily for 6–12 weeks. In patients who do not require hospitalization, itraconazole 200 mg once or twice daily for 6–12 weeks, can be used.
Inflammatory/fibrotic disease	0.02	*Fibrosing mediastinitis*: Antifungal therapy has not been proven to be effective but should be considered, especially in patients with elevated ESR[e] or CF[f] titers ≥1:32. Surgery may be of benefit if disease is detected early; late disease may not respond to therapy. *Sarcoid-like*: NSAIDs or corticosteroids may be of benefit for some patients.
Chronic pulmonary histoplasmosis	0.05	Antifungal therapy generally recommended for all patients. Itraconazole 200–400 mg po daily × 12–24 months, is the treatment of choice. Itraconazole and ketoconazole (200–800 mg/day orally for 1 year) are effective in 75% to 85% of cases, but relapses are common. Fluconazole 200–400 mg daily is less effective (64%) than ketoconazole or itraconazole. AmB 0.7 mg/kg/day for a minimum total dose of 35 mg/kg is effective in 59% to 100% of cases, and should be used in patients who require hospitalization or who are unable to take itraconazole because of drug interactions, allergies, failure to absorb drug, or failure to improve clinically after a minimum of 12 weeks of itraconazole therapy.
Immunosuppressed host		
Disseminated histoplasmosis	0.02–0.05	*Disseminated histoplasmosis:* Untreated mortality 83% to 93%; Relapse 5% to 23% in non-AIDS patients.
Acute (Infantile)		*Nonimmunosuppressed patients:* Ketoconazole 400 mg/day orally × 6–12 months or AmB total dose of 35 mg/kg IV
Subacute		*Immunosuppressed patients (non-AIDS) or + endocarditis or CNS disease:* AmB total dose of >35 mg/kg
Progressive histoplasmosis (immunocompetent patients and immunosuppressed patients without AIDS)		*Life-threatening disease:* AmB 0.7–1 mg/kg/day IV, for a total dosage of 35 mg/kg over 2–4 months. After the patient is afebrile, able to take oral medications, and no longer requires blood pressure or ventilatory support, therapy can be changed to itraconazole 200–400 mg orally daily for 6–18 months. *Non–life-threatening disease:* Itraconazole 200–400 mg orally daily for 6–18 months. Fluconazole therapy (400–800 mg daily) should be reserved for patients intolerant to itraconazole; the development of resistance may lead to relapses.
Progressive disease of AIDS	25–50[g]	AmB for a total dose of 15–30 mg/kg (1–2 g over 4–10 weeks) or itraconazole 200 mg three times daily for 3 days, then twice daily for 12 weeks, followed by lifelong suppressive therapy with itraconazole 200–400 mg orally daily.

[a]As a percentage of all patients presenting with histoplasmosis.
[b]AmB, desoxycholate amphotericin B.
[c]NSAIDs, nonsteroidal anti-inflammatory drugs.
[d]Effectiveness of corticosteriods is controversial.
[e]ESR, erythrocyte sedimentation rate.
[f]CF, complement fixation.
[g]As a percentage of AIDS patients presenting with histoplasmosis as the initial manifestation of their disease.
(*Compiled from Refs. 17, 19, 20, and 48.*)

usually indicative of recent infection, although some patients with severe disease or profound immunosuppression may demonstrate a weaker antibody response. Because the ID test is not as sensitive as CF, it should be used to assess the importance of weakly reactive results obtained by CF rather than as a screening procedure. Radioimmunoassay (RIA), which measures immunoglobulin M (IgM) and IgG antibodies against a histoplasmin extract, is the most sensitive test, but it may show a large number of false-positive reactions in patients living in an endemic area.[14,17,20]

In the AIDS patient with PDH, the diagnosis is best established by bone marrow biopsy and culture, which yield positive cultures in >90% of patients, although blood cultures and histopathologic exam and culture of pulmonary tissue, sputum, skin, and lymph nodes may also be helpful. Detection of *H. capsulatum* polysaccharide antigen (HPA) in urine, blood, or cerebrospinal fluid (CSF) by enzyme-linked immunosorbent assay (ELISA) or by modified radioimmunoassay assay are promising new techniques for the rapid diagnosis of histoplasmosis. The HPA (RIA) levels have also been used successfully to monitor the course of therapy and detect relapses in patients with AIDS, and the clearance of antigen from serum and urine correlates with clinical efficacy during maintenance therapy with itraconazole. Unfortunately, these tests are not yet available for clinical use.[14,17,20]

▶ TREATMENT: Histoplasmosis

NON–HIV-INFECTED PATIENT

Table 119–2 summarizes the recommended therapy for the treatment of histoplasmosis. In general, asymptomatic or mildly ill patients and patients with sarcoid-like disease do not benefit from antifungal therapy. Patients with mild, self-limited disease, chronic disseminated disease, or chronic pulmonary histoplasmosis who have no underlying immunosuppression can usually be treated with either oral ketoconazole or IV amphotericin B. The goals of therapy are resolution of clinical abnormalities, prevention of relapse, and eradication of infection whenever possible, although chronic suppression of infection may be adequate in immunosuppressed patients, including those with HIV.[19,20]

HIV-INFECTED PATIENT

In AIDS patients, intensive 12-week primary antifungal therapy (induction and consolidation therapy) is followed by lifelong suppressive (maintenance) therapy with itraconazole. Amphotericin B dosages of 50 mg/day (up to 1 mg/kg/day) should be administered to a cumulative dose of 15–35 mg/kg (1–2 g) in patients who require hospitalization. Amphotericin B can be replaced with itraconazole 200 mg orally twice daily, when the patient no longer requires hospitalization or intravenous therapy, to complete a 12-week total course of induction therapy. In patients who do not require hospitalization, itraconazole therapy for 12 weeks may be used.

Fluconazole 800 mg orally daily as induction, followed by 400 mg daily, was effective in 88% of patients, but relapses occurred in approximately one-third of patients, and *in vitro* resistance developed in ≈50% of patients who relapsed.

In regions experiencing high rates of histoplasmosis (>5 cases/100 patient years), itraconazole 200 mg daily is recommended as prophylactic therapy in HIV-infected patients. Fluconazole is not an acceptable alternative because of its inferior activity against *H. capsulatum* and its lower efficacy for treatment of histoplasmosis.[19]

EVALUATION OF THERAPEUTIC OUTCOMES

Response to therapy should be measured by resolution of radiologic, serologic, and microbiologic parameters, and by improvement in signs and symptoms of infection. Although investigators are limited by the lack of standardized criteria to quantify the extent of infection, degree of immunosuppression, or treatment response, response rates (based on resolution or improvement in presenting signs and symptoms) of >80% have been reported in case series in AIDS patients receiving varied dosages of amphotericin B. Rapid responses are reported, with the resolution of symptoms in 25% and 75% of patients by day 3 and day 7 of therapy, respectively.

After the initial course of therapy for histoplasmosis is complete, lifelong suppressive therapy with oral azoles or amphotericin B (1–1.5 mg/kg weekly or biweekly) is recommended, because of the frequent recurrence of infection.[24,25] Relapse rates in AIDS patients not receiving maintenance therapy range from 50% to 90%.[19]

Antigen testing may be useful for monitoring therapy in patients with disseminated histoplasmosis. Antigen concentrations decrease with therapy, and increase with relapse. Some investigators recommend that treatment should continue until antigen concentrations revert to negative or <4 units. If treatment is discontinued before antigen concentrations in serum and urine revert to negative, patients should be followed closely for relapse, and antigen levels should be monitored every 3 to 6 months until they become negative.[19]

BLASTOMYCOSIS

North American blastomycosis is a systemic fungal infection caused by *Blastomyces dermatitidis* a dimorphic fungus that infects primarily the lungs. Patients, however, may present with a variety of pulmonary and extrapulmonary clinical manifestations. Pulmonary disease may be acute or chronic and can mimic infection with tuberculosis, pyogenic bacteria, other fungi, or malignancy. Blastomycosis can disseminate to virtually every other body organ, and approximately 40% of patients with blastomycosis present with skin, bone and joint, or genitourinary tract involvement without any evidence of pulmonary disease.[21]

EPIDEMIOLOGY

Blastomycosis was renamed "North American blastomycosis" in 1942, when Conant and Howell named a similar fungus endemic to South America *Blastomyces braziliensis* and the disease it caused "South American blastomycosis." The disease had previously been called paracoccidioidomycosis. Although the disease is now recognized to be endemic to the southeastern and south central states of the United States (especially those bordering on the Mississippi and Ohio river basins), and the midwestern states and Canadian provinces bordering on the Great Lakes, numerous cases of North American blastomycosis have been diagnosed in Africa, northern parts of South America, India, and Europe. Endemic areas have primarily been defined by analysis of sporadic cases and epidemics or clusters of disease, because the lack of a dependable skin or laboratory test makes wide-scale epidemiologic testing to determine the incidence of infection unfeasible at present.[20,21] Although initial review of sporadic cases suggested that males with outdoor occupations that exposed them to soil were at greatest risk for blastomycosis, more recent data suggest that there is no sex, age, or occupational predilection for blastomycosis.[20,21]

Although *B. dermatitidis* is generally considered to be a soil inhabitant, attempts to isolate the organism in nature have frequently been unsuccessful. *Blastomyces dermatitidis* has been isolated from soil containing decayed vegetation, decomposed wood, and pigeon manure, frequently in association with warm moist soil of wooded areas that is rich in organic debris.[20,21]

PATHOPHYSIOLOGY AND CLINICAL PRESENTATION

Pulmonary infection probably occurs by inhalation of conidia, which convert to the yeast form in the lung. A vigorous inflammatory response ensues, with neutrophilic recruitment to the lungs followed by the development of cell-mediated immunity and the formation of noncaseating granulomas.[12,20,21]

Acute pulmonary blastomycosis is generally an asymptomatic or self-limited disease characterized by fever, shaking chills, and productive, purulent cough, with or without hemoptysis, in immunocompetent individuals. The clinical presentation may be difficult to differentiate from other respiratory infections, including bacterial pneumonia, on the basis of clinical symptoms alone. Sporadic (nonepidemic) cases of pulmonary blastomycosis may present as a more chronic or subacute disease, with low-grade fever, night sweats, weight loss, and productive cough that resembles tuberculosis rather than bacterial pneumonia.[20,21]

Chronic pulmonary blastomycosis is characterized by fever, malaise, weight loss, night sweats, chest pain, and productive cough. Patients are often thought to have tuberculosis. Unlike patients with chronic pulmonary histoplasmosis, patients with chronic pulmonary blastomycosis often have evidence of disseminated disease that may appear 1 to 3 years after the primary pneumonia has resolved. Reactivation of disease may occur in the lungs or as the foci of new infection in other organs. In approximately 40% of patients, however, dissemination is not accompanied by reactivation of pulmonary disease. The most common sites for disseminated disease include the skin and bony skeleton, although less commonly the prostate, oropharyngeal mucosa, and abdominal viscera are involved. Central nervous system disease, while exceedingly uncommon, is associated with the highest mortality rate.[20,21]

DIAGNOSIS

The simplest and most successful method of diagnosing blastomycosis is by direct microscopic visualization of the large, multinucleated yeast with single, broad-based buds in sputum or other respiratory specimens, following digestion of cells and debris with 10% potassium hydroxide, because, like *Histoplasma,* colonization does not occur with *Blastomyces.*[14,21] Histopathologic examination of tissue biopsies and culture of secretions should also be used to identify *B. dermatitidis,* although it may require up to 30 days to isolate and identify a small inoculum. Unfortunately, no reliable skin test exists to determine the incidence and prevalence of disease in endemic populations. Reliable serologic diagnosis of blastomycosis has long been hampered by the lack of specific and standardized reagents, and, unfortunately, serologic response does not always correlate with clinical improvement, although some investigators have noted that a decline in the number of precipitins or CF titers may offer evidence of a favorable prognosis in patients with established disease.[20,21]

▶ TREATMENT: Blastomycosis

NON–HIV-INFECTED PATIENT

In patients with mild pulmonary blastomycosis, the clinical presentation of the patient, the immune competence of the patient, and the toxicity of the antifungal agents are the main determinants of whether or not to administer antifungal therapy. All immunocompromised patients and patients with progressive pulmonary disease or with extrapulmonary disease should be treated (Table 119–3). In the case of disease limited to the lungs, cure may have occurred before the diagnosis is made and without treatment. Regardless of whether or not the patient receives treatment, however, they must be followed carefully for many years for evidence of reactivation or progressive disease.[20–22]

Some authors recommend ketoconazole therapy for the treatment of self-limited pulmonary disease, with the hope of preventing late extrapulmonary disease; however, data supporting the efficacy of these regimens are lacking.[20,21] Ketoconazole appears to be as effective as amphotericin B for nonlife-threatening, nonmeningeal, mild-to-moderate blastomycosis in immunocompetent hosts. In a prospective, randomized, multicenter study conducted by the National Institute of Allergy and Infectious Diseases (NIAID) Mycoses Study Group,[23] high-dose (800 mg/day) oral therapy with ketoconazole was associated with a significantly higher cure rate than was low-dose (400 mg/day) therapy (85% vs 70%, respectively) in 80 patients with blastomycosis. The increased frequency of adverse effects (primarily intolerable nausea and vomiting) associated with high-dose therapy, however, prompted the NIAID's recommendation of low-dose ketoconazole therapy for patients with nonmeningeal, nonlife-threatening disease.[23] More recently, itraconazole has demonstrated efficacy as a first-line agent in the treatment of nonlife-threatening non-CNS blastomycosis, although it is more costly. Itraconazole 200–400 mg daily was effective in 90% of patients, and for compliant patients who completed at least 2 months of therapy, a success rate of 95% was noted. No therapeutic advantage was noted with the higher (400 mg) dosage as compared with those patients treated with 200 mg. Patients with CNS disease, progressive or life-threatening disease, or those experiencing toxicity while on ketoconazole should receive amphotericin B (0.7–1 mg/kg/day until a total dosage of 1.5–2.5 g is achieved).

All patients with disseminated blastomycosis, as well as those patients with extrapulmonary disease, require therapy. Ketoconazole 400 mg orally per day for 6 months cures more than 80% of patients with chronic pulmonary and nonmeningeal disseminated blastomycosis. Amphotericin B is more efficacious but more toxic, and, therefore, is reserved for noncompliant patients and patients with overwhelming or life-threatening disease, CNS infection, and treatment failures. Cumulative dosages of >1 g have resulted in cure without relapse in 70% to 91% of patients with blastomycosis. Relapse rates depend on the total dosage of amphotericin B administered.[20–22] Patients with genitourinary tract disease should be treated initially with 600–800 mg/day of ketoconazole because of the low concentrations of drug achieved in the urine and prostate tissue.

Patients should be monitored carefully for signs of clinical failure, and those who fail or are unable to tolerate itraconazole therapy, or who develop CNS disease, should be treated with amphotericin B for a total dose of 1.5–2.5 g.[20,21,23]

TABLE 119–3. Therapy of Blastomycosis

Type of Disease	Preferred Treatment	Comments
Pulmonary[a]		
Life-threatening	AmB[b] IV 0.7–1 mg/kg/day IV (total dose 1.5–2.5 g)	Patients may be initiated on AmB and changed to oral itraconazole 200–400 mg orally daily after patient is clinically stabilized and a minimum dose of 500 mg of amphotericin B has been administered.
Mild to moderate	Itraconazole 200 mg orally daily × ≥6 months	*Alternative therapy*: Ketoconazole 400–800 mg orally daily × ≥6 months or fluconazole 400–800 mg orally daily × ≥6 months. *In patients intolerant to azoles or in whom disease progresses during azole therapy*: AmB 0.5–0.7 mg/kg/day IV (total dose 1.5–2.5 g).
Disseminated or Extrapulmonary		
CNS[c]	AmB 0.7–1 mg/kg/day IV (total dose 1.5–2.5 g)	For patients unable to tolerate a full course of AmB, consider lipid formulations of AmB or fluconazole ≥ 800 mg orally daily.
Non-CNS		
Life-threatening	AmB 0.7–1 mg/kg/day IV (total dose 1.5–2.5 g)	Patient may be initiated on AmB and changed to oral itraconazole 200–400 mg orally daily after patient is stabilized.
Mild to moderate	Itraconazole 200–400 mg orally daily × ≥6 months	Ketoconazole 400–800 mg orally daily or fluconazole 400–800 mg orally daily × ≥6 months. *In patients intolerant to azoles or in whom disease progresses during azole therapy*: AmB 0.5–0.7 mg/kg/day IV (total dose 1.5–2.5 g). *Bone disease*: Therapy with azoles should be continued for 12 months.
Immunocompromised Host		
Acute disease	AmB 0.7–1 mg/kg/day IV (total dose 1.5–2.5 g)	Patients without CNS infection may be switched to itraconazole after clinically stabilized and a minimum dose of 1 g of amphotericin B has been administered.
Suppressive therapy	Itraconazole 200–400 mg orally daily	For patients with CNS disease or those intolerant to itraconazole, consider fluconazole 800 mg orally daily.

[a]Some patients with acute pulmonary infection may have a spontaneous cure. Patients with progressive pulmonary disease should be treated.
[b]AmB, desoxycholate amphotericin B.
[c]CNS, central nervous system.
(*Compiled from Refs. 20–23.*)

Lipid preparations of amphotericin B are effective in animal models of blastomycosis, but they have not been adequately evaluated in humans. Limited clinical experience suggests that these preparations may provide an alternative for patients unable to experience standard therapy with amphotericin B because of toxicity. Surgery has only a limited role in the treatment of blastomycosis.

HIV-INFECTED PATIENT

For unclear reasons, blastomycosis is an uncommon opportunistic disease among immunocompromised individuals, including AIDS patients; however, blastomycosis may occur as a late (CD4 lymphocytes

<200/mm^3) and frequently fatal complication of HIV infection. In this population, overwhelming disseminated disease with frequent involvement of the CNS is common.[20] Following induction therapy with amphotericin B (total dose of 1 g), HIV-infected patients should receive chronic suppressive therapy with an oral azole antifungal. Despite its higher cost, itraconazole has become the drug of choice for nonlife-threatening histoplasmosis (mild-to-moderate disease) in HIV-infected patients.[21]

COCCIDIOIDOMYCOSIS

EPIDEMIOLOGY

Coccidioidomycosis is caused by infection with *Coccidioides immitis,* a dimorphic fungus found in the southwestern and western United States, as well as in parts of Mexico and South America. In North America, the endemic regions encompass the semiarid regions of the southwestern United States from California to Texas known as the Lower Sonoran Zone, where there is scant annual rainfall, hot summers, and sandy, alkaline soil. *Coccidioides immitis* grows in the soil as a mold, and mycelia proliferate during the rainy season. During the dry season, resistant arthroconidia form and become airborne when the soil is disturbed.

Although generally considered to be a regional disease, coccidioidomycosis has increased in importance in recent years because of the increased tourism and population in endemic areas, the increased use of immunosuppressive therapy in transplantation and oncology, and the AIDS epidemic. Although there is no racial, hormonal, or immunologic predisposition for acquiring primary disease, these factors affect the risk of subsequent dissemination of disease.[24]

PATHOPHYSIOLOGY

When individuals come in contact with contaminated soil during ranching, dust storms, or proximity to construction sites or archaeologic excavations, arthroconidia are inhaled into the respiratory tree, where they transform into spherules, which reproduce by cleavage of the cytoplasm to produce endospores. The endospores are released when the spherules reach maturity. Similar to histoplasmosis, an acute inflammatory response in the tissue leads to infiltration of mononuclear cells, ultimately resulting in granuloma formation.[24]

CLINICAL PRESENTATION

Coccidioidomycosis encompasses a spectrum of illnesses ranging from primary uncomplicated respiratory tract infection that resolves spontaneously to progressive pulmonary or disseminated infection.[25,26] Initial or primary infection with *C. immitis* almost always involves the lungs. Although approximately one-third of the population in endemic areas is infected, the average incidence of symptomatic disease is only approximately 0.43%. Sixty percent of subjects are asymptomatic or have nonspecific symptoms that are often indistinguishable from ordinary upper respiratory infections, including fever, cough, headache, sore throat, myalgias, and fatigue. A fine diffuse rash may appear during the first few days of the illness. "Valley fever" is a syndrome characterized by erythema nodosum and erythema multiforme of the upper trunk and extremities in association with diffuse joint aches or fever. Valley fever occurs in approximately 25% of patients, although, more commonly, a diffuse mild erythroderma or maculopapular rash is observed. Patients may have pleuritic chest pain and peripheral eosinophilia. Radiographic features tend to be quite variable; hilar adenopathy with alveolar infiltrates, tissue excavation of an infiltrate (resulting in a thin-walled cavity), or small pleural effusions are all commonly seen. The development of erythema nodosum is thought to indicate the development of hypersensitivity to *C. immitis*.[24]

Some patients present with an acute pneumonia as the primary manifestation of disease. They have a productive cough that may be blood-streaked, as well as single or multiple soft or dense homogeneous hilar or basal infiltrates on chest roentgenogram. The disease usually lasts a few days to a few weeks and usually resolves spontaneously without therapy, although it can be fatal, particularly in patients who are immunocompromised.[24]

Although most primary pneumonias follow a benign course, pulmonary coccidioidomycosis can also develop into a chronic, persistent pneumonia complicated by hemoptysis, pulmonary scarring, and the formation of cavities or bronchopleural fistulas. Necrosis of pulmonary tissue with drainage and cavity formation occurs commonly in coccidioidal pneumonia. Most parenchymal cavities close spontaneously or form dense nodular scar tissue that may become superinfected with bacteria or spherules of *C. immitis*. These patients often have persistent cough, fevers, and weight loss. Primary disease lasting more than 6 weeks is termed persistent pulmonary coccidioidomycosis. Rarely, chronic pulmonary (also known as chronic progressive) pneumonia occurs, in which patients usually experience persistent cough, weight loss, chest pain, and intermittent fevers and hemoptysis. *Coccidioides immitis* can often be cultured from the sputum for a period of several years. Chest radiographs usually demonstrate apical fibronodular lesions or slowly progressive cavitation.[24]

Disseminated infection with *C. immitis* occurs in less than 1% of infected patients. The most common sites for dissemination are the skin, lymph nodes, bone, and meninges, although the spleen, liver, kidney, and adrenal gland may also be involved.[24] Occasionally, miliary coccidioidomycosis occurs, with rapid, widespread dissemination, often in concert with positive blood cultures for *C. immitis*. Patients with AIDS frequently present with miliary disease. Coccidioidomycosis in AIDS patients appears to be caused by reactivation of disease in most patients.[24,26]

Risk factors for severe, disseminated infection include race (blacks, Hispanics, Native Americans, and Filipinos) and pregnancy, although these data have been disputed by several investigators. Older data suggest that race-related differences in the incidence of severe disease exist, while newer studies suggest that an exposure to dust containing high inocula of *C. immitis* played a more important role. Pregnancy may lead to a general depression in cell-mediated immunity (particularly during the third trimester) or to an increase in sex hormones that stimulate the growth of the fungus. Immunocompromised hosts, particularly patients with AIDS and those receiving corticosteroids or immunosuppressive agents, are also at an increased risk for disseminated disease.[26] For unclear reasons, males appear to be at higher risk than females for disseminated disease, as are neonates and patients with type B or AB blood type. Surprisingly, the risk of disseminated disease does not appear to increase with age or the presence of diabetes mellitus.[24,26]

Central nervous system infection with *C. immitis* is a particularly devastating complication that develops in approximately 16% of patients with disseminated coccidioidomycosis.[26] Left untreated, coccidioidal meningitis is invariably fatal within 1 to 2 years. Early diagnosis is important, because early treatment appears to correlate with improved outcome. Patients may present with meningeal disease without previous symptoms of primary pulmonary infection, although disease usually occurs within 6 months after the primary infection. Signs of meningeal irritation common in bacterial meningitis are often absent. The signs and symptoms of coccidioidal meningitis are often subtle and nonspecific, including headache, weakness, changes in mental status (lethargy and confusion), neck stiffness, low-grade fever, weight loss, and occasionally hydrocephalus. Space-occupying lesions are rare, and the main areas of involvement are the basilar meninges. Analysis of the CSF generally reveals a lymphocytic pleocytosis with elevated protein and a decreased glucose. Although serum is usually positive for coccidioidal CF antibodies, the coccidioidal skin test is often negative.[24,26]

Infection of the genitourinary system is an increasingly recognized site of disseminated disease. Although patients tend to have chronic disease at these sites, including endometritis, prostatitis, epididymitis, and coccidioidouria, these do not necessarily indicate disseminated disease or a poor prognostic sign. Therapy is generally not necessary, except in the AIDS population, in whom chronic suppressive therapy is usually required.[24,26]

DIAGNOSIS

A number of tests have been developed to detect past or present infection with *C. immitis*. Most patients develop a positive skin test within 3 weeks of the onset of symptoms. Baseline evaluation of skin test reactivity and serology is essential in order to assess cell-mediated immunity. Patients who develop early positive skin test reactivity or whose coccidioidin skin test reactivity turns from negative to positive during therapy have an improved prognosis versus patients whose skin test reactivity develops later or does not change during therapy.[24,26] Patients with disseminated coccidioidomycosis whose skin tests are persistently negative are more likely to require prolonged therapy, and they are more likely to relapse after completion of therapy. The coccidioidal skin test also affects serologic tests for histoplasmosis but not those for coccidioidomycosis.[26]

Antibody production can be used to follow the course of disease because most patients produce antibodies in response to infection with *C. immitis*. Early infection is characterized by the development of the IgM antibody, which peaks within 2 to 3 weeks of infection then declines rapidly. The IgM antibody can be detected by either tube precipitin or immunodiffusion techniques.[24,26]

The IgG antibody levels rise between 4 and 12 weeks after infection and decrease slowly over months to years, and IgG can be detected in many body fluids, including serum, CSF, and pleural fluid by CF and ID techniques. Higher titers (>1:16 or 1:32) occur more frequently with severe disease. Titers can be followed serially to evaluate the efficacy of antifungal therapy.[24]

Recovery of *C. immitis* from infected tissues or secretions for direct examination and culture provides an accurate and rapid method of diagnosis. Because the spherule-endospore phase of coccidioidomycosis found in tissue is not infective, transmission of coccidioidomycosis from person to person does not occur. The mycelial-arthroconidia phase of *C. immitis* is extremely infective, however, and laboratory-acquired disease because of inhalation of aerially transmitted infective arthroconidia has been documented in more than 200 cases. In the past, inoculation of laboratory animals to produce spherule-containing abscesses was used to diagnose coccidioidomycosis definitively. This has largely been replaced by detection of antigen from an extract of the mold phase. Direct microscopic examination and histopathologic studies of infected tissues will reveal the large, mature endosporulating spherules. Young spherules without endospores may be confused, however, with other fungi. Silver stains of body fluids or tissue biopsies are also helpful.[13,24]

▶ TREATMENT: Coccidioidomycosis

GENERAL GUIDELINES

Therapy for coccidioidomycosis is difficult, and the results are unpredictable. The efficacy of antifungal therapy for coccidioidomycosis is often less certain than that for other fungal etiologies, such as blastomycosis, histoplasmosis, or cryptococcus, even when *in vitro* susceptibilities and the sites of infections are similar. The refractoriness of coccidioidomycosis may relate to the ability of *C. immitis* spherules to release hundreds of endospores, maximally challenging host defenses.[24,26] Fortunately, only approximately 5% of infected patients require therapy.[26]

SPECIFIC AGENTS USED FOR THE TREATMENT OF COCCIDIOIDOMYCOSIS

Specific antifungals (and their usual dosages) for the treatment of coccidioidomycosis include amphotericin B IV (0.5–0.7 mg/kg/day), ketoconazole (400 mg orally daily), IV or oral fluconazole (400–800 mg daily), and itraconazole (200 mg orally twice daily).[25,26] If itraconazole is used, measurement of serum concentrations may be helpful to ascertain whether oral bioavailability is adequate. Amphotericin B is generally preferred as initial therapy in patients with rapidly progressive disease, whereas azoles are generally preferred in patients with subacute or chronic presentations.[25,26]

PRIMARY RESPIRATORY INFECTION

Although most patients with symptomatic primary pulmonary disease recover without therapy, management should include follow-up visits for 1 to 2 years to document resolution of disease or to identify as early as possible, evidence of pulmonary or extrapulmonary complications. Management of primary respiratory infections is very controversial because of the lack of prospective, controlled trials. Patients with severe infections or concurrent risk factors (e.g., HIV infection, organ transplant, or high doses of corticosteroids) should probably be treated, particularly in patients with high CF titers in whom incipient or occult dissemination is likely. Because some racial or ethnic populations have a higher risk of dissemination, some clinicians advocate their inclusion in the high-risk group. Common indicators used to judge the severity of infection include weight loss (>10%); intense night sweats persisting >3 weeks; infiltrates involving more than one-half of one lung or portions of both lungs; prominent or persistent hilar adenopathy; CF antibody titers of >1:16; failure to develop dermal sensitivity to coccidial antigens; inability to work; or symptoms that persist for >2 months.[25,26]

Commonly prescribed therapies include currently available oral azole antifungals at their recommended doses, for courses of therapy ranging from 3 to 6 months.[25,26] In patients with diffuse pneumonia with bilateral reticulonodular or miliary infiltrates, therapy is usually initiated with amphotericin B; several weeks of therapy are generally required to produce clear evidence of improvement; consolidation therapy with oral azoles can be considered at that time. The total duration of therapy should be at least 1 year, and in patients with underlying immunodeficiency, oral azole therapy should be continued as secondary prophylaxis.

INFECTIONS OF THE PULMONARY CAVITY

Many pulmonary infections that are caused by *C. immitis* are benign in their course and do not require intervention. In the absence of controlled clinical trials, we lack evidence of the benefit of antifungal therapy, and asymptomatic infections are generally left untreated. Symptomatic patients may benefit from oral azole therapy, although recurrence of symptoms may occur in some patients once therapy is discontinued. Surgical resection of localized cavities provides resolution of the problem in patients in whom the risks of surgery are not too high.[25,26]

EXTRAPULMONARY (DISSEMINATED) DISEASE

NONMENINGEAL DISEASE

Almost all patients with disease located outside the lungs should receive antifungal therapy; therapy is usually initiated with 400 mg daily of an oral azole. Amphotericin B is an alternative therapy, and may be necessary in patients with worsening lesions or with disease in particularly critical locations such as the vertebral column. Approximately 50% to 75% of patients treated with amphotericin B for nonmeningeal disease achieve a sustained remission, and therapy is usually curative in patients with infections localized strictly to skin and soft tissues without extensive abscess formation or tissue damage. The efficacy of local injection into joints or the peritoneum, as well as intra-articular or intradermal administration, remains poorly studied. Amphotericin B appears to be most efficacious when cell-mediated immunity is intact (as evidenced by a positive coccidioidin or spherulin skin test or low CF antibody titer). Controlled trials that document these clinical impressions are lacking, however.[25,26]

MENINGEAL DISEASE

Fluconazole has become the drug of choice for the treatment of coccidioidal meningitis.[10,11,27] A minimum dose of 400 mg orally daily leads to a clinical response in most patients and obviates the need for intrathecal amphotericin B. Some clinicians will initiate therapy with 800 or 1,000 mg daily, and itraconazole dosages of 400–600 mg daily are comparably effective. It is also clear, however, that fluconazole only leads to remission rather than curing the infections; thus, suppressive therapy must be continued for life. Ketoconazole cannot be routinely recommended for the treatment of coccidioidal meningitis because of its poor CNS penetration following oral administration. Patients who do not respond to fluconazole or to itraconazole therapy are candidates for intrathecal amphotericin B therapy, with or without continuation of azole therapy. The intrathecal dose of amphotericin B ranges from 0.01 to 1.5 mg, given at intervals ranging from daily to weekly. Therapy is initiated with a low dosage and titrated upward as patient tolerance develops.[10,11,25–27]

CRYPTOCOCCOSIS

EPIDEMIOLOGY

Cryptococcosis is a noncontagious, systemic mycotic infection caused by the ubiquitous encapsulated soil yeast *Cryptococcus neoformans,* which is found in soil, particularly in pigeon droppings, although disease occurs throughout the world, even in areas where pigeons are absent. Infection is acquired by inhalation of the organism. The incidence of cryptococcosis has risen dramatically in recent years, reflecting the increased numbers of immunocompromised patients, including those with malignancies, diabetes mellitus, chronic renal failure, and organ transplants, or those receiving immunosuppressive agents. The AIDS epidemic has also contributed to the increased numbers of patients; cryptococcosis is the fourth most common infectious complication of AIDS and the second most common fungal pathogen.[28]

Although *C. neoformans* produces no toxins and evokes only a minimal inflammatory response in tissue, the polysaccharide capsule appears to allow the organism to resist phagocytosis by the host. The capsular polysaccharide of *C. neoformans* appears to comprise the major virulence factor for this pathogen. Four serotypes of *C. neoformans* (A through D) have been identified; they vary in their polysaccharide content, virulence, geographic foci, and response to antifungal therapy. Serotypes A and D are commonly associated with pigeon droppings and other environmental sites, and generally require shorter therapy than do infections caused by serotypes B or C, which have been found only in infected humans and animals. Serotypes B and C appear more resistant to antifungal agents *in vitro*. Patients with AIDS are almost always infected with serotypes A and D, even in areas endemic for serotypes B and C. There is no particular geographic area of endemic focus for *C. neoformans*.

Cell-mediated immunity appears to play a major role in host defense against infection with *C. neoformans;* 29% to 55% of patients with cryptococcal meningitis have a predisposing condition. Many patients with disseminated cryptococcosis demonstrate defects in cell-mediated immunity. The predilection of *C. neoformans* for the CNS appears to be caused by the lack of immunoglobulins and complement and the excellent growth media afforded by CSF.[28]

CLINICAL PRESENTATION

Primary cryptococcosis in humans almost always occurs in the lungs, although the pulmonary focus usually produces a subclinical infection. Symptomatic infections are usually manifested by cough, rales, and shortness of breath that generally resolve spontaneously. Disease may remain localized in the lungs or it may disseminate to other tissues, particularly the CNS, although the skin can also be affected. Hematogenous spread generally occurs in the immunocompromised host although it has also been seen in individuals with intact immune systems. Cryptococcemia is the most common symptomatic extraneural infection associated with *C. neoformans*. Cryptococcemia can be documented in 5% to 22% of non-AIDS patients, and CNS involvement of *C. neoformans* can be found in 18% to 50% of AIDS patients. In the non-AIDS patient, the symptoms of cryptococcal meningitis are nonspecific. Headache, fever, nausea, vomiting, mental status changes, and neck stiffness are generally observed. Less common symptoms include visual disturbances (photophobia and blurred vision), papilledema, seizures, and aphasia. In AIDS patients, fever and headache are common, but meningismus and photophobia are much less common than in non-AIDS patients. Approximately 10% to 12% of AIDS patients have asymptomatic disease, similar to the rate observed in non-AIDS patients. Cryptococcal disease is present in 7.5% to 10% of AIDS patients. Therefore, patients with evidence of extraneural cryptococcosis should be evaluated for CNS disease.[28]

DIAGNOSIS

Examination of CSF in patients with cryptococcal meningitis generally reveals an elevated opening pressure, CSF pleocytosis (usually lymphocytes), leukocytosis, a decreased CSF glucose, an elevated CSF protein, and a positive cryptococcal antigen. Antigens to *C. neoformans* can be detected by latex agglutination. The test is rapid, specific, and extremely sensitive, but false-negatives can occur. False-positive tests can result from cross-reactivity with rheumatoid factor and *T. beigelii*. *C. neoformans* can be detected in approximately 60% of patients by India ink smear of CSF, and it can be cultured in more than 96% of patients. Occasionally, large volumes of CSF are required in order to confirm the diagnosis. The CSF parameters in patients with AIDS are similar to those seen in non-AIDS patients with the exception of a decreased inflammatory response to the pathogen, resulting in a strikingly low number of leukocytes in CSF and extraordinarily high cryptococcal antigen titers.[13,28]

▶ TREATMENT: Cryptococcosis

The choice of treatment for disease caused by *Cryptococcus neoformans* depends on both the anatomic sites of involvement and the host's immune status.

NONIMMUNOCOMPROMISED PATIENTS

For asymptomatic, immunocompetent hosts with isolated pulmonary disease and no evidence of CNS disease, careful observation may be warranted; in the case of symptomatic infection, fluconazole or amphotericin B is warranted (Table 119–4). In those individuals with non-CNS cryptococcemia, a positive serum cryptococcal antigen titer (>1:8), cutaneous infection, a positive urine culture, or prostatic disease, the clinician must decide whether to follow the regimen for isolated pulmonary disease or the more aggressive regimen for patients with CNS (disseminated) disease.[16]

Prior to the introduction of amphotericin B, cryptococcal meningitis was an almost uniformly fatal disease; approximately 86% of patients died within 1 year. The use of large (1–1.5 mg/kg) daily doses of amphotericin B resulted in cure rates of approximately 64%. When amphotericin B is combined with flucytosine, a smaller dose of amphotericin B can be employed because of the *in vitro* and *in vivo* synergy between the two antifungal agents. Resistance develops to flucytosine in up to 30% of patients treated with 5-flucytosine alone, limiting its usefulness as monotherapy.[29,30] Combination therapy with amphotericin B and flucytosine will sterilize CSF within 2 weeks of treatment in 60% to 90% of patients, and most immunocompetent patients will be treated successfully with 6 weeks of combination therapy.[28] However, because of the need for prolonged IV therapy and the potential for renal and hematologic toxicity with this regimen, alternative regimens have been advocated. Despite a lack of clinically controlled trials in this population, amphotericin B induction therapy for 2 weeks, followed by consolidation therapy with fluconazole for an additional 8 to 10 weeks is frequently recommended, based on data extrapolated from studies conducted in HIV-infected patients. Suppressive therapy with fluconazole 200 mg daily for 6 to 12 months after the completion of induction and consolidation therapy is optional.[16,30–32]

Pilot studies evaluating combination therapy with fluconazole plus flucytosine as initial therapy yielded unsatisfactory results, and is discouraged even in "low-risk" patients. Ketoconazole has been used successfully in the treatment of cutaneous cryptococcosis, but it is not useful in the treatment of CNS disease, probably because of its poor penetration into the CNS.[16]

Despite low CSF concentrations of amphotericin B (2% to 3% of those observed in plasma), the use of intrathecal amphotericin B is not recommended for the treatment of cryptococcal meningitis except in very ill patients, or in those patients with recurrent or progressive disease despite aggressive therapy with IV amphotericin B. The dosage of amphotericin B employed is usually 0.5 mg administered via the lumbar, cisternal, or intraventricular (via an Ommaya reservoir) route two or three times weekly. Side effects of intrathecal amphotericin B include arachnoiditis and paresthesias. Intrathecal amphotericin B therapy should be administered in combination with IV amphotericin B.[32]

IMMUNOCOMPROMISED PATIENTS

Immunocompromised hosts with isolated pulmonary and extrapulmonary disease without CNS disease should be treated similar to nonimmunocompromised patients with CNS disease. Immunocompromised patients with CNS infection require more prolonged therapy; treatment regimens are based on those utilized in the HIV-infected population and follow induction and consolidation therapy followed by 6 to 12 months of suppressive therapy with fluconazole.[16]

HIV-INFECTED PATIENTS

There are no controlled clinical trials evaluating the therapy of isolated pulmonary infection; thus, the specific treatment of choice is unclear. However, because these patients are at high risk for disseminated infection, antifungal therapy is warranted in all patients. Lifelong therapy with fluconazole is recommended; in cases where fluconazole is not an option, itraconazole can be used.

Fluconazole is beneficial for both acute and chronic maintenance therapy for cryptococcal meningitis. Amphotericin B 0.4–0.5 mg/kg IV daily was compared to oral fluconazole 200 mg daily. Although the overall 10 week mortality was the same in both groups, the time until the CSF culture became negative was longer, and there were more deaths in the first 2 weeks of therapy in the fluconazole group.[31]

TABLE 119–4. Therapy of Cryptococcosis[a,b]

Type of Disease and Common Clinical Manifestations	Therapy/Comments
Nonimmunocompromised Host	
Isolated pulmonary disease (without evidence of CNS infection)	Comparative trials for AmB[c] vs azoles not available. *Asymptomatic disease:* Drug therapy generally not required; observe carefully or fluconazole 400 mg orally daily × 3–6 months. *Mild to moderate symptoms:* Fluconazole 200–400 mg orally daily × 3–6 months. *Severe disease or inability to take azoles:* amphotericin B 0.4–0.7 mg/kg/day (total dose of 1–2 g).
Cryptococcemia with positive serum antigen titer (>1:8), cutaneous infection, a positive urine culture, or prostatic disease	Clinician must decide whether to follow the pulmonary therapeutic regimen or the CNS (disseminated) regimen.
Recurrent or progressive disease not responsive to AmB	AmB[d] IV 0.5–0.75 mg/kg/day +/− IT AmB 0.5 mg 2–3 times weekly.
CNS disease	AmB[d] IV 0.7–1 mg/kg/day + 5-FC 100 mg/kg/day orally × 2 weeks, followed by fluconazole 400 mg orally daily for a minimum of 10 weeks (in patients intolerant to fluconazole substitute itraconazole 200–400 mg orally daily); *or* AmB[d] IV 0.7–1 mg/kg/day + 5-FC 100 mg/kg/day orally × 6–10 weeks; *or* AmB[d] IV 0.7–1 mg/kg/day × 10 weeks. *Refractory disease:* Intrathecal or intraventricular amphotericin B.
Immunocompromised Patients	
Non-CNS pulmonary and extrapulmonary disease	Same as nonimmunocompromised patients with CNS disease.
CNS disease	AmB[d] IV 0.7–1 mg/kg/day × 2 weeks; followed by fluconazole 400–800 mg orally daily 8–10 weeks; followed by fluconazole 200 mg orally daily × 6–12 months (in patients intolerant to fluconazole substitute itraconazole 200–400 mg orally daily). *Refractory disease:* Intrathecal or intraventricular amphotericin B.
HIV-Infected Patients	
Isolated pulmonary disease (without evidence of CNS infection)	*Mild to moderate symptoms or asymptomatic with a positive pulmonary specimen:* Fluconazole 200–400 mg orally daily × lifelong; *or* Itraconazole 200–400 mg orally daily × lifelong; *or* Fluconazole 400 mg orally daily + 5-FC 100–150 mg/kg/day orally × 10 weeks. *Severe disease:* Amphotericin B until symptoms are controlled, followed by fluconazole.
CNS disease	
Acute (induction/consolidation therapy) [follow all regimens with suppressive therapy]	AmB[d] IV 0.7–1 mg/kg/day + 5-FC 100 mg/kg/day orally × ≥2 weeks, then fluconazole 400 mg orally daily × ≥8 weeks;[e] *or* AmB[d] IV 0.7–1 mg/kg/day + 5-FC 100 mg/kg/day orally × 6–10 weeks;[e] *or* AmB[d] IV 0.7–1 mg/kg/day × 6–10 weeks;[e] *or* Fluconazole 400–800 mg orally daily × 10–12 weeks; *or* Itraconazole 400–800 mg orally daily × 10–12 weeks; *or* Fluconazole 400–800 mg orally daily + 5-FC 100–150 mg/kg/day orally × 6 weeks;[e] *or* Lipid formulation of amphotericin B IV 3–6 mg/kg/day × 6–10 weeks. *Note: Induction therapy with azoles alone is discouraged.*
Suppressive/maintenance therapy	Fluconazole 200–400 mg orally daily × lifelong; *or* Itraconazole 200 mg orally twice daily × lifelong; *or* Amphotericin B IV 1 mg/kg 1–3 times weekly × lifelong.

[a]When more than one therapy is listed, they are listed in order of preference.
[b]See text for definitions of induction, consolidation, suppressive/maintenance therapy, and prophylactic therapy.
[c]AmB, deoxycholate amphotericin B; IV, intravenous; IT, intrathecal; 5-FC, flucytosine; CNS, central nervous system.
[d]In patients with significant renal disease, lipid formulations of amphotericin B can be substituted for deoxycholate AmB during the induction phase.
[e]Or until CSF cultures are negative.
(*Compiled from Refs. 28–32.*)

In later trials,[32] amphotericin B 0.7 mg/kg IV daily for 2 weeks (with or without oral flucytosine 100 mg/kg/day), followed by consolidation therapy with either itraconazole 400 mg po qd or fluconazole 400 mg po qd led to markedly improved outcomes in comparison to earlier regimens. This study confirmed the benefit of early high dose (0.7 mg/kg/day) amphotericin B use, the utility of flucytosine added to amphotericin B for induction therapy, and the slight superiority of fluconazole over itraconazole for consolidation therapy.

Amphotericin B, combined with flucytosine, is the initial treatment of choice. In patients who cannot tolerate flucytosine, amphotericin B alone is an acceptable alternative. After the initial successful 2-week induction period, consolidation therapy with fluconazole can be administered for 8 weeks or until CSF cultures are negative. In cases in which fluconazole cannot be given, itraconazole is an acceptable, albeit less effective, alternative. Combination therapy with fluconazole plus flucytosine is effective; however, it is recommended as an alternative to the above therapies because of its potential for toxicity. Lipid formulations of amphotericin B are effective, but the optimal dosage is unknown.[16]

In HIV-infected patients with elevated intracranial pressure at the initiation of antifungal therapy, lumbar drainage should remove enough CSF to reduce the opening pressure by 50%. Patients should initially undergo daily lumbar punctures to maintain CSF opening pressure in the normal range. When the CSF pressure is normal for several days, the procedure can be suspended. Adjunctive steroid treatment is not recommended as therapy has resulted in mixed results and its impact on outcome is unclear. Similarly, neither mannitol nor acetazolamide therapy provide any clear benefit in the management of elevated intracranial pressure.[16]

SUPPRESSIVE (MAINTENANCE) THERAPY FOR CRYPTOCOCCAL MENINGITIS IN HIV-INFECTED PATIENT

Relapse of *C. neoformans* meningitis occurs in approximately 50% of AIDS patients after completion of primary therapy. Persistence of asymptomatic urinary *C. neoformans* has been documented in a high percentage of AIDS patients despite seemingly adequate courses of therapy for primary meningeal disease. The prostate appears to act as a sequestered reservoir of infection in these patients, resulting in systemic relapse. Fluconazole is recommended for chronic suppressive therapy of cryptococcal meningitis in AIDS patients. The AIDS Clinical Trials Groups (ACTG) 026 study demonstrated that oral fluconazole 200 mg daily was superior to IV administration of amphotericin B 1 mg/kg weekly in preventing relapse. In addition, the fluconazole-treated group showed a lower incidence of adverse drug reactions and bacterial infections.[32] Randomized comparative trials also demonstrated the superiority of fluconazole versus itraconazole as maintenance therapy. Thus, itraconazole should be reserved for patients intolerant to fluconazole. Ketoconazole is not effective as maintenance therapy.

Although some preliminary studies suggest lower relapse rates of opportunistic infections when patients have been successfully treated with potent antiretroviral therapy, until proven otherwise, maintenance therapy for cryptococcal meningitis should be continued for life. For selected patients who have responded very well to highly active antiretroviral therapy (HAART), the clinician may consider discontinuation of maintenance therapy following 12 to 18 months of successful suppression of HIV viral replication.[16,30–32]

EVALUATION OF THERAPEUTIC OUTCOMES

Once the CNS is involved, the usual course is weeks to months of progressive deterioration with 80% of untreated patients dying within the first year. The prognosis of cryptococcal meningitis depends largely on the underlying predisposing factors of the host. Although cryptococcal antigen is positive in 90% of patients with cryptococcal meningitis, fewer than half of the patients with cryptococcal meningitis develop antibody to capsular polysaccharide. Those who produce antibody have a slightly improved prognosis. In contrast, the presence of headache is a favorable symptom, presumably because it leads to an earlier diagnosis. A favorable outcome is also associated with a normal mental status upon diagnosis, and a CSF white blood cell (WBC) count of $<20/mm^3$. A poor outcome is predicted, however, by the presence of one or more underlying diseases (including hematopoietic disorders and AIDS), corticosteroid or immunosuppressive therapy, pretreatment serum cryptococcal antigen titers of 1:32, and posttherapy serum antigen titers of 1:8. In non-AIDS patients, the cryptococcal antigen titer can be followed during therapy to assess response to antifungal therapy. In AIDS patients, decreasing titers are not necessarily predictive of success, and titers rarely become negative at the completion of therapy.[10,11]

CANDIDA INFECTIONS

Candida spp. are yeasts that exist primarily as small (4–6 μm), unicellular, thin walled, ovoid cells that reproduce by budding. On agar media, they form smooth, white, creamy colonies resembling staphylococci. Although there are more than 150 species of *Candida,* eight species—*C. albicans, C. tropicalis, C. parapsilosis, C. krusei, C. stellatoidea, C. guilliermondi, C. lusitaniae,* and *C. glabrata*—are regarded as clinically important pathogens in human disease.[8,12] Yeast forms, hyphae, and pseudohyphae may be found in clinical specimens. Until recently, a rapid presumptive identification of *C. albicans* could be made by incubation of the organism in serum; formation of a germ tube within 1 to 2 hours offered a positive identification of *C. albicans.*[8] Unfortunately, *C. dubliniensis,* a new species of *Candida* which was recently identified as an important cause of mucosal colonization and infection in HIV-infected individuals, is also germ tube positive. A negative germ tube test does not rule out the possibility of *C. albicans,* but further biochemical tests must be performed in order to differentiate between other non-*albicans* species.[8,33]

EPIDEMIOLOGY

C. albicans is a normal commensal of the skin, female genital tract, and the entire GI tract of humans. Therefore, the mere presence of hyphae or pseudohyphae in a clinical specimen is insufficient for the diagnosis of invasive disease. The majority of infections with *C. albicans* are acquired endogenously, although human-to-human transmission can also occur. Oral candidiasis in the newborn is probably acquired during passage through the birth canal, and balanitis in the uncircumcised male may be acquired through contact with a female with vaginal candidiasis.[8] Although the term *fungemia* refers to the presence of fungi in the blood, the most commonly isolated organism is *C. albicans.* Candidiasis may cause mucocutaneous or systemic infection, including endocarditis, peritonitis, arthritis, and infection of the CNS. (Mucocutaneous infections caused by *Candida* are discussed in further detail in Chap. 118.)

PATHOPHYSIOLOGY

The role of an intact integument is crucial in the prevention of mucocutaneous or hematogenous candidiasis. After *Candida* invades the dermis or enters the bloodstream, polymorphonuclear leukocytes (PMNs) play a major role in the defense of the patient, because PMNs are capable of damaging pseudohyphae and can phagocytize and kill blastoconidia.[8] In addition to neutrophils, lymphocytes, monocytes, macrophages, complement, and eosinophils play a role in the prevention of infection. Adherence of *C. albicans* is important in the pathogenesis of oral candidiasis and subsequent colonization of the GI tract. Because evidence suggests that the GI tract is often the portal of entry for *Candida* in disseminated disease, factors that alter the adherence of *Candida* are crucial in the development of local and systemic infection. *Candida tropicalis* adheres to intravascular catheters at a higher rate than *C. albicans,* a factor that may help to account for the increased incidence of systemic infections caused by this pathogen.

HEMATOGENOUS CANDIDIASIS

EPIDEMIOLOGY

The term *systemic candidiasis* describes any candidal infection that invades beyond the membranes of the skin or mucosa. This term does not differentiate hematogenously disseminated candidiasis (in a neutropenic transplant patient) from infections arising from the urinary tract. Accordingly, some clinicians have proposed that systemic candidiasis be eliminated, and the term *hematogenous candidiasis* be used to describe the clinical circumstances in which hematogenous seeding to deep organs, such as the eye, brain, heart, and kidney, occurs in a patient.[10,11] Specific anatomic reference should be made to the site of the infection. For example, *Candida* infection of the peritoneum would be termed *Candida* peritonitis.

Hematogenous candidiasis is reported in significantly higher frequency because of the increased numbers of immunosuppressed patients, including those with lymphoreticular or hematologic malignancies, diabetes, immunodeficiency diseases, or those receiving immunosuppressive therapy with high-dose corticosteroids, immunosuppressants, antineoplastic agents, or broad-spectrum antimicrobial agents.[8,10,11] Patients who have undergone surgery (particularly surgery of the GI tract) are increasingly susceptible to disseminated candidal infections.[34,35]

The Centers for Disease Control and Prevention's (CDC) National Nosocomial Infection Survey implicated fungi as the cause of 8% of nosocomial infections. Although *C. albicans* accounted for 53% of *Candida* species,[11] non-*albicans* species of *Candida* are increasingly frequent causes of invasive candidal infections.[36,37] The SENTRY antimicrobial surveillance program conducted in 34 medical centers throughout the United States, Canada, and Latin America, reported that of 634 bloodstream infections in 1997–1998 caused by *Candida* species, 54% were caused by *C. albicans,* 16% by *C. glabrata,* and 15% by *C. parapsilosis*. However, *C. lusitaniae* infections are a cause of breakthrough fungemia in cancer patients.[36]

PATHOPHYSIOLOGY

Candida is generally acquired via the GI tract, although organisms may also enter the bloodstream via indwelling IV catheters. Risk factors for hematogenous disease include prior therapy with antibiotics, the presence of indwelling urinary or IV catheters, recent surgery, concomitant bacterial infections, extensive burns, and the administration of total parenteral nutrition. In the postoperative group, patients undergoing organ transplants, heart surgery, or GI tract surgery are at the greatest risk of infection.[8,35] A case-controlled study in patients with acute lymphocytic leukemia found previous bacteremia, prolonged neutropenia, prolonged fever, prolonged administration of antimicrobial agents, treatment with multiple antimicrobial agents, and a relatively high concentration of *Candida* in the stool to be significant risk factors for candidemia. In a logistic regression analysis, however, only administration of vancomycin, imipenem, or both was identified as an independent risk factor for candidemia. Further analysis showed that administration of vancomycin promoted proliferation of *Candida* in the GI tract and that this proliferation was associated with an increased risk of candidemia.[10,11]

Recognition of the role of the GI tract in invasive *Candida* infections has led to efforts to decrease infections by prophylactic administration of topical or systemically absorbed antifungal agents in immunocompromised patients. The use of systemically absorbable agents, such as azole antifungal agents, appears to decrease the risk of invasive fungal infections. Numerous investigators have raised concerns, however, regarding the potential for selection of intrinsically resistant pathogens or the development of resistant strains with widespread use of these agents. For example, although administration of oral fluconazole appears to decrease the incidence of invasive *Candida* infections in patients undergoing bone marrow transplantation, some centers have reported an increase in the number of infections caused by *C. krusei,* a species of *Candida* that is intrinsically resistant to fluconazole.[38,39]

Dissemination of *C. albicans* can result in infection in single or multiple organs, particularly the kidney, brain, myocardium, skin, eye, bone, and joints. Three distinct presentations of disseminated *C. albicans* have been recognized. In the first (and most common) type, patients present with the acute onset of fever, tachycardia, tachypnea, and occasionally chills or hypotension. The clinical presentation is generally indistinguishable from that seen with sepsis of bacterial origin. The second group of patients develops intermittent fevers and are ill only when febrile. A third group of patients manifests progressive deterioration of their condition with or without fever.[12] In most patients, multiple, micro, and macroabscesses are formed. Infection of the liver and spleen is becoming recognized as a particularly common and difficult-to-treat site of infection that characteristically occurs in patients undergoing chemotherapy for acute leukemia or lymphoma. Hepatosplenic candidiasis, which has been termed *chronic systemic candidiasis* by some investigators in order to distinguish this syndrome from acute, disseminated disease, is often manifested only as fever while the patient remains neutropenic ($<1{,}000$ WBC/mm^3). As the WBC count increases to $>1{,}000$ cells/mm^3, imaging studies can detect the presence of abscess or microabscesses in the liver and spleen, often found with acute suppurative and granulomatous reactions. Infection may persist for months and ultimately cause the patient's death despite aggressive systemic therapy with antifungal agents.[9]

DIAGNOSIS

The diagnosis of hematogenous candidiasis remains a major stumbling block in the treatment of infectious diseases. Although a variety of serologic tests have been proposed for the detection of *Candida* protein antigens, serum antibodies to *Candida,* and antibodies to cell wall components such as mannan, no test has demonstrated reliable accuracy in the clinical setting for the diagnosis of disseminated infection with *Candida*.[8,13] The problem is often confounded by the absence of positive blood cultures; only 25% to 45% of neutropenic patients with disseminated candidiasis at autopsy have a positive blood culture with *C. albicans* prior to death. The interpretation of positive surveillance cultures of the skin, mouth, sputum, feces, or urine is hampered by their occurrence as commensal pathogens and in distinguishing colonization from invasive disease. Patients with positive blood cultures for *C. tropicalis* should, however, receive serious consideration as candidates for systemic antifungal therapy.

▶ TREATMENT: Hematogenous Candidiasis

Both amphotericin B and the azoles have a role in the treatment of hematogenous candidiasis, and the choice of therapy is guided by weighing the greater activity of amphotericin B for some non-*albicans* species (e.g., *Candida krusei*) against the lower toxicity and ease of administration of the azole antifungal agents. Controlled clinical trials are available to guide therapy for the treatment of hematogenous candidiasis in the nonneutropenic adult. Susceptibility testing can be useful in dealing with infections caused by non-*albicans* species of *Candida*. In this setting, particularly if the patient has been treated previously with an azole antifungal agent, the possibility of microbiologic resistance must be considered.

NONIMMUNOCOMPROMISED PATIENT

The clinical management of suspected or documented candidemia poses significant clinical dilemmas (Table 119–5).[41,42] Fraser and colleagues[34] documented the high rate of mortality in nonneutropenic patients with fungal blood cultures. Mortality was highest in patients with sustained positive blood cultures, those who did not receive antifungal therapy, and those infected with non-albicans strains of *Candida*. This study clearly documented the importance of early recognition and treatment of positive fungal blood cultures.

Few data are available for assessing the role of fluconazole as empiric therapy for suspected fungemia or for isolates other than *C. albicans*. Because fluconazole has poor activity against *Aspergillus* spp. and some non-*albicans* strains of *Candida*, many clinicians advocate amphotericin B as the therapy of choice in patients with suspected fungemia. If therapy is given, its use should be limited to patients with (a) *Candida* colonization at multiple sites, (b) multiple other risk factors, and (c) absence of any other uncorrected causes of fever.

Administration of fluconazole 400 mg daily IV or orally is as efficacious as IV amphotericin B 0.5–0.6 mg/kg/day in nonneutropenic patients with blood cultures with *C. albicans*.[40,42] Studies evaluating the utility of the recently licensed intravenous formulation of itraconazole (200 mg IV every 12 hours for 4 doses, followed by 200 mg daily) are currently underway. Initial nonmedical management should include removal of all existing central venous catheters. In patients intolerant to amphotericin B or fluconazole, one of the lipid formulations may be used. Treatment should continue until 2 weeks following the last positive blood culture and resolution of signs and symptoms of infection.

Because *C. glabrata* often has reduced susceptibility to both fluconazole and amphotericin B, optimal therapy is unclear. Larger doses of fluconazole (800 mg daily in a 70-kg patient) have been used in less critically ill patients, or amphotericin B (≥0.7 mg/kg/day). *C. krusei* infections should be treated with large doses of amphotericin B (≥1 mg/kg/day).

IMMUNOCOMPROMISED PATIENTS

In immunocompromised patients, the presence of candidemia is associated with evidence of disseminated disease in >70% of patients and with a 70% to 80% fatality rate. Therapy should include removal of the catheter and administration of systemic antifungal therapy.[9] The optimal agent, dose, and duration of therapy is unclear, and patients must be carefully monitored with serial blood cultures and careful physical examinations, particularly of the retina. Most clinicians recommend amphotericin B in total dosages of 0.5–1 g administered over approximately 1 to 2 weeks in patients with *Candida* endophthalmitis and in all neutropenic patients with candidemia.[8,12,40] Longer courses of therapy may be needed in some patients.[12] Observational studies suggest that fluconazole and amphotericin B are similarly effective for the treatment of *C. albicans* bloodstream infections in the neutropenic patient; controlled data, however, are lacking. In patients intolerant to amphotericin B or fluconazole, one of the lipid formulations may be used. In a randomized trial, amphotericin B lipid complex (ABLC) was found to be equivalent to 0.6–1 mg/kg/day amphotericin B, and open-label therapy with amphotericin B colloid dispersion (ABCD) has been successful.

The decision to add flucytosine to therapy with amphotericin B for bloodstream infections remains controversial; although *in vitro* studies document synergy with these agents against *C. albicans,* the *in vivo* efficacy has not been well studied at this time. Similarly, the clinical use of combinations of azole antifungal agents (ketoconazole, fluconazole, itraconazole) with amphotericin B or flucytosine is also under investigation.

Many clinicians advocate early institution of empiric IV amphotericin B in patients with neutropenia and persistent (>5 to 7 days) fever.[40] Only two prospective randomized studies have examined the use of this practice. Pizzo and coworkers[43] evaluated neutropenic patients with fever of unknown origin after receiving broad-spectrum antimicrobial therapy with cephalothin, carbenicillin, plus gentamicin. After 1 week, patients were randomly assigned to discontinue antimicrobial therapy, to continue antimicrobial therapy until resolution of fever and granulocytopenia, or to continue antimicrobial therapy with the addition of amphotericin B (0.5 mg/kg/day). The results clearly favored administration of amphotericin B. The European Organization for Research on Treatment of Cancer (EORTC) conducted a prospective, randomized trial to evaluate the efficacy of empiric amphotericin B 1.2 mg/kg every other day or 0.6 mg/kg/day in febrile neutropenic cancer patients. The investigators concluded that empiric amphotericin B reduced the early mortality from fungal infection but appeared to have little effect on established infections, particularly in patients with progressive underlying diseases. Empiric therapy with amphotericin B was of particular benefit in patients who did not receive antifungal prophylaxis, those who were severely granulocytopenic, febrile patients with a clinically documented infection, and patients older than 15 years of age.[40,41]

Although empiric amphotericin B is clearly indicated for some patients, the potential toxicities (particularly nephrotoxicity) of this agent preclude its routine use in all patients. Suggested criteria for the empiric use of amphotericin B include (a) fever of 5 to 7 days duration that is unresponsive to antibacterial agents; (b) neutropenia of >7 days duration; (c) no other obvious cause for fever; (d) progressive debilitation; (e) chronic adrenal corticosteroid therapy; and (f) indwelling intravascular catheters. In patients who fail therapy with amphotericin B, lipid formulations of

TABLE 119–5. Therapy of Invasive Candidiasis

Type of Disease and Common Clinical Manifestations	Therapy/Comments
Prophylaxis of candidemia	
Neutropenic patients[a]	Fluconazole IV/po 400 mg daily during the period of neutropenia
Solid organ transplantation	
Liver transplantation	Patients with ≥2 key risk factors[b] AmB[c] IV 10–20 mg daily *or* Liposomal AmB (AmBisome) 1 mg/kg/day *or* Fluconazole 400 mg orally daily
Pancreatic transplantation	Fluconazole IV/po 400 mg daily × 7 days after transplantation
Empiric antifungal therapy (unknown *Candida* species)	
Clinically stable patient, no previous azole therapy	Fluconazole IV/po ≥6 mg/kg/day[d] *or* AmB IV ≥0.7 mg/kg/day
Clinically unstable patient	AmB IV ≥0.7 mg/kg/day
Suspected disseminated candidiasis in febrile nonneutropenic patients	None recommended; data are lacking defining subsets of patients who are appropriate for therapy. Refer to text.
Febrile neutropenic patients with prolonged fever despite 4 to 6 days of empiric antibacterial therapy	AmB IV 0.5–0.7 mg/kg/day or Liposomal AmB (AmBisome) IV 3 mg/kg/day
Treatment of candidemia and acute hematogenously disseminated candidiasis	
Nonimmunocompromised host[e]	*Treatment duration:* 2 weeks after the last positive blood culture and resolution of signs and symptoms of infection *Removal of existing venous catheters when feasible, plus:*
C. albicans, C. tropicalis, C. parapsilosis	AmB IV 0.6 mg/kg/day or Fluconazole IV/po 6 mg/kg/day *Patients intolerant or refractory to other therapy:*[f] ABLC IV 5 mg/kg/day Liposomal AmB IV 3–5 mg/kg/day ABCD IV 2–6 mg/kg/day
C. krusei	AmB IV ≥1 mg/kg/day
C. lusitaniae	Fluconazole IV/po 6 mg/kg/day
C. glabrata	AmB IV ≥0.7 mg/kg/day Some less critically ill patients have been successfully treated with fluconazole IV/po 12 mg/kg/day (800 mg/day in a 70-kg patient)
Neutropenic host	AmB IV 0.5–0.75 mg/kg/day (total dosages 0.5–1 g) or *Patients failing therapy with traditional AmB:* Lipid formulation of AmB IV 3–5 mg/kg/day
Chronic disseminated candidiasis (hepatosplenic candidiasis)	*Stable patients:* Fluconazole IV/po 6 mg/kg/day *Acutely ill or refractory patients:* AmB IV 0.6–0.7 mg/kg/day
Urinary candidiasis	*Asymptomatic disease:* Generally no therapy is required *Symptomatic or high-risk patients:*[g] Removal of urinary tract instruments, stents, and Foley catheters, + 7–14 days therapy with: Fluconazole 200 mg orally daily *or* AmB IV 0.3–1 mg/kg/day.

[a]Patients at significant risk for invasive candidiasis include those receiving standard chemotherapy for acute myelogenous leukemia, allogeneic bone-marrow transplants, or high-risk autologous bone-marrow transplants. However, among these populations, chemotherapy or bone-marrow transplant protocols do not all produce equivalent risk and local experience should be used to determine the relevance of prophylaxis.

[b]Risk factors include: retransplantation, creatinine of >2 mg/dL, choledochojejunostomy, intraoperative use of ≥40 units of blood products, fungal colonization detected within the first 3 days after transplantation.

[c]AmB, deoxycholate amphotericin B; IV, intravenous; PO, orally; ABLC, amphotericin B lipid complex; ABCD, amphotericin B colloid dispersion.

[d]400 mg/day in a 70-kg patient.

[e]Therapy is generally the same for AIDS/non-AIDS patients except where indicated and should continue for 2 weeks after the last positive blood culture and resolution of signs and symptoms of infection.

[f]Often defined as failure of ≥500 mg AmB, initial renal insufficiency (creatinine ≥2.5 mg/dL or creatinine clearance <25 mL/min), a significant increase in creatinine (to 2.5 mg/dL for adults or 1.5 mg/dL for children) or severe acute administration-related toxicity.

[g]Patients at high risk for dissemination include neutropenic patients, low-birth-weight infants, patients with renal allografts, and patients who will undergo urologic manipulation.

(*Compiled from Refs. 5 and 9.*)

amphotericin B may be used (3–5 mg/kg/day). Although fluconazole has been used successfully in the clinically unstable patient infected with an isolate of unknown species, most experts would initiate amphotericin B because of its broader spectrum of activity.

Itraconazole has a broader spectrum of activity, including *Aspergillus*, but extensive data evaluating its use in this setting are lacking. If used, the intravenous formulation should be used because the bioavailability of the oral formulations (including the solution) is unreliable.[40,41]

CANDIDURIA

Within the urinary tract, most common lesions are either *Candida* cystitis or hematogenously disseminated renal abscesses. *Candida* cystitis often follows catheterization or therapy with broad-spectrum antimicrobial therapy. The diagnosis of *Candida* cystitis may be problematic because of the frequent presence of *Candida* pseudohyphae and yeast cells in urine specimens secondary to urethral colonization. The usefulness of urine colony counts or antibody coating techniques is of questionable value. The recovery of 10,000 organisms or visualization of both yeast and pseudohyphae from fresh midstream urine or from bladder urine obtained by single catheterization (not indwelling) is suggestive of genitourinary candidiasis.[8] In most patients, the infection is asymptomatic and clears spontaneously without specific antifungal therapy.

Initial therapy of candidal cystitis should focus on removal of urinary catheters whenever possible. Changing the catheter will eliminate candiduria in only 20% of patients, while discontinuation will eradicate *Candida* in 40% of patients. Asymptomatic candiduria rarely requires therapy. Therapy should be used in symptomatic patients and in neutropenic patients, as well as in those patients with renal allografts and in those patients who will undergo urologic manipulation, because of the risk of dissemination.[44,45]

Fluconazole 200 mg daily for 14 days hastens the time to a negative urine culture as compared to placebo treatment, but 2 weeks after the end of therapy the frequency of a negative urine culture remains the same with both treatments.[45] Short courses of therapy are not recommended; treatment should include removal of catheters and stents whenever possible, plus 7 to 14 days therapy. Bladder irrigation with amphotericin B (50 mg in 500 mL of sterile water instilled twice daily into the bladder via a three-way catheter) is only transiently effective. Minimal quantities (<3%) of amphotericin B are absorbed systemically from the bladder.[18,45]

ASPERGILLOSIS

EPIDEMIOLOGY

Aspergillus is an ubiquitous mold that grows well on a variety of substrates, including soil, water, decaying vegetation, moldy hay or straw, and organic debris. Although more than 300 species of *Aspergillus* have been characterized, three species are most commonly pathogenic: *A. fumigatus, A. flavus,* and *A. niger*. The varying degrees of pathogenicity of each species depend on their relative geographic prevalence, conidial size and shape, thermotolerance, and production of mycotoxins. For example, transport of *A. fumigatus* conidia into the lungs is facilitated by their smaller diameter in comparison to *A. flavus* and *A. niger*.

The term *aspergillosis* may be broadly defined as a spectrum of diseases attributed to allergy, colonization, or tissue invasion caused by members of the fungal genus *Aspergillus*. A single satisfactory classification system for these disease entities is difficult because different populations of patients may develop the same type of infection. For example, osteomyelitis may result from local trauma or hematogenous dissemination in an immunocompromised host. Colonization in normal hosts can lead to allergic diseases ranging from asthma to allergic bronchopulmonary aspergillosis or, rarely, invasive disease.[48]

PATHOPHYSIOLOGY

Aspergillosis is generally acquired by inhalation of airborne conidia that are small enough (2.5–3 μm) to reach alveoli or the paranasal sinuses. Each conidiophore releases 10^4 conidia that remain suspended for long periods and are viable for months in dry locations. Although some authors advocate monitoring of hospital air for *Aspergillus* conidia, guidelines for interpreting results do not exist. The use of high-efficiency particulate air (HEPA) filters in operating rooms and laminar flow rooms and removal of immunocompromised patients from hospital renovation sites may be helpful in preventing infection in this population. Although the fate of *Aspergillus* conidia in the GI tract has not been closely studied, limited evidence suggests that this route may provide an important portal of entry for disseminated infections in humans.[46]

SUPERFICIAL INFECTION

Superficial or locally invasive infections of the ear, skin, or appendages can often be managed with topical antifungal therapy. Skin infections in patients with burn wounds, although uncommon, may progress to deep-tissue invasion despite the use of topical or parenteral antifungal agents. Risk factors for deep infection include extensive thermal injuries, malnutrition, cirrhosis, and previous infection with *Pseudomonas aeruginosa*.[46]

ALLERGIC BRONCHOPULMONARY ASPERGILLOSIS

Allergic manifestations of *Aspergillus* range in severity from mild asthma to allergic bronchopulmonary aspergillosis (BPA). Bronchopulmonary aspergillosis, which is almost always caused by *A. fumigatus,* is characterized by severe asthma with wheezing, fever, malaise, weight loss, chest pain, and a cough productive of blood-streaked sputum. Following recurrent episodes of severe asthma, the disease usually progresses to fibrosis and bronchiectasis with granuloma formation. When *Aspergillus* conidia become trapped in the viscous mucus of asthmatic patients, BPA develops. The fungus grows, releasing toxins and antigens. The resulting host sensitization results in a variety of immune reactions. Early in the course of disease, an IgE-mediated (type I) immune reaction results in bronchospasm, eosinophilia, and immediate skin reactivity. The ensuing fibrosis and pulmonary infiltrates appear to be mediated by circulating or precipitating antibody complexes of IgG antibody, followed by granuloma formation and mononuclear infiltration because of a type IV delayed hypersensitivity reaction. Therapy is aimed at minimizing the quantity of antigenic material released in the tracheobronchial tree. Management of acute asthma attacks minimizes trapping of *Aspergillus* by bronchial secretions, and administration of parenteral corticosteroids clears lung infiltrates.[46,47] Antifungal therapy is generally not indicated in the management of allergic manifestations of aspergillosis, although some patients have demonstrated a decrease in their corticosteroid dose following therapy with itraconazole. A recent double-blind, randomized, placebo-controlled trial showed that itraconazole 200 mg twice daily for 16 weeks resulted in significant differences in the amelioration of disease, as measured by the reduction in corticosteroid dose, and improvement in exercise tolerance and in pulmonary function.[48]

ASPERGILLOMA

In the nonimmunocompromised host, *Aspergillus* infections of the sinuses most commonly occur as saprophytic colonization (aspergillomas or "fungus balls") of previously abnormal sinus tissue. An aspergilloma is composed of intertwined *Aspergillus* hyphae matted together with fibrin, mucus, and cellular debris. Infection is usually localized in the maxillary sinus and is rarely associated with local invasion of adjacent bone or brain tissue. Sinus aspergillosis can also present as allergic sinusitis with nasal drainage of brownish mucous plugs. Therapy with corticosteroids and surgery is generally successful. In the immunocompromised host, subacute, chronic, or fulminant invasive disease can be seen, and a combination of antifungal and surgical therapy is generally required.[46,47,49,50]

Pulmonary aspergillomas are fungus balls arising in preexisting cavities because of tuberculosis, histoplasmosis, lung tumors, or radiation fibrosis, although occasionally no previous pulmonary disease is present. The diagnosis of aspergilloma is generally made on the basis of chest radiographs, on which aspergillomas appear as a solid rounded mass, sometimes mobile, of water density, within a spherical or ovoid cavity, and separated from the wall of the cavity by an airspace of variable size and shape. Patients generally experience chest pain, dyspnea, and sputum production. Hemoptysis is observed in 50% to 80% of patients, probably because of ulceration of the epithelial lining of the cavity with formation of granulation tissue, and hemoptysis is the cause of death in up to 26% of patients with aspergilloma. A poor prognosis is associated with increasing size or number of aspergillomas, immunosuppression (including corticosteroids), increasing *Aspergillus*-specific titers, underlying sarcoidosis, and HIV infection. Although *Aspergillus* can only be cultured in 50% to 60% of patients, precipitating antibodies are positive in virtually 100% of patients.

Invasive disease rarely occurs, and therapy is therefore controversial. There are no controlled clinical trials with which to guide therapy, and recommendations for treatment have been generated from uncontrolled trials and case reports.[50] Concern regarding the risk of severe hemorrhage has led some clinicians to use aggressive surgical excision of aspergillomas or pulmonary resection in patients with hemoptysis. Complications, including bronchopulmonary fistulas, hemorrhage, empyema, and persistent air space problems, have, however, led to the recommendation that surgical intervention be reserved for patients with severe (>500 mL/24 h) hemoptysis. Bronchial artery embolization (BAE) has been used to occlude the vessel that supplies the bleeding site in patients experiencing hemoptysis. Unfortunately, BAE is generally unsuccessful or only temporarily effective. Collateral circulation eventually develops, supplying blood flow to the affected area, and hemoptysis often recurs; consequently, reembolization is often unsuccessful. BAE should be used as a temporizing procedure in a patient with life-threatening disease, who might respond to more definitive therapy if hemoptysis is stabilized. Mild-to-moderate hemoptysis should be managed conservatively. Although IV amphotericin B is generally not useful in eradicating aspergillomas, inhaled or intracavitary instillation of amphotericin B has been employed successfully in a limited number of patients. Itraconazole has been efficacious in uncontrolled studies; however, the dose and duration of therapy have not been standardized. Hemoptysis generally ceases when the aspergilloma is eradicated.[46,47,50]

INVASIVE ASPERGILLOSIS

Although exposure to *Aspergillus* conidia is nearly universal, impaired host defenses are required for the development of invasive disease. Phagocytes (neutrophils, monocytes, macrophages) rather than antibodies or lymphocytes constitute the primary host defense system against invasive disease with aspergillosis. Macrophages prevent germination of conidia and also eradicate conidia, providing the first line of defense against invasive disease. Administration of corticosteroids appears to impair the killing of conidia by macrophages and to impair mobilization of neutrophils. Neutrophils halt hyphal growth and dissemination and kill mycelia, constituting a second line of defense. Prolonged neutropenia appears to be the most important predisposing factor to the development of invasive aspergillosis, accounting for the high frequency of disease in patients with acute leukemia. Complement provides a source of chemotactic factor, and facilitates neutrophil damage to hyphae and monocyte killing of conidia. Complement is not necessary for the attachment or ingestion of conidia by human alveolar macrophages.[46,47,51]

Until recently, aspergillosis was an uncommon fungal infection in patients with AIDS. AIDS patients may be at less risk for aspergillosis than other fungal infections because the primary cellular defect in AIDS patients is in the T lymphocytes, whereas neutrophils and macrophages constitute the primary lines of defense to infection with aspergillosis. Until recently, aspergillosis was reported as a late complication of disease in AIDS patients with additional risk factors for aspergillosis, such as corticosteroid use, neutropenia, previous *Pneumocystis carinii* or cytomegalovirus pneumonia, marijuana smoking, or the use of broad-spectrum antibiotics. One study reported, however, that approximately 50% of patients with aspergillosis had no classic risk factors. The majority of these patients had CD4 counts <50/mm^3. Although some patients diagnosed early in their infection responded to treatment, most patients do not respond to therapy with amphotericin B 0.5 mg/kg/day or itraconazole 200–600 mg daily.[56,57]

Invasive disease with *Aspergillus* can arise *de novo* or from any of the allergic or colonizing forms of aspergillosis. Predisposing factors to the development of invasive aspergillosis include glucocorticoid therapy, particularly following chronic administration or with higher dosages (30–200 mg of prednisone daily), cytotoxic agents, and recent or concurrent therapy with broad-spectrum antimicrobial agents. Patients with chronic hepatitis, alcoholism, diabetes mellitus, chronic granulomatous disease, leukopenia (<1,000 cells/mm^3), leukemia (particularly acute lymphocytic or myelogenous leukemia), lymphoma, and acute rejection of an organ transplant are also at a higher risk of invasive disease. Although rare, invasive aspergillosis has been reported in apparently normal hosts.[46,47]

CLINICAL PRESENTATION

Although the lung is the most common site of invasive disease, followed by the central nervous system, the liver, spleen, heart, GI tract, pericardium, and other body sites are involved in a substantial minority of cases. In neutropenic patients with *Aspergillus* pneumonia, hyphae invade the walls of bronchi and surrounding parenchyma, resulting in an acute necrotizing, pyogenic pneumonitis. As a result, patients often present with classic signs and symptoms of acute pulmonary embolus: pleuritic chest pain, fever, hemoptysis, and friction rubs. Late findings on radiographic studies include wedge-shaped pleural-based infiltrates or cavities on chest radiographs. Findings on CT scans include the "halo sign" (an area of low attenuation surrounding a nodular lung lesion) initially (caused by edema or bleeding surrounding an ischemic area) and, later, the "crescent sign" (an air crescent near the periphery of a lung nodule, caused by contraction of infarcted tissue). The CT abnormalities are best documented in neutropenic marrow transplant recipients. CT abnormalities commonly precede plain chest radiograph abnormalities.

Invasion of blood vessels causes thrombosis with resultant infarction, necrosis, and dissemination to other tissues and organs in the body. Survival beyond 2 or 3 weeks is uncommon. If bone marrow function returns, cavitation of the pulmonary lesion generally occurs and the spread of infection may be halted. The progressive nature of the disease and its refractoriness to therapy are, in part, caused by the organism's rapid growth and its tendency to invade blood vessels.[46,47]

DIAGNOSIS

The diagnosis of aspergillosis is complicated by the presence of *Aspergillus* as a normal commensal in the human GI tract and respiratory secretions, and establishment of a definitive diagnosis of disease is difficult. Though suggestive of infection, the presence of hyphae in a smear or biopsy specimen is not diagnostic. Demonstration of *Aspergillus* by repeated culture and microscopic examination of tissue provides the most firm diagnosis.[13,14,46,47] The appearance of *Aspergillus* in tissues varies with increasing host resistance from the normal vegetative hyphae found with necrotic tissue and exudate in the alveoli of immunocompromised hosts to the compact tangled filaments ("granules") observed in fungal balls. Identification of *Aspergillus* is generally based on the appearance of 2–4 μm wide septate hyphae that are dichotomously branched at 45° angles. Sporulation is rarely observed in tissue.[13,14]

In the immunocompromised host, aspergillosis is characterized by vascular invasion leading to thrombosis, infarction, and necrosis of tissue. Abundant hyphae in radially branching clusters can be observed in tissue. In contrast, vascular invasion is uncommon, and there are sparse numbers of hyphae in patients with chronic granulomatous disease. Although growth on Sabouraud dextrose or brain-heart infusion agar may be used for primary culture, bronchoscopy or bronchoalveolar lavage cultures are positive in only 40% of histopathologically identified specimens.[8] Blood, CSF, and bone marrow cultures are rarely positive for *Aspergillus*.

Many clinicians treat positive respiratory cultures of *Aspergillus* as a common contaminant and argue that a minimum of two to three positive cultures is necessary before antifungal therapy is indicated. Any positive culture, however, may be indicative of true infection in the immunocompromised host, and the positive predictive value may be as high as 80% to 90% in patients with leukemia or bone marrow transplants. In a large series (98 patients) reported by the National Institutes for Health, 82% of patients had positive fungal cultures at some point during the course of their terminal illness. Despite these vigorous culturing methods, only 34% of patients had one antemortem culture positive for *Aspergillus* and only 9% had more than one positive culture.[46] Isolation of *Aspergillus* from respiratory tract cultures correlated with proven aspergillosis in 100% of patients with acute leukemia, 94% of neutropenic patients, and 65% of patients receiving adrenal corticosteroids, but only 40% of patients receiving parenteral antibiotics.

Serologic tests (immunoprecipitation, ID, and counterimmunoelectrophoresis) to detect antibody production to *Aspergillus* are generally helpful only in the diagnosis of allergic BPA and aspergilloma. Unfortunately, their usefulness in invasive aspergillosis is limited because of the inability of these patients to elaborate antibodies. Although serum precipitins are positive in 70% to 80% of patients with invasive pulmonary aspergillosis, the specificity and predictive value of single antibody titers is relatively low. Serum antigen detection has shown promise in animal models of *Aspergillus* infection; however, results cannot be directly extrapolated to humans because these models employed IV injection of *Aspergillus* rather than acquisition via the respiratory tract, as occurs in human hosts.[8,46] Several promising assays have been developed to detect *Aspergillus* galactomannan in urine, sera, CSF, and bronchoalveolar lavage specimens by enzyme immunoassay (EIA), enzyme-linked immunosorbent assay (ELISA), and immunoblot. Studies with an EIA system commercially available in Europe for detection of galactomannan reported positive predictive values of 54% and negative predictive values of 95%, largely among bone marrow transplant recipients. However, no antigen tests are currently approved for use in the United States.[49,50]

▶ TREATMENT: Invasive Aspergillosis

Therapy for invasive aspergillosis is far from optimal at this time, in part because of the difficulties in establishing a diagnosis, and in part because of a lack of truly effective antifungal agents. Administration of amphotericin B appears to decrease mortality from >90% to approximately 45%. These data, however, are difficult to interpret because many patients were diagnosed postmortem or amphotericin B therapy was not administered until the patient had very advanced disease. Mortality from pulmonary aspergillosis in bone marrow transplant recipients exceeds 94% regardless of therapy.[46] Although early diagnosis and administration of antifungal therapy may result in higher response rates, correction of underlying immune deficits (in particular, return of neutrophil counts) is of paramount importance in eradication of infection.[49,50]

Until the diagnosis of aspergillosis can be more rapidly and definitively determined, empiric therapy must be instituted when invasive disease is suspected. In patients at highest risk for invasive disease (acute leukemia and bone marrow transplant recipients), the most important predisposing factors include prolonged severe neutropenia (<100 cells/mm^3 for >1 week), graft rejection, chronic administration of corticosteroids, and tissue damage from preexisting infection. In these patients, antifungal therapy should be instituted in any of these conditions: (a) persistent fever or progressive sinusitis unresponsive to antimicrobial therapy; (b) an eschar over the nose, sinuses, or palate; (c) the presence of characteristic radiographic findings, including wedge-shaped infarcts, nodular densities, and new cavitary lesions; or (d) any clinical manifestation suggestive of orbital or cavernous sinus disease or an acute vascular event associated with fever. Isolation of *Aspergillus* spp. from nasal or respiratory tract secretions should be considered confirmatory evidence in any of the previously mentioned clinical settings.[46,47]

NON-HIV-INFECTED PATIENT

Intravenous therapy with amphotericin B remains the preferred therapy, at least initially, in acutely ill patients. Because *Aspergillus* is only moderately susceptible to amphotericin B, full doses (1–1.5 mg/kg/day) are generally recommended, with response measured by defervescence and radiographic clearing. To treat microfoci, therapy should be continued after resolution of clinical and radiographic abnormalities until cultures (if they can be obtained) are negative, and reversible underlying predispositions have abated. Clinical response rather than any arbitrary total dose should guide duration of therapy. The optimal dosage or duration of amphotericin B therapy for the treatment of invasive disease is unknown and dependent on the extent of disease, the response to therapy, and the patient's underlying disease(s) and immune status. Unfortunately, the response rate averages only 37% (range, 14% to 83%) and the response to therapy is largely related to the extent of aspergillosis at the time of diagnosis, and host factors, such as resolution of neutropenia and the return of neutrophil function, lessening immunosuppression, and the return of graft function from a bone marrow or organ transplant.

Lipid formulations of amphotericin B may be indicated in patients with impaired renal function, and in those patients who develop nephrotoxicity while receiving deoxycholate amphotericin B. The lipid-based formulations may be preferred as initial therapy in patients with marginal renal function or in patients receiving other nephrotoxic drugs. Although these preparations appear less toxic than standard preparations, only limited data regarding their relative efficacy for invasive aspergillosis are available at this time, as the studies with the lipid preparations have been open-label or with historical conventional amphotericin B controls.[53–56] Although most studies in animals suggest that larger doses of the lipid preparations are required to produce therapeutic effects equivalent to deoxycholate amphotericin, a recent clinical trial questions whether the larger lipid doses are needed.[56]

Even though older azole antifungal agents (miconazole and ketoconazole) possess poor *in vitro* activity against *Aspergillus* spp., newer triazoles demonstrate improved activity both *in vitro* and in animal models of infection.[57] Itraconazole (100–500 mg daily for 11 to 192 days) shows therapeutic benefit in patients with pulmonary, skeletal, and pericardial aspergillosis, particularly in those patients who are less immunocompromised.[46–50] The wide range of dosages, durations of therapy, and degree of immunosuppression in these trials makes selection of an appropriate regimen difficult. Jennings and Hardin[47] reviewed the role of itraconazole for aspergillosis and recommended that itraconazole be reserved as a second-line agent for patients intolerant or not responding to high-dose amphotericin B. If itraconazole is used, a loading dose of 200 mg three times daily for 2 to 3 days should be employed, followed by itraconazole 200 mg twice daily for a minimum of 6 months. Although early studies employing relatively low dosages (50–100 mg daily) of fluconazole demonstrated some activity against less-invasive forms of aspergillosis, including chronic pulmonary disease and aspergillomas, data regarding the use of higher dosages (>100 mg daily) in patients with invasive disease are not available. Oral itraconazole is an alternative for patients who can take oral medication, are likely to be adherent, can be demonstrated (by serum level monitoring) to absorb the drug, and are unlikely to experience interactions with other medications, and as follow-up therapy in patients who respond to initial IV therapy.[50]

Caspofungin was approved by the FDA for use as salvage therapy in patients who are intolerant or who fail therapy with one of the amphotericin B formulations.[57–59] Caspofungin has *in vitro* activity against *Aspergillus* species, and is indicated for the treatment of invasive aspergillosis in patients who are refractory or intolerant to other therapies such as conventional amphotericin B, lipid formulations of amphotericin B, and/or itraconazole. Caspofungin has not yet been studied for first-line therapy for patients with aspergillosis. Because of the high risk of mortality from invasive aspergillosis even following treatment with standard therapy such as amphotericin B or itraconazole, caspofungin may offer a new mechanism for salvage therapy for patients with this disease. Voriconazole, an investigational triazole, has been used in open-label studies of invasive aspergillosis with >50% complete or partial response rates in ongoing studies.[57,58]

The use of adjuvant therapies, such as granulocyte transfusions or recombinant colony-stimulating factors remains controversial, and controlled trials are lacking at this time. Although some authors advocate combination therapy with azoles, flucytosine, or rifampin plus amphotericin B controlled clinical studies verifying the efficacy of these combination therapies are lacking.

The use of prophylactic antifungal therapy to prevent primary infection or reactivation of aspergillosis during subsequent courses of chemotherapy is controversial.[19,47] Studies assessing the utility of IV administration of amphotericin B in low doses (0.1 mg/kg/day) as prophylactic therapy or with higher dosages of 0.5–0.6 mg/kg/day as empiric therapy for invasive fungal infections in patients with granulocytopenia have not included sufficient numbers of patients to enable detection of differences in the number of *Aspergillus* infections.[47] The prophylactic use of intranasal amphotericin B aerosol sprays (5 or 10 mg daily in three divided doses) appeared beneficial in small studies in human and animal models. A larger randomized trial found, however, that amphotericin B sprays reduced colonization of the nasal mucosal without any reduction in the frequency of invasive pulmonary infections with aspergillosis. Because failure of amphotericin B sprays may be a result of the ability of small airborne conidia to access the alveolar spaces directly and to establish infection, use of aerosolized forms of amphotericin B capable of reaching the alveolar spaces may be required.[47]

In granulocytopenic patients who recover from an episode of invasive aspergillosis, the risk of relapse of aspergillosis during subsequent courses of chemotherapy is >50%. Secondary prophylaxis of aspergillosis with empiric administration of high-dose amphotericin B decreases the risk of relapse. Amphotericin B 1 mg/kg/day is started 24 to 48 hours prior to the start of chemotherapy and continued throughout the period of granulocytopenia. Some investigators recommend the addition of flucytosine (dosed to achieve peak serum concentrations of 30–60 μg/mL) to the amphotericin B regimen. Although the use of itraconazole (alone or in combination with amphotericin B or flucytosine) may be beneficial in this patient population, little is known regarding its efficacy in this setting. If itraconazole is administered, serum levels should be monitored to assess absorption, because poor absorption of drug has been documented in this patient population.[58]

ANTIFUNGAL THERAPY

The antifungal armamentarium for the treatment of invasive fungal infections includes (a) inhibitors of the fungal cell membrane, such as polyenes (e.g., amphotericin B) and azole antifungals; (b) inhibitors of DNA (5-flucytosine); and, more recently (c) inhibitors of cell wall biosynthesis such as the recently approved agent caspofungin.

Antifungal therapy generally uses one or more of these agents, depending on the severity of infection, and the patients' immune status. Rarely are the agents used in combination. Often, therapy is initiated with an intravenous agent such as amphotericin B, and therapy is changed to an oral (azole) regimen as the patient's clinical status improves and oral therapy is tolerated. The most widely used combination therapy consists of 5-flucytosine plus amphotericin B. The role of combination therapy is unclear at this time; controlled trials are lacking and the possibility of therapeutic antagonism when using azoles in combination with amphotericin B remains debated. Controlled trials are needed to define the role of azoles plus amphotericin B, and azoles or amphotericin B plus caspofungin.

AMPHOTERICIN B

Amphotericin B remains the therapy of choice for many systemic fungal infections despite a lack of controlled clinical trials documenting the optimal dosage, duration of therapy, or relative efficacy of this agent in comparison to newer azole antifungal agents, such as ketoconazole, itraconazole, or fluconazole. During pregnancy, amphotericin B remains the treatment of choice for most fungal infections because azole antifungals are teratogenic.[18,60]

Recommendations for the administration of amphotericin B are largely empiric and, in general, have not been tested in a controlled fashion. Most clinicians recommend administration of a 1 mg test dose of amphotericin B in 25–50 mL of 5% dextrose in water or as an aliquot of the initial daily dose infused over 1 to 2 hours in order to detect the rare patient likely to experience an anaphylactic reaction to the drug. If tolerated, the remaining daily dose is prepared in a concentration of 0.1 mg/mL of 5% dextrose and infused over 2 to 4 hours. Amphotericin B is usually administered in gradually increasing dosages; most guidelines suggest daily increments of 5 mg or 0.1 mg/kg until the maximum daily dose of 0.5–0.75 mg/kg daily is achieved. Many clinicians, however, advocate the rapid escalation of doses in patients with documented infections or highly suspicious clinical symptoms; often therapy is instituted with 0.25 mg/kg on the first day of therapy, followed by full-dose therapy on subsequent days of treatment.[18]

Infusion of amphotericin B over 2 hours is safe and may result in a lower incidence of fever and chills. The use of rapid infusions of amphotericin B should be avoided in patients with renal impairment because they may be unable to tolerate the increased intracellular potassium released secondary to high serum concentrations of amphotericin B.[18]

The optimal total dosage or duration of amphotericin B therapy has not been determined for most fungal infections. For most deep-seated infections, therapy is often continued for 6 to 12 weeks. In severe infections, in those infections caused by less-susceptible pathogens (*Aspergillus* or *C. tropicalis*), in those infections in sites that are difficult to penetrate, or in immunocompromised hosts, however, the daily dosage of amphotericin B may range up to 1 mg/kg and total dosages of 2–4 g of amphotericin B may be administered over a period of months to years.

The side effects of amphotericin B are generally categorized as acute (infusion-related) or long-term. Shaking chills, fever, myalgias, arthralgias, and headache are reported in >50% of patients receiving amphotericin B. Evidence suggests that some of the infusion-related side effects may be caused by induction of prostaglandins. A variety of premedications are routinely used in an effort to decrease the incidence and severity of these reactions; however, few have been studied in a controlled fashion. Administration of oral ibuprofen (10 mg/kg) 30 minutes prior to administration of amphotericin B reduces the incidence of chills from 87% to 49%. Meperidine has also been successful in terminating fever and chills in a randomized, double-blind trial. In another study, the administration of IV hydrocortisone (25 mg) at the beginning of amphotericin B infusions was significantly more effective than aspirin and diphenhydramine in reducing the incidence of fever, chills, and vomiting. Larger doses of hydrocortisone do not appear to offer any additional benefit.[18]

Thrombophlebitis is commonly reported in patients receiving amphotericin B therapy, probably as a result of the acidic pH of the reconstituted solution. Methods to reduce the problem include infusion into distal hand veins or in central venous lines in patients receiving long-term therapy, use of dilute solutions (>0.1 mg/mL), and the addition of 500–1,000 units of heparin per liter of solution. The efficacy of heparin in reducing the incidence of phlebitis has not been studied in a controlled fashion.[18]

The relatively nonselective affinity of amphotericin B for ergosterol versus cholesterol is thought to provide the basis for many of the long-term side effects of amphotericin B. The most significant side effect of amphotericin B administration is renal toxicity. Although the exact mechanism of this adverse effect is unclear, amphotericin B appears to alter membrane permeability and activate an intrarenal tubuloglomerular feedback mechanism that alters proximal and distal tubule delivery of ions, resulting in a decreased glomerular filtration and renal blood flow. Hypokalemia and hypomagnesemia may occur in association with decreased renal function, and the administration of supplemental potassium and magnesium may be required. Reversible impairment of renal function occurs within the first 2 weeks of amphotericin B therapy in up to 80% of patients. Irreversible renal dysfunction, while rare, occurs in some patients. It is unclear whether this effect is related to the total cumulative dosage of amphotericin B or individual patient susceptibility. Amphotericin B can also produce a reversible renal tubular acidosis in patients receiving total dosages of 0.5–1 g or more.[18] In an effort to decrease the incidence of nephrotoxicity, clinicians have tried several therapeutic modalities, including sodium loading, alternate-day therapy, and mannitol administration.

Amphotericin B can also produce a normochromic, normocytic anemia that is thought to result from a direct inhibition of erythrocyte or erythropoietin production. Hemoglobin concentrations generally return to normal within 2 to 3 months following discontinuation of amphotericin B. Thrombocytopenia has been rarely reported.

Combination therapy with amphotericin B and flucytosine may result in enhanced bone marrow suppression. The increased toxicity may result from enhanced cellular penetration of flucytosine or accumulation of flucytosine resulting from amphotericin B-induced renal dysfunction. Serum concentrations of flucytosine should be monitored carefully to maintain peak concentrations (2 hours after oral administration) of <100 g/mL.[10]

The association between increased pulmonary toxicity with the concomitant use of amphotericin B and granulocyte transfusions remains controversial. Nevertheless, slow administration of amphotericin B and avoidance of concomitant administration of amphotericin B and granulocytes is recommended in order to minimize the potential interaction.

LIPOSOMAL AMPHOTERICIN B

Interest has been focused on the use of lipid preparations of amphotericin B. In these preparations, amphotericin B is incorporated into the phospholipid bilayer membrane, rather than in the enclosed aqueous phase. The preparation consists of both sheets and multilamellar spherical liposomes, ranging in size from 0.5 μm to 6 μm. The sheets contain more amphotericin B than do the spheres. The optimal preparation and sterol composition of these compounds is still unknown (Table 119–6).[53,60]

The majority of liposomally encapsulated drug appears to be cleared by the reticuloendothelial system; amphotericin B is taken up by macrophages in the lung, liver, spleen, bone marrow, and circulating monocytes in plasma. In the lung, liposome-loaded monocytes migrate to alveoli to become alveolar macrophages. The various lipid formulations of amphotericin B exhibit markedly different pharmacokinetics; however, the clinical implications of these differences remain unclear.[53] Although larger doses of these preparations are required to achieve similar pharmacologic effects as the deoxycholate form of amphotericin B, the toxicity appears to be much lower.[60]

The use of liposomal preparations of amphotericin B has resulted in decreased toxicity in animal models of infection and in early human clinical trials.[53]

FLUCYTOSINE

Flucytosine (also known as 5-flucytosine or 5-FC) is a fluorinated pyrimidine analog that is highly water-soluble. Flucytosine

TABLE 119–6. Pharmacology of Lipid Preparations of Amphotericin B

	Deoxycholate Amphotericin	Amphotericin B Lipid Complex	Amphotericin B Colloid Dispersion	Liposomal Amphotericin B
Brand name (manufacturer)	Fungizone	Abelcet	Amphocil	Ambisome
	(Bristol Myers Squibb, Lyphomed)	(The Liposome Company)	(Sequus)	(Fujisawa/Nexstar)
Molecular weight	416	306	531	706
Size (nm)	<10	1,600–11,000	120–140	80–120
Drug formulation	Micelles	Lipid complex	Colloid dispersion	Lyophilized powder
Appearance	Suspension	Ribbons, sheets	Disks	Small unilamellar vesicles
mol % amphotericin	34	35	50	<10
Protein binding (%)	High (90)	Low (12)	High (99)	High (99.8)
Water solubility	Poor	Excellent	Poor	Poor
Dosage (mg/kg/day)	0.3–1	5	7	5
CSF penetration	Poor	Excellent	Poor	Poor
(CSF/serum)	(<10%)	(> 80%)	(<10%)	(<10%)
Elimination half-life (h)	20	30	8	21–64

CSF, cerebrospinal fluid.
(*Adapted from Refs. 8, 11, 53, and 55.*)

is transported into the cell and transformed into 5-fluorouracil (an antimetabolite) by cytosine deaminase, which then inhibits DNA synthesis by incorporation into RNA. Patients with creatinine clearances <40 mL/min should receive 100–150 mg/kg daily in four divided doses. The dosage should be reduced by 50% in patients with a creatinine clearance of 25–50 mL/min, and by 75% in patients with a clearance of 13–25 mL/min. Peak serum concentrations (2 hours after an oral dose) should be monitored in all patients (particularly those with a creatinine clearance of <10 mL/min) to maintain peak serum concentrations >100 mg/L.[29,30]

Flucytosine is generally associated with very few side effects in patients with normal renal, GI, and hematologic function, although rash, GI discomfort, diarrhea (5% to 10%), and reversible elevations in hepatic enzymes are occasionally observed. In patients with renal dysfunction or with concomitant amphotericin B therapy, leukopenia, thrombocytopenia, and (rarely) enterocolitis may occur. Although studies have suggested that little or no conversion of flucytosine to 5-fluorouracil occurs *in vitro,* serum concentrations of >1,000 ng/mL (therapeutic for the treatment of malignancies) have been documented in some patients. Investigators have theorized that flucytosine may be secreted into the GI tract, deaminated by intestinal bacteria, and reabsorbed as 5-fluorouracil.[29,30]

Flucytosine is used in the treatment of cryptococcosis, candidiasis, and chromomycosis. The rapid development of resistance to flucytosine, however, precludes its use as single-agent therapy except perhaps in the treatment of chromomycosis. Mechanisms for drug resistance may include loss of deaminase and decreased permeability to the drug.[29,30]

PNEUMOCANDINS

The pneumocandins are a new class of antifungal agents which appear to act by inhibiting the synthesis of β(1,3)-D-glucan, an essential component of the cell wall of susceptible filamentous fungi that is absent in mammalian cells. Caspofungin is the first of this class of agents approved in the United States; clinical trials are currently evaluating several other agents from this class, including FK463 and LY303366.[58,59,61,62]

CASPOFUNGIN

Caspofungin is metabolized by hydrolysis and *N*-acetylation, and the excretion of the drug and its metabolites in humans is 35% of dose in feces and 41% of dose in urine. Renal clearance of caspofungin is low and total clearance of the drug is 12 mL/min. Therefore, there is no dosage adjustment is necessary for patients with renal insufficiency. Becasue caspofungin is not dialyzable, supplementary dosing is not required following hemodialysis.

In clinical trials, concomitant use of cyclosporine and caspofungin resulted in elevated liver function tests two to three times the upper limit of normal. Therefore, it is generally not recommended to use these two drugs in combination. Additionally, when caspofungin was administered concurrently with tacrolimus, tacrolimus levels were reduced by 20% as compared to when the healthy volunteers received tacrolimus alone. The mechanism for these interactions is not yet known. Caspofungin is not a cytochrome P450 inducer of enzyme 3A4, and is considered a poor substrate of P450 enzymes. Overall, caspofungin was found to show no cytochrome P450 inhibition in clinical studies, and did not interact when administered concomitantly with amphotericin B, itraconazole, or mycophenolate.[58]

Caspofungin may cause histamine release resulting in rash, facial swelling, and itchiness in up to approximately 2.9% of patients. Additional events reported infrequently in the open-label noncomparative study include pulmonary edema, acute respiratory distress syndrome, and radiographic infiltrates. Caspofungin does not appear to affect renal function significantly; however, liver function tests should be monitored. Caspofungin has not been studied in patients with severe hepatic dysfunction or in pediatric patients. Additionally, safety data for use in bone marrow transplantation patients with hepatic dysfunction who may require multiple immunosuppressants such as cyclosporine, the patient population most likely to receive the agent, are very limited.[58]

The recommended dose for an adult patient is a 70-mg loading dose administered on day 1 of therapy, followed by subsequent doses of 50 mg once daily. Duration of treatment should be based upon the severity of the patients' underlying disease, recovery from immunosuppression, and clinical response. Caspofungin should be administered slowly via intravenous infusion over 1 hour.[58]

AZOLE ANTIFUNGAL AGENTS

The introduction of the azole antifungal agents has rapidly expanded the armamentarium of agents useful in the treatment of systemic fungal infections. Clotrimazole, an early imidazole antifungal, proved inadequate for the treatment of systemic infections because it was found to induce its own metabolism rapidly after oral or IV administration. Its use is now largely confined to topical therapy, primarily for the treatment of vulvovaginal candidiasis and the treatment and prophylaxis of mucocutaneous candidiasis. N-Substitution of imidazoles, such as miconazole, clotrimazole, and ketoconazole, has resulted in the triazole antifungal agents itraconazole and fluconazole. Although these agents have the same mechanism of action and spectrum of activity as imidazoles, they appear to interact much less with human cytochrome P450. Consequently, they have less effect on human sterol metabolism.[63]

MICONAZOLE

Miconazole was the first systemically available imidazole antifungal agent (Table 119–7). Miconazole is poorly soluble in aqueous solutions and is, therefore, administered in a polyethoxylated castor oil vehicle (Cremaphor EL) for IV administration. This vehicle appears to be responsible for many of the adverse effects associated with miconazole therapy, which include phlebitis and pruritus in more than 20% of patients; nausea, fever, and chills in 10% to 20%; and vomiting and anemia in >5%. With higher dosages of the drug, thrombocytosis, rouleaux formation of erythrocytes, and hyperlipidemia are reported. Rapid infusions of miconazole have resulted in cardiorespiratory arrest and anaphylactoid reactions, which are theorized to result from massive histamine release triggered by the solvent vehicle.

Although miconazole has been widely used for a variety of systemic fungal infections, including cryptococcosis, coccidioidomycosis, candidiasis, and paracoccidioidomycosis, its IV use has been largely supplanted by newer azoles. At this time, it remains the drug of choice for the treatment of infections caused by *Pseudallescheria boydii*. Miconazole is generally administered in dosages of 600–3,600 mg daily in three or four doses as an IV infusion over 30 to 60 minutes. Miconazole is widely used in topical formulations for the treatment of vulvovaginal candidiasis and superficial skin infections.[10,11]

KETOCONAZOLE

Ketoconazole is an orally available imidazole with a broad spectrum of activity against most fungal pathogens with the exception of *Aspergillus* spp. Ketoconazole is poorly soluble in aqueous fluids; it is soluble only in acidic (pH < 3) media. Consequently, the dissolution and absorption of ketoconazole is impaired in patients with elevated gastric pH. Patients with achlorhydria because of drugs (antacids or H_2-receptor antagonists) or disease (including AIDS patients) may not adequately absorb the drug. In addition, sucralfate appears to interfere with the absorption of ketoconazole when they are administered simultaneously. This interaction can be avoided by separating the doses by 2 hours. For unclear reasons, some bone marrow transplant patients have also demonstrated a decreased absorption of ketoconazole. In achlorhydric patients, ketoconazole may be dissolved in 0.1 N HCl and the solution sipped through a straw (to avoid erosion of tooth enamel). Alternatively, administration of oral glutamic acid capsules (360–720 mg) may be employed to increase absorption.[10,11]

TABLE 119–7. Pharmacology of Azole Antifungal Agents

Feature	Miconazole	Ketoconazole	Itraconazole	Fluconazole
Molecular weight	416	531	706	306
Water solubility	Poor	Poor	Poor	Excellent
Protein binding (%)	High (90)	High (99)	High (99.8)	Low (12)
CSF penetration (CSF/serum)	Poor (<10%)	Poor (<10%)	Poor (<10%)	Excellent (>80%)
Affinity for mammalian cytochrome P450	High	High	Low	Low
Elimination half-life (h)	20	8	21–64	30
Excretion in urine (%)	<5	<5	<1	80
Reduction of dose in renal failure	Not necessary	Not necessary	Not necessary	>50 mL/min: no reduction 20–50 mL/min: reduce by 50% 10–20 mL/min: reduce by 75%
Oral bioavailability (%)	<10%	~75[a]		90[b]
With meal		(See text)	~20[b] (capsule)	
Without meal			~55[b] (solution)	
Influence of food on oral bioavailability	Not applicable	Variable	Increase (capsule) Decrease (solution)	None
Effect of ↑ gastric pH on oral bioavailability	Not applicable	Decrease	Decrease (capsule) No effect (solution)	None
Dosage formulations	IV 20 mg/mL IV solution in 1% Cremophor EL	Oral 200-mg tabs	IV/oral 100-mg capsules, 10 mg/mL suspension, IV solution	IV/oral 50-, 100-, 150-, 200-mg tabs, 2 mg/mL IV solution, 50 mg or 200 mg/5 mL suspension
Usual daily dose	200–2400 mg	200–800 mg	100–400 mg	100–800 mg
Dosing regimen	Every 8 hours	Once daily	≤200 mg: once daily >200 mg: twice daily	Once daily

[a]As compared to aqueous oral solution.
[b]As compared to intravenous solution.
CSF, cerebrospinal fluid.
(Compiled from Refs. 10, 11, and 64.)

The most common adverse effect of ketoconazole is dose-related GI discomfort. Nausea, vomiting, and anorexia have been reported in more than 20% of patients receiving 200 mg daily; the incidence rises to >50% of patients when the dosage is increased to 400 mg daily. As many patients experience GI discomfort with ketoconazole, administration with food is generally recommended.

Ketoconazole inhibits adrenal steroid synthesis by reversible, dose-dependent inhibition of the cytochrome P450-dependent 11-β-hydroxylation of steroids. Although precipitation of adrenal crisis is exceedingly rare, patients should be considered potentially unable to mount an adrenal stress response. Administration of ketoconazole as a single (rather than multiple) daily dose appears to minimize adrenal axis suppression. Gynecomastia, decreased libido, oligospermia, azoospermia, and impotence secondary to decreased testosterone synthesis have been reported in men following high (>600 mg) daily dosages and during prolonged administration of lower dosages. Ketoconazole is teratogenic in rats and should not be used in pregnant women.[10,11,23]

ITRACONAZOLE

Itraconazole is triazole antifungal with a broad spectrum of antifungal activity. Despite its marked structural similarity to ketoconazole, itraconazole differs in several important respects. Itraconazole appears to have greater specificity against fungal versus mammalian cytochrome P450, resulting in greater potency and a decrease in P450-mediated side effects. In addition, itraconazole possesses excellent *in vitro* activity against *Aspergillus* and *Sporothrix* spp. Recently, two new formulations of the drug were made available; both use cyclodextrin as a solubilizing vehicle to increase the solubility of the drug.[64]

Like ketoconazole, itraconazole depends on the availability of low gastric pH for dissolution and absorption of the capsule formulation. Administration with food appears to enhance significantly the bioavailability of itraconazole capsules, while it decreases the bioavailability of the oral solution. Because itraconazole exhibits pH-dependent dissolution and absorption, absorption of the capsule formulation is impaired in patients receiving antacids or H_2-receptor antagonists and in patients with achlorhydria. The earlier (capsule) formulation of itraconazole exhibits unpredictable oral bioavailability, particularly in subjects with hypochlorhydria, and in patients with enteropathy caused by mucositis or graft-versus-host gut disease. Plasma concentrations of itraconazole following a single oral dose (capsules) in HIV-infected patients are approximately 50% lower than concentrations observed in healthy volunteers. The oral bioavailability of the solution is unaffected by alterations in gastric pH or in patients with enteropathy.[8,9,64]

Adverse effects of itraconazole appear to be similar to those observed with ketoconazole, but they occur with lower frequency. Gastrointestinal disturbances (primarily nausea, vomiting, epigastric pain, and diarrhea) have been the most common complaints, occurring in up to 20% of patients receiving the capsule formulation, and are more common with dosages >400 mg/day. The gastrointestinal disturbances appear to be more common in patients receiving the solution formulation of itraconazole. Although there are no data in humans, itraconazole, similar to the other azoles, is potentially teratogenic and should be avoided in pregnant women. Although cyclodextrin is not absorbed following oral administration, use of the intravenous formulation of itraconazole is limited to 2 weeks because of concerns for potential nephrotoxicity secondary to accumulation of the cyclodextrin vehicle.[10,11,64]

FLUCONAZOLE

Fluconazole is a triazole antifungal agent with markedly different pharmacologic features than previously marketed azole antifungals. The small molecular weight, low protein binding, and increased water solubility of fluconazole results in rapid, essentially complete absorption of drug following oral administration.

Fluconazole is excreted primarily (>80%) as unchanged drug in the urine, with the remainder of the dose excreted as glucuronide and N-oxide metabolites in the urine and as unchanged drug in the feces.

Side effects of fluconazole suggest that the drug is well tolerated in most patients. Gastrointestinal complaints are the most frequently reported, followed by headaches and rash. Unlike ketoconazole, fluconazole does not inhibit testicular or adrenal steroidogenesis in healthy volunteers or hospitalized patients. Reversible alopecia occurs not infrequently and usually appears after several months of treatment with higher doses of fluconazole. Fluconazole has been associated with several well-described cases of fetal malformations and should not be used in pregnant women.[10,11,64]

INVESTIGATIONAL ANTIFUNGALS

Three investigational triazoles are currently under clinical development. Voriconazole, ravuconazole (BMS-207147), and posaconazole (SCH56592) have activity against *Aspergillus* species and fluconazole-resistant strains of *Candida,* including *C. albicans, C. krusei,* and *C. glabrata.*[56,57,65,66]

Lipid-complex nystatin, and two new pneumocandin derivatives (LY303366 and FK463) are also under development.[56,57,61,62,66]

DRUG INTERACTIONS WITH AZOLE ANTIFUNGAL AGENTS

Drug interactions with azole antifungals can generally be placed into three broad categories: (a) decreases in azole bioavailability because of chelation or secondary to increases in gastric pH; (b) interactions with other cytochrome P450-metabolized drugs; and (c) interactions caused by inhibition of *p*-glycoprotein. Drug interactions in the second categories may result in increases or decreases in the azole antifungal, in the interacting drug, or in both drugs.[10,11]

Simultaneous administration of sucralfate and ketoconazole (and probably itraconazole but not fluconazole) results in a significant decrease in oral bioavailability, probably via a chelation interaction at acidic pHs. This interaction can be avoided by separation of doses by 2 hours.

The interaction of azole antifungal agents with other cytochromes P450-metabolized drugs is well recognized. The azoles appear to be metabolized almost entirely via the cytochrome P450 3A4 subfamily. As expected, they interact with other drugs metabolized partly or wholly via this enzyme pathway. Decreases in the metabolism of warfarin and cyclosporine because of administration of IV miconazole results in increased plasma concentrations and toxicity of both drugs. Although older agents, such as miconazole, have been poorly studied, numerous clinically significant interactions have been documented with ketoconazole, itraconazole, and fluconazole with a variety of other drugs (Tables 119–8 and 119–9). In most cases, the azole interferes with the metabolism of the other cytochromes P450-metabolized drug.[10,11]

Particularly noteworthy are the interactions between azoles and cisapride, terfenadine, astemizole, or loratadine. Cisapride, terfenadine, and astemizole are metabolized almost entirely via the

TABLE 119–8. Effects of Common Concomitantly Administered Drugs on Azole Antifungal Drug Concentrations

Drug Affecting Azole Concentration	Azole Antifungal Drug Concentration[a]		
	Ketoconazole	***Itraconazole***	***Fluconazole***
Alterations in cytochrome P450			
Carbamazepine	None known[b]	↓	None known
Phenytoin	↓	↓	None known
Isoniazid	↓	None known	None known
Rifampin	↓	↓	↓
Rifabutin	None known	↓	No effect[c]
Protease inhibitors	None known	None known	None known
Inhibition of absorption from the gastrointestinal tract			
Sucralfate	↓	No effect	No effect
Histamine 2 receptor antagonists	↓	↓	No effect
Omeprazole	↓	↓	No effect
Antacids	↓	↓	No effect
Didanosine (DDI)	None known	↓	None known

[a]Reductions in plasma azole concentrations have led to therapeutic failure for some fungal infections.
[b]None known: Interaction has not been studied in human subjects; however, caution should be used in using this combination until further information is available.
[c]No effect: Drug combination has been studied in human subjects and no clinically significant pharmacokinetic or pharmacodynamic interaction was detected.

TABLE 119–9. Effects of Azole Antifungal Drugs on Serum Concentrations of Common Concomitantly Administered Drugs

Drug Affected by Azole	Azole Antifungal Drug		
	Ketoconazole	***Itraconazole***	***Fluconazole***
Alterations in cytochrome P450			
Warfarin	↑[a]	↑	↑[a]
Cyclosporine	↑[a]	↑[a]	↑[a]
Phenytoin	↑[a]	None known[c]	↑[a]
Triazolam, alprazolam, midazolam	↑	None known	None known
Diltiazem	↑	None known	None known
Lovastatin	None known	None known	↑
Zidovudine	None known	None known	↑
Carbamazepine	None known	None known	↑[a]
Loratidine	↑	None known	None known
[Terfenadine]	↑[b]	↑[b]	No effect[d]
[Astemizole]	↑[b]	↑[b]	None known
[Cisapride]	↑[b]	↑[b]	↑
Oral hypoglycemics	↑	None known	↑
Isoniazid	↓[a]	None known	None known
Rifampin	↓[a]	None known	None known
Rifabutin	None known	None known	↑
Tacrolimus	None known	None known	↑[a]
Quinidine	↑	None known	None known
Protease inhibitors	↑	↑	↑
Inhibition of p-glycoprotein			
Digoxin	None known	↑[a]	None known

[a]Clinically significant interaction; serum concentrations of drug and/or clinical status of patient should be monitored.
[b]Life-threatening interaction causing arrhythmias; avoid use of combination.
[c]None known: Interaction has not been studied in human subjects, however, caution should be used in using in this combination until further information is available.
[d]No effect: Drug combination has been studied in human subjects and no clinically significant pharmacokinetic or pharmacodynamic interaction was detected.
[ ], drug has been removed from the US market.
(*Adapted from Refs. 10, 11, and 64.*)

cytochrome P450 3A4 subfamily; inhibition of metabolism by azoles results in accumulation of the cardiotoxic parent drug. Torsade de pointes and fatal arrhythmias have been described as consequences of the interactions between azoles (ketoconazole and itraconazole) and terfenadine. Although no published reports are available, the manufacturer reports similar toxicities in patients receiving cisapride and itraconazole, ketoconazole, fluconazole, or miconazole (manufacturer's package insert for cisapride, September 1995). Syncope and torsade de pointes have been reported in a patient receiving erythromycin (which also inhibits cytochrome P450 3A4), ketoconazole, and astemizole (manufacturer's package insert for astemizole, July 1993). Recently, terfenadine, astemizole, and cisapride were withdrawn from the US market because of the potential for these toxicities.[10,11]

The interaction between ketoconazole and cyclosporine has been exploited in order to reduce drug costs associated with administration of cyclosporine following organ transplantation. Relative to ketoconazole and itraconazole, fluconazole appears to be intermediate in its ability to inhibit human cytochromes P450. The magnitude of fluconazole-induced inhibition of cyclosporine metabolism appears, however, to depend on the dosage of fluconazole.

Predictably, drugs, such as rifampin, rifabutin, isoniazid, phenytoin, and carbamazepine, which are known to induce the activity of cytochromes P450, result in increased metabolism of the azole antifungals and may result in therapeutic failures. Increased dosages of azole antifungals may be required in patients receiving these combinations of drugs.[10,11]

Itraconazole is an inhibitor of intestinal *p*-glycoprotein. Significant increases in digoxin (a *p*-glycoprotein substrate) have been observed in patients receiving both agents concurrently. Interactions with other substrates of *p*-glycoprotein would be expected to occur.

PLASMA CONCENTRATION MONITORING OF ANTIFUNGAL AGENTS

Routine monitoring of plasma concentrations of antifungal agents to assess efficacy or toxicity of these agents is generally not available. Correlations between plasma concentrations of antifungal agents and therapeutic outcomes have been poorly studied. Under certain circumstances, serum or plasma concentration monitoring is warranted; for example, in patients susceptible to 5-flucytosine toxicity, or to document adequate oral absorption of ketoconazole or itraconazole in cases of suspected treatment failure, concern about compliance or absorption, or when drug interactions that might reduce the solubility or accelerate the metabolism of azoles are suspected. Although "therapeutic" levels have not been defined, some investigators recommend maintenance of serum concentrations of itraconazole (2 to 4 hours after administration) of 1 μg/mL, measured by bioassay.[6,19] Among AIDS patients, patients receiving a dosage of 200 mg once or twice daily achieved median plasma concentrations of ≈ 3 μg/mL or 6 μg/mL, respectively.[19]

▶ PRINCIPLES OF PHARMACOTHERAPY

- Systemic mycoses may be caused by pathogenic fungi, including histoplasmosis, coccidioidomycosis, cryptococcosis, blastomycosis, paracoccidioidmycosis, and sporotrichosis, or opportunistic fungi, such as *C. albicans, Aspergillus* spp., *Trichosporon, C. glabrata, Fusarium, Alternaria,* and *Mucor*.
- The diagnosis of fungal infection is generally accomplished by careful evaluation of clinical symptoms, results of serologic tests, and histopathologic examination and culture of clinical specimens.
- Histoplasmosis is caused by *H. capsulatum* and is endemic in parts of the central United States along the Ohio and Mississippi River valleys. Although most patients experience asymptomatic infection, some may experience chronic, disseminated disease.
- Asymptomatic patients with histoplasmosis are not treated, although non-AIDS patients with evident disease are treated with either oral ketoconazole or intravenous amphotericin B; AIDS patients are treated with amphotericin B, and then receive lifelong suppression.
- Blastomycosis is caused by *B. dermatitidis* and is generally an asymptomatic, self-limited disease; however, reactivation can lead to chronic disease. Although treatment for self-limited disease is controversial, patients with chronic pulmonary disease or extrapulmonary disease should be treated with ketoconazole and those with CNS, progressive, or life-threatening disease should receive amphotericin.
- Coccidioidomycosis is caused by *C. immitis* and is endemic in some parts of the southwest United States. It may cause nonspecific symptoms, acute pneumonia, chronic pulmonary, or disseminated disease. Primary pulmonary disease (unless severe) is often not treated, while extrapulmonary disease is treated with amphotericin B, and meningitis is treated with fluconazole.
- Cryptococcus is caused by *C. neoformans* and occurs primarily in immunocompromised patients. Nonimmunocompromised patients with acute meningitis are treated with amphotericin B with flucytosine. Patients infected with HIV require long-term treatment with fluconazole or itraconazole.
- A variety of *Candida* spp. (including *C. albicans, C. glabrata, C. tropicalis, C. krusei*) may cause diseases, such as mucocutaneous, oral, esophageal, vaginal, and hematogenous candidiasis, as well as candiduria.
- Aspergillosis may be caused by a variety of *Aspergillus* spp. that may cause superficial infections, pneumonia, allergic bronchopulmonary aspergillosis, or invasive infection. Treatment with amphotericin B is generally instituted but often not successful.

REFERENCES

1. Bennett JE. Introduction to mycoses. In: Mandell GL, Bennett JE, Dolin R, eds. Principles and Practice of Infectious Diseases, 5th ed. Philadelphia, Churchill Livingstone, 2000:2654–2656.
2. Pfaller MA, Jones RN, Messer SA, et al. National surveillance of nosocomial blood stream infection due to *Candida* albicans: Frequency of occurrence and antifungal susceptibility in the SCOPE program. Diagn Microbiol Infect Dis 1998;31:327–332.
3. Pfaller MA, Jones RN, Doern GV, et al. International surveillance of blood stream infections due to Candida species in the European SENTRY Program: Species distribution and antifungal susceptibility including the investigational triazole and echinocandin agents. SENTRY Participant Group (Europe). Diagn Microbiol Infect Dis 1999;35(1): 19–25.
4. Singh N. Invasive mycoses in organ transplant recipients: Controversies in prophylaxis and management. J Antimicrob Chemother 2000;45(6):749–755.
5. National Committee for Clinical Laboratory Standards (NCCLS). Reference method for broth dilution antifungal susceptibility testing of yeasts:

Approved standard. NCCLS document M27-A. Wayne, PA, NCCLS, 1997.
6. Summers KK, Hardin TC, Gore SJ, Graybill JR. Therapeutic drug monitoring of systemic antifungal therapy. J Antimicrob Chemother 1997;40:753–764.
7. Sobel JD. Practice guidelines for the treatment of fungal infections. Clin Infect Dis 2000;30:652.
8. Bennett JE. Pathogenic fungi. In: Sherris JC, ed. Medical Microbiology, 2nd ed. New York, Elsevier, 1991:440.
9. Rex JH, Walsh TJ, Sobel JD, et al. Practice guidelines for the treatment of candidiasis. Clin Infect Dis 2000;30:662–678.
10. Kauffman CA, Carver PL. Antifungal agents in the 1990s: Current status and future developments. Drugs 1997;53:539–549.
11. Kauffman CA, Carver PL. Use of azoles for systemic antifungal therapy. Adv Pharmacol 1997;39:143–189.
12. Edwards JE. Candida species. In: Mandell GL, Bennett JE, Dolin R, eds. Principles and Practice of Infectious Diseases, 5th ed. Philadelphia, Churchill Livingstone, 2000:2656–2671.
13. de Repentigny L. Serodiagnosis of candidiasis, aspergillosis, and cryptococcosis. Clin Infect Dis 1992;14(suppl 1):S11–S22.
14. Kaufman L. Laboratory methods for the diagnosis and confirmation of systemic mycoses. Clin Infect Dis 1992;14(suppl 1):S23–S29.
15. Perfect JR. Antifungal prophylaxis: To prevent or not. Am J Med 1993;94:233–234.
16. Saag MS, Graybill RJ, Larsen RA, et al. Practice guidelines for the management of cryptococcal disease. Clin Infect Dis 2000;30:710–718.
17. Deepe GS. Histoplasma capsulatum. In: Mandell GL, Bennett JE, Dolin R, eds. Principles and Practice of Infectious Diseases, 5th ed. Philadelphia, Churchill Livingstone, 2000:2718–2733.
18. Gallis HA, Drew RH, Pickard WW. Amphotericin B: 30 years of clinical experience. Rev Infect Dis 1990;12:308–329.
19. Wheat J, Sarosi G, McKinsey D, et al. Practice guidelines for the management of patients with histoplasmosis. Clin Infect Dis 2000;30:688–695.
20. Bradsher RW. Histoplasmosis and blastomycosis. Clin Infect Dis 1996;22(suppl 2):S102–S111.
21. Chapman SW. Blastomyces dermatitidis. In: Mandell GL, Bennett JE, Dolin R, eds. Principles and Practice of Infectious Diseases, 5th ed. Philadelphia, Churchill Livingstone, 2000:2741–2746.
22. Chapman SW, Bradsher RW Jr, Campbell GD Jr, et al. Practice guidelines for the management of patients with blastomycoses. Clin Infect Dis 2000;30:679–683.
23. National Institute of Allergy and Infectious Diseases Mycoses Study Group. Treatment of blastomycosis and histoplasmosis with ketoconazole: Results of a prospective randomized clinical trial. Ann Intern Med 1985;103:861–872.
24. Galgiani J. Coccidioides immitis. In: Mandell GL, Bennett JE, Dolin R, eds. Principles and Practice of Infectious Diseases, 5th ed. Philadelphia, Churchill Livingstone, 2000:2747–2757.
25. Galgiani JN, Ampel NM, Catanzaro A, et al. Practice guidelines for the treatment of coccidioidomycoses. Clin Infect Dis 2000;30:658–661.
26. Stevens DA. Current concepts: Coccidioidomycosis. N Engl J Med 1995;332:1077–1082.
27. Galgiani JN, Catanzaro A, Cloud GA, et al. Fluconazole therapy for coccidioidal meningitis. Ann Intern Med 1993:119:28–35.
28. Bennett JE, Dismukes WE, Duma RJ, et al. A comparison of amphotericin B alone and combined with flucytosine in the treatment of cryptococcal meningitis. N Engl J Med 1979;301:126–131.
29. Francis P, Walsh TJ. Evolving role of flucytosine in immunocompromised patients: New insights into safety, pharmacokinetics, and antifungal therapy. Clin Infect Dis 1992;15:1003–1018.
30. Powderly WG, Saag MS, Cloud GA, et al. A controlled trial of fluconazole or amphotericin B to prevent relapse of cryptococcal meningitis in patients with the acquired immunodeficiency syndrome. N Engl J Med 1992;326:793–798.
31. Saag MS, Powderly WG, Cloud GA, et al. Comparison of amphotericin B with fluconazole in the treatment of acute AIDS associated cryptococcal meningitis: The NIAID Mycoses Study Group and the AIDS Clinical Trials Group. N Engl J Med 1992;326:83–89.
32. van der Horst CM, Saag MS, Cloud GA, et al. Treatment of cryptococcal meningitis associated with the acquired immunodeficiency syndrome. N Engl J Med 1997;37:15–21.
33. Sullivan DJ, Westerneng TJ, Haynes KA, et al. *Candida dubliniensis sp. nov:* Phenotyping and molecular characterization of a novel species associated with oral candidosis in HIV-infected individuals. Microbiology 1995:141;1507–1521.
34. Fraser VJ, Jones M, Dunkel J, et al. Candidemia in a tertiary care hospital: Epidemiology, risk factors, and predictors of mortality. Clin Infect Dis 1992;15:414–421.
35. Wey SB, Mori M, Pfaller MA, et al. Risk factors for hospital-acquired candidemia: A matched case-control study. Arch Intern Med 1989;149:2349–2353.
36. Minari A, Hachem R, Raad I. *Candida lusitaniae:* A cause of breakthrough fungemia in cancer patients. Clin Infect Dis 2001;32:186–190.
37. Pfaller MA, Jones RN, Doern GV, et al. International surveillance of bloodstream infections due to Candida species: Frequency of occurrence and antifungal susceptibilities of isolates collected in 1997 in the United States, Canada, and South America for the SENTRY program. J Clin Microbiol 1998;36:1886–1889.
38. Winston DJ, Chandrasekar PH, Lazarus HM, et al. Fluconazole prophylaxis of fungal infections in patients with acute leukemia: Results of a randomized placebo-controlled, double-blind, multicenter trial. Ann Intern Med 1993;118:495–503.
39. Goodman JL, Winston DJ, Greenfield RA, et al. A controlled trial of fluconazole to prevent fungal infections in patients undergoing bone marrow transplantation. N Engl J Med 1992;326:845–851.
40. Edwards DE. International conference for the development of a consensus on the management and prevention of severe candidal infections. Clin Infect Dis 1997;25:43–59.
41. Pfaller MA. Nosocomial candidiasis: Emerging species, reservoirs, and modes of transmission. Clin Infect Dis 1996;22(suppl 2):S89–S94.
42. Rex JH, Bennett JE, Sugar AM, et al. A randomized trial comparing fluconazole with amphotericin B for the treatment of candidemia in patients without neutropenia. N Engl J Med 1994;331:1325–1330.
43. Pizzo PA, Robichaud KJ, Gill FA, Witebsky FG. Empiric antibiotic and antifungal therapy for cancer patients with prolonged fever and granulocytopenia. Am J Med 1982;72:101–111.
44. Kauffman CA, Vazquez JA, Sobel JD, et al. Prospective multicenter surveillance study of funguria in hospitalized patients. Clin Infect Dis 2000;30:14–18.
45. Sobel JD, Kauffman CA, McKinsey D, et al. Candiduria: A randomized, double-blind study of treatment with fluconazole and placebo. Clin Infect Dis 2000;30:19–24.
46. Denning DW, Stevens DA. Antifungal and surgical treatment of invasive aspergillosis: Review of 2,121 published cases. Rev Infect Dis 1990;12:1147–1181.
47. Jennings TS, Hardin TC. Treatment of aspergillosis with itraconazole. Ann Pharmacother 1993;27:1206–1211.
48. Stevens DA, Schwartz HJ, Lee JT, et al. A randomized trial of itraconazole in allergic bronchopulmonary aspergillosis. N Engl J Med 2000;342:756–762.
49. Harari S. Current strategies in the treatment of invasive *Aspergillus* infections in immunocompromised patients. Drugs 1999;58(4):621–631.
50. Stevens DA, Kan VL, Judson MA, et al. Practice guidelines for diseases caused by *Aspergillus*. Clin Infect Dis 2000;30:696–709.
51. Lin SJ, Schranz J, Teutsch SM. Aspergillus case fatality rate: Systematic review of the literature. Clin Infect Dis 2001;32:358–366.
52. Holding KJ, Dworkin MS, Wan PCT, et al. Aspergillosis among people infected with human immunodeficiency virus: Incidence and survival. Clin Infect Dis 2000;31:1253–1257.
53. Wong-Beringer A, Jacobs RA, Guglielmo BJ. Lipid formulations of amphotericin B: Clinical efficacy and toxicities. Clin Infect Dis 1998;27:603–618.
54. Ellis M, Spence D, de Pauw B, et al. An EORTC international multicenter randomized trial (EORTC no. 19923) comparing two dosages of liposomal amphotericin B for treatment of invasive aspergillosis. Clin Infect Dis 1998;27:1406–1412.

55. Wingard JR, White ML, Anaissie E, et al. A randomized, double-blind, comparative trial evaluating the safety of liposomal amphotericin B versus amphotericin B lipid complex in the empirical treatment of febrile neutropenia. Clin Infect Dis 2000;31:1155–1163.
56. Mills W, Chopra R, Linch DC, et al. Liposomal amphotericin B in the treatment of fungal infections in neutropenic patients: A single-centre experience of 133 episodes in 116 patients. Br J Haematol 1994;86:754–760.
57. Pfaller MA, Messer SA, Hollis RJ, et al. In vitro susceptibilities of *Candida* bloodstream isolates to the new triazole antifungal agents BMS-207147, Sch 56592, and voriconazole. Antimicrob Agents Chemother 1998;42(12):3242–3244.
58. Caspofungin Package Insert.
59. Espinel-Ingroff A. Comparison of in vitro activities of the new triazole SCH56592 and the echinocandins MK-0991 (L-743,872) and LY303366 against opportunistic filamentous and dimorphic fungi and yeasts. J Clin Microbiol 1998;36(10):2950–2956.
60. King CT, Rogers PD, Cleary JD, et al. Antifungal therapy during pregnancy. Clin Infect Dis 1998;27(5):1151–1160.
61. Andriole VT. Current and future antifungal therapy: New targets for antifungal therapy. Int J Antimicrob Agents 2000;16:317–321.
62. Maesaki S, Hossain MA, Miyazaki Y, et al. Efficacy of FK463, a (1,3)-beta-D-glucan synthase inhibitor, in disseminated azole-resistant candida albicans infection in mice. Antimicrob Agents Chemother 2000;44(6):1728–1730.
63. Como JA, Dismukes WE. Oral azole drugs as systemic antifungal therapy. N Engl J Med 1994;330:263–272.
64. Stevens DA. Itraconazole in cyclodextrin solution. Pharmacotherapy 1999;19(5):603–611.
65. Kappe R. Antifungal activity of the new azole UK-109, 496 (voriconazole). Mycoses 1999;43(suppl 2):83–86.
66. De Pauw BE. New antifungal agents and preparations. Int J Antimicrob Agents 2000;16:147–150.

120

INFECTIONS IN IMMUNOCOMPROMISED PATIENTS

Douglas N. Fish

An immunocompromised host is a patient with intrinsic or acquired defects in host defenses that predispose to infection. Advances in modern medicine are creating more immunocompromised hosts than ever before. Historically, many of these patients died from their underlying diseases. Dramatic improvements in survival have been achieved by more aggressive therapy of underlying diseases and improved supportive care. Because aggressive therapy often renders patients profoundly immunosuppressed for long periods, however, opportunistic infections remain important causes of morbidity and mortality. This chapter focuses on risk factors for infection, common pathogens and infection sites, and prevention and management of suspected or documented infections in hematology and oncology patients (including bone marrow transplant [BMT] patients), and solid organ transplant recipients. Chapter 123 discusses infectious complications associated with human immunodeficiency virus (HIV) infection.

RISK FACTORS FOR INFECTION

GRANULOCYTOPENIA

Granulocytopenia is an abnormally reduced number of granulocytes (primarily neutrophils) circulating in peripheral blood. Although exact definitions of granulocytopenia often vary, an absolute neutrophil count (ANC) of <1,000 cells/mm^3 indicates a reduction sufficient to predispose patients to infection.[1] The ANC is the sum of the absolute numbers of both mature neutrophils (polymorphonuclear cells [PMNs], also called "polys" or "segs") and immature neutrophils ("bands"). The absolute number of PMNs and bands is determined by dividing the percentage of these cells (obtained from the white blood cell [WBC] differential) by 100, and then multiplying the quotient obtained by the total number of WBCs.

The degree or severity of granulocytopenia is an important risk factor for infection. All granulocytopenic patients are considered to be at risk for infection; however, those with an ANC of <500 cells/mm^3 are at greater risk than those with ANCs of 500–1,000 cells/mm^3. Most treatment guidelines use an ANC of <500 cells/mm^3 as the critical value in making therapeutic decisions regarding the management of infections.[1–3] Risk of infection and death is greatest among patients with <100 granulocytes/mm^3.[1]

In addition to the degree of granulocytopenia, both the rate of neutrophil decline and the duration of neutropenia are important risk factors for infection.[1–3] In patients with chemotherapy-induced neutropenia, the risk of infection is increased according to the rapidity of ANC decline. Patients whose ANCs are falling rapidly and are expected to be <500/mm^3 within 24 hours are already considered to be severely neutropenic and are treated accordingly. Infection risk also increases as the duration of neutropenia increases; patients with severe neutropenia of >7 to 10 days' duration are considered to be at especially high risk.[1,4] The duration of chemotherapy-induced neutropenia varies considerably among subsets of cancer patients according to the specific chemotherapeutic agents used and the intensity of treatment. Patients undergoing BMT may have no detectable granulocytes in peripheral blood for up to 3 to 4 weeks and are at particular risk for severe infections with a variety of pathogens.

Bacteria and fungi commonly cause infections in neutropenic patients. Gram-positive cocci (*Staphylococcus aureus, S. epidermidis,* streptococci, and enterococci) have emerged as the most common cause of acute bacterial infections among granulocytopenic patients. Gram-negative bacilli (*Escherichia coli, Klebsiella pneumoniae, Pseudomonas aeruginosa*) were traditionally the most common cause of bacterial infection and remain frequent pathogens, although now not as common as gram-positive bacteria.[3,5] Patients who are neutropenic for extended periods of time and who receive broad-spectrum antibiotics are at risk for fungal infection, usually because of *Candida* or *Aspergillus* spp.[3,6] Viral infections, although not as common as bacterial and fungal infections, may also cause severe infection in the granulocytopenic patient.[5–7] Successful treatment of infections in neutropenic patients is dependent on resolution of neutropenia.[1–3]

Patients with granulocytopenia can be divided into low- and high-risk groups based on the projected duration of granulocytopenia and resultant risk of infection.[3] Patients who have been granulocytopenic for no more than 10 days are considered to be at relatively low risk of severe infection and usually have excellent clinical outcomes. High-risk patients are those with granulocytopenia for more than 10 days; these patients are at increased risk for severe infection from bacteria, as well as from fungi, viruses, and parasites.

Although not readily quantifiable, abnormalities may exist in granulocyte function, as well as in cell numbers. Defects in phagocyte function may be caused by underlying disease (e.g., leukemias) or its treatment (e.g., corticosteroids, antineoplastic agents, radiation). Leukemic patients with relapsing disease are at increased risk of infection, even in the absence of neutropenia.[2]

IMMUNE SYSTEM DEFECTS

In addition to granulocytopenia, defects in T-lymphocyte and macrophage function (cell-mediated immunity), B-cell function (humoral immunity), or both predispose patients to infection. Cellular immune dysfunction is the result of underlying disease or immunosuppressive drug therapy; these defects result in a reduced ability of the host to defend against intracellular pathogens. Patients with Hodgkin's disease and transplant patients receiving immunosuppressive drugs, such as cyclosporine, tacrolimus, mycophenolate, corticosteroids, antineoplastic agents, or azathioprine, are at risk for a variety of bacterial,

TABLE 120–1. Risk Factors and Common Pathogens in Immunocompromised Patients

Risk Factor	Patient Conditions	Common Pathogens
Neutropenia	Acute leukemia Chemotherapy	Bacteria: *Escherichia coli, Klebsiella pneumoniae, Pseudomonas aeruginosa, Staphylococcus aureus, Staphylococcus epidermidis*, streptococci, enterococci Fungi: *Candida, Aspergillus, Zygomycetes* Viruses: Herpes simplex
Impaired cell-mediated immunity	Lymphoma Immunosuppressive therapy (steroids, cyclosporine, chemotherapy)	Bacteria: *Listeria, Nocardia, Legionella,* Mycobacteria Fungi: *Cryptococcus neoformans, Candida, Aspergillus, Histoplasma capsulatum* Viruses: Cytomegalovirus, varicella-zoster, herpes simplex Protozoal: *Pneumocystis carinii*
Impaired humoral immunity	Multiple myeloma Chronic lymphocytic leukemia Splenectomy Immunosuppressive therapy (steroids, chemotherapy)	Bacteria: *S. pneumoniae, H. influenzae, N. meningitidis*
Loss of protective barriers		
Skin	Venipuncture, bone marrow aspiration, urinary catheterization, vascular access devices, radiation, biopsies	Bacteria: *S. aureus, S. epidermidis, Bacillus* spp. Fungi: *Candida*
Mucous membranes	Respiratory support equipment, endoscopy, chemotherapy, radiation	Bacteria: *S. aureus, S. epidermidis,* Enterobacteriaceae, streptococci, *P. aeruginosa, Bacteroides* spp. Fungi: *Candida* Viruses: Herpes simplex
Surgery	Solid organ transplantation	Bacteria: *S. aureus, S. epidermidis,* Enterobacteriaceae, *P. aeruginosa, Bacteroides* spp. Fungi: *Candida* Viruses: Herpes simplex
Alteration of normal microbial flora	Antimicrobial therapy Chemotherapy Hospital environment	Bacteria: Enterobacteriaceae, *P. aeruginosa, Legionella, S. aureus, S. epidermidis* Fungi: *Candida, Aspergillus*
Blood products, donor organs	Bone marrow transplantation Solid organ transplantation	Fungi: *Candida* Viruses: Cytomegalovirus, Epstein-Barr virus, hepatitis B, hepatitis C Protozoal: *Toxoplasma gondii*

(Compiled from Refs. 1–4, 5, 8, and 27.)

fungal, viral, and protozoal infections (Table 120–1). While some of these pathogens are associated with asymptomatic or mild disease in normal hosts, they can cause disseminated, life-threatening infections in immunocompromised hosts.

Underlying disease frequently causes defects in humoral immune function. Patients with multiple myeloma and chronic lymphocytic leukemia have progressive hypogammaglobulinemia that results in defective humoral immunity. Splenectomy performed as a part of the staging process for Hodgkin's disease places patients at risk for infectious complications. Disease states with humoral immune dysfunction predispose the patient to serious, life-threatening infection with encapsulated organisms, such as *Streptococcus pneumoniae, Haemophilus influenzae,* and *Neisseria meningitidis.*

DESTRUCTION OF PROTECTIVE BARRIERS

Loss of protective barriers is a major factor predisposing immunocompromised patients to infection. Damage to skin and mucous membranes by surgery, venipuncture, intravenous (IV) and urinary catheters, radiation, and chemotherapy disrupts major host defense systems, leaving patients at high risk for infection. Chemotherapy-induced mucositis may erode mucous membranes of the oropharynx and gastrointestinal (GI) tract and establish a portal for subsequent infection by bacteria, herpes simplex, and *Candida*. Medical and surgical procedures, such as transplant surgery, indwelling IV catheter placement, bone marrow aspiration, biopsies, and endoscopy further damage the integument and predispose patients to infection. Infections resulting from disruption of protective integumentary barriers are usually a result of skin flora, such as *S. aureus, S. epidermidis,* and various streptococci.[3,4]

ENVIRONMENTAL CONTAMINATION/ALTERATION OF MICROBIAL FLORA

Infections in immunocompromised patients are caused by organisms either colonizing the host or acquired from the environment. Microorganisms may easily be transferred from patient-to-patient on the hands of hospital personnel unless strict infection control guidelines are followed. Contaminated equipment, such as nebulizers or ventilators, and contaminated water supplies have been responsible for outbreaks of *P. aeruginosa* and *Legionella pneumophila* infections, respectively. Foods, such as fruits and green leafy vegetables, that are often heavily colonized with gram-negative bacteria and fungi are also sources of microbial contamination and subsequent infection in immunocompromised hosts.[2,8]

Most infections in cancer patients are caused by organisms colonizing body sites, such as the skin, oropharynx, and GI tract.[8] The GI tract is the most common site from which infections in immunocompromised hosts originate. Periodontitis, pharyngitis, esophagitis, colitis, perirectal cellulitis, and bacteremias are predominantly caused by normal flora of the gut; bloodstream infections are thought to arise from microbial translocation across injured GI mucosa.[8] Normal flora may also be significantly disrupted and altered; oropharyngeal flora rapidly changes to primarily gram-negative bacilli in hospitalized patients. Many cancer patients may already be colonized with gram-negative bacilli upon admission, perhaps the result of frequent hospitalizations and clinic visits. In hospitalized cancer patients, 50% of infections, however, are caused by colonizing organisms acquired after admission.[8]

Although hospitalization and severity of illness are risk factors for colonization by gram-negative bacilli, administration of broad-spectrum antimicrobial agents has the greatest impact on flora of immunocompromised hosts. Use of these agents disrupts the delicate balance of GI tract flora and predisposes patients to infection with more virulent pathogens. Antineoplastic drugs (e.g., cyclophosphamide, doxorubicin, fluorouracil) and acid-suppressive therapy (e.g., H_2-receptor antagonists, antacids) may also result in changes in GI flora and possibly predispose patients to infection.[9]

Numerous factors, such as underlying disease, immunosuppressive drug therapy, and antimicrobial administration, determine the immunocompromised host's risk of developing infection. Several risk factors are present concomitantly in many patients (Table 120–1).

INFECTIONS IN NEUTROPENIC CANCER PATIENTS

Infection remains the leading cause of autopsy-determined death in neutropenic cancer patients (ANC < 1,000/mm^3); 6% to 30% of deaths are caused by infection.[10,11] Patients with profound neutropenia are at greatest risk for systemic infection. Areas of impaired or damaged host defenses, such as the oropharynx, lungs, skin, sinuses, and GI tract, are common sites of infection. These local infections may also progress to cause systemic infection and bacteremia.[8,10] Febrile episodes in granulocytopenic cancer patients can be attributed to microbiologically or clinically documented infection in only about 30% to 40% of cases.[2,4,12]

ETIOLOGY

Table 120–1 lists organisms commonly infecting immunocompromised patients. About 55% to 60% of bacteremic episodes in cancer patients are the result of gram-positive organisms, as compared to only 9% to 18% of episodes documented during the 1970s and 1980s.[3,4] This shift is thought to have been caused by the frequent use of indwelling IV catheters (e.g., Hickman, Broviac) and broad-spectrum antibiotics with excellent gram-negative activity but relatively poor gram-positive coverage.[3,4,8,12–14] *S. aureus* and coagulase-negative staphylococci (especially *S. epidermidis*) are the most common organisms, but *Bacillus* spp. and *Corynebacterium jeikeium* may also cause indwelling catheter infections.[4,5] Viridans streptococci have also emerged as important pathogens, particularly in patients with chemotherapy-induced mucositis of the oropharynx.[4,12,15] Enterococci, including vancomycin-resistant strains, may also be problematic in many institutions.[3]

Gram-positive infections do not always cause immediately life-threatening infections and are associated with somewhat lower mortality rates as compared to gram-negative infections (15% vs 30% to 75%, respectively). However, gram-positive infections may also cause severe complications, such as disseminated intravascular coagulation (DIC) and adult respiratory distress syndrome (ARDS).[4,5,12] Thus, prevention and timely treatment of gram-positive infections are clearly of great importance in the management of neutropenic cancer patients.

Gram-negative infections remain important causes of morbidity and mortality in immunocompromised cancer patients, and the relative frequency of infection due to specific pathogens has been shifting among gram-negative infections as well. *Escherichia coli* and *Klebsiella* spp. remain the most common isolates at many centers. The frequency of infections resulting from other organisms, however, such as *Enterobacter, Serratia,* and *Citrobacter,* has been increasing.[4,5,11] *Enterobacter* spp. have emerged as important causes of bacteremias; the use of broad spectrum antibiotics, particularly third-generation cephalosporins, is thought to have played a major role in this trend. Infections due to *Enterobacter, Serratia,* and *Citrobacter* may be difficult to treat because of the ease of β-lactamase induction and the more frequent development of resistance to multiple antibiotics.[4,5,12] Infections caused by *P. aeruginosa* have decreased in frequency during the past decade; however, morbidity and mortality associated with these infections remain very high.[3,8,11] In addition, the frequency of infection caused by difficult-to-treat organisms, such as *Stenotrophomonas maltophilia* and *Burkholderia cepacia,* appears to be increasing at many centers, probably because of selective pressures of broad-spectrum antimicrobial use.[4,5,8,11,12] Although the GI tract is a common site of bacterial infection, severe infections caused by anaerobic organisms are relatively infrequent.[16] Anaerobes are most frequently found in mixed infections, such as perirectal cellulitis and mucositis-associated oropharyngeal infections.[4]

In addition to bacterial infections, neutropenic cancer patients are at risk for invasive fungal infections. Patients with extended periods of profound neutropenia who have been receiving broad-spectrum antibiotics, corticosteroids, or both, are at the highest risk for invasive fungal infection. A large international autopsy study revealed that 12% to 25% of patients with hematologic malignancies had deep fungal infections that had not been diagnosed prior to the time of death. Approximately 65% of these infections were the result of *Candida* spp., and another 30% were caused by *Aspergillus* species.[17]

Candida albicans is the most common fungal pathogen in neutropenic cancer patients, accounting for approximately 50% of all fungal isolates. Because candidal species are normal flora, alteration of body host defenses is an important risk factor for the development of these infections. Oral thrush is the most common clinical manifestation of fungal infection, occurring in as much as 60% of all patients.[5] Mucous membranes damaged from chemotherapy and radiation serve as areas of candidal surface colonization and subsequent entry into the bloodstream; disease may then disseminate throughout the body. Organs, such as the liver, spleen, kidney, and lungs, are commonly involved in disseminated disease.[5,17,18] Hepatosplenic candidiasis, also known as chronic disseminated candidiasis, is an important infection in patients with hematologic malignancies.[19] *Candida* is isolated from the blood in less than 25% of these patients; therefore, histopathologic identification from biopsy specimens is often required.[3] Other species of *Candida,* such as *C. tropicalis, C. parapsilosis,* and *C. krusei,* are being isolated with increasing frequency. An increase has also been noted in infections caused by *Torulopsis glabrata, Trichosporon* spp., *Fusarium* spp., and *Curvularia*.[3,5,8]

Infections resulting from *Aspergillus* spp. are usually acquired via inhalation of airborne spores. After colonizing the lungs, *Aspergillus* invades the lung parenchyma and pulmonary vessels, resulting in hemorrhage, pulmonary infarcts, and a high mortality rate. Invasive pulmonary disease is the dominant manifestation of infection (80% to 90% of cases). However, *Aspergillus* spp. may also cause other infections in neutropenic patients including sinusitis, cutaneous infection, and disseminated disease involving multiple organs including the central nervous system.[20] Prolonged granulocytopenia is the primary risk factor for invasive pulmonary aspergillosis in neutropenic patients with acute leukemia; use of corticosteroids may also predispose patients to disease.[5,20] Invasive aspergillosis should be suspected in those neutropenic cancer patients colonized with *Aspergillus* who remain persistently febrile despite a week or more of broad-spectrum antibiotic therapy.[1,3,5,20]

Chemotherapy-induced mucous membrane damage may predispose neutropenic cancer patients to the reactivation of herpes simplex virus (HSV), manifesting as gingivostomatitis or recurrent genital infections. Untreated oropharyngeal HSV infections may spread to involve the esophagus and often coexist with candidal infections. Clinical disease resulting from HSV occurs most often in patients with serologic evidence (e.g., serum antibodies to HSV) of prior infection. Both HSV-seropositive BMT patients and HSV-seropositive leukemics receiving intensive chemotherapy are at high risk for recurrent HSV disease during periods of immunosuppression.[21–24]

Pneumocystis carinii and *Toxoplasma gondii* are the most common parasitic pathogens in immunocompromised cancer patients. Patients with hematologic malignancies (acute lymphocytic leukemia, lymphoma, Hodgkin's disease) and those receiving high-dose corticosteroids as part of chemotherapy regimens are at the greatest risk of infection.[5,22–24] Routine use of trimethoprim-sulfamethoxazole (TMP/SMX) prophylaxis has, however, substantially reduced the incidence of these infections.[22–24]

Because the majority of infecting organisms in cancer patients are from the host's own flora, some centers have employed routine surveillance cultures in an attempt to prospectively identify causes of fever and suspected infection. In a typical surveillance culture program, cultures of the nose, mouth, axillae, and perirectal area are performed twice weekly, and culture results are correlated with the clinical status of the patient. Because these cultures are costly and of low diagnostic yield, the utility of surveillance culture programs is felt to be limited. Surveillance cultures are, however, useful as research tools and in certain clinical situations; these situations include patients with prolonged profound neutropenia and in institutions with high rates of antimicrobial resistance or that have problems with virulent pathogens, such as *P. aeruginosa* or *Aspergillus flavus*. Surveillance cultures should be limited to the anterior nares for detecting colonization with methicillin-resistant *S. aureus* and *Aspergillus* and to the rectum for detecting *P. aeruginosa,* multiple-antibiotic-resistant gram-negative rods, *Candida,* or *Salmonella*.[1–4]

CLINICAL PRESENTATION

Because neutropenic cancer patients are at high risk for serious infections, frequent clinical assessments and physical examinations must be performed to search for possible signs of infection. The most important clinical finding in the neutropenic patient is the presence of fever. Fever in this setting is variously defined as a single oral temperature of ≥38.3°C (100.9°F), multiple oral temperatures of ≥38.0°C (100.4°F) persisting for over 1 hour, or three oral temperatures of >38.0°C (100.4°F) during a 24-hour period in the absence of other causes.[1–4] Because of the significant morbidity and mortality associated with infection in the neutropenic cancer patient, fever should be considered to be the result of infection until proven otherwise. The site of infection can be documented clinically or microbiologically in only 30% to 40% of febrile neutropenic cancer patients.[3,4,12] Other causes of fever unrelated to infection in this patient population include reactions to blood products, chemotherapeutic agents, and other drugs, including biologics, cell lysis, and the underlying malignancy itself.

At the appearance of fever, the patient should be carefully evaluated for other signs and symptoms of infection. Physical assessment should include examination of all common sites of infection including respiratory tract, urinary tract, gastrointestinal tract, mucous membranes, sinuses, and intravascular catheter insertion sites. The usual clinical signs and symptoms of infection may, however, be absent or altered in neutropenic patients because of their relative reduction in leukocytes and inability to mount an appropriate inflammatory response. For example, cough, sputum production and purulence, were less commonly found with pneumonia, and dysuria, frequency, urgency, and pyuria less commonly found with urinary tract infections in granulocytopenic patients.[25] Even patients with bacteremia commonly exhibit no signs of infection other than fever.[4,25] At the onset of fever, at least two sets of blood cultures should be obtained, including cultures both from peripheral veins and vascular access devices. These cultures should be evaluated for bacteria and fungi. Urine cultures should be obtained if a urinary catheter is in place or the urinalysis is abnormal. Other cultures (e.g., diarrheal stools, sputum) should be obtained as clinically indicated according to the presence of signs or symptoms. Because the lungs are a common site of systemic infection in this patient population, a chest radiograph should be performed at the onset of febrile episodes. Other laboratory tests should include serum chemistries, complete blood cell count, liver function tests, and any other tests as clinically indicated based on physical examination and other points of assessment.[1–4]

▶ TREATMENT: Infections in Neutropenic Cancer Patients

FEBRILE EPISODES IN NEUTROPENIC CANCER PATIENTS

The goals of antimicrobial drug use in neutropenic patients (including BMT recipients) include prevention of bacterial, fungal, viral, and protozoal infections during periods of neutropenia and effective treatment of established infections to reduce patient morbidity and mortality and allow for administration of optimal neoplastic therapy. All of these goals must be achieved at the lowest possible toxicity and cost. Guidelines for management of febrile episodes and documented infections in neutropenic patients are presented in Fig. 120–1[1] (from the Infectious Diseases Society of America [IDSA], revised in 1997). Although many controversies remain regarding optimal management of these patients, the IDSA guidelines remain the basis for antimicrobial management of febrile neutropenia.

Because fever in the neutropenic cancer patient is considered a result of infection until proven otherwise, high-dose, parenteral, broad-spectrum, bactericidal, empiric antibiotic therapy should be initiated at the onset of fever or at the first signs or symptoms of infection. Withholding antibiotic therapy until isolation of an organism results in unacceptably high mortality rates.[1] In immunocompromised patients, undiagnosed infection can rapidly disseminate and result in death if left untreated or if treated improperly. Failure to initiate appropriate antibiotic therapy for *P. aeruginosa* bacteremia at the onset of fever in granulocytopenic cancer patients resulted in mortality rates of 15% and 70% within 12 and 48 hours, respectively.[26] Empiric antibiotic therapy reduced early morbidity and mortality by at least 50% as compared to the pre-1970s.[11] Therapy must be appropriate, however, and promptly initiated.

The goal of empiric antibiotic therapy is to protect the neutropenic patient from early death caused by undiagnosed infection.

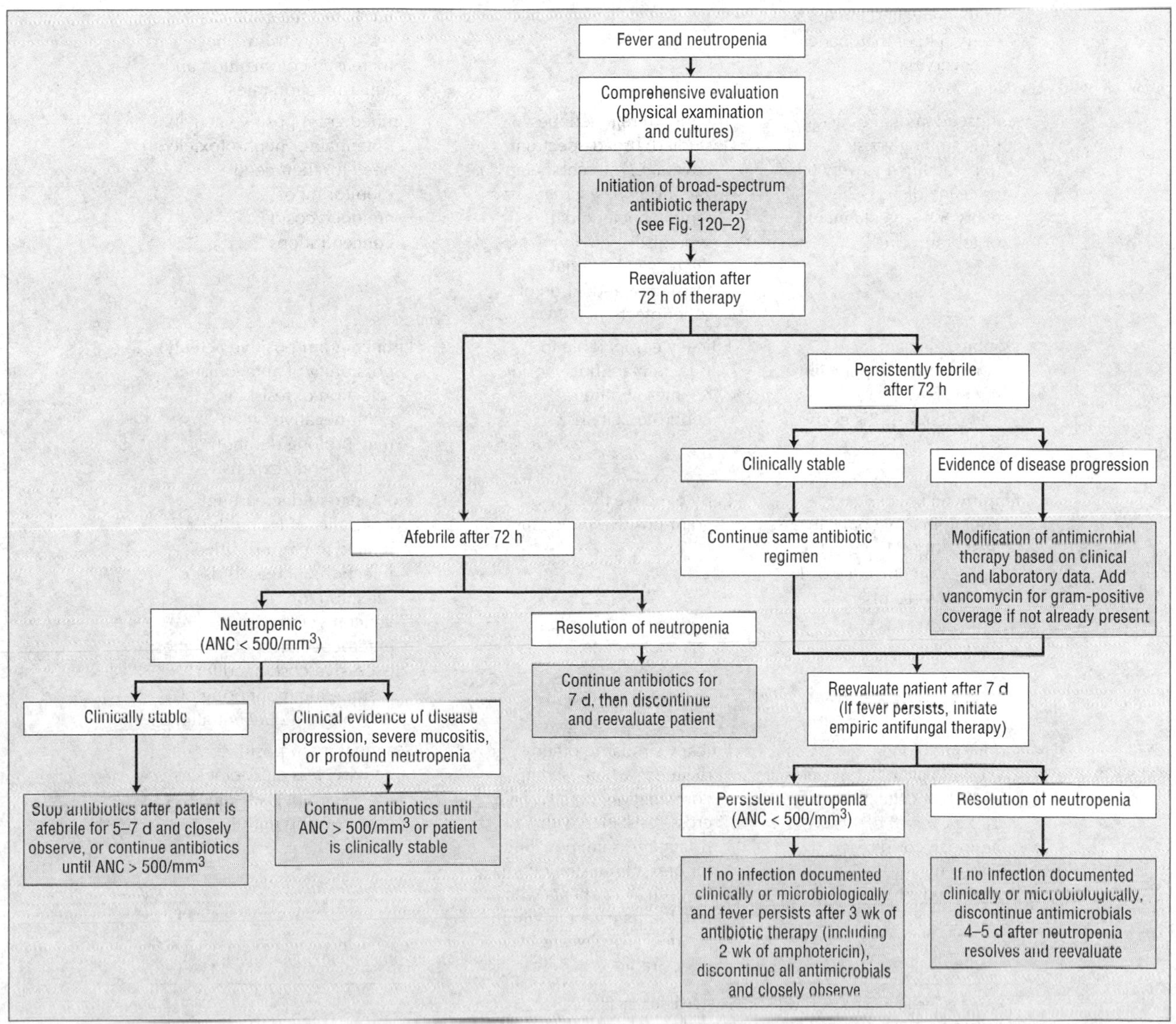

FIGURE 120–1. Management of febrile episodes in neutropenic cancer patients. ANC, absolute neutrophil count. *(Adapted from Ref. 1.)*

The optimal antibiotic regimen for empiric therapy in febrile neutropenic cancer patients remains controversial; however, because of their frequency and relative pathogenicity, *P. aeruginosa,* other gram-negative bacilli, and *S. aureus* remain the primary targets of empiric antimicrobial therapy. Although *P. aeruginosa* infections appear to have decreased in frequency relative to other bacterial organisms, adequate antipseudomonal antibiotic coverage must still be included in empiric regimens because of the high mortality associated with this pathogen.[1–4,12,27]

At least five different types of empiric antibiotic regimens are in use: (a) monotherapy with an antipseudomonal β-lactam, aztreonam, or carbapenem (imipenem/cilastatin, meropenem); (b) aminoglycoside plus an antipseudomonal penicillin (e.g., piperacillin), an antipseudomonal cephalosporin (ceftazidime, cefepime), or carbapenem; (c) double antipseudomonal β-lactam therapy; (d) addition of vancomycin to β-lactam regimens; and (e) fluoroquinolone (ciprofloxacin, levofloxacin) in combination with antipseudomonal β-lactam, aminoglycoside, or vancomycin.[1–4,12,27] Each of these regimens has advantages and disadvantages, which are summarized in Table 120–2. There is no overwhelming evidence that any one of these regimens is superior to the others. The overall response to empiric antibiotic regimens in febrile neutropenic cancer patients is about 75%

TABLE 120–2. Comparative Advantages and Disadvantages of Various Antibiotic Regimens for Empiric Therapy of Febrile Neutropenic Cancer Patients

Regimen	Potential Advantages	Potential Disadvantages
β-Lactam monotherapy (ceftazidime 1–2 g every 8 h, cefepime 1–2 g every 12 h, piperacillin/tazobactam 4.5 g every 6 h, imipenem/cilastatin 0.5 g every 6 h, or meropenem 1 g every 8 h)[a]	Efficacy apparently comparable to combination regimens; decreased drug toxicities; ease of administration; possibly less expensive	Possibly less efficacy in profound neutropenia or prolonged neutropenia; limited gram-positive activity; no potential for additive/synergistic effects; increased selection of resistant organisms; increased colonization and superinfection rates
Antipseudomonal β-lactam plus aminoglycoside (piperacillin 4 g every 6 h or ceftazidime 1–2 g every 8 h + gentamicin or tobramycin)[a,b]	Traditional regimen, best studied; broad-spectrum coverage; optimal therapy of *Pseudomonas aeruginosa;* rapidly bactericidal; synergistic activity; decreased bacterial resistance; reduction of superinfections	Limited gram-positive activity; potential for nephrotoxicity; need for therapeutic monitoring of aminoglycoside concentrations
Double β-lactam combination (piperacillin 4 g every 6 h + ceftazidime 1–2 g every 8 h)[a]	Efficacy comparable to β-lactam/aminoglycoside regimens without nephrotoxicity risk	Limited gram-positive activity; possibility of antagonism; selection of resistant gram-negative organisms; may prolong duration of neutropenia; expensive
Empiric regimens containing vancomycin (ceftazidime 1–2 g every 8 h + vancomycin 0.5–1 g every 6–12 h)[a]	Early effective therapy of gram-positive infections	No apparent decrease in morbidity or mortality related to gram-positive infection; increased risk of selection for vancomycin-resistant enterococci; risk of toxicities; excessive cost; need for therapeutic monitoring of vancomycin concentrations
Fluoroquinolones (ciprofloxacin 0.4 g every 8–12 h + ceftazidime 1–2 g every 8 h, aminoglycoside, or vancomycin 0.5–1 g every 6–12 h)[a]	Efficacy similar to other regimens when used in combination therapy; no cross-resistance with β-lactams; safe; possibility for oral administration; may be useful in patients with renal impairment in whom aminoglycosides are undesirable	Marginal gram-positive activity; less efficacious as monotherapy; resistance may develop rapidly

[a]Dosing guidelines in patients with normal renal function.

[b]Gentamicin or tobramycin 2 mg/kg loading dose, followed by maintenance dose determined by serum concentrations. Choice of specific agent determined according to institutional susceptibilities to individual drugs.

(Adapted from Refs. 1, 3, 4, 12, and 27.)

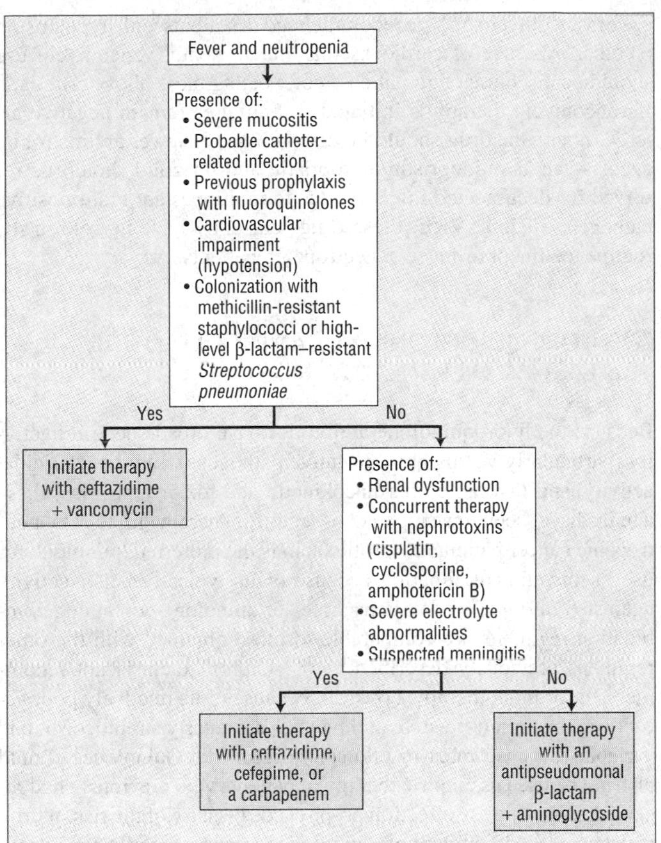
Fever and neutropenia
Presence of:
• Severe mucositis
• Probable catheter-related infection
• Previous prophylaxis with fluoroquinolones
• Cardiovascular impairment (hypotension)
• Colonization with methicillin-resistant staphylococci or high-level β-lactam–resistant Streptococcus pneumoniae
Yes
No
Initiate therapy with ceftazidime + vancomycin
Presence of:
• Renal dysfunction
• Concurrent therapy with nephrotoxins (cisplatin, cyclosporine, amphotericin B)
• Severe electrolyte abnormalities
• Suspected meningitis
Yes
No
Initiate therapy with ceftazidime, cefepime, or a carbapenem
Initiate therapy with an antipseudomonal β-lactam + aminoglycoside

FIGURE 120–2. Guide to selection of initial empiric antibiotic therapy in neutropenic cancer patients. *(Adapted from Ref. 1.)*

to 90%, regardless of whether or not a pathogen is isolated or which antimicrobial regimen is used.[12]

When designing optimal empiric antibiotic regimens, clinicians must consider infection patterns and antimicrobial susceptibility trends in their respective institutions. Also, patient factors, such as drug allergies and concomitant nephrotoxins, must be considered. Regardless of initial antibiotic selection, empiric regimens must be appropriately revised on the basis of documented infections, susceptibilities of bacterial isolates, development of more defined clinical signs and symptoms of infection, or a combination of these. The IDSA guidelines recommend three general empiric antibiotic regimens, selected as shown in Fig. 120–2. Other alternative regimens may also be appropriate, however, based on specific patient characteristics.

β-LACTAM MONOTHERAPY

Several β-lactam antibiotics have been evaluated as monotherapy for the management of febrile episodes in neutropenic cancer patients including antipseudomonal cephalosporins (cefoperazone, ceftazidime, cefepime), antipseudomonal penicillins (ticarcillin/clavulanic acid, piperacillin, piperacillin/tazobactam, mezlocillin), and carbapenems (imipenem/cilastatin, meropenem).[1–4] Although the ureidopenicillins (e.g., piperacillin, mezlocillin) have good activity against *E. coli, K. pneumoniae,* and *P. aeruginosa,* response rates in febrile neutropenic cancer patients have been only about 50%, much lower than the 75% to 90% response rates usually noted.[11] Regimens with ceftazidime, cefepime, and the carbapenems have been much more successful.[27–33] A more recent study demonstrated piperacillin/tazobactam monotherapy to be comparable to monotherapy with cefepime.[32] A landmark early study compared ceftazidime monotherapy with a three-drug combination (cephalothin, gentamicin, carbenicillin) in 550 episodes of fever and neutropenia.[28] Ceftazidime monotherapy was as effective as combination therapy in initial empiric management (first 72 hours); 78% of febrile patients with undocumented infections were managed successfully with one antibiotic, and no morbidity or mortality resulted from adding other antimicrobial agents only when clinically indicated. Ceftazidime monotherapy was more recently compared with the combination of piperacillin plus tobramycin in 876 febrile episodes.[12] Both regimens were similar in efficacy, even in patients with prolonged, profound neutropenia. Similar favorable results have been reported with cefepime and the carbapenems.[27,30,33–35]

The use of monotherapy has many potential advantages and disadvantages (Table 120–2). Perhaps the most common concerns are those regarding the selection of resistant strains of organisms, such as *P. aeruginosa, Enterobacter* spp., and *Serratia spp.,* through β-lactamase induction.[1,4,12,36] Activity against gram-positive organisms, such as coagulase-negative staphylococci, methicillin-resistant *S. aureus,* and enterococci, is poor with single β-lactams. Also, colonization and superinfection with both gram-positive and gram-negative organisms may occur more often with β-lactam monotherapy than when β-lactams are administered in combination with an aminoglycoside.[1]

Use of monotherapy may not be appropriate in institutions with high rates of gram-positive infections or infections caused by gram-negative pathogens such as *P. aeruginosa* and *Enterobacter* spp. Imipenem/cilastatin and meropenem, however, are less susceptible to inducible β-lactamases and may often be effectively used in these institutions. Monotherapy should usually be limited to patients with an ANC of 500–1,000/mm^3 or only for brief periods of more severe neutropenia;[1] however, patients with more severe, protracted neutropenia may also be successfully treated with monotherapy.[1,3,4,12,28]

AMINOGLYCOSIDE PLUS ANTIPSEUDOMONAL β-LACTAM

Regimens consisting of an aminoglycoside plus an antipseudomonal penicillin, antipseudomonal cephalosporin, or carbapenem have traditionally been the most commonly used for empiric treatment of febrile neutropenia, although many such regimens may have inadequate gram-positive activity (Table 120–2). This relative lack of activity remains a concern because of the increasing incidence of gram-positive infections. The choice of aminoglycoside and β-lactam for inclusion in empiric regimens should be based on institutional epidemiology and antimicrobial susceptibility patterns. If *P. aeruginosa* is a common institutional pathogen, use of empiric tobramycin or amikacin may be strongly considered because they are generally more active than gentamicin against this organism. However, gentamicin is still an appropriate choice in many institutions based on known susceptibility patterns in those locations. Piperacillin and ceftazidime are the best-studied β-lactams for *P. aeruginosa;* cefepime and piperacillin/tazobactam have also been recently studied.[37,38]

Combinations of broad-spectrum β-lactams and aminoglycosides often provide synergistic activity against bacteria commonly infecting neutropenic patients. The exact role of synergy in the outcome of febrile neutropenic patients treated with empiric antibiotic therapy, however, remains somewhat controversial, particularly in light of the efficacy of single drug regimens. Data from the European Organization for Research in the Treatment of Cancer (EORTC) demonstrate that response to combinations of β-lactam plus aminoglycoside is primarily related to the activity of the β-lactam agent; thus, the need for synergy with highly active agents, such as ceftazidime, is unclear.[4,12] Nevertheless, synergistic combinations of antibiotics appear to be beneficial in patients with persistent profound neutropenia.

Aminoglycoside toxicity may be a concern in patients receiving these regimens because they may already be receiving other nephrotoxic drugs, such as cisplatin and cyclosporine. Administration of aminoglycosides in large single daily doses (once-daily dosing) may be as effective, less costly, and no more toxic than conventional dosing methods.[39] A number of randomized, prospective trials involving approximately 800 patients have now been conducted to evaluate the efficacy of once-daily dosing in febrile neutropenia. A review of these studies failed to find significant differences in either efficacy or toxicity between once-daily dosing and traditional dosing of aminoglycosides.[40] Although once-daily dosing regimens appear to be safe and efficacious in these patients, there is not yet sufficient data to recommend once-daily dosing for routine use at this time.

DOUBLE β-LACTAM THERAPY

Double β-lactam therapy remains a controversial regimen for empiric management of febrile episodes in neutropenic patients. Several combinations of antipseudomonal β-lactams have been studied; all have included a penicillin (e.g., piperacillin) in combination with a cephalosporin (e.g., ceftazidime).[1] Combinations of broad-spectrum β-lactams are as effective as aminoglycoside/antipseudomonal β-lactam regimens.[1] Although double β-lactam combinations may be less toxic than aminoglycoside-containing regimens, these regimens are expensive and have relatively poor activity against gram-positive organisms. Also, theoretical concerns exist regarding possible antibiotic antagonism and the emergence of resistant organisms.[4,12,41] Double β-lactam regimens are not commonly used at most institutions.

EMPIRIC REGIMENS CONTAINING VANCOMYCIN

There has been considerable debate over the inclusion of vancomycin in initial empiric therapy of febrile neutropenia. This controversy continues because of the increasing incidence of gram-positive infections in these patients. One approach is to include vancomycin in the initial empiric antibiotic regimen, thereby providing early effective treatment of possible gram-positive infections. A second approach is to withhold vancomycin from initial empiric regimens, later adding the drug if gram-positive organisms are isolated from cultures or if there is no response to initial therapy. Support for both of these approaches can be found in the medical literature.[1–4,12] Several prospective studies, however, indicate that there is no advantage to adding vancomycin to initial empiric regimens routinely.[42,43] In addition to increased costs of therapy, there is overwhelming evidence that the selection of vancomycin-resistant enterococci (VRE) is associated with excessive vancomycin use.[44]

Vancomycin is recommended for inclusion in initial empiric regimens only in patients at high risk of gram-positive infection, particularly because of methicillin-resistant *S. aureus* and coagulase-negative staphylococci[1–4,12,27,43] including those with evidence of infection of central venous catheters and other indwelling lines, severe mucositis, or pneumonitis in hospitals with high rates of methicillin-resistant staphylococcal infections. Empiric vancomycin use may also be justified in institutions employing empiric antibiotic regimens without good activity against streptococci (e.g., ciprofloxacin) and in patients known to be colonized with methicillin-resistant staphylococci or *S. pneumoniae* with high-level resistance to β-lactams. Lastly, empiric use of vancomycin may be recommended in patients with hypotension or other evidence of cardiovascular impairment.[1] Vancomycin use should be discouraged in patients not meeting these above criteria.[44] If vancomycin therapy is initiated and cultures remain negative after 72 hours, the drug should be discontinued.[4] Newer antimicrobial agents such as quinupristin/dalfopristin and linezolid should be reserved for documented infection due to multiresistant gram-positive pathogens such as VRE; these drugs currently have no role in the routine treatment of fever in neutropenic patients.

FLUOROQUINOLONE PLUS AMINOGLYCOSIDE, β-LACTAM, OR VANCOMYCIN

Because the fluoroquinolone antibiotics have broad-spectrum activity (particularly versus gram-negative pathogens), rapid bactericidal activity, and favorable pharmacokinetic and toxicity profiles, these agents have been investigated as empiric therapy in febrile neutropenic cancer patients. Ciprofloxacin is the preferred quinolone for use in this clinical situation because of its typically better activity against *P. aeruginosa*. Response rates of quinolone-containing combination regimens are comparable to those obtained with the other regimens previously described.[1,4,27,45] Ciprofloxacin is not recommended for monotherapy, however, because of its relatively poor activity against gram-positive pathogens, particularly streptococci, and variable response rates in clinical studies.[1,4,27] Quinolones should also not be used as empiric therapy in patients who previously had received quinolones as infection prophylaxis because of the risk of drug resistance.[1,4] Although fluoroquinolones are not generally considered first-line empiric therapy, they may be useful as one component of combination regimens in patients with poor renal function.

ORAL ANTIBIOTIC THERAPY FOR INPATIENT AND OUTPATIENT MANAGEMENT OF FEBRILE NEUTROPENIA

Because of the excellent spectrum of activity and favorable pharmacokinetics of newer oral antibiotics, particularly the fluoroquinolones, conversion of IV therapy to oral therapy is possible and may allow for less expensive hospitalizations and earlier patient discharges. Carefully selected neutropenic patients may be safely switched from broad-spectrum parenteral therapy to oral antibiotics (usually ciprofloxacin) with response rates comparable to patients remaining on IV therapy.[46–49] Patient selection criteria often included defervescence within 72 hours after initiation of parenteral therapy, hemodynamic stability, absence of positive cultures or discernible site of infection, and ability to take oral medications. Many of these patients were able to complete their course of therapy at home.[1,46–49] Oral ofloxacin has also been studied as initial therapy of febrile neutropenic episodes; there was no difference in efficacy compared to patients receiving initial therapy with parenteral β-lactam/aminoglycoside regimens.[46–49] Changing parenteral antimicrobials to oral regimens in carefully selected patients is now relatively common in practice.

The availability of oral antibiotics with broad spectra of activity has even made possible the treatment of febrile neutropenia completely in the outpatient setting. Patients undergoing chemotherapy with an expected duration of neutropenia of less than 7 days, or those patients with prolonged neutropenia who are without fever and who are clinically stable, may safely self-administer antibiotics at home on first becoming febrile, without examination by a physician or laboratory evaluation.[46–49] Fluoroquinolones, either as monotherapy or in combination with clindamycin or amoxicillin/clavulanate for enhanced gram-positive coverage, have been most commonly studied. Oral cephalosporins, such as cefixime, may also be suitable for outpatient treatment.[1] Careful patient selection is obviously required for such management strategies; important patient characteristics include a history of medication compliance, good caregiver support, and close proximity to medical care in the event of failure to respond to home therapy. Outpatient therapy of low-risk patients is now in widespread practice in many institutions.

ANTIMICROBIAL THERAPY AFTER INITIATION OF EMPIRIC THERAPY

After the administration of 72 hours of empiric antimicrobial therapy, the clinical status and culture results of febrile neutropenic patients should be reevaluated to determine whether or not therapeutic modifications are necessary. Additions or modifications to the initial antimicrobial regimen will likely be required in patients with ANC $<500/mm^3$ for greater than a week. Modifications of antimicrobial therapy should be based on clinical and laboratory data; antibiotic therapy should be optimized based on culture results. During periods of neutropenia, however, patients should generally continue to receive broad-spectrum therapy because of the risk of secondary infections or breakthrough bacteremias when antimicrobial coverage is too narrow.[1–4,12,27]

The most appropriate management of patients who remain febrile in the absence of microbiologic or clinical documentation of infection is still highly controversial. It important to note that the persistence of fever does not necessarily mean failure of a given antimicrobial regimen. This is particularly true if patients are otherwise clinically stable. Even patients with documented infection who are receiving appropriate antimicrobial therapy (based on in vitro susceptibility tests) will often remain febrile until resolution of neutropenia occurs. Persistently febrile patients should be carefully evaluated and modifications to existing antimicrobial not generally made within the first 4 to 7 days of therapy unless evidence of clinical deterioration is present (Fig. 120–1).[1,43]

INITIATION OF ANTIFUNGAL THERAPY

A high percentage of febrile patients who die during prolonged neutropenia have evidence of invasive fungal infection on autopsy, even though many had no evidence of fungal disease before death.[17] Persistence of fever or development of a new fever during broad-spectrum antibiotic therapy may indicate the presence of fungal infection in approximately 33% of patients.[50] The lack of rapid, sensitive diagnostic tests for fungi and the high morbidity and mortality associated with waiting for isolation of fungal organisms justify the empiric addition of antifungal therapy in this clinical setting.[50] Therefore, empiric antifungal therapy should be initiated after 4 to 5 days of broad-spectrum antibiotic therapy to prevent fungal superinfection or treat undiagnosed fungal infection.

The optimal empiric antifungal regimen is not presently known. Amphotericin B or fluconazole are, however, the antifungals most commonly used. *Aspergillus* is particularly common in patients with hematologic malignancies and BMT patients; therefore, amphotericin B is usually preferred in these patients.[4,17] Concerns regarding the emergence of azole-resistant fungi have also prevented fluconazole and itraconazole from replacing amphotericin B as the gold standard in persistently febrile neutropenic patients in spite of the high rate of amphotericin B toxicities.[4,17] Lipid-associated amphotericin B products in the setting of febrile neutropenia have efficacy that is similar to conventional amphotericin B, while causing substantially reduced toxicities.[51,52] Although lipid-associated amphotericin B products are promising because of the potential for reduced toxicities, the relative lack of experience with these products and significantly higher cost in comparison to conventional amphotericin B makes their role in the empiric therapy of febrile neutropenia uncertain at this time.[4]

Antifungal therapy should be continued for at least 2 weeks in the absence of signs and symptoms of active fungal disease, but many clinicians continue empiric antifungal therapy until resolution of granulocytopenia. In addition to fungal infections, other causes of persistent fever of unknown origin include resistant bacterial infection, tissue necrosis as a result of underlying tumor, nonbacterial and nonfungal infection (e.g., viral, mycobacterial, parasitic), and drug or blood product administration.

INITIATION OF ANTIVIRAL THERAPY

Febrile neutropenic patients with vesicular or ulcerative skin or mucosal lesions should be carefully evaluated for infection resulting from herpes simplex or varicella-zoster virus (VZV). If viral infection is presumed or documented, these patients should receive aggressive acyclovir therapy to aid healing of primary lesions and prevent disseminated disease. Routine use of antiviral agents in the management of patients without mucosal lesions or other evidence of viral infection is not generally recommended.[1,4]

MANAGEMENT OF CATHETER INFECTIONS

Cancer patients are at high risk for development of catheter-related infections (incidence of 9% to 80%, depending on the series), most often because of *S. aureus* or coagulase-negative staphylococci.[1,2] The diagnosis of catheter-related bacteremia is made when blood cultures from both peripheral blood and the catheter itself are positive. Three types of infections have been identified: exit-site infection, subcutaneous tunnel infection, and catheter-related bacteremia/fungemia.[50] Indwelling catheters are invaluable for providing continued vascular access in these patients; attempts at controlling infections with antimicrobial therapy should be made in most cases prior to removing the catheter. Indications for catheter removal include subcutaneous tunnel infection, failure of bacteremia to clear within 72 hours after initiation of antibiotic therapy, persistence of fever, septic emboli, hypotension associated with catheter use, a nonpatent catheter, or bacteremia caused by *Bacillus* spp., *Corynebacterium jeikeium, P. aeruginosa,* and fungus (*Candida* spp.).[1,53] Removal of catheters in patients with fungemia may be adequate to achieve resolution of fungal infection; however, 10 to 14 days of antifungal therapy with amphotericin B or fluconazole may avoid development of fungal abscesses or disseminated disease. When multilumen catheters are involved, administration of antimicrobial agents should be rotated among the ports to ensure eradication of the infecting organism from all catheter sites.

DURATION OF THERAPY

The optimal duration of antimicrobial therapy in the neutropenic cancer patient remains controversial. Decisions regarding discontinuation of empiric antimicrobial therapy often are more difficult and complex than those regarding initiation of therapy (Fig. 120–1). One point on which most authorities agree, however, is that the most important determinant of the total duration of antibiotic therapy is the patient's ANC.[1–4] If the ANC is $\geq$500/mm^3, if the patient is afebrile for 48 to 72 hours and clinically stable, and if no pathogen has been isolated, then antibiotics may be discontinued after 7 days of therapy. Patients with ANCs of <500/mm^3 should be maintained on antibiotics until resolution of neutropenia, even if afebrile.[1] Prolonged antibiotic use has been associated with superinfections resulting from resistant bacteria and fungi, and increases the risk of antibiotic-related toxicities.[4] If patients are clinically stable but the ANC is still <500/mm^3, antibiotics may be discontinued after a total of 5 to 7 afebrile days. Patients, however, who remain profoundly neutropenic (ANC of <100/mm^3), have mucosal lesions, or have unstable vital signs should continue to receive antibiotics until the ANC has increased to $\geq$500/mm^3 or the patient is clinically stable. Patients who are persistently neutropenic and febrile, but who are clinically stable with negative blood cultures, may often be successfully discontinued from antimicrobial therapy. These patients, however, must be carefully monitored as reinstitution of antibiotics is necessary in approximately 50% of cases.[1–4] Patients with documented infections should receive antimicrobial therapy until the infecting organism is eradicated and signs and symptoms of infection have resolved (at least 10 to 14 days of therapy).

COLONY-STIMULATING FACTORS

Because resolution of granulocytopenia is the most important determinant of patient outcome from both febrile episodes and documented infections, many studies have evaluated hematopoietic colony-stimulating factors (CSFs) (sargramostim, granulocyte-macrophage colony-stimulating factor [GM-CSF], filgrastim, granulocyte colony-stimulating factor [G-CSF], and macrophage colony-stimulating factor [M-CSF]) as adjunct therapy to antimicrobial treatment of febrile neutropenic cancer patients.[54–56] These studies consistently found that the use of CSFs reduces the total duration and severity of chemotherapy-related neutropenia. Compared to placebo, however, these studies failed to demonstrate consistent benefits of CSFs related to important outcome variables, such as total febrile days, days of hospitalization, infectious complications, or mortality.[54–56] An expert panel of the American Society of Clinical Oncology (ASCO) has concluded that there is no clear support for the routine use of CSFs in febrile neutropenic patients.[54] The ASCO panel further concluded that the use of CSFs may be useful in patients with pneumonia, fungal sepsis, multiorgan dysfunction, hypotension, or other factors likely to cause rapid clinical deterioration. It was clearly stated, however, that even under these severe circumstances the benefits of CSF therapy were not substantiated. Although CSFs are not recommended for routine therapy of febrile neutropenia, clinical judgment may be exercised in determining which patients may likely benefit from judicious use of these expensive agents.

The direct transfusion of neutrophils has also been studied for the treatment of febrile neutropenia or other opportunistic infections. The overall efficacy of neutrophil transfusions has been quite variable with response rates ranging from 29% to 83% in neutropenic patients. The routine use of neutrophil transfusions is thus considered experimental and is not recommended for routine treatment of febrile neutropenic patients.[57]

PROPHYLAXIS

INFECTIONS IN NEUTROPENIC CANCER PATIENTS

Efforts are routinely made to prevent infectious complications in neutropenic patients through a number of environmental modifications and prophylactic antimicrobial regimens. The goal of antimicrobial prophylaxis in cancer patients is to decrease the number and severity of systemic infections during prolonged periods of neutropenia.

General Measures

Because approximately 50% of pathogens infecting neutropenic cancer patients are acquired in the hospital,[8] reducing acquisition of infectious organisms from the environment is a basic component in controlling nosocomial infection rates. Neutropenic patients should be placed in reverse isolation (isolation to protect patients from contracting infections after exposure to others) with strict adherence to infection control guidelines by hospital personnel. Proper, meticulous hand washing by hospital personnel is a simple, yet very effective infection control measure. Fresh fruits and vegetables are frequently colonized with bacteria and fungi; therefore, most centers exclude these foods from the diets of neutropenic patients.[8,24,43]

To reduce the risk of infection caused by airborne pathogens, such as *Aspergillus* spp., laminar air flow rooms are in use at some cancer centers. Laminar air flow rooms work by directing filtered air away from the patient, thus minimizing the risk of infection from airborne or environmental pathogens. When laminar air flow rooms are combined with dietary restrictions, infection control practices, and nonabsorbable antibiotics, rates of infection in neutropenic cancer patients are reduced by at least 50%.[24,43] Laminar air flow rooms are expensive, however, and use of these protective environments does not improve overall survival in BMT recipients.[8,24,43]

Bacterial Infections

Early attempts at pharmacologic reduction of flora colonizing the GI tract used combinations of nonabsorbable antibiotics, including gentamicin, nystatin, vancomycin, polymyxin B, and colistin. If anaerobic flora are preserved within the GI tract, risk of infection and subsequent bacteremia from virulent gram-negative bacilli is decreased; this is referred to as *colonization resistance*. These combinations of nonabsorbable antibiotics, however, destroy resident anaerobic flora as well as aerobic gram-negative rods. Therefore, colonization resistance is not preserved, and patients may be at risk for gram-negative infections because of translocation of virulent pathogens, such as *P. aeruginosa,* into the bloodstream.

Although clinical trials have demonstrated that oral nonabsorbable antibiotics successfully reduce infections, these regimens are not routinely recommended for infection prophylaxis[8,43] because of several problems associated with these regimens, including unpalatability, high cost, and frequent adverse effects (e.g., nausea, vomiting, diarrhea). Poor compliance inherent with these regimens may lead to abrupt discontinuation of antibiotics, which, in turn, may enable rapid repopulation of the GI tract with more virulent organisms and subsequent infection. Use of nonabsorbable antibiotic regimens has also been associated with the development of resistance to aminoglycosides among gram-negative bacilli, making the aminoglycosides useless as treatment alternatives for the ensuing infections.[8,43]

Recognition of the value of preservation of colonization resistance has prompted numerous studies of orally administered absorbable antibiotics, particularly TMP/SMX and the fluoroquinolones. Unlike nonabsorbable regimens, these antibiotics theoretically provide protection against systemic infections in addition to preserving colonization resistance and being well tolerated. Data from most placebo-controlled studies indicate that TMP/SMX significantly reduces infection rates in cancer patients.[1] Although TMP/SMX is also effective as prophylaxis against *P. carinii,* its lack of activity against *P. aeruginosa* is worrisome, particularly in institutions in which pseudomonal infections are frequent. Other concerns with TMP/SMX prophylaxis include selection of resistant organisms, predisposition to development of fungal infections, and delay in bone marrow recovery resulting in prolonged neutropenic episodes.[8]

Numerous studies show that oral fluoroquinolones are more effective than placebo, nonabsorbable antibiotics, and TMP/SMX in preventing gram-negative infections in neutropenic cancer patients.[8,43,58] There are, however, several limitations to their injudicious use. In particular, quinolone prophylaxis has clearly led to an increase in the frequency of gram-positive infections. As a result, combination of a quinolone with a second agent providing enhanced gram-positive activity (e.g., Rifampin, penicillin, or a macrolide) may be required for effective prophylaxis.[43,59–61] Fluoroquinolone prophylaxis has been associated with the development of resistant gram-negative organisms.[8,43,58] In addition, fluoroquinolone prophylaxis has apparently not changed infectious mortality among cancer patients in spite of efficacy in preventing gram-negative infections. Patients experiencing breakthrough infection during fluoroquinolone prophylaxis should not be subsequently placed on a fluoroquinolone for empiric therapy, thus removing a valuable class of drugs from the available list of alternatives. The use of fluoroquinolones for prophylaxis of bacterial infections is generally discouraged, although the exact role of these drugs in this indication remains controversial even after extensive study.[43,58]

The use of antibacterial prophylaxis remains somewhat controversial because of poor patient tolerance, lack of consistent efficacy, potential for development of resistant bacteria, high cost, and lack of impact on patient survival.[1,4] Prophylaxis, however, is generally indicated for patients expected to be profoundly neutropenic for greater than 1 week, such as BMT patients. Additional risk factors that may provide justification for prophylaxis include extensive mucous membrane or skin lesions, presence of indwelling catheters, need for instrumentation, or severe periodontal disease.[1] Granulocyte recovery eliminates the need for continued prophylaxis, and recovery may be facilitated via use of CSFs.[54–56] In contrast to their unclear role in the treatment of febrile neutropenia, CSFs have been formally recommended by the ASCO for prevention of febrile neutropenia in high-risk patients. Such patients include those receiving chemotherapy regimens that produce a high rate of febrile neutropenia (>40% incidence) or those with active tissue infection at the time of chemotherapy, history of febrile neutropenia with previous courses of chemotherapy, or underlying bone marrow compromise.[54]

Fungal Infections

Because most neutropenic patients are at risk for mucocutaneous candidal infections that may disseminate and cause serious systemic illness, antifungal prophylaxis is administered during high-risk periods. Antifungal agents administered for both local effects (nystatin suspension, clotrimazole troches) and systemic activity (ketoconazole, fluconazole, itraconazole) have been employed to prevent fungal infections. Although the choice of antifungal prophylaxis agents remains controversial, azole compounds (clotrimazole, ketoconazole, fluconazole, itraconazole) appear to be more effective and better tolerated than nystatin suspension.[43,62–64] Fluconazole prophylaxis (400 mg/day) has been particularly well studied and reduces the incidence of both superficial and systemic fungal infections, as well as significantly decreases the mortality from fungal infections in BMT recipients.[64,65] The use of fluconazole prophylaxis has resulted in emergence of infections caused by *C. krusei* and *T. glabrata,* pathogens that are frequently resistant to fluconazole and other azole-type antifungal agents.[64,65] Routine fluconazole prophylaxis (400 mg/day) should, therefore, be limited to patients undergoing BMT.[64] Prophylaxis against fungal infection is beneficial in leukemic patients, although the choice of either fluconazole, itraconazole, or amphotericin B should be determined by the types of fungal isolates at individual institutions.[64]

Strategies being investigated for *Aspergillus* prophylaxis in neutropenic patients include the oral azole itraconazole, reduced doses of amphotericin B, and intranasal/aerosolized amphotericin B.[66] None of these interventions can be routinely recommended in clinical practice at this time.

Other Infections

The use of TMP/SMX in cancer patients at risk for *P. carinii* pneumonia has substantially reduced the incidence of this infection.[8] Acyclovir prophylaxis is employed in most centers to reduce risk of HSV reactivation in patients with acute leukemia undergoing intensive chemotherapy. Varicella vaccine provides good protection (90%) in leukemic children and may also be useful in seronegative adults, although the vaccine has been less well studied in this population.

EVALUATION OF THERAPEUTIC OUTCOMES

Close monitoring of febrile neutropenic patients, including both clinical and laboratory data, is essential for early detection and treatment of infectious complications. In addition, because many of the drugs that may be used in this setting have significant toxicity potential (aminoglycosides, amphotericin B), careful attention must be paid to the prevention and management of drug-related adverse effects. The reader is referred to individual chapters within this book for more detailed discussions of monitoring parameters related to specific types of infections (e.g., pneumonia, urinary tract infections).

INFECTIONS IN BONE MARROW TRANSPLANT PATIENTS

Along with graft-versus-host disease (GVHD), infection remains a major barrier to successful bone marrow transplantation. Recipients of BMT share risk factors discussed previously with other cancer patients. These patients, however, are at enhanced risk of infection because of prolonged periods of neutropenia. In addition, patients receiving allogeneic transplants have added immune system insults imposed by often prolonged immunosuppressive drug therapy for the prevention and treatment of GVHD. Pretransplant conditioning regimens

TABLE 120–3. Infectious Complications after Bone Marrow and Solid Organ Transplantation: Syndromes of Disease and Treatment Guidelines

Pathogen	Syndromes of Disease	Treatment
Bacterial		
Gram-negative aerobic bacilli (Enterobacteriaceae, *Pseudomonas aeruginosa, Haemophilus influenzae*)	Blood, urinary tract, pulmonary, abdomen	*Empiric:* Ceftazidime 1–2 g every 8 h + Aminoglycoside;[a,b] cefepime 1–2 g every 12 h + aminoglycoside;[a,b] piperacillin 3–4 g every 6 h + aminoglycoside[a,b] *Definitive:* According to culture and sensitivity results
Gram-positive cocci (*Staphylococcus aureus, S. epidermidis, Streptococcus pneumoniae, Enterococcus fecaelis*)	Skin, blood, urinary tract, pulmonary, abdomen	*Empiric:* Nafcillin 1–2 g every 4–6 h; vancomycin 0.5–1 g every 6–12 h *Definitive:* According to culture and sensitivity results
Legionella spp.	Pulmonary	Erythromycin 0.5–1 g every 6 h
Listeria monocytogenes	Central nervous system	Ampicillin 1–2 g every 4–6 h with gentamicin;[a] TMP/SMX 4 mg/kg every 12 h[b]
Nocardia spp.	Skin, pulmonary, central nervous system	Sulfadiazine 1 g every 4–6 h; TMP/SMX 4 mg/kg every 12 h[b]
Fungal		
Candida spp.	Blood, urinary tract, mucous membranes, skin	Clotrimazole 10 mg five times daily; nystatin 100,000 U every 6 h; ketoconazole 200 mg daily; fluconazole 100–400 mg daily; itraconazole 200–400 mg daily; amphotericin B 0.5–0.7 mg/kg/day ± 5-flucytosine 100–150 mg/kg/day divided every 6 h
Aspergillus spp.	Skin, pulmonary, central nervous system	Amphotericin B 1 mg/kg/day ± 5-flucytosine; itraconazole 200–400 mg daily; lipid-associated amphotericin B 4–5 mg/kg daily;[e] caspofungin 50 mg daily[e]
Cryptococcus neoformans	Skin, pulmonary, central nervous system	Amphotericin B 0.5 mg/kg/day ± 5-flucytosine; fluconazole 400 mg daily
Zygomycetes (Mucor)	Rhinocerebral disease	Amphotericin B 1 mg/kg/day; lipid-associated amphotericin B 4–5 mg/kg daily[e]
Viral		
Herpes simplex virus	Skin, central nervous system, mucous membranes, pulmonary	Acyclovir 5–10 mg/kg every 8 h; foscarnet 40 mg/kg every 8 h
Cytomegalovirus	Pulmonary, blood, urinary tract, GI tract	Ganciclovir 5 mg/kg every 12 h; foscarnet 60 mg/kg every 8 h; hyperimmune globulins 100–500 mg/kg every 1–2 wk
Varicella-zoster virus	Skin, disseminated disease	Acyclovir 10 mg/kg every 8 h; foscarnet 40 mg/kg every 8 h
Epstein-Barr virus	Lymphoproliferative disease	No effective treatment
Papovaviruses (BK, JC)	Skin, central nervous system	No effective treatment
Protozoal/parasitic		
Pneumocystis carinii	Pulmonary	TMP/SMX 15–20 mg/kg/day divided every 6 h;[c] atovaquone 750 mg every 12 h; pentamidine 4 mg/kg daily; dapsone 100 mg daily + TMP 15–20 mg/kg/d divided every 6 h; clindamycin 450–600 mg every 6 h + primaquine 15 mg daily
Toxoplasma gondii	Central nervous system	Pyrimethamine 50–100 mg daily + sulfadiazine 1 g every 4–6 h;[d] pyrimethamine 50–100 mg daily + clindamycin 450–600 mg every 6 h[d]
Strongyloides stercoralis	Pulmonary, central nervous system	Thiabendazole 25 mg/kg every 12 h (max 3g/day)

[a]Gentamicin or tobramycin 2 mg/kg loading dose, followed by maintenance dose determined by serum concentrations. Choice of specific agent determined according to institutional susceptibilities to individual drugs.
[b]For penicillin-allergic adults, use ciprofloxacin 0.4 g every 8–12 h plus an aminoglycoside.
[c]Based on the trimethoprim component of the combination.
[d]Folinic acid (5–10 mg/day) often recommended in conjunction with pyrimethamine-containing regimens for prevention of bone marrow toxicity.
[e]For use in cases refractory to amphotericin B or itraconazole.
TMP/SMX = trimethoprim/sulfamethoxazole

(high-dose chemotherapy and total body irradiation), as well as GVHD itself, often disrupt protective barriers, such as mucous membranes, skin, and the GI tract, placing patients at further risk of infection. Patients experiencing marrow graft failure have extended periods of profound neutropenia, often resulting in death due to infectious causes. The Food and Drug Administration (FDA) approved sargramostim (GM-CSF) for marrow graft failure in both autologous and allogeneic transplants.

ETIOLOGY AND CLINICAL PRESENTATION OF INFECTIONS

After the administration of intensive conditioning regimens to eliminate malignant cells and prevent rejection of donor marrow, patients may remain profoundly neutropenic for 3 to 4 weeks. During this period, they are at risk for the same types of infectious complications noted in other granulocytopenic cancer patients (e.g., bacterial and fungal infections) and should be managed accordingly (Table 120–1). Table 120–3 lists regimens for the treatment of specific infections.

Fungal infections, especially those caused by *Candida* and *Aspergillus* species, are serious and often fatal complications associated with BMT. Fungi remain a serious cause of infection, particularly in allogeneic BMT recipients, for up to 1 to 2 years following transplantation and may occur in as many as 10% of patients.[24,67] Mortality rates associated with invasive aspergillosis infections may be as high as 90%.[67,68]

In addition to bacterial and fungal infections, BMT recipients also are at risk for serious HSV infections manifesting as severe gingivostomatitis, esophagitis, genital lesions, and, rarely, pneumonia during the first month posttransplant. Clinical disease is more common in patients with serologic evidence (e.g., serum antibodies) of prior exposure and latent HSV infection pretransplant. Therefore, reactivation of latent disease during periods of immunosuppression is the most common etiology of HSV infection. Without prophylaxis, as many as 80% of HSV-seropositive patients experience mucocutaneous disease after intensive chemotherapy, as compared to fewer than 25% of seronegative patients.[22,53] The HSV infections often coexist with candidal infection and mucositis secondary to chemotherapy, radiation, or both.[23] Acyclovir-resistant HSV infections also occur following BMT but are not common.[24] Painful swallowing associated with these conditions makes it difficult for patients to take oral medications and maintain adequate nutritional intake. Because of the considerable morbidity associated with reactivation of HSV posttransplant, the HSV serologic status of patients should be determined prior to transplant.

Recipients of BMT remain at high risk for infection after bone marrow engraftment has occurred. Significant defects in neutrophil function and cell-mediated and humoral immunity, persisting for several months posttransplant, predispose patients to infectious complications. Acute and chronic GVHD result in prolonged periods of immunosuppression and increased infection rates.

Bone marrow transplant patients are at high risk for cytomegalovirus (CMV) infections during the early postengraftment period. These range in severity from asymptomatic viral shedding (urine, throat, lungs) to life-threatening disseminated disease and interstitial pneumonia.[23,24]

As with HSV, patients seropositive for CMV pretransplant are at high risk for recurrent disease during periods of immunosuppression; about 70% of seropositive patients develop recurrent CMV disease after transplantation.[22–24,53,69] Other risk factors for CMV disease in BMT patients include advanced age, human lymphocyte antigen (HLA) mismatch, total body irradiation, multiagent conditioning regimens, and presence of GVHD.[53] Patients without evidence of latent CMV infection (CMV seronegative) pretransplant may develop primary CMV disease after receiving bone marrow or blood products from CMV-seropositive donors. Onset of both primary and recurrent CMV infection is 1 to 2 months posttransplant; patients receiving allogeneic transplants are at highest risk for CMV disease.[22–24,53]

The most serious clinical manifestation of CMV disease and the leading cause of infectious death in BMT recipients is interstitial pneumonia (IP), which is associated with an 85% mortality rate if untreated.[22,24,53] This clinical syndrome manifests as fever, dyspnea, hypoxia, nonproductive cough, and diffuse pulmonary infiltrates. As many as 40% of allogeneic BMT patients will develop IP of; these patients with IP, up to 40% of cases are the result of CMV.[22,53] Interstitial pneumonia also may be caused by other infectious (*P. carinii*, varicella-zoster virus) and noninfectious causes (pulmonary damage by radiation and chemotherapy).[24]

During the late transplant period (beginning about 4 months posttransplant), infections remain a major problem in patients suffering from chronic GVHD. Additional immunosuppressive therapy for treatment of GVHD places these patients at added risk for infection. Infections common during the late transplant period include those caused by encapsulated organisms, such as *S. pneumoniae* and *H. influenzae;* infections resulting from staphylococci and gram-negative bacilli are less common.[22,53] Patients not suffering from chronic GVHD generally have few infections in this period.

Up to 50% of all patients surviving up to 10 months posttransplant develop an infection caused by VZV. Infection with VZV is most common in patients receiving allogeneic transplants with acute or chronic GVHD.[22–24] Both primary (varicella) or recurrent disease (herpes zoster) usually present as skin lesions, most of which remain contained to local areas; however, 30% to 45% of these infections may disseminate to other cutaneous areas or body organs, causing mortality as high as 50%.[22–24,53]

▶ PROPHYLAXIS AND MANAGEMENT: Infection in Bone Marrow Transplant Recipients

The goals of antimicrobial drug use in BMT patients include (a) prevention of bacterial, fungal, viral, and protozoal infections during periods of neutropenia and postengraftment and (b) effective treatment of established infections. The overall goal of prophylaxis and treatment of infection in BMT patients is the prevention of infectious morbidity and mortality. These goals must be achieved at the lowest possible toxicity and cost. Prophylactic therapy should be specifically aimed at pathogens known to cause a high incidence of infection within the BMT population, the specific institution, or both. In addition, prophylactic therapy should be limited to those regimens proven to be effective through well-designed clinical trials.

BACTERIAL INFECTIONS

Prophylaxis of infections in BMT patients is in many ways similar to that used in other neutropenic patients. Selective decontamination with oral antimicrobials is commonly used; considerations are the same as those previously discussed. Fluoroquinolones have become the most frequently used agents, often combined with another agent (e.g., macrolides, rifampin) for enhanced gram-positive activity.[22,59,60] These regimens are usually begun within 72 hours of beginning the chemotherapy conditioning regimens and continued throughout the neutropenic period. Patients who become febrile while receiving prophylaxis should be managed according to general guidelines for febrile neutropenic patients.

Because of the high incidence of gram-positive infections following transplantation, some centers employ prophylactic parenteral vancomycin. Studies of this practice have produced conflicting data. Vancomycin prophylaxis appears to decrease the overall incidence of gram-positive bacterial infections, number of days of empiric antimicrobial therapy, and cost of therapy.[24] However, important mortality benefits were not consistently demonstrated, and there are significant concerns regarding the selection of vancomycin-resistant enterococci. Prophylactic vancomycin use is thus not generally recommended except in institutions with high rates of infection with methicillin-resistant staphylococci among BMT recipients.[22,24] There is currently no role for linezolid or quinupristin/dalfopristin except in documented infections caused by VRE.

VIRAL INFECTIONS

Prophylaxis of recurrent HSV infection was evaluated in a number of clinical studies using various dosage regimens of acyclovir.[24] Depending on the series, 0% to 10% of HSV-seropositive patients receiving acyclovir experienced viral shedding, clinical symptoms of viral reactivation, or both, as compared to 60% to 80% of patients receiving placebo. Acyclovir doses commonly used for prophylaxis are 250 mg/m^2 (5 mg/kg) IV every 8 hours or 200–400 mg orally four to five times daily.[22,24] Intravenous therapy will eventually be necessary in most patients because of the development of severe mucositis from conditioning regimens. Oral acyclovir, however, is effective and considerably less expensive in those patients who can take oral medications. Although the duration of antiviral prophylaxis differs between centers, acyclovir is usually begun at the time of the conditioning regimen and continued for about 6 weeks or until resolution of neutropenia. Besides preventing recurrence of HSV disease, acyclovir prophylaxis also may reduce the incidence of CMV reactivation.[70] High-dose oral acyclovir given for 6 months posttransplant also significantly reduces reactivation of VZV infections; however, routine use of long-term acyclovir is controversial and not generally used specifically for this indication.[24,53] Patients developing active HSV or VZV infection should be treated with high-dose acyclovir (10 mg/kg IV every 8 hours).

Acyclovir-resistant HSV has occasionally been reported in BMT patients receiving acyclovir prophylaxis. Foscarnet is the drug of choice for treatment of acyclovir-resistant HSV. Foscarnet, however, has not been well studied for HSV prophylaxis.[22,24]

Prevention of CMV disease has been extensively studied in BMT patients because of the great potential for morbidity and mortality. If possible, CMV-seronegative patients should receive donor marrow and supportive blood products from seronegative donors only; however, CMV-seropositive patients are not at additional risk by receiving blood or marrow from seropositive donors.[25] Although acyclovir has relatively poor *in vitro* activity versus CMV, a decrease in CMV infection and an improvement in overall survival was reported in HSV- and CMV-seropositive allogeneic BMT recipients receiving IV acyclovir.[70] Although acyclovir prophylaxis is commonly used in many transplant centers, this practice is somewhat controversial and is not universally recommended because of the intrinsically poor activity of acyclovir against CMV.[24]

Ganciclovir has also been studied for prophylaxis because of its superior activity against CMV compared to acyclovir. Although administration of prophylactic ganciclovir to CMV-seropositive patients may significantly decrease the occurrence of CMV disease, studies found no clear survival benefit, and ganciclovir-related bone marrow suppression was frequently problematic. Ganciclovir prophylaxis is recommended by some authorities for all seropositive patients, although this practice is not universally accepted.[22,24] Perhaps a more appropriate role for ganciclovir is in early or preemptive therapy, in which ganciclovir is administered at first isolation of CMV from the blood or bronchoalveolar lavage (BAL) fluid. Detection of CMV may be accomplished through use either of a monoclonal antibody-based test for viral antigens or by detection of viral DNA through polymerase chain reaction (PCR)-based tests. Preemptive therapy was evaluated in several studies and was shown to significantly reduce the occurrence of CMV disease (including CMV pneumonia), as well as improve survival significantly up to 180 days posttransplant.[24] Because CMV viremia and BAL cultures are highly predictive of subsequent CMV disease, preemptive ganciclovir therapy should be considered for patients in whom CMV is detected by either antigen-detection or PCR-based methods. Colony-stimulating factors are beneficial in this setting, providing benefits similar to those noted in neutropenic AIDS patients receiving ganciclovir therapy for CMV retinitis.

Pharmacologic prevention of CMV disease with either intravenous immunoglobulin (IVIG) or hyperimmune CMV-IVIG produced variable and inconclusive results.[22,71] The benefits of immunoglobulins for CMV prophylaxis in BMT patients have not been conclusively demonstrated and their use is not currently recommended.[24]

Ganciclovir is the drug of choice in the treatment of active CMV infection in BMT patients (Table 120–3). Foscarnet is effective in the treatment of severe CMV disease in AIDS patients and may also be of benefit for treatment or prevention of infections in BMT patients. Foscarnet may be used as an alternative to ganciclovir because of its relative lack of bone marrow toxicity. Foscarnet-related nephrotoxicity may be problematic, however, especially in the posttransplant period when patients may be receiving other nephrotoxic agents. Use of cidofovir is also limited by risk of nephrotoxicity, and this agent has not been well studied in BMT patients.

Numerous single-agent treatments, such as vidarabine, interferon, and ganciclovir, have been unsuccessfully employed as treatment for CMV pneumonitis. The combination of high-dose IVIG and ganciclovir may, however, decrease the mortality of this syndrome from 85% to only 30% to 50%.[72,73] Ganciclovir plus hyperimmune CMV-IVIG is also considered to be effective for the treatment of CMV disease, although this regimen has not been as extensively studied in this population in a controlled fashion. The potential for ganciclovir-associated bone marrow suppression prior to marrow engraftment and in patients who are just recovering from granulocytopenia remains a concern, especially in patients with unstable renal function. Ganciclovir plus CMV-IVIG is widely employed as the treatment regimen of choice for severe or life-threatening CMV disease. Ganciclovir plus IVIG is also frequently used although CMV-IVIG is replacing IVIG in many institutions.[22,71]

FUNGAL INFECTIONS

Fluconazole prophylaxis, as previously discussed for neutropenic patients, is safe and efficacious for prevention of mucocutaneous and disseminated candidal infections in BMT patients and is usually continued throughout the period of granulocytopenia. The variable activity of fluconazole against non-*albicans* species of *Candida* may be problematic in this population, as is lack of activity against *Aspergillus*. Prophylaxis with fluconazole (as well as itraconazole), although effectively reducing colonization and infection with yeasts, has not been consistently demonstrated to reduce overall mortality or invasive infections such as aspergillosis in BMT recipients.[65] Low-dose amphotericin B (0.10–0.25 mg/kg/day) is occasionally used in institutions with high rates of *Aspergillus* infection after BMT. Low-dose liposomal amphotericin B (1 mg/kg/day) has also been studied.[74] As with the azoles, amphotericin B prophylaxis has not been clearly demonstrated to provide benefits in either overall or infection-related mortality following BMT.[8,22,64,65] Despite the controversies regarding absolute benefits of prophylaxis, fluconazole is generally recommended for most patients undergoing BMT.[24] Low-dose amphotericin B prophylaxis should be reserved for those institutions with high rates of infection due to azole-resistant yeasts (e.g., *Candida krusei*) or high rates of invasive disease such as aspergillosis.[24] Fluconazole and other azole antifungals may cause significant elevations in serum cyclosporine concentrations and predispose to cyclosporine toxicities; this interaction should be closely monitored in BMT patients receiving these agents concurrently.[64]

PROTOZOAL INFECTIONS

Pulmonary infection with *P. carinii* is a relatively infrequent complication of BMT. Mortality rates in this population, however, are approximately 60% and are especially high in patients with GVHD.[22] Prophylactic use of TMP/SMX (one double-strength tablet three times/week or one single-strength tablet daily) is commonly employed in this setting. Toxoplasmosis is not a common infection in BMT patients; nevertheless, its occurrence should also be prevented by TMP/SMX prophylaxis.[24]

USE OF COLONY-STIMULATING FACTORS

Several studies have evaluated the use of filgrastim (G-CSF) and sargramostim (GM-CSF) in BMT patients in an effort to speed bone marrow recovery, to reduce the period of neutropenia, and to decrease infectious complications. Although the time to neutrophil recovery was consistently decreased, these studies failed to show significant differences in infection rates, transplant-related mortality, or overall survival. The use of CSFs appears to be safe, but their use in BMT patients has not been formally recommended because of lack of clear benefits.[54]

EVALUATION OF THERAPEUTIC OUTCOMES

Close monitoring of BMT patients, including both clinical and laboratory data, is essential for early detection and treatment of infectious complications. In addition, because many of the drugs that may be commonly used in this setting have significant toxicity potential in BMT patients (e.g., ganciclovir, amphotericin B, TMP/SMX), careful attention must be paid to the prevention and management of drug-related adverse effects. Monitoring parameters related to specific types of infections (e.g., pneumonia, urinary tract infections) should be applied as appropriate. The reader is referred to other chapters within this book for more specific information.

INFECTIONS IN SOLID ORGAN TRANSPLANT RECIPIENTS

Since the introduction of cyclosporine in 1980, solid organ transplantation has become an established mode of treatment for end-stage diseases of the kidney, liver, heart, lungs, and pancreas; small-bowel transplantation is also now becoming more common. Both patient and allograft survival rates greatly exceed those of the past. Reasons for improved survival include improvements in immunosuppressive drug therapy, candidate selection, transplant surgery techniques, and more experience in the management of complications (including infection) in these patients. Major hindrances to successful transplantation and extended long-term survival include problems with allograft dysfunction and rejection and infectious complications. Despite advances in diagnostic techniques and antimicrobial therapy, infection remains an important cause of morbidity and mortality.

RISK FACTORS

Many of the risk factors for infection discussed at the beginning of this chapter are present in solid organ transplant patients (Table 120–1). The most important risk factor in this population is the immunosuppressive drug therapy that patients receive for prevention and treatment of allograft rejection. Risk of infection is dependent on specific immunosuppressive drug regimens as well as on the intensity (dose) and duration of immunosuppression. Most opportunistic infections in transplant patients occur during the first 6 months posttransplant when the intensity and total cumulative doses of immunosuppressive therapy are very high.[75,76]

Since the introduction of cyclosporine-containing regimens, the incidence, types, and severity of infectious complications associated with these regimens have been compared with those of past regimens.[75,76] Tacrolimus may be associated with lower rates of serious bacterial and viral infections than are seen with cyclosporine-based immunosuppressive regimens,[76,77] possibly because of a steroid-sparing effect of tacrolimus that enables patients to be maintained on greatly reduced doses of corticosteroids; in many cases, steroids are completely unnecessary.[77,78] When evaluating published literature on infection patterns after solid organ transplantation, one must always consider the organ being transplanted and the nature of the immunosuppressive drug regimens in use at reporting centers.

Immunosuppressive drugs, often in escalated doses, are also used to treat episodes of graft rejection. Drugs used to treat rejection include immunoglobulins directed against T cells (e.g., antithymocyte globulin [ATG]), murine monoclonal antibodies (muromonab, OKT3), and high- dose IV or oral corticosteroids. Rejection episodes often occur during the posttransplant period when the overall cumulative dose of net state of immunosuppression is highest (2 to 4 months).[76] Therefore, patients already at risk for infection are placed at even higher risk if additional immunosuppressive therapy is needed to treat one or more episodes of graft rejection. Immunosuppressive drug therapy must be carefully evaluated when infections occur because, in many cases, immunosuppression may have to be reduced in order for the patient to survive the infectious episode; this is done at the expense of increased risk of graft rejection.

Risk of increased infectious complications from immunosuppressive therapy used to treat rejection episodes is also determined, at least in part, by the specific therapy employed. The many drug combinations used to prevent and treat allograft rejection, however, make it difficult to determine the contribution of each specific agent to the overall infection risk. Use of ATG appears to be associated with significantly higher infection rates, particularly CMV infections.[75,76] Although the risk of infection with muromonab use is less well defined, patients receiving this agent may have increased rates of viral (HSV, CMV) and *P. carinii* infections.[75,76] Because much of the data concerning muromonab for treatment of rejection are from patients who failed standard antirejection therapy (steroids ± ATG), however, prior immunosuppression may have played a role in infection development. High-dose corticosteroids are often used in the treatment of rejection and place patients at further risk for infections.

ETIOLOGY

As with cancer patients, microorganisms infecting solid organ transplant patients are present pretransplant or acquired from exogenous sources. All transplant recipients are at risk for mucocutaneous candidiasis from species colonizing body sites. Invasive fungal infection may also occur in 30% to 40% of heart, lung, pancreas, and liver transplant recipients; rates are highest following liver transplantation and are associated with mortality rates of up to 60% to 70%.[67,68,80,81] Abdominal surgery, especially the demanding operations required for liver transplantation, predispose patients to serious fungal disease, most likely as a consequence of entering an area highly colonized with *Candida spp.*[79] Lung transplant recipients are particularly at risk for invasive aspergillosis; these infections may occur in up to 10% of patients.[67] Liver and lung transplant recipients are also at particularly high risk for serious gram-negative bacterial infections as a result of the technically difficult surgical procedures.[76]

Organisms present as latent tissue infections may reactivate and cause clinical disease posttransplant after the administration of immunosuppressive drug therapy. Disease resulting from infection reactivation has been noted with viral (HSV I and II, CMV, VZV, Epstein-Barr virus [EBV]), protozoal *(T. gondii, P. carinii),* and mycobacterial *(Mycobacterium tuberculosis)* organisms. Serologic or immunologic tests are performed prior to transplantation to assess the risk for infection because of reactivation and identify other subclinical infections (hepatitis B, *Legionella*). Many patients with reactivated disease have no clinical symptoms; often the only evidence of active infection is a rise in antibody titer from the pretransplant baseline, a positive culture, or histologic evidence. Reactivation of latent infection may also result in severe, life-threatening disease in immunosuppressed hosts.

Exogenous sources of infection in transplant patients include environmental contamination and transmission of microorganisms via transplanted organs and blood products. Environmental sources of infection are similar to those noted in other immunocompromised hosts, such as cancer patients. Airborne pathogens, especially fungi, such as *Aspergillus* and *Cryptococcus neoformans,* may cause infections in transplant patients; this is thought to be a direct cause of increased *Aspergillus* infections among lung transplant patients.[67] Transplant patients are also at risk for common nosocomial infections and infections occurring as hospital outbreaks *(P. aeruginosa* and *Legionella).* Optimal prevention and management of nosocomial infections in transplant patients requires knowledge of current epidemiology of infections and susceptibility patterns in the institution.

Infections transmitted via donor organs or blood products are major causes of morbidity and mortality in transplant patients and may include HSV, *T. gondii,* and hepatitis B and C. The most important infections transmitted from the donor, however, are caused by CMV. These infections may cause serious disease (pneumonia, hepatitis, hematologic disorders, chorioretinitis), as well as predisposing patients to other opportunistic infections and contributing to allograft dysfunction.[76,82] In contrast to reactivation disease, transplant patients contracting primary CMV disease are at increased risk for serious, life-threatening infections.[75,76] The most important source of primary CMV infection in transplant patients is the donor organ. Efforts are made to avoid transplanting organs from CMV-seropositive donors into CMV-seronegative recipients because of the potentially severe consequences. With the scarcity of suitable organs and the rapidity with which transplant decisions must often be made, however, this is not always possible. The consequences of transplanting an organ from a CMV-seropositive donor into an already CMV-seropositive recipient are less clear. Evidence exists that CMV reinfection (as well as reactivation) syndromes may occur in these patients.[83] Organs from donors seropositive for *T. gondii* or HSV are generally not withheld from seronegative patients. Organs from known HIV-infected donors, however, are not used for transplantation. Asymptomatic HIV-seropositive individuals with a $CD4^+$ lymphocyte count greater than 400/mm^3 may be considered for liver, heart, or lung transplantation without prohibitively high risk of acceleration of HIV disease.[84] However, this practice is not widespread because of the shortage of donor organs. The impact of protease inhibitors and highly active antiretroviral therapy (HAART) on long-term outcome of HIV-infected patients following transplantation is also not known.

In addition to transmission from donor organs, primary CMV disease may also be transmitted from seropositive blood products, although this is a much less common mode of transmission. Risk of such transmission increases with the administration of large numbers of blood products.

Table 120–3 contains information on microbiology, clinical presentation, and treatment of infections in solid organ recipients. Although opportunistic viral, fungal, and protozoal infections may commonly occur, bacterial infections remain the most frequent infectious complications after transplantation in all allograft recipients.

TIMING OF INFECTIONS AFTER TRANSPLANTATION

Although risk of infection with specific pathogens varies with the type of transplant, the time course of infections is similar in all transplant recipients. The overall risk of infection is greatest during the first 6 months posttransplant when the greatest number of risk factors are present. Both daily doses and cumulative doses of immunosuppressive drugs are at high levels, and additional agents may be necessary for treatment of acute rejection episodes.[75,76]

The overall time course for infections can be divided into three periods posttransplant. During the first month posttransplant, patients are at risk for infections already present and brought forward from the pretransplant period (e.g., hepatitis B); postoperative infections, such as surgical wound and catheter infections; infection resulting from colonized donor organs (pneumonia following lung transplant); and reactivation of HSV.[75,76] From 2 to 6 months posttransplant, risk is highest for viral infections, including CMV, EBV, and hepatitis B

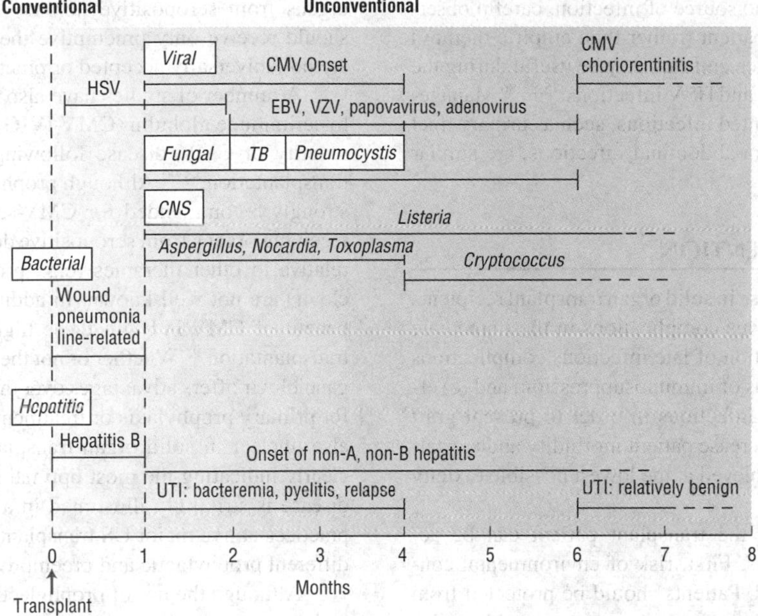

FIGURE 120–3. Timetable for the occurrence of infection in the renal transplant patient. CMV, cytomegalovirus; CNS, central nervous system; EBV, Epstein-Barr virus; HSV, herpes simplex virus; TB, tuberculosis; UTI, urinary tract infection; VZV, varicella-zoster virus. *(From Ref. 85, with permission.)*

and C. The combination of these "immunomodulating" viruses plus sustained immunosuppressive therapy leads to a high risk for opportunistic infections with pathogens such as *P. carinii, Aspergillus,* and *Nocardia asteroides*.[67,75,76] After 6 months, the patient is at risk for persistent infections (particularly viral) from earlier posttransplant periods, reactivation of VZV and *C. neoformans,* and routine infections affecting the general population.[76] In addition, patients who have required additional immunosuppression therapy for acute or chronic rejection are at continued high risk for opportunistic infections *(Aspergillus, P. carinii)*.[67,75,76] Although Fig. 120–3 illustrates infection patterns after kidney transplantation, this time course can be applied to other types of solid organ transplants. The relative incidence and importance of a particular pathogen will vary, however, according to the type of transplant.

TYPES OF INFECTIONS AND CLINICAL PRESENTATION

Transplant patients are at risk for infections occurring at a variety of sites, including skin, surgical wound, urinary tract, lungs, blood, abdomen, and central nervous system; however, most infections occur at or near the site of the transplanted organ. For example, heart transplant and heart and lung transplant recipients are most often infected within the lungs or thoracic cavity. Urinary tract infections remain an important cause of morbidity in renal transplant patients, especially in the early posttransplant period. Administration of prophylactic antibiotics, such as TMP/SMX, to these patients has, however, reduced the incidence and severity of urinary tract infections.[75,76] Serious, life-threatening bacterial and fungal infections originating from the abdomen and GI tract are most common after liver transplantation and are related to variables such as length of surgery and surgical procedures performed. Risk of bacteremia, usually originating from the gut, is highest in liver transplant patients. Renal transplant recipients are at the lowest risk of infections and infectious deaths, while patients receiving heart and lung transplants are at the highest risk of infection-related morbidity and mortality.[75,76]

Clinical presentation of infection in transplant patients is variable and depends on the infecting organism, site of infection, host immune status, time after transplantation, and dose and duration of immunosuppressive therapy. History of prior exposure is important, because primary disease is usually more symptomatic and severe than disease caused by reactivation. As in neutropenic patients, fever is the single most important clinical sign indicating the presence of infection.[75,76] At the onset of fever, patients should be evaluated for other signs and symptoms of infection, especially at sites near the surgical incision and transplanted organ. Physical assessment should include examination of all common sites of infection including respiratory tract, urinary tract, gastrointestinal tract, mucous membranes, sinuses, and intravascular catheter insertion sites. Febrile responses to infection may be blunted by the administration of high-dose corticosteroids. At least two sets of blood cultures should be obtained, including cultures both from peripheral veins and any vascular access devices. These cultures should be evaluated for bacteria and fungi. Urine cultures should be obtained if a urinary catheter is in place or the urinalysis is abnormal. Other cultures should be obtained as clinically indicated according to the presence of signs or symptoms. Because the lungs are a common site of systemic infection in this patient population, a chest radiograph should be performed. Other laboratory tests should include serum chemistries, complete blood cell count, liver function tests, and any other tests as clinically indicated based on physical examination and other points of assessment.

Signs of allograft dysfunction may be related to infection; distinguishing fever resulting from allograft rejection versus infection is often difficult and must be determined via allograft biopsy. Noninfectious sources of fever may include drug therapy and medical or surgical problems, such as embolic events and ischemic injury.

In contrast to febrile neutropenic patients, the threshold for initiating empiric antimicrobial therapy is higher in febrile transplant patients. As seen in Table 120–3, appropriate therapy for the large numbers of pathogens that may cause infections in transplant patients varies greatly from organism to organism. Therefore, careful attempts at definitive diagnosis of suspected infections must be made. If comprehensive workup reveals no source of infection, careful observation of the febrile transplant patient (rather than empiric therapy) is a common practice. Surveillance cultures may be useful during the first 3 months for detecting CMV and HSV infections.[75,82,86] Management and monitoring of documented infections, such as urinary tract infections, pneumonias, and intra-abdominal infections, are similar to that in other types of patients.

PREVENTION

The goals of antimicrobial drug use in solid organ transplant recipients include (a) prevention of infectious complications in the immediate postoperative period; (b) prevention of late infectious complications associated with prolonged periods of immunosuppression; and (c) effective treatment of established infections in order to prevent graft dysfunction and rejection and decrease patient morbidity and mortality. All of these goals must be achieved at the lowest possible toxicity and cost.

Prevention of infection in the transplant patient can be accomplished in a number of ways. First, risk of environmental contamination should be minimized. Patients should be protected from institutional infectious outbreaks. Transplant patients should receive the pneumococcal vaccine once and the influenza vaccine yearly; however, their immunologic responses to these vaccines may be blunted by immunosuppressive therapy.[75,87]

Because the most important source of primary CMV disease is an infected donor organ, CMV-seronegative patients should not receive organs or blood products from seropositive donors if possible. A number of pharmacologic strategies have also been studied in an attempt to prevent CMV infection. Prophylactic ganciclovir (usually 5 mg/kg every 12 hours) has been demonstrated effective in reducing the incidence of both primary and reactivated CMV disease in solid organ transplantation.[82,86,88] Ganciclovir prophylaxis may also significantly reduce reactivation of CMV disease in seropositive patients receiving ALG for treatment of acute rejection.[82,89] High-dose oral acyclovir effectively reduces the incidence of CMV infection and disease following renal transplantation.[90] However, acyclovir is less efficacious in high-risk renal transplant patients (donor-positive, recipient-negative for CMV serum antibodies) and other nonrenal transplant types.[82,86,88,91,92] Preemptive ganciclovir (initiated following actual isolation of CMV from blood, urine, BAL fluid, or other site) is more effective than acyclovir in the prevention of both primary and reactivation disease in liver transplant recipients. Preemptive ganciclovir effectively prevents CMV disease in other types of solid organ transplants as well.[82,86,88] Ganciclovir-related bone marrow suppression is not as problematic in solid organ transplant recipients as in BMT patients; most studies report the drug as being reasonably well tolerated.[88]

Whether prophylaxis or preemptive therapy is the best approach to prevention of CMV disease is still controversial.[82,86] Prophylaxis is effective and easy to administer without need for careful discrimination among suitable patients. However, universal prophylaxis results in unnecessary exposure of low-risk individuals to adverse effects of drugs and there are concerns that prolonged exposure may increase the risk of viral resistance to drugs. Preemptive therapy is effective and results in exposure of fewer patients to drugs. However, this strategy requires the availability and routine use of sensitive and specific diagnostic tests in order to identify high-risk individuals at an early stage of CMV infection. Although currently available PCR-based methods make this latter consideration less of an issue, PCR testing is not available at all centers. Prophylactic therapy should be used in patients at highest risk of disease (i.e., seronegative patients receiving organs from seropositive donors), while other lower-risk patients should receive only preemptive therapy.[86] These recommendations are not universally accepted or practiced, however.[82]

A number of studies have also demonstrated the value of CMV hyperimmune globulin (CMV-IVIG) in decreasing the incidence and severity of CMV disease following kidney, heart, lung, and liver transplantation.[88,90] Although prophylaxis with CMV-IVIG has been strongly recommended for CMV-seronegative transplant recipients receiving organs from seropositive donors, the benefits of CMV-IVIG relative to other therapies (e.g., prophylactic or preemptive ganciclovir) are not well known. In addition, one study demonstrated no benefit of CMV-IVIG in these high-risk patients undergoing liver transplantation.[93] Whether or not the combination of CMV-IVIG plus ganciclovir offers advantages over the use of either agent alone, either for primary prophylaxis or treatment of established CMV disease, is also unclear in solid organ transplantation.[82,86,87] The lack of data clearly indicating the most optimal regimen for prevention of CMV disease is strikingly illustrated in a review in which a summary of practices at five major US transplant centers revealed a wide array of different prophylactic and preemptive regimens in use.[88]

Although the use of prophylactic acyclovir in HSV-seropositive patients undergoing bone marrow transplantation is well accepted, prophylaxis in solid organ transplant recipients remains controversial. Acyclovir is being used at some centers because of the high incidence of clinical HSV infection, including pneumonias, after transplantation.

Prophylactic antimicrobial agents are of benefit to transplant patients in certain clinical situations. Antibiotic prophylaxis, with agents such as cefazolin begun perioperatively and continued for less than 24 hours, is considered to effectively reduce wound infection rates effectively following renal transplantation.[87,94] Surgical prophylaxis is considered mandatory in liver, heart, and lung transplant patients because of the high risk of perioperative bacterial infections. In addition, posttransplant antibiotic prophylaxis is effective in decreasing the number of bacterial infections in renal transplant patients. Prophylactic TMP/SMX has been traditionally used because it is inexpensive and well tolerated; other antibiotics, such as the fluoroquinolones, have been evaluated.[87] Administration of oral low-dose TMP/SMX (one double-strength tablet daily) for 6 to 12 months for prevention of *P. carinii* infection following heart and lung transplantation is common, although the efficacy and optimal duration are still somewhat controversial.[75,76] Selective bowel decontamination with nonabsorbable antibiotics in combination with a low bacterial diet (no fresh fruits and vegetables) effectively reduces oropharyngeal and GI colonization with gram-negative aerobes and *Candida* in liver transplant patients.[75,76]

Because immunosuppressed transplant recipients are at risk for mucocutaneous fungal infections, prophylactic oral or topical antifungal agents may be indicated in these patients. Liver transplant patients are clearly at high risk for invasive fungal infections and should be prophylaxed with fluconazole (400 mg/d).[64] It has also been suggested that lung and heart and lung transplant recipients receive high-dose fluconazole prophylaxis, although data for this recommendation are lacking.[64] Cyclosporine concentrations should be closely monitored in transplant patients receiving fluconazole and other azole antifungal agents.[64]

Transplant patients, especially heart and heart and lung recipients, without serologic evidence of prior exposure to *T. gondii* who receive organs from seropositive donors are at high risk for toxoplasmosis.[75,76] Many of these patients will be receiving TMP/SMX for prophylaxis of *P. carinii* infection; this agent will also provide effective prophylaxis against *T. gondii,* as well as against

Nocardia asteroides. Although prophylaxis is not routinely given at all centers, this therapy may be justified in high-risk patients because of the delays in diagnosis and serious infections associated with toxoplasmosis.[75,76]

The use of prophylactic isoniazid (INH) therapy for transplant patients with evidence of exposure to *M. tuberculosis* (those with a positive purified protein derivative skin test) remains controversial. Risk of reactivation and development of clinical tuberculosis is enhanced with posttransplant immunosuppression. Some clinicians believe, however, that the risk of INH-induced hepatotoxicity, especially in liver transplant recipients, outweighs the benefits of treatment.

EVALUATION OF THERAPEUTIC OUTCOMES

Close monitoring of transplant recipients, including both clinical and laboratory data, is essential for early detection and treatment of potentially severe opportunistic infections.

▶ PRINCIPLES OF PHARMACOTHERAPY

- An *immunocompromised host* is a patient with defects in host defenses that predispose to infection. Risk factors include granulocytopenia, immune system defects (including immunosuppressive drug therapy), compromise of natural host defenses, environmental contamination, and changes in normal flora of the host.
- Immunocompromised patients are at high risk for a variety of bacterial, fungal, viral, and protozoal infections. Infection is documented in only 30% to 40% of febrile episodes in neutropenic patients.
- Risk of infection in granulocytopenic patients is associated with both the severity and duration of neutropenia. Patients with severe neutropenia (ANC < 500 cells/mm^3) for greater than 7 to 10 days are considered to be at high risk of infection.
- Bacterial infections caused by gram-positive cocci (staphylococci and streptococci) occur most frequently, followed by gram-negative bacterial infections caused by Enterobacteriaceae and *P. aeruginosa*. Fungal infections caused by *Candida* and *Aspergillus,* as well as certain viral infections (herpes simplex virus, cytomegalovirus), are also particularly important causes of morbidity and mortality.
- Fever (>38°C [100.4°F]) is the most important clinical finding in neutropenic patients and is usually the stimulus for further diagnostic workup and treatment. Infection should be considered as the cause of fever until proven otherwise. Appropriate antimicrobial therapy must be rapidly instituted and patients aggressively treated to prevent excessive morbidity and mortality.
- Initial antimicrobial regimens for treatment of febrile neutropenia must have good activity against *P. aeruginosa* and Enterobacteriaceae. Regimens most commonly recommended for initial treatment include monotherapy with an antipseudomonal β-lactam or carbapenem, or a combination regimen consisting of an antipseudomonal β-lactam plus an aminoglycoside.
- Neutropenic patients who remain febrile after 72 hours should be reevaluated to determine whether antimicrobial modifications are necessary. Common modifications to regimens include addition of vancomycin (if not already present), and antifungal therapy (fluconazole or amphotericin B).
- The optimal duration of therapy for febrile neutropenia is controversial. The decision to discontinue antimicrobials is based on resolution of granulocytopenia, persistent fever, culture results, and clinical stability of the patient.
- Prophylactic antimicrobials are commonly administered to cancer patients with anticipated prolonged neutropenia, as well as to both bone marrow and solid organ transplant recipients. Common prophylactic regimens may include antibacterial, antifungal, antiviral, or antiprotozoal agents, or a combination of these, selected according to risk of infection with specific pathogens in each patient population. Optimal prophylactic regimens are controversial for most types of infection.
- Patients undergoing bone marrow transplantation are at an extremely high risk of infection because of prolonged neutropenia following intensive chemotherapy ± irradiation, while solid organ transplant recipients are at risk because of prolonged administration of immunosuppressive drugs. Fungal *(Aspergillus)* and viral (CMV) infections are particularly troublesome in these patients and prophylactic regimens directed against these pathogens are commonly used. When documented, these infections must be treated very aggressively in order to optimize patient outcome. Nevertheless, associated mortality rates are often very high despite appropriate and aggressive antimicrobial therapy.
- Immunocompromised patients must be continuously assessed for evidence of infection and response to antimicrobial therapy. Because a large number of antimicrobials may potentially be used, including many with significant toxicities, the occurrence of drug-related adverse effects must also be carefully assessed.

REFERENCES

1. Hughes WT, Armstrong D, Bodey GP, et al. Guidelines for the use of antimicrobial agents in neutropenic patients with unexplained fever. Clin Infect Dis 1997;25:551–573.
2. Pizzo PA. Management of fever in patients with cancer and treatment-induced neutropenia. N Engl J Med 1993;328:1323–1332.
3. Pizzo PA. Current concepts: fever in immunocompromised patients. N Engl J Med 1999;341:893–900.
4. Giamarellou H. Empiric therapy for infections in the febrile, neutropenic, compromised host. Med Clin North Am 1995;79:559–580.
5. Koll BS, Brown AE. Changing patterns of infections in the immunocompromised patient with cancer. Hematol Oncol Clin North Am 1993;7:753–769.
6. Groll A, Shah PM, Mentzel C, et al. Trends in the post-mortem epidemiology of invasive fungal infections at a University hospital. J Infect 1996;33:23–32.
7. Rabella N, Rodriguez P, Labeaga R, et al. Conventional respiratory viruses recovered from immunocompromised patients: Clinical considerations. Clin Infect Dis 1999;28:1043–1048.
8. Hathorn JW. Critical appraisal of antimicrobials for prevention of infections in immunocompromised hosts. Hematol Oncol Clin North Am 1993;7:1051–1099.
9. Bonten MJM, Gaillard CA, van der Geest S, et al. The role of intragastric acidity and stress ulcus prophylaxis on colonization and infection in mechanically ventilated ICU patients: A stratified, randomized, double-blind study of sucralfate versus antacids. Am J Respir Crit Care Med 1995;152:1825–1834.
10. Talcott JA, Finberg R, Mayer RJ, Goldman L. The medical course of cancer patients with fever and neutropenia. Arch Intern Med 1988;148:2561–2568.

11. Hathorn JW, Rubin M, Pizzo PA. Empirical antibiotic therapy in the febrile neutropenic cancer patient: Clinical efficacy and impact of monotherapy. Antimicrob Agents Chemother 1987;31:971–977.
12. De Pauw BE, Donnelly JP. Controversies in the antibacterial treatment of patients with neutropenia: A matter of comprehension or apprehension. Cancer Invest 1997;15:37–46.
13. Bow EJ, Loewen R, Vaughan D. Reduced requirement for gram-negative antibiotic therapy in febrile, neutropenic patients with cancer who are receiving antibacterial chemoprophylaxis with oral quinolones. Clin Infect Dis 1996;20:907–912.
14. Cruciani M, Rampazzo R, Malena M, et al. Prophylaxis with fluoroquinolones for bacterial infections in neutropenic patients: A meta-analysis. Clin Infect Dis 1996;23:795–805.
15. Bochud PY, Eggiman PH, Calandra TH, et al. Bacteremia due to viridans streptococcus in neutropenic patients with cancer: Clinical spectrum and risk factors. Clin Infect Dis 1994;18:25–31.
16. Brown EA, Talbot GH, Provencher M, Cassileth P. Anaerobic bacteremia in patients with acute leukemia. Infect Control Hosp Epidemiol 1989;10:65–69.
17. Bodey GP, Bueltmann B, Duguid W, et al. Fungal infections in cancer patients: An international autopsy survey. Eur J Clin Microbiol Infect Dis 1992;11:99–109.
18. Meurman JH, Pyrhonen S, Teerenhovi L, Lindqvist C. Oral sources of septicaemia in patients with malignancies. Oral Oncol 1997;33:389–397.
19. Thaler M, Pastakia B, Shawker TH, et al. Hepatic candidiasis in cancer patients: The evolving picture of the syndrome. Ann Intern Med 1988;108:88–100.
20. Denning DW. Invasive aspergillosis. Clin Infect Dis 1998;26:781–805.
21. Kibbler CC. Infections in solid organ transplant recipients. Curr Topics Pathol 1999;92:19–35.
22. Momin F, Chandrasekar PH. Antimicrobial prophylaxis in bone marrow transplantation. Ann Intern Med 1995;123:205–215.
23. Ketterer N, Espinouse D, Chomarat M, et al. Infections following peripheral blood progenitor cell transplantation for lymphoproliferative malignancies: Etiology and potential risk factors. Am J Med 1999;106:191–197.
24. Serody JS, Shea TC. Prevention of infections in bone marrow transplant recipients. Infect Dis Clin North Am 1997;11:459–477.
25. Sickles EA, Greene WH, Wiernik PH. Clinical presentation of infection in granulocytopenic patients. Arch Intern Med 1975;135:715–719.
26. Bodey GP, Jadeja L, Elting L. *Pseudomonas* bacteremia: Retrospective analysis of 410 episodes. Arch Intern Med 1985;145:1621–1629.
27. Kibbler CC. Neutropenic infections: Strategies for empirical therapy. J Antimicrob Chemother 1995;36(suppl B):107–117.
28. Pizzo PA, Hathorn JW, Hiemenz J, et al. A randomized trial comparing ceftazidime alone with combination antibiotic therapy in cancer patients with fever and neutropenia. N Engl J Med 1986;315:552–558.
29. Egerer G, Goldschmidt H, Salwender H, et al. Efficacy of continuous infusion of ceftazidime for patients with neutropenic fever after high-dose chemotherapy and peripheral blood stem cell transplantation. Int J Antimicrob Agents 2000;15:119–123.
30. Engervall P, Kalin M, Dornbusch K, Bjorkholm M. Cefepime as empirical monotherapy in febrile patients with hematological malignancies and neutropenia: A randomized, single-center phase II trial. J Chemother 1999;11:278–286.
31. Cometta A, Calandra T, Gaya H, et al. Monotherapy with meropenem versus combination therapy with ceftazidime plus amikacin as empiric therapy for fever in granulocytopenic patients with cancer. Antimicrob Agents Chemother 1996;40:1108–1115.
32. Bohme A, Shah PM, Stille W, Hoelzer D. Piperacillin/tazobactam versus cefepime as initial empirical antimicrobial therapy in febrile neutropenic patients: A prospective randomized pilot study. Eur J Med Res 1998;3:324–330.
33. Winston DJ, Ho WG, Bruckner DA, Champlin RE. Beta-lactam antibiotic therapy in febrile, granulocytopenic patients: A randomized trial comparing cefoperazone plus piperacillin, ceftazidime plus piperacillin, and imipenem alone. Ann Intern Med 1991;115:849–859.
34. Fish DN, Singletary TJ. Meropenem: A new carbapenem antibiotic. Pharmacotherapy 1997;17:644–669.
35. Ramphal R, Gucalp R, Rotstein C, et al. Clinical experience with single agent and combination regimens in the management of infection in the febrile neutropenic patient. Am J Med 1996;100(suppl 6A): 83S–89S.
36. Rains CP, Bryson HM, Peters DH. Ceftazidime: An update on its antibacterial activity, pharmacokinetic properties and therapeutic efficacy. Drugs 1995;49:577–617.
37. Chastagner P, Plouvier E, Eyer D, et al. Efficacy of cefepime and amikacin in the empiric treatment of febrile neutropenic children with cancer. Med Pediatr Oncol 2000;34:306–308.
38. Marie JP, Marjanovic Z, Vekhoff A, et al. Piperacillin/tazobactam plus tobramycin versus ceftazidime plus tobramycin as empiric therapy for fever in severely neutropenic patients. Suppport Care Cancer 1999;7: 89–94.
39. Hatala R, Dinh TT, Cook DJ. Single daily dosing of aminoglycosides in immunocompromised adults: A systematic review. Clin Infect Dis 1997;24:810–815.
40. Hatala R, Dinh TT, Cook DJ. Single daily dosing of aminoglycosides in immunocompromised adults: A systematic review. Clin Infect Dis 1997;24:810–815.
41. Gutmann L, Williamson R, Kitzis MD, Acar JF. Synergism and antagonism in double β-lactam antibiotic combinations. Am J Med 1986;80 (suppl 5C):21–29.
42. EORTC International Antimicrobial Therapy Cooperative Group and the National Cancer Institute of Canada—Clinical Trials Group. Vancomycin added to empirical combination antibiotic therapy for fever in granulocytopenic cancer patients. J Infect Dis 1991;163:951–958.
43. Viscoli C, Castagnola E. Planned progressive antimicrobial therapy in neutropenic patients. Br J Haematol 1998;102:879–888.
44. Centers for Disease Control and Prevention. Recommendations for preventing the spread of vancomycin resistance: Recommendations of the Hospital Infection Control Practices Advisory Committee (HICPAC). MMWR Morb Mortal Wkly Rep 1995(Sept 22);44(No. RR-12):1–13.
45. Antabli BA, Bross P, Siegel RS, et al. Empiric antimicrobial therapy of febrile neutropenic patients undergoing haematopoietic stem cell transplantation. Int J Antimicrob Agents 1999;13:127–130.
46. Rolston KVI, Rubenstein EB, Freifeld A. Early empiric antibiotic therapy for febrile neutropenia patients at low risk. Infect Dis Clin North Am 1996;10:223–237.
47. Escalante CP, Rubenstein EB, Rolston KVI. Outpatient antibiotic therapy for febrile episodes in low-risk neutropenic patients with cancer. Cancer Invest 1997;15:237–242.
48. Freifeld A, Pizzo P. Use of fluoroquinolones for empirical management of febrile neutropenia in pediatric cancer patients. Pediatr Infect Dis J 1997;16:140–146.
49. Freifeld A, Marchigiani D, Walsh T, et al. A double-blind comparison of empirical oral and intravenous antibiotic therapy for low-risk febrile patients with neutropenia during cancer chemotherapy. N Engl J Med 1999;341:305–311.
50. Pizzo PA, Robichaud KJ, Gill FA, Witebsky FG. Empiric antibiotic and antifungal therapy for cancer patients with prolonged fever and granulocytopenia. Am J Med 1982;72:101–111.
51. White MH, Anaissie EJ, Kusne S, et al. Amphotericin B colloidal dispersion vs. amphotericin B as therapy for invasive aspergillosis. Clin Infect Dis 1997;24:635–642.
52. Walsh TJ, Finberg RW, Arndt C, et al. Liposomal amphotericin B for empirical therapy in patients with persistent fever and neutropenia. N Engl J Med 1999;340:764–771.
53. Sable CA, Donowitz GR. Infections in bone marrow transplant recipients. Clin Infect Dis 1994;18:273–284.
54. American Society of Clinical Oncology. American Society of Clinical Oncology recommendations for the use of hematopoietic colony-stimulating factors: Evidence-based, clinical practice guidelines. J Clin Oncol 1994;12:2471–2508.
55. Geller RB. Use of cytokines in the treatment of acute myelocytic leukemia: A critical review. J Clin Oncol 1996;14:1371–1382.
56. Dix SP, Gilmore CE. Cytokine therapy after bone marrow transplantation. Pharmacotherapy 1996;16:593–608.

57. Huebel K, Dale DC, Engert A, Liles WC. Current status of granulocyte (neutrophil) transfusion therapy for infectious diseases. J Infect Dis 2001;183:321–328.
58. Cruciani M, Rampazzo R, Malena M, et al. Prophylaxis with fluoroquinolones for bacterial infections in neutropenic infections: A meta-analysis. Clin Infect Dis 1996;23:795–805.
59. Gilbert C, Meisenberg B, Vredenburgh J, et al. Sequential prophylactic oral and empiric once-daily parenteral antibiotics for neutropenia and fever after high-dose chemotherapy and autologous bone marrow support. J Clin Oncol 1994;12:1005–1011.
60. Kern WV, Hay B, Kern P, et al. A randomized trial of roxithromycin in patients with acute leukemia and bone marrow transplant recipients receiving fluoroquinolone prophylaxis. Antimicrob Agents Chemother 1994;38:465–472.
61. Munoz L, Martino R, Subira M, et al. Intensified prophylaxis of febrile neutropenia with ofloxacin plus rifampin during severe short-duration neutropenia in patients with lymphoma. Leuk Lymphoma 1999;34: 585–589.
62. Reents S, Goodwin SD, Singh V. Antifungal prophylaxis in immunocompromised hosts. Ann Pharmacother 1993;27:53–60.
63. Young GA, Bosly A, Gibbs DL, Durrant S. A double-blind comparison of fluconazole and nystatin in the prevention of candidiasis in patients with leukaemia. Antifungal Prophylaxis Study Group. Eur J Cancer 1999;35:1208–1213.
64. Edwards JE Jr, Bodey GP, Bowden RA, et al. International conference for the development of a consensus on the management and prevention of severe candidal infections. Clin Infect Dis 1997;25:43–59.
65. Gubbins PO, Bowman JL, Penzak SR. Antifungal prophylaxis to prevent invasive mycoses among bone marrow transplantation patients. Pharmacother 1998;18:549–564.
66. Beyer J, Schwartz S, Heinemann V, Siegert W. Strategies in prevention of invasive pulmonary aspergillosis in immunocompromised or neutropenic patients. Antimicrob Agents Chemother 1994;38:911–917.
67. Paterson DL, Singh N. Invasive aspergillosis in transplant recipients. Medicine 1999;78:123–138.
68. Lin S-J, Schranz J, Teutsch SM. Aspergillosis case-fatality rate: Systematic review of the literature. Clin Infect Dis 2001;32:358–366.
69. Meyers JD, Flournoy N, Thomas ED. Risk factors for cytomegalovirus infection after human marrow transplantation. J Infect Dis 1986;153:478–488.
70. Meyers JD, Reed EC, Shepp DH, et al. Acyclovir for prevention of cytomegalovirus infection and disease after allogeneic marrow transplantation. N Engl J Med 1988;318:70–75.
71. Barnes RA. Immunotherapy and immunoprophylaxis in bone marrow transplantation. J Hosp Infect 1995;30(suppl):223–231.
72. Schmidt GM, Kovacs A, Zaia JA, et al. Ganciclovir/immunoglobulin combination therapy for the treatment of human cytomegalovirus-associated interstitial pneumonia in bone marrow allograft recipients. Transplantation 1988;46:905–907.
73. Emanuel D, Cunningham I, Jules-Elysee K, et al. Cytomegalovirus pneumonia after bone marrow transplantation successfully treated with the combination of ganciclovir and high-dose intravenous immune globulin. Ann Intern Med 1988;109:777–782.
74. Kibbler CC. Infections in solid organ transplant recipients. Curr Top Pathol 1999; 92:19–35.
75. Kontoyiannis DP, Rubin RH. Infection in the organ transplant recipient: An overview. Infect Dis Clin North Am 1995;9:811–822.
76. Hooks MA. Tacrolimus, a new immunosuppressant—A review of the literature. Ann Pharmacother 1994;28:501–511.
77. The U.S. Multicenter FK506 Liver Study Group. A comparison of tacrolimus (FK506) and cyclosporine for immunosuppression in liver transplantation. N Engl J Med 1994;331:1110–1115.
78. Kusne S, Dummer JS, Singh N, et al. Infections after liver transplantation: An analysis of 101 consecutive cases. Medicine 1988;67:132–143.
79. Hibberd PL, Rubin RH. Clinical aspects of fungal infection in organ transplant recipients. Clin Infect Dis 1994;19(suppl 1):S33–S40.
80. Singh N, Gayowski T, Wagener MM, et al. Invasive fungal infections in liver transplant recipients receiving tacrolimus as the primary immunosuppressive agent. Clin Infect Dis 1997;24:179–184.
81. Paya CV. Prevention of cytomegalovirus disease in recipients of solid-organ transplants. Clin Infect Dis 2001;32:596–603.
82. Chou S. Neutralizing antibody responses to reinfecting strains of cytomegalovirus in transplant recipients. J Infect Dis 1990;160:16–21.
83. Rubin RH, Tolkoff-Rubin NE. The impact of infection on the outcome of transplantation. Transplant Proc 1991;23:2068–2074.
84. Singh N. Preemptive therapy versus universal prophylaxis with ganciclovir for cytomegalovirus in solid organ transplant recipients. Clin Infect Dis 2001;32:742–751.
85. Rubin RH, Wolfson JS, Cosimi AB, Tolkoff-Rubin NE. Infection in the renal transplant recipient. Am J Med 1981;70:405–411.
86. Patel R, Snydman DR, Rubin RH, et al. Cytomegalovirus prophylaxis in solid organ transplant recipients. Transplantation 1996;61:1279–1289.
87. Rubin RH, Tolkoff-Rubin NE. Antimicrobial strategies in the care of organ transplant recipients. Antimicrob Agents Chemother 1993;37:619–624.
88. Hibberd PL, Tolkoff-Rubin NE, Conti D, et al. Preemptive ganciclovir therapy to prevent cytomegalovirus disease in cytomegalovirus antibody-positive renal transplant recipients: A randomized controlled trial. Ann Intern Med 1995;123:18–26.
89. Dickinson BI, Gora-Harper ML, McCraney SA, et al. Studies evaluating high-dose acyclovir, intravenous immune globulin, and cytomegalovirus hyperimmunoglobulin for prophylaxis against cytomegalovirus in kidney transplant recipients. Ann Pharmacother 1996;30:1452–1462.
90. Singh N, Yu VL, Mieles L, et al. High-dose acyclovir compared with short-course preemptive ganciclovir therapy to prevent cytomegalovirus disease in liver transplant recipients. Ann Intern Med 1994;120:375–381.
91. Goral S, Ynares C, Dummer S, et al. Acyclovir prophylaxis for cytomegalovirus disease in high-risk renal transplant recipients: Is it effective? Kidney Int 1996;50(suppl 57):S62–S65.
92. Snydman DR, Werner BG, Dougherty NN, et al. Cytomegalovirus immune globulin prophylaxis in liver transplantation: A randomized, double-blind, placebo-controlled trial. Ann Intern Med 1993;119:984–991.
93. Barone GW, Hudec WA, Sailors DM, et al. Prophylactic wound antibiotics for combined kidney and pancreas transplants. Clin Transplant 1996;10:386–388.
94. Menichetti F. Prevention of candidiasis in the immunocompromised host: What are the best strategies? Int J Infect Dis 1997;1(suppl 1):S52–S55.

121

ANTIMICROBIAL PROPHYLAXIS IN SURGERY

John W. Devlin, Salmaan Kanji, Stephen W. Janning, and Michael J. Rybak

According to the National Center for Health Statistics, approximately 46 million surgical procedures are performed annually in the United States, the majority of which are done in an outpatient setting.[1] Infection is the most common complication of surgery.[2] Surgical site infections (SSIs) occur in approximately 3% to 6% of patients and prolong hospitalization by an average of 7 days at a direct annual cost of 5 to 10 billion dollars.[3,4] SSIs are the third (14% to 16%) most frequent cause of nosocomial infections among hospitalized patients and the primary (40%) cause of nosocomial infection in surgical patients.[3] Prophylactic administration of antibiotics decreases the risk of infection after many surgical procedures and thus represents an important component of care for the surgical population.

Antibiotics administered prior to the contamination of previously sterile tissues or fluids are deemed *prophylactic* antibiotics. The goal of therapy is to *prevent* an infection from developing. Although eradication of distal (preexisting, unrelated to surgery) infections lowers the risk for subsequent postoperative infections, it does not, per se, constitute a prophylactic regimen. In fact, surgical prophylaxis may be prescribed concurrently with antibiotics to treat distal site infections because of important antimicrobial spectrum and timing-related concerns. Both SSIs and distal site infections not directly related to the surgical site are termed nosocomial (e.g., urinary tract infections, pneumonia, and so on). Prevention of these surgical site infections is a major goal of antibiotic prophylaxis.

Presumptive antibiotic therapy is administered when an infection is suspected, but not yet proven. Clinical scenarios where presumptive therapy is commonly employed include acute cholecystitis, open compound fractures, and acute appendicitis of less than 24 hours' duration. In these situations, if signs of perforation or infection are absent during surgery, then routine prophylactic rather than presumptive therapy is warranted. An operative finding of a gangrenous gallbladder or a perforated appendix, however, is suggestive of an established infectious process and thus a *therapeutic* antibiotic regimen is required.[3]

According to the Centers for Disease Control and Prevention's (CDC) National Nosocomial Infections Surveillance System (NNIS)[3] (Fig. 121–1), SSIs can be categorized as either incisional (e.g., cellulitis of the incision site) or organ/space (e.g., meningitis). Incisional SSIs are further subcategorized into superficial (involving only the skin or subcutaneous tissue) and deep (fascial and muscle layers) infections. Organ/space SSIs can involve any anatomic area other than the incision site. For example, a patient who develops bacterial peritonitis after bowel surgery would have an organ/space SSI. By definition, SSIs must occur within 30 days of surgery. If a prosthetic implant is involved, however, a deep incisional or organ/space SSI can still be reported up to 1 year from the date of surgery. Although microbiologic testing of surgical drainage material or sites may help guide care, the specificity of a negative culture is poor and generally does not rule out a SSI.[3]

SURGICAL SITE INFECTION RISK FACTORS

SSI incidence depends on both procedure and patient-related factors. Traditionally, the risk for SSIs has been stratified by surgical procedure in a classification system developed by the National Research Council (NRC)[5] (Table 121–1). The NRC classification system proposes that the risk of a SSI depends on the microbiology of the surgical site, the presence of a preexisting infection, the likelihood of contaminating previously sterile tissue during surgery, and events during and after surgery.[5,6] A patient's NRC procedure classification is the primary determinant of whether antibiotic prophylaxis is warranted. It should be emphasized, however, that because a patient's NRC wound classification is influenced by surgical findings (e.g., gangrenous gallbladder) and perioperative events (e.g., major technique breaks), categorization generally occurs intraoperatively.[7]

INHERENT PATIENT RISK

The NRC classification system does not account for the influence of underlying patient risk factors for SSI development, instead categorizing the risks for SSIs simply based on a specific surgical procedure. Table 121–2 lists disease states and conditions known to increase SSI risk. Preexisting distal infections increase SSI rates and should be resolved prior to surgery whenever possible. Diabetic patients have an increased risk of SSIs if perioperative blood glucose exceeds 200 mg/dL. Perioperative insulin infusions in uncontrolled diabetics undergoing coronary artery bypass graft surgery will significantly reduce the risk of deep wound infections.[8] Preoperative smoking has been identified as an independent risk factor for SSI because of the deleterious effects of nicotine on wound healing. Preoperative immunosuppression, including corticosteroid use, may increase infection risk. Although malnutrition is associated with a higher frequency of SSI, clinical trials have not shown that perioperative nutritional supplementation decreases the incidence of infection.[9]

Colonization of the nares with *Staphylococcus aureus* is a well described SSI risk factor.[3] Two small prospective trials suggest that eradication of nasal *S. aureus* with mupirocin significantly reduces the incidence of SSI when compared to historical controls in patients undergoing both cardiac[10] and upper gastrointestinal surgery.[11] Larger prospective trials, however, are needed before this therapy can be routinely advocated. Other factors shown to increase the risk of SSI include age, length of preoperative hospital stay, and obesity.[3]

IDENTIFYING RISK FACTORS FOR SURGICAL SITE INFECTIONS

Two large epidemiologic studies have been published that objectively quantify SSI risk based on specific patient and procedure-related

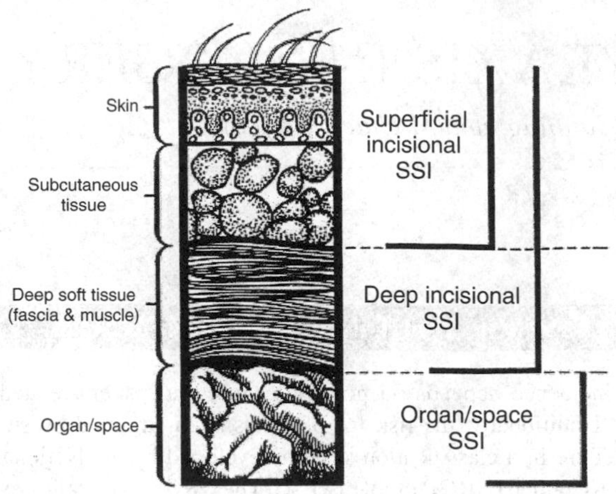

FIGURE 121–1. Cross-section of abdominal wall depicting CDC classifications of surgical site infections.[3]

factors. The Study on the Efficacy of Nosocomial Infection Control (SENIC) analyzed more than 100,000 surgery cases to identify and validate risk factors for SSI.[12] Abdominal operations, operations lasting longer than 2 hours, contaminated or dirty procedures (as per NRC classification), and more than three underlying medical diagnoses were each associated with an increased incidence of SSI. When NRC classification was stratified by number of SENIC risk factors present, SSI incidence varied by as much as a factor of 15 within the same NRC operative category[13] (Table 121–3).

The NNIS, in a subsequent analysis of more than 84,000 surgical cases, attempted to simplify and refine the SENIC system by quantifying intrinsic patient risk using the American Society of Anesthesiologists (ASA) preoperative assessment score[14,15] (Table 121–4). An ASA score of ≥3 was found to be a strong predictor for the development of a SSI. Other factors associated with increased SSI incidence include contaminated or dirty operations (NRC criteria) and surgical procedures lasting longer than average.

Although evidence-based recommendations for antimicrobial prophylaxis during surgery are best established using the results of randomized clinical trials, many studies have small sample sizes and do not stratify patients according to overall SSI risk. Future studies, particularly those involving clean procedures, should be stratified by SSI risk so that the subset of high-risk patients who might benefit the most from prophylaxis is clearly established.

All hospitals should implement a comprehensive infection control program to minimize SSIs.[16] Although prophylactic antibiotic therapy is a crucial strategy in reducing SSI risk, other measures also reduce the risk of infection. Length of hospitalization is associated with increased colonization and infection with nosocomial bacteria, and leads to a higher incidence of SSI. Elective surgery is routinely postponed should a patient be hospitalized for an unrelated medical problem prior to surgery. Shaving the incision site with a razor the day before surgery is also associated with higher infection rates; instead, clipping the operative site just prior to the procedure is preferred. Preoperative showering with chlorhexidine soap, while reducing bacterial colony counts, has not definitively been shown to reduce SSI risk.[3]

BACTERIOLOGY

The most important consideration when choosing antibiotic prophylaxis is the bacteriology of the surgical site. Organisms involved in a SSI are acquired one of two ways: endogenously (from the patient's own normal flora) and exogenously (from contamination during the surgical procedure). Based on the type and anatomic location of the procedure, and the NRC classification (Table 121–1), resident flora can be anticipated and appropriate antibiotic choices can be made. According to NNIS data, *S. aureus,* coagulase negative staphylococci, *Enterococcus* spp., *Escherichia coli,* and *Pseudomonas aeruginosa* are the pathogens most commonly isolated[3] (Table 121–5). With the widespread use of broad-spectrum antibiotics, however, *Candida* spp. and methicillin-resistant *S. aureus* are becoming more prevalent.[3]

TABLE 121–1. NRC Wound Classification, Risk of SSI, and Indication for Antibiotics

	SSI Rate (%)			
Classification	*Preop Antibiotics*	*No Preop Antibiotics*	Criteria	Antibiotics
Clean	5.1	0.8	No acute inflammation or transection of gastrointestinal, oropharyngeal, genitourinary, biliary, or respiratory tracts. Elective case, no technique break.	Not indicated unless high-risk procedure*
Clean-contaminated	10.1	1.3	Controlled opening of aforementioned tracts with minimal spillage/minor technique break. Clean procedures performed emergently or with major technique breaks.	Prophylactic antibiotics indicated.
Contaminated	21.9	10.2	Acute, nonpurulent inflammation present. Major spillage/technique break during clean-contaminated procedure.	Prophylactic antibiotics indicated.
Dirty	N/A	N/A	Obvious preexisting infection present (abscess, pus, or necrotic tissue present).	Therapeutic antibiotics required.

*High-risk procedures include implantation of prosthetic materials and other procedures where surgical site infection (SSI) is associated with high morbidity (see text).
NRC, National Research Council; SSI, Surgical Site Infection;
(Adapted from Refs. 5 and 120.)

TABLE 121–2. Patient and Operation Characteristics that May Influence the Risk of SSI

Patient	Operation
Age	Duration of surgical scrub
Nutritional status	Preoperative skin preparation
Diabetes	Preoperative shaving
Smoking	Duration of operation
Obesity	Antimicrobial prophylaxis
Coexisting infections at distal body sites	Operating room ventilation
Colonization with resistant microorganisms	Sterilization of instruments
Altered immune response	Implantation of prosthetic materials
Length of preoperative stay	Surgical drains
	Surgical technique

(Adapted from Ref. 3.)

Factors affecting the ability of an organism to induce a SSI depend on organism count, organism virulence, and host immunocompetency. Organisms in the commensal flora are generally not pathogenic. These organisms often serve the host as a form of protection against invasive organisms that would otherwise colonize the tissue site. Opportunistic organisms are usually kept in check by normal flora and are rarely problematic unless they are found in large numbers. Loss of this protective flora, through the use of broad-spectrum antibiotics, can upset this balance, thus allowing pathogenic bacteria to proliferate and infection to occur.[17]

If translocated to a normally sterile tissue site or fluid during a surgical procedure, normal flora can become pathogenic. For example, *S. aureus* or *S. epidermidis* may be translocated from the surface of the skin to deeper tissues or *E. coli* from the colon to the peritoneal cavity, bloodstream, or urinary tract. Studies in animals and healthy volunteers show that the number of acquired organisms is an important factor in the development of secondary infections.[18,19] Animal models of infection demonstrate that although more than 1,000,000 *S. aureus* per square centimeter or gram of tissue are required to produce infection, less than 100,000 *S. pyogenes* per square centimeter or gram of tissue would be required at the same site.[19,20]

Impaired host defense reduces the number of bacteria required to establish an infection. A breach of normal host defenses through surgical intervention (e.g., insertion of a prosthetic device) may potentiate the ability of organisms to cause infection. In addition, the loss of specific immune factors, such as complement activation, tissue-

TABLE 121–3. Surgical Site Infection Incidence (%) Stratified by National Research Council Wound Classification and SENIC Risk Factors[a]

No. of SENIC Risk Factors	Clean	Clean-Contaminated	Contaminated	Dirty
0	1.1	0.6	N/A	N/A
1	3.9	2.8	4.5	6.7
2	8.4	8.4	8.3	10.9
3	15.8	17.7	11.0	18.8
4	N/A	N/A	23.9	27.4

[a]The Study on the Efficacy of Nosocomial Infection Control (SENIC) risk factors include abdominal operation, operations lasting ≥2 hours, contaminated or dirty procedures by National Research Council (NRC) classification, and more than three underlying medical diagnoses.
(Adapted from Ref. 13.)

TABLE 121–4. American Society of Anesthesiologists Physical Status Classification

Class	Description
1	Normal healthy patient
2	Mild systemic disease
3	Severe systemic disease that is not incapacitating
4	Incapacitating systemic disease that is a constant threat to life
5	Not expected to survive 24 hours with or without operation

From Ref. 15.

derived inhibitors (e.g., pro-inflammatory cytokines), cell-mediated response (e.g., T-cell function), and granulocytic or phagocytic function (e.g., neutrophils, macrophages) can greatly increase the risk for SSI development.[21,22] Vascular occlusive states related to the surgical procedure, or those occurring from hypovolemic shock, can greatly affect blood flow to the surgical site, thus diminishing host defense mechanisms against microbial invasion.[23] Traumatized tissue, hematomas, and the presence of foreign material also increase the risk for infections.[23,24] When a foreign body is introduced during a surgical procedure, fewer than 100 bacterial colony-forming units (CFUs) are required to cause a SSI.[24] Studies examining *S. aureus*-contaminated wound infections on the skin of healthy volunteers demonstrate a 10,000-fold reduction in the number of organisms required to establish a wound infection if sutures are not present.[18]

ANTIMICROBIAL RESISTANCE

Colonization of the host with antibiotic-resistant hospital flora prior to or during surgery may lead to a SSI that is unresponsive to routine antibiotic therapy. Epidemiologic studies demonstrate that the most common cause for nosocomially acquired multiresistant organisms is transmission from hospital personnel.[25] Concomitant treatment with broad-spectrum antibiotics also increases the risk for colonization with hospital flora.

With cephalosporins established as first-line agents for prophylaxis over the past decade, organisms resistant to cephalosporins represent the majority of pathogens causing SSIs. The CDC recently

TABLE 121–5. Major Pathogens in Surgical Wound Infections

Pathogen	Percent of Infections*
Staphylococcus aureus	20
Coagulase-negative staphylococci	14
Enterococcus spp.	12
Escherichia coli	8
Pseudomonas aeruginosa	8
Enterobacter spp.	7
Proteus mirabilis	3
Klebsiella pneumoniae	3
Other *Streptococcus* spp.	3
Candida albicans	3
Group D streptococci	2
Other gram-positive aerobes	2
Bacteroides fragilis	2

*Data reported by the NNIS from 1990–1996.
(Adapted from Ref. 5.)

reported an alarming increase in the incidence of vancomycin-resistant enterococci (VRE) infections, particularly those with *Enterococcus faecium*.[3] Risk factors for VRE colonization include severe concomitant diseases, immunosuppression, admission to the intensive care unit, previous intra-abdominal or cardiothoracic surgery, indwelling catheters, and prolonged courses of antimicrobials, including vancomycin.[26] In an effort to control the spread of VRE, the CDC has published recommendations that include strict criteria for the use of vancomycin as surgical prophylaxis.[27] The guidelines suggest vancomycin substitution for cefazolin as SSI prophylaxis only when there is a high prevalence of methicillin-resistant *S. aureus* or in patients who have a documented history of a life-threatening allergy to penicillins or cephalosporins. Other limitations to vancomycin use, besides the risk of inducing resistant organisms, include its narrow spectrum of activity, its poor penetration into some tissues, and the potential for infusion-related reactions. The emergence of *S. aureus* displaying intermediate resistance (minimal inhibitory concentration [MIC] $\geq 8\ \mu$g/mL) further underscores the need to limit routine use of vancomycin for prophylaxis.[28]

Although cefazolin remains a mainstay in cardiovascular SSI prophylaxis, its failure has been reported in cases involving methicillin-sensitive *S. aureus* (MSSA). In a comparison trial between cefamandole and cefazolin, significantly more failures were attributed to cefazolin even though the primary pathogen was MSSA.[29] A similar trial comparing cefazolin versus cefuroxime, however, did not show any difference in SSI incidence between the two regimens.[30] It has been proposed that the β-lactamase expressed by some MSSA is capable of hydrolyzing cefazolin more readily than cefuroxime or cefamandole. Although this trend is disturbing, the overall incidence of cefazolin failure remains low and cefazolin remains the drug of choice for SSI prophylaxis in cardiovascular surgery.[31]

Lastly, the increase in frequency of fungal infections in surgical patients is of increasing concern. In hospitalized patients the incidence of nosocomial candida infections has approximately doubled from 1991 to 1996.[32] Overzealous use of broad-spectrum antibiotics is the most likely cause for this increase. A recent study in patients undergoing cardiovascular surgery identified sex (female), length of stay in the intensive care unit, and duration of central venous catheterization as risk factors for postoperative Candida infections.[33] Although presurgical Candida colonization is associated with a higher risk of fungal SSIs, the routine preoperative use of prophylactic antifungal agents is not being advocated at this time.[32,34]

SCHEDULING ANTIBIOTIC ADMINISTRATION

Basic principles for the use of antimicrobial surgical prophylaxis include (a) the agents should be delivered to the surgical site prior to the initial incision, and (b) bactericidal antibiotic concentrations should be maintained at the surgical site throughout the surgical procedure. Although animal and human models demonstrate the efficacy of a single dose of an antibiotic administered just prior to bacterial contamination,[35,36] long operations often require intraoperative doses of antibiotics to maintain adequate concentrations at the surgical site for the duration of the surgery.[36,37] Even though most studies that compared single versus multiple doses of prophylactic antibiotics failed to show a benefit of multidose regimens,[38] the durations of operations in these studies may not be as long as those frequently observed in clinical practice, and more research needs to be done with longer procedures.

Proponents of administering a second antibiotic dose during lengthy operations suggest that the risk for SSI is just as great at the end of surgery, during wound closing, as it is during the initial incision.[39] One study in patients undergoing clean-contaminated operations suggests that procedures longer than 3 hours require a second intraoperative dose of cefazolin or the substitution of cefazolin with a longer-acting antimicrobial agent.[40] Studies in patients undergoing cardiac surgery have demonstrated a higher infection rate among patients with undetectable antibiotic serum concentrations at the conclusion of the procedure.[41]

Antibiotics should be administered with anesthesia just prior to the initial incision. Administration of antibiotics too early may result in concentrations below the MIC toward the end of the operation, and administration too late leaves the patient unprotected at the time of the initial incision. In a study examining the timing of antibiotics in 2,847 patients receiving prophylaxis, Classen et al.[37] evaluated patients who received prophylaxis early (2 to 24 hours before surgery), preoperatively (0 to 2 hours prior to surgery), perioperative (up to 3 hours after first incision), and postoperatively (>3 hours after the first incision). The risk of infection was lowest (0.6%) for those patients who received preoperative prophylaxis, moderate (1.4%) for those who received perioperative antibiotics, and greatest for those who received either postoperative antibiotics (3.3%) or preoperative antibiotics too early (3.8%). These results indicate that the risk for a SSI increases dramatically with each hour that elapses from the initial incision, to the time when antibiotics are eventually administered. For these reasons, prophylactic antibiotics should not be prescribed to be given "on call to the OR," which can occur 2 hours or more prior to the initial incision, nor should concurrent therapeutic antibiotics be relied on to provide adequate protection. In both situations the chance for improperly timed doses is high.

Despite the importance of appropriately timed prophylactic antibiotic therapy, few patients receive antibiotics at the optimal time in relation to surgery. Potential barriers include antibiotics ordered after the patient has arrived in the operating room, delayed antibiotic preparation or delivery, and the use of antibiotics that require long infusion times. A recent study assessed the timing of prophylactic antibiotics in 100 patients and found that only 26% of patients received an antibiotic dose within 2 hours of the initial surgical incision.[42] Underlying disease states that may affect antibiotic metabolism and/or elimination should be considered when developing a prophylactic regimen. For example, patients with thermal burn and spinal cord injuries have been shown to eliminate certain classes of antibiotics, primarily the aminoglycosides and β-lactams, at unusually high rates as compared to controls.[43] Individuals undergoing cardiac bypass may have altered antibiotic disposition related to increased volume of distribution and reduced total body clearance and thus require special dosing consideration.[44]

ANTIMICROBIAL CHOICE

The choice of prophylaxis depends on the type of surgical procedure, the most frequent pathogens seen with this procedure, the safety and efficacy profile of the antimicrobial agent, the current literature evidence to support its use, and cost. Although most SSIs involve the patient's normal flora, antimicrobial selection must also consider the susceptibility patterns of nosocomial pathogens within each institution. Typically, gram-positive coverage should be included in the choice of surgical prophylaxis because organisms such as *S. aureus* and *S. epidermidis* are commonly encountered as skin flora. The decision to broaden antibiotic prophylaxis to agents with gram-negative and anaerobic spectra of activity depends on both the surgical site (e.g., upper respiratory tract, gastrointestinal tract, genitourinary tract), and whether the operation will transect a hollow viscous or mucous membrane that may contain resident flora.[3]

Although antimicrobial prophylaxis may be administered through a variety of routes (e.g., oral, topical, intramuscular), the parenteral route is favored because of the reliability by which adequate tissue concentrations may be acheived.[45] Cephalosporins are the most commonly prescribed agents for surgical prophylaxis because of their broad antimicrobial spectrum, their favorable pharmacokinetic profile, their low incidence of adverse side effects, and low cost. First-generation cephalosporins such as cefazolin are the preferred choice for surgical prophylaxis, particularly for clean surgical procedures.[3,7,17,31] In cases in which broader gram-negative and anaerobic coverage is desired, antianaerobic cephalosporins, such as cefoxitin or cefotetan, are appropriate choices. Although third-generation cephalosporins (e.g., ceftriaxone) have been advocated for prophylaxis because of their increased gram-negative coverage and prolonged half-lives, their inferior gram-positive and anaerobic activity, in addition to their high cost, has discouraged the widespread use of these agents.[3,7,17,31]

Allergic reactions are the most common side effects associated with cephalosporin use. These can range from minor skin manifestations at the site of infusion, to rash, pruritus, and on rare occasions, anaphylaxis (<0.02%). The structural similarity between penicillins and cephalosporins (each containing a β-lactam ring) has led to considerable confusion about the cross-allergenicity between these two classes of drugs. Twenty percent of the general population is labeled "penicillin-allergic," yet studies suggest that of the "penicillin-allergic"-labeled patients, only 2% to 20% will have positive results in a penicillin skin test.[46] Current literature suggests that the rate of cross-reactivity is approximately 2%, but because only 20% of all "penicillin-allergic" patients are truly penicillin-allergic, the true incidence of cross-reactivity is likely less than 1%.[47] Routine penicillin skin testing is not cost effective.[48] In summary, the administration of cephalosporins is both safe and cost-effective for many patients who are labeled "penicillin allergic," and they may be used in patients who have not experienced an immediate or type I penicillin allergy.

Vancomycin may be considered for prophylactic therapy in surgical procedures involving implantation of a prosthetic device in which the rate of methicillin-resistant *S. aureus* (MRSA) is high.[27] If the risk of MRSA is low and a β-lactam hypersensitivity exists, clindamycin can be used for many procedures instead of cefazolin in order to limit vancomycin use. Infusion-related side effects, such as thrombophlebitis and hypotension, particularly with vancomycin, can usually be controlled by adequate dilution and slower administration rates.[49,50]

Pseudomembranous colitis related to cephalosporin use is infrequent and generally easily treated with a short course of oral metronidazole, although infrequent, bleeding abnormalities related to cephalosporin use have been reported.[51] The primary hematologic effect appears to be an inhibition of vitamin K-dependent clotting factors that results in a prolongation of the prothrombin time. The mechanism for this effect, most commonly seen with cefotetan, is related to the methylthiotetrazole (NMTT) side chain of the β-lactam molecule. Most data indicate that patients at greatest risk for this hypoprothrombinemic effect have received a prolonged course of these agents and have underlying risk factors for vitamin K deficiency, such as malnutrition.[52]

Inappropriate prophylactic antibiotic use not only may induce antibiotic resistance but can also negatively affect an institution's antibiotic budget, and thus initiatives to curtail inappropriate antibiotic use have become the focus of many drug use evaluation efforts. Potential sources of inappropriate antibiotic prophylaxis include the use of broad spectrum antimicrobials when a narrow spectrum agent is warranted, extending prophylaxis for durations beyond that recommended in published guidelines, and using expensive antibiotics when equivalent, cheaper agents are available. The most effective tools to ensure appropriate prophylactic antibiotic prescribing are knowledge of one's institutional postsurgical infection rate for each type of surgical procedure, and the bacterial epidemiology patterns for each surgical population. Individualized institutional guidelines that take into account best literature evidence, institution-based antibiotic susceptibility data, and surgeon preference are also important tools to rationalize antibiotic prophylaxis use.[53,54]

RECOMMENDATIONS FOR SPECIFIC TYPES OF SURGERY

Guidelines for surgical prophylaxis are usually structured according to the affected tissues during an operation. While many different surgical procedures may be performed at any one anatomic site, this method of categorization is still optimal because the factors related to the success of a prophylactic regimen, such as the endogenous flora that is expected and the pharmacokinetics, pharmacodynamics, and spectrum of selected antimicrobials, are generally constant for a particular surgical site (see section "Antimicrobial Choice" earlier in chapter). The choice of antimicrobial prophylaxis is always best evaluated using the results of properly conducted clinical trials. In the absence of studies specific to the procedure in question, extrapolation from data on regimens for different procedures in the same anatomic site in question can usually be made. Subsequent modifications to each prophylactic regimen should be based on intraoperative findings or events.

While a comprehensive review of the surgical prophylaxis literature is beyond the scope of this chapter, there are important factors that should be reviewed for each type/site of surgery. Table 121–6 summarizes specific recommendations. The reader is also referred to recently published guidelines and review articles.[3,7,17,31]

GASTRODUODENAL SURGERY

Insignificant numbers of bacteria are usually found in the stomach and duodenum because of their acidity. The rate of SSIs in gastroduodenal surgery is generally low; thus, procedures in this region can be classified as clean procedures. The risk for a SSI in this population increases with any condition that will increase the pH of gastroduodenal secretions and subsequently lead to bacterial overgrowth, such as obstruction, hemorrhage, malignancy, or concomitant acid suppression therapy.[55] Antimicrobial prophylaxis is of clinical benefit only in this high-risk population. In most cases, a single dose of IV cefazolin will provide adequate prophylaxis.[56] For patients with a β-lactam allergy, oral ciprofloxacin is as efficacious as parenteral cefuroxime as prophylactic therapy for gastroduodenal surgery.[57] Postoperative therapeutic antibiotics may be indicated if perforation is detected during surgery, depending on whether an established infection is present.

The use of antibiotic prophylaxis for percutaneous endoscopic gastrostomy (PEG) is controversial. Although postoperative peristomal infection can occur in up to 30% of patients, clinical trials with cefazolin given 30 minutes preoperatively in this population are conflicting.[58] Recently, a pharmacoeconomic study using a meta-analysis of available studies to determine efficacy[59] suggested that antibiotic prophylaxis cost was effective for patients undergoing PEG placements.

TABLE 121–6. Most Likely Pathogens and Specific Recommendations for Surgical Prophylaxis

Type of Operation	Likely Pathogens	Recommended Prophylaxis Regimen*	Comments
Gastroduodenal	Enteric gram-negative bacilli, gram-positive cocci, oral anaerobes	Cefazolin 1 g × 1 (see text for recommendations for percutaneous endoscopic gastrostomy)	High-risk patients only (obstruction, hemorrhage, malignancy, acid suppression therapy, morbid obesity)
Biliary tract	Enteric gram-negative bacilli, anaerobes	Cefazolin 1 g × 1 for high-risk patients Laparoscopic: none	High-risk patients only (acute cholecystitis, common duct stones, previous biliary surgery, jaundice, age > 60 years, obesity, diabetes mellitus)
Colorectal	Enteric gram-negative bacilli, anaerobes	PO: neomycin 1 g + erythromycin base 1 g at 1 PM, 2 PM, and 11 PM 1 day preop plus mechanical bowel prep. IV: cefoxitin or cefotetan 1 g × 1	Benefits of oral plus IV is controversial except for colostomy reversal and rectal resection
Appendectomy	Enteric gram-negative bacilli, anaerobes	Cefoxitin or cefotetan 1 g × 1	A second intraoperative dose of cefoxitin may be required if procedure lasts longer than 3 hours
Urologic	*E. coli*	Cefazolin 1 g × 1	Generally not recommended in patients with sterile preop urine cultures
Caesarean section	Enteric gram-negative bacilli, anaerobes, group B streptococci, enterococci	Cefazolin 2 g × 1	Give after cord is clamped
Hysterectomy	Enteric gram-negative bacilli, anaerobes, group B streptococci, enterococci	Vaginal: Cefazolin 1 g × 1 Abdominal: Cefotetan 1 g × 1 or Cefazolin 1 g × 1	Antibiotic prophylaxis should not exceed 24 hours
Head and neck	*S. aureus*, streptococci, oral anaerobes	Cefazolin 2 g or clindamycin 600 mg at induction and q8h × 2 more doses	Addition of gentamicin to clindamycin is controversial
Cardiothoracic	*S. aureus, S. epidermidis*, corynebacterium, enteric gram-negative bacilli	Cefazolin 1 g q8h × 48 h	Second-generation cephalosporins have also been advocated In areas with high prevalence of *S. aureus* resistance, vancomycin should be considered
Vascular	*S. aureus, S. epidermidis*, enteric gram-negative bacilli	Cefazolin 1 g at induction and q8h × 2 more doses	Abdominal and lower extremities have the highest infection rates
Orthopedic	*S. aureus, S. epidermidis*	Joint replacement: cefazolin 1 g × 1 preop, then q8h × 2 more doses Hip fracture repair: same as above except continue for 48 hours	Open fractures assumed contaminated with gram-negative bacilli; aminoglycosides often used—see text
Neurosurgery	*S. aureus, S. epidermidis*	CSF shunt procedures: cefazolin 1 g × 1 or ceftriaxone 2 g × 1 Craniotomy: cefazolin 1 g × 1 or cefotaxime 1 g × 1 or trimethoprim-sulfamethoxazole (160/800) IV × 1	No agents have been shown better than cefazolin in randomized control comparative trials

*One-time doses are optimally infused at induction of anesthesia except as noted. Repeat doses may be required for long procedures. See text for references.

HEPATOBILIARY SURGERY

Although the bile is normally sterile, and the SSI rate after biliary surgery is low, antibiotic prophylaxis has been proven to be of benefit in this population. This is likely a result of bile contamination (bactibilia) increasing the frequency of SSIs and being present in many patients (e.g., acute cholecystitis, biliary obstruction, and advanced age).[60] In general, however, the correlation between bactibilia in surgical specimens and the subsequent pathogens implicated in a SSI is poor. The most frequently encountered organisms include *E. coli*, *Klebsiella* spp., and *Enterococcus* spp. *Pseudomonas* is an uncommon finding in the absence of cholangitis. Trials comparing first-, second-, and third-generation cephalosporins have not demonstrated benefit over single-dose cefazolin prophylaxis, even in high-risk patients (e.g., age >60, previous biliary surgery, acute cholecystitis, jaundice, obesity, diabetes, common bile duct stones).[61] Ciprofloxacin is an effective alternative for β-lactam allergic patients undergoing open cholecystectomy.[62] For low-risk patients undergoing elective laparoscopic cholecystectomy, antibiotic prophylaxis has not been shown to be of benefit and is not recommended.[63] The risk for SSIs in cirrhotic patients undergoing transjugular intrahepatic portosystemic shunt (TIPS) surgery may be reduced with a single prophylactic dose of ceftriaxone,[64] but not with single doses of shorter acting cephalosporins.[65] Antibiotic prophylaxis is not currently recommended prior to endoscopic retrograde cholangiopancreatography (ERCP).[66]

Although surgeons may use presumptive antibiotic therapy for patients with acute cholecystitis or cholangitis and defer surgery until the patient is afebrile in an effort to decrease the risk of subsequent infections, this practice is controversial. Detection of an active infection during surgery (e.g., gangrenous gallbladder, suppurative cholangitis) is an indication for a course of postoperative therapeutic antibiotics. In either case, antibiotics with additional antianaerobic activity (e.g., cefoxitin or cefotetan) are indicated.[67]

COLORECTAL SURGERY

In the absence of adequate prophylactic therapy, the risk for SSI after colorectal surgery is large because of the significant bacterial counts in fecal material present in the colon (it frequently exceeds 10^9 per gram). Anaerobes and gram-negative aerobes predominate, although gram-positive aerobes may also play an important role. Risk factors for SSIs include age >60 years, hypoalbuminemia, poor preoperative bowel preparation, corticosteroid therapy, malignancy and operations lasting longer than 3.5 hours.[7] Antimicrobial prophylaxis reduced mortality from 11.2% to 4.5% in a pooled analysis of trials comparing antimicrobial prophylaxis to no prophylaxis for colon surgery.[68] Reducing this bacteria load with a thorough bowel preparation regimen (4 L of polyethylene glycol solution or 90 mL of sodium phosphate solution administered orally the day before surgery) is the single most important method of SSI prevention.[69]

Effective antibiotic prophylaxis reduces the risk for a SSI risk even further. Several oral regimens designed to reduce bacterial counts in the colon have been studied.[70] The combination of 1 g of neomycin and 1 g of erythromycin base given orally 19, 18, and 9 hours preoperatively is the most commonly used regimen in the United States.[70] Neomycin, although poorly absorbed, provides intraluminal concentrations that are high enough to effectively kill most gram-negative aerobes. Oral erythromycin, although partially absorbed, still produces concentrations in the colon that are sufficient to suppress common anaerobes. If surgery is postponed, the antibiotics must be readministered to maintain efficacy. Optimally, the bowel preparation regimen should be completed prior to starting the oral antibiotic regimen. This is of particular concern because most procedures are now performed electively on a "same day surgery" basis. In this case, the bowel preparation regimen is self-administered by the patient at home, on the day prior to hospital admission, and thus compliance cannot be carefully monitored.

Patients who cannot take oral medications should receive parenteral antibiotics. Cefoxitin or cefotetan are most commonly used but a variety of other second generation and some third-generation cephalosporins are also effective.[71] The addition of metronidazole to cephalosporin therapy has not resulted in additional benefit in most comparative studies.[72] For β-lactam-allergic patients, perioperative doses of gentamicin and metronidazole have been used.[73] It remains controversial whether the addition of preoperative parenteral antibiotics, to the standard preoperative oral antibiotic regimen described above, will decrease SSI rates lower than oral prophylaxis alone, however, combination therapy is superior to parenteral therapy alone.[74,75] Postoperative antibiotics are generally unnecessary in the absence of any untoward events or findings during surgery. Intravenous antibiotics are required for colostomy reversal and rectal resection, because enterally administered antibiotics will not reach the distal segment that is to be reanastomosed or resected.[74,76] The role for supplemental perioperative oxygen during colorectal resection was recently studied.[77] Patients who received 80% inspired oxygen perioperatively had half (5%) the incidence of SSIs as compared to patients receiving 30% inspired oxygen (11%). The authors concluded that oxygen augmented the bactericidal activity of neutrophils by boosting superoxide radical production and oxidative killing and recommended its routine use.

APPENDECTOMY

Suspected appendicitis is a frequent cause for abdominal surgery. Numerous antibiotic regimens, all with activity against gram-positive, gram-negative aerobes and anaerobic pathogens have been studied and found to be effective in reducing SSI incidence. A cephalosporin with antianaerobic activity, such as cefoxitin or cefotetan, is recommended as first-line therapy; however, a comparative trial of cefoxitin and cefotetan suggests that cefotetan may be superior, possibly because of its longer duration of action.[78] In the case of β-lactam allergy, metronidazole in combination with gentamicin is also an effective regimen.[79] Broad-spectrum antibiotics covering nosocomial pathogens (i.e., *Pseudomonas*) have not been shown to further reduce SSI risk,[80] and, instead, may increase the cost of therapy and promote bacterial resistance. Although single-dose therapy with cefotetan is adequate, prophylaxis with cefoxitin may require intraoperative dosing if the procedure extends beyond 3 hours in duration. Established intra-abdominal infections (e.g., gangrenous or perforated appendix) require an appropriate course of postoperative therapeutic antibiotics. Laparoscopic appendectomy is reported to produce lower postoperative infection rates than open appendectomy; however, antimicrobial prophylaxis was used in all patients in these studies, thus the role for prophylaxis in this population remains unstudied.[81]

UROLOGIC PROCEDURES

Preoperative bacteruria is the most important risk factor for development of a SSI after urologic surgery. All patients should have a pre operative urinalysis prior to surgery and should receive *therapeutic* antibiotics if bacteruria is detected. Patients with sterile urine preoperatively are at low risk for developing a SSI and the benefit of *prophylactic* antibiotics in this setting is controversial.[82] Recent reviews suggest that antibiotic prophylaxis is warranted in high-risk patients (e.g., prolonged indwelling catheterization, positive urine cultures, neutropenia) undergoing transurethral, perineal, or suprapubic resection of the prostate, resection of bladder tumors, or cystoscopy.[82] The exact incidence of SSIs in this population is obscured, however, by the frequent use of postoperative urinary catheters and the subsequent risk of bacteriuria. *E. coli* is the most frequently encountered organism. Routine use of broad-spectrum antibiotics such as third-generation cephalosporins and fluoroquinolones do not decrease SSI rates more than cefazolin and are not recommended. A recent comparative trial determined that a single dose of oral ciprofloxacin was as effective as intravenous cefazolin and suggested that this may be a cheaper and easier alternative for outpatient urologic surgery.[83] Regimens longer than a single dose have not been shown to improve outcome. Urologic procedures requiring an abdominal approach, such as a nephrectomy or cystectomy, require antibiotic prophylaxis similar to that which would be used for a clean-contaminated abdominal procedure.[82]

CAESAREAN SECTION

Caesarean section is the most frequently performed surgical procedure in the United States.[7] Prophylactic antibiotics are given to avoid endometritis, the most commonly occurring SSI. In the past, antibiotics were recommended only for "high-risk" patients, including those with premature membrane rupture, or those not receiving prenatal care. Recently, several large trials, as well as a meta-analysis, have shown benefit in administering prophylactic antibiotics to all women undergoing emergent caesarean section regardless of their underlying risk factors.[84] Cefazolin remains the drug of choice despite a wide spectrum of potential pathogens.[85] Providing a broader spectrum of coverage with cefoxitin (for anaerobes) or piperacillin (for *Pseudomonas* or enterococci), does not appear to lower postoperative infection rates further.[84] For patients with a β-lactam allergy, preoperative metronidazole is an acceptable alternative.[86]

Unlike most other surgical procedures, a single 2-g dose of cefazolin is superior to a 1-g dose and should therefore be used.[87] During a caesarean section, unlike other surgical procedures, antibiotics should be administered *after* the initial incision is made and after the umbilical cord is clamped. This minimizes infant drug exposure and potentially decreases the incidence of neonatal sepsis. Longer durations of prophylactic therapy have not been shown to result in lower infection rates.[88]

HYSTERECTOMY

The most important factor affecting the incidence of SSI after hysterectomy is the type of procedure that is performed. Vaginal hysterectomies are associated with a high rate of postoperative infection when performed without the benefit of prophylactic antibiotics because of the polymicrobial flora normally present at the operative site.[89] As with caesarean sections, cefazolin is the drug of choice for vaginal hysterectomies despite the wide spectrum of possible pathogens.[89] Single-dose therapy should be adequate, but most reports use a 24-hour regimen. The American College of Obstetricians and Gynecologists (ACOG) recommends the use of a first-, second-, or third-generation cephalosporin.[90] For patients with a β-lactam allergy, a single preoperative dose of doxycycline is also effective.[91]

Prophylactic antibiotics are recommended for abdominal hysterectomy despite the lack of bacterial contamination from the vaginal flora. Both cefazolin and antianaerobic cephalosporins (e.g., cefoxitin, cefotetan) have been studied extensively.[92] Single-dose cefotetan has been shown to be superior to single-dose cefazolin,[93] and the investigators suggest that cefotetan should be the drug of choice for abdominal hysterectomies; other authors, however, suggest that either agent is appropriate provided that 24 hours of antimicrobial coverage is not exceeded.[7] ACOG guidelines suggest that first-, second-, or third-generation cephalosporins can be used for prophylaxis.[90] Metronidazole is also effective and may be used if patients are allergic to β-lactam antibiotics.[92] Recent evidence suggests that antibiotic prophylaxis may not be required in laparoscopic gynecologic surgery or tubal microsurgery.[94] Similar to other surgical procedures, perioperative events and findings may require the use of *therapeutic* antibiotics after surgery.

HEAD AND NECK SURGERY

Use of prophylactic antibiotics during head and neck surgery depends on the procedure type. Clean procedures (as per NRC definition), such as parotidectomy or simple tooth extraction, are associated with a very low incidence of SSI. Head and neck procedures involving an incision through a mucosal layer, carry with them a higher risk for SSI. The normal flora of the mouth is polymicrobial; both anaerobes and gram-positive aerobes predominate. Although typical doses of cefazolin are usually ineffective for anaerobic infections, a 2-g dose produces concentrations high enough to inhibit these organisms. A recent pharmacokinetic study suggests that a single dose of clindamycin is adequate for prophylaxis in maxillofacial surgery unless the procedure lasts longer than 4 hours, in which event, a second dose should be administered intraoperatively.[95] A combination of clindamycin plus gentamicin has also been described, but was found to offer no advantage over clindamycin alone.[96] There is no additional benefit in extending therapy beyond 24 hours.[31] Topical therapy with clindamycin, amoxicillin/clavulanate, and ticarcillin/clavulanate have been described in small trials, but the exact role for topical antibiotics has yet to be defined.[97]

CARDIOTHORACIC SURGERY

Although cardiac surgery is generally considered a clean procedure, antibiotic prophylaxis does lower SSI incidence. The substantial morbidity related to a SSI in this population coupled with the routine implementation of prosthetic devices in this population further justifies the routine use of prophylaxis.[98] Patients who develop SSIs after coronary artery bypass graft (CABG) surgery have a mortality rate of 22% at 1 year as compared to 0.6% for those patients who do not develop a SSI.[99] Risk factors for developing a SSI after cardiac surgery include obesity, renal insufficiency, connective tissue disease, reexploration for bleeding, and poorly timed administration of antibiotics.[98] Skin flora pathogens predominate; gram-negative organisms are rare.

Cefazolin has been extensively studied and is considered the drug of choice.[30] Although several studies and a meta-analysis have been published that advocate the use of second-generation cephalosporins (e.g., cefuroxime) rather than cefazolin, various methodologic flaws in these studies have limited the extrapolation of these results to practice. Cefazolin has been shown to be as effective as cefuroxime in a large randomized trial of 702 patients undergoing open heart surgery and thus remains the standard of care.[100] Both patient weight and timing of cefazolin administration relative to surgery must be considered when developing a dosing strategy. Patients weighing more than 80 kg should receive 2 g of cefazolin rather than 1 g. Doses should be administered no earlier than 60 minutes before the first incision and no later than at the beginning of induction.[98] Extending therapy beyond 48 hours does not lower SSI rates further.[101] Recent evidence suggests that single dose cefazolin therapy may in fact be sufficient.[102]

Routine vancomycin administration is potentially justified in hospitals having a high incidence of MRSA or when sternal wounds are to be explored surgically for possible mediastinitis. In this latter situation, mediastinitis constitutes a failure of a prior prophylactic regimen. Continued postoperative vancomycin should be guided by culture and sensitivity data.[48] Subsequent antibiotic therapy is guided by intraoperative findings.

Pulmonary resection is associated with significant SSI risk and prophylactic antibiotics have an established role in preventing postoperative infectious morbidity. First-generation cephalosporins are inadequate; 48 hours of cefuroxime is preferred.[103] A regimen of ampicillin/sulbactam is superior to first-generation cephalosporins; however, further studies are required before this agent can be recommended as first-line prophylactic therapy.[104]

VASCULAR SURGERY

Vascular surgery, like cardiac surgery, is generally considered a "clean" surgery by NRC criteria. A SSI in this setting, however, may result in extensive morbidity and mortality, particularly when a prosthetic graft is involved. Prophylactic antibiotics are of benefit, particularly for procedures involving the abdominal aorta and the lower extremities. Cefazolin is regarded as the drug of choice.[105] Twenty-four hours of prophylaxis with IV cefazolin is adequate; longer courses may lead to bacterial resistance.[106] For patients with β-lactam allergy, 24 hours of oral ciprofloxacin has also been shown to be effective.[107]

ORTHOPEDIC SURGERY

Most orthopedic surgery is clean by definition and thus prophylactic antibiotics are generally indicated only when prosthetic materials (e.g., pins, plates, artificial joints) are implanted.[108] A late-occurring infectious complication in this surgical population can result in substantial morbidity and may lead to prosthesis failure and subsequent removal. Staphylococci are the most frequently encountered pathogens; gram-negative aerobes are infrequent. Similar to many other surgical sites, cefazolin use is supported by substantial literature evidence and is, therefore, the prophylactic agent of choice. Vancomycin, although effective, is not recommended for routine use unless a patient has a documented history of a serious allergy to β-lactams or the propensity for MRSA infections at a particular institution necessitates its use. The current recommended duration of treatment for joint replacement and hip fracture surgery is 24 hours.[7] Antibiotic-impregnated cement and beads have been used to lower SSI rates but conclusive data regarding their efficacy are lacking.[108]

Patients suffering open (compound) fractures are particularly susceptible to infection because bacterial contamination has almost always already occurred. The use of antibiotics is *presumptive* under these circumstances. Cefazolin is often combined with an aminoglycoside in this setting, but controlled trials are lacking.[109] A recent clinical trial comparing clindamycin and cloxacillin suggest that clindamycin is superior and may be appropriate as monotherapy for Gustilo Type I and Type II open fractures, but not for Gustilo Type III fractures for which added gram-negative activity is recommended.[110] Duration of antibiotic therapy is highly variable and depends on surgical findings during débridement, results of intraoperative cultures, and clinical status.[111] Established joint infections and osteomyelitis require an extended course of *therapeutic* antibiotics.

NEUROSURGERY

Definitive recommendations on the role of antibiotic prophylaxis in neurosurgery cannot yet be made at this time.[112] While the rates of SSI after these generally clean operations are low, the morbidity and mortality of SSI, should it occur, is high. Procedures involving cerebrospinal fluid (CSF) shunt placement should be considered separately as this involves placement of a foreign body and is associated with higher infection rates. When choosing an antibiotic, one must not only consider the spectrum of activity, but also the penetration of the agent into the site of action (CSF). A meta-analysis suggests that single doses of cefazolin or, where required, vancomycin appear to lower SSI risk after craniotomy.[113] The largest prospective randomized trial to date of 826 patients undergoing clean neurosurgical procedures suggested that a single dose of ceftizoxime was as effective as a combination regimen of single-dose vancomycin and gentamicin. The authors also report that ceftizoxime was better tolerated and more consistently achieved adequate CSF levels to inhibit the most common organisms.[114] A more recent study of 780 patients undergoing neurosurgical procedures, that include shunt surgery, reported that single doses of cefotaxime and trimethoprim-sulfamethoxazole are equally effective in preventing SSIs.[115] Studies performed on procedures involving a shunt have been small in size and do not consistently show lower infection rates with antibiotic prophylaxis, although the results of two meta-analysis suggests they may.[116,117] Because no trials have shown superiority of any one agent, single doses of cefazolin appears to be an acceptable choice.[113]

SSIs associated with spinal surgery are rare but devastating when they occur. Large randomized, controlled trials are lacking but cefazolin is the antibiotic most commonly recommended.[118] Recently, it was suggested that the cefazolin's penetration into both intervertebral disks and CSF may be inadequate and that a combination of cefuroxime and gentamicin may be better. There is a paucity of clinical trials comparing these two regimens.[119]

PHARMACOECONOMIC IMPLICATIONS

It is paramount to consider the cost implications of pharmacotherapy guidelines that affect a large number of patients. Although investigators have incorporated basic financial analysis into the results of antibiotic prophylaxis comparative trials,[48,54,59,99] robust pharmacoeconomic studies of various regimens of antimicrobial prophylaxis in surgery are lacking. Most of these studies are cost-minimization studies because only drug acquisition costs were considered. Studies that incorporate all relevant drug and treatment costs in relation to pertinent patient outcomes such as incidence of SSIs, hospital length of stay, and antibiotic-related adverse events are needed.

THERAPEUTIC OUTCOME EVALUATION

When evaluating the outcome of surgical antibiotic prophylaxis, it is important to differentiate any potential SSI from other postoperative infection(s) or complication(s). While fever and leukocytosis are common in the immediate postoperative period, they typically resolve with prompt ambulation, timely removal of invasive devices, prevention and/or resolution of atelectasis through optimal respiratory care, and effective analgesia. It is also important to remember that the emergence of distal infections, such as pneumonia, do not constitute a failure of surgical prophylaxis. Prophylaxis should be as short as possible as prolonged prophylactic regimens may contribute to the selection of resistant organisms and make any infection more difficult to treat.

Surgical site appearance is the most important determinant of the presence of an infection. Drainage of pus from the incision accompanied by redness, warmth, and pain or tenderness are highly suggestive of an SSI. By definition, any surgical site that requires incision and drainage by the surgeon is considered infected regardless of appearance. Failure to heal and wound dehiscence are also commonly seen with SSIs, although surgical technique and nutritional status may be important contributing factors.

The presentation of signs and symptoms consistent with a SSI, in relation to previous surgery, is an important consideration when evaluating therapeutic outcomes after surgical prophylaxis. Many SSIs will not be evident during acute hospitalization. In fact, surgical site infections may not become evident until up to 30 days later, or in the case of prosthesis implantation, up to 1 year later. Thus the true incidence of SSI, can only be determined by completing comprehensive postdischarge surveillance. All studies investigating the efficacy of surgical prophylaxis must include adequate postdischarge follow-up in order to be able to thoroughly assess the success of any prophylactic regimen.

▶ PRINCIPLES OF PHARMACOTHERAPY

Antimicrobial prophylaxis is a key component of surgical care. The incidence of SSIs can be substantially reduced with the appropriate use of prophylaxis. Indiscriminate use, however, may lead to increased antimicrobial resistance and unnecessary cost. The following principles should be considered when designing an antimicrobial prophylactic regimen for patients undergoing surgery:

- Prophylaxis with antimicrobials is only one component of perioperative infection prevention. A definitive surgical procedure employing optimal aseptic technique is the best defense against SSI.
- The choice of antibiotics depends on intrinsic patient risk, and type of surgical procedure. First-generation cephalosporins (cefazolin), because of their spectrum of activity, safety, and cost, remain the mainstay for antimicrobial prophylaxis for the most procedures.
- Appropriate timing of prophylactic antibiotic administration is crucial. Optimally, doses should be administered within 1 hour of incision. The use of "on call to OR" regimens or relying on current therapeutic antibiotic therapy results in improperly timed doses and leads to increased SSI risk.
- Broad-spectrum antibiotics administered over a prolonged period will increase costs and adverse effects without lowering SSI incidence.
- Postdischarge surveillance is necessary to determine true SSI incidence.
- Vancomycin as a prophylactic agent should be limited to those cases in which there is a documented history of life-threatening β-lactam hypersensitivity or where the incidence of infections with organisms resistant to cefazolin (e.g., MRSA) is high enough to justify use.
- Single-dose prophylactic regimens are effective for many types of surgery.

REFERENCES

1. Mitka M. Preventing surgical infection is more important than ever. JAMA 2000;283:44–45.
2. de Lalla F. Antimicrobial chemotherapy in the control of surgical infectious complications. J Chemother 1999;11:440–445.
3. Mangram AJ, Horan TC, Pearson ML, et al. Guideline for prevention of surgical site infection, 1999. Centers for Disease Control and Prevention (CDC) Hospital Infection Control Practices Advisory Committee. Am J Infect Control 1999;27:97–132.
4. Polk HC, Christmas AB. Prophylactic antibiotics in surgery and surgical wound infections. Am Surg 2000;66:105–111.
5. National Academy of Sciences—National Research Council. Postoperative wound infections: The influence of ultraviolet irradiation of the operating room and of various other factors. Ann Surg 1964;160: 32–135.
6. Cruse PJE, Foord R. A five-year prospective study of 23,649 surgical wounds. Arch Surg 1973;107:206–210.
7. American Society of Health-System Pharmacists Commission on Therapeutics. ASHP therapeutic guidelines on antimicrobial prophylaxis in surgery. In: Deffenbaugh J, ed. Best Practices for Health System Pharmacy. Bethesda, MD, ASHP, 1999:349–396.
8. Furnary AP, Zerr KJ, Grunkemeier GL, Starr A. Continuous intravenous insulin infusion reduces the incidence of deep sternal wound infection in diabetic patients after cardiac surgical procedures. Ann Thorac Surg 1999;67:352–360.
9. The Veterans Affairs Total Parenteral Nutrition Cooperative Study Group. Perioperative total parenteral nutrition in surgical patients. N Engl J Med 1991;325:525–532.
10. Kluytmans JA, Mouton JW, VandenBergh MF, et al. Reduction of surgical-site infections in cardiothoracic surgery by elimination of nasal carriage of *Staphylococcus aureus*. Infect Control Hosp Epidemiol 1996;17:780–785.
11. Masahiko Y, Yuichiro D, Masatoshi I, et al. Preoperative intranasal mupirocin ointment significantly reduces postoperative infection with *Staphylococcus aureus* in patients undergoing upper gastrointestinal surgery. Surg Today 2000;30:16–21.
12. Haley RW, Culver DH, Morgan WM, et al. Identifying patients at high risk of surgical wound infection: A simple multivariate index of patient susceptibility and wound contamination. Am J Epidemiol 1985;121: 206–215.
13. Weigelt JA, Dryer D, Haley RW. The necessity and efficiency of wound surveillance after discharge. Arch Surg 1992;127:77–82.
14. Culver DH, Horan TC, Gaynes RP, et al. Surgical wound infection rates by wound class, operative procedure, and patient risk index. Am J Med 1991;91(suppl 3B):152S–157S.
15. Owens WD, Felts JA, Spitznagel EL. ASA physical status classifications: A study of consistency of ratings. Anesthesiology 1978;49:239–243.
16. McConkey SJ, L'Ecuyer PB, Murphy DM, et al. Results of a comprehensive infection control program for reducing surgical-site infections in coronary artery bypass surgery. Infect Control Hosp Epidemiol 1999;20:533–538.
17. Gyssens IC. Preventing postoperative infections: Current treatment recommendations. Drugs 1999;57:175–185.
18. Elek SD, Conen PE. The virulence of *Staphylococcus pyogenes* for man: A study of the problems of wound infection. Br J Exp Pathol 1958;38:573–586.
19. Burke JF. Identification of the sources of staphylococci contaminating the surgical wound during operation. Ann Surg 1963;158:898–904.
20. Kaiser AB, Kernodle DS, Parker RA. Low-inoculum model of surgical wound infection. J Infect Dis 1992;166:393–399.
21. Meakins JL, Pietsch JB, Bubenick O, et al. Delayed hypersensitivity: Indicator of acquired failure of host defenses in sepsis and trauma. Ann Surg 1977;186:241–250.
22. Christou NV, McLean APH, Meakins JL. Host defense in blunt trauma: Interrelationships of kinetics of anergy and depressed neutrophil function, nutritional status and sepsis. J Trauma 1980;20:833–841.
23. Richet HM, Chidiac C, Prat A, et al. Analysis of risk factors for surgical wound infections following vascular surgery. Am J Med 1991;91: (suppl 3b):170S–172S.
24. Zimmerli W, Waldvogel FA, Vaudaux P, et al. Pathogenesis of foreign body infection: Description and characteristics of an animal model. J Infect Dis 1987;146:487–497.
25. Schaberg D. Major trends in the microbial etiology of nosocomial infection. Am J Med 1991;91(suppl 3B):72S–75S.
26. Murray BE. Vancomycin-resistant enterococcal infections. N Engl J Med 2000;342:710–721.
27. Hospital Infection Control Practices Advisory Committee. Recommendations for preventing the spread of vancomycin resistance. MMWR Morb Mortal Wkly Rep 1995;44:1–13.

28. Centers for Disease Control and Prevention. Interim guidelines for prevention and control of *Staphylococcus aureus* infection associated with reduced susceptibility to vancomycin. MMWR Morb Mortal Wkly Rep 1997;46:626–635.
29. Kaiser AB, Petracek, MR, Lea JW IV, et al. Efficacy of cefazolin, cefamandole, and gentamicin as prophylactic agents in cardiac surgery. Ann Surg 1987;206:791–797.
30. Ariano RE, Zhanel GG. Antimicrobial prophylaxis in coronary bypass surgery: A critical appraisal. DICP 1991;25:478–484.
31. Anonymous. Antimicrobial prophylaxis in surgery. Med Lett Drugs Ther 1997;39:97–102.
32. Munoz P, Burrillo A, Bouza E. Criteria used when initiating antifungal therapy against *Candida* spp. in the intensive care unit. Int J Antimicrob Agents 2000;15:83–90.
33. Tran LT, Auger P, Marchand R, et al. Epidemiological study of *Candida* spp. colonization in cardiovascular surgical patients. Mycoses 1997;40:169–173.
34. Pittet D, Monod M, Suter PM, et al. Candida colonization and subsequent infections in critically ill surgical patients. Ann Surg 1994;220:751–758.
35. Burke JF. The effective period of preventive antibiotic action in experimental incisions and dermal lesions. Surgery 1961;50:161–168.
36. DiPiro JT, Cheung RPF, Bowden TA, Mansberger JA. Single-dose systemic antibiotic prophylaxis of surgical wound infections. Am J Surg 1986;152:552–559.
37. Classen DC, Evans RS, Pestotnik SL, et al. The timing of prophylactic administration of antibiotics and the risk of surgical wound infection. N Engl J Med 1992;326:281–286.
38. Novelli A. Antimicrobial prophylaxis in surgery: The role of pharmacokinetics. J Chemother 1999;11:565–572.
39. Esposito S. Is single-dose antibiotic prophylaxis sufficient for any surgical procedure? J Chemother 1999;11:556–564.
40. Scher KS. Studies on the duration of antibiotic administration for surgical prophylaxis. Am Surg 1997;63:59–62.
41. Goldman DA, Hopkins CC, Karchmer AW. Cephalothin prophylaxis in cardiac valve surgery: A prospective, double-blind comparison of two-day and six-day regimen. J Thorac Cardiovasc Surg 1977;73:470–479.
42. Collier PE, Rudolph M, Ruckert D, et al. Are preoperative antibiotics administered preoperatively? Am J Med Qual 1998;13:94–97.
43. Weinbren MJ. Pharmacokinetics of antibiotics in burn patients. J Antimicrob Chemother 1999;44:319–327.
44. Lewis DR, Longman RJ, Wisheart JD, et al. The pharmacokinetics of a single dose of gentamicin (4 mg/kg) as prophylaxis in cardiac surgery requiring cardiopulmonary bypass. Cardiovasc Surg 1999;7:398–401.
45. Dellinger EP, Gross PA, Barrett TL, et al. Quality standard for antimicrobial prophylaxis in surgical procedures. Clin Infect Dis 1994;18:422–427.
46. Gadde J, Spence M, Wheeler B, Adkinson NF Jr. Clinical experience with penicillin skin testing in a large inner-city STD clinic. JAMA 1993;270: 2456–2463.
47. Kishiyama JL, Adelman DC. The cross-reactivity and immunology of beta-lactam antibiotics. Drug Saf 1994;10:318–327.
48. Phillips E, Louie M, Knowles SR, et al. Cost-effectiveness analysis of six strategies for cardiovascular surgery prophylaxis in patients labeled penicillin allergic. Am J Health Syst Pharm 2000;57:339–345.
49. Romanelli VA, Howie MB, Myerowitz PD, et al. Intraoperative and postoperative effects of vancomycin administration in cardiac surgery patients: A prospective, double-blind, randomized trial. Crit Care Med 1993;21:1124–1131.
50. Polk RE. Anaphylactoid reactions to glycopeptide antibiotics. J Antimicrob Chemother 1991;27(suppl B):17–29.
51. Sattler FR, Weitekamp MR, Ballard JO. Potential for bleeding with the new beta-lactam antibiotics. Ann Intern Med 1986;105:924–931.
52. Williams KJ, Bax RP, Brown H, Machin SJ. Antibiotic treatment and associated prolonged prothrombin time. J Clin Pathol 1991;44:738–741.
53. Welch L, Teague AC, Knight BA, et al. A quality management approach to optimizing delivery and administration of preoperative antibiotics. Clin Perform Qual Health Care 1998;6:168–171.
54. Frighetto L, Marra CA, Stiver HG, et al. Economic impact of standardized orders for antimicrobial prophylaxis program. Ann Pharmacother 2000;34:154–160.
55. LoCicero J, Nichols RL. Sepsis after gastroduodenal operations: Relationship to gastric acid, motility, and endogenous microflora. South Med J 1980;73:878–880.
56. Lewis RT, Goodall RG, Marien B, et al. Efficacy and distribution of single-dose preoperative antibiotic prophylaxis in high-risk gastroduodenal surgery. Can J Surg 1991;34:117–122.
57. McArdle CS, Morran CG, Anderson JR, et al. Oral ciprofloxacin as prophylaxis in gastroduodenal surgery. J Hosp Infect 1995;30:211–216.
58. Jain NK, Larson DE, Schroeder KW, et al. Antibiotic prophylaxis for percutaneous endoscopic gastrostomy. A prospective, randomized, double-blind clinical trial. Ann Intern Med 1987;107:824–828.
59. Kulling D, Sonnenberg A, Fried M, Bauerfeind P. Cost analysis of antibiotic prophylaxis for PEG. Gastrointest Endosc 2000;51:152–156.
60. Meijer WS, Schmitz PIM, Jeekel J. Meta-analysis of randomized controlled clinical trials of antibiotic prophylaxis in biliary tract surgery. Br J Surg 1990;77:283–290.
61. Jewesson PJ, Stiver G, Wai A, et al. Double-blind comparison of cefazolin and ceftizoxime for prophylaxis against infections following elective biliary tract surgery. Antimicrob Agents Chemother 1996;40:70–74.
62. Agrawal CS, Sehgal R, Singh RK, Gupta AK. Antibiotic prophylaxis in elective cholecystectomy: A randomized, double blinded study comparing ciprofloxacin and cefuroxime. Indian J Physiol Pharmacol 1999; 43:501–504.
63. Tocchi A, Lepre L, Costa G, et al. The need for antibiotic prophylaxis in elective laparoscopic cholecystectomy: A prospective randomized study. Arch Surg 2000;135:67–70.
64. Gulberg V, Deibert P, Ochs A, et al. Prevention of infectious complications after transjugular intrahepatic portosystemic shunt in cirrhotic patients with a single dose of ceftriaxone. Hepatogastroenterology 1999; 46:1126–1130.
65. Deibert P, Schwartz S, Olschewski M, et al. Risk factors and prevention of early infection after implantation or revision of transjugular intrahepatic portosystemic shunts: Results of a randomized study. Dig Dis Sci 1998;43:1708–1713.
66. Harris A, Chan AC, Torres-Viera C, et al. Meta-analysis of antibiotic prophylaxis in endoscopic retrograde cholangiopancreatography (ERCP). Endoscopy 1999;31:718–724.
67. Sheen-Chen SM, Chen WJ, Eng HL, et al. Bacteriology and antimicrobial choice in hepatolithiasis. Am J Infect Control 2000;28:298–301.
68. Baum ML, Anish DS, Chalmers TC, et al. A survey of clinical trials of antibiotic prophylaxis in colon surgery: Evidence against further use of no-treatment controls. N Engl J Med 1981;305:795–799.
69. Oliveira L, Wexner SD, Daniel N, et al. Mechanical bowel preparation for elective colorectal surgery. A prospective, randomized, surgeon-blinded trial comparing sodium phosphate and polyethylene glycol-based oral lavage solutions. Dis Colon Rectum 1997;40:585–591.
70. Solla JA, Rothenberger DA. Preoperative bowel preparation. A survey of colon and rectal surgeons. Dis Colon Rectum 1990;33:154–159.
71. Jewesson P, Chow A, Wai A, et al. A double-blind, randomized study of three antimicrobial regimens in the prevention of infections after colorectal surgery. Diagn Microbiol Infect Dis 1997;29:155–165.
72. Zanella E, Rulli F. A multicenter randomized trial of prophylaxis with intravenous cefepime + metronidazole or ceftriaxone + metronidazole in colorectal surgery. The 230 Study Group. J Chemother 2000;12: 63–71.
73. McDonald PJ, Karran SJ. A comparison of intravenous cefoxitin and a combination of gentamicin and metronidazole as prophylaxis in colorectal surgery. Dis Colon Rectum 1983;26:661–664.
74. DiPiro JT. Short-term prophylaxis in clean-contaminated surgery. J Chemother 1999;11:551–555.
75. Song F, Glenny AM. Antimicrobial prophylaxis in colorectal surgery: A systematic review of randomized controlled trials. Br J Surg 1998; 1232–1241.

76. Ghorra SG, Rzeczycki TP, Natarajan R, Pricolo VE. Colostomy closure: Impact of preoperative risk factors on morbidity. Am Surg 1999;65:266–269.
77. Greif R, Akca O, Horn EP, et al. Supplemental perioperative oxygen to reduce the incidence of surgical-wound infection. N Engl J Med 2000; 342:161–167.
78. Liberman MA, Greason KL, Frame S, Ragland JJ. Single-dose cefotetan or cefoxitin versus multiple-dose cefoxitin as prophylaxis in patients undergoing appendectomy for acute nonperforated appendicitis. J Am Coll Surg 1995;180:77–80.
79. Lau WY, Fan ST, Chu KW, et al. Cefoxitin versus gentamicin and metronidazole in prevention of post-appendicectomy sepsis: A randomized, prospective trial. J Antimicrob Chemother 1986;18:613–619.
80. Lau WY, Fan ST, Chu KW, et al. Randomized, prospective, and double-blind trial of new β-lactams in the treatment of appendicitis. Antimicrob Agents Chemother 1985;28:639–642.
81. Chung RS, Rowland DY, Li P, Diaz J. A meta-analysis of randomized controlled trials of laparoscopic versus conventional appendectomy. Am J Surg 1999;177:250–256.
82. Olson ES, Cookson BD. Do antimicrobials have a role in preventing septicaemia following instrumentation of the urinary tract? J Hosp Infect 2000;45:85–97.
83. Christiano AP, Hollowell CM, Kim H, et al. Double-blind randomized comparison of single-dose ciprofloxacin versus intravenous cefazolin in patients undergoing outpatient endourologic surgery. Urology 2000;55:182–185.
84. Smaill F, Hofmeyr GJ. Antibiotic prophylaxis for cesarean section. Cochrane Database Syst Rev 2000;(2):CD000933.
85. Rouzi AA, Khalifa F, Ba'aqeel H, et al. The routine use of cefazolin in cesarean section. Int J Gynaecol Obstet 2000;69:107–112.
86. Elyan A, Mahran M, el Maraghy M, Abou-Seeda M. Prophylactic intravenous metronidazole in cesarean section. Chemioterapia 1984;3:67–70.
87. Faro S, Martens MG, Hammill HA, et al. Antibiotic prophylaxis: Is there a difference? Am J Obstet Gynecol 1990;162:900–909.
88. Hopkins L, Smaill F. Antibiotic prophylaxis regimens and drugs for cesarean section. Cochrane Database Syst Rev 2000;(2):CD001136.
89. Giuliani B, Periti E, Mecacci, F. Antimicrobial prophylaxis in obstetric and gynecological surgery. J Chemother 1999;11:577–580.
90. American College of Obstetricians and Gynecologists. Antibiotics and gynecologic infections. Int J Gynaecol Obstet 1997;58:333–340.
91. Hemsell DL, Hemsell PG, Nobles BJ. Doxycycline and cefamandole prophylaxis for premenopausal women undergoing vaginal hysterectomy. Surg Gynecol Obstet 1985;161:462–464.
92. Mittendorf R, Aronson MP, Berry RE, et al. Avoiding serious infections associated with abdominal hysterectomy: A meta-analysis of antibiotic prophylaxis. Am J Obstet Gynecol 1993;169:1119–1124.
93. Hemsell DL, Johnson ER, Hemsell PG, et al. Cefazolin is inferior to cefotetan as single-dose prophylaxis for women undergoing elective total abdominal hysterectomy. Clin Infect Dis 1995;20:677–684.
94. Sturlese E, Retto G, Pulia A, et al. Benefits of antibiotic prophylaxis in laparoscopic gynaecological surgery. Clin Exp Obstet Gynecol 1999;26:217–218.
95. Meuller SC, Henkel KO, Neumann J, et al. Perioperative antibiotic prophylaxis in maxillofacial surgery: Penetration of clindamycin into various tissues. J Craniomaxillofac Surg 1999;27:172–176.
96. Johnson JT, Yu VL, Myers EN, Wagner RL. An assessment of the need for gram-negative bacterial coverage in antibiotic prophylaxis for oncological head and neck surgery. J Infect Dis 1987;155:331–333.
97. Grandis JR, Vickers RM, Rihs JD, et al. Efficacy of topical amoxicillin plus clavulanate/ticarcillin plus clavulanate and clindamycin in contaminated head and neck surgery: Effect of antibiotic spectra and duration of therapy. J Infect Dis 1994;170:729–732.
98. Roy MC. Surgical-site infections after coronary artery bypass graft surgery: Discriminating site-specific risk factors to improve prevention efforts. Infect Control Hosp Epidemiol 1998;19:229–233.
99. Hollenbeak CS, Murphy DM, Koenig S, et al. The clinical and economic impact of deep chest surgical site infections following coronary artery bypass graft surgery. Chest 2000;118:397–402.
100. Curtis JJ, Boley TM, Walls JT, et al. Randomized prospective comparison of first- and second-generation cephalosporins as infection prophylaxis for cardiac surgery. Am J Surg 1993;166:734–737.
101. Harbath S, Samore MH, Lichtenberg D, Carmeli Y. Prolonged antibiotic prophylaxis after cardiovascular surgery and its effect on surgical site infections and antimicrobial resistance. Circulation 2000;101:2916–2921.
102. Bucknell SJ, Mohajeri M, Low J, et al. Single-versus multiple-dose antibiotics prophylaxis for cardiac surgery. Aust N Z J Surg 2000;70: 409–411.
103. Bernard A, Pillet M, Goudet P, Viard H. Antibiotic prophylaxis in pulmonary surgery. A prospective randomized double-blind trial of flash cefuroxime versus forty-eight-hour cefuroxime. J Thorac Cardiovasc Surg 1994;107:896–900.
104. Boldt J, Piper S, Uphus D, et al. Preoperative microbiologic screening and antibiotic prophylaxis in pulmonary resection operations. Ann Thorac Surg 1999;68:208–211.
105. Marroni M, Cao P, Fiorio M, et al. Prospective, randomized, double-blind trial comparing teicoplanin and cefazolin as antibiotic prophylaxis in prosthetic vascular surgery. Eur J Clin Microbiol Infect Dis 1999;18: 175–178.
106. Terpstra S, Noorkhoek GT, Voesten HG, et al. Rapid emergence of resistant coagulase-negative staphylococci on the skin after antibiotic prophylaxis. J Hosp Infect 1999;43:195–202.
107. Risberg B, Drott C, Dalman P, et al. Oral ciprofloxacin versus intravenous cefuroxime as prophylaxis against postoperative infection in vascular surgery: A randomised double-blind, prospective multicentre study. Eur J Vasc Endovasc Surg 1995;10:346–351.
108. Hanssen AD, Osmon DR. The use of prophylactic antimicrobial agents during and after hip arthroplasty. Clin Orthop 1999;369:124–138.
109. Patzakis MJ, Wilkins J, Wiss DA. Infection following intramedullary nailing of long bones. Clin Orthop 1986;212:182–191.
110. Vasenius J, Tulikoura I, Vainionpaa S, Rokkanen P. Clindamycin versus cloxacillin in the treatment of 240 open fractures. A randomized prospective study. Ann Chir Gynaecol 1998;87:224–228.
111. Dellinger EP, Caplan ES, Weaver LD, et al. Duration of preventive antibiotic administration for open extremity fractures. Arch Surg 1988;123: 333–339.
112. Hosein IK, Hill DW, Hatfield RH. Controversies in the prevention of neurosurgical infection. J Hosp Infect 1999;43:5–11.
113. Barker FG. Efficacy of prophylactic antibiotics for craniotomy: A meta-analysis. Neurosurgery 1994;35:484–492.
114. Pons VG, Denlinger SL, Guglielmo BJ, et al. Ceftizoxime versus vancomycin and gentamicin in neurosurgical prophylaxis: A randomized, prospective, blinded clinical trial. Neurosurgery 1993;33:416–422.
115. Whitby M, Johnson BC, Atkinson RL, Stuart G. The comparative efficacy of intravenous cefotaxime and trimethoprim/sulfamethoxazole in preventing infection after neurosurgery: A prospective, randomized study. Brisbane Neurosurgical Infection Group. Br J Neurosurg 2000;14:13–18.
116. Haines SJ, Walters BC. Antibiotic prophylaxis for cerebrospinal fluid shunts: A meta-analysis. Neurosurgery 1994;34:87–93.
117. Langley JM, Leblanc JC, Drake J, Milner R. Efficacy of antimicrobial prophylaxis in placement of cerebrospinal fluid shunts: Meta-analysis. Clin Infect Dis 1993;17:98–103.
118. Rimoldi RL, Haye W. The use of antibiotics for wound prophylaxis in spinal surgery. Orthop Clin North Am 1996;27:47–52.
119. Riley LH 3rd. Prophylactic antibiotics for spine surgery: Description of a regimen and its rationale. J South Orthop Assoc 1998;7:212–217.
120. Olson M, O'Connor M, Schwartz ML. Surgical wound infection: A 5-year prospective study of 20,193 wounds at the Minneapolis VA Medical Center. Ann Surg 1984;199:253–259.

122
VACCINES, TOXOIDS, AND OTHER IMMUNOBIOLOGICS

Joseph S. Bertino, Jr., and Mary S. Hayney

The discovery and introduction of vaccines, toxoids, and immunoglobulins has resulted in a significant decline in worldwide morbidity and mortality because of their respective diseases. In addition, they have been shown to be generally safe and cost-effective.[1] This chapter introduces the reader to three groups of agents: vaccines, toxoids, and immune sera (together known as immunobiologics). These groups are defined, and related agents are dealt with concurrently to illustrate total immunotherapy. Obscure agents and agents used only by the military (i.e., protection from bioterrorism) have been eliminated from this discussion in the interest of brevity.

The process of inducing or providing immunity artificially by administering an immunobiologic agent is known as immunization. The term *immunization* is considered more specific than the term *vaccination*.

PRODUCTS TO PRODUCE IMMUNIZATION

Vaccines and toxoids are separate and distinct products. Both types of products, however, act to induce active immunity; that is, immunity generated by a natural immunologic response to an antigen. Vaccines are derived from the infecting organism itself. Viral vaccines can be live attenuated or killed. Killed viral vaccines may consist of whole or split viral particles, specific viral fragments (subunits), or virus-like particles. Bacterial vaccines are generally killed whole bacteria or specific bacterial wall antigens or conjugates. Live attenuated vaccines induce an immunologic response more consistent with that occurring with natural infection. Because the organisms in live attenuated vaccines multiply in the body after injection, they may confer lifelong immunity with one dose (as does a primary natural infection). Most killed vaccines, on the other hand, do not induce permanent immunity and require additional doses at varying time intervals (booster doses). Killed vaccines can also differ in immunity potential depending on their composition. For example, polysaccharide vaccines tend to be poorly immunogenic in infants, whereas conjugated vaccines of the same antigen tend to be highly immunogenic (e.g., pneumococcal polysaccharide vaccine vs pneumococcal conjugated vaccine). Vaccines may also contain adjuvant agents to increase their immunogenicity.

Toxoids are inactivated bacterial toxins that are generally combined with aluminum salts (alum) to enhance their antigenicity by prolonging antigen absorption and exposure. These adjuvants also increase local tissue irritation when injected. Toxoids retain the ability to stimulate the formation of antitoxin.

Immune sera are sterile solutions containing antibody derived from human (immunoglobulin) or equine (horse antitoxin) sources. Immunoglobulins are derived from donor pools of blood plasma and are processed using cold ethanol fractionation in order to inactivate any potentially infecting agent. Antitoxins are made by immunizing animals with an antigen and then harvesting the antibodies (antitoxins) made against the antigens. These sera are indicated for induction of passive immunity (temporary immunity to infection as a result of the administration of antibodies not produced by the host). Human immune sera is preferred because of its lower incidence of serum sickness and other allergic reactions as compared to equine derived sera (see the section "Other Immunobiologics" later in this chapter).

In addition to the active component in an immunobiologic, other active and inert ingredients are often present. Suspending agents, such as water, saline, or complex fluids containing proteins (such as albumin) or antigens, are used as the vehicle for the immunobiologic agent. Preservatives, stabilizers, and antibiotics are often added to help maintain sterility. It must be kept in mind that patients may respond with allergic reactions, not to the immunobiologic agent itself, but to the other components of the pharmaceutical preparation. Different manufacturers of the same immunobiologic may have different active and inert ingredients or different quantities of these ingredients in their product.

Certain vaccines manufactured by various companies are considered interchangeable. Hepatitis B vaccine produced by two different companies (Merck & Co., Inc., West Point, PA, and SmithKline Beecham, Collegeville, PA) are considered interchangeable.[1] Human diploid cell vaccine, chicken fibroblast vaccine and rabies vaccine adsorbed are fully interchangeable with intramuscular (IM) use only. Diphtheria, acellular pertussis, and tetanus (DaPT Hepatitis A), and inactivated polio vaccines are interchangeable between manufacturers. Finally, all licensed *H. influenzae* type b conjugate vaccines are considered interchangeable for the primary series of three doses of vaccine.

In general, vaccines and toxoids must be kept refrigerated, as breaking the "cold chain" may result in loss of potency. Certain vaccines, such as measles-mumps-rubella (MMR), may also be frozen. Immune sera generally should be kept refrigerated and not frozen except for lyophilized intravenous (IV) human immunoglobulin, which can be stored at room temperature. Certain vaccines, such as yellow fever and varicella, are very sensitive to increased temperature. While some vaccines may be stored below 0°C (32°F), toxoids in general tend to aggregate upon freezing, leading to increased adverse local effects. On the other hand, some vaccines, when stored under incorrect conditions, may not be easily distinguished from potent vaccines.

FACTORS AFFECTING RESPONSE TO IMMUNIZATION

Various factors are known to affect response to vaccines and toxoids. Viability of the antigen is an important factor (live attenuated vs killed) as previously discussed. Total dose is also important, as there seems to exist a threshold dose above which no further increase in antibody titer is seen. The use of split doses or multiple reduced doses of a vaccine (such as those used in patients with allergies to some immunobiologic component as both a desensitization and an immunization program), however, may result in inadequate protection. In such instances, serologic testing should be performed to ascertain whether or not protection to the antigen had been attained. The interval between immunization doses, the number of doses given, or both may change immune response to an agent. For hepatitis B vaccine, giving the third dose (in a three-dose series) at 12 months (after the first dose) results in increased antibody titers, as compared to giving the third dose at 6 months.[2] Alternatively, additional doses of influenza vaccine are minimally effective in immunocompetent, nonhuman immunodeficiency virus (HIV)-infected patients, HIV-infected patients, and patients with acquired immunodeficiency syndrome (AIDS)-related complex (ARC).[3] Generally, intervals longer than those recommended between vaccine doses do not reduce immune response.[4]

The route and site of administration of the immunobiologic is also important. This is best illustrated by the hepatitis B vaccine, which elicits a satisfactory antibody response when given in the deltoid muscle but not consistently when administered in the gluteal area.[5] Injections should be administered in a site where there is little likelihood of site damage. Immunobiologics containing adjuvants should be given into muscle mass because they can cause irritation when given subcutaneously or intradermally.

VACCINE ADMINISTRATION

Subcutaneous injections should be administered into the thigh of infants and in the deltoid area of older children and adults. A five-eighths- to three-quarter-inch, 23- to 25-gauge needle should be used, being careful not to administer the dose intradermally or intramuscularly. For IM injection, the anterolateral aspect of the upper thigh (infants and toddlers) or the deltoid muscle of the upper arm (children and adults) should be used. When giving an IM injection to an adult, at least a 1-inch needle should be used for persons <90 kg and a 1.5-inch needle for persons ≥90 kg to assure injection in the muscle.[6] The buttock should not be used because of the potential for inadequate immunologic response and because of the potential risk of injury to the sciatic nerve. When the buttock must be used (as for large doses of immunoglobulin), only the upper, outer quadrant should be used with the needle being inserted anteriorly. Intradermal injections should be administered on the volar surface of the forearm except for human diploid cell (rabies) vaccine (HDCV), which should be given into the deltoid area to reduce reactions. A three-eighths- to three-quarter-inch, 25- or 27-gauge needle should be used, with care being taken to not inject the immunobiologic substance into the subcutaneous tissue.

Jet injectors are considered safe and effective for multiple-person immunization despite the fact that the nozzle tip is reused repeatedly. No reports exist in the United States of transmission of blood-borne pathogens (HIV or hepatitis B or C) with the use of jet injectors.[1] Generally, it is suggested that if a jet injector is used, the device should be cleaned or the tip changed if contamination of the nozzle is noted. In addition, the swabbing of the nozzle with alcohol or acetone between patients is routinely suggested.

For orally administered vaccines the general recommendation is to readminister the vaccine at the same visit if the vaccine is regurgitated within 5 to 10 minutes of administration. If the second dose is not retained, neither dose should be counted, and the vaccine should be readministered at the next visit.

Questions often arise concerning the simultaneous administration of vaccines. In general, inactivated vaccines can be simultaneously administered at separate sites. If single-site administration must be done, the thigh muscle is the preferred site of injection. If two or more killed antigens cannot be administered simultaneously, they may be administered with no regard to spacing between doses. Killed and live antigens may be administered simultaneously, or, if they cannot be administered simultaneously, at any interval between doses, with the exception of cholera (killed) and yellow fever (live) vaccine, which should be given at least 3 weeks apart. Simultaneous administration of live attenuated vaccines should be avoided if possible, unless specified (MMR). Theoretically, live vaccines should be given at least 1 month apart. The data on simultaneous administration of live attenuated viral vaccines should be prefaced with the knowledge that simultaneous administration of these vaccines has been performed with no resultant decrease in immunity to any of the agents used, when compared to single vaccine administration alone. Live viral vaccines may interfere with purified protein derivative (PPD) response; thus, tuberculin testing should be postponed 4 to 6 weeks after live virus vaccine administration.

The simultaneous administration of immunoglobulin (general or disease specific) and live attenuated vaccines (but not inactivated vaccines) may inhibit host antibody response because of impairment of viral replication. Guidelines state that there is a dose relationship between administration of immunoglobulin and inhibition of immune response to a vaccine (Table 122–1). Whole blood and other blood products containing antibodies may interfere with the response to the MMR vaccine. For women who have experienced a birth and have received a blood product in the last trimester or anti-RhoD immunoglobulin (IG) at the time of delivery, vaccination with MMR should be done immediately, with antibody testing at least 3 months later to determine response. In any patient, if vaccination with MMR and immunoglobulin administration must be done, separate injection sites are recommended with seroconversion to the viral antigens confirmed at 3 months and reimmunization if necessary. Immunoglobulin does not interfere with the response to oral vaccines or yellow fever vaccine.

Simultaneous administration of killed vaccines along with immunoglobulins is not contraindicated. Different sites are recommended, however, for killed vaccine and immunoglobulin administration. It is not recommended to increase the dose or number of vaccines used in this circumstance.

IMMUNIZATION OF SPECIAL POPULATIONS

NEONATES, INFANTS, AND PREGNANT WOMEN

The age of the recipient is another important determining factor in vaccine and toxoid response. In the first few months of life, passive immunity (temporary immunity to infection as a result of the acquisition of antibodies via maternal-fetal passage) both protects an infant and prevents adequate vaccine and toxoid response to certain agents.

Premature infants should be vaccinated at the same chronologic age using the same schedule and precautions as full-term infants. The full recommended doses of vaccines should be used, regardless of age or birth weight. Hepatitis B vaccine should be administered if the infant weighs 2,000 g, or it should be held until the infant is 2 months of age. Breast-fed infants should be vaccinated according to standard pediatric schedules.

Pregnant women present a particularly difficult problem in deciding on vaccination. In general, administration of live attenuated vaccines should not be done during pregnancy, and inactivated vaccines should not be given until the second trimester; however, inactivated vaccines have not been shown to be teratogenic during the first trimester.[7,8] Administration of the rubella vaccine during pregnancy is not a reason to interrupt pregnancy routinely.[7] Diphtheria and tetanus vaccination should be carried out with the use of a booster dose or a complete series of vaccines in unimmunized women. Hepatitis B, inactivated polio, and pneumococcal vaccines are all recommended

TABLE 122–1. Suggested Intervals Between Administration of Immunoglobulin Preparations for Various Indications and Vaccines Containing Live Measles Virus[a]

Indication	Dose (Including mg IgG/AG)	Suggested Interval Before Vaccination (mo)
Tetanus (TIG)	250 units (10 mg IgG/kg) IM	3
Hepatitis A (IG)		
Contact prophylaxis	0.02 mL/kg (3.3 mg IgG/kg) IM	3
International Travel	0.06 mL/kg (10 mg IgG/kg) IM	3
Hepatitis B prophylaxis (HBIg)	0.06 mL/kg (10 mg IgG/kg) IM	3
Rabies prophylaxis (HRIg)	20 IU/kg (22 mg IgG/kg) IM	4
Varicella prophylaxis (VZIg)	125 units/10 kg (20–40 mg IgG/kg) IM (max 625 units)	5
Measles prophylaxis (Ig)		
Normal contact	0.25 mL/kg (40 mg IgG/kg) IM	5
Immunocompromised contact	0.50 mL/kg (80 mg IgG/kg) IM	6
Blood Transfusion		
Red blood cells (RBCs) washed	10 mL/kg (negligible IgG/kg) IV	0
RBCs adenine-saline added	10 mL/kg (10 mg IgG/kg) IV	3
Packed RBCs (Hct 65%)[b]	10 mL/kg (60 mg IgG/kg) IV	6
Whole blood (Hct 35%–50%)[b]	10 mL/kg (80–100 mg IgG/kg) IV	6
Plasma/platelet products	10 mL/kg (160 mg IgG/kg) IV	7
Replacement of humoral immune deficiencies	300–400 mg/kg IV[c] (as IgIV)	8
Treatment of		
ITP[d]	400 mg/kg IV (as IgIV)	8
ITP[d]	1000 mg/kg IV (as IgIV)	10
Kawasaki's disease	2 g/kg IV (as IgIV)	11

[a]This table is not intended for determining the correct indications and dosage for the use of immunoglobulin preparations. Unvaccinated persons may not be fully protected against measles during the entire suggested interval and additional doses of immunoglobulin measles vaccine for both may be indicated following measles exposure. The concentration of measles antibody in a particular immunoglobulin preparation can vary by lot. The rate of antibody clearance following receipt of an immunoglobulin preparation can also vary. The recommended intervals are extrapolated from an estimated half-time of 30 days for passively acquired antibody and an observed interference with the immune response to measles vaccine for 5 months following a dose of 80 mg IgG/kg.
[b]Assumes a serum IgG concentration of 16 mg/mL.
[c]Measles vaccination is recommended for children with HIV infection but is contraindicated in patients with congenital disorders of the immune system.
[d]Immune (formally, idiopathic) thrombocytopenic purpura.
IGIV, immunoglobulin intravenous
(Adapted from Ref. 49.)

in pregnant women, if indicated. All pregnant women who are in the second or third trimester during influenza season should receive an influenza vaccine.

IMMUNOCOMPROMISED HOSTS

Vaccination in compromised hosts (those with chronic disease, such as diabetes, connective tissue disease, or alcoholics, or those with cancer or HIV disease) must be individualized based on the disease state and its treatment. The Centers for Disease Control and Prevention (CDC) has classified persons with immunocompromised conditions into three groups:[8]

1. Persons with a condition that causes limited immune deficiency (renal disease, diabetes, liver disease, asplenia).
2. Individuals who are severely immunocompromised but not as a result of HIV infection (congenital immunodeficiency, drug- or radiation-induced disease, hematologic or solid tumor).
3. Persons with HIV infection.

Patients with chronic pulmonary, renal, hepatic, or metabolic disease who are not receiving immunosuppressants may receive both live attenuated and killed vaccines and toxoids to induce active immunity. These patients often need higher doses of vaccines or more frequent dosing to induce immunity. Generally, immunization should be considered early in the course of the disease in an attempt to induce immunity at a point when the disease is less severe.

Those patients with active malignant disease may receive killed vaccines or toxoids but should not be given live vaccines. The MMR vaccine is not contraindicated for close contacts, however. Live virus vaccines may be administered to persons with leukemia who have not received chemotherapy for at least 3 months. Vaccines should be timed to avoid coinciding with the start of chemotherapy or radiation therapy (at least 2 weeks in advance of the start of these therapies). If vaccines cannot be given at least 2 weeks or more before the start of these therapies, immunization should be postponed until 3 months after the therapy has been completed. Passive immunization with immunoglobulin may be used in place of active immunization, regardless of the history of immunization.

Glucocorticoids may cause suppressed responses to vaccines. When steroid therapy duration is ≤ 2 weeks (low to-moderate dose, that is <20 mg or 2 mg/kg/day, whichever is less), then no contraindication to immunization exists.[8] In addition, long-term, alternate-day steroid therapy with short-acting agents, maintenance physiologic doses, topical, aerosol, intra-articular, bursal, or tendon injections are not considered contraindications to immunization. If patients have been receiving high-dose corticosteroids or have had a course lasting >2 weeks, then a 3-month period of time should pass before immunization with live virus vaccines.

The patient with HIV infection requires special consideration. Responses to live and killed antigens are generally suboptimal and decreases as the disease progresses because HIV produces defects in cell-mediated immunity and humoral immunity.

The CDC has developed three categories for immunologic classification of HIV infection:[9] (a) patients with no evidence of immunosuppression; (b) patients with moderate immunosuppression; and (c) patients with severe immunosuppression. For children up to age 16 years with HIV infection, immunization following the standard schedules is recommended for hepatitis B, DaPT, HIB, IPV, and influenza. MMR is not suggested in severely immunosuppressed children. Varicella vaccine is recommended only in children with no evidence of immunosuppression. Pneumococcal vaccine is recommended for HIV-infected persons >2 years of age. There is no suggestion that larger doses or more frequent vaccine dosing is of benefit. Other killed vaccines may be used without concern for increased risk. Live typhoid vaccine should be avoided. Yellow fever vaccine may be used if absolutely necessary, but it may pose a theoretical risk of encephalitis.

MISCONCEPTIONS ABOUT THE USE OF IMMUNIZATION

There are very few contraindications to the use of vaccines except as those outlined earlier. These contraindications include a history of anaphylactic reactions to the vaccine or a component of the vaccine, immunosuppression (as specified for each group), pregnancy (for MMR), and administration of immunoglobulin or blood products. For agents such as DaPT, unexplained encephalopathy occurring within 7 days of a dose of pertussis vaccine or an anaphylactic reaction are contraindications. Precautions include hypotonic, hyporesponsive episode; fever of ≥40.5°C (104.9°F) or crying lasting ≥3 hours within 48 hours of a previous dose; or seizures with or without fever within 3 days after a dose. Generally, history of mild-to-moderate local reactions, mild acute illnesses, concurrent antibiotic use, prematurity, family history of adverse events, diarrhea, and breast feeding are not contraindications to immunization.

OBTAINING AN IMMUNIZATION HISTORY

An immunization history should be obtained from every patient, regardless of the reason for the health care visit. Ideally, any history provided by the patient from memory should be verified by reviewing the patient's personal, written "shot record" or a database that contains the complete immunization history. If an official, written record is not available, patient characteristics (military service, travel history, occupation) may provide clues as to the immunization history. Serologic testing for immunity against certain diseases can provide specific information, but it is routinely employed for only a few selected diseases (measles, rubella, hepatitis A and B, varicella) and selected circumstances (employment in a health care facility). If a written record does not exist, one should be generated at the time of initiation of immunization. Patients without a written record should be considered susceptible and an immunization program started and completed unless a serious adverse reaction occurs. As a general rule, the risks associated with overimmunization are minimal relative to the risks associated with contracting vaccine-preventable diseases.[1]

VACCINE DELIVERY

Shortfalls in vaccine coverage exist in both the adult and pediatric populations.[10,11] Among children, those of preschool age historically have been the most neglected.[12] Entry into public school is contingent on receipt of certain required immunizations, resulting in vaccine coverage rates above 97% in children 6 years of age and older. The lack of a similar enforcement mechanism in younger patients, however, has contributed to exceptionally low immunization rates (<50%), particularly in children younger than 2 years of age. From 1989 to 1991, the United States experienced a national measles epidemic, largely caused by inadequately immunized preschool-aged children. Additionally, other segments of the population (adolescents and senior citizens) have been identified as needing better vaccine coverage.[13]

In many instances, unvaccinated individuals have been seen by health care providers, but they have not received the indicated vaccines either because of oversight, inappropriate "contraindications" to vaccination, or a reluctance to administer multiple vaccines at the same visit. These missed opportunities to immunize patients occur in patients of all ages and in a variety of practice settings.[14]

According to the CDC, every health care visit, regardless of its purpose, should be viewed as an opportunity to review a patient's immunization status and to administer needed vaccines. Immunization is perhaps the most cost-effective medical practice available. Pharmaceutical care should encompass assessment of individuals' vaccine needs, administration of indicated agents, and documentation of immunization histories. The outcome measurement of what percentage of patients in a particular practice site is completely immunized is extremely important because the benefits of optimal vaccine use extend beyond the individual patient to the public as a whole. Pharmacists can provide important interventions in vaccine therapy.[15]

COMBINATION VACCINES

The problem of numerous vaccine injections is being addressed through the development of combination vaccines.[16] The combining of several antigens that normally would be administered as separate entities can reduce the number of injections required. Several combination vaccines have been approved for use in the United States, and each has an HIB conjugate as one component. Problems encountered include chemical incompatibility and immunologic interference.

NATIONAL VACCINE INJURY COMPENSATION ACT

In 1986, the National Vaccine Injury Compensation Act (NVICA) was passed by the United States Congress.[17] The act consists of four parts. Part A outlines compensation for vaccine-related injuries, per a Vaccine Injury Table, and limits the size of compensatory awards to injured individuals. Part B is the "no-fault" provision, which frees the manufacturer from liability for damage if adequate warnings for vaccine use are provided. Part C provides that health care providers and vaccine manufacturers must report adverse reactions to vaccines to the Food and Drug Administration (FDA) within 7 days of their occurrence. Part D gives legal recourse against the Secretary of the Department of Health and Human Services for not performing duties as outlined by the act.[17,18] The bill also instituted mandatory record keeping by health care providers in the permanent medical record. Specifically, the manufacturer and lot number of the vaccine, date of administration, and name, address, and title of the person giving the vaccine must be recorded. Additionally, the Act mandates that health care providers report to their local health department or to the FDA any occurrence of adverse reactions. To facilitate reporting of any adverse events suspected of being vaccine-related, the Vaccine Adverse Event Reporting System (VAERS) was established. The VAERS toll-free telephone number for obtaining information or report forms is 1-800-822-7967.[18]

USE OF VACCINES AND TOXOIDS

Appendixes 121–1 and 121–2 show the recommended schedules for routine immunization of children and adults. Appendix 121–3 lists the minimum age for initial vaccination and minimum interval between vaccine doses. Many states require children to be fully immunized prior to entering elementary school; however, optimal protection is achieved by giving the recommended vaccines at the recommended ages, which means special attention should be devoted to children younger than 2 years of age. Adults and adolescents also require vaccination, and are often unaware of this need. All adults should be fully immunized against diphtheria, tetanus, measles, mumps, and rubella. Certain high-risk individuals should be vaccinated against other agents as outlined in Appendix 121–3.

TOXOIDS

DIPHTHERIA TOXOID ADSORBED AND DIPHTHERIA ANTITOXIN

Diphtheria toxoid adsorbed is a sterile suspension of modified toxins of *Corynebacterium diphtheriae,* which induce immunity against the exotoxin of this organism. Two strengths of diphtheria toxoid are available in the United States: the pediatric strength (D) and the adult strength (d), which contains less antigen because of the higher rate of adverse effects seen when the pediatric strength is used in adult patients.[19] The widespread use of diphtheria toxoid has essentially eliminated diphtheria from the United States.

Primary immunization with D is indicated for children older than 6 weeks of age. The usual dose is 0.5 mL IM at rotating sites. Generally, the toxoid is given in combination with tetanus toxoid and acellular pertussis vaccine (as DaPT) at ages 2, 4, and 6 months of age. Additional doses are given at 15 to 18 months of age and again at 4 to 6 years of age.[20,21] Completing the primary D immunization series usually induces immunity of at least 10 years' duration in 90% of persons. Booster doses should be given every 10 years. Adverse effects of diphtheria toxoid include mild to moderate tenderness, erythema, and induration at the injection site. Rarely do systemic reactions occur.[19]

If primary immunization is given to an immunosuppressed patient, an additional dose of D should be administered 1 month following the return to normal immune status. Diphtheria toxoid may be administered to persons with mild febrile illnesses and with other live or killed vaccines.[20]

For nonimmunized adults, a complete three-dose series of diphtheria toxoid should be administered with the first two doses given at least 4 weeks apart and the third dose given 6 to 12 months after the second. The combined preparation, diphtheria-tetanus (Td) is recommended in adults because it contains less diphtheria toxoid than DT or DPT and is associated with fewer reactions to the diphtheria component. It also includes the recommended tetanus toxoid, but it omits the pertussis component, which is not used in patients older than 7 years of age. All adults should receive booster doses of Td every 10 years.

Diphtheria antitoxin (DA) is a sterile antitoxin derived from hyperimmunized horses and is indicated for immediate use in patients with diphtheria. It should be stored at 2°C (35.6°F) to 8°C (46.4°F), but may be frozen without affecting potency. It is rarely indicated for diphtheria prophylaxis. The DA vaccine is given IM or IV in a dosage related to the site and size of the diphtheric membrane, severity of illness, and duration of illness. Sensitivity testing by performing an intradermal or scratch test and a conjunctival test should be performed before administration. These tests do not rule out systemic allergic reactions in 100% of the cases.

The usual dose of DA is 20,000–40,000 U for pharyngeal disease, 40,000–60,000 U for nasopharyngeal lesions, and 80,000–120,000 U for extensive disease of 3 days or more. When given IV, the dose should be diluted 1:20 in 0.9% saline or dextrose 5% in water and infused at 1 mL/min after being warmed to 32°C (89.6°F) to 34°C (93.2°F).

Adverse reactions to DA include anaphylactic reactions in 7% of patients, serum sickness occurring 12 days postadministration, or both. Serum sickness may be accelerated (7 to 12 days) in persons previously sensitized. Fortunately, the widespread use of diphtheria toxoid has greatly reduced the incidence of the disease and, thus, the use of DA.

TETANUS TOXOID, TETANUS TOXOID ADSORBED, AND TETANUS IMMUNOGLOBULIN

Tetanus toxoid and tetanus toxoid adsorbed (adsorbed onto aluminum hydroxide, phosphate, or potassium sulfate to increase antigenicity) are sterile suspensions of the toxoid derived from *Clostridium tetani.* Both toxoids are used to promote active immunity against tetanus; however, tetanus toxoid adsorbed (T) is the preferred agent, because it elicits a greater immune response and is associated with fewer adverse reactions.

Although single doses of T in a nonimmunized individual do not produce sufficient antibody response, a series of three 0.5-mL doses results in protection for 90% of vaccinees. Primary vaccination provides protection for at least 10 years. Additional doses of T (combined with diphtheria toxoid Td) are recommended as part of traumatic wound management if a patient has not received a dose of T over the preceding 5 years. For minor or clean wounds, no dose is given. Table 122–2 summarizes these recommendations. In certain situations, tetanus immunoglobulin (TIg) should also be given. It can be administered with T, provided separate syringes and separate injection sites are used.

In children, primary immunization against tetanus is usually offered in conjunction with diphtheria and pertussis vaccination (using DTaP). A 0.5-mL dose is recommended at 2, 4, 6, and 15 to 18 months of age, but the first dose can be administered as early as 6 weeks of age.[21,22] In children 7 years old and older, and in adults who have not previously been immunized, a series of three 0.5-mL doses of Td are administered IM initially. The first two doses are given 1 to 2 months apart, and the third dose is recommended at 6 to 12 months after the second dose. Boosters are recommended every 10 years, and unless there is contraindication to diphtheria toxoid, Td should be used. Tetanus toxoid may be simultaneously given with other killed and live vaccines, and if indicated, it may be given to immunosuppressed patients.

Adverse reactions to tetanus toxoid include mild-to-moderate local reactions at the injection site, such as warmth, erythema, and induration. Rarely, fever, malaise, aches and pains, or neurologic disorders have been reported. In general, major local reactions occur

TABLE 122–2. Summary Guide to Tetanus Prophylaxis in Routine Wound Management[a]

History of Tetanus Toxoid	Clean Minor Wounds		All Other Wounds[b]	
	Td[c]	*TIg*[d]	*Td*[d]	*TIg*[d]
Uncertain or <3 doses	Yes	No	Yes	Yes
≥3 doses[e]	No[f]	No	No[g]	No

[a]Refer also to text on specific vaccines or toxoids for contraindications, precautions, dosages, side effects, adverse reactions, and special considerations. Important details are in the text and in the ACIP recommendations on diptheria, tetanus, and pertussis (DTP).
[b]Such as, but not limited to, wounds contaminated with dirt, feces, and saliva; puncture wounds; avulsions; and wounds resulting from missiles, crushing, burns, and frostbite.
[c]Td tetanus and diptheria toxoids absorbed (for adult use). For children younger than 7 years old, DPT (DT, if pertussis vaccine is contraindicated) is preferred to tetanus toixoid alone. For persons 7 years old and older, Td is preferred to tetanus toxoid alone.
[d]TIg, tetanus immunoglobulin.
[e]If only three doses of fluid toxoid have been received, a fourth dose of toxoid, preferably an absorbed toxoid, should be given.
[f]Yes if >10 years since last dose.
[g]Yes if >5 years since last dose. (More frequent boosters are not needed and can accentuate side effects.)
(From Ref. 21.)

within 2 to 8 hours after administration to patients with high serum tetanus antitoxin levels. This type of reaction suggests a high level of protection. Local reactions do not limit the use of the toxoid for further dosing. Although safe use during pregnancy has not been definitely established, tetanus toxoid has been administered to pregnant women for the prevention of neonatal tetanus. Generally, waiting until the second trimester is suggested.

Tetanus immunoglobulin is a sterile, concentrated, nonpyrogenic solution of immunoglobulins prepared from hyperimmunized humans. It is used to provide passive immunity to tetanus following the occurrence of traumatic wounds in nonimmunized or suboptimally immunized persons (see Table 122–2). A dose of 250–500 U IM should be administered. When administered with tetanus toxoid adsorbed (TTA), separate sites for administration should be used. Also, TIg is used for the treatment of tetanus. In this setting, a single dose of 3,000–6,000 U IM is administered.

Adverse effects of TIg include pain, tenderness, erythema, and muscle stiffness at the injection site, which may persist for several hours. Rarely do systemic reactions occur. Intravenous administration has been associated with severe adverse reactions and is not recommended.

VACCINES

BACILLE CALMETTE-GUÉRIN VACCINE

The increased incidence of TB has led the CDC to recommend greater use of bacille Calmette-Guérin (BCG) vaccine.[23] All available BCG vaccines are derived from a live attenuated strain of *Mycobacterium bovis*. Because many brands are available throughout the world, and because subculture of *M. bovis* can alter the immunologic properties, immunogenicity varies with the brand of vaccine. In the United States, the Tice strain of *M. bovis* is used to produce the vaccine. This heterogeneity of BCG vaccine immunogenicity and the fact that the majority of TB prevention trials with the vaccine have examined different at-risk populations in different geographic areas, have led to some questions concerning the efficacy of BCG vaccine in TB prevention. Multiple meta-analyses of these BCG trials lead to the conclusion that the vaccine is efficacious (>80%) in preventing serious illness in children. Data are not conclusive, however, in clarifying vaccine efficacy for preventing pulmonary TB in adolescents and adults, or in health care workers. Additionally, the protective effects of BCG vaccine based on different vaccine strains, the age of initial vaccination, or the use of vaccine in HIV-infected individuals are still indeterminate.

The CDC has issued guidelines recommending which persons are candidates for BCG vaccine.[23] These guidelines cover children, high- and low-risk health care workers, and persons with HIV infection. When using BCG vaccine, a negative Mantoux skin test should be assured before vaccination because of the difficulty in using the skin test for a prolonged period of time following immunization.

In the pediatric population, generally, acquisition of tuberculosis (TB) in a child is a result of exposure from infected adults who often reside in the same household. Vaccination with BCG should be considered for an infant or child who has a negative tuberculin skin test but who is continually exposed to an untreated or ineffectively treated patient with infectious pulmonary TB, especially if the infection is caused by isoniazid- and rifampin-resistant strains of *M. tuberculosis*.

While infection control measures are paramount in reducing the transmission of TB in health care facilities, there are certain situations in which use of BCG may be considered. Another important consideration for using BCG in health care workers is the potential interference with diagnosing a newly acquired TB infection in a vaccinated person. Generally, BCG vaccination of health care workers should be considered when infection control precautions have been implemented but have not been effective in preventing the spread of TB, especially multidrug-resistant strains. Vaccination with BCG should not be required for employment or assignment of health care workers in specific work areas. In areas where the TB risk is low, vaccination of health care workers with BCG is unnecessary.

In HIV-infected persons, the data are inconsistent to address safety issues with this live vaccine. In addition, the efficacy of BCG vaccine in HIV-infected persons is unknown. Therefore, even in high-risk groups, such as children with continuous household exposure and health care workers in the high-risk category, BCG vaccination is not recommended by the CDC, although the World Health Organization (WHO) does recommend BCG use in asymptomatic HIV-positive children in a high-risk situation. In addition, the vaccine is contraindicated in persons who are immunocompromised because of leukemia, lymphoma, and generalized malignancy, and in those who are receiving corticosteroids, alkylating agents, antimetabolites, or radiation therapy.

Adverse effects of the vaccine are usually local in nature. These include moderate axillary or cervical lymphadenopathy and induration and subsequent pustule formation at the injection site (with intradermal use) persisting for up to 3 months. Permanent scarring generally does occur. When subcutaneous injection is used, higher rates of local reactions are seen, including muscle soreness, erythema, and purulent drainage. For the treatment of BCG adenitis (adherent or fistulated lymph nodes), treatment ranges from no treatment to surgical drainage and administration of anti-TB drugs, or both. These local reactions are approximately 15-fold more common in infants younger than 1 year of age versus children 1 to 20 years of age. Little incidence data are available in older age groups. More uncommon are severe reactions, including suppurative lymphadenitis, caseous lesions at the injection site (occurring within 5 months of vaccination), and disseminated BCG infection. Occasional reports of erythema multiforme in adults have been reported. Although Vaccination with BCG has not been shown to cause harm to the fetus, it is not recommended during pregnancy.[23]

It is generally believed that BCG induces a positive Mantoux TB test. Some individuals who receive BCG, however, may have no induced reactivity to the TB skin test. Tuberculin reactivity develops 6 to 12 weeks after vaccination. Tuberculin reactivity induced by BCG does not persist longer than 10 years after immunization. In addition, the presence or size of a postvaccination-positive TB skin test reaction does not predict protection by BCG. Tuberculin skin testing is not contraindicated for persons who have been vaccinated with BCG, and the skin test results of such persons are used to support or exclude the diagnosis of *M. tuberculosis* infection. A diagnosis of *M. tuberculosis* infection and the use of preventive therapy should be considered for any BCG-vaccinated person who has a tuberculin skin test reaction of >10 mm of induration, especially if any of the following circumstances are present: (a) the vaccinated person is a contact of another person who has infectious TB, particularly if the infectious person has transmitted *M. tuberculosis* to others; (b) the vaccinated person was born or has resided in a country in which the prevalence of TB is high; or (c) the vaccinated person is exposed continually to populations in which the prevalence of TB is high (some health care workers, employees and volunteers at homeless shelters, and workers at drug-treatment centers). Studies have demonstrated that persons who are infected with HIV have decreased tuberculin skin test responses after BCG vaccination compared to uninfected persons.

Vaccination with BCG should be reserved for persons who have a reaction of <5 mm induration after skin testing with 5 TU of PPD tuberculin. The Tice strain of BCG is administered percutaneously; 0.3 mL of the reconstituted vaccine is usually placed on the skin in the lower deltoid area (the upper arm) and delivered through a multiple-puncture disk. Infants younger than 30 days of age should receive one-half the usual dose, prepared by increasing the amount of diluent added to the lyophilized vaccine. If the indications for vaccination persist, these infants should receive a full dose of the vaccine after they are 1 year of age, if they have an induration of <5 mm when tested with 5 TU of PPD tuberculin. Normal reactions to the vaccine are characterized by the formation of a bluish-red pustule within 2 to 3 weeks after vaccination. After approximately 6 weeks, the pustule ulcerates, forming a lesion approximately 5 mm in diameter. Draining lesions resulting from vaccination should be kept clean and bandaged. Scabs form and heal usually within 3 months after vaccination. Tuberculin reactivity resulting from BCG vaccination should be documented. A vaccinated person should be tuberculin skin tested 3 months after BCG administration, and the induration size documented. Vaccinated persons whose skin test results are negative (<5 mm of induration) and who are enrolled in ongoing periodic skin testing programs (health care workers) should continue to be included in ongoing testing programs if their skin test results are <5 mm induration. Those vaccinees who have positive tuberculin skin test reactions (>5 mm of induration) after vaccination should not be retested except after exposure to a case of infectious TB; an increase in induration (>10 mm increase for persons younger than 35 years of age and >15 mm increase for persons older than 35 years of age) from a previous to the current skin test may indicate a newly acquired *M. tuberculosis* infection.

Although the major use of BCG vaccine has been as immunoprophylaxis of tuberculosis, other uses of the agent in neoplastic disease have been studied. In these circumstances, the agent has been used in various dosages and routes of administration. Specific protocols are generally followed. This form of immunotherapy in neoplastic disease has been met with limited success.

HEPATITIS A VACCINE

Two interchangeable vaccines are available for use in the United States to induce active immunity, Havrix (Glaxo Smith Kline) and Vaqta (Merck & Co.). Available vaccines are killed whole-virus vaccines that are propagated through the use of cell culture in human fibroblasts. The live virus is then formalin-inactivated and adsorbed to aluminum. Havrix is formulated with 2-phenoxyethanol as a preservative, whereas Vaqta contains no preservatives. For Havrix, the final vaccine potency (per dose) is expressed as enzyme-linked immunosorbent assay (ELISA) units (ELU). For Vaqta, the antigen content is expressed as units (U) of hepatitis A antigen. These vaccines should be stored and shipped at temperatures of 2°C (35.6°F) to 8°C (46.4°F) and not frozen. Storage at 37°C (98.6°F) for 1 week does not affect immunogenicity.

The CDC has issued guidelines on active and passive immunization against hepatitis A virus (HAV), and the reader is referred to this publication for a complete discussion of the material that follows.[24]

A number of groups have been determined to be at risk for HAV infection; thus, the CDC has suggested that they receive active immunization with hepatitis A vaccine. These groups include (a) travelers to areas that are not developed (even if the traveler is staying in a luxury hotel); (b) men who have sex with men; (c) persons working with primates; (d) persons who have clotting factor disorders; (e) illegal drug users; (f) persons with chronic liver disease; (g) food handlers where the vaccine is cost-effective; and (h) children in highly endemic areas. Other groups who may not be at risk but who may serve to expose large numbers of people to HAV include those working in a daycare center, those working in a home for the disabled, and those working in food service. The CDC has stated that to eradicate HAV effectively, children 2 years of age or younger would ideally be vaccinated. In fact, CDC recommends immunizing children when the annual hepatitis A rate is ≥20 per 100,000 persons. In areas where the hepatitis A rate is ≥10 per 100,000 persons, immunization should be considered.

While no lower limit of anti-HAV titer has been defined to prevent HAV infection, *in vitro* data suggest that anti-HAV levels of ≥20 mIU/mL (measured with an enzyme immunoassay) or ≥10 mIU/mL (measured with a modified radioimmunoassay) may be protective.

Both commercially available hepatitis A vaccines are highly immunogenic over a wide age and weight range. In persons older than 18 years of age, Havrix (1440 ELU dose) anti-HAV levels of ≥20 mIU/mL were seen in 88% of adults within 15 days of the first dose and in 99% to 100% after 30 days. After a second dose, all persons had seroconversion with high geometric mean antibody titers (GMTs) for anti-HAV. Results with Vaqta were similar, with 95% seroconversion 1 month after a 50 U dose and 100% conversion 1 month after a second dose 6 months later. In children and adolescents, both commercially available vaccines have been shown to be highly immunogenic with 100% seroconversion 1 month after two doses were given at 0 and 6 months.

In addition, hepatitis A vaccine has been shown to be effective in stopping outbreaks of the disease during an epidemic.[24]

ROUTE OF ADMINISTRATION, VACCINATION SCHEDULE, AND DOSAGE

The vaccine should be administered intramuscularly into the deltoid muscle. Havrix is licensed in three formulations, with the formulation and number of doses differing according to the vaccinee's age. For persons 2 to 18 years of age 720 ELU (0.5 mL) per dose in a two-dose schedule (0 and 6 to 12 months) is recommended. For persons older than 18 years of age, 1,440 ELU (1 mL) per dose in a two-dose schedule (0 and 6 to 12 months) is recommended. Vaqta is licensed in two formulations, and the formulation and number of doses differ according to the person's age. For persons 2 to 17 years of age, 25 U (0.5 mL) in a two-dose schedule (0 and 6 to 18 months) is recommended, while for persons older than 17 years of age, 50 U per dose in a two-dose schedule (0 and 6 months) is used. Because seroconversion rates are so high, obtaining anti-HAV titers is not recommended.

The vaccine is highly effective in the prevention of hepatitis A infections, particularly in children and adolescents.[24] In addition, data exist to suggest that in outbreak settings, vaccination of susceptible individuals with HAV results in a substantial decrease in hepatitis A infections.[24]

Unlike hepatitis B vaccine, factors such as body size, age, smoking status, and sex do not appear to affect the development of seroconversion. The vaccine can be given with immunoglobulin and although the levels of anti-HAV are blunted, they still are 100-fold higher than levels that are considered protective.

There is only limited data about the persistence of protective levels of anti-HAV because the vaccine has only been available for a limited time period. It is estimated, however, that protective levels of anti-HAV may be present for 20 years or longer.[24] In addition, the effect of immune memory on the duration or protection is unknown.

Adverse effects of HAV have been mild and generally local in nature. Within 3 days of injection, injection site soreness, redness, or pain is reported in approximately 50% of vaccinees, and headache in 5% to 10% of vaccinees. Adverse effect rates may be less in children than adults. Although the vaccine is an inactivated virus and its potential risk to the fetus is low, its use in pregnancy is not recommended. The vaccine may be used in immunocompromised individuals with safety.

HEPATITIS B VACCINE

Hepatitis B vaccine is an inactivated vaccine, consisting of hepatitis B surface antigen (HBsAg) subunit particles, and it does not include the preS1 or preS2 particles. Recombinant hepatitis B vaccine was introduced in the United States in the 1980s. Currently, two brands of hepatitis B vaccine, Recombivax-HB and Energix-B, are available for use in the United States. These recombinant vaccines are approximately equally effective (albeit they produce lower GMTs) as compared to human plasma-derived vaccine. The vaccine induces only antihepatitis B surface antibody (anti-HBs) in recipients.[25,26]

Clinical trials in healthy individuals have demonstrated antibody conversion rates of approximately 90% after completion of the three-dose series[26] and a protective effect in vaccinees subsequently exposed to hepatitis B virus (HBV). The 10% of patients who are considered unprotected fall into the categories of nonresponders (anti-HBs <2.1 mIU/mL) and hyporesponders (anti-HBs 2.1–9.9 mIU/mL). Of persons who do not develop protective levels of anti-HBs, approximately 50% are nonresponders and 50% hyporesponders. Lack of development of a protective response is seen in older individuals, with nonresponse rates increasing with increasing age (older than 50 years of age).[27] Other factors that have been identified as leading to poor vaccine response include increased body mass index, being a smoker, and male sex.[28–30] Smoking status is the most important factor in determining nonresponse in normal individuals. Nonsmokers have an approximate sevenfold increased chance of developing protective levels of anti-HBs as do smokers.[28,29] Although the two available vaccines are considered equivalent in inducing protection to hepatitis B, some data suggest that Recombivax-HB may have a higher failure rate than Engerix-B.[28–32] (The true significance of this is still unclear.) A normal immune response has also been seen in patients with Down's syndrome.[27] Response rates in hemodialysis and immunocompromised patients have been lower, requiring higher vaccine dosages to achieve protective levels. The vaccine protects against all hepatitis B serotypes, including delta viroid, but does not cross-react with other hepatitis viruses.

In the preexposure setting, the vaccine has been recommended for persons with occupational risk (health care workers, public safety workers), persons in training for health care fields, clients and staff of institutions for the developmentally disabled, hemodialysis patients, recipients of clotting factor concentrate, household contacts and sex partners of hepatitis B carriers, adoptees from countries where hepatitis B is endemic, international travelers (those spending more than 6 months in areas with high rates of hepatitis B infection or high-risk, short-term travelers), injecting drug users, sexually active homosexual/bisexual men, sexually active heterosexual men and women, and inmates of long-term correctional facilities.[25–27] In addition, the American Academy of Pediatrics recommends universal immunization of all newborns using thimerosal-free vaccine.[26]

Hepatitis B vaccine is also used with hepatitis B immunoglobulin (HBIg) in the postexposure setting. Persons for whom this regimen is recommended include susceptible individuals having percutaneous or permucosal exposure to blood containing HBsAg, sexual contacts of HBsAg carriers who will continue to be exposed, and infants born to mothers who are HBsAg carriers.[27,32,33] HBIg does not interfere with the induction of neutralizing antibody, and the combination is more protective than when two doses of HBIg alone are given (85% to 90% efficacy vs 70% to 75%).[34]

For neonates born to mothers who are not positive for HBsAg, the primary vaccination series is 5 μg of Recombivax-HB or 10 μg of Engerix-B. The first dose should be given at 0 to 2 days of age, the second dose at 1 to 2 months of age, and the third dose at 6 to 18 months of age. An alternative schedule of the three doses administered at 2, 4, and 6 to 18 months of age may be used. In addition, the appropriate pediatric dose of either brand of hepatitis B vaccine may be used at 2, 4, and 6 months of age for primary immunization.[35] This schedule corresponds more closely with the immunization schedule for other vaccines in infancy. In infants born to HBsAg-positive mothers, immunization should proceed on a different dosing regimen. In addition to administration of HBIg, vaccination with 5 μg of Recombivax-HB or 10 μg of Engerix-B should be given at 12 hours after birth (but no more than 7 days after birth), at 1 month, and at 6 months of age. These infants should be tested for anti-HBs at 9 months of age or later. A fourth dose of vaccine should be administered to infants who are anti-HBs nonresponders or hyporesponders (this is very uncommon) and who are HBsAg negative. These children should be tested 1 month after the fourth dose for anti-HBs. If titers of <10 mIU/mL are still not achieved, two additional doses, 1 month apart, may be given with testing for anti-HBs 1 month after the last dose.

For persons younger than 19 years old, 5 μg of Recombivax-HB or 10 μg of Engerix-B should be administered at 0, 1, and 6 months. Children and adolescents ages 11 to 15 years may also receive 10 μg of Recombivax-HB (only) at 0 and 6 months. Adults 19 years of age and older should receive 10 μg of Recombivax-HB or 20 μg of Engerix-B at 0, 1, and 6 months.

Hemodialysis patients are considered poor responders to hepatitis B vaccine; thus, the dose of vaccine is escalated in this population. These patients should receive either 40 μg of Recombivax-HB in a 0-, 1-, and 6-month schedule or 40 μg of Engerix-B in a 0-, 1-, 2-, and 6-month schedule. Anti-HBs should be determined and if the value is <10 mIU/mL, one to three booster doses should be administered.

In addition, these persons should be tested yearly and boosted with a single dose of 40 μg if anti-HBs is <10 mIU/mL.[27]

The preferred site of administration is the deltoid muscle in adults (immunogenicity is significantly lower in adults who receive injection in the buttock) and the anterolateral thigh in infants.

Patients who should receive postvaccination serologic testing include immunocompromised patients (because of any cause), persons at occupational risk of exposure, and infants born to HBsAG-positive mothers. Data have questioned the cost-effectiveness of postvaccination anti-HBs testing in health care workers; however, the CDC continues to recommend this.[29]

Approximately 5% to 15% of normal persons will not mount a sufficient antibody titer. In some instances, this may be because of measuring the anti-HBs level too long after the last vaccination in the primary series. Generally, although measurement of anti-HBs is suggested 1 to 6 months after the last dose of vaccine, in reality, measurement of anti-HBs 1 to 3 months after the last dose is probably wiser.[31] Data in gay men suggest that 15% to 25% respond (with development of protective anti-HBs levels) to a single additional dose of vaccine with 30% to 50% responding to three additional doses.[36] These data were generated, using the plasma-derived vaccine.

Our data suggest that three doses of 40 μg Recombivax-HB results in development of protective antibody response in 100% of normal hypo- and nonresponders.[37] Thus, our suggestion (and what we believe is cost-effective) for a person who has not mounted a protective anti-HBs titer after a standard vaccine series is to administer a standard dose at 0, 1, and 2 months with anti-HBs testing 1 to 2 months after the last dose. Approximately 65% of non- and hyporesponders will develop a protective anti-HBs titer with this regimen. If a protective anti-HBs titer is still lacking, the person should be checked for HBsAG (which can cause a lack of response). If HBsAG is negative, then 40 μg of Recombivax-HB should be administered at 0, 1, and 2 months with an anti-HBs titer obtained 1 to 2 months after the last dose. If this strategy does not work, we do not recommend any additional doses of vaccine. Non- and hyporesponse may be determined genetically (on the HLA locus); however, the data to assure this are limited.

The need for booster doses of vaccine has not been established.[38,39] Of persons who develop protective antibody ($\geq$10 or more sample ratio units by radioimmunoassay or positive antibody by enzyme immunoassay), 10% to 15% will have lost detectable antibody within 4 years with 40% to 75% of patients having a protective antibody level after 6 to 10 years. Protection against serious infection and liver inflammation appears to persist.[39,40] Controversy continues, however, for individuals with normal immune function. Some authors recommend checking antibody status 3 to 5 years after initial vaccination and administering a single booster dose if antibody concentration is less than 10 mIU/mL. Other authors note that data suggest that protection is in force for at least 7 to 9 years, and thus, they do not recommend repeat doses before then.[25,41] World Health Organization information suggests that no cases of hepatitis B have been reported in individuals who have mounted a protective level of anti-HBs after a vaccine series, even with the progression of time. Immune memory may play a function in this regard. Further studies are needed to elucidate this, and thus, no booster doses are recommended for normal individuals.

The same dosage schedule used for primary immunization is used in the postexposure setting. The hepatitis B vaccine series should be initiated as soon as possible after HBIg administration.

Side effects following vaccine administration have been minimal, with soreness at the injection site being the primary complaint in approximately 25% of vaccinees. Arthralgias and neurologic side effects are exceedingly rare.[27] The incidence of Guillain-Barré syndrome temporally related to administration of the vaccine does not appear to be above the expected case rate in adults, and no etiologic association with the vaccine has been made. The vaccine does not adversely or therapeutically affect hepatitis B carriers or persons who are already antibody positive.[42]

HEPATITIS B IMMUNOGLOBULIN

Hepatitis B immunoglobulin is used for postexposure, and rarely preexposure, prophylaxis for hepatitis B infection. The product is prepared from pooled plasma obtained from a small group of healthy donors who have high titers of hepatitis B surface antibody (anti-HBs) as a result of hyperimmunization with hepatitis B vaccine. Immune serum globulin is not indicated for hepatitis B postexposure prophylaxis.

Indications for the use of HBIg include passive immunization following exposure to hepatitis B virus via percutaneous, permucosal, or oral ingestion routes (needlesticks, accidental splash, sexual contact, mouth pipetting) and for infants born to mothers who are hepatitis B carriers. It has also been used for preexposure prophylaxis in the dialysis setting. With the advent of hepatitis B vaccine and the use of erythropoietin, however, a decline in the incidence of hepatitis B in dialysis units has been noted, and thus, HBIg is not generally recommended.

Reports on the use of HBIg have confirmed a significant protective effect of this product (70% to 75% efficacy) and, in general, superior efficacy when compared to standard immunoglobulin.[27,42,44] There is evidence, however, that HBIg may prolong the incubation period in situations where protective efficacy is not achieved.[45]

The timing of HBIg prophylaxis—regarding both frequency of dosing and proximity to the time of exposure—has not been completely defined. The CDC recommends that HBIg be given as soon as possible after acute exposures (percutaneous, permucosal, oral ingestion), preferably within 24 hours. It is not recommended that HBIg be given beyond 14 days after acute exposure. Variations in the recommendations reflect the relative risk associated with the type of exposure that exists.[46] Generally, the use of HBIg (single dose) with initiation of the hepatitis B vaccine series is thought to be 70% to 95% effective in preventing infection with hepatitis B.[47]

HAEMOPHILUS INFLUENZAE TYPE B VACCINES

Before 1995, *H. influenzae* type b (HIB) was responsible for thousands of cases of serious illnesses (meningitis, epiglottitis, pneumonia, sepsis, septic arthritis). The incidence of HIB disease has declined by 95%, however, since the introduction of the conjugate vaccines based on the organism's capsular substance, polyribosyl ribitol phosphate (PRP).[48]

The HIB vaccines in use are conjugate products, consisting either of a polysaccharide or oligosaccharide of PRP covalently linked to a protein carrier. The protein carrier is important because it provides for T-lymphocyte-dependent immunologic response, whereas earlier HIB vaccines that consisted of only unconjugated PRP elicited a response that was T-cell independent. T-cell involvement in the response provides for (a) a greater antibody response, regardless of the age of the patient receiving the vaccine; (b) immunologic response at an earlier age (including infants); and (c) a booster effect on subsequent exposure to the HIB capsule, whether through revaccination or natural exposure. The protein carrier is not considered a vaccine and should not be substituted for immunization against tetanus, diphtheria, or *Neisseria meningitidis*.

The HIB conjugate vaccines are stable at 2°C (35.6°F) to 8°C (46.4°F) and should not be frozen. They are indicated for routine use in all infants and children younger than 5 years of age. All of the conjugate products are immunogenic, but only three of the four commercially available products are sufficiently immunogenic for use in infants. Additionally, these three products differ in their immunogenicity and schedule of administration. The primary series of HIB vaccination consists of a 0.5-mL IM dose at ages 2, 4, and 6 months, if HbOC (HibTITER) or PRP-T (OmniHIB) is used. If PRP-OMP is being used, the primary series consists of doses given at 2 and 4 months of age. The series should not be initiated in an infant younger than 6 weeks of age. Although use of one product for the entire primary series is desirable, adequate protection is achieved even when different products are used during the initial doses. Following the primary series, a booster dose is recommended at age 12 to 15 months. Any of the four HIB conjugate products, including PRP-D (ProHIBiT), are suitable for the booster dose, regardless of which conjugate was used for the primary series of doses.[1,48] Additionally, the DTaP-Hib combination can be used for this booster dose.

Schedules become more complex for infants who do not begin their HIB immunization at the recommended age or who have fallen behind in the immunization schedule. For infants 7 to 11 months of age who have not been vaccinated, three doses of HbOC, PRP-OMP, or PRP-T should be given: two doses, spaced 8 weeks apart, and then a booster dose at age 12 to 18 months (but at least 8 weeks since dose two). For unvaccinated children ages 12 to 14 months, two doses should be given, with an interval of 2 months between them. In a child older than 15 months, a single dose of any of the four conjugate vaccines is indicated. The American Academy of Pediatrics has made recommendations for children with lapsed immunization. For infants 7 to 11 months who have received one or two doses of HIB vaccine, one dose of vaccine with a booster dose give at least 8 weeks later at age 12 to 15 months should be given. For children 12 to 14 months who received two doses, a single dose is indicated. If the child received only one dose before 12 months, two additional doses separated by 8 weeks should be given. A single dose of vaccine is needed for a child who is 15 to 59 months of age and who has received any incomplete schedule.[49]

Vaccines for HIB are recommended for routine use only for patients up through 59 months of age; beyond this age, most individuals will have natural immunity to HIB infection. Patients with certain underlying conditions (HIV infection, IgG_2 subclass deficiency, sickle cell disease, splenectomy, bone marrow transplants, and those receiving chemotherapy for malignancies) are at higher-than-normal risk for HIB infection, and use of at least one dose of vaccine in these patients should be considered, although efficacy data are lacking in most of these situations.

Adverse reactions to the HIB vaccine are uncommon. Erythema and induration at the injection site occur in approximately 25% of children and resolve within 24 hours. Fever, diarrhea, and vomiting are occasionally reported. Fever of greater than 38°C (100.4°F) is reported in 2.4% of children.

INFLUENZA VIRUS VACCINE

Influenza is respiratory illness that is characterized by abrupt onset of fever, myalgia, headache, severe malaise, cough, sore throat, and rhinitis. The illness typically resolves in several days, but can exacerbate a chronic medical condition or lead to secondary bacterial pneumonia. Influenza activity each winter results in increased numbers of physician visits, hospitalizations, and deaths.

The Advisory Committee on Immunization Practices (ACIP) makes yearly recommendations concerning the use and composition of influenza virus vaccine. These are published in Morbidity and Mortality Weekly Report annually. The reader should refer to these annual guidelines as a supplemental update to this chapter.

Influenza is classified as type A or B, with influenza A further subtyped based on hemagglutinin (H) and neuraminidase (N) surface antigens. Influenza A causes significant disease in humans, and the virus is subject to mutation by a phenomenon known as antigenic drift and shift, resulting in the development of different influenza strains. Previous exposure to or vaccination against one strain does not confer protection against other strains. Influenza B, also a significant cause of human disease, is less likely to mutate. The antigenic composition of influenza vaccine is determined from year-to-year by the predominant circulating strains worldwide and generally, changes on a yearly basis.[50]

Influenza vaccine is an inactivated (killed), trivalent whole- or split-virus vaccine. Available preparations generally contain 45 μg of antigen, in 15-μg trivalent units per 0.5 mL and are administered by intramuscular injection. Split-virus vaccine must be used for children from 6 months to 12 years of age. Children 6 to 35 months old receive 0.25 mL of split-virus vaccine. Two doses of vaccine administered at least 1 month apart are necessary for all children younger than 9 years old who are receiving the vaccine for the first time. Split-virus vaccine is less reactogenic than whole-virus vaccine, particularly in children.[51] Whole- or split-virus vaccine can be administered to individuals older than 12 years of age.

Response to influenza vaccine is generally measured in terms of antibody response and, more importantly, efficacy. The elderly and individuals with chronic diseases are less likely to develop antibody levels that are considered protective and may remain susceptible to influenza infection. However, vaccination confers protection from secondary complications and reduces the risk of hospitalization or pneumonia by 50% to 60% and death by 80%. Influenza vaccine is cost-effective in nursing home populations, in the elderly who live in the community, and in healthy working adults.[51,54]

Annual influenza vaccination is strongly recommended for individuals over the age of 6 months with chronic medical conditions, that make them at increased risk for the complications of influenza. Annual influenza vaccination should be given to (a) all individuals 50 years of age and older; (b) residents of nursing homes; (c) adults and children with chronic cardiovascular or pulmonary diseases, including asthma; (d) adults and children with chronic metabolic disease, renal dysfunction, hemoglobinopathies, or immunosuppression (including immunosuppression from medications and HIV); (e) children and teenagers receiving chronic aspirin therapy; and (f) pregnant women who will be in the second or third trimester during the influenza season. In addition, the influenza vaccination should be recommended for these groups which can transmit influenza to high-risk groups: (a) health care workers in both inpatient and outpatient settings; (b) employees of residential care facilities for high-risk patients; and (c) household members (including children) of persons in high-risk groups. Finally, influenza vaccination should be offered to anyone wishing to avoid influenza infection.[55] The optimal time period for influenza vaccination administration is October through mid-November. However, the vaccine can be administered to unvaccinated individuals in high-risk groups throughout the influenza season, which typically lasts until April. Administration of the influenza vaccination is contraindicated in persons with known anaphylactic reaction to eggs or another component of the vaccine. Adults with acute febrile illness should be vaccinated when their symptoms have abated. Vaccination need not be delayed in individuals with minor illness with or without fever.

Antiviral prophylaxis should be considered in individuals for whom the vaccine is contraindicated or for unvaccinated high-risk individuals as a bridge until a response to the vaccine has been mounted. Both amantadine and rimantadine are highly effective in preventing influenza A infection. Rimantadine is much better tolerated in the nursing home population.[56] The neuraminidase inhibitors, zanamivir and oseltamivir, have been shown to be effective for infection prophylaxis, but neither is approved for this use.[57,58]

Adverse reactions to the vaccine include local tenderness or low-grade fever in 3% to 5% of vaccinees beginning 6 to 12 hours postimmunization and lasting 1 to 2 days. Treatment with salicylates or acetaminophen is recommended. A slight increase in the risk of Guillain-Barré syndrome may follow in the weeks following influenza vaccination. The risk is estimated to be one case of Guillain-Barré syndrome per million doses of influenza vaccine administered.[59]

LYME DISEASE VACCINE

Lyme disease is the most common tickborne illness in the United States. It is caused by *Borrelia burgdorferi* infection transmitted by the Ixodes tick. Lyme disease is endemic in the northeast and north-central United States. In northern California, *B. burgdorferi* infection is transmitted by the *Ixodes pacificus* tick. Early Lyme disease is characterized the erythema migrans rash (a target-shaped rash present in 70% to 90% of patients) and flu-like symptoms. Early disseminated disease occurs 1 to several months after infection. Lymphocytic meningitis, cranial neuropathy, migratory joint pain, muscle pains, myocarditis or transient heart block may be present in this stage. Migratory polyarthritis, typically in weightbearing joints, chronic axonal polyneuropathy, or encephalopathy is characteristically present in late disseminated Lyme disease.

The antigen in the Lyme disease vaccine is recombinant outer-surface protein A (OspA). Antibodies to OspA are protective against infection. A three-dose series scheduled at 0, 1, and 12 months is required. Alternative compressed schedules are being investigated.

In clinical trials, the vaccine was 76% effective in preventing definite Lyme disease after the complete series, but only 49% effective after the first two doses.[60] Currently, the vaccine is only approved for use in individuals aged 15 to 70 years of age. The Lyme disease vaccine series is recommended for individuals at high risk for contracting the infection—individuals who reside, work, or recreate in areas of high or moderate risk, including people who have had Lyme disease previously.[60] Because the vaccine series take 12 months to complete with partial protection conferred by the first two doses, travelers to endemic areas should be advised to practice personal protection measures, such as application of pesticides, tucking pants into boots, wearing long-sleeved shirts, and frequent self-inspection. The Lyme disease vaccine is associated with local reactions and some systemic effects. These are generally mild and last 3 or 4 days.[60,61] Limitations of this vaccine include (a) an unknown duration of protection and need for booster doses; (b) unknown safety in individuals with joint diseases; (c) unknown efficacy in individuals older than 70 years; and (d) unknown safety and efficacy in children, though clinical trials of the vaccine in children are nearing completion.

MEASLES VACCINE

Measles (rubeola) is a highly contagious viral illness that is characterized by rash and high fever. Complications of measles infections include severe diarrhea, otitis media, pneumonia, and encephalitis. Measles results in 1–2 deaths per 1,000 cases, with the death rate much higher in developing countries. With widespread vaccination, measles has been targeted for elimination in the Americas in the next few years.

The measles vaccine is a live attenuated viral vaccine that produces a subclinical, noncommunicable infection. Approximately 95% of vaccine recipients seroconvert after a single dose, and most are protected for life.[62] Most persons failing to respond to the initial dose of measles vaccine will seroconvert following a second dose, and this forms the basis for the two-dose vaccine strategy that was implemented in the United States in 1989. The second dose is not harmful to individuals who seroconverted after the first dose, because it merely reinforces their immunity. Important genetic determinants of measles vaccine response are being elucidated.[63]

The measles vaccine is administered subcutaneously as a 0.5-mL dose in the arm (or in the thigh, if the patient is younger than 15 months of age). The vaccine is routinely administered for primary immunization to persons 12 to 15 months of age, usually as the MMR vaccine. The measles vaccine is not administered earlier than 12 months (except in certain outbreak circumstances) because persisting maternal antibody that was acquired transplacentally late in gestation can neutralize the vaccine virus and deprive the opportunity for immune response. A second dose of MMR is recommended when children are aged 4 to 6 years.[64] The second dose of vaccine results in seroconversion in 95% of those individuals who were first-dose nonresponders.[65]

Measles-containing vaccine should not be given to pregnant women or immunosuppressed patients. The one exception is HIV-infected patients, who are at very high risk for severe complications if they develop measles.[66,67] Persons with HIV who have never had measles or been vaccinated against it should be given measles-containing vaccine, unless there is evidence of severe immunosuppression.[9] The second dose should be given 1 month later rather than waiting for entry to school.[64]

Recent administration of immunoglobulin interferes with measles vaccine response,[68] so the recommended interval between the immunoglobulin and vaccine is determined by the dose of immunoglobulin.[1] The administration of other live vaccines not administered on the same day should be delayed for at least 30 days following measles or MMR vaccine. Live measles vaccine may suppress a positive tuberculin skin test for up to 6 weeks postadministration.[1] Historically, persons with a history of anaphylactic reaction to egg protein were considered to be at high risk for serious reactions to measles vaccine, a product derived from chick embryo fibroblasts. As a precaution, skin testing of egg-allergic persons and possible egg-desensitization was recommended prior to measles vaccination. Skin test results poorly predict adverse reactions, however, and the risk of measles vaccination to egg-allergic patients has been shown to be exceedingly low. Therefore, individuals in need of measles vaccine should receive it, regardless of the history of egg allergy.[64] A history of serious neomycin hypersensitivity remains a contraindication to measles vaccine use, as each 0.5-mL dose contains 25 μg of neomycin. Finally, mild febrile illness and upper respiratory tract infections are not contraindications to vaccination.[69–72]

Measles vaccination is indicated in all persons born after 1956 or in those who lack documentation of wild virus infection either by history or antibody titers. Persons who received killed measles vaccine alone, or who were given live vaccine within 3 months of receiving killed vaccine, or who received a vaccine of unknown type between 1963 and 1967 should be revaccinated. Revaccination should be considered for students entering college, because of outbreaks on college campuses. It is also important to vaccinate health care workers who have no documentation of vaccination and who were born in 1957 or later, because of the possibility of becoming infected by patients and transmitting the disease to their patients.[64] If two doses are needed (the person has never been vaccinated), the doses should be given at least 1 month apart. Following vaccination, antibodies may be detected within 2 to 3 weeks in patients 12 months of age or older.

For postexposure prophylaxis, the vaccine is effective if given within 72 hours of exposure. In addition, immunoglobulin may be administered at a dose of 0.25 mg/kg IM (maximum dose, 15 mL), if given within 6 days of exposure. In infants, postexposure vaccination may be given as early as 6 months of age, but it should be repeated at 12 to 15 months of age.

The measles vaccine has an excellent safety record. The most common side effect following vaccination is fever, which occurs in 5% to 15% of vaccinees. Transient rash (generalized) may also occur in about 5% of vaccine recipients. These reactions generally appear 5 to 12 days postvaccination and last 2 to 5 days. Febrile seizures rarely occur, and there is no association between MMR vaccination and development of a subsequent seizure disorder. Other adverse effects, such as headache, cough, sore throat, eye pain, malaise, and transient thrombocytopenia, occur less frequently. Local reactions at the injection site, while rare, may occur in subjects who have previously been vaccinated with killed vaccine.

MENINGOCOCCAL POLYSACCHARIDE VACCINE

Neisseria meningitidis is a leading cause of meningitis and sepsis in children and young adults in the United States. The vast majority of cases are sporadic, although the frequency of outbreaks, most often involving serogroup C, is increasing.

A quadrivalent vaccine containing capsular polysaccharides for serotypes A, C, Y, and W-135 has been available since the early 1970s. Although serogroup B causes approximately one-third of all cases, it has not been incorporated into the vaccine because group B polysaccharide is not immunogenic. The meningococcal polysaccharide vaccine is indicated in high-risk populations, such as those exposed to the disease, those in the midst of uncontrolled outbreaks, travelers to an area with epidemic or hyperendemic meningococcal disease, or individuals who have terminal complement component deficiencies or asplenia.

College freshmen, particularly those living in dormitories or residence halls, are at modestly increased risk of invasive meningococcal disease as compared to the rest of the population in this age group.[73–76] The ACIP recommends that health care providers inform students and parents about the increased risk and that a safe effective vaccine is available. The meningococcal polysaccharide vaccine should be made easily available for those college freshmen wishing to decrease their risk for meningococcal disease.[73]

Meningococcal polysaccharide vaccine is administered subcutaneously as a single 0.5-mL dose. Vaccinees should be older than 2 years of age because of the difficulty younger patients have responding to polysaccharide antigens. Younger children may produce sufficient antibody levels against serogroup A, however, if given two doses 3 months apart.[73] Antibody levels thought to be protective are attained within 10 to 14 days. Revaccination may be considered in 2 to 3 years in high-risk children, who are younger than 4 years old, on initial vaccination because of rapid antibody decline. Older children and adults who remain at high risk should be revaccinated after 3 to 5 years.[73] The vaccine shows documented effectiveness in preventing meningococcal disease in 85% to 95% of recipients for serotypes A and C. Efficacy of the vaccine for serotypes Y and W-135 is presumed but not documented. Adverse effects of meningococcal polysaccharide vaccine include fever and erythema at the injection site lasting 1 to 2 days.

MUMPS VACCINE

Mumps is a viral illness that classically causes bilateral parotitis 16 to 18 days after exposure. Fever, headache, malaise, myalgia, and anorexia may precede the parotitis. Serious complications are rare, although more common in adults.

The mumps vaccine is a lyophilized live attenuated vaccine prepared from chick embryo cultures. Each 0.5-mL dose of the vaccine also contains 25 μg of neomycin. The vaccine is available alone or in combinations with measles and rubella vaccines.

The mumps vaccine is used to produce active immunity while producing a subclinical, noncommunicable infection. A single dose induces antibody formation in 97% of children older than 12 months of age and 93% of adults. Clinical efficacy ranges from 75% to 95%. The duration of immunity following vaccination is unknown, but data collected in the 30 years of use indicate that the efficacy persists.[64]

The vaccine is usually given in combination with measles and rubella vaccines (as MMR) and is administered as a 0.5-mL subcutaneous injection in the upper arm. Dosing recommendations coincide with those for measles vaccine, with the first dose being administered at age 12 to 15 months, and the second dose prior to entry into elementary school. If the vaccine is given before 12 months of age, revaccination is necessary and should be given after reaching 1 year of age. The vaccine is also indicated in previously unvaccinated adults, in those who have previously been vaccinated with killed mumps vaccine (an older product no longer available), and in those with an uncertain history of wild virus infection. Postexposure vaccination is of no benefit.[64]

Mumps vaccine should not be given to pregnant women or immunosuppressed patients. Additionally, conception should be avoided for 3 months following vaccination. Anaphylactic reactions to mumps-containing vaccines are very rare and generally not associated with hypersensitivity to eggs. Therefore, egg allergy is not a contraindication to vaccination. The effect of immunoglobulin preparations on mumps vaccine response is unknown, but the response to measles and rubella is compromised if administered after immunoglobulins. The recommended interval between the immunoglobulin and vaccine is determined by the dose of immunoglobulin.[64] Finally, the vaccine should not be given to individuals with anaphylactic reactions to neomycin.

Serious adverse reactions to the vaccine are rarely reported. Parotitis, rash, pruritus, and purpura rarely occur. Local reactions, including soreness, burning, and stinging, may occur at the injection site.

PERTUSSIS VACCINE

Pertussis is a caused by a bacterial infection with *Bordetella pertussis*. The illness is characterized by paroxysms of coughing to expel thick mucous. In the early part of this century, pertussis was a common childhood infection and was a significant cause of childhood mortality. In recent years, the incidence of disease has been increasing in all age groups. Although infants and young children remain at highest risk for infections and its complications, investigators recently determined that older adults also are at increased risk of complications from pertussis.[77]

Acellular pertussis vaccines contain selective components of the *B. pertussis* organism. All acellular vaccines contain pertussis toxin (PT), and some contain one or more additional bacterial components (filamentous hemagglutinin [FHA], pertactin [a 69-kDa outer membrane protein], and fimbriae types 2 and 3). Acellular pertussis vaccine is recommended for all doses of the pertussis schedule at 2, 4, 6, and 15 to 18 months of age. A fifth dose of pertussis vaccine is given to children 4 to 6 years old.[78,79] Pertussis vaccine is administered in combination with diphtheria and tetanus (DTaP). Although the pertussis vaccine is not recommended for individuals 7 years of age and older, booster doses for adolescents and adults may be incorporated into future recommendations because members of these groups are important reservoirs of infection.

Local administration site reactions occur relatively commonly. Systemic reactions, such as moderate fever, occur in 3% to 5% of vaccinees. Very rarely, high fever, febrile seizures, persistent crying spells, hypotonic hyporesponsive episodes occur following vaccination. Allergy to a vaccine component and encephalopathy without known cause within 7 days of a pertussis vaccine are contraindications to future doses of vaccine. Efficacy of the vaccine is estimated to be about 80%.[78]

POLIOVIRUS VACCINES

Poliomyelitis is a contagious viral infection that usually causes asymptomatic infection, but in its serious form, causes acute flaccid paralysis. Poliovirus is spread via the fecal oral route. The virus replicates in the upper respiratory tract, gastrointestinal tract, and local lymphatics. The vast majority of polio infections are subclinical and asymptomatic. Indigenous polio has been absent from the United States since 1979, and the last case in the Americas was reported in 1991. Global eradication efforts are entering the final stages, and the eradication of polio should be accomplished in the next few years.

Two types of trivalent poliovirus vaccines are licensed for distribution in the United States. An inactivated vaccine, developed by Salk, was licensed for use in 1955. In 1987, an enhanced-potency inactivated polio vaccine (eIPV) was introduced, which has replaced the original inactivated vaccine. Since 1962, a live attenuated, oral polio vaccine (OPV), developed by Sabin, has been the primary immunizing agent for poliovirus infection. Currently, eIPV is the recommended vaccine for the primary series and booster dose for children in the United States, but OPV will continue to be used in the areas of the world that have circulating poliovirus, and in rare circumstances in the United States, such as an outbreak.[80]

The eIPV series is administered routinely to children at ages 2, 4, and 6 to 18 months and 4 to 6 years. Protective antibodies to all three serotypes develop in 90% to 100% of children after two doses of vaccine. After three doses, 99% to 100% develop protective immunity, and the fourth dose results in long-term immunity.[80]

Primary poliomyelitis immunization is recommended for all children up to age 18. Primary immunization of adults over the age of 18 is not routinely recommended because a high level of immunity already exists in this age group and the risk of exposure in developed countries is small. Unimmunized adults who are at increased risk for exposure because of travel, residence, or occupation should, however, receive eIPV series.

Allergies to any component of eIPV, including streptomycin, polymyxin B, and neomycin, are contraindications to vaccine use. There are no serious side effects attributable to eIPV, and the only other contraindication is pregnancy, in which case eIPV should be given only if there is a clear need, such as women who will be traveling or living in an area with endemic or epidemic poliovirus. eIPV is recommended for immunodeficient individuals and their household contacts. However, the response may be compromised, but some protection against infection may be conferred.[80]

The routine use of OPV in the United States has been discontinued, because OPV is very rarely associated with vaccine-associated paralytic poliomyelitis (VAPP) in vaccinees (1 in 6.2 million doses) or contacts (1 in 7.6 million doses). Individuals with primary immune deficiency are at increased risk for this adverse reaction, and for this reason, OPV is not recommended for persons who are immunodeficient or for normal individuals who reside in a household with an immunocompromised person.[79] The use of OPV is reserved for polio outbreak control.[80]

Incompletely immunized adults or children should complete the series of IPV regardless of the interval since initiation of primary immunization. Adults do not routinely need a booster dose unless there is an increased risk of exposure (travel), in which case, a single dose of IPV can be given.[80]

PNEUMOCOCCAL POLYSACCHARIDE VACCINE

Pneumococcal vaccine (Pneumovax 23 and Pnu-Immune 23) is a mixture of highly purified capsular polysaccharides from 23 of the 83 most prevalent or invasive types of *Streptococcus pneumoniae* seen in the United States. The serotypes included are 1, 2, 3, 4, 5, 6B, 7F, 8, 9N, 9V, 10A, 12F, 14, 15B, 17F, 18C, 19A, 20, 22F, 23F, and 33F. These 23 types represent 85% to 90% of all blood isolates and 85% of pneumococcal isolates from other generally sterile sites seen in the United States. Each 0.5-mL dose of vaccine contains 25 μg of each polysaccharide type dissolved in isotonic saline solution (for a total of 575 μg of polysaccharide) and 0.25% phenol as preservative. Significant cross-reactivity with other pneumococcal capsular antigens not represented in the vaccine does not occur.[82]

Pneumococcal vaccine efficacy has been debated in the literature. In nonbacteremic disease, although prelicensure trials in young healthy gold miners in South Africa showed reduction in disease rates,[83] in the postmarketing period, randomized clinical trials performed in elderly persons with chronic disease did not confirm these findings.[82] A meta-analysis of various trials also has not confirmed protection in nonbacteremic disease with pneumococcal vaccine.[82] In addition, the vaccine has not been shown to be effective for the prevention of sinusitis or acute otitis media in children caused by the lack of immunogenicity of polysaccharide vaccines.

For invasive disease, reduction rates of 56% to 81% have been shown with the vaccine. In adults, vaccine efficacy was shown for persons with chronic disease and immunocompromised individuals ≥65 years of age. A meta-analysis of nine randomized controlled trials concluded that the vaccine was efficacious in reducing the frequency of bacteremic pneumococcal pneumonia among adults in low-risk groups. Cost-effectiveness has also been shown.[82] The vaccine is only effective for the serotypes included.

Pneumococcal vaccine induces type-specific antibodies (T-cell independent mechanisms) with a twofold rise within 2 to 3 weeks in 80% of young healthy adults. No correlation of antibody levels and protection has been defined. Antibody levels to these strains remain elevated for at least 5 years. In certain individuals, these levels decline within 10 years. Children may be protected for only 3 to 5 years. Elderly individuals and patients with chronic disease may have lower antibody levels produced with the vaccine. Children younger than 2 years of age do not respond adequately to the vaccine.

A number of other groups including immunocompromised patients (leukemia, lymphoma, multiple myeloma), dialysis patients, and AIDS patients, have reduced antibody production with the vaccine. Asymptomatic HIV-infected patients respond sufficiently to the vaccine. Patients with Hodgkin's disease respond to the vaccine better before splenectomy, chemotherapy, or radiation therapy.

Pneumococcal vaccine is recommended for the following immunocompetent persons.[82]

- Persons 65 years of age or older. If an individual received vaccine more than 5 years earlier and was younger than age 65 at the time of administration, revaccination should be given.
- Persons ages 2 to 64 years of age with a chronic illness.
- Persons ages 2 to 64 of age with functional or anatomic asplenia. When splenectomy is planned, pneumococcal vaccine should be given at least 2 weeks prior to surgery. A single revaccination is recommended at ≥5 years in subjects older than 10 years of age and at 3 years in subjects younger than 10 years of age.
- Persons ages 2 to 64 years of age living in environments where the risk of invasive pneumococcal disease or its complications are increased. This does not include day care center employees and children.

Pneumococcal vaccine is recommended for immunocompromised persons 2 years of age or older with: (a) HIV infection; (b) leukemia; (c) lymphoma; (d) Hodgkin's disease; (e) multiple myeloma; (f) generalized malignancy; (g) chronic renal failure or nephrotic syndrome; (h) patients receiving immunosuppressive therapy including corticosteroids; or (i) organ and bone marrow transplant recipients. A single revaccination should be given if 5 years or more has passed since receipt of the first dose in subjects older than 10 years of age. In subjects 10 years of age or older, revaccination should be given 3 years after the previous dose.

While the safety of pneumococcal vaccine during the first trimester of pregnancy has not been evaluated, no adverse effects have been seen in newborns whose mothers received the vaccine during pregnancy.[82]

Pneumococcal vaccine safety is well documented. Local reactions occur frequently within the first 48 hours and are generally mild. Local erythema and induration (30%), local discomfort (40%), and local swelling (3%) are the side effects most commonly observed. Revaccination has been associated with no more local adverse effects than after the first dose.[82,83] Rarely, severe systemic reactions can occur, and they consist of weakness, myalgia, headache, photophobia, chills, and fever. Guillain-Barré syndrome has not been reported. In patients with HIV infection, pneumococcal vaccine may cause a transient increase in viral replication, however, the importance of this is unknown.

The vaccine should be administered intramuscularly or subcutaneously as a single 0.5-mL dose. The vaccine may be given simultaneously as influenza vaccine (in separate arms) and with DaPT or poliovirus vaccine.

PNEUMOCOCCAL CONJUGATE VACCINE

Because of the lack of immune responsiveness in children younger than 2 years of age when exposed to polysaccharide vaccines, manufacturers have been developing conjugate vaccines to offer children protection from certain strains of *S. pneumoniae*. Formation of serotype conjugates to assure stability and immunogenicity of each strain is complex and difficult. Thus, work has progressed slowly.

Currently, a heptavalent vaccine (Prevnar) is available for use in children. This vaccine contains the conjugated capsular polysaccharides of serotypes 4, 6B, 9V, 14, 18C, 19F, and 23F, which cause approximately 80% of pediatric pneumococcal bacteremias in the United States.[84] The vaccine elicits a primary T-cell-dependent antibody response with the first dose and an immunologic memory effect after 4 doses. The vaccine is administered as 0.5 ml IM at 2, 4, and 6 months of age, and between 12 and 15 months of age. Erythema, swelling, and tenderness at the injection site occur in 10% to 20% of children and fever >38°C (100.4°F) occurs in 15% to 20% of children.

The vaccine reduces invasive pneumococcal disease caused by the serotypes in the vaccine by 100%. In addition, the vaccine appears to reduce the incidence of recurrent otitis media by 23%.[84]

RABIES VACCINE

HDCV, rabies vaccine adsorbed (RVA), and purified chick embryo cell culture rabies vaccine (PCEC) are killed vaccines used for preexposure and postexposure rabies virus prophylaxis. Transmission of rabies can occur via percutaneous, permucosal, or airborne exposure to the rabies virus. Circumstances favoring such transmission include animal bites or attacks and contamination of scratches, cuts, abrasions, or mucous membranes with saliva or other infectious material (brain tissue). Unprovoked attacks and daytime attacks by nocturnal animals are considered highly suspect. Common wild animal transmitters include skunks, foxes, and raccoons. Dog rabies is very common in certain foreign countries (India, African nations). Rodents, rabbits, and hares are rarely infected. There have been a few reports of a person-to-person transmission.[85] Reports of rabid animals have increased over the past decade in the United States.

Preexposure indications for using HDCV, RVA, or PCEC include persons whose vocation or avocation place them at high risk for rabies exposure, for example, veterinarians, animal handlers, laboratory workers in rabies research laboratories, and field personnel (trappers, hunters, cave explorers). Travelers who will be in a country or area of a country where there is a constant threat of rabies, whose stay is likely to extend beyond 1 month, and who may not have readily available medical services (Peace Corps workers, missionaries) should also be considered for preexposure prophylaxis. The population at large need not be vaccinated.[85] The vaccine is not recommended for persons who are immunocompromised because of inadequate response. If the vaccine is used in immunocompromised persons, it should be given by the IM route only and antibody titers should be checked postimmunization. Completion of a course of immunization should be completed with the same product as no data exists on interchangeability of products.

Postexposure prophylaxis should be given after percutaneous or permucosal exposure to saliva or other infectious material from a high-risk source. Each case needs to be considered individually. Consideration needs to be given to the geographic area, species of animal, circumstances of the incident, and type of exposure. Local or state health departments may be able to provide guidelines.

The HDCV for preexposure prophylaxis is administered in three doses of 1 mL IM or 0.1 mL intradermally on days 0 and 7 and once between days 21 and 28.[85] For intradermal prophylaxis HDCV must be given using the specific intradermal dosage form and syringe. Although the literature suggests that intradermal vaccine gives protective titers in an equal number of patients compared to IM dosing,[86,88] field reports suggest that intradermal HDCV may give a nonprotection rate of 7.5%.[89,90] This observation has lead the New York State Department of Health to recommend the routine use of IM rabies vaccine.[88] If intradermal injection is used, it is suggested that rabies antibody titers be checked 30 days after the last dose of vaccine. Rabies vaccine adsorbed and PCEC may be used intramuscularly but not intradermally for preexposure prophylaxis. Pregnancy is not a contraindication if the risk of rabies is great.

An IM booster dose every second year is recommended for persons who will have continued exposure. Some authors recommend testing rabies antibody with booster doses deferred if the rapid fluorescent focus inhibition test (RFFIT) is >1:5. Intradermal booster doses, although recommended the CDC,[85] is not recommended by the New York State Department of Health.[90] Suboptimal responses have been documented in persons receiving chloroquine chemoprophylaxis for malaria;[85] thus, the vaccine should be administered 1 month prior to the institution of chloroquine therapy. If this is not possible, IM HDCV, RVA, or PCEC should be used. For individuals who have received the duck-embryo vaccines in the past, a single IM booster dose of HDCV, RVA, or PCEC may be used.

Preexposure prophylaxis does not eliminate the need for postexposure prophylaxis. The regimen for postexposure prophylaxis is determined by whether or not a person has previously received HDCV, RVA, or PCEC. Persons previously immunized with HDCV, RVA, or PCEC or those who have received postexposure prophylaxis previously should receive two 1-mL IM doses of HDCV, RVA, or PCEC on postexposure days 0 and 3. Rabies immunoglobulin should not be given to this group. Individuals who have not been previously immunized should receive the recommended regimen of rabies immunoglobulin (see Rabies Immunoglobulin section) and five doses of HDCV, RVA, or PCEC, 1-mL IM on days 0, 3, 7, 14, and 28 after exposure.[85] The intradermal route should not be used for postexposure prophylaxis.

Intramuscular vaccine should be given in the deltoid muscle in adults and the anterolateral thigh in children. The gluteal region should not be used.

Adverse reactions to HDCV, RVA, and PCEC are not uncommon. Approximately 20% of vaccinees will experience pain, erythema, swelling, and itching at the injection site. Another 20% of vaccinees may have headache, nausea, abdominal pain, muscle aches, dizziness, or a combination of these.[85] Systemic allergic reactions ranging from hives to anaphylaxis occur in a very small number of subjects. It is recommended that persons exposed to rabies who do have adverse reactions continue the vaccine series in a setting with medical support services. In persons receiving booster doses of HDCV an immune complex-like disease has been seen 2 to 21 days later in as many as 7% of vaccinees. The incidence of serum sickness-like reactions 7 to 14 days later with RVA booster doses is <1%.

Antibody conversion occurs in virtually 100% of HDCV or RVA recipients by 7 to 10 days following immunization. The CDC considers titers of 1:5 by RFFIT testing as being protective. The World Health Organization (WHO) uses a value of 0.5 IU/mL as evidence of protective antibody. Persons who are receiving corticosteroids or other immunosuppressant agents and who receive postexposure prophylaxis should have their antibody status determined. Chloroquine or mefloquine may weaken the antibody response to HDCV when it is administered intradermally. In patients receiving these agents, the IM route is recommended.

RABIES IMMUNOGLOBULIN

Human rabies immunoglobulin is an immunoglobulin used in conjunction with rabies vaccine as part of postexposure rabies management for previously unvaccinated individuals. The product is derived from plasma obtained from donors who have been hyperimmunized with rabies vaccine and have high titers of circulating antibody.

In persons who have not been previously immunized against rabies, rabies immunoglobulin is given simultaneously with rabies HDCV, RVA, or PCEC to provide optimal coverage in the interval before immune response to the vaccine occurs. The efficacy of this regimen has been clearly demonstrated. In situations in which a vaccine has been used alone, mortality rates of 50% to 60% have been observed. Mortality after the combination vaccine and rabies immunoglobulin regimens is an exceedingly rare event; however, failures have been reported when the wound was not infiltrated with rabies immunoglobulin.[91]

Rabies immunoglobulin does not interfere with vaccine-induced antibody formation. Its use is not recommended beyond 8 days after initiation of the vaccine series nor in persons previously immunized to rabies, however.

Human rabies immunoglobulin is administered in a dose of 20 IU/kg (0.133 mL/kg), half to be given intramuscularly and the other half infiltrated around the wound site. This product should never be administered by the intravenous route. Because other antibodies in the rabies immunoglobulin may interfere with the response to live virus vaccines (MMR), it is recommended that these immunizations be delayed for 3 months.

Side effects are rare but may include local soreness at the wound or IM injection site and mild temperature elevations. Caution is advised when administering this product to persons with known systemic allergies to immunoglobulin or thimerosal. Pregnancy is not a contraindication for its use.

RUBELLA VACCINE

An erythematous rash, lymphadenopathy, arthralgia, and low-grade fever characterize rubella (German Measles). As many as 25% to 50% of rubella infections are subclinical. The most important consequence of rubella infection occurs during pregnancy, particularly during the first trimester. Congenital rubella syndrome is associated with auditory, ophthalmic, cardiac, and neurologic defects. Rubella infection during pregnancy can also result in miscarriage or stillbirth. The primary goal of rubella immunization is to prevent congenital rubella syndrome.

Rubella vaccine contains lyophilized live attenuated rubella (German measles) virus grown in human diploid cell culture. The vaccine is available alone or in combination with measles or mumps vaccine, or both. Each 0.5-mL dose also contains 25 μg of neomycin.

Rubella vaccine induces antibodies to the virus that are protective against wild-virus infection. Following a single 0.5-mL subcutaneous dose, 95% of children 1 year of age or older become rubella antibody positive within 2 to 6 weeks.[93] The duration of immunity has not been established, and booster doses are not recommended. A second dose is recommended, however, at the same time measles vaccine is administered (as a second dose of MMR). The vaccine is indicated for children older than 1 year of age. Although individuals born before 1957 are assumed to be immune to rubella, this is not sufficient for women who could become pregnant. Therefore, all women of childbearing potential should have documentation of receiving at least one dose of a rubella-containing vaccine or laboratory evidence of immunity.[93] Recent administration of immunoglobulin interferes with rubella vaccine response,[91] so the recommended interval between the immunoglobulin and vaccine is determined by the dose of immunoglobulin.[1] The vaccine should not be given to immunosuppressed individuals, although MMR vaccine should be administered to infants with HIV without severe immunosuppression as soon as possible after their first birthday.[62] The vaccine should not be given to individuals with anaphylactic reactions to neomycin.[62]

Adverse effects of the rubella virus vaccine tend to increase with the age of the recipient. Symptoms are similar to wild-virus infection and include lymphadenopathy, rash, urticaria, fever, malaise, sore throat, headache, myalgias, and paresthesias of the extremities. These occur 7 to 12 days after vaccination and last 1 to 5 days. Joint symptoms occur more often in susceptible postpubertal females. Arthralgia occurs in 25% of such vaccinees and 10% will have arthritis-like symptoms. These symptoms usually begin 1 to 3 weeks after vaccination and persist for 1 day to 3 weeks. A very small excess risk of chronic arthropathy exists.[93] The vaccine may cause suppression of tuberculin skin tests for up to 6 weeks postvaccination. While the vaccine virus may be excreted in nose and throat secretions, it is not contagious.

Although the rubella vaccine has never been associated with congenital rubella syndrome, its use during pregnancy is contraindicated. However, routine pregnancy testing prior to vaccination in not recommended. Women should be counseled not to become pregnant for 3 months following vaccination. Termination of pregnancy is not indicated in women who are accidentally given the vaccine or they become pregnant during the 3 months after vaccination.

VARICELLA VACCINE

Varicella is a highly contagious disease caused by varicella zoster virus. The clinical illness is characterized by the appearance of successive waves of pruritic vesicles that rapidly crust over. Malaise and fever are common and last for 2 to 3 days. The virus remains dormant in the dorsal ganglia and reactivates as herpes zoster, also known as shingles. Although the exact stimulus for reactivation is unknown, a decrease in varicella-specific cell mediated immunity associated with age or immunosuppression appears to be necessary, but not sufficient for reactivation.

Live attenuated varicella vaccine contains the Oka-Merck strain of varicella virus, which was attenuated by propagation through several different cell culture lines. Varicella vaccine is a lyophilized product that must be kept frozen and protected from light. Once reconstituted, it must be administered subcutaneously within 30 minutes. Each 0.5-mL dose contains a minimum of 1,350 plaque-forming units of virus, as well as 12.5 mg of hydrolyzed gelatin and trace amounts of neomycin, fetal bovine serum, and residual components from cell culture.[94]

The varicella vaccine is safe and immunogenic in healthy children and adults.[95] A single dose results in seroconversion in greater than 94% of healthy children, and over 90% have persisting antibodies 1 year later. Studies in normal, healthy adults have shown lower seroconversion rates (as low as 80%) following a single dose, but this increases to 95% when a two-dose regimen is used. In clinical studies, Varicella vaccine has been 70% to more than 95% effective in preventing chickenpox. Vaccinated individuals who develop chickenpox typically experience milder disease, with less fever and fewer skin lesions, many of which do not vesiculate.[94] Similarly, the secondary spread of virus following vaccination occurs at a low rate and has resulted in mild disease, confirming attenuation of the virus.[96]

The duration of protection provided by varicella vaccine is unknown, but it is of concern because chickenpox typically is more severe in adults than children. Recent findings reveal a potential self-boosting of vaccinated individuals as the latent vaccine virus reactivates in those with the lowest varicella antibody titers.[97] Humoral and cell-mediated immunity persists for a minimum of 6 years in vaccinated children, suggesting that protection is long-lasting.[98] Additionally, children who are immunized against varicella and then exposed to wild-virus experience an immunologic boost.[99] As varicella vaccine use becomes more widespread, the circulation of wild-virus can be expected to diminish, and the opportunity for immunologic boosting because of natural exposure will also decline. It is not known whether booster doses will be needed under these circumstances. Long-term studies assessing the duration of protection and the advisability of booster doses are ongoing.

The varicella vaccine is recommended for all children at 12 to 18 months of age. It is also recommended for patients above this age, if they have not already had chickenpox. Individuals who are 12 months to 12 years of age require one dose. Persons 13 years of age and older should receive two doses, separated by 4 to 8 weeks.[100] Varicella vaccine can be used for postexposure prophylaxis. The vaccine has been shown to be effective in the prevention or modification of varicella infection when given within 3 days, and possibly 5 days, of exposure.[101–104] Because the varicella vaccine is a live vaccine, it is contraindicated in pregnant or immunosuppressed individuals. An exception is that children with asymptomatic or mildly symptomatic HIV should receive two doses of varicella vaccine 3 months apart. Varicella vaccination is also contraindicated in individuals with a history of anaphylactic reaction to any component of the vaccine. Persons who have received blood, plasma, or immunoglobulin products within the past 5 months should not receive varicella vaccine, because of concern that passively acquired antibody will interfere with response to the vaccine. Although no adverse events associated with salicylate use after vaccination have been reported, salicylates should be avoided for 6 weeks postvaccination because of the association of salicylate use and Reye's syndrome following varicella infection.[100]

The varicella vaccine has an excellent safety record. Pain, local swelling, and erythema at the injection site occurs in up to 32% of patients and fever in 10% to 15%. A varicella-like rash occurs in approximately 4% of vaccinees, accompanied by few if any systemic symptoms. The rash may be localized at the injection site or generalized. Lesions are usually few in number (2 to 10) and often papular rather than vesicular. Transmission of vaccine virus to susceptible close contacts has occurred, but it is very rare and is believed to occur only when the vaccinee develops a rash. Because the risk of vaccine virus transmission is very low and primary infection can be very severe, vaccination of household contacts of immunosuppressed patients is recommended to prevent introduction of varicella into the household.[94,100]

Acquisition of either wild-virus or the vaccine strain of varicella renders an individual susceptible to zoster (shingles) at a later date because of reactivation of latent virus. Data indicate that following varicella vaccination, zoster occurs less frequently than following natural infection. In fact, the varicella vaccine is being investigated as a means to boost cellular immunity in the elderly to prevent shingles.[105]

VARICELLA-ZOSTER IMMUNOGLOBULIN

Varicella-zoster immunoglobulin (VZIg) is used for passive immunization of susceptible immunodeficient patients exposed to varicella infection. VZIg is prepared from plasma found in routine screening of normal volunteer blood donors to contain high titers of varicella antibody. On average, VZIg contains 10 to 20 times more varicella antibody than immunoglobulin.[100]

Postexposure prophylaxis with VZIg is indicated for the following susceptible individuals: (a) children with primary or acquired immunodeficiency, with neoplastic disease, or who require immunosuppressive therapy; (b) neonates whose mothers develop varicella within 5 days before or 2 days after delivery; (c) preterm infants

(<28 weeks gestation or who weigh <1,000 g) who are exposed to varicella while hospitalized; (d) susceptible pregnant women; (e) immunosuppressed adults and adolescents. Because healthy adults and adolescents who develop varicella are at increased risk for severe disease, complications, and death, VZIg could be considered in this population with disease modification rather than prevention being the goal. If varicella is prevented, vaccination should be offered at a later date. Exposure to varicella is defined as direct indoor contact for more than 1 hour with an infectious person. A negative history of clinical disease is not a reliable indicator of varicella susceptibility. The majority of those with a negative clinical history will have detectable antibody upon laboratory testing. Caution is warranted when interpreting a low positive result in an immunosuppressed patient who has received blood products or immunoglobulin as the circulating antibody may be acquired passively.

The clinical efficacy of VZIg can be measured by the rate at which it prevents infection, modifies disease, or prevents subclinical disease. Following household exposure, 30% to 50% of immunocompromised children who receive VZIg will develop disease. Neonates receiving VZIg exposed *in utero* will develop infection at about the same rate as neonates who did not receive VZIg, but the complication rate is substantially reduced among the infants treated with VZIg.[100]

For maximum effectiveness, VZIg must be given within 48 hours and not more than 96 hours following exposure. Because this agent may only attenuate infection, patients who receive VZIg may still have a period of communicability, and VZIg may prolong the incubation period to 28 days. Exact duration of antibody protection is not known, but is assumed to be at least one half-life of the immunoglobulin or approximately 3 weeks.

Varicella zoster immunoglobulin is distributed by the American Red Cross Services. Contact with the distribution centers must be made within 72 hours of exposure and specific criteria met in order for the product to be released.

Administration of VZIg is by the intramuscular route (never intravenously) at doses of 125 U/10 kg of body weight up to 625 U (five vials) for patients weighing more than 40 kg. The dose for newborn infants is 125 U. Side effects include local soreness at the site of injection. Although VZIg should be avoided in persons with bleeding diathesis, there are no other contraindications for the use of this product.

OTHER IMMUNOBIOLOGICS

IMMUNOGLOBULIN

Immunoglobulin is available as both intramuscular (IGIM) and intravenous preparations (IGIV). The IGIM preparation, or the Cohn fraction II, is prepared from pooled plasma of several thousand donors by cold ethanol fractionation. It typically contains greater than 95% IgG and trace amounts of IgM, IgA, and other plasma proteins. Because Ig is harvested from a large donor pool, it contains a wide spectrum of IgG antibodies to the pathogens prevalent in the area from which the donors were obtained. In the fractionation process, high-molecular-weight IgG aggregates are formed, which can activate complement in the absence of antigen and precipitate anaphylactoid reactions. For this reason, IGIM is unsuitable for IV administration. Intramuscular Ig typically contains 15% to 18% protein and not less than 90% IgG. A number of IV preparations of Ig are commercially available in the United States. Generally, these preparations contain greater than 90% IgG monomers and trace to small amounts of IgA. These products are available as lyophilized powders or solutions.

When administered either IV or IM, IG distributes in approximately 5% of the body weight of the recipient. The plasma half-life of Ig averages 18 to 32 days. This range of half-life is probably attributable to the variation in the half-life of IgG subclasses. Peak serum concentrations occur relatively immediately with IGIV, whereas IGIM produces peak concentrations within 2 days. After the initial period of equilibration, circulating IgG levels are superimposable between IV and IM equivalent dosages. No dosage adjustment is necessary in patients with renal or hepatic insufficiency, or both, dialysis patients, or geriatric patients.

Immunoglobulin is indicated in a wide variety of circumstances to provide passive immunity to individuals.[106] The indications for IGIM differ from that for IGIV. Intramuscular IG is indicated for providing passive immunity in hepatitis A infections, hepatitis B exposures (however, HBIg is significantly more effective), measles, varicella, and primary immunodeficiency diseases. Although IGIM is indicated for the treatment of primary immunodeficiency, IGIV is better tolerated and more effective. Intramuscular IG is not indicated for prevention of rubella, mumps, or poliomyelitis. Table 122–3 lists the suggested dosages for IGIM for the prevention or attenuation of various infectious diseases.

TABLE 122–3. Suggested Dosages for IGIM

Indications and Dosage of Intramuscular Immune Globulin in Infectious Diseases	
Primary immunodeficiency states	1.2 mL/kg IM then 0.6 mL/kg every 2–4 weeks
Hepatitis A exposure	0.02 mL/kg IM within 2 weeks
Hepatitis A prophylaxis	0.02 mL/kg IM for exposure <3 months duration 0.06 mL/kg IM for exposure up to 5 months duration
Hepatitis B exposure	0.06 mL/kg (HBIg preferred in known exposures)
Measles exposure	0.25 mL/kg (maximum dose 15 mL) as soon as possible 0.5 mL/kg (maximum dose 15 mL) as soon as possible for immunocompromised individuals
Varicella exposure	0.6–1.2 mL/kg as soon as possible when VZIg is not available

There are many approved indications, as well as nonapproved indications, for IGIV. The therapeutic dose of IGIV is empirically set at 2 g/kg. Often this dose is given in five daily doses of 400 mg/kg each, but it may be preferable to divide the total dose into two daily doses of 1 g/kg if the patient can tolerate the volume of the infusion.[107]

- *Primary immunodeficiency states:* In primary immunodeficiency states, monthly doses of between 100 and 800 mg/kg are administered, with the average dose being 200–400 mg/kg. The immunodeficiency states for which IGIV is indicated include both antibody deficiencies and combined immune deficiencies. In patients with immune deficiency who are candidates for IGIV, those with IgA deficiency should receive Gammagard brand because it has the lowest amount of IgA. Significant reactions can occur in patients with low intrinsic levels of IgA given IGIV with greater amounts of IgA. Intravenous IG is indicated for some patients with HIV; however, the data to support its use are better in the pediatric population.[108] With the advent of new antiretroviral agents and combination therapies, the usefulness of IGIV may be even more limited.
- *Idiopathic thrombocytopenic purpura:* For the treatment of idiopathic (or immune) thrombocytopenic purpura (ITP), doses of 400 mg/kg daily for 2 to 5 days are indicated. Some manufacturers recommend 1 g/kg for 1 to 2 days. Adults tend to respond less well to IGIV than do children. Intravenous IG is acceptable for treatment of both chronic and acute ITP, and IGIV has been used in ITP associated with pregnancy without adverse effects on the fetus.[106] Corticosteroids remain the drugs of choice for adult ITP. In thrombotic thrombocytopenia purpura, IGIV is reported to be effective in patients who do not respond to plasmapheresis. Other platelet disorders in which IGIV may be useful include neonatal immune thrombocytopenia, perinatal autoimmune thrombocytopenia, drug-induced thrombocytopenia, thrombocytopenia secondary to infection, and transfusion refractory thrombocytopenia; however, the data to support these uses are minimal.
- *Chronic lymphocytic leukemia (CLL):* IGIV is used as a prophylaxis measure in CLL patients who have had a serious bacterial infection. Doses of 400 mg/kg every 3 to 4 weeks are used.
- *Kawasaki disease (mucocutaneous lymph node syndrome):* This disease, which generally occurs in children, carries the hallmark of development of coronary artery abnormalities. Generally, it is recommended by the American Academy of Pediatrics that if the strict criteria for Kawasaki disease is met, an IGIV dose of 400 mg/kg/day for 4 consecutive days be used, or, preferably, 2 g/kg as a single dose. The dose should be administered within 10 days of disease onset. Aspirin therapy should also be initiated.[109]
- *Bone marrow transplant:* IGIV is approved for reducing graft-versus-host disease and infections in patients over the age of 20 years. Patients receive 500 mg/kg 7 and 2 days before transplantation and weekly up to 3 months after. At 100 days posttransplant, patients receive a monthly dose of IGIV for 1 year. Following this regimen, infection (CMV, fungal, bacterial, and interstitial pneumonia) decreased from 51% to 34% in bone marrow transplant patients. Intravenous IG is not indicated in patients younger than 20 years of age.
- *Varicella zoster:* Another approved indication for IGIV is in the prophylaxis of varicella zoster if VZIg is not available.

A number of other proposed uses of IGIV can be identified. It is important to note that generally these are not approved indications and are not generally accepted in the medical community for routine treatment. These uses include:

- *Neonatal sepsis:* Neonatal sepsis can cause significant morbidity within 24 hours of birth. While group B streptococcus and *E. coli* remain the primary infecting organisms, other bacteria and fungi may be associated with sepsis. IVIG appears to be effective in neonates <34 weeks' gestational age or who weigh <1,500 g. Routine use is not recommended; however, IGIV may be useful in neonates with recurrent infections.[110]
- *Guillain Barré syndrome:* In controlled clinical trials, IGIV was shown to be effective and is considered an alternative to plasmapheresis.[111]
- *Autoimmune diseases:* IGIV may be effective in self-limited immunoregulatory diseases but less effective in chronic diseases, such as systemic lupus erythematosus. Overall, there is little evidence that IGIV is useful in the management of autoimmune diseases, except for patients with severe active disease who have not responded to or tolerated other interventions.[110]
- *Intractable epilepsy:* In patients who have confirmed IgG deficiency, IGIV may be useful. For certain syndromes, such as West or Lennox-Gastaut, IGIV may be considered.[110]
- *Chronic inflammatory demyelinating polyneuropathy:* Although steroids are the first-line therapy, IGIV may be used in patients who fail steroids or do not tolerate steroids.[112]
- *Cytomegalovirus infection:* The use of CMV-IVIG is recommended instead of the use of IGIV.

Other diseases for which IGIV has been used in an uncontrolled setting include amyotrophic lateral sclerosis, rheumatoid arthritis, and factor VIII inhibition because of autoantibody.[106]

Adverse effects of IG vary with the route of administration. Following IGIM, pain, tenderness, and muscle stiffness persisting for hours or days are common. Repeat courses may cause sensitization with resultant allergic reactions. With IGIV, adverse effects occur in less than 1% of immunocompetent patients and in less than 10% of others. Most adverse effects are related to the rate of the infusion. Infusion should be given at a rate of 0.01–0.02 mL/kg/min for 30 minutes and then, if no reactions occur, increased to 0.02–0.04 mL/kg/min. Although infusion rate recommendations vary slightly depending on the preparation, the guidelines presented can be followed for the various IV preparations.

Immunoglobulin products are derived from human blood. Precautions such as donor screening and fractionation procedures and solvent-detergent treatment during the manufacture process render the IGIV products free of HIV, hepatitis B, and hepatitis C viruses. Although no manufacturing process can guarantee that there is no viral contamination, the potential infection risk from immunoglobulin preparations is very small.[110]

RH_O(D) IMMUNOGLOBULIN

Rh_o(D) immunoglobulin (RDIg) is a sterile solution of immunoglobulins prepared from human sera with high titers of Rh_o(D) antibody. Plasma or serum used to prepare RDIg is negative for hepatitis B surface antigen.

Rh_o(D) immunoglobulin suppresses the antibody response and formation of anti-Rh_o(D) in Rh_o(D)-negative, D^u-negative women exposed to Rh_o(D)-positive blood. Administration of RDIg prevents erythroblastosis fetalis in subsequent pregnancies with a Rh_o(D)-positive fetus. When administered within 72 hours of delivery of a full-term infant, RDIg reduces active antibody formation from 12% to 1% to

2%. The reduction in antibody formation is lower when RDIg is given beyond 72 hours postpartum. Smaller doses of RDIg are used after abortion, miscarriage, amniocentesis, or abdominal trauma. In addition, RDIg is also used in the case of a premenopausal woman who is Rh_o(D)-negative or D^u-negative and who has inadvertently received Rh_o(D)-positive or D^u-positive blood or blood products.

The dosage of RDIg varies with the indication. A standard dose of 300 μg is given within 72 hours of a term delivery. Occasionally, where the fetus is known to be Rh_o(D)-positive, a 300-μg dose is given at 28 weeks' gestation and within 72 hours after delivery. For postpregnancy termination occurring up to 13 weeks' gestation, one microdose (50 μg) vial is given within 72 hours. For pregnancy termination after 13 weeks, one standard dose (300 μg) is given within 72 hours. In other circumstances, such as in abdominal trauma, amniocentesis, or transfusion accidents, the dosage (number of standard dose vials) is based on the estimated packed red blood cell volume of the fetal/maternal hemorrhage divided by 15. Rh_o(D) immunoglobulin is administered intramuscularly only.

When considering RDIg for use, one must be certain of the mother's Rh_o(D) and D^u antigen status; RDIg should not be given to individuals positive for either of these antigens or to those with anti-Rh_o(D) antibodies. Occasionally, a large fetal bleed of Rh_o(D)-positive or D^u-positive blood may make cross-matching of the mother difficult. In these cases, RDIg should only be given if previous tests have shown the mother to be Rh_o(D)-negative and D^u-negative with no anti-Rh_o(D) antibody.

Adverse reactions to RDIg include injection site tenderness and fever.

CYTOMEGALOVIRUS IMMUNOGLOBULIN

Cytomegalovirus immunoglobulin intravenous (CMV-IGIV) contains IgG antibodies obtained from healthy persons with high titers of antibodies to cytomegalovirus (CMV).[113]

Attenuation of primary CMV disease associated with solid organ transplantation in seronegative recipients of seropositive organs is the indication for CMV-IGIV.[112] It is dosed using a tapering schedule. Dosage is 150 mg/kg preoperatively or within 72 hours postoperatively; 100 mg/kg at 2, 4, 6, and 8 weeks; and 50 mg/kg at weeks 12 and 16. These doses are for all ages. The use of CMV-IVIG has resulted in a significant decrease in CMV-related syndromes. Further studies are needed to determine the efficacy of CMV-IGIV in bone marrow transplantation. CMV-IGIV has been effective in some studies, but ineffective in others.

Adverse effects of CMV-IGIV are seen in fewer than 5% of recipients and include flushing, chills, muscle cramps, back pain, chest tightness, fever, nausea, vomiting, hypotension, and tachycardia. These adverse events may be related to the infusion rate and can be managed by temporarily discontinuing the infusion. The infusion may be restarted at a decreased rate. Anaphylaxis rarely occurs, and should be considered if hypotension develops during the infusion. Because CMV-IVIG contains other antibodies, live viral vaccines should be withheld until 3 months after CMV-IVIG administration.

VACCINES FOR TRAVEL

CHOLERA VACCINE

The available vaccine for cholera consists of a suspension of killed whole-cell *Vibrio cholerae* bacteria from two bacterial strains: Ogawa and Inaba.

Cholera vaccine is approximately 50% effective in reducing the incidence of disease but does not prevent transmission of infection. The vaccine provides greater efficacy in persons who have previously had the disease. The duration of antibody following vaccination is 3 to 6 months, as compared to 3 years following natural infection. Frequent booster doses (every 6 months) are needed to sustain protection. The vaccine may be used in immunocompromised individuals.[114]

The primary use of cholera vaccine is in travelers who will be visiting highly endemic areas under less-than-adequate hygienic conditions. The risk of cholera to tourists is exceedingly low and does not warrant routine vaccination.[117]

The primary immunization series in adults consists of two 0.5-mL IM or subcutaneous doses administered 1 week to 1 month apart. Doses in children younger than 10 years of age are modified accordingly: 0.2 mL for ages 6 months to 4 years and 0.3 mL for ages 5 to 10 years of age. The intradermal route may be used in individuals 5 years of age or older with a 0.2-mL dose. Similar sized booster doses are recommended every 6 months.[114]

Side effects are common and consist of local reactions (pain, erythema, induration, tenderness), fever, malaise, and headache. The systemic reactions, such as fever, malaise, and headache, occur in <1% of individuals and may last 1 to 2 days. Serious reactions, including neurologic complications, are rare. No data are available on its use in pregnancy. The only contraindication is a history of previous severe systemic reaction to the vaccine. A 3-week interval between administrations of cholera and yellow fever vaccine is recommended because of reported decreased antibody response with their simultaneous administration. There is no evidence, however, that protection is affected by simultaneous administration, and when necessary, it may be done.[114]

JAPANESE ENCEPHALITIS VIRUS VACCINE

Japanese encephalitis is an arboviral infection spread by mosquitoes. It affects 50,000 people annually in Asia and Oceania, causing viral encephalitis. Transmission is seasonal, with the highest times of transmission occurring in the summer and early fall. Although the risk for the most travelers is quite low, the risk for individuals depends on the season, location, and duration of travel. It is estimated that the risk of acquiring Japanese encephalitis is less than 1 person per 1 million travelers; however, this may be a low estimate.[114]

Monovalent inactivated Japanese encephalitis virus vaccine has been commercially available in the United States since 1992. Three doses are needed to provide protective levels of neutralizing antibodies. The vaccine is more immunogenic when administered in a 0-, 7-, 30-day schedule rather that in a 0-, 7-, 14-day regimen (GMTs are higher at 6 months for the 30-day schedule). Duration of antibody protection is unknown. Protective titers have been reported for up to 3 years after primary immunization. Additionally, single booster doses given 1 year after primary immunization have resulted in substantial rises in antibody titers.

Adverse reactions include pain and tenderness at the injection site (20%) and systemic side effects, such as fever, headache, malaise, rash, chills, dizziness, myalgia, nausea, vomiting, and abdominal pain in 10%.[114] In addition, there are sporadic reports of hypersensitivity reactions to the vaccine. The manifestations of this type of reaction include urticaria, angioedema, and respiratory distress. These reactions generally have occurred after a median of 12 hours after the first dose of vaccine with 88% of reactions within 3 days. After a second dose, these hypersensitivity reactions may occur 3 to 14 days after injection.

The Japanese encephalitis virus vaccine is recommended for US expatriates residing in areas where Japanese encephalitis is endemic or epidemic. The vaccine is not routinely recommended for travelers to Asia.

The Japanese encephalitis vaccine is administered to individuals 3 years of age as 1-mL doses given subcutaneously on days 0, 7, and 30. The 0-, 7-, and 14-day schedule can be used if time is a constraint. In addition, a 0-, 7-day schedule can be used if absolutely necessary, and it will provide protection for 80% of persons. The last dose should be administered at least 10 days before traveling to observe for adverse reactions. For children ages 1 to 3 years, 0.5 mL of vaccine is administered subcutaneously using the schedules already listed. No data are available for infants. Booster doses are recommended every 36 months with 1-mL booster doses being given to children who are 3 years of age or older, even if they received 0.5 mL as initial dose. Pregnant women who travel to an epidemic or endemic area should be vaccinated. No data are available for immunocompromised patients. The Japanese encephalitis vaccine can be administered simultaneously with the DPT vaccine. No data are available for concurrent administration with other vaccines or antimalarial agents.

TYPHOID VACCINE

Typhoid fever is an illness caused by infection with *Salmonella typhi*. Typhoid is spread via the fecal-oral route. Clinical illness in its severe form is characterized by gradually rising fever that reaches 39°C (102.2°F) to 41°C (105.8°F) and persists for up to 2 weeks. Headaches, abdominal discomfort, malaise, myalgia, and anorexia are usually present. Older children and adults usually have constipation while diarrhea is common in infants. Complications include intestinal perforation and hemorrhage. Two percent to 5% of patients become chronic gallbladder carriers of *S. typhi*.

Although rare in developed countries, typhoid is common in Africa, Asia, Central America, and South America. Travelers to these areas should be advised that careful selection of food and beverages is the most effective means of preventing infection, but should be offered immunization if the itinerary puts the travelers at high risk for typhoid.

Three typhoid vaccines are available in the United States. The oral typhoid vaccine is a live attenuated preparation that is given as a four-dose series with one capsule administered every other day. The capsules should be taken on an empty stomach with cool or lukewarm liquid. The series should be completed 1 week prior to travel and should not be used in anyone younger than 6 years old. The oral vaccine should not be administered during a course of antibiotics. The injectable typhoid vaccine (ViCPS) is a polysaccharide vaccine given as a single intramuscular dose at least 2 weeks before travel. This polysaccharide vaccine should not be given to children younger than 2 years old. Another injectable typhoid vaccine is also available (Typhoid vaccine USP). It is a heat-phenol inactivated bacterial vaccine. This vaccine can be used in adults and children as young as 6 months of age. The vaccine series consists of two doses at least 4 weeks apart. This inactivated typhoid vaccine should be used only when the other two preparations cannot be used because typhoid vaccine USP is associated with significantly more adverse effects and is no more effective.[115]

Booster doses of all three vaccine preparations are recommended if continued or repeated exposure is expected. The entire four-dose oral vaccine series should be repeated every 5 years. The ViCPS preparation requires revaccination every 2 years, whereas the typhoid vaccine USP should be readministered every 3 years. A single dose is required even if more than 3 years have elapsed since the primary series.

The oral typhoid vaccine is well tolerated with rare reports of gastrointestinal discomfort, fever, headache, or rash. Local injection site reactions are the most commonly reported adverse event following the injectable typhoid vaccine, ViCPS. Systemic symptoms, such as fever, flu-like symptoms, gastrointestinal discomfort, tremor, or neck pain, are occasionally reported. Most vaccinees will report injection site reactions after the injectable typhoid vaccine USP. Malaise, headache, muscle aches, and fever may also occur. Very rarely, serious adverse events, such as chest paint, hypotension, and shock, have been reported.

Because the oral vaccine is a live attenuated preparation, its use in the immunocompromised should be avoided. Both parenteral vaccines can be administered to immunocompromised persons because they are inactivated. None of the vaccines should be given to febrile individuals. Pregnancy is not an absolute contraindication to use of any of the vaccines, but the benefits versus the risks must be weighed.[115]

YELLOW FEVER VACCINE

Live attenuated yellow fever virus vaccine is recommended for persons who will be traveling or living in areas where yellow fever infection occurs (parts of Africa and South America) and is required for entry into certain countries.[114] Vaccination should also be considered for laboratory workers who may be exposed to the virus. The reconstituted vaccine is thermolabile, and unused portions must be discarded 1 hour after reconstitution.

The recommended dose is 0.5 mL subcutaneously given once with similar booster doses recommended every 10 years. The vaccine, however, has been shown to be highly immunogenic with antibodies persisting for at least 40 years and perhaps for life. Mild side effects consisting of headache, myalgias, and low-grade fever 1 to 2 weeks after vaccination occur in less than 10% of vaccinees; treatment should be symptomatic. Immediate hypersensitivity reactions are rare (1 per 1 million doses) and occur primarily in persons who have anaphylactic reactions to eggs. Neurologic accidents are rare (20 cases to date) and have occurred primarily in infants younger than 4 months of age in whom the vaccine is not recommended.

On theoretical grounds, the vaccine should be avoided during pregnancy unless travel to a high-risk area is imperative. It may be given to breast-feeding mothers. The vaccine may be used in immunocompromised patients if the risk of infection in an endemic area outweighs the potential vaccine risk. Additionally, it should not be given to infants younger than 4 months of age and, in general, should be used only if a child is 9 months of age or older. Children 4 to 9 months must be considered on an individual basis. It is contraindicated in persons with a history of an anaphylactic reaction to eggs. Where the history is in question, intradermal testing consisting of 0.02-mL doses of vaccine and normal saline control applied to the volar surface of the forearm should be done. The demonstration of an erythematous, urticarial wheal and negative control constitutes a positive response and contraindicates vaccination. This intradermal testing may be sufficient to produce antibodies, however, serologic testing should be done to confirm this.

Yellow fever vaccine may be simultaneously administered with all other vaccines except cholera; a 3-week interval between vaccines is recommended. Simultaneous administration of immunoglobulin does not interfere with the immune response to this agent.

REFERENCES

1. Advisory Committee on Immunization Practices. General recommendations on immunization. MMWR Morb Mortal Wkly Rep 1994;43 (RR-1):1–38.
2. Jilg W, Schmidt M, Deinhardt F. Prolonged immunity after late booster doses of hepatitis B vaccine. J Infect Dis 1988;157:1267–1269.
3. Miotti P, Nelson KE, Dallabetta GA, et al. The influence of HIV infection on antibody response to a two-dose regimen of influenza vaccine. JAMA 1989;262:779–783.
4. Immunization Practices Advisory Committee. General recommendations on immunization. MMWR Morb Mortal Wkly Rep 1989;38:205–228.
5. Centers for Disease Control. Suboptimal response to hepatitis B vaccine given by injection into the buttock. MMWR Morb Mortal Wkly Rep 1985;34:105–113.
6. Poland, GA, Borrud, A, Jacobson, RM, et al. Determination of deltoid fat pad thickness. Implications for needle length in adult immunization. JAMA 1997;277:1709–1711.
7. Centers for Disease Control. Adult immunization: Recommendations of the Immunization Practices Advisory Committee. MMWR Morb Mortal Wkly Rep 1991;40:1–94.
8. Advisory Committee on Immunization Practices. Use of vaccines and immune globulins in persons with altered immunocompetence. MMWR Morb Mortal Wkly Rep 1993;42(RR-4):1–19.
9. Centers for Disease Control. 1999 USPHS/IDSA guidelines for the prevention of opportunistic infections in persons infected with human immunodeficiency virus. MMWR Morb Mortal Wkly Rep 1999;48 (RR-10):1–82.
10. Centers for Disease Control. Physician vaccination referral practices and vaccines for children—New York, 1994. MMWR Morb Mortal Wkly Rep 1995;44:3–6.
11. Fedson DS. Adult immunization: Summary of the National Vaccine Advisory Committee Report. JAMA 1994;272:1133–1137.
12. Centers for Disease Control. State and national vaccination coverage levels among children aged 19–35 months—United States, April-December 1994. MMWR Morb Mortal Wkly Rep 1995;44:613–623.
13. Centers for Disease Control. Immunization of adolescents: Recommendations of the Advisory Committee on Immunization Practices, the American Academy of Pediatrics, the American Academy of Family Physicians, and the American Medical Association. MMWR Morb Mortal Wkly Rep 1996;45(RR-13):1–19.
14. Szilagyi PG, Rodewald LE, Humiston SG, et al. Missed opportunities for childhood vaccinations in office practices and the effect on vaccination status. Pediatrics 1993;91:1–7.
15. Vondracek, TG, Pham, TP and Huycke, MM. A hospital-based pharmacy intervention program for pneumococcal vaccination. Arch Int Med 1998;158:1543–47.
16. Immunization Practices Advisory Committee. Combination vaccines for childhood immunization. MMWR Morb Mortal Wkly Rep 1999;48 (RR-5):1–30.
17. Bartell LH, Charney SA. National Vaccine Injury Compensation Act: A viable alternative to litigation? J Pharm Pract 1989;2:36–44.
18. Centers for Disease Control. Vaccine Adverse Event Reporting System—United States. MMWR Morb Mortal Wkly Rep 1990;39:730–733.
19. Middaugh JP. Side effects of diphtheria-tetanus toxoid in adults. Am J Public Health 1979;69:246–249.
20. Peter G. Diphtheria. In: 1997 Red Book: Report of the Committee on Infectious Diseases, 4th ed. Elk Grove Village, IL, American Academy of Pediatrics, 1997:191–195.
21. Centers for Disease Control. Recommendation of the Immunization Practices Advisory Committee: Diphtheria, tetanus and pertussis: Guidelines for vaccine prophylaxis and other preventive measures. MMWR Morb Mortal Wkly Rep 1981;30:392–396, 401–407.
22. Peter G. Tetanus. In: 1997 Red Book: Report of the Committee on Infectious Diseases, 24th ed. Elk Grove Village, IL, American Academy of Pediatrics, 1997:518–523.
23. A Joint Statement by the Advisory Council for the Elimination of Tuberculosis and the Advisory Committee on Immunization Practices. The role of BCG vaccine in the prevention and control of tuberculosis in the United States. MMWR Morb Mortal Wkly Rep 1996;45(No. RR-4): 1–27.
24. Advisory Committee on Immunization Practices. Prevention of hepatitis A through active or passive immunization. MMWR Morb Mortal Wkly Rep 1999;48(RR-12):1–54.
25. Advisory Committee on Immunization Practices. Hepatitis B virus: A comprehensive strategy for eliminating transmission in the United States through universal childhood vaccination. MMWR Morb Mortal Wkly Rep 1991;40(RR-13):1–25.
26. Committee on Infectious Diseases. Universal hepatitis B immunization. Pediatrics 1992;89:795–800.
27. Centers for Disease Control. Recommendations for protection against viral hepatitis. MMWR Morb Mortal Wkly Rep 1985;34:313–327.
28. Roome AJ, Walsh SJ, Cartter ML, Hadler JL. Hepatitis B vaccine responsiveness in Connecticut public safety personnel. JAMA 1993;270:2931–2934.
29. Alimonos KA, Murray J, Nafziger AN, Bertino JS Jr. Prediction of response to hepatitis B vaccine in health care workers: Whose titers of antibodies to hepatitis B surface antigen should be determined after a 3-dose series and what are the implications of cost-effectiveness? Clin Infect Dis 1998;26:566–571.
30. Wood RC, MacDonald KL, White KE, et al. Risk factors for lack of detectable antibody following hepatitis B vaccination of Minnesota health care workers. JAMA 1993;270:2935–2939.
31. Margolis HS, Presson AC. Host factors related to poor immunogenicity of hepatitis B vaccine in adults. JAMA 1993;270:2971–2972.
32. Treadwell TL, Keeffe EB, Lake J, et al. Immunogenicity of two recombinant hepatitis B vaccines in older individuals. Am J Med 1993;95: 584–588.
33. Tada H, Mosohiko Y, Mishira J, et al. Combined passive and active immunization for preventing perinatal transmission of hepatitis B virus carrier state. Pediatrics 1982;70:613–619.
34. Seef L, Koff D. Passive and active immunoprophylaxis of hepatitis B. Gastroenterology 1984;86:958–981.
35. Centers for Disease Control. Recommendations of the Immunization Practices Advisory Committee: Hepatitis B virus: A comprehensive strategy for eliminating transmission in the United States through universal childhood vaccination. MMWR Morb Mortal Wkly Rep 1992;40: 1–25.
36. Hadler SC, Francis DP, Maynard JE, et al. Long-term immunogenicity and efficacy of hepatitis B vaccine in homosexual men. N Engl J Med 1986;315:209–214.
37. Bertino JS Jr, Tirrell P, Greenberg R, et al. A comparative trial of standard or high-dose recombinant hepatitis B vaccine versus a vaccine containing S subunit, PreS1 and PreS2 particles for revaccination of healthy adult nonresponders. J Infect Dis 1997;337:256–260.
38. Troisi C, Heiberg D, Hollinger F. Normal immune response to hepatitis B vaccine in patients with Down's syndrome: A basis for immunization guidelines. JAMA 1985;254:3196–3199.
39. Wainwright RB, McMahon BJ, Bulkow LR, et al. Duration of immunogenicity and efficacy of hepatitis B vaccine in a Yupik Eskimo population. JAMA 1989;261:2362–2366.
40. Lo KJ, Lee SD, Tsai YT, et al. Long-term immunogenicity and efficacy of hepatitis B vaccine in infants born to HBeAG-positive HBsAG-carrier mothers. Hepatology 1988;8:1647–1650.
41. Lanphear BP. Hepatitis B immunoprophylaxis: Developing a cost-effective program in the hospital setting. Infect Control Hosp Epidemiol 1990;11:47–50.
42. Dienstag JL, Stevens CO, Bhan AK, et al. Hepatitis B vaccine administered to chronic carrier of hepatitis B surface antigen. Ann Intern Med 1982;96:575–579.
43. Prince AM. Hepatitis B immune globulin: Final report of a controlled multicenter trial of efficacy in prevention of dialysis-associated hepatitis. J Infect Dis 1978;137:131–144.

44. Seef LB. Type B hepatitis after needle-stick exposure: Prevention with hepatitis B immune globulin. Ann Intern Med 1978;88:285–293.
45. Grady GF, Lee VA. Hepatitis B immune globulin-prevention of hepatitis from accidental exposure among medical personnel. N Engl J Med 1975;293:1067–1070.
46. Perillo R, Campbell C, Strang S, et al. Immune globulin and hepatitis B immune globulin: Prophylactic measures for intimate contacts exposed to acute type B hepatitis. Arch Intern Med 1984;144:81–85.
47. Centers for Disease Control. Update on hepatitis B prophylaxis. MMWR Morb Mortal Wkly Rep 1987;36:353–360.
48. Centers for Disease Control and Prevention. Progress toward eliminating Haemophilus influenzae type b disease among infants and children—United States, 1987–1997. MMWR Morb Mortal Wkly Rep 1998;47(46):993–998.
49. American Academy of Pediatrics. *Haemophilus influenzae* infections. In: Peter G, ed. 1997 Red Book: Report of the Committee on Infectious Diseases. Elk Grove Village, IL, American Academy of Pediatrics, 1997:220–231.
50. LaMontagne JR, Noble GR, Quinnan GV, et al. Summary of clinical trials of inactivated influenza vaccine—1978. Rev Infect Dis 1983;5:723–736.
51. Gross RA, Ennis FA. Influenza vaccine: Split product versus whole virus types: How do they differ? N Engl J Med 1977;296:567–568.
52. Nichol K L, Margolis K L, Wuorenma J, Von Sternberg T. The efficacy and cost effectiveness of vaccination against influenza among elderly persons living in the community. N Engl J Med 1994;331:778–784.
53. Nichol KL, Lind A, Margolis K L, et al. The effectiveness of vaccination against influenza in healthy, working adults. N Engl J Med 1995;333:889–893.
54. Nichol KL,Wuorenma J, von Sternberg T. Benefits of influenza vaccination for low-, intermediate-, and high-risk senior citizens. Arch Intern Med 1998;158:1769–1776.
55. Centers for Disease Control and Prevention. Prevention and control of influenza. Recommendations of the Advisory Committee on Immunization Practices (ACIP). MMWR Morb Mortal Wkly Rep 2000;49(No. RR-3):1–38.
56. Keyser LA, Karl M. Nafziger AN, Bertino JS Jr. Comparison of central nervous system adverse effects of amantadine and rimantadine used as sequential prophylaxis of influenza A in elderly nursing home patients. Arch Intern Med 2000;160:1485–1488.
57. Hayden FG, Atmar RL, Schilling M, et al. Use of the selective oral neuraminidase inhibitor oseltamivir to prevent influenza. N Engl J Med 1999;341:1336–1343.
58. Monto AS, Robinson DP, Herlocher ML, et al. Zanamivir in the prevention of influenza among healthy adults. JAMA 1999;282:31–35.
59. Lasky T, Terracciano GJ, Magder L, et al. The Guillain-Barré syndrome and the 1992–1993 and 1993–1994 influenza vaccines. N Engl J Med 1998;339:1797–1802.
60. Centers for Disease Control and Prevention. Recommendations for the use of Lyme disease vaccine. Recommendations of the Advisory Committee on Immunization Practices (ACIP). MMWR Morb Mortal Wkly Rep 1999;48(No. RR-7):1–25.
61. Sigal LH, Zahradnik JM, Lavin P, et al. A vaccine consisting of recombinant *Borrelia burgdorferi* outer-surface protein A to prevent Lyme disease. N Engl J Med 1998;339:216–222.
62. Markowitz LE, Preblud SR, Fine PE, Orenstein WA. Duration of live measles vaccine-induced immunity. Pediatr Infect Dis J 1990;9: 101–110.
63. Poland GA. Immunogenetic mechanisms of antibody response to measles vaccine: The role of HLA genes. Vaccine 1999;17(13–14SI): 1719–1725.
64. Centers for Disease Control and Prevention. Measles, mumps, and rubella—Vaccine use and strategies for elimination of measles, rubella, and congenital rubella syndrome and control of Mumps: Recommendations of the Advisory Committee on Immunization Practices (ACIP). MMWR Morb Mortal Wkly Rep 1998;47(No. RR-8):1–57.
65. Cote TR, Sivertson D, Horan JM et al. Evaluation of a two-dose measles, mumps, and rubella vaccination schedule in a cohort of college athletes. Public Health Rep 1993;108:431–435.
66. Palumbo P, Hoyt L, Demasio K, et al. Population-based study of measles and measles immunization in human immunodeficiency virus-infected children. Pediatr Infect Dis J 1992;11:1008–1014.
67. Kaplan LJ, Daum R, Smaron M, et al. Severe measles in immunocompromised patients. JAMA 1992;267:1237–1241.
68. Siber GR, Werner BC, Halsey NA. Interference of immune globulin with measles and rubella immunization. J Pediatr 1993;122:204–211.
69. King GE, Markowitz LE, Heath J, et al. Antibody response to measles-mumps rubella vaccine of children with mild illness at the time of vaccination. JAMA 1996;275:704–707.
70. Dennehy PH, Saracen CL, Peter G. Seroconversion rates to combined measles mumps-rubella-varicella vaccine of children with upper respiratory tract infection. Pedatrics 1994;94:514–516.
71. Ratnam S, West R, Gadag V. Measles and rubella antibody response after measles mumps-rubella vaccination in children with afebrile upper respiratory tract infection. J Pediatr 1995;127:432–434.
72. Edmonson MB, Davis JP, Hopfensperger DJ, Berg JL, Payton LA. Measles vaccination during the respiratory virus season and risk of vaccine failure. Pediatrics 1996;98:905–910.
73. Centers for Disease Control and Prevention. Prevention and control of meningococcal disease and meningococcal disease and college students. Recommendations of the Advisory Committee on Immunization Practices (ACIP). MMWR Morb Mortal Wkly Rep 2000;49(RR-7):1–20.
74. Froeschel J. Meningococcal disease in college students. Clin Infect Dis 1999;29:215–216.
75. Bruce M, Rosenstein NE, Capparella J, et al. Meningococcal disease in college students. In: Abstracts of the 39th Annual Meeting of the Infectious Diseases Society of America, Philadelphia, PA, November 18–21, 1999:63.
76. Neal KR, Nguyen-Van-Tam J, Monk P, et al. Invasive meningococcal disease among university undergraduates: Association with universities providing relatively large amounts of catered hall accommodations. Epidemiol Infect 1999;122:351–357.
77. De Serres G, Shaddmani R, Duval B, et al. Morbidity of pertussis in adolescents and adults. J Infect Dis 2000;182:174–179.
78. Centers for Disease Control and Prevention. Pertussis vaccination: Use of acellular pertussis vaccines among infants and young children. Recommendations of the Advisory Committee on Immunization Practices (ACIP). MMWR Morb Mortal Wkly Rep 1997;46(No. RR-7):1–25.
79. Centers for Disease Control and Prevention. Notice to Readers: Recommended Childhood Immunization Schedule—United States, MMWR Morb Mortal Wkly Rep 2000;49(02);35–38, 47.
80. Centers for Disease Control and Prevention. Poliomyelitis prevention in the United States: Updated recommendations of the Advisory Committee on Immunization Practices (ACIP). MMWR Morb Mortal Wkly Rep 2000;49(No. RR-5):1–22.
81. Strebel PM, Sutter RW, Cochi SL, et al. Epidemiology of poliomyelitis in the United States on decade after the last reported case of indigenous wild virus-associated disease. Clin Infect Dis 1992;14:568–579.
82. Recommendations of the Immunization Practices Advisory Committee. Prevention of pneumococcal disease. MMWR Morb Mortal Wkly Rep 1997;46(RR-8):1–31.
83. Hilleman M, Carlson A, McLean A, et al. *Streptococcus pneumoniae* polysaccharide vaccine: Age and dose responses, safety, persistence of antibody, revaccination, and simultaneous administration of pneumococcal and influenza vaccines. Rev Infect Dis 1981;3:S31–S42.
84. A pneumococcal conjugate vaccine for infants and children. Med Lett 2000;42:25–27.
85. Advisory Committee on Immunization Practices. Rabies prevention. MMWR Morb Mortal Wkly Rep 1999;48(RR-1):1–41.
86. Bernhard KW, Roberts MA, Samner J, et al. Human diploid cell rabies vaccine: Effectiveness of immunization with small intradermal or subcutaneous doses. JAMA 1982;247:1138–1142.
87. Bernard KW, Mallonnee J, Wright JC, et al. Preexposure immunization with intradermal human diploid cell rabies vaccine. JAMA 1987;257: 1059–1063.

88. Fishbein DB, Pacer RE, Holmes DF, et al. Rabies preexposure prophylaxis with human diploid cell rabies vaccine: A dose-response study. J Infect Dis 1987;156:50–55.
89. Trimarchi CV, Safford M Jr. Poor response to rabies vaccination by the intradermal route. JAMA 1992;268:874.
90. State of New York, Department of Health Memorandum, Public Health Series H-28, PH-11, Series 92–93. Rabies control update. November 25, 1992.
91. Wilde H, Sirikawin S, Sabcharoen A, et al. Failure of postexposure treatment of rabies in children. J Infect Dis 1997;22:228–232.
92. Balfour HH, Groth KE, Edelman CK. RA27/3 rubella vaccine. Am J Dis Child 1990;134:350–353.
93. Tingle AJ, Mitchell LA, Grace M, et al. Randomised double-blind placebo controlled study on adverse effects of rubella immunisation in seronegative women. Lancet 1997;349:1277–1281.
94. Centers for Disease Control and Prevention. Prevention of varicella: Update recommendations of the Advisory Committee on Immunization Practices (ACIP). MMWR Morb Mortal Wkly Rep 1999;48(RR-6):1–5.
95. Watson BM, Piercy SA, Plotkin SA, Starr SE. Modified chickenpox in children immunized with the Oka/Merck varicella vaccine. Pediatrics 1993;91:17–22.
96. Krause PR, Klinman DM Efficacy, immunogenicity, safety, and use of live attenuated chickenpox vaccine J Pediatr 1995;127:518–525.
97. Krause PR, Klinman DM. Varicella vaccination: Evidence for frequent reactivation of the vaccine strain in healthy children. Nat Med 2000;6(4):451–454.
98. Watson B, Gupta R, Randall R, Starr S. Persistence of cell-mediated and humoral immune responses in healthy children immunized with live attenuated varicella vaccine. J Infect Dis 1994;169:197–199.
99. Johnson C, Rome LP, Stancin T, Kumar ML. Humoral immunity and clinical reinfections following varicella vaccine in healthy children. Pediatrics 1989;84:418–421.
100. Centers for Disease Control and Prevention. Prevention of varicella: Recommendations of the Advisory Committee on Immunization Practices (ACIP). MMWR Morb Mortal Wkly Rep 1996;45(RR-11):1–36.
101. Asano Y, Nakayama H, Yazaki T, Kato R, Hirose S. Protection against varicella in family contacts by immediate inoculation with varicella vaccine. Pediatrics 1977;59:3–7.
102. Arbeter AM, Starr SE, Plotkin SA. Varicella vaccine studies in healthy children and adults. Pediatrics 1986;78(suppl):748–756.
103. Salzman MB, Garcia C. Postexposure varicella vaccination in siblings of children with active varicella. Pediatr Infect Dis J 1998;17(3):256–257.
104. Watson B, Seward J, Yang A, et al. Postexposure effectiveness of varicella vaccine. Pediatrics 2000;105:84–88.
105. Raeder CK, Hayney MS. Immunology of varicella immunization in the elderly. Ann Pharmacother 2000;34:228–234.
106. Steere AC, Sikand V, Meurice F, et al. Vaccination against lyme disease using recombinant *Borrelia burgdorferi* outer-surface lipoprotein a with adjuvant. N Engl J Med 1998;339:209–215.
107. Berkman SA, Lee ML, Gale RP. Clinical uses of intravenous immunoglobulins Ann Intern Med 1990;112(4):278–292.
108. Dalakas MC. Intravenous immune globulin therapy for neurologic diseases. Ann Intern Med 1997;126:721–730.
109. Working Group on Antiretroviral Therapy: National Pediatric HIV Resource Center. Antiretroviral therapy and medical management of the human immunodeficiency virus-infected child Pediatr Infect Dis J 1993;12:513–522.
110. American Academy of Pediatrics. Kawasaki disease. In: Peter G, ed. 1997 Red Book: Report of the Committee on Infectious Diseases. Elk Grove Village, IL, American Academy of Pediatrics, 1997:316–319.
111. Ratko TA, Burnett DA, Foulke GE, et al. Recommendations for off-label use of intravenously administered immunoglobulin preparations. JAMA 1995;273:1865–1870.
112. Plasma Exchange/Sandoglobulin Guillain-Barré Syndrome Trial Group. Randomised trial of plasma exchange, intravenous immunoglobulin, and plasma exchange followed by intravenous immunoglobulin in Guillain-Barré syndrome. Lancet 1997;349:225–230.
113. Dyck PJ, Litchy WJ, Dratz KM, et al. A plasma exchange versus immune globulin infusion trial in chronic inflammatory demyelinating polyradiculoneuropathy. Ann Neurol 1994;6:838–845.
114. Snydman DR. Cytomegalovirus immunoglobulins in the prevention and treatment of cytomegalovirus disease. Rev Infect Dis 1990;12(suppl 7): S839–S848.
115. Centers for Disease Control and Prevention. Typhoid immunization. Recommendations of the Advisory Committee on Immunization Practices (ACIP). MMWR Morb Mortal Wkly Rep 1994;43(No. RR-14):1–7.
116. Centers for Disease Control. Health Information for International Travel. Atlanta, GA, DHHS, 2000.
117. Harrison LH, Dwyer DM, Maples CT, Billmann L. Risk of meningococcal infection in college students. JAMA 1999;281:1906–1910.

122
Childhood Immunization Schedule

Immunization	Birth	1 month	2 months	4 months	6 months	12 months	15 months	18 months	24 months	4–6 years	11–12 years	14–16 years
Hepatitis B[2]		#1	#2				#3				Hep B	
Hepatitis B (Recombivax only[3])											Hep B	
Diptheria, Tetanus & Pertussis[4]			#1	#2	#3		B1[4]			B2		
Tetanus & Diptheria											B3	
H. influenzae Type b[5]			#1	#2	#3		B1					
Polio[6]			IPV #1	IPV #2			IPV #3[6]			IPV #4[6]		
Measles, Mumps & Rubella[7]							#1			BI[7]	MMR[7]	
Varicella[8]							#1				Var[8]	
Hepatitis A[9]								Hepatitis A[9] – in selected areas				
Pneumococcal[10]			#1	#2	#3		B1					

Adapted from material approved by the Advisory Committee on Immunization Practices (ACIP), the American Academy of Pediatrics (AAP), and the American Academy of Family Physicians (AAFP).

1. This schedule indicates that recommended ages for routine administration of currently licensed childhood vaccines as of November 1, 1999. Additional vaccines may be licensed and recommended during the year. Licensed combination vaccines may be used whenever any components of the combination are indicated and its other components are not contraindicated. Providers should consult the manufacturers' package inserts for detailed recommendations.
2. ***Infants born to HBsAg-negative mothers*** should receive the first dose of hepatitits B (Hep B) vaccine by age 2 months. The second dose should be at least 1 month after the first dose. The third dose should be administered at least 4 months after the first dose and at least 2 months after the second dose, but not before 6 months of age.
   Infants born to HBsAg-positive mothers should receive hepatitis B vaccine and 0.5 mL of hepatitis B immune globulin (HBIg) within 12 hours of birth at separate sites. The second dose is recommended at 1 month of age and the third dose at 6 months of age.
   Infants born to mothers whose HBsAg status is unknown should receive hepatitis B vaccine within 12 hours of birth. Maternal blood should be drawn at the time of delivery to determine the mother's HBsAg status; if the HBsAg test is positive, the infant should receive HBIg as soon as possible (no later than 1 week of age).
   All children and adolescents (through 18 years of age) who have not been immunized against hepatitis B may begin the series during any visit. Special efforts should be made to immunize children who were born in, or whose parents were born in, areas of the world with moderate or high endemicity of hepatitis B virus infection.
3. You now have the option to vaccinate adolescents 11 to 15 years of age according to either a two- or a three-dose hepatitis B immunization schedule. In September 1999, Merck Vaccine Division received approval for an optional two-dose schedule of Recombivax HB (10 μg) for adolescents aged 11 to 15 years. ***The dose schedule is only available using Recombivax 10 μg, given at 0 and 4 to 6 months, and only for adolescents 11 through 15 years of age.*** Adolescents who have already begun the three-dose series with Recombivax (5 μg) may *not* be switched to the new two-dose series. Adolescents immunized according to the alternative schedule appear to develop immunity levels similar to those immunized with the three-dose schedule; however, data on long-term immunity is not yet available.
   The newly approved two-dose schedule will be available through the public-funded vaccine distribution program following the CDC's negotiation of a vaccine contract for this alternative schedule. Health care providers will receive information in The Vac Scene when the new schedule becomes available. (From The Vac Scene, Vol. 6 No. 2 Mar/Apr 2000, Public Health Seattle & King County.)

4. The fourth dose of DTaP (diptheria and tetanus toxoids and acellular pertussis vaccine) may be administered as early as 12 months of age, provided 6 months have elapsed since the third dose and the child is unlikely to return at age 15 to 18 months. **Td** (tetanus and diptheria toxoids) is recommended at 11 to 12 years of age if at least 5 years have elapsed since the last dose of DTP, DTaP, or DT. Subsequent routine Td boosters are recommended every 10 years.
5. Three ***Haemophilus influenzae*** type b (Hib) conjugate vaccines are licensed for infant use. If PRP-OMP (pedvax HIB or ComVax [Merck]) is administered at 2 and 4 months of age, a dose at 6 months is not required. Because clinical studies in infants demonstrate that using some combination products may induce a lower immune response to the Hib vaccine component, DTaP/Hib combination products should not be used for primary immunization in infants at 2, 4, or 6 months of age, unless FDA-approved for these ages.
6. To eliminate the risk of vaccine-associated paralytic polio (VAPP), an all-IPV schedule is now recommended for routine childhood polio vaccination in the United States. All children should receive four doses IPV at 2 months, 4 months, 6 to 18 months, and 4 to 6 years. OPV (if available) may be used only in these circumstances:

    a. Mass vaccination campaigns to control outbreaks of paralytic polio.
    b. Unvaccinated children who will be traveling in less than 4 weeks to areas where polio is endemic or epidemic.
    c. Children of parents who do not accept the recommended number of vaccine injections. These children may receive OPV only for the third and fourth dose or both; in this situation, health care providers should administer OPV only after discussing the risk for VAPP with the parents or caregivers.
    d. During the transition to an all-IPV schedule, recommendations for the use of remaining OPV supplies in physicians' offices and clinics have been issued by the American Academy of Pediatrics (see *Pediatrics,* December 1999).

7. The second dose of ***measles, mumps, and rubella*** *(MMR)* vaccine is recommended routinely at 4 to 6 years of age but may be administered during any visit, provided at least 4 weeks have elapsed since receipt of the first dose and that both doses are administered beginning at or after 12 months of age. Those who have not previously received the second dose should complete the schedule by the 11 to 12-year-old visit.
8. ***Varicella*** (Var) vaccine is recommended at any visit on or after the first birthday for susceptible children; that is, those who lack a reliable history of chickenpox (as judged by a health care provider) and who have not been immunized. Susceptible persons 13 years of age or older should receive two doses, given at least 4 weeks apart.
9. ***Hepatitis A*** (Hep A) is shaded to indicate its recommended use in selected states and/or regions (these include Arkansas, Arizona, California, Idaho, New Mexico, Nevada, Oklahoma, Oregon, South Dakota, Utah, and Washington); consult your local public authority. (Also see MMWR Morb Mortal Wkly Rep. 1999; 48 (RR-12):1–37.)
10. The first multivalent conjugate ***pneumococcal vaccine*** to prevent invasive disease caused by *Streptococcus pneumoniae* (pneumococcus) in infants and toddlers was approved by the FDA in February 2000. It is known as Prevnar (dubbed "PCV7") and is manufactured by Wyeth-Lederle Vaccines. The vaccine contains the seven most common strains for pneumococcus that account for approximately 80% of invasive disease (e.g., bacteremia and meningitis) in infants.

    With the decline of invasive Hib disease (since the advent of Hib conjugate vaccine), *S. pneumoniae* has become the leading cause of bacterial meningitis among children younger than 5 years of age in the United States. Infants have the highest rates of pneumococcal meningitis, approximately 10 cases per 100,000 population.

    Clinical trials included a large multicenter safety and efficacy study conducted at Northern California Kaiser Permanente. The controlled, double-blind trial enrolled approximately 38,000 children, about half of whom received Prevnar. In this trial, the vaccine was 100% effective in preventing invasive pneumococcal disease caused by the seven strains of pneumococcus in the vaccine. The vaccine was shown to be 90% effective in preventing invasive disease from illnesses caused by all pneumococcal subtypes. Children who received PCV7 had 8% fewer visits of tympanostomy tube placements. The duration of protection following PCV7 is currently unknown. Also, the effect of PCV7 on nasopharyngeal carriage of pneumococci is not clear at this time.

    Side effects in the trials were generally mild and included local injection site reactions, irritability, drowsiness, and decreased appetite. Approximately 21% of the children had fevers greater than 37.9°C (100.3°F) as compared to about 14% in the control group not receiving Prevnar.

    See MMWR 2000;49(RR09):1–38. The primary series consist of three IM injections routinely given at 2, 4, and 6 months of age with the fourth (booster) dose at 12 to 15 months of age. Until the vaccine is included on the federal contract, providers who purchase Prevnar may give the vaccine without a VIS. The cost per five-dose box is approximately $290. (From The Vac Scene, Vol. 6 No.2, Public Health-Seattle & King County).

APPENDIX 122–2
Immunization Schedules in Healthy Adults

	Vaccine/Toxoid[a]					
Age Group (y)	*Td*[b]	*Measles*	*Mumps*	*Rubella*	*Influenza*	*Pneumococcal*
18–24	X	X	X	X		
25–49	X	X[c]	X[c]	X		
50–64	X				X	X
≥65	X				X	X

[a]Refer to sections in text on specific vaccines or toxoids for indications, contraindications, precautions, dosages, side effects, adverse reactions, and special considerations. Additional vaccines may be suggested for adults with special circumstances.

[b]Td, tetanus and diptheria toxoids, absorbed (for adult use), which is a combined preparation containing <2 flocculation units of diptheria toxoid.

[c]Indicated for persons born after 1956.

(From Refs. 7, 56, and 83 with permission.)

APPENDIX 122–3
Minimum Age for Pediatric Vaccination

Vaccine	Minimum Age for First Dose	Minimum Interval from Dose 1 to 2[a]	Minimum Interval from Dose 2 to 3[a]	Minimum Interval from Dose 3 to 4[a]
DTaP[b]	15 mo[c]			6 mo
HIB (primary series)				
HbOC	6 wk	1 mo	1 mo	[d]
PRP-T	6 wk	1 mo	1 mo	[d]
PRP-OMP	6 wk	1 mo	[d]	
Pneumococcal conjugate	2 mo	2 mo	2 mo	6 mo
eIPV[e]	6 wk	4 wk	6 mo[f]	
MMR	12 mo[g]	1 mo		
Hepatitis B	Birth	1 mo	2 mo[h]	

DTaP, diptheria-tetanus-acellular pertussis; HIB, *Haemophilus influenzae* type b conjugate; eIPV, enhanced-potency inactivated poliovirus vaccine; MMR, measles-mumps-rubella

[a]These minimum acceptable ages and intervals may not correspond with the optimal recommended ages and intervals of vaccination.

[b]Children who have received all four primary vaccination doses before their fourth birthday should receive a fifth dose of DT or DTaP at 4 to 6 years of age, before entering kindergarten or elementary school, and at least 6 months after the fourth dose. The total number of doses of diptheria and tetanus toxoid should not exceed six each before the seventh birthday.

[c]The American Academy of Pediatrics permits DTaP and OPV to be administered as early as 4 weeks of age in areas with high endemicity and during outbreaks.

[d]The booster dose of HIB vaccine that is recommended following the primary vaccination series should be administered no earlier than 12 months of age and at least 2 months after the previous dose of HIB vaccine.

[e]See text to differentiate conventional inactivated poliovirus vaccine from enhanced-potency IPV.

[f]For unvaccinated adults at increased risk of exposure to poliovirus with <3 months but >2 months available before protection is needed, three doses of IPV should be administered at least 1 month apart.

[g]Although the age for measles vaccination may be as young as 6 months in outbreak areas where cases are occurring in infants, infants initially vaccinated before the first birthday should be revaccinated at 12 to 15 months of age, and an additional dose of vaccine should be administered at the time of school entry or according to local policy. Doses of MMR or other measles-containing vaccines should be a separated by at least 1 month.

[h]This final dose is recommended no earlier than 4 months of age.

(From Ref. 49 with permission.)

123

HUMAN IMMUNODEFICIENCY VIRUS INFECTION

Courtney V. Fletcher, Thomas N. Kakuda, and Ann C. Collier

The acquired immunodeficiency syndrome (AIDS) was first recognized by the medical community as a distinct clinical entity in 1981. This syndrome was initially described in a cohort of young homosexual men with profound immunologic deficits, *Pneumocystis carinii* pneumonia (PCP), and Kaposi's sarcoma.[1,2] A retrovirus, human immunodeficiency virus type 1 (HIV-1) (formerly called lymphadenopathy-associated virus [LAV] or human T lymphotropic virus type III [HTLV-III]) is the major cause of AIDS.[3,4] A second retrovirus, HIV-2, is also recognized to cause AIDS, although it is far less prevalent than HIV-1. These retroviruses are transmitted by sexual contact and by contact with contaminated blood or blood products. Several risk behaviors for acquisition of HIV infection have been identified, most notably the practice of anorectal intercourse and the sharing of blood-contaminated needles by injection-drug users. Transmission of HIV between heterosexuals and from childbearing women to their offspring is an increasing problem worldwide. Global statistics on the prevalence and incidence of this disease remain grim, and all treatments to date have been unsuccessful in eradicating HIV. However, potent combinations of antiretroviral agents, also known as highly active antiretroviral therapy (HAART), have been able to suppress HIV replication, delay the onset of AIDS, and prolong patient survival in adults and children.[5,6] Unfortunately, this success is tempered by the long-term toxicities that may arise from using these agents.[7] This chapter discusses the epidemiology and manifestations of HIV disease, therapeutic strategies directed at inhibiting the virus, and management of HIV-associated opportunistic infections.

EPIDEMIOLOGY

Persons infected with HIV and AIDS cases in the United States conform to the Centers for Disease Control and Prevention (CDC) surveillance case definition and are reported by health care providers to a public health department.[8,9] The CDC case definition for AIDS was first established in 1981, at the outbreak of the disease and has undergone modifications in 1985, 1987, and 1993. The latest version expanded the definition of AIDS to include not only persons with serious symptomatic disease, but also all HIV-infected individuals who have <200 CD4 lymphocytes/μL or a percentage of CD4 lymphocytes <14% of the total lymphocytes. Table 123–1 presents the classification system for adult and adolescent HIV infection and a listing of clinical conditions included in the 1993 definition.[9] Beginning January 1, 2000 the CDC also recommended statewide surveillance of HIV infection.[8]

The cumulative number of reported AIDS cases in the United States at the end of December 1999 was 733,374; 430,441 have already died. Reported cases in men outnumbered women by approximately 5 to 1. AIDS is a leading cause of death among men between the ages of 25 and 44 years living in the United States. Compared with their distribution in the overall population, African American and Hispanic populations are disproportionately affected by AIDS (37% and 18%, respectively). The estimated prevalence of HIV in the United States in 1999 was 800,000 to 900,000 individuals. Approximately two-thirds were diagnosed with either HIV infection or AIDS. Each year, approximately 40,000 new cases of HIV are reported in the United States; many more remain undiagnosed. Men who have sex with men account for the majority of cases. However, women account for a growing proportion (32%) of those newly infected.[8,10] HIV infection, however, is a worldwide epidemic. The World Health Organization (WHO) estimates that 34.3 million adults and children are infected with HIV worldwide—primarily in sub-Saharan Africa (24.5 million) and Southeast Asia (5.6 million). Children younger than 15 years old account for 1.3 million infections worldwide. Approximately 5.4 million additional infections occur each year, mainly (95%) in developing countries. Most of these infections will be acquired through heterosexual transmission.[11]

ETIOLOGY

HIV is a member of the *Lentivirinae* (lenti = slow) subfamily of retroviruses. Lentiviruses are characterized by their indolent infectious cycle. There are two related but distinct types of HIV: HIV-1 and HIV-2. HIV-2, found mostly in Western Africa, is comprised of six distinct phylogenetic lineages designated as subtypes (clades) A to F. HIV-1 can also be categorized based on phylogeny. Three groups of HIV-1 are currently recognized: M (main), N (new or non-M, non-O), and O (outlier). The 11 subtypes of HIV-1 group M are identified as A to K. HIV-1 subtype B is primarily responsible for the epidemic in North America and Western Europe. The origin of these viruses is of considerable interest. The accumulated evidence suggests HIV in humans was the result of a cross-species transmission (zoonosis) from primates infected with simian immunodeficiency virus (SIV). Phylogenetic and geographic relationships suggest HIV-2 arose from SIV that infects sooty mangabeys. The origin of HIV-1 is less clear but similarities exist between SIVcpz, a virus that infects chimpanzees (*Pan troglodytes troglodytes*), and HIV-1. Cultural practices such as the preparation and eating of bushmeat or keeping chimpanzees as pets may have allowed the virus to jump from primate to man. The earliest known human infection with HIV has been traced to central Africa in 1959. Modern transportation, promiscuity, and drug abuse have caused the rapid spread of the virus within the United States and throughout the world.[12] This chapter focuses on HIV-1 because this is the predominant strain likely to be encountered in the United States.

DETECTION OF HIV AND SURROGATE MARKERS OF DISEASE PROGRESSION

When HIV-1 infection is suspected, whether owing to symptoms or high-risk behavior, it should be confirmed by laboratory methods. The most common method is an enzyme linked immunosorbent assay (ELISA) that detects antibodies against HIV-1. The ELISA test is both highly sensitive (>99%) and specific (>99%) but false-positives can occur in multiparous women; in recent recipients of

TABLE 123–1. Centers for Disease Control and Prevention 1993 Revised Classification System for HIV Infection in Adults and AIDS Surveillance Case Definition

CD4+ T-cell Categories (Absolute Number and Percentage)	(A) Asymptomatic, Acute (Primary) HIV or PGL*	(B) Symptomatic, not (A) or (C) Conditions	(C) AIDS-Indicator Conditions
≥500/μL or ≥29%	A1	B1	C1
200–499/μL or 14–28%	A2	B2	C2
<200/μL or <14%	A3	B3	C3
AIDS-indicator conditions			
Candidiasis of bronchi, trachea, or lungs		Lymphoma, Burkitt's	
Candidiasis, esophageal		Lymphoma, immunoblastic	
Cervical cancer, invasive		Lymphoma, primary, of brain	
Coccidioidomycosis, disseminated or extrapulmonary		*Mycobacterium avium* complex or *M. kansasii*, disseminated or extrapulmonary	
Cryptococcosis, extrapulmonary		*Mycobacterium tuberculosis*, any site (pulmonary or extrapulmonary)	
Cryptosporidiosis, chronic intestinal (duration >1 month)		*Mycobacterium*, other species or unidentified species, disseminated or extrapulmonary	
Cytomegalovirus disease (other than liver, spleen, or nodes)		*Pneumocystis carinii* pneumonia	
Cytomegalovirus retinitis (with loss of vision)		Pneumonia, recurrent	
Encephalopathy, HIV-related		Progressive multifocal leukoencephalopathy	
Herpes simplex: chronic ulcer(s) (duration >1 month); or bronchitis, or pneumonitis, or esophagitis		*Salmonella* septicemia, recurrent	
Histoplasmosis, disseminated or extrapulmonary		Toxoplasmosis of brain	
Isosporiasis, chronic intestinal (duration >1 month)		Wasting syndrome caused by HIV	
Kaposi's sarcoma			

*PGL, persistent generalized lymphadenopathy.

hepatitis B, HIV, influenza, or rabies vaccine; in patients with multiple blood transfusion, liver disease, renal failure; or in those patients on chronic hemodialysis. False-negatives may occur if the patient is newly infected and the test is performed before antibody production is adequate. The minimum time to develop antibodies is 3 to 4 weeks from initial exposure, with greater than 95% of individuals developing antibodies after 6 months. Convenient methods for obtaining an ELISA sample have been developed including an oral collection device (OraSure), an over-the-counter home finger-stick blood-collection test system (Home Access), and a urine test (Calpyte). Positive ELISAs are repeated in duplicate, and if one or both tests are reactive, a confirmatory test is performed for final diagnosis. Western blot is the most commonly used confirmatory test, although an indirect immunofluorescence assay (IFA) is also available. A reactive ELISA and positive confirmatory test indicates an established HIV infection. If the confirmatory test is indeterminate, the dilemma can be resolved by retesting the individual after 30 days or by performing a viral load assay if the patient is at high risk or symptomatic.[13]

The viral load test quantifies the degree of viremia by measuring the amount of viral RNA (HIV RNA). There are four methods for determining HIV RNA: reverse transcriptase-coupled polymerase chain reaction (RT-PCR), branched DNA (bDNA), transcription-mediated amplification, and nucleic acid sequence-based assay (NASBA). RT-PCR and bDNA are more widely used than the other techniques. Irrespective of the method used, viral load is reported as the number of viral RNA copies per milliliter. Because each assay has its own lower limit of sensitivity, sensitivity to viral subtypes and results can vary from one assay method to the other; therefore, it is recommended that the same assay method be used consistently within patients. Reductions in viral load are often reported in base 10 logarithm. For example, if a patient initially presents with a viral load of 100,000 copies/mL (10^5 copies/mL) and subsequently has a viral load of 10,000 copies/mL (10^4 copies/mL), the decrease in viral load is 1 $\log_{10}$. Viral load assays have greater than 99% specificity and can be used to detect most strains of HIV. More importantly, viral load can be used as a prognostic factor to monitor disease progression and the effects of treatment.[13]

Because HIV attacks and destroys cells bearing the CD4 receptor, the number of CD4 lymphocytes in the blood is a surrogate marker of disease progression. The normal adult CD4 lymphocyte count ranges from 500 to 1600 cells/μL or 40% to 70% of all lymphocytes. CD4 counts in children are age-dependent, with younger children having higher CD4 counts. Depletion of CD4 cells has been associated with the development of opportunistic infection and other AIDS malignancies.[14] Viral load is a better predictor of disease progression than the absolute CD4 lymphocyte count, but prognosis is much more accurate when the two are used together.[13]

TRANSMISSION OF HIV

Infection with HIV occurs through three primary modes: sexual, parenteral, and perinatal. Sexual intercourse, primarily receptive anal and vaginal intercourse, is the most common method for transmission.[10] HIV can be found in semen and cervical secretions, and exposure to either of these infected body fluids may transmit the virus. Male-to-male transmission of HIV accounted for 34% of AIDS cases in the United States in 1999. Women infected by their male partner are increasingly common.[10] No sexual act between individuals can be considered absolutely safe. The probability of HIV transmission from receptive anorectal intercourse is 0.1% to 3% per sexual contact; for receptive vaginal intercourse, the risk is approximately 0.1% to 0.2%.[15] In general, the probability of infection is increased when the index partner is in an advanced stage of disease. Persons at highest risk for heterosexual transmission include persons with ulcerative sexually transmitted diseases, individuals with multiple sex partners, and sexual partners of injection-drug users. Risk of transmission is elevated when women experience vaginal bleeding during intercourse. Individuals with genital ulcers, such as from syphilis, chancroid, or herpes, are at a fourfold greater risk of contracting HIV. Gonorrhea, chlamydia, and trichomoniasis increase the risk two- to three-fold. Sexual partners of circumcised males are less likely to acquire HIV infection when compared with sex partners of uncircumcised males, suggesting that the absence of the foreskin has a protective effect for the partner. Infections can also occur from artificial insemination with infected semen. The risk of acquiring HIV infection from oral intercourse is less-well established. Casual contact with AIDS patients or persons with HIV is not a significant risk factor for HIV transmission. Prevention of sexual transmission in adults has primarily been focused on encouraging the use of condoms, reducing high-risk behavior (anal intercourse and promiscuity), and the treatment of sexually transmitted diseases. A combined approach has been advocated for successful prevention. Abstinence is encouraged among adolescents. Future interventions under developments such as HIV vaccines and topical vaginal microbicides may further limit the spread of sexually transmitted HIV.[16]

Parenteral transmission of HIV broadly encompasses infections caused by contaminated blood exposure, such as from needlesticks, intravenous injection with used needles, receipt of blood products, or organ transplants. The use of contaminated needles or other injection-related paraphernalia by drug abusers is the main cause of parenteral transmissions and currently accounts for a quarter of AIDS cases reported in the United States. Cases in which receipt of infected blood transfusion, blood components, or organ transplant was involved, currently are less than 1% of reports.[10] This low incidence is attributable to blood- and organ-donor screening and viral inactivation procedures for many clotting factors. These preventative measures have reduced the estimated risk for receiving tainted blood or blood products to 1 in 493,000.[17] Health care workers have a small but definite occupational risk of contracting HIV through accidental injury. Most cases of occupationally acquired HIV have been the result of a percutaneous needlestick injury. Studies indicate that the risk of HIV infection following this route is approximately 0.3%. Significant risk factors for seroconversion include deep injury, injury with a device visibly contaminated with blood, and exposure from a source whom later died of AIDS. Guidelines for health care and public safety workers have been developed to minimize the hazard of occupational exposure.[18]

Perinatal infection or vertical transmission, is the most common cause of pediatric HIV infection. Most infections occur during or near to the time of birth and therefore treatment of the infected mother is important. The risk of mother-to-child transmission is approximately 25% in the absence of breast feeding and antiretroviral therapy. Factors that increase the likelihood of vertical transmission include prolonged rupture of membranes; chorioamnionitis; genital infections during pregnancy; preterm delivery, vaginal delivery; birth weight below 2,500 g; illicit drug use during pregnancy; and a high maternal viral load.[19] Breast-feeding can also transmit HIV. The estimated frequency of breast milk transmission in one study was 16.2% with the majority of infections developing within the first 6 months. Formula feeding prevented 44% of infections and was associated with a higher HIV-free survival rate after 2 years.[20] In countries in which safe and available alternatives to breast-feeding exist, HIV-infected mothers are strongly urged not to breast feed.

PATHOGENESIS

The life cycle of HIV (Fig. 123–1) is complicated but necessary to understand because the current strategies employed in the treatment of HIV target various points in this cycle. Once HIV enters a human body, the outer glycoprotein (gp160) expressed on the virus allows HIV to bind to CD4 receptors. These receptors are present on the surface of T helper cells (Th lymphocytes), and to monocytes, macrophages, and dendritic cells. The glycoprotein consists of two subunits: gp120 and gp41. The gp120 subunit has high affinity for CD4 receptor and is responsible for the initial binding of the virus to the cell. Once initial binding occurs, the intimate association of HIV with the cell is enhanced further by chemokine coreceptors. There are two major chemokine receptors involved in HIV infection, CXCR4 and CCR5, but other receptors, such as CCR2b and CCR3, may also play a role. Genetic defects in the expression of chemokine receptors appear to protect some individuals from developing AIDS despite their being exposed to the virus.[21] Attachment of HIV to the cell promotes fusion and internalization (adsorption) of the virus—a process mediated by the gp41 subunit.

After internalization, the virus is uncoated in preparation for replication. The genetic material of HIV is positive-sense, single-strand RNA (ssRNA); the virus must transcribe this RNA into DNA to optimally replicate in human cells (transcription normally occurs from DNA to RNA—HIV works backward, hence the name retrovirus). To do so, HIV is equipped with a unique enzyme, RNA-dependent DNA polymerase (reverse transcriptase). Reverse transcriptase first synthesizes a complementary strand of DNA using the viral RNA as a template. The RNA portion of this DNA-RNA hybrid is then partially removed by ribonuclease H (RNase H) allowing reverse transcriptase to complete the synthesis of a double-stranded DNA (dsDNA) molecule. Unfortunately, the fidelity of reverse transcriptase is poor and many mistakes are made during the process. These errors in the final DNA product contribute to the rapid mutation of the virus and allow drug resistance to evolve. Following reverse transcription, the final dsDNA product migrates into the nucleus and is integrated into the host cell chromosome by integrase, another enzyme unique to HIV.

The integration of HIV into the host chromosome is troublesome for several reasons. First, HIV can establish a chronic and persistent infection, particularly in long-lived cells of the immune system such as memory T lymphocytes.[22] Second, integration is random, thus making it difficult to target and extract integrated HIV. Last, random integration of HIV may cause cellular abnormalities leading to cancer.

Activation of the infected cell by antigens, cytokines, or other factors induces the cell to produce nuclear factor κB (NF-κB), an enhancer-binding protein. NF-κB normally regulates the expression of T-lymphocyte genes involved in growth, but can also inadvertently activate replication of HIV. When HIV replication is induced, the host DNA polymerase transcribes the integrated proviral DNA into messenger RNA (mRNA) with subsequent translation of the mRNA into viral proteins. At first, transcription and translation are done at a low level, yielding various regulatory HIV proteins such as Tat, Nef, and Rev. The Tat protein is a potent amplifier of HIV gene expression;

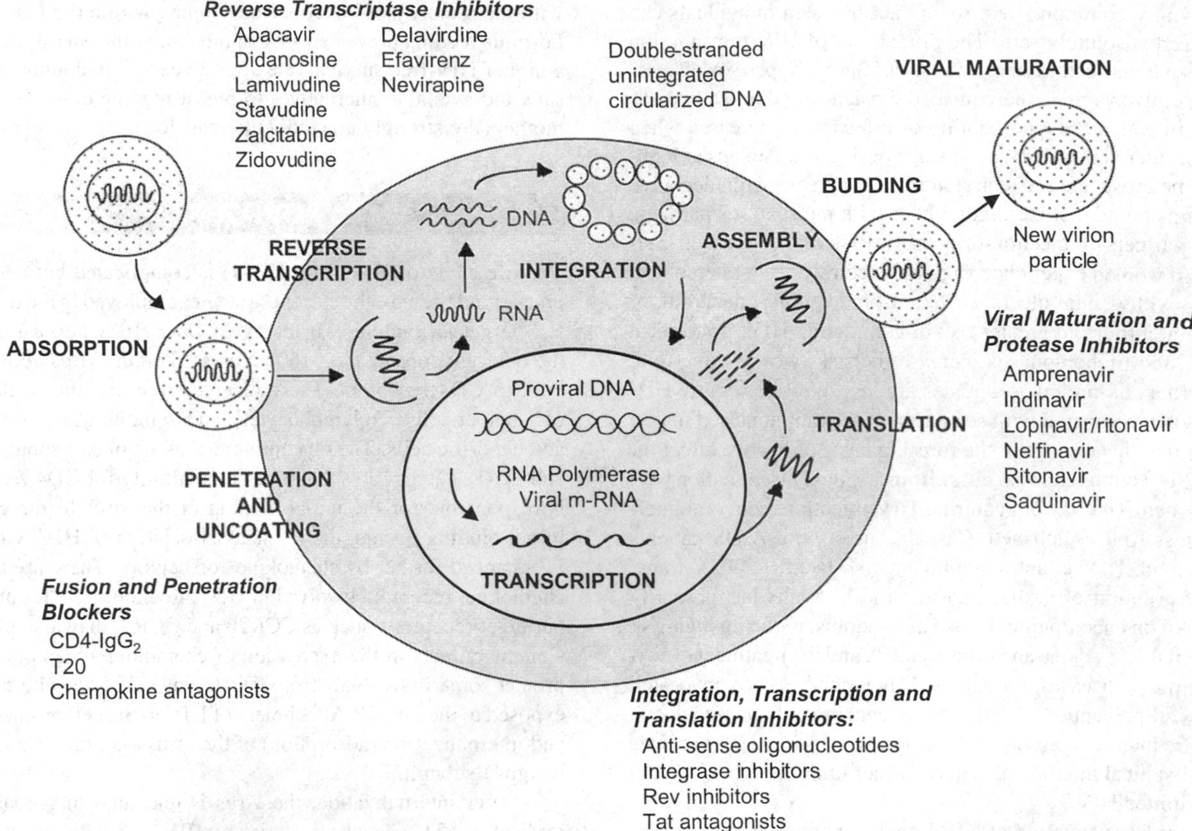

FIGURE 123–1. Life cycle of HIV with potential targets where replication may be interrupted and known or putative antiretroviral agents. *(Reprinted with permission; copyright Courtney V. Fletcher, 2001.)*

it binds to a specific RNA sequence of HIV that initiates and stabilizes transcription elongation. There is no evident function for Nef, although it appears to down-regulate class I molecules and to protect infected cells from cytotoxic T lymphocytes.[23] Deletion of the Nef gene has been noted in HIV strains that have infected a cohort of long-term nonprogressors.[24] The Rev protein regulates posttranscriptional activity and like Tat is essential for HIV replication. Rev essentially shifts synthesis of HIV regulatory proteins to structural proteins (e.g., gp120) by inhibiting viral mRNA splicing and exporting the mRNA outside the nucleus.[23]

Assembly of new virion particles occurs in a stepwise manner, beginning with the coalescence of HIV proteins beneath the host cell lipid bilayer. The nucleocapsid is subsequently formed with viral ss-RNA and other components packaged inside. Once packaged, the virion then buds through the plasma membrane, acquiring the characteristics of the host lipid bilayer. After the virus buds, the maturation process begins. Within the virion, HIV protease begins cleaving a large precursor polypeptide into functional proteins that are necessary to produce a complete virus. Without this enzyme, the virion is immature and unable to adequately infect cells.[25]

HIV-1 exhibits a very high turnover rate, with an estimated 10 billion new viruses produced each day. More than 99% of these viruses are produced in newly infected cells. Ultimately, most infected cells will be destroyed from a number of mechanisms, including cell lysis by newly budding virions, cytotoxic T-lymphocyte-induced cell killing, syncytia formation, or apoptosis. Syncytia formation occurs when viral protein expressed on the surface of the infected cell act as ligands for receptors expressed on uninfected cells. Uninfected cells clump onto the infected cell and fuse into a giant multinucleated cell. The syncytium-inducing virus phenotype may develop later in disease and is associated with more rapid disease progression.

CLINICAL PRESENTATION

Clinical presentation of primary HIV infection may vary but patients often have an acute retroviral syndrome or mononucleosis-like illness. The most common symptoms are fever, sore throat, fatigue, weight loss, and myalgia.[26] Approximately 40% to 80% of patients also exhibit a morbilliform or maculopapular rash, usually involving the trunk. Other common manifestations (>50%) include diarrhea, lymphadenopathy, nausea, night sweats, and vomiting.[27] Aseptic meningitis (fever, headache, photophobia, and stiff neck) may be present in a quarter of presenting cases. Symptoms often last 2 weeks and hospitalization may be required for 15% of patients.[26] Primary infection is often associated with a high viral load >100,000 and development of an immune response that for a period of time suppresses, but does not eliminate, viral replication. During this period, HIV is trapped by follicular dendritic cells in lymphoid tissue and replicates in the germinal center. The amount of HIV RNA in plasma falls substantially at that point and symptoms gradually resolve. This decline coincides with the development of an immune response to HIV. The clinically latent period, however, is not virologically latent because HIV replication and immune system deterioration are ongoing. A persistent decrease in CD4 lymphocytes is the most measurable aspect of this immune system destruction.[22] Plasma viral load on the other hand, will appear to have stabilized at a particular level or "set point." The set point that is established correlates directly with progression to AIDS and

TABLE 123–2. Centers for Disease Control and Prevention 1994 Revised Classification System for HIV Infection in Children Younger than 13 Years of Age

Immunologic Categories	< 12 Months cells/μL (%)[a]	1–5 years cells/μL (%)*	6–12 years cells/μL (%)*
1. No evidence of suppression	≥1500 (≥25%)	≥1000 (≥25%)	≥500 (≥25%)
2. Evidence of moderate suppression	750–1499 (15%–24%)	500–999 (15%–24%)	200–499 (15%–24%)
3. Severe suppression	<750 (<15%)	<500 (<15%)	<200 (<15%)

Immunologic Categories	N: No Signs/Symptoms	A: Mild Signs/Symptoms	B: Moderate Signs/Symptoms	C: Severe Signs/Symptoms
1. No evidence of suppression	N1	A1	B1	C1
2. Evidence of moderate suppression	N2	A2	B2	C2
3. Severe suppression	N3	A3	B3	C3

*Percentage of total lymphocytes.

morbidity. The Multicenter AIDS Cohort Study (MACS) measured viral load in 181 HIV-positive men and followed them for as long as 11 years. Only 8% of patients with fewer than 4,530 copies/mL progressed to AIDS within 5 years, whereas the 5-year progression rate for those with initial viral loads above 36,270 copies/mL was 62%. The mortality rates within 5 years were 5% and 49%, respectively. Those with viral loads between 4,531 and 13,020 progressed to AIDS at a rate of 26%, with a mortality rate of 10%; and those with viral loads from 13,021 to 36,270 progressed to AIDS at a rate of 49%, with a mortality rate of 25%. Clearly, a higher level of viremia at the onset is associated with poorer prognosis.[28]

Most neonates born with HIV are asymptomatic. Upon physical exam, they often present with unexplained physical signs such as lymphadenopathy, hepatomegaly, splenomegaly, failure to thrive and weight loss or unexplained low birth weight (in prenatally exposed infants), and fever of unknown origin. Laboratory findings include anemia, hypergammaglobulinemia (primarily IgA and IgM), altered mononuclear cell function, and altered T-cell subset ratios.[29] Of note, the normal range for CD4 cell counts in children <13 years is much different than in adults (Table 123–2). Bacterial infections, including streptococcus pneumonia, *Salmonella* species, and mycobacterium tuberculosis may be more prevalent in children with AIDS than in adults with the disease. Kaposi's sarcoma is rare in children. Children with HIV infection may develop lymphocytic interstitial pneumonitis without evidence of *P. carinii* or other pathogens on lung biopsy. Some children present with progressive, unexplained, neurologic deterioration, including late-onset seizures, loss of developmental milestones, cessation of brain growth, and diffuse, unexplained encephalopathy. A history of recurrent or persistent bacterial, fungal, or viral infections, which may be chronic, and initially subclinical or slowly progressive, has been observed. Included in this group are children with recurrent bacterial sepsis, meningitis, and chronic otitis media, and children with chronic oral candidiasis and presumed disseminated histoplasmosis. The CDC's current pediatric AIDS surveillance definition (Table 123–2) excludes children with congenital or perinatally acquired cytomegalovirus or other identified causes of congenital immunodeficiency.[30] Management of the HIV-infected child involves similar principles as the adult: antiretroviral therapy, treatment and prophylaxis of opportunistic infections, and supportive care.[31] Pediatric treatment recommendations are often categorized as neonatal, child, adolescent, and adult. While there is no universal definition of the age ranges for these categories, the following are usually accepted: neonate, first month of life; infant; 1–12 months; child, 1–12 years; adolescent, 12–18 years; and adults, greater than 18 years.

▶ TREATMENT: Human Immunodeficiency Virus Infection

DESIRED OUTCOME

The goal of antiretroviral therapy is to achieve maximum suppression of HIV replication. This is commonly interpreted to be an HIV RNA level in plasma that is less than the lower limit of quantitation (i.e., undetectable). Studies show that long-term response to therapy (i.e., durability) is determined by the viral load nadir achieved.[32,33] Secondary goals include an increase in CD4 lymphocytes and an improved quality of life. The ultimate goal, however, is decreased morbidity and mortality.

GENERAL APPROACH TO TREATMENT

In mid-1997 the National Institutes of Health Office of AIDS Research convened a panel to define the scientific principles that would serve as a guide for the clinical use of antiretroviral agents.[34] The 11 principles presented below are an amalgamation of knowledge of the life cycle of HIV, the consequences of HIV replication, clinical trials of antiretroviral agents, and scientific opinion.

1. Ongoing HIV replication leads to immune-system damage and progression to AIDS. HIV infection is always harmful, and true long-term survival free of clinically significant immune dysfunction is unusual.
2. Plasma HIV RNA levels indicate the magnitude of HIV replication and its associated rate of CD4 cell destruction, whereas CD4 cell counts indicate the extent of HIV-induced immune damage already suffered. Regular, periodic measurement of plasma HIV RNA levels and CD4 cell counts is necessary to determine the risk of disease progression in an HIV-infected individual and to determine when to initiate or modify antiretroviral treatment regimens.
3. Because rates of disease progression differ among individuals, treatment decisions should be

individualized by level of risk indicated by plasma HIV RNA levels and CD4 cell counts.

4. The use of potent combination antiretroviral therapy to suppress HIV replication to below the levels of detection of sensitive plasma HIV RNA assays limits the potential for selection of antiretroviral-resistant HIV variants, the major factor limiting the ability of antiretroviral drugs to inhibit virus replication and delay disease progression. Therefore, maximum achievable suppression of HIV replication should be the goal of therapy.
5. The most effective means to accomplish durable suppression of HIV replication is the simultaneous initiation of combinations of effective anti-HIV drugs with which the patient has not been previously treated and that are not cross-resistant with antiretroviral agents with which the patient has been treated previously.
6. Each of the antiretroviral drugs used in combination therapy regimens should always be used according to optimum schedules and dosages.
7. The available effective antiretroviral drugs are limited in number and mechanism of action, and cross-resistance between specific drugs has been documented. Therefore, any change in antiretroviral therapy increases future therapeutic constraints.
8. Women should receive optimal antiretroviral therapy regardless of pregnancy status.
9. The same principles of antiretroviral therapy apply to both HIV-infected children and adults, although the treatment of HIV-infected children involves unique pharmacologic, virologic, and immunologic considerations.
10. Persons with acute primary HIV infections should be treated with combination antiretroviral therapy to suppress virus replication to levels below the limit of detection of sensitive plasma HIV RNA assays.
11. HIV-infected persons, even those with viral loads below detectable limits, should be considered infectious and should be counseled to avoid sexual and drug-use behaviors that are associated with transmission or acquisition of HIV and other infectious pathogens.

The extent to which these principles will stand the test of time is unknown; new information on the pathogenesis of HIV accrues constantly. The field of antiretroviral therapy is also rapidly evolving. Several of the clinical trials used in formulating the principles of therapy enrolled small numbers of participants and had limited followup. Sixteen agents are now FDA approved and more are certain to come. Health care professionals involved in care of the HIV-infected person must always consult the most current literature with respect to the principles and strategies for therapy. At this time, a particularly excellent source for information on treatment guidelines can be found at: http://www.hivatis.org. With these caveats, Table 123–3 presents the state-of-the-art for treatment of the HIV-infected individual at the time of the writing of this chapter. Treatment is recommended for all HIV-infected persons with symptomatic disease or CD4 lymphocyte counts <200 cell/μL. Treatment should be considered in patients with CD4 counts between 200 and 350 cell/μL. Treatment should also be considered in individuals with plasma HIV RNA $>30{,}000$ copies/mL by bDNA or $>55{,}000$ copies/mL by RT-PCR, as the 3-year risk of developing AIDS if left untreated is $>30\%$ in this cohort.[35] Many experts would defer therapy in persons with HIV RNA in plasma $<30{,}000$ (bDNA) or $<55{,}000$ (RT-PCR) and CD4 cells $>$ 350 cells/μL. However, a more aggressive treatment approach recommends treatment if HIV RNA is $>5{,}000$ copies/mL.[36] The available data do not permit an absolute treatment threshold to be established based on plasma HIV RNA level. Therefore, the relative merits of a cautious approach that delays therapy for patients with values $<5{,}000$ copies/mL, and considers therapy for patients with values between 5,000 and 10,000 copies/mL, is as valid as an aggressive approach of offering therapy to any patient who requests it and is committed to lifelong medication compliance.

PHARMACOLOGIC THERAPY

Conceptually, there are three primary methods of therapeutic intervention against HIV: inhibition of viral replication, vaccination to stimulate a more effective immune response, and restoration of the immune system with immunomodulators. Several approaches for an HIV vaccine are in development, including whole-killed virus, subunit and peptide vaccination, recombinant live vector, and naked DNA delivery. Although clinical studies of vaccines have been done, at this point, optimal vaccine strategies are still being explored. Genetic variability in HIV and a nascent understanding the role of the immune system in suppressing viral replication are significant barriers to the development of an effective HIV vaccine with long-lasting and protective immunity.[37] Among immunomodulators, interleukin-2 (aldesleukin or IL-2) appears to be the most promising. Several methods of dosing and administration have been attempted—the most common is subcutaneous administration for five consecutive days in 2-month cycles. The main benefit of IL-2 is increased CD4 cells; unfortunately, it is also associated with significant toxicities. Studies to assess clinical end points are underway.[38]

ANTIRETROVIRAL AGENTS

Inhibiting viral replication with HAART has been the most clinically successful strategy. Thus far, there have been two primary groups of drugs used: reverse transcriptase inhibitors and protease inhibitors (Table 123–4). Reverse transcriptase inhibitors are of two types: those that are chemical derivatives of purine- and pyrimidine-based nucleosides and nucleotides (nucleoside/nucleotide reverse transcriptase inhibitors or NRTIs), and those that are not (nonnucleoside reverse transcriptase inhibitors or NNRTIs). Nucleoside reverse transcriptase inhibitors include thymidine analogs such as stavudine (d4T), zidovudine (AZT or ZDV), and phosphonavir (phosphazid); cytosine analogs such as emtricitabine (FTC), lamivudine (3TC), and zalcitabine (ddC); the inosine derivative didanosine (ddI); and the guanosine analogs abacavir sulfate (ABV) and andoxovir guanosine (DXG). Tenofovir disoproxil fumarate (TDF) is an adenosine-derived nucleotide reverse transcriptase inhibitor. As a class, the NRTIs require phosphorylation to the 5′-triphosphate moiety to be active. Intracellular phosphorylation occurs by cytoplasmic or mitochondrial kinases and phosphotransferases. Following prodrug activation, the 5′-triphosphate moiety acts in two ways: (a) it competes with endogenous deoxynucleotides for reverse transcriptase and (b) it prematurely terminates DNA elongation due to the modified 3′-hydroxyl group. Hydroxyurea, a ribonucleotide reductase inhibitor, depletes intracellular deoxynucleotides and has been used in combination with nucleoside/nucleotide reverse transcriptase inhibitors with some success.

TABLE 123–3. Treatment of HIV Infection*

Recommended Antiretroviral Agents for Initial Therapy		
Strongly recommended	An antiretroviral regimen is comprised of one choice from column A and from column B. The drugs are not listed in priority order	
	Column A	*Column B*
	Indinavir	Zidovudine + lamivudine
	Indinavir + ritonavir	Didanosine + lamivudine
	Lopinavir + ritonavir	Stavudine + lamivudine
	Nelfinavir	Stavudine + didanosine*
	Saquinavir (sgc or hgc) + ritonavir	Zidovudine + didanosine
	Efavirenz	
Recommended as alternatives	*Column A*	*Column B*
	Abacavir	Zidovudine + zalcitabine
	Amprenavir	
	Delavirdine	
	Nelfinavir + saquinavir-sgc	
	Nevirapine	
	Ritonavir	
	Saquinavir-sgc	
No recommendation: Insufficient data	Hydroxyurea in combination with antiretroviral agents	
	Ritonavir + amprenavir	
	Ritonavir + nelfinavir	
Not recommended: Should not be offered	All monotherapies, whether from column A or B	
	Column A	*Column B*
	Saquinavir-hgc	Stavudine + zidovudine
		Zalcitabine + didanosine
		Zalcitabine + lamivudine
		Zalcitabine + stavudine

Possible Regimens for Patients Who Have Failed Antiretroviral Therapy	
Prior Regimen	*New Regimen (not listed in priority order)*
2 NRTIs +	2 new NRTIs +
Nelfinavir	Ritonavir; or indinavir; or saquinavir + ritonavir; or NNRTI + ritonavir; or NNRTI + indinavir
Ritonavir	Saquinavir + ritonavir; or nelfinavir + NNRTI; or nelfinavir + saquinavir
Indinavir	Saquinavir + ritonavir; or nelfinavir + NNRTI; or nelfinavir + saquinavir
Saquinavir	Saquinavir + ritonavir; or NNRTI + indinavir
2 NRTIs + NNRTI	2 new NRTIs + a protease inhibitor
2 NRTIs	2 new NRTIs + a protease inhibitor
	2 new NRTIs + saquinavir + ritonavir
	1 new NRTI + 1 NNRTI + a protease inhibitor
	2 protease inhibitors + NNRTI
1 NRTI	2 new NRTIs + a protease inhibitor
	2 new NRTIs + NNRTI
	1 new NRTI + 1 NNRTI + a protease inhibitor

*Pregnant women may be at increased risk for lactic acidosis and liver damage when treated with the combination of stavudine and didanosine. This combination should be used in pregnant women only when the potential benefit clearly outweighs the potential risk.

Abbreviations: sgc, soft gelatin capsule; hgc, hard gelatin capsule; NRTI, nucleoside reverse transcriptase inhibitor; NNRTI, nonnucleoside reverse transcriptase inhibitor.

Adapted from: Panel on Clinical Practice for Treatment of HIV Infection. Guidelines for the use of antiretroviral agents in HIV-infected adults and adolescents. Living document, August 13, 2001. http://www.hivatis.org. Accessed November 26, 2001.

Presumably, the reduction of endogenous triphosphates by hydroxyurea shifts the competition for reverse transcriptase in favor of the exogenous triphosphate (i.e., nucleoside/nucleotide reverse transcriptase inhibitor). Mycophenolic acid, an inosine monophosphate dehydrogenase inhibitor, can cause similar shifts in endogenous nucleotide pools. Although nucleoside and nucleotide reverse transcriptase inhibitors are specific for HIV reverse transcriptase, their adverse effects may in part be owing to some inhibition of human DNA polymerases, particularly mitochondrial DNA polymerase γ.[39]

Nonnucleoside reverse transcriptase inhibitors are a chemically heterogeneous group of agents that bind noncompetitively to reverse transcriptase close to the catalytic site. Unlike nucleoside and nucleotide reverse transcriptase inhibitors, nonnucleoside reverse transcriptase inhibitors do not require intracellular activation, do not compete against endogenous deoxynucleotides, and do not have strong antiviral activity against HIV-2. Available nonnucleosides include efavirenz (EFV), delavirdine (DLV), and nevirapine (NVP).[40] Capravirine and calanolide A are two agents in clinical development under this class.

The protease inhibitors (PIs) are a potent class of antiretrovirals that include amprenavir (APV), indinavir (IDV), lopinavir (LPV), nelfinavir (NFV), ritonavir (RTV), saquinavir (SQV), and tipranavir (TPV). The pharmacology, safety and efficacy of these drugs are reviewed elsewhere.[41] Briefly, protease inhibitors block the maturation process, thereby resulting in the production of immature, noninfectious virions.[25]

Novel antiviral agents are currently in development and exploit other areas of HIV replication. Pentafuside (T-20) and its derivative

TABLE 123–4. Pharmacologic Parameters of Antiretroviral Compounds

Drug	*In Vitro* Susceptibility (μM IC_{50} range)	F (%)	V_d (L/kg)	$T_{1/2}$ (h)	CL/F (L/h)	Adult Dose[a]	Plasma C_{max}/C_{min} (μM)	Ratio fetal:maternal conc.	Ratio CSF:plasma conc.
Nucleoside Reverse Transcriptase Inhibitors									
Abacavir	0.07–5.8	83	0.86	1.5	49.8	300 mg bid	10.7/0.04	?	0.3
Didanosine	0.01–10	40	0.83	1.4	26.9	200 mg bid 400 mg qd	4/0.02	0.3–0.5	0.22
Lamivudine	0.002–15	86	1.3	5	23.1	150 mg bid	7.5/0.22	>0.7	0.12
Stavudine	0.009–4	86	0.53	1.4	34	40 mg bid	4/0.004	>0.7	0.02
Zalcitabine	0.03–0.5	85	0.53	2	12	0.75 mg tid	0.05/0.001	0.3–0.5	0.2
Zidovudine	0.01–0.048	64	1.6	1.1	112	200 mg tid 300 mg bid	2/0.2	>0.7	0.6
Nonnucleoside Reverse Transcriptase Inhibitors									
Delavirdine	0.05–0.1[c]	85	0.48[b]	5.8	4	400 mg tid	35/14	?	0.004
Efavirenz	0.0017–0.025[c]	43	10.2[b]	48	10.3	600 mg qd	12.9/5.6	?	0.007
Nevirapine	0.010–0.1	50	1.21	25	2.6	200 mg bid[d]	5.5/3.0	1	0.45
Protease Inhibitors									
Amprenavir	0.012–0.41	?	6.1[b]	9	64.9	1200 mg bid	10.7/0.56	?	0.02
Indinavir	0.025–0.1[c]	60	1.2[b]	1.5	43	800 mg q8h	13/0.25	?	0.07
Lopinavir[e]	0.004–0.027	?	0.74[b]	5.5	6.5	400 mg bid	15.4/8.8	?	?
Nelfinavir	0.009–0.06	?	2[b]	2.6	37.4	750 mg tid 1,250 mg bid	5.6/0.7	?	IND
Ritonavir	0.0038–0.154	60	0.41[b]	3–5	8.8	600 mg bid[d]	16/5	?	IND
Saquinavir[f]	0.001–0.03	12	10	3	80	1,200 mg tid	0.4/0.15	?	IND

CL, total body clearance; C_{max}, maximum plasma concentration; C_{min}, minimum plasma concentration; CSF, cerebrospinal fluid; F, bioavailability; IC_{50-90}, concentration required to produce 50% or 90% inhibition of HIV strains *in vitro*; IND, indeterminate with standard analytic techniques; $T_{1/2}$, elimination half-life; V_d, distribution volume.

[a]Dose adjustment may be required for weight, renal or hepatic disease, and drug interactions.

[b]V_d/F.

[c]Range given is for IC_{90} or IC_{95}.

[d]Initial dose escalation recommended to minimize side effects.

[e]Available as coformulation 4:1 lopinavir:ritonavir.

[f]Soft-gel formulation.

T-1249 are polypeptides designed to bind gp41, blocking the fusion process. Fusion can also be aborted by chemokine receptor antagonists such as AMD-3100, a bicyclam inhibitor of the CXCR4 receptor, and the anti-CCR5 monoclonal antibody PRO-140. Integrase represents another HIV-specific enzyme that can be targeted for inhibition. Although development of integrase inhibitors has been problematic, *in vitro* studies appear promising.[42]

DRUG INTERACTIONS

The clinical use of antiretroviral agents is complicated by the significant drug-drug interactions that can occur with many of these agents. Some interactions are beneficial and purposely used, others may be harmful, leading to inadequate drug concentrations. Clinicians involved in the pharmacotherapy of HIV must maintain a current knowledge of drug interactions for these reasons. Efavirenz and nevirapine are inducers of drug metabolism, whereas delavirdine and the protease inhibitors inhibit drug metabolism.[43] Ritonavir is a potent inhibitor of cytochrome P450 3A-mediated metabolism and is now primarily used as a pharmacokinetic enhancer of other protease inhibitors.[44] Lopinavir is coformulated with ritonavir (LPV/r) for this reason. Nucleoside reverse transcriptase inhibitors may also have interactions amongst themselves. Zidovudine and stavudine, for example, are phosphorylated by the same kinases; because antagonism occurs between these two drugs both *in vitro* and *in vivo*, the two should never be given together.[45] Complicating matters is the drug interaction potential of antituberculosis agents, particularly rifamycins. Rifampin is contraindicated with most protease inhibitors because drug concentrations of the protease inhibitors are substantially reduced. If patients require simultaneous treatment for both HIV and tuberculosis, a regimen consisting of efavirenz, ritonavir, or ritonavir/saquinavir should be considered.[46] The herbal product Saint John's wort (*Hypericum perforatum*) is also a potent inducer of metabolism and is contraindicated with protease inhibitors. Among healthy volunteers, St. John's wort decreased indinavir area under the curve on average 57%.[47]

PIVOTAL DEVELOPMENTS IN TREATMENT STRATEGIES

The pharmacotherapy of HIV infection has rapidly changed over the years, as newer agents became available and treatment paradigms evolved. Initially (circa 1985), treatment of HIV began with zidovudine monotherapy, as this was the first drug to demonstrate a survival benefit in patients infected with HIV. Individuals with AIDS or AIDS-related complex were randomized to receive either zidovudine 1,500 mg/day or placebo. In this trial, zidovudine reduced the probability of developing an opportunistic infection (23% vs 43%, $P < 0.001$) and significantly improved survival. After 12 weeks of treatment, zidovudine recipients had a higher CD4 count (68 cells/μL) as compared to placebo recipients (33 cells/μL).[48] A subsequent study of zidovudine, however, showed that the durability of zidovudine effect was limited.[49] Since these initial studies, the dosing of zidovudine has been refined to reflect the intracellular half-life of triphosphorylated zidovudine; zidovudine is now dosed 600 mg/day, typically given bid.

The introduction of didanosine and zalcitabine in 1991 and 1992, respectively, allowed experimentation with various NRTI combinations. One of the most significant milestones in the evolution of antiretroviral therapy was the finding that combining two NRTIs had a synergistic effect and provided better immunologic and virologic improvements than a single nucleoside analog alone. The AIDS Clinical Trials Group (ACTG) protocol 175 was a randomized, double-blind, placebo-controlled study comparing four treatment arms: zidovudine (200 mg tid), didanosine (200 mg bid), zidovudine plus didanosine, and zidovudine plus zalcitabine (0.75 mg tid). This study enrolled 2,467 HIV-infected adults (1,067 antiretroviral-naive patients and 1,400 with previous therapy) with CD4 counts between 200 and 500 cells/μL. The median duration of treatment was 118 weeks. Primary end points for this study were a greater than 50% decline in CD4 count, development of AIDS, or death. Of patients receiving zidovudine monotherapy, 32% progressed to the primary end point as compared to 22% on didanosine monotherapy, 18% for zidovudine plus didanosine, and 20% zidovudine plus zalcitabine. When zidovudine was used alone, the incidence of AIDS-defining events was 16% as compared to 11% to 12% in the other three arms. The mortality rate in the zidovudine-only group was 9% as compared to 7% in the zidovudine plus zalcitabine group and 5% in the two didanosine-containing arms. Mean CD4 counts at week 8 were substantially higher in the group receiving zidovudine and didanosine (63 cells/μL) than didanosine alone (49 cells/μL), zidovudine plus zalcitabine (41 cells/μL), or zidovudine alone (14 cells/μL) in treatment-naive patients.[50] Viral load data from a subset of patients revealed a mean decrease in viral load of 0.26 $\log_{10}$ copies/mL for zidovudine monotherapy, 0.65 for didanosine monotherapy, 0.93 for zidovudine and didanosine, and 0.89 for zidovudine with zalcitabine after 8 weeks. A higher baseline viral load, less suppression of viral load by treatment, and syncytium-inducing virus were significantly associated with an increased risk for progression of disease.[51] Taken together, ACTG protocol 175 demonstrated that the combined regimen of zidovudine and didanosine or zalcitabine was superior to zidovudine monotherapy in immunologic and virologic parameters, particularly in patients with no previous antiretroviral therapy.

Dual therapy gave way to triple therapy as newer agents (i.e., nonnucleosides and protease inhibitors) were introduced after 1996. The potency and durability of triple therapy was exemplified in a double-blind, placebo-controlled study (protocol 035) of zidovudine, lamivudine, and indinavir. Zidovudine-experienced, lamivudine-naive patients were randomized to receive either indinavir monotherapy, zidovudine in combination with lamivudine, or all three drugs. Triple therapy resulted in viral load reduction to less than 500 copies/mL in 78% of patients after 2 years versus 30% to 45% in the other two study arms (intention-to-treat analysis).[52] After 3 years, more than two-thirds of patients originally starting triple therapy had remained below 500 copies/mL. The median increase in CD4 cell count was greater than 200 cells/μL in this cohort.[53] A reduction in mortality with a regimen of zidovudine, lamivudine, and indinavir was demonstrated in ACTG protocol 320, which compared triple therapy to zidovudine and lamivudine.[54] A total of 1,156 lamivudine and protease inhibitor-naive patients with <200 CD4 cells/μL were enrolled in this multicenter, randomized, placebo-controlled study. Progression of disease to AIDS or death was lower in the group given indinavir as compared to the group given placebo (6% and 11%, respectively). Moreover, indinavir reduced the incidence of mortality by half: mortality was 3.1% in the two-drug regimen and 1.4% in the three-drug regimen. The effects of treatment were similar regardless of whether the CD4 count was below 50 cells/μL or between 51 and 200 cells/μL. The use of triple therapy or HAART is clearly associated with a reduced incidence of opportunistic infections and improved survival.[5,6] Therefore, current recommendations for treating HIV advocate a minimum of three antiretroviral agents.[31,35,36] The typical regimen consists of two nucleoside analogs with either a protease inhibitor (often pharmacologically enhanced with ritonavir), nonnucleoside, or a third nucleoside analog such as abacavir. The initial choice in drugs is critical to long-term success, and factors such as adherence, efficacy (virologic and immunologic), durability, which drugs to start with and what to change to (i.e., sequencing), and tolerability are paramount to success. Brief comments on these factors follow below.

The simplest definition of adherence is the patient's ability to take medication as directed. Antiretroviral therapy is complex and long-term, and the risk for virologic failure increases as adherence decreases. Patients with greater than 95% adherence on a protease inhibitor regimen had better virologic and immunologic outcomes and a lower hospitalization rate than those patients with adherence below this threshold.[55] As clinicians, it is important to communicate to the patient the importance of proper medication taking with specific education aimed at understanding the disease process, monitoring, and goals of therapy. An individual's "readiness" to take medications should be clearly established before any treatment is initiated.[35] Caregivers, friends, and/or family members should be included in this process as social and psychological support are among the most important factors that influence adherence in this patient population.[56]

Several clinical trials have demonstrated the virologic and immunologic efficacy of antiretrovirals; the results are succinctly summarized elsewhere.[57–59] Unfortunately, only a few have been large, randomized, comparative (head-to-head) trials. Nevertheless, these trials provide insight on the subtle differences in efficacy among antiretrovirals. The first randomized comparative trial of protease inhibitors was the CHEESE (Comparative trial in HIV-infected persons Evaluating Efficacy and Safety of saquinavir-Enhanced oral formulation and indinavir as part of triple therapy) study. A total of 70 antiretroviral-naive patients were randomized to take either saquinavir soft-gel 1,200 mg tid or indinavir 800 mg tid with zidovudine 200 mg tid and lamivudine 150 mg bid. The proportion of patients with HIV RNA < 400 copies/mL was 82.9% and 85.7% on intention-to-treat analysis for saquinavir soft-gel and indinavir, respectively. Although there was a greater increase in CD4 cell counts at week 24 for patients receiving soft-gel saquinavir, this difference later disappeared. Both regimens were well tolerated.[60] A second study, PROAB 3006, compared amprenavir 1,200 mg bid with indinavir 800 mg q8h in protease inhibitor-naive patients. At week 48, 30% of patients achieved HIV RNA < 400 copies/mL on amprenavir versus 46% in the indinavir arm (intention-to-treat analysis). Overall tolerability was similar between the two drugs.[61] Superior virologic efficacy was seen with lopinavir/ritonavir 400/100 mg bid compared with nelfinavir 750 mg tid in antiretroviral-naive patients concomitantly treated with 40 mg bid of stavudine and lamivudine 150 mg bid. This double-blind, randomized, placebo-controlled trial involving 637 patients resulted in 75% of lopinavir/ritonavir treated patients achieving viral load <400 copies/mL versus 63% of nelfinavir treated patients after 48 weeks. The mean increases in CD4 cell counts were similar for both agents, 195 cells/μL with nelfinavir and 207 cells/μL with lopinavir/ritonavir. Overall tolerability was similar between the two agents.[62] Significantly more patients achieved viral suppression at 48 weeks with the nonnucleoside agent efavirenz given in combination with zidovudine/lamivudine than regimens of indinavir/zidovudine/lamivudine or indinavir/efavirenz in a multicenter, randomized, open-label study involving 432 patients. Both zidovudine and lamivudine were dosed bid, 300 and 150 mg, respectively. The administered dose for efavirenz was 600 mg qd and that for indinavir was 800 mg q8h. For the indinavir/efavirenz arm, efavirenz was given 600 mg qd with indinavir 1,000 mg q8h to account for the drug interaction. The proportion of patients achieving HIV RNA < 400 copies/mL was 70% for those receiving treatment with efavirenz/zidovudine/lamivudine, 53% for those receiving treatment with indinavir/efavirenz, and 48% for those receiving treatment with indinavir/zidovudine/lamivudine; mean increases in CD4 cell counts were 201, 180, and 185 respectively.[63]

The durability and sequencing of a regimen is equally important as its efficacy. Since the advent of HAART, patients have been living longer with improved quality of life. The consequence of this is that patients will have to rely on their treatment for years to come, not months. Data on the long-term durability of HAART are scarce. The initiation of antiretroviral therapy in a treatment-naive person must come with consideration for what agents will be available should the first regimen fail. Unfortunately, the limited number of antiretrovirals and the development of drug resistance are significant obstacles to the ideal sequencing of antiretrovirals.

As with any medication, adverse effects occur with antiretroviral agents, which may limit the patient's ability to tolerate medication. Several important adverse effects have been recognized with the currently available antiretrovirals, including mitochondrial toxicity with nucleoside and nucleotide reverse transcriptase inhibitors, rash with nonnucleosides, and metabolic perturbations with protease inhibitors. A discussion on the specific presentation and management of these adverse effects is beyond the scope of this chapter but can be found elsewhere.[7,39]

TREATMENT IN SPECIAL POPULATIONS

PREGNANCY

Treatment recommendations have been made to address the specific requirements for HIV-infected pregnant women and the prevention of vertical transmission.[64] Therapy is warranted particularly in light of the dramatic reduction in transmission seen with zidovudine monotherapy (ACTG protocol 076). ACTG protocol 076 randomized 477 HIV-infected pregnant women (14 to 34 weeks' gestation) to either zidovudine or placebo. The zidovudine regimen consisted of antepartum zidovudine (100 mg five times daily) plus a continuous infusion of zidovudine during labor (2 mg/kg IV over 1 hour followed by 1 mg/kg/h), and zidovudine for the newborn (2 mg/kg orally q6h for 6 weeks). The HIV transmission rate was 25.5% among those that received placebo, but was 8.3% when the mothers and their babies received zidovudine. This difference corresponds to a two-thirds reduction in the risk of maternal-to-infant HIV transmission. Adverse reactions associated with zidovudine therapy in the study were minimal: hemoglobin concentrations were significantly lower at birth in infants whose mothers received zidovudine, but this difference disappeared by 12 weeks of age; there was no difference in minor or major structural abnormalities in the two groups.[65] An abbreviated course of zidovudine (i.e., given during labor or in the first 48 hours of life) can also substantially reduce transmission and may be easier for the patient to take.[66] Alternatively, single-dose nevirapine given to the mother during labor and to the baby within 3 days of birth can also reduce transmission of HIV.[67] Unfortunately, little is known about the use of other antiretrovirals in pregnant women and the effect these drugs may have on the developing fetus. Protease inhibitor use among 89 pregnancies appeared generally safe to both mother and baby in a retrospective multicenter survey.[68] In general, pregnant women should be treated similarly as nonpregnant adults; if possible, zidovudine should be used for both mother and infant.[64]

POSTEXPOSURE PROPHYLAXIS

Protection of health care workers from accidental exposure to HIV is an important concern. The CDC has issued guidelines governing treatment for occupational HIV exposure. Postexposure prophylaxis with a triple-drug regimen consisting of two nucleoside reverse transcriptase inhibitors and a protease inhibitor (indinavir or nelfinavir) is recommended for percutaneous blood exposure involving significant risk (large volume of blood or blood from patients with advanced AIDS). Two nucleoside reverse transcriptase inhibitors may be offered to the health care worker with a lower risk of exposure, such as those involving the mucous membrane or skin. Treatment is not necessary if the source of exposure is urine or saliva. The optimal duration of treatment is unknown but at least 4 weeks of therapy is advocated. Treatment should ideally be initiated within 1 to 2 hours of exposure.[18] Guidelines have also been developed for postcoital and postinjection-drug use prophylaxis.[69]

EVALUATION OF THERAPEUTIC OUTCOMES

Following the initiation of therapy, patients are usually monitored at 3-month intervals with immunologic (CD4 count), virologic (HIV RNA), and clinical assessments. There are two general indications to change therapy: significant toxicity or treatment failure. Each of the available antiretroviral agents has its own set of drug-limiting adverse reactions;[7] fortunately, alternatives with nonoverlapping adverse effects are available. For example, the patient who experiences significant peripheral neuropathy on the combination of didanosine and stavudine could be changed to a combination of zidovudine and lamivudine. Specific criteria to indicate treatment failure have not been established through controlled clinical trials. As a general guide, the following events should prompt consideration for changing therapy:

- Less than 1 $\log_{10}$ reduction in HIV RNA 1 month after the initiation of therapy or a failure to achieve maximal suppression of HIV replication within 4 to 6 months
- A persistent decline in the CD4 cell count or a return to pretreatment value or an increase in HIV RNA of 0.3–0.5 $\log_{10}$ copies/mL from nadir
- Clinical disease progression, usually the development of a new opportunistic infection

THERAPEUTIC FAILURE

Therapeutic failure in HIV therapy may be the result of nonadherence to medication, development of drug resistance, intolerance to one or more medications, adverse drug-drug interactions, or pharmacokinetic-pharmacodynamic variability. Few clinical data are available to indicate what alternative strategies should be employed for patients who fail their initial regimen. Moreover, the data that are available are confounded by the heterogeneity in the patients and their infecting viruses, which makes the results difficult to interpret. In general, patients failing their first regimen should be treated with a drug representing a new class (e.g., if the patient was initially treated with a protease inhibitor, the protease inhibitor can be switched to a nonnucleoside reverse transcriptase inhibitor). The guiding principles (numbers 5 and 7) recommend changing to at least two new antiretroviral drugs that are not cross-resistant with agents the patient has received previously. Table 123–3 presents some examples of alternative regimens. Virologic resistance testing may help guide the health care provider in selecting appropriate agents.[70] In addition to an alternative antiretroviral regimen, other investigational strategies suggested for therapeutic failure include drug holidays, structured or strategic treatment interruptions (STIs), and structured intermittent therapy (SIT). Although there are subtle differences between these strategies, the overall premise is similar: stop all antiretrovirals and allow the patient time off medication. Undoubtedly, any strategy that discontinues antiretroviral therapy will allow viral replication to occur with subsequent declines in CD4 lymphocytes. Reinitiation of therapy is then intended to reestablish control of the disease. For example, the COMET study treated 10 patients with zidovudine, lamivudine, and indinavir for 28 days and then temporarily withdrew treatment for another 28 days. Viral load declined while on treatment but rapidly rebounded within 7 days of treatment interruption in all 10 patients. Upon reinitiation of the same regimen, viral load once again declined. No resistance was detected and half of the patients were able to maintain HIV-RNA below 200 copies/mL for 1 year.[71] There remain numerous uncertainties about these discontinuation strategies, including how long the patient can remain off medications, how often this cycle can be done, and, most importantly, the ability of the strategy to reduce morbidity and mortality as conventional HAART therapy has done. Prospective studies are necessary to answer these questions.

INFECTIOUS COMPLICATIONS OF AIDS

It is not HIV itself that produces most of the morbidity and mortality associated with AIDS. Rather, opportunistic infections, many caused by organisms that are common in the environment, are responsible for almost 90% of deaths.[72] These opportunistic diseases often represent the reactivation of quiescent infections and thus are overt manifestations of the loss of cell-mediated immunity. The development of certain opportunistic infections is directly or indirectly related to the level of CD4 lymphocytes (Fig. 123–2) and can be predicted with some degree of accuracy.[73] Until the immunosuppression induced by HIV can be prevented, the prevention and management of opportunistic infections will remain an essential component of the comprehensive care of HIV-infected individuals.

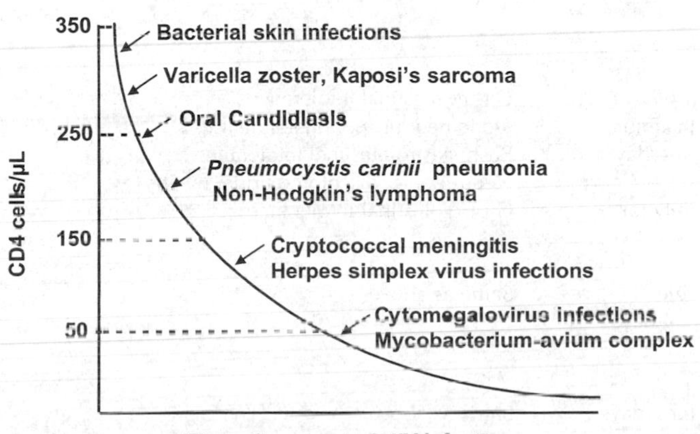

FIGURE 123–2. Natural history of opportunistic infections associated with HIV infection. *(Reprinted with permission; copyright Courtney V. Fletcher, 1995.)*

Surveillance data indicate that the incidence of certain opportunistic infections in HIV-infected persons in the United States continues to change. In particular, since the introduction of combination antiretroviral therapy, especially regimens that include an HIV-protease inhibitor, the incidence of PCP, toxoplasmic encephalitis, cryptococcal meningitis, esophageal candidiasis, herpes zoster, and *Mycobacterium avium* complex (MAC) have decreased.[74] For example, the incidence of PCP declined 21.% per year during the period 1996–1998 versus a 3.4% reduction during the period 1992–1995.[75] Similarly, MAC disease declined 39.9% per year and candidal esophagitis declined 16.7% per year as compared to decreases of 4.7% per year and 0.2% per year, respectively, during these same periods. Potent antiretroviral regimens and prophylactic strategies for opportunistic infections are major factors associated with these decreases. Nevertheless, opportunistic diseases continue to be relatively frequent complications of HIV disease and occur at low CD4 lymphocyte counts. For example, the risk of an opportunistic infection was almost sixfold higher in persons receiving highly active antiretroviral therapy with a baseline CD4 count <50 cells/μL as compared to >200 cells/μL.[76] The most common opportunistic diseases and their frequencies found before death in 1,883 patients with AIDS between the years 1990 and 1994 were PCP, 45%; MAC, 25%; wasting syndrome, 25%; bacterial pneumonia, 24%; cytomegalovirus (CMV) disease, 23%; and candidiasis, 22%.[77] A CDC surveillance study of >49,000 HIV-infected persons found that 46% of the cases of PCP that occurred were in persons not previously receiving medical care, and 32% were in persons receiving prophylaxis. These data illustrate the importance of the early identification of HIV infection and provision of medical care and continued research on preventative strategies.

Table 123–5 lists the spectrum of infectious diseases observed in HIV-infected individuals and recommended first-line regimens for treatment, and Table 123–6 lists the recommended therapies for primary prophylaxis. An exhaustive review of all opportunistic infections associated with HIV infection is beyond the scope of this chapter. The major opportunistic infections include *Pneumocystis carinii* pneumonia, candidal esophagitis (discussed elsewhere in this text), central nervous system toxoplasmosis, cryptococcosis, mycobacterial disease, and herpes group virus infections. The following discussion emphasizes these pathogens and provides an overview of the epidemiology, diagnosis, clinical manifestations, and results of treatment for these infections. Readers desiring more specific information, either for the diseases or agents mentioned, need to consult additional references.

PNEUMOCYSTIS CARINII

PCP is the most common life-threatening opportunistic infection in patients with AIDS. Early in the AIDS epidemic approximately 60% of patients with AIDS had PCP as their AIDS-defining event and 80% experienced PCP at some point during their lifetime.[78] The advent of effective prophylaxis for PCP has decreased the relative incidence of PCP. However, PCP prophylaxis has not eliminated the disease because of persons unaware of their HIV infection, breakthrough PCP in those receiving prophylaxis, and variable compliance with prophylaxis. The taxonomy of the organism is unclear, having been classified as both protozoan and fungal. Recent evidence based on genomic sequences suggests that *P. carinii* is a fungus.[79] Exposure to *P. carinii* is widespread, as 80% of the population have developed serum antibodies by age 2 or 3 years.[80] The organism appears to reside without

TABLE 123–5. Therapies for Common Opportunistic Pathogens in HIV-Infected Individuals

Clinical Disease	Selected Initial Therapies for Acute Infection in Adults	Common Drug or Dose-Limiting Adverse Reactions
FUNGI		
Candidiasis, oral	Fluconazole 200 mg po single dose or 100 mg po for 5 days	Taste, patient acceptance
	or	
	Nystatin 500,000 units po swish 4–6 times daily for 7–10 days	
	or	
	Clotrimazole 10 mg (1 troche) po 5 times daily for 7–10 days	
Candidiasis, esophageal	Fluconazole 200 mg po or iv on the first day then 100 mg/day for 10–14 days	Elevated liver function tests, hepatotoxicity, nausea, and vomiting
	or	Elevated liver function tests, hepatotoxicity, rash,
	Ketoconazole 400 mg/day po for 10–14 days	nausea, and vomiting
Pneumocystis carinii pneumonia	Trimethoprim-sulfamethoxazole iv or po 12–20 mg/kg/day as TMP component in 3–4 divided doses for 21 days*	Skin rash, fever, leukopenia Thrombocytopenia
	or	
	Pentamidine iv 3–4 mg/kg/day for 21 days*	Azotemia, hypoglycemia Hyperglycemia
	Mild Episodes	
	Atovaquone suspension 750 mg (5 mL) po twice daily with meals for 21 days*	Rash, elevated liver enzymes, diarrhea
Cryptococcal meningitis	Amphotericin B iv 0.5–1 mg/kg/day for minimum of 2 weeks *with or without* flucytosine 100–150 mg/kg/day po in 4 divided doses *followed by* fluconazole 100–200 mg/day po*	Nephrotoxicity, hypokalemia, anemia, fever, chills Bone marrow suppression, elevated liver enzymes Same as above
Histoplasmosis	Amphotericin B 0.5–1 mg/kg/day iv for 6–8 weeks*	Same as above
	or	
	Itraconazole 200–400 mg/day po for 3 months*	Elevated liver function tests, hepatotoxicity, nausea, vomiting, hypertension
Coccidioidomycosis	Amphotericin B 0.5–1 mg/kg/day iv for ≥6–8 weeks*	Same as above
PROTOZOA		
Toxoplasmic encephalitis	Pyrimethamine 200 mg po once then 50–100 mg/day	Bone marrow suppression
	plus	
	Sulfadiazine 1–1.5 g po four times daily	Allergy, rash, drug fever
	and	
	Folinic acid 10–20 mg po daily for a minimum of 28 days*	
Isosporiasis	Trimethoprim and sulfamethoxazole 1–2 double-strength tablets (160 mg TMP and 800 mg SMX) po twice daily for 2–4 weeks	Same as above
BACTERIA		
Organisms associated with T-cell defects		
Mycobacterium avium complex	Clarithromycin 500 mg po twice daily, *plus* ethambutol 15 mg/kg/day po to a maximum of 1,000 mg/day, *and* rifabutin 300 mg/day[a]	Gastrointestinal intolerance Optic neuritis, peripheral neuritis Rash, gastrointestinal intolerance Neutropenia, discolored urine, uveitis
Salmonella enterocolitis or bacteremia	Ciprofloxacin 500–750 mg po twice daily for 14 days	Gastrointestinal intolerance
	or	
	Trimethoprim (160 mg)-sulfamethoxazole (800 mg) 1 tablet po twice daily for 14 days	Same as above
Organisms associated with B-cell defects		
Campylobacter enterocolitis	Ciprofloxacin 500 mg po twice daily for 7 days	Same as above
	or	
	Erythromycin 250–500 mg po four times daily for 7 days	Gastrointestinal intolerance, colitis, ototoxicity
Shigella enterocolitis	Ciprofloxacin 500 mg po twice daily for 5 days	Same as above

TABLE 123–5. (continued)

Clinical Disease	Selected Initial Therapies for Acute Infection in Adults	Common Drug or Dose-Limiting Adverse Reactions
VIRUSES		
Mucocutaneous herpes simplex	Acyclovir 1–2 g/day po in 3–5 divided doses for 7–10 days	Gastrointestinal intolerance
	or	
	Valacyclovir 500 mg po q12 h for 7–10 days	Gastrointestinal intolerance
	or	
	Famciclovir 500 mg po q12 h for 7–10 days	Headache, gastrointestinal intolerance
Varicella zoster	Acyclovir 30 mg/kg/day iv in 3 divided doses *or* 4 g/day po for 7–10 days	Obstructive nephropathy, CNS symptomatology
	or	
	Valacyclovir 1 g po q8h for 7–10 days	Gastrointestinal intolerance
	or	
	Famciclovir 500 mg po q8h for 7–10 days	Same as above
Cytomegalovirus	Ganciclovir 7.5–10 mg/kg/day in 2–3 divided doses for 14 days*	Neutropenia, thrombocytopenia
	or	
	Foscarnet 180 mg/kg/day in 2 or 3 divided doses for 14 days*	Nephrotoxicity, hypo/hypercalcemia, hypo/hyperphosphatemia, anemia
Cytomegalovirus retinitis	Ganciclovir intraocular implant	

*Maintenance therapy is recommended.

consequence in the human unless the host becomes immunologically compromised; immunosuppression allows the organism to multiply, giving rise to clinical disease.

PCP in patients with AIDS differs in clinical presentation from patients with other immunosuppressive conditions, such as malignant neoplasms. In AIDS patients, the presentation is often more subacute. Characteristic symptoms include fever and dyspnea; clinical signs are tachypnea with or without rales or rhonchi, and a nonproductive or mildly productive cough. Chest radiographs may show florid or subtle infiltrates or occasionally be normal. Infiltrates are usually interstitial and bilateral. Arterial blood gases may show minimal hypoxia (PaO_2 80–95 mm Hg), but in more advanced disease may be markedly abnormal. The onset of PCP is often insidious, occurring over a period of weeks, although more fulminant presentations can occur. The diagnosis of PCP is usually made by identification of the organism in induced sputum or in specimens obtained from bronchoalveolar lavage. Less commonly, transbronchial biopsy is used for diagnosis.

Untreated PCP has a mortality of nearly 100%. Treatment with agents such as trimethoprim-sulfamethoxazole (TMP/SMX or cotrimoxazole) or parenteral pentamidine is associated with a 60% to 100% response rate. Historically, pentamidine was the drug of choice for PCP until the 1970s when Hughes and colleagues compared the efficacy and tolerance of TMP/SMX and pentamidine in children with PCP.[81] Both agents were found to be equally efficacious, however, TMP/SMX was less toxic. TMP/SMX became the regimen of choice for treatment and subsequently prophylaxis of PCP in patient with and without HIV.[82]

TMP/SMX, when used for the treatment of PCP, is usually given in doses of 15–20 mg/kg/day (based on the TMP component) as three to four divided doses. Doses of 12–15 mg/kg/day may be as effective and perhaps might reduce the incidence of toxicity. TMP/SMX is usually initiated by the intravenous route, although oral therapy (as oral absorption is high) may suffice in mildly ill and reliable patients, or to complete a course of therapy after a response has been achieved with intravenous administration. If oral therapy is used, it would be prudent to document absorption with serum concentrations of TMP or SMX as gastrointestinal disturbances or a malabsorption syndrome are known to alter drug absorption in patients with AIDS. Target concentrations for TMP are between 5 and 8 μg/mL.

For treatment of HIV-associated PCP, pentamidine isethionate is administered intravenously, usually in doses of 4 mg/kg/d, although a pilot study has reported successful treatment with 3 mg/kg/d.[83,84] Aerosolized pentamidine should not be used for treatment of PCP as comparative studies with intravenous pentamidine indicate that aerosolized treatment is associated with a slower clinical response, higher rates of therapeutic failure and PCP relapse.[84,85]

The efficacy of TMP/SMX or pentamidine for treatment of an initial episode of PCP in HIV-infected individuals is similar, with published response rates between 60% and 80%. Although comparative studies between the two regimens are few, one prospective, randomized trial found that oxygenation improved more quickly and survival was better in those who received TMP/SMX.[86] The optimum length of therapy for treatment of PCP with either agent is not known, but 21 days is commonly recommended. Clinical improvement in patients with AIDS is often slower than in non-AIDS patients. One study demonstrated improvement in chest radiograph or gallium scan in only two-thirds of patients at the end of treatment.[87] Thus, the lack of prompt clinical improvement is not necessarily an indication of no response. In fact, patients frequently may worsen before they improve. However, continued worsening after 4 days, or lack of improvement after 7 to 10 days, is an indication for a change in therapy, regardless of which agent was started initially. There are no data regarding the utility of concurrent therapy with both TMP/SMX and pentamidine, and this approach is not recommended.

Adverse reactions to both TMP/SMX and pentamidine are common and range between 20% and 85% in this setting. The more common adverse reactions seen with TMP/SMX are rash, fever, leukopenia, elevated transaminases, and thrombocytopenia. Mild rashes should be watched closely for progression to more severe reactions, but are not an absolute contraindication to continuing therapy. The incidence of these adverse reactions is higher in HIV-infected individuals than in those not infected with HIV.[88] For pentamidine,

TABLE 123–6. Therapies for Prophylaxis of First Episode Opportunistic Diseases in Adults and Adolescents

Pathogen	Indication	First Choice
I. Standard of care		
Pneumocystis carinii	CD4+ count <200/μL or oropharyngeal candidiasis *or* unexplained fever ≥ 2 weeks	Trimethoprim-sulfamethoxazole (TMP/SMX) 1 DS tablet po qd
Mycobacterium tuberculosis		
Isoniazid-sensitive	TST reaction ≥ 5 mm *or* prior positive TST result without treatment *or* contact with case of active tuberculosis	Isoniazid 300 mg po *plus* pyridoxine, 50 mg po qd for 9 mo, *or* Isoniazid 900 mg po *plus* pyridoxine 50 mg po twice weekly × 12 mo
Isoniazid-resistant	Same; high probability of exposure to isoniazid-resistant tuberculosis	Rifampin 600 mg po qd *plus* pyrazinamide, 200 mg/kg po qd for 2 mo
Toxoplasma gondii	IgG antibody to *Toxoplasma* and CD4+ count < 100/μL	TMP/SMX 1 DS tablet po qd
Mycobacterium avium complex	CD4+ count < 50/μL	Azithromycin 1,200 mg po once weekly *or* Clarithromycin 500 mg po bid
Varicella-zoster virus (VZV)	Significant exposure to chickenpox or shingles for patients who have no history of either condition or, if available, negative antibody to VZV	Varicella zoster immunoglobulin (VZIG), 5 vials (1.25 mL each) im, administered ideally within 48 h of exposure, but ≤ 96 h
II. Generally recommended		
Streptococcus pneumoniae	All patients	Pneumococcal vaccine 0.5 mL im × 1
Hepatitis B virus	All susceptible (anti-HBc-negative) patients	Engerix B 20 μg im × 3 doses *or* Recombivax HB 10 μg im × 3 doses
Influenza virus	All patients (annually, before influenza season)	Whole or split virus 0.5 mL im/y
Hepatitis A virus	All susceptible (anti-HAV-negative) patients with chronic hepatitis C	Hepatitis A vaccine 2 doses
III. Indicated for use only in selected circumstances		
Bacteria	Neutropenia	Granulocyte-colony-stimulating factor (G-CSF) 5–10 μg/kg sc qd × 2–4 wk *or* granulocyte-macrophage colony-stimulating factor (GM-CSF) 250 μg/m² iv over 2 h qd × 2–4 wk
Cryptococcus neoformans	CD4+ count < 50/μL	Fluconazole 100–200 mg po qd
Histoplasma capsulatum	CD4+ count < 100/μL, endemic geographic area	Itraconazole capsule 200 mg po qd
Cytomegalovirus	CD4+ count < 50/μL and CMV antibody positivity	Oral ganciclovir 1 g po tid

From Centers for Disease Control and Prevention. 1999 USPHS/IDSA guidelines for the prevention of opportunistic infections in persons infected with human immunodeficiency virus. MMWR, Morb Mortal Wkly Rep 1999;48:1–59.

side effects include hypotension; tachycardia; nausea; vomiting; severe hypoglycemia or hyperglycemia; pancreatitis; irreversible diabetes mellitus; elevated transaminases; nephrotoxicity; leukopenia; and cardiac arrhythmias. Some of these reactions appear infusion-rate related (hypotension, tachycardia) and can be minimized by infusing pentamidine over 1 hour or more. The overall incidence of adverse reactions to pentamidine appears similar between individuals infected with HIV and those not infected. Dosage modification or pharmacokinetic monitoring can reduce somewhat the toxicity of both pentamidine and TMP/SMX.[87] Dose reductions of pentamidine from 4 to 3 mg/kg/day appears successful in minimizing further rises in serum creatinine. Maintenance of serum TMP concentrations between 5 and 8 μg/mL may help prevent severe myelosuppression.

The early addition of adjunctive corticosteroid therapy to anti-PCP regimens decreases the risk of respiratory failure and improve survival in patients with AIDS and moderate to severe PCP (PaO_2 ≤70 mm Hg or A-a gradient ≥35 mm Hg).[89,90] The adverse effects associated with corticosteroid therapy in these patients were minimal, primarily an increased incidence of herpetic lesions, although some concerns exist about the potential for reactivation of tuberculosis. The optimal dose and duration of corticosteroid therapy have not been identified. The regimen currently recommended is 40 mg of prednisone orally twice daily during days 1 through 5; 40 mg once daily days 6 through 10; and 20 mg once daily on days 11 through 21, or for the duration of therapy.[91] Methylprednisolone at 75% of the prednisone dose can be used if parenteral therapy is necessary. In general, adjunctive corticosteroid therapy should be initiated when antipneumocystis therapy is started, as the data supporting the use of corticosteroids are based on initiation within the first 24 to 72 hours of the start of antipneumocystis therapy.

HIV-infected individuals who have had PCP are at high risk for recurrent PCP if no prophylactic measures are taken. Even though the treatment of PCP is becoming increasingly successful, the mortality rate from first episode PCP is still between 5% and 20%, and therapy is often complicated by adverse reactions. Prevention of PCP is clearly a preferable strategy to treatment. The relative risk of PCP in 1,665 HIV-infected participants who did not have AIDS was 4.9 in those participants with CD4 lymphocyte counts <200/μL.[92] These data indicate that HIV-infected adults with a CD4 count <200 cells/μL or whose CD4 cells are <20% of total lymphocytes, are at high risk to develop PCP and are especially likely to benefit from prophylactic therapy. Currently, in the United States, PCP prophylaxis is recommended for all HIV-infected individuals who have already had previous PCP. Prophylaxis is also recommended for any HIV-infected person who has a CD4 lymphocyte count <200 cells/μL, or whose CD4 cells are <20% of total lymphocytes, or who have unexplained fever (>100°F/37.7°C) for ≥2 weeks, or who have a history of oropharyngeal candidiasis.[93]

TMP/SMX is the preferred therapy for both primary and secondary prophylaxis of PCP in adults and adolescents. TMP/SMX is the most effective and least expensive agent for prophylaxis; it also appears to confer cross-protection against toxoplasmosis and many bacterial infections. A study comparing TMP/SMX, dapsone, and aerosolized pentamidine for primary PCP prophylaxis in 843 patients with HIV infection and <200 CD4 cells found that all three treatment strategies had similar efficacy.[94] However, the lowest rates of PCP breakthrough among all subgroups were in those individuals currently taking TMP/SMX. Dapsone failures were more common with the 50-mg/day than the 100-mg/day dose. TMP/SMX and dapsone were more effective than aerosolized pentamidine in patients with fewer than 100 CD4 cells. These data provide additional support for the selection of TMP/SMX as the first-line agent for PCP prophylaxis. The recommended dose in adults and adolescents is one double-strength tablet daily, although other regimens, such as one double-strength tablet thrice weekly or one single-strength tablet daily, and gradual dose escalation using liquid TMP/SMX, have been used in an attempt to reduce the incidence of adverse reactions and to improve compliance. If TMP/SMX cannot be tolerated, alternative prophylactic regimens include dapsone, dapsone plus pyrimethamine and leucovorin, aerosolized pentamidine, and atovaquone. Issues to be considered with the use of aerosolized pentamidine include the potential for upper lobe pneumonia, presumably secondary to decreased drug deposition in these areas; late breakthrough disseminated disease (extrapulmonary pneumocystosis);[95] and cost, as aerosolized pentamidine is considerably more expensive than TMP/SMX.

TMP/SMX is also the recommended drug of choice for PCP prophylaxis in children.[96] As previously described, the normal range for CD4 lymphocytes is very different for children than for adults. Both the absolute CD4 count and CD4 cells as a percentage of the total should be determined. A CD4 percentage less than 25% is an indication of immunosuppression. The utility of TMP/SMX for prophylaxis is well established for children who are not HIV-infected and who are receiving myelosuppressive therapy.[97] The TMP/SMX regimen recommended (although other acceptable alternatives exist) is 150 mg/m^2/day of TMP and 750 mg/m^2/day of SMX given in divided doses twice daily, three times weekly on consecutive days (e.g., Monday-Tuesday-Wednesday). The total daily dose of TMP/SMX in children should not exceed 320 mg of TMP with 1,600 mg of SMX. PCP prophylaxis in HIV-exposed/infected children is strongly recommended as follows: (a) all HIV-exposed infants beginning at 4–6 weeks of age and continuing to 12 months of age if infection status is unknown; (b) all HIV-infected infants beginning at 4–6 weeks of age to 12 months of age; and (c) all HIV-infected children older than 1 year with severe immunosuppression.[96]

TOXOPLASMA GONDII

The seroprevalence of *Toxoplasma gondii* in HIV-infected individuals from major urban areas of the United States varies from 10% to 45%, but is considerably higher in countries such as France. The parasite is passed to humans from raw or undercooked meat, and contact with feces from infected cats. *T. gondii* can infect any organ of the body and cause an acute infection; it has a predilection for the brain and the eye. Once infected, the organism can replicate forming tissue cysts that persist for the life of the host. Many individuals will not have symptoms of disease. Immunosuppression, however, allows the release of tachyzoites from tissue cysts that produce a necrotic foci of infection, most often the brain. In the patient with AIDS, *T. gondii* is an important opportunistic pathogen, responsible for most focal intracerebral lesions.[98] A retrospective study suggested that 30% of AIDS patients seropositive for *T. gondii* will ultimately develop toxoplasmic encephalitis.[99]

The clinical signs and symptoms of toxoplasmosis are most frequently associated with involvement of the central nervous system (CNS) and, less commonly, the lungs and eyes, although any organ can be affected. Clinical presentation often includes fever, headache, seizures (in approximately 10% to 25% of patients), focal neurologic abnormalities (in approximately 60% to 90%), and mental status changes. Brain biopsy is required to make a definitive diagnosis of toxoplasmic encephalitis although presumptive diagnosis is commonly made in *T. gondii*-seropositive patients with typical CNS lesions. Characteristic radiographic abnormalities found by computerized axial tomography (CAT) or magnetic resonance imaging (MRI) have also been useful in the diagnosis of CNS toxoplasmosis.

The initial treatment of CNS toxoplasmosis is usually empiric. Brain biopsy in the patient with AIDS may be complicated by potential morbidity, location of lesion(s), or thrombocytopenia. Antitoxoplasma therapy is usually initiated in patients with AIDS who are seropositive for *Toxoplasma*, have clinical symptoms suspicious for toxoplasmosis, and have characteristic findings on neuroradiographic studies (multiple ring-enhancing lesions). In this setting, brain biopsy is usually not undertaken unless the patient either fails to respond clinically or radiologically to 10 to 14 days of therapy, or clinically deteriorates. Brain biopsy is an initial consideration in the *T. gondii*-seronegative patient or in patients with atypical lesions.

The combination of pyrimethamine and sulfadiazine is considered the most effective regimen for acute therapy of AIDS-related CNS toxoplasmosis.[100] This regimen works synergistically by sequentially inhibiting two steps in folic acid synthesis of the proliferative form of *T. gondii*. There is no widespread agreement on the optimal doses of pyrimethamine and sulfadiazine. Pyrimethamine loading doses of 75 mg orally on the first day, followed by 25 mg/day thereafter have been commonly used. The erratic concentrations of pyrimethamine found in patients with AIDS and toxoplasmic encephalitis at lower doses (25 mg/day) have prompted some investigators to use larger doses.[101] Loading doses of 100–200 mg followed by daily oral doses of 1–1.5 mg/kg/day (50–100 mg/day) have been recommended.[102] The usual dose of sulfadiazine is 1–1.5 g every 6 hours (4–8 g/day). Folinic acid, in doses of 10–20 mg/day (although doses as high as 50 mg/day have been used), is usually added

MAC prophylaxis is now strongly recommended for all HIV-infected adults and adolescents with a CD4 count <50 cells/μL.[96] The first-line choices are either azithromycin (1,200 mg once weekly) or clarithromycin (500 mg bid); rifabutin is an alternative. Persons considered for prophylaxis should be evaluated to be sure that they do not have active disease caused by MAC or *M. tuberculosis*.

HERPESVIRUS INFECTIONS

HERPES SIMPLEX VIRUS

Herpes simplex viruses (HSV) types 1 and 2 cause significant morbidity in patients with AIDS. Seropositivity for HSV is widespread among adults with AIDS, and clinical disease is usually the result of reactivation of latent virus. The manifestations of HSV disease observed in persons with AIDS include orolabial, genital, anorectal mucocutaneous disease, esophagitis, and, less commonly, encephalitis. Ulcerative HSV lesions present for longer than 1 month in an individual with laboratory evidence for HIV infection, or no other apparent cause for immunodeficiency, are considered an AIDS-defining condition.

Anorectal lesions are common clinically evident HSV disease causing morbidity in homosexual men with AIDS, and likely reflect the common risk factors, for acquisition (sexual contact) of both HSV and HIV. Chronic perianal HSV lesions were among the first opportunistic infections associated with AIDS.[123] Symptoms include pain, itching, and painful defecation. The clinical presentation of anal, orolabial and genital herpes in the patient with AIDS are similar to that in other immunosuppressed individuals. The severity of the episode can range from mild to severely destructive. The severity of mucocutaneous HSV disease increases with progressive immunosuppression. Other HSV manifestations, such as encephalitis, are rare in the patient with AIDS, but are life threatening. Differentiation from other central nervous system infections such as those caused by *C. neoformans* or *T. gondii* is important, and prompt treatment is essential.

Acyclovir is the drug of choice for treatment of HSV disease. For mild to moderate mucocutaneous disease oral acyclovir in doses of 200 mg five times daily or 400 mg tid are used, although regimens of 400 mg 5 times daily have occasionally been described as clinically necessary. Intravenous acyclovir (15 mg/kg/day) should be used in those settings in which absorption of oral drug is questionable, or oral tolerance is unlikely (HSV esophagitis), or perhaps when severe mucocutaneous disease is present. Treatment of mucocutaneous disease should be continued until all lesions have crusted. Intravenous acyclovir (30 mg/kg/day) should also be used for viscerally disseminated disease and for HSV encephalitis. Famciclovir or the oral prodrug of acyclovir, valacyclovir, are alternatives to oral acyclovir.

Recurrent HSV disease is common in many patients with AIDS following discontinuation of therapy. These individuals can often be managed with low-dose suppressive oral acyclovir therapy, as have other immunosuppressed patients at risk for frequently recurring HSV diseases.[124] Regimens commonly used include acyclovir 200 mg qid, 400 mg bid, or 800 mg qd.

Acyclovir-resistant HSV has been isolated from patients with AIDS.[125] The primary mechanism of resistance appears to be a deficiency in viral thymidine kinase. Strategies that have been employed for management of severe, acyclovir-resistant HSV infections include increasing the dose of acyclovir, discontinuation of acyclovir, or use of an alternative antiviral agent. Vidarabine and foscarnet, because they do not require phosphorylation by thymidine kinase, are examples of potential alternative agents.[126,127] A randomized comparison of foscarnet and vidarabine indicate that foscarnet is more effective and associated with fewer adverse reactions than vidarabine.[128]

VARICELLA-ZOSTER VIRUS

Most adults with AIDS have been previously infected with varicella-zoster virus (VZV) and thus are not susceptible to primary infection (chickenpox) but may develop recurrent infection (zoster). The prevalence of zoster in HIV-infected individuals appears higher than in other age-matched immunocompetent persons, and seems to reliably herald the loss of cell-mediated immunity and progression to AIDS.[129]

Zoster usually begins as radicular pain followed by localized erythematous rash and characteristic vesicles. Zoster will usually remain confined to a limited number of dermatomes, but complications such as widespread cutaneous involvement and disseminated visceral zoster may occur. Like the treatment of HSV infections, acyclovir is the drug of choice for VZV infections. Although an oral acyclovir regimen of 4 g/day is effective for the treatment of zoster in immunocompetent adults, the drug has not been fully evaluated in immunocompromised patients such as those with AIDS.[130] For practical reasons, oral acyclovir or famciclovir is often used for localized zoster. However, careful monitoring for signs of progression of zoster is essential. AIDS patients with disseminated cutaneous or visceral zoster should receive treatment with intravenous acyclovir in doses of 30 mg/kg/d for at least 7 days or until all lesions are crusted. Acyclovir-resistant VZV infections have been reported in patients with AIDS.[131]

CYTOMEGALOVIRUS

CMV is the most common life-threatening viral infection in patients with AIDS. Like other herpes group viruses, infection with CMV is ubiquitous; seropositivity among homosexual men with AIDS approaches 100%.[132] There are numerous manifestations of CMV infection, including retinitis, esophagitis, hepatitis, gastrointestinal involvement, and, less commonly, radiculopathy, encephalitis, and pneumonitis. CMV end-organ disease occurs in as many as 44.9% of AIDS patients, particularly when their CD4 cell count is below 50 cells/μL. The incidence, however, has decreased in the era of HAART.[75]

CMV retinitis, the most commonly recognized CMV disease associated with AIDS, occurs in approximately 29% to 32% of patients with AIDS.[133] CMV retinitis is usually associated with a painless progressive loss of vision. Patients may initially complain of blurry vision, loss of visual acuity, or "floaters." CMV retinitis usually begins unilaterally, but bilateral involvement may occur. Untreated, CMV retinitis invariably leads to blindness. The diagnosis of CMV retinitis is made by funduscopic examination and identification of characteristic findings. Lesions characteristic of CMV retinitis include a fluffy white perivascular exudate frequently associated with hemorrhage. Early diagnosis and treatment is crucial to prevent further visual deterioration.

The first approved agent of treatment for CMV diseases was ganciclovir. Structurally ganciclovir differs from acyclovir only by a single hydroxyl side chain, but it is 30 to 50 times more active *in vitro* against CMV. The use of ganciclovir therapy has traditionally been divided into two phases—induction and maintenance—because high relapse rates are found after discontinuation of the drug following successful completion of a 2- to 3-week course of initial therapy. Induction regimens are typically 7.5–10 mg/kg/day intravenously in two or three equally divided doses for 14 days or longer if there is a slow clinical response. Maintenance therapy is usually 5–6 mg/kg once daily, although doses of 10 mg/kg have been used, 5 to 7 days per week for an indefinite period of time. Initial response rates for retinal CMV disease range from 60% to 90%.[134] Unfortunately, even with intravenous maintenance therapy, relapse of CMV retinitis is common and occurs at a median of approximately 55 to 80 days.

Despite the poor oral bioavailability of ganciclovir (6% to 9%), oral regimens have been evaluated as a possible alternative to long-term intravenous maintenance administration. Two randomized trials have evaluated intravenous or oral ganciclovir as maintenance therapy for CMV retinitis. In both studies, oral ganciclovir maintenance therapy was associated with a slightly more rapid rate of disease progression. The differences in mean time to progression ranged from 5 to 11 days.[135,136] The convenience of oral administration, however, may favor use of oral drug in certain individuals. The recommended dose of oral ganciclovir for maintenance therapy of CMV retinitis is 1,000 mg tid taken with food. CMV isolates resistant to ganciclovir have been recovered from immunocompromised patients.

Neutropenia and thrombocytopenia are the most common drug- or dose-limiting adverse reactions associated with use of intravenous ganciclovir. Up to 50% of patients with AIDS receiving ganciclovir (alone) may need a dose reduction or interruption of therapy as a result of hematologic toxicity. Filgrastim (G-CSF), erythropoietin, or sargramostim (GM-CSF) offers some potential amelioration of the adverse hematologic effects of ganciclovir. Intravitreal administration has also been used as salvage therapy in an attempt to circumvent these adverse reactions.[133] Sustained-release intraocular ganciclovir implants represent another strategy developed not only to overcome systemic toxicity but also to avoid the need for intravitreal injections. One hundred seventy-three patients representing 222 eyes were randomized to receive either ganciclovir implant 1 μg/h (75 eyes), 2 μg/h (71 eyes), or intravenous ganciclovir (76 eyes). Median progression to CMV retinitis was similar in the 1 and 2 μg/h implant groups, 221 days and 191 days, respectively; however, median time to progression in the patients treated with intravenous ganciclovir was 71 days ($p < 0.001$). Intravenous ganciclovir was associated with an almost threefold risk of progression as compared to ganciclovir implants.[137] Ganciclovir implants, however, do not protect patients from CMV occurring elsewhere including the initial uninvolved eye. Intravenous ganciclovir cuts the risk of CMV retinitis in the initially uninvolved eye by half. Extraocular involvement of CMV did not occur in patients receiving intravenous ganciclovir as compared to 10.3% of patients who received an implant only. Therefore, patients having an implant should also receive systemic therapy such as oral ganciclovir.

Foscarnet is a pyrophosphate analog with both anti-HIV and anti-CMV activity. Controlled trials to evaluate immediate versus delayed foscarnet therapy of CMV retinitis in HIV infected individuals found immediate foscarnet therapy more effective than delayed therapy in preventing progression of CMV disease.[138] Furthermore, prolonged survival and an anti-HIV effect (as assessed by a decline in HIV or p24 antigen) was observed.[139] An unblinded randomized trial comparing ganciclovir with foscarnet therapy of CMV retinitis was conducted in 234 patients with AIDS.[140] Both drugs were administered in standard 14-day induction regimens followed by maintenance therapy. Ganciclovir and foscarnet were equally effective in delaying the progression of CMV disease. The median time to progression of retinitis was 56 days in the ganciclovir groups and 59 days in the foscarnet group. There was a difference, however, in survival between these two groups. Median survival was 8.5 months for ganciclovir recipients whereas it was 12.6 months for those who received foscarnet. The explanation for this survival difference is unknown. It is conceivable that the difference in mortality was a result of the anti-HIV effect of foscarnet. Adverse reactions that necessitated a switch in therapy were more common among the foscarnet recipients. The choice of therapy for CMV retinitis is largely dictated by the adverse reaction profiles of the two agents, convenience, concomitant medications being taken by the patient, and underlying disease states.

While foscarnet appears less likely to cause neutropenia than ganciclovir, it has a variety of potential adverse effects. The most common side effects are renal insufficiency and metabolic disturbances (both increases and decreases) in calcium and phosphorus. Other adverse reactions include anemia, thrombocytopenia, infusion site reactions, nausea and vomiting, penile ulcerations, and seizures. Hydration reduces the incidence of serum creatinine elevations from 66% in a nonhydrated control group to 13% in hydrated individuals.[141] Foscarnet, like ganciclovir, is currently administered in two phases: induction and maintenance. Induction doses are 180 mg/kg/d intravenously in two or three divided doses for 14 days, followed by maintenance therapy in doses of 90–120 mg/kg intravenously once daily; foscarnet doses must be adjusted in individuals with renal insufficiency.

Other approaches to the treatment of CMV disease include the combination of ganciclovir and foscarnet, and cidofovir. In patients who have relapsed CMV retinitis, the ganciclovir-foscarnet combination was compared with retreatment with either drug alone.[142] The median times to retinitis progression were foscarnet, 1.3 months; ganciclovir, 2.0 months; and ganciclovir-foscarnet, 4.3 months. Adverse events among the three groups were similar. However, the combined use of ganciclovir-foscarnet had the greatest negative impact on quality of life, most likely because of the time-intensive and complex administration requirements. Cidofovir is a nucleotide analog shown to delay the progression of CMV retinitis. In a study of 64 patients with AIDS and previously untreated CMV retinitis, the median time to progression was 21 days in the deferred-therapy group versus 64 days in those patients who received low-dose cidofovir.[143] While cidofovir has certain advantages over ganciclovir and foscarnet, including a less-frequent dosing schedule, the drug is nephrotoxic and can cause irreversible damage to the proximal renal tubules. Cidofovir must be given with aggressive IV hydration and concomitant probenecid, although these efforts only reduce, not prevent nephrotoxicity. Also concerning is the finding that cidofovir did not show a significant effect on CMV viremia at the 3-week assessment point in the trial previously mentioned; this finding is in contrast to ganciclovir or foscarnet that both suppress CMV viremia.

CMV infection of the gastrointestinal tract can involve sites ranging from the esophagus and stomach to the colon and rectum. In one series of AIDS patients with gastrointestinal tract infection, the colon was the most common site of infection followed by the stomach or esophagus.[144] CMV colitis may be characterized by abdominal pain, fever, weight loss, and diarrhea—symptoms that are quite common among patients with HIV disease even in the absence of CMV infection. Characteristic symptoms of CMV esophagitis are dysphagia and substernal chest pain. Barium contrast studies may demonstrate abnormalities, but will not distinguish between other etiologic agents such as *Candida* or HSV, both of which are more common. The definitive diagnosis of CMV gastrointestinal infection requires endoscopy and biopsy with histologic identification of CMV inclusions or in situ antigen detection.

The therapy of CMV gastrointestinal disease is more controversial. Few randomized, controlled trials have been conducted.

A small randomized comparison of ganciclovir and foscarnet for AIDS-associated gastrointestinal disease found both therapies equally effective.[145] Judged by endoscopy, 83% of foscarnet recipients and 85% of ganciclovir recipients showed a response. Survival, however, was poor at less than 40 weeks for both groups. Although this study did not include a randomization to subsequent maintenance therapy, it is interesting that there was no difference in the time to progression of disease between those patients who received maintenance therapy and those who did not. Symptomatic CMV gastrointestinal disease warrants treatment and it appears that ganciclovir and foscarnet are equivalent. The role of maintenance therapy is less clear.

Various strategies have been evaluated to determine whether CMV disease in HIV-infected individuals can be prevented. High-dose oral acyclovir is effective in reducing the incidence of CMV infection and disease in bone marrow and renal transplant recipients but not in patients infected with HIV.[146–148] Valacyclovir is an oral prodrug of acyclovir that achieves three- to fourfold higher concentrations following an equivalent dose. Valacyclovir given 2 g qid reduced the relative risk of CMV disease by 33% as compared to acyclovir given either as 3.2 g or 800 mg per day.[146] The delay in developing disease was also longer in the valacyclovir-treated group. A randomized, double-blind, placebo-controlled study of oral ganciclovir (1,000 mg q8h) in CMV seropositive patients with AIDS found that oral ganciclovir significantly reduced the incidence of CMV disease.[149] CMV disease occurred in 26% of placebo recipients versus 14% of ganciclovir recipients ($p < 0.001$). However, there was no difference in survival between the two groups: the 1-year mortality rate was 26% for placebo versus 21% for ganciclovir recipients. A study of oral ganciclovir for prevention in patients with a slightly higher CD4 lymphocyte count did not find any protective benefit. Currently, prophylaxis with oral ganciclovir should be considered in HIV-infected adults and adolescents who have a CD4 cell count <50 cells/μL; ganciclovir prophylaxis is not a recommended standard of care.

DISCONTINUATION OF PROPHYLAXIS FOR OPPORTUNISTIC INFECTIONS

The ability of highly active antiretroviral regimens to restore the CD4 cell count to levels rarely associated with the development of opportunistic infections has raised the question of whether primary and secondary prophylaxis can be safely discontinued. To date, this question has been best addressed for the primary prophylaxis of PCP and MAC disease, and secondary prophylaxis of CMV retinitis. The current recommendations are as follows:[14] For PCP, prophylaxis can be discontinued in patients receiving and responding to HAART who have had a sustained increase in their CD4 cell count from <200 cells/μL to >200 cells/μL for at least 3 to 6 months. As most of the patients in the studies that have evaluated primary prophylaxis discontinuation had undetectable levels of HIV RNA in plasma, an additional criterion should probably be a sustained reduction in viral load for the 3- to 6-month period as well. Prophylaxis should be reinstated if the CD4 count drops to <200 cells/μL. Data from observational studies indicates that primary prophylaxis for MAC disease can be discontinued in patients who have CD4 counts >100 cells/μL for a period of 3 to 6 months; ideally, these individuals should have a sustained suppression in HIV RNA in plasma for this same period. Prophylaxis should be restarted if the CD4 count returns to <50 cells/μL. Maintenance therapy (secondary prophylaxis) for CMV retinitis can be discontinued in patients whose CD4 cells have increased to >100–150 cells/μL for 3 to 6 months and whose HIV RNA in plasma is suppressed for this same period. Additional considerations should include the anatomic location of the CMV lesion (sight-threatening or not), adequate vision in the other eye, and the availability of regular eye examinations.

EPILOGUE

Irrefutable progress has been made in the management of HIV: disease progression can be delayed, survival can be prolonged, and the risk of maternal-to-fetal HIV transmission reduced. Sixteen antiretroviral agents are now available for clinical use and additional compounds are likely to follow. However, therapy is still suboptimal in that complete suppression of viral replication has not been achieved. There remain significant deficits in our understanding of the virologic and immunologic processes associated with HIV infection and the clinical pharmacology of anti-HIV compounds. Critical issues include the need for simpler and more potent regimens, emergence of drug-resistant viral isolates, and the inexorably progressive nature of HIV infection in some patients despite antiretroviral therapy. There is a clear need for more selective and potent inhibitors of HIV. The medical management of opportunistic infections associated with HIV disease has also changed dramatically since the recognition of AIDS early in the 1980s, and has improved survival. The approach to PCP is most illustrative. The transition from an era marked by only treatment of established disease to one in which primary and secondary prophylaxis based on CD4 lymphocyte count are standards of care, reflects both progress in understanding the risk factors for opportunistic infections and in pharmacologic therapy. Collectively, three important lessons have been learned from the treatment of HIV and associated opportunistic infections: the need for prospective immunologic and virologic monitoring and early recognition of HIV infection; the use of potent combinations of antiretroviral agents to maximally inhibit viral replication; and primary and secondary prophylaxis of opportunistic infections. Emphasis on these principles coupled with carefully controlled investigations of novel agents and therapeutic strategies will continue to offer definite benefit and improve the quality of life for HIV-infected individuals, and yield an advantage over this pernicious virus that causes AIDS.

▶ PRINCIPLES OF PHARMACOTHERAPY

Infection with HIV causes a spectrum of diseases, the end stage manifestation of which is AIDS.

- Ongoing replication of HIV has a primary role in the onset and progression of disease.
- The replication of HIV can be suppressed with a potent combination of antiretroviral agents, which, for a period of time, can prevent further progression of disease.
- General principles for the management of opportunistic infections include prospective monitoring, primary prophylaxis, treatment, and secondary prophylaxis.

ACKNOWLEDGMENTS

Grant Support: RO1 AI33835, UO1 AI41089, UO1 AI38858, UO1 AI27551, UO1 AI27661, AI27757, and AI27664 from the National Institute of Allergy and Infectious Disease.

REFFRENCES

1. Centers for Disease Control and Prevention. *Pneumocystis* pneumonia—Los Angeles. MMWR Morb Mortal Wkly Rep 1981;30:250–252.
2. Centers for Disease Control and Prevention. Kaposi's sarcoma and *Pneumocystis* pneumonia among homosexual men—New York and California. MMWR Morb Mortal Wkly Rep 1981;30:305–308.
3. Barre-Sinoussi F, Chermann J, Rey F, et al. Isolation of a T-lymphotropic retrovirus from a patient at risk for acquired immunodeficiency syndrome (AIDS). Science 1983;220:868–871.
4. Gallo R, Salahuddin S, Popovic M, et al. Frequent detection and isolation of cytopathic retroviruses (HTLV-III) from patients with AIDS and at risk for AIDS. Science 1984;224:500–503.
5. Palella FJ Jr, Delaney KM, Moorman AC, et al. Declining morbidity and mortality among patients with advanced human immunodeficiency virus infection. N Engl J Med 1998;338:853–860.
6. de Martino M, Tovo P A, Balducci M, et al. Reduction in mortality with availability of antiretroviral therapy for children with perinatal HIV-1 infection. JAMA 2000;284:190–197.
7. Carr A, Cooper DA. Adverse effects of antiretroviral therapy. Lancet 2000;356:1423–1430.
8. Centers for Disease Control and Prevention. Guidelines for national human immunodeficiency virus case surveillance, including monitoring for human immunodeficiency virus infection and acquired immunodeficiency syndrome. MMWR Morb Mortal Wkly Rep 1999;48(RR- 13): 1–31.
9. Centers for Disease Control and Prevention. 1993 revised classification system for HIV infection and expanded surveillance case definitions for AIDS among adolescents and adults. MMWR Morb Mortal Wkly Rep 1992;41(RR-17):1–19.
10. Centers for Disease Control and Prevention. HIV/AIDS Surveillance Report 1999;11(2):1–44.
11. Joint United Nations Programme on HIV/AIDS. AIDS epidemic update: December 2000.
12. Hahn BH, Shaw GM, De Cock KM, et al. AIDS as a zoonosis: Scientific and public health implications. Science 2000;287:607–614.
13. Mylonakis E, Paliou M, Lally M, et al. Laboratory testing for infection with the human immunodeficiency virus: Established and novel approaches. Am J Med 2000;109:568–576.
14. Kovacs JA, Masur H. Prophylaxis against opportunistic infections in patients with human immunodeficiency virus infection. N Engl J Med 2000;342:1416–1429.
15. Mastro TD, de Vincenzi I. Probabilities of sexual HIV-1 transmission. AIDS 1996;10(suppl A):S75–S82.
16. Royce RA, Sena A, Cates W Jr, et al. Sexual transmission of HIV. N Engl J Med 1997;336:1072–1079.
17. Schreiber GB, Busch MP, Kleinman SH. The risk of transfusion-transmitted viral infections. N Engl J Med 1996;26:1685–1690.
18. Centers for Disease Control and Prevention. Public Health Service guidelines for the management of health-care worker exposures to HIV and recommendations for postexposure prophylaxis. MMWR Morb Mortal Wkly Rep 1998;47(RR-7):1–33.
19. Van Dyke RB, Korber BT, Popek E, et al. The Ariel project: A prospective cohort study of maternal-child transmission of human immunodeficiency virus type 1 in the era of maternal antiviral therapy. J Infect Dis 1999;179:319–328.
20. Nduati R, John G, Mbori-Ngacha D, et al. Effect of breast-feeding and formula feeding on transmission of HIV-1. JAMA 2000;283:1167–1174.
21. Dean M, Carrington M, Winkler C, et al. Genetic restriction of HIV-1 infection and progression to AIDS by a deletion allele of the CKR5 structural gene. Science 1996;273:1856–1862.
22. Pierson T, McArthur J, Siliciano RF. Reservoirs for HIV-1: Mechanisms for viral persistence in the presence of antiviral immune responses and antiretroviral therapy. Annu Rev Immunol 2000;18:665–708.
23. Frankel AD, Young JAT. HIV-1: Fifteen proteins and an RNA. Annu Rev Biochem 1998;67:1 25.
24. Learmont JC, Geczy AF, Mills J, et al. Immunologic and virologic status after 14 to 18 years of infection with an attenuated strain of HIV-1: A report from the Sydney blood bank cohort. N Engl J Med 1999;340:1715–1722.
25. Kohl NE, Emini EA, Schleif WA, et al. Active human immunodeficiency virus protease is required for viral infectivity. Proc Natl Acad Sci U S A 1988(85):4686–4690.
26. Schacker T, Collier AC, Hughes J, et al. Clinical and epidemiologic features of primary HIV infection. Ann Intern Med 1996;125:257–264.
27. Kahn JO, Walker BD. Acute human immunodeficiency virus type 1 infection. N Engl J Med 1998;339:33–39.
28. Mellors JW, Rinaldo CR Jr, Gupta P, et al. Prognosis in HIV-1 infection predicted by the quantity of virus in plasma. Science 1996;272:1167–1170.
29. Love JT Jr, Shearer WT. Prevention, diagnosis, and treatment of pediatric HIV infection. Compr Ther 1996;22:719–726.
30. Centers for Disease Control and Prevention. 1994 Revised classification system for human immunodeficiency virus infection in children less than 13 years of age. MMWR Morb Mortal Wkly Rep 1994;43(RR-12): 1–10.
31. Working Group on Antiretroviral Therapy and Medical Management of AIDS. Guidelines for the use of antiretroviral agents in pediatric HIV infection. 2001. Living document: August 8, 2001. http://www.hivatis.org.
32. Kempf DJ, Rode RA, Xu Y, et al. The duration of viral suppression during protease inhibitor therapy for HIV-1 infection is predicted by plasma HIV-1 RNA at the nadir. AIDS 1998;12:F9–F14.
33. Raboud JM, Montaner JS, Conway B, et al. Suppression of plasma viral load below 20 copies/mL is required to achieve a long-term response to therapy. AIDS 1998;12:1619–1624.
34. NIH Panel to Define Principles of Therapy of HIV Infection. Report of the NIH panel to define principles of therapy of HIV infection. 1997. Guidelines for the use of antiretroviral agents in HIV-infected adults and adolescents. Living document: February 5, 2001. http://www.hivatis.org.
35. Panel on Clinical Practices for the Treatment of HIV Infection. Guidelines for the use of antiretroviral agents in HIV-infected adults and adolescents. 2001. Living document: August 13, 2001. http://www.hivatis.org.
36. Carpenter CCJ, Cooper DA, Fischl MA, et al. Antiviral therapy in adults: Updated recommendations of the International AIDS Society—USA Panel. JAMA 2000;283:381–390.
37. Voss G, Villinger F. Adjuvanted vaccine strategies and live vector approaches for the prevention of AIDS. AIDS 2000;14(suppl 3):S153–S165.
38. Piscitelli SC, Bhat N, Pau A. A risk-benefit assessment of interleukin-2 as an adjunct to antiviral therapy in HIV infection. Drug Saf 2000;22(1): 19–31.
39. Kakuda TN. Pharmacology of nucleoside and nucleotide reverse transcriptase inhibitor- induced mitochondrial toxicity. Clin Ther 2000;22(6):685–708.
40. Harris M, Montaner JS. Clinical uses of non-nucleoside reverse transcriptase inhibitors. Rev Med Virol 2000;10:217–229.
41. Eron JJ Jr. HIV-1 protease inhibitors. Clin Infect Dis 2000;30(suppl 2):S160–S170.
42. Murphy RL. New antiretroviral drugs in development. AIDS 2000; 14(suppl 3):S227–S234.
43. Barry M, Mulcahy F, Merry C, et al. Pharmacokinetics and potential interactions amongst antiretroviral agents used to treat patients with HIV infection. Clin Pharmacokinet 1999;36(4):289–304.
44. Flexner C. Dual protease inhibitor therapy in HIV-infected patients: Pharmacologic rationale and clinical benefits. Annu Rev Pharmacol Toxicol 2000;40:649–674.
45. Havlir DV, Tierney C, Friedland GH, et al. In vivo antagonism with zidovudine plus stavudine combination therapy. J Infect Dis 2000;182:321–325.
46. Centers for Disease Control and Prevention. Updated guidelines for the use of rifabutin or rifampin for the treatment and prevention of tuberculosis among HIV-infected patients taking protease inhibitors or non-nucleoside reverse transcriptase inhibitors. MMWR Morb Mortal Wkly Rep 2000;49(9):185–189.

47. Piscitelli SC, Burstein AH, Chaitt D, et al. Indinavir concentrations and St John's wort. Lancet 2000;355:547–548.
48. Fischl MA, Richman DD, Grieco MH, et al. The efficacy of azidothymidine (AZT) in the treatment of patients with AIDS and AIDS-related complex. N Engl J Med 1987;317:185–191.
49. Volberding PA, Lagakos SW, Grimes JM, et al. The duration of zidovudine benefit in persons with asymptomatic HIV infection. JAMA 1994;272(6):437–442.
50. Hammer SM, Katzenstein DA, Hughes MD, et al. A trial comparing nucleoside monotherapy with combination therapy in HIV-infected adults with CD4 cell counts from 200 to 500 per cubic millimeter. N Engl J Med 1996;335:1081–1090.
51. Katzenstein DA, Hammer SM, Hughes MD, et al. The relation of virologic and immunologic markers to clinical outcomes after nucleoside therapy in HIV-infected adults with 200 to 500 CD4 cells per cubic millimeter. N Engl J Med 1996;335:1091–1098.
52. Sabin CA, Cozzi-Lepri A, Phillips AN. A practical guide to applying the intention-to-treat principle to clinical trials in HIV infection. HIV Clin Trials 2000;1:31–38.
53. Gulick RM, Mellors JW, Havlir D, et al. 3-Year suppression of HIV viremia with indinavir, zidovudine, and lamivudine. Ann Intern Med 2000;133:35–39.
54. Hammer S, Squires K, Hughes M, et al. A controlled trial of two nucleoside analogues plus indinavir in persons with human immunodeficiency virus infection and CD4 cell counts of 200 per cubic millimeter or less. AIDS Clinical Trials Group 320 Study Team. N Engl J Med 1997;337:725–733.
55. Paterson DL, Swindells S, Mohr J, et al. Adherence to protease inhibitor therapy and outcomes in patients with HIV infection. Ann Intern Med 2000;133:21–30.
56. Singh N, Berman SM, Swindells S, et al. Adherence to human immunodeficiency virus-infected patients to antiretroviral therapy. J Infect Dis 1999;29:824–830.
57. Spooner KM, Lane HC, Masur H. Antiretroviral therapy: Reference guide to major clinical trials in patients infected with human immunodeficiency virus. Clin Infect Dis 1995;20(5):1145–1151.
58. Spooner KM, Lane HC, Masur H. Guide to major clinical trials of antiretroviral therapy administered to patients infected with human immunodeficiency virus. Clin Infect Dis 1996;23:15–27.
59. Tavel JA, Miller KD, Masur H. Guide to major clinical trials of antiretroviral therapy in human immunodeficiency virus-infected patients: Protease inhibitors, non-nucleoside reverse transcriptase inhibitors, and nucleotide reverse transcriptase inhibitors. Clin Infect Dis 1999;28:643–676.
60. Cohen-Stuart JWT, Schuurman R, Burger DM, et al. Randomized trial comparing saquinavir soft gelatin capsules versus indinavir as part of triple therapy (CHEESE study). AIDS 1999;13:F53–F58.
61. Noble S, Goa KL. Amprenavir: A review of its clinical potential in patients with HIV infection. Drugs 2000;60:1383–1410.
62. Hurst M, Faulds D. Lopinavir. Drugs 2000;60:1371–1379.
63. Staszewski S, Morales-Ramirez J, Tashima KT, et al. Efavirenz plus zidovudine and lamivudine, efavirenz plus indinavir, and indinavir plus zidovudine and lamivudine in the treatment of HIV-1 infection in adults. N Engl J Med 1999;341:1865–1873.
64. United States Public Health Services. Public Health Service Task Force recommendations for the use of antiretroviral drugs in pregnant HIV-1 infected women for maternal health and interventions to reduce perinatal HIV-1 transmission in the United States. 2000. Living document. January 24, 2001. http://www.hivatis.org.
65. Connor EM, Sperling RS, Gelber R, et al. Reduction in maternal-infant transmission of human immunodeficiency virus type 1 with zidovudine treatment. N Engl J Med 1994;331:1173–1180.
66. Wade NA, Birkhead GS, Warren BL, et al. Abbreviated regimens of zidovudine prophylaxis and perinatal transmission of the human immunodeficiency virus. N Engl J Med 1998;339:1409–1414.
67. Guay LA, Musoke P, Fleming T, et al. Intrapartum and neonatal single-dose nevirapine compared with zidovudine for prevention of mother-to-child transmission of HIV-1 in Kampala, Uganda: HIVNET 012 randomised trial. Lancet 1999;354:795–802.
68. Morris AB, Cu-Uvin S, Harwell JI, et al. Multicenter review of protease inhibitors in 89 pregnancies. J Acquir Immune Defic Syndr 2000;25:306–311.
69. Centers for Disease Control and Prevention. Management of possible sexual, injecting-drug-use, or other nonoccupational exposure to HIV, including considerations related to antiretroviral therapy. MMWR Morb Mortal Wkly Rep 1998;47(RR-17):1–15.
70. Hirsch MS, Brun-Vezinet F, D'Aquila RT, et al. Antiretroviral drug resistance testing in adult HIV-1 infection: Recommendations of an international AIDS society—USA panel. JAMA 2000;283:2417–2426.
71. Neumann AU, Tubiana R, Calvez V, et al. HIV-1 rebound during interruption of highly active antiretroviral therapy has no deleterious effect on reinitiated treatment. AIDS 1999;13:677–683.
72. Masur H, Ognibene F, Yarchoan R, et al. CD4 counts as predictors of opportunistic pneumonias in human immunodeficiency virus (HIV) infection. Ann Intern Med 1989;111:223–231.
73. Centers for Disease Control and Prevention. Public Health Service Task Force on antipneumocystis prophylaxis in human immunodeficiency virus-infected individuals. MMWR Morb Mortal Wkly Rep 1989;38:1–9.
74. Moore R, Chaisson R. Natural history of opportunistic disease in an HIV-infected urban clinical cohort. Ann Intern Med 1996;124:633–642.
75. Kaplan JE, Hanson D, Dworkin MS, et al. Epidemiology of human immunodeficiency virus-associated opportunistic infections in the United States in the era of highly active antiretroviral therapy. Clin Infect Dis 2000;30:S5–14.
76. Ledergerber B, Egger M, Erard V, et al. AIDS-related opportunistic illnesses occurring after initiation of potent antiretroviral therapy. JAMA 2000;282:2220–2226.
77. Chan I, Neaton J, Saravolatz L, et al. Frequencies of opportunistic diseases prior to death among HIV-infected persons. AIDS 1995;9:1145–1151.
78. Centers for Disease Control and Prevention. Public Health Service Task Force on antipneumocystis prophylaxis in human immunodeficiency virus-infected individuals. MMWR Morb Mortal Wkly Rep 1989;38:1–9.
79. Davey RJ, H. M. Recent advances in the diagnosis, treatment, and prevention of *Pneumocystis carinii* pneumonia. Antimicrob Agents Chemother 1990;34:499–504.
80. Santamauro J, Stover D. *Pneumocystis carinii* pneumonia. Med Clin North Am 1997;81:299–318.
81. Hughes W, Feldman S, Chaudary S, et al. Comparison of pentamidine isethionate and trimethoprim-sulfamethoxazole in the treatment of *Pneumocystis carinii* pneumonia. J Pediatr 1978;92:285–291.
82. Masur H. Prevention and treatment of *Pneumocystis* pneumonia. N Engl J Med 1992;327:1853–60.
83. Conte J, Chernoff D, Feigal D, et al. Intravenous or inhaled pentamidine for treating *Pneumocystis carinii* pneumonia in AIDS. Ann Intern Med 1990;113:203–209.
84. Conte J Jr, Hollander H, Golden J, et al. Inhaled pentamidine or reduced dose intravenous pentamidine for *Pneumocystis carinii* pneumonia: A pilot study. Ann Intern Med 1987;107:495–498.
85. Soo Hoo G, Mohsenifar Z, Meyer R. Inhaled or intravenous pentamidine therapy for *Pneumocystis carinii* pneumonia. Ann Intern Med 1990;113:195–202.
86. Sattler F, Cowan R, Nielsen D, et al. Trimethoprim-sulfamethoxazole compared with pentamidine for treatment of *Pneumocystis carinii* pneumonia in the acquired immunodeficiency syndrome. Ann Intern Med 1988;109:280–287.
87. Wharton J, Coleman D, Wofsy C, et al. Trimethoprim-sulfamethoxazole or pentamidine for *Pneumocystis carinii* pneumonia in the acquired immunodeficiency syndrome. Ann Intern Med 1986;105:37–44.
88. Wofsy C. Use of trimethoprim-sulfamethoxazole in the treatment of *Pneumocystis carinii* pneumonitis in patients with acquired immunodeficiency syndrome. Rev Infect Dis 1987;9(suppl 2):S184–S194.
89. Bozzette S, Sattler F, Chiu J, et al. A controlled trial of early adjunctive treatment with corticosteroids for *Pneumocystis carinii* pneumonia in the acquired immunodeficiency syndrome. N Engl J Med 1990;323:1451–1457.

90. Gagnon S, Boota A, Fischl M, et al. Corticosteroids as adjunctive therapy for severe *Pneumocystis carinii* pneumonia in the acquired immunodeficiency syndrome. N Engl J Med 1990;323:1444–1450.
91. The National Institutes of Health-University of California Expert Panel for Corticosteroids as Adjunctive Therapy for *Pneumocystis carinii* Pneumonia. Consensus statement on the use of corticosteroids as adjunctive therapy for *Pneumocystis* pneumonia in the acquired immunodeficiency syndrome. N Engl J Med 1990;323:1500–1504.
92. Phair J, Munoz A, Detels R, et al. The risk of *Pneumocystis carinii* pneumonia among men infected with human immunodeficiency virus type 1. N Engl J Med 1990;322:161–165.
93. Centers for Disease Control and Prevention. Recommendation for prophylaxis against *Pneumocystis carinii* pneumonia for adults and adolescents infected with human immunodeficiency virus. MMWR Morb Mortal Wkly Rep 1992;41:1–11.
94. Bozzette S, Finkelstein D, Spector S, et al. A randomized trial of three antipneumocystis agents in patients with advanced human immunodeficiency virus infection. NIAID AIDS Clinical Trials Group. N Engl J Med 1995;332:693–699.
95. Northfelt D, Clement M, Safrin S. Extrapulmonary pneumocystosis: Clinical features in human immunodeficiency virus infection. Medicine 1990;69:392–398.
96. Centers for Disease Control and Prevention. 1999 USPHS/IDSA guidelines for the prevention of opportunistic infections in persons infected with human immunodeficiency virus. MMWR Morb Mortal Wkly Rep 1999;48(RR-10):1–59.
97. Hughes W, Kuhn S, Chaudhary S, et al. Successful chemoprophylaxis for *Pneumocystis carinii* pneumonitis. N Engl J Med 1977;297:1419–1426.
98. Tuazon C. Toxoplasmosis in AIDS patients. J Antimicrob Chemother 1989;23(suppl A):77–82.
99. Grant I, Gold J, Rosenblum M, et al. *Toxoplasma gondii* serology in HIV-infected patients: the development of central nervous system toxoplasmosis. AIDS 1990;4:519–521.
100. Katlama C, Wit S, O'Doherty E, et al. Pyrimethamine-clindamycin vs. pyrimethamine-sulfadiazine as acute and long-term therapy for toxoplasmic encephalitis in patients with AIDS. Clin Infect Dis 1996;22: 268–275.
101. Weiss L, Harris C, Berger M, et al. Pyrimethamine concentrations in serum and cerebrospinal fluid during treatment of acute *Toxoplasma* encephalitis in patients with AIDS. J Infect Dis 1988;157:580–583.
102. Wong S, Remington J. Toxoplasmosis in the setting of AIDS. Baltimore, MD, Williams & Wilkins, 1994.
103. Luft B, Remington J. Toxoplasmic encephalitis. J Infect Dis 1988;157: 1–6.
104. Herald A, Flepp M, Chave J-P, et al. Treatment for cerebral toxoplasmosis protects against *Pneumocystis carinii* pneumonia in patients with AIDS. Ann Intern Med 1991;115:760–763.
105. Jacobson M, Besch C, Child C, et al. Toxicity of clindamycin as prophylaxis for AIDS-associated toxoplasmic encephalitis. Lancet 1992;339:333–334.
106. Chuck S, Sande M. Infections with *Cryptococcus neoformans* in the acquired immunodeficiency syndrome. N Engl J Med 1989;321: 794–799.
107. Bennett J, Dismukes W, Duma R, et al. A comparison of amphotericin B alone and combined with flucytosine in the treatment of cryptococcal meningitis. N Engl J Med 1979;301:126–131.
108. Robinson P, Knirsch A, Joseph J. Fluconazole for life-threatening fungal infections in patients who cannot be treated with conventional antifungal agents. Rev Infect Dis 1990;12(suppl 3):S349–S363.
109. Larsen R, Leal M, Chan L. Fluconazole compared with amphotericin B plus flucytosine for cryptococcal meningitis in AIDS. Ann Intern Med 1990,113:183–187.
110. Saag M, Powderly W, Cloud G, et al. Comparison of amphotericin B with fluconazole in the treatment of acute AIDS-associated cryptococcal meningitis. N Engl J Med 1992;326:83–89.
111. van der Horst C, Saag M, Cloud G, et al. Treatment of cryptococcal meningitis associated with the acquired immunodeficiency syndrome. National Institute of Allergy and Infectious Diseases Mycoses Study Group and AIDS Clinical Trials Group. N Engl J Med 1997;337:15–21.
112. Bozzette S, Larsen R, Chiu J, et al. A placebo-controlled trial of maintenance therapy with fluconazole after treatment of cryptococcal meningitis in the acquired immunodeficiency syndrome. N Engl J Med 1991;324:580–584.
113. Powderly W, Saag M, Cloud G, et al. A controlled trial of fluconazole or amphotericin B to prevent relapse of cryptococcal meningitis in patients with the acquired immunodeficiency syndrome. N Engl J Med 1992;326:793–798.
114. Powderly W, Finkelstein D, Feinberg J, et al. A randomized trial comparing fluconazole with clotrimazole troches for the prevention of fungal infections in patients with advanced human immunodeficiency virus infection. N Engl J Med 1995;332:700–705.
115. Benson C, Ellner J. Mycobacterium avium complex infection and AIDS: Advances in theory and practice. Clin Infect Dis 1993;17:7–20.
116. Horsburgh C *Jr. Mycobacterium avium* complex infection in the acquired immunodeficiency syndrome. N Engl J Med 1991;324:332–338.
117. Peloquin C. *Mycobacterium avium* complex infection. Pharmacokinetic and pharmacodynamic considerations that may improve clinical outcomes. Clin Pharmacokinet 1997;32:132–144.
118. Shafran S, Singer J, Zarowny D, et al. A comparison of two regimens for the treatment of *Mycobacterium avium* complex bacteremia in AIDS: Rifabutin, ethambutol, and clarithromycin versus rifampin, ethambutol, clofazimine, and ciprofloxacin. N Engl J Med 1996;335:377–383.
119. Ward T, Rimland D, Kauffman C, et al. Randomized, open-label trial of azithromycin plus ethambutol vs. clarithromycin plus ethambutol as therapy for *Mycobacterium avium* complex bacteremia in patients with human immunodeficiency virus infection. Clin Infect Dis 1998;27:1278–1285.
120. Lundgren J, Masur H. New approaches to managing opportunistic infections. AIDS 1999;13:S227–S234.
121. Pierce M, Crampton S, Henry D, et al. A randomized trial of clarithromycin as prophylaxis against disseminated *Mycobacterium avium* complex infections in patients with advanced acquired immunodeficiency syndrome. N Engl J Med 1996;335:383–391.
122. Havlir D, Dube M, Sattler F, et al. Prophylaxis against disseminated *Mycobacterium avium* complex with weekly azithromycin, daily rifabutin, or both. N Engl J Med 1996;335:392–398.
123. Siegel F, Lopez C, Hammer B, et al. Severe acquired immunodeficiency in male homosexuals, manifested by chronic perianal ulcerative herpes simplex lesions. N Engl J Med 1981;305:1439–1444.
124. Wade J, Newton B, Flournoy N, et al. Oral acyclovir for prevention of herpes simplex virus reactivation after marrow transplantation. Ann Intern Med 1984;100:823–828.
125. Erlich K, Mills J, Chatis P, et al. Acyclovir-resistant herpes simples virus infections in patients with the acquired immunodeficiency syndrome. N Engl J Med 1989;320:293–296.
126. Erlich K, Jacobson M, Koehler J, et al. Foscarnet therapy for severe acyclovir-resistant herpes simples virus type-2 infections in patients with the acquired immunodeficiency syndrome. Ann Intern Med 1989;110:710–713.
127. Fletcher C, Englund J, Bean B, et al. Continuous infusion high-dose acyclovir for serious herpesvirus infections. Antimicrob Agents Chemother 1989;33:1375–1378.
128. Safrin S, Crumpacker C, Chatis P, et al. A controlled trial comparing foscarnet with vidarabine for acyclovir-resistant mucocutaneous herpes simplex virus in the acquired immunodeficiency syndrome. N Engl J Med 1991;325:551–555.
129. Melbye M, Grossman R, Goedert J, et al. Risk of AIDS after herpes zoster. Lancet 1987;1:728–731.
130. Huff J, Bean B, Balfour H Jr, et al. Therapy of herpes zoster with oral acyclovir. Am J Med 1988;85(suppl 2A):84–89.
131. Jacobson M, Berger T, Fikrig S, et al. Acyclovir-resistant varicella-zoster virus infection after chronic oral acyclovir therapy in patients with the acquired immunodeficiency syndrome. Ann Intern Med 1990;112: 187–191.
132. Quinnan G, Masur H, Rook A, et al. Herpesvirus infections in the acquired immunodeficiency syndrome. JAMA 1984;252:72–77.
133. Smith C. Local therapy for cytomegalovirus retinitis. Ann Pharmacother 1998;32:248–255.

134. Fletcher C, Balfour H Jr. Evaluation of ganciclovir for cytomegalovirus disease. Ann Pharmacother 1989;23:5–12.
135. Drew L, Ives D, Lalezari J, et al. Oral ganciclovir as maintenance treatment for cytomegalovirus retinitis in patients with AIDS. N Engl J Med 1995;333:615–620.
136. The Oral Ganciclovir European and Australian Cooperative Study Group. Intravenous versus oral ganciclovir: European/Australian comparative study of efficacy and safety in the prevention of cytomegalovirus retinitis recurrence in patients with AIDS. AIDS 1995;9:471–477.
137. Musch D, Martin D, Gordon J, et al. Treatment of cytomegalovirus retinitis with a sustained-release ganciclovir implant. N Engl J Med 1997;337:83–90.
138. Palestine A, Polis M, de Smet M, et al. A randomized controlled trial of foscarnet in the treatment of cytomegalovirus retinitis in patients with AIDS. Ann Intern Med 1991;115:665–673.
139. Polis M, de Smet M, Bard B, et al. Increased survival of a cohort of patients with acquired immunodeficiency syndrome and cytomegalovirus retinitis who received sodium phosphonoformate (foscarnet). Am J Med 1993;94:175–180.
140. Studies of the Ocular Complications of AIDS Research Group. Mortality in patients with the acquired immunodeficiency syndrome treated with either foscarnet or ganciclovir for cytomegalovirus retinitis. N Engl J Med 1992;326:213–220.
141. Deray G, Katlama C, Dohin E. Prevention of foscarnet nephrotoxicity. Ann Intern Med 1990;113:332.
142. Studies of Ocular Complications of AIDS Research Group in Collaboration with the AIDS Clinical Trial Group. Combination foscarnet and ganciclovir therapy vs monotherapy for the treatment of relapsed cytomegalovirus retinitis in patients with AIDS. Arch Ophthalmol 1996;114:23–33.
143. Studies of Ocular Complications of AIDS Research Group in Collaboration with the AIDS Clinical Trials Group. Parenteral cidofovir for cytomegalovirus retinitis in patients with AIDS: the HPMPC peripheral cytomegalovirus retinitis trial. Ann Intern Med 1997;126:264–274.
144. Dietrich D, Chachoua A, LaFleur F, et al. Ganciclovir treatment of gastrointestinal infections caused by cytomegalovirus in patients with AIDS. Rev Infect Dis 1988;10(suppl 3):S532–S537.
145. Blanshard C, Benhamou Y, Dohin E, et al. Treatment of AIDS-associated gastrointestinal cytomegalovirus infection with foscarnet and ganciclovir: A randomized comparison. J Infect Dis 1995;172:622–628.
146. Feinberg J, Hurwitz S, Cooper D, et al. A randomized, double-blind trial of valacyclovir prophylaxis for cytomegalovirus disease in patients with advanced human immunodeficiency virus infection. J Infect Dis 1998;177:48–56.
147. Fletcher C, Englund J, Edelman C, et al. Pharmacologic basis for high-dose oral acyclovir prophylaxis of cytomegalovirus disease in renal allograft recipients. Antimicrob Agents Chemother 1991;35:938–943.
148. Meyers J, Reed E, Shepp D, et al. Acyclovir for prevention of cytomegalovirus infection and disease after allogeneic marrow transplantation. N Engl J Med 1988;318:70–75.
149. Spector S, McKinley G, Lalezari J, et al. Oral ganciclovir for the prevention of cytomegalovirus disease in persons with AIDS. N Engl J Med 1996;334:1491–1497.

124

CANCER TREATMENT AND CHEMOTHERAPY

Carol McManus Balmer and Amy Wells Valley

Cancer is a group of more than 100 different diseases, characterized by uncontrolled cellular growth, local tissue invasion, and distant metastases.[1] It is second only to cardiovascular disease in causes of mortality in Americans. More than 1.2 million cases of cancer are diagnosed annually, and cancer claims about 553,000 lives in the United States each year.[2] The estimated incidence of common cancers and cancer-related deaths is illustrated in Fig. 124–1. The four most common cancers are prostate, breast, lung, and colorectal cancer. The most common cause of cancer-related deaths in the United States is lung cancer, which claims about 157,000 lives each year. These cancers are discussed in further detail in the chapters that follow.

The role of the pharmacist in the management of the cancer patient can be very diverse. Thorough knowledge of antineoplastic drug pharmacology and pharmacokinetics is essential to prevent and to manage many drug-induced toxicities. Supportive-care issues such as nutritional support, pain management, infection, and nausea and vomiting require application of both clinical and pharmacologic principles. Provision of drug information is another critical role for the oncology pharmacist. This service is provided to other health professionals and to patients and their families. Experienced pharmacists are able to fulfill these roles and to make valuable contributions to patient care in the oncology setting.

This chapter introduces the basic concepts of carcinogenesis, tumor growth, and cancer treatment, provides general information on the pharmacology and clinical use of the antineoplastic agents, and presents an overview of supportive care issues in the oncology patient.

ETIOLOGY OF CANCER

CARCINOGENESIS

The mechanism by which cancers occur is incompletely understood. A cancer, or neoplasm, is thought to develop from a cell in which the normal mechanisms for control of growth and proliferation are altered. Current evidence supports the concept of carcinogenesis as a multistage process that is genetically regulated (Fig. 124–2).[3–6] The first step in this process is *initiation,* which requires exposure of normal cells to carcinogenic substances. These carcinogens produce genetic damage that, if not repaired, results in irreversible cellular mutations. This mutated cell has an altered response to its environment and a selective growth advantage, giving it the potential to develop into a clonal population of neoplastic cells. During the second phase, known as *promotion,* carcinogens or other factors alter the environment to favor growth of the mutated cell population over normal cells. The primary difference between initiation and promotion is that promotion is a reversible process. In fact, because it is reversible, the promotion phase may be the target of future chemoprevention strategies, including changes in lifestyle and diet. At some point, however, the mutated cell becomes cancerous (*conversion or transformation*). Depending on the type of cancer, 5 to 20 years may elapse between the carcinogenic phases and the development of a clinically detectable cancer. The final stage of neoplastic growth, called *progression,* involves further genetic changes leading to increased cell proliferation. The critical elements of this phase include tumor invasion into local tissues and the development of metastases.

Substances that may act as carcinogens or initiators include chemical, physical, and biologic agents.[6,7] Exposure to chemicals may occur by virtue of occupational and environmental means, as well as lifestyle habits. The association of aniline dye exposure and bladder cancer is one such example. Benzene is known to cause some leukemias. Some drugs and hormones used for therapeutic purposes are also classified as carcinogenic chemicals (Table 124–1). Physical agents that act as carcinogens include ionizing radiation and ultraviolet light. These types of radiation induce mutations by forming free radicals that damage deoxyribonucleic acid (DNA) and other cellular components. Viruses are biologic agents that are associated with certain cancers. The Epstein-Barr virus is believed to be an important factor in the initiation of African Burkitt's lymphoma. Likewise, infection with hepatitis B virus is known to be a major cause of hepatocellular cancer. All the previously mentioned carcinogens, as well as age, gender, diet, growth factors, and chronic irritation, are among the factors considered to be promoters of carcinogenesis.

GENETIC BASIS OF CANCER

Cancer has been described as "a malady of genes, arising from genetic damage of diverse sorts and leading to distortions of either expression or biochemical function of genes."[8] In recent years, there has been marked progress in the understanding of the genetic changes that lead to the development of cancer, largely because of improvements in research techniques and new information generated as part of the human genome project.[3,6,7,9] There are two major classes of genes involved in carcinogenesis: oncogenes and tumor-suppressor genes. Figure 124–3 illustrates the effects of oncogenes and tumor-suppressor genes on normal cellular function. Oncogenes develop from normal genes, called protooncogenes, and may have important roles in all phases of carcinogenesis. Protooncogenes are present in all cells and are essential regulators of normal cellular functions, including the cell cycle. Genetic alteration of the protooncogene through point mutation, chromosomal rearrangement or gene amplification activates the oncogene. These genetic alterations may be caused by carcinogenic agents such as radiation, chemicals, or viruses (*somatic mutations*), or they may be inherited (*germ-line mutations*). Once activated, the oncogene produces either excessive amounts of the normal gene product or an abnormal gene product. The result is dysregulation of normal cell growth and proliferation, which imparts a distinct growth advantage to the cell and increases the probability of neoplastic

Leading Sites of New Cancer Cases and Deaths—2001 Estimates*

Cancer cases by site and sex: Male	Cancer cases by site and sex: Female	Cancer deaths by site and sex: Male	Cancer deaths by site and sex: Female
Prostate 198,100 (31%)	Breast 192,200 (31%)	Lung & bronchus 90,100 (31%)	Lung & bronchus 67,300 (25%)
Lung & bronchus 90,700 (14%)	Lung & bronchus 78,800 (13%)	Prostate 31,500 (11%)	Breast 40,200 (15%)
Colon and rectum 67,300 (10%)	Colon and rectum 68,100 (11%)	Colon and rectum 27,700 (10%)	Colon and rectum 29,000 (11%)
Urinary bladder 39,200 (6%)	Uterine corpus 38,300 (6%)	Pancreas 14,100 (5%)	Pancreas 14,800 (6%)
Non-Hodgkin's lymphoma 31,100 (5%)	Non-Hodgkin's lymphoma 25,100 (4%)	Non-Hodgkin's lymphoma 13,800 (5%)	Ovary 13,900 (5%)
Melanoma of the skin 29,000 (5%)	Ovary 23,400 (4%)	Leukemia 12,000 (4%)	Non-Hodgkin's lymphoma 12,500 (5%)
Oral cavity 20,200 (3%)	Melanoma of the skin 22,400 (4%)	Esophagus 9,500 (3%)	Leukemia 9,500 (4%)
Kidney 18,700 (3%)	Urinary bladder 15,100 (2%)	Liver 8,900 (3%)	Uterine corpus 6,600 (2%)
Leukemia 17,700 (3%)	Pancreas 15,000 (2%)	Urinary bladder 8,300 (3%)	Brain 5,900 (2%)
Pancreas 14,200 (2%)	Thyroid 14,900 (2%)	Kidney 7,500 (3%)	Stomach 5,400 (2%)
All sites 643,000 (100%)	All sites 625,000 (100%)	All sites 286,100 (100%)	All sites 267,300 (100%)

* Excludes basal and squamous cell skin cancers in situ carcinomas, except urinary bladder, American Cancer Society, Inc., Surveillance Research, 2001.

FIGURE 124–1. 2001 Cancer incidences (*left*) and deaths (*right*) in the United States for males and females. *(From American Cancer Society. Cancer Facts and Figures–2001. Atlanta, GA, American Cancer Society, 2001, with permission.)*

transformation. An example is the *myc* family of oncogenes. The normal gene product of *myc* acts as a signal for cellular proliferation. As an oncogene, the gene product is overexpressed or amplified, resulting in excessive cellular proliferation. Table 124–2 lists examples of other oncogenes and their classification by mechanism.

In contrast, tumor-suppressor genes regulate and inhibit inappropriate cellular growth and proliferation.[3,4,6,9] Gene loss or mutation results in loss of control over normal cell growth (see Fig. 124–3). Two common examples of tumor-suppressor genes are the retinoblastoma (Rb) and *p*53 genes. Mutation of *p*53 is one of the most common genetic changes associated with cancer, and is estimated to occur in half of all malignancies.[9] The normal gene product of *p*53 is responsible for negative regulation of the cell cycle, allowing the cell cycle to halt for repairs, corrections, and responses to other external signals. Inactivation of *p*53 removes this checkpoint, allowing mutations to occur. Mutation of *p*53 has been linked to a variety of

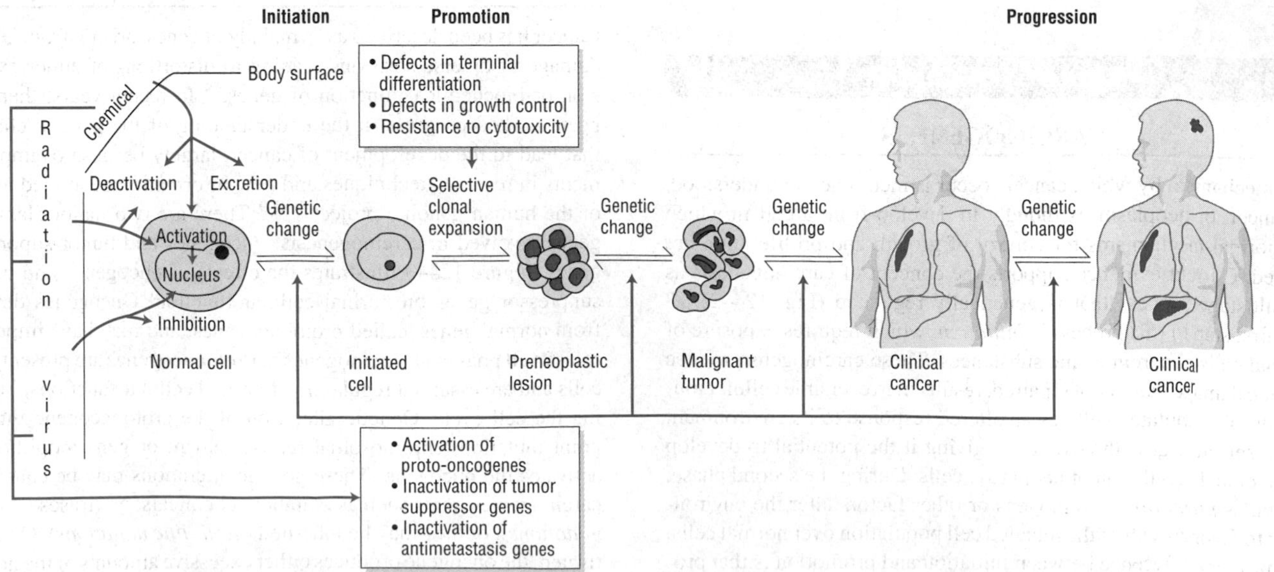

FIGURE 124–2. Multistage model of carcinogenesis. *(Adapted from Weston A, Harris CC. Chemical carcinogenesis. In: Bast RC, Kufe DW, Pollock RE, Weichselbaum RR, Holland JF, Frei E eds. Cancer Medicine, 5th ed. Lea & Febiger, 2000:186, with permission.)*

TABLE 124–1. Selected Drugs and Hormones Known to Cause Cancer in Humans

Drug or Hormone	Type of Cancer Caused
Alkylating agents (e.g., chlorambucil, mechlorethamine, melphalan, nitrosoureas)	Leukemia
Anabolic steroids	Liver
Analgesics containing phenacetin	Renal, urinary bladder
Anthracyclines (e.g., doxorubicin)	Leukemia
Antiestrogens (tamoxifen)	Endometrium
Coal tars (topical)	Skin
Estrogens	
Nonsteroidal (diethylstilbesterol)	Vagina/cervix, endometrium, breast, testes
Steroidal (estrogen replacement therapy, oral contraceptives)	Endometrium, breast, liver
Epipodophyllotoxins (etoposide, teniposide)	Leukemia
Immunosuppressive drugs (cyclosporine, azathioprine)	Lymphoma, skin
Oxazaphosphorines (cyclophosphamide, ifosfamide)	Urinary bladder, leukemia

Compiled from Refs. 5, 6, and 10.

malignancies, including brain tumors (astrocytoma); carcinomas of the breast, colon, lung, cervix and anus; and osteosarcoma. Another important function of *p*53 may be modulation of cytotoxic drug effects. Loss of *p*53 has been associated with antineoplastic drug resistance.

Another group of genes important in carcinogenesis is the DNA repair genes.[6] The normal function of these genes is to repair DNA that is damaged by environmental factors, or errors in DNA that occur during replication. If not corrected, these errors can result in mutations that activate oncogenes or inactivate tumor suppressor genes. As mutations in the genome accumulate, the risk for malignant transformation increases. The DNA repair genes have been classified as tumor suppressor genes, because a loss in their function results in increased risk for carcinogenesis. Deficiencies in DNA repair genes have been discovered in familial colon cancer (hereditary nonpolyposis colon cancer, or HNPCC) and breast cancer syndromes.

Oncogenes and tumor-suppressor genes provide the stimulatory and inhibitory signals that ultimately regulate the cell cycle.[9–11] These signals converge on a molecular system in the nucleus known as the cell cycle clock (see Fig. 124–3). The function of the clock in normal tissue is to integrate the signal input and to determine if the cell cycle should proceed. The clock is composed of a series of interacting proteins, the most important of which are cyclins and cyclin-dependent kinases (CDKs). Cyclins (especially cyclin D1) and CDKs promote entry into the cell cycle and are overexpressed in several cancers, including breast cancer. Inhibitors of CDK have been identified as important negative regulators of the cell cycle.

When the normal regulatory mechanisms for cellular growth fail, backup defense systems may be activated. The secondary defenses include apoptosis (programmed cell death or suicide) and cellular senescence (aging). Apoptosis (pronounced "ay-puh-TOE-sis") is a normal mechanism of cell death required for tissue homeostasis.[9–11] This process is regulated by oncogenes and tumor-suppressor genes and is also a mechanism of cellular death after exposure to cytotoxic agents. Overexpression of oncogenes responsible for apoptosis may produce an "immortal" cell, which has increased potential for malignancy. The *bcl*-2 oncogene is an example. The most common chromosomal abnormality found in lymphoid malignancies is the t(14;18) translocation. The *bcl*-2 protooncogene is normally located on chromosome 18. Translocation of this protooncogene to chromosome 14 in proximity to the immunoglobulin heavy chain gene leads to overexpression

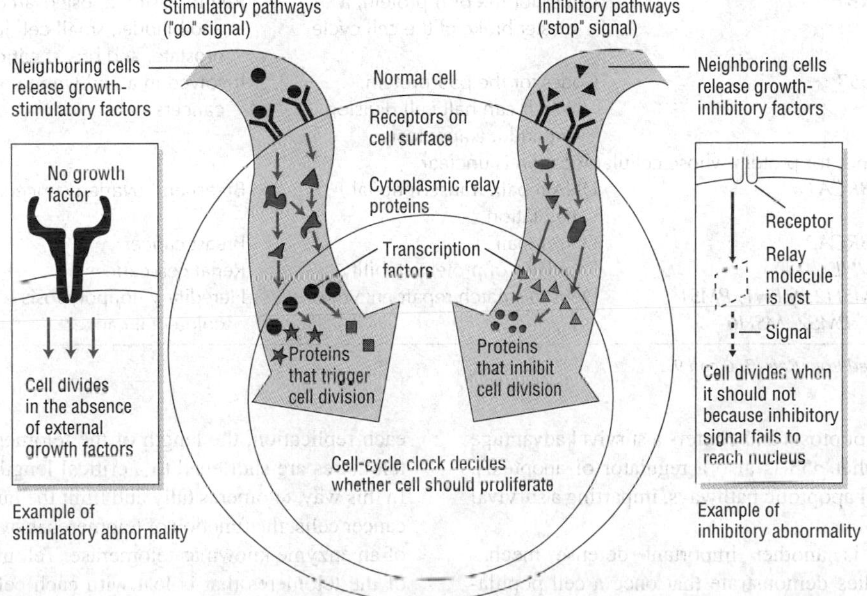

FIGURE 124–3. The effects of oncogenes and tumor-suppressor genes on cellular function. Signaling pathways in normal cells relay growth-controlling messages from the outer surface to the nucleus, where the cell-cycle clock receives these messages and decides whether the cell should divide. In cancer cells, genetic mutations can either activate oncogenes, resulting in excessive stimulation (too many "go" signals) or inactivate tumor-suppressor genes, resulting in loss of cell-cycle inhibition (no "stop" signals). Examples of abnormal stimulatory or inhibitory processes are provided in the boxes. *(Adapted from Ref. 7. with permission.)*

TABLE 124–2. Examples of Oncogenes and Tumor-Suppressor Genes

Gene	Function	Associated Human Cancers
ONCOGENES		
Genes for growth factors or their receptors		
EGFR or *ERB-B1*	Codes for epidermal growth factor (EGFR)	Glioblastoma, breast cancer, receptor squamous carcinoma
HER-2/NEU or *ERB-B2*	Codes for a growth factor receptor	Breast, salivary gland, prostate, bladder, and ovarian cancers
Genes for cytoplasmic relays in stimulatory signaling pathways		
K-RAS	Code for guanine nucleotide-proteins with GTPase activity	Lung, ovarian, colon, pancreatic binding cancers
N-RAS		Neuroblastoma, acute leukemia
Genes for transcription factors that activate growth-promoting genes		
c-MYC		Leukemia and breast, colon, gastric, and lung cancers
N-MYC		Neuroblastoma, small cell lung cancer, and glioblastoma
Genes for cytoplasmic kinases		
BCR-ABL	Codes for a nonreceptor tyrosine kinase	CML
Genes for other molecules		
BCL-2	Codes for a protein that blocks apoptosis.	Low grade B-cell lymphomas
CYCD-1	Codes for cyclin D1, a cell cycle clock stimulator.	Breast, head, and neck cancers
TUMOR-SUPPRESSOR GENES		
Genes for proteins in the cytoplasm		
APC		Colon and gastric cancer
NF-1	Codes for a protein that inhibits the stimulatory Ras protein	Neurofibroma, leukemia, and pheochromocytoma
NF-2		Meningioma, ependymoma, and schwannoma
Genes for proteins in the nucleus		
P16/INK4A	Codes for the cyclin-dependent kinase inhibitor	Involved in a wide range of cancers
RB1	Codes for the pRB protein, a master brake of the cell cycle	Retinoblastoma, osteosarcoma, and bladder, small cell lung, prostate, and breast cancers
p53	Codes for the p53 protein, which can halt cell division and induce apoptosis	Involved in a wide range of cancers
Genes for protein whose cellular location is unclear		
BRCA1	DNA repair, transcriptional regulation	Breast and ovarian cancers
BRCA2	DNA repair	Breast cancer
VHL	Regulator of protein stability	Renal cell cancer
MSH2, MLH1, PMS1, PMS2, MSH6	DNA mismatch repair enzymes	Hereditary nonpolyposis colorectal cancer

Adapted from Refs. 3, 6 and 9.

of *bcl*-2, which decreases apoptosis and confers a survival advantage to the cell. Studies show that *p*53 is also a regulator of apoptosis. Loss of *p*53 disrupts normal apoptotic pathways, imparting a survival advantage to the cell.

Cellular senescence is another important defense mechanism.[6,9,10] Laboratory studies demonstrate that once a cell population has undergone a preset number of doublings, growth stops and cells die. This is known as senescence. Subsequent research has determined that this process is regulated by telomeres. Telomeres are the DNA segments or caps at the end of chromosomes. They are responsible for protecting the end of the DNA from damage. With each replication, the length of the telomeres is shortened. After the telomeres are shortened to a critical length, senescence is triggered. In this way, telomeres tally and limit the number of cell doublings. In cancer cells, the function of telomeres is overcome by overexpression of an enzyme known as telomerase. Telomerase replaces the portion of the telomeres that is lost with each cell division, thereby avoiding senescence and permitting an infinite number of cell doublings. Telomerase is a target for antineoplastic drug development.

As information regarding the role of oncogenes and tumor-suppressor genes accumulated, it became evident that a single mutation was probably not sufficient to initiate cancer.[5–7,9] Scientists

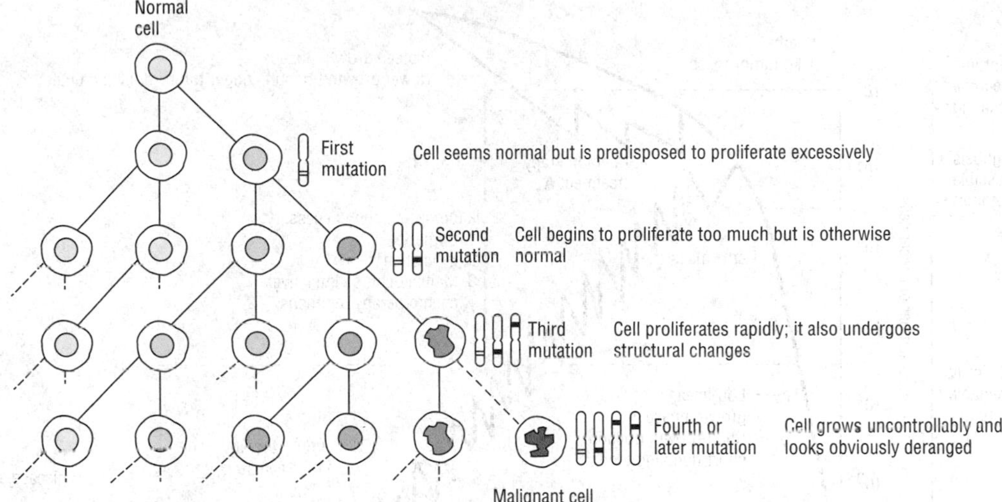

FIGURE 124–4. Emergence of a cancer cell from a normal cell is thought to occur through a process known as clonal evolution. First, one daughter cell inherits or acquires a cancer-promoting mutation and passes the defect to its progeny and all future generations. At some point, one of the descendants acquires a second mutation, and a later descendant acquires a third, and so on. Eventually, some cell accumulates enough mutations to cross the threshold to cancer. *(From Cavanee WK, White RL. The genetic basis of cancer. Sci Am 1995;72–79, with permission.)*

postulated that combinations of mutations were required for carcinogenesis and that each mutation was inherited by the next generation of cells (Fig. 124–4). Thus, in an established tumor there may be several detectable genetic mutations. Early mutations are found in both premalignant lesions and in established tumors, whereas later mutations are found only in the established tumor. This theory of sequential genetic mutations resulting in cancer has been best demonstrated in colon cancer and in brain tumors. In colon cancer, the initial genetic mutation is believed to be loss of the APC (adenomatous polyposis coli) gene, which results in formation of a small benign polyp. Oncogenic mutation of the *ras* gene is often the next step, leading to enlargement of the polyp. Loss of function of DNA mismatch repair enzymes may occur at many points in the progression of malignant transformation. Loss of the *p*53 gene and another gene, believed to be the "deleted in colorectal cancer" (DCC) gene, complete the transformation into a malignant lesion. Loss of p53 is thought to be a late event in the development and progression of the malignancy.

Identification of genes and other proteins involved in carcinogenesis has several important clinical implications. In the future, they may be used in cancer screening to identify individuals at increased risk for cancer and in cancer treatment to design new anticancer agents and gene therapies. Specific genetic abnormalities are so commonly associated with some types of cancers that the presence of that abnormality aids in the diagnosis of that cancer. If the presence of these genes (i.e., gene expression profile) can reliably predict the clinical course of a cancer or response to certain cancer therapies, then genetic analysis may also become an important prognostic and treatment decision tool.[12]

PRINCIPLES OF TUMOR GROWTH

The study of tumor growth forms the foundation for many of the basic principles of modern cancer chemotherapy. The growth of most tumors is illustrated by the Gompertzian tumor growth curve (Fig. 124–5).[6,11,13] Gompertz was a German insurance actuary who described the relationship between age and expected death. This mathematical model also approximates tumor-cell proliferation. In the early stages, tumor growth is exponential, which means that the tumor takes a constant amount of time to double its size. During this early phase, a large portion of the tumor cells is actively dividing. This population of cells is called the *growth fraction.* The doubling time, or time required for the tumor to double in size, is very short. Because most anticancer drugs have greater effect on rapidly dividing cells, tumors are most sensitive to the effects of chemotherapy when the tumor is small and the growth fraction is high. However, as the tumor grows, the doubling time is slowed.[11,13] The growth fraction is decreased, probably owing to the tumor outgrowing its blood and nutrient supply or the inability of blood and nutrients to diffuse throughout the tumor mass. Wide variability exists in measured doubling times for different cancers. The doubling time of most solid tumors is approximately 2 to 3 months. However, some tumors have doubling times of only days (e.g., high-grade or aggressive lymphomas) and others have even longer doubling times (e.g., some salivary gland tumors).[6]

Figure 124–5 also illustrates the impact of tumor burden. It takes about 10^9 cancer cells (1-g mass, 1 cm in diameter) for a tumor to be clinically detectable by palpation or radiography. Such a tumor has undergone approximately 30 doublings in cell number. It only takes 10 additional doublings for this 1-g mass to reach 1 kg in size. A tumor possessing 10^{12} cancer cells (1-kg mass) is considered lethal. Thus, a tumor is clinically undetectable for most of its life span. Tumor burden also impacts response to chemotherapy. The cell kill hypothesis states that a certain percentage of cancer cells (not a certain number of cells) will be killed with each course of chemotherapy. For example, if a tumor consists of 1,000 cancer cells and the chemotherapy regimen kills 90% of the cells, then 10% or 100 cancer cells would remain. The second chemotherapy course kills another 90% of cells, and again only 10% or 10 cells remain. According to this hypothesis, the tumor burden will never reach absolute zero. Tumors consisting of less than 10^4 cells are believed to be small enough for elimination by host factors, including immunologic mechanisms, and these

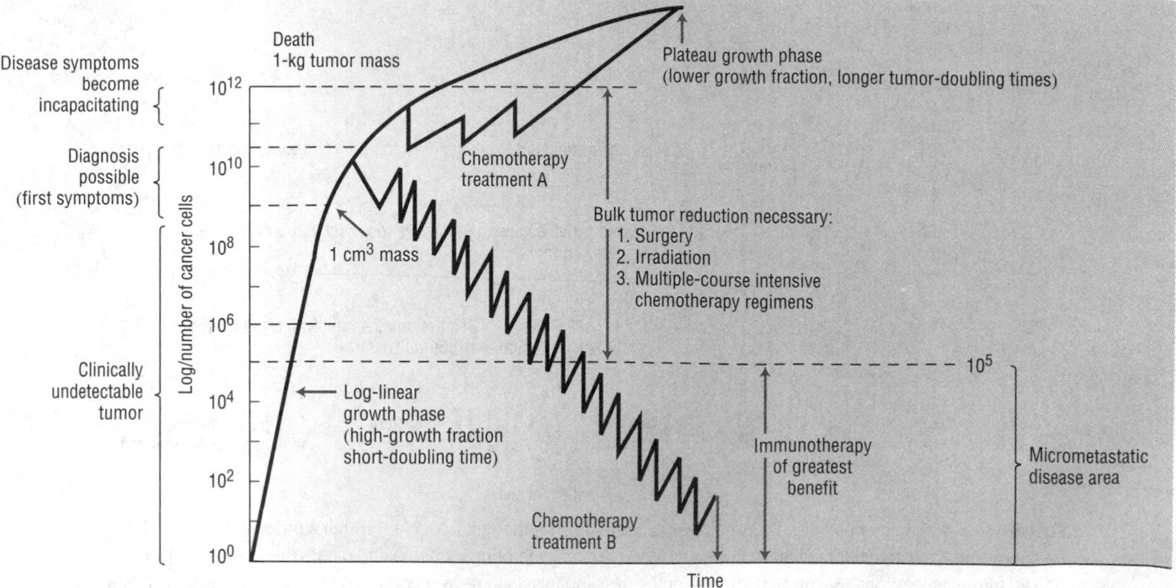

FIGURE 124–5. Gompertzian kinetics tumor-growth curve. Relationship to symptoms, diagnosis, and various treatment regimens. *(From Buick RN. Cellular basis of chemotherapy. In: Dorr RT, Von Hoff DD, eds. Cancer Chemotherapy Handbook, 2nd ed. New York, Elsevier, 1994:8, with permission.)*

factors must be in place for a cure to be possible. The limitations of this theory are that it assumes all cancers are equally responsive and that drug resistance and metastases do not occur.[1,6,11,13]

INVASION AND METASTASIS

Metastasis is the spread of neoplastic cells from the primary tumor site to distant sites.[6,14] Despite advances in diagnostic techniques and screening for cancer, many patients have detectable metastatic disease at diagnosis. Once clinically evident distant metastases are present, cancers are seldom curable. Newly diagnosed cancer patients may also have microscopic cancer metastases. Although clinically undetectable, these small clusters of diseased cells must be present, because many patients subsequently relapse at distant sites despite removal of the primary tumor. Some patients with micrometastatic disease may be cured with systemic chemotherapy.

The two primary pathways of metastasis are hematogenous and lymphatic. Other, less-common, modes of disease spread include dissemination via cerebrospinal fluid and transabdominal spread within the peritoneal cavity. Tumors are constantly shedding neoplastic cells into the systemic circulation or surrounding lymphatics. This process may begin early in the life of the tumor and often increases with time. The time course for metastasis depends largely on the biology of the tumor. Breast cancer, for example, tends to metastasize very early. Not all of the shed cancer cells, or "seeds," result in a metastatic lesion. The "seed" must first find the appropriate "soil," or an environment suitable for growth.[14] This process is illustrated in the diverse patterns of metastasis that are characteristic of individual types of cancer. An example is prostate cancer, which commonly metastasizes to bone, but rarely to the brain.

The process of invasion and metastasis involves several essential steps (Fig. 124–6). After neoplastic transformation, the malignant cells and surrounding host tissue secrete substances that stimulate the formation of new blood vessels to provide oxygen and nutrients. This process is known as *angiogenesis* or *neovascularization.*[15] Tumor cells must then detach from the primary mass and invade surrounding blood and lymph vessels. The tumor cells or cell aggregates detach and embolize through these vessels, but most do not survive circulation. The disseminated cells must then attach to the vascular endothelium. The cells may proliferate within the lumen of the vessel, but most commonly extravasate into the surrounding tissue. The local microenvironment may provide growth factors that can serve as "fertilizer" to potentiate the proliferation of the metastasis. At every step of the way, the potential metastatic cell must fight the host immune system. Last, the metastasis must again initiate angiogenesis to ensure

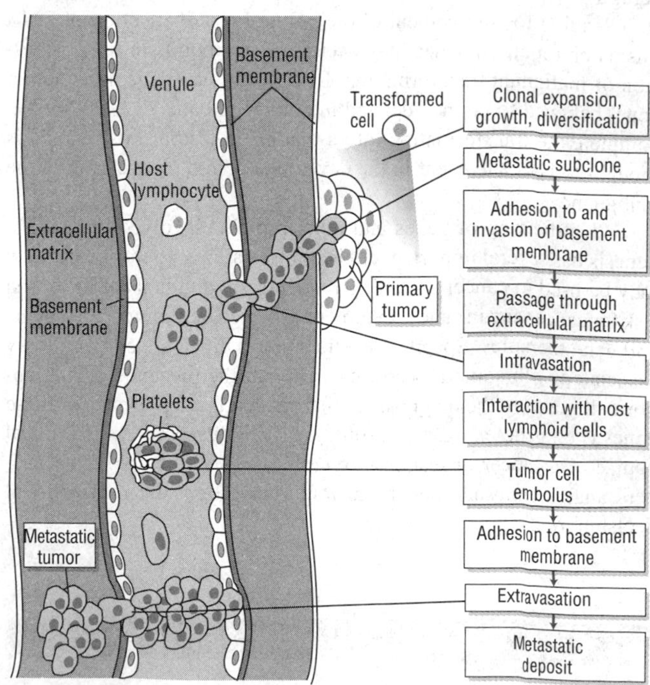

FIGURE 124–6. The process of developing a cancer metastasis. *(From Kumar V, Cotran RS, Robbins SL. Neoplasia. In: Kumar V, Cotran RS, Robbins SL, eds. Robbins' Pathologic Basis of Disease. Philadelphia, WB Saunders, 1997:303, with permission.)*

continued growth and proliferation. Because angiogenesis has been recognized as a critical element in primary tumor growth as well as metastasis, it has become a target for development of new anticancer agents.

PATHOLOGY OF CANCER

TUMOR CHARACTERISTICS

Tumors may be either benign or malignant. Benign tumors are noncancerous growths that are often encapsulated, localized, and indolent. Cells of benign tumors resemble the cells from which they developed. These masses seldom metastasize and, once removed, they rarely recur. In contrast, malignant tumors invade and destroy the surrounding tissue. The cells of malignant tumors are genetically unstable, and loss of normal cell architecture results in cells that are atypical of their tissue or cell of origin. These cells lose the ability to perform their usual functions. This loss of structure and function is defined as anaplasia. In contrast to benign tumors, malignant tumors tend to metastasize and, consequently, recurrences are common after removal or destruction of the primary tumor.

TUMOR ORIGIN

Tumors may arise from any of four basic tissue types: epithelial tissue, connective tissue (i.e., muscle, bone, and cartilage), lymphoid tissue, and nerve tissue. Although some malignant cells are atypical of their cells of origin, the involved cells usually retain enough of their parent's traits to identify their origin. Benign tumors are named by adding the suffix *-oma* to the name of the cell type. Hence, adenomas are benign growths of glandular origin, or growths that exhibit a glandular pattern. Table 124–3 lists common tumor nomenclature by tissue type.[6]

Some cancers are preceded by cellular changes that are abnormal, but not yet malignant. Correction of these early changes could potentially prevent the occurrence of a cancer. Precancerous lesions may be described as consisting of either hyperplastic or dysplastic cells. Hyperplasia is an increase in the number of cells in a particular tissue or organ, which results in an increased size of the organ. It should not be confused with hypertrophy, which is an increase in the size of the individual cells. Hyperplasia occurs in response to a stimulus and reverses when the stimulus is removed. Dysplasia is defined as an abnormal change in the size, shape, or organization of cells or tissues. Hyperplasia and dysplasia may precede the appearance of a cancer by several months or years.

Malignant cells are divided into those of epithelial origin or the other tissue types. Carcinomas are malignant growths arising from epithelial cells. Malignant growths of muscle or connective tissue are called sarcomas. Therefore, an adenocarcinoma is a malignant tumor arising from glandular tissue. Another term used frequently in the description of malignancy is *carcinoma in situ*. In this instance, the cancer is limited to the epithelial cells of origin; it has not yet invaded the basement membrane. Carcinoma *in situ* is a preinvasive stage of malignancy, and most tumors have progressed well beyond this stage at diagnosis. Like all classification systems, there are exceptions to these rules. Malignancies of hematologic origin are classified separately. Leukemias and lymphomas are discussed in later chapters.

DIAGNOSIS AND STAGING

SCREENING

Because cancers are most curable with surgery or radiation before they have metastasized, early detection and treatment have obvious potential benefit. In addition, small tumors are more responsive to chemotherapy, as discussed previously. Early diagnosis is difficult for many cancers because they do not produce clinical signs or symptoms until they have become large or have metastasized. Lack of effective screening methods for some cancers and inaccessibility of some anatomic sites further complicate the process. Education of the public on the early warning signs of common cancers is extremely important for facilitating early detection. For some cancers, effective screening procedures do exist. The Papanicolaou (Pap) smear test, for example, is an effective tool to detect cervical cancer in its early stages. Self-examination of the breasts in women and of the

TABLE 124–3. Tumor Classification by Tissue Type

Tissue of Origin	Benign	Malignant
Epithelial		
Surface epithelium	Papilloma	Carcinoma (squamous, epidermoid)
Glandular tissue	Adenoma	Adenocarcinoma
Connective tissue		
Fibrous tissue	Fibroma	Fibrosarcoma
Bone	Osteoma	Osteosarcoma
Smooth muscle	Leiomyoma	Leiomyosarcoma
Striated muscle	Rhabdomyoma	Rhabdomyosarcoma
Fat	Lipoma	Liposarcoma
Lymphoid tissue and hematopoietic cells		
Bone marrow elements		Leukemias
Lymphoid tissue		Hodgkin's disease, non-Hodgkin's lymphoma
Plasma cell		Multiple myeloma
Neural tissue		
Glial tissue	"Benign" gliomas	Glioblastoma multiforme, astrocytoma
Nerve sheath	Neurofibroma	Neurofibrosarcoma
Melanocytes	Pigmented nevus (mole)	Malignant melanoma
Mixed tumors		
Gonadal tissue	Teratoma	Teratocarcinoma

Adapted from Ref. 6.

TABLE 124–4. Recommendations for Early Detection of Cancer in Average Risk, Asymptomatic Persons

Disease	Test or Procedure	Sex	Age (y)	Frequency
Breast cancer	Breast self-examination	F	20 and older	Monthly
	Clinical breast examination	F	20–39	Every 3 years
			40 and older	Every year
	Mammography	F	40 and older	Every year
Cervical cancer	Pap test and pelvic examination	F	18 and older; younger than 18 if sexually active	Every year[a]
Colon and rectum cancer	Fecal occult blood test and	M and F	50 and older	Every year
	Flexible sigmoidoscopy[b] OR	M and F	50 and older	Every 5 years
	Colonoscopy, OR	M and F	50 and older	Every 10 years
	Double contrast barium enema	M and F	50 and older	Every 5 years
Prostate cancer	Digital rectal exam and	M	50 and older	Every year[c]
	Prostate-specific antigen (PSA) blood test	M	50 and older	Every year[c]
Cancer-related check-up	Health counseling and physical exam[d]	M and F	20–40	Every 3 years
			40 and older	Every year

[a]After three negative annual examinations, the Pap test may be done at less frequent intervals, as determined by the physician.

[b]Flexible sigmoidoscopy together with fecal occult blood test (FOBT) is preferable to either test alone, although annual FOBT alone and flexible sigmoidoscopy every 5 years without FOBT has some benefit. Digital rectal examination should be performed prior to insertion of sigmoidoscope or colonoscope.

[c]Beginning at age 50, men with a life expectancy of at least 10 years should discuss the need for Prostate-specific antigen (PSA) testing and digital rectal examination (DRE) with their health care provider. Information should be provided on benefits and limitations of testing.

[d]To include examination for cancers of the mouth, thyroid, testicles, skin, lymph nodes, prostate, and ovaries, as well as health counseling about tobacco, sun exposure, diet and nutrition, risk factors, sexual practices, and environmental and occupational exposures.

From The American Cancer Society recommendations for the early detection of cancer in average risk, asymptomatic people. CA Cancer J Clin 2001;51:40.

testicles in men may lead to early diagnosis of cancers in these organs. The American Cancer Society has published guidelines for routine screening examinations. Table 124–4 lists its recommendations.[16]

DIAGNOSIS

The presenting signs and symptoms of cancer vary widely and depend on the type of cancer. The presentation in adults may include any of cancer's seven warning signs (Table 124–5), as well as pain or loss of appetite.[17] The warning signs of cancer in children are different, and reflect the types of tumors more common in this patient population (Table 124–6).[18] Even with increased public awareness, the fear of a cancer diagnosis can deter patients from seeking medical attention. The definitive diagnosis of cancer relies on the procurement of a sample of the tissue or cells suspected of malignancy and pathologic assessment of this sample. This sample can be obtained by numerous methods, including biopsy, exfoliative cytology, or fine-needle aspiration. A tissue diagnosis is essential, because many benign conditions can masquerade as cancer. Definitive treatment should not begin without a pathologic diagnosis.

TABLE 124–5. Cancer's Seven Warning Signs

Change in bowel or bladder habits
A sore that does not heal
Unusual bleeding or discharge
Thickening or lump in breast or elsewhere
Indigestion or difficulty in swallowing
Obvious change in wart or mole
Nagging cough or hoarseness

If YOU have a warning signal, see your doctor!

STAGING

In addition to tissue diagnosis, tumors should be staged to determine the extent of disease before any definitive treatment is initiated.[19] The process is dictated by knowledge of the biology of the tumor and by the signs and symptoms elicited in the history and physical examination. Staging provides information on prognosis and guides treatment selection. After treatment is implemented, the staging workup is usually repeated to evaluate the effectiveness of the treatment. Uniform staging criteria are imperative in clinical research aimed at evaluating cancer treatment regimens. Staging has been valuable in learning more about the biology of various tumor types. A staging workup may involve x-rays, computed tomography (CT) scans, magnetic resonance imaging (MRI), ultrasounds, bone-marrow biopsies, bone scans,

TABLE 124–6. Cancer's Warning Signs in Children

Continued, unexplained weight loss
Headaches with vomiting in the morning
Increased swelling or persistent pain in bones or joints
Lump or mass in abdomen, neck, or elsewhere
Development of a whitish appearance in the pupil of the eye
Recurrent fevers not caused by infections
Excessive bruising or bleeding
Noticeable paleness or prolonged tiredness

From Ref. 18.

lumbar puncture, and a variety of laboratory tests, including appropriate tumor markers. Some cancers produce antigens, or other substances, that are characteristic of that particular cancer. These so-called tumor markers are often nonspecific and may be elevated in many different cancer types, or in patients with nonmalignant diseases. As a result, tumor markers are generally more useful for monitoring response and detecting recurrence than as diagnostic tools. Examples are the measure of human chorionic gonadotropin (hCG) and α-fetoprotein in patients with testicular cancer, or prostate-specific antigen (PSA) in prostate cancer.[6]

The most commonly applied staging system for solid tumors is the TNM classification, where T = tumor, N = node, and M = metastases. A numerical value is assigned to each letter to indicate the size or extent of disease. The designated rating for tumor describes the size of the primary mass and ranges from T_1 to T_4. Carcinoma *in situ* is designated T_{is}. Nodes are described in terms of the extent and quality of nodal involvement (N_0 to N_3). Metastases are scored depending on their presence or absence (M_0 or M_1). To simplify the staging process, most cancers are classified according to extent of disease by a numerical system involving stages I through IV. Stage I usually indicates localized tumor, stages II and III represent local and regional extension of disease, and stage IV denotes the presence of distant metastases. The assigned TNM rating translates into a particular stage classification. For example, $T_3N_1M_0$ tumor describes a moderate- to large-sized primary mass, with regional lymph node involvement and no distant metastases, and for most cancers is stage III. The criteria for classifying disease extent are quite specific for each different type of cancer. For some tumors, alternative alphabetical systems (stage A, B, C, or D) are used in clinical practice. Table 124–7 provides an example of the staging system for colorectal cancer.[19]

TABLE 124–7. TNM Staging Classification System for Colorectal Cancer

Primary Tumor (T)
- T_x Primary tumor cannot be assessed
- T_0 No evidence of primary tumor
- T_{is} Carcinoma *in situ:* intraepithelial or invasion of lamina propria
- T_1 Tumor invades submucosa
- T_2 Tumor invades muscularis propria
- T_3 Tumor invades through the muscularis propria into the subserosa, or into nonperitonealized pericolic or perirectal tissues
- T_4 Tumor perforates the visceral peritoneum, or directly invades other organs or structures

Regional Lymph Nodes (N)
- N_x Regional lymph nodes cannot be assessed
- N_0 No regional lymph node metastasis
- N_1 Metastasis in one to three pericolic or perirectal lymph nodes
- N_2 Metastasis in four or more pericolic or perirectal lymph nodes

Distant Metastasis (M)
- M_x Presence of distant metastasis cannot be assessed
- M_0 No distant metastasis
- M_1 Distant metastasis

Stage	Grouping			Dukes	Modified Astler-Collier
Stage 0	T_{is}	N_0	M_0		
Stage I	T_1	N_0	M_0	A	A
	T_2	N_0	M_0	A	B1
Stage II	T_3	N_0	M_0	B	B2
	T_4	N_0	M_0	B	B2, B3
Stage III	Any T	N_1	M_0	C	C1-3
	Any T	N_2	M_0	C	C1-3
Stage IV	Any T	Any N	M_1	"D"	D

From Ref. 19.

▶ TREATMENT: Modalities of Cancer Treatment

Four primary modalities are employed in the approach to cancer treatment: surgery, radiation, chemotherapy, and biologic therapy.[20] The oldest of these is surgery, which plays a major role in the diagnosis and treatment of cancer. Surgery remains the treatment of choice for most solid tumors diagnosed in the early stages. Radiation therapy was first used for cancer treatment in the late 1800s and remains a mainstay in the management of cancer. Although very effective for treating many types of cancer, surgery and radiation are local treatments. These modalities are likely to produce a cure in patients with truly localized disease. But because most patients with cancer have metastatic disease at diagnosis, localized therapies often fail to completely eliminate the cancer. In addition, systemic diseases such as leukemia cannot be treated with a localized modality. Chemotherapy (including hormonal therapy) accesses the systemic circulation and can theoretically treat the primary tumor, as well as any metastatic disease. Biologic therapy, also known as immunotherapy, provides another means to deliver systemic anticancer therapy. This modality usually involves stimulating the host's immune system to fight the cancer. Many of the agents in this category are naturally occurring cytokines, which have been produced with recombinant-DNA technology. Examples of agents used in biologic therapy include tumor vaccines, interferons (IFNs), interleukins (ILs), and monoclonal antibodies.

Many cancers appear to be eliminated by surgery or radiation. However, the high incidence of later recurrence implies that the primary tumor began to metastasize before it was removed. These early metastases are too small to detect with currently available diagnostic tests and are known as micrometastases. Adjuvant therapy is defined as the use of systemic agents to eradicate micrometastatic disease following localized modalities such as surgery or radiation or both. The hope is that systemic therapy given in this setting will reduce subsequent recurrence rates and prolong long-term survival. Thus, adjuvant therapy is given to patients with potentially curable malignancies, who have no clinically detectable disease after surgery or radiation. Because adjuvant therapy is given at a time that the cancer is undetectable, its effectiveness cannot be measured by response rates; instead, it is evaluated by recurrence rates and survival. The value of adjuvant therapy is best established in colorectal and breast cancers. Chemotherapy may also be given in the neoadjuvant or preoperative setting. The goals in this instance are to make other treatment modalities more effective by reducing tumor burden, as well as to destroy micrometastases. For example, in head and neck cancer, neoadjuvant chemotherapy is employed in an attempt to shrink large tumors and to make them more amenable to later surgical resection, and possibly spare critical organs, such as the larynx.

The management of most types of cancer involves the use of combined modalities. Early stage breast cancer is a good example of the use of a combined-modality approach. The primary tumor is removed surgically, and radiation therapy is delivered to the remaining breast (after lumpectomy) or to the axilla (if there is marked lymph node involvement). Adjuvant chemotherapy and/or hormonal therapy is then administered to eradicate any micrometastatic disease.

▶ TREATMENT: Principles of Chemotherapy

PURPOSES OF CHEMOTHERAPY

The era of modern cancer chemotherapy was born in 1941, when Goodman and Gilman first administered nitrogen mustard to patients with lymphoma.[21] Since that time, numerous antineoplastic agents have been developed, and a variety of chemotherapy regimens have been investigated in every type of cancer. Table 124–8 lists tumors and their responsiveness to chemotherapy.[13,22] Cancer chemotherapy may be indicated as a primary, palliative, adjuvant, or neoadjuvant treatment modality. Treatment with cytotoxic drugs is the primary curative modality for a few diseases, including leukemias, choriocarcinomas, and testicular cancer. Most solid tumors are not curable with chemotherapy alone, either because of the biology of the tumor or because of advanced disease at presentation. Chemotherapy in this setting is often initiated for palliative purposes. It is often possible to decrease tumor size or to retard growth enough to reduce untoward symptoms caused by the tumor. Adjuvant and neoadjuvant chemotherapy are defined in the previous section.

RESPONSE CRITERIA

The response to chemotherapy and other treatment modalities may be described as a cure, complete response, partial response, stable disease, or progression.[22,23] These terms are used routinely in oncology to define the response to chemotherapy and other treatment modalities. A cure implies that the patient is entirely free of disease and has the same life expectancy as a cancer-free individual. Although there is no way to be absolutely certain that an individual patient is cured, a stable plateau in the survival curve after cancer treatment is taken as evidence of cure. For most cancers, the survival curves have plateaued by about 5 years. Thus, 5 years of survival without disease recurrence is equated with a cure. However, there are some malignancies, such as breast cancer and melanoma, for example, in which patients are still at significant risk for relapse after 5 years.

Complete response (CR) means complete disappearance of all cancer without evidence of new disease for at least 1 month after treatment. The terms "cure" and "CR" are not synonymous. Although an individual must have a CR to be cured, many individuals who achieve a CR will eventually relapse. *A partial response* (PR) is defined as a 50% or greater decrease in the tumor size or other objective disease markers, and no evidence of any new disease for at least 1 month. Overall objective response rates for a given treatment are determined by adding the CR and PR rates. Despite the small changes in tumor size, some patients may experience subjective improvement in the symptoms caused by their cancer. Although clinically important, this does not indicate an objective response. The term *clinical benefit response* was recently coined; it refers to patients who have clinical

TABLE 124–8. The Role of Chemotherapy in the Treatment of Cancer

Chemotherapy used alone with curative intent	
Acute lymphocytic leukemia	Acute nonlymphocytic (myelogenous) leukemia
Burkitt's lymphoma	Diffuse large cell lymphoma
Hodgkin's disease	Testicular cancer
Choriocarcinoma (gestational trophoblastic neoplasm)	
Chemotherapy used as adjuvant therapy with curative intent	
Breast cancer	Colorectal cancer
Ewing's sarcoma	Osteosarcoma
Wilm's tumor	Ovarian cancer
Chemotherapy used as neoadjuvant therapy	
Anal carcinoma*	Bladder cancer
Breast cancer (locally advanced)*	Cervical cancer
Esophageal cancer	Head and neck cancers*
Osteosarcoma*	Rectal cancer
Soft tissue sarcoma*	
Chemotherapy used to palliate symptoms in advanced disease	
Bladder cancer	Brain tumors
Breast cancer*	Carcinoid tumors
Cervical cancer	Chronic lymphocytic leukemia
Chronic myelogenous leukemia*	Colorectal cancer
Endometrial cancer	Esophageal cancer
Gastric cancer	Head and neck cancers
Hairy cell leukemia*	Kaposi's sarcoma
Low grade lymphomas	Metastatic melanoma
Multiple myeloma*	Mycosis fungoides
Neuroblastoma*	Nonsmall cell lung cancer
Osteosarcoma	Ovarian cancer*
Pancreatic cancer	Prostate cancer
Small cell lung cancer*	Soft tissue sarcoma
Chemotherapy has little or no effect on palliation	
Hepatocellular cancer	Renal cell carcinoma
Thyroid cancer	

*Significant increase in survival is achieved.
Adapted from Refs. 6, 13, and 22.

benefit as measured by decreases in pain or analgesic consumption, or improved quality of life or performance status. A patient whose tumor size neither grows nor shrinks by more than 25% has stable disease. Progression of disease is defined as a 25% increase in the tumor size or the development of any new lesions while receiving treatment. These response definitions are applicable to solid tumors, but diseases such as leukemias and multiple myeloma are not characterized by discrete, measurable masses. Responses in these diseases are measured by elimination of abnormal cells (e.g., return to normal hematology parameters and normal bone marrow in leukemia), return of tumor markers to normal levels (e.g., normal serum protein electrophoresis in multiple myeloma), disappearance of pleural or peritoneal effusions, or improved function of affected organs (e.g., improved renal function after obstructive uropathy).

FACTORS AFFECTING RESPONSE TO CHEMOTHERAPY

These include tumor burden, tumor-cell heterogeneity, drug resistance, dose intensity, and patient-specific factors. The significance of tumor burden has been discussed earlier. Tumors consist of a heterogeneous population of cell types. Because of the genetic instability of cancer cells compared to normal cells, mutations commonly occur during cell division. Large tumors have undergone many cell divisions and express multiple cell mutations resulting in genetically varied cell populations.[6,13,22] In 1979, Goldie and Coldman proposed that these cytogenetic changes were not completely random and were highly associated with the development of the ability of tumors to resist drug action.[1,6,13] The probability of developing resistant cell populations increases as tumor size increases. It is believed that a small percentage of resistant cancer cells may survive initial chemotherapy. Resistant populations later proliferate and eventually become the dominant cell types. This explains the common pattern of an initial response to chemotherapy, followed by progressive tumor regrowth despite continuing the same treatment regimen.

Drug resistance may be either an acquired or inherited property of a neoplastic cell. Mechanisms of drug resistance include decreased activation of prodrugs, decreased uptake of drugs secondary to alterations in drug transport systems, changes in target enzymes, alterations in the cell's ability to repair drug-induced damage, and increased drug inactivation.[6,13,20] Research in the area of drug resistance currently focuses on pleiotropic drug resistance or multidrug resistance (MDR).[13,20,24,25] When some cancer cells are exposed to increasing concentrations of a specific antineoplastic agent *in vitro*, they become resistant to that agent. Surprisingly, these same cells also become resistant to other structurally unrelated antineoplastic agents; that is, they are multidrug resistant. Cytotoxic agents derived from natural products, such as the anthracyclines, actinomycin D, mitomycin C, the vinca alkaloids, the epipodophyllotoxins, and the taxanes, produce MDR. The resistant cancer cells possess a membrane-associated protein known as P170 or P-glycoprotein, which appears to enhance the export of toxins, such as chemotherapy agents, out of the cell (Fig. 124–7). The gene that encodes for P-glycoprotein is known as the *mdr-1* gene. Expression of this gene is amplified in cells that are resistant to the natural products listed previously. P-glycoprotein is also found in high concentrations in tumors that are traditionally resistant to chemotherapy (e.g., renal cell and non–small cell lung cancers) and thus may also be an important mechanism of intrinsic or inherited drug resistance. Several drugs have been investigated as possible inhibitors of this efflux pump, such as the calcium channel blockers, quinidine, cyclosporine, and the phenothiazines. Another efflux pump, known as the multidrug resistance-associated protein (MRP) was also recently identified. Other potential mechanisms of drug

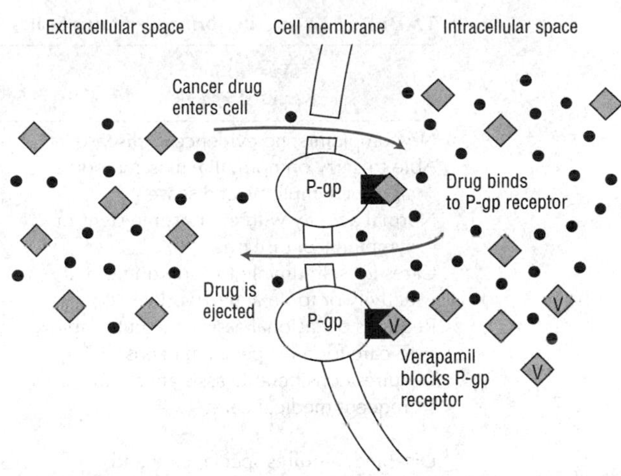

FIGURE 124–7. P-glycoprotein (P-gp) is a membrane-associated protein that acts as a drug efflux pump. Anticancer agents enter the cell, bind to the P-gp receptor, and are ejected. Some agents that modify multidrug resistance, like verapamil, block the P-gp receptor, allowing the anticancer agent to remain in the cell.

resistance include inactivation of chemotherapy agents by glutathione metabolism, upregulation of target enzymes such as topoisomerases or dihydrofolate reductase, and decreased apoptosis after exposure to chemotherapy.[24] The last mechanism can be mediated by *bcl*-2 oncogene overexpression or loss of the *p*53 gene, as discussed in the oncogene section.

The relationship between dose and response has been extensively explored in the arena of cancer chemotherapy. Dose is believed to be a critical factor in determining response for many types of cancers. Dose intensity is defined as the dose delivered to the patient over a specified period of time.[1,26] The delivery of optimal dose intensity is compromised by the toxicities of the oncologic drugs. Treatment cycles are commonly delayed owing to inadequate recovery from drug toxicity, especially myelosuppression. Subsequent doses of chemotherapy are often reduced to prevent or reduce the severity of these toxicities. The impact of this issue on patient outcome has been proven in studies showing reduced rates of response and survival in individuals receiving less-than-optimal chemotherapy doses.[26] The development of drug- and toxicity-specific chemoprotective agents may aid in the application of dose-intensity principles.[27] The colony-stimulating factors avert neutropenia and permit delivery of dose-intensive regimens that are usually dose-compromised by neutropenia. Monitoring of antineoplastic drug concentrations may also improve the therapeutic index. Pharmacokinetic and pharmacodynamic modeling is associated with improved responses and decreased toxicity in children with acute leukemia.[28] The issue of dose intensity is brought into a new light in the era of high-dose chemotherapy with autologous hematopoietic stem cell support. Although lethal myelosuppression is avoided by administering hematopoietic stem cells, other severe end-organ toxicities emerge as antineoplastic doses are increased.

Patient-specific factors create unpredictable variability in response to chemotherapy. The biology of cancer is strongly affected by host characteristics and genetics. The pathway of genetic mutations that resulted in malignancy can also affect response to therapy. For example, breast cancers that overexpress the HER-2/neu (EGFR-2) oncogene are often refractory to regimens like CMF (cyclophosphamide, methotrexate, and 5-fluorouracil), but sensitive to anthracycline-based regimens.[29] Interindividual variations in drug absorption or metabolism may lead to sub- or supertherapeutic levels of antineoplastic agents and their metabolites.[30] As a result, both drug efficacy and drug toxicity can be affected. Underlying

TABLE 124–9. Performance Status Scales

Description: Karnofsky Scale	Karnofsky Scale (%)	Zubrod Scale (ECOG)	Description: ECOG Scale
No complaints; no evidence of disease	100	0	Fully active, able to carry on all predisease activity
Able to carry on normal activity; minor signs or symptoms of disease	90		
Normal activity with effort, some signs or symptoms of disease	80	1	Restricted in strenuous activity, but ambulatory and able to carry out work of a light or sedentary nature
Cares for self; unable to carry on normal activity or to do active work	70		
Requires occasional assistance but is able to care for most personal needs	60	2	Out of bed more than 50% of time; ambulatory and capable of self-care, but unable to carry out any work activities
Requires considerable assistance and frequent medical care	50		
Disabled; requires special care and assistance	40	3	In bed more than 50% of time; capable of only limited self-care
Severely disabled; hospitalization indicated, although death not imminent	30		
Very sick; hospitalization necessary; requires active supportive treatment	20	4	Bedridden; cannot carry out any self-care; completely disabled
Moribund; fatal processes progressing rapidly	10		
Dead	0		

ECOG, Eastern Cooperative Oncology Group.
Adapted from Ref. 22.

nononcologic disease states may also affect response to treatment by limiting treatment options. The overall functional status of a patient may be assessed using performance status scales, such as the Karnofsky and Eastern Cooperative Oncology Group (ECOG) scales (Table 124–9).[22] These scales can be used to predict patient tolerance of chemotherapy, as well as to assess the effects of chemotherapy on the patient's level of activity and quality of life. In many cancers, performance status at diagnosis is the most important prognostic indicator.

COMBINATION CHEMOTHERAPY

Although single-agent therapy is sometimes employed, more commonly the approach to chemotherapy involves administration of multiple agents.[1,20,22] This approach is based on the Goldie-Coldman hypothesis, which addresses the issue of tumor cell heterogeneity and the inevitable development of drug resistance. Combination chemotherapy is employed to target as many types of cells in the tumor as possible. Selection of agents for combination chemotherapy regimens involves consideration of drug-specific factors such as mechanism of action, antitumor activity, and toxicity profile. Drugs that possess minimally overlapping mechanisms of action and toxicities are combined, when possible. Myelosuppressive combinations are sometimes alternated with nonmyelosuppressive combinations to allow bone marrow recovery, while gaining additive antitumor effects. The selected agents should each have significant activity against the tumor that is to be treated. If a synergistic reaction is known to exist for two agents, they may be combined in various treatment regimens.

CELL CYCLE

Both cancer cells and normal cells reproduce in a series of steps known as the cell cycle. Figure 124–8 depicts the cell cycle and the phases of activity for commonly used antineoplastic agents.[11,13] The first phase is mitosis (M). Mitosis lasts for approximately 30 to 60 minutes and during this phase, cell division occurs. After mitosis, the cell might enter a dormant phase (G_0), or might proceed to the first gap phase (G_1). G_0 is the largest variable in the cell cycle, and during this resting phase, the cell is not actively committed to cell division. Some stimulus results in the cell entering the first gap phase (G_1). During G_1, the cell prepares for DNA synthesis by manufacturing necessary enzymes. DNA synthesis (S) occurs next, and this phase lasts 10 to 20 hours. The percentage of cells in the S phase can be measured by flow cytometry and is an indicator of the rate of tumor-cell proliferation. Tumors with a high percentage of S-phase cells are aggressively growing. The synthesis phase is followed by a second gap or premitotic phase (G_2), lasting 2 to 10 hours. During this second gap, the cell prepares for mitosis by producing ribonucleic acid (RNA) and specialized proteins, as well as the mitotic spindle apparatus. The cycle then begins again with the M phase. Most normal human cells exist in the G_0 phase, and most cancer cells are not sensitive to the effects of chemotherapy when in this stage. The cell cycle is regulated by external mitogens, including cytokines, hormones, and growth factors. As mentioned earlier, some of the genes that regulate the cell cycle are known to be protooncogenes and tumor-suppressor genes.

All cancer cells do not proliferate faster than normal cells; some cancer cells reproduce more rapidly, and others are more indolent. Many anticancer drugs target rapidly proliferating cells (both normal and cancerous cells) and these agents may act at selective or multiple sites of the cell cycle. Agents with major activity in a particular phase of the cell cycle are known as cell cycle phase-specific agents. The antimetabolites exert their major effect during the S phase. Cell cycle phase-specific agents may also be active to a lesser extent in

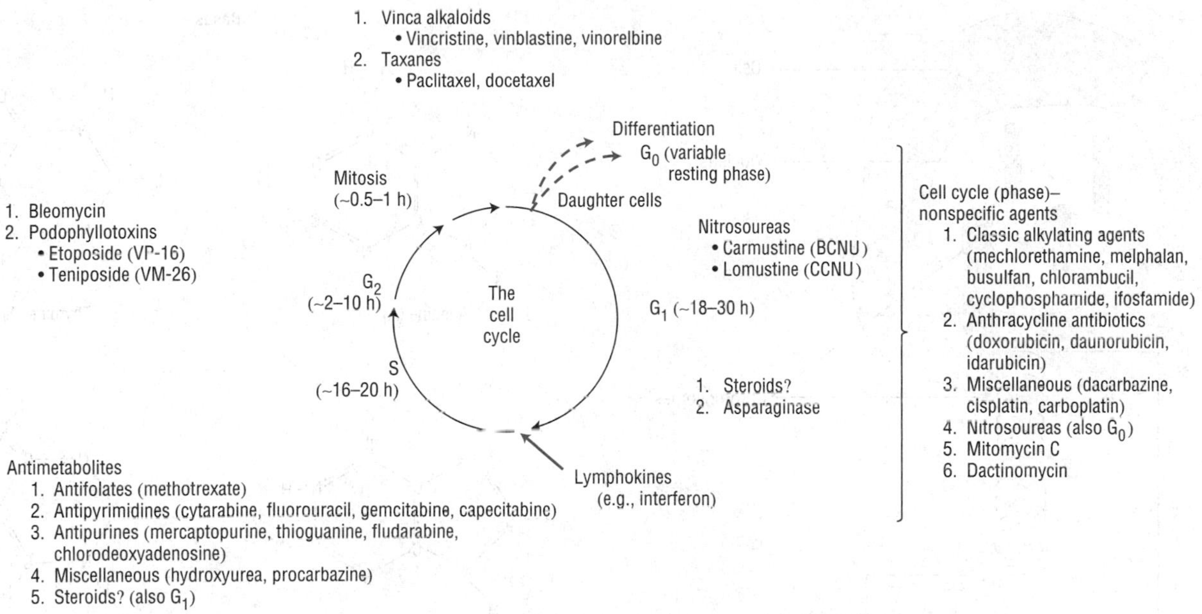

1. Vinca alkaloids
   • Vincristine, vinblastine, vinorelbine
2. Taxanes
   • Paclitaxel, docetaxel

Differentiation
G_0 (variable resting phase)
Mitosis (~0.5–1 h)
Daughter cells

1. Bleomycin
2. Podophyllotoxins
   • Etoposide (VP-16)
   • Teniposide (VM-26)

Nitrosoureas
• Carmustine (BCNU)
• Lomustine (CCNU)

G_2 (~2–10 h)
The cell cycle
G_1 (~18–30 h)
S (~16–20 h)

1. Steroids?
2. Asparaginase

Lymphokines (e.g., interferon)

Cell cycle (phase)–nonspecific agents
1. Classic alkylating agents (mechlorethamine, melphalan, busulfan, chlorambucil, cyclophosphamide, ifosfamide)
2. Anthracycline antibiotics (doxorubicin, daunorubicin, idarubicin)
3. Miscellaneous (dacarbazine, cisplatin, carboplatin)
4. Nitrosoureas (also G_0)
5. Mitomycin C
6. Dactinomycin

Antimetabolites
1. Antifolates (methotrexate)
2. Antipyrimidines (cytarabine, fluorouracil, gemcitabine, capecitabine)
3. Antipurines (mercaptopurine, thioguanine, fludarabine, chlorodeoxyadenosine)
4. Miscellaneous (hydroxyurea, procarbazine)
5. Steroids? (also G_1)

FIGURE 124–8. Cell cycle activity for anticancer drugs. Cell cycle (phase)-specific agents appear to be most active during a particular phase, but may also be active in another phase. Cell cycle (phase)-nonspecific agents may have greater activity in one phase than another, but not to the degree of cell cycle (phase)-specific agents. In many cases, it is likely that drug cytotoxicity involves multiple intracellular sites of action and may not be linked to specific cell-cycle events.

other phases of the cycle. Cell cycle phase-nonspecific agents are those with significant activity in multiple phases. The alkylating agents, such as nitrogen mustard, are examples. In many cases, the cytotoxic effects of a drug may result from interactions with other intracellular activities and are not related to specific cell cycle events. Hormones are an example of this type of drug.

Knowledge of cell cycle specificity has been applied to the scheduling of chemotherapy administration. By definition, phase-specific agents exert their major activity when cells are in a particular phase of the cell cycle. At any given time, the heterogeneous cell populations within a tumor are at various phases in the cell cycle. By giving phase-specific agents as a continuous infusion or in multiple repeated fractions, it is theoretically possible to target more cells as they progress in to the drug-sensitive phase. Thus, phase-specific agents are also termed *schedule dependent.* In contrast, cell cycle phase-nonspecific drugs are active in many phases and, consequently, are not schedule dependent. The activity of this group of drugs is dependent on the magnitude of the dose, and these drugs are termed *dose dependent.*

MOLECULAR BIOLOGY

Because many antineoplastic agents interfere with the cellular synthesis of DNA, RNA, and proteins, it is important to review the basic principles of molecular biology.[3,31] Each normal human cell contains 46 chromosomes, which are composed of DNA (deoxyribonucleic acid) (Fig. 124–9). DNA carries hereditary information in units called genes. A single chromosome can contain 20,000 or more genes. Genes code for specific proteins that regulate cellular activity and inherited traits. The genetic information is encoded in DNA by precise sequencing of subunits known as nucleotides. Each nucleotide consists of a sugar (deoxyribose), phosphoric acid, and a base. Four bases exist in DNA: adenine, thymine, guanine, and cytosine. Adenine and guanine are purine-type bases; thymine and cytosine are pyrimidine-type bases (Fig. 124–10). These nucleotides are connected linearly to form a chain. Each DNA molecule is made up of two chains of nucleotides, which wind around each other to form a double helix (see Fig. 124–9). The two strands are held together by chemical bonding between the bases. The bonding process is very specific; adenine binds only with thymine, and guanine binds only with cytosine. This is known as complementary base pairing. RNA (ribonucleic acid) is important in the DNA-directed synthesis of proteins or enzymes. RNA differs from DNA in that it is composed of a single strand of nucleotides, the sugar is ribose, and the base uracil is substituted for thymine. There are three known types of RNA: messenger RNA (mRNA), transfer RNA (tRNA), and ribosomal RNA (rRNA).

DNA SYNTHESIS

During the DNA synthesis phase, which takes place in the cell nucleus, the DNA unwinds and exposes its nucleotides. When DNA unwinds for replication or protein synthesis, only the portion of the molecule containing the needed nucleotides needs to be exposed. Rather than unwinding the entire strand, topoisomerase I and II enzymes cleave the DNA strands to facilitate unwinding of the section that is needed. The enzyme DNA polymerase matches free complementary nucleotides from the environment to the exposed nucleotides of the DNA (see Fig. 124–9). The newly created strands rewind, resulting in two complete double helices. The topoisomerase enzymes are also responsible for resealing the cleaved DNA strands.

PROTEIN SYNTHESIS

The synthesis of proteins is a more complex process (Fig. 124–11). Proteins consist of chains of amino acids in very specific sequences. As in DNA synthesis, the double helix must unwind. However, in protein synthesis, only the portion of the DNA molecule that codes for the desired protein is exposed. The enzyme RNA polymerase

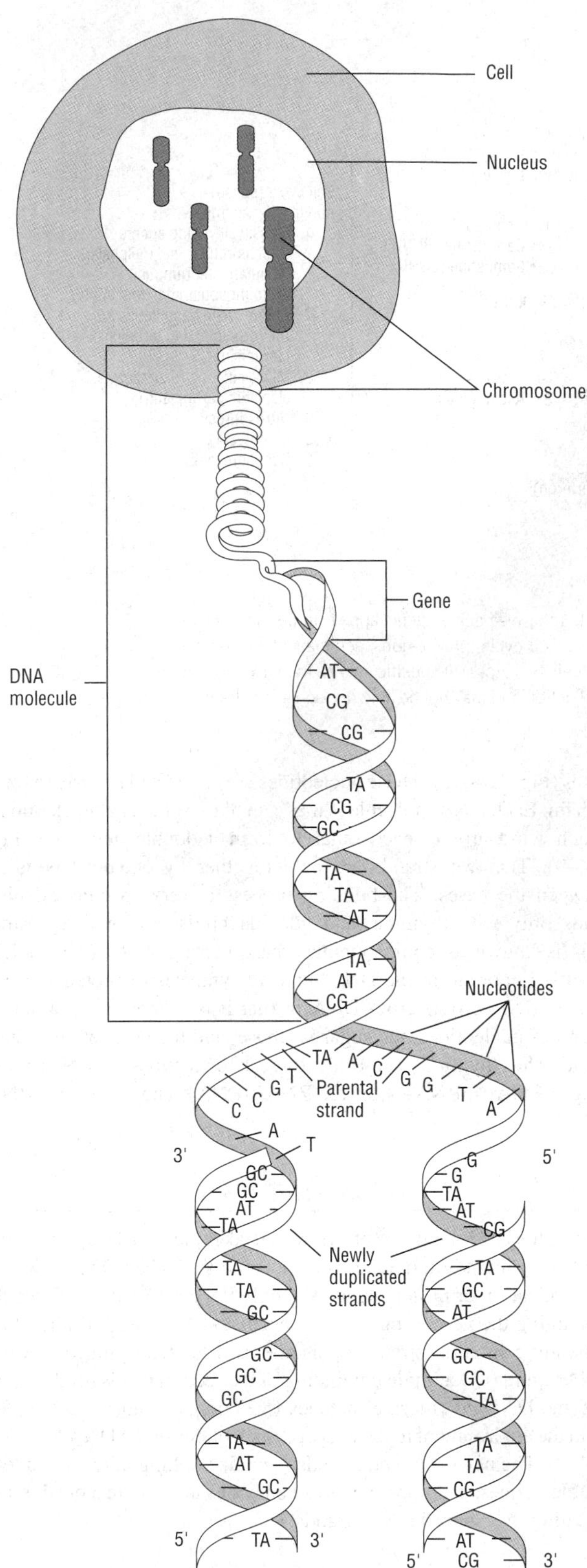

FIGURE 124–9. Structure and function of DNA. Within the cellular nucleus, tightly coiled strands of DNA are packaged in units called chromosomes. Working subunits of chromosomes are called genes. During DNA replication, the double-stranded DNA helix unwinds, exposing individual nucleotides. Complementary nucleotides are retrieved and assembled by DNA polymerases to form new strands of DNA.

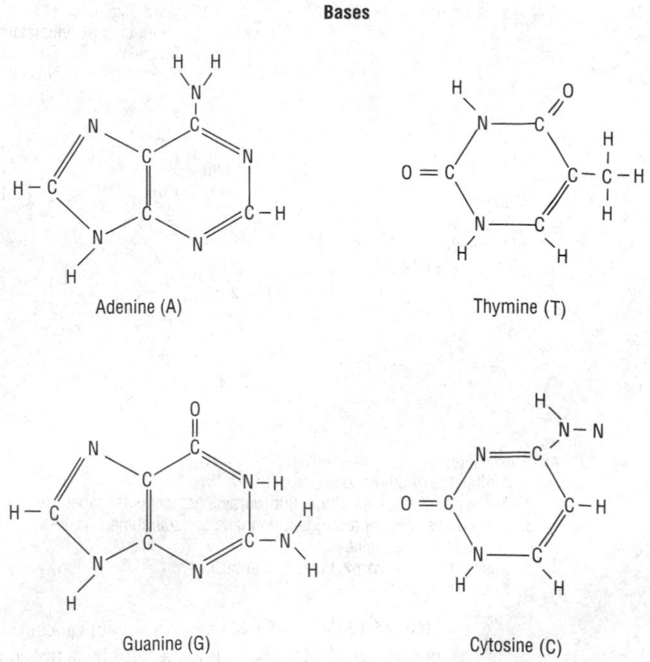

Bases

Adenine (A)

Thymine (T)

Guanine (G)

Cytosine (C)

FIGURE 124–10. Structures of DNA constituents.

matches free complementary RNA nucleotides to the exposed DNA nucleotides, and the resultant chain of nucleotides is called mRNA. This process is called transcription. The mRNA travels to ribosomes in the cytoplasm, where protein synthesis occurs. Each three nucleotides of the mRNA chain compose a codon, whose sequence is specific for a particular amino acid. The codon is recognized by tRNA, which then carries the amino acid to the ribosome, where it is added to the growing peptide chain. This process is known as translation. The completed protein is then ready for its intended use as an enzyme or as a structural component.

CLINICAL PHARMACOLOGY OF ANTICANCER AGENTS

Agents used in cancer chemotherapy are commonly categorized by their mechanism of action or by their origin. The alkylating agents exert their effects on DNA and protein synthesis by binding to DNA and preventing the unwinding of the DNA molecule. The antimetabolites resemble naturally occurring nuclear structural components ("metabolites"), such as the nucleotide bases, or inhibit enzymes involved in the synthesis of DNA and proteins. Antitumor antibiotics gain their name from their source of derivation; they are fermentation products of *Streptomyces* species. Fig. 124–12 depicts the sites of activity of common categories of antineoplastic agents.[21] The following section discusses these classes of agents and the most commonly used cytotoxic agents in the treatment of cancer. Table 124–10 summarizes the clinical uses of these agents.

ANTIMETABOLITES

FLUORINATED PYRIMIDINES

Fluorouracil

Fluorouracil (5-FU) is a fluorinated analog of the naturally occurring pyrimidine uracil that was originally synthesized in the late 1950s (Fig. 124–13). It is a prodrug and must be metabolized to the

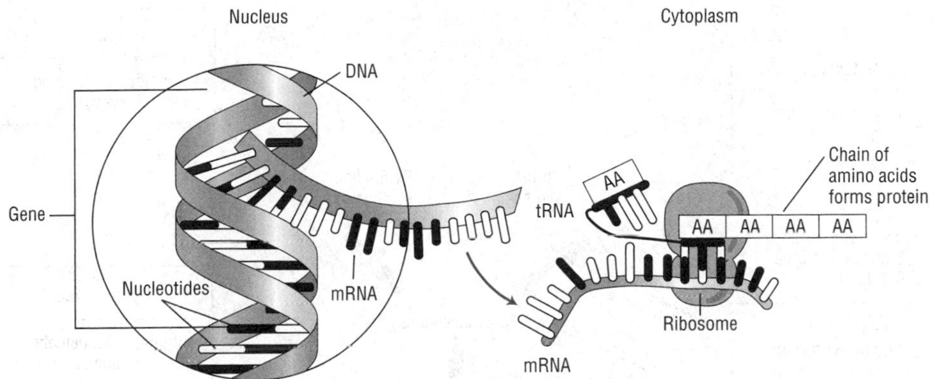

FIGURE 124–11. Protein synthesis. When a specific protein is needed, the portion of DNA responsible for that protein unwinds, exposing the necessary nucleotide sequence. Complementary nucleotides are assembled to form messenger RNA (mRNA), which travels to ribosomes in the cytoplasm. There, transfer RNA (tRNA) matches amino acids to the nucleotide sequence on the mRNA. The amino acids are assembled to form proteins.

nucleotide form, fluorodeoxyuridine monophosphate (FdUMP), to be active. In the presence of folates, FdUMP binds tightly to and interferes with the function of thymidylate synthase. This enzyme is required for synthesis of thymidine, one of the four essential building blocks of DNA. Another metabolite of 5-FU, the triphosphate nucleotide, is incorporated into RNA as a false base, and interferes with its function. Interference with both thymidine formation and RNA function is important in producing the cytotoxic effects of 5-FU. Although 5-FU nucleotides can also be incorporated directly into DNA and affects its stability, the contribution to cell damage remains unclear. The method of administration influences the mechanism of action, with thimidylate-synthesis inhibition playing a greater role in continuous-infusion regimens, and incorporation into RNA being more important for intermittent-bolus schedules.[36]

Several pharmacologic strategies have been attempted to increase the cytotoxicity of 5-FU against tumor cells and to decrease its toxicity to normal cells. The most successful of these attempts at biochemical modulation are combinations of fluorouracil and the reduced folate leucovorin. Folates increase the stability of the FdUMP-thymidylate synthase complex, and, in turn, increase the cytotoxicity and clinical usefulness of the drug.[34,36] Newer modulation strategies focus on inhibition of the enzyme dihydropyrimidine dehydrogenase (DPD), which is responsible for breakdown of 5-FU, or diversion of DPD to the related pyrimidine uracil. Interfering with the effects of DPD may increase or prolong systemic exposure to 5-FU, and even permit oral dosing.[37]

Pharmacokinetics. Fluorouracil distributes rapidly throughout the body and also is cleared rapidly from the plasma. Its elimination pattern is dependent on the dose and schedule of administration. After IV bolus, 90% of 5-FU is metabolized, mainly in the liver by the enzyme DPD, with a half-life of 8 to 14 minutes. Deficiency of DPD correlates with increased toxicity of 5-FU. In continuous infusion regimens, clearance exceeds hepatic blood flow, indicating that extrahepatic metabolism occurs. Clearance rates vary widely from patient to patient.[34,35] Because some of the clearance of 5-FU is extrahepatic and only small amounts of drug are excreted unchanged in the urine, dose adjustment is not necessary in patients with hepatic or renal dysfunction.[39]

Toxicity. Clinical toxicity of 5-FU is a function of the schedule, dose, and route of administration. It is most typically administered either as an intravenous bolus or as continuous intravenous infusion. Higher total doses are tolerated by continuous infusion compared with bolus regimens. The dose-limiting toxicity after bolus administration is myelosuppression, which especially affects neutrophils and platelets. In continuous-infusion regimens, and in combination regimens with leucovorin, gastrointestinal mucosal damage becomes dose limiting, and myelosuppression is less prominent. Diarrhea and stomatitis secondary to mucosal damage can be life-threatening, with elderly women at greatest risk. Severe diarrhea necessitates dose reduction on subsequent cycles of 5-FU. Conventional antidiarrheal agents, such as loperamide, and also octreotide are useful in the treatment of 5-FU-induced diarrhea. Oral cryotherapy, consisting of ice chips in the mouth for 30 minutes before and during bolus 5-FU administration, can decrease the incidence of mucositis. Dermatologic toxicities, including hyperpigmentation, alopecia, photosensitivity, and nail banding, can also occur. Ocular toxicity manifests as excessive tearing, itching, and burning. Application of ocular ice packs before and during the 5-FU bolus administration may decrease the severity of this toxicity.[34] Nausea and vomiting are generally mild and easily controlled. Hand-foot syndrome (palmar-plantar erythrodysesthesia), which produces painful erythema and swelling, occurs with continuous infusion regimens. Major organ toxicities have been increasingly recognized with higher doses of 5-FU. Myocardial ischemic symptoms such as chest pain or arrhythmia occur in approximately 2% of patients receiving 5-FU and may exceed 5% in patients receiving high-dose continuous infusions. Neurotoxicity, in the form of cognitive dysfunction and cerebellar ataxia, is rare in monthly schedules of administration, but emerges in high dose weekly schedules of 5-FU.[35,38] A clinically important drug interaction between 5-FU and warfarin has been recognized. Patients receiving warfarin require careful monitoring and are likely to need dose reductions during 5-FU chemotherapy.[40]

Capecitabine

Capecitabine is an orally active pyrimidine analog. Despite the similarity of its name to cytidine derivatives such as cytarabine and gemcitabine, capecitabine is an analog of uracil (Fig. 124–13) and is a prodrug of 5-FU. Because capecitabine is converted to 5-FU, it shares the same mechanisms of action. It was designed to generate 5-FU selectively within tumors.[41,42]

Pharmacokinetics. Capecitabine is absorbed as an intact molecule, and is converted to 5 FU through a cascade of three enzymatic reactions. It is metabolized in the liver by a carboxyesterase to

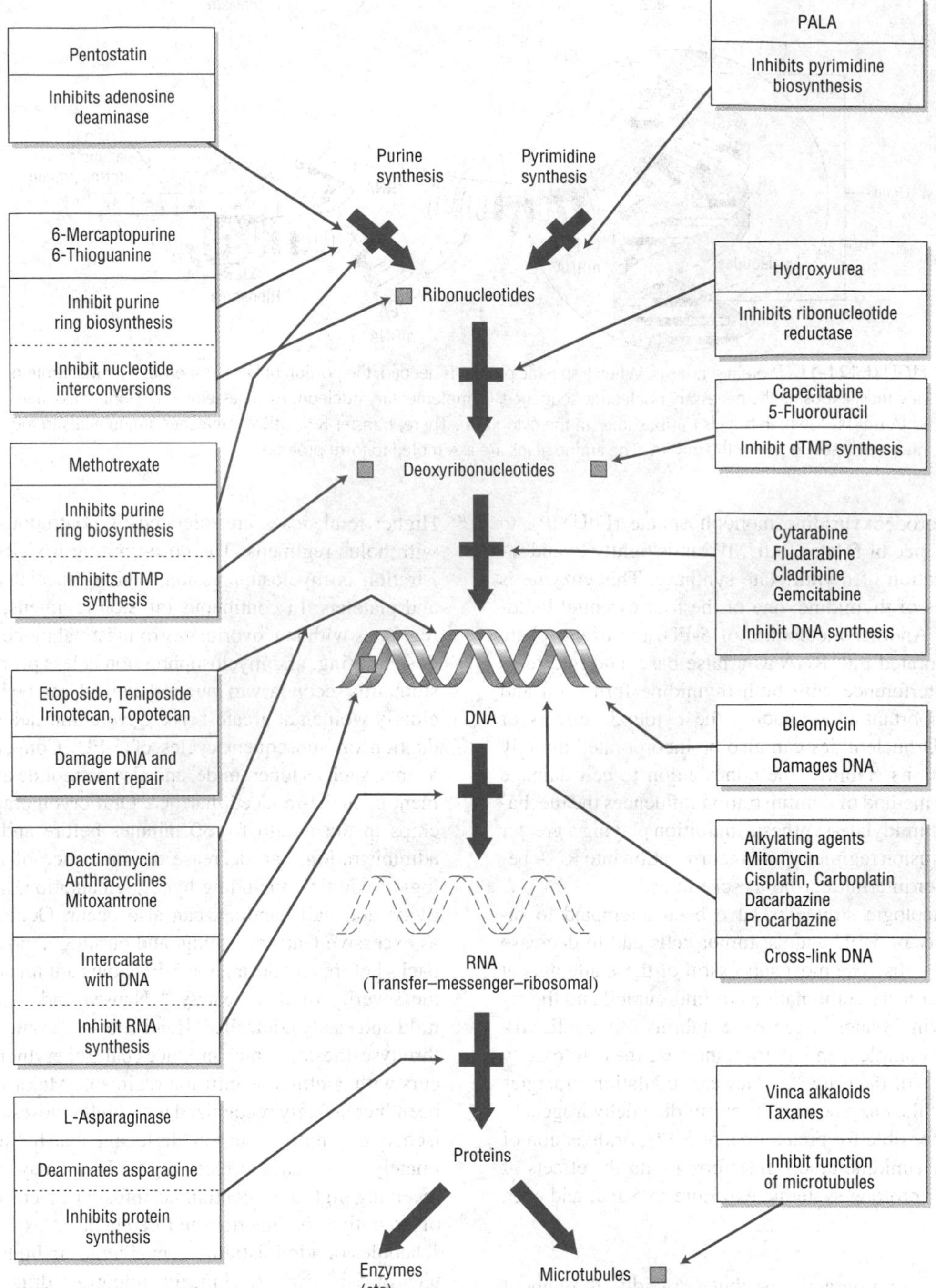

FIGURE 124–12. Mechanisms of action of commonly used antineoplastic agents. *(Adapted from Calabresi P, Chabner BA. Chemotherapy of neoplastic diseases. In: Hardman JG, Limbird LE, Molinoff PB, Ruddon RW, Gilman AC eds. Goodman & Gilman's The Pharmacologic Basis of Therapeutics, 9th ed. New York, McGraw-Hill, 1996:1226.)*

5-deoxy-5-fluorocytidine, then to 5-deoxy-5-fluorouridine (5-DFUR) by cytidine deaminase in the liver and tumor tissues. 5-FU is next released from 5-DFUR by activation at the tumor site through the action of tumor-associated thymidine phosphorylase.[41,42] The concentration of this enzyme is several times higher in some, but not all, tumor tissues than in healthy tissues, producing selectively higher 5-FU concentrations from capecitabine in these tumors.[43]

Peak plasma concentrations of 5-FU are reached approximately 2 hours after oral capecitabine administration. Although food reduces the rate and extent of absorption, capecitabine should be given with food to minimize nausea. Pharmacokinetics of capecitabine are dose proportional and do not change over time. Concentrations decline exponentially with a half-life of 30 to 60 minutes, with more than 70% of the capecitabine dose recovered in urine as drug-related species.[39] Although capecitabine depends on the liver for metabolism, initial dose modifications are not required for patients with mild to moderate liver dysfunction.[42,44] However, renal insufficiency has clinically important effects on capecitabine elimination (Table 124–11).[44]

TABLE 124–10. Selected Clinical Uses of Anticancer Agents

Agent	Approved Indications	Other Clinical Uses
Antimetabolites		
Capecitabine	Breast cancer, colorectal cancer	Indolent
Cladribine	Hairy cell leukemia	NHL
Cytarabine	ANLL, ALL, CML* CNS leukemia (IT), Lymphomatous meningitis (liposomal)	NHL
Fludarabine	CLL	Indolent NHL, Waldenstrom's macroglobulinemia
Fluorouracil	Colorectal, breast, gastric, and pancreatic cancers	Esophageal, head and neck, and cervical cancers, cataract surgery
Gemcitabine	Pancreatic cancer, NSCLC	Bladder, head and neck, and ovarian cancers
6-Mercapturine	ALL	—
Methotrexate	ALL, CNS leukemia (IT) GTN	NHL, bladder, breast, gastric, head and neck cancers, osteosarcoma, HSCT, rheumatoid arthritis, SLE, ectopic pregnancy
Pentostatin	Hairy cell leukemia	—
6-Thioguanine	ANLL	—
Plant alkaloids		
Docetaxel	Breast cancer, NSCLC	SCLC, gastric, head and neck, and ovarian cancers, melanoma, soft tissue sarcomas
Etoposide	Testicular cancer, SCLC	ANLL, HD, NHL, NSCLC, gastric cancer, HSCT, KS
Irinotecan	Colorectal cancer	NSCLC, cervical, gastric, and ovarian cancers
Paclitaxel	Breast and ovarian cancers, KS, NSCLC	SCLC, bladder, esophageal, head and neck, and testicular cancers
Teniposide	ALL	—
Topotecan	Ovarian cancer	SCLC
Vincristine	ALL	HD, NHL, myeloma, SCLC, brain tumors, breast cancer, KS, soft tissue sarcoma, osteosarcoma, neuroblastoma, Wilm's tumor
Vinblastine	HD, NHL, testicular cancer, KS	NSCLC, bladder, breast, prostate, and renal cell cancers
Vinorelbine	NSCLC	HD, breast, ovarian, and prostate cancers
Alkylating agents		
Altretamine	Ovarian cancer	—
Busulfan	CML	HSCT
Carmustine	Brain tumors, myeloma, HD, NHL	HSCT, melanoma
Chlorambucil	CLL, NHL, HD	—
Cyclophosphamide	NHL, CLL, CML*, ANLL, ALL, myeloma, neuroblastoma, breast and ovarian cancers retinoblastoma	HD, NSCLC, SCLC, bladder and endometrial cancers, HSCT, soft-tissue sarcoma, SLE
Dacarbazine	Melanoma, HD	Soft-tissue sarcoma, brain tumors
Ifosfamide	Testicular cancer	NSCLC, SCLC, NHL, soft-tissue sarcoma
Mechlorethamine	HD, CML*, CLL*, NSCLC*	NHL (topically in cutaneous T-cell NHL)
Melphalan	Myeloma, ovarian cancer*	HSCT, melanoma (regional limb perfusion)
Procarbazine	HD	Brain tumors, NSCLC
Temozolamide	Brain tumors	Melanoma
Thiotepa	Breast and ovarian* cancers, intracavitary effusions*, bladder cancer (BI)	BMT
Antitumor antibiotics		
Bleomycin	Testicular cancer, HD, NHL, squamous cell cancer of the head and neck, cervix, skin, penis or vulva, malignant pleural effusions	KS
Dactinomycin	Wilm's tumor, soft-tissue sarcoma, GTN, testicular cancer	—
Daunorubicin	ANLL, ALL, KS (liposomal)	—
Doxorubicin	ALL, ANLL, NHL, HD Wilm's tumor, bladder, breast, gastric, ovarian, and thyroid cancers, neuroblastoma, SCLC, osteosarcoma, soft-tissue sarcoma, KS (liposomal)	NSCLC, myeloma, endometrial cancer
Epirubicin	Breast cancer	
Idarubicin	ANLL	—
Mitomycin C	Gastric and pancreatic* cancers	Bladder (BI), breast, colorectal, and esophageal cancers, NSCLC, pterygium
Mitoxantrone	ANLL, prostate cancer	NHL, HD, breast cancer, multiple sclerosis
Valrubicin	Bladder cancer (BI)	—

TABLE 124–10. (Continued)

Agent	Approved Indications	Other Clinical Uses
Heavy metal compounds		
Carboplatin	Ovarian cancer	NSCLC, SCLC, bladder, head and neck, and testicular cancers
Cisplatin	Bladder, ovarian, and testicular cancers	NHL, NSCLC, SCLC, cervical, endometrial, esophageal, head and neck, and gastric cancers, melanoma, osteosarcoma
Immune therapies		
Aldesleukin	Renal cell cancer	Melanoma
Interferon-α	KS, hairy-cell leukemia, melanoma, hepatitis B and C condyloma acuminata	CML, NHL, myeloma, renal cell cancer
Monoclonal antibodies		
Alemtuzumab	B-cell CLL	—
Gemtuzumab ozogamicin	CD33-positive AML	—
Rituximab	Indolent NHL	Aggressive NHL, CLL
Trastuzumab	Breast cancer	—
Retinoids		
Alitretinoin	Cutaneous AIDS-KS lesions	—
Bexarotene	Cutaneous T-cell lymphoma	
Tretinoin	APL	—
Other		
Arsenic trioxide	APL	—
L-Asparaginase	ALL	—
Denileukin diftitox	Cutaneous T-cell lymphoma	
Estramustine	Prostate cancer	—
Hydroxyurea	CML, melanoma*, ovarian* and head and neck* cancers, sickle cell anemia	—
Imatinib	CML	—

*Although an FDA-approved indication, the drug is no longer used for this disease.
ALL, acute lymphocytic leukemia; ANLL, acute nonlymphocytic leukemia; APL, acute promyelocytic leukemia; BI, bladder instillation; CLL, chronic lymphocytic leukemia; CML, chronic myelogenous leukemia; GTN, gestational trophoblastic neoplasm; HD, Hodgkin's disease; HSCT, hematopoietic stem cell transplantation; IT, intrathecal; KS, Kaposi's sarcoma; NHL, non-Hodgkin's lymphoma; NSCLC, Non–small cell lung cancer; SCLC, small cell lung cancer; SLE, systemic lupus erythematosis.

Toxicity. Because chronic twice-daily oral dosing of capecitabine produces sustained 5-FU levels, similar to continuous intravenous infusions of 5-FU, the toxicity pattern is similar to that of 5-FU infusions. Myelosuppression is uncommonly dose limiting, and alopecia is rare, but diarrhea can be severe. The usual onset of diarrhea is approximately 1 month, but it may begin from 1 day to nearly a year after initiation of capecitabine therapy. As with 5-FU, the elderly are at greater risk for severe diarrhea and its complications. Diarrhea can usually be managed with antidiarrheals such as loperamide. Nausea is common but is usually mild.[41]

Another toxicity similar to continuous 5-FU infusion is hand-foot syndrome (palmar-plantar erythrodysesthesia), which can be dose limiting. More than half of patients on capecitabine will experience some degree of painless or painful erythema and swelling of the hands and/or feet that can desquamate, blister, or ulcerate. Severe hand-foot syndrome occurs in 10% to 15% of patients and necessitates treatment interruption followed by dose reduction. Topical emollients may provide symptomatic relief.[41]

Altered coagulation parameters, with or without bleeding, may occur in patients receiving coumarin anticoagulants with capecitabine. Caution and careful monitoring are required.[40,44]

CYTIDINE ANALOGS

Cytarabine

Cytarabine (arabinosyl cytosine, cytosine arabinoside, ara-C) is an arabinose analog of cytosine. Arabinose nucleosides differ from normal human nucleosides only by the orientation of one hydroxyl group in the sugar portion of the nucleoside (see Fig. 124–13). Cytarabine was originally isolated from sponges, but is now produced synthetically.

Ara-C has many effects on DNA synthesis. It penetrates cells by a carrier-mediated process and is phosphorylated to its active triphosphate form (ara-CTP) within tumor cells. Ara-CTP inhibits DNA polymerase, an enzyme responsible for strand elongation. It is also incorporated directly into DNA, where it inhibits the replication of DNA and acts as a chain terminator to prevent DNA elongation. Activation of ara-C is opposed by deaminase enzymes, particularly cytidine deaminase, which degrades ara-C to an inactive form, ara-U.[33,34]

Pharmacokinetics. Ara-C distributes rapidly into total body water. It enters the central nervous system (CNS) readily and achieves concentrations equal to 20% to 40% of simultaneous plasma levels. Cytidine deaminase is widely present in the liver, plasma, white blood cells, and gastrointestinal (GI) tract; consequently, ara-C disappears rapidly from plasma after intravenous administration, with a half-life of only a few minutes. Increased concentrations of deaminase enzymes in tumor cells may account for the resistance of some cancers to the antitumor effects of ara-C. Other important mechanisms of resistance are reduced levels of the activating kinase enzymes, and short retention of Ara-C within tumor cells. Cytarabine is well absorbed after subcutaneous injection, but has very low oral bioavailability, since it is rapidly destroyed by deaminase enzymes in the gastrointestinal tract.[34,38,45]

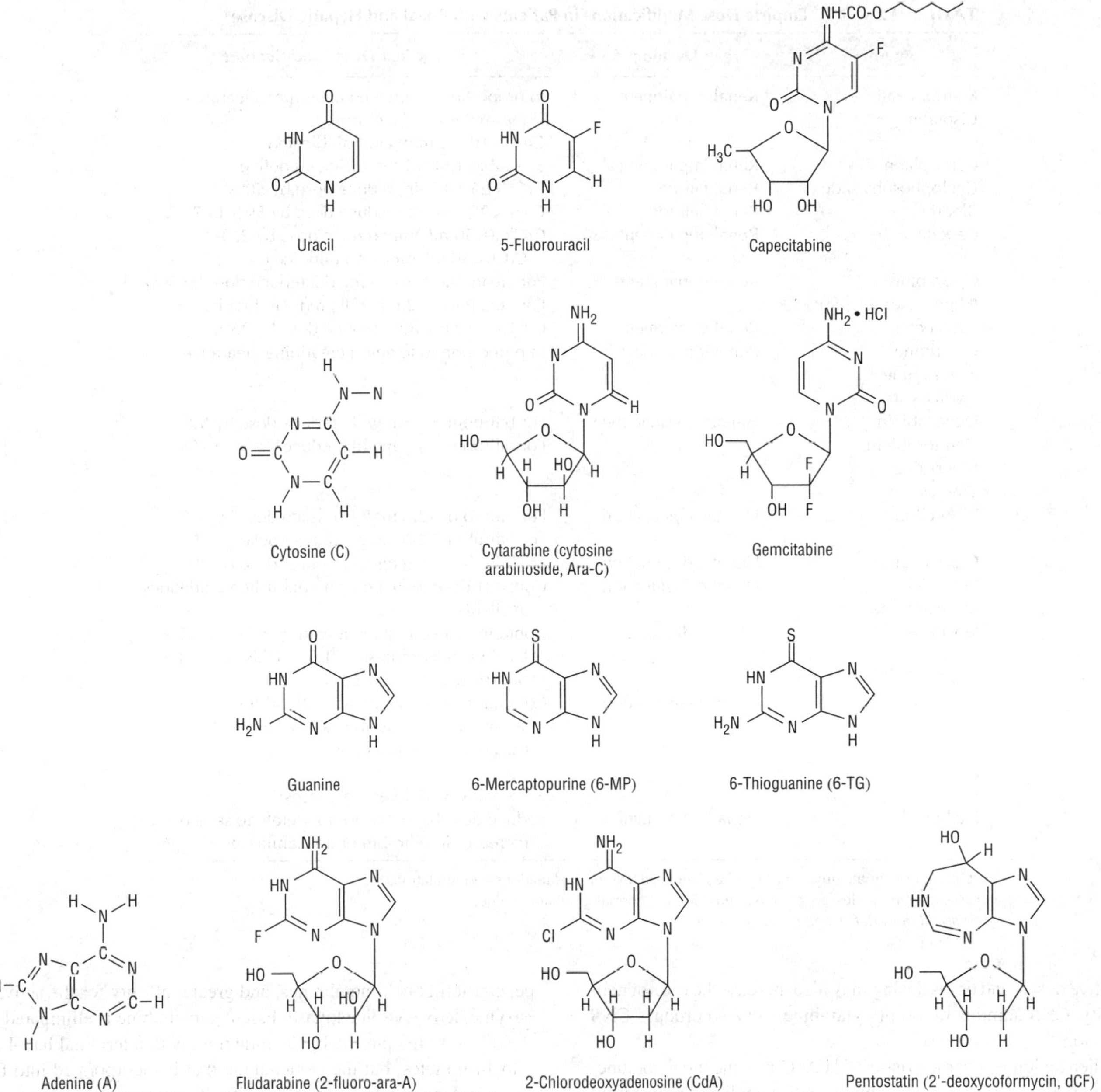

FIGURE 124–13. Structures of natural purines and pyrimidines and their structural analogs.

Cytidine deaminase levels are very low in the brain and cerebral spinal fluid, resulting in a longer half-life of ara-C elimination (2 to 3 hours) in the CNS after CNS administration of traditional formulations of cytarabine. Cytotoxic concentrations are maintained in the CNS for more than 2 weeks following CNS administration of depot formulated cytarabine (Depocyte), permitting much less frequent dosing.[46]

Toxicity. The dose-limiting toxicity of cytarabine in conventional schedules is myelosuppression, which particularly affects neutrophils. Alopecia is common, but nausea is mild and major organ damage is rare. At high doses (>1g/m^2 per dose), a very different pattern of toxicity is seen. In addition to profound myelosuppression and severe nausea, characteristic CNS, ocular, hepatic, dermatologic, and pulmonary toxicities emerge. The most characteristic toxicity of high-dose ara-C (HDAC) regimens is neurotoxicity, typically manifesting as a cerebellar syndrome of dysarthria, nystagmus, and ataxia, often with dysdiadochokinesia and dysmetria. Cerebral dysfunction, with generalized encephalopathy and seizures, may accompany the cerebellar syndrome or occur independently. CNS toxicity has been documented in up to 40% of patients receiving HDAC, with severe toxicity in about 10% with the dose-intense regimens used during the 1980s and early 1990s. Cerebellar toxicity is usually reversible, resolving over several days after cytarabine discontinuation, but may be permanent, and is occasionally fatal.[47] Risk of CNS toxicity is strongly correlated with advanced age and renal dysfunction. Renal insufficiency permits accumulation of high levels of ara-CTP, which is believed to be neurotoxic. A combination of dose reduction and once-daily rather than twice-daily dosing is recommended in patients with renal insufficiency (Table 124–11).[48] Hepatic dysfunction, high

TABLE 124–11. Empiric Dose Modifications in Patients with Renal and Hepatic Disease*

Agent	Organ Dysfunction	Suggested Dose Modification
Methotrexate Cisplatin	Renal impairment	In proportion to lowered creatinine clearance (normal 60 mL/min/m²) CrCl <10 mL/min, contraindicated
Carboplatin	Renal impairment	See Table 124–14 for dosing guideline
Cyclophosphamide	Renal failure	CrCl <25 mL/min; reduce dose by 50%
Bleomycin	Renal failure	CrCl <25 mL/min; reduce dose by 50% to 75%
Capecitabine	Renal impairment	CrCl 30–50 mL/min; reduce dose by 25% CrCl <30 mL/min; contraindicated
Cytarabine (High dose: >1 g/m²)	Renal impairment	For creatinine 1.5–1.9 mg/dL, reduce dose by 50% For creatinine >2.0 mg/dL, reduce dose by 95%
Topotecan	Renal impairment	CrCl 20–39 mL/min; reduce dose by 25%
Cladribine Fludarabine Hydroxyurea	Renal impairment	In proportion to lowered creatinine clearance
Doxorubicin Daunorubicin Vincristine Vinblastine	Hepatic dysfunction	For bilirubin >1.5 mg/dL, reduce dose by 50% For bilirubin >3.0 mg/dL, reduce dose by 75%
Vinorelbine	Hepatic dysfunction	For bilirubin >2.0 mg/dL, reduce dose by 50% For bilirubin >3.0 mg/gL, reduce dose by 75%
Gemcitabine	Hepatic dysfunction	For bilirubin >1.6 mg/dL, reduce dose by 20%
Idarubicin Mitoxantrone	Hepatic dysfunction	Consider dose reductions; no published guidelines available
Docetaxel	Hepatic dysfunction	Contraindicated in patient with bilirubin >1.5 × ULN or transaminases >1.5 × ULN or alkaline phosphtases >2.5 × ULN
Irinotecan	Hepatic dysfunction	Contraindicated in patients with bilirubin >2 mg/dL, or transaminases >3 × ULN (without liver metastases)
and		>5 × ULN (with liver metastases)
Paclitaxel	Hepatic dysfunction	Reduce dose by ≥50% for moderate to severe increases in bilirubin or transaminases

*Only approximate guidelines can be given. See text for explanations and limitations.
CrCl, creatinine clearance; ULN, upper limit of normal laboratory values.
Adapted from Ref. 1 and package inserts.

cumulative doses, and bolus dosing may also increase the risks of neurotoxicity. CNS administration of cytarabine can also produce CNS dysfunction.[46,47]

Other toxicities characteristic of HDAC are chemical conjunctivitis, which can be prevented or managed by application of steroid eye drops or saline eye washes; intrahepatic cholestasis; and dermatologic toxicity consisting most characteristically of either palmar-plantar or acral erythema. Pulmonary toxicity may be related to a capillary-leak syndrome. Respiratory distress and noncardiogenic pulmonary edema typically present suddenly, a few days to a month after treatment with HDAC.[33,49]

Gemcitabine

Gemcitabine is a fluorine-substituted deoxycytidine analog related structurally to cytarabine (Fig. 124–13). Its activation and mechanism of action are similar to those of cytarabine, with phosphorylation to the active diphosphate and triphosphate forms necessary for antitumor effect. Gemcitabine is incorporated into DNA, where it inhibits DNA polymerase activity. It also inhibits ribonucleotide reductase, blocking conversion of ribonucleotides to their deoxy forms and inhibiting *de novo* nucleotide production. Gemcitabine demonstrates important differences from ara-C in schedule dependency and activity. With comparable exposure, gemcitabine achieves intracellular concentrations about 20 times higher than does ara-C, secondary to increased penetration of cell membranes, and greater affinity for the activating enzyme deoxycytidine kinase. Parent gemcitabine is eliminated very rapidly from the plasma by deamination, with a terminal half-life of 8 to 14 minutes, but the gemcitabine that is incorporated into DNA has a prolonged intracellular half-life. Its stereoconfiguration causes another normal base pair to be added next to the fraudulent gemcitabine base pair in the DNA strand. This "masked chain termination" protects the gemcitabine from excision and elimination.[35,45,50]

Toxicity. Gemcitabine's dose-limiting side effect is myelosuppression, predominantly neutropenia. Elevations in liver transaminases are common. Although these hepatic abnormalities rarely necessitate stopping treatment, dose reductions are recommended in patients with elevated bilirubin levels. Patients with increased serum creatinine levels are also at risk of increased toxicities (Table 124–11).[51] Mild proteinuria and hematuria occur in about half of patients, but are rarely clinically significant. Generalized rashes occur in about 25% of patients. The rashes are typically erythematous, pruritic, and maculopapular and develop 2 to 3 days after drug administration. They are reversible, respond to local therapy, and only rarely require discontinuation of drug. Fevers and flu-like symptoms, which usually occur within 6 to 12 hours of drug administration, are also common, especially following administration of the first dose. Nausea and vomiting are mild, but peripheral edema may be clinically important. In contrast to cytarabine, gemcitabine is not neurotoxic.[45,50]

PURINES AND PURINE ANTIMETABOLITES

6-Mercaptopurine and 6-Thioguanine

Some of the oldest and newest anticancer agents are synthetic analogs of the naturally occurring purines guanine and adenine (see Fig. 124–13). 6-Mercaptopurine (6-MP) was the first purine analog to be used in cancer chemotherapy. Thioguanine (6-TG) is the two-amino analog of 6-mercaptopurine. Both drugs are rapidly converted to ribonucleotides that inhibit purine biosynthesis. They also undergo purine interconversion reactions needed to supply purine precursors for synthesis of nucleic acids. 6-TG may be incorporated into DNA as a "false" purine. Clinical cross-resistance is generally observed.[29,35]

Pharmacokinetics. Both compounds are rapidly activated and widely distributed Their oral bioavailability is variable, incomplete, and reduced by food intake. Variability in absorption results in significant differences in systemic exposure to a given dose of 6-MP and is an important prognostic consideration affecting the risk of relapse in children with ALL.[48]

6-MP and 6-TG are eliminated primarily by metabolism in the liver and other tissues.[49] Metabolites are eliminated renally, and consideration should be given to decreasing doses for patients with hepatic or renal disease. No guidelines are available.

An important difference between these agents is the pathway of metabolic inactivation. 6-MP depends on xanthine oxidase for an initial oxidation step. Because of this dependence, its metabolism is markedly decreased by concomitant administration of the xanthine oxidase inhibitor allopurinol, and serious toxicity may result. This drug interaction is of major clinical significance, and oral 6-MP doses must be reduced by at least 50% when allopurinol is administered together with 6-MP. Because xanthine oxidase is not involved in the elimination of 6-TG, no interaction with allopurinol occurs, and no dose reduction is necessary.[33,35]

Toxicity. Both 6-MP and 6-TG are relatively well tolerated. Gastrointestinal toxicity occurs more commonly with 6-MP than 6-TG, but is rarely severe Bone marrow suppression is mild with typical oral doses of 6-MP, but is dose limiting for 6-TG. Chronically administered 6-MP produces dose-related hepatic injury in 6% to 40% of patients, which typically manifests as jaundice after 1 to 2 months of treatment.[35,38] Genetic differences in thiopurine methyltransferase, an enzyme involved in methylation of 6-MP and 6-TG, have recently been correlated with occurrence of dose- limiting toxicities, and can potentially guide dose adjustments.[52]

Fludarabine Monophosphate

Fludarabine monophosphate (FAMP) is an analog of the purine adenine that incorporates two structural changes from the parent molecule (see Fig. 124–13). The arabinose analog of adenine (ara-A or vidarabine) was first developed in an attempt to design new antineoplastics using the same structural alterations that resulted in the effective anticancer drug cytarabine. Ara-A demonstrated some antineoplastic activity but was rapidly inactivated by deaminase enzymes. The fluorinated analog, fludarabine or F-ara-A, proved to be both resistant to deamination and to have significant antitumor activity.[35,38,53]

Pharmacology and Pharmacokinetics. Fludarabine monophosphate is rapidly dephosphorylated in plasma to F-ara-A; it then enters cells where the enzyme deoxycytidine kinase rephosphorylates F-ara-A to its active triphosphate form (F-ara-ATP). The intracellular accumulation of F-ara-ATP inhibits DNA synthesis. Like cytarabine, fludarabine interferes with DNA polymerase, causing chain termination. Unlike ara-C, fludarabine is also incorporated into RNA, resulting in inhibited transcription. It is inactivated by deaminase enzymes and is eliminated with a terminal half-life of about 10 hours. Renal excretion accounts for the major clearance of metabolites, and renal failure predisposes patients to increased toxicity (Table 124–11).[45,53]

Toxicity. Fludarabine in high doses was an extremely effective antileukemic agent during phase I trials, but its use was limited by a syndrome of delayed CNS toxicity, characterized by blindness, paralysis, and coma. Fortunately, severe CNS toxicity is rare at the lower doses that are required for treatment of patients with chronic lymphocytic leukemia (25 mg/m^2/day × 5 days). About 15% of patients treated with this dose of fludarabine experience some degree of neurotoxicity, most commonly somnolence, mild peripheral neuropathy, paresthesias, and mild visual disturbances. The usual dose-limiting toxicity at these lower doses is myelosuppression. Fludarabine is also immunosuppressive, with associated opportunistic infections. Interstitial pneumonitis may occur after several courses of therapy, and is slowly reversible. Nausea and vomiting are mild and easily controlled.[35,38,53]

Cladribine

Cladribine (2-chlorodeoxyadenosine, 2-CDA) is a purine nucleoside analog (Fig. 124–13) that is resistant to inactivation by adenosine deaminase. Like fludarabine, it is sequentially phosphorylated intracellularly by deoxycytidine kinase. The triphosphate form of this agent is incorporated into DNA, resulting in inhibition of DNA synthesis and early chain termination. Cladribine's antitumor activity is unusual in that it affects both actively dividing and resting cancer cells. It also induces apoptosis.[48,53]

Pharmacokinetics. In contrast to the other purine nucleoside analogs, cladribine is well absorbed orally, with a bioavailability of approximately 50%, although it is not yet available in an oral preparation. The terminal elimination half-life approaches 7 hours. The metabolic fate of cladribine is unknown, although approximately 20% of the drug is eliminated unchanged in the urine.[45,54]

Toxicity. The dose-limiting toxicity of cladribine is myelosuppression. Like fludarabine, cladribine possesses immunosuppressive effects that place patients at risk for serious opportunistic infections. The most common serious toxicity is culture-negative fever, usually beginning on the fifth to seventh day of therapy.[45,54]

METHOTREXATE

Folate vitamins are essential cofactors in DNA synthesis. They carry one-carbon groups in transfer reactions that are required for purine and thymidylic acid synthesis and, in turn, for formation of DNA and for cell division. Natural folates circulating in the blood have a single glutamic acid group, but within cells they are converted to polyglutamates, which are more efficient cofactors and which are preferentially retained inside the cells.[29,35,55,56]

Dietary folates must be chemically reduced to their tetrahydro forms, with four hydrogens on the pteridine ring, to be active. The enzyme responsible for this reduction is dihydrofolate reductase, and it is this enzyme whose actions methotrexate and other antifolates inhibit. The result of this inhibition is depletion of intracellular pools of reduced folate (tetrahydrofolates) essential for thymidylate and purine

drug interactions may occur if the vincas are given in conjunction with substrates and inhibitors of the 3A subfamily of cytochrome P450.[64]

PACLITAXEL AND DOCETAXEL

Paclitaxel and docetaxel are taxane plant alkaloids with antimitotic activity. Paclitaxel (Taxol) was isolated from the bark of the Pacific yew tree, *Taxus brevifolia,* but is now produced semisynthetically from the needles of the European yew, *Taxus baccata.* Docetaxel (Taxotere) is a semisynthetic taxoid extracted from 10-deacetyl baccatin III, a noncytotoxic precursor found in the renewable needle biomass of yew plants.[58–60]

Clinical Pharmacology

Paclitaxel and docetaxel both act by binding to tubulin but, unlike the vincas, do not interfere with tubulin assembly. Instead, the taxanes promote microtubule assembly and interfere with microtubule disassembly. They induce tubulin polymerization, resulting in formation of inappropriately stable, nonfunctional microtubules. The stability of the microtubles damages cells, because the dynamics of microtubule-dependent structures required for mitosis and other cellular functions are disrupted. Taxanes also have some nonmitotic actions, such as inhibition of angiogensis, that can promote cell death. Resistance to the antitumor effects of the taxanes is attributable to alterations in tubulin or tubulin binding sites, or to P-glycoprotein-mediated multidrug resistance. Although paclitaxel and docetaxel have very similar mechanisms of action, cross-resistance between the two agents is incomplete.[58–60,65]

Pharmacokinetics

The taxanes bind extensively to plasma and tissue proteins, resulting in large volumes of distribution and plasma protein binding >90%. Elimination half-lives range from 1.3 to 8.6 hours for paclitaxel and 11.4 to 18.5 hours for docetaxel, and are not dose dependent. Elimination is primarily through hepatic metabolism and biliary excretion; less than 10% of parent drug is found unchanged in the urine. Dose reductions are necessary for patients with moderate or severely elevated bilirubin or serum aminotransferase concentrations (Table 124–11). The pharmacodynamics of paclitaxel are nonlinear; docetaxel shows a linear pharmacodynamic pattern.[59,60,65]

Toxicity

The dose-limiting side effect of the taxanes is myelosuppression, particularly neutropenia. For paclitaxel, the incidence of neutropenia is related to the duration of infusion, with longer durations producing more profound neutropenia. Neutropenia produced by docetaxel is not schedule dependent. Both drugs produce cumulative peripheral neuropathy. Other common shared toxicities include mucositis, total alopecia, mild nausea and vomiting, and hypersensitivity reactions.[58–60,65]

Hypersensitivity reactions are very common from paclitaxel, and occur in 30% to 60% of unprotected patients. Pretreatment with corticosteroids and H_1- and H_2-receptor antagonists (Table 124–12) reduces the incidence of serious hypersensitivity reactions to 2% to 4%. It is also safe and effective to substitute a single-dose of dexamethasone just prior to paclitaxel administration.[66] Hypersensitivity reactions may be caused, in part, by the Cremophor EL (castor oil and absolute ethanol) vehicle used in its formulation. Docetaxel is much more water soluble than paclitaxel and is formulated in a polysorbate 80 vehicle. However, docetaxel is also associated with hypersensitivity reactions, suggesting that the taxane ring structure contributes

TABLE 124–12. Prophylactic Regimens for Patients Receiving Taxanes

Paclitaxel (Taxol)
Dexamethasone 20 mg PO at 12 and 6 hours *or* 20 mg IV 30 to 60 minutes prior to paclitaxel
Diphenhydramine 50 mg IV 30 to 60 minutes prior to paclitaxel
Cimetidine 300 mg or ranitidine 50 mg IV 30 to 60 minutes prior to paclitaxel
Docetaxel (Taxotere)
Dexamethasone 8 mg PO bid × 3 days, starting 24 hours prior to docetaxel

to the hypersensitivity risk. The risk of hypersensitivity reactions is decreased in weekly dosing regimens.[59,63,65]

Docetaxel, but not paclitaxel, causes cumulative fluid retention, producing edema, weight gain, and pleural effusions. Corticosteroids are recommended with docetaxel to delay the onset, and reduce the incidence and severity of fluid retention. Concurrently, the steriods decrease the risk of hypersensitivity reactions to docetaxel (see Table 124–12).[63,65] Docetaxel also commonly causes dermatologic reactions, usually a maculopapular rash affecting the hands and feet, with occasional desquamation.

Toxicities unique to paclitaxel include myalgias and cardiac toxicity. Asymptomatic bradycardia is the most common adverse cardiac effect, although heart block and ventricular arrhythmias can also occur. Serious cardiac effects are uncommon.[59–61]

Drug Interactions

Administration of paclitaxel after cisplatin reduces paclitaxel clearance and produces more severe neutropenia than when paclitaxel precedes cisplatin. Toxicity of doxorubicin-paclitaxel regimens is also affected by sequence of drug administration. Because hepatic P450 enzymes (CYP3A4) mediate taxane metabolism, agents that interact with these enzymes can alter taxane pharmacokinetics and clinical effects.[61]

TOPOISOMERASE-TARGETING DRUGS

ETOPOSIDE AND TENIPOSIDE

Etoposide (VP-16) and teniposide (VM-26) are semisynthetic podophyllotoxin derivatives. Podophyllin is extracted from the mayapple or mandrake plant. Like the vincas, it binds to tubulin and interferes with microtubule formation. Unlike the parent compound, however, etoposide and teniposide damage tumor cells by causing strand breakage, through inhibiting the DNA repair enzyme topoisomerase II.[60,67,68]

Pharmacology

Topoisomerases are essential enzymes involved in maintaining DNA topologic structure during replication and transcription. As shown in Fig. 124–16, DNA topoisomerase enzymes relieve torsional strain during DNA unwinding by producing strand breaks. They cleave DNA strands and form intermediates with the strands, producing a gap through which DNA strands can pass, then they reseal the strand breaks. Topoisomerase I produces single-strand breaks; topoisomerase II produces double-strand breaks. Etoposide and teniposide both form complexes with topoisomerase II and DNA that inhibit strand resealing. Teniposide is much more potent than etoposide in stimulating DNA cleavage. Resistance may be caused by differences in topoisomerase II levels, by increased cell ability to

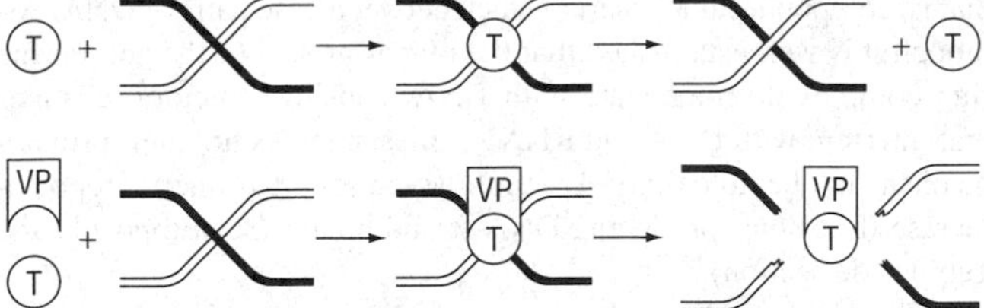

FIGURE 124–16. Topoisomerase II (T) interaction with DNA and etoposide (VP). T normally interacts with DNA to produce breakage–cleavage reactions required for normal cellular function (*upper panel*). The epipodophyllotoxins seem to cause DNA strand breakage by forming a complex with DNA and T (*lower panel*). *(From Bender RA, Hamel F, Hande KR. Plant alkaloids. In: Chabner BA, Collins JM eds. Cancer Chemotherapy: Principles and Practice. Philadelphia, Lippincott, 1990;253–275, with permission.)*

repair strand breaks, or by increased levels of P-glycoproteins. They are usually clinically cross-resistant. Etoposide and teniposide are cell-cycle phase specific and arrest cells in the S or early G2 phase. As a result, activity is much greater when they are administered in divided doses over several days, rather than in large single doses.[60,67,68]

Pharmacokinetics

Etoposide and teniposide are not soluble in water. Etoposide is formulated in a polyethylene glycol (PEG) solution, and teniposide is solubilized in polyoxyethylated castor oil (Cremophor EL). These formulations result in concentration-dependent stability, and contribute to hypotension with rapid infusions and to hypersensitivity reactions. Etoposide phosphate is a water-soluble derivative that is rapidly converted to etoposide. This formulation permits bolus dosing and treatment at high drug concentrations. It is pharmacokinetically and biologically equivalent to etoposide. Etoposide is available for oral use in liquid-filled gelatin capsules. Oral bioavailability is dose dependent; mean bioavailabilities of 76% to 86% have been reported after administration of a 100-mg oral dose, as compared to 45% following a 400-mg dose. Interpatient variability is marked.[67,68]

Both renal and hepatic function contribute to etoposide elimination. Approximately 40% to 60% of a delivered dose can be recovered in the urine, primarily as unchanged drug. Fecal elimination accounts for up to 16% of a dose, but biliary excretion is minimal. The disposition of much of an administered etoposide dose is still unknown. Patients with normal renal and hepatic function show terminal half-lives of approximately 4 to 8 hours. Etoposide is highly (approximately 95%) protein bound, primarily to albumin. The unbound fraction, and consequently the pharmacologic effects, are much greater in patients with low serum albumin, as commonly occurs in cancer patients. Elevated serum bilirubin levels may also alter binding.[67–69] The pharmacologic effects resulting from a particular etoposide dose depend on a complex interplay of protein binding and renal and hepatic function. Unfortunately, no prospectively validated guidelines for dose changes in patients with abnormal organ function or hypoalbuminemia are available.[67]

Teniposide is even more highly protein bound than is etoposide (>97%). It has a lower systemic clearance, a longer elimination half-life of about 9 hours, and less urine elimination of parent drug than etoposide. Renal elimination accounts for only about 10% of teniposide clearance. Hepatic metabolism is the predominant route of teniposide elimination, but validated dose modification guidelines are not available for patients with impaired hepatic function. As with etoposide, serum albumin and factors that affect protein binding must be taken into consideration in dosing decisions.[39,67–69]

Toxicity

Both etoposide and teniposide are well tolerated. Their dose-limiting toxicity is myelosuppression. Nausea and vomiting are usually mild, although more likely after oral administration of etoposide than parenteral. Alopecia is common, and mucositis may be limiting at high doses. Orthostatic hypotension can occur with either drug, but is generally preventable by a slow infusion time over 30 minutes to 1 hour. Etoposide phosphate may be administered as a rapid bolus without producing cardiovascular effects. Hypersensitivity reactions have occasionally been reported. Major organ toxicity is rare, but both agents can cause secondary leukemias.[60,67,68]

IRINOTECAN AND TOPOTECAN

Camptothecin, a plant alkaloid derived from *Camptotheca acuminata,* is a potent inhibitor of DNA topoisomerase I. Clinical trials failed to show expected antitumor activity, and the drug produced severe, unpredictable toxicity. The camptothecin analogs irinotecan (CPT-11) and topotecan were synthesized in very successful efforts to reduce toxicity and improve therapeutic effects.[66]

Clinical Pharmacology

Both irinotecan and topotecan poison the actions of the topoisomerase I enzymes. The actions of topoisomerase enzymes have been described above (see Etoposide and Teniposide). Topoisomerase I enzymes stabilize DNA single-strand breaks and inhibit strand resealing (Fig. 124–17).[66,70–72] Topotecan's active metabolite SN-38 causes cell damage by producing intermediate forms of drug-stabilized DNA-topoisomerase I complexes ("cleavable complexes") that collide with moving replication forks. This leads to replication arrest, disassembly of the replication forks, and fragmentation of the chromosomes.[72]

Pharmacokinetics

Irinotecan is rapidly converted by carboxylesterases to the active metabolite SN-38, which has 100- to 1,000-fold greater antitumor

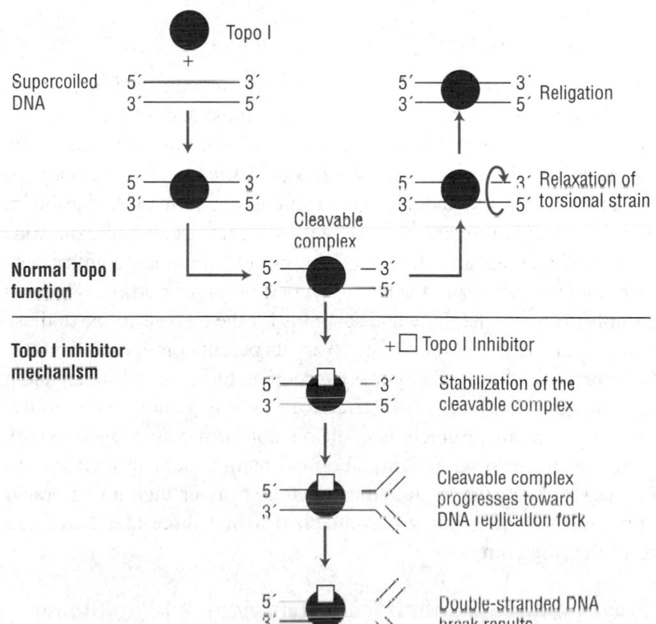

FIGURE 124–17. Topoisomerase I (Topo I) function (*top*) and mechanism of topoisomerase I inhibitors (*bottom*).

activity than irinotecan. Irinotecan, SN-38, and topotecan all undergo pH-dependent hydrolysis of their E-ring lactone to an open-ringed hydroxy acid. Only the closed lactone form, which is favored in acidic environments, exerts antitumor effects. The preferred diluent for these agents is 5% dextrose, which has a more acidic pH than saline and slows hydrolysis of the lactone ring. However, once administered systemically, hydrolysis occurs rapidly. The major route of elimination of irinotecan and SN-38 is biliary excretion, and elevated total bilirubin levels have been associated with increased gastrointestinal toxicity and myelosuppression. Dosage reductions should be considered in patients with elevated total bilirubin. In contrast, topotecan undergoes renal excretion, with approximately 50% eliminated in the urine in the first 24 hours. Dosage reductions are recommended for renal insufficiency (see Table 124–11).[66,71–73]

Toxicity

The dose-limiting toxicity of both irinotecan and topotecan agents is myelosuppression. For irinotecan, diarrhea can also be dose limiting, with grade 4 diarrhea occurring in 20% of patients. The diarrhea has two different presentations-an acute onset form that begins during or immediately after irinotecan administration, and a chronic form with onset several days after drug administration. The acute form is a cholinergic process that is often accompanied by facial flushing, diaphoresis, and abdominal cramping. It can be managed or prevented with atropine. The chronic form is a secretory diarrhea, which may result in life-threatening dehydration. Prompt initiation of high-dose loperamide at the first sign of diarrhea has reduced the incidence of grade 4 diarrhea to 2% of courses. Loperamide 4 mg should be given orally at the onset of diarrhea or abdominal cramping and continued at a dose of 2 mg every 2 hours until no bowel movement has occurred for 12 hours. Diarrhea is not commonly observed with topotecan and is mild when it occurs.

Nausea and vomiting from irinotecan can be severe, but are usually preventable. In contrast, nausea and vomiting from topotecan are mild. Side effects common to both agents include alopecia, rash, low-grade fevers, malaise, mucositis, and mild elevations in liver function tests.[66,70–72]

ANTHRACENE DERIVATIVES

The anthracene derivatives are very useful anticancer drugs with a broad spectrum of anticancer activity. The most widely used and best understood of the group is doxorubicin, also commonly known by its earliest trade name, Adriamycin or "Adria". Other members of the anthracene group include daunorubicin (daunomycin), idarubicin, epirubicin, and mitoxantrone. All of these agents except mitoxantrone are anthracyclines and share a common, four-membered anthracene ring complex with an attached aglycone or sugar portion. The ring complex is a chromophore and accounts for the intense colors of these compounds. Doxorubicin differs from its parent compound daunorubicin by the addition of a hydroxyl group on the attached sugar, and it is sometimes consequently referred to as hydroxydaunorubicin. A hydroxyl group on epirubicin is in the epi conformation compared with doxorubicin (epidoxorubicin), and idarubicin is demethoxydaunorubicin. Mitoxantrone is an anthracenedione rather than an anthracycline and has no sugar group attached to the three-membered anthracene ring complex.[33,68,74]

Doxorubicin, Daunorubicin, Idarubicin, and Epirubicin

Anthracyclines have been classified as antitumor antibiotics, but it is more accurate to refer to them as intercalating topoisomerase inhibitors. Traditionally they have been considered intercalating agents, that is, compounds that insert or stack between base pairs of DNA. Although it is well established that the planar groups of the anthracene ring complex do intercalate with DNA, causing structural changes that interfere with DNA and RNA synthesis, this is not their primary mechanism of cytotoxicity. The anthracyclines are primarily topoisomerase II poisons, producing DNA strand breaks (see Etoposide and Teniposide section).[68,74]

The anthracyclines also undergo electron reductions to reactive compounds that can damage DNA and cell membranes. Free radicals formed from reduction of the anthracyclines first donate electrons to oxygen to make superoxide, which can react with itself to make hydrogen peroxide. Cleavage of hydrogen peroxide produces the highly reactive and destructive hydroxyl radical. This last step requires iron, and the anthracyclines are potent iron binders. Iron-anthracycline complexes can bind to DNA and react rapidly with hydrogen peroxide to produce the hydroxyl radicals that actually cleave DNA. Human cells have natural defenses against oxygen radical damage, in the form of enzymes that can convert the radicals to less reactive compounds, or that can repair DNA damage. Differences in distribution of these defensive enzymes may account for characteristic sites of toxicities of the anthracyclines. For example, cardiac muscle has low levels of defensive enzymes and high levels of enzymes that activate anthracyclines (see Toxicity discussion). Oxygen free radical formation is firmly established as a cause of cardiac damage and extravasation injury, but is not a major mechanism of tumor-cell kill. Resistance to the anthracyclines is usually secondary to P-glycoprotein-dependent multidrug resistance, causing the anthracyclines to be actively pumped out of tumor cells. Altered topoisomerase II activity may also be clinically important.[68,74]

Pharmacokinetics

The most important factor in the pharmacokinetic behavior of the anthracyclines is their extensive tissue binding. They distribute rapidly to all body tissues except those of the CNS. When circulating in plasma, they are about 75% bound to plasma proteins, but within tissues, are bound very tightly to DNA. This binding accounts for their large volumes of distribution; ranging from 200 to 2,500 L/m^2. Anthracyclines are released slowly from tissues, with half-lives of 20 to 30 hours, and may be detected in tissue even months after administration. All are metabolized in the liver to alcohol metabolites: doxorubicinol, idarubicinol, daunorubicinol, and epirubicinol. Idarubicinol is the most active, with cytotoxic activity comparable to the parent compound. Epirubicin is also metabolized to glucuronide aglycone conjugates. Metabolites are excreted in the bile. Less than 10% of any anthracycline dose is eliminated in the urine, although this is enough of these highly colored drugs to discolor the urine a characteristic orange-red color.

The ability of the liver to metabolize anthracyclines is much greater than the rate of release of drug from tissues, which brings into question the validity of empiric guidelines for dose modification based on elevated liver function tests (see Table 124–11). Dose modifications are clearly necessary for patients with severe liver impairment; the evidence supporting dose reductions of anthracyclines for patients with mild to moderately elevated bilirubins is less consistent. The presence of large or diffuse liver metastases may alter anthracycline pharmacokinetics, even in the absence of bilirubin elevations. There is some evidence that aspartate aminotransferase levels may be more useful than bilirubin in adjustment of anthracycline doses. In the absence of prospectively validated dosing guidelines, dose reduction in patients with elevated bilirubin remains the accepted recommendation.[39,68,74]

Toxicity

The anthracyclines are very active and very toxic drugs. The most common acute dose-limiting toxicity is myelosuppression. They also cause moderate to severe dose-related nausea and vomiting, alopecia, and mucositis. Mucositis may be dose limiting in doxorubicin infusion protocols.[33,68,74] Secondary acute myeloid leukemia with chromosome translocations similar to epipodophyllotoxin-associated leukemia has been recognized.[68] However, the anthracyclines are most famous for their cardiac toxicity and for extravasation injuries.

All anthracyclines produce acute, chronic, and late-onset patterns of cardiac damage. Doxorubicin's cardiac damage is most thoroughly characterized. Acute toxicity consists primarily of rhythm disturbances, especially nonspecific ST-T wave changes, sinus tachycardia, and increased frequency of ventricular premature beats. Typically, these occur within the first 24 hours after drug administration. They are usually self-limited and do not appear to increase the risks of future cardiac events. A rare subacute pericarditis-myocarditis syndrome of fever, pericarditis, and congestive heart failure can also occur at low cumulative doses and may be fatal.[49,75,76]

Much more serious than the acute cardiac changes are the risks of chronic congestive cardiomyopathy, which limit the cumulative dose of anthracyclines that can be administered. Cardiomyopathy is attributed to free radical formation within the heart muscle, producing damage to the sarcoplasmic reticulum and gradual loss of myofibrils from the cells. The damaged sarcoplasmic membrane loses its ability to bind calcium, disrupting the link between electrical excitation and muscle contraction. Clinical evidence of cardiac damage is dose related and depends on the extent of myofibril loss. Although there is a real but very low incidence of clinically evident damage in patients with cumulative doxorubicin doses less than 550 mg/m^2 by IV bolus, the incidence approaches 50% by 1,000 mg/m^2. The risk is greater and deterioration occurs at lower cumulative doses in patients with previous cardiac irradiation. The elderly, the very young, females, and those with preexisting hypertension or cardiac disease are also at increased risk.[49,68,74–76]

Long-term cancer survivors who received anthracyclines are at risk for late cardiotoxicity, with an onset of 5 to 20 years or more after drug administration. Late toxicity is characterized by delayed progressive left ventricular dysfunction. Arrhythmias, occasionally resulting in sudden death, may occur.

The incidence of congestive cardiomyopathy is closely associated with dose schedule. The risk estimates outlined above refer to traditional doxorubicin dosing, that is, 60 mg/m^2 by intravenous bolus every 3 to 4 weeks. It has been established that cardiac damage correlates with peaks of drug concentration achieved, rather than with total exposure to the drug (AUC, area under the concentration-time curve). Administering the same total dose in small weekly doses or by continuous infusion over 2 to 4 days markedly improves the cardiology risk-benefit ratio of doxorubicin administration, but produces more severe stomatitis. Serial endomyocardial biopsies or evaluations of left ventricular ejection fraction may be useful in assessing the extent of cardiac muscle injury. This information is used to estimate the risk of continuing anthracycline therapy for patients who are responding to treatment, but approaching the recommended maximum dose. Unfortunately, the appearance of cardiac toxicity is typically delayed until months or years after completion of therapy, which decreases the utility of prospective monitoring.[49,68,74–76]

Although many different pharmacologic interventions to prevent cardiac damage have been attempted, the only FDA approved cardiac chemoprotective agent is dexrazoxane (ICRF 187). Its carboxylamine metabolite is a potent chelator of iron in its ferric state. Anthracycline complexation with iron is essential for the free radical formation that initiates cardiac damage. Dexrazoxane disrupts the iron-anthracycline complex and prevents reactive radical formation, reducing the incidence and severity of doxorubicin-induced cardiomyopathy. Formulation of anthracyclines in liposomal delivery systems also decreases their cardiotoxicity, because liposomes are not taken up as readily by cardiac tissue as free anthracyclines.[49,68,74–77]

Daunorubicin and doxorubicin have similar potential for cardiac toxicity, but because of the limited use of daunorubicin and the rarity of high cumulative doses in the leukemic population, clinically important cardiomyopathy is uncommonly seen. Doses of 900–1,000 mg/m^2 are approximately equivalent in risk to doxorubicin doses of 550 mg/m^2. Idarubicin is less cardiotoxic than doxorubicin or daunorubicin in equivalent doses. Epirubicin is about half as cardiotoxic as doxorubicin on an equimolar basis, with an equivalent cardiotoxic epirubicin dose of about 900 mg/m^2. However, clincally useful doses of epirubicin are approximately double the equivalent doxorubicin doses, which may prove to make the differences in cardiac toxicity clinically insignificant.[33,49,75,78]

The other classic toxicity of the anthracycline drugs is tissue damage on extravasation. Deep ulceration with tissue necrosis may occur and progress over many weeks. Ulcers typically have raised red edges and necrotic centers, and heal very slowly if at all. Drug may be detected in the ulcer tissue for months after extravasation. No remedy has been proven to prevent or reverse tissue damage, although application of ice to the extravasation site is the current standard of care. Topical application of dimethylsulfoxide (DMSO) to the extravasation site is anecdotally useful in humans.[63,79] Doxorubicin may also cause a dermatologic "flare" reaction that presents during or immediately after injection, with redness and urticaria extending up the vein. It is self-limiting and usually subsides within 30 minutes. Doxorubicin may also reactivate skin damage in sites of previous radiation therapy, the so-called "radiation recall" reaction.[33,74]

Both doxorubicin and daunorubicin are available in liposomal formulations. Drug within liposomes is protected from systemic degradation and can be delivered in higher amounts to target tissues. The toxicity of liposomal anthracyclines differ from the parent compounds in that the risks of cardiac toxicity and extravasation injuries are substantially lessened.[68,77,80]

Mitoxantrone

The anthracenedione mitoxantrone was synthesized in an attempt to develop agents with comparable antitumor activity to doxorubicin but with an improved safety profile. Like the anthracyclines, mitoxantrone is an intercalating topoisomerase II inhibitor, but its potential for free radical formation is much less than that of the anthracyclines. Pharmacokinetics are characterized by extensive tissue binding and slow elimination, with metabolism and biliary excretion accounting for most of the known elimination (Table 124–11). Perhaps because of the decreased tendency for free radical formation, the risks of cardiac toxicity and ulceration after extravasation, although still present, are markedly reduced. Other nonmarrow toxicities of mitoxantrone are also less than the traditional anthracyclines. Nausea and vomiting, mucositis, and alopecia are less common and severe than with doxorubicin. Mitoxantrone's intense blue color produces a blue-green discoloration of urine and may give a blue tint to sclera and skin.[68,74]

ALKYLATING AGENTS

The alkylating agents are among the oldest and most useful of antineoplastic drugs. Their clinical use evolved from the observation of bone marrow suppression and lymph node shrinkage in soldiers exposed to sulfur mustard gas warfare during World War I. On the possibility

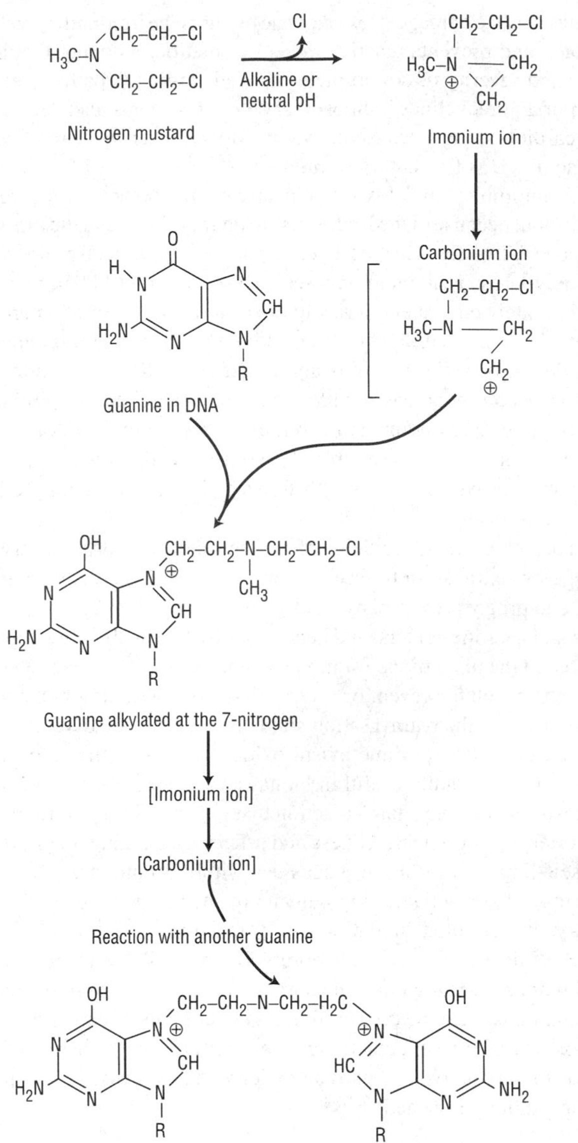

FIGURE 124–18. Alkylation reaction of nitrogen mustard. In solution, the drug forms a reactive cyclic intermediate that reacts with the 7-nitrogen of a guanine residue in DNA to form a covalent linkage. The second arm can then cyclize and react with nucleophilic groups such as a second guanine moiety in an opposite DNA strand or in the same strand. Reactions between DNA and RNA and between DNA and protein also occur.

that similar agents might be useful in treating cancerous overgrowths of lymphoid tissues, less-reactive derivatives were synthesized. Their effectiveness as anticancer agents was confirmed by clinical trials in the middle 1940s.[81]

All of the alkylating agents work through the covalent bonding of highly reactive alkyl groups or substituted alkyl groups with nucleophilic groups of proteins and nucleic acids (Fig. 124–18). Some alkylating agents react directly with biologic molecules; others form an intermediate compound that reacts with the targets. The most common binding site for alkylating agents is the seven-nitrogen group of guanine. These covalent interactions result in cross-linking between two DNA strands or between two bases in the same strand of DNA. Reactions between DNA and RNA and between drug and proteins may also occur, but the main insult that results in cell death is inhibition of DNA replication, because the interlinked strands do not separate as required. Because the alkylating agents can damage DNA during any phase of the cell cycle, they are considered cell-cycle nonphase specific. However, their greatest effect is seen in rapidly dividing cells.

All alkylators are cytotoxic, mutagenic, teratogenic, carcinogenic, and myelosuppressive. Resistance to these agents can occur from increased DNA repair capabilities, from decreased entry into or accelerated exit from cells, from increased inactivation of the agents inside cells, or from lack of cellular mechanisms to result in cell death following DNA damage. They react with water and are inactivated by hydrolysis, making spontaneous degradation an important component of their elimination.

The pharmacology, pharmacokinetics, and toxicities of the most commonly used alkylating agents are detailed below. Table 124–13 outlines the characteristics of alkylating agents with more limited use.

CYCLOPHOSPHAMIDE AND IFOSFAMIDE

Cyclophosphamide is a nitrogen mustard derivative, and is one of the most widely used alkylating agents. Ifosfamide is closely related in structure, clinical use, and toxicity. Neither agent is active in its parent form and must be activated by mixed hepatic oxidase enzymes. The active metabolite of cyclophosphamide is phosphoramide mustard. Another metabolite, 4-hydroxycyclophosphamide is cytotoxic, but is not an alkylating agent, and probably acts as a transport form to deliver phosphoramide mustard into cells. Ifosfamide is hepatically activated to ifosfamide mustard, but activation to the alkylating form occurs more slowly than with cyclophosphamide. Acrolein, a metabolite of both cyclophosphamide and ifosfamide, has little antitumor activity, but is responsible for some of their toxicity.[33,81–83]

Pharmacokinetics

Cyclophosphamide is well absorbed orally, with a systemic bioavailability approaching 100%. The terminal-phase half-life is about 7 hours, and the major metabolic site is the liver. About 15% of unchanged drug and most of the inactive metabolites are eliminated in the urine. Empiric dose reductions have been recommended for patients with creatinine clearances below 25 mL/min (Table 124–11) However, spontaneous degradation is likely more important than renal excretion in cyclophosphamide clearance. Although cyclophosphamide is largely metabolized, dose reductions are unnecessary for patients with hepatic dysfunction. Significant amounts of cyclophosphamide can be cleared by dialysis. It does not enter the CNS in significant concentrations.[81–83]

Pharmacokinetics of ifosfamide are similar. Because of the slower rate of activation, ifosfamide must be used in greater doses (approximately three to four times) than the cyclophosphamide dose required to achieve similar alkylating activity. More unchanged drug is excreted in the urine (20% to 50%) than is true for cyclophosphamide. The half-life is schedule dependent and is about 6 hours when divided daily doses are administered, but increases to 16 hours with single large doses. One important difference is that unchanged ifosfamide is detectable in the CNS in significant quantities, although only very small amounts of the active metabolites are detectable. This penetration may account for ifosfamide's CNS toxicity.[76–78]

Toxicity

Myelosuppression occurs with both agents and is dose limiting for cyclophosphamide. White blood cells are particularly sensitive to these drugs, but they are relatively platelet sparing. Recovery from leukopenia is rapid, indicating little stem-cell damage. Emetogenicity is dose dependent; in high-dose regimens, both agents are severe emetogens.

TABLE 124–13. Comparison of Less-Commonly Used Alkylating Agents

Agent (Brand Name)	Pharmacokinetics	Characteristic Toxicities*	Comments
Busulfan (Myleran)	Oral bioavailability: 100% Selective toxicity for myeloid cells Hepatic metabolism with half-life of 2 to 3 hours CYP 3A3/4 substrate 10% to 50% excreted in urine as metabolites Crosses blood-brain barrier	Myelosuppression (dose limiting) Nausea and vomiting (mild at standard doses, more severe with high doses) Hyperpigmentation Pulmonary fibrosis Hepatic venoocclusive disease (HSCT) Seizures (HSCT) Oral mucositis (HSCT)	Prophylactic anticonvulsants used to prevent seizures with high dose regimens High dose regimens use adjusted ideal body weight for morbidly obese patients Administer IV busulfan via central venous catheter
Chlorambucil (Leukeran)	Oral bioavailability: 50% to 80% Selective toxicity for lymphocytes Food decreases absorption Hepatic metabolism with half-life of 1.5 to 2 hours 60% excreted in urine as inactive metabolites	Myelosuppression (dose limiting) Nausea and vomiting (mild) Secondary leukemia	
Mechlorethamine or nitrogen mustard (Mustargen)	Rapidly degraded within minutes of administration	Myelosuppression (dose limiting) Nausea and vomiting (severe) Vesicant Secondary leukemia Infertility	Highly unstable in aqueous solution Administer within 15 minutes of admixture
Melphalan, or L-phenylalanine mustard, L-PAM (Alkeran)	Oral bioavailability variable, but approximately 70% Food decreases absorption Degraded in bloodstream with half-life of 1 to 2 hours; 10% to 30% of drug excreted unchanged in the urine	Myelosuppression (dose limiting) Nausea and vomiting (mild)	Although only 10% to 30% of drug eliminated in urine in first 24 hours, toxicity increased in patients with renal insufficiency. Dose reduction indicated in these patients. Used in HSCT as preparative regimen.
Procarbazine (Matulane)	Oral bioavailability: 100% Monoamine oxidase inhibitor; counsel patients on tyramine-free diet; multiple drug interactions Prodrug converted to active form by hepatic P450 enzymes Rapid metabolism with half-life of 1 hour Crosses blood-brain barrier	Myelosuppression (dose limiting) Nausea and vomiting (moderate to severe, may be dose limiting) Anorexia Disulfuram-like reaction CNS (depression, headache, mania, Insomnia, hallucinations, and so on) Secondary leukemia Infertility	
Thiotepa	Hepatic metabolism with half-life of 1 to 2 hours Active metabolite, TEPA, has half-life of 3 to 21 hours Crosses blood-brain barrier	Myelosuppression (dose limiting) Nausea and vomiting (mild at standard doses, severe with high doses)	Used intravenously in HSCT as preparative regimens, intravesically for bladder cancer, and intrathecally for carcinomatous meningitis

Adapted from Refs. 33, 76, and 81–83.

The nausea and vomiting from cyclophosphamide, but not ifosfamide, are characterized by a delay in onset of up to 8 hours. Alopecia is also dose related.[33,81,82]

The classic toxicity of these drugs, and the dose-limiting toxicity for ifosfamide, is hemorrhagic cystitis. This is a syndrome of damage to the bladder mucosa, producing hematuria, frequency, and irritation. It can also cause fibrosis of the bladder, massive hemorrhage, and bladder carcinoma. The toxic metabolite acrolein produces cystitis by binding to critical thiols in the bladder wall. Damage may be minimized by hydration and by frequent voiding, to decrease acrolein contact with the bladder mucosa. Patients receiving conventional doses of cyclophosphamide should be counseled to drink 3 L of fluids on the day of cyclophosphamide administration, and for 2 days after dosing. In most cases, this will prevent mucosal damage. However, with ifosfamide, hydration alone is inadequate. The sulfhydryl compound "mesna" (*m*ercapto *e*thane *s*ulfonate *s*odium [*Na*]) must be used in conjunction with hydration. The sulfhydryl groups of mesna bind preferentially to acrolein in the bladder, forming a nontoxic complex that can be voided, and preventing mucosal acrolein attachment and damage. Mesna does not interfere with the cytotoxic activity of cyclophosphamide or ifosfamide. For high-dose cyclophosphamide regimens (>2 g/m^2/dose), hyperhydration, mesna, or continuous bladder irrigations have been used successfully to prevent hemorrhagic cystitis.[84]

Although bladder toxicity is most characteristic of these compounds, damage to the renal tubules may also occur. Nephrotoxicity has been best documented in children receiving ifosfamide and in patients receiving high-dose cyclophosphamide regimens. Toxicity may be mediated by acrolein, similar to bladder toxicity, or through the effects of the ifosfamide metabolite chloroacetaldehyde. Mesna may not maintain a high enough concentration the renal tubules to prevent acrolein-induced nephrotoxicity.[84,85]

CNS toxicity is common with ifosfamide but does not occur with cyclophosphamide. It typically presents as decreased level of arousal, occasionally with progression to somnolence, coma, and death. Confusion, hallucinations, and seizures may also occur. CNS toxicity is more common from single large ifosfamide doses, and may be caused by the chloroacetaldehyde metabolite. Rare toxicities from cyclophosphamide include pulmonary fibrosis and cardiac toxicity, especially in bone marrow transplant doses. Cyclophosphamide can also cause SIADH.[81,82]

NITROSOUREAS

The nitrosoureas are alkylating agents characterized by lipophilicity and ability to cross the blood-brain barrier. Carmustine or bischloroethylnitrosourea (BCNU) and lomustine (CCNU) are commercially available. BCNU is available as an intravenous preparation and as a drug-impregnated biodegradable wafer (Gliadel) for direct application to residual tumor tissue following surgical resection of brain tumors. The nitrosoureas decompose to reactive alkylating metabolites and to isocyanate compounds that have several effects on reproducing cells.[33,81,82]

Pharmacokinetics

The nitrosoureas are extensively and rapidly biotransformed after administration, and the degradation products demonstrate a prolonged elimination, perhaps from binding to cellular components. Metabolites and a small percentage of intact drug are excreted in urine. Because of the lipophilic nature of these compounds, they enter the CNS readily and achieve concentrations of about 30% of plasma levels. This has made them useful agents in the treatment of patients with brain tumors. Lomustine is administered orally and is well absorbed.

Toxicity

Myelosuppression is the dose-limiting toxicity of the nitrosoureas in conventional doses. The myelosuppression is unusually delayed and prolonged, and complete recovery typically takes 6 to 8 weeks. Thrombocytopenia occurs earlier but is generally more pronounced than leukopenia. The nitrosoureas cause severe nausea and vomiting. They are also renal toxins and produce dose-related cumulative glomerulosclerosis, severe tubular loss, and interstitial fibrosis. Carmustine commonly causes facial flushing and pain along the vein during infusion, which may be related to its alcohol vehicle. In long-term treatment or in the high doses of carmustine used with bone marrow transplantation, interstitial pneumonitis and pulmonary fibrosis can be dose limiting. Incidence may be as high as 30%. Patients typically present with shortness of breath, tachypnea, and nonproductive cough, and may improve clinically with administration of corticosteroids. Lomustine has also occasionally produced pulmonary damage.[33,81,82]

NONCLASSIC ALKYLATING AGENTS

Several other cytotoxic agents appear to act as alkylators, although their structures do not include the classic alkylating groups. They are capable of binding covalently to cellular components and include procarbazine (Table 124–13), dacarbazine, temazolamide, and some antitumor antibiotics.[33,81,82]

Dacarbazine and Temozolomide

Dacarbazine, or dimethyl triazeno imidazole carboxamide (DTIC), and temozolomide (dihydro methyl oxoimidaso tetrazino carboxamide) are nonclassic alkylating agents. Both compounds undergo demethylation to the same active intermediates (monomethyl triazeno imidazole carboxamide [MTIC]) that interrupts DNA replication by causing methylation of guanine. Unlike dacarbazine, temozolomide does not require the liver for activation, and is chemical degraded to MTIC at physiologic pH. Both drugs inhibit DNA, RNA, and protein synthesis.[81,86,87]

Pharmacokinetics. Important pharmacokinetic differences exist between the two drugs. Dacarbazine is poorly absorbed, and must be administered by intravenous infusion; temozolomide is rapidly absorbed after oral administration, and is approximately 100% bioavailable when given on a completely empty stomach. Darcarbazine penetrates the CNS poorly, but temozolomide readily crosses the blood-brain barrier, achieving therapeutically active concentrations in cerebral spinal fluid and brain tumor tissues. Both drugs disappear from the plasma biphasically with α-phase half-lives of about 19 minutes for dacarbazine, and 1 hour for temozolomide. Dacarbazine's β-phase half-life is 5 hours as compared to 1.8 hours for temazolomide. About half of an administered dacarbazine dose is recoverable in urine as parent drug, but only very small amounts of temozolomide metabolites are excreted renally.[81,86,87]

Toxicity. Toxicity to dacarbazine is characterized by nausea and vomiting, which tends to decrease with successive doses on multiple-day schedules, and by mild to moderate myelosuppression. It can also produce a flu-like syndrome, which occurs after several days of dacarbazine treatment; burning pain along the injection path; constipation; and photosensitivity. Temozolomide's toxicities are similar: mild to moderate myelosuppression, nausea and vomiting, constipation, and fatigue. An important exception is headache, which occurs in about one-fourth of patients receiving temozolomide, and which can be severe. Elevation of liver function tests can occur with either drug.[81,86,87]

HEAVY METAL COMPOUNDS

CISPLATIN

Cisplatin is a platinum complex with a broad spectrum of antitumor activity and remarkable usefulness in cancer treatment. Recognition of its cytotoxic activity was the result of a serendipitous observation that bacterial growth in culture was altered when an electric current was delivered to the media through platinum electrodes. The growth change was noted to be similar to that produced by alkylating agents and radiation, and it was found that a platinum-chloride complex, now known as cisplatin, generated by the current was responsible for the changes. In early clinical trials, cisplatin had desirable efficacy but unacceptable serious toxicity, especially gastrointestinal and renal toxicities. Later, successful attempts were made to improve the therapeutic index by hydration and vigorous antiemetic therapy, which led to cisplatin's approval for commercial use in the late 1970s.[33,81]

Clinical Pharmacology

Cisplatin's cytotoxicity depends on platinum binding to DNA and the formation of intrastrand cross-links or adducts between neighboring

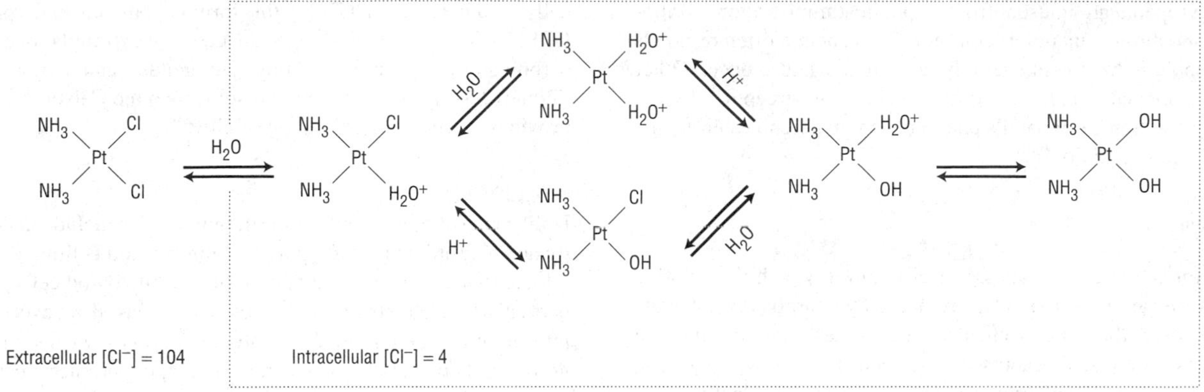

Extracellular $[Cl^-] = 104$ Intracellular $[Cl^-] = 4$

FIGURE 124–19. The aquation reaction of cisplatin. *(From Loehrer PJ, Einhorn LH. Cisplatin. Ann Intern Med 1984;100:705, with permission.)*

guanines. These intrastrand links cause a major bending of the DNA. They may cause cellular damage by distorting the normal DNA conformation and preventing bases that are normally paired from lining up with each other. Interstrand cross-links also occur.[81,88]

The cytotoxic form of cisplatin is the aquated or aquo species, in which hydroxyl groups or water molecules replace the two chloride groups (Fig. 124–19). This reaction occurs readily in low concentrations of chloride, such as the concentrations present within cells, and produces a positively charged compound that can react with DNA. The aquated species is responsible for both the efficacy and toxicity of cisplatin. Resistance to the therapeutic effects of cisplatin may occur through several mechanisms. The ability to repair cisplatin-induced DNA damage may be increased, or cisplatin may be inactivated by increased levels of intracellular glutathione, metallothioneins, or other thiol-containing proteins. Altered uptake of cisplatin compounds into cells may also affect sensitivity to platinum compounds.[81,89]

Pharmacokinetics

Assessment of cisplatin's pharmacokinetics following intravenous infusion is complicated by the existence of three major compartments: free or unbound drug, protein-bound drug, and drug bound to erythrocytes. Its removal pattern is triphasic. The first two phases represent removal of free drug, with elimination half-lives of 20 to 30 minutes and of about 1 hour. This elimination is primarily renal and represents a combination of glomerular filtration and tubular secretion. Protein-bound drug is removed much more slowly, with a terminal half-life of 1 to 3 days. Although renal excretion is important in elimination of protein-bound drug, protein catabolism and biliary excretion also contribute. In addition to depending on renal function for its elimination, cisplatin is also nephrotoxic; thus dose reduction is recommended for patients with preexisting or therapy-induced renal dysfunction (see Table 124–11). Clearance decreases, and exposure to drug (AUC) to increases, with successive cisplatin courses, even in the absence of significant changes in creatinine clearance. These changes correlate with increased drug toxicity and make guidelines for dose changes based on serum creatinine or creatinine clearance unreliable.[81,90]

Toxicity

Cisplatin is a highly toxic antineoplastic agent, with potential for serious nephrotoxicity, ototoxicity, peripheral neuropathy, emesis, and anemia. The significant efficacy of cisplatin against many tumor types makes it a valuable agent despite these toxicities, most of which can be prevented or managed with aggressive supportive care measures. Nephrotoxicity and emesis, which were originally dose limiting, can be successfully prevented.

Cisplatin is well established as a renal tubule poison. The proximal renal tubules are most sensitive to cisplatin-induced damage, but distal tubular function is also affected. Nephrotoxicity is characterized clinically by reduced glomerular filtration rates (GFRs); electrolyte losses, especially potassium and magnesium; and renal failure, which may occur acutely, even in the first day after drug administration. Hypomagnesemia and reduced filtration rate are most characteristic of the acute phase of toxicity. Reduction in creatinine clearance, which may not produce elevated serum creatinine, occurs chronically. Renal damage from cisplatin is often slowly reversible, although hypomagnesemia and reduced creatinine clearance may persist in one-third or more of patients for many years. Risk of nephrotoxicity correlates with high single doses, cumulative doses, dehydration, preexisting renal impairment, and administration of other renal toxins.[49,81,91]

The incidence of nephrotoxicity can be decreased by careful diuresis and by aggressive hydration with chloride-containing solutions, which help to keep the cisplatin in the renal tubules in the nonaquated and therefore nontoxic form. Mannitol may protect the kidney by delaying cisplatin binding onto renal tubular proteins. Furosemide has not been convincingly shown to decrease nephrotoxicity, but diuretics are useful for patients with cardiovascular compromise to prevent fluid overload. Amifostine (WR-2721) is a thiol ester that can protect normal tissues against radiotherapy and alkylating agent-induced damage. It is moderately effective as a chemoprotectant for cisplatin nephrotoxicity, but is not widely used because it increases the emetogenicity of the regimen, and also produces hypotension.[49,81,91,92]

Cisplatin is one of the most severe emetogens among marketed antineoplastic agents. Acute nausea and vomiting can be prevented or limited with corticosteroids and serotonin-receptor antagonists. Approximately 60% of patients who receive cisplatin will also experience delayed nausea and vomiting 2 to 4 days after drug administration, which is less easily prevented, and which can have a serious impact on fluid and nutritional status.[93]

Neuropathy, which includes ototoxicity, peripheral neuropathy, and, rarely, ocular toxicity, has emerged as a dose-limiting toxicity of cisplatin with effective management of renal damage and emesis. Ototoxicity most commonly affects the high-frequency hearing ranges and may be associated with loss of outer hair cells from the cochlea. Hearing loss is usually permanent, but vestibular toxicity generally reverses over time. Effective means of preventing ototoxicity are not known. Peripheral neuropathy is characteristically distal, in a "stocking-and-glove" distribution, and may begin and progress after cisplatin is discontinued. Common symptoms include paresthesias and mild to severe pain. Peripheral neuropathy is associated with cumulative doses and is usually reversible, although complete resolution may take more than a year.[49,81] Although significant neutropenia or thrombocytopenia are unusual from cisplatin administration, normocytic, normochronic anemia is common. This anemia often responds to erythropoietin treatment. Hemolytic anemia can also occur. Other toxicities of cisplatin include disturbances in color perception, hypersensitivity reactions, Raynaud's phenomenon, hypercholesterolemia, and rare hepatic toxicity.[49,81]

CARBOPLATIN

Carboplatin is a structural analog of cisplatin in which the chloride groups of the parent compound are replaced by a carboxycyclobutane moiety. It shares the same mechanism of action as cisplatin, although it generates an aquated reactive form much more slowly than cisplatin. The spectrum of activity is similar, although not identical, and cross-resistance between the two agents is common. Carboplatin differs markedly from cisplatin, however, in its pharmacokinetics and toxicity.[33,81]

Pharmacokinetics

Many pharmacokinetic differences between carboplatin and cisplatin are explained by differences in plasma protein binding. Carboplatin binds to plasma protein more slowly and less extensively than does cisplatin, resulting in a much longer plasma half-life of unbound carboplatin platinum. Carboplatin's pharmacokinetics are linear, with a steady-state volume of distribution approximately equal to total body water, and clearance of ultrafilterable carboplatin platinum is more than double that of creatinine clearance. The reduced protein binding also results in a much larger percentage of carboplatin than cisplatin being excreted in urine (60% to 80%). Patients with compromised renal function require dose reductions to limit myelosuppressive toxicity. Several guidelines for dose modification for patients with impaired renal function have been developed,[94,95] but the most widely used dosage schema uses a target AUC and renal function parameters to estimate the carboplatin dose.[94] This schema was developed by Calvert and colleagues and is referred to as the Calvert formula (Table 124–14). Estimated or measured creatinine clearance is typically used to represent GFR in this formula, but may underpredict the GFR.[96] Chatelut et al. developed an alternative formula for estimating carboplatin doses based on body size, gender, and serum creatinine (Table 124–14). It is more cumbersome than the Calvert formula, but provides a better approximation of GFR.[95,96]

TABLE 124–14. Carboplatin Dose Modifications in Patients with Impaired Renal Function

Calvert Formula
  Dose = AUC × (GFR + 25)
  where
  Dose = Total dose in milligrams
  AUC = Desired area under the curve in mg/mL × min:
    Target AUC is 5–7 for single-agent carboplatin.
    Target AUC is 4–5 for carboplatin in combination with other myelosuppressive drugs.
  GFR = Glomerular filtration rate (not normalized for surface area).
    Estimated or measured creatinine clearance is usually substituted for true GFR, but may underestimate carboplatin dose.
  25 = Average nonrenal clearance for adults

From Ref. 94.

Chatelut Formula
  Dose = AUC × Estimated Carboplatin Clearance
  where
  Estimated Carboplatin Clearance = 0.134 × weight + [218 × weight × (1 − 0.00457 × age) × (1 − 0.314 × sex]/creatinine expressed in micromolar concentration
  Note: weight in kilogram, age in years, and sex = 0 for males and 1 for females

From Ref. 95.

Toxicity

Unlike cisplatin, whose dose-limiting toxicities include nephrotoxicity and neurotoxicity, carboplatin administration is limited by hematologic toxicity. It causes suppression of white blood cells, and more particularly, platelets, with characteristic delayed recovery that can prevent retreatment more frequently than every 4 weeks. In contrast, however, its potential to cause renal damage, peripheral neuropathy, and ototoxicity is much less than that of comparable cisplatin doses, making it is a very useful alternative to cisplatin therapy in patients with preexisting compromise to these organs, or at high risk of damage. The emetogenic potential of carboplatin is also substantially less than that of cisplatin, although it is still a moderate to severe emetogen.[81,97] Carboplatin's efficacy, low risk of major organ toxicity, and simple administration have made it the most commonly used platinum agent. With its extensive use, however, have come greater problems with hypersensitivity reactions. Carboplatin-associated hypersensitivity reactions develop in about one quarter of patients who receive more than seven courses of platinum drug therapy. Reactions are rare with initial drug administration. Symptoms range from itching and erythema to respiratory arrest.[97] Skin testing with the carboplatin infusion solution prior to premedications can predict most patients to whom carboplatin can be safely administered.[98]

MISCELLANEOUS AGENTS

BLEOMYCIN

Bleomycin or "bleo" is an antitumor antibiotic. It is a mixture of peptides from fungal *Streptomyces* species, and, as such, its strength is expressed in units of drug activity. One unit is roughly equal to 1 mg of polypeptide protein.[99] The predominant peptide is bleomycin A2, which makes up approximately 70% of the commercial product. Bleomycin's cytotoxicity is secondary to DNA strand breakage, or scission, which it produces via free radical formation. Cytotoxicity depends on binding of an iron-bleomycin complex to DNA. The bleomycin-iron complex then reduces molecular oxygen to free oxygen radicals that cause primarily single-strand breaks in DNA. Bleomycin has greatest effect on cells in the G2 phase of the cell cycle and in mitosis.[33,99,100]

Pharmacokinetics

Bleomycin is taken up slowly by cells and is inactivated within cells by the enzyme aminohydrolase. This enzyme is widely distributed but is present in only low concentrations in the skin and the lungs, explaining the predominant toxicities of bleomycin to those sites. The presence of hydrolase enzymes in tumor cells is the primary mechanism of resistance to bleomycin. Cells can also become resistant by repairing the DNA breaks produced by bleomycin. Bleomycin is eliminated renally; 45% to 70% of the dose is excreted in the urine within 24 hours. Half-life of elimination is 2 to 4 hours in patients with normal renal function but may increase to more than 20 hours in patients with renal failure. Increased toxicity, especially pulmonary toxicity, is associated with renal impairment. Dose reduction proportional to the degree of impairment is recommended in patients with severely compromised renal function (see Table 124–11).[33,99,100]

Following intrapleural administration, cavitary levels are about 10 to 20 times higher than corresponding plasma levels, although nearly half of an intracavitary dose eventually reaches the systemic circulation.[101]

Toxicity

Bleomycin is not myelosuppressive. Nausea and vomiting are also mild. Bleomycin does produce fevers within hours to 2 days of administration in 25% to 50% of patients. Fevers may be prevented or managed with antipyretics. Rarely, high fevers occur, which can produce tachypnea, hypotension, delirium, and even death. These reactions are not true hypersensitivity reactions. They are likely caused by the direct release of pyrogens. Lymphoma patients with disease-related fevers are most susceptible to hyperpyrexial episodes. Administering a test dose before the first dose has only limited utility in predicting which patients are at risk for this reaction.[33,99,100]

The most important toxicities of bleomycin are to the lungs and the skin. Interstitial pneumonitis can progress to fibrosis and cause death from hypoxia. Incidence is related both to high single doses (greater than 30 U) and to cumulative dose, with an incidence of approximately 3% up to a total dose of 450 U, and of 10% in patients receiving higher doses. Advanced age, preexisting pulmonary disease, previous chest irradiation, exposure to high oxygen concentrations, and renal impairment also increase risk. The clinical features are usually dyspnea with pulmonary infiltrates. Deterioration may be sudden and severe and may occur months after completing therapy. Lung biopsy is required for definitive diagnosis. The only established treatment of pulmonary damage is drug discontinuation, but pulmonary symptoms may continue to progress after bleomycin is stopped. The value of corticosteroids has not been proven. Pulmonary symptoms may gradually reverse in patients who survive bleomycin pneumonitis.[49,99,100]

Mucocutaneous toxicity is less serious than pulmonary damage, but more common. It includes mild stomatitis; hyperpigmentation over the elbows, knees, and small joints of the hands; thickening of the nail beds; alopecia; and a syndrome of skin erythema and edema.[99,100]

HYDROXYUREA

Hydroxyurea is a unique drug that inhibits ribonucleotide reductase, the enzyme required to convert ribonucleotides into the deoxyribonucleotide forms required for both DNA synthesis and repair. Cells accumulate in the S phase because DNA synthesis is inhibited, and only abnormally short DNA strands are produced. Hydroxyurea is well absorbed orally. The main route of elimination is renal excretion, although the percentage detected in urine varies markedly from patient to patient. It distributes rapidly to tissues and enters both the CNS and "third-space" fluids readily. Toxicity is primarily marrow suppression of rapid onset, which is sometimes a desired therapeutic effect of the drug. Chronic therapy produces skin hyperpigmentation, erythema especially of the face and hands, and rashes.[33,35]

L-ASPARAGINASE

L-Asparaginase is unique among cytotoxic drugs in its unusual mechanism of action, patterns of toxicity, and source. It is an enzyme produced by bacteria. It is commercially available in two forms, both of *Escherichia coli* origin. The first is an unconjugated form of the enzyme, available under the trade name Elspar, which is sometimes called native protein. L-Asparaginase is also marketed as pegaspargase (Oncospar), in which L-asparaginase is covalently conjugated to PEG.

Clinical Pharmacology

L-Asparagine is a nonessential amino acid that can be synthesized by most mammalian cells, except for those of certain lymphoid human malignancies, which lack or have very low levels of the synthetase enzyme required for L-asparagine formation. L-Asparagine is normally degraded by the enzyme L-asparaginase, which depletes existing supplies and inhibits protein synthesis. Increased L-asparagine synthetase activity within tumor cells causes resistance to L-asparaginase treatment.[33,101,102]

Pharmacokinetics

The metabolic fate and elimination of L-asparaginase are are believed to be mediated by antibody formation against L-asparaginase. The half-life of elimination of the native protein form of L-asparaginase is about 1 day. Conjugation with PEG reduces uptake by the reticuloendothelial system and antibody formation, prolonging the half-life to about 6 days. PEG protection of L-asparaginase permits both lower doses and less-frequent drug administration. Clearance of either preparation is accelerated in patients who develop hypersensitivity to the drug. Asparaginase distributes within the intravascular space and achieves low but useful levels within the CNS. No L-asparaginase activity is detectable in urine.[101,102]

Toxicity

Hypersensitivity reactions occur in about 25% of patients receiving unconjugated L-asparaginase and are most common in those receiving intravenous doses, single-agent therapy, or repeated courses of treatment. True anaphylaxis occurs in 5% to 9% of patients, and is fatal in about 1%, mandating allergic precautions during administration. Skin testing is helpful in selecting patients at high risk for allergic reactions. PEG-asparaginase is indicated for patients with hypersensitivity reactions to conventional L-asparaginase. Although hypersensitivity reactions are still common in patients receiving the PEG-conjugated form of L-asparaginase, they are rarely severe.[101,102]

L-Asparaginase's inhibition of protein synthesis produces several toxicities, particularly hemorrhage or thrombosis from impaired synthesis of clotting factors and/or naturally occurring anticoagulants, such as protein C and antithrombin III. Hyperglycemia secondary to decreased insulin synthesis is also common and can be abrupt in onset. Acute pancreatitis and liver toxicity are common, and are sometimes dose limiting. Cerebral dysfunction, which most typically manifests as somnolence or confusion but which may progress to coma, occurs in about 25% of patients. This may be secondary to low amino acid levels within the CNS. Nausea occurs in more than half of patients. L-Asparaginase, however, does not produce myelosuppression, mucositis, or alopecia. The incidence of nonhypersensitivity-related adverse reactions is not affected by conjugation of L-asparaginase with PEG.[101,102]

ESTRAMUSTINE

Estramustine is an unusual drug in that it structurally combines the alkylating agent nor-nitrogen mustard with the hormone estradiol. It was designed with the intent that the estradiol portion of the molecule would facilitate uptake of the alkylating agent into hormone-sensitive prostate cancer cells. Despite the inclusion of an alkylator, estramustine does not function *in vivo* as an alkylating agent. Estrogens are released after its administration, but all of estramustine's pharmacologic effects cannot be attributed to estrogenic hormones. In the mid-1980s, estramustine was redefined as an antimicrotubule agent. It binds covalently to microtubule-associated proteins (MAPs) that are part of the structural support for microtubules. The binding causes the separation of MAPs from the microtubules, inhibiting microtubule assembly and eventually causing their disassembly.[58]

Pharmacokinetics

Estramustine is administered orally and is well absorbed, with a bioavailability of at least 75%. Milk and calcium-containing antacids can decrease absorption. Metabolites of both nor-nitrogen mustard and estradiol are excreted into the bile, feces, and urine.[58]

Toxicity

Nausea and vomiting are the dose-limiting effects of oral estramustine. Despite the presence of the alkylator, myelosuppression is very uncommon. Although the estrogenic component of estramustine is not believed to contribute significantly to its cytotoxic effects, it does contribute to toxicity. Most patients develop gynecomastia and nipple tenderness. Cardiovascular effects that are attributable to the estrogenic component include edema, thromboembolism, myocardial infarction, and cerebrovascular events.[58]

ARSENIC TRIOXIDE

Arsenic is an organic element and a well-known poison that was recently marketed as a treatment for acute promyelocytic leukemia (APL). Although its medicinal uses date back thousands of years, its current clinical role is attributed to successful use in the 1970s of a traditional Chinese medication that contained arsenic trioxide. As an antineoplastic, arsenic trioxide acts as a differentiating agent, inducing the growth progression of cancerous cells into mature, more normal cells. It also induces programmed cell death or apoptosis.[104,105]

Pharmacokinetics

Arsenic is eliminated in the feces, urine, sweat, hair, skin, and lungs, although most arsenic eventually is eliminated in the urine. The half-life of elimination is 3 to 5 days after oral administration.[104]

Toxicity

Dose-limiting adverse effects of arsenic trioxide are weight gain secondary to fluid retention, and peripheral neuropathy. Although the neuropathy is slowly reversible, it has occasionally been severe enough to produce paralysis. Its most common side effects are dizziness during infusion, prolonged QTc interval on electrocardiogram, skin reactions, hyperglycemia, and musculoskeletal pain.[104] About 30% to 50% of patients with APL who are treated with arsenic develop the "retinoic acid syndrome" (see discussion on Retinoids), a syndrome of pulmonary infiltrates, progressive respiratory distress, and hypotension that must be treated promptly with corticosteroids.[104,106] Environmental arsenic ingestion is associated with an increase in cancer incidence, but it is not objectively proven to be a carcinogen.[104]

BIOLOGICS AND BIOLOGICALLY DIRECTED THERAPIES

The conventional anticancer drugs are relatively indiscriminate cellular poisons. Although a few, such as methotrexate, capecitabine, and L-asparaginase demonstrate some degree of selectivity for malignant cells, the selectivity is incomplete, and dose-limiting damage to normal cells also occurs. Recently, anticancer research has focused on development of anticancer agents that have been designed to target malignant cells more specifically, or the biochemical processes that control cancerous cell growth. Many have produced clinical successes and are now commercially available. Many more agents, using a variety of increasingly specific therapeutic approaches, are under clinical development.

BIOLOGIC RESPONSE MODIFIERS

INTERFERONS

The interferons (IFN) are a family of proteins produced by nucleated cells and by recombinant-DNA technology, which have antiviral, antiproliferative, and immunoregulatory activities. They are classified as α, β, or γ interferons based on antigenic, biologic, and pharmacologic properties. Many subtypes of IFN-α are known. IFN-α-2a and -α-2b, approved for anticancer indications, are very similar single-species recombinant products.

The mechanisms of IFN-α's antitumor action are complex. IFN increases the activity of cytotoxic cells within the immune system, but direct antiproliferative effects also play a role. IFNs prolong the cell cycle, which results in cytostasis, an increase in cell size, and apoptosis. They can inhibit new blood vessel formation in tumors and can increase the expression of antigens on tumor-cell surfaces, making the cancerous cells more easily recognized by the cells of the immune system. They also inhibit or block certain oncogenes that can direct the unregulated cell growth that is characteristic of cancerous cells. Alterations in gene expression may change the levels of receptors for other cytokines, or the concentration of regulatory proteins on immune cells, or may activate enzymes that alter cellular growth and function.[107,108]

Pharmacokinetics

The interferons are not absorbed orally, because they are proteins destroyed by digestive enzymes. The bioavailability of IFN-α after intramuscular or subcutaneous administration is nearly complete, however. Total body clearance is nearly double normal creatinine clearance, suggesting that renal secretion and catabolism or extrarenal elimination occur. Little or no IFN is excreted into the urine, and hepatic metabolism of IFN-α is minor. Animal data indicate that proteolytic degradation in renal tubules is the major method of elimination. The plasma half-life of elimination is 4 to 5 hours, but biologic effects peak at 24 to 48 hours, and may persist for several days.[107,108]

Toxicity

The most characteristic toxicity of IFN is an acute flu-like syndrome of fever, chills, malaise, myalgias, and headaches that begins within a few hours after administration. These symptoms can be managed with antipyretics. Tolerance to the flu-like effects develops over 1 to 2 weeks but does not develop to fatigue, which is dose related and is the most common dose-limiting toxicity of IFN-α. Gastrointestinal toxicities, myelosuppression, increased liver function tests, and proteinuria are rarely troublesome at low doses, but increase in incidence and severity as doses increase.[63,107,108] Neurologic or psychiatric side effects have become increasingly important with chronic use of IFNs. Typically, patients begin to complain of depression, mental slowing, and memory loss after several weeks of therapy. In a few patients, high dose IFN therapy produces confusion, severe depression, lethargy, mania, and suicidal behaviors. Prophylactic antidepressant therapy may help prevent or manage depressive symptoms.[109]

INTERLEUKIN-2 (ALDESLEUKIN)

Interleukin-2 (IL-2, aldesleukin) is a lymphokine produced recombinantly that has diverse immunologic effects. IL-2 promotes B- and T-cell proliferation and differentiation and initiates a cytokine cascade with multiple interacting immunologic effects. The IL-2 receptor is expressed in increased amounts on activated T cells and mediates most of the effects of IL-2. Antitumor effects depend on proliferation of a variety of cytotoxic cells that can recognize and destroy tumor cells without damaging normal cells. Some of these cytotoxic cells are natural killer (NK) cells, lymphokine-activated killer (LAK) cells, and tumor-infiltrating lymphocytes (TIL).[110,111]

Pharmacokinetics

Like the interferons, IL-2 preparations are proteins that are not absorbed after oral administration. Bioavailability after intramuscular injection is approximately 35%. Serum concentrations following intravenous administration are proportional to dose and decline biexponentially, with a terminal half-life of 30 to 120 minutes. Elimination is slower after subcutaneous administration, and peak concentrations achieved are lower. Clearance is estimated at 120 mL/min, suggesting that renal tubular filtration is the major means of elimination.[111]

Toxicity

The toxicity of IL-2 is related to dose, route, and duration of therapy, but, in general, IL-2 is toxic therapy that requires vigorous supportive care. Low doses may be well tolerated, even in outpatient administration.[112,113]

The most common dose-limiting toxicities are hypotension, fluid retention, and renal dysfunction. IL-2 decreases peripheral vascular resistance, producing peripheral vasodilation, tachycardia, and hypotension. A characteristic vascular- or capillary-leak syndrome (VLS) produces fluid retention, which in turn can cause respiratory compromise. These toxicities require administration of vasopressors in most patients, judicious use of fluid support and diuretics, and supplemental oxygen. Patients with underlying cardiovascular or renal abnormalities are more susceptible to these adverse effects, making careful patient selection important.[63,110–112]

In addition to the hemodynamic and renal effects, most patients treated with IL-2 in full doses experience thrombocytopenia, anemia, eosinophilia, reversible cholestasis, and skin erythema with burning and pruritus. Neuropsychiatric changes, hypothyroidism, and bacterial infections, particularly staphylococcal infections, are also common. Bacterial infections are attributed to an IL-2 associated neutrophil chemotactic defect.[110–113] In general, the toxicities from IL-2 therapy reverse quickly once therapy is stopped, and can be managed or prevented by careful prospective monitoring and pharmacologic supportive care. Although most acute IL-2 adverse effects can be ameliorated by corticosteroid administration, steroids potentially decrease the antitumor effects of IL-2. Their concurrent use is not recommended.[110–112]

DENILEUKIN DIFTITOX

Denileukin diftitox (DAB_{389}IL-2, Ontak) is the first commercially available immunotoxin, a recombinant fusion protein that combines the active sections of both IL-2 and diphtheria toxin. Unconjugated diphtheria toxin is much too toxic to administer to humans. As the "payload" of the fusion protein however, its cytotoxic effects are directed to cells that express the high affinity form of IL-2 receptor, such as cancer cells of some patients with cutaneous T-cell lymphoma. Once denileukin diftitox interacts with the IL-2 receptors, the immunotoxin inhibits protein synthesis in the cancer cells and causes cell death.[114]

Pharmacokinetics

Denileukin diftitox is administered intravenously and rapidly distributed. The terminal half-life is approximately 70 to 80 minutes. It is metabolized by proteolytic degradation. Development of antibodies to the fusion protein accelerates its clearance.[115]

Toxicity

Although denileukin diftitox is directed therapy, its target of cells that express high affinity IL-2 receptors is not a specific target, that is, these receptors are expressed on cells other than cancer cells. Denileukin diftitox produces acute hypersensitivity reactions in about 60% of patients within 24 hours of drug infusion. Hypotension, back pain, dyspnea, and chest pain or tightness are the most common hypersensitivity reactions. Anaphylaxis occurs in 1 to 2% of patients. Symptoms usually respond to temporarily stopping or decreasing the rate of the infusion. Premedication with antihistamines and acetaminophen is recommended, but routine use of steroids should be avoided. Flu-like symptoms, sometimes with prominent diarrhea, occur in most patients, and respond to symptomatic management. Denileukin diftitox also produces a vascular leak syndrome, with symptoms of hypotension, edema, and hypoalbuminemia, in about 25% of patients. At least two of these symptoms must be present simultaneously within the first 2 weeks of a treatment cycle for diagnosis of VLS. It differs from the VLS produced by high dose IL-2 in that it occurs in fewer patients, is delayed in onset, is usually self-limited, and does not consistently recur on retreatment. Thrombotic events and infections are also problematic, but myelosuppression, with the exception of lymphopenia, is uncommon.[114,115]

ENDOCRINE THERAPIES

Perhaps the earliest successful approach to target the growth processes of cancerous cells was the use of endocrine therapies. Endocrine manipulation is an option for management of cancers from tissues whose growth is under gonadal hormonal control, especially breast, prostate, and endometrial cancers. These cancers may regress if the "feeding" hormone is eliminated or antagonized. Major organ system toxicity is uncommon from hormonal treatment, making it the least toxic of systemic anticancer therapies. Increasingly specific agents such as the selective estrogen receptor modulators (SERMs) and aromatase inhibitors have recently been marketed. The clinical applications and toxicity of individual agents are detailed in the breast and prostate cancer chapters.

Corticosteroids are also useful anticancer agents because of their lymphocytotoxic effects. Their primary use is in management of hematologic malignancies, especially lymphomas, lymphocytic leukemias, and the plasma cell cancer multiple myeloma. In addition to their cytotoxic effects, corticosteroids have many other applications in supportive care of cancer patients, as outlined in Table 124–15. The corticosteroids have diverse toxicities in chronic or high-dose use but

TABLE 124–15. Application of Corticosteroids in Supportive Care of Cancer Patients

Nausea and vomiting
Cerebral edema secondary to brain metastases or cranial irradiation
Spinal cord compression
Hypercalcemia
Transfusion reactions
Appetite stimulation
Radiation or drug-induced pneumonitis
Prevention and treatment of anaphylactic reactions
Graft-versus-host disease after bone marrow transplantation
Pain secondary to nerve compression or edema
Fluid retention from docetaxel

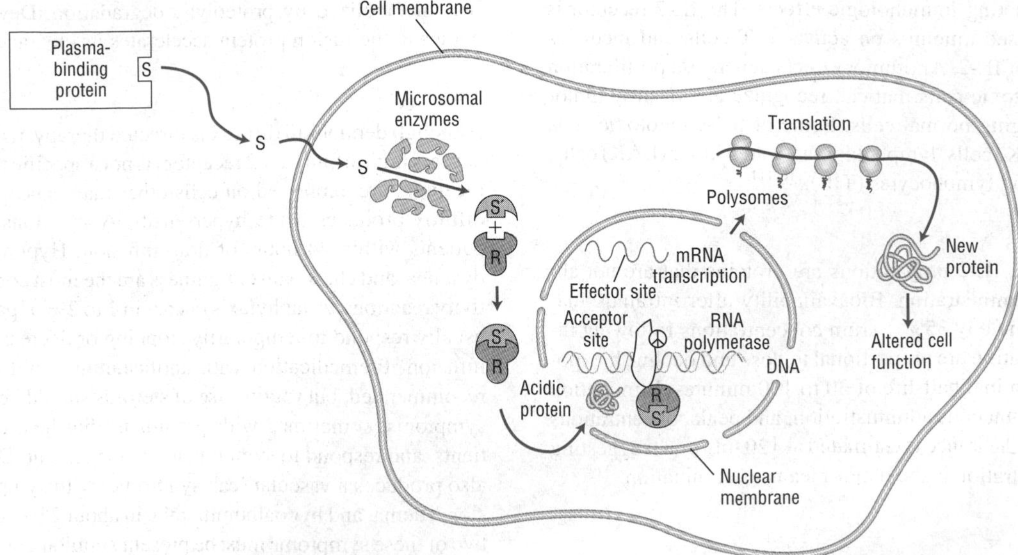

FIGURE 124–20. Representation of the mechanism of steroid hormone action. Hormones (S) diffuse into cells, bind to receptors (R), and are translocated to the nucleus, where they bind to DNA and alter expression of specific genes and, in turn, change protein production and alter cell function. *(From Lipman ME, Eil C. Steroid therapy of cancer. In: Chabner BA ed. Pharmacologic Principles of Cancer Treatment. Philadelphia, Saunders, 1982:132–182, with permission.)*

are generally well tolerated in the short-term therapies usually used in cancer treatment.[116]

All steroid hormones share the same four-ring cyclopentaneperhydrophenanthrene structure, and all are derived from cholesterol. Despite their greatly diverse actions, all steroid hormones are believed to act by a similar mechanism (Fig. 124–20).

RETINOIDS

Vitamin A and its metabolites, collectively referred to as the retinoids, play important roles in numerous biologic processes, including normal cellular differentiation. Because cancerous growth is characterized by abnormal cellular differentiation, retinoids are proving to have important therapeutic roles in the treatment and perhaps prevention of cancers. All-*trans*-retinoic acid (ATRA, tretinoin) is a naturally occurring derivative of vitamin A (retinol). Other retinoids indicated for treatment of cancers include alitretinoin (9-*cis*-retinoic acid, Panretin) which is available in gel form for topical management of Kaposi's sarcoma lesions and bexarotene (Targretin) gel or capsules for treatment of cutaneous T-cell lymphoma.[117]

CLINICAL PHARMACOLOGY

Retinoids are classed as morphogens, small molecules released from one type of cells that can affect the growth and differentiation of neighboring cells. Their normal roles in the human body are to induce differentiation of some cells, stop the differentiation of others, and both suppress and induce apoptosis in different cell types. Their diverse actions come from the diversity of their receptors. The two classes of retinoid receptors are retinoid X receptors (RXRs), and retinoic acid receptors (RARs), each with α, β, and γ subclasses. RXRs are versatile; they bind to RARs and to other nuclear receptors such as thyroid hormone receptors. Once activated, the receptors act as transcription factors that in turn regulate the expression of genes that control cellular growth and differentiation.[117]

All-*trans*-retinoic binds primarily to the RAR-α receptors and produces high complete-remission rates in patients with APL. The genetic defect in APL is a 15;17 chromosomal translocation. The gene for nuclear retinoic acid receptor α (RAR-α) is located on chromosome 17, and the translocation produces an abnormal RAR-α fusion protein. ATRA reverses these effects and promotes terminal myeloid cellular differentiation.[118]

Alitretinoin, or 9-*cis*-retinoic acid, is considered a panagonist; that is, it binds to all known retinoid receptors, producing diverse regulatory effects. Bexarotene is synthetic and is classed as a rexinoid. It is the first RXR-selective retinoid agonist. The exact mechanism of action of alitretinoin and bexarotene as anticancer agents is unknown.[120]

PHARMACOKINETICS

Following oral administration, both ATRA and bexarotene reach peak plasma concentrations at 1 to 2 hours. Both are heavily protein bound. ATRA is rapidly cleared from the systemic circulation, with a half-life of approximately 1 hour. Bexarotene is cleared more slowly; its terminal half-life is 2 to 5 hours. P450 enzymes hydroxylate both compounds; bexarotene also produces oxidative metabolites. Their metabolites are conjugated and excreted through the hepatobiliary system. Over time, plasma concentrations of ATRA produced by a given dose markedly diminish, which may be associated with loss of clinical response. Topical bexarotene and alitretinoin are not significantly absorbed.[118–121]

TOXICITY

ATRA's most commonly reported adverse effect is headache, which usually responds to mild analgesics. However, intracranial hypertension (pseudotumor cerebri) also occurs. These patients present with severe headache, nausea, and papilledema. Other toxicities are common to vitamin A derivatives in general and affect the skin and mucous membranes (xerostomia, cheilitis, skin desquamation), the eyes (dryness, blepharoconjunctivitis, corneal erosion), musculoskeletal system (myalgias, arthralgias, bone pain), and hypertriglyceridemia. Dry skin and mucous membranes respond well to topical emollients. Tolerance usually develops to headache and musculoskeletal symptoms with continued dosing. Reversible elevations in serum transaminases and bilirubin may occur. ATRA also shares the teratogenic properties of the retinoids, and all patients should be counseled to avoid pregnancy.[118]

Hyperleukocytosis occurs in up to 50% of APL patients who receive ATRA. This requires no specific intervention if unaccompanied by other symptoms but may be an early indicator of the "retinoic-acid syndrome." This syndrome is not specific to retinoic acid, because it also occurs with arsenic treatment of APL patients. It may be linked instead to therapy-mediated leukocyte differentiation in APL patients. It occurs in up to 25% of patients and is characterized by fever and respiratory distress in addition to hyperleukocytosis. Patients may develop pulmonary infiltrates, pleural or pericardial effusions, weight gain, edema, and hypotension, similar to vascular leak syndrome seen with IL-2 administration. Progressive respiratory deterioration, multiorgan failure, and death are common, without prompt institution of high-dose corticosteroids.[118]

Oral bexarotene's most common toxicities are hyperlipidemia (primarily hypertriglyceridemia) in most patients; hypercholesteremia; hypothyroidism; weakness; itching, skin disorder and rash. Typical Vitamin A toxicities are uncommon, since bexarotene is a selective retinoid agonist.[119,120] Topical bexarotene and alitretinoin primarily produce skin irritation as toxicity.[121]

IMATINIB MESYLATE

Imatinib mesylate (STI-571, Gleevec) is the first tyrosine kinase inhibitor to be approved for treatment of cancer. It inhibits the deregulated BCR-ABL tyrosine kinase that is the molecular abnormality in patients with chronic myelogenous leukemia (CML), and that results from the "Philadelphia chromosome" translocation that is characteristic of CML. The deregulated tyrosine kinase constantly drives leukemic cell proliferation. Imatinib inhibits cell proliferation and induces apoptosis in the Philadelphia chromosome-positive cells. It is relatively, but not completely, selective for these cells.[122–124]

PHARMACOKINETICS

Imatinib is administered orally and is well absorbed, with peak levels achieved within 2 to 4 hours. It is highly protein bound, and metabolized in the liver, primarily by the cytochrome P450 enzyme CYP3A4. Drug interactions are expected with CYP34A inhibitors or inducers. Unchanged drug and metabolites are eliminated in the feces, with half-lives of about 18 hours and 40 hours, respectively. Data on the dosing of patients with impaired hepatic function are not available. Dose modifications are not expected to be necessary for patients with renal impairment.[122,123]

TOXICITY

Imatinib mesylate is generally well tolerated. The most common side effects are mild to moderate nausea and vomiting in about half of patients. To reduce nausea, it should be taken with a meal and a full glass of water. The most troublesome side effect has been periorbital or lower limb edema in about half of patients, that responds to diuretics or dose reduction. Pleural effusion, ascites, or pulmonary edema occur in up to 5% of patients. Muscle cramps, rash, diarrhea, neutropenia, and thrombocytopenia are also common. Severe increases in liver function tests occur in up to 5% of patients.[122–124]

THALIDOMIDE

Thalidomide, the infamous drug that caused severe limb deformities (phocomelia or "seal limbs") when used by pregnant women as an over-the-counter sedative in the 1960s, is approved for treatment of leprosy and has orphan drug status for multiple myeloma. It has documented clinical activity in several other cancers as well. Thalidomide is a glutamic acid derivative, and broadly classed as an immunomodulatory agent. It has many potential mechanisms of action as an anticancer agent. It is an angiogenesis inhibitor, interfering with the growth of new blood vessels needed for tumor growth. This action is also linked to its teratogenic effects. Other possible mechanisms include: direct inhibition of cancer cells, free radical oxidative damage to DNA, interfering with adhesion of cancer cells, inhibiting tumor necrosis factor-α production, or altering secretion of cytokines that affect the growth of cancer cells.[125,126]

PHARMACOKINETICS

Thalidomide is poorly soluble and unstable in water, so it is administered orally. Peak levels are reached in about 4 hours, and it is widely distributed, with a large volume of distribution. Once absorbed, it is rapidly degraded by spontaneous cleavage to multiple metabolites, which are then excreted in the urine, with an elimination half-life of about 8 hours. Half-lives increase with increasing doses. The effects of impaired renal or hepatic function on thalidomide clearance are not established.[126]

TOXICITY

Dose-related sedation, depression, weakness or fatigue, and constipation are the most common adverse effects, but are usually mild to moderate in severity. Peripheral neuropathy occurs in up to one-fourth of patients. Great care must be taken to prevent thalidomide's use during pregnancy.[126,127]

MONOCLONAL ANTIBODIES

The monoclonal antibodies have become important biologic response modifiers used in the treatment of cancer. There are currently four agents approved for use as anticancer agents within the United States: trastuzumab, rituximab, gemtuzumab, and alemtuzumab. These agents consist of specific immunoglobulin sequences that are known to recognize a specific antigen or protein on the surface of cells. There are several mechanisms by which monoclonal antibodies may induce death of cancer cells. Direct mechanisms include induction of apoptosis, blockade of a growth factor receptor, or induction of anti-idiotype antibodies. Important indirect mechanisms include antibody-dependent cellular toxicity (ADCC) and complement-mediated cellular toxicity.[128,129] Gemtuzumab is unique in that it is combined with a cytotoxic antibiotic, calicheamicin. Once gemtuzumab binds to its cellular surface receptor, the complex is internalized. The cytotoxic antibiotic is liberated into the cytoplasm by lysozymes, where it can interfere with DNA synthesis and cause cell death.[130] Table 124–16 summarizes the characteristics of the monoclonal antibodies, and Table 124–10 presents their uses.[130–134]

Although monoclonal antibodies are designed to be specific to a particular target antigen, that target antigen may also be expressed on normal tissue to some degree, decreasing their selectivity. Thus, toxicity often occurs when the monoclonal antibodies bind to normal cells, or are recognized by the immune system. All of the monoclonal antibodies are associated with some degree of infusion-related reactions. The severity of these reactions can range from mild (e.g., fever,

TABLE 124–16. Summary of Monoclonal Antibodies Used in the Treatment of Cancer

Agent (Brand Name)	Molecular Target	Mechanism of Action	Adverse Effects	Comments
Alemtuzumab (Campath)	Targeted to CD52 antigen, which is expressed on the surface of normal and malignant B and T lymphocytes, NK cells, monocytes, macrophages	Binds to CD52, causing antibody-dependent lysis of leukemic cells	Severe infusion-related reactions*	Premedicate with diphenhydramine and APAP. Start doses low and gradually increase to full dose. Must be infused over 2 hours.
			Immunosuppression and increased risk for infection* (grades 3 or 4, 37%; fatal in 18%)	Monitor blood pressure closely during infusion especially in patients with ischemic heart disease and those on antihypertensive medication*.
			Severe, prolonged myelosuppression*, including neutropenia (64%), anemia (38%), and thrombocytopenia (50%)	Patients should receive prophylaxis against PCP and HSV infection during therapy and afterwards until $CD4^+$ counts ≥200.
			Others: mucositis, diarrhea, edema	
Gemtuzumab Ozogamicin (Mylotarg)	Monoclonal antibody conjugated to a cytotoxic antitumor antibiotic, calicheamicin. The antibody is targeted to CD33 antigen, which is expressed on leukemic blasts and immature normal cells, but not on normal hematopoietic stem cells	Binds to CD33, forming complex that is internalized. Calicheamicin is released in cell, causing DNA double-strand breaks and cell death	Severe myelosuppression* occurs in all patients with febrile neutropenia (21%), and bleeding (grades 3 or 4; 15%)	Patients frequently require RBC and platelet transfusions
			Severe infusion-related reactions*, including anaphylaxis and pulmonary toxicity	Premedicate with diphenhydramine and APAP. Most reactions occur after end of 2-hour infusion and resolve within 4 hours.
			Pulmonary toxicity*, usually following infusion-reaction, and consisting of dyspnea, pleural effusions, pulmonary edema, and ARDS	Patients with WBCs >30,000/mm^3 may be at increased risk.
			Increased risk for infection (grade 3 or 4 infection in 28%), most commonly sepsis, pneumonia and HSV	
			Hepatic toxicity*, including severe VOD	Risk is increased if drug is given with other cytotoxics, before or after HSCT, or to those with hepatic insufficiency.
			Tumor lysis syndrome	
			Others: mucositis, diarrhea, rhinitis and hypokalemia	
Rituximab (Rituxan)	Targeted to CD20 antigen, which is expressed on normal and malignant B lymphocytes	Binds to CD20 and causes cell lysis by either antibody-dependent or complement-dependent mechanisms	Severe infusion-related reactions*, including anaphylaxis, and cardiopulmonary toxicity	Start infusion slowly and increase rate as tolerated. Reactions usually occur 30–120 minutes into the infusion.
			Tumor lysis syndrome*	Take measures to prevent tumor lysis syndrome in patients with high tumor burden
			Severe mucocutaneous reactions*	Patients with severe mucocutaneous reactions should not receive further therapy
			Myelosuppression, mostly lymphopenia	
			Increased risk for infection (grades 3 or 4; 2%)	
			Others: Immune/ autoimmune events, rash, diarrhea, rhinitis	

TABLE 124–16. (Continued)

Agent (Brand Name)	Molecular Target	Mechanism of Action	Adverse Effects	Comments
Trastuzumab (Herceptin)	Targeted to EGFR-2 or HER-2 receptor protein, which is overexpressed in 25% to 30% of breast cancers	Binds to HER-2 causing antibody-dependent cell lysis	Infusion-related reactions*, including anaphylaxis and pulmonary toxicity	Infuse loading dose over 90 minutes. Subsequent infusions over 30 minutes as tolerated.
			Cardiomyopathy	Patients should undergo baseline and periodic evaluation of cardiac function. Risk is increased with concurrent anthracyclines.
			Pulmonary toxicity, including dyspnea, pulmonary infiltrates, effusions, pulmonary edema, and ARDS	
			Others: Diarrhea, minor infections, rash, rhinitis	

*Boxed warnings in the package insert; potentially lethal toxicities.
APAP, acetaminophen; EGFR-2, epidermal growth factor receptor, type 2; HER-2, human epidermal growth factor receptor, type 2; HSCT, hematopoietic stem cell transplant; HSV, herpes simplex virus; NK, natural killer; PCP, *Pneumocystis carinii* pneumonia; RBC, red blood cells; VOD, venoocclusive disease.

chills, nausea, rash) to severe, life-threatening anaphylaxis with cardiopulmonary collapse. Many patients also experience chest or back pain during the infusion. Patients with circulating tumor cells in the bloodstream are at highest risk for more severe reactions. For these reasons, patients must be monitored closely during drug infusion. The reactions tend to be more severe with the initial infusions, and subside with subsequent treatment. Most agents require premedication with antihistamines and acetaminophen. Recommended infusion rates are usually lower for the initial doses, with incremental increases as tolerated by the patient. In the case of alemtuzumab, a low starting dose is recommended, with progressive increases to full dose over a 2-week period. For patients experiencing signs or symptoms of infusion-related reactions, the infusion should be interrupted and prompt treatment with antihistamines, corticosteroids, and other supportive measures should be initiated. Pulmonary toxicity may occur as part of the infusion-related reaction or may occur as a distinct entity.[63,128–134]

GENERAL SUPPORTIVE CARE ISSUES

The treatment of cancer with antineoplastic drugs is complicated by the incidence of multiple serious toxicities, many of which are life-threatening. Drug-specific toxicities, such as doxorubicin-induced cardiotoxicity and bleomycin-related pulmonary toxicity, were discussed in the previous sections. Several adverse effects are common to many antineoplastic agents. These include nausea and vomiting, myelosuppression, mucositis, alopecia, infertility, and carcinogenesis. Nutritional support and pain management are also important supportive care issues, although malnutrition and pain are not usually direct results of drug toxicity. The management of chemotherapy-induced nausea and vomiting and the basic principles of nutritional support and pain management are discussed in detail in other sections of this text.

Because many antineoplastic drugs affect DNA synthesis, any cell with a high turnover rate will be more sensitive to the toxic effects of chemotherapy. Cancer cells do not necessarily proliferate faster than normal cells. Normal tissues that consist of rapidly proliferating cells are targets for the toxicities of many anticancer drugs.[13] The bone marrow, intestinal mucosa, and hair follicles are such tissue sites where drug effects are manifested.

MYELOSUPPRESSION

Although not seen with all antineoplastic agents, myelosuppression is the most common dose-limiting side effect of cytotoxic agents. Bone marrow suppression does not usually occur immediately after chemotherapy administration. Blood components that have already been produced must be consumed before the effect is evident. WBCs, especially neutrophil precursors, are most significantly affected because of their rapid proliferation and short life span (6 to 12 hours). Platelets (5- to 10-day life span) are also affected, but to a much less degree than neutrophil. Erythrocytes, with a 120-day life span, are affected the least. Usual nadirs, or lowest blood cell counts, occur at 10 to 14 days following chemotherapy administration, with recovery by 3 to 4 weeks. There are some exceptions to this general rule. The nitrosoureas and mitomycin C exhibit a delayed pattern of nadir (4 to 6 weeks) and recovery (6 to 8 weeks). Planned courses of chemotherapy may have to be delayed while waiting for the granulocyte count to return to normal. For a patient to safely receive another cycle of chemotherapy, a WBC count $>3{,}000/mm^3$ or an absolute neutrophil count (ANC) of $\geq 1{,}500/mm^3$ and a platelet count of $\geq 100{,}000/mm^3$ are usually required.

Myelotoxicity is a desired therapeutic effect in leukemia patients during induction chemotherapy. However, myelosuppression is an undesirable side effect during chemotherapy for other malignancies. If significant myelosuppression has occurred with prior courses of chemotherapy, the doses of the offending agent(s) in subsequent courses may be reduced. However, dosage reduction may also compromise antitumor response. The magnitude of dose reduction is dictated by the degree of myelosuppression incurred and the incidence and severity of infection or bleeding. Empiric dosage reductions may be made or hematopoietic growth factors initiated for the first chemotherapy treatment if the patient has a low baseline WBC or platelet count, has diminished bone marrow reserve, has impaired drug-elimination capabilities, or is to receive a combination of several drugs that cause myelosuppression. Patients who have received multiple prior courses of other myelotoxic chemotherapy regimens or extensive radiation therapy, especially to the pelvis, may have a decreased bone marrow reserve. They are more sensitive to the myelosuppressive effects of chemotherapy, and normal doses may produce profound marrow toxicity. The pharmacokinetic profile of a myelosuppressive agent is also important in determining the appropriate dose. For example, the anthracyclines produce bone marrow suppression as an acute dose-limiting toxicity, and these agents depend on biliary excretion as their primary route of elimination. A patient with biliary obstruction may have compromised elimination of anthracyclines and is at increased risk for severe bone marrow suppression.

NEUTROPENIA

When the ANC falls below 500, infection risk increases.[134–136] The ANC may be calculated by multiplying the percentage of neutrophils (segmented plus banded neutrophils) by the total WBC count. The risk of infection is also directly proportional to the duration of neutropenia. Other risk factors for infection include alteration in the integrity of physical defense barriers and the functional integrity of WBCs. The patient's underlying cancer, as well as treatment with cytotoxic drugs and radiation, can affect neutrophil function. The diagnosis of infection in the neutropenic patient is complicated by the lack of WBCs. Usual signs and symptoms of infection, such as pus, abscesses, and infiltrates on chest x-ray, depend on the presence of WBCs. The only reliable indication of infection in these patients is fever. Definitive culture results may take days, and a septic neutropenic cancer patient can die within hours if not treated. Therefore, the basic approach to the management of the febrile neutropenic cancer patient is prompt initiation of empiric antibiotics. The antibiotics are chosen based on reliable coverage of the most likely organisms, antibiotic sensitivities at the institution, the patient's signs and symptoms (if present), side-effect profiles, and cost.[136] The most common source of infection in these patients is self-infection with body flora, which includes both gram-positive and gram-negative bacteria. Although bacteria cause most early infections, fungi become important pathogens as the course of neutropenia is prolonged. Traditionally, all febrile neutropenic cancer patients have received intravenous antibiotics in the hospital setting until full recovery of neutrophils. However, it is possible to identify patients at low risk for infectious complications who are candidates for alternative treatment strategies, including early discharge from the hospital and outpatient oral or intravenous antibiotics.[137] Specific treatment of infections in immunocompromised hosts is discussed elsewhere in this text.

Numerous methods have been explored to prevent infections in cancer patients.[134,135] Colony-stimulating factors (CSFs) are commonly employed for this reason.[138–140] These hormones are naturally occurring proteins that are essential for the normal growth and maturation of blood cell components (Fig. 124–21). The CSFs have the ability to enhance the production and also the function of their target cells. Two agents, G-CSF (granulocyte colony-stimulating factor) and GM-CSF (granulocyte-macrophage colony-stimulating factor) are commercially available in the United States. G-CSF (filgrastim, Neupogen) specifically stimulates the production of neutrophilic

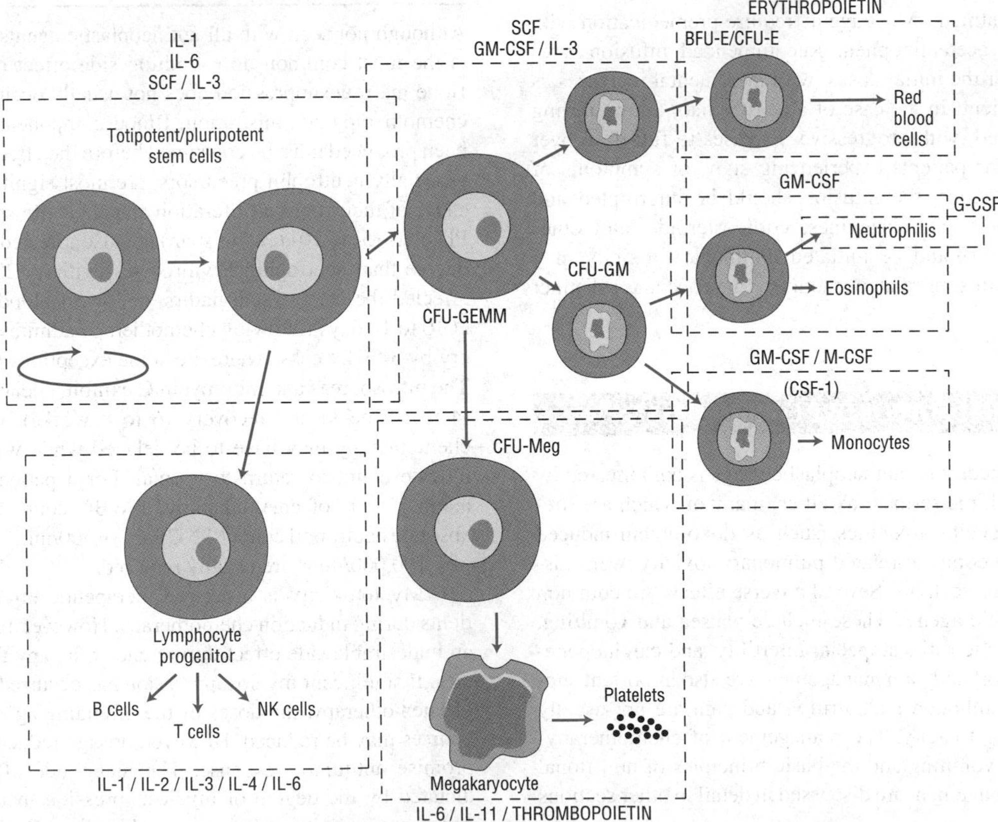

FIGURE 124–21. Regulation of hematopoietic cell development. A self-sustaining pool of marrow stem cells differentiates under the influence of specific growth factors to form a variety of myeloid and lymphoid cells. SCF, stem cell factor; GM-CSF, granulocyte–macrophage colony-stimulating factor; G-CSF, granulocyte colony-stimulating factor; M-CSF, macrophage colony-stimulating factor; and IL-1, IL-2, IL-3, IL-4, IL-6, IL-11, interleukins 1–6, and 11, respectively. *(Adapted from Hillman RS. Hematopoietic agents: Growth factors, minerals and vitamins. In: Hardman JG, Limbird LE, Molinoff PB, Ruddon RW, Gilman AG eds. Goodman & Gilman's The Pharmacologic Basis of Therapeutics, 9th ed. New York, McGraw-Hill, 1996:1312.)*

TABLE 124–17. Granulocyte Colony-stimulating Factor (G-CSF) and Granulocyte–Macrophage Colony-stimulating Factor (GM-CSF) Products and Sources

CSF	Generic Name	Brand Name	Manufacturer	Recombinant-DNA Source
G-CSF	Filgrastim	Neupogen	Amgen	*Escherichia coli*
	Lenograstim	Neutrogin[b] Investigational	Chugai-Rhone Poulenc	CHO[a] cells
GM-CSF	Sargramostim	Leukine	Immunex	*Saccharomyces cerevisiae* Yeast
	Molgramostim	Leucomax[b]	Schering-Plough/Sandoz	*E. coli*

[a]Chinese hamster ovary.
[b]Available outside the United States.

granulocytes. GM-CSF (sargramostim, Leukine) promotes the proliferation of granulocytes (neutrophils and eosinophils), as well as monocytes/macrophages. Although GM-CSF stimulates megakaryocytes, no consistent effect on platelet production has been defined in clinical trials. Both agents initially enhance demargination and mobilization of mature cells from the marrow and then provide constant stimulation of stem cell progenitors. Several host sources have been employed in the recombinant-DNA technology used to produce CSFs, including bacteria (*E. coli*), yeast, and mammalian cells (Chinese hamster ovary or CHO cells) (Table 124–17). Products derived from yeast or mammalian sources are glycosylated to varying degrees, as are naturally occurring CSFs, whereas those derived from *E. coli* are nonglycosylated. This difference does not result in any clinically significant effects on neutrophil production.

The CSFs reduce the incidence, magnitude, and duration of neutropenia when used as preventive therapy following a variety of myelosuppressive chemotherapy regimens.[138–140] These effects have been accompanied by a modest decrease in febrile days, fewer infections, and fewer days on antibiotics. An unexpected benefit in some G-CSF studies has been a decrease in the incidence of mucositis. Growth factors have also permitted the administration of subsequent chemotherapy courses on schedule, resulting in enhanced dose intensity. However, the increased dose intensity provided by the CSFs has not yet been found to translate into improved tumor response or survival. Because of lack of impact on response rates and survival, decisions regarding appropriate use of growth factors are based on weighing proven clinical benefits against economic considerations. The American Society of Clinical Oncology has developed evidence-based clinical practice guidelines to promote appropriate use of the CSFs.[139,140]

Growth factors may be used in either the primary or secondary prophylaxis of neutropenia. Primary prophylaxis refers to the use of CSFs to prevent neutropenia with the first cycle of chemotherapy. This strategy is only clinically and economically appropriate for patients who are receiving a chemotherapy regimen associated with febrile neutropenia in more than 40% of patients.[140] Secondary prophylaxis refers to the use of growth factors to prevent recurrent neutropenia in patients who experienced neutropenia with the prior cycle of chemotherapy. Because this method of using CSFs has not been demonstrated to improve disease-free or overall survival, it is recommended that secondary prophylaxis be reserved for patients with curable malignancies where dose should not be compromised.[140]

Although there is experience with both G-CSF and GM-CSF in prevention of febrile neutropenia after administration of standard doses of chemotherapy, at this time only G-CSF is FDA approved for this indication. One exception is in the induction treatment of acute myelogenous leukemia, in which both GM-CSF and G-CSF have demonstrated a reduction in the duration of neutropenia, often accompanied by modest decrease in hospitalization and infectious complications. Benefits have been most clearly documented in patients older than age 55 years. Similar data are available for G-CSF in the treatment of patients with acute lymphoblastic leukemia. These beneficial effects, however, have not resulted in improved response rates or overall survival.[140]

Only a few studies have addressed the role of CSFs in the treatment of established neutropenia.[139,140] These studies suggest no or only minimal clinical benefit from use of CSFs. At this time, the CSFs should not be routinely employed in patients with established neutropenia, regardless of the presence of fever. Both CSFs have also proven effective in acceleration of hematopoietic engraftment and in treatment of graft failure following bone marrow transplantation. Other uses for the CSFs include peripheral blood stem cell (PBSC) mobilization, neutropenia in AIDS patients, myelodysplastic syndromes, congenital neutropenia, and aplastic anemia. Growth factors should not be used in patients receiving concomitant chemotherapy and radiotherapy, especially if the radiation involves the mediastinum. These patients appear to experience more significant thrombocytopenia when administered CSFs.

At currently recommended doses, the CSFs are well tolerated. Side effects are more commonly seen with GM-CSF and may be related to the drug's ability to enhance binding of neutrophils to endothelial cells or to activation of monocytes/macrophages, which may stimulate the release of cytokines, such as IL-1 and tumor necrosis factor.[138] The most common toxicity of the CSFs is bone pain (20% to 25% of patients), which can be treated with acetaminophen or NSAIDs. Bone pain was the most significant toxicity seen in clinical trials with G-CSF. Other side effects of G-CSF include an increase in lactate dehydrogenase, alkaline phosphatase, and uric acid levels. Additional toxicities of GM-CSF include constitutional symptoms, such as low-grade fever, myalgias, arthralgias, lethargy, and mild headache. GM-CSF may also produce an elevation in liver transaminase enzymes. At higher doses of GM-CSF, pleural and pericardial effusions, capillary-leak syndrome, and thrombus formation may occur. A first-dose reaction described after GM-CSF administration has been reported more commonly with the *E. coli*-derived product (molgramostim), which is investigational in the United States. This reaction is more common after intravenous infusion and consists of dyspnea, facial flushing, hypotension, hypoxia, and tachycardia. Both G-CSF and GM-CSF may produce mild erythema at subcutaneous injection sites, as well as a generalized maculopapular rash with either subcutaneous or intravenous administration.

For prophylaxis of chemotherapy-induced neutropenia, CSF therapy should not begin sooner than 24 hours after the last dose of chemotherapy and should be continued until the ANC exceeds a safe level following the expected chemotherapy nadir. In the setting of bone marrow transplantation, CSFs should not begin sooner than 24 hours after the last dose of chemotherapy or 12 hours after the last radiotherapy treatment. The recommended starting dose of G-CSF is

5 μg/kg/day in all settings except for PBSC mobilization, where doses of 10 μg/kg/day are used. The recommended dose of yeast-derived GM-CSF is 250 μg/m²/day. Pharmacokinetic data favor subcutaneous injection as the most effective route. However, in patients in whom subcutaneous injections are not feasible (e.g., where there is anasarca), the drugs may be given intravenously. Because of the high cost associated with CSF use, alternative dosing regimens have been explored. These regimens attempt to decrease the total amount of CSF used by either delaying the start of CSFs (e.g., to day 3 after chemotherapy), decreasing the dose (e.g., to 3 μg/kg/day G-CSF), or decreasing the duration of CSF therapy. Specifically, the posttreatment target ANC of 10,000/mm³ recommended by product information is often reduced to an ANC of greater than 2,000 or 5,000/mm³ in clinical practice. Standardized doses of 300 μg or 480 μg of G-CSF and 500 μg of GM-CSF, based on product vial sizes, are often used to minimize waste.

THROMBOCYTOPENIA

Chemotherapy-induced thrombocytopenia puts the patient at risk for significant bleeding. To date, platelet transfusions remain the mainstay of management.[141] Typically, platelet transfusion is indicated for patients with a platelet count of <10,000/mm³, or for patients with lesser degrees of thrombocytopenia with signs or symptoms of hemorrhage. Patients with thrombocytopenia who must undergo a surgical procedure are also appropriate candidates for transfusion. For patients with nonmyeloid malignancies who experienced significant thrombocytopenia with a prior cycle of chemotherapy, oprelvekin (IL-11, Neumega) may be considered as secondary prophylaxis. When used after chemotherapy regimens associated with a high risk for thrombocytopenia, oprelvekin decreased the need for platelet transfusions, as well as the numbers of platelets required for transfusion.[142,143] Unfortunately, oprelvekin is associated with some significant adverse effects, mostly related to fluid retention (e.g., edema, dilutional anemia, dyspnea, pleural effusions). Cardiac toxicity, especially tachycardia, and atrial fibrillation/flutter have also been observed. Milder side effects include skin rashes and conjunctival redness. Considering the modest clinical benefit, the adverse effects and the high cost, oprelvekin use should be reserved for patients at high risk for severe thrombocytopenia from chemotherapy where dose reduction is known to compromise disease response. The dose of oprelvekin is 50 μg/kg SQ qd starting 6 to 24 hours after completion of chemotherapy. Start of therapy may be delayed until day 3 without compromising results. Oprelvekin is continued until the postnadir platelet count exceeds 50,000/mm³. Duration of therapy should not exceed 21 days and should be discontinued 2 days prior to the next cycle of chemotherapy.[143] Other CSFs, such as interleukins-1, -3, and -6, have also been studied, but significant impact on platelet counts within an acceptable adverse-effect profile has not been demonstrated. The recent discovery and development of thrombopoietin may represent the most significant factor in the future of thrombocytopenia treatment.

ANEMIA

Anemia is a common hematologic complication of cancer chemotherapy.[144] The incidence of anemia depends on several factors, including the type and duration of therapy, and the type and stage of the underlying malignancy. For example, cisplatin and carboplatin are more commonly associated with anemia than many other chemotherapeutic agents. Multiple conditions are known to cause anemia in cancer patients, including chronic gastrointestinal blood loss, nutrient deficiency (e.g., iron, folate), chemotherapy and radiation therapy, bone marrow invasion by the tumor, hemolysis, renal dysfunction, and anemia of chronic disease. Of all the signs and symptoms of anemia, fatigue is most common in cancer patients.[145] In fact, fatigue is the most commonly reported symptom overall in patients undergoing chemotherapy. The presence of fatigue is correlated with the severity of anemia; treatment of anemia results in improvement in fatigue and quality of life. Anemia is only one of many possible causes of fatigue in patients with cancer. Other common causes of fatigue include insomnia, depression, unrelieved pain, and the underlying malignancy.

Previously, the only option for the treatment of chemotherapy-related anemia was red blood cell transfusions. This intervention is still the mainstay of acute management, but the availability of human recombinant erythropoietin (rHuEPO, epoetin alfa) has provided another therapeutic tool.[146,147] Several studies have documented the efficacy of rHuEPO in the anemia associated with chemotherapy.[147–149] Epoetin alfa increases hemoglobin and hematocrit, decreases transfusion requirements, and improves quality of life. Several early indicators of response have been derived, including an increase in hemoglobin of 0.5–1.0 g/dL above baseline, a decline in ferritin, or an increase in the absolute reticulocyte count after 2 to 4 weeks of therapy. These surrogate end points can be used to identify nonresponders early, so that therapy may be modified or discontinued, as indicated. Serum erythropoietin levels have minimal utility in predicting response or monitoring therapy.

Clinical practice guidelines to guide the appropriate use of rHuEPO have been developed.[148,150] The first step is to evaluate the underlying cause of the anemia and initiate specific therapy, as indicated. For example, patients with iron deficiency anemia should receive iron supplementation. Patients with chronic bleeding or hemolysis are not appropriate candidates for epoetin alfa therapy. For patients who are receiving chemotherapy, and for whom no otherwise treatable cause is identified, rHuEPO may be started at 150 U/kg or 10,000 units subcutaneously three times a week. Alternatively, doses of 40,000 units subcutaneously once a week have been employed. After 4 weeks, the hemoglobin should be reassessed. In patients who do not achieve at least a 1 g/dL rise in hemoglobin, the dose should be increased to 300 U/kg or 20,000 units three times a week, or 60,000 units once a week. Patients who do not respond after 4 weeks at the higher dose with a 1 g/dL increase in hemoglobin should be taken off of rHuEPO. Iron deficiency should be ruled out as a cause of treatment failure prior to discontinuing epoetin alfa. Treatment with rHuEPO should also be discontinued in patients who complete planned chemotherapy or in those who have resolution of their anemia (hemoglobin ≥12–13 g/dL). New formulations of rHuEPO with prolonged duration of action permit less frequent dosing.

MUCOSITIS

The gastrointestinal (GI) mucosa is composed of epithelial cells with a high mitotic index and rapid turnover rate, making it a common site of chemotherapy-induced toxicity.[93,151] The subsequent inflammation, or mucositis, can lead to painful ulcerations, local infection, and inability to eat, drink, or swallow. Disruption of the GI mucosal barrier may also provide an avenue for systemic microbial invasion. The time course for development and resolution of mucositis often parallels that of neutropenia. Agents most commonly associated with mucositis include 5-FU, doxorubicin, and methotrexate. The most effective means of preventing mucositis is through good oral hygiene. Patients at high risk for this toxicity (with poor dentition, high-dose chemotherapy, or radiation therapy involving the oropharynx) should be evaluated by a dentist prior to chemotherapy and should be instructed to rinse their mouths frequently with baking soda and salt water or plain saline rinses during and between courses of chemotherapy.[93] The benefit of chlorhexidine (Peridex) rinses over saline rinses is unclear. In patients undergoing radiation therapy to the head and neck region, chlorhexidine rinses have detrimental effects on the oral mucosa. For patients receiving 5-FU treatment, the use of ice (oral cryotherapy) may decrease the risk for mucositis by decreasing drug delivery to the oral mucosa.[93,151] After mucositis has developed, treatment is mainly supportive, including use of topical or systemic analgesics and oral hygiene (including the rinses described). Viscous lidocaine, diphenhydramine liquid, and dyclonine are topical anesthetics commonly employed. Severe cases of mucositis may lead to dehydration and require intravenous hydration. Local infections caused by *Candida* species and reactivation of herpes simplex viruses are common in these patients. Suspicious lesions should be cultured, and appropriate antifungal and/or antiviral treatment should then be instituted. Antifungal therapy may be delivered topically for mild infections (thrush), using clotrimazole (Mycelex) troches or nystatin (Nilstat, others) oral suspension. For more severe oral or esophageal fungal infections, systemic treatment with oral ketoconazole (Nizoral), fluconazole (Diflucan), or intravenous amphotericin B is indicated.[93,151]

Mucosal damage can occur at any point along the entire length of the GI tract. In the lower portion of the GI tract, this damage is usually manifested as diarrhea (mild to life-threatening in nature) and abdominal pain. Support with intravenous fluids and electrolyte supplementation should be initiated promptly in severe cases. After infectious causes have been ruled out, diarrhea can safely be treated with antispasmodics such as Lomotil or loperamide (Immodium). The somatostatin analog octreotide has also been used successfully to treat severe cases of chemotherapy-induced diarrhea.[93] The specific treatment of early and late diarrhea from irinotecan (CPT-11) was discussed previously.

ALOPECIA

Although not a life-threatening side effect of chemotherapy, the toxicity that many patients find most distressing is alopecia. Alopecia from chemotherapy is usually temporary, and the degree of hair loss varies widely.[152] The loss of hair is not limited to the scalp; any area of the body may be affected. Patients receiving a taxane as part of their chemotherapy regimen are especially prone to total body alopecia. Hair loss usually begins 1 to 2 weeks after chemotherapy, and regrowth may begin before the chemotherapy courses are completed. Cryotherapy (local application of ice) and scalp tourniquets have both been investigated as methods of preventing alopecia. Both techniques produce vasoconstriction, resulting in decreased exposure of hair follicles to the chemotherapy agents. These techniques are not uniformly effective and are contraindicated in patients with cancers that may metastasize to the scalp, such as leukemia and lymphoma.

EXTRAVASATION

Vesicants are antineoplastic agents that may cause severe tissue damage if they escape from the vasculature.[63,79] These agents include the anthracyclines, actinomycin D, the vinca alkaloids, mitomycin C, and nitrogen mustard. The anthracyclines are the most notorious agents, and most extensively investigated. The tissue damage may result in prolonged pain, tissue sloughing, infection, and loss of mobility. Prompt initiation of the appropriate interventions is important to minimize morbidity. Unfortunately, most information on extravasation management is anecdotal; few controlled clinical studies have been conducted to determine optimal intervention strategies. Therefore, prevention has become the focus of extravasation management. The most important method of prevention is good administration technique,[63] but even then, extravasations may occur. The vein selected for administration should be on the distal portion of the arm. The large veins of the forearm are desirable because if a drug does extravasate, there is adequate soft-tissue coverage to protect crucial structures like nerves and tendons, and joint function is not risked. Peripherally administered vesicants should be given slowly via intravenous injection (IV push) through the side arm of a running IV. The person administering the vesicant should verify needle stability and adequate blood return after each 1–2 mL of drug is injected. Vesicants should not be administered by intravenous infusion unless the patient has a central venous catheter. For extravasation of vesicants, one of the most important interventions is the application of ice packs to the affected area. One exception to this rule is the vinca alkaloids, which are better managed with application of heat. Only a few antidotes to vesicant agents are employed clinically. Sodium thiosulfate is used to neutralize nitrogen mustard extravasations, and hyaluronidase (if available) can improve the outcome after extravasation of vinca alkaloids, etoposide, and taxanes. Topical application of DMSO may be an effective method for managing anthracycline and mitomycin C extravasations.[79]

INFERTILITY

Advances in the treatment of some cancers, such as Hodgkin's disease and testicular cancer, have produced long-term survivors and the opportunity to examine the late consequences of chemotherapy administration. Infertility and secondary cancers have emerged as important late effects. The gonadal toxicities of chemotherapy have not received much attention in the past because they are not life-threatening. High rates of fertility deficits and sexual dysfunction have been noted for both men and women.[153,154] In men, the antitumor drugs have been shown to produce severe oligospermia or azoospermia as well as infertility. Serum testosterone levels are only rarely altered. The recovery of spermatogenesis after completion of chemotherapy is unpredictable. Men receiving combination chemotherapy appear to have more long-lasting adverse effects on fertility than men receiving single-agent therapy. Age, total dose, duration of therapy, and type of drug are other important variables. In women, toxic effects on the ovaries result clinically in amenorrhea, vaginal epithelial atrophy, and menopausal symptoms. These effects are related to dose and age. Younger patients are more resistant to the effects on the ovaries. As with men, the recovery of fertility is unpredictable, but women younger then 25 years of age appear to have the best outcomes. The effects of the alkylating agents on fertility have been extensively studied. This group of drugs exerts profound and consistently detrimental effects on reproductive function. Less is known about commonly used agents such as doxorubicin, taxanes, and platinum compounds. Patients with potentially curable tumors, who desire to have children in the future, should be informed about the risk for infertility and sperm or oocyte banking options.

SECONDARY MALIGNANCIES

Secondary cancers induced by chemotherapy and radiation are a serious long-term complication.[155] Although many types of solid tumors have been reported as chemotherapy-induced malignancies, acute nonlymphocytic leukemia (ANLL) is the most common secondary cancer. ANLL has been reported following successful treatment of Hodgkin's disease, acute leukemias, non Hodgkin's lymphomas, multiple myeloma, breast cancer, and advanced ovarian cancer. For curable cancers, the relatively small risk for occurrence of secondary malignancies is far outweighed by the benefits of survival in large numbers of patients. However, for cancers such as ovarian cancer, the risk of leukemia is not offset by improved survival in chemotherapy recipients. The issue of secondary malignancies is of particular concern in patients receiving adjuvant chemotherapy. As with the late complication of infertility, the antineoplastic agents primarily associated with secondary cancers are the alkylating agents. Etoposide, teniposide, and the anthracyclines have also been linked to secondary leukemias. Solid tumors as secondary malignancies occur more commonly after treatment with radiation than with chemotherapy.

SAFETY AND HANDLING ISSUES

As discussed previously, the cytotoxic drugs used to treat cancer are carcinogenic, mutagenic, and teratogenic. Consequently, these drugs should be handled with care to avoid inadvertent exposure of health care professionals.[156] All pharmacies should have written procedures for handling these drugs safely, and all personnel should be oriented to these procedures. The most common avenue of exposure is via inhalation of aerosolized drug. Individuals preparing chemotherapy should work in a Class II biologic safety cabinet and wear gowns and powder-free disposable latex gloves. The gowns should be made of lint-free, low-permeability fabric with a solid front, long sleeves, and tight-fitting elastic cuffs. Negative-pressure techniques should be employed in drug preparation to minimize aerosolization. Health care workers administering these agents should take similar precautions to avoid exposure. Kits for cleaning up chemotherapy spills should be located in all areas of the institution in which chemotherapy is handled. Cytotoxic waste should be disposed of properly, and patients should be informed of proper methods of disposing of potentially contaminated body excreta and cytotoxic waste.

CANCER PREVENTION

DIET

The relationship between diet and cancer is the subject of intense investigation. There is evidence that suggests that up to one-third of cancer deaths in the United States are attributable to dietary factors.[149] Although controversy exists over the true role of diet in carcinogenesis, some general recommendations have been developed by the American Cancer Society (Table 124–18).[157] There is strong evidence that increased consumption of fruits and vegetables lowers the risk for many cancers, especially those of the gastrointestinal and respiratory tracts. Consumption of a high-fat diet appears to increase the risk for breast, colorectal, and prostate cancers. The average American consumes 36% to 38% of daily calories as fat. A decrease in fat intake to less than 30% of daily calories may decrease the risk for developing cancer, as well as heart disease. Obese individuals have increased risk of several cancers, including colorectal, breast, biliary, and uterine cancers. The inverse relationship between dietary fiber and colon cancer has received much attention. The American diet is typically low in fiber (11 g/day). High fiber intake (20–30 g/day) may decrease the risk of colon cancer. A high alcohol intake has been shown to increase the risk for many upper aerodigestive tract malignancies, especially in smokers.

TABLE 124–18. American Cancer Society Dietary Recommendations

Choose most of the foods you eat from plant sources
- Eat five or more servings of fruits and vegetables daily
- Eat other foods from plant sources, such as breads, cereals, grain products, rice, pasta, or beans several times each day

Limit your intake of high-fat foods, particularly from animal sources
- Choose foods low in fat
- Limit consumption of meats, especially high-fat meats

Be physically active: achieve and maintain a healthy weight
- Be at least moderately active for 30 minutes or more most days of the week
- Stay within your healthy weight range

Limit consumption of alcoholic beverages, if you drink at all

From Ref. 157.

CHEMOPREVENTION

This is defined as the systemic use of natural or synthetic products to reverse, suppress, or prevent carcinogenesis. Several agents have been studied in chemoprevention. There is evidence that vitamins and trace elements such as vitamin A and related retinoids, vitamins C and E, and selenium may prevent, halt, or reverse the carcinogenic process. These vitamins are present in fresh fruits and vegetables. The known effects of these agents on the cancer process have resulted in several trials to determine their effectiveness as chemoprotective agents.[158] To date, some of the most encouraging results have been seen with use of retinoids in a variety of malignancies, including squamous cell skin cancer, head and neck cancer, and cervical cancer. There is also evidence that retinoids may reverse oral leukoplakia, a premalignant lesion of the oral mucosa associated with tobacco use. Patients with smoking-related malignancy have acquired a so-called field cancerization defect, meaning that any part of the aerodigestive tract exposed to the tobacco carcinogens is at risk for development of cancer. For example, patients cured of head and neck cancer commonly present several years later with a second primary cancer of the upper aerodigestive tract. Clinical trials of vitamin A and the retinoids have shown significant activity against oral leukoplakia and the development of second primary tumors in patients with head and neck cancer. In addition to smoking cessation, patients cured of their head and neck malignancy should be considered candidates for chemoprevention. In contrast, β-carotene has no benefit in prevention of lung cancer; in fact, one large trial suggested it caused an increased risk of cancer.[159] These results emphasize the importance of evaluating chemoprevention strategies in a systematic fashion before they are used widely in clinical practice.

The role of calcium as a chemopreventive agent for colorectal cancer has also been studied. Calcium is thought to inhibit mucosal injury and hyperproliferation of the gastrointestinal lining that is induced by bile acids and other carcinogens. In a large clinical trial, calcium supplementation was found to confer a modest decrease in the risk for formation of colonic adenomas, a known precursor to cancer.[160] These study results have been eclipsed by data on the selective inhibitors of the cyclooxygenase type-2 (COX-2) enzymes.[161] Expression of COX-2 is increased in colon cancers, and appears to act as a tumor promoter. Nonselective COX inhibitors, such as aspirin and other NSAIDs, have previously demonstrated a reduction in risk for colon cancer. The selective COX-2 inhibitor celecoxib was approved by the FDA as a chemoprevention agent in 1999, based on its ability to decrease the number of precancerous polyps in individuals with the inherited colon cancer syndrome known as familial adenomatous polyposis (FAP). Future studies will explore the ability of selective COX-2 inhibitors to prevent colorectal cancer in average risk persons and in the prevention of other malignancies.

Hormonal therapy may represent another effective mechanism of chemoprevention. It is known that certain hormones play a role in the initiation, promotion, and progression of malignancy. For example, estrogen is known to stimulate breast cancer cell growth and testosterone stimulates prostate cancer growth. The antiestrogen tamoxifen effectively blocks this stimulatory effect in breast cancer. A large clinical trial sponsored by the National Surgical Adjuvant Bowel and Breast Project (NSABP) assessed tamoxifen's efficacy in breast cancer prevention in high-risk individuals. The trial was stopped prematurely in 1998 after demonstrating a 45% reduction in the risk of developing breast cancer among patients receiving tamoxifen compared with placebo.[162] However, there was also a mild increase in risk for endometrial cancer and thromboembolic disease. The ultimate role and appropriate patients for tamoxifen prevention remain to be determined. The Study of Tamoxifen and Raloxifene (STAR) is currently underway and will compare the effects of tamoxifen to another SERM, raloxifene, in breast cancer prevention. The nationwide Prostate Cancer Prevention Trial is assessing the efficacy of the 5-α-reductase inhibitor finasteride, which inhibits the conversion of testosterone to its active form, dihydrotestosterone, in preventing prostate cancer. The results of these trials will provide valuable information on the utility of hormonal manipulation on cancer prevention.

TOBACCO

Cigarette smoking remains the most preventable cause of premature death in the United States. More than 400,000 deaths per year and 30% of all cancers in the United States are due to smoking.[163] For many types of cancer, the underlying etiology is unknown. One notable exception is lung cancer; cigarette smoking is the major cause of this disease. More than 90% of all cases of lung cancer are diagnosed in smokers. Tobacco smoking also increases the relative risk for development of many other types of cancer, including cancers of the mouth, pharynx, larynx, esophagus, and bladder. Passive inhalation of exhaled tobacco byproducts and cigarette smoke represents a significant risk factor for lung cancer in the nonsmoking population. Smokeless tobacco has been connected to the development of oral cancers. Abstinence from chewing and smoking tobacco is believed to be a major factor in the prevention of these malignancies.

SUN EXPOSURE

The association between sun exposure and skin neoplasms is also well established. The incidence of both nonmelanomatous skin cancer and melanoma has steadily increased in past decades, paralleling the increase in recreational sun exposure.[164] During this same time period, protection from ultraviolet light exposure normally provided by the ozone layer has been compromised. Fair-skinned individuals who sunburn easily are particularly at high risk. Melanoma and skin cancers can be largely prevented by minimizing exposure to the sun and by applying strong sunscreens and sunblocks to sun-exposed areas (SPF-15 or greater).

REFERENCES

1. Kaufman D, Chabner BA. Clinical strategies for cancer treatment: The role of drugs. In: Chabner BA, Longo DL, eds. Cancer Chemotherapy and Biotherapy: Principles and Practice. Philadelphia, Lippincott-Raven, 1996:1–16.
2. American Cancer Society. Cancer facts and figures—2001. Atlanta, GA, American Cancer Society, 2001.
3. Liotta LA, Liu ET. Essentials of molecular biology: Genomics and cancer. In: DeVita VT, Hellman S, Rosenberg SA, eds. Cancer: Principles and Practice of Oncology, 6th ed. Philadelphia, Lippincott Williams & Wilkins, 2000:17–30.
4. Cavanee WK, White RL. The genetic basis of cancer. Sci Am 1995; 72–79.
5. Compagni A, Christofori G. Recent advances in research on multistage tumorigenesis. Br J Cancer 2000;83:1–5.
6. Kumar V, Cotran RS, Robbins' SL. Neoplasia. In: Kumar V, Cotran RS, Robbins SL, eds. Robbins' Pathologic Basis of Disease. Philadelphia, WB Saunders, 1997:260–327.
7. Weston A, Harris CC. Chemical carcinogenesis. In: Bast RC, Kufe DW, Pollock RE, Weichselbaum RR, Holland JF, Frei E, eds. Cancer Medicine, 5th ed. Lea & Fabiger 2000:185–194.
8. Bishop JM. The molecular genetics of cancer. Science 1987;235:305–311.
9. Weinberg RA. How cancer arises. Sci Am 1996;275:62–70.
10. Lundberg AS, Weinberg RA. Control of the cell cycle and apoptosis. Eur J Cancer 1999;35:531–539.
11. Gilewski TA, Dang C, Sarbone A, Norton L. Principles of chemotherapy: Cytokinetics. In: Bast, RC, Kufe DW, Pollock RE, Weichselbaum RR, Holland JF, Frei E, eds. Cancer Medicine, 5th ed. Lea & Fabiger 2000:511–538.
12. Marx J. DNA arrays reveal cancer in its many forms. Science 2000;289: 1670–1672.
13. Buick RN. Cellular basis of chemotherapy. In: Dorr RT, Von Hoff DD, eds. Cancer Chemotherapy Handbook, 2nd ed. New York, Elsevier, 1994: 3–14.
14. Stetler-Stevenson WG, Kleiner DE Jr. Molecular biology of cancer: Invasion and metastasis. In: DeVita VT, Hellman S, Rosenberg SA, eds. Cancer: Principles and Practice of Oncology, 6th ed. Philadelphia, Lippincott Williams & Wilkins, 2000:123–136.
15. Folkman J. Tumor angiogenesis. In: Bast, RC, Kufe DW, Pollock RE, Weichselbaum RR, Holland JF, Frei E, eds. Cancer Medicine, Lea & Fabiger 5th ed. 2000:132–152.
16. American Cancer Society. Recommendations for the early detection of cancer in average risk, asymptomatic people. CA Cancer J Clin 2001; 51:40.
17. American Cancer Society. Seven warning signs of cancer. Atlanta, GA, American Cancer Society.
18. American Cancer Society. Eight warnings signs of cancer in children. Atlanta, GA, American Cancer Society.
19. Fleming ID, Cooper JS, Henson DE, Hutter RVP, Kennedy BJ, Murphy GP, O'Sullivan B. AJCC Cancer Staging Manual, 5th edition. Philadelphia, Lippincott Williams and Wilkins, 1997.
20. Yaeger TE, Brady LW. Basis for major current therapies for cancer. In: Lenhard RE, Osteen RT, Gansler T, eds. Clinical Oncology. Atlanta, GA, American Cancer Society, 2001:159–230.
21. Calabresi P, Chabner BA. Chemotherapy of neoplastic diseases. In: Hardman JG, Limbird LE, Molinoff PB, Ruddon RW, Gilman AG, eds. Goodman & Gilman's The Pharmacologic Basis of Therapeutics, 9th ed. New York, McGraw-Hill, 1996:1225–1232.
22. Haskell CM. Principles of cancer chemotherapy. In: Haskell CM, ed. Cancer Treatment, 5th ed. Philadelphia, WB Saunders, 2001: 62–86.
23. Balmer CB, Finley RS. Principles of cancer treatment. In: Finley RS, Balmer CM, eds. Concepts in Oncology Therapeutics. 1998: 15–32.
24. Safa AR. Multidrug resistance. In: Schilsky RL, Milano GA, Ratain MJ, eds. Principles of Antineoplastic Drug Development and Pharmacology. New York, Marcel Dekker, 1996:457–486.
25. Tan B, Piwnica-Worms D, Ratner L. Multidrug resistance transporters and modulation. Curr Opin Oncol 2000;12:450–458.
26. Hryniuk WM. Dose intensity. In: Schilsky RL, Milano GA, Ratain MJ, eds. Principles of Antineoplastic Drug Development and Pharmacology. New York, Marcel Dekker, 1996:263–280.
27. Links M, Lewis C. Chemoprotectants. A review of their clinical pharmacology and therapeutic efficacy. Drugs 1999;57:293–308.

28. Burke GA, Estlin EJ, Lowis SP. The role of pharmacokinetic and pharmacodynamic studies in the planning of protocols for the treatment of childhood cancer. Cancer Treat Rev 1999;25:13–27.
29. Ravdin P. The use of HER2 testing in the management of breast cancer. Semin Oncol 2000;27(5 suppl 9):33–42.
30. Collins JM. Pharmacokinetics and clinical monitoring. In: Chabner BA, Longo DL, eds. Cancer Chemotherapy and Biotherapy: Principles and Practice. Philadelphia, Lippincott-Raven, 1996:17–29.
31. Klausner R, Collins F. Understanding gene testing. Rockville, MD, US Department of Health and Human Services, Public Health Service, National Institutes of Health, National Cancer Institute, NIH Publication No. 96–3905, December 1995.
32. Ross J. Structure and function of the gene. In: Abeloff MD, Armitage JO, Lichter AS, Niederhuber JE, eds. Clinical Oncology, 2nd edition. Philadelphia, Churchill Livingstone, 2000:3–9.
33. Pratt WB, Ruddon RW, Ensminger WD, Maybaum J. The Anticancer Drugs, 2nd ed. New York, Oxford University Press, 1994:69–107.
34. Pizzorno G, Handschumacher RE, Cheng Y-C. Pyrimidines and purine antimetabolites. In: Bast RC Jr, Kufe DW, Pollock RE, Weichselbaum RR, Holland JF, Frei E III, eds. Holland-Frei Cancer Medicine, 5th ed. Hamilton, Ontario, BC Decker, 2000:625–647.
35. 5-Fluorouracil: Forty-plus and still ticking. A review of its preclinical and clinical development. Invest New Drugs 2000;18:299–313.
36. Sobrero AF, Aschele C, Bertino JR. Fluorouracil in colorectal cancer—A tale of two drugs: Implications for biochemical modulation. J Clin Oncol 1997;15:368–381.
37. Ignoffo RJ. Novel oral fluoropyrimidines in the treatment of metastatic colorectal cancer. Amer J Health Syst Pharm 1999;56:2417–2428.
38. Dutcher JP, Novik Y, O'Boyle K, Marcoullis G, Secco Ch, Wiernik PH. 20th Century advances in drug therapy in oncology—Part I. Clin Pharmacol 2000;40:1007–1024.
39. Donelli MG, Zucchetti M, Munzone E, D'Incalci M, Crosignani A. Pharmacokinetics of anticancer agents in patients with impaired liver function. Eur J Cancer 1998;34;33–46.
40. Kolesar JM, Johnson CL, Freeberg BL, Berlin JD, Schiller JH. Warfarin-5-FU interaction—A consecutive case series. Pharmacotherapy 1999;19:1445–1449.
41. Dooley M, Goa KL. Capecitabine. Drugs 1999;58:69–76.
42. Reigner B, Blesch K, Weidekamm E. Clinical pharmacokinetics of capecitabine. Clin Pharmacokinet 2001;40:85–104.
43. Schuller J, Cassidy J, Dumont E, et al. Preferential activation of capecitabine in tumor following oral administration to colorectal cancer patients. Cancer Chemother Pharmacol 2000;45:291–297.
44. Roche Laboratories. Xeloda (capecitabine) product information. 2000.
45. Johnson SA. Clinical pharmacokinetics of nucleoside analogues: Focus on haematological malignancies. Clin Phamacokinet 2000;39:5–26.
46. Glantz MJ, LaFollette S, Jaeckle KA, et al. Randomized trial of a slow-release versus a standard formulation of cytarabine for the intrathecal treatment of lymphomatous meningitis. J Clin Oncol 1999;17:3110–3116.
47. Baker WJ, Royer GL Jr, Weiss RB. Cytarabine and neurologic toxicity. J Clin Oncol 1991;9:679–693.
48. Smith GA, Damon LE, Rugo HS, Ries CA, Linker CA. High-dose cytarabine dose modification reduces the incidence of neurotoxicity in patients with renal insufficiency. J Clin Oncol 1997;15:833–839.
49. Balmer C, Mahay H. Major organ toxicity. In: Finley RS, Balmer C, eds. Concepts in Oncology Therapeutics, 2nd ed. Bethesda, MD, ASHP, 1998:121–145.
50. Gucchelaar HJ, Richel DJ, van Knapen A. Clinical, toxicological and pharmacological aspects of gemcitabine. Cancer Treat Rev 1996;22:15–31.
51. Venook AP, Egorin MJ, Rosner GL, et al. Phase I and pharmacokinetic trial of gemcitabine in patients with hepatic or renal dysfunction: Cancer and leukemia group B 9565. J Clin Oncol 2000;18:2780–2787.
52. Evans WE, Hon YY, Bomgaars L, et al. Preponderance of thiopurine S-methyltransferase deficiency and heterozygosity among patients intolerant to mercaptopurine or azathoprine. J Clin Oncol 2001;19:2293–2301.
53. Kolesar JM, Morris AK, Kuhn JG. Purine nucleoside analogs: Fludarabine, pentostatin and cladribine. Part 1: Fludarabine. J Oncol Pharm Prac 1996;2:160–181.
54. Morris AK, Kolesar J, Kuhn JG. Purine nucleoside analogs: Fludarabine, pentostatin and cladribine. Part 3: Cladribine. J Oncol Pharm Prac 1997;3:94–109.
55. Chu E, Allegra CJ. Antifolates. In: Chabner BA, Longo DL, eds. Cancer Chemotherapy and Biotherapy: Principles and Practice. Philadelphia, Lippincott-Raven, 1996:109–148.
56. Kamen BA, Cole PD, Bertino JR. Folate antagonists. In: Bast RC Jr, Kufe DW, Pollock RE, Weichselbaum RR, Holland JF, Frei E III, eds. Holland-Frei Cancer Medicine, 5th ed. Hamilton, Ontario, BC Decker, 2000:612–624.
57. Madden T, Eaton VE. Methotrexate. In: Schumacher GE, ed. Therapeutic Drug Monitoring. Norwalk, CT, Appleton & Lange, 1995:527–552.
58. Rowinsky EK, Donehower RC. Antimicrotubule agents. In: Chabner BA, Longo DL, eds. Cancer Chemotherapy and Biotherapy: Principles and Practice. Philadelphia, Lippincott-Raven, 1996:263–296.
59. Beck WT, Cass CE, Houghton PJ. Microtubule-targeting anticancer drugs derived from plants and microbes: Vinca alkaloids, taxanes, and epothilones. In: Bast RC Jr, Kufe DW, Pollock RE, Weichselbaum RR, Holland JF, Frei E III, eds. Holland-Frei Cancer Medicine, 5th ed. Hamilton, Ontario, BC Decker, 2000:680–698.
60. Dutcher JP, Novik Y, O'Boyle K, Marcoullis G, Secco C, Wiernik PH. 20th Century advances in drug therapy in oncology—Part II. Clin Pharmacol 2000;40:1079–1092.
61. Dumontet C, Sikic BI. Mechanisms of action of and resistance to antitubulin agents: Microtubule dynamics, drug transport, and cell death. J Clin Oncol 1999;17:1061–1070.
62. McCune JS, Lindley C. Appropriateness of maximum dose-guidelines for vincristine. Am J Health Syst Pharm 1997;54:1755–1758.
63. Albanell J, Baselga J. Systemic therapy emergencies. Semin Oncol 2000;27:347–361.
64. Chan JD. Pharmacokinetic drug interactions of vinca alkaloids: Summary of case reports. Pharmacotherapy 1998;18:1304–1307.
65. Figgitt DP, Wiseman LR. Docetaxel: An update of its use in advanced breast cancer. Drugs 2000;59:621–651.
66. Markman M, Kennedy A, Webster K, et al. Simplified regimen for the prevention of paclitaxel-associated hypersensitivity reactions. J Clin Oncol 1997;15:3517. Letter.
67. Hande KR. Etoposide: Four decades of development of a topoisomerase II inhibitor. Eur J Cancer 1998;34:1514–1521.
68. Rubin EH, Hait WN. Anthracyclines and DNA intercalators/epipodophyllotoxins/DNA topoisomerases. In: Bast RC Jr, Kufe DW, Pollock RE, Weichselbaum RR, Holland JF, Frei E III, eds. Holland-Frei Cancer Medicine, 5th ed. Hamilton, Ontario, BC Decker, 2000: 670–679.
69. Stewart CF. Use of etoposide in patients with organ dysfunction: Pharmacokinetic and pharmacodynamic considerations. Cancer Chemother Pharmacol 1994;34(suppl):S76–S83.
70. Wiseman LR, Markham A. Irinotecan. A review of its pharmacological properties and clinical efficacy in the management of advanced colorectal cancer. Drugs 1996;52:606–623.
71. Vanhoefer U, Harstrick A, Achterrath W, et al. Irinotecan in the treatment of colorectal cancer: Clinical overview. J Clin Oncol 2001;19:1501–1518.
72. Dennis MJ, Beijnen JH, Grochow LB, van Warmerdam LJ. An overview of the clinical pharmacology of topotecan. Semin Oncol 1997;24 (suppl 5):S5–S18.
73. Gallo JM, Laub PB, Rowinsky EK, Grochow LB, Baker SD. Population pharmacokinetic model for topotecan derived from phase I trials. J Clin Oncol 2000;18:2459–2467.
74. Doroshow JH. Anthracyclines and anthracenediones. In: Chabner BA, Longo DL, eds. Cancer Chemotherapy and Biotherapy: Principles and Practice. Philadelphia, Lippincott-Raven, 1996:409–434.
75. Shan K, Lincoff M, Young JB. Anthracycline-induced cardiotoxicity. Ann Intern Med 1996;125:47–58.

76. Singal PK, Li T, Kumar D, Danelisen I, Iliskovic N. Adriamycin-induced heart failure: Mechanism and modulation. Mol Cell Biochem 2000; 207:77–85.
77. Batist G, Ramakrishnan G, Rao CS, et al. Reduced cardiotoxicity and preserved antitumor efficacy of liposome-encapsulated doxorubicin and cyclophosphamide compared with conventional doxorubicin and cyclophosphamide in a randomized, multicenter trial of metastatic breast cancer. J Clin Oncol 2001;19:1444–1454.
78. Ryberg M, Nielsen D, Skovsgaard T, Hansen J, Jensen BV, Dombernowsky P. Epirubicin cardiotoxicity: An analysis of 469 patients with metastatic breast cancer. J Clin Oncol 1998;16:302–3508.
79. Dorr RT. Pharmacologic management of vesicant chemotherapy extravasations. In: Dorr RT, Von Hoff DD, eds. Cancer Chemotherapy Handbook, 2nd ed. Stamford, CT, Appleton & Lange, 1994:109–118.
80. Patel J. Liposomal doxorubicin: Doxil[R]. J Oncol Pharm Pract 1996;2:201–210.
81. Colvin DM. Alkylating agents and platinum antitumor compounds. In: Bast RC Jr, Kufe DW, Pollock RE, Weichselbaum RR, Holland JF, Frei E III, eds. Holland-Frei Cancer Medicine, 5th ed. Hamilton, Ontario, BC Decker, 2000:648–669.
82. Tew K, Colvin M, Chabner BA. Alkylating agents. In: Chabner BA, Longo DL, eds. Cancer Chemotherapy and Biotherapy: Principles and Practice. Philadelphia, Lippincott-Raven, 1996:297–332.
83. Boddy AV, Yule SM. Metabolism and pharmacokinetics of oxazaphosphorines. Clin Pharmacokinet 2000;38:291–304.
84. West NJ. Prevention and treatment of hemorrhagic cystitis. Pharmacotherapy 1997;17:696–706.
85. Witte RS, Elson P, Bono B, et al. Eastern cooperative oncology group phase II trial of ifosfamide in the treatment of previously treated advanced urothelial carcinoma. J Clin Oncol 1997;15:589–593.
86. Yung WK, Prados MD, Yaya-Tur R, et al. Multicenter phase II trial of temozolomide in patients with anaplastic astrocytoma or anaplastic oligoastrocytoma at first relapse. Temodal Brain Tumor Group. J Clin Oncol 1999;17:2762–2771.
87. Middleton MR, Grob JJ, Aaronson N, et al. Randomized phase III study of temozolamide versus dacarbazine in the treatment of patients with advanced metastatic malignant melanoma. J Clin Oncol 2000;18:158–166.
88. Jordan P, Carmo-Fonseca M. Molecular mechanisms involved in cisplatin cytotoxicity. Cell Mol Life Sci 2000;7:1229–1235.
89. Giaccone G. Clinical perspectives on platinum resistance. Drugs 2000;59 (suppl 4):9–17.
90. O'Dwyer PJ, Stevenson JP, Johnson SW. Clinical pharmacokinetics and administration of established platinum drugs. Drugs 2000;59 (suppl 4):19–27.
91. Pinzani V, Bressolle F, Haug IJ, et al. Cisplatin-induced renal toxicity and toxicity-modulating strategies: A review. Cancer Chemother Pharmacol 1994;35:1–9.
92. Foster-Nora JA, Siden R. Amifostine for protection from antineoplastic drug toxicity. Am J Health Syst Pharm 1997;54:787–800
93. Valley AW. Gastrointestinal complications of cancer chemotherapy. In: Finley RS, Balmer C, eds. Concepts in Oncology Therapeutics, 2nd ed. Bethesda, MD, American Society of Health-Systems Pharmacists 1998:147–171
94. Calvert AH. Dose optimisation of carboplatin in adults. Anticancer Res 1994;14:2273–2278.
95. Chatelut E, Canal P, Brunner V, et al. Predication of carboplatin clearance from standard morphological and biological patient characteristics. J Natl Cancer Inst 1995;87:573–580.
96. Donahue A, McCune JS, Faucette S, et al. Measured versus estimated glomerular filtration rate in the Calvert equation: Influence on carboplatin dosing. Cancer Chemother Pharmacol 2001;47:373–379.
97. Markman M, Kennedy A, Webster K, et al. Clinical features of hypersensitivity reactions to carboplatin. J Clin Oncol 1999;17:1141–1145.
98. Zanotti KM, Rybicki LA, Kennedy AW, et al. Carboplatin skin testing: A skin-testing protocol for predicting hypersensitivity to carboplatin chemotherapy. J Clin Oncol 2001;19:3126–3129.
99. Lazo JS, Chabner BA. Bleomycin. In: Chabner BA, Longo DL, eds. Cancer Chemotherapy and Biotherapy: Principles and Practice. Philadelphia, Lippincott-Raven, 1996:379–394.
100. Laso JS. Bleomycin. Cancer Chemother Biol Response Modif 1999;18: 39–45.
101. Andrews CO, Gora ML. Pleural effusions: Pathophysiology and management. Ann Pharmacother 1994;28:894–902.
102. Chabner BA. Enzyme therapy: L-Asparaginase. In: Chabner BA, Longo DL, eds. Cancer Chemotherapy and Biotherapy: Principles and Practice. Philadelphia, Lippincott-Raven, 1996:485–492.
103. Kurtzberg J. Asparaginase. In: Bast RC Jr, Kufe DW, Pollock RE, Weichselbaum RR, Holland JF, Frei E III, eds. Holland-Frei Cancer Medicine, 5th ed. Hamilton, Ontario, BC Decker, 2000:699–705.
104. Novick SC, Warrell RP Jr. Arsenicals in hematologic cancers. Semin Oncol 2000;27:495–501.
105. Chen Z, Chen G-Q, Shen Z-X, Chen S-J, Wang Z-Y. Treatment of acute promyelocytic leukemia with arsenic compounds: *In vitro* and *in vivo* studies. Semin Hematol 2001;38:26–36.
106. Camacho LH, Soignet SL, Chanel S, et al. Leukocytosis and the retinoic acid syndrome in patients with acute promyelocytic leukemia treated with arsenic trioxide. J Clin Oncol 2000;18:2630–2625.
107. Borden EC, Williams BRG. Interferons. In: Bast RC Jr, Kufe DW, Pollock RE, Weichselbaum RR, Holland JF, Frei E III, eds. Holland-Frei Cancer Medicine, 5th ed. Hamilton, Ontario, BC Decker, 2000:815–824.
108. Witt PL, Lindner DJ, D'Cunha J, Borden EC. Pharmacology of interferons: Induced proteins, cell activation, and antitumor activity. In: Chabner BA, Longo DL, eds. Cancer Chemotherapy and Biotherapy: Principles and Practice. Philadelphia, Lippincott-Raven, 1996:585–608.
109. Trask PC, Esper P, Riba M, Redman. Psychiatric side effects of interferon therapy: prevalence, proposed mechanisms, and future directions. J Clin Oncol 2000;18:2316–2326.
110. Grimm EA. Cytokines: Biology and applications in cancer medicine. In: Bast RC Jr, Kufe DW, Pollock RE, Weichselbaum RR, Holland JF, Frei E III, eds. Holland-Frei Cancer Medicine, 5th ed. Hamilton, Ontario, BC Decker, 2000:826–834.
111. Bruton JK, Koeller JM. Recombinant interleukin-2. Pharmacotherapy 1994;14:635–656.
112. Atkins MB, Lotze MT, Dutcher JP, et al. High-dose recombinant interleukin 2 therapy for patients with metastatic melanoma: Analysis of 270 patients treated between 1985 and 1993. J Clin Oncol 1999;17:2105–2116.
113. Sundin DJ, Wolin MJ. Toxicity management in patients receiving low-dose aldesleukin therapy. Ann Pharmacother 1998;32:1344–1352.
114. Olsen E, Duvic M, Frankel A, et al. Pivotal phase III trial of two dose levels of denileukin diftitox for the treatment of cutaneous T-cell lymphoma. J Clin Oncol 2001;19:376–388.
115. Ligand Pharmaceuticals. Ontak (denileukin diftitox) product information. San Diego, 1999.
116. McKay LI, Cidlowki JA. Corticosteroids. In: Bast RC Jr, Kufe DW, Pollock RE, Weichselbaum RR, Holland JF, Frei E III, eds. Holland-Frei Cancer Medicine, 5th ed. Hamilton, Ontario, BC Decker, 2000:730–742.
117. Davies PJA, Lippman SM. Biologic basis of retinoid pharmacology: Implications for cancer prevention and therapy. Adv Oncol 1996;12(2): 2–10.
118. Frankel SR, Eardley A, Heller G, et al. All-trans-retinoic acid for acute promyelocytic leukemia. Ann Intern Med 1994;120:278–286.
119. Duvic M, Hymes K, Heald P, et al. Bexarotene is effective and safe for treatment of refractory advanced-state cutaneous T-cell lymphoma: Multinational phase II-III trial results. J Clin Oncol 2001;19:2456–2471.
120. Ligand Pharmaceuticals. Targretin (bexarotene) product information. San Diego, 1999.
121. Duvic M, Friedman-Kien AE, Looney DJ, et al. Topical treatment of cutaneous lesions of acquired immunodeficiency syndrome-related Kaposi sarcoma using alitretinoin gel: Results of phase 1 and 2 trials. Arch Dermatol 2000;136:1461–1469.

122. Anonymous. Gleevec (STI-571) for chronic myeloid leukemia. Med Lett 2001;43:49–50.
123. Novartis Pharma AG. Gleevec (imatinib mesylate) product information. East Hanover, NJ, 2001.
124. Goldman JM, Melo JV. Targeting the bcr-abl tyrosine kinase in chronic myeloid leukemia. N Engl J Med 2001;344:1084–1086. Editorial.
125. Richardson P, Hideshima T, Anderson K. Thalidomide: The revival of a drug with therapeutic promise in the treatment of cancer. PPO Updates 2001;15(2):1–18.
126. Raje N, Anderson K. Thalidomide—A revival story. N Engl J Med 1999;341:1606–1609. Editorial.
127. Singhal S, Mehta J, Desikan R, et al. Antitumor activity of thalidomide in refractory multiple myeloma. N Engl J Med 1999;341:1565–1571.
128. Green MC, Murray JL, Hortobagyi GN. Monoclonal antibody therapy for solid tumors. Cancer Treat Rev 2000;26:269–286.
129. White CA, Weaver RL, Gillo-Lopez AJ. Antibody-targeted immunotherapy for treatment of malignancy. Annu Rev Med 2001;52:125–145.
130. Anonymous. Gemtuzumab for relapsed acute myeloid leukemia. Med Lett 2000;42:67–68.
131. Wood AM. Rituximab: An innovative therapy for non-Hodgkin's lymphoma. Am J Health Syst Pharm 2001;58:215–229.
132. Colomer R, Shamon LA, Tsai MS, Lupu R. Herceptin: From the bench to the clinic. Cancer Invest 2001;19:49–56.
133. Flynn JM, Byrd JC. Campath-1H monoclonal antibody therapy. Curr Opin Oncol 2000;12:574–581.
134. DePauw BE, Donelly JP. Infections in the immunocompromised host: General principles. In: Mandell GP, Bennett JE, Dolin R, eds. Principles and Practice of Infectious Disease, 5th ed. Philadelphia, Churchill Livingstone, 2000:3079–3090.
135. Pizzo PA. Empirical therapy and prevention of infection in the immunocompromised host. In: Mandell GP, Bennett JE, Dolin R, eds. Principles and Practice of Infectious Disease, 5th ed. Philadelphia, Churchill Livingstone, 2000:3102–3112.
136. Hughes WT, Armstrong D, Bodey GP, et al. 1997 Guidelines for the use of antimicrobial agents in neutropenic patients with unexplained fever. Clin Infect Dis 1997;25:551–573.
137. Rolston KV, Talcott JA. Ambulatory antimicrobial therapy for hematologic malignancies. Oncology (Huntingt) 2000;14:17–22.
138. Nemunaitis J. A comparative review of the colony-stimulating factors. Drugs 1997;54:709–729.
139. ASCO Ad Hoc Colony-Stimulating Factor Guideline Expert Panel. American Society of Clinical Oncology recommendations for the use of hematopoietic colony-stimulating factors: Evidence-based, clinical practice guidelines. J Clin Oncol 1994;12:2471–2508.
140. ASCO Ad Hoc Colony-Stimulating Factor Guideline Expert Panel. 2000 Update of recommendations for the use of hematopoietic colony-stimulating factors: Evidence-based, clinical practice guidelines. J Clin Oncol 2000;3558–3585.
141. Schiffer CA, Anderson KC, Bennett CL, et al. Platelet transfusion for patients with cancer: Clinical practice guidelines of the American Society of Clinical Oncology. J Clin Oncol 2001;19:1519–1538.
142. Demetri GD. Pharmacologic treatment options in patients with thrombocytopenia. Semin Hematol 2000;37(2 suppl 4):11–18.
143. Adams VR, Brenner TL. Oprelvekin (Neumega). J Oncol Pharm Pract 1999;5:117–24.
144. Johnston E, Crawford J. The hematologic support of the cancer patient. In: Berger A, Portenoy RK, Weissman DE, eds: Principles and Practice of Supportive Oncology. Philadelphia, Lippincott- Raven Publishers, 1998:549–555.
145. Cella D. Factors influencing quality of life in cancer patients: Anemia and fatigue. Semin Oncol 1998;25 (suppl 7):43–46.
146. Cazzola M, Mercuriali F, Brugnara C. Use of recombinant human erythropoietin outside the setting of uremia. Blood 1997;89:4248–4267.
147. Jilani SM, Glaspy JA. Impact of epoetin alfa in chemotherapy-associated anemia. Semin Oncol 1998;25:571–576.
148. Glaspy J, Bukowski R, Steinberg D, Taylor C, Tchekmedyian S, Vadhan-Raj S. Impact of therapy with epoetin alfa on clinical outcomes in patients with nonmyeloid malignancies during cancer chemotherapy in community oncology practice. J Clin Oncol 1997;15:1218–1234.
149. Demetri GD, Kris M, Wade J, Degos L, Cella D. Quality of life benefit in chemotherapy patients treated with epoetin alfa is independent of disease response or tumor type: Results from a prospective community oncology study. J Clin Oncol 1998;16:3412–3425.
150. Koeller JM. Clinical guidelines for the treatment of cancer-related anemia. Pharmacotherapy 1998;18:156–169.
151. Berger AM, Kilroy TJ. Oral complications. In: DeVita VT Jr, Hellman S, Rosenberg SA, eds. Cancer: Principles and Practice of Oncology, 6th ed. Philadelphia, Lippincott Williams & Wilkins, 2001:2881–2893.
152. Siepp CA. Hair loss. In: DeVita VT Jr, Hellman S, Rosenberg SA, eds. Cancer: Principles and Practice of Oncology, 6th ed. Philadelphia, Lippincott Williams & Wilkins, 2001:2922–2923.
153. Howell S, Shalet S. Gonadal damage from chemotherapy and radiotherapy. Endocrin Metab Clin North Am 1998;27:927–943.
154. Lenz KL, Valley AW. Infertility after chemotherapy: A review of the risks and strategies for prevention. J Oncol Pharm Pract 1996;2:75–100.
155. Green DM, D'Angio GJD. Second malignant neoplasms. In: Abeloff MD, Armitage JO, Lichter AS, Niederhuber JE, eds. Clinical Oncology, 2nd ed. Philadelphia, Churchill Livingstone, 2000:1082–1100.
156. ASHP technical assistance bulletin on handling cytotoxic and hazardous drugs. Am J Hosp Pharm 1990;47:1033–1049.
157. American Cancer Society Guidelines for Nutrition and Cancer Prevention. Atlanta, GA, American Cancer Society, 1999 (Publication No. 99–75M-No.2021–CC).
158. Lippman SM, Lee JJ, Sabichi AL. Cancer chemoprevention: Progress and promise. J Natl Cancer Inst 1998;90:1514–1528.
159. Siegfried JM. Biology and chemoprevention of lung cancer. Chest 1998; 113(suppl):40S–45S.
160. Baron JA, Beach M, Mandel JS, et al. Calcium supplements for the prevention of colorectal adenomas. N Engl J Med 1999;340:101–107.
161. Steinbach G, Lynch PM, Phillips RKS, et al. The effect of celecoxib, a cyclooxygenase inhibitor, in familial adenomatous polyposis. N Engl J Med 2000;342:1946–1952.
162. Lippman SM, Brown PH. Tamoxifen prevention of breast cancer: An instance of the fingerpost. J Natl Cancer Inst 1999;91:1809–1819.
163. Bergen AW, Caporaso N. Cigarette smoking. J Natl Cancer Inst 1999; 91:1365–1375.
164. Gilchriest BA, Eller MS, Geller AC, Yaar M. The pathogenesis of melanoma induced by ultraviolet radiation. N Engl J Med 1999;340:48.

125
BREAST CANCER

Celeste Lindley

Breast cancer is the most common site of cancer and is second only to lung cancer as a cause of cancer death in American women. It is estimated that 192,200 new cases of breast cancer will be diagnosed and that 40,200 women will die of breast cancer in 2001.[1] These projections are based on the Surveillance, Epidemiology, and End Results (SEER) program of the National Cancer Institute (NCI). Since 1973, the SEER program has collected cancer incidence, mortality, and survival data each year for residents in nine metropolitan areas (or entire states), comprising about 10% of all the cancers diagnosed in the United States.

A great deal of public and health professional concern currently surrounds the increasing incidence of breast cancer. According to SEER registry data, the incidence of breast cancer increased by more than 40% from 1973 to 1998—that is, from 82.6 to 118.1 per 100,000.[2] In 1980, the breast cancer incidence rate started to rise more sharply. Between 1980 and 1987, cancer incidence rate grew from 85.5 to 113.3 per 100,000, which represents an increase of 32.5% or about 4% per year. From 1987 to 1998, breast cancer incidence rates have increased an average of only 0.5% per year (Fig. 125–1).

The increased incidence of breast cancer is believed to be a result of three factors.[3] Approximately 30% of the increase is because of the slow, but steady increase in breast cancer that has been observed over the last 50 years. It is likely that this gradual increase is related to dietary, body habitus, hormonal, and reproductive factors that will be discussed in detail in the upcoming section on epidemiology. About 60% of the increase is attributable to the detection of cases that were present in the population, but were often not detected without the use of mammographic screening and regular examinations. About 10% of the new cases occur because women are living longer and the mortality from other causes is decreasing.

The increase in breast cancer incidence in the 1980s is characterized by an increase in the detection of small-sized lesions as well as carcinoma *in situ*.[4] The incidence rate for invasive cancers smaller than 1 cm grew from 9 per 100,000 in 1982 to 36 per 100,000 in 1988. The number of cancers 1–1.9 cm detected increased from 40 per 100,000 in 1982 to 84 per 100,000 in 1988. On the other hand, the rate of detection for tumors 2–2.9 cm remained about the same from 1982 to 1989, while the number of large cancers found at diagnosis (those of 3 cm) decreased. Although not reflected in the SEER data, the rate of detection of carcinoma *in situ* increased greatly from 4 per 100,000 in 1973 to a high of 15 per 100,000 in 1987. Ductal carcinoma *in situ,* which often manifests solely as microcalcifications seen on screening mammography, is estimated to account for 10% to 20% of all breast cancer diagnoses in screened populations.[5] Increased public awareness and increased use of screening mammography are largely responsible for increased detection of breast cancers in the small or localized stage.

It is well recognized that breast cancer in the early stages is potentially curable in most patients and that metastatic breast cancer is incurable. Thus, increased detection of localized and small breast cancer seen in the 1980s should have an impact on mortality rate from breast cancer. Age-adjusted mortality rates in the United States were relatively stable in the period from the 1950s and to the late 1980s, when an overall decline was first noted. From 1989 to 1995, mortality rates from breast cancer decreased an average of 1.6% annually; the decrease then accelerated to a decline of 3.4% annually from 1995 to 1998 (Fig. 125–1).[2] The decline in breast cancer mortality rate has been observed in white women, and the decrease was proportionately greater in women younger than 50 years of age than in older women. From 1973 to 1998, the cumulative decline in mortality rates for white women younger than age 50 was more than 35% with much of this decline occurring since 1988. In contrast to those trends among younger women, mortality rates for white women age 50 years and older increased slowly during the 1970s and 1980s, although since the late 1980s, mortality has also begun to decline in this group. The trends in breast cancer mortality among African American women have been unfavorable. Mortality rates increased by an average of 1.3% per year for African American women in all age groups from 1973 to 1991, but have not increased over the past few years. The recent overall decline of breast cancer mortality has been attributed to changes in screening practices and effectiveness of adjuvant systemic therapy following primary local-regional therapy.[7]

EPIDEMIOLOGY AND ETIOLOGY

The two variables most strongly associated with the occurrence of breast cancer are gender and age. Although one commonly thinks of breast cancer as a disease confined to women, about 1,500 cases of male breast cancer were projected to be diagnosed in the United States in 2001.[1] Although male gender had been considered a poor prognostic factor in some investigations, it is now believed that higher mortality rates in men are attributable to more advanced disease at the time of diagnosis. When stage and other known prognostic factors are controlled for, men do not fare differently from their female counterparts. Similarly, treatment of male breast cancer is not different from treatment of breast cancer in females.

The incidence of breast cancer increases with advancing age. Perhaps the most frequently quoted breast cancer statistic is that one in eight women will develop breast cancer during their lifetime.[3] It should be emphasized that this is a cumulative lifetime risk of developing the disease from birth to age 110 and that the estimates are weighted by the probability of surviving through each decade of life. Women older than 90 years of age contribute very little to the overall risk statistic because their numbers are so small. The "one in eight women" figure has created fear of a breast cancer epidemic, with some women assuming that it translates to one in eight women being diagnosed with breast cancer each year. Feuer et al. developed a more useful method of presenting the risk data based on age intervals.[3] As Table 125–1 demonstrates, the risk of a woman developing breast cancer before the age of 40 years is 1 in 257. It is apparent from this table that although the cumulative probability of developing breast cancer increases with increasing age, more than half of the risk occurs after age 60 years.

Aside from female gender and age, a number of additional risk factors have been identified. Complex experimental and

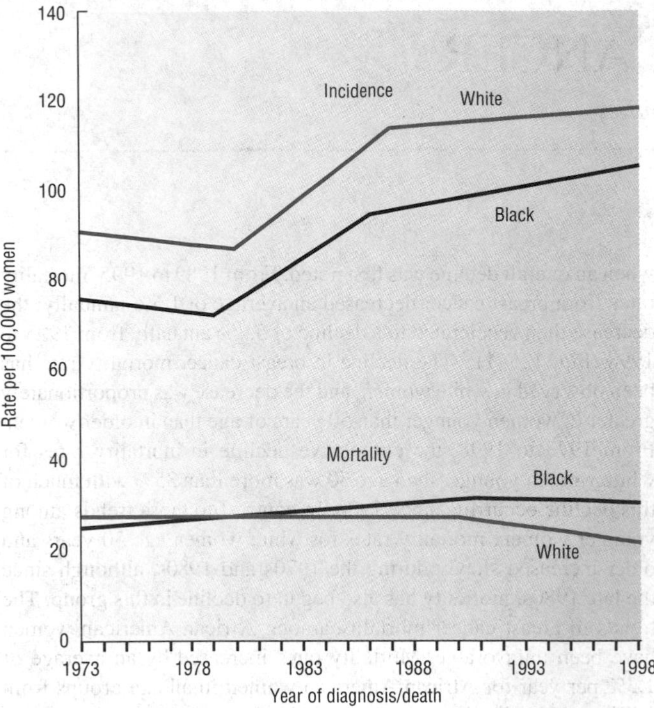

FIGURE 125–1. Breast cancer incidence and mortality rates by race, SEER, 1973–1998.

epidemiologic evidence points to an association between breast cancer and endocrine factors, environment, and genetics. Although the exact nature of the association is unclear, most factors recognized as increasing a woman's risk above the average are related to one or more of these influences. The strength of the association between a given risk factor and the development of breast cancer is indicated by a "relative risk ratio" or "odds ratio." These are derived from epidemiologic, case control, or cohort studies in which the incidence of disease among persons possessing a characteristic in question is divided by the incidence of disease among otherwise similar persons without the characteristic. Computation of "relative risk ratios" through epidemiologic research is complex and inexact. This area of research is hindered by many fundamental methodologic problems such as selection bias, recall bias, incomplete data, and, most important, the presence of confounding factors. A large number of case control and cohort studies that examine the relationship between certain factors and risk of developing breast cancer have been conducted and often have yielded conflicting results. However, it is important to review established and probable risk factors for cancer and to continue to conduct research in this area. Through these efforts, the etiology of breast cancer can be further elucidated, women who would benefit from intensified surveillance or prophylactic treatment may be identified, and recommendations for modifiable risk factors that will ultimately reduce the incidence of breast cancer can be established.

TABLE 125–1. Risk of Developing Breast Cancer in SEER Areas, Women, All Races 1995–1997

Age Interval (y)	Probability (%) of Developing Invasive Breast Cancer During the Interval
30–40	0.40 or 1 in 257
40–50	1.49 or 1 in 67
50–60	2.75 or 1 in 36
60–70	3.49 or 1 in 28
70–80	4.13 or 1 in 24
From birth to death	12.83 or 1 in 8

From NCI SEER Data.

An understanding of the relationship between age and the incidence of breast cancer is particularly relevant when one discusses "risk factors" or factors other than age that increase a woman's probability of developing breast cancer. The "relative risk" (RR) of developing breast cancer for an individual woman in a defined risk group is usually multiplied by the probability of a woman developing breast cancer during her lifetime, and this figure is taken as the cumulative lifetime risk of that individual developing breast cancer. However, the risk of developing breast cancer is age dependent. Therefore, a more meaningful way to counsel patients regarding their risk of developing breast cancer based on the presence of a known risk factor incorporates an age-specific incidence rate, not cumulative lifetime risk. For example, if a 40-year-old woman with a strong family history of breast cancer is thought to have a "relative risk ratio" of 2.0, her risk of developing breast cancer by the age of 50 is only 2.98% (2 × 1.49) not 25.66% (2 × 12.83) (see Table 125–1). It is also important to note that recognized risk factors are not "additive" in a simple mathematical sense and that the observed cumulative lifetime risk associated with nongenetic risk factors has rarely exceeded 30% (1 in 3) in any study, regardless of the number and significance of individual risk factors. Finally, it should be emphasized that more than 60% of women with breast cancer have no identifiable major risk factor, indicating that the search for the etiology of this disease is largely incomplete.[5]

ENDOCRINE FACTORS

A number of endocrine factors have been linked to the incidence of breast cancer.[8] Many of these relate to the total duration of menstrual life. Early menarche, generally defined as menstruation beginning before age 12, has been shown by a number of investigators to increase the cumulative lifetime risk of breast cancer development compared to menarche at age 16 or greater. Conversely, early age of natural menopause has been shown to result in a reduction of risk. Similarly, investigators have reported that bilateral oophorectomy prior to age 35 reduces the relative risk of developing breast cancer.

Nulliparity and a late age at first birth (greater or equal to 30 years) have been reported to increase the lifetime risk of developing breast cancer twofold. Women who have their first child after the age of 35 have a slightly higher risk than a nulliparous woman. It has been suggested that the period between the onset of menses and the age of first pregnancy provides a "window of initiation" for the development of breast cancer. This is a time when an unbalanced hormonal environment reacts with the abundant and highly responsive breast tissue. Investigators have postulated that international differences in age of menarche, age at menopause, and childbearing may account for a substantial part of the international differences in the incidence of breast cancer. In underdeveloped countries where the incidence of breast cancer is low compared to the United States, a late onset of menarche is the rule and frequently there is a decreased interval between puberty and first pregnancy followed by several pregnancies and early menopause.

Many studies have evaluated the relationship between exogenous hormones and development of breast cancer. Postmenopausal estrogen replacement therapy has been the subject of several recent meta-analyses. A report from investigators from the Harvard School of Public Health concluded that women who have used estrogens in the past are not at an increased risk of breast cancer, but that current use may be associated with a 40% increased risk (i.e., RR = 1.4). This meta-analysis also suggested that long-term use might lead to a slight increase in risk.[9] Another meta-analysis has suggested that the combined results from multiple studies provide evidence that menopausal therapy (consisting of 0.625 mg or less of conjugated estrogen per day) does not increase breast cancer risk.[10] A study from the Centers for Disease Control and Prevention reported that the risk did not appear to increase until after at least 5 years of estrogen use.[11] These data are encouraging and suggest that a large effect of hormone therapy on breast cancer risk may be excluded and that the use of low doses of estrogen for short periods as replacement therapy in postmenopausal women is relatively safe. The important question is how the benefits of estrogen replacement therapy (lowered cardiovascular mortality, decreased bone loss, relief of menopausal symptoms) weigh against the risks (increased endometrial cancer, if used without progesterone, and slight increase in breast cancer). The Women's Health Initiative, a study sponsored by the National Cancer Institute, will randomize 80,000 women to take or not take postmenopausal estrogen replacement therapy and should provide important answers regarding the benefits and risks associated with this therapy.

The use of postmenopausal estrogen replacement therapy in women with a history of breast cancer is generally considered contraindicated. Because of the association of estrogen and risk of breast cancer, many physicians believe that patients with a strong family history or other risk factors for breast cancer should not receive postmenopausal estrogen replacement therapy. This dogma has recently been challenged in the medical literature.[12] Proponents of estrogen replacement therapy in patients with successfully treated operable breast cancer often state that the benefits of replacement therapy in terms of cardiovascular risk reduction and reduction of morbidity and mortality from osteoporosis and subsequent fractures outweigh an unknown but potential increased risk of breast cancer development. At the current time, there is not enough information to state confidently that estrogen replacement therapy has any significant impact, positive or negative, on prognosis in women with a personal or family history of breast cancer and all recommendations are based on speculation and circumstantial evidence.

There are more than 20 epidemiologic studies of the potential carcinogenic effect of oral contraceptives, most of which have not shown a relationship between birth control pills and breast cancer incidence. But results are conflicting and assessment of the studies necessitates consideration of the particular oral contraceptive products involved, daily and cumulative doses of the hormones administered, and the latency for development of breast cancer. A review and meta-analyses suggest that there has been no overall increase in the risk of breast cancer for women who had ever received oral contraceptive drugs. But women who had used these agents for a prolonged period of time or prior to a first pregnancy were at a higher risk (RR = 1.5–2) of developing breast cancer until the age of 45 years.[13] It should be pointed out that early use of oral contraceptives may be associated with early menarche and may result in late age of first birth, both of which are recognized risk factors for breast cancer. Although it is not entirely possible to rule out a promotional effect of oral contraceptives on breast cancer development in young patients, most experts believe that the safety and benefits of low-dose oral contraceptives currently outweigh the potential risks and that changes in the prescribing practice for the use of oral contraceptives are not warranted. Oral contraceptives are known to reduce the risk of ovarian cancer by about 40% and the risk of endometrial cancer by 60%.[5]

GENETIC FACTORS

Both personal and family histories influence a woman's risk of developing breast cancer. A past medical history for breast cancer is associated with the relative risk of 5.0 for the development of a contralateral breast cancer. Cancer of the uterus and ovary have also been associated with an increased risk of the development of breast cancer. Breast cancer is observed as part of cancer family syndromes in association with other tumors. Only 5% of breast cancer patients are thought to have a pedigree consistent with hereditary breast cancer.

A topic that bears some discussion because of its prevalence in the general population is the relationship of fibrocystic breast disease to the development of invasive breast cancer. As many as 85% of American women have "lumpy breasts" and may bear a clinical diagnosis of fibrocystic breast disease or benign breast disease. The relative risk of breast cancer in patients with a history of fibrocystic breast disease has ranged from 1.5 to 2.0 in reported studies. But fibrocystic disease involves a heterogeneous group of pathologic changes associated with various degrees of breast cancer risk. Thus, a clinical diagnosis of fibrocystic or benign breast disease has little practical significance for counseling patients regarding individual risk of breast cancer. A useful system for classifying benign breast disease was recently adapted by the American College of Pathologists.[14] Benign breast conditions were classified as nonproliferative or proliferative, and on the basis of review of more than 10,000 breast biopsies, relative risks of breast cancer were determined. Women with proliferative disease were found to have a relative risk of 1.9 and the subcategory of women with atypical hyperplasia had a relative risk of 4.4. Nonproliferative breast disease was not associated with an excess risk of breast cancer. About 80% of the reviewed biopsies were found to have nonproliferative breast disease, and of those demonstrating proliferation, only 3.6% were "atypical." These data suggest that in most women, benign breast disease or fibrocystic disease is most often not associated with proliferation and the women are not at an increased risk for developing breast cancer. However, it must be noted that "lumpy breasts" may lead to a delay in diagnosis of breast cancer owing to the inability of the patient or physician to detect a true malignant lesion.[14]

It has been recognized for some time that a family history of breast cancer is associated rather strongly with a woman's own risk for developing the disease. Empirical estimates of the risks associated with particular patterns of family history of breast cancer indicate the following:[15]

1. Having any first-degree relative with breast cancer increases a woman's risk of breast cancer 1.5- to 3-fold, depending on age.
2. The higher relative risk is associated with breast cancer with onset younger than age 45 years in one or more first-degree relatives.
3. Having multiple first-degree relatives affected has been inconsistently associated with elevated risks
4. Having a second-degree relative affected increases a woman's risk of developing breast cancer by approximately 50% (relative risk = 1.5).
5. Affected family members on the maternal side and the paternal side contribute similarly to the risk.

Although certain patterns of family history are associated with substantial elevations in the risk of breast cancer, these high-risk patterns occur infrequently in the general population (Table 125–2). The percentage of all breast cancers in the population that can be attributed to family history range between 6% and 12%. Thus, it appears that genetically transmitted susceptibility contributes to their etiology of breast cancer in a sizable minority of patients.

In the early 1990s, pedigree analysis of 23 high-risk families for breast and ovarian cancer provided evidence for a rare autosomal dominant allele.[5,16] From these families, a gene on the long arm of chromosome 17 (17q21) was identified as abnormal in a large percentage of these hereditary breast and ovarian cancer patients. Isolation of the BRCA1 gene was initially reported in 1994. Already a

TABLE 125–2. Established and Probable Risk Factors for Breast Cancer

Risk Factor	Comparison Category	Risk Category	Typical Relative Risk
Family history of breast cancer	No first-degree relatives affected	Mother affected before the age of 60 y	2.0
		Mother affected after the age of 60 y	1.4
		Two first-degree relatives affected	4–6
		Breast cancer in one or more second-degree relatives	1.36
		Ovarian cancer in one or more first-degree relatives	1.59
Age at menarche	16 y	11 y	1.3
Age at birth of first child	Before 20 y	20–24 y	1.3
		25–29 y	1.6
		≥ 30 y	1.9
Age at menopause	45–54 y	After 55 y	1.5
		Before 45 y	0.7
		Oophrectomy before 35 y	0.4
Benign breast disease	No biopsy or aspiration	Proliferation only	1.5
		Atypical hyperplasia	3.5
		Lobular carcinoma *in situ*	7.2
Obesity	10th percentile	90th percentile	
		Age, 30–49 y	0.8
		Age ≥ 50 y	1.2
Oral contraceptive use	Never used	Ever used	1.0
		≥ 4 y before first pregnancy	1.7
Postmenopausal estrogen replacement	Never used	Current use all ages	1.4
		15+ y	1.3
		Past use	1.0
Alcohol use	Nondrinker	1 drink/day	1.10
		2 drinks/day	1.25
		3 drinks/day	1.50

Adapted from Ref. 8.

second breast cancer gene, called BRCA2, has been mapped to chromosome 13. From these data, a woman with a strong family history of breast or ovarian cancer, or both, who carries a germ-line mutation of BRCA1 faces roughly an 85% lifetime risk of breast cancer and a 60% risk of ovarian cancer. Carriers of the BRCA2 mutation have similar risks for breast cancer but much lower risks for ovarian cancer. An interesting and exciting development in this area concerns genetic counseling for women in high-risk families. Now that BRCA1 and BRCA2 germ-line mutations can be identified, many women in high-risk and lower-risk groups are seeking genetic testing. This has resulted in a large number of issues that are currently unresolved. Perhaps of most importance, the risk of breast and ovarian cancer in BRCA1 and BRCA2 carriers was derived from studies of high-risk families and may not apply to all carriers of these mutations. It has been reported that Jewish people of Eastern European decent (Ashkenazi Jews) have an unusually high (2%) carrier rate of germ-line mutations in BRCA1 and BRCA2 as compared to the normal US population. A recent study that examined carriers of BRCA1 and BRCA2 in Ashkenazi Jews in the Washington, DC, area found that more than 2% of the population carried these germ-line mutations, and that these mutations increase the risks of breast, ovarian, and prostate cancer in Ashkenazi Jews as compared to the SEER data from the general population.[17] But the risks of these cancers, and breast cancer in particular, fell well below previous estimates based on subjects from high-risk families; the risks were 50% for breast cancer and 16% for ovarian cancer, rather than the 85% and 60% estimates on the basis of studies in patients who were BRCA-positive and had strong family histories for these cancers. In addition, Ashkenazi Jewish families with breast cancer have a far higher probability of being carriers of the BRCA1 mutation (48%) than do non-Ashkenazi Jewish families with breast cancer (17%), which suggests that the BRCA1 mutation is a more important predictor of breast carrier development in Ashkenazi Jewish families than in non-Ashkenazi Jewish families. These observations, taken together, underscore the role of other modifying factors in determining whether a given BRCA mutation causes cancer. Furthermore, new genes are still being discovered that contribute to the risk of breast cancer through different mechanisms. Without facts about these other variables, it is difficult to predict one's likelihood of developing disease based on the presence of a specific mutation. The question of who should receive screening for BRCA is unresolved. The probability of being a carrier of the gene is related to ethnicity and family history. Important factors in family history include the number of affected and unaffected family members, age at which cancer is diagnosed, and the presence of ovarian cancer. Current estimates are that if breast and ovarian cancer occur concurrently in one or more family members, the risk of a BRCA1 mutation increases 20-fold.

To date, there are no clear recommendations for carriers of BRCA1 and BRCA2 from high-risk families. Bilateral total mastectomy does reduce the risk of breast cancer occurrence; however, both breast and ovarian cancer have been reported in patients who have had prophylactic removal of these organs.[15,16] Current recommendations for BRCA carriers who do not opt for surgical prophylaxis is mammography every 6 months. Because no effective screening for ovarian cancer exists, most experts recommend bilateral oophorectomy at completion of childbearing and estrogen replacement therapy until the age of 50 years. Estrogen replacement therapy provides approximately one-third of physiologic estrogen concentrations and, although controversial, most feel that the benefits in terms of cardiovascular disease and osteoporosis outweigh the risk of cancer.

Most importantly, isolation and cloning of BRCA1 and BRCA2 should ultimately lead to a greater understanding of the biology of malignant transformation of mammary epithelium, and to major advances in diagnostics and therapeutics benefiting all breast cancer patients. It is hoped that an improved basic understanding of the molecular mechanisms involved in breast cancer development and the discovery of novel approaches to reverse or prevent these processes will ultimately lead to the ability to cure this extremely common and often fatal disease.

ENVIRONMENTAL AND LIFESTYLE FACTORS

The observation that breast cancer incidence rates vary 10-fold between countries suggests that environmental factors play an important role in the etiology of breast cancer. Perhaps the most compelling evidence is derived from studies of Asian women who migrated from Japan to the San Francisco Bay area. Although the incidence of breast cancer in Asian women is quite low (10 to 15 per 100,000 women), the incidence of breast cancer in Asian women who were US born, or who migrated from Asia to the United States, gradually increases to equal that of the white population in the same area.[5]

Diet is an obvious environmental factor, and possible relations between fat or cholesterol intake and steroid hormone metabolism have led to an emphasis on dietary fat as a possible etiologic agent. International studies demonstrate a positive correlation between age-adjusted cancer mortality rate and national per capita fat intake.[18] The correlation is stronger in postmenopausal than in premenopausal women. Studies in laboratory animals provide further evidence of a relationship between dietary fat intake and breast cancer.[19] Despite these compelling indirect data, case control and prospective studies performed in the United States have generally failed to show an association between dietary fat and breast cancer risk. There was no relation between the relative risk of breast cancer and calorie-adjusted total fat, saturated fat, linoleic acid, or cholesterol intake. In fact, the relative risk of developing breast cancer among the women with the highest quintile of total fat intake was 0.85 as compared to women in the lowest quintile. However, the difference in fat intake among women in these two extremes was only 25%.[20] Practically, this suggests that women who reduce fat intake in the context of the usual American diet are not likely to reduce their breast cancer risk. The possible benefits of lowering fat intake to levels substantially below 30% of caloric intake will need to be tested in randomized trials.

Additional investigated dietary factors include micronutrients and food-derived heterocyclic amines. Many of the studies that have examined the relative risk for breast cancer for high fat intake have also examined the association between breast cancer and intake of fiber, β-carotene, and vitamins C, E, and A. The relationship between vitamin A and breast cancer risk is unclear. In contrast, most studies support some benefit from β-carotene, vitamin C, and/or dietary fiber.[18] It should be cautioned that these studies are limited by very small numbers of breast cancer cases, as well as the many difficulties inherent in cohort and case control studies. Experimental and epidemiologic evidence suggests an association between breast cancer and the Western diet, which typically includes a high amount of cooked meats and fat, as well as a high caloric intake. One group of compounds that may play a role in human breast cancer is heterocyclic amines found in commonly cooked beef, fish, and chicken. At least 19 heterocyclic amines with mutagenic activity have been identified in grilled, broiled, and fried meat and fish. Among these heterocyclic amines, 10 were examined for long-term carcinogenicity and all proved to be positive.[21] Experimental studies examining the interaction between heterocyclic amines and other dietary factors with respect to mammary carcinogenesis are warranted.

Both body weight and height are associated with breast cancer. Indices of obesity are related to breast cancer risks in a complex way that differs by age and menopausal status. Most studies of premenopausal women show either no relationship with body weight or slightly declining breast cancer risks with increasing body weight. One plausible biologic mechanism to explain this phenomenon is reduced ovarian activity in obese women. Most studies in postmenopausal women, however, show increasing breast cancer risks with increasing body weight. In addition to obesity, the distribution of body fat also may play an independent role in breast cancer. Upper body (central or abdominal) adiposity increases the risk of breast cancer independent of overall obesity. This association may be related to the excess levels of free-circulating estrogen resulting from the conversion of androstenedione to estradiol in peripheral adipose tissue in conjunction with suppressed levels of circulating sex hormone binding globulin in women with central adiposity.[22]

Reports of more than 50 epidemiologic investigations of the relationship between alcohol and breast cancer have appeared in the literature. A recent meta-analysis[23] of these studies indicates both a modest positive association between alcohol and breast cancer and a dose-response relationship. Data suggest that risk increases with consumption of alcohol in general, regardless of the beverage type. Several factors, including age, weight, and estrogen usage, have been shown to modify this relation in some studies. The mechanism of the alcohol-breast cancer hypothesis may include increased levels of estradiol or other reproductive steroid hormones; altered hepatic mechanism of carcinogens; production of cytotoxic protein products; diminished immunologic surveillance; impaired DNA repair; or possibly an influencing effect of alcohol on cell membrane integrity and/or metabolism of conjugers.[23] A series of methodologic issues in the study of alcohol and breast cancer are apparent from the meta-analysis, and these include inherent errors in alcohol assessment, the relatively small relative risk demonstrated, the presence of confounding variables in women who drink alcohol, and the lack of consistency of positive findings for the relationship between alcohol and the development of breast cancer. In addition, animal studies have yielded mixed results regarding the influence of alcohol on the incidence of breast cancer. Although a causal relationship between alcohol consumption and breast cancer has not been proven in a prospective trial, the weight of the epidemiologic and preclinical evidence suggests that a relationship, direct or indirect, may exist.

Radiation is associated with an increased risk of breast cancer in survivors of the atomic bomb, in patients given radiation for postpartum mastitis, in women receiving multiple fluoroscopes during therapy for tuberculosis, and in animal models. Interestingly, this risk appears to be confined to exposure to radiation prior to the age of 40, which again suggests that a "window of initiation" for breast cancer occurs at a relatively early age. Exposure to diagnostic x-rays including annual screening mammography does not impart a sufficient dose of radiation for clinical concern. A critical reassessment of benefits versus risks from screening mammography found recently that for a woman beginning annual screening mammography at age 50 years and continuing to age 75 years, the benefit exceeds the radiation risk by a factor of 100. Even for a woman who begins annual screening at age 35 years and continues until age 75 years, the benefit of reduced mortality is projected to exceed the radiation risk by a factor of more than 25.[24]

Cigarette smoking and augmentation mammoplasty do not appear to increase the risk of breast cancer. Blood pressure medications, reserpine, and other drugs that increase prolactin levels have not been shown to increase the risk of breast cancer. Caffeine also has no predisposing effect on breast cancer, but may play a role in exacerbation of benign breast disease. The role of environmental carcinogens has not been systematically evaluated.

CLINICAL PRESENTATION

A painless lump is the initial sign in more than 90% of women with breast cancer. The typical malignant mass is solitary, unilateral, solid, hard, irregular, and nonmobile. In approximately 10% of cases, stabbing or aching pain is the first symptom. Less commonly, nipple discharge, retraction, or dimpling may herald the onset of the disease. In more advanced cases, prominent skin edema, redness, warmth, and induration of the underlying tissue may be observed.

The breast is a complex organ composed of skin, subcutaneous tissue, fatty tissue, and branching ductal and glandular structures. Various diseases that affect these structures can produce a palpable mass. In addition, the physiologic changes associated with the menstrual cycle can cause abnormalities of the breast that produce a three-dimensional mass. The foremost common causes of breast masses in young women are fibroadenoma, fibrocystic disease, carcinoma, and fat necrosis.

Approximately 80% of women first detect some breast abnormalities themselves, underscoring the importance of breast self-examination. In the United States, it is increasingly common for breast cancer to be detected during routine screening mammography in asymptomatic women. It is widely accepted that the smaller the mass, the higher the likelihood of cure, and the more conservative the treatment options offered to the patient. Thus, as the number of breast cancer cases found by screening mammography increases, overall survival of breast cancer patients is expected to improve significantly.

Breast cancer that is confined to a localized breast lesion is often referred to as *early, primary, localized,* or *curable*. Unfortunately, as is discussed shortly, breast cancer cells often spread by contiguity, lymph channels, and through the blood to distant sites. As discussed in subsequent sections, this often occurs early in the breast cancer growth, and deposits of tumor cells form in distant sites (micrometastases) that cannot be detected with current diagnostic methods and equipment. When breast cancer cells can be detected clinically or radiologically in sites distant from the breast, the disease is referred to as *advanced* or *metastatic* breast cancer. Tissues most commonly involved with metastases are lymph nodes (other than axillary or internal mammary), skin, bone, liver, lungs, and brain. Symptoms of bone pain, difficulty breathing, abdominal enlargement, jaundice, and mental status changes may herald the clinical presentation of metastatic breast cancer. Approximately 10% of women have signs and symptoms of distant metastases when they first seek treatment. In virtually all of them, a breast mass has been present for several months to years. In addition, approximately one-half of all patients who initially are treated for localized disease develop signs and symptoms of metastatic breast cancer, most commonly 3 to 5 years following local potentially curative therapy with surgery, radiation, and systemic adjuvant therapy.

DIAGNOSIS

Initial workup for a woman presenting with a lesion or symptoms suggestive of breast cancer should include a careful history, physical examination of the breast, three-dimensional mammography, and possibly other breast imaging techniques such as ultrasound. Most (80% to 85%) breast cancers can be visualized on a mammogram as a mass, a cluster of calcifications, or a combination of both. The detection of a mass smaller than 2 mm is considered ideal, but it is difficult in practice to detect tumors smaller than 5 mm. Large, noncalcified masses may be difficult to detect in the dense glandular breast, which is common in premenopausal women. The threshold for the detection of a cancer is variable and depends on the radiographic abnormality, the fat-to-glandular tissue ratio of the breast, the technical quality of the examination, and the diligence and expertise of the radiologist.

Interpretations of mammography obtained either for screening or to evaluate a new breast mass generally fall into one of three categories: (a) the radiologist notes nothing suspicious for malignancy; (b) something of concern is seen and followup or further testing is advised; or (c) something clearly suspicious is present and a biopsy is indicated. A detailed discussion of abnormal mammogram radiographic findings and their significance is beyond the scope of this chapter, although excellent references are available.[25,26] It should be noted, however, that well-circumscribed x-ray masses are benign in 98% of cases; such lesions may not require a biopsy, but may be followed radiographically at 6-month intervals. Masses interpreted as "suspicious and a biopsy should be performed" have a 20% to 30% probability of malignancy. Masses interpreted as "highly suspicious radiographically" are malignant in 75% to 90% of cases. The overall probability of malignancy when a biopsy is performed on a nonpalpable mammographic abnormality ranges from 20% to 35%.[27]

Breast biopsy is indicated for a mammographic abnormality that suggests malignancy or for a palpable mass on physical examination. The type of biopsy depends on the mass size and characteristics. Excisional biopsy is the standard biopsy technique for clinically benign lesions or for malignant lesions less than 2 cm in diameter. This term indicates the complete removal of the abnormal tissue. Excisional biopsy may be performed with either a local or general anesthesia, and is usually done as an outpatient operative procedure.

Mammographically, and less commonly ultrasonographically, guided-needle biopsy is a promising technique for the diagnosis of breast lesions. This procedure is associated with minimal discomfort and anxiety, few complications, and no disfigurement and could represent significant cost-savings when compared to conventional surgical excisional biopsy. Needle biopsies have included both core-needle biopsy (which removes a core of tissue) and fine-needle aspiration (which removes cells from the suspicious site). These procedures require experienced mammographers and cytopathologists. Numerous studies show that the accuracy of core-needle biopsy is at least equal to that of traditional localization and open-surgical excisional breast biopsy. The accuracy of fine-needle aspiration is quite good in experienced hands, but its limitations include false negatives (range 1% to 10%) and specimens with insufficient material for diagnosis (1% to 10%). Results of a fine-needle aspiration can be used as the basis for mastectomy when the physical examination and mammographic abnormality coincide with the cytologic diagnosis. It should be pointed out that excisional biopsy, as well as needle localization biopsy, with fine-needle or core, is used only to establish the diagnosis. Following confirmation of malignancy, subsequent surgical procedures are performed to assure complete removal of the abnormal tissue.[5]

STAGING AND PROGNOSIS

Few malignant diseases illustrate the importance of stage (anatomic extent of disease) at the time of diagnosis and overall survival more clearly than breast cancer. Stage is defined on the basis of the primary tumor size (T_{1-4}), presence and extent of lymph node involvement (N_{1-3}), and presence or absence of distant metastases (M) (Fig. 125–2

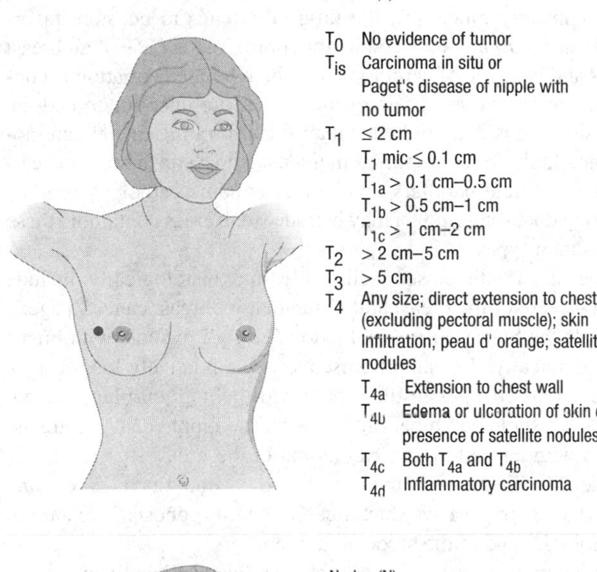

Tumor (T)

- T_0 No evidence of tumor
- T_{is} Carcinoma in situ or Paget's disease of nipple with no tumor
- T_1 ≤ 2 cm
  - T_1 mic ≤ 0.1 cm
  - $T_{1a} > 0.1$ cm–0.5 cm
  - $T_{1b} > 0.5$ cm–1 cm
  - $T_{1c} > 1$ cm–2 cm
- T_2 > 2 cm–5 cm
- T_3 > 5 cm
- T_4 Any size; direct extension to chest wall (excluding pectoral muscle); skin infiltration; peau d' orange; satellite nodules
  - T_{4a} Extension to chest wall
  - T_{4b} Edema or ulceration of skin or presence of satellite nodules
  - T_{4c} Both T_{4a} and T_{4b}
  - T_{4d} Inflammatory carcinoma

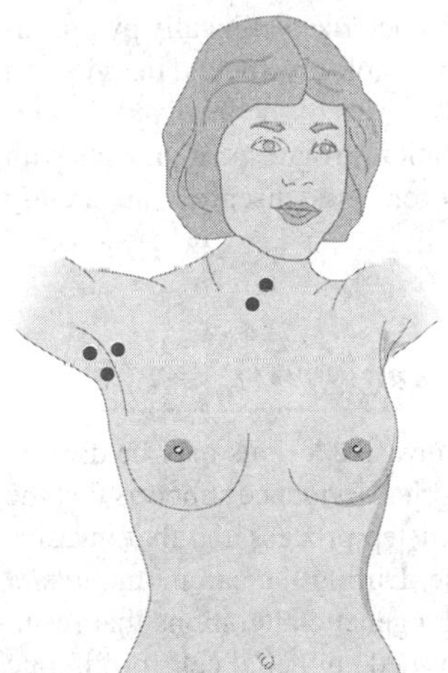

Nodes (N)

- N_0 No regional lymph node metastasis
- N_1 Metastasis to movable ipsilateral axillary lymph node or nodes
- N_2 Metastasis to ipsilateral axillary node that are fixed to one another or other structures
- N_3 Metastasis to ipsilateral internal lymph node(s)

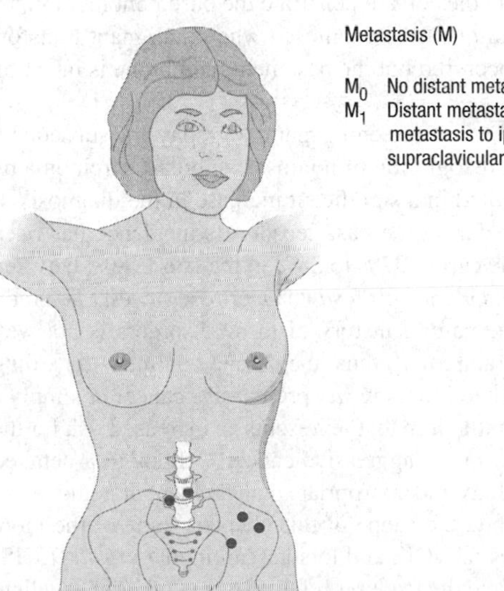

Metastasis (M)

- M_0 No distant metastases
- M_1 Distant metastasis, including metastasis to ipsilateral supraclavicular lymph node(s)

FIGURE 125–2. TNM four-stage system. *(Adapted from Davidson NE. Breast cancer. In: Dale DC, Federman DD, eds. Scientific American Medicine. New York, Scientific American, 2001:1.)*

TABLE 125–3. Stages of Primary Breast Cancer*

	T	N	M
Stage 0	T_{is}	N_0	M_0
Stage I	T_1	N_0	M_0
Stage IIA	T_0	N_1	M_0
	T_1	N_1	
	T_2	N_0	
Stage IIB	T_2	N_1	M_0
	T_3	N_0	
Stage IIIA	T_0	N_2	M_0
	T_1	N_2	
	T_2	N_2	
	T_3	N_1, N_2	
Stage IIIB	T_4	Any N	M_0
	Any T	N_3	
Stage IV	Any T	Any N	M_1

*See Figure 125–3.

Adapted from Davidson NE. Breast cancer. In: Dale DC, Federman DD, eds. Scientific American Medicine. New York, Scientific American, 2001:1–13.

and Table 125–3). Although many possible combinations of T and N are possible within a given stage, simplistically, stage 0 represents carcinoma *in situ* or disease that has not invaded the basement membrane. Stage I represents small primary tumor without lymph node involvement, and the majority of stage II disease involves regional lymph nodes. Stages 0, I, and II are often referred to as *early breast cancer*. It is in these early stages that the disease is curable. Stage III, also referred to as *locally advanced disease,* usually represents a large tumor with extensive nodal involvement in which either node or tumor is fixed to the chest wall. Stage IV disease is characterized by the presence of metastases to organs distant from the primary tumor. Stages III and IV are often referred to as *advanced disease*. Although a small number of patients with stage III disease may be cured, most patients with locally advanced breast cancers are incurable with currently available standard treatment approaches.

Table 125–4 shows the approximate percentage of patients presenting with each stage of breast cancer and an estimate of their 5-year disease-free survival (DFS). Five-year DFS is not synonymous with cure and 10-year DFS rates are on average 20% lower for each stage. It is important to recognize that many subsets exist within each stage. Both detection and treatment approaches for breast cancer are evolving at a rapid rate, and therefore these estimates may vary among reference sources. Current estimates suggest that most women present with early breast cancer and that most of these women can be cured with today's treatment approaches. As discussed in subsequent sections, adjuvant (postsurgery) systemic therapy has improved absolute survival rates by up to 10% in selected populations of patients with

TABLE 125–4. Estimated Stage at Presentation and 5-year Disease-Free Survival (DFS): Breast Cancer

	Percent of Total Cases	5-Year DFS[a] (%)
Stage I	40	70–90
Stage II	40	50–70
Stage III	15	20–30
Stage IV	5	0–10[b]

[a]With current conventional local and systemic therapy.

[b]Patients in stage IV are rarely free of disease; however, 10% to 20% of these patients may survive with minimal disease for 5 to 10 years.

early breast cancer (stages I and II). Combined modality approaches with neoadjuvant chemotherapy (before surgery), surgery and/or radiation, followed by adjuvant chemotherapy have resulted in benefits of a similar magnitude in patients with locally advanced breast cancer (stage III). Unfortunately, many women with early breast cancer and locally advanced breast cancer eventually experience recurrence, usually manifested in lungs, bone, liver, skin, or brain following treatment of the primary disease.[5]

PATHOLOGY

The pathologic evaluation of breast lesions serves to establish the histologic diagnosis and to confirm the presence or absence of other factors believed to influence prognosis. These nonhistologic prognostic factors include the presence of necrosis, lymphatic or vascular invasion, nuclear grade, hormone receptor status, proliferative index, amount of aneuploidy, presence or absence of oncogenes, presence or absence of mutations in the tumor suppressor *p53* gene, and, perhaps, presence or absence of elevated growth factor levels, as well as enzymes (cathepsin D), proteins, and angiogenesis factors.

INVASIVE CARCINOMA

Invasive breast cancers are a histologically heterogeneous group of lesions. Most breast carcinomas are adenocarcinomas and are classified on the basis of their microscopic appearance as either ductal or lobular corresponding to the ducts and lobules of the normal breast. The various histologic types of breast cancer have different prognoses, but it is unknown whether their response to therapy differs, because patients in therapeutic trials are not typically stratified according to histologic type. The five most common types of invasive breast cancer are briefly described.

Invasive or *infiltrating ductal carcinoma* is the most common histology. The other histologic patterns can occur alone or with infiltrating ductal carcinoma. These tumors are generally referred to as infiltrating ductal carcinoma "not otherwise specified" and account for approximately 75% of all invasive breast cancers. These tumors commonly spread to the axillary lymph nodes and their prognosis is poorer than for other histologic types (specifically tubular, medullary, mucinous/colloid). *Infiltrating lobular carcinoma* accounts for 5% to 10% of breast tumors. Typical presentation is an area of ill-defined thickening in the breast, in contrast to a prominent lump characteristic of infiltrating ductal carcinoma. A greater proportion of infiltrating lobular carcinomas are multicentric tumors, either in the same or opposite breast, as compared with infiltrating ductal carcinoma. Overall, infiltrating lobular carcinoma and infiltrating ductal carcinoma have similar likelihoods of axillary node involvement and prognosis, yet the sites of metastases tend to differ. Ductal carcinoma more frequently metastasizes to the bone or to the liver, lung, or brain, whereas lobular carcinoma more commonly metastasizes to meningeal and serosal surfaces and other unusual sites.

The three most common special types of invasive cancer are *tubular, medullary,* and *mucinous. Medullary carcinoma* is a well-defined lesion with a characteristic microscopic appearance that includes a well-circumscribed border, intense infiltration with small lymphocytes, and other factors. It accounts for 5% to 7% of all breast carcinomas and is believed to have a better prognosis than infiltrating ductal carcinoma. *Mucinous (or colloid) carcinoma* constitutes approximately 3% of all breast carcinomas and is characterized by the abundant accumulation of extracellular mucin around clusters of tumor cells. It is slow growing and can be bulky. When the tumor is predominantly mucinous, the prognosis tends to be more favorable. *Tubular carcinoma* accounts for approximately 2% of all breast cancers and is a type of carcinoma in which tubule formation is conspicuous on pathology. Axillary metastases are uncommon and the prognosis is considerably better than for infiltrating ductal carcinomas. Histologies rarely reported include adenocystic carcinoma, carcinosarcomas, and papillary carcinoma. In some pathology reports, infiltrating ductal carcinoma may include small areas containing these special tumor types.

Special situations seen clinically and histologically include Paget's disease of the breast and inflammatory breast cancer. Paget's disease of the breast occurs in 1% to 4% of all patients with breast cancer. Clinically, the patient presents with a relatively long history of eczematous changes in the nipple with itching, burning, oozing, bleeding, or some combination of these. The nipple changes are associated with an underlying carcinoma in the breast that is usually palpable. The histology of the tumor type is either ductal carcinoma *in situ* (DCIS) or invasive ductal carcinoma. Prognosis is related to the histologic type of the associated tumor.

Inflammatory breast cancer is characterized clinically by prominent skin, edema, redness and warmth, visible erysipeloid margin, and induration of the underlying tissue. Biopsies of the involved skin reveal cancer cells in the dermal lymphatics. Prognosis of patients with inflammatory breast cancer is poor, even if the disease is apparently localized.[5]

NONINVASIVE CARCINOMA

As with invasive carcinoma, the noninvasive lesions may be divided broadly into ductal and lobular categories. Evidence supports that the development of malignancy is a multistep process and that invasive breast cancer has a preinvasive phase. During the carcinoma *in situ* phase, normal epithelial cells undergo genetic alterations that result in malignant transformation. Transformed epithelial cells proliferate and pile up within lobulars or ducts, but lack the required genetic alterations that enable the cells to penetrate the basement membrane. Therefore, carcinoma *in situ* is diagnosed when malignant transformation of cells has occurred but the basement membrane is intact by light microscopy.

The widespread use of screening mammography and subsequent biopsy coupled with recognition of noninvasive breast carcinoma by pathologists has resulted in a significant increase in the diagnosis of *in situ* breast cancer during the past decade. Its incidence has risen from 1% to 5% in the early 1970s to 28% in the late 1980s; between 1988 and 1996, the incidence of *in situ* cancer rose steadily at a ratio of 6% per year.[6] The natural history of these disorders is not well described in the literature and, thus, the debate continues regarding carcinoma *in situ*: Is carcinoma *in situ* preinvasive cancer or simply a marker of unstable epithelium that represents an increased risk for the development of subsequent aggressive cancer? Although a detailed discussion of the biology and appropriate management of noninvasive breast cancer is beyond the scope of this chapter, some of the more salient characteristics of DCIS and lobular carcinoma *in situ* (LCIS) are described below and the reader is referred to a number of excellent reviews for a more comprehensive discussion.[5,28,29]

DCIS is seen more frequently than LCIS at a rate of about 6 to 3:1. Most DCIS cases diagnosed currently are small nonpalpable lesions, unlike its presentation as a palpable mass in more than half of cases in years prior to mammography. Most cases of DCIS today are found by biopsies performed for clustered calcifications seen on screening mammography. There are four distinct histologic patterns of DCIS, which probably represent successive steps in its evolution toward invasive carcinoma. The biologic characteristics are consistent with its role as a direct precursor to invasive carcinoma, which appears to develop in the most cases if left untreated within 10 years of diagnosis. The peak incidence of DCIS is 51 to 59 years, which closely parallels that of invasive carcinoma. Treatment of DCIS is dependent on its presentation, size, and pathology. The patient and physician have the following options: (a) excision with negative margins, preferably 1–2 cm; (b) excision followed by breast irradiation; and (c) traditional total mastectomy with reconstruction. It is important to note, however, that in all cases, carcinoma *in situ* is treated as cancer. Mastectomy had been the standard treatment of DCIS for several decades. The combined data from 1,061 women who underwent mastectomy for DCIS, reported in 14 published studies, with followup ranging from 2 years to more than 15 years, show an overall local recurrence rate of only 0.75% and overall cancer mortality rate of less than 1%. Breast conservation, that is, wide local excision followed by irradiation of breast tissue, may be an effective alternative to mastectomy. The recently completed NASBP B17 trial randomized 808 women with DCIS to receive lumpectomy alone or lumpectomy with radiation.[30] The results of this trial demonstrated an advantage for radiation plus lumpectomy in terms of fewer local recurrences. Although radiation following lumpectomy does not appear to change the survival of patients with DCIS, it significantly reduces the incidence of local recurrences and enhances the breast preservation rate in these women. If more than one area of the breast is involved with DCIS, a mastectomy is the preferred option. It has also been suggested that breast conservation may not be appropriate for younger women whose lifetime risk of breast cancer is high given a diagnosis of DCIS. Axillary dissection is generally not indicated. There is currently no proven benefit for the use of cytotoxic chemotherapy or hormonal manipulation in this disease. Followup of women who have been treated for DCIS should be as comprehensive as that of a woman with invasive carcinoma to facilitate early detection of any subsequent malignancy.

LCIS is a microscopic diagnosis, not a gross abnormality. Therefore, it is always nonpalpable and it is virtually impossible to make the diagnosis of LCIS by clinical examination. Unlike DCIS, LCIS does not demonstrate calcifications on mammography and, in fact, is not associated with mammographic abnormalities. LCIS is most frequently diagnosed in biopsy specimens that were obtained because of symptoms or mammography findings consistent with benign lesions. Multicentricity is common (>30%) with LCIS and the opposite breast is affected in up to 50% of patients. It is unclear whether LCIS proceeds to invasive carcinoma or serves as a marker for a high probability of invasive carcinoma developing elsewhere in the breast. Thus, the management of LCIS is very controversial. Some experts favor a program of breast examination, periodic physician examination, and mammography as management of LCIS. In selected patients who are particularly anxious about the development of cancer, bilateral total mastectomies and prompt reconstruction represent a reasonable approach. Radiation, systemic chemotherapy, or hormonal therapy has no role in the management of LCIS.

PROGNOSTIC FACTORS

The natural history of breast cancer varies between patients, with some having an extremely aggressive disease that progress rapidly, whereas others follow a more indolent course. The ability to predict which patients have a better disease prognosis is extremely important in designing treatment recommendations to maximize quantity and quality of life. A number of potential pathologic prognostic and predictive factors have been identified and intense research in this area is ongoing. Prognostic factors are measurements available at diagnosis or time of surgery that, in the absence of adjuvant therapy, are associated with recurrence rate, death rate, or other clinical outcome. Predictive factors are measurements available at diagnosis that are associated with the response to a specific therapy. Prognostic and predictive factors fall into three categories: patient characteristics that are independent of the disease such as age; disease characteristics such as tumor size or histologic type; and biomarkers that are measurable parameters in tissues, cells, or fluids, such as hormone receptor status.

The median age for the diagnosis of breast cancer is between the ages of 60 and 65 years. Younger women, particularly women younger than 35 years of age, have a more aggressive form of the disease, and elderly women, particularly those older than 70 years of age with breast cancer, frequently have hormone receptor protein in their malignant tissue, suggesting a more indolent tumor pattern and a higher likelihood of response to hormonal therapy. Race appears to be prognostic but not predictive. Black breast cancer patients are generally younger and often have larger tumors at diagnosis, and a smaller percentage have hormone receptors in their tumor tissue. These factors contribute to a poorer prognosis. It should be emphasized that for both age and race, in cases of similar clinical presentation, adjuvant treatment confers similar benefits to black and white women.

Tumor size and the presence and number of involved axillary lymph nodes are established primary factors in assessing the risk for breast cancer recurrence and subsequent metastatic disease. Table 125–5 shows the 5-year relapse rate according to size of primary tumor and axillary node involvement from results of three investigations.[31–33] These data clearly demonstrate that the major factor that influences the likelihood of recurrence is the presence of positive axillary nodes. But regardless of axillary node studies, the size of the primary tumor remains an independent prognostic factor for disease recurrence. In axillary node-negative patients, a tumor size of less than 2 cm is associated with a very favorable prognosis. However, there does not appear to be a large difference between prognosis in patients with large (greater than 5 cm) tumors and negative nodes, as compared to patients with 2- to 5-cm tumors and negative nodes. Thus, the size of the primary tumor in patients with negative axillary lymph nodes may not provide as much information regarding prognosis as in node-positive patients. The number of affected nodes is directly related to disease recurrence. Estimates are that 35% of patients with one to three positive nodes will relapse within 5 years, as compared to 75% of patients with greater than or equal to four positive nodes.[34,35]

TABLE 125–5. Five-Year Relapse Rate (%) Based on Size of Primary Tumor and Axillary Nodal Status

	Size of Primary Tumor (cm)		
Axillary Status	*<2*	*2–5*	*>5*
Axillary nodes negative			
Fisher et al.[31]	12	24	27
Nemoto et al.[32]	13	19	25
Valagussa et al.[33]	8	24	19
Axillary nodes positive			
Fisher et al.[31]	50	60	79
Nemoto et al.[32]	39	50	65
Valagussa et al.[33]	37	64	74

Aside from the stage (TNM) of the disease, hormone receptor studies have received the most attention in the characterization of primary breast cancer. Hormone receptors are used clinically as indicators of prognosis and to predict response to hormone therapy. Hormone receptors are cytoplasmic proteins that transmit signals to the nucleus of the cell for growth and proliferation. The hormone receptors clinically useful in discussions of breast cancer include the estrogen receptor (ER) and the progesterone receptor (PR). The presence of these proteins in the primary tumor (or less often metastases) is routinely measured by enzyme-linked immunochemical assays and radioassays (enzyme-linked immunosorbent assay [ELISA]). Concentrations of hormone receptors less than 3 femptomole (fmol) per milligram of cytosol protein are considered negative, 3–10 fmol/mg of cytosol protein are "intermediate," and concentrations of hormone receptors greater than 10 fmol/mg of cytosol protein are positive. The level (i.e., quantitative) of hormone receptor and the methodology used to assess hormone receptors are important for predictive ability. Although the estrogen receptor has received the most attention to date, more recent data suggest that the presence of the progesterone receptor protein is required for the functional effects of the estrogen receptor protein to occur. This is evidenced by studies that have reported that response to hormonal manipulation and prognosis are highly correlated with the presence of both positive estrogen receptor protein and positive progesterone receptor protein. Hormone receptors are most valuable in predicting response to hormone therapy. Approximately 70% to 80% of patients who are ER-positive and PR-positive will respond to hormonal manipulation. ER-negative patients rarely respond to hormonal manipulation. The response rate in patients who are ER-negative and PR-positive is somewhere between.

Approximately 50% to 70% of patients with primary or metastatic breast cancer have hormone receptor-positive tumors. The median level and frequency of hormone receptor-positive tumors are higher in postmenopausal patients as compared to premenopausal patients. This difference is likely responsible for the different recommendations for adjuvant and metastatic treatment of breast cancer between premenopausal and postmenopausal patients discussed in later sections of this chapter. Many experts suggest that breast cancer in postmenopausal women is substantively different than that occurring in premenopausal women. Breast cancer is predominantly a disease of the elderly. When it occurs in younger patients, the course of the disease is more aggressive. This is observed with many of the other common tumor types. Hormone receptor positivity, more common in postmenopausal women, is associated with a superior response to hormone therapy and a longer disease-free interval between primary and subsequent metastatic disease, and overall a more favorable prognosis. The presence of hormone receptors in tumors is associated with a favorable disease-free interval and perhaps an overall survival difference of 5% to 10% (as compared to hormone receptor-negative patients). But the value of hormone receptors as a prognostic factor is being eroded by increasing knowledge of newer prognostic factors such as epidermal growth factor receptor, proliferative capacity, nuclear grade, and expression of the HER-2/neu oncogene.[36–42]

The rate of tumor cell proliferation also has prognostic significance in breast cancer recurrence. Rate of cell proliferation can be determined with either the tritiated thymidine-labeling index (TLI) or DNA flow cytometry, which determines the percentage of tumor cells actively dividing (S-phase fraction). Both techniques have shown that patients with rapidly proliferating tumors have a decreased DFS as compared to patients with slowly proliferating tumors.[38] S-phase fraction has been disappointing as a predictor of response to cytotoxic chemotherapy. Flow cytometry can also detect abnormal DNA content, or aneuploidy, in breast cancer cells. Although there are conflicting reports regarding the clinical significance of ploidy status, some studies report that patients with aneuploid tumors have significantly shorter relapse-free survival times than do patients with diploid tumors.[38]

Nuclear grade and tumor (histologic) differentiation are known, independent prognostic indicators. Several histologic grading systems have been developed and shown to have prognostic value in the evaluation of breast cancer. Fisher et al.[39] have shown a 5-year survival of 93% for patients with good nuclear grade as compared to 79% for patients with poor nuclear grade. However, interobserver lack of concordance between pathologist grading has thwarted the use of this prognostic indicator in clinical trials.

A number of additional potential prognostic factors have been identified in the past five years. These include overexpression of the erbB-2 (or HER-2/neu) oncogene, cathepsin D, angiogenic growth factors, mutations in the tumor suppresser *p53* gene, and others.[36–40] Many of the new potential prognostic factors have been shown to be strongly correlated with established risk factors. For example, ER-positive tumors are commonly HER-2-negative and cathepsin D-negative as well, making it difficult to discern from clinical trials the relative importance of potential prognostic factors. Thus, it is unclear which of these is truly an independent prognostic factor. Identification of these numerous factors and correlations between these and known prognostic factors that affect clinical outcome is of interest because each correlation allows basic mechanistic insights into disease processes. Practically, they allow prediction of probable clinical outcomes that can guide therapeutic decision making. Several of these new prognostic factors, specifically the HER-2 oncogene overexpression and *p53* mutations, have shown early promise as predictors of efficacy of adjuvant chemotherapy.

The HER-2/neu gene is located on 17q21 and is transcribed into a 4.5-kda mRNA, which is translated into a 185-kda glycoprotein. The HER-2/neu protein is expressed at low levels in the epithelial cells of normal breast tissue. HER-2/neu is a member of the growth factor receptor family and its overexpression is associated with transmission of growth signals that control aspects of normal cell growth and division. Preclinical and clinical studies indicate that HER-2 overexpression may have prognostic and predictive value. Ross and Fletcher reviewed 52 published studies of the prognostic value of HER-2 overexpression in breast cancer.[41] Most of the studies retrospectively assessed HER-2 overexpression by using tissue blocks from patients who participated in clinical trials. In 46 (88%) of the studies, HER-2 gene amplification or protein overexpression independently predicted decreased disease-free survival time and lower overall survival rates. These findings were demonstrated by univariate but not multivariate analysis in 13 of the studies (25%) and by multivariate analysis in 33 (63%). Six studies (12%) showed no correlation between HER-2 status and outcome. Failure to corroborate findings with multivariate analysis may result from the influence of other variables that have negative prognostic value. Thor et al. reported the results of a Cancer and Leukemia Group B trial confirming HER-2 as an independent prognostic factor.[42] Significantly shorter disease-free survival (risk ratio = 1.58, 95% confidence interval [CI] = 1.25–2.00, $p < 0.001$) and significantly shorter overall survival (risk ratio = 1.84, 95% CI = 1.43–2.38, $p < 0.001$) were shown by univariate analysis in patients with HER-2 gene amplification. Similar results were reported with multivariate analysis of survival time and HER-2 gene or protein overexpression. In the same study, HER-2 status was shown to predict for prolonged survival as a result of anthracycline-based therapy. The data were obtained from an extension of an earlier trial that had found greater disease-free and overall survival times in HER-2 positive patients receiving dose-intensive CAF (cyclophosphamide

600 mg/m^2, doxorubicin hydrochloride 60 mg/m^2, and fluorouracil 600 mg/m^2). The results of this study varied with the statistical methods employed; the authors concluded that the presence of multiple negative prognostic indicators may have confounded the results. The best evidence supporting HER-2 status as a predictor of survival time in patients receiving anthracycline-based therapy was provided by the National Surgical Adjuvant Breast and Bowel Project (NSABP).[43] The project's B-11 trial examined the value of adding doxorubicin to melphalan and fluorouracil as adjuvant therapy for node-positive, hormone-receptor-negative breast cancer. Disease-free and overall survival times were significantly extended with the addition of doxorubicin. Further analysis showed that the benefit of doxorubicin-based therapy was limited to patients in whom HER-2 was overexpressed. Of note, studies performed in node-negative women did not support the prognostic value of HER-2 overexpression.

Although there is a growing understanding of the prognostic significance of individual factors, it is not clear how to practically use multiple prognostic factors in concert. The development of decision-making systems for clinical applications will require improvements in the areas of (a) standardization of methodologies and interlaboratory quality control for prognostic factor determinations, (b) definition of a limited set of prognostic markers that are independently predictive, and (c) staging systems that integrate this information. The NIH convened an expert panel to develop a consensus statement on adjuvant therapy for breast cancer.[44] One question addressed by the Consensus Development Panel was which factors should be used to select systemic adjuvant therapy. The panel identified age, tumor size, axillary node status, histologic tumor type, standardized pathologic grade, and hormone receptor status as the only currently accepted prognostic and predictive factors.

▶ TREATMENT: Breast Cancer

EARLY BREAST CANCER

LOCAL-REGIONAL THERAPY

Most patients presenting with breast cancer today have either an *in situ* tumor—a small tumor with negative lymph nodes (stage I)—or a small stage II cancer. Surgery alone can cure most, if not all, patients with *in situ* cancers and approximately half of all patients with stage II cancers. The choice of surgical procedures has changed drastically over the past 50 years. This is in part a result of our changing understanding of the biology of breast cancer and in part a result of a series of well-conducted trials performed over this time period.

The Halstedian theory and concept of tumor growth, formulated at the end of the 19th century, held that breast cancer was a local-regional disease that spread to involve larger contiguous areas of the breast, chest wall, and adjacent lymph nodes. This hypothesis gave rise to emphasis throughout most of the 20th century on the Halsted radical mastectomy, the hallmark of an approach holding that cure of early diseases could best be achieved with expansive, meticulously performed surgical procedures. The *radical mastectomy* involves removal of the breast and both major and minor pectoralis muscles. The axillary nodes on the same side (ipsilateral) as the breast lesion are also removed. Substantial morbidity is associated with this procedure. Muscle resection decreases strength and range of motion, and removal of axillary lymph nodes can produce edema of the arm and resected breast area. This procedure was often followed by external beam radiation therapy to the involved area.

During the 1960s, it was recognized that breast cancer is often microscopically disseminated at the time of initial diagnosis. The evolutionary concept that breast cancer is not only a local, but also a systemic disease has resulted in major changes in local and systemic therapy. In 1980, the Commission on Cancer of the American College of Surgeons reported that there had been an apparent gradual shift from a radical to modified radical mastectomy since December of 1972.[45] The modified radical mastectomy, also termed *total mastectomy with axillary lymph node dissection*, is not as precisely defined or standardized as the radical mastectomy. The pectoralis minor muscle may be excised, divided, or left intact, and, more importantly, there may be variation in the extent of axillary lymph node dissection ranging from sampling to full dissection. It was recognized during this time period that a major factor in prognosis was involvement of axillary lymph nodes rather than the type of initial surgical procedure performed.

Results of a large trial conducted in the United States by the NSABP repudiated the Halsted theory and supported the alternative systemic hypothesis. NSABP B-04, published in 1977, randomized nearly 2,000 women among three treatment regimens: radical mastectomy, simple mastectomy with local-regional irradiation, and simple mastectomy and removal of nodes if they later became clinically positive.[46] Forty percent of patients who underwent the radical mastectomy had pathologically positive lymph nodes; thus, it can be assumed that 40% of patients in the other two groups had positive axillary nodes that were not removed. Despite the disparity in local-regional treatment, no significant difference in treatment failure, distant metastases, or overall survival was observed through more than 14 years of followup.

With negation of the primacy radical mastectomy, the NSABP instituted a second trial (B-06) in which patients with stage I or stage II breast cancer with a tumor size 4 cm or less, were treated with either modified radical mastectomy or lumpectomy with or without radiation therapy.[47] Lumpectomy followed by radiation resulted in a 5-year survival of 85% as compared to 76% for modified radical mastectomy with consistent findings at the 8-year results of the study. This study also found that radiation therapy reduced the probability of local tumor recurrence by approximately 30% in patients treated with lumpectomy. The local failure rate of modified radical mastectomy was 8.1% as compared to 7.2% for lumpectomy alone and 1.1% for lumpectomy and radiation therapy. Neither the rate nor development of distant metastases nor contralateral breast cancer was different in the treatment groups.

The National Institutes of Health (NIH) Consensus Conference on the Treatment of Early Stage Breast Cancer addressed the roles of modified radical mastectomy versus breast conservation and concluded that primary therapy for breast cancer stages I and II should be *breast conservation*.[44] Breast conservation consists of lumpectomy, also referred to as segmental mastectomy or partial mastectomy, and is defined as excision of the primary tumor and adjacent breast tissue, followed by radiation therapy to reduce the risk of local recurrence. Removal of level I–II axillary lymph nodes is recommended for completeness of staging and prognostic information. The reason given for favoring breast conservation therapy is that it achieved similar results to more extensive surgical procedures with cosmetically superior results.

Most patients with breast cancer can be treated by lumpectomy and radiation therapy. Several factors should be considered in selecting patients for breast conservation therapy. Multiple sites of cancer within the breast and the inability to attain negative pathologic margins on the excised breast specimen are predictive for an increased risk of recurrence with breast-conserving therapy and indications for mastectomy. Preexisting collagen vascular disease is a contraindication for the use of breast-conserving radiation and surgery. Although local recurrence following breast-conservation therapy is not associated with increased mortality, it is distressing to the patient and requires surgical removal of the breast. In addition, reconstructive therapy is often not feasible in a breast that has previously received irradiation. Another major consideration in selecting patients for breast-conserving therapy is the expected cosmetic result. Although the size of the tumor is not an important consideration for breast cancer recurrence, the relationship of the size of the tumor to the total breast volume is an important cosmetic consideration. If the volume of the tissue removed is large in a woman with small breasts, better results can often be obtained with mastectomy and reconstruction. Despite the desire of the patient and the willingness of the surgeon to avoid mastectomy, in some circumstances, a lumpectomy will approximate so closely a mastectomy that both the patient and the physician will agree that preservation of a very limited amount of breast tissue would not justify the inconvenience of radiation therapy. Aside from the probability of local recurrence and the ability to achieve a satisfactory cosmetic result, consideration must be given to the availability of an external beam radiation facility and the patient's willingness to comply with the prescribed course of radiotherapy. In most instances, external beam radiation therapy used in conjunction with breast-conserving procedures involves 4 to 6 weeks of radiation therapy directed to the breast tissue (a total of 5,000 cGy administered in 200-cGy doses daily to eradicate residual disease). Complications associated with radiation therapy to the breast are minor and include reddening and erythema of the breast tissue and subsequent shrinkage of total breast mass beyond that predicted on the basis of breast tissue removal.

Simple or total mastectomy involves removal of the entire breast without dissection of the underlying muscle or axillary nodes. The major disadvantage of this procedure is that axillary nodal status is not determined and, thus, important prognostic information may be lost. This procedure is used in patients with carcinoma *in situ,* in whom there is a 1% incidence of axillary node involvement, or in cases of local recurrence following breast-conservation therapy. But the importance of determining axillary lymph node involvement is being challenged by the identification of new prognostic pathologic factors that bear concordance with axillary nodal status and with the new and evolving recommendations for systemic adjuvant therapy for all patients regardless of nodal status. However, at present axillary lymph node dissection with histopathologic study of the axillary specimen is the gold standard for detecting axillary nodal involvement and determining the number of nodes-contained tumor. Although highly accurate, its morbidity is significant with an acute complication rate as high as 20% to 30% and rates of chronic lymphedema also in the order of 20% to 30%.[48,49] A new procedure involving intraoperative lymphatic mapping and sentinel lymph node biopsy is undergoing evaluation at many centers across the United States.[50] Intraoperative lymphatic mapping using a vital blue dye can identify the first axillary node to receive emphatic drainage from a primary breast carcinoma. Focal histopathologic assessment of this sentinel node can be used to determine the tumor status of the entire axillary basin. A number of large multicenter prospective trials sponsored by the American College of Surgeons and the NSABP are currently examining sentinel lymph node biopsy versus axillary lymph node dissection. The results of these trials will validate the clinical utility of sentinel lymph node biopsy in the management of patients with breast cancer. Thus, simple mastectomy may be a reasonable alternative for women who wish to avoid the inconvenience of radiation therapy and preserve their option for breast reconstruction in the future. The NSABP B-04 and B-06 trials are widely credited with the finding that breast conservation is an appropriate primary therapy for the majority of women with stages I and II disease, and is preferable in that it provides survival rates equivalent to those of modified radical mastectomy. But these trials were also important for the valuable information they provided regarding the natural history of the disease and the identification of pathologic prognostic factors associated with early cancer spread. The preponderance of information available regarding predicting women most likely to benefit from systemic adjuvant therapy was derived from pathologic evaluation of the archives of these trials.

SYSTEMIC ADJUVANT THERAPY

Systemic adjuvant therapy is defined as the administration of systemic therapy following definitive therapy (surgery, radiation, or a combination of these) when there is no evidence of metastatic disease, but a high likelihood of disease recurrence. The concept of breast cancer being a systemic disease and the rationale of adjuvant chemotherapy was based on a series of laboratory and clinical investigations conducted during the 1960s and 1970s that were directed primarily toward achieving a better understanding of tumor metastases. Table 125–6 illustrates the laboratory findings, clinical abnormalities, and biologic hypothesis that lead to recognition of breast cancer as a systemic disease and documented the value of adjuvant chemotherapy. The very earliest adjuvant trials in breast cancer consisted of perioperative administration of alkylating agents with the intent of eradicating micrometastases that were disseminated at the time of surgical excision of the tumor. Many collaborative research groups have conducted stepwise series of studies designed to identify appropriate candidates for systemic adjuvant therapy, as well as optimal regimens and duration of systemic adjuvant therapy. Several hundred randomized clinical trials evaluating various systemic adjuvant modalities have been reported. Most published results confirmed that chemotherapy, hormonal therapy, or a combination of the two, result in advantages in DFS or overall survival for all treated patients, or more commonly for patients in specific prognostic subgroups (nodal involvement,

TABLE 125–6. Laboratory Findings, Clinical Observations, and Biologic Hypothesis of Breast Cancer as a Systemic Disease and the Value of Adjuvant Chemotherapy

- By the time cancer becomes clinically detectable, it is advanced (about 30 doublings) and has had ample opportunity to establish distant micrometastases.
- There is no orderly pattern of tumor cell dissemination, and the bloodstream is of considerable importance in tumor spread.
- Operable breast cancer is often a systemic disease and variations in local-regional therapy have not substantially affected survival. Only by control of distant disease can there be an improvement in the outcome of breast cancer patients.
- Likelihood of disease recurrence is related to size of tumor mass and axillary node involvement at diagnosis.
- Recurrence of breast cancer following local-regional therapy is most commonly at sites distant from the breast.
- Tumor growth fraction is inversely related to tumor population site. Therefore, optimal kinetic conditions to achieve cure with chemotherapy exist in the setting of micrometastatic disease.
- Efficacy of chemotherapy is dose dependent and optimal doses of combination chemotherapy can be more safely and effectively administered in the adjuvant setting as opposed to the setting of advanced disease.

TABLE 125–7. Ten-Year Results of the Overview Analysis

	Hormonal		Chemotherapy	
	Reduction in Annual Odds		*Reduction in Annual Odds*	
	Recurrence (%)	*Death (%)*	*Recurrence (%)*	*Death (%)*
All patients	47 ± 3	26 ± 4	24 ± 2	15 ± 2
< 40	54 ± 13	52 ± 17	37 ± 7	27 ± 5
40–99	41 ± 10	22 ± 13	34 ± 5	27 ± 5
50–59	37 ± 6	11 ± 8	22 ± 4	14 ± 4
60–69	54 ± 5	33 ± 6	18 ± 4	8 ± 4
≥ 70	54 ± 13	34 ± 13	NS	NS

NS, not significant
From Refs. 52–54.

menopausal status, hormonal receptor status, growth fraction, nuclear grade). The huge amount of data generated by these trials has resulted in a great deal of controversy, with different conclusions being reached by various experts.

A number of factors make interpretation of results of systemic adjuvant therapy trials difficult. These include differences in the patient populations studied, the variation in natural history of breast cancer, the absence of information regarding pathologic prognostic factors in many studies, and differences in treatment approach and methods of analysis. It is important to remember that the goal of systemic adjuvant therapy is cure. Therefore, patients in these studies must be followed for long periods of time before results can be determined. In addition, because most patients with early breast cancer (50% to 90%) in the various trials are cured with local-regional therapy alone, large numbers of patients are required to show a statistically significant difference that can be attributed to systemic adjuvant therapy. For these reasons, combined analysis, or meta-analysis, of all breast cancer trials has been conducted and is the most frequently referred to information regarding systemic adjuvant therapy. This effort, organized by the Early Breast Cancer Trialists' Collaborative Group, is based on a worldwide collaboration involving 133 randomized trials conducted between 1957 and 1985. The results of the Early Breast Cancer Trialists' Collaborative Group meta-analysis were published in 1988, 1992, and 1998. Many important questions regarding the optimal way to administer adjuvant chemotherapy[50,52–54] and hormonal therapy and the degree of benefit to in terms of disease-free and absolute survival to clinically relevant subsets of patients have been answered by these meta-analysis. In the 1998 analysis, many trials had more than 15 years of followup, giving the analysis more statistical power. The analysis of tamoxifen versus no tamoxifen included 55 trials with 37,000 patients.[52] The analysis of chemotherapy plus tamoxifen versus tamoxifen is based on data from nine studies including 3,920 patients, age 50 years or older.[54] The analysis of chemotherapy versus no chemotherapy is based on 47 trials that contained 17,723 patients.[53] *Simply stated, the results of the meta-analysis support the use of adjuvant hormonal therapy in all patients with positive hormone-receptor status, and this finding is reflected in the 2000 NIH Consensus Conference Statement*[44] *that adjuvant hormonal therapy should be recommended to women whose tumors contain hormone receptor protein regardless of age, menopausal status, involvement of axillary lymph nodes, or tumor size. The results of the meta analysis also support a benefit to adjuvant chemotherapy again reflected in the 2000 NIH Consensus Conference Statement that it is accepted practice to offer cytotoxic chemotherapy to most women with lymph node metastases or with primary breast cancers larger than 1 cm in diameter (both node-negative and node positive).*[44] It is important to understand the magnitude of the benefit associated with adjuvant therapy in breast cancer. Table 125–7 shows the proportional reduction in the annual odds of recurrence and death by age for adjuvant polychemotherapy and adjuvant tamoxifen given for 5 years in women with positive hormone receptors tumors based on the results of the meta-analysis. Throughout these reports, the results are presented as they are in Table 125–7, as proportional benefits that compares the effects of two groups, in this case, chemotherapy or hormonal therapy versus no chemotherapy or hormonal therapy. A proportional reduction of one quarter might equivalently be described as an odds ratio or hazard ratio of 0.75, an odds reduction of 25%, or a 25% reduction in the death rate. For a given proportional reduction in death rate, the absolute improvement in 10-year survival will depend on the risk of death with no treatment which, for breast cancer, is known to vary based on prognostic factors that include patient characteristics, disease characteristics and biomarkers identified earlier in this chapter. Table 125–8 shows the number of deaths avoided per 100 patients treated in several hypothetical subsets of patients with different estimated 10-year survivals without adjuvant therapy as a function of different estimates of treatment benefit shown as the proportional reductions in mortality if they did receive adjuvant therapy. Approximately 12 of every 100 patients benefited at 10 years from adjuvant therapy when a 30% proportional reduction in mortality is observed in the highest risk subgroups (50% death rate with no adjuvant therapy). In contrast, the same 30% proportional reduction in mortality translated to a benefit for three of 100 patients in the lowest risk subset (10% death rate with no adjuvant therapy). Thus, the absolute benefit of adjuvant therapy is dependent on both the proportional reduction in mortality and the risk of disease recurrence with the greatest benefit observed in the highest risk treatment groups given a fixed proportional reduction in mortality. Table 125–9 further demonstrates this using data from the meta-analysis by showing absolute benefits of adjuvant chemotherapy in terms of age and nodal status. In the highest risk group, node-positive women younger than 50 years of age, only

TABLE 125–8. Absolute Reduction in Mortality at 10 Years per 100 Patients Treated

Estimated 10-yr death rate with no therapy	Hypothetical proportional reduction in mortality due to treatment				
	50%	*40%*	*30%*	*20%*	*10%*
50% (5-cm tumor, negative nodes)	21	16	12	7	4
30% (average tumor diameter, negative nodes)	14	11	8	5	3
10% (< 1-cm tumor, negative nodes)	5	4	3	2	1

Adapted from Ref. 23 (with permission).

TABLE 125–9. Absolute Benefits of Adjuvant Chemotherapy by Age and Nodal Status

	With Polychemotherapy (%)	With No Polychemotherapy (%)	Absolute Benefit (%)
Disease-free survival			
Age < 50 y			
Node negative	68.3	58.0	10.3
Node positive	47.6	32.2	15.4
Age 50–69 y			
Node negative	65.6	59.9	5.7
Node positive	43.4	39.0	5.4
Overall survival			
Age < 50 y			
Node negative	77.6	71.9	5.7
Node positive	53.8	41.4	12.4
Age 50–69 y			
Node negative	71.2	64.8	6.4
Node positive	48.6	46.3	2.3

Adapted from Ref. 23 (with permission).

41.4% were alive at 10 years with no polychemotherapy as compared to 53.8% with polychemotherapy, which translates to an absolute survival benefit of 12.4%; however, in the node-negative, fewer than 50 subsets of patients where survival with no polychemotherapy was highest (i.e., 71.9) polychemotherapy produced an absolute benefit of only 5.7%. It should be pointed out that all of these differences in survival are highly statistically significant and forms the basis of the 2000 NIH Consensus Development Group recommendation that it is accepted medical practice to offer cytotoxic chemotherapy to most women with early stage breast cancer. However, the absolute benefit in node-positive women age 50 to 69 years is quite small (2.3%), and depending on other disease characteristics and comorbid conditions, patients may elect not to pursue treatment. Although a 2% absolute reduction in death attributable to polychemotherapy may appear small, at least two investigators have reported that most patients with breast cancer would accept severe toxicity from treatment to achieve as little as a 1% to 5% improvement in survival.[55,56]

Several international and national groups have development guidelines for treatment of early stage breast cancer based on specific patient and disease characteristics and the results of the meta-analysis. In February 1998, an international group of research met at St. Gallen in Switzerland for the Sixth International Conference of Adjuvant Therapy of Primary Breast Cancer.[57] At the conclusion of the conference, a consensus panel of experts reviewed and modified its previous guidelines and recommendations for selection of adjuvant systemic therapies in specific patient populations outside of the framework of clinical trials (Table 125–10). Criteria used to construct Table 125–10 included risk of relapse, predicted response, results of treatment from randomized clinical trials and patient preferences concerning risks and benefits of effective therapy. Patient populations are defined based on risk of relapse. The panel defined minimal/low risk as patients with all of the following: negative lymph nodes, tumor <1 cm, ER-positive grade 1, and age <35 years. High-risk node-negative patients have one of the following: tumor >2 cm, ER-negative grade 2–3, age <35 years. Intermediate risk includes all patients that fall outside of criteria for minimal or high risk. Node-positive patients are by definition at high risk. Elderly patients are listed separately because specific considerations are required regarding toxicity and competing cause of morbidity and mortality. Therapies for which high-level evidence of benefit has been demonstrated are noted in bold text and therapies that are still investigational or require special consideration are noted as described in the footnotes.

The National Comprehensive Cancer Network (NCCN) developed practice guidelines for the treatment of breast cancer. Figure 125–3 illustrates the NCCN guidelines for adjuvant treatment of stages I to IIIA breast cancer following total mastectomy or lumpectomy. These more recent guidelines reflect the increasing trend toward the use of chemotherapy in postmenopausal (older than age 50 years), as well as the well established premenopausal (younger than age 50 years) patient, hormonal therapy in all hormone receptor-positive women regardless of age or menopausal status, and the combination of both chemotherapy and hormonal therapy.[58]

Intensive research efforts are directed toward identifying those characteristics of the primary tumor (pathologic prognostic factors) that may predict for a higher or lower likelihood of metastases and death in node-negative patients. Although a multitude of prognostic factors are being investigated, no single factor or combination of factors sufficiently identifies those at risk of metastases or is sufficiently standardized to be reproducibly applicable to all patients. Furthermore, it cannot be assumed that patients with a poor prognosis have the same or greater likelihood of benefiting from adjuvant therapy. Certainly, decisions regarding adjuvant therapy, particularly in node-negative patients, should be individualized based on the estimated risk of relapse and death, the expected benefits of treatment, the toxicity of treatment, and the impact of therapy on quality of life. There is an increasing trend in clinical decision making to take hormone receptor status, nuclear grade, and tumor size into consideration in recommending adjuvant therapy. HER-2 is gaining acceptance as a predictor of poor prognosis and indicator of benefit from systemic adjuvant therapy. For a more in-depth discussion of the issues and controversies regarding adjuvant therapy of breast cancer, the reader is referred to several excellent references.[59–60]

Adjuvant Chemotherapy

Cytotoxic drugs that have been used alone and in combination as adjuvant therapy in breast cancer include doxorubicin, epirubicin, cyclophosphamide, methotrexate, fluorouracil, melphalan, prednisone, and vincristine. The most common combination chemotherapy regimens employed in the adjuvant and metastatic setting are listed in Table 125–11.

Combination chemotherapy regimens used in the adjuvant setting are essentially the same as regimens used for metastatic breast

TABLE 125–10. Adjuvant Treatment for Patients With Node-Negative (A) and Node-Positive (B) Breast Cancer[a]

A. Node Negative			
Patient Group	***Minimal/Low Risk***	***Intermediate Risk***	***High Risk***
Premenopausal, ER or PR positive	**None or tamoxifen**	**Tamoxifen ± chemotherapy[b]** Ovarian ablation[c] GnRH analog[c]	**Chemotherapy + tamoxifen[b]** Ovarian ablation[c] GnRH analog[c]
Premenopausal, ER and PR negative	Not applicable	Not applicable	**Chemotherapy[d]**
Postmenopausal, ER or PR positive	**None or tamoxifen**	**Tamoxifen ± chemotherapy[b]**	**Tamoxifen + chemotherapy[b]**
Postmenopausal, ER and PR negative	Not applicable	Not applicable	**Chemotherapy[d]**
Elderly	**None or tamoxifen**	**Tamoxifen** ± chemotherapy	**Tamoxifen** If no ER and PR expression: chemotherapy

B. Node Positive	
Patient Group	***Treatments***
Premenopausal, ER or PR positive	**Chemotherapy + tamoxifen** **Ovarian ablation** (or GnRH analog) ± tamoxifen[c] Chemotherapy ± ovarian ablation or (GnRH analog) ± tamoxifen[c]
Premenopausal, ER and PR negative	**Chemotherapy[d]**
Postmenopausal, ER or PR positive	**Tamoxifen + chemotherapy[b]**
Postmenopausal, ER and PR negative	**Chemotherapy[d]**
Elderly	**Tamoxifen** If no ER and PR expression: **chemotherapy**

[a]ER = estrogen receptor; PR = progesterone receptor; GnRH = gonadotropin releasing hormone. Bold entries are treatments accepted for routine use or baseline in clinical trials.
[b]The addition of chemotherapy is considered an acceptable option based on evidence from clinical trials. Considerations about a low relative risk of relapse, age, toxic effects, socioeconomic implications, and information on patient's preference might justify the use of **tamoxifen alone.**
[c]Indicates treatments still being tested in randomized clinical trials.
[d]The addition of tamoxifen following chemotherapy might be considered for patients whose tumors are classified as ER and PR negative but which exhibit minimal/trace levels of either ER or PR.

cancer. One important exception exists with respect to adjuvant treatment of breast cancer at the current time. During the past several years, a number of recently marketed agents, the most notable being the taxanes paclitaxel and docetaxel, demonstrated significant single-agent activity in metastatic breast cancer. Combination therapy with a taxane and anthracycline, cyclophosphamide, cisplatin, fluorouracil, vinorelbine or trastuzumab showed high activity in phase II trials in treatment of metastatic disease. Some of these newer combinations are being investigated in randomized clinical trials in the adjuvant setting. However, it would be premature to move these newer combination regimens into the adjuvant setting in routine clinical practice at the current time.

The basic principle of adjuvant therapy for any cancer type is that the regimen with the highest response rate in advanced disease is the optimal regimen for use in the adjuvant setting. Early administration of effective combination chemotherapy at a time when the tumor burden is low should increase the likelihood of cure and minimize the emergence of drug-resistant tumor cell clones. Doxorubicin has historically been referred to as the most active single agent in the treatment of metastatic breast cancer. This has led to the assumption that doxorubicin-containing regimens are associated with a higher cure rate than nondoxorubicin-containing regimens when used in the adjuvant setting. An indirect comparison of the effects of adjuvant chemotherapy in 12 trials that used doxorubicin-containing regimens with results of trials in which cyclophosphamide, methotrexate, fluorouracil (CMF)-type regimens did show a significant advantage for the doxorubicin regimens.[53] In the meta-analysis, anthracycline containing regimens were modestly superior in reducing recurrence and death compared to regimens without anthracyclines. A 12 ± 4% reduction in annual odds of recurrence and a 11 ± 5% reduction in annual odds of death was reported in the 1998 update, and this translated to an absolute difference in overall mortality at 5 years of 3%. Doxorubicin-containing regimens have grown in popularity, not only because they are somewhat more effective but also because most trials have used only four cycles (whereas, trials with cyclophosphamide, methotrexate and fluorouracil have traditionally administered six cycles), and are well tolerated. Epirubicin is an anthracycline that has been available in Europe for more than a decade but was first introduced to the US market in late 1999 with an indication for adjuvant therapy of breast cancer.

A recently reported large randomized trial suggests that the sequential use of paclitaxel after doxorubicin and cyclophosphamide (four cycles) offers an advantage over doxorubicin and cyclophosphamide alone.[61] In this trial, lymph node positive pre- and postmenopausal patients were randomized to one of three dose levels of doxorubicin in the doxorubicin plus cyclophosphamide and then either no additional therapy or four additional cycles of paclitaxel. Women who received paclitaxel had a statistically significant improvement in disease-free survival (90% vs 86%) and overall survival (97% vs 95%) at a median followup time of only 2 years. This represents a 22% reduction in the odds of relapse and a 26% reduction in odds of death. Subgroup analysis demonstrated that the survival benefit almost exclusively occured in patients with hormone receptor negative disease. Although the results of this trial was adequate to gain paclitaxel an FDA approved indication for adjuvant therapy of women with four or more positive nodes, many experts, including the 2000 NIH Consensus Development Panel, feel that it is premature to incorporate paclitaxel routinely into adjuvant treatment regimens.

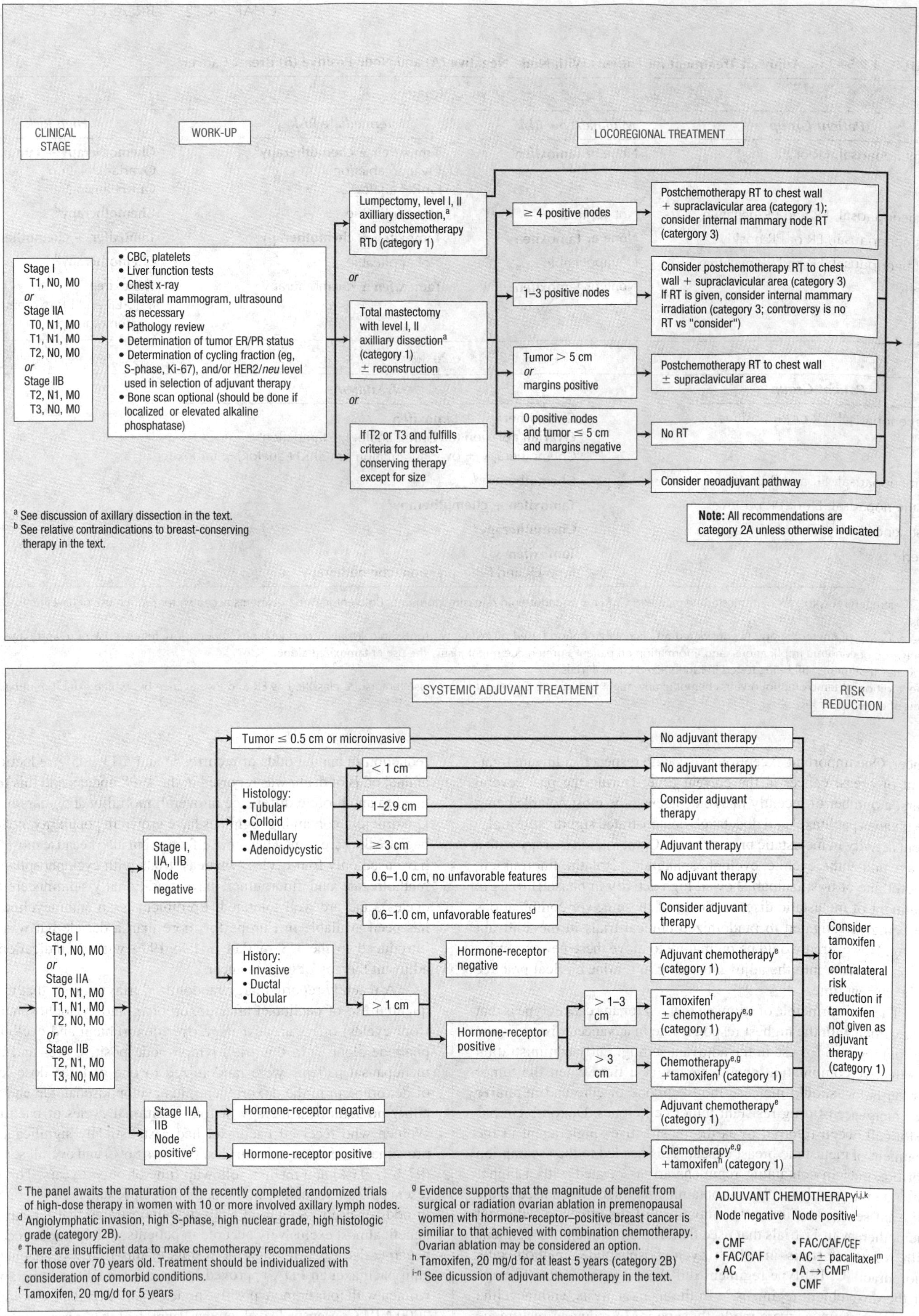

CLINICAL STAGE

WORK-UP

LOCOREGIONAL TREATMENT

Stage I
T1, N0, M0
or
Stage IIA
T0, N1, M0
T1, N1, M0
T2, N0, M0
or
Stage IIB
T2, N1, M0
T3, N0, M0

- CBC, platelets
- Liver function tests
- Chest x-ray
- Bilateral mammogram, ultrasound as necessary
- Pathology review
- Determination of tumor ER/PR status
- Determination of cycling fraction (eg, S-phase, Ki-67), and/or HER2/*neu* level used in selection of adjuvant therapy
- Bone scan optional (should be done if localized or elevated alkaline phosphatase)

Lumpectomy, level I, II axillary dissection,[a] and postchemotherapy RTb (category 1)

or

Total mastectomy with level I, II axillary dissection[a] (category 1) ± reconstruction

or

If T2 or T3 and fulfills criteria for breast-conserving therapy except for size

$\geq$ 4 positive nodes → Postchemotherapy RT to chest wall + supraclavicular area (category 1); consider internal mammary node RT (category 3)

1–3 positive nodes → Consider postchemotherapy RT to chest wall + supraclavicular area (category 3) If RT is given, consider internal mammary irradiation (category 3; controversy is no RT vs "consider")

Tumor > 5 cm *or* margins positive → Postchemotherapy RT to chest wall ± supraclavicular area

0 positive nodes and tumor $\leq$ 5 cm and margins negative → No RT

Consider neoadjuvant pathway

[a] See discussion of axillary dissection in the text.
[b] See relative contraindications to breast-conserving therapy in the text.

Note: All recommendations are category 2A unless otherwise indicated

SYSTEMIC ADJUVANT TREATMENT

RISK REDUCTION

Stage I
T1, N0, M0
or
Stage IIA
T0, N1, M0
T1, N1, M0
T2, N0, M0
or
Stage IIB
T2, N1, M0
T3, N0, M0

Stage I, IIA, IIB Node negative

Tumor $\leq$ 0.5 cm or microinvasive → No adjuvant therapy

Histology:
- Tubular
- Colloid
- Medullary
- Adenoidcystic

< 1 cm → No adjuvant therapy

1–2.9 cm → Consider adjuvant therapy

$\geq$ 3 cm → Adjuvant therapy

History:
- Invasive
- Ductal
- Lobular

0.6–1.0 cm, no unfavorable features → No adjuvant therapy

0.6–1.0 cm, unfavorable features[d] → Consider adjuvant therapy

> 1 cm → Hormone-receptor negative → Adjuvant chemotherapy[e] (category 1)

> 1 cm → Hormone-receptor positive → > 1–3 cm → Tamoxifen[f] ± chemotherapy[e,g] (category 1)

> 3 cm → Chemotherapy[e,g] +tamoxifen[f] (category 1)

Stage IIA, IIB Node positive[c]

Hormone-receptor negative → Adjuvant chemotherapy[e] (category 1)

Hormone-receptor positive → Chemotherapy[e,g] +tamoxifen[h] (category 1)

Consider tamoxifen for contralateral risk reduction if tamoxifen not given as adjuvant therapy (category 1)

[c] The panel awaits the maturation of the recently completed randomized trials of high-dose therapy in women with 10 or more involved axillary lymph nodes.
[d] Angiolymphatic invasion, high S-phase, high nuclear grade, high histologic grade (category 2B).
[e] There are insufficient data to make chemotherapy recommendations for those over 70 years old. Treatment should be individualized with consideration of comorbid conditions.
[f] Tamoxifen, 20 mg/d for 5 years
[g] Evidence supports that the magnitude of benefit from surgical or radiation ovarian ablation in premenopausal women with hormone-receptor–positive breast cancer is similiar to that achieved with combination chemotherapy. Ovarian ablation may be considered an option.
[h] Tamoxifen, 20 mg/d for at least 5 years (category 2B)
[i-n] See dicussion of adjuvant chemotherapy in the text.

ADJUVANT CHEMOTHERAPY[i,j,k]	
Node negative	Node positive[l]
• CMF • FAC/CAF • AC	• FAC/CAF/CEF • AC ± pacalitaxel[m] • A → CMF[n] • CMF

FIGURE 125–3. NCNN treatment guidelines for invasive breast cancer. *(Reproduced with permission from the National Comprehensive Cancer Network, Inc., version 2000)*

TABLE 125–11. Chemotherapy of Breast Cancer

AC
Doxorubicin 60 mg/m^2 IV, day 1
Cyclophosphamide 600 mg/m^2 IV, day 1
Repeat cycle every 21 days times 4 cycles followed by Paclitaxel 175 mg/m^2 IV Day 1q 21 days for four additional courses
1. In: DeVita VT, Hellman S, Rosenberg SA, eds. Cancer: Principles & Practice of Oncology, 5th ed. Philadelphia, Lippincott, 1997:1557.
2. Casciato DA, Lowitz BB, eds. Manual of Clinical Oncology, 3rd ed. Boston, Little, Brown, 1995:596.
3. Taxol® (Paclitaxel) product information. Bristol Myers: Illinois, July 2000.

CAF (FAC)
Cyclophosphamide 100 mg/m^2 PO, days 1–14 or 600 mg/m^2 IV, day 1
Doxorubicin 25 mg/m^2 IV, days 1 and 8 or 60 mg/m^2 IV, day 1
Fluorouracil 500–600 mg/m^2 IV, days 1 and 8
Repeat cycle every 28 days
1. Facts and Comparisons. May 1996:643a.
2. Chemotherapy Sourcebook, 2nd ed. 1996:845.
3. Smalley RV, Carpenter J, Bartolucci A, Vogel C, Krauss S. A comparison of cyclophosphamide, adriamycin, 5-fluorouracil (CAF) and cyclophosphamide, methotrexate, 5-fluorouracil, vincristine, prednisone (CMFVP) in patients with metastatic breast cancer. Cancer 1977;40:625–632.

OR
Cyclophosphamide 500 mg/m^2 IV, day 1
Doxorubicin 50 mg/m^2 IV, day 1
Fluorouracil 500 mg/m^2 IV, day 1[a]
Repeat cycle every 21 days
1. Finley RS. Neoplastic disorders. In: Young LL, Koda-Kimble MA, eds. Applied Therapeutics: The Clinical Use of Drugs, 6th ed. Vancouver, Applied Therapeutics, 1995:90–116.
2. Lindley CM. Breast cancer. In: DiPiro JT, Talbert RL, Yee GC, et al., eds. Pharmacotherapy, 3rd ed. Stanford, Appleton & Lange, 1996:2485.

CFM (CNF, FNC)
Cyclophosphamide 500–600 mg/m^2 IV, day 1
Fluorouracil 500–600 mg/m^2 IV, day 1
Mitoxantrone 10–12 mg/m^2 IV, day 1
Repeat cycle every 21 days
1. Casciato DA, Lowitz BB, eds. Manual of Clinical Oncology, 3rd ed. Boston, Little, Brown, 1995:596.
2. Alonso MC, Tabernero JM, Ojeda B, et al. A phase III randomized trial of cyclophosphamide, mitoxantone, and 5-fluorouracil (CNF) versus cyclophosphamide, adriamycin, and 5-fluorouracil (CAF) in patients with metastatic breast cancer. Breast Cancer Res Treat 1995;24:15–24.

CMF
Cyclophosphamide 100 mg/m^2 PO, days 1–14 or 600 mg/m^2 IV, days 1 and 8
Methotrexate 40 mg/m^2 IV, days 1 and 8
Fluorouracil 600 mg/m^2 IV, days 1 and 8
Repeat cycle every 28 days
OR
Cyclophosphamide 600 mg/m^2 IV, day 1
Methotrexate 40 mg/m^2 IV, day 1
Fluorouracil 600 mg/m^2 IV, day 1
Repeat cycle every 21 days
1. Chemotherapy Sourcebook, 2nd ed. 1996:1146.
2. Hall PD, Lesher BA, Hall RK. Adjuvant therapy of nodenegative breast cancer. Ann Pharmacother 1995;29:292.

NFL
Mitoxantrone 12 mg/m^2 IV, day 1
Fluorouracil 350 mg/m^2 IV, days 1–3, given after leucovorin
Leucovorin 300 mg IV, over 1 hour, days 1–3
Repeat cycle every 21 days
1. Hainsworth JD, Andrews MB, Johnson DH, et al. Mitoxantrone, fluorouracil, and high-dose leucovorin: An effective, well-tolerated regimen for metastatic breast cancer. J Clin Oncol 1991;9:1732.

Sequential DOX-CMF
Doxorubicin 75 mg/m^2 IV, every 21 days for 4 cycles followed by 21 or 28 days CMF for 8 cycles
1. Bonadonna G, Zambetti M, Valagussa P. Sequential or alternating doxorubicin and CMF regimens in breast cancer with more than three positive nodes. JAMA 1995;273:542–543.

VATH
Vinblastine 4.5 mg/m^2 IV, day 1
Doxorubicin 45 mg/m^2 IV, day 1
Thiotepa 12 mg/m^2 IV, day 1
Fluoxymesterone 10 mg PO tid
Repeat cycle every 21 days
1. Skeel RT. Carcinoma of the breast. In: Skeel RT, Lachant NA, eds. Handbook of Cancer Chemotherapy, 4th ed. Boston, Little, Brown, 1995:283.
1. Chemotherapy Sourcebook, 2nd ed. 1996:848.

Vinorelbine
Doxorubicin
Vinorelbine 25 mg/m^2 IV, days 1 and 8
Doxorubicin 50 mg/m^2 IV, day 1
Repeat cycle every 21 days
1. Spielman M, Dorval T, Turpin F, et al. Phase II trial of vinorelbine/doxorubicin as first-line therapy of advanced breast cancer. J Clin Oncol 1994;12:1764–1770.

Single-Agent Regimens

Anastrozole
Anastrozole 1 mg PO daily
1. Anastrozole, a potent and selective aromatase inhibitor, versus megestrol acetate in postmenopausal women with advanced breast cancer: Results of overview analysis of two phase III trials. J Clin Oncol 1996;14:2000–2011.

Docetaxel
Docetaxel 60–100 mg/m^2 IV, over 1 hour, every 21 days
Concomitant dexamethasone 8 mg PO bid for 5 days, begin 1 day before docetaxel
1. Taxotere® (docetaxel) product information. Rhone Poulenc Rorer. Collegeville, PA, May 1996.

Gemcitabine
Gemcitabine 725 mg/m^2 IV, over 30 minutes, weekly for 3 weeks, followed by 1-week rest
Repeat cycle every 28 days
1. Carmichael J, Possinger K, Phillip P, et al. Advanced breast cancer: A phase II trial with gemcitabine. J Clin Oncol 1995;13:2731–2736.
2. Carmichael J, Walling J. Phase II activity of gemcitabine in advanced breast cancer. Semin Oncol 1996;23(suppl 10):77–86.

Megestrol
Megestrol 40 mg PO qid
1. Bozdar A, Jonat W, Howell A, et al. Anastrozole, a potent and selective aromatase inhibitor, versus megestrol acetate in postmenopausal women with advanced breast cancer: Results of overview analysis of two phase III trials. J Clin Oncol 1996;14:2000–2011.

Paclitaxel[b]
Paclitaxel[b] 250 mg/m^2 IV, over 3 or 24 hours, every 21 days
OR
Paclitaxel[b] 175 mg/m^2 IV, over 3 hours, every 21 days
1. Seidman AD, Tiersten A, et al. Phase II trial of paclitaxel by 3 hour infusion as initial and salvage chemotherapy for metastatic breast cancer. J Clin Oncol 1995;13:2575–2581.
2. Taxol® (Paclitaxel) product information. Bristol Myers: Illinois, April 1994.

Tamoxifen
Tamoxifen 20 mg PO daily
1. Nolvadex® (Tamoxifen) product information. Zeneca Pharmaceuticals.

Vinorelbine
Vinorelbine 30 mg/m^2 IV, every 7 days
1. Fumoleau P, Delozier T, Extra JM, et al. Vinorelbine in the treatment of breast cancer. Semin Oncol 1995;22:(suppl 5):22.
2. Navelbine® (Vinorelbine) product information. Glaxo Wellcome; Research Triangle Park, December 1994.

[a]Also given day 8 with FAC.

No validated predictive factors exist for response to chemotherapy, but evidence is accumulating that HER-2/neu may be the first to make the list. The first studies that examined the potential role of HER-2/neu status for predicting response to adjuvant chemotherapy concentrated on regimens that contained cyclophosphamide, methotrexate, and fluorouracil. The general trend reported in these and subsequent studies is that patients whose tumors have little or no detectable levels of HER-2/neu derive considerable benefit from these regimens, but patients whose tumors have amplified HER-2/neu genes or overexpressed HER-2/neu do not benefit from these therapies. The conclusions, however, are based on retrospective analysis and have not been validated in prospective studies with sufficient statistical power to detect interactions between treatment and HER-2/neu status. Three large cooperative group studies, one conducted by the Cancer and Leukemia Group B, another by the National Surgical Adjuvant Breast and Bowel Project, and the third by the Southwestern Oncology Group, were retrospective analyses of HER-2/neu status, other tumor characteristics, and response to adjuvant therapy containing anthracycline-based regimens.[42,43,62] Although the designs were different, all three groups found that patients whose tumor overexpressed the HER-2/neu oncogene clearly benefitted from anthracycline-based regimens. An issue in interpretation of these findings is the possibility that it was not overexpression of HER-2/neu but a coexisting variable, either known ones such as the estrogen receptor or an unknown one, that accounted for these findings. In addition, HER-2/neu overexpression is correlated with a number of negative prognostic factors and, therefore, the relative importance of HER-2/neu as compared to other negative prognostic factors was unclear. These studies, together with other results that have been presented at national and international meetings and preclinical data, strongly suggest that the hypothesized interaction between HER-2/neu overexpression and adjuvant doxorubicin therapy is real. A major issue with interpreting the data and reaching a consensus regarding the value of doxorubicin-containing adjuvant chemotherapy for patients who are HER-2/neu-positive has been questioned regarding the most reliable reproducible and predictive method to determine HER-2/neu status. Most of the clinical trials have employed an immunohistochemical staining method to determine HER-2/neu status in breast cancer tissue. A recent publication compared immunohistochemical with fluorescence *in situ* hybridization (FISH), and concluded that FISH was significantly better than immunohistochemical in predicting response to trastuzumab therapy.[63] The immunohistochemical methods that are commercially available are not standardized and, particularly, when reported as 2+ are frequently not positive by FISH analysis. Although experts are calling for consensus regarding the most reliable reproducible and predictive method to determine HER-2/neu status as well as prospective clinical studies with anthracycline-based regimens, where patients are randomized based on HER-2/neu status, before overexpression of HER-2/neu is accepted and is used for determining adjuvant therapy for women with breast cancer. Current clinical practice strongly suggests that these determinations are being made in decisions regarding anthracycline-based regimens based on HER-2/neu status.

Although the optimal duration of adjuvant chemotherapy administration is unknown, it appears to be on the order of 12 to 16 weeks. Chemotherapy is usually initiated within 3 weeks of surgical removal of the primary tumor. The use of "neoadjuvant chemotherapy" or "primary chemotherapy" prior to surgery and radiation, as discussed in the section on locally advanced breast cancer (stage III), is predominantly confined to clinical trials in stage I and stage II breast cancer. "Dose intensity" and "dose density" appear to be critical factors in achieving optimal outcomes in adjuvant breast cancer therapy. *Dose intensity* is defined as the amount of drug administered per unit of time and is typically reported in milligrams per square meter of body surface per week ($mg/m^2/wk$). Increasing dose, decreasing time, or both can increase dose intensity. *Dose density* is equivalent to the concept of increasing dose intensity, but not by increasing the numerator of the fraction mg/m^2/time, as occurs with dose escalation, but by decreasing the denominator of time. The issue of dose intensity first received wide attention in 1981, when the Milan group reported a retrospective analysis of their original CMF adjuvant study suggesting that only those patients who received at least 85% of their planned CMF dose benefitted significantly from adjuvant therapy, whereas those receiving less than 65% of the planned dose had the same disease-free survival and overall survival as the group of controlled patients treated by surgery alone. Another technique to analyze dose intensity retrospectively was reported by Hryniuk and Levine. An analysis of the planned dose intensity of a variety of CMF-based adjuvant regimen showed that it significantly correlated with disease-free survival independent of other factors. Although these retrospective analyses provided support for the hypothesis, the dose intensity might be important in the adjuvant therapy of breast cancer. Three more recent studies that have escalated the dose of cyclophosphamide or doxorubicin in the standard anthracycline-containing regimens reported that this intervention offers no therapeutic advantage and is associated with greater toxicity. A study by the Cancer Leukemia Group B that is often discussed assigned 1,572 women to three treatment groups given different doses and schedules of CAF. The high-dose arm had twice the dose intensity and twice the drug dose as the low-dose arm. Moderate-dose arm had two-thirds the dose intensity as the high-dose arm but the same total drug dose. None of these schedules is really dose intensive by today's standards. At a median followup of 9 years, disease-free and overall survival for patients on the moderate- and high-dose arms were superior to those for the patients on the low-dose arm. There was no difference in disease-free survival or overall survival between the moderate and the high-dose arms. Therefore, it would appear that reducing the dose for standard treatment regimens should be avoided, unless necessitated by severe toxicity. But increasing doses beyond that contained in standard treatment regimens does not appear to be beneficial.

A major focus in clinical investigation is the use of more high-dose chemotherapy regimens as adjuvant therapy. Because bone marrow suppression is the dose-limiting toxicity for most chemotherapeutic agents, high-dose chemotherapy regimens followed by colony-stimulating factors (CSFs) or reinfusion of autologous hematopoietic stem cells have been developed. Trials to define the specific usefulness of high-dose regimens, as well as autologous hematopoietic stem cell transplantation (HSCT) in conjunction with dose-intense regimens, are justified given the positive response rates seen in the metastatic breast cancer setting and the very poor prognosis associated with stage II disease with four to nine and, particularly, 10 or more positive axillary lymph nodes. Several cooperative groups are conducting trials of high-dose chemotherapy versus conventional adjuvant therapy, although none of the trials have shown a significant difference to date and preliminary results suggest that a benefit of high-dose therapy is unlikely to be found.

The short-term toxic effects of chemotherapy used in the adjuvant setting are generally well tolerated. Although a number of investigators have demonstrated a reduction in quality of life, most patients are able to maintain a reasonable level of function and emotional and social well-being during treatment.[64] In general, supportive therapy of the patient receiving systemic adjuvant chemotherapy has improved in the past decade. Increased attention to the impact of symptoms on quality of life may account for some of this improvement. In addition, serotonin-antagonist antiemetics have become available to assist in managing chemotherapy-induced nausea and vomiting, and CSFs are often helpful in preventing febrile neutropenia, particularly in elderly patients or patients receiving high-dose and dose-intense chemotherapy regimens. However, a number of side effects are common with the regimens employed and patients should be appropriately counseled regarding the likelihood of alopecia, weight gain, and fatigue. Patients who are menstruating will experience a cessation of menses that may or may not return. Along with cessation of menses are accompanying signs and symptoms of menopause. Deep-vein thrombosis has been reported in women receiving combination chemotherapy regimens.[65] A recent study estimated that 1 to 10 of 10,000 patients treated for 6 months with cyclophosphamide-based regimens might be expected to have leukemia within 10 years of diagnosis of breast cancer.[66]

Cardiomyopathy induced by doxorubicin occurs less than 1% of the time in women whose total dose is less than 320 mg/m^2 of body surface area.[66] Toxicities associated with the chemotherapy regimens employed in the experimental autologous HSCT programs are likely to be greater than those incurred with the standard adjuvant chemotherapy regimens described.

A final note before leaving the topic of adjuvant chemotherapy in stage I and stage II breast cancer. As discussed previously, the magnitude of survival benefit for chemotherapy appears to be small, with an absolute odds reduction in mortality of only 5% at 10 years for patients with negative axillary lymph nodes and 10% for patients with positive axillary lymph nodes. In addition, there is currently no means to identify patients who will attain this survival benefit. However, two investigators report that most patients with breast cancer would accept severe toxicity from treatment to achieve as little as a 1% to 5% improvement in survival.[67,68] Therefore, in the absence of the ability to predict who will benefit, it is likely that most patients with stage I and stage II breast cancer will choose adjuvant chemotherapy treatment.

Adjuvant Endocrine Therapy

Hormonal therapies that have been studied in the treatment of primary or early breast cancer include oophorectomy, ovarian irradiation, tamoxifen, and luteinizing hormone-releasing hormone (LHRH) agonists.

Tamoxifen is currently the adjuvant hormonal therapy of choice. Tamoxifen has been used in the adjuvant setting for three decades. Tamoxifen is antiestrogenic in breast cancer cells, but it appears to have estrogenic properties in other tissues and organs.[69,70] Newer information confirms that tamoxifen and other similar drugs have many estrogenic and antiestrogenic effects that depend on the tissue and the gene in question and they are more appropriately called selective estrogen receptor modulators. Although tamoxifen's major mechanism of action has been attributed to its ability to block hormone receptors, studies have shown that the drug is capable of stimulating the production of transforming growth factor β, an inhibitory growth factor that could in fact inhibit the growth of estrogen receptor-positive and -negative cancer cells. Tamoxifen has also been shown in laboratory studies to reduce angiogenesis, possibly by decreasing local stimulatory growth factors, thus creating a hostile environment for tumor cells. Women receiving adjuvant tamoxifen therapy have a reduced incidence of development of contralateral breast cancer compared to women not receiving adjuvant tamoxifen therapy.[52,72] This observation, coupled with evidence of tamoxifen's beneficial estrogenic effects on the cardiovascular system and bone density, has led to tamoxifen being the hormonal agent of choice, not only in the adjuvant setting but also in the treatment of metastatic disease. An exception to this is premenopausal patients who may derive equivalent benefit from ovarian ablation via surgery or administration of LHRH agonists.

The optimal dose of tamoxifen is unclear and seems to depend on the country of origin of the original trials. For example, in the United Kingdom, 20 or 40 mg/day is usually recommended.[71] In Canada and Denmark,[72] 30 mg/day is used, but in the United States, 20 mg/day is used exclusively. The Early Breast Cancer Trialist Group showed that more is not necessarily better for response rates.[52] Decensi compared the standard 20 mg/day dose of tamoxifen with 10 mg/day and 10 mg every other day and measured certain end points that were related to the estrogenicity of tamoxifen and checked the circuiting levels of tamoxifen and metabolites.[73] All of the markers of tamoxifen action were essentially unchanged, despite an 80% decrease in circulating tamoxifen levels. Although this suggests that lower doses may be effective, no clinical trials have addressed this question. Therefore, the current recommended dose for tamoxifen in both the adjuvant, as well as the metastatic, and preventative settings is 20 mg/day. Because tamoxifen has a long biologic half-life, it can be administered as a single daily dose. Adjuvant tamoxifen therapy is generally initiated shortly after surgery or as soon as pathology results are known and the decision to administer tamoxifen as adjuvant therapy is made. An interesting theory with some laboratory and clinical support holds that tamoxifen antagonizes the beneficial effect of chemotherapy in women aged 50 years or younger. Chemotherapy acts by inhibiting (DNA) synthesis, thereby, causing death of tumor cells, whereas, tamoxifen is believed to have a static effect on tumor cell growth. The growth inhibitory effect of tamoxifen may therefore diminish the cytotoxic effect of chemotherapy, resulting in subsequent recurrence of disease in women who received the two agents together. This led to controversy regarding the optimal way to administer chemoendocrine therapy in the adjuvant setting with some experts favoring sequential use (chemotherapy followed by tamoxifen), while others continue to use concurrent (chemotherapy plus tamoxifen) therapy. The optimal duration of tamoxifen therapy in the adjuvant setting is currently defined as 5 years. Data currently do not exist to support the use of more prolonged (greater than 5 years) courses of tamoxifen in the adjuvant setting.

The best information regarding the side effects of tamoxifen come from the National Surgical Adjuvant Breast and Bowel Project, Breast Cancer Prevention Trial.[74] This trial randomized 13,388 women at increased risk for breast cancer, 35 years of age or older, to placebo (n = 6,707) or 20 mg/day of tamoxifen (n = 6,681) for 5 years. Although the primary finding of this study was that tamoxifen reduced the risk of invasive breast cancer by 49%, this study also provides an excellent opportunity to objectively quantitate side effects associated with tamoxifen. Information was collected with regard to the occurrence of hot flashes, vaginal discharge, irregular menses, fluid retention, nausea, skin changes, diarrhea, and weigh gain or loss. The self-administered depression scale and a global quality of life and a sexual function scale were administered at each follow-up visit. The only symptomatic differences noted between the placebo and tamoxifen group were related to hot flashes and vaginal discharge, both of which occurred more often in the later group. The proportion of women who reported hot flashes as being quite a bit or extremely bothersome were 45.7% in the tamoxifen group as compared to 28.7% in the placebo group. The proportion reporting vaginal discharge that was moderately bothersome or worse was 29% in the tamoxifen group as compared with 13% in the placebo group. There were no notable differences between the two groups relative to any of the find ings obtained from the various self-reporting instruments. Tamoxifen administration did not alter the average annual rate of ischemic heart disease, but a reduction in hip radius and spine fractures was observed. Of note, the rates of stroke, pulmonary embolism and deep-vein thrombosis were elevated in the tamoxifen group (risk ratio: stroke, 1.59, 95% confidence interval 0.93–2.77; pulmonary embolism, 3.01, 95% confidence interval 1.15–9.27; and deep-vein thrombosis, 1.60, 95% confidence interval 0.91–2.86). These events occurred more frequently in women age 50 years or older. The rate of endometrial cancer was increased in the tamoxifen group (risk ratio = 2.53, 95% confidence interval 1.35–4.97), and this increased risk occurred predominately in women age 50 years or older. The increased risk in endometrial carcinoma is similar in magnitude to that associated with postmenopausal estrogen replacement therapy and is likely a consequence of an estrogenic effect of tamoxifen on the endometrium. Some experts argue that this risk is acceptable because the endometrial cancer induced by tamoxifen is low-stage, low-grade, and easily treated with surgery or other means and does not pose a life-threatening risk to women. Toremifene is a recently marketed antiestrogen whose primary advantage is a lower estrogenic to antiestrogenic ratio as compared to tamoxifen.[75] Toremifene has been found to have efficacy similar to that of tamoxifen in metastatic disease and a generally similar side effect profile. Currently, toremifene is indicated as an alternative to tamoxifen in patients with metastatic breast cancer, but studies are ongoing that evaluate its safety and efficacy in the adjuvant setting.[76] In the NSABP-P1 trial, no increase in liver, colon, rectal, ovarian, or other tumors was observed in the tamoxifen group as compared to the group who received placebo. Currently, routine endometrial biopsy is not recommended for women receiving tamoxifen therapy. However, gynecologic exams and education regarding the importance of immediately reporting vaginal bleeding to primary physicians for further evaluation are important counseling points to women receiving tamoxifen therapy.

LOCALLY ADVANCED BREAST CANCER (STAGE III)

Locally advanced cancer of the breast refers to breast carcinomas with significant primary tumor and nodal disease, but in which distant metastases cannot be documented. This stage of breast cancer has been shown to be poorly controlled by surgery alone and to have a poor prognosis. Patients may present with a wide spectrum of disease, ranging from large tumors to skin or chest wall involvement, sometimes associated with advanced regional lymph node tumor involvement. Many patients with stage III breast cancer have disease that is technically unresectable at diagnosis. Inflammatory breast cancer with pathologic evidence of dermal lymphatic tumor permeation with clinical findings of diffuse erythema induration and edema of at least 30% of the breast usually without a palpable mass is a special type of locally advanced breast cancer.

Local-regional therapy of locally advanced breast cancer consists of surgery, radiation, or a combination of the two. The reported local recurrence rate ranges from 6% to 40% with mastectomy alone, and with radiation alone, 25% to 50%. Survival with either modality is approximately 40% to 50% at 5 years and 30% at 10 years.[5] Radiation therapy can be effective in controlling these locally advanced cancers, but doses greater than those used to treat early stage tumors are required. Although 5,000 cGy is effective in eradicating microscopic amounts of tumor in breast-conservation techniques, doses in excess of 6,000 cGy are required for gross tumor. These higher doses of radiation therapy are associated with moderate to severe arm edema, brachial plexopathy, and adverse cosmetic effects such as breast retraction and telangiectasia. The results from a number of trials suggest that there is no advantage for mastectomy over primary radiation therapy in patients with stage III disease. The benefit of combining mastectomy and postoperative radiation for patients with locally advanced breast cancer is controversial. Retrospective studies of patients treated with a combination of mastectomy and radiation show excellent local tumor control (local-regional recurrence 10% to 20%) in 5 years as compared to mastectomy or radiation alone (15% to 40%), but demonstration of a definitive impact on survival is lacking. Addition of radiation to mastectomy to improve local tumor control must be balanced against the possible increase and likelihood of complications. Unfortunately, similar to early breast cancer, distant metastases are the ultimate cause of death.

In the early 1980s, reports began to appear in the literature describing improvement in local-regional tumor control, DFS, and sometimes overall survival with combinations of multiagent chemotherapy, surgery, and radiation.[5] The natural history of locally advanced breast cancer suggested that even when local-regional control was accomplished, systemic relapse and death from breast cancer were eventually observed in the majority of patients. This led to interest in the use of "neoadjuvant" or "primary" chemotherapy in locally advanced breast cancer. Neoadjuvant or primary chemotherapy is the administration of systemic chemotherapy prior to a definitive local-regional procedure. Early aggressive systemic therapy has been used to control micrometastases, reduce tumor bulk, and allow for more limited procedures for local control. Primary or neoadjuvant chemotherapy followed by surgery with radiation therapy or both, and adjuvant systemic therapy has become the treatment choice for locally advanced breast cancer, including inflammatory breast cancer. Most tumors respond with more than a 50% decrease in tumor size; about 70% of patients experience downstaging through neoadjuvant chemotherapy. Breast conservation is possible for many patients with locally advanced breast cancer, and almost all patients initially are rendered disease free.

Although it is clear that neoadjuvant chemotherapy should be the initial choice of treatment for patients with locally advanced breast cancer, it is unclear what the optimal sequence of subsequent therapies should be, whether one or two local treatment modalities are necessary, and whether the addition of hormonal therapy to chemotherapy has significant benefit. The use of neoadjuvant treatment strategies for early breast cancer is currently under evaluation. One of the research directions to improve the survival of patients with locally advanced breast cancer is dose intensification of neoadjuvant or postoperative (adjuvant) chemotherapy. Several reports of open phase II trials have suggested an early benefit in DFS, comparative trials are necessary to assess the relative value of dose intensification in this group of patients.

METASTATIC BREAST CANCER (STAGE IV)

The goal of therapy with early and locally advanced breast cancer is to cure the disease. But breast cancer is currently incurable after it has advanced beyond a local-regional disease. The goal of treatment of metastatic breast cancer is to improve symptoms and quality of life. Thus, it is important to choose therapy with good activity while minimizing toxicities. Treatment of metastatic breast cancer with either cytotoxic or endocrine therapy often results in regression of disease and improvements in quality of life. In patients who respond to therapy, duration of survival is also increased. The choice of therapy for metastatic disease is based on the site of disease involvement and

TABLE 125–12. Endocrine Therapies Used for Metastatic Breast Cancer

Class	Drug	Dose	Side Effects
Antiestrogens	Tamoxifen Toremifene	20 mg PO qd 60 mg qd	Disease flare, hot flashes, nausea, vomiting, edema, thromboembolism, endometrial cancer
LHRH analogs	Leuprolide Goserelin	7.5 mg SC q28days 3.6 mg SC q28days	Amenorrhea, hot flashes, occasional nausea
Progestins	Medroxyprogesterone acetate Megestrol acetate	400–1000 mg IM qwk 40 mg tid	Weight gain, hot flashes, vaginal bleeding, edema, thromoembolism
Aromatase inhibitors	Anastrazole Letrozole Aminoglutethimide Exemestane 25 mg PO qd	1 mg qd 2.5 mg qd 250 mg PO qid w/hydrocortisone 40 mg/day	Lethargy, rash, postural dizziness, ataxia, nystagmus, nausea
Estrogens	Ethinylestradiol Conjugated estrogens	1 mg PO tid 2.5 mg PO tid	Nausea/vomiting, fluid retention, hot flashes, anorexia, thromboembolism, hepatic dysfunction
Androgens	Fluoxymesterone	10 mg PO bid	Deepening voice, alopecia, hirsutism, facial/truncal acne, fluid retention, menstrual irregularities, cholestatic jaundice

presence or absence of certain characteristics. For example, patients who experience a long DFS following local-regional therapy, or have disease that is primarily located in the bone or soft tissue, or are late premenopausal or postmenopausal will likely respond to endocrine therapy. The most important factor predicting response to endocrine therapy is the presence of estrogen and progesterone receptors in the primary tumor tissue. Fifty percent to 60% of ER-positive patients and 75% to 80% of ER- and PR-positive patients will respond to hormonal therapy, while those with ER- and PR-negative tumors have a less than 10% response rate. Thus, the largest factor determining choice of endocrine versus cytotoxic chemotherapy is the presence of hormone receptors in the primary breast tumor. Site of disease is also important in that numerous studies have shown that endocrine therapy is more likely to be effective in patients with bone and soft tissue metastases. Patients with visceral involvement (e.g., liver) and central nervous system involvement usually do not respond to hormonal therapy and seldom respond to chemotherapy. Endocrine therapy is the treatment of choice for patients who are hormone receptor positive and exhibit the first sign of metastatic disease in soft tissue, bone, or pleura owing to the equal probability of response to hormonal compared to chemotherapy and the lower toxicity profile of endocrine therapy.

Patients who respond to initial endocrine therapy often respond to a second hormonal manipulation. Response rate is lower and duration of response is shorter with second hormonal manipulations. Patients are sequentially treated with endocrine therapy until they have progressive symptoms resulting from advancing metastatic disease, at which time cytotoxic chemotherapy can be given. Combinations of hormonal therapies or chemotherapy plus hormones are not employed in the setting of metastatic breast cancer. Women with hormone receptor-negative tumors, with rapidly progressive lung, liver, or bone marrow involvement, or having failed initial endocrine therapy are not likely to benefit from endocrine therapy and are usually treated initially with cytotoxic chemotherapy.

ENDOCRINE THERAPY

In general, there is little evidence that the response or survival benefit from one endocrine therapy is clearly superior to that achieved with other therapies. Antiestrogens, aromatase inhibitors, progestins, estrogens, and androgens, as well as surgical procedures including oophorectomy, adrenalectomy, and hypophysectomy, are equivalent in many randomized trials in patients with metastatic breast cancer. Because most endocrine therapies are equally effective, the choice of a particular one is based primarily on toxicity (Table 125–12). In women who received tamoxifen as adjuvant therapy, tamoxifen is still usually the preferred initial agent when metastases are present. An exception to this occurs when the patient is receiving adjuvant tamoxifen at the time or within 1 year of occurrence of metastatic disease. In these cases, either a progestin or an aromatase inhibitor is generally employed.

Tamoxifen is generally considered to be the agent of choice in both premenopausal and postmenopausal women with metastatic breast cancer who are also hormone receptor positive. Tamoxifen is usually administered in 20 mg once-daily doses. There is no advantage for higher doses of tamoxifen. Moreover, long-term administration of very-high doses of tamoxifen (e.g., 12 months of 60–100 mg/m^2 twice daily) are associated with decreased visual acuity and retinopathy.

A dose schedule of tamoxifen 20 mg/day reaches a steady-state concentration after about 4 months of therapy. The half-life of tamoxifen during chronic dosing is 7 days. Serum tamoxifen concentrations can be detected 6 weeks after discontinuation of therapy. Thus, the maximum beneficial effects of tamoxifen are not observed for at least 2 months following initiation of therapy and it is unlikely that symptoms of metastatic disease will return if patients miss several doses. The toxicities of tamoxifen are described in the Adjuvant Endocrine Therapy section of this chapter. The only additional toxicity that one might expect to find in the setting of metastatic breast cancer is a tumor flare or hypercalcemia, which occurs in approximately 5% of patients following the initiation of any endocrine therapy and is not an indication to discontinue tamoxifen therapy. It is generally accepted that this is a positive indication that the patient will respond to endocrine therapy.

No difference has been found in two randomized trials of the overall response rate between tamoxifen and oophorectomy in premenopausal women. However, the secondary response rate to oophorectomy after tamoxifen treatment was somewhat higher than the response to tamoxifen after primary oophorectomy (33% vs 11%).[76] Some experts interpret this as suggesting that tamoxifen does not completely antagonize estrogen production, particularly in premenopausal women. Ovarian ablation (surgically or chemically) is still commonly used in some parts of the United States and is considered by many specialists to be the endocrine therapy of choice in premenopausal women. The mortality rate with surgical oophorectomy is low, usually less than 2% to 3% in appropriately selected patients. Chemical castration with LHRH analogs is increasingly used in lieu of oophorectomy in premenopausal women. In postmenopausal patients, response rate to surgical oophorectomy was inferior to tamoxifen and, thus, oophorectomy is not employed in this group.

Medical castration with LHRH analogs has been used in premenopausal metastatic breast cancer patients and induces remission in about one-third of unselected cases. The mechanism of action of LHRH analogs in breast cancer is thought to result from down-regulation of LHRH receptors in the pituitary. Decreased levels of luteinizing hormone subsequently lead to a decrease in estrogen to castrated levels. Thus, the effect of LHRH analogs on circulating estrogen levels in premenopausal breast cancer simulates oophorectomy. The two agents available in the United States are leuprolide and goserelin. Both of these agents are administered as a subcutaneous injection every 4 weeks and are associated with minimal side effects including amenorrhea, hot flashes, and occasional nausea. A recent meta-analysis reported on combined tamoxifen and LHRH agonists versus LHRH agonists-alone in premenopausal patients with metastatic breast cancer.[77] With a median followup of 6.8 years, there was a significant survival benefit and progression-free survival benefit in favor of the combined treatment. The overall response rate was significantly higher on combined endocrine treatment. The meta-analysis concluded that if a premenopausal woman with metastatic breast cancer is thought to be suitable for endocrine treatment, the combination of LHRH agonists plus tamoxifen should be considered as the new standard treatment.

A number of antiestrogens are currently in development for the treatment of breast cancer.[65,66] The goal of these newer compounds is to maintain the beneficial effects of tamoxifen's antagonism at breast cells, as well as its estrogenic properties on bone density and lipid profile, while avoiding the estrogenic effect of tamoxifen on the endometrium. There are currently two types of antiestrogens in development, the triphenylethylenes, which include toremifene, droloxifene, idoxifene, and raloxifene, and the pure antiestrogens. The pure antiestrogens differ from the triphenylethylene (tamoxifen-like) antiestrogens in their chemical structure, pharmacology, and biologic activity. Toremifene was approved in May 1997 for the treatment of metastatic breast cancer in postmenopausal women with estrogen receptor-positive or unknown tumors. Efficacy was based on three trials in a total of 1,500 postmenopausal metastatic breast cancer patients. The trials compared 60 mg of toremifene to either 20 mg or 40 mg of tamoxifen. The primary efficacy variables included response rate and time to progression. Survival was also determined. Two of the three studies showed similar results for all effectiveness end points, although one study did show a longer time to progression for tamoxifen. Incidences of adverse effects were comparable between the two medications. Data to support the use of toremifene in the adjuvant setting, or in premenopausal women, are currently lacking. Data are insufficient to allow evaluation of the long-term toxicity of toremifene, and it is still unknown if toremifene will differ from tamoxifen with respect to endometrial cancer and bone mineralization. Cross-resistance to toremifene has been demonstrated in patients with tamoxifen-refractory disease. Therefore, at the current time, toremifene appears to be an alternative to tamoxifen in postmenopausal patients with positive or unknown hormone receptor status with metastatic breast cancer. Costs of the two products are equivalent.

Raloxifene, also a member of the triphenylethylene-type of antiestrogen, received approval in December 1997 for prevention of osteoporosis in postmenopausal women. The manufacturer of raloxifene refers to this agent as a selective estrogen receptor modulator based on its estrogenic agonist activity in the skeleton and on lipid metabolism and estrogen antagonist action in the breast and uterus. This product is being marketed as an alternative to hormone replacement therapy for patients concerned about breast and endometrial cancer. Conjugated estrogen administration is associated with increased risk of breast cancer, endometrial hypoplasia, and endometrial cancer. Preliminary data indicate that raloxifene is not associated with development of breast or endometrial cancer. The role of raloxifene in the treatment of patients with metastatic breast cancer is currently unknown.

Antiestrogens bind to estrogen receptors and prevent receptor-mediated gene transcription and are therefore used to block the effect of estrogen on the end target. In postmenopausal and castrated women, the main source of estrogen is derived from the peripheral conversion of androstenedione, produced by the adrenal gland, into estrone and estradiol. This conversion requires the aromatase enzyme. Aromatase also catalyzes the conversion of androgens to estrogens in the ovary in premenopausal women and in extraglandular tissue, including the breast itself, in postmenopausal women. Therefore, aromatase inhibitors would effectively reduce the level of circulating estrogens, as well as that in the target organ. Aminoglutethimide is the prototype aromatase inhibitor. Aminoglutethimide has been compared to tamoxifen, adrenalectomy, and hypophysectomy in randomized trials. In general, response rates are equivalent, but in several trials, aminoglutethimide appeared to be more effective than tamoxifen. Aminoglutethimide has been demonstrated to produce secondary response rates equivalent or superior to progestational agents and surgical procedures in women who have become refractory to tamoxifen. Although effective, a significant limitation of aminoglutethimide is its toxicity profile. Aminoglutethimide inhibits the adrenal conversion of cholesterol to pregnenolone, resulting in a decrease in androstenedione and, thus, glucocorticoids. For this reason, aminoglutethimide has been traditionally administered concurrently with hydrocortisone, 40 mg/day divided into three doses at 3 PM, 6 PM, and 10 PM. The rationale behind this dosage administration of hydrocortisone is that it mimics the natural cortisol production and thereby prevents the suppression of hypothalamic-pituitary axis. Side effects of aminoglutethimide include nystagmus, ataxia, lethargy, dizziness, nausea, and rash. Although aminoglutethimide has historically been very effective in the treatment of women with metastatic breast cancer, its use has been considered third-line owing to its toxicity profile.

In 1997, two nonsteroidal aromatase inhibitors—anastrozole and letrozole—were introduced to the US market. Both have far greater selectivity and higher potency for the aromatase enzyme than does aminoglutethimide. Additional agents are in development. The major advantage of these newer compounds is their reduced toxicity profile, which consists mainly of nausea, hot flashes, and mild fatigue. Supplemental corticosteroids are not necessary with these newer agents. The new inhibitors have been compared with megestrol as second-line therapy in postmenopausal women with positive or unknown hormone receptor status who have failed tamoxifen therapy. Response rates throughout these studies have varied widely between 10% and 30% and have typically shown antitumor activity similar to that of megestrol, as well as improved tolerability. In one study, a higher response rate and an improved time to treatment failure were documented for letrozole.[78] Toxicity patterns showed more nausea, vomiting, and hot flashes with the aromatase inhibitor and more weight gain and fluid retention with progesterone. Studies that have compared anastrozole and letrozole to tamoxifen in first-line therapy of patients with metastatic disease have been conducted.

Both anastrozole and letrozole are approved for first-line therapy for advanced breast cancer in postmenopausal women. Large trials have compared these agents to tamoxifen and found similar response rates and a longer median time to progression for patients receiving the selective aromatase inhibitor.[79] A consistent finding in these trials was lower incidence of thromboembolic events and vaginal bleeding in patients who received selective aromatase inhibitors, which, together with the advantage in terms of time to progression, led to the conclusion that the new aromatase inhibitors may be superior to tamoxifen as first-line therapy for advanced breast cancer in postmenopausal women. Although difficult to tell from the published trials, this may be particularly true in patients who received tamoxifen as adjuvant therapy. As an increasing number of women receive 5 years of adjuvant tamoxifen therapy, it will be more common to see failures on tamoxifen converted to selective aromatase inhibitors as first-line hormonal therapy for metastatic disease. A selective irreversible, steroidal aromatase inactivator, exemestane (Aromasin), was introduced to the US market in 2000.[80] Exemestane is an irreversible, steroidal aromatase inactivator structurally related to the natural substrate anderstame diome and acts as a false substrate for the aromatase enzyme in its process to an intermediate that binds irreversibly to the active site of the enzyme causing its inactivation (also known as "suicide inhibition"). Exemestane is indicated for the treatment of advanced breast cancer in postmenopausal women whose disease has progressed following tamoxifen therapy.

Progestins such as megestrol acetate (Megace) and medroxyprogesterone acetate (Provera) have been compared with tamoxifen in randomized trials and have been found to yield equal response rates. Although there were no direct comparisons of these two forms of progestational therapy, they appear to be equally effective. Medroxyprogesterone acetate is more frequently used in Europe, and megestrol acetate is more frequently used in the United States. Several recent trials suggest that progestins may be an alternative to first-line therapy with tamoxifen. The most common dose used for medroxyprogesterone is 160 mg/day; the most common side effect is weight gain, occurring in 20% to 50% of patients. Patients experiencing weight gain may have fluid retention, but fluid retention is not totally responsible for total weight gain. In cachectic cancer patients, the weight gain may be desirable, but this is not uniformly true of all patients with metastatic breast cancer. Additional side effects associated with progestins include vaginal bleeding in 5% to 10% of patients either while patients are taking the progestational agent or when it is discontinued, and somewhat less than a 10% incidence of hot flashes.

Estrogens and androgens are used rarely today because these agents are more toxic than the other hormonal agents discussed thus far. About one-third of patients placed on estrogens will discontinue them because of side effects, the most important of which are vomiting and fluid retention. Less-common side effects include areolar hyperpigmentation, breast tenderness and engorgement, vaginal discharge, incontinence, hot flashes, and phlebitis. All the effective androgens have masculinizing effects, including hirsutism and acne, in more than 50% of patients. In addition to their toxicities, the mechanism by which these agents exert a therapeutic effect in breast cancer is unknown. About 20% response rates were reported in clinical trials conducted in the 1960s and 1970s in unselected groups of breast cancer patients. Given the recent availability of the aromatase inhibitors, use of androgens and estrogens will likely become obsolete.

CYTOTOXIC THERAPY

Cytotoxic chemotherapy is eventually required in most patients with metastatic breast cancer. Patients with hormone receptor-negative tumors require chemotherapy as initial therapy of symptomatic metastases. Patients who initially respond to hormonal manipulations eventually cease to respond and go on to require chemotherapy. Combination chemotherapy results in an objective response in about 40% of patients previously unexposed to chemotherapy. Most patients have partial responses, and complete disappearance of disease occurs in fewer than 10% of patients treated. The median duration of response is 5 to 12 months, but some patients will have an excellent response to an initial course of chemotherapy and may live 5 to 10 years or longer without evidence of disease. In general, median survival of patients after treatment with commonly used drug combinations for metastatic breast cancer is 14 to 33 months. The median time to response has ranged from 2 to 3 months in most studies, but this period depends in large part on the site of measurable disease. The median time to appearance of response is between 3 and 6 weeks in patients whose disease is primarily in the skin and lymph nodes, 6 and 9 weeks for patients with metastatic lung involvement, 15 weeks with hepatic involvement, and nearly 18 weeks in patients with bone involvement. Thus, it is oftentimes the case that an immediate response to therapy is not apparent and, in general, once a chemotherapy regimen has been initiated, it is continued until there is unequivocal evidence of progressive disease.

There are no well-defined clinical characteristics or established tests to identify patients likely to benefit from chemotherapy. Factors associated with an increased probability of response that have been identified include a good performance status, a limited number (one to two) of disease sites, and patients who respond to chemotherapy or hormonal therapy with a long disease-free interval. Patients whose disease progresses during chemotherapy have a lower probability of response to a different type of chemotherapy. However, this is not necessarily true for patients who are given chemotherapy after some interval during which they have received no chemotherapy. Patients who do not respond to endocrine therapy are as likely to respond to chemotherapy as patients who are treated with chemotherapy as their initial treatment modality. Age, menopausal status, and receptor status have not been associated with favorable or unfavorable response to chemotherapy. Although site of disease is not generally a predictor of response to chemotherapy, patients with visceral disease involvement typically respond poorly to all forms of therapy, including chemotherapy.

A number of chemotherapeutic agents have demonstrated activity in the treatment of breast cancer, including doxorubicin, cyclophosphamide, fluorouracil, methotrexate, mitoxantrone, vinblastine, mitomycin-C, thiotepa, and melphalan. The objective response rates reported with these drugs as single-agent therapy range from 20% to 40%. The drug discovery program of the National Cancer Institute and the pharmaceutical industry recently provided oncologists with a wide array of new chemotherapeutic agents that have considerable potential for breast cancer treatment. Foremost among these new agents are paclitaxel and docetaxel, which have impressive single-agent response rates as high as 50% to 60% in patients with metastatic breast disease who have not received prior chemotherapy for metastatic disease.[81] Paclitaxel (Taxol) was approved by the FDA in 1994 for single-agent treatment of metastatic breast cancer for patients who had relapsed following therapy with a doxorubicin-containing regimen. The recommended dose of paclitaxel is 175 mg/m^2 every 21 days, which is considerably higher than the dose used for treatment of ovarian cancer, the other disease for which paclitaxel has obtained FDA approval for use. Efforts are now being directed toward optimizing dose and schedule of single-agent paclitaxel in the metastatic setting. Recent reports describe a dose-dense regimen of 175 mg/m^2/wk (6 weeks, rest 2 weeks) with exceptional response rates.[82] Docetaxel (Taxotere) has also demonstrated high single-agent activity against metastatic breast cancer. The FDA approved it in 1995 for treatment of metastatic breast cancer for patients with relapse following therapy with doxorubicin-containing regimens. The approved dose is 60–100 mg/m^2 administered every 3 weeks. Impressive overall response rates of 54% to 68% were reported in four studies of docetaxel 100 mg/m^2 as first-line chemotherapy. Although randomized controlled studies comparing doses in the 60–100 mg/m^2 range have not been performed, a dose-response relationship with docetaxel has been demonstrated indirectly and, therefore, the importance of maintaining dose intensity with this agent is recognized. Myelosuppression is the major dose-limiting toxicity of docetaxel. Nonhematologic toxicities include fatigue, mucosal toxicity, mild to moderate nausea/vomiting, diarrhea, and neurosensory complaints. Although results from randomized trials are not yet available, docetaxel seems to be associated with less neuropathy, myalgia, and hypersensitivity than paclitaxel; but febrile neutropenia, fluid retention, and skin reactions appear to occur more frequently with the newer taxane. The median cumulative docetaxel dose to the onset of fluid retention is 400 mg/m^2 in nonpremedicated patients. Recent data demonstrate that the prophylactic use of dexamethasone 8 mg orally, twice a day for 3 to 5 days, starting 24 hours before docetaxel infusion can significantly delay the onset and reduce the severity of fluid retention.

Vinorelbine (Navelbine), a microtubule interactive agent, has also shown impressive response rates in metastatic breast cancer.[83] Vinorelbine was approved by the FDA in 1994 for the treatment of nonsmall cell lung cancer. It is not yet approved for breast cancer, but response rates in patients with advanced breast cancer to weekly IV doses of 30 mg/m^2 of vinorelbine range from 30% to 50% with an overall 5% complete response rate in the phase I and phase II studies reported. As has been observed with paclitaxel and docetaxel, patients with less prior treatment have a higher response rate than those who are more heavily pretreated. Importantly, paclitaxel, docetaxel, and vinorelbine do not appear to be cross-resistant with anthracyclines, which are currently considered first-line in treatment of metastatic breast cancer.

Combination chemotherapy regimens are associated with higher response rates than is single-agent therapy in the treatment of metastatic breast cancer. The chemotherapy regimens frequently used first-line in the metastatic setting are similar to the ones previously described for the adjuvant setting. As discussed above, the taxanes and vinorelbine have demonstrated unusually high activity as single agents in metastatic disease. Initial clinical trials of new cytotoxic agents involve patients who have experienced disease progression after treatment with the best available therapy. If the new drugs prove efficacious in these very poor-prognosis patients, trials will progress to patients with no prior treatment. Docetaxel, paclitaxel, and vinorelbine are currently moving into first-line treatment of metastatic breast cancer, oftentimes in combination with anthracyclines. When cytotoxic drugs are used in combination, it is important to consider the dose-response relationship and the toxicity profiles of the agents involved. It often is necessary to reduce the dose of drugs given in combination to avoid excessive toxicity, which may also inadvertently result in the administration of suboptimal doses. The emerging role of the taxanes and their optimal integration into new combination treatment strategies for patients with metastatic breast cancers is a major focus of research. Specific information regarding the most promising combination regimens and their attendant toxicities can be found only in the primary literature. In addition to determining the combination chemotherapy regimen of first, second, and third choice, other issues that remain to be determined in the management of metastatic breast cancer with systemic chemotherapy include optimal duration of treatment. Recognizing that complete response is not frequently observed, typically patients will receive one chemotherapy regimen until evidence of disease progression, at which time a second regimen may be initiated.

There is a clear dose-response effect for most of the drugs used to treat breast cancer. Research innovations designed to improve the efficacy of combination chemotherapy have included the use of high doses of drugs. Very high doses of single agents or combinations have been used with autologous HSCT to circumvent dose-limiting myelosuppression. Autologous HSCT was developed as a treatment for solid tumors responsive to, but not currently cured by, chemotherapy. Metastatic breast cancer has been the model for solid tumors in a number of large autologous HSCT research programs. Peripheral blood progenitor cells have largely replaced autologous bone marrow cells in most transplant programs because of their lower cost, greater convenience, and shortened time to engraftment. A recent review of the results of these programs suggests that patients with refractory metastatic disease treated with autologous HSCT have a high response rate, but the duration of response is brief.[84,85] But patients with metastatic breast cancer who obtain a complete response or a near complete response to conventional combination chemotherapy regimens may derive a far greater benefit from participation in high-dose chemotherapy with stem cell support. From the limited data available, it would appear that approximately 10% to 20% of patients with metastatic breast cancer who receive high-dose chemotherapy with stem cell support following a complete or near complete response to conventional chemotherapy may actually be cured of their disease or at least derive the benefit of a prolonged disease-free interval. Current controversy surrounds when to administer high-dose therapy in the small percentage of patients with metastatic disease who are complete responders to conventional chemotherapy (i.e., immediately following response to conventional therapy or at relapse). Ongoing work in this field includes the use of multicycle high-dose therapy, modulation of drug resistance, and use of maintenance therapy with biologic agents.

BIOLOGIC THERAPY

Trastuzumab (Herceptin) is a humanized monoclonal antibody that binds with a specific epitope of the HER-2/neu protein. The parent antibody (monoclonal antibody, 4D5) induces a specific biologic response through activation of HER-2/neu; this response includes autophosphorylation of the tyrosine kinase internal domain leading to inhibition of cellular growth, decreased malignant potential, and possibly reversal of resistance to endocrine therapy and certain chemotherapies. Single-agent treatment with trastuzumab has a response rate of 15% to 20% of patients with HER-2/neu overexpressing cancers.[86] Moreover, the results of a large randomized trial demonstrated that trastuzumab is at least additive and, perhaps, synergistic with other chemotherapeutic agents.[87] In combination with first-line doxorubicin and cyclophosphamide, trastuzumab modestly increased response rates and time to progression when compared to doxorubicin and cyclophosphamide alone. In a second part of the same clinical trial, patients with doxorubicin refractory metastatic breast cancer were randomly assigned to treatment with either trastuzumab and paclitaxel or paclitaxel alone. The patients treated with the combination experienced nearly a doubling in response (paclitaxel 25% response rate, paclitaxel and trastuzumab 57% response rate) time to progression (paclitaxel 4.2 months, paclitaxel plus trastuzumab 7.1 months) and even survival (paclitaxel 18.4 months and paclitaxel plus trastuzumab 22.1 months) when compared to those treated with paclitaxel alone. The studies also suggest that trastuzumab is reasonably well tolerated. Although trastuzumab does not appear to enhance hematopoietic, hepatic or renal toxicity of standard chemotherapy, an increase in congestive heart failure was observed in both of the large studies. The common adverse effects are infusion-related, primarily fever and chills, and occur in about 40% of patients during the initial infusion.[88] Other infusion-related reactions include nausea, vomiting, pain at tumor site, rigors, headaches, dizziness, dyspnea, hypotension, rash, and asthenia. These reactions are usually mild to moderate and rarely require discontinuation of therapy. Acetaminophen and diphenhydramine may be used, alone or in combination with, reducing the trastuzumab infusion rate to treat these reactions. If infusion-related symptoms occur, subsequent doses should be infused over 90 minutes. Infusion over 30 minutes is appropriate if symptoms subside. Trastuzumab is administered as an initial loading dose of 4 mg/kg; this is followed by a 2-mg/kg dose administered weekly. Trastuzumab, when used in combination with paclitaxel, paclitaxel is administered every 3 weeks. Many studies are ongoing that are evaluating different combinations of trastuzumab and promising results have been reported with the combination of trastuzumab plus vinorelbine.[89] Although trastuzumab is currently indicated only for the treatment of metastatic breast cancer, several cooperative groups are evaluating its safety and efficacy in women with HER-2/neu overexpressing breast cancer in the adjuvant setting. It should be noted that only 20% to 30% of patients with metastatic breast cancer overexpress HER-2/neu and commercially available immunohistochemical tests that are reported back as HER-2/neu-2+ positive are often negative by the more sensitive and specific FISH technique. To date, there is no benefit associated with the administration of trastuzumab to the subset of patients who are HER-2/neu-negative and a very questionable benefit associated with administration of trastuzumab to women who are HER-2neu-positive by immunohistochemical staining.

RADIATION THERAPY

Radiation is an important modality in the treatment of symptomatic metastatic disease. The most common indication for the treatment with radiation therapy is painful bone metastases or other localized sites of disease refractory to systemic therapy. Radiation therapy gives significant pain relief to approximately 90% of patients who are treated for painful bone metastases. Radiation is also an important modality in the palliative treatment of metastatic brain lesions and spinal cord lesions, which respond poorly to systemic therapy, as well as eye or orbit lesions and other sites where significant accumulation of tumor cells occurs.

PREVENTION AND EARLY DETECTION

Current efforts at breast cancer prevention are directed toward the identification and removal of risk factors. Unfortunately, a number of risk factors associated with development of breast cancer, such as family history of breast cancer or personal history of breast or other gynecologic malignancies, cannot be modified. Isolation and cloning of breast cancer susceptibility genes now allows screening of women with histories suggestive of "breast cancer families" and identification of appropriate candidates for prophylactic bilateral mastectomy. There are currently no absolute indications for prophylactic bilateral mastectomy. This surgery is considered for women at very high risk for the development of breast cancer, particularly if the women's breasts are difficult to evaluate by both physical examination and mammography, and they have persistent disabling fears that they will have the disease.

In the past 5 years, there has been increasing interest in "chemoprevention" of breast cancer. This includes interventions directed at inhibiting neoplastic development through pharmacologic measures. Two important agents being studied in research on breast cancer chemoprevention are retinoids and tamoxifen. Retinoids (all vitamin A [Retinol] and its isomer derivatives and synthetic analogs) are biologic regulators of orderly epithelial cell development and are therefore potentially ideal agents for controlling abnormal epithelial proliferation that occurs in carcinogenesis. The agent that is currently receiving the most attention as a chemoprevention agent is tamoxifen. As previously described, tamoxifen is useful as an adjunct after treatment of primary breast cancer, especially in postmenopausal women. In randomized trials of tamoxifen as an adjuvant treatment for breast cancer, women who received tamoxifen were also found to have a reduced incidence of contralateral primary breast carcinomas.

The NSABP recently conducted a trial in the United States comparing 5 years of tamoxifen therapy to placebo in 16,000 women aged 35 years and older who were at increased risk for breast cancer (the Breast Cancer Prevention Trial [BCPT]). This trial was the first large chemoprevention trial conducted in the United States and generated a great deal of controversy. Controversy largely surrounded the unknown benefit of tamoxifen therapy as a chemoprevention agent, and the potential for toxicity associated with its administration. Tamoxifen has been repeatedly shown to be a relatively safe drug with an acceptable toxicity profile when used to treat patients with breast cancer. But its estrogenic effects on the uterus and possibly the coagulation system renders increases the risk of serious adverse effects. The results of the NSABP breast cancer prevention trial were published in the Journal of the National Cancer Institute in September 1998.[74] The design of this trial included women ($n = 13{,}388$) at increased risk for breast cancer because they were 60 years of age or older, with women 35 to 59 years of age with a 5-year predicted risk for breast cancer of at least 1.66%, or who had a history of lobular carcinoma *in situ* were randomly assigned to receive placebo ($n = 6{,}707$) or 20 mg/day of tamoxifen ($n = 6{,}681$) for 5 years. Gail's algorithm, based on a multivariate logistic regression model using combinations of risks factors, was used to estimate the probability of occurrence of breast cancer over time. Tamoxifen reduced the risk of invasive breast cancer by 49% ($p < 0.001$) with cumulative incidence through 69 months of followup of 43.4 versus 22.0/1,000 women in the placebo and tamoxifen group, respectively. The decreased risk occurred in women aged 49 years or younger (44%), 50 to 59 years (51%), and 60 years or older (55%). Risk was also reduced in women with a history of lobular carcinoma *in situ* (56%), with atypical hyperplasia (86%) in those in any category of predicted 5-year risk. Tamoxifen also reduced the risk of noninvasive breast cancer by 50% ($p < 0.002$). Tamoxifen reduced the recurrence of estrogen receptor positive tumors by 69% but no difference in occurrence of estrogen receptor negative tumors was seen. Toxicities associated with tamoxifen were described in the section on adjuvant endocrine therapy. A recent report by the American Society of Clinical Oncology technology assessment on breast cancer risk reduction comparing tamoxifen and raloxifene concluded that for women with a defined 5-year projected risk of breast cancer of greater than 1.66, tamoxifen may be offered to reduce their risk.[90]

TABLE 125–13. Guidelines for Early Detection of Breast Cancer

	U.S. Preventive Task Force	American Cancer Society	National Cancer Institute
Breast self-exam (BSE)	NR	Monthly (20+)	NR
Clinical breast exam (CBE)	Annual 50–69 with mammography	Every 3 years (20–40)	Every 3 years (20–40) Annual (40+)
Mammogram	NR (40–49) 1–2 years (50–69)	Annual (40+)	NR (40–49) Annual (50+)

NR = not recommended.

Although raloxifene was shown to reduce the risk of invasive breast cancer by similar percentage, in clinical trials where it was evaluated for its benefits for osteoporosis, the task force concluded the use of raloxifene to currently be reserved for its approved indication which is to prevent bone loss in post-menopausal women. The ongoing STAR trial directly compares the efficacy and safety of tamoxifen and raloxifene in chemoprevention of breast cancer. Use of raloxifene for this indication should await the results of this trial. At the present time, the effect of using tamoxifen or raloxifene with other medications, such as hormone replacement therapy and using tamoxifen and raloxifene in combination or sequentially, has not been adequately studied.

The rationale for early detection of breast cancer is based on the clear relationship between stage of breast cancer at diagnosis and the probability for cure. Thus, if all breast cancer could be detected at a very early stage of the disease (i.e., small primary tumor and negative lymph nodes), then more patients with the disease could be cured. Screening guidelines for early detection of breast cancer have been put forward by the American Cancer Society, the US Preventive Task Force, and the National Cancer Institute (Table 125–13).[91,92] Currently, the American Cancer Society recommends that all women over the age of 20 years perform monthly breast self-examinations. There is evidence to support this recommendation, and at least one investigator demonstrated that women who perform breast self-examinations were generally diagnosed with an earlier stage of the disease and had a higher 5-year survival rate when compared to women who did not perform self-examinations.[93] However, the results of a recently reported randomized clinical trial in 267,040 women, conducted by the NCI in Shanghai, found that the group of women trained and performing monthly breast self-exams did not have earlier stage disease at diagnosis and underwent more biopsies for benign conditions, as compared to the group who were not trained to perform monthly breast self-exams.[94] Although the results of this study have dampened enthusiasm, most US experts continue to promote the value of breast self-exam as an effective screening procedure. Numerous brochures are available that outline the current methodology for performing breast examinations. It is generally agreed that for this to be an effective screening tool, the examination should be thorough and conducted at approximately the same time in a woman's monthly cycle. Recommendations for breast examination by a physician (clinical breast exam) vary among the three groups. Patients discover most breast cancers during regular self-examinations. Therefore, the value of the clinical breast exam recommendation for women who perform regular self-examinations is questionable. However, an annual physician examination may be of value to the many women who fail to perform monthly self-examinations.

Clearly, the largest area of controversy in screening recommendations for breast cancer surrounds annual mammography. Most, if not all, guidelines recommend annual mammography for women 50 years of age and older. Nearly 75% of all breast cancer occurs in women 50 years of age or older and it has been conclusively demonstrated that regular use of screening mammography can reduce mortality from breast cancer by 20% to 40% in this age group. Controversy regarding the use of screening mammography is largely confined to women younger than 50 years of age. The American Cancer Society recommends that a baseline mammography be performed in women who are between 35 and 40 years of age, and that screening mammography occur every 1 to 2 years in the 40- to 50-year-old age group. However, in December 1993, the National Cancer Institute (NCI) withdrew its support of the use of screening mammography in women younger than 50 years of age. This was based on a report of the NCI's International Workshop on Screening for Breast Cancer held in February 1993.[95] Data from eight major randomized control trials of breast cancer screening performed over the previous 30 years were reviewed and it was concluded that no benefit from screening women between the ages of 40 and 49 years was apparent 5 to 7 years after enrollment into any of these studies. Possible reasons for these findings include the much lower incidence of breast cancer in women 40 to 49 years of age and the increased density of breast tissue found in menstruating women, which renders detection of lesions by mammography more difficult.

Opponents of screening women younger than 50 years of age suggest that multiple studies have failed to prove a benefit. However, proponents for screening women 40 to 49 years of age claim that the studies were not designed to detect a difference of a 25% to 30% decrease in mortality. A recent review of these trials concluded that none of these trials included in the NCI analysis had enough statistical power to be able to provide clear proof of benefit for screening women ages 40 to 49 years because none of the trials involved sufficient numbers of women in these age groups.[96] These authors suggest that the conclusion from these trials is that a benefit from screening was demonstrated that lacked statistical significance. Even with all their performance and design flaws (insufficient numbers of women ages 40 to 49 years, poor-quality mammography, single-view mammography, 2-year screening interval, high contamination rate, and high intervention threshold), five of the eight trials suggest a benefit, which indicates the benefit would be significant if the number of women in these trials had been sufficiently large to permit statistical significance. The debate regarding the value of screening mammography in women younger than 50 years of age continues among various health care providers and is the source of great confusion for the health care consumer.

The NIH conducted another Consensus Development Panel to address cancer screening for women ages 40 to 49 in January 1997.[97] The NIH Consensus Statement on Breast Cancer Screening of Women Ages 40 to 49 contains two reports: a majority report and a minority report. Although the entire panel initially achieved consensus at the end of the consensus conference, 2 of the 12 panel members subsequently differed on the draft document in the weeks that followed and ultimately did not agree entirely with the majority statement. It should be emphasized that the January 1997 press release of the panel's report created a great deal of public and political pressure on the NCI to reverse its conclusion, which, once again, found that data currently available do not warrant a universal recommendation for mammography for all women in their forties. The panel went on to state that "each woman should decide for herself whether to undergo mammography. . . . Her decision may be based, not only on objective analysis of the scientific evidence and consideration of her individual medical history, but also on how she perceives and weighs each potential risk and benefit, the value she places on each, and how she deals with uncertainty."[97] The report further states that information should be developed and provided to women in their forties regarding potential benefits and risks to enable each woman to make the most appropriate decision. Educational materials for physicians were also recommended in the report. The minority report believed that risks of mammography were overemphasized by the majority and concluded that the data did support the recommendation for mammography screening for all women in this age group, and that survival benefit and diagnosis at an earlier stage outweighed the potential risks.

Significant advances in the safety and efficacy of screening mammography have occurred during the past two decades. These advances have enabled superior visualization of breast and breast tissue with a concurrent reduction in the dose of radiation that is delivered. Approximately 10% of all palpable masses are not detected by mammography. This is most commonly observed in premenopausal women, and may be directly related to the increased density of breast tissue in this estrogen-rich environment. Radiation from yearly mammograms during the ages 40 to 49 has been estimated as possibly causing one additional death per 10,000 women.[97] As women age, incidence for developing mammography-related breast cancer is lower because of the lower carcinogenic effects of radiation in older women. Although the safety and efficacy of screening mammography in terms of image quality and dosimetry are very acceptable, the American College of Radiology (ACR) has recognized for some years the need for greater quality control in mammography. A voluntary accreditation program developed by this organization and adopted by various state and federal agencies has greatly improved the overall quality of mammography in the majority of facilities in this country. Many of the details of the accreditation process have recently been adopted for use by governmental agencies, culminating in the Mammography Quality Standards of 1992. This act, which essentially codifies the ACR program, assures that all mammographic facilities will now be required to achieve a common high standard of quality assurance. Responsibility for operation of the act has been given to the FDA. As of October 1, 1994, all facilities that offer mammography must be FDA-certified to remain open. Passage of this landmark legislation, as well as provision of appropriate levels of funding to conduct this program, represents an important contribution to the health of women.

EVALUATION OF THERAPEUTIC OUTCOMES

The desired therapeutic outcome of adjuvant therapy of breast cancer differs significantly from that of metastatic disease. Adjuvant therapy—chemotherapy, hormonal therapy, or both—is administered with curative intent. The rationale for adjuvant therapy in breast cancer is that breast cancer, even when diagnosed in early stages when clinical evidence of distant spread is not apparent, is a systemic disease that spreads early to distant sites. Adjuvant therapy is intended to eradicate these micrometastases and thus cure the patient of breast cancer. Therefore, the overall goal of adjuvant therapy is to cure the disease, which is something that cannot be fully evaluated for years following initial diagnosis and treatment. In addition, because there is no clinical evidence of disease at the time adjuvant therapy is administered, assessment of disease response is not possible. Instead, a predetermined number of cycles of adjuvant therapy and/or years of hormonal therapy is administered. Adjuvant chemotherapy is often associated with significant toxicity. Maintaining dose intensity has been demonstrated to be important in the cure of disease and, therefore, optimizing supportive care measures such as antiemetics and growth factors is highly recommended.

Palliation is the therapeutic outcome in treatment of metastatic breast cancer. In general, the least-toxic therapies are used initially with increasingly aggressive therapies applied in a sequential fashion and in a manner that does not significantly compromise the quality of the patient's life. Tumor response to a particular treatment regimen may be measured by clinical chemistry such as liver enzyme elevation in a patient with hepatic metastases, or imaging techniques such as bone scans or chest x-rays. However, assessment of the patient's clinical status and symptom control is often adequate to evaluate response to the therapy administered. In the patient with metastatic breast cancer, it is common to initiate hormonal therapy or chemotherapy and continue administration until signs and symptoms of disease progress or new signs and symptoms present. Optimizing quality of life is the therapeutic end point in the treatment of patients with metastatic breast cancer. A number of valid and reliable tools are available for objective assessment of quality of life in patients with breast cancer.

CONCLUSIONS

Breast cancer is the most commonly occurring cancer in women in the United States, and is second only to lung cancer as the most common cancer cause of death. The incidence of breast cancer has been increasing during the past 50 years and has increased rapidly since the early 1980s. It is unclear whether the recent increase in the incidence of breast cancer reflects a true increase in the new cases of this disease, or, instead, increased detection of the disease by screening mammography. The etiology of breast cancer is unknown, but a number of factors that increase a woman's chances of developing the disease have been identified. These risk factors, as well as information regarding the biology of the disease, suggest that a complex interplay between hormones, genetic factors, and environmental and life-style influences all contribute to the etiology of this disease. The recent identification of the BRCA1 and BRCA2 genes, tumor-suppresser genes important in the development of inherited and perhaps sporadic breast and ovarian cancer, holds promise in identifying patients at high risk, as well as improving our basic understanding of the causes of breast and ovarian cancer.

Most breast cancers are diagnosed in early stages before the disease has disseminated to sites distant from the breast. Treatment consists of local management, as well as systemic adjuvant therapy with either chemotherapy, hormonal therapy, or a combination of these. Breast-conservation therapy, which consists of complete removal of the tumor (lumpectomy), combined with breast irradiation and axillary lymph node sampling, is currently the preferred method of treatment for most patients with localized breast cancer. Patients who are not candidates for breast conservation or who do not choose this local therapy will generally receive the modified radical mastectomy.

It is apparent from clinical and laboratory experiments and observation that the spread of breast cancer via the bloodstream occurs early in the course of the disease. This results in patients relapsing with systemic metastatic disease following local curative therapy. The likelihood of later development of metastatic disease is related to the size of the primary tumor, presence of lymph node involvement and number of nodes affected, and a number of additional pathologic prognostic factors, which include proliferative capacity, nuclear grade, hormone receptor status, and presence or absence of oncogenes and other protein products. Systemic adjuvant therapy is commonly administered to patients with localized breast cancer following surgical procedures to diminish the risk of or delay disease recurrence. Specific recommendations for adjuvant therapy are determined by stage of the disease, age of the patient, presence of hormone receptors in the primary tumor, as well as other pathologic prognostic factors. An NIH consensus conference, as well as an international consensus group, has developed adjuvant therapy treatment recommendations, and these treatment recommendations continue to evolve as new data become available.

Advanced breast cancer includes locally advanced breast cancer (stage III) and metastatic breast cancer (stage IV). Treatment of stage III breast cancer generally consists of a combination of surgery, radiation, and chemotherapy administered in an aggressive approach. Although response rates and survival have improved, there is still much progress to be made in stage III breast cancer. Metastatic breast cancer is usually incurable. The only exception to this is that some promising long-term response rates have been observed in a subset of patients with metastatic disease who have a complete or near complete response to conventional chemotherapy and then receive high-dose chemotherapy with stem cell support. Unfortunately, this represents a small number of the total population of patients with metastatic breast cancer. Metastatic breast cancer is treated with endocrine therapy or combination chemotherapy. Patients who are hormone receptor-positive will generally receive initial endocrine therapy followed by combination chemotherapy when endocrine therapy fails. Patients who are hormone receptor-negative or who have disease involving the liver or central nervous system will generally receive combination chemotherapy as first-line therapy of metastatic disease. Combination chemotherapy will result in an objective response in about 50% of patients previously unexposed to chemotherapy. Most patients have partial response, and complete disappearance of disease occurs in fewer than 20% of patients treated. Median duration of response is 5 to 12 months; although some patients will have an excellent response to an initial course of chemotherapy and may live 5 to 10 years without evidence of disease. In general, survival of patients after treatment with commonly used drug combinations for metastatic breast cancer is a median of 14 to 33 months. Response to second- and third-line combination chemotherapy has been on the order of 20% to 40%. This is in large part dependent on previous chemotherapy regimens the patient has received. The availability of paclitaxel, docetaxel, and vinorelbine offers the promise of more successful second- and third-line treatment of metastatic breast cancer in the future.

Current efforts at breast cancer prevention are directed toward the identification and removal of risk factors. In addition, two agents, the retinoids and tamoxifen, are being evaluated for their ability to prevent breast cancer. Any statement regarding the value of these modalities awaits the results of ongoing clinical trials. Early detection of breast cancer remains an important modality for decreasing breast cancer mortality. The rationale for early detection of breast cancer is based on the clear relationship between stage of breast cancer at diagnosis and the probability of a cure. The American Cancer Society, the US Preventive Task Force, and the National Cancer Institute have developed screening guidelines for early detection of breast cancer. Although all these agencies agree that annual clinical breast exam and screening mammographies should be performed in women older than 50 years of age, controversy exists regarding the value of screening women in the 40- to 50-year-old age group. This controversy has, unfortunately, created a great deal of confusion in the general public.

Intensive research efforts are ongoing in all aspects of breast cancer etiology, detection, prevention, and treatment. Efforts in the past have resulted in substantial reduction in mortality in selected patient subsets. The information obtained in the next decade will hopefully result in the knowledge required to significantly reduce mortality from breast cancer for all women.

▶ PRINCIPLES OF PHARMACOTHERAPY

- Breast cancer is most commonly diagnosed in early stages, when it is a highly curable malignancy.
- Local therapy of early stage breast cancer consists of either modified radical mastectomy or lumpectomy plus external beam radiation therapy.
- Adjuvant systemic therapy with tamoxifen (20 mg/day) for 5 years reduces the risk of breast cancer recurrence by 50% and risk of death by 25% in all estrogen receptor-positive women.
- Adjuvant systemic therapy with combination chemotherapy reduces mortality from breast cancer in all patient subsets but is of greatest benefit in estrogen receptor-negative premenopausal patients.
- Initial therapy of metastatic breast cancer in women with hormone receptor-positive tumors should consist of hormonal therapy.
- Women with metastatic breast cancer who are hormone receptor positive and respond to an initial hormonal manipulation will usually respond to a second hormonal manipulation.
- Twenty-five percent to 50% of women with metastatic breast cancer will respond to chemotherapy regimens; doxorubicin- and taxane-containing regimens are the most active.
- The goal of adjuvant chemotherapy is curative, while the goal of chemotherapy in the metastatic setting is palliative. Therefore, dose intensity is more important in the adjuvant setting than in the metastatic setting.
- Although experts do not agree on the benefits of annual screening mammography in women younger than 50 years of age, a large number of national and international studies demonstrate a 20% to 40% reduction in breast cancer mortality from annual or biannual screening mammography in women aged 50 to 70 years.

REFERENCES

1. Greenlee RT, Hill-Harmon MB, Murray T, Thun D. Cancer Statistics 2001. CA Cancer J Clin 2001;51:15–38.
2. Ries LAG, Eisner MP, Kosary CL, et al, eds. SEER Cancer Statistics Review: 1973–1998. Bethesda, MD, National Cancer Institute, 2001.
3. Feuer EJ, Wun LM, Boring CC, et al. The lifetime risk of developing breast cancer. J Natl Cancer Inst 1993;85:892–897.
4. Miller BA, Feuer EJ, Hankey BF. Recent incidence trends for breast cancer in women and the relevance of early detection: An update. CA Cancer J Clin 1993;43:27–41.

5. Abeloff MD, Lichter AS, Niederhuber JE, Pierce LJ, Aziz DC. Breast. Management of specific malignancies. In: Clinical Oncology. Churchill Livingstone, 1995:1617–1714.
6. American Cancer Society home page. Available at: http://www.cancer.org. Accessed February 28, 2001.
7. Harris JR, Lippman ME, Veronesi U, Willett W. Breast cancer. Part 1. N Engl J Med 1992;327:319–328.
8. Colditz GA, Stampfer MJ, Willett WC. Prospective study of estrogen replacement therapy and risk of breast cancer in postmenopausal women. JAMA 1990;264:2648–2653.
9. Dupont WD, Page DL. Menopausal estrogen replacement therapy and breast cancer. Arch Intern Med 1991;151:67–72.
10. Steinberg KK, Thacker SB, Smith SJ, et al. A meta-analysis of the effect of estrogen replacement therapy on the risk of breast cancer. JAMA 1991;265:1985–1990.
11. DiSaia PJ. Hormone-replacement therapy in patients with breast cancer. Cancer 1993;71:1490s–1500s.
12. Romieu I, Berlin JA, Colditz G. Oral contraceptives and breast cancer: Review and meta-analysis. Cancer 1990;66:2253–2263.
13. Harris JR, Morrow M, Bonadonna G. Cancer of the breast. In: DeVita VT Jr, Hellman S, Rosenberg SA, eds. Cancer: Principles of Oncology, 4th ed. Philadelphia, Lippincott, 1993:1264–1324.
14. Thompson WD. Genetic epidemiology of breast cancer. Cancer 1994;74: 279–287.
15. Weber BL, Abel JK, Brody LC, et al. Familial breast cancer. Cancer 1994; 74:1013–1020.
16. Struewing JP, Hartge P, Wacholder S, et al. The risk of cancer associated with specific mutations of BRCA1 and BRCA2 among Ashkenazi Jews. N Engl J Med 1997;336:1401–1408.
17. Byers T. Nutritional risk factors for breast cancer. Cancer 1994;74: 288–295.
18. Howe GR. Dietary fat and breast cancer risks. Cancer 1994;74:1078–1084.
19. Howe GR, Friedenreich CM, Jain M, Miller AB. A cohort study of fat intake and risk of breast cancer. J Natl Cancer Inst 1991;83:336–340.
20. Nagao M, Ushijima T, Wakabayashi K, et al. Dietary carcinogens and mammary carcinogenesis. Cancer 1994;74:1063–1069.
21. Schapira DV, Kumar NB, Lyman GH. Obesity, body fat distribution and sex hormones in breast cancer patients. Cancer 1991;67:2215–2218.
22. Longnecker MP. Alcohol consumption in relation to risk of breast cancer. Cancer Causes Control 1994;5:73–82.
23. Feig SA, Ehrlich SM. Estimation of radiation risk from screening mammography: Recent trends and comparison with expected benefits. Radiology 1990;174:639–647.
24. McKenna RJ. The abnormal mammogram radiographic findings, diagnostic optional, pathology, and stage of cancer diagnosis. Cancer 1994;79: 244–255.
25. Baines CJ, Miller AB, Kopans DB. Canadian national breast screening study: Assessment of technical quality by external review. Am J Radiol 1990;155:743–747.
26. Kopans DB. The Breast Imaging Report. Philadelphia, Lippincott, 1989:351–353.
27. Frykberg ER, Bland KI. Overview of the biology and management of ductal carcinoma *in situ* of the breast. Cancer 1994;74:350–361.
28. Frykberg ER, Ames FC, Bland KI. Current concepts for management of early (*in situ* and occult invasive) breast carcinoma. In: Bland KI, Copeland EM, eds. The Breast: Comprehensive Management of Benign and Malignant Diseases. Philadelphia, WB Saunders, 1991:731–751.
29. Fisher B, Constantio J, Redmond C, et al. Lumpectomy compared with lumpectomy and radiation therapy for the treatment of intraductal breast cancer. N Engl J Med 1993;328:1581–1586.
30. Fisher B, Slack NH, Bross IDJ. Cancer of the breast: Size of neoplasm and prognosis. Cancer 1969;24:1071–1080.
31. Nemoto T, Vana T, Bedwani RN, et al. Management and survival of female breast cancer. Cancer 1980;45:2917–2924.
32. Valagussa P, Bonadonna G, Veronesi U. Patterns of relapse and survival in operable breast carcinoma with positive and negative axillary nodes. Tumori 1978;64:241–258.
33. McGuire WL, Clark GM. Prognosis in breast cancer. Recent Results Cancer Res 1989;115:170–174.
34. Osborne CK. Prognostic factors in breast cancer. Princ Pract Oncol Updates 1990;4:1–11.
35. Mansour EG, Ravdin PM, Dressler L. Prognostic factors in early breast cancer. Cancer 1994;74:381–400.
36. Osborne CKO, Ravdin PM. Adjuvant systemic therapy of primary breast cancer. In: Harris JR, Lippman ME, Morrow M, Osborne CK, eds. Diseases of the Breast, 2nd ed. Philadelphia, Lippincott-Williams & Wilkins, 2000:599–632.
37. Hedley DW, Clark GM, Cornelisse CJ, et al. Consensus review of the clinical utility of DNA cytometry in carcinoma of the breast. Cytometry 1993;14:482–485.
38. Fisher B, Redmond C, Fisher E, et al. Relative worth of estrogen or progesterone receptor and pathologic characteristics of differentiation as indicators of prognosis in node-negative breast and Bowel Project Protocol B 06. J Clin Oncol 1988;6:1076–1087.
39. Gasparini G, Pozza F, Harris AL. Evaluating the potential usefulness of new prognostic and predictive indicators in node-negative breast cancer patients. J Natl Cancer Inst 1993;85:1206–1219.
40. Ross JS, Fletcher JA. HER-2/neu (c-erb-B2) gene and protein in breast cancer. Am J Clin Pathol 1999;112(suppl):S53–S67.
41. Thor AD, Berry DA, Budman DR, et al. erbB-2, p53, and efficacy of adjuvant therapy in lymph node-positive breast cancer. J Natl Cancer Inst 1998;90:1346–1360.
42. Paik S, Bryant J, Park C, et al. erbB-2 and response to doxorubicin in patients with axillary lymph node-positive, hormone receptor-negative breast cancer. J Natl Cancer Inst 1998;90:1361–1370.
43. NIH Consensus Development Conference Statement. Adjuvant therapy for breast cancer 2000, November 1–3:1–23. www.NIH.GOV webset. Accessed February 28, 2001.
44. Nemoto T, Vana J, Bedwani RN, et al. Management and survival of female breast cancer: Results of a national survey by the American College of Surgeons. Cancer 1980;45:2917–2924.
45. Fisher B, Redmond C, Fisher ER, et al. Ten-year results of a randomized clinical trial comparing radical mastectomy and total mastectomy with or without radiation. N Engl J Med 1985;312:674–681.
46. Fisher B, Redmond C, Poisson R, et al. Eight-year results of a randomized clinical trial comparing total mastectomy and lumpectomy with or without irradiation in the treatment of breast cancer. N Engl J Med 1989;320:822–828.
47. Ivens D, Hoe AL, Podd TJ, et al. Assessment of morbidity from complete axillary dissection. Br J Cancer 1992;66:136–138.
48. Keramopoulos A, Tsionou C, Minaretzis D, et al. Arm morbidity following treatment of breast cancer with total axillary dissection: A multivariated approach. Oncology 1993;50:445–449.
49. Hsueh EC, Hansen N, Giuliano A. Intraoperative lymphatic mapping and sentinel lymph node dissection in breast cancer. CA Cancer J Clin 2000; 50:279–291.
50. Early Breast Cancer Trialists' Collaborative Group T. Systemic treatment of early breast cancer by hormonal, cytotoxic, or immune therapy: 133 randomized trials involving 31,000 recurrences and 24,000 deaths among 75,000 women. Lancet 1992;339:1–15.
51. Early Breast Cancer Trialists' Collaborative Group. Tamoxifen for early breast cancer: An overview of the randomized trials. Lancet 1998;351: 1451–1467.
52. Breast Cancer Trialists' Collaborative Group. Polychemotherapy for early breast cancer: An overview of the randomized trials. Lancet 1998;351: 1451–1467.
53. Gelber RD, Cole BF, Goldhirsch A, Roso C, Fisher B, Osborne CR, Boccardo F, Gray R, Gordon NH, Bengtsson NO, Suelda P: Adjuvant chemotherapy plus tamoxifen compared with tamoxifen alone for postmenopausal breast cancer. Lancet 1996;347(9008):1066–1071.
54. Ravidin PM, Siminoff IA, Harvey JA. Survey of breast cancer patients concerning their knowledge and expectations of adjuvant therapy. J Clin Oncol 1998;16:515–521.

55. Lindley C, Vasa S, Sawyer WT, Winer EP. Quality of life and preferences for treatment following systemic adjuvant therapy for early stage breast cancer. J Clin Oncol 1998;16:380–387.
56. Goldhirsch A, Glick JH, Gelber RD, et al. Meeting highlights: International Consensus Panel on the Treatment of Primary Breast Cancer. J Natl Cancer Inst 1998;90:1601–1608.
57. NCCN Guidelines. Oncology 2000.
58. Hortobagyi G. Adjuvant therapy for breast cancer. Annu Rev Med 2000;51:377–392.
59. Buzdar AU, Hortobagyi GN. Recent advances in adjuvant therapy of breast cancer. Semin Oncol 1999;26(suppl 12):21–27.
60. Taxol (Paclitaxel) Product Information. Bristol Myers, Illinois, July 2000.
61. Ravdin PM, Green S, Albain KS, et al. Initial report of the SWOG biological correlative study of c-erbB-2 expression as a predictor of outcome in a trial comparing adjuvant CAF T with tamoxifen (T) alone. Proc Am Soc Clin Oncol 1998;17:97a.
62. Comparison of fluorescence *in situ* hybridization and immunohistochemistry for the evaluation of HER-2/neu in breast cancer. J Clin Oncol 1999;17:1974–1982.
63. Winer EP. Quality-of-life research in patients with breast cancer. Cancer 1994;74:410–415.
64. Levine MN, Gent M, Hirsh J, et al. The thrombogenic effect of anticancer drug therapy in women with stage II breast cancer. N Engl J Med 1988;318:404–407.
65. Curtis RE, Boice JD Jr, Stovall M, et al. Risk of leukemia after chemotherapy and radiation treatment for breast cancer. N Engl J Med 1992;326:1745–1751.
66. Henderson IC, Sloss JL, Jaffe N, et al. Serial studies of cardiac function in patients receiving adriamycin. Cancer Treat Rep 1978;62:923–929.
66. Slevin ML, Stubbs L, Plant HJ, et al. Attitudes to chemotherapy: Comparing views of patients with cancer: Attitudes of doctors, nurses, and the general public. BMJ 1990;300:1458–1460.
67. Lindley C, Vasa S, Sawyer WT, Winer EP. Quality of life and preferences for treatment following systemic adjuvant therapy for early stage breast cancer. J Clin Oncol 1998;16:1380–1387.
68. Love RR, Mazess RB, Barden HS, et al. Effects of tamoxifen on bone mineral density in postmenopausal women with breast cancer. N Engl J Med 1992;326:852–856.
69. Love RR, Wiebe DA, Newcomb PA, et al. Effects of tamoxifen on cardiovascular risk factors in postmenopausal women. Ann Intern Med 1992;115:860–864.
70. Ward HWC. Antiestrogen therapy for breast cancer: A trial of tamoxifen at two dose levels. Br Med J 1973;1:13–14.
71. Jordan VC. Tamoxifen: Too much of a good thing? J Clin Oncol 1999;17:2629.
72. Decensi A, Gandini S, Guerrieri-Gonzaga A, et al. Effect of blood tamoxifen concentrations on surrogate biomarkers in a trial of dose reduction in healthy women. J Clin Oncol 1999;17:2633–2638.
73. Fisher B, Costantino JP, Wickerham DL, et al. Tamoxifen for prevention of breast cancer: Report of the national surgical adjuvant breast and bowel project P-1 study. J Natl Cancer Inst 1998;90:1371–1388.
74. Fareston (Toremifene) Product Information. Roberts Pharmaceutical Company, Eatontown, NJ 1999.
75. Holli K, Valavaara R, Blanco G, et al. Safety and efficacy results of a randomized trial comparing adjuvant toremifene and tamoxifen in postmenopausal patients with node-positive breast cancer. J Clin Oncol 2000;18:3487–3494.
76. Ingle JN, Krook JE, Green SJ, et al. Randomized trial of bilateral oophorectomy versus tamoxifen in premenopausal women with metastatic breast cancer. J Clin Oncol 1986;4:178–185.
77. Klijn JGM, Blamey RW, Boccardo F, et al. Combined tamoxifen and luteinizing hormone-releasing hormone (LHRH) agonist versus LHRH agonist alone in premenopausal advanced breast cancer: A meta-analysis of four randomized trials. J Clin Oncol 2001;19:343–353.
78. Femara (Letrozole) Product Information. Novartis Pharmaceuticals Corporation, East Hanover, NJ Jan 2001.
79. Nabholtz JM, Buzdar A, Pollak M, et al. Anastrozole is superior to tamoxifen as first-line therapy for advanced breast cancer in postmenopausal women: Results of a North American multicenter randomized trial. J Clin Oncol 2000;18:3758–3767.
80. Aromasin (Exemestane) Product Information. Pharmacia and UpJohn, Kalama 200, Michigan, October 1999.
81. D'Andrea GM, Seidman A. Docetaxel and paclitaxel in breast cancer therapy: Present status and future prospects. Semin Oncol 1997;24 (suppl 13):S13-27–S13-44.
82. Akerley W, Sikov W, Cummings F, et al. Weekly high-dose paclitaxel in metastatic and locally advanced breast cancer: A preliminary report. Semin Oncol 1997;24(suppl 17):S17-87–S17-90.
83. Hortobagyi GN. New cytotoxic agents for the treatment of breast cancer. Oncology 1996;10(suppl 6):21–29.
84. Burtness B. High-dose chemotherapy for breast cancer. PPO Updates 1997;11:1–13.
85. Peters WP, Dansey R. New concepts in the treatment of breast cancer using high-dose chemotherapy. Cancer Chemother Pharmacol 1997;40 (suppl):S88–S93.
86. Cobleigh MA, Vogel CL, Tripathy D et al. Multinational study of the efficacy and safety of humanized anti-HER2 monoclonal antibody in women who have HER2-overexpressing metastatic breast cancer that progressed after chemotherapy for metastatic disease. J Clin Oncol 1999;17:2639–2648.
87. Slamon DJ, Leyland-Jones B, Shak S, et al. Use of chemotherapy plus a monoclonal antibody against HER2 for metastatic breast cancer that overexpresses HER2. N Engl J Med 2001;344:783–792.
88. CE. Pharmacology and therapeutic use of trastuzumab in breast cancer. Am J Health Syst Pharm 2000;57:2077–2079.
90. Chlebowski RT, Collyar DE, Somerfield MR, et al. American Society of Clinical Oncology Technology assessment on breast cancer risk reduction strategies: Tamoxifen and raloxifene. J Clin Oncol 1999;17:1939.
91. Leitch AM, Dodd GD, Costanza M, et al. American Cancer Society guidelines for the early detection of breast cancer: Update 1997. CA Cancer J Clin 1997;47:150–153.
92. Guide to Clinical Preventive Sciences, 2nd ed. Report of the US Preventive Services Task Force. Washington, DC, Department of Health and Human Services, 1995.
93. Huguley CM, Brown RL, Greenberg RS, Clark WS. Breast self-examination and survival from breast cancer. Cancer 1988;62:1389–1396.
94. Thomas DB, Gao DL, Self SG, et al. Randomized trial of breast self-examination in Shanghai: Methodology and preliminary results. J Natl Cancer Inst 1997;89:355–365.
95. Fletcher SW, Black W, Harris R, et al. Report of the international workshop on screening for breast cancer. J Natl Cancer Inst 1993;85:1644–1656.
96. Kopans DB, Halpern E, Hulka CA. Statistical power in breast cancer screening trials and mortality reduction among women 40–49 years of age with particular emphasis on the National Breast Screening Study of Canada. Cancer 1994;74:1196–1203.
97. National Institutes of Health Consensus Development Panel. National Institutes of Health consensus development conference statement: Breast cancer screening for women Ages 40–49, January 21–23, 1997. J Natl Cancer Inst 1997;89:1015–1026.

126
LUNG CANCER

Sally A. Felton and Rebecca S. Finley

Lung cancer is a major cause of morbidity and mortality that has reached epidemic proportions in many industrialized countries and is the most frequently fatal malignancy in the world. The American Cancer Society estimates that 184,600 new cases of lung cancer will be diagnosed in the United States during 2001, resulting in approximately 162,500 deaths.[1] Despite major advances in the understanding and management of lung cancer, the overall 5-year survival rate for all types of lung cancer remains a dismal 14%.[2]

Lung cancer is estimated to account for 13% of all newly diagnosed cancers in adults.[1] It remains the leading cause of cancer death in men aged 35 years and older (accounting for 32% of all cancer deaths) and the leading cause of cancer death in women (25% of all cancer deaths).[1] In 1987, for the first time, lung cancer surpassed breast cancer as the primary cause of cancer death among American women.[1] Although the death rate from lung cancer increased for the past several decades, it now appears to be declining in the United States. The incidence of lung cancer increases with age; the peak age of diagnosis is between 55 and 65 years. Among patients 40 years of age and older, the likelihood that a solitary pulmonary nodule seen on chest x-ray is a carcinoma is high and this probability increases proportionally with age. Patients with lung cancer may undergo surgery, chemotherapy, radiation, or multimodality therapy, depending on the histologic type of the tumor, its size and location, and the presence of metastases at diagnosis.

ETIOLOGY

Lung carcinomas arise from normal bronchial epithelial cells that have acquired multiple genetic lesions and are capable of expressing a variety of phenotypes.[3] The natural history of lung cancer begins with exposure of these normal cells to carcinogens, which cause chronic inflammation eventually leading to the genetic and cytologic changes that progress to carcinoma. Activation of protooncogenes, inhibition or mutation of tumor-suppressor genes, and production of autocrine growth factors also contribute to cellular proliferation and malignant transformation.[3,4] Under normal circumstances, cell surface peptidases produced by epithelial cells degrade and regulate these growth factors, but these enzymes are expressed at low or undetectable levels by most lung cancer cells, thus facilitating uncontrolled growth.[5] Although individual lung carcinomas may have multiple molecular abnormalities, some specific changes have been associated with the various types of lung cancer. For example, *p53* mutations have been observed in approximately 90% of small cell lung cancers but in only about 50% of nonsmall cell lung cancers, and this type of mutation appears to be more frequent in the squamous cell and large cell subtypes of nonsmall cell lung cancers than in adenocarcinomas.[6,7] Evidence is accumulating that such molecular changes not only influence the transformation from normal to malignant cell but also may have an impact on the progression of the disease and its response to therapy and therefore strongly influence the patient's prognosis (Table 126–1). As in many other malignant diseases, further elucidation of molecular attributes of lung cancer are likely to provide insight regarding improved preventive, diagnostic, prognostic, and therapeutic strategies.

Numerous studies have established the relationship between tobacco exposure and lung cancer. The American Cancer Society estimates that cigarette smoking is responsible for about 83% of all lung cancer cases, and studies have established a dose-response relationship between the number of cigarettes smoked, the number of years an individual has smoked, the tar and nicotine content of cigarettes, and the development of lung cancer.[2] Likewise, smokers with obstructive airway disease or chronic bronchitis have a three- to five-fold greater risk of developing lung cancer than do smokers with normal pulmonary function.[14] Mattson et al. estimated that a 35-year-old man who smokes 25 cigarettes per day or more has a 13% risk of dying of lung cancer before age 75.[15] The increased rate of lung cancer deaths among women has also been attributed to increased smoking.[1] Cessation of smoking is associated with a gradual decrease in the risk, but a long period of time (more than 6 years) is necessary before an appreciable decline of the risk occurs.[16] Antismoking campaigns, increased tobacco taxes, and smoke-free areas in many public areas and businesses along with societal pressures have been somewhat successful in reducing the number of adult Americans who smoke. However, the high number of lung cancers in ex-smokers emphasizes the need to prevent individuals from ever smoking. Passive exposure to cigarette smoke is believed to contribute to the increased risk of lung cancer in nonsmokers living with smokers. Other carcinogens also increase the risk of lung cancer and may act synergistically with cigarette smoking.[2] Occupational or environmental exposure to asbestos, chloromethyl ethers, various heavy metals, polycyclic aromatic hydrocarbons, and radon has also been associated with the development of lung cancer.[2] In addition, the incidence of lung cancer is higher in urban than in rural areas, and air pollution has been implicated as a possible causative agent.[17]

Observational epidemiologic data suggest that intake of β-carotene and carotene (vitamin A) is inversely associated with lung cancer risk.[18,19] The first prospective randomized chemoprevention trial with antioxidants in a large, well-nourished population was reported in 1994.[20] In this trial, more than 29,000 middle-aged male smokers were randomized to receive dietary supplementation with β-carotene, α-tocopherol, or both for 6 years. Interestingly, the trial failed to detect any significant protective effect of either vitamin and, in fact, there were significantly more new cases of lung cancer in the group treated with β-carotene. Other prospective trials have also failed to demonstrate significant positive effects of carotenoids, vitamin C, or vitamin E against lung cancer. Conversely, several other trials and case-control studies show a significant difference in relative risk related to intake of one of these antioxidants.[2,18] Additional studies are necessary to define the role of antioxidants in lung cancer prevention.

HISTOLOGIC CLASSIFICATION

The World Health Organization lung cancer classification is accepted worldwide (Table 126–2).[21] Four major cell types of carcinomas

TABLE 126–1. Examples of Relationship of Molecular Changes in Lung Cancer to Clinical Outcomes

Molecular Changes	Impact on Clinical Outcome	Reference
Microsatellite alterations	Reduced survival	3
Overexpression of BCL2	Decreased response to chemotherapy and radiation therapy	3
Expression of gastrin-releasing peptide and other bombesin-like peptides (SCLC)	Promote tumor growth	3
Overexpression of MYC (SCLC)	Reduced survival	3
Overexpression of HER2/neu (NSCLC)	Shorter survival, multidrug resistance	8
High hepatocyte growth factor levels (NSCLC)	Poor outcome	9
K-ras mutations (NSCLC)	Poor prognosis	10, 11
Absent RB expression (NSCLC)	Poor prognosis	3
Reduced E-cadherin expression (NSCLC)	Increased lymph node metastases; poor survival	12
Decreased α_3-integrin expression (NSCLC)	Poor prognosis	13

SCLC, small cell lung cancer; NSCLC, nonsmall cell lung cancer

(squamous cell, adenocarcinoma, large cell, and small cell carcinomas) account for more than 90% of all lung tumors. Histologic confirmation of cell type is usually made by light microscopy and is essential in treatment planning because of differences in the natural histories, clinical features, and response to therapy of the various types. As noted earlier, several additional biologic and cytogenetic characteristics (e.g., secretion of peptide hormones, autocrine growth factor receptors, specific mutations, or chromosomal deletions of lung tumors) are currently being evaluated for their prognostic significance. In terms of management strategy and overall prognosis, adenocarcinoma, squamous cell, and large cell carcinomas are frequently grouped together and referred to as nonsmall cell lung cancer (NSCLC).

TABLE 126–2. World Health Organization Classification of Lung Cancer

I. Benign
II. Dysplasia and carcinoma *in situ*
III. Malignant
- A. Squamous cell carcinoma (epidermoid)
- B. Small cell carcinoma
  1. Oat cell
  2. Intermediate cell
  3. Combined oat cell
- C. Adenocarcinoma
  1. Acinar
  2. Papillary
  3. Bronchoalveolar
  4. Mucus secreting
- D. Large cell carcinoma
  1. Giant cell
  2. Clear cell

From Ref. 3.

Although once the most common type of NSCLC, squamous cell (or epidermoid) carcinoma now accounts for less than 30% of all lung cancers and is distinguished histologically by evidence of squamous differentiation. This tumor tends to be central in origin, arising from metaplastic bronchial epithelium, and frequently extends into the bronchial lumen, resulting in obstruction. Squamous cell carcinomas (along with small cell lung cancers [SCLC]) have a much higher incidence among smokers and among males and appear to have a strong dose-response relationship to tobacco exposure.[2,22] Although they can grow rapidly, most squamous cell carcinomas tend to be slow growing and confined to the lungs (especially early in the disease course). Such tumors may eventually metastasize to the hilar and mediastinal lymph nodes, liver, adrenal glands, kidneys, bone, and gastrointestinal tract.

Adenocarcinoma is now the most common type of lung cancer in the United States, accounting for about 40% of cases. This is partly a result of the increased incidence of lung cancer in women, who tend to have more adenocarcinomas than epidermoid cancers. Interestingly, it does not have a dose-response relationship to tobacco exposure. These tumors are usually located in the peripheral sections of the lung and are distinguished pathologically by a glandular or papillary pattern and mucin production.[2] The presentation and natural history of adenocarcinomas are quite variable. These tumors can present as a single nodule, multifocal nodules, or rapidly progressing, bilateral, diffuse processes. They are likely to metastasize at an early stage (often before the diagnosis of the primary tumor) and spread widely to distant sites including the contralateral lung, liver, bone, adrenal glands, kidneys, and central nervous system. As a result, adenocarcinoma has a worse prognosis than squamous cell carcinoma.

Large cell carcinomas are anaplastic tumors that show no evidence of differentiation. These tumors account for only about 15% of all lung cancers.[2] These tumors tend to be large and bulky tumors arising in the periphery of the lung, to have a propensity to metastasize in a pattern quite similar to adenocarcinomas, and to be associated with a similar poor prognosis.

Small cell carcinomas account for about 20% of all lung tumors. Almost all cases are associated with a history of smoking. They are distinguished by a proliferation of neoplastic cells with round to oval nuclei. These tumors tend to arise in the central portion of the lung but may also be found in the lung periphery. SCLC is a very aggressive and rapidly growing tumor with approximately 60% to 70% of patients initially presenting with disseminated disease outside of the hemithorax.[22] These tumors commonly express neuroendocrine differentiation that may account for some of the paraneoplastic syndromes frequently associated with this disease. SCLC secretes gastrin-releasing peptide that acts as an autocrine growth factor.[23] Secretion of other peptide hormones, cytogenetic abnormalities, and amplification and increased expression of oncogenes are also common. This disease has a propensity to metastasize to the lymph nodes, opposite lung, liver, adrenal glands and other endocrine organs, bone, bone marrow, and central nervous system.

Lung tumors frequently exhibit more than one histology and it is now evident that all types of lung cancer share a common pluripotent stem cell. Studies of lung cancer cells have also shown that cell lines may spontaneously change phenotype, which may explain the mixed histology.[5] Occasionally patients can also have multiple lung nodules arising in different lobes or the contralateral lung. This is referred to as *synchronous tumors,* and the nodules may be of similar or different cell types. This usually worsens the patient's overall prognosis.

CLINICAL PRESENTATION

Location and extent of the tumor determines the presenting signs and symptoms. If the lesion is in the central portion of the bronchial tree, it is likely to cause symptoms at an earlier stage than will a lesion in the periphery of the lung, which may remain asymptomatic until the lesion is quite large or has spread to other areas. The most common initial signs and symptoms include cough, dyspnea, chest pain, sputum production, and hemoptysis. Unfortunately, many patients with lung cancer also have chronic pulmonary and/or cardiovascular diseases (usually related to smoking), and such symptoms may go unnoticed or be attributed to the concomitant disease. Many patients also exhibit systemic symptoms such as anorexia, weight loss, and fatigue that are suggestive of a malignancy.[2,22] Table 126–3 lists other signs and symptoms that may be associated with the primary tumor or its spread within the thorax. Such symptomatology may occur at the tumor's initial presentation or at any point during its recurrence or progression.

Disseminated disease also may be responsible for extrapulmonary signs and symptoms such as neurologic deficits resulting from central nervous system metastases, bone pain or pathologic fractures secondary to bone metastases, or liver dysfunction resulting from tumor involvement in the liver.

Paraneoplastic syndromes are signs and symptoms that occur at sites away from the primary tumor or its metastases and are not associated with "direct" tumor involvement. They may be caused by the production of biologically active substances (e.g., peptide hormones) or antibodies, or by other undefined mechanisms. Paraneoplastic syndromes occur more frequently with lung cancer than with any other tumor. These syndromes may be the first signs of a tumor and may prompt the search for an underlying malignancy. Paraneoplastic syndromes that commonly occur in association with lung cancers include cachexia, hypercalcemia, syndrome of inappropriate antidiuretic hormone secretion, and Cushing's syndrome.[2,22]

TABLE 126–3. Common Signs and Symptoms of Lung Cancer

Local signs and symptoms associated with primary tumor or regional spread within the thorax
- Cough
- Hemoptysis
- Dyspnea
- Rust-streaked or purulent sputum
- Chest, shoulder, or arm pain
- Wheeze and stridor
- Superior vena caval obstruction
- Pleural effusion or pneumonitis
- Dysphagia (secondary to esophageal compression)
- Hoarseness (secondary to laryngeal nerve paralysis)
- Horner's syndrome
- Phrenic nerve paralysis
- Pericardial effusion/tamponade
- Tracheal obstruction

Extrapulmonary signs and symptoms associated with metastatic involvement
- Bone pain and/or pathologic fractures
- Liver dysfunction
- Neurologic deficits
- Spinal cord compression

Paraneoplastic syndromes
- Weight loss
- Cushing's syndrome
- Hypercalcemia
- Syndrome of inappropriate antidiuretic hormone (SIADH)
- Pulmonary hypertrophic osteoarthropathy
- Clubbing
- Anemia
- Eaton-Lambert myasthenic syndrome

SCREENING

At the time of initial diagnosis, many patients with lung cancer have advanced disease and, unfortunately, the prognosis is poor. In an attempt to detect lung tumors earlier and to improve the cure rate, screening studies have been conducted in high-risk populations (e.g., men older than age 40 who smoke).[24–26] Chest x-rays and sputum cytology are the most commonly used screening techniques in these studies. Although several of these studies have reported that lung cancers may be detected at an earlier stage, actual mortality rates are not affected.[25,26] Furthermore, chest x-rays and sputum cytology are associated with false-positive results in approximately 5% and 0.5% of these high-risk individuals, respectively, leading to unnecessary and costly work-ups and anxiety.[27] Currently, no biochemical markers (tumor markers) have been identified with sufficient sensitivity and specificity to reliably screen for early lung cancer.

DIAGNOSIS

Once signs and symptoms of lung cancer have been recognized, chest x-rays, computed tomography scans (CT), and positron emission tomography (PET) scans are the most valuable diagnostic tests. Chest x-ray is the primary method of lung cancer detection and may also be useful in measuring tumor size, establishing gross lymph node enlargement, and aiding in detection of other tumor-related findings, such as pleural effusion, lobar collapse, and metastatic bone involvement of ribs, spine, and shoulders. CT is helpful in all of the foregoing, as well as in evaluation of parenchymal lung abnormalities, detection of masses only suspected on the chest x-ray, and assessment of mediastinal and hilar lymph nodes. PET scans, however, are reportedly more accurate than CT scans in distinguishing malignant from benign lesions and identifying metastatic spread.[28]

Clinical characteristics of a lung nodule may also help to differentiate benign from malignant nodules and thus determine when invasive diagnostic tests are warranted. For example, benign lesions usually have sharp borders, whereas malignant lesions usually have irregular or radiating borders.

When there is clinical and radiologic evidence of a tumor, pathologic confirmation must be established. This may be accomplished by examination of sputum cytology and/or tumor biopsy by fiberoptic bronchoscopy, percutaneous needle biopsy, or open-lung biopsy. All patients must also have a thorough history and physical examination with emphasis on detecting signs and symptoms of the primary tumor, regional spread of the tumor, distant metastases, and paraneoplastic syndromes. The physical examination also aids in determining whether or not a patient may be able to withstand aggressive surgery or chemotherapy.

Unfortunately, by the time the tumor is diagnosed, dissemination has already occurred in many patients. Determination of the extent (or stage) of the tumor involvement is important because it will aid in the selection of treatment, and estimation of the probability of cure and survival, as well as facilitating comparison of the individual patient to large-scale clinical trials.

STAGING

NONSMALL CELL LUNG CANCER

The American Joint Committee[29] has established a TNM staging classification for lung cancer based on the primary tumor size and extent (T), regional lymph node involvement (N), and the presence or absence of distant metastases (M). Table 126–4 outlines this staging system. For comparison of various therapeutic modalities, a more simple stage grouping system is also used in which stage I refers to tumors confined to the lung without lymphatic spread; stage II refers to large tumors with ipsilateral peribronchial or hilar lymph node involvement; stage III includes other lymph node and regional involvement; and stage IV includes any tumor with distant metastases.[29]

The primary tumor is assessed with chest x-rays and fiberoptic bronchoscopy, whereas lymphatic spread is usually assessed by mediastinoscopy, gallium-67 citrate scanning, CT and/or PET scans.[2] If the history and physical examination or other routine clinical studies (e.g., complete blood cell count [CBC], liver functions tests) suggest the possibility of metastatic disease, then special scans (e.g., bone, brain, or liver) or biopsies (e.g., bone marrow or liver) may be necessary for staging.[2]

SMALL CELL LUNG CANCER

A two-stage classification established by the Veterans Administration Lung Cancer Study Group is widely used in the United States to stage SCLC.[22] Limited disease is classified as disease confined to one hemithorax and to the regional lymph nodes. All other disease is classified as extensive. Approximately 70% of patients initially present with extensive disease. Because of this high frequency of disseminated disease at diagnosis (bone 38%; liver 22% to 28%; bone marrow 17% to 23%; central nervous system [CNS] 8% to 14%), radionuclide scans of the bone and liver, CT scans of the brain, and bone marrow biopsies are generally recommended prior to initiation of therapy.[22] In addition, any suspicious signs or symptoms detected during the physical examination should be carefully investigated.

TABLE 126–4. Tumor (T), Node (N), Metastasis (M) Staging for Lung Cancer

T_X	Positive malignant cell; no lesion seen
T_1	≤ 3 cm surrounded by lung or visceral pleura
T_2	> 3 cm or involvement of main bronchus 2 cm or more distal to the carina, or invasion of visceral pleura, or associated atelectasis or obstructive pneumonitis extending to hilar region
T_3	Direct invasion of chest wall, diaphragm, mediastinal pleura, or parietal pericardium; or tumor in main bronchus less than 2 cm distal to the carina; or associated atelectasis or obstructive pneumonitis of the entire lung
T_4	Invasion of mediastinum, heart, great vessel, trachea, esophagus, vertebral body, carina; or tumor with a malignant pleural effusion
N_0	No regional lymph node involvement
N_1	Metastasis in ipsilateral peribronchial and/or ipsilateral hilar lymph node(s), including direct extension
N_2	Metastasis in ipsilateral mediastinal and/or subcarinal lymph node(s)
N_3	Metastasis in contralateral mediastinal, contralateral hilar, ipsilateral or contralateral scalene, or supraclavicular lymph node(s)
M_0	No distant metastases
M_1	Distant metastases

Stage Groupings

Stage IA	T_1	N_0	M_0
Stage IB	T_2	N_0	M_0
Stage IIA	T_1	N_1	M_0
Stage IIB	T_2	N_1	M_0
	T_3	N_0	M_0
Stage IIIA	T_1–T_3	N_2	M_0
	T_3	N_1	M_0
Stage IIIB	Any T	N_3	M_0
	T_4	Any N	M_0
Stage IV	Any T	Any N	M_1

From Ref. 23.

▶ TREATMENT: Lung Cancer

NONSMALL CELL LUNG CANCER

Currently only surgery and, to a lesser extent, radiation therapy offer an opportunity for long-term survival in a significant percentage of patients, although only about 30% of unselected patients have localized disease (stage I or II) that is amenable to local therapy.[2] Curative therapy in this disease is determined by the anatomic stage of the disease (it must be localized with no evidence of distant metastases) and the ability of the patient to tolerate aggressive therapy. If left untreated, most patients with NSCLC die within 1 year of diagnosis.

SURGERY

Surgical resection is the treatment of choice for NSCLC patients with clinical stage I and II (disease that by all evidence is stage I or II prior to surgical resection and examination of lymph nodes) disease. Overall, more than 50% of patients with stage I and 35% of patients with stage II disease who undergo complete surgical resection survive 5 years without disease recurrence.[30] The single most important prognostic factor for patients undergoing surgical resection is the presence or absence of lymph node involvement. One early series of 216 patients with clinical stage I disease (based on evaluation of all presurgery data) before surgical resection reported that only 125 patients were found to have stage I disease after resection and pathologic examination of lymph nodes.[30] The addition of spiral CT and PET scanning of the chest to the initial preoperative staging plan have markedly improved the accuracy of clinical staging. However, mediastinal lymph node sampling via mediastinoscopy or dissection at the time of surgery, is important to confirm the presence or absence of lymph node involvement.

The size of the tumor is of prognostic importance in stage I and stage II disease. Martini and colleagues reported an 82% 5-year survival and a 74% 10-year survival for 291 patients with stage IA (T_1N_0) versus a 68% 5-year survival and a 60% 10-year survival for 307 patients with stage IB (T_2N_0); this is statistically significant ($P < 0.0004$).[31] As expected, survival was better for patients with small tumors ≤2 cm than for those with tumors ≥5 cm. Disease recurred in 206 of these patients (34%), with 60% of the recurrences documented within 2 years of initial treatment. Typically, removal of the involved lobe of the lung (e.g., lobectomy) is the recommended surgical procedure for Stage IA tumors, but there is some evidence that pneumonectomy may reduce the rate of local recurrences for patients with larger size stage IB tumors.[30,31]

Stage II (T_1N_1) disease has a poorer prognosis with the 5-year survival rate after complete surgical resection of approximately 40%.[2] Pneumonectomy or removal of the entire lung (vs lobectomy) is the recommended surgical procedure for stage II disease with lymph node involvement ($T_{1-3}N_1$). Despite complete resection (no apparent residual disease remaining), as many as 50% of patients with stage II disease develop recurrent disease and die within 2 years.[2] It is therefore postulated that many of these patients may benefit from postoperative radiotherapy to improve local control, as well as from chemotherapy to decrease the risk of undiagnosed systemic micrometastasis.[30] Ongoing clinical trials are attempting to more clearly define the role of such adjuvant therapy in stage II disease.

Management of locally advanced NSCLC stage IIIA ($T_{1-3}N_2$, T_3N_1) tumors is more controversial. Although many stage IIIA tumors are resectable or potentially resectable, the prognosis is poorer, with 5-year survival rates ranging from 10% to 30% depending on tumor size and lymph node involvement.[2] For patients with surgically resectable, locally advanced stage IIIA and more advanced IIIB (any TN_3 or T_4 any N) disease, recent trials indicate that neoadjuvant (before surgery) chemotherapy with or without concurrent radiotherapy, followed by surgery, improves local and regional control and overall survival when compared to preoperative radiation followed by surgery.[32] Preoperative chemotherapy may also increase the likelihood that an advanced local tumor may be completely resected at the time of surgery.[2] Large-scale phase III trials are underway to evaluate various combinations of neoadjuvant chemotherapy with or without radiotherapy versus initial surgery followed by adjuvant therapy. Accurate disease staging, consistent eligibility criteria, and multidisciplinary communication will be essential to the success of these trials in elucidating the role of future neoadjuvant therapy in locally advanced NSCLC. Stage IV disease with systemic metastasis is, by definition, not surgically resectable for cure and is therefore classified as nonresectable.

RADIOTHERAPY

Radiation therapy (radiotherapy) is used in a variety of settings for the treatment of NSCLC. Thoracic radiotherapy may be administered with curative intent for treatment of small localized tumors in some patients. Most commonly radiotherapy is administered postsurgically (adjuvant therapy) for prevention of local disease recurrence, as well as in advanced disease for the palliation of tumor-related symptoms (i.e., control of pain from bone metastases, hemoptysis, or obstructive symptoms).

Stage I or II NSCLC

Adjuvant thoracic radiotherapy is given postoperatively when surgical margins indicate that there is residual disease.[33] The goal of radiotherapy in this setting is curative, by eliminating the residual disease and reducing the risk of local disease recurrence. Radiotherapy alone (without chemotherapy or surgery) is the treatment of choice for stage I and II patients who refuse surgery or who are considered high surgical risks because of concomitant illness or restrictive pulmonary reserve.[2] It is also used when the tumor is unresectable because of fixation to a major blood vessel, the trachea, or the esophagus. Of those patients, the 2- and 5-year survival rates appear to be highest for patients whose tumors would otherwise be considered resectable.

Stage III NSCLC

Thoracic radiotherapy may be given in the neoadjuvant (preoperative) and/or adjuvant (postoperative) setting. For locally advanced disease that is surgically resectable, adjuvant radiotherapy has been used to reduce the risk of local disease recurrence. However, when given without chemotherapy it does not impact overall survival rates because many of these patients develop systemic (distant) metastases.[2] Guidelines published by the American Society of Clinical Oncology (ASCO) recommend that patients with locally advanced nonresectable stage III disease and good performance status should receive thoracic radiotherapy plus chemotherapy to optimize local tumor control and diminish or eradicate systemic micrometastatic disease.[34] The use of radiotherapy alone or postoperatively (without chemotherapy) in stage III disease should be reserved for those patients with a poor performance status who are at high risk for significant chemotherapy-induced toxicity.

Stage IV NSCLC

Palliative radiotherapy with chemotherapy may be used in selected patients to control local and systemic disease and to reduce disease-related symptoms. Brain metastases are also commonly treated with radiotherapy; in the case of a solitary brain lesion, surgical resection may be used.

When thoracic radiotherapy is used with curative intent, high total-dose fractions ≥60 Gy are required (there appears to be a linear correlation between dose and local control of NSCLC).[35] These higher dosages of radiotherapy frequently result in severe esophagitis, pneumonitis, and pulmonary toxicity in the surrounding normal tissues. Improved radiotherapy delivery techniques, such as multiple daily radiation fractions (hyperfractionated radiotherapy) and three-dimensional treatment planning, allow delivery of greater dosage fractions specifically to the tumor site while decreasing the toxicity to surrounding normal tissues, as compared to standard radiotherapy. However, concurrent radiotherapy plus chemotherapy with radiosensitizing agents, such as cisplatin, paclitaxel, and gemcitabine, further complicate the risks for severe toxicity, often necessitating dose reductions in one or both treatment modalities.[36] Numerous randomized combined modality trials have been initiated to evaluate the optimal delivery method, schedule, and dosages for radiotherapy in concert with cisplatin and the newer chemotherapy agents.

CHEMOTHERAPY

Response rates for chemotherapy in advanced stage NSCLC have historically been disappointingly low, with a poor long-term survival rate. Until recently the use of chemotherapy was considered controversial. But studies consistently show that patients with advanced stage NSCLC who respond to chemotherapy are more likely to have a survival benefit and reduced symptoms as compared to patients who did not respond to chemotherapy.[2] In addition, combination chemotherapy regimens that include newer active agents are demonstrating higher response rates and longer median survival durations than ever before.

Metastatic or Recurrent Disease

Although surgery and radiation therapies have been the mainstay of treatment options for patients with localized or regional disease, about 70% of NSCLC patients present with advanced, poor prognosis stage III and IV disease at the time of diagnosis. The majority of these advanced tumors are not surgically resectable. Patients with advanced stage disease who initially respond to radiotherapy, with or without surgery, relapse quickly and die from disease-related complications within 1 year. Likewise, patients who have recurrent disease following surgical resection are usually not candidates for further surgical interventions. Although chemotherapy (single-agent and combination regimens) has been used for treatment of NSCLC for more than three decades, the overall survival benefits were not clearly established until just a few years ago. Several studies have compared chemotherapy to the best supportive care and have shown a consistently better outcome for chemotherapy.[2,37–39] However, many of the early trials produced conflicting results, some of which may have been a result of study design flaws, including inadequate sample size or use of ineffective chemotherapy agent(s) or regimens.[2] In 1995, the Non-Small Cell Lung Cancer Collaborative Group released the results of a large meta-analysis encompassing over 25 years of clinical trials of chemotherapy in the management of NSCLC.[40] This meta-analysis included data for 9,387 patients from 52 randomized clinical trials that compared chemotherapy alone versus best supportive care and chemotherapy plus radiotherapy or surgery versus either single treatment modality. Best supportive care generally consists of symptom management with palliative radiotherapy, corticosteroids, pain management, and antibiotics as required. The results of the meta-analysis showed that chemotherapy, when combined with either surgery and or radiotherapy, improved survival for patients with advanced stage NSCLC and may also have a role in the treatment of early stage disease.[40] Cisplatin-containing chemotherapy regimens appear to be superior to older noncisplatin-containing regimens, and regimens containing alkylating agents generally produced inferior outcomes. The roles of individual chemotherapy agents/regimens were not compared in this particular meta-analysis and require further evaluation.

Subsequently, ASCO released Treatment Guidelines for Unresectable NSCLC in 1997, confirming the role of chemotherapy in advanced stage III and stage IV disease, and further recommending that a platinum-based combination regimen (cisplatin or carboplatin) should be used.[34] Duration of treatment with combination chemotherapy plus radiotherapy for advanced stage NSCLC should be a minimum of two cycles to a maximum of eight cycles in most cases.[34]

Over the past 30 years, thousands of clinical trials have evaluated chemotherapy for the treatment of advanced NSCLC. Often the results have seemed inconsistent or even conflicting. Direct comparison of study results between clinical trials is difficult and requires critical assessment of the study design, inclusion criteria (performance status, history of prior weight loss and staging criteria), exclusion criteria, and assessment methodology. An excellent example is the importance of enrollment criteria for stage III locally advanced disease. Subset analysis is particularly important for stage III disease, because IIIA includes locally advanced disease while stage IIIB includes more bulky regional disease with an overall poorer prognosis. Also, whether or not pathologic documentation of stage IIIA (N_2) disease was required is important because, if it was not, then some stage II (N_1) patients with a better prognosis may have been erroneously enrolled. Poorly defined stage III patient enrollment, with or without documented N_2 disease, may have contributed to the wide ranges reported in long-term survival rates and response rates between study arms in many of the early clinical trials.

Standardized response criteria are also important for the comparison of clinical trial results. The standard definition of a complete response (CR) is the complete disappearance of all evidence of the tumor as verified by two scans at least 4 weeks apart, whereas a partial response (PR) is defined as a reduction in measurable tumor mass of more than 50% for ≥4 weeks. Because many lung tumors do not have definite margins and are difficult to measure, the term *objective response* (OR) has been used to describe disease in which there has been a definite decrease in the size of the lesion without the appearance of any new lesions.[2] Tumor response to chemotherapy is generally evaluated at the end of the second or third cycle and at the end of every second cycle thereafter. Patients with stable disease (SD), with OR, or with measurable decrease in tumor size (CR, PR) should continue with the same chemotherapy regimen. The chemotherapy regimen should be discontinued for documented progressive disease (PD) and an alternative regimen or investigational protocol should be considered.

Several prognostic factors have important implications in terms of response and survival for NSCLC patients selected to receive chemotherapy. These factors include the patient's current performance status, percentage of weight loss from baseline, and extent of disease (stage).[2] Among these factors, an initial favorable performance status (Eastern Cooperative Oncology Group [ECOG] 0-2) appears to be the most consistent factor predicting a better response and improved survival after chemotherapy. There is little evidence to support the usefulness of chemotherapy in persons with an ECOG performance status of ≥3 (Karnofsky performance status of less than 50%).[2,40] Patients with an unfavorable prognosis (poor performance status, elevated lactate dehydrogenase [LDH], weight loss >5%, and/or significant concomitant diseases) should receive supportive care and palliative radiation when necessary.

Currently, phase II and phase III randomized trials with subset selection and disease documentation are ongoing to evaluate the efficacy of various combinations of chemotherapy, radiation, and surgery. Clinicians must refrain from extrapolating the results from early clinical trials into their general daily practice and should continue, whenever possible, to refer patients to carefully designed randomized trials to define the optimal therapy for the various subsets of NSCLC.

Chemotherapy for stage IV NSCLC is not curative, despite significant advances in available treatment options. But improved response rates, a modest increase in survival, and decreased toxicity profiles observed with many of the newer chemotherapy agents and combination regimens have led most experts to agree that most patients with stage IV disease should receive at least one chemotherapy regimen.[2,34]

The cost-effectiveness ratio for the use of chemotherapy versus best supportive care in advanced stages III and IV NSCLC has also been evaluated. Jaakimainen et al. demonstrated a modest increase in survival, improved symptom management, and decreased medical costs for patients receiving chemotherapy versus those receiving best supportive care.[41] The potentially high costs of chemotherapy, especially with the newer agents, are generally offset by using outpatient oncology clinics for drug administration and by the decreased costs incurred from best supportive care for symptom management and hospitalization (often prolonged). Cost calculations for cisplatin plus one of the new agents given in a combination regimen for advanced stage

TABLE 126–5. Traditional Combination Chemotherapy in Non-Small Cell Lung Cancer

Combination (Reference)	Dosages	Schedule	Overall Response Rate
CE (2)			
DDP	60–100 mg/m² IV day 1	Repeat course every 3 to 4 weeks	19% to 30%
ETOP	80–120 mg/m² IV days 1 through 3		
DDP/VIN (2)			
DDP	120 mg/m² IV days 1 and 29	Repeat every 6 weeks	30%
VIN	3 mg/m² IV every week × 6 weeks	Then repeat course every 2 weeks	
MVP (48)			
MT	8 mg/m² IV days 1 and 29		43%
VIN	3 mg/m² IV days 1, 8, 29, and 36		
DDP	80 mg/m² IV 1 and 29		
ICE (2)			
IFOS	1.5 g/m² IV × 3 days	Repeat every 3 weeks	43%
CARBO	300–350 mg/m² day 1		
ETOP	60–100 mg/m² × 3 days		

CARBO, carboplatin; DDP, cisplatin; ETOP, etoposide; IFOS, ifosfamide; MT, mitomycin; VIN, vindesine.

NSCLC is less than $20,000 per life-year gained, which is in the range of other widely accepted interventions.[42] New information is forthcoming comparing the cost of therapy between the various new single-agent and combination chemotherapy regimens.[43–45] These data will enable decision makers to analyze the cost-effectiveness of regimens with similar response rates, survival, and quality of life.

Single-agent Chemotherapy

Single-agent chemotherapy has generally demonstrated objective response rates of 5% to 25% with no significant effect on overall survival. When responses do occur with single-agent chemotherapy, the duration of the response is usually brief (2 to 4 months) and complete responses are rare.[2] Among the most active single agents in NSCLC are cisplatin, carboplatin, docetaxel, etoposide, gemcitabine, ifosfamide, irinotecan, mitomycin, paclitaxel, topotecan, vinblastine, and vinorelbine. Numerous investigational agents, including LY231514, a thymidylate synthase inhibitor; Marimastat, a matrix metalloproteinase inhibitor (cytostatic agent); tirapazamine, a cytotoxic that targets hypoxic cells; ZD-1839 (Iressa) and CI-1033, epidermal growth factor receptor (EGFR) inhibitors are currently undergoing evaluation as single agents and in combination therapy in phase II and phase III clinical trials.

Combination Chemotherapy

Combination of two or more chemotherapy agents has been used in the management of NSCLC since the late 1960s. Response rates for combination chemotherapy regimens generally have been better than single-agent therapy, but improvement in overall survival rates has not been consistently observed.[46,47] Active combination chemotherapy regimens that have consistently reported response rates exceeding 30% have used various combinations of cisplatin, carboplatin, gemcitabine, ifosfamide, mitomycin, and vinblastine, vindesine or vinorelbine (Tables 126–5 and 126–6). Evidence suggests that cisplatin dose may have an impact on tumor response.

Newer chemotherapeutic agents in four distinct classes have shown single-agent activity of greater than 20% in NSCLC. The plant alkaloids (vinorelbine), taxanes (antimicrotubule agents; paclitaxel and docetaxel), antimetabolites (gemcitabine), and topoisomerase I inhibitors (topotecan and irinotecan) are being extensively studied in various combinations with platinum compounds (cisplatin or carboplatin). In addition to evaluation in advanced disease, various combinations of multimodality regimens using these chemotherapy regimens with concurrent or sequential radiation therapy including neoadjuvant (prior to surgery) and adjuvant therapy (postsurgery) are also being studied. Whereas earlier studies of chemotherapy focused primarily on response rates, newer studies focus on survival (disease-free and overall), quality of life, toxicity (short- and long-term), and cost-effectiveness. Results from many recently published trials combining these new chemotherapy agents with platinum-based regimens have suggested improved 1-year survival rates in advanced NSCLC of 30% to 40% versus 15% to 25% with the older cisplatin-based combination regimens (Table 126–6).

Vinorelbine (Navelbine) is a semisynthetic vinca alkaloid. Single-agent activity has been demonstrated in advanced NSCLC, with response rates of up to 33%, median survivals of 40 weeks, and 1-year survival rates of 24% to 30%.[51] The combination of vinorelbine plus cisplatin has demonstrated superior efficacy to either agent alone, and to vindesine plus cisplatin in randomized phase III trials.[51,56]

Neutropenia is the dose-limiting toxicity for vinorelbine therapy. Thrombocytopenia and moderate to severe anemia have occurred in less than 1% and 10% of patients, respectively. Mild to moderate non-hematologic adverse effects include nausea and vomiting, peripheral neuropathy, and transient elevations in liver function tests. Vinorelbine is easily administered in the outpatient oncology setting by peripheral or central venous access over 6 to 10 minutes, followed by a 75–100-mL intravenous flush. Longer infusions of vinorelbine are

TABLE 126–6. Single-Agent and Combination Regimens Using Newer Agents for Non-Small Cell Lung Cancer

Reference	Evaluable/Total Patients (Stage)	Regimen	Overall Response Rates (%)	Median Survival Duration	Median 1-Year Survival (%)	Time to Disease Progression
Cisplatin + Paclitaxel or Gemcitabine or Docetaxel versus Carboplatin + Paclitaxel						
ECOG trial 1594 Phase III Schiller (49)	1146/1207 (1083 PS 0-1) (63 PS 2) 98 Stage IIIB 968 Stage IV	**CP** (*reference arm for trial*) Cisplatin 75 mg/m² IV day 1 Paclitaxel 175 mg/m²/24 h CIV Day 1 Cycle: Every 21 days	21.3	7.8 mo	31	3.5 mo
		GC Gemcitabine 1,000 mg/m² IV Days 1, 8, 15 Cisplatin 100 mg/m² IV day 1 Cycle: Every 28 days	21.0	8.1 mo	36	4.5 mo*
		DC Docetaxel 75 mg/m² IV day 1 Cisplatin 75 mg/m² IV day 1 Cycle: Every 21 days	17.3	7.4 mo	31	3.3 mo
		PCb Paclitaxel 225 mg/m²/3 h IV day 1 Carboplatin AUC 6 IV day 1 Cycle: Every 21 days	15.3	8.2 mo	34	3.3 mo
Paclitaxel + Carboplatin versus Vinorelbine + Cisplatin						
SWOG Phase III Kelly (50)	408/444 chemonaive (PS 0-1) 12% stage IIIB n = 207	**PCb** Paclitaxel 225 mg/m²/3 h IV day 1 Carboplatin AUC 6 IV day 1 Cycle: Every 21 days	PR 27	8.0 mo	36	NR
	11% stage IIIB n = 201	**VC** Vinorelbine 25 mg/m² IV weekly Cisplatin 100 mg/m² IV day 1 Cycle: Every 28 days	PR 27	8.0 mo	33	NR
Cisplatin + Vinorelbine or Vindestine versus Vinorelbine						
LeChavalier (51)	192/206 chemonaive (PS ≤ 2) 23 Stage IIIA 58 Stage IIIB 102 Stage IV	**VC** Vinorelbine 30 mg/m² IV weekly Cisplatin 120 mg/m² IV days 1 and 29, then every 6 weeks	30	9.2 mo*	35*	NR
	183/200 21 Stage IIIA 49 Stage IIIB 109 Stage IV	**VIND/C** *versus* Vindesine 3 mg/m² IV every week × 6 weeks then every 2 weeks thereafter Cisplatin 120 mg/m² IV days 1 and 29, then every 6 weeks	19	7.4 mo	27	NR
	199/206 20 Stage IIIA 65 Stage IIIB 97 Stage IV	**V** *versus* Vinorelbine 30 mg/m² IV weekly	14	7.2 mo	30	NR
Cisplatin + Gemcitabine or Etoposide						
Abratt (52)	50/53 chemonaive (PS 0 = 1, 1 = 34, 2 = 18) 14 Stage IIIA 19 Stage IIIB 20 Stage IV	**GC** Gemcitabine 1,000 mg/m² IV weekly on days 1, 8, 15 Cisplatin 100 mg/m² IV day 15 Cycle: Every 28 days	52 (CR 4%) (PR 48%)	13 mo	61	NR
Cardenal (53)	135/135 chemonaive (PS 0-1) 67 Stage IIIB 68 Stage IV	**GC** Gemcitabine 1,250 mg/m² IV weekly on days 1 and 8 Cisplatin 100 mg/m² IV day 1 Cycle: Every 21 days	40.6* ($P = 0.02$)	8.7 mo	NR	8.7 mo* ($P = 0.01$)
		EC Etoposide 100 mg/m² IV days 1, 2, 3 Cisplatin 100 mg/m² IV day 1 Cycle: Every 21 days	21.9	7.2 mo	NR	7.2 mo

TABLE 126–6. (Continued)

Reference	Evaluable/Total Patients (Stage)	Regimen	Overall Response Rates (%)	Median Survival Duration	Median 1-Year Survival (%)	Time to Disease Progression
Irinotecan + Cisplatin						
DeVore (54)	52 chemonaive (PS 0 = 12, 1 = 32, 2 = 8) 11 Stage IIIB 44 Stage IV	**IC** Irinotecan 60 mg/m^2 IV days 1, 8, 15 • Required ≤ 40 mg/m^2 in 60% of patients Cisplatin 80 mg/m^2 IV day 1 Cycle: Every 28 days	28.8	9.9 mo	37	NR
Masuda (55)	378/398 chemonaive (PS 0-1 93%, 2% to 7%) 37% Stage IIIB 63% Stage IV	**IC** Irinotecan 60 mg/m^2 IV days 1, 8, 15 Cisplatin 80 mg/m^2 IV day 1 Cycle: Every 28 days	43	50.3 wk	47.5	
		C/VIND Cisplatin 80 mg/m^2 IV day 1 Vindesine 3 mg/m^2 IV days 1, 8, 15 Cycle: Every 28 days	31	47.4 wk	37.9	
		I (CPT-11) Irinotecan 100 mg/m^2 IV days 1, 8, 15	21	46.1 wk	40.7	

*Statistically significant difference.
NR, not reported.

associated with an increased frequency of peripheral injection site reactions.[57] Based on the survival advantage and minimal added toxicity of vinorelbine combined with cisplatin, some experts consider this regimen to be a standard against which future combination chemotherapy regimens should be measured. For example, the Southwest Oncology Group (SWOG 9509) is currently conducting a randomized phase III trial of cisplatin plus vinorelbine versus carboplatin plus paclitaxel in chemotherapy-naive patients with advanced NSCLC.

The **taxanes**, paclitaxel (Taxol) and docetaxel (Taxotere), are antimicrotubular agents that bind to the microtubules and promote and stabilize microtubular assembly, resulting in the inhibition of mitosis and cell death. Paclitaxel as a single agent and in combination regimens has been evaluated in patients with advanced NSCLC with positive results. Regimens have included paclitaxel administered by 1-hour, 3-hour, and 24-hour continuous infusion schedules at low doses (175 mg/m^2) and high doses (250 mg/m^2) with granulocyte colony-stimulating factor (G-CSF) support. Neutropenia is the dose-limiting toxicity of paclitaxel, but nonhematologic adverse reactions occur with differing frequencies based on the duration of infusion.[58] Hypersensitivity reactions (possibly caused by the Cremophor EL base) were frequent in the early phase I trials, leading to the current recommendations for pretreatment with corticosteroids and histamine H_1 and H_2 antagonists. Paclitaxel, because of its aqueous insolubility, is formulated in Cremophor EL and dehydrated alcohol, requiring non-PVC administration systems.

Bonomi and colleagues[59] of ECOG reported the preliminary results of 560 evaluable patients enrolled in a three-arm randomized trial with improved 1-year survival rates of 37% and 39% in the cisplatin plus paclitaxel 175 mg/m^2/24h infusion and the cisplatin plus paclitaxel 250 mg/m^2/24h infusion with G-CSF support, respectively, versus the standard regimen of cisplatin plus etoposide, which yielded a 1-year survival rate of 31%. Although no difference in efficacy was observed between the low- and high-dose paclitaxel arms, the high-dose arm resulted in significantly greater toxicity (neutropenia and peripheral neuropathy) and was more costly.

Langer and colleagues,[60] also of ECOG, reported the results from a phase II trial of 53 patients with stage IIIB or IV NSCLC treated with paclitaxel (135–215 mg/m^2) via 24-hour continuous infusion plus carboplatin dosed to an area under the curve (AUC) 7.5 on day 2 and given every 3 weeks. The regimen resulted in significant myelosuppression, with moderate to severe neutropenia in 57% of patients after the first cycle, necessitating the addition of G-CSF for the second and subsequent cycles. Significant thrombocytopenia and anemia were also reported in 47% and 33% of patients, respectively. Despite initially high response rates of 62% and an encouraging 1-year survival rate of 54%, the 2-year and 3-year survival rates remain dismal at 15% and 4%, respectively. A subsequent trial by Langer and colleagues[61] compared a 1-hour versus a 24-hour infusion of paclitaxel plus carboplatin, using identical dosage escalation. The 1-hour regimen resulted in an increased rate of peripheral neuropathy and minimal myelosuppression, but the response rate decreased to 27% (overall survival rates are not yet available). The shorter (<3 hours) infusions of paclitaxel are easily administered in the outpatient oncology setting and rarely require G-CSF support, making them more convenient and acceptable to patients than the 24-hour infusions. However, the results of ongoing cooperative trials in advanced NSCLC are required to clarify the most appropriate infusion schedule and the role of paclitaxel in combination with platinum compounds and the other newer agents.

Docetaxel (Taxotere) is an active semisynthetic taxoid, without the schedule-dependent efficacy and somewhat different toxicity issues than associated with paclitaxel administration. Most of the early docetaxel clinical trials used dosages of 60, 75, or 100 mg/m^2 infused intravenously over 1 hour every 3 weeks. Initial phase II single-agent docetaxel studies reported response rates from 25% to 38%, median survivals of 9 months and a 1-year survival rate of about 38% in chemotherapy-naive patients with advanced NSCLC.[2,62] Docetaxel is also active as a second-line agent against previously platinum-treated NSCLC with response rates of 15% to 21%, median survival of 7 months, and 1-year survival of 25%.[2,62,63]

Myelosuppression, primarily dose-dependent grade IV neutropenia, is the dose-limiting toxicity for docetaxel when given on an every 3-week cycle in single-agent and combination regimens.[62,63] However, when docetaxel is infused on a weekly schedule (36–43 mg/m^2 for 6 weeks followed by 2 weeks off), it is well tolerated with a different toxicity profile.[64,65] Nonhematologic moderate to severe fatigue and asthenia then emerge as the dose-limiting toxicity.

Myelosuppression on the weekly infusion schedule is generally mild and infrequent.

Nonhematologic adverse effects reported with all docetaxel dosing schedules include hypersensitivity reactions, rash, asthenia, fatigue, mucositis, alopecia, nail changes, conjunctival toxicity, peripheral neuropathy, and occasional symptomatic fluid retention syndrome (often a cumulative effect, with increasing risk at dosages $\geq$400 mg/m^2 resulting in peripheral edema and occasional pleural effusions). Patients should be premedicated with an oral corticosteroid regimen (i.e., dexamethasone 8 mg po twice daily) beginning 12 to 24 hours prior to the docetaxel infusion and continuing for a minimum of three doses for a total of 3 to 5 days to prevent or reduce the symptoms and severity of fluid retention syndrome and hypersensitivity reactions.[63,64]

Docetaxel received FDA approval in 1999 for the treatment of advanced stage IIIB and stage IV metastatic NSCLC after failure of a platinum-based chemotherapy regimen. Approval was granted based on the preliminary analysis presented from two randomized trials. The first trial compared docetaxel to best supportive care in 204 patients previously treated with platinum. The initial dose of docetaxel of 100 mg/m^2 (D 100) IV over 1 hour every 3 weeks was decreased to 75 mg/m^2 (D 75) after an interim study analysis reported a greater risk of severe neutropenia with the higher dose. The D 75 dose level was active and reported a significant advantage to best supportive care in terms of time-to-disease progression (10.6 weeks vs 6.7 weeks), median survival (7.5 months vs 4.6 months; $P = 0.047$) and 1-year survival 37% vs 11%; $P = 0.003$).[66] In the second trial, 373 patients previously treated with platinum were randomized to receive docetaxel 100 mg/m^2 or 75 mg/m^2 on day 1, or vinorelbine 30 mg/m^2 (V) on days 1, 8, and 15, or ifosfamide 2 g/m^2/day (I) plus mesna on days 1 through 3. All regimens were repeated intravenously every 3 weeks. The docetaxel arms reported higher partial response rates (D 100 10.8% vs D 75 6.7% vs V or I 0.8%) and minimal differences in median time-to-disease progression (7.9 months to 8.5 months) and median survival (5.5 months to 5.7 months). However, the 1-year survival rate for the D 75 regimen was 32%; the rate was 21% for the D 100 regimen ($P =$ NS) arm versus 19% for the vinorelbine and ifosfamide regimens (32% vs 19%; $P = 0.025$).[67]

Docetaxel has been successfully administered to chemotherapy-naive patients in combination regimens with both cisplatin and carboplatin. Docetaxel 75 mg/m^2 plus cisplatin (75–100 mg/m^2) infused on day 1 every 3 weeks is active and well tolerated with neutropenia being the dose-limiting toxicity.[62] Based on phase II data, this combination was included as one of the four arms in the randomized phase III ECOG 1594 trial (see discussion of this trial in gemcitabine section).[49] The addition of filgrastim (Neupogen) allowed a greater dose intensity in one phase II docetaxel plus cisplatin trial, resulting in a higher initial response rate and a slightly increased median survival. Investigators are currently evaluating combinations of docetaxel (65–80 mg/m^2) plus carboplatin (AUC 5 to 6) administered every 3 weeks.[62] The docetaxel plus carboplatin combination is also active, with neutropenia reported as the dose-limiting toxicity. Decreasing the carboplatin AUC to 5 while maintaining a higher docetaxel dose-intensity appears to maintain efficacy and to cause less neutropenia, and is thus being further investigated. However, the results of these encouraging studies must be confirmed in larger phase III trials. Numerous phase II and III multi-institutional and cooperative group trials are ongoing to evaluate the efficacy and toxicity of docetaxel with carboplatin, cisplatin, vinorelbine, gemcitabine, irinotecan, and thoracic radiation therapy.

Gemcitabine (Gemzar) is a nucleoside analog (antimetabolite) that is phosphorylated intracellularly by deoxycytidine kinase. It has an increased membrane permeability and affinity for deoxycytidine kinase, yielding higher intracellular concentrations of the active metabolite and prolonged inhibition of DNA, as compared to its structurally related predecessor cytarabine. Phase I and II trials of gemcitabine have demonstrated antitumor activity against a variety of solid tumors, including lung, breast, ovarian, and pancreatic cancers. Gemcitabine has been shown in numerous phase I and phase II trials to exhibit schedule-dependent toxicity.[68] Two slightly different gemcitabine treatment schedules are used in both single-agent and combination regimens for treatment of NSCLC in the outpatient setting. Gemcitabine 1,000 mg/m^2 is given IV over 30 minutes on days 1, 8, and 15 with cycles repeated every 28 days,[69] or gemcitabine 1,000–1,250 mg/m^2 on days 1 and 8 with cycles repeated every 21 days. Myelosuppression, primarily thrombocytopenia, is the dose-limiting toxicity for single-agent gemcitabine regimens and it frequently necessitates dosage reductions in the three consecutive weeks schedule (followed by 1 week off). Less thrombocytopenia is seen with the days 1 and 8 (every 21 days) regimen.[70] The overall toxicity profile for single-agent gemcitabine is modest. Toxicities include reversible elevations of aspartate transaminase (AST) and alanine transaminase (ALT) (hepatotoxicity), myelosuppression, anemia, mild nausea and vomiting, rash, flu-like symptoms, edema, fatigue, and anorexia.

Gemcitabine was approved in the United States in 1998 for use in first-line combination therapy with cisplatin for the treatment of nonresectable, locally advanced or metastatic NSCLC.[68] The FDA approved this new indication for gemcitabine based on data presented from 657 patients who participated in two randomized clinical trials with cisplatin. In one trial, gemcitabine 1,000 mg/m^2 IV on days 1, 8, and 15 plus cisplatin 100 mg/m^2 IV on day 1 every 28 days was compared to single-agent cisplatin.[71] The second registration trial compared gemcitabine 1,250 mg/m^2 IV on days 1 and 8 plus cisplatin 100 mg/m^2 IV on day 1 every 21 days to cisplatin 100 mg/m^2 IV on day 1 plus etoposide 100 mg/m^2 IV on days 1, 2, and 3[53] (Table 126–6). In both studies the objective response rates (26% vs 10% and 33% vs 14%, respectively), median survival (9.0 months vs 7.6 months and 8.7 months vs 7.0 months, respectively), and time-to-disease progression was significantly better for the gemcitabine plus cisplatin combinations.

The much anticipated preliminary results of a randomized phase III trial in patients with advanced NSCLC were reported in May 2000. This Eastern Cooperative Oncology Group (ECOG 1594) trial compared three platinum-containing regimens (cisplatin plus either gemcitabine (GC) or docetaxel (DC) vs paclitaxel plus carboplatin (PCb)) to the standard reference arm of cisplatin plus paclitaxel (CP).[49] Of the 1,207 patients enrolled from October 1996 through May 1999, 1,146 were eligible for data analysis. Enrollment included patients with stage IIIB with a poorer prognosis, which included a pleural or pericardial effusion (disease not responsive to radiotherapy), and patients with stage IV NSCLC. Patients were stratified by performance status (PS) and baseline weight loss. Patients with PS 0–2 were initially eligible for the trial, but an interim analysis revealed that patients with a PS 2 experienced increased toxicity with the cisplatin containing regimens and the study was subsequently limited to patients with PS 0–1 only. There were no significant differences between the paclitaxel plus cisplatin control arm and the other three regimens in response rate, median survival, or 1-year survival (Table 126–6). However, the GC regimen resulted in a modest 1 month advantage in time-to-disease progression ($P = 0.002$).

As expected, different toxicity patterns were reported for the four regimens. The PCb regimen was the best-tolerated regimen, but it also had the lowest response rate and time-to-disease progression.

The GC regimen had a higher incidence of severe thrombocytopenia and moderate to severe renal dysfunction, but had the lowest incidence of severe neutropenia and febrile neutropenia. Moderate nausea was a problem for all of the cisplatin-containing regimens and was the greatest in the GC regimen with higher dosage of cisplatin (100 mg/m^2 vs 75 mg/m^2). Overall, the results of the four regimens were quite similar in this trial, and no clear significant advantage for one regimen over another was evident.[49] The high proportion of patients with stage IV disease in this trial is probably responsible for the disappointingly low overall response rates and median survival. In the community setting, the PCb regimen may be slightly easier to administer and monitor. Both the GC and DC regimens warrant further investigation in advanced NSCLC with varying dosages and infusion schedules to evaluate efficacy and improve toxicity. Altering the gemcitabine dose and schedule to days 1 and 8 only, eliminating the day 15 dose, has successfully improved the toxicity profile in other gemcitabine containing regimens.

A randomized follow-up trial, ECOG 1599, opened for enrollment in late May 2000 to compare a modified version of PCb to GC. The doses and administration schedules were altered slightly in an attempt to equilibrate the toxicity profile between the arms while maintaining efficacy. The paclitaxel dose was decreased to 200 mg/m^2 in PCb arm, while in the GC arm the gemcitabine schedule was changed to day 1 and 8 only (no day 15) and the cisplatin dose was decreased to 60 mg/m^2.

Irinotecan (Camptosar, CPT-11) and **topotecan** (Hycamtin) are water-soluble analogs of camptothecin, which are potent inhibitors of topoisomerase I, the nuclear enzyme responsible for maintaining DNA topologic structure. Inhibition of topoisomerase I stabilizes single-strand DNA breaks and prevents religation (resealing), resulting in DNA dysfunction and apoptosis.[72] The role of irinotecan in the treatment of NSCLC is well documented, while the use of topotecan remains unclear, with conflicting data from early, small-scale trials.[73]

Single-agent irinotecan studies reported initial response rates of up to 35% in chemotherapy-naive advanced-stage NSCLC patients.[2,73] Unfortunately, response rates were low for previously treated patients with refractory disease. The primary dose-limiting toxicities associated with irinotecan-containing regimens are neutropenia and potentially severe late-onset diarrhea (see the discussion of treatment guidelines for irinotecan-induced acute and late-onset diarrhea included in Chap. 127).

Combination chemotherapy with irinotecan plus cisplatin yielded preliminary response rates of 40% to 54% in patients with chemotherapy-naive advanced-stage NSCLC. The irinotecan-cisplatin combination produced modest improvements in 1-year survival rates of 35% to 47%.[54,55,74] Irinotecan plus cisplatin is currently being evaluated as the reference arm for a four-arm Japan Cooperative Group study for advanced NSCLC and worldwide in numerous combination regimens combined with gemcitabine, docetaxel, and/or vinorelbine.

Preclinical data indicate that radiotherapy increases the proportion of cells in the S-phase, which may enhance the efficacy of topoisomerase I inhibitors. Thus, trials evaluating irinotecan as a single agent in combination chemotherapy regimens plus radiotherapy have been undertaken. A phase I/II trial of bimodality therapy for locally advanced NSCLC with single-agent irinotecan 60 mg/m^2 weekly for 6 weeks plus concurrent thoracic radiotherapy to the tumor site and regional lymph nodes resulted in an objective response rate of 77% (survival data not available for phase I).[75] The combined modality therapy resulted in dose-limiting esophagitis, severe pneumonitis, and diarrhea. The combination initially appears to be promising and a phase II continuation trial with irinotecan decreased to 45 mg/m^2 weekly plus concurrent radiotherapy will provide further toxicity evaluation and survival data for the regimen.

Guidelines

Stage I and Stage II NSCLC. The role of chemotherapy in early stage disease has not been clearly defined. Surgery, with or without radiotherapy, remains the "curative" treatment of choice for stage I and stage II NSCLC. Presently, trials are ongoing to evaluate the addition of postoperative adjuvant chemotherapy in combined regimens for a high-risk subset of stage I_b and stage II disease. The rationale for this research is based on the principle of eradicating undiagnosed micrometastases and preventing the onset of systemic disease by the addition of adjuvant chemotherapy with or without radiotherapy. This approach has been successful in locally advanced stage III disease.

Stage III and Stage IV NSCLC. For stage III disease that is surgically resectable, neoadjuvant chemotherapy, with or without radiotherapy, is given prior to surgery in an effort to (a) provide immediate systemic therapy to eradicate undetectable micrometastases and thereby prevent or delay the development of systemic disease; (b) decrease local tumor burden and thereby increase the potential for complete surgical resection; (c) take advantage of the treatment-naive tumors that may be more chemosensitive because of smaller size (earlier treatment vs after surgery), higher growth rate, and smaller hypoxic areas (traditionally chemoresistant areas); and (d) administer chemotherapy to patients who may have a better performance status prior to surgery and who are able to tolerate full-dose therapy. Conversely, potential disadvantages of neoadjuvant chemotherapy include (a) risk that toxicity resulting from the chemotherapy may decrease the patient's ability to tolerate subsequent surgery and/or radiation; (b) risk that if the tumor does not respond to the chemotherapy it will continue to grow and become nonresectable; and (c) a significant prolongation of the duration of treatment.

The rationale described above and the availability of newer chemotherapy regimens with apparent increased activity in NSCLC stimulated several pilot studies of neoadjuvant chemotherapy for patients with advanced stage III disease. The highest response rates have been observed with regimens that include a platinum agent combined with a second or third new chemotherapy agent. Results of these studies indicate that most patients with stage III disease are able to tolerate two or three courses of aggressive chemotherapy followed by definitive surgery and/or radiation. Although several of these early studies reported encouraging response rates (>50%), survival advantages could not be appropriately addressed in most of these nonrandomized trials.

The benefits of combined chemotherapy and radiotherapy has been clearly demonstrated for stage III nonresectable disease. The Cancer and Leukemia Group B (CALGB 8433) randomized 155 patients patient's with newly diagnosed nonresectable stage III NSCLC, a good performance (PS 0–1), no evidence of pleural effusions, and no prior treatment, to receive either radiation (RT) alone or two courses of cisplatin and vinblastine followed by radiation (CT-RT). Response rate in the combined modality therapy (CT-RT) was 56% versus 43% for the RT alone (P = NS). However; after 7 years of followup the median survival in CT-RT arm (13.7 months) remains significantly better than the RT arm (9.6 months) ($P = 0.012$), with 13 long-term survivors in CT-RT arm and only half as many in the RT group.[76] A meta-analysis of 11 trials including 1,780 patients with locally advanced stage III NSCLC receiving thoracic radiotherapy, with or without cisplatin-based chemotherapy, also concluded that mortality was reduced by 13% in patients randomized to receive chemotherapy.[77] Overall, evidence strongly suggests that chemotherapy with or without radiotherapy increases the likelihood that tumors may be completely resected and is superior to radiotherapy alone followed by surgery. Subsequently, in 1997, the American Society of Clinical Oncology (ASCO) released Treatment Guidelines for Unresectable NSCLC, confirming the role of chemotherapy in advanced stage III and stage IV disease and further recommending that a platinum-based combination regimen be used.[34] Duration of treatment with combination chemotherapy plus radiotherapy for advanced stage NSCLC should be two to eight cycles.[34]

SMALL CELL LUNG CANCER

CHEMOTHERAPY

In contrast to NSCLC, the use of aggressive combination chemotherapy regimens in SCLC has demonstrated a four- to fivefold increase in median survival. Without treatment, survival is generally less than 5 to 7 weeks for patients with metastatic disease (extensive-disease SCLC) and less than 12 weeks for patients with regional disease (limited-disease SCLC). Because SCLC has the propensity to disseminate early on in the disease, surgery is rarely indicated, except possibly in the occasional patients who present with a small, isolated lesion. A number of factors have been identified that appear to have prognostic importance in SCLC.[78,79] Patients who initially present with limited disease and are treated with aggressive chemotherapy regimens demonstrate a significantly longer median survival than do patients presenting with extensive disease treated with the same regimens.[22,80] Patients with a better performance status (PS–0, able to carry out all normal activity without restriction) and no weight loss at the time of initial diagnosis also have an improved prognosis.[22,81] Females appear to have a better prognosis than do males, as do patients younger than age 60 to 70 years. Patients with normal pretreatment serum LDH are also more likely to have limited disease, higher complete response rates, and longer median survivals.[81,82] A simple prognostic model for SCLC has been developed and verified; it uses LDH levels in concert with performance status and extent of disease.[83] In addition, LDH levels have been shown to be an independent prognostic factor for SCLC, correlating with disease stage, response to therapy, and survival.[81,82] A European study also reported that serum neuron-specific endolase (S-NSE), a biologic marker, may be substituted for LDH levels in the simple prognostic model for SCLC.[84]

A number of cytotoxic agents have demonstrated significant single-agent activity in chemotherapy-naive patients with limited- and extensive-disease SCLC, but the activity in recurrent or refractory SCLC is modest. Among the more commonly used chemotherapy agents in the United States are cisplatin, carboplatin, cyclophosphamide, ifosfamide, doxorubicin, etoposide (intravenous and oral regimens), and vincristine. Newer agents currently being investigated in the treatment of SCLC include docetaxel, epirubicin, gemcitabine, irinotecan, paclitaxel, topotecan (intravenous and oral regimens), and vinorelbine. Table 126–7 describes selected single-agent and combination chemotherapy regimens that use these newer agents.

Both paclitaxel and topotecan show promising activity as second-line agents, and these agents are currently being evaluated in combination chemotherapy regimens. A single-agent phase II trial of paclitaxel in heavily pretreated patients with drug-resistant SCLC reported partial responses in seven patients (29%) and stable disease in five patients, with a median overall survival of 100 days.[85] Topotecan administered as a second-line agent in drug-resistant patients, produced objective responses and decreased symptoms in 25% to 38% of patients.[87,88]

Combination Chemotherapy

Combination chemotherapy is clearly superior to single-agent therapy. Aggressive regimens appear to produce the highest response rates, longest median survivals, and the greatest percentage of long-term survivors.[22] Despite the apparent benefit of combination chemotherapy, the higher incidence of acute toxicity, neutropenic fever, and toxic death in the palliative (metastatic disease, noncurable) treatment setting must be considered.

In the United States, the most frequently used regimens include: (a) PE (EP): cisplatin (P) + etoposide (E); (b) CAV: cyclophosphamide (C) + doxorubicin (A) + vincristine (V); (c) CAE: cyclophosphamide (C) + doxorubicin (A) + etoposide (E); (d) EC: etoposide (E) + carboplatin (C); and (e) ICE: ifosfamide (I) + carboplatin (C) + etoposide (E). Table 126–8 describes selected combination chemotherapy regimens for SCLC. Overall response rates (80% to 90% vs 60% to 80%) and survival durations (12 to 20 months vs 7 to 11 months) are generally superior for patients with limited-disease versus extensive-disease stage (Table 126–9). The 2-year disease-free survival rate for patients with limited-disease stage at diagnosis is 15% to 40%. In comparison, very few patients with extensive-disease stage at diagnosis are alive at 2 years without disease. Unfortunately, when disease recurs, it is usually less sensitive to chemotherapy. SCLC that progresses during, or that recurs within ≤3 months of the initial chemotherapy is considered drug resistant. Restaging to determine the efficacy of induction therapy is done after two to three cycles of treatment. At this point, therapy is continued for patients with a complete or partial response or stable disease and discontinued or changed to a non-cross-resistant regimen in patients demonstrating evidence of progressive disease.

The optimal choice of combination chemotherapy regimen and scheduling continues to be the focus of ongoing clinical investigations. A recent meta-analysis of 19 randomized trials (4,054 evaluable patients) compared cisplatin-based to noncisplatin chemotherapy regimens.[100] Of these 19 trials, 10 trials randomized patients to cisplatin plus etoposide (PE) versus a regimen without either drug, and 9 trials compared PE to a regimen without cisplatin, but which may have included etoposide. Both the overall and subset analysis concluded that cisplatin-containing regimens yield a higher response rate, improved overall survival, lower incidence of life-threatening myelosuppression, and no increased risk of treatment-related mortality versus the non-cisplatin-containing regimens.

In a three-arm trial, the Southeastern Cancer Study Group compared four cycles of cisplatin and etoposide (PE) to six cycles of cyclophosphamide, doxorubicin, and vincristine (CAV) or CAV alternating with PE (total of six cycles) in a phase III trial of 437 patients with limited or extensive-disease stage SCLC.[95] The results of this study showed that four cycles of PE had equivalent efficacy to six cycles of CAV and CAV/PE with no significant difference in response rate or median survival (Table 126–8). Toxicity differed between the arms, with the PE regimen causing more severe nausea and vomiting and the CAV regimen more frequent severe myelosuppression, neurotoxicity, and cardiac toxicity. Carboplatin has been substituted for cisplatin in numerous SCLC regimens and has been shown to have similar efficacy

TABLE 126–7. Selected Single-Agent and Combination Trials of Newer Agents in Small Cell Lung Cancer

Study Author	Evaluable/Total Patients (Stage)	Drug Regimen/Dose	Overall Response Rate	Median Survival Duration (wk)	1-Year Survival
Smit (85) 1998	21/24 (9 LD) (15 ED) Drug resistant	**Paclitaxel** 175 mg/m² IV Day 1 over 3 hours every 3 weeks	29% (7 PR) (+ 5 SD)	14	NR
Glisson (86) 1999	38/41 ED Chemonaive	**TEP** Cisplatin 75 mg/m² IV day 1 Etoposide 80 mg/m² IV days 1 to 3 **Paclitaxel** 130 mg/m² IV day 1 over 3 h every 3 weeks × 6 cycles	90% (6 CR) (28 PR)	47	NR
Ardizzoni (87) 1997	92/101 (47 Drug res.) (45 Drug sens.)	**Topotecan** 1.5 mg/m² IV qd × 5, every 3 weeks	Drug res. 6.4% (1 CR) (2 PR)	33	NR
			Drug Sens. 37.8% (6 CR) (11 PR)	48	NR
Perez-Soler (88) 1996	28/32 Drug res. (VP-16 + CP)	**Topotecan** 1.25 mg/m² IV qd × 5, every 3 weeks (Cycle 2, ↓ 1.0 mg/m²)	11% (3 PR) (+ 5 SD)	20	3.5%
Eckardt (89) 1996 (Abstract) *Pooled analysis*	168 Drug Sens.	**Topotecan** 1.5 mg/m² IV qd × 5, every 3 weeks	18% (10 CR) (20 PR)	30	21%
Masuda (90) 1992	15/16 (5 LD) (10 ED) (Drug Res. + Drug Sens.)	**Irinotecan** 100 mg/m² IV over 90 min every week (median 7 cycles; range, 2–13)	47% (7 SD)	27	NR
Noda (91) 2000 (Abstract) Phase III trial Japan Clinical Oncology Group	ED 77	**CP** Irinotecan 60 mg/m² IV days 1, 8, 15 Cisplatin 60 mg/m² IV day 1 Cycle: every 4 weeks × 4 cycles *vs*	89% (13% CR) (P=0.013)	420 days	1 y: 60% (P=0.0047) 2 y: 19%
	ED 77	**PE** Cisplatin 60 mg/m² IV day 1 Etoposide 100 mg/m² IV days 1, 2, and 3 Cycle: every 3 weeks × 4 cycles	67% (2% CR)	300 days	1 y: 40% 2y: 6.5%
Cormier (92) 1994	26/29 ED Chemonaive	**Gemcitabine** 1000 mg/m² IV every week × 3, every 28 days (patients 1 to 17) followed by: **Gemcitabine** 1,250 mg/m² IV every week × 3, every 28 days (patients 18 to 26)	27% (1 CR) (6 PR) (12 SD)	52	NR
DePierre (93) 1995 (Abstract)	30 Chemonaive	**Vinorelbine** 30 mg/m² IV every week × 10 weeks	26.7% (8 PR) (7 SD)	NR	NR
Furuse (94) 1996	24/24 Drug sens.	**Vinorelbine** 25 mg/m² IV every week × ≥4 weeks	12.5% (3 PR) (9 SD)	NR	NR

Drug res, drug-resistant tumors, progressing during first-line therapy or within 3 months from response to chemotherapy; Drug Sens, drug-sensitive tumors, progressing > 3 months from initial response to chemotherapy; ED, extensive-disease stage; LD, limited-disease stage.

with somewhat less toxicity, particularly for patients with preexisting renal dysfunction or severe neuropathy.[22] A randomized trial with 143 evaluable patients (82 limited-disease stage and 62 extensive-disease stage) compared carboplatin and etoposide (CE) versus PE. The overall survival was 11.8 months for CE group and 12.5 months for the PE group.[98] Based on these data, PE, or, alternatively, CE, have become one of the most commonly used regimens to treat SCLC in the United States.

Combination chemotherapy regimens that include irinotecan have shown promise in both chemotherapy-naive and previously treated limited-disease stage and extensive-disease stage SCLC.[22,90] Noda et al. reported preliminary data from a Japanese Clinical Oncology Group phase III trial in extensive-disease stage SCLC. One hundred fifty-four (77 per arm) patients were randomized to CP (irinotecan [CPT-11] 60 mg/m² IV on days 1, 8, and 15 combined with cisplatin 60 mg/m² IV day 1 given every 4 weeks for

TABLE 126–8. Selected Combination Chemotherapy Regimens for Small Cell Lung Cancer

Study Author	Evaluable and Total Patients and Characteristics	Drug Regimen/Dose	Overall Response Rates (CR + PR)	Median Survival Duration (months)
Roth (95) 1992	437 ED	Arm A: **PE** Cisplatin 20 mg/m²/day IV days 1 to 5 Etoposide 80 mg/m²/day IV days 1 to 5 Cycle: every 3 weeks × **4 cycles**	51% (CR 10%)	ED 8.3
		vs Arm B: **CAV** Cyclophosphamide 1,000 mg/m² IV day 1 Doxorubicin 40 mg/m² day 1 Vincristine 1 mg/m² day 1 Cycle: every 3 weeks × **6 cycles**	61% (CR 7%)	ED 8.6
		vs Arm C: **CAV/PE** **CAV** on day 1 followed by **PE** on days 22 to 26 Cycle: every 6 weeks × **3 cycles**	59% (CR 7%)	ED 8.1
Fukuoka[1] (96) (1991)	288/300 **Chemonaive** **32% PS ≥ 2** LD ED 49 46	Arm A: **CAV** Cyclophosphamide 1,000 mg/m² IV day 1 Doxorubicin 50 mg/m² IV day 1 Vincristine 1.4 mg/m² (max 2 mg) IV day 1 Cycle: every 3 weeks × **6 cycles**	LD + ED 52 (55%) 25/51% (LD) 27/59% (ED)	LD + ED 9.9 LD ED 12.4 8.7
	LD ED 44 51	*vs* Arm B: **PE** Cistplatin 80 mg/m² IV day 1 Etoposide 100 mg/m² IV days 1, 3, and 5 Cycle: every 3 weeks × **4 cycles**	LD + ED 74 (78%) 34/77% (LD) 40/78% (ED)	LD + ED 9.9 LD ED 11.7 8.3
	LD ED 49 40	*vs* Arm C: **CAV/PE** **CAV** on day 1 followed by **PE** on days 22 to 26 Cycle: every 6 weeks × **3 cycles**	LD + ED 68 (76%) 43/88% (LD) 25/63% (ED)	LD + ED 11.8 LD ED 16.8 9
Hainsworth[2] (97) 1997	79 **Chemonaive** LD ED 41 79	**TCE** Paclitaxel 200 mg/m² IV over 1 hour, day 1 Carboplatin—AUC 6 IV, day 1 Etoposide 50 mg alternating with 100 mg orally, days 1 to 10 Cycle: every 21 days × 4 cycles	LD ED 98% 84% CR% 71% 21%	LD ED > 16 10
Skarlos[3] (98) 1994 Hellenic Cooperative Oncology Group	141 **Chemonaive** LD ED 41 31	Arm A: **CE** Carboplatin 300 mg/m² IV day 1 Etoposide 100 mg/m² IV days 1 to 3	LD ED 86% 64% CR% 37% 16%	LD + ED 11.8
	LD ED 41 30	Arm B: **PE** Cisplatin 50 mg/m² IV days 1 and 2 Etoposide 100 mg/m² IV days 1 to 3	LD ED 73% 50% CR% 44% 10%	LD + ED 12.5
Mavroudis[4] (99) (2000)	118/133 **Chemonaive** LD ED 29 33 (Evauable 49/62)	Arm B: **TEP** Cisplatin 80 mg/m² IV day 1 Etoposide 120 mg/m² IV day 1 and then lowered to 80 mg/m² IV on days 2 and 4 Paclitaxel 175 mg/m² IV + GCSF 5 μg/kg/day on days 5 to 15 Cycle: every 4 weeks	LD + ED CR 5% (3) PR 45% (28)	LD + ED 10.5
	LD ED 30 41 (Evauable 69/71)	Arm A: **PE** Cisplatin 80 mg/m² IV day 1 Etoposide 120 mg/m² IV days 1 to 3	LD + ED CR 4% (3) PR 42% (30)	LD + ED 11.5

ED, extensive-disease stage; LD, limited-disease stage.

1. LD patients with CR or PR after induction chemotherapy received thoracic radiotherapy only.
2. LD patients with CR or PR after induction chemotherapy received concurrent thoracic radiotherapy with cycles 3 and 4.
3. LD patients with CR or PR, and ED patients with CR after induction chemotherapy received concurrent thoracic radiotherapy and prophylactic cranial irradiation beginning with cycle 3.
4. Study was stopped prematurely because of high rate of severe toxicity and death (eight toxic deaths vs zero) in the TEP arm.

TABLE 126–9. SCLC Responses to Optimal Chemotherapy Regimens Based on Stage of Disease

	Limited Disease	Extensive Disease
Overall response (CR + PR)	80% to 95%	60% to 85%
Complete response	50% to 60%	15% to 30%
Median survival (months)	12% to 20%	7% to 11%
2-year disease-free survival	15% to 40%	Rare

Adapted from Ref. 22.

four cycles) versus EP (etoposide and cisplatin given every 3 weeks for four cycles).[91] Study enrollment was halted after the interim analysis results showed a statistically significant difference in median survival and 1-year survival in the CP arm (Table 126–7). CP was well tolerated, with significantly less moderate to severe neutropenia (66% vs 92%) and thrombocytopenia (5% vs 19%) versus the EP arm, respectively. As expected, moderate to severe diarrhea was reported in 16% of patients receiving irinotecan. But the improved overall survival, although it was statistically significant, represents only a modest improvement. Additional studies are ongoing, combining irinotecan with various conventional and newer agents.

Duration of Treatment

Induction followed by maintenance chemotherapy for limited-disease stage and extensive-disease stage SCLC was evaluated in a randomized trial with 585 evaluable patients who received cyclophosphamide, doxorubicin, and etoposide (CAE) regimen for 5 cycles versus 12 cycles.[101] The extended chemotherapy regimen did not significantly improve long-term survival (median survival: 325 days; limited-disease stage disease: 396 days vs extensive-disease stage disease: 267 days, with a 3.2% overall survival in both arms at 5 years). In addition, patients who received the extended duration (12 cycles) of chemotherapy experienced an increased incidence of acute toxicity and second malignancies. ECOG demonstrated an overall median survival of approximately 20 months in a comparative study of cisplatin and etoposide (PE) for four cycles plus concurrent once-daily or twice-daily thoracic radiotherapy.[102] This trial reported the longest overall median survival for SCLC observed to date in a cooperative trial group, which further supports the recommendation for a short course of induction therapy. These data have been confirmed by several randomized trials, comparing induction with or without maintenance chemotherapy regimens and versus supportive care, with most studies reporting similar survival outcomes.[22] Most experts currently recommend that chemotherapy be administered for four to six cycles in SCLC patients who respond (CR, PR) to initial induction chemotherapy.

Dose Intensity

Experimental animal and human tumor data suggest that the amount of drug administered over a unit of time may be critical to the degree of tumor cell kill.[103] The importance of "dose-intensity" has been evaluated in many types of human cancer, particularly those like SCLC, which are initially responsive to chemotherapy, but are not usually curable with conventional therapies. Randomized trials comparing dose-intensive (high-dose) CAE, CAVE, PE, and CEEP (CTX, epirubicin, etoposide, and cisplatin) versus standard-dose regimens have failed to demonstrate significant differences in overall survival.[104–108] In some studies, however, a significant difference was observed in patients with limited-disease stage SCLC.[108] A meta-analysis of 60 reported clinical trials failed to establish a consistent relationship between dose intensity and survival for most SCLC chemotherapy regimens.[109] Dose intensity can also be increased by giving weekly chemotherapy versus standard 3-week intervals. Numerous trials have explored weekly chemotherapy with a variety of combination regimens, and most of these trials failed to demonstrate a survival advantage for weekly chemotherapy in SCLC.[110,111]

The incidence and severity of toxicities such as granulocytopenia, febrile neutropenia, mucositis, and weight loss are significantly higher in patients who receive dose-intensive treatment regimens. Currently, dose-intensive chemotherapy regimens should not be considered as standard oncology practice and should be reserved for clinical trials, in patients with limited-disease stage SCLC and for the evaluation of newer agents.

Alternating Noncross-resistant Regimens

Because the duration of response is usually brief (less than 1 year) for patients achieving a complete response, it appears that drug-resistant cells continue to grow during treatment and eventually constitute a major portion of the tumor. The Goldie-Coldman theory predicts that cycling of two active, non-cross-resistant chemotherapy regimens may overcome this problem.[112] Although theoretically it would seem ideal to administer all the drugs simultaneously, the treatment-related toxic effects would be prohibitive. Several phase III clinical trials have used alternating, non-cross-resistant regimens in the management of SCLC and most have failed to demonstrate substantial benefits.[113,114] It should be noted, however, that the second regimen was not cross-resistant and subtherapeutic doses were administered in many of these early trials.[115] In one large trial of patients with extensive-disease stage SCLC, the National Cancer Institute of Canada demonstrated a higher overall response rate ($n = 285$, 80% vs 63%, $P < 0.002$) and longer progression-free survival and overall survival (9.6 vs 8.0 months, $P = 0.03$) for patients randomized to receive six cycles of CAV alternating with CE versus CAV only.[116] In contrast, Fukuoka et al. compared CAV versus CE versus alternating cycles of CAV/CE in limited- and extensive-disease stage SCLC patients.[95] Although no difference in survival was observed between the regimens for patients with extensive-disease stage SCLC, an overall survival advantage was demonstrated in the patients with limited-disease stage SCLC receiving alternating CAV/CE regimen versus either the CE or CAV regimens (16.8 months CAV/CE versus 11.7 months CAV and 12.4 months CE arms, respectively). After adjusting for prognostic factors, the investigators found that CAV/PE versus PE was significantly superior ($P = .032$), but the difference between the CAV/PE versus CAV did not reach statistical significance.

In summary, limited-disease stage SCLC patients appear to have a greater response rate to alternating non-cross-resistant regimens than do extensive-disease stage SCLC patients. The recent availability of new cytotoxic agents with novel mechanisms of action, such as the taxanes, paclitaxel and docetaxel, and the topoisomerase I inhibitors, irinotecan and topotecan, provide new opportunities for exploring alternating noncross-resistant regimens.

Combination Chemotherapy Plus Colony-stimulating Factor

Most SCLC chemotherapy regimens are associated with a significant degree of toxicity, especially severe neutropenia, which increases the risk of serious and life-threatening infections. Therefore, the more aggressive SCLC regimens have been combined with a colony-stimulating factor such as filgrastim (G-CSF, Neupogen) or sargramostim (GM-CSF, Leukine) to reduce the incidence and severity of infectious complications. When patients receiving CAE therapy were randomized to receive either filgrastim or placebo, those receiving the colony-stimulating factor experienced shorter duration's of severe neutropenia (5.2 vs 1.8 days), fewer febrile neutropenic episodes, and required fewer days of antibiotic therapy and hospitalization.[117]

Hematopoietic Stem Cell Transplantation

High-dose chemotherapy followed by bone marrow or peripheral blood stem-cell transplant has been evaluated in numerous small phase I and phase II trials of patients with limited-disease stage or extensive-disease stage SCLC, with inconsistent results.[22,118–121] Promising results were reported from an early randomized phase III trial of selected patients younger than 65 years of age with a good performance status and no serious concurrent medical conditions. One hundred one patients initially received conventional chemotherapy with methotrexate, cyclophosphamide, vincristine, doxorubicin plus prophylactic cranial irradiation (PCI) for three cycles, followed by two cycles of cisplatin and etoposide. Patients ($n = 45$) with either limited-disease in CR or PR or extensive-disease in CR were randomized to receive either an additional cycle of conventional chemotherapy with carmustine, cyclophosphamide, etoposide or the same agents at high dosages followed by autologous bone marrow transplantation. Disease-free survival was significantly increased in the patients receiving high-dose chemotherapy plus autologous bone marrow transplantation (28 weeks vs 10 weeks, $P = 0.002$) measured from the time of randomization. But no significant difference was noted in the median overall survival, measured from the date of the first cycle of induction chemotherapy (68 weeks vs 55 weeks respectively, including four deaths as a consequence of complications attributed to high-dose plus peripheral blood stem-cell transplant therapy; $P = 0.13$).[119]

Because there exists a small, but definite, cure rate in SCLC, extensive research efforts to evaluate potential new treatment modalities are crucial. Thus, further evaluation of high-dose chemotherapy plus hematopoietic stem cell transplantation continues to be investigated in select cohorts of younger SCLC patients with good performance status and minimal concurrent disease states.

RADIOTHERAPY

SCLC, a rapidly proliferating tumor, is considered very radiosensitive. Radiotherapy has been used alone and in combination with chemotherapy to treat tumors limited to the thoracic cavity. The rationale for combined modality therapy is based on the premise that the addition of radiotherapy to chemotherapy will better control bulky disease within the chest primary tumor site.[22] This combined-modality therapy may decrease the incidence and delay the onset of local tumor recurrences.[122] In most randomized trials, combined modality therapy has only modestly improved disease-free survival (e.g., 1 to 4 months) and 2-year survival (7% vs 17%) over that achieved with chemotherapy alone. A meta-analysis of 13 randomized studies of more than 2,100 patients with limited-disease stage SCLC reported that chemotherapy plus radiation significantly reduced the death rate by 14% and improved the 3-year survival by 5.4%.[123] The optimal dose and scheduling of thoracic radiotherapy (once-daily vs twice-daily) plus chemotherapy has not been fully defined by large-scale randomized clinical trials. But it appears that thoracic radiotherapy given concurrently with cycle one of chemotherapy versus later cycles or alternating with chemotherapy are more likely to produce favorable responses than when radiotherapy is administered following chemotherapy.[22,124,125] Unfortunately, many studies of combined-modality therapy have been associated with increased morbidity when compared to chemotherapy alone or radiotherapy after chemotherapy. Patients who receive twice-daily radiotherapy experience a greater incidence of severe esophagitis. When radiation therapy is combined with radiosensitizing drugs (e.g., doxorubicin), the incidence of radiation esophagitis and pneumonitis increases. Factors that are associated with a higher risk for severe radiation pneumonitis include PS $\geq$ 1, female > male, and forced expiratory volume of the lung in 1 second (FEV_1) < 2 L.[126] Interestingly, chemotherapy regimen, radiotherapy dose, and field size were not predictors of severe radiation pneumonitis. Combined-modality clinical trials currently underway are evaluating various dosages, schedules, and new techniques as three-dimensional radiotherapy in combination with a variety of chemotherapeutic agents in an attempt to maximize tumor control with an acceptable degree of toxicity.

Brain Metastases

Brain metastases are present at the time of diagnosis in 10% of SCLC patients. The cumulative incidence of brain metastasis rises to 50% in patients alive at 2 years, which is consistent with the rate previously documented in autopsy review series.[22,127] The role of prophylactic cranial irradiation (PCI) is based on the theory that eradication of microscopic or subclinical brain metastases would prevent or delay the onset of brain metastases. Early small-scale trials evaluated the addition of PCI to chemotherapy and thoracic radiotherapy, resulting in a decrease in the rate of brain metastases, but no discernible difference in overall survival in most studies. Neurologic and cognitive impairment and abnormalities on brain CT scans have been reported in long-term survivors receiving PCI.[128,129] A retrospective analysis of these data confirmed that the use of PCI should be restricted to selected SCLC patients who achieve a complete remission after initial chemotherapy and thoracic radiotherapy. Patients with residual systemic disease should not receive PCI because of the continued high risk for seeding the CNS with metastases, negating any potential benefits and denying the patients a future chance of palliative irradiation for acute CNS symptoms.[130] Based on the potential toxicity of PCI and the unconfirmed survival advantage, the role of PCI has been a point of controversy for many years.[22,131,132] However, the Prophylactic Cranial Irradiation Overview Collaborative Group recently published meta-analysis results from seven SCLC trials enrolling patients from 1985 onward. The analysis included data from 987 patients with SCLC in complete remission after initial therapy and compared overall survival with the addition of PCI to an observation group. The pooled relative rate of death in the patients receiving PCI compared to the observation group was 0.84, which corresponded to a modest 5.4% absolute increase in overall survival at 3 years (15.3% alive in observation group vs 20.7% alive in the PCI group, $P = 0.01$).[132] In addition, PCI increased the rate of disease-free survival and decreased the incidence of brain metastases with a trend toward greater benefit with earlier delivery of PCI.

For patients with symptomatic brain metastases, therapeutic dosages of cranial irradiation usually control the CNS disease. Dexamethasone (to decrease intracranial pressure) and anticonvulsants are routinely administered to patients with brain metastases for symptomatic control and seizure prevention. Patients generally die because of complications from systemic disease progression.

Topotecan crosses the intact blood-brain barrier resulting in drug concentrations in the cerebrospinal fluid of 30% to 40% of plasma levels.[133,134] Several trials of intravenous topotecan recently reported a reduction in the size of brain metastases.[135,136] As this agent becomes more widely used in the treatment of newly diagnosed SCLC, it will be important to evaluate whether or not it has an impact on the frequency of brain metastases in later stages of the disease.

COMPLICATIONS AND SUPPORTIVE CARE

Patients with lung cancer frequently have numerous concurrent medical problems. Such problems may be related to invasion of the primary tumor and its metastases, paraneoplastic syndromes (see Clinical Presentation), chemotherapy and radiotherapy toxicity, or concomitant disease states (e.g., cardiac disease, renal dysfunction, chronic obstructive pulmonary disease, asthma, diabetes). Depression is also common in patients with SCLC and NSCLC; it may be persistent and should be treated.[137] Identification, diagnosis, and treatment of the patient as a whole may improve the patient's overall quality of life and tolerance to cancer treatments.

The chemotherapy regimens used in the management of lung cancer are intensive and are associated with a wide variety of toxic effects. Nausea and vomiting may be severe. Cisplatin-containing regimens require the use of aggressive acute and delayed antiemetic regimens containing a 5-HT_3 antagonist plus dexamethasone. Patients experiencing protracted nausea and vomiting may require intravenous hydration and nutritional support. Myelosuppression is often the dose-limiting toxicity associated with chemotherapy. Granulocytopenia places patients at a high risk for serious infections. Other toxic effects associated with these chemotherapy regimens include mucositis, nephrotoxicity, peripheral neuropathies, and ototoxicity.

Likewise, patients receiving radiation therapy may experience complications including severe esophagitis, fatigue, radiation pneumonitis, and cardiac toxicity. When combined with chemotherapy, these toxicities are often enhanced.[138] The patient's baseline performance status and the degree of pulmonary dysfunction (e.g., chronic obstructive pulmonary disease from years of tobacco use/smoking) must be considered in the decision of radiation dosage and fractionation.

It is readily apparent that many lung cancer patients receive complex pharmacologic regimens that may include chemotherapeutic agents, antiemetics, antibiotics, analgesics, anticoagulants, bronchodilators, corticosteroids, anticonvulsants, and cardiovascular agents. Such regimens necessitate intensive therapeutic monitoring in order to avoid drug-related and radiotherapy-related toxic effects and to optimize therapeutic outcome for individual patients.

▶ PRINCIPLES OF PHARMACOTHERAPY

- Lung cancer is the leading cause of cancer deaths in both men and women in the United States. The overall 5-year survival rate for all types of lung cancer is approximately 14%. Cigarette smoking is responsible for about 83% of all lung cancers.
- Four major histologic types account for > 90% of all lung cancers; these include adenocarcinoma, large cell and squamous cell carcinoma, and small cell lung cancer. Small cell cancer is the most rapidly growing and, in general, the most sensitive to cytotoxic chemotherapy.
- Although early detection strategies have been very effective in reducing mortality of other common cancers such as cervical and breast cancers, efforts to detect lung tumors at an earlier stage (e.g., sputum cytology or chest x-rays) have not reduced the mortality rates associated with lung cancer.
- Many lung cancers go undetected until they are advanced because individuals who have a long history of cigarette smoking are unlikely to notice the early symptoms of cough or dyspnea. It is often symptoms associated with large tumors or metastatic disease that prompt medical attention.
- Surgery is the treatment of choice for NSCLC that are early stage (stage I or II). If the tumor is deemed inoperable owing to its anatomic location, or if the patient is a poor surgical risk, radiation therapy may be used, although 5-year survival rates are usually inferior to those with surgery.
- For patients with locally advanced NSCLC (stage III), recent evidence suggests that chemotherapy with or without radiation followed by surgery improves survival over radiation followed by surgery.
- Although, historically, NSCLC has not been considered to be amenable to cytotoxic chemotherapy, regimens developed in recent years demonstrate improved response and survival rates. Several randomized trials have demonstrated that combination chemotherapy was superior to best supportive care. Patients who are most likely to benefit from chemotherapy include those with a good baseline performance status, no (or minimal) weight loss prior to treatment, and less-extensive disease spread. Regimens that demonstrate the highest response rates include cisplatin plus either etoposide, vinorelbine, paclitaxel, docetaxel, or gemcitabine.
- No single regimen is considered the standard first-line treatment for NSCLC. The most appropriate chemotherapy regimen for a patient with NSCLC should be selected based on the patient's ability to tolerate the expected toxicities and consideration of whether concomitant radiation will be administered (and how that will impact toxicities). For example, single-agent vinorelbine is an acceptable alternative for elderly or debilitated patients who cannot tolerate the side effects of cisplatin.
- Combination chemotherapy will prolong the survival of most patients with SCLC. Patients with limited disease are more likely to have a complete response to chemotherapy and longer survival than those who have extensive disease at the time of diagnosis. Patients with no weight loss and a better performance status at diagnosis also have an improved prognosis.
- The most widely used chemotherapy regimens for SCLC include cyclophosphamide, doxorubicin, and etoposide; cisplatin and etoposide; and ifosfamide, carboplatin, and etoposide.
- Despite very high response rates to chemotherapy, most patients with SCLC eventually have disease progression and die from this disease. In most studies, alternative strategies, such as alternating non-cross-resistant chemotherapy regimens or high-dose chemotherapy with hematopoietic stem cell transplantation, have not improved long-term survival rates.
- Radiation therapy to the involved lung field given concurrently or alternating with chemotherapy appears to improve survival, but may also significantly increase the risk of toxicities, including myelosuppression and esophagitis.
- Over the past decade, supportive care therapies such as hematopoietic growth factors to attenuate myelosuppression and

5-HT_3 antagonist antiemetics have drastically improved patients' abilities to tolerate the toxicities associated with cytotoxic regimens commonly used to treat lung cancer.

REFERENCES

1. Greenlee RT, Hill-Harmon MB, Murray T, Thun M. Cancer statistics, 2001. CA Cancer J Clin 2001;51:15–36.
2. Ginsberg RJ, Vokes EE, Rosenzweig K. Non-small cell lung cancer. In: DeVita VT, Hellman S, Rosenberg SA, eds. Cancer. Principles and Practice of Oncology, 6th ed. Philadelphia, Lippincott-Williams and Wilkins, 2001:925–983.
3. Sekido Y, Fong KM, Minna JM. Molecular biology of lung cancer. In: DeVita VT, Hellman S, Rosenberg SA, eds. Cancer. Principles and Practice of Oncology, 6th ed. Philadelphia, Lippincott-Williams and Wilkins, 2001:917–925.
4. Aaronson SA. Growth factors and cancer. Science 1991;254:1146–1153.
5. Miller YE, Franklin WA. Molecular events in lung carcinogenesis. Hematol Oncol Clin North Am 1997;11:215–234.
6. Bennett WP, Hussein SP, Vahakangas KH et al. Molecular epidemiology of human cancer risk: Gene-environment interactions and p53 mutations spectrum in human lung cancer. J Pathol 1999;187:8–18.
7. Tammemagi MC, McLaughlin JR, Bull SB. Meta-analysis of p53 tumor-suppressor gene alternations and clinicopathological features in resected lung cancers. Cancer Epidemiol Biomarkers Prev 1999;8:625–634.
8. Tsai CM, Chang KT, Wu LH, et al. Correlations between intrinsic chemoresistance and HER-2/neu gene expression, p53 gene mutations, and cell proliferation characteristics in non-small cell lung cancer cell lines. Cancer Res 1996;56:206–209.
9. Siegfried JM, Weissfeld LA, Singh-Kaw P, et al. Association of immunoreactive hepatocyte growth factor with poor survival in resectable non-small cell lung cancer. Cancer Res 1997;57:433–439.
10. Rosell R, Li S, Skacel Z, et al. Prognostic impact of mutated *K-ras* gene in surgically resected non-small cell lung cancer patients. Oncogene 1993;8:2407–2412.
11. Huncharek M, Muscat J, Geschwind JF. *K-ras* oncogene mutation as a prognostic marker in non-small cell lung cancer: A combined analysis of 881 cases. Carcinogenesis 1999;20:1507–1510.
12. Sulzer MA, Leers MP, van Noord JA, Bollen EC, Theunissen PH. Reduced E-cadherin expression is associated with increased lymph node metastasis and unfavorable prognosis in non-small cell lung cancer. Am J Res Crit Care Med 1998;157:1319–1323.
13. Adachi M, Taki T, Huang C, et al. Reduced integrin alpha-3 expression as a factor of poor prognosis in patients with adenocarcinoma of the lung. J Clin Oncol 1998;16:1060–1067.
14. Islam SS, Schottenfeld D. Declining FEV_1 and chronic productive cough in cigarette smokers: A 25-year prospective study of lung cancer incidence in Tecumseh, Michigan. Cancer Epidemiol Biomarkers Prev 1994;3:289–298.
15. Mattson ME, Pollack ES, Cullen JW. What are the odds that smoking will kill you? Am J Public Health 1987;77:425–431.
16. Damber LA, Larson LG. Smoking and lung cancer with special regard to type of cancer: A case-control study in north Sweden. Br J Cancer 1986;53:673–681.
17. Menck HR, Casagrande JT, Henderson BE. Industrial air pollution. Possible effect on lung cancer. Science 1974;183:210–212.
18. Menkes MS, Comstock GW, Vulleumier JP, et al. Serum beta-carotene, vitamin A and E, selenium and the risk of lung cancer. N Engl J Med 1986;315:1250–1254.
19. Ziegler RG, Mason TJ, Stemhagen A, et al. Carotenoid intake, vegetables, and the risk of lung cancer among white men in New Jersey. Am J Epidemiol 1986;123:1080–1093.
20. The Alpha-Tocopherol, Beta Carotene Cancer Prevention Study Group. The effect of vitamin E and beta carotene on the incidence of lung cancer and other cancers in male smokers. N Engl J Med 1994;330:1029–1035.
21. Sobin LH. The World Health Organization's histological classification of lung tumors: A comparison of the first and second editions. Cancer Detect Prev 1982;5:391–406.
22. Murren J, Glatstein E, Pass HI. Small cell lung cancer. In: DeVita VT, Hellman S, Rosenberg SA, eds. Cancer. Principles and Practice of Oncology, 6th ed. Philadelphia, Lippincott-Williams and Wilkins, 2001: 983–1018.
23. Cuttitta F, Carney DN, Mulshine J, et al. Bombesin-like peptides can function as autocrine growth factors in human small-cell lung cancer. Nature 1985;316:823–826.
24. Fontana RS, Sanderson DR, Woolner LB, et al. Lung cancer screening: The Mayo program. J Occup Med 1986;28:746–750.
25. Melamed MR, Flehinger BJ, Zaman MB, et al. Screening for early lung cancer. Results of the Memorial Sloan-Kettering study in New York. Chest 1984;86:44–53.
26. Tockman MS. Survival and mortality from lung cancer in a screened population. The Johns Hopkins study. Chest 1986;89(suppl):324S–325S.
27. Eddy DM. Screening for lung cancer. Ann Intern Med 1989;111: 232–237.
28. Saunders CA, Dussek JE, O'Doherty MJ, et al. Evaluation of fluorine-18-fluorodeoxy-glucose whole-body positron emission tomography imaging in the staging of lung cancer. Ann Thorac Surg 1999;67:790–797.
29. American Joint Committee on Cancer (AJCC). Manual for Staging of Cancer, 4th ed. Philadelphia, Lippincott, 1997:127–137.
30. Deslauriers J, Grégoire J. Surgical therapy for early non-small cell lung cancer. Chest 2000;177(suppl 4):104S–109S.
31. Martini N, Bains MS, Burt ME, et al. Incidence of local recurrence and second primary tumors in resected stage I lung cancer. J Thorac Cardiovasc Surg 1995;109(1):120–129.
32. Langer CJ. Induction or neoadjuvant therapy in resectable non-small cell lung cancer. Semin Oncol 1999;26(suppl 5):34–39.
33. National Comprehensive Cancer Network. NCCN non-small-cell lung cancer practice guidelines. Oncology 1996;10(suppl):81–111.
34. Non-Small-Cell Lung Cancer Expert Panel for the American Society of Clinical Oncology. Clinical practice guidelines for the treatment of unresectable non-small-cell lung cancer. J Clin Oncol 1997;15: 2996–3018.
35. Sause WT, Turrisi AT. Principles and applications of preoperative and standard radiotherapy for regionally advanced non-small cell lung cancer. In: Pass HI, Mitchell JB, Johnson DH, et al., eds. Lung Cancer: Principles and Practice. Philadelphia, Lippincott-Raven, 1996:697–710.
36. Johnson DH. Locally advanced unresectable non-small cell lung cancer: New treatment strategies. Chest 2000;117:123S–125S.
37. Cormesir Y, Bergeron D, LaForge J, et al. Benefits of polychemotherapy in advanced non-small-cell bronchogenic carcinoma. Cancer 1982; 50:845–849.
38. Rapp E, Pater J, Willan A, et al. Chemotherapy can prolong survival in patients with advanced non-small cell lung cancer: Report of a Canadian multicenter randomized trial. J Clin Oncol 1988;6:633–641.
39. Cartei G, Cartei F, Cantone A, et al. Cisplatin-cyclophosphamide-mitomycin combination chemotherapy with supportive care versus supportive care alone for treatment of metastatic non- small-cell lung cancer. J Natl Cancer Inst 1993;85:794–800.
40. Non-Small Cell Collaborative Group. Chemotherapy in non-small cell lung cancer: A meta-analysis using updated data on individual patients from 52 randomized clinical trials. BMJ 1995;311:899–909.
41. Jaakimainen L, Goodwin J, Pater J, et al. Counting the costs of chemotherapy in a National Cancer Institute of Canada randomized trial in non-small cell lung cancer. J Clin Oncol 1990;8:1301–1309.
42. Evans WK, Will BP, Berthelot JM, et al. The cost of managing lung cancer in Canada. Oncology 1995;9:147–153.
43. Ramsey SD, Moinpour M, Lovato LC, et al. An economic analysis of Southwest Oncology Group Trial S9509: Cisplatin/vinorelbine vs. carboplatin/paclitaxel for advanced non-small cell lung cancer. Proc Am Soc Clin Oncol 2000;19:1913. Abstract.
44. Evans WK, Will BP, Berthelot JM, Earle CC. Cost of combined modality interventions for stage III non-small-cell lung cancer. J Clin Oncol 1997;15(9):3038–3048.

45. Sacristan JA, Kennedy-Martin T, Roswell R, et al. Economic evaluation in a randomized phase III clinical trial comparing gemcitabine/cisplatin and etoposide/cisplatin in non-small cell lung cancer. Lung Cancer 2000;28:97–107.
46. Marino P, Preatoni A, Cantoni A, et al. Single-agent chemotherapy versus combination chemotherapy in advanced non-small cell lung cancer: A quality and meta-analysis study. Lung Cancer 1995;13:1–12.
47. Lilenbaum RC, Langenberg P, Dickersin K. Single agent versus combination chemotherapy in patients with advanced nonsmall cell lung carcinoma. Cancer 1998;82:116–126.
48. Fukuoka M, Masuda N, Furuse K, et al. A randomized trial in inoperable non-small cell lung cancer: Vindesine and cisplatin versus mitomycin, vindesine, and cisplatin versus etoposide and cisplatin alternating with vindesine and mitomycin. J Clin Oncol 1991;9:606–613.
49. Schiller JH, Harrington D, Sandler A. A randomized phase III trial of four chemotherapy regimens in advanced non-small cell lung cancer (NSCLC). Proc Am Soc Clin Oncol 2000;19:A-2. Abstract.
50. Kelly K, Crowley J, Bunn RB, et al. A randomized phase III trial of paclitaxel plus carboplatin (PC) versus vinorelbine plus cisplatin (VC) in untreated advanced non-small cell lung cancer (NSCLC): A Southwest Oncology Group (SWOG) trial. Proc Am Soc Clin Oncol 1999;18: A-1777. Abstract.
51. LeChevalier T, Brisgand D, Douillard J, et al. Randomized study of vinorelbine and cisplatin versus vindesine and cisplatin versus vinorelbine alone in advanced non-small-cell lung cancer: Results of a European multicenter trial including 612 patients. J Clin Oncol 1994:12;360–367.
52. Abratt RP, Bezwoda WR, Falkson G, et al. Efficacy and safety profile of gemcitabine in non- small cell lung cancer: A phase II study. J Clin Oncol 1994;12:1535–1540.
53. Cardenal F, Lopez-Cabrerizo MP, Anton A, et al. Randomized phase III study of gemcitabine-cisplatin versus etoposide-cisplatin in the treatment of locally advanced or metastatic non-small-cell lung cancer. J Clin Oncol 1999;17:12–18.
54. DeVore RF, Johnson DH, Crawford J, et al. Phase II study of irinotecan plus cisplatin in patients with advanced non-small-cell lung cancer. J Clin Oncol 1999;17(9):2710–2720.
55. Masuda N, Fukoka M, Negro S, et al. Randomized trial comparing cisplatin (CDDP) and irinotecan (CPT-11) versus CDDP and vindesine (VDS) versus CPT-11 alone in advanced non- small cell lung cancer (NSCLC), a multicenter phase III study. Proc Am Soc Clin Oncol 1999;18:1774. Abstract.
56. Wozniak AJ, Crowley JJ, Balcerzak SP, et al. Randomized trial comparing cisplatin with cisplatin plus vinorelbine in the treatment of advanced non-small cell lung cancer: A Southwestern Oncology Group study. J Clin Oncol 1998;16:459–465.
57. Rittenberg CN, Gralla RJ, Rehmeyer TA. Assessing and managing venous irritation associated with vinorelbine tartrate (Navelbine). Oncol Nurs Forum 1995;22:707–710.
58. Rowinsky EK, Donehower RC. Antimicrotubule agents. In: Chabner BA, Longo DL, eds. Cancer Chemotherapy and Biotherapy, Principles and Practice, 2nd ed. Philadelphia, Lippincott-Raven, 1996:263–296.
59. Bonomi P, Kim K, Chang A, et al. Phase III trial comparing etoposide (E), cisplatin (C) versus Taxol (T) with cisplatin-G-CSF (G) versus Taxol-cisplatin in advanced non-small cell lung cancer. The Eastern Cooperative Oncology Group (ECOG) trial. Proc Am Soc Clin Oncol 1996;15:382. Abstract.
60. Langer C, Leighton J, Comis RL, et al. Paclitaxel and carboplatin in combination in the treatment of advanced non-small-cell-lung cancer: A phase II toxicity, response, and survival analysis. J Clin Oncol 1995;13:1860–1870.
61. Langer CJ, Rosvold E, Millenson M,, et al. Paclitaxel by 1- or 24-hour infusion combined with carboplatin in advanced non-small cell lung cancer (NSCLC): A comparative analysis. Proc Am Soc Clin Oncol 1997;16:A-1625. Abstract.
62. Belani, CP. Paclitaxel and docetaxel combination in non-small cell lung cancer. Chest 2000;17(4):144S–151S.
63. Gandara DR, Vokes E, Green M,, et al. Docetaxel (Taxotere) in platinum-treated non-small cell lung cancer (NSCLC): Confirmation of prolonged survival in a multicenter trial. Proc Am Soc Clin Oncol 1997;16:A-1632. Abstract.
64. Hainsworth JD, Burris HA, Erland JB. Phase 1 trial of docetaxel administered by weekly infusion in patients with advanced refractory cancer. J Clin Oncol 1998;16:2164–2168.
65. McKay CE, Hainsworth JD, Burria HA. Weekly docetaxel in the treatment of elderly patients with advanced non-small cell lung cancer (NSCLC): A Minnie Pearl Cancer Research Network phase II trial. Proc Am Soc Clin Oncol 2000;19:A-1964. Abstract.
66. Shepherd FA, Dancey J, Ramlau R. Prospective randomized trial of docetaxel versus best supportive care in patients with non-small cell lung cancer previously treated with platinum-based chemotherapy. J Clin Oncol 2000;18:2095–2103.
67. Fossella FV, DeVore R, Kerr RN. Randomized phase III trail of docetaxel versus vinorelbine or ifosfamide in patients with advanced non-small-cell lung cancer previously treated with platinum containing chemotherapy regimens. J Clin Oncol 2000;18:2354–2362.
68. Gemzar package insert. Indianapolis, IN, Eli Lilly and Company, May 1996.
69. Fossella FV, Lippman SM, Shin DM, et al. Maximum-tolerated dose defined for single-agent gemcitabine: A phase I dose-escalation study in chemotherapy-naive patients with advanced non-small cell lung cancer. J Clin Oncol 1997;15:310–316.
70. Carrato A, Garcia gomez J, Alberola V, et al. Carboplatin (CARBO) in combination with gemcitabine (GEM) in advanced non-small cell lung cancer (NSCLC). Comparison of two consecutive phase II trials using different schedules. Proc Am Soc Clin Oncol 1999;18:A-19225. Abstract.
71. Sandler AB, Nemunaitis J, Denham C, et al. Phase III trial of gemcitabine plus cisplatin versus cisplatin alone in patients with locally advanced or metastatic non-small cell lung cancer. J Clin Oncol 2000;18(1):122–130.
72. Takimoto CH, Arbuck SG. The camptothecins. In: Chabner BA, Longo DL, eds. Cancer Chemotherapy and Biotherapy, Principles and Practice, 2nd ed. Philadelphia, Lippincott-Raven, 1996:463–484.
73. Natale RB. Experience with new chemotherapeutic agents in non-small cell lung cancer. Chest 1998;113(suppl 1):32S–39S.
74. Masuda N, Fukuoka M, Fujita A, et al. A phase II trial of combination CPT-11 and cisplatin for advanced non-small cell lung cancer. CPT-11 Lung Cancer Study Group. Br J Cancer 1998;78(2):251–256.
75. Takeda K, Negoro S, Kudoh S, et al. Phase I/II study of weekly irinotecan and concurrent radiation therapy for locally advanced non-small cell lung cancer. Br J Cancer 1999;79(9–10):1462–1467.
76. Dillman RO, Herndon J, Seagren SL, et al. Improved survival in stage III non-small lung cancer: Seven-year followup of cancer and leukemia group B (CALGB) 8433 trial. J Natl Cancer Inst 1996;88(17):1210–1215.
77. Pignon JP, Stewart RL, Souhami R, et al. A meta-analysis using individual patient data from randomized clinical trials of chemotherapy in non-small cell lung cancer: (3) Survival in the locally advanced setting. Proc Am Soc Clin Oncol 1994;13:334. Abstract.
78. Armstrong JG. Long-term outcome of small cell lung cancer. Cancer Treat Rev 1990;17:1–13.
79. Lassen U, Osterlind K, Hansen M, et al. Long-term survival in small-cell lung cancer; Post treatment characteristics in patients surviving 5 to 18+ years—An analysis of 1,714 consecutive patients. J Clin Oncol 1995;13(5):1215–1220.
80. Spiegelman D, Maurer L, Ware J, et al. Prognostic factors in small-cell carcinoma of the lung: An analysis of 1251 patients. J Clin Oncol 1989;7:334–354.
81. Albain K, Crowley JJ, LeBlanc M, Livingston RB. Determinants of improved outcome in small-cell lung cancer: an analysis of the 2,580-patient Southwest Oncology Group Database. J Clin Oncol 1990;8:1563–1574.
82. Sagman U, Feld R, Evans WK, et al. The prognostic significance of pretreatment serum lactate dehydrogenase in patients with small-cell lung cancer. J Clin Oncol 1991;9:954–961.
83. Sagman U, Leblanc M, Maki E, et al. Verification of a multi-center prognostic model for small-cell lung carcinoma (SCLC). For the Consensus Group for Prognostic Factors. Proc Am Soc Clin Oncol 1993;12:337. Abstract.

84. Jorgensen LG, Osterlind K, Genolla J, et al. Serum neuron-specific enolase (S-NSE) and the prognosis in small-cell lung cancer (SCLC). A combination multivariable analysis on data from nine centers. Br J Cancer 1996;74:463–467.
85. Smit EF, Fokkema E, Biesma B, et al. A phase II study of paclitaxel in heavily pretreated patients with small-cell lung cancer. Br J Cancer 1998;77(2):347–351.
86. Glisson BS, Kurie JM, Perez-Soler R, et al. Cisplatin, etoposide and paclitaxel in the treatment of patients with extensive small-cell lung carcinoma. J Clin Oncol 1999;17(8):2309–2315.
87. Ardizzani A, Hansen H, Dombernowsky P, et al. Topotecan, a new active drug in the second-line treatment of small-cell lung cancer: A phase II study in patients with refractory and sensitive disease. J Clin Oncol 1997;15(5):2090–2096.
88. Perez-Solar R, Glisson BS, Lee JS, et al. Treatment of patients with small-cell lung cancer refractory to etoposide and cisplatin with the topoisomerase I poison topotecan. J Clin Oncol 1996;14:2785–2790.
89. Eckardt J, Depierre A, Ardizzoni A, et al. Pooled analysis of topotecan (T) in the second-line treatment of patients (pts) with sensitive small-cell lung cancer (SCLC). Proc Am Soc Clin Oncol 1997;17:1624. Abstract.
90. Masuda N, Fukuoka M, Kusunoki Y, et al. CPT-11: A new derivative of camptothecin for the treatment of refractory or relapsed small-cell lung cancer. J Clin Oncol 1992;10:1225–1229.
91. Noda K, Nishiwaki Y, Kawahara M, et al. Randomized phase III study of irinotecan (CPT-11) and cisplatin versus etoposide and cisplatin in extensive-disease small cell lung cancer: Japan Clinical Oncology Group Study (JCOG9511). Proc Am Soc Clin Oncol 2000;19:1887. Abstract.
92. Cormier Y, Eisenhauer E, Muldal A. Gemcitabine is an active new agent in previously untreated extensive small-cell lung cancer, a study of the National Cancer Institute of Canada clinical trials group. Ann Oncol 1994;5:283–285.
93. DePierre A, LeChevalier T, Quoix E, et al. Phase II study of Navelbine (NVB) in small-cell lung cancer (SCLC). Proc Am Soc Clin Oncol 1995;14:A1050. Abstract.
94. Furuse K, Kubota K, Kawahara M, et al. Phase II study of vinorelbine in heavily pretreated small cell lung cancer. Oncology 1996;53:169–172.
95. Roth BJ, Johnson DH, Einhorn LH, et al. Randomized study of cyclophosphamide, doxorubicin, and vincristine versus etoposide and cisplatin versus alternation of these two regimens in extensive small-cell lung cancer: A Phase III trial of the Southeastern Cancer Study Group. J Clin Oncol 1992;10:282–291.
96. Fukuoka M, Furuse K, Saijo N, et al. Randomized trail of cyclophosphamide, doxorubicin, and vincristine versus cisplatin and etoposide versus alteration of these regimens in small-cell lung cancer. J Natl Cancer Inst 1991;83:855–856.
97. Hainsworth JD, Gray JR, Stroup SL, et al. Paclitaxel, carboplatin, and extended-schedule etoposide in the treatment of small-cell lung cancer: Comparison of sequential Phase II trials using different dose intensities. J Clin Oncol 1997;15(12):3464–3470.
98. Skarlos, DV, Samantas E, Kosmidis P, et al. Randomized comparison of etoposide-cisplatin versus etoposide-carboplatin and irradiation in small cell lung cancer: A Hellenic Cooperative Group study. Ann Oncol 1994;5:601–607.
99. Mavroudis D, Papadakis E, Veslemes M, et al. A multicenter randomized trial phase III study comparing paclitaxel-cisplatin-etoposide (TEP) versus cisplatin-etoposide (EP) as front-line treatment in patients with small cell lung cancer (SCLC). The Greek Lung Cancer Cooperative Group. Proc Am Soc Clin Oncol 2000;19:1894. Abstract.
100. Pujol JL, Carestia L, Daures JP. Is there a case for cisplatin in the treatment of small-cell lung cancer? A meta-analysis of randomized trials of a cisplatin-containing regimen versus a regimen without this alkylating agent. Br J Cancer 2000;83(1):8–15.
101. Giaccone G, Dalesio O, McVie GJ. Maintenance chemotherapy in small-cell-lung cancer: Long-term results of a randomized trial, EORTC. J Clin Oncol 1993;11(7):1230–1234.
102. Johnson DH, Kim K, Sauuse W, et al. Cisplatin (P) and etoposide (E) + thoracic radiotherapy (TRT) administered once or twice daily (bid) in limited stage IIs) small-cell lung cancer (SCLC): Final report of intergroup trial 0096. Proc Am Soc Clin Oncol 1996;15:374 Abstract.
103. Schabel FM, Griswold DP, Corbett TH, et al. Increasing the therapeutic response rates to anticancer drugs by applying the basic principles of pharmacology. Cancer 1984;54:1160–1167.
104. Johnson DH, Einhorn LH, Birch R, et al. A randomized comparison of high-dose versus conventional-dose cyclophosphamide, doxorubicin, and vincristine for extensive stage small cell lung cancer. J Clin Oncol 1987;5:1731–1738.
105. Ihde DC, Johnson BE, Mulshine JL, et al. Randomized trial of high-dose versus standard-dose etoposide and cisplatin in extensive stage small cell lung cancer. Proc Am Soc Clin Oncol 1987;6:181.
106. Pujol JL, Douillard JY, Riviere A, et al. Dose-intensity of a four-drug chemotherapy regimen with or without recombinant human granulocyte-macrophage colony-stimulating factor in extensive-stage small-cell lung cancer: A multicenter randomized Phase III study. J Clin Oncol 1997;15(5):2082–2089.
107. Ihde DC, Mulshine JL, Kramer BS, et al. Prospective randomized comparison of high-dose etoposide and cisplatin chemotherapy in patients with extensive-stage small-cell lung cancer. J Clin Oncol 1994;12: 2022–2034.
108. Arriagada R, Le Chevalier T, Pierrce PJ, et al. Initial chemotherapeutic doses and survival in patients with limited small-cell lung cancer. N Engl J Med 1993;325:1848–1852.
109. Klasa RJ, Murray N, Coldman AJ. Dose-intensity meta-analysis of chemotherapy regimens in small-cell carcinoma of the lung. J Clin Oncol 1991;9:499–508.
110. Sculier JP, Pasemans M, Bureau G, et al. Multiple drug weekly chemotherapy versus combination regimen in small-cell lung cancer: A phase III randomized study conducted by the European Lung Cancer Working Party. J Clin Oncol 1993;11:1858–1865.
111. Furuse K, Kubota K, Nishiwaki Y, et al. Phase III study of dose intensive weekly chemotherapy with recombinant human granulocyte-colony stimulating factor (G-CSF) versus standard chemotherapy in extensive disease small cell lung cancer (SCLC). Proc Am Soc Clin Oncol 1996;15:117 Abstract.
112. Goldie JH, Coldman AJ, Gudauskas GA. Rationale for the use of alternating non-cross-resistant chemotherapy. Cancer Treat Rep 1982;66:439–449.
113. Goodman GE, Crowley JJ, Blasko JC, et al. Treatment of limited small-cell lung cancer with etoposide and cisplatin alternating with vincristine, doxorubicin, and cyclophosphamide versus concurrent etoposide, vincristine, doxorubicin, and cyclophosphamide and chest radiotherapy: A Southwest Oncology Group study. J Clin Oncol 1990;8:39–47.
114. Wolf M, Pritsch M, Drings P, et al. Cyclic-alternating versus response-oriented chemotherapy in small-cell lung cancer: A German multicenter randomized trial of 321 patients. J Clin Oncol 1991;9:614–624.
115. Greco FA, Johnson DH, Hainsworth JD, Wolff SN. Chemotherapy of small-cell lung cancer. Semin Oncol 1985;4(suppl 6):31–37.
116. Evans WK, Feld R, Murray N, et al. Superiority of alternating non-cross-resistant chemotherapy in extensive small cell lung cancer: A multicenter, randomized clinical trial by the National Cancer Institute of Canada. Ann Intern Med 1987;107:451–458.
117. Crawford J, Ozer H, Stoller R, et al. Reduction by granulocyte colony-stimulating factor of fever and neutropenia induced by chemotherapy in patients with small-cell lung cancer. N Engl J Med 1991;325(3):164–170.
118. Sandler, AB. Current management of small cell lung cancer. Semin Oncol 1997;24(4):463–476.
119. Humblet Y, Symann M, Bosly A, et al. Late intensification chemotherapy with autologous bone marrow transplant in selected small-cell carcinoma of the lung: A randomized study. J Clin Oncol 1987;5:1864–1873.
120. Elias AD, Ayash L, Frei E III, et al. Intensive combined modality therapy for limited-stage small-cell lung cancer. J Natl Cancer Inst 1993;85: 559–566.

121. Leyvraz S, Rosti G, Lange A, et al. Early intensification chemotherapy for the treatment of small-cell lung cancer (SCLC). Proc Am Soc Clin Oncol 1997;16:1626. Abstract.
122. Wilson HE, Stanley K, Vincent RG, et al. Comparison of chemotherapy alone versus chemotherapy and radiation therapy of extensive small cell carcinoma of the lung. J Surg Oncol 1983;23:181–184.
123. Johnson DH, Arriagada R, Ihde DC, et al. Meta-analysis of randomized trials evaluating the role of thoracic radiotherapy in limited-stage small cell lung cancer. Proc Am Soc Clin Oncol 1992;11:288. Abstract.
124. Murray N, Coy P, Pater JL, et al. Importance of timing for thoracic irradiation in the combined modality treatment of limited-stage small-cell-lung cancer. J Clin Oncol 1993;11:336–344.
125. Turrisi AT, Kyungmann K, Blum R, et al. Twice-daily compared with once-daily thoracic radiotherapy in limited small-cell lung cancer treated concurrently with cisplatin and etoposide. N Engl J Med 1999;340(4):265–271.
126. Robnett TJ, Machtay M, Vines EF, et al. Factors predicting severe radiation pneumonitis in patients receiving definitive chemoradiation for lung cancer. Int J Radiat Oncol Biol Phys 2000;48:89–94.
127. Arriagada R, LeChevalier T, Borie F, et al. Prophylactic cranial irradiation for patients with small-cell lung cancer in complete remission. J Natl Cancer Inst 1995:87:187–190.
128. Fleck JF, Einhorn LH, Lauer RC, et al. Is prophylactic cranial irradiation indicated in small-cell lung cancer? J Clin Oncol 1990;8:209–214.
129. Johnson BE, Becker B, Goff WB, et al. Neurologic, neuropsychologic, and cranial computed tomography scan abnormalities in 2–10-year survivors of small cell lung cancer. J Clin Oncol 1985;3:1659–1667.
130. Kristensen CA, Kristjansen P, Hansen HH, Systemic chemotherapy of brain metastases from small-cell lung cancer: A review. J Clin Oncol 1992;10:1498–1502.
131. Shaw EG, Su JQ, Eagan RT, et al. Prophylactic cranial irradiation in complete responders with small-cell lung cancer: Analysis of the Mayo Clinic and North Central Cancer Treatment Group data bases. J Clin Oncol 1994;12:2327–2332.
132. Auperin A, Arriagada R, Pignon J-P, et al. for the Prophylactic Cranial Irradiation Overview Collaborative Group. Prophylactic cranial irradiation for patients with small-cell lung cancer in complete remission. N Engl J Med 1999;341(7):476–84.
133. Rothenberg ML. Topoisomerase I inhibitors: Review and update. Ann Oncol 1997;8:837–855.
134. Sung C, Blaney SM, Cole DE, et al. A pharmacokinetic model of topotecan clearance from plasma and cerebrospinal fluid. Cancer Res 1994;54:5118–5122.
135. Ardizzoni A, Wanders J, Hansen H, et al. Activity of topotecan in the treatment of small-cell lung cancer patients with brain metastases. Eur Ann Neuro Oncol 1996.
136. Manegold C, von Pawel J, Scheilthauer W, et al. Response of SCLC brain metastases on topotecan therapy. Proc Eur Soc Med Oncol 1997;7(suppl 5):5100. Abstract.
137. Hopewood P, Stephens RJ for the British Medical Research Council Lung Cancer Working Party. Depression in patients with lung cancer: Prevalence and risk factors derived from quality-of-life data. J Clin Oncol 2000;18:893–903.
138. Payne DG, Feld R. Concurrent radiotherapy and chemotherapy in lung cancer at the Princess Margaret Hospital. Antibiot Chemother 1988;41:96–101.

127

COLORECTAL CANCER

Lisa E. Davis

Colorectal cancer involves the colon, rectum, and the anal canal. It is one of the three most common cancers occurring in adult men and women in the United States, and accounts for approximately one of nine cancer diagnoses. In 2001, an estimated 135,400 new cases were diagnosed, of which 98,200 involve the colon and 37,200 the rectum.[1]

For both adult men and women, colorectal cancer is the third leading cause of cancer-related deaths in the United States. An estimated 56,700 deaths occurred during 2001.[1] Mortality associated with colorectal cancer has decreased during the past 30 years; the rate of decline is greatest for females.

Mortality rates associated with colorectal cancer in the United States are comparable to those of other industrialized areas in North America, certain areas of Northern and Western Europe, Australia, New Zealand, and Japan.[2] Deaths attributed to cancer of the colon or rectum in less-developed areas such as South America and Middle Africa are less frequent than in the United States.

Multiple factors are associated with the development of these malignancies, including acquired and inherited genetic susceptibility, environmental elements, and lifestyle. Overall, approximately 37% of affected individuals undergo a surgical procedure alone intended for cure. An additional 37% of individuals can potentially be cured by undergoing surgery followed by radiation therapy (XRT), chemotherapy, or both. Curability is influenced primarily by extent of tumor invasion into adjacent tissues or organs and presence of metastatic disease. Five-year survival rates are close to 92% and 86% for persons with early stages of colon and rectal cancer, respectively.[3] After tumor has spread regionally to adjacent organs or lymph nodes, survival rates drop to 68% for colon cancer and to 57% for cancer of the rectum. Five-year survival for individuals with metastatic disease is approximately 8%.

Treatment modalities include surgery, XRT, chemotherapy, and immunotherapy. Surgery is the most important and definitive procedure associated with cure; radiation therapy can be used to improve curability following surgical resection and to reduce symptoms and complications associated with advanced disease. Chemotherapy is used in adjuvant treatment regimens. Chemotherapy, either a single agent or a combination of agents, is used for advanced stages of disease. Although the efficacy of a standard postoperative monitoring program for patients with resected colorectal cancer has not been established, elements of such a program may include clinical history and physical examination, colonoscopy, serum carcinoembryonic antigen (CEA) measurements, and chest x-ray.

EPIDEMIOLOGY

Incidence rates worldwide vary by as much as 20-fold. The highest incidence rates occur in highly industrialized areas such as North America, Northern and Western Europe, Australia, and New Zealand. The lowest incidence rates are seen in India and in less-developed areas such as South America and rural Africa.[4] Rates have increased substantially, however, in previously lower-risk countries such as Japan and China, as well as among persons migrating from low-risk areas to the United States. Within one or two generations, the incidence rates among migrating groups approximate those of the new host country, suggesting that environmental and dietary factors may influence a late stage in colorectal carcinogenesis. However, colorectal cancers are known to develop more frequently in certain families and genetic predisposition to this disease is also well-recognized.

The incidence of colon cancer is greatest among males, who have an age-adjusted incidence rate of 36.7 per 100,000, as compared to females for whom the rate is 27.6 per 100,000.[3] Cancer of the rectum occurs less frequently; the incidence rate is 16.2 and 9.5 per 100,000 for males and females, respectively. Cancer of the colon and rectum is the third most frequent malignancy among US men and white and African American women, but is second next to breast cancer for Hispanic, American Indian/Alaskan Native, and Asian/Pacific Islander women. The overall incidence of colon and rectal cancers in the United States has declined steadily since 1985 at an average rate of 1.6% per year.[5] However, this decline is attributable primarily to decreasing rates among white males and females because incidence rates in African American males and females have remained level since about 1980. Because of large year-to-year variations in colorectal cancer incidence rates in minority population groups, it is difficult to compare trends; however, downward trends in colorectal cancer incidence appear to be greater for African-Americans and whites than for Hispanics, Asian Pacific Islanders, and American Indian/Alaskan Native Americans. Trends for incidence and mortality rates among white males and females in the United States can be compared in Fig. 127–1.

The median age at diagnosis is about 72 years.[3] Fewer than 3% of affected persons are younger than age 44 years. An individual's risk, however, increases with increasing age. Seventy-one percent of cases develop in adults older than 65 years of age. The stage of disease at presentation is similar among different ethnic groups, although the tendency to present with later-stage disease is slightly higher for African Americans.

Approximately 11% of all cancer deaths are a result of cancer of the colon or rectum. Roughly 56,700 deaths were estimated in 2001, despite a decline in overall combined mortality for both colon and rectal cancer observed during the last 20 years. For women, the decline in colorectal cancer mortality rates have been evident since 1950, whereas death rates among men did not start to decline until the late 1970s.[5] These trends in mortality rates are similar to those observed in other countries. Overall mortality rates remain higher among African American males and females and the rates of decline are lower as compared to those for white males and females. Colorectal cancer mortality rates are lower for Hispanics, American Indians/Alaskan Natives, and Asian Pacific Islanders than for whites or African Americans. Factors contributing to the overall decline in colorectal cancer mortality likely include decreasing incidence rates, screening programs with early polyp removal, and more effective and better-tolerated treatments.

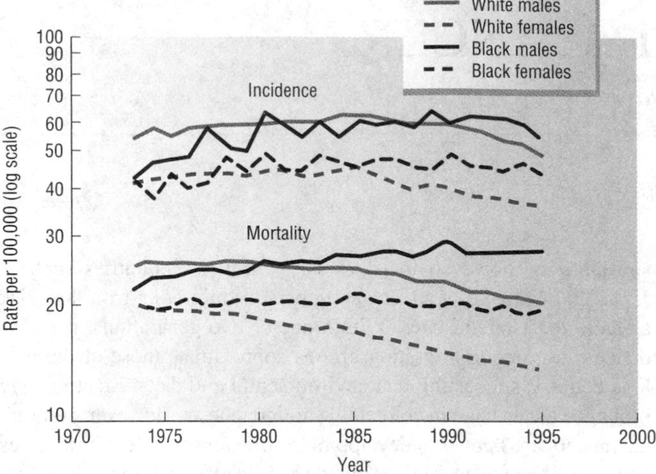

FIGURE 127–1. SEER incidence and mortality rates age-adjusted and age-specific. Colon and rectum cancer, 1973–1997. (*From Ref. 3.*)

ETIOLOGY

Numerous studies suggest that the development of colorectal cancer can be caused or promoted by dietary or environmental factors that affect the bowel, in addition to host physical and genetic susceptibilities. An understanding of these processes has formed the basis for several interventional and preventive trials, which are discussed later in this chapter. Key areas of study have included dietary fiber, fat, and micronutrient intake.

DIETARY INTAKE AND NUTRIENTS

Epidemiologic studies of worldwide incidence of colorectal cancer suggest that economic development and dietary habits strongly influence its development. An inverse correlation between dietary fat and fiber intake exists within most diets; inhabitants of affluent societies are more likely to have more fat and less fiber in their diets. Although findings based on epidemiologic data are subject to potential recall and selection bias, as well as inconsistencies in how dietary fibers are categorized and measured, numerous studies have attempted to ascertain the true contribution of dietary fiber alone toward cancer development. The confounding effects of micronutrients that are contained in fruits and vegetables have been less well-studied.

FIBER

Dietary fiber is the part of ingested plant material that is not processed by normal human digestive enzymes. Fibers are frequently classified as either water soluble (pectins, gums, mucilages) or insoluble (celluloses, hemicellulose, lignins). The insoluble fibers have been most consistently associated with reduced cancer risk. Foods that are high in fiber include vegetables, fruit, grains, and cereals. Numerous studies clearly demonstrate an inverse association between dietary fiber intake and colorectal cancer development.[6] The degree of colorectal cancer risk reduction associated with increased consumption of vegetables and fruit is variable but generally modest. No single category of dietary fiber appears superior, although the findings with vegetable consumption are more consistent than those of fruit. Also, fiber from fruit and vegetable sources may be more desirable than cereal fiber.[7] Postulated protective effects of dietary fiber include dilution or absorption of carcinogens in the bowel, reduced fecal pH, reduced bowel transit time, alterations in bile acid metabolism, or increased production of short-chain fatty acids.[8] These effects may also reflect an associated concomitant reduction in dietary fat intake.

In a meta-analysis of six case-control studies of vegetable consumption and colon cancer risk, a combined odds ratio of 0.48 (95% confidence interval [CI], 0.41–0.57) was observed between the highest and lowest quintiles of consumption.[7] Findings from a pooled analysis of 13 case-control studies of dietary fiber and colorectal cancer were similar; however, relative risk estimates approximated 1.00 after the analysis was restricted to use of validated dietary questionnaires and quantitative estimates of nutrient intake.[9] Although five case-control studies found inverse associations that were not all significant, a prospective study of dietary factors and risk of colorectal adenomas in men using data from the Health Professionals Follow-Up Study showed an increased intake in vegetables and fruit was associated with significant risk reduction. In contrast, a larger prospective, cohort study of women, using data from the Nurses's Health Study, found no association between fiber intake and risk of colorectal adenoma or cancer, although a weak association existed between dietary fiber and colorectal cancer with respect to folate consumption.[10] Thus, the evidence that increased dietary fiber consumption reduces colorectal cancer risk is suggestive, but not conclusive.

FAT

Numerous epidemiologic studies also suggest that a relationship exists between dietary fat intake and colorectal cancer risk.[6] Although estimates from 16 cohort studies of meat consumption and colorectal cancer show an elevated risk, these findings are not strong or consistent.[6] Whether the source of the fat is important is unclear, because most of the fat in many of these studies was derived from ingested animal meat. Studies conducted in countries where colorectal cancer incidence is high suggest significantly elevated odds ratios with higher meat consumption. The association between red meat consumption and colorectal cancer is strongest. However, whether the risk is associated with the fat source or the cooking or processing methods is unclear. Findings from studies comparing saturated and unsaturated fat are also conflicting.

The role of dietary fat in cancer development may be a result of its influence on fecal bile acid concentrations. The release of bile acids is stimulated following ingestion of dietary fat. These acids are then converted by colonic flora to secondary bile acids, which are associated with bowel mucosal irritation and cell proliferation responses and may promote tumor growth.[11] The effects of carcinogenic heterocyclic amines, formed when meat is cooked, may also be important, although the risks associated with heterocyclic amine exposure appear to be greatest for genetically susceptible individuals.[12] Therefore, while data indicate that animal meat and saturated fat intake and processing appear to be associated with an increased risk of colorectal cancer, the magnitude of risk has not been determined.

CALCIUM AND MICRONUTRIENTS

The role of calcium intake on colorectal cancer risk has been investigated in cohort and case-control studies but the results of these studies are inconsistent.[6] Calcium's protective effect may be related to a reduction in mucosal cell proliferation rates or through its binding to bile salts in the intestine. High levels of dietary folate, a key constituent of vegetables, are associated with decreased colorectal cancer and adenoma risk.[6] Folate availability influences DNA methylation, which is an important process in maintaining normal bowel mucosa. However, the level of folate intake and any associated level of colorectal cancer risk has yet to be elucidated. Additional micronutrient deficiencies that have been demonstrated through several studies to increase colorectal cancer risk include selenium, vitamin C, vitamin E, and β-carotene; however, the benefit of dietary supplementation does not appear to be substantial.[13]

LIFESTYLE FACTORS

NONSTEROIDAL ANTI-INFLAMMATORY DRUG AND ASPIRIN USE

Several lifestyle factors are known to affect colorectal cancer risk (Table 127–1). Studies have consistently demonstrated that regular (at least two doses per week) nonsteroidal anti-inflammatory drug (NSAID) and aspirin use is associated with a reduced risk of colorectal cancer.[6] In the Nurse's Health Study, a decreased risk of colorectal cancer was seen in women who took aspirin regularly for at least 10 consecutive years, with the greatest reduction occurring with an intake of four to six tablets per week.[14] In a population-based study of nonaspirin NSAID users who had taken NSAIDs for at least 48 months of the previous 5 years, the relative risk of colorectal cancer was 0.49 (95% CI, 0.24–1.00) for users as compared to nonusers.[15] Additional studies support these findings that regular aspirin or NSAID use may decrease the risk of colorectal cancer by as much as 50%. The potential mechanisms by which these agents exert their protective effects appear to be linked primarily to their inhibition of cyclooxygenase-2 (COX-2) and free radical formation. Increased COX-2 levels are elevated in colorectal adenocarcinomas and may act as a promoter of neoplasia by increasing the expression of bcl-2. COX-2 overexpression is associated with prolonged abnormal cell survival, chronic inflammation-associated carcinogenesis, increased tumor cell invasiveness, and enhanced production of angiogenesis-promoting factors.[16] NSAIDs may also inhibit carcinogenesis via COX-independent mechanisms. 15-LOX-1, a lipoxygenase, is the key enzyme responsible for metabolizing colonic linoleic acid to 13-S-hydroxyoctadecadienoic acid, an inducer of apoptosis. NSAIDs increase the expression of 15-LOX-1, thereby inducing apoptosis in colorectal cancer cells.[17]

TABLE 127–1. Lifestyle Factors Associated with Colorectal Cancer Risk

Factor	Comments
Aspirin and nonaspirin NSAID use	Regular use associated with risk reduction perhaps as much as 50%
Postmenopausal hormone use	Exogenous hormone intake decreases colorectal cancer risk 19% to 34%
Alcohol intake	Heavy use increases colorectal risk two- to threefold
Physical inactivity and obesity	Elevated body mass index and physical inactivity associated with increased risk
Tobacco use	Use of tobacco products estimated to contribute up to 12% of colorectal cancer deaths annually
Diabetes	Hyperinsulinemia may increase colorectal cancer risk
Serum lipid levels	Elevated serum triglycerides associated with increased risk of adenomatous polyps

EXOGENOUS HORMONE USE

Exogenous hormone use, particularly postmenopausal hormone replacement therapy, is associated with a significant reduction in colorectal cancer risk.[6,18] A meta-analysis of 18 epidemiologic studies of postmenopausal hormone replacement therapy showed a 20% reduction (RR = 0.80, 95% CI, 0.74–0.86) in risk of colon cancer, and a 19% reduction (RR = 0.81, 95% CI, 9.72–0.92) in risk of rectal cancer, in women who received hormone replacement therapy as compared to women who never used hormone replacement therapy.[18] The risk is reduced in postmenopausal women receiving both estrogen only and combined estrogen and progestin therapy, and persists for approximately 10 years after therapy is discontinued. Risk reduction appears greatest among women who are currently receiving hormone replacement therapy; colorectal cancer risk is 34% lower in women who are currently receiving hormone replacement therapy than in women who have never received hormone replacement therapy. Although a prospective study of oral contraceptive use suggests a protective effect, other studies do not support this association.

Several mechanisms for a protective effect of estrogens on the bowel have been identified.[6,18] Declining estrogen levels associated with aging are associated with estrogen receptor hypermethylation, resulting in reduced expression of the estrogen receptor gene and dysregulated colonic mucosal cell growth. In addition, estrogen use may reduce serum levels of insulin-like growth factor-I (IGF-I), an important mitogen that influences cell-cycle progression in certain cells. Both normal and cancerous colorectal cells express IGF-I receptors.[18]

OBESITY AND PHYSICAL INACTIVITY

Physical inactivity and elevated body mass index (BMI), independent of level of physical activity, are associated with an elevated risk of colon cancer and colon adenoma.[13,19] Individuals with a total higher level of activity throughout life have the lowest risk. There is less evidence that physical inactivity or obesity influences risk of rectal cancer.[6] The risk of colon cancer may be increased as much as twofold in men who are in the highest quintile of body size. Furthermore, a high body mass may also be a risk factor for increased colon cancer mortality. The evidence linking elevated BMI with increased colon cancer risk is less consistent for women; however, the Iowa Women's Health Study showed that cancer risk was 40% higher in women who were in the highest quintile of BMI as compared to the cancer risk of women in the lowest quintile. Hypotheses for these relationships include the observation that physical activity stimulates bowel peristalsis, resulting in decreased bowel transit time, and the possibility that exercise-induced alterations in body glucose, insulin levels, and perhaps other hormones may reduce tumor cell growth.[6]

Type 2 diabetes mellitus, independent of body mass size and physical activity level, is also associated with an increased risk of colorectal cancer in women. Data from the Nurses's Health Study suggest that colon cancer risk may be increased by 49% in diabetic women as compared to nondiabetic women.[20] These and other findings support a role for hyperinsulinemia as a possible link between obesity, sedentary lifestyle, and diabetes mellitus and colon cancer.

ALCOHOL AND TOBACCO USE

High alcohol consumption increases risk of rectal and colon cancer, perhaps as much as two- to threefold, although some studies have found no significant increase in risk.[6,13] No single source of alcohol is associated with any greater risk. The evidence is strongest in men; however, alcohol consumption is generally greater in men than in women. Smoking tobacco products, including cigarettes, cigars, and pipes, may contribute to as much as 12% of all colorectal cancer deaths.[21] Although a link between smoking and colorectal cancer in earlier studies has been controversial, a prospective cohort study of approximately 1.2 million Americans showed that long-term cigarette smoking is associated with a multivariate-adjusted colorectal cancer mortality rate ratio of 1.32 (95% CI, 1.16–1.49) and 1.41 (95% CI, 1.26–1.58) for men and women smokers, respectively, as compared to men and women who had never smoked. The cancer-promoting effects of alcohol and tobacco may be through generation of carcinogens or their direct toxic effects on bowel tissue.

CLINICAL RISK FACTORS

CHRONIC INFLAMMATORY BOWEL DISEASES

Several clinical conditions and genetic disorders increase one's risk of developing colorectal cancer. Chronic ulcerative colitis, particularly when it involves the entire large intestine, predisposes individuals to colorectal cancer at a rate that is 4- to 20-fold greater than average.[13] The risk is even greater for young individuals and increases for all affected individuals with increasing extent of bowel involvement and disease duration. The cumulative risk of colorectal cancer is low early in life, and increases to about 14% to 17% at age 30. Although a precise causative link has not been established, chronic underlying inflammation may be a significant predisposing factor. The progressive dysplastic changes that the bowel mucosa undergo are similar to those observed in adenomatous polyps. Similarly, patients with Crohn's disease are also at increased risk, although the relative risk is slightly lower than that of patients with ulcerative colitis. This difference may be related to the decreased length of bowel affected by the chronic inflammatory process in individuals with Crohn's disease. Overall, persons diagnosed with either disease constitute approximately 1% to 2% of all new cases of colorectal cancer each year. Additional risk factors include age greater than 40 years, history of colorectal polyps, prior colorectal carcinoma, pelvic irradiation, or noncancer surgery (cholecystectomy or ureterosigmoidostomy).

GENETIC SUSCEPTIBILITY

HEREDITARY

Although most cases of colorectal cancer are sporadic in nature, as many as 10% of cases are thought to be hereditary. First-degree relatives of patients diagnosed with colorectal cancer have an increased risk of the disease that is at least two to four times that of persons in the general population without a family history.[22] Approximately 10% to 15% of patients who develop colorectal cancer will also have a family history of colorectal cancer. The two most common forms of hereditary cancer are familial adenomatous polyposis (FAP) and hereditary nonpolyposis colorectal cancer (HNPCC). FAP is a rare autosomal dominant trait that is caused by inherited inactivating mutations of the adenomatous polyposis coli (APC) gene and accounts for 0.5% to 1% of all colorectal cancers. The disease is manifested by hundreds to thousands of tiny sessile adenomatous polyps that carpet the colon and rectum, typically arising during adolescence.[6,23,24] Symptoms generally present between the ages of 25 to 35 years, at which time cancer is already present in about half of patients. The risk of developing colorectal cancer for individuals with untreated FAP is virtually 100%; most will develop colorectal cancer by their fourth decade of life. Several variants of FAP exist and are associated with different extracolonic manifestations.[6]

HNPCC, also referred to as Lynch syndrome I or II, is an autosomal dominantly inherited syndrome that accounts for 1% to 5% of colon cancer cases.[6,24] In contrast to FAP, adenomatous polyps generally number only up to 100 and tend to be located primarily in the proximal (cecum, ascending, transverse) colon. Type I or Lynch syndrome I is characterized by the aggregation of colorectal cancer at an early age within a particular family, whereas type II (Lynch syndrome II, family cancer syndrome) represents multiple colon and extracolonic adenocarcinomas as well.[25] Common extracolonic sites include endometrial carcinoma and carcinomas of the breast, stomach, ovary, pancreas, small bowel, and urinary tract. The age at onset of colorectal cancer on average is 40 to 44 years of age. Because the clinical presentation of HNPCC is difficult to distinguish from "sporadic" forms of colorectal cancer, the diagnosis of HNPCC can be confirmed by the presence of germ-line mutations in a family of genes responsible for DNA mismatch-repair (MMR). Carriers of a germ-line mutation have an 80% to 85% risk of developing colorectal cancer over their lifetime.[25]

ENZYME POLYMORPHISMS

Increasing evidence suggests that certain high-prevalence genetic polymorphisms, such as *N*-acetyltransferases (NAT1, NAT2), certain cytochrome P450 enzymes, and methylenetetrahydrofolate reductase (MTHFR) enzymes, may confer genetic susceptibility to colorectal cancer.[6] Individuals with certain variations in NAT1, NAT2, and CYP1A2 enzyme genotypes may be particularly susceptible to carcinogenic effects of a high dietary intake of meat or tobacco smoke. Variants of MTHFR, another polymorphic enzyme, may influence the association of colorectal cancer risk with dietary folate or vitamin B_{12} intake.

PATHOPHYSIOLOGY

ANATOMY AND BOWEL FUNCTION

The large intestine consists of the cecum; ascending, transverse, descending, and sigmoid colon; and the rectum (Fig. 127–2). In adults,

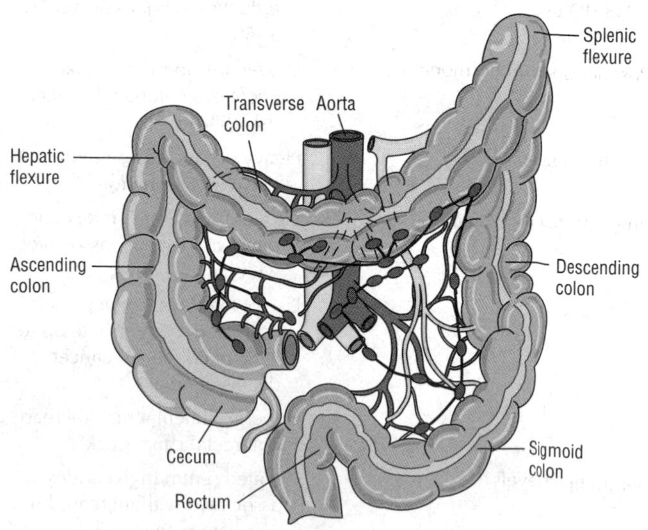

FIGURE 127–2. Colon and rectum anatomy.

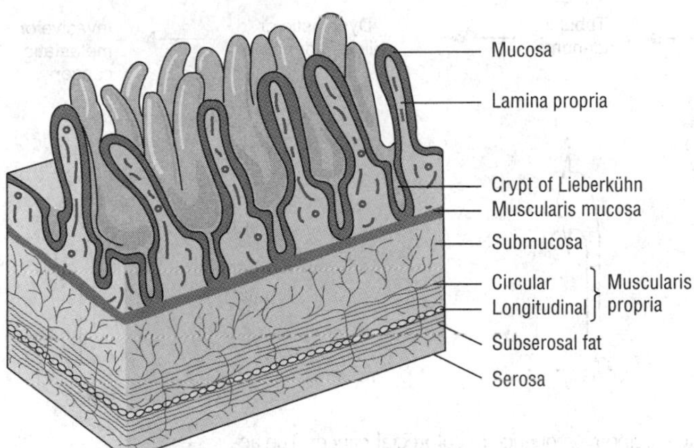

FIGURE 127–3. Cross section of bowel wall.

it extends approximately 1.5 m and has a diameter ranging from 8 cm in the cecum to 2 cm in the sigmoid colon. The function of the large intestine is to receive 500–2000 mL of ileal contents per day. Absorption of fluid and solutes occurs in the right colon or the segments proximal to the middle of the transverse colon, with movement and storage of fecal material in the left colon and distal segments of the colon. Mucus secretion from goblet cells into the intestinal lumen lubricates the mucosal surface and facilitates movement of the dehydrated feces. It also serves to protect the luminal wall from bacteria and colonic irritants such as bile acids.

Four major tissue layers, from the lumen outward, form the large intestine: the mucosa, submucosa, muscularis externa, and serosa (Fig. 127–3). Embedded in the submucosa and muscularis externa is a rich lymphatic capillary system. Lymphatic channels do not extend into the mucosa. The muscularis externa consists of circular smooth muscle and three outer longitudinal smooth muscle bands. Contraction of these muscle groups moves colonic material toward the anal canal. The outermost layer of the colon, the serosa, secretes a fluid that allows the colon to slide easily over nearby structures within the peritoneum. The serosa covers only the anterior and lateral aspects of the upper third of the rectum. The lower third lies completely extraperitoneal and is surrounded by fibrofatty tissue as well as adjacent organs and structures.

The surface epithelium of the colonic mucosa undergoes continual renewal, and complete replacement of epithelial cells occurs every 4 to 8 days. Cell replication normally takes place within the lower third of crypts, the tubular glands located within the intestinal mucosa. The cells then mature and differentiate to either goblet or absorptive cells as they migrate toward the bowel lumen. The total number of epithelial cells remains relatively constant as the number of cells migrating from the crypts is balanced by the rate of exfoliation of cells from the mucosal surface. This two-phase process is critical to the malignant transformation of the epithelial cells. The number of dysplastic and hyperplastic aberrant crypt foci increases with increasing age; as the mass of abnormal cells accumulates at the top of the crypt and starts to protrude into the stream of fecal matter, their contact with fecal mutagens can lead to further cell mutations and eventual adenoma formation.[6]

COLORECTAL TUMORIGENESIS

The development of a colorectal neoplasm is a multistep process of several genetic and phenotypic alterations of normal bowel epithelium structure and function. Since the majority of colorectal cancers develop sporadically, efforts have been directed toward identifying these alterations, determining whether they develop in any type of sequential order, and learning whether discovery of the presence of such changes may lead to improved cancer detection and/or treatment outcomes.

A genetic model has been proposed for colorectal tumorigenesis that describes a process of transformation from adenoma to carcinoma.[26] However, at least three separate additional molecular pathways to developing colorectal cancer have been identified.[6] These include a pathway for HNPCC, an ulcerative-colitis dysplasia-carcinoma sequence, and a pathway involving loss of function of the ER gene through hypermethylation. Some of the molecular processes are common to more than one pathway.

Fig. 127–4 is an overview of the adenoma-carcinoma model. The adenoma–carcinoma sequence of tumor development reflects an accumulation of mutations within colonic epithelium, each of which results in cellular replication or enhanced invasiveness. Key elements of this process include hyperproliferation of epithelial cells to form a small benign neoplasm or adenoma in conjunction with cellular gene mutations.[27,28] These mutations occur early and frequently in sporadic cases of both adenomas and colorectal cancer. Genetic changes include mutational activation of oncogenes as well as inactivation of tumor-suppressor genes. Both types of genetic alterations are required to produce the malignant tumor.

Oncogenes are mutated forms of normal cellular genes, or protooncogenes, that induce many of the aberrant features of malignant cells. Activating mutations of ras protooncogenes, primarily involving the K-*ras* and N-*ras* genes, occur frequently in colorectal cancer.[26–28] The *ras* family of genes is responsible for encoding proteins involved in signal transduction. Although the complete effects of these mutated genes are not completely understood, their activation is believed to be important for cellular proliferation and tumor progression.

Tumor-suppressor genes are normal cellular genes that are capable of transforming normal cells to cancerous cells through their deletion or inactivation. One of the earliest genetic changes in colorectal tumorigenesis involves the mutation or loss of the *APC* gene, a tumor-suppressor gene, localized on the long arm of chromosome 5q21. The *APC* gene encodes for a protein that binds to α- and β-catenin, which belong to a family of proteins associated with intracellular adhesion.[28] β-Catenin binds to the cytoplasmic domain of E-cadherin, an important molecule responsible for cell–cell adhesion. These activities among others are believed to be involved in regulation of cell shape and cell-to-cell communication and may affect cell-cycle regulation or apoptosis. These alterations lead to abnormal epithelial proliferation and differentiation of cells. Inactivation of the *APC* gene is the single gene defect responsible for FAP, and is frequently, but not always, seen in sporadic colorectal cancer cases. A single mutation of the *APC* gene is capable of creating conditions of abnormal cell adhesion, migration, and replication, leading to polyp formation.[6]

Mutational inactivations of two additional important tumor-suppressor genes, *p53*, located on chromosome 17p, and the *DCC* (deleted in colorectal carcinoma) gene, located on chromosome 18q, occur later during the adenoma-carcinoma sequence.[26–28] Normal *p53* gene expression is responsible for apoptosis, an irreversible cell process resulting in cell death. Loss of *p53* activity through mutation is the most common genetic abnormality associated with human tumors and may contribute toward their growth advantage by allowing for uninhibited cellular proliferation, despite damaged DNA.[28] The protein encoded by the normal *DCC* gene is believed to share similar structural features to certain types of cell-adhesion molecules, and as such may interact with various proteins to control cell–cell interaction and cellular proliferation. Loss of specific

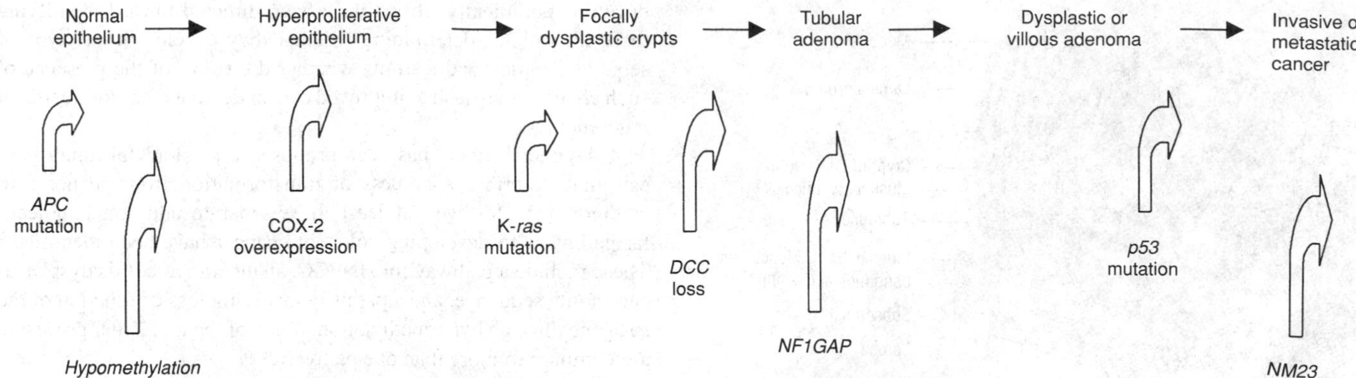

FIGURE 127–4 Genetic changes associated with the adenoma to carcinoma sequence in colorectal cancer. The accumulation of genetic changes in the pathogenesis of colorectal cancer includes DNA hypomethylation across the genome, COX-2 (cyclooxygenase-2) overexpression, mutation or deletion of tumor-suppressor genes (*APC* [adenomatous polyposis coli], *DCC* [deleted in colorectal cancer], *NFIGAP, p53*), activation of oncogenes (K-*ras*), and presence of metastasis genes (*NM23*). *(Adapted from Ref. 27.)*

cell-adhesive properties could contribute toward tumor invasion and metastasis.

A distinct group of genetic traits has also been identified for individuals with HNPCC but occur in "sporadic" cases of colorectal cancer, as well. "Replication errors" occur frequently and represent widespread alterations in the length of a series of repeated nucleotides, or microsatellites, within tumor DNA.[27] Mutations of those genes that appear to recognize and regulate DNA mismatch replication errors, or MMR genes, *MSH2, MLH1, PMS1, PMS2,* and *MSH6,* contribute to microsatellite instability and colorectal tumorigenesis.[24,28] Although mutations of *MLH1* and *MSH2* account for most cases of HNPCC, mutations of *PMS1* and *PMS2* have also been documented. Failure to repair DNA mismatches results in microsatellite instability, which accelerates further gene mutations, leading to oncogene activation or tumor-suppressor gene inactivation. Tumor progression may then be facilitated through a link between DNA repair defects and mutations of critical growth regulatory genes. Inactivation of a receptor for type II transforming growth factor-β (TGF-β), a protein that has antiproliferative effects on colonic epithelial cell growth, has been demonstrated in cells with replication errors.[29]

HISTOLOGY

Adenocarcinomas account for more than 90% of tumors of the large intestine.[30] Other histologic types such as mucinous adenocarcinoma, signet-ring adenocarcinoma, carcinoid simplex, and carcinoid tumors occur less frequently. Adenocarcinomas are assigned one of three tumor grade designations based on the degree of cellular differentiation, the degree to which the tumor resembles the structure, and function of its cell of origin. The most differentiated adenocarcinomas, or grade I tumors, generally resemble adenomas, whereas grade III tumors are considered "high grade," the most undifferentiated, and have frequently lost the characteristics of mature normal cells. Features of well-differentiated tumors include relatively normal tubule and glandular formation and low numbers of mitoses. Poorly differentiated or high-grade tumors contain few or no glandular structures and have an increased nuclear-to-cytoplasmic ratio, large nuclei, and dark staining caused by increased DNA content. Poorly differentiated tumors are associated with a worse prognosis than those that are better differentiated.[30]

Mucinous adenocarcinomas possess the same basic structure as adenocarcinomas but differ in that they secrete an abundant quantity of extracellular mucus. They account for only about 10% of colorectal carcinomas but tend to be frequent in patients with HNPCC and patients with coexisting ulcerative colitis.[23] Signet-ring adenocarcinomas have a characteristic appearance because of the displacement of the nucleus to one side by large vacuoles of intracellular mucin. Patients tend to present with a more advanced stage of disease and have a highly invasive tumor. Both mucinous and signet-ring adenocarcinoma histologies confer a poor prognosis.

DNA content of the tumor is also related to overall prognosis.[30] This is easily and reliably measured with flow cytometry. Tumors with DNA content equal to normal are referred to as diploid; tumors with abnormal DNA content are referred to as aneuploid. Aneuploid tumors are more likely to recur following primary resection, and patients with aneuploid tumors have decreased survival compared to patients with diploid tumors.

MANIFESTATIONS AND COMPLICATIONS

The signs and symptoms associated with colorectal cancer can be extremely varied, subtle, and nonspecific. Patients with early stage colorectal cancer are often asymptomatic and usually found as a result of screening studies. Rectal bleeding and persistent changes in bowel habits, generally increased frequency or looser stools, are the most common signs of colorectal cancer. Any change in bowel habits (e.g., constipation, diarrhea, alteration in size or shape of stool), vague abdominal discomfort, abdominal pain, or distention may all be warning signs of a malignant process.

Colorectal lesions tend to involve the bowel in a circular rather than longitudinal fashion, thereby narrowing and compressing the lumen. The presence or absence of symptoms is therefore often related to the location and size of the primary tumor and extent of disease involvement.[31] Tumors of the cecum and ascending colon are usually not associated with significant changes in bowel habits; although, watery diarrhea sometimes develops. In contrast, obstructive symptoms and changes in bowel habits frequently develop with tumors located in the transverse and descending colon. This is where the stool is the driest.

Nausea, vomiting, and abdominal discomfort are often secondary signs of a larger underlying problem such as obstruction, perforation, and/or bleeding. Bleeding may be acute or chronic and most commonly appears as bright, red blood mixed with stool. Iron deficiency anemia, presenting as weakness and occasionally high-output congestive heart failure, frequently develops as a result of chronic occult blood loss.

Approximately 20% of patients with colorectal cancer present with metastatic disease.[3] Metastatic spread occurs as a result of direct tumor invasion of adjacent tissues or by lymphatic or hematogenous spread. The venous drainage of the colon and rectum influences the pattern of metastases most commonly seen. The most common site of metastasis is the liver, often the only site of metastatic disease in 40% of patients, followed by the lungs and then bones, specifically the sacrum, coccyx, pelvis, and lumbar vertebrae. Hepatomegaly, obstruction, weight loss, and jaundice are indicative of liver metastases, which are present in 5% to 10% of patients at presentation. Other evidence of widespread disease may include leg edema as a consequence of lymph node involvement, thrombophlebitis, fistula formation, jaundice, weight loss, or pain, especially in the lower back or radiating down the legs. Pain associated with hepatic metastases is sometimes localized in the right upper quadrant of the abdomen, right posterior chest, or right shoulder, and characterized as a continuous ache.

COLORECTAL CANCER PREVENTION

Cancer prevention efforts can be considered as either primary or secondary. Primary prevention strategies are aimed at preventing the development of colorectal cancer in a population at risk. Secondary prevention approaches are undertaken to prevent malignancy in a population that has already manifested an initial disease process. The basis for primary prevention depends on identification of etiologic factors followed by eradication or alteration of their effects on carcinogenesis. Primary prevention also includes lifestyle and diet modification. Several primary preventive measures have undergone or are currently undergoing study; Table 127–2 lists some of the most promising strategies.

TABLE 127–2. Prevention Strategies for Colorectal Cancer

Prevention Strategy	Proposed Mechanism of Protective Effect
High-fiber diet supplementation*	Decreases fecal bile acids; decreases bowel transit time, direct binding to fecal mutagens, dilution of fecal material
Dietary fat reduction*	Decreases fecal bile acids; reduces consumption of heterocyclic amines and other carcinogens that are produced through meat preparation and processing techniques
Nonsteroidal anti-inflammatory agents	Inhibits COX-2; induces apoptosis via 15-LOX-1
Folic acid	Increases levels of intracellular folate
Calcium	Direct binding to bile and fatty acids; inhibits epithelial-cell proliferation
Estrogens	Decreases synthesis of secondary bile acids; decreases production of IGF-I; direct antiproliferative effects on colorectal epithelium
Ursodiol	Modulates bile acid composition
Eflornithine	Inhibits cellular proliferation through alterations in polyamine metabolism
Oltipraz	Induces glutathione *S*-transferase, a mutagen-detoxification enzyme

COX-2, cyclooxygenase-2; 15-LOX-1, 15-lipoxygenase-1; IGF-I, insulin-like growth factor I.
*To date, findings from randomized trials have failed to demonstrate a protective effect of low-fat and high fiber fruits, and vegetable dietary intake, in reducing risk of recurrence of colorectal adenomas or colorectal cancer.
Adapted from Reference 36.

HIGH-FIBER, LOW-FAT DIET

Although early studies suggest that a substantial increase in daily dietary fiber and/or decrease in dietary fat intake might reduce colorectal cancer risk significantly, results from recent randomized trials are inconsistent.[32] The Polyp Prevention Trial, a multicenter, randomized, controlled trial of low-fat, high-fiber diet intervention in 2,079 men and women who had had at least one colorectal adenomas removed within the preceding 6 months, found that a low-fat diet that is high in fiber, fruit, and vegetables has no effect on risk of recurrence of colorectal adenomas.[33] The influence of fruit and vegetable consumption alone on colorectal cancer incidence was prospectively evaluated in two large cohorts of individuals enrolled in the Nurses' Health Study and the Health Professionals' Follow-up Study.[34] A difference in vegetable and fruit consumption of one additional serving each day had no influence on colorectal cancer risk. Furthermore, a trial of high-fiber dietary supplementation in 1,429 men and women who had had one or more colorectal adenomas removed within 3 months prior to study randomization, also failed to show any protection for wheat-bran fiber dietary supplementation against recurrent colorectal adenomas.[35] However, because diets that are low in fat and high in fiber have potentially beneficial and protective effects for other chronic diseases such as coronary heart disease, these dietary recommendations remain appropriate.

CHEMOPREVENTION

The most widely studied agents for the chemoprevention of colorectal cancer are aspirin and the NSAIDs. Although COX-2 expression is not elevated in normal colonic epithelium, up to 40% of colorectal adenomas and 90% of sporadic colon carcinomas have elevated levels of COX-2.[36] In randomized studies of individuals with FAP, sulindac and celecoxib, a selective COX-2 inhibitor, have been shown to reduce the size and number of adenomatous polyps.[17,36] In 1999, the Food and Drug Administration (FDA) approved the use of celecoxib to reduce the number of adenomatous colorectal polyps in FAP, as an adjunct to usual care. This approval was based primarily on results from a trial of 77 patients with FAP who received celecoxib, 400 mg orally twice daily, or placebo, for 6 months. Celecoxib administration resulted in a statistically significant reduction in mean polyp number (28% vs 4.5%) and polyp burden (30.7% vs 4.9%) compared to placebo.[37] The efficacy of celecoxib to other agents has not been compared. In addition, its effects are likely to be transient, because patients receiving sulindac were noted to experience an increase in size and number of polyps within 3 months after the sulindac was discontinued.[36] Although epidemiologic data suggest a potential benefit for aspirin or other NSAID use in the general population, any protective effect of these agents against colorectal cancer and their associated risks have not been evaluated adequately in a prospective trial.

The Calcium Polyp Prevention Study evaluated the effect of calcium carbonate supplementation on risk of recurrence of colorectal adenomas in 930 subjects with a recent history of colorectal adenomas randomized to receive calcium carbonate 3 g (1,200 mg of elemental calcium) or placebo daily.[38] Followup colonoscopies were performed at 1 and 4 years after initial evaluation. In 832 subjects who underwent both followup colonoscopic examinations, calcium supplementation was associated with a moderate reduction in risk of recurrent colorectal adenomas (adjusted risk ratio, 0.85; 95% CI, 0.74–0.98, $P = 0.03$). Before recommendations for calcium supplementation can be made for the general population, however, further studies are

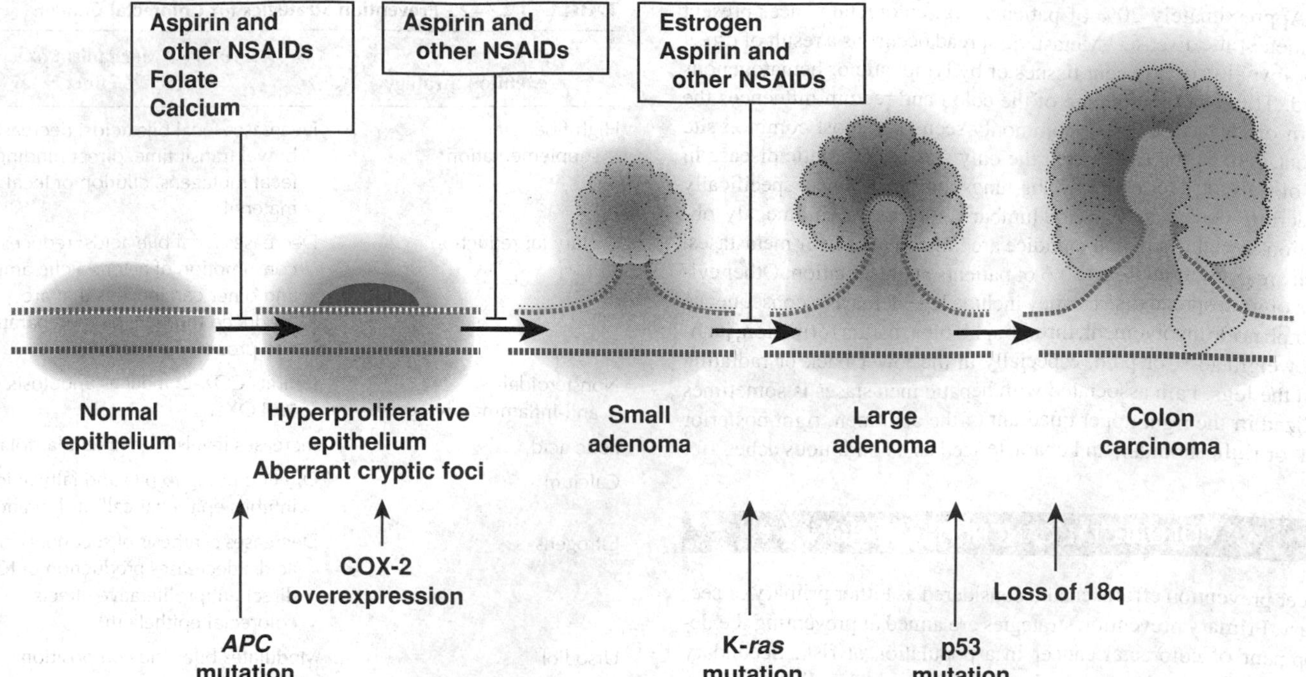

FIGURE 127–5. Sites of chemopreventive effects of various agents on colon carcinogenesis. *(Modified from Ref. 36.)*

needed to confirm these findings to determine risk-benefit ratios in individuals with different baseline levels of colorectal cancer risk.

Additional intervention trials of various micronutrients, including selenium and folic acid, and other chemopreventive agents have been completed or are ongoing.[32,36] A particular challenge for studies of chemoprevention is the lack of definitive associations between intermediate biomarkers commonly employed in chemoprevention trials (e.g., tritiated thymidine incorporation for colonic epithelial proliferation, presence of abnormal crypts, premalignant adenomas) and frank cancer development. Because of their different mechanisms of action and sites of influence on the process of colorectal carcinogenesis, certain populations of individuals may benefit most from selected agents. Fig. 127–5 depicts sites where selected chemopreventive agents may influence colon carcinogenesis.

SURGICAL RESECTION

Despite the potential for NSAIDs to reduce adenoma development and to induce adenoma regression in individuals with FAP, their effects are incomplete and therefore inadequate to replace surgical resection as an important means of cancer prevention for these high-risk individuals. Individuals with FAP who are found to have polyposis on lower endoscopy screening examinations should undergo total proctocolectomy and ileal-pouch-anal anastomosis or total abdominal colectomy with an ileorectal anastomosis.[23,24] Because of the high incidence of metachronous cancers (25% to 40%) in patients with HNPCC, prophylactic total colectomy with an ileorectal anastomosis is recommended for those individuals.[24] Colonoscopic polypectomy, removal of polyps detected during screening colonoscopy, is considered standard of care for all individuals to prevent the progression of premalignant adenomatous polyps to adenocarcinomas.

SCREENING TECHNIQUES FOR COLORECTAL POLYPS AND CANCER

Based on the recognized incidence of colorectal cancer, identification of high-risk individuals, and the high rate of curability associated with localized lesions, screening recommendations for early detection of colorectal cancer have been established.[39] Table 127–3 outlines the current American Cancer Society guidelines for screening and surveillance for early detection of colorectal polyps and cancer. Men and women who are 50 years of age and older and have no personal history of inflammatory bowel disease and no personal or family history of colorectal cancer are considered at average-risk. More rigorous screening recommendations are recommended for high-risk individuals.

DIGITAL RECTAL EXAMINATION

The digital rectal examination has been a traditional part of the annual physical examination in patients older than 40 years of age and accounts for the detection of approximately 10% of all cancers that are within reach of 7–10 cm of the anus. By itself, the digital rectal examination is not an effective screening tool; it should be used in combination with other screening examinations.[39]

FECAL OCCULT BLOOD TESTING

The use of fecal occult blood tests annually or biennially results further in an increased number of asymptomatic individuals with early stages of disease discovered and has been shown to significantly reduce the incidence of colorectal cancer.[40] Furthermore, this is the only test that has been demonstrated through randomized trials to reduce colorectal cancer mortality. Three major methods are available to detect occult blood in the feces: guaiac dye or derivative, heme-porphyrin, and immunochemical methods. Guaiac-based tests use paper impregnated with a guaiac resin that contains α-guaiaconic acid, a phenolic compound that responds to peroxidases in the blood. When a solution containing hydrogen peroxide is poured over paper that was previously exposed to absorbed peroxidases from blood in the stool, the phenolic compound is oxidized and a blue colorization develops.

The sensitivity of the test, a positive result in the setting in which blood is present, can be influenced by several factors. Because hemoglobin is degraded by bacteria in the stool, test sensitivity is diminished when samples are stored or when the lesion is located

TABLE 127–3. American Cancer Society Guidelines for Screening and Surveillance for Early Detection of Colorectal Polyps and Cancer

Risk Category	Recommendation[a]	Age to Begin (years)	Interval
Average Risk	FOBT plus: Flexible sigmoidoscopy *or* TCE[b]	Age 50	FOBT every year Flexible sigmoidoscopy every 5 years Colonoscopy every 10 years or DCBE every 5 years
Moderate Risk			
People with single, small (< 1 cm) or multiple adenomatous polyps of any size	Colonoscopy	At time of initial polyp diagnosis	TCE within 3 years after initial polyp removal; if normal, as per average risk recommendations
People with large (≥ 1 cm) or multiple adenomatous polyps of any size	Colonoscopy	At time of initial polyp diagnosis	TCE within 3 years after initial polyp removal, if normal, TCE every 5 years
Personal history of curative-intent resection of colorectal cancer	TCE	Within 1 year after resection	If normal, TCE in 3 years If still normal, TCE every 5 years
Colorectal cancer or adenomatous polyps in first-degree relative younger than 60 years of age or in two or more first-degree relatives of any age	TCE	Age 40 or 10 years before youngest case in family, whichever is earlier	Every 5 years
Colorectal cancer in other relatives (not included above)	As per average risk recommendations (above); may consider beginning screening before age 50 years		
High Risk			
Family history of familial adenomatous polyposis	Early surveillance with endoscopy, counseling to consider genetic testing, and referral to specialty center	Puberty	If genetic test positive or polyposis confirmed, consider colectomy; otherwise, endoscopy every 1 to 2 years
Family history of hereditary nonpolyposis colon cancer	Colonoscopy and counseling to consider genetic testing	Age 21	If genetic test positive, or if patient has not had genetic testing, colonoscopy every 2 years until age 40 years, then every year
Inflammatory bowel disease	Colonoscopies with biopsies for dysplasia	8 years after the start of pancolitis; 12 to 15 years after the start of left-sided colitis	Every 1 to 2 years

DCBE, double-contrast barium enema; FOBT, fecal occult blood testing; TCE, total colon examination.
[a]Digital rectal examination should be done at the time of each sigmoidoscopy, colonoscopy, or DCBE.
[b]TCE includes either colonoscopy or DCBE. The choice of procedure should depend on the medical status of the patient and the relative quality of the medical examinations available in a specific community. Flexible sigmoidoscopy should be performed in those instances in which the rectosigmoid colon is not well visualized by DCBE. DCBE would be performed when the entire colon has not been adequately evaluated by colonoscopy.
From Ref. 39.

in the proximal area of the bowel. Although the sensitivity can be improved by rehydrating the stool sample, the procedure is more costly and time consuming and the specificity of the test is reduced. Ascorbic acid ingestion in excess of 250 mg/day, failure to ingest a high-residue diet for several days prior to testing, and assays of dry stools may also yield false-negative results.[41] Conversely, foods containing pseudoperoxidase or peroxidase activity can cause a false-positive reaction: rare red meat and uncooked fruits and vegetables such as broccoli, turnips, cauliflower, cantaloupe, and radishes. These foods should be avoided for 3 days prior to and during testing. Other sources of potential false-positive results include the use of iron supplements, rectal medications, or any medications that may potentially alter the integrity of the gastrointestinal lining. Anti-inflammatory agents should be avoided for 7 days prior to and during testing. Because tumors bleed intermittently, multiple stool specimens should be sampled to minimize false-negative results.

Heme porphyrin and immunochemical assays were developed to reduce the rate of false-positive results associated with fecal guaiac blood tests. The heme-porphyrin assay quantifies the conversion of heme to fluorescent porphyrins. Because it also measures fecal heme that has been degraded by bacteria, the site of bleeding or fecal storage does not alter test sensitivity significantly. Immunochemical tests react with the globin moiety of hemoglobin and are therefore affected less by dietary influences. However, test sensitivity is influenced by bleeding site and stool storage. Both of these assays are more complex and labor intensive to perform. A particular advantage of the immunochemical tests is that dietary restrictions are unnecessary. Several comparative trials of fecal occult blood tests have been performed.[41] The HemeSelect, Hemoccult II SENSA, and FlexSure OBT appear to provide the best combination of sensitivity and specificity. A two-step approach in which a combination of the HemeSelect and the Hemoccult II SENSA tests are both used improves overall screening sensitivity without compromising test specificity. Clinical guidelines have been developed for performing and interpreting results of fecal occult blood tests.[41]

The limitations associated with fecal occult blood screening remain an issue of active concern. Many early stage tumors do not bleed, and therefore the false-negative rates are approximately 70% for cancer and 90% for polyps. Between 1% and 5% of unselected individuals will have a positive test result and approximately 2% to 17% of those individuals will be found to have colorectal cancer.[41] Even though false-positive rates are only between 2% and 10%, a false-positive result can prove to be very expensive and inconvenient for a patient because of the follow-up tests required for a positive result. Nevertheless, studies evaluating the effects of fecal occult blood screening tests have established that their annual use reduces colorectal cancer mortality by approximately 33%.[41,42]

FLEXIBLE SIGMOIDOSCOPY

Sigmoidoscopy is useful for examining the lower 35% to 60% of the bowel, depending on the instrument, and thus increases the detection rate by approximately two- to threefold. A 60-cm flexible sigmoidoscope can be used to reach the splenic flexure in order to detect 50% to 60% of cancers, but it requires more operator training, is associated with increased risk, and patient tolerance is less than with the 35-cm instrument.[43] The combination of sigmoidoscopy plus fecal occult blood testing improves sensitivity for lesions that will be missed by sigmoidoscopy alone, but not nonbleeding lesions such as polyps. Findings from the Kaiser-Permanent Medical Care Program show that screening sigmoidoscopy could effectively reduce mortality from colorectal cancer by 60%.[44] These data, however, have yet to be validated through randomized trials.

TOTAL COLONIC EXAMINATION

Total colonic examination can be accomplished with colonoscopy or double-contrast barium enema. A colonoscope facilitates examination of the bowel to the cecum in the majority of patients, and allows for simultaneous removal of premalignant lesions. Although it allows for greater visualization of the colon, colonoscopy involves greater risk and inconvenience to patients. However, it is preferred by many professionals based on its superior ability to detect lesions in the proximal colon as compared to sigmoidoscopy.[45] This may be increasingly important as the proportion of tumors occurring in the proximal or right (cecum, ascending, and transverse colon) side of the colon has increased over the past 30 years with fewer occurring in the rectum and distal or left (descending and sigmoid colon) side. It remains controversial whether this observation reflects a change in the biology of the disease or the nature of screening techniques. The majority of lesions, however, still occur in the distal colon.

A double-contrast barium enema produces an image of the entire colon in most examinations, and the retained barium outlines small polyps and mucosal lesions. This approach is the least expensive method of examining the entire colon but is considered inferior to colonoscopy for detecting polyps and colorectal cancer.[45] The combination of double-contrast barium enema with flexible sigmoidoscopy provides greater sensitivity for detecting a colorectal malignancy but is less convenient than colonoscopy alone. Because it takes approximately 10 years for normal mucosa to evolve into an invasive carcinoma, the use of double-contrast barium enemas in routine screening practices for average-risk individuals is recommended only every 5 to 10 years.

MOLECULAR SCREENING

Molecular screening strategies include the analysis of stool samples for presence of K-*ras* oncogene or mutant DNA mismatch-repair genes in cells that are shed from adenomas or adenocarcinomas in the bowel. Although available tests have reliable sensitivity and specificity, the cost and complexity associated with their analysis make them unlikely screening tools for the general population at present. Genetic testing is an important cancer-screening approach for family members of individuals diagnosed with FAP or HNPCC, and is appropriate for selected individuals, but should only be offered in conjunction with genetic counseling.

WORKUP AND DIAGNOSIS

When a patient is suspected of having colorectal carcinoma, a careful history and physical examination should be performed. The patient history should include a past medical history and family history, especially noting the presence of inflammatory bowel disease, colorectal cancer, polyps, and cancers of the breast, ovary, and endometrium. A complete physical examination includes careful abdominal examination for the presence of masses or ascites, a rectal examination, and an assessment for possible hepatomegaly and lymphadenopathy. In all women, a breast and pelvic examination is recommended, especially in women with a history of breast, ovarian, or endometrial cancer. Table 127–4 summarizes the recommended tests for pretreatment evaluation of patients with potentially curable colorectal cancer.

An unexplained anemia in an older patient requires surveillance of the entire large bowel, especially the right colon. Red blood cell indices (e.g., hemoglobin, hematocrit, mean corpuscular volume, reticulocyte count) and a workup of iron status (e.g., serum ferritin, serum iron, and total iron-binding capacity) may be useful to confirm acute or chronic blood loss and/or iron-deficiency anemia. An evaluation of the entire large bowel is undertaken with either colonoscopy or sigmoidoscopy and a double-contrast barium enema. A barium enema may be preferred in situations in which a partially obstructing lesion prohibits passage of the endoscope; however, it should be avoided if complete obstruction or perforation of the bowel is suspected. A characteristic finding indicative of colon cancer seen on barium enema is an apple core-shaped lesion with tumor involving the circumference of the bowel. When possible, the endoscope is used to collect tissue for a histologic evaluation and provide a preliminary diagnosis following the procedure.

Baseline laboratory tests should be obtained and include a complete blood cell (CBC) count, platelet count, prothrombin time (PT), activated partial thromboplastin time (aPTT), liver function tests, and

TABLE 127–4. Recommended Pretreatment Evaluation for Patients with Potentially Curable Colorectal Cancer

Personal medical history and family history of colorectal polyps, cancer, or other malignancies
Physical examination, including evaluation for lymphadenopathy, hepatomegaly, and ascites. Women should undergo appropriate evaluations to rule out breast, ovarian, or endometrial cancers
Complete blood count, liver chemistries, and serum carcinoembryonic antigen
Total colonic evaluation with colonoscopy or proctosigmoidoscopy with double-contrast barium enema
Chest x-ray
Abdominal CT scan
Additional studies as indicated

From Refs. 30 and 48.

serum CEA. Abnormal liver function tests may suggest liver involvement with tumor. However, patients with metastatic disease to the liver may have normal liver function tests, and abnormal liver function tests are not always indicative of metastatic disease.

CEA belongs to a group of cell-surface glycoproteins, termed "oncofetal proteins," which are expressed during embryonic development and reexpressed on the cell surfaces of many carcinomas, particularly those of the gastrointestinal tract. Although the function of CEA is not well understood, it is proposed to be a cellular adhesion molecule and possibly contributes toward tumor invasion and metastasis.

The concentration of CEA can be measured in the blood and can therefore potentially serve as a "marker" for colorectal cancer. However, not all colorectal cancers produce CEA. Approximately 28% of patients with stage A and 45% of patients with stage B colorectal cancer have an elevated serum CEA level at time of diagnosis.[46] Elevated concentrations are even more frequent in patients with metastatic disease. It is important to recognize, however, several concomitant disease states that elevate CEA: alcoholic and chronic hepatitis, diverticulitis, renal failure, cholelithiasis, fibrocystic breast disease, smoking, and other carcinomas.[46] Most commercially available assays list a normal range of less than 3.0 ng/mL and 5.0 ng/mL for nonsmokers and smokers, respectively. Although CEA measurement is too insensitive and nonspecific to be used as a screening test for early stage colorectal cancer, it may be useful for monitoring colorectal cancer response to treatment, particularly if the pretreatment concentration is elevated. The CEA test also has preoperative prognostic implications because it has been shown to correlate with the size and degree of differentiation of the carcinoma. Elevated preoperative CEA levels correlate with a poor survival, regardless of tumor stage upon diagnosis. After a potentially curative resection, CEA levels should return to normal within 4 to 6 weeks.[46] Persistently elevated CEA levels may indicate residual or recurrent disease. Although additional tumor markers are frequently elevated in patients with colorectal cancer, there is insufficient evidence to recommend their routine use in patients with newly diagnosed disease.

Radiographic imaging studies help evaluate the extent of disease involvement. A chest x-ray should be performed to rule out the presence of metastatic spread to the lungs. A bone scan can also be helpful in evaluating the extent of disease involvement in a symptomatic patient. A computed tomography (CT) scan or ultrasound of the abdomen is often performed to evaluate hepatic and retroperitoneal involvement and occult abdominal and pelvic disease, and to determine the depth of tumor penetration into the bowel wall and/or invasion to adjacent organs. Detection of lymph node involvement with either study is limited by the difficulty of distinguishing inflammatory or reactive lymph nodes from those infiltrated with tumor. Because CT scans may not adequately detect peritoneal seeding, small distant lymph node metastasis, or liver metastasis in colon cancer, an occasional patient may need to undergo a laparotomy in order to confirm metastatic disease. This is infrequent, however, because most patients eventually undergo surgical resection for colorectal cancer unless the procedure is contraindicated. Positron emission tomography (PET) imaging can be useful in discriminating between benign and malignant disease by detecting tumor-related metabolic alterations in affected tissues.[47] However, its utility in the evaluation and management of patients with colorectal cancer is still undergoing study.

Intrarectal or transrectal ultrasonography is a technique that is becoming more widely available for the evaluation of patients with rectal cancer. It is excellent for detecting the depth of tumor penetration and, like pelvic CT scans, is fair to good in determining lymph node involvement.[48] Cystoscopy or IV pyelography studies are rarely indicated except for very large rectal tumors found on examination, if the patient exhibits symptoms, or if a CT scan suggests bladder involvement. Intraluminal and hepatic MRI studies may also provide useful information.

Immunodetection of tumors using tumor-directed antibodies is receiving greater recognition as an imaging technique for the early detection and imaging of colorectal cancers. Several tumor-associated proteins have been identified within or on the surface membrane of colorectal malignant cells to which monoclonal antibodies have been targeted. Of these, CEA and TAG-72 antigen have undergone the greatest amount of study. Radiolabeled monoclonal antibodies directed against these antigens have been used in clinical studies for both external immunoscintigraphy as well as intraoperative localization of tumor. OncoScint, an indium-111-labeled monoclonal antibody targeted to the TAG-72 antigen (^{111}In-Satumomab pendetide), is an FDA-approved diagnostic imaging agent available for determining the location and extent of extrahepatic disease in patients with colorectal cancer. OncoScint is generally reserved for use in detecting clinically occult disease that is suggested by rising CEA levels but is undetectable using conventional imaging studies. CEA-Scan arcitumomab (IMMU-4^{99m}Tc Fab′), a radiolabeled murine monoclonal immunoglobulin directed against the human CEA molecule, and HumaSPECT-Tc (^{99m}Tc 88BV59), a radiolabeled human monoclonal immunoglobulin that recognizes a tumor-associated antigen (CTAA 16.88, CTA #1), can also provide useful information regarding the presence, extent, and location of colorectal cancer.[49] The use of these agents is generally reserved for those patients who have completed standard diagnostic imaging tests but may still require additional information regarding the extent of disease. However, they may play an important role in identifying metastatic or recurrent disease in individuals with negative standard radiographic studies. Although these approaches are helpful for addressing some of the limitations of current radiographic techniques, they are limited somewhat by the heterogeneity associated with antigen expression at different sites of tumor within individual patients and because they tend to localize nonspecifically to sites of inflammation, benign colonic polyps, and in normal bone marrow, spleen, and hepatic tissues.

STAGING

The purpose of the staging examinations is to describe precisely the malignancy at a point in its natural history that is germane to patient treatment options and overall prognosis. Traditionally, the Dukes' classification, originally published in 1932, has been used in the staging of colorectal cancers.[30] Since its original publication, it has undergone several modifications; a modified Astler–Coller (MAC) version is used more extensively. Prognosis and survival data associated with each stage of disease in this classification system have been collected extensively. However, because multiple staging systems exist and have been used for various clinical trials, the literature is often difficult to evaluate. Therefore, in an effort to standardize the staging system for colorectal cancer, the American Joint Committee on Cancer (AJCC) and the International Union Against Cancer (IUAC) jointly agreed to use and recommend the TNM classification system. This classification takes three aspects of cancer growth—T (tumor size), N (lymph node involvement), and M (presence or absence of metastases)—into account for determining the disease stage. The TNM classification also allows for various subdivisions within each of the three categories (Table 127–5). Stage 0 disease is defined as a TNM grouping of Tis, N0, M0 whereas stage I tumors include those that are T1 or T2, N0, M0; stage II disease includes T3 or T4, N0, M0; stage III

TABLE 127–5. TNM Staging Definitions for Colorectal Cancer

Criteria	Classification	Definition
Primary tumor (T)	TX	Primary tumor cannot be assessed
	T0	No evidence of primary tumor
	Tis	Carcinoma *in situ:* intraepithelial or invasion of the lamina propria*
	T1	Tumor invades submucosa
	T2	Tumor invades muscularis propria
	T3	Tumor invades through the muscularis propria into the subserosa, or into the nonperitonealized pericolic tissues
	T4	Tumor directly invades other organs or structures and/or perforates the visceral peritoneum
Regional lymph nodes (N)	NX	Regional nodes cannot be assessed
	N0	No regional lymph node metastasis
	N1	Metastasis in one to three pericolic lymph nodes
	N2	Metastasis in four or more pericolic lymph nodes
Distant metastasis (M)	MX	Presence of distant metastasis cannot be assessed
	M0	No distant metastasis
	M1	Distant metastasis

*Tis includes cancer cells confined within the glandular basement membrane (intraepithelial) or lamina propria (intramucosal) with no extension through the muscularis mucosae into the submucosa.

From American Joint Committee on Cancer. Colon and rectum. In: AJCC Cancer Staging Manual, 5th ed. Philadelphia, PA: Lippincott-Raven, 1997, pp 83–90.

tumors are defined as any T, N1 to N3, M0, and tumors that are any T, any N, M1 are stage IV. Future modifications may include additional subcategories to provide further staging discrimination and account for serum CEA measurements.[50] Fig. 127–6 is a representation of the relationship between the MAC and AJCC/IUAC staging systems.

The stage of colorectal cancer upon diagnosis, identified primarily by depth of tumor invasion of the bowel wall and presence or absence of involved lymph nodes, is the most important independent prognostic factor for survival and disease recurrence. Table 127–6 compares the stage of disease upon presentation and relative survival rates for individuals with colon and rectum cancer. The stage

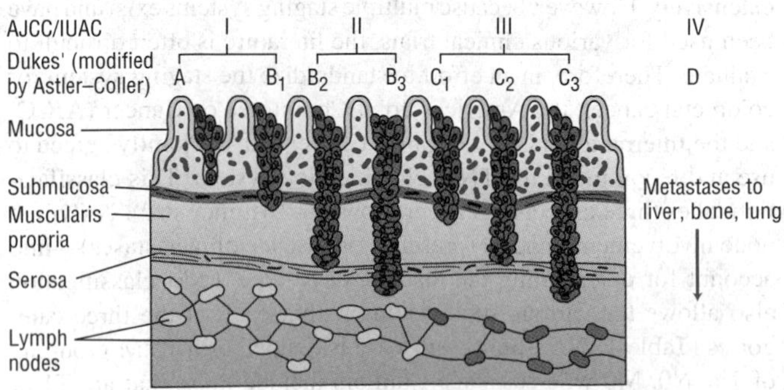

FIGURE 127–6. Staging system for colorectal cancer.

TABLE 127–6. Colon and Rectum Cancer Disease Stage and Survival Rates (SEER Data, 1989–1996)

Tumor Stage at Diagnosis	Stage Distribution (%)*		5-Year Relative Survival (%)	
	Colon	Rectum	Colon	Rectum
Localized	35	42	91.7	86.4
Regional	38	35	68.2	56.9
Distant	21	16	8.8	6.6
All stages	—	—	61.8	60.0

*Approximately 5% and 8% of cancers of the colon and rectum, respectively, were unstaged.

From Ref. 3.

of disease also provides the basis for determining the most appropriate initial treatment. However, additional clinical and pathologic variables may affect the prognosis of patients with colorectal cancer. Consideration of these factors plays an important role in determining optimal strategies for treatment as well as appropriate follow-up. The patient's overall health status will also influence treatment tolerability and therapeutic options. Clinical factors present at time of diagnosis that are associated with a poor prognosis and decreased survival include bowel obstruction or perforation, rectal bleeding, high preoperative CEA level, distant metastases, and location of the primary tumor in the rectum or rectosigmoid area.[30,46]

Pathologic variables associated with a negative influence on prognosis include increasing depth of muscular invasion; presence of venous, lymphatic, or perineural invasion; increasing number of involved lymph nodes; presence of peritumoral lymphoid reaction, mucinous or signet-ring histology; high proliferation indices; tumor aneuploidy; and presence of certain tumor tissue molecular markers (18q/*DCC* mutation or loss, K-*ras* mutations, microsatellite instability, elevated thymidylate synthase (TS) expression, lack of *p27* expression, *bcl-2* overexpression, and *p53* mutation or loss).[30,50]

Allelic loss of chromosome 18q, which is located on the *DCC* gene, is predictive of mortality, independent of tumor differentiation, vascular invasion, and TNM stage. Five-year survival rates of approximately 93% are associated with stage II colorectal cancer; survival rates for patients with stage II disease and allelic loss of chromosome 18q drop to approximately 54%, similar to that for patients with stage III disease and intact chromosome 18q. In individuals with stage III disease, the presence of chromosome 18q allelic loss is associated with a 5-year disease-free survival rate of 38%, as compared to 76% among individuals without loss of heterozygosity.[51] Tumors that overexpress TS, which is responsible for converting deoxyuridine monophosphate (dUMP) to deoxythymidine monophosphate (dTMP), an essential step for DNA synthesis, are less sensitive to 5-fluorouracil (5-FU) chemotherapy. Although the 10-year overall survival for individuals with TS-positive tumors was no different from that with TS-negative tumors, survival in a subset of patients who received chemotherapy was only 42.9% for TS-positive tumors as compared to 85.7% for TS-negative tumors.[52] Similarly, tumors that overexpress mutant *p53* demonstrate a high degree of resistance to radiation, 5-FU, and certain other chemotherapeutic agents and are associated with a poorer prognosis.[53] In contrast, colorectal cancers that demonstrate microsatellite instability appear to be associated with a more favorable outcome.[54] Evaluation of these factors may provide important clues as to which patients will benefit most from more aggressive therapy and those individuals who may not require systemic chemotherapy. A large number of additional pathologic factors appear to have prognostic significance but have been studied less sufficiently to date.[50,53]

▶ TREATMENT: Colorectal Cancer

DESIRED OUTCOME

Treatment goals for cancer of the colon or rectum are based on the stage of disease at presentation. Stages I, II, and III disease are considered potentially curable and, as such, are managed ideally with the intent of eradicating known and micrometastatic sites of tumor to achieve remission and avoid disease recurrence. Because stage IV disease is not curable, treatments are offered to reduce symptoms, to avoid disease-related complications, and to prolong survival. Treatment strategies for individuals who manifest premalignant forms of the disease (e.g., adenomatous polyps) should be undertaken to prevent polyp progression and transformation to malignancy.

GENERAL APPROACH TO TREATMENT

Although advanced age is not an absolute contraindication for relatively aggressive therapies, a consideration of the age of the patient, concomitant disease states, lifestyle factors, and the patient's wishes are incorporated into the treatment planning process. Special or emergent conditions, such as bowel perforation, spinal cord compression, and severe pain, anemia, or other symptomatic problems, need to be addressed acutely, after which time a more long-term disease-specific plan can be developed. The treatment approaches for colorectal cancer reflect two primary treatment goals: curative therapy for localized disease or palliative therapy for metastatic cancer. For patients for whom treatment intent is curative, surgical resection of the primary tumor is the most important component of therapy. Depending on the extent of disease and whether the tumor originated in the colon or rectum, further adjuvant chemotherapy or chemotherapy plus XRT may be appropriate. Surgery, with few exceptions, is used infrequently for metastatic disease. In this setting, systemic chemotherapy is the mainstay of treatment; XRT may also be useful for disease palliation of localized symptoms or when chemotherapy is no longer effective. Patients with metastatic disease who are asymptomatic may benefit from initiation of therapy and treatment should not be withheld until they develop symptoms.

NONPHARMACOLOGIC THERAPY

SURGERY

Surgical removal of the primary tumor is the treatment of choice for patients with potentially curable colorectal cancer. Patients with advanced, metastatic colorectal cancer may also require surgery for palliation of bleeding, obstruction, or localized abdominal pain caused by a bulky tumor mass.[48] Surgical resection of a limited number of metastases that are isolated to the liver, lungs, or brain may offer improved survival to selected individuals. This approach is addressed in greater detail in the discussion of the management of metastatic colorectal cancer.

The surgical approach for colon cancer generally involves a complete resection of the tumor with an appropriate margin of tumor-free bowel and a regional lymphadenectomy. In the elective setting, a temporary colostomy is rarely required.[30] A total colectomy is frequently, however, indicated for selected patients with FAP or chronic ulcerative colitis. Laparoscopic-assisted colectomy may offer patients the potential for reduced pain and hospitalization associated with an open resection colectomy; however, the results of ongoing studies are necessary to determine whether this newer approach provides an acceptable rate of surgery-related morbidity and mortality.

Surgery for rectal cancer depends on the region of tumor involvement. A low anterior resection is the procedure of choice in patients with lesions in the mid- to upper rectum.[55] Patients with lesions in the lower portion of the rectum may require an abdominoperineal resection if either the amount of unaffected bowel is insufficient for a resection far enough away from the tumor or too close to areas that cannot permit an anastomosis. Newer surgical techniques have been developed in an attempt to retain function of the rectal sphincter and still achieve complete tumor resection. Individuals who are not candidates for sphincter-sparing resections or have extensive local spread of tumor will require an abdominoperineal resection. This involves removal of the distal sigmoid, rectosigmoid, rectum, and anus with the establishment of a permanent sigmoid colostomy. Fewer than one-third of patients will require a permanent colostomy for rectal cancer.[55] The American Cancer Society and several national and international ostomy associations offer patient education materials and ostomy rehabilitation services. Surgery for colorectal cancer is associated with a morbidity and mortality rate of 8% to 15% and 1% to 2%, respectively, depending on the type and extent of procedure.[48] Other complications associated with colorectal surgery can include infection, anastomotic leakage, obstruction, adhesion formation, and malabsorption syndromes. Other complications that occur more frequently with surgery for rectal cancer include urinary retention, incontinence, impotence, and locoregional recurrence.

RADIATION THERAPY

XRT can be administered in conjunction with curative surgical resection and in the setting of advanced or metastatic disease. In patients undergoing surgery for rectal cancer, XRT is used to reduce risk of local tumor recurrence. Symptom reduction is the primary goal of XRT for patients with advanced or metastatic disease. Radiation therapy is given prior to or following surgery and can be delivered using a variety of dosing regimens, administration schedules, and techniques that expose different amounts of body surface area.[55]

Accumulating data suggest that preoperative XRT may be used to reduce the initial size of the tumor to such an extent that the tumor could be reclassified to a lower stage, or "downstaged," and therefore rendered more resectable. This might then lead to improved patient survival or result in the need for a less extensive surgical procedure. Preoperative XRT is also administered to reduce the amount of tumor seeding that can occur during surgery; however, this approach is more likely to affect a greater area than is necessary.[55] Postoperative administration of XRT may more adequately treat a defined area, but is associated with more toxicity because of a greater amount of bowel being present in the treatment field.

Adverse effects associated with XRT can be acute or chronic. Acute effects primarily include hematologic depression, dysuria, diarrhea, abdominal cramping, and proctitis. Chronic symptoms that sometimes persist for months following discontinuation of XRT may involve persistent diarrhea, proctitis or enteritis, small bowel obstruction, perineal tenderness, and impaired wound healing.

PHARMACOLOGIC AGENTS USED FOR COLORECTAL CANCER

CYTOTOXIC CHEMOTHERAPY

For more than 40 years, 5-FU has been the most widely used chemotherapeutic agent for colorectal cancer. Most recently, irinotecan, also an active agent against colorectal cancer, has been recognized to provide further antitumor effects when administered with 5-FU. This observation, in addition to the discovery of other active agents with different mechanisms of action, provides patients with greater pharmacologic treatment options than ever previously available. The pharmacology of key agents used for colorectal cancer is discussed briefly in the next section.

5-Fluorouracil and 5-Fluoro-2′-Deoxyuridine

As a prodrug, 5-FU undergoes anabolism to two primary products, 5-fluorouridine-5′-triphosphate (FUTP) and 5-fluorodeoxyuridine-5′-monophosphate (FdUMP), to exert its antitumor effects (Fig. 127–7).[56,57] 5-Fluoro-2′-deoxyuridine (FUDR, Floxuridine) produces the same cytotoxic effects as 5-FU through its conversion in a single-step reaction by deoxyuridine kinase to the active metabolite FdUMP. FUTP is incorporated into RNA, thereby impairing protein synthesis. FdUMP forms a tight but reversible covalent bond with TS in the presence of methylenetetrahydrofolate (CH_2FH_4), one of the intracellular metabolites of folinic acid. TS is the key enzyme necessary for *de novo* biosynthesis of thymidylate through conversion of deoxyuridine monophosphate (dUMP) to 2′-deoxythymidine-5′-monophosphate (dTMP). The lack of available TS reduces the rate of DNA synthesis, replication, and repair. When combined with folinic acid, the antitumor effects of 5-FU are enhanced through stabilization of the ternary complex of TS, FdUMP, and CH_2FH_4.

5-FU is typically administered as an intravenous (IV) bolus injection, generally once weekly or daily for 5 days each month, or via a continuous IV infusion. Although the duration of continuous IV infusions is usually 1 to 5 days, it can extend for many weeks. FUDR can be administered intravenously but intrahepatic use is more common. It is preferable to 5-FU for intrahepatic administration because a much greater percentage of FUDR is removed from the systemic circulation with one pass through the liver.

Clinical studies comparing efficacy of bolus and continuous infusion schedules generally favor continuous infusion of 5-FU. This is consistent with evidence that suggests that the duration of infusion may be an important determinant of the biologic activity of 5-FU, particularly because of its short plasma half-life and S-phase specificity for optimal TS inhibition.[57,58] Whereas the primary cytotoxic effect associated with bolus 5-FU is on RNA synthesis, interference with DNA is the predominant effect of continuous 5-FU infusion. Thus, 5-FU can be considered to act as two different drugs, depending on the schedule of administration. Continuous IV infusions also permit increased 5-FU dose intensity; this factor may also account for higher response rates that are observed with prolonged infusions of 5-FU. Because of the more costly and cumbersome nature of continuous IV infusions, however, in the United States, 5-FU is most commonly administered as an IV bolus injection.

Toxicity patterns also differ based on the dose, route, and schedule of 5-FU administration. Leukopenia is the primary dose-limiting toxicity of IV bolus 5-FU, although diarrhea, stomatitis, and nausea and vomiting can also occur.[57,59] The incidence and severity of stomatitis can be significantly reduced with the use of oral cryotherapy. In this approach, the patient is required to chew and hold ice chips in the mouth during the period between 5 minutes prior to and

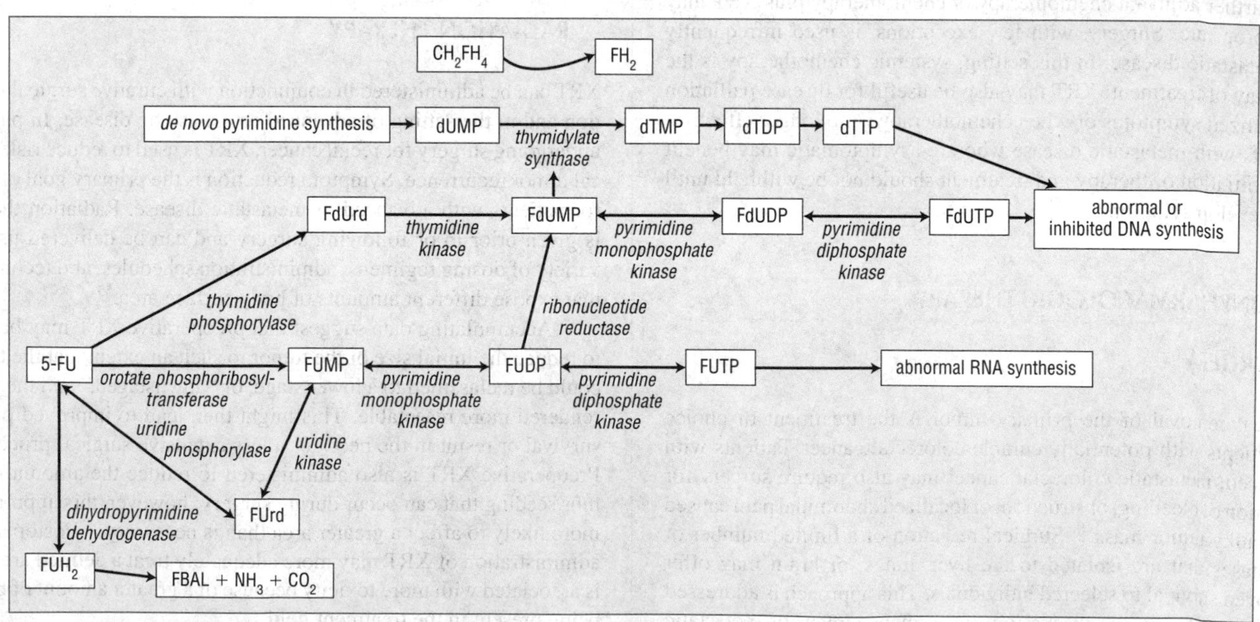

FIGURE 127–7. Pathways of 5-FU metabolic activation and inactivation. CH_2FH_4, methylenetetrahydrofolate; CO_2, carbon dioxide; FH_2, dihydrofolate; dUMP, deoxyuridine monophosphate; dTMP, deoxythymidine monophosphate; dTDP, deoxythymidine diphosphate; dTTP, deoxythymidine triphosphate; FdUrd, fluorodeoxyuridine; FdUMP, fluorodeoxyuridine monophosphate; FdUDP, fluorodeoxyuridine diphosphate; FdUTP, fluorodeoxyuridine triphosphate; 5-FU, 5-fluorouracil; FUMP, fluorouridine monophosphate; FUDP, fluorouridine diphosphate; FUTP, fluorouridine triphosphate; FUrd, fluorouridine; FUH_2, dihydrofluorouracil; FBAL, α-fluoro-β-alanine; NH_3, urea. *Modified from Ref. 56 and Benson AB. Therapy for advanced colorectal cancer. Semin Oncol 1998;(5 suppl 11):2–11.*

TABLE 127–7. Examples of Combination 5-FU Plus Leucovorin Treatment Regimens for Colorectal Cancer

	5-Fluorouracil		Leucovorin		
Regimen	*Duration*	*mg/m²/day*	*Duration*	*mg/m²/day*	Comments
Daily × five 5-FU + LDLV; repeat every 3 to 5 weeks	IVP	370–425	IVP	20	Mayo regimen
Daily × five 5-FU + HDLV; repeat every 3 to 5 weeks	IVP	370–400	IVP	200	Modified Machover regimen
Weekly 5-FU + HDLV; weekly × 6 with 2-week rest	IVP	600	2-h CIV	500	Roswell Park regimen
Weekly 5-FU + LDLV; weekly × 6 with 2-week rest	IVP	500–600	IVP	20–25	
Biweekly 5-FU + HDLV; days 1 and 2; repeat every 2 weeks	IVP, then 22-h CIV	300–400 300–600	2-h CIV	200	de Gramont regimen
Weekly 24-h CIV 5-FU + HDLV; repeat weekly	24-h CIV	2,600	2- to 24-h CIV	500	

CIV, continuous intravenous infusion; HDLV, high-dose leucovorin; IVP, intravenous bolus; LDLV, low-dose leucovorin.
Adapted from Ref. 61.

30 minutes following the bolus injection of 5-FU. The basis for the protective effect of this procedure is based on the premise that local vasoconstriction caused by the ice chips temporarily reduces blood flow to the oral mucosa, thereby reducing drug exposure to the oral mucosa.

Although continuous IV infusion 5-FU is generally well tolerated, dose-limiting toxicities can be substantial. A distinct toxicity, palmar-plantar erythrodysesthesia ("hand-foot syndrome") and stomatitis occur most frequently with this route of administration.[59] Hand-foot syndrome occurs in 24% to 40% of patients receiving extended continuous IV infusions and is characterized by painful swelling and erythroderma of the soles of the feet, palms of the hands, and distal fingers. This type of skin toxicity is fully reversible upon interruption of therapy or dose reduction, and is not life-threatening; however, it can be significant and acutely disabling. The incidence of stomatitis, diarrhea, and hematologic toxicity is not substantial at standard doses but increases with increasing doses of 5-FU. In a meta-analysis of six randomized trials, no significant difference was noted in the incidence of mucositis, diarrhea, nausea and vomiting, or alopecia between continuous and bolus IV 5-FU administration.[59]

Biochemical Modulation of 5-FU

The nature of the pharmacology of 5-FU provides several opportunities to increase its antitumor activity, the most common of which is accomplished by using concomitant calcium leucovorin. Other promising strategies have included the use of 5-FU with other modulators such as methotrexate, trimetrexate, interferon-α, dipyridamole, and PALA (*N*-(phosphonacetyl)-L-aspartate).[56] However, none of these combinations have proven more effective or less toxic than the combination of 5-FU plus leucovorin. The sequential administration of methotrexate provides a modest improvement to 5-FU efficacy but is more complex to deliver and is thus given infrequently.[56,60] With the exception of continuous IV infusion treatment regimens, 5-FU is almost always administered in combination with leucovorin.

Leucovorin is generally nontoxic in therapeutic doses, although hypersensitivity reactions such as anaphylaxis and urticaria have been reported. The combination of 5-FU plus leucovorin, however, produces greater toxicity to the gastrointestinal epithelium, the primary dose-limiting toxicity. An increase in the incidence and severity of stomatitis and mucositis, diarrhea, and leukopenia is most commonly observed.[61,62] Serious toxic effects develop in 3% to 6% of patients.[63,64] Seizures have infrequently developed in association with combination 5-FU plus leucovorin regimens. The mechanism may be similar to that between anticonvulsants and folic acid.

Several different leucovorin dosage regimens are used; they are most typically referred to as either "high dose" (≥ 200 mg/m²/day) or "low dose" (≤ 25 mg/m²/day) leucovorin. Table 127–7 lists examples of some of these regimens. Although comparative trials have ascertained no significant differences among these regimens regarding efficacy, the nature and severity of toxicities differ. Diarrhea is more frequent in a weekly high-dose leucovorin (HDLV) for the 6-week regimen (23% to 40%) as compared to a daily for 5 days low-dose leucovorin (LDLV) regimen (9% to 11%) or weekly (9% to 14%) and biweekly (2.2% to 16%) continuous infusion regimens using high-dose leucovorin and 5-FU.[61]

Severe diarrhea develops in 25% of patients receiving high-dose leucovorin regimens, and has resulted in a 5% mortality rate as a result of diarrhea-related events or cardiovascular collapse.[65] Early treatment of diarrhea-related dehydration with bowel rest, IV fluids, and discontinuation of chemotherapy until resolution of all symptoms is recommended. Loperamide and diphenoxylate can be used for symptomatic treatment if an infectious etiology has been excluded. For those patients who do not respond to these treatment measures, the use of octreotide acetate should be considered. Several studies have demonstrated the safety and efficacy of octreotide acetate, administered subcutaneously at a starting dosage of 100–150 μg three times daily, or 50 to 150 μg/h via continuous IV infusion.[66] Some patients may require higher doses of octreotide; doses up to 2,000 μg three times daily for 5 days have been used safely in patients with 5-FU-induced diarrhea.

Stomatitis and mucositis and leukopenia are the most frequent dose-limiting toxicities for LDLV regimens as compared to HDLV regimens.[61,62] The incidence of stomatitis using a daily for 5 days regimen of LDLV ranges from 15% to 31%. A significant increase in leukopenia and stomatitis was noted in the daily for 5 days LDLV plus 5-FU arm as compared to a weekly arm of 5-FU plus LDLV administered as an IV bolus or continuous infusion (7.9% to 29% vs 1.4% to 4%) and (9.9% to 28% vs 0%), respectively.[61] More treatment-related deaths caused by sepsis occur with the daily for 5 days LDLV plus 5-FU, which could be explained by higher doses of 5-FU given as IV bolus infusions. Continuous or intermittent administration of 5-FU permits use of higher doses of 5-FU to be administered with significantly less myelosuppression, stomatitis, and diarrhea.

Irinotecan

Irinotecan (CPT-11, Camptosar) is a water-soluble camptothecin derivative that inhibits topoisomerase I, thereby interfering with the relegation step of the process of DNA replication and transcription.[67] Irinotecan itself is a weak inhibitor of topoisomerase I and therefore must be converted to an active metabolite, 7-ethyl-10-hydroxy camptothecin (SN-38), which is 100- to 1,000-fold more potent than the parent drug.[68]

Irinotecan has been administered using a variety of IV dosing schedules ranging from 100–150 mg/m^2 weekly, or 150–250 mg/m^2 biweekly, or 125 mg/m^2 weekly for 4 weeks, followed by a 2-week rest period, to 300 to 350 mg/m^2 IV every 3 weeks.[67,69] In each of these regimens, neutropenia and diarrhea are the dose-limiting toxicities. The most common administration schedules in the United States are 125 mg/m^2 IV given weekly for 4 consecutive weeks followed by a rest period, with therapy repeated every 6 weeks based on patient tolerance or the regimen or 350 mg/m^2 given IV every 3 weeks.[67,69]

The most common adverse effects of irinotecan are diarrhea, neutropenia, nausea and vomiting, asthenia, abdominal pain, and alopecia; diarrhea and neutropenia are dose limiting.[67] Two distinct patterns of diarrhea have been described. Early onset diarrhea occurs during or within 2 to 6 hours after irinotecan administration and is characterized by lacrimation, diaphoresis, abdominal cramping, flushing, and/or diarrhea. These cholinergic symptoms, thought to be due to inhibition of acetylcholinesterase, respond to atropine 0.25–1 mg given intravenously or subcutaneously. Approximately 12% of patients experience the acute symptoms during or shortly following the irinotecan.[67] More commonly, late-onset diarrhea appears, 1 to 12 days or more after irinotecan administration and may last for 3 to 5 days.[69,70] A few patients have required hospitalization or discontinuation of therapy, and fatalities have been reported. The incidence of late-onset diarrhea has been as high as 39% in some studies, but is now much lower with aggressive antidiarrheal intervention.[67,69,70] Aggressive intervention with high-dose loperamide therapy should consist of 4 mg taken at the first sign of soft or watery stools, followed by 2 mg orally every 2 hours until symptom free for 12 hours. This regimen can be modified to 4 mg every 4 hours taken during the night. Of note, a significant correlation has been identified between the severity of diarrhea, CPT-11, and SN-38 area under the concentration-versus-time curve (AUC).[67,68]

Bone marrow suppression due to irinotecan is not cumulative and affects primarily the neutrophils, with a median nadir at 8 to 15 days followed by prompt recovery. The incidence of febrile neutropenia and sepsis requiring hospitalization is more common at higher dosage levels.[69,70] The use of granulocyte colony-stimulating factors is generally not required unless the patient has persistent myelosuppression despite a dose reduction. An idiosyncratic pulmonary-induced toxicity and drug interaction with phenothiazines has been reported with irinotecan. Discontinuation of irinotecan has resulted in symptomatic improvement of dyspnea, pulmonary infiltrates, and/or fever.[69] At this time however, routine pulmonary function testing is not recommended.

Trials with other topoisomerase I inhibitors, topotecan, and 9-aminocamptothecin have also been performed in patients with colorectal cancer. Despite promising antitumor activity against colorectal carcinomas in preclinical studies, tumor response rates in phase II clinical trials have not been meaningful.[67] It is therefore unlikely that either agent will play a significant role in colorectal cancer management.

Capecitabine

Capecitabine (Xeloda) is an oral, tumor-activated and tumor-selective fluoropyrimidine carbamate. As a prodrug, it passes through the intestines as an intact molecule and is converted to 5-FU through three sequential conversion steps: first by hepatic carboxylesterase, next, by hepatic and tumor cytidine deaminase, and finally by thymidine phosphorylase, which is present in greatest concentrations at the tumor site.[71] These activation steps lead to an approximate threefold increase in tumor and 1.4-fold increase in hepatic 5-FU levels. Because capecitabine first passes through the intestines as an intact molecule, the incidence of diarrhea is significantly reduced. However, diarrhea, nausea and vomiting, hand-foot syndrome, and abdominal pain are the most common dose-limiting toxicities with its use. Capecitabine has been studied against colorectal cancer using a variety of dosing schedules, the most common consisting of 2,500 mg/m^2/day given orally in two divided doses on an intermittent schedule for 2 weeks on and 1 week off. Important potential advantages with capecitabine chemotherapy include its oral administration and minimal myelosuppression. In 2001, the FDA approved capecitabine for use in metastatic colorectal carcinoma when treatment with a fluoropyrimidine alone is preferred.

Mitomycin C

Mitomycin C (Mutamycin) in combination with 5-FU, with or without leucovorin has been used to induce tumor responses in patients with metastatic disease, primarily rectal cancer. Mitomycin C acts primarily as an alkylating agent to inhibit DNA and RNA synthesis by causing DNA cross-linking and strand breaks. The treatment schedules for mitomycin C vary, but most commonly involve mitomycin C 10–20 mg/m^2 as an IV bolus injection every 6 to 8 weeks. Mitomycin C causes nausea and vomiting; myelosuppression is most typically dose-limiting. Infrequently, interstitial pneumonitis and hemolytic uremic syndrome are associated with its use.

Trimetrexate

Trimetrexate (Neutrexin) is a folic acid antagonist that offers several advantages over methotrexate, including a broader range of *in vitro* and *in vivo* antitumor activity, greater lipophilicity, receptor-independent cellular uptake, and it does not require folypolyglutamyl synthetase for polyglutamation to become active.[72] Although the activity of trimetrexate as a single agent against colorectal cancer is modest, the combination of 5-FU, leucovorin, and trimetrexate shows significant activity. The rationale for this combination is based on an attempt to maximize the accumulation of 5-phosphoribosyl-1-pyrophosphate (PRPP), which promotes the conversion of 5-FU to FUMP. Diarrhea and myelosuppression are the most common dose-limiting toxicities.

LEVAMISOLE

Levamisole (Ergamisol) is a synthetic, oral anthelmintic drug with immunomodulatory properties. Some of its stimulatory effects on the immune system include T-cell activation, augmentation of macrophage

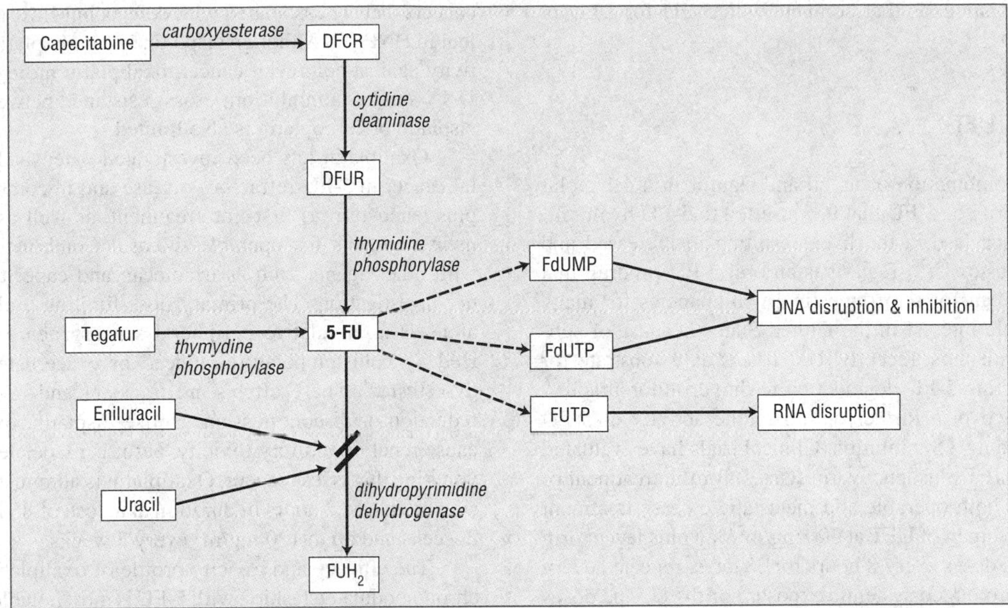

FIGURE 127–8. Comparative pharmacology of oral fluoropyrimidines. DFCR, 5′-deoxy-5-fluorocytidine; DFUR, 5′-deoxy-5-fluorouridine; 5-FU, 5-fluorouracil; FdUMP, fluorodeoxyuridine monophosphate; FdUTP, fluorodeoxyuridine diphosphate; FUTP, fluorouridine triphosphate; FUH_2, dihydrofluorouracil.

activity, and enhancement of the chemotactic response of polymorphonuclear cells and monocytes. Levamisole alone does not produce direct cytotoxicity against colorectal cancer cells but may act by restoring cellular immune response activity following reduction of tumor burden by 5-FU.[73] Levamisole is used with concomitant 5-FU in an adjuvant treatment regimen for stage III colon cancer and is given as 50 mg orally every 8 hours for 3 days every 2 weeks.

Toxicities caused by levamisole are generally mild, infrequent, and clinically tolerable. Levamisole is associated with taste abnormalities (described as metallic and occasionally associated with an altered sense of smell), arthralgias, and myalgias.[74] Central nervous system (CNS) toxicities expressed as anxiety, irritability, somnolence, depression, insomnia, agitation, confusion, or cerebellar ataxia occur in fewer than 5% of patients and resolve upon discontinuation of therapy. Significant hematologic depression develops in less than 1% of patients receiving levamisole alone; however, agranulocytosis has been reported which, in a few cases, has been fatal. Up to 40% of patients treated with levamisole plus 5-FU show laboratory abnormalities consistent with hepatic toxicity noted by elevations in liver function enzymes (alkaline phosphatase, transaminases, or serum bilirubin) or CT-documented fatty infiltration of the liver.[75] These laboratory changes are mild, rarely symptomatic, and reversible on discontinuation of therapy.

INVESTIGATIONAL AGENTS FOR COLORECTAL CANCER

At present, 5-FU plus leucovorin and irinotecan are the most frequently used chemotherapeutic agents for cancer of the colon and rectum. Newer agents, such as oral fluorinated pyrimidines, oxaliplatin, a platinum analog, thymidylate synthase inhibitors, and monoclonal antibodies, have been studied in an attempt to further improve antitumor efficacy and reduce treatment toxicities. Additional strategies are targeted toward augmenting the host immune system response, regulating tumor growth, and altering microenvironmental factors that support angiogenesis and tumor metastases.

Oral Fluorinated Pyrimidines

Extensive understanding of the pharmacology of 5-FU has led to the investigation of agents that would prolong *in vivo* 5-FU exposure and enhance antitumor effects without the use of continuous IV infusions. Key strategies include administration of 5-FU prodrugs and inhibitors of 5-FU catabolism. Potential advantages of oral forms of 5-FU include prolonged 5-FU exposure at lower peak concentrations, patient convenience, lower treatment costs, and decreased toxic effects. Fig. 127–8 depicts the comparative pharmacology of these agents. An understanding of the role of dihydropyrimidine dehydrogenase (DPD) in 5-FU catabolism is essential.

DPD is the rate-limiting enzyme responsible for 5-FU catabolism to dihydrofluorouracil, which is further catabolized to CO_2, urea, and α-fluoro-β-alanine (FBAL).[68,76] Patients with normal DPD activity excrete greater than 80% of a dose of 5-FU as FBAL, with a 5-FU elimination half-life that is variable but generally between 8 and 20 minutes.[77] In contrast, patients with deficient or lower levels of DPD eliminate greater than 90% of a dose of 5-FU as unchanged drug, with a mean elimination half-life greater than 2.5 hours.[76] These individuals also develop extreme toxicities following 5-FU administration.[68] Although found primarily in the liver, the presence of intestinal DPD contributes to wide variability in oral 5-FU absorption, and the circadian pattern of its activity might account for the variability in 5-FU systemic clearance among individuals. DPD inactivation increases the bioavailability and reduces systemic clearance of oral 5-FU to produce comparable systemic levels achieved with IV 5-FU. Furthermore, the production of FBAL, which is believed to contribute to 5-FU-associated neurotoxicity and hand-foot syndrome, is also reduced with DPD inhibition.[77] Moreover, DPD expression in tumor cells appears to confer some degree of tumor resistance to 5-FU. Several studies have demonstrated in a variety of tumor types that an inverse correlation exists between tumor DPD expression and tumor response to therapy. Thus, the inactivation of DPD may improve the therapeutic index and clinical activity of 5-FU, in addition to facilitating reliable oral administration. This can be achieved through administration of compounds that compete with 5-FU for DPD or directly inhibit DPD.

Uracil-Tegafur (UFT)

UFT (Ftorafur), a combination of uracil and tegafur in a 4:1 molar ratio, is an oral prodrug of 5-FU that is converted to 5-FU by thymidine/uridine phosphorylase in the liver, resulting in increased and sustained 5-FU exposure.[68,76] Tegafur is an oral 5-FU prodrug that has been used in Japan for gastrointestinal malignancies for many years but gained little interest in the United States because of substantial toxicities until most recently. Uracil acts as a substrate for DPD, thereby inhibiting 5-FU degradation to dihydrofluorouracil.[76] The addition of leucovorin further optimizes the activity of 5-FU from UFT by enhancing TS inhibition. Clinical trials have evaluated the combination of UFT plus leucovorin (Orzel) for the treatment of colorectal cancer in both operable and metastatic disease treatment settings. A dosing regimen of UFT at 300 mg/m^2/day plus leucovorin given in divided oral doses every 8 hours for 28 days, repeated every 35 days, results in prolonged systemic exposure of 5-FU. The doses of leucovorin used have ranged from 15 to 150 mg/m^2/day. Treatment combinations are generally well tolerated with diarrhea manifesting as the dose-limiting toxicity.

Eniluracil

Eniluracil (776C85, 5-Ethynyluracil) is a potent DPD inactivator that first binds to it in a reversible manner and then irreversibly inactivates the enzyme. It is administered with oral 5-FU in a 10:1 ratio. Doses of 10–40 mg/day of eniluracil provide maximal inhibition of DPD.[78] Eniluracil itself does not possess any antitumor activity but when given with oral 5-FU, markedly improves the therapeutic index of 5-FU by improving its bioavailability, reducing the variability in 5-FU pharmacokinetic disposition, and decreasing formation of toxic 5-FU catabolites.[68,76,77] A single 20-mg/m^2 dose of oral 5-FU, when given with eniluracil, has a bioavailability that is comparable to a 600-mg/m^2 IV bolus injection of 5-FU.[78] The majority of regimens studied have administered eniluracil with oral 5-FU, given twice daily, for 28 consecutive days and repeated every 35 days. Steady-state 5-FU concentrations achieved with these oral regimens approximate those observed with continuous IV 5-FU infusion.[77,78] Diarrhea is the principal dose-limiting toxicity of eniluracil plus 5-FU; other adverse effects include mild to moderate nausea and vomiting, mucositis, and liver function test abnormalities. While the efficacy and toxicity of eniluracil plus 5-FU appears similar to IV 5-FU plus leucovorin, the results of comparative trials will be important to assess how these eniluracil-containing regimens affect patient survival.

Oxaliplatin

Oxaliplatin (Eloxatin, L-OHP) is an investigational 1,2-diaminocyclohexane (DACH) platinum carrier ligand with a different mechanism of action compared to that of cisplatin.[68,79] Both drugs bind to two close or adjacent guanine or adenine base pairs leading to the formation of DNA adducts or cross-links, thereby resulting in the inhibition of DNA synthesis; however, the spatial DNA structural binding of nonleaving DACH adducts is hypothesized to lead to nonrecognition by the DNA MMR complex.[79] Thus, oxaliplatin-induced DNA damage may play a particularly important role in colorectal cancers that are associated with defects in MMR genes, as are prevalent in HNPCC. Although cisplatin and carboplatin possess some activity against colorectal cancer, oxaliplatin more effectively inhibits DNA synthesis inhibition; cross-resistance between oxaliplatin and cisplatin or carboplatin is also limited.[79]

Oxaliplatin has been investigated extensively against colorectal cancer in 5-FU-refractory disease and in combination with 5-FU plus leucovorin as first-line treatment, as well as in adjuvant treatment regimens for operable disease. Combinations of oxaliplatin with other agents such as irinotecan and capecitabine are also under investigation. The primary dose-limiting toxicity of oxaliplatin alone is a cumulative peripheral sensory neurotoxicity, characterized by cold temperature-induced or exacerbated paresthesia and dysesthesia.[79] These effects are transient and reversible upon dose reduction or discontinuation. Unlike cisplatin, oxaliplatin does not cause renal or auditory toxicity, but it is associated with nausea and vomiting that is less severe. Oxaliplatin is administered as an IV infusion of at least 2 hours in duration at a dose of 85 mg/m^2 given every 2 weeks and up to 130 mg/m^2 every 3 weeks.

The efficacy and toxicity profile of oxaliplatin when given in a chronomodulated fashion with 5-FU is most notable. The chronomodulated regimen takes advantage of the diurnal variation associated with several key enzymes involved in 5-FU metabolism, and delivers drugs in a schedule that provides peak drug levels at times when the tumor is most susceptible. Chronomodulation allows for an increase in median dose intensity of 5-FU with a significant decrease in the incidence and severity of bone marrow suppression, neurotoxicity, and stomatitis. Overall patient survival, however, does not appear to be significantly greater with chronomodulated 5-FU. Furthermore, the ability of oxaliplatin to improve patient survival beyond that with 5-FU plus leucovorin alone will be an important determinant for the role of oxaliplatin in colorectal cancer management.

Raltitrexed

Raltitrexed (ZD1694, Tomudex) is a quinazoline water-soluble, folate analog that acts as a potent and selective inhibitor of TS.[76] Raltitrexed is transported by a reduced-folate carrier into the cell and is rapidly metabolized by folylpolyglutamate synthase (FPGS) to higher-chain polyglutamates, which are 60- to 100-fold more potent than the parent compound. The intracellular polyglutamates bind to the folate substrate site of TS and accumulate, resulting in sustained TS inhibition and cell death. Several other folate-based TS inhibitors that are in clinical development differ from raltitrexed in chemical structure, degree of lipophilicity, method of entry into the cell, degree of polyglutamylation, dosing schedule, route of administration, and toxicity profile.[68,76] These agents, due to differences in intracellular polyglutamylation and folate carrier transport, may also differ with regard to spectrum of antitumor activity. In comparison to 5-FU, these specific TS inhibitors are more selective, potent, and may be less toxic. Because the extent and duration of TS inhibition is associated with antitumor efficacy, these agents offer a potential therapeutic advantage compared to 5-FU. In addition, determinations of FPGS, tissue TS expression, and *p53* gene status, as well as posttreatment polyglutamates and TS expression, may help identify patients who would be most likely to benefit from TS inhibitors, as well as aid in dosage adjustments.[68,76]

Raltitrexed has been evaluated as a single agent dosed at 3 mg/m^2 IV every 3 weeks and in combination with other agents at different dosage schedules against colorectal cancer. The most frequent toxicities with raltitrexed are transient leukopenia, diarrhea, nausea and vomiting, asthenia, and clinically insignificant increases in hepatic transaminase enzymes. Raltitrexed appears to have a more convenient dosing schedule, similar efficacy, and a favorable toxicity profile compared to 5-FU plus leucovorin.[80]

IMMUNOTHERAPY

A variety of agents with immunomodulating effects have undergone or are currently under study for colorectal cancer, including bacillus Calmette–Guérin (BCG), levamisole, autologous tumor cell vaccines, IFN-α, and monoclonal antibodies. Of these, monoclonal antibodies and tumor cell vaccines demonstrate the most promising activity.

Monoclonal Antibodies

Edrecolomab. Edrecolomab (17-1A MoAb, Panorex) is a murine 17-1A monoclonal antibody directed against a tumor-specific 34-kDa glycoprotein located on the cell membrane of colorectal tumor cells. Although the primary mechanism for its antitumor activity is believed due to initiation of antibody-dependent cytotoxicity (ADCC) on antibody-coated tumor cells, other mechanisms may also be important. Edrecolomab has been studied alone and in combination with 5-FU following curative surgery for stage III colorectal cancer.[81] It is administered as a 500-mg IV infusion given postoperatively that is followed by four monthly infusions of 100 mg. Although the most common toxicities are gastrointestinal and general flu-like symptoms, they are infrequent. Anaphylactic reactions are rare and can be managed with IV steroids. The formation of human antimouse antibodies (HAMA) is frequent with edrecolomab, and may positively affect its efficacy. Because some of these antibodies interact with the idiotype of the 17-1A mouse antibody and induce additional antibodies against themselves that also react against the 17-1A antigen, this phenomenon is being exploited in trials of anti-idiotype tumor vaccines against colorectal cancer.[82]

Cetuximab. Cetuximab (IMC-C225, Erbitux) is a chimerized monoclonal antibody directed against an epidermal growth factor receptor (EGFR) that is undergoing evaluation for treatment for refractory colorectal cancer, both alone and in combination with other chemotherapeutic agents. The current dosing regimen consists of a 400-mg/m^2 IV loading dose that is followed by weekly maintenance IV doses of 250 mg/m^2. Side effects observed thus far include an acneiform rash that resolves with discontinuation of therapy, anaphylaxis that occurs infrequently with the first treatment dose, asthenia, nausea, and fever.[83]

Tumor Vaccines

Four general types of vaccines are undergoing evaluation for colorectal cancer: autologous tumor vaccines, anti-idiotype vaccines, genetically modified vaccines, and vaccines comprised of purified tumor peptides, proteins, or other molecules.[84] OncoVax is a vaccine prepared from autologous tumor cells mixed with BCG that has been evaluated as adjuvant treatment for stage II or III colon cancer. Randomized trials have not demonstrated a benefit in clinical outcome for all treated individuals but there is a trend toward improved survival for a subset of patients who received the intended treatment with vaccine and demonstrated an immune response to the tumor.[85] Anti-idiotype vaccines are developed by first producing antibodies against a specific tumor-associated antigen (Ab1) and subsequently generating anti-idiotype antibodies against the Ab1 antibodies, referred to as Ab2. Some of the anti-idiotype antibodies (Ab2) mimic the structure of the tumor-associated antigen and can serve as an immunogen for additional antibodies (Ab3), which recognize the tumor-associated antigen. Thus, the anti-idiotype antibodies can be used as a vaccine to evoke cellular and humoral immune responses against a specific tumor-associated antigen. CeaVac is a murine anti-idiotype antibody that mimics the CEA epitope and has been shown to generate anti-CEA humoral and immune responses in vaccinated patients. Early studies indicate that this vaccine does not induce tumor regression but may be useful as adjuvant therapy for individuals with early stage disease.

Vaccines that use genetically modified viral vectors to express a tumor antigen, such as CEA, or mutant genes, or cytokines, are also being studied. Vaccines of specific whole tumor proteins, peptides, and other molecules that are expressed on colorectal cancer cells can be used to produce an antitumor response.[84] However, the immunogenicity of these vaccines is variable, depending on the type of molecule used, how it is recognized and processed by the immune system, and how it activates the immune system.

TUMOR GROWTH REGULATION TARGETS

Many potential molecular targets that influence tumor growth in colorectal cancer and other malignancies are undergoing intensive investigation.[68,86] Farnesyl transferase inhibitors, which inhibit cell signal transduction processes, antibodies or other compounds that block overexpressed growth factor receptors such as EGFR or HER2/neu, and strategies to introduce wild-type, or normal *p53* gene into target cells are aimed toward inhibiting aberrant tumor cell stimulation and growth.

TUMOR MICROENVIRONMENTAL TARGETS

Processes that support tumor metastases and angiogenesis, or neovascularization, provide further opportunity to block colorectal cancer spread and growth.[68,86] Many antiangiogenic agents are in clinical trials; angiogenesis inhibitors of particular interest for colorectal cancer involve those directed toward vascular endothelial growth factor (VEGF), which is commonly expressed in colorectal cancer liver metastases.[86] Matrix metalloproteinases (MMP), zinc-containing enzymes responsible for extracellular matrix protein turnover and remodeling, play an important role in angiogenesis and tumor metastases. Tumor spread is facilitated by the presence of these enzymes, which are activated and expressed to a greater degree during tumor progression and metastasis. Clinical trials of inhibitors of VEGF, MMP, and other growth factors and tumor-associated degradative enzymes are underway.

TREATMENT OF COLORECTAL CANCER

TREATMENT OF OPERABLE COLORECTAL CANCER

Individuals with operable—stages I, II, and III—colorectal cancer should undergo a complete surgical resection of the primary tumor mass with a regional lymphadenectomy as a curative approach for their disease. Adjuvant therapy in colorectal cancer is administered to selected individuals after complete tumor resection in an attempt to eliminate residual local or metastatic microscopic disease, thereby decreasing tumor relapse and improving patient survival. Adjuvant XRT plus chemotherapy is considered standard treatment for patients with stage II/III rectal cancer, and adjuvant chemotherapy is standard therapy for patients with stage III colon cancer. The approach to adjuvant therapy requires different treatment strategies for colon and rectal cancer because the natural history and patterns of recurrence following resection are uniquely different. Because tumors arising in the rectum are technically more difficult to resect with wide circumferential margins, local recurrences occur more frequently than with colon cancers. Therefore, XRT is an important aspect of adjuvant therapy for rectal cancer to reduce risk of local tumor recurrence.

The stage of disease is the most important prognostic factor for risk of relapse and survival, and is, therefore, the primary determinant for the selection of patients into adjuvant treatment trials. Because more than 90% of patients with stage I colorectal cancer are cured by surgical resection alone, adjuvant therapy is not indicated.[30] Also, by definition, adjuvant therapy is not given to patients with metastatic disease. The administration of cytotoxic agents with proven activity at maximally tolerated doses is most effective when the tumor burden is minimal and tumor growth kinetics is optimal. An additional factor, the risk-to-benefit ratio for therapy, must be favorable for individuals who remain asymptomatic for their natural life expectancy after tumor resection. For adjuvant therapy to be beneficial for a specific malignancy, clinical trials need to demonstrate a significant improvement in the rates of local recurrence, survival, or quality of life.

Adjuvant Therapy for Colon Cancer

The presence of lymph node involvement with tumor places patients with stage III colon cancer at highest risk for relapse and the risk of death within 5 years of surgical resection alone is as high as 70%.[30,87] In this population of patients, adjuvant chemotherapy significantly decreases risk of cancer recurrence and death and is considered standard of care. The value of adjuvant therapy is less clear for patients with stage II colon cancer. Although there is no lymph node involvement, these tumors can penetrate through the muscle wall, into surrounding structures, or through the visceral peritoneum. Consequently, an intermediate risk of relapse still exists because of the invasive nature of stage II disease. Results of studies that have attempted to determine whether patients with stage II disease benefit from adjuvant therapy are conflicting.[87–90] Furthermore, results from trials that suggest that adjuvant therapy improves survival for stage II disease frequently enrolled individuals with a high risk of relapse and failed to include untreated control groups. Therefore, at present, various tumor molecular genetic factors (e.g., chromosome 18q deletion, tumor ploidy, mutations of protooncogenes or tumor-suppressor genes, and tumor TS expression) are being studied in an effort to identify subsets of patients with stage II disease who have an increased risk of relapse. Subsequent studies can then determine whether these patients with certain "high risk" genetic abnormalities will respond adequately to adjuvant chemotherapy and benefit clinically. Fig. 127–9 summarizes current practice guidelines for adjuvant therapy of colon cancer from the National Comprehensive Cancer Network (NCCN), a not-for-profit alliance of US cancer centers.

Radiation Therapy. There is currently no definitive role for adjuvant XRT in colon cancer because most recurrences are extrapelvic and occur in the abdomen.[30,87] Although local recurrence and debilitating pelvic pain is uncommon, a subset of patients with T3 or T4 tumors located in the cecum, hepatic and splenic flexures, and sigmoid are at increased risk of local recurrence and may benefit from postoperative XRT and chemotherapy. Early trials using effective doses of whole abdominal XRT were limited by considerable

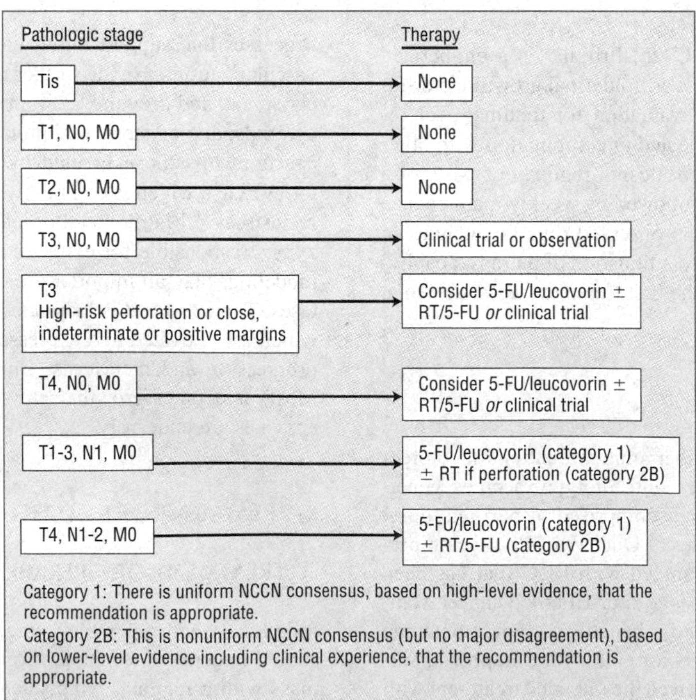

FIGURE 127–9. NCCN practice guidelines for adjuvant therapy for early stage cancer of the colon. *(Reproduced from Version 2000. Revision date: June 1, 2000. ©2000 National Comprehensive Cancer Network, Inc. These guidelines and this illustration may not be reproduced in any form without the express written permission of NCCN.)*

toxicity.[91] However, results from studies combining abdominal XRT plus 5-FU are promising. To date, postoperative local XRT may reduce the risk of local recurrence and improve survival compared to adjuvant chemotherapy alone but should only be considered for select patients with colon cancer.[30]

Single-Agent Chemotherapy. Alkylating agents such as nitrogen mustard and thiotepa were the first chemotherapeutic drugs used in the adjuvant setting in the late 1950s.[30] Their use, however, failed to improve results associated with surgery alone, perhaps as a result of suboptimal drug doses and schedules, and flaws in study design. During the 1970s, interest centered around the use of single-agent chemotherapy with 5-FU and FUDR, based on their activity against metastatic colorectal cancer, and immunotherapy. In 1988, a meta-analysis of 5-FU-based adjuvant therapy was published that evaluated phase III trials that compared adjuvant 5-FU to surgery alone.[92] A small but statistically insignificant improved survival was noted with 5-FU-based regimens. These findings questioned the value of the standard use of IV bolus 5-FU alone as adjuvant therapy for colon cancer, but results from recent studies suggest that protracted, continuous IV 5-FU infusion treatment schedules are effective adjuvant therapy.[93,94] Subsequent randomized trials have since confirmed that adjuvant 5-FU in combination with levamisole or leucovorin improves survival.

Combination Chemotherapy

5-FU PLUS LEVAMISOLE

In 1990, the National Institutes of Health Consensus Development Conference recommended that the use of 5-FU and levamisole be considered standard therapy for patients with surgically treated stage III colon cancer. In a study sponsored by the Mayo Clinic and the North Central Cancer Treatment Group (NCCTG), surgery alone was compared with postoperative levamisole and postoperative levamisole plus 5-FU in patients with surgically treated stage II and stage III colorectal cancer.[95] 5-FU, 450 mg/m^2/day, was administered by IV bolus injection for 5 consecutive days, starting within 21 to 35 days following surgery. Starting 1 month later, patients received 5-FU, 450 mg/m^2, as a single IV bolus injection each week for 48 weeks. Levamisole was administered 50 mg orally every 8 hours each day for 3 consecutive days. Each 3-day cycle was repeated every 2 weeks and continued for 1 year. Although the combination of levamisole and 5-FU significantly reduced recurrence rates, it did not confer a statistically significant survival advantage. A small but significant survival benefit for patients with stage III disease was, however, identified through subset analysis of the data. Results of a larger Intergroup trial, first published in 1990 and later updated in 1995 after a median followup of 6.5 years, demonstrated that the combination of 5-FU plus levamisole following surgical resection in patients with stage III colon cancer reduced the recurrence rate by 40% and the death rate by 33%.[73] Levamisole alone provided no significant reduction in either recurrence or deaths. Toxicities from postoperative levamisole or levamisole plus 5-FU were clinically tolerable. This combination is recognized as highly cost-effective adjuvant therapy for stage III colon cancer, as the cost per year of life saved, less than $5,000, is considered to be favorable for a medical intervention.[87,96]

The role of 5-FU plus levamisole as adjuvant therapy for patients with stage II colon cancer remains inconclusive. An analysis of the data from the Intergroup trial, with a median follow-up of 7 years, found a 31% reduction in recurrence rate that was not statistically significant and no improvement in overall survival.[89] Compared to patients with stage III colon cancer, the relative reduction in recurrence was similar, although the absolute reduction was less than 10%. In addition, only one of the four NSABP adjuvant studies that were analyzed to determine the comparative efficacy of adjuvant therapy in patients with stage II and stage III colon cancer contained a 5-FU plus levamisole treatment arm.[88] Moreover, a pooled analysis of adjuvant therapy trials for stage II colon cancer revealed no improvement in event-free or overall survival with treatment.[90]

5-FU PLUS LEUCOVORIN

Combinations of 5-FU plus leucovorin have undergone extensive study in the adjuvant setting, based on the observation that 5-FU plus leucovorin substantially improves response rates compared to 5-FU alone for metastatic disease. Since the mid-1980s, several large randomized trials have evaluated the efficacy of 5-FU plus leucovorin as adjuvant therapy for patients with stage II or III colon cancer. In each of the studies, rates of recurrence and survival improved substantially for patients receiving 5-FU plus either high-dose or low-dose leucovorin compared to surgery alone.[87] Surgery alone treatment arms were dropped from study designs after results from the Intergroup trial of the efficacy of adjuvant 5-FU plus levamisole became available. Most recently, trials compared the efficacy of levamisole versus leucovorin and 6 versus 12-month adjuvant treatment regimens of 5-FU (Table 127–8).

In light of previous data confirming the efficacy of postoperative adjuvant 5-FU, semustine (methyl-CCNU), and vincristine (MOF), patients with stage II and III colorectal cancer were randomized to receive either MOF chemotherapy or weekly 5-FU (500 mg/m^2) plus high-dose leucovorin (500 mg/m^2) given in 6-week cycles for 48 weeks.[63] The benefit of adding high-dose leucovorin to 5-FU produced a significant survival advantage in terms of both disease-free survival and overall survival (Table 127–8). An Intergroup study that compared an intensive regimen of six cycles of 5-FU (425 mg/m^2/day) plus low-dose leucovorin (20 mg/m^2/day) given daily for 5 consecutive days and repeated every 4 to 5 weeks to surgery alone in 317 patients with high-risk stage II or stage III colon cancer also showed significant improvement in relapse-free and overall survival.[97] This study was discontinued prematurely when results of the survival benefit associated with 5-FU plus levamisole became available, which suggested that an untreated control arm was no longer appropriate. The International Multicentre Pooled Analysis of Colon Cancer Trials (IMPACT) analyzed pooled data from three ongoing trials comparing surgery alone to adjuvant 5-FU (370–400 mg/m^2/day) plus high-dose leucovorin (200 mg/m^2/day) administered also in a 5-consecutive-day fashion for 6 months in patients with stage II and stage III colon cancer.[64] Fifty-six percent of patients were diagnosed with stage II disease. The recurrence and death rates were reduced by 35% and 22%, respectively. The results of these trials indicate that comparable benefit can be achieved using 5-FU-based regimens that use intense 6-month courses of adjuvant 5-FU plus low- or high-dose leucovorin or weekly 5-FU plus high-dose leucovorin given for 1 year. However, none of these regimens were compared to an acknowledged standard of care treatment, the combination of 5-FU plus levamisole.

Most recently, three large trials were conducted in an attempt to determine whether the combination of 5-FU plus leucovorin is superior to the standard 5-FU plus levamisole regimen or whether a combination of all three agents in patients with high-risk stage II and stage III colon cancer is superior to a two-drug regimen.[98–100] In

TABLE 127–8. Selected Trials of Adjuvant 5-FU Plus Leucovorin for Colon Cancer

Trial	Total No. Patients	Regimen	Duration (months)	DFS (%)	OS (%)	Endpoint (years)
NSABP C-03[63]	1081	5-FU + HD-LV	6	73	84	3
		MOF	6	64	77	
NSABP C-04[96]	2151	5-FU + LEV	12	60	70	5
		5-FU + HD-LV	6	65	74	
		5-FU + HD-LV + LEV[a]	6	64	73	
Intergroup[95]	317	5-FU + LD-LV	6	74	74	6
		Observation		58	63	
NCCTG 894651[97]	915	5-FU + LEV	6	58	60	5
		5-FU + LEV	12	63	68	
		5-FU + LD-LV + LEV	6	63	70	
		5-FU + LD-LV + LEV	12	57	63	
IMPACT[64]	1526	5-FU + HD-LV	6	71	83	3
		Observation		62	78	
INT-0089[98]	3759	5-FU + LD-LV	6	60	66	5
		5-FU + HD-LV	6	59	65	
		5-FU + LD-LV	6	59	66	
		5-FU + LEV	12	56	63	
		5-FU + HD-LV	6	60	65	
		5-FU + LEV	12	56	63	
		5-FU + LD-LV	6	59	66	
		5-FU + LD-LV + LEV	6	60	67	
		5-FU + LEV	12	56	63	
		5-FU + LD-LV + LEV	12	60	67	
SWOG 9415/INT-0153[93]	1078	CIFU[b] + LEV	6	—	76	3
		5-FU + LD-LV + LEV	6	—	77	
RMH[94]	716	PVI[c] 5-FU	3	69	75	5
		5-FU + LD-LV	6	60	74	

CIFU, continuous infusion 5-FU; DFS, disease-free survival; 5-FU, 5-fluorouracil; HD-LV, high-dose leucovorin (200–500 mg/m^2); LD-LV, low-dose leucovorin (20 mg/m^2); LEV, levamisole; MOF, semustine, vincristine, 5-fluorouracil; OS, overall survival; PVI, protracted venous infusion.

[a]HD-LV for 6 months, LEV administered for 12 months.

[b]CIFU 250 mg/m^2/d × 56 days every 9 weeks for 3 cycles.

[c]PVI 5-FU 300 mg/m^2/d × 12 weeks.

addition, these trials also attempted to assess the impact of 6 versus 12 months of adjuvant chemotherapy on efficacy. In the NSABP C-04 trial, patients with stage II and III colon cancer were randomized to one of three study arms consisting of weekly 5-FU plus high-dose leucovorin (5-FU + HD-LV) for 6 months, 5-FU plus levamisole (5-FU + LEV) for 12 months, or the combination of 5-FU plus high-dose leucovorin and levamisole (5-FU + HD-LV + LEV).[98] The 5-FU and leucovorin were administered for 6 months; the levamisole was continued for a total of 12 months. In a pairwise comparison between 5-FU + HD-LV versus 5-FU + LEV, there was a significant prolongation in disease-free survival (65% vs 60%) and a trend toward improved survival (74% vs 70%, $P = 0.07$) with HD-LV. In a comparison between 5-FU + HD-LV and 5-FU + HD-LV + LEV, there were no differences in disease-free or overall survival.

A second trial conducted by the NCCTG and the Canada Clinical Trials group was a comparison of 5-FU plus leucovorin and 5-FU plus leucovorin plus levamisole and 6 versus 12 months' duration of treatment.[99] Nine hundred fifteen patients with poor prognosis stage II or III colon cancer were randomized to receive 6 or 12 months of standard 5-FU plus levamisole or the daily times 5-consecutive-day regimen of 5-FU (370 mg/m^2/day) plus low-dose leucovorin (20 mg/m^2/day) and levamisole, resulting in four treatment arms. With a median follow-up of 5 years, there was no significant improvement in relapse rates or survival between a 12- and 6-month course of the three drugs. Treatment with 6 months of 5-FU plus levamisole was inferior to a 6-month course of therapy with all three drugs.

A third adjuvant trial (INT-0089) randomized high-risk stage II and III patients with colon cancer to receive 12 months of 5-FU plus levamisole or 6 months of 5-FU plus low-dose leucovorin, 5-FU plus high-dose leucovorin, or 5-FU plus low-dose leucovorin and levamisole.[100] Patients with stage II disease represented approximately 20% of the study population. With a median follow-up in excess of 4 years, 6 months of 5-FU plus leucovorin appeared as effective as the standard 12-month 5-FU plus levamisole regimen. No difference in response rates was observed between the low-dose and high-dose leucovorin arms. Regardless of the leucovorin dose, a slight trend toward improved overall survival was observed in both leucovorin arms compared to 5-FU plus levamisole. The addition of levamisole did not appear to significantly add to the efficacy of 5-FU plus leucovorin. The percentages of disease-free (56% to 60%) and overall (63% to 66%) survival are comparable to those achieved in other trials. Based on these findings, many clinicians would choose to administer adjuvant therapy with 5-FU plus leucovorin for 6 months in preference to the 12-month regimen of 5-FU plus levamisole. Also, with the exception of diarrhea, the weekly high-dose leucovorin regimen may be less toxic and is the preferred treatment regimen by many practitioners. However, specific differences in the toxicity profiles of these regimens and patient compliance issues should be considered to

TABLE 127–9. Treatment Toxicities in Intergroup Trial 0089

	Percentage of Grade III Toxicity or Worse			
Toxicity	*5-FU/LD-LV*	*5-FU/HD-LV*	*5-FU/LEV*	*5-FU/LV/LEV*
Leukopenia	11.9	2.8	9.0	14.9
Neutropenia	24.1	3.9	18.8	35.1
Stomatitis	18.2	1.4	3.6	22.6
Diarrhea	21.1	30.0	11.4	17.9

5-FU, 5-fluorouracil; HD-LV, high-dose leucovorin; LD-LV, low-dose leucovorin; LEV, levamisole.
Reproduced from Ref. 87.

help determine the optimal adjuvant chemotherapy regimen for an individual patient. Table 127–7 gives examples of 5-FU plus leucovorin regimens used as adjuvant therapy.

An analysis of the treatment-related toxicities in the INT-0089 trial reveals several important differences (Table 127–9). Grade 3 or worse toxicities, consisting of diarrhea, leukopenia, and stomatitis, usually occurred during the first month of therapy. Toxicities were most prevalent in the low-dose leucovorin arms with or without levamisole. The incidence of diarrhea occurred more frequently in the high-dose leucovorin arm, followed by low-dose leucovorin with or without levamisole, and was least with levamisole alone. Granulocytopenia and stomatitis were more commonly observed with low-dose leucovorin as compared to high-dose leucovorin or levamisole, although the addition of levamisole to the low-dose leucovorin arm further augmented the risk of granulocytopenia and stomatitis. A similar pattern of increased toxicity was observed with the addition of levamisole to low and high doses of leucovorin.[98,99] In a preliminary analysis of toxicity based on patient age, the risk of stomatitis and leukopenia appears greater in patients older than 70 years as compared to those between the ages of 40 and 70 years and those younger than 40 years of age. Results from other studies also suggest that the incidence of neutropenia and stomatitis is increased in women, particularly elderly women, and is associated with a decrease in 5-FU clearance.[101] Therefore, differences in the relative frequency of these important toxicities may guide treatment selection between 6-month regimens using low- or high-dose leucovorin or the 12-month regimen with 5-FU plus levamisole.

Over the last 10 years, studies of 5-FU plus levamisole or 5-FU plus leucovorin have demonstrated a 30% to 40% reduction in relapse rates in patients with stage III colon cancer. Results from most recent studies demonstrate that 6 months of adjuvant 5-FU plus low- or high-dose leucovorin is at least as effective than 12 months of 5-FU plus levamisole in patients with stage III colon cancer. Shorter treatment schedules of continuous IV infusion of 5-FU alone have a different toxicity profile and may be as effective as 6 months of 5-FU plus leucovorin; however, trials included a heterogeneous population of patients with Dukes' B and C cancer of the colon and rectum.[93,94] At this time, patients with stage III colon cancer should receive adjuvant treatment with either 5-FU plus low- or high-dose leucovorin, 5-FU plus levamisole, or a regimen under investigation in clinical trials.

The addition of levamisole to the combination of 5-FU plus leucovorin does not appear to be of additional benefit and increases toxicity. The impact of adjuvant therapy on patients with stage II colon cancer is currently unknown, although high-risk individuals (e.g., greater depth of muscle invasion, venous or lymphatic invasion, chromosome 18q allelic loss, tumor aneuploidy, mucinous or signet-ring histology, poor tumor differentiation, or mutant *p53* gene overexpression) probably benefit from adjuvant therapy. Those individuals should be offered adjuvant chemotherapy, preferably in the setting of a randomized clinical trial based on individual clinical, pathologic, and biologic prognostic factors. Despite the lack of a consensus regarding the use of adjuvant chemotherapy for individuals with high-risk stage II colon cancer, many practitioners offer this therapy to selected patients. Optimal dosing, administration schedule, and duration of therapy have yet to be determined. Although efficacy of high- and low-dose leucovorin with each of the regimens is similar, the costs of leucovorin doses ranging from 20 to 500 mg/m^2 are significantly different, and compliance issues regarding daily or weekly drug administration should be considered. Treatment toxicities, overall treatment costs, and the effect of treatments on overall quality of life will also play a role in influencing therapeutic decisions.

Investigational Adjuvant Therapy Regimens. Despite the significant reduction in cancer recurrence and increased survival afforded with 5-FU-based adjuvant chemotherapy, the results obtained thus far indicate need for continued improvement. Several strategies are underway, utilizing protracted 5-FU infusion, oral fluorinated pyrimidines, and immunotherapy, and evaluating irinotecan and oxaliplatin in the adjuvant treatment setting.[87] The potential of the monoclonal antibody edrecolomab has been most recognized to date. After 7 years of follow-up, antibody treatment with edrecolomab in 189 patients with stage III cancer of the colon or rectum resulted in a 23% reduction in cancer recurrence and a 32% reduction in overall mortality as compared to observation alone.[81] Recent findings from a Phase III trial comparing edrecolomab to standard adjuvant therapy, however, indicate that adjuvant edrecolomab may be inferior. Results from preliminary studies of the anti-idiotype antibody vaccine against CEA, CeaVac, in patients with resected colorectal cancer also appear promising.[84]

Perioperative Portal Vein Infusion. Because the liver is the site of recurrence in approximately 40% of patients, infusion of chemotherapy via the portal vein provides an additional adjuvant treatment approach. The rationale for this is based on a belief that intraoperative manipulation of the tumor provides emboli of tumor that travel directly into the portal vein circulation, ultimately developing into hepatic micrometastasis.[30] Historically, 5-FU has been the most common agent used for hepatic portal vein infusion. Because greater than 80% of a dose of 5-FU administered systemically is metabolized by the liver, direct hepatic infusion of 5-FU provides high local concentrations of the drug at the most common site of recurrence and minimizes systemic toxicity. Perioperative portal vein chemotherapy administration might then destroy cells before they can establish tumor growth.

An early trial evaluated the effect of a postoperative infusion of 1 g of 5-FU infused via the portal vein daily for 7 days as compared to no further therapy following surgical resection in patients with stages I to III colorectal cancer. Heparin was also infused to reduce thrombosis.[102] Those patients who received 5-FU and heparin experienced a significant benefit in the reduction of hepatic metastasis and a dramatic improvement in survival. Results from a trial of 1,158 patients with stages I to III colon cancer, who were randomized to receive either a continuous infusion of 5-FU 600 mg/m^2/day for 7 days with heparin via the portal vein or no therapy following surgical resection are also encouraging.[103] Although there was no significant difference in hepatic metastases between the two groups, a modest but statistically significant improvement in disease-free survival (68% vs 60%) and overall survival (76% vs 71%) was observed in the chemotherapy group. There was no significant difference in the frequency of hepatic metastases between the two treatment groups and therefore the clinical benefit is likely due to its effect on systemic micrometastases. However, its success may in fact be related to the timing of drug administration.[87] In contrast to other studies where portal vein infusion has been started 30 to 40 days postoperatively, the 5-FU was administered immediately in this trial. This concept is currently being evaluated in additional phase III trials.

Results of other trials evaluating postoperative portal vein infusions and 5-FU or other agents are mixed. A meta-analysis of 4,000 patients in 10 randomized trials of portal vein infusion suggests a small (about 4%) but absolute improvement in 5-year survival with portal vein infusion.[104] However, these authors acknowledge that the flaws in some study designs and inadequate data to date require additional evidence from large randomized trials to determine whether this approach improves patient outcome. At this time, therefore, the value of portal vein infusion of 5-FU for colon cancer remains unproven and controversial and should be considered only in the setting of a controlled clinical trial.

Adjuvant Therapy for Rectal Cancer

Rectal cancer involves those tumors found below the peritoneal reflection in the most distal 15 cm of the large bowel and, as such, is very distinct from colon cancer in that it has a propensity for both local and distant recurrence. The higher incidence of local failure and poorer overall prognosis associated with rectal cancer is due to anatomic limitations in excising adequate radial margins around the rectal tumor. Although an abdominoperitoneal surgical resection of the tumor and adjacent tissues results in a high probability of local control and long-term survival, the sequelae, including need for a permanent colostomy and high incidence of sexual and genitourinary dysfunction, have led to investigation of approaches that use multimodal therapies which preserve the integrity of the anal sphincter. In addition, because treatment with surgery, XRT, or systemic chemotherapy at the time of the recurrence is often suboptimal, adjuvant therapy after tumor resection is an important aspect of treatment of the primary tumor.

Radiation Therapy Plus 5-FU-Based Chemotherapy. The effectiveness of postoperative irradiation and 5-FU-based chemotherapy for stage II or III rectal cancer is well-established. Although T1 tumors with a favorable histology may be treated successfully with local excision alone, adjuvant irradiation plus chemotherapy should be offered for larger lesions. Similar to adjuvant therapy for colon cancer, 5-FU provides the basis for chemotherapy regimens for rectal cancer. The radiation therapy decreases the rate of local pelvic recurrences whereas the 5-FU decreases the risk of distant tumor recurrence and enhances the effectiveness of the radiation. The optimal delivery schedule for these two therapies is the subject of ongoing investigation; however, many trials have demonstrated improved local control and survival for patients who receive a combination of postoperative XRT and chemotherapy as compared to surgery alone. In 1990, based on results from the Gastrointestinal Tumor Study Group (GITSG) and the Mayo/NCCTG studies, the National Cancer Institute Consensus Conference recommended that standard postoperative adjuvant treatment for patients with stage II or III rectal tumors should consist of six cycles of 5-FU-based chemotherapy with concurrent pelvic XRT.[105]

The GITSG trial was designed to evaluate patients with stage II or III rectal cancer who were randomized into one of four groups: (a) observation only (control); (b) postoperative XRT alone; (c) postoperative chemotherapy consisting of 5-FU and semustine (methyl-CCNU) for 18 months; or (d) postoperative combination of XRT and chemotherapy.[106] The XRT was administered over 4 to 5.5 weeks. Despite a substantial number of protocol violations and a median follow-up of only 80 months, the study finished earlier than anticipated because of the statistically significant results that favored the combined modality treatment. The patients receiving the combination therapy had a reduction in both local (11% vs 24%) and distant (26% vs 34%) recurrence rates as compared to the control group. Local and distant recurrence rates for patients receiving chemotherapy or XRT were similar between groups. Although overall survival did not differ significantly among the four treatment groups at the time of initial data analysis, a subsequent reestimate of survival probabilities at a median followup of 94 months demonstrated that the combination treatment was associated with a 24% survival advantage over the control group.[107] As expected, combined modality therapy resulted in severe hematologic toxicity, enteritis, and diarrhea as compared to either chemotherapy or XRT alone.

The Mayo/NCCTG trial compared postoperative XRT alone, postoperative XRT with concurrent 5-FU plus semustine chemotherapy, and pre- and postirradiation chemotherapy in a similar population of 204 patients with rectal cancer.[108] The decision to consider XRT as the control group was based on the acknowledgment that, in many centers, XRT alone was considered standard therapy. This was the first randomized trial in which one cycle of combination chemotherapy was given before and after XRT in addition to the administration of 5-FU during XRT. This is sometimes referred to as a "sandwich" treatment regimen. The use of combined chemotherapy and XRT significantly affected local recurrence, relapse-free survival, and overall survival as compared to XRT alone. Patients receiving combined therapy experienced a 42% recurrence rate at 5 years, as compared to a 63% recurrence rate in the XRT-only group for an overall relative reduction by 34%. Similarly, reductions of 46% and 37% in local and distant recurrence rates were seen in the combined group compared to XRT alone. A 36% improvement in disease-free and 29% improvement in overall survival at 5 years was observed in the combined group.

Acute complications such as severe hematologic toxicity (leukopenia and thrombocytopenia), enteritis, and diarrhea were commonly observed in the combined group. Hematologic toxicity was more noticeable during postirradiation chemotherapy, despite reduced doses. Although small bowel complications were uncommon, four deaths were reported as a result of complications as a consequence of small bowel obstruction, fistulas, septicemia resulting from perforation, and hemorrhage. There was a 6% incidence of primary cancers, equally divided between the XRT and combined groups. Because of the leukemogenic potential associated with semustine and results from prospective comparative trials that demonstrate that it does not contribute to overall treatment efficacy, semustine is no longer included in standard adjuvant treatment regimens. This regimen without semustine represents a popular adjuvant treatment regimen for rectal cancer.

Additional trials have sought to determine optimal combinations of concurrent radiation and 5-FU. Based on preclinical studies that suggest continuous infusions of 5-FU provide more effective radiosensitization than IV bolus injections, the Gastrointestinal Intergroup compared continuous IV 5-FU infusion to intermittent bolus injections.[109] Six hundred sixty patients with stage II or III rectal cancer received either continuous infusion or IV bolus 5-FU with postoperative pelvic XRT, in addition to pre- and postirradiation

5-FU. At a median follow-up of 46 months, patients who received continuous infusion 5-FU experienced a reduction in distance metastases and improved disease-free and overall survival. The incidence of leukopenia (WBCs < 2,000/mm^3) was greater in the IV bolus 5-FU group, whereas diarrhea was more frequent in the protracted infusion group. Many treatment centers now employ continuous infusion 5-FU throughout the 5- or 6-week schedule of postoperative XRT for rectal cancer. Despite evidence that leucovorin improves efficacy of 5-FU in other treatment settings, the role of this and other 5-FU modulators in adjuvant treatment for rectal cancer remain to be determined.[110] Use of oral alternatives to 5-FU that are also known to enhance radiation effects, such as capecitabine, is under investigation as well.

Preoperative (Neoadjuvant) Versus Postoperative Therapy. Interest in preoperative or neoadjuvant therapy has increased based on advances in imaging techniques to more accurately stage rectal tumors preoperatively and the success of combined XRT plus 5-FU administered in the postoperative setting. Both pre- and postoperative XRT administered in conventional doses effectively decrease local recurrence rates for rectal cancer by up to 50% as compared to rates with surgery alone.[104] Preoperative XRT, by shrinking and thereby "downstaging" the tumor prior to surgical resection, improves sphincter preservation but the primary concern with this approach is potential over treatment with XRT. While this is a common treatment strategy in some European countries, the issue of pre- versus postoperative XRT is a subject of debate and investigation in the United States. Furthermore, the way that XRT and 5-FU are delivered varies widely. Some practitioners deliver XRT as 45–55 Gy in small fractions of 1.8–2.0 Gy over a period of 5 to 6 weeks, whereas short, intensive courses deliver therapy in five fractions over a period of 1 week. 5-FU might be administered as IV bolus injections for 3 or 4 days during the first and last weeks of XRT or via a continuous IV infusion. Although concurrent XRT plus 5-FU continuous infusion is theoretically more efficacious, based or the results from postoperative chemoradiation therapies, short intensive-course chemoradiation strategies are less expensive and more convenient for the patient. Preliminary results of NSABP Trial R-03 suggest that pre- and postoperative chemoradiation therapies are similarly safe and efficacious, but long-term survival and toxicity data will be needed to make a definitive conclusion.

Several trials that have compared preoperative therapy to surgery alone have failed to show a survival benefit with preoperative XRT; however, the Swedish Rectal Cancer Trial, a randomized trial of 1,168 patients with resectable rectal cancer who underwent a short course of intensive preoperative XRT followed by surgery within 1 week or surgery alone, was able to demonstrate improved local recurrence rates (11% vs 27%, $P < 0.001$) and 5-year survival for those patients who received XRT plus surgery versus surgery alone (58% vs 48%, $P = 0.004$).[111,112] These findings will need to be verified in future trials before this therapy can be considered standard of care. Moreover, the short-course therapy is unlikely to sufficiently downstage the tumor because it will have only been completed 1 week prior to surgery. Whether 5-FU can be safely incorporated into such a regimen will also require further evaluation.

Results from the GITSG, NSABP, and Intergroup trials indicate that survival benefits can be achieved with the addition of 5-FU to postoperative XRT for resectable rectal cancer.[106–110] Adjuvant chemotherapy plus XRT decreases local tumor recurrence after surgery and increases the probability of sphincter preservation in patients with clinically resectable disease. Neoadjuvant therapy may provide similar benefits and additionally improve the rate of resectability in patients with locally advanced disease by downstaging the tumor, but regimens have not been investigated sufficiently to be considered standard therapy at this time. The NCCN Practice Guidelines for rectal cancer indicate that postoperative 5-FU plus XRT is considered appropriate adjuvant therapy for resectable T2 or larger lesions (Fig. 127–10). Neoadjuvant 5-FU chemoradiation followed by abdominoperineal or low anterior resection or surgery alone plus postoperative 5-FU or 5-FU plus XRT should be considered for locally unresectable tumors.

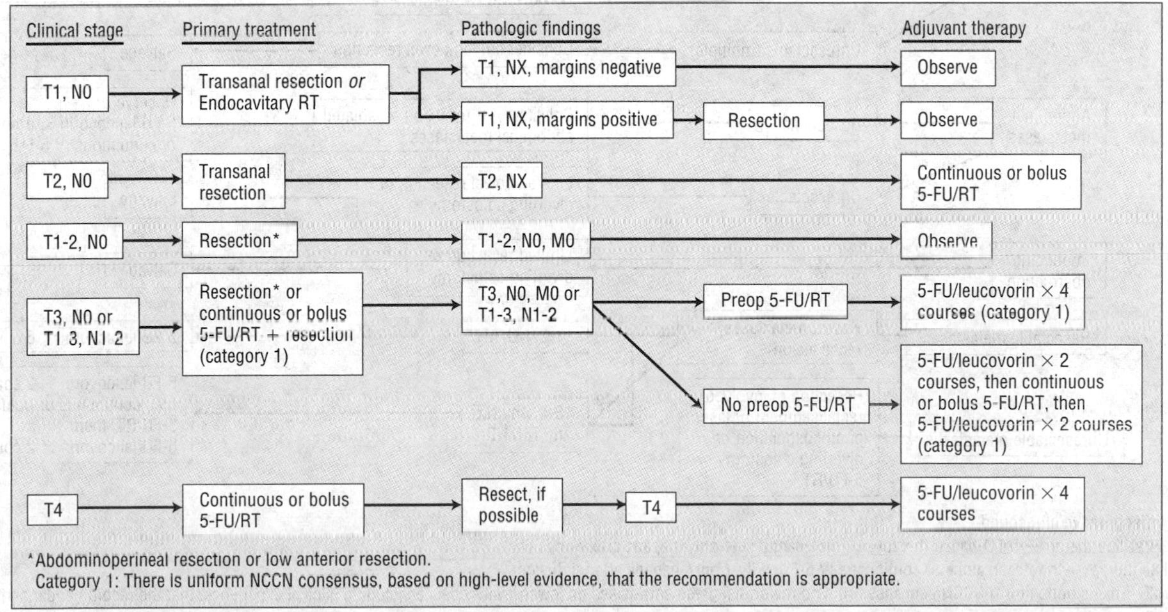

FIGURE 127–10. NCCN practice guidelines for adjuvant therapy for early stage cancer of the rectum. *(Reproduced from Version 2000. Revision date: June1, 2000. ©2000 National Comprehensive Cancer Network, Inc. These guidelines and this illustration may not be reproduced in any form without the express written permission of NCCN.)*

TREATMENT OF METASTATIC COLORECTAL CANCER

Several advances have been made most recently in developing efficacious treatment options for metastatic colorectal cancer. Whereas surgery and XRT are most often used to manage isolated sites of tumor, chemotherapy is most useful for patients with disseminated disease and is the primary treatment modality for unresectable metastatic colorectal cancer. Accepted standard initial therapies for metastatic cancer of the colon or rectum consist of irinotecan plus 5-FU and leucovorin or 5-FU plus leucovorin. Upon disease progression following standard initial therapy, appropriate treatment options may include continuous infusion 5-FU, irinotecan, intrahepatic therapy for selected patients, supportive care, or participation in a clinical trial. The site(s) of tumor involvement and history of prior chemotherapy help to define an appropriate management strategy. Fig. 127–11 describes the NCCN Practice Guidelines for initial therapy of metastatic disease. In general, treatment options are similar for metastatic cancer of the colon and rectum. Treatment goals for metastatic disease are to reduce patients' symptoms and extend survival.

Initial Therapy for Metastatic Disease

Surgery. Surgical resection of discrete hepatic, pulmonary, abdominal, or brain metastases in patients with colorectal cancer that can be accomplished may offer selected patients an opportunity to experience extended disease-free survival.[113] Patients who have from one to three small nodules isolated to the liver, lungs, or abdomen have the most favorable outcome. Up to 25% of patients will present with hepatic metastases at time of diagnosis and 60% of patients with colorectal cancer will develop hepatic metastases sometime during the course of their disease. Five-year survival for patients who undergo surgical resection of metastases isolated to the liver ranges from 20% to 39%, with a median survival duration of 28 to 40 months, and is associated with an operative mortality rate less than 5%.[114] These results differ significantly from those in unresectable metastatic colorectal cancer in which 5-year survival is uncommon and median survival is about 12 months. Patients with no significant general medical risk factors, fewer than four hepatic lesions, CEA levels less than 200 ng/mL, small tumor size, lack of extrahepatic tumor, and adequate surgical margins have the best opportunity for an improved long-term

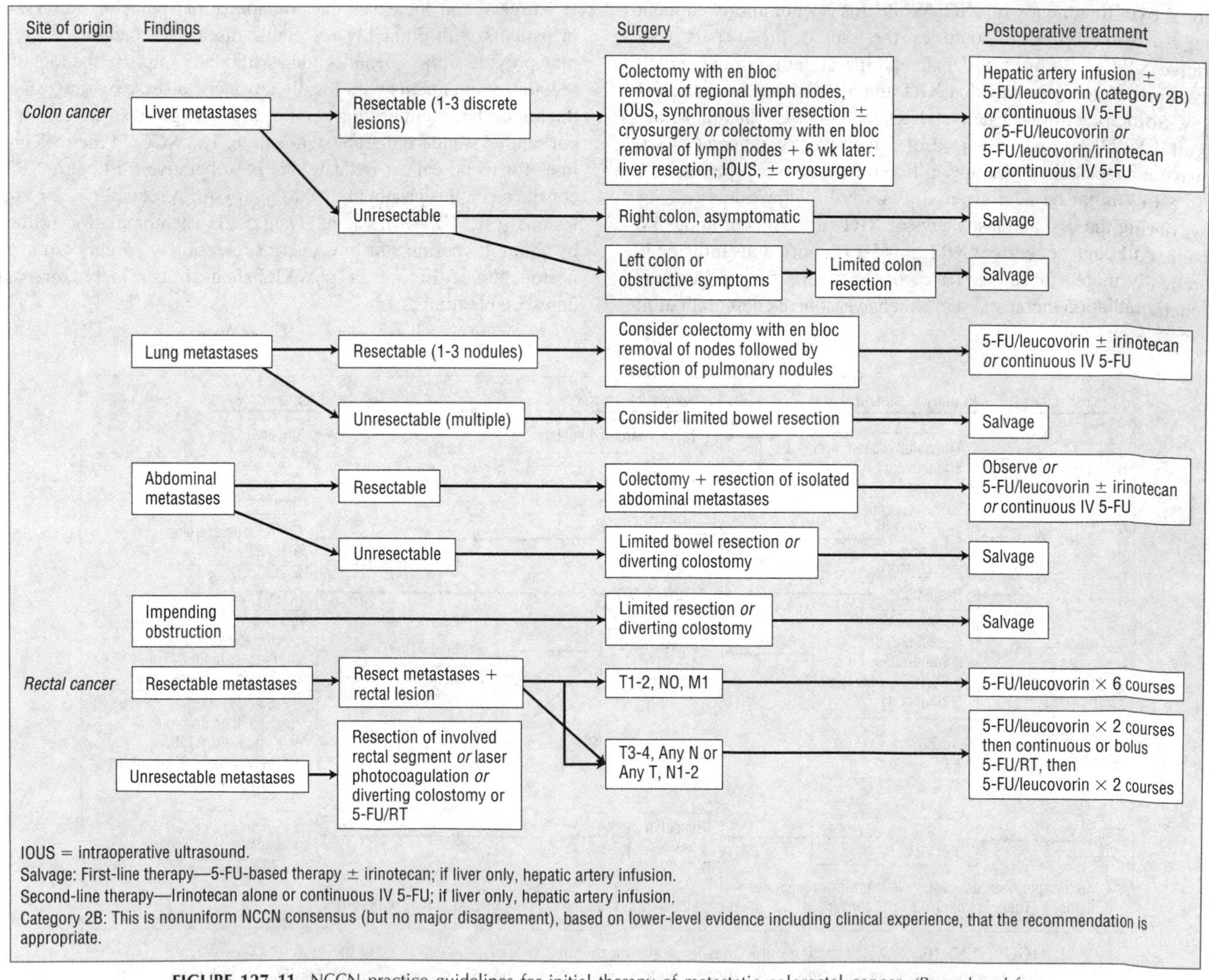

FIGURE 127–11. NCCN practice guidelines for initial therapy of metastatic colorectal cancer. *(Reproduced from Version 2000. Revision date: June 1, 2000 ©2000 National Comprehensive Cancer Network, Inc. These guidelines and this illustration may not be reproduced in any form without the express written permission of NCCN.)*

outcome. Ablative therapies that involve destroying the tumor through freezing and thawing (cryoablation), heat (radiofrequency), or alcohol injection, are less potentially curable but may be useful for patients who have very small hepatic lesions and are unable to undergo liver resection surgery.[114] Outcomes associated with resection of isolated pulmonary, abdominal, and brain metastases have been less studied; however, this approach is potentially curative and should be considered for patients with resectable disease who are appropriate surgical candidates.

Because approximately two-thirds of patients who undergo liver resection of hepatic metastases will have disease recurrence, adjuvant systemic and hepatic arterial infusion chemotherapy have been studied in an attempt to improve long-term outcome. A randomized trial that compared hepatic floxuridine plus IV 5-FU to IV 5-FU alone following resection of hepatic metastases in 156 patients showed improved 2-year survival (86% vs 72%, $P = 0.03$) and hepatic recurrence-free survival at 2 years (90% vs 60%, $P < 0.001$) with the combined therapy.[115] Many practitioners offer adjuvant chemotherapy to select patients following potentially curative hepatic resection but further studies are needed to determine an optimal treatment regimen.

Systemic Chemotherapy. Two recent meta-analyses were performed to estimate the magnitude of benefit and harms associated with palliative chemotherapy for metastatic colorectal cancer. In a pooled analysis of randomized trials comparing chemotherapy to observation or supportive care alone, a total of nine trials that included 614 patients were evaluated.[116] All trials used 5-FU-based chemotherapy but three trials where hepatic arterial or portal vein administration was used were also included. Several trials allowed delayed or discretionary use of chemotherapy in patients assigned to observation or supportive care alone; 12% to 57% of control patients received at least one course of chemotherapy. Despite these discrepancies, chemotherapy was associated with a significant reduction in mortality at 1 (risk ratio 0.69; 95% CI 0.60–0.81, $P < 0.00001$) but not 2 years (risk ratio 0.93; 95% CI 0.87–1.00, $P = 0.053$).

A larger meta-analysis analyzed individual patient data and summary statistics when individual patient data were not available from 13 randomized trials that included 1,365 patients.[117] Eligible trials compared palliative chemotherapy given via any route of administration to supportive care alone or treatments not involving chemotherapy. Trials that allowed chemotherapy use in control patients were not excluded. In the analysis of seven trials where individual patient data was available, palliative chemotherapy was shown to reduce risk of death by 35% (95% CI, 24% to 44%), which translates to a prolongation in median survival by 3.7 months. The investigators were unable to determine the extent to which treatment resulted in significant toxicities or affected quality of life because of inadequate data. However, the results of both analyses suggest that palliative chemotherapy is beneficial and improves survival in metastatic colorectal cancer. Because many patients assigned to control arms eventually received chemotherapy, the magnitude of survival benefit associated with chemotherapy could be underestimated.

5-FU continues to be incorporated into current first-line chemotherapy regimens used for metastatic colorectal cancer. When administered in bolus injection treatment schedules, 5-FU is given most frequently with leucovorin, which improves response rates but has minimal impact on overall survival. The addition of irinotecan to 5-FU plus leucovorin significantly improves response rates, progression-free survival, and median survival, without adversely affecting quality of life. This three-drug combination is considered the standard reference treatment as first-line therapy for metastatic colorectal cancer. Ongoing trials are evaluating this regimen, as well as standard combinations of 5-FU plus leucovorin, to investigational treatments with oral fluoropyrimidines and newer agents. Table 127–10 summarizes potentially useful chemotherapeutic treatments for metastatic colorectal cancer.

5-FU

5-FU has been administered as a single agent by IV bolus injection but response rates are only 10% to 20%.[30,57] Typical regimens consist of 5-FU at a dose of 450–500 mg/m^2/day for 5 consecutive days as an IV bolus injection administered over 5 to 10 minutes. This is repeated every 4 to 5 weeks. Alternatively, 5-FU may be administered as a bolus IV injection in doses ranging up to 600 mg/m^2 administered weekly for 6 of 8 weeks. Unfortunately, no significant survival improvement has been gained with IV bolus 5-FU alone, although a small survival benefit (12 to 18 months vs 6 to 8 months) has been documented for patients receiving weekly 5-FU IV bolus injections who were able to achieve an objective response.[30] However, because response rates are greater with 5-FU given via continuous IV infusion or in combination with other agents, bolus IV 5-FU alone is considered ineffective for metastatic colorectal cancer.

A variety of continuous IV infusion 5-FU regimens have been developed to increase the duration of drug exposure during the S phase and increase DNA-dependent cell cytotoxicity. Some of these schedules involve short (24- to 48-hour) weekly or biweekly or protracted continuous 5-FU infusions for up to 12 weeks.[62] The de Gramont regimen (Table 127–7) incorporates a leucovorin-modulated bolus IV 5-FU dose into a two-weekly administration regimen of 5-FU continuous infusion. Doses of 5-FU employed in 24- to 48-hour infusions generally range from 1,000 to 2,000 mg/m^2 per day. A regimen utilizing 300 mg/m^2/day for 10 weeks is considered the maximally tolerated dose for protracted continuous infusion. This approach is one of the most efficacious methods of dose intensification, based on the assumption that a dose-response relationship exists for colorectal cancer. The maximum cumulative 5-FU dose that can be administered via continuous IV infusion in a 28-day period is approximately 4,000–7,400 mg/m^2 as compared to 2,400–2,500 mg/m^2 with IV bolus 5-FU.[118]

Despite differences in dose intensity among the different regimens, no clear survival advantages or trends are obvious for any particular regimen. However, in comparison to IV bolus 5-FU, response rates with continuous infusion are increased approximately twofold. In a meta-analysis of six randomized trials evaluating 1,219 patients with advanced colorectal cancer that compared efficacy of continuous infusion and bolus IV 5-FU, a significantly higher tumor response rate (22% vs 14%, $P = 0.0002$) was observed in patients receiving 5-FU by continuous IV infusion.[58] Although continuous infusion 5-FU was also associated with a significant survival benefit (overall hazard ratio 0.88, $P = 0.04$), this effect is generally considered as marginal. Therefore, until future studies demonstrate a clinical benefit with continuous infusion 5-FU with respect to the added expense and complications associated with venous access devices and portable infusion pumps, current practices continue to favor IV bolus schedules for initial therapy of metastatic disease.

5-FU PLUS LEUCOVORIN

Numerous studies have evaluated various doses and administration schedules of 5-FU plus leucovorin in an attempt to improve treatment response rates and survival in metastatic colorectal cancer. Response

TABLE 127–10. Chemotherapeutic Regimens for Metastatic Colorectal Cancer

Regimen	Major Dose-Limiting Toxicities
Initial Therapy	
Weekly: irinotecan (80 mg/m^2) + 24-hour 5-FU infusion (2,300 mg/m^2) + leucovorin (500 mg/m^2)[124]	Diarrhea, neutropenia
Every 2 weeks: irinotecan (180 mg/m^2 on day 1) + IV bolus 5-FU (400 mg/m^2) followed by a 22-hour IV 5-FU infusion (600 mg/m^2) + leucovorin (200 mg/m^2 given on days 1 and 2)[124]	Neutropenia, diarrhea
Weekly 5-FU (600 mg/m^2) + HDLV (500 mg/m^2); weekly × 6 with 2-week rest, repeated every 8 weeks (Roswell Park regimen)[65]	Diarrhea, mucositis
Daily x 5 consecutive days: 5-FU (425 mg/m^2/day) + LDLV (20 mg/m^2/day); repeated every 3 to 5 weeks (Mayo Clinic regimen)[119,125]	Mucositis, neutropenia
Capecitabine 1,250 mg/m^2 PO twice daily for 14 days, repeated every 3 weeks[127]	Diarrhea, hand-foot syndrome
Second-Line Therapy*	
Irinotecan 125 mg/m^2 IV every week for 4 weeks, followed by a 2-week rest period, repeated every 6 weeks[125]	Neutropenia, diarrhea
Irinotecan 350 mg/m^2 IV every 3 weeks[133,134]	Neutropenia, diarrhea
5-FU 250–300 mg/m^2/day continuous IV infusion until disease progression[134]	Mucositis, hand-foot syndrome
Trimetrexate + 5-FU + leucovorin[75]	Diarrhea, neutropenia
5-FU 300 mg/m^2/day continuous IV infusion until disease progression (maximum 24 weeks) + mitomycin-C 7 mg/m^2 IV every 6 weeks[138]	Myelosuppression, mucositis, hemolytic uremic syndrome
Investigational	
Two-weekly regimen of IV bolus and 22-hour continuous infusion 5-FU + leucovorin + oxaliplatin 85 mg/m^2 IV infusion on day 1[129]	Neutropenia, peripheral sensory neuropathy
Chronomodulated 5-FU + leucovorin + oxaliplatin 125 mg/m^2 IV infusion[128]	Diarrhea, peripheral sensory neuropathy
Raltitrexed 3–4 mg/m^2 IV every 3 weeks[80]	Neutropenia, hepatic transaminase elevations

*Depending on first-line therapy; if 5-FU plus leucovorin, then single-agent irinotecan. If 5-FU plus leucovorin plus irinotecan, then continuous IV infusion 5-FU or investigational agents/clinical trial or supportive care.

rates of 14% to 58% have been observed with a variety of doses of 5-FU with leucovorin doses between 20 and 500 mg/m^2.[61] Leucovorin can be given by IV bolus, continuous infusion, and orally. The administration sequence and timing of leucovorin may be important factors in evaluating the efficacy of biochemical modulation with leucovorin. A schedule for administering leucovorin prior to 5-FU is the most effective approach to enable the level of intracellular-reduced folates to accumulate prior to 5-FU administration. Prolonged exposure of low levels of leucovorin increases the intracellular concentration of reduced long-chain polyglutamates, which, in turn, stabilize the FdUMP-thymidylate synthase complex, resulting in increased 5-FU cytotoxicity. However, the maximum tolerated dose of 5-FU when given in combination with leucovorin is lower than that when given alone. In addition, a qualitative alteration of the toxicity pattern has been noted.

Despite significantly higher response rates and improved progression-free survival achieved with leucovorin-modulated 5-FU regimens, their effect on overall survival is only modest. The lack of any clear survival benefit detected in clinical trials might be explained by the generally short duration of tumor responses, the large number of patients who do not respond to treatment, or the effects of crossover administration of 5-FU plus leucovorin in patients who fail single-agent 5-FU.[61] Phase III trials evaluating 5-FU and leucovorin for metastatic colorectal cancer have been criticized because doses of 5-FU used in control groups have been below the maximum-tolerated dose.[65] As a result, the addition of leucovorin may appear to produce a greater antitumor effect when in fact it is being compared to a suboptimal control group. Thus, the dose of 5-FU must also be evaluated.

The most practical issue at present, however, is whether a weekly or monthly high- or low-dose leucovorin-containing regimen is most preferable. The most commonly used regimens in the United States involve weekly IV bolus 5-FU administered at the midpoint of a 2-hour IV infusion of high-dose leucovorin (Roswell Park regimen) or a monthly regimen of low-dose IV bolus leucovorin followed by IV bolus 5-FU given daily for 5 consecutive days and repeated every 4 to 5 weeks (Mayo Clinic regimen) (Table 127–7). These regimens have been compared in randomized trials.

In a phase III trial conducted by the GITSG, a 5-day course of IV bolus 5-FU (500 mg/m^2) repeated every 4 weeks was compared to a combination of 5-FU (600 mg/m^2) and low-dose (25 mg/m^2) or high-dose (500 mg/m^2) leucovorin, administered for 6 of 8 weeks.[65] The 5-FU and low-dose leucovorin regimen was no more effective than 5-FU alone (19% vs 12% response rate), whereas a 30% response rate was observed in patients who received weekly 5-FU and high-dose leucovorin. A trend toward improved survival was also observed with the high-dose leucovorin regimen. Conflicting results were published by the Mayo Clinic and NCCTG, which found 5-FU (425 mg/m^2/day by IV bolus injection for 5 days, repeated every 4 to 5 weeks) and low-dose leucovorin (20 mg/m^2) to be more effective than either 5-FU alone or 5-FU (370 mg/m^2/day for 5 days) with high-dose leucovorin (200 mg/m^2/day) (42%, 10%, and 31% response rate, respectively).[119] Although the low-dose leucovorin regimen was more effective than the high-dose regimen, the difference in response could be attributed to the higher doses of 5-FU that were administered in combination with low-dose leucovorin. Median survival, 12.7 months, was no different between low- or high-dose leucovorin regimens. A subsequent collaborative trial by the Mayo Clinic and NCCTG compared daily 5-FU (425 mg/m^2/day) plus low-dose leucovorin (20 mg/m^2) to weekly 5-FU (600 mg/m^2) plus high-dose (500 mg/m^2) leucovorin in 372 patients with metastatic disease.[120] There were no differences in tumor response (35% vs 31%), median survival (9.3 months vs 10.7 months) or palliative responses between the low- and high-dose leucovorin regimens. Low-dose leucovorin was, however, associated with significantly more leukopenia and stomatitis whereas high-dose leucovorin caused more diarrhea and a greater hospitalization requirement to manage toxicity. In a separate trial comparing high- (500 mg/m^2) and low-dose (20 mg/m^2) leucovorin plus 5-FU at equal doses (500 mg/m^2) in 291 patients with inoperable or metastatic colorectal cancer, there were no differences in median response duration, progression-free, or overall survival.[121] While the incidence of mucositis was similar for both groups (9.8% vs 11.5%), grade 3 or 4 diarrhea was more common with high-dose leucovorin (27% vs 16.1%).

Overall, response rates and survival outcomes with weekly and daily regimens of 5-FU plus low- or high-dose leucovorin appear comparable. Leucovorin doses greater than 20 mg/m^2 when administered on a daily schedule do not appear advantageous whereas high-dose leucovorin (500 mg/m^2) is more effective than low-dose leucovorin in a weekly treatment regimen.[122] The toxicity profiles of these regimens differ, however. Weekly (high-dose leucovorin) treatment schedules are associated with a higher incidence of diarrhea, the primary dose-limiting toxicity, and mucositis and leukopenia are relatively infrequent.[121] Mucositis tends to be dose-limiting and leukopenia is more common with the daily (low-dose leucovorin) treatment schedule. An increased frequency and severity of toxicities have been observed in women and in patients older than 70 years of age; however, there are no differences in survival benefit with treatment and dosage adjustments are not recommended.[122,123]

5-FU plus low-dose leucovorin is currently recommended, but remains controversial, as the preferred 5-FU plus leucovorin regimen for metastatic colorectal cancer based on response rates, toxicity, lower estimated drug costs, and quality of life indices such as performance status, weight gain, and symptoms.[61,62,120,121] However, the weekly schedule of high-dose leucovorin plus 5-FU may be more convenient for the patient in terms of fewer scheduled clinic appointments, less interference with work schedules, and ease in dose adjustments based on toxicity. The optimal dose and schedule of administration of 5-FU in combination with leucovorin for metastatic disease still remains to be defined. Higher response rates of 24% to 54% have been noted in biweekly regimens of 5-FU administered first as an IV bolus infusion followed by a 22-hour continuous infusion in combination with high doses of leucovorin administered over 2 hours.[61] However, in subsequent trials, the response rates with these regimens were lower. High response rates (39% to 58%) have also been observed in previously untreated and treated patients receiving weekly 5-FU as a continuous 24-hour infusion in combination with high doses of leucovorin given over 2 to 24 hours. However, median survival rates have not changed significantly since the pivotal trials were published, although weekly continuous infusions of 5-FU plus leucovorin have produced a prolongation in survival, in some cases by greater than 22 months.[61,65,119] The incorporation of newer agents into treatment regimens rather continual adjustments of 5-FU and leucovorin doses and administration schedules will most likely result in the greatest advances in drug therapy for metastatic colorectal cancer.

IRINOTECAN PLUS 5-FU/LEUCOVORIN

In recognition of irinotecan's activity against untreated and 5-FU-resistant colorectal cancer, in addition to its unique mechanism of action, several investigations have been initiated to determine whether the addition of irinotecan to 5-FU plus leucovorin as initial therapy for metastatic disease could further improve survival. In a randomized trial of 387 previously untreated patients with advanced colorectal cancer, irinotecan plus 5 FU and leucovorin was compared to 5-FU plus leucovorin with regard to tumor response, survival, and quality of life.[124] The choice of one of two 5-FU plus leucovorin regimens was left to the discretion of participating investigators. Patients randomized to 5-FU plus leucovorin could receive weekly 5-FU 2600 mg/m^2 as a 24-hour IV infusion plus leucovorin 500 mg/m^2 or as an every 2-week regimen of IV bolus 5-FU (400 mg/m^2) followed by a 22-hour IV infusion (600 mg/m^2) with leucovorin (200 mg/m^2 given on days 1 and 2). For the three-drug treatment, a weekly regimen of irinotecan (80 mg/m^2) with a 24-hour infusion of 5-FU (2300 mg/m^2) plus leucovorin 500 mg/m^2 or an every 2-week treatment consisting of irinotecan (180 mg/m^2) on day 1 with IV bolus 5-FU (400 mg/m^2) followed by a 22-hour IV infusion (600 mg/m^2) plus leucovorin (200 mg/m^2 given on days 1 and 2) could be used. Tumor response was greater in the irinotecan group (49% vs 31%, $P < 0.001$) as was median time to disease progression (6.7 months vs 4.4 months, $P < 0.001$) and median survival (17.4 months vs 14.1 months, $P = 0.031$). Diarrhea and neutropenia were the most common toxicities and were worse in the irinotecan-containing groups. Diarrhea was the most common reason for dose reduction or treatment discontinuation with the weekly regimens and led to hospital admission for 32% of patients receiving irinotecan compared to 12% of patients who received only 5-FU plus leucovorin. Neutropenia was the most common cause of dose reductions with the 2-weekly regimens. Results from questionnaires indicated that a definite deterioration in quality of life developed consistently later in the irinotecan group.

A second randomized trial compared the addition of irinotecan (125 mg/m^2) to weekly 5-FU plus leucovorin (5-FU 500 mg/m^2 IV bolus plus leucovorin 20 mg/m^2 IV bolus, each given weekly for 4 weeks, repeated every 6 weeks) to the Mayo Clinic regimen (5-FU 425 mg/m^2 IV bolus plus leucovorin 20 mg/m^2 IV bolus, each given daily for 5 consecutive days, repeated every 4 weeks) and to irinotecan alone (125 mg/m^2 IV weekly for 4 weeks, repeated every 6 weeks) as first-line therapy in 683 patients with metastatic colorectal cancer.[125] The combination of irinotecan, 5-FU, and leucovorin resulted in significantly longer median progression free survival (7.0 months vs 4.3 months vs 4.2 months), greater tumor response (39% vs 21% vs 18%), and longer median overall survival (14.8 months vs 12.6 months vs 12.0 months) as compared to 5-FU plus leucovorin and irinotecan alone, respectively. The incidence of grade 3 or 4 diarrhea was 22.7% with the three-drug combination as compared to 13.2% with 5-FU plus leucovorin and 31% with irinotecan alone. However, the incidence of grade 3 diarrhea was almost threefold greater with triple-drug therapy as compared to the two-drug regimen. Midcycle dose reductions caused by neutropenia, which were more common with the three-drug treatment, could potentially have lowered subsequent risk of grade 4 diarrhea. Mucositis was more frequent in the 5-FU plus leucovorin group. Quality of life analyses did not indicate that the addition of irinotecan to 5-FU plus leucovorin compromised quality of life.

The results of this study support findings from the previous study that the addition of irinotecan to 5-FU plus leucovorin (IFL) as first-line therapy for metastatic colorectal cancer increases survival. In addition, the results are clinically meaningful because they reflect a comparison of triple-drug therapy to a standard 5-FU plus leucovorin treatment regimen that is used commonly in the United States. These findings support the current consensus that the three-drug treatment regimen with irinotecan, 5-FU, and leucovorin be considered as standard first-line therapy for metastatic colorectal cancer. Irinotecan received approval from the FDA in 2000 as first-line therapy for metastatic colorectal cancer in combination with 5-FU and leucovorin. However, whether a similar palliative effect could be obtained with sequential, rather than concomitant drug administration remains to be determined. Furthermore, an evaluation of early treatment-related deaths that occurred during NCI-sponsored cooperative studies of IFL indicates that rates of treatment-induced or treatment-exacerbated deaths due to IFL are 3-fold higher compared to control regimens.[126] Two distinct syndromes are apparent: a gastrointestinal syndrome characterized by severe diarrhea, nausea, vomiting, anorexia, and abdominal cramping; and, a vascular syndrome consisting of acute, fatal myocardial infarction, pulmonary embolus, or cerebrovasular accident. Patients who have died from these complications tended to be older. Therefore, patients who receive IFL should be monitored closely to recognize any of these toxicities early so that aggressive therapeutic interventions can be made and therapy withheld to avoid serious sequelae. The use of 5-FU plus leucovorin without irinotecan as first-line therapy when a less toxic regimen is desirable is still considered appropriate for selected patients.

CAPECITABINE

Capecitabine has been compared to 5-FU plus leucovorin as first-line therapy for metastatic colorectal cancer in two randomized phase III trials. In a pooled analysis of 1207 patients randomized to capecitabine (1,250 mg/m^2 PO twice daily for 14 days, repeated every 3 weeks) or the Mayo Clinic regimen (5-FU 450 mg/m^2 plus leucovorin 20 mg/m^2 for 5 consecutive days, repeated every 4 weeks), tumor response to capecitabine was superior to that with 5-FU plus leucovorin (25.7% vs 16.7%, $P < 0.0002$).[127] Time to tumor progression (median, 4.6 months vs 4.7 months) and median survival (12.9 months), however, were not different. Hand-foot syndrome was more common with capecitabine whereas grade 3 or 4 neutropenia and stomatitis was more common with 5-FU plus leucovorin. Despite comparable efficacy to IV 5-FU plus leucovorin, the convenience of oral administration and a different toxicity profile makes capecitabine a potentially useful alternative to IV 5-FU regimens in the setting of metastatic disease. Since, however, the IV treatment arm in these comparative studies could be considered more toxic than the weekly IV 5-FU/leucovorin treatment schedule, it is premature to conclude that capecitabine is as efficacious and less toxic than all parenteral 5-FU-based regimens.

Investigational 5-FU-Based Treatment Regimens

OXALIPLATIN PLUS 5-FU PLUS LEUCOVORIN

Incorporation of oxaliplatin into flat and chronomodulated 5-FU-based regimens as first-line therapy for metastatic colorectal cancer is associated with higher response rates and improved progression-free survival but has no significant impact on overall survival. In a comparison of chronomodulated 5-FU plus leucovorin, with and without oxaliplatin (125 mg/m^2 as a 6-hour IV infusion), given every 21 days to 200 patients with previously untreated metastatic colorectal cancer, 5-FU plus leucovorin was associated with a 16% objective response rate (95% CI, 9% to 24%) as compared to a 53% response rate (95% CI, 42% to 63%) in patients who received oxaliplatin ($P < 0.001$).[128] Median progression-free survival was also improved (6.1 months vs 8.7 months), but median overall survival (19.9 months vs 19.4 months) was no different. However, the study was not designed to assess survival differences; furthermore, the effect of second-line oxaliplatin in patients who failed first-line 5-FU plus leucovorin may have also invalidated treatment survival differences. The addition of oxaliplatin to 5-FU plus leucovorin was associated with grade 3 or 4 diarrhea in 43% of patients and 13% of patients experienced moderate functional impairment because of peripheral sensory neuropathy. The chronomodulated 5-FU administration schedule appeared to facilitate the addition of oxaliplatin without compromising dose intensity or incurring an unacceptable level of toxicity.

A comparison of a 2-weekly regimen of IV bolus and 22-hour continuous infusion 5-FU plus leucovorin (LV5FU2), with or without oxaliplatin (85 mg/m^2 as a 2-hour infusion on day 1) was designed to evaluate progression-free survival as a primary endpoint in 420 previously untreated patients.[129] Tumor response (50.7% vs 22.3%, $P = 0.0001$) and progression-free survival (median, 9.0 months vs 6.2 months, $P = 0.0003$) were improved with oxaliplatin compared to LV5FU2 alone; an observed improvement in overall survival did not reach statistical significance (median, 16.2 months vs 14.7 months, $P = 0.12$). Although the three-drug regimen was associated with higher frequencies of grade 3 and 4 toxicities, primarily neutropenia, diarrhea, and neurosensory toxicity, they did not significantly impair quality of life.

These two trials were reviewed in March 2000 by the Oncologic Drugs Advisory Committee (ODAC), which voted not to recommend that the FDA approve oxaliplatin for the first-line treatment of patients with advanced colorectal cancer in combination with 5-FU-based chemotherapy on the basis that neither trial adequately demonstrated a survival advantage. Whether oxaliplatin becomes available in the future will depend on the results of additional data and survival analyses.

OTHER AGENTS

Comparisons of 5-FU-based regimens alone and in combination with other agents, including trimetrexate, raltitrexed, methotrexate, interferon-α, and PALA, have also been investigated in previously untreated patients with metastatic colorectal cancer.[30,56] Trimetrexate, raltitrexed, and methotrexate improve response rates and have small effects on progression-free intervals with minimal or no effect on overall survival. These agents are all undergoing study in combination with other active agents against colorectal cancer. The addition of interferon-α or PALA to 5-FU plus leucovorin increases toxicities and does not improve overall efficacy.

Newest Strategies. Observation that various tumor characteristics (e.g., TS expression), patient drug-metabolizing enzymes (e.g., DPD, plasma uracil/dihydrouracil ratio), and molecular markers (e.g., chromosome 18q allelic loss, microsatellite instability, p53 mutation or loss) may predict prognosis and response to certain therapies; may lead to opportunities to select optimal first-line therapies for individual patients. Patients who are deficient in DPD experience severe and potentially life-threatening toxicities with conventional doses of 5-FU. However, determination of DPD activity is relatively time-consuming and the techniques are not amenable to routine clinical practice. As an alternative, plasma ratio determinations of uracil and dihydrouracil, which are more easily obtainable, appear to identify individuals with DPD deficiency and who are therefore at risk of developing significant toxicities.[130] Of factors predictive for tumor sensitivity to 5-FU, TS expression has been most studied.[56] Results from *in vitro* studies demonstrate that pretreatment intratumoral TS levels are inversely correlated to tumor response to 5-FU. Whether increased tumor TS expression reflects a biologically more aggressive tumor or is directly related to 5-FU resistance is unknown. Studies are underway to use this and other information to identify rational therapeutic approaches for select patients.

Hepatic Artery Infusion. The rationale for hepatic artery infusion (HAI) is based on the principle that normal liver hepatocytes and early micrometastases obtain their primary blood supply from the portal vein. In contrast, tumors in the liver are thought to receive most of their blood supply via the hepatic artery.[131] Floxuridine (FUDR) and 5-FU have undergone the most study for hepatic artery infusion either via continuous infusion or IV bolus injection. The majority of trials of hepatic arterial infusions have been directed at patients with unresectable liver metastases or as adjuvant therapy following curative resection of isolated metastases.

The pharmacokinetic properties of FUDR in particular provide for rapid systemic clearance and high liver drug extraction (94% to 99%).[131] Delivery of FUDR via the hepatic artery therefore results in increased local drug concentrations at the tumor site that produce higher tumor response rates. 5-FU has a much lower extraction rate but is also used frequently. Because a significant amount of an administered dose of these agents is metabolized by the liver, systemic toxicity caused by exposure of normal extrahepatic tissues is minimized. FUDR is typically administered as a continuous 24-hour infusion at a dose of 0.1–0.3 mg/kg/day for a total of 14 days. This is in contrast to a comparable IV dose equal to 0.125 mg/kg/day. Heparin, in doses ranging from 10,000 to 17,500 U/50 mL of solution, is often added to the HAI mixture in an attempt to decrease the incidence of arterial thromboses.

Regional HAI can be accomplished using a hepatic arterial port, a totally implantable pump, or a percutaneously placed catheter into the hepatic artery that is connected to an external pump. The volume of drug required to administer FUDR can be contained within an implantable pump whereas 5-FU administration generally requires use of an external pump. Early trials of HAI revealed objective response rates ranging from 30% to 80%, many of which were observed in previously treated patients. The greatest problems encountered were related to complications of external catheters such as arterial thrombosis, catheter dislodgement, bleeding, bulky pump equipment limiting patient mobility, and hospitalization. The availability of implantable, portable infusion devices has significantly decreased complications and renewed interest in hepatic arterial infusion chemotherapy. As a result, randomized trials comparing HAI with systemic therapy in patients with liver metastases were initiated in the 1980s. Results of these trials demonstrate that HAI consistently produces higher tumor response rates compared to systemic chemotherapy.[113,131] However, the majority of studies have allowed patients in the systemic therapy treatment groups to crossover to HAI upon tumor progression; therefore, the impact of these treatments on survival is difficult to interpret.

Several prospective, randomized trials have compared FUDR via HAI to systemic infusion of FUDR and 5-FU but the numbers of patients studied (41 to 168) have been relatively small. Response rates with HAI range are approximately threefold higher compared to systemic therapy (range, 42% to 62% vs 10% to 38%).[131] Median survival rates are slightly higher for patients receiving HAI compared to systemic therapy (13 to 20 months vs 6.3 to 16 months) but differences are not statistically significant. In general, a trend toward a superior survival rate at 1 or 2 years appears to exist for patients who receive HAI, whether it is administered initially or following failure with systemic therapy. In some trials, the systemic therapy for the control groups has been criticized as being suboptimal, however. Most recently, 5-FU plus leucovorin (5-FU/LV), administered via HAI or IV, was compared to HAI FUDR in 168 patients with unresectable liver metastases. Median survival times for patients treated with HAI 5-FU/LV, IV 5-FU/LV, and HAI FUDR (18.7 months vs 17.6 months vs 12.7 months, respectively) were no different. Although there were no significant differences between treatments in time to disease progression, a trend favored HAI 5-FU plus leucovorin. Further studies are needed to evaluate whether the addition of leucovorin to HAI provides significant benefit.

Patients with minimal liver involvement and lack of extrahepatic disease are most suitable for HAI therapy. Because extrahepatic disease eventually develops in 40% to 70% of patients who undergo HAI for isolated liver metastases, the addition of systemic therapy to treatment represents a potential opportunity to improve outcome. In a study of systemic 5-FU plus leucovorin administered following completion of a 14-day continuous HAI infusion of FUDR in 40 patients with unresectable liver metastases, however, 45% of patients experienced extrahepatic disease progression.[132] Although this was not a comparative trial, these results suggest that the addition of systemic therapy did not reduce extrahepatic disease. Trials of combined HAI and systemic therapy, including IV irinotecan, are in progress.

The primary limitations of HAI include development and/or progression of extrahepatic disease and treatment toxicities. Common toxicities include hepatobiliary toxicity and gastric ulceration, which can be life-threatening. The degree of hepatobiliary toxicity ranges from an elevation in hepatic enzymes resulting in a chemical hepatitis to sclerosing cholangitis (bile duct strictures). Elevation of liver function enzymes occurs in 26% to 79% of patients and is manifested by an elevation of transaminase enzymes or increased serum bilirubin levels, noted in 25% of patients. Bile duct toxicity resulting in biliary sclerosis occurs in fewer than 10% of patients with careful monitoring and is thought to result from ischemia and inflammation caused by the exposure of the bile ducts to high drug concentrations. Therefore, serum glutamic-oxaloacetic transaminase (SGOT), alkaline phosphatase, and bilirubin should be monitored closely during HAI, and dose reduction or discontinuation of therapy should occur until serum bilirubin levels return to normal. Biliary sclerosis often resolves upon discontinuation of therapy within 2 to 4 weeks, although irreversible damage can occur. In an attempt to reduce inflammation and ischemia of bile ducts, dexamethasone is frequently added to HAI FUDR and appears to decrease the extent of liver function test abnormalities that occur in patients who experience hepatobiliary toxicity. Another approach is to alternate HAI FUDR with hepatic arterial bolus 5-FU, which does not cause hepatobiliary toxicity.

Gastritis and gastrointestinal ulceration with risk of gastric hemorrhage can also develop, which are reversible upon discontinuation of therapy. These effects are believed due to perfusion of chemotherapy into the stomach and duodenum via small vessels branching from the hepatic artery. These toxicities may be ameliorated by surgical ligation of the blood vessels supplying the stomach and duodenum or H_2-antagonist therapy. Cholecystitis, which occurs in approximately one-third of patients, can be avoided through removal of the gallbladder at the time of catheter placement.[131]

Because of toxicities associated with HAI, most patients require some transient interruption of therapy, a decrease in dosage, or discontinuation of therapy. Furthermore, extrahepatic disease progression

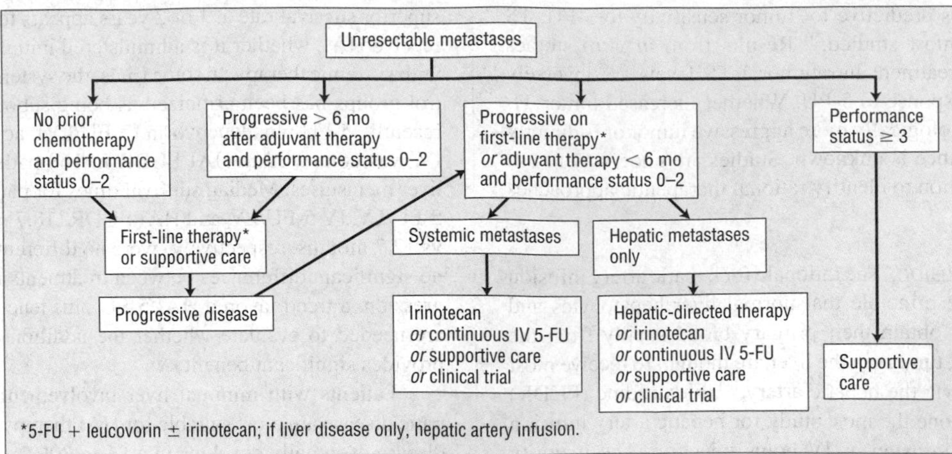

FIGURE 127–12. Algorithm for treatment of unresectable metastatic colorectal cancer.

with HAI therapy alone remains a clinical problem. Although increased response rates and a trend toward improved survival have been reported, the costs and toxicities with this approach are significant. However, an estimated cost of $22,160 for 1 year of HAI using an internal pump is much lower than an estimated cost of $54,000 for 1 year of IV irinotecan.[131] Therefore, for the minority of patients who present with unresectable disease to the liver only, HAI may represent a reasonable therapeutic option but should not be considered standard therapy until the results of ongoing trials comparing HAI and systemic therapy, as well as combined HAI and systemic therapy, which do not allow crossover treatment, become available.

Second-Line Therapy

Systemic chemotherapy represents the mainstay of therapy for patients whose disease progresses following initial treatment for metastatic disease. Figure 127–12 depicts an algorithm for treatment of refractory metastatic disease. Treatment options are based on type of and response to prior treatments, the site and extent of disease, and patient factors and treatment preferences.

Systemic Chemotherapy. Two important trials have delineated appropriate standard of care for patients who experience disease progression with 5-FU therapy for metastatic colorectal cancer.[133,134] The results of these trials demonstrate a survival benefit associated with irinotecan, which was approved by the FDA in 1996, as second-line therapy for recurrent or progressive disease following 5-FU. In phase II studies of previously treatment patients with metastatic colorectal cancer, objective response rates of 13% to 27% have been observed.[135]

In a phase III trial of 189 patients with metastatic colorectal cancer that had progressed within 6 months of treatment with 5-FU, irinotecan was compared to supportive care alone with regard to survival, quality of life, and other clinical variables.[133] Irinotecan was administered as 350 mg/m^2 IV every 3 weeks; the dose was reduced to 300 mg/m^2 for individuals who were 70 years of age or older, had a World Health Organization performance status of 2, or who had clinical risk factors for developing excessive treatment toxicity. Supportive care could include any symptomatic therapy with the exception of irinotecan or any other topoisomerase I inhibitor. With the exception of more patients with poor performance status being in the supportive care group, baseline patient characteristics were similar between groups. Median survival was 9.2 months (range, 0–18.9 months) with irinotecan, as compared to 6.5 months (range, 0.7–19.3 months) with supportive care alone. One-year survival was significantly greater with irinotecan (36.2% vs 13.8%, $P = 0.0001$) and was not associated with significantly worse quality of life scores except for diarrhea. Clinical variables such as cognitive functioning, pain, dyspnea, and appetite loss were in favor of irinotecan therapy. The most common grade 3 or 4 side effects with irinotecan included leukopenia and neutropenia (22%), diarrhea (22%), nausea (14%), and vomiting (14%). Seventy-two percent of patients receiving irinotecan required hospital admission for adverse events compared to 63% of supportive care patients. Thus, irinotecan was associated with an improved survival and quality of life compared to supportive care alone that appeared to balance treatment-related toxicities.

A comparison of irinotecan to continuous infusion 5-FU in a similar population of 267 patients allocated patients to irinotecan, 300–350 mg/m^2 IV every 3 weeks, or one of three continuous infusion 5-FU regimens: leucovorin 200 mg/m^2 IV over 2 hours followed by IV bolus 5-FU (400 mg/m^2) and 22-hour continuous infusion 5-FU (600 mg/m^2), given the first 2 days of every 2-week period; 5-FU 250–300 mg/m^2 as prolonged continuous IV infusion until disease progression; or 5-FU 2,600–3,000 mg/m^2/day IV over 24 hours, with or without leucovorin (20–500 mg/m^2 IV), given weekly for 6 weeks, with a 2-week rest period between cycles.[134] Median follow-up after 15 months revealed a longer 1-year survival (45% vs 32%) and median survival (10.8 months, range 1.2–18.7 months vs 8.5 months, range 0.8–20.9 months) with irinotecan, as compared to 5-FU. The median pain-free survival was approximately 2 months greater with irinotecan, but this difference was not statistically significant. Sixty-nine percent of patients receiving irinotecan experienced at least one grade 3 or 4 toxicity as compared to 54% of patients receiving 5-FU ($P = 0.013$). The most common toxicities with irinotecan were diarrhea, neutropenia, pain, vomiting, and asthenia, whereas pain, asthenia, diarrhea, and dermatologic toxicities were most common with 5-FU. There was no difference in hospitalization requirement for adverse effects between treatments.

Based on the results of these trials, irinotecan should be considered standard second-line therapy for patients who have failed prior treatment with 5-FU-based regimens. Either dosage regimen (irinotecan 125 mg/m^2 IV weekly for 4 weeks followed by a 2-week rest period or 300–350 mg/m^2 IV every 3 weeks) is acceptable. For the every 3-week regimen, initial administration of irinotecan at the lower dose should be considered for patients who have received significant prior pelvic or abdominal irradiation. Protracted continuous infusion 5-FU could be considered for those individuals with disease that no longer responds to bolus IV 5-FU plus leucovorin or irinotecan. Alternatively, patients may be suitable candidates for participation in a clinical trial. One interesting subject of debate is whether treatment could be suspended once disease stabilization occurs and restarted upon disease progression. In a small number of patients who achieved a partial response or disease stabilization with 5-FU plus leucovorin, chemotherapy was discontinued and then restarted upon disease progression.[136] Reinstitution of therapy resulted in partial tumor response and disease stabilization in 18% and 53% of patients, respectively. While the efficacy of this approach requires confirmation from randomized trials, these preliminary data support the inclusion of 5-FU in salvage treatment regimens with other agents.

Despite the lack of activity of oxaliplatin alone against 5-FU-refractory disease, when oxaliplatin has been administered in a bimonthly regimen with high-dose leucovorin and continuous 5-FU infusion, a 20.6% response rate with a median overall survival in excess of 10 months has been observed.[137] Mitomycin C, also in combination with continuous infusion 5-FU, produced a higher response rate (54% vs 38%) and significantly longer median failure free survival (7.9 months vs 5.4 months, $P = 0.033$) with no decrease in quality of life, as compared to 5-FU alone.[138] Thus, these agents may act synergistically with 5-FU, particularly when it is administered as a continuous IV infusion, and these combinations deserve further study. Synergistic clinical activity between raltitrexed and 5-FU has also been observed. Pilot studies of higher doses of single-agent raltitrexed and different treatment schedules of raltitrexed plus 5-FU demonstrate modest activity as second-line therapy.

Hepatic-Directed Therapies. Patients with hepatic-predominant disease whose disease progresses with systemic therapy may be candidates for palliative HAI, chemoembolization, intralesional injection of ethanol or cytotoxic agents, cryoablation or radiation therapy. Response rates to HAI therapy in patients that are refractory to 5-FU-based therapy may be as high as 33%.[139] Although HAI has not been compared to IV irinotecan as second-line therapy, tumor response rates from historical data are similar. Future applications of HAI may include hepatic-targeted therapy with antiangiogenic factors, small molecules designed to interfere with molecular targets, or attenuated genetically modified viruses.

The largest experience with hepatic arterial chemoembolization has been seen in patients with metastatic carcinoid tumors or primary hepatocellular carcinomas. Most recently, small trials have been expanded to include hepatic metastases caused by colorectal cancer.[140,141] Hepatic arterial chemoembolization delivers high concentrations of cytotoxic agents directly to the tumor and results in the embolization or devascularization of the liver, which blocks perfusion of the tumor and eliminates its blood supply. This procedure involves the instillation of a mixture that incorporates chemotherapeutic agents, radioactive contrast dye, and/or an embolic agent directly into the hepatic artery. Agents and doses most commonly studied include doxorubicin (40–60 mg), mitomycin (10–20 mg), and cisplatin (100–150 mg), which are usually dissolved in approximately 10–15 mL of a radiographic contrast dye.[140] Addition of an embolic agent to the mixture, such as a gelatin sponge (Gelfoam), polyvinyl alcohol particles, bovine collagen, or iodized poppy-seed oil (Lipiodol, Ethiodol), results in either a temporary or permanent occlusion of the hepatic artery. Although approximately 80% of patients in one trial experienced a response, the number of patients with colorectal cancer who have undergone this procedure thus far is relatively low. In addition, patients still experience eventual disease progression. However, preliminary results from small series suggest that the high tumor responses may be associated with a survival benefit and randomized trials comparing systemic therapy to hepatic chemoembolization for unresectable disease are ongoing.

PHARMACOECONOMIC CONSIDERATIONS

The estimated costs of treating colorectal cancer in the United States alone exceeds 6.5 billion dollars per year.[142,143] The total cost for managing a patient with cancer of the colon cancer is estimated to be approximately $45,000 to $61,000. Costs for patients with rectal cancer are approximately 15% higher because of the added expense of radiation therapy. These cost estimates are higher than estimated lifetime attributable costs for treating other common tumors such as cancer of the breast, prostate, and lung.[142] In addition, medical care costs vary, depending on the stage of disease. Medicare claims data reveal greater costs are incurred during the initial phase of care as compared to the terminal stage of disease.[143] For all stages of disease, initial care accounted for approximately one-half of the long-term cancer-related cost. Thus, a long-term approach is needed to accurately estimate the cost of treating patients diagnosed with colorectal cancer. The impact of changes in clinical practice on treatment costs, such as increased use of adjuvant therapy, changes in duration of hospital stay and outpatient delivery of health services, and incorporation of costly agents into standard treatment regimens, must also be continually considered.

An evaluation of the cost-effectiveness of adjuvant therapy for stage III colon cancer determined that 12 months of adjuvant therapy of 5-FU plus levamisole resulted in 1.88 years of life expectancy for each treated patient, using a 6% discounted rate of $2,094 per life-year saved.[144] However, a more accurate estimate of cost-effectiveness of current adjuvant therapy will need to evaluate 6-month courses of 5-FU plus leucovorin and consider patients with both stage III and high-risk stage II disease. In an economic evaluation of medical care consumption in the phase III trial comparing irinotecan with continuous infusion of 5-FU for 5-FU-refractory metastatic disease, costs associated with hospital care consumption for toxicity and disease-related complications were similar for both treatments.[145] However, the findings of this study are limited by the variable costs associated with different 5-FU treatment regimens, retrospective data collection, and lack of statistical power.

Although several investigations have evaluated cost-effectiveness of various screening procedures, published data regarding costs associated with colorectal cancer prevention are not currently available. In a cost-effectiveness analysis of various screening procedures for average-risk individuals, using an estimation of compliance of 60%, the use of annual rehydrated fecal occult blood testing plus sigmoidoscopy every 5 years was determined to be the most effective strategy for white males and was associated with an incremental cost-effectiveness ratio of $92,900 per year of life-gained.[146] Colonoscopy was less effective. However, a separate comparison of the cost-effectiveness of fecal occult blood testing, flexible sigmoidoscopy, and colonoscopy found colonoscopy to be the most cost-effective screening strategy when performed every 10 years.[147] These evaluations are sensitive to the impact of uncertainty about actual compliance rates in different clinical practice settings, which must be considered in the interpretation of these data. Most accepted screening strategies, however, have cost-effectiveness ratios that are well below the accepted benchmark of $50,000 per life-year saved.[142]

EVALUATION OF THERAPEUTIC OUTCOMES

The goal of monitoring is to evaluate whether the patient is receiving any benefit from the management of the disease or to detect recurrence. Similarly, follow-up examinations help to determine whether preventive interventions or screening studies effectively reduce an individual's risk for developing colorectal cancer or presenting with an advanced stage of disease. During treatment for active disease, patients should undergo monitoring for measurable tumor response, progression, or new metastases; these tests may include chest CT scans or x-rays, abdominal or pelvic CT scans or x-rays, depending on the site of disease being evaluated for response, and CEA measurements every 2 to 3 months if the CEA is or was previously elevated. In addition, a CBC should be obtained prior to each course of chemotherapy administration to ensure that hematologic indices are adequate. Baseline liver function tests and an assessment of renal function should be evaluated prior to and periodically during therapy. These tests and other selected serum chemistries should also be evaluated with the development of any new symptoms or significant change in disease status. Patients should be evaluated during every treatment visit for the presence of anticipated side effects, which generally include loose stools or diarrhea, nausea or vomiting, mouth sores, fatigue, and fever.

Symptoms of recurrence such as pain syndromes, changes in bowel habits, rectal or vaginal bleeding, pelvic masses, anorexia, and weight loss develop in fewer than 50% of patients. A greater percentage of recurrences are detected in asymptomatic patients because of increased serum CEA levels that lead to further examination. Although the value of CEA monitoring for asymptomatic disease recurrence is questioned by some because of the related expense and emotional stress associated with false-positive elevations, CEA monitoring plays an important role in postoperative follow-up studies for most individuals. Patients who undergo curative surgical resection, with or without adjuvant therapy, require close follow-up based on the premise that early detection and treatment of recurrence could still render them cured. In addition, early treatment for asymptomatic metastatic colorectal cancer appears superior to delayed therapy. Specific practice guidelines for postoperative surveillance examinations have been developed by the NCCN (Table 127–11). Colorectal cancer surveillance guidelines published by the American Society of Clinical Oncology recommend against routinely monitoring liver function tests, CBC, fecal occult blood testing, CT scans, annual chest x-rays, or pelvic imaging in asymptomatic patients.[148]

Recent advances in the treatment for cancer of the colon and rectum now offer the potential to improve patient survival but for many patients, improved disease- and progression-free survival represent equally important therapeutic outcomes. Table 127–12 summarizes current treatment options. Although treatment approaches for metastatic colorectal cancer have been historically assessed by their ability to produce a measurable objective tumor response, which is generally believed necessary for any treatment to improve survival, the effects of therapies on survival are clinically more meaningful than their ability to induce a tumor response. In the absence of the ability of a specific treatment to improve survival, important outcome measures should include the effects of the treatment on patient symptoms, daily activities and performance status, and other quality-of-life indicators. Because metastatic colorectal cancer is incurable, a specific decision regarding an individual patient's care will ultimately be required; this should be based on a careful assessment of the balance between risks associated with treatment (or lack thereof) and benefits of treatment. Effort should also be made to ensure that the costs of screening, diagnostic tests, treatments, and follow-up procedures for colorectal cancer are consistent with their value in improving patient outcomes.

TABLE 127–11. NCCN Postoperative Surveillance Practice Guidelines for Colon and Rectal Cancer

- Physical exam, including digital rectal examination every 3 months for 2 years, then every 6 months for 3 years
- CEA every 3 months for 2 years, then every 6 months for 3 years*
- Colonoscopy in 1 year; repeat in 1 year if abnormal or every 3 years if negative for polyps

*For colon cancer, T2 or greater lesions.

Reproduced from Version 2000. Revision date: June 1, 2000©2000 National Comprehensive Cancer Network, Inc. These guidelines and this illustration may not be reproduced in any form without the express written permission of NCCN.

TABLE 127–12. Summary of Current Treatment Options for Cancer of the Colon and Rectum

Stage I	Surgical resection of primary tumor and regional mesenteric lymph nodes
Stage II	
Colon	Surgical resection; consider adjuvant therapy or clinical trial for individuals with high-risk disease
Rectum	Surgical resection, then postoperative 5-FU-based chemotherapy and 5-FU-chemosensitized radiotherapy; preoperative 5-FU-chemosensitized radiotherapy, then surgical resection
Stage III	
Colon	Surgery + adjuvant chemotherapy[a]
Rectum	Surgical resection, then postoperative 5-FU-based chemotherapy and 5-FU-chemosensitized radiotherapy; preoperative 5-FU-chemosensitized radiotherapy, then surgical resection + adjuvant 5-FU-based chemotherapy
Stage IV	Systemic chemotherapy;[b] radiation therapy; hepatic artery infusion chemotherapy (liver disease only); surgical resection of isolated hepatic, pulmonary, abdominal, or brain metastases ± adjuvant chemotherapy; symptom management

[a]5-FU + leucovorin for 6 months or 5-FU + levamisole for 12 months.
[b]First-line therapy: 5-FU plus leucovorin ± irinotecan.

► PRINCIPLES OF PHARMACOTHERAPY

- Maintaining a diet with high-fiber and low-fat intake has not been proven to reduce colorectal cancer risk but is beneficial for reducing risk of other chronic diseases. Hormone replacement therapy significantly reduces risk in postmenopausal women, and aspirin and other NSAIDs reduce colorectal cancer incidence and mortality, although choice of optimal agent(s), doses, and duration of administration are undefined. Celecoxib, 400 mg po twice daily, reduces polyp number and burden in individuals with familial adenomatous polyposis, but these effects do not persist upon drug discontinuation.
- Effective colorectal cancer screening programs incorporate regular physical examinations including digital rectal exam and fecal occult blood testing, starting at age 50 years for average-risk individuals, in combination with colonoscopy every 10 years or flexible sigmoidoscopy or double-contrast barium enema every 5 years.

- The stage of colorectal cancer upon diagnosis—determined by depth of bowel invasion, lymph node involvement, and presence of metastases—is the most important prognostic factor for disease recurrence and survival. Newer prognostic factors include tumor *p*53 status, chromosome 18q allelic loss, and tumor thymidylate synthase expression, which may also be important determinants of tumor response to specific chemotherapeutic agents and help identify those individuals likely to benefit from adjuvant therapy.
- Surgical removal of tumor is the treatment of choice for patients with resectable colorectal cancer. Adjuvant chemotherapy, consisting of 6-month treatment with 5-FU plus leucovorin or 12-month treatment with 5-FU plus levamisole, should be offered to patients with stage III colon cancer and considered for patients with high-risk stage II disease. Adjuvant 5-FU regimens incorporate a schedule of high- or low-dose leucovorin; neither has proven superior. Adjuvant chemotherapy significantly reduces risk of cancer recurrence and overall mortality compared to observation alone.
- Adjuvant therapy consisting of 5-FU-based chemosensitized radiation therapy should be offered to patients with stage II or III cancer of the rectum. Although a postoperative schedule of adjuvant treatment has been standard practice in the United States, preoperative or neoadjuvant chemotherapy and/or radiation therapy may be considered but is not currently considered standard care. Adjuvant 5-FU chemotherapy plus radiation decreases risk of local and distant disease recurrence as compared to observation alone.
- Tumor resection for metastatic colorectal cancer is generally reserved for selected individuals with fewer than four isolated hepatic, pulmonary, or abdominal lesions. Patients with isolated unresectable hepatic metastases may benefit from hepatic intra-arterial chemotherapy, which has not been proven to, but may, offer a survival benefit.
- Palliative 5-FU-based chemotherapy regimens for metastatic colorectal cancer provide a modest improvement in survival and can be highly beneficial in reducing patient symptoms and their effects on daily activities and general sense of well-being. Intravenous 5-FU forms the basis for chemotherapy regimens for initial treatment of metastatic colorectal cancer. Effective regimens incorporate 5-FU as an IV bolus or short infusion in combination with low-dose (20 mg/m^2) or high-dose (200–500 mg/m^2) leucovorin administered 5 days weekly, once weekly, or biweekly. Dose-limiting toxicities associated with low-dose leucovorin regimens consist primarily of mucositis and leukopenia, whereas diarrhea is most often dose limiting for high-dose leucovorin regimens. Triple-drug therapy consisting of irinotecan, 5-FU, and leucovorin improves survival compared to 5-FU plus leucovorin alone, and is considered by many practitioners as standard first-line therapy for metastatic disease. Selection of a specific regimen should be based on anticipated side effects, patient convenience, and cost considerations.
- Irinotecan improves survival in patients with tumor progression within 6 months following or during treatment with 5-FU therapy, as compared to continuous IV infusion 5-FU or supportive care alone, without detrimental effects on quality of life. Patients who fail irinotecan or bolus 5-FU therapies may benefit from continuous IV infusion 5-FU, alone or in combination with leucovorin. Mucositis and hand foot syndrome can be dose limiting with continuous IV infusion 5-FU.
- Capecitabine is an acceptable alternative to parenteral 5-FU/leucovorin for metastatic colorectal cancer. Although it provides no greater benefit with regard to tumor progression, duration of response, or overall survival, its oral dosing may offer greater patient convenience. Ultimately, toxicity, patient compliance, and cost issues will likely determine its role in the management of metastatic disease.
- Several monoclonal antibodies are under investigation for colorectal cancer treatment. Cetuximab, an anti-epidermal growth factor receptor (EGFR) monoclonal antibody, has significant activity in 5-FU- and irinotecan-resistant colorectal cancer and appears beneficial to patients with refractory disease.

REFERENCES

1. Cancer facts figures 2001. Atlanta, GA, American Cancer Society, Inc; 2001.
2. Pisani P, Parkin DM, Bray F, Ferlay J. Estimates of the worldwide mortality from 25 cancers in 1990. Int J Cancer 1999;83:18–29.
3. Ries LAG, Eisner MP, Kosary CL, et al., eds. SEER Cancer Statistics Review, 1973–1997. Bethesda, MD, National Cancer Institute, 1997.
4. Parkin DM, Pisani P, Ferlay J. Estimates of the worldwide incidence of 25 major cancers in 1990. Int J Cancer 1999;80:827–841.
5. Ries LAG, Wingo PA, Miller DS, et al. The annual report to the nation on the status of cancer, 1973–1997, with a special section on colorectal cancer. Cancer 2000;88:2398–2424.
6. Potter JD. Colorectal cancer: Molecules and populations. J Natl Cancer Inst 1999;91:916–932.
7. Trock B, Lanza E, Greenwald P. Dietary fiber, vegetables, and colon cancer: Critical review and meta-analyses of the epidemiologic evidence. J Natl Cancer Inst 1990;82:650–661.
8. Kritchevsky D. Epidemiology of fibre, resistant starch and colorectal cancer. Eur J Cancer Prev 1995;4:345–352.
9. Friedenreich CM, Brant RF, Riboli E. Influence of methodologic factors in a pooled analysis of 13 case-control studies of colorectal cancer and dietary fiber [erratum appears in Epidemiology 1994;5:385]. Epidemiology 1994;5:66–79.
10. Fuchs CS, Giovannucci EL, Colditz GA. Dietary fiber and the risk of colorectal cancer and adenoma in women. N Engl J Med 1999;340:169–176.
11. Peipins LA, Sandler RS. Epidemiology of colorectal adenomas. Epidemiol Rev 1994;16:273–297.
12. Augustsson K, Skog K, Jägerstad M, et al. Dietary heterocyclic amines and cancer of the colon, rectum, bladder and kidney: A population-based study. Lancet 1999;353:703–707.
13. Kroser JA, Bachwich DR, Lichtenstein GR. Risk factors for the development of colorectal carcinoma and their modification. Hematol Oncol Clin North Am 1997;11:547–577.
14. Giovannucci E, Egan KM, Hunter DJ, et al. Aspirin and the risk of colorectal cancer in women. N Engl J Med 1995;333:609–614.
15. Smalley W, Ray WA, Daugherty J, Griffin MR. Use of nonsteroidal anti-inflammatory drugs and incidence of colorectal cancer. Arch Intern Med 1999;159:161–166.
16. Dannenberg AJ, Zakim D. Chemoprevention of colorectal cancer through inhibition of cyclooxygenase-2. Semin Oncol 1999;26:499–504.
17. Hong WK, Spitz MR, Lippman SM. Cancer chemoprevention in the 21st century: Genetics, risk modelling, and molecular targets. J Clin Oncol 2000;18(Nov 1 suppl):9s–18s.
18. Grodstein F, Newcomb PA, Stampfer MJ. Postmenopausal hormone therapy and the risk of colorectal cancer: A review and meta-analysis. Am J Med 1999;106:574–582.
19. Giovannucci E, Ascherio A, Rimm EB, et al. Physical activity, obesity, and risk for colon cancer and adenoma in men. Ann Intern Med 1995;12:327–334.

20. Hu FB, Manson JE, Liu S, et al. Prospective study of adult onset diabetes mellitus (Type 2) and risk of colorectal cancer in women. J Natl Cancer Inst 1999;91:542–547.
21. Chao A, Thun MJ, Jacobs EJ, et al. Cigarette smoking and colorectal cancer morality in the Cancer Prevention Study II. J Natl Cancer Inst 2000;92:1888–1896.
22. Fuchs CS, Giovannucci EL, Colditzs GA, et al. A prospective study of family history and the risk of colorectal cancer. N Engl J Med 1994; 331:1669–1674.
23. Rustgi AK. Hereditary gastrointestinal polyposis and nonpolyposis syndromes. N Engl J Med 1994;331:1694–1702.
24. Vasen HFA. Clinical diagnosis and management of hereditary colorectal cancer syndromes. J Clin Oncol 2000;18(Nov 1 suppl):81s–92s.
25. Lynch HT, Lynch J. Lynch syndrome: Genetics, natural history, genetic counseling, and prevention. J Clin Oncol 2000;18(Nove 1 suppl): 19s–31s.
26. Fearon ER, Vogelstein B. A genetic model for colorectal tumorigenesis. Cell 1990;61:759–767.
27. Midgley R, Kerr D. Colorectal cancer. Lancet 1999;353:391–399.
28. Hoops TC, Traber PG. Molecular pathogenesis of colorectal cancer. Hematol Oncol Clin North Am 1997;11:609–633.
29. Markowitz S, Wang J, Myeroff L, et al. Inactivation of the type II TGF-β receptor in colon cancer cells with microsatellite instability. Science 1995;268:1336–1338.
30. Cohen AM, Minsky BD, Schilsky RL. Cancer of the colon. In: DeVita VT, Hellman S, Rosenberg SA, eds. Cancer: Principles and Practice of Oncology, 5th ed. Philadelphia, Lippincott, 1997:1144–1197.
31. Silverman AL, Desai TK, Dhar R, et al. Clinical features, evaluation and detection of colorectal cancer. Gastroenterol Clin North Am 1988; 17:713–725.
32. Alberts DS, Slatery ML, Giovannucci E, et al. Primary prevention of colon cancer with dietary and micronutrient interventions. Cancer 1998; 83:1734–1739.
33. Schatzkin A, Lanza E, Corle D, et al. Lack of effect of a low-fat, high-fiber diet on the recurrence of colorectal adenomas. N Engl J Med 1999; 342:1149–1155.
34. Michels KB, Giovannucci E, Joshipura KJ. Prospective study of fruit and vegetable consumption and incidence of colon and rectal cancers. J Natl Cancer Inst 2000;92:1740–1752.
35. Alberts DS, Martinez ME, Roe DJ, et al. Lack of effect of a high-fiber cereal supplement on the recurrence of colorectal adenomas. N Engl J Med 2000;342:1156–1162.
36. Jänne PA, Mayer RJ. Chemoprevention of colorectal cancer. N Engl J Med 2000;324:1960–1968.
37. Steinbach G, Lynch PM, Phillips RK, et al. The effect of celecoxib, a cyclooxygenase-2 inhibitor, in familial adenomatous polyposis. N Engl J Med 2000;342:1946–1952.
38. Baron JA, Beach M, Mandel JS, et al. Calcium supplements for the prevention of colorectal adenomas. N Engl J Med 1999;340:101–107.
39. Byers T, Levin B, Rothenberger D, et al. American Cancer Society guidelines for screening and surveillance for early detection of colorectal polyps and cancer: Update 1997. CA Cancer J Clin 1997;47:154–160.
40. Mandel JS, Church TR, Bond JH. The effect of fecal occult-blood screening on the incidence of colorectal cancer. N Engl J Med 2000;343: 1603–1607.
41. Ransohoff DF, Lang CA. Screening for colorectal cancer with the fecal occult blood test: A background paper. Ann Intern Med 1997;126: 811–822.
42. Mandel JS, Bond JH, Church TR, et al. Reducing mortality from colorectal cancer by screening for fecal occult blood. Minnesota Colon Cancer Control Study [erratum appears in N Engl J Med 1993;329:672]. N Engl J Med 1993;328:1365–1371.
43. Ferrante JM. Colorectal cancer screening. Med Clin North Am 1996; 80:27–43.
44. Selby JV, Friedman GD, Quesenberry CP, Weiss NS. A case-control study of screening sigmoidoscopy and mortality from colorectal cancer. N Engl J Med 1992;326:653–657.
45. Rex DK, Johnson DA, Lieberman DA, et al. Colorectal cancer prevention 2000: Screening recommendations of the American College of Gastroenterology. Am J Gastroenterol 2000;95:868–877.
46. American Society of Clinical Oncology. Clinical practice guidelines for the use of tumor markers in breast and colorectal cancer. J Clin Oncol 1996;14:2843–2877.
47. Akhurst T, Larson SM. Positron emission tomography imaging of colorectal cancer. Semin Oncol 1999;26:577–583.
48. Bertagnolli MM, Mahmoud NN, Daly JM. Surgical aspects of colorectal carcinoma. Hematol Oncol Clin North Am 1997;11:655–677.
49. Moffat FL, Gulec SA, Serafini AN, et al. A thousand points of light or just dim bulbs? Radiolabeled antibodies and colorectal cancer imaging. Cancer Invest 1999;17:322–334.
50. Compton C, Fenoglio-Preiser CM, Pettigrew N, Fielding LP. American Joint Committee on Cancer Prognostic Factors Consensus Conference Colorectal Working Group. Cancer 2000;88:1739–1757.
51. Ogunbiyi OA, Goodfellow PJ, Herfarth K, et al. Confirmation that chromosome 18q allelic loss in colon cancer is a prognostic indicator. J Clin Oncol 1998;16:427–433.
52. Yamachika T, Nakanishi H, Tsukamoto T, et al. A new prognostic factor for colorectal carcinoma, thymidylate synthase, and its therapeutic significance. Cancer 1998;82:70–77.
53. McLeod HL, Murray GI. Tumour markers of prognosis in colorectal cancer. Br J Cancer 1999;79:191–203.
54. Gryfe R, Kim H, Hsieh ETK, et al. Tumor microsatellite instability and clinical outcome in young patients with colorectal cancer. N Engl J Med 2000;342:69–77.
55. Cohen Am, Minsky BD, Schilsky RL. Cancer of the rectum. In: DeVita VT, Hellman S, Rosenberg SA, eds. Cancer: Principles and Practice of Oncology, 5th ed. Philadelphia, Lippincott, 1997:1197–1234.
56. Schmoll HJ, Büchele T, Grothey A, Dempke W. Where do we stand with 5-fluorouracil? Semin Oncol 1999;26:589–605.
57. Sobrero AF, Aschele C, Bertino JR. Fluorouracil in colorectal cancer—A tale of two drugs: Implications for biochemical modulation. J Clin Oncol 1997;15:368–381.
58. The Meta-Analysis Group in Cancer. Efficacy of intravenous continuous infusion of fluorouracil compared with bolus administration in advanced colorectal cancer. J Clin Oncol 1998;16:301–308.
59. The Meta-Analysis Group in Cancer. Toxicity of fluorouracil in patients with advanced colorectal cancer: Effect of administration schedule and prognostic factors. J Clin Oncol 1998;16:3537–3541.
60. Advanced Colorectal Cancer Meta-Analysis Project. Meta-analysis of randomized trials testing the biochemical modulation of fluorouracil by methotrexate in metastatic colorectal cancer. J Clin Oncol 1994;12:960–969.
61. Machover D. A comprehensive review of 5-fluorouracil and leucovorin in patients with metastatic colorectal carcinoma. Cancer 1997;80:1179–1187.
62. Vincent M, Labianca R, Harper P. Which 5-fluorouracil regimen? The great debate. Anticancer Drugs 1999;10:337–354.
63. Wolmark N, Rockette H, Fisher B, et al. The benefit of leucovorin-modulated fluorouracil as postoperative adjuvant therapy for primary colon cancer: Results from National Surgical Adjuvant Breast and Bowel Project Protocol C-03. J Clin Oncol 1993;11:1879–1887.
64. International Multicentre Pooled Analysis of Colon Cancer Trials (IMPACT) Investigators. Efficacy of adjuvant fluorouracil and folinic acid in colon cancer. Lancet 1995;345:939–944.
65. Petrelli N, Douglass HO, Herrera L, et al. The modulation of fluorouracil with leucovorin in metastatic colorectal carcinoma: A prospective randomized phase III trial. J Clin Oncol 1989;7:1419–1426.
66. Wadler S, Benson AB, Engelking C, et al. Recommended guidelines for the treatment of chemotherapy-induced diarrhea. J Clin Oncol 1998; 16:3169–3178.
67. Rothenberg ML, Blanke CD. Topoisomerase I inhibitors in the treatment of colorectal cancer. Semin Oncol 1999;26:632–639.
68. O'Reilly S, Rowinsky EK. Experimental chemotherapeutic agents for the treatment of colorectal carcinoma. Hematol Clin North Am 1997; 11:721–758.

69. Cersosimo RJ. Irinotecan: A new antineoplastic agent for the management of colorectal cancer. Ann Pharmacother 1998;32:1324–1333.
70. Rougier P, Douillard JY, Culine S, et al. Phase II study of irinotecan in the treatment of advanced colorectal cancer in chemotherapy-naive patients and patients pretreated with fluorouracil-based chemotherapy. J Clin Oncol 1997;15:251–260.
71. Cassidy J. Potential of Xeloda in colorectal cancer and other solid tumors. Oncology 1999;57(suppl 1):27–32.
72. Blanke CD, Messenger M, Taplin SC. Trimetrexate: Review and current clinical experience in advanced colorectal cancer. Semin Oncol 1997; 24(5 suppl 18):S18-57–S18-63.
73. AbdAlla EE, Blair GE, Jones RA, et al. Mechanism of synergy of levamisole and fluorouracil: Induction of human leukocyte antigen class I in a colorectal cancer cell line. J Natl Cancer Inst 1995;87:489–496.
74. Moertel CG, Fleming TR, Macdonald JS, et al. Fluorouracil plus levamisole as effective adjuvant therapy after resection of stage III colon carcinoma: A final report. Ann Intern Med 1995;122:321–326.
75. Vaughn DJ, Haller DG. The role of adjuvant chemotherapy in the treatment of colorectal cancer. Hematol Clin North Am 1997;11:699–719.
76. Rustum YM, Harstrick A, Cao S, et al. Thymidylate synthase inhibitors in cancer therapy: Direct and indirect inhibitors. J Clin Oncol 1997;15: 389–400.
77. Baker SD, Diasio RB, O'Reilly S, et al. Phase I and pharmacologic study of oral fluorouracil on a chronic daily schedule in combination with the dihydropyrimidine dehydrogenase inactivator eniluracil. J Clin Oncol 2000;18:915–926.
78. Brito RA, Medgyesy D, Zukowski TH, et al. Fluoropyrimidines: A critical evaluation. Oncology 1999;57(suppl 1):2–8.
79. Cvitkovic E, Bekradda M. Oxaliplatin: A new therapeutic option in colorectal cancer. Semin Oncol 1999;26:647–662.
80. Cocconi G, Cunningham D, Van Cutsem E, et al. Open, randomized, multicenter trial of raltitrexed versus fluorouracil plus high-dose leucovorin in patients with advanced colorectal cancer. J Clin Oncol 1998;16:2943–2952.
81. Riethmüller G, Holz E, Schlimok G, et al. Monoclonal antibody therapy of Dukes' C colorectal carcinoma: Seven-year outcome of a multicenter randomized trial. J Clin Oncol 1998;16:1788–1794.
82. Dillman RO. Unconjugated monoclonal antibodies for the treatment of hematologic and solid malignancies. ASCO Educational Book Spring 1999:461–468.
83. Cohen RB, Falcey JW, Paulter VJ, et al. Safety profile of the monoclonal antibody (MoAb) IMC-C225, an anti-epidermal growth factor receptor (EGFR) used in the treatment of EGFR-positive tumors. Proc Am Soc Clin Oncol 2000;19:474a. Abstract.
84. Foon KA, Yannelli J, Bhattacharya-Chatterjee M. Colorectal cancer as a model for immunotherapy. Clin Cancer Res 1999;5:225–236.
85. Harris JE, Ryan L, Hoover HC, et al. Adjuvant active specific immunotherapy for stage II and III colon cancer with an autologous tumor cell vaccine: Eastern Cooperative Oncology Group Study E5283. J Clin Oncol 2000;18:148–157.
86. Meropol NJ. Novel targets in colorectal cancer. ASCO Educational Book Spring 2000;631–638.
87. Macdonald JS. Adjuvant therapy of colon cancer. CA Cancer J Clin 1999; 49:202–219.
88. Mamounas E, Wieand S, Wolmark N, et al. Comparative efficacy of adjuvant chemotherapy in patients with Dukes' B versus Dukes' C colon cancer: Results from four National Surgical Adjuvant Breast and Bowel Project adjuvant studies (C-01, C-02, C-03, and C-04). J Clin Oncol 1999;17:1349–1355.
89. Moertel CG, Fleming TR, Jacdonald JS, et al. Intergroup study of fluorouracil plus levamisole as adjuvant therapy for stage II/Dukes' B2 colon cancer. J Clin Oncol 1995;13:2936–2943.
90. International Multicentre Pooled Analysis of B2 Colon Cancer Trials (IMPACT B2) Investigators. Efficacy of adjuvant fluorouracil and folinic acid in B2 colon cancer. J Clin Oncol 1999;17:1356–1363.
91. Minsky BD. The role of adjuvant radiation therapy in the treatment of colorectal cancer. Hematol Clin North Am 1997;11:679–697.
92. Buyse M, Zeleniuch-Jacquotte A, Chalmers TC. Adjuvant therapy of colorectal cancer—Why we still don't know. JAMA 1988;259:3571–3578.
93. Poplin E, Benedetti J, Estes N, et al. Phase III randomized trial of bolus 5-FU/leucovorin/levamisole versus 5-FU continuous infusion/levamisole as adjuvant therapy for high-risk colon cancer (SWOG 9415/INT-0153). Proc Am Soc Clin Oncol 2000;19:240a. Abstract.
94. Saini A, Cunningham D, Norman AR, et al. Multicentre randomized trial of protracted venous infusion (PVI) 5-FU compared to 5-FU/folinic acid (5FU/FA) as adjuvant therapy for colorectal cancer. Proc Am Soc Clin Oncol 2000;19:240a. Abstract.
95. Laurie JA, Moertel CG, Fleming TR, et al. Surgical adjuvant therapy of large bowel carcinoma: An evaluation of levamisole and combination of levamisole and 5-fluorouracil. The North Central Cancer Treatment Group and the Mayo Clinic. J Clin Oncol 1989;7:1447–1456.
96. Brown ML, Nayfield SG, Shibley LM. Adjuvant therapy for stage III colon cancer: Economics returns to research and cost-effectiveness of treatment. J Natl Cancer Inst 1994;86:424–430.
97. O'Connell MJ, Mailliard J, Kahn MJ, et al. Controlled trial of fluorouracil and low-dose leucovorin given for 6 months as postoperative adjuvant therapy for colon cancer. J Clin Oncol 1997;15:246–250.
98. Wolmark N, Rockette H, Mamounas E, et al. Clinical trial to assess the relative efficacy of fluorouracil and leucovorin, fluorouracil and levamisole, and fluorouracil, leucovorin, and levamisole in patients with Dukes' B and C carcinoma of the colon: Results from National Surgical Adjuvant Breast and Bowel Project C-04. J Clin Oncol 1999;17:3553–3559.
99. O'Connell MJ, Laurie JA, Kahn M, et al. Prospectively randomized trial of postoperative adjuvant chemotherapy in patients with high-risk colon cancer. J Clin Oncol 1998;16:295–300.
100. Haller DG, Catalano PJ, Macdonald JS, Mayer RJ. Fluorouracil (FU), leucovorin (LV) and levamisole (LEV) adjuvant therapy for colon cancer: Five-year final report of INT-0089. Proc Am Soc Clin Oncol 1998; 17:256a. Abstract.
101. Weinerman B. Increased incidence of toxicity in elderly females treated with 5FU, leucovorin. Proc Am Soc Clin Oncol 1996;15:225.
102. Taylor I, Machin D, Mullee M, et al. A randomized controlled trial of adjuvant portal vein cytotoxic perfusion in colorectal cancer. Br J Surg 1985;72:359–363.
103. Wolmark N, Rockette H, Petrelli N, et al. Long-term results of the efficacy of perioperative portal vein infusion of 5-FU for treatment of colon cancer: NSABP C-02. Proc Am Soc Clin Oncol 1994;13:194. Abstract.
104. Liver Infusion Meta-analysis Group. Portal vein chemotherapy for colorectal cancer: A meta-analysis of 4000 patients in 10 studies. J Natl Cancer Inst 1997;89:497–505.
105. National Institutes of Health Consensus Development Conference. Adjuvant therapy for patients with colon and rectal cancer. JAMA 1990; 264:1444–1450.
106. Gastrointestinal Tumor Study Group. Prolongation of the disease-free interval in surgically treated rectal carcinoma. N Engl J Med 1985;312: 1465–1472.
107. Douglass HO, Moertel CG, Mayer RJ, et al. Survival after postoperative combination treatment of rectal cancer. N Engl J Med 1986;315: 1294–1295.
108. Krook JE, Moertel CG, Gunderson LL, et al. Effective surgical adjuvant therapy for high-risk rectal carcinoma. N Engl J Med 1991;324:709–715.
109. O'Connell MJ, Martenson JA, Wieand HS, et al. Improving adjuvant therapy for rectal cancer by combining protracted infusion fluorouracil with radiation therapy after curative surgery. N Engl J Med 1994;331:502–507.
110. Tepper JE, O'Connell MJ, Petroni GR, et al. Adjuvant postoperative fluorouracil-modulated chemotherapy combined with pelvic radiation therapy for rectal cancer: Initial results of Intergroup 0114. J Clin Oncol 1997;15:2030–2039.
111. Swedish Cancer Rectal Trial. Improved survival with preoperative radiotherapy in resectable rectal cancer. N Engl J Med 1997;336:980–987.

112. Swedish Cancer Rectal Trial. Correction to improved survival with preoperative radiotherapy in resectable rectal cancer. N Engl J Med 1997; 336:1539.
113. VanderMeer TJ, Callery MP, Meyers WC. The approach to the patient with single and multiple liver metastases, pulmonary metastases, and intra-abdominal metastases from colorectal carcinoma. Hematol Clin North Am 1997;11:721–758.
114. Fong Y, Salo J. Surgical therapy of hepatic colorectal metastasis. Semin Oncol 1999;26:514–523.
115. Kemeny N, Huang Y, Cohen AM, et al. Hepatic arterial infusion of chemotherapy after resection of hepatic metastases from colorectal cancer. N Engl J Med 1999;341:2039–2048.
116. Jonker DJ, Maroun JA, Kocha W. Survival benefit of chemotherapy in metastatic colorectal cancer: A meta-analysis of randomized controlled trials. Br J Cancer 2000;82:1789–1794.
117. Colorectal Cancer Collaborative Group. Palliative chemotherapy for advanced colorectal cancer: Systematic review and meta-analysis. BMJ 2000;321:531–535.
118. Leichman CG. Prolonged infusion of fluorinated pyrimidines in gastrointestinal malignancies: A review of recent clinical trials. Cancer Invest 1994; 12:166–175.
119. Poon MA, O'Connell MJ, Wieand HS, et al. Biochemical modulation of fluorouracil with leucovorin: Confirmatory evidence of improved therapeutic efficacy in advanced colorectal cancer. J Clin Oncol 1991;9:1967–1972.
120. Buroker TR, O'Connell MJ, Wieand HS, et al. Randomized comparison of two schedules of fluorouracil and leucovorin in the treatment of advanced colorectal cancer. J Clin Oncol 1994;12:14–20.
121. Jüger E, Heike M, Bernhard H, et al. Weekly high-dose leucovorin versus low-dose leucovorin combined with fluorouracil in advanced colorectal cancer: Results of a randomized multicenter trial. J Clin Oncol 1996;14:2274–2279.
122. Grem JL. Systemic treatment options in advanced colorectal cancer: Perspectives on combination 5-fluorouracil plus leucovorin. Semin Oncol 1997;24(5 suppl 18):S18-8–S18-18.
123. Popescu RA, Norman A, Ross PJ, et al. Adjuvant or palliative chemotherapy for colorectal cancer in patients 70 years or older. J Clin Oncol 1999; 17:2412–2418.
124. Douillard JY, Cunningham D, Roth AD, et al. Irinotecan combined with fluorouracil compared with fluorouracil alone as first-line treatment for metastatic colorectal cancer: A multicentre randomized trial. Lancet 2000;355:1041–1047.
125. Saltz LB, Cox JV, Blanke C, et al. Irinotecan plus fluorouracil and leucovorin for metastatic colorectal cancer. N Engl J Med 2000;343:905–914.
126. Rothenberg ML, Meropol NJ, Poplin EA, et al. Mortality associated with irinotecan plus bolus fluorouracil/leucovorin. Summary findings of an independent panel. J. Clin Oncol 2001;19:3801–3807.
127. Hoff P. Capecitabine as first-line treatment for colorectal cancer (CRC): Integrated results of 1207 patients (pts) from 2 randomized, phase III studies. On behalf of the Capecitabine CRC Study Group. Ann Oncol 2000;11(suppl 4):60.
128. Giaccheti S, Perpoint B, Zidani R, et al. Phase III multicenter randomized trial of oxaliplatin added to chronomodulated fluorouracil-leucovorin as first-line treatment of metastatic colorectal cancer. J Clin Oncol 2000;18:136–147.
129. de Gramont A, Figer A, Seymour M, et al. Leucovorin and fluorouracil with or without oxaliplatin as first-line treatment in advanced colorectal cancer. J Clin Oncol 2000;18:2938–2947.
130. Gamelin E, Boisdron-Celle M, Guérin-Meyer V, et al. Correlation between uracil and dihydrouracil plasma ratio, fluorouracil (5-FU) pharmacokinetic parameters, and tolerance in patients with advanced colorectal cancer: A potential interest for predicting 5-FU toxicity and determining optimal 5-FU dosage. J Clin Oncol 1999;17:1105–1110.
131. Kemeny NE, Ron IG. Hepatic arterial chemotherapy in metastatic colorectal patients. Semin Oncol 1999;26:524–535.
132. Lorenz ML, Müller HH. Randomized, multicenter trial of fluorouracil plus leucovorin administered either via hepatic arterial or intravenous infusion versus fluorodeoxyuridine administered via hepatic arterial infusion in patients with nonresectable liver metastases from colorectal carcinoma. J Clin Oncol 2000;18:243–254.
133. Cunningham D, Pyrhönen S, James RD, et al. Randomised trial of irinotecan plus supportive care versus supportive care alone after fluorouracil failure for patients with metastatic colorectal cancer. Lancet 1998;352:1413–1418.
134. Rougier P, Van Cutsem E, Bajetta E, et al. Randomised trial of irinotecan versus fluorouracil by continuous infusion after fluorouracil failure in patients with metastatic colorectal cancer. Lancet 1998;352:1407–1412.
135. Rothenberg ML. Efficacy and toxicity of irinotecan in patients with colorectal cancer. Semin Oncol 1998;25(5 suppl 11):39–46.
136. Goldberg RM. Is repeated treatment with a fluorouracil-based regimen useful in colorectal cancer? Semin Oncol 1998;25(5 suppl 11):21–28.
137. André T, Bensmaine MA, Louvet C, et al. Multicenter phase II study of bimonthly high-dose leucovorin, fluorouracil infusion, and oxaliplatin for metastatic colorectal cancer resistant to the same leucovorin and fluorouracil regimen. J Clin Oncol 1999;17:3560–3568.
138. Ross P, Norman A, Cunningham D, et al. A prospective randomized trial of protracted venous infusion 5-fluorouracil with or without mitomycin C in advanced colorectal cancer. Ann Oncol 1997;8:995–1001.
139. Patt YZ, Hoque A, Lozano R, et al. Phase II trial of hepatic arterial infusion of fluorouracil and recombinant human interferon alfa-2b for liver metastases of colorectal cancer refractory to systemic fluorouracil and leucovorin. J Clin Oncol 1997;15:1432–1438.
140. Soulen MC. Chemoembolization of hepatic malignancies. Oncology 1994; 8:77–84.
141. Tellez C, Benson AB, Lyster MT, et al. Phase II trial of chemoembolization for the treatment of metastatic colorectal carcinoma to the liver and review of the literature. Cancer 1998;82:1250–1259.
142. Schrag D, Weeks J. Costs and cost-effectiveness of colorectal cancer prevention and therapy. Semin Oncol 1999;26:561–568.
143. Brown ML, Riley GF, Potosky AL, Etzioni RD. Obtaining long-term disease specific costs of care. Application to Medicare enrollees diagnosed with colorectal cancer. Med Care 1999;37:1249–1259.
144. Brown ML, Nayfield SG, Shibley LM: Adjuvant therapy for stage III colon cancer: Economics returns to research and cost-effectiveness of treatment. J Natl Cancer Inst 1994;86:424–430.
145. Schmitt C, Blijham G, Jolain B, et al. Medical care consumption in a phase III trial comparing irinotecan with infusional 5-fluorouracil (5-FU) in patients with metastatic colorectal cancer after 5-FU failure. Anticancer Drugs 1999;10:617–623.
146. Frazier AL, Colditz GA, Fuchs CS, Kuntz KM. Cost-effectiveness of screening for colorectal cancer in the general population. JAMA 2000; 18:1954–1961.
147. Sonnenberg A, Delco F, Inadomi JM. Cost-effectiveness of colonoscopy in screening for colorectal cancer. Ann Intern Med 2000;133:573–584.
148. Desch CE, Benson AB, Smith TJ, et al. Recommended colorectal cancer surveillance guidelines by the American Society of Clinical Oncology. J Clin Oncol 1999;17:1312–1321.

128
PROSTATE CANCER

Jill M. Kolesar

Prostate cancer is the most frequent cancer among American men and represents the second leading cause of cancer-related deaths in all males.[1] In the United States alone, it is estimated that 198,100 new cases of prostatic carcinoma will be diagnosed and more than 31,500 men will die from this disease in 2001.[1] Although prostate cancer incidence increased during the late 1980s and early 1990s owing to widespread prostate specific antigen (PSA) screening, recent data suggest a continuing decline in prostate cancer incidence and mortality.[1]

Localized prostate cancer can be cured by surgery or radiation therapy; however, advanced prostate cancer is not yet curable. Treatment for advanced prostate cancer can provide significant disease palliation for many patients for several years after diagnosis. The endocrine dependence of this tumor is well documented, and hormonal manipulation to decrease circulating androgens remains the basis for the treatment of advanced disease.

EPIDEMIOLOGY AND ETIOLOGY

Table 128–1 summarizes the possible factors associated with prostate cancer.[2–4] The only widely accepted risk factors for prostate cancer are age, race, and family history of prostate cancer.[3] The disease is rare under the age of 40, but the incidence sharply increases with each subsequent decade, most likely because the individual has had a lifetime exposure to testosterone, a known growth signal for the prostate.[3]

The incidence of clinical prostate cancer varies across geographic regions. Scandinavian countries and the United States report the highest incidence of prostate cancer, whereas the disease is relatively rare in Japan and other Asian countries.[5] African-American men have the highest rate of prostate cancer in the world, and in the United States, overall 5-year survival is approximately 15% less for African-Americans compared with whites.[1] Hormonal, genetic, and dietary differences may contribute to the altered susceptibility to prostate cancer in these populations.[3] Testosterone, commonly implicated in the pathogenesis of prostate cancer, is 15% higher in African-American men compared with white males. Activity of 5-α-reductase, the enzyme that converts testosterone to its more active form, dihydrotestosterone (DHT), in the prostate, is decreased in Japanese men compared with African-Americans and whites.[3] In addition, genetic variations in the androgen receptor exist. Activation of the androgen receptor is inversely correlated with CAG repeat length. Shorter CAG repeat sequences have been found in African-Americans. Therefore, the combination of increased testosterone and increased androgen receptor activation may account for the increased risk of prostate cancer for African-American men.[3] The Asian diet generally is considered to be low in fat and high in fiber with a high concentration of phytoestrogens. Phytoestrogens, consisting of isoflavinoids, flavonoids, and lignans, are potential chemoprotectants.[6] Combining the protection from a low-fat diet with decreased DHT activity may explain the decreased risk of prostate cancer found in Asian men.

A positive family history for prostate cancer is associated with a two- to threefold risk elevation. Three other factors, the age of the man at risk, the age of the affected relative, and the number of relatives diagnosed with prostate cancer, modify the magnitude of the excess risk. In general, younger age (< 65) of the man at risk, younger age of affected relatives, and increased number of relatives with prostate cancer increase the risk of prostate cancer beyond two- to threefold.[3] Carter and colleagues[2] have demonstrated that familial clustering of prostate cancer can be explained by Mendelian inheritance of a rare, autosomal dominant allele, which accounts for 9% of all prostate cancer and 45% of disease reported in men under the age of 55.[2] Genome-wide scans have identified potential prostate cancer susceptibility loci on chromosome 1, 2q, 12p, 15q, 16p, and 16q.[7,8]

Other factors thought to be associated with prostate cancer include occupational exposure, diet, benign prostatic hyperplasia (BPH), and vasectomy.[3] Workers exposed to alkaline batteries come into contact with cadmium, a trace mineral that may be antagonistic to zinc. Zinc is found in very high levels in the prostate and is required in several enzymes involved in DNA and RNA repair and synthesis. Farm and rubber-industry workers also may be at increased risk for prostate cancer.

A number of epidemiologic studies support an association between high fat intake and risk of prostate cancer. A strong correlation between national per capita fat consumption and national prostate cancer mortality has been reported, and prospective case-control studies suggest that a high-fat diet doubles the risk of prostate cancer.

Other dietary factors implicated in prostate cancer include retinol, carotenoids, lycopene, and vitamin D consumption.[3,9] Retinol, or vitamin A, intake, especially in men older than 70, is correlated with an increased risk of prostate cancer, whereas intake of its precursor, β-carotene, has a protective or neutral effect. Lycopene, obtained primarily from tomatoes, decreases the risk of prostate cancer in small cohort studies.[9] The antioxidant vitamin E also may decrease the risk of prostate cancer. Men who developed prostate cancer in one cohort study had lower levels of 1,25$(OH)_2$-vitamin D than matched controls, although a prospective study did not support this.[3] Clearly, dietary risk factors require further evaluation, but because fat and vitamins are modifiable risk factors, dietary intervention may be promising in prostate cancer prevention.

Vasectomy was evaluated as a risk factor for prostate cancer in 5 original cohort studies and 10 case-control studies. Some case-control studies have shown an increased incidence of prostate cancer in men who have had vasectomies, although similarly designed studies also have shown no association. It seems unlikely that prostate cancer and vasectomy are causally linked, and small elevations in risk may be explained by increasing age in the study group and detection bias. BPH is one of the most common problems of elderly men, affecting more than 40% of men over the age of 70. BPH results in the urinary symptoms hesitancy and frequency. Since prostate cancer affects a similar age group and often has similar presenting symptoms, the presence of BPH often complicates the diagnosis of prostate cancer, although it does not appear to increase the risk of developing prostate cancer.[3]

TABLE 128–1. Risk Factors Associated with Prostate Cancer

Factor	Possible Relationship
Probable Risk Factors	
Age	Median incidence in men greater than 50 years old
Race	African-Americans have higher incidence and death rate
Genetic	Familial prostate cancer inherited in an autosomal dominant manner
	Mutations in *p53*, Rb, E-cahedrin, α-catenin, androgen receptor, KIA1, microsatellite instability, loss of heterozygocity at 1, 2q, 12p, 15q, 16p, and 16q
	Candidate prostate cancer gene locus identified on chromosome 1
Possible Risk Factors	
Environmental	Clinical carcinoma incidence varies worldwide
	Latent carcinoma similar between regions
	Nationalized males adopt intermediate incidence rates between that of the United States and their native country
Occupational	Increased risk associated with cadmium exposure
Diet	Increased risk associated with high-meat and -fat diets
	Decreased intake of 1,25-dihydroxyvitamin D, vitamin E, lycopene, and β-carotene increases risk
Hormonal	Does not occur in eunuchs
	Low incidence in cirrhotic patients
	Up to 80% are hormonally dependent
	African-Americans have 15% increased testosterone
	Japanese have decreased 5-α-reductase activities
	Polymorphic expression of the androgen receptor

Compiled from Refs. 3 and 4.

Smoking has not been associated with an increased risk of prostate cancer, however, smokers with prostate cancer have an increased mortality resulting from the disease when compared with nonsmokers with prostate cancer (relative risk 1.5 to 2.0).[3] In addition, in a prospective cohort analysis, alcohol consumption was not associated with the development of prostate cancer.[11]

PATHOPHYSIOLOGY

MOLECULAR GENETICS

A familial association in prostate cancer has been recognized and generally is accepted to be genetically determined, although the precise genetic mechanism has not been identified. In addition, a number of genes are mutated in sporadic cases of prostate cancer, although the relative contribution and interrelationship of these genes are still unknown.

E-cadherin gene inactivation via hypermethylation has been reported frequently in prostate cancer.[4] E-cadherin is a prognostic marker in prostate cancer, with aberrant E-cadherin expression associated with high-grade tumors and poor outcome in terms of disease progression and overall survival.[4] P-cadherin expression is absent in most prostate cancers; however, in prostate cancers where P-cadherin is expressed, PSA is characteristically absent. The cadherin-catenin pathway may be inactivated by gene mutations or hypermethylation and is thought to be an early event in prostate carcinogenesis.

In cells with DNA damage, *p53* is thought to function by halting cell-cycle progression, resulting in cell death via apoptotic pathways. The loss of functional *p53* may result in replication of damaged DNA and subsequently unregulated cell growth. Point mutations in *p53* thought to be caused by environmental toxins have been identified in 42% of prostate carcinomas. Mutations were present in stages B to D, although not in latent prostate carcinomas studied.[12] *Rb* mutations, also thought to be important in cell-cycle regulation, have been reported in prostate cancer patients.[4] Abnormal *p53* and *Rb,* as measured by immunohistochemistry, may be independent predictors of survival. In one study,[13] 15-year survival was 38% in patients with abnormal *p53* compared with 87% for those with normal *p53.* Aberrant *p53* also predicts radiation failure and is mutated in approximately 60% of metastatic bone marrow lesions.[14]

KAI1, or *Kang ai,* which is Chinese for anticancer, is an antimetastatic gene. The gene codes for a protein belonging to a family of leukocyte surface glycoproteins that function in cell-cell interactions and cell–extracellular matrix interactions and that is downregulated, without mutation, during the progression of prostate cancer.[15]

There are currently 374 different reported mutations in the androgen receptor gene.[16] Mutations in the androgen receptor gene appear to occur more frequently in advanced and hormone-refractory prostate cancer.[16] Mutated androgen receptors may be activated not only by testicular androgens but also by several androgens, steroids, and nonsteroidal antiandrogens, promoting subsequemt prostate cancer growth. Androgen receptor mutations are speculated to explain the antiandrogen withdrawal syndrome.[17]

An additional hormonal mechanism may be mutation in 5-α-reductase; the enzyme responsible for converting testosterone to active DHT. In one series, mutations were identified in 57% of prostate cancer patients.[18] While the function of the mutated enzyme has not been identified, it is hypothesized to be an activation, where increased amounts of DHT are formed. A significant number of latent prostatic carcinomas in Japanese men contain an inactivating mutation in the androgen receptor, whereas no such mutations were found in latent carcinomas of white American men.[19] It appears that the stage in which an androgen receptor mutation occurs (latent versus metastatic), as well as the functional significance of the mutation, can alter the clinical course of prostate cancer. Additional genetic analysis has identified mutations in H-*ras* in less than 4% of American prostate carcinomas and up to 25% of Japanese carcinomas. Mutations in late-stage clinical carcinoma were identified in Ha-*ras;* however, latent prostate carcinoma had mutations in K-*ras,* possibly indicating a protective mutation.[4]

Although the molecular characterization of prostate cancer is evolving, this area of study represents a major advance in our understanding of disease pathology and may represent future avenues for diagnosis, staging, and treatment of prostate cancer.

RATIONALE FOR HORMONAL MANAGEMENT

The prostate gland is a solid, rounded, heart-shaped organ positioned between the neck of the bladder and the urogenital diaphragm (Fig. 128–1). The organ consists of single anterior, posterior, and median lobes and two lateral lobes. The posterior lobe is palpable by anterior rectal examination at 2 to 5 cm from the anal verge. Within the four morphologically defined areas of the prostate gland, 95%

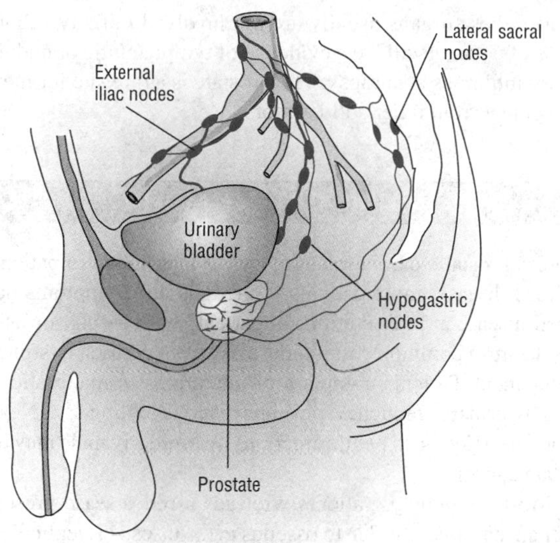

FIGURE 128–1. The prostate gland.

of the carcinomas arise from the glandular epithelium of the peripheral zone.[20] In contrast, benign prostatic hyperplasia arises from the central or periurethral regions of the prostate gland.

Normal growth and differentiation of the prostate depends on the presence of androgens, specifically DHT.[21] The testes and the adrenal glands are the major sources of circulating androgens. Hormonal regulation of androgen synthesis is mediated through a series of biochemical interactions between the hypothalamus, pituitary, adrenal glands, and testes (Fig. 128–2). Luteinizing hormone–releasing hormone (LH-RH) released from the hypothalamus stimulates the release of luteinizing hormone (LH) and follicle-stimulating hormone (FSH) from the anterior pituitary gland. LH complexes with receptors on the Leydig cell testicular membrane and stimulates the production

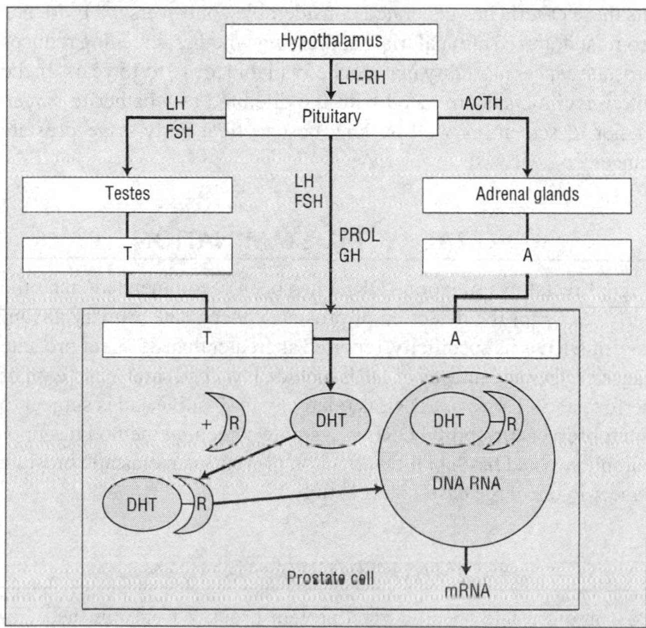

FIGURE 128–2. Hormonal regulation of the prostate gland. LH-RH = luteinizing hormone releasing hormone; LH = luteinizing hormone; FSH = follicle-stimulating hormone; PROL = prolactin; ACTH = adrenocorticotropic hormone; GH = growth hormone; A = androgens; T = testosterone; R = receptor; DHT = dihydrotestosterone.

of testosterone and small amounts of estrogen. FSH acts on the Sertoli cells within the testes to promote the maturation of LH receptors and to produce an androgen-binding protein. Circulating testosterone and estradiol influence the synthesis of LH-RH, LH, and FSH by a negative-feedback loop operating at the hypothalamic and pituitary level.[21] Prolactin, growth hormone, and estradiol appear to be important accessory regulators for prostatic tissue permeability, receptor binding, and testosterone synthesis.

Testosterone, the major androgenic hormone, accounts for 95% of the androgen concentration. The primary source of testosterone is the testes; however, 3% to 5% of the testosterone concentration is derived from direct adrenal cortical secretion of testosterone or C19 steroids such as androstenedione.[18,22]

Only 2% of total plasma testosterone is present in the physiologically active unbound state. The remaining testosterone is reversibly bound to a steroid hormone–binding globulin. The unbound testosterone or androgen precursors penetrate the prostatic cell by passive diffusion and are converted to DHT by 5-α-reductase.[23] DHT subsequently binds with a specific cytoplasmic receptor. This DHT-receptor complex is then transported to the nucleus of the cell, where transcription and ultimately translation of stored genetic material occur.[21]

Huggins and Hodges[24] observed that both normal and malignant prostatic tissue contains a high level of acid phosphatase, suggesting that prostatic malignancy represents an overgrowth of prostate tissue. They then demonstrated that a decrease in serum acid phosphatase along with symptomatic relief occurred in patients with metastatic prostate cancer treated with either estrogens or orchiectomy therapies known to reduce circulating androgens.[24] Androgen ablation is used in the treatment and palliation of advanced prostate cancer because prostatic epithelium undergoes atrophy when the normal physiologic effect of androgens is reduced.[12]

Hormonal manipulations to ablate or reduce circulating androgens can occur through several mechanisms[21,23,26] (Table 128–2). The organs responsible for androgen production can be removed surgically (orchiectomy, hypophysectomy, adrenalectomy). Hormonal pathways that modulate prostatic growth can be interrupted at several steps (see Fig. 128–2). Interference with LH-RH or LH can reduce testosterone secretion by the testes (estrogens, LH-RH agonists, progestogens, and cyproterone acetate). Estrogen administration reduces androgens by directly inhibiting LH release, by acting directly on the prostate cell, or by decreasing free androgens by increasing steroid-binding globulin levels.[21]

Isolation of the naturally occurring hypothalamic decapeptide hormone gonadotropin hormone–releasing hormone or LH-RH has

TABLE 128–2. Hormonal Manipulations in Prostate Cancer

Androgen source ablation	Antiandrogens
Orchiectomy	Flutamide
Adrenalectomy	Bicalutamide
Hypophysectomy	Nilutamide
LH-RH or LH inhibition	Cyproterone acetate[b]
Estrogens	Progesterones
LH-RH agonists	5-α-Reductase inhibition
Progesterones[a]	Finasteride[b]
Cyproterone acetate[b]	
Androgen synthesis inhibition	
Aminoglutethimide	
Ketoconazole	
Progesterones[a]	

[a]Minor mechanisms of action.
[b]Investigational compounds or use.

provided another group of effective agents for advanced prostate cancer treatment.[25–27] The physiologic response to LH-RH depends on both the dose and the mode of administration. Intermittent pulsed LH-RH administration, which mimics the endogenous release pattern, causes sustained release of both LH and FSH, whereas high-dose or continuous intravenous administration of LH-RH inhibits gonadotropin release due to receptor downregulation.[27] Structural modification of the naturally occurring LH-RH and innovative delivery have produced a series of LH-RH agonists that cause a similar downregulation of pituitary receptors and a decrease in testosterone production.[25–27]

Androgen synthesis can be inhibited in the testes or in the adrenal gland. Aminoglutethimide inhibits the desmolase-enzyme complex in the adrenal gland, thereby preventing the conversion of cholesterol to pregnenolone. Pregnenolone is the precursor substrate for all adrenal-derived steroids, including androgens, glucocorticoids, and mineralocorticoids.[28] Ketoconazole, an imidazole antifungal agent, causes a dose-related reversible reduction in serum cortisol and testosterone concentration by inhibiting both adrenal and testicular steroidogenesis.[29] As a secondary mechanism to its antiandrogen action, megestrol acetate inhibits the synthesis of androgens. This inhibition appears to occur at the adrenal level, but circulating levels of testosterone also are reduced, suggesting that inhibition at the testicular level also may occur.[30]

Antiandrogens inhibit the formation of the DHT-receptor complex and thereby interfere with androgen-mediated action at the cellular level.[31–34] Megestrol acetate, a progestational agent, also is available and has antiandrogen actions.[30] Finally, the conversion of testosterone to DHT may be inhibited by 5-α-reductase inhibitors.[34]

PATHOLOGY

The normal prostate is composed of acinar secretory cells arranged in a radial shape and surrounded by a foundation of supporting tissue. The size, shape, or presence of acini is almost always altered in the gland that has been invaded by prostatic carcinoma. Adenocarcinoma, the major pathologic cell type, accounts for more than 95% of prostate cancer cases.[35] Much rarer tumor types include small cell neuroendocrine cancers, sarcomas, and transitional cell carcinomas.

Prostate cancer can be graded systematically according to the histologic appearance of the malignant cell and then grouped into well, moderately, or poorly differentiated grades.[36] Gland architecture is examined and then rated on a scale of 1 (well-differentiated) to 5 (poorly differentiated). Two different specimens are examined, and the score for each specimen is added. Groupings for total Gleason score are 2 to 4 for well-differentiated, 5 or 6 for moderately differentiated, and 7 to 10 for poorly differentiated. Poorly differentiated tumors grow rapidly (poor prognosis), whereas well-differentiated tumors grow slowly (better prognosis).

Metastatic spread can occur by local extension, lymphatic drainage, or hematogenous dissemination.[37] Lymph node metastases are more common in patients with large, undifferentiated tumors that invade the seminal vesicles. The pelvic and abdominal lymph node groups are the most common sites of lymph node involvement (see Fig. 128–1). Skeletal metastases from hematogenous spread are the most common sites of distant spread. Typically, the bone lesions are osteoblastic or a combination of osteoblastic and osteolytic. The most common site of bone involvement is the lumbar spine. Other sites of bone involvement include the proximal femurs, pelvis, thoracic spine, ribs, sternum, skull, and humerus. The lung, liver, brain, and adrenal glands are the most common sites of visceral involvement; however, these organs usually are not involved initially. About 25% to 35% of patients will have evidence of lymphangitic or nodular pulmonary infiltrates at autopsy. The prostate is a rare site for metastatic involvement from other solid tumors.

CLINICAL PRESENTATION

Whereas prostatic carcinoma may be asymptomatic in patients with localized disease, most patients with signs and symptoms have advanced disease at presentation. In patients with locally invasive disease, the most common complaints arise from ureteral dysfunction or impingement. Patients complain of alterations in micturation manifested by urinary frequency, hesitancy, and dribbling.[35,37] New-onset impotence or less firm penile erections in an elderly male may indicate prostate cancer.

Most commonly, patients with advanced disease present with back pain and stiffness due to osseous metastases.[38] Eventually, spinal cord lesions may lead to cord compression if not treated properly.[38] Rarely, pathologic fractures can occur. Lower extremity edema can occur as a result of lymphatic obstruction. Anemia and weight loss are nonspecific signs of advanced disease.

CURRENT SCREENING RECOMMENDATIONS

Since prostate cancer is not curable in advanced stages, prevention efforts are under intensive evaluation. Primary prevention with finasteride is being evaluated in the Prostate Cancer Prevention Trial (PCPT), with completion projected in 2004. Until results from this trial are available, primary prevention with finasteride cannot be recommended. Early detection of potentially curable prostate cancers is the goal of prostate cancer screening. For cancer screening to be beneficial, it must reliably detect cancer in an early stage, when intervention would decrease mortality. Whether prostate cancer screening fits these criteria has generated considerable controversy.[40] Evidence from randomized clinical trials addressing whether screening reduces prostate cancer mortality may not be available for 10 to 15 years. In the interim, clinicians are faced with the dilemma of whether to screen or not to screen, as well as how best to treat early-stage prostate cancer.

DIGITAL RECTAL EXAMINATION

Digital rectal examination (DRE) has been recommended since the early 1900s for the detection of prostate cancer. The primary advantage of DRE is its specificity, reported at greater than 85%, for prostate cancer. Other advantages of DRE include low cost, safety, and ease of performance. However, DRE is relatively insensitive and is subject to interobserver variability. DRE as a single screening method has poor compliance and has had little effect on preventing metastatic prostate cancer in one large case-control study.[41]

PROSTATE-SPECIFIC ANTIGEN

PSA is a prostate-specific glycoprotein produced only in the cytoplasm of benign and malignant prostate cells.[42] PSA functions as a serine protease, which liquefies seminal fluid after ejaculation. In addition to its biologic activity, PSA also may enhance cellular growth by its ability to cleave insulin-like growth factor–binding proteins. Cleavage activates insulin-like growth factor (IGF), which can then bind to IGF receptors and stimulate growth in the prostate.[42]

Unlike acid phosphatase, PSA levels are not influenced by ambient conditions or subject to diurnal variation but are influenced by sedentary conditions. Therefore, it is recommended that all PSA measurements be made on sera collected from ambulatory patients.[39] PSA levels not only rise with prostatic manipulation such as transrectal ultrasound (TRUS) and/or biopsy but also remain above normal for several weeks thereafter. PSA has a serum half-life of 2 to 3 days.[42]

PSA is used widely for prostate cancer screening in the United States, with simplicity its major advantage and low specificity its primary limitation. PSA may be elevated in men with acute urinary retention, acute prostatitis, prostatic ischemia, infarction, as well as BPH, a nearly universal condition in men at risk for prostate cancer. PSA elevations between 4.1 and 10 ng/mL cannot distinguish between BPH and prostate cancer, limiting the utility of PSA alone for the early detection of prostate cancer. Additionally, only 38% to 48% of men with clinically significant prostate cancer have a serum PSA outside the reference range.[42]

Neither DRE nor PSA is sensitive or specific enough to be used alone as a screening test.[42] Although the relative predictability of DRE and PSA is similar, the tumors identified by each method are different. Catalona and associates[43] confirmed that the combination of a DRE plus PSA determination is a better method of detecting prostate cancer than DRE alone.

Efforts to increase PSA specificity include the use of free PSA measurements, age- and race-specific PSA levels, PSA density, and PSA velocity.[44] An increase in serum PSA with increasing age in the absence of clinically detectable prostate cancer has been documented by a number of investigators. The proposed age-specific PSA reference ranges (upper limit defined by the 95th percentile) for white and African-American men are provided in Table 128–3.[44]

CURRENT SCREENING RECOMMENDATIONS

The common approach to prostate cancer screening today involves offering PSA measurements beginning at age 50 to all men of normal risk with a 10-year or greater life expectancy. Despite this common practice, the benefits of prostate cancer screening are unproven. PSA measurements can identify small, subclinical prostate cancers, where no intervention may be required. Detecting prostate cancer in those not needing therapy not only increases the cost of care through unecessary screening and workups but also increases the toxicity of therapy, by subjecting some patients to unecessary therapy.[45]

TABLE 128–3. Diagnostic Algorithm for Prostate Cancer

PSA[a]	DRE[b]	Diagnostic Action
≤Age-specific range[c]	Neg	Offer annual PSA and DRE
>Age-specific range[c]	Neg	TRUS: Biopsy-visible lesions. Sextant biopsy of remaining prostate, with two cores containing transition zone tissue
Any value	Pos	TRUS: Biopsy-palpable and -visible lesions; sextant biopsy of remaining prostate

[a]Tandem-R or IMx PSA.
[b]Digital rectal exam.
[c]

Age Range (yr)	Normal PSA Range (ng/mL) White	African-American
40–49	0–2.5	0–2.0
50–59	0–3.5	0–4.0
60–69	0–4.5	0–4.5
70–79	0–6.5	0–5.5

Compiled from Ref. 42.

Currently, the American College of Physicians recommends that rather than screening all men for prostate cancer as a matter of routine, physicians should describe the potential benefits and known harms of screening, diagnosis, and treatment, listen to the patient's concerns, and then decide on an individual's course of therapy. In a randomized, controlled trial of an educational videotape describing the advantages and disadvantages of prostate cancer screening, patients who viewed the videotape had an increase of 78% ($P = .001$) in prostate cancer knowledge and a decrease of 18.5% ($P = .009$) in requests for screening over control patients.[46] The American Cancer Society (ACS) currently recommends that DRE and PSA be offered annually to men beginning at age 50 years with at least a 10-year life expectancy and to younger men (45 years old) who are considered to be at high risk for prostate cancer development (strong familial predisposition or African-American).[44] The ACS defines an abnormal PSA value to be above 4.0 ng/mL. If both tests are normal, no further diagnostic action is required; however, if either is abnormal, further workup by TRUS is indicated.

Two ongoing national randomized trials will provide important data to help resolve the prostate cancer screening controversies. The first is the Prostate, Lung, Colon, and Ovarian (PLCO) Trial, which is designed to test the efficacy of prostate cancer screening in 74,000 men age 60 to 74.[41] The second is the Prostate Cancer Intervention Versus Observation (PIVOT) Trial, which is a randomized study comparing radical prostatectomy with expectant management. These trials, when completed likely will provide key information regarding the costs and benefits of prostate cancer screening and the most appropriate early management.[47]

DIAGNOSIS

Transperianal or transrectal prostate biopsy is necessary to confirm a prostate cancer diagnosis and to grade the tumor specimen. TRUS-guided biopsies of hypoechoic areas may help define extraprostatic extension.[37] For patients with visceral or lytic metastases, these lesions should be biopsied, because this presentation is common for one of the variant histologies (small cell neuroendocrine) that requires a treatment strategy different from that for adenocarcinomas.[48]

Table 128–4 summarizes the diagnostic staging workup. When DRE is performed, prostatic carcinoma is classically characterized

TABLE 128–4. Diagnostic and Staging Workup for Prostate Cancer

Initial tests	Digital rectal examination (DRE) Prostate-specific antigen (PSA) Transrectal ultrasonography (TRUS) if either DRE positive or PSA elevated Biopsy
Staging tests	Gleason score on biopsy specimen Bone scan Complete blood count Liver function tests Serum phosphatases (acid/alkaline) Excretory urogram Chest x-ray
Additional staging tests (depends on T classification, PSA, and Gleason score)	Skeletal films Lymph node evaluation Pelvic CT scan ^{111}In-labeled capromab pendetide scan Bipedal lymphangiogram Transrectal MRI

by a rock-hard nodule or mass in the gland, whereas the gland is smooth and rubbery in BPH. Recent studies have demonstrated that elevated PSA values may predict for pelvic lymph node and bone involvement.[42] If these findings are confirmed, it might be possible to avoid some staging tests (pelvic lymph node dissection, bone scans) in some patients.

STAGING

The information obtained from the diagnostic tests is used to stage the patient. There are two commonly recognized staging classification systems (Table 128–5). The formal international classification system (TNM), adopted by the International Union Against Cancer (UICC) in 1974, was updated in 1992 in an effort to provide congruence with the classical American Urologic System (AUS) staging system for prostate cancer.[49] The AUS classification is the most commonly used staging system in the United States (see Table 128–5). Patients are assigned to stages A through D and corresponding subcategories based on size of the tumor (T), local or regional extension, presence of involved lymph node groups (N), and presence of metastases (M).[49] Some studies classify patients who have progressed after hormonal therapy as stage D_3.[37,49] Based on National Cancer Database figures from 1993 including over 84,400 prostate cancer diagnoses, 25%, 49%, 15%, and 12% are initially diagnosed as stage 0 to I, II, III, and IV, respectively.[54] Localized prostate cancer (stages 0 to I and II) was diagnosed more frequently (74% versus 65%) and advanced disease (stages III and IV) was diagnosed less frequently (26% versus 34%) when comparing the 1990 to the 1986 incidence rates.

PROGNOSIS

The prognosis for patients with prostate cancer depends on the histologic grade, the tumor size, and the local extent of the primary tumor.[36] The most important prognostic criterion appears to be the histologic grade, because the degree of differentiation ultimately determines the stage of disease. Poorly differentiated tumors are highly associated with both regional lymph node involvement and distant metastases.[36] Other prognostic factors that are being explored include DNA content, cell proliferative activity, epidermal growth factor (EGF), transforming growth factor α, EGF receptor, *ERBB2* oncogene, *ras* oncogene, *RB1* tumor-suppressor gene, *p53* tumor-suppressor gene, and change in PSA.[51]

During 1986 to 1993, 5-year overall survival rates were estimated at 90% for whites and 75% for African-Americans.[1] For this same

TABLE 128–5. Staging and Classification Systems for Prostate Cancer

AUS[a] Stage (A–D)	AJC-UICC[b] Classification (TNM)
A (occult, nonpalpable)	$T_XN_XM_X$ (cannot be assessed)
	$T_0N_0M_0$ (nonpalpable)
A_1: Focal	T_0: Focal or diffuse
A_2: Diffuse	
B (confined to prostate)	$T_1N_0M_0$, $T_2N_0M_0$
B_1: Single nodule in one lobe, <1.5 cm	T_1 (Clinically inapparent tumor not palpable or visible by imaging)
	T_{1a}: Tumor incidental histologic finding in 5% or less of tissue resected
	T_{1b}: Tumor incidental histologic finding in 5% or more of tissue resected
	T_{1c}: Tumor identified by needle biopsy (e.g., because of elevated PSA)
B_2: Diffuse involvement of whole gland, >1.5 cm	T_2: (Tumor confined within the prostate[c])
	T_{2a}: Tumor involves half of a lobe or less
	T_{2b}: Tumor involves more than half a lobe, but not both lobes
	T_{2c}: Tumor involves both lobes
C (localized to periprostatic area)	$T_3N_0M_0$, $T_4N_0M_0$
C_1: No seminal vesicle involvement, <70 g	T_3: (Tumor extends through the prostatic capsule[d])
	T_{3a}: Unilateral extracapsular extension
	T_{3b}: Bilateral extracapsular extension
	T_{3c}: Tumor invades the seminal vesicle(s)
C_2: Seminal vesicle involvement, >70 g	T_4: (Tumor is fixed or invades adjacent structures other than the seminal vesicles)
	T_{4a}: Tumor invades any of bladder neck, external sphincter, or rectum
	T_{4b}: Tumor invades levator muscles and/or is fixed to the pelvic wall
D (metastatic disease)	Any T, N_{1-4}, M_0, or N_{0-4}, M_1
D_1: Pelvic lymph nodes or ureteral obstruction	N_1: Metastasis in a single lymph node, 2 cm or less in greatest dimension
D_2: Bone, distant lymph node, organ, or soft tissue metastases	N_2: Metastasis in single lymph node more than 2 cm but not more than 5 cm in greatest dimension; or multiple lymph node metastases, none more than 5 cm in greatest dimension
	N_3: Metastasis in lymph node more than 5 cm in greatest dimension
	M_{1a}: Nonregional lymph node(s)
	M_{1b}: Bone(s)
	M_{1c}: Other site(s)

[a]American Urologic System.
[b]American Joint Committee–International Union Against Cancer.
[c]Note: Tumor found in one or both lobes by needle biopsy, but not palpable or visible by imaging, is classified as T_{1c}.
[d]Note: Invasion into the prostatic apex or into (but not beyond) the prostatic capsule is not classified as T_3 but as T_2.
From Ref. 49, with permission.

period, the survival rates for localized disease (100%), regional disease (95%), and distant disease (31%) in white males were higher than the survival rates for localized disease (91%), regional disease (85%), and distant disease (26%) in African-American males.[1] A 6.3% decline in age-adjusted mortality has been documented for the period 1991 to 1995.[52] Ten-year cancer-specific survival is estimated as 95% for stage A_1, 80% for stages A_2 to B_2, 60% for stage C, 40% for stage D_1, and 10% for stage D_2.[53] It is estimated that more than 85% of patients with stage A_1 can be cured, whereas fewer than 1% of patients with stage D_2 will be cured.

▶ TREATMENT: Prostate Cancer

DESIRED OUTCOME

Localized prostate cancer is curable, and treatment modalities (surgery and radiation) should be performed with an effort to reduce any postprocedure complications (impotence, stricture, and incontinence).[35] Advanced prostate cancer (stage D) is not currently curable, and treatment should focus on providing symptom relief and maintaining quality of life.[50]

GENERAL APPROACH TO TREATMENT

The initial treatment for prostate cancer depends primarily on the disease stage.[35,48] Figure 128–3 shows the National Comprehensive Cancer Network (NCCN) consensus-based practice guidelines for initial prostate cancer management.[48] All the treatment options were considered "category 1" by the panel of experts that developed these guidelines; this means that the recommendations were uncontested and generally accepted by all panel members.

Patients with incidental carcinoma found at the time of a transurethral resection for BPH (stage A_1 or T_{1a} or T_{1b}) usually require only careful observation because the 10-year survival rate for these patients is very high.[35] The patient's life expectancy and the probability of having organ-confined disease, as judged by clinical stage, PSA levels, and Gleason score, may alter the treatment decision for patients with stage T_1 or T_2 prostate cancer.[35,48,55] More aggressive therapy is used when the patient's life expectancy exceeds 10 years.[35,48] Patient preference is also important to consider.

Radical prostatectomy and radiation therapy generally are considered therapeutically equivalent for localized prostate cancer,

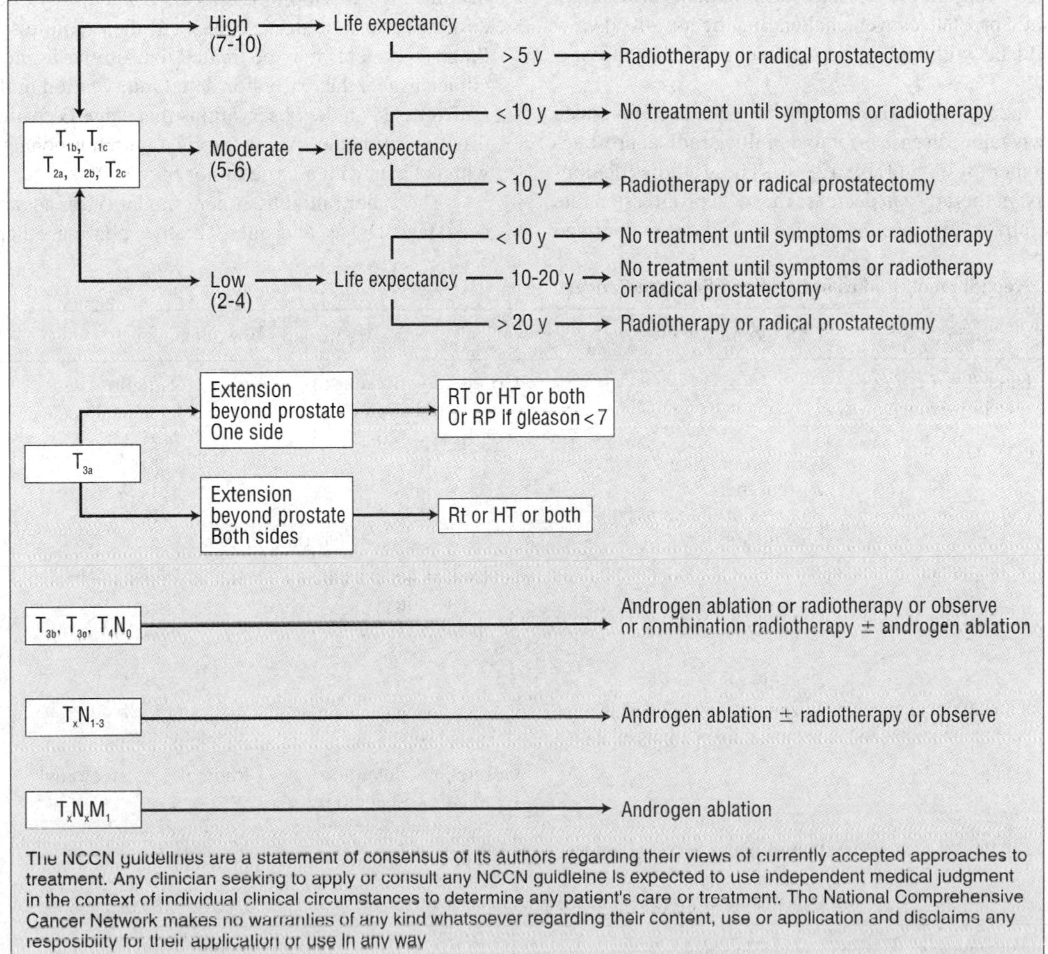

FIGURE 128–3. Initial therapy for prostate cancer. *(Copyrighted by the National Comprehensive Cancer Network. All rights reserved. These guidelines and illustrations may not be reproduced in any form without the express written permission of the NCCN.)*

although neither have been proven better than observation alone.[48,55] A prospective, randomized trial comparing the two treatments showed a cause-specific survival of 81.2% in the surgery group and 84.6% ($p = 0.024$) in the radiation group. Patients in the surgery group also had an increased incidence of incontinence and a poorer quality of life, suggesting that radiation therapy may be preferred.[56] Complications from radical prostatectomy include blood loss, stricture formation, incontinence, lymphocele, fistula formation, anesthetic risk, and impotence.[57] Nerve-sparing radical prostatectomy can be performed in many patients; 50% to 80% regain sexual potency within the first year.[58] Acute complications from radiation therapy include cystitis, proctitis, hematuria, urinary retention, penoscrotal edema, and impotence (30% incidence).[35,37] Chronic complications include proctitis, diarrhea, cystitis, enteritis, impotence, urethral stricture, and incontinence.[35,37] Since radiation and prostatectomy have significant and immediate morbidity when compared with observation alone, many patients may elect to postpone therapy until symptoms develop. There are ongoing studies to define the best treatment for patients with stage B_2 or C disease.[35,37] The failure rate for stage C patients is much higher than for either stage A or B patients, and better diagnostic techniques have demonstrated that some stage C patients have occult disease dissemination at presentation. Although external beam radiotherapy has been the primary treatment option, some investigators feel there is also a role for androgen deprivation prior to definitive local treatment (neoadjuvant hormonal therapy). Recent evidence suggests that immediate initiation of androgen-ablation therapy after radiation therapy improves survival in patients with node-positive or metastatic prostate cancer, challenging the long-held view that therapy should be withheld in these patients until symptoms develop.[59]

Neoadjuvant androgen-ablative therapy has been used to reduce tumor size or "downstage" disease prior to definitive radical prostatectomy or radiation therapy[60–62] (Table 128–6). These studies demonstrate that neoadjuvant therapy can decrease the local progression rate after radiation therapy or increase the chance to find organ-confined disease at surgery in clinical stage T_1 and T_2 prostate cancers.[61,63] In a prospective evaluation with more than 5 years of follow-up, neoadjuvant hormonal therapy prior to radical prostatectomy resulted in disease downstaging and a decrease in PSA failure, but only in patients receiving combined androgen blockade (CAB) for longer than 3 months.[64] These preliminary studies provide encouraging results, and flutamide (in combination with an LH-RH agonist) has been approved for use prior to and during the period of radiation therapy for patients with stage B_2 or C prostate cancer. However, the optimal duration of neoadjuvant therapy and optimal regimen need to be more fully evaluated.[63]

Cryosurgery[65] or brachytherapy (interstitial radiotherapy)[66] has been used for localized prostate cancer, however, there is not long enough follow-up to recommend these modalities over radical prostatectomy or radiotherapy as primary therapy.

The treatment of patients with localized prostate cancer remains less than optimal because many of the studies used inadequate methods to define the patient populations treated and assess outcomes.[67] No intermediate end points, including PSA levels, are known to be valid surrogate markers, so investigation using compounds such as ^{111}In-labeled capromab pendedite[68] to help determine disease extent should continue.[67]

There is controversy about the best approach to treating patients with stage D prostate cancer because therapy is palliative and cure is not possible. Patients with stage D_0 prostate cancer may be watched carefully, and appropriate local therapy (surgery or radiation) may be instituted when symptoms appear. The majority of these patients will develop metastatic disease and will then require systemic therapy.[35] Stage D_1 patients may be treated in a similar fashion; however, some clinicians feel that early hormonal intervention in these cases is warranted based on the observations that stage D_2 patients with minimal disease have better overall survival with hormonal therapy compared with patients with a large tumor burden.[69]

The major initial treatment modality for advanced prostate cancer (stage D_2) is androgen-ablative pharmacotherapy using either

TABLE 128–6. Neoadjuvant Studies in Localized Prostate Cancer

Reference	Stage(s)	Outcome Parameter(s)	Treatment Outcome		Significance
60	Large T_2, T_3, T_4 No bone mets. (B_2–C)		Goserelin + flutamide[a] + radiation $N = 226$	Radiation $N = 230$	
		Local progression[b]	46%	71%	$P < .001$
		Distant mets.[b]	34%	41%	$P = .09$
		Progression-free survival[b]	36%	15%	$P < .001$
		Overall survival[b]	No difference		$P = .7$
62	$T_{2b}N_XM_0$ (B_2)		Leuprolide + flutamide + radical prostatectomy[c] $N = 138$	Radical prostatectomy $N = 144$	
		Capsule penetration	47%	78%	$P < .001$
		Tumor at urethral margin	6%	17%	$P < .01$
		Tumor at inked margin	18%	48%	$P < .001$
61	T_1, T_2, T_3		Goserelin + flutamide[c] + radical prostatectomy $N = 69$	Radical prostatectomy[d] $N = 72$	
		Pathologic organ confined	73%	56%	
		Positive margins	17%	36%	
		PSA disease-free rate	89%	84%	

[a]Given for 2 months before radiation, then for 2 months during radiation.
[b]Evaluated at 5 years.
[c]Given for 3 months prior to radical prostatectomy.
[d]Nonrandomized control group.

orchiectomy or LH-RH agonists either alone or combined with antiandrogens.[21,35] Estrogens also have been used; however, the primary estrogen, diethylstilbesterol (DES), was withdrawn from the U.S. market in 1997. Recently, there is a renewed interest in intramuscular estrogen.[70] Secondary hormonal manipulations, cytotoxic chemotherapy, or supportive care is used for the patient who progresses after initial therapy.

ORCHIECTOMY

Bilateral orchiectomy rapidly reduces circulating androgens to castrate levels (< 50 ng/dL).[35] Unfortunately, many patients are not surgical candidates owing to their advanced age, and other patients find this procedure psychologically unacceptable.[35] Orchiectomy is probably the preferred initial treatment in patients with impending spinal cord compression or ureteral obstruction.

LH-RH AGONISTS

LH-RH agonists are a reversible method of androgen ablation and are as effective as orchiectomy in treating prostate cancer.[69] Currently available LH-RH agonists include leuprolide,[25] leuprolide depot,[25,70] and goserelin acetate implant.[26] Leuprolide acetate is administered once daily, whereas leuprolide depot and goserelin acetate implant can be administered either once monthly, once every 12 weeks, or once every 16 weeks (leuprolide depot, 4 months). A leuprolide implant administered annually is in clinical trials and is effective in suppressing testosterone.[72] The leuprolide depot formulation contains leuprolide acetate in coated pellets. The dose is administered intramuscularly, and the coating dissolves at different rates to allow sustained leuprolide levels throughout the dosing interval. Goserelin acetate implant contains goserelin acetate dispersed in a plastic matrix of D, L-lactic and glycolic acid copolymer and is administered subcutaneously. Hydrolysis of the copolymer material provides continuous release of goserelin over the dosing period.

Several randomized trials have demonstrated that leuprolide and goserelin are effective agents when used alone in patients with advanced prostate cancer.[25,26] Response rates around 80% have been reported, with a lower incidence of adverse effects compared with estrogens.[25,26] There are no direct comparative trials of the currently available LH-RH agonists, but a recent meta-analysis reported that there is no difference in efficacy or toxicity between leuprolide and gosrelin. Therefore, the choice between the two is usually made based on cost and patient and physician preference for a dosing schedule.

The most common adverse effects reported with LH-RH agonist therapy include a disease flare-up during the first week of therapy, hot flashes, erectile impotence, decreased libido, and injection-site reactions.[25,26] The disease flare-up is thought to be caused by initial induction of LH and FSH by the LH-RH agonist and manifests clinically as either increased bone pain or increased urinary symptoms.[25,26] This flare reaction usually resolves after 2 weeks and has a similar onset and duration pattern for the depot LH-RH products.[70,71]

LH-RH agonist monotherapy can be used as initial therapy, with similar response rates to orchiectomy and estrogen administration expected. There is a lower incidence of cardiovascular related adverse effects associated with LH-RH therapy than with estrogen administration. Patients should be counseled to expect worsening symptoms during the first week of therapy, and caution should be exercised when initiating LH-RH agonist therapy in patients with widely metastatic disease involving the spinal cord or having the potential for ureteral obstruction because irreversible complications may occur.

TABLE 128–7. Antiandrogens

Antiandrogen	Usual Dose	Adverse Effects
Flutamide	750 mg/day	Gynecomastia Hot flushes Gastrointestinal disturbances (diarrhea) Liver function test abnormalities Breast tenderness Methemoglobinemia
Bicalutamide	50 mg/day	Gynecomastia Hot flushes Gastrointestinal disturbances (diarrhea) Liver function test abnormalities Breast tenderness
Nilutamide	300 mg/day for 1st month then 150 mg/day	Gynecomastia Hot flushes Gastrointestinal disturbances (nausea or constipation) Liver function test abnormalities Breast tenderness Visual disturbances (impaired dark adaptation) Alcohol intolerance Interstitial pneumonitis

ANTIANDROGENS

Three antiandrogens, flutamide,[31] bicalutamide,[33,72] and nilutamide,[32] are currently available (Table 128–7).

Antiandrogens have been used as monotherapy in previously untreated patients, but a recent meta-analysis determined that monotherapy with antiandrogens is less effective than LH-RH agonist therapy.[71] Efficacy of the antiandrogens was similar. Flutamide has a response rate of 50% to 87%,[31] bicalutamide has a response rate of 54% to 70%,[73] and nilutamide has a response rate of approximately 40%.[74] Objective responses are manifested as decreased bone pain, decreased prostate size, decreased PSA, and/or improved performance status. However, for advanced prostate cancer, all currently available antiandrogens are indicated only in combination with androgen-ablation therapy; flutamide and bicalutamide are indicated in combination with an LH-RH agonist, and nilutamide is indicated in combination with orchiectomy.[31–33]

The most common antiandrogen-related adverse effects are listed in Table 128–7. In the only randomized comparison of bicalutamide plus an LH-RH agonist versus flutamide plus an LH-RH agonist, diarrhea was more common in flutamide-treated patients.[75,76] Antiandrogens can reduce the symptoms from the flare phenomenon associated with LH-RH agonist therapy.

COMBINED HORMONAL BLOCKADE

Although up to 80% of patients with advanced prostate cancer will respond to initial hormonal manipulation, almost all patients will relapse within 2 to 4 years after initiating therapy.[35] Two mechanisms have been proposed to explain this tumor resistance.[77] The tumor could be heterogeneously composed of cells that are hormone-dependent and hormone-independent, or the tumor could be stimulated by extratesticular androgens that are converted intracellularly to DHT. The rationale for combination hormonal therapy is to interfere with multiple hormonal pathways to completely eliminate androgen action. In clinical trials, combination hormonal therapy, sometimes also referred to as *maximal androgen deprivation* or *total androgen blockade,* has been used. The combination of LH-RH agonists or orchiectomy with antiandrogens is the most extensively studied combined androgen-deprivation approach.

Labrie and colleagnes[78] provided information for the initial reports combining an LH-RH agonist with flutamide and subsequently have provided follow-up for 363 patients. Response rates, the main end point of these studies, have been greater than 90% in previously untreated patients.[78] However, response rates of less than 35% have been observed with this combination in patients previously treated with initial hormonal manipulation.

These studies, although quite encouraging, have been criticized for lack of a concurrent control arm and for using response rather than survival as the final end point. For these reasons, the National Cancer Institute (NCI) sponsored a randomized, placebo-controlled, double-blind multicenter trial comparing leuprolide with leuprolide plus 250 mg flutamide orally three times a day in newly diagnosed patients with stage D prostate cancer.[69,78]

Both median progression-free survival (16.5 versus 13.9 months) and overall median survival (35.6 versus 28.3 months) were significantly longer in the 303 evaluable patients treated with leuprolide plus flutamide than in the 300 evaluable patients treated with leuprolide alone. The best response to combination therapy was observed in patients with minimal disease (no disease in ribs, long bones, or soft tissue other than lymph nodes) and a good performance status. An update of this trial has demonstrated that median survival was 61 months in the combination arm and 41 months in the leuprolide-alone arm in patients with minimal disease.[79] The addition of flutamide to leuprolide reduced the symptoms from the flare phenomenon associated with LH-RH agonist therapy. Patients in both groups experienced common adverse effects associated with LH-RH agonist treatment. Diarrhea was the only additional adverse effect attributable to flutamide administration. In a comparison of goserelin with goserelin and flutamide conducted in 589 patients and with 10 years of follow-up, CAB showed no benefit over goserelin alone.[80]

Several other studies comparing CAB with conventional medical or surgical castration have been performed[76,81–84] (Table 128–8). In studies with LH-RH agonists, the results have varied, with no consistent benefit demonstrated for CAB.

A recently completed NCI intergroup trial involving 1371 evaluable stage D_2 prostate cancer patients failed to show any significant survival benefits for the combination of orchiectomy plus flutamide over orchiectomy alone.[84] Like other studies of CAB, overall survival was longest in patients with minimal disease. Diarrhea, elevated liver function tests, and anemia were more common in those patients who received flutamide.

A meta-analysis of 22 randomized trials in 5710 patients comparing maximal androgen blockade with conventional medical or surgical castration failed to show any additional survival benefit for maximal androgen blockade.[85]

In one of the few combination androgen-deprivation studies comparing two different antiandrogens (bicalutamide versus flutamide), the time to treatment failure (the main study end point), time to progression (as defined by appearance of new or worsening bone or extraskeletal lesions), and time to death were equivalent, suggesting that the two treatments are equally effective.[86]

Although some investigators now consider CAB to be the initial hormonal therapy of choice for newly diagnosed patients, the clinician is left to weigh the costs of combined therapy against potential benefits in light of conflicting results in the randomized trials.[21] For those trials which did show an advantage for CAB, whether these effects are specific to the testosterone-deprivation method (orchiectomy versus leuprolide versus goserelin), the antiandrogen (flutamide versus bicalutamide versus nilutamide), the duration of therapy, or patient selection is not clear. Until further carefully designed studies that use survival, time to progression, quality of life, patient preference, and cost as end points are conducted, it is appropariate to use either LH-RH agonist monotherapy or CAB as initial therapy for metastatic prostate cancer. CAB may be most beneficial for improving survival

TABLE 128–8. Summary of Randomized Combined Androgen Blockade Trials

Reference	Treatment	*N*	Disease-free Survival (mo)		Overall Median Survival (mo)	
69	Leuprolide	300	13.9		28.3	
	Leuprolide + flutamide	303	16.5	*P* = .039	35.6	*P* = .035
81	Orchiectomy	133	16.8		27.6	
	Goserelin + flutamide	129	16.5	NS	22.7	NS
82	Orchiectomy	148			27.1	
	Goserelin + flutamide	149			34.4	*P* = .02
84	Goserelin	282			26.9	
	Goserelin + flutamide	287			29	NS
74	Orchiectomy	208	14.7		29.8	
	Orchiectomy + nilutamide	202	20.8	*P* = .0041	37.1	*P* = .0041
79	Orchiectomy	681	19		30	
	Orchiectomy + flutamide	690	20	NS	32	NS
76	Goserelin + bicalutamide	404	0.9 (0.75–1.08)[a]		0.87 (0.754–1.03)[a]	
	Goserelin + flutamide	409				

[a]Reported as the hazard ratio for goserelin + bicalutamide compared to goserelin + flutamide.
NS = not significant.

in patients with minimal disease and for preventing tumor flare, particularily in those with advanced metastatic disease. All other patients may be started on LH-RH monotherapy, and an antiandrogen may be added after several months if androgen ablation is incomplete.

There is still considerable debate concerning when to start hormonal-deprivation therapy in patients with advanced prostate cancer.[87] The original recommendation to start therapy when symptoms appeared was based on the Veterans Administration Cooperative Urologic Research Group (VACURG) trials, in which no overall survival difference was demonstrated in patients who either started DES initially or crossed over to active treatment when symptoms appeared; the excess mortality was attributed to estrogen administration.[88] Because LH-RH agonists and antiandrogens are considered suitable alternatives with less cardiovascular toxicity, it is not clear whether delaying therapy is justified. Reanalysis of the original VACURG data[89] and recent combined androgen deprivation trials[83,90] demonstrate a survival advantage for young, good-performance-status, minimal-disease patients treated initially with hormonal therapy, suggesting that early intervention before symptoms appear may be appropriate.[87] The issue of when best to start hormonal therapy is the subject of several clinical trials.[87]

ESTROGENS

DES was once a mainstay of prostate cancer therapy. While very effective in androgen ablation, DES-treated patients experienced increased cardiovascular mortality.[88] LH-RH agonists, with equivalent efficacy and decreased cardiovascular toxicity, supplanted DES as a mainstay of therapy. Recent evidence suggesting that parenteral estrogen reduces or negates the adverse cardiovascular effects of estrogen has renewed interest in estrogen androgen ablation. Hedlund and colleagues compared monthly intramuscular injections of polyestradiol phosphate with total androgen blockade by orchiectomy or CAB in 915 men, showing no difference in survival or cardiovascular mortality.[70] Other available estrogenic substances, such as ethinyl estradiol, conjugated estrogens, chlorotrianisene, and polyestradiol phosphate, cost more than DES and have not been studied as extensively.[21]

SECONDARY TREATMENTS

Secondary or salvage therapies for patients who progress after their initial therapy depend on what was used for initial management[48] (Fig. 128–4). For patients initially diagnosed with localized prostate cancer, radiotherapy can be used in the case of failed radical prostatectomy. Alternatively, androgen ablation can be used in patients who progress after either radiation therapy or radical prostatectomy.

Secondary hormonal manipulations, such as adding an antiandrogen to a patient who incompletely suppresses testosterone secretion with an LH-RH agonist, or withdrawing antiandrogens in a patient receiving combination therapy, or using agents that inhibit androgen synthesis, can be attempted in patients initially treated with one hormonal modality. Supportive care, chemotherapy, or local radiotherapy can be used in patients who have failed all forms of androgen-ablation manipulations because these patients are considered to have androgen-independent disease.

For patients who initially received an LH-RH agonist alone, castrate testosterone levels should be documented. Patients with inadequate testosterone suppression (> 20 ng/dL) can be treated by adding an antiandrogen or performing an orchiectomy. If castrate testosterone levels have been achieved, the patient is considered to have androgen-independent disease, and palliative androgen-independent salvage therapy can be used.

If the patient initially received combined androgen blockade with an LH-RH agonist with an antiandrogen, then androgen withdrawal would be the first salvage manipulation. Objective and subjective responses have been noted following the discontinuation of flutamide,[92] bicalutamide,[72,93] or nilutamide[94] in patients receiving these agents as part of combined androgen ablation with an LH-RH agonist. Mutations in the androgen receptor have been demonstrated that allow antiandrogens such as flutamide, bicalutamide, and nilutamide (or their metabolites) to become agonists and activate the androgen receptor.[95] Patient responses to androgen withdrawal manifest as significant PSA reductions and improved clinical symptoms. Androgen withdrawal responses lasting 3 to 14 months have been noted in up to 35% of patients, and predicting response seems to be most closely related to longer androgen exposure times.[17] Incomplete cross-resistance has

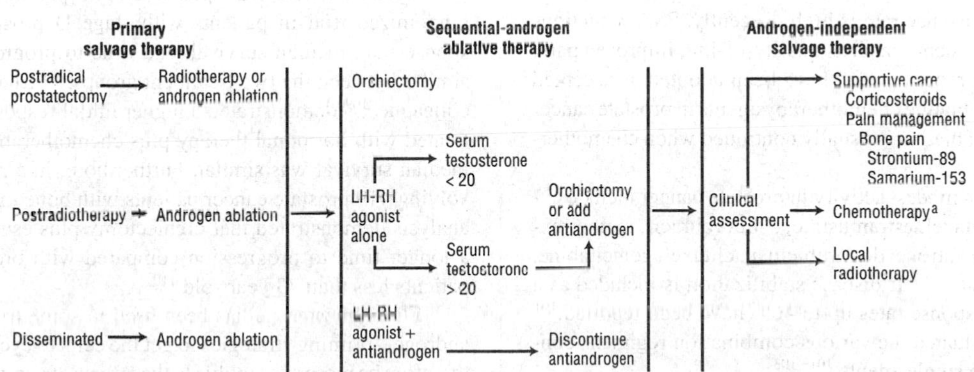

The NCCN guidelines are a statement of consensus of its authors regarding their views of currently accepted approaches to treatment. Any clinician seeking to apply or consult any NCCN guideline is expected to use independent medical judgment in the context of individual clinical circumstances to determine any patient's care or treatment. The National Comprehensive Cancer Network makes no warranties of any kind whatsoever regarding their content, use or application and disclaims any responsibility for their application or use in any way.

FIGURE 128–4. Secondary therapy for prostate cancer. *(Adapted from Ref. 48.) (Copyrighted by the National Comprehensive Cancer Network. All right reserved. These guidelines and illustrations may not be reproduced in any form without the express written permission of the NCCN.)*

been noted in some patients who received bicalutamide after they had progressed while receiving flutamide.[72] Adding an agent that blocks adrenal androgen synthesis, such as aminoglutethimide, at the time that androgens are withdrawn may produce a better response than androgen withdrawal alone.[96] Because of the potential for response immediately after antiandrogen withdrawal, a sufficient observation and assessment period (usually 4 to 6 weeks) is usually required before a patient can be enrolled on a clinical trial evaluating a new agent or therapy for advanced prostate cancer.

Androgen synthesis inhibitors, such as aminoglutethimide[28] or ketoconazole,[29,35] can provide symptomatic relief for a short time in approximately 50% of patients with progressive disease despite previous androgen-ablation therapy. Adverse effects during aminoglutethimide therapy occur in approximately 50% of patients.[28] Central nervous system effects that include lethargy, ataxia, and dizziness are the major adverse reactions. A generalized morbiliform, pruritic rash has been reported in up to 30% of patients treated. The rash is usually self-limiting and resolves within 5 to 8 days with continued therapy. Adverse effects from ketoconazole include gastrointestinal intolerance, transient rises in liver and renal function tests, and hypoadrenalism.

After all hormonal manipulations are exhausted, the patient is considered to have androgen-independent disease. At this point, palliative supportive therapy is appropriate.[48,97] Palliation can be achieved by pain management, using radioisotopes such as strontium-89[98] or samarium-153 lexidronam[99] for bone-related pain, analgesics, corticosteroids, bisphosphonates,[97] or local radiotherapy.[48] While phase III clinical trials evaluating the efficacy of bisphosphonates in prostate cancer have not been completed, bisphosphontes are used routinely in breast cancer and multiple myleoma and are safe for use in prosate cancer patients. The usual dose of pamidronate is 90 mg every month. A trial of pamidronate can be initiated in prostate cancer patients with bone pain; if no benefit is observed, the drug may be discontinued. Chemotherapy with approved agents that have demonstrated palliative activity or in the context of a clinical research trial is another option.[48]

Despite extensive testing of both single agents, combination chemotherapy regimens, and combination chemotherapy/hormonal regimens, no currently approved antineoplastic agent or combinations prolong survival in patients with advanced prostate cancer.[48] This might be so in part because the majority of chemotherapy trials have been done in patients with hormone-refractory prostate cancer when the expected resistance rate is high. Recently, PSA reductions and/or clinical improvements, such as quality-of-life, improved pain, and reduced analgesic requirements, have been adopted as accepted end points for trials evaluating chemotherapy agents in prostate cancer patients.[101] Androgen ablation is usually continued when chemotherapy is initiated.[35]

Single agents with modest activity in prostate cancer include cyclophosphamide, docetaxel, estramustine, 5-fluorouracil, methotrexate, dacarbazine, mitoxantrone, doxorubicin, paclitaxel, gemcitabine, vinorelbine, and cisplatin.[101] If disease stabilization is included as a favorable response, response rates up to 46% have been reported.[101] Several trials have evaluated the various combination regimens containing the most active single agents.[101–103]

Both estramustine combined with vinblastine[102,104] and mitoxantrone combined with prednisone are active combination regimens for refractory prostate cancer.[105] Although estramustine as a single agent[104,106] produced similar response rates to other available chemotherapy agents, development of estramustine combinations (such as estramustine plus vinblastine or estramustine plus docetaxel) continued when its mechanism of action was discovered to involve inhibition of microtubule proteins rather than alkylation.[103,104]

Estramustine and vinblastine combinations have been evaluated in several trials.[103,104] Response is manifested as objective tumor regression (partial response rate up to 50%), PSA declines, pain relief, and delay in bone scan progression. The toxicities of estramustine combined with vinblastine are nausea, gynecomastia, fatigue, and fluid retention. When vinblastine monotherapy was compared with estramustine plus vinblastine in a large phase III intergroup trial for men with metastatic androgen-independent prostate cancer, patients receiving the combination had improved time to progression and PSA improvement, although overall survival did not reach statistical significance.[107]

Mitoxantrone plus prednisone is another combination regimen that can palliate hormone-refractory prostate cancer.[105] One hundred and sixty-one patients with hormone-refractory prostate cancer with pain were randomized to receive either 10 mg/day prednisone alone or this same prednisone dose with mitoxantrone. The primary end point was a palliative ("clinical benefit") response, as assessed by a pain scale and analgesic requirements. Quality of life was assessed with a series of linear analog health-assessment scales and the Prostate Cancer-Specific Quality of Life Instrument.

Palliative responses were noted in 29% of patients in the mitoxantrone plus prednisone group and 12% of patients in the prednisone-alone group ($P = .01$). The duration of palliative response was greater and quality-of-life scores for pain, physical activity, constipation, and mood were better in patients who received mitoxantrone plus prednisone. Overall survival was the same in both groups. Patients treated with mitoxantrone plus prednisone experienced tolerable adverse effects; however, five patients did develop some cardiac-related adverse effects. Mitoxantrone plus corticosteroids is approved by the Food and Drug Administration (FDA) for hormone-refractory prostate cancer.

Other possible chemotherapeutic regimens suggested by the National Comprehensive Cancer Network (NCCN) guidelines and clinical trials include ketoconazole plus doxorubicin, estramustine plus etoposide, or estramustine plus paclitaxel.[48]

Although it would seem rational that prostate cancer is a heterogeneous disease composed of cells sensitive to hormonal therapy, chemotherapy, both therapies, or neither therapy, attempts to combine endocrine therapy and chemotherapy to produce an additive effect have not produced significant response rates. When orchiectomy was compared with DES plus cyclophosphamide in a prospective, randomized trial in patients with stage D prostate cancer, the response rate, median survival, and time to progressive disease were similar between the two treatment groups.[108] Likewise, Osborne and colleagues[109] demonstrated a higher initial response rate for patients treated with hormonal therapy plus chemotherapy; however, overall median survival was similar. Furthermore, in a randomized trial involving 419 prostate cancer patients with bone metastases, subgroup analysis demonstrated that orchiectomy plus estramustine produced a longer time to progression compared with orchiectomy alone in patients less than 73 years old.[110]

Fluoxymesterone has been used in some trials designed to test androgen-priming strategies to get the cells to cycle more rapidly and therefore be more susceptible to the effects of cytotoxic chemotherapy. However, the response rates have been inconsistent and spinal cord compression has occurred in some patients, so it appears that the risks of androgen priming outweigh the benefits.[109]

Whenever possible, cytotoxic chemotherapy for hormone-refractory prostate cancer should be offered to the patient as part of the clinical trial. To make the results of a clinical trial applicable to the majority of hormone-refractory prostate cancer patients, the patient populations need to be clearly defined with regard to disease extent and hormone sensitivity.[111] Likewise, responses should be quantified by accepted disease-regression measures. If surrogate markers, such as PSA changes, are used, the response needs to be described in terms of the percentage decline, the number of times the decline is documented, and the period during which the decline is maintained.[111,112] Quality-of-life end points are also appropriate outcome parameters to measure.[50]

Many new drugs and new combinations are in development for prostate cancer management.[101] Docetaxel has been evaluated as both a single agent and in combination with estramustine, with PSA responses of more than 50%[115] reported for the single agent and up to 75% for the combination.[116] The first 38-patient trial of suramin demonstrated a 42-week median survival and significant PSA declines (greater than 75%).[114] Suramin also shows promise in combination with hydrocortisone.[117] Other efforts include agents with novel anticancer targets and mechanisms (apoptosis inhibitors, growth factor inhibitors, and antimetastasis agents), targeted therapy (vaccines, monoclonal antibodies, or growth receptor antibodies), oncogene regulation (farnesyl transferase inhibitors), matrix metalloproteinase inhibitors, and gene therapy.

CHEMOPREVENTION EFFORTS

Prostate cancer is a significant health concern with few modifiable risk factors. Because androgens are involved in prostate cancer development, it would seem that prolonged administration of drugs that block androgens may prevent subclinical disease from becoming clinically apparent.[118] In testing strategies for prostate cancer prevention, valid surrogate markers need to be identified. Currently, PSA, nuclear morphology, apoptotic bodies, proliferation indices, microvessel density, and genetic expression, as intermediate end points to monitor cancer prevention efforts, are under investigation.[7] As part of an NCI chemoprevention effort, a large double-blind, randomized trial comparing 5 mg/day finasteride for 7 years with placebo has been initiated. This trial has met its target accrual goal of 18,000 participants 55 years of age or older with a normal PSA and DRE. All patients will be biopsied after 7 years or sooner if prostate cancer is diagnosed before this time point. Long-term follow-up is needed before any conclusions can be drawn. In addition to determining whether this intervention will reduce the prostate cancer incidence, it also will provide information about the epidemiology, risk factors, natural history, screening, and diagnosis of prostate cancer and will collect important quality-of-life data. Other potential prostate cancer prevention efforts include tyrosine kinase inhibitors, differentiation inducers, and angiogenesis inhibitors.[118]

ECONOMIC CONSIDERATIONS

The main economic concerns for prostate cancer focus on prostate cancer screening for asymptomatic men and the use of combined hormonal blockade as treatment for advanced disease. Prostate cancer screening remains highly controversial because the survival benefits and the associated costs are not well defined.[119] Krahn and collegues[120] determined that annual screening of all eligible men would cost 45 million Canadian dollars, or 0.15% of total health care expenditures. Available cost-utility studies estimate that the cost per crude or quality-adjusted life-year gained from prostate cancer screening ranges from \$3000 to \$729,000.[119–122] Since the cost-effectiveness of prostate cancer screening cannot be determined until the benefits are documented, it is important to incorporate economic analysis into the large ongoing screening studies.

TABLE 128–9. Comparative Costs of Hormonal Therapy for Advanced Prostate Cancer

Drug	Dose	Average Wholesale Price per Month of Therapy
Leuprolide depot	7.5 mg/mo	\$566.85
Leuprolide depot	22.5 mg/12 wk	\$1700.63
Leuprolide depot	30 mg/16 wk	\$2267.50
Goserelin implant	3.6 mg every 28 days	\$439.24
Goserelin implant	10.8 mg/12 wk	\$1317.74
Flutamide	750 mg/day	\$315.70
Bicalutamide	50 mg/day	\$319.74
Nilutamide	300 mg/day for 1st mo then 150 mg/day	\$467.16 then \$233.58
		Average Wholesale Price per 3 Months of Therapy
Combined Androgen Blockade		
Leuprolide depot 22.5 mg/12 wk		
+flutamide	750 mg/days	\$2647.97
+bicalutamide	50 mg/days	\$2659.85
+nilutamide	150 mg/days	\$2401.37 (\$2634.95 1st month)
Goserelin depot 10.8 mg/12 wk		
+flutamide	750 mg/day	\$2265.08
+bicalutamide	50 mg/day	\$2270.96
+nilutamide	150 mg/day	\$2018.48 (\$2252.06 1st month)

Compiled from Ref. 124.

Table 128–9 lists the costs for the initial hormonal therapies for stage D_2 prostate cancer. Using a societal perspective and data from the original leuprolide plus flutamide versus leuprolide alone trial to calculate the incremental cost per life-year gained, Hillner and colleagues[121] concluded that CAB has an incremental cost-effectiveness of \$25,300 per life-year gained, which is within current accepted benchmarks. The cost dropped to \$13,700 per life-year gained in patients with minimal disease.

In a follow-up study, this same group used physician focus group estimates to generate quality-of-life factors and incorporated these factors into an economic model.[122] The incremental cost per quality-adjusted life-year gained seemed reasonable when data from the original CAB were used[10]: \$25,000 for patients with minimal disease and \$18,000 for patients with severe disease. However, these incremental costs increased dramatically to \$53,700 for patients with minimal disease and \$41,000 for patients with severe disease when the same model was applied to survival data from a meta-analysis.

Because there is considerable debate about the value of using CAB for advanced prostate cancer, continued economic assessments of this therapy will be crucial to help policymakers and physicians decide on the most appropriate therapy. It also will become very important to incorporate economic analyses into chemotherapy trials because these efforts move toward including clinical benefit response as a main endpoint.

EVALUATION OF THERAPEUTIC OUTCOMES

Clinical trials in prostate cancer should include homogeneous populations[123] and adequate staging criteria. Age-adjusted overall survival and disease-free survival should be the ultimate outcome measures, although standardized subjective and objective response criteria also should be included. Objective parameters include assessment of the primary tumor size, evaluation of involved lymph nodes, and the response of tumor markers to treatment. There is still no agreement about which surrogate marker(s), such as PSA, is(are) most useful and how to best quantify the changes in these surrogates to predict a meaningful response.[112] Efforts to better identify markers, such as PSA or ^{111}In-labeled capromab pendetide scanning to predict or diagnose recurrence, may improve overall outcome.[68] Clinical benefit responses can be documented by evaluating performance status changes, weight changes, and analgesic requirements. Quality-of-life assessments should be included in all clinical trials.[50]

FUTURE DIRECTIONS

Prostate cancer occurs in older males and is curable when local disease is present. Efforts are under way to better define screening and early detection approaches and how best to use PSA as a screening, diagnostic, and therapeutic monitoring test. Proper staging at initial patient presentation is essential because the therapy intensity will depend on the disease stage. Patients with localized prostate cancer can be managed effectively with surgery or radiation therapy. For patients with advanced disease, there are many treatment options. Androgen-ablative therapy is very effective for symptom palliation. Initial androgen-ablative measures include orchiectomy or an LH-RH agonist. CAB using an antiandrogen with either orchiectomy or an LH-RH agonist is used routinely despite equivocal studies and its cost. The effects of androgen ablation seem most pronounced in patients with minimal disease. Studies are still ongoing to define the best initial therapy, to determine when to start initial therapy, to identify which patient subpopulation might benefit best from a given treatment modality, and to identify which surrogate markers should be used to monitor disease activity.

Secondary therapies, including alternate hormonal therapies, antiandrogen withdrawal in a patient receiving CAB, chemotherapy, local radiotherapy, or supportive care can provide disease palliation. Continued efforts to develop new agents with novel mechanisms of action that prolong survival are ongoing. Further insight into the molecular basis for prostate cancer development may provide new therapeutic approaches.

▶ PRINCIPLES OF PHARMACOTHERAPY

- Prostate cancer is the most frequent cancer in U.S. men. African-American ancestry, family history, and increased age are the primary risk factors for prostate cancer.
- Mutations in E-cadherin, *p53*, and the androgen receptor are important in prostate carcinogenesis and may affect treatment outcomes.
- PSA is a useful marker for detecting prostate cancer at early stages, predicting outcome for localized disease, defining disease-free status, and following response to androgen-deprivation therapy or chemotherapy for advanced- stage disease.
- Prostate cancer screening is controversial. The American Cancer Society currently recommends that digital rectal examination and PSA be offered annually to men beginning at age 50 years with at least a 10-year life expectancy and to younger men (45 years old) who are considered to be at high risk for prostate cancer development (strong familial predisposition or African-American).
- The prognosis for prostate cancer patients depends on the histologic grade, the tumor size, and disease stage. More than 85% of patients with stage A_1 disease but less than 1% of those with stage D_2 can be cured.
- Localized prostate cancer is curable by surgery or radiation therapy. Advanced prostate cancer (stage D) is not currently curable, and treatment should focus on providing symptom relief and maintaining quality of life.
- Androgen-deprivation therapy, such as using an LH-RH agonist plus an antiandrogen, can be used prior to radiation therapy for patients with locally advanced (stage B_2 or C) prostate cancer to improve outcomes over radiation therapy alone.
- Androgen-deprivation therapy, with either orchiectomy, an LH-RH agonist alone or an LH-RH agonist plus an antiandrogen (combined hormonal blockade), can be used to provide palliation for patients with advanced (stage D_2) prostate cancer. The effects of androgen deprivation seem most pronounced in patients with minimal disease at diagnosis.
- Antiandrogen withdrawal, for patients having progressive disease while receiving combined hormonal blockade with an LH-RH agonist plus an antiandrogen, can provide additional symptomatic relief. Mutations in the androgen receptor have been documented that cause antiandrogen compounds to act like receptor agonists.
- Chemotherapy, with regimens such as mitoxantrone plus corticosteroids (prednisone) or estramustine plus vinblastine, have been shown to provide a clinical benefit response in patients with hormone-refractory prostate cancer. Patients with hormone-refractory prostate cancer should be considered for entry on clinical trials investigating new therapies for prostate cancer.

REFERENCES

1. Greenlee RT. Murray T. Bolden S. Wingo PA. Cancer statistics, 2001. CA 2001;51:15–36.
2. Carter BS, Beaty TH, Steinberg GD, et al. Mendelian inheritance of familial prostate cancer. Proc Natl Acad Sci USA 1992;89:3367–3372.
3. Giovannucci E. How is individual risk for prostate cancer assessed? Hematol Oncol Clin North Am 1996;10:537–548.
4. Isaacs WB, Bova SG, Morton RA, et al. Molecular genetics and chromosomal alterations in prostate cancer. Cancer 1995;75:2004–2012.
5. Ross R, Coetzee GA, Reichardt J, et al. Does the racial-ethnic variation in prostate cancer have a hormonal basis? Cancer 1995;75:1778–1882.
6. Denis L, Morton MD, Griffiths K. Diet and its preventative role in prostate cancer. Eur Urol 1999;35:377–387.
7. Smith JR, Freije D, Carpten JD, et al. Major susceptibility locus for prostate cancer on chromosome 1 suggested by a genome-wide search. Science 1996;274:1371–1374.
8. Suarez BK, Lin J, Burmester JK, et al. A genome screen of multiplex sibships with prostate cancer. Am J Hum Genet 2000;66:933–934.
9. Norrish AE, Jackson RT, Sharpe SJ, Skeaff CM. Prostate cancer and dietary carotenoids. Am J Epidemiol 2000;15:124–127.
10. Schwingl PJ, Guess HA, Safety and effectiveness of vasectomy. Fertil Steril 2000;73:923–936.

11. Schuurman AG, Goldbohm RA, van den Brandt PA. A prospective cohort study on consumption of alcoholic beverages in relation to prostate cancer incidence. Cancer Causes Control 1999;10:597–605.
12. Chi SG, deVere RW, White FJ. p53 in prostate cancer: Frequent expressed transition mutations. Natl Cancer Inst Monogr 1994;86:926–933.
13. Theodorescu D, Broder SR, Boyd JC, et al. p53, bcl-2 and retinoblastoma proteins as long-term prognostic markers in localized carcinoma of the prostate. J Urol 1997;158:131–137.
14. Rakozy C, Grignon DJ, Li Y, et al. p53 gene alteration in prostate cancer after radiation failure and their association with clinical outcome: A molecular and immunohistochemical analysis. Pathol Res Pract 1999;195: 129–135.
15. Dong JT, Suzuki H, Pin SS, et al. Down-regulation of the KAI1 metastasis suppressor gene during the progression of human prostatic cancer infrequently involves gene mutation or allelic loss. Cancer Res 1996;56:4387–4390.
16. Gottlieb B, Beitel LK, Lumbrosso R, et al. Update of the androgen receptor gene mutations database. Hum Mutat 1999;14:103–114.
17. Taplin ME, Bubley GJ, Shuster TD, et al. Mutation of the androgen receptor gene in metastic androgen independent prostate cancer. N Engl J Med 1995;332:1334–1342.
18. Kelly WK, Slovin S, Scher HI. Steroid hormone withdrawl syndromes: Pathophysiology and clinical significance. Urol Clin North Am 1997;24:421–431.
19. Takahashi H, Furusato M, Allsbrook WC, et al. Prevalence of androgen receptor gene mutations in latent prostatic carcinomas from Japanese men. Cancer Res 1995;55:1621–1624.
20. Balducci L, Pow-Sang J, Friedland J, Diaz JI. Prostate cancer. Clin Geriatr Med 1997;13:283–306.
21. Garnick MB. Hormonal therapy in the management of prostate cancer: From Huggins to the present. Urology 1997;49:5–15.
22. Lalani N, Lanaido ME, Abel PD. Molecular and cellular biology of prostate cancer. Cancer Metastasis Rev 1997;16:29–66.
23. Garnick M, Fair W. First international conference on neoadjuvant hormonal therapy of prostate cancer: Overview consensus statement. Urology 1997;39(Suppl 3):1–4.
24. Huggins C, Hodges CV. Studies on prostatic cancer: 1. The effect of castration, of estrogen, and of androgen injection on serum phosphatases in metastatic carcinoma of the prostate. Cancer Res 1941;1:293–297.
25. Plosker GL, Brogden RN. Leuprorelin: A review of its pharmacology and therapeutic use in prostatic cancer, endometriosis and other sex hormone-related disorders. Drugs 1994;48:930–967.
26. Brogden RN, Faulds D. Goserelin. A review of its pharmacodynamic and pharmacokinetic properties and therapeutic efficacy in prostate cancer. Drugs Aging 1995;6:324–343.
27. Conn PM, Crowley WF. Gonadotropin-releasing hormone and its analogues. N Engl J Med 1991;324:93–103.
28. Crawford ED, Ahmann FR, Davis MA, et al. Aminoglutethimide in metastatic adenocarcinoma of the prostate. Prog Clin Biol Res 1987;243A:283–288.
29. Trump DL, Havlin KH, Messing EM, et al. High-dose ketoconazole in advanced hormone-refractory prostate cancer: Endocrinologic and clinical effects. J Clin Oncol 1989;7:1093–1098.
30. Geller J. Megestrol acetate plus low-dose estrogen in the management of advanced prostatic carcinoma. Urol Clin North Am 1991;18:83–91.
31. Labrie F. Mechanism of action and pure antiandrogenic properties of flutamide. Cancer 1993;72:3816 3827.
32. Dole EJ, Holdsworth MT. Nilutamide: An antiandrogen for the treatment of prostate cancer. Ann Pharmacother 1997;31:65–75.
33. Blackledge GR, Cockshott ID, Furr BJ. Casodex (bicalutamide): Overview of a new antiandrogen developed for the treatment of prostate cancer. Eur Urol 1997;31(Suppl 2):30–39.
34. Rittmaster RS. Finasteride. N Engl J Med 1994;330:120–125.
35. Frydenberg M, Stricker PD, Kaye KW. Prostate cancer diagnosis and management. Lancet 1997;349:1681–1687.
36. Gleason DF. Histologic grade, clinical stage, and patient age in prostate cancer. Natl Cancer Inst Mongr 1988;7:15–18.
37. Garnick MB. Prostate cancer: Screening, diagnosis, and management. Ann Intern Med 1993;118:804–818.
38. Osborn JL, Getzenberg RH, Trump DL. Spinal cord compression in prostate cancer. J. Neurooncol 1995;23:135–147.
39. Coltman CA, Thompson IM, Feigl P. Prostate Cancer Prevention Trial update. Eur Urol 1999;35:544–547.
40. Collins MM, Barry MJ. Controversies in prostate cancer screening: Analogies to the early lung cancer screening debate. JAMA 1996;276:1976–1979.
41. Gohagan JK, Prorok PC, Kramer BS, et al. The prostate, lung, colorectal, and ovarian cancer screening trial of the National Cancer Institute. Cancer 1995;75:1869–1873.
42. Oesterline JE. Prostate specific antigen: Its role in diagnostics and staging of prostate cancer. Cancer 1995;75(Suppl):1795–1804.
43. Catalona WJ, Smith DS, Ratliff TL, et al. Measurement of prostate-specific antigen in serum as a screening test for prostate cancer. N Engl J Med 1991;324:1156–1161.
44. Meyer F, Fradet Y. Clinical basics: What's new in prostate cancer? CMAJ 1998;159:968–972.
45. Ross KS, Carter HB, Pearson JD, Guess HA. Comparative efficacy of prostate specific antigen screening strategies for prostate cancer detection. JAMA 2000;284:1399–1405.
46. Volk R, Cass AR, Spann SJ. A randomized controlled trial of shared decision making for prostate cancer screening. Arch Fam Med 1999;8: 333–340.
47. Wilt TJ, Brawer MK. Early intervention or expectant management for prostate cancer. The Prostate Cancer Intervention Versus Observation Trial (PIVOT): A randomized trial comparing radical prostatectomy with expectant management for the treatment of clinically localized prostate cancer. Semin Urol 1995;13:130–136.
48. National Comprehensive Cancer Network. The Complete Library of NCCN Oncology Practice Guidelines, Rockledge, PA Version 2000.
49. Montie JE. Staging of prostate cancer: Current TNM classification and future prospects for prognostic factors. Cancer 1995;75(Suppl):1814–1818.
50. Fossa SD. Quality of life in advanced prostate cancer. Semin Oncol 1996;23:32–34.
51. Visakorpi T, Kallioniemi OP, Kaivula T, Isola J. New prognostic factors in prostatic carcinoma. Eur Urol 1993;24:438–449.
52. Hoeksema M, Law C. Cancer mortality rates fall: A turning point for the nation. J Natl Cancer Inst 1996;88:1706–1707.
53. Scardino PT, Weaver R, Hudson MA. Early detection of prostate cancer. Hum Pathol 1992;23:211–222.
54. Partin AW, Kattan MW, Subong EN, et al. Combination of prostate-specific antigen, clinical stage, and Gleason score to predict pathological stage of localized prostate cancer. A multi-institutional update [published erratum appears in JAMA 1997;278:118]. JAMA 1997;227: 1445–1451.
55. Wilt TJ. Uncertainty in prostate cancer care: The physician's role in clearing the confusion. JAMA 2000;283:3258–3260.
56. Akakura A, Isaka S, Akimoto S, et al. Long-term results of a randomized trial for the treatment of stages B_2 and C prostate cancer: Radical prostatectomy versus external beam radiation with a common endocrine therapy in both modalities. Urology 1999;54:313–318.
57. Goldenberg LS, Ramsey EW, Jewett MA. Clinical basics: Prostate cancer: Surgical treatment of localized disease. CMAJ 1998;159:1265–1271.
58. Walsh PC, Partin AW, Epstein JI. Cancer control and quality of life following anatomical radical retropubic prostatectomy: Results at 10 years. J Urol 1994;152:1831–1836.
59. Messing EM, Manola J, Sarosdy M, et al. Immediate hormonal therapy compared with observation after radical prostatectomy and pelvic lymphadenopathy in men with node positive cancer. N Engl J Med 1999;341:1781–1788.
60. Pilepich M, Krall J, al Saraff M, et al. Androgen deprivation with radiation therapy compared with radiation therapy alone for locally advanced prostatic carcinoma: A randomized comparison trial of the Radiation Therapy Oncology Group. Urology 1995;45:616–623.

61. Fair WR, Cookson MS, Stroumbakis N, et al. The indications, rationale, and results of neoadjuvant androgen deprivation in the treatment of prostatic cancer: Memorial Sloan-Kettering Cancer Center results. Urology 1997;49:46–55.
62. Soloway M, Sharafi R, Wajsman Z, et al. Randomized prospective study comparing radical prostatectomy alone versus radical prostatectomy preceded by androgen blockade in clinical stage B2 ($T_{2b}N_xM_0$) prostate cancer. The Leupron Depot Neoadjuvant Prostate Cancer Study Group. J Urol 1995;154:424–428.
63. Roach M. Neoadjuvant total androgen suppression and radiotherapy in the management of locally advanced prostate cancer. Semin Urol 1996;14:32–38.
64. Meyer F, Moore L, Bairati I, et al. Neoadjuvant hormonal therapy before radical prostatectomy and risk of prostate specific antigen failure. J Urol 1999;162:2024–2028.
65. Wong WS, Chinn DO, Chinn M, et al. Cryosurgery as a treatment for prostate carcinoma: Results and complications. Cancer 1997;79:963–974.
66. D'Amico AV, Coleman CN. Role of interstitial radiotherapy in the management of clinically organ-confined prostate cancer: The jury is still out. J Clin Oncol 1996;14:304–315.
67. Schellhammer P, Cockett A, Boccon-Gibod L, et al. Assessment of end points for clinical trials for localized prostate cancer. Urology 1997;49: 27–38.
68. Troyer JK, Beckett ML, Wright GL Jr. Detection and characterization of the prostate-specific membrane antigen (PSMA) in tissue extracts and body fluids. Int J Cancer 1995;62:552–558.
69. Prostate Cancer Trialist's Collaborative Group. Maximum androgen blockade in advanced prostate cancer: An overview of the randomised trials. Lancet 2000;355:1491–1498.
70. Hedlunf PO, Henriksson P. Parenteral estrogen versus total androgen blockade in the treatment of advanced prostate carcinoma: Effects of overall survival and cardiovascular mortality. Urology 2000;55:328–333.
71. Seidenfield J, Samson DJ, Hasselblad V, et al. Single therapy androgen suppression in men with advanced prostate cancer: A systematic review and meta analysis. Ann Intern Med 2000;132:566–577.
72. Scher H, Leibertz C, Kelly W, et al. Bicalutamide for advanced prostate cancer: The natural history versus treated history of disease. J Clin Oncol 1997;15:2928–2938.
73. Bales G, Chodak G. A controlled trial of bicalutamide versus castration in patients with advanced prostate cancer. Urology 1996;47:38–43.
74. Decensi A, Bocardo F, Guarneri D, et al. Monotherapy with nilutamide, a pure nonsteroidal antiandrogen, in untreated patients with metastatic carcinoma of the prostate. J Urol 1991;146:377–381.
75. Boccardo F, Rubagotti A, Barichello M, et al. Bicalutamide monotherapy versus flutamide plus gosrelin in prostate cancer patients: Results of an Italian Prostate Cancer Project study. J Clin Oncol 1999;17:2027–2038.
76. Schellhammer P, Sharifi R, Block N, et al. A controlled trial of bicalutamide versus flutamide, each in combination with luteinizing hormone-releasing hormone analogue therapy, in patients with advanced prostate cancer. Casodex Combination Study Group. Urology 1995;45:745–752.
77. Labrie F, Dupont A, Simard J, et al. Intracrinology: The basis for the rational design of endocrine therapy at all stages of prostate cancer. Eur Urol 1993;2:94–105.
78. Labrie F, Dupont A, Cusan L, et al. Combination therapy with flutamide and medical (LH-RH agonist) or surgical castration in advanced prostate cancer: 7-year clinical experience. J Steroid Biochem Mol Biol 1990;37:943–950.
79. Eisenberger M, Crawford ED, Blumenstein B, et al. National Cancer Institute Integroup Study 0036. Prognostic factors in stage D_2 prostate cancer: Important implications for future trials: Results of a cooperative intergroup study (INT 0036). Semin Oncol 1994;21:613–619.
80. Tyrell CJ, Altwein JE, Klippel F, et al. Comparison of an LH-RH analogue with combined androgen blockade in advanced prostate cancer. Eur Urol 2000;37:205–211.
81. Iversen P, Rasmussen F, Klarskov P, Christensen IJ. Long-term results of Danish Prostatic Cancer Group Trial 86: Goserelin acetate plus flutamide versus orchiectomy in advanced prostate cancer. Cancer 1993;72:3851–3854.
82. Tyrell CJ, Altwein JE, Klippel F, et al. Multicenter randomized trial comparing Zoladex with Zoladex plus flutamide in the treatment of advanced prostate cancer: Survival update. International Prostate Cancer Study Group. Cancer 1993;72:3878–3879.
83. Denis LJ, Carnelro de Moura JL, Bono A, et al. Goserelin acetate and flutamide versus bilateral orchiectomy: A phase III EORTC trial (30853). EORTC GU Group and EORTC Data Center. Urology 1993;42:119–129.
84. Eisenberger M, Crawford ED, McLeod D, et al. A comparison of bilateral orchiectomy (orch) with or without flutamide in stage D_2 prostate cancer (PC) (NCI INT-0105 SWOG/ECOG) [Abstract]. Proc ASCO 1997;16:2a.
85. Prostate Cancer Trialists' Collaborative Group. Maximum androgen blockade in advanced prostate cancer: An overview of 22 randomised trials with 3283 deaths in 5710 patients. Lancet 1995;346:265–269.
86. Schellhammer P, Sharifi R, Block N, et al. A controlled trial of bicalutamide versus flutamide, each in combination with luteinizing hormone-releasing hromone analogue therapy, in patients with advanced prostate carcinoma: Analysis of time to progression. Cancer 1996;78:2164–2169.
87. Mazeman E, Bertrand P. Early versus delayed hormonal therapy in advanced prostate cancer [Discussion 49]. Eur Urol 1996;30(Suppl 1): 40–43.
88. The Veterans Administration Cooperative Urological Research Group. Carcinoma of the prostate: Treatment comparisons. J Urol 1967;98:516–522.
89. Byar DP, Corle DK. Hormone therapy for prostate cancer: Results of the Veterans Administration Cooperative Urologic Research Group studies. Natl Cancer Inst Monogr 1988;7:165–170.
90. Denis L, Murphy GP. Overview of phase III trials on combined androgen treatment in patients with metastatic prostate cancer. Cancer 1993;72:3888–3895.
91. Blackard CE. The Veterans' Administration Cooperative Urological Research Group. Studies of carcinoma of the prostate: A review. Cancer Chemother Rep 1975;59:225–227.
92. Scher HI, Kelly WK. Flutamide withdrawal syndrome: Its impact on clinical trials in hormone refractory prostate cancer. J Clin Oncol 1993; 11:1566–1572.
93. Small E, Srinivas S. The androgen withdrawal syndrome: Experience in a large cohort of unselected patients with advanced prostate cancer. Cancer 1995;76:1428–1434.
94. Huan SD, Gerridzen RG, Yau JC, Stewart DJ. Antiandrogen withdrawal syndrome with nilutamide. Urology 1997;49:632–634.
95. Scher HI, Kolvenbag GJ. The antiandrogen withdrawal syndrome in relapsed prostate cancer [Discussion 24–27]. Eur Urol 1997;31 (Suppl 2): 3–7.
96. Sartor O, Cooper M, Weinberger M, et al. Surprising activity of flutamide withdrawal, when combined with aminoglutethimide, in treatment of hormone-refractory prostate cancer. J Natl Cancer Inst 1994;86:222–227.
97. Esper PS, Pienta KJ. Supportive care in the patient with hormone refractory prostate cancer. Semin Urol Oncol 1997;15:56–64.
98. Crawford ED, Kozlowski JM, Debruyne FM, et al. The use of strontium 89 for palliation of pain from bone metastases associated with hormone-refractory prostate cancer. Urology 1994;44:481–485.
99. Resche I, Chatal JF, Pecking A, et al. A dose-controlled study of ^{153}Sm-ethylenediaminetetramethylenephosphonate (EDTMP) in the treatment of patients with painful bone metastases. Eur J Cancer 1997; 33:1583–1591.
100. Adami S. Bisphosphonates in prostate cancer. Cancer 1997;80:1686–1690.
101. Siu LL, Moore MJ. Other chemotherapy regimens including mitoxantrone and suramin. Semin Urol Oncol 1997;15:20–27.

102. Seidman AD, Scher HI, Petrylak D, et al. Estramustine and vinblastine: Use of prostate specific antigen as a clinical trial end point for hormone refractory prostatic cancer. J Urol 1992;147:931–934.
103. Hudes G. Estramustine-based chemotherapy. Semin Urol Oncol 1997; 15:13–19.
104. Perry CM, McTavish D. Estramustine phosphate sodium: A review of its pharmacodynamic and pharmacokinetic properties, and therapeutic efficacy in prostate cancer. Drugs Aging 1995;7:49–74.
105. Tannock If, Osoba D, Stockler Mr, Et Al. Chemotherapy with mitoxantrone plus prednisone or prednisone alone for symptomatic hormone-resistant prostate cancer: A Canadian randomized trial with palliative end points. J Clin Oncol 1996;14:1756–1764.
106. Iversen P, Rasmussen F, Asmussen C, et al. Estramustine phosphate versus placebo as second line treatment after orchiectomy in patients with metastatic prostate cancer. DAPROCA study 9002. Danish Prostatic Cancer Group. J Urol 1997;157:929–934.
107. Hudes G, Einhorn L, Ross E, et al. Vinblastine versus vinblastine plus oral estramustine phosphate for patients with hormone refractory prostate cancer. J Clin Oncol 1999;17:3160–166.
108. Murphy GP, Beckley S, Brady MF, et al. Treatment of newly diagnosed metastatic prostate cancer patients with chemotherapy agents in combination with hormones versus hormones alone. Cancer 1983;51:1264–1272.
109. Osborne CK, Blumenstein B, Crawford ED, et al. Combined versus sequential chemo-endocrine therapy in advanced prostate cancer: Final results of a randomized southwest oncology group study. J Clin Oncol 1990;8:1675–1682.
110. Janknegt RA, Boon TA, van de Beek C, Grob P. Combined hormono/chemotherapy as primary treatment for metastatic prostate: A randomized, multicenter study of orchiectomy alone versus orchiectomy plus estramustine phosphate. The Dutch Estracyt Study Group. Urology 1997; 49:411–420.
111. Scher HI, Mazumdar M, Kelly WK. Clinical trials in relapsed prostate cancer: Defining the target. J Natl Cancer Inst 1996;88:1623–1634.
112. Kelly WK, Slovin S, Scher HI. Clinical use of posttherapy prostate-specific antigen changes in advanced prostate cancer. Semin Oncol 1996;23:8–14.
113. Roth BJ. New therapeutic agents for hormone-refractory prostate cancer. Semin Oncol 1996;23:49–55.
114. Sanda MG. Biological principles and clinical development of prostate cancer gene therapy. Semin Urol Oncol 1997;15:43–55.
115. Petrylak DP, Macarthur R, O'Connor J, et al. Phase I/II studies of docetaxel combined with estramustine in men with hormone refractory prostate cancer. Semin Oncol 1999;26:28–33.
116. Picus J, Schultz M. Docetaxel as monotherapy in the treatment of hormone refractory prostate cancer. Semin Oncol 1999;26:14–18.
117. Hussain M, Fisher EI, Petrylak DP, et al. Androgen deprivation and four course of fixed-schedule suramin treatment in patients with newly diagnosed metastatic prostate cancer. J Clin Oncol 2000;18:1043–1049.
118. Karp JE, Chiarodo A, Brawley O, Kelloff GJ. Prostate cancer prevention: Investigational approaches and opportunities. Cancer Res 1996;56:5547–5556.
119. Benoit RM, Naslund MJ. The economics of prostate cancer screening. Oncology (Huntingt) 1997;11:1533–1543.
120. Krahn MD, Coombs AB, Levy IG. Current and projected annual direct costs of screening asymptomatic men for prostate cancer using prostate specific antigen. CMAJ 1999;160:49–57.
121. Hillner BE, McLeod DG, Crawford ED, Bennett CL. Estimating the cost-effectiveness of total androgen blockade with flutamide in M_1 prostate cancer. Urology 1995;45:633–640.
122. Bennett CL, Matchar D, McCrory D, et al. Cost-effective models for flutamide for prostate carcinoma patients: Are they helpful to policy makers? Cancer 1996;77:1854–1861.
123. Scher HI, Steineck G, Kelly WK. Hormone-refractory (D_3) prostate cancer: Refining the concept. Urology 1995;46:142–148.
124. Drug Topics: Annual Pharmacists' Reference (Redbook). Oradell, NJ, Medical Economics, 1998.

129
LYMPHOMAS

Val R. Adams and Gary C. Yee

Lymphomas are a heterogeneous group of malignancies that arise from malignant transformation of immune cells that reside predominantly in lymphoid tissues. They most commonly present as a solid tumor, but can sometimes present as circulating tumor cells in peripheral blood. The differing histology of lymphoma cells has led to classification of Hodgkin's disease (Reed-Sternberg cells) or non-Hodgkin's lymphoma (B- or T-cell lymphocyte markers). Non-Hodgkin's lymphomas (NHLs) are further classified into distinct clinical entities, which are defined by a combination of morphology, immunophenotype, genetic features, and clinical features. Chemotherapy is the mainstay of treatment in patients with lymphoma, especially those with widespread disease. Overall cure rates are high for many subtypes of lymphomas, even when patients present with advanced disease.

HODGKIN'S DISEASE

Thomas Hodgkin first described the mysterious disease of the lymph system that bears his name in 1932. Hodgkin's disease is a form of lymphoma, the cause of which is still unknown, and is invariably fatal if left untreated. Studies demonstrate the orderly spread of this disease. Hodgkin's disease is classified into one of four histologic subtypes that differ in their natural history. These differences can also influence the staging workup and treatment. The stage of Hodgkin's disease influences prognosis and is the primary factor that guides therapy. The pathologic stage is an indicator of the extent of disease and is based on histopathologic examination of the specimen obtained from biopsy of appropriate tissue during staging procedures. Dramatic advances have been made in the understanding and treatment of Hodgkin's disease during the past four decades. Today, most newly diagnosed patients with Hodgkin's disease will be cured with modern therapy. This extraordinary success has not been without cost. The treatment programs are intense, technically demanding, and associated with considerable acute toxicity and long-term complications. The long-term effects of standard chemotherapy regimens have been more fully documented in recent years and could shape therapy in the future.[1–3]

EPIDEMIOLOGY AND ETIOLOGY

It is estimated that nearly 7,400 new cases of Hodgkin's disease will be diagnosed in the United States in 2001, which represents less than 1% of all known cancers. It is expected that there will be 1,300 deaths associated with Hodgkin's disease during this same time period. This disease occurs slightly more frequently in males than in females.[1] Once thought to be only a disease of the young, it is now recognized that Hodgkin's disease exhibits a bimodal distribution in industrialized countries. The first peak occurs between the ages of 15 and 40 years (usually 25 to 30 years) and again in those older than 55 years.[4] In recent years, there has been an increasing incidence in younger patients and a declining incidence in those over 40 years of age, which may be a result of more accurate diagnosis of lymphoid malignancies in this age group.[5] When only deaths caused by Hodgkin's disease are considered, the 5- and 10-year survival rate for all stages is 82% and 72%, respectively.[6] Death rates owing to recurrent Hodgkin's disease are less than death rates from other causes 15 years after treatment.[3]

The etiology of Hodgkin's disease has not been fully elucidated. Environmental risk factors have been linked with Hodgkin's disease, but only appear to play a minor role. Farmers, wood workers, and meat workers appear to be at a slightly increased risk. Infection has been considered a potential cause ever since the disease was first described. Viruses have emerged as the leading candidates for an infectious etiology. Studies have suggested an increased risk of Hodgkin's disease in patients who have had mononucleosis caused by the Epstein-Barr virus (EBV). Reed-Sternberg cells, which are large, bilobate, multinuclear cells associated with Hodgkin's disease, have been found in mononucleosis patients. Both serologic and molecular methods have linked EBV to Hodgkin's disease.[2,4,7,8] Homosexual men infected with HIV are also at a slightly increased risk of developing Hodgkin's disease. Occasional geographic clusters of cases further support the linkage between Hodgkin's disease and an infectious agent. Genetic factors also predispose people to Hodgkin's disease. There has been a small increased risk associated with certain HLA types and in people with ataxia telangiectasia. The strongest evidence suggesting that genes are important in the etiology of Hodgkin's disease comes from identical twin studies, which show that the unaffected identical twin has about a 100-fold increase in risk.[4]

HISTOPATHOLOGY AND CLASSIFICATION

Lymphocytes, the principal cellular component of lymphoid tissue, are widely distributed throughout the body and in aggregated centers. The bone marrow and thymus are the primary organs of lymphopoiesis, with secondary sites being the lymph nodes, spleen, lamina propria of the gastrointestinal tract, and Waldeyer's ring.

Hodgkin's disease is unique among the lymphomas because only a small percentage of cells from the involved tissue are malignant; the vast majority of cells are normal reactive hematopoietic cells. The exact cellular origin of the malignant cell has yet to be determined. It is believed that the Reed-Sternberg cell and its variants are derived from either B-lymphocytes or a macrophage/reticulum cell lineage. More recent availability of monoclonal antibodies and molecular biology tools has greatly improved our understanding of the immunohistology and histopathology of Hodgkin's disease. Although the bcl-2 oncogene has been identified in Hodgkin's tissue samples (which would indicate a B cell origin), there is evidence to suggest that the t(14:18) chromosomal translocation is associated with a bystander normal lymphocyte and not the Reed-Sternberg cell. Alterations in the expression of *p*53, a tumor-suppressor gene, have been observed in all types of Hodgkin's disease except lymphocyte-predominance disease. An explanation for the apparent multilineage origin of the Reed-Sternberg cell is that the malignant cell represents an *in vivo* clonal population that occurs in response to viral stimuli (EBV) that promotes fusion of the interdigitating reticular cell, B cells, T cells, or both lymphocytes.[2,4,7,8]

Lukes, Hicks, and Butler introduced a histopathologic classification of Hodgkin's disease (known as the Lukes-Butler classification) that was modified at the 1965 Rye conference and is referred to today as the Rye classification.[9] This classification is still widely accepted by both pathologists and clinicians, although a new classification system has been proposed. In 1994, the International Lymphoma Study Group (ILSG) published a Revised European-American Classification of Lymphoid Neoplasms called the REAL classification.[10] The Rye classification divides Hodgkin's disease into four subtypes: lymphocyte-predominance, nodular sclerosis, mixed cellularity, and lymphocyte-depletion whereas the REAL classification makes a distinction between nodular lymphocyte predominance Hodgkin's disease and lymphocyte-rich classic Hodgkin's disease. The subtypes in these classification systems are based on characteristics of the Reed-Sternberg cell, the surrounding cells, and connective tissue. Nodular sclerosis has features that make it distinct from the other three subtypes, which represent a continuum of background cellularity, with lymphocyte-predominance being the most cellular and lymphocyte-depletion being the least cellular.[4,9] With the introduction of extensive staging, sophisticated megavolt radiotherapy, and effective combination chemotherapy, the true prognostic value of these subtypes is becoming less clear.[4]

NODULAR SCLEROSIS

Nodular sclerosis Hodgkin's disease (NSHD) has two features that distinguish it from all other forms: the presence of the lacunar cell, which is a variant of the Reed-Sternberg cell, and the presence of a capsule that divides the lymphoid tissue into distinct nodules. Reed-Sternberg cells are actually rare. This subtype can represent up to slightly more than one-half of all Hodgkin's disease and is equally divided between females and males. NSHD is associated with a more favorable prognosis because it is often localized, although involvement of the mediastinum is common.[5,8]

LYMPHOCYTE-PREDOMINANCE

Lymphocyte-predominance Hodgkin's disease (LPHD) has characteristic benign-appearing lymphocytes that have a more diffuse growth pattern. The lymph nodes are usually partially to completely destroyed. Reed-Sternberg cells are uncommon, while the predominant cell appears to be a B-lymphocyte. Fibrosis is also uncommon. This subtype can account for about 10% of all Hodgkin's disease and is slightly more common in males than females. LPHD is an indolent disease similar to B-cell non-Hodgkin's lymphoma and commonly presents as a localized tumor and has a more favorable prognosis. However, patients with this tumor have an increased risk of late relapse or a secondary non-Hodgkin's lymphoma.[5,8]

MIXED CELLULARITY

Mixed cellularity Hodgkin's disease (MCHD) occupies a position between the lymphocyte-predominance and lymphocyte-depletion subtypes with regard to the number of neoplastic cells present. It can be mistaken for high-grade non-Hodgkin's lymphoma. Reed-Sternberg cells are more common in this subtype. Diffuse fibrosis is uncommon. This subtype can account for about 30% of all Hodgkin's disease, is slightly more common in males than females, and is associated with an intermediate prognosis.[5,8]

LYMPHOCYTE-DEPLETION

Lymphocyte-depletion Hodgkin's disease (LDHD) is associated with an abundance of Reed-Sternberg cells and their variants. It also can be easily mistaken for high-grade non-Hodgkin's lymphoma. Diffuse fibrosis and necrosis are commonly seen. This subtype accounts for 7% of all Hodgkin's disease, is more common in males than females, is often widespread at the time of diagnosis and may be associated with a less favorable prognosis. This category is also most commonly associated with AIDS for which the prognosis is very poor.[5,8]

TABLE 129–1. Clinical Features of the Lymphomas

	Hodgkin's Disease	Non-Hodgkin's Lymphoma
Lymph node disease	Centripetal	Centrifugal
Contiguous spread	Common	Uncommon
Mediastinal disease	50%	20%[a]
Abdominal disease	Uncommon	Common
Bone marrow	Uncommon involvement	Common
Liver involvement	Uncommon (if present, spleen usually involved)	Common in follicular, uncommon in diffuse
Extranodal disease	Uncommon	Gastrointestinal tract, Waldeyer's ring, testes, epitrochlear nodes, brain
Systemic "B" symptoms	40%	20%

[a]With the exception of T-cell lymphoblastic lymphoma.

CLINICAL PRESENTATION

Most patients with lymphoma present with some form of adenopathy. The clinical presentations of Hodgkin's disease and the non-Hodgkin's lymphomas have some striking differences (Table 129–1). It is generally not possible to differentiate between the various lymphomas by the physical characteristics of the lymph node itself, but the distribution can offer useful information.

Patients with Hodgkin's disease may have adenopathy that waxes and wanes for an average of 5 months before diagnosis. This adenopathy is usually localized to the cervical region and is painless and rubbery. Adenopathy of the inguinal and axillary regions may be present at diagnosis but is less common, whereas involvement of Waldeyer's ring and the epitrochlear nodes occurs in roughly 1% of patients (Fig. 129–1). Other common sites of nodal involvement include the mediastinal, hilar, and retroperitoneal regions. As many as 40% of patients with Hodgkin's disease may also present with constitutional symptoms (B symptoms) including fever, drenching night sweats, and weight loss. Pruritus is also commonly noted in patients with Hodgkin's disease, but its presence does not appear to have significant prognostic value.[2,4]

DIAGNOSIS AND STAGING

The diagnosis and pathologic classification of Hodgkin's disease can only be made by biopsy (preferably an excisional biopsy) of the enlarged node and histopathologic examination under a microscope. Full evaluation of extent of disease, or staging, is necessary with Hodgkin's disease. Staging determines appropriate treatment of the disease and provides useful information regarding prognosis. In addition, specific knowledge of the involved sites can be used to determine response.

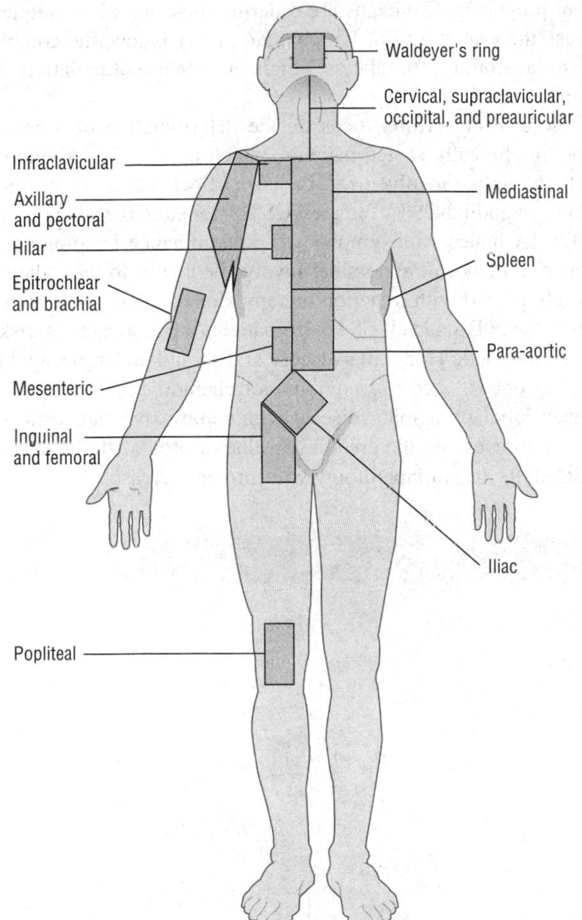

FIGURE 129–1. Representation of the anatomic regions used in the staging of Hodgkin's disease. *(From Rosenberg SA. Staging of Hodgkin's disease. Radiology 1966;87:146 (Letter), with permission.)*

TABLE 129–2. The Cotswolds Staging Classification of Hodgkin's Disease

Stage I	Involvement of a single lymph node region or structure (I) or of a single extralymphatic organ or site (I_E)
Stage II	Involvement of two or more lymph node regions on the same side of the diaphragm (II) or localized involvement of an extralymphatic organ or site and of one or more lymph node regions on the same side of the diaphragm (II_E). The number of nodal regions involved should be indicated by a subscript (e.g., II_2)
Stage III	Involvement of lymph node regions on both sides of the diaphragm (III), which may also be accompanied by localized involvement of an extralymphatic organ or site (III_E) or by involvement of the spleen (IIIS) or both ($IIIS_E$). III_1: with or without splenic, hilar, celiac, or portal node involvement. III_2: with para-aortic, iliac, or mesenteric node involvement
Stage IV	Diffuse or disseminated involvement of one or more extralymphatic organs or tissues with or without associated lymph node enlargement
	A—No symptoms
	B—Fever, night sweats, weight loss (>10%)
	X—Bulky disease
	> one-third the width of the mediastinum
	> 10 cm maximal dimension of nodal mass
	E—Involvement of extralymphatic tissue on one side of the diaphragm by limited direct extension from an adjacent, involved lymph node region
	S—Involvement of the spleen
	CS—Clinical stage
	PS—Pathologic stage

Adapted from Refs. 11 and 12.

Presence of advanced stage, extensive B symptoms, and massive mediastinal involvement implies a poorer prognosis for a given patient.

The Ann Arbor staging classification, which was developed at the 1970 Ann Arbor conference, has proven to be a good workable scheme.[11] At the Cotswold meeting in 1989, the Ann Arbor classification was modified to account for new diagnostic techniques (e.g., computed tomography (CT) and magnetic resonance imaging (MRI)) and the realization that prognosis is associated with the bulk of the disease and the number of involved nodal sites (Table 129–2).[12] After careful staging, about one-half of patients have localized disease (stages I, II, and IIE) and the remainder has advanced disease (stages III or IV). Approximately 10% to 15% of patients present with metastatic disease (stage IV). It is important to note that Hodgkin's disease appears to follow a predictable pattern of nodal spread that is not seen with the non-Hodgkin's lymphomas.

Diagnostic and staging procedures are based on recommendations made at the Ann Arbor and Cotswolds conferences and new scientific advances as outlined in the NCCN guidelines.[11–13] Table 129–3 lists the mandatory workup procedures and those that are useful in selected cases.

TABLE 129–3. Workup for Hodgkin's Disease

Mandatory	Reserved for Selected Patients (Indications)
Biopsy (confirm diagnosis and subtype	Lymphangiogram (CS I or II and intent to treat with radiation alone)
History (age, gender, fever, night sweats, weight loss, pruritus, performance status, fatigue)	Gallium scan (equivocal CT)
Physical exam (evaluate for lymphadenopathy, size of liver and spleen)	Staging laparotomy (supradiaphragmatic disease treated with RT alone; except with LPHD)
Laboratory tests (CBC with differential, ESR, LDH, LFTs, SCr, BUN, albumin, alkaline phosphatase)	Counseling on fertility concerns and options (child-bearing potential and receiving sterilizing therapy)
Radiographic exams (chest x-ray, CT chest/abdomen/pelvis)	Laboratory tests (HIV, pregnancy if at risk)
Bone marrow biopsy (stage IIB or higher)	

Adapted from Refs. 11–13.

Staging can be based on clinical or pathologic findings. Clinical staging (CS) is based on all noninvasive procedures (history, physical exam, laboratory tests, and radiologic findings), whereas pathologic staging (PS) is based on the biopsy findings of strategic sites (muscle, bone, skin, spleen, abdominal nodes) with an invasive procedure such as a laparoscopy or laparotomy. Those patients with extranodal disease (muscle, skin, bone, Waldeyer's ring) contiguous to involved nodes are classified with the subscript "E" in the Cotswolds staging system.[12]

Invasive staging procedures such as laparotomy and lymphangiogram are being used less frequently during staging. These tests can detect occult disease in the abdomen, which would require systemic chemotherapy in addition to radiation for patients with early stage supradiaphragmatic disease. Therefore, these tests should only be considered for patients who will be treated with radiation alone if the results are negative. When the treatment plan includes systemic therapy, the use of these tests does not impact treatment decisions or patient prognosis. Clinicians are ordering these tests less frequently because the availability of lymphangiography is low, the complications of laparotomy are relatively high, and the use of radiation alone is decreasing.[2,4,8]

More recent efforts focus on the determination of prognostic factors in clinically staged patients, which predict the likelihood of occult abdominal involvement. Because select subgroups of CS I-II patients, including CS IA females, CS IIA females age 26 or younger, and CS IA males with lymphocyte predominance histology are at lowest risk of occult abdominal involvement (6% to 9%), they can be safely treated with radiation therapy alone. The remainder of patients with CS IIA and all CS IB-IIB patients are at substantial risk for subdiaphragmatic Hodgkin's disease and should undergo staging laparotomy or be treated with combination chemotherapy. As the ability to detect subdiaphragmatic disease with noninvasive diagnostic techniques improves and the predictive value of prognostic indicators is validated, the use of laparotomy will further decrease.[2,4,8,14]

▶ TREATMENT: Hodgkin's Disease

The current goal in the treatment of Hodgkin's disease is to maximize curability while minimizing short- and long-term treatment-related complications. The development of effective therapies for all stages of Hodgkin's disease remains one of the most remarkable achievements in modern cancer care. The introduction of modern linear accelerators providing radiation beams in the range of <10 MeV, effective combination chemotherapy regimens, and new methods of combining these two modalities have all contributed to high cure rates.

In general, early stage Hodgkin's disease is usually treated with radiation therapy; advanced-stage disease is usually treated with combination chemotherapy; and bulky disease, regardless of stage, is usually treated with combined chemotherapy and radiation therapy. However, some clinicians prefer combined modality therapy for nonbulky early and advanced-stage disease, and there is evidence that chemotherapy is an acceptable alternative to radiation therapy for some patients with early-stage disease. This section reviews treatment of early stage favorable disease, early stage unfavorable disease, advanced-stage disease, and salvage therapy.[2,8,15]

Analysis of early studies lead to the identification of prognostic factors that could predict poor treatment outcomes of early stage Hodgkin's disease. Patient characteristics that have been determined as unfavorable prognostic factors include: advanced age ($\geq$50 years), male gender, MCHD histology, presence of B-symptoms, number of involved nodal regions ($\geq$3 or 4), large mediastinal mass, extranodal disease, elevated erythrocyte sedimentation rate (ESR), presence of anemia, and low serum albumin.[8] Some clinical trials performed by large cancer groups (e.g., European Organization for Research and Treatment of Cancer [EORTC] and German Hodgkin's Lymphoma Study Group [GHSG]) have used combinations of these prognostic factors to stratify patients into unfavorable or favorable disease.[2]

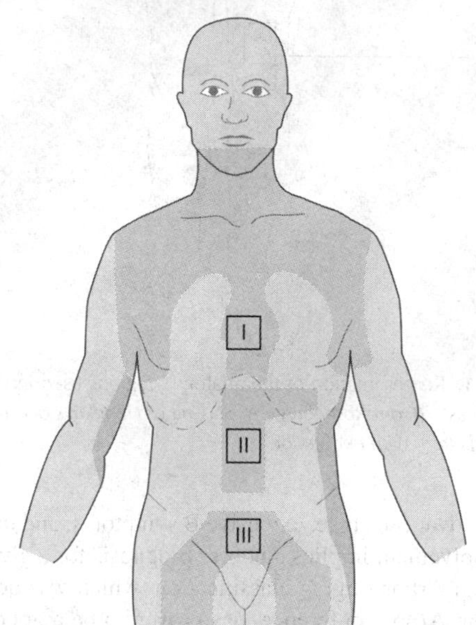

FIGURE 129–2. Radiation fields (shaded areas) commonly employed in Hodgkin's disease. I, mantle; II, para-aortic–splenic pedicle; III, pelvic; I + II, subtotal nodal irradiation; I + II + III, total nodal irradiation. *(From Eyre HJ, Farver ML. Hodgkin's disease and non-Hodgkin's lymphomas. In: Holleb AI, Fink, DJ, Murphy GP, eds. Textbook of Clinical Oncology. Atlanta, GA, American Cancer Society, 1991:382, with permission.)*

TREATMENT OF EARLY STAGE FAVORABLE DISEASE

RADIATION THERAPY ALONE

Patients with stage IA or IIA disease can be successfully treated with radiation therapy alone. The types of fields used are shown in Fig. 129–2. Mantle irradiation with doses ranging from 40 Gy to 44 Gy is usually employed. This may be followed with treatment of the para-aortic splenic pedicle field alone, or including the area below the bifurcation of the aorta including the iliac nodes (which is called the spade field), with radiation doses ranging from 30 Gy to 40 Gy. Treatment of these additional uninvolved areas is called extended-field radiotherapy. Extended-field radiotherapy (also called subtotal nodal irradiation) is still considered by many to be the treatment of choice for stage IA and IIA disease (see Fig. 129–2).[3,4] This treatment produces disease-free survival rates ranging from 65% to 85% and overall survival rates ranging from 75% to 93%, although some studies have reported no significant difference in both disease-free survival and overall survival when involved-field (mantle) radiation is given versus extended-field radiation. These studies also revealed pelvic relapse rates of less than 5%, indicating that total nodal irradiation may not be necessary.[16–19] A recent meta-analysis conducted by Specht and colleagues[20] indicates that more extensive radiotherapy may reduce the risk of treatment failure at 10 years (31% vs 43%), although there was no improvement in overall 10-year survival (77.0% vs 77.1%).

Because laparotomy is associated with complications, the EORTC tested its necessity in a randomized controlled trial. Patients with supradiaphragmatic CS I or II Hodgkin's disease without bulky disease or B symptoms were randomized to receive radiation or have a laparotomy and then to receive radiation and/or chemotherapy as deemed appropriate. There was no statistical difference in freedom from progression or overall survival rates at 6 years, with or without laparotomy (78% vs 83% and 91% vs 85%, respectively).[21] Therefore, laparotomy is not necessary to treat patients with radiation if they have a favorable prognosis, supradiaphragmatic disease, and CS I or II disease (low risk of abdominal disease).

Nodal involvement below the diaphragm (subdiaphragmatic) is seen in only about 10% of patients with stage I and II disease. Patients who do not have splenic involvement (60% of patients) can receive extended-field or total nodal irradiation (see Fig. 129–2). With these approaches, the outcome will be similar to patients treated for supradiaphragmatic disease.[22]

CHEMOTHERAPY IN COMBINATION WITH RADIATION

Over the last 10 to 15 years, most trials have evaluated treatment regimens that minimize long-term complications, while maintaining high cure rates. The combination of chemotherapy and radiation holds the promise of decreasing the number of patients who relapse as well as minimizing toxicity, depending on the volume of radiation and chemotherapy regimen selected.[3]

Several early studies compared a "non toxic chemotherapy regimen" consisting of vinblastine, bleomycin, and methotrexate (VBM), combined with involved field radiation in CS I or II disease to subtotal nodal radiation. The recurrence rates were less with the combination, but survival was not different between the two groups. Investigators also discovered that this was a toxic regimen, with as many as 16% of patients experiencing pulmonary toxicity.[2,23,24] A similar trial (EORTC H7F) was conducted in patients with favorable CS I to stage IIA Hodgkin's disease comparing six cycles of epirubicin, bleomycin, vinblastine, and prednisone (EBVP) plus involved-field radiation to subtotal nodal and splenic irradiation. After 6 years of followup, the relapse-free survival rate was higher for the EBVP plus radiation arm as compared to radiation (92% vs 81%, respectively), but the overall survival rates did not differ (98% vs 96%, respectively).[2]

To minimize toxicity, most current studies are focusing on determining how many cycles of chemotherapy and the volume of radiation that must be used to obtain optimal patient outcomes. Traditionally, a minimum of six cycles have been used; although some data suggest that as few as four cycles of chemotherapy can cure occult abdominal disease. Based on this knowledge, investigators have compared four cycles of ABVD with subtotal nodal radiation with four cycles of ABVD and involved field radiation.[2] After a median followup of 87 months, no significant difference was noted in freedom from progression or overall survival (97% vs 94% and 93% vs 94%, respectively), which indicates that with four cycles of ABVD, the volume of radiation can be reduced from subtotal nodal to involved field. Some investigators currently administer as few as two cycles of chemotherapy with radiation. A study done by GHSG randomized 643 patients with favorable CS IA to stage IIB disease to subtotal nodal and splenic irradiation alone or to two courses of ABVD and the same radiation protocol. Preliminary results show that freedom from treatment failure with the combined treatment modality was superior to radiation alone (96% vs 87%, respectively), but no difference was observed in overall survival (98% vs 97%, respectively).[2] The current standard therapy in British Colombia for early stage Hodgkin's disease is two cycles of ABVD chemotherapy followed by extended field or involved field radiation. By using this approach, these investigators recently reported their 10-year failure-free survival as 90% and overall survival at 96%.[25]

CHEMOTHERAPY ALONE

There are limited data evaluating chemotherapy alone versus radiation or chemoradiotherapy in patients with early stage favorable disease. Two large studies have compared six cycles of MOPP chemotherapy to subtotal nodal radiation. One study, which was primarily comprised of unfavorable early stage Hodgkin's disease patients, reported no difference in disease-free survival or overall survival.[26] In the second study, no difference in disease-free survival was detected, but a significant difference in overall survival was observed in patients receiving radiation (56% vs 93%).[27] This difference was attributed to the inefficiency of salvage chemotherapy.

A study comparing CVPP to CVPP plus involved field radiation has been completed. After 7 years of followup in the subset of favorable disease patients, no difference was seen in the chemotherapy group as compared to the chemoradiotherapy group in terms of disease-free survival or overall survival.[2] Further studies are ongoing to determine if chemotherapy alone is a viable option for early stage disease.

TREATMENT OF EARLY STAGE UNFAVORABLE DISEASE

RADIATION THERAPY ALONE

The exact criteria used to define unfavorable prognosis varies between studies, but most include patients with bulky disease, B-symptoms, and advanced age. Patients with early stage disease and massive mediastinal involvement (mediastinal masses larger than one-third the greatest chest diameter on x-ray) have very high relapse rates if treated with radiation alone.[8,28] Patients with B symptoms are also at a high risk of relapse if treated with radiation alone.[8,28] Studies comparing radiation alone to combined modality treatment show that radiation alone is associated with higher relapse rates, but overall survival rates are not different.[28] The overall survival was not different because of the effectiveness of salvage chemotherapy. Although radiation provides the same survival rate as chemoradiotherapy, most clinicians use combined modality therapy to reduce the relapse rate.

CHEMOTHERAPY IN COMBINATION WITH RADIATION

The combination of chemotherapy and radiation therapy can significantly decrease relapse rates as compared with radiation alone. In a meta-analysis, Specht and colleagues[20] indicated that the addition of chemotherapy to radiotherapy can reduce the risk of failure by about 50% at 10 years, but does not significantly improve survival. The primary conclusion from this analysis is that the use of chemotherapy allows for less intensive radiation (a reduction in radiotherapy fields) and appears to achieve similar survival rates. Because of improved relapse rates and the ability to avoid laparoscopy, most oncologists treat unfavorable early disease with chemoradiotherapy.

The current questions evolve around choosing the best chemotherapy regimen to combine with radiation as well as duration of therapy. Two large trials done in the 1970s and 1980s compared MOPP to ABVD in a split-course treatment (three cycles of chemotherapy, followed by radiation, then three more cycles of chemotherapy). The first study found no difference in freedom from progression, but the second study found ABVD to be superior in terms of freedom from treatment failure (68% vs 90%).[2] These differences lead to early closure of the trial. However, after 10 years of followup the overall survival rates did not differ between groups (87% vs 87%).[29] The use of the less-toxic regimen EBVP, which is effective in favorable disease, was found to be inferior to MOPP/ABV in patients with unfavorable disease.[2] Other regimens that are effective include CVPP in combination with mantle irradiation.[2] A relatively new regimen, Stanford V, has generated a great amount of interest because in patients with bulky early stage disease and advanced stage disease, it has produced a projected 6-year survival of 93% and freedom from progression rate of 89%.[30] Because ABVD has become the standard in advanced stage Hodgkin's disease, it has also become the standard in unfavorable early stage disease.[2] The guidelines published by NCCN in 1999, however, list the Stanford V and MOPP/ABVD regimens as alternatives to be used with radiation.[13]

CHEMOTHERAPY ALONE

Similar to early stage disease with a favorable prognosis, there are limited data with chemotherapy alone in unfavorable early stage disease. A randomized controlled trial that compared six cycles of CVPP to six cycles of CVPP plus radiation found chemotherapy alone to be inferior. The 7-year freedom from relapse rates for CVPP alone and CVPP plus radiation were 34% versus 75%, and overall survival rates of 66% versus 84%, respectively.[31] When patients with bulky mediastinal disease and other risk factors (except B symptoms) received CVPP alone or CVPP plus radiation, no significant difference in 7-year overall survival (81% vs 89%, respectively) was noted, although disease-free survival was lower in the CVPP alone arm (62% vs 71%).[31] Currently, there is little support for using chemotherapy alone in patients with early stage unfavorable disease.

TREATMENT OF ADVANCED STAGE DISEASE

Advanced stage disease consists of stage III and IV disease. It is almost always wide spread and mandates systemic chemotherapy. However, there is a subset of patients who are classified with stage $IIIA_1$ disease (limited spleen, celiac, splenic, or portal nodes), who have a favorable disease outcome and respond well to total nodal irradiation. The disease-free and overall survival rates compare favorably to earlier stage disease; 20-year disease-free survival is 65%.[32] However, more recent retrospective data suggest that stage $IIIA_1$ disease is better managed with combined modality therapy or combination chemotherapy alone.[33] Bulky mediastinal and stage $IIIA_2$ disease is similar to stage IV disease in that combination chemotherapy is the mainstay of treatment.

CHEMOTHERAPY

One of the initial combination chemotherapy regimens introduced in the early 1960s that was shown to produce cures in advanced Hodgkin's disease was the MOPP regimen (Table 129–4).[34] MOPP chemotherapy has been the mainstay of treatment for patients with stage III and stage IV advanced Hodgkin's disease. According to the 20-year followup of the National Cancer Institute trial, MOPP has produced complete remissions (disappearance of all measurable disease) in 84% of patients and has a 10-year cure rate of 54%. Forty-six percent of the original patients are still alive at a median of 14 years (19% died as a result of other illness).[35] This is in contrast to the results of single-agent therapy, in which remissions occur less rapidly and are not as durable. Several other trials reviewed by Longo reported similar results, with complete response rates ranging from 80% to 95% and cure rates ranging from 55% to 65%.[36] These studies indicate that patients should receive two cycles of therapy beyond that required to produce a complete response; a minimum of six cycles should be administered. Maintenance therapy has not been shown to increase survival and may contribute to the long-term complications seen with therapy. The delivery of full or nearly full doses of chemotherapy is extremely important (e.g., dose intensity). Dose reduction within the various studies is probably the single most important factor explaining the differences in response rates between institutions administering seemingly similar regimens.[36] Dosage reductions based on toxicity may be made, but significant reductions can alter response and survival.[35]

MOPP VARIATIONS AND OTHER ALTERNATIVE REGIMENS

Ever since MOPP therapy was created and the efficacy confirmed, researchers have been modifying the regimen in an attempt to improve efficacy and possibly decrease toxicity. Table 129–4 lists some MOPP variations and other commonly used regimens.[36] MVPP (vinblastine substituted for vincristine), CVPP (cyclophosphamide substituted

TABLE 129–4. Combination Chemotherapy Regimens for Hodgkin's Disease

Drug	(mg/m²)	Route	Days
MOPP			
Mechlorethamine	6	IV	1, 8
Vincristine	1.4	IV	1, 8
Procarbazine	100	PO	1–14
Prednisone	40	PO	1–14
ABVD			
Doxorubicin	25	IV	1, 15
Bleomycin	10	IV	1, 15
Vinblastine	6	IV	1, 15
Dacarbazine	375	IV	1, 15
ChlVPP			
Chlorambucil	6	PO	1–14
Vinblastine	6	IV	1, 8
Procarbazine	100	PO	1–14
Prednisone	40	PO	1–14
MOPP/ABVD			
Alternating months of MOPP and ABVD			
MOPP/ABV Hybrid			
Mechlorethamine	6	IV	1
Vincristine	1.4	IV	1
Procarbazine	100	PO	1–7
Prednisone	40	PO	1–14
Doxorubicin	35	IV	8
Bleomycin	10	IV	8
Vinblastine	6	IV	8

Adapted from Ref. 36.

for mechlorethamine), BCVPP (carmustine, cyclophosphamide, vinblastine, procarbazine, and prednisone), and ChlVPP (chlorambucil substituted for mechlorethamine, vinblastine substituted for vincristine) are attractive alternatives to MOPP because they offer equal efficacy and differing or less severe toxicities. ChlVPP is especially attractive because of its equivalent activity and less-severe emetogenicity and neurotoxicity. The various combination chemotherapy regimens appear to produce initial complete response rates in more than 80% of the patients treated and to result in a 55% to 65% cure rate for advanced Hodgkin's disease.

One of the first alternative regimens was ABVD (doxorubicin, bleomycin, vinblastine, dacarbazine) developed by Bonadonna (Table 129–4). ABVD was initially shown to be effective in MOPP failures,[37] and was later compared directly to MOPP in advanced disease, and produced an 82% complete response rate in contrast to a 67% complete response rate with MOPP. Despite these differences in response, no major differences in 5-year survival were noted.[38] The difference in response is most likely a result of excessive dosage reductions, which occurred in the MOPP arm. Improved failure-free survival was demonstrated with ABVD in a subgroup with poor prognostic factors.

ALTERNATING AND HYBRID REGIMENS

The Goldie-Coldman hypothesis regarding spontaneous mutation rates and the development of resistant clones can explain many clinical findings related to cancer chemotherapy, including chemotherapy failure.[39] This hypothesis has led to the investigation of alternating non–cross-resistant drug combinations.[40] A key requirement in such a concept is that each regimen possesses equal activity. A major reason for using alternating or hybrid regimens is to decrease cumulative toxicities. In alternating and hybrid regimens such as MOPP and ABVD, the sterilizing and leukemogenic doses of procarbazine and nitrogen mustard are reduced by 50%, and the cardiotoxic dose of doxorubicin is reduced by 50% in the alternating regimen and by 33% in the hybrid regimen. In addition, the potential for pulmonary toxicity from bleomycin should also be reduced.

Several trials have been performed to evaluate various ways of administering noncross-resistant MOPP and ABVD regimens. Table 129–5 summarizes the results of selected trials representing different approaches. The Milan Cancer Institute found MOPP alternating with ABVD to be superior to MOPP alone.[41] This is one of the few randomized trials that reported a true advantage for the alternating regimen. But the conclusions from this study are questionable because of the high dropout rate in the alternating regimen (22%) and the dose attenuation of the MOPP regimen. CALGB compared the ABVD regimen with alternating the MOPP and ABVD regimens and found no difference in efficacy.[38] Alternating MOPP and ABVD appears to provide minimal if any improvement over MOPP or ABVD. Studies have also evaluated alternating regimens with combining both regimens in a monthly cycle (known as hybrid regimens). The National Cancer Institute of Canada[42] compared the MOPP/ABVD alternating regimen to the MOPP/ABV hybrid regimen (omitting the dacarbazine and increasing doxorubicin from 25 mg/m^2 to 35 mg/m^2) and the Milan Cancer Institute[43] compared the MOPP/ABVD alternating regimen to the MOPP/ABVD hybrid regimen. Neither of these studies detected a difference in freedom from progression or overall survival. However, both the Canadian NCI[42] and the Milan group[43] found that patients treated with the hybrid regimen were more likely to develop neutropenic fever and stomatitis. It has also been reported that the MOPP/ABV hybrid regimen is more toxic than the ABVD regimen.[44] Finally, some investigators attempted to improve efficacy with the sequential use of MOPP and ABVD. Results of an intergroup trial[45] showed sequential MOPP and ABVD to be inferior to the MOPP/ABV hybrid regimen in terms of response and survival. They also reported a lower rate of secondary malignancies in the hybrid arm.

None of the alternating, hybrid, or sequential regimen trials have clearly demonstrated an advantage over fully dosed four-drug (e.g., MOPP or ABVD) regimens. Because MOPP has more toxicity when dose intensity is maintained, ABVD is the standard four-drug regimen. Until further data are available, the more complex hybrid or alternating regimens are unlikely to replace the well-established four-drug regimens.

CHEMOTHERAPY IN COMBINATION WITH RADIATION

The role of radiotherapy when added to chemotherapy for the treatment of Hodgkin's disease is controversial. In settings in which radiation therapy alone demonstrated poor results (disease with large mediastinal involvement, bulky disease, stage IIIA$_2$ disease, stage IV disease), chemotherapy alone or a combination of chemotherapy and radiation therapy remains the only other option.

Loeffler and colleagues[46] conducted a meta-analysis of chemotherapy versus combined modality treatment trials in intermediate- or advanced-stage Hodgkin's disease. In studies that compared standard chemotherapy to the same chemotherapy plus radiation, no overall survival advantage could be detected after 10 years of followup,

TABLE 129–5. Randomized Trials Evaluating Various Methods of Delivering Both MOPP and ABVD

Regimen	CR (%)	FFP	OS	Reference
MOPP versus MOPP	74	36% (8 y)	64% (8 y)	Milan Cancer Institute
alternating with ABVD	89	65% (8 y)	84% (8 y)	
ABVD versus MOPP	82	61% (5 y)	73% (5 y)	Cancer and Leukemia
alternating with ABVD	83	65% (5 y)	75% (5 y)	Group B (CALGB)
MOPP alternating with	51	67% (5 y)	81% (5 y)	National Cancer Institute
ABVD versus MOPP/ ABV hybrid	54	71% (5 y)	83% (5 y)	of Canada
MOPP alternating with	91	67% (10 y)	74% (10 y)	Milan Cancer Institute
ABVD versus MOPP/ ABV hybrid	89	69% (10 y)	72% (10 y)	
Sequential MOPP then	75	54% (8 y)	71% (8 y)	Intergroup trial
ABVD versus MOPP/ABVD hybrid	83	64% (8 y)	79% (8 y)	

CR, complete response rate; FFP, freedom from progression; OS, overall survival.

although the addition of radiation improved tumor control. These trials included approximately equal numbers of early stage and advanced stage patients. The meta-analysis also evaluated studies that compared prolonged chemotherapy treatments (additional cycles of the same chemotherapy or a different regimen) and standard chemotherapy combined with radiation therapy. Surprisingly, there was no difference in tumor control rates, but a survival advantage favoring the prolonged chemotherapy group was observed. Most of the patients in the latter trials had advanced disease. There were several limitations of this meta-analysis: limited data were available regarding the presence of bulky mediastinal disease and cause of death; and trials differed in their design and the type and number of cycles of chemotherapy, and dose and field size of radiation therapy. Overall, results from this analysis suggest that combined modality therapy should be reserved for patients with nodular sclerosis Hodgkin's disease, for patients without stage IV disease, and for patients with bulky nodal involvement.

Future directions for the treatment of advanced stage Hodgkin's disease include new regimens with or without radiation therapy. Two new treatment regimens, Stanford V and BEACOPP, have shown very high complete remission rates, and early analysis of these trials show high disease-free survival rates. However, longer followup is required before these regimens can become the standard of care.[2] Although the Stanford V regimen has not been directly compared with ABVD (the current standard) and the followup is relatively short, the NCCN expert panel included it as an option in their treatment guideline.[13]

SALVAGE CHEMOTHERAPY

Patients who relapse after radiation therapy alone have a good chance of being cured with combination chemotherapy.[36] MOPP or one of its variants can cure 55% to 65% of patients treated for advanced Hodgkin's disease. The remaining 35% to 45% of patients will either not respond initially, or will relapse after achieving a complete response.[36] For patients who relapse after an initial complete response to MOPP, reinduction is possible. The NCI has reported on its long-term followup of MOPP-retreated patients.[47] Patients with long initial remissions had a 45% disease-free survival rate at 10 years. However, it is doubtful whether a regimen that was unable to cure when used as first-line therapy should be used for salvage when other effective regimens with a lower likelihood of cross-resistance are available. The choice of salvage treatment should be guided by the estimation of the patient's tolerance for a particular set of agents. Examples of salvage regimens and their response data can be found in the review of chemotherapy in Hodgkin's disease.[36] Although approximately 40% of patients will achieve a complete response, only 10% to 15% of those treated will eventually be cured by their salvage regimen.

Patients who relapse after salvage chemotherapy are candidates for high-dose therapy with hematopoietic stem cell transplantation (HSCT). High-dose therapy should also be considered in patients who relapse within 12 months of initial remission or in those who are refractory to first line chemotherapy. The role of HSCT in Hodgkin's disease is reviewed in Chap. 134.

COMPLICATIONS

A variety of acute and chronic toxicities may occur as a result of staging procedures or treatment for Hodgkin's disease.[36] Immunologic dysfunction may result from the Hodgkin's disease process itself, but further impairment may be induced following staging laparotomy and splenectomy, radiation therapy, and/or chemotherapy. This impairment in cellular immunity predisposes the patient to infection with encapsulated organisms. Therefore, vaccination against *Pneumococcus*, *H. influenzae* type B, and *Meningococcus* is recommended 10 to 14 days prior to initiation of therapy for Hodgkin's disease.

Radiation therapy commonly causes anorexia, xerostomia, odynophagia, skin burns, and changes in taste perception, which is usually transient and seldom produces significant morbidity. Hypothyroidism and myelosuppression can also be seen. More serious toxic effects involving the mantle and the heart can occur during radiation therapy for Hodgkin's disease. Radiation pneumonitis and fibrosis, pericarditis, and cardiomyopathy have been reported. Neurologic complications of radiotherapy include rare spinal cord transections with overlap of mantle and para-aortic fields or Lhermitte's syndrome (consisting of numbness and tingling caused by head flexion) in up to 15% of patients. Pelvic irradiation may cause infertility in males and females. In addition, growth retardation may result from radiotherapy in pediatric patients. As the techniques for radiation therapy improve, the risk of serious complications associated with its use will be reduced.

Side effects of chemotherapy can be acute or long-term. Acute toxic effects seen with the treatment of Hodgkin's disease are similar to those seen with most combination regimens. Myelosuppression is the major dose-limiting toxicity of most of these regimens. Hematopoietic growth factors, such as granulocyte colony-stimulating factor (G-CSF) or granulocyte-macrophage colony-stimulating factor (GM-CSF), can decrease the neutropenia associated with these regimens and allow for the delivery of optimal drug doses on schedule.

Nausea and vomiting are frequently seen with the use of dacarbazine, doxorubicin, and mechlorethamine, although the severity of this complication has been diminished with the use of 5-HT_3 antagonists. Many patients experience neurotoxicity secondary to vincristine. Other acute adverse effects include alopecia, dermatitis, mucositis, phlebitis, malaise and fatigue, and renal dysfunction. Bleomycin or nitrosoureas may cause pneumonitis and doxorubicin may lead to the development of cardiomyopathy. Patients receiving radiation with chemotherapy have a higher risk of toxicities than do those patients not receiving radiation.

Long-term complications of radiation therapy, chemotherapy, and combined modality therapy are more evident as the curability and long-term survival of Hodgkin's disease patients improves.[3] Gonadal dysfunction and secondary malignancies are important considerations in the treatment of this malignancy. Almost all men and up to 50% of premenopausal women treated with six full cycles of regimens containing alkylating agents will become sterile. This appears to be a dose-related phenomenon. For men, there does not appear to be a safe nonsterilizing dose of nitrogen mustard or chlorambucil, so if fertility is a major concern, ABVD may be the best alternative.[2,3,8]

Now that 10-, 15-, and 20-year survival data are available, evaluation of secondary malignancies can be made. Recent reports show that 20 years after treatment for Hodgkin's disease, the risk of developing a secondary cancer can be as high as 38%.[25] The tumors most commonly diagnosed include female breast cancer, lung cancer, digestive cancers, and buccal cancers. Radiation therapy is associated with the highest risk of developing a solid tumor (relative risk = 4.6).[48] Other observed secondary malignancies include a variety of solid tumors, non-Hodgkin's lymphomas, acute leukemias, and associated myelodysplastic syndromes. The overall risk of developing acute leukemia (most commonly acute nonlymphocytic leukemia) ranges from 3% to 6%, but may be significantly higher in certain subsets of patients. There is a higher risk of developing acute leukemia in patients treated with MOPP as compared to ABVD; combined modality therapy further increases the risk of developing secondary leukemias.[49]

An international collaborative group of cancer registries and hospitals recently reported on 163 cases of leukemia in 29,552 patients with Hodgkin's disease.[15] This is the largest report of its kind. They presented their results in terms of relative risk rather than percent chance of developing acute leukemia. Chemotherapy alone had a ninefold increased risk of developing leukemia as compared to radiation therapy alone. For patients treated with more than six cycles of combination chemotherapy containing mechlorethamine or procarbazine, the risk of leukemia was 14 times higher than for radiation alone. For patients in this series treated with chemotherapy and radiation, the relative risks were 7.7, or roughly equal to that of chemotherapy alone. The incidence of leukemia peaked at 5 years following chemotherapy, with development lasting for at least 8 years after completion of therapy. Future trials must focus on maintaining high cure rates in Hodgkin's disease while decreasing the number and severity of long-term complications.

CURRENT RECOMMENDATIONS

With radiation therapy, chemotherapy, and salvage HSCT, more than 75% of patients with advanced Hodgkin's disease can now be cured. Although the special circumstances of the patient, available resources, technologies, and the skill of the practitioners influence specific treatment recommendations, the following general recommendations can be made (Table 129–6).

TABLE 129–6. General Treatment Recommendations for Hodgkin's Disease[a,b]

Early Stage Disease	
Favorable Prognosis (CS I or II with no risk factors)	Extended field radiation or 4–6 cycles of ABVD or EBVP plus involved field radiation
Unfavorable Prognosis (CS I or II with risk factors)	4–6 cycles of ABVD or MOPP/ABV plus involved field radiation
Advanced Stage Disease (CS III or IV)	6–8 cycles of ABVD, or MOPP/ABV, or ChlVPP, or MOPP plus radiation to residual lymphoma or sites of bulky disease
Relapsed Disease	
Relapse after radiation	6–8 cycles of chemotherapy with or without radiation (treat as if this were primary advanced disease)
Relapse after primary chemotherapy[c,d]	Salvage chemotherapy at conventional doses or high-dose chemotherapy and autologous hematopoietic stem cell transplantation

[a]Patients should be considered for clinical trials when possible.
[b]In general, patients with large mediastinal adenopathy should be treated with chemotherapy followed by radiation to the mediastinum.
[c]A standard regimen or approach does not exist.
[d]Highly selected patients may be treated with radiation alone.

For patients with favorable early stage disease, either extended field radiation alone or four to six cycles of chemotherapy plus involved field radiation should be used. If exploratory laparotomy or radiation is not desirable, combination chemotherapy can be recommended. Patients who have unfavorable early stage disease should be treated with four to six cycles of chemotherapy plus involved field radiation. Ongoing trials in early stage disease are evaluating the role of combination chemotherapy alone, modified chemotherapy regimens or shorter courses of standard chemotherapy combined with radiation therapy, and limited radiation field sizes.

Radiation therapy alone may not be appropriate for stage IIIA disease, except in the instance of pathologic stage $IIIA_1$ disease with few splenic nodes. For all other (clinical or pathologic) stage III patients and stage IV patients, combination chemotherapy is the recommended treatment. The chemotherapy regimen selected should be based on expected toxicity, which vary between regimens. Based on the recent CALGB data (discussed earlier) and issues related to sterility, ABVD is a reasonable initial regimen (although the cardiopulmonary toxicities of doxorubicin and bleomycin must be considered). If fertility is not an issue, the MOPP alternative, ChlVPP, should be considered because it is very well tolerated and does not generally cause alopecia or neuropathy. Its leukemogenic effects are likely less than those seen with MOPP, but higher than ABVD. Adverse effects such as nausea and vomiting and neurotoxicity generally lead to larger dosage reductions of MOPP than with ABVD, which can reduce efficacy. Alternating MOPP/ABVD or hybrid MOPP/ABV may be used, although neither has been definitively proven to provide benefit over standard four drug regimens. In addition, MOPP/ABV hybrid has been shown to cause more serious toxicity, including a higher rate of secondary malignancies, when compared to ABVD. The routine use of radiation therapy following combination chemotherapy (combined modality therapy) cannot be recommended with currently available data. Only in the instance of large bulky mediastinal disease is this appropriate.

Early stage patients who relapse after radiation therapy alone respond well to combination chemotherapy. Patients with advanced disease who fail or have relapsed following combination chemotherapy may be treated with conventional salvage therapy or with salvage chemotherapy followed by high dose therapy with hematopoietic stem cell support (Chap. 134). The decision to use salvage chemotherapy alone versus high-dose therapy with stem cell support depends on the patient's risk factors for relapse following salvage chemotherapy.

NON-HODGKIN'S LYMPHOMA

The NHLs are a heterogeneous group of lymphoproliferative disorders that affect people from early childhood to late adulthood. Advances in molecular biology techniques and our understanding of the human immune system have led to major progress in understanding the pathogenesis and treatment of the lymphomas. NHLs are classified into distinct clinical entities that are defined by a combination of morphology, immunophenotype, genetic features, and clinical features. These differences influence the natural history, and approach and response to treatment. The use of extensive combination chemotherapeutic regimens has shown dramatic improvement in survival and cure in patients with a disease that once was considered incurable. The 5-year survival rate for patients with NHL has increased from 47% to 53% over the past 25 years.[1,50] Further improvement in survival is anticipated with the continued expansion of our therapeutic armamentarium, including high-dose chemotherapy and biologic therapy.

EPIDEMIOLOGY AND ETIOLOGY

NHL is the fifth most common cause of newly diagnosed cancer in the United States and accounts for approximately 4% of all cancers. An estimated 56,200 new cases will be diagnosed in 2001 (55% male and 45% female), and it is estimated that 26,300 people will die from NHL during this same period.[1] Although the average age of patients at the time of diagnosis is about 65 years, NHL can occur at any age.[51] The incidence generally increases with age, and is higher in men than in women, and is higher in whites than in blacks.[50] The incidence of NHL has increased by more than 80% in the United States since the early 1970s, from 8.6 cases per 100,000 in 1973 to about 16 cases per 100,000 in the mid-1990s, with an average increase of approximately 3% to 4% per year.[50] The incidence of NHL appears to have plateaued since reaching its peak in 1994, but it is not clear whether this observation is a long-term trend. The increase in the incidence of NHL over the past three decades is second only to melanoma and has been referred to as an epidemic of NHL. Although the increased incidence has been particularly noted among the elderly and patients with AIDS, much of this increase cannot be explained by known risk factors.[51]

The etiology of NHL is unknown, although several genetic diseases, environmental agents, and infectious agents have been associated with the development of NHL. An increased incidence of NHL is seen in many congenital and acquired immunodeficiency states, supporting the role of immune dysregulation in the etiology of NHL. Patients with congenital immunodeficiency disorders (Wiskott-Aldrich syndrome, ataxia, telangiectasia), acquired immunodeficiency disorders (AIDS, acquired hypogammaglobulinemia, graft-versus-host disease), and chronic pharmacologic immunosuppression (solid organ transplantation) are predisposed to the development of NHL.[51] Autoimmune diseases (Hashimoto's thyroiditis, Sjögren's syndrome) cause chronic inflammation in the mucosa-associated lymphoid tissue (MALT), which predisposes patients to subsequent lymphoid malignancies. Other autoimmune diseases such as systemic lupus erythematosus and rheumatoid arthritis are also associated with the development of NHL, but the use of immunosuppressive agents in these diseases makes the pathologic cause less clear.[51]

Certain infections have been associated with the development of lymphoma.[51,52] EBV was discovered in cell lines from tumors of patients with African (endemic) Burkitt's lymphoma, and EBV DNA is associated with 95% of endemic Burkitt's lymphoma. However, EBV is associated with sporadic Burkitt's lymphoma in about 30% of cases. EBV is also associated with posttransplant lymphoproliferative disorders (PTLDs) and some lymphomas in patients with AIDS or congenital immunodeficiencies. The human T-cell lymphotropic virus type 1 (HTLV-1) was the first human retrovirus associated with a malignancy. This type C RNA virus is strongly associated with an aggressive form of T-cell lymphoma, known as adult T-cell leukemia/lymphoma (ATL).[51] HTLV-1 is endemic in southern Japan, Africa, and the Caribbean. In endemic areas, more than 50% of all NHL cases are ATL. A third virus associated with NHL is human herpes virus 8 (HHV-8).[51] This virus was originally isolated from Kaposi's sarcoma lesions in AIDS patients. Finally, gastric infection with *Helicobacter pylori,* a gram-negative bacteria that leads to chronic gastritis, is associated with gastric MALT lymphomas.[51]

A number of physical agents have also been associated with the development of NHL.[51,52] Exposure to herbicides, particularly exposure to phenoxy herbicides, is associated with the development of NHL. These observations may explain why certain occupations, such as farmers, forestry workers, and agricultural workers, are associated with a higher risk of NHL. A higher risk of NHL is also associated with exposure to other chemical solvents and dyes, exposure to radiation from nuclear explosions, and high intake of meats and dietary fats.

GENETIC ABNORMALITIES

Chromosomal translocations are a hallmark of many lymphoid malignancies.[53,54] The presence of these specific translocations can be helpful in the diagnosis and classification of lymphoid malignancies. The mechanisms leading to the translocations are unknown, but they usually involve the antigen receptor loci. In contrast to most myeloid and some lymphoid leukemias, NHL usually place a structurally intact cellular protooncogene under the regulatory influence of the highly expressed immunoglobulin (Ig) or T-cell receptor (TCR) genes, leading to effects on cell growth, cellular differentiation, or apoptosis. The most common chromosomal translocations involve t(8;14), t(14;18), and t(11;14); each translocation involves the immunoglobulin heavy-chain gene locus on chromosome 14 at 14q32. The translocation t(8;14) that involves c-myc, a well-characterized oncogene clearly associated with malignancy, is implicated in nearly all cases of Burkitt's lymphoma. The translocation t(14;18) that involves bcl-2, one of several putative B-cell lymphoma-associated oncogenes, is found in about 85% of human follicular B-cell lymphomas. The translocation t(11;14) that involves bcl-1, is found in most patients with mantle cell lymphoma. Another putative B-cell lymphoma-associated oncogene, bcl-6, is found in about a third of diffuse, large cell lymphomas.

Although mutations in the *p*53 tumor-suppressor gene have been recognized in many human neoplasms, such mutations have not been consistently found in patients with lymphoma, which suggests that it may occur late in malignant evolution.

Detection of translocations, such as bcl-2 in follicular lymphomas, can be used clinically to monitor for minimal residual disease. In patients with follicular lymphoma who received monoclonal antibody-purged autologous bone marrow transplantation, those whose bone marrow was negative by polymerase chain reaction (PCR) for the bcl-2 rearrangement after purging had significantly longer freedom from recurrence than those whose bone marrow remained PCR positive.[55]

PATHOLOGY AND CLASSIFICATION

NHLs are neoplasms derived from the monoclonal proliferation of malignant B or T lymphocytes and their precursors. More than 80% of malignant lymphomas in the United States are of B-cell origin. Proliferation of malignant cells results in the replacement of the normal cells and architecture of lymph nodes or bone marrow with a relatively uniform population of lymphoid cells. The classification of NHLs has evolved over the last five decades, as advances in immunology and genetics have allowed scientists to recognize a number of previously unrecognized subtypes of NHLs (Table 129–7). The current classification schemes characterize the NHLs according to the cell of origin (B cell vs T cell), clinical features, and morphologic features. Additional immunohistochemical markers, cytogenetic features, and genotypic characteristics may also help to further classify NHL into subtypes.

MORPHOLOGY

The macroscopic and microscopic appearance of the involved tissue remains one of the most important factors in the diagnosis and classification of NHLs. In the 1950s, Rappaport and coworkers proposed a morphologic classification of malignant lymphomas based on two features: (a) that the malignant cell would disrupt the nodal architecture in a *nodular* or *diffuse* manner, and (b) that lymphomas of histiocytic origin existed.[56] The Rappaport classification gained rapid acceptance in the United States because of its precision, simplicity, and prognostic

TABLE 129–7. Evolution in the Classification of Non-Hodgkin's Lymphomas

Time	Classification System	Basis for Classification
1950s–1960s	Rappaport	Morphology
1970s–1980s	Luke and Collins	Morphology and immunophenotype
1970s–1980s	Kiel	Morphology and immunophenotype
1980s–1990s	International Working Formulation	Morphology
1990s	REAL	Disease entities
2001	Revised REAL/WHO	Disease entities

REAL, Revised European-American Classification Lymphoid Neoplasms developed by the International Lymphoma Study Group (ILSG); WHO, World Health Organization

significance (Table 129–7). Application of the system divided NHLs into those with large (i.e., incorrectly called "histiocytes") or small cells, with or without a nodular (i.e., follicular) growth pattern.

IMMUNOLOGY

In the 1970s, it became apparent that NHLs were tumors of the immune system and were derived from B or T lymphocytes. The availability of techniques using antibodies to antigens on the surface of lymphoid cells (i.e., immunophenotype) and cytochemical assays lead to the following conclusions: (a) most NHLs were of B-cell origin; (b) all follicular or nodular lymphomas were of follicle center cell origin; and (c) most lymphomas previously classified as reticulum cell sarcoma, clasmatocytic lymphoma, or histiocytic lymphoma had the immunologic characteristics of transformed lymphocytes. Using this new information, a number of expert pathologists independently developed new classification schemes for NHL in the 1970s and 1980s. The Kiel classification was based primarily on the work of Lennert and became widely used in Europe.[57] In North America, the Lukes and Collins classification scheme[58] was used briefly, but was soon superseded by the consensus Working Formulation (Table 129–7).[59] Like the Rappaport classification, divisions within the Working Formulation were based largely on cell size (large ["histiocytic"] vs small [lymphocytic]), cell shape (round vs not round), and growth pattern (follicular [nodular] vs diffuse). Both the Kiel and Working Formulation classification schemes also considered the histologic grade of the tumor, which correlated with the natural history of patients with the various subtypes of NHL. "Low grade" indicated longer median survival (i.e., indolent), whereas "high grade" indicated shorter median survival (i.e., aggressive). In the 1980s and early 1990s, the Working Formulation became the most widely used classification scheme in North America, whereas the Kiel classification was widely used in Europe. It was based on the premise that NHL was a single disease with a range of histologic grade and clinical aggressiveness.

NEW DISEASE ENTITIES

In the 1980s and early 1990s, rapid advances in immunology and genetics allowed scientists to recognize a number of previously unrecognized subtypes of NHL. Cytogenetic and molecular genetic analyses identified the presence of many chromosomal translocations, oncogenes, and their gene products in patients with NHL (see Genetic Abnormalities section). In addition, diseases that would have been lumped together as "low grade" or "intermediate/high grade" in the Working Formulation showed marked differences in survival, prompting scientists to reevaluate lymphoma classification schemes.

Information from these studies have allowed scientists to further classify B-cell lymphomas as malignant expansions of cells from either the germinal center, mantle zone, or marginal zone of normal lymph nodes. Germinal centers are complex structures that form in spleen and lymph nodes in response to antigenic challenge. In addition to B-cells, germinal centers contain antigen-presenting cells and helper T-cells that cooperate in mediating the B-cell changes that result in a more potent secondary immune response. Malignant transformation often occurs or is initiated in germinal center B cells. Follicular, Burkitt's, and most large cell lymphomas are believed to be tumors of germinal center B cells. Three histologically distinct microenvironments have been described within the germinal center: a mantle zone surrounding interior dark, and light zones. The mantle zone contains small resting B cells that have not been exposed to antigen ("naive"). Tumors of cells from the mantle zone are usually clinically indolent and histologically low grade. Antigen-triggered activation of the densely packed B cells of the dark zone causes cells to proliferate and subjects genomic DNA to somatic hypermutation. Surviving clones from within the dark zone then enter the light zone where proliferation slows and affinity selection occurs. Antigen-specific B cells generated in the germinal center reaction leave the follicle and reappear in the outer mantle zone, to form a marginal zone. Marginal zones are particularly prominent in mesenteric lymph nodes, Peyer's patches, and the spleen. These postgerminal center B cells include memory B cells of the marginal zone and plasma cells. Marginal cell B-cell lymphomas tend to be indolent and may be either extranodal or nodal; extranodal marginal cell B-cell lymphomas are also referred to as MALT lymphomas.

T-cell lymphomas can be classified on the basis of antigen expression as either precursor (thymic) or mature (peripheral) in origin. These classifications clinically translate to precursor lymphoblastic lymphomas or to a heterogeneous group of peripheral T-cell lymphomas. Tumors of natural killer (NK) or NK-like T cells are uncommon.

The International Lymphoma Study Group (ILSG), an informal group of 19 hematopathologists from the United States, Europe, and Asia, adopted a new approach to lymphoma classification in 1993. Because it represented a revision of current or prior European and American lymphoma classifications, it was called the Revised European-American Classification of Lymphoid Neoplasms (REAL). The REAL classification system is based on the principle that a classification is a list of "real" disease entities, which are defined by a combination of morphology, immunophenotype, genetic features, and clinical features.[60] The relative importance of each of these criteria for both definition and diagnosis differs among different diseases. Morphology is always important, and some diseases are primarily defined by morphology alone (e.g., follicular lymphoma), although immunophenotype can be helpful in difficult cases. Some diseases have a specific immunophenotype (e.g., mantle cell lymphoma, small lymphocytic lymphoma) that is virtually diagnostic of that disease. A specific genetic abnormality is important in some lymphomas—t(11;14) in mantle cell lymphoma, t(8;14) in Burkitt's lymphoma, and t(14;18) in follicular lymphoma whereas other lymphomas lack specific genetic abnormalities (e.g., MALT lymphoma, diffuse large

B-cell lymphoma). Finally, other lymphomas consider clinical features (e.g., extranodal versus nodal presentation in marginal zone lymphoma and peripheral T-cell lymphoma). A recent retrospective study of the REAL classification confirmed the clinical relevance of this approach.[61]

The REAL classification categorizes lymphoid malignancies into three major categories: B-cell lymphomas, T-cell (and putative NK cell) lymphomas, and Hodgkin's disease (Table 129–8). Within the B-cell and T-cell neoplasm category, there are two major categories: "precursor" neoplasms, corresponding to lymphoblastic lymphomas and leukemias, and "peripheral" neoplasms, comprising the remainder of B- and T-cell lymphomas and leukemias. The REAL classification uses the term "grade" to refer to histologic parameters such as cell and nuclear size, density of chromatin, and proliferation fraction and the term "aggressiveness" to denote clinical behavior of a tumor. This classification scheme includes both lymphomas and lymphoid leukemias because there is no distinction between the solid and circulating forms of these diseases. The REAL classification includes several previously unrecognized types of lymphomas, including mantle cell lymphoma, monocytoid B cell lymphoma, extranodal lymphoma of MALT, splenic marginal zone lymphoma, primary mediastinal large B cell lymphoma, and a variety of T cell lymphomas. New entities not specifically recognized in the Working Formulation account for about 20% to 25% of the cases.

Since 1995, members of the European and American Hematopathology societies have been working to develop a new World Health Organization (WHO) classification of hematologic malignancies. A Clinical Advisory Committee consisting of expert hematologists and oncologists was formed to ensure that the classification would be clinically useful. It will use an updated version of the REAL classification and will expand the principles of the REAL classification to the classification of myeloid and histiocytic malignancies. Although the final WHO classification is not yet available, the Clinical Advisory Committee has agreed that clinical groupings of lymphoid neoplasms into prognostic categories are neither necessary nor desirable because such arbitrary groupings could hamper understanding of the specific features of some of the diseases. It was concluded that there are no groups of diseases that require identical treatment, and treatment must be individualized to a specific disease.[62] When completed, the WHO classification will represent the first true consensus on the classification of hematologic malignancies and will hopefully replace existing classifications.

TABLE 129–8. Revised European-American Classification of Lymphoid Malignancies

- B-Cell Neoplasms
  - Precursor B-Cell Neoplasms
    - Precursor B-lymphoblastic leukemia/lymphoma (B-LBL)
  - Peripheral B-Cell Neoplasms
    - B-cell chronic lymphocytic leukema (B-CLL)/small lymphocytic lymphoma (B-SLL)
    - Lympoplasmacytoid lymphoma (LPL)/immunocytoma
    - Mantle cell lymphoma (MCL)
    - Follicle center lymphoma, follicular
      - Provisional cytologic grades: I (small cell), II (mixed small and large cell), III (large cell)
      - Provisional subtype: diffuse, predominantly small cell type
    - Marginal zone B-cell lymphoma, extranodal mucosa-associated lymphoid tissue (MALT) type (with or without monocytoid B cells)
      - Provisional subtype: nodal marginal zone lymphoma (with or without monocytoid B cells)
      - Provisional entity: splenic marginal zone lymphoma (with or without villous lymphocytes)
    - Hairy cell leukemia (HCL)
    - Plasmacytoma/plasma cell myeloma
    - Diffuse large B-cell lymphoma (DLBCL)[a]
      - Subtype: primary mediastinal (thymic) B-cell lymphoma (PMBL)
    - Burkitt's lymphoma
    - Provisional entity: high-grade B-cell lymphoma, Burkitt-like[a]
- T-Cell and Putative Natural Killer Cell Neoplasms
  - Precursor T-Cell Neoplasms
    - Precursor T-lymphoblastic lymphoma/leukemia (T-LBL)
  - Peripheral T-Cell Neoplasms
    - T-cell chronic lymphocytic leukemia (T-CLL)/prolymphocytic leukemia (T-PLL)
    - Large granular lymphocyte leukemia (LGL)
      - T-cell type
      - Natural killer cell type
    - Mycosis fungoides/Sézary syndrome (MF/SS)
    - Peripheral T-cell lymphoma, unspecified[a]
      - Provisional cytologic categories: medium-sized cell, mixed medium and large cell, large cell, lymphoepitheloid cell
      - Provisional subtype: hepatosplenic ?? T-cell lymphoma
      - Provisional subtype: subcutaneous panniculitic T-cell lymphoma
    - Angioimmunoblastic T-cell lymphoma (AILD)
    - Angiocentric lymphoma
    - Intestinal T-cell lymphoma (with or without enteropathy associated)
    - Adult T-cell lymphoma/leukemia (ATL/L)
    - Anaplastic large cell lymphoma (ALCL), CD30+, T- and null-cell types
    - Provisional entity: anaplastic large cell lymphoma, Hodgkin's-like

[a]These categories are thought likely to include more than one disease entity.

CLINICAL PRESENTATION

Patients with NHL present with a wide variety of symptoms, depending on the site of involvement and whether tumor involvement is nodal or extranodal. Sites of involvement and dissemination of the malignant cells can sometimes be predicted based on the cell of origin and the observation that the tumor frequently disseminates to areas where the normal counterparts of the lymphoma cells are located. For example, B-cell lymphomas involve areas of the lymphoid system normally populated by B lymphocytes, such as lymph nodes, spleen, and bone marrow. T-cell lymphomas commonly disseminate to various extranodal sites, such as the skin and lungs. In contrast to Hodgkin's disease, the bone marrow is commonly involved in NHL.

In general, patients may have either localized or generalized adenopathy, with the involved nodes being painless, rubbery, and discrete, and usually located in the cervical and supraclavicular regions as in Hodgkin's disease. The liver or spleen may be enlarged in patients with generalized adenopathy. Patients with mesenteric or gastrointestinal involvement may present with signs and symptoms of nausea, vomiting, obstruction, abdominal pain, a palpable abdominal mass, or gastrointestinal bleeding. Patients with bone marrow involvement may have symptoms related to anemia, neutropenia, or thrombocytopenia. NHL has a greater tendency to involve the testes, epitrochlear nodes, and Waldeyer's ring than Hodgkin's disease. The incidence of solitary brain lymphoma is increasing, especially in patients with AIDS. Infrequently, patients with NHL may present with

TABLE 129–9. Patient Characteristics of the Common Histologic Types of Non-Hodgkin's Lymphoma

Histologic Type	% of Total	% Male	Median Age	% Stage I or II	% Marrow Positive	% IPI 0/1	% IPI 4/5
Small B-lymphocytic (B-CLL/B-SLL)	6.7	53	65	6	73	17	10
Lymphoplasmacytoid (LPL)	1.2	53	63	20	73	20	13
Mantle cell (MCL)	6.0	74	63	19	63	19	19
Follicular, all grades	22.1	42	59	33	42	39	6
Marginal zone, B cell, MALT	7.6	45	61	66	14	38	5
Marginal zone B cell, nodal	1.8	41	58	18	41	36	9
Diffuse large B cell (DLBCL)	30.6	55	64	51	17	31	16
Primary mediastinal large B cell (PMBL)	2.4	34	37	66	3	44	9
Burkitt's	<1.0	89	31	56	33	44	22
High-grade B cell, Burkitt-like	2.1	59	55	50	21	25	18
Precursor T-lymphoblastic (T-LBL)	1.7	74	25	13	43	35	22
Peripheral T cell, all types	7.0	56	61	18	37	14	27
Anaplastic large T/null cell (ALCL)	2.4	69	33	50	12	50	19

IPI, International Prognostic Index; MALT, mucosa-associated lymphoid tissue

acute renal failure from retroperitoneal adenopathy causing ureteral obstruction or from metabolic abnormalities such as hyperuricemia with uric acid nephropathy.

In contrast to Hodgkin's disease, only about 20% of patients with NHL have the constitutional symptoms of fever, night sweats, and weight loss of greater than 10%. The clinical features of Hodgkin's disease and NHLs are compared in Table 129–1.

DIAGNOSIS, STAGING, AND PROGNOSTIC SYSTEMS

As with Hodgkin's disease, the diagnosis of NHL must be established by pathologic review of tissue obtained by biopsy. The preferred procedure is an excisional biopsy, where the entire involved lymph node is removed for review by an experienced hematopathologist. This procedure should be done carefully to prevent distortional artifact of the architecture, which could lead to an inaccurate diagnosis. Needle biopsy of the node can sometimes provide adequate tissue for pathologic diagnosis if an excisional biopsy cannot be performed. When adenopathy is not present, diagnosis may be established by biopsy of cutaneous lesions, bone marrow biopsy and aspiration in patients with unexplained myelosuppression, liver biopsy in patients with hepatomegaly or elevated liver function transaminases, or biopsy of involved extranodal organs, such as bone, Waldeyer's ring, lung, and testis.

After the diagnosis is established, further workup is required to determine the extent of involvement.[51] Clinical staging always begins with a thorough history and physical examination. Patients should be questioned about the presence or absence and extent of fever, night sweats, and weight loss. A detailed history of lymphadenopathy should also be obtained, including when and where the lymph nodes were first noted, and their rate of growth. A complete physical examination is performed to assess the extent of disease involvement, with special attention given to all nodal areas. All patients should have a complete blood count, serum chemistries including liver and renal profiles, a chest x-ray, and bone marrow aspiration and biopsy. The likelihood of bone marrow involvement varies among the different histologic types of lymphoma (Table 129–9). Lumbar puncture to evaluate the cerebrospinal fluid (CSF) is recommended in patients who have histologic types of lymphoma that often spread to the CNS.

Imaging studies are usually important in the staging work up.[51] CT scanning can identify both nodal and extranodal sites of disease, and has largely replaced lymphangiography for the evaluation of retroperitoneal lymphadenopathy. The abdominal and pelvic CT scan can identify mesenteric and retrocrural node involvement. CT scans can also detect tumor involvement of organs, including the kidneys, ovary, spleen, and liver. MRI is of limited usefulness in the staging of NHL. Gallium scans are sometimes used as part of the staging work up. Other tests, such as liver-spleen scan, bone scan, upper gastrointestinal series, and intravenous pyelogram, are sometimes useful in patients with organ symptomatology or serum chemistry abnormalities.

Staging laparotomy was widely used in the late 1960s and 1970s as part of the staging work up in patients with lymphoma. But it is rarely used today because of technical improvements in imaging studies and the morbidity and potential mortality associated with the procedure.

The Ann Arbor staging classification developed for the clinical staging of Hodgkin's disease is also used to stage patients with NHL (see Table 129–2). After completion of the staging workup, most patients will be found to have advanced disease (stages III and IV). The frequency of localized disease at the time of diagnosis varies depending on the histologic type of lymphoma (Table 129–9). Stage is a more important prognostic factor in Hodgkin's disease than in NHL.

The Ann Arbor system emphasizes the distribution of nodal disease sites because Hodgkin's disease usually spreads through contiguous lymph nodes and does not involve extranodal sites (Table 129–1). But NHL is a disease with tremendous heterogeneity that does not spread through contiguous lymph nodes, and that often involves extranodal sites. As a result of these clinical differences between Hodgkin's disease and NHL, there is poor correlation between Ann Arbor stage and prognosis.

This lack of accuracy with the Ann Arbor classification system in NHL has lead to an international effort to develop a consensus regarding prognostic factors in the diffuse, large cell lymphomas. This effort, which was referred to as the International Non-Hodgkin's Lymphoma Prognostic Factors Project, was based on more than 2,000 patients with diffuse aggressive lymphomas treated with an anthracycline-containing combination chemotherapy regimen in the United States, Europe, and Canada. Five risk factors correlated with low response to chemotherapy and poor survival: (a) age >60 years; (b) advanced tumor stage (Ann Arbor stages III or IV); (c) reduced performance status ≥2; (d) abnormal serum lactate dehydrogenase (LDH) levels; and (e) two or more extranodal sites of disease.[63] It is unclear whether the effect of serum LDH level is related to a tumor or a host event. LDH likely measures cellular catabolism (the enzyme is released from injured cells), or the product of tumor burden and proliferation. Because each of the factors has approximately the same impact (e.g., relative risk) on prognosis, the number of adverse risk factors is summed to provide the International Prognostic Index (IPI). Patients could therefore have a score of 0 to 5. Table 129–10 shows the correlation between the IPI score and complete response rate and 5-year survival. For patients younger than 60 years old, a simplified IPI score can be developed based on Ann Arbor stage, serum LDH, and performance status.

The IPI system was initially developed only for patients with diffuse aggressive lymphomas treated with an anthracycline-containing combination chemotherapy regimen. Although the prognostic factors for other histologic subtypes of NHL have not been studied as extensively, the system applies to most other NHL subtypes (Table 129–11).

TABLE 129–10. Risk Factors and Survival According to the International Non-Hodgkin's Lymphoma Prognostic Factors Project

All Patients	Patients ≤ 60 Years of Age
Age ≥ 60 years of age	LDH > normal
LDH > normal	Performance status ≥ 2
Performance status ≥2	Ann Arbor stage III or IV
Ann Arbor stage III or IV	
Extranodal involvement ≥ 2 sites	

Risk Group	Number of Risk Factors	Complete Response Rate (%)	5-Year Survival Rate (%)
Patients of all ages			
Low	0,1	87	73
Low–intermediate	2	67	51
High–intermediate	3	55	43
High	4,5	44	26
Patients ≤ 60 years of age			
Low	0	92	83
Low–intermediate	1	78	69
High–intermediate	2	57	46
High	3	46	32

LDH, lactic dehydrogenase
Adapted from Ref. 63.

▶ TREATMENT: Non-Hodgkin's Lymphoma

SPECIFIC DISEASE ENTITIES

GENERAL TREATMENT PRINCIPLES

The primary goals in the treatment of NHL are to relieve symptoms, to cure patients of their disease whenever possible, and to minimize the risk of serious acceptable toxicities. The treatment strategy depends on many factors including a patient's age, concomitant disease, histologic subtype, and stage of disease.

Historically, both the clinical behavior and degree of aggressiveness are often used to describe NHLs. The term *favorable* is used to describe indolent lymphomas because of their relatively slow growing behavior. Patients with an indolent lymphoma usually have a relatively long survival, with or without aggressive chemotherapy. Although these lymphomas respond to a wide range of therapeutic approaches, there is no evidence of a survival plateau, which indicates that patients are rarely cured of their disease. In contrast, aggressive lymphomas are termed *unfavorable* because of their rapid growth

TABLE 129–11. Survival by Histologic Type and the International Prognostic Index

Histologic Type	% of Total	5-year Failure-Free Survival (%)			5-year Overall Survival (%)		
		All Patients	*IPI 0/1*	*IPI 4/5*	*All Patients*	*IPI 0/1*	*IPI 4/5*
Small B-lymphocytic (B-CLL/B-SLL)	6.7	25	35	13	51	76	38
Lymphoplasmacytoid (LPL)	1.2	25	NA	NA	59	NA	NA
Mantle cell (MCL)	6.0	11	27	0	27	57	0
Follicular, all grades	22.1	40	55	6	72	84	17
Marginal zone, B cell, MALT	7.6	60	83	0	74	89	40
Marginal zone B cell, nodal	1.8	29	30	0	57	76	50
Diffuse large B cell (DLBCL)	30.6	41	63	19	46	73	22
Primary mediastinal large B cell (PMBL)	2.4	48	69	0	50	77	0
Burkitt's	<1.0	44	NA	NA	44	NA	NA
High-grade B cell, Burkitt-like	2.1	43	71	0	47	71	0
Precursor T-lymphoblastic (T-LBL)	1.7	24	29	40	26	29	40
Peripheral T cell, all types	7.0	18	27	10	25	36	15
Anaplastic large T/null cell (ALCL)	2.4	58	49	83	77	81	83

CLL, chronic lymphocytic leukemia; FFS, failure-free survival; IPI, International Prognostic Index; MALT, mucosa-associated lymphoid tissue; NA, not available; OS, overall survival rate and short survival (measured in weeks to months), if appropriate therapy is not initiated. Although these unfavorable lymphomas are generally more aggressive than indolent lymphomas, many patients with aggressive lymphomas who respond to chemotherapy can experience prolonged disease-free survival and some are cured of their disease. Therefore, the terminology for the NHLs represents a paradox, where "favorable" is bad and "unfavorable" is good in terms of the likelihood for cure.

Therapeutic approaches to NHL include radiation therapy, chemotherapy, and biologic agents. The role of radiation therapy in the treatment of NHL differs from its role in the treatment of Hodgkin's disease. Although the disease is responsive to radiation therapy, only a small percentage of patients with NHL present with truly localized disease that can be treated with local or regional radiation therapy. Radiation therapy is used more commonly in advanced disease, primarily as a palliative measure to control local bulky disease.

Effective chemotherapy for NHL ranges from single-agent therapy in indolent lymphomas to aggressive, complex combination chemotherapy regimens in aggressive lymphomas. The most active agents used in the treatment of NHL include the alkylating agents (e.g., cyclophosphamide, chlorambucil), bleomycin, doxorubicin, purine analogs, etoposide, methotrexate, vincristine, and corticosteroids (e.g., prednisone, dexamethasone). With the availability of monoclonal antibodies for the therapy of lymphoma, there is increasing interest in adding monoclonal antibodies to combination chemotherapy regimens.

Appropriate therapy for NHL depends on the patient's age, histologic type, stage of disease, site of disease, and IPI score (or presence of adverse prognostic factors). In general, treatment of lymphoma can be divided into limited disease and advanced disease. Limited disease includes those patients with localized disease (Ann Arbor stages I and II). Advanced disease is defined as all Ann Arbor stage III or IV patients, and also frequently includes Ann Arbor stage II patients with one or more of the poor prognostic features listed in Table 129–10.[63]

The following sections discuss the clinical characteristics and therapy of the some of the most common disease entities.

B-CELL NEOPLASMS

B-Cell Chronic Lymphocytic Leukemia (B-CLL)/Small Lymphocytic Lymphoma (B-SLL)

B-CLL accounts for more than 90% of chronic lymphocytic leukemia in the United States and Europe. This type of lymphoma is classified in the Working Formulation as *small lymphocytic lymphoma, consistent with CLL.*[60] In the International Lymphoma Classification Project, B-CLL/B-SLL accounted for 6.7% of all cases.[61] Most cases occur in older adults and most patients have stage IV disease, including marrow involvement (Table 129–9). The 5-year overall and failure-free survival was 51% and 25%, respectively. Therapy of disseminated B-CLL/B-SLL is similar to that of chronic lymphocytic leukemia (see Chap. 132).

Lymphoplasmacytoid Lymphoma (LPL)

LPL is an uncommon type of lymphoma, comprising only 1.2% of cases in the REAL clinical study.[61] Most cases of LPL are classified in the Working Formulation as *small lymphocytic plasmacytoid lymphoma.*[60] The clinical characteristics of LPL are similar to those of B-CLL/B-SLL (Table 129–9). The clinical course of LPL is indolent, and survival in patients with LPL is similar to that of B-CLL/B-SLL. Transformation to large cell lymphoma may occur. Therapy of advanced LPL is similar to that of chronic lymphocytic leukemia (see Chap. 132).

Mantle Cell Lymphoma (MCL)

MCL is one of the new disease entities previously unrecognized by other classification systems. This histologic type was found in 6% of cases in the International Lymphoma Classification Project.[61] Most cases of MCL are classified in the Working Formulation as *diffuse small cleaved cell lymphoma,* although some cases would be classified in other categories.[60] The chromosomal translocation t(11;14) occurs in most cases of MCL. MCL usually occurs in older adults, particularly in men, and most patients have advanced disease at the time of diagnosis (Table 129–9). The course of the disease is moderately aggressive; the median overall survival is about three years, with no evidence of a survival plateau.

Patients with disseminated MCL are usually treated with the same intensive combination chemotherapy regimens that are used in diffuse aggressive lymphomas. Overall response rates to these regimens is about 80%, with about one-half of patients achieving a complete response.[64] Median progression-free and overall survival was 20 and 36 months, respectively. In patients who respond to initial therapy, interferon-α may have a role as maintenance or consolidation therapy.[65] Despite the high response rates, MCL is not considered curable with standard chemotherapy. Therefore, younger patients who have an initial response to chemotherapy often undergo autologous or allogeneic HSCT as consolidation therapy.[65] Because MCL usually expresses CD20, rituximab has been used with some success in patients with newly diagnosed and relapsed MCL.[65,66]

Follicular Lymphomas

The combined group of follicular lymphomas makes up the second most common histologic type of NHL in the United States, comprising about 20% of all NHLs in the International NHL Classification Project and up to 70% of low-grade lymphomas reported in American and European clinical trials.[51,61] These lymphomas are classified as *follicular small cleaved cell, follicular mixed cell, and follicular large cell lymphoma* in the Working Formulation.[60] In the study that lead to the development of the Working Formulation, patients with follicular small cleaved cell and mixed cell lymphomas had significantly better survival than did those with follicular large cell lymphoma.[59] Therefore, follicular small cleaved cell and mixed cell lymphomas were considered as low-grade lymphomas whereas follicular large cell lymphomas were considered as intermediate-grade. However, it is difficult to divide cases of follicular lymphoma into distinct subtypes because there is a continuous gradation in the number of large cells, and there are no uniform criteria for assignment of follicular lymphoma into the various subtypes. As a result, there is major disagreement, even among expert hematopathologists, on the subtype in many cases. In the International NHL Classification Project, the percent agreement for the various grades of the follicular lymphomas was only 61% to 73%.[61] Therefore, the REAL classification does not include subclassification of follicular lymphomas, although provisional categories based on the prominence of large cells are included (Table 129–8). Numerous criteria have been proposed for grading follicular lymphoma, but no consensus has been reached among the expert hematopathologists. Because some studies suggest that follicular large cell lymphoma has a different clinical course and may respond differently to chemotherapy than the other subtypes (discussed below), some experts believe that it is important to develop uniform criteria in order to identify this subgroup of patients.

Follicular lymphomas tend to occur in older adults, with a slight female predominance (Table 129–9). Most patients have advanced disease at diagnosis, but about 25% to 33% of patients have localized disease (stage I or stage II) at diagnosis.[61,67] Extranodal disease, bulky disease, and B symptoms are uncommon features at diagnosis. Most patients with follicular lymphoma have the chromosomal translocation t(14;18) at the time of diagnosis.

The clinical course is generally indolent, with median survivals of 8 to 10 years. Most patients have dramatic responses to initial therapy, and their disease course is characterized by multiple relapses, with responses to salvage therapy becoming progressively shorter after every relapse, eventually leading to death from disease-related causes.[68] The natural history of follicular lymphoma shows a pattern of constant relapses over time (i.e., no evidence of a survival plateau), which suggests that patients are not cured of their disease. But the natural history of follicular lymphoma can be unpredictable. Spontaneous regression of disease has been noted in as many as 20% to 30% of patients.[68] There is also a high conversion rate of follicular lymphoma to a more aggressive histology over time that steadily increases after diagnosis and reaches 40% to 70% at 8 to 10 years.[68]

Certain subsets of patients with follicular lymphoma have a much better or worse prognosis. Some studies suggest that the natural history of follicular large cell lymphoma is similar to that of other aggressive lymphomas and that treatment with intensive combination chemotherapy regimens may result in long-term disease-free survival, including a possible plateau in the survival curve.[69] It would be clinically helpful to identify patients in different prognostic groups based on disease characteristics at the time of diagnosis.[68] Patients who are predicted to have a poor prognosis (i.e., high-risk) could then be offered aggressive or experimental therapy, while those who are predicted to have a good prognosis (i.e., low-risk) could be treated with standard therapy, therefore avoiding unnecessary toxicity.

Several studies have attempted to develop a prognostic system for patients with follicular lymphoma. In the International NHL Classification Project, IPI score correlated with both failure-free and overall survival in patients with follicular lymphoma (Table 129–11). In that analysis, fewer than 20% of patients with IPI scores of 4/5 were alive at 5 years, as compared to more than 80% of patients with IPI scores of 0/1. But the IPI was originally based on a study of patients with diffuse aggressive lymphomas and this system has limited discriminating power in follicular lymphoma because more than 90% of patients were allocated in the favorable (i.e., 0/1) or intermediate risk (i.e., 2/3) groups. Italian investigators recently developed a predictive model based on nearly 1,000 cases of follicular lymphoma.[67] In that model, six factors were found to independently correlate with overall survival: age >60 years, female sex, two or more extranodal sites, elevated serum LDH levels, presence of B symptoms, and erythrocyte sedimentation rate ≥30. Three of the factors (age, number of extranodal sites, and serum LDH levels) were also identified as important predictive factors in the IPI. Because the relative risk associated with each factor was similar, the investigators developed a risk score by summing the number of risk factors present in a patient at the time of diagnosis. Because none of the cases presented with all six risk factors, patients were grouped into one of three risk groups, based on the number of risk factors present: low-risk (0/1), intermediate-risk (2), and high-risk (3-5). Five- and 10-year survival rates were, respectively, 90% and 65% for low-risk patients; 75% and 54% for intermediate-risk patients; and 38% and 11% for high-risk patients. The new system appeared to have higher discriminating power among groups as compared to the IPI system.

Therapy of Localized Disease (Stages I and II). Radiation therapy is the standard treatment for early stage follicular lymphoma. Involved field, extended-field, and total nodal irradiation have been used. Carefully staged patients with either stage I or contiguous stage II disease treated with radiation therapy can achieve high disease-free survival rates at 10 years. In a retrospective study from Stanford University, 44% of patients with stage I or II follicular lymphoma treated with radiation therapy were alive relapse-free after 10 years of followup.[70] Patients who received radiation to both sides of the diaphragm (total and subtotal lymphoid irradiation) had significantly longer relapse-free survival as compared to those who received radiation to only one side of the diaphragm (involved and extended-field irradiation), but overall survival was similar regardless of the extent of radiation therapy. Late relapses are uncommon; only 10% of patients who reached ten years without relapse subsequently experienced a recurrence.

Chemotherapy is not recommended in most patients with localized follicular lymphoma, but it may be helpful in some patients with high-risk stage II disease (e.g., multiple sites of involvement or bulky disease).

Most patients with stage I or II follicular lymphoma are cured of their disease with radiation therapy alone. Most centers use radiation at a dose of 30–40 Gy to either involved or regional fields, which would consist of irradiation to the involved nodal region plus one additional uninvolved region on each side of the involved nodes. Extended-field irradiation is not usually used because of the absence of a survival benefit and possible increased risk of secondary malignancies. In addition, previous use of extended-field irradiation compromises the ability of that patient to receive subsequent chemotherapy.

Therapy of Advanced Disease (Stages III and IV). The management of stage III and IV indolent lymphomas remains controversial, as standard therapeutic approaches have not been shown to be curative despite the high complete remission rates to initial therapy. Therapeutic options for these patients are diverse and include watchful waiting, radiation therapy, single-agent chemotherapy, combination chemotherapy, biologic therapy, and combined-modality therapy.[51,71] Although complete remission can be achieved in 50% to 80% of patients with various treatments, the median time to relapse is usually only 18 to 36 months. Approximately 20% of patients who have a complete response remain in remission for longer than 10 years. After relapse, patients are retreated and again high remission rates can be achieved (see below). Unfortunately, the response rates and duration of response both decrease with each retreatment.

Two different initial treatment approaches exist and are described as conservative or aggressive. Patients treated with the conservative approach receive no initial therapy followed by single-agent chemotherapy or radiation therapy when treatment is needed. With the aggressive approach, patients usually receive aggressive combination chemotherapy, extensive radiation therapy, or both, early in the disease course, even if they are asymptomatic. There are no convincing data to indicate that immediate aggressive therapy significantly improves survival as compared with conservative therapy. More than 80% of patients with stage III or IV follicular lymphoma are alive at 5 years, and the median survival is approximately 7 to 8 years.

At the time of relapse, many treatment options are available.[72] At the time of relapse, the following factors must be considered:

(a) age; (b) symptomatic status of the patient; (c) tumor burden; (d) rate of regrowth (based on previous assessment of active disease sites); (e) presence or absence of characteristics suggesting transformation or biologic progression; (f) prior therapy; (g) degree and duration of response to prior therapy; and (h) availability of clinical trials.

No Initial Therapy. Because there are no convincing data that standard treatment approaches have improved survival, some oncologists have adopted a "watch and wait" approach for asymptomatic patients.[68] Therapy was initiated for rapidly progressive or bulky adenopathy, systemic symptoms, anemia, thrombocytopenia, or disease in threatening sites such as the orbit or spinal cord. The median time until treatment was required was 3 to 5 years, and approximately 20% of patients do not require therapy for as long as 10 years. The 10-year survival rate was 73%, which was not significantly different from patients who received therapy at the time of diagnosis. As described above, patients with follicular lymphoma who are followed without therapy sometimes have spontaneous regressions that can be complete, while the disease in other patients can convert to a more aggressive histology. If a watch and wait approach is chosen, the patient should be evaluated at least every 2 months for the first year and quarterly thereafter, so that intervention can occur before serious problems occur.

Radiation. Follicular lymphoma is sensitive to radiation therapy, and total lymphoid irradiation or whole-body irradiation has been used to treat patients with advanced follicular lymphoma. Although the results with total lymphoid irradiation have been excellent in selected patients with limited stage III follicular lymphoma,[73] extensive radiation therapy is rarely used for patients with advanced follicular lymphoma requiring systemic therapy because of concerns regarding prolonged myelosuppression and difficulties in administering future treatments. Total lymphoid irradiation has been given in combination with chemotherapy, but studies fail to show a survival advantage for combined modality treatment.[51] As a result, new high-dose chemotherapy regimens usually do not include the use of total lymphoid irradiation.

Alkylating Agents. Oral alkylating agents, given either alone or in combination, have been the mainstay of treatment for follicular lymphoma. In a randomized trial of oral chlorambucil (0.1–0.2 mg/kg/day), oral cyclophosphamide (1.5–2.5 mg/kg/day), or CVP (cyclophosphamide, vincristine, and prednisone) in patients with indolent lymphoma, no significant difference in overall survival or freedom from relapse between the three groups was observed.[68] The dosage of single-agent chlorambucil or cyclophosphamide is usually adjusted to maintain a platelet count above 100,000/mm^3 and a white blood cell count above 3,000/mm^3. Although single-agent alkylating agents have a high initial complete remission rate, the time required to achieve a complete response is slow (median time is 12 months). Complete responses occur more rapidly with combination chemotherapy. There is no benefit of maintenance therapy. After the "best" response is achieved, many experts will discontinue therapy and observe.

Both single-agent alkylating agents and CVP are well tolerated by most patients. The advantages of oral chlorambucil are no hair loss, little or no nausea, and minimal myelosuppression. Because of its mild side effect profile, oral chlorambucil is usually recommended for older patients who are minimally symptomatic or who have other comorbidities. There are some concerns with the risk of secondary acute leukemia in patients receiving continuous exposure to alkylating agents.

Purine Analogs. Several studies have reported encouraging results with two adenosine analogues, fludarabine phosphate and 2-chlorodeoxyadenosine (2-CdA, cladribine), in previously untreated and relapsed advanced follicular lymphoma. The mechanism of action for both drugs is not well understood, but both agents accumulate in lymphocytes and are resistant to adenosine deaminase. In patients with relapsed or refractory indolent lymphoma, single-agent fludarabine has an overall response rate of almost 50% and a complete response rate of 10% to 15%. Response rates are higher in previously untreated patients, with overall and complete response rates of 70% and almost 40%, respectively.[71] The median time to progression is less than 6 months for relapsed disease and more than 12 months for previously untreated patients. Although the response rates to 2-CdA in previously untreated patients is similar to those with fludarabine, the duration of response appears to be shorter with 2-CdA. Combination regimens that include one of these purine analogs are also being investigated.[71] Fludarabine, mitoxantrone, and dexamethasone (FND) is one example of a fludarabine-containing regimen that has shown encouraging results in relapsed patients with indolent lymphoma.[74]

Purine analogs usually do not cause nausea and vomiting or hair loss, but they are associated with cumulative and prolonged myelosuppression and profound immunosuppression, which increases the risk of opportunistic infections, such as fungal infections, *Pneumocystis carinii* pneumonia, and viral infections.

Interferon-α. Single-agent interferon-α (IFN-α) is active in the treatment of follicular lymphoma, with objective response rates of 30% to 50% in patients with relapsed disease.[75] About 10% of patients have a complete response to IFN-α. Based on these encouraging results, several randomized controlled trials have evaluated the potential benefit of adding IFN-α to combination chemotherapy. Based on the results of one of these trials, IFN-α-2b (INTRON A) was granted FDA approval as initial treatment for patients with clinically aggressive follicular lymphoma and a large tumor burden, in combination with an anthracycline-containing regimen. Its approval was based on the Groupe d'Etude des Lymphomes Folliculaires (GELF) trial, which compared CHVP (cyclophosphamide, doxorubicin, teniposide, and prednisone) to CHVP and IFN-α-2b.[76] CHVP was given monthly for six cycles, then every two months for six more cycles, while IFN-α-2b was given at a dose of 5 million units three times a week for 18 months. Patients who received concurrent IFN-α-2b had a significantly higher response rate (85% vs 69%), which translated into significant differences in median progression-free interval (2.9 years vs 1.5 years) and overall survival (not reached vs 5.6 years).

At least 10 randomized controlled trials in the United States and Europe have evaluated the role of IFN-α either during induction, as maintenance therapy, or in both settings. The results of these trials are inconsistent.[71,77] In a meta-analysis of more than 1,500 newly diagnosed patients from the various randomized trials, the efficacy of IFN-α depended on the intensity of the chemotherapy regimen and response to induction chemotherapy. The major conclusion of the meta-analysis was that IFN-α was probably beneficial in responsive patients (had a partial response (PR) or complete response (CR) to induction chemotherapy) who were receiving more intensive chemotherapy (anthracycline- or anthracene-containing regimen).

In the most recent randomized controlled trial, 571 patients with stage III or IV indolent NHLs (mostly follicular) were studied as part of a Southwest Oncology Group (SWOG) trial. Patients who responded to intensive chemotherapy that consisted of six to eight cycles of prednisone, methotrexate, doxorubicin, cyclophosphamide, and etoposide/mechlorethamine, vincristine, procarbazine, and prednisone (ProMACE-MOPP) or chemotherapy plus irradiation therapy were randomized to receive either consolidation IFN-α-2b (2 million units/m^2 given three times weekly SQ) for 2 years or observation.[78] With a median followup of more than 6 years, no difference in progression-free or overall survival was observed.

The reasons for the divergent results are not easily explained.[77] Based on these negative results, some experts question whether physicians should recommend IFN-α to patients, particularly given the significant cost and toxicities associated with this agent and the recent availability of other treatment options (see below).

Monoclonal Antibodies. B-cell lymphomas have served as a model for immunotherapy with monoclonal antibodies for more than 20 years, beginning with the successful use of custom-made monoclonal antibodies targeted against the idiotype present on the patient's cancer cells.[79] These encouraging results lead to the development of monoclonal antibodies against a more "generic" target, a molecule on the surface of B cells that would be present on tumor cells.[80] One potential target, the CD20 molecule, was present only on cells in the B-lymphocyte lineage. It is expressed on the surface of both normal and malignant B cells, but not on other normal tissues. Rituximab (Rituxan) is a chimeric monoclonal antibody directed at the CD20 molecule. Since rituximab was approved in November 1997 to treat relapsed or refractory indolent or follicular CD20$^+$ lymphomas, it has become one of the most widely used therapies for follicular lymphomas. Its approval was based on an open-label multicenter study that enrolled 166 patients with relapsed or recurrent indolent lymphoma.[81] Rituximab, given intravenously at a dose of 375 mg/m^2 weekly × 4, resulted in an overall response rate of 48% (CR: 6%, PR: 42%). Median time to progression for responders was 13.2 months and median duration of response was 11.6 months. Most of the adverse effects are infusion-related, particularly after the first infusion, and consist of fever, chills, respiratory symptoms, fatigue, headache, pruritus, and angioedema.

Although rituximab is usually given in patients who have relapsed, it is also being used as first-line therapy, either alone or in combination with chemotherapy. In a study of 50 patients with previously untreated follicular lymphoma with a low tumor burden, 73% of patients had an objective response (CR: 20%) to single-agent rituximab (375 mg/m^2 weekly × 4).[82] It is interesting to note that many of these patients remain in molecular remission (i.e., PCR-negative) at 12 months. Investigators have evaluated different dosages and dosage schedules of single-agent rituximab, including higher dosages (up to 2 g/m^2), more frequent administration (three times per week), and more doses (weekly × 8). Although these alternative dosages or dosage schedules have been well tolerated (i.e., no dose-limiting toxicity was observed), they do not appear to increase the antitumor activity of rituximab.

Another advantage of rituximab is that it can be safely used as a retreatment option. Approximately 40% of patients who relapsed after a response to rituximab have an objective response to retreatment with rituxumab.[83] Interestingly, patients who respond the second time usually have longer durations of remission than they did to the first course. Therefore, many clinicians will consider retreatment with rituximab for patients who have a sustained (i.e., more than 6 months) first remission and if their tumor has continued expression of CD20 antigen.

Because of its activity and non-overlapping toxicities with other chemotherapy agents, rituximab is being evaluated in combination with other chemotherapy agents earlier in treatment.[80] In a phase II trial of six courses of rituxumab and cyclophosphamide, doxorubicin, vincristine, and prednisone (CHOP) chemotherapy, the overall and complete response rate in 40 patients with previously untreated or relapsed indolent lymphoma was 95% and 55%, respectively.[84] More than 70% of patients are progression-free after 4 years of follow up. Table 129–12 shows the CHOP regimen that is widely used in the treatment of NHL. In the CHOP and rituximab regimen, two doses of rituximab are given before the start of CHOP therapy; two more doses are given in the middle of the six cycles of CHOP; and two additional doses are given at the end of CHOP therapy. No significant additional toxicity was observed in patients who received CHOP and rituximab.

TABLE 129–12. CHOP Regimen

Drug	Dose (mg/m^2)	Route	Treatment Days
Cyclophosphamide	750	IV	1
Doxorubicin	50	IV	1
Vincristine	1.4	IV	1
Prednisone	100	PO	1–5
One cycle is 21 days			

Note: Another name for doxorubicin is hydroxyldaunomycin
Adapted from Ref. 88.

Other monoclonal antibody based therapies being investigated in indolent lymphomas include immunotoxins and radiolabeled antibodies.[72,85] Encouraging results have been reported for two anti-CD20 radioimmunoconjugates, and both are currently awaiting FDA approval for clinical use in indolent lymphomas: ^{131}I-tositumomab (Bexxar) and ^{90}Y-ibritumomab tiuxetan (Zevalin). Encouraging results have been reported with combinations of radioimmunoconjugates and chemotherapy.

Based on these encouraging results, the current SWOG study randomizes patients with advanced indolent lymphomas to three arms: (a) CHOP alone; (b) CHOP and rituximab (given concurrently); and (c) CHOP and ^{131}I-tositumomab (given sequentially).

Hematopoietic Stem Cell Transplantation. High-dose chemotherapy, followed by autologous or allogeneic (HSCT), is another option for patients with relapsed follicular lymphoma (see Chap. 134).[72,86] In patients who are transplanted at the time of initial treatment failure, 5-year event-free survival is approximately 40% to 50%. There is a continuing risk of relapse after autologous HSCT, but the presence of a survival plateau after allogeneic HSCT suggests that some patients may be cured of their disease. High-dose myeloablative transplants are usually reserved for younger patients without serious comorbidities, but nonmyeloablative allogeneic transplants may be an option for older patients who would not otherwise be eligible for autologous or allogeneic HSCT.

Investigational Therapies. As discussed above, the idiotype present on the patient's tumor cells can serve as a potential target for immunotherapy. This idiotype can be used to manufacture a patient-specific vaccine.[79] Vaccines would potentially produce both humoral and cellular immune responses, and would also be longer acting than passive immunotherapy. Various approaches are being tested to improve the immune response to vaccines.

Marginal Zone B-cell Lymphoma, Malt and Nodal Types

Marginal zone B-cell lymphomas, MALT (extranodal) and nodal types, are two of the new forms of NHL not previously recognized in the Working Formulation. In the Working Formulation, these types of lymphomas were most commonly diagnosed as *small lymphocytic lymphoma or small lymphocytic lymphoma, with plasmacytoid characteristics,* although some were classified as diffuse lymphomas.[60] Extranodal and nodal types of marginal zone B-cell lymphomas represent approximately 7.6% and 1.8% of new cases of NHLs.[61] Clinically, MALT lymphomas tend to be indolent. Most patients present with localized disease involving extranodal sites, which involves glandular epithelial tissues of various sites, such as the stomach, lungs, parotid gland, thyroid, and orbit (Table 129–9). The stomach is the most frequent site and gastric MALT lymphomas are frequently associated with chronic gastritis and *Helicobacter pylori* infection. Because MALT lymphomas tend to remain localized for long periods, local treatment (surgery or local/regional radiation therapy) is effective and offers the opportunity for cure. Patients with gastric MALT lymphomas who are positive for *H. pylori* should be treated for their infection (e.g., antibiotics). Patients with disseminated MALT lymphoma should be treated with the same type of chemotherapy used in patients with indolent lymphoma.

The nodal type of marginal zone B-cell lymphoma is sometimes referred to as monocytoid B-cell lymphoma. There is a strong association between this type of lymphoma and Sjögren's syndrome and other collagen vascular disease. Because many patients also have extranodal MALT-type lymphoma, some experts believe that this type of lymphoma represents nodal spread of the lymphoma. Treatment is similar to that of follicular lymphoma.

Diffuse Large B-cell Lymphoma (DLBCL)

DLBCLs are the most common lymphoma in the International NHL Classification Project, accounting for about 30% of all NHLs.[61] Most DLBCLs are classified as *diffuse large cell cleaved, noncleaved, or immunoblastic or diffuse mixed cell* in the Working Formulation.[60] DLBCLs are characterized by the presence of large cells, which are usually at least twice the size of small lymphocytes. The median age at the time of diagnosis is in the sixth decade, but DLBCL can affect individuals of all ages, from children to the elderly. Patients often present with a rapidly enlarging symptomatic mass, with B symptoms in about one-third of the cases.[51] About one-half of patients present with localized (stage I or II) disease. Approximately one-third of patients with DLBCL present with extranodal disease; common sites include the head and neck, gastrointestinal tract, skin, bone, testis, and CNS. DLBCL is the most common type of diffuse aggressive lymphomas, which share in common an aggressive clinical behavior that leads to death within weeks to months if the tumor is not treated. Diffuse aggressive lymphomas are also sensitive to many chemotherapeutic agents, and some patients treated with chemotherapy can be cured of their disease.

Several factors correlate with response to chemotherapy and survival in patients with aggressive lymphoma. Because the IPI was originally developed based on patients with aggressive lymphoma, IPI score correlates with prognosis (Table 129–10).[63] Although IPI is a clinically useful tool to estimate prognosis, the factors used to calculate the IPI score probably represent clinical surrogates for the biologic heterogeneity among DLBCL and many researchers are interested in determining the prognostic importance of certain phenotypic and molecular characteristics of DLBCL.[87] For example, markers of apoptosis, cell-cycle regulation, cell lineage, and cell proliferation are being evaluated as potentially clinically useful prognostic factors. Gene expression profiling with biochips may also correlate with survival. Gene expression profiling identified two molecularly distinct forms of DLBCL, based on gene expression patterns indicative of different stages of B-cell differentiation.[88] One type expressed genes characteristic of germinal center B-cells, while the second type expressed genes normally induced during *in vitro* activation of peripheral blood B cells. Patients with germinal center B-like DLBCL had a significantly better overall survival than those with activated B-like DLBCL. These results suggest that molecular classification of tumors on the basis of gene expression may allow identification of clinically significant subtypes of cancer.

Therapy of Localized Disease (Stages I and II).

Before 1980, radiation therapy was the primary treatment for patients with localized DLBCL. Five-year disease-free survival with radiation therapy alone was approximately 50% and 20% in patients with stage I and stage II disease, respectively.[51] Randomized trials in the 1980s showed that radiation therapy followed by chemotherapy resulted in significantly longer disease-free and overall survival as compared with radiation therapy alone. Other studies reported excellent results with a short course of chemotherapy (three cycles) followed by involved-field radiotherapy or six to eight cycles of CHOP chemotherapy, with or without consolidation radiotherapy. With either of these approaches, 5-year progression-free survival was >90% for patients with stage I disease and about 70% for patients with stage II disease.[51]

Because it was not clear which approach was more effective, SWOG performed a randomized trial that compared three cycles of CHOP and involved field radiotherapy or eight cycles of CHOP in patients with localized aggressive lymphoma.[89] Patients treated with three cycles of CHOP plus radiotherapy had significantly better 5-year progression-free (77% vs 64%) and overall (82% vs 72%) survival than patients who were treated with CHOP alone. The incidence of life-threatening toxicity was higher in patients who received CHOP alone. Based on the results of this trial, the current standard for therapy of localized aggressive lymphoma is three cycles of CHOP followed by involved field radiation therapy. The optimal dose of involved field radiation is not known, but 30 Gy is recommended for patients with favorable presentations and 35–40 Gy for patients with initial bulky disease.[51]

Therapy of Advanced Disease (Bulky Stages II, III, and IV).

It has been known since the late 1970s that intensive combination chemotherapy can cure some patients with disseminated DLBCL. Initial studies with COP (same as CVP) produced a plateau on the survival curve of just 10%, with a median survival of less than 1 year. Based on the activity of single-agent doxorubicin, McKelvey et al. developed the CHOP regimen (Table 129–12).[90] A few years later, a SWOG study showed that CHOP was more active than COP, and CHOP chemotherapy rapidly became the treatment of choice for patients with aggressive lymphomas.[91] Studies in larger numbers of patients showed that approximately 50% of patients had a complete remission to CHOP chemotherapy, and 50% to 75% of the patients who had a complete response (about one-third of all the patients) experienced long-term disease-free survival and cure of their disease.

In an effort to improve these results, many investigators used several general approaches to develop second- and third-generation regimens in the 1980s and early 1990s.[52] The first approach was to add a nonmyelotoxic drug, most often bleomycin, to the 3-week cycle (e.g., CHOP-Bleo, BACOP). The second approach was to add nonmyelosuppressive agents *between* cycles of CHOP or BACOP. One example of this strategy was the M-BACOD (methotrexate, bleomycin, doxorubicin, cyclophosphamide, vincristine, and dexamethasone) regimen, in which high-dose methotrexate, with leucovorin rescue, was administered on day 10. M-BACOD was later modified to m-BACOD, which included the same drugs but had a lower methotrexate dosage. Another variation on this strategy was to give semicontinuous or weekly therapy; relatively small doses of myelosuppressive agents are administered, alternating, over a 12-week period with nonmyelosuppressive agents. An example of this strategy is MACOP-B (methotrexate with leucovorin rescue, doxorubicin, cyclophosphamide, vincristine, prednisone, and bleomycin). The third approach was to give as many drugs as possible, as flexibly as possible (e.g., ProMACE-MOPP). ProMACE-MOPP was later modified to ProMACE-CytaBOM (prednisone, doxorubicin, cyclophosphamide, and etoposide, followed by cytarabine, bleomycin, vincristine, and methotrexate with leucovorin rescue). Results of phase II trials suggested that these second- and third-generation regimens were more active than CHOP, with slightly higher complete response rates and improved disease-free survival rates.[51,52] However, they were also more difficult to administer, more toxic, and more expensive. Based on these results, oncologists generally adopted one of these second- or third-generation combination regimens as their standard regimen for patients with advanced aggressive lymphomas.

Several randomized studies have compared different combination regimens in patients with aggressive lymphoma.[51,52] Although the results of these studies show that no one regimen is clearly superior to another, they show the superiority of anthracycline-containing regimens over those that do not contain an anthracycline. In the largest and most widely quoted study, the SWOG initiated a randomized trial in 1986 that compared CHOP to three of the most commonly used third-generation regimens (m-BACOD, ProMACE/CytaBOM, and MACOP-B) in nearly 900 patients with bulky stage II, stage III, or stage IV aggressive lymphoma. At the time of the initial publication (median followup = 35 months), no differences in disease-free and overall survival was observed between the four groups.[92] Furthermore, no significant difference in disease-free or overall survival was observed in any subgroup of patients. The risk of treatment-related mortality, however, was higher in patients receiving one of the third-generation regimens. Extended followup of that trial (i.e., 10 years) shows that 38% of patients who participated in that trial are probably cured of their disease, regardless of the initial combination chemotherapy regimen. Interestingly, the overall survival is about 10% higher than the disease-free survival, which probably reflects the effectiveness of salvage high-dose chemotherapy with autologous HSCT (see below).

Based on the lack of survival benefit with the newer combination chemotherapy regimens, the less complicated and less expensive CHOP regimen should be considered as the treatment of choice for DLBCL and other aggressive lymphomas. Unfortunately, the major conclusion from these studies is not that all of these regimens are extremely effective, but that all of these regimens are equally bad. Fewer than 50% of patients with DLBCL are currently cured of their disease with combination chemotherapy and most patients who relapse after an initial response do so in the first 2 years. New treatment approaches are clearly needed.[87]

The IPI score should be calculated for every patient with DLBCL and incorporated into treatment decisions for individual patients (Table 129–10). Patients with a low IPI score should be treated with conventional CHOP therapy. But patients with a high-intermediate or high-risk IPI score should be identified as candidates for more aggressive treatments. One approach is to add biologic therapy to standard chemotherapy. In a pilot study of 33 patients with previously untreated CD20$^+$ aggressive NHL, the addition of rituximab to six cycles of CHOP chemotherapy produced a 94% objective response rate, with 61% of patients achieving a complete response.[93] Rituximab was given at a dosage of 375 mg/m^2 on day 1 of each cycle; cyclophosphamide, doxorubicin, and vincristine were given intravenously on day 3, and oral prednisone was given on days 3 to 7. With short follow-up, only one patient who had a complete response has relapsed. In the 18 patients with an IPI score of ≥ 2, the combination of rituximab and CHOP achieved an objective response rate of 89% and complete response rate of 56%. No significant additional toxicity was noted. Based on these encouraging results, randomized studies are in progress, including a large United States study in elderly patients (see below).

Another approach in high-risk patients is to give high-dose chemotherapy (HDC) with autologous HSCT as intensive consolidation in high-risk patients with DLBCL who achieve a remission with standard chemotherapy (see Chap. 134). Several randomized controlled trials have been conducted in patients with aggressive NHLs, and the results of these trials have been critically reviewed recently by two independent panels of experts.[94,95] Based on a review of the available evidence, it was concluded that HDC with autologous HSCT is effective in high-risk (i.e., high-intermediate/high-risk based on IPI score) patients who have a complete remission to conventional therapy (first complete remission in high-risk patients) and in untreated high-risk patients (high-dose sequential therapy in untreated high-risk patients).[95] There was inadequate evidence to make a treatment recommendation for the other possible clinical situations, such as in patients who do not respond to standard induction therapy (primary refractory disease) or in patients who have a partial remission to standard induction therapy (first partial remission after full-course induction therapy).

Unfortunately, the available evidence has lead to a discussion of when HDC with autologous HSCT should be offered to high-risk patients with aggressive NHLs: early (i.e., when patients are in their first complete remission) or later (i.e., after patients have relapsed). To address this question, the various cooperative groups in the United States have agreed to conduct a randomized clinical trial or early versus delayed HDC for patients with high-risk (high-intermediate or high-risk based on IPI score) DLBCL. In this trial, referred to as the North American High-Dose Therapy Trial, patients younger than 65 years old will receive five courses of CHOP chemotherapy. Patients who have a partial or complete response will then be randomized to receive either three more cycles of CHOP or one additional cycle of CHOP followed by HDC with autologous HSCT. Patients on the standard CHOP treatment who relapse will then receive the same HDC therapy.

In summary, all patients with bulky stage II, stage III, or stage IV disease should be treated with chemotherapy until a complete response is achieved; a rapid response to chemotherapy (i.e., a complete response achieved in the first three treatment cycles) is associated with a more durable remission when compared to patients who require longer treatment. Two or more cycles of chemotherapy should be given following attainment of a complete response. Most patients are treated for 6 to 9 months. The use of long-term maintenance therapy following a complete response does not improve survival. HDC with autologous HSCT should be considered in high-risk patients who respond to standard chemotherapy. Results with the combination of rituximab and chemotherapy have been encouraging. Patients should be enrolled in clinical trials of new treatment approaches, whenever possible.

Therapy of Elderly Patients with Advanced Disease. More than one-half of patients with NHL are older than 60 years of age at diagnosis, and about one-third are over the age of 70 years. The

International Non-Hodgkin's Lymphoma Prognostic Factors Project showed that patients older than 60 years of age had a significantly lower complete response rate and overall survival.[63] The reasons for the poorer outcome in elderly patients are not clear. Older patients do not tolerate intensive chemotherapy as well as younger patients, and some studies report that older patients have a higher risk of treatment-related mortality. As a result, many oncologists treat elderly patients with reduced dose or less aggressive chemotherapy regimens. In general, these less-intensive regimens have used anthracyclines with less cardiotoxicity than doxorubicin, have substituted mitoxantrone for doxorubicin, or have used short-duration weekly therapy.[51]

Over the past few years, several nonrandomized and randomized trials have evaluated different treatment approaches in older patients with aggressive NHL.[51] The results of these studies suggest that carefully selected elderly patients with good performance status and without significant comorbidities may tolerate aggressive anthracycline-containing regimens as well as younger patients. These patients should be treated initially with full-dose CHOP or similar regimens; dosages can be reduced later if severe toxicity occurs. Hematopoietic growth factors may allow elderly patients to maintain dose intensity.

The combination of rituximab and CHOP is being studied in a large cooperative group trial in the United States. In that trial, elderly patients with aggressive NHL are randomized to either rituximab and CHOP or CHOP alone; patients who achieve a complete or partial response are then randomized to receive rituximab as maintenance therapy versus no maintenance therapy.

Salvage Therapy. Although many patients with aggressive NHL experience long-term survival and cure with intensive chemotherapy, nearly 50% of patients fail to achieve a complete remission and, of those patients who do achieve a complete remission, approximately 20% to 30% subsequently relapse. Therefore, approximately 60% to 70% of all patients with aggressive NHL will require salvage therapy at some time during their disease course. Response to salvage therapy depends on the initial responsiveness of the tumor to chemotherapy. Patients who achieve an initial complete remission and then relapse generally have a better response to salvage therapy than those who are primarily or partially resistant to chemotherapy.

Many conventional-dose salvage chemotherapy regimens have been used in patients with relapsed or refractory NHL. Many patients who respond to salvage therapy (i.e., chemosensitive relapse) will then receive HDC with autologous HSCT. In an effort to avoid cross-resistance, most salvage regimens incorporate drugs that are not used in the initial therapy. Some of the more commonly used salvage regimens include MIME (mitoguazone, ifosfamide, methotrexate, etoposide), DHAP (cisplatin, high-dose cytarabine, dexamethasone), ESHAP (etoposide, methylprednisolone, high-dose cytarabine, cisplatin), and MINE followed by ESHAP, and no one regimen appears to be clearly superior to any other regimen.[51,52,96] With these salvage regimens, approximately 25% to 35% of patients achieve a complete response, with a median duration of remission of 1 to 2 years. Only 5% to 10% of patients will have long-term disease-free survival.

ICE (ifosfamide, carboplatin, and etoposide) chemotherapy is a newer regimen that has been used in patients with refractory disease.[97] Some experts believe that ICE is better tolerated than older cisplatin-based regimens, particularly in older patients. The combination of ICE and rituximab is currently being evaluated as a salvage regimen; rituximab is given before the first dose of ICE and then weekly during the regimen. SWOG is currently comparing ICE plus rituximab with ICE alone in a randomized trial of salvage therapy.

To improve the cure rate, many studies have evaluated HDC with autologous HSCT as intensive consolidation therapy in patients who respond to salvage therapy (see Chap. 134).[94,95] In the PARMA study, 215 patients with relapsed aggressive NHL who had a response to DHAP salvage therapy were randomized to receive either HDC or continued DHAP therapy.[98] Patients who received HDC had significantly longer 5-year disease-free survival (46% vs 12%) and overall survival (53% vs 32%) than those treated with conventional salvage therapy. Further analysis of that study showed that patients who relapsed within 12 months of their initial diagnosis were less likely to benefit from HDC than were patients who relapsed after 12 months. Based on a review of the available evidence, including the PARMA study, it was concluded that HDC with autologous HSCT is effective in patients who relapse for the first time and who have responded to salvage therapy (first chemotherapy-sensitive relapse).[94,95] Unfortunately, there was inadequate evidence to make a treatment recommendation for patients who relapse and have not responded to salvage therapy (chemotherapy-resistant relapse). Based on these studies, HDC with autologous HSCT is considered to be the treatment of choice in younger patients with chemotherapy-sensitive relapse.[51,52] HDC with autologous HSCT is not recommended in patients with untested or chemotherapy-refractory relapse.

Primary Mediastinal Large B-cell Lymphoma

Primary mediastial large B-cell lymphoma (PMBL) is a distinct clinicopathologic entity, accounting for approximately 7% of all DLBCLs and 2.4% of all NHLs in the International NHL Classification Project.[61] This type of lymphoma tends to occur in younger patients (median age at presentation is 30 years old) and has a female predominance (Table 129–9).[99] Patients present with a locally invasive mediastinal mass originating in the thymus, with frequent airway compromise and superior vena cava syndrome. Although the disease course is similar to that of other aggressive lymphomas, the biologic features of PMBL clearly differentiate PMBL from other types of DLBCL.[99] Patients with PMBL should be treated similar to other patients with localized DLBCL.

Burkitt's Lymphoma and High-Grade B-cell Lymphoma, Burkitt-like

Burkitt's lymphoma is a rare and highly aggressive lymphoma that occurs primarily in young men (Table 129–9). It is classified as *small noncleaved cell, Burkitt's type* in the Working Formulation. Although it has different clinical forms, each requiring different treatment approaches, Burkitt's lymphoma is potentially curable, with overall and disease-free survival rates similar to that of DLBCL.[51] Patients with a large tumor burden can develop potentially life-threatening tumor lysis syndrome during treatment. Burkitt-like lymphoma is also an aggressive lymphoma that shares certain characteristics with Burkitt's lymphoma and DLBCL (Table 129–9). It is classified as *small noncleaved, non-Burkitt* in the Working Formulation. A recent study of the biologic and clinical characteristics of Burkitt-like lymphoma suggests that Burkitt-like lymphoma should continue to be a separate category in a lymphoma classification system or be classified as a variant of Burkitt's lymphoma.[100] Some oncologists treat Burkitt-like lymphoma as they treat Burkitt's lymphoma, whereas others treat Burkitt-like lymphomas as they treat DLBCL. In patients with Burkitt-like lymphoma treated with second- or third-generation doxorubicin-containing regimens, 5-year survival rates were nearly identical.[100]

T-CELL NEOPLASMS

Precursor T-lymphoblastic Lymphoma

Precursor T-lymphoblastic lymphoma (T-LBL) is an uncommon aggressive lymphoma that typically occurs in young adult males (Table 129–9). T-LBL is classified as *lymphoblastic, convoluted or nonconvoluted* in the Working Formulation.[60] It constitutes approximately 40% of childhood lymphomas and 15% of childhood acute lymphoblastic leukemias. Patients often present with a rapidly enlarging symptomatic mediastinal mass or peripheral lymphadenopathy. T-LBL is potentially curable with intensive combination chemotherapy regimens similar to those used in patients with DLBCL or acute lymphoblastic leukemia.[51]

Peripheral T-cell Lymphomas, all Types

Peripheral T-cell lymphomas represents the largest group of T-cell lymphomas in the REAL classification, comprising approximately 7% of all NHLs in the International NHL Classification Project.[61] They are classified as *diffuse small cleaved cell, diffuse mixed cell, diffuse large cell, and immunoblastic* in the Working Formulation.[60] Patients are usually adults with generalized disease. The disease is usually aggressive, but potentially curable with the same regimens used to treat DLBCL.[51] In the International NHL Classification Project, patients with peripheral T-cell lymphoma had among the lowest 5-year failure-free and overall survival rates.[61]

Anaplastic Large T/null-cell Lymphoma

Anaplastic large T/null-cell lymphoma (ALCL) represents the second most common type of T-cell lymphoma in the REAL classification.[61] ALCL is one of the newly recognized subtypes of lymphoma. In children, ALCL is often advanced at the time of diagnosis, but it exhibits a good response to therapy with a high likelihood of cure.[51] In adults, the tumor is aggressive but potentially curable with the same chemotherapy regimens used to treat DLBCL.

NON-HODGKIN'S LYMPHOMA IN AIDS

The risk of NHL for patients with AIDS is increased approximately 150- to 250-fold as compared to the risk to the general population.[101] AIDS-related lymphoma arises as a consequence of long-term stimulation and proliferation of B lymphocytes from HIV and the reactivation of prior EBV infection caused by HIV-induced immunosuppression.[51,52,102] AIDS-related lymphoma usually occurs late in the course of HIV infection and is the cause of death in approximately 15% of HIV-infected individuals. Although HIV infects T-cells, more than 95% of AIDS-related lymphomas are B-cell neoplasms. Most AIDS-related lymphomas are classified as small noncleaved cell histology (Burkitt's or Burkitt-like), diffuse large cell type, or immunoblastic subtype. The latter two entities are classified as DLBCL in the REAL classification (Table 129–8).

The clinical presentation is similar to that observed in other immunocompromised states. Most patients with AIDS-related lymphoma present with "B" symptoms and have advanced stage (III or IV) disease at the time of diagnosis.[51,52,103] Involvement of extranodal sites is common. The clinical course of AIDS-related lymphoma is aggressive; median survival is about 6 months and 2-year survival is only 10% to 20%. Factors associated with decreased survival include age greater than 35 years, history of injection drug use, poor performance status, CD4 cell count $<100/\mu L$, a history of AIDS prior to the diagnosis of lymphoma, stage III or IV disease, and elevated LDH levels.[103] The IPI has also been validated for use in patients with AIDS-related lymphoma.

The treatment of patients with AIDS-associated lymphomas is difficult because the immunocompromised state of these patients increases their risk of significant toxicity due to myelosuppressive therapy. Except for primary CNS lymphoma, AIDS-related lymphoma is never considered truly localized and systemic chemotherapy is indicated. For patients with adequate immune function and without a history of an opportunistic infection, chemotherapy regimens similar to that used for aggressive lymphomas may be used.[51,52] However, many patients with AIDS-related lymphoma are treated with less-intensive regimens because of the increased risk of treatment-related toxicity. The results of treatment with standard chemotherapy regimens, including CHOP and other third-generation regimens, have been disappointing. In a randomized comparison of m-BACOD (bleomycin, doxorubicin [Adriamycin], cyclophosphamide, vincristine, and dexamethasone) versus reduced-dose m-BACOD, the complete response rate (52% vs 41%) and median survival (31 weeks vs 35 weeks) were not significantly different.[104] Despite routine use of GM-CSF, grade 3 or higher toxicity was more common in patients who received standard-dose therapy (70% vs 51%). The results of this study suggest that low-dose chemotherapy is equivalent to standard-dose chemotherapy. Newer approaches, such as the EPOCH regimen developed at the National Cancer Institute, appear promising.[103] Intrathecal chemotherapy should be administered to prevent CNS relapses. Antiretroviral therapy and prophylactic antibiotics should be continued during chemotherapy.

CONCLUSIONS

Several decades ago, lymphomas were considered a fatal disease. Today, most patients with Hodgkin's disease and many patients with aggressive NHLs can be cured with radiation therapy, chemotherapy, or a combination of radiation and chemotherapy. Our ability to achieve long-term survival and cure in these patients is the result of many factors, including development of accurate and reproducible classification systems; a more uniform approach to the staging of lymphoma; and advances in treatment strategies, especially the use of intensive combination chemotherapy. The routine use of hematopoietic growth factors allows oncologists to maintain dose intensity, which may be important for the treatment of Hodgkin's disease and aggressive lymphomas. The use of HDC with autologous HSCT as intensive consolidation therapy for selected patients with aggressive NHL who respond to initial induction therapy or to salvage therapy after relapse has also contributed to increased cure rates.

New treatment approaches are needed, particularly for indolent lymphomas. Although many new therapies have been developed recently for indolent lymphomas, there is no convincing evidence that any of these therapies have changed the natural history of the disease. One of the most exciting new therapies is biologic therapy with anti-CD20 monoclonal antibodies. Investigational radiolabeled anti-CD20 antibodies (i.e., radioimmunoconjugates) are also in clinical development, and may be commercially available soon. As these new biologic therapies become available, it will be important to better understand how to use these agents, either alone or combined with standard chemotherapy. Although approximately one-third of patients with aggressive lymphomas can be cured of their disease, most patients will relapse and eventually die of their disease. More effective induction chemotherapy regimens are needed for newly diagnosed patients, and more active salvage therapy is needed for patients with relapsed aggressive NHL.

The goal for the future is to develop treatment modalities to achieve cure in a larger number of patients. But the acute and chronic toxicities associated with treatment must also be considered, particularly in elderly patients and those with significant comorbidities. Anti-CD20 monoclonal antibodies, which can be safely added to combination chemotherapy, are particularly attractive in patients who are not candidates for intensive anthracycline-containing chemotherapy regimens or HSCT.

Finally, a better understanding of the pathogenesis of NHL through continued research in molecular biology and immunology will hopefully allow for the development of specific therapies aimed at molecular targets. In addition, gene expression profiling may also allow researchers to identify new clinically important subtypes of NHL.

▶ PRINCIPLES OF PHARMACOTHERAPY

- Lymphomas are a heterogeneous group of malignancies that arise from malignant transformation of immune cells that reside predominantly in lymphoid tissues.
- Lymphomas can be divided into Hodgkin's disease and non-Hodgkin's lymphoma, based on the histopathologic examination of the tumor tissue.
- Hodgkin's disease is curable, even when patients present with advanced disease.
- Prognosis for Hodgkin's disease depends on histology, stage, patient age, performance status, presence or absence of extensive B symptoms, and serum LDH level.
- Patients with early stage Hodgkin's disease should be treated with radiation therapy alone.
- Patients with advanced-stage Hodgkin's disease should be treated with combination chemotherapy.
- The current classification system for non-Hodgkin's lymphoma is the REAL classification system, which is based on the principle that a classification is a list of specific disease entities, which are defined by a combination of morphology, immunophenotype, genetic features, and clinical features.
- The International Prognostic Index (IPI) score can be used to predict prognosis for many patients with non-Hodgkin's lymphoma.
- Patients with localized follicular lymphoma can be cured with radiation therapy alone.
- Although advanced follicular lymphoma is not curable, there are many treatment options, including watchful waiting, extended-field radiation therapy, single-agent alkylating agents, anthracycline-containing combination chemotherapy, purine analogues, interferon-α, anti-CD20 monoclonal antibodies, and high-dose chemotherapy with autologous hematopoietic stem cell rescue.
- Patients with bulky stage II, stage III, or stage IV aggressive lymphomas can be cured of their disease with intensive combination chemotherapy.
- Based on the lack of survival benefit with the newer combination chemotherapy regimens, the less complicated and less expensive CHOP regimen should be considered as the treatment of choice for diffuse large B-cell lymphoma.
- Conventional-dose salvage therapy can induce responses in patients with aggressive lymphomas who relapse, but long-term survival and cure is uncommon.
- Some patients with aggressive lymphoma who relapse and respond to salvage therapy can be cured with high-dose chemotherapy and autologous hematopoietic stem cell transplantation.
- Supportive care, including management of chemotherapy-related toxicities, is important to maintain dose intensity for the treatment of aggressive lymphomas.

REFERENCES

1. Greenlee RT, Hill-Harmon MB, Murray T, Thun M. Cancer statistics, 2001. CA Cancer J Clin 2001;51:15–36.
2. Diehl V, Mauch P, Harris NL. Hodgkin's disease. In: DeVita VT Jr, Hellman S, Rosenberg SA, eds. Cancer: Principles & Practice of Oncology, 6th ed. Philadelphia, Lippincott Williams & Wilkins, 2001:2339–2387.
3. Donaldson SS, Hancock SL, Hoppe RT. The Janeway lecture. Hodgkin's disease—Finding the balance between cure and late effects. Cancer J Sci Am 1999;5:325–333.
4. Kaufman D, Longo DL. Hodgkin's disease. In: Abeloff MD, Armitage JO, Lichter AS, Niederhuber JE, eds. Clinical Oncology, 2nd ed. Philadelphia, Churchill Livingstone, 2000:2620–2657.
5. Glaser SL, Swartz WG. Time trends in Hodgkin's disease incidence. The role of diagnostic accuracy. Cancer 1990;66:2196–2204.
6. Kennedy BJ, Loeb V Jr, Peterson VM, Donegan WL, Natarajan N, Mettlin C. National survey of patterns of care for Hodgkin's disease. Cancer 1985;56:2547–2556.
7. Haluska FG, Brufsky AM, Canellos GP. The cellular biology of the Reed-Sternberg cell. Blood 1994;84:1005–1019.
8. Eghbali H, Soubeyran P, Tchen N, de Mascarel I, Soubeyran I, Richaud P. Current treatment of Hodgkin's disease. Crit Rev Oncol Hematol 2000;35:49–73.
9. Lukes RJ, Butler JJ, Hicks ED. Natural history of Hodgkin's disease as related to its pathological picture. Cancer 1966;26:319.
10. Harris NL, Jaffe ES, Stein H, et al. A revised European-American classification of lymphoid neoplasms: A proposal from the International Lymphoma Study Group. Blood 1994;84:1361–1392.
11. Carbone PP, Kaplan HS, Musshoff K, Smithers DW, Tubiana M. Report of the Committee on Hodgkin's Disease Staging Classification. Cancer Res 1971;31:1860–1861.
12. Lister TA, Crowther D, Sutcliffe SB, et al. Report of a committee convened to discuss the evaluation and staging of patients with Hodgkin's disease: Cotswolds meeting. J Clin Oncol 1989;7:1630–1636.
13. NCCN practice guidelines for Hodgkin's disease. National Comprehensive Cancer Network. Oncology (Huntingt) 1999;13:78–110.
14. Leibenhaut MH, Hoppe RT, Efron B, Halpern J, Nelsen T, Rosenberg SA. Prognostic indicators of laparotomy findings in clinical stage I–II supradiaphragmatic Hodgkin's disease. J Clin Oncol 1989;7:81–91.
15. Kaldor JM, Day NE, Clarke EA, et al. Leukemia following Hodgkin's disease. N Engl J Med 1990;322:7–13.
16. Mauch P, Tarbell N, Weinstein H, et al. Stage IA and IIA supradiaphragmatic Hodgkin's disease: Prognostic factors in surgically staged patients treated with mantle and para-aortic irradiation. J Clin Oncol 1988; 6:1576–1583.
17. Zagars G, Rubin P. Hodgkin's disease stages IA and IIA. A long-term follow-up study on the gains achieved by modern therapy. Cancer 1985;56:1905–1912.

18. Hoppe RT, Coleman CN, Cox RS, Rosenberg SA, Kaplan HS. The management of stage I–II Hodgkin's disease with irradiation alone or combined modality therapy: The Stanford experience. Blood 1982;59:455–465.
19. Hellman S, Mauch P. Role of radiation therapy in the treatment of Hodgkin's disease. Cancer Treat Rep 1982;66:915–923.
20. Specht L, Gray RG, Clarke MJ, Peto R. Influence of more extensive radiotherapy and adjuvant chemotherapy on long-term outcome of early-stage Hodgkin's disease: A meta-analysis of 23 randomized trials involving 3,888 patients. International Hodgkin's Disease Collaborative Group. J Clin Oncol 1998;16:830–843.
21. Carde P, Hagenbeek A, Hayat M, et al. Clinical staging versus laparotomy and combined modality with MOPP versus ABVD in early-stage Hodgkin's disease: The H6 twin randomized trials from the European Organization for Research and Treatment of Cancer Lymphoma Cooperative Group. J Clin Oncol 1993;11:2258–2272.
22. Krikorian JG, Portlock CS, Mauch PM. Hodgkin's disease presenting below the diaphragm: A review. J Clin Oncol 1986;4:1551–1562.
23. Horning SJ, Hoppe RT, Hancock SL, Rosenberg SA. Vinblastine, bleomycin, and methotrexate: An effective adjuvant in favorable Hodgkin's disease. J Clin Oncol 1988;6:1822–1831.
24. Horning SJ, Hoppe RT, Mason J, et al. Stanford-Kaiser Permanente G1 study for clinical stage I to IIA Hodgkin's disease: Subtotal lymphoid irradiation versus vinblastine, methotrexate, and bleomycin chemotherapy and regional irradiation. J Clin Oncol 1997;15:1736–1744.
25. Connors JM, Fairey R, Gascoyne RD, et al. Optimized combined modality treatment for early stage Hodgkin's lymphoma (HL) reduces relapses and risk of 2nd neoplasms (2nd CA's). Annual Meeting of the American Society of Clinical Oncology, San Francisco, CA, 2001. Vol. 20.
26. Longo DL, Glatstein E, Duffey PL, et al. Radiation therapy versus combination chemotherapy in the treatment of early-stage Hodgkin's disease: Seven-year results of a prospective randomized trial. J Clin Oncol 1991;9:906–917.
27. Biti GP, Cimino G, Cartoni C, et al. Extended-field radiotherapy is superior to MOPP chemotherapy for the treatment of pathologic stage I–IIA Hodgkin's disease: Eight-year update of an Italian prospective randomized study. J Clin Oncol 1992;10:378–382.
28. Crnkovich MJ, Leopold K, Hoppe RT, Mauch PM. Stage I to IIB Hodgkin's disease: The combined experience at Stanford University and the Joint Center for Radiation Therapy. J Clin Oncol 1987;5:1041–1049.
29. Bonfante V, Viviani S, Devizzi L, et al. Ten-years experience with ABVD plus radiotherapy: Subtotal nodal (STNI) vs involved field (IFRT) in early stage Hodgkin's disease (Hd). Annual Meeting of the American Society of Clinical Oncology, San Francisco, CA, 2001.
30. Horning SJ, Williams J, Bartlett NL, et al. Assessment of the Stanford V regimen and consolidative radiotherapy for bulky and advanced Hodgkin's disease: Eastern Cooperative Oncology Group pilot study E1492. J Clin Oncol 2000;18:972–980.
31. Pavlovsky S, Maschio M, Santarelli MT, et al. Randomized trial of chemotherapy versus chemotherapy plus radiotherapy for stage I–II Hodgkin's disease. J Natl Cancer Inst 1988;80:1466–1473.
32. Hoppe RT, Cox RS, Rosenberg SA, Kaplan HS. Prognostic factors in pathologic stage III Hodgkin's disease. Cancer Treat Rep 1982;66:743–749.
33. Marcus KC, Kalish LA, Coleman CN, et al. Improved survival in patients with limited stage IIIA Hodgkin's disease treated with combined radiation therapy and chemotherapy. J Clin Oncol 1994;12:2567–2572.
34. DeVita VT Jr, Simon RM, Hubbard SM, et al. Curability of advanced Hodgkin's disease with chemotherapy. Long-term follow-up of MOPP-treated patients at the National Cancer Institute. Ann Intern Med 1980;92:587–595.
35. Longo DL, Young RC, Wesley M, et al. Twenty years of MOPP therapy for Hodgkin's disease. J Clin Oncol 1986;4:1295–1306.
36. Longo DL. The use of chemotherapy in the treatment of Hodgkin's disease. Semin Oncol 1990;17:716–735.
37. Santoro A, Bonfante V, Bonadonna G. Salvage chemotherapy with ABVD in MOPP-resistant Hodgkin's disease. Ann Intern Med 1982; 96:139–143.
38. Canellos GP, Anderson JR, Propert KJ, et al. Chemotherapy of advanced Hodgkin's disease with MOPP, ABVD, or MOPP alternating with ABVD. N Engl J Med 1992;327:1478–1484.
39. Goldie JH, Coldman AJ. The genetic origin of drug resistance in neoplasms: Implications for systemic therapy. Cancer Res 1984;44:3643–3653.
40. Goldie JH, Coldman AJ, Gudauskas GA. Rationale for the use of alternating non-cross-resistant chemotherapy. Cancer Treat Rep 1982;66:439–449.
41. Bonadonna G, Valagussa P, Santoro A. Alternating non-cross-resistant combination chemotherapy or MOPP in stage IV Hodgkin's disease. A report of 8-year results. Ann Intern Med 1986;104:739–746.
42. Connors JM, Klimo P, Adams G, et al. Treatment of advanced Hodgkin's disease with chemotherapy—Comparison of MOPP/ABV hybrid regimen with alternating courses of MOPP and ABVD: A report from the National Cancer Institute of Canada clinical trials group. J Clin Oncol 1997;15:1638–1645.
43. Viviani S, Bonadonna G, Santoro A, et al. Alternating versus hybrid MOPP and ABVD combinations in advanced Hodgkin's disease: Ten-year results. J Clin Oncol 1996;14:1421–1430.
44. Duggan D, Petroni G, Johnson J, et al. MOPP/ABV versus ABVD for advanced Hodgkin's disease—A preliminary report of CALGB 8952 (with SWOG, ECOG, NCIC). Annual Meeting of the American Society of Clinical Oncology, 1997. Vol. 16.
45. Glick JH, Young ML, Harrington D, et al. MOPP/ABV hybrid chemotherapy for advanced Hodgkin's disease significantly improves failure-free and overall survival: The 8-year results of the intergroup trial. J Clin Oncol 1998;16:19–26.
46. Loeffler M, Brosteanu O, Hasenclever D, et al. Meta-analysis of chemotherapy versus combined modality treatment trials in Hodgkin's disease. International Database on Hodgkin's Disease Overview Study Group. J Clin Oncol 1998;16:818–829.
47. Longo DL, Duffey PL, Young RC, et al. Conventional-dose salvage combination chemotherapy in patients relapsing with Hodgkin's disease after combination chemotherapy: The low probability for cure. J Clin Oncol 1992;10:210–218.
48. Dores G, Curtis R, Travis L. Second cancer risk following Hodgkin's disease (HD): An analysis of 15,465 patients reported to the National Cancer Institute's Surveillance, Epidemiology and End Results (SEER) program. Annual Meeting of the American Society of Clinical Oncology, San Francisco, CA, 2001. Vol. 20.
49. Zarrabi MH, Rosner F. Second neoplasms in Hodgkin's disease: Current controversies. Hematol Oncol Clin North Am 1989;3:303–318.
50. Ries L, Eisner M, Kosary C, et al. SEER Cancer Statistics Review, 1973–1998. Bethesda, MD, National Cancer Institute, 2001.
51. Armitage JO, Mauch PM, Harris NL, Bierman P. Non-Hodgkin's lymphoma. In: DeVita VT, Hellman S, Rosenberg SA, eds. Cancer: Principles & Practice of Oncology. Philadelphia, Lippincott Williams & Wilkins, 2001:2256–2316.
52. Lister TA, Armitage JO. Non-Hodgkin's lymphoma. In: Abeloff MD, Armitage JO, Lichter AS, Niederhuber JE, eds. Clinical Oncology. New York, Churchill Livingstone, 2000:2658–2719.
53. Vanasse G, Concannon P, Willerford DM. Regulated genomic instability and neoplasia in the lymphoid lineage. Blood 1999;94:3997–4010.
54. Kuppers R, Klein U, Hansmann ML, Rajewsky K. Cellular origins of human B-cell lymphomas. N Engl J Med 1999;341:1520–1529.
55. Freeman AS, Neuberg D, Mauch P, et al. Long-term follow-up of autologous bone marrow transplantation in patients with relapsed follicular lymphoma. Blood 1999;94:3325–3333.
56. Rappaport H, Winter WI, Hicks EB. Follicular lymphoma: A reevaluation of its position in the scheme of malignant lymphoma, based on a survey of 253 cases. Cancer 1956;9:792–821.

57. Lennert K, Mohri N, Stein H. The histopathology of malignant lymphoma. Br J Haematol 1975;31(suppl):1488–1503.
58. Lukes RF, Collins RD. Immunologic characterization of human malignant lymphomas. Cancer 1974;34:1488–1503.
59. The Non-Hodgkin's Lymphoma Classification Project: National Cancer Institute-sponsored study of classifications of non-Hodgkin's lymphomas. Summary and description of a working formulation for clinical usage. Cancer 1982;49:2112–2135.
60. Harris NL, Jaffe ES, Stein H. A revised European-American classification of lymphoid neoplasms: A proposal from the International Lymphoma Study Group. Blood 1994;84:1361–1392.
61. The Non-Hodgkin's Lymphoma Classification Project: A clinical evaluation of the International Lymphoma Study Group classification of non-Hodgkin's lymphoma. Blood 1997;89:3909–3918.
62. Harris NL, Jaffe ES, Diebold J, et al. World Health Organization Classification of neoplastic diseases of the hematopoietic and lymphoid tissues: Report of the Clinical Advisory Committee meeting—Airlie House, Virginia, November 1997. J Clin Oncol 1999;17:3835–3849.
63. The International Non-Hodgkin's Lymphoma Prognostic Factors Project: A predictive model for aggressive non-Hodgkin's lymphoma. N Engl J Med 1993;329:987–994.
64. Fisher RI. Mantle cell lymphoma: Prognostic factors and treatment results. In: Schechter GP, Hoffman R, Schrier S, eds. Hematology 1999. New Orleans, American Society of Hematology Education Book, 1999:325–328.
65. Coiffier B. Mantle cell lymphoma: New treatment possibilities. In: Schechter GP, Hoffman R, Schrier S, eds. Hematology 1999. New Orleans, American Society of Hematology Education Book, 1999:329–334.
66. Foran JM, Rohatiner AZS, Cunningham D, et al. European phase II study of rituximab (chimeric anti-CD20 monoclonal antibody) for patients with newly diagnosed mantle-cell lymphoma and previously treated mantle-cell lymphoma, immunocytoma, and small B-cell lymphocytic lymphoma. J Clin Oncol 2000;18:317–324.
67. Federico M, Vitolo U, Zinzani PL, et al. Prognosis of follicular lymphoma: A predictive model based on a retrospective analysis of 987 cases. Blood 2000;95:783–789.
68. Horning SJ. Natural history of and therapy for the indolent non-Hodgkin's lymphomas. Semin Oncol 1993;20(suppl 5):75–88.
69. Rodriguez J, McLaughlin P, Hagenmeister FB, et al. Follicular large cell lymphoma: An aggressive lymphoma that often presents with favorable prognostic features. Blood 1999;93:2202–2207.
70. Mac Manus MP, Hoppe RT. Is radiotherapy curative for stage I and II low-grade follicular lymphomas? Results of a long-term follow-up study of patients treated at Stanford University. J Clin Oncol 1996;14:1282–1290.
71. Cheson BD. New therapeutic strategies for the treatment of indolent non-Hodgkin's lymphoma. In: Schechter GP, Hoffman R, Schrier S, eds. Hematology 1999. New Orleans, American Society of Hematology Education Book, 1999:291–298.
72. Cabanillas F, Horning S, Kaminski M, Champlin R. Managing indolent lymphomas in relapse: Working our way through a plethora of options. In: Schechter GP, Berliner N, Telen MJ, eds. Hematology 2000. San Francisco, American Society of Hematology Education Book, 2000: 166–179.
73. Murtha AD, Knox SJ, Hoppe RT, Rupnow BA, Hanson J. Long-term follow-up of patients with stage III follicular lymphoma treated with primary radiotherapy at Stanford University. Int J Radiat Oncol Biol Phys 2001;49:3–15.
74. McLaughlin P, Hagemeister F, Romaguera J, et al. Fludarabine, mitoxantrone, and dexamethasone. An effective new regimen for indolent lymphoma. J Clin Oncol 1996;14:1262–1268.
75. Parkinson DR, Sznol M, Cheson BD. Biologic therapies for low-grade lymphomas. Semin Oncol 1993;20(suppl 5):111–117.
76. Solal-Céligny P, Lepage E, Brousse N, et al. Doxorubicin-containing regimen with or without interferon alfa-2b for advanced follicular lymphoma: final analysis of survival and toxicity in the Groupe d'Etude des Lymphomes Folliculaires 86 Trial. J Clin Oncol 1998;16:2332–2338.
77. Cheson BD. The curious case of the baffling biological. J Clin Oncol 2000;18:2007–2009.
78. Fisher RI, Dana BW, LeBlanc M, et al. Interferon-alfa consolidation after intensive chemotherapy does not prolong the progression-free survival of patients with low-grade non-Hodgkin's lymphoma: Results of the Southwest Oncology Group Randomized Phase III Study 8809. J Clin Oncol 2000;18:2010–2016.
79. Levy R. Karnofsky lecture: Immunotherapy of lymphoma. J Clin Oncol 1999;17(Nov suppl):7–13.
80. Grillo-Lopez AJ, White CA, Varns C, et al. Overview of the clinical development of rituximab: First monoclonal antibody approved for treatment of lymphoma. Semin Oncol 1999;26(suppl 14):66–73.
81. McLaughlin P, Grillo-Lopez AJ, Link BK, et al. Rituximab chimeric anti-CD20 monoclonal antibody therapy for relapsed indolent lymphoma: Half of patients respond to a four-dose treatment program. J Clin Oncol 1998;16:2825–2833.
82. Colombat P, Salles G, Brousse N, et al. Rituximab (anti-CD20 monoclonal antibody) as single first-line therapy for patients with follicular lymphoma with a low tumor burden: Clinical and molecular evaluation. Blood 2001;97:101–106.
83. Davis TA, Grillo-Lopez AJ, White CA, et al. Rituximab anti-CD20 monoclonal antibody therapy in non-Hodgkin's lymphoma: Safety and efficacy of re-treatment. J Clin Oncol 2000;18:3135–3143.
84. Czuczman MS, Grillo-Lopez AJ, White CA, et al. Treatment of patients with low-grade B-cell lymphoma with the combination of chimeric anti-CD20 monoclonal antibody and CHOP chemotherapy. J Clin Oncol 1999;17:268–276.
85. Press OW. Monoclonal antibody therapy for indolent non-Hodgkin's lymphoma. In: Schechter GP, Hoffman R, Schrier S, eds. Hematology 1999. New Orleans, American Society of Hematology Education Book, 1999:305–311.
86. Freedman AS. Bone marrow transplantation for indolent lymphoma. In: Schechter GP, Hoffman R, Schrier S, eds. Hematology 1999. New Orleans, American Society of Hematology Education Book, 1999:298–304.
87. Horning SJ, Gascoyne ER, Fisher RI. Large-cell lymphomas: Let's chop down barriers to progress. ASCO Educational Book, Spring, 1999:319–331.
88. Alizadeh AA, Eisen MB, Davis RE, et al. Distinct types of diffuse large B-cell lymphoma identified by gene expression profiling. Nature 2000;403:503–511.
89. Miller TP, Dahlberg S, Cassady JR, et al. Chemotherapy alone compared with chemotherapy plus radiotherapy for localized intermediate- and high-grade non-Hodgkin's lymphoma. N Engl J Med 1998;339: 21–26.
90. McKelvey EM, Gottleib JA, Wilson HE, et al. Hydroxyldaunomycin (Adriamycin) combination chemotherapy in malignant lymphoma. Cancer 1976;38:1484–1493.
91. Jones SE, Grozea PN, Metz EN, et al. Superiority of adriamycin-containing combination chemotherapy in the treatment of diffuse lymphoma: A Southwest Oncology Group study. Cancer 1979;43:417–425.
92. Fisher RI, Gaynor ER, Dahlberg S, et al. Comparison of a standard regimen (CHOP) with three intensive chemotherapy regimens for advanced non-Hodgkin's lymphoma. N Engl J Med 1993;328:1002–1006.
93. Vose JM, Link BK, Grossbard ML, et al. Phase II study of rituximab in combination with CHOP chemotherapy in patients with previously untreated, aggressive non-Hodgkin's lymphoma. J Clin Oncol 2001;19:389–397.
94. Shipp MA, Abeloff MD, Antman KH, et al. International consensus conference on high-dose therapy with hematopoietic stem cell transplantation in aggressive non-Hodgkin's lymphomas: Report of the jury. J Clin Oncol 1999;17:423–429.
95. Hahn T, Wolff SN, Czuczman M, et al. The role of cytotoxic therapy with hematopoietic stem cell transplantation in the therapy of diffuse large cell B cell non-Hodgkin's lymphoma: An evidence-based review. Biol Blood Marrow Transplant 2001;7:308–331.

96. Rodriguez-Monge EJ, Cabanillas F. Long-term follow-up of platinum-based lymphoma salvage regimens. The M.D. Anderson Cancer Center experience. Hematol Oncol Clin North Am 1997;11: 937–947.
97. Fields KK, Zorsky PE, Hiemenz JW, et al. Ifosfamide, carboplatin, and etoposide: A new regimen with broad spectrum of activity. J Clin Oncol 1994;12:544–552.
98. Philip T, Guglielmi C, Hagenbeek A, et al. Autologous bone marrow transplantation as compared with salvage chemotherapy in relapses of chemotherapy-sensitive non-Hodgkin's lymphoma. N Engl J Med 1995;333:1540–1545.
99. van Besien K, Kelta M, Bahaguna P. Primary mediastinal B-cell lymphoma: A review of pathology and management. J Clin Oncol 2001;19: 1855–1864.
100. Braziel RM, Arber DA, Slovak ML, et al. The Burkitt-like lymphomas: A Southwest Oncology group study delineating phenotypic, genotypic, and clinical features. Blood 2001;97:3713–3720.
101. Goedert JJ. The epidemiology of acquired immunodeficiency syndrome malignancies. Semin Oncol 2000;27:390–401.
102. Tulpule A, Levine AM. Acquired immunodeficiency syndrome-related lymphoma. In: Haskell CM, ed. Cancer Treatment. Philadelphia, WB Saunders, 2001:1550–1554.
103. Levine AM. Acquired immunodeficiency syndrome-related lymphomas: Clinical aspects. Semin Oncol 2000;27:442–453.
104. Kaplan LD, Straus DJ, Testa MA, et al. Low dose compared with standard dose m-BACOD chemotherapy for non-Hodgkin's lymphoma associated with human immunodeficiency virus infection. N Engl J Med 1997;336:1641–1648.

130
OVARIAN CANCER

William C. Zamboni, Laura L. Jung, and Margaret E. Tonda

Ovarian cancer is the fifth most common noncutaneous malignancy diagnosed in women.[1] Overall, it is the fifth leading cause of cancer-related death and the most common death from gynecologic malignancy.[1] The incidence of ovarian cancer is highest in the United States, Europe, and Israel, and lowest in Japan and developing countries.[2] In the United States alone, it is estimated that 23,400 new cases of ovarian cancer will be diagnosed and 13,900 women will die from this disease in 2001.[1] Based on Surveillance, Epidemiology, and End Results (SEER) data collected from 1989 to 1996, 5-year survival in white females for all stages approximates 50%; however, survival dramatically increases to 95% in patients with localized disease.[1] Unfortunately, most patients have disseminated disease at diagnosis because symptoms usually do not appear until late in the disease course.[1] Overall survival is slightly higher for whites (50%) than for African Americans (48%), as is survival for patients with localized disease (whites: 95% vs blacks: 91%).[1] Surgery is an integral part of ovarian cancer management. Chemotherapy, primarily the combination of a taxane plus a platinum analog, plays an important role for adjuvant therapy of localized and advanced disease.

EPIDEMIOLOGY

Ovarian cancer usually occurs in postmenopausal white women during the sixth decade of life.[2] Only 5% to 10% of ovarian cancer is familial; the majority of ovarian cancer occurs sporadically. For women in the United States, the overall lifetime risk of developing ovarian cancer is 1.4% to 1.8%.[2] The most important risk factor appears to be family history of ovarian cancer. The lifetime risk for developing ovarian cancer markedly increases to 7% to 9% in women with a family history involving two or more first-degree relatives.[2,3] The risk for ovarian cancer is decreased to 0.6% in women who have had several pregnancies, especially in women who first became pregnant before age 25, and is increased to 3.4% in nulliparous women, suggesting that uninterrupted ovulation may be a contributing factor.[2] Prolonged oral contraceptive use or breast-feeding lowers the risk for developing ovarian cancer.[2,4] An increased risk has been associated with environmental exposure to asbestos or talc.[2,3]

Several hereditary ovarian cancer syndromes have been described, which include the development of breast and ovarian cancers or ovarian, endometrial, and nonpolyposis colon cancers.[2,5] These syndromes tend to occur at an earlier age than the usual development for each of the individual malignancies and account for about 5% of the total ovarian cancer incidence.[2,5]

A number of genetic abnormalities have been detected in patients with ovarian cancer.[6–8] These include alterations in BRCA1, BRCA2, p21, Her2Neu, p53, OVAC1, OVAC2, and Rb gene function, and loss of heterozygosity on chromosomes 6, 9, 13q, 17, 18q, 19p, and 22q. Alterations in these genes can be hereditary following an autosomal dominant pattern of inheritance for BRCA1 and BRCA2.

BRCA1 gene is presumed to function as a tumor-suppressor gene and is located on chromosome 17q12-21. BRCA2 gene is located on chromosome 13q12-13. Current risk estimates for the development of ovarian cancer in women with mutations in BRCA1 are 26% to 85% by 70 years of age, whereas mutations in BRCA2 appear to confer a lesser risk of developing this disease with an estimated risk of <10% by 70 years of age.[9,10] These estimates of ovarian cancer need to be interpreted with caution as they are limited by selection bias of the study populations for families with large numbers of breast and ovarian cancer.

Identification of BRCA1 mutations in patients may confer some survival benefit. Rubin and colleagues reported an improved overall survival (77 months vs 29 months, respectively) in patients with ovarian cancer with BRCA1 mutations than their matched controls not known to have hereditary cancer.[8] Inheritance of BRCA1 gene mutations may also be linked with other risk modifiers. Pregnancy is associated with reduction in the number of ovulations and therefore, ovarian stimulation. However, Narod and colleagues reported an increased risk of ovarian cancer with parity, yet a protective effect of late birth was also seen.[11]

Despite the progress made in understanding the genetic mechanisms and implications of ovarian cancer, much of this information is currently too premature to be clinically useful. Given current guidelines for the followup care of individuals at high genetic risk of ovarian cancer and the lack of clinically useful information, especially with BRCA mutations, additional clinical trials and research programs to further determine screening mechanisms for early detection, chemoprevention, and improved treatment are necessary.[9,10]

PATHOLOGY

Most ovarian tumors (85% to 90%) are derived from the epithelial surface of the ovary.[2] The histologic types (percent incidence) of epithelial ovarian cancer are serous cystadenocarcinoma (40%), endometrioid (15%), mucinous cystadenocarcinoma (12%), clear cell (6%), and undifferentiated carcinoma (17%).[2,12] Epithelial ovarian cancers can be classified as benign, malignant, or borderline (low malignant potential). The remaining ovarian tumors are derived from germ, sex chord, and stromal cell origin.[12]

CLINICAL PRESENTATION

The majority of women with ovarian cancer have no symptoms until the malignancy has spread outside the pelvis.[2,12] Patients with early ovarian cancer can present with nonspecific, vague abdominal symptoms such as nausea, discomfort, dyspepsia, flatulence, bloating, fullness, early satiety, and digestive disturbances.[2,12] These symptoms can easily be confused with symptoms that happen normally throughout the menstrual cycle. Late symptoms can include pain, abdominal distention, ascites, and abdominal or pelvic masses.[2,12] A palpable ovary in a postmenopausal woman should be promptly evaluated because functional cysts do not usually occur in this age group.[12]

DIAGNOSIS

The diagnostic workup for suspected ovarian cancer includes a careful physical examination including a thorough breast examination, a pap smear, and a rectovaginal examination.[12,13] A detailed family history should be taken, especially noting the rate and pattern of relatives with malignancies.

A complete blood count, chemistry profile (including liver and renal function tests), and a CA-125 assay should be performed.[2,3] CA-125 is an antigen common to most nonmucinous epithelial ovarian cancers and is detected in the laboratory by using OC-125, a monoclonal antibody directed at this antigen.[14,15] CA-125 is a useful tumor marker because it is found in more than 80% of ovarian tumors and rising (or falling) titers correlate with disease extent.[14,15] Normal CA-125 values are less than 35 U/mL.[14,15]

Refractory disease is often associated with a CA-125 level that does not return to normal or that remains elevated after completion of chemotherapy.[14,15] A new elevation in the CA-125 level may be the first sign of relapse.[15]

Other diagnostic tests should include a chest x-ray, an intravenous pyelogram, cystoscopy, proctoscopy, and a barium enema. Depending on clinical evaluation, computed tomography (CT), magnetic resonance imaging (MRI), or ultrasound may be indicated. An upper GI series is indicated in patients with gastrointestinal symptoms or with bowel obstruction.

The approach to diagnosing an adnexal mass discovered on pelvic examination depends on several factors, including the patient's reproductive age, adnexal mass size, menopausal status, and symptoms.[16] Exploratory laparotomy is indicated in premenarchal women, women with masses greater than 8 cm, women with masses that increase or persist through several menstrual cycles or that are fixed to peritoneal surfaces, women with bilateral masses, or women with intra-abdominal pain or ascites.[16]

SCREENING

Ovarian cancer is an ideal malignancy for early screening efforts because greater than 65% of cases are currently diagnosed with advanced disease.[17–19] However, for screening efforts to be successful, suitable sensitive, specific, cost-effective screening tests with an adequate positive predictive value must be available. Also, there must be a detectable preclinical phase, and the disease must be amenable to therapy.[17–19] Three screening tests have been used to detect ovarian cancer: bimanual rectovaginal pelvic examination; CA-125 determination; and transvaginal sonography (TVS).[3,19] Bimanual rectovaginal pelvic examination is inadequate for screening purposes because it lacks useful sensitivity and specificity.[17–19] CA-125 is elevated in only 50% of stage I cases and a significant number of women with benign ovarian disease have abnormal CA-125 values.[17–19] TVS is not specific enough to use as the sole screening modality.

The following screening guidelines were developed at a National Institutes of Health (NIH) consensus conference:[20]

- All women should have a comprehensive family history taken focusing on all the known ovarian cancer risk factors. Rectovaginal pelvic exam should be performed as part of ordinary medical care.
- For women without a family history of ovarian cancer or with a family history of ovarian cancer in one relative, routine screening with ultrasound or CA-125 is not recommended because current evidence does not support any benefit. Participation in ovarian cancer screening trials is appropriate.
- In women with a family history of ovarian cancer in two or more relatives, the risk for developing ovarian cancer is 7%. No conclusive data show that screening in these patients will produce additional benefit. However, because this situation carries a 3% risk of having a hereditary ovarian cancer syndrome, these women should be counseled by a gynecologic oncologist or other qualified specialist regarding their individual risk.
- Women from families with hereditary ovarian cancer syndromes (i.e., Lynch II syndrome) have a 40% lifetime risk of developing ovarian cancer. Although no data indicate that screening will reduce mortality, annual rectovaginal pelvic examination, CA-125 determinations, and TVS are recommended in these women until age 35 or when childbearing is complete. Prophylactic bilateral oophorectomy should then be considered to reduce the overall risk.

With regard to possible ovarian cancer development, current recommendations for followup care for individuals with BRCA1 and/or possibly BRCA2 mutations include genetic counseling and annual or semiannual transvaginal ultrasound with color flow Doppler and serum CA-125 beginning at age 25 to 35 years.[13] There is not enough information to recommend for, or against, prophylactic oophorectomy or prophylactic use of oral contraceptives in BRCA1 carriers. Participation in ongoing ovarian cancer screening trials should be encouraged.

STAGING

The stage of ovarian cancer depends on the extent of disease found at surgical exploration (Table 130–1). Epithelial ovarian cancer spreads by peritoneal surface shedding and lymphatic dissemination (Fig. 130–1).[12] A careful and accurate surgical staging laparotomy is necessary to properly stage the patient; it is therefore recommended that a gynecologic-oncologic surgeon do this procedure to prevent understaging.[21,22] Total abdominal hysterectomy, bilateral salpingo-oophorectomy, and partial omentectomy are performed.[3,12,13] A careful examination of all serosal surfaces is done and biopsies of any grossly involved areas are taken. Ovarian capsule rupture, if present, is noted. Ascites is collected and peritoneal washings are done. Integral to the initial surgical staging procedure, the surgeon attempts to debulk as much gross tumor as possible because the amount of residual disease in patients with stage III ovarian cancer correlates with survival.[3]

TABLE 130–1. FIGO* Staging for Epithelial Ovarian Cancer

I: Confined to the ovaries
- IA: One ovary, no ascites, intact capsule
- IB: Both ovaries, no ascites, intact capsule
- IC: Ruptured capsule, capsular involvement, positive peritoneal washings, or malignant ascites

II: Ovarian tumor with pelvic extension
- IIA: Extension to uterus or tubes
- IIB: Extension to other pelvic organs (bladder, rectum, or vagina)
- IIC: Pelvic extension, plus findings for IC

III: Tumor outside the pelvis or with positive nodes
- IIIA: Microscopic seeding outside true pelvis
- IIIB: Gross deposits ≤2 cm
- IIIC: Gross deposits >2 cm or positive nodes

IV: Distant organ involvement, including liver parenchyma or pleural space

*International Federation of Gynecologic Oncologists.

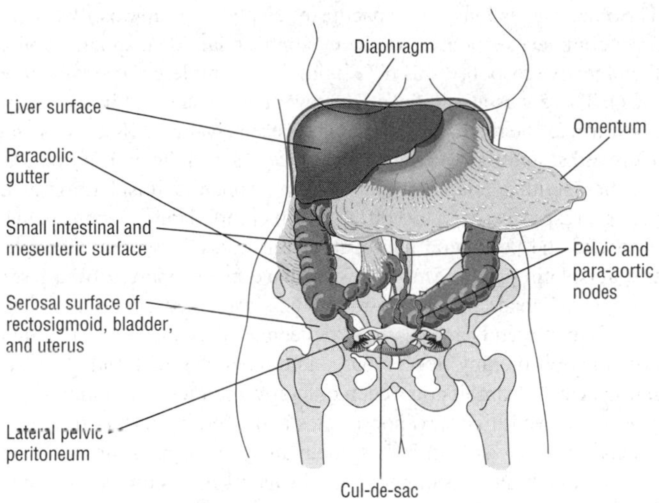

FIGURE 130–1. Staging laparotomy for ovarian cancer.

PROGNOSIS

The prognosis for patients with epithelial ovarian cancer is related to disease stage, pathologic grade, and cell histology. Patients with well-differentiated stage IA or IB tumors have a 5-year survival rate of greater than 90% with no additional benefit derived from adjuvant therapy.[3,13,20,23] With adjuvant therapy, patients with any poorly differentiated stage I, stage IC, or stage II disease have an 80% 5-year survival rate.[3,13,24] Survival in patients with stage III disease is poorer than in earlier stages, and is directly related to the size of residual tumors present after debulking surgery. Patients with implants less than 0.5 cm have a median survival of 40 months, those with implants 0.5–2 cm have a median survival of 18 months, and those with residual tumor greater than 2 cm have a median survival of 6 to 12 months.[25–27] The 5-year survival rate for stage IV patients is only 5% to 10%.[2] Patients with borderline ovarian cancer have an excellent prognosis, with a 5-year survival rate of 93% and a 10-year survival rate of 91%.[2]

▶ TREATMENT: Ovarian Cancer

Ovarian cancer management is based on the histologic type, pathologic grade, and the stage of disease at initial presentation (Fig. 130–2). In general, the treatment of patients with ovarian cancer initially involves surgical debulking at the time of staging laparotomy followed by adjuvant chemotherapy.[28] However, the effect of debulking on outcome in stage IV disease patients is unclear.[29] Second-line therapy is recommended if residual disease is found after adjuvant chemotherapy. Although response rates are high, many patients with ovarian cancer still die from their disease, so it is appropriate to enter patients with any disease stage into clinical research studies.

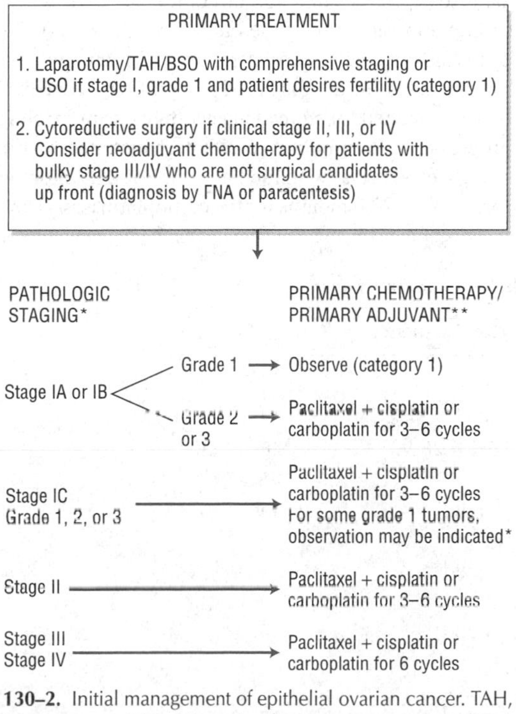

PRIMARY TREATMENT

1. Laparotomy/TAH/BSO with comprehensive staging or USO if stage I, grade 1 and patient desires fertility (category 1)
2. Cytoreductive surgery if clinical stage II, III, or IV
   Consider neoadjuvant chemotherapy for patients with bulky stage III/IV who are not surgical candidates up front (diagnosis by FNA or paracentesis)

↓

PATHOLOGIC STAGING*		PRIMARY CHEMOTHERAPY/ PRIMARY ADJUVANT**
Stage IA or IB	Grade 1 →	Observe (category 1)
	Grade 2 or 3 →	Paclitaxel + cisplatin or carboplatin for 3–6 cycles
Stage IC Grade 1, 2, or 3	→	Paclitaxel + cisplatin or carboplatin for 3–6 cycles For some grade 1 tumors, observation may be indicated*
Stage II	→	Paclitaxel + cisplatin or carboplatin for 3–6 cycles
Stage III Stage IV	→	Paclitaxel + cisplatin or carboplatin for 6 cycles

FIGURE 130–2. Initial management of epithelial ovarian cancer. TAH, total abdominal hysterectomy, BSO, bilateral salpingo-oophorectomy; USO, unilateral salpingo-oophorectomy. *Clear cell pathology is considered high grade regardless of the stage. **Acceptable regimens include (a) cisplatin, 75 mg/m^2, + paclitaxel, 135 mg/m^2, over 24 h *or* carboplatin, AUC 7.5, + paclitaxel, 175 mg/m^2, over 3 h for six cycles for stage III or stage IV disease and for three to six cycles for lower-stage disease; (b) whole abdominopelvic RT for low-bulk disease (category 3). *(From Ref. 28, with permission. See Figure 130–3 for National Comprehensive Cancer Network guidelines.)*

TREATMENT BY STAGE

LOCAL/LIMITED DISEASE (STAGES I AND II)

Approximately one-third of ovarian cancer patients present with localized disease (stage I or II) at initial diagnosis.[3,20] In patients with apparent early stage disease, comprehensive surgical staging is of utmost importance because approximately one-third of patients will have metastatic disease that is not apparent on gross total resection.[3,30] During laparotomy, the patient should undergo comprehensive staging, total abdominal hysterectomy, and bilateral salpingo-oophorectomy.[28] Women with stage IA, grade 1 ovarian tumors who wish to preserve ovarian and reproduction function can undergo a unilateral salpingo-oophorectomy without significant risk of decreased survival.[3,28,31] The beneficial effects of adjuvant chemotherapy in localized disease depend on the stage and the disease subtype. Postoperative adjuvant chemotherapy is not required in grade 1, stage IA or IB ovarian cancer, whereas patients with grade 2 or 3, stage IA or IB, and stage IC ovarian cancer benefit from adjuvant chemotherapy.[3,12,20,28] All patients with stage II disease should receive adjuvant treatment.[12,20,23,28] The role of adjuvant chemotherapy for patients with stage I is controversial. Recent data suggests that the outcome of patients with stage I disease who relapse following no adjuvant chemotherapy is similar to patients with stage III disease who relapse following chemotherapy.[32] For localized ovarian cancer (stage I or II), the recommended adjuvant regimen is paclitaxel plus cisplatin or carboplatin given for 3 to 6 cycles.[28]

ADVANCED DISEASE (STAGES III AND IV)

The majority of women with ovarian cancer present with stage III or IV disease.[3] The approach to the treatment of advanced ovarian cancer is initial surgical debulking followed by adjuvant/consolidative paclitaxel plus cisplatin or carboplatin for six cycles[28] (Fig. 130–2). Overall survival is a function of the initial disease stage (stage III vs IV) and the amount of residual disease left after surgical debulking.

PRIMARY CYTOREDUCTIVE SURGERY

The surgical removal of ovarian tumors should be as complete as possible to increase the likelihood of response to chemotherapy. The amount of residual disease after debulking is also a strong prognostic factor. Stage III disease patients with optimal debulking (≤2 cm of residual tumor) have a 4-year survival rate of approximately 30%.[2,3] Patients with stage III or IV disease who have undergone suboptimal debulking (>2 cm of residual tumor) have less than a 10% chance of long-term survival.[3,25,27]

PRIMARY/ADJUVANT CHEMOTHERAPY

Systemic chemotherapy following optimal surgical debulking is the cornerstone of first-line treatment of advanced epithelial ovarian cancer. Although there have been only modest improvements in long-term survival, there have been significant improvements in the relative 5-year survival of patients with advanced ovarian cancer. Table 130–2 summarizes the chemotherapeutic regimens used as the initial treatment of newly diagnosed ovarian cancer.

The combination of cyclophosphamide and cisplatin or carboplatin was once the first-line adjuvant therapy of choice in women with advanced-stage ovarian cancer.[26,27,33] However, paclitaxel alone, and in combination with platinum analogs, has shown significant activity in ovarian cancer.[34–36] McGuire et al. reported that the combination of paclitaxel 135 mg/m^2 over 24 hours and cisplatin 75 mg/m^2 achieved better response rates and survival outcomes than did cyclophosphamide 750 mg/m^2 and cisplatin 75 mg/m^2 in patients with newly diagnosed suboptimally debulked stages III and IV ovarian cancer.[37] The objective response in the paclitaxel/cisplatin group was 73%, with 51% complete responses; in the cyclophosphamide/cisplatin group, the objective response was 60%, with 31% complete responses ($p = 0.01$). There was a significant improvement in survival in the paclitaxel arm as the median progression-free survival was 18 months and 13 months, and the median survival was 38 months and 24 months for the paclitaxel/cisplatin- and cyclophosphamide/cisplatin-treated groups, respectively ($p < 0.001$ for both comparisons). Neutropenia, alopecia, and peripheral neuropathy were more severe in the paclitaxel/cisplatin group. Similar results have been reported by a large European-Canadian Phase III randomized trial study.[38]

Cisplatin and carboplatin have been used as single-agent and in combination therapy in previously untreated stage III and IV ovarian cancer.[39] Combination chemotherapy regimens containing cisplatin achieved higher response rates and overall survival than regimens without cisplatin.[13,40] A meta-analysis comparing treatment with platinum analogs either as single agents or in combination regimens reported a greater overall response and longer survival in the combination treatment group.[40]

Carboplatin has been used in place of cisplatin in combination therapy for patients with advanced ovarian cancer because of better tolerability, ease of administration, and apparent equivalent survival.[41–44] Reviews from pilot Phase I/II trials report favorable results with paclitaxel plus carboplatin combinations.[12,45] Three prospective, randomized Phase III trials comparing carboplatin/paclitaxel versus cisplatin/paclitaxel in patients with advanced ovarian cancer have been conducted.[46–48] Preliminary results concluded that carboplatin/paclitaxel is the preferred regimen because of equal efficacy and less toxicity. In the US study (Gynecologic Oncology Group [GOG] 158), 840 previously untreated patients with stage III optimal disease (no residual tumor nodule >1 cm) were randomized to carboplatin (area under the curve [AUC] = 7.5) plus paclitaxel 175 mg/m^2 over 3 hours or cisplatin 75 mg/m^2 plus paclitaxel 135 mg/m^2 over 24 hours administered every 21 days for 6 cycles.[46,49] The study was designed for equivalence with the primary end point as time to progression. Preliminary results demonstrated no difference in recurrence-free survival with median times of 21.7 months for the cisplatin arm versus 22.0 months for the carboplatin arm. The survival

TABLE 130–2. Initial Chemotherapeutic Regimens for Epithelial Ovarian Cancer

Drug(s)	Dose(s)	Cycle Frequency	Ref.
Cisplatin	100 mg/m^2 IV day 1	q28d	44
Carboplatin	400–800 mg/m^2 IV day 1	q28–35d	39
Cisplatin Cyclophosphamide	50–100 mg/m^2 IV day 1 500–1000 mg/m^2 IV day 1	q21–28d	26, 27, 33
Carboplatin Cyclophosphamide	200–300 mg/m^2 IV day 1 500–1000 mg/m^2 IV day 1	q28d	43, 44
Cisplatin Carboplatin	50 mg/m^2 IV day 1 300 mg/m^2 IV day 1	q28d	52
Cisplatin Doxorubicin Cyclophosphamide	50–60 mg/m^2 IV day 1 40–50 mg/m^2 IV day 1 500–750 mg/m^2 IV day 1	q28d	27, 33
Paclitaxel Cisplatin	135 mg/m^2 IV (24 h infusion) day 1 75 mg/m^2 IV day 1	q21d	37
Paclitaxel Carboplatin	175 mg/m^2 IV (3 h infusion) day 1 Dosed to AUC 5–7.5 IV day 1	q21d	28, 45, 46, 50
Docetaxel Carboplatin	75 mg/m^2 IV day 1 Dosed to AUC 5 IV day 1	q21d	51

AUC, area under the curve.

analysis is still ongoing. More toxicity was observed in the cisplatin arm. The incidence of grade 4 leukopenia, grade 3/4 gastrointestinal toxicity, grade 1–4 fever, and grade 1–4 metabolic toxicity were more common for patients in the cisplatin arm, whereas, patients in the carboplatin arm experienced more grade 3/4 thrombocytopenia and grade 1/2 pain. Neurotoxicity was similar between the two treatment arms, which may be related to the carboplatin dose (AUC = 7.5).[49] Additionally, this study also addressed the issue of second-look surgery in patients with optimal stage III disease. Preliminary results indicate second-look surgery does not influence the recurrence-free survival in this patient population. These results suggest carboplatin/paclitaxel is preferred over cisplatin/paclitaxel because of the apparent equivalent efficacy, better tolerability, and ease of administration. The Contemporary Management of Ovarian Cancer Workshop recommended carboplatin (AUC = 5–7.5) and paclitaxel (135 mg/m^2 over 3 hours), with cycles repeated every 21 days, as treatment for patients with advanced ovarian cancer.[50] Recent results from a large randomized trial of paclitaxel/carboplatin versus docetaxel/carboplatin in more than 1,000 patients with stage IC to stage IV epithelial ovarian cancer showed similar response rates between the two arms.[51] The main differences observed between the two arms were in treatment-related toxicities; patients in the paclitaxel group experienced more neurotoxicity, whereas patients in the docetaxel group experienced more myelosuppression. Preliminary data suggests similar survival between the two groups; however, long-term followup is still ongoing.

Cisplatin has also been studied in combination with carboplatin. In a phase II study, patients with advanced ovarian cancer received low doses (50 mg/m^2) of cisplatin plus moderate doses (300 mg/m^2) of carboplatin.[52] The overall response rate was 71%, with 57% achieving a complete response (CR). This platinum analog combination may be a practical alternative to high-dose cisplatin in the initial treatment of advanced ovarian cancer.

Dose intensity, or the amount of drug delivered over a specified time interval (expressed as mg/m^2/wk) may be an important factor in determining treatment outcomes with platinum-based regimens in patients with ovarian cancer.[53] However, a retrospective review of 45 randomized trials found no correlation between cisplatin dose and treatment outcome.[40] In addition, a prospective randomized trial in patients with suboptimally debulked stage III (>1-cm residual masses) and any stage IV disease, randomized patients to receive cyclophosphamide 500 mg/m^2 IV plus either cisplatin 50 mg/m^2 IV($n = 235$) or 100 mg/m^2 IV ($n = 223$) every 3 weeks.[54] Patients in the cisplatin 50 mg/m^2 group received eight cycles and patients in the cisplatin 100 mg/m^2 group received four cycles (same total cisplatin dose). Clinical and pathologic response rates, response duration, and survival were similar in both groups. Hematologic and gastrointestinal effects, febrile episodes, septic events, and renal toxicities were significantly more common and severe in the patients receiving the higher cisplatin dose. Similarly, Kaye et al. reported no survival difference in patients receiving six cycles of cyclophosphamide plus cisplatin 100 mg/m^2 IV or 50 mg/m^2 IV.[55] Neurotoxicity persisted in more patients in the high-dose arm (10 of 31), as compared to the low-dose arm (1 of 24). Likewise, dose-intensity analyses with carboplatin have demonstrated equivocal results.[56–58] Accumulating evidence seems to indicate that the dose response curve for the platinum compounds levels off within the clinically useful dosage range.[56] However, it is not clear that providing higher cumulative platinum doses confers any survival advantage over the standard cisplatin 75 mg/m^2 IV dose.

The duration of consolidative chemotherapy has been evaluated in several studies. In a study by Hainsworth et al., the administration of a cisplatin-containing regimen repeated at 4-week intervals for 6 months produced results comparable to prolonged treatment.[27] In advanced ovarian cancer, the administration of five cycles of cyclophosphamide, cisplatin, and doxorubicin was equally effective and less toxic as compared to 10 cycles of chemotherapy.[59] Six to nine cycles of chemotherapy have become the standard approach and result in clinical response rates of approximately 60% to 70% with 5-year survival rates of 10% to 20%. Because approximately 50% of patients with a confirmed pathologic response will ultimately relapse,[12] chemotherapy may be extended for two or three cycles beyond best response.[3,17] The National Comprehensive Cancer Network (NCCN) guidelines recommend three to six cycles of treatment for lower stage tumors and at least six cycles of treatment for patients with stage III or IV disease.[28] These results are also supported by the faculty at the Contemporary Management of Ovarian Cancer Workshop.[50] Ongoing studies are evaluating the use of maintenance dose paclitaxel and longer durations of primary chemotherapy in patients with advanced ovarian cancer.

Many questions still need to be answered about initial therapy for advanced stages of ovarian cancer. Ongoing clinical trials are addressing whether some of the paclitaxel-containing regimens are better than current regimens for early stage disease. There are also several comparative trials for advanced-stage ovarian cancer. These studies include determining the optimal paclitaxel dose, schedule, and treatment duration, and determining whether dose intensification aided by growth factor support will achieve higher response rates and improve survival. In addition, low-dose weekly carboplatin/paclitaxel, new triplet combinations of carboplatin/paclitaxel with agents such as gemcitabine or topotecan, sequential doublets such as cisplatin/topotecan followed by cisplatin/paclitaxel, are also under investigation.[60,61]

RECURRENT/REFRACTORY DISEASE

Approximately 20% to 50% of patients without evidence of residual disease on second-look laparotomy will relapse.[3] The choices for effective treatment of recurrent ovarian cancer are limited. Options include secondary cytoreductive surgery, salvage chemotherapy, hormonal therapy, radiotherapy, intraperitoneal chemotherapy, and high-dose chemotherapy with stem-cell support. Patients who respond to initial chemotherapy and whose response last the longest, have the greatest likelihood of achieving a response to the same first-line regimen or to second-line treatment.[63] Also, patients with recurrent or refractory disease after initial chemotherapy historically have a poor overall prognosis. Improved outcomes have been achieved in recurrent and refractory ovarian cancer with the use of high-dose chemotherapeutic agents such as cisplatin, carboplatin, and paclitaxel and the use of combination regimens containing these agents. In addition, topotecan, pegylated liposomal doxorubicin, and gemcitabine have shown antitumor activity in patients with relapsed-refractory ovarian cancer.[63–71] Table 130–3 summarizes the chemotherapeutic regimens used in the treatment of recurrent or refractory ovarian cancer.

SECONDARY CYTOREDUCTIVE SURGERY/INTERVAL SURGICAL DEBULKING

Operative reexploration (or secondary laparotomy) was once an integral part of the management of advanced ovarian carcinoma.[72] However, the role of secondary cytoreduction (or interval debulking) after consolidative chemotherapy is currently unclear. A

TABLE 130–3. Chemotherapeutic Regimens for Relapsed or Refractory Ovarian Cancer

Drug(s)	Dose(s)	Cycle Frequency	Ref.
Gemcitabine	800–1,200 mg/m^2 IV days 1, 8, and 15	q28d	69, 70, 71
Docetaxel	100 mg/m^2 IV day 1	q21d	91, 92, 93
Liposomal doxorubicin	40–50 mg/m^2 IV day 1	q28d	67, 68
Paclitaxel	80 mg/m^2 IV (1-h infusion) day 1	q wk	89
Paclitaxel Carboplatin	135–250^a mg/m^2 IV^b day 1 400–800 mg/m^2 IV day 1	q21d q28–35d	87, 88 39
Paclitaxel Cisplatin	135 mg/m^2 IV day 1 75 mg/m^2 IV day 1	q21d	37
Topotecan	1.5 mg/m^2 IV qd × 5 days	q21d	64
Tamoxifen	20 mg po bid	Continuous	76
Etoposide	50 mg/m^2 po qd × 21 days	q28d	106
Altretamine	260 mg/m^2 po (total daily dose divided in four doses) × 14–21 days	q28d	104, 105

^{a}Filgrastim used with 250 mg/m^2 dose.
^{b}3-h or 24-h infusion.

Gynecologic Oncology Group (GOG) symposium debated the role of secondary cytoreduction.[73] Several conflicting studies exist with regard to the survival advantages of secondary cytoreduction. A nonrandomized GOG study evaluated 112 International Federation of Gynecology and Obstetrics (FIGO) stage I or II ovarian cancer patients who first underwent initial surgical staging and then underwent a restaging operation following adjuvant therapy. The study reported that only 5% of the patients who were asymptomatic prior to surgery had disease confirmed by second-look laparotomy, as compared to half of the patients who were symptomatic prior to second-look laparotomy.[74] These data suggest that second-look laparotomy may not be warranted in asymptomatic patients with early-stage disease. In addition, the National Cancer Institute (NCI) consensus conference recommends that second-look operations should be performed only when the results will change management or as part of a clinical trial.[20]

Recent data suggest that interval surgical debulking may improve outcomes. In a randomized trial, van der Burg et al. performed interval debulking surgery on 140 stage IIb to stage IV suboptimally debulked (>1 cm of residual disease) ovarian cancer patients after receiving three cycles of cisplatin plus cyclophosphamide.[75] Patients then received an additional three cycles of these same drugs after surgery. Patients randomized to the nonsurgical treatment arm received six cycles of chemotherapy. Interval debulking surgery significantly prolonged overall and progression-free survival and reduced the death risk by 33%. The additional surgery was not associated with excessive morbidity.

The overall effect of interval debulking is influenced by several factors including initial response to chemotherapy, the amount of residual disease before and after second-look surgery, and the presence of microscopic residual disease. Ongoing trials will help define which patients should benefit most from interval debulking surgery.

SALVAGE CHEMOTHERAPY

The NCCN guidelines for salvage therapy for recurrent or refractory disease include several treatment options (Fig. 130–3).[28] Patients with prior low-stage, low-grade disease who have disease recurrence and who have never received chemotherapy should be treated as if they are newly diagnosed advanced-stage patients, undergoing surgical debulking and adjuvant chemotherapy with the combination of paclitaxel and a platinum agent. The NCCN guidelines suggest that tamoxifen is an appropriate therapy in patients with stage I or II ovarian cancer with a rising CA-125 as their only manifestation of disease progression.[28,76]

The choice of retreatment with platinum-containing chemotherapy depends on the time frame in which the disease recurs.[3] Patients with advanced ovarian cancer who experience disease recurrence following initial chemotherapy, are divided into two therapeutic groups. Patients who do not respond to the initial platinum-containing chemotherapy or who have recurrence within 6 months after discontinuing treatment are defined as *platinum-refractory*. These patients are unlikely to benefit from additional platinum or paclitaxel therapy and would be candidates for treatment with second-line salvage chemotherapy.[28] Patients who respond to the initial chemotherapy and relapse more than 6 months after discontinuation of chemotherapy are termed *platinum-sensitive*. These patients often benefit from secondary treatment with paclitaxel alone, a platinum alone, or paclitaxel in combination with a platinum analog.[77–82] Patients who had a long disease-free interval with a locally recurrent tumor might benefit from a second cytoreductive surgery.

A useful guideline when treating a patient with refractory or relapsed disease is to administer a salvage regimen for two courses and then to evaluate for response.[63] If no response is observed, then an alternative salvage regimen may be selected. In the case of topotecan or liposomal doxorubicin, evidence suggests continuation of treatment for four cycles and then to evaluate for response.

Cisplatin has shown a steep dose-response curve in ovarian carcinoma, where increasing the dose of cisplatin may achieve greater antitumor response.[53,83] The major cisplatin-associated toxicities when administered at doses of 50–100 mg/m^2 per cycle are nausea, vomiting, and electrolyte disturbances, including prolonged magnesium wasting and nephrotoxicity. Increasing the dose of cisplatin to 200 mg/m^2 per cycle results in myelosuppression and significant, long-lasting neurotoxicity.[83] Amifostine, a thiol chemoprotective agent, reduces the cumulative hematologic, renal, and neural toxicities associated with cyclophosphamide plus cisplatin in ovarian cancer patients.[84]

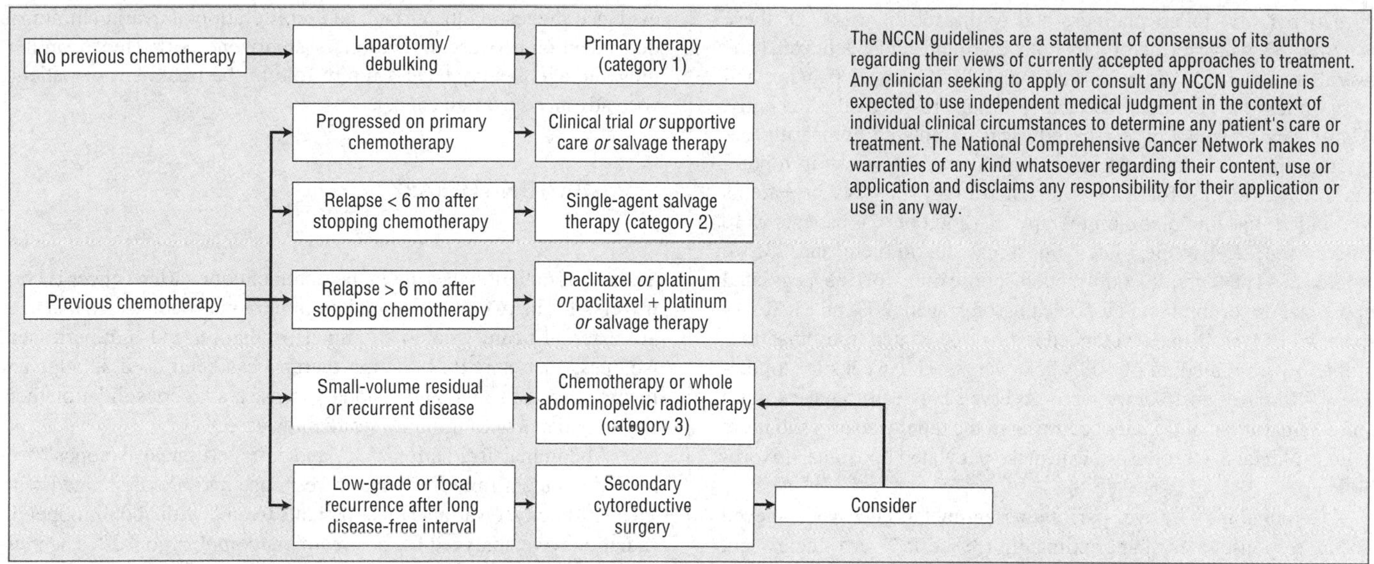

FIGURE 130–3. Management of recurrent/relapsed/progressive epithelial ovarian cancer. The following categories are used in the NCCN guidelines; Category 1, recommendations that are uncontested and generally accepted by all authorities in the field; Category 2, recommendations that are somewhat controversial; Category 3, recommendations that caused real disagreements among members of the NCCN panel. *(From Ref. 28, with permission. Copyrighted by the National Comprehensive Cancer Network. All rights reserved. These guidelines and illustrations may not be reproduced in any form without the express written permission of the NCCN.)*

Additionally, carboplatin has been used in the treatment of platinum-refractory ovarian cancer. Kavanagh et al. treated 33 platinum-refractory ovarian cancer patients with disease progression after taxane salvage therapy with carboplatin 300 mg/m^2 every 28 days.[85] These investigators noted a 21% partial response (PR) rate, a 39% stabilization rate, and a median response duration greater than 7 months. However, all responding patients had a platinum-free interval of at least 12 months.

Paclitaxel has also shown significant activity in platinum-refractory ovarian cancer.[35,86–88] At the approved dose of 175 mg/m^2 over 3 hours every 21 days, the response rate was 15% in patients with relapsed ovarian cancer.[86] Dose-intense paclitaxel regimens (250 mg/m^2 over 24 hours every 21 days plus filgrastim support) appear to produce higher objective response rates compared to conventional-dose regimens.[87,88] Altering infusion schedules of paclitaxel have been explored to maximize the cytotoxic activity of paclitaxel against ovarian cancer cells.[62] Weekly infusions may increase the dose-intensity of paclitaxel while minimizing bone marrow suppression and other toxicities associated with paclitaxel administration.[62,89–91] Paclitaxel can be safely administered weekly at a dose of 80 mg/m^2 over 1 hour to heavily pretreated patients with advanced ovarian cancer resulting in clinical response rates of approximately 30% in patients with relapsed ovarian cancer.[89–91] Ongoing and future clinical trials will help define the role of weekly paclitaxel in the treatment of patients with advanced ovarian cancer.

Docetaxel offers an alternative taxane treatment in patients with platinum-refractory ovarian cancer.[91–93] Preclinical studies show that docetaxel has more potent *in vitro* activity than does paclitaxel.[94] Docetaxel has produced overall response rates of 20% to 40% in patients with platinum-sensitive and platinum-refractory advanced ovarian cancer.[91–93,95] The response rates ranged from 17% to 20% in patients who were platinum-refractory, defined as a treatment free interval of 0 to 4 months.[92,95] Neutropenia is the dose-limiting toxicity of docetaxel and fluid retention appears to be a cumulative toxicity, which can be managed with diuretics and steroids. Docetaxel is active in patients who have received prior platinum therapy, but it is important to assess the activity of docetaxel after paclitaxel failure, particularly because paclitaxel is considered a standard in front-line regimens. Further studies are also indicated to determine if docetaxel has a role as part of initial chemotherapy.

As most patients will receive a taxane in combination with a platinum agent as initial therapy, there is a need for effective noncross-resistant agents for use as second-line and salvage chemotherapy. Topotecan, an analog of the plant alkaloid 20(S)-camptothecin, is active in patients with metastatic ovarian cancer and is noncross-resistant with platinum-based chemotherapy.[64,65,96,97] Preclinical studies suggest that protracted schedules of administration using low doses of topotecan achieve the greatest antitumor response.[98] Topotecan has demonstrated efficacy in phase II trials as second-line and salvage therapy in patients who have relapsed after, or progressed during, platinum-based therapy.[64,65,96,97] A randomized phase III trial compared topotecan and paclitaxel in patients with advanced ovarian cancer who had failed one platinum-based regimen.[64] Patients were randomized to receive topotecan 1.5 mg/m^2/day as a 30-minute infusion for 5 days repeated every 21 days or paclitaxel 175 mg/m^2 as a 3-hour infusion every 21 days. The overall response rate was 20.5% and 13.2% for the topotecan and paclitaxel treated groups, respectively. The median time to progression for topotecan-treated patients (32 weeks) was not significantly different than for paclitaxel-treated patients (20 weeks). Median survival was 61 weeks in the topotecan-treated group and 43 weeks in the paclitaxel-treated group. Topotecan was well tolerated with minimal nonhematologic toxicities.[64,65,96,97]

Pegylated liposomal doxorubicin is an emerging option for patients with recurrent ovarian cancer.[66–68] In an early Phase II study, 35 patients with progressive disease after at least one platinum and paclitaxel-based regimen received pegylated liposomal doxorubicin 50 mg/m^2 every 3 weeks (with a dose reduction to 40 mg/m^2 in the event of grade 3 or 4 toxicities or a lengthening of the interval to 4 weeks);[66] the overall response rate was 25.7%. Another Phase II study assessed the efficacy of pegylated liposomal doxorubicin in

89 patients who failed platinum and paclitaxel therapy.[67] Of these patients, 82 were refractory to both platinum and paclitaxel. The overall response rates were 16.9% and 18.3% in all patients and in the platinum/paclitaxel refractory group, respectively. Recently, a large randomized Phase III study was completed comparing pegylated liposomal doxorubicin 50 mg/m^2 every 4 weeks to topotecan 1.5 mg/m^2/day for 5 days repeated every 21 days in patients who failed first-line platinum therapy.[68] A total of 474 patients were randomized; 239 to pegylated liposomal doxorubicin and 235 to topotecan. The overall confirmed response rate for the pegylated liposomal doxorubicin and topotecan groups were 20% and 17%, respectively. Overall survival tended to favor pegylated liposomal doxorubicin with a median of 108 weeks versus 71.1 weeks for topotecan. Differences in toxicity were observed between the arms, with more hematological toxicity occurring in the topotecan arm and more palmar-plantar erythrodysesthesia in the pegylated liposomal doxorubicin arm.

Gemcitabine, a novel pyrimidine antimetabolite, has achieved overall response rates of approximately 13% to 19% as a single agent in patients with platinum-sensitive and platinum-refractory recurrent ovarian cancer.[69–71] The main toxicities include myelosuppression, fatigue, myalgias, and skin rash. Gemcitabine is a promising agent in combination with other agents in previously untreated and treated patients with advanced ovarian cancer.[99] Because of the noncross-resistant activity and *in vivo* synergy with platinum agents, the NCI is sponsoring clinical studies evaluating gemcitabine in doublet regimens in patients with refractory disease and with carboplatin/taxane regimens in previously untreated patients.[100,101]

Other agents that have shown an overall response rate of 15% to 25% in patients with recurrent ovarian cancer include altretamine, etoposide, ifosfamide, 5-fluorouracil, tamoxifen, vinorelbine, gemcitabine, and oxaliplatin.[76,102–109] Response rates tend to be higher in the platinum-sensitive subgroups. There is limited data in the scientific literature in well-defined refractory patient populations. Of these agents, altretamine, etoposide, and tamoxifen are available in oral formulations, allowing for easy administration. Altretamine (hexamethylmelamine) is a chemotherapeutic agent that undergoes metabolic activation to form alkylating intermediates.[103] Altretamine is approved as single-agent therapy at doses of 260 mg/m^2/day administered in four divided doses for 14 to 21 days given every 28 days.[104,105] When altretamine is administered in combination with other bone marrow suppressive agents, the dose is reduced to 150 mg/m^2/day for 14 days repeated every 28 days. Oral etoposide, 50 mg/m^2/day for 21 days every 28 days, has a response rate of 27% and 34% in patients with platinum-refractory and platinum-sensitive ovarian cancer, respectively.[106] However, secondary acute myeloid leukemia is a risk after high cumulative doses. Tamoxifen has also been used in the salvage setting and usually produces responses in patients with tumors expressing positive estrogen receptors.[76,107]

Much progress has been made in the treatment of refractory and relapsed ovarian cancer. However, because most patients will receive paclitaxel and platinum combinations as first-line adjuvant therapy, there is still a need to develop noncross-resistant agents that are active in patients who have progressed on, or relapsed after, this combination regimen. Management of advanced ovarian cancer that is refractory to first-line therapy is not well defined. Selection of salvage regimens is based on the mechanism of actions and toxicity profiles of the particular agents. Additionally, there are a variety of innovative treatment options that may have a role in the treatment of patients with advanced ovarian cancer including antitumor vaccines, gene therapy, and angiogenesis inhibitors. Preclinical studies suggest that adenovirus-based p53 therapy combined with cisplatin and/or paclitaxel may work against ovarian tumors.[110,111] There is also evidence suggesting the growth and proliferation of ovarian tumors is dependent on neovascularization, or angiogenesis.[112] Hence, antiangiogenic agents may have a future role in the treatment of patients with advanced ovarian cancer.

RADIATION THERAPY

The use of radiation therapy in the treatment of ovarian cancer is controversial. The two forms of radiation therapy used in ovarian cancer are external beam whole-abdominal irradiation and intraperitoneal isotopes, such as ^{32}P. Radiation therapy has been used as adjuvant therapy in patients with no residual disease and as consolidation therapy in patients with minimal residual disease.

Abdominal irradiation[113,114] and intraperitoneal isotopes[115,116] have not shown improvements in response and are associated with greater toxicity. Ovarian cancer patients treated with abdominopelvic radiation were analyzed for postreatment complications.[114] The incidence of acute complications associated with treatment were vomiting (61%) and diarrhea (68%). Serious late complications included bowel obstruction in 4.2% of patients; 64% required surgical intervention. The incidence of bowel obstruction was significantly higher in the intraperitoneal ^{32}P- versus the cisplatin-treated groups (11% and 2%, respectively; $p = 0.004$).[116] There is currently no study reporting the use of radiation therapy to be superior to chemotherapy for ovarian cancer in any treatment setting.

INTRAPERITONEAL CHEMOTHERAPY

Significant advances have occurred in understanding the advantages, limitations, and administration methods of intraperitoneal (IP) chemotherapy for ovarian cancer treatment.[117–119] Following initial treatment of advanced ovarian cancer, many patients who achieve a complete clinical response will have persistent disease or will develop recurrent disease. Overall, the proportion of patients achieving long-term survival is small.[40] Ovarian cancer is an ideal disease for IP chemotherapy because the bulk of the disease remains in the peritoneal cavity.[117–119] The theoretical advantage of IP administration is to increase the dose intensity and total drug exposure directly to the tumor, while decreasing the systemic exposure and possible toxicity. With IP administration, cytotoxic agents are instilled directly into the peritoneal cavity in large volumes to allow these agents to reach all sites within the peritoneal cavity. Studies show potential value in IP administration for initial, consolidation, and salvage therapy. Data suggest that patients with small-volume tumors (<2 cm) are best suited for IP administration as initial therapy or as salvage therapy in relapsed disease. Therefore, IP administration is a theoretically attractive approach taking into account the biology of the disease, the anatomic characteristics of the peritoneal cavity, and the pharmacokinetic advantage of drugs when administered intraperitoneally versus intravenously. Drugs that have been administered IP include cisplatin, carboplatin, cytarabine, etoposide, doxorubicin, mitoxantrone, paclitaxel, 5-fluorouracil, thiotepa, melphalan, methotrexate and topotecan.[117–126] Table 130–4 summarizes IP chemotherapeutic regimens.

Of particular interest are the agents that appear to be the most effective against ovarian cancer, which include the platinum analogs and paclitaxel. These agents appear to have a pharmacologic advantage when administered intraperitoneally. Peritoneal exposure of cisplatin or carboplatin after IP administration is approximately 10- to 20-fold

TABLE 130–4. Intraperitoneal (IP) Chemotherapeutic Regimens for Ovarian Cancer

Drug(s)	Dose(s)	Cycle Frequency	Ref.
Topotecan	3 mg/m^2 (24-h infusion) day 1	q21d	120
Cisplatin	50–100 mg/m^2 IP day 1	q21–28d	127, 133
Cisplatin Cyclophosphamide	100 mg/m^2 IP day 1 600 mg/m^2 IV day 1	q21d	127
Etoposide Cisplatin Sodium Thiosulfate	200–350 mg/m^2 IP day 1 100 200 mg/m^2 IP day 1 12–16 mg/m^2 IV day 1	q28d	128, 130
Cisplatin Cytarabine	100–150 mg/m^2 IP day 1 600–1200 mg/m^2 IP day 1	q28d	131
Paclitaxel	125 mg/m^2 IP day 1	q28d	126
Mitoxantrone	20–30 mg/m^2 IP day 1	q28d	118

greater than after systemic administration.[123,124] The exposure of the peritoneal cavity to paclitaxel after IP administration is approximately 30 times higher than plasma exposure.[125,126] Additionally, cytotoxic concentrations of paclitaxel may persist within the peritoneal cavity for 5 to 7 days after a single dose. Therefore, weekly administration may result in continuous exposure of peritoneum surface to the drug.[117]

Multicenter, randomized trials using IP chemotherapy as first-line therapy have been conducted.[127–129] In a phase III trial, women with previously untreated, stage III ovarian carcinoma with residual tumors of <2 cm were randomized to receive cyclophosphamide 600 mg/m^2 in combination with IP cisplatin 100 mg/m^2 or IV cisplatin 100 mg/m^2.[127] Median survival was significantly longer in the IP cisplatin treated group (49 months) as compared to the IV cisplatin-treated group (41 months). In addition, moderate-to-severe tinnitus, hearing loss, and neuromuscular toxicities were significantly more frequent in the IV cisplatin-treated group. These data suggest that IP cisplatin is more effective and less toxic than IV cisplatin. However, further studies are needed to confirm the advantage of IP cisplatin over IV cisplatin.

The combination of IP cisplatin, IP etoposide, and IV sodium thiosulfate has been evaluated in patients with newly diagnosed stage III and IV ovarian cancer.[128] The complete response rate in evaluable patients was 48% in the IP group and 52% in the IV group. There was no difference in response rates between the groups as a function of size of residual disease (<1 cm or >1 cm). At a median followup of 46 months, there was no difference between IP and IV therapy with regard to time to recurrence (12 and 14 months, respectively) or survival (44% and 50%, respectively). Both regimens were well tolerated with similar hematologic and nonhematologic toxicities.

A Phase III trial examined a total of 462 eligible patients with small (<1 cm in maximal diameter), residual, advanced ovarian cancer who were randomized to receive 2 courses of either carboplatin (AUC = 9) followed by IV paclitaxel 135 mg/m^2 over 24 hours and IP cisplatin 100 mg/m^2 every 21 days for six cycles, or IV paclitaxel 135 mg/m^2 over 24 hours and IV cisplatin 75 mg/m^2 every 21 days for six cycles.[129] Progression-free survival was superior in the IP arm versus the IV arm (median 27.9 months vs 22.2 months, respectively). Overall survival was 63.2 months in the IP arm versus 52.2 months in the IV arm. Although a significant improvement in progression-free survival was observed, toxicity was much greater in the experimental arm. Results from this study provide future direction for clinical studies in patients with small-volume disease.

Intraperitoneal therapy has also been evaluated as salvage therapy in patients with relapsed and refractory ovarian cancer in many Phase I and II clinical trials.[117–119] Intraperitoneal cisplatin and carboplatin have achieved documented complete responses in relapsed patients initially treated with systemic platinum containing regimens.[130,131] In the salvage setting, most of the IP experience has been with cisplatin either alone or in combination. The primary toxicity associated with IP cisplatin was bone marrow suppression; neurotoxicity and nephrotoxicity have also been observed.[119] At doses greater than 125 mg/m^2, the dose-limiting toxicity of paclitaxel IP is abdominal pain.[126] Mitoxantrone IP is associated with a high incidence of severe abdominal pain, abdominal adhesions, and bowel obstructions that require surgical treatment.[118] Large volumes of 0.9% sodium chloride can reduce the severity and frequency of local mitoxantrone IP-related adverse effects. The impact of IP chemotherapy on survival in the salvage setting is limited because of the absence of randomized trials; however, there is some indirect evidence suggesting a positive influence.[119] Several studies have evaluated factors that influence the response to IP therapy.[117–119] A retrospective study evaluated the results of IP cisplatin with etoposide or cytarabine as salvage therapy.[130] Of patients with microscopic disease at the time of IP therapy, 41% achieved a surgically defined complete response, whereas only 29% of patients with macroscopic disease (largest residual tumor mass less than 0.5 cm in diameter) had a surgically defined complete response. Patients whose largest residual tumor mass was greater than 1 cm had less than a 5% complete response rate. This is consistent with data showing a 1–2-cm depth of penetration of IP cisplatin into tumor or normal tissue.[132] An objective response rate of less than 10% is anticipated for IP cisplatin in patients who fail to demonstrate at least a partial response to initial systemic cisplatin.[119] Thus, IP cisplatin should not be used in cisplatin-refractory patients. In addition to platinum sensitivity and tumor size, extent of tumor spread must also be considered. IP therapy is most beneficial when the tumor is confined to the abdomen.[117–119] IP therapy is unlikely to have an advantage in patients with bulky disease because drug penetration into larger tumor nodules is limited. Additionally, patients best suited for IP administration should have limited IP adhesions with free fluid distribution.

Complications from IP therapy may be related to catheter function, infection, or bowel problems.[119,133] Mechanical obstruction to fluid inflow has been reported in approximately 5% of patients. Most commonly this results from fibrin sheath formation around the catheter tip.[134] In some cases, peritoneal adhesions obstruct fluid entry into the abdominal cavity, causing uneven distribution of the chemotherapeutic agent. Infectious complications, such as superficial cellulitis around the catheter entry site, deep tissue infections, and peritonitis, are the most prevalent IP-related complications and are reported in approximately 10% of patients.[133,134] Bowel-related complications (approximately 3% incidence) include obstruction, ileus, and perforation. IP administration may also result in a false CA-125 elevation.[133]

Currently, IP chemotherapy outcomes for ovarian cancer treatment have been very encouraging, but additional well-designed comparative trials are needed to define the role of IP versus systemic chemotherapy. The NCCN guidelines consider intraperitoneal therapy an investigational approach to ovarian cancer management.

AUTOLOGOUS HEMATOPOIETIC STEM CELL TRANSPLANTATION

Ovarian cancer is initially very chemosensitive; however, drug resistance is a major issue. Increased drug exposure to chemotherapeutic agents is a likely way of overcoming resistance and of possibly increasing response rates and survival. The use of high-dose myeloablative chemotherapy followed by bone marrow or peripheral blood progenitor cell rescue has been used as salvage therapy in hematologic and solid tumor malignancies. The most common ablative regimens used in ovarian cancer contain platinum analogs (i.e., cisplatin or carboplatin), alkylating agents (i.e., melphalan, thiotepa, or cyclophosphamide), and/or etoposide.[135–139]

Shpall et al. evaluated the use of IP cisplatin and high-dose systemic cyclophosphamide and thiotepa followed by autologous bone marrow support in advanced ovarian cancer.[135] Of patients evaluated, 75% had pathologically documented partial response (i.e., >75% reduction in tumor mass). Legros et al. treated poor-prognosis ovarian cancer patients with either high-dose melphalan or high-dose carboplatin plus cyclophosphamide followed by autologous stem-cell transplantation after receiving cisplatin induction therapy and second-look operations.[138] They reported an overall 60% 5-year survival rate and a 73% 5-year survival rate in patients with a pathologic complete response at second-look laparotomy. In patients with persistent or recurrent ovarian cancer treated with high-dose chemotherapy plus autologous stem-cell transplantation, tumor bulk and chemosensitivity to prior regimens were the most important prognostic factors.[139] The use of high-dose chemotherapy in the setting of ovarian cancer has been reviewed.[140,141] The data demonstrate increased response rates with limited survival advantages.

Recently, Stiff et al. analyzed data from 421 women who were reported to the Autologous Blood and Marrow Transplant registry from 1989 to 1996.[142] This project was undertaken to assess the effectiveness of high-dose chemotherapy and autotransplantation. More than 80% of the patients analyzed had stage III or IV disease at diagnosis and approximately 50% were in a clinical complete response before transplantation. Because of the limitations of this study, such as center-specific differences in selection of patients for transplant, varied timings of transplant, and varied high-dose chemotherapy regimens, the authors suggest data from this study can only be used to identify groups of patients that should or should not be studied further. The results indicate that patients with platinum-refractory disease have a 2.24 times higher mortality rate than do patients with platinum-sensitive disease. The probability of a 2-year survival after transplantation was 23% and 39% for patients with platinum-refractory and platinum-sensitive disease, respectively. The results from this study suggest better outcomes with autotransplantation than with conventional chemotherapy. However, there are inherent biases because of the relatively small numbers of patients studied in this trial that must be considered. Randomized trials are needed to fully understand the role of transplantation in patients with ovarian cancer.

A large, randomized Phase III trial (GOG 164) study comparing standard-dose chemotherapy to high-dose chemotherapy plus peripheral blood progenitor cell transplantation was recently closed in the United States because of slow accrual.[140] Currently, investigators in Europe are conducting randomized trials using high-dose chemotherapy and stem-cell transplantation. Until the results from this and other ongoing trials are available, the role of bone marrow or peripheral blood progenitor cell transplantation in the initial and subsequent treatment of advanced refractory ovarian cancer is unclear and should be considered an investigational approach.

BORDERLINE OVARIAN CANCER

Borderline (low malignant potential) ovarian cancers account for approximately 15% of all epithelial ovarian cancers; the majority (75%) are stage I at the time of diagnosis.[143] These tumors must be recognized, because their prognosis and treatment are clearly different from those of malignant invasive carcinomas. Trimble and Trimble reviewed 953 patients with a mean followup of 7 years and found a survival rate of 92% for advanced-stage tumors with the usual cause of death being benign disease complications (e.g., small-bowel obstruction) and therapy-related complications. Malignant transformation was rarely the cause of death. In one series, the 5-, 10-, 15-, and 20-year survival rates of patients with all stages of low malignant-potential tumors were 97%, 95%, 92%, and 89%, respectively.[143]

In patients with stage I or II disease, no additional chemotherapy or radiation treatment is indicated for a completely resected tumor of low malignant potential.[144,145] In the presence of bilateral ovarian cystic neoplasms or a single ovary involvement, partial oophorectomy, or a unilateral salpingo-oophorectomy can be performed if childbearing potential is to be maintained. When childbearing is not a consideration, a total abdominal hysterectomy and bilateral salpingo-oophorectomy is appropriate therapy because most clinicians favor removing the remaining ovarian tissue, which is at risk for recurrence of a borderline tumor or rarely developing invasive carcinoma.

Patients with advanced disease should undergo a total hysterectomy, bilateral salpingo-oophorectomy, omentectomy, node sampling, and aggressive cytoreductive surgery. However, there is little evidence that adjuvant chemotherapy or radiotherapy improves outcome.[143,145] There have been no controlled studies comparing postoperative treatment with no treatment.

NONEPITHELIAL OVARIAN CANCER

OVARIAN STROMAL TUMORS

Ovarian stromal tumors normally have an indolent natural history and rarely occur bilaterally. They are managed by unilateral salpingo-oophorectomy and usually do not require additional treatment.[3,12] Stage II stromal tumors require more extensive surgery owing to the lack of effective adjuvant therapy. Because this tumor is relatively rare, the role of chemotherapy is unclear.

OVARIAN GERM-CELL TUMORS

Ovarian-derived germ-cell tumors are rare and may have a mixed histology. Thus, treatment should be directed toward the most malignant component of the tumor. Surgery alone has not been very effective, producing 2-year survival rates of 13% to 16%.[146] Combination chemotherapy has produced high cure rates and improved prognosis in patients with germ-cell tumors.

Endodermal sinus and dysgerminoma are two subtypes of germ-cell tumors. Endodermal sinus tumors are aggressive tumors that usually occur unilaterally. Without chemotherapy, most patients die from their disease; thus, patients with all stages of disease should receive combination chemotherapy. The most common combination chemotherapeutic regimens used are vincristine, dactinomycin, and cyclophosphamide in combination, and cisplatin plus bleomycin in combination with vincristine or etoposide.[146] Dysgerminoma tumors have a high cure rate and are highly sensitive to radiation therapy; however, the sterility associated with abdominal irradiation has resulted in systemic chemotherapy becoming first-line therapy. The treatment of choice for newly diagnosed disease is a platinum-containing regimen.[146–148] The combination of bleomycin, etoposide, and cisplatin (BEP) demonstrated a 97% remission rate at 10 to 54 months in 35 patients with germ-cell tumors.[149] Also, two GOG trials demonstrated that 89 of 93 patients with stages I, II, and III disease and completely resected tumors were disease-free after three BEP cycles.[147–149] Patients with recurrent or refractory disease after cisplatin-based chemotherapy can be treated with radiation therapy.[146]

PHARMACOECONOMIC CONSIDERATIONS

The majority of economic analyses in ovarian cancer management have focused on the cost effectiveness of paclitaxel combinations as initial treatment regimens because the combination of paclitaxel and cisplatin has increased the median survival of newly diagnosed patients with advanced-stage disease compared to the combination of cisplatin and cyclophosphamide.[37] In the United States, incremental costs per life-year gained of $19,820 (inpatient) or $21,222 (outpatient)[150] and $19,603[151,152] have been calculated for patients treated with paclitaxel plus cisplatin compared to cyclophosphamide plus cisplatin. In comparison, the incremental costs per life-year gained of $20,355[153] and $32,213[154] have been reported for patients treated with paclitaxel plus cisplatin as compared to cyclophosphamide plus cisplatin in Canada. In addition, Messori et al. reported an $18,200 cost per quality-adjusted life-year gained.[151,152] The results of these studies suggest that the additional cost for the combination of paclitaxel and cisplatin compares favorably to costs for other medical interventions that are considered cost-effective. Cost considerations should be an important factor in the decision-making process of using a particular treatment strategy or deciding whether to pursue a "new" strategy in randomized trials.

EVALUATION OF TREATMENT OUTCOMES

When applied mainly to clinical trials, CR is defined as complete resolution of all disease and is further categorized either as a pathologic or clinical complete response.[3] A pathologic CR is defined as no detectable disease on second-look laparotomy. A clinical CR is defined as no detectable disease by radiologic imaging techniques. The recent NIH consensus conference on ovarian cancer concluded that second-look laparotomy should be performed only in clinical trials.[20] Partial response (PR) is defined as a greater than 50% decrease in all measurable disease. Stable disease is defined as disease maintenance without progression. In addition, general definitions for response duration and survival apply to ovarian cancer. Disease-free survival is defined from the point of achieving a complete response to the time of disease recurrence. Recent studies have evaluated percent CA-125 declines as a surrogate marker for response.[155,156]

Localized ovarian cancer is highly curable by surgery and, if appropriate, chemotherapy. The goals of therapy should be to maintain the patient's quality of life and, if possible and desired, to preserve reproductive capabilities. Newly diagnosed advanced ovarian cancer is highly responsive to surgical debulking and subsequent consolidative chemotherapy; however, cure rates are much lower than with localized disease. The goals of therapy in advanced ovarian carcinoma are to cure the disease, to extend disease-free survival, and to prolong overall survival. Patients with recurrent or refractory disease are generally not curable and have a poor long-term prognosis. Thus, the primary direction of therapy may be symptom management, quality of life maintenance, and treatment-related toxicity minimization.[156]

FUTURE DIRECTIONS

Although the number of women in the United States dying from ovarian cancer continues to increase, substantial treatment progress has been made. However, there are still several therapeutic questions that need to be asked and problems that need to be solved. New approaches to the treatment of advanced primary as well as recurrent and refractory ovarian cancer, such as agents to overcome resistance, should be studied. The optimum adjuvant and consolidation treatment modalities should be determined. The role of IP chemotherapy in all stages of disease is unclear, as is the most appropriate salvage therapy. Answering these therapeutic questions and solving these therapeutic problems may prolong the long-term survival in patients with local and advanced ovarian cancer.

▶ PRINCIPLES OF PHARMACOTHERAPY

- Ovarian cancer usually occurs in postmenopausal women in the sixth decade of life; the risk of developing ovarian cancer is increased in women with a family history involving two or more first-degree relatives.
- Patients with local disease have a 5-year survival rate greater than 90%; however, most patients present with disseminated disease, because symptoms do not appear until late in the disease course, and have a 5-year survival rate of 5% to 10%.
- CA-125 is an antigen common to most nonmucinous epithelial ovarian carcinoma and is a useful marker for ovarian cancer; rising or falling CA-125 titers correlate with the disease extent.
- Ovarian cancer management is based on the histologic type, pathologic grade, and disease stage at initial presentation. In general, the treatment of patients with ovarian cancer involves surgical debulking at the time of staging laparotomy and primary or adjuvant chemotherapy.
- The beneficial effects of adjuvant chemotherapy in the treatment of local disease depend on the stage and disease subtype. Postoperative adjuvant chemotherapy is not required in stage IA or IB grade 1, whereas patients with stage IA or IB grade 2 or 3, and stage IC do require adjuvant chemotherapy. All patients with stage II disease require adjuvant treatment. Paclitaxel plus

cisplatin or carboplatin for three to six cycles is the current recommended adjuvant therapy for these patients.

- Survival of patients with advanced ovarian cancer is a function of stage at initial diagnosis and the amount of residual after surgical debulking. Patients with stage III disease treated with optimal debulking (≤2 cm of residual tumor) have a 4-year survival rate of 30%, whereas patients with stage III or IV disease who have undergone suboptimal debulking (>2 cm of residual disease) have less than a 10% long-term survival.
- Current recommended treatment of advanced ovarian cancer (stage III or IV) is based on initial surgical debulking followed by paclitaxel plus carboplatin for six cycles.
- Approximately 20% to 50% of patients without evidence of disease on second-look laparotomy will relapse. In addition, patients who were initially sensitive to chemotherapy and whose response lasted the longest have the greatest likelihood of achieving a response to retreatment with the initial treatment regimen or treatment with salvage therapy.
- Patients with disease that is refractory to the initial platinum-containing chemotherapy or that recurs within 6 months after treatment (platinum-refractory) are unlikely to benefit from standard dose platinum therapy. However, patients who relapse more than 6 months after the initial platinum-containing regimen (platinum-sensitive) have a response rate of 27% to 59% with a standard-dose second-line platinum regimen.
- The NCCN guidelines recommend retreatment with either paclitaxel or platinum, or the combination of paclitaxel and a platinum compound if disease recurs more than 6 months after the initial treatment with paclitaxel in combination with a platinum analog. Treatment options for patients with refractory disease or disease recurrence within 6 months after treatment include topotecan, altretamine, oral etoposide, liposomal doxorubicin, gemcitabine, tamoxifen, referral for a clinical trial, or supportive care therapy.

REFERENCES

1. Greenlee RT, Hill-Harmon MB, Murray T, Thun M. Cancer statistics, 2001. CA Cancer J Clin 2001;51:15–36.
2. Holschneider CH and Berek JS. Ovarian cancer: Epidemiology, biology, and prognostic factors. Semin Surg Oncol 2000;19:3–10.
3. Cannistra SA. Cancer of the ovary [published erratum appears in N Engl J Med 1994;330:448]. N Engl J Med 1993;329:1550–1559.
4. Woutersz TB. Benefits of oral contraception: Thirty years' experience. Int J Fertil 1991;3:26–31.
5. Lynch HT, Watson P, Lynch JF, et al. Hereditary ovarian cancer: Heterogeneity in age at onset. Cancer 1993;71(suppl 2):573–581.
6. Lancaster JM, Wiseman RW. Recent advances in the molecular genetics of hereditary breast and ovarian cancer. Prog Clin Biol Res 1997;396: 31–51.
7. Lynch HT, Casey MJ, Lynch J, White T, Godwin AK. Genetics and ovarian carcinoma. Semin Oncol 1998;25(3):265–280.
8. Rubin SC, Benjamin I, Behbakht K. Clinical and pathological features in women with germ-line mutations of BRCA1. N Engl J Med 1996;335:1413–1416.
9. Eisinger F, Alby N, Bremond A, et al. Recommendations for medical management of hereditary breast and ovarian cancer: the French National Ad Hoc Committee. Ann Oncol 1998;9:939–950.
10. Burke W, Daly M, Garber J, et al. Recommendations for followup of individuals with an inherited predisposition to cancer, BRCA1 and BRCA2. Cancer genetics studies consortium. JAMA 1997;277:997–1003.
11. Narod SA, Goldgar D, Cannon-Albright L, et al. Risk modifiers in carriers of BRCA1 mutations. Int J Cancer 1995;64:394–398.
12. Ozols RF, Vermorken JB. Chemotherapy of advanced ovarian cancer: Current status and future directions. Semin Oncol 1997;24:S2-1–S2-9.
13. Hand R, Fremgen A, Chmiel JS, et al. Staging procedures, clinical management, and survival outcome for ovarian carcinoma. JAMA 1993;269:1119–1122.
14. Kenemans P, Yedema CA, Bon GG, von Mensdorff-Pouilly S. CA-125 in gynecologic oncology—A review. Eur J Obstet Gynecol Reprod Biol 1993;49:115–124.
15. Hempling RE. Tumor markers in epithelial ovarian cancer. Obstet Gynecol Clin North Am 1994;21:41–61.
16. Ozols RF, Schwartz PE, and Eifel PJ. Ovarian cancer, fallopian tube carcinoma, and peritoneal carcinoma. In: Devita VT, Hellman S, Rosenberg SA, eds. Cancer: Principles and Practice of Oncology, 6th ed. Philadelphia, Lippincott-Williams & Wilkins, 2001:1597–1632.
17. Mackey SE, Creasman WT. Ovarian cancer screening. J Clin Oncol 1995;13:783–793.
18. van Nagell JR, DePriest PD, Gallion HH, Pavlik EJ. Ovarian cancer screening. Cancer 1993;71:1523–1528.
19. Carlson KJ, Skates S, Singer DE. Screening for ovarian cancer. Ann Intern Med 1994;121:124–132.
20. NIH Consensus Conference. Ovarian cancer. Screening, treatment, and followup. NIH Consensus Development Panel on Ovarian Cancer [see comments]. JAMA 1995;273:491–497.
21. Nguyen HN, Averette HE, Hoskins W, et al. National survey of ovarian carcinoma. Part V. The impact of physician's specialty on patients' survival. Cancer 1993;72:3663–3670.
22. Boente MP, Yek K, Hogan VM, Ozols RF. Current status of staging laparotomy in colorectal and ovarian cancer. Cancer Treat Res 1996;82:337–357.
23. Young RC, Walton LA, Ellenberg SS, et al. Adjuvant therapy in stage I and stage II epithelial ovarian cancer: Result of two prospective randomized trials. N Engl J Med 1990;322:1021–1027.
24. Kawai M, Kikkawa F, Hattori S, et al. Long-term followup of patients with epithelial carcinoma of the ovary. Int J Gynaecol Obstet 1994;44:259–266.
25. Louie KG, Ozols RF, Myers CE, et al. Long-term results of a cisplatin-containing combination chemotherapy regimen for the treatment of advanced ovarian carcinoma. J Clin Oncol 1986;4:1579–1585.
26. Omura GA, Brady MF, Homesley HD, et al. Long-term followup and prognostic factor analysis in advanced ovarian carcinoma: The Gynecologic Oncology Group experience. J Clin Oncol 1991;9:1138–1150.
27. Hainsworth JD, Grosh WW, Burnett LS, et al. Advanced ovarian cancer: Long-term results of treatment with intensive cisplatin-based chemotherapy of brief duration. Ann Intern Med 1988;108:165–170.
28. Morgan RJ Jr, Copeland L, Gershenson D, et al. Update of the NCCN ovarian cancer practice guidelines. Oncology 1997;11:95–105.
29. Goodman HM, Harlow BL, Sheets EE, et al. The role of cytoreductive surgery in the management of stage IV epithelial ovarian carcinoma. Gynecol Oncol 1992;46:367–371.
30. Hoskins W, Rice L, Rubin S. Ovarian cancer surgical practice guidelines. Society of surgical oncology practice guidelines: Ovarian cancer. Oncology 1997;11:896–900, 903–904.
31. Miyazaki T, Tomoda Y, Ohta M, et al. Preservation of ovarian function and reproductive ability in patients with malignant ovarian tumors. Gynecol Oncol 1988;30:329–341.
32. Kolomainen DF, A'Hern R, Gore M. Can patients with relapsed previously untreated stage I epithelial ovarian cancer (EOC) be salvaged? Proc Am Soc Clin Oncol 2001;20:201a. Abstract.
33. Neijt JP, ten Bokkel Huinink WW, van der Burg ME, et al. Randomized trial comparing two combination chemotherapy regimens (CHAP-5 v CP) in advanced ovarian carcinoma. J Clin Oncol 1987;5: 1157–1168.
34. McGuire WP. Taxol: A new drug with significant activity as a salvage therapy in advanced epithelial ovarian carcinoma. Gynecol Oncol 1993;51:78–85.

35. Rowinsky EK, Donehower RC. Paclitaxel (Taxol) [published erratum appears in N Engl J Med 1995;333:75]. N Engl J Med 1995;332:1004–1014.
36. Kohler DR, Goldspiel BR. Paclitaxel (Taxol). Pharmacotherapy 1994; 14:3–34.
37. McGuire WP, Hoskins WJ, Brady MF, et al. Cyclophosphamide and cisplatin compared with paclitaxel and cisplatin in patients with stage III and stage IV ovarian cancer. N Engl J Med 1996;334:1–6.
38. Stuart G, Bertelsen K, Mangioni C, et al. Updated analysis shows a highly significant improved overall survival for cisplatin-paclitaxel as first line treatment of advanced ovarian cancer. Mature results of EORTC-GCCG, NOCOVA, NCIC, CTG and Scottish Intergroup trial. Proc Am Soc Clin Oncol 1999;17: 361a. Abstract.
39. Taylor AE, Wiltshaw E, Gore ME, Fryatt I, Fisher C. Long-term followup of the first randomized study of cisplatin versus carboplatin for advanced epithelial ovarian cancer. J Clin Oncol 1994;12:2066–2070.
40. Group AOCT. Chemotherapy in advanced ovarian cancer: An overview of randomized clinical trials. BMJ 1991;303:884–893.
41. Aabo K, Adams M, Adnitt P, et al. Chemotherapy in advanced ovarian cancer: Four systematic meta-analyses of individual patient data from 37 randomized trials. Br J Cancer 1998;78:1479–1487.
42. Go RS, Adjei AA. Review of the comparative pharmacology and clinical activity of cisplatin and carboplatin. J Clin Oncol 1999;17:409–422.
43. Alberts DS, Green S, Hannigan EV, et al. Improved therapeutic index of carboplatin plus cyclophosphamide versus cisplatin plus cyclophosphamide: Final report by the Southwest Oncology Group of a phase III randomized trial in stages III and IV ovarian cancer [published erratum appears in J Clin Oncol 1992;10:1505]. J Clin Oncol 1992;10:706–717.
44. Swenerton K, Jeffrey J, Stuart G, et al. Cisplatin-cyclophosphamide versus carboplatin-cyclophosphamide in advanced ovarian cancer: A randomized phase III study of the National Cancer Institute of Canada Clinical Trials Group. J Clin Oncol 1992;10:718–726.
45. Ozols RF. Carboplatin and paclitaxel in ovarian cancer. Semin Oncol 1995;22:78–83.
46. Ozols RF, Bundy RN, Fowler J, et al. Randomized phase III study of cisplatin/paclitaxel versus carboplatin/paclitaxel in optimal stage III epithelial ovarian cancer. Gynecologic Oncology Group Trial (GOG 158). Proc Am Soc Clin Oncol 1999:18:356a. Abstract.
47. du Bois A, Lueck HJ, Meier W, et al. Cisplatin/paclitaxel vs. carboplatin/paclitaxel in ovarian cancer: Update of an Arbeitsgemeinschaft Gynaekologische Onkologie (AGO) Study Group Trial. Proc Am Soc Clin Oncol 1999;18:356a. Abstract.
48. Neijt JP, Hansen M, Hansen SW, et al. Randomized phase III study in previously untreated epithelial ovarian cancer FIGO stage IIB, IIC, III, IV, comparing paclitaxel-cisplatin and paclitaxel-carboplatin. Proc Am Soc Clin Oncol 1997;16:352a. Abstract.
49. Ozols RF. Paclitaxel (Taxol)/carboplatin combination chemotherapy in the treatment of advanced ovarian cancer. Semin Oncol 2000;27(suppl 7): 3–7.
50. Ozols RF. Management of advanced ovarian cancer consensus summary. Semin Oncol 2000;27(suppl 7):47–49.
51. Vasey R. Preliminary results of the SCOTROC trial: A phase III comparison of paclitaxel-carboplatin (PC) and docetaxel-carboplatin (DC) as first-line chemotherapy for stage Ic-IV epithelial ovarian cancer (EOC). Proc Am Soc Clin Oncol 2001;20:202a. Abstract.
52. Segelov E, Stuart-Harris R, Bell D, et al. A phase II study of carboplatin and cisplatin in advanced ovarian cancer. Eur J Gynaecol Oncol 1994;15:277–282.
53. Levin L, Hryniuk WM. Dose intensity analysis of chemotherapy regimens in ovarian carcinoma. J Clin Oncol 1987;5:756–767.
54. McGuire WP, Hoskins WJ, Brady MF, et al. Assessment of dose-intensive therapy in suboptimally debulked ovarian cancer: A Gynecologic Oncology Group study. J Clin Oncol 1995;13:1589–1599.
55. Kaye SB, Paul J, Cassidy J, et al. Mature results of a randomized trial of two doses of cisplatin for the treatment of ovarian cancer. Scottish Gynecology Cancer Trials Group. J Clin Oncol 1996;14:2113–2119.
56. McGuire WP. How many more nails to seal the coffin of dose intensity? Ann Oncol 1997;8:311–313. Editorial.
57. Jakobsen A, Bertelsen K, Andersen JE, et al. Dose-effect study of carboplatin in ovarian cancer: A Danish Ovarian Cancer Group study. J Clin Oncol 1997;15:193–198.
58. Gore M, Mainwaring P, Macfarlane V, et al. Randomized trial of dose-intensity with single-agent carboplatin in patients with epithelial ovarian cancer. J Clin Oncol 1998;16:2426–2434.
59. Hakes TB, Chalas E, Hoskins WJ, et al. Randomized prospective trial of 5 versus 10 cycles of cyclophosphamide, doxorubicin, and cisplatin in advanced ovarian carcinoma. Gynecol Oncol 1992;45:284–289.
60. Hansen SW, Anderson H, Boman K, et al. Gemcitabine, carboplatin and paclitaxel (GCP) as first-line treatment of ovarian cancer FIGO stages IIB-IV. Proc Am Soc Clin Oncol 1999;18:357a. Abstract.
61. Hoskins P, Eisenhauer E, Fisher B, et al. Sequential couplets of cisplatin/topotecan and cisplatin/paclitaxel as first-line therapy for advanced epithelial ovarian cancer (EOC): An NCIC Clinical Trials Group Phase II study. Proc Am Soc Clin Oncol 1999;18:357a. Abstract.
62. Markman M. Weekly paclitaxel in the management of ovarian cancer. Semin Oncol 2000;27:37–40.
63. Dunton CJ. New options for the treatment of advanced ovarian cancer. Semin Oncol 1997;23:S5-2–S5-11.
64. ten Bokkel Huinink W, Gore M, Carmichael J, et al. Topotecan versus paclitaxel for the treatment of recurrent epithelial ovarian cancer [see comments]. J Clin Oncol 1997;15:2183–2193.
65. Swisher EM, Mutch DG, Rader JS, Elbendary A, Herzog TJ. Topotecan in platinum- and paclitaxel resistant ovarian cancer. Gynecol Oncol 1997;66:480–486.
66. Muggia FM, Hainsworth JD, Jeffers S, et al. Phase II study of liposomal doxorubicin in refractory ovarian cancer: Antitumor activity and toxicity modification by liposomal encapsulation. J Clin Oncol 1997;15:987–993.
67. Gordon AN, Granai CO, Rose PG, et al. Phase II study of liposomal doxorubicin in platinum- and paclitaxel refractory epithelial ovarian cancer. J Clin Oncol 2000;18:3093–3100.
68. Gordon AN, Fleagle JT, Guthrie D, et al. Recurrent epithelial ovarian carcinoma: A randomized phase III trial of pegylated liposomal doxorubicin versus topotecan. J Clin Oncol 2001;19:3312–3322.
69. Lund B, Hansen P, Theilade K, et al. Phase II study of gemcitabine (2′,2′-difluorodeoxycytidine in previously treated ovarian cancer patients. J Natl Cancer Inst 1994;6:1530–1533.
70. Shapiro JD, Millward MJ, Rischin D, et al. Activity of gemcitabine in patients with advanced ovarian cancer: Responses seen following platinum and paclitaxel. Gynecol Oncol 1996;63:89–93.
71. Friedlander M, Milward MJ, Bell D, et al. A phase II study of gemcitabine in platinum pre-treated patients with advanced epithelial ovarian cancer. Ann Oncol 1998;9:1343–1345.
72. Walton L, Ellenberg SS, Major F Jr, et al. Results of second-look laparotomy in patients with early stage ovarian carcinoma. Obstet Gynecol 1987;70:770–773.
73. Potter ME. Secondary cytoreduction in ovarian cancer: Pro or con? Gynecol Oncol 1993;51:131–135.
74. Schilder RJ, Boente MP, Corn BW, et al. The management of early ovarian cancer. Oncology (Huntingt) 1995;9:171–182; discussion 185–187.
75. van der Burg ME, van Lent M, Buyse M, et al. The effect of debulking surgery after induction chemotherapy on the prognosis in advanced epithelial ovarian cancer. Gynecological Cancer Cooperative Group of the European Organization for Research and Treatment of Cancer [see comments]. N Engl J Med 1995;332:629–634.
76. Hatch KD, Beecham JB, Blessing JA, Creasman WT. Responsiveness of patients with advanced ovarian carcinoma to tamoxifen. A Gynecologic Oncology Group study of second-line therapy in 105 patients. Cancer 1991;68:269–271.
77. Markman M, Rothman R, Hakes T, et al. Second-line platinum therapy in patients with ovarian cancer previously treated with cisplatin. J Clin Oncol 1991;9:389–393.
78. Seltzer V, Vogl S, Kaplan B. Recurrent ovarian carcinoma: retreatment utilizing combination chemotherapy including cis-diamminedichloroplatinum in patients previously responding to this agent. Gynecol 1989; 21:167–176.

79. Rose PG, Fusco N, Fluellen L, et al. Second-line therapy with Paclitaxel and carboplatin following recurrent disease following first-line therapy with paclitaxel and platinum in ovarian or peritoneal carcinoma. J Clin Oncol 1998;16:1494–1497.
80. Gershenson DM, Kavanagh JJ, Copeland LJ, et al. Retreatment of patients with recurrent epithelial ovarian cancer with cisplatin-based chemotherapy. Obstet Gynecol 1989;73:798–802.
81. Colombo N, Marzola M, Parma G, et al. Paclitaxel vs CAP in recurrent platinum sensitive ovarian cancer: a randomized Phase II study. Proc Am Soc Clin Oncol 1996;15:279. Abstract.
82. Belinson JL, Markman M, Webster KD, et al. Treatment of relapsed carcinoma of the ovary with single agent paclitaxel following exposure to paclitaxel and platinum employed as initial therapy. Proc Am Soc Clin Oncol 2000;19:392a. Abstract.
83. Rothenberg ML, Ozols RF, Glatstein E, et al. Dose-intensive induction therapy with cyclophosphamide, cisplatin, and consolidative abdominal radiation in advanced-stage epithelial ovarian cancer [see comments]. J Clin Oncol 1992;10:727–734.
84. Kemp G, Rose P, Lurain J, et al. Amifostine pretreatment for protection against cyclophosphamide-induced toxicities: Results of a randomized control trial in patients with advanced ovarian cancer. J Clin Oncol 1996;14:2101–2112.
85. Kavanagh J, Tresukosol D, Edwards C, et al. Carboplatin reinduction after taxane in patients with platinum-refractory epithelial ovarian cancer. J Clin Oncol 1995;13:1584–1588.
86. Eisenhauer EA, ten Bokkel Huinink WW, Swenerton KD, et al. European-Canadian randomized trial of paclitaxel in relapsed ovarian cancer: High-dose versus low-dose and long versus short infusion. J Clin Oncol 1994;12:2654–2666.
87. Kohn EC, Sarosy G, Bicher A, et al. Dose-intense Taxol: High response rate in patients with platinum-resistant recurrent ovarian cancer. J Natl Cancer Inst 1994;86:18–24.
88. Einzig AI. Review of phase II trials of Taxol (paclitaxel) in patients with advanced ovarian cancer. Ann Oncol 1994;5:S29–S32.
89. Fennelly D, Aghajanian C, Schapiro F, et al. Phase I and pharmacologic study of paclitaxel administered weekly in patients with relapsed ovarian cancer. J Clin Oncol 1997;51:187.
90. Abu-Rustum NR, Aghajanian C, Barakat RR, et al. Salvage weekly paclitaxel in recurrent ovarian cancer. Semin Oncol 1997;24:S15-62–S15-67.
91. Kavanagh JJ, Kudelka AP, Gonzalez de Leon C, et al. Phase II study of docetaxel in patients with epithelial ovarian carcinoma refractory to platinum. Clin Cancer Research 1996:2;837–842.
92. Piccart MJ, Gore M, Ten Bokkel Huinink W, et al. Docetaxel: An active new drug for treatment of advanced epithelial ovarian cancer. J Natl Cancer Inst 1995:87;676–681.
93. Francis P, Schneider J, Hann L, et al. Phase II trial of docetaxel in patients with platinum-refractory advanced ovarian cancer. J Clin Oncol 1994;12:2301–2308.
94. Kellard LR, Abel G. Comparative in vitro cytotoxicity of Taxol and Taxotere against cisplatin-sensitive and resistant human ovarian carcinoma cell lines. Cancer Chemother Pharmacol 1992;30:444–450.
95. Aapro M, Pujade-Lauraine E, Lhomme C, et al. Phase II study of Taxotere in ovarian cancer. Proc Am Soc Clin Oncol 1993;12;258. Abstract.
96. Markman M. Topotecan: An important new drug in the management of ovarian cancer. Semin Oncol 1997;24:S5–S11.
97. Creemers GJ, Bolis G, Gore M, et al. Topotecan, an active drug in the second-line treatment of epithelial ovarian cancer: Results of a large European phase II study [see comments]. J Clin Oncol 1996;14:3056–3061.
98. Stewart CF, Zamboni WC, Crom WR, et al. Topoisomerase I interactive drugs in children with cancer. Invest New Drugs 1996;14:37–47.
99. Ozols RF. The role of gemcitabine in the treatment of ovarian cancer. Semin Oncol 2000;27:40–47.
100. Trimble EL. Innovative therapies for advanced ovarian cancer. Semin Oncol 2000;27;24–30.
101. Bergman AM, Ruiz van Haperen VWT, Veerman G, et al. Synergistic interaction between cisplatin and gemcitabine *in vivo.* Clin Cancer Res 1996;2;521–530.
102. McGuire WP. Primary treatment of epithelial ovarian malignancies. Cancer 1993;71:1541–1550.
103. Lee CR, Faulds D. Altretamine. A review of its pharmacodynamic and pharmacokinetic properties, and therapeutic potential in cancer chemotherapy. Drugs 1995;49:932–953.
104. Manetta A, MacNeill C, Lyter JA, et al. Hexamethylmelamine as a single second-line agent in ovarian cancer. Gynecol Oncol 1990;36:93–96.
105. Rosen GF, Lurain JR, Newton M. Hexamethylmelamine in ovarian cancer after failure of cisplatin-based multiple-agent chemotherapy. Gynecol Oncol 1987;27:173–179.
106. Rose P, Blessing J, Mayer A, Homesley H. Prolonged oral etoposide as second-line therapy for platinum-resistant and platinum-sensitive ovarian carcinoma. A Gynecologic Oncology Group Study. J Clin Oncol 1998;16:405–410.
107. Gelmann EP. Tamoxifen for the treatment of malignancies other than breast and endometrial carcinoma. Semin Oncol 1997;24:S1-65–S1-70.
108. Bougnoux P, Dieras V, Petit T, et al. A multicenter phase II of oxaliplatin as a single agent in platinum and/or taxanes pretreated advanced ovarian cancer: Final results. Proc Am Soc Clin Oncol 1999;18:368. Abstract.
109. Chollet P, Bensmaine MA, Brienza S, et al. Single agent activity of oxaliplatin in heavily advanced epithelial ovarian cancer. Ann Oncol 1996;7:1065–1070.
110. Gurnani M, Lipari P, Dell J, et al. Adenovirus-mediated p53 gene therapy has greater efficacy when combined with chemotherapy against human head and neck, ovarian, prostate, and breast cancer. Cancer Chemother Pharmacol 199;44:143–151.
111. Song K, Cowan KH, Sinha BK. In vivo studies of adenovirus-mediated p53 gene therapy for cis-platinum-resistant human ovarian tumor xenografts. Oncol Res 1999;11:153–159.
112. Alvarez AA, Krigman HR, Whitaker RS, et al. The prognostic significance of angiogenesis in epithelial ovarian carcinoma. Clin Cancer Res 1999;5:587–591.
113. Chiara S, Conte P, Franzone P, et al. High-risk early-stage ovarian cancer. Randomized clinical trial comparing cisplatin plus cyclophosphamide versus whole abdominal radiotherapy. Am J Clin Oncol 1994;17:72–76.
114. Fyles AW, Dembo AJ, Bush RS, et al. Analysis of complications in patients treated with abdominopelvic radiation therapy for ovarian carcinoma. Int J Radiat Oncol Biol Phys 1992;22:847–851.
115. Soper JT, Berchuck A, Dodge R, Clarke-Pearson DL. Adjuvant therapy with intraperitoneal chromic phosphate (32P) in women with early ovarian carcinoma after comprehensive surgical staging. Obstet Gynecol 1992;79:993–997.
116. Vergotte IB, Vergote-De Vos LN, Abeler VM, et al. Randomized trial comparing cisplatin with radioactive phosphorus or whole-abdomen irradiation as adjuvant treatment of ovarian cancer. Cancer 1992;69:741–749.
117. Markman M. Intraperitoneal chemotherapy. Crit Rev Oncol Hematol 1999;31:239–246.
118. Vermorken JB. The role of intraperitoneal chemotherapy in epithelial ovarian cancer. Int J Gynecol Cancer 2000;10(suppl 1):26–32.
119. Markman M. Intraperitoneal therapy of ovarian cancer. Semin Oncol 1998;25:356–360.
120. Plaxe SC, Christen RD, O'Quigley J, et al. Phase I and pharmacokinetic study of IP topotecan. Invest New Drugs 1998;16:147–153.
121. Feun LG, Blessing JA, Major FR, et al. A Phase II study of intraperitoneal cisplatin and thiotepa in residual ovarian carcinoma: A gynecologic oncology group study. Gynecol Oncol 1998;71:410–415.
122. Morgan RJ, Braly P, Leong L, et al. Phase II trial of combination intraperitoneal cisplatin and 5-fluorouracil in previously treated patients with advanced ovarian cancer: Long-term follow-up. Gynecol Oncol 2000;77:433–438.
123. Casper ES, Kelsen DP, Alcock NW, et al. IP cisplatin in patients with malignant ascites: Pharmacokinetics evaluation and comparison with the IV route. Cancer Treat Rep 1983;67:325–328.
124. Elferink F, van der Viigh WJF, Klein I, et al. Pharmacokinetics of carboplatin after intraperitoneal administration. Cancer Chemother Pharmacol 1988;21:57–60.

125. Markman M, Francis P, Rowinsky E, Hoskins W. Intraperitoneal paclitaxel: A possible role in the management of ovarian cancer? Semin Oncol 1995;22:84–87.
126. Markman M, Francis P, Rowinsky E, et al. Intraperitoneal Taxol (paclitaxel) in the management of ovarian cancer. Ann Oncol 1994;5:S55–S58.
127. Alberts DS, Liu PY, Hannigan EV, et al. Intraperitoneal cisplatin plus intravenous cyclophosphamide versus intravenous cisplatin plus intravenous cyclophosphamide for stage III ovarian cancer. N Engl J Med 1996;335:1950–1955.
128. Kirmani S, Braly PS, McClay EF, et al. A comparison of intravenous versus intraperitoneal chemotherapy for the initial treatment of ovarian cancer. Gynecol Oncol 1994;54:338–344.
129. Markman M, Bundy B, Akberst DS, et al. Phase III trial of standard-dose of intravenous cisplatin plus paclitaxel versus moderately high-dose carboplatin followed by intravenous paclitaxel and intraperitoneal cisplatin in small-volume stage III ovarian carcinoma: An intergroup study of the Gynecologic Oncology Group, Southwestern Oncology Group and Eastern Cooperative Oncology Group. J Clin Oncol 2001;19:1001–1007.
130. Markman M, Reichman B, Hakes T, et al. Responses to second-line cisplatin-based intraperitoneal therapy in ovarian cancer: Influence of a prior response to intravenous cisplatin. J Clin Oncol 1991;9:1801–1805.
131. Piver MS, Recio FO, Baker TR, Driscoll D. Evaluation of survival after second-line intraperitoneal cisplatin-based chemotherapy for advanced ovarian cancer. Cancer 1994;73:1693–1698.
132. Los G, Mutsaers PH, Vijgh WJ. Direct diffusion of cis-diamminedichloroplatinum(II) in intraperitoneal rat tumors after intraperitoneal chemotherapy: A comparison with systemic chemotherapy. Cancer Res 1989;49:3380–3384.
133. Schneider JG. Intraperitoneal chemotherapy. Obstet Gynecol Clin North Am 1994;21:195–212.
134. Brandner P, Neis KJ. Use of an implantable catheter system for intraperitoneal chemotherapy in ovarian cancer. Artif Organs 1994;18:328–330.
135. Shpall EJ, Clarke-Pearson D, Soper JT, et al. High-dose alkylating agent chemotherapy with autologous bone marrow support in patients with stage III/IV epithelial ovarian cancer. Gynecol Oncol 1990;38:386–391.
136. Shpall EJ, Jones RB, Bearman S. High-dose therapy with autologous bone marrow transplantation for the treatment of solid tumors. Curr Opin Oncol 1994;6:135–138.
137. Mulder PO, Willemse PH, Aalders JG, et al. High-dose chemotherapy with autologous bone marrow transplantation in patients with refractory ovarian cancer. Eur J Cancer Clin Oncol 1989;25:645–649.
138. Legros M, Dauplat J, Fleury J, et al. High-dose chemotherapy with hematopoietic rescue in patients with stage III to IV ovarian cancer: Long-term results [see comments]. J Clin Oncol 1997;15:1302–1308.
139. Stiff PJ, Bayer R, Kerger C, et al. High-dose chemotherapy with autologous transplantation for persistent/relapsed ovarian cancer: A multivariate analysis of survival for 100 consecutively treated patients [see comments]. J Clin Oncol 1997;15:1309–1317.
140. McGuire WP. High-dose chemotherapeutic approaches to ovarian cancer. Semin Oncol 2000;27(suppl 7):41–46.
141. Herrin VE, Thigpen JT. High-dose chemotherapy in ovarian carcinoma. Semin Oncol 1999;26:99–105.
142. Stiff PJ, Veum-Stone J, Lazarus HM, et al. High-dose chemotherapy and autologous stem cell transplantation for ovarian cancer: An autologous blood and marrow transplant registry report. Ann Intern Med 2000;133:504–515.
143. Trimble CL, Trimble EL. Management of epithelial ovarian tumors of low malignant potential. Gynecol Oncol 1994;55:S52–S61.
144. Leake JF. Tumors of low malignant potential. Curr Opin Obstet Gynecol 1992;4:81–85.
145. Trope C, Kaern J, Vergote IB, Kristensen G, Abeler V. Are borderline tumors of the ovary over-treated both surgically and systemically? A review of four prospective randomized trials including 253 patients with borderline tumors. Gynecol Oncol 1993;51:236–243.
146. Williams SD. Chemotherapy of ovarian germ cell tumors. Hematol Oncol Clin North Am 1991;5:1261–1269.
147. Segelov E, Campbell J, Ng M, et al. Cisplatin-based chemotherapy for ovarian germ cell malignancies: The Australian experience. J Clin Oncol 1994;12:378–384.
148. Williams S, Blessing JA, Liao SY, Ball H, Hanjani P. Adjuvant therapy of ovarian germ cell tumors with cisplatin, etoposide, and bleomycin: A trial of the Gynecologic Oncology Group. J Clin Oncol 1994;12:701–706.
149. Gershenson DM. Update on malignant ovarian germ cell tumors. Cancer 1993;71:1581–1590.
150. McGuire W, Neugut AI, Arikian S, Doyle J, Dezii CM. Analysis of the cost-effectiveness of paclitaxel as alternative combination therapy for advanced ovarian cancer. J Clin Oncol 1997;15:640–645.
151. Messori A, Trippoli S, Becagli P, Tendi E. Pharmacoeconomic profile of paclitaxel as a first-line treatment for patients with advanced ovarian carcinoma. A lifetime cost-effectiveness analysis. Cancer 1996;78:2366–2373.
152. Messori A, Cecchi M, Becagli P, Trippoli S. Pharmacoeconomic profile of paclitaxel as a first-line treatment for patients with advanced ovarian carcinoma. A lifetime cost-effectiveness analysis. Cancer 1997;79:2264–2266. Letter.
153. Covens A, Boucher S, Roche K, et al. Is paclitaxel and cisplatin a cost-effective first-line therapy for advanced ovarian carcinoma? Cancer 1996;77:2086–2091.
154. Elit LM, Gafni A, Levine MN. Economic and policy implications of adopting paclitaxel as first-line therapy for advanced ovarian cancer: An Ontario perspective. J Clin Oncol 1997;15:632–639.
155. Rustin GJ, Nelstrop AE, McClean P, et al. Defining response of ovarian carcinoma to initial chemotherapy according to serum CA-125. J Clin Oncol 1996;14:1545–1551.
156. Montazeri A, McEwen J, Gillis CR. Quality of life in patients with ovarian cancer: Current state of research. Support Care Cancer 1996;4:169–179.

131
ACUTE LEUKEMIAS

Suzanne D. Day and David W. Henry

The leukemias are heterogeneous hematologic malignancies characterized by unregulated proliferation of the blood-forming cells of the bone marrow. These immature proliferating leukemia cells (blasts) physically "crowd out" or inhibit normal cellular maturation in bone marrow, resulting in anemia, granulocytopenia, and thrombocytopenia. Leukemic blasts may also leave the bone marrow and infiltrate a variety of tissues such as lymph nodes, skin, liver, spleen, kidney, and the central nervous system.

The term *leukemia* was coined by Virchow to describe the "white blood" of some patients that he saw under the microscope in 1845.[1] Historically, leukemia has been classified as acute or chronic based on differences in cell of origin and cell line maturation, patient life expectancy, clinical presentation, rapidity of progression of the untreated disease, and response to therapy. Using these categories, four major leukemias are recognized: acute lymphocytic (or lymphoblastic) leukemia (ALL), acute myeloid (or nonlymphocytic) leukemia (AML), chronic lymphocytic leukemia (CLL), and chronic myeloid leukemia (CML). Undifferentiated, immature cells that autonomously proliferate characterize acute leukemias. Chronic leukemias also autonomously proliferate, but the cells are more differentiated and mature.[1] Untreated, the acute leukemias are rapidly progressive, resulting in death in 2 to 3 months.

INCIDENCE AND EPIDEMIOLOGY

Approximately 13,500 new cases of acute leukemias—10,000 cases of AML and 3,500 cases of ALL—are diagnosed per year in the United States, accounting for less than 3% of the total cancer incidence. The incidence has been relatively stable for two decades. An estimated 8,600 deaths per year, and 1.6% of all cancer deaths, are caused by acute leukemias. The acute leukemias are an uncommon cause of cancer-related death after age 35 years, but they are the leading cause of cancer-related deaths in persons younger than age 35.[1,2] In adults, acute and chronic leukemias occur at equal rates. More than 90% of the cases of acute and chronic leukemia occur in adults. There are approximately 2.5 cases of AML and 1.3 cases of ALL per 100,000 individuals. The median age at diagnosis of patients with AML is 65 years while the median age for ALL patients is age 10 years.[1,2] The incidence of AML rises with age from 1 in 100,000 individuals younger than age 40 years to 15 per 100,000 older than age 75 years.[1] Acute leukemia is slightly more common in males than in females. In the United States, acute leukemia is more common among whites than among African Americans.[1,3]

Despite the low incidence rate, the acute leukemias are the most common malignancy in children younger than 15 years of age.[4–6] Of the 12,400 new cancer diagnoses in children each year, 2,400 of them are ALL.[4] AML accounts for 15% to 20% of all childhood leukemias, and the chronic leukemias account for less than 5%.[5] The annual incidence of childhood acute leukemias is 44 and 25 per million in white and African American children younger than 15 years of age, respectively. Childhood ALL has a slight male dominance and peaks at age 4 years.[6] AML in children has not displayed any gender or racial preference, and occurs throughout childhood without any peak age periods. Acute leukemia during the first 4 weeks of life (congenital leukemia) is usually AML.[6]

Chemotherapy has dramatically improved the outlook of patients with acute leukemia. Over 85% of children and young adults with acute leukemia achieve an initial complete remission from their disease. Overall, 65% to 85% of adults achieve an initial complete remission.[1,6] Long-term survival in children ranges from 30% to 90% depending on the type of leukemia and patient risk factors.[4] The prognosis of adult acute leukemia is generally worse than that of childhood leukemia, with only 20% to 40% of patients becoming long-term survivors.[1,6]

ETIOLOGY

The exact cause of the acute leukemias is unknown. A multifactorial process involving genetics, environmental factors, toxins, immunologic status, and viral exposures is likely. Table 131–1 summarizes the major factors that are linked to acute leukemias.[1,2,7,8] In pediatric ALL, a number of environmental factors have been investigated as possible causes: exposure to ionizing radiation, toxic chemicals, diagnostic radiography materials, herbicides and pesticides; maternal use of alcohol, contraceptives, diethylstilbestrol, or cigarettes; parental exposure to drugs or chemicals; and chemical contamination of groundwater.[6] Although there have been several reports of a possible link of electromagnetic fields of high-voltage power lines to the development of leukemia, a recent report by Linet and colleagues provides little evidence to support this association.[9] This study was a blinded comprehensive case-control study of 638 children with ALL and 620 controls. The magnetic field in each child's bedroom was measured and the distance from the home to any power lines was determined, but no correlation to the occurrence of childhood ALL could be made. In most patients who develop leukemia, a causative agent cannot be identified.

PATHOGENESIS

A basic understanding of normal hematopoiesis is needed before one can understand the pathogenesis of leukemia. The reader is referred to Chap. 98 for a detailed discussion of hematopoiesis. Normal hematopoiesis consists of multiple, well-orchestrated steps of cellular development. A pool of pluripotent stem cells undergoes differentiation, proliferation, and maturation, to form the mature blood cells seen in the peripheral circulation. These pluripotent stem cells initially differentiate to form two distinct stem cell pools. The myeloid stem cell gives rise to six types of blood cells (erythrocytes, platelets, monocytes, basophils, neutrophils, and eosinophils); while the lymphoid stem cell differentiates to form circulating B and T lymphocytes. Leukemia may develop at any stage and within any cell line.

TABLE 131–1. Conditions Associated With an Increased Frequency of Acute Leukemia

Drugs	Kostman's syndrome
Alkylating agents	Neurofibromatosis
Epipodophyllotoxins	**Chemical**
Genetic Conditions	Benzene
Down's syndrome	**Radiation**
Bloom's syndrome	Ionizing radiation
Fanconi's anemia	**Virus**
Kleinfelter's syndrome	HTLV-1 and HTLV-2
Ataxia telangiectasia	**Social Habits**
Langerhans' cell histiocytosis	Cigarette smoking
Schwachman's syndrome	Maternal marijuana use
Severe combined immunodeficiency	Maternal ethanol use

Figure 131–1 illustrates sites in the development of blood cells at which leukemias arise.

Two features are common to both AML and ALL: First, both arise from a single leukemic cell that proliferates (monoclonality). Second, there is a failure to maintain a relative balance between proliferation and differentiation, so that the cells do not differentiate past a particular stage of hematopoiesis. Cells (lymphoblasts or myeloblasts) then proliferate uncontrollably. Proliferation and differentiation are under genetic control, and when the balance between the two is altered in favor of proliferation, leukemia occurs. New antileukemia drug therapies are being developed that are specifically targeted to the biologic processes involved in proliferation and differentiation.[1]

AML probably arises from a defect in the pluripotent stem cell or a more committed myeloid precursor resulting in partial differentiation and proliferation of immature precursors of the myeloid blood-forming cells. In older patients, trilineage leukemic involvement is seen because the cell of origin is probably a very early stem cell. In younger patients, a more differentiated stem cell becomes malignant, allowing maturation of some granulocytic and erythroid populations. These two forms of AML exhibit different patterns of resistance to chemotherapy, with resistance more evident in the elderly population of AML.[10] The French–American–British (FAB) classification system outlined in Table 131–2 identifies nine different morphologic subtypes of AML. As an example, in acute promyelocytic leukemia (APL, M3 FAB classification), the leukemia cells mature and differentiate up to the stage of the promyelocyte, but no further. They then proliferate as promyelocytes without differentiation or maturation into mature neutrophils.

ALL is a disease characterized by proliferation of immature lymphoblasts. In this type of acute leukemia, the defect is probably at the level of the lymphopoietic stem cell or at the level of a very early lymphoid precursor.[1,6] Markers on the cell surface or membrane of the lymphoblast can be used to classify ALL (Table 131–3). Advances in the use of monoclonal antibodies for surface markers led to the recognition of subclasses of B- and T-cell lineages.[4] ALL may also be described by cytogenetic abnormalities. Chromosomes may be too many (hyperploidy) or too few (hypoploidy) or exhibit specific translocations.[4,6]

Leukemic cells have a growth advantage over normal cells, leading to a "crowding out" phenomenon in the bone marrow. This growth advantage is not caused by more rapid proliferation as compared with normal cells, but is probably caused by a factor produced by leukemic cells that inhibits normal cellular proliferation and differentiation, or to a lower rate of leukemic cell loss as compared with normal blood cells (loss of programmed cell death).[10]

The types of genetic alterations that lead to leukemia have only recently become evident. The genetic defects may include (a) activation of a normally suppressed gene (protooncogene) to create an oncogene which produces a protein product that signals increased proliferation; (b) loss of signals for the blood cell to differentiate; (c) loss of tumor-suppressor genes that control normal proliferation; and (d) loss of signals for programmed cell death (apoptosis). Most normal cells are programmed to die eventually through apoptosis, but in cancer cells, the appropriate programmed signal is often interrupted, leading to continued survival, replication, and drug resistance. Signal transduction, RNA transcription, cell-cycle control factors, cell differentiation, and programmed cell death may all be affected.

One example of a genetic defect leading to acute leukemia is abnormal activation of the *ras* gene.[11] These genes produce G proteins (guanine nucleotide-binding proteins) that couple activation of outer

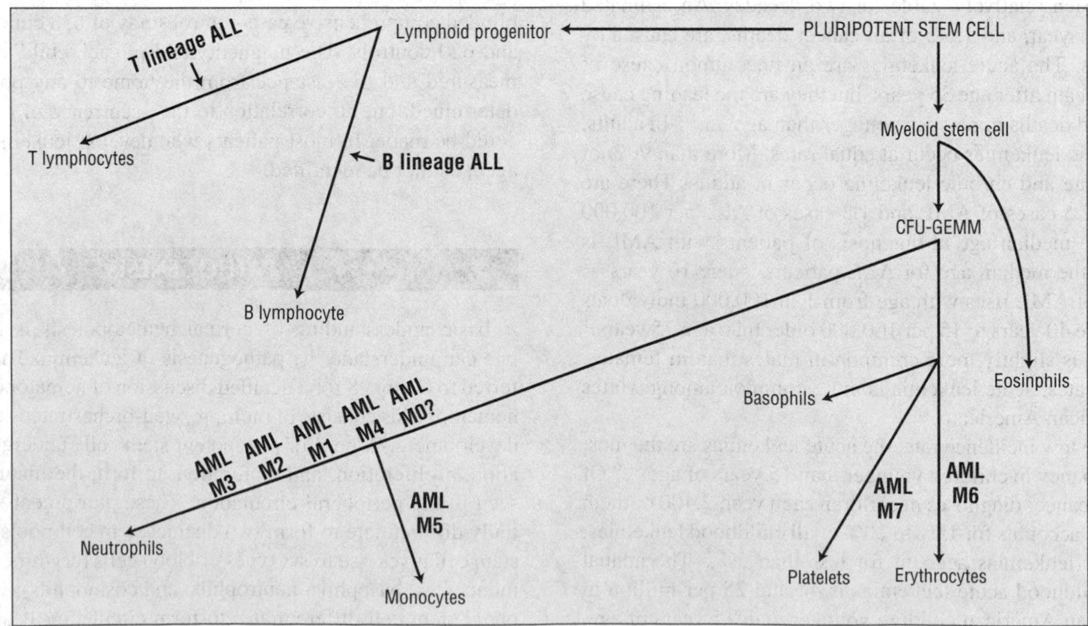

FIGURE 131–1. Simplified schema of blood cell development and approximate level of differentiation for the acute leukemias.

TABLE 131–2. Morphologic (FAB) Classification of Acute Nonlymphocytic Leukemia

		Frequency of FAB Subtype[a]		
	Subtype	*Adults (%)*	*Children <2 yr (%)*	*Children >2 yr (%)*
M_0	Acute myeloblastic leukemia undifferentiated	low	low	low
M_1	Acute myeloblastic leukemia with minimal differentiation	15	17	25
M_2	Acute myeloblastic leukemia with maturation	25		27
M_3	Acute promyelocytic leukemia	10		5
M_4	Acute myelomonocytic leukemia	25	30	26
M_{5a}	Acute monoblastic leukemia without differentiation	5	52	16
M_{5b}	Acute monoblastic leukemia with differentiation	5		
M_6	Acute erythroleukemia	5		2
M_7	Megakaryocytic leukemia	10		5–7

FAB = French–American–British.
[a]Percentages should be compared vertically and not horizontally.
Adapted from Refs. 1 and 7.

cell membrane receptors to activation of signal transduction. The abnormal activation of these signal transduction pathways can lead to increased cell proliferation. Point mutations in the *ras* gene lead to unregulated proliferation and differentiation. Defects in this gene are present in 25% to 44% of AML patients, and in 6% to 18% of ALL patients. Disruption of *ras* signaling may lead to clinically useful therapies. The investigational agents called farnesyl transferase inhibitors block an early part of the *ras* pathway, and are undergoing evaluation in various types of cancer, including leukemias.

Another example of a genetic cause of leukemia is the loss or mutation of genes that suppress cancer development. These genes are referred to as tumor suppressor genes. The tumor suppressor gene *p53* is found in some hematologic malignancies. Alterations in *p53* are found in 5% to 10% of AML patients, and in 3% of childhood ALL patients.[10] Leukemia cells from patients with relapsed T-cell ALL have a mutant *p53* frequency of 50%.[6] Normal *p53* allows cells to stop in the G_1 phase of the cell cycle to repair damaged DNA. Mutant *p53* does not stop the cells in G_1, but allows cells to proliferate without DNA repair, ultimately accumulating chromosomal aberrations that cause cancer. Mutant *p53* also impairs apoptosis, resulting in drug resistance. The net effect of these genetic changes is to give either the leukemia cell a proliferative advantage over normal hematopoietic cells or to prevent normal differentiation and cell death of the leukemia cell.[12] Certain antileukemia drugs such as doxorubicin may induce normal *p53* production.[13]

TABLE 131–3. Morphologic (FAB) Classification and Immunophenotypes of Acute Lymphocytic Leukemia

		Frequency of FAB Subtype[a]	
Subtype	Cells of Origin	*Adults (%)*	*Children (%)*
L_1	Early pre-B cell Pre-B cell B cell T cell	30	85
L_2	Early pre-B cell Pre-B cell B cell T cell	65	14
L_3	B cell	5	1

FAB = French–American–British.
[a]Percentages should be compared vertically and not horizontally.
Adapted from Refs. 1 and 6.

A long list of molecular abnormalities involved in leukemic cells was recently compiled.[16] The exact mechanisms for most of these abnormalities are not fully understood, but there has been much progress in understanding the biology of cancer in recent years.[14,15]

CLINICAL PRESENTATION

SIGNS AND SYMPTOMS

The signs and symptoms of acute leukemia are nonspecific and can be attributed to replacement of normal functional blood cells with immature dysfunctional leukemic cells and to leukemic infiltration of a specific organ or site.[1] In general, signs and symptoms of acute leukemia are indistinguishable between AML and ALL at presentation. Diagnosis requires a combination of history of illness, physical exam, and laboratory evaluation.

Commonly patients present with a 1- to 3-month history of symptoms. Anemia often manifests as fatigue, malaise, and pallor. Less commonly, palpitations or dyspnea on exertion may be noted. Granulocytopenia may present as fever with or without frank infection. Thrombocytopenia may manifest as simple petechiae or frank bleeding or bruising, often involving the gums, skin, or gastrointestinal tract. Menorrhagia may be seen in premenopausal women. As leukemic infiltrates may involve any organ, unusual presenting symptoms such as gum hypertrophy, loss of vision, the presence of an abnormal mass, or bone pain may also be observed. Leukemic meningitis occurs at presentation in less than 5% of patients. With meningeal involvement, seizures, headache, diplopia, nausea, or vomiting may be reported or the patient may be asymptomatic. As is frequently seen with many types of cancer, mild weight loss may be present. Approximately 10% of cases of acute leukemia can be diagnosed by routine blood analysis without any significant history of physical findings.[1,3]

PHYSICAL AND LABORATORY FINDINGS

Physical findings are compatible with anemia (pallor, tachycardia, cardiac murmurs); granulocytopenia (infection, fever with or without sepsis); thrombocytopenia (bruising, frank bleeding, petechiae, ecchymoses, purpura, menorrhagia); and leukemic infiltration (lymphadenopathy, splenomegaly, hepatomegaly, sternal tenderness). Petechiae and ecchymoses are more common in AML. Bone pain, hepatomegaly, and splenomegaly are more common in ALL. Lymphadenopathy is rare in AML but is common in ALL. Although infrequent at presentation, neurologic signs and symptoms are most often associated with ALL and include cranial palsies or neuropathies, nausea/vomiting, and headache. Other physical findings related to leukemia cell infiltration include gingival hypertrophy and skin manifestations. Skin or soft-tissue infiltration by myeloid leukemia creates a chloroma, so named because intracellular enzymes create a greenish discoloration similar to chlorophyll.[1–3]

At diagnosis, laboratory evaluations reveal a normocytic, normochromic anemia with decreased reticulocytes nearly always present because of decreased red blood cell production.[3] Severe thrombocytopenia (platelet counts <50,000/μL) is present at diagnosis in more than one-half of patients. The white blood cell (WBC) count is greatly elevated (>100,000/μL) in 20% of cases and reduced (<5,000/μL) in another 20% of cases.[3,6] Hyperleukocytosis can be life-threatening and require emergent leukapheresis, especially in AML, because blasts can occlude small vessels in the brain, heart, lungs, or elsewhere.[3] A high white blood cell count is often associated with T-cell ALL and acute monocytic leukemia.[1,3] The peripheral blood smear usually demonstrates a decrease in normal granulocytes, with an increase in blasts.[1,3]

Serum uric acid is mildly elevated in approximately one-half of patients with adult leukemia caused by presence of rapid cell kill and tumor lysis syndrome at presentation. Additionally patients may present with associated hyperkalemia, hyperphosphatemia, and hypocalcemia.[1,3] Occasionally, patients may present with renal failure secondary to uric acid nephropathy. Hypercalcemia can also occur and is often caused by ectopic parathyroid hormone production by leukemic cells, or rapid destruction of large numbers of leukemic cells.

APL, or AML-M_3, is characterized by many of the same signs and symptoms as other types of AML. One important difference is the propensity of APL to cause disseminated intravascular coagulation. This syndrome is characterized by thrombocytopenia, hypofibrinogenemia, depletion of clotting factors resulting in prolonged prothrombin and partial thromboplastin times, and a bleeding diathesis. These specific laboratory values and physical findings are helpful to identify this subtype of AML so that appropriate therapy may be instituted (discussed later in the chapter).

Initial and serial bone marrow aspirates and biopsies are necessary to establish a diagnosis and to follow disease progression and response to therapy. Critical evaluations of the marrow include morphologic examination, cytochemical staining, immunophenotyping, and cytogenetic, or chromosomal, analysis. At diagnosis, the marrow is usually hypercellular with a predominance of blasts. Leukemia is diagnosed if more than 30% of the marrow cells are blasts. If the percentage is below 5%, then the marrow is considered normal. If the marrow has between 5% and 30% leukemic blasts, the term *myelodysplastic syndrome* is used. This condition is considered a preleukemic state that will eventually evolve into frank AML.[3] Cytochemical stains are often beneficial in helping to determine if the acute leukemia is of myeloid or lymphoid lineage. Immunophenotyping involves the analysis of 160 antigen groups, known as clusters of differentiation, present on the surface of hematopoietic cells. While no leukemia-specific antigens have been identified, absence or presence of certain antigen groups distinguish lymphoid or myeloid lineage of the leukemia.[1] Cytogenetic analysis of the marrow to determine the presence of nonrandom chromosomal abnormalities, oncogene mutations, and tumor-suppressor genes in leukemic cells are also helpful for diagnosis, establishing prognosis, and evaluating response to therapy. Identifying chromosomal translocations is important because they have been linked to rearrangement and altered regulation of cellular oncogenes.[6] Unique translocations often identify the type of acute leukemia. For example, APL is characterized by the translocation of chromosomes 15 and 17, t(15;17). Recently, technically difficult cytogenetic analysis has been supplemented with fluorescent *in situ* hybridization (FISH) that allows for quick, sensitive analysis of samples that might be inadequate for karyotyping.[16] FISH is a process in which specific genes in an intact cell are visualized using fluorescent-labeled probes.

RISK FACTORS

Many clinical and laboratory features at diagnosis are associated with response to treatment. Identification of these risk factors may allow the oncologist to better understand the disease and to tailor treatment according to the predicted response. Such factors aid in identifying patients most likely to attain a complete remission, to maintain that remission, and to experience long-term survival. For example, if a patient has many clinical and laboratory features that are associated with a good response to chemotherapy ("good risk"), then the oncologist may choose to give less-intensive therapy to reduce the risk of long-term toxic effects. Conversely, if a patient is unlikely to respond well to therapy ("high risk" or "poor risk"), then the oncologist may choose to give more intensive chemotherapy.

In both adults and children with ALL, recent studies have identified several risk factors that correlate with prognosis (Table 131–4). Poor prognostic factors primarily involve high WBC at presentation, very young or old age at presentation, delayed remission induction, male sex, and the presence of specific chromosomal cytogenetic abnormalities.[17] As most patients with ALL achieve a complete clinical remission, these factors refer to the risk of leukemic relapse rather than the risk of not achieving a complete remission. It was once thought that the presence of any chromosomal translocation in the leukemic cells was an adverse prognostic factor. A study of 139 children with ALL revealed that the outcome for patients with a chromosomal translocation is not inferior to the group lacking a translocation.[18] The more important consideration is the specific rearrangement. Several specific chromosomal translocations have been identified and are now being routinely used in risk assessment and, subsequently, to direct therapy (Table 131–4).

Adult patients generally have a poorer prognosis than children due to disease biology and treatment tolerance. Adults typically have more cytogenetic abnormalities, particularly the presence of the Philadelphia chromosome or t(9;22), which confer higher risk disease. Other poor prognostic factors more common in adults include an increased incidence of expression of myeloid antigens, less frequent pre-B immunophenotype, increased incidence of chemotherapy

TABLE 131–4. Prognostic Factors in ALL Risk for Leukemia Relapse

Factor	Low	High
Morphology	L1	L2, L3
Immunologic phenotype	Early pre-B cell	Null cell, T cell, pre-B cell, B cell
WBC at diagnosis	<10,000/μL	>50,000/μL
Platelets	>100,000/μL	<30,000/μL
Patient age	3–7 years	<1 year or >10 years
Cytogenetics	Normal karyotype	t(9;22); t(4;11); −7; +8
Myeloid markers	Absent	Present
CNS leukemia	Absent	Present
Node/liver/spleen enlargement	Absent	Massive
Mediastinal mass	Absent	Present
Time to remission	<4 weeks	>4 weeks

resistance, slower response to chemotherapy, increased incidence of high WBC at presentation, and increased frequency of a mediastinal mass or extramedullary involvement.

To create a standard of comparison, a definition of "standard risk" ALL was developed: patients aged 1 to 9 with a presenting WBC count of 50,000/μL^3 or less.[19] The risk category of a patient may be modified by consideration of additional prognostic factors including DNA index (ratio of leukemia cell to normal cell DNA concentrations), cytogenetics, early response to treatment, immunophenotype, and central nervous system (CNS) involvement.[19]

Prognostic factors in adult AML were recently defined. The most important patient factor is age, with younger patients more likely to achieve a complete remission than older patients (older than age 70).[1,3] The lower complete remission rate in older patients appears to result from increased frequency of fatal infectious and bleeding complications as well as chemotherapy resistance.[3] The duration of remission is also shorter in older patients as compared to younger patients. Other patient-specific prognostic factors include concurrent infection and any major organ impairment.[3] FAB morphologic subtype may be a factor, with types M_0, M_5, M_6, and M_7 having the worst outcome.[1,3] Patients with extramedullary disease, CNS involvement, or underlying myelodysplastic syndrome have a worse prognosis.[1,3] Certain cytogenetic abnormalities are also known to worsen the response rate and survival of patients with AML (Table 131–5).[1,6,16] In addition, patients who develop a "secondary" leukemia after treatment of another malignancy usually have a very poor response to antileukemic chemotherapy.[1]

TABLE 131–5. Prognostic Factors for AML

Characteristic	Prognosis
Older age	Poor
Antecedent hematologic disorder	Poor
Secondary leukemia	Poor
Cytogenetics:	
Abnormalities of chromosome 5 or 7	Poor
Trisomy 8	Poor
t(9;11)	Poor
t(15;17)	Favorable
t(8;21)	Favorable
Inv(16)	Favorable

Adapted from Scheinberg DA, Maslak P, Weiss M. Acute leukemias In: DeVita VT, Hellman S, Rosenberg SA, eds. Cancer: Principles and Practice of Oncology, 6th ed. Philadelphia, Lippincott Williams & Wilkins, 2001:2404–2433.

Prognostic factors associated with pediatric AML have been reported; although few factors are consistently identified and predictive of outcome from therapy. Factors that reduce the chances of a complete remission include an initial WBC count greater than 100,000/μL, FAB classification M_1 without Auer rods present, certain chromosome abnormalities (Table 131–5), AML evolving from myelodysplastic syndrome, and having AML secondary to prior chemotherapy or radiation therapy.[7] Remission duration may be influenced negatively by the same factors as well as age <2 years and having FAB classifications M_4 or M_5.[7]

▶ TREATMENT: Acute Leukemia

DESIRED OUTCOME

The short-term goal of treatment for acute leukemia is to rapidly achieve a complete clinical and hematologic remission. In the absence of a complete remission, a rapid and fatal outcome is inevitable. Complete remission is defined as the disappearance of all clinical and bone marrow evidence (normal cellularity with less than 5% blasts) of leukemia, with restoration of normal hematopoiesis. Partial remission is a significant response to treatment, although evidence of residual disease (5% to 25% blasts) in the bone marrow remains.

After a complete remission is achieved, the goal is to maintain the patient in continuous complete remission. As discussed later, the occurrence of leukemic relapse in the bone marrow significantly reduces the likelihood of curing the disease. Most patients who will die from acute leukemia die within the first 6 years; the survival curve (percentage alive vs time) beyond the sixth year after therapy does not continue to decline as rapidly.[1] When the survival curve achieves a plateau, the patients still alive are likely to be cured.

TREATMENT OF ACUTE LYMPHOBLASTIC LEUKEMIA

Successful treatment in ALL was first developed in children. Current regimens induce remission in greater than 95% of children with ALL. Cure rates in children have risen from approximately 10% with treatments used in the 1960s to approximately 80% in the 1990s.[4] Although treatment results with adult ALL are worse than those with childhood ALL, recent use of aggressive chemotherapy in adult ALL has increased the complete remission rate to 70% to 85%. The proportion of 5-year disease-free survivors is approximately 35% to 50%, with the higher rates in younger adults receiving allogeneic stem-cell transplants.[1,20] In adults, T-cell ALL and mature B-cell ALL have 5-year disease-free survival rates of approximately 50%.[20]

Therapy for ALL has historically been divided into four phases: (a) remission induction; (b) central nervous system prophylaxis; (c) consolidation therapy; and (d) maintenance therapy (Fig. 131–2). Recently, more complex regimens have been explored, and the lines between phases of therapy are less clear. All patients still receive some form of initial induction therapy to yield a complete remission. Some form of postremission therapy is needed to treat microscopic disease and may include some intensive inpatient therapy (consolidation or intensification therapy) followed by less aggressive outpatient therapy (maintenance or continuation). Central nervous system prophylaxis is needed at some time during therapy in all ALL patients to prevent leukemic meningitis. Tables 131–6 and 131–7 illustrate several representative treatment regimens for adult and pediatric ALL.

REMISSION INDUCTION

The goal of remission induction is to rapidly induce a complete clinical and hematologic remission. The combination of vincristine and prednisone induces complete remission in about 50% of adults and 85% of children with ALL.[1,6] The addition of an anthracycline (daunorubicin or doxorubicin) to vincristine and prednisone in adults increases the complete remission rate to 83% and carries a treatment-related mortality rate of only 3% to 17%.[1,25] The addition of an anthracycline or L-asparaginase in children increases the complete remission rate to >95% and prolongs the duration of remission.[6] The addition of a

TABLE 131–6. Representative Chemotherapy Regimens for Adult Acute Lymphocytic Leukemia

Remission Induction		CNS Prophylaxis		Consolidation		Maintenance
Drug and Dose	*Days*	*Prophylaxis*	*Days*	*Drug and Dose*	*Days*	*Drug, Dose, and Timing*
German or Hoelzer Regimen (Adult)[21]						
PRED (PO) 60 mg/m^2	1–28	Cranial irradiation		DEX (PO) 10 mg/m^2	1–28	MP (PO) 60 mg/m^2 qd
VCR (IV) 1.5 mg/m^2[a]	1, 8, 15, 22	MTX (IT) 10 mg/m^2[b]	31, 38, 45, 52	VCR (IV) 1.5 mg/m^2[a]	1, 8, 15, 22	and
DNR (IV) 25 mg/m^2	1, 8, 15, 22			DOX (IV) 25 mg/m^2	1, 8, 15, 22	MTX (PO/IV) 20 mg/m^2
ASP (IV) 5,000 U/m^2	1–14					weekly, weeks 10–18
						and 29–130
CTX (IV) 650 mg/m^2[c]	29, 43, 57			CTX (IV) 650 mg/m^2[c]	29	
Ara-C (IV) 75 mg/m^2	31–34, 38–41, 45–48, 52–55			Ara-C (IV) 75 mg/m^2	31–34, 38–41	
				TG (PO) 60 mg/m^2	29–42	
MP (PO) 60 mg/m^2	29–57					
CALGB 8811 (Adult)[22]						
Course I				**Course II: Early Intensification**		**Course V**
CTX (IV) 1,200 mg/m^2	1			MTX (IT) 15 mg	1	VCR (IV) 2 mg
DNR (IV) 45 mg/m^2	1, 2, 3			CTX (IV) 1,000 mg/m^2	1	day 1 monthly
VCR (IV) 2 mg	1, 8, 15, 22			MP (PO) 60 mg/m^2	1–14	PRED (PO) 60 mg/m^2
PRED (PO) 60 mg/m^2	1–21			Ara-C (SQ) 75 mg/m^2	1–4, 8–11	days 1–5 monthly
ASP (SC) 6,000 U/m^2	5, 8, 11, 15, 18, 22			VCR (IV) 2 mg	15, 22	MTX (PO) 20 mg/m^2 days
				ASP (SQ) 6,000 U/m^2	15, 18, 22, 25	1, 8, 15, 22 monthly
						MP (PO) 60 mg/m^2
						days 1–28 monthly
Induction chemotherapy for patients ≥60 yr old, use:						
CTX (IV) 800 mg/m^2	1					
DNR (IV) 30 mg/m^2	1–3					
PRED (PO) 60 mg/m^2	1–7					
		Course III		**Course IV: Late Intensification**		
		Cranial irradiation		DOX (IV) 30 mg/m^2	1, 8, 15	
		MTX (IT) 15 mg	1, 8, 15, 22, 29	VCR (IV) 2 mg	1, 8, 15	
		MP (PO) 60 mg/m^2	1–70	DEX (PO) 10 mg/m^2	1–14	
		MTX (PO) 20 mg/m^2	36, 43, 50, 57, 64	CTX (IV) 1,000 mg/m^2	29	
				TG (PO) 60 mg/m^2	29–42	
				Ara-C (SQ) 75 mg/m^2	29–32, 36–39	

Ara-C, cytarabine; ASP, asparaginase; CALGB, Cancer and Leukemia Group B; CNS, central nervous system; CTX, cyclophosphamide; DEX, dexamethasone; DNR, daunorubicin; DOX, doxorubicin; MP, mercaptopurine; MTX, methotrexate; PRED, prednisone; TG, thioguanine; VCR, vincristine.

[a]Maximum single dose, 2 mg.

[b]Maximum single dose, 15 mg.

[c]Maximum single dose, 1,000 mg.

TABLE 131–7. Representative Chemotherapy Regimens for Pediatric Acute Lymphocytic Leukemia

Remission Induction			Consolidation		Maintenance
Drug and Dose	*Timing*	*CNS Prophylaxis*	*Drug and Dose*	*Days*	*Drug, Dose, and Timing*
Children's Cancer Group 1882 (Pediatric)[23]					
			Consolidation I		**Interim Maintenance**
PRED (PO) 60 mg/m²/day	28 d	Cranial irradiation	CTX (IV) 1 g/m²	0, 28	VCR (IV) 1.5 mg/m², days 0, 10, 20, 30, 40
VCR (IV) 1.5 mg/m²/wk	4 wk	MTX (IT) throughout protocol			
DNR (IV) 25 mg/m²/wk	4 wk		Ara-C (SQ/IV) 75 mg/m²	1–4, 8–11, 29–32, 36–39	MTX (IV) 100 mg/m², days 0, 10, 20, 30, 40
ASP (IM) 6000 U/m²	3x weekly 9 doses		MP 60 mg/m² PO	0–13, 28–41	ASP (IM) 15,000 U/m², days 1, 11, 21, 31, 41
			VCR 1.5 mg/m²	14, 21, 42, 49	
			ASP (IM) 6000 U/m²	14, 16, 18, 21, 23, 25, 42, 44, 46, 49, 51, 53	
			Reinduction–Reconsolidation I, II		**Maintenance (3-month cycles)**
			VCR 1.5 mg/m²	0, 7, 14, 42, 49	VCR (IV) 1.5 mg/m², days 0, 28, 56
			DEX 10 mg/m² PO qd	0–20, then taper	PDN 60 mg/m², days 0–4, 28–32, 56–60
			DOX 25 mg/m²	0, 7, 14	MP 75 mg/m², days 0–83
			ASP (IM) 6000 U/m²	3, 5, 7, 10, 12, 14, 42, 44, 46, 49, 51, 53	MTX 20 mg/m², PO, days 7, 14, 21, 28, 35, 42, 49, 56, 63, 70, 77
			CTX (IV) 1 g/m²	28	
			Ara-C (SC/IV) 75 mg/m²/day	29–32, 36–39	
			TG (PO) 60 mg/m²/day	28–41	
POG 9904 (Pediatric)[24]					**Overlapping VCR/DEX Pulse Therapy**
PRED (PO) 40 mg/m² (Maximum dose 60 mg/day)	1–29	MTX (IT), throughout protocol	MTX (IV) 1 g/m² (with leucovorin rescue)	44, 65, 86, 107, 128, 149	Weeks 8, 17, 25, 41, 57, 73, 89, 105: VCR (IV) 1.5 mg/m² x 2 doses
VCR (IV) 1.5 mg/m²	1, 8, 15, 22		MP (PO) 50 mg/m²/day	29–171	DEX (PO) 6 mg/m²/day x 7 days
ASP (IM) 6,000 U/m²	2, 5, 8, 12 15, 19				
					Maintenance Weeks 25–130: MP (PO) 75 mg/m²/day MTX (PO) 20 mg/m²/wk

Ara-C, cytarabine; ASP, asparaginase; CTX, cyclophosphamide; DEX, dexamethasone; DNR, daunorubicin; DOX, doxorubicin; HCT, hydrocortisone; MP, mercaptopurine; MTX, methotrexate; PRED, prednisone; TG, thioguanine; VCR, vincristine.

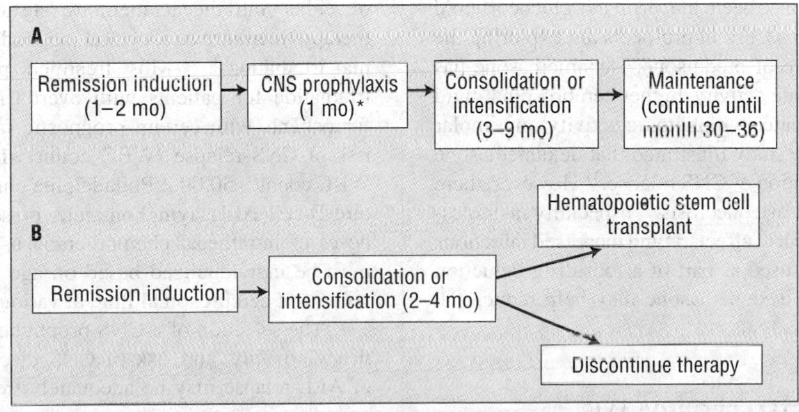

FIGURE 131–2. Treatment algorithm for **(A)** acute lymphocytic and **(B)** nonlymphocytic leukemias. *In pediatric ALL, CNS prophylaxis is given throughout induction, intensification, and maintenance.

fourth induction agent may further prolong the duration of remission, but also increases the risk of toxicity. In children, four-drug induction regimens are generally used only for higher-risk patients. In adults, most patients are higher-risk, and four- to seven-drug induction regimens are commonly used.

Few prospective studies have compared remission induction regimens. The value of adding more drugs to the basic three- or four-drug induction regimen is unclear. Equally unclear is the value of higher doses of the standard combination of drugs for remission induction. Data suggest that high-dose methotrexate and cytarabine alternating with fractionated cyclophosphamide plus vincristine, doxorubicin, and dexamethasone (hyper-CVAD) may improve response and survival in patients with B-cell ALL,[26] as well as that for nonselected adult ALL patients.[27] However, this treatment may be associated with significant cerebellar toxicity.[28,29] Higher doses of cyclophosphamide may be indicated for patients with T-cell ALL.[20]

In pediatric ALL, therapy is based upon the risk of relapse. Low- and standard-risk patients are generally begun on a three-drug induction regimen with a glucocorticoid, vincristine, and asparaginase. High-risk patients require more aggressive therapy. It has been suggested that most treatment failures in childhood ALL result from inadequate initial reduction of the leukemic clone and the acquisition of drug resistance by residual lymphoblasts.[30] This is the basis upon which many trials have incorporated four-drug (or more) induction remission regimens and aggressive intensification or consolidation regimens in the management of higher-risk patients. Many centers now add an anthracycline such as doxorubicin or daunorubicin to the basic glucocorticoid, vincristine, and asparaginase induction regimen backbone. Other agents that have been used up front in remission induction therapy include cyclophosphamide, methotrexate, cytarabine, and teniposide. Table 131–6 provides examples of remission induction regimens.

Three clinically useful sources of asparaginase exist: *Escherichia coli* (gram-negative bacteria), *Erwinia caratovora* (plant parasite), and pegaspargase (asparaginase covalently conjugated to polyethylene glycol). Only *E. coli* asparaginase and polyethylene glycol (PEG)-asparaginase are available through normal commercial channels, but *Erwinia* asparaginase can be ordered from the manufacturer for patients who have had allergic reactions to the other products. Conventional *E. coli* asparaginase can cause severe hypersensitivity reactions depending upon dose, frequency of administration, and route of administration. Pegaspargase has less immunogenicity and a longer half-life, allowing administration every 14 days instead of three times per week.[31]

Historically, prednisone has been the primary glucocorticoid used in pediatric ALL regimens. Current protocols are exploring the role of dexamethasone in place of prednisone. Dexamethasone has an increased duration of biologic activity, higher cerebrospinal fluid (CSF)-to-plasma ratio, and greater lymphotoxic activity on a molar basis than prednisone.[32,33] One study illustrated that dexamethasone is associated with better prevention of CNS relapse.[34] However, there is some evidence for increased osteonecrosis,[29] especially in adolescents, increased neurocognitive late effects,[35] and increased infectious morbidity and mortality when used as part of a four-drug induction regimen.[36] Shorter courses of dexamethasone may help reduce the risk of these adverse effects.

CENTRAL NERVOUS SYSTEM PROPHYLAXIS

In pediatric ALL patients, CNS prophylaxis is generally begun early in induction and continued throughout consolidation and maintenance. As seen in Table 131–6, adults often receive their CNS prophylaxis after achieving complete remission. This phase may overlap with or be incorporated into induction, consolidation, or maintenance. The difference in adults and children probably reflects the lower percentage of adults that achieve remission and long-term disease-free survival.

The rationale for CNS prophylaxis is based on two observations. First, many chemotherapeutic agents do not readily cross the blood-brain barrier. Second, many patients with ALL with no evidence of CNS involvement at diagnosis experience a relapse of their leukemia in the CNS. The CNS relapse rate without prophylaxis in adult ALL patients is approximately 21% to 50%, and in children it exceeds 50%.[25] Current treatment approaches have reduced the incidence to 10% or less.[1,6] These observations indicate that the CNS is a potential sanctuary for leukemic cells and that undetectable leukemic cells are present in the CNS in many patients. Detectable CNS involvement at the time of diagnosis is relatively uncommon (5% to 10%) in ALL.[1] Factors that are associated with an increased risk of CNS involvement at diagnosis include a high initial white blood cell count, T-cell phenotype, and B-cell phenotype.[6,20]

The goal of CNS prophylaxis is to eradicate undetectable leukemic cells present in the CNS. Leukemic meningitis is more easily prevented than treated. Once CNS relapse has occurred, patients are at increased risk of bone marrow relapse and death from refractory leukemia. In early studies, CNS prophylaxis was shown to significantly decrease the risk of CNS relapse in adults, but it had no impact on survival.[37] As survival improves, CNS prophylaxis may become more important for adults.

Initial trials in childhood ALL, in the 1960s, established cranial irradiation and intrathecal methotrexate as the standard for prevention of CNS relapse. Subsequent efforts have examined the need for radiation because of its potential long-term sequelae. Cranial irradiation is associated with headache, meningismus, neuropsychological deficits, endocrine dysfunction, greater susceptibility to brain tumors (in children exposed at age 5 years or younger), short stature, and obesity.[6] Furthermore, it has been reported that about 50% of the children receiving cranial irradiation will develop a "somnolence syndrome" characterized by some degree of lethargy, irritability, or low-grade fever at a median onset of 4 to 8 weeks.[6] Adults may experience similar problems.

In the 1980s, trials were conducted examining intrathecal chemotherapy alone or combined with radiation therapy at lower doses than previously used in children. The majority of children with good-prognosis ALL can be treated with age-adjusted doses of either intrathecal methotrexate or triple intrathecal chemotherapy (methotrexate, cytarabine, and hydrocortisone), without cranial irradiation.[38,39] Most treatment protocols now reserve cranial irradiation for patients with overt CNS leukemia at diagnosis or for patients with certain prognostic factors placing them at higher risk of CNS relapse (WBC count $>100{,}000/\mu L$; T-cell ALL with WBC count $>50{,}000$; Philadelphia chromosome-positive ALL; mature B-cell ALL; lymphomatous presentation; and infants).[1,6] The doses of intrathecal chemotherapy used in pediatric ALL patients must be individualized based on age because of differences in the volume of cerebrospinal fluid at various ages (Table 131–8).

The selection of a CNS prophylaxis regimen must consider efficacy, toxicity, and risk of CNS disease. Patients with a low risk of ALL relapse may be adequately treated with intrathecal therapy or high-dose systemic therapy alone. Those with intermediate-risk ALL may need a combination of intrathecal and high-dose systemic chemotherapy. High-risk patients generally receive cranial irradiation and intrathecal therapy, but in the future may not need the cranial

TABLE 131–8. Intrathecal Therapy in Pediatric ALL

Age (y)	Cytarabine (mg)	Methotrexate (mg)	Hydrocortisone (mg)
≥1	16	8	8
≥2	20	10	10
3–8	24	12	12
≥9	30	15	15

ALL, acute lymphocytic leukemia.

irradiation if current studies show that high-dose systemic therapy plus intrathecal therapy is adequate.[6]

CONSOLIDATION THERAPY

Consolidation (or intensification) therapy in ALL is started after a complete remission has been achieved, and refers to continued intensive chemotherapy in an attempt to eradicate clinically undetectable disease. Regimens usually incorporate either noncross-resistant drugs different from the induction regimen or else more dose-intensive use of the same drugs.

Randomized trials have been equivocal in demonstrating a survival benefit for adults, but the importance to overall survival is more clear in children.[1,6] The specific benefit of any one regimen is difficult to demonstrate because of the overall complexity of therapy in ALL. The adult regimens listed in Table 131–6 offer two different approaches to consolidation with similar results. The German regimen mostly imitates the induction regimen, but substitutes dexamethasone for prednisone (better CNS penetration to prevent leukemic meningitis), doxorubicin for daunorubicin, and thioguanine for mercaptopurine.[21]

The CALGB (Cancer and Leukemia Group B) trial uses a consolidation regimen far more complicated than the induction regimen. The latter includes different drugs and higher doses, at least with the cyclophosphamide dose.[22] The outcomes from these distinctly different trials are similar. The German investigators found a median survival duration of 27.5 months and an estimated 5-year survival rate of 39%.[21] The CALGB study reported a short followup time (median, 43 months) so that only 3-year estimates were available; however, the results included a median survival duration of 36 months and an overall survival rate of 39% for those 30 to 59 years old.[22] A consolidation phase in adult ALL therapy appears necessary, although specific questions remain about drug selection, duration of therapy, dosing, and timing of administration.

Current pediatric studies vary the intensity of consolidation therapy based on the risk factors identified for the patient. Age between 2 and 10 years old, white blood cells below 50,000/μL, and DNA index greater than or equal to 1.16 would start a patient as standard-risk. If the patient does not meet any one of those criteria, they are high risk. If high-risk chromosomal translocations such as t(9;22) (Philadelphia chromosome) are present, the patient would be high-risk or very-high-risk even if age, white blood cell count, and DNA index are standard risk. If the patient has the above standard-risk features plus low-risk chromosomal aberrations, such as t(12;21) or trisomies at chromosomes 4, 10, and 17, they might be considered low-risk for relapse. Additionally, patients who respond slowly to therapy (slow early response; >25% blasts in the bone marrow at day 7) are at higher risk of relapse if they are not treated on more aggressive regimens such as the Children's Cancer Group (CCG) augmented-Berlin–Frankfurt Munster (BFM) regimen (CCG 1882, Table 131–7).[23]

In the United States, prior to the year 2000, there were two multi-institutional research groups, the Pediatric Oncology Group (POG) and the Children's Cancer Group (CCG). They have now joined forces as the Children's Oncology Group (COG). These two groups have taken different approaches to the consolidation phase of treatment. POG has based consolidation regimens on antimetabolites (methotrexate, mercaptopurine, or cytarabine), whereas CCG has used more intensive consolidation regimens that add anthracyclines, cyclophosphamide, and asparaginase to the antimetabolites. The CCG regimens incorporate either one or two intensification (interim maintenance-reinduction-reconsolidation) phases. Table 131–7 gives examples of the POG and CCG types of regimens. The antimetabolite-based regimens may have a reduced risk of late toxicities; however, the more intensive consolidation regimens appear to result in better survival for some patients, especially those at higher risk of relapse.

The ongoing final POG and CCG studies, plus the new COG studies, are designed to continue the assessment of the intensity of consolidation needed for patients with different levels of risk. For example, the continuing CCG studies use the augmented-BFM regimen (CCG 1882, Table 131–7) with double intensification for higher-risk patients. The same regimen with only one intensification is used for lower-risk patients, and standard-risk patients are being tested with one versus two intensification phases. Ongoing POG studies for low-risk patients compare an antimetabolite-based consolidation to the CCG low-risk consolidation with one intensification. For standard-risk POG patients, the CCG low-risk regimen is used with additional methotrexate dose-intensity during the first half of the maintenance phase. For higher-risk patients, the regimen is essentially the same as the CCG 1882 augmented-BFM regimen (two intensifications). Both groups consider patients who are Philadelphia chromosome-positive (t(9;22)) or those with hypodiploidy (low number of chromosomes) to be very high risk, and these patients proceed to allogeneic stem-cell transplant for consolidation, if available.

Pediatric patients with T-cell ALL have also been treated differently by POG and CCG in the past. CCG includes T-cell patients along with pre-B cell patients, and places them on protocols based on standard risk factors, which usually places them on high-risk regimens. POG has used a separate protocol for T-cell ALL and T-cell lymphoblastic lymphoma patients. Combinations of drugs are rotated for approximately 24 months, with minimal difference between induction, consolidation, and maintenance. The current regimen includes prednisone, mercaptopurine, high-dose methotrexate, L-asparaginase, vincristine, and doxorubicin. Drugs that target T-cells, such as the investigational agent Compound 506U78, may influence investigators to continue to treat T-cell leukemia and lymphoma patients on separate protocols. Adults with T-cell ALL are placed on protocols by risk factor, similar to the CCG method.

Children and adults with mature B-cell ALL are treated with the hyper-CVAD regimen mentioned earlier under remission induction, or similar protocols. The regimens were developed for pediatric Burkitt's lymphoma protocols.

MAINTENANCE THERAPY

Many adult ALL patients relapse shortly after completion of remission induction and consolidation therapy, presumably because of residual disease. Maintenance therapy allows long-term drug exposure to slowly dividing cells, allows the immune system time to eradicate leukemia cells, and promotes apoptosis (programmed cell death).[25] The goal of maintenance therapy is therefore to further eradicate residual leukemic cells and prolong remission duration. Although maintenance therapy is clearly beneficial in childhood ALL, the possible benefit in adults has only recently been suggested. In some adult ALL trials that included induction and consolidation, but omitted maintenance, the disease-free survival at 2 years was only 18% to 35% as compared to a survival rate of almost 40% in trials that included maintenance.[1,40,41]

Maintenance therapy usually consists of mercaptopurine and methotrexate, at doses that produce relatively little myelosuppression, with intermittent "pulses" of vincristine and prednisone. Tables 131–6 and 131–7 list the typical doses for these agents in this phase. The optimal duration of maintenance therapy in adults and children is unknown, but most treatment programs continue maintenance therapy for at least 30 months. Decisions about maintenance therapy are also based upon what subtype of ALL is found. Common pre-B-cell ALL does benefit from conventional maintenance therapy with methotrexate and mercaptopurine. Patients with B-cell ALL or Philadelphia chromosome-positive ALL probably gain greater benefit from intensive induction and consolidation and little from maintenance.[20]

An additional issue in maintenance therapy of pediatric ALL has been interpatient variability in the pharmacokinetics of oral methotrexate and mercaptopurine. Slow absorbers and rapid eliminators are at higher risk of treatment failure because of decreased exposure to methotrexate or mercaptopurine.[42] Furthermore, patients who take their oral methotrexate and mercaptopurine on an evening versus a morning schedule appear to have a superior outcome.[43] To account for the interpatient variability, some clinicians titrate the dose of either agent to maintain a WBC count of 1,500 to 4,000/μL. Some protocols circumvent bioavailability and poor compliance problems for methotrexate by parenteral administration. The importance of these pharmacokinetic issues in adults is less well defined.

In an effort to determine the long-term outcome of the duration and intensity of maintenance therapy, the Childhood ALL Collaborative Group recently published findings from a large meta-analysis involving 12,000 randomized children from 42 trials initiated prior to 1987.[44] The analysis revealed that longer maintenance, pulses of vincristine and prednisone, and the inclusion of one or two intensive reinduction courses significantly reduced total number of deaths or relapse. However, only intensive reinduction could improve overall survival.

ALL IN INFANTS

ALL and AML in infants are <5% of the reported acute leukemias in childhood, but they are associated with poor outcomes.[45] Typically, event-free survival is in the 20% to 40% range. Low survival rates for the ALL patients are probably related to the number of high-risk features found in these patients and to greater drug resistance associated with the primitive nature of the lymphoblasts.[46] Recent CCG studies using intensive systemic chemotherapy with intrathecal plus high-dose methotrexate have shown improved survival rates as compared to historical controls.[45] CNS relapses were not increased and patients appeared to be having fewer neurologic abnormalities. Stem-cell transplants have often been used for infants who have t(4;11) MLL rearrangements, which in many studies has been the majority of patients.[46]

ALL IN THE ELDERLY

A significant number of ALL cases occur in patients older than age 60 years but no specific treatment recommendations can be made. The response to therapy and durability of response seem less than in younger adults or children. Older patients have a higher incidence than younger patients of the Philadelphia chromosome and a lower occurrence of T-cell ALL.[25] Recent trials that included patients over age 60 demonstrated that the 3-year survival rate could be up to 20%.[55] For example, in CALGB 8811 (Table 131–6), 9% of the patients were older than age 60 years. The complete remission rate was approximately 65%, but the 3-year survival rate was only 17%.[23] In general, older patients have a lower complete remission rate and, when achieved, the duration of remission is shorter than with younger patients.

TREATMENT OF RELAPSED ALL

The most common site for relapse is the bone marrow, although isolated relapses can occur in the CNS or testicles. Marrow relapse usually follows isolated CNS or testicular relapses. Therefore, patients with isolated relapses are treated with aggressive systemic chemotherapy just as patients with a marrow relapse are treated, in addition to use of localized radiation (cranial or testicular).[1,6]

Patients who have completed treatment and who have stayed in remission for longer periods are more likely to go into remission again.[6] Patients with more favorable risk factors initially, and those who received less intensive initial treatments are more likely to respond well to relapse regimens. In general, long-term survival after relapse is very poor, and aggressive therapies are used. For patients with longer first remissions, the current POG relapse protocol uses chemotherapy with an induction containing prednisone, vincristine, doxorubicin, and asparaginase, followed by consolidation with ifosfamide and etoposide, and then cytarabine and idarubicin. Continuation (maintenance) uses the same combinations as consolidation plus thioguanine and methotrexate, and vincristine, dexamethasone, and asparaginase. For patients with shorter initial remissions or who relapse on therapy (including most adults), once a second remission is induced (CR2), chemotherapy is not likely to result in as long of survival as allogeneic hematopoietic stem cell transplantation (HSCT).[1,4,6,48] Patients who undergo HSCT are less likely to relapse, but are more likely to experience treatment-related morbidity and mortality. Some newer data suggest that relapsed pediatric patients may have better 5-year disease-free survival after allogeneic transplants as compared to chemotherapy alone in CR2, regardless of duration of remission, white blood cell count at diagnosis, or number of agents used in initial induction.[49] Very-high-risk patients, such as those whose leukemic cells are Philadelphia chromosome-positive (Ph+, t(9;22)) or infants with t(4;11) MLL, are exceptions that are thought to have better survival rates if they are transplanted in first remission.[1,6] For children, if no very-high-risk features are identified, patients in first remission fare just as well with chemotherapy as with transplants.[6] In adults, the literature is more controversial,[1] but if the patient is not too old, and an allogeneic matched-sibling donor is available, many treatment centers would transplant in first remission. Autologous HSCT have not been demonstrated to be superior to chemotherapy. Placental blood transplants, matched unrelated donor transplants, and mismatched related donor transplants are under investigation. These types of transplants may still be important because many patients do not have matched sibling donors available.

ROLE OF COLONY STIMULATING FACTORS IN ALL

Researchers have studied the use of granulocyte colony-stimulating factor (G-CSF) in children and adults with ALL in attempts to improve outcomes. In a large randomized trial of 164 patients with ALL (aged 2 months to 17 years) at St. Jude Children's Research Hospital, patients received either G-CSF (10 μg/kg/day SQ) or placebo after remission induction therapy.[50] G-CSF failed to significantly lower the rate of hospitalization for febrile neutropenia, to decrease the number of severe infections, or to increase the likelihood of event-free survival at 3 years. Patients treated with G-CSF did have shorter median hospital days (6 days compared to 10 days) and fewer documented infections. Unfortunately, this did not translate to a reduction in total costs of supportive care. Welte[51] administered G-CSF after each course of therapy during consolidation in pediatric high-risk ALL patients. Febrile neutropenia, culture-positive infections, and duration of intravenous antibiotics were reduced, while increasing adherence to the treatment schedule. Similar results were found in one adult ALL study[52] and in a third pediatric study.[53] In the latter study of high-risk pediatric ALL patients, the benefits were only apparent after one of the two chemotherapy combinations that were alternated during consolidation. As with the St. Jude study, 3-year event-free survival was not improved. Although neutropenic ALL patients may derive some clinical benefits from the use of G-CSF, overall costs and event-free survival are not improved.

TREATMENT OF ACUTE MYELOID LEUKEMIA

AML accounts for the majority of acute leukemia in adults and occurs with increasing frequency in elderly patients. It accounts for only 20% of the acute leukemias in children, but is responsible for 30% of leukemia-related mortality.[60] With recent advances in chemotherapy and supportive care, 65% to 85% of all patients achieve complete remission and 20% to 40% become long-term survivors.[1] In children, the long-term survival with chemotherapy may be 30% to 45%.[6] Overall, the median duration of remission is 1 to 2 years.[1] In patients older than age 60 years, the median duration of remission is shorter than 1 year. In contrast to ALL, active drugs in AML are marrow suppressive, with the exception of all-*trans*-retinoic acid (ATRA). As a result, patients with AML, particularly elderly patients (older than age 60 years), are at greater risk for treatment-related fatal infectious and bleeding complications.

Treatment of AML, unlike that of ALL, usually only consists of induction and intensive postremission therapy (see Fig. 131-2). Central nervous system prophylaxis is not routinely given in adult AML, but is generally administered to pediatric patients. Table 131-9 presents several representative induction regimens for treatment of AML.[54-60]

REMISSION INDUCTION

As with ALL, the goal of remission induction for AML is to rapidly induce a complete remission. Compared to ALL, however, fewer patients with AML achieve complete remission. The lower complete remission rate in AML is related in part to differences in the toxicity of the drugs in remission induction regimens. In ALL, several active agents are relatively nonmyelosuppressive (prednisone, vincristine, L-asparaginase), whereas in AML, active agents (except all-*trans*-retinoic acid) are myelosuppressive. As a result, patients with ALL may achieve complete remission without severe and prolonged marrow hypoplasia. In contrast, because the complete remission rate in AML is related to the intensity of the remission induction regimen, the drugs used in AML are given at doses that uniformly cause severe marrow hypoplasia. One reason for the lower complete remission rate in AML as compared to ALL is the inability to give optimal doses of chemotherapy because of marrow toxicity. With continued improvement of supportive care for patients undergoing chemotherapy, more intensive treatment regimens are being given in an effort to reduce the high rate of leukemic relapse and increase the proportion of long-term survivors. Most patients achieve a complete remission after one or two courses of chemotherapy. Patients who require additional chemotherapy to achieve a complete remission have been reported to have a poor prognosis, even if remission is ultimately achieved.[1]

The most active single agents in AML are the anthracycline antibiotics (daunorubicin, doxorubicin, and idarubicin) and the antimetabolite cytarabine. The most common regimen ("7+3") combines daunorubicin administered as a short infusion of 45–60 mg/m²/day on days 1 to 3 along with cytarabine administered as a continuous 24-hour infusion of 100 mg/m²/day on days 1 to 7. The complete remission rate with the 7+3 regimen is 60% to 80% in younger patients.[61] The remission rate decreases to 40% to 50% in patients older than age 60 years.[61] In terms of overall survival, a retrospective review from the Eastern Cooperative Oncology Group (ECOG) evaluating data from over 1,400 newly diagnosed AML patients receiving a standard anthracycline and cytarabine induction regimen reports overall survival rates of 15% at 5 years.[62] Several trials have attempted to improve upon conventional 7+3 therapy, but have shown no improvement by (a) increasing cytarabine to 10 days, (b) shortening cytarabine to 5 days, (c) substituting doxorubicin for daunorubicin, (d) adding thioguanine, or (e) increasing cytarabine to 200 mg/m²/day continuous infusion.[3]

Other trials have evaluated idarubicin or mitoxantrone as alternatives to daunorubicin in combination with standard continuous infusion cytarabine.[55,62-68] Initial data from the majority of trials suggested idarubicin or mitoxantrone had an advantage over

TABLE 131-9. Representative Chemotherapy Regimens for Adult AML

Induction Therapy	
Yates/CALGB[54] ("7+3")	Daunorubicin 45 mg/m² IV qd on days 1 to 3 Cytarabine 100 mg/m² CIV qd on days 1 to 7
Weirnik[55]	Idarubicin 13 mg/m² IV qd on days 1 to 3 Cytarabine 100 mg/m² CIV qd on days 1 to 7
Weick[56]	Daunorubicin 45 mg/m² IV qd on days 1 to 3 Cytarabine 2,000 mg/m² IV q12h × 12 doses on days 1 to 6
Mitus[57]	Cytarabine 100 mg/m² CIV qd on days 1 to 7 Daunorubicin 45 mg/m² IV qd on days 1 to 3 Cytarabine 2,000 mg/m² IV q12h × 6 doses on days 8 to 10
Bishop/ALSG[58] ("7+3+7")	Cytarabine 100 mg/m² CIV qd on days 1 to 7 Daunorubicin 50 mg/m² IV qd on days 1 to 3 Etoposide 75 mg/m² IV qd on days 1 to 7
Bishop[59] ("HIDAC+3+7")	Cytarabine 3,000 mg/m² IV q12h on days 1, 3, 5, and 7 Daunorubicin 50 mg/m² IV qd on days 1 to 3 Etoposide 75 mg/m² IV qd on days 1 to 7
Postremission Chemotherapy*	
Mitus[57]	*Cycles 1 and 3* Cytarabine 200 mg/m² CIV qd on days 1 to 5 Daunorubicin 60 mg/m² IV qd on days 1 and 2 *Cycle 2* Cytarabine 2,000 mg/m² IV q12h × 6 doses on days 1 to 3 Etoposide 100 mg/m² IV qd on days 4 and 5
Mayer[60]	Cytarabine 3,000 mg/m² IV q12h on days 1, 3, and 5 (6 doses) × 1 to 4 cycles

*Number of postremission chemotherapy cycles is dependent on patient characteristics and inclusion of HSCT in treatment plan.

standard therapy in terms of either increased complete remission rates in patients younger than 60 years of age or increased survival durations.[55,64,68] Conversely, another trial in patients with a median age of 62 years showed no difference in complete remission rates or survival, but did report an increased number of patients entered a complete remission with only one course of idarubicin plus cytarabine as compared daunorubicin plus cytarabine.[62] Berman et al. reviewed long-term followup results from three previously reported randomized trials evaluating idarubicin versus daunorubicin.[65] While two of the trials initially reported advantages in the idarubicin arms, only one trial maintained a significant difference favoring idarubicin after long-term followup analysis. A recent randomized trial in AML patients older than 55 years of age compared standard doses of cytarabine combined with either daunorubicin, idarubicin, or mitoxantrone and reports no difference in response or toxicity between the three regimens.[66] Thus, the anthracycline of choice for a standard 7+3 regimen remains controversial with many investigators adopting idarubicin into the induction regimen in younger AML patients.

Bishop et al. in conjunction with Australian Leukemia Study Group studied the impact of etoposide in remission induction regimens for AML.[58] In a randomized comparison of standard 7+3 with or without etoposide on days 1 to 7 (7+3+7) in newly diagnosed AML patients ages 15 to 70 years, the complete remission rate and overall survival rates were no different between arms when evaluating all patients. A subset analysis in patients younger than age 55 years showed the duration of remissions and overall survival doubled in the etoposide-containing arms. The 7+3+7 regimen was more toxic in patients older than 55 years of age. A small trial in relapsed or refractory patients younger than 70 years of age also reported an increased duration of remission in patients receiving etoposide combined with high-dose cytarabine as compared to high-dose cytarabine alone, thus, confirming the activity of etoposide in the treatment of AML.[69]

Experimental tumor models suggest a steep dose-response curve for cytarabine; thus, higher doses of cytarabine have also been evaluated as a means to enhance the outcome of remission induction therapy.[70] Mitus and colleagues added high-dose cytarabine on days 8 to 10 following conventional 7+3 therapy.[57] The remission rate after induction therapy in this trial was 89%, which is higher than that achieved in the Southeastern Cancer Study Group or the CALGB trial reported in Table 131–9. In patients younger than 60 years of age, Bishop et al. reported high-dose cytarabine (3,000 mg/m^2 q12h on days 1, 3, 5, and 7) combined with daunorubicin and etoposide resulted in improved durations of CR but similar complete remission rates and overall survival as compared to the combination with standard dose of cytarabine.[59] Weick et al., in conjunction with the Southwest Oncology Group (SWOG), compared standard- or high-dose cytarabine (2,000 mg/m^2 q12h × 12 doses) combined with daunorubicin.[56] The increase in cytarabine dose during induction alone did not significantly impact complete remission rates or overall survival, but did improve relapse-free survival. In this study, high-dose cytarabine was associated with more toxicity. Of note, a recent retrospective review conducted by the European Group for Blood and Marrow Transplantation demonstrated the dose of cytarabine administered during induction and/or consolidation did not influence the outcome in patients who ultimately went on to receive allogeneic or autologous stem-cell transplant.[71] These data suggest that high doses of cytarabine during induction may not be needed in patients planned to receive a stem cell transplant during postremission therapy. In summary, the role of high-dose cytarabine during induction remains controversial. If used during induction, high-dose cytarabine is more appropriate in younger patients than in elderly patients because of poor tolerance by elderly patients.

The National Comprehensive Cancer Network (NCCN) published guidelines for the treatment of AML.[72] The classic 7+3 regimen may be a disservice to patients younger than age 60 because the long-term durability is less than some recent studies that employed high-dose cytarabine in induction.[72] The NCCN committee actually recommended more aggressive chemotherapy as compared to historical approaches, using high-dose cytarabine with an anthracycline if the patient was younger than age 60 years in order to improve survival. In patients older than age 60 years, or in patients with a generally poor performance status, conventional 7+3 should be used.

As with adult AML, the most effective remission regimens for children have included an anthracycline with cytarabine with or without thioguanine, yielding a remission rate of 70% to 85%. Recent trials examined the combination of noncross-resistant drugs used simultaneously in an effort to overcome possible induction failure as a result of selection and growth of drug-resistant clones arising by spontaneous mutation. One trial compared cytarabine, daunorubicin, etoposide, thioguanine, and dexamethasone with standard 7+3 therapy with cytarabine and daunorubicin and found them to be equally effective.[73]

POSTREMISSION THERAPY

Although most adults with AML achieve a complete remission, the duration of remission is short (4 to 8 months) if no further treatment is given. Relapse is presumably a consequence of the presence of residual, but clinically undetectable, leukemic cells after remission induction therapy. The goal of intensive postremission therapy is to eradicate these residual leukemic cells and to prevent the emergence of drug-resistant disease. The need for postremission therapy is based on postmortem analysis and cell kinetic data suggesting that nearly 10^9 residual leukemic cells remain after effective remission induction therapy.[3] Strategies evaluated as postremission therapy include (a) low dose, prolonged maintenance therapy; (b) short-course intensive chemotherapy-alone regimens; and (c) high-dose chemotherapy with or without radiation therapy followed by allogeneic or autologous HSCT.

Chemotherapy

In the treatment of AML, postremission therapy is often referred to as consolidation or maintenance therapy. Two randomized trials clearly demonstrated that maintenance therapy following remission induction therapy prolongs survival versus no therapy.[74,75] Cassileth et al., in conjunction with ECOG, demonstrated that one course of more intensive chemotherapy, termed consolidation therapy, increased survival as compared to lower-dose maintenance therapy administered for 2 years.[76] The event-free survival rate at 4 years was significantly higher in the group receiving one course of high-dose cytarabine combined with amsacrine as compared to the group receiving prolonged cytarabine and 6-thioguanine (27% vs 16%). Of note, the mortality rate approached 60% in patients age 60 years or older who were receiving the intensive consolidation arm, indicating alternate consolidation regimens may be warranted in older patients.

Increasing the intensity of chemotherapy consolidation regimens was evaluated in a large trial conducted by the CALGB.[60] In this trial of more than 1,000 patients who received standard 7+3 induction, 569 patients entered a complete remission and were randomized to receive one of three cytarabine-based consolidation regimens: 100 mg/m^2/day or 400 mg/m^2/day as a continuous 24-hour infusion or

3,000 mg/m^2 q12h on days 1, 3, and 5. For patients younger than age 60 years, the results indicated the probability of remaining in a complete remission after 4 years was significantly greater in the patients receiving the high-dose cytarabine arm. Patients older than age 60 years had lower response rates in all arms and did not benefit from the administration of higher doses of cytarabine, probably because they were unable to tolerate the high-dose regimen. Dose-limiting neurotoxicity in the high-dose arm was greater in elderly patients and occurred in 32% of patients older than 60 years of age. Only 29% of patients older than 60 years of age tolerated all four courses of therapy as compared 56% of patients of all ages. In this trial, patients with favorable cytogenetics fared particularly well, with 84% of patients exhibiting a long-term disease-free survival.

Table 131–9 lists other approaches to intensive chemotherapy consolidation. One common consolidation regimen, known as the 5+2 regimen, employs a modified version of the 7+3 induction regimen, administering 5 days of standard-dose cytarabine and 2 days of the same anthracycline used in the induction regimen. In the study from Boston, postremission therapy included a combination of standard-dose cytarabine and daunorubicin for two cycles with a combination of intensified cytarabine with etoposide given between the cycles.[57] Many of the patients later underwent HSCT. The overall survival at 5 years was 55%.

It is not clear whether the same agents (cytarabine and an anthracycline) given for remission induction should be used for postremission therapy in higher doses, or whether different agents altogether should be given. If leukemic relapse is caused by a resistant cell line, then the use of different agents that are noncross-resistant with drugs used in induction would appear to be beneficial.

High-dose cytarabine appears to be a key part of postremission therapy today, especially if not used in induction therapy. How many g/m^2 of cytarabine to give, how many doses per cycle, or how many cycles of cytarabine to give, remain unanswered questions. The only generally accepted practice is that induction alone is insufficient and that some form of postremission therapy prolongs survival. The NCCN guidelines recommend four cycles of high-dose cytarabine for patients younger than 60 years of age and with good cytogenetics.[81] If a patient is older than age 60 years, a dose-reduced high-dose cytarabine regimen or enrollment in a clinical trial is recommended. Patients with unfavorable cytogenetics, underlying myelodysplastic syndrome, or secondary AML should be referred for an HSCT.[72]

Children with AML should also receive postremission therapy if an HSCT is not available. The event-free survival is again about 30% to 40%. Drugs given as consolidation therapy for pediatric AML usually include cytarabine, thioguanine, daunorubicin, doxorubicin, mitoxantrone, etoposide, fludarabine, or dexamethasone. A survival advantage has been shown for those patients who have an HLA-compatible sibling donor and who go on to receive an allogeneic transplantation, yielding a 5-year disease-free survival rate of 50% to 54%.[73,77] There appears, however, to be no survival advantage for autologous transplant over intensive chemotherapy for AML in first remission (event-free survival at 3 years of 36% to 38%).[78]

Allogeneic Hematopoietic Stem Cell Transplantation

Blood and bone marrow transplantation, appropriately termed *hematopoietic stem cell transplant,* involves the administration of myeloablative regimens of chemotherapy with or without total body irradiation followed by the infusion of hematopoietic stem cells obtained from the blood or marrow of a donor or the patient. BMT represents the most aggressive approach to postremission therapy in the management of AML. Much controversy surrounds this treatment approach, specifically the appropriateness, timing, treatment design, and selection of the donor.

When managing AML, allogeneic HSCT (alloHSCT) is designed around three principles: (a) administration of a myeloablative preparative regimen that provides immunosuppression to allow the donor cells to engraft and maximizes leukemic cell kill; (b) infusion of healthy, appropriately HLA-matched allogeneic stem cells to help the patient recover more promptly from the preparative regimen; and (c) establishment of a posttransplant immune-based antileukemic response. The immune-based response, referred to as a graft-versus-leukemia effect, often accompanies the graft-versus-host disease (GVHD) reaction. The immune-based benefit of alloHSCT has been demonstrated through the observation of consistently lower relapse rates with alloHSCT as compared to autologous or syngeneic HSCT. This potential benefit of alloHSCT can be offset by an increased number of complications, such as GVHD and infections, leading to a higher mortality rate following alloHSCT.

AlloHSCT was first evaluated as a treatment modality for AML in refractory patients, but because of initial successes in small numbers of patients, it has also been evaluated as intensive postremission therapy in AML patients in first or subsequent remission. Nonrandomized trials of alloHSCT performed in AML patients in first complete remission report 5-year survival rates of 45% to 60% with relapse rates of 10% to 20%.[79,80] Transplant-related mortality following alloHSCT is generally reported as 20% to 30%. As clinicians have gained more experience in this intensive form of therapy and been provided with more effective immunosuppressive and antibiotic regimens, transplant-related mortality rates have decreased and survival rates have increased. Bone marrow registry data indicate that long-term survival rates in AML patients in first remission receiving an alloHSCT have increased from approximately 45% in the early 1980s to approximately 60% in the mid 1990s.[1]

Table 131–10 presents randomized comparisons of alloHSCT to autologous HSCT (autoHSCT) or intensive consolidation

TABLE 131–10. Comparative Trials of Allogeneic HSCT or Autologous HSCT or Chemotherapy Alone as Postremission Therapy for AML In First Complete Remission

	Disease-Free Survival at 4 Years			Overall Survival at 4 Years		
	AlloHSCT	*AutoHSCT*	*Chemo*	*AlloHSCT*	*AutoHSCT*	*Chemo*
Zittoun et al.[81] (EORTC-GIMEMA)	55%	48%	30%	59%	56%	46%
Harrousseau et al.[92] (GOELAM)	44%	44%	40%	53%	50%	54%
Cassileth et al.[83] (Intergroup)	43%	35%	35%	46%	43%	52%

chemotherapy alone.[81–83] Although results vary, in general, alloHSCT from an HLA-matched sibling donor in AML patients in first complete remission results in long-term disease-free survival in 40% to 70% of patients. Several published comparisons report higher disease-free survival rates and lower relapse rates with alloHSCT in AML in first complete remission as compared to chemotherapy-alone postremission regimens.[84]

Despite any potential advantages that alloHSCT may offer, this therapy is still generally restricted to patients younger than 60 years of age, limiting the number of patients eligible for treatment of this disease which primarily affects the elderly. One new approach, termed nonmyeloablative stem-cell transplant (alloNST), uses less toxic, nonmyeloablative preparative regimens and is now being evaluated in AML patients, particularly older patients or those with comorbid illnesses limiting eligibility for conventional alloHSCT. Allogeneic NST was designed to provide enough immunosuppression in the preparative regimen to allow for engraftment of donor cells and depends heavily on the development of a graft-versus-leukemia effect as a means to treat and prevent relapse of AML. Initial results of small studies evaluating alloNST in AML patients indicate the procedure is well tolerated in a wide age range of patients, and that it is associated with low rates of regimen-related toxicity.[85] Evaluations in larger numbers of patients are necessary to determine the comparative impact of alloNST on GVHD and disease-free and overall survival. Because only 30% of patients will have an HLA-matched sibling donor, alloHSCT is further restricted as a treatment alternative for AML patients. Matched unrelated donor transplantation using a phenotypically HLA-matched donor identified from the bone marrow registries is considered as a treatment alternative for young adults and pediatric AML patients. This approach is associated with long-term disease-free survival rates of 30% to 40% and generally lower overall survival rates than in AML patients undergoing HLA-matched sibling donor alloHSCT because of higher complication rates with the procedure. Anasetti reported a 50% long-term response rate among a small number of high-risk AML patients receiving unrelated donor transplantation.[86]

Autologous Hematopoietic Stem Cell Transplantation

Autologous HSCT (autoHSCT) involves the collection and storage of peripheral blood or bone marrow from the patient prior to administration of a myeloablative preparative regimen. The autologous stem cells are then infused following the preparative regimen in order to rescue the patient from the complications of the high dose therapy. Advantages of autoHSCT over alloHSCT include decreased complication rates because of lack of immunosuppression and GVHD, and more broad applicability because of a lack of donor limitations and fewer age restrictions. While the preparative regimen still provides antileukemic activity, autoHSCT is associated with higher incidences of relapse because of a lack of a graft-versus-leukemia effect and potential tumor contamination of autologous stem cells. Long-term survival following autoHSCT for AML in first complete remission ranges from 35% to 50%.[76,81,87,88] Long-term response rates decrease proportionally as autoHSCT is employed in second or subsequent complete remission.

A number of trials have evaluated *ex vivo* purging of autologous stem cells collected from the bone marrow with chemotherapy agents or monoclonal antibodies as a means to decrease tumor contamination.[89–92] Although inconsistent, the majority of data suggest no survival or relapse advantage, but more prolonged neutrophil recovery or immunosuppression in the patients receiving purged bone marrows. Because normal progenitors repopulate the peripheral blood following myelosuppressive therapy preferentially over leukemic progenitors, there is much interest and evaluation underway using peripheral blood as the source of donor stem cells in attempt to decrease contamination and speed recovery.[1] Other controversies in autoHSCT include the optimal timing of therapy, the amount of consolidation therapy needed, the dose of stem cells needed, and the impact of post-transplant therapy.[93] Table 131–10 compares autoHSCT versus other postremission therapies; they are discussed below.

Comparisons of Postremission Therapy Options

Several randomized trials in AML patients in first complete remission have compared outcomes following alloHSCT, autoHSCT, and/or intensive consolidation chemotherapy. Table 131–10 summarizes these trials.[81–83] In most trials, eligible patients based on age and donor availability received an alloHSCT and the remaining patients were randomized between autoHSCT and chemotherapy alone. Zittoun et al. noted a disease-free survival advantage for alloHSCT or autoHSCT as compared to chemotherapy alone, but no differences in overall survival.[81] Survival rates were comparable because of a higher relapse rate in the chemotherapy group as compared to a higher treatment-related mortality rate in the alloHSCT group. Harrousseau et al. reported similar disease-free and overall survival rates between alloHSCT, autoHSCT, and chemotherapy alone, and noted that consolidation with a second course of chemotherapy is less toxic than HSCT.[82] Cassileth et al. also reported comparable disease-free and overall survival rates between postinduction high-dose cytarabine, autoHSCT, and alloHSCT.[83]

According to the NCCN guidelines, the decision to proceed to HSCT depends on cytogenetics.[60] If the patient has a low-risk cytogenetic profile and is younger than age 60 years, then high-dose cytarabine for four cycles is preferred over autologous or allogeneic HSCT. If the patient has a poor-risk cytogenetic profile and is younger than age 60 years, then allogeneic or matched unrelated donor transplant should be considered early after remission induction. Autologous marrow can be used if a hematologic and cytogenetic remission is achieved. For patients older than age 60 years, the NCCN guidelines do not favor HSCT and recommend either enrollment into a clinical trial or conventional high-dose cytarabine should be considered. Despite this recommendation, many clinicians consider autoHSCT and possibly alloNST in selected patients older than age 60 years. For the AML patient who relapses early after induction therapy, if a sibling or matched unrelated donor is available, then HSCT is the primary reinduction therapy because conventional chemotherapy offers little help. If the relapse occurred late, then HSCT can be used as postremission consolidation after conventional induction therapy.[72]

AML IN THE ELDERLY

As the median age at diagnosis is 65 years of age, AML is a disease of the elderly. Unfortunately, long-term cure rates are lower in older patients, ranging from 5% to 8%.[94,95] In patients older than age 55 years, an ECOG review reported the median duration of survival to be 6 to 9 months as compared to 11 months in patients younger than age 55 years. The actual response and survival rates may be even lower as many elderly patients with AML are not included in clinical trials because of a lack of eligibility and poor performance status.[96]

Elderly patients with AML have a poor outcome as a result of the presence of unfavorable prognostic factors in the majority of patients, including poor-risk cytogenetic features, preceding myelodysplasia, and a higher incidence of inherent drug resistance. Greater than 70% of *de novo* AML patients older than age 55 years will express the multidrug resistance (MDR) phenotype associated with chemotherapy resistance including resistance to the leukemia-active anthracyclines and etoposide.[97] Older patients with AML may also have poor outcome because of the inability to withstand aggressive therapy as a result of poor organ function, poor performance status, or existing comorbidities. Although older patients with AML may be able to tolerate aggressive induction therapy, intensive postremission therapy is often too toxic, thus, increasing the likelihood of patient relapse.[98] Older AML patients have also been reported to have an impaired capacity to recover from intensive therapy as a consequence of leukemic involvement of earlier hematopoietic cells.[96]

With standard 7+3 induction therapy, the complete response rate in older AML patients ranges from 40% to 50%. Half of the remaining patients are likely to die during induction therapy from infection or other complication and the other half often has refractory disease.[98] More elderly patients than younger patients will require two courses of induction therapy to achieve a remission. While initially accepted in older patients, palliative care approaches in older patients with AML with moderate to good performance status and organ function are now considered inappropriate. Löwenberg and colleagues prospectively randomized patients to either a conventional chemotherapy arm or to an observation arm on which patients could receive modest doses of chemotherapy for symptom palliation. The chemotherapy group survived a median of 21 weeks versus 11 weeks for the observation group. The quality of life of each group was similar, each spending approximately 50% of the study time in the hospital.[99] Chemotherapy may prolong survival without significantly decreasing the quality of life for elderly patients. Thus, chemotherapy is the treatment of choice for elderly patients; the best chemotherapy regimen and overall treatment approach are controversial.

In an effort to improve response rates, trials have tried to determine the best anthracycline and the appropriate dose. Unlike younger patients, comparative data in elderly patients do not suggest any significant efficacy or toxicity advantages of idarubicin or mitoxantrone over daunorubicin for AML induction therapy.[66,100] Early noncomparative trials suggested the morbidity and mortality rates during induction were higher than desired in elderly AML patients receiving aggressive doses of daunorubicin (>45 mg/m^2/day × 3 d). More recent trials suggest that older AML patients can safely withstand higher doses of daunorubicin (60–70 mg/m^2/day), which may be a result of enhancements in supportive care.[94,101,102] Unlike younger patients, older patients with AML do not experience added benefit when etoposide is incorporated into an anthracycline and cytarabine-containing regimen.[58] Higher doses of cytarabine during induction are also not beneficial in the elderly. Postremission strategies in elderly AML patients are less-well defined. Even though high-dose cytarabine has become a standard component of postremission therapy in younger patients, its role is controversial. In the elderly, attenuated-dose cytarabine during induction decreases remission and survival rates while decreasing treatment-related mortality rates. This raises concerns that attenuated-dose cytarabine during postremission therapy may cause similar outcome. In the trial comparing postremission cytarabine doses, Mayer et al. reported less benefit of higher doses of cytarabine (3,000 mg/m^2) in patients older than age 60 years as compared to younger patients.[60] Mayer et al. noted no improvement in response rate in patients older than age 60 years who were receiving high-dose cytarabine during induction, primarily because only 29% of older patients were able to tolerate the regimen as compared to 62% of younger patients.[60] Toxicity, particularly neurotoxicity, was more frequent in the elderly, and significantly limited the ability to deliver the planned four courses of therapy. A recent ECOG review of more than 300 older AML patients reported cytarabine doses of 1,500 mg/m^2 × 12 doses in patients younger than age 70 years, or six doses in patients older than age 70 years, were well tolerated with a treatment-related mortality rate of only 2% and median survival at 2 years of 30%.[101] Thus, some clinicians question the need for doses of cytarabine as high as 3,000 mg/m^2 and suggest attenuated high-dose regimens (such as 1,500/mg/m^2) may be sufficient and beneficial. The appropriate number of cycles of postremission consolidation therapy is unknown and currently under investigation in a randomized ECOG trial.[98]

While maintenance therapy is considered inferior to intensive consolidation chemotherapy in younger patients, its role in older patients with AML is still undefined and not given appropriate consideration given the published outcomes. Data from the German Acute Leukemia Group demonstrated a disease-free survival advantage among patients receiving maintenance therapy following consolidation as compared to no maintenance therapy.[103] Because older patients may not be able to tolerate more aggressive postremission strategies such as HSCT, maintenance therapy may play an important role in improving outcomes. A recent EORTC trial demonstrated higher disease-free survival in elderly patients receiving prolonged low-dose cytarabine maintenance therapy as compared to patients undergoing observation only.[94] Unfortunately, disease-free survivals were low in both groups, 13% and 7%, and overall survival was similar between groups.

More novel approaches to postremission therapy targeted at immune modulation have been the subject of recent clinical trials in the elderly in an effort to enhance long-term outcomes. Nonrandomized data that used interleukin-2 (IL-2) as a means to enhance immune-mediated prevention of relapse have been promising.[104] The CALGB is currently conducting a randomized trial in the elderly comparing 90 days of postremission low-dose, subcutaneous IL-2 versus observation. FLT-3 ligand is another immunomodulatory cytokine that enhances recovery and activity of hematopoietic and dendritic cells and is currently under investigation as postremission therapy in elderly AML patients.

TREATMENT OF RELAPSED OR REFRACTORY AML

The most common cause of treatment failure in AML patients receiving chemotherapy alone or undergoing HSCT is relapse. In addition, a substantial number of patients, especially elderly patients, experience refractory disease as defined by the inability to achieve a complete remission after two courses of induction therapy. In most cases, the preferred method of treatment for relapse or refractory disease is HSCT. Prolonged disease-free survivals are observed in 30% to 40% of patients receiving allogeneic or autologous HSCT in first relapse or second complete remission.[105,106] Unfortunately, only a small percentage of relapsed or refractory patients will be eligible for HSCT, particularly allogeneic HSCT, because of age and donor restrictions.

The timing of HSCT to treat relapse is controversial. Data from the Fred Hutchinson Cancer Research Center suggest that outcome of HLA-matched, related allogeneic HSCT performed at the time of first relapse is comparable to that observed when performed in second complete remission.[105] While performing the allogeneic HSCT in first relapse eliminates the need for and toxicity of salvage chemotherapy, the feasibility of this approach can be limited by the logistics required to prepare and activate a donor. A comparison conducted by the International Bone Marrow Transplant Registry demonstrated the superiority of allogeneic HSCT over chemotherapy as treatment of relapse occurring 1 to 2 years following induction.[107] In patients younger than age 30 years, prolonged leukemia-free survival occurred in 41% of allogeneic HSCT recipients as compared to 17% of patients receiving chemotherapy; similar advantages were observed in patients older than age 30 years, but unfortunately leukemia-free survivals were low in both groups. In the treatment of refractory disease, allogeneic HSCT is superior to autologous HSCT in patients younger than age 55 years.[108,109]

If patients relapse following allogeneic HSCT, the outcome is poor with a median survival approaching 3 to 4 months.[1] In this scenario, treatment options depend on performance status, clinical condition, and the time since allogeneic HSCT. Patients relapsing less than 100 days following allogeneic HSCT are unlikely to respond to current strategies and salvage attempts are often associated with a high treatment-related mortality. For patients relapsing more than 1 year after allogeneic HSCT, second allogeneic HSCT may be an alternative in selected young patients, but prolonged survival is generally less than 10% with this approach.[1] Other strategies investigated for AML relapsing after allogeneic HSCT, but demonstrating only limited, short-lived success include immune manipulation to stimulate a graft-versus-leukemia effect through donor lymphocyte infusions or premature discontinuation of cyclosporine and other immunosuppressives.

Autologous HSCT is an option at the time of first relapse if cells have been previously collected and stored during first remission. If such cells were not collected, then it is necessary to achieve a second complete remission in order to proceed to autologous HSCT. Prolonged disease-free survivals of 30% and 20% are reported when autologous HSCT is performed in second and third complete remission, respectively.[89,110] The advantages of autologous HSCT are the lack of donor limitations and fewer age-based restrictions; the disadvantage is the need to achieve a complete remission, which requires exposure to more cytotoxic chemotherapy. If patients relapse following autologous HSCT, allogeneic HSCT from a related or unrelated donor is preferred in selected younger patients. For older patients, investigational strategies should be considered for high-performance status patients relapsing after autologous HSCT.

If patients with relapsed or refractory disease are not candidates for HSCT, the primary mode of treatment, until recently, was salvage chemotherapy. The ability to achieve a second complete remission with salvage chemotherapy is proportionally related to the duration of the first remission. Approximately 50% to 60% of patients relapsing greater than 2 years after induction therapy will achieve a second complete remission often with the same induction regimen.[111] On the other hand, only 10% to 20% of patients relapsing within 6 to 12 months following induction are able to achieve a second complete remission with alternate salvage chemotherapy regimens. The most commonly used salvage regimens are high-dose cytarabine-based regimens with doses of 2,000–3,000 mg/m^2 q12h for 8 to 12 doses. High-dose cytarabine schedules that use once-daily doses or alternate-day doses have also been used in an attempt to minimize toxicity.[1] Cytarabine has been administered alone or in combination with various agents, including etoposide, fludarabine, topotecan, and an anthracycline, as treatment of relapsed or refractory AML. Response rates to such salvage regimens range from 30% to 50%, but are often short-lived.[1] Patients receiving high-dose cytarabine during induction may be less likely to benefit from such a regimen for treatment of relapse and thus require alternate salvage strategies. As treatment of relapsed disease following high-dose cytarabine, near myeloablative doses of etoposide and cyclophosphamide are associated with a response rate of 30%, but with an associated unfortunate short duration of remission.[112]

Approximately 70% of relapsed or refractory AML expresses the MDR phenotype conferring a high degree of chemotherapy resistance because of its encoding and overexpression of the P-glycoprotein protein.[113] P-glycoprotein is a membrane protein capable of removing certain antineoplastics from the intracellular to extracellular space.[113] Antagonists of the P-glycoprotein, such as cyclosporine or the cyclosporine analog PSC 833, have been investigated as a strategy to overcome resistance in these patients. In addition to inhibiting P-glycoprotein, cyclosporine may also affect the disposition of agents such as anthracyclines and thus increase the exposure to cytotoxic agents. List et al. reported a slightly higher complete remission rate in relapsed or refractory AML patients receiving high-dose cytarabine and daunorubicin with cyclosporine as compared to the same regimen without cyclosporine (40% vs 33%).[114] The relapse-free survival at 2 years was higher in patients receiving the cyclosporine-containing regimen (34% vs 9%). Conversely, Estey et al. observed decreased survival in relapsed or refractory patients older than age 60 years receiving cyclosporine to inhibit P-glycoprotein with chemotherapy.[115] PSC 833 is 10-fold more effective in inhibiting P-glycoprotein than cyclosporine and lacks cyclosporine's renal toxicity. Unfortunately, randomized trials conducted by ECOG and CALGB observed no advantages among relapsed or refractory patients receiving PSC 833 with chemotherapy and more regimen-related deaths in patients older than age 60 years receiving the MDR modulator.[116,117] Other MDR inhibitors with limited interference with hepatic metabolism are currently under investigation.

Monoclonal antibodies have been the subject of recent investigations in the treatment of relapsed or refractory AML and have the ability to deliver targeted therapy to the malignant cell. Gemtuzumab (Mylotarg®, formerly known as CMA-676) is an anti-CD33 antibody complexed to the antitumor antibiotic calicheamicin that was recently approved by the FDA for treatment of relapsed disease in AML patients older than age 60 years. CD33 is expressed in 90% of leukemic blasts; thus, this anti-CD33-directed product provides targeted cell kill to leukemic cells. In a phase II trial, 142 patients with AML in first untreated relapse received gemtuzumab 9 mg/m^2 for two doses separated by 14 days.[118] Complete remission occurred in 16% of patients and another 13% of patients had normalization of blood counts with the exception of persistent platelet counts $<100,000/\mu L$. Toxicity can be problematic with gemtuzumab. Reported adverse effects include infusion-related fever and chills in 80% of patients, prolonged neutropenia and thrombocytopenia in 89% of patients, transient elevations in hepatic enzymes in 20% of patients, and infrequent, but severe, hypotension and shortness of breath. Because gemtuzumab lacks specific dose-limiting organ toxicities it is also being investigated in combination with other chemotherapy agents. Other antibodies under investigation in salvage regimens and high-dose preparative regimens for AML include radiolabeled anti-CD45 agents and HuM195, a humanized mouse monoclonal targeted against the CD33 antigen.

Numerous classes of new agents are being investigated as alternate treatment approaches for relapsed or refractory AML including the antiangiogenesis agents thalidomide and SU 5416. Hypomethylating agents such as decitabine, and histone deacetylase inhibitors such as phenylbutyrate, are also under investigation.[119,120] Arsenic trioxide, which is effective in the treatment of APL, is also under investigation for treatment of AML via its modulation of apoptotic and chromatin remodeling pathways.[121] STI-571, the tyrosine kinase inhibitor exhibiting efficacy in the treatment of chronic myelogenous leukemia, also inhibits AML cell lines and is currently undergoing clinical trials in AML.[122]

TREATMENT OF ACUTE PROMYELOCYTIC LEUKEMIA

APL is a subclass of AML that accounts for 10% of all cases. It has historically been diagnosed by the distinctive cytoplasmic granules seen on light microscopy. APL is clinically unique from the other subclasses because of the common occurrence of severe coagulopathy at diagnosis and during induction therapy. In APL, differentiation and maturation arrest are caused by alterations in the retinoic acid receptor because of the translocation of chromosomes 15 and 17. The discovery of the t(15;17) now provides a cytogenetic marker of the disease and is a prognostic marker in favor of response to differentiation therapy with ATRA.[123]

Historically, treatment of APL involved combination chemotherapy regimens used in the treatment of other subclasses of AML. Such standard regimens produced complete remission rates of 50% to 60%, but were associated with high treatment-related mortality rate caused by hemorrhagic complications.[124] The introduction of differentiation therapy with ATRA allows for high complete remission rates without life-threatening pancytopenia or exacerbated bleeding complication as a result of the characteristic coagulopathy.[123] The pharmacology, pharmacokinetics, and toxicity of ATRA are reviewed in Chap. 115.

ATRA was first reported in 1987 to induce remission in patients with APL and was subsequently approved by the FDA for treatment of APL.[125] ATRA is usually given orally in a dose of 45 mg/m^2, as a single dose or divided into two doses, given after a meal. ATRA-based regimens can achieve complete remission rates as high as 95% in APL patients. The time to achieve remission is 1 to 3 months. ATRA does not cross the blood-brain barrier; therefore, leukemic meningitis should be treated with conventional intrathecal chemotherapy.

While being devoid of myelosuppressive effects, ATRA therapy is associated with headache, skin and mucous membrane reactions, bone pain, nausea, and the retinoic acid syndrome. When ATRA is started, rapid onset of differentiation of promyelocytes occurs, which can lead to leukocytosis and/or retinoic acid syndrome. The retinoic acid syndrome (fever, respiratory distress, interstitial pulmonary infiltrates, and weight gain), also referred to as differentiation syndrome, has been reported initially to be fatal in one-third of cases. Combination of chemotherapy with ATRA induction decreases the incidence of retinoic acid syndrome and rapid initiation of dexamethasone, 10 mg IV twice daily for 3 days, at presentation of retinoic acid syndrome decreases associated mortality. Various guidelines regarding the initial WBC count have been used to signal the need for chemotherapy, such as a WBC count of 3,000–10,000/μL. Investigators agree that if the WBC count exceeds 20,000/μL, then the patient needs combination therapy. In addition, other investigators add chemotherapy to ATRA if the WBC count rises more than 4,000/μL over the first 2 days of ATRA therapy.

A number of clinical trials have evaluated the time course for administration of ATRA. Fenaux et al. determined that ATRA as induction followed by two cycles of consolidation chemotherapy produced similar complete remission, but decreased relapse and increased event-free and overall survival as compared to chemotherapy alone for induction and consolidation.[126] Tallman et al. similarly demonstrated ATRA followed by chemotherapy consolidation increased disease free and overall survival as compared to chemotherapy induction and consolidation.[127] Of concern, Fenaux et al. reported 30% of patients receiving ATRA as induction relapsed at 4 years and 25% of patients experience the retinoic acid syndrome.[126]

In an effort to extend the duration of remission and decrease ATRA-associated toxicity, other trials have evaluated the outcome of simultaneous administration of ATRA with chemotherapy during induction therapy. Burnett et al. compared concurrent administration of ATRA with chemotherapy during induction to ATRA given 5 days before anthracycline-based induction chemotherapy with the hope of reducing coagulopathy-related complications by giving ATRA before chemotherapy.[128] Interestingly, concurrent administration was superior in terms of complete response rates, early death, and overall survival at 3 years. In a subsequent study, Fenaux et al. demonstrated similar complete response rates with concurrent or sequential ATRA and standard induction chemotherapy, but noted decreased relapse rates at 2 years in the concurrent administration group (suggesting a synergistic or additive effect for the combination).[129] The overall incidence of retinoic acid syndrome in the study was low (15%), probably because of concurrent administration and because the study design allowed for early initiation of chemotherapy in the sequential arm if the white blood cell count increased during ATRA induction.

Unlike other subtypes of AML, the role of maintenance therapy is better defined in APL. Nonrandomized trials support a benefit of continuous low-dose methotrexate and 6-mercaptopurine in prevention of relapse of APL.[130] Fenaux et al. also demonstrated increased event-free and overall survival in patients receiving continuous low-dose chemotherapy maintenance after achieving a complete remission as compared to no maintenance therapy in APL patients.[129] Continuous ATRA maintenance was also associated with decreased relapse rates and improved survival in a US intergroup study.[127] Concerns have been raised about clinical resistance with continuous prolonged ATRA therapy because of hypercatabolism of the drug leading to inability to maintain adequate serum levels of ATRA.[131] To address this concern, Fenaux et al. evaluated ATRA maintenance therapy administered on an intermittent basis in an effort to overcome the autoinduction of metabolism problem. Fenaux et al. demonstrated that such therapy was associated with a decreased relapse rate.[129] Furthermore, Fenaux et al. reported an additive effect of maintenance chemotherapy and intermittent ATRA with only 7.6% of patients relapsing at 2 years on the combination maintenance therapy.[129]

Relapsed APL can also be effectively treated with ATRA therapy in a large number of cases. Fenaux et al. reported that patients relapsing after ATRA-based therapy were able to achieve second complete remission with ATRA-based reinduction.[126] For patients resistant to induction or reinduction with ATRA-based regimens alternative strategies include allogeneic or autologous HSCT. Outcomes with autologous HSCT are dependent on the pretransplant extent of disease and include remissions of over 28 months in patients who are able to achieve a second complete remission before autologous transplant.

Recent data also suggest arsenic trioxide can induce clinical remissions in relapsed APL patients through its induction of apoptosis and differentiation.[132] Given these data, arsenic trioxide is now FDA-approved for the treatment of APL patients who have not responded to or have relapsed following first-line therapy with ATRA and anthracycline-based chemotherapy. The recommended dose is 0.15 mg/kg/day IV until bone marrow remission, not to exceed 60 doses, followed by consolidation beginning 3 to 6 weeks after completion of induction at the same dose for a total of 25 doses over a period up to 5 weeks. Arsenic trioxide was unexpectedly associated with a high incidence of hepatotoxicity in newly diagnosed patients, but was associated with tolerable hepatotoxicity in relapsed patients. Following induction of a complete remission with arsenic trioxide in relapsed patients, postremission therapy with combination arsenic trioxide and chemotherapy was associated with molecular remissions and improved disease-free survival as compared to chemotherapy or arsenic trioxide alone following remission.[132] Additional investigations are underway to evaluated the role of arsenic trioxide in multidrug postremission regimens.

USE OF COLONY-STIMULATING FACTORS IN AML

In AML, colony-stimulating factors, or hematopoietic growth factors, have been evaluated as a means to enhance chemotherapy cytotoxicity and to minimize neutropenic complications following induction and consolidation chemotherapy. No benefit has been demonstrated using colony-stimulating factors as priming agents administered during induction therapy in an effort to recruit leukemia cells into the cycle to enhance susceptibility to cell-cycle-specific chemotherapy agents. Thus, use of colony-stimulating factors during chemotherapy administration is discouraged outside the setting of a clinical trial.

Both filgrastim (*Escherichia coli*-derived G-CSF) and sargramostim (yeast-derived GM-CSF) are approved by the FDA to treat neutropenia after antileukemia therapy. The original package inserts listed myeloid malignancies as contraindications to the use of filgrastim or sargramostim. Myeloid blast cells carry receptors for G-CSF and GM-CSF, and the fear initially existed that using these factors would stimulate regrowth of the myeloid leukemia. Subsequent studies show this not to be true.

A number of randomized trials, primarily in elderly patients, consistently demonstrate reduction in neutropenia when G-CSF or GM-CSF is administered following AML induction chemotherapy.[66,133–139] While neutropenia can be reduced from 2–12 days depending on the trial, results vary in terms of improvements in infectious morbidity and mortality, resource utilization, and disease response rates (see Table 131–11). Comparison of outcomes between trials is difficult because of differences in study design and ages of patients evaluated. The use of colony-stimulating factors in elderly AML patients has received particular attention because complications related to prolonged neutropenia, particularly infection, are the major causes of failure to achieve remission. In a randomized, blinded, placebo-controlled trial, Rowe et al. evaluated sargramostim following induction and consolidation therapy in AML patients older than age 55 years.[66] There was a statistically significant reduction in infection and an increase in overall survival in the patients receiving GM-CSF. To date, only one randomized trial evaluating *E. coli*-derived GM-CSF during and after chemotherapy has shown a negative impact of colony-stimulating factor therapy by reporting an unexplained decreased complete remission rate in the GM-CSF arm.[138] Heil et al. is the only trial thus far to report reductions in the duration of hospitalization associated with G-CSF use following AML induction chemotherapy.[134]

As a result of these trials, the American Society of Clinical Oncology's *Guidelines for the Use of Hematopoietic Colony-Stimulating Factors* recommends colony-stimulating factors after initial induction therapy in patients older than age 55 years as acceptable clinical practice.[140] Routine use in younger patients remains controversial. Other controversial issues surrounding colony-stimulating factor use in AML include which colony-stimulating factor to use, what dose, which day to start after chemotherapy, how long to continue, and should the marrow be examined for leukemia prior to starting a colony-stimulating factor. One economic analysis evaluating several studies of colony-stimulating factors in acute leukemia reports cost savings of $2,200 to $2,300 in two studies using colony-stimulating factors following AML induction therapy.[141]

SUPPORTIVE CARE

The most common and significant toxic effect of antileukemic agents is marrow suppression. With the exception of prednisone, L-asparaginase, and vincristine, antineoplastic agents used to treat acute leukemias cause myelosuppression. During AML remission induction therapy, daily monitoring of the complete blood count and the absolute neutrophil count is necessary to determine when red cell and platelet transfusions are needed and when neutropenia is achieved. Less frequent monitoring than daily may be sufficient during ALL induction. Marrow hypoplasia from the myelosuppressive regimens usually reaches its lowest point (nadir) after 1 to 2 weeks of therapy and lasts for another 1 to 2 weeks. During this period of hypoplasia, infectious and bleeding complications are major causes of death in leukemic patients. As typical signs and symptoms of infection may be absent in the neutropenic host, frequent monitoring of vital signs (especially fever) and daily physical examination are important. Infection control strategies often include routine hand washing; dietary restrictions; reverse isolation and laminar-airflow rooms; routine surveillance cultures; fungal, pneumocystis, and bacterial prophylaxis; and the empiric use of broad-spectrum antibiotics when fever occurs (see Chap. 111). The NCCN guidelines, in contrast to those of many institutions, do not recommend prophylactic antimicrobials unless there is a documented recurrent problem at the institution.[72] Patients are often seen by a dentist prior to induction therapy to identify and treat potential infectious sources in the mouth. Chlorhexidine mouthwash may be used to maintain good oral hygiene. Pediatric ALL patients on standard induction regimens, which generally are minimally myelosuppressive, often have recovered blood counts earlier and do not require as aggressive of measures. However, they do require close monitoring of vital signs and blood counts until their counts recover. *Pneumocystis carinii* prophylaxis (usually trimethoprim-sulfamethoxazole) is begun on all patients by the end of induction and continues until 6 months after therapy is discontinued.

TABLE 131–11. Colony-Stimulating Factors Following Induction Therapy for AML

Reference	Drug	Enhanced Neutrophil Recovery	Other Benefits Related to Colony-Stimulating Factor Therapy
Godwin et al.[133]	G-CSF	Yes	Fewer days of fever and antibiotics
Heil et al.[134]	G-CSF	Yes	Decreased duration of hospitalization
Dombret et al.[135]	G-CSF	Yes	Increased complete remission rate
Rowe et al.[66]	GM-CSF (yeast)	Yes	Decreased incidence of infection and increased survival
Stone et al.[136]	GM-CSF (*E. coli*)	Yes	None
Witz et al.[137]	GM-CSF (*E. coli*)	Yes	Increased disease-free survival
Zittoun et al.[138]	GM-CSF (*E. coli*)	No	Decreased complete remission rate
Lowenberg et al.[139]	GM-CSF (*E. coli*)	Yes	None

Acute leukemia patients, particularly those with an initial elevated white blood cell count, should receive allopurinol, good hydration, and possibly sodium bicarbonate prior to and during chemotherapy to prevent the development of urate nephropathy from rapid destruction of white cells. In adults, 300 mg of allopurinol once daily, started 1 to 2 days prior to chemotherapy, is usually adequate. Children should receive 10 mg/kg/day of allopurinol on the same schedule. Urine pH should be raised to approximately 7 if sodium bicarbonate is used. Once marrow hypoplasia ensues, these measures may be discontinued. Tumor lysis syndrome may lead not only to hyperuricemia but also to hyperkalemia, hyperphosphatemia, and hypocalcemia. Hypercalcemia has been observed in some patients secondary to ectopic parathyroid production by leukemia cells.

Hematologic support consists primarily of platelet and packed red cell transfusions. Platelet transfusions are often given for peripheral counts below 5,000/μL or clinical signs of bleeding. Transfusions of packed red cells may also be indicated for a hematocrit under 25%, profound fatigue, shortness of breath, tachycardia, or chest pain. Promyelocytic leukemia can release procoagulants that can cause disseminated intravascular coagulation, necessitating close monitoring and heparin or antithrombin III therapy. Because of the gastrointestinal toxic effects of chemotherapy, parenteral nutrition may be required. Patients are frequently receiving infusions of antibiotics, fluids, hyperalimentation, and blood products simultaneously. To provide the total support needed for these patients, a multiple-lumen central venous access device such as a Hickman catheter is placed at the start of therapy.

EVALUATION OF PATIENT OUTCOMES

Appropriate development of a pharmaceutical care plan for the acute leukemia patient begins with establishing the diagnosis and prognosis for the patient. Long-term therapeutic goals for the patient may include long-term disease-free survival, although palliative care is a possibility in rare patients. The short-term outcome initially is the establishment of remission. The return of hematologic values to normal and a repeat bone marrow biopsy that demonstrates no evidence of disease serve as documentation that remission has been achieved. Monitoring guidelines for induction or consolidation are similar. After the appropriate postremission therapy has been completed, the patient may return monthly for 1 year and then every 3 months, to check hematologic values. If no evidence of disease exists after 5 years from the diagnosis and the patient has been in continuous complete remission, the patient is considered cured.

Intense monitoring of fevers, hematologic and chemistry laboratory values, microbiology reports, and the patient's physical condition are necessary to identify infection, risk of bleeds, and tumor lysis syndrome early. A coagulation-screening panel will identify patients with ongoing disseminated intravascular coagulation, a particular risk with acute promyelocytic leukemia.

During therapy, the pharmacist can be an important agent in patient education. Patients should receive information regarding acute and chronic toxicities of the chemotherapy being administered as well as possible treatments for those toxicities. The pharmacist can also be an important resource for information regarding antibiotics, antiemetics, nutritional support, colony-stimulating factors, and other supportive care issues.

Pharmacists need to be involved in checking drug doses and any dose modifications for organ dysfunction or prior toxicity. Pharmacists are often in the best position to recognize the potential for medication errors and to help avoid them. Similarly, pharmacists are often able to identify the possibility that patient problems are secondary to drug treatments. For standard-risk pediatric ALL patients, drug-induced problems such as hyperglycemia, behavioral changes, hypertension, pancreatitis, and coagulation defects are not uncommon. In AML induction regimens, fever may be cytarabine-induced, as well as leukemia- or infection-induced. Mucositis is common during AML induction, and may be symptomatically treated.

Numerous late sequelae from leukemia therapy have been recognized.[4,6] CNS irradiation may lead to several different neurologic problems; most common are cortical atrophy and other endocrine dysfunctions resulting in obesity, short stature, precocious puberty, and osteoporosis. Intellectual function and perceptual motor function can be disturbed. Reduced growth hormone production from the pituitary in children may decrease the rate and extent of growth. Secondary gliomas after cranial radiation have been reported. Long-term cardiomyopathy with symptomatic congestive heart failure has been observed months or years later in some patients receiving anthracyclines during acute leukemia therapy, especially in pediatrics or after high cumulative doses.[91,142] Most recently has been the observation that secondary AML can occur in pediatric ALL patients after receiving etoposide or teniposide.[7] Pharmacists caring for leukemia patients after acute therapy is completed should monitor for these effects and initiate any necessary follow-up. The long-term consequences of HSCT are discussed in Chap. 134.

▶ PRINCIPLES OF PHARMACOTHERAPY

Although not a common malignancy in patients older than age 35 years, the acute leukemias are the most common malignancy in children and the leading cause of cancer-related death in patients younger than age 35 years.

- The genetic alterations leading to acute leukemia are quickly being discovered and offer targets for future drug therapy. In contemporary practice, the t(15;17) is a specific indicator for initiation of all-*trans*-retinoic acid in acute promyelocytic leukemia.
- Therapeutic choices for both ALL and AML are now based on specific risk factors such as age or WBC count at time of diagnosis in ALL. For both ALL and AML, cytogenetic reports offer significant information regarding risk stratification.
- For children with ALL, the foundation of therapy is vincristine, prednisone, and asparaginase. An anthracycline is sometimes added. For adults with ALL, vincristine, prednisone, and an anthracycline are given, and asparaginase is sometimes added.
- Because the risk of CNS relapse is so great in ALL, all patients receive prophylaxis, but the choice of therapy can include radiation therapy and single-agent intrathecal administration, triple-drug intrathecal chemotherapy alone, or combinations of high-dose systemic chemotherapy and intrathecal single-agent chemotherapy.
- Postremission ALL therapy is given for up to 3 years to eradicate microscopic disease. Hematopoietic stem-cell transplant is a more aggressive strategy in ALL patients with very-high-risk features.
- AML therapy usually includes induction therapy with an anthracycline and cytarabine. Postremission therapy can include

either consolidation chemotherapy with or without maintenance therapy, or hematopoietic stem cell transplantation.

- Colony-stimulating factors can now be safely and effectively used with myelosuppressive chemotherapy for acute leukemias. The benefits can include reduced incidence of serious infections, reduced hospital stays, and fewer treatment delays, but do not include prolonged disease-free survival.
- Acute leukemia is a life-threatening illness for most patients. In pediatric ALL, long-term survival can be 60% to 80%. In pediatric AML, fewer than 50% of patients achieve long-term survival. In adults with ALL, fewer than half survive 5 years. In adult AML, only 20% to 40% can expect to live beyond 5 years.

REFERENCES

1. Scheinberg DA, Maslak P, Weiss M. Acute leukemias In: DeVita VT, Hellman S, Rosenberg SA, eds. Cancer: Principles and Practice of Oncology, 6th ed. Philadelphia, Lippincott-Williams & Wilkins, 2001: 2404–2433.
2. Greenlee RT, Hill-Haimon MB, Murray T, Thun M. Cancer statistics, 2001. CA Cancer J Clin 2001;51:15–36.
3. Schiffer CA. Acute myeloid leukemia in adults. In: Holland JF, Frei E, Bast RC, et al., eds. Cancer Medicine, 4th ed. Philadelphia, Williams & Wilkins, 1997:2617–2649.
4. Pui CH, Evans WE. Acute lymphoblastic leukemia. N Engl J Med 1998;339:605–615.
5. Weinstein HJ, Tarbell NJ. Leukemias and lymphomas of childhood. In: Devita VT, Hellman S, Rosenberg SA, eds. Cancer: Principles and Practice of Oncology, 5th ed. Philadelphia, Lippincott-Raven, 1997: 2145–2165.
6. Margolin JF, Poplack DG. Acute lymphoblastic leukemia. In: Pizzo PA, Poplack DG, eds. Principles and Practice of Pediatric Oncology, 3rd ed. Philadelphia, Lippincott-Raven, 1997:409–462.
7. Golub TR, Weinstein HJ, Grier HE. Acute myelogenous leukemia. In: Pizzo PA, Poplack DG, eds. Principles and Practice of Pediatric Oncology, 3rd ed. Philadelphia, Lippincott-Raven, 1997:463–482.
8. Sandler DP, Ross JA. Epidemiology of acute leukemia in children and adults. Semin Oncol 1997;24:3–16.
9. Linet MS, Hatch E, Kleinerman RA, et al. Residential exposure to magnetic fields and acute lymphoblastic leukemia in children. N Engl J Med 1997;337:1–7.
10. Russell NH. Biology of acute leukaemia. Lancet 1997;349:118–122.
11. Beaupre DM, Kurzrock R. RAS and leukemia: From basic mechanisms to gene-directed therapy. J Clin Oncol 1999;17:1071–1079.
12. Cline MJ. The molecular basis of leukemia. N Engl J Med 1994;330:328–336.
13. Prokocimer M, Rotter V. Structure and function of p53 in normal cells and their aberrations in cancer cells: Projection on the hematologic cell lineages. Blood 1994;84:2391–2411.
14. Bloomfield CD, Caligiuri MA. Molecular biology of leukemias. In: DeVita VT, Hellman S, Rosenberg SA, eds. Cancer: Principles and Practice of Oncology, 6th ed. Philadelphia, Lippincott-Williams & Wilkins, 2001:2389–2404.
15. Rubnitz JE, Camitta BM, Mahmoud H, et al. Childhood acute lymphoblastic leukemia with the MLL-ENL fusion and t(11;19)(q23;p13.3) translocation. J Clin Oncol 1999;17:191–196.
16. Rubnitz JE, Crist WM. Molecular genetics of childhood cancer: Implications for pathogenesis, diagnosis, and treatment. Pediatrics 1997;100: 101–108.
17. Dietz-Lovett K. An overview of acute and chronic leukemias. Dev Support Cancer Care 1998;2:66–72.
18. Rubin CM, LeBeau MM, Mick R, et al. Impact of chromosomal translocations on prognosis in childhood acute lymphoblastic leukemia. J Clin Oncol 1991;9:2183–2192.
19. Smith M, Arthur D, Camitta B, et al. Uniform approach to risk classification and treatment assignment for children with acute lymphoblastic leukemia. J Clin Oncol 1996;14:18–24.
20. Hoelzer D, Gokbuget N. New approaches to acute lymphoblastic leukemia in adults: Where do we go? Semin Oncol 2000;27:540–559.
21. Hoelzer D, Thiel E, Löffler H, et al. Prognostic factors in a multicenter study for treatment of acute lymphoblastic leukemia in adults. Blood 1988;71:123–131.
22. Larson RA, Dodge RK, Burns CP, et al. A five-drug remission induction regimen with intensive consolidation for adults with acute lymphoblastic leukemia: Cancer and Leukemia Group B study 8811. Blood 1995;85:2025–2037.
23. Nachman J, Sather HN, Gaynon PS, et al. Augmented Berlin-Frankfurt-Munster therapy abrogates the adverse prognostic significance of slow early response to induction chemotherapy for children and adolescents with acute lymphoblastic leukemia and unfavorable presenting features: A report from the Children's Cancer Group. J Clin Oncol 1997;15:2222–2230.
24. Land VJ, Shuster JJ, Crist WM, et al. Comparison of two schedules of intermediate-dose methotrexate and cytarabine consolidation therapy for childhood B-precursor cell acute lymphoblastic leukemia: A Pediatric Oncology Group study. J Clin Oncol 1994;12:1939–1945.
25. Laport GF, Larson RA. Treatment of adult acute lymphoblastic leukemia. Semin Oncol 1997;24:70–82.
26. Thomas DA, Cortes J, O'Brien S, et al. Hyper-CVAD program in Burkitt's-type adult acute lymphoblastic leukemia. J Clin Oncol 1999;17:2461–2470.
27. Kantarjian HM, O'Brien S, Smith TL, et al. Results of treatment with hyper-CVAD, a dose-intensive regimen, in adult acute lymphocytic leukemia. J Clin Oncol 2000;18:547–561.
28. Koh LP, Lim LC. Cerebellar toxicity following hyper-CVAD regimen for acute lymphoblastic leukemia. Br J Haematol 1999;104:644–645.
29. Mattano LA, Sather HN, Trigg ME, Nachman JB. Osteonecrosis as a complication of treating acute lymphoblastic leukemia in children: A report from the children's cancer group. J Clin Oncol 2000;18:3262–3272.
30. Rivera GK, Raimondi SC, Hancock ML, et al. Improved outcome in childhood acute lymphoblastic leukaemia with reinforced early treatment and rotational combination chemotherapy. Lancet 1991;337:61–66.
31. Ettinger LJ, Kurtzberg J, Voute PA, et al. An open-label multicenter study of polyethylene glycol-L-asparaginase for the treatment of acute lymphoblastic leukemia. Cancer 1998;75:1176–1181.
32. Gaynon PS, Lustig RH. The use of glucocorticoids in acute lymphoblastic leukemia of childhood. Molecular, cellular, and clinical considerations. J Pediatr Hematol Oncol 1995;17:1–12.
33. Ito C, Evans WE, McNinch L, et al. Comparative cytotoxicity of dexamethasone and prednisolone in childhood acute lymphoblastic leukemia. J Clin Oncol 1996;14:2370–2376.
34. Jones B, Freeman AI, Shuster JJ, et al. Lower incidence of meningeal leukemia when prednisone is replaced by dexamethasone in the treatment of acute lymphocytic leukemia. Med Pediatr Oncol 1991;19:269–275.
35. Waber DP, Carpentieri SC, Klar N, et al. Cognitive sequelae in children treated for acute lymphoblastic leukemia with dexamethasone or prednisone. J Pediatr Hematol Oncol 2000;22(3):206–213.
36. Hurwitz CA, Silverman LB, Schorin MA, et al. Substituting dexamethasone for prednisone complicates remission induction in children with acute lymphoblastic leukemia. Cancer 2000;88:1964–1969.
37. Omura GA, Raney M. Long-term survival in adult acute lymphoblastic leukemia: Follow-up of a Southeastern Cancer Study Group trial. J Clin Oncol 1985;3:1053–1058.
38. Pullen J, Boyett J, Shuster J. Extended triple intrathecal chemotherapy trial for prevention of CNS relapse in good-risk and poor-risk patients with B-progenitor acute lymphoblastic leukemia: A Pediatric Oncology Group study. J Clin Oncol 1993;11:839–849.
39. Tubergen DG, Gilchrist GS, O'Brien RT, et al. Prevention of CNS disease in intermediate-risk acute lymphoblastic leukemia: Comparison of cranial radiation and intrathecal methotrexate and the importance

of systemic therapy. A Children's Cancer Group report. J Clin Oncol 1993;11:520–526.

40. Cassileth PA, Anderson JW, Bennett JM, et al. Adult acute lymphocytic leukemia: The Eastern Cooperative Oncology Group experience. Leukemia 1992;6(suppl 2):178–181.
41. Dekker AW, van't Veer MB, Sizoo W, et al. Intensive postremission chemotherapy without maintenance therapy in adults with acute lymphoblastic leukemia. J Clin Oncol 1997;15:476–482.
42. Koren G, Ferrazini G, Sulhlt D, et al. Systemic exposure to mercaptopurine as a prognostic factor in acute lymphoblastic leukemia in children. N Engl J Med 1990;323:17–21.
43. Schmiegelow K, Glomstein A, Kristinsson J, et al. Impact of morning versus evening schedule for oral methotrexate and 6-mercaptopurine on relapse risk for children with acute lymphoblastic leukemia. J Pediatr Hematol Oncol 1997;2:102–109.
44. Richards S, Gray R, Peto R, et al. Childhood ALL Collaborative Group. Duration and intensity of maintenance chemotherapy in acute leukemia: Overview of 42 trials involving 12,000 randomised children. Lancet 1996;347:1783–1788.
45. Reamon GH, Sposto R, Sensel MG, et al. Treatment outcome and prognostic factors for infants with acute lymphoblastic leukemia treated on two consecutive trials of the Children's Cancer Group. J Clin Oncol 1999;17:445–455.
46. Pui CH, Evans WE. Acute lymphoblastic leukemia in infants. J Clin Oncol 1999;17:43 8–440.
47. Ong ST, Larson RA. Current management of acute lymphoblastic leukemia in adults. Oncology 1995;9:433–441.
48. Barrett AJ, Horowitz MH, Pollock BH, et al. Bone marrow transplants from HLA-identical siblings as compared with chemotherapy for children with acute lymphoblastic leukemia in a second remission. N Engl J Med 1994;331:1253–1258.
49. Boulad F, Steinherz P, Reyes B, et al. Allogeneic bone marrow transplantation versus chemotherapy for the treatment of childhood acute lymphoblastic leukemia in second remission: A single-institution study. J Clin Oncol 1999;17:197–207.
50. Pui CH, Boyett JM, Hughes WT, et al. Human granulocyte colony-stimulating factor after induction chemotherapy in children with acute lymphoblastic leukemia. N Engl J Med 1997;336:1781–1787.
51. Welte K, Reiter A, Mempel K, et al. A randomized phase III study of the efficacy of granulocyte colony-stimulating factor in children with high-risk acute lymphoblastic leukemia. Berlin-Frankfurt-Munster Study Group. Blood 1996;87:3143–3150.
52. Ottmann O, Hoelzer D, Gracien E, et al. Concomitant granulocyte colony-stimulating factor and induction chemoradiotherapy in adult acute lymphoblastic leukemia: A randomized phase III trial. Blood 1995;86:444–450.
53. Michel G, Landman-Parker J, Auclerc MF, et al. Use of recombinant human granulocyte colony-stimulating factor to increase chemotherapy dose-intensity: A randomized trial in very high-risk childhood acute lymphoblastic leukemia. J Clin Oncol 2000;18:1517–1524.
54. Yates J, Gildewell O, Wiernik, et al. Cytosine arabinoside with daunorubicin or adriamycin for therapy of acute myelocytic leukemia: A CALGB study. Blood 1982;60:454–462.
55. Weirnik PH, Banks PLC, Case DC Jr, et al. Cytarabine plus idarubicin or daunorubicin as induction and consolidation therapy for previously untreated adult patients with acute myeloid leukemia. Blood 1992;79:1924.
56. Weick JK, Kopecky KJ, Appelbaum FR, et al. A randomized investigation of high dose versus standard-dose cytosine arabinoside with daunorubicin in patients with previously untreated acute myeloid leukemia: A Southwest Oncology Group study. Blood 1996;88:2841–2851.
57. Mitus AJ, Miller KB, Schenkein DP, et al. Improved survival for patients with acute myelogenous leukemia. J Clin Oncol 1995;13:560–569.
58. Bishop JF, Lowenthal RM, Joshua D, et al. Etoposide in acute nonlymphocytic leukemia. Blood 1990;75:27.
59. Bishop JF, Matthews JP, Young GA, et al. A randomized study of high-dose cytarabine in induction in acute myeloid leukemia. Blood 1996;87:1710–1717.
60. Mayer RJ, Davis RB, Schiffer CA, et al. Intensive postremission chemotherapy in adults with acute myeloid leukemia. N Engl J Med 1994;331:896–903.
61. Mastrianni DM, Tung NM, Tenen DG. Acute myelogenous leukemia: Current treatment and future directions. Am J Med 1992;92:286–295.
62. Bennett JM, Young ML, Andersen JW, et al. Long-term survival in acute myeloid leukemia: The Eastern Cooperative Oncology Group experience. Cancer 1997;8:2205–2209.
63. Mandelli F, Petti MC, Ardia A, et al. A randomised clinical trial comparing idarubicin and cytarabine to daunorubicin and cytarabine in the treatment of acute non-lymphoid leukaemia: A multicentric study from the Italian Co-operative Group GIMEMA. Eur J Cancer 1991;27:750–755.
64. Berman E, Heller G, Santorsa J, et al. Results of a randomized trial comparing idarubicin and cytosine arabinoside with daunorubicin and cytosine arabinoside in adult patients with newly diagnosed acute myelogenous leukemia. Blood 1991;77:1666–1674.
65. Berman E, Wiernik P, Vogler R, et al. Long-term follow-up of three randomized trials comparing idarubicin and daunorubicin as induction therapies for patients with untreated acute myeloid leukemia. Cancer 1997;80:2181–2185.
66. Rowe JM, Neuberg W, Friedenberg W, et al. A phase III study of daunorubicin vs idarubicin vs mitoxantrone for older adult patients (>55 yrs) with acute myelogenous leukemia (AML): A study of the Eastern Cooperative Oncology Group (E3993). Blood 1998;92:313a.
67. Arlin Z, Case DC Jr, Moore J, et al. Randomized multicenter trial of cytosine arabinoside with mitoxantrone or daunorubicin in previously untreated adult patients with acute nonlymphocytic leukemia (AML). Leukemia 1990;4:177–183.
68. Vogler WR, Velez-Garcia E, Omura G, et al. A phase 3 trial comparing daunorubicin or idarubicin combined with cytosine arabinoside in acute myelogenous leukemia. J Clin Oncol 1992;10:1103–1111.
69. Vogler WR, McCarley DH, Stagg M, et al. A phase III trial of high dose cytosine arabinoside with or without etoposide in relapsed and refractory acute myelogenous leukemia. Leukemia 1994;9:1847–1853.
70. Plunkett W, Iacoboni S, Keating MJ. Cellular pharmacology and optimal therapy concentrations of 1-β-D-arabinofuranosylcytosine 51-triphosphate in leukemic blasts during treatment of refractory leukemia with high-dose 1-β-D-arabinofuranosylcytosine. Scand J Haematol 1986;44:51–59.
71. Cahn JY, Labopin M, Sierra J, et al. No impact of high-dose cytarabine on the outcome of patients transplanted for acute myeloblastic leukaemia in first remission. Acute Leukaemia Working Party of the European Group for Blood and Marrow Transplant (EBMT). Br J Haematol 2000;110:308–314.
72. National Comprehensive Cancer Network Acute Leukemia Practice Guidelines Committee. NCCN acute leukemia practice guidelines. Oncology 1996;11(suppl):205–221.
73. Wells RJ, Woods WG, Buckley JD, et al. Treatment of newly diagnosed children and adolescents with acute myeloid leukemia: A Children's Cancer Group study. J Clin Oncol 1994;12:2367–2377.
74. Buchner T, Urbanitz D, Hiddeman W, et al. Intensified induction and consolidation with and without maintenance chemotherapy for acute myeloid leukemia: Two multicenter studies of the German AML Cooperative Group. J Clin Oncol 1985;3:1583.
75. Cassileth PA, Harrington DP, Hines JD, et al. Maintenance chemotherapy prolongs remission duration in adult acute nonlymphocytic leukemia. J Clin Oncol 1988;6:583.
76. Cassileth PA, Lynch E, Hines JD, et al. Varying intensity of postremission therapy in acute myeloid leukemia. Blood 1992;79:1924–1930.
77. Nesbit ME, Buckley JD, Feig SA, et al. Chemotherapy for induction of remission of childhood acute myeloid leukemia followed by marrow transplantation or multiagent chemotherapy: A report from the Children's Cancer Group. J Clin Oncol 1994;12:127–135.
78. Ravindranath Y, Yeager AM, Chang MN, et al. Autologous bone marrow transplantation versus intensive consolidation chemotherapy for acute myeloid leukemia in childhood. N Engl J Med 1996;334:1428–1434.

79. Clift RA, Buckner CD, Appelbaum FR, et al. Allogeneic bone marrow transplantation in patients with acute myeloid leukemia in first remission. A randomized trial of two irradiation regimens. Blood 1990;76:1867.
80. Geller RB, Saral R, Pianadosi S, et al. Allogeneic bone marrow transplantation after high-dose busulfan and cyclophosphamide in patients with acute nonlymphocytic leukemia. Blood 1989;73:3380.
81. Zittoun RA, Mandelli F, Willemze R, et al. Autologous or allogeneic bone marrow transplantation compared with intensive chemotherapy in acute myelogenous leukemia in first remission. N Engl J Med 1995;332:217–223.
82. Harrousseau JL, Cahn JY, Pignon B, et al. Comparison of autologous bone marrow transplantation and intensive chemotherapy as postremission therapy in adult acute myeloid leukemia. The Groupe Ouest Est Leucemies Aigues Myeloblastiques (GOELAM). Blood 1997;90:2978–2986.
83. Cassileth PA, Harrington DP, Appelbaum FR, et al. Chemotherapy compared with autologous or allogeneic bone marrow transplantation in the management of acute leukemia in first remission. N Engl J Med 1998;339:1649–1656.
84. Reiffers J. HLA-identical sibling hematopoietic stem cell transplantation for acute myeloid leukemia. In: Atkinson K, ed. Clinical Bone Marrow and Stem Cell Transplantation, 2nd ed. New York, Cambridge University Press, 2000:433–445.
85. Sandmaier BM, McSweeney P, Yu C, et al. Nonmyeloablative transplants: Preclinical and clinical results. Semin Oncol 2000;27:78–81.
86. Anasetti C. Transplantation of hematopoietic stem cells from alternate donors in acute myelogenous leukemia. Leukemia 2000;14:502–504.
87. Archimbaud E, Thomas X, Michallet M, et al. Prospective genetically randomized comparison between intensive post-induction chemotherapy and bone marrow transplantation in adults with newly diagnosed acute myeloid leukemia. J Clin Oncol 1994;12:262.
88. Schiller GJ, Nimer SD, Territo MC, et al. Bone marrow transplantation versus high-dose cytarabine-based consolidation chemotherapy for acute myelogenous leukemia in first remission. J Clin Oncol 1992;10:41.
89. Yeager AM, Kaizer H, Santos GW, et al. Autologous bone marrow transplantation in patients with acute non-lymphoblastic leukemia using ex vivo marrow treatment with 4-hydroperoxycyclophosphamide. N Engl J Med 1986;315:141–147.
90. Rowley SD, Jones RJ, Piantadosi S, et al. Efficacy of *ex vivo* purging for autologous bone marrow transplantation in the treatment of acute nonlymphoblastic leukemia. Blood 1989;74:501–506.
91. Lapore JP, Douay L, Lopez M, et al. One hundred twenty-five adult patients with primary acute leukemia autografted with marrow purged by Mafosfamide: A 10-year single institution experience. Blood 1994;84:3810.
92. Korbling M, Fliedner TM, Holle R, et al. Autologous blood stem cell (ABSCT) versus purged bone marrow transplantation (pABMT) in standard risk AML: Influence of source and cell composition of the autograft on hematopoietic reconstitution and disease-free survival. Bone Marrow Transplant 1991;7:343.
93. Burnett AK. Autologous hematopoietic stem cell transplantation for acute myeloid leukemia. In: Atkinson K, ed. Clinical Bone Marrow and Blood Stem Cell Transplantation, 2nd ed. New York, Cambridge University Press, 2000:252–266.
94. Lowenberg B, Sucieu S, Archimbaud E, et al. Mitoxantrone versus daunorubicin in induction and consolidation therapy: The value of low-dose cytarabine for maintenance of remission, and an assessment of prognostic factors in acute myeloid leukemia in the elderly: Final report of the Leukemia Organization for the Research and Treatment of Cancer and the Dutch-Belgium Hemato-Oncology Cooperative Hovon Group randomized phase III study AML-9. J Clin Oncol 1998;16:872–880.
95. Stone RM. Therapy of older adults with AML: CALGB studies. In: Hiddeman W, Buchner T, Wormann B, et al., eds. Acute Leukemias VIII: Prognostic Factors and Treatment Strategies. Berlin, Springer-Verlag, 1999.
96. Hiddeman W, Kern W, Schoch C, et al. Management of acute myeloid leukemia in elderly patients. J Clin Oncol 1999;17:3569–3576.
97. Leith CP, Kopecky KJ, Godwin J, et al. Acute myeloid leukemia in the elderly: Assessment of multidrug resistance (MDR) and cytogenetics distinguishes biologic subgroups with remarkably distinct responses to standard chemotherapy: A Southwest Oncology Group study. Blood 1997;89:3323–3329.
98. Rowe JM. Treatment of acute myelogenous leukemia in older adults. Leukemia 2000;14:480–487.
99. Löwenberg B, Zittoun R, Kerkhofs H, et al. On the value of intensive remission-induction chemotherapy in elderly patients of 65? years with acute myeloid leukemia: A randomized phase III study of the European Organization for Research and Treatment of Cancer Leukemia Group. J Clin Oncol 1989;7:1268–1274.
100. AML Collaborative Group. A systematic collaborative review of randomized trials comparing idarubicin with daunorubicin (or other anthracyclines) as induction therapy for acute myeloid leukemia. Br J Haematol 1998;103:100–109.
101. Rowe JM, Andersen JW, Mazza JJ, et al. Randomized placebo-controlled phase III study of granulocyte-macrophage colony stimulating factor in adult patients (>55–70 years) with acute myelogenous leukemia: A study of the Eastern Cooperative Oncology Group (E1490). Blood 1995;86:457–462.
102. Hewlett J, Kopecky KJ, Head D, et al. A prospective evaluation of the roles of allogeneic marrow transplantation and low-dose monthly maintenance chemotherapy in the treatment of adult acute myelogenous leukemia (AML): A Southwest Oncology Group study. Leukemia 1995;9:562–569.
103. Buchner T, Urbanitz D, Hiddeman W, et al. Intensified induction and consolidation with or without maintenance chemotherapy for acute myeloid leukemia (AML): Two multicenter studies of the German AML Cooperative Group. J Clin Oncol 1985;3:1583–1589.
104. Hellstrand K, Mellqvist U, Wallhut E, et al. Histamine and interleukin-2 in acute myelogenous leukemia. Leuk Lymphoma 1997;27:429–439.
105. Clift RA, Buckner CD, Appelbaum FR, et al. Allogeneic marrow transplantation during untreated first relapse of acute myeloid leukemia. J Clin Oncol 1992;10:1071.
106. Petersen FB, Lynch MHE, Clift RA, et al. Autologous marrow transplantation for patients with acute myeloid leukemia in untreated first relapse or in second complete remission. J Clin Oncol 1991;11:1353.
107. Gale RP, Horowitz MM, Rees JKH, et al. Chemotherapy versus transplants for acute myelogenous leukemia in second remission. Leukemia 1996;10:13–19.
108. Forman SJ, Schmidt GM, Nademanne AP, et al. Allogeneic bone marrow transplantation as therapy for primary, induction failure for patients with acute leukemia. J Clin Oncol 1991;9:1570–1574.
109. Biggs JC, Horowitz MM, Gale RP, et al. Bone marrow transplants may cure patients with acute leukemia never achieving remission with chemotherapy. Blood 1992;80:1090–1093.
110. Chopra R, Goldstone AH, McMillan AK, et al. Successful treatment of acute myeloid leukemia beyond first remission with autologous bone marrow transplantation using busulfan/cyclophosphamide and unpurged marrow: The British autograft group experience. J Clin Oncol 1991;9:1840–1847.
111. Tallman MS, Mocharnuk RS. Acute myeloid leukemia: New avenues for treatment and supportive care? In: Medscape: Hematology-Oncology Clinical Management, vol. 4: Acute Myeloid Leukemia. 2001:1–31.
112. Brown RA, Herzig RH, Wolff SN, et al. High-dose etoposide and cyclophosphamide without bone marrow transplantation for resistant hematologic malignancy. Blood 1990;76:473.
113. Maslak P, Hegewisch-Becker S, Godfrey L, et al. Flow cytometric determination of the multidrug resistant phenotype in acute leukemia. Cytometry 1994;17:84.
114. List AF, Kopecky KJ, Willman CL, et al. Benefit of cyclosporine (CsA) modulation of anthracycline resistance in high-risk AML: A Southwest Oncology Group study. Blood 1998;92(suppl 1):312a. Abstract.
115. Estey E. New agents and new targets for the treatment of AML. In: American Society of Hematology Educational Program Book, 2000. San Francisco, American Society of Hematology Annual Meeting, 2000: 70–74.

116. Greenberg P, Advani R, Tallman M, et al. Treatment of refractory/relapsed AML with PSC833 plus mitoxantrone, etoposide, cytarabine (PBSC-MEC) vs MEC: Randomized phase III trial (E2995). Blood 1999;94(suppl 1):383a. Abstract.
117. Baer MR, George SL, Dodge RK. Phase III study of PSC-833 modulation of multidrug resistance (MD) in previously untreated acute myeloid leukemia (AML) patients (PTS) >60 years (CALGB 9720). Blood 1999; 94(suppl 1):383a. Abstract.
118. Sievers EL, Larson RA, Estey E, et al. Efficacy and safety of CMA-676 in patients with AML in first relapse. Blood 1999;94(suppl 1):696a. Abstract.
119. Kantarjian HM, O'Brien SM, Estey E, et al. Decitabine studies in chronic and acute myelogenous leukemia. Leukemia 1997;11(suppl 1):S35–S36.
120. Warrell RP, He LZ, Richon V, et al. Therapeutic targeting of transcription in acute promyelocytic leukemia by use of an inhibitor of histone deacetylase. J Natl Cancer Inst 1998;90:1621.
121. Perkins C, Kim CN, Fang G, et al. Arsenic induces apoptosis of multidrug-resistant human myeloid leukemia cells that express bcr-abl or overexpress MDR, MRP, Bcl, or Bcl-xL. Blood 2000;95:1014–1022.
122. Heinrich M, Zigler A, Griffith D, et al. Selective pharmacological inhibition of wild-type and mutant c-kit receptor tyrosine kinase activity in hematopoietic cells. Blood 1999;94(suppl 1):265a. Abstract.
123. Warrell RP, de Thè H, Wang Z, Degos L. Acute promyelocytic leukemia. N Engl J Med 1993;329:177–189.
124. Head D, Kopecky KJ, Weick J, et al. Effect of aggressive daunomycin therapy on survival in acute promyelocytic leukemia. Blood 1995;86:1717.
125. Meng er H, Yu-chun Y, Shu-rong C, et al. All-*trans*-retinoic acid with or without low-dose cytosine arabinoside in acute promyelocytic leukemia. Chin Med J (Engl) 1987;100:949–953.
126. Fenaux P, Chevret S, Guierci A, et al. Long-term follow-up confirms the benefit of all-trans-retinoic acid in acute promyelocytic leukemia. European APL group. Leukemia 2000;14:1371–1377.
127. Tallman MS, Andersen JW, Schiffer CA, et al, All-*trans*-retinoic acid in acute promyelocytic leukemia. N Engl J Med 1997;337:1021–1028.
128. Burnett AK, Goldstone AH, Gray RG, et al. All-*trans*-retinoic acid given concurrently with induction chemotherapy improves the outcomes of APL: Results of the UK MRC ATRA trial. Blood 1997;90(suppl 1): 1474.
129. Fenaux P, Chastang C, Chevret S, et al. A randomized comparison of All-*trans*-retinoic acid (ATRA) followed by chemotherapy and ATRA plus chemotherapy and the role of maintenance therapy in newly diagnosed acute promyelocytic leukemia. Blood 1999;94:1192–1200.
130. Kantarjian H, Keating M, Walters RS, et al. Role of maintenance chemotherapy in acute promyelocytic leukemia. Cancer 1987;59:1258.
131. Delva L, Cornic M, Balitrand N, et al. Resistance to All-*trans*-retinoic acid (ATRA) therapy in relapsing acute promyelocytic leukemia: Study of in vitro ATRA sensitivity and cellular retinoic acid binding protein levels in leukemic cells. Blood 1993;82:2175.
132. Niu C, Yan H, Yu T, et al. Studies of treatment of acute promyelocytic leukemia with arsenic trioxide: Remission induction, follow-up, and molecular monitoring in 11 newly diagnosed and 47 relapsed acute promyelocytic leukemia patients. Blood 1999;94:3315–3324.
133. Godwin JE, Kopecky KJ, Head DR, et al. A double-blind placebo-controlled trial of granulocyte colony-stimulating factor in elderly patients with previously untreated acute myeloid leukemia: A Southwest Oncology Group Study (9031). Blood 1998;91:3607–3615.
134. Heil G, Hoelzer D, Sanz MA, et al. A randomized, double-blind, placebo-controlled, phase III study of filgrastim in remission induction and consolidation therapy for adults with *de novo* acute myeloid leukemia. Blood 1997;90:4710–4718.
135. Drombert H, Chastang C, Fenaux P, et al. A controlled study of recombinant human granulocyte colony-stimulating factor in elderly patients after treatment for acute myelogenous leukemia. AML Cooperative Study Group. N Engl J Med 1995;332:1678–1683.
136. Stone RM, Berg DT, George SL, et al. Granulocyte-macrophage colony-stimulating factor after initial chemotherapy for elderly patients with primary acute myelogenous leukemia. N Engl J Med 1995;332:1671–1677.
137. Witz F, Sadoun A, Perrin MC, et al. A placebo-controlled study of recombinant human granulocyte-macrophage colony-stimulating factor administered during and after induction treatment for *de novo* acute myelogenous leukemia in elderly patients. Blood 1998;91:2722–2730.
138. Zittoun R, Suciu S, Mandelli F, et al. Granulocyte-macrophage colony-stimulating factor associated with induction treatment of acute myelogenous leukemia: A randomized trial by the European Organization for Research and Treatment of Cancer Leukemia Cooperative Group. J Clin Oncol 1996;14:2150–2159.
139. Lowenberg B, Boogaerts MA, Daenen SMGJ, et al. Value of different modalities of granulocyte-macrophage colony-stimulating factor applied during or after induction therapy of acute myeloid leukemia. J Clin Oncol 1997;15:3496–3506.
140. Ozer H, Armitage JO, Bennett CL, et al. 2000 Update of recommendations for the use of hematopoietic colony-stimulating factors: Evidence-based, clinical practice guidelines. J Clin Oncol 2000;18:3558–3585.
141. Bennett CL, Stinson TJ, Laver JH, et al. Cost analyses of adjunct colony stimulating factors for acute leukemia: Can they improve clinical decision making. Leuk Lymphoma 2000;37:65–70.
142. Lipshultz S, Lipsitz S, Sallan S, et al. Chronic progressive left ventricular systolic dysfunction and afterload excess years after doxorubicin therapy for childhood acute lymphoblastic leukemia. Proc ASCO 2000;19:580a (#2281).

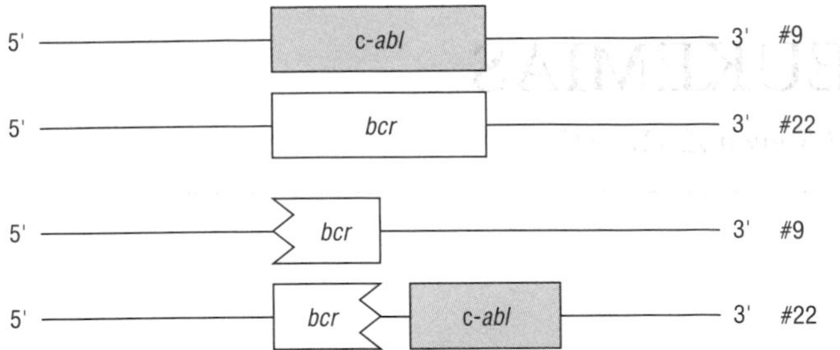

FIGURE 132–1. Diagram of the chromosomal translocation that results in the Philadelphia chromosome. This abnormality is encountered in 90% to 95% of patients who have chronic myelogenous leukemia.[89]

additional divisions by CML progenitor cells before reaching a nonproliferative stage; the resulting number of circulating granulocytes may be many times higher than normal. Immature CML progenitors are also less responsive to cellular and molecular controls that inhibit growth and proliferation in normal hematopoietic cells, such as the induction of apoptosis. Later in the clinical course of CML, cytopenias may occur corresponding to fibrotic changes in the bone marrow.[3] The chronic phase is not simply a period of increasing granulocytosis; it is common for the white blood cell count to oscillate, and the immature myeloid cells begin to lose the ability to differentiate into mature functioning cells.[2,3] At this stage, therapeutic intervention can effectively control the expansion of these clonal cells and normalize the white blood cell count. As CML progresses, the malignant clone becomes more genetically unstable, and chromosomal abnormalities other than Ph may occur. Clinical evidence of the accelerated phase of CML begins to emerge as the patient's white blood cell count becomes increasingly difficult to manage. The rate of progression of CML is subject to wide variability, and blastic phase can sometimes erupt without any apparent accelerated phase. The relative mass of the chronic phase cell populations, genetic predetermination, and differences in either genetic stability or proliferative state of the leukemic cells are possible explanations for this variability.[2,3]

The final stage of CML, known as the acute phase or blastic phase, is marked by the presence of rapidly proliferating blast cells that have lost the ability to differentiate into nonproliferating cells.[2,3] The proliferative advantage of blast cells over normal hematopoietic cells is even greater than that of chronic phase leukemic cells. CML in blastic phase is relatively resistant to treatment. The poor response to chemotherapy is not exclusively a result of drug resistance; it also results from the high proliferative rate of blastic phase CML and the replacement of malignant cells eliminated by chemotherapy.[3,8] The increased proliferative rate of blastic phase CML is the consequence of a number of factors, one of which may be the high levels of cytokines produced by CML cells. For example, interleukin-1β is produced in large quantities by CML cells in culture, and antibodies against interleukin-1β have been shown to inhibit the clonal expansion of blastic phase CML cells *in vitro*. Interleukin-1β may also indirectly stimulate blastic phase CML cells by inducing endothelial cells and fibroblasts to secrete hematopoietic growth factors.[9]

bcr-abl AS A THERAPEUTIC TARGET

The *bcr-abl* fusion gene produces a mutant tyrosine kinase that is involved in both the increased proliferation of the CML clone and in the reduction in FAS-mediated apoptosis. The characterization of the ATP binding site on the tyrosine kinase has led to a new class of inhibitors. The first of these inhibitors, STI571 (Gleevec), was recently approved for the treatment of CML. The early results of clinical trials suggest that this will be a very important agent in the treatment of CML, and is discussed in more detail under the treatment section of this chapter.[10,11]

CLINICAL PRESENTATION AND PROGNOSIS

The diagnosis of CML is usually made during the chronic phase following an abnormal peripheral blood smear. Occasionally, the blood sample is obtained during a routine physical examination or, more commonly, after the patient presents with symptoms such as weight loss, fatigue, malaise, night sweats, and fever. Splenomegaly and hepatomegaly are found in 30% to 40% of patients. Typical laboratory findings of the peripheral blood during the chronic phase include leukocytosis, thrombocytosis, basophilia, and low leukocyte alkaline phosphatase. In one series of newly diagnosed CML, the most common feature of the peripheral blood was a highly elevated white blood cell (WBC) count (>100,000/μL) occurring in about 70% of patients.[3,12]

Before the advent of modern therapeutic strategies, CML patients had a median survival after diagnosis of about 3 years, with only about 20% of patients alive at 5 years. With the use of current therapies, including single-agent and combination chemotherapy, interferon, and hematopoietic stem cell transplantation (HSCT), 5-year survival ranges between 40% and 80%.[13] To date, only allogeneic HSCT has been able to cure patients by permanently eliminating the Ph-positive clone. There are no long-term follow-up data for STI571, but it is likely that it will further improve 5-year survival rates without permanent elimination of Ph.

Important prognostic factors include age, spleen size, platelet number, and percent blasts at diagnosis. Although these factors have prognostic importance, they often fail to accurately predict the risk for disease progression in an individual patient. One recently identified molecular marker for disease progression is the methylation of the *abl* gene. The *abl* gene has an inhibitory effect on *bcr-abl* oncogene and its methylation reverses that inhibitory effect leading to progression to blast crisis.[14]

The accelerated phase is clinically the least distinct of the three phases of CML and may be difficult to recognize in some patients. Hematologic signs and symptoms reflect a progression in myeloproliferative acceleration and the approach of fatal blast crisis. Physical symptoms of acceleration include a resurgence of splenic enlargement, unexplained fever, and persistent bone pain. WBC counts and other signs and symptoms begin to be increasingly difficult to control with conventional oral chemotherapeutic agents. Recently, shortening of telomer length in CML cells was reported to be associated with shorter time to accelerated phase.[15]

The clinical course of CML terminates in blastic phase in which patients have peripheral blood and bone marrow findings very similar to acute leukemia. The one laboratory test that is used by most clinicians to confirm this phase is the presence of greater than 30% blasts in the bone marrow or peripheral blood.[3] The median survival for patients in blastic phase is 4 to 6 months, with most treatment options providing no survival advantage. STI571 has shown interesting activity in blastic phase CML.[11]

Cure of CML can be achieved only by eradication of the Ph-positive cells. Conventional cytotoxic chemotherapy can be used in chronic-phase CML to attain hematologic remission, which is defined as normalization of the white blood cell count. However, conventional chemotherapy used in chronic phase does not eliminate the Ph-positive clone and has only marginally improved median survival in CML. Interferon can produce hematologic and cytogenetic responses that lead to longer median survivals, but only rarely has been able to eliminate the malignant clone, as evidenced by recurrence of the Ph clone after stopping interferon therapy.[3] Cytogenetic remission has been defined as the elimination of Ph from bone marrow, whereas major cytogenetic response is defined as fewer than 35% Ph-positive cells in the bone marrow. Although bone marrow aspirates are the conventional method of determining response, it may be possible to use polymerase chain reaction (PCR) in peripheral blood buffy coat to measure *bcr* gene rearrangements to monitor disease status.[16] To date, only allogeneic HSCT has been shown to permanently eliminate the Ph-positive malignant clone. Table 132–1 illustrates the effect of various treatment modalities on survival in chronic-phase CML.[17]

TABLE 132–1. Effect of Therapy on Survival in Patients With Early Chronic-Phase CML

Therapy	5-year Survival (%)	Median Survival (months)
Busulfan	30–40	40–50
Hydroxyurea	40–50	50–60
Interferon	50–70	60–80
Interferon + Ara-C	60–80	NA[b]
Allogeneic Transplant[a]		
Sibling	60–80	NA[b]
Unrelated	50–70	NA[b]

[a]Results from experienced centers.
[b]Not available.
(Adapted from Refs. 17 and 26.)

▶ TREATMENT: Chronic Myelogenous Leukemia

CONVENTIONAL CHEMOTHERAPY

Although many chemotherapeutic agents have been used to manage chronic-phase CML, two have been used most frequently: busulfan (Myleran) and hydroxyurea (Hydrea). These agents can be taken orally, are inexpensive, have reasonable side-effect profiles, and are able to rapidly normalize elevated white blood cell counts in chronic-phase CML. Although both agents produce predictable declines in white blood cell count and in hematologic remissions in 70% to 80% of chronic-phase CML patients, busulfan and hydroxyurea have very little effect on Ph-positive cells in bone marrow.[2,3] Despite the fact that busulfan is still commonly used, results from a randomized study of nearly 500 CML patients by the German CML Study Group showed that hydroxyurea treatment provided a significant survival advantage of about 1 year over busulfan therapy and thus hydroxyurea has become the most commonly used agent to maintain target white cell counts in chronic phase CML.[18] More intense combination chemotherapy has not been shown to provide any improvement in survival over single-agent therapy.

Hydroxyurea inhibits the enzyme ribonucleotide reductase, leading to suppression of DNA synthesis, elimination of cells in the S phase of the cell cycle, and synchronization in the G_1 or pre-DNA synthesis phase.[19] Hydroxyurea is administered either daily or intermittently. In the daily schedule, hydroxyurea is initiated at 40–50 mg/kg/day in divided doses until the white blood cell count falls below 10,000/μL. At this point, the dose can be decreased to a maintenance level of 20 mg/kg/day, or temporarily discontinued and reinitiated at the daily maintenance dose when the white blood cell count begins to climb. With hydroxyurea therapy, the white blood cell count rarely continues to fall if the drug is discontinued. Because prolonged daily administration of hydroxyurea has been associated with adverse dermatologic effects, an intermittent maintenance dose of 20 mg/kg twice daily (40 mg/kg/day) 2 days each week is effective in controlling the white blood cell count while minimizing cutaneous toxicity.[19] Occasional dose adjustments may be required in both maintenance dose schedules. To demonstrate the variability in hydroxyurea dosing, Table 132–2 presents an alternative regimen that uses a sliding scale dose of hydroxyurea based on white blood cell count.

Initial doses of busulfan are 4–8 mg/day; this regimen is continued until the white blood cell count approaches 20,000/μL, at which time it is discontinued. The white blood cell count will continue to fall after the drug is discontinued and appropriate white blood cell counts can be maintained for several weeks without continuous drug therapy. Toxicities include prolonged myelosuppression, pulmonary fibrosis, and skin hyperpigmentation. Patients who received busulfan therapy prior to allogeneic HSCT appear to have a greater incidence of complications.[20] For this reason, and because of the possibility of inducing drug resistance in the malignant clone, busulfan is not recommended in patients who are candidates for HSCT.[3]

INTERFERONS

The interferons are a family of glycoproteins involved in many of the functional aspects of the hematopoietic system. Interferon-alpha (IFN-α) and interferon-beta (IFN-β) bind to the same cell-surface receptor on target cells, whereas interferon-gamma (IFN-γ) binds to a separate receptor. Although all have been studied in the treatment of chronic-phase CML, IFN-α has been most extensively investigated in the management of CML and is FDA approved for this indication.[3] IFN-α was first isolated from leukocytes after viral exposure. Two recombinant forms are presently marketed: IFN-α_{2a} (Roferon A) and IFN-α_{2b} (Intron A). In addition, a polyethylene glycol conjugate (PEG-IFN-α) approved for the treatment of hepatitis C is currently being evaluated in CML and may allow for less-frequent dosing and possibly improved tolerability. Fibroblasts are the primary source of IFN-β and although this form has potent inhibitory activity on CML cells *in vitro*, no effect has been shown in normalizing blood counts *in vivo*.[21] IFN-γ, originally found in T lymphocytes, has been

TABLE 132–2. Sliding Scale Dosing of Hydroxyurea

White Blood Cell Count ($\times 10^3/\mu$L)	Hydroxyurea Dosing Range (g)
>100	5–7
80–100	4–5
50–80	3–4
30–50	2–3
20–30	1.5–2
10–20	1.0–1.5
5–10*	0.5–1.0

*Desired maintenance white blood cell count.
(Adapted from Ref. 3.)

used in combination with IFN-α in the treatment of chronic-phase CML, with disappointing results.[22]

The exact mechanism of IFN-α activity in CML is unknown but may involve the binding of IFN-α to its receptor, which initiates a biochemical cascade that can result in direct cytotoxicity to leukemic cells. For example, synthesis of the enzyme 2′-5′-oligoadenylate-synthetase is enhanced by IFN-α receptor binding and results in the activation of RNAse, which leads to degradation of CML growth factors and oncogene transcripts required for growth of the malignant clone.[3,23] Another theory is that IFN-α receptor binding results in an increased expression of histocompatibility antigens, correcting a down-regulation of histocompatibility expression in the leukemic clone and resulting in the recognition of CML cells as "foreign" and improved immune surveillance.[3,24] Alternatively, a reduced expression of cell-adhesion molecules on CML progenitor cells may be responsible for their propensity to enter the circulation rather than adhering to the bone marrow stroma as do normal cells. This decreased adhesion could also be a mechanism by which the leukemic cells escape normal hematopoietic regulation. In coculture experiments performed with bone marrow-derived stromal cells and CML cells, it was found that cell adhesion was increased sixfold in the presence of IFN-α over control.[3,24,25]

The enthusiasm regarding the use of human IFN-α in the treatment of chronic-phase CML is based on the observation that some patients achieve cytogenetic response (a decrease or loss of Ph-positive cells), which leads to prolonged survival.[3,26] Studies performed with the two forms of recombinant IFN-α (IFN-α_{2a} and IFN-α_{2b}) demonstrate similar results. Long-term follow-up results from MD Anderson Cancer Center in early chronic-phase CML patients with partially pure human IFN-α, recombinant IFN-α_{2a}, and IFN-α_{2b} showed complete hematologic remissions (normalization of blood count) in about 80% of patients and major cytogenetic responses (suppression of Ph-positive metaphases to $<35\%$ of total) occurred in about 40%. Estimated median survival was 89 months.[27] Other groups have generally confirmed the MD Anderson experience, reporting that 50% to 70% of patients achieve a hematologic remission and about 30% to 50% obtain some form of cytogenetic response.[3,28,29] The doses used in these studies ranged from 2×10^6 U/m^2 to 5×10^6 U/m^2 administered daily either subcutaneously or intramuscularly.[27–29] Several smaller studies have used three-times-weekly dosing and have generally reported lower remission rates. The importance of IFN-α dose is discussed later in this section.[30–33]

Perhaps the most compelling evidence of IFN-α efficacy comes from four prospective, randomized studies compaeing IFN-α to chemotherapy. All of the studies show an improved survival rate in patients receiving IFN-α. Five-year survival rates in patients receiving IFN-α were about 50% to 60% as compared with 30% to 40% in patients receiving busulfan or hydroxyurea.[28,34,35,36] An updated review suggests that while 10-year survival may be as high as 40% to 50%, there is no clear survival plateau, which suggests that these patients are not cured of their disease.[37]

Although it is difficult to compare IFN-α studies because of variation in prior therapy, IFN-α dosing, and disease status at the time of treatment, several observations regarding IFN-α therapy can be made. First, patients who achieve any cytogenetic response have a distinct survival advantage over those with no decrease in the percentage of Ph-positive cells. Second, patients who have been previously treated with other agents, who have been diagnosed greater than 1 year prior to the start of therapy, or who are in accelerated-phase CML respond poorly to IFN-α. Third, the optimal dose schedule appears to be 5×10^6 U/m^2/day; doses above 5×10^6 U/m^2/day are likely to increase the incidence of toxicities while doses below 5×10^6 U/m^2/day may compromise response.[3,26]

TABLE 132–3. Recommended Dosing and Monitoring of IFN-α Therapy in CML

Cytoreduction	*Monitoring/Comments*
Hydroxyurea started	Reduces IFN-α toxicity
IFN-α started when WBC count drops to 10,000–20,000/μL	
IFN-α titration	
IFN-α start at 3×10^6U/day for 3–7 days	Premedicate with acetaminophen
Increase to 5×10^6U/day for 3–7 days	Elderly may not tolerate high doses SE: fatigue, depression, insomnia Hold and restart at 50% for severe SE
IFN-α maintenance	
IFN-α 5×10^6U/m^2/day	Maintain WBC above 2000/μL Platelets above 50,000/μL Cytogenetics every 3–6 months

SE, side effect.
(Adapted from Ref. 3.)

Because of the risk of intolerable toxicity and the importance of dose, IFN-α dosing regimens usually start low and are gradually increased. For example, one method of dosing IFN-α is 3×10^6 U/day for 3 to 7 days, followed by 5×10^6 U/day for 3 to 7 days, and followed by, if tolerated, 5×10^6 U/m^2/day as a maintenance dose.[3] Table 132–3 shows this IFN-α dosing regimen in chronic-phase CML along with toxicity and monitoring guidelines.

A cost-utility analysis performed in Europe and converted into US dollars shows that the use of low-dose IFN-α would cost less than \$20,000 per quality-adjusted life-year (QALY) gained as compared with \$50,000 to \$100,000 per QALY with higher-dose regimens.[38] The use of IFN-α in CML is easily justified on a cost-utility basis if the lower dosing regimens are equivalent to higher dose regimens. Because the results of most studies suggest that low-dose regimens are inferior, the cost of the higher dose regimen is more realistic. Another study performed in the United States found that the incremental cost effectiveness of IFN-α was \$34,800 per QALY. The dosing regimen of IFN-α used to develop the cost-effectiveness model was 5×10^6 U/m^2/day until a complete hematologic response and then changed to three-times-weekly maintenance dosing.[39] Because of the inability of IFN-α to cure CML, a cost-effectiveness study comparing IFN-α with matched unrelated allogeneic HSCT was performed. These investigators found an intermediate cost-effectiveness ratio between \$50,000 and \$100,000 per QALY in patients receiving HSCT.[40]

Adverse effects of IFN-α therapy may limit the administration of optimal doses of IFN-α and consist of both short-term constitutional effects and potentially dose-limiting long-term effects. The most predictable early toxicity is a flu-like syndrome characterized by fever, chills, myalgias, headache, and anorexia. These dose-dependent effects are a result of IFN-α-induced leukocytosis and release of cytokines. This acute flu-like syndrome can be ameliorated by starting IFN-α dosing at 50% of the final dose during the first week, giving the drug at bedtime, and coadministering acetaminophen or indomethacin. Reduction of initial white blood cell counts to around 10,000/μL with hydroxyurea may also reduce these symptoms.[3] Despite these methods of ameliorating toxicity, the flu-like syndrome is an important source of morbidity, occasionally requiring termination of therapy. Cardiovascular toxicities (tachycardia, hypotension) are seen in about 15% of patients in the first few weeks. Long-term adverse effects include weight loss, alopecia, neurologic effects (paresthesias, cognitive impairment, depression), and immune-mediated complications (hemolysis, thrombocytopenia, nephrotic syndrome, systemic lupus erythematosus, hypothyroidism), which can be dose limiting in about 5% to 20% of patients.[3]

There are an increasing number of studies evaluating combinations of IFN-α and chemotherapy, including busulfan, hydroxyurea, and cytosine arabinoside (Ara-C). Results from IFN-α plus busulfan studies reported cytogenetic responses at least as frequently as with IFN-α alone, but at the price of myelosuppression as a dose-limiting toxicity.[3,41] Three cycles of intensive chemotherapy consisting of daunorubicin, Ara-C, vincristine, and prednisone followed by daily maintenance IFN-α resulted in significant cytogenetic responses. These responses proved to be transient in most patients and survival rates were equivalent to patients treated with IFN-α alone.[2] Hydroxyurea is frequently used to lower white blood cell counts prior to administering IFN-α. While there are no data reporting improved response with combination hydroxyurea and IFN-α, it does not appear to have the toxicity associated with combination IFN-α and busulfan.[2,3]

Contrary to the experience with busulfan, hydroxyurea, or intensive chemotherapy, favorable outcomes have been reported from a combination of low-dose Ara-C and IFN-α. Two common methods of dosing Ara-C are 10 mg/m^2 subcutaneously for 10 days of each month or 15 mg/m^2 subcutaneously daily in divided doses for 2 weeks during the first cycle then for 7 days of each month thereafter. Studies have generally demonstrated a superior cytogenetic response in the combination regimen, as compared to IFN-α alone. Cytogenetic response in the combination group were in the range of 40% to 50% in early chronic phase as compared to 30% to 40% in the IFN-α alone groups.[42–44] In the largest study to date, 745 previously untreated patients in chronic phase were randomized to receive either hydroxyurea (50 mg/kg) and IFN-α (5×10^6 U/m^2), or the same combination plus Ara-C at 20 mg/m^2 for 10 days repeated monthly.[45] Patients who received Ara-C plus IFN-α therapy were found to have significantly improved survival, and the trial was prematurely terminated for that reason. The major cytogenetic response rate was 41% for the IFN-α plus Ara-C group versus 24% for the IFN-α group. It is generally thought that low-dose Ara-C will increase response rates in chronic phase CML patients being managed with IFN-α. This increased response may lead to improved survival compared to patients managed with IFN-α alone, but at the expense of increased myelotoxicity.[3,26]

The addition of polyethylene glycol to the IFN-α molecule produces a product with a longer half-life that allows once weekly instead of daily dosing.[3] In 43 heavily pretreated patients, CML dose ranging was performed with monotherapy PEG-IFN-α and a maximally tolerated dose of 630 μg every week was determined. Maximum tolerated dose for combined low-dose Ara-C and IFN-α was reached at 540 μg weekly.[46] More than 80% of patients had a complete hematologic remission and nearly 20% had a major cytogenetic response, both of which were encouraging results in these relatively high-risk patients. PEG-IFN-α is likely to be an important new formulation because of its improved toxicity profile and the importance of IFN-α dose in achieving cytogenetic response.

TYROSINE KINASE INHIBITOR

The tyrosine kinase inhibitors inhibit the p210 tyrosine kinase, which leads to differentiation and apoptosis in the CML clone. These agents competitively bind to the ATP-binding site of the tyrosine kinase, which leads to inhibition of the phosphorylation of kinase substrates and growth factor signals in the CML clone. The first agent of this class is a recently marketed agent STI571 (imatinib mesylate, Gleevec), which was approved by the FDA based upon important activity described in studies in chronic phase and blastic phase CML. A Phase I trial in chronic phase CML patients who failed IFN-α produced very impressive results. In this dose-escalation study of 54 patients, those patients who received at least 300 mg daily had a rate of complete hematologic remission of nearly 100% and a major cytogenetic remission rate greater than 30%. Hematologic responses were seen within 4 weeks of starting the drug. Major cytogenetic response occurred as early as 2 months and as late as 10 months after the start of treatment. A complete cytogenetic remission was obtained in seven patients (13%) and two of the seven patients had a molecular remission. The lack of a clear dose-limiting toxicity and the high response rates in these high-risk chronic phase CML patients makes STI571 unique among various therapies for CML.[10]

STI571 has also been studied in patients with blast crisis. Patients with blast crisis CML (n = 48) and Ph positive acute lymphoblastic leukemia (n = 10) were given 300–1,000 mg daily of STI571. The overall hematologic response rate was 79%. Major cytogenetic responses occurred in 7 of 58 patients (12%) with five of the seven being complete responses.[11]

Toxicity of STI571 includes nausea and vomiting, myalgias, and diarrhea. These toxicities are dose related and generally mild. In patients with blast crisis CML, neutropenia and thrombocytopenia can be severe, which may be related to disease response in a highly involved marrow.

These encouraging results suggest that STI571 may allow prolonged maintenance of patients in chronic phase, making CML a disease that can be managed indefinitely. In patients with blast crisis CML, it may allow conversion back to chronic phase where HSCT can be considered.

INVESTIGATIONAL AGENTS

Homoharringtonine (HHT) is a highly active plant alkaloid that is administered as a low-dose continuous infusion. Cytogenetic response is in the range of 30% to 40%, with many of these patients being IFN-α resistant.[3,47] In a recent evaluation of the combination of HHT and low-dose cytarabine in chronic phase CML, there was about a 70% complete hematologic remission and a 30% cytogenetic response. These results were similar to HHT alone, but survival was better in the combination group. The major limitation of HHT was cardiotoxicity associated with short infusion.

Decitabine is a hypomethylating cytidine analog. It produces response rates of 25% in blast crisis and 53% in accelerated phase. A recent report of 162 patients in CML blast crisis were treated with intermittent chemotherapy (n = 90), decitabine (n = 31), or other single agents (n = 41). Decitabine produced a small survival advantage in older patients as compared to intermittent chemotherapy.[3,48]

NONPHARMACOLOGIC THERAPY

Nondrug therapy for CML includes leukapheresis and splenectomy. Leukapheresis can be used to maintain safe white blood cell counts when pregnancy prevents the use of potentially teratogenic chemotherapy. Leukapheresis may be used when white blood cell counts become high enough (>100,000/μL) to cause symptoms of hyperleukocytosis and rapid reduction of WBC count is required. Leukapheresis is accompanied by allopurinol (300 mg/m^2/day) and, when possible, by hydroxyurea (1,000 mg/m^2 every 8 hours).[3]

Because splenomegaly is often a painful consequence of the disease, splenectomy has occasionally been a useful therapeutic intervention in CML. But controlled studies show that splenectomy does not delay the appearance of blastic phase, does not provide any benefit over chemotherapy alone and does not improve survival.[49] If performed before allogeneic HSCT, splenectomy may speed hematopoietic recovery, but may also increase the incidence of graft-versus-host disease (GVHD).[50] The role of splenectomy is limited and should be reserved for symptomatic relief in patients unresponsive to other treatments (chemotherapy, radiation).[3]

HEMATOPOIETIC STEM CELL TRANSPLANTATION

After reviewing all of the treatment modalities used for CML, the clinician is left with the fact that with conventional chemotherapy or IFN-α CML is ultimately a fatal disease. The only therapeutic option that can result in cure—defined as eradication of the Ph-positive clone—is allogeneic HSCT. INF-α can produce long-term survival but survival curves do not show a survival plateau consistent with cure. In contrast, HSCT has a distinct survival plateau with relapse rates being uncommon 5 years after transplant. Generally, HSCT is reserved for younger patients with an HLA-identical sibling donor. Although HSCT is discussed in detail in Chap. 134, this chapter discusses special aspects of HSCT that relate to the treatment of CML.

Approximately 60% of CML patients in chronic phase undergoing allogeneic HSCT from an HLA-identical sibling donor can be cured of their disease. Results with this type of transplant can be improved by transplanting patients within the first year of diagnosis, with 5-year survival rates approaching 80% at experienced centers.[3,51] In younger patients (< 50 years) with an HLA-matched sibling donor, allogeneic HSCT is considered the treatment of choice by most clinicians and should be performed shortly after diagnosis. Unfortunately, fewer than 30% of patients eligible for HSCT will have this ideal donor, and alternative donors must be considered.

The most common alternative donor is an unrelated individual who is HLA matched. Recent results from two studies are promising, with the studies reporting 50% to 60% of young patients undergoing transplantation within the first year of diagnosis being alive and in remission at 5 years.[52,53] These results and a prior decision analysis suggest that patients who are candidates for unrelated transplant, similar to patients undergoing HLA-matched sibling transplants, should be transplanted within the first year of diagnosis to optimize outcomes.[54]

In addition to age and length between diagnosis and transplant, another factor that may influence patient outcome following HSCT is the prior use of IFN-α. Beelen et al. reported that use of IFN-α prior to allogeneic HSCT is deleterious to outcomes.[55] There was a higher graft failure rate and slower engraftment time in patients receiving IFN-α therapy before transplant, leading to reduced 5-year survival rates. This study led to a series of reports evaluating the effect of pretransplant IFN-α on outcomes in patients undergoing allogeneic HSCT. In a group of unrelated HSCT patients, the use of IFN-α for greater than 6 months was associated with an increased risk of severe acute GVHD.[56] In a reanalysis of their data, Beelen et al. reported that patients receiving 12 months or more of pretransplant IFN-α were at significantly higher risk of transplant-related mortality.[57] A recent study reported an increased mortality in patients who received pretransplant IFN-α. A short period between the last dose of IFN-α and transplantation appeared to be the critical risk factor.[58] If IFN-α was discontinued at least 90 days before transplant, no effect on survival was observed. Finally, in a recent study by the International Bone Marrow Transplant Registry (IBMTR) in matched sibling donors, IFN-α for less than 6 months did not affect survival.[59] These studies in combination with the recent report that IFN-α response within the first 3 months of diagnosis predicts for good outcome has led to a recommendation by some experts to use IFN-α for 3 to 6 months at which time a decision can be made either to continue IFN-α or to proceed with a matched related or unrelated HSCT.[60]

While allogeneic HSCT can produce cure it is associated with early mortality. Given that many patients treated with INF-α are alive at 5 years, strategies to reduce the early mortality associated with HSCT are critical. One method of reducing the morbidity and mortality associated with acute GVHD in patients undergoing allogeneic HSCT is T-cell depletion of the donor stem cell product. Unfortunately, T-cell depletion increases the relapse rates in CML patients because of the loss of a graft-versus-leukemia (GVL) effect. The recognition that GVL is required to cure many patients with CML led to a series of studies evaluating methods to stimulate GVL after HSCT. Low-dose IL-2 ($2–6 \times 10^5$ U/m^2/day) has been used to produce a GVL effect starting a median of 60 days after transplant in a group of patients without acute GVHD. IL-2 effectively stimulated immune-related tumor surveillance, leading to significantly lower rates of disease relapse without high rates of severe acute GVHD. Immunostimulants such as IL-2 may be useful in reducing relapses in patients with minimal residual disease after HSCT.[61]

The use of donor lymphocyte infusion is another form of cellular immunotherapy. The infusion of lymphocytes from the stem cell donor stimulates a graft-versus-host reaction accompanied by a beneficial GVL effect. In relapsed CML, donor lymphocytes have been very successful in obtaining durable responses. These responses strongly correlate with the development of GVHD.[3] A recent study compared escalating doses of donor lymphocytes to single-dose lymphocytes. There was a significantly lower incidence of GVHD with escalating doses rather than single-dose donor lymphocytes with a similar 70% to 90% complete cytogenetic remission rate.[62] This study suggests that by administering donor lymphocytes in fractionated doses rather than a single large dose and waiting until after recovery from tissue damage caused by the preparative regimen, it may be possible to initiate a GVL effect while minimizing GVHD.

The importance of detecting the *bcr-abl* fusion gene product after allogeneic HSCT is controversial. A large study has clarified this issue in patients undergoing allogeneic HSCT for CML. Radich et al. studied 346 patients and collected 634 blood samples for PCR analysis of *bcr-abl*. This group found that a positive PCR 3 months or 36 months after transplant did not predict for relapse of their CML, but that a positive PCR at 6 or 12 months after transplant was highly predictive.[63] With this tool it may be possible to identify patients who are at high risk for clinical relapse after transplant and to treat them with donor lymphocyte infusion or IFN-α in an attempt to suppress or eradicate residual disease.[3]

The use of autologous HSCT has received attention as a result of the observation that there is a reduction in the Ph clone in marrow harvested in chronic phase and stored prior to transplantation. The use of IFN-α to obtain a cytogenetic remission followed by HSCT has resulted in prolonged relapse free survival with 50% disease-free at 5 years. Although this report is encouraging, it must be interpreted cautiously given the short follow-up.[64] Longer follow-up is required to determine whether patients who undergo autologous HSCT after achieving IFN-α–induced cytogenetic complete remission have been cured.

In general, relapse rates remain very high with autologous HSCT, and methods for successfully purging CML marrow have been elusive because of the similarity between CML cells and normal stem cells.

It is likely that purging CML cells would also eliminate normal marrow stem cells required for bone marrow engraftment. New molecular methods of purging, such as the *in vitro* use of antisense oligonucleotide directed against *bcr-abl* mRNA, may be more successful. Antisense oligonucleotides with sequences that are "antisense" and complementary to mRNA for the p210 BCR-ABL have been shown to suppress leukemic cell growth by 95% with no effect on the growth of normal and immature bone marrow cells. In addition to purging techniques, the use of posttransplant IFN-α and IL-2 in order to reduce relapse may be useful.[3,65]

CHRONIC LYMPHOCYTIC LEUKEMIA

Chronic lymphocytic leukemia is a lymphoproliferative disorder resulting in a progressive accumulation of functionally incompetent lymphocytes. CLL is an indolent disease that usually results from malignant transformation of a B lymphocyte with subsequent clonal proliferation. CLL is a common form of leukemia in the United States, but is rare in Japan and China. It is estimated that about 8,100 new cases of CLL will be diagnosed in the United States in 2001.[1] Occasional family clusters have been recognized, and first-degree relatives of patients with CLL are at three times the risk of developing a lymphoid malignancy as compared to the general population. CLL is a disease of the elderly, with a median age of onset in the sixth decade of life, although about 10% of CLL occurs in patients who are younger than 50 years of age and there is a slight male predominance. Etiologic factors have not been identified in CLL, and there are no data supporting either radiation or viral oncogenesis.[3]

CLINICAL PRESENTATION AND STAGING

The diagnosis of CLL is often made incidentally during a routine blood draw or after the patient complains of various constitutional symptoms (fatigue, fever). These symptoms result from reduction in normal hematopoiesis and the production of dysfunctional lymphocytes.[3] Often an abnormal CBC is characterized by high numbers of mature-looking small lymphocytes. Lymphocytosis is nearly always present, and a bone marrow aspirate usually shows an infiltration of mature-appearing lymphocytes making up 30% of nucleated cells. Diagnosis can be confirmed by analyzing phenotypic characteristics of the peripheral blood lymphocytes. If there is a monoclonal B lymphocytosis, this is often sufficient to confirm the diagnosis. Rarely, it becomes difficult to differentiate between CLL and a leukemic phase of indolent non-Hodgkin's lymphoma, which explains the occasional misdiagnosis of these disease entities. In about 60% of patients, there is lymphadenopathy, usually in the cervical, axillary, or inguinal areas. Intra-abdominal nodes may also be palpable, and about 50% of patients have spleen and liver enlargement. In addition to these relatively common presentations, lymphoid infiltrates can uncommonly be detected at other anatomic sites, including skin, lung, gastrointestinal tract, and central nervous system.[3]

A number of laboratory abnormalities can be identified at the time of diagnosis. As stated above, lymphocytosis in the peripheral blood and lymphocytic infiltration of the bone marrow are usually seen at diagnosis. Frequently, anemia, thrombocytopenia, and neutropenia are evident either at the time of diagnosis or some time during the course of the disease. The underlying reason for these cytopenias is not clear but most likely results from infiltration of the bone marrow by malignant lymphocytes. Other potential causes of cytopenias include autoimmune consumption of red blood cells and platelets and excessive T-suppressor cell or diminished T-helper cell function.[3] Hypogammaglobulinemia is often present at diagnosis and develops in nearly all patients as the disease progresses. Unlike the Ph in CML, there is no single cytogenetic marker for CLL. Although no single chromosomal rearrangement identifies CLL, more than 80% of patients with CLL have cytogenetic abnormalities. A number of the chromosomal rearrangements have predictive value in determining prognosis for a given patient.[3]

There is a wide variability in survival times, with some patients dying within a year of diagnosis and others living two decades with CLL. The Rai staging system has helped to design appropriate management strategies for CLL. The difference between stage I CLL and stage II CLL is the involvement of abdominal organs rather than more superficial lymph nodes. Prognosis is poorer with increasing stage, and it can be concluded that duration of survival is related to tumor burden at diagnosis. There remains variability in disease course within each stage so that one patient may have an indolent course with long survival time, whereas another patient may have more aggressive disease and a relatively short survival time. The Rai staging system has been combined into a risk classification scheme, low risk being stage 0, intermediate risk being stages I and II, and high risk being stages III and IV with median survivals of greater than 10 years, 7 years, and 2–4 years, respectively.[3]

▶ TREATMENT: Chronic Lymphocytic Leukemia

There are no curative treatments for CLL and therapy is designed to improve quality of life.[3] Without a method to cure this disease, it is not surprising that management of CLL patients is highly variable. Some clinicians delay drug therapy after diagnosis to obtain several weeks of baseline information on signs and symptoms of the disease.[3] The decision on whether drug therapy should be initiated after this baseline period is based on several parameters. Treatment is often instituted for the following indications: if there are signs and symptoms of progressive disease, worsening of blood dyscrasias, autoimmune complications, symptomatic splenomegaly, bulky lymph nodes, severe lymphocytosis (greater than 100,000–200,000/μL), and increased infectious complications.

Most stage 0 patients do not require treatment and are usually managed with close observation. In patients with stage I or II disease, management is controversial because the results of studies in this group of patients have not found a consistent survival benefit from drug therapy.[3] The use of cytotoxic chemotherapy in early stage CLL is usually reserved for patients who have disease characteristics consistent with more aggressive disease such as short lymphocyte doubling times and diffuse lymphocytic infiltrates in the bone marrow biopsy. In stage III and IV disease, treatment is required with the goal of achieving a partial or complete remission. Median survival times for patients who achieve some form of remission exceed 4 years, whereas those who do not achieve remission have a median survival of less than 2 years.[3] Historically, drug therapy is begun with chlorambucil and corticosteroids; chlorambucil can be replaced with cyclophosphamide without compromising response rates. Splenic radiation or splenectomy is often recommended in patients with stage III and IV disease to reduce symptoms and to improve autoimmune blood dyscrasia.[3]

CYTOTOXIC CHEMOTHERAPY

In a recent meta-analysis the controversies surrounding CLL management were evaluated.[66] The issue of deferred treatment was evaluated with delayed treatment having no adverse effect on 10-year survival. If only deaths caused by CLL are considered, there was a statistically significant improvement in survival when treatment was deferred. Chlorambucil with prednisone continues to be a common initial treatment for CLL. The use of this combination is based on a small number of studies. In the same meta-analysis discussed above, three small studies reported no advantage in the treatment of CLL with the addition of prednisone.[66] However, prednisone may be valuable in CLL associated autoimmune blood dyscrasias.[67] Chlorambucil is dosed either daily or intermittently every 2 to 4 weeks. One study showed that chlorambucil given intermittently reduced marrow toxicity without compromising response rates.[68]

Cyclophosphamide produces a similar response rate as chlorambucil and can be used in patients who have difficulty tolerating chlorambucil or in whom response is not optimal. Some patients refractory to chlorambucil will respond to cyclophosphamide. Cyclophosphamide is less commonly used because of its risk of hemorrhagic cystitis with prolonged treatment.[3]

Inadequate initial response to chemotherapy or the development of refractory disease after chronic treatment results in subsequent response rates that are half those seen with chlorambucil and prednisone in newly diagnosed patients. In these patients, more intensive combination chemotherapy resulted in response rates that range between 30% and 40% with median durations of response of less than 1 year.[3] The purine nucleoside analogs, fludarabine, 2-chlorodeoxyadenosine (2-Cda), and 2-deoxycoformycin (Pentostatin), have an important role in the management of patients who have become resistant to chlorambucil and increasingly in initial therapy for patients who have not received chemotherapy.

Fludarabine was initially studied in patients refractory to standard chlorambucil and prednisone. In a study of 369 patients with previously treated CLL, Keating et al.[69] reported that fludarabine produced about a 30% complete remission rate, and a 15% partial remission rate for an overall response rate of 45%. Sorensen et al. reported similar results with fludarabine in patients with refractory CLL.[70] In general, responses of significant duration occurred in patients with lower-stage disease. Patients receiving prior alkylating therapy who do not respond to the purine nucleosides have a poor survival. With these promising response rates in patients with refractory disease, fludarabine began to be studied in chemotherapy-naive patients, resulting in response rates of about 60% to 80%.[71] This high response rate was also reported in a randomized study comparing fludarabine to combination chemotherapy. Patients in the fludarabine arm had an overall response rate of 71% versus 60% for combination therapy. Fludarabine treatment also led to improvement in the duration of complete and partial remissions.[72] The most recent randomized study compared fludarabine to chlorambucil in the setting of primary therapy. Patients on fludarabine had a five times higher complete remission rate (5% to 20%). Despite the higher complete remission rate, no difference in overall survival and a higher rate of severe neutropenia and infection was observed in those treated with fludarabine.[73] There continues to be concern about the cost of fludarabine and its potent effects on $CD4^+$ lymphocytes and resulting infectious risk.[3,74]

Pentostatin and 2-Cda inhibit adenosine deaminase, leading to lethal accumulation of deoxyadenosine in lymphocytes. Pentostatin has only moderate activity in CLL, with a response rate of less than 30%. It is unlikely that Pentostatin alone will have a significant role in the treatment of CLL,[3,75] 2-Cda does have good activity in CLL, with overall response rates in the range of 45% in previously treated patients.[3,76] Despite equivalent overall response to fludarabine, complete remission with 2-Cda was only 4%, lower than that reported with fludarabine therapy. A small study in previously untreated patients suggested similar activity as with fludarabine, with an overall response rate of 85% and complete response rate of 25%.[77] Larger studies are required to investigate 2-Cda in the treatment of CLL to determine whether complete remission rates are comparable to fludarabine.

Cross-resistance between 2-Cda and fludarabine was evaluated in 28 fludarabine-resistant CLL patients. Only two patients had a partial remission with 2-Cda without normalization of anemia or thrombocytopenia. It is unlikely that patients who fail fludarabine therapy will benefit from 2-Cda.[78]

BIOLOGIC THERAPY

The current role of IFN-α is limited. Unlike low-grade non-Hodgkin's lymphoma or hairy cell leukemia, in which IFN-α responses range from 50% to 90%, the response in advanced CLL is less than 20%.[79] In one study, there was a 50% response with low-dose IFN-α (2×10^6 U/m^2 three times per week) in patients with untreated low-risk CLL.[3] The relevance of this finding is unclear given the good quality of life and long-term survival of these patients with supportive care alone.

A potentially useful application of low-dose IFN-α is following cytotoxic chemotherapy to increase the duration of response. Ferrara et al.[80] demonstrated a significant reduction in relapse in patients given IFN-α after cytotoxic chemotherapy. In addition, two patients who received a partial remission with chemotherapy subsequently had a complete remission with IFN-α therapy. This experience is consistent with observations that IFN-α works best in patients with low tumor burden.

There is limited information on monoclonal antibody therapy in CLL. CLL is a B-cell cancer with the lymphocytes usually expressing CD20, CD52, and other B-cell antigens. Alemtuzumab (Campath) has been recently approved for the treatment of refractory CLL. It binds to the CD52 molecule, which is highly expressed on the CLL clone. There seems to be a high partial response rate at the expense of both immunosuppression and myelosuppression.[81] The recent approval by the FDA was based on studies which showed about a 20% to 30% response rate in patients refractory to alkylating therapy and fludarabine. This response rate is encouraging given that these patients are usually unresponsive to any current therapy. There is a high risk of mortality from infection as a result of the potent immunosuppressive activity of Campath. Other toxicities include infusion-related reactions and myelosuppression.

Results with anti-CD20 antibody (Rituxan) have been disappointing despite its good activity in other B-cell cancers such as indolent NHL. One possible explanation for this poor activity is the low level of CD20 expression in CLL.[82]

Infection as a result of hypogammaglobulinemia is a major cause of morbidity and mortality in patients with CLL.[3] Low immunoglobulin levels have been reported in up to 70% of unselected patients with CLL. The decline in immunoglobulin concentrations correlates with the stage and duration of disease; patients with advanced disease or disease of long duration have the lowest immunoglobulin levels. CLL has the greatest effect on IgM followed by IgA and finally IgG.[83] The efficacy of administering intravenous IgG preparations to CLL patients with hypogammaglobulinemia was reported in a randomized, placebo-controlled, double-blind clinical trial of intravenous IgG dosed at 400 mg/kg every 3 weeks for 1 year.[84] There was a significant reduction in bacterial infections in the intravenous IgG group, with 14 bacterial infections versus 36 infections in the placebo arm. However, no significant difference in mortality from infections was observed. A cost-effectiveness study based on this experience demonstrated that its routine use is difficult to justify on a cost-utility basis.[85] The implications from these two studies are that intravenous IgG reduces non–life-threatening infections, but does not modify the risk of severe potentially fatal infections. Additionally, the value of giving only an IgG antibody when IgM and IgA deficiencies are most common must also be questioned.

Severe and persistent autoimmune-related decline in red blood cells and platelets is a significant source of morbidity and mortality in about 20% to 30% of CLL patients.[3] Although corticosteroids are considered the therapy of choice for autoimmune blood disorders associated with CLL, intravenous IgG may be helpful in patients who are not receiving benefit from prednisone or who are unable to receive prednisone.[3]

HEMATOPOIETIC STEM CELL TRANSPLANTATION

There is an increasing experience with the use of HSCT in CLL.[86] Early mortality with autologous and allogeneic HSCT is less than 10% and 15% to 40%, respectively. Those patients who achieve molecular remission as determined by PCR seem to have longer disease-free survival.[87] Cure is not currently achievable in CLL, but some experts believe that allogeneic HSCT is the most likely method of producing cure by initiating a GVL effect.[86]

Allogeneic HSCT for CLL is an area of growing interest. Although this modality of treatment holds promise of cure, difficulties will continue to arise given the advanced age of most CLL patients and high treatment-related mortality. The median age of onset of 60 years of age eliminates standard allogeneic transplant as an acceptable option for most CLL patients. Because cures are elusive in CLL and the best chance for cure may be the use of allogeneic HSCT, CLL may be a disease in which to evaluate low-intensity allogeneic HSCT.[3] Preliminary data suggest that low-intensity allogeneic HSCT with fludarabine-based preparation reduces transplant-related mortality while maintaining comparable disease remission as compared with standard allogeneic HSCT, although this is based on a small number of patients with short follow-up.[88]

EVALUATION OF THERAPEUTIC OUTCOMES

Chemotherapy in chronic-phase CML is used to maintain a normal WBC count and usually consists of oral hydroxyurea therapy. Although combination chemotherapy can produce hematologic remissions, it is unable to produce permanent cytogenetic responses. For the past several decades, allogeneic HSCT has been the only curative therapy for CML. Cytogenetic responses have been obtained with IFN-α, leading to an improved duration of survival. However, there are no convincing data to show that IFN-α can permanently eliminate the malignant clone. STI571 is an exciting new relatively nontoxic oral drug that is likely to replace IFN-α as initial therapy for patients who are not candidates for HSCT. It is likely that improved cure rates in CML will come by increasing the number of patients who can receive allogeneic HSCT. The use of low-dose intensity HSCT may allow the use of allogeneic transplant in older patients. Donor lymphocyte infusions may prolong survival in patients who have relapsed after HSCT. Because CLL is often an indolent disease that occurs in older patients, an important goal should be to optimize quality of life rather than to use aggressive, relatively toxic, therapy. Chemotherapy increasingly involves the administration of fludarabine with the intent of obtaining complete remission. However, in the older patient, the use of chlorambucil may still be preferred to decrease infectious risk. In younger patients with more aggressive CLL, autologous or allogeneic HSCT may offer long-term disease-free survival.

► PRINCIPLES OF PHARMACOTHERAPY

- Hydroxyurea has become the drug of choice to maintain white blood cell counts in CML patients in chronic phase.
- Busulfan should be avoided in patients who are being considered for HSCT.
- Allogeneic HSCT is the only method currently available that cures patients with CML.
- In patients younger than 50 years of age with a matched related or unrelated donor, allogeneic HSCT should be considered within the first year of diagnosis.
- Interferon-α was the first nontransplant therapy capable of inducing patients into cytogenetic remission.
- The recently approved drug STI571 is a well-tolerated orally administered drug that has been shown to produce cytogenetic remissions.
- Patients who achieve cytogenetic remission have improved survival.
- CLL is managed by reducing tumor load and preventing and treating infectious and hematologic complications.
- Fludarabine is now used initially for younger patients and chlorambucil is used initially in older patients or patients at high risk for infections.
- Fludarabine resistance predicts for resistance to other nucleoside drugs including 2-Cda and pentostatin.
- Campath is an effective salvage therapy in fludarabine resistant patients but at the expense of increased infectious mortality.
- Allogeneic or autologous HSCT may have a role in younger patients with CLL, although it is not clear whether these patients are cured of their disease.

REFERENCES

1. Greenlee RT, Hill-Harmon MB, Murray T, Thun M. Cancer statistics, 2001. CA Cancer J Clin 2001;51:15–36.
2. Faderl S, Talpaz M, Estrov Z, Kantarjian H. Chronic myelogenous leukemia: Biology and therapy. Ann Intern Med 1999;131:207–219.
3. Kantarjian H, Faderl S, Talpaz M. Chronic leukemias. In: Devita VT, Hellman S, Rosenberg SA, eds. Cancer: Principles and Practice of Oncology, 6th ed. Philadelphia, Lippincott, 2001:2433–2447.
4. Rowley JD. Molecular cytogenetics: Rosetta stone for understanding cancer—Twenty-ninth G.H.A Clowes Memorial Award Lecture. Cancer Res 1990;50:3816–3825.

5. Butturini A, Gale RP. Age of onset and type of leukemia. Lancet 1989;2: 789–791.
6. Waller CF, Fetscher S, Lange W. Treatment-related CML. Ann Hematol 1999;78:341–344.
7. Daley GQ, Van Etten RA, Baltimore D. Induction of chronic myelogenous leukemia in mice by the p210 *bcr-abl* gene of the Philadelphia chromosome. Science 1990;247:824–830.
8. Preisler H, Raza A. An overview of some studies of chronic myelogenous leukemia: Biological-clinical observations and viewing the disease as a chaotic system. Leuk Lymphoma 1993;11:145–150.
9. Estrov Z, Kurzrock R, Talpaz M. Role of interleukin-1 inhibitory molecules in therapy of acute and chronic myelogenous leukemia. Leuk Lymphoma 1993;10:407–411.
10. Druker BJ, Talpaz M, Resta DJ, et al. Efficacy and safety of a specific inhibitor of the *bcr-abl* tyrosine kinase in chronic myelogenous leukemia. N Engl J Med 2001;344:1031–1037.
11. Druker BJ, Sawyers CL, Kantarjian H, et al. Activity of a specific inhibitor of the *bcr-abl* tyrosine kinase in the blast crisis of chronic myelogenous leukemia and acute lymphocytic leukemia with the Philadelphia chromosome. N Engl J Med 2001;344:1038–1042.
12. Sawyers CL. Chronic myelogenous leukemia. N Engl J Med 1999;340: 1330–1340.
13. Hehlmann R, Hochhaus A, Berger U, et al. Current trends in the management of chronic myelogenous leukemia. Ann Hematol 2000;79:345–354.
14. Asimakopoulos FA, Shteper PJ, Krichevsky S, et al. ABL methylation is a distinct molecular event associated with clonal evolution of chronic myelogenous leukemia. Blood 1999;94:2452–2460.
15. Boultwood J, Peniket A, Watkins et al. Telomere length shortening in chronic myelogenous leukemia is associated with reduced time to accelerated phase. Blood 2000;96:358–361.
16. Stock W, Westbrook CA, Petersen B, et al. Value of molecular monitoring during the treatment of chronic myelogenous leukemia: A Cancer and Leukemia Group B study. J Clin Oncol 1997;15:26–36.
17. Hill JM, Meehan KR. Chronic myelogenous leukemia. Postgrad Med 1999;106:149–159.
18. Hehlmann R, Heimpel H, Hasford J, et al. Randomized comparison of busulfan and hydroxyurea in chronic myelogenous leukemia and prolongation of survival by hydroxyurea. Blood 1993;82:398–407.
19. Kennedy BJ. The evolution of hydroxyurea therapy in chronic myelogenous leukemia. Semin Oncol 1992;19:21–26.
20. Goldman JM, Szydlo R, Horowitz MM, et al. Choice of pretransplant treatment and timing of transplant for chronic myelogenous leukemia in chronic phase. Blood 1993;82:2235–2238.
21. Aulitzky WE, Despres D, Rudolf G, et al. Recombinant interferon beta in chronic myelogenous leukemia. Semin Hematol 1993;30:14–16.
22. Kloke O, Wandl U, Opalka B, et al. A prospective randomized comparison of single-agent interferon-alpha with the combination of interferon-alpha and low-dose interferon-gamma in CML. Eur J Hematol 1992;48:93–98.
23. Freund M, Huber C. Interferon alpha has become a standard in the treatment of chronic myelogenous leukemia. Semin Hematol 1993;30:1–5.
24. Dowding C, Gordon M, Guo A, et al. Potential mechanisms of action of interferon-alpha in CML. Leuk Lymphoma 1993;11:185–191.
25. Guilhot F, Lacotte-Thierry L. Interferon-alpha: Mechanisms of action in chronic myelogenous leukemia in chronic phase. Hematol Cell Therapy 1998;40:237–239.
26. Silver RT, Woolf SH, Hehlmann R, et al. An evidence-based analysis of the effect of busulfan, hydroxyurea, interferon, and allogeneic bone marrow transplantation in treating the chronic phase of chronic myelogenous leukemia: Developed for the ASH. Blood 1999;94:1517–1536.
27. Kantarjian HM, Smith TL, O'Brien, et al. Prolonged survival in chronic myelogenous leukemia after cytogenetic response to interferon-alpha therapy. The Leukemia Service. Ann Intern Med 1995;122:254–261.
28. The Italian Cooperative Study Group on Chronic Myeloid Leukemia. Interferon-alpha-2a as compared with conventional chemotherapy for the treatment of CML. N Engl J Med 1994;330:820–825.
29. Morra E, Alimena G, Lazzarino M, et al. Evolving approaches with interferon alpha in chronic myelogenous leukemia. Semin Hematol 1993;30:26–27.
30. Schofield JR, Robinson WA, Murphy JR, et al. Low doses of interferon-alpha are as effective as higher doses in inducing remissions and prolonging survival in chronic myelogenous leukemia. Ann Intern Med 1994;121:736–744.
31. Alimena G, Morra E, Lazzarino, et al. Interferon-alpha 2a as therapy for Philadelphia chromosome positive chronic myelogenous leukemia: A study of 82 patients treated with intermittent or daily administration. Blood 1988;72:642–647.
32. Freund M, von Wussow P, Diedrich H, et al. Recombinant human interferon-alpha 2b in chronic myelogenous leukemia: Dose dependency of response and frequency of neutralizing interferon antibodies. Br J Haematol 1989;72:350–356.
33. Anger B, Porzolt F, Leichte R, et al. A phase I/II study of recombinant interferon-alpha 2a for chronic myelogenous leukemia. Blut 1989;58:275–278.
34. Hehlmann R, Heimpel H, Hasford J, et al. Randomized comparison of interferon-alpha with busulfan and hydroxyurea in CML. Blood 1994;84:4064–4077.
35. Ohniski K, Ohno R, Tomonaga N, et al. A randomized trial comparing interferon-alpha with busulfan for newly diagnosed chronic myelogenous leukemia in chronic phase. Blood 1995;86:906–916.
36. Allan NC, Richards SM, Shepard PC, et al. UK Medical Research Council: Randomized, multicenter trial of interferon-alpha for chronic myelogenous leukemia: Improved survival irrespective of cytogenetic response. Lancet 1995;345:1392–1397.
37. Kantarjian HM, Gilles FJ, O'Brien S, et al. Therapeutic choices in younger patients with chronic myelogenous leukemia. Cancer 2000;89:1647–1658.
38. Liberato NL, Quaglini S, Barosi J. Cost effectiveness of interferon-alpha in chronic myelogenous leukemia. J Clin Oncol 1997;15:2673–2682.
39. Kattan MW, Inoue Y, Giles FJ, et al. Cost effectiveness of interferon-alpha and conventional chemotherapy in chronic myelogenous leukemia. Ann Intern Med 1996;125:541–548.
40. Lee SJ, Anasetti C, Kuntz KM, et al. The costs and cost-effectiveness of unrelated donor bone marrow transplantation for chronic phase chronic myelogenous leukemia. Blood 1998;92:4047–4052.
41. Freund M, Hild F, Grote-Metke A, et al. Combination of chemotherapy and interferon alpha-2b in the treatment of chronic myelogenous leukemia. Semin Hematol 1993;30:11–13.
42. Guilhot F. Interferon alpha and low-dose cytosine arabinoside for the treatment of patients with chronic myelogenous leukemia in chronic phase. Semin Hematol 1993;30:24–25.
43. Kantarjian HM, O'Brien S, Smith TL, et al. Treatment of Philadelphia chromosome positive early chronic phase chronic myelogenous leukemia with daily doses of interferon-alpha and low-dose Ara-C. J Clin Oncol 1999;17:284–292.
44. Rosti, Bonifaz F, DeVivo A, et al. Cytarabine increases karyotypic response in interferon-treated chronic myelogenous leukemia patients: Results of a national prospective randomized trial of the Italian Cooperative Study Group on chronic myelogenous leukemia. Blood 1999;94: 600a.
45. Guilhot F, Cahstang C, Michallet M, et al. Interferon-alpha 2a combined with cytosine arabinoside versus interferon alone in chronic myelogenous leukemia. N Engl J Med 1997;337:223–229.
46. Talpaz M, Cortes J, O'Brien S, et al. Peg-interferon-α2a (Pegasys) with or without Ara-C in patients with relapsed or refractory chronic phase chronic phase myelogenous leukemia. Blood 2000;96:736a.
47. Kantarjian HM, Talpaz M, Smith TL, et al. Homoharringtonine and low-dose cytarabine in the management of late chronic phase chronic myelogenous leukemia. J Clin Oncol 2000;18:3513–3521.
48. Sacchi S, Kantarjian HM, O'Brien S, et al. Chronic myelogenous leukemia in non-lymphoid blastic-phase. Cancer 1999;86:2632–2641.
49. The Italian Cooperative Study Group on Chronic Myeloid Leukemia. Results of a prospective randomized trial of early splenectomy in chronic myeloid leukemia. Cancer 1984;54:333–338.
50. Gratwohl A, Goldman J, Gluckman E, et al. Effect of splenectomy before bone marrow transplantation on survival in chronic granulocytic leukemia. Lancet 1985;2:1290–1291.

51. Lichtin AE, Woolf SH, Silver RT, Hehlmann R. Chronic myeloid leukemia—ASH Practice Guidelines and Beyond. Blood 1998, Educational Materials.
52. McGlave P, Shu XO, Wen W, et al. Unrelated donor marrow transplantation therapy for chronic myelogenous leukemia: 9 years' experience of the National Marrow Donor Program. Blood 2000;95:2219–2225.
53. Hansen J, Goolby TA, Martin PJ, et al. Bone marrow transplantation from unrelated donors for patients with chronic myelogenous leukemia. N Engl J Med 1998;338:962–968.
54. Lee SJ, Kuntz KM, Horowitz MM, et al. Unrelated donor bone marrow transplantation for chronic myelogenous leukemia: A decision analysis. Ann Intern Med 1997;127:1080–1088.
55. Beelen DW, Graeven U, Elmaagacli, et al. Prolonged administration of interferon-alpha in patients with chronic phase Philadelphia chromosome positive CML before allogeneic bone marrow transplantation may adversely affect transplant outcome. Blood 1995;85:2981–2990.
56. Morton AJ, Gooley T, Hansen JA, et al. Association between pretransplant interferon-alpha and outcome after unrelated donor marrow transplantation for chronic myelogenous leukemia in chronic phase. Blood 1998;92:394–401.
57. Beelan DW, Elmaagachi AH, Schaefer UW. The adverse influence of pre-transplant interferon-alpha on transplant outcome after marrow transplantation for chronic phase chronic myelogenous leukemia increases with the duration of interferon-alpha. Blood 1999;93:1779–1780. Letter.
58. Hehlmann R, Hochhaus A, Kolb HJ, et al. Interferon-alpha before allogeneic bone marrow transplantation in chronic myelogenous leukemia does not affect outcome adversely provided it is discontinued at least 90 days before the procedure. Blood 1999;94:3668–3677.
59. Giralt S, Szydlo R, Goldman JM, et al. Effect of short-term interferon therapy on the outcome of subsequent HLA-identical sibling bone marrow transplantation for chronic myelogenous leukemia: An analysis from the IBMTR. Blood 2000;90:410–415.
60. Mahon FX, Faberes C, Pueyo S, et al. Response at 3 months is a good predictive factor for newly diagnosed chronic myelogenous leukemia patients treated with recombinant interferon-alpha. Blood 1998;92:4059–4065.
61. Soiffer R, Murray C, Fairclough D, et al. Low-dose IL-2 following T-cell-depleted allogeneic bone marrow transplantation for chronic myelogenous leukemia. Blood 1994;84:213a.
62. Dazzi F, Szydlo M, Craddock C, et al. Comparison of single dose and escalating dose regimens of donor lymphocyte infusion for relapse after allografting for chronic myelogenous leukemia. Blood 2000;95: 67–71.
63. Radich JP, Gehly G, Gooley T, et al. Polymerase chain reaction detection of the BCR-ABL fusion transcript after allogeneic bone marrow transplantation for chronic myelogenous leukemia: Results and implications in 346 patients. Blood 1995;85:2632–2638.
64. Bhatia R, Verfaillie M, Miller JS, McGlave FB. Autologous transplantation therapy for chronic myelogenous leukemia. Blood 1997;89:2623–2634.
65. DeFabritiis P, Amadori S, Calabretta B, Mandelli F. Elimination of clonogenic Philadelphia positive cells using BCR-ABL antisense oligodeoxynucleotides. Bone Marrow Transplant 1993;12:261–265.
66. CLL Trialists' Collaborative Group: Chemotherapeutic options in chronic lymphocytic leukemia: A meta-analysis of the randomized trials. J Natl Cancer Inst 1999;91:861–868.
67. Mauro FR, Foa R, Cerretti R, et al. Autoimmune hemolytic anemia in chronic lymphocytic leukemia: Clinical, therapeutic, and prognostic factors. Blood 2000;95:2736–2792.
68. Sawitsky A, Rai KR, Glidewell O, et al. Comparison of daily versus intermittent chlorambucil and prednisone therapy in the treatment of patients with chronic lymphocytic leukemia. Blood 1977;50:1049–1059.
69. Keating MJ, O'Brien S, Kantarjian H, et al. Nucleoside analogs in treatment of chronic lymphocytic leukemia. Leuk Lymphoma 1993;10:139–145.
70. Sorensen JM, Vena DA, Fallavollita, et al. Treatment of refractory chronic lymphocytic leukemia with fludarabine phosphate via the group C protocol mechanism of the National Cancer Institute: Five-year follow-up report. J Clin Oncol 1997;15:458–465.
71. Keating MJ, O'Brien S, Lerner S, et al. Long-term follow-up of patients with CLL receiving fludarabine regimens as initial therapy. Blood 1998;92:1165–1171.
72. Johnson S, Smith AG, Loffler H, et al. Multicenter prospective randomized trial of fludarabine versus CAP for advanced stage chronic lymphocytic leukemia. N Engl J Med 1996;347:1432–1438.
73. Rai KR, Bercedis LP, Appelbaum FR, et al. Fludarabine compared with chlorambucil as primary therapy for chronic lymphocytic leukemia. N Engl J Med 2000;343:1750–1757.
74. Dighiero G, Binet JL. When and how to treat chronic lymphocytic leukemia. N Engl J Med 2000;343:799–801.
75. Pott-Hoeck, Hiddemann W. Purine analogs in the treatment of low-grade lymphomas and chronic lymphocytic leukemia. Ann Oncol 1995;6:421–433.
76. Saven A, Carrera CJ, Carson DA, et al. 2-Chlorodeoxyadenosine treatment of refractory chronic lymphocytic leukemia. Leuk Lymphoma 1991;5:133–138.
77. Saven A, Lemon RH, Kosty M, et al. 2-Cda activity in patients with untreated chronic lymphocytic leukemia. J Clin Oncol 1995;13:570–574.
78. O'Brien S, Kantarjian H, Estey E, et al. Lack of effect of 2-chlorodeoxyadenosine therapy in patients with chronic lymphocytic leukemia refractory to fludarabine therapy. N Engl J Med 1994;330:319–322.
79. Montserrat E, Villamor N, Urbano-Ispizua A, et al. Alpha interferon in chronic lymphocytic leukemia. Eur J Cancer 1991;27:S74–S77.
80. Ferrara F, Rametta V, Mele G, et al. Recombinant interferon-α-2A as maintenance treatment for patients with advanced stage chronic lymphocytic leukemia responding to chemotherapy. Am J Hematol 1992;41:45–49.
81. Rai KR. New biologic therapies. Semin Hematol 1999;26:107–114.
82. Keating MJ. Chronic lymphocytic leukemia. Semin Oncol 1999;26:107–114.
83. Morrison VA. The infectious complications of chronic lymphocytic leukemia. Semin Oncol 1998;25:98–106.
84. Cooperative Group for the Study of Immunoglobulin in Chronic Lymphocytic Leukemia. Intravenous immunoglobulin for the prevention of infection in chronic lymphocytic leukemia. A randomized, controlled clinical trial. N Engl J Med 1988;319:902–907.
85. Weeks JC, Tierney MR, Weinstein MC. Cost effectiveness of prophylactic intravenous immune globulin in chronic lymphocytic leukemia. N Engl J Med 1991;325:81–86.
86. Pavletic ZS, Arrowsmith ER, Bierman PJ, et al. Outcome of allogeneic stem cell transplantation for B-cell CLL. Bone Marrow Transplant 2000;7:717–722.
87. Provan D, Bartlett-Pandite L, Zwicky C, et al. Eradication of PCR detectable chronic lymphocytic leukemia cells is associated with improved outcome after bone marrow transplantation. Blood 1996;88:2228–2235.
88. Schetelig J, Held TK, Bornhauser M, et al. Non-myeloablative allogeneic stem cell transplants in chronic lymphocytic leukemia from related and unrelated donors. Blood 2000;96:200a.
89. Fishleder AJ. Oncogenes and cancer: clinical applications. Cleve Clin J Med 1990;57:721–726.

133
MELANOMA

Rowena N. Schwartz

Cutaneous melanoma is becoming an increasingly more common disease. It is estimated that about 51,400 new cases of melanoma will be diagnosed in 2001; this projection may represent an underestimation, however, as many superficial and *in situ* melanomas are probably underreported. In the late 1970s, the incidence of cutaneous melanoma in the United States took a dramatic leap; it is estimated that the risk of developing melanoma for someone born in the United States in the year 2000 may be as high as 1 in 85.[1,2] During the past decade, the incidence of melanoma has increased in the United States at a rate faster than that of any other malignancy except for lung cancer in women.

Worldwide, the incidence of cancer varies. The incidence is about 1 per 100,000 per year in the non-Caucasian population, but is as high as 40 per 100,000 per year for fair-skinned people living in the Queensland province of Australia.[3] The increase in the incidence of melanoma has most affected industrialized countries. Not only has the incidence of this malignancy increased dramatically—by over 80% between 1973 and 1987—but also the mortality has increased by almost 30%.[4] Melanoma is one of the few cancers in which both the incidence and the mortality are increasing every year.

ETIOLOGY

The etiology of melanoma, like that of most other malignancies, is not fully understood. A number of host factors and environmental factors have been identified, and it is likely that these factors alone or in combination increase the occurrence of cutaneous melanomas. These factors are listed in Table 133–1.

Genetic factors have been strongly linked to the development of melanoma, but appear to account for only a small percentage of the overall incidence. Familial atypical multiple mole syndrome (FAMMS) or hereditary dysplastic nevus syndrome (HDNS) is a hereditary disease characterized by a predisposition to develop dysplastic nevi and cutaneous melanoma. About 8% to 10% of cases of melanoma are associated with family history or HDNS. The $p16^{INK4a}$ gene localized on the 9p21 locus is affected through germline mutations or deletions in approximately 50% of patients with familial melanoma. In individuals with dysplastic nevus and a family history of cutaneous melanoma, the cumulative lifetime incidence approaches 100%,[5] whereas dysplastic nevi are thought to be precursors of 20% to 40% of sporadic melanoma.

Sunlight is one of the most important environmental factors in the pathogenesis of melanoma. It was once thought that only radiation in the ultraviolet B (UVB) range (280 to 320 nm) was important in the etiology of melanoma. It now appears that prolonged exposure to radiation in the ultraviolet A (UVA) range (320 to 400 nm) is also an important risk factor for the development of sporadic melanoma. This has created a concern about recommendations for UVB-blocking sunscreens as a method for preventing melanoma. When used correctly, these sunscreens prevent the physical symptoms of a sunburn including erythema and pain and the prevention of burn symptoms may allow individuals to sustain a more prolonged sun exposure, ultimately resulting in intense irradiation of the skin by UVA light.

The incidence of melanoma has been associated with the latitude and the intensity of solar exposure among susceptible populations. Whites with fair hair (red or blond) and light-colored eyes (blue, gray, or green) who have a tendency to burn and/or rarely tan with exposure to sunlight are especially at risk. The risk of developing non-melanoma skin cancers, such as squamous cell and basal cell cancer, is directly related to total sun exposure, and it was thought that melanoma was similarly related to lifetime exposure to the sun. Epidemiologic research has not been able to demonstrate a similar relationship between cumulative exposure to sunlight and the occurrence of cutaneous melanoma. In fact, studies have demonstrated that the risk for the development of melanoma is lower in outdoor workers than in indoor workers.[6] These findings suggest that the relationship of the sun to cutaneous melanoma is more complex than that of total exposure. Intermittent overexposure to sunlight, blistering sunburns, and the time of life of exposure to the sun are now believed to be the more critical factors for development of cutaneous melanoma.[3] Individuals who have a history of severe sunburns appear to have a higher risk of developing melanoma than those individuals who have had chronic sun exposure without a history of sunburn. The risk with sunlight and ultraviolet radiation seems to be most active during childhood and adolescence. Intensive exposure to sunlight during infancy and early adolescence is more hazardous than exposure during adult life.

Immunocompromised patients are at increased risk for the development of cutaneous melanoma. Immunodeficiency affects those individuals with ataxia telangiectasia, chronic lymphocytic leukemia, Hodgkin's disease, and immunosuppression following organ transplant. Acquired immunodeficiency syndrome (AIDS) also has been shown to increase the risk of developing cutaneous melanoma.

PATHOGENESIS

The pathogenesis of melanoma is not fully understood, but advances in immunology and molecular biology of melanoma provide a number of potential new avenues for the development of novel treatment strategies. Human melanocytes are dendritic pigmented cells that arise from the neural-crest tissue during early fetal development and migrate by 4 to 6 weeks to a variety of sites within the body, such as the skin, uveal tract, meninges, and ectodermal mucosa. In the adult, the majority of melanocytes are located at the epidermal-dermal junction of the skin and the choroid of the eye, but they can be found in a variety of other tissues, such as the meninges and the alimentary and respiratory tract. Primary melanoma can therefore arise in any area of the body with melanocytes. The skin is the most frequent site of melanoma; cutaneous melanoma constitutes 90% of all melanoma. Primary melanoma can also arise in the eye (ocular melanoma) and, less frequently, in the meninges, respiratory tract, and gallbladder.

TABLE 133–1. Risk Factors for Melanoma

Host Risk Factors	External Risk Factors
• Adulthood (>15 years) • History of cutaneous melanoma • Dysplastic nevi • Cutaneous melanoma in first-degree relative • Immunodeficiency/immunosuppression • High density of nevi • High degree of freckling • Sunburn easily/tan rarely • Blond or red hair • Blue or green or gray eyes • Socioeconomic status (higher > lower) • White (vs. black) race	• Intense intermittent sun exposures • History of sunburn • More than 4 painful sunburns before the age of 15 • Outdoor leisure

Compiled from Refs. 1 and 4.

Normal melanocytes arise from melanoblasts and undergo a series of differentiation events before reaching a final end-cell differentiation state. They can be arrested in their differentiation process at any given state of maturation without loss of their proliferation capacity. Melanocytes adhere to the basement membrane of the epidermis and, despite a resting state, maintain a lifelong proliferation potential. Melanocytes synthesize melanin to protect various tissues, such as the skin, from ultraviolet radiation-induced damage, and reach the keratinocytes in the upper layers of the epidermis via dendrites. Tyrosinase is an essential enzyme used within the melanosomes to synthesize melanin.

There is a malignant transformation of skin melanocytes or of preexisting nevocellular nevi in the development of melanoma, and the development and progression of melanoma from melanocytes follow a series of distinct steps. The pathologic components of the progression in human melanoma appear to involve a series of morphologic stages: (1) an acquired or congenital melanocytic nevus, (2) melanocytic nevus with architectural atypia, (3) histologically dysplastic nevus with cytologic atypia and architectural atypia, (4) primary melanoma in radial growth phase in which limited growth and radial expansion of the nevus may occur without metastatic competence (nontumorigenic melanoma), (5) primary melanoma in vertical growth phase with or without transit metastases in which proliferation and increased angiogenesis appear to be uncontrolled, (6) regional lymph node metastatic melanoma (lymphatic), and (7) distant metastatic melanoma (hematogenous).[7,8] Individual melanomas can omit steps in this development. The progression from the melanocyte to the melanoma likely involves genetic aberrations.

Primary melanoma is characterized by radial growth and limited vertical thickness (<0.75 mm). Although primary melanoma demonstrates little tendency to metastasize, it has a potential for metastasis with the onset of a vertical growth phase. Metastatic melanoma is seen with an increase in vertical thickness. Therefore, the thickness of a primary melanoma is an important prognostic indicator that is used in the staging classification of cutaneous melanoma.

Normal melanocytes require growth factors for proliferation, but melanoma cells are able to proliferate in the absence of growth factor supplementation. Melanoma cells secrete a variety of growth autocrine and paracrine factors that facilitate their proliferation. Additionally, with progression, melanoma cells increase production of certain growth factors and cytokines. Basic fibroblast growth factors are thought to be an important mediator of growth stimulation and cell survival, and they act as a motility factor for melanoma cells. They up-regulate serine proteinases and metalloproteinases. Melanoma cells are strong producers of chemoattractive proteins such as interleukin-8 (IL-8). Vascular endothelial growth factor can be triggered in the vertical growth phase. Most of these changes occur between the radial growth phase and the vertical growth phase of primary melanoma, and metastatic cells often show the highest productions of cytokines.

The types of products that have been isolated from melanoma include various growth factors, proteases, protease inhibitors, cell adhesion proteins, and host response modifiers.[9] Melanoma cells express all major types of adhesion receptors, including integrins and cadherins. Expression of these receptors increases with melanoma progression.

The understanding of the biology of melanoma has provided potential targets for drug therapy. For example, the understanding of hematopoietic and dendritic cell growth factors, has led to the clinical investigation of granulocyte-macrophage colony-stimulating factor in melanoma. The identification of potential targets for therapy, such as fibroblast growth factors has led to investigations of antisense oligonucleotides to block the role of the basic fibroblast growth factors in modulating melanoma.

Immune factors appear to be involved in the progression of melanoma more than in most other solid tumors. Spontaneous cancer regressions are rare, but are a well-documented phenomenon seen in melanoma.[1] Focal regression in primary melanoma has also been reported. The regression of tumor appears to be associated with host immunity.

The use of monoclonal antibodies has made it possible to identify a number of different tumor antigens on melanoma cells in both human and murine models. Melanoma-associated antigens have been identified in the cellular membrane and cytoplasm of melanoma cells. Ganglioside antigens have been of particular interest in the development of immunotherapy for melanoma. A large number of murine monoclonal antibodies to melanoma-associated antigens have been developed and are currently being used in clinical trials for the diagnosis and the treatment of melanoma.

The humoral and cellular responses of individuals with melanoma-associated antigens offer an insight into the potential of immunotherapy in the management of metastatic disease. Melanoma-directed antibodies have been isolated in the sera of patients with melanoma. The presence of antimelanoma antibodies in the sera of patients correlates with the clinical status of the patients, and the antibodies disappear from the serum as the disease progresses. This phenomenon may be explained by the possible formation of anti-idiotype antibody directed against the antimelanoma antibody, by the increase in the circulation of soluble tumor antigens that saturate all the antibody combining sites, by the elevation in the levels of immunosuppression, or by the absorption of the antibodies on the tumor mass.

In recent years, interest has focused on the role of the cell-mediated immune response in melanoma. Specific cell-mediated responses may play a role in tumor regression, but the role of specific cells such as cytotoxic T lymphocytes is not fully understood. Tumor-infiltrating lymphocytes have been shown *in vivo* and *in vitro* to possess antitumor reactivity. Because many of these tumor-infiltrating lymphocytes are tumor-specific, they have been a target for manipulation in immunotherapeutic approaches for melanoma.

Specific genetic alterations have been demonstrated in the pathogenesis of melanoma. At least six genes with loci showing random deletions, rare translocations, and rare amplifications on chromosome 1, 6, 7, 9, 10, and 11 have been identified in melanoma cells.

Alterations in other genes located on other chromosomes may also contribute to the progression of melanoma. Alterations of chromosome 1 are seen in many forms of human cancer. The region of chromosome 1 that is involved in melanoma involves the tumor suppressor gene. The alterations seen in chromosome 6 potentially link melanoma and the major histocompatibility complex. As noted earlier, melanoma frequently affects the 9p21 locus. In sporadic melanoma, sporadic mutations are found in the *ras* gene; this mutation is seen more commonly in melanomas related to sun exposure. A number of oncogenes can be activated in melanoma. The genetic influence to melanoma progression appears to involve a series of complex interactions. As these interactions are understood, the potential for gene therapy in melanoma expands.

HISTOLOGIC SUBTYPES

Cutaneous melanomas are categorized by growth patterns. The four histologic subtypes of cutaneous melanoma are distinctive in developmental phases and clinical features. The four major subtypes of cutaneous melanoma are superficial spreading melanoma, nodular melanoma, lentigo maligna melanoma, and acral lentiginous melanoma.[10] There is no difference in the clinical outcome of the four subtypes, if the comparison is controlled for depth of penetration. Uveal melanoma is considered a separate disease from cutaneous melanoma.

Superficial spreading melanoma is the most common morphologic type of cutaneous melanoma and accounts for about 60% to 70% of all melanoma. The lesions usually arise from a preexisting nevus and evolve slowly over 1 to 5 years. At some point, superficial spreading melanoma may progress to a more rapid growth phase. Early in the lesion development, the superficial spreading melanoma is a flat macule or barely raised plaque with color variations that are black or blue. As the lesion develops, the surface becomes irregular and asymmetric. The lesion enlarges when it enters a vertical growth phase, and the edges appear notched, scalloped, or lacy. Patches of regression may appear within the lesion, signified by amelanotic or depigmented areas. Superficial spreading melanoma usually occurs after puberty and is more common in women.

Nodular melanoma is the second most common growth pattern of melanoma and occurs in 15% to 30% of patients. It has no radial growth phase; it is a "pure" vertical growth phase disease. In nodular melanoma, a small, expansive nodule in the papillary dermis invades the reticular dermis and subcutis. Nodular melanoma is more aggressive and develops more rapidly than superficial spreading melanoma. These lesions are dark blue-black or bluish-red and often uniform in color, although a small percentage of nodular melanomas are amelanotic and have a fleshy appearance. Nodular melanomas are raised and often symmetric. They occur at any age and are most common on the trunk, head, and neck. Nodular melanomas are more common in men.

Lentigo maligna melanoma represents a small percentage of melanomas. It is unique in that it does not have the same propensity to metastasize that the other histologic subtypes have. Lentigo maligna melanomas are generally large (>3 cm), flat, and tan-colored lesions with shades of brown and black. This subtype of melanoma occurs in an older age group, typically appearing on the face of elderly Caucasians. Lentigo maligna melanoma is uncommon before the age of 30 and may have been present for over 5 years before it is recognized.

Acral lentiginous melanoma is characteristically seen on the palms of the hands, soles of the feet, and beneath the nailbeds. Most acral lentiginous melanomas are located on the sole of the foot and look like a large (>3 cm) tan or brown stain. The lesions often have irregular, convoluted borders. Acral lentiginous melanoma includes subungual melanoma and may present as a brown or black line in the great toe or the thumbnail. About half of the subungual melanoma result in nail destruction, and a majority ulcerate. Acral lentiginous melanoma occurs in less than 10% of Caucasians with melanoma, but is the most common type of melanoma reported in African Americans (70%), Asians (46%), and Hispanics.

Uveal melanoma is the most common primary intraocular malignancy seen in adults, but is an uncommon tumor. Unlike cutaneous melanoma, the frequency and mortality of uveal melanoma has remained steady. This melanoma arises from the pigmented epithelium of the choroid. Iris melanoma is a subset of uveal melanoma and tends to have a more benign course. The risk of metastasis varies with the histologic type and size of the tumor, as well as the location in the eye. Metastases occur most frequently in the liver, but have been documented in a variety of tissues.

CLINICAL PRESENTATION

The initial clinical presentation of melanoma is often a melanoma lesion, as more than 90% of all primary melanomas are grossly visible. The lesion can be located anywhere on the body, but is most common on the lower extremities in women and on the back and trunk of men. The clinical features used to describe or evaluate a questionable lesion are called the ABCDs of melanoma. Unlike benign pigmented lesions, the shape of a melanoma lesion is often (A) *asymmetric*. Benign lesions tend to have regular margins, whereas melanoma lesions often have irregular (B) *borders*. The (C) *color* of melanoma lesions is often variegated, ranging from tan to blue-black, and at times, the lesion is intermingled with colors of red, purple, and white. The size or (D) *diameter* of a melanoma lesion is frequently 6 mm or greater when it is identified, whereas benign lesions are usually smaller. Early melanoma lesions may be diagnosed at a smaller size. Another warning sign of a potential melanoma is a change in a preexisting nevus. Some clinicians use the ABCDEs of melanoma, adding (E) for *evolution* or *enlargement* of a mole. Changes such as a sudden or continuous enlargement of a lesion, an elevation of a lesion, or any change in the skin surrounding a nevus, including redness or swelling, are important clinical signs. Uncommonly, the sensation of the lesion may become itchy, or tender and painful. Friability of the lesion, resulting in bleeding or oozing, is also a danger sign.[11] Perhaps the most important warning sign of danger is the evolution in any characteristic of a lesion.

The clinical appearance of a melanoma depends on the histogenesis and the stage of development of the lesion. It is usually possible to distinguish three variants of cutaneous melanoma, including flat melanoma, nodular melanoma, and a flat melanoma with a nodular area. Flat melanoma usually corresponds to the histologic classification of superficial spreading melanoma.

The number of pigmented moles (melanocytic nevi) and non-melanocytic lesions that resemble melanoma complicate the identification of melanoma. White adults average between 10 and 40 ordinary nevi on their skin. These lesions are usually absent at birth, increase in number through adult life, then gradually decline in number. They appear as tiny pinpoint macules and are usually uniform in color, but increase in size to a maximum of 4 to 6 mm. The appearance of non-melanocytic pigmented lesions, such as seborrheic keratoses, pigmented basal cell carcinoma, and vascular lesions can also be similar to that of a melanoma lesion.

TABLE 133–2. Self-Examination of Suspicious Moles

- Examine your body front and back in the mirror, and then right and left sides, arms raised.
- Bend elbows and look carefully at forearms and upper arms and palms.
- Look at the backs of the legs and feet. Look specifically in the spaces between toes and at the soles of the feet.
- Examine the back of the neck and scalp with the help of a hand-held mirror; part hair (or use blow dryer) to lift hair and give you a closer look.
- Check the back and buttocks with a hand-held mirror.

Derived from publications of the American Academy of Dermatology.

SCREENING

Improved survival rates for melanoma are thought to result from the treatment of lesions diagnosed at an earlier stage of development. Efforts to improve survival are concentrated on the diagnosis and treatment of the primary lesion. The identification of early melanoma allows the opportunity to treat the lesions when they are thin and curable. The cost-effectiveness of massive screening for all adults by a physician has never been demonstrated. A number of agencies, such as the American Academy of Dermatology and the American Cancer Society, have sponsored free annual screenings. Routine examination of the skin by physicians is recommended for individuals at high risk. The entire cutaneous surface should be examined, including the scalp.

Self-examination of the skin places the responsibilities of identification on the individual. Educational pamphlets describing the method of self-examination for the public are available through the American Cancer Society, the American Academy of Dermatology, and the Skin Cancer Foundation (Table 133–2). If a newly discovered pigmented lesion appears or if a preexisting pigmented lesion changes, the individual should see a physician immediately.

DIAGNOSIS

A biopsy is critical in establishing the diagnosis of melanoma. The subsequent histologic interpretation of the biopsy determines the therapy and prognosis. An excisional biopsy with a margin of normal-appearing skin is recommended for a suspicious lesion, with a section of underlying subcutaneous fat included for microstaging.[12] When an excisional biopsy is impractical, an incisional biopsy can be performed, but it should include a core of full thickness of skin and subcutaneous tissue. When excisional biopsies may be inappropriate, as with the face or palmar surface of the hands, a full-thickness incisional or punch biopsy is preferable to a shave biopsy.

Examination of any individual with a suspected melanoma includes a complete history and total body skin evaluation. The focus of the patient history is to identify potential risk factors, and it must include a complete family history. Total dermatologic examination is necessary for staging. For patients with melanomas of 1 mm or more in thickness, baseline chest x-ray examination and liver chemistries are generally recommended, despite the fact that they are relatively insensitive in detecting clinically occult distant disease. Any clinical indication of regional lymph node involvement should be confirmed by means of fine needle aspiration or biopsy of the enlarged lymph node. Additionally, any other signs or symptoms suggestive of metastatic disease should be completely evaluated.

TABLE 133–3. Clark Level

Clark Level	Anatomic Landmark
N	Epidermis
I	Dermo-epidermal junction
II	Papillary dermis
III	Interface between papillary dermis and reticular dermis
IV	Reticular dermis and subcutaneous fat

STAGING

The size of a primary melanoma lesion correlates with the likelihood of metastases. The prognostic factor originally used to determine survival was based on the cross-sectional profile of the primary tumor; the cross-sectional profile could be evaluated if the deepest invasive tumor cells lay above or below the sweat glands.[13] Clark further clarified this assessment, describing the relationship between the depth of invasion of the cancer cells and the standard anatomic landmarks of the skin (Table 133–3).[14] Clark's classification is a practical approach for patients with more superficial tumors, because tumors classified as Clark's levels I through III seldom metastasize. Criticism of the Clark classification system is related to problems associated with practical measurements. Melanoma lesions that occur in the presence of lymphoid infiltration, fibrosis, or even the cells of preexisting nevi are difficult to assess with classic reference landmarks.

Breslow replaced Clark's classification of reference landmarks, using instead the thickness of the primary melanoma lesion for classification.[15] Tumor thickness is quantified to the nearest tenth of a millimeter with an ocular micrometer, measuring from the top of the granular layer of the overlying epidermis to the deepest contiguous invasive melanoma cell. The correlation between tumor thickness and probability of tumor metastases is strong, but does not take into account aspects such as tumor satellites and vascular invasion. There are a number of prognostic factors, in addition to tumor thickness and level of invasion, that have been associated with a patient's probability of developing metastatic disease, although tumor thickness is often the only variable that is routinely used clinically to predict a patient's probability of survival.[16]

The American Joint Committee on Cancer (AJCC) developed a staging system that divides localized melanoma into four stages according to the microstaging criteria of Breslow and Clark.[17] In addition to consideration of the primary lesion, the AJCC staging system addresses aspects of the tumor satellite, the extent of lymph node involvement, and the presence of metastatic disease. Recent analysis of several large databases worldwide has identified areas in which the current AJCC staging system (1997) may not reflect the natural history of melanoma. Issues such as the appropriate cut-off values for primary tumor thickness, ulceration of the melanoma, and the satellite lesions of the primary tumor may warrant reevaluation. The cut-off values initially proposed by Breslow for primary tumor thickness were initially used in the AJCC staging system, but it appears that cut-off depths of 1, 2, and 4 mm of thickness may better predict overall survival. The presence of ulceration of the primary lesion has been correlated with poorer survival for patients with very thin or thick lesions, but ulceration of the melanoma was not included in the 1997 AJCC staging system.

The AJCC and the International Union Against Cancer Tumor-Node-Metastasis Committee recently approved a revised staging system for cutaneous melanoma and presented it at the 2001 American Society of Clinical Oncology meeting. Revisions of the new melanoma staging system include criteria that involve (1) melanoma thickness and ulceration for all tumors (except T1 tumors); (2) the number of metastatic lymph nodes versus gross dimensions, and the delineation of clinically occult versus clinically apparent nodal metastases; (3) the site of distant metastases and the presence of elevated serum lactate dehydrogenase for metastatic disease; (4) upstaging of all patients with stage I, II, and III disease when a primary melanoma is ulcerated; and (5) a new convention for separating clinical and pathologic staging to include information obtained from intraoperative lymphatic mapping and sentinel node biopsy.[18,19] Clinical staging includes microstaging of the primary melanoma, as well as clinical and radiologic evaluation. It is used after complete excision of the primary melanoma with clinical assessment for regional and distant metastasis. Pathologic staging includes the microstaging of the primary melanoma and pathologic information about the regional nodes after partial or complete lymphadenectomy. At this time, it appears that patients with very limited disease (stage 0 or 1A disease) do not require pathologic evaluation of lymph nodes (Table 133–4 and Table 133–5).

As with other solid tumors, the involvement of the regional lymph nodes is a powerful predictor of tumor burden and patient outcome. Until recently, the primary method to determine nodal status was by surgical resection and analysis of the lymph nodes via a regional lymph node dissection. In recent years, preoperative lymphoscintigraphy and intraoperative sentinel node mapping have become more prevalent methods to evaluate lymph nodes associated with the primary cutaneous melanoma.[20,21] Lymphatic mapping and subsequent sentinel node biopsy is based on the theory that regions of the skin have patterns of lymphatic drainage to specific lymph nodes in the regional lymphatic basin. The sentinel lymph node is believed to be the first node in the lymphatic basin into which the primary melanoma drains.

Unlike other solid tumors, melanoma appears to progress in an orderly nodal distribution. The evaluation of sentinel nodes has been used for detection of micrometastases in breast cancer and is gaining popularity in the detection of metastases in melanoma. Sentinel lymph node biopsy provides an avenue for a more thorough examination of a single sentinel node than is possible when examining multiple lymph nodes with a lymph node dissection, and it may be most useful in melanomas located in ambiguous drainage sites such as the head and neck areas. Additionally, the detection of clinically undetectable disease in a lymph node basin that is not directly adjacent to the primary lesion may allow for the upstaging of patients who are initially believed to have node-negative disease. Currently, there is increased interest in developing mechanisms to refine the detection of occult micrometastases in biopsied lymph nodes through the more sensitive reverse transcriptase-polymerase chain reaction (RT-PCR) assays to detect the presence of tyrosinase messenger RNA; the hope is to eventually refine this technique for the detection of occult melanoma cells in the blood of patients with small clinical lesions.[22]

TABLE 133–4. Melanoma TNM Classification

T Classification	Thickness	Ulcerative Status
T1	≤1.0 mm	A: without ulceration and level II/III B: with ulceration or level IV/V
T2	1.01–2.0 mm	A: without ulceration B: with ulceration
T3	2.01–4.0 mm	A: without ulceration B: with ulceration
T4	>4 mm	A: without ulceration B: with ulceration
N Classification	**No. Metastatic Nodes**	**Nodal Metastatic Mass**
N1	1 node	A: micrometastasis[a] B: macrometastasis[b]
N2	2–3 nodes	A: micrometastasis B: macrometastasis C: in-transit metastases/satellite(s) without metastatic nodes
N3	4 or more metastatic lymph nodes, matted nodes, ulcerated melanoma, metastatic lymph nodes, or intransit metastatic or satellite lesions	
M Classification	**Site**	**Serum Lactate Dehydrogenase**
M1a	Distant skin, subcutaneous, or nodal metastatic disease	Normal
M1b	Lung metastases	Normal
M1c	All other visceral metastases Any distant metastasis	Normal elevated

[a]Micrometastases are diagnosed after sentinel or elective lymphadenectomy.
[b]Macrometastases are defined as clinically detectable lymph node metastases confirmed by therapeutic lymphadenectomy or when any lymph node metastasis exhibits extracapsular extension.
Compiled from Refs. 18 and 19.

TABLE 133–5. American Joint Committee on Cancer Tumor (T), Node (N), Metastasis (M) Stage Grouping for Cutaneous Melanoma

Pathologic Stage	T	N	M	Clinical Stage	T	N	M
0	Tis	N0	M0	0	Tis	N0	M0
IA	T1a	N0	M0	IA	T1a	N0	M0
IB	T1b	N0	M0	IB	T1b	N0	M0
	T2a	N0	M0		T2a	N0	M0
IIA	T2b	N0	M0	IIA	T2b	N0	M0
	T3a	N0	M0		T3a	N0	M0
IIB	T3b	N0	M0	IIB	T3b	N0	M0
	T4a	N0	M0		T4a	N0	M0
IIC	T4b	N0	M0	IIC	T4b	N0	M0
IIIA	T1-4a	N1a	M0	IIIA	Any T1-4a	N1b	M0
IIIB	T1-4a	N1b	M0	IIIB	Any T1-4a	N2b	M0
	T1-4a	N2a	M0				
IIIC	Any T	N2b, N2c	M0	IIIC	Any T	N2c	M0
	Any T	N3	M0		Any T	N3	M0
IV	Any T	Any N	M1	IV	Any T	Any N	M1

Compiled from Refs. 18 and 19.

The stage of the melanoma at the time of diagnosis is one of the primary indicators of the natural history of the disease; other factors have also been shown to influence the survival of patients with primary melanoma. Factors such as tumor growth phase, mitotic rate, density of tumor-infiltrating lymphocytes in the tumor tissue, anatomic site of the primary tumor, gender, and age have all been demonstrated to have an impact on survival (Table 133–6).[16] In a recently published analysis of a series of trials for patients with metastatic disease,[23] a number of additional prognostic factors were identified for patients with advanced disease. The number of metastatic sites; disease involvement of the gastrointestinal tract, liver, pleura, or lung; or an Eastern Cooperative Oncology Group (ECOG) performance status equal to or greater than 1 were associated with poor prognosis. Females and patients with prior immunotherapy were associated with prolonged survival in this analysis.

TABLE 133–6. Prognostic Factors for Cutaneous Melanoma

Tumor-Related Factors
- Tumor thickness
- Level of tumor invasion
- Anatomic site of primary tumor (increased survival in tumors of extremities versus axial, neck, head, and trunk)
- Mitotic rate (correlated with decreased survival)
- Angiogenesis
- Occurrence of microsatellites
- Area of tumor regression
- Presence of tumor-infiltrating lymphocytes (correlated with increased survival)

Patient-Related Factors
- Age (decreased survival in patients > 60 yrs of age)
- Gender (survival: female > male)

From Ref. 16.

▶ TREATMENT: Melanoma

The appropriate treatment and management of a patient with cutaneous melanoma are determined primarily by the extent or stage of the disease. Local disease can be cured with surgical ablation. Regional disease involves the surgical resection of the primary lesion and, depending on the risk of recurrence, adjuvant therapy with interferon-alfa-2b (IFN-α-2b). Treatment for disseminated melanoma remains a challenge. Although the literature provides numerous clinical trials of single-agent or combination chemotherapy, immunotherapy, and biochemotherapy regimens, there is not a single standard treatment regimen for metastatic melanoma.

SURGERY

Cutaneous melanoma that is localized can be cured, in most cases, with surgical excision. The extent of margin excised is important in the prevention of local recurrence and ultimate survival. Primary tumors less than 1 mm thick require a 1-cm margin,[24] a significant reduction from the 5-cm margin recommended in the past. Large primary tumors between 1 and 4 mm thick can also be surgically excised, but appear to require a more extensive margin of up to 2 cm.[25] Primary tumors more than 4 mm thick require at least a 2-cm margin, but it is not clear if a larger margin is beneficial. Management of lentigo maligna melanoma may be problematic, as subclinical extension of atypical junctional melanocytic hyperplasia may extend beyond the visible margins; it is important to excise these lesions completely.

When there is no distant disease, but involvement in isolated regional lymph nodes is detected via physical exam, therapeutic lymphadenectomy is recommended. The extent of therapeutic lymph node dissection is often modified according to the anatomic area of the lymphadenopathy. The role of lymphadenectomy is not as well established when the clinical examination shows no apparent involvement of the regional lymph nodes. Prophylactic regional lymph node dissection has not been shown to prolong survival or decrease time to relapse in randomized clinical trials, although a subgroup of patients with stage

I melanoma will have microscopic metastatic disease in nonpalpable lymph nodes.[26,27]

Selective regional lymphadenectomy performed after scintigraphic and dye lymphographic identification of the affected sentinel draining lymph node(s) is becoming increasingly common in major melanoma centers.[28] If the sentinel node is found to have micrometastatic melanoma, regional dissection of the involved nodal basin is performed. If lymphatic mapping with sentinel node biopsy is available, it should be considered in patients with melanomas that are more than 1 mm thick or Clark's level IV.

One of the most important aspects of the surgical management of cutaneous melanoma is the role of patient follow-up. Postsurgical follow-up of patients who have had a melanoma excised is essential. Even after excision, there remains a risk of undetected metastatic disease, a risk of a second primary cutaneous melanoma, and a risk of a non-melanoma primary malignancy. Scheduled screening in addition to routine surgical follow-up is required for any patient who has had a melanoma; the frequency and duration recommended depend on the stage of melanoma. The optimal duration of follow-up is controversial. Most patients who develop recurrent disease do so in the first 5 years following treatment, but late recurrences in patients over 10 years following surgery have been documented, and the increased lifetime risk of developing a second primary melanoma supports lifetime dermatologic surveillance for all patients.

The role of curative surgery is limited to early-stage disease in cutaneous melanoma. Beyond that, its role is less defined, for surgery may offer a mechanism of palliation of isolated metastases. Resection of isolated lesions in the brain[29] and the lungs[30] may be appropriate in certain cases, and this approach warrants evaluation based on the individual patient's comfort and quality of life. Surgery can be an option when the lesion is accessible and when the lesion may cause problems if not removed. Melanoma in the gastrointestinal tract can lead to bowel obstruction, and appropriate resection or bypass may allow the patient significant relief of symptoms. On the other hand, surgery may constitute a significant physical challenge or financial burden to a patient with a limited life expectancy. The clinical scenarios involving surgical resection should be fully evaluated in terms of overall quality of life.

The risk of relapse and death after the resection of a local or regional cutaneous melanoma is the primary determinant for the use of adjuvant therapy after primary resection. Adjuvant trials have focused on patients at intermediate or high risk of recurrence.

PHARMACOLOGIC THERAPY

IMMUNOTHERAPY

Melanoma is one of the most immunogenic solid tumors; it appears to interact with and respond to the immune system of the host in which it arises. Spontaneous regressions of melanoma suggest the importance of the immune system in disease modulation. Lymphoid infiltration into the primary melanoma also suggests that immunomodulation may have an impact on the biology of melanoma. Early work in melanoma with nonspecific immunomodulators, such as levamisole and the Calmette-Guérin bacillus, demonstrated that tumor regression could occur with these therapies, although many of these regressions proved to be limited and short-lived. Coupled with the fact that melanoma is one of the tumors most resistant to other standard systemic treatment modalities used for cancer, radiation, chemotherapy, and immunotherapy offer an avenue of treatment if surgery fails or is not an option. Although the complete response rate in patients with melanoma treated with biotherapy has been low, the durability of the responses can be significant. This has led to increasing research in the optimization of biotherapeutic approaches for patients with metastatic melanoma and to the establishment of biotherapy in the adjuvant setting.

Interferon Therapy

The *interferons* consist of a group of antigenically and genetically distinct species and subspecies; the interferons have immunomodulatory activity and are directly cytostatic and cytotoxic. A number of studies have focused on various doses and schedules of recombinant interferon for the treatment of metastatic melanoma (Table 133–7). Response rates in metastatic melanoma range from 10% to 30%, but overall response rates are approximately 15% for IFN-α and IFN-β. Unfortunately, the optimal dose, treatment schedule, and treatment combination/regimens have not yet been established for the management of metastatic melanoma.

In initial clinical trials with interferon therapy for patients with metastatic cutaneous melanoma, response rates were highest in those patients with minimal disease. Responses occurred in all sites of disease, but were most frequent in subcutaneous, lymph node, and pulmonary metastases. The success of interferon in patients with

TABLE 133–7. Interferon-α Therapy of Metastatic Melanoma

Interferon	Dose (mU/m²)	Route	Weekly Schedule	Response Rate (%)	Reference
α2a	12	IM	3 × week	20	31
α2a	50	IM	3 × week	23	32
α2a	20	IV	Daily × 5	0	33
α2a	50	IM	3 × week	11	34
α2a	3–36	IM	Daily × 7	10	35
α2a	18	IM	—	14	36
α2a	18	IM	Daily × 7	8	37
α2b	10–100	IM/IV	Daily × 7	22	38
α2b	10	SC	3 × week	27	39
α2b	30	SC/IV	3 × week	25	40
α2b	10	IM	3 × week	14	41

IM = intramuscular; IV = intravenous; SC = subcutaneous.

minimal disease has encouraged investigators to evaluate the benefit of interferon in patients who had undergone curative surgical resection, but were at risk for recurrent disease (e.g., because of bulky disease or regional lymph node involvement). Early trials of short-term and/or low-dose regimens of IFN-α did not demonstrate a survival benefit in the adjuvant setting.[42]

In an attempt to optimize response in the adjuvant setting, a strategy was developed to deliver what is considered maximum tolerated doses of IFN-α for 1 month, and then provide prolonged therapy with IFN-α at more tolerable doses for 48 weeks. The rationale for the induction phase was to provide peak levels of interferon sufficient to inhibit tumor growth and provide both antiangiogenic and immunomodulatory effects while avoiding the production of anti-interferon antibodies. A large, multicenter, cooperative group trial of IFN-α-2b versus observation was designed for patients with high-risk (stage IIb and III disease) melanoma following curative surgical resection. IFN-α-2b was given intravenously (IV) as an induction therapy at maximum tolerated doses of 20 million IU/m^2/dose 5 days per week for 4 weeks; treatment was continued for 48 weeks with IFN-α-2b, 10 million IU/m^2/dose given subcutaneously three times per week. This therapy is now often referred to as high-dose interferon (HDI) treatment. Induction therapy was given in an outpatient setting, and maintenance therapy could be self-administered at home by patients or their caregivers. Analysis of the course for the 280 patients demonstrated a disease-free survival and an overall survival advantage with interferon treatment for patients with stage IIb and III disease following surgical resection.[43] The prolongation of overall survival was about 1 year, and the most significant reduction in melanoma recurrence was during the early treatment period. Subgroup analysis of this study indicated that patients with large primary tumors and node-negative disease (T4N0M0) did not receive the same benefit from therapy, but the small number of patients in this group made it difficult to draw definite conclusions about the role of interferon treatment for adjuvant therapy in this subgroup. Whether the information from this trial should be extrapolated to patients with local recurrences, satellite lesions, or in-transit metastases is not known and should be evaluated on an individual case basis.

Toxicities to the IFN-α therapy were common and severe in most patients at some point during therapy, necessitating dose reductions and/or delays during both the induction and maintenance phases of the study. Dose modifications were required for dose-limiting constitutional symptoms, hematologic toxicity, and hepatic toxicities, but 74% of the patients were able to complete the year of therapy in an outpatient setting. Guidelines for interferon dose modifications, based on the criteria used in the cooperative trial and the experience of investigators, are shown in Table 133–8. The frequency and severity of toxicity seen with HDI treatment in the adjuvant setting have raised several important questions: (1) Are the toxic reactions associated with HDI treatment worth the potential benefits of HDI for patients? (2) What are the mechanism(s) and best standard(s) of care for patients who experience interferon toxicity? (3) Is the regimen/schedule of interferon used in the initial positive trial (HDI) necessary to achieve the benefits seen in this study?

One of the categories of toxicities seen with interferon therapy is actually a diverse group of side effects referred to as constitutional symptoms. Some of these symptoms are acute, such as fever, chills, myalgia, and fatigue, while others are more chronic, such as fatigue, anorexia, and depression. Acetaminophen can help to prevent or minimize acute dose-related symptoms, but opiates such as meperidine are necessary when patients experience severe chills or rigors, most commonly during the IV induction phase of HDI treatment. Nonsteroidal anti-inflammatory agents (NSAIDs) have been used to manage interferon-related myalgia, but may have overlapping side effects with interferon; for example, they may decrease renal blood flow or lead to nausea. Like acetaminophen, NSAIDs may mask fevers that occur in patients who experience neutropenia while on therapy.

TABLE 133–8. Interferon-α Dose Modification Guidelines

Sign/Symptom	Evaluation	Dose Modification
Anorexia	Calorie counts	33%–50% with nutrition consult
Weight loss	>10% weight loss	33%–50% with nutrition consult
Fatigue	Thyroid function	33%–50% after dose delay of 1–2 weeks
Depression	Beck's inventory	33%–50% with psychiatric evaluation
↑ AST	LFTs	33%–50% when LFTs are <3× normal limits
↓ WBC	ANC	33%–50% when ANC < 250/mm^3

AST = aspartate transaminase; LFT = liver function test; WBC = white blood cell count; ANC = absolute neutrophil count.
From Ref. 44.

Fatigue is one of the most frequently observed dose-limiting toxic reactions seen with interferon therapy. The mechanisms of interferon-induced fatigue are not fully understood at this time and are often multifactorial in individual patients. It appears that interferon-induced fatigue is dose-related and may be exacerbated by continued therapy. Pharmacologic (e.g., amantadine) and nonpharmacologic (e.g., exercise, psychosocial techniques, distraction, energy management, dietary modifications) interventions are currently being evaluated in the treatment of both cancer-related fatigue and interferon-related fatigue.[45]

Anorexia was reported in about 70% of patients receiving adjuvant interferon therapy for melanoma and is thought to be mediated through direct effects on hypothalamic neurons, modification of normal hypothalamic neurotransmitter/neuropeptides, or effects from stimulation of other cytokines.[46] Taste alterations may contribute to anorexia. Investigational strategies for ameliorating interferon-induced anorexia include nutritional intervention, use of appetite stimulants such as megestrol acetate, and patient education. Glucocorticoids should not be used as an appetite stimulant or as part of an antiemetic therapy, as they may have an adverse impact the immunomodulatory effects of the interferon. Depression is not uncommon and warrants evaluation and treatment based on patient symptoms. Other toxic reactions, such as hematologic or hepatic toxic reactions, require monitoring and appropriate dose modification.

Because of the associated toxicity and adverse effects seen with IFN-α therapy, there has been worldwide concern about the usefulness of this intensive adjuvant therapy for melanoma—despite the benefits in relapse-free and overall survival. A subsequent report from the ECOG study demonstrated a quality-of-life benefit with interferon therapy based on a quality of life-adjusted survival analysis (Q-TWIST).[47] This analysis calculates the number of quality-adjusted life years gained as a result of IFN-α treatment, or the clinical benefit of time without toxic reactions and without disease.

Many questions remain concerning the optimal use of interferon in the adjuvant setting. A subsequent ECOG trial designed to evaluate the impact of lower doses of interferon, 3 MU given subcutaneously daily three times weekly (called low-dose interferon [LDI]) for 24 months, compared with the HDI regimen described earlier versus observation did not demonstrate a survival advantage of HDI versus observation. At a median follow-up of 52 months, the 5-year estimated relapse-free survival for HDI treatment was 44%; LDI treatment, 40%; and observation, 35%. HDI treatment was shown to be statistically superior for relapse-free survival, prolonging median time to relapse by 10 months compared with observation and LDI treatment. Suprisingly, there was no overall survival benefit for HDI or LDI treatment compared with observation, although investigators speculated that the number of patients in the observation arm that received interferon therapy after disease progression affected this analysis of survival.[48]

Because of the success of the HDI treatment in disease-free and overall survival in early studies,[43,48] a number of current trials are addressing the issues of dose and duration of therapy. Current studies are focusing on an HDI regimen for short (4 weeks) or intermediate duration (3 months). Less promising are studies that have evaluated prolonged therapy with LDI regimens without the induction therapy. Recently, investigators have combined interferon with other potential treatment approaches in the adjuvant setting for high-risk patients. For example, HDI has been combined with melanoma vaccines such as GM2-KLH/QS-21 in an attempt to capitalize on the success of HDI treatment alone.[49]

The role of interferon in advanced disease is not clear, especially for those patients who have recurrent disease after adjuvant IFN-α-2b therapy. IFN-α has been used as a single agent in patients with metastatic disease who have not received adjuvant therapy and in combination with other biotherapy ± chemotherapy for metastatic melanoma. One of the challenges with combination therapy is the possible exacerbation of toxic reactions (e.g., nausea, vomiting, renal insufficiency, and neurologic difficulties) that may result from concomitant chemotherapy. Hematologic toxicity is generally not dose-limiting and correlates with dosage, schedule, and route of administration. In an attempt to limit systemic toxicity and to optimize local benefit, the regional administration of interferon has been evaluated in a variety of settings. Intralesional and perilesional application of interferon has been shown to have some efficacy in small lesions and appears to be well tolerated.[50]

Interleukin Therapy

Interleukin-2 (IL-2), a glycoprotein produced by activated lymphocytes, has been extensively studied in the management of metastatic melanoma. The precise mechanism of cytotoxicity of IL-2 is unknown; high concentrations of IL-2 have not been shown to have a direct antitumor effect on cancer cells *in vitro*. Both *in vitro* and *in vivo*, IL-2 stimulates the production and release of many secondary monocyte-derived and T cell-derived cytokines—including IL-4, IL-5, IL-6, IL-8, tumor necrosis factor-α, granulocyte-macrophage colony-stimulating factor, and IFN-γ—which may have direct or indirect antitumor activity. In addition, IL-2 appears to stimulate the cytotoxic activities of natural killer cells, monocytes, lymphokine-activated killer (LAK) cells, and cytotoxic T lymphocytes. Although the clinical significance is not currently understood, preliminary studies have shown that several human melanoma cell lines express both α and β chains of the rIL-2 receptor that specifically binds to rIL-2.

Preclinical studies demonstrated a dose-response relationship between IL-2 and tumor responses; therefore, the initial clinical trials that evaluated the use of IL-2 in the treatment of patients with melanoma involved relatively high doses of the drug as a single agent or in combination with LAK cells (Table 133–9). The response rates seen in these trials ranged from 15% to 25%, and 2% to 5% of patients achieved complete responses, some of which were durable. Responses were seen at a number of metastatic sites, such as lung, liver, bone, lymph node, and subcutaneous tissue. Particularly encouraging were the responses in patients with large tumor burdens.[61] Based on the reevaluation of early clinical trials, the Food and Drug Administration (FDA) has approved the use of high-dose rIL-2 (aldesleukin) for the treatment of metastatic melanoma.

TABLE 133–9. Aldesleukin ± LAK Cells in Metastatic Melanoma

Reference	Route	Number	CR	CR + PR (%)
51	Bolus	26	0	12
52	Bolus	46	2	22
53	Bolus	42	0	10
54	Bolus	27	0	26
55	Bolus	134	9	17
56	CI	10	0	50
57	CI	33	0	3
58	CI	33	0	12
59	CI	17	0	6
60	CI	15	0	0

LAK = lymphokine-activated killer; CR = complete response; PR = partial response; CI = continuous infusion.

The high doses of IL-2 used in the initial clinical trials and recommended in the labeling of the drug are associated with significant and frequent toxic reactions and may limit the practicality of therapy for individual patients. At the high doses (600,000 IU/kg/dose every 8 hours for 14 doses) approved for treatment of metastatic melanoma, cytokine-induced capillary leak syndrome is a common problem, including hypotension, supraventricular tachycardia, visceral edema, dyspnea, and arrhythmias. The increased permeability of capillary walls allows for a fluid shift from the intravascular space into tissue. As the patient becomes intravascularly dehydrated, hypotension occurs, resulting in reflex tachycardia and arrhythmias. In addition, the decrease in blood volume may decrease renal blood flow and urine output, which become evident as an increase in the blood urea nitrogen and serum creatinine levels, edema, weight gain, and a decrease in urine output (input > output). Visceral edema can result in pulmonary congestion, pleural effusions, and edema. The management of patients receiving high-dose rIL-2 requires careful monitoring and a staff trained in critical care, such as hypotension management. Although some institutions manage patients receiving high-dose rIL-2 in an intensive care unit, these patients can be managed with intensive care on designated oncology units. Additional side effects seen with rIL-2 include constitutional symptoms; pruritus and eosinophilia; bone marrow suppression, including thrombocytopenia; increase in liver function test findings; and nausea.

In an attempt to provide the benefit of IL-2 therapy without the limiting side effects, several investigators have evaluated continuous infusion IL-2 therapy, and lower dose IL-2 alone[53] or with chemotherapy[62] and interferon therapy.[63–65] Response rates have been promising, but there has been no significant effect on survival. At this time, direct head-to-head comparisons of various dosing schedules and regimens are needed to determine the optimum approach to rIL-2 therapy in metastatic melanoma.

The co-administration of LAK cells with IL-2 does not appear to significantly improve clinical response. Although some studies have suggested an improved response with the co-administration of tumor-infiltrating lymphocytes with rIL-2, the therapy is technically difficult and costly, and an overall clinical benefit has not been clearly demonstrated.

One of the greatest challenges in the management of patients with metastatic melanoma with immunotherapy is to determine on a patient-by-patient basis if the potential benefits of rIL-2 outweigh the substantial risk. It is obvious by the reports of long-term responses (>10 years) in some patients that the risk is certainly worth the benefit for some individuals. A number of parameters such as HLA expression and pretreatment immunologic status have been evaluated as potential predictors to therapy. Unfortunately, at this time it is difficult to determine which patients will respond to IL-2 therapy, as no biologic or immunologic parameters have been found to correlate consistently with response.

Immunization

Active specific immunization has become one of the most studied strategies for immunomodulation for melanoma. Specific cellular immune responses to melanoma antigens occur through the recognition of the foreign peptide on a self major histocompatibility complex molecule by a T-cell receptor. Current melanoma vaccines stimulate the antibody response of cytotoxic T lymphocytes to these specific tumor antigens. Melanoma antigens are either tumor-associated antigens or melanoma-associated antigens. The former are common to melanoma cells and other tumor cells, whereas the latter are usually proteins or glycoproteins found predominantly in melanomas and, at times, in normal melanocytes. Predominant melanocytic antigens include Melan-A/MART-1, tyrosinase, and gp100. The use of tumor-associated or melanoma-associated antigens for melanoma vaccines can be difficult, as the expression of antigens in melanoma cells is often heterogeneous and may change in response to the patient's immune response. Unfortunately, tumor-associated and melanoma-associated antigens tend to be weak immunogenics, although physical alterations can increase immunogenicity.

Melanoma vaccines range from complex antigen mixtures to purified antigens (Table 133–10). Complex vaccines are polyvalent, can stimulate an immune response to a number of tumor antigens, and are less susceptible to antigenic modulation by the cancer cells. Single-antigen vaccines can be problematic if a single antigen-resistant antigen-negative tumor cell develops.

Melanoma vaccines can be prepared from a patient's own tumor (autologous preparations); in this case, the vaccine targets antigens from the patient's melanoma cell. Autologous vaccines may involve modification of the tumor cells with a hapten to increase the immunogenicity of the preparation. Allogeneic preparations do not require patient tissue to prepare the vaccine. Allogeneic preparations often include a number of cell lines to increase the content of immunogenic tumor-associated and melanoma-associated antigens. Early results with one polyvalent whole cell melanoma vaccine suggest a potential role in the adjuvant setting; currently, a phase III clinical trial is under way to compare the efficacy of the polyvalent whole cell melanoma vaccine to that of IFN-α-2b for patients with surgically resected stage III melanoma.[66]

Melanoma vaccines may also be prepared with tumor cell lysate. Such vaccines can be prepared from the whole cells or from the cellular elements most likely to contain the antigens important for the induction of protective immune responses. Material shed from the melanoma cells is believed to be rich in cell surface antigens and has been used for the preparation of a melanoma vaccine. Melacine is a lysate vaccine prepared from two human melanoma cell lines administered with an adjuvant immunostimulant monophosphoryl lipid A and purified mycobacterial cell wall skeleton called DETOX. Initial reports from uncontrolled clinical trials with melacine have suggested that it may have a role in treatment of metastatic melanoma.[67]

An alternative approach to vaccine construction is to develop a vaccine from a single, highly specific antigen. Preparations currently in clinical trials include vaccines prepared from gangliosides, peptides such as MAGE or MART, and anti-idiotype monoclonal antibodies. Gangliosides GM_2, GD_2, GM_3, GD_3, and O-acetyl-GD_3 are present on the surface of many melanoma cells, but GM_2 is the most consistently expressed and immunogenic antigen. The vaccines from a single antigen can be prepared in a reproducible manner on a large scale, which gives them an advantage. It is unclear, however, if a single antigen or peptide will be sufficient to result in tumor cell kill.

TABLE 133–10. Melanoma Vaccines

Whole Melanoma Cells
Autologous cells
Allogeneic cells
Haptenized cells
Melanoma Cell Lysates
Viral oncolysates
Shed melanoma cell supernatant
Purified Antigens
Gangliosides (GM2, GD2)
Anti-idiotype Monoclonal Antibodies
Anti-GD3 gangliosides

Monoclonal Antibodies

In the diagnosis and treatment of melanoma, two strategies have involved monoclonal antibodies: treatment with a monoclonal antibody to activate the host immune system[68,69] and treatment with a conjugated monoclonal antibody. Initial trials of monoclonal antibodies, which have been conjugated to cytotoxic agents, radioisotopes, and toxins (e.g., ricin A), were limited secondary to the production of the monoclonal antibody. A problem seen in current studies is the development of neutralizing antibodies to the murine monoclonal antibodies. Humanized murine or pure human monoclonal antibodies against melanoma-associated antigens could potentially avoid the problem with the human antimouse antibody.

Ferrone has developed a purified melanoma vaccine from an anti-idiotype mouse monoclonal antibody.[70] This vaccine is composed of three monoclonal anti-idiotype antibodies that include the internal image of several determinants of the melanoma-associated antigen. One of the problems with this antibody is the inability to directly induce a cell-mediated antitumor effect; therefore, adjuvants are now being used to increase the ability of the anti-idiotype antibodies to induce a greater immune response.

Gene Therapy

Although still experimental, several strategies for gene therapy are currently under investigation for the treatment of melanoma.[71] One approach to gene therapy for melanoma is to modify melanoma cells with the insertion of one or more cytokine genes and then to administer these altered allogeneic or autologous cells as a vaccine. Cytokine gene transduction has been accomplished with a number of cytokines including IL-2, tumor necrosis factor-α, IL-4, and interferon. It is hoped that the insertion of cytokine genes into melanoma cells will significantly increase the cells' immunogenicity.

Genes can also be transferred *in vitro* into tumor-infiltrating lymphocytes associated with melanoma in an attempt to potentiate the cytotoxicity of these cells. Rosenberg and colleagues were the first to attempt to transduce the gene coding for resistance to neomycin into human tumor-infiltrating lymphocytes.[72,73] This approach has since been used to transfer the tumor necrosis factor gene into tumor-infiltrating lymphocytes.

CHEMOTHERAPY

Single-Agent Chemotherapy

A number of cytotoxic agents have demonstrated *in vitro* activity to melanoma; however, only a few drugs have shown a response rate greater than 10% consistently in patients with melanoma. Because chemotherapy has rarely cured a patient with melanoma, the aim of chemotherapy is palliation. The results of clinical trials are generally expressed in terms of response rates, which generally indicate the fraction of patients who experience a partial response plus the fraction who experience a complete response. Partial response criteria vary, but usually require a 50% reduction in the size of the tumor for a minimum of 1 month. A complete response would require a total regression of all metastases for at least 1 month and is uncommon (<5%). It is essential to realize that these response rates do not reflect survival and do not evaluate benefit to the patient. Response rates also do not represent the toxicities and the complications of therapy.

Dacarbazine (DTIC), a cytotoxic drug thought to exert its antitumor effect through alkylation, is currently the most effective single agent for the treatment of melanoma. It is the only FDA-approved chemotherapeutic agent for the treatment of metastatic melanoma in the United States. In prospective controlled clinical trials, the response rates were 20% to 25%,[74] with an average duration of response of 5 to 7 months. Early clinical trials show that patients with skin, subcutaneous tissue, and lymph node involvement respond most frequently, whereas metastatic disease to the liver, bone, and central nervous system is often unresponsive.[10] Complete responses are uncommon, with a dismal 2% of patients treated with single-agent dacarbazine sustaining long-term complete responses.[75] The optimum dose schedule of dacarbazine has never been determined; therefore, single-dose regimens are often preferred for patient convenience. Common side effects of dacarbazine therapy include moderate myelosuppression, severe nausea and vomiting, and a flu-like syndrome after large doses. Available antiemetics can prevent and manage the nausea and vomiting, so it is not a major complication. At this time, there is no known role for DTIC in the adjuvant setting.

Temozolomide is one of a series of imidazoletetrazine derivatives that was developed as a potential alternative to dacarbazine. Temozolomide is a prodrug of the active metabolite of dacarbazine. DTIC requires hepatic transformation to its active intermediate, whereas at physiologic pH, temozolomide chemically degrades to the cytotoxic triazene monomethyl 5-triazeno imidazole carboxamide (MTIC). Temozolomide is an attractive alternative to dacarbazine, as it is administered orally and appears to be less emetogenic than dacarbazine. In addition, temozolomide can cross into the central nervous system to achieve approximately 50% of circulating blood concentrations in the central nervous system and, therefore, may be beneficial for patients with metastases in the central nervous system.[76]

Temozolomide has been directly compared to dacarbazine in a phase III trial in patients with advanced melanoma.[77] Temozolomide was administered orally at starting doses of 200 mg/m^2/day for 5 days every 28 days, while dacarbazine was administered IV at doses of 250 mg/m^2/day for 5 days every 21 days. Systemic MTIC levels were higher in patients who received DTIC, but a slight survival advantage was seen in patients treated with temozolomide (7.7 months versus 6.4 months). Quality of life was also improved in patients receiving temozolomide, but the dosing regimen used in the study could have biased this perception. Dacarbazine is often administered IV as a single monthly dose, which would eliminate the need for patients to receive treatment for 5 days every month.

The *nitrosoureas* have also been shown to be active against melanoma. Again, response rates for this group of alkylating agents tend to fall between 10% and 20%. Sites of responses are similar to those seen with dacarbazine.[78] It was initially thought that there might be an added benefit to the use of the lipophilic nitrosoureas in a malignancy that can metastasize to the brain. Unfortunately, despite the ability of these agents to cross the blood-brain barrier, the commercially available nitrosoureas have not been shown to produce an increased response in melanoma in the central nervous system. Fotemustine, an investigational nitrosourea, has induced preliminary responses in a limited number of patients with cerebral metastases.[79] The most common toxic reaction to the nitrosoureas is myelosuppression that can be delayed. Leukopenia and thrombocytopenia may be seen as long as 3 to 5 weeks after drug administration and may limit the application of these agents in multidrug regimens.

Cisplatin and related compounds have also been evaluated in the management of metastatic melanoma.[80–82] The effectiveness of platinum compounds as single agents is limited, with response rates reported to be less than 10%.[83] The toxicities of cisplatin can be problematic; they include acute and delayed nausea and vomiting, renal toxicity, and neurotoxicity.

Combination Chemotherapy

In an attempt to extend the efficacy of dacarbazine, DTIC has been combined with other chemotherapeutic agents and, most recently, with immunotherapy. The combination of dacarbazine with other chemotherapy, most commonly cisplatin, has increased the response rates reported with dacarbazine alone, but the survival benefit has been minimal.[83–85] Again, responses were often limited to metastases in soft tissue, lymph nodes, and the lung—the sites most likely to respond to single-agent dacarbazine therapy. The concern with combination chemotherapy is increased toxicity, and any reports of an increase in response rates should be weighed with overall quality of life.

The Dartmouth regimen is a combination chemotherapy regimen that includes carmustine, dacarbazine, cisplatin, and tamoxifen. Initial reports from uncontrolled phase II trials of this combination suggested high response rates of 20% to 50%; however, few patients have achieved long-term survival. The benefit of tamoxifen to this regimen has been controversial, but a controlled clinical trial from the National Cancer Institute of Canada showed no benefit from tamoxifen in this combination.[86] Careful analysis of the initial studies reveals that the criteria used to measure response were not consistent with standards used in large multicenter studies. A Phase III multicenter study that compared the Dartmouth regimen to single-agent dacarbazine therapy found no difference in survival between the two treatment groups.[87] A small increase, one that was not statistically significant, in tumor response occurred with the combination therapy. At this time, dacarbazine remains the standard for comparison of new regimens.

ENDOCRINE THERAPY

The role of endocrine therapy in the management of melanoma has been debated over the last decade. Initial reports that described high-affinity cytoplasmic estrogen receptors in patients with metastatic melanoma led to speculation about the possible benefits of antiestrogens in modulating the biology of melanoma.[88] Additionally, estrogens have been shown to suppress T-lymphocyte activity and to suppress or stimulate the activities of B-lymphocytes, macrophages, and natural killer cells. All these activities support a hypothesis that estrogens may influence the immunologic mechanisms that appear to be important in melanoma.

Tamoxifen was shown to have a response and survival benefit in one randomized trial when combined with dacarbazine in 117 patients with metastatic melanoma; this benefit was most pronounced in women.[89] As discussed previously, subsequent trials have not been able to confirm the initial reported benefit of the antiestrogen when combined with chemotherapy, and tamoxifen is no longer routinely included in chemotherapy regimens.

Megestrol acetate, a synthetic progestin, has also been combined with chemotherapy in an attempt to enhance patient responses and survival. In a small study of 19 patients with melanoma, the addition of megestrol, 160 mg/day, to dacarbazine, cisplatin, and carmustine suggested a response benefit.[90] Unfortunately, the trial was small, and further investigation has not supported the routine use of progestins in the management of melanoma.

BIOCHEMOTHERAPY

Low overall response rates and toxicity have limited the use of chemotherapy alone or immunotherapy alone in the management of metastatic melanoma. A new generation of multidrug combinations includes IFN-α and/or IL-2 with chemotherapy (biochemotherapy). Results from initial trials suggest higher response rates than those seen with either chemotherapy or biotherapy alone. Biochemotherapy approaches include combinations of interferon and chemotherapy;[91,92] IL-2 and chemotherapy;[54,93–96] or the combination of IL-2, chemotherapy, and interferon.[97–101] Results to date suggest response rates in the 30% to 60% range, with 10% to 20% complete remissions.

Several randomized phase III trials have compared IL-2-based biochemotherapy with chemotherapy or chemotherapy plus interferon to help determine if biochemotherapy should be considered standard therapy for stage IV disease.[102–104] Benefits seen in these trials include increased response rates or increased time-to-treatment failure, but these relatively small trials have not demonstrated a consistent statistical benefit. Currently, an Intergroup trial is comparing the effects of cisplatin, vinblastine, and dacarbazine (CVD) chemotherapy to the effects of CVD chemotherapy plus IL-2 plus interferon for patients with metastatic melanoma to determine if there is a benefit of combined treatment that outweighs the cost, toxicities, and patient inhospital time associated with the biochemotherapy regimen.

One of the problems that appears in preliminary studies with biochemotherapy is the relatively short duration of response. Recurrence rates among patients who respond to therapy is as high as 50% within 18 to 24 months.[105] Strategies such as the administration of subcutaneous low-dose IL-2 are being investigated in an effort to prolong overall survival and time to progression in the patients who respond to treatment. The initial response rates, durable complete remission, and activity in those patients in which HDI therapy has failed has stimulated interest in evaluating biochemotherapy in the adjuvant setting for patients with high-risk node-positive disease.

LIMB PERFUSION

For recurrent melanoma of the limbs, one approach to therapy is regional isolated perfusion with cytostatic drugs.[106–108] After regional perfusions, objective response rates have been reported to be as high as 80%. The role of hyperthermia (39°C to 40°C) with regional isolated perfusion is not clearly defined. Although most clinical trials have used melphalan, it is not known whether the combination of melphalan with other agents may improve results. Initial work with the biologic response modifiers, such as tumor necrosis factor, has been encouraging.[109]

PREVENTION AND DETECTION

The success of early treatment emphasizes the need for early detection and prevention.[110,111] The American Academy of Dermatology recommends monthly self-examination of skin as a mechanism of recognizing moles or marks on the skin that may be melanoma. Patients with a strong family history should have a clinical examination and, in some cases, screening photography to document size, shape, and location of moles.

Education and re-education about the importance of sun protection can help decrease the rising incidence of this disease. Historically, patients have been counseled that the use of sunscreens with a sun protection factor (SPF) of 15 or greater can limit the risk of skin cancer. It is important to include counseling about the appropriate use of sunscreens to optimize benefits from these products.[112] A recent study noted that most consumers typically apply less sunscreen than is necessary to establish the SPF number on the bottle; the actual SPF received is 20% to 50% of that number.[113]

Sunscreen lotions are more efficient in protecting against shorter ultraviolet wavelengths that lead to sunburns than in protecting against the longer wavelengths in the UVA range that may lead to skin damage and skin cancers, such as melanoma. It is not clear what impact the use of high-potency sunscreens will have on the incidence of melanoma, as the lag time for melanoma is about two decades and the high-potency sunscreens have been popular only for about 10 years.

It is important to educate the public that sunscreens do not make it possible to increase the time in the sun. The slogan "Slip! Slop! Slap!" ("slip on a shirt, slop on the sunscreen, and slap on a hat") initially developed for public health campaigns in Australia provides a more comprehensive approach to sun protection. Avoiding the sun, especially during the peak hours of the sun intensity (10 AM to 4 PM); using protective clothing and head coverings; and staying in the shade when outdoors are important education concepts for those individuals who are in the sun for prolonged periods of time and/or who are at high risk of sunburn.

► PRINCIPLES OF PHARMACOTHERAPY

- Cutaneous melanoma is becoming a common cancer, but it can be prevented and cured if detected early. Public education about screening, early detection, and prevention provide one strategy for curbing the steady increase in this disease.

- Early-stage melanoma has excellent complete response rates with surgical resection.
- Patients with locally advanced disease are at increased risk of recurrence of cutaneous melanoma after surgical resection. High-dose interferon therapy is the current standard for adjuvant treatment of these patients. The toxicities with this therapy are significant and require close patient monitoring and dose delay and/or reduction in a large percentage of the patients.
- Metastatic melanoma remains a clinical challenge. At this time, there is no standard therapy. Dacarbazine is considered one of the most active agents; the use of combination chemotherapy has not been shown in head-to-head comparative trials to be superior to single-agent therapy with dacarbazine.
- High-dose IL-2 is associated with response rates of only about 16%, but some of these responses are durable. The toxicities with this regimen are high, but the potential benefit is that a small subset of patients may have a durable response.
- The treatment of patients with metastatic melanoma with biochemotherapy appears promising, but the definitive drug combination and/or schedules have not been defined. The role of biochemotherapy continues to be explored in the treatment of patients with metastatic melanoma.

REFERENCES

1. Koh HK. Cutaneous melanoma. N Engl J Med 1991;325:171–182.
2. Greenlee RT, Hill-Harmon MB, Murray T, et al. Cancer statistics, 2001. CA Cancer J Clin 2001;51:15–36.
3. Autier P. Epidemiology of melanoma. In: Lejeune FJ, Chaudhuri PK, Das Gupta TK, eds. Malignant Melanoma: Medical and Surgical Management. New York: McGraw-Hill, 1994:1–7.
4. Rigel DS, Kopf AW, Friedman RJ. The rate of malignant melanoma in the United States: are we making an impact? J Am Acad Dermatol 1987;17:1050–1053.
5. Greene MH, Clark WH, Tucker M, et al. Acquired precursors of cutaneous malignant melanoma. N Engl J Med 1985;312:91–94.
6. Gallagher RP, Elwood JM, Yang P. Is chronic sunlight exposure important in accounting for increases in melanoma incidence? Int J Cancer 1989;44:813–815.
7. Kirkwood JM, Lotze MT. Melanoma. In: Kirkwood JM, Lotze MT, Yasko JM, eds. Current Cancer Therapeutics. Philadelphia: Current Medicine, 1994:131.
8. Clark WH, Elder DE, Guerry DT, et al. A study of tumor progression: the precursor lesions of superficial spreading and nodular melanoma. Hum Pathol 1984;15:1147–1165.
9. Dore JF, Carrel S. Biology of melanoma differentiation and progression. In: Lejeune FJ, Chaudhuri PK, Das Gupta K, eds. Malignant Melanoma: Medical and Surgical Management. New York: McGraw-Hill, 1994: 9–26.
10. Balch CM, Houghton AN, Peters LJ. Cutaneous melanoma. In: DeVita, Hellman S, Rosenberg SA, eds. Cancer: Principles and Practice of Oncology. 4th ed. Philadelphia: JB Lippincott, 1993:1613–1614.
11. Friedman RJ, Rigel DS, Silverman MK, et al. Malignant melanoma in the 1990s: the continued importance of early detection and the role of physician examination and self-examination of the skin. Ca Cancer J Clin 1991;41:201–227.
12. NIH Consensus Development Panel on Early Melanoma. Diagnosis and treatment of early melanoma. NIH Consensus Conference. JAMA 1992;268:1314–1319.
13. Cochran AJ. Histology and prognosis in malignant melanoma. J Pathol 1969;97:459–468.
14. Clark WH Jr. A classification of malignant melanoma in man correlated with histogenesis and biologic behavior. In: Montagna W, Hu F, eds. Advances in Biology of the Skin: The Pigmentary System. London: Pergammon, 1967:621–645.
15. Breslow A. Thickness, cross-sectional areas and depth of invasion in the prognosis of cutaneous melanoma. Ann Surg 1970;172:1902–1908.
16. Halpern AC, Schuchter LM. Prognostic models in melanoma. Semin Oncol 1997;24(suppl 4):2–7.
17. Flemming ID, Cooper JS, Henson DE, et al., eds. AJCC Cancer Staging Manual. 5th ed. Philadelphia: Lippincott-Raven, 1997:163–167.
18. Balch CM, Buzaid AC, Atkins MB, et al. A new American Joint Committee on Cancer staging system for cutaneous melanoma. Cancer 2000;88:1484–1491.
19. Balch C, Buzaid AC, Soong SJ, et al. Final version of the AJCC staging system for cutaneous melanoma. J Clin Oncol 2001;19:3635–3648.
20. Morton DL, Wen DR, Wong JH, et al. Technical details of intraoperative lymphatic mapping for early stage melanoma. Arch Surg 1992;127: 392–399.
21. Ross MI, Reintgen D, Balch CM. Selective lymphadenectomy: emerging role of lymphatic mapping and sentinel node biopsy in the management of early stage melanoma. Semin Surg Oncol 1993;9:219–223.
22. Hoon DS, Wang Y, Dale PS, et al. Detection of occult melanoma cells in blood with a multiple-marker polymerase chain reaction assay. J Clin Oncol 1995;13:2109–2116.
23. Manola J, Atkins M, Ibrahim J, Kirkwood J. Prognostic factors in metastatic melanoma: a pooled analysis of Eastern Cooperative Oncology Group trials. J Clin Oncol 2000;18:3782–3793.
24. Veronesi U, Cascinelli N. Narrow excision (1-cm margin): a safe procedure for thin cutaneous melanoma. Arch Surg 1991;126:438–441.
25. Balch CM, Urist MM, Karakousis CP, et al. Efficiency of 2-cm surgical margins for intermediate-thickness melanomas (1–4 mm): results of a multi-institutional randomized surgical trial. Ann Surg 1993;218: 262–269.
26. Balch CM, Soong SJ, Bartolucci AA, et al. Efficacy of elective regional lymph node dissection of 1 to 4 mm thick melanomas for patients 60 years of age and younger. Ann Surg 1996;224:255–266.
27. Cay CL, Sober AJ, Lew RA, et al. Malignant melanoma patients with positive nodes and relatively good prognosis: microstaging retains prognostic significance in clinical stage I melanoma patients with metastases to regional nodes. Cancer 1981;47:955–962.
28. Morton DL, Thompson JF, Essner R, et al. Validation of the accuracy of intraoprative lymphatic mapping and sentinel lymphadenectomy for early-stage melanoma: a multicenter trial. Multicenter Selective Lymphadenectomy Trial Group. Ann Surg 1999;230(4):453–463.
29. Somoza S, Kondziolka D, Lansford D, et al. Stereostatic radiosurgery for cerebral metastatic melanoma. J Neurosurg 1993;79:661–666.
30. Harpole DH, Johnson CM, Wolfe, et al. Analysis of 945 cases of pulmonary metastatic melanoma. J Thorac Cardiovasc Surg 1992;103: 743–750.
31. Creagan ET, Ahmann DL, Green SJ, et al. Phase II study of low dose recombinant leukocyte A interferon in disseminated malignant melanoma. J Clin Oncol 1984;2:1002–1005.
32. Creagan ET, Ahmann DL, Green SJ, et al. Phase II study of recombinant leukocyte A interferon (rIFN-alpha A) in disseminated malignant melanoma. Cancer 1984;54:2844–2849.
33. Coates A, Rallings M, Hersey P, Swanson C. Phase II study of recombinant alpha 2-interferon in advanced malignant melanoma. J Interferon Res 1986;6:1–4.
34. Hersey P, Hasic E, MacDonald M, et al. Effects of recombinant leukocytes interferon (rIFN-alpha a) on tumor growth and immune responses in patient with metastatic melanoma. Br J Cancer 1985;51:815–826.
35. Legha SS, Papadopoulos NE, Plager C, et al. Clinical evaluation of recombinant interferon alfa-2a (Roferon-a) in metastatic melanoma using two different schedules. J Clin Oncol 1987;5:1240–1246.
36. Elsasser-Beile U, Drews H. Interferon in the treatment of malignant melanoma: results of clinical studies. Fortschr Med 1987;105:401.
37. Steiner A, Wolf C, Pehamberger H. Comparison of the effects of three different treatment regimens of recombinant interferons (r-IFN alpha, r-IFN gamma, and r-IFN-alpha + cimetidine) in disseminated malignant melanoma. J Cancer Res Clin Oncol 1987;113:459–465.

38. Kirkwood JM, Ernstoff MS, Davis CA, et al. Comparison of intramuscular and intravenous recombinant alpha-2 interferon in melanoma and other cancers. Ann Intern Med 1985;103:32–36.
39. Dorval T, Palangie T, Jouve M, et al. Clinical phase II trial of recombinant DNA interferon (interferon alfa 2b) in patients with metastatic malignant melanoma. Cancer 1986;58:215–218.
40. Robinson WA, Mughal TI, Thomas MR, et al. Treatment of metastatic malignant melanoma with recombinant interferon alpha-2. Immunobiology 1986;172:275–282.
41. Sertoli MR, Bernengo MG, Ardizzoni A, et al. Phase II trial of recombinant alfa-2b interferon in the treatment of metastatic skin melanoma. Oncology 1989;46:96–98.
42. Cascinelli N. Evaluation of efficacy of adjuvant rIFN alfa 2A in melanoma patients with regional node metastases. Proc Am Soc Clin Oncol 1995;14:1410.
43. Kirkwood JM, Straderman MH, Ernstoff MS, et al. Interferon alfa-2b adjuvant therapy of high-risk resected cutaneous melanoma: the Eastern Cooperative Oncology Group trial EST 1684. J Clin Oncol 1996;14: 7–17.
44. Borden EC, Parkinson D. A perspective on the clinical effectiveness and tolerance of interferon-alfa. Semin Oncol 1998;25(suppl 1):3–8.
45. Dalakas MC, Mock V, Hawkins MJ. Fatigue: definitions, mechanisms, and paradigms for study. Semin Oncol 1998;25(suppl 1):48–53.
46. Plata-Salaman CR. Cytokines and anorexia: a brief overview. Semin Oncol 1998;25(suppl 1):64–72.
47. Cole BF, Gelber RD, Kirkwood JM, et al. A quality-of-life-adjusted survival analysis of interferon alfa-2b adjuvant treatment for high-risk resected cutaneous melanoma: an Eastern Cooperative Oncology Group study (E1684). J Clin Oncol 1996;14:2666–2673.
48. Kirkwood JM, Ibrahim JG, Sondak VK, et al. High- and low-dose interferon alfa 2 b in high risk melanoma: first analysis of Intergroup Trial E1690/S9111/C9190. J Clin Oncol 2000;18:2444–2458.
49. Kirkwood JM, Ibrahim J, Lawson DH, et al. High-dose interferon alfa-2 b does not diminish antibody response to GM2 vaccination in patients with resected melanoma: results of the multicenter Eastern Cooperative Oncology Group Phase II trial E2696. J Clin Oncol 2001:19:1430–1436.
50. Von Wussow P, Bock B, Hartmann F, Deicher H. Intralesional interferon-alpha therapy in advanced malignant melanoma. Cancer 1988; 61:1071–1074.
51. Hersh EM, Murray JL, Kong WK, et al. Phase I study of cancer therapy with recombinant interleukin-2 administered by intravenous bolus injection. Biotherapy 1989;1:215–216.
52. Parkinson DR, Abrams JS, Wiernik PH, et al. Interleukin-2 therapy in patients with metastatic malignant melanoma: a phase II study. J Clin Oncol 1990:8:1650–1656.
53. Whitehead RP, Kopecky KJ, Samson MK, et al. Phase II study of intravenous bolus recombinant interleulun-2 in advanced malignant melanoma: Southwest Oncology Group study. J Natl Cancer Inst 1991; 83:1250–1252.
54. Demchak PA, Mier JW, Robert NJ, et al. Interleukin-2 and high-dose cisplatin in patients with metastatic melanoma: a pilot study. J Clin Oncol 1991;9:1821–1830.
55. Rosenberg SA, Yang JC, Topalian SL, et al. Treatment of 283 consecutive patients with metastatic melanoma or renal cell cancer using high-dose bolus interleukin-2. JAMA 1994;271:907–913.
56. West WH, Tauer KW, Yannelli JR, et al. Constant-infusion recombinant interleukin-2 in adoptive immunotherapy of advanced cancer. N Engl J Med 1987;316:898–905.
57. Dutcher JP, Gaynor ER, Boldt DH, et al. A phase II study of high-dose continuous infusion interleukin-2 with lymphokine-activated killer cells in patients with metastatic melanoma. J Clin Oncol 1991;9:641–648.
58. Dillman RO, Oldham RK, Tauer KW, et al. Continuous interleukin-2 and lymphokine-activated killer cells for advanced cancer: a National Biotherapy Study Group trial. J Clin Oncol 1991;9:1233–1240.
59. Perez EA, Scudder SA, Meyers FA, et al. Weekly 24-hour continuous infusion interleukin-2 for metastatic melanoma and renal cell carcinoma: a phase I study. J Immunother 1991;10:57–62.
60. Vlasveld LT, Horenblas S, Hekman A, et al. Phase II study of intermittent continuous infusion of low-dose recombinant interleukin-2 in advanced melanoma and renal cell carcinoma. Ann Oncol 1994;5:179–181.
61. Atkins MB, Lotze MT, Dutcher JP, et al. High dose recombinant interleukin-2 therapy for patients with metastatic melanoma: analysis of 270 patients treated between 1985–1993. J Clin Oncol 1999;17:2105–2116.
62. Flaherty LE, Redman BG, Chabot G, et al. A phase I-II study of dacarbazine in combination with outpatient interleukin-2 in metastatic malignant melanoma. Cancer 1990;65:2471–2477.
63. Richards JM, Mehta N, Schroeder L, et al. Sequential chemotherapy in the treatment of metastatic melanoma. J Clin Oncol 1992;10:1338–1343.
64. Keilholz U, Scheibenbogen C, Tilgen W, et al. Interferon-alpha and interleukin-2 in the treatment of metastatic melanoma. Cancer 1993; 72:607–614.
65. Atzpodien J, Korfer A, Fanks CR, et al. Home therapy with recombinant interleukin-2 and interferon-alpha 2b in advanced human malignancies. Lancet 1990;335:1509–1512.
66. Conforti AM, Ollila DW, Kelley MC, et al. Update on active specific immunotherapy with melanoma vaccines. J Surg Oncol 1997;66: 55–64.
67. Wallack MK, Sicanandham M, Balch CM, et al. A phase III randomized, double-blind, multi-institutional trial of vaccinia melanoma oncolysate-active specific immunotherapy for patients with stage II melanoma. Cancer 1995;75:34–42.
68. Carrasquillo JA, Abrams PG, Schroff RW, et al. Effect of antibody dose on the imaging and biodistribution of indium-111 9.2.27 anti-melanoma monoclonal antibody. J Nucl Med 1988;29:39–47.
69. Murray JL, Rosenblum MG, Lamki L, et al. Clinical parameters related to optimal tumor localization of indium-111-labeled mouse antimelanoma monoclonal antibody ZME-018. J Nucl Med 1987;28:25–33.
70. Ferrone S. Human tumor associated antigen mimicry by anti-idiotypic antibodies. Ann N Y Acad Sci 1993;690:214–221.
71. Parmiani G, Colombo MP. Somatic gene therapy of human melanoma: preclinical studies and early clinical trials. Melanoma Res 1995;5: 295–301.
72. Rosenberg ST, Aebersold P, Cornetta K. Gene transfer into human—immunotherapy of patients with advanced melanoma, using tumor-infiltrating lymphocytes modified by retroviral gene transduction. N Engl J Med 1990;323:570–578.
73. Rosenberg SA, Anderson F, Blaese M, et al. The development of gene therapy for the treatment of cancer. Ann Surg 1993;218:455–464.
74. Comis RL. DTIC in malignant melanoma: a perspective. Cancer Treat Rep 1976;64:1123.
75. Hill GJ, Krementz ET, Hill HZ. Dimethyl traiazenoimidazole carboxamide and combination therapy for melanoma: IV. Late results after complete responses to chemotherapy. Cancer 1984;53:1299–1305.
76. Newlands ES, Stevens MF, Wedge SR, et al. Temozolomide: a review of its discovery, chemical properties, pre-clinical development and clinical trials. Cancer Treat Rev 1997;23:35–61.
77. Middleton MR, Grob JJ, Aaronson N, et al. Randomized phase III study of temozolomide versus dacarbazine in the treatment of advanced metastatic melanoma. J Clin Oncol 2000;18:158–163.
78. Ahmann DL. Nitrosoureas in the management of disseminated malignant melanoma. Cancer Treat Rep 1976;60:747.
79. Jacquillat C, Khayat D, Banzet P, et al. Final report of the French multicenter phase II study of the nitrosourea fotemustine in 153 evaluable patients with disseminated malignant melanoma including patients with cerebral metastases. Cancer 1990;66:1873–1878.
80. Mechl Z, Kreja P. Cis-diamminedichloroplatinum in the treatment of disseminated malignant melanoma. Neoplasia 1983;30:371–377.
81. Olver I, Green M, Peters W, et al. A phase II trial of zeniplatin in metastatic melanoma. Am J Clin Oncol 1995;18:56–58.
82. Evans L, Casper ES, Rosenbluth R. Phase II trial of carboplatin in advanced melanoma. Cancer Treat Rep 1987;71:171.
83. Steffens TA, Bajorin D, Chapman PB, et al. A phase II trial of high-dose cisplatin and dacarbazine: lack of efficacy of high-dose, cisplatin-based therapy for metastatic melanoma. Cancer 1991;68:1230-1237.

84. Luger SM, Kirkwood JM, Ernstoff MS, Vlock DR. High-dose cisplatin and dacarbazine in the treatment of metastatic melanoma. J Natl Cancer Inst 1990;82:1934–1937.
85. Murren JR, DeRosa W, Durivage HJ, et al. High-dose cisplatin plus DTIC in the treatment of metastatic melanoma. Cancer 1991;67:1514–1517.
86. Rusthoven JJ, Quirt IC, Iscoe NA, et al. Randomized, double-blind, placebo-controlled trial comparing the response rates of carmustine, dacarbazine, and cisplatin with and without tamoxifen in patients with metastatic melanoma. National Cancer Institute of Canada clinical trials group. J Clin Oncol 1996;14:2083–2090.
87. Chapman PB, Einhorn LH, Meyers ML, et al. Phase III multicenter randomized trial of Dartmouth regimen versus dacarbazine in patients with metastatic melanoma. J Clin Oncol 1999;17:2745–2751.
88. Adami HO, Bergstrom R, Holmberg L, et al. The effect of female sex hormones on cancer survival. JAMA 1990;263:2189–2193.
89. Cocconi G, Bella M, Calabresi F, et al. Treatment of metastatic malignant melanoma with dacarbazine plus tamoxifen. N Engl J Med 1992;327:516–523.
90. Nathanson L, Meelu MA, Losada R. Chemohormone therapy of metastatic melanoma with megestrol acetate plus dacarbazine, carmustine, and cisplatin. Cancer 1994;73:98–102.
91. Margolin KA, Doroshow JH, Akman ST. Phase II trial of cisplatin and alpha-interferon in advanced malignant melanoma. J Clin Oncol 1992; 10:1574–1578.
92. Pyrhonen S, Hahka-Kemppinen M, Muhonen T. A promising interferon plus four-drug chemotherapy regimen for metastatic melanoma. J Clin Oncol 1992;10:1919–1926.
93. Mitchell MS, Kempf RA, Harel W, et al. Effectiveness and tolerability of low-dose cyclophosphamide and low-dose intravenous interleukin-2 disseminated melanoma. J Clin Oncol 1988;6:409–424.
94. Shiloni E, Pouillart P, Janssens J, et al. Sequential dacarbazine chemotherapy followed by recombinant interleukin-2 in metastatic melanoma: a pilot multicenter phase I-II study. Eur J Cancer Clin Oncol 1989: 25(suppl 3):S45–S49.
95. Stoter G, Aamdal S, Rodenhuis S, et al. Sequential administration of recombinant human interleukin-2 and dacarbazine in metastatic melanoma: a multicenter phase II study. J Clin Oncol 1991;9:1687–1691.
96. Flaherty LE, Robinson W, Redman BG, et al. A phase II study of dacarbazine and cisplatin in combination with outpatient administered interleukin-2 in metastatic malignant melanoma. Cancer 1993;71:3520–3525.
97. Richards JM, Mehta N, Ramming K, Skosey P. Sequential chemoimmunotherapy in the treatment of metastatic melanoma. J Clin Oncol 1992;10:1338–1343.
98. Khayat D, Tourani JM, Benhammouda A, et al. Sequential chemoimmunotherapy with cisplatin, interleukin-2, and interferon alfa-2a for metastatic melanoma. J Clin Oncol 1993;11:2173–2180.
99. Bajetta E, Negretti E, Giannotti B, et al. Phase II study of interferon-2a and dacarbazine in advanced melanoma. Am J Clin Oncol 1990;13: 405–409.
100. Falkson CI, Falkson G, Falkson HC. Improved results with the addition of recumbent interferon alpha-2b to dacarbazine in treatment with patients with metastatic malignant melanoma. J Clin Oncol 1991;9:1403–1408.
101. Smith KA, Green JA, Eccles JM. Interferon alpha-2a and vindesine in the treatment of advanced malignant melanoma. Eur J Cancer 1992;28: 438–441.
102. Keiholz U, Goey SH, Punt CJ, et al. Interferon alfa-2a and interleukin-2 with or without cisplatin in metastatic melanoma: a randomized trial of the European Organization for Research and Treatment of Cancer Melanoma Cooperative Group. J Clin Oncol 1997;15:2579–2588.
103. Rosenberg SA, Yang JC, Schwartzentruber DJ, et al. Prospective randomized trial of the treatment of patients with metastatic melanoma using chemotherapy with cisplatin, dacarbazine, and tamoxifen alone or in combination with interleukin-2 and interferon alfa-2b. J Clin Oncol 1999;17:968–975.
104. Eton O, Legha S, Bedikian A, et al. Phase III randomized trial of cisplatin, vinblastine and dacarbazine (CVD) plus interleukin-2 and interferon-alfpha-2b versus CVD in patients with metastatic melanoma. Proc ASCO 2000;19:552(abstract 2174).
105. Legha SS, Ring S, Eton O, et al. Development of biochemotherapy regimen with concurrent administration of cisplatin, vinblastine, dacarbazine, interferon alfa, and interleukin-2 for patients with metastatic melanoma. J Clin Oncol 1998;16:1752–1759.
106. Kroon BBR. Regional isolation perfusion in melanoma of the limbs: accomplishments, unsolved problems, future. Eur J Surg Oncol 1998; 14:101–110.
107. Klaase JM, Kroon BBR, van Geel AN, et al. Prognostic factors for tumor response and limb recurrence-free interval in patients with advanced melanoma of the limbs treated with regional isolated perfusion with melphalan. Surgery 1994;115:39–45.
108. Klaase JM, Kroon BBR, van Geel AN, et al. A retrospective comparative study evaluating the results of a single perfusion versus double-perfusion schedule with melphalan in patients with recurrent melanoma of the lower limb. Cancer 1993;71:2990–2994.
109. Lejeuene FJ, Lienard D. Isolation perfusion of the limbs for in transit melanoma metastasized with cytokines and chemotherapy. In: Lejeune FJ, Chaudhuri PK, Das Gupta TK, eds. Malignant Melanoma: Medical and Surgical Management. New York: McGraw-Hill, 1994:233–240.
110. Lober CW, Dysplastic (atypical) nevi: significance and management. South Med J 1992;85:870–877.
111. Koh HK, Geller AC, Miller DR, Lew RA. Screening for melanoma and skin cancer in the United States. In: Miller AB, Chamberlain J, Day NE, et al., eds. Cancer Screening. New York: Cambridge University Press, 1990.
112. Westerdahl J, Olsson H, Masback A, et al. Is the use of sunscreens a risk factor for malignant melanoma? Melanoma Res 1995;5:59–65.
113. Stokes R, Diffey B. How well are sunscreen users protected? Photodermatol Photoimmunol Photomed 1997;13:186–188.

134
HEMATOPOIETIC STEM CELL TRANSPLANTATION

Janelle B. Perkins and Gary C. Yee

Hematopoietic stem cell transplantation (HSCT) is a process that involves intravenous infusion of hematopoietic stem cells from a compatible donor into a recipient usually following administration of high-dose chemotherapy. Hematopoietic stem cells can be derived from the bone marrow, from peripheral blood, or from umbilical cord blood. The rationale for HSCT in the treatment of malignant disease is based on studies that show that most anticancer drugs have a steep dose-response relationship and that bone marrow suppression limits the chemotherapy dosage that can be safely administered. Although standard-dose chemotherapy can prolong survival in many cancer patients, most patients are not cured of their disease (Fig. 134–1). The infusion of hematopoietic stem cells allows oncologists to administer very-high chemotherapy doses (as much as 10-fold higher). If tumor cells that are resistant to standard doses are sensitive to higher doses of chemotherapy, then tumor cell kill will be greatly increased, and the likelihood of cure would be higher with HSCT. The chemotherapy dose cannot be escalated indefinitely, however, because of the risk of death caused by nonhematopoietic toxicity. High-dose chemotherapy followed by HSCT has become an important treatment modality for a variety of malignant and nonmalignant diseases. Approximately 50,000 transplants are performed worldwide each year, primarily for malignant diseases. Historically the most common type of donor was a genetically nonidentical individual such as a histocompatible sibling (referred to as allogeneic HSCT). But the number of autologous transplants—in which the patient serves as his or her own donor—has increased dramatically, and the number of autologous transplants performed each year currently exceeds the number of allogeneic transplants. Although this chapter focuses on the application of HSCT in the treatment of malignant disease, it is important to note that many nonmalignant diseases—including aplastic anemia, thalassemia, sickle cell anemia, immunodeficiency disorders, and other genetic disorders—are potentially curable with allogeneic HSCT. Transplantation is also being investigated as a treatment modality in patients with life-threatening autoimmune diseases such as rheumatoid arthritis, systemic and multiple sclerosis, and systemic lupus erythematosus.

This chapter summarizes the procedures involved in HSCT, and current issues in the field of HSCT, as well as the application of HSCT in the treatment of malignant diseases. More detailed information on HSCT can be found in recently published reviews and books.[1–5] Information on HSCT can also be found on several Web sites (www.Bmtinfo.org; www.IBMTR.org; and www.Marrow.org)

DONORS AND HISTOCOMPATIBILITY TESTING

Different types of donors are used in HSCT. In autologous transplants, patients receive their own hematopoietic stem cells that were collected and stored before intensive cytotoxic therapy. In syngeneic transplants, an identical twin serves as the donor. In allogeneic transplants, the donor is genetically not identical to the recipient but shares some common tissue antigens. Immunologic compatibility is evaluated with studies of cell surface antigens encoded by genes of the major histocompatibility complex (MHC), which, in humans, is located on the sixth chromosome and is referred to as the HLA (human leukocyte antigen) complex.[6] The genes of the HLA system are clustered in three distinct regions designated class I, class II, and class III. Class I and class II antigens function as major transplantation antigens, while products of class III genes play other important roles in the immune system. The major class I loci in humans are referred to as HLA-A, HLA-B, and HLA-C. There is one major class II locus (HLA-D); this region is comprised of three sets of genes encoding HLA-DR, HLA-DQ, and HLA-DP molecules. Class I and class II antigens differ in their tissue distribution, structure, and function. Class I antigens are expressed on virtually all nucleated cells and serve as the primary targets for cytotoxic T lymphocytes. In contrast, class II antigens are normally expressed only on macrophages, B lymphocytes, and activated T lymphocytes, and serve as the primary targets for helper T lymphocytes.

Historically, the most important HLA loci in allogeneic transplantation were HLA-A, HLA-B, and HLA-D (specifically, HLA-DR).[7] Typing for HLA-A, HLA-B, and HLA-DR has been traditionally performed by serologic typing with standard microcytotoxicity assays. HLA types determined by this method are reported as the loci (A, B, or DR), followed by a number (e.g., HLA-A2). A lowercase "w" is sometimes added before the number to indicate "workshop" or tentative designation based on American or international histocompatibility workshops. Typing for the HLA-D region also can be performed with cellular typing methods, such as the mixed lymphocyte reaction (MLR) or mixed lymphocyte culture (MLC). A "positive" MLR or MLC indicates incompatibility somewhere in the HLA-D region. Individuals who have a low degree of reactivity in the MLR or MLC (expressed as a low percent relative response), and who meet other selection criteria, could serve as donors. However, recent studies indicate that MLR or MLC reactivity does not correlate significantly with the risk of acute graft-versus-host disease (GVHD) or graft failure, and most HSCT centers no longer use this method alone to determine HLA compatibility.[7] In addition to serologic typing, HSCT centers now use DNA-based molecular typing techniques, such as polymerase chain reaction (PCR), for HLA-DR typing because of the extensive polymorphism in the HLA-D region and the high error rate in serologic typing. For example, although there are more than 100 DRB1 alleles, serologic reagents can distinguish no more than 15 different DR serotypes. DNA-based techniques in matching HLA-DR alleles to select unrelated donors may reduce the risk of severe acute GVHD in that setting. And some studies show that matching the other HLA alleles by molecular typing may affect outcomes in matched unrelated donor transplantation.[8–10]

The most common donor for allogeneic transplants is an HLA-identical sibling. However, only about 30% of Americans have an

could increase the risk of GVHD. Concerns were also raised over the safety and ethics of administering G-CSF to normal individuals volunteering as donors. Short-term effects are similar to those seen in cancer patients (e.g., bone pain, headache, fever). Because the potential long-term effects related to G-CSF are unknown, prolonged follow-up of donors is recommended.[31]

In early investigations of allogeneic PBPC transplants, patients experienced more rapid hematopoietic recovery and required fewer transfusions when compared to historical control patients receiving bone marrow. Although these studies have not reported an increased risk of acute GVHD, relapse, or transplant-related mortality in patients receiving allogeneic PBPC transplants, a higher incidence of chronic GVHD was observed.[32] As seen in the autologous setting, allogeneic PBPC transplants may offer an economic benefit over bone marrow transplants because of a reduced use of resources (e.g., transfusions, total parenteral nutrition, and supportive care medications).[33] Results of other studies, including a randomized controlled trial, confirm that the recovery of both neutrophils and platelets is faster with peripheral blood from HLA-identical siblings than with bone marrow.[34,35] Although results of the randomized study showed that the incidence of acute or chronic GVHD was not significantly different between the two groups, patients who received allogeneic PBPCs tended to have a higher incidence of chronic GVHD as compared with those who received bone marrow. These studies also show that disease-free and overall survival rates are at least equivalent and possibly improved in patients receiving allogeneic PBPCs. Use of PBPCs from unrelated donors is also being investigated.[36]

In addition to bone marrow and peripheral blood, hematopoietic stem cells are also found in umbilical cord blood (UCB). UCB is an attractive source for several reasons. Because the stem cells are collected from placental blood, there is no risk to the mother or the baby. There is also very low risk of transmissible infectious diseases, such as cytomegalovirus and Epstein-Barr virus. In addition, the cells are available immediately because the donor does not have to be located and harvested. Initially, UCB was obtained from siblings but now recipients of transplants from unrelated donors account for almost all patients who receive UCB transplants. Worldwide, about 200 transplantations of UCB from related donors and 1,000 from unrelated donors have been performed. In data pooled from the Eurocord-Cord Blood Transplant Group and the International Bone Marrow Transplant Registry, 113 children who had received UCB transplants were compared to 2,052 children who had received bone marrow transplants during the same time period. All donors were HLA-matched siblings. A multivariate analysis showed that patients who received UCB transplants had a lower risk of acute and chronic GVHD, but the UCB group also had a higher risk of delayed neutrophil and platelet engraftment. The mortality rate in the two groups was similar.[37]

UCB can also be used as a source of hematopoietic stem cells in patients who do not have a HLA-matched sibling donor. In some series, recipients of unrelated UCB have experienced delayed engraftment as compared to recipients of MUD bone marrow or PBPC transplants, which may be related to the low numbers of infused $CD34^+$ cells. The incidence of GVHD appears to be similar or slightly less with unrelated UCB, even when donors are not completely HLA-matched, as compared with MUD marrow transplants.[38,39] Although not directly compared, survival rates in children with acute leukemias are similar to those seen after a bone marrow transplant.[40]

A major limitation to UCB transplants is the limited volume of blood collected, usually 60–150 mL. Although the relatively low numbers of hematopoietic cells may be adequate for hematopoietic engraftment in children and small adults, it may not be adequate for larger recipients. Efforts to expand the number of hematopoietic stem cells include culturing them *ex vivo* with combinations of HGF or "pooling" several units of UCB for one recipient. More experience is needed with larger and older recipients before this procedure can be recommended as a standard procedure in that population.

APPROACHES TO ERADICATE MALIGNANT CELLS

PRETRANSPLANT CHEMOTHERAPY

Nearly all patients who receive HSCT must be prepared (or "conditioned") before infusion of hematopoietic stem cells.[41,42] In patients with malignant disease, the goal of the preparative or conditioning regimen is to kill as many malignant cells as possible. Preparative regimens usually include commonly used anticancer drugs given at very high doses—doses that would be associated with severe and life-threatening bone marrow suppression if hematopoietic stem cells were not infused. In patients undergoing allogeneic HSCT, another purpose of the preparative regimen is to suppress the immune system of the recipient so that the graft is not rejected.

In some preparative regimens, the only drug given is cyclophosphamide, a drug with both immunosuppressive and cytotoxic effects. Because of the inadequate antitumor activity of cyclophosphamide in some types of cancers, other drugs are often added. Examples of drugs that often are included in preparative regimens are cytarabine (ara-C), busulfan, thiotepa, etoposide (VP-16), carboplatin, cisplatin, carmustine (BCNU), melphalan, ifosfamide, mitoxantrone, and paclitaxel.

Total body irradiation (TBI) is also commonly used in pretransplant preparative regimens. In patients with malignant disease, the rationale is to eradicate malignant cells located in areas inaccessible to the systemic circulation and thus, to the cytotoxic agents. TBI also has significant immunosuppressive activity. Historically, the standard TBI regimen involved the administration of a midline tissue dose of about 1000 cGy (1 cGy = 1 rad), which is more than twice the lethal dose of radiation for a normal person. Many centers currently give fractionated (split over several days, once or twice a day) rather than single-dose TBI to patients with malignant disease. The rationale for this approach is an improved therapeutic ratio—destruction of more leukemic cells and marrow stem cells while sparing other normal tissues. The acute toxicities of TBI consist of fever, nausea, vomiting, diarrhea, mucositis, and tender swelling of the parotid gland. Long-term complications of TBI-containing regimens include cataract formation, growth retardation, carcinogenesis, permanent reproductive sterility, and secondary malignancies.

LEUKEMIA

Most patients with leukemia undergoing allogeneic HSCT receive the combination of cyclophosphamide and TBI (CyTBI). When given with TBI, cyclophosphamide is usually given first, as two 60 mg/kg/day doses, followed by TBI. TBI can be given as a single dose or fractionated over several days. One variation of that regimen is to give hyperfractionated TBI first, followed by cyclophosphamide. In that regimen, 11 TBI doses of 120 cGy are given; doses are given three times a day on days −7 to −5 (*note:* day 0 is designated as the day of transplant), and twice a day on the last day (day −4). After TBI, two doses of cyclophosphamide are given intravenously once a day at a dosage of 60 mg/kg on days −3 and −2. This regimen appears to be more effective than the standard CyTBI regimen in patients with acute lymphocytic leukemia (ALL). It is not clear whether the increased effectiveness is related to the hyperfractionated TBI or the change in the sequence of TBI and cyclophosphamide administration.

Because of the many acute and chronic toxicities of TBI, it would be advantageous to omit it from the preparative regimen. One widely used preparative regimen that does not include TBI is busulfan and cyclophosphamide (BuCy). In the original regimen (BuCy4), busulfan was given orally at a dosage of 1 mg/kg every 6 hours (4 mg/kg/day) for 16 doses on days −9 to −6, followed by four doses of cyclophosphamide, given intravenously once daily at a dosage of 50 mg/kg on days −5 to −2. In one widely used modification of that regimen (BuCy2), the total cyclophosphamide dosage is reduced from 200 (50 × 4) to 120 (60 × 2) mg/kg. Busulfan blood levels are monitored at some centers because some studies suggest that systemic exposure may correlate with outcome.[43] An intravenous (IV) form of busulfan is also available commercially and may reduce some of the interpatient variability in systemic exposure. The dose of IV busulfan approved for pretransplant conditioning regimens is 0.8 mg/kg every 6 hours for 4 days. Once-a-day dosing regimens have also been developed, which may facilitate outpatient administration of intravenous busulfan.

Prospective randomized studies have compared CyTBI to BuCy in patients with various forms of leukemia. In patients with CML in first chronic phase, BuCy had similar or greater antileukemic activity and was better tolerated than CyTBI.[44,45] But in patients with acute nonlymphocytic leukemia (ANLL) in first remission or advanced leukemia (e.g., patients beyond first remission or first chronic phase), the CyTBI regimen was associated with significantly better disease-free survival rates than BuCy.[46,47] BuCy has also been associated with more regimen-related toxicity than CyTBI in some studies.[48]

Other drugs have been evaluated in addition to or instead of cyclophosphamide in the preparative regimen, particularly in patients with ALL. Examples include cytarabine or etoposide in combination with TBI. There are no convincing data to indicate that any of these regimens are superior to CyTBI or BuCy. The same preparative regimens are usually given to patients undergoing autologous HSCT for leukemia.

LYMPHOMA

Based on experience in patients with leukemia, the initial regimen used in many patients with lymphoma was CyTBI, particularly in allogeneic HSCT. Most preparative regimens used in autologous transplantation for lymphoma include cyclophosphamide and at least one other drug. TBI is usually not included in the conditioning regimen. One widely used regimen in autologous transplantation is the CBV regimen, which consists of cyclophosphamide, carmustine (BCNU), and etoposide (VP-16). In that original regimen, cyclophosphamide was given at a dosage of 1.5 g/m^2 on days −6 to −3, carmustine was given at a dosage of 300 mg/m^2 on day −6, and etoposide was given at a dosage of 100 mg/m^2 every 12 hours for six doses on days −6 to −4. Some centers have modified the original CBV regimen by changing the dosage of some of the drugs or adding or substituting other drugs including cytosine arabinoside, etoposide, melphalan, lomustine, and thioguanine. Other widely used regimens are BEAC (BCNU, etoposide, ara-C, and cyclophosphamide) and BEAM (BCNU, etoposide, ara-C, and melphalan). No one preparative regimen is clearly superior to other regimens in the treatment of lymphoma.

Although TBI is usually not included in the conditioning regimen, some form of radiation therapy is often given, depending on the type, location, and extent of disease. Instead of TBI, some patients receive localized radiation in high doses to areas of residual or bulky disease. Many patients with Hodgkin's disease have received thoracic radiation as primary therapy for their disease, so TBI is usually avoided in patients with Hodgkin's disease. Conversely, most patients with indolent non-Hodgkin's lymphoma receive TBI as part of their preparative regimen because of the known sensitivity of these tumors to low doses of radiation.

SOLID TUMORS

Most conditioning regimens in autologous transplantation include at least one alkylating agent because of their steep dose-response curve and other favorable characteristics previously discussed. Many regimens include more than one alkylating agent, based on preclinical studies that show that resistance to a specific alkylating agent does not impart cross-resistance to other alkylating agents. Other anticancer drugs that modulate the activity of alkylating agents in a synergistic manner, such as etoposide, are also attractive drugs to include in high-dose preparative regimens. The dose of nonalkylating agents with antitumor activity has also been escalated in patients with solid tumors based on tumor-specific activity. Examples include mitoxantrone, paclitaxel, and topotecan. It is not clear whether these regimens offer any clinical advantages to those that include only alkylating agents.

PURGING THE STEM CELL PRODUCT

One disadvantage of autologous HSCT is that the stem cell product (graft) may be contaminated with malignant cells. Infusion of these malignant cells may contribute to tumor relapse. Many approaches have been developed to eliminate ("purge") the marrow of these tumor cells.[49] The most common approach is to add substances, such as chemicals or monoclonal antibodies, to the stem cell product while it is outside of the body *(ex vivo)* (Fig. 134–3). Because the substances are removed before infusion of the stem cells, nonhematopoietic tissues are not exposed to the substances and therefore are not damaged. However, these substances can remove or damage hematopoietic stem cells, which are essential for complete and rapid engraftment, and purging has been associated with a delay in marrow recovery. *Ex vivo* marrow purging also is performed in allogeneic HSCT in an attempt to eliminate T lymphocytes believed to be responsible for acute GVHD (Fig. 134–3). Results with this approach are discussed in the "Graft-Versus-Host Disease" section later in the chapter.

One approach is to add one or more monoclonal antibodies that are directed against specific antigens present on the tumor cells, but which are absent on nearly all other cells.[50] Although this approach is theoretically attractive, it is limited because not all cells from patients with the same type of cancer will express a specific antigen. Furthermore, for some types of cancers, it has been difficult to identify antigens distinct from those present on normal hematopoietic stem cells. To date, this strategy has been used most commonly in patients with lymphoid malignancies, either ALL or non-Hodgkin's lymphoma.

Another method of purging is to add chemicals or drugs to kill the tumor cells.[51] The advantage of this technique is that it can be used for a broader range of tumor types. However, chemical purging is not completely selective for tumor cells, and it is therefore important to add the precise amount of chemical or drug that kills sufficient numbers of tumor cells while sparing the largest number of hematopoietic stem cells. The chemical that is most commonly used for purging is 4-hydroperoxycyclophosphamide (4-HC), a congener of cyclophosphamide. A stable compound, 4-HC enters cells and is rapidly reduced to 4-hydroxycyclophosphamide, which serves as the precursor to the reactive phosphoramide mustard. The level of aldehyde dehydrogenase, the enzyme that inactivates 4-hydroxycyclophosphamide, appears to be highest in early hematopoietic progenitors and decreases as these cells differentiate. This observation may explain why 4-HC appears to have an acceptable therapeutic index. Other analogs of

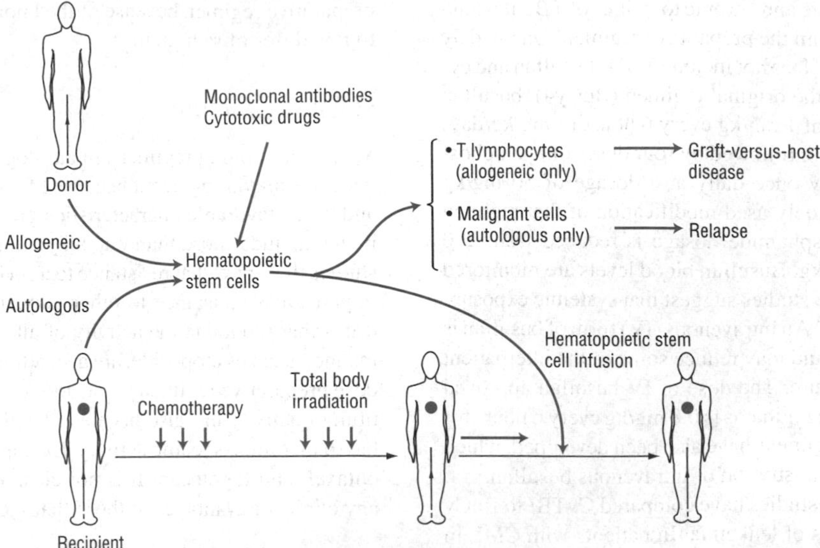

FIGURE 134–3. The use of *ex vivo* marrow purging to remove or destroy T lymphocytes (allogeneic only) or residual malignant cells (autologous only).

cyclophosphamide (e.g., Mafosfamide) also are being investigated as chemical purging agents.

Another method to purge malignant cells is to identify, select, and concentrate hematopoietic stem cells, a process known as positive selection.[49] In this process, cells collected from marrow or peripheral blood are treated *ex vivo* with monoclonal antibodies against CD34. $CD34^+$ cells are therefore separated from those that are $CD34^-$, including most malignant cells. Although preliminary results with one of these techniques show that a one- to four-log depletion of tumor cells can be achieved, no significant difference in neutrophil recovery, immune reconstitution, or progression-free survival rate was observed.[52,53]

Although purging has been extensively studied, there is a lack of convincing evidence that it improves transplant outcomes. These techniques can be cumbersome and add cost to the transplant procedure. Therefore their use should be restricted to randomized trials that evaluate not only efficiency of tumor cell removal but also relapse-free and overall survival rates.[54]

POSTTRANSPLANT IMMUNOTHERAPY

The rationale for posttransplant immunotherapy is based on observations that T lymphocytes responsible for GVHD can be directed toward malignant cells. This is referred to as the "graft-versus-leukemia" (GVL) or "graft-versus-tumor" (GVT) effect. Evidence for GVT is based on retrospective studies that show that patients who developed GVHD had a lower risk of leukemic relapse than those who did not develop GVHD; the overall survival rate, however, was not different because of the increased nonrelapse mortality associated with GVHD. Other anecdotal evidence supporting a GVT effect was the increased risk of relapse found with T-cell-depleted transplants as compared to unmodified transplants, and the difference in relapse rates between recipients of syngeneic and HLA-identical sibling transplants.

Based on these retrospective studies, a prospective randomized study was done to determine whether a reduction in the intensity of acute GVHD prophylaxis or infusion of donor leukocytes (e.g., T lymphocytes) would reduce the risk of relapse in patients with advanced hematologic malignancies treated with allogeneic HSCT.[55] Although the risk of acute GVHD was increased in patients randomized to receive short methotrexate or long methotrexate plus donor buffy coat cells, the risk of relapse was not decreased and the survival rate was not improved.

Donor lymphocyte/leukocyte infusions, either alone or in combination with interferon-α (IFN-α), have also been given to induce a GVT effect in patients who have relapsed after allogeneic HSCT.[56,57] In a report of 140 patients who received donor lymphocyte/leukocyte infusions for treatment of posttransplant relapse, complete responses were observed in 60% of CML patients, with higher response rates in patients with cytogenetic and chronic phase relapse than in patients with more advanced disease.[58] Response rates in patients with acute leukemia and myelodysplasia were lower, which may be related to the rapid proliferation of acute leukemia versus the often prolonged time to response after donor lymphocyte/leukocyte infusions or to the lack of suitable target antigens on non-CML cells for recognition by donor cytotoxic T lymphocytes. The most serious complications of donor lymphocyte/leukocyte infusions are GVHD and pancytopenia, which contribute to a 14% nonrelapse mortality at 1 year. Investigators are evaluating other strategies such as T lymphocyte dose escalation, selective depletion of $CD8^+$ cells or transduction of donor T lymphocytes with suicide genes.[56,57]

Based on reports that GVHD developed after cyclosporine was withdrawn in rats after syngeneic or autologous HSCT, some investigators have induced GVHD after autologous transplant in an attempt to induce a GVT effect.[59] In human studies, GVHD after autologous transplant is induced with administration of low doses of cyclosporine (1 mg/kg, given intravenously) for 28 days, beginning on the day of marrow infusion. With this regimen, about two-thirds of patients develop autologous GVHD of the skin while receiving the drug. The skin rash either resolved spontaneously or with systemic corticosteroids. Preliminary results with this approach have been encouraging but randomized studies are needed to determine a correlation between development of GVHD and an improved disease-free survival rate.[59]

Another approach is to administer a cytokines with immunomodulatory activity, such as interleukin-2 (IL-2) or interferon.[60–62] Some beneficial effects have been observed with the use of these agents and studies are ongoing to further define their role in prolonging relapse-free survival after HSCT. Other investigators have evaluated the use of posttransplant adoptive cellular immunotherapy which consists of the infusion of specific effector cells such as T lymphocytes or NK cells.[59] In this approach, a tumor-specific target (i.e., a tumor-specific antigen that is expressed exclusively or preferentially by tumor cells) is identified, and then T lymphocytes are stimulated by the antigen *ex vivo* with the addition of cytokines such as IL-2. These stimulated T lymphocytes are subsequently infused back into the patient after transplant during a time of low tumor burden. If a tumor-specific antigen is identified, another approach is to develop a vaccine to that antigen and then administer it in the posttransplant period. Preliminary vaccine studies have been done in breast and ovarian cancer and in myeloma.[63,64]

NONMYELOABLATIVE TRANSPLANTS

The newest approach to take advantage of the immunoreactivity between healthy donor T-lymphocytes and host tumor cells is the use of nonmyeloablative transplants (NMT, "mini" transplants, or transplant "lite"). The use of NMT is based on the assumption that most of the antitumor activity associated with allogeneic transplants is the result of the donor T lymphocyte-mediated GVT effect, and not the result of the myeloablative doses of chemotherapy or radiation (as was previously thought). If this assumption is correct, the major role of the conditioning regimen is to suppress the host immune system, thus allowing engraftment of donor hematopoietic stem cells and donor T lymphocyte cytotoxicity. In that model, regimens that consist of myeloablative doses of chemoradiotherapy would be replaced with those that include lower, less-intensive doses of the same drugs or new anticancer drugs that are immunosuppressive. A major advantage of this approach is that transplants could be potentially offered to patients who would not typically be considered for allogeneic HSCT because of their unacceptably high risk of transplant-related complications (e.g., increased age or those with moderately compromised organ function).

NMTs are now being evaluated in patients with hematologic malignancies and solid tumors.[65–68] Regimens have included combinations of fludarabine, antithymocyte globulin (ATG), cyclophosphamide, and/or low dose TBI. NMT is often followed by donor lymphocyte/leukocyte infusions posttransplant to prevent graft failure and to further augment immune-mediated cytotoxicity. Preliminary results show that the nonmyeloablative regimens are well tolerated with less-severe myelosuppression and organ toxicity. Graft rejection is seen in approximately 10% of patients. Although GVHD is delayed as compared with historical controls treated with standard myeloablative regimens, it continues to be a major clinical problem. In addition, because the GVT effect is not immediate (onset of response may take 2 to 6 months), slower growing, more indolent diseases such as CML, chronic lymphocytic leukemia (CLL), or indolent non-Hodgkin's lymphomas are more likely to benefit than fast-growing or bulky tumors. Longer followup is required to determine whether patients treated with NMT will have an improved survival rate as compared with other treatments.

CLINICAL RESULTS

Because of the relative high cost and the morbidity and mortality associated with the procedure, HSCT should only be performed in cancer patients who have little chance of long-term survival with standard-dose chemotherapy. Table 134–1 lists the most common types of cancer treated with HSCT. HSCT can be used at different times in the disease course (Table 134–2). Although HSCT can cure a few patients with refractory disease, it is most effective when the tumor burden is low (i.e., when the patient is in remission) and still responding to chemotherapy. HSCT is currently most often used as intensive consolidation therapy in patients who have responded to standard-dose chemotherapy but who have a low likelihood of long-term survival or cure. HSCT is also commonly used in patients who experience relapse or recurrence of their cancer and respond to salvage chemotherapy (i.e., sensitive relapse). These patients undergo HSCT during their remission.

ACUTE NONLYMPHOCYTIC LEUKEMIA

In ANLL, HCST is the only curative option for patients who fail initial induction therapy, or for patients who have experienced leukemic relapse. The proportion of long-term survivors after autologous or allogeneic HSCT when patients receive transplantation while in untreated first relapse or in second remission is approximately 20% to 35% (Table 134–3).[69] Patients who receive transplantation while in

TABLE 134–1. Use of Hematopoietic Stem Cell Transplantation in Selected Malignant Diseases

	Bone Marrow Transplantation		
Disease	*Preferred Type*	*Potentially Curative in Advanced Disease*	*Standard Therapy*[a]
Acute leukemia	Allogeneic in most cases	Yes	Yes
Chronic myelogenous leukemia	Allogeneic	Yes	Yes
Chronic lymphocytic leukemia	Controversial	Uncertain	No
Multiple myeloma	Controversial	Uncertain	No
Non-Hodgkin's lymphoma			
Histologically aggressive	Autologous in most cases	Yes	Yes
Histologically indolent	Autologous in most cases	Uncertain	Yes
Hodgkin's disease	Autologous in most cases	Yes	Yes
Breast cancer	Autologous	Uncertain	No
Testicular cancer	Autologous	Yes	Yes
Neuroblastoma	Uncertain	Probably	Yes

[a]Standard therapy is defined as treatment that is widely accepted by physicians and routinely reimbursed by most third-party payers at some point in the course of the disease. As noted in the text, the designation of hematopoietic stem cell transplantation as standard therapy is controversial.

Reprinted from Armitage JO. Bone marrow transplantation. N Engl J Med 1994;330:827–838.

TABLE 134–2. Possibilities for Timing of Hematopoietic Stem Cell Transplantation in the Treatment of Cancer

Primary treatment
Partial responders or slow responders (before progression)
Initial complete remission (i.e., consolidation)
Nonresponders (primary treatment failure)
Relapse
  Untested (i.e., no other salvage therapy)
  Tested (i.e., after other salvage therapy)
    Sensitive relapse (i.e., complete or partial remission)
    Resistant relapse (i.e., no response or progression)
End-stage patients

Modified from Armitage JO. Bone marrow transplantation in the treatment of patients with lymphoma. Blood 1989;73:1750.

second complete remission have longer survival than those treated with standard chemotherapy, especially patients who are younger than 30 years of age and those who had first complete remissions greater than 1 year in duration. The proportion of long-term survivors decreases to about 20% when patients receive transplantation while in chemotherapy-resistant first relapse, or to 10% to 15% when HSCT is performed after patients have had multiple relapses.

For patients who achieve a complete remission with standard remission-induction therapy, the role of HSCT is less clear. Response rates and median survival rates have steadily improved in patients with ANLL treated with intensive consolidation chemotherapy. Of these patients with ANLL, 20% to 40% survive for more than 5 years and are probably cured of their disease (see Chap. 131). In contrast, long-term survival is observed in 40% to 60% of patients with ANLL treated with allogeneic HSCT from an HLA-identical sibling while in first remission (Table 134–3).[69] This improvement in disease-free survival rate with allogeneic HSCT has been confirmed in several prospective studies, but the difference is not statistically significant in all studies. In a series of more than 600 patients in first remission (mostly adults), the allogeneic HSCT group had significantly better disease-free survival rate at 4 years than did those in the intensive chemotherapy group (55% vs 30%).[70] Similar findings were reported in a United States intergroup trial.[71] A significant difference favoring allogeneic HSCT over conventional consolidation was seen in patients with either good or poor prognosis cytogenetics. The overall survival rate, however, was not significantly different between the two groups in either study.

TABLE 134–3. Long-Term Results of High-Dose Chemotherapy with Allogeneic Transplantation Versus Intensive Chemotherapy in the Treatment of Leukemias

		Long-Term Survival (%)	
Disease	Status	*BMT*	*Chemotherapy*
ANLL	1st remission	40–60	20–30
	2nd remission	20–30	0
	Multiple relapses	10–15	0
ALL	1st remission (high risk)	30–50	30–50
	2nd remission	25–40	<10
	Multiple relapses	10–15	0
CML	Chronic phase	50–60	0
	Accelerated/blast phase	15–30	0

ANLL, acute nonlymphocytic leukemia; ALL, acute lymphoblastic leukemia; CML, chronic myelogenous leukemia.

The Children's Cancer Study Group randomized 652 children and adolescents to receive allogeneic or autologous HSCT or aggressive consolidation chemotherapy following remission induction.[72] The overall survival rates at 8 years were 60%, 48%, and 53% in the allogeneic HSCT, autologous HSCT, and chemotherapy groups, respectively. The only significant difference in survival rate was between the allogeneic HSCT group and the other two groups. The superiority of allogeneic HSCT over chemotherapy has not been a consistent result in other studies in children with ANLL in first remission, which may be related to variability in the comparison chemotherapy regimens.[73]

Because some studies show that patients treated with allogeneic HSCT as intensive postremission therapy have a longer disease-free survival than do patients treated with standard intensive chemotherapy, some clinicians argue that all eligible patients should be offered allogeneic HSCT during first remission. Others believe that allogeneic HSCT should be delayed until the patient relapses, which would spare patients cured with standard chemotherapy from the risks of HSCT. Because 20% to 35% of patients who receive transplantation while in first relapse or second remission can be cured with HSCT, the overall proportion of patients cured of their ANLL is similar, regardless of whether HSCT is offered to all patients as intensive postremission therapy or only after they have experienced leukemic relapse. Identification of factors that would accurately predict relapse would aid in selecting patients who would benefit most from allogeneic HSCT when done in first remission.

Another controversy in the use of HSCT as treatment for ANLL is whether patients should undergo allogeneic or autologous HSCT and the source of hematopoietic stem cells for autologous transplants. The use of autologous HSCT in patients with ANLL has been reviewed by Gorin.[74] Both of the prospective studies discussed previously also included groups of patients treated with autologous HSCT.[70,71] Disease-free survival at 4 years favored allogeneic over autologous HSCT, but statistical significance was not reached. The causes of death differed depending on the type of transplant. The risk of death as a consequence of leukemic relapse was higher in the autologous HSCT group, while the risk of nonrelapse mortality—primarily related to GVHD—was higher in the allogeneic HSCT group. Most of the patients in the autologous HSCT group did not receive purged marrow. When compared to conventional chemotherapy, results of autologous transplant were superior in most of the trials thus making autologous transplant an acceptable option in patients without HLA matched donors.[75] The leukemia-free survival rate is similar in patients who receive autologous PBPC transplants to those who receive unpurged bone marrow transplants.[76]

MYELODYSPLASTIC SYNDROME

Myelodysplastic syndrome (MDS) is a heterogeneous group of disorders associated with an increased risk of transformation to AML. Hormones, chemotherapy, and differentiating agents (including HGF) have been used as treatment for MDS. None of these therapies is curative or increases the survival rate. Allogeneic HSCT is the only curative treatment for patients with this syndrome.[77] Long-term survival after allogeneic HSCT is approximately 50%, but varies with the subtype of disease, presence of cytogenetic abnormalities, patient age, and percentage of blasts in the bone marrow. Patients who receive transplantation early in their disease course have a lower risk of disease recurrence. A perceived limitation to the use of allogeneic HSCT is patient age. The median age at the time of diagnosis of MDS is in the seventh decade of life, at which time the frequency and severity of transplant-related complications often preclude eligibility. Researchers from the Fred Hutchinson Cancer Research Center published their experience in 55- to 65-year-old patients with MDS.[78]

Their results indicate that allogeneic HSCT is feasible for patients in this age group and age alone should not exclude patients from receiving this potentially curative therapy.

ACUTE LYMPHOBLASTIC LEUKEMIA

With improvements in the therapy of ALL, most children and adolescents with ALL achieve long-term disease-free survival with chemotherapy. Although the cure rate in adults with ALL is lower than in children, many adults also can be cured of their disease with conventional chemotherapy (see Chap. 131). Therefore, HSCT is usually reserved for patients with ALL who have experienced relapse, particularly if the duration of the first remission is short (less than 18 months) or in patients who do not respond to initial remission induction therapy.[79–81] Although many studies show that chemotherapy can often induce a second or subsequent remission, the duration of remission is usually short and long-term survival is uncommon. In comparison, 25% to 40% of patients with ALL who receive transplantation while in second remission become long-term survivors (Table 134–3). In a large matched-pair analysis of children with ALL in second remission, children who received allogeneic HSCT had significantly better disease-free survival rates at 5 years than did those children who received continued chemotherapy (40% vs 17%).[82] The difference in survival rate was related to a marked difference in the risk of relapse. Long-term survival rate after allogeneic HSCT decreases to 10% to 15% in patients who have had multiple relapses.

The application of allogeneic HSCT as intensive consolidation during first remission in patients with ALL who are at high risk for relapse is controversial. Examples of patients in this high-risk group are most adults and some children with high-risk features, such as those with high white blood cell counts or certain genetic abnormalities, or those who require repeated courses to induce a complete remission. The long-term, disease-free survival rate is approximately 60% in children and 40% in adults with high-risk features who received transplantation while in first remission (Table 134–3).[80,81] In a prospective comparison of chemotherapy versus allogeneic HSCT for adults with ALL in first remission, the disease-free survival rate was higher in the HSCT group (45% vs 31%), although the difference was of borderline statistical significance.[83] In that study, a significantly better survival rate was observed in those patients with high-risk ALL (39% vs 14%), which suggests that allogeneic HSCT may be preferred over chemotherapy in certain patient groups. Results from the NMDP for adult patients with high-risk ALL receiving HSCT from MUDs compares favorably to chemotherapy and matches those seen with HLA-identical sibling donor transplants.[84] In this series, patients who received transplantation in first complete remission had an overall survival rate at 2 years of 40%.

In results published by the British Medical Research Council, children with high-risk ALL received HSCT after achieving complete remission with intensive induction therapy.[85] Their data were compared to children receiving the same induction but who did not receive HSCT because of lack of a donor or refusal to receive HSCT. Although there was a trend suggesting benefit with transplant, neither the event-free or overall survival rate at 10 years was significantly different between those children who received transplantation and those who did not. The relapse rate was lower in the HSCT group, but there were also more nonrelapse-related deaths. The investigators concluded that unless nonrelapse-related mortality can be reduced or a subset of patients is identified in whom the benefit is clear, HSCT should not be considered standard therapy for children with ALL in first remission.

Although there is less experience with autologous transplants, studies suggest that long-term survival rate with autologous transplants is slightly lower as compared to allogeneic HSCT.[81] The long-term survival rate is 20% to 30% in children and adults with ALL treated with autologous HSCT while in remission (primarily second or subsequent remission). High-dose chemotherapy with autologous HSCT has also been used as intensive postremission therapy in adults with ALL, but its role cannot be established until more comparative data is available.

CHRONIC MYELOGENOUS LEUKEMIA

Many studies indicate that high-dose chemotherapy with allogeneic HSCT from HLA-identical sibling donors can cure 60% to 70% of patients with chronic-phase CML (Table 134–3).[86] As a result, CML is currently the most common indication for allogeneic HSCT, and allogeneic HSCT is considered to be the treatment of choice for patients younger than age 50 years. In some series, the best results are achieved when HSCT is performed early after diagnosis and in younger patients. For example, the long-term survival rate in patients who receive transplantation within 1 year of diagnosis is approximately 80%, as compared to 40% to 50% when HSCT is performed 1 to 3 years from diagnosis. Because busulfan may increase the risk of posttransplant interstitial pneumonitis and hepatic venoocclusive disease, it has been recommended that standard doses of busulfan be avoided if patients are eligible for and considering HSCT. Prolonged IFN-α therapy for more than 6 months before HSCT may adversely affect transplant outcome. When allogeneic HSCT is delayed until the patient is in accelerated or blast phase, the survival rate is worse, but 15% to 30% of patients still can be cured (Table 134–3).[86]

Because of the relatively long duration of the chronic phase, there is usually adequate time to perform a search for a fully or closely matched unrelated donor for those patients with CML who lack an HLA-identical sibling donor. Therefore, CML has become the most common indication for allogeneic HSCT from unrelated donors. In a report of 196 patients with Philadelphia chromosome-positive CML treated with allogeneic HSCT from unrelated donors, overall survival rate at 5 years was 57%.[87] In a multivariate analysis, the survival rate was worse in patients who had an interval from diagnosis to transplantation of 1 year or more, an HLA-DRB1 mismatch, a high body-weight index, or were older than 50 years of age. Patients younger than 50 years old who received transplants from unrelated donors matched for HLA-A, B, and DRB1 within 1 year of diagnosis had a survival rate of 74% at 5 years, which compared favorably with patients who received transplantation at the same center with grafts from HLA-matched siblings. Graft failure occurred in 5% of patients and grade III or IV acute GVHD was observed in 35% of patients receiving 6/6 HLA-matched grafts. Nearly 40% of patients died without recurrent disease; the most common cause of death was GVHD. These results were confirmed in a larger series of 1,423 patients reported by the NMDP.[88]

Experience with autologous HSCT is limited but it appears that autologous HSCT is less effective in eradication of the malignant clone than allogeneic HSCT.[89] Because the major cause of treatment failure is leukemic relapse, many HSCT centers are investigating new preparative regimens, pharmacologic or immunologic approaches to purge stem cells of malignant cells, or posttransplant therapies.

CHRONIC LYMPHOCYTIC LEUKEMIA

HSCT is being evaluated in patients with CLL because this form of leukemia is considered incurable with conventional chemotherapy.[90] Four-year overall survival rates are reported to be 60% to 90% after autologous HSCT. In most series, however, relapses up to 5 years posttransplant are observed. Allogeneic transplant has been used in younger patients with CLL and studies provide encouraging evidence that this may be a curative modality in some patients.[91] Relapse rates are <20% in the first 3 years, but transplant-related mortality rates as high as 40% have been reported. Because of the higher median age of patients with CLL and because of the evidence of GVT seen with allogeneic HSCT, CLL is an excellent malignancy in which to test the feasibility and efficacy of NMT. These studies are ongoing.[65,66]

LYMPHOMA

Although most patients with Hodgkin's disease and some with aggressive non-Hodgkin's lymphoma are cured with combination chemotherapy, for those who relapse and for those who never achieve a complete remission, the prognosis is poor. Similarly, most patients with indolent non-Hodgkin's lymphoma are not cured of their disease with chemotherapy. Although lymphoma is currently the second most common indication for HSCT, it is estimated that only a small proportion of the eligible patients are currently treated with this procedure.[92]

Based on the success of allogeneic HSCT in leukemia, allogeneic or syngeneic HSCT was used initially as salvage therapy in patients with relapsed or refractory Hodgkin's disease or aggressive non-Hodgkin's lymphoma. Long-term results of these early studies show that some of these patients can be cured with HSCT.[92] Although a graft-versus-lymphoma effect has been reported, there is no convincing evidence that the survival rate is higher with allogeneic HSCT as compared to autologous HSCT, probably because of the higher risk of transplant-related complications that are associated with allogeneic HSCT. As a result, most eligible patients with lymphoma currently are treated with autologous HSCT.

High-dose chemotherapy with autologous HSCT can be used at different times in the disease course of lymphoma (Table 134–2).[93–95] It is most commonly used as salvage therapy in patients with Hodgkin's disease or aggressive non-Hodgkin's lymphoma who initially obtain a complete remission with conventional therapy but then relapse. In that setting, high-dose chemotherapy with HSCT produces a complete remission rate of 25% to 80%, with many patients in unmaintained, continuous complete remission for more than 5 years. The best results have been observed in patients who receive transplantation after responding to conventional-dose salvage therapy. Results indicate that more than one-half of patients who received transplantation at a time when minimal disease was present are alive; many of these patients are likely to be cured of their disease. Patients with newly diagnosed non-Hodgkin's lymphoma responding to conventional therapy but who fail to obtain a complete response may also benefit from HSCT. In a report from the Autologous Blood and Marrow Transplant Registry of 184 patients who never achieved a complete remission with conventional chemotherapy (but were still chemotherapy-sensitive), 44% experienced a complete response after autologous HSCT. The progression-free survival rate at 5 years was 37%, indicating that some of these patients may achieve long-term benefit from this procedure.[96] Patients with refractory disease have a poor long-term survival rate even with HSCT.

Results from uncontrolled trials with the use of high-dose chemotherapy as intensive consolidation therapy (i.e., during first complete remission) in patients who are at high-risk for relapse are encouraging. In a large prospective randomized trial of patients with aggressive non-Hodgkin's lymphoma in first complete remission at high risk for relapse, disease-free and overall survival rates were longer in patients treated with HSCT as compared to those who were treated with standard therapy.[97] The disease-free survival rate at 8 years was 55% for those receiving HSCT and 39% for those who were treated with conventional chemotherapy ($p = 0.02$). Other investigators report similar results.[98,99]

Fewer patients with indolent non-Hodgkin's lymphoma have been treated with high-dose chemotherapy autologous HSCT and most of these were patients who relapsed following primary induction therapy. Early results are encouraging, and most patients have achieved a complete remission, although these remissions are generally not durable.[94] Several factors are associated with prolonged survival after HSCT: transplant while in first remission, previous exposure to fewer courses of chemotherapy, and sensitive disease at the time of transplant.[100] Because of the indolent nature of the disease, longer followup is required before high-dose chemotherapy with autologous HSCT can be recommended for this group of patients. In addition, because these lymphomas tend to be slow-growing, they have become an indication for the study of NMT.

A major problem in lymphoma patients is disease relapse posttransplant. Prognosis for these individuals is poor; treatment options include further chemotherapy, allogeneic HSCT, biologic therapy, or investigational agents. Rituximab has been investigated in this setting with encouraging results reported.[101] Posttransplant immunotherapy to prevent relapse is an area of active investigation.

Another issue concerning HSCT for lymphoma that was recently reported is an apparent increase in risk of secondary malignancies and MDS posttransplant.[102] Patients with lymphoma may be at higher risk for this complication because of intensive therapy with alkylating agents and etoposide prior to transplant. The risk may be reduced if patients are transplanted earlier in the course of their disease.

MULTIPLE MYELOMA

Multiple myeloma is a relatively rare hematologic malignancy characterized by uncontrolled proliferation of plasma cells derived from a single malignant clone. Although combination chemotherapy induces a response in most patients, complete responses are uncommon and the disease is not curable with standard-dose chemotherapy. High-dose chemotherapy with autologous rescue induces a complete or partial response in 70% to 80% of newly diagnosed patients with multiple myeloma, and some of these patients may be cured of their disease. In a randomized trial, patients randomized to high-dose melphalan and autologous HSCT had significantly longer survival than did those patients treated with standard-dose chemotherapy plus IFN-α.[103] However, patients in the autologous HSCT group continued to relapse after 3 years of followup, which suggests that few, if any, patients will be cured. Several factors are predictive of response to high-dose chemotherapy with autologous rescue: response to standard therapy; younger than 50 years of age; β_2-microglobulin levels below 2.5 mg/L; and time from diagnosis less than 12 months. The most commonly used preparative regimen is high-dose melphalan, given either alone or combined with other cytotoxic agents or TBI. Some aggressive protocols include two transplants.[104] As previously discussed, vaccination strategies posttransplant to maintain responses is also being investigated.[64]

To take advantage of the GVT effect, allogeneic transplant has been used in patients with myeloma. Although transplant-related mortality is high, either because of the advanced age of myeloma patients or characteristics of prior therapy, this treatment option should be considered in younger patients who are not heavily pretreated because of the long-term survival seen in many patients treated with allogeneic transplants.[105] Newer strategies include NMT and donor lymphocyte/leukocyte infusions.[106–108]

BREAST CANCER

Several thousand women have received high-dose chemotherapy with HSCT for the treatment of breast cancer. The rationale of this therapy was originally based on preclinical studies that supported a steep dose-response curve for alkylating agents in mammary tumor cell lines. Early phase II studies in patients with metastatic disease resulted in high response rates and prolonged disease-free survival as compared to historical controls. Because of this data, patients with early stage disease but with high risk for relapse were also treated with HSCT. The role of high-dose chemotherapy and autologous HSCT was recently reviewed.[109,110]

METASTATIC BREAST CANCER

Response rates reported in early phase II studies of autologous HSCT in women with metastatic breast cancer were 60% to 80%; median survival was superior to historical controls and 5% to 10% of patients with metastatic breast cancer were alive and progression free 3 to 5 years after transplant. Treatment-related mortality was also high (25%). With the introduction of HGFs, more widespread use of PBPC transplants, more rapid engraftment, and better supportive care, mortality rates associated with high-dose chemotherapy have dropped to less than 5% at experienced centers.

The Autologous Blood and Marrow Transplant Registry (ABMTR) of North America reported results of more than 5,800 consecutively treated women who received high-dose chemotherapy with autologous rescue for breast cancer at more than 130 centers between 1989 and 1995. The combination of cyclophosphamide, thiotepa, and carboplatin (STAMP V) was used in more than 25% of all patients.[111] Transplant-related mortality declined from 22% in 1989 to 5% in 1995. Median survival in the patients with metastatic breast cancer (n = 3,450) was 19 months; overall and progression-free survival rates at 3 years were 30% and 18%, respectively. Most patients had chemotherapy-sensitive disease (complete or partial response before transplant), and women who achieved a complete response pretransplant had better survival (overall and progression-free survival rates at 3 years of 46% and 32%, respectively) than did those women in partial remission or with resistant disease. Evaluation of phase II and registry data, although encouraging, was difficult because of small sample size, selection bias, and reporting bias.

Because of biases inherent in comparisons involving historical controls, randomized trials were necessary to determine the safety and efficacy of high-dose chemotherapy in contrast to standard chemotherapy. Such trials have been difficult to perform, especially in the United States, because of the public and medical community's perception of the value of high-dose chemotherapy in breast cancer. For patients with metastatic breast cancer, several randomized trials have been initiated, some of which have been presented in abstract form at international meetings. Only two trials have been completed and published in peer reviewed journals. One trial was discredited because of fraudulent research practices of the principal investigator.[112] The other trial was sponsored by the National Cancer Institute and recently published by Stadtmauer and colleagues.[113] In that trial, 553 patients with metastatic or locally recurrent breast cancer were enrolled and 199 patients were randomized to high-dose chemotherapy with cyclophosphamide, thiotepa, and carboplatin followed by HSCT or "maintenance" therapy with cyclophosphamide, methotrexate, and 5-fluorouracil (CMF) for 2 years. One hundred and eighty-four women were included in the primary analysis. All patients received standard induction therapy prior to randomization. Results showed no difference in overall survival rates at 3 years: 32% for the transplant arm and 38% in the maintenance therapy arm. Serious adverse events were more common in the transplant group but there was no difference in treatment-related mortality. The study was powered to detect a doubling of the median survival with high-dose chemotherapy assuming a median survival of 2.5 years in the standard-dose group; given the data, transplant would be unlikely to be associated even with a moderate improvement in survival. The results strongly suggest that women with metastatic breast cancer treated with high-dose chemotherapy and transplant do not have improved survival as compared to those women who receive standard-dose "maintenance" therapy. Most experts agree that the benefit (or lack thereof) cannot be decided based on data from one trial. Published results from other randomized trials when completed are necessary before a definitive conclusion can be made about the role of high-dose chemotherapy in the treatment of metastatic breast cancer.

LOCALLY ADVANCED BREAST CANCER

Women with breast cancer that has spread outside of the breast into multiple axillary lymph nodes (but not beyond) are at an increased risk of relapse and, with current standard adjuvant therapy, have an overall survival rate of 50% to 60% at 5 years. These patients are also considered candidates for high-dose chemotherapy. Based on the initially encouraging results seen with metastatic disease, high-dose chemotherapy with autologous stem-cell rescue is also being used in patients with high-risk primary disease. Patients usually receive several courses of standard-dose adjuvant chemotherapy, followed by high-dose chemotherapy with autologous rescue as intensive consolidation. In the ABMTR report discussed earlier, more than 1,700 women with high-risk primary disease (e.g., stage II with at least four positive axillary lymph nodes, stage III, or inflammatory breast cancer) received high-dose chemotherapy. Overall and progression-free survival rates at 3 years were 74% and 65% for stage II, 70% and 60% for stage III, and 52% and 42% for inflammatory disease, respectively.[111] These promising results prompted multiple phase III randomized trials.

Although several randomized trials are in progress, results of only two have been published in peer-reviewed journals.[114,115] In both studies, women with extensive lymph node metastasis were treated with standard adjuvant or neoadjuvant therapy and then randomized to high-dose chemotherapy or no additional chemotherapy. High-dose regimens consisted of cyclophosphamide, thiotepa, and carboplatin in one study,[114] and in another study, two cycles of cyclophosphamide, etoposide, and cisplatin, with each cycle followed by stem-cell infusion.[115] No significant differences in overall or disease-free survival rates were noted in patients receiving high-dose chemotherapy. Other larger cooperative group studies are either ongoing or undergoing analysis and the final results of these trials will hopefully determine the role of high-dose chemotherapy in the treatment of locally advanced breast cancer.

With the lack of definitive evidence of benefit from high-dose chemotherapy in the treatment of breast cancer, research has now shifted to the use of posttransplant immunotherapy in an effort to treat residual disease. Approaches include vaccination strategies posttransplant, enhancement of the immune activity of the stem-cell product, and even allogeneic transplantation.[65,116,117]

OTHER SOLID TUMORS

High-dose chemotherapy with autologous HSCT has been used as salvage therapy for many adults with solid tumors, particularly

TABLE 134–4. Dose-Limiting Nonhematologic Toxicities for Selected Chemotherapeutic Agents Included in Conditioning Regimens in Hematopoietic Stem Cell Transplantation

Drug	Conventional Dose[a] (mg/m²)	ABMT[b] Dose (mg/m²)	Dose-limiting Toxicity
Busulfan	2	450	Hepatic
Carboplatin	400	2000	Hepatic, renal
Carmustine	200	1200	Pulmonary, hepatic
Cisplatin	100	200	Renal, peripheral neuropathy
Cyclophosphamide	1000	7500	Cardiomyopathy
Etoposide	300–600	2400	Mucositis
Ifosfamide	5000	18000	Renal
Melphalan	40	225	Mucositis
Thiotepa	20–50	1125	Mucositis, CNS

[a]Doses are approximate and are for drugs as single agents. When combinations are used, doses may need to be decreased.
[b]ABMT, autologous bone marrow transplantation.
Modified from Eder JP, Elias A, Shea TC, et al. A phase I–II study of cyclophosphamide, thiotepa, and carboplatin with autologous bone marrow transplantation in solid tumor patients. J Clin Oncol 1990;8:1242.

chemotherapy-responsive tumors such as germ cell tumors, ovarian cancer, and small cell lung cancer. Many children with neuroblastoma, Ewing's sarcoma, rhabdomyosarcoma, and brain tumors also have received transplantation with varying success. The reader is referred to detailed reviews regarding the role of high-dose chemotherapy in these tumors.[3–5]

TRANSPLANT-RELATED COMPLICATIONS

Although many patients with cancer who are treated with high-dose chemotherapy and autologous or allogeneic transplantation experience long-term survival and cure of their disease, this modality is associated with many serious and potentially life-threatening complications. In the early 1970s, early posttransplant mortality was extremely high, and most HSCT patients did not survive beyond 100 days. During those early years of allogeneic HSCT, death was usually related to infection, GVHD, interstitial pneumonia, and leukemic relapse. Today, largely because of the availability of improved broad-spectrum antibiotics, immunosuppressive drugs, antiviral drugs, and HGF and other biotechnology drugs, transplant-related mortality after allogeneic HSCT with HLA-matched sibling donors has been reduced to 20% to 30% at most centers. Until recently, allogeneic HSCT was usually restricted to patients younger than 50 years old with an HLA-identical sibling donor. With advances in the prevention and treatment of transplant-related complications and the availability of nonmyeloablative transplants, allogeneic HSCT is now being offered to patients older than 50 years of age. The risk of transplant-related mortality after high-dose chemotherapy with autologous HSCT is less than 5% at many centers, depending on patient population and conditioning regimen.

Most patients treated with HSCT experience some degree of transplant-related toxicity in nonhematopoietic tissues and some patients experience early death as a result of these toxicities. In this setting, these nonhematologic toxicities are dose limiting. Because of the severity and uniqueness of these transplant-related toxicities, toxicity-grading scales were developed specifically for grading toxicities in HSCT patients.

Transplant-related toxicity is usually more severe in allogeneic HSCT recipients as compared to autologous HSCT recipients, because of GVHD and posttransplant immunosuppression. Severe toxicities are also more common in patients with advanced disease at the time of HSCT. In the setting of autologous HSCT, transplant-related toxicity is usually related to the drugs in the conditioning regimen or infection. Table 134–4 lists the dose-limiting nonhematologic toxicity for several drugs that are commonly included in conditioning regimens. These toxicities may be uncommon or rare with the administration of conventional doses of a specific drug. Several unusual and severe manifestations of regimen-related toxicities are discussed in detail below.

HEPATIC VENOOCCLUSIVE DISEASE

Hepatic venoocclusive disease occurs as a result of chemotherapy-induced damage and obliteration of the small intrahepatic central venules leading to necrosis of hepatocytes, portal hypertension, and hepatic failure.[118,119] Clinical signs of hepatic venoocclusive disease include fluid retention leading to sudden weight gain and ascites, hepatomegaly (sometimes painful), and hyperbilirubinemia usually occurring within the first 3 weeks after transplant. The incidence of hepatic venoocclusive disease ranges from 5% to 20% in most series. Severe hepatic venoocclusive disease is fatal in 50% to 75% of patients who develop it. Factors reported to increase the risk of hepatic venoocclusive disease include the use of TBI-containing conditioning regimens and the presence of elevated liver function tests pretransplant. The use of some drugs, such as busulfan or carmustine, also may increase the risk of hepatic venoocclusive disease. Busulfan concentrations have been correlated with the risk of hepatic venoocclusive disease.[120] Patients with a high area-under-the-curve (AUC) for busulfan concentration had a greater risk of hepatic venoocclusive disease than did those patients with a low AUC. Based on these studies, some HSCT centers adjust busulfan doses based on plasma concentrations. Some studies suggest that prostaglandin E1, unfractionated and low-molecular-weight heparin, or ursodiol may be partially effective in the prevention of hepatic venoocclusive disease.[118,119] Treatment is generally supportive. Recombinant tissue plasminogen activator is sometimes given to patients with severe venoocclusive disease because of the possible role of the coagulation cascade in the pathogenesis of venoocclusive disease.[121]

PULMONARY COMPLICATIONS

Pulmonary complications following HSCT can be categorized as infectious and noninfectious; infections are discussed in Chap. 120; noninfectious complications are described as early (<3 months posttransplant) and late (>3 months posttransplant). Early complications include diffuse alveolar hemorrhage and idiopathic interstitial pneumonitis.[122] Diffuse alveolar hemorrhage is diagnosed by examination of bronchoalveolar lavage fluid. Although it can be severe and life-threatening, prompt treatment with high doses of corticosteroids is reportedly beneficial. Idiopathic interstitial pneumonitis also is a severe form of regimen-related toxicity. Patients with idiopathic interstitial pneumonitis are clinically indistinguishable from those with interstitial pneumonitis related to infection. The risk is similar in recipients of autologous or allogeneic HSCT, but appears higher in patients who are conditioned with a TBI-containing regimen or who have acute GVHD. Mortality has been reported to be as high as 70% and treatment is supportive care only.

Late pulmonary complications cover a wide spectrum of disorders and include both obstructive and restrictive lung diseases. Included in these disorders are bronchiolitis obliterans with or without organizing pneumonia, diffuse alveolar damage, and lymphocytic interstitial pneumonia.[123] Therapy consists of steroids, which are about 50% effective; patients with mild to moderate airflow impairment appear to have the best response. Mortality from these disorders is about 40%.

GRAFT FAILURE

Initial engraftment usually occurs in the first 2 to 4 weeks posttransplant and is evidenced by rising peripheral blood counts and the presence of hematopoietic precursor cells in the marrow. In allogeneic HSCT, the presence of donor cells is confirmed with cytogenetic markers (chimerism). In most patients, engraftment is sustained with complete recovery of hematopoiesis.

Graft failure can occur after autologous, syngeneic, and allogeneic hematopoietic stem cell transplantation and can be a result of an immunologic reaction between donor and host, and infusion of low numbers of stem cells, a viral infection, or drug reaction. Two syndromes have been observed: Early graft failure occurs when the rate of neutrophil recovery is delayed (primary graft failure or delayed engraftment), whereas late graft failure is characterized by a decline in the neutrophil count after initial engraftment (secondary graft failure). With widespread use of PBPCs and posttransplant growth factors, graft failure is rare after autologous transplantation. When graft failure occurs after allogeneic HSCT and is characterized by the regrowth of immunocompetent host cells and a simultaneous loss of donor cells, it is referred to as graft rejection. Graft rejection occurs rarely in recipients of unmodified marrow from HLA-identical sibling donors. An increased risk of graft rejection has been observed in recipients of marrow from partially HLA-mismatched donors, recipients of T-cell-depleted marrow recipients of marrow from matched unrelated donors, and patients with severe aplastic anemia.[124]

The long-term prognosis in patients with graft failure is poor. Despite supportive care, death may result from infection or bleeding. In some patients with an HLA-identical sibling donor, a second infusion of stem cells can be attempted. The most effective therapy for graft failure is G-CSF or GM-CSF. The 2000 American Society of Clinical Oncology (ASCO) guidelines recommend that patients with graft failure after HSCT be treated with GM-CSF 250 μg/m^2/day for 14 days followed by a 7-day break. Up to three such courses with dose escalation to 500 μg/m^2/day in the last course is advised.[125]

The prophylactic use of G-CSF or GM-CSF posttransplant dramatically reduces the incidence of early graft failure and accelerated the rate of myeloid recovery posttransplant. The usual dosage of GM-CSF is 250 μg/m^2/day. Higher dosages (e.g., 10 μg/kg/day) of G-CSF can be given because of its more favorable adverse effect profile as compared to GM-CSF. HGFs also accelerate the rate of hematopoietic recovery in patients undergoing allogeneic HSCT without increasing the risk of GVHD, and both G-CSF and GM-CSF have received FDA approval for this indication.

The role of HGFs is less clear in patients who receive mobilized PBPCs instead of bone marrow as a source of hematopoietic stem cells. Some investigators believe that PBPCs are primarily responsible for the rapid neutrophil and platelet recovery observed after high-dose chemotherapy, and that posttransplant administration of recombinant G-CSF or GM-CSF might be unnecessary. However, in a prospective randomized trial, patients who received mobilized PBPCs and posttransplant recombinant G-CSF had significantly more rapid neutrophil recovery than did those patients who received mobilized PBPCs alone.[126] Similar findings were reported in the allogeneic PBPC setting.[127,128] Neither of the studies done in the allogeneic setting showed a significant improvement in clinical outcomes (e.g., reduced antibiotic usage, decreased number of hospital days) despite a more rapid neutrophil recovery.

Many different dosages and schedules of G-CSF have been used after PBPC transplantation. Originally, G-CSF was given at a dose of 5–10 μg/kg/day beginning on the day of or the day after infusion of PBPCs and continued until neutrophil recovery to greater than an arbitrary number of neutrophils (500–1,000/μL). In one study of three different G-CSF dosages (5, 10, and 16 μg/kg/day), there was no difference in the rate of hematopoietic recovery between the different dosages.[129] In another study, delayed initiation of G-CSF at a dosage of 5 μg/kg/day until day 5 posttransplant did not impair hematopoietic recovery after PBPC transplantation.[130]

None of the commercially available HGFs has a significant effect on platelet recovery. Results of studies with investigational platelet growth factors given posttransplant, such as thrombopoietin and interleukin-11, have been disappointing.[131,132]

GRAFT-VERSUS-HOST DISEASE

GVHD is caused by immunocompetent donor T lymphocytes reacting against antigens on host tissues.[133] In that setting, donor T lymphocytes recognize histocompatibility antigens of the host as genetically foreign, become activated, proliferate, and attack recipient tissue, thereby producing the clinical syndrome of GVHD. Excessive or dysfunctional production of inflammatory cytokines such as interleukin-1 (IL-1) and tumor necrosis factor-α (TNF-α) (referred to as the "cytokine storm") by the activated T lymphocytes result in the recruitment of other cell types (e.g., macrophages, NK cells) that also contribute to the pathology associated with GVHD. Two different clinical syndromes have been recognized, depending on the onset of GVHD. Acute GVHD occurs early, while chronic GVHD occurs late in the posttransplant course.

ACUTE GRAFT-VERSUS-HOST DISEASE

Acute GVHD usually becomes clinically evident during the first 60 days posttransplant and is characterized by selective epithelial damage of target organs. The principal target organs for acute GVHD are the skin, liver, and gastrointestinal tract. Acute GVHD is classified into four grades, depending on the number of organs involved and the degree of involvement of each organ (Fig. 134-4). Grade I disease involves only the skin, while grades II through IV involve the skin and either the liver, or gastrointestinal tract, or both. The initial sign of acute GVHD is usually a generalized maculopapular rash. Acute GVHD usually progresses, involving the liver, the gastrointestinal

is higher in recipients of marrow from HLA-nonidentical related or unrelated donors, and in patients who had prior acute GVHD. Twenty percent to 30% of patients develop the disease *de novo* (without prior acute GVHD).

If no functional impairment is present, patients with limited disease are not treated. Many patients with extensive chronic GVHD, if left untreated, will die of infections or become disabled. The long-term survival rate is worse in certain subgroups of patients, such as patients with thrombocytopenia or progressive onset of chronic GVHD, and those who fail to respond to immunosuppressive therapy. Initial treatment in patients with standard risk chronic GVHD (platelet count $> 100{,}000/\mu L$) consists of prednisone alone. Those patients with high-risk disease (platelet count $< 100{,}000/\mu L$) appear to benefit from combined alternate-day therapy with prednisone and cyclosporine.[146,147] Treatment is continued until signs and symptoms of the disease have resolved, usually over a period of several months. As chronic GVHD improves, immunosuppressive therapy is gradually tapered and finally discontinued provided there is no flare of GVHD. Patients who fail initial therapy have a very poor prognosis and several therapies have been investigated with varying degrees of success: thalidomide, ultraviolet A irradiation after oral treatment with β-methoxypsoralen (PUVA), extracorporeal photophoresis, tacrolimus, total lymphoid irradiation, mycophenolate mofetil, and others.[146,147] Infection is the primary cause of death in patients with chronic GVHD, and antimicrobial prophylaxis is an important component of the care of patients being treated for chronic GVHD. Patients should receive oral trimethoprim-sulfamethoxazole, penicillin, and acyclovir to prevent those infections commonly seen in immunocompromised patients.

INFECTION

Patients undergoing high-dose chemotherapy with autologous or allogeneic transplantation are severely immunocompromised and therefore at high risk for bacterial, fungal, and viral infection. Management of these infections is discussed in detail in Chap. 120.

LATE COMPLICATIONS

With the success of HSCT, the number of long-term survivors has grown. Many survivors experience delayed complications of transplantation. Major late complications include restrictive and obstructive pulmonary disease; cataract formation; endocrine dysfunction, including sterility; impaired growth; infections; and secondary malignancies.[148,149]

REFERENCES

1. Lennard AL, Jackson GH. Stem cell transplantation. BMJ 2000;321: 433–437.
2. Shea TC. Introduction: Current issues in high-dose chemotherapy and stem cell support. Bone Marrow Transplant 1999;23(suppl 2):s1–s5.
3. Thomas ED, Blume KG, Forman SJ, eds. Hematopoietic Cell Transplantation, 2nd ed. Malden, MA, Blackwell Science, 1999.
4. Armitage JO, Antman KH, eds. High-Dose Cancer Therapy: Pharmacology, Hematopoietins, Stem Cells, 3rd ed. Philadelphia, Lippincott-Williams & Wilkins, 2000.
5. MacNeil M, Eisenhauer EA. High-dose chemotherapy: Is it standard management for any common solid tumor? Ann Oncol 1999;10:1145–1161.
6. Klein J, Sato A. Advances in immunology: The HLA system (first of two parts). N Engl J Med 2000;343:702–709.
7. Mickelson EM, Petersdorf E, Anasetti C, et al. HLA matching in hematopoietic cell transplantation. Hum Immunol 2000;61:91–100.
8. Petersdorf EW, Gooley TA, Anasetti C, et al. Optimizing outcome after unrelated marrow transplantation by comprehensive matching of HLA class I and II alleles in the donor and recipient. Blood 1998;92:3515–3520.
9. Scott I, O'Shea J, Tiercy J, et al. Molecular typing shows a high level of HLA class I incompatibility in serologically well-matched donor/patient pairs: Implications for unrelated bone marrow donor selection. Blood 1998;92:4864–4871.
10. Sasazuki T, Juji T, Morishima Y, et al. Effect of matching of class I HLA alleles on clinical outcome after transplantation of hematopoietic stem cells from an unrelated donor. N Engl J Med 1998;339:1177–1185.
11. Kernan NA, Bartsch G, Ash RC, et al. Analysis of 462 transplantations from unrelated donors facilitated by the National Marrow Donor Program. N Engl J Med 1993;328:593–602.
12. Szydlo R, Goldman JM, Klein JP, et al. Results of allogeneic bone marrow transplants for leukemia using donors other than HLA-identical siblings. J Clin Oncol 1997;15:1767–1777.
13. Heslop H. Haematopoietic stem cell transplantation from unrelated donors. Br J Haematol 1999;105:2–6.
14. Siena S, Schiavo R, Pedrazzoli T, Carlo-Stella C. Therapeutic relevance of $CD34^+$ cell dose in blood cell transplantation for cancer therapy. J Clin Oncol 2000;18:1360–1377.
15. Weaver CH, Hazelton B, Birch R, et al. An analysis of engraftment kinetics as a function of the CD34 content of peripheral blood progenitor cell collections in 692 patients after the administration of myeloablative chemotherapy. Blood 1995;86:3961–3969.
16. Glaspy JA. Economic considerations in the use of peripheral blood progenitor cells to support high-dose chemotherapy. Bone Marrow Transplant 1999;23(suppl 2):s21–s27.
17. Schulman KA, Birch R, Zhen B, Pania N, Weaver CH. Effect of $CD34^+$ cell dose on resource utilization in patients after high-dose chemotherapy with peripheral blood stem cell support. J Clin Oncol 1999;17:1227–1233.
18. Koc ON, Gerson SL, Cooper BW, et al. Randomized cross-over trial of progenitor cell mobilization: High-dose cyclophosphamide plus granulocyte colony stimulating factor (G-CSF) versus granulocyte-macrophage colony-stimulating factor plus G-CSF. J Clin Oncol 2000;18:1824–1830.
19. Weaver CH, Schulman KA, Wilson-Relyea B, et al. Randomized trial of filgrastim, sargramostim, or sequential sargramostim and filgrastim after myelosuppressive chemotherapy for the harvesting of peripheral blood stem cells. J Clin Oncol 2000;18:43–53.
20. Bolwell BM, Goormastic M, Yanssen T, et al. Comparison of G-CSF with GM-CSF for mobilizing peripheral blood progenitor cells and for enhancing marrow recovery after autologous bone marrow transplant. Bone Marrow Transplant 1994;14(6):913–918.
21. Shpall EJ, Wheeler CA, Turner SA, et al. A randomized phase 3 study of peripheral blood progenitor cell mobilization with stem cell factor and filgrastim in high-risk breast cancer patients. Blood 1999;93:2491–2501.
22. Facon T, Harousseau J, Maloisel F, et al. Stem cell factor in combination with filgrastim after chemotherapy improves peripheral blood progenitor cell yield and reduces apheresis requirements in multiple myeloma patients: A randomized, controlled trial. Blood 1999;94:1218–1225.
23. Lyman SD, Jacobsen SEW. c-*Kit* ligand and FLT3 ligand: Stem/progenitor cell factors with overlapping yet distinct activities. Blood 1998; 91:1101–1134.
24. Murray LJ, Luens KM, Estrada MF, et al. Thrombopoietin mobilizes $CD34^+$ cell subsets into peripheral blood and expands multilineage progenitors in bone marrow of cancer patients with normal hematopoiesis. Exp Hematol 1998;26:207–216.
25. DiPersio JF, Schuster MW, Abboud CM, et al. Mobilization of peripheral blood stem cells by concurrent administration of daniplestim and granulocyte colony-stimulating factor in patients with breast cancer or lymphoma. J Clin Oncol 2000;18:2762–2771.
26. Stiff PJ. Management strategies for the hard-to-mobilize patient. Bone Marrow Transplant 1999;23(suppl 2):s29–s33.
27. Beyer J, Schwella N, Zingsem J, et al. Hematopoietic rescue after high-dose chemotherapy using autologous peripheral blood progenitor cells or

bone marrow: A randomized comparison. J Clin Oncol 1995;13:1328–1335.
28. Schmitz N, Linch DC, Dreger P, et al. Filgrastim-mobilized peripheral blood progenitor cell transplantation in comparison with autologous bone marrow transplantation: Results of a randomized phase III trial in lymphoma patients. Lancet 1996;347:353–357.
29. Smith TJ, Hillner BE, Schmitz N, et al. Economic analysis of a randomized clinical trial to compare filgrastim-mobilized peripheral blood progenitor cell transplantation with autologous bone marrow transplantation in patients with Hodgkin's and non-Hodgkin's lymphoma. J Clin Oncol 1997;15:5–10.
30. Meisenberg BR, Ferran K, Hollenbach K, et al. Reduced charges and costs associated with outpatient autologous stem cell transplantation. Bone Marrow Transplant 1999;21:927–932.
31. Rubia J, Martinez C, Solano S, et al. Administration of recombinant human granulocyte colony-stimulating factor to normal donors: Results of the Spanish National Donor Registry. Bone Marrow Transplant 1999;24:723–728.
32. Van Hoef MEHM. HLA-identical sibling peripheral blood progenitor cell transplants. Bone Marrow Transplant 1999;24:707–714.
33. Bennett CL, Waters TM, Stinson TJ, et al. Valuing clinical strategies early in development: A cost analysis of allogeneic peripheral blood stem cell transplantation. Bone Marrow Transplant 1999;24:555–560.
34. Champlin RE, Schmitz N, Horowitz MM, et al. Blood stem cells compared with bone marrow as a source of hematopoietic cells for allogeneic transplantation. Blood 2000;95:3702–3709.
35. Bensinger WI, Martin PJ, Storer B, et al. Transplantation of bone marrow as compared with peripheral blood cells from HLA-identical relatives in patients with hematologic cancers. N Engl J Med 2001;34:175–181.
36. Ringden O, Remberger M, Runde V, et al. Peripheral blood stem cell transplantation from unrelated donors: A comparison with marrow transplantation. Blood 1999;94:455–464.
37. Rocha V, Wagner JE, Sobocinski KA, et al. Graft-versus-host disease in children who have received a cord-blood or bone marrow transplant from an HLA-identical sibling. N Engl J Med 2000;342:1846–54.
38. Barker JN, Davies SM, DeFor T, et al. Survival after transplantation of unrelated donor umbilical cord blood is comparable to that of human leukocyte antigen-matched unrelated donor bone marrow: Results of a matched-pair analysis. Blood 2001;97:2957–2961.
39. Rubinstein P, Carrier C, Scaradavou A, et al. Outcomes among 562 recipients of placental-blood transplants from unrelated donors. N Engl J Med 1998;339:1565–1577.
40. Rocha V, Cornish J, Sievers EL, et al. Comparison of outcomes of unrelated bone marrow and umbilical cord blood transplants in children with acute leukemia. Blood 2001;97:2962–2971.
41. Bensinger WI, Buckner CD. Preparative regimens. In: Thomas ED, Blume KG, Forman SJ, eds. Hematopoietic Cell Transplantation, 2nd ed. Malden, MA, Blackwell Science, 1999.
42. Colvin OM, Petros W. Pharmacologic strategies for high-dose therapy. In: Armitage JO, Antman KH, eds. High-Dose Cancer Therapy: Pharmacology, Hematopoietins, Stem Cells, 3rd ed. Philadelphia, Lippincott-Williams & Wilkins, 2000.
43. Slattery JT, Clift RA, Buckner CD, et al. Marrow transplantation for chronic myeloid leukemia: The influence of plasma busulfan levels on the outcome of transplantation. Blood 1997;89:3055–3060.
44. Clift RA, Buckner CD, Thomas ED, et al. Marrow transplantation for chronic myeloid leukemia: A randomized study comparing cyclophosphamide and total body irradiation with busulfan and cyclophosphamide. Blood 1994;84:2036–2043.
45. Devergie A, Blaise D, Attal M, et al. Allogeneic bone marrow transplantation for chronic myeloid leukemia in first chronic phase: A randomized trial of busulfan-cytoxan versus cytoxan-total body irradiation as preparative regimen: A report from the French society of bone marrow graft. Blood 1995;85:2263–2268.
46. Blaise D, Maraninchi D, Michallet M, et al. Long-term follow-up of a randomized trial comparing the combination of cyclophosphamide with total body irradiation or busulfan as conditioning regimen for patients receiving HLA-identical marrow grafts from acute myeloblastic leukemia in first complete remission. Blood 2001;97:3669–3671.
47. Appelbaum FR. Is there a best transplant conditioning regimen for acute myeloid leukemia? Leukemia 2000;14:497–501.
48. Davies SM, Ramsay NKC, Klein JP, et al. Comparison of preparative regimens in transplants for children with acute lymphoblastic leukemia. J Clin Oncol 2000;18:340–347.
49. Roman-Unfer S, Cook B, Nieto Y, Shpall E. Negative and positive stem cell selection. In: Armitage JO, Antman KH, eds. High-Dose Cancer Therapy: Pharmacology, Hematopoietins, Stem Cells, 3rd ed. Philadelphia, Lippincott-Williams & Wilkins, 2000.
50. Gribben JG. Antibody-mediated purging. In: Thomas ED, Blume KG, Forman SJ, eds. Hematopoietic Cell Transplantation, 2nd ed. Malden, MA, Blackwell Science, 1999.
51. Colvin OM. Pharmacological purging of bone marrow. In: Thomas ED, Blume KG, Forman SJ, eds. Hematopoietic Cell Transplantation, 2nd ed. Malden, MA, Blackwell Science, 1999.
52. Vescio R, Schiller G, Stewart AK, et al. Multicenter phase III trial to evaluate $CD34^+$ selected versus unselected autologous peripheral blood progenitor cell transplantation in multiple myeloma. Blood 1999; 93(6):1858–1868.
53. Shpall EJ, LeMaistre CF, Holland K, et al. A prospective randomized trial of buffy coat versus CD34-selected autologous bone marrow support in high-risk breast cancer patients receiving high-dose chemotherapy. Blood 1997;90:4313–4320.
54. Bensinger WI. Should we purge? Bone Marrow Transplant 1998;21: 113–115.
55. Sullivan KM, Storb R, Buckner CD, et al. Graft-versus-host disease as adoptive immunotherapy in patients with advanced hematologic malignancies. N Engl J Med 1989;320:828–834.
56. Mackinnon S. Who may benefit from donor leucocyte infusions after allogeneic stem cell transplantation? Br J Haematol 2000;110:12–17.
57. Locatelli F. The role of repeat transplantation of haemopoietic stem cells and adoptive immunotherapy in treatment of leukaemia relapsing following allogeneic transplantation. Br J Haematol 1998;102:633–638.
58. Collins RH, Shpilberg O, Drobyski WR, et al. Donor leukocyte infusions in 140 patients with relapsed malignancy after allogeneic bone marrow transplantation. J Clin Oncol 1997;15:433–444.
59. Guillaume T, Rubinstein DB, Symann M. Immune reconstitution and immunotherapy after autologous hematopoietic stem cell transplantation. Blood 1998;92:1471–1490.
60. Nagler A, Ackerstein A, Or R, Naparstek E, Slavin S. Immunotherapy with recombinant human interleukin-2 and recombinant α interferon in lymphoma patients post autologous marrow or stem cell transplantation. Blood 1997;89:3951–3959.
61. Robinson N, Benyunes MC, Thompson JA, et al. Interleukin-2 after autologous stem cell transplantation for hematologic malignancies: A phase I/II study. Bone Marrow Transplant 1997;19:425–442.
62. Cunningham D, Powles R, Malpas J, et al. A randomized trial of maintenance interferon following high dose chemotherapy in multiple myeloma: Long-term follow-up results. Br J Haematol 1998;102:495–502.
63. Holmberg LA, Oparin DV, Gooley T, et al. Clinical outcome of breast and ovarian cancer patients treated with high-dose chemotherapy, autologous stem cell rescue and THERATOPE STn-KLH cancer vaccine. Bone Marrow Transplant 2000;25:1233–1241.
64. Reichardt VL, Okada CY, Liso A, et al. Idiotype vaccination using dendritic cells after autologous peripheral blood stem cell transplantation for multiple myeloma—A feasibility study. Blood 1999;93:2411–2419.
65. Carella AM, Champlin R, Slavin S, McSweeney P, Storb R. Mini-allografts: Ongoing trials in humans. Bone Marrow Transplant 2000;25: 345–350.
66. McSweeney PA, Niederwieser D, Shizuru JA, et al. Hematopoietic cell transplantation in older patients with hematologic malignancies: Replacing high-dose cytotoxic therapy with graft-versus-tumor effects. Blood 2001;97:3390–3400.
67. Giralt S, Thall PF, Khouri I, et al. Melphalan and purine analog-containing preparative regimens: Reduced-intensity conditioning for patients with hematologic malignancies undergoing allogeneic progenitor cell transplantation. Blood 2001;97:631–637.

68. Childs R, Chernoff A, Contentin N, et al. Regression of metastatic renal cell carcinoma after nonmyeloablative allogeneic peripheral blood stem cell transplantation. N Engl J Med 2000;343:750–758.
69. Clift RA, Buckner CD. Marrow transplantation for acute myeloid leukemia. Cancer Invest 1998;16:53–61.
70. Zittoun RA, Mandelli F, Willemze R, et al. Autologous or allogeneic bone marrow transplantation compared with intensive chemotherapy in acute myelogenous leukemia. N Engl J Med 1995;332:217–223.
71. Cassileth PA, Harrington DP, Appelbaum FR, et al. Chemotherapy compared with autologous or allogeneic bone marrow transplantation in the management of acute myeloid leukemia in first remission. N Engl J Med 1998;339:1649–1656.
72. Woods WG, Neudorf S. Gold S, et al. A comparison of allogeneic bone marrow transplantation, autologous bone marrow transplantation, and aggressive chemotherapy in children with acute myeloid leukemia in remission: A report for the Children's Cancer Group. Blood 2001;97:56–62.
73. Creutzig U, Reinhardt D, Zimmermann M, Klingebiel T, and Gadner H. Intensive chemotherapy versus bone marrow transplantation in pediatric acute myeloid leukemia: A matter of controversies. Blood 2001;97:3671–3672.
74. Gorin NC. Autologous stem cell transplantation in acute myelocytic leukemia. Blood 1998;92:1073–1090.
75. Burnett AK, Goldstone AH, Stevens RMF, et al. Randomized comparison of addition of autologous bone marrow transplantation to intensive chemotherapy for acute myeloid leukemia in first remission: Results of MRC AML 10 trial. Lancet 1998;351:700–708.
76. Reiffers J, Labopin M, Sanz M, et al. Autologous blood cell vs marrow transplantation for acute myeloid leukemia in complete remission: An EBMT retrospective analysis. Bone Marrow Transplant 2000;25:1115–1119.
77. Heaney ML, Golde DW. Medical progress: Myelodysplasia. N Engl J Med 1999;340:1649–1660.
78. Deeg HJ, Shulman HM, Anderson JE, et al. Allogeneic and syngeneic marrow transplantation for myelodysplastic syndrome in patients 55–66 years of age. Blood 2000;95:1188–1194.
79. Chessells JM. Relapsed lymphoblastic leukaemia in children: A continuing challenge. Br J Haematol 1998;102:423–438.
80. Martin TG, Gajewski JL. Allogeneic stem cell transplantation for acute lymphocytic leukemia in adults. Hematol Oncol Clin North Am 2001;15:91–120.
81. Martin TG, Linker CA. Autologous stem cell transplantation for acute lymphocytic leukemia in adults. Hematol Oncol Clin North Am 2001;15:121–143.
82. Barrett AJ, Horowitz MM, Pollock BH, et al. Bone marrow transplants from HLA-identical siblings as compared with chemotherapy for children with acute lymphoblastic leukemia in a second remission. N Engl J Med 1994;331:1253–1258.
83. Sebban C, Lepage E, Vernant JP, et al. Allogeneic bone marrow transplantation in adult acute lymphoblastic leukemia in first complete remission: A comparative study. J Clin Oncol 1994;12:2580–2587.
84. Cornelissen JJ, Carston M, Kollman C, et al. Unrelated marrow transplantation for adult patients with poor-risk acute lymphoblastic leukemia: Strong graft-versus-leukemia effect and risk factors determining outcome. Blood 2001;97:1572–1577.
85. Wheeler KA, Richards SM, Bailey CC, et al. Bone marrow transplantation versus chemotherapy in the treatment of very high risk childhood acute lymphoblastic leukemia in first remission: Results from Medical Research Council UKALL X and XI. Blood 2000;96:2412–2418.
86. Passweg JR, Rowlings PA, Horowitz MM. Related donor bone marrow transplantation for chronic myelogenous leukemia. Hematol Oncol Clin North Am 1998;12:81–93.
87. Hansen JA, Gooley TA, Martin PJ, et al. Bone marrow transplants from unrelated donors for patients with chronic myeloid leukemia. N Engl Med 1998;338:962–968.
88. McGlave PB, Shu XO, Wen W, et al. Unrelated donor marrow transplantation for chronic myelogenous leukemia: 9 years experience of the National Marrow Donor Program. Blood 2000;95:2219–2225.
89. Bhatia R, Forman SJ. Autologous transplantation for the treatment of chronic myelogenous leukemia. Hematol Oncol Clin North Am 1998;12:151–172.
90. Dreger P, Michallet M, Schmitz N. Stem cell transplantation for chronic lymphocytic leukemia: The 1999 perspective. Ann Oncol 2000;11 (Suppl 1):49–53.
91. Pavletic ZS, Arrowsmith ER, Bierman PJ, et al. Outcome of allogeneic stem cell transplantation for B cell chronic lymphocytic leukemia. Bone Marrow Transplant 2000;25:717–722.
92. Bishop MR, Kessinger A. Blood stem cell transplantation in non-Hodgkin's lymphoma. Cancer Invest 1997;15:138–142.
93. Shipp MA, Abeloff MD, Antman KH, et al. International consensus conference on high-dose therapy with hematopoietic stem cell transplantation in aggressive non-Hodgkin's lymphomas: Report of the Jury. J Clin Oncol 1999;17:423–429.
94. Armitage JO. High-dose therapy and ABMT for follicular lymphoma. Blood 2001;97:337.
95. Aisenberg AC. Problems in Hodgkin's disease management. Blood 1999;93:761–779.
96. Vose JM, Zhang M, Rowlings PA, et al. Autologous transplantation for diffuse aggressive non-Hodgkin's lymphoma in patients never achieving remission: A report from the Autologous Blood and Marrow Transplant registry. J Clin Oncol 2001;19:406–413.
97. Haioun C, Lepage E, Gisselbrecht C, et al. Survival benefit of high dose therapy in poor-risk aggressive non-Hodgkin's lymphoma: Final analysis of the prospective LNH87–2 protocol—A Groupe d'Etude des Lymphomes de l'Adulte Study. J Clin Oncol 2000;18:3025–3030.
98. Gianni AM, Bregni M, Siena S, et al. High dose chemotherapy and autologous bone marrow transplantation compared with MACOP-B in aggressive B-cell lymphoma. N Engl J Med 1997;336:1290–1297.
99. Sweetenham JW, Santini G, Qian W, et al. High-dose therapy and autologous stem cell transplantation versus conventional dose consolidation/maintenance therapy as postremission therapy for adult patients with lymphoblastic lymphoma: Results of a randomized trial of the European Group for Blood and Marrow Transplantation and the United Kingdom Lymphoma Group. J Clin Oncol 2001;19:2729–2736.
100. Horning SJ, Negrin RS, Hoppe RT, et al. High-dose therapy and autologous bone marrow transplantation for follicular lymphoma in first complete or partial remission: Results of a phase II clinical trial. Blood 2001;97:404–409.
101. Tsai ED, Moore HCF, Hardy CL, et al. Rituximab (anti-CD20 monoclonal antibody) therapy for progressive intermediate-grade non-Hodgkin's lymphoma after high-dose therapy and autologous peripheral stem cell transplantation. Bone Marrow Transplant 1999;24:521–526.
102. Pedersen-Bjergaard J, Andersen M, and Christiansen DH. Therapy-related acute myeloid leukemia and myelodysplasia after high-dose chemotherapy and autologous stem cell transplantation. Blood 2000;95:3273–3279.
103. Attal M, Harousseau JL, Stoppa AM, et al. A prospective, randomized trial of autologous bone marrow transplantation and chemotherapy in multiple myeloma. N Engl J Med 1996;335:91–97.
104. Barlogie B, Jagannath S, Desidan KR, et al. Total therapy with tandem transplants for newly diagnosed multiple myeloma. Blood 1999;93:55–65.
105. Martinelli G, Terragna C, Zamagni E, et al. Molecular remission after allogeneic or autologous transplantation of hematopoietic stem cells for multiple myeloma. J Clin Oncol 2000;18:2273–2281.
106. Lokhorst GM, Schattenberg A, Cornelissen JJ, et al. Donor lymphocyte infusions for relapsed multiple myeloma after allogeneic stem cell transplantation: Predictive factors for response and long-term outcome. J Clin Oncol 2000;18:3031–3937.
107. Badros AA, Barlogie B, Morris C, et al. High response rate in refractory and poor-risk multiple myeloma after allotransplantation using a nonmyeloablative conditioning regimen and donor lymphocyte infusions. Blood 2001;97:2574–2579.
108. Salama M, Nevill T, Marcellus D, et al. Donor leukocyte infusions for multiple myeloma. Bone Marrow Transplant 2000;26:1179–1184.

109. Zujewski J, Nelson A, Abrams J. Much ado about not . . . enough data: high-dose chemotherapy with autologous stem cell rescue for breast cancer. J Natl Cancer Inst 1998;90:200–209.
110. Gluck S, Stewart D. High-dose therapy in breast cancer: Out of favor but not out of promise. Bone Marrow Transplant 2000;25:1017–1019.
111. Antman KH, Rowlings PA, Vaughan WP, et al. High-dose chemotherapy with autologous hematopoietic stem cell support for breast cancer in North America. J Clin Oncol 1997;15:187–1879.
112. Weiss RB, gill GG, Hudis CA. An on-site audit of the South African trial of high-dose chemotherapy for metastatic breast cancer and associated publications. J Clin Oncol 2001;19:2771–2777.
113. Stadtmauer EA, O'Neill A, Goldstein LJ, et al. Conventional-dose chemotherapy compared with high-dose chemotherapy plus autologous hematopoietic stem-cell transplantation for metastatic breast cancer. N Engl J Med 2000;342:1069–1076.
114. Rodenhuis S, Richel DJ, van der Vall E, et al. Randomised trial of high-dose chemotherapy and haemopoietic progenitor-cell support in operable breast cancer with extensive axillary lymph-node involvement. Lancet 1998;352:515–521.
115. Hortobagyi GN, Buzdar AU, Theriault RL, et al. Randomized trial of high-dose chemotherapy and blood cell autografts for high-risk primary breast carcinoma. J Natl Cancer Inst 2000;92:225–233.
116. Sosman JA, Stiff P, Moss SM, et al. Pilot trial of interleukin-2 with granulocyte colony-stimulating factor for the mobilization of progenitor cells in advanced breast cancer patients undergoing high-dose chemotherapy: Expansion of immune effectors within the stem-cell graft and post-stem-cell infusion. J Clin Oncol 2001;19:634–644.
117. Ueno NT, Fondon G, Mirza NQ, et al. Allogeneic peripheral-blood progenitor-cell transplantation for poor-risk patients with breast cancer. J Clin Oncol 1998;16:986–993.
118. Bearman SI. The syndrome of hepatic veno-occlusive disease after marrow transplantation. Blood 1995;85:3005–3020.
119. Carreras E, Bertz H, Arcese W, et al. Incidence and outcome of hepatic veno-occlusive disease after blood or marrow transplantation: A prospective cohort study of the European Group for Blood and Marrow Transplantation. Blood 1998;92:3599–3604.
120. Dix SP, Wingard JR, Mullins RE, et al. Association of busulfan area under the curve with veno-occlusive disease following BMT. Bone Marrow Transplant 1996;17:225–230.
121. Bearman SI, Lee JL, Baron AE, McDonald GB. Treatment of hepatic venoocclusive disease with recombinant human tissue plasminogen activator and heparin in 42 marrow transplant patients. Blood 1997;89:1501–1506.
122. Soubani AO, Miller KB, Hassoun PM. Pulmonary complications of bone marrow transplantation. Chest 1996;109:1066–1077.
123. Palmas A, Tefferi A, Myers JL, et al. Late-onset noninfectious pulmonary complications after allogeneic bone marrow transplantation. Br J Haematol 1998;100:680–687.
124. Davies SM, Kollman C, Anasetti C, et al. Engraftment and survival after unrelated-donor bone marrow transplantation. Blood 2000;96:4096–4102.
125. Ozer H, Armitage JO, Bennett CL, et al. 2000 Update of recommendations for the use of hematopoietic colony-stimulating factors: Evidence-based, clinical practice guidelines. J Clin Oncol 2000;18:3558–3585.
126. Klumpp TR, Mangan KF, Goldberg SL, et al. Granulocyte colony-stimulating factor accelerates neutrophil engraftment following peripheral blood stem cell transplantation: A prospective, randomized trial. J Clin Oncol 1995;13:1323–1327.
127. Bishop MR, Tarantolo SR, Geller RB, et al. A randomized, double blind trial of filgrastim (granulocyte colony-stimulating factor) versus placebo following allogeneic blood stem cell transplantation. Blood 2000;96: 80–85.
128. Przepiorka D, Smith TL, Folloder J, et al. Controlled trial of filgrastim for acceleration of neutrophil recovery after allogeneic blood stem cell transplantation from human leukocyte antigen-matched related donors. Blood 2001;97:3405–3410.
129. Bolwell B, Goormastic M, Dannley R, et al. G-CSF post-autologous progenitor cell transplantation: a randomized study of 5, 10, and 16 μg/kg/day. Bone Marrow Transplant 1997;19:215–219.
130. Bolwell B, Pohlman B, Andresen S, et al. Delayed G-CSF after autologous progenitor cell transplantation: Prospective randomized trial. Bone Marrow Transplant 1998;21:369–373.
131. Fields KK, Crump M, Bence-Bruckler, et al. Use of PEG-rHuMGDF in platelet engraftment after autologous stem cell transplantation. Bone Marrow Transplant 2000;29:1083–1088.
132. Vrendenburgh JJ, Hussein A, Fisher D, et al. A randomized trial of recombinant human interleukin-11 following autologous bone marrow transplantation with peripheral blood progenitor support in patients with breast cancer. Biol Blood Marrow Transplant 1998;4:134–141.
133. Lazarus HM, Vogelsang GB, Rowe JM. Prevention and treatment of acute graft versus host disease: The old and the new. A report from the Eastern Cooperative Oncology Group (ECOG). Bone Marrow Transplant 1997;19:577–600.
134. Przepiorka D, Smith TL, Folloder J, et al. Risk factors for acute graft-versus-host disease after allogeneic blood stem cell transplantation. Blood 1999;94:1465–1470.
135. Kernan NA. T-cell depletion for prevention of graft-versus-host disease. In: Thomas ED, Blume KG, Forman SJ, eds. Hematopoietic Cell Transplantation, 2nd ed. Malden, MA, Blackwell Science, 1999.
136. Storb R, Pepe M, Anasetti C, et al. What role for prednisone in prevention of acute graft-versus-host disease in patients undergoing marrow transplants? Blood 1990;76:1037–1345
137. Sayer HG, Longton G, Bowden R, et al. Increased risk of infection in marrow transplant patients receiving methylprednisolone for graft-versus-host disease prevention. Blood 1994;84:1328–1332.
138. Chao NJ, Schmidt GM, Niland JC, et al. Cyclosporine, methotrexate, and prednisone compared with cyclosporine and prednisone alone for prophylaxis of acute graft-versus-host disease. N Engl J Med 1993; 329:1225–1230.
139. Ruutu T, Volin L, Parkkali T, Juvonen E, Elonen E. Cyclosporine, methotrexate, and methylprednisolone compared with cyclosporine and methotrexate for the prevention of graft-versus host disease in bone marrow transplantation from HLA-identical sibling donor: A prospective randomized study. Blood 2000;96:2391–2398.
140. Jacobson P, Uberti J, Davis W, Ratanatharathorn V. Tacrolimus: A new agent for the prevention of graft-versus-host disease in hematopoietic stem cell transplantation. Bone Marrow Transplant 1998;22:217–225.
141. Ratanatharathorn V, Nash RA, Przepiorka D, et al. Phase III study comparing methotrexate and tacrolimus (Prograf, FK506) with methotrexate and cyclosporine for graft-versus-host disease prophylaxis after HLA-identical sibling bone marrow transplantation. Blood 1998;92:2303–2314.
142. Nash RA, Antin JH, Karanes C, et al. Phase 3 study comparing methotrexate and tacrolimus with methotrexate and cyclosporine for prophylaxis of acute graft-versus-host disease after marrow transplantation from unrelated donors. Blood 2000;96:2062–2068.
143. Blaise D, Olive D, Michallet M, et al. Impairment of leukaemia-free survival by addition of interleukin-2 antibody to standard graft-versus-host prophylaxis. Lancet 1995;345:1144–1146.
144. Bass EB, Powe NR, Goodman SN et al. Efficacy of immune globulin in preventing complications of bone marrow transplantation: A meta-analysis. Bone Marrow Transplant 1993;12:273–282.
145. Barrett AJ, Mavroudis D, Tisdale J, et al. T cell-depleted bone marrow transplantation and delayed T cell add-back to control acute GVHD and conserve a graft-versus-leukemia effect. Bone Marrow Transplant 1998;21:543–551.
146. Gaziev J, Galimberti M, Lucarelli G, Polchi P. Chronic graft-versus-host disease: Is there an alternative to the conventional treatment. Bone Marrow Transplant 2000;25:689–696.
147. Vogelsang GB. How I treat chronic graft-versus-host disease. Blood 2001;97:1196–1201.
148. Duell T, Van Lint MT, Ljungman P, et al. Health and functional status of long-term survivors of bone marrow transplantation. Ann Intern Med 1997;126:184–192.
149. Buchsel PC, Leum EW, Randolph SR. Delayed complications of bone marrow transplantation: An update. Oncol Nurs Forum 1996;23:1267–1291.

135

ASSESSMENT OF NUTRITION STATUS AND NUTRITION REQUIREMENTS

Katherine Hammond Chessman and Kathleen M. Teasley-Strausburg

A thorough nutrition assessment is the first step in formulating a patient-specific nutrition care plan. Nutrition assessment has three major goals: (1) to identify the patient who has or is at risk for developing malnutrition, including disorders resulting from nutrient deficiencies (undernutrition), either protein-energy malnutrition (PEM) or obesity (overnutrition), or impaired metabolism (under- or overnutrition), (2) to determine a person's risk of malnutrition-associated complications, and (3) to establish a baseline against which to measure the outcome of nutrition therapy.[1]

The assessment of a patient's nutrition status initially involves identification of the presence of risk factors for malnutrition typically through a nutrition screening process. If the patient is determined to be at risk for malnutrition by established screening parameters, a comprehensive nutrition assessment is performed to identify the type and extent of malnutrition present. This comprehensive nutrition assessment should include a nutrition-focused medical and dietary history, physical examination including anthropometric measurements, and laboratory measurements and provides a basis for determining the patient's nutrition requirements and the optimal type and timing of nutrition intervention.

Nutrition requirements depend on an individual's clinical condition and the need for continued maintenance of adequate nutrition or whether starvation or ongoing metabolic stress dictate a need for repletion. For patients who are obese, usual nutrition requirements may be altered due to the need for weight loss. In children, there is the added consideration of sustaining normal growth and development. Organ function (e.g., renal or hepatic function) may affect nutrient use. Nutrition assessment requires physical assessment skills, knowledge of objective measurements of nutrition status, and the ability to apply general guidelines for nutrition requirements in the context of patient-specific factors.

This chapter reviews the current tools used for nutrition screening and assessment. It also provides guidelines for accurate, relevant, and cost-effective nutrition assessment, including the determination of patient-specific nutrition requirements.

CLASSIFICATION OF NUTRITION DISEASE

Undernutrition usually is the result of starvation (inadequate nutrition intake) or altered metabolism (inappropriate use of ingested nutrients). Pure starvation occurs when inadequate amounts of appropriate nutrients are available to support tissue repair or synthesis, and changes can be reversed by adequate feeding.[2] An alteration in nutrient metabolism exists when the cell has altered substrate demands or use such as cachexia associated with inflammatory or neoplastic conditions. In such situations, enhancing nutritional intake may not be able to meet the increased demand.[2] Regardless of the cause, undernutrition results in changes in subcellular, cellular, and/or organ function that expose the individual to increased risks of morbidity and mortality. In general, deficiency states can be categorized as those involving protein and calories (PEM) or those involving single nutrients such as individual vitamins or trace minerals. PEM may be classified as marasmus, kwashiorkor, or and mixed marasmus/kwashiorkor[4,5]:

Marasmus is a chronic condition resulting from a prolonged deficiency in total intake and/or nutrient utilization. Somatic protein (skeletal muscle) and adipose tissue (subcutaneous fat) wasting occurs, but visceral protein production (e.g., albumin, transferrin) is preserved. Weight loss usually exceeds 10% of usual or expected weight. When severe, cell-mediated immunity (measured by delayed cutaneous hypersensitivity) and muscle function are impaired. Patients with wasting diseases such as cancer commonly have marasmus and a starved, wasted appearance.

Kwashiorkor develops when there is adequate calorie but a relatively inadequate protein intake. These patients generally are well nourished but are extremely catabolic, usually secondary to trauma, infection, or burns. There is depletion of visceral (and to some degree somatic) protein pools with relative preservation of adipose tissue. Kwashiorkor is characterized by hypoalbuminemia and edema. In the setting of metabolic stress and protein deprivation, kwashiorkor may develop rapidly and may result in impaired immune function.

Mixed marasmus/kwashiorkor is a form of severe PEM that develops in chronically ill, starved patients undergoing hypermetabolic stress. There is reduced visceral protein synthesis superimposed on wasting of somatic protein and energy (adipose tissue) stores. Immunocompetence is lowered, increasing the incidence of infection, and wound healing is compromised.

Single-nutrient deficiencies can occur, especially in patients with PEM. Depletion of individual nutrients leads to symptoms related to that nutrient's function. Therefore, all potential deficiency states should be evaluated before an acute or chronic nutrition care plan is developed. Overnutrition (obesity) is a major health care concern in the United States today with a prevalence of 22.5%.[3] Nutrition assessment allows identification of obese individuals or those at risk of becoming obese and the numerous consequences related to overnutrition, including type II diabetes mellitus, cardiovascular disease, and stroke (see Chapter 140).

NUTRITION SCREENING

Since a thorough nutrition assessment on every patient is not practical (or warranted), nutrition screening provides a systematic way of identifying individuals at risk for malnutrition or PEM. Risk factors for undernutrition include any disease state, complicating condition, treatment, or socioeconomic condition that may result in a decreased nutrient intake, altered metabolism, and/or malabsorption. Nutrition screening can be done in the home by the patient or home health care professional, in long-term care facilities, in ambulatory care clinics, or in the hospital. Various rating and classification systems have been proposed to assess nutrition risk and guide subsequent interventions.[4–6] Checklists are used in many clinical settings to quantify a person's food and alcohol consumption habits; ability to buy, prepare, and eat food; weight history; diagnoses; or medical/surgical procedures. Depending on the specific criteria evaluated, three to four risk factors may put a person "at risk" for malnutrition. Pediatric screening programs most often evaluate growth parameters against the National Center for Health Statistics (NCHS)—a part of the Centers for Disease Control and Prevention—growth charts[7] and conditions known to increase nutrition risk.[8] Hospital screening programs also should identify patients receiving specialized nutrition support (enteral or parenteral nutrition) prior to admission.

The Joint Commission on Accreditation of Healthcare Organizations (JCAHO) hospital standards requires that "in its initial patient assessment, the hospital identifies patients at risk for nutritional problems."[9] For patients found to be at risk for malnutrition, a nutrition assessment and nutrition care plan are required.[9] A nutrition screening process needs to take place within an institution-designated period of time (usually 24 to 72 hours) of hospital admission. In the hospital setting, patients initially determined to be not at risk should be reevaluated every 7 to 14 days to detect deterioration in nutrition status secondary to changes in food intake or clinical condition. By identifying at-risk individuals, nutrition screening can be a cost-effective way to help decrease complications and length of hospital stay.[10]

NUTRITION ASSESSMENT

Nutrition assessment is the first step in the development of a nutrition care plan. Components of a thorough nutrition assessment include a medical and dietary history, physical examination, and laboratory studies.

CLINICAL EVALUATION

Clinical evaluation with a nutrition-focused medical and dietary history and physical examination (PE) remains the oldest, simplest, and most widely used method of evaluating nutrition status. Clinical evaluation of nutrition status correlates well with objective evaluations (e.g., laboratory parameters, anthropometric measurements). The medical and dietary history components of the clinical evaluation will provide information about factors that predispose the patient to developing malnutrition (e.g., prematurity, chronic diseases, gastrointestinal malfunction, alcohol abuse). The clinician should direct the interview to elicit any history of weight loss, anorexia, vomiting, diarrhea, and decreased or unusual food intake (Table 135–1).

The nutrition-focused PE consists of an assessment of lean body mass (LBM) and the physical findings of vitamin deficiency, trace mineral deficiency, and essential fatty acid deficiency (EFAD). The assessment should characterize the presence and degree of muscle wasting, edema, loss of subcutaneous fat, dermatitis, glossitis, cheilosis, and/or jaundice[11] (Table 135–2).

TABLE 135–1. Pertinent Data from Medical and Dietary History for Nutrition Assessment

Nutrition Intake and Dietary Habits
Anorexia, unusual or absent taste
Dietary intake, special diets including enteral or parenteral nutrition
Formula or breastfeeding, age at initiation of solid foods
Supplemental vitamin, mineral, or herbal intake
Food allergies or intolerance
Underlying Pathology with Nutritional Effects
Chronic infections or inflammatory states
Neoplastic diseases
Endocrine disorders
Chronic illness including pulmonary disease, cirrhosis, renal failure
Hypermetabolic states such as trauma, burns, sepsis
Digestive or absorptive disease, nausea, vomiting, diarrhea
Hyperlipidemia
Prematurity
End-Organ Effects
Weight change, failure to thrive
Skin or hair changes
Activity and energy level, exercise tolerance, fatique
Obesity
Gastrointestinal tract symptoms: diarrhea, vomiting, constipation
Miscellaneous
Catabolic medications or therapies: corticosteroids, immunosuppressive agents, radiation, or chemotherapy
Other medications: diuretics, laxatives, anabolic steroids
Genetic background: body habitus of parents, siblings, and family
Alcohol or drug abuse

Subjective global assessment (SGA) uses selected parameters from the clinical evaluation alone (history, PE) to identify nutrition-related disease. SGA includes an evaluation of weight changes, dietary intake changes, gastrointestinal (GI) symptoms, functional capacity, and diseases. PE findings evaluated in the SGA include subcutaneous fat, muscle wasting, edema, and ascites.[11]

TABLE 135–2. Physical Findings Suggestive of Malnutrition

General Appearance
Edema (especially ankle and sacral)
Cachexia
Ascites
Signs and symptoms of dehydration: poor skin turgor, sunken eyes, orthostasis, dry mucous membranes
Muscle-wasting, loss of subcutaneous fat
Obesity
Skin and Mucous Membranes
Thin, shiny, or scaling skin
Decubitus ulcers
Ecchymoses, perifollicular petechiae
Poorly healing surgical or traumatic wounds
Pallor or redness of gums, fissures at mouth edge
Glossitis; stomatitis; cheilosis
Musculoskeletal
Retarded growth
Bone pain or tenderness, epiphyseal swelling
Muscle mass less than expected for habitus, genetic history, and level of exercise
Neurologic
Ataxia, positive Romberg test, decreased vibratory or position sense
Nystagmus
Convulsions, paralysis
Encephalopathy
Failure to meet age-appropriate developmental milestones
Hepatic
Jaundice
Hepatomegaly

ANTHROPOMETRIC MEASUREMENTS

Anthropometric measurements, gross measurements of body cell mass, are used to evaluate LBM and fat stores. The most common measurements are stature (height or length, depending on age), weight, head circumference (for children younger than 3 years of age), and measurements of limb size, such as skinfold thickness, midarm muscle circumference (MAMC), and wrist circumference. Bioelectrical impedance analysis (BIA) is also an anthropometric assessment tool. These parameters are used to compare an individual with a population and as repeated measurements in an individual to monitor the response to a nutrition care plan. In adults, nutrition-related changes in anthropometric measurements occur slowly; several weeks or more often are required before detectable changes are noted. In infants and young children, changes may occur more quickly. Acute changes in anthropometric measurements, specifically weight and skinfold thickness, usually reflect changes in hydration status, and this must be considered when one interprets these parameters.

WEIGHT, STATURE, AND HEAD CIRCUMFERENCE

Body weight is a nonspecific measure of body cell mass, representing skeletal mass, body fat, and the energy-using component referred to as LBM. Changes in weight over time, particularly in the absence of edema, ascites, and voluntary losses, are an important indicator of altered LBM. Interpretation of any actual body weight (ABW) measurement should take into consideration ideal weight for height [ideal body weight (IBW)], usual body weight (UBW), fluid status, and age (Table 135–3). Dehydration from nausea, vomiting, diarrhea, other fluid losses and decreased fluid intake may result in decreased ABW but not a loss in LBM. The presence of edema or ascites indicates excess total body water, which will increase ABW. More subtle changes in fluid status may be detected by monitoring the patient's daily fluid intake and output, which should be evaluated along with weight changes.

The IBW provides a population reference standard against which the ABW can be compared to detect both over- and undernutrition states. The IBW for a given height is that weight correlating with maximum longevity. Numerous reference tables have been generated based on various population statistics.[11] In clinical practice, mathematical equations based on gender and height are used commonly to estimate IBW. Commonly used equations for adults (age 18 years and older) and children are:[12]

TABLE 135–3. Evaluation of Actual Body Weight[11]

Actual Body Weight (ABW) Compared with Ideal Body Weight (IBW)	
Undernutrition	
ABW < 69% IBW	Severe malnutrition
ABW 70–79% IBW	Moderate malnutrition
ABW 80–90% IBW	Mild malnutrition
Normal	
ABW 90–120% IBW	Normal
Overnutrition	
ABW > 120% IBW	Overweight
ABW ≥ 150% IBW	Obese
ABW ≥ 200% IBW	Morbidly obese
Actual Body Weight (ABW) Compared with Usual Body Weight (UBW)	
ABW 85–95% UBW	Mild malnutrition
ABW 75–84% UBW	Moderate malnutrition
ABW ≤ 74% UBW	Severe malnutrition

Males:

$$\text{IBW (kg)} = 50 + (2.3 \times \text{height in inches over 5 ft})$$

Females:

$$\text{IBW (kg)} = 45.5 + (2.3 \times \text{height in inches over 5 ft})$$

Children (1–18 years):

$$\text{IBW (kg)} = [(\text{height in cm})^2 \times 1.65]/1000$$

IBW in children also can be determined by identifying the 50th percentile weight, which corresponds to the child's stature on the appropriate NCHS growth chart.[7] Adjusted body weight for obesity can be calculated as:

$$\text{Adjusted weight} = [(\text{ABW} - \text{IBW}) \times 0.2] + \text{IBW}$$

EXAMPLES OF IBW CALCULATION AND ASSESSMENT

Male: Weight: 165 lb (75 kg); height: 6 ft 2 in:

$$\text{IBW} = 50\text{ kg} + (2.3 \times 14) = 82.2\text{ kg}$$

ABW = 91% IBW. Interpretation: Normal.

Female: Weight: 198 lb (90 kg); height: 5 ft 6 in:

$$\text{IBW} = 45.5\text{ kg} + (2.3 \times 6) = 59.3\text{ kg}$$

ABW = 152% IBW. Interpretation: Obese.
Child: Weight: 28.6 lb (13 kg); height: 3 ft 2 in (96.5 cm):

$$\text{IBW} = [(96.5)^2 \times 1.65]/1000 = 15.4\text{ kg}$$

ABW = 84% IBW. Interpretation: Mild malnutrition.

Change in weight over time can be calculated as the percentage of UBW, where percent change = (ABW/UBW) × 100. Use of the UBW as a reference point provides a more accurate reflection of clinically and nutritionally significant weight changes. Determining a patient's UBW, however, depends on patient or family recall, which may be inaccurate. The use of UBW avoids the problems of normative tables, and it documents comparative changes in body weight. The change in weight should be interpreted relative to time. In adults, unintentional weight loss of more than 10% in less than 6 months has been correlated with a poor clinical outcome.[1]

The best indicator of adequate nutrition in a child is appropriate growth.[1] Weight, height, and head circumference should be plotted on the appropriate NCHS gender- and age-based growth curve at each medical encounter.[7] These growth charts were developed initially in 1977 from a large population of normal children and revised recently through a cooperative effort of many agencies, including the National Center for Chronic Disease Prevention and Health Promotion. Special growth charts are available for assessment of short- and long-term growth of premature infants[13,14] and children with Down syndrome.[15] For premature infants with corrected postnatal age of 40 weeks or more, the NCHS growth charts can be used; however, weight for age and length for age should be plotted according to corrected postnatal age until 2 and 3.5 years of age, respectively.[16]

Appropriate minimum time intervals between measurements for meaningful evaluation of growth are weight, 7 days; length, 4 weeks; height, 8 weeks; and head circumference, 7 days in infants and every 4 weeks in children up to 3 years of age.[17] Usual growth velocities for weight, height, and head circumference that can be used to assess adequacy of growth between intervals too close to plot accurately on a growth chart are shown in Table 135–4. For newborns, it is also useful

TABLE 135–4. Expected Growth Velocities in Children[7]

Age	Weight (g/d)	Height (cm/mo)	Head Circumference (cm/wk)
0–3 mos	24–35	2.8–3.4	0.5
3–6 mos	15–21	1.7–2.4	0.5
6–12 mos	10–13	1.3–1.6	0.5
1–3 yr	5–9	0.6–1.0	—
4–6 yr	5–6	0.5–0.6	—
7–10 yr	7–11	0.4–0.5	—

to know that average weight gain is 10–20 g/kg per day (20–30 g/day in term infants and 10–25 g/day in preterm infants).[18] Weight gain declines considerably after 2 to 3 months of age. Head growth (measured by head circumference) can be compromised during periods of critical illness or malnutrition. Sustained head growth during these periods suggests hydrocephalus.

EXAMPLE OF GROWTH ASSESSMENT

Infant: Age: 2 months; weight: 3.9 kg; weight at 1 month of age, 3.1 kg; days since last weight: 30:

$$\text{Growth velocity} = [(3.9\text{ kg} - 3.1\text{ kg}) \times 1000\text{ g/kg}]/30\text{ days} = 26.7\text{ g/d}$$

Interpretation: Normal growth.

Growth failure or failure to thrive is defined as weight for age or weight for height (or length) below the 5th percentile or a falloff of two or more major percentiles (major percentiles are defined as 95th, 90th, 75th, 50th, 25th, 10th, and 5th). Weight-for-height evaluation is age-independent and helps differentiate the stunted child (chronic malnutrition) from the wasted child (acute malnutrition). Short stature, which is associated with many chronic diseases, is a manifestation of chronic undernutrition.

BODY MASS INDEX

Body mass index (BMI), defined as body weight in kilograms divided by height in meters squared, is another way to assess appropriateness of weight for height. BMI can be used to categorize both obesity and undernutrition in adults and children. Tables listing BMI stratified by height and weight are available for quick reference.[19] Values greater than 27 are associated with overweight, and values less than 18.5 are indicative of mild malnutrition. This index is not a reflection of body composition, as demonstrated in the situation of a very muscular person who has a high BMI but a low percentage of total body fat. In this setting, the person may be falsely categorized as obese based solely on BMI. Suggested interpretation of BMI values is shown in Table 135–5.[20,21]

EXAMPLES OF BMI CALCULATION AND ASSESSMENT

Male: Age: 40 years; weight: 180 lb (81.8 kg); height: 5 ft 10 in (177.8 cm, 1.778 m):

$$\text{BMI} = 81.1/(1.78)^2 = 25.8\text{ kg/m}^2$$

Interpretation: Healthy.

TABLE 135–5. Interpretation of Body Mass Index Values[20,21]

BMI (kg/m^2)	Nutrition Status
Adults	
<16	Severe malnutrition
16–17	Moderate malnutrition
17–18.5	Mild malnutrition
19–25	Healthy (19–34 years of age)
21–27	Healthy (over 35 years of age)
25–30	Overweight (19–34 years of age)
27.5–30	Overweight (over 35 years of age)
30–40	Moderate obesity
>40	Severe or morbid obesity
Children	
BMI for age < 5th percentile	Underweight
BMI for age 5th–85th percentile	Healthy
BMI for age > 85th percentile	At risk for overweight
BMI for age ≥ 95th percentile	Overweight

Female: Age: 25 years; weight: 160 lb (72.7 kg); height: 5 ft 5 in (165.1 cm, 1.651 m):

$$\text{BMI} = 72.7/(1.65)^2 = 26.7\text{ kg/m}^2$$

Interpretation: Overweight.

Although guidelines for BMI have not yet been universally accepted, in general, healthy weights are those associated with a reduction in disease risk. While BMI correlates strongly with total body fat, individual variation, especially in very muscular persons, may lead to erroneous classification of either obesity or malnutrition when BMI alone is used to assess nutrition status. A major advantage of the revised NCHS growth charts for children is the addition of charts for assessment of BMI based on age and gender. It is hoped that such charts will heighten parental and health care provider awareness of those children whose BMI and family history put them at risk for obesity and its associated risks in adulthood.

SKINFOLD THICKNESS AND MAMC

Skinfold thickness measurement provides an estimate of subcutaneous fat, whereas MAMC estimates skeletal muscle mass. These simple, noninvasive anthropometric measurements are not used commonly in clinical practice but are appropriate for both population analysis and individual long-term monitoring. Triceps skinfold thickness (TSF) is the most commonly used of the skinfold measurements, although reference standards also exist for subscapular and iliac sites. More than half the total body fat is subcutaneous, and changes in subcutaneous fat have been assumed to reflect changes in total body fat. Careful technique in the use of pressure-regulated calipers is essential for reproducibility and reliability in measuring TSF. MAMC is a calculated value based on the measurement of the midarm circumference and TSF.

Individual anthropometric measurements should be interpreted cautiously because standards do not account for individual variations in bone size, large muscle mass, hydrational status, or skin compressibility; reference standards do not account for obesity, ethnicity, illness, and increased age; technique is critical and interobserver error may be as high as 30%. Furthermore, in adults, these parameters are slow to change, often requiring weeks before significant alterations from baseline can be detected.

BIA is a simple, noninvasive, and relatively inexpensive technique used to measure LBM.[22–24] It is based on the fact that lean tissue has a higher electrical conductivity (less resistance) because of its greater fluid and electrolyte content than does fat, which is a poor conductor of current. By placing electrodes on the wrist and ankle and applying a very small electric current, impedance (resistance) to flow can be measured. Assessment of LBM, total body water (TBW), and the distribution of TBW into compartments can be determined with BIA. Increased TBW decreases impedance; therefore, it is important to evaluate fluid status along with BIA data. Other potential limitations of BIA include variability with electrolyte imbalance, interference by large fat masses (obesity), and the need for good reference standards that reflect variations in individual body sizes and clinical conditions. While BIA equations have high validity when used in the population in which they were developed initially (mostly young, healthy adults), BIA equations are subject to errors that cannot be determined a priori unless they are validated in the specific population in which they are applied.[25–27]

BIOCHEMICAL ASSESSMENT OF LBM

LBM includes skeletal muscle, somatic protein, and functional proteins such as circulating proteins and the visceral proteins. It can be assessed by creatinine-height index and serum visceral protein concentrations in addition to body weight and MAMC measurements.

CREATININE-HEIGHT INDEX

Creatinine-height index (CHI) is based on the excretion of creatinine (Cr), the metabolic end product of creatine, a complex molecule synthesized in the liver and concentrated in body muscle. Cr is excreted at a constant rate unchanged in the urine; therefore, collection of a timed urine with measurement of total Cr excreted indirectly reflects the total muscle mass. For clinical assessment, the Cr production of an adult patient (obtained by the measurement of Cr in a 24-hour urine collection) is compared with the expected Cr excretion of a healthy gender-matched individual of similar height. CHI is calculated as the actual 24-hour Cr excretion divided by expected Cr excretion multiplied by 100, where expected Cr excretion for males is IBW (kg) × 23 mg/kg and for females is IBW (kg) × 18 mg/kg.[28] CHI is interpreted as mild LBM depletion if the CHI is 80% to 90% of expected, moderate depletion if CHI is 60% to 80% of predicted, and severe depletion if the CHI is less than 60% of predicted.

Example of CHI Calculation

Female: IBW: 50 kg; 24-hour Cr excretion: 750 mg:

CHI = 750 mg (actual excretion)/
900 mg (expected excretion, 18 mg/kg × 50 kg) = 78%

Interpretation: Moderate depletion.

The CHI will not reflect muscle mass accurately in individuals with impaired renal function or dehydration and also may be affected by dietary protein intake, steroids, exercise, age, or stress. The most common source of error is an incomplete 24-hour urine collection. The clinical utility of CHI has been questioned,[29] and variations of the index have been suggested.[30]

VISCERAL PROTEINS

Measuring serum concentrations of transport proteins synthesized by the liver can assess the visceral protein compartment. It is assumed that a low serum protein concentration in states of undernutrition reflects the hepatic protein synthetic mass and therefore indirectly the functional protein mass of other organs such as heart, lung, kidney, and intestines. The visceral proteins currently thought to be of greatest relevance for nutrition assessment are serum albumin, transferrin, retinol-binding protein, and prealbumin (thyroxine-binding prealbumin, transthyretin). Many factors other than nutrition affect the serum concentration of these proteins, such as age, abnormal renal (nephrotic syndrome) or GI tract (protein-losing enteropathy) losses, hydration status (dehydration may result in hemoconcentration, overhydration in hemodilution), renal and hepatic function (since this is the primary synthesis site), and metabolic stress (sepsis, trauma, surgery, and/or infection). Therefore, visceral protein data must be interpreted relative to the individual's clinical status[31–34] (Table 135–6).

Albumin (ALB) was one of the first identified biochemical markers of malnutrition and has long been used in population studies. Due to its large body pool size (4–5 g/kg of body weight), high extravascular distribution (60%), and long biologic half-life (18–20 days), ALB is a relatively insensitive index of early protein malnutrition.[34] However, chronic protein deficiency in the setting of adequate nonprotein calorie intake leads to marked hypoalbuminemia because of a net loss of ALB from the intravascular and extravascular compartments (kwashiorkor malnutrition). Serum ALB concentrations also are affected by calorie deficiency; hepatic, renal, and GI disease; and infection, trauma, stress, and burns. In many cases, interpretation of serum ALB concentrations is difficult; however, data consistently indicate a positive correlation between decreased serum ALB concentrations and poor clinical outcome in a variety of settings.[1] Additionally, low serum ALB (≤2.5 g/dL) can be expected to exacerbate ascites and peripheral, pulmonary, and gut edema due to decreased colloid oncotic pressure.[28]

Transferrin (TFN) is a glycoprotein that binds and transports ferric iron to the liver and reticuloendothelial system for storage. As a surrogate marker of nutrition status, it is more likely to respond to protein depletion before changes in serum ALB concentrations are manifest because of its shorter biologic half-life (8 days) and smaller body pool (<100 mg/kg of body weight).[34] Serum TFN concentrations may be determined by direct measurement or can be estimated indirectly from measurement of total iron-binding capacity (TIBC), where TFN = (TIBC × 0.8) − 43. Critical illness, hydration status, and iron stores affect the serum TFN concentration. In iron deficiency, the hepatic synthesis of TFN is increased, resulting in increased serum concentrations.

Thyroxine-binding prealbumin is also referred to as *prealbumin or transthyretin*. It is the transport protein for thyroxine and a carrier protein for retinol-binding protein. It has a short biologic half-life (1–2 days) and a small body pool (10 mg/kg of body weight).[34] Prealbumin may be reduced in as few as 3 days after calorie and protein intake is decreased or when hypercatabolism or severe metabolic stress (trauma, burns) is present. Because of its short half-life, it is most useful in monitoring the short-term, acute effects of nutrition support.[35] As with ALB and TFN, serum prealbumin concentrations are depressed with liver disease because of decreased hepatic synthesis. Increased concentrations have been noted in patients with renal disease and are thought to result from impaired renal degradation.

Retinol-binding protein (RBP) is a specific transport protein for vitamin A alcohol (retinol). It is filtered by the glomeruli and metabolized by the kidney. RBP has a very short biologic half-life (12 hours) and a very small body pool (2 mg/kg of body weight).[34] Serum RBP concentrations decrease with metabolic stress, liver disease, and vitamin A deficiency and increase with chronic renal failure and vitamin A supplementation.[34] These serum proteins (ALB, TFN, prealbumin, RBP) are of greatest value in assessing uncomplicated semistarvation

TABLE 135–6. Summary of Visceral Proteins Used for Assessment of Lean Body Mass[31–34]

Serum Protein	Function	Factors Resulting in Increased Values	Factors Resulting in Decreased Values
Albumin	Maintain plasma oncotic pressure; carrier for small molecules	Dehydration, anabolic steroids, insulin, infection	Overhydration, edema, renal insufficiency, nephrotic syndrome, poor dietary intake, impaired digestion, burns, congestive heart failure, cirrhosis, thyroid/adrenal/pituitary hormones, trauma, sepsis
Transferrin	Binds Fe in plasma and transports to bone	Fe deficiency, pregnancy, hypoxia, chronic blood loss, estrogens	Chronic infection, cirrhosis, burns, enteropathies, nephrotic syndrome, cortisone, testosterone
Prealbumin (transthyretin)	Binds T_3 and to a lesser extent T_4; carrier for RBP	Renal dysfunction	Cirrhosis, hepatitis, stress, surgery, inflammation, hyperthyroidism, cystic fibrosis, renal dysfunction, Zn deficiency
Retinol-binding protein	Transports vitamin A in plasma; binds noncovalently to prealbumin	Renal dysfunction, vitamin A supplementation	Same as prealbumin; also vitamin A deficiency
Fibronectin	Glycoprotein with opsonic activity; may exert chemotactic activity and facilitate wound healing	None currently described	Trauma, shock, burns, sepsis, disseminated intravascular coagulation, inappropriate specimen handling
Somatomedin C	Insulin-like peptide with anabolic actions on fat, muscle, cartilage, and cultured cells	None currently described	Growth hormone deficiency, psychosocial growth failure, hypothyroidism, renal failure, cirrhosis, drugs (estrogens, corticosteroids)

and recovery. In the setting of acute stress (e.g., trauma, burn injury, sepsis), these proteins become poor markers of nutrition status. Their synthesis is downregulated as the liver reprioritizes hepatic protein synthesis in response to systemic injury. In this setting, the liver produces acute-phase reactants such as C-reactive protein, α_1-acid glycoprotein, and α_1-antitrypsin. Other serum proteins, such as fibronectin (an opsonic protein) and somatomedin-C (insulin-like growth factor-1), which have a very short half-life of less than 12 to 24 hours, have been suggested as indicators of nutrition status.[33] However, the clinical availability of these alternative tests is limited, and their relevance to nutrition status and the outcome of patients is debatable.

Plasma amino acid (AAs) concentrations also have been used to assess LBM. Altered AA patterns have been identified in the setting of PEM and are characterized by a slight decrease in essential AA concentrations and an increase or no change in the concentration of nonessential AAs. Consequently, the ratio of essential to nonessential AA concentrations decreases and has been used to characterize PEM. However, unless the nutrition depletion is severe, plasma AA concentrations are maintained fairly constant by the body's homeostatic mechanisms. The depletion state is often clinically apparent before changes in AA concentrations become significant. Furthermore, plasma AA concentrations are altered in various disease states, such as hepatic and renal failure and sepsis. In addition to the lack of sensitivity and specificity, the measurement of plasma AA concentrations is not widely available and is expensive. Therefore, plasma AA concentrations are of limited usefulness in the routine assessment of LBM. Plasma AA concentrations have been used to develop and evaluate pediatric enteral and parenteral nutrition products.

INDICES OF IMMUNE FUNCTION

The frequency with which immunocompetence is impaired and the high incidence of infection in patients with malnutrition suggests that certain tests of immune function could be used as nutrition status markers[36] and as predictors of outcome.[37] Nutrition factors interact with immune status either directly, affecting primarily the lymphoid system, or indirectly, affecting cellular metabolism or another organ system that is in turn involved with the regulation of immunocompetence. Indicators of immune function that frequently are part of nutrition assessment are the total lymphocyte count (TLC) and delayed cutaneous hypersensitivity (DCH) reactions. Both are simple, readily available, and inexpensive. TLC reflects the number of circulating lymphocytes, T and B cells. Tissues that generate T cells are very sensitive to malnutrition and undergo involution with a decrease in T-cell production[36] and eventually lymphopenia. TLC is calculated from a complete blood count (CBC) with differential: TLC = (percent lymphocytes × total number of white blood cells). Values of less than 1500 cells/mm^3 and 900 cells/mm^3 have been associated with moderate nutrition depletion and severe depletion, respectively.[11]

DCH is commonly assessed using antigens to which the patient has been previously sensitized. The recall antigens used most frequently in nutrition assessment are mumps, *Candida albicans*, streptokinase-streptodornase, *Trichophyton*, coccidioidin, and purified protein derivative (PPD). Anergy is associated with malnutrition and may be restored with nutrition repletion. Other more sophisticated tests of immune function may be used to evaluate nutrition status. These include lymphocyte surface antigens (CD4 and CD8 counts, CD4/CD8 ratio), T-lymphocyte responsiveness, and serum interleukin concentrations.[37] The impact of the timing of nutrition intervention has been evaluated using these tests.[38]

Immune function indicators may be affected by many nonnutrition factors; therefore, they are nonspecific indicators of malnutrition. Nonnutrition factors that affect TLC include infection (e.g., HIV/AIDS, pertussis, viruses, tuberculosis), immunosuppressive drugs (e.g., corticosteroids, cyclosporine, chemotherapy, antilymphocyte globulin), and the presence of leukemia and lymphoma. DCH can be affected by fever, viral illness, recent live virus vaccination, critical illness, irradiation, immunosuppressive drugs, diabetes mellitus, HIV/AIDS, cancer, and surgery. This lack of specificity currently limits the usefulness of these tests as markers of nutrition status and outcome predictors. There may be a role for these tests as indices of response when a nutrition regimen includes immunotherapy.[39] Nutrients such as arginine, omega-3 fatty acids, and nucleic acids given in pharmacologic doses have been shown to improve immune function in a variety of settings.[40–42] Monitoring the efficacy of a nutrition care plan that includes these potentially immunomodulating nutrients may need to include assessment of immune function with these or other immune function indicators.

SPECIFIC NUTRIENT DEFICIENCIES

The assessment of nutrition status should include an evaluation of possible trace mineral, vitamin, and essential fatty acid deficiencies. Because of their key role in metabolic processes (as coenzymes and cofactors), a deficiency of any of these nutrients may result in altered metabolism and cell dysfunction and may interfere with processes necessary for repletion of PEM. The assessment of single-nutrient-deficiency states includes an accurate history to evaluate symptoms and identify factors that may predispose the patient to developing a deficiency state. A focused PE for signs of deficiencies and biochemical assessment to confirm a suspected diagnosis also should be done. Ideally, biochemical assessment should be based on the nutrient's function (e.g., metalloenzyme activity) rather than simply measuring the serum concentration of the nutrient. Unfortunately, few practical methods to assess micronutrient function are available currently, and most assays measure tissue or fluid concentrations of a nutrient.

TRACE MINERALS

The trace minerals essential to humans for which deficiency states have been described include zinc, copper, manganese, selenium, chromium, iodine, fluoride, molybdenum, and iron.[43] Each of these minerals participates in a variety of biologic functions and is necessary for normal metabolism as a coenzyme and/or has a role in hormonal metabolism and erythropoiesis.[44] Other trace minerals essential to humans but for which deficiency states have not been recognized include tin, nickel, vanadium, cobalt, gallium, aluminum, arsenic, boron, bromine, cadmium, germanium, and silicon. Toxicities can occur with excess intake of some trace elements. With the current public focus on alternative and complementary medicine, care should be taken to assess for signs and symptoms of toxicities as well as deficiencies (Table 135–7).

Zinc deficiency is characterized clinically by the development of a moist eczematous dermatitis most apparent in the nasolabial folds and around orifices. Other presenting signs and symptoms of zinc deficiency may include hypogeusia (blunted sense of taste), alopecia, diarrhea, rash (which may vary from papular, scaly lesions to weeping, open erosions), apathy, and depression.[32,43–45] Zinc deficiency occurs most frequently in the setting of abnormal GI losses, such as in Crohn's disease, malabsorptive states, and extensive ostomy or fistula losses, or from prolonged inadequate intake, such as with zinc-free or inadequately zinc supplemented parenteral nutrition (PN). Zinc deficiency can be documented by the presence of low plasma zinc concentrations. However, plasma zinc concentration decreases in acute stress states such as trauma, surgery, or sepsis and will remain depressed until the stress resolves. Also, since zinc is a normal contaminant of most blood collection tubes, special zinc-free collection tubes must be used for plasma assays. Hair zinc analysis by atomic absorption spectroscopy or neutron activation analysis may be a good indicator of zinc status in children.[46] Lymphocyte 5′-nucleotidase activity and leukocyte zinc content are better indicators of zinc status but are not widely available.

Copper deficiency may present as hypochromic, microcytic hematologic changes (e.g., anemia, leukopenia, neutropenia), skeletal demineralization, and hypercholesterolemia[43,47] (see Table 135–7). In severe cases, such as in Menkes' syndrome, copper deficiency is further manifested as hypothermia, hair and skin depigmentation, progressive mental deterioration, and growth retardation. Factors predisposing to copper deficiency include malabsorption states, protein-losing enteropathy, nephrotic syndrome, copper deficient enteral nutrition, and copper-free PN.[42,43,49,50] Excess copper ingested on a chronic basis can result in liver cirrhosis (Wilson's disease). Copper deficiency is assessed most frequently on the basis of plasma copper or ceruloplasmin concentrations.[45] As with zinc, plasma copper concentrations may not accurately reflect total body copper status because it may be altered by a variety of conditions and may even be normal when hepatic stores are deficient (see Table 135–7). Copper function also may be assessed by measuring activity of cuproenzymes (erythrocyte superoxide dismutase activity or cytochrome-C oxidase in platelets or leukocytes). Enzyme activity is decreased significantly in copper deficiency.[45,47] However, measurements of the activity of these enzymes are method- and technique-sensitive and not available routinely.[43]

Chromium is important primarily as a cofactor for insulin. Chromium deficiency is characterized by glucose intolerance and impaired protein use, but patients also may present with increased free fatty acid concentrations and a low respiratory quotient (see Table 135–7). Chromium deficiency has been identified only in patients receiving long-term PN in whom chromium intake was inadequate.[44,45,50] Plasma concentrations do not accurately reflect a person's chromium nutritional status presumably because the biologically active form of chromium is an organic substance known as the *glucose tolerance factor*. Chromium toxicity is not a common clinical concern and has been reported only with contaminated drinking water or industrial exposure.

Manganese is important in the functions of many enzymes, including arginase (urea production), pyruvate carboxylase (glucose synthesis), and superoxide dismutase (antioxidant). Manganese deficiency has been reported only in association with chemically defined manganese-deficient oral diets.[42] The symptoms of manganese deficiency include nausea, vomiting, dermatitis, color changes in hair, hypocholesterolemia, and growth retardation (see Table 135–7). Manganese toxicity is of more concern, however, and has been described in several patients receiving long-term PN.[51–53] Manganese appears to accumulate in brain tissue, especially in the setting of chronic cholestasis and short bowel syndrome. Clinical toxicity is evidenced primarily by extrapyramidal symptoms mimicking Parkinson's disease. Serum manganese concentrations do not correlate well with the clinical presentation, but magnetic resonance imaging (MRI) of the basal ganglia may show hyperintensity areas, especially in the globus pallidus. In most cases, discontinuation of manganese in the

TABLE 135–7. Assessment of Trace Mineral Status

Trace Mineral	Signs of Deficiency	Signs of Toxicity	Clinical Factors that Alter Plasma Concentrations
Chromium	Glucose intolerance, peripheral neuropathy, increased free fatty acid levels, low respiratory quotient, weight loss, increased LDL cholesterol, glucosuria, impaired protein utilization	Industrial exposure: skin/nasal septal lesions, allergic dermatitis, increased incidence of lung cancer	Decreased: long-term inadequate intake
Copper	Neutropenia, leukopenia, hypochromic anemia, osteoporosis, hair and skin depigmentation, dermatitis, anorexia, diarrhea, mental deterioration, hypercholesterolemia	Wilson's disease: liver cirrhosis, diarrhea, vomiting, metallic taste	Decreased: serum ceruloplasmin, corticosteroids, Wilson's disease Increased: infection, rheumatoid arthritis, pregnancy, oral contraceptives
Iodine	Hypothyroid goiter, neuromuscular impairment, deaf-mutism, increased embryonic and postnatal mortality, cognitive impairment, deaf-mutism, impaired fertility, cretinism (severe cases)	Thyrotoxicosis: nodular goiter, weight loss, tachycardia, muscle weakness, warm skin	Decreased: long-term decreased intake
Iron	Microcytic, hypochromic anemia, fatigue, weakness, pallor, glossitis, headache, dysphagia, fingernail changes, gastric atrophy, paresthesias	Liver cirrhosis, cardiomyopathy, pancreatic damage, skin pigmentation	Increased: blood transfusion Decreased: blood loss of any kind
Manganese	Nausea, vomiting, dermatitis, hair color changes, hypocholesterolemia, growth retardation, defective carbohydrate and protein metabolism	Parkinsonian-like symptoms, hyperirritability, hallucinations, libido disturbances, ataxia	Decreased: not known Increased: decreased biliary excretion
Molybdenum	Tachycardia, tachypnea, altered mental status, visual changes, headache, nausea, vomiting	Goutlike syndrome, increased urinary copper	
Selenium	Muscle weakness and pain, cardiomyopathy	Nausea, vomiting, hair and nail loss, tooth decay, skin lesions, irritability, fatigue, peripheral neuropathy	Decreased: malignancy, liver failure, pregnancy Increased: reticuloendothelial neoplasia
Zinc	Dermatitis, hypogeusia, alopecia, diarrhea, apathy, depression, growth retardation, impaired wound healing, immunosuppression	Acute: gastric distress, nausea, dizziness, death with large intravenous doses Chronic: immunosuppression, decreased HDL cholesterol, copper deficiency	Decreased: infection, hypoalbuminemia, corticosteroids, stress, pregnancy, burns, inflammation Increased: tissue injury, hemolysis, contaminated collection tube

PN solution resulted in resolution of neurologic symptoms in 6 months with partial or total normalization of the MRI after 1 to 2 years. Other methods of evaluating manganese status include measuring the manganese content of mononuclear blood cells[54] and the activity of manganese superoxide dismutase, a mitochondrial antioxidant enzyme.[55] While these methods are good indicators of manganese status, they are not widely available.

Selenium, as selenocysteine, is incorporated into glutathione peroxidase, iodothyronine deiodinase, and selenoprotein P, making it an important antioxidant. Prematurity, acute illness, chronic GI losses, and long-term selenium-free PN are associated with low selenium levels and decreased glutathione peroxidase activity.[45,56–58] The clinical significance of reduced selenium levels is unclear. Selenium deficiency has been described in patients receiving long-term selenium-free PN. Muscle pain and weakness are the most frequently observed signs and symptoms (see Table 135–7), but severe biochemical deficiency is not always accompanied by these symptoms.[59] Fatal cardiomyopathy has been reported in several cases. Selenium toxicity may occur when patients receive prolonged therapy at doses exceeding 200 μg/kg per day.[60] Selenium status may be assessed by measuring plasma concentrations, which will reflect recent selenium intake. Decreased concentrations may indicate selenium deficiency, but reductions also have been observed in patients with malignancies, liver failure, and pregnancy. Measurement of the activity of the selenium-containing enzyme glutathione peroxidase in erythrocytes or the plasma concentration of selenoprotein P may be more sensitive measurements of selenium status because they reflect chronic ingestion, but neither is widely available.[59]

Molybdenum is a cofactor for aldehyde, xanthine, and sulfite oxidases.[61] There is only one known case of molybdenum deficiency in a patient receiving long-term home PN who presented with symptoms that included tachycardia, tachypnea, headache, night blindness, nausea, vomiting, central scotomas, lethargy, disorientation, and ultimately coma.[62] Symptoms were reversed when molybdenum was added to the PN solution. Predisposing factors to molybdenum deficiency appear to be low birth weight,[63] excessive loss via the GI tract, such as with short bowel syndrome, and long-term inadequate intake, such as with molybdenum-free PN. Symptoms of molybdenum toxicity can be found in Table 135–7. Urine xanthine can be used to assess molybdenum status but is not readily available.[45]

Deficiency of iodine, a component of thyroid hormones, may result in goiter formation (see Chapter 75). However, not everyone with an iodine-deficient diet will develop a goiter. Thyroxine (T_4) and triiodothyronine (T_3) can be used to assess iodine status[64] (see Table 135–7). Intravenous iodine supplements typically are not necessary except during long-term PN with minimal enteral intake. Iodine needs generally are met by cutaneous absorption of iodine from germicides (e.g., povidone-iodine) used in catheter care or consumption of iodized salt.[65,66] Patients not using povidone-iodine may need iodine supplementation. Iodine excess is rarely a clinical concern when thyroid function is normal.

Iron is an important component of hemoglobin, myoglobin, and cytochrome enzymes. Therefore, it is important in oxygen transport, muscle iron storage, and production of cellular energy. Patients with iron deficiency anemia generally present with fatigue, weakness, and pallor, but they also may have other symptoms[45,67] (see Chapter 99). Inadequate iron intake, malabsorption, and blood loss are the principal causes of iron deficiency anemia. Iron toxicity (overload) including organ damage can occur when chronic intake exceeds requirements. Iron deficiency is confirmed by assessment of body iron stores, as reflected indirectly by measurement of hemoglobin, serum iron, TIBC, and serum ferritin or directly by marrow staining and liver biopsy[67] (see Table 99–2). Although the direct methods are the most accurate, they are invasive, and indirect measurements are used more commonly. Indirect parameters may be altered, however, by chronic illness independent of iron stores; thus concomitant illness must be considered in their interpretation.[32]

VITAMINS

A thorough, nutrition-focused history and PE is the most valuable means of screening patients for findings that suggest vitamin deficiency or toxicity[11,32,68] (Table 135–8). It is uncommon to see a single vitamin deficiency; usually multiple vitamin deficiencies occur with general malnutrition. However, single vitamin deficiencies do occur; thiamine deficiency may result in lactic acidosis and encephalopathy,[69] wherease pernicious anemia due to vitamin B_{12} deficiency also has been reported.

Laboratory assessment may be useful to confirm the clinical suspicion of a deficiency state. The first indication of a deficiency is usually a fall in circulating serum concentrations of the vitamin or its coenzyme. Subsequently, there is a decrease in urinary excretion of the vitamin, which, in turn, is followed by diminished tissue concentrations of the vitamin. The most common measurements of vitamin status are assays of circulating amounts in plasma or serum. Assays of biochemical or metabolic function of the vitamin are more likely to reflect body stores than are serum concentrations. Most of these functional assays use erythrocyte or leukocyte extracts to determine apoenzyme activity, which is dependent on the vitamin coenzyme (see Table 135–8).

ESSENTIAL FATTY ACIDS

The body can synthesize most fatty acids except for linoleic acid (an omega-6 fatty acid) and linolenic acid (an omega-3 fatty acid). Therefore, intake of approximately 2% to 4% of total calories as these fatty acids is essential. EFAD is rare in adults and children but can occur with prolonged use of lipid-free PN, with severe fat malabsorption, with very-low-fat enteral formulas, or with severe PEM, especially in stressed patients.[70] In critically ill adults and older children with increased metabolic demands, EFAD has been reported to occur within 1 week of starting lipid-free PN.[70,71] Newborns, especially those born preterm, have limited fat stores; therefore, they may develop EFAD more rapidly than adults. Biochemical EFAD has been noted within 72 hours after birth in preterm infants receiving fat-free intravenous solutions.[72] Symptoms of EFAD include dermatitis (e.g., dry, cracked, scaly skin), alopecia, impaired wound healing, growth failure, thrombocytopenia, and anemia.

Linoleic acid normally is converted to arachidonic acid (a tetraene fatty acid). If linoleic acid is unavailable, oleic acid will be substituted, which results in production of eicosatrienoic acid (a triene fatty acid) as the metabolic end product. Therefore, EFAD can be detected on the basis of decreased tetraene production and increased triene production. Normally, the ratio of trienes to tetraenes is less than 0.4; when this ratio becomes greater than 0.4, the diagnosis of EFAD is established. Analysis of plasma fatty acids, however, is expensive and not widely available.

CARNITINE

Carnitine, a quaternary amine required for transport of long-chain fatty acids into the mitochondria for β-oxidation and energy production, is available from a wide variety of dietary sources (especially meats) and can be synthesized from lysine and methionine. Synthesis is decreased in premature infants, and low plasma carnitine concentrations and/or overt carnitine deficiency have been documented in premature infants receiving PN or carnitine-free diets in the setting of severe PEM, as well as in those with inborn errors of metabolism.[73–75] Other predisposing factors to carnitine deficiency include chronic kidney or liver disease, vitamin C deficiency, and a vegetarian diet.[75,76] The clinical presentation of carnitine deficiency includes generalized skeletal muscle weakness, fatty liver, and fasting hypoglycemia. Carnitine status can be assessed by measurement of plasma, urine, or red blood cell carnitine concentrations.[76]

MUSCLE FUNCTION TESTS

One of the newest approaches to nutrition assessment is to evaluate muscle function as an end-organ response. Hand-grip strength (forearm muscle dynamometry), respiratory muscle strength, and muscle response to electrical stimulation have been used.[1,77] Hand-grip strength has been shown to correlate with patient outcome.[1] Forearm muscle dynamometry is a relatively simple, noninvasive, and inexpensive procedure. Stimulation of the ulnar nerve causes measurable muscle contraction. In the setting of malnutrition, increased fatigue and a slowed muscle relaxation rate have been noted; these indices return to normal after refeeding. Both these parameters have the advantage of being indicators of tissue function rather than composition. Their utility in clinical practice is currently hampered by a

TABLE 135–8. Assessment of Vitamin Status

Vitamin	Signs of Deficiency	Laboratory Assay	Comments
Water-Soluble Vitamins			
Thiamine (B_1)	Paresthesias, nystagmus, impaired memory, lactic acidosis, congestive heart failure, Wernicke-Korsakoff syndrome	Red blood transketolase activity	
Riboflavin (B_2)	Mucositis, dermatitis, cheilosis, photophobia, corneal vascularization, lacrimation, decreased vision, impaired wound healing, normocytic anemia	Urinary riboflavin	Varies with age, pregnancy, exercise, nitrogen balance
Pantothenic acid (B_3)	Fatigue, malaise, headache, insomnia, vomiting, abdominal cramps	Serum pantothenic acid	
Niacin (B_5)	Pellagra: dermatitis, dementia, glossitis, diarrhea, loss of memory, headaches	Urinary niacin metabolites	Varies with age, gender, blood levels not done
Pyridoxine (B_6)	Dermatitis, neuritis, convulsions, microcytic anemia	Plasma B_6	Varies with age, gender, pregnancy
Folate (B_9)	Megaloblastic anemia, diarrhea, glossitis	Serum folate	Decreased in cases of increased cellular or tissue turnover (pregnancy, malignancy, hemolytic anemia)
Cyanocobalamin (B_{12})	Pernicious anemia, glossitis, spinal cord degeneration, peripheral neuropathy	Serum B_{12}	Decrease in elderly, distal ileal resection, loss of gastric intrinsic factor
Biotin	Dermatitis, depression, lassitude, somnolence	Urinary biotin	
Ascorbic acid	Enlargement and keratosis of hair follicles, impaired wound healing, anemia, lethargy, depression, bleeding ecchymosis	Plasma ascorbic acid	
Fat-Soluble Vitamins			
A	Dermatitis, night blindness, keratomalacia, xerophthalmia	Serum vitamin A	
D	Rickets, osteomalacia, muscle weakness	Plasma 25-hydroxyvitamin D	Decreased in uremia, cirrhosis, elderly, may be decreased in winter
E	Hemolysis	Serum vitamin E	Low blood lipoprotein
K	Bleeding	Prothrombin time	Hepatic disease, anticoagulation

lack of appropriate reference standards and limited data confirming their sensitivity and specificity as nutrition assessment tools.

OTHER NUTRITION ASSESSMENT TOOLS

Various methods to determine body composition have been used in the research setting. These methods generally are complex, require expensive technology, and at present are limited to research centers. One of the most promising for clinical practice is dual-energy x-ray absorptiometry (DEXA). This procedure is now available in many hospitals and clinics for measuring bone density. DEXA can be used to quantify the mineral, fat, and lean tissue compartments. Ultrasound and infrared interactance can be used to measure subcutaneous fat. The latter uses an inexpensive and portable device, but the results of measurements have not been used extensively for nutrition assessment. Magnetic resonance imaging (MRI) and computed tomography (CT) can measure subcutaneous, intraabdominal, and regional fat distribution. Neutron activation is a means of measuring body nitrogen, calcium, sodium, chloride, and phosphorus. These measurements can then be used to calculate total body fat, bone, and protein. Isotope dilution methods determine TBW and underwater weighing determines density. In addition, these methods can be used to estimate LBM and body fat. Furthermore, LBM also can be estimated via total body conductivity (TOBEC) and by measuring the naturally occurring isotope ^{40}K.

ASSESSMENT OF NUTRIENT REQUIREMENTS

Nutrient requirements vary with age, gender, size, disease state, clinical condition, nutrition status, and physical activity level. An assessment of nutrient requirements therefore must be made using guidelines interpreted in the context of these patient-specific factors. As a general reference point, the U.S. Recommended Dietary Allowances (RDAs) should be considered.[78] However, these RDAs were intended initially to prevent nutritional deficiencies in a healthy population of individuals and have been criticized for not accommodating the variability of health conditions in the U.S. population. Currently, the Dietary Reference Intakes (DRIs) are being developed by the National Academy of Sciences to address these concerns. The full set of DRIs will be released by the end of 2001 at a total cost of $5.4 million.[79] The four categories of the new DRIs are Estimated Average Requirements

(EARs), Recommended Dietary Allowances (RDAs), Adequate Intakes (AIs), and Tolerable Upper Intake Level (UL). EARs can be used for planning recommended nutrient intake for groups because they are defined as the amount of the nutrient that meets the needs of 50% of persons in a given group. The RDA is designated as nutrient intake that meets the needs of almost all persons in the designated group. The RDA is approximately 2 standard deviations above the EAR for nutrients where the requirement is well defined and 1.2 times the EAR for nutrients where there is more variability. AI is defined as the average intake by a designated group that appears to sustain a particular nutritional state, growth, or other functional indication of health. This category is reserved for nutrients for which no EAR or RDA has been determined. Finally the UL is the maximum intake of a nutrient that is unlikely to pose adverse affects in almost all persons in a designated group. DRIs have been established for seven nutrient groups: (1) calcium, phosphorus, magnesium, vitamin D, and fluoride, (2) folate and other B vitamins, (3) antioxidants (e.g., selenium, vitamins C and E), (4) trace elements, (5) macronutrients (e.g., protein, fat), (6) electrolytes and water, and (7) other food components (e.g., fiber, phytoestrogens). Reports from four of the seven working groups have been published.[80–83]

ENERGY REQUIREMENTS

There are numerous methods for determining an individual's energy or calorie (kcal) requirement. The most commonly used methods to determine energy requirements are calories per body weight (kcal/kg), equations that estimate energy expenditure, or indirect calorimetry.

The simplest method to assess energy requirements is to use population estimates of calories per body weight. This method assumes standard values for the energy requirements associated with various disease states or clinical conditions as well as the additional requirements for repletion of a malnourished individual. It does not take into consideration age- or gender-related differences in energy metabolism. Adult requirements determined by this method, using ABW or adjusted body weight in kilograms, generally are accepted to be:

Healthy, normal nutrition status	≈ 25 kcal/kg
Malnourished or mildly metabolically stressed	≈ 30 kcal/kg
Critically ill, hypermetabolic	≈ 30–35 kcal/kg
Major burn injury	≥ 40 kcal/kg

Suggested caloric intakes for maintenance and normal growth of healthy infants and children (RDAs) are shown in Table 135–9.[78] These maintenance energy requirements are approximately 150% of basal metabolic rate (BMR). Caloric requirements increase with fever, sepsis, major surgery, trauma, burns, and long-term growth failure and in the presence of chronic conditions such as bronchopulmonary dysplasia and congenital heart disease. Caloric needs may decrease with obesity and neurologic disability (e.g., cerebral palsy). Clinical judgment and close monitoring are essential to ensure that the desired nutrition therapy outcomes are attained.

TABLE 135–9. Suggested Daily Caloric and Protein Intake for Healthy Children: Recommended Dietary Allowances[78]

Age (years)	Total Calories (per kg/d)	Protein (g/kg/d)
0–0.5	108	2.2
0.5–1.0	98	1.6
1–3	102	1.2
4–6	90	1.1
7–10	70	1.0
Boys		
11–14	55	0.9
15–18	45	0.8
Girls		
11–14	47	1.0
15–18	40	0.8

EXAMPLES OF CALORIE CALCULATIONS USING PER-KILOGRAM METHOD

Male: Age: 31 years; weight: 130 lb (59.1 kg); height: 5 ft 6 in (167.6 cm); burns over 70% of body:

$$\text{kcal/d required} = 40\ \text{kcal/kg} \times 59.1\ \text{kg} = 2364$$

Child: Age: 2 years; weight: 20 lb (9.1 kg); weight is 50th percentile for height on NCHS chart:

$$\text{kcal/day required} = 102\ \text{kcal/kg/d (RDA)} \times 9.1\ \text{kg} = 928$$

Various equations can be used to estimate energy needs[84–88] (Table 135–10). The Harris-Benedict equations (HBEs) are the most popular means to assess energy requirements. They have the advantage of taking into consideration the age, height, weight, gender, and clinical condition of the patient. The HBEs were derived from oxygen consumption measurements made on normally nourished individuals who were in a fasting and resting state. While these equations are commonly referred to as the basal energy expenditure (BEE) equations, they actually estimate resting energy expenditure (REE). This is the amount of energy expended by an awake individual to perform only basal functions such as breathing, circulating blood, and fasting metabolic processes. The original HBE along with modifications for adults over age 60 years are shown in Table 135–10. Since these equations approximate REE, their results must be modified by a factor that is most representative of the individual's clinical condition. For

TABLE 135–10. Equations to Estimate Basal Energy Expenditure in Adults and Children

Harris-Benedict[84] (kcal/d)
Males: BEE = 66 + [13.7W(kg)] + [5H(cm)] – (6.8A)
Females: BEE = 655 + [9.6W(kg)] + [1.8H(cm)] – (4.7A)

Modified Harris-Benedict[85] (kcal/d)
Males: BEE = [8.8W(kg)] + [1128H(m)] – 1071
Females: BEE = [9.2W(kg)] + [637H(m)] – 302

Caldwell-Kennedy[86] (kcal/d)
Infants (<3 years of age): BEE = 22 + (31W) + [1.2H(cm)]

Schofield[87] (MJ/d) (to convert to kcal/d multiply by 239.2)
3–10 years of age
Males: BMR = (0.08W) + [0.55H(m)] + 1.74
Females: BMR = (0.07W) + [0.68H(m)] + 1.55
10–18 years of age
Males: BMR = (0.07W) + [0.57H(m)] + 2.16
Females: BMR = (0.04W) + [1.95H(m)] + 0.84

FAO/WHO/UNU[88] (kcal/d)
3–10 years of age
Males: BMR = 22.7W + 495
Females: BMR = 22.5W + 499
10–18 years of age
Males: BMR = 17.5W + 651
Females: BMR = 12.2W + 746

Key: W = weight in kilograms; H = height in centimeters (cm) or meters (m), as indicated; A = age in years; BEE = basal energy expenditure; BMR = basal metabolic rate; FAO/WHO/UNU = Food and Agriculture Organization/World Health Organization/United Nations University.

TABLE 135–11. Stress Factors for Use in Children and Adults

Condition	Factor
No Stress	
Confined to bed	1.2
Out of bed—normal activity	1.3
Mild Stress	
Postoperative recovery, uncomplicated surgery	1.0
Trauma, mild (e.g., long bone fracture)	1.2
Moderate Stress	
Sepsis (moderate)	1.3
Trauma, central nervous system (sedated)	1.3
Trauma, moderate to severe	1.5
Severe Stress	
Sepsis (severe)	1.6
Trauma, central nervous system (severe)	Up to 2.0
Burns (proportionate to burned area)	Up to 2.0

example, an individual who is confined to bed may require a calorie intake that is 20% above the REE, whereas a person who is suffering from a severe burn injury may require a 150% to 200% increase over the calculated REE. The response to stress in children is similar to that seen in critically ill adults,[89] and the "stress factors" used in adults can be used in children[90,91] (Table 135–11).

EXAMPLES OF CALORIE CALCULATIONS USING ENERGY EXPENDITURE EQUATIONS

Male: Age: 31 years; weight: 130 lb (59.1 kg); height: 5 ft 6 in (167.6 cm); burns over 70% of body:

$$\text{REE using HBE (kcal/day)} = 66 + (13.7 \times 59.1) + (5 \times 167.6) - (6.8 \times 31) = 1503$$

$$\begin{aligned}\text{Calorie needs per day} &= \text{REE} \times \text{stress factor}\\ &= 1500 \times (1.5 - 2)\\ &= 2250 - 3000\end{aligned}$$

Controversy exists over the accuracy and reliability of predicting energy expenditure based on these equations because clinical judgments will vary with each clinician.[92–94] Additionally, in validation studies in healthy subjects, these equations have been shown to overestimate REE by 5% to 15%.[94] It is also important to note that ABW (up to a BMI of 57 kg/m^2 in men and 40 kg/m^2 in women) not lean body weight was used to generate the original data with these equations.[94]

The most accurate clinical tool for determining energy requirements is to measure them using indirect calorimetry, also referred to as metabolic gas monitoring.[95] Indirect calorimetry is based on the fact that when substrates (carbohydrates, fat, protein) are oxidized, oxygen (O_2) is consumed and carbon dioxide (CO_2) is produced. O_2 consumption and CO_2 production vary depending on the substrate being oxidized. Indirect calorimetry is a noninvasive procedure in which oxygen consumption (VO_2, mL/min) and carbon dioxide production (VCO_2, mL/min) are measured. Using the abbreviated Weir equation, REE (kcal/day) can be calculated: REE = $(3.9VO_2 + 1.1VCO_2) \times 1.44$.[95]

The measured energy expenditure represents the actual energy expended by the patient during the time period when the measurement was taken. It is often extrapolated to a 24-hour period to approximate daily energy requirements. Measurement of REE reflects alterations in energy requirements due to disease or clinical condition but does not include energy required for nutritional repletion of a malnourished individual or growth in a child. The energy intake required for these functions can be calculated as follows depending on nutrition goals: maintenance, 1.0 to 1.3 × REE; repletion, 1.3 to 1.5 × REE; and depletion, less than 1.0 × REE.

The data obtained from indirect calorimetry also can be used to determine a respiratory quotient (RQ). The RQ reflects substrate oxidation, which characterizes substrate use, and is calculated as follows: RQ = VCO_2/VO_2. RQ values for nutrient substrates are: fat, 0.7; carbohydrate, 1.0; protein, 0.80; and mixed substrate (fat, carbohydrate, and protein), 0.85. An RQ value of greater than 1.0 represents either lipogenesis or hyperventilation; an RQ value of less than 0.7 may indicate a ketogenic diet, fat gluconeogenesis, or ethanol oxidation. Values outside the 0.67 to 1.3 range should raise doubts as to the test's validity. Clinically, the RQ is used to determine if a patient is being overfed, which is indicated by an RQ value greater than 1.0.

EXAMPLE OF INDIRECT CALORIMETRY INTERPRETATION

Male: Age: 31 years; weight: 130 lb (59.1 kg); IBW: 63.8 kg; ABW: 93% IBW; height: 5 ft 6 in (167.6 cm); burns over 70% of body:

Indirect calorimetry results:

$$\text{REE} = 2250 \text{ kcal/day} \qquad \text{RQ} = 0.85$$

Interpretation: Since repletion is not necessary, calorie requirements are 1.0 to 1.3 × REE which yields an estimated intake of 2250 to 2925 kcal/d. Intake should be increased to meet this goal. RQ shows oxidation of a mixed fuel source, which is desirable. No changes needed in substrate ratios.

There are limitations to the use of indirect calorimetry.[94,95] Not all institutions have metabolic carts available or personnel trained to use them. Calibration errors are common, and this process overestimates REE for patients with hyperventilation, metabolic acidosis, overfeeding, and air leaks in the system. Underestimates of REE are likely with hypoventilation, metabolic alkalosis, underfeeding, and gluconeogenesis. While mechanically ventilated patients may be technically easier to study (i.e., the indirect calorimeter circuit can be plugged into the ventilator circuit), to get a steady-state reading, the patient must be at complete rest for 1 hour, must not receive bolus feedings either by tube or orally for 4 hours, should have no changes in substrate delivery for 12 hours, must be on an FiO_2 of less than 0.6, and the positive end-expiratory pressure (PEEP) must be less than 5 cm H_2O. Unfortunately, many of the patients in whom indirect calorimetry would be desirable will not meet these requirements.

PROTEIN

Daily protein requirements are based on age, nutrition status, disease state, and clinical condition. The RDA for protein for children is shown in Table 135–9 and for individuals over 18 years of age is 0.8 g/kg per day.[78] In adults older than 60 years of age, protein needs are increased to 1 g/kg per day to help reduce the LBM loss that occurs with aging, and up to 1.5–2.0 g/kg per day may be needed in states of metabolic stress such as infection, trauma, and surgery to prevent LBM loss.[78,96] In general, protein intake should be approximately 12% to 14% of total calories in the normal diet.

Protein metabolism depends on both kidney and liver function. Therefore, protein requirements will be altered with decreased kidney or liver function (see Chapter 139). Critical illness (e.g., sepsis, burns, trauma) will result in a hypercatabolic state in which there is increased protein synthesis and degradation. Consequently, protein requirements will be increased to 1.5–2.0 g/kg per day. In burn patients, protein requirements may be as high as 3.0 g/kg per day. Liver failure typically results in the need for protein restriction (0.5 g/kg/day) except if a hypercatabolic state is also present, in which case the requirement may be increased to 1.5 g/kg per day. Protein needs in renal failure are variable and affected by renal replacement therapies. The application of these guidelines requires both clinical judgment and frequent monitoring of renal and liver function, serum chemistries, clinical condition, and nutrition outcomes (see Chapter 139).

Nitrogen is found only in protein and at a relatively constant ratio of 1 g nitrogen per 6.25 g protein. This ratio may vary somewhat for commercial enteral and parenteral formulations depending on the biologic value of the protein source. Adequacy of protein intake can be assessed clinically by measuring urinary nitrogen excretion and comparing it with nitrogen intake—a nitrogen balance study. Nitrogen balance indirectly reflects an individual's protein use or protein catabolic rate (PCR), which increases in states associated with hypercatabolism.[97] As the stress level increases, the concomitant increase in protein catabolism results in an increase in urinary nitrogen excretion.[98] Usually, the amount of urea nitrogen is measured in a 24-hour urine collection (24-h UUN). The quantity of UUN accounts for 80% to 90% of the total urinary nitrogen (TUN) excreted. Therefore, total nitrogen output (TNO) can be approximated as TNO (g/day) = UUN + 4, where the factor 4 represents estimated skin, fecal, and respiratory nitrogen losses.[99] Alternatively, if available, TUN can be measured and may be more accurate, but it is more expensive.[99] If TUN is used, then the best estimate of TNO is TUN × 1.05.[99] In the setting of renal failure, where neither measured UUN nor TUN represents nitrogen generation, protein turnover can be approximated by using equations based on urea kinetics to estimate the rate of urea production.[100]

EXAMPLE OF NITROGEN BALANCE CALCULATION

Patient is receiving 75 g protein per day (1 g/kg/day); results from 24-h urine urea nitrogen: 10 g nitrogen per day:

$$\text{Nitrogen balance} = (75\text{ g protein}/6.25\text{ g nitrogen per gram of protein}) - (10 + 4) = -2\text{ g/day}$$

Interpretation: Patient is in negative nitrogen balance; more protein and/or more calories may be needed to meet current needs.

FLUID

The daily fluid requirement for adults depends on many factors and is approximately 30–35 mL/kg. It also can be estimated as 1 mL/kcal or as 1500 mL/m^2/24 h. Fluid requirements per kilogram are higher for children and even higher for preterm infants due to their higher percentage of TBW and basal energy expenditure (BEE). Additionally, premature neonates have increased fluid requirements due to greater insensible losses and the kidney's inefficiency in concentrating urine. The Holliday-Segar method is a commonly employed, quick, and simple method for estimating minimum daily fluid needs of children that also can be applied to adults. Children who weigh less than 10 kg should receive at least 100 mL/kg per day. An additional 50 mL/kg per day should be provided for each kilogram body weight between 11 and 20 kg and 20 mL/kg per day for each kilogram above 20 kg. Thus maintenance fluid needs for a child weighing 8 kg would be 800 mL/d, whereas 1350 ml/d would be the projected need for a 17-kg child.

Factors that alter fluid needs for both adults and children are shown in Table 135–12. When determining daily fluid intake for an individual, all sources of fluid intake must be taken into consideration (e.g., fluid vehicles for intravenous medications, intravenous or feeding tube flushes). Fluid status is assessed by monitoring urine output and specific gravity, serum electrolytes, and weight changes. A urine output of at least 1.0 mL/kg per hour (in children) or approximately 50 mL/h (in adults) is considered adequate to ensure tissue perfusion. Urine output should be higher if large fluid volumes or high renal solute loads are being administered. Urine specific gravity depends on the kidney's concentrating and diluting capabilities. Concomitant diuretic therapy due to increased solute excretion will limit the usefulness of urine specific gravity as an index of fluid status.

TABLE 135–12. Factors that Alter Fluid Requirements

Increased Requirements	Decreased Requirements
Fever	Fluid overload
Radiant warmers	Cardiac failure
Diuretics	Decreased urinary output
Vomiting	Heat shields
Nasogastric suction	Relatively high humidity
Ostomy/fistula drainage	Humidified air via endotracheal tube
Diarrhea	Renal failure
Glycosuria	Hypoproteinemia with starvation
Phototherapy	
Increased Ambient Temperature	
Hyperventilation	
Prematurity	
Excessive sweating	
Increase metabolism	

MICRONUTRIENTS

Requirements for micronutrients (e.g., electrolytes, trace minerals, and vitamins) vary with the route by which the nutrient is ingested[78–83,101–103] (Table 135–13). The variability between oral and parenteral requirements is due to the nutrient's bioavailability. Micronutrients poorly absorbed via the GI tract usually will be required in greater doses enterally than parenterally. However, many water-soluble micronutrients are excreted more rapidly via the kidneys when administered intravenously. In these situations, the intravenous dose will be greater than the oral dose. Other factors that affect micronutrient requirements include GI losses via diarrhea, vomiting, or high-output fistula; wound healing; and hypermetabolism/catabolism. Cutaneous micronutrient losses (e.g., zinc, copper, and selenium) also may be significant after major burn injury.[104,105] Sodium, potassium, magnesium, and phosphorus are particularly dependent on renal function, and in the setting of renal failure, intake may need to be restricted. Calcium needs, on the other hand, may be increased in these patients. Patients who are severely malnourished will have increased electrolyte requirements during early refeeding owing to preexisting deficiencies and/or rapid intracellular uptake with anabolism.[106] Failure to provide adequate electrolytes during refeeding has resulted in death from the refeeding syndrome.[107]

DRUG-NUTRIENT INTERACTIONS

Drug nutrient interactions can be clinically significant and include drug-induced nutrient deficiencies, poor therapeutic response to a drug, enhanced drug toxicity, and interference with nutrition regimens if nutrition support is discontinued or withheld due to adverse

TABLE 135–13. Recommended Daily Maintenance Intakes for Electrolytes, Trace Minerals, and Vitamins

	ADULT		PEDIATRIC	
Nutrient	*Enteral*[78–83]	*Parenteral*[101]	*Enteral*[78–83, 102]	*Parenteral*[103]
Electrolytes/Minerals				
Acetate[a]	—	—	—	—
Calcium	1000–1200 mg	0–15 mEq	0–12 mo: 210–270 mg 1–3 yr: 500 mg 4–8 yr: 800 mg 9–18 yr: 1300 mg	Premature: 2–4 mEq/kg/day Other: 2–3 mEq/kg/day
Chloride[a]	—	—	—	2–6 mEq/kg/day
Fluoride	1.5–4 mg	—	0–6 mo: 0.01 mg 6–12 mo: 0.5 mg 1–8 yr: 0.7–1 mg 9–18 yr: 2–3 mg	—
Magnesium	M: 400–420 mg F: 210–320 mg	10–20 mEq	0–6 mo: 30 mg 6–12 mo: 75 mg 1–3 yr: 80 mg 4–8 yr: 130 mg 9–13 yr: 240 mg 14–18 yr: 360–410 mg	0.25–1 mEq/kg/day
Phosphorus	700 mg	20–45 mmol	0–6 mo: 100 mg 6–12 mo: 275 mg 1–8 yr: 460–500 mg 9–18 yr: 1250 mg	Premature: 1.5–2 mmol/kg/day Others: 1–2 mmol/kg/day
Potassium[b,c]	1875–5625 mg	60–100 mEq	2–5 mEq/kg/day	2–5 mEq/kg/day
Sodium[b,c]	1100–3300 mg	60–100 mEq	2–6 mEq/kg/day	2–6 mEq/kg/day
Trace Minerals				
Chromium[d]	50–200 mcg	10–15 mcg	Infants: 10–40 mcg Other: 20–200 mcg	0.14–0.2 mcg/kg/day (max 5 mcg)
Copper[e]	1.5–3 mg	0.5–1.5 mg	Infants: 0.5–1 mg Other: 1–5 mg	20 mcg/kg/day; max 300 mcg/day
Iodine[f]	150 mcg	70–140 mcg	0–12 mo: 40–50 mcg 1–6 yr: 70–90 mcg 7–18 yr: 120–150 mcg	1 mcg/kg/day
Iron	10–15 mg	Varies	0–6 mo: 6 mg 6 mo–10 yr: 10 mg 11–18 yr: 12–15 mg	Not established
Manganese[e]	2–5 mg	0.15–0.8 mg	Infants: 0.01–0.06 mg Other: 1–5 mg	1 mcg/kg/day (max 50 mcg)
Molybdenum	75–250 mcg	100–200 mcg	Infants: 30–80 mcg Other: 50–300 mcg	0.25 mcg/kg/day (max 5 mcg)
Selenium	55 mcg	40–80 mcg	0–12 mo: 15–20 mcg 1–8 yr: 20–30 mcg 9–18 yr: 40–55 mcg	1.5–3 mcg/kg/day (max
Zinc[g]	12–15 mg	2.5–4 mg	0–12 mo: 5 mg 1–10 yr: 10 mg 11–18 yr: 12–15 mg	Premature: 300–400 mcg/kg/day Other: 50–250 mcg/kg/day
Vitamins				
Ascorbic acid	75–90 mg	100 mg	0–12 mo: 40–50 mg 1–8 yr: 15–25 mg 9–18 yr: 40–55 mg	80 mg
Biotin	30 mcg	60 mcg	0–12 mo: 5–6 mcg 1–8 yr: 8–12 mcg 9–12 yr: 20–25 mcg	20 mcg
Cyanocobalamin (B_{12})	2.4 mcg	5 mcg	0–12 mo: 0.4–0.5 mcg 1–8 yr: 0.9–1.2 mcg 9–12 yr: 1.8–2.4 mcg	1 mcg
Folic acid	400 mcg	400 mcg	0–12 mo: 65–80 mcg 1–3 yr: 150 mcg 4–8 yr: 200 mcg	140 mcg

TABLE 135–13. (*Continued*)

	ADULT		PEDIATRIC	
Nutrient	*Enteral*[78–83]	*Parenteral*[101]	*Enteral*[78–83, 102]	*Parenteral*[103]
Niacin	M: 16 mg NE F: 14	40 mg NE	0–12 mo: 2–4 mg NE 1–3 yr: 6–8 mg NE 4–8 yr: 12 mg NE 9–18 yr: 14–16 mg NE	17 mg NE
Pantothenic acid	5 mg	15 mg	0–12 mo: 1.7–1.8 mg 1–8 yr: 2–3 mg 9–18 yr: 4–5 mg	5 mg
Pyridoxine (B_6)	1.3–1.7 mg	4 mg	0–12 mo: 0.1–0.3 mg 1–8 yr: 0.9–1.2 mg 9–18 yr: 1–1.3 mg	1 mg
Riboflavin	1.1–1.3 mg	3.6 mg	0–12 mo: 0.3–0.4 mg 1–8 yr: 0.5–0.6 mg 9–18 yr: 0.9–1.3 mg	1.4 mg
Thiamine	1.1–1.2 mg	3 mg	0–12 mo: 0.2–0.3 mg 1–8 yr: 0.7–1 mg 9–18 yr: 2–3 mg	1.2 mg
Vitamin A	800–1000 mcg RE	600 mcg RE 3300 IU	0–12 mo: 375 mcg RE 1–10 yr: 400–700 11–18 yr: 800–1000	700 mcg RE 2300 IU
Vitamin D	5–15 mcg (200–600 IU)	5 mcg (200 IU)	5 mcg (200 IU)	5 mcg (200 IU)
Vitamin E	15 mg TE	10 IU	0–12 mo: 4–6 mg TE 1–3 yr: 6 mg TE 4–8 yr: 7 mg TE 9–18 yr: 11–15 mg TE	7 IU
Vitamin K	60–80 mcg	0.7–2.5 mg	0–6 mo: 5 mcg 6–12 mo: 10 mcg 1–6 yr: 15–20 mcg 7–18 yr: 45–65 mcg	200 mcg

[a]As needed to maintain acid base balance.
[b]Newborns and low-birth-weight or very-low-birth-weight infants or with concomitant disease (e.g., necrotizing enterocolitis) may have higher requirements. Intake in nonhealthy children must be individualized.
[c]No RDA has been established.
[d]An additional 20 μg chromium per day is recommended in patients with intestinal losses.
[e]May accumulate in cholestasis.
[f]Long-term PN only; if no topicals containing iodide or table salt are used.
[g]An additional 12.2 mg zinc per liter of small bowel fluid lost and 17.1 mg zinc per kilogram of stool or ileostomy output is recommended; an additional 2 mg zinc per day for acute catabolic stress.
Abbreviations: NE = niacin equivalents; PN = parenteral nutrition; RE = retinal equivalents; TE = tocopherol equivalent.

effects.[108–112] Patient outcomes may be enhanced if a program for counseling and a method for screening medication profiles for significant drug-nutrient interactions is established.[9] As part of the screening process, it is important to recognize the risk factors that influence drug-nutrient interactions. The potential for drug-nutrient interactions is greater in pediatric and elderly individuals, those with poor nutrition status (obesity and marasmus), and those with chronic and/or multiple drug therapies.

Mineral and electrolyte serum concentrations may change due to drug therapy. For example, urine sodium, potassium, and magnesium wasting may occur, causing a reduction in the respective serum concentrations (see Chapters 51 and 52). Serum electrolyte concentrations also may increase as a direct result of the mechanism of the drug (e.g., potassium-sparing diuretics) or due to the drug's salt form. Corticosteroids and cyclosporine are known to cause hyperglycemia, whereas other drugs are prescribed to pharmacologically lower blood glucose concentrations (e.g., insulin and oral hypoglycemics; see Chapter 74).

Vitamin status also may be affected by drug therapies (Table 135–14). For example, sulfasalazine therapy has been noted to cause a decrease in folic acid, isoniazid therapy causes pyridoxine deficiency, and furosemide therapy may result in decreased concentrations of thiamin. Furthermore, some drug therapy outcomes may be affected by vitamins. Large doses of folic acid will decrease the therapeutic effect of methotrexate, whereas changes in an individual's usual vitamin K intake have the potential to cause variability in the anticoagulation effects of warfarin.

Drug delivery systems also may contain nutrients. Most intravenous therapies (maintenance intravenous fluids, drugs, electrolyte replacements) are delivered using either dextrose (e.g., dextrose 5% in water, D_5W) or sodium (e.g, 0.9% NaCl, normal saline) in the admixture. There are also drug delivery systems that use 10% lipid emulsion formulations (e.g., propofol) that may provide a large amount of calories to an individual. In these instances, nutrition support regimens must be varied to accommodate the increase in calories from other sources.

TABLE 135–14. Drug Effects on Vitamin Status

Drug	Possible Vitamin Effect
Antacids	Thiamine deficiency
Antibiotics	Vitamin K deficiency
Anticonvulsants	Vitamin D and folic acid impaired absorption
Antineoplastics	Folic acid antagonism and malabsorption
Antipsychotics	Decreased riboflavin
Cathartics	Increased requirements for vitamins D, C, and B_6
Cholestyramine	Vitamins A, D, E, and K, β-carotene malabsorption
Colestipol	Vitamins A, D, E, and K, β-carotene malabsorption
Corticosteroids	Decreased vitamins A and C
Diuretics (loop)	Thiamin deficiency
Histamine2-antagonists	Vitamin B_{12} deficiency
Isoniazid	Vitamin B_6 deficiency
Mineral oil	Vitamins A, D, E, and K malabsorption
Orlistat	Vitamins A, D, E, and K malabsorption
Pentamidine	Folic acid deficiency
Proton pump inhibitors	Vitamin B_{12} deficiency

PRACTICAL GUIDELINES FOR NUTRITION ASSESSMENT

The value of any given marker or group of markers used for nutrition assessment is only as great as its ability to accurately identify the patient with malnutrition and to correlate with malnutrition-associated complications. Most of the currently available markers of nutrition status were first used in epidemiologic studies to define large populations suffering from malnutrition caused by famine. The response of the various markers of nutrition status to nutrition therapy and the correlation between improvement in these markers and decreased morbidity and mortality further support their validity. However, when applied to an individual, most of these markers lack specificity and sensitivity, which makes the development of a clinically useful, cost-effective approach to individual patient nutrition assessment challenging.

The importance of the nutrition-focused history and PE in both nutrition screening and nutrition assessment cannot be overemphasized. The least amount of objective data that can further substantiate the clinical impression and provide a baseline for subsequent monitoring are those markers which show the best correlation with outcome: weight and serum albumin concentration. The cost-effectiveness of the addition of further biochemical parameters is yet to be determined. The assessment of other anthropometric measures probably is most useful in the setting of anticipated long-term nutrition support in which these measurements will serve as a longitudinal marker of an individual's response to the nutrition care plan.

Initially, nutrition requirements are determined on the basis of assumptions made about the patient's clinical condition and the nutrition needs associated with repletion or growth, if needed. Once a nutrition intervention has been initiated, periodic reassessment of nutrition status will determine the accuracy of the initial estimate of nutrition requirements. Also, nutrition requirements may be dynamic in the setting of acute or critical illness—as the patient's clinical status changes, so may protein and energy requirements. This further emphasizes the need for continued reassessment.

Better markers of nutrition status and methods for determining patient-specific nutrition requirements are needed. Functional tests and simple, noninvasive tests for body composition analysis hold promise for the future. However, until better methods of assessment become available clinically and are demonstrated to be cost-effective, the currently available battery of tests will continue to be the mainstay of nutrition assessment.

▶ PRINCIPLES OF NUTRITION ASSESSMENT

- Nutrition screening programs in institutions should identify those at risk for poor nutrition-related outcomes.
- Nutrition assessment is the first step in formulating a patient-specific nutrition care plan.
- A nutrition-focused medical history will reveal the likelihood of malnutrition and nutrient deficiencies.
- A nutrition-focused PE will help to identify the severity of malnutrition and the potential existence of nutrient deficiencies.
- Biochemical and anthropometric parameters should be chosen based on findings in the history and PE to support the nutrition assessment and should be practical and cost-effective.
- Anthropometric parameters should be assessed based on published standards.
- Laboratory tests used for nutrition assessment must be interpreted in the context of the physical findings and medical history as well as the limitations of each test.
- When determining patient-specific nutrition requirements, goals should be established based on the level of stress and the need for maintenance or repletion in adults as well as for continued growth and development in children.
- Determination of nutrition requirements requires consideration of patient- and disease-specific factors known to affect nutrition status.
- The practitioner must recognize that an initial nutrition assessment and determination of nutrition requirements defines an empirical starting point for a nutrition care plan.
- Close monitoring is required so that timely adjustments to the nutrition care plan may be made based on patient-specific responses to ensure appropriate nutrition-related outcomes.

REFERENCES

1. Klein S, Kinney J, Jeejeebhoy K, et al. Nutrition support in clinical practice: Review of published data and recommendations for future research directions. J Parenter Enter Nutr 1997;21:133–156.
2. Kotler DP. Cachexia. Ann Intern Med 2000;133:622–634.
3. Flegal KM, Carroll MD, Kuczmarski RJ, Johnson CL. Overweight and obesity in the United States: Prevalence and trends, 1960–1994. Int J Obes Relat Metab Disord 1998;22:39–47.
4. American Academy of Family Physicians, American Dietetic Association, and National Council on the Aging, Inc. Nutrition Interventions Manual for Professionals Caring for Older Americans. Washington, Nutrition Screening Initiative, 1992. *http://www.aafp.org/nsi/*.
5. Council on Practice, Quality Management Committee. Identifying patients at risk: ADA's definitions for nutrition screening and nutrition assessment. J Am Diet Assoc 1994;94:838–839.
6. Kovacevich DS, Boney AR, Braunschweig CL, et al. Nutrition risk classification: a reproducible and valid tool for nurses. Nutr Clin Pract 1997;12:20–25.
7. Centers for Disease Control and Prevention, National Center for Health Statistics. CDC growth charts: United States, 2000. *http://www.cdc.gov/growthcharts/*.

8. A.S.P.E.N. Board of Directors. Definition of terms used in A.S.P.E.N. guidelines and standards. Nutr Clin Pract 1995;10:1–3.
9. Joint Commission on Accreditation of Healthcare Organizations. 2000 Hospital Accreditation Standards. Oakbrook Terrace, IL, Joint Commission Resources, 2000.
10. McClave SA, Mitoraj TE, Thielmeier KA, Greenburg RA. Differentiating subtypes (hypoalbuminemic versus marasmic) of protein-calorie malnutrition: incidence and clinical significance in a university hospital setting. J Parenter Enter Nutr 1992;16:337–342.
11. Shopbell JM, Hopkins B, Shronts EP. Nutrition screening and assessment. In: Gottschlich MM, ed. The Science and Practice of Nutrition Support: A Case-Based Core Curriculum, America Society for Parenteral and Enteral Nutrition. Dubuque, IO, Kendall/Hunt, 2001:107–140.
12. Taketomo CK, Hodding JH, Kraus DM. Pediatric Dosage Handbook, 7th ed. Cleveland, Lexi-Comp, 2000:1091.
13. Shaffer SG, Quimoro CL, Anderson JV, Hall RT. Postnatal weight changes in low birth weight infants. Pediatrics 1987;79:702–705.
14. Lair CS, Kennedy KA. Monitoring postnatal growth in the neonatal intensive care unit. Nutr Clin Prac 1997;12:124–129.
15. Cronk C, Crocker AC, Pueschel SM, et al. Growth charts for children with Down syndrome: 1 month to 18 years of age. Pediatrics 1988;81:102–110.
16. Reimers KJ, Carlson SJ, Lombard KA. Nutritional management of infants with bronchopulmonary dysplasia. Nutr Clin Pract 1992;7:127–132.
17. Klish WJ. Nutritional assessment. In: Wyllie R, Hyams JS, eds. Pediatric Gastrointestinal Disease: Pathophysiology, Diagnosis, Management. Philadelphia, Saunders, 1993:1090–1109.
18. Crouch JB. Anthropometric assessment. In: Groh-Wargo S, Thompson M, Cox JH, eds. Nutritional Care for High-Risk Newborns, rev. ed. Chicago, Precept Press, 1994:9–14.
19. Dickey RA, Baluska DG, Bray GW, et al. AACE/ACE Position Statement on the Prevention, Diagnosis, and Treatment of Obesity, 1998 revision. *http://www.aace.com/clinguideindex.htm.*
20. Meisler JG, St. Jeor. Summary and recommendations from the American Health Foundation's expert panel on healthy weight. Am J Clin Nutr 1996;63:474S–477S.
21. Himes JH, Dietz WH. Guidelines for overweight in adolescent preventive services: Recommendations from an expert committee. Am J Clin Nutr 1994;59:307–316.
22. Chumlea WC, Guo S. Bioelectrical impedance and body composition: Present status and future directions. Nutr Rev 1994;52:123–131.
23. Kyle UG, Pichard C. Dynamic assessment of fat free mass during catabolism and recovery. Curr Opin Clin Nutr Metab Care 2000;3:317–322.
24. Elia M, Ward LC. New techniques in nutritional assessment: Body composition methods. Proc Nutr Soc 1999;58:33–38.
25. Pichard C, Kyle UG, Janssens JP, et al. Body composition by x-ray absorptiometry and bio-electrical impedance in chronic respiratory insufficiency patients. Nutrition 1997;13:952–958.
26. Roubenoff R, Baumgartner RN, Harris TB, et al. Application of bioelectrical impedance analysis to elderly population. J Gerontol 1997;52A:M129–M136.
27. Kyle UG, Genton L, Mentha G, et al. Reliable bioelectrical impedance analysis estimate of fat-free mass in liver, lung, and heart transplant patients. J Parenter Enter Nutr 2001;25:45–51.
28. Shronts EP, Fish JA, Hammond KP. Nutrition assessment. In: Merritt RJ, Souba WW, eds. The A.S.P.E.N. Nutrition Support Practice Manual. Silver Spring, MD, American Society for Parenteral and Enteral Nutrition, 1998:1–17.
29. Rosenfalck AM, Snorgaard O, Almdal T. Creatinine height index and lean body mass in adult patients with insulin-dependent diabetes mellitus followed for 7 years from onset. J Parenter Enter Nutr 1994; 18:50–54.
30. Van Hoeyweghen RJ, De Leeuw IH, Vandewoude FJ. Creatinine arm index as alternative for creatinine height index. Am J Clin Nutr 1992; 56:611–615.
31. Veldee MS. Nutrition. In: Burtin CA, Ashwood ER, eds. Tietz Textbook of Clinical Chemistry, 2d ed. Philadelphia, Saunders, 1994:1236–1274.
32. Painter PC, Cope JY, Smith JL. Appendix: Table 41–20, Clinical chemistry and toxicology. In: Burtis CA, Ashwood ER, eds. Tietz Textbook of Clinical Chemistry, 2d ed. Philadelphia, Saunders, 1994:2176–2211.
33. Mattox TW, Brown RO, Boucher BA, et al. Use of fibronectin and somatomedin-C as markers of enteral nutrition support in traumatized patients using a modified amino acid formula. J Parenter Enter Nutr 1988;12:592–596.
34. Spiekerman AM. Proteins used in nutritional assessment. Clin Lab Med 1993;13:353–369.
35. Erstad BL, Campbell DJ, Rollins CJ, Rappaport WD. Albumin and prealbumin concentrations in patients receiving postoperative parenteral nutrition. Pharmacotherapy 1994;14:458–462.
36. Chandra RK, Sarchielli P. Nutritional status and immune response. Clin Lab Med 1993;13:455–461.
37. Peck MD, Alexander JW. The use of immunologic tests to predict outcome in surgical patients. Nutrition 1990;6:16–19.
38. Sacks GS, Brown RO, Teague D, et al. Early nutrition support modifies immune function in patients sustaining severe head injury. J Parenter Enter Nutr 1995;19:387–392.
39. Alexander JW, Peck MD. Future prospects for adjunctive therapy: Pharmacologic and nutritional approaches to immune system modulation. Crit Care Med 1990;18:S159–S164.
40. Moore FA, Moore EE, Kudsk KA, et al. Clinical benefits of an immune-enhancing diet for early postinjury enteral feeding. J Trauma 1994;37:607–615.
41. Kudsk KA, Minard G, Croce MA, et al. A randomized trial of isonitrogenous enteral diets after severe trauma: An immune-enhancing diet reduces septic complications. Ann Surg 1996;224:531–543.
42. Barton RG. Immune-enhancing enteral formulas: Are they beneficial in critically ill patients. Nutr Clin Prac 1997;12:51–62.
43. Baumgartner TG. Trace elements in clinical nutrition. Nutr Clin Pract 1993;8:251–263.
44. Nielson FH. Other trace elements. In: Ziegler EE, Filer LJ, eds. Present Knowledge in Nutrition, 7th ed. Washington, ILSI Press, 1996:353–377.
45. Shenkin A. Micronutrients. In: Rombeau JL, Rolandelli RH, eds. Clinical Nutrition: Enteral and Tube Feeding, 3d ed. Philadelphia, Saunders, 1997:96–111.
46. Weber CW, Nelson GW, Vasquez-de-Vaquera M, et al. Trace elements in the hair of healthy and malnourished children. J Trop Pediatr 1990;36:230–234.
47. Stoeker BJ. Chromium. In: Ziegler EE, Filer LJ, eds. Present Knowledge in Nutrition, 7th ed. Washington, ILSI Press,1996:344–352.
48. Tamura H, Hirose S, Watanabe O, et al. Anemia and neutropenia due to copper deficiency in enteral nutrition. J Parenter Enter Nutr 1994;18:185–189.
49. Wasa M, Satani M, Tanano H, et al. Copper deficiency with pancytopenia during parenteral nutrition. J Parenter Enter Nutr 1994;18:190–192.
50. Verhage AH, Cheong WK, Jeejeebhoy KN. Neurologic symptoms due to possible chromium deficiency in long term parenteral nutrition that closely mimic metronidazole-induced syndromes. J Parenter Enter Nutr 1996;20:123–127.
51. Alves G, Thiebot J, Tracqui A, et al. Neurologic disorders due to brain manganese deposition in a jaundiced patient receiving long-term parenteral nutrition. J Parenter Enter Nutr 1997;21: 41–45.
52. Fell JME, Reynolds AP, Meadows N, et al. Manganese toxicity in children receiving long term parenteral nutrition. Lancet 1996;347:1218–1221.
53. Keen CL, Zidenbery-Cherr S, Lonnerdal B. Nutritional and toxicological aspects of manganese intake: An overview. In: Mertz W, Abernathy CO, Olin SS, eds. Risk Assessment of Essential Elements. Washington, ILSI Press, 1994:221–235.
54. Matasuda A, Kimura M, Takeda T, et al. Changes in manganese content of mononuclear blood cells in patients receiving total parenteral nutrition. Clin Chem 1994;40:829–832.

55. Malecki EA, Lo HC, Yang H, et al. Tissue manganese concentrations and antioxidant enzyme activities in rats given total parenteral nutrition with and without supplemental manganese. J Parenter Enter Nutr 1995;19:222–226.
56. Abrams CK, Siram SM, Galsim C, et al. Selenium deficiency in long-term total parenteral nutrition. Nutr Clin Pract 1992;7:175–178.
57. Lockitch G, Jacobson B, Quigley G, et al. Selenium deficiency in low birth weight neonates: An unrecognized problem. J Pediatr 1989; 114:865–870.
58. Rannem T, Ladefoged K, Hylander E, et al. The effect of selenium supplementation on skeletal and cardiac muscle in selenium-depleted patients. J Parenter Enteral Nutr 1995;19:351–355.
59. Rannem T, Persson-Moschos M, Huang W, et al. Selenoprotein P in patients on home parenteral nutrition. J Parenter Enteral Nutr 1996;20: 287–291.
60. Levander OA, Burk PF. Selenium. In: Ziegler EE, Filer LJ, eds. Present Knowledge in Nutrition, 7th ed. Washington, ILSI Press, 1996:320–328.
61. Sardesi VM. Molybdenum: An essential trace element. Nutr Clin Prac 1993;8:277–281.
62. Abumrad NN, Schneider AJ, Steel D, Rogers LS. Amino acid intolerance during prolonged parenteral nutrition reversed by molybdenate therapy. Am J Clin Nutr 1981;34:2551–2559.
63. Friel JK, MacDonald AC, Mercer CN, et al. Molybdenum requirements in low-birth-weight infants receiving parenteral and enteral nutrition. J Parenter Enter Nutr 1999;23:155–159.
64. Clugston GA, Hetzel. Iodine. In: Shils ME, Olson JA, Shike M, eds. Modern Nutrition in Health and Disease, 8th ed. Philadelphia, Lea & Febiger, 1994:252–263.
65. Nichoalds GE. Iodine. In: Baumgartner TG, ed. Clinical Guide to Parenteral Micronutrition, 3d ed. Deerfield, IL, Fujisawa USA, 1997:361–374.
66. Moukarzel AA, Buchman AL, Salas JS, et al. Iodine supplementation in children receiving long-term parenteral nutrition. J Pediatr 1992;121:252–254.
67. Jordan NS. Hematology: Red and white blood cells. In: Traub SL, ed. Basic Skills in Interpreting Laboratory Date, 2d ed. Bethesda, MD, American Society of Health-System Pharmacists, 1996:297–320.
68. McCormick DB, Greene HL. Vitamins. In: Burtis CA, Ashwood ER, eds. Tietz Textbook of Clinical Chemistry, 2d ed. Philadelphia, Saunders, 1994:1275–1316.
69. Centers for Disease Control and Prevention. Lactic acidosis traced to thiamin deficiency related to nationwide shortage of multivitamins for total parenteral nutrition—United States, 1997. JAMA 1997;278:109–111.
70. Adolph M, Hailer S, Echart J. Serum phospholipid fatty acids in severely injured patients on total parenteral nutrition with medium chain/long chain tryglyceride emulsions. Ann Nutr Metab 1995;39:251–260.
71. Sacks GS, Brown RO, Collier P, Kudsk KA. Failure of tropical vegetable oils to prevent essential fatty acid deficiency in a critically ill patient receiving long-term parenteral nutrition. J Parenter Enter Nutr 1994;18:274–277.
72. Foote KD, MacKinnon MJ, Innis SM. Effect of early introduction of formula versus fat-free parenteral nutrition on essential fatty acid status of preterm infants. Am J Clin Nutr 1991;54: 93–97.
73. Tibboel D, Delemarre FMC, Przyrembel H, et al. Carnitine deficiency in surgical neonates receiving total parenteral nutrition. J Pediatr Surg 1990;25:418–421.
74. Borum PR. Carnitine in neonatal nutrition. J Child Neurol 1995;10 (Suppl 2):S25–S31.
75. Broquist HP. Carnitine. In: Shils ME, Olson JA, Shike M, eds. Modern Nutrition in Health and Disease, 8th ed. Philadelphia, Lea & Febiger, 1994:459–465.
76. Borum PR. Carnitine. In: Baumgartner TG, ed. Clinical Guide to Parenteral Micronutrition, 3d ed. Deerfield, IL, Fujisawa USA, 1997:629–641.
77. Cerra FB, Benitez MR, Blackburn GL, et al. Applied nutrition in ICU patients: A consensus statement of the American College of Chest Physicians. Chest 1997;111:769–778.
78. Food and Nutrition Board, National Research Council. Recommended Dietary Allowances, 10th ed. Washington, National Academy of Sciences, 1989.
79. Food and Nutrition Board, Institute of Medicine, National Academy of Sciences. Dietary Reference Intakes Series. Washington, National Academy Press, 2001. *http://ww4.nas.edu.*
80. Food and Nutrition Board, Institute of Medicine. Dietary Reference Intakes for Thiamin, Riboflavin, Niacin, Vitamin B_6, Folate, Vitamin B_{12}, Pantothenic Acid, Biotin, and Choline. Washington, National Academy Press, 1999.
81. Food and Nutrition Board, Institute of Medicine. Dietary Reference Intakes for Calcium, Phosphorus, Magnesium, Vitamin D, and Fluoride. Washington, National Academy Press, 1999.
82. Food and Nutrition Board, Institute of Medicine. Dietary Reference Intakes for Vitamin C, Vitamin E, Selenium, and Carotenoids. Washington, National Academy Press, 2000.
83. Food and Nutrition Board, Institute of Medicine. Dietary Reference Intakes for Vitamin A, Vitamin K, Arsenic, Boron, Chromium, Copper, Iodine, Iron, Manganese, Molybdenum, Nickel, Silicon, Vanadium, and Zinc. Washington, National Academy Press, 2001.
84. Harris JA, Benedict FG. A Biometric Study of Basal Metabolism in Man. Publication 279. Washington, Carnegie Institute, 1919.
85. Young VR. Macronutrient needs in the elderly. Nutr Rev 1992;50:454–462.
86. Caldwell MD, Kennedy CC. Normal nutritional requirements. Surg Clin North Am 1981;61:489–507.
87. Schofield C. Predicting basal metabolic rate, new standards and review of previous work. Hum Nutr Clin Nutr 1985;39(Suppl 1):5–41.
88. World Health Organization. Energy and Protein Requirements: Report of a Joint FAO/WHO/UNU Expert Consultation. WHO Technical Report Series No. 724. Geneva, World Health Organization, 1985.
89. Weise K, Zaritsky A. Endocrine manifestations of critical illness in the child. Pediatr Clin North Am 1987;34:119–130.
90. Dimand RJ. Parenteral nutrition in the critically ill infant and child. In: Baker RD, Baker SS, Davis AM, eds. Pediatric Parenteral Nutrition. New York, Chapman & Hall, 1997:273–300.
91. Pollack MM. Nutritional support of children in the intensive care unit. In: Suskind RM, Lewinter-Suskind L, eds. Textbook of Pediatric Nutrition, 2d ed. New York, Raven Press, 1993:207–216.
92. Garrel DR, Jobin N, DeJonge LHM. Should we still use the Harris and Benedict equations? Nutr Clin Pract 1996;11:99–103.
93. Osborne BJ, Saba AK, Wood SJ, et al. Clinical comparison of three methods to determine resting energy expenditure. Nutr Clin Pract 1994;9:241–246.
94. Frankenfield D. Energy and macrosubstrate requirements. In: Gottschlich MM, ed. The Science and Practice of Nutrition Support: A Case-Based Core Curriculum, America Society for Parenteral and Enteral Nutrition. Dubuque, IO, Kendall/Hunt, 2001:31–52.
95. McClave SA, Snider HL. Use of indirect calorimetry in clinical nutrition. Nutr Clin Pract 1992;7:207–221.
96. McGee M, Binkley J, Jensen GL. Geriatric Nutrition. In: Gottschlich MM, ed. The Science and Practice of Nutrition Support: A Case-Based Core Curriculum, America Society for Parenteral and Enteral Nutrition. Dubuque, IO, Kendall/Hunt, 2001:373–389.
97. Long CL, Lowry SR. Hormonal regulation of protein metabolism. J Parenter Enter Nutr 1990;14:555–562.
98. Barton RG. Nutrition support in critical illness. Nutr Clin Pract 1994; 9:127–139.
99. Velasco N, Long CL, Otto DA, et al. Comparison of three methods for the estimation of total nitrogen losses in hospitalized patients. J Parenter Enter Nutr 1990;14:517–522.
100. Russell MK, McAdams MP. Laboratory monitoring of nutritional status. In: Matarese LE, Gottschlich MM. Contemporary Nutrition

Support Practice: A Clinical Guide. Philadelphia, Saunders, 1998:47–63.

101. American Medical Association Department of Foods and Nutrition. Multivitamin preparations for parenteral use: A statement by the Nutrition Advisory Group. J Parenter Enter Nutr 1979;3:258–262.
102. Kleinman RE, ed. Committee on Nutrition, American Academy of Pediatrics. Pediatric Nutrition Handbook, 4th ed. Elk Grove Village, IL, American Academy of Pediatrics, 1998.
103. Greene HL, Hambidge KM, Schanler R, Tsang RC. Guidelines for the use of vitamins, trace elements, calcium, magnesium, and phosphorus in infants and children receiving total parenteral nutrition: Report of the Subcommittee on Pediatric Parenteral Nutrient Requirements from the Committee on Clinical Practice Issues of the American Society for Clinical Nutrition. Am J Clin Nutr 1988;48:1324–1342.
104. Berger MM, Cavadini C, Bart A, et al. Cutaneous copper and zinc losses in burns. Burns 1992;18:373–380.
105. Berger MM, Cavadini C, Bart A, et al. Selenium losses in 10 burned patients. Clin Nutr 1992;11:75–82.
106. Solomon SM, Kirby DF. The refeeding syndrome: A review. J Parenter Enter Nutr 1990;14:90–97.
107. Weinsier R, Krumdieck C. Death resulting from overzealous total parenteral nutrition: The refeeding syndrome revisited. Am J Clin Nutr 1981;34:393–399.
108. Jefferson JW. Drug and diet interactions: Avoiding therapeutic paralysis. J Clin Psychiatry 1998;59:31–39.
109. Fuhr U. Drug interactions with grapefruit juice: Extent, probable mechanism and clinical relevance. Drug Saf 1998;18:251–272.
110. Kirk JK. Significant drug-nutrient interactions. Am Fam Physician 1995;51:1175–82.
111. Singh BN. Effects of food on clinical pharmacokinetics. Clin Pharmacokinet 1999;37: 213–55.
112. Thomas JA, Burns RA. Important drug-nutrient interactions in the elderly. Drugs Aging 1998;13:199–209.

136

PREVALENCE AND SIGNIFICANCE OF MALNUTRITION

Pamela D. Reiter and Gordon Sacks

The term *malnutrition* has been used to characterize a broad range of altered nutritional states. *Overnutrition* is the term used to describe excess nutrient intake, whereas *undernutrition* is used to describe insufficient intake or substrate use. Both nutritional states can contribute to the poor outcome of many disease states. Unless specifically stated, this chapter will use the nomenclature of malnutrition as synonymous with undernutrition (refer to Chapter 140 for a discussion on overnutrition/obesity). In children, malnutrition can be defined by a variety of criteria. Stages (e.g., Waterlow stages) have been developed to define the severity of protein-energy malnutrition. Anthropometric evaluations, using established age-based growth curves, can define acute and chronic malnutrition using either Z-scores or height and weight percentiles. In general, malnutrition in children is defined as growth that declines below the 5th percentile for age or less than 90% to 95% of the median value for age. In this chapter, the prevalence of malnutrition as defined by a variety of nutrition assessment parameters is documented, and the significant impact of abnormalities in these nutrition assessment parameters on the morbidity and mortality of selected disease states is presented. Interventional strategies for the prevention and management of malnutrition and the economic consequences of malnutrition are also presented.

PREVALENCE

Although malnutrition occurs throughout the world, it is most prevalent in underdeveloped countries, where food supply, ignorance, poverty, overcrowding, and poor sanitation are contributing factors. The most susceptible individuals in developed and underdeveloped countries are infants (especially premature infants), pregnant or lactating women, and the elderly. The factors that contribute to malnutrition in developed countries include a decline in breast-feeding, poor maternal nutrition before and during pregnancy, misconceptions about the use of certain foods, fad diets, and alcohol or drug abuse. In the United States, poor nutrition in the community occurs mostly in lower socioeconomic groups but may be present throughout society when fad diets and alcohol or drug abuse are factors.

Malnutrition is associated most commonly with exacerbations of chronic disease and acute illness and thus is prevalent in the hospital setting. Recognition of the scope of the problem coincides with the systematic application of nutrition assessment techniques to hospitalized individuals in the last two decades. The prevalence of previously unrecognized malnutrition is 40% to 55% among adult patients from varying socioeconomic backgrounds hospitalized in a variety of institutions.[1] The prevalence of malnutrition has declined and there has been a heightened awareness of nutritional disease and better in-hospital nutrition management since the mid-1970s.[2] Worldwide, nearly 200 million children are moderately to severely underweight, and 70 million are severely malnourished.[3] Over one half of global childhood deaths under 5 years of age can be attributed directly or indirectly to malnutrition.[4] Chronic malnutrition in children less than 2 years of age is an independent predictor of poor cognitive development lasting up to 11 years of age.[5] Unfortunately, children have both limited body stores and high metabolic demands. These characteristics place them at particular risk for developing malnutrition, especially during illness.

While the majority of undernourished children are from underdeveloped countries, malnutrition is also common in the United States and other industrial countries. In 1974, a publicly funded health and nutrition program known as the Pediatric Nutrition Surveillance System (PedNSS) was established in the United States.[6] This system generates data on the prevalence of malnutrition in children generally younger than 5 years of age enrolled in a variety of federal and state programs. The prevalence of shortness (height for age) in children younger than 24 months of age during 1980 to 1991 was 10%, which is more than twice the expected value. However, in older children aged 2 to 5 years, the prevalence was only slightly higher than expected. Thinness, or weight for height, has been stable at 2.5% to 5% since 1980 and indicates that the prevalence of acute or severe malnutrition is low. Anemia, hematologic evidence of poor nutrition status, and/or iron deficiency was high between 1980 and 1985 (20% to 30%) but has declined rapidly and now approaches 5%.

Children with chronic disease and those in periods of rapid growth have the highest prevalence of malnutrition. Hendricks and colleagues described the change in prevalence of protein-energy malnutrition in hospitalized children over a 15-year period.[7] Overall prevalence was high, but significant reductions were detected in acute malnutrition (weight for height <90% of median) from 33.6% to 24.5% and chronic malnutrition (weight for height <95% of median) from 46.8% in 1976 to 27.3% in the 1990s.

EFFECT ON ORGAN AND CELLULAR FUNCTION

The outcome of malnutrition is an inappropriate reduction in lean body mass resulting in loss of structure and/or function (Table 136–1). Essentially every organ system is affected by malnutrition. The clinical significance of the effect will depend on the specific anatomic structure or system and on the degree of malnutrition. For example, with mild malnutrition, loss of skeletal muscle mass may be apparent as weakness or a decreased level of physical activity. However, alterations in cardiac function usually are not apparent until severe malnutrition is present.

Alterations in the immune system (Table 136–2) represent an end-organ or functional response to malnutrition and may reflect a decline in lean body mass as well as a deficiency in specific nutrients such as zinc.[8] Clinically, this is manifested as an increased incidence of infection.

TABLE 136–1. End-Organ Responses in Malnutrition

Organ	Anatomic Responses	Physiologic Responses
Heart	Four-chamber dilation; atrophic degeneration with necrosis and fibrosis; myofibrillar disruption	QT prolongation, low voltage, bradycardia; decreased cardiac output, stroke volume, and contractility; preload intolerance; diminished responsiveness to drugs
Lung	Emphysematous changes; pulmonary infarcts; reduced bacterial clearance; muscle atrophy	Pneumonia; decreases in functional residual capacity, vital capacity, and maximum breathing capacity; depressed hypoxic/hypercarbic drives
Hematologic	Failure of stem-cell production; decreased PMN chemotaxis; decreased lymphocyte count with reduced helper T and increased suppressor T and killer cells; decreased blastogenesis to phytohemagglutinin	Anemia; anergy; decreased granuloma formation; impaired response to chemotherapy; increased infection rate
Renal system	Epithelial swelling; atrophy; mild cortical calcification; depressed erythropoietin synthesis	Reduced glomerular filtration rate and inability to handle sodium loads; polyuria; metabolic acidosis
Gastrointestinal system	Disproportionate mass loss; hypoplastic and atrophic changes; decrease in total mucosal height	Depressed enzymatic activity; shortened transit time; impaired motility; propensity for bacterial overgrowth; maldigestion and malabsorption
Liver	Mass loss; periportal fat accumulation	Decreased visceral protein synthesis; depressed microsomal activity; eventual hepatic insufficiency

From Cerra FB (ed.). Manual of Surgical Nutrition. St Louis, MO, CV Mosby, 1984, p 6, with permission.

Malnourished patients have an increased likelihood of developing wound infections from altered immunity. Although wound healing occurs at the expense of other tissues, in the setting of protein-energy malnutrition (PEM), the rate at which wounds heal and the tensile strength of the wound are decreased.[9] Deficiency of arginine, copper, vitamin C, vitamin A, or zinc also may contribute to decreased wound healing (Table 136–3). Supplemental vitamin A can promote wound healing in animal models,[9] and arginine has improved markers of wound healing (i.e., protein and hydroxyproline in the wound bed) in elderly healthy human volunteers.[10] Other nutrients, when ingested in excessive amounts, may impair wound healing. For example, excess vitamin E antagonizes the promotion of wound healing by vitamin A, and excess zinc will displace copper and interfere with lysyl oxidase (the enzyme necessary for collagen cross-link formation).[9]

TABLE 136–2. Immune Response Mechanisms in Malnutrition

Parameter	Observation in Malnutrition
Cell-mediated immune response	
Delayed cutaneous hypersensitivity	Decreased
Lymphocyte transformation	Decreased
Polymorphonuclear leukocyte response	
Phagocytosis	Normal or decreased
Metabolism	Decreased
Bactericidal capacity	Decreased
Chemotaxis	Decreased
Total lymphocyte count	Decreased
T cells	
$CD4^+$	Decreased
$CD8^+$	Decreased
Helper to suppressor ratio	Decreased
Humoral response	
Complement activity (CH50)	Decreased
Secretory IgA	Decreased
Serum complement	Decreased or normal
Serum immunoglobulins	Normal
Serum opsonization	Normal

DISEASE-SPECIFIC CONSEQUENCES

Malnutrition seldom exists as an isolated disease state but rather is usually found in patients with other preexisting illnesses. Often the primary disease or complications of the disease predispose an individual to the development of malnutrition. The primary factors that enhance the likelihood of developing malnutrition include decreased dietary intake (e.g., due to nausea, vomiting, anorexia), malabsorption (e.g., due to short bowel syndrome, severe diarrhea, high-output fistula), and altered metabolism (hypermetabolic and catabolic states due to sepsis, trauma, cancer, or AIDS). Malnutrition is also associated with major organ failure: renal, hepatic, cardiac, and pulmonary failure and multisystem organ failure (see Chapter 139).

CANCER

Patients with cancer have many factors that contribute to the likelihood of developing malnutrition (Table 136–4). The frequency is

TABLE 136–3. Nutritional Disorders and Wound Healing

Nutritional Disorder	Effect on Wound Healing
Arginine deficiency	Altered collagen formation
Copper deficiency	Impaired lysyl oxidase activity
Protein-energy malnutrition	Decreased wound strength because of reduced hydroxyproline content of wound; decreased rate of wound healing; increased incidence of wound infection
Vitamin C deficiency	Decreased fibroblast maturation with failure of collagen synthesis; decreased angiogenesis
Vitamin A deficiency	Decreased collagen accumulation; formation of abnormal collagen
Zinc deficiency	Impaired DNA and protein synthesis; impaired mitosis and cell proliferation

TABLE 136–4. Risk Factors for Malnutrition in Cancer Patients

Risk Factor	Nutrition Consequence
Primary disease	
Tumor type	Weight loss, anorexia, altered taste, altered metabolism
Complicating conditions	
Malabsorption	Impaired absorption of all or selected nutrients, diarrhea
Bowel obstruction	Nausea and vomiting, inability to ingest nutrients orally or by enteral nutrition
Infection	Increased energy expenditure and protein requirements, altered metabolism, anorexia, malabsorption
Psychological response	Anorexia, food aversion
Treatments	
Chemotherapy	Taste and appetite alterations, nausea and vomiting, mucositis, esophagitis, diarrhea, constipation
Surgery	
Radical resection of oropharyngeal region	Problems with chewing and swallowing
Esophageal reconstruction	Gastric stasis and hypochlorhydria secondary to vagotomy; diarrhea and steatorrhea
Gastrectomy	Dumping syndrome, malabsorption, lack of intrinsic factor, hypoglycemia
Intestinal resection	Malabsorption, renal oxalate stones, metabolic acidosis, diarrhea
Pancreatectomy	Malabsorption, diabetes mellitus
Radiation	
Head and neck	Stomatitis, dysgeusia, xerostomia
Abdomen and pelvis	Bowel obstruction, fistulae, radiation enteritis (diarrhea, protein-losing enteropathy, malabsorption)

highest (>80%) in patients with gastric and pancreatic tumors and lowest in patients with hematologic malignancies.[11] Weight loss, a sign of malnutrition, occurs in 30% to 80% of adult cancer patients. A significant relationship between weight loss and reduced survival has been demonstrated for some (lung, prostate, colon cancer) but not all tumor types.[11] The degree of reduction in median survival is statistically significant for some cancers and ranges from 49% to 79%. Malnutrition in children with cancer is common, and the prevalence is highest in those with Ewing's sarcoma (67%) and neuroblastoma (47%) and lowest in those with acute leukemias (6%) and non-Hodgkin's lymphomas (10% to 15%).[12] The stage of disease progression and chemotherapy-related complications also have been associated with an increased prevalence.[13] Theoretically, early recognition and management of malnutrition in cancer patients may minimize the nutritional consequences, improve tumor response and reduce side effects of therapy, and improve survival. Cancer patients treated with bone marrow transplantation have shown improved tumor response and clinical outcome with parenteral nutrition (PN) compared with control groups not receiving PN.[14]

Improved nutrition status enhances survival and improves treatment tolerance in many but not all children.[13,15,16] PN has been shown to be of benefit to malnourished children undergoing radiation therapy but failed to benefit well-nourished children.[17] Conversely, well-nourished children treated with PN at the initiation of therapy for metastatic neuroblastoma appeared to have longer remission and improved survival compared with their malnourished cohorts.[12] Malnutrition in cancer patients due to simple starvation, characterized by normal metabolism but inadequate nutrient intake or malabsorption, appears to be responsive to nutrition intervention.[18] However, malnutrition due to cancer cachexia, characterized by altered nutrient use despite adequate supply, does not.[19,20] Treatment of malnutrition due to cancer cachexia is controversial, especially in the absence of data showing an improved quality of life with nutrition therapy.

AIDS

Generalized wasting and malnutrition are common characteristics of HIV/AIDS. The etiology and risk factors of AIDS-associated malnutrition are multifactorial[21–24] (Table 136–5). In many patients, weight loss and wasting may be one of the earliest symptoms along with opportunistic infection. The malnutrition is often progressive and may lead to death in some patients.[25,26] Poor nutrition status as indicated by weight loss and decreased serum albumin concentrations has been shown to be a predictor of survival in adult AIDS patients.[27–29]

TABLE 136–5. Risk Factors for Malnutrition in AIDS

Risk Factor	Nutrition Consequence
General factors: decreased oral intake, malabsorption	Anorexia, poor diet, esophageal/oral lesions, emotional stress, HIV wasting syndrome, diarrhea, enteropathy, medication side effects
Opportunistic infections: bacterial (MAI, TB); viral (CMV, herpes); fungal (*Candida albicans,* cryptococcus); protozoal (*Pneumocystis carinii,* microsporidia, isospora belli, cryptosporidia, *Giardia lamblia*)	Fever, hypermetabolism, anorexia, malabsorption
Malignancies: Kaposi's sarcoma, lymphoma	Anorexia, hypermetabolism, medication side effects
Medications: antibiotics, anticancer chemotherapy, antidepressants	Nausea, vomiting, diarrhea, anorexia, mucositis
Neuropsychiatric disorders: dementia, depression, anxiety, encephalopathy	Poor oral intake, anorexia, poor diet
Socioeconomic factors: IV drug abuse, low income	Poor oral intake, anorexia, poor diet

Furthermore, micronutrient deficiencies such as vitamin A or vitamin B_{12} have been associated with a decline in CD4 cell count and HIV disease progression.[30] Over the past several years, however, nutritional problems have shifted from the characteristic lethal wasting associated with opportunistic infections to a syndrome of subcutaneous fat atrophy, visceral fat accumulation, hypertriglceridemia, and insulin resistance.[31] The etiology is unclear but may be related to new protease inhibitor therapy.[32] The implications of these metabolic and body compositional changes on outcome and development of comorbidities (i.e., atherosclerosis) are unclear at this time.

In HIV-positive children, a number of growth patterns exist, but most will experience nutritional deficits and growth abnormalities.[22] Infants with perinatally acquired AIDS have normal birth weights but show signs of growth delay as early as 4 months.[33] Failure to thrive has been reported in up to 33% of HIV-infected children.[23] Impaired linear growth also appears to correlate with periods of rapid viral replication during the first 18 months of life.[34] There is a direct relationship between these growth abnormalities and morbidity and mortality.[35] Up to 80% of older infants and children (4 months to 11 years) with AIDS or advanced HIV disease demonstrate evidence of retarded growth velocity with weight below the 25th percentile.[36] Growth velocity and survival can be improved markedly with aggressive nutritional therapy and antiviral therapy.[22,24,36,37]

The response to nutrition intervention in adults with AIDS has been variable. Supplemental dietary intake of selected micronutrients has been shown to have an impact on mortality in HIV-1 seropositive homosexual/bisexual men. High intakes of B-group vitamins (B_1, B_6, niacin) and β-carotene were associated with improved survival, whereas an increased intake of zinc was associated with poorer survival.[38] In a retrospective review of home PN in 22 AIDS patients with weight loss greater than 10% of usual body weight, 15 patients gained weight, 6 stabilized, and 2 continued to lose weight.[39] Lean body mass repletion in AIDS patients with weight loss and inadequate food intake has been reported when enteral nutrition was the sole source of nutrient intake.[40] Kotler and associates compared the effects of PN and an oral semi-elemental diet on body weight, body composition, survival, quality of life, and medical costs in AIDS outpatients with malabsorption syndromes.[41] At the end of 3 months, the PN group gained more weight and significantly more fat, but body cell mass measurements and survival did not differ between the groups. However, the group receiving an oral diet scored significantly better on a physical functioning subscale of quality of life. The most dramatic differences were in medical costs, with a fourfold cost increase in patients receiving PN versus oral diet therapy.[41]

With earlier diagnosis and initiation of treatment for HIV-positive status prior to the onset of AIDS, the prevalence of malnutrition may decline. New treatment modalities for AIDS are also being developed that may affect the prevalence of malnutrition and the response to nutrition intervention in this patient population (see Chapter 123).

CRITICAL ILLNESS/TRAUMA/BURN INJURY

One of the characteristics of critical illness is hypermetabolism. Trauma, burn injury, and sepsis are all catalysts for the release of mediators that initiate and regulate the hypermetabolic response. The metabolic consequences of this response include altered carbohydrate metabolism, increased protein synthesis and degradation, and increased lipid oxidation, which ultimately result in loss of protein and lean body mass.[42,43] In a previously well-nourished individual, critical illness can result in the rapid onset of kwashiorkor-like malnutrition within 5 to 7 days. In a previously malnourished individual, critical illness can precipitate severe mixed marasmus-kwashiorkor in 3 to 5 days. In a prospective study of 129 patients admitted to the intensive care unit (ICU), 43% were malnourished.[44] The malnourished patients had an increased length of stay in the ICU (a mean of 27 versus 19 days) and a statistically significant increased incidence of complications (55% versus 40%) compared with well-nourished patients with a similar severity of illness.

The goal of nutrition support in critically ill patients is to prevent the development or worsening of malnutrition. Patient outcomes related to tissue repair and organ function may be improved through nutrition support in these patients.[43] Enteral nutrition (EN) initiated within 24 to 48 hours of injury may attenuate the hypermetabolic response.[45,46] Enteral nutrition also has been shown to result in fewer septic complications when compared with PN.[47,48] Two recent meta-analyses suggest that critically ill patients may derive the greatest benefit when enterally fed an immune-enhanced formula that contains pharmacologic doses of immune-modulating nutrients such as arginine, glutamine, nucleic acids, and omega-3 fatty acids.[49,50]

INFLAMMATORY BOWEL DISEASE

Malnutrition has been reported in 20% to 45% of patients with inflammatory bowel disease (IBD). Malabsorption, increased gastrointestinal losses, or poor oral intake are the predominant causes.[51] Decreased food intake may be due to pain, anorexia, or altered taste; malabsorption may be due to mucosal abnormalities, bacterial overgrowth, or diminished absorptive surface after surgical resection of diseased bowel, and hypermetabolism may be a consequence of fever and infection.[52] Various nutrient abnormalities, such as anemia and vitamin and trace mineral deficiencies, have been observed in IBD patients.[51] Growth failure occurs in 15% to 40% of prepubertal patients and is characterized by retarded skeletal maturation (which may be irreversible) and delayed development of secondary sex characteristics.[53] The nutrition consequences of ulcerative colitis tend to be less severe than those of Crohn's disease. Approximately 25% to 50% of patients with ulcerative colitis are hypoalbuminemic, and 2% to 20% experience growth failure.

Nutrition management of IBD may be achieved with enteral nutrition and/or PN.[54] Enteral is the preferred route except in patients with a high-output fistula or obstruction or if enteral feeding exacerbates pain. EN or PN nutrition is likely to facilitate remission in 60% to 80% of patients with acute Crohn's disease. However, the course of ulcerative colitis is not influenced by the use of nutrition support, although nutrition status may be maintained in an acute exacerbation.

CHRONIC INTESTINAL PSEUDO-OBSTRUCTION

Pseudo-obstruction, a hypomotility or dysmotility disorder of the gastrointestinal tract that is thought to be a neuromuscular disorder of the smooth muscle and/or its innervation, often presents with the symptoms of bowel obstruction. Prolonged dysmotility can result in malnutrition as well as growth failure in children.[55] The primary factors contributing to a risk of malnutrition are anorexia, nausea, vomiting, and obstruction, which may recur over years. Approximately 15% to 30% of patients with pseudo-obstruction require nutrition support with either PN or EN.[55]

SHORT BOWEL SYNDROME

Short bowel syndrome (SBS) is the result of the surgical resection of a large portion of the intestinal tract. The degree of nutrition impairment depends on the amount and location of excised bowel. Malabsorption is present to some extent immediately following surgery and may be temporary or permanent.[56] Bowel adaptation will occur over time (6 to 12 months) but may not result in restoration of the full absorptive capacity of the intestine. Intestinal adaptation occurs more frequently in children than in adults.[57] In fact, the premature infant may have the best adaptive response to SBS owing to normal rapid intestinal growth during late gestation when the jejunum, ileum, and colon more than double in length.[58]

Adults who have 600 to 700 cm of ileum remaining after surgical resection (i.e., 100 to 200 cm of ileum resected) will require vitamin B_{12}, calcium, and magnesium supplementation. Massive resection of the small bowel leaving less than 60 cm in adults and 10 to 20 cm in children will result in severe malabsorption of all nutrients and will require total or supplemental PN for months or years postoperatively.[57,59,60] In the absence of nutrition support, malnutrition is inevitable and can be life-threatening. For those children with extensive bowel loss or life-threatening complications from prolonged PN, innovative surgical procedures including bowel lengthening and transplantation can improve the gut's adaptive process and reduce the need for PN.[57,61–63]

SURGICAL PATIENTS

Malnourished patients tend to have a greater risk of postoperative morbidity and mortality than well-nourished patients. Several nutrition assessment parameters predict morbidity and mortality in surgical patients. Mullen and colleagues examined the value of 16 nutritional and immunologic variables and found serum transferrin and albumin concentrations and delayed cutaneous hypersensitivity reaction to be the most reliable predictors of outcome.[64] These factors have been confirmed by several authors to correlate with morbidity and mortality.[65–68] A comprehensive study by Buzby and associates[69] confirmed the findings of Mullen and colleagues[64] and suggested that the measurement of triceps skinfold thickness also was a useful predictor. They developed a linear continuous quantitative predictive outcome assessment tool, the prognostic nutritional index (PNI). The PNI accurately identified 87% of the patients who ultimately developed significant complications and 96% of the postoperative deaths. This predictive index has been validated in prospective studies of different patient groups by comparing the risk of morbidity and mortality predicted by the model with actual outcome.[70–72] The Subjective Global Assessment (SGA), developed by Detsky and colleagues, is a clinical method that can aid in the recognition of undernutrition by evaluating a patient's nutritional status based on features of the medical history and physical examination.[73] In prospective studies, SGA has been shown to be very successful in predicting complications in surgical patients. One study demonstrated SGA to be a better predictor of postoperative infectious complications than serum albumin, serum transferrin, delayed hypersensitivity skin testing, anthropometry, creatinine-height index, and the PNI.[73]

No studies have evaluated the effect of nutrition support on the PNI and the subsequent patient outcome. However, the use of preoperative PN in patients with malnutrition, particularly when associated with a low serum albumin concentration, has been demonstrated to reduce the incidence of major postoperative complications in several patient populations.[74] Furthermore, early postoperative PN has been shown to improve convalescence coincident with improvement in nutrition status after esophagogastrectomy[75] and radical bladder cystectomy.[76] Conflicting data were found in the multi-institutional VA Cooperative Study.[77] This prospective, randomized clinical trial in 395 malnourished patients evaluated the impact of perioperative PN on mortality and the rate of postoperative complications at 30 and 90 days. Differences in mortality at 30 and 90 days were not statistically significant, and there was no significant reduction in complication rate. The types of complications in the two groups were different. The PN group had a higher incidence of infectious complications and a lower incidence of noninfectious complications. The incidence of noninfectious complications was higher in those with the greatest degree of malnutrition (determined by calculation of a nutrition risk index using serum albumin concentration and weight). In the PN group, the highest incidence of infectious complications was in the borderline or mildly malnourished patients. The investigators concluded that perioperative PN did not result in an improved postoperative course except in patients who were severely malnourished preoperatively . In patients who were mildly to moderately malnourished, the incidence of infectious complications associated with the use of PN outweighed the benefits. As with critically ill patients, enteral feeding with immune-enhanced formulas appears to promote the best nutrition and clinical outcome with fewer metabolic and infectious complications.[49,50]

PEDIATRIC DISEASES

Regardless of the disease process, pediatric patients in general are at greater risk for nutrition disorders and develop the most severe consequences more frequently. Nutrition deficiency in the young affects existing organs and cells, may impair normal development, and may result in permanent, irreversible damage. Pharmacologic and technologic advances in neonatal medicine have improved the survival of extremely premature infants (<750 g). However, the prevalence of neonatal diseases such as bronchopulmonary dysplasia and necrotizing enterocolitis also has increased, which may further complicate the infant's nutrition status.

BRONCHOPULMONARY DYSPLASIA

Bronchopulmonary dysplasia (BPD) or chronic lung disease (CLD) is a clinical, pathologic, and radiographic disease of the newborn resulting from prolonged exposure to positive-pressure ventilation and elevated oxygen concentrations.[78] Risk factors for developing BPD include extent of prematurity, nutrition status, and immunologic status. Characteristics of BPD include pulmonary edema and tissue destruction with subsequent repair, fibrosis, and inflammation. These infants also have an elevated metabolic rate and growth failure.

Early evidence of growth failure and altered body composition is common in infants with BPD when compared with their peers without BPD.[79] The origin of this growth failure is multifactorial. Elevations in both resting and total energy expenditure have been reported.[80,81] Given that pulmonary edema is common, fluid restriction is often necessary. This restriction further impedes provision of adequate calories and may contribute to poor growth.[82] Futhermore, there exists a direct relationship between growth retardation and severity of lung disease and energy expenditure.[83] When infants with BPD receive appropriate oxygen therapy during the first year of life, growth patterns of matched infants without BPD can be attained.[84,85] Although early growth failure is a common finding in infants with BPD, the persistence of growth failure beyond the neonatal period is disputable and complex. Growth failure during the first 2 years of life, early childhood, and beyond has been reported,[78] but it appears that prematurity and sociodemographic factors rather than BPD are most predictive of future growth.[86,87] Catch-up growth can be attained faster when infants are fed higher intakes of protein, calcium, phosphorus, and zinc.[88]

NECROTIZING ENTEROCOLITIS

Necrotizing enterocolitis (NEC) is a complex disorder characterized by intestinal mucosal injury secondary to ischemia, bacterial overgrowth, and/or the presence of nutrients within the gut lumen. NEC typically occurs in premature infants (<38 weeks' gestational age), low-birth- weight infants (<2500 g), and in the first 1 to 10 days of life. The severe inflammation of the intestinal tract caused by the mucosal injury results in malabsorption of nutrients. Total bowel rest is the treatment of choice; hence, to prevent malnutrition, PN is indicated.[89] If NEC results in bowel perforation, necrosis, or stricture, surgery is required to resect the injured portion of the bowel. SBS may be a consequence if more than 70% of the bowel is resected, and long-term home PN will then be required.[89] Additionally, infants with advanced disease who require surgery are at increased risk of growth failure.[90] Fortunately, the survival rate of NEC has improved over the past decade to 50% to 80% depending on gestational age at the time of diagnosis. If significant intestinal resection can be avoided, growth and nutrient absorption in these children ultimately may be normal.[91]

CYSTIC FIBROSIS

The predominant clinical findings of cystic fibrosis (CF) are related to altered pulmonary function and pancreatic exocrine function. Growth retardation and failure to thrive are classic features of CF. According to the National Cystic Fibrosis Patient Registry data, malnutrition (height for age or weight for age <5th percentile) is very prevalent in infants (47%), adolescents (34%), and children with newly diagnosed CF (44%).[92] The occurrence of malnutrition is closely related to the deterioration of lung function and contributes to the patient's poor clinical outcome.[93] Factors that contribute to the nutrition disorders associated with CF include an increased energy expenditure, malabsorption, anorexia, pharmacotherapy, and inadequate pulmonary toilet.[94] Increased energy requirements in CF patients are the result of the increased amount of work required to breathe and an elevated resting energy expenditure (REE) during pulmonary exacerbation. Recent data suggest that children with only mild to moderate lung disease may be spared from this rise in REE during an acute exacerbation.[95] It is also theorized that the genetic defect that causes CF affects metabolism, causing an increase in energy requirements.

As life expectancy of patients with CF increased, the recognition of CF-associated diseases has also increased. CF-related diabetes mellitus is now a well-recognized problem and further complicates the nutritional status in those individuals.[96] Altered pancreatic function occurs in about 85% of patients with CF. Insufficiency of pancreatic enzyme secretion into the intestine reduces the absorption of fat and fat-soluble vitamins. Consequently, more than two-thirds of the CF centers in North America use a hydrolyzed (semi-elemental) enteral formula for infants with CF. However, the nutrition benefits of this expensive hydrolyzed formula over a conventional cow's milk formula have been challenged recently. These recent investigations do not support the use of a hydrolyzed formula as part of routine nutrition care.[97,98] The physical pounding on the back of the patient while in a partially inverted position, i.e., pulmonary toilet, is designed to loosen the thickened bronchial secretions that impair breathing. It may be performed numerous times throughout the day and may result in an increase in energy expenditure. It also interferes with the feeding schedule, which needs to be designed to ensure that the stomach is empty or nearly empty before the pulmonary toilet process begins to prevent pulmonary aspiration of stomach contents. Finally, the disease itself contributes to the development of anorexia in patients with CF. Nutritional management typically focuses on the use of oral pancreatic enzymes (e.g., Viokase, Pancrease), supplemental fat-soluble vitamins, and a high-protein, high-calorie diet.[92] If nutrition status cannot be maintained with these measures, supplemental EN or PN may be indicated.

SOLID-ORGAN FAILURE IN CHILDHOOD

Malnutrition with growth impairment is a well-recognized complication of renal, hepatic, and cardiac failure in children. Mechanisms responsible for malnutrition include both reduced energy intake and increased energy requirements.[99–101] Early clinical onset of organ failure can have profound effects on growth and development. Among children diagnosed with hereditary renal disorders, 50% had marked growth retardation (mean age at observation 10 yrs).[99] Prevalence of malnutrition in hospitalized children with cardiac disease varies with age and type of cardiac lesion. Seventy-nine percent of infants with heart disease had evidence of acute malnutrition compared with less than 30% in all other age groups. Chronic malnutrition was common in all age groups with a prevalence of 82%, 84%, 61%, 58%, and 38% in infants, toddlers, preschool children, school-age children, and adolescents, respectively.[102] Children with complex cardiac disease or left-to-right intracardiac shunts had the highest prevalence of both acute and chronic malnutrition (38% to 80%). Catch-up growth in children with chronic renal failure, complex congenital heart lesions, and advanced cirrhosis can be attained with aggressive feeding regimens, including tube feedings.[100,101,103] Optimizing nutritional status can improve outcomes and reduce morbidity.[104,105]

MANAGEMENT

The increased awareness of the prevalence and significance of untreated protein-calorie malnutrition has provided a strong incentive for a more rigorous evaluation of abnormalities of nutrition status and prompt nutrition support of malnourished patients. If nutrition assessment (see Chapter 135) reveals no malnutrition, then the patient should be counseled on appropriate maintenance goals for nutrition intake. If mild to moderate malnutrition is present, an anabolic feeding regimen should be initiated using oral supplements. If anorexia is a major contributing factor, enteral tube feeding may be indicated. Intact nutrients can be administered enterally when normal bowel function is present, but a specially designed formula that has a modified fat content, is lactose-free, contains fiber, and/or is calorie or protein enriched may be indicated if intestinal function is compromised (see Chapter 138). If malabsorption is a major contributing factor, tube feeding using a disease-specific formula or, alternatively, supplemental or total PN may be indicated. In the presence of severe malnutrition, an anabolic feeding regimen should be initiated either enterally or parenterally depending on intestinal function and malabsorption[106] (Fig. 136–1). When bowel obstruction, SBS, or hypoperfusion of the gut is present, PN is indicated. The anticipated duration of the need for parenteral support will dictate the use of peripheral versus central vein administration of PN (see Chapter 137). Routine reevaluation of the response to nutrition therapy and attainment of nutrition goals should be incorporated into the overall patient care plan.

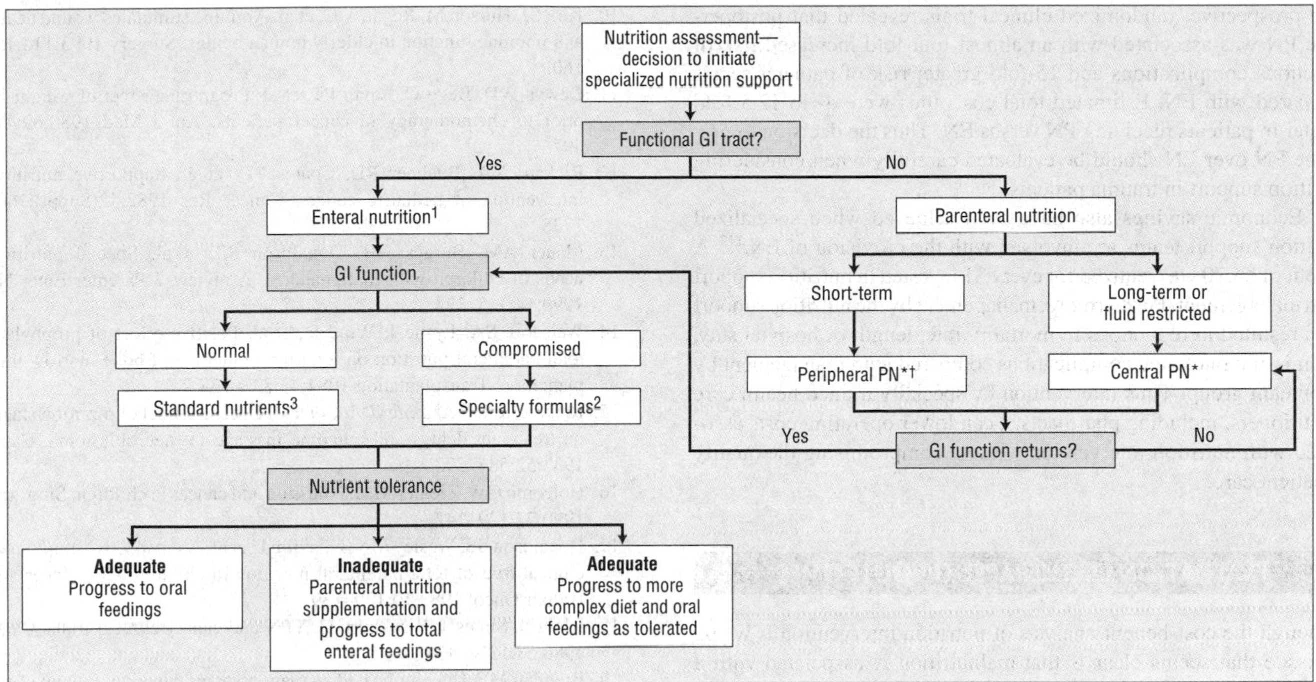

FIGURE 136–1. Routes to deliver nutrition support to adults: Clinical decision algorithm. *Formulation of enteral and parenteral solution should be made considering organ function (e.g., cardiac, renal, respiratory, hepatic). †In selected patients, peripheral parenteral nutrition may be considered to provide partial or total nutrition support for up to 2 weeks in patients who cannot ingest or absorb oral or enteral-tube-delivered nutrients or when central vein parenteral nutrition is not feasible. [1]Short-term: nasogastric, nasojejunal. Long-term: gastrostomy, jejunostomy. Feeding may be more appropriate distal to the pylorus if patient has increased risk of aspiration. [2]Formulas should be tailored to patient GI tolerance and include elemental low/high fat content, lactose-free, fiber-rich, and modular formulas. [3]Polymeric, complete formulas are appropriate.

PHARMACOECONOMIC CONSIDERATIONS

Malnourished patients have increased complications during their hospital course, an increased length of stay (LOS), and thereby increased health care costs.[2,107–109] They are among the 10% of patients who disproportionately consume health care resources.[110] Robinson and associates conducted a prospective study of 100 general medical patients with similar "diagnosis severity" to determine the relationship between nutrition status on admission to the hospital and length of stay and hospital costs.[107] Nutrition status was defined using diet history, history of weight loss, anthropometrics, visceral protein measurements, and delayed cutaneous hypersensitivity. Of the 100 patients, 40 were identified as malnourished, 44 were well nourished, and 16 were borderline. The diagnoses of malnutrition included kwashiorkor (12 patients), marasmus (1 patient), and mixed kwashiorkor-marasmus (27 patients). Malnourished patients had a significantly prolonged LOS compared with normal or borderline patients (15.6 ± 2.2, 8.2 ± 0.7, and 10.2 ± 1.7, mean ± SEM, respectively). Hospital charges also were significantly greater in the malnourished patients than in the normal patients ($16,691 ± $4389 versus $7692 ± $687, mean ± SEM).

In a retrospective study, Reilly and associates evaluated the effect of the likelihood of malnutrition (LOM) at admission on hospital length of stay, costs, and charges in medical and surgical patients.[108] LOM was determined from diet history, physical examination, height-for-weight measurement, serum albumin concentration, and total lymphocyte count. LOM, defined as an abnormality in any one of the preceding criteria, was present in 59% of the medical patients and 48% of the surgical patients on admission. Across all major medical and surgical diagnosis- related groups (DRGs), patients with an LOM had a greater LOS. Consequently, hospital charges, which also were converted to direct variable costs, were greater for patients with LOM.

Although the evidence is strong that malnutrition is associated with increased health care costs, it has been more difficult to establish the cost-benefit or cost savings of nutrition intervention. Based on assumptions derived from the literature, Twomey and Patching[111] concluded that preoperative PN could be cost saving in patients undergoing surgery for gastrointestinal cancer. A similar conclusion applied to a broader patient population is supported by a model that examines the financial implications of malnutrition and nutrition therapy.[110] This model takes into consideration the increased costs associated with an increased LOS, morbidity and mortality caused by malnutrition, as well as the costs of identifying patients at risk for malnutrition, providing nutrition support, and managing the complications associated with the nutrition support. Tucker and Miguel confirmed the association between poor nutritional status and prolonged length of hospital stay and also determined that when nutrition intervention occurred (oral, enteral, or parenteral nutrition), the average LOS was decreased by 2.1 days.[109]

Trauma patients are at an unusually high risk for developing malnutrition due to the hypermetabolic and hypercatabolic state associated with underlying injury. Although several clinical trials have compared the efficacy of EN versus PN, little data are available regarding the cost-effectiveness of these two routes of administration. Trice and colleagues[112] assessed the economic impact of the delivery of EN versus PN to trauma patients. Their evaluation of the data from nine prospective, randomized clinical trials revealed that postoperative PN was associated with an almost four-fold increased risk of infectious complications and 15-fold greater risk of catheter sepsis compared with EN. Estimated total costs thus were 4- to 12.5-fold greater in patients receiving PN versus EN. Thus the decision to prescribe PN over EN should be evaluated carefully when considering nutrition support in trauma patients.

Economic savings also have been achieved when specialized nutrition support teams are involved with the provision of EN.[113] A benefit of $4.20 was realized for every $1 invested in nutrition support team management. Furthermore, management by the nutrition support team resulted in reductions in mortality rate, length of hospital stay, readmission rates, and complications compared with management by a nonteam group. Thus intervention by specially trained health care practitioners, including pharmacists, can lower operating costs associated with nutrition intervention without compromising the quality of patient care.

EVALUATION OF THERAPEUTIC OUTCOMES

Although the cost-benefit analysis of nutrition intervention is weak, the issue that seems clear is that malnutrition is associated with a significant morbidity and mortality in numerous disease states and clinical settings. Furthermore, it is likely that improved patient outcomes can be achieved by a systematic approach to identify the presence of risk factors for malnutrition, quantitate the degree of malnutrition, and initiate nutrition management.[114] The clinician's responsibilities in the management of nutrition disease include the following:

1. Assist in identifying patients at risk for malnutrition and/or candidates for nutrition intervention.
2. Assist in the design of patient-specific nutrition-support regimens.
3. Evaluate and manage all drug-nutrient interactions.
4. Evaluate laboratory data, especially parameters used to determine safety and efficacy of nutrition support.

REFERENCES

1. Gallagher-Allred DR, Voss AC, Finn SC, et al. Malnutrition and clinical outcomes: The case for medical nutrition therapy. J Am Diet Assoc 1996;96:361–366.
2. Coats KG, Morgan SL, Bartolucci AA, Weinsier RL. Hospital-associated malnutrition: A re-evaluation 12 years later. J Am Diet Assoc 1993;93: 27–33.
3. Iyengar GV, Nair PP. Global outlook on nutrition and the environment: Meeting challenges of the next millennium. Sci Total Environ 2000;249:331–346.
4. The state of the world's children 1998: A UNICEF report. Malnutrition: Causes, consequences, and solution. Nutr Rev 1998;56:115–123.
5. Mendez MA, Adair LS. Severity and timing of stunting in the first two years of life affect performance on cognitive tests in late childhood. J Nutr 1999;129:1555–1562.
6. CDC, Pediatric Nutrition Surveillance System—United States, 1980–1991. MMWR Morb Mortal Wkly Rep 1992;41(SS7):1–24.
7. Hendricks KM, Duggan C, Gallagher L, et al.. Malnutrition in hospitalized pediatric patients. Arch Pediatr Adolesc Med 1995;149:1118–1122.
8. Prasad AS. Zinc: An overview. Nutrition 1995;11:93–99.
9. Albina JE. Nutrition and wound healing. J Parenter Enter Nutr 1994;18:367–376.
10. Kirk SJ, Hurson M, Regan MC, et al. Arginine stimulates wound healing and immune function in elderly human beings. Surgery 1993;114:155–160.
11. Dewys WD, Begg C, Lavin PT, et al. Prognostic effect of weight loss prior to chemotherapy in cancer patients. Am J Med 1980;69:491–497.
12. Rickard KA, Baehner RL, Coates TD, et al. Supportive nutritional intervention in pediatric cancer. Cancer Res 1982;42(Suppl):766S–773S.
13. Mauer AM, Burgess JB, Donaldson SS, et al. Special nutritional needs of children with malignancies: A review. J Parenter Enter Nutr 1990;14:315–324.
14. Weisdorf SA, Lysne J, Wind D, et al. Positive effect of prophylactic total parenteral nutrition on long-term outcome of bone marrow transplantation. Transplantation 1987;43:833–838.
15. Rickard KA, Detamore CM, Coates TD, et al. Effect of nutrition staging on treatment delays and outcome in stage IV neuroblastoma. Cancer 1983;52:587–598.
16. Holcomb GW, Ziegler MM. Nutrition and cancer in children. Surg Annu 1990:22:129–142.
17. Donaldson SS, Wesley MN, Ghavimi F, et al. A prospective, randomized clinical trial of total parenteral nutrition in children with cancer. Med Pediatr Oncol 1982;10:129–139.
18. Klein S, Simes J, Blackburn G. TPN and cancer clinical trials. Cancer 1986;58:1378–1386.
19. Brennan MF. Uncomplicated starvation versus cancer cachexia. Cancer Res 1977;37:2359–2364.
20. Kern KA, Norton JA. Cancer cachexia. J Parenter Enteral Nutr 1988;12:286–298.
21. Raiten DJ. Nutrition and HIV. Nutr Clin Pract 1991;6(3 Suppl):1S–94S.
22. Miller TL. Malnutrition: Metabolic changes in children, comparisons with adults. J Nutr 1996;126:2623S–31S.
23. Winter H. Gastrointestinal tract function and malnutrition in HIV-infected children. J Nutr 1996;126:2620S–2622S.
24. Oleske JM, Rothpletz-Puglia PM, Winter H. Historical perspectives on the evolution in understanding the importance of nutritional care in pediatric HIV infection. J Nutr 1996;126:2616S–19S.
25. ASPEN Board of Directors. Acquired immune deficiency syndrome. J Parenter Enter Nutr 1993;17(Suppl):13SA–14SA.
26. Kotler D, Tierney A, Wang J, et al. Magnitude of body-cell-mass depletion and the timing of death from wasting in AIDS. Am J Clin Nutr 1989;50:444–447.
27. Chlebowski RT, Grosvenor MB, Bernhard NH, et al. Nutritional status, gastrointestinal dysfunction, and survival in patients with AIDS. Am J Gastroenterol 1989;84:1288–1292.
28. Trujillo EB, Borlase BC, Bell SJ, et al. Assessment of nutritional status, nutrient intake, and nutrition support in AIDS patients. J Am Diet Assoc 1992;92:477–478.
29. Guenter P, Muurahainen N, Simons G, et al. Relationships among nutritional status, disease progression, and survival in HIV infection. J Acquir Immune Defic Syndr 1993;6:1130–1138.
30. Baum MK, Shor-Posner G, Lu, et al. Micronutrients and HIV-1 disease progression. AIDS 1995;9:1051–1056.
31. Kotler DP, Rosenbaum K, Wang J, et al. Studies of body composition and fat distribution in HIV-infected and control subjects. J Acquir Immune Defic Syndr Hum Retrovirol 1999;20:228–237.
32. Carr A, Semaras K, Chisholm DJ, et al. Pathogenesis of HIV-1 protease inhibitor-associated peripheral lipodystrophy, hyperlipidemia, and insulin resistance. Lancet 1998;351:1881–1883.
33. McKinney RE, Robertson JWR. Effect of human immunodeficiency virus infection on the growth of young children. J Pediatr 1993;123: 579–582.
34. Pollack H, Glasberg H, Lee E, et al. Impaired early growth of infants perinatally infected with human immunodeficiency virus: Correlation with viral load. J Pediatr 1997;130:915–922.
35. Brettler DB, Forsberg A, Bolivar E, et al. Growth failure as a prognostic indicator for progression to acquired immunodeficiency syndrome in children with hemophilia. J Pediatr 1990;117:584–588.

36. McKinney RE, Maha MA, Connor EM, et al. A multicenter trial of oral zidovudine in children with advanced human immunodeficiency virus disease. N Engl J Med 1991;324:1018–1025.
37. Beisel WR. Nutrition and immune function: Overview. J Nutr 1996;126:2611S–2615S.
38. Tang AM, Graham NMH, Saah AJ. Effects of micronutrient intake on survival in human immunodeficiency virus type 1 infection. Am J Epidemiol 1996;143:1244–1256.
39. Singer P, Rothkopf MM, Kvetan V, et al. Risks and benefits of home parenteral nutrition in the acquired immunodeficiency syndrome. J Parenter Enter Nutr 1991;15:75–79.
40. Kotler DP, Tierney AR, Ferraro R, et al. Enteral alimentation and repletion of body cell mass in malnourished patients with acquired immunodeficiency syndrome. Am J Clin Nutr 1991;53:149–154.
41. Kotler DP, Fogleman L, Tierney AR. Comparison of total parenteral nutrition and an oral, semielemental diet on body composition, physical function, and nutrition-related costs in patients with malabsorption due to acquired immunodeficiency syndrome. J Parenter Enter Nutr 1998;22:120–126.
42. Barton RG. Nutrition support in critical illness. Nutr Clin Pract 1994; 9:127–139.
43. Cerra FB, Benitez MR, Blackburn GL, et al. Applied nutrition in ICU patients: A consensus statement of the American College of Chest Physicians. Chest 1997:111:769–778.
44. Giner M, Laviano A, Meguid MM, Gleason JR. In 1995 a correlation between malnutrition and poor outcome in critically ill patients still exists. Nutrition 1996;12:23–29.
45. Peterson VM, Moore EE, Jones TN, et al. Total enteral nutrition versus total parenteral nutrition after major torso injury: Attenuation of hepatic protein reprioritization. Surgery 1988;104:199–207.
46. Chiarelli A, Enzi G, Casadei A, et al. Very early nutrition supplementation in burned patients. Am J Clin Nutr 1990;51:1035–1039.
47. Moore FA, Feliciano DV, Andrassy RJ, et al. Early enteral feeding, compared with parenteral, reduces postoperative septic complications: The results of a meta-analysis. Ann Surg 1992;216:172–183.
48. Kudsk KA, Croce MA, Fabian TC, et al. Enteral versus parenteral feeding: Effects on septic morbidity after blunt and penetrating abdominal trauma. Ann Surg 1992;215:503–513.
49. Heys SD, Walker LG, Smith I, et al. Enteral nutritional supplementation with key nutrients in patients with critical illness and cancer: A meta-analysis of randomized controlled clinical trials. Ann Surg 1999;229:467–477.
50. Beale RJ, Bryg DJ, Bihari DJ. Immunonutrition in the critically ill: A systematic review of clinical outcome. Crit Care Med 1999;27: 2799–805.
51. Bowling TE. Inflammatory bowel disease. Eur J Gastroenterol Hepatol 1995;7:521 527.
52. Afonso JJ, Rombeau JL. Parenteral nutrition for patients with inflammatory bowel disease. In: Rombeau JL, Caldwell MD, eds. Clinical Nutrition: Parenteral Nutrition, 2d ed. Philadelphia, Saunders, 1993:427–441.
53. Seidman EG, LeLeiko N, Ament M, et al. Nutritional issues in pediatric inflammatory bowel disease: Symposium report. J Pediatr Gastroenterol Nutr 1991;12:424–438.
54. ASPEN Board of Directors. Inflammatory bowel disease. J Parenter Enteral Nutr 1993;17(Suppl):18SA–20SA, 45SA.
55. Vargas JH, Sachs P, Ament ME. Chronic intestinal pseudo-obstruction syndrome in pediatrics: Results of a national survey by members of the North American Society for Pediatric Gastroenterology and Nutrition. J Pediatr Gastroenterol Nutr 1988;7:323–332.
56. Thompson JS. Management of the short bowel syndrome. Gastroenterol Clin North Am 1994;23:403–419.
57. Thompson JS, Langnas AN, Pinch LW, et al. Surgical approach to short-bowel syndrome: Experience in a population of 160 patients. Ann Surg 1995;222:600–607.
58. Touloukian RJ, Walker Smith GJ. Normal intestinal length in preterm infants. J Pediatr Surg 1983;18:720–723.
59. Bernard DKH, Shaw MJ. Principles of nutrition therapy for short-bowel syndrome. Nutr Clin Pract 1993;8:153–162.
60. ASPEN Board of Directors. Short bowel syndrome. J Parenter Enter Nutr 1993;17(Suppl):19SA–20SA.
61. Figueroa-Colon R, Harris PR, Birdsong E, et al. Impact of intestinal lengthening on the nutritional outcome for children with short bowel syndrome. J Pediatr Surg 1996;31:912–916.
62. Thompson JS, Pinch LW, Vanderhoof JA, et al. Experience with intestinal lengthening for the short-bowel syndrome. J Pediatr Surg 1991;26: 721–724.
63. Langnas AN, Shaw BW, Antonson DL, et al. Preliminary experience with intestinal transplantation in infants and children. Pediatrics 1996;97: 443–448.
64. Mullen JL, Gertner MH, Buzby GP, et al. Implications of malnutrition in the surgical patient. Arch Surg 1979;114:121–125.
65. Rudman D, Feller AB, Nagraj HS, et al. Relation of serum albumin concentration to death rate in nursing home men. J Parenter Enter Nutr 1987;11:360–363.
66. Meakins JL, Pietsch JB, Bubenick O, et al. Delayed hypersensitivity: An indicator of acquired failure of host defenses in sepsis and trauma. Ann Surg 1977;186:241–250.
67. Harvey KB, Ruggiero JA, Regan CS, et al. Hospital morbidity-mortality risk factors using nutritional assessment. J Clin Nutr 1978;26:251–257.
68. Kaminsky MV, Fitzgerald MJ, Murphy RJ, et al. Correlation of mortality with serum transferrin and anergy. J Parenter Enter Nutr 1977;1:27A.
69. Buzby GP, Mullen JL, Mathews DC, et al. Prognostic nutritional index in gastrointestinal surgery. Am J Surg 1980;139:160–166.
70. Yamanaka H, Nishi M, Kanemaki T, et al. Preoperative nutritional assessment to predict postoperative complication in gastric cancer patients. J Parenter Enter Nutr 1989;13:286–291.
71. Smale BF, Mullen JL, Buzby GP, Rosato EF. The efficacy of nutritional assessment and support in cancer surgery. Cancer 1981;47:2375–2381.
72. Dempsey DT, Buzby GP, Mullen JL. Nutritional assessment in the seriously ill patient. J Am Coll Nutr 1983;2:15–23.
73. Detsky AS, Baker JP, O'Rourke K, et al. Predicting nutrition-associated complications for residents undergoing gastrointestinal surgery. J Parenter Enter Nutr 1987;11:440–446.
74. Klein S, Kinney J, Jeejeebhoy K, et al. Nutrition support in clinical practice: Review of published data and recommendations for future research directions. J Parenter Enter Nutr 1997;21:133–156.
75. Moghissi K, Hornshaw J, Teasdale PR, Dawes EA. Parenteral nutrition in carcinoma of the oesophagus treated by surgery: Nitrogen balance and clinical studies. Br J Surg 1977;64:125–128.
76. Askanazi J, Hensle TW, Starker PM, et al. Effect of immediate postoperative nutritional support on length of hospitalization. Ann Surg 1986;203:236–239.
77. The Veterans Affairs Total Parenteral Nutrition Cooperative Study Group. Perioperative total parenteral nutrition. N Engl J Med 1991;325: 525–532.
78. Northway WH. Bronchopulmonary dysplasia: Then and now. Arch Dis Child 1990;65:1076–1081.
79. deRegnier RA, Guilbert TW, Mills MM, Georgieff MK. Growth failure and altered body composition are established by one month of age in infants with bronchopulmonary dysplasia. J Nutr 1996;126: 168–175.
80. de Gamarra E. Energy expenditure in premature newborns with bronchopulmonary dysplasia. Biol Neonate 1992;61:337–344.
81. Thureen PJ, Hay WW. Conditions requiring special nutritional management. In: Tsang RC, Lucas A, Uauy R, Zlotkin S, eds. Nutritional Needs of the Preterm Infant: Scientific Basis and Practical Guidelines. Baltimore, Williams & Wilkins, 1993:243 265.
82. Wilson DC, McClure G, Halliday HL, et al. Nutrition and bronchopulmonary dysplasia. Arch Dis Child 1991;66:37–38.
83. Kurzner SI, Garg M, Bautista DB, et al. Growth failure in bronchopulmonary dysplasia: Elevated metabolic rates and pulmonary mechanics. J Pediatr 1988;112:73–80.
84. Chye JK, Gray PH. Rehospitalization and growth of infants with bronchopulmonary dysplasia: A matched control study. J Paediatr Child Health 1995;31:105–111.
85. Tammela OKT, Koivisto ME. A 1-year followup of low birth weight infants with and without bronchopulmonary dysplasia: Health, growth,

clinical lung disease, cardiovascular and neurological sequelae. Early Hum Dev 1992;30:109–120.

86. Robertson CMT, Etches PC, Goldson E, Kyle JM. Eight-year school performance, neurodevelopmental, and growth outcome of neonates with bronchopulmonary dysplasia: A comparative study. Pediatrics 1992;89:365–372.
87. Vrienich LA, Bozynski MEA, Shyr Y, et al. The effect of bronchopulmonary dysplasia on growth at school age. Pediatrics 1995;95:855–859.
88. Brunton JA, Saigal S, Atkinson SA. Growth and body composition in infants with bronchopulmonary dysplasia up to 3 months corrected age: A randomized trial of high-energy nutrient-enriched formula fed after hospital discharge. J Pediatr 1998;133:340–345.
89. ASPEN Board of Directors. Necrotizing enterocolitis. J Parenter Enter Nutr 1993;17(Suppl):SA37.
90. Walsh MC, Kliegman RM, Hack M. Severity of necrotizing enterocolitis: Influence on outcome at 2 years of age. Pediatrics 1989;84:808–814.
91. Abbasi S, Pereira GR, Johnson L, et al. Long-term assessment of growth, nutritional status, and gastrointestinal function in survivors of necrotizing entercolitis. J Pediatr 1984;104:550–554.
92. Lai H, Kosorok MR, Sondel SA, et al. Growth status in children with cystic fibrosis based on the national Cystic Fibrosis Patient Registry data: Evaluation of various criteria used to identify malnutrition. J Pediatr 1998:132:478–485.
93. Roulet M. Protein-energy malnutrition in cystic fibrosis patients. Acta Paediatr Suppl 1994;83:43–48.
94. Ramsay BW, Farrell PM, Penchartz P, et al. Consensus report: Nutritional assessment and management of cystic fibrosis. Am J Clin Nutr 1992;55:108–116.
95. Stallings VA, Fung EB, Hofley PM, Scanlin TF. Acute pulmonary exacerbation is not associated with increased energy expenditure in children with cystic fibrosis. J Pediatr 1998;132:493–499.
96. Wilson DC, Kalnins D, Stewart C et al. Challenges in the dietary treatment of cystic fibrosis related diabetes mellitus. Clin Nutr 2000;19: 87–93.
97. Erskine JM, Lingard CD, Sontage MK, Accurso FJ. Enteral nutrition for patients with cystic fibrosis: Comparison of a semi-elemental and non-elemental formula. J Pediatr 1998;132:265–269.
98. Ellis L, Kalnins D, Corey M, et al. Do infants with cystic fibrosis need a protein hydrolystate formula? A prospective, randomized, comparative study. J Pediatr. 1998;132:270–276.
99. Haffner D, Weinfurth A, Manz F et al. Long-term outcome of paediatric patients with hereditary tubular disorders. Nephron 1999;83:250–260.
100. Schwarz SM, Gewitz MH, See CC et al. Enteral nutrition in infants with congenital heart disease and growth failure. Pediatrics 1990;86:368–373.
101. Charlton CP, Buchanan E, Holden CE et al. Intensive enteral feeding in advanced cirrhosis: Reversal of malnutrition without precipitation of hepatic encephalopathy. Arch Dis Child 1992;67:603–607.
102. Cameron JW, Rosenthal A, Olson AD. Malnutrition in hospitalized children with congenital heart disease. Arch Pediatr Adolesc Med 1995;149:1098–1102.
103. Claris-Appiani A, Ardissino GL, Dacco V, et al. Catch-up growth in children with chronic renal failure treated with long-term enteral nutrition. J Parenter Enter Nutr 1995;19:175–178.
104. Varan B, Tokel K, Yilmaz G. Malnutrition and growth failure in cyanotic and acyanotic congenital heart disease with and without pulmonary hypertension. Arch Dis Child 1999;81:49– 52.
105. Unger R, DeKleermaeker M, Gidding SS, Christoffel KK. Calories count: Improved weight gain with dietary intervention in congenital heart disease. Am J Dis Child 1992;146:1078–1084.
106. ASPEN Board of Directors. Routes to deliver nutrition support to adults: Clinical decision algorithm. In: Clinical Pathways and Algorithms for Delivery of Parenteral and Enteral Nutrition Support in Adults. Silver Spring, MD, ASPEN, 1998:5.
107. Robinson G, Goldstein M, Levine GM. Impact of nutritional status on DRG length of stay. J Parenter Enter Nutr 1987;11:49–51.
108. Reilly JJ, Hull SF, Albert N, et al. Economic impact of malnutrition: A model system for hospitalized patients. J Parenter Enter Nutr 1988;12:371–376.
109. Tucker HN, Miguel SG. Cost containment through nutrition intervention (Review). Nutr Rev 1996;54:111–121.
110. Bernstein LH, Shaw-Stiffel TA, Schorow M, Brouillette R. Financial implications of malnutrition (Review). Clin Lab Med 1993;13:491–507.
111. Twomey PL, Patching SC. Cost-effectiveness of nutritional support. J Parenter Enteral Nutr 1985;9:3–10.
112. Trice S, Melnik G, Page CP. Complications and costs of early postoperative parenteral versus enteral nutrition in trauma patients. Nutr Clin Pract 1997;12:114–119.
113. Hassell JT, Games AD, Shaffer B, Harkins, LE. Nutrition support team management of enterally fed patients in a community hospital is cost-beneficial. J Am Diet Assoc 1994;94:993–998.
114. ASPEN Board of Directors. Rationale for adult nutrition support guidelines. J Parenter Enter Nutr 1993;17(Suppl):5SA–6SA.

137

PARENTERAL NUTRITION

Todd W. Mattox

Maintenance of adequate nutrition status during illness has been recognized for over 50 years as an integral part of the medical treatment plan for patients who are unable to use normal physiologic means of nourishment. Successful techniques for providing intravenous nutrition support were introduced to clinical practice in the early 1960s.[1] Dilute nutrient solutions containing glucose with or without hydrolyzed protein were infused peripherally along with intravenous fat emulsion to provide adequate calories. Metabolic complications associated with fluid overload and electrolyte imbalances stimulated the investigation of central venous access. The use of larger vessels permitted infusion of more concentrated formulas, which decreased the fluid volume required and avoided the phlebitis that occurred commonly when hypertonic infusions were given peripherally.

By the late 1960s, Rhoads and Dudrick had documented continued growth and improvement in nutritional markers in humans with the use of central intravenous nutrition.[1] By the early 1970s, intravenous nutrition was used to sustain growth and development in premature infants.[2]

During the subsequent 25 to 30 years, clinical experience and research resulted in the development of standard protocols that promoted better patient care and resulted in a decline in complications associated with parenteral nutrition (PN) therapy.[3] The scope of practice for nutrition support clinicians has broadened as a result of increasing knowledge regarding the metabolic consequences associated with acute injury and chronic disease states. The increase in the number of nutritional products, techniques, and equipment designed for use in providing nutritional care also has contributed to growth of the discipline. Depending on the level of nutritional intervention required, nutrition support clinicians may use specially formulated parenteral or enteral nutrients to maintain or restore optimal nutrition status.[4] The pharmacist's role in providing safe and effective nutrition-support care requires a clear understanding of the principles of patient selection, initial therapy design, preparation and dispensing of the nutritional formulations, and outcome monitoring[5–8] (Table 137–1). This chapter reviews indications for PN, components of PN formulations, routes of intravenous administration, practical aspects of regimen design, solution admixture, outcome monitoring, and management of complications for both adult and pediatric (neonates, infants, and children) patients.

DESIRED OUTCOMES

The overall objective of nutrition support therapy is to promote positive clinical outcomes of an illness or improve a patient's quality of life. Four fundamental steps are key to providing optimal care for patients who require nutrition support. They are definition of nutrition goals, determination of nutrient requirements for achievement of the nutrition goals, delivery of the required nutrients, and subsequent assessment of the nutrition regimen.[7,8]

A patient's nutrition goals can be established after a thorough nutritional assessment (see Chapter 135). Nutrient requirements and an appropriate route for delivery of the required nutrients then can be determined (see Chapters 135 and 136). Goals of nutrition support include correction of the patient's caloric and nitrogen imbalances, fluid or electrolyte abnormalities, and any known vitamin or trace element abnormalities without causing or worsening other metabolic complications. Specific caloric goals include energy equilibrium and preservation of fat calorie stores in well-nourished individuals and positive energy balance in malnourished patients with depleted endogenous fat stores. Obese patients with excess endogenous fat stores (>120% of ideal body weight) may require less caloric support than nonobese patients with the same clinical condition.[9] Specific nitrogen goals are positive nitrogen balance or nitrogen equilibrium and improvement in the serum concentration of visceral protein markers such as transferrin or prealbumin.

The gastrointestinal (GI) tract is the optimal route for providing nutrients unless obstruction, severe pancreatitis, or other GI complications are present[10] (see Fig. 136–1). Other considerations that may have an impact on determination of an appropriate route for nutrition support include expected duration of nutrition therapy and risk of aspiration. Patients who have a nonfunctional GI tract or are otherwise not a candidate for enteral nutrition (EN) may benefit from PN. Use of the intravenous route for nutrition support is also commonly referred to as total parenteral nutrition (TPN) or hyperalimentation. Routine monitoring is necessary to ensure that the nutrition regimen is suitable for a given patient as his or her clinical condition changes and to minimize or treat complications early.

INDICATIONS FOR NUTRITION SUPPORT

Although improvement in nutrition status as defined by various clinical nutrition markers has been reported in patients who received PN, the impact on clinical outcome has been difficult to demonstrate. Several investigations have reported a positive effect of PN on complications and mortality, whereas others have failed to demonstrate any difference.[11–13] Early studies have been criticized for defects in study design such as small sample sizes, inappropriate randomization, and inconsistent baseline nutrition status among the study group, which hindered demonstration of the effectiveness of PN therapy. However, the association between malnutrition and development of complications and mortality has been well documented.[14,15] These conflicting data have complicated identification of the patient who is most likely to benefit from PN. Guidelines regarding the candidates for PN are based on clinical experience and investigations in specific patient populations where PN therapy is often prone to misuse such as preoperative patients or patients receiving chemotherapy[16,17] (Table 137–2).

In a continuing effort to define appropriate candidates for specialized nutrition intervention, representatives from the National Institutes of Health, ASPEN, and the American Society of Clinical Nutrition authored a critical review of the clinical use of nutrition support. The group focused on nutrition assessment; nutrition support

TABLE 137–1. Scope of Practice for Nutrition Support Pharmacists

Assessment of the patient's nutrition care needs
- Determine nutrient requirements based on patient's data.
- Prevent and/or identify nutrient–nutrient, drug–nutrient, drug–drug, and drug–disease/condition interactions.
- Assess suitability for specialized nutrition support.

Development of a nutrition care plan
- Define goals and objectives of specialized nutrition support therapy.
- Select the preferred route for administration of nutrition support therapy.
- Design patient-specific feeding formulations.

Implementation of the nutrition care plan
- Obtain or write prescriptions for feeding formulations.
- Be proficient with techniques of compounding feeding formulations.
- Perform or supervise the compounding and dispensing of parenteral feeding formulations.

Monitoring the patient response to the nutrition therapy
- Evaluate laboratory data to determine the patient's clinical, nutritional, and metabolic responses to specialized nutrition support.
- Prevent and/or identify nutrient–nutrient, drug–nutrient, drug–drug, and drug–disease/condition interactions.
- Evaluate continued need for specialized nutrition support.

Administrative management
- Participate in development of policy and procedures for patient care and operational aspects of specialized nutrition support.

Quality of care
- Develop and implement quality improvement activities directed at the process of nutritional and metabolic care.

Advancement of nutrition support pharmacy practice
- Contribute to the professional development of pharmacists and other health care professionals and to the education of patients through presentations, publications, and research.

Adapted from Ref. 5.

in patients with GI diseases, wasting diseases, and critical illness; and perioperative nutrition support.[11,13] While the intent of the report was to identify future directions for research, it may serve as a means for an institution to evaluate its current practices.

Determining the most appropriate time to initiate PN is difficult. The decision to initiate PN is based on the assessment that the patient cannot meet his or her nutritional requirements with use of the GI tract. This assessment must include an evaluation of the potential risks of initiating therapy, such as infection and other metabolic abnormalities.[18] In general, the younger the patient, the sooner PN should be considered. For example, preterm and term infants who have failed EN support or have a dysfunctional GI tract may benefit from initiation of PN after 1 to 3 days of suboptimal nutritional intake.[19] Well-nourished children who are not candidates for EN should be considered candidates for PN after 5 to 7 days of suboptimal nutritional intake.[20] Children with preexisting malnutrition likely will require earlier intervention. Adults who are not candidates for EN should be considered candidates for PN after 7–10 days of suboptimal nutritional intake.[13,17] Guidelines for older children are similar to those in adults.

PN COMPONENTS

PN solutions should provide the optimal combination of macronutrients and micronutrients to meet the specific nutritional requirements of the patient. Macronutrients include water, protein, dextrose, and intravenous lipid emulsion. Micronutrients include vitamins, trace elements, and electrolytes. Both macronutrients and micronutrients are necessary for maintenance of normal metabolism. In general, macronutrients are used for energy (dextrose, fat) and as structural substrates (protein, fats). Micronutrients are required to support a variety of metabolic activities necessary for cellular homeostasis such as enzymatic reactions, fluid balance, and regulation of electrophysiologic processes. These components usually require individualized adjustments as the patient's clinical condition dictates changes in metabolic stress, organ function, fluid and electrolyte balance, and acid-base status.

AMINO ACIDS

Protein in PN solutions is provided in the form of crystalline amino acids (CAAs), which are used primarily for protein synthesis. Including the caloric contribution from protein when calculating calories provided by the PN regimen is controversial.[21] While sufficient energy substrate should be provided to allow use of amino acids for protein synthesis rather than as an energy source, oxidation of amino acids for energy has been demonstrated in critically ill patients and is thought to occur because of metabolic derangements seen during severe metabolic stress.[22] Hence some practice settings may differ in expressing calories provided by a PN regimen as total calories (protein, carbohydrate, and fat calories) or nonprotein calories (carbohydrate and fat calories). When oxidized for energy, 1 g of protein yields 4 kcal.

Commercially available CAA solutions may be categorized as standard amino acid solutions or modified amino acid solutions. Standard CAA solutions are designed for use in patients with "normal" organ function and nutritional requirements (Table 137–3). Although standard CAA solutions differ in the proportion of specific amino acids, they contain a balanced profile of essential, semiessential, and nonessential L-amino acids. Despite these differences, similar effects on markers of protein use have been reported.[22] These products also differ in protein concentration and total nitrogen (11% to 17%) and electrolyte content. Because the nitrogen concentration of dietary protein is approximately 16%, 6.25 (100 g protein/16 g nitrogen) is commonly accepted as the conversion figure for calculating the amount of nitrogen provided by CAA protein. Differences in nitrogen content per gram of amino acids among CAA products may affect calculation of nitrogen amounts infused when determining nitrogen balance.[22,23] The clinical significance of these differences in calculations of nitrogen balance for routine clinical use is not known.[23]

Electrolyte composition of standard CAA solutions varies from small, obligatory amounts to the provision of maintenance requirement of most electrolytes for an adult. The contribution of electrolytes from CAA solutions must be considered when determining a patient's individual requirements. The availability of CAA in several different concentrations facilitates compounding of patient-specific PN regimens. Highly concentrated products (10% and 15%) are attractive for use in critically ill patients who typically require fluid restriction but have large protein needs. Modified amino acid solutions are designed for use in patients who have altered protein requirements such as those with hepatic encephalopathy, renal failure, and metabolic stress/trauma, as well as neonates and pediatric patients (see Table 137–3). These solutions tend to be more expensive than standard CAA solutions. The rationale for and clinical efficacy of modified amino acids in disease-specific PN regimens is controversial (see Chapter 139).

Several commercially available CAA solutions are designed to provide conditionally essential amino acids (CEAAs). CEAAs are

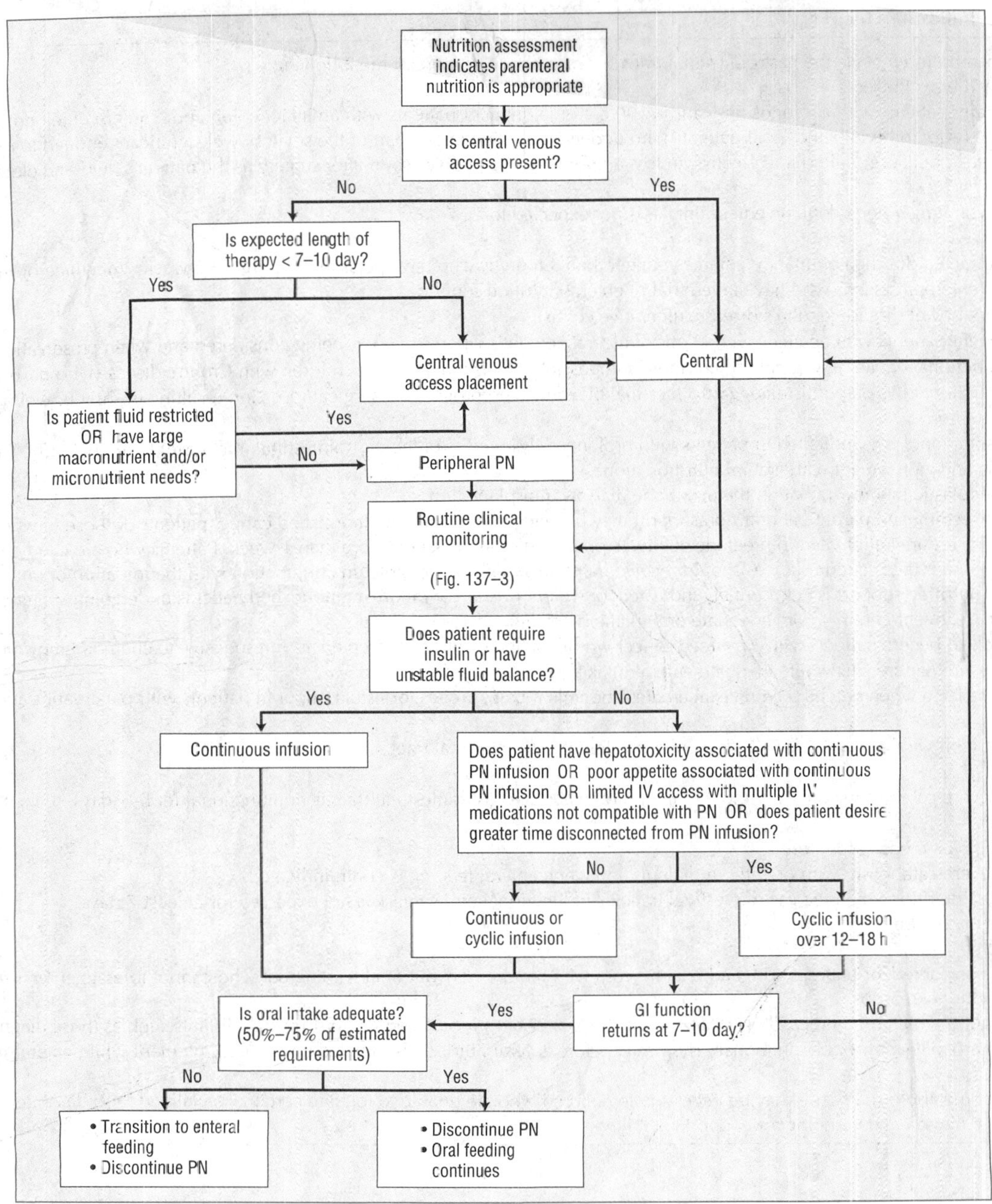

FIGURE 137–1. The route of PN and the infusion pattern (type) depend on the patient's clinical stature and the expected length of therapy

considered nonessential during health because they are produced from other amino acids. However, under certain physiologic conditions such as prematurity or sepsis, these amino acids cannot be synthesized in sufficient quantities.[22] CAA solutions specifically designed for use in neonates and some pediatric patients contain increased amounts of taurine, aspartic acid, and glutamic acid. Other CEAAs, such as cysteine, carnitine, and glutamine, are not available in commercial CAA solutions in pharmacologic amounts because they are relatively unstable or poorly soluble.[22]

PN solutions therefore may need to be modified by clinicians to provide supplemental amounts of CEAAs. Cysteine is a CEAA in preterm and term infants that may be added to PN solutions at the time of compounding. An additional benefit of including cysteine is that it enhances calcium and phosphate solubility in PN solutions by decreasing the solution pH.[24] Carnitine is a quarternary amine required for transport of free fatty acids into the mitochondria for β-oxidation and energy production.[25] Newborns are at risk for carnitine deficiency because of their immature synthetic and conservation mechanisms. Decreased plasma carnitine concentrations are associated with impaired lipid metabolism in patients receiving intravenous lipid emulsion (IVLE).[26,27] Supplemental carnitine may be added to the PN solution at the time of compounding. However, routine use in patients who are not receiving treatment for carnitine deficiency associated with an inborn error of metabolism is controversial.[26]

Glutamine is the most abundant free amino acid in the body and is an important intermediate for many metabolic processes. Glutamine is reported to have an important role in maintaining intestinal integrity, immune function, and protein synthesis during conditions of metabolic stress.[22,27] Investigations in humans and animals have reported positive effects on nutritional markers such as nitrogen balance, whereas others have reported significant improvement

TABLE 137–2. Indications for TPN

1. Inability to absorb nutrients via the gastrointestinal tract because of one or more of the following:
   a. Massive small bowel resection.
   Adults: Usually patients with a jejunostomy and <100 cm of jejunum or patients with an intact colon and <50 cm of jejunum or ileum.
   Pediatrics: PN should be initiated in all patients who undergo resection of any part of the small bowel significant enough to result in restriction of enteral intake because of fluid and electrolyte loss and/or malabsorption as soon after surgery as the patient's fluid and electrolyte balance stabilizes.
   b. Intractable vomiting when adequate enteral intake is not expected for 5–7 days.
   c. Severe diarrhea
   Chronic protracted diarrhea of infancy: Infants younger than 3 months who have persistent diarrhea >2 weeks with three or more stool cultures negative for enteropathogens who have failed trial of enteral nutrition support.
   d. Inflammatory bowel disease (Crohn's disease, ulcerative colitis)
   PN may benefit patients with acute exacerbations of ulcerative colitis when surgery is being considered and when preservation of lean body mass and functional capacity with enteral nutrition is impossible. PN is indicated for children with Crohn's disease who have near complete bowel obstruction, high-output fistulae, gastrointestinal bleeding, and progressive surgical resection resulting in short bowel syndrome.
   e. Bowel obstruction
   Pseudo-obstruction: PN is indicated in patients with prolonged dysmotility of the gastrointestinal tract distal to the pylorus or in patients who cannot grow and gain weight with enteral nutrition alone.
2. Cancer: antineoplastic therapy, radiation therapy, bone marrow transplantation
   a. Enteral tube feeding and parenteral nutrition support may benefit some severely malnourished cancer patients or those in whom gastrointestinal or other toxicities are anticipated to preclude adequate oral nutritional intake for more than 1 week. Patients who are candidates for nutrition intervention under these circumstances should receive nutrition support, if possible, in conjunction with the initiation of oncologic therapy.
   b. Specialized nutrition support is not routinely indicated for well-nourished or mildly malnourished patients undergoing surgery, chemotherapy, or radiation treatment and in whom adequate oral intake is anticipated.
   c. PN is unlikely to benefit patients with advanced cancer whose malignancy is documented as unresponsive to chemotherapy or radiation therapy.
3. Moderate to severe pancreatitis when adequate enteral intake is not expected for 5–7 days.
   PN should be used when enteral feeding exacerbates abdominal pain, ascites, or fistula ouput in patients with pancreatitis and limited oral intake.
4. Severe malnutrition with a temporary (5–7 days) nonfunctional gastrointestinal tract.
5. Critical care
   Moderate to severe catabolism with or without malnutrition when the gastrointestinal tract is nonfunctional for 5–7 days. (e.g., major surgery, trauma, sepsis).
6. Organ failures (liver, renal, respiratory)
   Moderate to severe catabolism with or without malnutrition when enteral feeding is contraindicated.
7. Preoperative malnutrition when the gastrointestinal tract is not functional and surgery is not expected for at least 7 days.
8. Hyperemesis gravidarum
9. Eating disorders
   PN should be considered for patients with anorexia nervosa who require nonvolitional feeding but who cannot tolerate enteral support for physical or emotional reasons.
10. Low birth weight (premature) infants: PN is indicated 1–2 days after birth in selected low birth weight infants such as those diagnosed with necrotizing enterocolitis or bronchopulmonary dysplasia, before enteral nutrition is initiated and as a supplement while enteral nutrition is being advanced.
11. Inborn errors of metabolism: PN use may be necessary in children who are unable to tolerate certain specialized formulas enterally because of disease-induced nausea and vomiting and poor palatability of the formulas.

Adapted from ref. 17.

in other outcome markers such as decreased length of hospitalization, incidence of infections, and GI toxicities associated with chemotherapy or radiation.[28] However, the best adult candidate for response to glutamine therapy has not been clearly identified.[28] The clinical utility of glutamine in neonates is less clear.[29] The clinical use of glutamine is further complicated because there is no commercially available intravenous glutamine formulation. Currently available CAA solutions do not contain glutamine because of poor solubility and instability.[29] Use of intravenous glutamine requires special manufacturing techniques not readily available in many institutional pharmacies.[30] The expense of extemporaneously preparing glutamine-containing PN solutions has been justified by some clinicians on the basis of the cost savings associated with improved clinical outcomes.[28] Additional controlled trials are warranted to clearly justify risks and costs associated with extemporaneous compounding before routine use of intravenous glutamine can be recommended.[22,28] Dipeptide amino acids are a potential parenteral source for CEAAs that may provide a solution to the instability and solubility limitations. Dipeptides are synthesized by combining two amino acids with a peptide bond. The resulting protein is more soluble and stable than the individual amino acids.[22] Intravenous dipeptide formulations would be advantageous clinically because they incorporate higher concentrations of some specific amino acids, as well as some low- solubility, low-stability amino acids that are omitted or present in small quantities in current CAA solutions. In addition, use of dipeptides would allow formulation of CAA solutions with a higher nitrogen content. Further studies are needed to assess long-term safety and optimal combinations of amino acids in different disease states. Examples of commercially available CAA products and some investigational amino acids are listed in Table 137–3.

DEXTROSE

The primary energy source in PN solutions is carbohydrate, usually in the form of dextrose monohydrate. This nutritional substrate is available in a variety of concentrations ranging from 5% to 70%. When oxidized, each gram of hydrated dextrose provides 3.4 kcal. Dextrose

TABLE 137–3. Macronutrient Components of Parenteral Nutrition Solutions

Nutritional Substrate	Intravenous Source	Commercial Product (Manufacturer)		Comments
Fluid	Sterile water for injection USP	Various manufacturers		
Nitrogen	Crystalline amino acids			
	• Standard solutions	Aminosyn	(Abbott)	Contain a balanced profile of essential, semi-essential, and non-essential L-amino acids
		Aminosyn II	(Abbott)	
		FreAmine III	(Braun)	
		Travasol	(Clintec)	
		Clinisol	(Clintec)	
		Novamine	(Clintec)	
	• Disease-specific solutions			
	Hepatic encephalopathy	Aminosyn HF	(Abbott)	Amino acid profile include higher concentrations of BCAA and lower concentrations of AAA and methionine.
		Hepatasol	(Clintec)	
		Hepatamine	(Braun)	
	Renal failure	Aminosyn RF	(Abbott)	Amino acid profile includes higher concentrations of EAA and histidine.
		RenAmine	(Clintec)	
		Aminess	(Clintec)	
		NephrAmine	(Braun)	
	Metabolic stress/trauma	Aminosyn HBC	(Abbott)	Amino acid profile provides standard essential, semi-essential, and non-essential amino acids with higher concentrations of BCAA
		BranchAmin[a]	(Clintec)	
		FreAmine HBC	(Braun)	
	Pediatrics	Aminosyn PF	(Abbott)	Amino acid profile includes standard essential, semi-essential, and non-essential amino acids with lower concentrations of methionine, phenylalanine, and glycine. These solutions also contain taurine, glutamate, and aspartate.
		Trophamine	(Braun)	
	• Conditional or essential amino acids[b]			
	Cysteine HCL		(GensiaSicor)	
	L-Carnitine	Carnitor	(SigmaTau)	
	L-Glutamine			Investigational
	• Intravenous dipeptides			
	• L-Alanyl-L-glutamine			Investigational
	• Glycyl-L-tyrosine			Investigational
	• L-Alanyl-L-tyrosine			Investigational
	• N-acetyl-L-tyrosine			Used in Trophamine (Braun)
Energy				
Carbohydrate	Dextrose	Various manufacturers		
	Glycerol			Used in ProcalAmine (Braun)
	Xylitol			Investigational
Fat	Intravenous fat emulsion			
	• LCT emulsions {oil source}	Liposyn II	(Abbott)	{soybean/safflower}
		Liposyn III	(Abbott)	{soybean}
		Intralipid	(Clintec)	{soybean}
	• LCT/MCT combination			Investigational
	• Short-chain fatty acids			Investigational
	• Omega-3 fatty acids			Investigational

BCAA = Branched-chain amino acids (leucine, isoleucine, valine); AAA = aromatic amino acids (includes phenylalanine and tyrosine).
EAA = essential amino acids (leucine, isoleucine, valine, phenylalanine, tryptophan, methionine, threonine, and lysine); LCT = long-chain triglycerides.
MCT = medium-chain triglyceride.
[a]Used as a supplement to a standard crystalline amino acid solution to increase BCAA content.
[b]Used as supplements to crystalline amino acid solutions.

is oxidized at a maximum rate of 4–7 mg/kg per minute in adults receiving intravenous dextrose infusions.[31] Premature infants have a higher rate of glucose oxidation and use because of their relatively large body proportion of metabolically active organs. Oxidation rates of 12–15 mg/kg per minute have been reported in very low-birth-weight neonates and term infants.[32 33] However, an investigation of critically ill children up to 11 years old reported glucose oxidation rates similar to those observed in adults.[33] The appropriate dose of intravenous dextrose depends on the patient's age and clinical condition. If the dextrose infusion rate exceeds the glucose oxidation rate metabolically expensive pathways such as glycogen repletion and lipid synthesis will be favored.

In addition, higher infusion rates also may contribute to the development of hyperglycemia, excess carbon dioxide production, and increased biochemical markers for liver function.[33] Although infusion rates of up to 11–12 mg/kg per minute have been recommended for young children, the recommended dose of dextrose for routine clinical care rarely exceeds 5 mg/kg per minute in older critically ill children and adults.[16,20,30,31,33]

Insulin is essential to transport dextrose into many cells such as skeletal muscle for oxidation to yield energy. Because many clinical conditions associated with impaired insulin secretion or activity my complicate provision of PN, non-insulin-dependent sources of carbohydrate have been investigated (see Table 137–3). Of these nutrients, only glycerol is available commercially for clinical use in humans as a carbohydrate source for PN. Glycerol is a sugar alcohol that provides 4.3 kcal/g and is available as a 3% solution in combination with 3% amino acids and supplemental electrolytes (ProcalAmine, B. Braun). This product is nearly isotonic, so it may be infused peripherally. A major disadvantage of this formula is the dilute concentrations of amino acids and carbohydrate. Most adult patients require up to 3–4 L/day of ProcalAmine solution together with lipid emulsion as a caloric source to provide minimum energy requirements.[34] Intravenous glycerol use in catabolic adults is safe and effective, but similar data are not available for infants and children.[35]

LIPID EMULSION

IVLE is used as a concentrated source of calories as well as a source of essential fatty acids. Commercially available IVLE products differ in source of triglycerides (soybean oil or a combination of soybean oil and safflower oil), fatty acid content, and commercially available concentrations (10%, 20% and 30%) (see Table 137–3). These products also contain egg phospholipids as an emulsifying agent and glycerol to make the emulsion isotonic. Although the caloric contribution of fat is 9 kcal/g, the caloric content of IVLE is 1.1 kcal/mL for 10% emulsion, 2 kcal/mL for 20% emulsion, and 3 kcal/mL for 30% emulsion because of the caloric contribution of the egg phospholipid and glycerol.[36] The sources of triglyceride in IVLEs differ in fatty acid composition. Soybean oil emulsions contain approximately 50% to 55% linoleic acid and 4% to 10% linolenic acid, whereas IVLEs that contain safflower oil are made of approximately 66% linoleic acid and 4% linolenic acid.[36] Linolenic acid, an omega-3 fatty acid, and linoleic acid, an omega-6 fatty acid, are both polyunsaturated long-chain triglycerides (LCTs).[37] IVLE products also differ in phospholipid and triglyceride concentrations. Higher-concentrated IVLEs (20%, 30%) have a lower phospholipid-to-triglyceride ratio compared with 10% IVLE.[38] Because higher amounts of circulating phospholipids have been associated with impaired triglyceride clearance in neonates and infants, 20% IVLE is the preferred product for this population.[19,20,30,38,39]

Both types of IVLEs are effective in the treatment or prevention of essential fatty acid deficiency (EFAD). EFAD is the result of a biochemical deficiency of linoleic acid and arachidonic acid, which are considered essential in humans.[40] Although linolenic acid may be essential, all commercially available IVLEs contain soybean oil as a predominant source of linolenic acid. These fatty acids are important for a variety of functions such as cellular integrity, platelet function, and wound healing.[20,37,40] Normally, linoleic acid is converted to the tetraene arachidonic acid. When linoleic acid is not present in sufficient amounts, oleic acid is converted to the triene 5,8,11-eicosatrienoic acid, a fatty acid of lesser physiologic integrity, and EFAD occurs. EFAD may be prevented by providing 2% to 5% of total calories as linoleic acid. This may be achieved in most adult patients by giving approximately 100 g IVLE weekly.[41] Neonates and infants require a minimum of 0.5–1 g/kg daily.[19,20]

As a caloric source, IVLE is most useful in metabolically stressed patients, those with pancreatitis or diabetes, and those with carbon dioxide-retaining ventilator dependency.[42] The use of IVLE may facilitate provision of adequate calories and minimize complications of nutrition therapy such as hyperglycemia, hepatotoxicity, or increased production of carbon dioxide. The IVLE dose is usually started at 0.5 g/kg per day in neonates and 0.5–1 g/kg per day in older children and increased daily by 0.5–1 g/kg per day to a maximum of 3–4 g/kg per day.[19,20,38] More conservative doses are warranted for jaundiced neonates because fatty acids released during hydrolysis can displace bilirubin from albumin- binding sites and thereby increase the risk of kernicterus.[16,38,39] The dose of IVLE in adults should not exceed 2.5 g/kg per day or 60% of total daily calories. However, some practitioners have recommended lower doses of approximately 1–1.5 g/kg per day, not to exceed 30% to 35% of total calories to minimize negative effects of long-chain fatty acids on immune function.[16,37,39,42] Plasma clearance of IVLE is directly related to gestational age of infants and appears to be influenced by rate of infusion.[20,38,39] Plasma lipid clearance is improved in infants when IVLE is given as continuous infusion.[38,39] In addition, data in animals and humans suggest that rapid infusion of the current long-chain fatty acid formulations may have a negative impact on immunocompetence by saturating the reticuloendothelial system.[37,39] Although manufacturer's information recommends IVLE infusion over 4 to 8 hours for adults and a rate of 50–100 mL/h in infants and older children, infusion over 16 to 24 hours or 0.15 g/kg per hour or less in adults and neonates, respectively, appears to be the best clinical strategy to promote IVLE clearance and minimize risk of negative effects on immune function.[16,38,39]

The manufacturer's guidelines recommend initiating IVLE in adults with a test dose of 0.5–1 mL/min for the first 15 to 30 minutes and 0.05–0.1 mL/min for 10 to 15 minutes in pediatric patients because of the potential for an immediate hypersensitivity reaction. In most patients, this is probably not necessary because of the relatively low incidence and benign nature of acute adverse reactions. In addition, infusion over 24 hours eliminates the need for a test dose because the infusion rate is less than the test-dose rate recommended by the manufacturer. Although the frequency of acute adverse effects is reported to be less than 1% with current formulations, patients receiving their first dose of IVLE should be monitored for dyspnea, chest tightness, palpitations, and chills. Headache, nausea, and fever also have been reported and may be associated with a rapid infusion rate. In general, the use of IVLE is contraindicated in patients with an impaired ability to clear lipid emulsion, such as patients with pathologic hyperlipidemia and hypertriglyceridemia associated with pancreatitis.[39] Finally, patients with a reported egg allergy should be evaluated carefully for the nature and severity of the reaction before deciding to initiate a lipid-based PN regimen. Hepatic abnormalities such as elevated transaminases, hepatomegaly, and intrahepatic cholestasis have been reported with multiple infusions, although these alterations are transient and usually are associated with excessive doses.[42]

Commercially available 10% and 20% IVLE products may be administered either by central or peripheral route. They may be added directly to the PN solution as a total nutrient admixture (TNA) or 3-in-1 system (lipids, protein, glucose, and additives), or they may be piggybacked with the CAA-dextrose solution.[42] The more concentrated 30% IVLE is only approved for use in the preparation of TNA and is not intended for direct intravenous administration.

The negative effects of LCTs on immune function have stimulated a search for new sources of lipids.[37,43] Medium-chain triglycerides (MCTs) may offer several advantages, especially for critically ill patients. MCTs are hydrolyzed and cleared more rapidly than LCTs, and they do not accumulate in the liver. In addition, MCTs do not require carnitine for entrance into mitochondria for oxidation.

However, MCTs are not a source of essential fatty acids. Subsequent studies of intravenous MCT-LCT mixtures in a number of patients have demonstrated safety and efficacy comparable with standard LCT emulsions.[37,43] Several MCT- LCT products are available in Europe, although no intravenous MCT formulations are currently available commercially in the United States. Other intravenous lipid formulations currently being investigated contain omega-3 polyunsaturated fatty acids (PUFAs).[44] Current IVLEs contain omega-6 PUFAs as linoleic acid and omega-3 PUFAs as linolenic acid. Omega-3 PUFAs are metabolized to cytokine mediators, which may be less inflammatory and immunosuppressive than those derived from omega-6 PUFAs. The effect of IVLE administration on immune function, as well as patient morbidity and mortality, is not clear.[45,46] However, investigations of enteral solutions with a higher concentration of omega-3 PUFAs have reported decreased infections and improvement in in vitro immunologic indices in critically ill patients.[47] Although IVLE products remain the most common source of parenteral lipids, a number of drugs have been introduced that contain lipid as either a vehicle for delivery or as a portion of the drug molecular formulation. Propofol, an intravenous anesthetic, is delivered in a soybean oil-in-water emulsion that is essentially the same as Intralipid 10%. This agent is used commonly for continuous sedation of ventilated patients and should be considered a potentially significant source of calories that may require adjustment of a patient's nutrition regimen.[48] The antifungal amphotericin B is available in several lipid-containing combinations such as liposomal and lipid complex formulations. The caloric contribution from these products when used in standard doses generally is small and is not relevant clinically.[49] While use of amphotericin B with IVLE admixtures is controversial, the caloric contribution from these mixtures is significant and should be considered when determining a patient's nutrition regimen.[49]

VITAMINS

Vitamins are necessary for the maintenance of normal metabolism and cellular function. Fat-soluble vitamins (i.e., A, D, E, and K) are stored extensively in the body's fat tissue, whereas water-soluble vitamins are stored in limited amounts by the body. Maintenance guidelines for daily parenteral vitamin supplements have been established by the Nutrition Advisory Group of the American Medical Association (NAG-AMA) for adults, children, and infants.[50] The NAG-AMA identified 13 essential vitamins that include four fat-soluble vitamins and nine water-soluble vitamins. These guidelines are based on the recommended daily allowances (RDAs), which are designed to meet requirements of healthy people. Vitamin requirements for preterm infants and patients with metabolic stress or specific organ failures are controversial.[16,51,52,53] Revised NAG-AMA recommendations for parenteral vitamin requirements in infants and children reflect data reported in pediatric patients who received currently available formulations.[53] In general, the revised recommendations focused on changes for preterm infants requiring PN.

Several adult and pediatric parenteral multiple vitamin products formulated to comply with the NAG-AMA guidelines are available commercially. Recently, MVI-Pediatric (NeoSan Pharmaceuticals) and Infuvite Pediatric (Baxter) were formulated to meet the revised NAG-AMA guidelines for infants weighing less than 1 kg to children up to 11 years old. However, there are no commercially available intravenous multivitamin products designed to specifically meet the unique requirements of premature infants including higher vitamin A and lower vitamin B_1, B_2, B_6, and B_{12} doses relative to recommendations for term infants and older children. Children older than 11 years of age should receive an adult vitamin formulation.

Parenteral multiple-vitamin formulations designed for use in pediatric patients provide 13 essential vitamins, including vitamin K. In the past, parenteral multiple-vitamin formulations for adults contained only 12 essential vitamins. Vitamin K was not included to minimize the risk of a drug-nutrient interaction in patients receiving anticoagulants, which antagonize vitamin K. However, in 2000, the Food and Drug Administration (FDA) mandated reformulation of adult parenteral multiple-vitamin products to include 150 μg vitamin K in addition to higher doses of vitamins B_1, B_6, and C.[54] The NAG-AMA recommendation for vitamin K in adults is 2–4 mg weekly. However, other practitioners have recommended larger doses of 5–10 mg weekly. An investigation of patients receiving long-term IVLE-containing PN at home suggests that supplemental vitamin K may not be necessary.[55] Vegetable oils such as soybean and safflower oils used in IVLEs are a natural source of phylloquinine (vitamin K_1). However, the vitamin K concentration depends on the type and concentration of vegetable oil in the IVLE.[55,56] Mean concentrations of 13.2 and 26.5 μg/100 mL were reported for 10% and 20% Liposyn II (Abbott), which contains both soybean and safflower oil.[56] Mean concentrations of 30.9 and 67.5 μg/100 mL were reported for 10% and 20% Intralipid (Kabivitrum), which contains only soybean oil. The bioavailability of vitamin K_1 from IVLEs is not known. While some have reported maintenance of normal plasma vitamin K_1 concentrations and normal prothrombin times in small numbers of patients receiving long-term IVLE-containing PN at home, use of PN without routine vitamin K supplementation in adults cannot be recommended at this time.

Vitamin K may be given intramuscularly or subcutaneously or added to the PN solution.[58] Vitamin requirements may be altered in malnutrition and other specific disease states or with certain drug therapies. Individual and combination products are available to provide additional or tailored supplementation, which may be necessary to prevent development of vitamin toxicities or deficiencies caused by altered metabolism or drug therapy.

TRACE ELEMENTS

Trace elements are minerals that are required in very small amounts for a variety of biochemical and physiologic functions. Many trace elements are an important part of metalloenzymes and also function as cofactors in a variety of regulatory metabolic pathways.[51,53] Although 17 trace elements have demonstrated biologic importance, clear deficiency syndromes in humans have been described only for iron, iodine, cobalt (as vitamin B_{12}), zinc, and copper.[53,58,59] The NAG-AMA recognized zinc, copper, and chromium as being essential for intravenous supplementation in patients receiving PN.[60] While a clear deficiency syndrome for manganese has not been reported in humans, the NAG-AMA considered manganese essential based on case reports of patients receiving PN with metabolic complications that corrected after manganese supplementation.[60] Recent reports of syndromes associated with selenium and molybdenum deficiency suggest that they also may be essential.[53,58,59] Recommendations for trace elements in pediatric patients receiving PN have been revised as well.[53]

Intravenous trace elements are available as single-mineral solutions and as multiple-mineral combinations with or without electrolytes. Most products provide the daily requirements for the trace minerals considered essential by the NAG-AMA (zinc, copper, chromium, and manganese), whereas some also include iodide, molybdenum, or selenium. Combination products are available for pediatric patients that provide manganese, copper, chromium, zinc, and selenium. Usual recommended intake is 0.3 mL/kg for children weighing less than 3 kg and 0.2 mL/kg (maximum 5 mL/d) for children weighing more than 3 kg. Children weighing more than 25 kg should receive an adult trace elements formulation.

Requirements for trace elements also change depending on the clinical condition of the patient. For example, higher doses of supplemental zinc likely are necessary in patients with high-output ostomies or diarrhea because the predominant route of excretion for zinc is via the GI tract. Manganese and copper are excreted through the biliary tract, whereas chromium, molybdenum, and selenium are excreted renally. Hence these trace elements should be restricted or withheld from PN solutions in patients with cholestatic liver disease and renal failure, respectively.

ELECTROLYTES

Electrolytes such as sodium, potassium, calcium, magnesium, phosphorus, chloride, and acetate are necessary components of PN for the maintenance of numerous cellular functions including acid-base balance and cellular growth. Electrolytes may be given to maintain normal serum concentrations or to correct deficits. Patients who have "normal" organ function and relatively normal serum concentrations of any electrolyte should receive normal maintenance doses of electrolytes on initiation of PN and daily thereafter. Requirements for specific electrolytes will vary according to the patient's age, disease state, organ function (see Chapter 139), previous and current drug therapy, nutrition status, and extrarenal losses such as nasogastric suction, vomiting, diarrhea, or fistulas (Table 137–4). Electrolytes are available commercially as single- and multiple-nutrient solutions. Multiple-electrolyte solutions are useful in stable patients with normal organ function who are receiving PN. Concentrated multiple-electrolyte solutions designed for addition to PN solutions generally contain only sodium, potassium, calcium, and magnesium. Phosphorus must be added as a separate additive. Further information regarding metabolism and requirements of vitamins, trace elements, and electrolytes is given elsewhere.[30,61,62]

DESIGNING A PARENTERAL NUTRITION REGIMEN

Several factors including available venous access, fluid status of the patient, and macronutrient and micronutrient requirements are important considerations when designing the PN regimen for an individual patient. A patient's venous access and fluid status will determine how concentrated the PN solution may be compounded and hence will have an impact on the amount of nutrient that may be provided. PN solutions may be administered by central or peripheral venous access. The clinical condition of the patient will determine which route is most appropriate (Fig. 137–1).

ROUTES OF PN ADMINISTRATION

PERIPHERAL ROUTE

Because of physical limitations of peripheral veins, peripheral parenteral nutrition (PPN) regimens usually are dilute solutions of amino acids, dextrose, and micronutrients. Although early PPN studies supported the use of amino acids alone as protein-sparing therapy, subsequent investigations have challenged this theory.[63,64] The rationale for protein-sparing PPN was based on the theory that the provision of dextrose in the setting of altered metabolism or stress would promote further increases in serum insulin concentrations and thereby hinder the use of endogenous fat stores and promote nitrogen catabolism.[63,64] Protein-sparing PPN is used for patients with marginal nutrition status and inadequate oral intake who are not candidates for central catheter placement and when the expected length of PN therapy is less than 1 week. However, two recent investigations of adults receiving postoperative PN suggest that some patients who meet criteria for protein-sparing PPN may not benefit from PN support.[11,13,17,65]

The addition of IVLEs to PPN is referred to as the lipid system. The lipid system is designed for use in mild to moderately stressed patients in whom central access is unavailable or undesirable and

TABLE 137–4. Fluid, Electrolyte, and Acid–Base Abnormalities

Problem	Possible Causes	Intervention
Hypovolemia	Gastrointestinal fluid losses, osmotic diuresis	Increase fluid intake
Hypervolemia	Renal failure, cardiac failure, excess fluid intake	Decrease fluid intake, diuretics
Hyponatremia	Gastrointestinal losses, fluid overload, diuretics	Varies with cause
Hypernatremia	Dehydration, net relative sodium excess	Increase fluid intake, decrease sodium intake
Hypokalemia	Gastrointestinal losses, diuretics, anabolism	Increase potassium intake
Hyperkalemia	Renal failure, potassium-sparing drug therapy, metabolic acidosis	Decrease potassium intake, correct metabolic acidosis
Hypophosphatemia	Phosphate-binding antacids, anabolism, phosphate-free dialysate	Discontinue phosphate binders, increase phosphorus intake
Hyperphosphatemia	Renal failure	Decrease phosphorus intake
Hypomagnesemia	Diarrhea, malabsorption, anabolism; magnesium-wasting drug therapy	Increase magnesium intake
Hypermagnesemia	Renal failure	Decrease magnesium intake
Hypocalcemia	Hypoalbuminemia, chronic renal failure	Calculate estimated serum calcium concentration corrected for hypoalbuminemia, or monitor serum ionized calcium concentrations to verify hypocalcemia; increase calcium intake if necessary
Hypercalcemia	Dehydration, malignancy	Decrease calcium intake, increase fluid intake
Metabolic acidosis	Diarrhea, high-output fistulae, renal failure	Treat underlying causes, increase acetate and decrease Cl in PN solution
Metabolic alkalosis	Gastric losses	Treat underlying cause, increase Cl and decrease acetate in PN solution

Adapted from Ref. 90, with permission.

function of the GI tract is expected to return within 7 to 10 days. The addition of IVLE increases caloric support to levels more consistent with PN regimens administered centrally. Advantages of PPN include a lower risk of infectious, metabolic, and technical complications that may occur with central vein catheterization. However, several other factors may complicate use of PPN in many patient populations. Patients who have received multiple courses of chemotherapy, malnourished patients, elderly patients, and others with an illness of long duration who have already been subjected to multiple venous accesses for administration of fluids and medications are likely to have limited peripheral venous access. Use of PPN is also limited by relatively poor tolerance of peripheral veins to hypertonic solutions. Thrombophlebitis is a commonly reported complication in patients receiving PPN. Although the risk of developing phlebitis is greater with solution osmolarities greater than 600–900 mosm/L,[63,64] peripherally administered total nutrient admixtures with much higher osmolarities have been associated with low infusion-site complications in some centers.[66] Efforts to minimize development of phlebitis in patients receiving PPN include addition of IVLEs to the regimen as a possible venous lumen protectant, subtherapeutic doses of heparin (1000 units/L) to prevent thrombus formation, and/or small doses of hydrocortisone (5 mg/L) to minimize inflammation of the access site.[64] The osmolarity of a PN solution may be estimated by using the guidelines for osmolarities of selected PN components in Table 137–5. Because lower-osmolarity solutions are relatively dilute, much larger volumes of solution generally are required to meet nutritional requirements. Finally, patients with large nutrition requirements who receive PPN likely will require the use of IVLEs as a caloric source, so these patients also should be evaluated for lipid tolerance.

In summary, PPN is a relatively safe and simple method of nutritional support when patients are selected appropriately. Candidates for PPN include patients who do not have large nutritional requirements, are not fluid restricted, and are expected to regain function of the GI tract within 7 to 10 days.[63]

CENTRAL ROUTE

Central parenteral nutrition (CPN) solutions are highly concentrated hypertonic solutions that must be administered through a large central vein. Unlike peripheral veins, central veins have a higher blood flow, which quickly dilutes the hypertonic solutions. There are multiple sites for obtaining central venous access in adult and pediatric patients. The choice of site depends on a number of factors, including the age and anatomy of the patient. Central venous catheters most commonly are inserted percutaneously into the subclavian vein and advanced so that the tip is at the superior vena cava. If this approach is not possible, the internal jugular vein may be used. Radiographic verification of correct placement is necessary prior to infusion of the CPN solution. Catheterization may be performed either in the operating suite or in the patient's hospital room. Strict adherence to established protocols and catheter placement by an experienced clinician lessen the risk of complications[67,68] (Table 137–6).

TABLE 137–5. Osmolarities of Selected Parenteral Nutrients

Nutrient	Osmolarity
Amino acid	100 mosm/%
Dextrose	50 mosm/%
Lipid emulsion	1.7 mosm/%
Sodium (acetate, chloride, phosphate)	2 mosm/mEq
Potassium (acetate, chloride, phosphate)	2 mosm/mEq
Magnesium sulfate	1 mosm/mEq
Calcium gluconate	1.4 mosm/mEq

TABLE 137–6. Complications of Central Venous Catheters

Complication	Description
Arterial injury	Puncture of subclavian or carotid artery during catheter insertion.
Pneumothorax	Perforation of the pleura or lung during insertion, which results in air collection in the pleural space.
Air embolism	Introduction of air into the catheter, which subsequently enters the venous circulation.
Catheter embolism	A portion of the catheter fragments and enters the venous circulation.
Venous thrombosis	Formation of thrombosis inside the lumen of the catheter and/or inside the vessel around the catheter, which may result in catheter or vessel occlusion.
Chylothorax	Injury to the thoracic duct during catheter insertion.
Brachial plexus injury	Injury to the nerve during catheter insertion, or injury secondary to catheter malposition or extravasation of a hypertonic solution.

Adapted from Ref. 67.

Central venous catheters vary in composition, lumen size, number of injection ports, and other special features that affect ease or convenience of care and maintenance. They may be placed for short- or long-term access. Frequently, short-term central venous access is obtained in critically ill neonates with an umbilical-placed catheter.[19] Other sites for central venous access in infants and older children are similar to those in adults.[19,20,67] When therapy is expected to last longer than 4 weeks, the catheter usually is tunneled subcutaneously before entering the central vessel, secured initially with retaining sutures, and anchored in place with a felt cuff that promotes the growth of subcutaneous fibrotic tissue around the catheter. The injection port may remain external or be concealed entirely beneath the skin. Implanted central venous catheters have a larger port or reservoir that is surgically placed beneath the skin surface and anchored in the muscle of the chest wall.

CPN is used predominantly for patients who require PN for periods of greater than 7 to 10 days during hospitalization or indefinitely at home. These patients may have large nutrient requirements, poor peripheral venous access, and/or fluctuating fluid requirements such as metabolically stressed patients with extensive surgery, trauma, sepsis, multiple-organ failure, or malignancy. Disadvantages of CPN include risks of catheter insertion, routine use of the catheter, and care of the access site. Relative to peripheral venous access, central venous catheter access is associated with a greater potential for infection. In addition, the risk of more serious catheter-induced trauma and related sequelae and other serious technical or mechanical problems is greater than with peripheral access.

ORDERING THE PN REGIMEN

Some health care systems may require the entire PN formula to be written in individual components and additives. More commonly, the ordering process has been simplified by the use of order forms designed specifically for PN. These standardized order forms promote education of practitioners by providing brief guidelines for initiating PN and foster cost-efficient nutrition support by minimizing errors in ordering, compounding, and administration.[69] Standardized order forms also may include options for ordering certain related procedures, laboratory tests, protocols for patient management, or consultations with other medical services related to the patient's nutrition support. Standardized forms and protocols should be reviewed and updated periodically to reflect changes in the practices and patient population of a practice setting and also advances in technology that may affect provision of nutrition support.

Once the route of delivery has been chosen, components of the PN regimen are decided based on the patient's nutritional assessment. The patient's clinical condition and the compounding practices of an institution will have an impact on decisions concerning PN infusion rates. For example, some institutions prepare PN solutions using a standard-formula format. This approach offers a variety of base formulas (CAA-dextrose combination) with a fixed nonprotein-calorie to nitrogen ratio (NPC:N). The standard formula format usually includes different formulas designed for mild to moderately stressed patients, renal failure patients, fluid-restricted patients, and liver failure patients. Because the NPC:N is fixed, the amount of nutrient delivered depends solely on the infusion rate. Other institutions may compound individualized formulas. This approach permits compounding of patient-specific solutions. Compounding of the PN solution is limited only by the concentrations of stock solutions and stability concerns. The amount of nutrient delivered depends on daily volume of the PN solution infused and the nutrient concentrations in the PN solution. The total daily amount of PN solution may be prepared in multiple 1-L bags or more cost effectively in a single container.[30]

Traditionally, PN solutions have been ordered by expressing the final concentrations of each component in the solution. For example, CAA and dextrose are ordered commonly in final percentage, electrolytes in milliequivalents per liter, and other additives in amount (milliliters or units) per day.

This inconsistency may promote confusion and misinterpretation of PN solution contents that may result in harm, especially when patients are transferred between health system environments. To ensure that PN labels in all health system environments clearly and accurately reflect the PN solution contents, guidelines for standardized PN labeling have been recommended.[30] In addition to including a variety of other information to the label such as dosing weight and route of administration, the guidelines suggest expressing PN ingredients in amounts per total volume, which minimizes need for pharmaceutical calculations to determine the nutrient value of the admixture. Computer software for calculating PN solutions is widely available, and several programs have adapted the recommended labeling guidelines. However, because some institutions may continue to follow traditional ordering practices, the steps for pharmaceutical calculations of a PN base solution will be reviewed briefly (Fig. 137–2).

There are several guidelines or clinical rules of thumb that may help the pharmacist calculate a PN regimen after a patient's nutritional requirements have been decided. For example, patients receiving only PN therapy likely will need larger volumes of fluid to provide maintenance requirements and replace extrarenal losses. However, patients requiring other intravenous drug therapy may receive adequate fluid in their intravenous maintenance solution (e.g., 0.45% NaCl in 5% dextrose) and/or piggybacked medications. Depending on individual institutional practices, maximally concentrating the PN solution and using an inexpensive maintenance fluid to manage hydration may provide a cost-effective regimen that requires fewer adjustments. Another guideline that may be helpful in designing a PN regimen where the CAA-dextrose base is infused separately from the IVLEs is to allow a volume of approximately 100–150 mL/L of base solution for electrolytes and other additives. Given this guideline, two clinically useful and highly concentrated base solutions are 7% CAA/15% dextrose (final concentration), which can be prepared from 10% CAA and 70% dextrose stock solutions, and 8% CAA/25% dextrose (final concentrations), compounded from 15% CAA and 70% dextrose stock solutions. PN regimens for patients who require very small amounts of additives, such as patients with renal failure, may be further concentrated.

COMPOUNDING, STORAGE, AND INFECTION CONTROL

Several considerations are necessary when preparing and storing PN solutions. In general, the type of solution being prepared will dictate methods of compounding, storage, and infusion. Currently, the two most commonly used types of PN solutions are the CAA-dextrose combination with or without IVLEs piggybacked into the PN line and TNAs. Use of TNA solutions offers several potential advantages, including reduced inventory (infusion pumps, tubing, and other related supplies), decreased time for compounding and administration, potential decrease in manipulations of the infusion line (which should correspond with a decreased risk of catheter contamination), and ease of delivery and storage for patients receiving home PN.[70] Potential disadvantages include increased risk of infections and stability and compatibility concerns. For example, stability of TNA solutions may be less predictable compared with CAA-dextrose solutions, which make their use less desirable in specific patient populations such as neonates and infants.[30] In addition, the opaque solution that results after the addition of IVLEs makes detection of particulate matter difficult, and TNA solutions cannot be filtered with a bacteria-retentive 0.22-μm filter.[30] Methods for compounding PN solutions vary based on a health care system's patient population and medical practices and the number of PN solutions that need to be prepared. PN base solutions may be prepared by using gravity-driven transfer of CAA stock solutions to partially filled bags of concentrated dextrose stock solutions.[71] Other practice settings may use commercially prepared CAA-dextrose products that are separated within a single bag and then mixed prior to use. Recent advances in compounding technology have facilitated use of automated compounders for preparing PN solutions. Automated compounders are computer-based systems that perform the calculations necessary to determine volumes of nutrient stock solutions for PN solutions. In addition, most automated compounder systems include software that communicates the determined calculations directly to a transfer pump device that delivers fluid from the source container to the final container by either a volumetric or gravimetric fluid pumping system.[71] Advantages associated with automated compounders include reduction in personnel time and compounding materials and improved accuracy of compounding. Disadvantages include the potential for equipment failure and power outages.

Assurance of solution sterility during compounding, storage, and administration is necessary to reduce the risk of infection and related complications.[72,73] Several studies have demonstrated that because of their acidic pH and hypertonicity, CAA-dextrose PN solutions are poor media for bacterial growth.[73] However, *Pseudomonas aeruginosa, Escherichia coli,* and fungi such as *Candida albicans* have been noted to grow in CAA-dextrose solutions.[42,73] Refrigeration at 4°C suppresses growth of both bacteria and *C. albicans* and should be the routine storage temperature.[73] The PN solution should be used within 24 hours after removal from refrigeration.[73,74] IVLEs support growth of gram-positive and gram-negative bacteria as well as fungi. Currently, the Centers for Disease Control and Prevention recommend a maximum hang time of 12 hours for IVLEs except when used within a TNA system based on reports of substantial microbial growth in contaminated IVLEs after 12 hours.[74] However, a clinical investigation of IVLE solutions infused for up to 24 hours in patients receiving PN demonstrated no correlation between risk of infection and length of hang time.[75] In view of these findings, many institutions now allow expiration times of up to 24 hours for IVLE infusions.

Results from investigations of microbial growth in TNA solutions do not agree.[76] In general, TNA solutions appear to support growth of bacteria less than IVLEs but more than CAA-dextrose solutions. However, investigations of TNAs hung for up to 24 hours have demonstrated that the risk of contamination was no greater than that reported with CAA-dextrose solutions.[42,74]

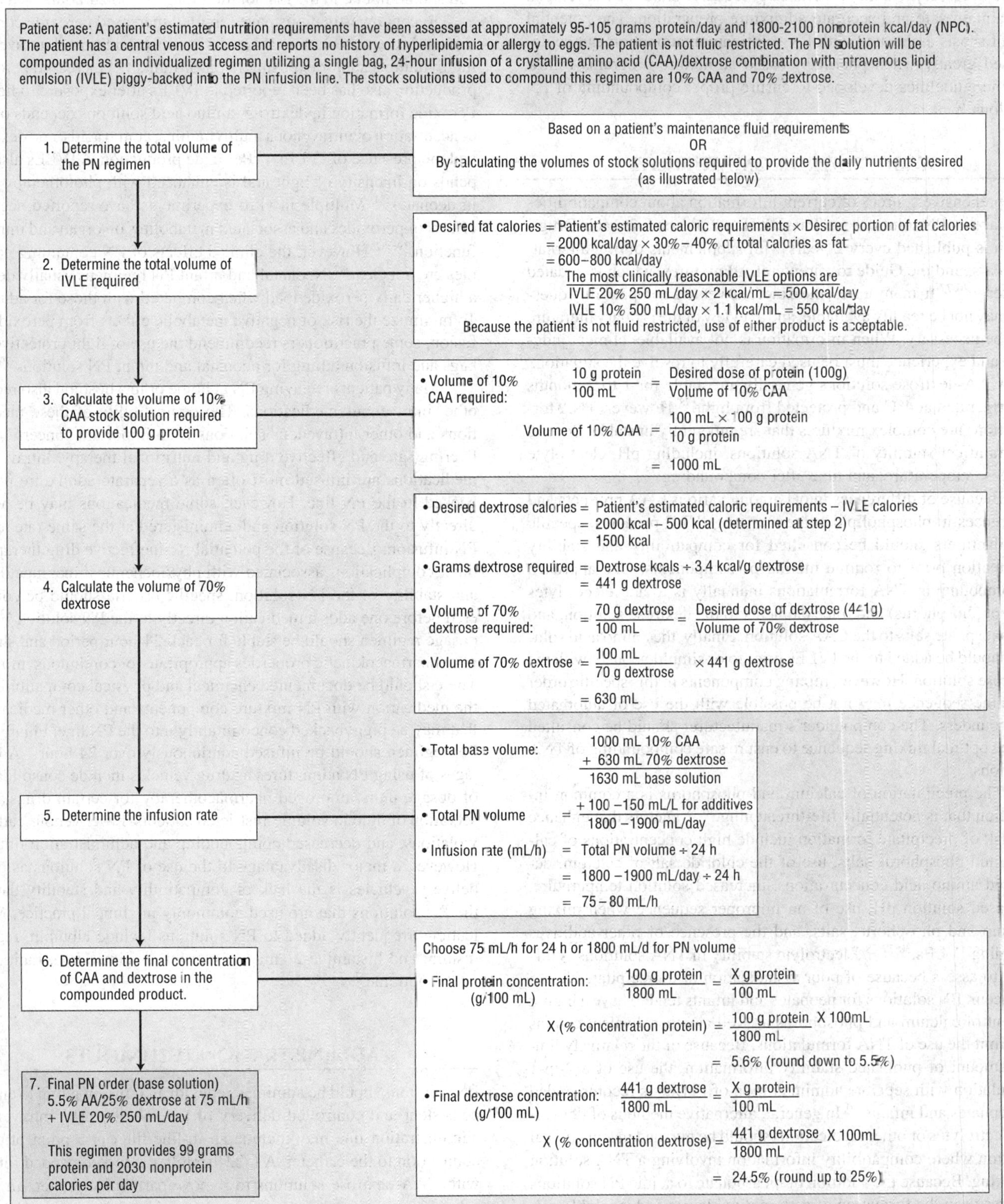

Patient case: A patient's estimated nutrition requirements have been assessed at approximately 95-105 grams protein/day and 1800-2100 nonprotein kcal/day (NPC). The patient has a central venous access and reports no history of hyperlipidemia or allergy to eggs. The patient is not fluid restricted. The PN solution will be compounded as an individualized regimen utilizing a single bag, 24-hour infusion of a crystalline amino acid (CAA)/dextrose combination with intravenous lipid emulsion (IVLE) piggy-backed into the PN infusion line. The stock solutions used to compound this regimen are 10% CAA and 70% dextrose.
1. Determine the total volume of the PN regimen
Based on a patient's maintenance fluid requirements
OR
By calculating the volumes of stock solutions required to provide the daily nutrients desired (as illustrated below)
2. Determine the total volume of IVLE required
• Desired fat calories = Patient's estimated caloric requirements × Desired portion of fat calories
= 2000 kcal/day × 30%–40% of total calories as fat
= 600–800 kcal/day
The most clinically reasonable IVLE options are
IVLE 20% 250 mL/day × 2 kcal/mL = 500 kcal/day
IVLE 10% 500 mL/day × 1.1 kcal/mL = 550 kcal/day
Because the patient is not fluid restricted, use of either product is acceptable.
3. Calculate the volume of 10% CAA stock solution required to provide 100 g protein
• Volume of 10% CAA required:
10 g protein / 100 mL = Desired dose of protein (100g) / Volume of 10% CAA
Volume of 10% CAA = 100 mL × 100 g protein / 10 g protein
= 1000 mL
4. Calculate the volume of 70% dextrose
• Desired dextrose calories = Patient's estimated caloric requirements – IVLE calories
= 2000 kcal – 500 kcal (determined at step 2)
= 1500 kcal
• Grams dextrose required = Dextrose kcals ÷ 3.4 kcal/g dextrose
= 441 g dextrose
• Volume of 70% dextrose required: = 70 g dextrose / 100 mL = Desired dose of dextrose (441g) / Volume of 70% dextrose
• Volume of 70% dextrose = 100 mL / 70 g dextrose × 441 g dextrose
= 630 mL
5. Determine the infusion rate
• Total base volume: 1000 mL 10% CAA
+ 630 mL 70% dextrose
1630 mL base solution
• Total PN volume = + 100 –150 mL/L for additives
1800 –1900 mL/day
• Infusion rate (mL/h) = Total PN volume ÷ 24 h
= 1800 –1900 mL/day ÷ 24 h
= 75–80 mL/h
6. Determine the final concentration of CAA and dextrose in the compounded product.
Choose 75 mL/h for 24 h or 1800 mL/d for PN volume
• Final protein concentration: (g/100 mL) = 100 g protein / 1800 mL = X g protein / 100 mL
X (% concentration protein) = 100 g protein X 100mL / 1800 mL
= 5.6% (round down to 5.5%)
• Final dextrose concentration: (g/100 mL) 441 g dextrose / 1800 mL = X g protein / 100 mL
X (% concentration dextrose) = 441 g dextrose X 100mL / 1800 mL
= 24.5% (round up to 25%)
7. Final PN order (base solution)
5.5% AA/25% dextrose at 75 mL/h
+ IVLE 20% 250 mL/day
This regimen provides 99 grams protein and 2030 nonprotein calories per day

FIGURE 137–2. Calculation of a compounding plan for a PN regimen.

PN solutions should be prepared using aseptic technique under a properly maintained laminar flow hood.[72,74] The hood should be situated such that the contaminant potential of normal work traffic and air currents is minimized. Personnel must be trained adequately and must practice strict aseptic technique. Supervision by a pharmacist experienced in compounding intravenous solutions and knowledgeable about stability, compatibility, and storage of PN solutions is also necessary. Quality assurance procedures should be developed to maintain safe and accurate admixture preparation. The potential risk of sepsis associated with PN solution contamination can be decreased greatly when pharmacy-based admixture programs follow specific guidelines developed to ensure proper compounding of PN solutions.[72]

STABILITY AND COMPATABILITY

Comprehensive sources of current information about compatibilities and stability PN solutions are Trissel's Handbook on Injectable Drugs, which is published every 2 years with supplements during alternating years, and the Guide to Parenteral Admixtures, which is updated quarterly.[76,77] In many cases, the exact answer to a compatibility question may not be readily available, and a review of the primary literature may be necessary. When information is not available, clinical judgment and experience must be used carefully to resolve the situation.

CAA-dextrose solutions generally are stable for 1 to 2 months if refrigerated at 4°C and protected from light.[78] However, TNA formulations are complex mixtures that are inherently unstable. Several factors affect stability of TNA solutions, including pH, electrolyte charges, temperature, and time after compounding.[78]

Because of differences in pH among various CAA products and differences in phospholipid content among IVLE products, specific manufacturers should be consulted for compatibility and stability information prior to routine mixing of components. One approach to compounding TNA formulations manually is to add electrolytes (except phosphorus) and trace elements to the dextrose solution, and add phosphate salts to the CAA solution. Finally, the amino acid solution should be added to the IVLEs prior to or simultaneously with the dextrose solution. However, mixing components in this specific order and time sequence may not be possible with the use of automated compounders. The compounder's manufacturer should be consulted for the optimal mixing sequence to ensure safe compounding of TNA solutions.

The precipitation of calcium and phosphorus is a common interaction that is potentially life-threatening.[30,78] Factors that enhance the risk of precipitate formation include high concentrations of calcium and phosphorus salts, use of the chloride salt of calcium, decreased amino acid concentrations, increased solution temperature, increased solution pH, use of an improper sequence when mixing calcium and phosphorus salts, and the presence of other additives including IVLEs.[30,77,78] Electrolyte stability in TNA solutions is difficult to assess because of poor visualization of a precipitate should one occur. PN solutions for neonates and infants tend to have a higher content of calcium and phosphorus as well as other divalent cations that limit the use of TNA formulations. Because of the relatively limited amount of published stability information, the use of a 2-in-1 formulation with separate administration of IVLEs is recommended for neonates and infants.[30] In general, alternative methods of delivering electrolytes or other medications should be pursued in any clinical situation where compatibility information involving a TNA solution is lacking. Because the addition of bicarbonate to acidic PN solutions may result in the formation of carbon dioxide gas and insoluble calcium and magnesium carbonates, the use of sodium bicarbonate in PN solutions is not recommended.[30] Use of a bicarbonate precursor salt such as acetate usually is preferred.

Vitamins may be affected adversely by changes in solution pH, presence of other additives, storage time, solution temperature, and exposure to light.[61,78] Because of variable stabilities of individual vitamins, intravenous vitamin solutions should be added to the PN solution as near to the time of administration as is clinically feasible and should not be in the PN solution longer than 24 hours.

Recent investigations have reported increased peroxide concentrations in dextrose–amino acid solutions after addition of intravenous multivitamins and/or exposure to air or light.[79,80] Increased peroxide production also has been reported in IVLEs after exposure to light.[81] Peroxide formation in dextrose–amino acid solutions depends on the concentration of intravenous multivitamins, amino acids, and dextrose and the presence of IVLEs.[79] Peroxide production in IVLEs also depends on intensity of light and is enhanced with phototherapy light in neonates.[81] Multiple in vitro experiments have reported negative effects of peroxides and associated metabolites on organ and immune function.[79–82] However, the clinical effects of PN containing peroxides are not clear.[82] Neonatal and infant PN regimens usually deliver a higher daily peroxide load when compared with those for adults.[79] To minimize the risk of negative metabolic effects from peroxide infusion, some practitioners recommend the use of light protective PN bags and infusion tubing for neonatal and infant PN solutions.[79,80]

Many patients receiving PN at home or in a hospital also receive other intravenous medications. The compatibility of these medications and other intravenous solutions is an important concern in delivering safe and effective drug and nutritional therapy. Intravenous medications are infused most often as a separate admixture piggybacked in the PN line. However, some medications may be added directly to the PN solution and administered at the same rate as the PN infusion. Because of the potential for ineffective drug therapy or other complications associated with physiochemical incompatibility and stability of the PN solution, specific criteria should be considered before one adds a medication directly to the PN solution.[83] The dosage regimen should be stable for each 24-hour period and should have pharmacokinetic properties appropriate for continuous infusion. There should be documented chemical and physical compatibility of the medication with PN mixture components and other medications that may be piggybacked concomitantly into the PN line. Finally, the PN regimen should be infused continuously over 24 hours. Advantages of using PN admixtures as drug vehicles include consolidation of dosage units, improved pharmacotherapy for certain drugs, conservation of fluid in volume-restricted patients, fewer venous catheter violations, and decreased compounding and administration times.[83] However, a major disadvantage to the use of PN solutions as drug-delivery vehicles is the lack of compatibility and stability data in the PN solutions that are used commonly in clinical practice. Medications frequently added to PN solutions include albumin, regular insulin, and histamine-2 antagonists such as cimetidine, ranitidine, and famotidine.[76,77,83]

ADMINISTRATION TECHNIQUES

PN solutions should be administered with an infusion pump to ensure consistent and controlled delivery of the solution. The intravenous administration line may include an in-line filter at a point prior to connection to the catheter. A 0.22-μm filter is recommended for use with CAA-dextrose solutions to remove particulate matter, air, and any microorganism that may be present in the solution from prior manipulations of the admixture or the administration line. Because the average size of IVLE particles is approximately 0.5 μm, IVLEs administered separately from the CAA-dextrose solution must be piggybacked into the PN line at a site beyond the in-line filter.[30] Routine use of in-line filters (>0.22 μm) with TNA solutions is controversial.[74,84] However, the FDA recommends use of a 1.2-μm filter, which may be effective in preventing catheter occlusion due to precipitates or lipid aggregates.[30] This filter size is also reported to remove *C. albicans*.

INITIATING THE PN INFUSION

The concentration of dextrose in the formula and the patient's history of glucose tolerance will dictate the infusion rate at which the PN solution should be initiated. Many institutions begin infusions slowly and increase the rate gradually over 24 to 48 hours to the desired rate. The infusion rate is likewise reduced in a stepwise fashion when the decision to end PN therapy is made. This approach should prevent development of hyperglycemia and rebound hypoglycemia, respectively. However, Krzyda and colleagues investigated 18 adult patients who were initiated on PN solutions at the desired rate and discontinued without a taper schedule.[85] None of the patients demonstrated clinical signs of hyperglycemia or hypoglycemia during the study. The blood glucose concentrations of patients who received insulin from the PN infusion were less predictable when the PN infusion was stopped compared with those from patients who did not require insulin. While these investigators observed no adverse effects from initiating and discontinuing PN infusions abruptly, tapered initiation and cessation has been recommended for patients receiving intermittent subcutaneous regular insulin, patients with severe renal or hepatic disease, patients with other disease states that may increase the risk for development of hypoglycemia such as severe diabetes or pancreatic malignancy, and patients who are receiving concurrent drug therapy that may predispose to development of hypoglycemia (oral hypoglycemics) or mask the cardiovascular symptoms of hypoglycemia (β-blockers).[86]

CONTINUOUS VERSUS INTERMITTENT INFUSIONS

PN solutions may be infused continuously or intermittently (see Fig. 137–1) Continuous infusions are attractive for use in patients with unstable fluid balance or glucose control. Cyclic PN is the infusion of PN over a period of time less than 24 hours, usually for 12 to 18 hours each day.[87] Cyclic PN is useful in hospitalized patients with limited venous access in whom administration of multiple other medications requires interruption of the PN infusion. Cyclic PN also may prevent or treat hepatotoxicities associated with continuous PN therapy. In addition, cyclic PN allows patients receiving PN at home the ability to resume a relatively normal lifestyle.[87] Recommendations for administration of cyclic PN are similar to those for continuous PN. Various protocols have been reported that suggest incremental increases to the maximum infusion rate for a desired period of time followed by a gradual taper to discontinue the solution. However, metabolically stable patients receiving lipid-based PN regimens are likely candidates for abrupt initiation and discontinuation of the cyclic PN regimen.[85,86] Cyclic PN may not be well tolerated by patients with severe glucose intolerance or diabetes or by those patients with unstable fluid balance.

EVALUATION OF OUTCOMES

Thorough and consistent monitoring of patients receiving PN is necessary to ensure that the desired nutritional outcomes are achieved and to prevent the occurrence of adverse effects or complications. Routine evaluation should include the assessment of the patient's clinical condition with a focus on nutritional and metabolic effects of the PN regimen. Serial documentation of a patient's response to a particular regimen is a helpful guide for determining appropriate adjustments in fluid, electrolyte, and nutrient therapies.

A number of biochemical and clinical measurements are necessary for effective monitoring of patients receiving PN. Important clinical laboratory measurements include serum concentrations of electrolytes, hematologic indices, and biochemical markers for renal function, liver function, and nutrition status. Other important clinical measurements include vital signs, weight, total fluid intake and losses, and nutritional intakes. The frequency of clinical laboratory measurements usually depends on the stability of a patient's clinical condition. Monitoring parameters considered important for patients receiving PN and the suggested frequency of measurement for each are outlined in Figure 137–3. Appropriate assessment and evaluation of patient data can identify impending complications that may be avoided or treated early. Monitoring protocols should be developed and tailored for the patient population, medical practices, and resources of individual practice settings.

COMPLICATIONS OF PN

PN can be a safe and effective therapy when appropriate patients have been selected and the course of therapy is monitored and adjusted correctly. However, PN support is a complex therapy that is associated with numerous complications. These complications may be divided into four categories: mechanical or technical, infectious, metabolic, and nutritional.

MECHANICAL/TECHNICAL

Mechanical or technical complications include malfunctions in the system used for intravenous delivery of the solution. Examples of such malfunctions include infusion pump failure, problems with administration sets or tubing, and problems with the catheter. Catheter-related complications are potentially life-threatening.

Pneumothorax, catheter misdirection into the wrong vein or ill-positioned within the cardiac chambers, arterial puncture, bleeding, and hematoma formation may occur during surgical placement of the catheter. Many of these complications, in addition to venous thrombosis and air embolism, may occur after insertion as well. Catheters occasionally occlude or break during use. If these problems cannot be rectified easily, the catheter may need to be surgically replaced.[67]

INFECTIONS

Infectious complications can be a major hazard in patients receiving CPN. Often these patients are predisposed to infection as a result of compromised immunity and/or concomitant infection already present in the urinary tract, wounds, or lungs. Frequent use of broad-spectrum antibiotic therapy and malnutrition are also predisposing factors for development of infection. Furthermore, bacterial translocation across the wall of the GI tract also has been implicated as a source of sepsis in patients receiving PN for prolonged periods without enteral feeding.[57] Infection may develop secondary to solution contamination.[74] However, strict adherence to specific protocols for preparation of PN solutions should minimized this occurrence.[72,73] A more common source of systemic infection is catheter-related infections. Catheter-related

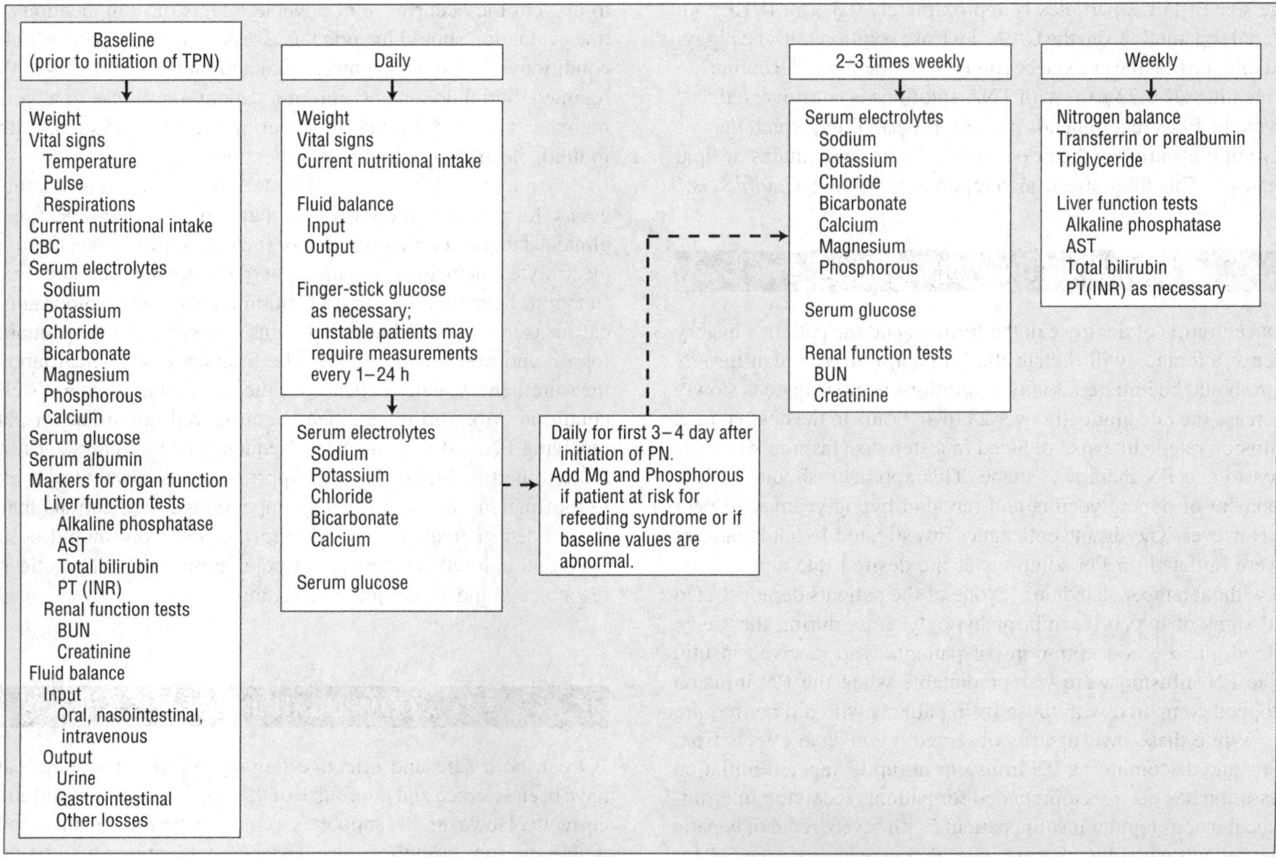

FIGURE 137–3. Monitoring strategy for patients receiving PN.

bloodstream infection is defined as the presence of bacterial or fungal growth from the catheter tip and peripheral blood cultures. Catheter infection or a colonized catheter is defined as microbial growth from the catheter tip or from a blood culture drawn from the catheter with no growth of the same organism in the peripheral blood culture.[74] Patients with catheter-related infections may exhibit signs of sepsis syndrome such as fever, chills, mental status changes, hypotension, or glucose intolerance. These infections occur when the catheter becomes colonized by direct microbial invasion of the skin at the insertion site or at the infusion site of the catheter. For example, colonization may occur after multiple manipulations of the line used for PN administration, which can occur when the PN line is used to administer other medications. Other examples include failure of in-line bacterial filters, poor placement technique, and poor care of the insertion site.[74]

When no other source of infection is apparent in symptomatic patients, the catheter should be evaluated as the potential source. Blood cultures are drawn from a peripheral site and from the central catheter. In many institutions the suspected catheter is removed, the tip is cultured quantitatively, and a new central catheter is inserted. If bacterial or fungal growth of the same organism occurs from the catheter tip and the peripheral blood culture, the exchanged catheter is removed, and another is placed in a different anatomic site. If bacterial or fungal growth occurs from the catheter tip or from a blood culture drawn from the catheter with no growth of the same organism in the peripheral culture, the catheter may be removed and replaced with another in the same anatomic location. However, because the clinical value of frequent central catheter replacement in patients with sepsis secondary to catheter-related infection is controversial, other treatment protocols have been suggested.[88]

METABOLIC/NUTRITIONAL

Metabolic complications associated with PN therapy are numerous and, if left untreated, may be potentially fatal. Common metabolic abnormalities related to substrate intolerance and fluid, electrolyte, and acid-base disorders are presented in Tables 137–4 and 137–7 along with predisposing factors and general strategies for intervention. The etiology, mechanisms, and implications of individual metabolic abnormalities are multifactorial and have been summarized in multiple reviews.[18–20,30,31,39,41,48,87–90]

PN-associated hepatic dysfunction, as evidenced by elevations in serum liver function measurements such as total bilirubin, AST, ALT, and alkaline phosphatase is well documented in the literature.[91,92] No single etiology has been identified, although several risk factors have been reported. Risk factors for children include degree of prematurity, sepsis, hypoxia, lack of enteral nutrition, small bowel bacterial overgrowth, GI conditions requiring surgical intervention, duration of PN therapy and long-term administration of excessive calories.[20,92–94] PN-associated hepatic dysfunction in infants is characterized clinically by a serum direct bilirubin concentration greater that 2 mg/dL.[93,94] Taurine deficiency has been proposed as the etiology of cholestasis in preterm infants and neonates.[20,92] Taurine is a CEAA not present in standard CAA solutions that is important in neonatal and infant bile metabolism. However, the effectiveness of PN regimens with CAA solutions containing supplemental taurine is unclear.[20,92] Risk factors for PN-associated hepatic dysfunction in adults include preexisting liver diseases, sepsis, preexisting malnutrition, extent of bowel resection, duration of PN therapy, lack of enteral intake, and long-term administration of excessive calories.[91,92,95,96] PN-associated hepatic dysfunction in adults typically presents as

TABLE 137–7. Substrate Intolerance in Parenteral Nutrition

Complication	Possible Causes	Intervention
Hyperglycemia	Stress, infection, corticosteroids, pancreatitis, diabetes mellitus, peritoneal dialysis, excessive dextrose administration	Decrease dextrose load by decreasing infusion rate or dextrose concentration (may substitute fat calories); administer insulin
Hypoglycemia	Abrupt withdrawal of dextrose, insulin overdose	Increase dextrose intake; decrease exogenous insulin; Taper infusion rate prior to discontinuing PN
Excess of carbon dioxide production	Excess dextrose intake	Decrease dextrose intake; balance calories from fat and dextrose
Hypertriglyceridemia	Stress, familial hyperlipidemia, pancreatitis; excess IVLE dose; rapid IVLE infusion rate	Decrease IVLE dose; decrease rate of IVLE infusion; discontinue IVLE if indicated
Abnormal liver function tests (elevated AST, alkaline phosphatase, and bilirubin)	Stress, infection. cancer, excess carbohydrate intake, excess caloric intake, essential fatty acid deficiency	Decrease dextrose load (substitute fat); decrease total calories; provide essential fatty acids; cycle PN infusion; transition to enteral nutrition regimen

AST = aspartate aminotransferase (SGOT).
IVLE = intravenous lipid emulsion.
PN = parenteral nutrition.
Adapted from Ref. 90, with permission.

steatosis and steatohepatosis on biopsy.[91,92] Clinically, PN- associated hepatic dysfunction is characterized by mild elevations in serum liver enzymes, usually less than three times the upper limit of normal, with peak enzyme levels usually occurring between 1 and 4 weeks after initiating PN.[91,92] In many cases, the liver abnormalities improve or resolve with manipulation of substrate intake or discontinuation of PN therapy. However, death from PN-associated liver failure in adults and pediatric patients receiving long-term home PN has been reported.[95,96]

Hypertriglyceridemia, defined as serum triglyceride concentrations of 400–500 mg/dL in adults and 150–200 mg/dL in preterm infants, neonates, and older pediatric patients, may occur in patients receiving IVLE-based PN. Risk factors include preexisting liver or pancreatic dysfunction, sepsis, multiple-organ failure, degree of prematurity, rate of IVLE infusion, and dose.[32,38,39]

IVLE-associated hypertriglyceridemia generally is thought to be due to defective lipid clearance.[38] Premature infants and neonates have relatively slower lipid clearance compared with adults because of immature metabolic pathways, including decreased lipoprotein lipase activity.[32,38,39] Reducing the infusion rate or IVLE dose or withholding IVLE therapy should be considered when patients present with hypertriglyceridemia or lipemic serum.[38,39] Use of heparin to stimulate lipoprotein lipase activity has been suggested as a potential therapeutic intervention to treat IVLE-associated hypertriglyceridemia.[16,38,39] The role of carnitine for treatment of IVLE-associated hypertriglyceridemia is not clear.[26,38,39]

The refeeding syndrome (RS) is a nutritional complication reported most frequently in severely malnourished adults with significant weight loss who receive PN.[97] RS is associated primarily with hypophosphatemia, although hypokalemia, hypomagnesemia, and life-threatening cardiac dysfunction have been reported as well. The mechanism of the electrolyte abnormalities appears to be related to acute provision of macronutrient substrates that promote anabolism in an environment of depleted total body stores of phosphorus, potassium, and magnesium. Cardiac dysfunction is thought to occur because of an acute volume expansion that increases cardiac demand. Recommendations for initiating PN in adults at risk for RS include providing less than 50% of the calculated nonprotein caloric requirements initially. The dextrose dose should be initiated at approximately 150–200 g/day. Calories should be advanced over 3 to 4 days to the desired goal. Because the metabolic abnormalities described with RS appear to be related primarily to acute provision of large amounts of dextrose, the goal protein dose may be provided with the initial PN infusion.[97] RS has not been as well described in pediatric patients receiving PN. However, similar guidelines adjusted for age would seem to be a sensible approach to initiating PN in severely malnourished pediatric patients.

Other nutritional complications of PN therapy may develop over a prolonged course of therapy (weeks to months) as a result of inappropriate intake of a particular nutrient. Certain conditions, such as metabolic stress in a previously malnourished patient, may elicit symptoms of deficiency much earlier if a nutrient is not appropriately provided. For example, lactic acidosis and other life-threatening complications associated with severe thiamine deficiency have been reported in patients who received PN solutions without multivitamin supplementation.[98] At least maintenance doses of vitamins, trace elements, and essential fatty acids should be provided to all patients with normal age-related organ function receiving PN.

Patients receiving PN regimens without IVLEs for extended periods (weeks to months) are at risk for development of EFAD. Clinical signs of EFAD include hair loss, desquamative dermatitis, thrombocytopenia, and malabsorption and diarrhea resulting from changes in intestinal mucosa.[40,41] EFAD also may be diagnosed by evaluating plasma fatty acid profiles. A triene-tetraene ratio more than 0.4 is biochemical evidence for EFAD. These manifestations may occur 1 to 3 weeks after initiation of fat-free PN in adults and within 72 hours in premature infants.[32]

Metabolic bone disease is a complication usually reported in adults and children receiving long-term home PN.[99] This disorder in adults is characterized by osteomalacia with or without osteoporosis that may present without associated clinical, radiologic, or biochemical abnormalaties. The diagnosis may not be made in premature infants until after the development of bone fractures or overt rickets. The etiology is poorly understood and likely multifactorial. Treatment options include pharmacologic intervention, calcium and vitamin D supplementation, and exercise.

Clinical symptoms of trace element deficiencies, although rare, have been reported in patients receiving PN. More commonly, decreased serum trace element concentrations have been reported in a variety of patient populations. However, the clinical significance of decreased concentrations of many trace elements is not known because serum concentrations often do not correlate with total body stores.[58,59] Clinical signs and symptoms of trace element deficiencies have been reviewed elsewhere.[50]

Occasionally, patients may develop nutrient-induced toxicities, most commonly as a result of the accumulation of fat-soluble vitamins or trace elements due to either excessive intake or decreased excretion. Certain disease states (e.g., severe renal or hepatic failure) may necessitate reduction in vitamin and trace element intake.

Many trace elements are present in PN components as contaminants.[50,100,101] The content varies among components and manufacturers. Some investigations of patients with normal organ function receiving PN have reported concern with elevated serum concentrations of particular trace elements.[58,101] Aluminum is a common contaminant of many sterile intravenous solutions including PN components that accumulates during long-term PN therapy, especially in patients with renal insufficiency.[101,102] Calcium and phosphorus solutions are among those components with higher levels of aluminum contamination.[102] Aluminum accumulation is associated with abnormal neurologic and hematologic function and metabolic bone disease in adults and premature infants.[58,98,101,102] However, the role of aluminum in the development of metabolic bone disease is controversial. Preterm infants are at higher risk of aluminum accumulation because they receive larger doses (micrograms per kilogram) from PN solutions than adults.[98,101,102] Preterm infants are more likely to retain aluminum because of premature renal function. In addition, preterm infants tend to have relatively larger calcium and phosphorus requirements. The FDA has proposed to restrict the aluminum contamination of large-volume PN solutions to a maximum of 25 μg/L and require statement of aluminum content on the label of small-volume PN solutions.[103] Final action is forthcoming.

HOME PN

Advances in technology for the delivery of intravenous solutions have allowed medically stable patients who require extended PN therapy to be maintained indefinitely on intravenous nutrition. An increasing concern for cost containment of health care services has fostered use of sophisticated infusion devices to provide PN at home. Numerous programs are now available to support patients with various long-term or permanent medical conditions outside the traditional health care setting. Standards have been developed to promote safe and effective care.[8] Home PN services may be coordinated and administered through a hospital, by a commercially operated corporation, or through a joint venture between the two.

Many factors are considered in selecting candidates for home PN therapy. Significant benefit must be expected from placing a patient into the program. Additionally, the patient and his or her caregiver must be willing to complete training successfully and assume numerous other responsibilities that are important for managing a new daily routine in the home. Other logistics such as funding, procurement of solutions and supplies, and clinical management and follow-up must be evaluated, resolved, and implemented for each patient in order to achieve the desired outcomes.[104,105]

Patients with Crohn's disease, ischemic bowel disease, severe GI motility disorders, extensive intestinal obstruction, and congenital bowel dysfunction have been maintained successfully with home PN.[104] However, patients with active cancer are the largest group of patients receiving home PN in the United States.[104] In the past, patients or their caregivers may have been trained to mix PN solutions in the home. Today, patients commonly receive premixed PN solutions from the hospital or a commercial vendor. Intravenous vitamins or other additives may be added daily by the patient or caregiver depending on the arrangement with the PN provider. The solution generally is administered through the night by infusion pump over 10 to 18 hours. A cycled regimen allows the patient time away from the pump during daylight hours and provides many patients with the freedom to have a reasonably normal daily routine. Clinical management and follow-up are performed periodically according to the needs of the patient and the protocol of the care provider. A coordinated effort among several health care professionals including physicians, pharmacists, nurses, social workers, and the patient and his or her caregiver, as well as the suppliers, is paramount to providing safe and effective management. Home PN affords some patients the potential for an ambulatory lifestyle while maintaining an intravenous feeding regimen previously only available in the hospital setting. For others, home PN may contribute to a better quality of life in the comfort of their home.

PHARMACOECONOMIC CONSIDERATIONS

Because numerous variables have an impact on the provision of PN support and the response to therapy, determining the true cost of PN is difficult.[106–108] In general, PN is an expensive intervention, and cost likely varies depending on the underlying indication for treatment and whether PN is provided at home or in an acute care setting.[104,106–108] Expenses associated with PN therapy may be categorized as direct and indirect costs[109] (Table 137–8). Direct costs may be further categorized as fixed or variable costs. Fixed costs do not depend on the volume of patients receiving therapy. For example, an automatic compounder and the tubing sets required to transfer volumes of stock solutions to the administration bag would be considered fixed costs in many practice settings. These costs per patient tend to be highest in low-volume environments. Variable costs such as PN administration bags are depend directly on the number of patients receiving PN. Other direct costs include ancillary services required by patients receiving PN and costs related to the management of nutritionally associated complications.

Benefits and other clinical effects of PN (i.e., length of stay, frequency of complications) in specific patient populations have been evaluated.[11,17] Few investigations have reported an economic assessment of the therapy. However, economic data from many of these reports would not necessarily reflect current costs. Indeed, the direct cost of PN solution components generally has declined over the past decade. Attempting to measure the cost or cost savings associated with reported benefits of PN therapy and other clinical effects based on results of controlled clinical trials is difficult.[107,108] Clinical outcomes measurements and hence economic outcomes are influenced by multiple factors, including experimental design, sample size, and specific health system practices. Several investigations used for determining costs and benefits of PN therapy have been criticized for such biases.[12,108]

While the results of economic analyses of PN remain controversial, similarities among several reports provide a basis for methods of limiting the costs of PN therapy. These include the following: (1) Use of PN only for appropriate patients as described by institution-specific criteria based on current consensus statements.[109] The costs and complications associated with EN have been demonstrated to be less than those associated with PN.[111,112] (2) Frequent evaluation of the need for standing laboratory measurements used for monitoring PN therapy. In general, the level of laboratory monitoring should decrease as

TABLE 137–8. Costs Associated With PN Therapy

Type of Cost	Description
Direct	
• PN solution	
Components	Dextrose, AA, IVLE, other additives
Preparation	Dependent on system used for compounding: solution transfer sets, bags, syringes, technician time, pharmacist time
Administration	Administration sets, solution filter, pump, nursing time
• Catheter placement and site management	Venous access device *Central catheter:* site of procedure (bedside vs operating room), radiographic confirmation of placement, supplies used for site care *Peripheral line:* nursing time, supplies used for site care
• Monitoring	Routine laboratory and clinical measurements, changes in therapy to prevent complications or toxicities, nutrition support clinician time
• Complications	Mechanical: treatment of specific complication Infectious: cost of antibiotic therapy or venous access replacement Metabolic: increased clinical and laboratory measurements, possible waste of PN solution
Indirect	
• Morbidity	Quality-of-life expenses such as cost of patient discomfort, time lost from work or other activities as a result of PN therapy
• Mortality	Cost of premature death based, for example, on expected future wages

a patient's clinical condition stabilizes (see Fig. 137–3). (3) Minimize cost of PN by using efficient purchasing practices for PN solutions and compounding supplies through contract purchasing, streamlined compounding procedures, standardize administration times and 24-hour hang times to reduce waste, single-bag PN solutions, and optimized monitoring plans.

CONCLUSIONS

Appropriate patient selection, assessment, and monitoring are key to successful nutritional therapy and prevention of unnecessary complications or harm to the patient. Standardized order forms and monitoring protocols are useful tools to ensure appropriate administration and monitoring of PN therapy. Because pharmacists have been actively involved in the provision of PN at many levels, including direct patient care, education, and research, nutrition support has been recognized as a pharmacy practice speciality.[113] In addition, standards of practice have been defined for pharmacists providing nutrition support care.[6] The future of PN therapy and the role of the nutrition-support pharmacist will be affected primarily by new insights from clinical research and economic challenges in the health care environment.

▶ PRINCIPLES OF PHARMACOTHERAPY

- Four steps to developing a successful nutrition plan include definition of nutrition goals, determination of nutrition requirements, determination of appropriate route of delivery of nutrients, and subsequent monitoring of the nutrition regimen to evaluate suitability of the regimen as a patient's clinical condition changes and to minimize or treat complications early.
- The appropriate route of nutrition support depends on the functional condition of the patient's GI tract, risk of aspiration, expected duration of nutrition therapy, and the clinical condition of the patient.
- Identifying the patient who is most likely to benefit from PN therapy is difficult. Indications for use of PN should be specific to a practice setting and based on current consensus statements.
- PN may be administered by peripheral or central venous access. PPN is useful in patients who do not have large nutrient requirements, are not fluid restricted, and are expected to regain function of the GI tract within 7 to 10 days. PPN is limited by the tolerance of peripheral veins to hypertonic solutions. CPN is useful in patients who have large nutrient requirements, fluctuating fluid status, and are likely to require PN support for more than 7 to 10 days. CPN is limited by the technical and infectious complications associated with establishing and maintaining central vascular access.
- PN solutions may be infused continuously or intermittently. Continuous infusions are useful in patients with unstable fluid balance or poor blood glucose control. Intermittent or cyclic PN is useful for patients with limited intravenous access who also require multiple intravenous medications not compatible with PN, those who developed hepatotoxicity while receiving continuous PN, or patients who desire more time disconnected from the PN infusion.
- Non-catheter-related complications of PN therapy are minimized with application of age-appropriate nutrient dosing guidelines, frequent monitoring, and rational adjustments to the PN regimen when metabolic abnormalities occur.
- Biochemical and clinical measurements considered necessary for effective monitoring of patients receiving PN include serum concentrations of electrolytes, hematologic indices, and biochemical markers for renal function, liver function, and nutrition status. Other important clinical measurements include vital signs, weight, total fluid intake and losses, and nutritional intakes. The frequency of clinical laboratory measurements usually depends on the stability of a patient's clinical condition.
- Expenses associated with PN therapy may be minimized by using PN usage guidelines based on current consensus statements, frequent evaluation of the need for standing laboratory measurements used for monitoring PN therapy, maximizing efficient purchasing practices for PN solutions and compounding supplies usually through contract purchasing, streamlining compounding procedures, and minimizing PN waste by standardizing administration times and using 24-hour, single-bag PN solutions.

ACKNOWLEDGMENT

The author would like to thank Pam Reiter, PharmD, for her valuable suggestions and review of the pediatric portions of this manuscript.

REFERENCES

1. Kinney JM. History of parenteral nutrition, with notes on clinical biology. In Rombeau JL, Rolandelli RH, eds. Clinical Nutrition: Parenteral Nutrition, 3d ed. Philadelphia, Saunders, 2001:1–20.
2. Driscoll JM, Heird WC, Schullinger JN, et al. Total intravenous alimentation in low birth weight infants: A preliminary report. J Pediatr 1972;81:145–153.
3. Wesley JR. Nutrition support teams: Past, present and future. Nutr Clin Pract 1995;10:219–228.
4. ASPEN Board of Directors. Definitions of terms used in ASPEN guidelines and standards. J Parenter Nutr 1995;19:1–2.
5. Holcombe BJ, Thorne DB, Strausburg KM, et al. Pharmacy practice insights: Analysis of the practice of nutrition support pharmacy specialists. Pharmacotherapy 1995;15:806–813.
6. American Society for Parenteral and Enteral Nutrition. Standards of practice for nutrition support pharmacists. Nutr Clin Pract 1993;8:124–127.
7. American Society for Parenteral and Enteral Nutrition. Standards for nutrition support: Hospitalized patients. Nutr Clin Pract 1995;10:208–219.
8. American Society for Parenteral and Enteral Nutrition. Standards for home nutrition support. Nutr Clin Pract 1999;14:151–162.
9. Choban PS, Flancbaum L. Nourishing the obese patient. Clin Nutr 2000;19:305–311.
10. ASPEN Board of Directors. Routes to deliver nutrition support in adults. J Parenter Enter Nutr 1993;17:7SA–8SA.
11. Klein S, Kinney J, Jeejeebhoy K, et al. Nutrition support in clinical practice: Review of published data and recommendations for future research directions. Summary of a conference sponsored by the National Institutes of Health, American Society for Parenteral and Enteral Nutrition, and American Society for Clinical Nutrition. J Parenter Enter Nutr 1997;21:133–156.
12. Wolfe BM, Mathiesen KA. Clinical practice guidelines in nutrition support: Can they be based on randomized clinical trials? J Parenter Enter Nutr 1997;21:1–6.
13. Koretz RL, Lipman TO, Klein S. AGA technical review on parenteral nutrition. Gastroenterology 2001;121:970–1001.
14. Giner M, Laviano, Meguid MM, Gleason JR. In 1995, a correlation between malnutrition and poor outcome in critically ill patients still exists. Nutrition 1996;12:23–29.
15. Tucker HN, Miguel SG. Cost containment through nutrition intervention. Nutr Rev 1996;54:111–121.
16. Cerra FB, Benitez MR, Blackburn GL, et al. Applied nutrition in ICU patients: A consensus statement of the American College of Chest Physicians. Chest 1997;111:769–778.
17. ASPEN Board of Directors. Guidelines for the use of parenteral and enteral nutrition in adults and pediatric patients. J Parenter Enter Nutr 1993;17:(4 Suppl):155A–525A.
18. Maroulis J, Kalfarentzos F. Complications of parenteral nutrition at the end of the century. Clin Nutr 2000;19:295–304.
19. Koo WWK, Cepeda EE. Parenteral nutrition in neonates. In Rombeau JL, Rolandelli RH, eds. Clinical Nutrition: Parenteral Nutrition, 3d ed. Philadelphia, Saunders, 2001:463–475.
20. Falcone RA, Warner BW. Pediatric parenteral nutrition. In Rombeau JL, Rolandelli RH, eds. Clinical Nutrition: Parenteral Nutrition, 3d ed. Philadelphia, Saunders, 2001:476–496.
21. Miles JM, Klein JA. Should protein be included in caloric calculations for a TPN prescription? Point-counterpoint. Nutr Clin Pract 1996;11:204–206.
22. Furst P, Stehle P. Are intravenous amino acid solutions unbalanced? New Horizons 1994;2:215–223.
23. Miller SJ. The nitrogen balance revisited. Hosp Pharm 1990;25:61–65, 70.
24. Shatsky F, McFeely EJ, Takahashi D. A table for estimating calcium and phosphorus compatibility in parenteral nutrition formulas that contain trophamine plus cysteine. Hosp Pharm 1995;30:690–692, 793.
25. Scaglia F, Longo N. Primary and secondary alterations of neonatal carnitine metabolism. Semin Perinatol 1999;23:152–161.
26. Borum PR. Carnitine in neonatal nutrition. J Child Neurol 1995; 10(Suppl):S25–S31.
27. Lipsky CL, Spear ML. Recent advances in parenteral nutrition. Clin Perinatol 1995;22:141–155.
28. Sacks GS. Glutamine supplementation in catabolic patients. Ann Pharmacother 1999;33:348–354.
29. Tubman TR, Thompson SW. Glutamine supplementation for preventing morbidity in preterm infants. Cochrane Database Syst Rev 2000;(2):CD001457.
30. National Advisory Group on Standards and Practice Guidelines for Parenteral Nutrition. Safe practices for parenteral nutrition formulations. J Parenter Enter Nutr 1998;22:49–66.
31. Rosemarin DK, Wardlaw GM, Mirtallo JM. Hyperglycemia associated with high, continuous infusion rates of total parenteral nutrition dextrose. Nutr Clin Pract 1996;11:151–156.
32. Thureen PJ, Hay, Jr WW. Intravenous nutrition and postnatal growth of the micropremie. Clin Perinatol 2000;27:197–219.
33. Sheridan RL, Yu YM, Prelack K, et al. Maximal parenteral glucose oxidation in hypermetabolic young children: A stable isotope study. J Parenter Enter Nutr 1998;22:212–216.
34. Waxman K, Day AT, Stellin GP, et al. Safety and efficacy of glycerol and amino acids in combination with lipid emulsion for peripheral parenteral nutrition support. J Parenter Enter Nutr 1992;16:374–378.
35. Product information. ProcalAmine. Irvine, CA, B. Braun Medical, 1998.
36. Fat emulsions. In: McEvoy GK, ed. AHFS Drug Information 2000. Bethesda, MD, American Society of Hospital Pharmacists, 2000:2384–2385.
37. Adolph M. Lipid emulsions in parenteral nutrition. Ann Nutr Metab 1999;43:1–13.
38. Putet G. Lipid metabolism of the micropremie. Clin Perinatol 2000; 27:57–69.
39. Sacks GS, Mouser JF. Is IV lipid emulsion safe in patients with hypertriglyceridemia? Nutr Clin Pract 1997;12:120–123.
40. Sardesai VM. The essential fatty acids. Nutr Clin Pract 1992;7:179–186.
41. Dickerson RN. Essential fatty acid deficiency: An "old" disorder that should not be forgotten. Hosp Pharm 1998;33:1435–1440.
42. Warshawsky KY. Intravenous fat in clinical practice. Nutr Clin Prac 1992;7:187–196.
43. Lai HS, Chen WJ. Effects of medium-chain and long-chain triacylglycerols in pediatroc surgical patients. Nutrition 2000;16:401–406.
44. Furst P, Kuhn KS. Fish oil emulsions: what benefits can they bring? Clin Nutr 2000;19:7–14.
45. Battistella FD, Wildergren JT, Anderson JT, et al. A prospective, randomized trial of intravenous fat emulsion administration in trauma victims requiring total parenteral nutrition. J Trauma 1997;43(1):52–58.
46. McCowen KC, Friel C, Sternberg J, et al. Hypocaloric total parenteral nutrition: Effectiveness in prevention of hyperglycemia and infectious complications. A randomized clinical trial. Crit Care Med 2000;28:3606–3611.
47. Beale RJ, Bryg DJ, Bihari D. Immunonutrition in the critically ill: A systematic review of clinical outcome. Crit Care Med 1999;27:2799–2805.
48. Roth MS, Martin AB, Katz JA. Nutritional implications of prolonged propofol use. Am J Health Syst Pharm 1997;54:694–695.
49. Sacks GS, Cleary JD. Nutritional impact of lipid-associated amphotericin B formulations. Ann Pharmacother 1997;31:121–122.
50. American Medical Association Department of Foods and Nutrition. Multivitamin preparations for parenteral use: A statement by the nutritional advisory group. J Parenter Enter Nutr 1979;3:258–262.
51. Demling RH, DeBiasse MA. Micronutrients in critical illness. Crit Care Clin 1995;11:651–673.

52. Greer FR. Vitamin metabolism and requirements in the micropremie. Clin Perinatol 2000;27:95–118.
53. Green HL, Hambidge KM, Schanler R, Tsang RC. Guidelines for the use of vitamins, trace elements, calcium, magnesium, and phosphorus in infants and children receiving total parenteral nutrition: Report of the Subcommittee on Pediatric Parenteral Nutrient Requirements from the Committee on Clinical Practice Issues of the American Society for Clinical Nutrition. Am J Clin Nutr 1988;48:1324–1342.
54. Parenteral multivitamin products; Drugs for human use; Drug efficacy implementation; amendment. Fed Reg 2000;65:21200–21201.
55. Chambrier C, Lellerq M, Saudin F, et al. Is vitamin K_1 supplementation necessary in long-term parenteral nutrition? J Parenter Enter Nutr 1998;22:87–90.
56. Lennon C, Davidson KW, Sandowski JA, Mason JB. The vitamin K content of intravenous lipid emulsion. J Parenter Enter Nutr 1993;17:142–144.
57. Schepers GP, Dimitry AR, Eckhauser FE, et al. Efficacy and safety of low-dose intravenous versus intramuscular vitamin K in parenteral nutrition patients. J Parenter Enter Nutr 1988;12:174–177.
58. Misra S, Kirby DF. Micronutrient and trace element monitoring in adult nutrition support. Nutr Clin Pract 2000;15:120–126.
59. Aggett PJ. Trace elements of the micropremie. Clin Perinatol 2000; 27:119–129.
60. American Medical Association. Guidelines for essential trace element preparations for parenteral use: A statement by the Nutrition Advisory Group. J Parenter Enter Nutr 1979;3:263–267.
61. Baumgartner TG, ed. Clinical Guide to Parenteral Micronutrition, 3d ed. Deerfield, IL, Fujasawa USA, 1997.
62. Schmidt GL. Guidelines for managing electrolytes in total parenteral nutrition solutions. Nutr Clin Pract 2000;15:94–109.
63. Miller SJ. Peripheral parenteral nutrition: theory and practice. Hosp Pharm 1991;26:796–801.
64. Payne-James JJ, Khawaja HT. First choice for total parenteral nutrition The peripheral route. J Parenter Enter Nutr 1993;17:468–478.
65. Veterans Affairs Total Parenteral Nutrition Cooperative Study Group. Perioperative total parenteral nutrition in surgical patients. New Engl J Med 1991;325:525–532.
66. Kane KF, Cologiovanni L, McKiernan J, et al. High osmolality feedings do not increase the incidence of thrombophlebitis during peripheral IV nutrition. J Parenter Enter Nutr 1996;20:194–197.
67. Grant JP. Vascular access for total parenteral nutrition: techniques and complications. In: Handbook of Total Parenteral Nutrition, 2d ed. Philadelphia, Saunders, 1992:107–138.
68. Fischer JE. Metabolism in surgical patients: Protein, carbohydrate, and fat utilization by oral and parenteral routes. In: Sabiston DC Jr, ed. Textbook of Surgery: The Biological Basis of Modern Surgical Practice, 15th ed. Philadelphia, Saunders, 1997:137–175.
69. Cerulli J, Malone M. Can changes to a total parenteral nutrition order form improve prescribing? Nutr Clin Pract 2000;15:143–151.
70. Campos ACL, Paluzzi M, Meguid MM. Clinical use of total nutrient admixtures. Nutrition 1990;6:347–356.
71. American Society for Health-System Pharmacists. ASHP guidelines on the safe use of automated compounding devices for the preparation of parenteral nutrition admixtures. Am J Health Syst Pharm 2000;57:1343–1348.
72. American Society for Health System Pharmacists. ASHP guidelines on quality assurance for pharmacy-prepared sterile products. Am J Health Syst Pharm 2000;57:1150–1169.
73. Thompson B, Robinson LA. Infection control of parenteral nutrition solutions. Nutr Clin Pract 1991;6:49–54.
74. Pearson ML. The Hospital Infection Control Practices Advisory Group: Guideline for prevention of intravascular device-related infections. Am J Infect Control 1996;24:262–293.
75. Ebbert ML, Farraj M, Hwang LT. The incidence and clinical significance of intravenous fat emulsion contamination during infusion. J Parenter Enter Nutr 1987;11:42–45.
76. Trissel LA. Handbook on Injectable Drugs, 11th ed. Bethesda, MD, American Society for Hospital Pharmacists, 2000.
77. Catania P, ed. King Guide to Parenteral Admixtures. Napa, CA, King Guide Publications, 2000.
78. Trissel LA. Amino acid injection. In: Handbook on Injectable Drugs, 11th ed. Bethesda, MD, American Society for Hospital Pharmacists, 2000:40–84.
79. Laborie S, Lavoie JC, Pineault M, Chessex P. Contribution of multivitamins, air and light in the generation of peroxides in adult and neonatal parenteral nutrition solutions. Ann Pharmacother 2000:34;440–445.
80. Laborie S, Lavoie JC, Pineault M, Chessex P. Protecting solutions of parenteral nutrition from peroxidation. J Parenter Enter Nutr 1999;23: 104–108.
81. Neuzil J, Darlow BA, Inder TE, et al. Oxidation of parenteral lipid emulsion by ambient and phototherapy lights: Potential toxicity of routine parenteral feeding. J Pediatr 1995;126:785–790.
82. Helbock HJ, Ames BN. Use of intravenous lipids in neonates. J Pediatr 1995;126:747–748.
83. Driscoll DF, Baptista RJ, Mitrano FP, et al. Parenteral nutrient admixtures as drug vehicles: theory and practice in the critical care setting. DICP 1991;25:276–283.
84. Mirtallo JM. The complexity of mixing calcium and phosphate. Am J Hosp Pharm 1994;51:1535–1536.
85. Krzyda EA, Andris DA, Whipple JK, et al. Glucose response to abrupt initiation and discontinuation of total parenteral nutrition. J Parenter Enter Nutr 1993;17:64–67.
86. Dickerson RN. How fast can I taper a TPN in a hospitalized patient? Hosp Pharm 1985;20:620–621.
87. Bennett KM, Rosen GH. Cyclic total parenteral nutrition. Nutr Clin Pract 1990;5:163–165.
88. Grant JP. Septic and metabolic complications: recognition and management. In: Handbook of Total Parenteral Nutrition, 2d ed. Philadelphia, Saunders, 1992:239–274.
89. McMahon MM. Management of hyperglycemia in hospitalized patients receiving parenteral nutrition. Nutr Clin Pract 1997;12:35–38.
90. Teasley-Strausburg KM, Shronts EP. Metabolic and gastrointestinal complications. In: Teasley-Strausburg KM, ed. Nutrition Support Handbook: A Compendium of Products with Guidelines for Usage Cincinnati, Harvey Whitney Books, 1992:295–303.
91. Briones ER, Iber FL. Liver and biliary tract changes and injury associated with total parenteral nutrition: Pathogenesis and prevention. J Am Coll Nutr 1995;14:219–228.
92. Quigley EMM, Marsh MN, Shaffer JL, Markin RS. Hepatobiliary complications of total parenteral nutrition. Gastroenterology 1993;104:286–301.
93. Sondheim JM, Asturias E, Cadnapaphornchai M. Infection and cholestasis in neonates with intestinal resection and long-term parenteral nutrition. J Pediatr Gastroenterol Nutr 1998;27:131–137.
94. Beath SV, Davies P, Papadopoulou A, et al. Parenteral nutrition-releated cholestasis in postsurgical neonates: Multivariate analysis of risk factors. J Pediatr Surg 1996 31:604–606.
95. Chan S, McCowen KC, Bistrian BR, et al. Incidence, prognosis, and etiology of end-stage liver disease in patients receiving home total parenteral nutrition. Surgery 1999;126:28–34.
96. Cavicchi M, Beau P, Crenn P, et al. Prevalence of liver disease and contributing factors in patients receiving home parenteral nutrition for permanent intestinal failure. Ann Intern Med 2000;132:525–532.
97. Brooks MJ, Melnik G. The refeeding syndrome: An approach to understanding its complications and preventing its occurrence. Pharmacotherapy 1995;15:713–726.
98. Center for Disease Control. Lactic acidosis traced to thiamine deficiency related to nationwide shortage of multivitamins for total parenteral nutrition—United States, 1997. Morb Mortal Week Rep 1997;46:523–528.
99. Buchman AL, Moukarzel A. Metabolic bone disease associated with total parenteral nutrition. Clin Nutr 2000;19:217–231.
100. Mouser JF, Hak EB, Helms RA, et al. Chromium and zinc concentrations in pediatric patients receiving long-term parenteral nutrition. Am J Health Sys Pharm 1999;56:1950–1956.
101. Klein GL. Aluminum in parenteral nutrition solutions revisited—again. Am J Clin Nutr 1995;61:449–456.

102. Davis A, Spillane R, Zublena L. Aluminum: a problem trace metal in nutrition support. Nutr Clin Pract 1999;14:227–231.
103. Klein GL, Leichter AM, Heyman MB, and the Patient Care Committee of the North American Society for Pediatric Gastroenterology and Nutrition. Aluminum in large and small volume parenterals used in total parenteral nutrition: Response to the Food and Drug Administration notice proposed rule by the North American Society for Pediatric Gastroenterology and Nutrition. J Pediatr Gastroenterol Nutr 1998;27:457–460.
104. Howard L, Hassan N. Home parenteral nutrition: 25 years later. Gastroenterol Clin North Am 1998;27:481–512.
105. Evans MA, Liffrig TK, Nelson JK, Compher C. Home nutrition support patient education materials. Nutr Clin Prac 1993;8:43–47.
106. Lipman TO. The cost of TPN: Is the price right? J Parenter Enter Nutr 1993;17:199–200.
107. Eisenberg JM, Glick HA, Buzby GP, et al. Does perioperative total parenteral nutrition reduce medical care costs? J Parenter Enter Nutrition 1993;17:201–209.
108. Twomey PL, Patching SC. Cost effectiveness of nutritional support. J Parenter Enter Nutr 1985;9:3–10.
109. Trujillo EB, Young LS, Chertow GM, et al. Metabolic and monetary costs of avoidable parenteral nutrition use. J Parenter Enter Nutr 1999;23:109–113.
110. Eisenberg JM, Glick H, Hillman AL, et al. Measuring the economic impact of perioperative total parenteral nutrition: Principles and design. Am J Clin Nutr 1988;47:382–391.
111. Lipman TO. Grains or veins: Is enteral nutrition really better than parenteral nutrition? A look at the evidence. J Parenter Enter Nutr 1998; 22:167–182.
112. Trice S, Melnik G, Page C. Complications and costs of early postoperative parenteral versus enteral nutrition in trauma patients. Nutr Clin Pract 1997;12:114–119.
113. Task Force on Specialty Recognition and Certification of Nutritional Support Pharmacists. Executive summary of petition requesting recognition of nutritional support pharmacy as a specialty. Am J Hosp Pharm 1991;48:1284.

138

ENTERAL NUTRITION

Douglas D. Janson and Katherine Hammond Chessman

Oral ingestion of food and the delivery of a liquid formula through a tube placed beyond the oral cavity are forms of enteral nutrition. Enteral nutrition and tube feeding are often used interchangeably to describe an artificial feeding method that includes the use of specialized feeding formulas, tubes, and pumps. Patients who are unable to chew or swallow because of a gastrointestinal (GI) obstruction, advanced neurologic or psychiatric diseases, prolonged unconsciousness associated with critical illness, or extreme prematurity benefit from nutrient delivery to the gut by tube feedings. Additionally, patients who are unable to eat a sufficient amount of calories will benefit from tube feedings.

In this chapter the principles and practices related to the successful use of enteral nutrition support are described. Digestive and absorptive physiology is reviewed and the rationale for the use of the enteral feeding route whenever possible is presented. The indications for enteral nutrition, and descriptions of various enteral access and administration methods are also summarized. Characteristics of commercially available formulas are presented, as well as initiation and monitoring guidelines to prevent complications. In addition, issues of drug compatibility, drug-nutrient interactions, and drug administration during enteral nutrition are discussed. Last, the effectiveness of enteral nutrition to enhance nutrition and disease outcome goals is reviewed.

GASTROINTESTINAL TRACT PHYSIOLOGY

Digestion and absorption are important and inseparably associated GI processes that generate the usable fuels for the body. Digestion consists of the stepwise conversion of a complex chemical and physical nutrient form into a molecular form acceptable to the intestinal mucosa. Absorption from the GI tract (GIT) consists of transfer of a nutrient across an intestinal cell membrane. The nutrient ultimately reaches the systemic circulation through the portal venous or splanchnic lymphatic systems, provided that it is not excreted by the GI or biliary tract. Ingested nutrients are primarily large polymers that cannot be absorbed by the mucosal membrane unless they are broken down or transformed into an absorbable molecular form. In addition, a coordinated interplay of GI motility and neurohormonal secretion is required to facilitate adequate digestion and absorption.[1,2]

Nutrient digestion involves the complex coordination of multiple mechanical, enzymatic, and physicochemical processes. Mechanical dissolution of food occurs by chewing, mixing, and grinding of the stomach contents. Food stimulates the secretion of numerous neurohormones and enzymes from the salivary glands, stomach, liver and biliary system, pancreas, and intestines (Table 138–1). As food passes along the gut lumen, these neurohormones control GI motility and secretion among the organs of the digestive system. Nutrient digestion occurs within the gut lumen and also on the intestinal mucosal membrane. Absorption is a specific function of the intestinal mucosal membrane. The basic absorptive unit is a finger-like projection called the villus, which is made up of epithelial cells called enterocytes. The enterocyte surface contains special luminal projections called microvilli, which provide an increased surface area that is referred to as the brush border membrane.[1,2]

Digestible carbohydrates are presented to the small intestine as polysaccharides (starches) and oligosaccharides (sucrose and lactose). Enzymatic digestion within the gut lumen and at the surface of the brush border membrane produces simple sugars that are translocated across the membrane via active and passive transport mechanisms. These simple sugars eventually are released into the portal vein, as shown in Figure 138–1. Polysaccharides such as cellulose complexes and other fiber components are digested within the colon by bacterial hydrolases, disaccharidases, and enzymes to short-chain fatty acids (SCFAs). Subsequent to their rapid colonic absorption, SCFAs stimulate sodium and water reabsorption, serve as an energy source, and are trophic or nourishing to the cells of the intestinal mucosa.[3] Fat is presented primarily to the gut as long-chain triglycerides (LCTs) containing 14 to 24 carbon atoms. LCT digestion includes lipolysis and the formation of mixed bile salt micelles which facilitate solubility and absorption across the mucosal membrane. Within the enterocyte cytosol, triglycerides are re-esterified and packaged into chylomicrons for release into the lymphatic system, as shown in Figure 138–1. Chylomicrons eventually reach the venous system after transport through the thoracic duct. Medium-chain triglycerides (MCTs) containing 8 to 12 carbon atoms do not require luminal lipolysis and can be absorbed intact by the mucosal membrane. Within the enterocyte, MCTs are acted on by intracellular lipase, and the resulting free fatty acids pass directly into the portal vein.[4]

Protein is presented to the gut primarily as large polypeptides and to a small extent as amino acids owing to the denaturation of protein within the stomach. Subsequent to the luminal digestion of polypeptides to oligopeptides of two to eight amino acids, brush border membrane amino-oligopeptidases generate dipeptides and tripeptides. Membrane translocation of the resulting peptides occurs via a peptide transport system, and free amino acids are carried via specific amino acid transport systems. Amino acids and dipeptides are then passed into the portal vein, as shown in Figure 138–1. The digestive and absorptive physiology of these and other nutrients such as water, electrolytes, vitamins, and trace elements are discussed in detail elsewhere.[5] Under normal circumstances, almost 100% of carbohydrates and more than 80% of amino acids are absorbed within the proximal jejunum. The majority of fat absorption occurs within the jejunum and is completed in the ileum. The absorptive location of these and other nutrients within the GI tract is variable.[5]

Understanding the mechanisms of digestive and absorptive physiology can greatly enhance the rational use of enteral nutrition support during conditions of normal or altered GI function. Several circumstances may alter the efficacy of nutrient digestion and absorption (Table 138–2). In particular, the functional immaturity of the neonatal gut may lead to clinical problems associated with inadequate digestion and absorption of enteral nutrition. These factors, as they relate to successful enteral nutrition practice, are discussed in detail throughout this chapter.

TABLE 138–1. Gastrointestinal Enzymes and Hormones

Enzyme/Hormone	Site of Secretion	Main Actions
Amylase	Salivary glands	Converts carbohydrates, starch, and glycogen to simple disachharides
Cholecystokinin (CCK)	Duodenum, jejunum	Stimulates pancreatic enzyme secretion and gallbladder contraction
Chymotrypsinogen	Pancreas	Breaks down proteins into proteases and peptides
Enteroglucagon	Duodenum, small intestine	Inhibits pancreatic enzyme secretion and bowel motility
Gastric inhibitory peptide (GIP)	Small intestine	Decreases gastric motility and stimulates insulin secretion
Gastrin	Stomach, duodenum	Stimulates gastric acid secretion and mucosal growth
Glucagon	Pancreas	Stimulates hepatic glycogenolysis and inhibits motility
Lipase	Pancreas	Hydrolyzes short-chain and medium-chain triglycerides, involved in fat absorption
Pancreatic polypeptide	Pancreas	Inhibits gallbladder contraction and pancreatic and biliary secretion
Pepsinogen	Stomach	Converts large proteins into polypeptides
Secretin	Small intestine	Stimulates hepatic and pancreatic water and bicarbonate
Trypsinogen	Pancreas	Breaks down proteins into proteases and peptides
Vasoactive inhibitory peptide (VIP)	Small intestine, pancreas	Vasodilator; stimulates water and bicarbonate secretion, release of insulin and glucagon, and production of small intestinal juice

GUT HOST DEFENSE MECHANISMS

Besides digesting and absorbing nutrients to maintain nutritional health, the GIT is actively involved in defending the host from toxins and antigens by means of nonimmunologic and immunologic mechanisms (Table 138–3). These gut host defense mechanisms are also collectively referred to as the gut barrier function.[6,7] The gut barrier acts to prevent the spread of intraluminal bacteria and endotoxin to systemic organs and tissues. Hydrochloric acid secreted by the stomach kills the majority of the bacteria ingested with food. Under normal circumstances, a mucus gel layer coats the intestinal epithelium and thereby alters the adherence of bacteria to the cells of the GIT and provides a favorable environment for anaerobic bacteria. Anaerobic bacteria, which normally colonize the mucus layer, aid in preventing tissue colonization by potential pathogens. Small bowel peristalsis further prevents bacterial stasis and overgrowth. The gut barrier function is also maintained by the intestinal immune system, known as the gut-associated lymphoid tissue (GALT). GALT regulates the local immune response to antigens within the GIT. Specific immunoglobulins are secreted to kill remaining organisms and neutralize any toxins they produce. Last, the hepatic Kupffer's cells help to maintain gut barrier function by clearing the portal blood of gut-derived bacteria and endotoxin. The integrity of gut barrier function may be affected by numerous pathogenic insults such as physiologic stress, ischemia, and a variety of drugs, including chemotherapeutic agents. The nutritional aspects that influence the maintenance of the gut barrier are discussed in the next section.

RATIONALE FOR ENTERAL NUTRITION

Enteral nutrition is the preferred route of nourishment if the GIT is functioning and accessible. A considerable body of laboratory and clinical evidence supports the importance and potential advantages of using enteral over parenteral nutrition. Advantages of enteral nutrition include maintaining the structure and function of the GIT, fewer metabolic and infectious complications, and lower costs. Experimental

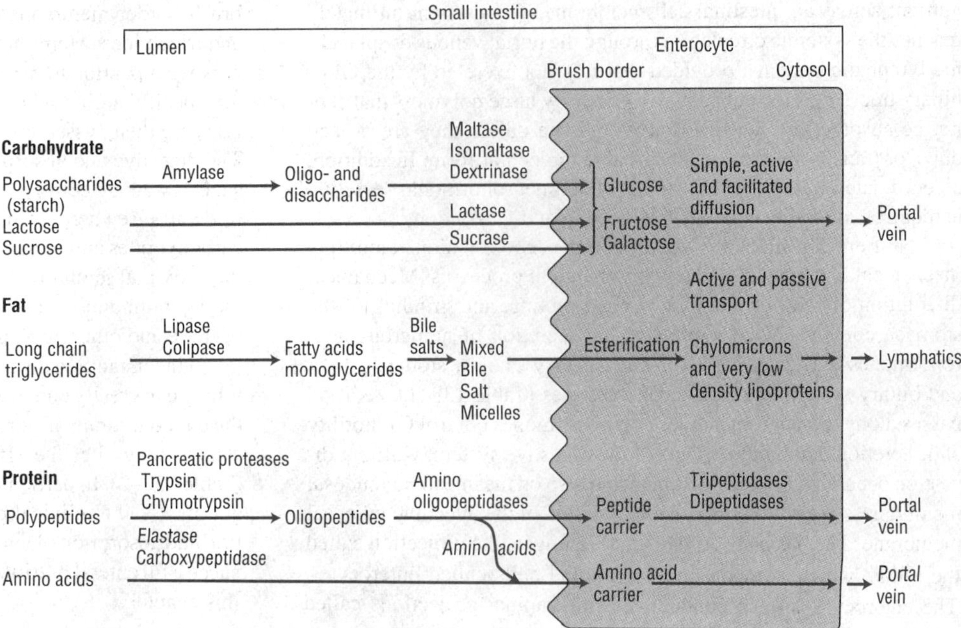

FIGURE 138–1. Schematic representation of carbohydrate, fat, and protein digestion and absorption within the small intestine. Subsequent to mechanical and enzymatic digestion of these substrates within the lumen and/or brush border of the enterocyte, smaller molecular forms are absorbed into the cytosol by numerous transport mechanisms. Then nutrients are released from the enteroctye into the systemic circulation.

TABLE 138–2. Factors Affecting Intestinal Nutrient Absorption

Method of ingestion
Digestibility
Gastric emptying
Intraluminal digestive capacity of the pancreas and the bile
Transit time
Contact surface
Length
Surface of villi
Brush border enzyme content
Carrier function
Diffusion barrier thickness (unstirred layer)

data derived predominantly from animal studies suggest that the maintenance of GIT structure and function depends on the presence and composition of luminal nutrients as well as the presence of trophic hormones. A frequently cited benefit of enteral nutrition is that it preserves the process of intestinal crypt cell renewal necessary for the support of normal villi structure and associated enzymatic functions that are required for normal digestion and absorption.[8–10] Mucosal atrophy and deficient disaccharidase and trypsin activities have been documented in small bowel biopsies obtained from malnourished infants with protracted diarrhea and malnutrition.[11] The data from these studies suggest that the absence of luminal nutrients induces gut atrophy, or mucosal hypoplasia, and decreased enzymatic activity. Clinically, the gut atrophy that occurs during a prolonged absence of enteral feeding may be responsible for the development of symptoms such as cramping and diarrhea when enteral nutrition is reintroduced.

The nutrient complexity of the enteral diet also appears to have an effect on the maintenance of intestinal mucosa mass. The weight of small intestinal mucosa segments and DNA and protein content of rats were best maintained when rats were fed a complex intact diet instead of an isocaloric hydrolyzed (partially digested) diet.[12,13] Furthermore, the colonic mucosal mass in rats fed a complex diet was better maintained than in those who received a hydrolyzed diet; this suggests that there may be some contribution of the fiber contained in the rat chow.[12] The presence of luminal nutrients in animals also has been shown to stimulate the production of enteric hormones such as gastrin and enteroglucagon, which are trophic to the gut mucosa.[14–16] These hormones are found in humans but have not been studied as intensively in humans as they have in animal models.

The intestine is an organ of protein synthesis as well as one of digestion and absorption. It therefore uses nutritional substrates directly. Glucose, glutamine, and L-leucine are examples of fuels used more efficiently when given via the enteral route as opposed to parenterally.[17,18] L-Leucine yields greater protein synthesis when given orally and is incorporated into the intestinal structure differently depending on the route of ingestion. Serum glutamine levels fall during stress, whereas intestinal uptake rises.[19] Glutamine and ketones are absent from parenteral solutions and may account for some of the intestinal structural deterioration seen during the administration of parenteral nutrition. The results from the aforementioned studies and others have stimulated several investigations into the effects of specific types of enteral diets, specific nutrients such as glutamine and fiber, and the interaction of trophic hormones on their ability to maintain the GI mucosa.

TABLE 138–3. Gut Host Defense Mechanisms

Nonimmunologic	Immunologic
Mechanical	Gut-associated lymphoid tissue (GALT)
Epithelial cell	Secretory immunoglobulin A
Epithelial mucus gel layer	Hepatic Kupffer's cells
Peristalsis	
Gastric acid	
Bile salts	
Salivary secretions	
Indigenous microflora	
Limits microbial proliferation	
Microbial antagonism	

Maintenance of the functional integrity of the GIT is intimately linked to proper gut barrier function. The immunologic and barrier functions listed in Table 138–3 prevent antigenic invasion of the gut mucosa, induction of local inflammation, and translocation of gut bacteria to the portal or lymphatic circulation. It has been suggested that bacterial translocation, the appearance of enteric organisms in the mesenteric lymph nodes, spleen, and liver, is promoted by parenteral nutrition and bowel rest. Since enteral nutrition better maintains the functional integrity of the gut, it also may prevent gut bacterial translocation. Animal studies comparing parenteral and enteral nutrient delivery supporting the theory of gut bacterial translocation include the following: Enteral nutrition resulted in higher secretary immunoglobulin A (IgA) and biliary tract secretions,[20] less bacterial leak through intestinal mucosa,[21] greater maintenance of mucosal weight and thickness with lower secretion of catabolic hormones following a burn injury,[22] and reduced mortality following septic[23] or hypotensive insult.[24] The results of one human study among healthy volunteers also suggest the potential role of enteral nutrition in maintaining the gut mucosal barrier and preventing bacterial translocation. Subjects receiving total parenteral nutrition (TPN) and complete bowel rest for 7 days, compared with subjects receiving enteral feedings, had significantly higher levels of arterial epinephrine, glucagon, and hepatic venous tumor necrosis factor when given an equivalent dose of enteral endotoxin. Additionally, the parenterally fed subjects also had enhancement of acute-phase protein response, increased peripheral amino acid mobilization, and increased peripheral lactate production, a metabolic response expected to occur with systemic endotoxin effect.[25] The 1990 summary guidelines for the scientific review of enteral food products by the Life Sciences Research Office, Federation of American Societies for Experimental Biology, concluded that although available human data are insufficient to establish whether the atrophic changes in the gut that are associated with a lack of enteral nutrition lead to clinically significant translocation of gut bacteria, endotoxins, and antigenic macromolecules, these considerations seem to justify the use of at least partial enteral nutrition as one means of maintaining the gut mucosa or reducing such complications.[26] Prospective, randomized clinical trials among critically ill patients comparing enteral and parenteral delivery are unable to substantiate a direct cause and effect between the parenteral route and gut bacterial translocation. However, critical reviews of the literature suggest that enteral nutrition may have a favorable impact on GI immunologic function and infectious morbidity.[27,28]

A metabolic advantage of enteral feeding compared with the parenteral route is improved glucose tolerance and markedly less hyperinsulinemia.[29,30] It has been proposed that better control of peripheral blood glucose levels occurs during enteral administration because the insulin released is absorbed with the glucose via the portal vein and is handled by the liver. The enteral feeding route is also as effective as the parenteral route in maintaining or promoting repletion of nutritional indices among several patient populations.[31] An additional physiologic benefit of enteral feeding is that it stimulates bile flow through the biliary tract and hence reduces the development

TABLE 138–4. Potential Indications for Enteral Nutrition

Neoplastic Disease	**Gastrointestinal Disease**
Chemotherapy	Inflammatory bowel disease
Radiotherapy	Short bowel syndrome
Upper gastrointestinal tumors	Esophageal motility disorder
Cancer cachexia	Pancreatitis
Organ Failure	Fistulas
Hepatic	Gastroesophageal reflux disease
Renal	Esophageal atresia
Cardiac cachexia	**Neurologic Impairment**
Pulmonary	Comatose state
Bronchopulmonary Dysplasia	Cerebrovascular accident
Congenital heart disease	Demyelinating disease
Hypermetabolic States	Severe depression
Closed head injury	Failure to thrive
Burns	Cerebral palsy
Trauma	**Other Indications**
Postoperative major surgery	Acquired immune deficiency syndrome
Sepsis	Anorexia nervosa
	Complications during pregnancy
	Geriatric patients with multiple chronic diseases
	Organ transplantation
	Inborn errors of metabolism
	Cystic fibrosis
	Extreme prematurity

of gallbladder sludge and stone formation, which has been associated with long-term parenteral nutrition and bowel rest.[32] Also, enteral nutrition removes the potential infectious or technical complications associated with the placement and use of a central venous access device required for parenteral nutrition. Finally, enteral nutrition is less costly than parenteral nutrition, as is discussed within the pharmacoeconomic considerations section of this chapter.

INDICATIONS FOR ENTERAL NUTRITION

Subsequent to assessing the patient's nutritional state and need for initiating specialized nutrition support, the clinician must assess the functional status of the GIT and the optimal access site for tube placement. An algorithmic approach to nutritional management is shown in Figure 136–1. Although enteral nutrition is indicated for many conditions or disease states (Table 138–4), its use is contraindicated for patients with a mechanical obstruction of the GIT, diffuse peritonitis, severe diarrhea that makes metabolic management difficult, severe GI hemorrhage, intractable vomiting, pseudo-obstruction, necrotizing enterocolitis, or severe malabsorption.

FUNCTIONAL STATUS OF THE GI TRACT

An assessment of the length, anatomy, and motility of the GIT is required prior to the initiation of enteral therapy. The minimum length of functional small bowel required for nutrient absorption in an adult is approximately 100 to 150 cm. In children, small bowel length of 20 cm with an intact ileocecal valve or 40 cm without the ileocecal valve is considered necessary for successful transition to enteral nutrition. Enteral nutrient delivery may effectively nourish some patients with less small bowel, especially if the ileocecal valve and the colon are present and intact.[33] Increased small bowel motility, results in a decrease in GI transit time. This may occur when the ileum and/or ileocecal valve are removed. The ileocecal valve acts as a brake and reduces the transit of the GI contents through the small bowel and into the colon. The colon maintains fluid and electrolyte balance in an enterally fed patient.

Hospitalized patients may have reduced gastric motility and emptying caused by sepsis, postoperative anesthetic agents, opioid analgesics, and underlying pathology such as diabetic gastroparesis. Reduced gastric motility can place a gastrically fed patient at risk for nausea, vomiting, and subsequent pulmonary aspiration of gastric contents. Successful enteral nutrition can be initiated by placing the tip of the feeding tube beyond the pylorus into the duodenum or, preferably, more distal into the jejunum. Early enteral feedings started within 12 to 24 hours for the postoperative patient via the small bowel are given frequently, even in the absence of bowel sounds. However, during states of shock, borderline tissue oxygenation, and unstable cardiopulmonary hemodynamics, initiation of early GI feedings should be withheld because nutrient delivery and its associated oxygen requirement can further compromise tissue perfusion. Anecdotal reports and animal studies suggest that early enteral nutrition can be provided to the GIT of a patient who has recently undergone a GI anastomosis without compromising the integrity of the anastomosis.[34] Placement of postanastomotic feeding tubes allows enteral nutrition to be used soon after surgery in infants with esophageal and duodenal atresia repairs and avoids protracted courses of parenteral nutrition.

Guidelines for the use of enteral nutrition have been published by the American Society of Parenteral and Enteral Nutrition.[35] Patients with neurologic impairment or psychological diseases who will not or cannot eat but have functioning GITs are candidates for enteral nutrition. Patients with organ failure or GI diseases and patients in hypermetabolic states such as burns or trauma frequently are candidates for enteral nutrition. Enteral feeding is indicated for those patients with colocutaneous or low-output ileal fistulas. Enteral nutrition is also favored for patients with an esophageal, gastric, duodenal, and proximal jejunal fistulas when distal GIT tube feeding access is possible. Extreme prematurity may also necessitate tube feeding because the suck-swallow mechanism has not developed.

The use of enteral nutrition during severe pancreatitis or associated complications has increased. The precise effect of enteral nutrition on exocrine pancreatic secretion when infused into the jejunum is unclear because of conflicting data from human and animal studies. Nonetheless, clinicians have administered specialized enteral formulas to patients with severe and complicated pancreatitis via the placement of a feeding tube into the jejunum. A prospective, randomized clinical trial that stratified patients with severe acute pancreatitis according to disease severity, compared TPN with total enteral nutrition (TEN) and demonstrated the clinical feasibility of TEN. In addition, TEN patients benefited by moderation of the acute-phase response and improvement in disease severity and clinical outcome despite unchanged pancreatic injury on computed tomography (CT) scan.[36] It has been recommended that TPN be used when enteral feeding exacerbates abdominal pain, ascites, or fistulous output in patients with pancreatitis and limited oral intake.[35] Several clinical trials have shown that enteral nutrition is effective in supporting Crohn's disease patients with exacerbations of their disease. However, enteral nutrition is contraindicated in Crohn's disease with concomitant high-output fistula or high-grade obstruction or when enteral feeding fails to normalize the nutritional status or results in unacceptable GI symptoms.[35] In patients with acquired immune deficiency syndrome (AIDS), enteral nutrition should be used unless situations of severe malabsorption develop because of GI infections such as cryptosporidium or cytomegalovirus or during complications of lymphoma involving the small bowel.[37]

ENTERAL ACCESS

Enteral nutrition support, distinguished from normal eating by the routes of nutrient intake and the equipment needed to administer it, should be used when oral intake is not adequate to meet needs. Because the conditions necessitating specialized nutrition support are varied, multiple options are available to provide this therapy. All routes involve placement of a tube through which a liquid formula is infused. As the site of nutrient delivery moves further away from the mouth, the tube insertion becomes more difficult and invasive but, at the same time, more permanent. The technique and selection of enteral routes and access devices have been reviewed extensively in the literature.[38,39] The indications, placement options, advantages, and disadvantages associated with the different tube feeding routes are summarized in Table 138–5.

The most frequently used short-term enteral feeding routes are those accessed by inserting a tube through the nose and threading it into the stomach or upper small bowel (Fig. 138–2). The names of these routes—nasogastric (NG), nasoduodenal (ND), and nasojejunal (NJ)—indicate both the tube insertion point and the termination point. The oral gastric (OG) route is reserved for patients in whom the nasopharyngeal area is unaccessible (e.g., those with choanal atresia, basilar skull fracture, or facial trauma) or in young infants because they are obligate nasal breathers. These routes do not require surgical intervention and therefore are the least invasive. They are also temporary because the tubes frequently are held in place by a piece of tape on the nose or face. One disadvantage is that they can be pulled out easily.

Dobbie and Hoffmeister[40] were the first to describe feeding through a flexible, weighted tube. Prior to their report, all enteral feedings were infused through heavy, large-bore, rigid rubber tubes. Use of a rigid tube was associated with loss of lower esophageal sphincter tone, otitis media, esophagitis, esophageal perforations, and mucosal injury.[41] Modern tubes patterned after Dr. Dobbie's prototype generally consist of small-bore, pliable silicone rubber or polyurethane, which makes them lightweight and comfortable for the patient. Modern feeding tubes are available in varying lengths of 16 to 60 inches and small-bore sizes of 6 to 12 French. This provides a broad range of options for pediatric and adult patients. A disadvantage of the small-bore tube is that it may become clogged, due to improper medication or formula administration or tube-flushing techniques.

TABLE 138–5. Options and Considerations in the Selection of Tube Feeding Access

Access	Indications	Tube Placement Options	Advantages	Disadvantages
Nasogastric or orogastric	Short-term Intact gag reflex Normal gastric emptying	Manually at bedside	Ease of placement Allows for intermittent bolus or continuous feeding Inexpensive Multiple commercially available tubes and sizes	Potential tube displacement Increased aspiration risk Small bore tube
Nasoduodenal or nasojejunal	Short-term Delayed gastric emptying (early postoperative period or diabetic neuropathy) High risk of gastroesophageal reflux or aspiration	Manually at bedside Fluoroscopic Endoscopic	Reduced aspiration risk Allows for early postoperative feeding Multiple commercially available tubes and sizes	Manual transpyloric passage requires greater skill Potential tube displacement Continuous (and cyclic) feeding only Attendant risks of complication for endoscopic placement Small bore tube
Esophagostomy or pharyngostomy	Long-term Nasopharyngeal access contraindicated Tumors of head or neck region	Bedside with local anesthesia or during surgery	Large-bore tube Easy tube placement	Dressing changes by patient more difficult owing to location Requires stoma site care
Gastrostomy	Long-term Normal gastric emptying Swallowing dysfunction owing to neuromuscular disease or central nervous system disorders Esophageal stricture or neoplasm	Surgically Endoscopically (percutaneous endoscopic gastrostomy [PEG]) Laparoscopically Fluoroscopically	Allows for intermittent, bolus, or continuous feeding Large-bore tube Multiple commercially available tubes and sizes Low-profile buttons available	Attendant risks for complication for each method of placement Higher cost, particularly with surgical placement Aspiration risk potential Requires stoma site care
Jejeunostomy	Long-term Impaired gastric emptying (diabetic neuropathy) Facilitate postoperative enteral feeding in trauma, malnourished or upper GIT surgery Inability to access upper GIT	Surgically Endoscopically (accessing jejunum via PEG) Laparoscopically Fluoroscopically	Allows for early postoperative feeding Reduced aspiration risk Multiple commercially available tubes and sizes	Attendant risks for complication for each method of placement Continuous (and cyclic) feeding only Requires stoma site care

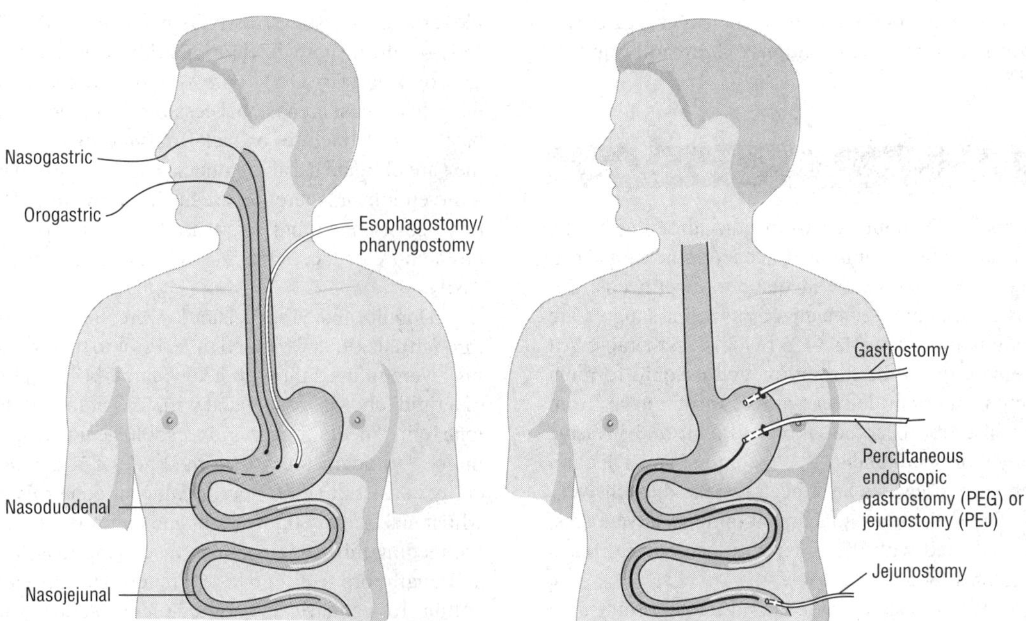

FIGURE 138–2. Access sites for tube feeding. NG, OG, ND, and NJ generally are short term (<6 weeks) enteral feeding routes. Esophagostomy/pharyngostomy, gastrostomy, PEG, PEJ, and jejunostomy are longer term (months to years) enteral feeding routes. If the patient is at increased aspiration risk, the location of the enteral tube tip can be selected to deliver the feedings beyond the pylorus.

In general, the stomach is the least expensive and the least labor-intensive access site to use for enteral feeding; however, it is not always the best. Patients who have delayed gastric emptying from complications of diabetes or gastric atony during the postoperative period or patients with severe gastroesophageal reflux disease or intractable vomiting are at a higher risk for aspiration of gastric contents into the pulmonary system. Therefore, postpyloric tube placement may be required to enable successful enteral feeding. Studies have yet to prove definitively whether postpyloric tube feedings actually do decrease the risk of aspiration and pneumonia. The NG, OG, ND, and NJ tubes can all be placed manually at the patient's bedside. Greater skill is required to place the feeding tube beyond the pylorus at the bedside. Several techniques have been described in the literature to help facilitate manual placement at the bedside. These include the use of a stylette (i.e., a wire placed in the tube to help guide its placement), weighted tubes, patient placement onto the right side, and/or use of metoclopramide or erythromycin. Even though success rates of 80% to 90% have been quoted in the literature using such techniques for postpyloric tube placement, this degree of success is not experienced by all clinicians.[38] Alternatively, it may be necessary to move the tube physically through the pylorus by using fluoroscopy or endoscopy, which also increases the cost of enteral therapy. Radiographic verification of NG or ND feeding tubes placed by manual techniques must be obtained routinely on all patients with altered consciousness or altered cough or gag reflex or those who are mechanically ventilated.[38]

More invasive yet more permanent enteral feeding access includes esophagostomy or pharyngostomy, gastrostomy, and jejunostomy placement (see Fig. 138–2). Pharyngostomies and esophagostomies are indicated in patients with head and neck malignancies or maxillofacial anomalies that contraindicate nasopharyngeal access. Cervical pharyngostomy and esophagostomy are invasive because the tube is located in the neck and passes through the skin into the esophagus or the pharynx. Therefore, they are generally considered long-term enteral access devices. These routes use large-bore tubes, and tube replacement can be accomplished quite easily. As with any ostomy, site care is required. Dressing changes may be difficult to perform by the patient owing to the location. Complications of these routes, though infrequent, include recurrent laryngeal nerve damage, aspiration, and infection.[39]

A feeding gastrostomy is another long-term enteral access device indicated for patients with adequate gastric emptying but esophageal obstruction, impaired swallowing, or inadequate oral intake due to neurologic impairment (e.g., cerebral palsy) or feeding aversion. A gastrostomy can be placed surgically under general anesthesia. The attendant risks of general anesthesia are hypotension and aspiration. However, if the patient requires surgery for another reason, a gastrostomy tube also can be placed at the time of surgery. The complication rates of surgical gastrostomy placement average less than 2% for such complications as wound infection (cellulitis) or dehiscence; tube-site problems including infection, continuous drainage, or fistula formation; tube dislodgment or subsequent peritoneal contamination; GI bleeding; and gastrocolic fistulas.[38]

The percutaneous endoscopic gastrostomy (PEG) is a popular nonoperative procedure that can be performed safely and cost-effectively using local anesthesia. PEGs generally are placed in an endoscopy suite, eliminating costly operating room time. However, small children will require general anesthesia for PEG placement. The results of a prospective, randomized comparison between PEG and operative gastrostomy placement demonstrated similar complication rates, but the PEG had a higher benefit-cost ratio. More recently, two other techniques for gastrostomy placement have been described in the literature. They are laparoscopically and fluoroscopically placed gastrostomy tubes. Further investigation will be required to define the role of these two techniques. Gastrostomies use large-bore tubes, are associated with less tube clogging, and allow for all methods of tube feeding administration.

Subsequent to the maturity of the surgical tract where the gastrostomy tube lies, a low-profile skin-level gastrostomy button may be placed for patient convenience and comfort. Gastrostomy sites require general stoma-site care to prevent inflammation and infection. When a gastrostomy tube is no longer needed, it is removed easily. In adults, a common practice is to cut off the tube at skin level and allow retained components to pass through the GI tract. This technique has been associated with serious complications in children, including esophageal perforation and death, and therefore is not recommended in children.[42–44] Gastrostomy removal by traction or endoscopy (if there is an internal bolster) is associated with few complications. The gastrocutaneous fistula closes spontaneously in more than 70% of patients. If leaking continues, most cases will respond to use of histamine-2-antagonist therapy and silver nitrate cautery. Surgical closure is required in up to 23% of those which do not close initially.[42] In general, the longer the tube is in place, the more likely it is that the fistulous tract will require surgical closure. Patients whose tubes are in place for less than 11 months are more likely to have spontaneous closure that those whose tubes are in for longer than 11 months.[42]

Jejunostomies are long-term enteral access devices indicated for stomach or duodenal obstruction, impaired gastric emptying from diabetic neuropathy, or the same situations as a gastrostomy tube. Frequently, jejunostomies are placed during a surgical procedure when the small bowel is readily accessible. This may allow for early postoperative enteral feeding because the small bowel is least affected by surgical manipulation, whereas gastric atony and colonic ileus may persist for a long time postoperatively. Delayed gastric emptying has been observed in 50% of patients undergoing pylorus-preserving pancreaticoduodenectomies.[45] Successful early enteral feeding of these patients requires gastric decompression while feeding into the small bowel through a jejunostomy tube. A jejunostomy tube may be placed surgically and has a complication rate of less than 1%, with intraperitoneal leakage of infusion as the major complication. Further, a jejunostomy tube may be created by conversion of a PEG to a percutaneous endoscopic jejunostomy (PEJ) by passing a feeding tube through the lumen of the PEG and then beyond the pylorus and into the jejunum. In addition, laparoscopically and fluoroscopically placed jejunostomies also are described in the literature.[33] Gastrojejunostomy tubes are available that allow gastric decompression and intestinal feeding via the same tube. Administration of enteral feeding into the jejunum should be done only by a continuous or a continuous-cyclic method of tube feeding due to GI bloating, cramping, and diarrhea that will result from formula bolused into the small intestinal lumen.

ADMINISTRATION METHODS

The administration methods for tube feeding are continuous, continuous cyclic, intermittent, and intermittent bolus (Table 138–6). The choice of administration method depends on the anatomic location of the feeding tube, the clinical condition of the patient, the environment in which the patient resides, the patient's intestinal function, and the patient's tolerance to the tube feeding.

CONTINUOUS FEEDING

Continuous tube feeding is characterized by the administration of enteral nutrition formula via a delivery system over 16 to 24 h/d. The delivery system includes a feeding reservoir or bag attached to an extension set that is connected to an infusion pump. The delivery system is then attached to the patient's enteral access tube. Continuous infusion may increase nursing time because routine checks of the enteral infusion are needed, but it may provide maximal tolerance by minimizing abdominal distension, vomiting, and diarrhea. Continuous delivery of nutrients is mandatory when the tube is placed in the small intestine. Continuous enteral feeding is practiced widely among critically ill patients.[45] Continuous feeding is also beneficial for patients who have limited absorption capacity because of a rapid GI transit or severely impaired digestion. Slow continuous administration in such patients allows greater time for digestion and absorption of nutrients as they pass through the intestine. For adults, infusion rates usually range from 50 to 125 mL/h, although rates of 150 mL/h

TABLE 138–6. Administration Methods for Tube Feeding

Method	Equipment	Indication	Infusion Example
Continuous	Infusion pump generally recommended Enteral formula container Administration set	Gastric tube feeding Postpyloric tube feeding Critically ill patient Limited absorption capacity Limited feeding tolerance via intermittent and bolus methods	Full strength isotonic formula infused at 20 mL/h, advanced by 20 mL/h increments every 8 h to desired goal rate as tolerated
Continuous cyclic	Infusion pump generally recommended Enteral formula container Administration set	Gastric or postpyloric tube feeding Home tube feeding Rehabilitation patient Nocturnal tube feeding Potential transition to oral intake during daytime Limited feeding tolerance via bolus or intermittent method	Formula infused over 10–14 h daily at desired goal rate to achieve nutrient requirements
Intermittent	Infusion pump or gravity flow Enteral formula container Administration set	Gastric tube feeding Home tube feeding Rehabilitation patient Patient unlikely to make transition to oral intake Limited feeding tolerance via bolus method	240–480 mL formula infused over 20–40 min 4–6 times daily
Intermittent bolus	Large syringe (60 mL)	Gastric tube feeding Home tube feeding Rehabilitation patient Patient unlikely to make transition to oral intake	240–480 mL formula infused over <10 min 4–6 times daily

have been reported without complications. In children, initial infusion rates of 1 to 2 mL/kg per hour or 20 to 25 mL/kg per day with similar rate advancements every 4 to 8 hours to the goal rate needed to meet caloric needs usually are tolerated well.

CONTINUOUS-CYCLIC FEEDING

Continuous-cyclic tube feeding uses the same delivery system as continuous feeding, but the formula is administered over 8 to 14 h/day at the desired rate which is a function of the tolerance of the patient and his or her nutrient requirements. Continuous-cyclic therapy generally is recommended for the non-critically ill patient, home tube feeding patient, or patients who are in rehabilitation settings. Cyclic enteral feedings allow a patient a physical and psychological break from being connected to the enteral infusion system and allow for greater rehabilitation and return to the activities of daily living. Frequently, continuous-cyclic enteral feeds are administered nocturnally, which may allow for transitioning a patient's diet to more oral intake during the daytime. Continuous-cyclic tube feedings may be administered into the stomach or small bowel. Cyclic feedings may require formulas of higher nutrient densities or higher infusion rates to compensate for the periods when the tube feedings are discontinued if other intake is not adequate to meet needs.[45] Therefore, monitoring for GI tolerance is particularly important when patients are being initiated on a continuous-cyclic enteral feeding protocol.

INTERMITTENT FEEDING

Intermittent feeding consists of the administration of 240 to 480 mL of formula in adults and older children and 90 to 300 mL in infants and younger children infused over 20 to 40 minutes four to eight times daily depending on the age of the patient and his or her nutrition requirements. This method of delivery should be administered only to patients with feeding tube tips that lie within the stomach because the stomach is capable of handling large and more rapid volumes of feeding formula. Since the stomach is the natural nutrient reservoir that controls the volume and osmolality reaching the small intestine, this prevents the dumping syndrome. The dumping syndrome occurs when a large quantity of a hyperosmolar solution is introduced too rapidly into the small bowel. Clinically, this syndrome manifests as nausea, cramping, light-headedness, and diarrhea. Intermittent enteral feeds may be administered by an infusion pump or via gravity flow with a roller clamp. Enteral pump-assisted infusion is preferred over manually adjusted roller clamps because of known inaccuracies and the acute sensitivity of some patients to small variances in infusion rates. However, gastric installation generally does not require meticulous titration as long as gastric motility and the pyloric sphincter are intact. Intermittent enteral feeding is indicated for home tube feeding patients or patients in rehabilitation-type settings. Intermittent feeding frequently is selected for patients who are not able to eat normally on their own, such as patients who have altered mental or cognitive function. Therefore, the tube feeding is given intermittently and is more consistent physiologically with normal eating patterns. Patients who receive intermittent feeding may be at higher risk for complications such as nausea, vomiting, and aspiration.

BOLUS FEEDING

Bolus feeding consists of the administration of volumes similar to those given with intermittent feedings but infused over less than 10 minutes four to eight times daily. It is used primarily for esophagostomy, pharyngostomy, or gastrostomy patients who have intact stomachs. The stomach then regulates the flow of formula into the intestine. Bolus feedings have the advantage of requiring little administration time and minimal equipment. Usually only a 60-mL syringe or bulb is needed to instill the feeding into the tube. Alternatively, bolus feedings can be infused via a complete infusion system consisting of an infusion reservoir, tubing, and possibly a feeding pump. In some patients, bolus feedings may not be tolerated and can result in cramping, nausea, vomiting, aspiration, and diarrhea. Bolus feedings during the day may be coupled with continuous nocturnal feedings to stimulate increased oral intake or to begin transitioning to bolus feedings.

FEEDING EQUIPMENT

Feeding containers, administration tubing, and infusion pumps all should be evaluated prior to their use. Feeding containers should be leakproof, unbreakable, and easy to clean. They should be equipped with a reliable closure and have easy-to-read volume markings. The adaptability of the container to multiple infusion sets, its volume capacity, and ease of distinguishing it from an intravenous container also should be examined. Administration sets consist of tubing that connects the feeding container to the feeding tube. These sets should be distinctly different from intravenous sets and adaptable to many feeding containers and feeding tubes. In addition, they should be long enough to connect the feeding container and patient easily. Last, the administration set should be equipped with an infusion control regulator that allows a reasonably accurate flow rate to within 20% of the expected rate. Pharmacists are asked to assist in evaluating enteral feeding pumps because of their familiarity with intravenous infusion pumps. Many considerations are the same for both types of pumps. They should be lightweight, easy to operate, have a reasonably long battery life, and require little maintenance. The pump should have a useful alarm system that indicates low battery power, an empty container, or rising pressure in the set. Rising pressure indicates set occlusion. Last, the pump should be easy to operate by hospital or nursing home personnel and patients alike. Additionally, for home use, portable pumps and enteral feeding bags that fit within a backpack can facilitate increased mobility, especially when feedings are continuous. Although delineation of the specific features of several manufacturers' enteral infusion pumps is beyond the scope of this chapter, they have been reviewed recently.[39]

CHARACTERISTICS OF ENTERAL FORMULAS

Since the introduction of the first infant formula in 1919 and enteral formulas intended for use in adults in the 1940s, the composition and nutrient profile of enteral formulas have become highly sophisticated. Initially, enteral formulas were created to provide essential nutrients, and formula enhancements were made, such as including fiber or modifying the specific amino acids, to optimize the biologic value and use. Enteral formulas also have been modified in nutrient composition by changing the content of the amino acids (such as glutamine and arginine), changing the omega-3 polyunsaturated fatty acid content, and adding ribonucleic acid to promote a favorable physiologic effect that improves disease outcome. Modifying the enteral formula's nutrient content to improve disease outcome for a patient has been coined *nutritional pharmacology*.[46] Currently, the U.S. Food and Drug Administration (FDA) considers enteral formulas to be medical foods. The use of a medical food product is based on a need to provide energy and/or specific nutrients because of an underlying medical condition.[47] A lack of consensus exists as to whether medical foods should be components of supportive care and/or whether they ought to be categorized as pharmacologic treatment.[48] The Life

TABLE 138–7. Enteral Formula Nutrient Complexity

Nutrient	Polymeric or Intact	Partially Hydrolyzed or Elemental
Carbohydrate	Starches Fruit, vegetable, cereal solids Glucose polymers Corn syrup solids Polysaccharides	Oligosaccharides Maltodextrins Disaccharides Maltose, sucrose, lactose Monosaccharides Glucose Galactose
Fat	Long-chain triglycerides Polyunsaturated fatty acids Corn oil Safflower oil Soybean oil Butter fat Menhaden Fish oils	Medium-chain triglycerides Coconut oil Palm kernel Free fatty acids Linoleic
Protein	Whole Egg, milk, wheat, whey Isolates Caseinate salts Lactalbumin	Oligopeptides Dipeptides Tripeptides L-Amino acids

Sciences Research Office has suggested that medical foods should "have documented evidence supporting claims of maintenance or improvement of nutritional status of patients . . . and/or improvement of one or more specific nutrient-related disease manifestations significantly more than that observed from use of commercially available nutritionally complete formulas."[26] Currently, the FDA has not developed any specific regulations for enteral formulas as to current food labeling requirements or to rules governing their health claims other than the regulatory statutes, which are designed to ensure good manufacturing practices for all processed foods. The macronutrient content of enteral formulas (namely, protein, carbohydrate, and fat) varies in nutrient complexity (Table 138–7). Nutrient complexity refers to the amount of hydrolysis and digestion a substrate source requires prior to intestinal absorption. Polymeric or intact substrates are of similar molecular form as the food we eat. Enteral formulas that contain partially hydrolyzed or elemental substrates are characterized as defined-formula diets. The caloric contribution of each of the macronutrients is as follows: carbohydrates, 4 kcal/g; protein, 4 kcal/g; and fat, 9 kcal/g. The micronutrients, including electrolytes, vitamins, trace elements, and water, do not contribute to caloric content.

PROTEIN COMPOSITION

Important factors concerning the protein within enteral formulas are the quantity, quality, and molecular form of protein. The essential amino acid content of the protein source determines the quality of the protein. The protein quality frequently is expressed in two standard ways, the biologic value and chemical score. It is desirable to have a protein source that is of high biologic value and chemical score because then less protein will be required to meet the patient's nitrogen requirements. Most of the readily available formulas contain proteins of high quality.[49] The molecular form of the protein source in enteral formulas will determine the amount of digestion that is required for adequate absorption within the small bowel. Polymeric or intact protein sources require complete digestion to smaller peptides and free amino acids before they are absorbed from the GIT. Therefore, enteral formula protein sources such as meat, milk, eggs, and caseinates require complete digestion by hydrochloric acid, specific protein enzymes, and pancreatic enzymes. Subsequent to these digestive processes, amino acids, oligopeptides, dipeptides, and tripeptides are presented to the enterocytes of the small bowel (see Fig. 138–1). The protein sources within enteral solutions also have been formulated with partially hydrolyzed proteins as peptides or elemental protein as L-amino acids (see Table 138–7). The carriers for the peptides have proven to be very efficient in that they do not depend on sodium to function properly. Free amino acids, on the other hand, are absorbed via sodium-dependent mechanisms that appear to be slower and less efficient than peptide ones. Therefore, partially digested protein entities are the most readily absorbable form of nitrogen substrate.[2,50] As the molecular form of protein is reduced in size, the osmotic load within the enteral formula is increased. Many commercially available enteral solutions contain combinations of intact and partially hydrolyzed protein sources.

CONDITIONALLY ESSENTIAL AMINO ACIDS

Glutamine and arginine also have been added to some enteral formulas. These amino acids normally are nonessential amino acids. However, during disease states of high physiologic stress, glutamine and arginine may become deficient and therefore have been characterized as conditionally essential. Glutamine is synthesized mostly in muscle and is used as the primary fuel for the enterocytes. Therefore, during glutamine-deficient states, the use of glutamine increases beyond the synthesis or release of glutamine from the muscle tissue. Since glutamine is the primary fuel for the enterocyte, it has undergone investigation to determine its role in maintaining the integrity of the gut mucosa. Furthermore, it has been postulated that glutamine may play a role in preventing bacterial translocation.[51] Since glutamine normally is not contained in TPN solutions, intravenous glutamine supplemented in TPN during nonfeeding of the GIT has been investigated. Two prospective, randomized clinical investigations of 0.57 g/kg intravenous glutamine supplemented in TPN among bone marrow transplant patients have demonstrated conflicting results relative to nutritional response and infectious complications. However, both demonstrated reduced length of hospital stay.[52,53] Glutamine-supplemented TPN in animals has been shown to increase the gut mass based on duodenal biopsies and reduced bowel permeability. Also in animal studies, glutamine-supplemented enteral amino acid diets have shown improved gut mass and function, whereas other investigators have found little benefit in supplementing glutamine to enteral diets.[3,54] However, there is little clinical research evaluating the benefit of enteral feeding solutions containing glutamine. The glutamine content of selected commercially available enteral formulas varies in the range of 1.8 to 14.2 g/L of formula.[55] Similar plasma amino acid profiles were reported from a prospective, randomized study of postoperative patients receiving either glutamine-enriched parenteral or enteral feedings.[56] Some investigators have raised concern as to whether glutamine actually may enhance some tumors in that it may act as a tumor stimulator. Obviously, further research and investigation are required to determine the potential benefits and harm associated with glutamine- enriched specialized nutrient formulas.[57]

Arginine is also a conditionally essential amino acid, in that it may not be synthesized in sufficient quantity during states of trauma or stress.[58] Data from animal investigations have demonstrated that arginine may have an antitumor effect, and among healthy subjects it has been shown to stimulate T-cell blastogenesis. In addition, supplemental arginine has been shown to decrease protein catabolism, enhance nitrogen retention following injury, and also accelerate wound healing. Arginine has been supplemented in selected enteral formulas in the range of 4.5 to 14 g/L of enteral formula. Diets enhanced with arginine have been studied in burn, cancer, and septic patients.

CARBOHYDRATE COMPOSITION

The carbohydrate component of enteral formulas usually provides the major source of nonprotein calories. Polymeric or intact enteral formulas contain starches and numerous types of glucose polymers, which require complete digestion to the monosaccharide moieties prior to intestinal absorption (see Fig. 138–1). As the hydrolysis of carbohydrate increases within an enteral formula, the osmolality of the formula is also further increased. Elemental carbohydrates such as glucose and galactose contribute significantly to the osmolality of enteral formulas, which is correlated directly with enteral feeding intolerance. Therefore, partially digested entities, rather than elemental sugars, are the choice for inclusion in enteral formulas. Glucose polymers provide an especially useful carbohydrate source that is tolerated by most individuals (see Table 138–7). The polymers are large chains that provide a minimal osmotic load yet are absorbed easily in the intestine. The one shortcoming of glucose polymers and oligosaccharides is that they are not as sweet as simple glucose and thus may decrease the palatability of orally consumed products. Finally, most commercially available enteral formulas are lactose-free because some ethnic populations are lactase deficient and disaccharidase production within the gut lumen is reduced during illness or bowel rest.

FAT COMPOSITION

Fat is an important constituent in the diet because it provides a concentrated calorie source and serves as a carrier for fat-soluble vitamins. Sufficient linoleic acid is required to prevent essential fatty acid deficiency (EFAD) and should approximate 1% to 3% of total daily calories.[59] The most frequent sources of polymeric intact fat are vegetable oils (soy or corn) rich in polyunsaturated fatty acids. The digestion and absorption of LCTs are more complicated than those of either protein or carbohydrates. Fat digestion requires pancreatic enzyme release and formation of mixed bile salt micelles, which then facilitate absorption across the intestinal enterocyte, as depicted in Figure 138–1. The concentration of fat in enteral feeding formulas varies from less than 2% to 45% of total calories. The LCT fat sources have carbon chain lengths of 12 carbon atoms. An alternative source of fat within enteral formulas is the MCTs, derived from palm kernel or coconut oils. MCTs are of 6 to 12 carbon atom lengths and have a caloric density between 8.2 and 8.4 kcal/g. MCTs do not contain the essential fats or linoleic acid. Therefore, most formulas contain some LCTs to provide essential fatty acids. Potential advantages of MCTs over LCTs are that they are more water soluble, they undergo rapid hydrolysis, they require little to no pancreatic lipase or bile salt for absorption, and they do not require carnitine to be used as energy. They also do not require chylomicron formation for small bowel enterocyte absorption. High fat content has been associated with delayed gastric emptying.

Also, some manufacturers have changed the source of long-chain fat (from omega-6 to omega-3 fatty acids) within enteral formulas to reduce the amount of the resulting physiologic products (i.e., prostaglandins, thromboxanes, and leukotrienes).[55,58] The omega-6 fatty acids are high in linoleic acid and are derived from vegetable oil, whereas the omega-3 fatty acids, derived from coldwater fish oils, are high in linolenic acid. The eicosanoid products of the omega-6 fatty acids have been shown to be potent inflammatory mediators and also decrease cell-mediated immunity. Therefore, if the fat content delivered from omega-3 fatty acids is increased, the patient should experience less inflammation and immunosuppression.

NUTRITIONALLY COMPLETE FORMULAS

Most commercially prepared formulas contain micronutrients, including electrolytes, vitamins, trace elements, and water, to make them nutritionally complete. Nutritionally complete commercial formulas provide the recommended daily allowances (RDAs) of micronutrients for a patient receiving a sufficient volume of formula to meet their daily energy and macronutrient needs. A given predetermined nutrient complement, however, may not fit an individual's need because electrolyte, vitamin, and trace element requirements vary with disease state and organ function. One common electrolyte abnormality associated with enteral nutrition is hyponatremia. Most formulas are made to mimic a low-salt diet, so hyponatremia could arise due to the limited sodium concentration. A low salt intake appears reasonable because many patients who receive enteral nutrition are elderly and may have compromised cardiac function. However, patients who do not receive a sufficient volume of enteral formula to meet their RDA for micronutrients as the result of complications of fluid restriction or volume intolerance may require supplemental minerals and vitamins. Based on the adequate or high levels of vitamins in the blood of patients who have received long-term enteral therapy, the stability and absorption of vitamins that are contained in complete enteral formulas are felt to be adequate.[60] Patients who are fed enterally and have significant fat malabsorption may, over a long-term period, develop deficiencies of fat-soluble vitamins and therefore may need further supplementation of these vitamins. Most enteral feeding formulas contain the RDA of trace elements including iron, zinc, copper, and iodine, again based on receiving a sufficient volume of formula to meet the macronutrient needs of the patient. Selected enteral formulas also contain the RDA of selenium, molybdenum, and chromium. During deficiency states, such as when diarrhea persists, supplementation of trace elements, namely, zinc, may be warranted.

FIBER CONTENT

Fiber, in the form of soy polysaccharide fiber, has been added to several enteral formulas in doses of 10 to 24 g of dietary fiber per liter. Subsequent to bacterial degradation of fiber within the colon, the end products of fiber ingestion are SCFAs. Potential benefits of fiber are the trophic effects on the large bowel mucosa as well as promotion of sodium and water absorption within the colon. In addition, the resulting SCFAs are an excellent energy source. Fiber also has the ability to regulate bowel function by moderating intestinal transit time in individuals with altered motility conditions. The experimental evidence and clinical implications of fiber-enhanced enteral nutrition among healthy volunteers and several patient populations has been reviewed recently.[61] These authors concluded that even though there is good experimental evidence that fiber may play an integral role in normal human nutrition, the results of clinical studies have been disappointing. Fiber supplementation may be beneficial in long-term tube feeding of constipated patients, especially those with minimal oral intake or those with neurologic impairment. In intensive care units, however, drugs and stress seem to be more powerful determinates of bowel function than the addition of fiber to formulas.

OSMOLALITY AND RENAL SOLUTE LOAD

Tolerance to enteral formulas can be affected by the osmolality and the renal solute load. The osmolality of a given enteral formula is a function of the size and quantity of ionic and molecular particles, primarily related to the protein, carbohydrate, electrolyte, and mineral content within a given volume of formula. The unit of measure of osmolality is milliosmoles per kilogram (mosm/kg). Enteral formulas with greater amounts of partially hydrolyzed or elemental substrates have a higher osmolality than formulas containing only polymeric or intact substrate forms. Therefore, formulas that contain sucrose or glucose, dipeptides and tripeptides, and amino acids are hyperosmolar. In general, enteral formulas range in osmolality from 300 to 900 mosm/kg. The American Academy of Pediatrics (AAP) recommends that enteral formulas for use in infants have an osmolality of approximately 450 mosm/kg. An extensive review of the osmolality of formulas and medications commonly used in neonatal intensive care units has been published.[62]

Increased caloric density increases the osmolality of an enteral formula. Symptoms of gastric retention, diarrhea, abdominal distension, nausea, and vomiting have been ascribed to the relative osmolality of the enteral feeding product. The results of clinical investigations to assess the relationship between osmolality and the incidence of GI side effects are conflicting.[63–65] Hospitalized patients administered hypotonic, isotonic, or hypertonic enteral formulas at a constant infusion rate demonstrated no significant differences in GI tolerance.[63] Other factors such as concurrent antibiotic therapy, which may alter the intestinal microflora; the method of delivery, such as continuous versus bolus; and the appropriate selection of an enteral feeding formula for its composition play as much a role in the associated tolerance to the formula as the osmolality of the formula alone.[66]

The renal solute load is made up collectively of the protein, sodium, potassium, and chloride content of the enteral formula. Formulas that contain a greater solute load increase the obligatory water loss via the kidney. It is estimated that 40 to 60 mL of water is the minimal amount necessary to excrete 1 g of nitrogen.[49] Those receiving high-nitrogen enteral formulas, such as a geriatric patient or a patient with altered mental status unable to ingest more water, may be at risk for significant dehydration. Dehydration may be detected clinically as thirst, dry mucous membranes, depressed skin turgor, or an increased serum blood urea nitrogen or sodium level.

The rapid administration of hyperosmolar formulas reduces the gastric emptying rate.[49] Continuous administration into the stomach allows the pylorus to regulate the delivery of nutrient content into the duodenum and hence reduce gastric retention and associated symptoms of nausea and vomiting. When administering enteral formulas into the small bowel, products that are iso-osmolar can be administered initially at slow rates and advanced incrementally based on tolerance. Hyperosmolar formulas may require slower advancement to prevent the development of the dumping syndrome. As the lumen of the small bowel receives hypertonic enteral feedings, the small bowel secretes water to effectively dilute the formula and make it iso-osmotic, hence contributing to the diarrhea and further fluid and electrolyte depletion.

SELECTING AN ENTERAL FORMULA

The selection of an appropriate enteral feeding formula requires knowledge of several patient characteristics. First, the patient's medical history should be obtained. The length of small bowel, nutrient digestibility, and functional capacity help determine the appropriate formula complexity. In addition, the patient's age, underlying diseases, nutritional status, and fluid tolerance are required to determine nutritional goals. Knowledge of the feeding site will allow the selection of the appropriate delivery method of enteral feeding and reduce potential complications of therapy.

CLASSIFICATION OF ENTERAL NUTRITION FORMULAS

It is easy to become overwhelmed with the variety of formulations available. Development of an enteral nutrition product formulary is cost-effective and minimizes confusion by identifying the rational use of prototype products. Different criteria have been proposed to evaluate and categorize enteral nutrition products based on their unique characteristics.[26,55,57] The enteral formulas listed in Tables 138–8 and 138–9 are categorized on the basis of the composition of the enteral formula and the intended patient population.

POLYMERIC FORMULAS

Polymeric solutions contain macronutrients in the form of intact protein, triglycerides, and carbohydrate polymers. They can be used orally or through a tube and provide complete nutrition.[57] An enteral formula is described as a complete product when it contains all the micro- and macronutrients necessary to meet the RDAs for a patient. The majority of enteral products available commercially are lactose-free, although enteral formulas are available as oral supplements that do contain lactose. Frequently, the polymeric lactose-free tube feeding products are referred to as complete, standard enteral products. Describing enteral products as standard implies that these products require normal GI digestive and absorptive function for maintaining the nutritional status of a patient. Polymeric enteral feeding products are used in numerous settings, including the critically ill, rehabilitation patients, and home enteral nutrition support patients.

These polymeric enteral or standard formulas intended for use in children older than 10 years of age and adults are manufactured with variable caloric and protein densities ranging from 1 to 2 kcal/mL and 35 to 60 g/L protein, respectively. Human breast milk and standard infant formulas provide 20 kcal/oz (0.67 kcal/mL) and 1 to 2 g protein per 100 mL. Human breast milk has less protein than commercial infant formulas, but the protein is of higher biologic value. Products that are calorically concentrated generally have higher osmolalities. Fiber also has been supplemented in some of the standard formulas. The commercially available blenderized diets are made from natural whole foods. They are complete products with variable amounts of fiber and lactose. These products, owing to the nature of their

TABLE 138–8. Enteral Formula Classification System

Category	Subcategories	Indication	Features	Adult Product Examples
Polymeric (normal GIT digestive and absroptive capacity required)	Lactose-free Lactose-containing Blenderized	Standard oral Supplement Complete tube feeding Oral supplement Lactose-intolerant Complete tube feeding	Iso-osmolar, high nitrogen, fiber-enhanced, and highly concentrated formulas available Palatable; hyperosmolar May contain lactose, high viscosity, and may require infusion pump	Osmolite (R) Resource (N) Iso Source VHN (N) Ultracal (MJ) Deliver 2.0 (MJ) Meritene (N) Complete modified (N)
Monomeric (less digestion and absorption required)	Chemically defined Elemental	Complete tube feeding and some use as oral supplements Disease states that alter digestive or absorptive surface capacity Complete tube feeding, rarely as an oral supplement Disease states that alter digestive or absorptive surface capacity Fat malabsorption	Nutrients hydrolyzed to varying degrees Osmolarity varies Free amino acids, >80% of kcal as oligosaccharides, <15% fat content as long-chain fat	Peptamen (C) Reabilan HN (C) Vivonex Plus (N) Tolerex (N)
Specialized (monomeric or polymeric)	Organ failure Immune support	Complete (±[a]) tube feeding, rarely as an oral supplement Specific products for pulmonary, renal, hepatic, and endocrine failure Complete tube feeding, rarely as an oral supplement Enhance immune competency during critical illness or sepsis	Composition varies; nutrient requirements modified to a specific disorder Specific nutrients modified for immunopharmacologic function	Pulmocare (R) Travasorb Renal (NE) Nutrihep (NE) DiabetiSource (N) Immun-Aid (MG) Impact (N)
Hydration	Glucose Electrolytes	Feeding tube or oral Dehydration, severe or chronic diarrhea		Equalyte (Ross) Pedialyte (Ross) Enfalyte (Mead Johnson)

[a]May or may not be complete nutrient composition.
Manufacturers: R = Ross, N = Novartis, MJ = Mead Johnson, C = Clintec, NE = Nestle, MG = McGaw.

composition, may have a higher viscosity and generally require an infusion pump and access through a large-bore feeding tube for successful administration.

MONOMERIC FORMULAS

Monomeric enteral formulas have partially hydrolyzed and/or elemental components of protein, carbohydrate, and fat and therefore require less digestive and absorptive capacity. The major difference between polymeric and monomeric formulas is that monomeric formulas contain protein in small molecular forms. The chemically defined enteral formulas are those in which the protein is in the form of oligopeptides, dipeptides, and tripeptides. The elemental products are those which generally contain L-amino acids as the protein source (see Tables 138–8 and 138–9). Carbohydrates frequently are in the form of oligosaccharides, sucrose, and glucose, whereas fat sources usually are in the form of MCTs with small amounts of LCTs to provide essential fatty acid requirements. In general, the osmolality of monomeric products is higher, ranging from 500 to 700 mosm/kg. The caloric density of monomeric formulas for adults generally is 1.0 kcal/mL with approximately 40 to 50 g protein per liter. The intact protein of polymeric products must be digested to lower-molecular-weight peptides and/or free amino acids prior to absorption, whereas the monomeric enteral products, which already contain dipeptides and tripeptides, are absorbed more readily by the enterocyte.

The physiologic basis and clinical relevance for the use of monomeric enteral formulas in the clinical setting have been reviewed extensively.[50,57] The results from human and animal intestinal perfusion studies indicate that the partially hydrolyzed sources of protein have an absorptive advantage over formulas that contain free amino

TABLE 138–9. Formulas for Infants and Children

Formula Type	Example Products (Mfg[a])	Indications
Polymeric		
Cow's milk–based	Enfamil 20, 24 kcal/oz, Enfamil Lactofree, Enfamil A.R. (MJ); Similac 20, 24 kcal/oz, Similac Lactose Free (R); Gerber Baby Formula (G); Carnation Good Start (C)	Normal, healthy infants
Soy-based	Isomil, Isomil DF[b] (MJ); Prosobee (R); Gerber Soy Formula (G)	Lactase deficiency or intolerance, galactosemia
Premature	Similac Special Care 20, 24 kcal/oz, Similac NeoSure 22 kcal/oz (R); Enfamil Premature 20, 24 kcal/oz, Enfamil EnfaCare 22 kcal/oz (MJ)	Preterm infant less than 2–3 kg
Transition	Similac 2, Isomil 2 (R); Carnation Follow-Up, Carnation Follow-Up Soy (C); Next Step, Next Step Soy (MJ)	Transition to cow's milk
Special diets	Similac PM 60/40 (R)	Renal, cardiac, or endocrine disorders
Children 1–10 years	PediaSure, PediaSure with Fiber (R); Kindercal[c] (MJ); Nutren Jr., Nutren Jr. with Fiber (N)	Functioning GI tract requiring tube feedings
Monomeric		
Infants	Nutramigen, Pregestimil, Portagen (MJ); Neocate (SHS); Alimentum (R)	Malabsorption, cow's milk protein allergy, chylothorax, cystic fibrosis, biliary atresia
Children 1–10 years	Vivonex Pediatric (No); Peptamen Junior (N); Neocate One + (SHS); EleCare (R)	Same as above

[a]Manufacturers: R = Ross Products Division, Abbott Laboratories; MJ = Mead Johnson Nutritionals; C = Carnation Nutritional Products; G = Gerber; S = Sandoz; SHS = SHS International Ltd; N = Nestlé Clinical Nutrition; No = Novartis.
[b]Diarrhea formula contains g/100 mL fiber.
[c]Contains soy fiber 5.9 g/1000 kcal.

acids. However, there are few controlled data on the nutritional efficacy of the protein hydrolysates or free amino acid formulations in humans. Even among pancreatectomized patients or those with severe short bowel, only slight differences in improved absorption have been shown to occur with the use of peptide-based diets. It has been hypothesized that the great reserve and adaptive capacity of the absorptive mucosa of the small bowel will still promote an adequate amount of nutrient absorption irrespective of the form of protein substrate delivered. Therefore, the relative indication for these products is currently controversial. Monomeric diets cannot be recommended for routine use in patients with normal GI function, those requiring early postoperative enteral feeding, or those with only mildly impaired pancreatic exocrine function, partial gastrectomy, and minor small intestinal resections. However, in pancreatectomized patients or those with markedly reduced GI surface area, the potential clinical benefit from the use of monomeric products warrants a therapeutic trial.[50,57] Monomeric products that have higher percentages of MCTs and small amounts of LCTs generally are recommended for patients with severe pancreatic insufficiency such as chronic pancreatitis and cystic fibrosis, severe abnormalities of the intestinal mucosa such as untreated celiac disease or extensive small bowel resection,[47] or chylothorax.

DISEASE STATE-SPECIFIC FORMULAS

A third descriptive category of enteral feeding formulas is the specialized formulas based on specific metabolic needs such as organ failure and immune dysfunction. These specialized enteral formulas vary in their nutrient complexity composition (see Table 138–8). Specific nutrient concerns during organ failure are discussed in Chapter 139. The specialized enteral formulas that have been formulated to enhance immune competency during critical illness or sepsis provide substrates in pharmacologic doses that have been shown experimentally to enhance immune function.[58,67] These products contain more arginine and ribonucleic acids and an increased proportion of omega-3 polyunsaturated fatty acids. Glutamine also has been supplemented in some of these formulas to promote intestinal mucosal integrity and reduce infectious complications. Two independent meta-analyses were conducted on prospectivel, randomized, and controlled trials involving critically ill or cancer patients receiving enteral nutrition support supplemented with immune-enhancing nutrients versus standard enteral nutrition support to determine the effects on morbidity, mortality, and length of hospital stay. A meta-analysis of 12 clinical trials (cumulative n = 1482) demonstrated a significant reduction in infection rate and length of hospital stay for trauma, septic, or surgical patients receiving immunonutrition formulations.[68] Likewise, a meta-analysis of 10 clinical trials (cumulative $n = 1009$) demonstrated significant reductions in infectious complications and overall length of hospital stay for critically ill or cancer patients receiving immunonutrition formulations.[69] No effect on mortality with immunonutrition was demonstrated from either of the meta-analyses. These data, however, provide no insight as to which nutrient(s) may have contributed to the improvement in clinical outcome. There are no disease-specific products currently marketed for use in infants or children younger than 10 years of age.

MODULAR FORMULAS

A fourth category of enteral products is the modular nutrient components (Table 138–10). Occasionally, especially in children, it is necessary to achieve a nutrient mix not supplied by a single commercially available product.[70] Formulas available in powder or concentrate can be mixed with less water than needed for the standard dilution to deliver more nutrients in less volume. Infant formulas generally are

TABLE 138–10. Modular Enteral Products

Primary Nutrient Supplied	Example Products (Mfg[a])
Carbohydrate	Moducal (MJ), Polycose (R)
Protein	ProMod (R), Propac (SM), Casec (MJ)
Fat	MCT Oil (MJ), Microlipid (SM)
Human milk fortifier	Enfamil Human Milk Fortifier (MJ), Similac Human Milk Fortifier (R)
Pectin/carbohydrate/potassium	Banana Flakes (K)
Carbohydrate and fat	Duocal (SHS)

[a]Manufacturers: R = Ross Products Division, Abbott Laboratories; MJ = Mead Johnson Nutritionals; SM = Sherwood Medical; K = Kanana; SHS = SHS International, Ltd.

concentrated to 24 kcal/oz in this way. Alternatively, a single nutrient component such as carbohydrate, protein, or fat can be added to ready-to-use solutions to enhance the specific substrate content. Protein modules may be added singularly to ready-made formulas when a higher nitrogen content is desired. These modules are marketed in powder form and may contain free amino acids, caseinates, or whole protein such as egg whites, solids, or whey. The module's nutrient complexity added to a commercial formula should be based on the patient's digestive capacity. Caloric enhancement of ready-made formulas also may be done by adding carbohydrate modules such as glucose polymers that are available in either solid or liquid forms. Human milk fortifiers are available for supplementation of premature human milk so that it meets the needs of a premature infant. Human milk fortifiers add additional calories, protein, and minerals and have been shown to improve nutritional outcomes in human milk-fed premature infants.[71–73]

HYDRATION FORMULAS

The last descriptive category of enteral products is hydration formulas. Oral hydration and rehydration formulas may be used in patients with diarrhea to prevent or treat dehydration or in patients with ostomies to replenish drainage fluid and subsequent electrolyte losses. Such formulas do not require intravenous access, are economical, and can be either purchased commercially or compounded extemporaneously. These formulas have been used successfully to manage mild to moderate dehydration in both children and adults. The oral rehydration solution is successful because of its glucose content. Glucose stimulates active transport systems, which in turn stimulate passive sodium and water uptake simultaneously with the glucose. Therefore, oral administration of several liters actually may decrease fecal water loss and generate a positive electrolyte balance.

FORMULARY AND DELIVERY SYSTEM CONSIDERATIONS

A practical issue that affects the enteral product selected for use in a patient is the product formulary of an institution. Obviously, the selection of product should be based on patient characteristics and product features, as discussed previously. However, such administrative concerns as cost, shelf life, ordering policies, product form, administration systems, and contract opportunities frequently are taken into account when an institution develops an enteral formulary. The majority of enteral products are available as ready-to-use, prepackaged liquids, whereas others are in a dehydrated, powdered state and require reconstitution prior to use. Advantages of ready-to-use liquid formulas are convenience and low susceptibility to microbiologic contamination. One of the disadvantages is that more storage space is required. The ease or convenience of packaging is especially important for patients involved in self-care, the disabled, and those who have difficulty receiving or following printed instructions.

Another practical issue that affects an institution's choice of an enteral delivery system is the potential complication of bacterial contamination. Both animal and human studies have demonstrated that contaminated enteral feeding formulas have been associated directly with infectious complications.[74–76] The GIT may serve as a port of entry for bacteria into the systemic circulation, especially in patients who are receiving multiple antibiotics or who have undergone a surgical procedure. The contamination of enteral feeding formulas has been associated with a lack of attention to proper handling techniques, inability to disinfect preparation equipment, and nonsterile or contaminating tube feeding additives. Stringent handling procedures are recommended to ensure that enteral feeding is safe for administration.[77] Sterile enteral diets have been available in the form of the closed-administration systems, which are prefilled containers in volumes of 1 to 1.5 L of ready-to-feed enteral formula. This is in contrast to the more conventional open systems, which require cans or mixed powders to be decanted into larger-volume delivery bags by institution personnel. The closed-administration system offers the advantage of requiring no mixing of formula and therefore lowers the risk of contamination and reduces time and labor required in preparing the formula. Numerous types of enteral formulas are now available in the closed-administration system. The closed-administration system also offers the advantage of allowing hang times beyond 24 to 36 hours, whereas the conventional delivery system necessitates hang times of generally 4 to 12 hours. A disadvantage of the closed-administration system is the inability to add minerals or color additives for diagnostic or preventive purposes without breaking the closed system.

INITIATING AN ENTERAL NUTRITION REGIMEN

After selecting the appropriate enteral access and feeding formula, the rate and strength of formula advancement must be determined. Schedules for progression of tube feeding from initial to target rates are important and may influence the maximum rate the patient can tolerate.[45] Frequently in the institutional setting, feeding into either the stomach or small bowel is begun with slow continuous feeding. Many patients will tolerate rapid advancement of a full-strength feeding formula from a rate of 20 to 25 mL/h with increments of 20 to 25 mL/h every 6 to 8 hours until the desired goal is achieved. In children, full-strength formulas are recommended initially at a rate of 1–2 mL/kg per hour or 20–25 mL/kg per day with advancement every 4 to 12 hours of similar volumes. The advancement of enteral feeding should be individualized for specific patient issues. Occasionally, half-strength dilution of the formula at a low rate (25 mL/h) may be necessary. This practice is used to prevent or treat GI complications of enteral feeding initiation such as diarrhea, abdominal cramping, bloating, and nausea. The rate is then increased in 25 mL/h increments every 6 to 8 hours to a maximal rate with subsequent increase of the formula strength in the next day(s).[45] Typically, rate progression should take no more than 3 days before the patient is at target feeding goals. Longer times to reach feeding goals frequently are required in patients with short bowel syndrome, in extremely premature infants, and in critically ill patients.

DRUG COMPATIBILITY WITH ENTERAL FORMULAS

Mixing of liquid medications with selected enteral nutrition products has been associated with several types of physical incompatibilities: granulation, gel formation, separation, and precipitation.[78,79] Not only can these physical incompatibilities inhibit drug absorption, gel formation potentially may clog small-bore enteral feeding tubes. Physical incompatibility with medications is more common in formulas that contain intact protein than in those with hydrolyzed protein. Also, medication and enteral formula incompatibilities are more common with the use of acidic pharmaceutical syrups. Liquid medications have osmolalities that range from 500–5000 mosm/kg.[80] Subsequent admixture of liquid medications into enteral formulas thus can greatly enhance the final osmolality and result in the development of diarrhea. The most prudent recommendation is to avoid the routine admixture whenever possible, especially for nonaqueous preparations and syrups. In the clinical setting, exceptions do exist, such as adding electrolyte injections of potassium or sodium to enteral formulas to assist in maintaining or repleting the electrolyte requirements for a patient.

COMPLICATIONS OF CONCOMITANT DRUG ADMINISTRATION

Enteral feeding tubes frequently are used as a route for the delivery of medications. However, the pharmacologic agent and its mode of delivery are modified when a feeding tube is placed. Concomitant administration of medications with enteral feedings delivered directly into the stomach through NG or gastrostomy tubes allows the stomach to function in its normal capacity for drug dissolution. However, placement of enteral tubes beyond the pylorus, such as with ND, NJ, and jejunostomy tubes, alters drug dissolution because the stomach is bypassed. Therefore, one must consider the anatomic location of the feeding tube tip when administering medications such as antacids or sucralfate because their therapeutic effect is designed to occur within the stomach. Because many drugs are best absorbed in the fasted state, medications should be administered on an empty stomach as much as possible. Patients receiving bolus intragastric feedings may receive medications appropriately spaced between the feedings.[81,82] For patients receiving continuous enteral feeding, the feedings may require interruption for drug administration, followed by prudent flushing of the tube with water. Pharmacists need to be aware of potential problems that may arise when medications are administered through

TABLE 138–11. General Considerations for Medication Administration by Enteral Feeding Tubes

1. Administer medications by mouth when feasible; consider enteral feeding tube as an alternative route.
2. Determine location of the feeding tube tip, because pre- or post-pyloric drug instillation can alter effectiveness.
3. Liquid dosage forms should be used if available. Dosage and frequency adjustment are required if changing from a sustained-release drug to administer a non-sustained-release liquid form.
4. Hyperosmolar medications require dilution.
5. The contents of hard or soft gelatin capsules reconstituted with 10–15 mL of water and crushed compressed tablets reconstituted with 15–30 mL of water can be administered when a liquid form is unavailable.
6. Do not crush and administer sustained-release or enteric-coated medications.
7. Flush the feeding tube with water prior to administering a medication. Do not mix medications. Administer each medication separately, flushing with water between medications. Flush with water after medication administration completed.
8. In general, do not add medications to the enteral formula. Exceptions exist for the adding of hypertonic electrolyte injection to enteral formulas. Be aware of specific drug-enteral product incompatibilities.

enteral feeding tubes, such as the degradation and/or inactivation of nutrient components or altered bioavailability of a drug that may compromise therapeutic efficacy[83–86] (Table 138–11).

Selecting the proper medication dosage form for administration by enteral feeding tubes is crucial to avoid drug inactivation and altered bioavailability (Table 138–12). Medications in sublingual form, sustained-released capsules or tablets, and enteric-coated tablets are designed not to be crushed and therefore should not be administered via enteral feeding tubes. An extensive list of oral dosage forms that should not be crushed is available in the literature.[87] For the most part, liquid drug preparations are the preferred dosage form when administering medications via enteral feeding tubes. In situations where a liquid medication is unavailable, compressed tablets or the contents of hard or soft gelatin capsules can be admixed with water (15–30 mL) and administered down enteral feeding tubes. Adherence to proper

TABLE 138–12. Guidelines for Medication Administration by Enteral Feeding Tubes

Dosage Form	Administered by Enteral Feeding Tube	Comment
Sublingual or buccal tablets	No	Low dosage of drug not designed for gastric or intestinal administration Altered drug bioavailability and potency owing to first-pass effect
Sustained-release capsules or tablets	Not preferred Do not crush	Crushing a sustained-release dosage form destroys its time-release effect Altered therapeutic drug response and gastrointestinal irritation can occur
Enteric-coated tablets	Not preferred Do not crush	Crushing can result in gastrointestinal irritation and drug inactivation
Compressed tablets (sugar or film coated)	Yes	May be crushed and administered without altering therapeutic drug response May clog small-bore feeding tubes
Hard or soft gelatin capsules	Yes	Powders from hard capsules and oils from soft capsules may be administered without altering therapeutic drug response
Liquid preparations Solutions Suspensions Elixirs Emulsions	Yes Preferred	Frequently recommended; however, drug form can be hyperosmolar, requiring dilution Strong acid syrups may interact with enteral formulas and clog tubes

TABLE 138–13. Medications with Special Considerations for Enteral Feeding Tube Administration

Drug	Interaction	Comments
Phenytoin	Reduced bioavailability demonstrated when administered during continuous tube feeding. Results of in vitro studies suggest that protein (caseinate salts) and calcium chloride may reduce phenytoin bioavailability.[89]	Limited data from clinical studies and case reports provide basis for suggestions to overcome incompatibility. Suggestions include holding tube feeding 2 h before and after phenytoin,[88] administering phenytoin capsules rather than the suspension during continuous feeding,[90] and using a meat-based enteral formula rather than a protein hydrolysate containing formula.[91] Monitor patient's clinical response and serum drug level closely.
Antibiotics (selected)	Reduced bioavailability demonstrated between food and penicillin, tetracycline, isoniazid, rifampin, enoxacin, norfloxacin, and ofloxacin.[92] Interaction also theoretically applied to continuous tube feeding.	Existence of clinical studies documenting enteral formula interaction with selected antibiotics is lacking. Holding tube feeding administration for specified time periods before and after drug administration has been recommended.[93] Monitor patient's clinical response closely.
Warfarin	Pharmacologic interaction demonstrated between warfarin and vitamin K contained in enteral feeding formulas, resulting in reduced anticoagulation effect.	Vitamin K is contained in most enteral products in doses less than 200 μg per 1000 kcal; adjust warfarin dose based on monitoring the INR and observing the vitamin K content of the enteral formula.
Antacids	Altered pharmacologic effect of antacid if administered into the small bowel. A physical incompatibility has been reported with aluminum-containing antacids causing an esophageal plug formation.	Administer antacids only into feeding tubes with the tip placed in the stomach. Administering aluminum-containing antacids after holding the tube feeding formula may prevent physical incompatibility formation.[94]

technique for administering the contents of tablets or capsules down feeding tubes, such as flushing of the tube with water prior to and following the administration of medication, is important to prevent clogging of the feeding tube.

DRUG-NUTRIENT INTERACTIONS

The most significant drug and nutrient interactions that can occur during continuous enteral nutrition are those in which the bioavailability of the drug is reduced and the desired pharmacologic effect is not achieved. Unfortunately, limited clinical studies are available to document the extent of this problem with enteral feeding. Most of the observations are anecdotal case reports among few patients. A reduction in the bioavailability of phenytoin has been demonstrated during continuous tube feeding, with subsequent subtherapeutic drug levels.[88] The exact cause for reduced phenytoin bioavailability during continuous enteral feeding is unclear; however, the results of in vitro studies suggest that protein and calcium chloride may bind the drug. A number of methods to minimize this interaction for patients receiving continuous tube feedings have been suggested (Table 138–13). Little consensus exists as to the best method to prevent or reduce the impact of this interaction. Pharmacists must be aware that patients may require higher than normal doses of phenytoin while on enteral nutrition. The patient's clinical response and serum phenytoin levels should be monitored closely during continuous enteral feeding and after the discontinuation of enteral feeds.

Clinical studies documenting altered bioavailability with antibiotics during continuous enteral feeding are lacking. However, based on case reports and theoretical concerns, holding the tube feeding for 30 minutes before and 30 minutes after a selected antibiotic is administered is recommended (see Table 138–13). Warfarin resistance also has been documented during enteral feeding owing to the vitamin K content of the enteral feeding products. Prior to 1980, it was thought that the content of vitamin K in dosages of up to 1330 μg/1000 kcal of enteral feeding formula was contributing to the pharmacologic interaction with warfarin. Subsequently, the vitamin K content within formulas intended for use in adults has been reformulated to less than 200 μg/1000 kcal. However, warfarin resistance has continued to be reported. Pharmacists should be observant of the vitamin K content within enteral formulas and adjust the warfarin dose based on the patient's international normalized ratio (INR).

COMPLICATIONS AND MONITORING OF ENTERAL NUTRITION

A major advantage of enteral nutrition over parenteral nutrition is a reduced complication rate.[66] Major complications and potential causes for GI, technical, and infectious complications associated with enteral tube feeding are listed in Table 138–14. Several of the factors responsible for the metabolic complications seen among enteral nutrition patients are similar to those seen during parenteral nutrition and are presented in Tables 137–4 and 137–7. However, the GI, technical, and infectious complications seen during enteral nutrition are unique to this route of therapy.

METABOLIC COMPLICATIONS

The metabolic complications related to hydration and electrolyte and glucose control are observed more frequently in patients with underlying illnesses that cause organ dysfunction. The micronutrient and water content within enteral feeding formulas are in fixed amounts (RDAs) intended for the average patient. Therefore, the frequency of clinical and laboratory assessment to monitor hydration, electrolyte, organ function, and glucose control adequately for a patient who is critically ill is greater than for a stable patient residing in a rehabilitation unit or at home (Table 138–15). Patients receiving long-term home enteral nutrition should have clinical and laboratory monitoring done weekly to every 2 to 3 months depending on clinical status. It is

TABLE 138–14. Complications of Tube Feeding

Complication	Causes
Gastrointestinal	
Diarrhea	Drug related
	Antibiotic-induced bacterial overgrowth
	Hyperosmolar medications administered via feeding tubes
	Antacids containing magnesium
	Malabsorption
	Hypoalbuminemia/gut mucosal atrophy
	Pancreatic insufficiency
	Inadequate GIT surface area
	Rapid GIT transit
	Radiation enteritis
	Tube feeding related
	Rapid formula administration
	Formula hyperosmolality
	Low residue (fiber) content
	Lactose intolerance
Nausea and vomiting	Bacterial contamination
	Gastric dysmotility (surgery, anticholinergic drugs, diabetic gastroparesis)
	Rapid infusion of hyperosmolar formula
Constipation	Dehydration
	Drug induced (anticholinergics)
	Inactivity
	Low residue (fiber) content
	Obstruction/fecal impaction
Abdominal distention/cramping	Too rapid formula administration
Technical	
Occluded feeding tube lumen	Insoluble complexation of enteral formula and medication(s)
	Inadequate flushing of feeding tube
	Undissolved feeding formula
Tube displacement	Self-extubation
	Vomiting or coughing
	Inadequate fixation (jejunostomy)
Aspiration	Improper patient position
	Gastroparesis/atony causing regurgitation
	Feeding tube malpositioned
	Compromised lower esophageal sphincter
	Diminished gag reflex
Peristomal excoriation	Improper skin and tube care
	GIT secretions leaking peristomally
Infectious	
Aspiration pneumonia	Same as technical—aspiration comments
	Prolonged use of large-bore polyvinylchloride tube

important to evaluate the actual content of water and micronutrients provided by the enteral formula for a patient at high risk for metabolic complications such as the critically ill. Additional hydration and electrolytes may need to be provided for patients being inadequately supported with an enteral formula. Conversely, for patients who have excessive fluid retention or increased serum electrolytes, the enteral formula may need to be changed to one that is more concentrated or provides less of a particular nutrient(s).

GI COMPLICATIONS

The GI complications associated with tube feeding include diarrhea, nausea and vomiting, constipation, abdominal distension, and cramping. In general, these side effects can be attributed to either drug-related, patient-related, or tube feeding-related factors. Diarrhea has been reported to occur in 2.3% to 30.6% of enterally fed patients.[66] It is speculated that the wide variability in incidence is caused, in part, by the multiplicity of clinical definitions for diarrhea. Monitoring of the patient for diarrhea includes evaluating stool frequency, consistency, and volume (see Table 138–15) and taking into consideration the patient's previous bowel habits and underlying disease state.[95] Drug-related causes of diarrhea include the administration of hyperosmolar medications or elixirs that contain high concentrations of sorbitol. Infectious causes, such as antibiotic-induced bacterial overgrowth by *Clostridium difficile* or other intestinal flora need to be considered when diarrhea develops. Diarrhea also may occur as a result of malabsorption, owing to such circumstances as severe malnutrition and related gut mucosal atrophy, exocrine failure such as chronic pancreatitis or cystic fibrosis, inadequate surface area or too rapid transit through the small bowel owing to radiation enteritis, short bowel syndrome, or celiac disease. During such clinical circumstances, a continuous infusion of chemically defined feeding formula may help improve the symptoms of malabsorption. Of the tube feeding-related factors that may contribute to diarrhea (see Table 138–14), the rate of infusion is a primary factor. Even hyperosmolar solutions can be infused without diarrhea or abdominal distension if the feeding is infused at a constant rate and titrated incrementally according to the tolerance of the patient.[66,95]

TABLE 138–15. Suggested Monitoring of Enteral Nutrition (EN) to Prevent Complications

Parameter	During Initiation of EN or for a Critically Ill Patient	During Stable EN Therapy or for a Rehabilitating Patient
Vital signs		
Temperature, respirations, pulse, blood pressure	Every 4–6 h	Every 12–24 h
Physical exam[a]		
Abdomen, lung fields, extremities, mucous membranes, skin turgor	Every 4–6 h	Every 12–24 h
Clinical assessment	Daily	Daily
Weight		
Total intake/output		
Urine, gastrointestinal and extraordinary fluid losses		
Stool frequency/consistency/volume		
Nausea or vomiting		
Concurrent medications and administration route	Daily	Daily
Verification of nasal or oral tube placement with x-ray	Done prior to initiating EN	N/A[b]
Ongoing assessment by tube placement	Every 6 h	Every 12 h
Gastric residual checks	Every 8–12 h	Every 8–12 h
Enterostomy tube site assessment for leakage and/or skin irritation/redness	Daily	Daily
Patient compliance with feeding procedures and feeding tube/ostomy care	N/A	Daily
Serum electrolytes, BUN/Cr, serum glucose[c]	Daily	2–3 times/wk
Serum calcium, magnesium, and phosphorous	4–5 times/wk	2–3 times/wk
Liver function tests	Weekly	Monthly
Urine glucose/acetone[c]	Every 6 h	Daily
Trace elements, vitamins	Frequently tailored to patient-specific situations	Frequently tailored to patient-specific situations

[a]Includes eyes, ear, nose, and throat exam for patients with nasoenteric feeding tubes.
[b]Not applicable.
[c]Frequency of glucose assessment is for the nondiabetic patient.

Occasionally, pharmacologic intervention is indicated to control severe diarrhea. The primary agents employed are opiates, diphenoxylate, and loperamide.[96] Diphenoxylate acts by the same mechanism as the opioids, by decreasing GI motility and secretions. These actions decrease the amount of fluid to be reabsorbed in the small intestine and colon and increase the transit time to allow more absorption of exogenous fluids. Loperamide decreases GI motility and decreases small bowel output via the ileum. It is two to three times as potent as diphenoxylate and thus may be administered less frequently. Use of these agents should be limited because overuse may produce constipation and paralytic ileus.

Nausea and vomiting in a patient receiving nasogastric tube feeding may be a result of gastric atony subsequent to recent surgery, the anticholinergic effects of drugs, and/or an underlying disease such as diabetic gastroparesis. Advancement of the feeding tube beyond the pylorus may reduce the associated symptoms of nausea and vomiting and enable successful enteral feeding. Constipation also may occur with tube feeding, particularly in the elderly and long-term enteral nutrition patients. Multiple causes may contribute to the constipation (see Table 138–14). Using enteral formulas with enhanced fiber may improve the symptoms of constipation; however, the exact amount and optimal source of fiber are yet to be established.[61,97]

TECHNICAL COMPLICATIONS

The technical complications of enteral nutrition frequently are associated with the feeding tube. Occluded feeding tubes have been reported to occur in 10% of patients.[66] It is a common cause for feeding tube replacement and increases the cost of enteral feeding. Different techniques for clearing obstructed tubes have included instillation of warm water, meat tenderizer, flat dark colas, and pancreatic enzymes[45] and passing of an endoscopic cytology brush.[66] Meat tenderizer (papain enzyme) should be avoided in patients at risk for aspiration due to the chemical pneumonitis induced by aspiration of the enzyme. Adherence to appropriate flushing protocols of the feeding tube during continuous tube feeding and medication administration is an extremely important variable in prevention of occluded feeding tubes (see Table 138–11). Inadvertent tube displacement has been reported to occur in greater than 50% of patients receiving enteral tube feeding.[66] Securing the tube and ongoing assessment of its appropriate placement may prevent tube displacement.

OTHER COMPLICATIONS

A unique complication of tube feedings in children, especially in the first year of life, is the development of feeding disorders due to oral hypersensitivity, poor oral/motor skills, and food aversion. Transitioning from tube to oral nutrition is often difficult and protracted. The involvement of an occupational or speech therapist, behavioral psychologist, or other trained individual often is necessary to improve oral intake. Avoidance of a strict nothing by mouth (NPO) status, if possible, and oral stimulation programs are recommended to avoid this complication.[98]

ASPIRATION OF GASTRIC CONTENTS

Bronchopulmonary aspiration of gastric contents is a potentially fatal complication of tube feeding. Patients who are mechanically ventilated or those with swallowing disorders are at higher risk for this complication. The incidence has been reported to be as high as 46%.[66] The use of small-bore feeding tubes may preserve lower esophageal sphincter function, and hence patients are less prone to develop reflux

TABLE 138–16. Suggested Monitoring of Enteral Nutrition (EN) to Promote Nutritional Efficacy

Parameter	During Initiation of EN or for a Critically Ill Patient	During Stable EN Therapy or for a Rehabilitating Patient	During Long-Term Home EN Therapy
Anthropometrics			
Weight	Daily	Weekly	Weekly
Triceps skinfold	N/A[a]	N/A	Every 1–2 mo
Midarm muscle circumference	N/A	N/A	Every 1–2 mo
Muscle function			
Level of physical endurance	N/A	Weekly	Weekly to monthly, then frequency tailored to the patient situation
Metabolic			
Albumin	Monthly	Monthly	Monthly, then frequently tailored to the patient situation
Transferrin	Weekly	Weekly	Once to twice monthly, then frequency tailored to the patient response
24-h urine urea nitrogen	Weekly	Once or twice monthly	Frequently tailored to patient-specific situations
Indirect calorimetry	Frequently tailored to patient-specific situations	Frequently tailored to patient-specific situations	Frequently tailored to patient-specific situations
Nutritional intake			
Calories	Daily	2–3 times weekly	Weekly, then tailored to the patient situation
Protein, fluid, electrolytes, trace elements, vitamins	Daily	2–3 times weekly	Weekly, then tailored to the patient situation
Skin integrity	Daily	Daily	Weekly
Wound healing			
Pressure sore(s)			

[a]Not applicable.

in the esophagus with potential for aspiration. Aspiration can be minimized further by not allowing a large volume to accumulate in the stomach. The amount of liquid residing in the stomach is called the gastric residual. After holding the tube feeding for at least 30 minutes, gastric residuals can be checked by attaching a syringe to the open end of the tube and filling it with the liquid. In adults, the residuals should be less than 200 mL.[99] In children, residuals greater than twice the bolus volume or twice the hourly infusion rate for continuous gastric feedings are considered excessive.[100] Small tubes often collapse easily when negative pressure is applied, making it difficult to measure residuals. The risk of aspiration also can be reduced by keeping the patient's head of the bed elevated to a 30- to 45-degree angle during feeding and for 30 to 60 minutes after intermittent boluses. This makes it more difficult for fluid to migrate up the esophagus against gravity.

Finally, the risk of aspiration may be reduced by infusion of feedings into the small intestine instead of the stomach. The inadvertent passage of a small-bore feeding tube into the tracheobronchial passage with subsequent infusion of an enteral diet can be fatal. Patients with a diminished gag reflex are at greatest risk for this complication. The small-bore tubes may not trigger the gag reflex, which indicates proper placement; therefore, the tube position always should be verified radiologicallly to reduce the chance of infusion into the lung. Alleviation or prevention of bronchopulmonary aspiration requires meticulous tube insertion and tube maintenance. Other infectious complications include acute otitis media and sinusitis. These complications have been associated with long-term use of polyvinylchloride tubes.[41]

THERAPEUTIC NUTRITION AND DISEASE OUTCOMES

Nutrition outcome goals of enteral tube feeding are to reverse protein-calorie malnutrition, promote growth and development of infants and children, or maintain an adequate nutritional state. Assessing the outcome of enteral nutrition includes monitoring objective measures of body composition, protein and energy balance, and subjective outcome for physiologic muscle function and wound healing (Table 138–16). These nutritional outcome indices have improved with enteral feedings among critically ill,[31] rehabilitation,[101] long-term home enteral patients,[102] and children with cancer.[103] Besides an improvement in nutrition outcome, another goal of enteral nutrition is to reduce disease-related morbidity and mortality. Measures of disease-related morbidity include the length of hospital stay, infectious complications, and the patient's sense of well-being. Such clinical outcome goals are extremely difficult to document with the use of enteral nutrition in part because other factors such as age, underlying comorbidities, extent of injury, immunocompetence, and end-organ complications also affect disease outcome.

Only a few prospective, randomized, controlled trials have demonstrated a change in disease outcome with the use of enteral nutrition. The results of clinical investigations of enteral nutrition in Crohn's disease suggest an improvement in some indices of clinical outcome. Historically, TPN and bowel rest were prescribed for patients with an active flare of their Crohn's disease. However, clinical investigation has established that for most patients with disease flare, bowel rest is not necessary to induce a clinical remission.[104] Short courses of nutrition support in hospitalized patients often demonstrate remission rates of 60% and 80% with either TPN or defined enteral diets, respectively. Polymeric and partially hydrolyzed formulas appear to be equivalent to the elemental formulas in clinical efficacy.[35,105] The contribution of enteral nutrition to the clinical outcome of patients with Crohn's disease will remain unanswered until prospective, randomized, controlled trials comparing enteral nutrition and placebo are performed.

The use of enteral nutrition over TPN has been evaluated for its effectiveness in reducing morbidity and mortality in critically ill patients. Heyland and colleagues[27] evaluated the role of enteral nutrition, particularly early enteral nutrition, on morbidity and mortality in critically ill patients. Of the eight randomized, nonblinded clinical trials, three studies used objective criteria to define infectious outcomes. Although no differences were seen in the incidence of multiple-organ failure syndrome or mortality in the enteral versus the parenteral group,[106] patients who received enteral nutrition had a 17% sepsis rate, which included a 3% rate of major septic complications, compared with the parenteral group, which had a septic complication rate of 37% and a 20% rate of major septic complications.[31] In the third study, the septic complication rate was 15.7% in the enteral nutrition group compared with 40% in the parenteral group.[107] The enteral and parenteral study groups were comparable with respect to age, injury type, and severity of illness scores.[31,107] Based on the results of the aforementioned studies and others reviewed, Heyland and colleagues conclude that sufficient data exist to suggest that critically ill patients benefit from early enteral nutrition and that enteral nutrition should be commenced as early as possible in the course of a patient's illness. Even if enteral nutrition may not meet all of the nutrient goals immediately, the role of tube feeding should be as a stimulant to the patient's GI immunologic function and mucosal integrity. Enteral nutrition thus may result in reduction of infectious complications in the critically ill patient. No prospective, randomized, controlled studies evaluating enteral nutrition in the critically ill have resulted in reduced mortality. Enteral formulas with altered nutrient composition that include different enhancements of hydrolyzed protein sources (dipeptides, tripeptides), ribonucleic acid, increased omega-3 fatty acids, arginine, and glutamine have demonstrated significant reduction in infectious rates and length of hospital stay.[68,69]

PHARMACOECONOMIC CONSIDERATIONS

Enteral nutrition has been shown to be consistently less expensive than TPN. A formal pharmacoeconomic analysis of nutrition support therapy should include an evaluation of therapeutic outcome relative to the cumulative cost associated with the nutrients; nonnutrient supplies; the time spent by professional staff in compounding, delivering, and managing therapy; laboratory monitoring; and management of complications that result from therapy. Although none of the existing analyses has addressed all these issues, selected comparisons of costs related to enteral and parenteral therapy derived from clinical research trials in institutional settings have been published. Nutritional support therapy costs can be divided into nutrient and nonnutrient supplies. Enteral nonnutrient supply costs include the specific enteral tube device, its related insertion technique, and infusion-related supplies, as described in Tables 138–5 and 138–6. The distribution of nutrient and nonnutrient costs was found to be 87% and 13% for enteral nutrition and 57% and 43% for parenteral nutrition among Veterans Administration Medical Center patients receiving nutrition support therapy.[108] The reported cost of enteral nutrition is approximately one-fourth to one-half that of parenteral nutrition.[108,109] This broad range in reported cost is largely owing to the extent of data that were included in the analysis. Including the cost of managing complications related to each therapy greatly increases the overall cost of parenteral nutrition as compared with enteral nutrition.[109]

▶ PRINCIPLES OF PHARMACOTHERAPY

- The GIT defends the host from toxins and antigens by both immunologic and nonimmunologic mechanisms, collectively referred to as the gut barrier function. Thus, when possible, enteral nutrition is preferred over TPN because it is as effective and may reduce infectious complications.
- Postpyloric placement of the feeding tube tip may prevent aspiration, and patients who are at high risk for aspiration (patients with gastric atony) should have the tube tip secured into the small bowel for successful feeding. Placement of a nasal feeding tube, at the bedside, requires an x-ray to verify that the tube is not within the lung.
- Patients fed via a gastric (stomach) tube may be fed continuously via an infusion pump or by bolus feeding. Gastric residual volumes should be checked to reduce the risk of aspiration. Patients with small bowel feeding tubes should only be fed continuously via an infusion pump to avoid dumping syndrome.
- Selection of the feeding formula depends on nutrition goals, the patient's primary disease state and related complications, and nutrient digestibility and absorption. Polymeric or standard products are used most commonly. Monomeric or partially hydrolyzed/elemental products are indicated for patients who have severe pancreatic insufficiency, have undergone a total pancreatectomy or a major small bowel resection, or have documented intolerance to polymeric formulas.
- Selection of a specialized product for patients with organ failure (pulmonary, renal, hepatic, endocrine) or immunologic impairment requires knowledge of the achievable nutritional and disease-related outcomes and the circumstances of the particular patient.
- Liquid medications should not be added to an enteral product without prior review of the compatibility literature. Medications that are nonaqueous or are contained within syrups often are incompatible with enteral products.
- Prior to administering medications through a feeding tube, one must determine where the feeding tube tip is located (stomach or small bowel) and whether the medication is in suitable dosage form. Suitable dosage forms include liquid preparations and gelatin capsules that may be opened and the contents administered through the tube. Medications that should not be crushed and administered through a tube include enteric-coated or sustained-release capsules or tablets and sublingual or buccal tablets.
- Enteral feeding products can alter the bioavailability and/or change the desired pharmacologic effect of several medications, including phenytoin, warfarin, and selected antibiotics and antacids.
- GI complications can be drug-related (hyperosmolar medication-induced diarrhea), patient-related (infection, malabsorption, dysmotility), or tube feeding-related (infusion rate and osmolality of the product). The risk of bronchopulmonary aspiration may be reduced by checking gastric residuals, keeping the head of the bed at a 30- to 45-degree angle, or by placing the feeding tube tip postpylorically.

REFERENCES

1. Cashman MD. Principles of digestive physiology for clinical nutrition. Nutr Clin Prac 1986;1:241–249.
2. Caspary WF. Physiology and pathophysiology of intestinal absorption. Am J Clin Nutr 1992;55:299S–308S.
3. O'Dwyer ST, Smith RJ, Kripke SA, et al. New fuels for the gut. In: Rombeau JL, Caldwell MD, eds. Clinical Nutrition: Enteral and Tube Feeding, 2d ed. Philadelphia, Saunders, 1990:548.

4. Record KE, Kolpek JH, Rapp RP. Long chain versus medium chain length triglycerides: A review of metabolism and clinical use. Nutr Clin Prac 1986;1:279–287.
5. Mirtallo JM. Nutrient metabolism. In: Dipiro JT, Talbert FL, Yee GL, et al., eds. Pharmacotherapy: A Pathophysiologic Approach, 3d ed. Stamford, CT, Appleton & Lange, 1997:2711–2734.
6. Mainous MR, Block EFJ, Dietch EA. Nutritional support of the gut: How and why. New Horizons 1994;2:193–201.
7. Langkamp-Henken B, Glezer JA, Kudsk KA. Immunologic structure and function of the gastrointestinal tract. Nutr Clin Pract 1992;7:100–108.
8. Gleeson MH, Dowling RH, Peters TJ. Biochemical changes in intestinal mucosa after experimental small bowel bypass in the rat. Clin Sci 1972;43:743–757.
9. Levine GM, Deren JJ, Steiger E, et al. Role of oral intake in maintenance of gut mass and disaccharide activity. Gastroenterology 1974;67:975–982.
10. Thompson JS, Vaughan WP, Forst CF, et al. The effect of route on nutrient delivery on gut structure and diamine oxidase levels. J Parenter Enter Nutr 1987;11:28–32.
11. Greene HL, McCabe DR, Merenstein GB. Protracted diarrhea and malnutrition in infancy: Changes in intestinal morphology and disaccharidase activities during treatment with total intravenous nutrition or oral elemental diets. J Pediatr 1975;87:695–704.
12. Morin CL, Ling V, Bourassa D. Small intestine and colonic changes induced by a chemically defined diet. Dig Dis Sci 1980;25:123–128.
13. Young EA, Cioletti LA, Winborn WB, et al. Comparative study of nutritional adaptation to defined formula diets in rats. Am J Clin Nutr 1980;33:2106–2118.
14. Johnson LR, Copeland EM, Dudrick SJ, et al. Structural and hormonal alterations in the gastrointestinal tract of parenterally fed rats. Gastroenterology 1975;68:1177–1183.
15. Sagor GR, Ghatei MA, Al-Mukhtar MYT, et al. Evidence for a humoral mechanism after small intestinal resection. Gastroenterology 1983;84:902–906.
16. Lickley HLA, Track NS, Vranic M, Bury KD. Metabolic responses to enteral and parenteral nutrition. Am J Surg 1978;135:172–176.
17. Adibi SA. Leucine absorption rate and net movements of sodium and water in human jejunum. J Appl Physiol 1970;28:753–757.
18. Souba WW, Scott TE, Wilmore DW. Intestinal consumption of intravenously administered fuels. J Parenter Enter Nutr 1985;9:18–22.
19. Souba WW, Wilmore DW. Postoperative alteration of arteriovenous exchange of amino acids across the gastrointestinal tract. Surgery 1983;94:342–350.
20. Alverdy J, Chi HS, Sheldon G. The effect of parenteral nutrition on gastrointestinal immunity: The importance of enteral immunity. Ann Surg 1985;202:681–684.
21. Alverdy JC, Aoys E, Moss GS. TPN promotes bacterial translocation from the gut. Surgery 1988;104:185–190.
22. Saito H, Trocki O, Alexander JW, et al. Effect of route of administration on the nutritional state, catabolic hormone secretion and gut mucosal integrity after burn injury. J Parenter Enter Nutr 1987;11:1–7.
23. Kudsk KA, Stone JM, Carpenter G, Sheldon GF. Enteral and parenteral feeding influences mortality after hemoglobin *E. coli* peritonitis in normal rats. J Trauma 1983;23:605–609.
24. Zaloga GP, Knowles R, Black KW, Prielipp R. Total parenteral nutrition increases mortality after hemorrhage. Crit Care Med 1991;19:54–59.
25. Fong Y, Marano MA, Barber A, et al. Total parenteral nutrition and bowel rest modify the metabolic response to endotoxin in humans. Ann Surg 1989;210:449–457.
26. Talbot JM. Guidelines for the scientific review of enteral food products for special medical purposes. J Parenter Enter Nutr 1991;15(Suppl):99S–174S.
27. Heyland DK, Cook DJ, Guyatt GH. Enteral nutrition in the critically ill patient: A critical review of the evidence. Intensive Care Med 1993;19:435–442.
28. Jolliet P, Pichard C, Biolo G, et al. Enteral nutrition in intensive care patients: A practical approach. Working Group on Nutrition and Metabolism, European Society of Intensive Care Medicine. Intensive Care Med 1998; 24(8):848–859.
29. Vernet O, Christin L, Schultz Y, et al. Enteral versus parenteral nutrition: Comparison of energy metabolism in healthy subjects. Am J Physiol 1986;250:E47–E54.
30. McArdle AH, Palmason C, Morency I, Brown RA. A rationale for enteral feeding as the preferable route for hyperalimentation. Surgery 1981;90:616–623.
31. Kudsk KA, Croce MA, Fabian TC, et al. Enteral versus parenteral feeding: Effects on septic morbidity after blunt and penetrating abdominal trauma. Ann Surg 1992;215:503–513.
32. Messing B, Bories C, Kunstlinger F, Bernier JJ. Does total parenteral nutrition induce gall bladder sludge formation and lithiasis? Gastroenterology 1983;84:1012–1019.
33. Carbonnel F, Cosnes J, Chevret S, et al. The role of anatomic factors in nutritional autonomy after extensive small bowel resection. J Parenter Enter Nutr 1996;20:275–280.
34. McClave SA, Lowen CC, Snider HL. Immunonutrition and enteral hyperalimentation of critically ill patients. Dig Dis Sci 1992;37:1153–1161.
35. American Society of Parenteral and Enteral Nutrition Board of Directors. Guidelines for the use of parenteral and enteral nutrition in adult and pediatric patients. J Parenter Enter Nutr 1993;17(Suppl):1SA–52SA.
36. Windsor ACJ, Kanwar S, Li AGK, et al. Compared with parenteral nutrition, enteral feeding attenuates the acute phase response and improves disease severity in acute pancreatitis. Gut 1998;42:431–435.
37. Bell SJ, Mascioli EA, Forse RA, Bistrian BR. Nutrition support and the human immunodeficiency virus (HIV). Parasitology 1993;107 (Suppl):S53–S67.
38. Minard G. Enteral access. Nutr Clin Pract 1994;9:172–182.
39. Lysen LK, Samour PQ. Enteral equipment. In: Matarese E, Gottschlich MM, eds. Contemporary Nutrition Support Practice: A Clinical Guide. Philadelphia, Saunders, 1998:202–215.
40. Dobbie RP, Hoffmeister JA. Continuous pump-tube enteric hyperalimentation. Surg Gynecol Obstet 1976;143:273–276.
41. Torosian MH, Rombeau JL. Feeding by tube enterostomy. Surg Gynecol Obstet 1980;150:918–927.
42. Kobak GE, McClenathan DT, Schurman SJ. Complications of removing percutaneious endoscopic gastrostomy tubes in children. J Pediatr Gastroenter Nutr 2000;30:404–407.
43. Yaseen M, Steele MI, Grunow JE. Nonendoscopic removal of percutaneous endoscopic gastrostomy tubes: Morbidity and mortality in children. Gastrointest Endosc 1996;44:235–238.
44. Peitersen-Oberndorff KE, Vos GD, Baeten CG. Sercus complications after incomplete removal of percutaneous endoscopic gastrostomy catheters. J Pediatr Gastroenterol Nutr 1999;2:230–232.
45. Clevenger FW, Rodriguez DJ. Decision-making for enteral feeding administration: The why behind where and how. Nutr Clin Pract 1995;10:104–113.
46. Cerra FB, Holman RT, Bankey PE, et al. Omega-3 polyunsaturated fatty acids as modulators of cellular function in the critically ill. Pharmacotherapy 1991;11:71–76.
47. Mueller C, Nestle M. Regulation of medical foods: Toward a rational policy. Nutr Clin Pract 1995;10:8–15.
48. Heymsfield SB. Enteral solutions: Is there a solution? Nutr Clin Prac 1995;10:4–7.
49. MacBurney MM, Russell C, Young LS. Formulas. In: Rombeau JL, Caldwell MD, eds. Clinical Nutrition: Enteral and Tube Feeding, 2d ed. Philadelphia, Saunders, 1990:149–173.
50. Silk DBA, Grimble GK. Relevance of physiology of nutrient absorption to formulation of enteral diets. Nutrition 1992;8:1–12.
51. Hall JC, Heel K, McCauley R. Glutamine. Br J Surg 1996;83(3):305–312.
52. Schloerb PR, Almar M. Total parenteral nutrition with glutamine in bone marrow transplantation and other clinical applications: A randomized, double-blind study. J Parenter Enter Nutr 1993;17:407–413.
53. Ziegler TR, Young LS, Benfell K, et al. Clinical and metabolic efficacy of glutamine-supplemented parenteral nutrition after bone marrow

transplantation: A randomized, double-blind, controlled study. Ann Intern Med 1992;116:821–828.
54. Zaloga GP, MacGregor DA. What to consider when choosing enteral or parenteral nutrition. J Crit Illness 1990;5:1180–1200.
55. Trujillo EB. Enteral nutrition: A comprehensive overview. In: Matarese E, Gottschlich MM, eds. Contemporary Nutrition Support Practice: A Clinical Guide. Philadelphia, Saunders, 1998:192–201.
56. Fish J, Sporay G, Beyer K, et al. A prospective randomized study of glutamine-enriched parenteral compared with enteral feeding in postoperative patients. Am J Clin Nutr 1997;65(4):977–983.
57. Shike M. Enteral feeding. In: Shils ME, Olson JA, Shike M, Ross AC, eds. Modern Nutrition in Health and Disease, 9th ed. Philadelphia, Lea & Febiger, 1999:1643–1656.
58. Kudsk KA. Clinical applications of enteral nutrition. Nutr Clin Prac 1994;9:165–171.
59. Mead J. Nutrients with special functions: Essential fatty acids. In: Alfin-Slater R, Kritchervsky D, eds. Human Nutrition, Vol. 3A. New York, Plenum Press, 1980:213–238.
60. Berner YN, Morse R, Frank D, et al. Vitamin plasma levels in long-term enteral feeding patients. J Parenter Enter Nutr 1989;13:525–528.
61. Scheppach WM, Bartram HP. Experimental evidence for and clinical implications of fiber and artificial enteral nutrition. Nutrition 1993;9:399–405.
62. Jew R, Owen D, Kaufman D, et al. Osmolality of commonly used medications and formulas in the neonatal intensive care unit. Nutr Clin Prac 1997;12:158–163.
63. Keohane PP, Attrill H, Love M, et al. Relation between osmolality of diet and gastrointestinal side effects in enteral nutrition. Br Med J 1984;288:678–680.
64. Zimmaro DM, Rolandelli RH, Koruda MJ, et al. Isotonic tube feeding formula induces liquid stool in normal subjects: Reversed by pectin. J Parenter Enter Nutr 1989;13:117–123.
65. Jones TN, Moore FA, Moore EE, McCroskey BL. Gastrointestinal symptoms attributed to jejunostomy feeding after major abdominal trauma: A critical analysis. Crit Care Med 1989;17:1146–1150.
66. Cabre E, Gassull MA. Complications of enteral feeding. Nutrition 1993;9:1–9.
67. Gottschlick MM, Jenkins M, Warden GD, et al. Differential effects of three enteral dietary regimens on selected outcome variables in burn patients. J Parenter Enter Nutr 1990;14:225–236.
68. Beale RJ, Bryg DJ, Bihari DJ. Immunonutrition in the critically ill: A systematic review of clinical outcome. Crit Care Med 1999;27:2799–2805.
69. Heys SD, Walker LG, Smith I, Eremin O. Enteral nutritional supplementation with key nutrients in patients with critical illness and cancer: A meta-analysis of randomized controlled clinical trials. Ann Surg 1999;229(4):467–477.
70. Davis A, Baker S. The use of modular nutrients in pediatrics. J Parenter Enter Nutr 1996;20:228–236.
71. Atkinson SA. Human milk feeding of the micropremie. Clin Perinatol 2000;27:235–247.
72. Porcelli P, Schanler R, Greer F, et al. Growth in human milk-fed very low birth weight infants receiving a new human milk fortifier. Ann Nutr Metab 2000;44:2–10.
73. Sankaran K, Papageorgiou A, Ninan A, Sankaran R. A randomized, controlled evaluation of two commercially available human breast milk fortifiers in health preterm neonates. J Am Diet Assoc 1996;96:1145–1149.
74. Levy J, Laethen T, Verhaegen G, et al. Contaminated enteral nutrition solutions as a cause of nosocomial bloodstream infection: A study using plasmid fingerprinting. J Parenter Enter Nutr 1989;13:228–234.
75. Thurn J, Crossley K, Gerdts A, et al. Enteral hyperalimentation as a source of nosocomial infection. J Hosp Infect 1990;15:203–217.
76. VanEnk R, Furtado D. Bacterial contamination of enteral nutrient solutions: Intestinal colonization and sepsis in mice after ingestion. J Parenter Enter Nutr 1986;10:503–507.
77. Beyer PL. Complications of enteral nutrition. In: Matarese E, Gottschlich MM, eds. Contemporary Nutrition Support Practice: A Clinical Guide. Philadelphia, Saunders, 1998:216–226.
78. Cutie AJ, Altman E, Lenkel L. Compatability of enteral products with commonly employed drug additives. J Parenter Enter Nutr 1983;7:186–191.
79. Hardin TC, Reed M, eds. Nutrition and Drug Therapy: Clinical Pharmacology Drug Compatability and Stability-An Annotated Bibliography. Silver Spring, MD, ASPEN, 1992.
80. Dickerson RN, Melnik G. Osmolality of oral drug solutions and suspensions. Am J Hosp Pharm 1988;45:832–834.
81. Kumpf VJ, Barber JR. Enteral nutrition. US Pharm 1987;June:H-1, 2, 5, 8–10, 15.
82. Bradley J. Principles of enteral nutrition. Hosp Pharm 1994;23:197–204.
83. Strom JG, Miller SW. Stability of drugs with enteral nutrient formulas. DICP 1990;24:130–134.
84. Gora ML, Tschampel MM, Visconti JA. Considerations of drug therapy in patients receiving enteral nutrition. Nutr Clin Pract 1989;4:105–110.
85. Thompson CA, Rollins CJ. Nutrient-drug interactions. In: Rombeau JL, Rolandelli RH, eds. Clinical Nutrition: Enteral and Tube Feeding, 3d ed. Philadelphia, Saunders, 1997:523–529.
86. Rollins CJ. General pharmacologic issues. In: Matarese E, Gottschlich MM, eds. Contemporary Nutrition Support Practice: A Clinical Guide. Philadelphia, Saunders, 1998:303–323.
87. Mitchell JF. Oral dosage forms that should not be crushed: 1996 revision. Hosp Pharm 1996;31:27–37.
88. Bauer LA. Interference of oral phenytoin absorption by continuous nasogastric feedings. Neurology 1982;32:570–572.
89. Melnick G. Pharmacologic aspects of enteral nutrition. In: Rombeau JL, Caldwell MD, eds. Clinical Nutrition: Enteral and Tube Feeding, 2d ed. Philadelphia, Saunders, 1990:472–509.
90. Nishimura LY, Armstrong RP, Plezia PM, Iacono RP. Influence of enteral feedings on phenytoin sodium absorption from capsules. Drug Intell Clin Pharm 1988;22:130–133.
91. Guidry JR, Eastwood TF, Curry SC. Phenytoin absorption in volunteers receiving selected enteral feeds. West J Med 1989;150:659–661.
92. Drug Facts and Comparisons. St. Louis, MO, Wolters Kluwer, 2001.
93. Gora ML, Tschampel MM, Visconti JA. Considerations of drug therapy in patients receiving enteral nutrition. Nutr Clin Pract 1989;4:105–110.
94. Valli C, Schulthess HK, Asper R, et al. Interaction of nutrients with antacids: A complication during enteral tube feeding. Lancet 1986;1 (8483):747–748.
95. Eisenberg PG. Causes of diarrhea in tube-fed patients: A comprehensive approach to diagnosis and management. Nutr Clin Pract 1993;8:119–123.
96. Mirtallo JM, Fabri PJ. Concurrent therapy for complications of enteral nutrition support. Hosp Formul 1982;17:545–549.
97. Shankardass K, Chuchmach S, Chelswick K, et al. Bowel function of long-term tube-fed patients consuming formulae with and without dietary fiber. J Parenter Enter Nutr 1990;14:508–512.
98. Bayzyk S. Factors associated with transition to oral feedings in infants fed by nasogastric tubes. Am J Occup Ther 1990;44:1070–1078.
99. McClave SA, Snider HL, Lowen CC, et al. Use of residual volume as a marker for enteral feeding intolerance: Prospective blinded comparison with physical examination and radiographic findings. J Parenter Enter Nutr 1992;16:99–105.
100. Davis AM. Pediatrics. In: Matarese LE, Gottschlich MM, eds. Contemporary Nutrition Support Practice: A Clinical Guide. Philadelphia: Saunders, 1998:347–364.
101. Hebuterne X, Broussard JF, Rampal P. Acute renutrition by cyclic enteral nutrition in elderly and younger patients. JAMA 1995;273:638–643.
102. Newmark SR, Simpson MS, Beskitt MP, et al. Home tube feeding for long-term nutritional support. J Parenter Enter Nutr 1981;5:76–79.
103. Matthew M, Bowman L, Williams R, et al. Complications and effectiveness of gastrostomy feedings in pediatric cancer patients. J Pediatr Hematol Oncol 1996;18:81–85.
104. Greenberg GR, Fleming CR, Jeejeebhoy KN, et al. Controlled trial of bowel rest and nutritional support in the management of Crohn's disease. Gut 1988;29:1309–1315.
105. Fleming CR. Nutrition in patients with Crohn's disease: Another piece of the puzzle. J Parenter Enter Nutr 1995;19:93.

106. Cerra FB, McPherson JP, Konstantinides FN, et al. Enteral nutrition does not prevent multiple organ failure syndrome (MOFS) after sepsis. Surgery 1988;104:727–733.
107. Moore FA, Moore EE, Jones TN, et al. TEN versus TPN following major abdominal trauma: Reduced septic morbidity. J Trauma 1989;29:916–923.
108. Hamaoui E, Lefkowitz R, Olender L, et al. Enteral nutrition in the early postoperative period: A new semielemental formula versus total parenteral nutrition. J Parenter Enter Nutr 1990;14:501–507.
109. McClave SA, Greene LM, Snider HL, et al. Comparison of the safety of early enteral vs parenteral nutrition in mild acute pancreatitis. J Parenter Enter Nutr 1996;21:14–20.

139

Nutritional Considerations in Major Organ Failure

Renee M. DeHart and Mary A. Worthington

Because organ failure may alter absorption, use, and excretion of nutrients, administration of standard nutrients to patients with organ dysfunction may be inappropriate. Individualization of a nutritional regimen for these patients often requires a planned, disease-specific approach. Different laboratory tests or more frequent monitoring of traditional markers may be necessary to ensure that the desired therapeutic goals are achieved. For example, it is impossible to collect a 24-hour urine specimen to measure urea nitrogen and nitrogen balance in an anuric patient. In this situation, an alternative method of calculating urea nitrogen appearance is required.

Patients with acute organ failure requiring nutrition support often are hospitalized in intensive care units (ICUs). With advances in treating chronic organ failure, increasing numbers of older, chronically ill patients will require nutritional support on a long-term basis. It therefore will become increasingly common for nutrition support to be provided in community and ambulatory settings. Regardless of the setting, the clinician needs a firm pathophysiologic foundation on which to build a pharmaceutical care plan to ensure appropriate outcomes for patients requiring nutritional support.

This chapter discusses the nutritional needs of patients with acute and chronic renal, hepatic, pulmonary, and gastrointestinal failure. The predominant approaches to ensure delivery of safe and efficacious nutrients to patients with these disorders are critically reviewed.

RENAL FAILURE

Patients with end-stage renal disease (ESRD) and concurrent malnutrition have an increased risk of morbidity and mortality.[1,2] The adequacy of dialysis and the serum albumin concentration are strong predictors of mortality in hemodialysis (HD) and peritoneal dialysis (PD) patients.[1–4] Energy expenditure in these patients appears to be similar to that in normal subjects.[5] Unfortunately, intake of nutrients often is decreased markedly (66% and 50% of recommended protein and energy intake).[6] The provision of appropriate nutrition is especially challenging in patients with oliguric or anuric renal failure due to the fluid intake limitations. Major differences exist between the metabolic, fluid, and electrolyte management of patients with acute versus chronic renal failure. For example, positive nitrogen balance is more difficult to achieve in patients with acute renal failure due to the increased rate of protein catabolism. Additionally, patients with acute renal failure are more likely to develop hyperglycemia during nutritional support and frequently are dialyzed by modalities that are not used commonly for the ESRD patient. Because of these differences, the nutritional management of patients with acute renal failure is discussed separately.[7,8]

ACUTE RENAL FAILURE

EPIDEMIOLOGY

Acute renal failure (ARF) occurs in approximately 5% of all hospitalized patients. The mortality rate of ARF patients who require renal replacement therapy ranges from 40% to as high as 80%.[9] Severe malnutrition has been found in 42% of patients with ARF and is an independent predictor of in-hospital mortality and increased morbidity from sepsis, shock, dysrhythmias, and acute respiratory failure.[10] The two main advances made in the treatment of ARF patients during the last 20 years are the introduction of continuous renal replacement therapy (CRRT) (see Chapter 43) and advances in the provision of nutritional support.[11]

PATHOPHYSIOLOGY

Energy Requirements

Patients with ARF typically require 30 to 35 kcal/kg per day.[11] Energy requirements in this patient population ideally should be measured by indirect calorimetry[12] (see Chapter 135). Energy expenditures of ARF patients are highly variable. In one study of mechanically ventilated ARF patients, measured energy expenditure ranged from 70% to 170% of predicted resting energy expenditure.[13]

Carbohydrate

Hyperglycemia and peripheral insulin resistance are common in ARF. These patients usually have a superimposed illness that may cause glucose intolerance. The etiology of glucose intolerance in ARF is thought to be due to increased levels of glucagon, growth hormone, and catecholamines, all known antagonists of insulin.[14] Other proposed mechanisms include an elevated glucagon-to-insulin ratio secondary to impaired degradation of these hormones and elevated secretion of inflammatory cytokines.

Fat

Intolerance to intravenous lipid emulsion (IVLE), evidenced by increased serum triglyceride concentrations, is common in ARF. Hypertriglyceridemia is thought to be caused by decreased catabolism of triglycerides and increased synthesis from free fatty acids (FFAs).[15] Hepatic triglyceride lipase and peripheral lipoprotein lipase activity may be reduced significantly in ARF patients.[16] Insulin resistance and metabolic acidosis may contribute to this process by inhibiting lipoprotein lipase.[17] Triglyceride concentrations therefore should be measured before administering IVLE to patients with ARF. FFA concentrations also are elevated in ARF. This aberration, however, is not appreciated by measurement of the triglyceride concentration.

Protein

Urea, the end product of nitrogen metabolism, accumulates rapidly in ARF. Most patients with ARF have a primary stressful illness that results in ureagenesis, and thus protein breakdown is accelerated markedly.[7,9] Protein catabolic rates (PCRs) of 1.4 to 1.8 g/kg per day are reported frequently.[18,19] Protein catabolism in ARF may be stimulated by insulin resistance, metabolic acidosis, circulating proteases, inflammatory mediators, and direct uremic toxin effects.[20] This stimulation may affect protein metabolism both directly (via modulation of protein synthesis) and indirectly (by inhibiting the action of anabolic hormones).[21] In addition to this increased catabolism of proteins, significant amounts of protein and amino acids are removed by dialysis. Amino acid losses of 5.2 g per conventional HD, 7.3 g per high-flux HD, and up to 13–16 g/d in children during continuous arteriovenous hemodialysis (CAVHD) or continuous venovenous hemofiltration (CVVH) have been reported.[22,23] The clearance of some amino acids are enhanced (histidine and tryptophan), whereas the clearance of phenylalanine and valine were reduced in nondialyzed patients with ARF.[24] In patients undergoing continuous venovenous hemodiafiltration (CVVHDF), glutamine represents 33% of all amino acid dialysate losses. Serum glutamine concentrations decrease significantly early during CVVHDF but return to baseline subsequently despite continued CVVHDF, suggesting altered glutamine metabolism early in the course of CVVHDF therapy.[25]

Fluid, Electrolyte, and Acid-Base Disorders

The volume status of patients with ARF depends primarily on residual urine output and the type of dialysis received, if any. The patient with oliguric ARF will have impaired excretion of sodium and water. In nonoliguric ARF, considerable sodium may be lost in the urine, necessitating replacement to maintain sodium balance. This also applies to the patient who is losing considerable gastric fluids. Patients on CRRT will lose sodium via hemofiltration or dialysis and should be given sodium as part of their CRRT replacement fluid regimen.

Hyperkalemia is observed frequently in ARF secondary to protein catabolism and intracellular potassium release. Hyperkalemia also results from the impaired secretion and excretion of potassium by the kidney and the endogenous release secondary to tissue breakdown. If this is severe, emergent dialysis may be indicated. Patients on CRRT, however, usually will require potassium replacement to avoid hypokalemia due to dialytic potassium losses.

Because phosphorus is excreted renally, hyperphosphatemia is common in ARF. Like potassium, large amounts of phosphorus are released into the circulation secondary to tissue breakdown during ARF. Control of hyperphosphatemia is important because as the calcium-phosphorus product (serum calcium in mg/dL multiplied by serum phosphorus in mg/dL) exceeds 55–70, the risk of developing metastatic calcification increases (see Chapter 51).[26] Conversely, with initiation of dialysis, particularly CRRT, patients must be monitored for dialysis-induced hypophosphatemia.

The net removal of calcium during the continuous dialysis modalities depends on the calcium concentration of the dialysate fluid.[27] Severe hypocalcemia has been reported when regional citrate anticoagulation has been used in a patient with ARF and hepatic failure who was treated with continuous venovenous hemodialysis (CVVHD).[28]

Hypermagnesemia is common in ARF secondary to impaired excretion and endogenous release from tissue breakdown. Serum magnesium concentrations do not decrease as quickly as potassium concentrations in patients receiving electrolyte-free nutrition regimens.

Patients with ARF usually have metabolic acidosis because of impaired excretion of organic acids. If potassium and sodium are needed in the parenteral nutrition (PN) regimen, they should be added as acetate salts, which will be converted to bicarbonate in the liver. This increase in bicarbonate will partially compensate their metabolic acidosis. Intermittent and continuous dialytic therapies also may help improve the metabolic acidosis accompanying ARF by increasing the removal of these endogenously generated acids as well as by increasing serum bicarbonate levels as the result of diffusion from the dialysate into the blood. Correction of acidosis was greatest when lactate buffers (lactate $>$ bicarbonate $\gg$ acetate) were used in one study employing CVVH.[29]

Trace Elements

The requirements for trace elements during nutritional support of ARF patients are not well established because trace element accumulation or losses during ARF have not been characterized rigorously. Zinc and chromium are excreted by the kidney and theoretically can accumulate due to reduced excretion and increased intake secondary to impurities in dialysate or intravenous fluids. This has been documented with chromium in patients on chronic dialysis.[30] Selenium concentrations are reduced in patients with ARF and may influence thyroid function, decreasing thyroxine concentrations.[31,32] Trace elements such as rubidium can be removed by dialysis if concentrations in the dialysate are adequately low; the clinical significance of this is unknown.[33] Because manganese and copper are excreted in bile and zinc and copper are removed by PD and HD,[34] most patients with ARF receiving PN should receive trace element supplementation.

Vitamins

Little information is available concerning alternations in vitamin requirements in ARF. Reduced plasma concentrations of vitamin A, ascorbate, vitamin D, and vitamin E have been reported in patients with ARF, whereas vitamin K concentrations are relatively increased.[35] Losses of vitamins via dialysis also must be considered. Traditional HD clears several water-soluble vitamins such as folic acid, vitamins C and B_{12}, and pyridoxine but not the highly protein-bound vitamins A and D.[34,36] The clinical significance of these findings in ARF is unknown. Currently, it seems prudent to administer vitamins at least in doses recommended by the Nutrition Advisory Group of the American Medical Association (NAG-AMA) for patients receiving PN (see Chapter 137) until additional information on specific dosage requirements is available. If the enteral route is used for nutritional support, vitamin adminstration should at least meet the recommended daily allowances (RDAs).

▶ TREATMENT: Acute Renal Failure

ADMINISTRATION ROUTES

Most patients with ARF have a superimposed illness that requires nutritional support by the parenteral route. Enteral nutrition (EN) should be considered when patients with ARF have functional gastrointestinal tracts. The products used frequently during EN in ARF are the calorically dense, electrolyte-free or electrolyte-reduced formulas (Table 139–1). These formulas are useful in patients with fluid overload, hyperkalemia, and hyperphosphatemia. Unfortunately, EN is impossible for many patients with ARF because they are critically ill and have an ileus.

TABLE 139–1. Enteral Nutrition Products for Patients with Renal Failure

Product	Flavors[a]	Caloric Density (kcal/mL)	Protein (g/L)	Potassium (mg/1000 kcal)	Phosphorus (mg/1000 kg)
Deliver 2.0 (Mead Johnson)	V	2.0	75	850	500
Magnacal Renal (Mead Johnson)	V	2.0	70	635	400
Nepro (Ross)	V, C, BP	2.0	70	523	340
NuBasics 2.0 (Nestlé)	V	2.0	80	960	670
Nutren 2.0 (Nestle)	V	2.0	80	960	670
NutriRenal (Nestlé)	V	2.0	70	628	350
Renalcal Diet (Nestlé)	C, L, G	2.0	34.4	N/A	N/A
Re/Neph (Ross)	V, S	2.0	68	N/A	160
Re/Neph HP/HC (Ross)	Ch, V, S	2.0	68	40	96
Re/Neph LP/HC (Ross)	V, S	2.0	21	104	150
Suplena (Ross)	V	2.0	30	510	160
TwoCal HN (Ross)	V, BP	2.0	84	1228	526

[a]V = vanilla; S = strawberry; C = cherry; L = lemonade; G = grape; Ch = chocolate; BP = butter pecan; N/A = not available.

SPECIALTY PRODUCTS

Improved survival and return of renal function were observed in the 1970s when essential amino acids (EAAs) plus glucose were compared with glucose alone in patients with ARF.[37] This led to the marketing of parenteral amino acids containing predominantly or solely EAAs (NephrAmine, RenAmin, Aminosyn-RF, and Aminess). These products were formulated on the hypothesis that significant nitrogen reuse (urea recycling) occurs during ARF to synthesize nonessential amino acids. Subsequently, several prospective, double-blinded studies indicated no significant reduction in mortality when the EAA formulations were used.[37] Thus urea recycling in the presence of uremia has been disproven. Based on the available data, it appears appropriate to use standard mixed amino acids rather than EAA solutions in ARF. An example of an initial PN solution to be used in ARF appears in Table 139–2.

DESIGN AND INITIATION OF NUTRITIONAL REGIMEN

Patients with ARF typically require 30 to 35 kcal/kg per day. In the absence of dialysis, the nutritional formula should be concentrated in a small volume and contain minimal sodium. In the oliguric patient receiving PD or HD, these restrictions may be lessened, but the formula generally will need to be concentrated (final dextrose concentration of 30%). When using these high-dextrose-concentration formulas,

TABLE 139–2. Examples of Initial Parenteral Nutrition Formulas for Patients with Organ Failure

	Acute Renal Failure	Chronic Renal Failure	Hepatic Failure	Hepatic Transplant	Pulmonary Failure	Short Bowel
Dextrose (%)[a]	40	30	25	15	20	20
CAAs (%)	Variable	4	5[b]	5	5	5
Lipids (%)	1	2	2	2	3	2
0.45 NaCl (L/d)	—	—	—	—	—	0.5–2
NaCl (mEq/L)	0	0	0	0	0	80[c]
Na acetate (mEq/L)	0	30	0	0	0	0
Na phosphate (mEq/L)	0[d]	7.5	15	15	30	7.5
K acetate (mEq/L)	0[d]	0	50	0	20	60
K chloride (mEq/L)	0	10	0	40	20	0
Ca gluconate (mEq/L)	5	5	5	10	5	10
Magnesium sulfate (mEq/L)	0	6	16	20	5	10
Multivitamins (mL/d)	10	10	10	10	10	10
Zinc (mg/d)	3	3–6	8	3–6	3	10
Copper (mg/d)	1.2	1.2	<1.2	1.2	1.2	1.2
Manganese (μg/d)	300	300	<300	300	300	≤300
Chromium (μg/d)	12	12	<12	12	12	20
Selenium (μg/d)	—	40	40	40	40	60

[a]Final concentrations after admixture.
[b]Hepatamine 4% when criteria for use are met.
[c]Does not include 0.45% sodium chloride injection or lipid.
[d]The continuous renal replacement therapies frequently require variable additions of potassium and phosphate salts.

careful monitoring of glucose homeostasis (every 6 hours) is important because of the predisposition toward hyperglycemia in ARF. Additionally, CRRT, which is increasingly popular in the treatment of ARF (see Chapter 43), contributes significant calories to a nutritional regimen. This is a direct result of the absorption of glucose from the dextrose-containing fluids frequently used as the dialysate or ultrafiltrate replacement fluids during CRRT. During continuous arteriovenous hemofiltration (CAVH), a net uptake of up to 300 g/d was reported when a 1.5% peritoneal dialysis fluid or 5% dextrose in saline was used as the ultrafiltrate replacement fluid at a mean rate of 1.39 L/h.[38] Other studies of CAVHD with dextrose-containing dialysates and blood flow rates of 150 mL/min reported glucose absorption of up to 45% (up to 355 g/d).[39] Thus these calories must be factored into the nutritional plan for the patient with ARF treated with these modalities.

Lipid administration during ARF is driven by serum triglyceride concentration monitoring. When the serum triglyceride level is less than 300 mg/dL, low doses of IVLE (3–7 kcal/kg/d over 24 hours) are recommended to prevent essential fatty acid deficiency and to provide a balanced caloric intake. IVLEs containing a combination of medium-chain triglycerides (MCTs) and long-chain triglycerides (LCTs) are available in Europe. MCTs are used readily for energy, not stored, and are carnitine-independent, all attractive features for a fuel source. MCT and LCT clearance when given parenterally is reduced by more than 60% in ARF.[40] Therefore, both LCT- and MCT-containing IVLEs need to be used with caution in ARF.

The question arises as to how much protein a patient with ARF requires. Although individual patient assessment of PCR and dialytic losses is necessary, it is not uncommon for patients to require 1.5 to 2.5 g/kg per day of protein or more to approach nitrogen balance. Noncatabolic patients not receiving dialysis who have a low urea nitrogen appearance (UNA) rate (<5 g/d) may be managed temporarily with a nutrition regimen low in protein (20–30 g/d or 0.6 g/kg/d) to minimize UNA from exogenous protein.[9] Once dialysis therapy is instituted, protein intake should be liberalized: 1 to 1.2 g/kg per day for HD patients and 1.2 to 1.5 g/kg per day for PD patients. CRRT removes large quantities of extracellular fluid and thereby allows infusion of the required substrates in a normal volume. Patients with ARF treated with CRRT should be provided with up to 2.5 g/kg per day of protein (as indicated by UNA plus nonurinary urea losses) as their blood chemistries tolerate. Although this can be done safely while providing a greater percentage of patients with a positive nitrogen balance, a reduction in mortality has not been documented conclusively.[41]

Several electrolytes (i.e., phosphorus, magnesium, and potassium) warrant special attention when designing the initial nutritional regimen/formula for the ARF patient. During early ARF, PN solutions should not contain potassium unless the patient is hypokalemic or undergoing CRRT. After several days, the serum potassium concentrations tend to decrease, often necessitating cautious addition of potassium to the PN solution. If the enteral route is used, formulas with minimal potassium may be needed. Serum potassium concentrations may decrease more rapidly in patients receiving continuous dialysis therapies. Potassium losses in CVVHD and CAVHD are proportional to the potassium gradient between blood and dialysate. Therefore, cautious additions of potassium may be considered earlier in the course of ARF for those patients treated by CAVHD or CVVHD. Serum magnesium concentrations do not decrease as quickly as potassium concentrations in patients receiving electrolyte-free nutrition regimens. As serum concentrations decrease toward normal and/or renal function returns, magnesium should be added to the PN solution in small amounts (4–6 mEq/L). An empirical PN formula for the patient with ARF is highlighted in Table 139–2.

Phosphorus can be omitted from the nutritional formula of patients receiving PN until the phosphorus level approaches normal (<5.0 mg/dL). It is prudent to monitor phosphorus concentrations daily and to add phosphorus in small doses once the serum concentration is below 4.0 mg/dL. Failure to do so can lead to severe hypophosphatemia despite continued renal failure, especially in the patient treated with CRRT. Patients with persistently high serum phosphorus levels who have a functional gastrointestinal tract can be prescribed phosphate-binding therapy (see Chapter 45) and enteral feedings low in phosphorus to minimize the absorption of exogenous phosphorus.

EVALUATION OF THERAPEUTIC OUTCOMES

ARF, despite recent advances in treatment, is still associated with a mortality rate of 39% to 69%.[10,41] The evaluation tools used in monitoring ARF patients are similar to other patients receiving PN and EN (see Chapters 137 and 138). However, there is no clear consensus on the benefit of nutritional supplementation on the outcome parameters of renal recovery or mortality. Some advocate protein malnutrition as a predictor of outcome in patients with multiple-organ dysfunction syndrome,[11] whereas others have not shown a survival benefit from aggressive nutritional support.[41] Recent data suggest that malnourished ARF patients experience a statistically significant higher mortality rate (odds ratio of in-hospital mortality of 7.21) compared with ARF patients without malnutrition.[10] While promising, these results need confirmation before it can be concluded that nutritional intervention significantly impacts patient survival in ARF.

CHRONIC RENAL FAILURE

Chronic renal insufficiency, as evidenced by the inability of the kidneys to excrete nitrogenous and other waste products, usually develops over months to years (see Chapter 44). Malnutrition secondary to reduced oral nutrient intake frequently is evident when the glomerular filtration rate (GFR) drops below 20 to 25 mL/min. Patients with chronic renal failure (CRF) are considered to have ESRD when the GFR falls below 10 mL/min or 15 mL/min in the patient with diabetic nephropathy (see Chapter 45). Malnutrition is also a common occurrence in ESRD not only because of decreased oral intake but also due to increased nutrient losses via the various renal replacement therapies. Because of its chronicity, malnutrition in these patients is treated most frequently in the ambulatory setting with EN.

EPIDEMIOLOGY

Protein-energy malnutrition is very common in the ESRD patient population. Significant malnutrition occurs in 20% to 36% of ESRD patients undergoing HD and 45% of patient commencing continuous ambulatory peritoneal dialysis (CAPD) or cycling peritoneal dialysis (CPD).[42,43] There appears to be a gender difference in nutritional status in patients with ESRD. In one study, women had a higher prevalence of malnutrition on initiation of CAPD.[43] Females also have poorer nutritional outcomes but appear to have a lower mortality rate.[44] Protein-energy malnutrition is a significant predictor of morbidity and mortality in most studies of patients with ESRD. In one study lasting 7 years, patients with a serum albumin concentration of less than 3.5 g/dL had a twofold increase in mortality risk relative to patients whose serum albumin concentration was greater than or equal to 4.0 g/dL.[45] In another study that compared long-term (10–15 years) and very long-term (15–30 years) with average (<5 years) ESRD survivors, expected survival was significantly greater in patients with baseline serum albumin concentrations greater than 3.5 g/dL. Serum albumin concentrations additionally increased in the long- and very long-term survivors during the study. Conversely, serum albumin concentrations decreased among patients who survived less than 5 years.[46]

Poor dietary intake of energy and protein contributes significantly to the prevalence of malnutrition in these patients. In one group of patients with CRF, mean caloric intake was 11 kcal/kg per day, and mean protein intake was 0.42 g/kg per day. Less than one-quarter of patients in this study met 75% or greater of their energy and protein needs.[47] In another study of nonexercising patients undergoing HD, mean protein intake was 58 g/d, again significantly lower than published recommendations for the majority of these patients.[48] Thus nutrition support appears to be a critical intervention in the care of the patient with ESRD.

PATHOPHYSIOLOGY

Carbohydrate

In general, ESRD patients are not as stressed as patients with ARF; however, more than one-half of ESRD patients have insulin resistance and hyperglycemia. This has been attributed to the increased glucagon-to-insulin ratio, resulting in protein breakdown and gluconeogenesis. In patients with normal peritoneal transport on CAPD, roughly 60% of glucose in the dialysate is absorbed. One method of estimating the quantity of glucose absorbed is: glucose absorbed (g/d) = $0.89x$ (g/d) − 43, where x is the total amount of dialysate glucose instilled daily.[49] This dialysate glucose absorption can worsen existing hyperglycemia and contribute significantly to the patient's energy intake. Therefore, kwashiorkor-type malnutrition is common. Although glucose control is not problematic unless the patient is diabetic, infected, or subjected to operative stress, insulin can be added to CAPD bags to control hyperglycemia (see Chapter 47).

Fat

Hypertriglyceridemia is common in ESRD patients.[50] This is mainly due to decreased catabolism of triglycerides secondary to decreased hepatic lipoprotein lipase activity.[15] Most ESRD patients receiving HD also receive heparin, which activates lipoprotein lipase and converts triglycerides to FFAs and glycerol. Carnitine, an amino acid necessary for the transport of long-chain fatty acids across mitochondria where oxidation results in energy production, is removed by HD and CAPD, and therefore, serum carnitine concentrations typically are reduced in ESRD.[51] The effect of carnitine supplementation on plasma lipid profiles is controversial. Recent guidelines do not advocate carnitine adminstration for the treatment of hypertriglyceridemia. Studies of carnitine for this indication have varied widely in duration (1 week to 15 months) and have used both oral and intravenous administration in varying doses (1 mg/kg to 2 g/d intravenously, 10 mg/kg/d to 3 g/d orally). Of 32 studies reviewed recently, 23 failed to find a change in triglyceride concentrations, whereas one actually demonstrated a 22% increase.[49] Patients receiving long-term dialysis treatment also have been shown to accumlate remnants of triglyceride-rich lipoproteins. This lipoprotein abnormality can result in type III hyperlipidemia with increased intermediate-density lipoprotein.

Leptin, which is produced and secreted by fat cells, appears to function as a lipostat mechanism via regulation of satiety (see Chapter 140). Leptin concentrations often are elevated in ESRD patients, particularly those undergoing CAPD.[52] Hyperleptinemia in ESRD patients may correlate positively with body fat mass[53] and negatively with lean body mass.[52] Further study is required to define the role of leptin on the body composition of patients with ESRD.

Protein

Secondary analysis of the Modifications of Diet in Renal Disease Study indicates that in nondiabetics, reduction of dietary protein intake may slow the rate of renal disease progression and ultimately delay the onset of dialysis[54] (see Chapter 44). Meta-analyses of diabetic as well as nondiabetic patients suggest that dietary protein restriction (range 0.5–0.85 g/kg/d) is weakly associated with slowing of the progression of renal disease.[55] The recent National Kidney Foundation Kidney Disease Outcomes Quality Initiative (K/DOQI) guidelines for nutrition in patients with chronic renal insufficiency recommend a diet providing 0.6 g/kg of protein per day for those with a GRF of less than 25 mL/min.[49] Although the safety of low-protein diets has been questioned, the recent analysis of Aparicis and colleagues strongly suggests that for carefully selected and monitored patients, protein intakes of as low as 0.3 g/kg per day supplemented with EAAs can be used safely.[56] Although it has been suggested that vegetable-based low-protein diets may further slow progession of renal failure beyond that of animal-based low-protein diets, not all studies have found this to be true.[57] Dietary protein intake can be estimated by calculating the protein equivalent of nitrogen appearance (PNA)[49] (Table 139–3).

ESRD patients receiving CAPD require special attention due to protein losses across the peritoneal membrane. Peritoneal protein losses average over 6 g/d in patients treated by CAPD.[58] PD protein losses, however, do not predict risk for malnutrition (as measured by serum albumin concentration) in all patients.[59] Nonetheless, these losses should be taken into consideration when designing the PN or EN formula for the CAPD patient. Recent guidelines suggest that dietary protein intake of at least 1.2 g/kg per day (at least 50% of high biologic value) is needed to consistently achieve neutral or positive nitrogen balance in nonacutely ill CAPD patients.[49]

Dialysate protein losses also must be examined for the ESRD patient undergoing HD. The amount of protein lost via HD depends on the dialysis membrane used and whether the membrane is being reused. Low-flux polymethylmethacrylate membranes on first use are associated with a loss of 6.1 g of amino acid per treatment. High-flux polysulfone membranes on first use are associated with an 8.0-g amino acid loss. Amino acid losses also increased by 50% after reuse of the

TABLE 139–3. Routine Nutritional Monitoring in Patients with ESRD[49]

Parameter	Frequency
Predialysis serum albumin	Monthly
Percent of usual postdialysis or postdrain body weight	Monthly
Subjective global assessment	Every 6 months
Protein equivalent of total nitrogen appearance (PNA)[a]	Monthly for HD, every 3–4 months for CAPD
Dietary interview and/or diary	Every 6 months
Predialysis prealbumin	As needed
Anthropometry	As needed
Dual energy x-ray absorptiometry	As needed

[a]Beginning of week PNA = Co/[36.3 + (5.48) (spKt/V) + (53.5/spKt/V)] = 0.168, where Co is predialysis BUN and spKt/V = Ln(R − 0.08 × t) + [4 − (3.5 × R)] × UF/W (R is postdialysis/predialysis BUN ratio, t is dialysis session in hours, UF is ultrafiltration in liters, W is postdialysis weight in kg).

high-flux polysulfone membrane.[60] As in the case with CAPD, these losses should be considered when designing the protein regimen of the ESRD patient treated with HD. Dietary protein intake of at least 1.2 g/kg per day (at least 50% of high biologic value) is recommended to attain neutral or positive nitrogen balance in clinically stable HD patients.[49]

Fluid and Electrolytes

Hyponatremia, often due to overhydration, is common in CRF but usually does not require additional administration of sodium. Regular dialysis is the principal means for control of body water and serum sodium concentration in the ESRD patient.

Patients with CRF or ESRD who develop hyperkalemia generally have ingested excessive potassium relative to the potassium-removing capacity of the failing kidney (and dialysis, in the case of ESRD). The undernourished CRF or ESRD patient receiving PN, however, may require considerable potassium as new body cell mass is synthesized. When inappropriately low amounts of potassium are given during refeeding, hypokalemia may develop.

Patients with CRF or ESRD often are treated for hyperphosphatemia with phosphorus-restricted diets and calcium-containing antacids as phosphate binders (see Chapters 44 and 45). When these patients receive aggressive nutritional support, the combination of refeeding (cellular uptake of phosphorus for synthesis of body cell mass) and vigorous phosphate-binding therapy can result in hypophosphatemia.

Clinically significant hypermagnesemia is less common in patients with CRF and ESRD compared with ARF. It is usually added to the PN solution in reduced doses (4 meq/L or less), and serum concentrations need to be monitored.

Metabolic acidosis, a common complication of ESRD, is associated with increased protein degradation and decreased synthesis of albumin.[49] Correction of acidosis in ESRD patients may be associated with increases in serum albumin, body weight, and midarm muscle circumference and fewer hospitalizations.[61,62] Appropriate stabilization of serum bicarbonate concentrations (>22 meq/L) via alteration of the dialysate bicarbonate levels or administration of oral bicarbonate salts thus seems a prudent nutritional intervention in these patients (see Chapter 45).

Trace Elements

There are considerable data regarding trace element requirements in patients with ESRD.[34] Decreased zinc concentrations in dialysis patients have been linked to taste disturbances and sexual dysfunction.[30] Zinc supplementation, however, has not universally reversed these anomalies. Although serum concentrations of this trace element are decreased, total body stores of zinc in ESRD often are increased.[30] This suggests a redistribution of zinc or increased need to maintain normal enzymatic function in ESRD.

Chromium serum concentrations are elevated in chronic HD and CAPD patients,[30] perhaps due to the fact that needles used during HD and the peritoneal and hemodialysates are sources of chromium. The clinical significance of these findings is unknown. Manganese serum concentrations are normal in the HD patient and patients undergoing PD.[63] Copper concentrations in erythrocytes have been reported to be decreased in HD and CAPD patients, but copper concentrations were unchanged in plasma and whole blood.[63] Both HD and CAPD patients have been found to have decreased selenium concentrations[64] that can be increased with oral selenium supplements of 135–140 μg/day in HD patients.[65] It appears that for patients undergoing HD, significant selenium losses occur through the pores of certain polysulfone dialysis membranes.[66]

The trace element with the most established significance in ESRD is aluminum. This toxicity is linked to aluminum in the dialysate or excessive use of aluminum-containing medications. Consequently, significant quantities of aluminum have been removed from currently available dialysis solutions, and calcium antacids have virtually replaced aluminum as phosphate binders. Aluminum toxicity can be treated with deferoxamine, as discussed in Chapter 45.

Vitamins

Vitamin status is better defined in patients with ESRD than in patients with ARF. CRF patients are prone to develop water-soluble vitamin deficiencies because of decreased dietary intake secondary to anorexia and restriction of certain foods because of their protein, potassium, or phosphorus content. Additionally, in the ESRD patient, HD losses of ascorbic acid, folic acid, and pyridoxine are common. Plasma ascorbic acid concentrations have been found to be normal in CAPD patients[67] but significantly reduced in HD patients unless given oral supplements of 200 mg/d in one study.[68] The highly protein-bound vitamins (A, D, and B_{12}) are not removed significantly by HD.[34] Vitamin D deficiency is correlated with decreased serum albumin concentrations, and supplementation of vitamin D has increased serum albumin concentrations significantly in deficient patients.[69] Vitamin A concentrations often are elevated in CRF and ESRD and can lead to hypervitaminosis A and its cirrhotic-like syndrome. Conversely, vitamin E supplementation may have a distinct benefit to patients with ESRD. Increased oxidative stress in ESRD may contribute to the accelerated atherosclerosis in these patients. Vitamin E in doses of 800 IU/d has been shown to decrease low-density lipoprotein oxidation in patients with ESRD, especially in patients undergoing CAPD.[70]

ESRD patients on HD have lower biotin intake and excretion than normal subjects, but plasma concentrations of biotin in HD patients are higher than in normal subjects, negating a need for biotin supplementation.[71] Thiamine concentrations decrease during dialysis; supplementation within the RDA recommendations are sufficient to keep concentrations in the normal range.[72] Elevated concentrations of homocysteine are associated with increased risk of cardiovascular disease. Hyperhomocysteinemia is common in patients with ESRD. Folate doses from 2.5 mg three times weekly to 60 mg/d have lowered homocysteine concentrations in ESRD patients but have not completely reduced concentrations to normal.[73,74]

▶ TREATMENT: Chronic Renal Failure

ADMINISTRATION ROUTES

CRF and ESRD patients who require nutritional support rarely need PN because their gastrointestinal tract usually is functional. The calorically dense low-electrolyte enteral formulas in Table 139–1 are particularly useful. Even though ESRD patients receive regular dialysis, many are anuric between dialysis sessions, so excess fluid intake is a potential problem. Nepro, Magnacal Renal, and Re/Neph are marketed specifically (due to their high caloric density and low electrolyte content) for the ESRD patient who receives regular dialysis. Suplena, Renalcal Diet, and Re/Neph LP/HC, which are lower in protein and some electrolytes than Nepro and others, can be used in CRF patients not yet undergoing HD or CAPD. If there is superimposed illness that precludes EN, standard mixed amino acids should be used as the protein component of the PN solution.

The association of poor nutritional status and increased morbidity and mortality in ESRD has led to the development of alternative nutritional delivery systems for the ESRD patient. One such approach is intradialytic parenteral nutrition (IDPN), or the provision of glucose–amino acid–lipid admixture during HD. IDPN typically allows for the infusion of 600–700 kcal per session. An evidence-based evaluation of 24 studies employing IDPN found that the use of IDPN was associated with decreased mortality, but only 3 of the 24 studies were randomized in nature.[75] Because of the weaknesses of the data, IDPN should be reserved for malnourished patients who have failed enteral feedings and other interventions. Charzot and colleagues[76] demonstrated that the addition of amino acid to the hemodialysate may prevent amino acid losses and, if provided in sufficient quantities, actually may be a means for nutritional supplementation. The future of this avenue of therapy remains to be determined.

Amino acid dialysate (AAD) is the IDPN counterpart for the CAPD patient. This technique entails using a 1.1% amino acid solution in place of one or two of the dextrose-containing PD exchanges per day. Improvements in serum transferrin and total protein concentrations have been observed; however, no beneficial effect has been noted on patient morbidity or mortality.[77] Adverse effects of this therapy have included exacerbations of uremic symptoms [due to increases in blood urea nitrogen (BUN)] and metabolic acidosis. Not all studies have demonstrated benefits from this intervention.[78] In summary, AAD may be useful in the treatment of malnourished CAPD patients, but better designed studies are needed.

Recombinant human growth hormone (rhGH) in doses of 0.2 IU/kg per day subcutaneously has been used experimentally in adults with ESRD to enhance anabolism.[79] Patients randomized to rhGH in one study demonstrated weight gains of 1.2 kg and increased transferrin concentrations after 4 weeks of therapy.[79] rhGH may play a future role in the treatment of ESRD patients who still have inadequate oral intake despite appropriate dietary counseling and oral supplements. Additional study is needed before this can be advocated in general practice.

DESIGN AND INITIATION OF NUTRITIONAL REGIMEN

Current recommendations that factor in concurrent illnesses and the likelihood of preexisting malnutrition advocate 35 kcal/kg per day and 1.2 g/kg per day of protein for chronic HD patients and 1.2–1.3 g/kg per day of protein for CAPD patients.[49] This is higher that the spontaneous dietary intake in most dialysis patients.[49] Therefore, dietary counseling of the chronic dialysis patient is important in the ambulatory setting.

Several electrolytes warrant special attention when providing PN or EN to a patient with CRF or ESRD. Generally, sodium should be administered to CRF patients during nutritional support only to replace losses in order to avoid overhydration. Although these patients also are predisposed to hyperkalemia, once anabolism is attained in CRF patients, potassium requirements may be as high as 40–80 mEq/d. This dose needs to be given carefully and requires serum potassium concentration monitoring. Clinically significant hypermagnesemia is less common in patients with CRF compared with ARF. It is usually added to the PN solution in reduced doses (4 meq/L).

Patients with CRF or ESRD often are treated for hyperphosphatemia. With agressive nutritional support, the combination of refeeding and phosphate-binding therapy can result in hypophosphatemia. Decreasing or temporarily discontinuing the phosphate-binding therapy is appropriate if this occurs. Thereafter, conservative amounts of phosphorus may need to be administered.

Some practitioners advocate withholding trace elements from CRF and ESRD patients receiving PN. There are no published guidelines specific for the use of trace elements in these patients. Because serum concentrations of certain trace elements are normal in ESRD patients (manganese) and others actually may be decreased (zinc and selenium), the standard dietary intake of these trace elements should be recommended, and standard trace element supplements should be added to PN regimens.[34] Additional zinc and selenium supplementation may be considered in documented cases of deficiency.

During PN in CRF or ESRD patients, elimination or reduction of the dose of vitamin A is recommended. Dialytic losses of ascorbic acid, folic acid, and pyridoxine are common. Thus ESRD patients should receive ascorbic acid 50–100 mg/d, pyridoxine 5–10 mg/d, and at least 1 mg/d folic acid in addition to the other essential vitamins.[34] An example of a PN solution for use in ESRD patients is presented in Table 139–2.

EVALUATION OF THERAPEUTIC OUTCOMES

The short- and long-term monitoring plan for the ESRD patient receiving PN or EN needs to be carefully tailored. Special attention should be paid to maintenance of fluid and electrolyte homeostasis. This can be achieved via frequent (daily) monitoring of serum electrolyte concentrations (e.g., sodium, potassium, phosphorus, magnesium, and calcium) and fluid balance. Serum glucose concentrations should be followed frequently (four times daily) in the ESRD patient who develops persistent hyperglycemia. UNA can be monitored to estimate nitrogen balance, with which protein provision can be adjusted to maintain a positive nitrogen balance.

Because protein-energy malnutrition is a significant predictor of morbidity and mortality in ESRD patients, monitoring to ensure the effectiveness of the long-term nutritional plan becomes critical. Albumin is perhaps the most studied marker of nutritional efficacy in this patient population. Increased serum albumin concentrations are correlated with increased survival. Thus monitoring of serum albumin concentrations should be considered a critical component of the monitoring plan to ensure patient longevity. Appropriate routine monitoring parameters to employ are listed in Table 139–3.[49] An algorithmic approach to improve nutritional status and ensure optimal outcomes is presented in Figure 139–1.[8]

HEPATIC FAILURE

The liver is the primary organ involved in the digestion, metabolism, and storage of nutrients. When functional capacity is depressed, profound nutrient intolerance (hyper- or hypoglycemia, hypertriglyceridemia, and hepatic encephalopathy) may result. Other sequelae that accompany the failing liver are fluid and electrolyte imbalances, vitamin deficiencies, and malnutrition. Nutritional supplementation provided to patients with alcoholic cirrhosis has reduced the frequency of hospitalizations.[80] Information is also available suggesting a survival benefit of nutritional supplementation in liver failure. In a study of oxandrolone and an enteral formula rich in branched-chain amino

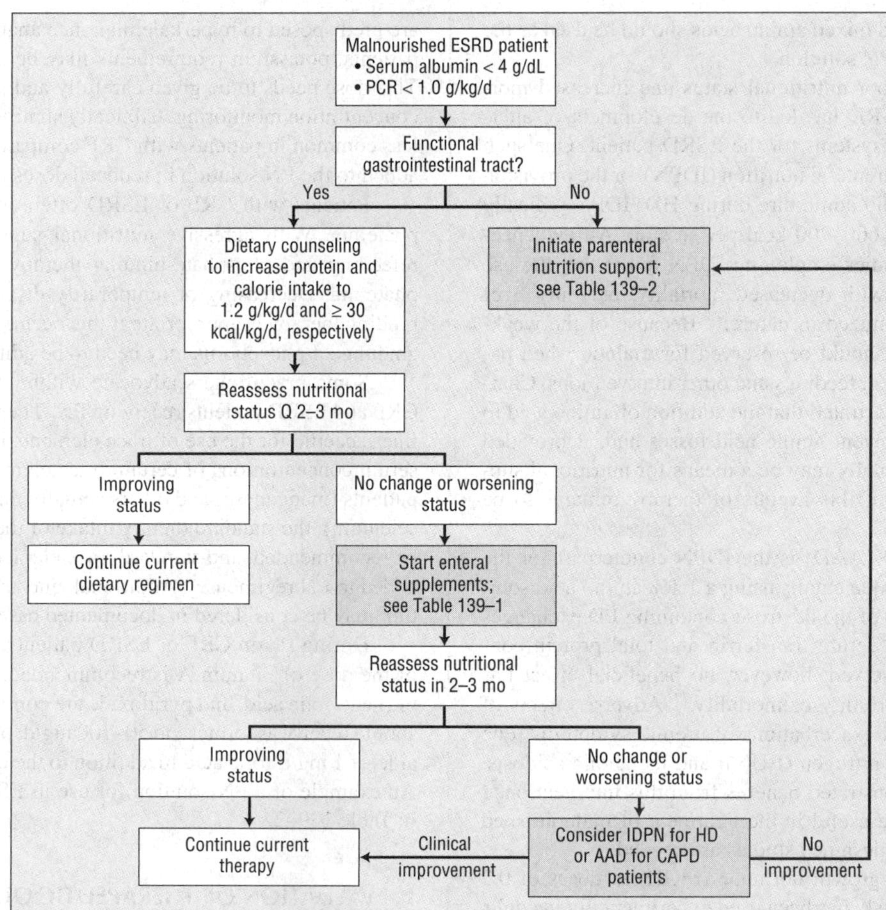

FIGURE 139–1. Algorithmic approach to nutritional support in the ESRD patient.

acids (BCAAs), severe protein-calorie malnutrition (PCM) was associated with a 6-month mortality rate of 45%, whereas moderate PCM was associated with a 6-month mortality rate of 29%.[81] Thus nutritional support has become an important component of the overall care of the patient with liver disease.

EPIDEMIOLOGY

Many patients with liver failure are in states of protein and/or energy malnutrition. It is estimated that 30% of cirrhotic patients have protein-energy malnutrition, 40% have protein malnutrition, and 10% have energy malnutrition.[82] In one study of alcoholic cirrhotic patients, 73% of patients had midarm muscle circumferences below the 5th percentile, and 51% had tricep skinfold thickness below the 25th percentile (see Chapter 135), which is indicative of protein and energy malnutrition, respectively.[83] This was despite caloric intake that averaged 40 kcal/kg per day. Aggressive support is thus imperative to optimize their care and to increase the likelihood of liver transplantation success.

PATHOPHYSIOLOGY

ENERGY

Patients with alcoholic hepatitis or cirrhosis frequently are hypermetabolic (up to 50% greater than expected) when their resting energy expenditure (REE) is normalized for lean body mass and compared with normal controls.[90] It must be emphasized, however, that providing excess calories should be avoided because this may promote liver dysfunction and increased production of carbon dioxide and an associated increased work of breathing. Indeed, in one study of 55 alcoholic cirrhotic patients, 34.5% were found to be hypermetabolic (measured/predicted REE > 1.1), 54.5% were normometabolic, and 11% were found to be hypometabolic.[89] This underscores the need for patient specific regimen design and monitoring.

CARBOHYDRATE

In healthy adults, approximately 60% of absorbed glucose is taken up by the liver and used for glycogen synthesis, triglyceride synthesis, and glycolysis. In general, glycogen synthesis and glycolysis are enhanced by insulin, whereas gluconeogenesis and glycogen breakdown are controlled by glucagon.

Hyperglycemia is common in cirrhosis as a result of peripheral insulin resistance, which is mediated by a decreased binding to insulin receptors and defective postreceptor signal handling in peripheral tissues. Plasma concentrations of insulin are elevated with or without a glucose stimulus. This makes administration of large doses of glucose problematic because administration of insulin to control hyperglycemia may not improve use substantially.

Patients with fulminant hepatitis are prone to hypoglycemia because hepatic glucose production is depressed secondary to decreased glycogen stores and diminished gluconeogenesis. Also, impaired degradation of insulin by the damaged liver may contribute to this disorder. A continuous intravenous infusion of glucose usually prevents hypoglycemia in acute hepatitis, but concentrations greater than 10% glucose may be needed in more severe cases.

FAT

The liver is responsible for synthesis of cholesterol, high-density lipoproteins, and very low-density lipoproteins. The enzymes lipoprotein lipase and lecithin-cholesterol acyltransferase also are synthesized in this organ. Increased serum triglyceride and FFA concentrations are encountered in patients with hepatic failure. Chronic alcohol ingestion is linked to increased circulating triglycerides and fatty infiltration of the liver.[85] Ingestion of high-fat diets may exacerbate these alterations in metabolism. The metabolism and safety of intravenous lipids in septic patients with hepatic failure has been evaluated.

Patients with severe liver failure may be at increased risk for essential fatty acid deficiency. The ratio of nonessential to essential fatty acids was found to be increased in patients with acute and chronic liver failure. These changes were due to decreased linoleic acid concentrations and increased concentrations of oleic acid.[86] Decreased levels of linoleic acid (but not longer-chain fatty acids) in liver failure can be increased with adminstration of an average of 33 g/d of IVLE supplementation.[87] Elimination and hydrolysis of triglycerides, as well as lipid oxidation, were not impaired significantly in these patients, and 4.5 mg/kg per minute infusions of 20% lipid emulsion for 2 hours did not result in side effects or impaired gas exchange.[88]

Diarrhea and steatorrhea are common in patients with hepatic cholestasis because of intestinal malabsorption (due in part to mucosal edema from hypoalbuminemia), inadequate bile acid delivery to the duodenum, and pancreatic dysfunction with decreased secretion of lipase.[85] Micelle formation is impeded, and thus the long-chain fatty acids pass through the colon, resulting in a foul-smelling, soapy diarrhea.

PROTEIN

Nitrogen requirements for the patient with liver failure are not unlike those of normal subjects, but intolerance to protein is well described in cirrhotic patients, and protein restriction has been used successfully as part of the therapy. A dilemma arises when the diet becomes so restrictive that malnutrition results, and the patient becomes susceptible to infection and other complications. Overzealous use of protein to correct nutritional deficits invariably results in hepatic encephalopathy.

Because the liver metabolizes the aromatic amino acids (i.e., phenylalanine, tyrosine, tryptophan), methionine, and glutamine, the plasma concentrations of these amino acids are elevated in cirrhotic patients. Plasma concentrations of the BCAAs (i.e., valine, leucine, isoleucine) often are depressed because these amino acids are metabolized by skeletal muscle. This altered plasma aminogram is thought to be involved in the etiology of hepatic encephalopathy. In health, the ratio of BCAAs to aromatic amino acids is approximately 3.5:1, whereas ratios of 1:1 have been associated with hepatic encephalopathy in patients with cirrhosis.[89]

FLUID AND ELECTROLYTES

Patients with severe cirrhosis often have ascites and peripheral edema. The excess of total body sodium in the presence of an even greater excess of total body water results in hyponatremia. Salt and fluid restrictions are required so as not to exacerbate this overhydrated state. Caution must be exercised, however, because severe sodium and fluid restriction may result in intravascular depletion, which may cause or exacerbate hepatic encephalopathy.

Hypokalemia is common in the patient with liver failure who has normal renal function. Poor nutritional intake and vomiting may initiate this disorder. Severe vomiting may lead to volume contraction metabolic alkalosis, with increased renal excretion of potassium. Secondary hyperaldosteronism, seen in the liver failure patient with intravascular depletion also increases renal excretion of potassium. Loop diuretic therapy causes increased renal excretion of potassium, whereas diarrhea from lactulose therapy increases fecal excretion of potassium. All these conditions can lead to profound hypokalemia. Therefore, potassium requirements in the liver failure patient receiving specialized nutritional support often are increased substantially.

Poor nutritional intake secondary to alcohol abuse and increased excretion of magnesium secondary to diuretic therapy contribute to hypomagnesemia. Even in cirrhotic patients with normal serum magnesium concentrations, muscle magnesium has been found to be depleted and independently associated with hepatic encephalopathy.[90] During nutrition support, requirements for phosphorus are also substantially supranormal because synthesis of body cell mass occurs. Therefore, this population is at risk for developing hypophosphatemia during refeeding.

TRACE ELEMENTS

Many patients with liver failure have a malabsorption syndrome and chronic diarrhea. Chronic diarrhea causes zinc deficiency because stool contains substantial quantities of zinc. Cytokines such as tumor necrosis factor (TNF), interleukin (IL)-1, and IL-6 may stimulate metallothionein, an intestinal zinc-binding protein, thereby inhibiting zinc absorption.[91] Considering the importance of zinc in metalloenzyme reactions, wound healing, immunocompetence, and the senses of taste and smell, patients with chronic diarrhea or large ostomy losses should be suspected of having zinc deficiency; measurement of serum concentrations may be used to confirm such deficiencies. Patients receiving a protein-restricted diet may be at additional risk because substantial amounts of zinc are found in red meat.

Because copper and manganese are excreted in the bile, it has been recommended that these two trace elements not be administered or be administered in reduced doses to patients with serious cholestasis[92] (see Table 139–2). Increased manganese whole blood concentrations have been associated with the magnetic resonance imaging (MRI) findings in chronic hepatic encephalopathy.[92] Direct measurements of manganese in brain globus pallidus of cirrhotic patients who died in hepatic coma were two- to seven-fold higher than expected.[93] It appears that brain manganese deposition is due to both liver failure and portal-systemic shunting based on animal models of hepatic failure.[94] These findings suggest that reduced quantities of manganese should be provided in the nutritional formulation to avoid exacerbating encephalopathy in the patient with chronic liver disease.

An association between alcoholism and low serum selenium concentrations has been reported. Serum concentrations of selenium were lowest in patients who had decompensated alcoholic cirrhosis. Because selenium is important in maintaining the enzyme glutathione peroxidase, a deficiency of this trace element has been implicated as a cause of hepatic injury in the alcoholic patient. However, because human serum contains at least three fractions of selenium, the use of serum selenium concentrations as an accurate marker for selenium deficiency is controversial. Therefore, care must be used in the interpretation of serum selenium concentrations.[91]

VITAMINS

Poor intake and malabsorption are the principal causes of vitamin deficiencies in patients with chronic liver disease. Depletion of hepatic stores of vitamin A, pyridoxine, folic acid, riboflavin, pantothenic acid, vitamin B_{12}, and thiamine have been reported in patients with hepatic failure. Folic acid deficiency, the most common vitamin deficiency, may lead to megaloblastic anemia, whereas thiamine deficiency may result in Wernicke's encephalopathy after rehydration with intravenous glucose.

Hepatic stores of vitamin A have been reported to be depleted in the patient with alcoholic liver injury.[95] Because vitamin D is metabolized to one of the active forms, 25-hydroxyvitamin D, in the liver, low concentrations of this vitamin are seen in patients with biliary cirrhosis. Impaired absorption of dietary vitamin D also may contribute to these low serum concentrations and the resulting osteoporosis. It is unclear whether vigorous supplementation of these fat-soluble vitamins should be provided during nutritional support, but clearly, therapeutic doses are indicated when a deficiency is documented.

▶ TREATMENT: Hepatic Failure

ADMINISTRATION ROUTE

If the gastrointestinal (GI) tract is functional and accessible, EN should be attempted. The indications for PN in the patient with liver failure are similar to those for general hospitalized patients. In most cases, PN in the patient with liver failure can be accomplished via the administration of standard mixed amino acids (Fig. 139–2).

Currently, two enteral products are marketed as supplements for patients with hepatic encephalopathy (Hepatic-Aid II and NutriHep). Both supplements have increased amounts of BCAAs and reduced amounts of aromatic amino acids (AAAs) and methionine but differ with regards to micronutrient composition. Hepatic-Aid II is virtually electrolyte- and vitamin-free, necessitating supplementation if tube feeding is used as the sole source of nutrient intake. NutriHep meets the U.S. RDA vitamin and mineral requirements, contains a high percentage of MCTs, and is supplemented with carnitine. The clinical trials using these products have yielded inconsistent outcomes.[96] At least two studies demonstrated improvements in hepatic encephalopathy with use of BCAA formulas. However, the remaining studies did not find improvement in hepatic encephalopathy.[89] Whether enteral feeding interventions improve mortality is perhaps even more controversial. At least three studies have demonstrated a significant improvement in early mortality, but one of these studies used a historical control,[97] and one used concurrent anabolic steroid therapy.[89]

There has been considerable interest in the use of vegetable-protein diets in the chronic management of patients with cirrhosis and hepatic encephalopathy. Enthusiasm for this therapy is based on the reduced amounts of AAAs and methionine in vegetable protein. The beneficial effects of vegetable protein also may result from decreased nitrogen absorption in response to decreased gastrointestinal transit time or an increased fecal nitrogen excretion by colonic bacterial flora. Compliance is more difficult to achieve with vegetable-based than animal-based protein diets in a large number of patients, however.

SPECIALTY PRODUCTS

The major controversy in nutritional support of the patient with liver failure has centered around the use of protein products. Modified amino acid solutions for PN (HepatAmine, others) are marketed for patients with liver failure and hepatic encephalopathy. They are enriched with BCAAs and have reduced amounts of AAAs and methionine. The products are formulated on the basis of the false neurotransmitter hypothesis, which concludes that hepatic encephalopathy may be due to increased AAA concentrations in the central nervous system.

BCAA products have not universally improved nitrogen balance. Standard amino acid mixtures can be used successfully without worsening encephalopathy. Studies examining improvement in encephalopathy or mortality rates with use of these modified amino acids have yielded conflicting results. This, coupled with the increased cost of these products, has led most clinicians to reserve these products for patients with severe encephalopathy who decompensate on standard amino acids despite continued lactulose-neomycin therapy.

DESIGN AND INITIATION OF NUTRITIONAL REGIMEN

Patients with alcoholic hepatitis or cirrhosis are frequently hypermetabolic. However, indirect calorimetry quantification may be preferred

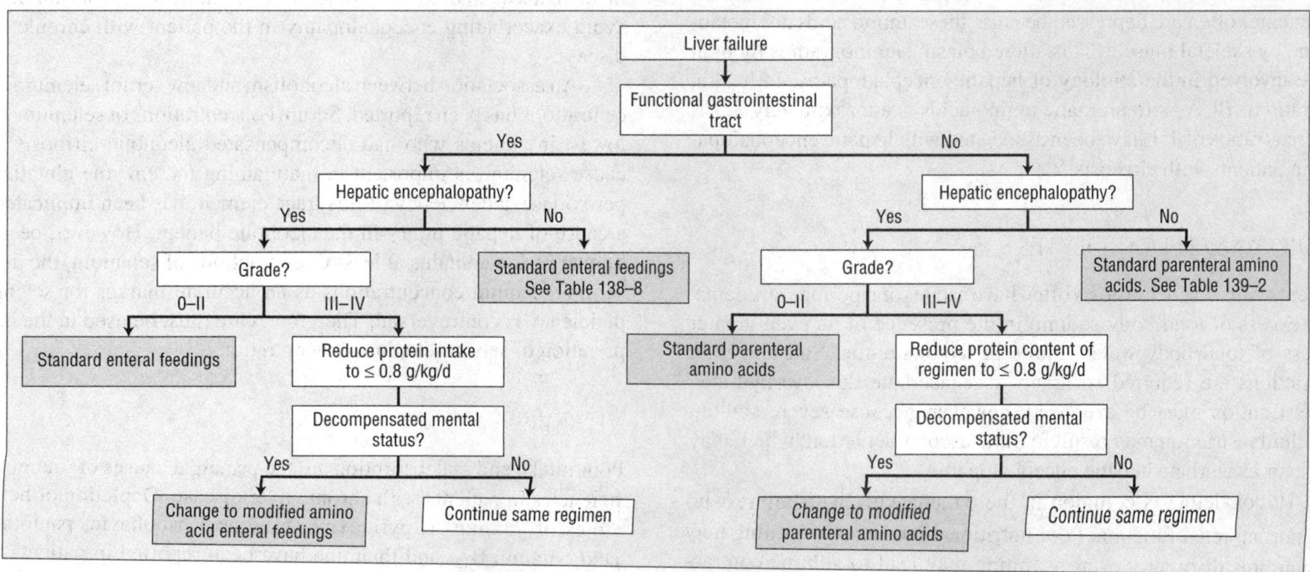

FIGURE 139–2. An algorithmic approach to nutritional support for the patient with hepatic failure.

to empirical estimates of caloric requirements in this setting to avoid providing excess calories. Excessive calorie provision actually may promote liver dysfunction and increased production of carbon dioxide with associated increased work of breathing. When dextrose-based PN is started in these patients, additional thiamine may be needed to prevent Wernicke's encephalopathy, especially if thiamine was not replaced after admission to the hospital.[89]

IVLE should be used in patients with liver failure only to prevent essential fatty acid deficiency (EFAD) when serum triglyceride concentrations exceed 300 mg/dL. If serum triglyceride concentrations are low or normal, IVLE also may be used as a calorie source. Monitoring serum triglyceride concentration and FFA oxidation (not available in all facilities) to ensure that lipid is both cleared and oxidized appropriately has been suggested. Triglyceride concentrations are the only available marker in most clinical practices at this time. Although not an indicator of use, this can help prevent marked hypertriglyceridemia and associated disorders (such as pancreatitis). Oral MCTs have been used occasionally with success because they do not require pancreatic enzymes or micelle formation before absorption. However, these products do not provide essential fatty acids.

Most clinicians routinely use standard mixed amino acids and reserve BCAA products for patients with severe encephalopathy who decompensate on standard amino acids despite continued lactulose-neomycin therapy. This is so because modified amino acid products containing only BCAAs have been shown not to improve nitrogen balance. Also, standard amino acid mixtures can improve plasma aminograms without worsening encephalopathy, as discussed previously.

The electrolytes that warrant the most careful monitoring in liver disease include sodium, potassium, phosphorus, and magnesium. During fluid and salt restriction, patients (especially those receiving concurrent lactulose therapy) should be observed for symptoms of volume depletion (e.g., pulse rate, blood pressure, dry mucus membranes). The magnesium dose should be individualized to maintain concentrations in the normal range. This often requires magnesium concentrations as high as 24 mEq/L in the PN solution, which is two to three times the standard daily dose.

Trace elements that warrant individual attention include zinc and chromium. Oral supplementation of zinc sulfate capsules or intravenous zinc chloride can be used to prevent deficiency or correct deficits. Oral supplementation with zinc sulfate 600 mg/d in cirrhotic patients has been reported to improve serum zinc concentrations and psychometric tests.[98] For patients receiving PN, withholding copper from the solution until a copper serum concentration in the normal range is documented or the cholestasis resolves, is appropriate. Patients who have chronic cholestasis may require copper in reduced doses (e.g., 0.6 mg/d); however, they should have serum copper concentrations checked regularly (once per month in the acute care setting and every 6 months in the ambulatory setting). Manganese restriction also may be required in these patients. For patients with liver failure secondary to cirrhosis and a nonfunctioning GI tract, Table 139–2 gives an example of an empirical central PN formula.

EVALUATION OF THERAPEUTIC OUTCOMES

The question arises which markers of nutritional adequacy are appropriate for the monitoring of nutritional status in patients with hepatic failure. Prealbumin and retinol-binding protein, traditionally sensitive markers of protein-energy malnutrition, may not be as reliable in patients with hepatic failure. Liver failure can cause decreased concentrations of both, independent of nutritional status.[99] Indeed, many of the commonly used markers of nutritional status correlate poorly with body cell mass in end-stage liver disease. Among anthropometry, handgrip dynamometry, laboratory tests, and body composition measured by dual-energy x-ray absorptiometry, midarm muscle circumference and handgrip strength were found to be the best predictors of body cell mass.[100] The poor correlation of other markers suggests that they are of limited value for patients with changing hepatic function.

QUALITY-OF-LIFE ISSUES

Nutritional supplementation provided to patients with alcoholic cirrhosis has been demonstrated to reduce the frequency of hospitalizations. Therefore, nutrition supplementation in liver failure should be viewed as a method of reducing nutrition-related complications, as well as improving quality of life by decreasing number of patient admissions to the hospital.

HEPATIC TRANSPLANTATION

Orthotopic liver transplantation (OLT) has become an important intervention for the patient with end-stage liver disease. Many patients receive PN support following this operation because of their poor preoperative nutritional status and the postoperative stress. Although hypermetabolism in the early postoperative period has been reported, a caloric intake of only 1.2 times basal energy expenditure (BEE) has met caloric needs immediately and for up to 28 days after transplantation.[101] Increased protein catabolism and urinary 3-methylhistidine levels also have been noted in response to the stress of liver transplantation and the administration of large doses of corticosteroids following surgical intervention.[101]

EPIDEMIOLOGY

The percentage of OLT patients requiring nutritional support has been well documented. In one report of 427 OLT patients, 32.7% received at least one form of nutritional support: 8.9% received tube feedings alone, 11.9% received PN alone, and a combination of tube feedings and PN was provided to 11.9%. In 102 consecutive patients undergoing elective OLT, 79% were at or below the 25th percentile of anthropometric measurements and 28% were below the 5th percentile.[102] This indicates a high prevalence of malnutrition in patients awaiting OLT. Patients below the 25th percentile for midarm circumference and tricep skinfold thickness in this study population experienced significantly more bacterial infections after OLT and had a nonsignificant increase in mortality rate. In a recent prospective study, enteral supplementation before OLT until transplantation improved midarm circumference and grip strength and was associated with a reduced number of deaths (although this did not reach statistical significance; $P = .075$).[103] Thus nutritional support is a frequently used and important therapy in the OLT patient population.

PATHOPHYSIOLOGY

CARBOHYDRATE, PROTEIN, AND FAT

Postoperative hyperglycemia is common during the first day after OLT. Cyclosporine, which is often given to these patients to prevent organ rejection, has been reported to suppress insulin synthesis and secretion.[104] Administration of this drug thus may contribute to the hyperglycemia observed during the postoperative period. Alterations in glucose uptake in peripheral tissue also may be present in these patients and thereby contribute to hyperglycemia after OLT.[105]

Most patients will tolerate standard amino acids following OLT because the new liver is functioning properly, and hepatic encephalopathy is not problematic. The excessive nitrogen losses associated with this procedure warrant the provision of at least 1.2 g/kg per day of protein.[101] One study demonstrated that at least 0.25 g/kg per day of nitrogen (1.38 g/kg/d of protein) is required to maintain a balanced plasma aminogram when OLT patients were fed 27 kcal/kg of ideal body weight per day.[106] Modified amino acids should be reserved for patients with marginal hepatic function associated with rejection or hepatic encephalopathy.

A combination of MCTs and LCTs has been studied in post-OLT patients. No significant differences in carbohydrate or lipid oxidation rates were seen, thus suggesting that MCT-specific emulsion is not the preferred lipid source for the PN regimen of the OLT patient.[107]

FLUID, ELECTROLYTE, AND ACID-BASE DISORDERS

Patients undergoing OLT receive a substantial amount of crystalloid and blood products during the operative procedure. This often results in an edematous state in the postoperative period, especially in patients who had ascites preoperatively. The large citrate load from administered blood products has been implicated in causing hypocalcemia (citrate binding of ionized calcium) and metabolic alkalosis (conversions of citrate to bicarbonate) in the postoperative period. Low serum concentrations of magnesium are common in the postoperative period. Reduced intake from restricted diets and increased urinary excretion secondary to cyclosporine therapy contribute to hypomagnesemia.

TRACE ELEMENTS AND VITAMINS

Low serum concentrations of zinc are common in the postoperative period. Restricted diets before surgery and hyperzincuria secondary to liver disease both contribute to hypozincemia in this population. These findings led investigators to recommend oral zinc supplementation before transplantation. Serum zinc concentrations have been found to recover rapidly after transplantation, obviating the need for further supplementation.[108] On the other hand, patients who have severe cholestasis before and after OLT should have copper and manganese restricted because they are excreted in the bile and thus serum concentrations may be elevated.

Low serum vitamin A concentrations are present in many patients with chronic liver disease. Mean serum vitamin A concentrations measure less than one-half normal in pre-OLT patients.[95] These abnormally low serum concentrations, however, were found to increase 1 week after transplantation and to normalize 2 weeks after transplantation.[95] Water-soluble vitamin E preparations have been used in an attempt to economically maintain therapeutic cyclosporine concentrations early in the posttransplant setting.[109]

Osteoporosis and fracture risk increase in patients after liver transplantation. Even patients awaiting OLT had a 43% incidence of osteoporosis in one study.[110] Serum 25-hydroxyvitamin D, 1,25-dihydroxyvitamin D, and parathyroid hormone concentrations were reduced in this cirrhotic patient population.[110] Three months after OLT, mean bone mineral density (BMD) expressed as a Z-score was −2.04 in one study and took a mean of 85 months to return to pre-OLT levels.[111] Single-dose bisphosphonate infusion did not alter bone formation or resorption in the early (30 days) post-OLT period.[112] It is likely that lowering steroid doses, BMD screening, preventive measures, and calcium and vitamin D supplementation will be the mainstay treatment options for this problem.[113]

▶ TREATMENT: Hepatic Transplantation

ADMINISTRATION ROUTES

Several studies have investigated the effect of route of feeding the OLT patient on patient outcome.[114] Hasse and colleagues compared nasointestinal feedings with maintenance intravenous fluids in the immediate postoperative period. Both groups were advanced to oral diets as tolerated after transplantation. Cumulative caloric and protein intakes were greater and nitrogen balance was better in the tube-fed patients. Additionally, 17.7% of patients given maintenance intravenous fluids developed viral infections compared with none in the tube-fed group.[114] Wicks and coworkers[115] demonstrated comparable efficacy between jejunal enteral feedings and PN in maintaining midarm muscle circumference and tricep skinfold thickness 10 days postoperatively. Another study demonstrated that patients fed via jejunostomy tube reached goal oral nutrition quicker and had less postoperative ileus than patients treated with PN after OLT.[116] Based on the current literature, OLT patients can be fed successfully enterally; however, small bowel access is needed for this to occur. This would necessitate placement of a nasoduodenal or nasojejunal tube during or immediately after surgery.

DESIGN AND INITIATION OF NUTRITIONAL REGIMEN

OLT patients should be given a nutritional formula that provides at least 1.2 times BEE per day. Because of the significant incidence of hyperglycemia immediately postoperatively, it is recommended to wait 24 hours before starting PN or to begin very slowly with a relatively low concentration of dextrose (e.g., $D_{10}W$ or $D_{15}W$). These patients also should be provided with at least 1.2 g/kg per day of protein. Because OLT patients frequently are edematous postoperatively, this can be achieved with higher concentrations of amino acids (using a 10% or 15% stock solution). Also, due to postoperative edema, sodium rarely needs to be added to the PN solution in these patients. Citrate-containing blood products bind ionized calcium, mandating supplemental doses of calcium. Additionally, OLT patients receiving cyclosporine therapy often will require magnesium in amounts that exceed standard doses during postoperative nutritional support. An example of a PN formula specific for OLT appears in Table 139–2.

EVALUATION OF THERAPEUTIC OUTCOMES

The monitoring plan of the OLT patient needs to be individualized. Patients receiving cyclosporine should be monitored closely (at least every 6 hours) for hyperglycemia. Following successful OLT, hepatic encephalopathy is no longer problematic. Thus nitrogen balance should be evaluated to determine the optimal amount of protein to be provided. Fluid balance (daily or more frequently) should be followed carefully to avoid volume overload, especially in patients who received large volumes of fluids intraoperatively. Daily (or more frequent if deficiency is documented) monitoring of magnesium is necessary, especially in patients receiving cyclosporine therapy. Zinc and vitamin A serum concentrations should return to normal after successful OLT, requiring less aggressive monitoring than was needed preoperatively.

The prognostic importance of pretransplant nutrition status perhaps has been overlooked in the past. A strong correlation between pretransplant nutrition status and posttransplant survival exists. Perhaps the most striking results are reported in a 1997 study by Selberg and colleagues.[117] Better nutrition status in this study was associated with an 88% (versus 54%) survival rate. Optimal nutrition status therefore should be ensured before transplantation as well as after transplantation. It appears that this will assist OLT patients in achieving the best therapeutic outcome possible.

Advances in nutritional support for the post-OLT patient additionally have led to restoration of nitrogen balance, enhancement of host defense mechanisms, and decreased time on the ventilator and in the ICU.[118] Therefore, the clinician should evaluate global outcome parameters throughly (e.g., time on mechanical ventilation and in the ICU), as well as more traditional parameters of nutrition efficacy (e.g., nitrogen balance and visceral protein markers). These global parameters should improve with the provision of more aggressive nutritional support in the post-OLT setting.

SHORT BOWEL SYNDROME

An intact functional gastrointestinal tract is essential for absorption and digestion of nutrients. Gastrointestinal failure secondary to the short bowel syndrome (SBS) is a disease state in which morbidity and mortality have been improved by PN. Both EN and PN have had major impacts on treatment of severe inflammatory bowel disease, enterocutaneous fistulas, and radiation enteritis. The goal of nutritional support in patients with SBS is to maintain nutritional status and/or correct nutritional deficiencies.

EPIDEMIOLOGY

SBS is a complex nutritional and metabolic condition that results from malabsorption following massive resection of the small intestine.[119,120] Patients who have less than 200 cm (or approximately one-third) of their jejunum-ileum remaining after resection can be categorized as having this disorder.[121 122] In adults, the most common etiologies of surgeries leading to SBS are Crohn's disease, mesenteric vascular disease, and malignancy.[120] This condition also may be functional as opposed to anatomic and occur in individuals who have not had resections but who have a decreased small bowel absorptive capacity due to etiologies such as radiation enteritis or severe inflammatory bowel disease.[121] Symptoms of SBS may vary between patients but generally include diarrhea, dehydration, electrolyte disturbances, and progressive malnutrition.[120,121]

Nutritional support is a major component of SBS management, and it is used to maintain a patient's nutritional status and/or correct nutritional deficiencies. Initially, after a major resection of the small intestine, PN is required. As the remaining small bowel adapts to improve its absorptive capacity, patients may transition slowly to EN and/or dietary therapy.[119] Some patients may require lifelong home PN based on such prognostic factors as a limited length of remaining small intestine and the absence of a functional colon. Wilmore and colleagues estimate that for adult patients to transition off of PN, the residual jejunum-ileum length needs to be greater than 120 cm for individuals without a colon or greater than 60 cm if a portion of the colon is in continuity with the remaining small intestine.[121] Additional factors that may predict a poor outcome include disease in the residual bowel and removal of the ileocecal valve, the physiologic sphincter that controls the rate of passage of intestinal contents from small to large bowel and prevents small bowel bacterial overgrowth.[120]

PATHOPHYSIOLOGY

INTESTINAL ADAPTATION

The adaptation process of the residual small intestine (absorptive capacity) begins within 12 to 24 hours after bowel resection.[121] The changes in the GI tract are gradual and may continue to occur for 1 to 2 years. Factors that act as stimuli for adaptation include luminal nutrients, pancreaticobiliary secretions, and intestinal hormones.[120,121] The ability of the remaining intestine to adjust after resection is also influenced by the area of bowel loss. The jejunum is the primary site for absorption of most nutrients, but if it is removed, the ileum usually can accommodate to take on its structural characteristics and functional roles. However, with ileal resection, the jejunum has a decreased capacity to adapt and perform the functions of the ileum.[123]

ENERGY REQUIREMENTS

Caloric intake and energy needs of SBS patients are variable. Individuals who have lost more than 50% of their small intestine typically require input of 30–40 kcal/kg of ideal body weight per day.[120] However, in a study of 10 stable ambulatory patients who consumed only an oral diet, a caloric intake equivalent to 2.5 times BEE was consumed and resulted in steady-state energy balance.[124]

CARBOHYDRATE, FAT, PROTEIN

Fat malabsorption is common in SBS, particularly after ileal resection.[123] The pathophysiology of this problem is complex and related to alterations in pancreatic enzyme secretion and bile salt absorption. The ileum is the major site of the latter process, and with its removal, bile salt malabsorption is common. Eventually, the total bile salt pool may be depleted, resulting in increased fat malabsorption and steatorrhea.[123] Some patients who are unable to absorb sufficient fat have been treated with MCTs, which do not require bile acids or pancreatic enzymes for absorption. However, MCTs do not provide essential fatty acids, which could lead to EFAD. Long-chain fatty acids would need to be given orally or parenterally to prevent this disorder. Even patients with SBS receiving chronic PN with intravenous LCT fat emulsion have been reported to have biochemical evidence of EFAD.[125] The patients developed SBS secondary to multiple intestinal resections from Crohn's disease, radiation enteritis, or vascular occlusion. Erythrocyte linoleic acid concentrations (essential fatty acid) were significantly lower, whereas erythrocyte palmitoleic and oleic acid concentrations were significantly higher in the patients supported by PN.[125]

Carbohydrate malabsorption plays a major role in the diarrhea associated with SBS. Unabsorbed carbohydrates are broken down by intestinal bacteria to short-chain fatty acids (SCFAs), producing an osmotic load in the distal small intestine and colon that can lead to this problem.[119] However, the colon is able to use these SCFAs as a source of energy, and thus they may provide a significant caloric source for patients with a massive resection and a preserved colon.[119,122,124]

Protein typically is well tolerated as a caloric source, although in EN patients it is controversial what molecular form of the macronutrient maximizes absorption. In the past, EN often was initiated with an elemental product that contained free amino acids as the protein source because the efficiency for protein uptake was perceived to be better. However, total protein absorption is faster and more complete from formulas that use dipeptides and tripeptides for protein.[119] It appears that the absorption of free amino acids by the enteral route is a saturable process, whereas the absorption of small peptides is not. These more complex protein sources also may stimulate intestinal adaptation.[119]

FLUID, ELECTROLYTE, AND ACID-BASE DISORDERS

After substantial resections of the small bowel, the postoperative course is complicated by fluid and electrolyte imbalances that typically last 1 to 3 weeks.[120] Patients may have high-volume gastric fluid loss from nasogastric tubes and small intestine fluid loss from ostomies. Sodium content usually is elevated in these secretions, with concentrations of approximately 80–100 mEq/L.[119] Acute gastric hypersecretion may occur after massive resection and contribute significantly to these deficits.[120] Secretory diarrhea also results in fluid and electrolyte losses that may be difficult to quantify.

Patients with end jejunostomies or proximal ileostomies can have recurrent dehydration and electrolyte deficiencies. A high jejunostomy can have output of 3 L/d of fluid, with sodium loss of 90 mEq/L.[122] These deficits occur in part because of the physiologic response of the upper GI tract and jejunum to oral intake of water and other low-sodium drinks.[122] To overcome the net secretion of sodium and water into the jejunum, the sodium content of fluids within the GI lumen must reach 90 mEq/L.[122] In patients who have small intestine in continuity with the colon, the malabsorbed bile and fatty acids stimulate sodium and water and excretion into the large bowel, but in general these patients are at less risk for sodium and water depletion.

Jejunal fluids contain approximately 15 mEq/L of potassium, but in some jejunostomy patients, concentrations can be higher and losses of this electrolyte more profound.[122,127] Other patients at risk for potassium deficiency include individuals with long-term sodium depletion, magnesium deficiency, or excessive loss from diarrhea.[122] Metabolic alkalosis, which may occur when a patient becomes dehydrated, accelerates the renal excretion of potassium as all hydrogen ions are conserved in an attempt to correct the acid-base disorder. As bicarbonate ions are excreted renally, potassium is taken with them to maintain osmotic balance.

Inadequate absorption of calcium may occur with SBS as a result of binding of calcium to unabsorbed fatty acids in the intestine. This also may result in hyperoxaluria and formation of calcium oxalate renal stones because dietary oxalate usually complexes with the intraluminal calcium and is excreted in the stool. As the result of decreased calcium available for binding, more oxalate is absorbed and available for renal excretion.[121] Vitamin D deficiency results in insufficient calcium absorption; thus SBS patients requiring long-term PN are at risk for metabolic bone disease. Other potential causes of this disorder include aluminum toxicity, suppression of parathyroid hormone by parenteral vitamin D, disruption of parathyroid hormone regulation, and cytokine effects on bone resorption.[128]

Magnesium deficiency is common in SBS patients with large ostomy or diarrheal losses. Due to the small percentage of total body magnesium found in the serum, urinary magnesium concentrations may decrease earlier with deficiency and may be a better estimate of total body stores than serum levels.[129] Sixteen outpatients with GI failure (12 with SBS, 4 with diffuse small bowel disease) had a mean serum magnesium concentration of 1.7 mg/dL, with a mean urinary excretion of 19 mg/24 h. The 16 age- and gender-matched controls had a mean serum magnesium concentration of 2 mg/dL, with a mean urinary excretion of 127 mg/24 h. These data suggest that urinary magnesium may be a superior way to assess magnesium status in outpatients who have GI failure.[129] Oral supplementation may be difficult because it can contribute to increased diarrhea or ostomy output.[121] However, repletion is necessary to correct calcium and potassium deficits in addition to magnesium losses[122] (see Chapter 52).

SBS patients can lose substantial amounts of chloride (60–140 mEq/L) in addition to sodium from ostomy output. Dehydration occurs when there are stable losses from an ostomy that are not replaced or when the patient is noncompliant with a restricted diet resulting in loss of more fluid than is taken in. These individuals have a high risk of developing hypochloremic metabolic alkalosis. Noncompliance with the infusion of appropriately prescribed fluids also can lead to dehydration. Patients who have SBS complicated by a pancreatic fistula and severe diarrhea lose considerable potassium and bicarbonate and may develop metabolic acidosis. Patients with severe diarrhea who have an intact colon will conserve sodium and chloride, resulting in considerable loss of potassium and bicarbonate and the development of metabolic acidosis. Quantifying fluid losses with particular attention to the sources of loss will aid in the acid-base management of these patients (see Chapter 53).

Lactic acidosis can occur in patients with SBS and may result in symptoms of ataxia and delirium.[130] D-Lactic acid is produced by the fermentation of malabsorbed carbohydrates by colonic bacteria, and increased concentrations are associated with small bowel bacterial overgrowth.[120,130] The diagnosis of D-lactic acidosis should be considered in patients with a functional colon who have an unexplained metabolic acidosis and an elevated anion gap.[120]

TRACE ELEMENTS

Patients with SBS are particularly prone to zinc deficiency as a result of excessive losses from stool, ostomy outputs, and fistula drainage. Signs of inadequate zinc include acrodermatitis and impaired wound healing. Although serum zinc concentrations are not always reflective of body zinc status, a low serum zinc concentration requires an adjustment in replacement amount.[122] Significant bowel resection and GI losses also contribute to imbalances of other trace elements, such as copper and chromium. Impaired intestinal absorption of selenium occurs with SBS, and cardiomyopathy related to its deficiency has occurred in patients on long-term PN without supplementation.[131] Therefore, selenium replacement is recommended for all patients on long-term PN. Monitoring for trace element deficiencies and the need for supplementation are essential for SBS patients, including those receiving PN, EN, or an adequate diet.

VITAMINS

Most water-soluble vitamins are absorbed in the proximal jejunum, and deficits of these vitamins are found only in more severe SBS.[120] Vitamin B_{12} is an exception due to its unique absorption in the ileum, and patients with ileal resection commonly develop vitamin B_{12} deficiency, necessitating therapy with parenteral cyanocobalamin. Small bowel bacterial overgrowth can contribute to diminished vitamin B_{12} because bacteria may metabolize the nutrient within the intestine, decreasing its availability for absorption.[121] SBS patients with fat malabsorption can acquire deficiencies in vitamins A, D, E, and K. These fat-soluble vitamins depend on bile salt micelles for effective absorption, and malabsorption with depletion of the bile salt pool can lead to their deficits.[123]

▶ TREATMENT: Short Bowel Syndrome

ADMINISTRATION ROUTES

After intestinal resection, the clinical course and nutritional management of SBS patients may be described in three stages.[132] The first stage, the initial postoperative period, is complicated by the fluid and electrolyte losses from ostomy and nasogastric tube outputs and/or massive diarrhea. This phase lasts 1 to 3 weeks, and the parenteral route should be used to supply nutritional needs.[120] The second stage lasts from a few months to over a year, and it is during this time that the bowel undergoes adaptive changes. Institution of enteral intake early during this stage is important because intraluminal nutrients are essential stimuli for intestinal adaptation.[120] As the amount of oral nutrition is advanced and tolerated slowly, the duration of the daily infusion of PN may be decreased.[119] In the final stage, adaptation is maximized, and the patient is maintained with nutritional support tailored for long-term ambulatory management. If patients are unable to achieve full oral nutrition, home PN may be used. However, PN may not be required on a daily basis. If PN is weaned, initially, one to two nights of PN may be eliminated each week. Eventually, some patients may be able to tolerate administration on an every-other or every-third-night basis.[119] During the different phases of management, PN is administered through a peripherally inserted central catheter or surgically placed indwelling central venous catheter[121] (see Chapter 137). Use of proper aseptic technique is vital in the care of these access sites because SBS patients have been shown to have significantly higher rates of catheter sepsis.[133]

DESIGN AND INITIATION OF NUTRITIONAL REGIMEN

The early phase of SBS is associated with a large day-to-day variation in fluid and electrolyte losses. Therefore, it is recommended to start a standard PN solution that meets the patient's maintenance metabolic, fluid, and electrolyte needs and a separate intravenous replacement solution based on actual fluid losses.[119] As fluid and electrolyte losses stabilize, it is sometimes possible to incorporate these replacement requirements into the PN solution. Because there are usually no substrate alterations in SBS patients, the PN solution typically is composed of standard crystalline amino acids, glucose, and intravenous lipids. An example of a PN formula for the patient with SBS is given in Table 139–2.

Careful monitoring of fluid and sodium status is warranted, with thorough attention given to all sources of fluid loss (e.g., from ostomies or diarrhea). Ideally, replacement should be provided so that patients are able to maintain a urine output of at least 1000 mL/d.[120] Patient evaluation should include regular weight checks and assessment of the physical examination for signs of postural hypotension, dehydration, or edema.[122] In addition to serum sodium concentrations, urinary sodium concentration is a valuable tool to assess sodium and water balance.[122] The amounts of chloride versus acetate salt forms chosen for cation delivery should be based on assessment of the acid-base balance of the patient and sources of GI losses. More proximal GI losses generally are associated with increased chloride needs and more distal outputs with increased bicarbonate (i.e., acetate) requirements. In addition, supplementation of potassium, calcium, magnesium, zinc, or other micronutrients over their maintenance amounts may be necessary to meet replacement needs.

Enteral intake is desirable and should be instituted as the patient recovers during the postoperative period.[120,121] However, oral input should be regulated carefully at this point. Small volumes (600–1000 mL/24 h) of oral electrolyte solutions (e.g., Pedialyte or Gatorade) may be given as frequent small portions with modest amounts of solid food composed primarily of complex carbohydrates and proteins (600–1000 kcal/24 h).[121] Currently, standard food diets usually are used over liquid formulas because they may be more effective in stimulating bowel adaptation.[120,121,134] However, in a patient who is intolerant of an oral diet, EN, given as a continuous infusion through a nasogastric or gastric feeding tube, should be tried.[120] Continuous administration of EN is advantageous over bolus feedings because it maximizes absorptive capacity and minimizes diarrhea.[119,120,122] Formulas with protein hydrolysates and a combination of MCTs and LCTs as well as elemental formulas have been suggested for these patients.[119,132] Because SBS may exacerbate lactose intolerance, lactose-free isotonic polymeric enteral formulas also have been recommended.[120]

Determination of appropriate content of a long-term oral diet for an SBS patient is individualized based on such factors as the site and length of remaining intestine, tolerance, and patient acceptance. Fat generally is not restricted in patients without a colon. However, patients with a colon may experience more diarrhea with a high-fat diet and may benefit from oral intake that has high-carbohydrate and low-fat content.[120] In addition to less diarrhea from a diet of this makeup, malabsorbed carbohydrates in the colon provide a source of energy as SCFAs.[119,122,126] The diet for patients with a functional colon also must account for oxalate content, and patients should avoid foods with high amounts of oxalate (e.g., spinach, parsley, rhubarb, cocoa, and tea).[122] Finally, oral diets in SBS patients often need to be supplemented to maintain electrolyte, mineral, vitamin, and trace element balance.

DRUG THERAPY

The delivery of medications to patients with SBS may present many challenges, including questionable absorption of oral therapies and for intravenous drugs the concerns of limiting the use of PN access sites and compatability issues.[135] It is also important to avoid oral products that contain sorbitol or mannitol as inactive ingredients to avoid medication-related diarrhea. However, pharmacologic interventions are very important in the management of SBS symptomatology. Loperamide and octreotide may be used to control diarrhea (see Chapter 36), and proton pump inhibitors and H_2-receptor antagonists are used to reduce gastric hypersecretion (see Chapter 33).

The use of specialized nutrients and growth factors to enhance small bowel adaptation has been a focus of recent research. The amino acid glutamine is a fuel for intestinal cells, and its necessity for maintaining intestinal structure in normal and stressed states has been identified recently.[121] Byrne and colleagues published an uncontrolled clinical study of patients who received glutamine in combination with rhGH plus a high-carbohydrate and low-fat diet.[135] The rhGH was added to the regimen because of its stimulant properties in bowel adaptation. Initial results showed that the use of the three treatment components resulted in significantly increased protein absorption and decreased stool output in eight PN-dependent SBS patients. Subsequently, 47 patients received this regimen for 4 weeks through a structured residential nutrition program. At the end of the treatment period,

57% of patients were able to discontinue PN. After a follow-up period of 1 year, 40% of patients were able to maintain nutrition status off PN with a continued high-carbohydrate and low-fat diet and glutamine supplementation.

Other researchers have investigated the effects of glutamine, rhGH, and a high-carbohydrate and low-fat diet on body composition and macronutrient absorption.[137,138] In these randomized, double-blind, placebo-controlled crossover studies in small numbers of patients, the treatment regimen increased body weight and lean body mass, but it did not significantly increase macronutrient or fluid absorption. The positive effects on body composition were not maintained when therapy was discontinued, and one investigator attributed the positive weight gain to increased extracellular fluid because all patients developed peripheral edema on therapy.[138] Results from larger, randomized clinical trials are needed to help clarify the effects of this three treatment regimen and to identify which patients may have the best benefit from its use.

SURGICAL THERAPY

Surgical management of SBS patients focuses on preventing GI resections by early diagnosis and, when possible, the use of conservative resections.[120] An evolving area of surgical treatment in SBS is intestinal transplantation. Currently, this procedure is considered a high-risk proposition, and it is reserved for patients with life-threatening complications of their intestinal failure (e.g., irreversible PN-related liver disease, recurrent sepsis, or lack of venous access).[119,120] Challenges of intestinal transplantation include development of better immunosuppressive regimens and early detection of rejection.[120] As improvements are made in these areas, use of this procedure will need to be assessed continually as an option for selected SBS patients.

EVALUATION OF THERAPEUTIC OUTCOMES

Long-term outcomes of adults with SBS have been examined. In a study of 124 patients with SBS unrelated to malignancy, survival rates at 2 and 5 years were 86% and 75%, respectively.[139] In these same patients, the probability of requiring continued PN support was 49% at 2 years and 45% at 5 years. Dependence on PN was related to residual intestinal length of less than 100 cm and absence of the terminal ileum and/or colon in continuity with the remaining small intestine.

The most comprehensive and thorough analysis of the clinical outcome of patients receiving home PN or EN comes from the Medicare and the North American Home Parenteral and Enteral Patient Registry.[140] It was estimated that 40,000 and 152,000 patients in the United States were receiving home PN and EN support, respectively. The number of patients receiving either PN or EN at home more than doubled between 1989 and 1992. Patients with GI failure, which included those with Crohn's disease, ischemic bowel disease, motility disorders, and congenital bowel defects, had relatively good outcomes, especially when compared with the groups with cancer or AIDS. The patients with GI failure had an 87% annual survival rate and a 50% to 75% likelihood of complete rehabilitation. Sepsis, metabolic disorders, and mechanical problems with catheters resulted in one to two hospitalizations per year for all patients.[140]

QUALITY-OF-LIFE ISSUES

Education of patients with SBS and their caregivers is essential, particularly in the setting of home PN and/or EN with its associated technology. In addition, quality-of-life issues should be addressed with these individuals. In a survey of 116 long-term home PN patients and their families, low quality of life was associated with increasing length of time on PN, fewer coping skills, and an inability to get along on their financial income.[141] Preparing patients and their caregivers for the possible stresses associated with this therapy (e.g., financial challenges, fatigue, depression, and social or emotional problems) may help to increase quality of life.

PULMONARY FAILURE

The provision of appropriate nutritional support plays a significant role in the management of patients with respiratory disease. The pathophysiology of acute or chronic pulmonary failure varies based on the underlying disease state. Optimization of nutritional therapy requires an understanding and consideration of the unique aspects of each disease process.[142] Grant describes three types of respiratory failure in relation to nutritional support: (1) depletion of respiratory muscles, (2) acute pulmonary parenchymal diseases, such as acute respiratory distress syndrome, and (3) chronic obstructive pulmonary disease.[143] Depletion of diaphragmatic or intercostal muscles may be due to malnutrition, prolonged mechanical ventilation, or dysfunction of respiratory chemoreceptors.[143] Inspiratory muscle fatigue is a major cause of pulmonary failure in patients with acute respiratory distress syndrome (ARDS) or chronic obstructive pulmonary disease (COPD).[142] Nutritional support plays a key role in optimizing respiratory muscle function in all these situations.

Although patients with pulmonary failure do not have the severe metabolic alterations observed in patients with renal or hepatic failure, there is substantial information to aid the practitioner in providing safe and efficacious nutritional support.[143,144]

EPIDEMIOLOGY

A significant percentage of patients with COPD have evidence of malnutrition, and weight loss often occurs as the disease progresses.[144–146] In a 1-year study of 126 stable COPD patients, Sahebjami and colleagues found that 46.8% had nutritional abnormalities based on body mass index (BMI) and other anthropometric measurements.[147] In their study, they found that BMI correlated with some pulmonary function tests, including diffusing capacity for carbon monoxide and forced expiratory volume in 1 second.[147] Patients with COPD frequently are hospitalized with exacerbations of their disease. In these individuals, a low BMI on admission and weight loss during the hospitalization have been associated with an increased risk for nonelective readmission within 14 days of discharge.[147]

The significance of body composition, in addition to body weight, in COPD has been reviewed.[145,146] Measurements of fat free mass (FFM) can be used to assess muscle mass, and depletion of FFM is related to impaired exercise performance.[149] Engelen and others studied body composition in patients with emphysema or chronic bronchitis.[150] They found a higher incidence of lean mass depletion in those with emphysema compared to those with chronic bronchitis (37% versus 12%).[150] In a further evaluation of these patients, the same investigators reported that skeletal muscle weakness was associated with wasting of extremity FFM that was independent of COPD subtype.[151]

PATHOPHYSIOLOGY

ENERGY

Several mechanisms have been proposed for the weight loss and malnutrition associated with COPD. First, patients with COPD have been shown to have an increased REE, with patients who are losing weight having significantly higher REE adjusted for FFM compared with weight-stable patients.[152] Total daily energy expenditure (TDE) also was found to be elevated in clinically stable COPD patients with both normal and increased REE.[153] Factors that may contribute to the increased REE include the oxygen cost of breathing, acute or chronic systemic inflammation, and medications.[146,153] The cause of elevated TDE despite a normal REE is still unknown. In addition to abnormal energy demands, patients with COPD may not consume adequate dietary intake to meet their needs, especially if they are more debilitated.[154]

Patients with acute respiratory failure also may have alterations in REE. Nonsurgical, septic patients who have acute respiratory failure requiring mechanical ventilation demonstrated a 20% increase in measured REE over the BEE predicted by the Harris-Benedict equation.[155] Other patients in this report who required mechanical ventilation and were not septic did not demonstrate hypermetabolism.[155] However, only small numbers of patients with the diagnosis of pneumonia or ARDS were studied, and their REE measurements also were increased at 200–300 kcal/d above BEE.[155] Thus nonseptic patients with acute respiratory failure may require only 10% to 20% above calculated BEE to meet nutrition needs. Patients with acute respiratory failure who are septic, however, may require energy at a level of 30% to 40% above the BEE.

CARBOHYDRATE

Early initiation of nutritional support, with the goal of meeting energy requirements, is beneficial in mechanically ventilated patients with acute pulmonary failure to limit ongoing wasting of respiratory muscles.[142] In addition, the ability of the respiratory system to respond to hypoxia and hypercapnia is decreased even early in semistarvation, but refeeding results in recovery of this respiratory drive.[143]

The benefits of refeeding patients with pulmonary failure must be weighed against the possible risks of increased carbon dioxide production and resulting hypercapnia.[143] This dilemma can be described based on respiratory quotient (RQ) values. The RQ is the ratio of the amount of CO_2 produced per amount of O_2 consumed in response to the oxidation of macronutrients by the human body. Thus oxidation of carbohydrate generates 1 mole of CO_2 for every mole of O_2 consumed, and the RQ for carbohydrate is 1.0.[144] Protein and fat oxidation produce RQs of 0.8 and 0.7, respectively.[144] The RQ for fat synthesis from carbohydrate is 8.0. These values demonstrate that when a subject is overfed with carbohydrate and net fat synthesis occurs, the amount of CO_2 produced markedly exceeds the amount of O_2 consumed, which can result in increased ventilatory demand.

Patients particularly at risk for nutrition-related increased CO_2 production are individuals with borderline ventilatory status who are not intubated.[143] In these patients, infusion of excessive carbohydrate-based intravenous nutrition can increase CO_2 production to the point where intubation may become necessary.[143] Overfeeding with glucose-based PN also has been associated with the inability to wean mechanical ventilation. Recommendations to reduce CO_2 production include (1) providing only the necessary caloric support, (2) substituting fat for some carbohydrate calories, and (3) changing to the enteral route to deliver nutritional needs.[143]

FAT

Administration of an intravenous fat emulsion to mechanically ventilated patients has the potential to adversely affect pulmonary gas exchange in some clinical conditions.[146] In a study of 48 mechanically ventilated patients with several types of respiratory failure, IVLE (500 mL of 10% solution) infused over 4 hours reduced oxygenation in patients with ARDS, but it had little effect in patients with COPD or infectious lung processes of less severity than ARDS.[156] When the IVLE administration rate was slowed to 8 hours in the ARDS patients, the adverse effects on oxygenation were reduced.[156] Initially, IVLE-related lung dysfunction was attributed to hyperlipemia. However, the clearance of triglycerides from IVLE actually is increased in critically ill patients compared with normal subjects. Intravenous infusions of fat have been shown to increase levels of prostaglandins E_2 and I_2, which have pulmonary vasodilatory effects, and elevated amounts of these substances could contribute to ventilation-perfusion inequalities associated with IVLE.[157] Studies of IVLE administration in septic patients with ARDS indicate a significant decrease in PO_2/FIO_2 (an index of oxygenation) and increases in mean pulmonary arterial pressure and pulmonary vasculature resistance.[158]

It is also important to consider the macronutrient composition of the diet in ambulatory COPD patients. In a review of nutritional intervention in COPD, studies investigating the effects of dietary intakes with varying percentages of fat content were evaluated.[159] Diets high in fat were found to place a lower demand on the respiratory system compared with diets with a higher carbohydrate content both immediately after a meal and when continued for a short duration ($\leq$2 weeks).[159]

PROTEIN

Undernourished patients have demonstrated a blunted response to hypercapnia that improves after as little as 1 week of adequate nutritional support. This response is thought to result from protein administration, as evidenced by decreased PCO_2, increased minute ventilation, and improved breathing patterns after the start of PN. Protein administration also may influence ventilatory demand by increased ventilatory response to hypoxia and hypercapnia.[146] This stimulation may be altered by the amino acid composition of the protein source, with increased amounts of BCAAs having a greater effect compared with standard amino acids.[144,146] Although this protein effect is potentially beneficial in some patients, it could lead to increased work of breathing and fatigue in individuals who already have an elevated respiratory drive (e.g., COPD or postoperative mechanical ventilation).[144]

FLUID AND ELECTROLYTES

In patients with ARDS or pulmonary edema, excessive fluid intake should be avoided, and it may be beneficial to restrict fluid intake.[144] An improved survival rate was reported in these patient groups if they did not have significant fluid gain in the ICU setting.[160] Patients in the ICU often receive substantial fluid loads from medication administration, and when possible, it is important to limit intake by concentrating these sources.

Alteration of micronutrient requirements in respiratory failure commonly is focused on phosphorus replacement. Phosphorus is essential in respiratory disease for its role in the synthesis of adenosine triphosphate (ATP) and 2,3-diphosphoglycerate (2,3-DPG).[144] Inadequate stores of ATP can lead to respiratory muscle weakness, and 2,3-DPG is essential for oxygen release from oxyhemoglobin.[144] In patients with acute respiratory failure, hypophosphatemia also has been shown to decrease diaphragmatic contractility.[161] In addition, mechanical ventilation actually can cause hypophosphatemia because the correction of respiratory acidosis will cause potassium and phosphorus to move intracellularly.[162] Finally, a significant percentage of critically ill patients can experience hypophosphatemia from refeeding.[163]

Most patients with moderate to severe hypophosphatemia and respiratory failure should be treated with intravenous sodium or potassium phosphate. Correction of hypophosphatemia using a graduated dosing scheme of phosphorus replacement for ICU patients receiving nutritional support has been reported (Table 139–4). In this study, use of the dosing regimen in ICU patients receiving nutritional support resulted in significant increases in serum phophorus at all levels of deficiency.[164]

ACID-BASE

Ventilator-dependent patients and those with stable COPD often have respiratory acidosis. A balanced mixture of chloride and acetate salts often is appropriate in these patients. The acid-base status of the ICU patient with pulmonary compromise should be monitored daily, whereas every 2 to 3 days may be adequate for the stable COPD patient.

TABLE 139–4. Acute Correction of Hypophosphatemia in the Critically Ill Patient

Serum Phosphorus Concentration (mg/dL)	Dose of Phosphorus (mmol/kg)
2.3–3.0	0.16
1.6–2.2	0.32
≤1.5	0.64

VITAMINS AND TRACE ELEMENTS

Patients with pulmonary disease usually do not have significant alterations in vitamin and trace element requirements, and they can receive standard doses of these micronutrients. Vitamins C and E, selenium, and β-carotene have been studied for their antioxidant properties in critically ill patients. In models for metabolic stress, antioxidants may decrease pentane production, but the role of supplementation of these compounds in ICU patients remains to be clarified.[165] COPD patients may have an increased burden of oxidants from cigarette smoke or release of oxygen free radicals from inflammatory leukocytes in the lungs, and deficiencies of antioxidants may contribute to oxidant/antioxidant imbalances in these individuals.[166] The value of supplementation of these substances in COPD will require further clarification.

► TREATMENT: Pulmonary Failure

ADMINISTRATION ROUTES

The enteral route is preferred for nutritional support in patients with acute and chronic respiratory failure.[143] The advantages of enteral feeding include preservation of gut integrity and immune function, reduction in infectious complications, and lower cost.[143,165] In acute pulmonary failure, PN support is recommended when the GI tract is not usable or as a supplement to EN if sufficient energy intake is not possible by the enteral route.[143,165]

SPECIALTY PRODUCTS

Most general EN formulas contain a balance of nonprotein energy between carbohydrate and fat. Elemental or chemically defined products are the exception because they are intended to be high-carbohydrate, low-fat formulas to enhance absorption and digestion. In general, administration of a high-carbohydrate formula will result in a significant increase in minute ventilation, heat production, and CO_2 production (V_{CO_2}) when compared with a high-fat formula. Because most general formulas contain balanced nonprotein calories, moderate doses of these products are appropriate in most patients with pulmonary disease.

Enteral formulas (e.g., *Pulmocare*, *NutriVent*, and Respalor) marketed for use specifically by patients with pulmonary disease are also available. In comparison with standard formulas, these products contain a higher percentage of nonprotein calories as fat. Several studies have evaluated the use of these products in patients with COPD and acute respiratory failure.[167–169]

The effects of a high-fat formula (Pulmocare) on respiratory demand and exercise tolerance were compared with a high-carbohydrate formula (Ensure Plus) and a noncaloric control liquid in 10 patients with severe stable COPD.[167] These patients underwent a 6-minute walk before and after consuming a 920-kcal meal of each formula or the control liquid in a randomized, crossover study design. Intake of the high-carbohydrate formula did result in significantly greater increases in minute ventilation, V_{CO_2}, O_2 consumption (V_{O_2}), RQ, and Pa_{CO_2} compared with the high-fat formula.[167] In addition to a higher demand on the respiratory system, the high-carbohydrate formula also resulted in a greater decline in the distance walked in 6 minutes and an increased perception of breathlessness.[167]

Akrabawi and colleagues compared the effects of two of these specialty products in patients with COPD.[168] In this study, the effect of a high-fat formula (55% fat calories; Pulmocare) versus a moderate-fat formula (41% fat calories; Respalor) on pulmonary function, gas exchange, RQ, and gastric emptying was determined. They found that V_{CO_2} and V_{O_2} were increased significantly at 30 and 90 minutes after ingestion of the moderate-fat formula, but at 150 minutes, the difference disappeared.[168] RQ was increased after ingestion of both products, with no significant difference in the values between formulas. The investigators noted that an increase in V_{CO_2} might exacerbate respiratory compromise; however, in stable patients, the clinical significance may be minimal due to the small effect.[168] They also reported that the higher rise in V_{CO_2} and V_{O_2} with the moderate-fat meal most likely was due to earlier gastric emptying found with this formula.[168] Delayed gastric emptying found with the higher-fat formula possibly could extend postingestion abdominal distension, affecting the diaphragm and lower thorax, which also could compromise respiratory status in COPD patients.[159]

In an investigation on acute respiratory failure, 32 patients weaning from mechanical ventilation were randomized to either a high-fat (Pulmocare) or high-carbohydrate (Ensure Plus) formula at 1.5 times BEE.[169] The patients receiving the high-fat formula demonstrated a significant decrease in RQ during mechanical ventilation and RQ and V_{CO_2} during weaning. The median time to receive mechanical ventilation was lower in the high-fat group (4 versus 6 days); however, this difference was not statistically significant.[169]

In summary, limited data now exist supporting the use of high-fat or moderate-fat enteral formulas in pulmonary patients. These specialized pulmonary EN products are calorically dense (1.5 kcal/mL), which may be helpful in feeding patients with severe ARDS or pulmonary edema and in others who may require fluid restriction.

An additional concentrated formula (Oxepa) has been marketed specifically for critically ill patients on mechanical ventilation. The macronutrient composition of Oxepa is similar to that of the other specialized pulmonary enteral formulas, with 55% of caloric content from fat. However, the lipid blend in the formula has been altered to potentially decrease the production of proinflammatory cytokines by including eicosapentaenoic acid (EPA) from fish oil and γ-linolenic acid (GLA) from borage oil. Nutrients with antioxidant properties (i.e., vitamin C, vitamin E, and β-carotene) also have been supplemented in the product. The effects of this formula when used as nutritional support in patients with ARDS was evaluated in a prospective, multicentered, double-blind, randomized, controlled trial.[170] In this study, Oxepa (EPA + GLA formula) was compared with a high-fat enteral product in 98 patients who received EN support at a caloric intake of 75% BEE times 1.3 for a minimum of 4 days. Patients who received the EPA + GLA formula had significantly decreased neutrophil counts in bronchoalveolar lavage fluid (a marker of pulmonary inflammation), fewer days of mechanical ventilation, and decreased length of ICU stay compared with those receiving the control formula.[170] The investigators concluded that use of the EPA + GLA formula would be beneficial for nutritional support and as adjuvant therapy in patients with ARDS or at risk for developing this disorder.[170] Further comparative studies will be valuable to determine the most appropriate use for this product and other EN formulas with potential immunomodulating properties.

There are some data addressing anabolic agents as adjunctive therapy to EN support in pulmonary patients. Improved lean body mass, maximal inspiratory pressure, and maximal exercise capacity have been reported in a small group of COPD patients receiving growth hormone plus EN.[171] Studies focusing on improved clinical outcome will need to be conducted before expensive biotechnology products can be used widely as adjunctive therapy to nutritional support in undernourished patients with respiratory disease.

DESIGN AND INITIATION OF NUTRITIONAL REGIMEN

In the patient with pulmonary failure, nutritional support should be given to meet energy and protein requirements and limit wasting of respiratory muscles.[142] No major alterations in substrate disposition have been noted in patients with pulmonary failure; thus moderate doses of intravenous carbohydrate, fat, and protein are appropriate in most conditions. In patients with borderline ventilatory status, the nutritional regimen should be monitored closely to prevent excessive CO_2 production, and adjustments of the proportion of nonprotein calories as fat and carbohydrate may be beneficial in some patients to decrease CO_2 production.[142] Ventilator-dependent patients in general can receive nonprotein calories administered within the following ranges, 55% to 80% carbohydrate and 20% to 45% lipid, because the oxidation of fat produces less CO_2 than glucose. Patients with sepsis and ARDS should be monitored closely during IVLE administration. Moderate doses of lipid (e.g., 1 g/kg/d) should be infused over a 24-hour period each day in these patients.[172] A reasonable protein dose is 1.0–1.5 g/kg per day for the patient with stable COPD. Patients who are mechanically ventilated with superimposed illness may require higher doses of protein (1.5–2.5 g/kg/d). An approach to the patient with respiratory failure requiring PN or EN support is shown in Figure 139–3.

Overfeeding with total calories in the pulmonary patient is probably as important to avoid as overfeeding with carbohydrates. Talpers and colleagues demonstrated a significant rise in V_{CO_2} in mechanically ventilated patients as total calories were increased from 1.0 to 1.5 and 2.0 times BEE.[173] When total calories were fixed at 1.3 times BEE, caloric composition (40% to 70% carbohydrate, 5% to 40% fat) had little effect on V_{CO_2}. In patients in whom fluid restriction is essential (e.g., severe ARDS) and PN is required, use of the more concentrated PN formulas with amino acids and IVLE is indicated. The use of dextrose 70%, amino acids 15%, and lipid 20% or 30% can deliver substantial calories in 1.5 L/d. An empirical PN formula for the patient with respiratory failure is shown in Table 139–2.

EVALUATION OF THERAPEUTIC OUTCOMES

It is clear that undernutrition is highly correlated with both impaired pulmonary function and mortality. Interventional studies of sufficient size and duration are needed to measure the impact of improvement in nutrition status on major clinical outcome indicators in patients with acute and chronic pulmonary failure. For patients with chronic respiratory failure (i.e., COPD), the effects of nutritional support on health-related quality of life and the ability to perform daily activities need to be ascertained.

▶ PRINCIPLES OF PHARMACOTHERAPY

- Carbohydrate calories absorbed via continuous renal replacement therapy must be accounted for when designing a PN/EN regimen of the patient with ARF.
- Lipid intolerance is common in ARF, requiring careful monitoring of serum triglyceride concentrations before and during IVLE administration.
- Protein requirements of the patient with ARF are highly variable and depend on PCR and dialytic losses of protein.
- Standard mixed amino acids should be used rather than EAA preparations in ARF.
- The nondialyzed patient with oliguric ARF should receive a PN/EN formula concentrated in a small volume.
- Empirical PN formulations for patients with ARF not on CRRT typically will contain minimal potassium, phosphorus, and

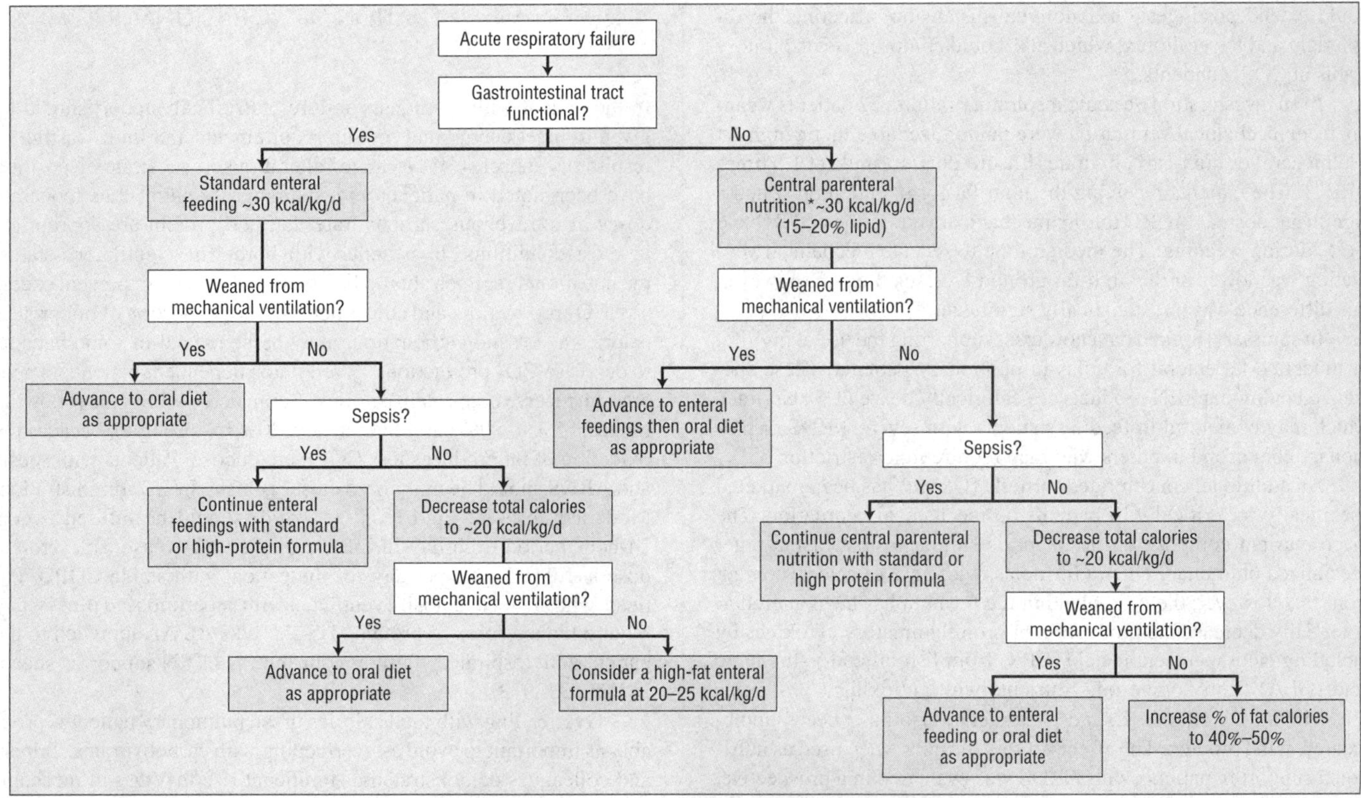

FIGURE 139–3. An algorithmic approach to nutritional support for the patient with acute respiratory failure. (*Some centers would consider peripheral PN, especially if the patient would require nutritional support for 1 week or less.)

magnesium. With refeeding, additional amounts of these electrolytes may need to be added.

- Sodium and potassium salts, if added to the PN formula for the patient with ARF, should be added as acetate salts.
- More than one-half of CRF patients experience hyperglycemia. Patients with ESRD who receive CAPD absorb substantial amounts (approximately 60%) of glucose from their peritoneal dialysate.
- Dialysate protein losses must be accounted for and added into the PN/EN nutritional plan for CRF patients. Peritoneal protein losses in patients treated by CAPD range from 6 to 7 g/d. The amount of protein lost via hemodialysis depends on membrane used and presence of reuse (typical range is from 6–12 g/dialysis).
- Although hyperkalemia and hyperphosphatemia are common early in the course of PN/EN with CRF patients, refeeding of these patients can result in hypokalemia and hypophosphatemia, warranting careful addition of these electrolytes to the PN/EN regimen.
- Calorically dense, low-electrolyte formulas may prove helpful in providing EN to the CRF or ESRD patient with preexisting electrolyte disturbances or volume overload. Likewise, the PN formula for these patients can be volume restricted by using higher concentrations of dextrose and amino acids ($D_{35}W$ and 7.5% amino acid final concentrations).
- Patients with alcoholic hepatitis or cirrhosis are frequently hypermetabolic.
- Hyperglycemia is common in cirrhosis. Patients with fulminant hepatitis are prone instead to hypoglycemia.
- Patients with liver disease may require zinc supplementation while receiving restricted amounts of copper and manganese.
- Folic acid and thiamine supplementation is important in patients with liver disease for the prevention of anemia and Wernicke's encephalopathy, respectively.
- For the OLT patient, energy provision of 1.2 times BEE with at least 1.2 g/kg per day of protein is appropriate.
- The high prevalence of postoperative hyperglycemia in the OLT patient mandates starting PN/EN slowly and with a low-dextrose-concentration formulation.
- Sodium rarely needs to be added to the PN solution of an OLT patient.
- Supplemental doses of calcium and magnesium are frequently required for the OLT patient.
- Pre-OLT patients frequently demonstrate depressed serum concentrations of zinc and vitamin A; these usually normalize after OLT, obviating the need for further supplementation.
- In SBS, PN should be used to meet nutritional needs in the postoperative period after intestinal resection.
- As small bowel adaptation occurs, some SBS patients receiving PN can be transitioned successfully to EN. Early initiation of enteral intake affects adaptation because intraluminal nutrients are a stimulus for this process.
- Increased fluid and electrolyte intake may be necessary in SBS patients to replace GI losses. In addition, patients may need increased calcium, magnesium, zinc, and other trace elements due to decreased absorption and/or excessive GI losses.
- SBS patients with a distal ileal resection are at risk for vitamin B_{12} deficiency and need PN replacement. Deficiencies of fat-soluble vitamins can occur in patients with fat malabsorption.
- Nonseptic patients with acute respiratory failure require only 10% to 20% above BEE to meet nutritional needs, whereas patients who are septic need to be given energy at 30% to 40% above BEE.

- Undernourished patients with pulmonary disease have a blunted response to hypercapnia that improves with nutritional support. However, excessive protein intake should be avoided because it may increase pulmonary workload.
- Excessive infusions of salt and water should be avoided in patients with pulmonary disease because they may exacerbate already compromised pulmonary function.
- The incidence of hypophosphatemia is higher in patients with pulmonary disease than in the general hospitalized population.
- Nutritional support is beneficial in optimizing respiratory muscle function in patients with pulmonary failure.
- In patients with pulmonary failure, overfeeding of total calories and carbohydrates should be avoided, particularly with PN, to prevent excessive CO_2 production.
- The incidence of hypophosphatemia is higher in patients with pulmonary disease than in the general hospitalized population.
- High-fat or moderate-fat EN formulas should be considered for use in patients with pulmonary disease.

REFERENCES

1. Kopple JD. Effect of nutrition of morbidity and mortality in maintenance dialysis patients. Am J Kidney Dis 1994;24:1002–1009.
2. Yang CS, Chen SW, Chiang CH, et al. Effect of increasing dialysis dose on serum albumin and mortality in hemodialysis patients. Am J Kidney Dis 1996;27:380–386.
3. Spiegel DM, Breyer JA. Serum albumin: A predictor of long-term outcome in peritoneal dialysis patients. Am J Kidney Dis 1994;23:283–285.
4. Struijk DG, Krediet RT, Koomen GC, et al. The effect of serum albumin at the start of CAPD treatment on patient survival. Perit Dial Int 1994;14:121–126.
5. Kopple JD. Dietary protein and energy requirements in ESRD patients. Am J Kidney Dis 1998;32(6 Suppl 4):S97–S104.
6. Ikizler TA, Greene JH, Yenicesu M, et al. Nitrogen balance in hospitalized chronic hemodialysis patients. Kidney Int 1996:50(Suppl): S53–S56.
7. Molina MF, Riella MC. Nutritional support in the patient with renal failure. Crit Care Clin 1995;11:685–704.
8. Ikizler TA, Hakim RM. Nutrition in end-stage renal disease. Kidney Int 1996;50:343–357.
9. Ikizler TA, Himmelfarb J. Nutrition in acute renal failure. Adv Ren Replace Ther 1997;4:54–63.
10. Fiaccadori E, Lombardi M, Leonardi S, et al. Prevalence and clinical outcome associated with pre-existing malnutrition in acute renal failure: A prospective cohort study. J Am Soc Nephrol 1999;10:581–593.
11. Kierdorf HP. The nutritional management of acute renal failure in the intensive care unit. New Horizons 1995;3:699–707.
12. Alvestrand A. Nutritional aspects in patients with acute renal failure/multiorgan failure. Blood Purif 1996;14:109–114.
13. Bouffard Y, Viale JP, Annat G, et al. Energy expenditure in the acute renal failure patient mechanically ventilated. Intensive Care Med 1987;13: 401–404.
14. Fougue D. Insulin-like growth factor 1 resistance in chronic renal failure. Miner Electrolyte Metab 1996;22:133–137.
15. Keane WF. Lipids and the kidney. Kidney Int 1994;46:910–920.
16. Gupta KL, Majumdar S, Sakhuja V. Postheparin lipolytic activity in acute and chronic renal failure. Ren Fail 1994;16:609–615.
17. Maheux P, Azhar S, Kern PA, et al. Relationship between insulin-mediated glucose disposal and regulation of plasma and adipose tissue lipoprotein lipase. Diabetologia 1997;40:850–858.
18. Ikizler TA, Greene JH, Wingard RL, et al. Nitrogen balance in acute renal failure (ARF) patients (Abstract). J Am Soc Nephrol 1995;6:466.
19. Macias WL, Alaka KJ, Murphy MH, et al. Impact of the nutritional regimen on protein catabolism and nitrogen balance in patients with acute renal failure. J Parenter Enter Nutr 1996;20:56–62.
20. Druml W. Protein metabolism in acute renal failure. Miner Electrolyte Metab 1998;24:47–54.
21. Cooney RN, Kimball SR, Vary TC. Regulation of skeletal muscle protein turnover during sepsis: Mechanisms and mediators. Shock 1997;7:1–16.
22. Hynote ED, McCamish MA, Depner TA, Davis PA. Amino acid losses during hemodialysis: Effects of high-solute flux and parenteral nutrition in acute renal failure. J Parenter Enter Nutr 1995;19:15–21.
23. Maxvold NJ, Smoyer WE, Custer JR, Bunchman TE. Amino acid loss and nitrogen balance in critically ill children with acute renal failure: A prospective comparison between classic hemofiltration and hemofiltration with dialysis. Crit Care Med 2000;28:1161–1165.
24. Druml W, Fischer M, Liebisch B, et al. Elimination of amino acids in renal failure. Am J Clin Nutr 1994;60:418–423.
25. Novak I, Sramek V, Pittrova H, et al. Glutamine and other amino acid losses during continuous venovenous hemodiafiltration. Artif Organs 1997;21:359–363.
26. Packman KS, Demeure MJ. Indications for parathyroidectomy and extent of treatment for patients with secondary hyperparathyroidism. Surg Clin North Am 1995;75:465–482.
27. Locatelli F, Pontoriero G, DiFilippo S. Electrolyte disorders and substitution fluid in continuous renal replacement therapy. Kidney Int Suppl 1998;66:S151–S155.
28. Meier-Kriesche HU, Finkel KW, Gitomer JJ, DuBose TD Jr. Unexpected severe hypocalcemia during continuous venovenous hemodialysis with regional citrate anticoagulation. Am J Kidney Dis 1999;33:e8.
29. Heering P, Ivens K, Thumer O, et al. The use of different buffers during continuous hemofiltration in critically ill patients with acute renal failure. Intensive Care Med 1999;25:1244–1251.
30. Gallieni M, Brancaccio D, Cozzolino M, Sabbioni E. Trace elements in renal failure: Are they clinically important? Nephrol Dial Transplant 1996;11:1232–1235.
31. Metnitz GH, Fischer M, Bartens C, et al. Impact of acute renal failure on antioxidant status in multiple organ failure. Acta Anaesthesiol Scand 2000;44:236–240.
32. Makropoulos W, Heintz B, Stefanidis I. Selenium deficiency and thyroid function in acute renal failure. Ren Fail 1997;19:129–136.
33. Gallieni M, Pietra R, Canavese C, et al. Trace elements in serum and tissues of dialysis patients (Abstract). J Am Soc Nephrol 1995;6:530.
34. Wolk R. Micronutrition in dialysis. Nutr Clin Prac 1993;8:257–276.
35. Druml W, Schwarzenhofer M, Apsner R, Horl WH. Fat-soluble vitamins in patients with acute renal failure. Miner Electrolyte Metab 1998;24:220–226.
36. Frankenfield DC, Reynolds HN. Nutritional effect of continuous hemodiafiltration. Nutrition 1995;11:388–393.
37. Seidner DL, Matarese LE, Steiger E. Nutritional care of the critically ill patient with renal failure. Semin Nephrol 1994;14:53–63.
38. Frankenfield DC, Reynolds HN, Badellino MM, Wiles CE. Glucose dynamics during continuous hemodiafiltration and total parenteral nutrition. Intensive Care Med 1995;21:1016–1022.
39. Bellomo R, Martin H, Parkin G, et al. Continuous arteriovenous haemodiafiltration in the critically ill: Influence on major nutrient balances. Intensive Care Med 1991;17:399–402.
40. Druml W, Fischer M, Sertl S, et al. Fat elimination in acute renal failure: Long chain versus medium chain triglycerides. Am J Clin Nutr 1992;55:468–472.
41. Bellomo R, Seacombe J, Daskalakis M, et al. A prospective comparative study of moderate versus high protein intake for critically ill patients with acute renal failure. Ren Fail 1997;1:111–120.
42. Aparicio M, Cano N, Chauveau P, et al. Nutritional status of haemodialysis patients: A French national cooperative study. French study group for nutrition in dialysis. Nephrol Dial Transplant 1999;14:1679–1686.
43. Chung SH, Lindholm B, Lee HB. Influence of initial nutritional status on continuous ambulatory peritoneal dialysis patient survival. Perit Dial Int 2000;20:19–26.
44. Sehgal AR. Outcomes of renal replacement therapy among blacks and women. Am J Kidney Dis 2000;35(4 Suppl 1):S148–S152.
45. Avram MM, Mittman N, Bonomini L, et al. Markers for survival in dialysis: A seven-year prospective study. Am J Kid Dis 1995;26:209–219.

46. Avram MM, Bonomini LV, Sreedhara R, Mittman N. Predictive value of nutritional markers (albumin, creatinine, cholesterol, and hematocrit) for patients on dialysis for up to 30 years. Am J Kidney Dis 1996;28:910–917.
47. Steiber AL. Clinical indicators associated with poor oral intake of patients with chronic renal failure. J Ren Nutr 1999;9:84–88.
48. Frey S, Mir AR, Lucas M. Visceral protein status and caloric intake in exercising versus nonexercising individuals with end-stage renal disease. J Ren Nutr 1999;9:71–77.
49. NKF-K/DOQI. Clinical practice guidelines for nutrition support in chronic renal failure. Am J Kidney Dis 2000;35(6 Suppl 2):S17–S104.
50. Gao H, Lew SQ, Bosch JP. Biochemical parameters, nutritional status and efficiency of dialysis in CAPD and CCPD patients. Am J Nephrol 1999;19:7–12.
51. Evans AM, Faull R, Fornasini G, et al. Pharmacokinetics of L-carnitine in patients with end-stage renal disease undergoing long-term hemodialysis. Clin Pharmacol Ther 2000;68:238–249.
52. Stenvinkel P, Lindholm B, Lonnqvist F, et al. Increases in serum leptin levels during peritoneal dialysis are associated with inflammation and a decrease in lean body mass. J Am Soc Nephrol 2000;11:1303–1309.
53. Nishikawa M, Takagi T, Yoshikawa N, et al. Measurements of serum leptin in patients with chronic renal failure on hemodialysis. Clin Nephrol 1999;51:296–303.
54. Levey AS, Adler S, Caggiula AW, et al. Effects of dietary protein restriction on the progression of advanced renal disease in the modification of diet in renal disease study. Am J Kidney Dis 1996;27:652–663.
55. Kasiske BL, Lakatua JD, Ma JZ, Louis TA. A meta-analysis of the effects of dietary protein restriction on the rate of decline in renal function. Am J Kidney Dis 1998;31(6):954–961.
56. Aparicio M, Chauveau P, Combe C. Are supplemented low-protien diets nutritionally safe? Am J Kidney Dis 2001;37(Suppl 2):S71–S76.
57. Soroka N, Silverberg DS, Greemland M, et al. Comparison of a vegetable-based (soy) and an animal-based low-protein diet in predialysis chronic renal failure patients. Nephron 1998;79:173–180.
58. Kabanda A, Goffin E, Bernard A, et al. Factors influencing serum levels and peritoneal clearances of low molecular weight proteins in continuous ambulatory peritoneal dialysis. Kidney Int 1995;48:1946–1952.
59. Harty JC, Boulton H, Venning MC, Gokal R. Is peritoneal permeability an adverse risk factor for malnutrition in CAPD patients? Miner Electrolyte Metab 1996;22:97–101.
60. Ikizler TA, Flakoll PJ, Parker RA, Hakim RM. Amino acid and albumin losses during hemodialysis. Kidney Int 1994;46:830–837.
61. Lofberg E, Wenerman J, Anderstam B, Bergstrom J. Correction of acidosis in dialysis patients increases branched-chain and total essential amino acid levels in muscle. Clin Nephrol 1997;48:230– 237.
62. Stein A, Moorhouse J, Iles-Smith H, et al. Role of an improvement in acid-base status and nutrition in CAPD patients. Kidney Int 1997;52:1089–1095.
63. Thomson NM, Stevens BJ, Humphrey TJ, et al. Comparison of trace elements in peritoneal dialysis, hemodialysis, and uremia. Kidney Int 1983;23:9–14.
64. Zima T, Mestek O, Nemecek K, et al. Trace elements in hemodialysis and continuous ambulatory peritoneal dialysis patients. Blood Purif 1998;16:253–260.
65. Temple KA, Smith AM, Cockram DB. Selenate-supplemented nutritional formula increases plasma selenium in hemodialysis patients. J Ren Nutr 2000;10:16–23.
66. Bogye G, Tompos G, Alfthan G. Selenium depletion in hemodialysis patients treated with polysulfone membranes. Nephron 2000;84:119–123.
67. Mydlik M, Derzsiova K, Svac J, et al. Peritoneal clearance and peritoneal transfer of oxalic acid, vitamin C, and vitamin B_6 during continuous ambulatory peritoneal dialysis. Artif Organs 1998;22:784–788.
68. Wang S, Eide TC, Sogn EM, et al. Plasma ascorbic acid in patients undergoing chronic haemodialysis. Eur J Clin Pharmacol 1999;55:527–532.
69. Yonemura K, Fujimoto T, Fujigaki Y, Hishida A. Vitamin D deficiency is implicated in reduced serum albumin concentrations in patients with end-stage renal disease. Am J Kidney Dis 2000;36:337–344.
70. Islam KN, O'Byrne D, Devaraj S, et al. Alpha-tocopherol supplementation decreases the oxidative susceptibility of LDL in renal failure patients on dialysis therapy. Atherosclerosis 2000;150:217–224.
71. Jung U, Helbich-Endermann M, Bitsch R, et al. Are patients with chronic renal failure (CRF) deficient in biotin and is regular biotin supplementation required? Z Ernahrungswiss 1998;37:363–367.
72. Frank T, Czeche K, Bitsch R, Stein G. Assessment of thiamin status in chronic renal failure patients, transplant recipients, and hemodialysis patients receiving a multivitamin supplementation. Int J Vitam Nutr Res 2000;70:159–166.
73. Dierkes J, Domrose U, Ambrosch A, et al. Response of hyperhomocysteinemia to folic acid supplementation in patients with end-stage renal disease. Clin Nephrol 1999;51:108–115.
74. Sunder-Plassmann G, Fodinger M, Buchmayer H, et al. Effect of high dose folic acid therapy on hyperhomocysteinemia in hemodialysis patients: Results of the Vienna multicenter study. J Am Soc Nephrol 2000;11:1106–1116.
75. Foulks CJ. An evidence-based evaluation of intradialytic parenteral nutrition. Am J Kidney Dis 1999;33:186–192.
76. Chazot C, Shahmir E, Matias B, et al. Dialytic nutrition: Provision of amino acids in dialysate during hemodialysis. Kidney Int 1997;52:1663–1670.
77. Kopple JD, Bernard D, Messana J, et al. Treatment of malnourished CAPD patients with an amino acid based dialysate. Kidney Int 1995; 47:1148–1157.
78. Jones CH, Smith M, Henderson MJ, et al. Fasting plasma amino acids are not normalized by 12-month amino acid-based dialysate in CAPD patients. Perit Dial Int 1999;19:174–177.
79. Iglesias P, Diez JJ, Fernandez-Reyes MJ, et al. Recombinant human growth hormone therapy in malnourished dialysis patients: A randomized, controlled study. Am J Kidney Dis 1998;32:454–463.
80. Hirsch S, Bunout D, Maza P, et al. Controlled trial on nutrition supplementation in outpatients with symptomatic alcoholic cirrhosis. J Parenter Enter Nutr 1993;17:119–124.
81. Mendenhall CL, Moritz TE, Roselle GA, et al. Protein energy malnutrition in severe alcoholic hepatitis: Diagnosis and response to treatment. J Parenter Enter Nutr 1995;19:258–265.
82. Moriwaki H, Tajika M, Miwa Y, et al. Nutritional pharmacotherapy of chronic liver disease: From support of liver failure to prevention of liver cancer. J Gastroenterol 2000;35(Suppl 12):13–17.
83. Campillo B, Bories PN, Pornin B, Devanley M. Influence of liver failure, ascites, and energy expenditure on the response to oral nutrition in alcoholic cirrhotic patients. Nutrition 1997;13:613–621.
84. Muller MJ, Loyal S, Schwarze M, et al. Resting energy expenditure and nutritional state in patients with liver cirrhosis before and after liver transplant. Clin Nutr 1994;13:145–152.
85. Schenker S, Halff GA. Nutritional therapy in alcoholic liver disease. Semin Liver Dis 1993;13:196–209.
86. Clemmesen JO, Hoy CE, Jeppesen PB, Ott P. Plasma phospholipid fatty acid pattern in severe liver disease. J Hepatol 2000;32:481–487.
87. Duerksen DR, Nehra V, Palombo JD, et al. Essential fatty acid deficiencies in patients with chronic liver disease are not reversed by short-term intravenous lipid supplementation. Dig Dis Sci 1999;44:1342–1348.
88. Druml W, Fischer M, Ratheiser K. Use of intravenous lipids in critically ill patients with sepsis without and with hepatic failure. J Parenter Enter Nutr 1998;22:217–223.
89. Marsano L, McClain CJ. Nutrition and alcoholic liver disease. J Parenter Enteral Nutr 1991;15:337–344.
90. Chacko RT, Chacko A. Serum and muscle magnesium in Indians with cirrhosis of liver. Indian J Med Res 1997;106:469–474.
91. McClain CJ, Marsano L, Burk RF, Bacon B. Trace metals in liver disease. Semin Liver Dis 1991;11:321–339.
92. Hauser RA, Zesiewicz TA, Rosemurgy AS, et al. Manganese intoxication and chronic liver failure. Ann Neurol 1994;36:871–875.

93. Layrargues GP, Rose C, Spahr L, et al. Role of manganese in the pathogenesis of portal-systemic encephalopathy. Metab Brain Dis 1998;13: 311–317.
94. Rose C, Butterworth FR, Zayed J, et al. Manganese deposition in basal ganglia structures results from both portal-systemic shunting and liver dysfunction. Gastroenterology 1999;117:640–644.
95. Janczewska I, Ericzon BG, Eriksson LS. Influence of orthotopic liver transplantation on serum vitamin A levels in patients with chronic liver disease. Scand J Gastroenterol 1995;30:68–71.
96. Nompleggi DJ, Bonkovsky HL. Nutritional supplementaion in chronic liver diease: An analytical review. Hepatology 1994;19:518–533.
97. Ichida T, Shibasaki K, Muto Y, et al. Clinical study of an enteral branched-chain amino acid solution in decompensated liver cirrhosis with hepatic encephalopathy. Nutrition 1995;11(Suppl 2):238–244.
98. Marchesini G, Fabbri A, Bianchi G, et al. Zinc supplementation and amino acid-nitrogen metabolism in patients with advanced cirrhosis. Hepatology 1996;23:1084–1092.
99. Calamita A, Dichi I, Papini-Berto SJ, et al. Plasma levels of transthyretin and retinol-binding protein in Child-A cirrhotic patients in relation to protein-calorie status and plasma amino acids, zinc, vitamin A, and plasma thyroid hormones. Arq Gastroenterol 1997;34:139–147.
100. Figueiredo FA, Dickson ER, Pasha TM, et al. Utility of standard nutritional parameters in detecting body cell mass depletion in patients with end-stage liver disease. Liver Transplant 2000;6:575–581.
101. Plevak DJ, DiCecco SR, Wiesner RH, et al. Nutritional support for liver transplantation: Identifying caloric and protein requirements. Mayo Clin Proc 1994;69:225–230.
102. Harrison J, McKiernan J, Neuberger JM. A prospective study on the effect of recipient nutritional status on outcome in liver transplantation. Transplant Int 1997;10:369–374.
103. LeCornu KA, McKiernan FJ, Kapadia SA, Neuberger JM. A prospective randomized study of preoperative nutritional supplementation in patients awaiting elective orthotopic liver transplantation. Transplantation 2000;69:1364–1369.
104. Dresner LS, Andersen DK, Kahng KU, et al. Effects of cyclosporine on glucose metabolism. Surgery 1989;106:163–170.
105. Konrad T, Steinmuller T, Vicini P, et al. Evidence for impaired glucose effectiveness in cirrhotic paitents after liver transplantation. Metabolism 2000;49:367–372.
106. Iapichino G, Radrizzani D, Bonetti G, et al. Early metabolic treatment after liver transplant: Amino acid tolerance. Intensive Care Med 1995;21:802–807.
107. Delafosse B, Viale JP, Pachiaudi C, et al. Long- and medium-chain triglycerides during parenteral nutrition in critically ill patients. Am J Physiol 1997;272:E550–E555.
108. Pescovitz MD, Mehta PL, Jindal RM, et al. Zinc deficiency and its repletion following liver transplantation in humans. Clin Transplant 1996;10: 256–260.
109. Pan SH, Lopez RR, Sher LS, et al. Enhanced oral cyclosporine absorption with water-soluble vitamin E early after liver transplantation. Pharmacotherapy 1996;16:59–65.
110. Monegal A, Navasa M, Guanabens N, et al. Osteoporosis and bone mineral metabolism disorders in cirrhotic patients referred for orthotopic liver transplantation. Calcif Tissue Int 1997;60:148–154.
111. Feller RB, McDonald JA, Sherbon KJ, McGaughan GW. Evidence of continuing bone recovery at a mean of 7 years after liver transplantation. Liver Transplant Surg 1999;5:407–413.
112. Bishop NJ, Ninkovic M, Alexander GJ, et al. Changes in calcium homeostasis in patients undergoing liver transplantation: Effects of a single infusion of pamidronate administered pre-operatively. Clin Sci 1999;97:157–163.
113. Ng TM, Bajjoka IE. Treatment options for osteoporosis in chronic liver disease patients requiring liver transplantation. Ann Pharmacother 1999;33:233–235.
114. Hasse JM, Blue LS, Liepa GU, et al. Early enteral nutrition in patients undergoing liver transplantation. J Parenter Enter Nutr 1995;19:437–443.
115. Wicks C, Somasundaram S, Bjarnason I, et al. Comparison of enteral feedings and total parenteral nutrition after liver transplantation. Lancet 1994;344:837–840.
116. Mehta PL, Alaka KJ, Filo RS, Leapman SB. Nutritional support following liver transplantation: Comparison of jejunal versus parenteral routes. Clin Transplant 1995;9:364–369.
117. Selberg O, Bottcher J, Tusch G, et al. Identification of high- and low-risk patients before liver transplantation: A prospective cohort study of nutritional and metabolic parameters in 150 patients. Hepatology 1997;25:652–657.
118. Reilly J, Mehta R, Teperman L, et al. Nutritional support after liver transplantation: A randomized, prospective study. J Parenter Enter Nutr 1990;14:386.
119. Vanderhoof JA, Langnas AN. Short bowel syndrome in children and adults. Gastroenterology 1997;113:1767–1778.
120. Scolapio JS, Fleming CR. Short bowel syndrome. Gastroenterol Clin North Am 1998;27:467–479.
121. Wilmore D, Byrne TA, Persinger RL. Short bowel syndrome: New therapeutic approaches. Curr Probl Surg 1997;34:391–444.
122. Forbes A, Chadwick C. Short bowel syndrome. In: Souba WW, Kohn-Keeth C, Mueller C, et al., eds. The A.S.P.E.N. Nutrition Support Practice Manuel, Vol 15. Silver Spring, MD, American Society for Parenteral and Enteral Nutrition, 1998:1–10.
123. Kvietys PR. Intestinal physiology relevant to short-bowel syndrome. Eur J Pediatr Surg 1999;9:196–199.
124. Messing B, Pigot F, Rongier M, et al. Intestinal absorption of free oral hyperalimentation in the very short bowel syndrome. Gastroenterology 1991;100:1502–1508.
125. Abushufa R, Reed P, Weinkove C, et al. Essential fatty acid status in patients on long-term home parenteral nutrition. J Parenter Enter Nutr 1995;19:286–290.
126. Royall D, Wolever TMS, Jeejeebhoy KN. Evidence for colonic conservation of malabsorbed carbohydrate in short bowel syndrome. Am J Gastroenterol 1992;87:751–756.
127. Nightingale JMD, Lennard-Jones JE, Walker ER, Farthing MJG. Jejunal efflux in short bowel syndrome. Lancet 1990;336:765–768.
128. Jeejeebhoy KN. Metabolic bone disease and total parenteral nutrition: a progress report. Am J Clin Nutr 1998;67:186–187.
129. Fleming CR, George L, Stoner GL, et al. The importance of urinary magnesium values in patients with gut failure. Mayo Clin Proc 1996;71: 21–24.
130. Vanderhoof JA, Young RJ, Murray N, Kaufman SS. Treatment strategies for small bowel bacterial overgrowth in short bowel syndrome. J Pediatr Gastroenterol Nutr 1998;27:155–160.
131. Rannem T, Hylander E, Ladefoged K, et al. The metabolism of [^{75}Se]selenite in patients with short bowel syndrome. J Parenter Enter Nutr 1996;20:412–416.
132. Shanbhogue LKR, Molenaar JC. Short bowel syndrome: Metabolic and surgical management. Br J Surg 1994;81:486–499.
133. Kurkchubasche AG, Smith SD, Rowe MI. Catheter sepsis in short-bowel syndrome. Arch Surg 1992;127:21–25.
134. McIntyre PB, Fitchew M, Lennard-Jones JE. Patients with a high jejuostomy do not need a special diet. Gastroenterology 1986;91: 25–33.
135. McFadden MA, DeLegge MH, Kirby DF. Medication delivery in the short-bowel syndrome. Parenter Enter Nutr 1993;17:180–186.
136. Byrne TA, Persinger RL, Young LS, et al. A new treatment for patients with short-bowel syndrome. Ann Surg 1995;222:243–255.
137. Ellegard L, Bosaeus I, Nordgren S, Bengtsson B. Low-dose recombinant human growth hormone increased body weight and lean body mass in patients with short bowel syndrome. Ann Surg 1997;225: 88–96.
138. Scolapio JS. Effect of growth hormone, glutamine, and diet on body composition in short bowel syndrome: A randomized, controlled study. J Parenter Enter Nutr 1999;23:309–313.
139. Messing B, Crenn P, Beau P, et al. Long-term survival and parenteral nutrition dependence in adult patients with the short bowel syndrome. Gastroenterology 1999;117:1043–1050.

140. Howard L, Ament M, Fleming CR, et al. Current use and clinical outcomes of home parenteral and enteral nutrition therapies in the United States. Gastroenterology 1995;109:355–365.
141. Smith CE. Quality of life in long-term total parenteral nutrition patients and their family caregivers. J Parenter Enter Nutr 1993;17:501–506.
142. ASPEN Board of Directors. Guidelines for the use of parenteral and enteral nutrition in adult and pediatric patients: Respiratory failure. J Parenter Enter Nutr 1993;17:17SA.
143. Grant JP. Nutrition care of patients with acute and chronic respiratory failure. Nutr Clin Prac 1994;9:11–17.
144. Mowatt-Larssen CA, Brown RO. Specialized nutritional support in respiratory disease. Clin Pharm 1993;12:276–292.
145. Wouters EF. Nutrition and metabolism in COPD. Chest 2000;117:274S–280S.
146. Donahoe M. Nutritional support in advanced lung disease: The pulmonary cachexia syndrome. Clin Chest Med 1997;18:547–561.
147. Sahebjami H, Doers JT, Render ML, Bond TL. Anthropometric and pulmonary function test profiles of outpatients with stable chronic obstructive pulmonary disease. Am J Med 1993;94:469–474.
148. Pouw EM, Ten Velde GP, Croonen BH, et al. Early nonelective readmission for chronic obstructive pulmonary disease is associated with weight loss. Clin Nutr 2000;19:95–99.
149. Baarends EM, Schols AM, Mostert R, Wouters EF. Peak exercise response in relation to tissue depletion in patients with chronic obstructive pulmonary disease. Eur Respir J 1997;10:2807–2813.
150. Engelen MP, Schols AM, Lamers RJ, Wouters EF. Different patterns of chronic tissue wasting among patients with chronic obstructive pulmonary disease. Clin Nutr 1999;18:275–280.
151. Engelen MP, Schols AM, Does JD, Wouters EF. Skeletal muscle weakness is associated with wasting of extremity fat-free mass but not with airflow obstruction in patients with chronic obstructive pulmonary disease. Am J Clin Nutr 2000;71:733–738.
152. Schols AM, Fredrix EW, Soeters PB, et al. Resting energy expenditure in patients with chronic obstructive pulmonary disease. Am J Clin Nutr 1991;54:983–987.
153. Baarends EM, Schols AM, Westerterp KR, Wouters EF. Total daily energy expenditure relative to resting energy expenditure in clinically stable patients with COPD. Thorax 1997;52:780–785.
154. Schols AM, Soeters PB, Mostert R, et al. Energy balance in chronic obstructive pulmonary disease. Am Rev Respir Dis 1991;143:1248–1252.
155. Liggett SB, Renfro AD. Energy expenditures of mechanically ventilated nonsurgical patients. Chest 1990; 98:682–686.
156. Hwang TL, Huang SL, Chen MF. Effects of intravenous fat emulsion on respiratory failure. Chest 1990;97:934–938.
157. Hageman JR, Hunt CE. Fat emulsions and lung function. Clin Chest Med 1986;7:69–77.
158. Venus B, Smith RA, Patel C, Sandoval E. Hemodynamic and gas exchange alterations during Intralipid infusion in patients with adult respiratory distress syndrome. Chest 1989;95:1278–1281.
159. Ferreira IM, Brooks D, Lacasse Y, Goldstein RS. Nutritional intervention in COPD: A systematic overview. Chest 2001;119:353–363.
160. Schuller D, Mitchell JP, Calandrino FS, Schuster DP. Fluid balance during pulmonary edema: Is fluid gain a marker or a cause of poor outcome? Chest 1991;100:1068–1075.
161. Aubier M, Murciano D, LecocguicY, et al. Effect of hypophosphatemia on diaphragmatic contractility in patients with acute respiratory failure. New Engl J Med 1985;313:420–424.
162. Laaban JP, Grateau G, Psychoyos I, et al. Hypophosphatemia induced by mechanical ventilation in patients with chronic obstructive pulmonary disease. Crit Care Med 1989;17:1115–1120.
163. Marik PE, Bedigian MK. Refeeding hypophosphatemia in critically ill patients in an intensive care unit. Arch Surg 1996;131:1043–1047.
164. Clark CL, Sacks GS, Dickerson RN, et al. Treatment of hypophosphatemia in patients receiving specialized nutrition support using a graduated dosing scheme: Results from a prospective clinical trial. Crit Care Med 1995;23:1504–1511.
165. Cerra FB, Benitez MR, Blackburn GL, et al. ACCP consensus statement: applied nutrition in ICU patients. Chest 1997;111:769–778.
166. MacNee W. Oxidants/antioxidants and COPD. Chest 2000;117:303S–317S.
167. Efthimiou J, Mounsey PF, Benson DN, et al. Effect of carbohydrate rich versus fat rich loads on gas exchange and walking performance in patients with chronic obstructive lung disease. Thorax 1992;47:451–456.
168. Akrabawi SS, Mobarhan S, Stoltz RR, Ferguson PW. Gastric emptying, pulmonary function, gas exchange, and respiratory quotient after feeding a moderate versus high fat enteral formula meal in chronic obstructive pulmonary disease patients. Nutrition 1996;12:260–265.
169. Van den Berg B, Bogaard JM, Hop WC. High fat, low carbohydrate, enteral feeding in patients weaning from the ventilator. Intensive Care Med 1994;20:470–475.
170. Gadek J, DeMichele SJ, Karlstad MD, et al. Effect of enteral feeding with eicosapentaenoic acid, γ-linolenic acid, and antioxidants in patients with acute respiratory distress syndrome. Crit Care Med 1999;27:1409–1420.
171. Burdet L, deMuralt B, Shutz Y, et al. Administration of growth hormone to underweight patients with chronic severe pulmonary disease: A prospective, ramdomized, controlled study. Am J Respir Crit Care Med 1997;156:1800–1806.
172. Skeie B, Askanazi J, Rothkopf MM, et al. Intravenous fat emulsion and lung function: A review. Crit Care Med 1988;16:183–194.
173. Talpers SS, Romberger DJ, Bunce SB, Pingleton SK. Nutritionally associated increased carbon dioxide production: Excess total calories vs. high proportion of carbohydrate calories. Chest 1992;102:551–555.

140

OBESITY

John V. St. Peter and Mehmood A. Khan

Obesity, a state of excess body fat stores, is considered a disease by some and predominantly a social problem by others. Each year millions of Americans—an estimated 15% to 35% of the population—resolve to lose weight, especially at the start of the calendar year.[1–4] Within months, weeks, or even days, the vast majority give up on this resolve without any weight loss. Many others ultimately will regain the weight that they lost initially. An estimated $30 to $50 billion is spent each year by Americans with little or no documented improvement.[5,6] Prospective evidence to support weight loss programs is scanty, inconclusive, and often controversial. Observational epidemiologic studies show that overall mortality parallels body weight increases above an optimal level.[7] This evidence is strongest for adults between the ages of 30 and 44 years. In older age groups, excess body weight increases the risk of death, but the degree of impact diminishes with age.[8] This chapter reviews the epidemiology, pathophysiology, and therapeutic approaches for obesity. Although nonpharmacologic treatment modalities are discussed, the pharmacotherapy of obesity is highlighted, and the role of pharmacotherapy relative to therapeutic options is discussed.[9]

DEFINITION OF CLINICAL OBESITY

Much of the confusion in interpreting studies by various investigators is due to their use of differing definitions and cutoff points to define obesity.[10] Furthermore, obesity can be defined epidemiologically based on health insurance data or physiologically based on body fat content. A clear distinction has been made between obesity and overweight by the National Center for Health Statistics (NCHS), yet researchers often use the two terms interchangeably.[11] *Overweight* refers to an excess body weight relative to a person's height. The body mass index (BMI) is a measure that attempts to correct weight changes for height. It is defined as weight in kilograms divided by height in meters squared (kg/m^2). In contrast, *obesity* refers to a state of excess body fat as determined by the various methods. These include measures of skinfold thickness, body density using underwater body weight, bioelectric impedance and conductivity, dual energy x-ray absorptiometry (DEXA), computed tomography (CT), and magnetic resonance imaging (MRI). Many of these measurement techniques that determine body fat directly are too expensive and time-consuming to be used in population studies.

It is not clear what the criterion for *normal* weight should be. Should normal weight be associated with low mortality, low morbidity, or both? In the absence of better sources, life insurance data were used in the past to develop tables of normality. These tables provide weight ranges for height and frame size (small, medium, and large) and are associated with the greatest longevity in individuals who were healthy at the time of initial examination when their height and weight were measured. These data predominantly represent information compiled from the upper-middle-class white population. They are specific for height and weight but not age. Indeed, they essentially predict longevity in young persons weighed in their early twenties. The weight range provided by these tables is known as desirable or ideal body weight. Overweight is then defined as a weight greater than 10% above the ideal weight for a person's height, and obesity is defined as greater than 20% above this ideal body weight.

The NCHS has conducted large national surveys in the United States of health including body habitus and nutrition over the past three decades.[12] These surveys have been conducted in three samples, known as the National Health and Nutrition Examination Surveys (NHANES). The data have been used to establish norms for BMI, height, weight, and gender in Americans of all ages. The normal BMI for males and females is 20 to 24.9. Overweight was defined as a BMI of 27.8 or more in men and 27.3 or more in women. The overweight criteria correspond to approximately 124% and 120% of the midpoints of the ranges of weights recommended, respectively, for men and women of medium frame in the 1983 Metropolitan Life Height and Weight tables as adjusted for clothing weight and heel height.[13] Severe overweight corresponds to a BMI of over 31.1 in men and over 32.3 in women.[14] The relationship between BMI and mortality is shown in Figure 140–1. Excess weight relative to height (BMI) is an acceptable measure of obesity; however, it does not always correspond to excess fat.

Neither the BMI nor the ideal body weight reflects true body composition or distribution of body fat. Body composition is a more direct measure of degree of adiposity and therefore mass of fat stores. The "gold standard" to determine body composition historically has been underwater weighing (body density). The formulas used in this technique were developed using healthy young males and therefore may not be applicable for obese and older individuals. Newer techniques have improved our ability to measure body composition. Wang and colleagues[15] have proposed five levels of modeling for body composition: atomic, molecular, cellular, tissue system, and whole body. Techniques have been developed to estimate body composition at all these levels. Body weight, BMI, body volume, body surface area, height, skin fold thickness, and body density are all measures of body composition at the whole body level.[15,16] In addition to the absolute excess fat mass, the distribution of this fat regionally in the body has an important effect on the mortality of obese individuals. A number of studies have demonstrated excess mortality associated with a central or android distribution of body fat.[16,17] Generally, central obesity reflects high levels of intraabdominal or visceral fat. Intraabdominal fat is best estimated by imaging techniques such as CT or MRI. More recent studies suggest that subcutaneous fat may be heterogeneous in its metabolic effects. In these studies, superficial subcutaneous fat had a weak association with metabolic markers of insulin resistance, whereas deep subcutaneous fat had a strong relationship with insulin resistance.[18] This pattern of obesity is associated with an increased prevalence of cardiovascular risk factors such as hyperlipidemia and glucose intolerance. These risk factors in part explain the high cardiovascular mortality rate of these individuals.[19] In contrast, a gynecoid (gluteofemoral) distribution of fat with low waist-to-hip ratios (WHRs) or low waist circumference (WC) has a lower risk of mortality for the same degree of adiposity. Clinically, WC is the narrowest circumference measured in the area between the last rib and the top of the iliac crest.[20] The hip measurement is the maximal circumference

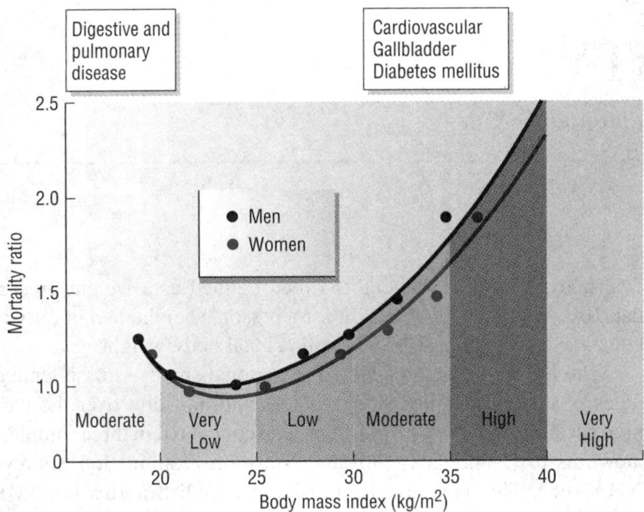

FIGURE 140–1. Mortality ratio and body mass index (BMI). This represents composite data for men and women demonstrating the relationship of body mass index to overall mortality. A J-shaped relationship exists wherein a BMI <20 kg/m^2 and <25 kg/m^2 correlates with an increase in relative mortality. The major causes of mortality are listed relative to BMI groupings. *(Adapted with permission from Bray GA. Obesity. In: Brown ML, et al, eds. Present Knowledge in nutrition, 6th ed. Washington, DC, International Life Sciences Institute–Nutrition Foundation, 1990.)*

around the buttocks.[20] Central obesity is associated with increased risks when WHR is 1.0 or more for men or 0.9 or more for females.[21] WC is an easier measurement to obtain in the clinical setting and is also independently associated with increased risks when 40 inches or more for males or 35 inches or more for females.[19]

EPIDEMIOLOGY

Obesity is increasing in prevalence in the United States. The NHANES II data (1976–1980) estimated a prevalence of overweight persons in the United States at 25.4% of adults, representing 34 million individuals. During NHANES III (1988–1991), the prevalence had increased to 33.3%, representing 55 million American adults.[22] The prevention of obesity therefore is a public health priority. This has been further emphasized by the current lack of any safe and effective long-term therapy for obesity. Individuals who were "fat" as children tend to remain overweight as adults.[23–25] Recent data from a large British study have provided further evidence for the relationship between an overweight childhood and subsequent excess weight as an adult.[26] In contrast to body weight, adult BMI was not well predicted from childhood weight. The fattest children had the highest risks of adult obesity. However, most obese adults had not been fat at earlier ages: Only 17% and 18% of obese 33-year-old men and women, respectively, had been fat at age 7 years. Thus most obese adults were not fat children. In contrast, early adulthood may be an important time for intervention to prevent future obesity. Of 4519 men and 4806 women in the study by Power and associates, obesity increased in prevalence from 2% to 11% in men and from 3% to 12% in women during the 10-year period between ages 23 and 33 years.[26] This is consistent with historical data from the U.S. Ten-State Nutrition Survey.[27]

The prevalence of overweight varies between races within the United States. Mexican-American women and black women had the highest prevalence, 48.1% and 49.1%, respectively. The prevalence of obesity also increases with age, reaching a maximum by the sixth decade in women and the seventh decade for men. Beyond this age, the prevalence progressively falls for both genders. Socioeconomic status also affects the prevalence of obesity in those between the ages of 25 and 54 years. The prevalence of overweight in nonpregnant women for each respective decade of life—25 to 34 years, 35 to 44 years, and 45 to 54 years—is 30.8%, 49.1%, and 54.1% of women with incomes below the poverty line versus 18.4%, 23.7%, and 30.3% of those above the poverty line.[26] Educational achievement, which is linked to socioeconomic status, is also correlated with the fraction of people who are overweight; prevalence of overweight is greatest in those with less than a high school education versus those with some college education.

ETIOLOGY

The etiology of obesity in the vast majority of individuals is unknown. It is likely multifactorial in origin, with environmental, genetic, and physiologic factors contributing to various degrees in different individuals. A definitive diagnosis of an underlying medical condition can be made in only a small minority of individuals. Even then, the diagnosed condition may or may not be treatable. One of the current controversies is the extent that genetic traits influence the risk of developing obesity as well as how these genetic traits interact with environmental factors to cause obesity.[28]

ENVIRONMENTAL FACTORS

Economic development is associated with lifestyle changes. Many of these societal changes may contribute to the observed rise in the prevalence of obesity throughout the world. Those which are most probably related to obesity include reduced physical activity or work (sedentary lifestyle), abundant and readily available food supply, increased fat intake, increased consumption of refined simple sugars, and decreased ingestion of vegetables, fruits, and complex carbohydrates. These changes in our environment likely contribute to a state of positive energy balance in many individuals[29] (Fig. 140–2). Observations from public health studies support this concept. For example, the prevalence of obesity in Copenhagen remained stable during the period between 1925 and 1942 at approximately 0.1%. However, since

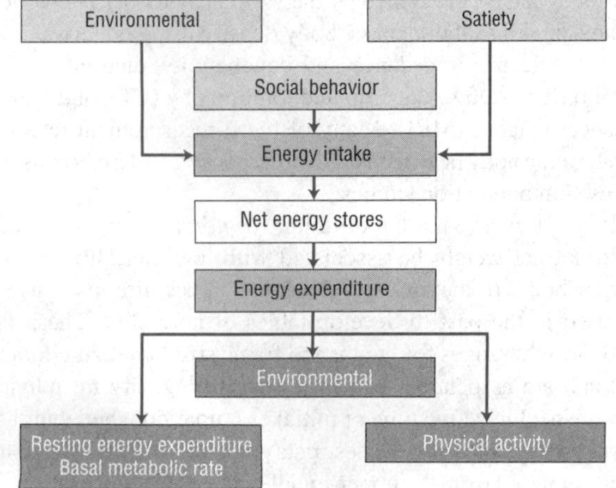

FIGURE 140–2. Net energy stores, determined by various inputs and outputs. Simply stated, obesity occurs when imbalance occurs between energy intake and expenditure.

the end of World War II, there has been a steady increase in the prevalence of obesity.[29] These observational data suggest an environmental role for the development of obesity.

NUTRITION

Decades of research have led to several thousand publications regarding nutrition therapy for obesity. Yet the appropriate diet that leads to long-term weight loss in ambulatory self-sufficient individuals is not known. The consensus is that weight regain is almost always inevitable. It is clear that excess caloric intake is a prerequisite to weight gain and obesity, but not all individuals with high caloric intake gain weight. There is an ongoing debate whether the primary consideration is total calorie intake or macronutrient composition of the diet (i.e., percent of calories as carbohydrates, protein, or fat). Of the three macronutrients, dietary fat has received the most attention. Both animals and humans prefer and often will seek out foods high in fat. High-fat foods have a desirable texture and sensory characteristic in the mouth. Although fat is itself tasteless, fats enhance the flavor of other foods. Clearly, one way that fatty foods promote weight gain is by increased energy intake because fat is more energy dense than other macronutrients. Furthermore, fats are stored with greater efficiency than protein or carbohydrates.[30] Nutritional management of obesity as discussed in this chapter is based on reducing calorie intake. Because the Western diet is high in fat, and because fat contains more than twice the calories per gram of carbohydrate and protein, in almost all diets the fat content is reduced by necessity.

APPETITE

CENTRAL RECEPTOR SYSTEMS

Multiple receptor systems, including those of the biogenic amines, are known to either stimulate or decrease food intake in both animals and humans. Serotonin, also known as 5-hydroxytryptamine (5-HT), and cells known to respond to 5-HT are found throughout the central nervous system and the periphery. At least seven distinct subfamilies of 5-HT receptors have been cloned to date, with each of these seven exhibiting one or more subtypes.[31] Currently, two major noradrenergic receptor subtypes are recognized (α and β), each with multiple subtypes.[32] Histamine and dopamine also demonstrate multiple receptor subtypes, but their role in regulation of human eating behaviors and food intake is less well documented. Direct stimulation of 5-HT_{1A} and noradrenergic α_2-receptors will increase food intake, whereas the opposite occurs with 5-HT_{2C} and noradrenergic α_1- or β_2-receptor activation. In animal models, stimulating histamine receptor subtypes 1 or 3 and dopamine receptor subtypes 1 or 2 results in lowering of food intake. Table 140–1 summarizes the major effects of direct receptor stimulation, inhibition, or changes in synaptic cleft amine concentrations on food intake.

PEPTIDES

Since the 1950s, it has been conjectured that weight is controlled via a hormone interaction at the level of the hypothalamus.[33] The protein product of the mouse obese gene (*ob*) described in 1994 appears to be the signaling mechanism between peripheral energy storage and hypothalamic feeding centers.[33,34] This protein was called *leptin* (after *leptos*, the Greek word for "thin"). The *ob/ob* genetically obese mouse does not produce leptin, and this animal's marked hyperphagia subsides with leptin supplementation. Adrenalectomy reverses the obese

TABLE 140–1. Effects of Various Neurotransmitters, Receptors, and Peptides on Food Intake

Neurotransmitter/ Receptor/Peptide	Action	Food Intake
Norepinephrine	Increase concentration	Decrease
α_1	Stimulate receptor	Decrease
α_2	Stimulate receptor	Increase
β_2	Stimulate receptor	Decrease
Serotonin	Increase concentration	Decrease
5-HT_{1A}	Stimulate receptor	Increase
5-HT_{1B}	Stimulate receptor	Decrease
5-HT_{2C}	Stimulate receptor	Decrease
Histamine		
H_1	Stimulate receptor	Decrease
H_3	Stimulate receptor	Decrease
Dopamine		
D_1	Stimulate receptor	Decrease
D_2	Stimulate receptor	Decrease
Leptin	Increase concentration	Decrease
Neuropeptide Y	Increase concentration	Increase
Galanin	Increase concentration	Increase

phenotype and restores the hypothalamic melanocortin tone in the *ob/ob* mouse, suggesting that glucocorticoids have a facilitative role in the development of obesity.[35] The human leptin homologue has been cloned, and various animal studies have demonstrated that leptin is produced in the periphery by white and possibly brown adipocytes.[36] Additionally, it appears that the sympathetic nervous system (SNS), via β_3-adrenoceptors, inhibits leptin expression[36] (Fig. 140–3). Unlike the leptin-deficient *ob/ob* mouse, obese human serum leptin levels increase as fat cell mass increases. There is a direct relationship between serum leptin concentrations and various markers of obesity such as percent body fat, BMI, and serum insulin concentrations.[37] Thus humans appear to be resistant to the satiety effects of leptin, and it is unknown whether leptin supplementation in humans will decrease obesity. Figure 140–3 shows the peripheral link that leptin appears to provide in signaling the central nervous system about the status of fat cell mass. A second peptide, neuropeptide Y (NPY), is being studied intensely for its effects on feeding. NPY elicits many effects both peripherally and centrally, including appetite stimulation. Messenger

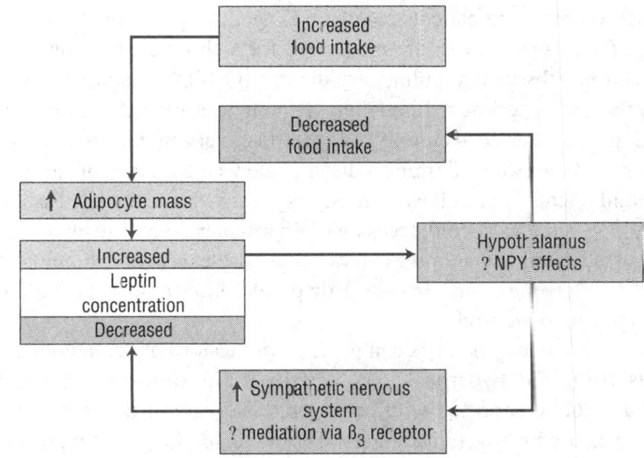

FIGURE 140–3. Effects of food intake on leptin concentrations and proposed feedback loops controlling food intake and leptin concentration. (NPY = neuropeptide Y.)

RNA for two new appetite-stimulating proteins called *orexins* has been observed to be concentrated in the lateral hypothalamus.[38] An understanding of the relationships between the sympathetic nervous system, leptin, NPY, orexins, and other hormones such as insulin and glucocorticoids is still evolving.[39] Exogenous manipulation of these proteins may provide future pharmacotherapeutic approaches to obesity management.

ACTIVITY

It is generally accepted that increased physical activity is an important component in the management of obesity. Similarly, a sedentary lifestyle predisposes to weight gain and obesity. Yet the question whether obese individuals are less physically active compared with age-matched lean individuals remains unanswered. Some studies show no difference in physical activity between lean and obese individuals, whereas others suggest that obese persons are less active.[40] Even when studies suggest that obese persons are less active, it cannot be determined whether less physical activity leads to obesity or physical inactivity is itself secondary to the physical effects of obesity. Physical activity includes voluntary work, recreational activity, and spontaneous physical activity including involuntary movements. Some authors have suggested that obese individuals have reduced levels of spontaneous physical activity leading to a lower daily energy expenditure.[41] However, results from studies designed to measure total daily energy expenditure remain controversial. A recent literature review found only a modest beneficial effect of exercise in preventing weight gain, with or without previous weight reduction.[42]

WEIGHT GAIN SECONDARY TO MEDICAL CONDITIONS

Occasionally patients present with obesity secondary to an identifiable acquired medical condition. The most common endocrine condition associated with weight gain is hypothyroidism[43] (see Chapter 75). These patients lose significant weight within weeks of thyroxin replacement therapy. However, many patients will not achieve a normal or ideal body weight despite adequate thyroid hormone replacement. Indeed, it is not uncommon for patients to request higher than physiologic replacement doses of thyroxin to artificially suppress their weight. It is important to remember that excess thyroid therapy can be associated with complications, including osteoporosis and cardiac disorders. Cushing's syndrome, another cause of obesity, is seen most commonly in patients receiving exogenous glucocorticoid therapy. These agents often are prescribed for a chronic condition such as chronic obstructive pulmonary disease (COPD), postorgan transplantation, or arthritis. Idiopathic Cushing's disease due to excess endogenous steroid secretion is, in contrast, very rare. In both iatrogenic and idiopathic Cushing's disease, the weight gain is in part due to fluid retention as well as increased adiposity. The adiposity associated with glucocorticoid excess has a particular body distribution in that it is central with relative loss of body muscle mass and thinning of the skin, leading to the characteristic purple skin striaie and a buffalo hump behind the neck.

Occasionally patients can present with lesions of the hypothalamus that lead to hyperphagia and obesity.[44] This disorder is rare and should not be confused with behavioral disorders of eating that are associated with psychopathology. These include binge eating disorders, which may respond to psychotherapy and in some cases pharmacotherapy (see Chapter 64). Obesity is itself associated with a higher prevalence of affective disorders, which if untreated may impair the success of any weight loss program. The clinician managing obesity must be aware of the presence of psychosocial disorders both as a cause and effect of obesity. Counseling strategies need to be incorporated into the management of selected obese individuals.[45] Furthermore, medications used to manage affective disorders, such as the serotonin reuptake inhibitors, have not been studied extensively with regard to combination use with appetite suppressant agents.

GENETIC SYNDROMES

Syndromes in which obesity is a major component are extremely rare. Prader-Willi's, Simpson-Goabi-Behmel's, Cohen's, Bardet-Biedl's, Carpenter's, Börjeson's, and Wilson-Turner's syndromes have all been associated with obesity.[20] Of these, Prader-Willi's syndrome is the most common and has a frequency of 1 in 20,000 live births. Other phenotypic features include changes in stature, mental retardation, and developmental abnormalities (e.g., hypogonadism). Because the incidence of these syndromes is rare, even collectively they contribute very little to the incidence of obesity. The clinician evaluating a patient for obesity needs to be aware of their existence, and the physical examination of obese patients always should include an assessment for secondary causes of obesity including genetic syndromes.

GENETIC PREDISPOSITION

Family studies show a clear correlation of body weight between parents and children. The correlation between siblings is even higher.[46,47] In monozygotic twins, BMI is almost always identical, and there is a strong correlation in the accumulation of visceral fat. These twin studies demonstrate the strong role of genetics in determining both obesity and distribution of body fat.[47] The incidence of obesity in adopted individuals relative to their adopted parents provides insight into the role of genetics versus family environment. These studies show a clear correlation between the BMI of adult adoptees and their biologic parents. This relationship does not exist between an adoptee and his or her adoptive parent. These observations further support the notion that genes are primarily responsible for determining adult body weight. The relative impact of genetic versus environmental factors varies between persons. In some individuals, genetic factors are the primary determinants of obesity, whereas in others, the obesity may be caused primarily by environmental factors. The actual variance in body fat between individuals determined by genes is not known. Estimates for this variance range from 20% to a high of almost 80%. Yet, clearly, without adequate caloric intake, obesity cannot occur. Thus the role of the environment is to facilitate expression of an underlying genetic trait for obesity. However, the specific gene or genes that code for obesity are unknown.[48] Most investigators would agree that more than one gene is involved in the development of human obesity.

PHYSIOLOGY

ENERGY BALANCE

The net balance of energy ingested relative to energy expended by an individual over time determines the degree of obesity. Figure 140–2 represents the interplay between energy intake and expenditure. Energy stores will increase if there is imbalance between intake and expenditure. An individual's metabolic rate is the single largest determinant of energy expenditure. *It is important to determine metabolic rate under standardized conditions, giving rise to terms such as resting* energy expenditure (REE) and basal metabolic rate (BMR). REE is defined as the energy expended by a person at rest under conditions of thermal neutrality. BMR is more precisely defined as the REE measured soon after awakening in the morning, at least 12 hours after the last meal. Metabolic rate increases after eating, based on the size and composition of the meal. It reaches a maximum approximately 1 hour after the meal is consumed and is essentially back to basal levels 4 hours after the meal. This increase in metabolic rate is known as the *thermogenic effect of food*.[49] The REE may include the residual thermic effect of a previous meal and may be lower than BMR during quiet sleep. In practice, BMR and REE differ by less than 10%, and the terms frequently are used interchangeably.

PERIPHERAL STORAGE AND THERMOGENESIS

Adipose tissue generally is divided into two major types, white and brown.[50] The primary function of white adipose tissue is lipid manufacture, storage, and release. Lipid storage occurs in response to insulin lipid release occurs during periods of calorie restriction, when insulin levels are suppressed. Brown type tissue is notable for its ability to dissipate energy via a process of uncoupled mitochondrial respiration.[46] Currently, the exact roles of each of these tissue subtypes are better defined in animal models than in humans. Adipose tissue is highly innervated by the sympathetic nervous system, and adrenergic stimulation is known to activate lipolysis in fat cells as well as increase energy expenditure in adipose tissue and skeletal muscle. These properties provide a potential pharmacologic avenue for altering energy balance and changing weight status. A major focus of research in obesity pharmacotherapy has centered on the activity of adrenergic receptors and their effect on adipose tissue with respect to energy storage and expenditure or thermogenesis.[50,51] All three subtypes of β-adrenergic receptors (β_1, β_2, and β_3) appear to be active in fat cell function. The β_3-receptor appears to be less responsive than β_1 and β_2 with respect to activation via norepinephrine. This has led to the development of specific β_3-adrenoceptor agonists. However, apparent differences in selectivity and responsiveness between animal and human β_3-receptors have complicated the drug development process. In vivo studies in humans suggest that the β_3-receptor may be largely responsible for adipose tissue adrenergic-mediated increases in thermogenesis.[52] Genetic polymorphisms have been identified in both the β_2- and β_3-receptor systems that are associated with obesity or excess weight gain.[53,54] Thus genetic susceptibility for excess weight status may in part be related to adrenergic dysfunction. The development of effective pharmacotherapies involving these receptor systems may be delayed pending definitive identification of receptor subtype contributions.

COMORBIDITIES

Obesity is associated with serious health risks and increased mortality (see Fig. 140–1). Several disease states and/or conditions are more prevalent in obese patients (Table 140–2). Increased body fat, increased total body weight, and a central distribution of body fat are all associated with an increased incidence of mortality, primarily due to cardiovascular disease. Hypertension, hyperlipidemia, insulin resistance, and glucose intolerance are all known cardiac risk factors that tend to cluster in obese individuals. Therefore, the obese individual is exposed to multiple risk factors. Epidemiologic studies have confirmed the relationship between obesity and increased risk of stroke and coronary heart disease in both men and women.[55,56] This increased mortality is seen even with modest excess body weight. The American Cancer Society study of 750,000 men and women found

TABLE 140–2. Obesity and Comorbid Conditions

Cardiovascular	**Musculoskeletal**
Hypertension	Degenerative joint disease
Left ventricular hypertrophy	**Skin**
Congestive heart failure	Acanthosis nigricans
Coronary artery disease	Stretch marks
Stroke	Hirsutism
Pulmonary	Skin tags
Obstructive airway disease	**Gastrointestinal**
Sleep apnea	Cholelithiasis
Pulmonary hypertension	Esophageal reflux
Metabolic	Hiatus hernia
Hypercholesterolemia	**Psychological**
Hypertriglyceridemia	Eating disorders
Low serum HDL	Depression
Diabetes mellitus and glucose intolerance	Affective disorders
Hyperinsulinemia	Social stigma
Polycystic ovary syndrome	**Neoplasm**
Increased serum urate	Breast cancer
	Colon cancer

an increased cardiac mortality even at body weights only 10% above average.[57] Blood pressure frequently is elevated in obese individuals and may in part explain the increased incidence of stroke and cardiovascular disease observed with obesity. Hypertension in lean individuals is associated with concentric hypertrophy due to an increased afterload, which increases the risk of cardiac ischemia. In contrast, with obesity eccentric dilatation is observed, leading to an increased volume load. This dilated cardiomyopathy is associated with a reduction in ventricular ejection fraction and a high-output cardiac state. The combination of obesity and hypertension is associated with thickening of the ventricular wall, ischemia, and increased heart volume. This leads more rapidly to heart failure.[58] Alterations in pulmonary function are common in patients with obesity. Most significant and costly in terms of morbidity and mortality is sleep apnea.[20] This disorder is more common in men. The exact mechanism by which obesity leads to sleep apnea is unknown, but weight loss often results in significant and sometimes dramatic improvements in sleep apnea.

Diabetes mellitus and impaired glucose tolerance are associated with insulin resistance and obesity. The cellular mechanism by which obesity causes insulin resistance is unknown. Proposed mechanisms include downregulation of insulin receptors, abnormal postreceptor signals, circulating antagonists to insulin such as fatty acids or cytokines, and impaired gene transcription in insulin-responsive cells. Regardless of the mechanism of the insulin resistance, as insulin response becomes impaired, the pancreatic β-cells respond by increasing insulin, resulting in a state of relative hyperinsulinemia. Although hyperinsulinemia is known to be associated with an increased risk of cardiovascular disease, it is not known whether the increased insulin levels contribute directly to cardiac disease or if they are just a marker for the underlying defect of insulin resistance and glucose intolerance. Insulin resistance in turn also frequently leads to impaired lipid metabolism (increased cholesterol, increased triglycerides, and a low high-density lipoprotein) and hypertension. As with cardiovascular disease, fat distribution is an important factor in determining the risk of developing type 2 diabetes. Central obesity has been shown to increase the risk of diabetes. Intentional weight loss has been shown to reduce mortality substantially in obese individuals with diabetes.[59]

Osteoarthritis in weight-bearing joints, such as the knees, may be related directly to the mechanical effects of excess body weight and the resulting forces exerted on these joint surfaces. The increase of osteoarthritis in non-weight-bearing joints, however, suggests that obesity may lead to altered cartilage, collagen, and even bone metabolism. Osteoarthritis and its symptoms, such as pain, are a significant barrier to physical activity and a key impediment to sustained weight loss.

Obesity affects the human reproductive system in a number of ways. Obesity is associated with earlier menarche in girls and hyperandrogenism, hirsutism, and anovulatory menstrual cycles in women. In some women this disorder manifests as overt polycystic ovary syndrome (PCOS).[20] Insulin resistance is common in these women. Weight loss, and more recently therapy with insulin-sensitizing drugs such as the thiazolidinediones and biguanides, can restore normal ovulation in some women.[60] These observations suggest that insulin resistance plays a part in the causation of PCOS-associated with obesity.

► TREATMENT: Obesity

GENERAL APPROACH TO TREATMENT

The success of obesity therapy has been measured most often as weight loss over study periods of up to 12 months. Successful obesity treatment plans have incorporated diet, exercise, behavior modification (with or without pharmacologic therapy), and/or surgical intervention. Figure 140–4 shows the sites of action of these therapies within the energy intake, storage, and expenditure cycle.

Patients seeking help for obesity do so for many reasons, including improvement in their quality of life, a reduction in associated morbidity, and to prolong their life. Yet numerous individuals seek therapy for obesity primarily for cosmetic purposes and often have unreasonable goals and expectations. Aggressive marketing of weight loss programs, therapies, and diets—parallel to the fashion industry's standards of desirable body profiles—has led many individuals to set impossible goals and expectations. In some cases these persons will go to extreme measures to achieve weight loss, even at the risk of injury to themselves. Clinicians therefore must be careful not only to fully discuss risks of therapies but also to clearly define achievable benefits and magnitude of weight loss. Criteria for weight loss vary from the most aggressive goal of trying to achieve an "ideal weight" to the more reasonable goals of modest (e.g., loss of 5% of body weight) but sustained weight loss. In practice, the goal has to be set based on many factors, including initial body weight, patient motivation and desire, presence of comorbid conditions, and age. For example, in patients with diabetes, even modest weight loss can improve glucose control and reduce mortality significantly,[59,61] yet in individuals with osteoarthritis, significantly more weight reduction may be required to improve symptoms. Indeed, dietary modification and exercise have been shown to ameliorate hyperglycemia, hyperlipidemia, and hypertension with weight loss of less than 5% of initial body weight.[62] These data emphasize the importance of defining end points and measures of success in any weight loss plan.

Most weight loss interventions consist of a combination of lifestyle changes, diet, drug therapy if indicated, and in some cases surgery. Prior to recommending any therapy, the clinician must evaluate the patient for the presence of secondary causes of obesity. If a

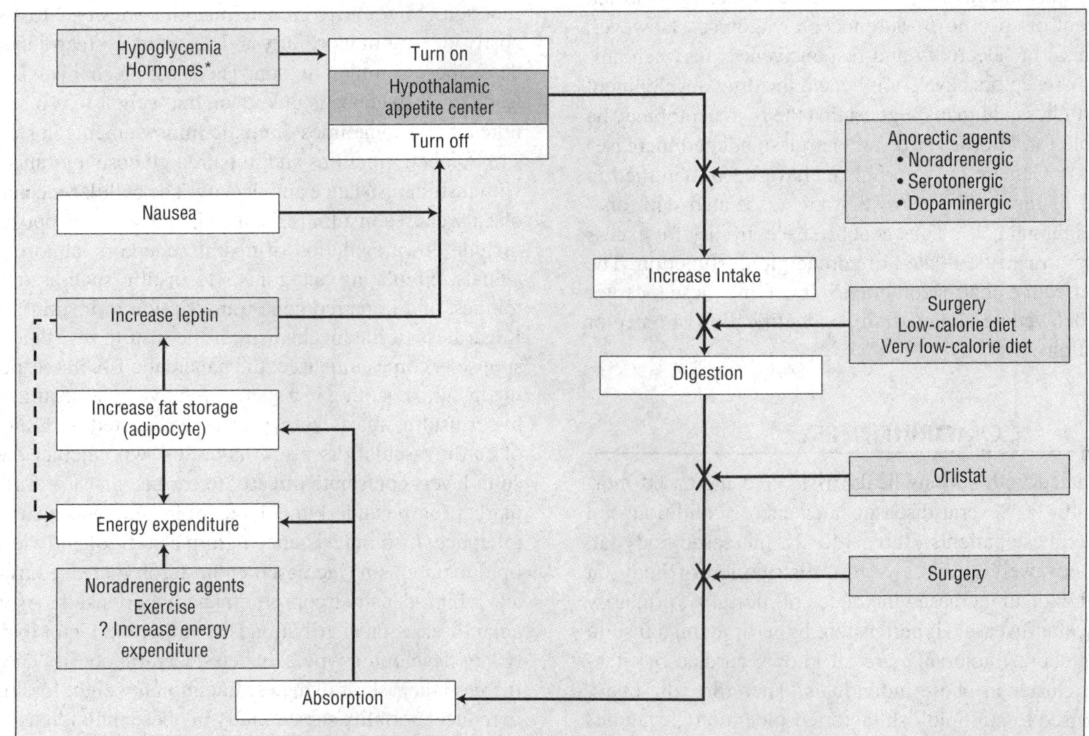

FIGURE 140–4. *Hypothalamic appetite centers in the brain modulate both central and peripheral signals. This figure demonstrates the sites of action for various obesity treatment modalities within the cycle of energy intake and storage.* Leptin, while signaling the central nervous system of the status of peripheral fat cell mass, may also have functions with regard to energy expenditure. Some appetite-suppressant agents, alone or in combination, also modulate energy expenditure. *Including insulin, thyroxine, glucocorticoids, and progesterones.

secondary cause is suspected, then a more complete diagnostic workup and appropriate therapy are paramount. The next step in the patient evaluation is to determine the presence and severity of other medical conditions either directly associated with obesity (e.g., diabetes) or which have an impact on therapeutic decision making (e.g., history of liver disease or cardiac arrhythmia). Appropriate laboratory tests to exclude and/or quantify the degree of specific conditions such as diabetes, liver dysfunction, and nephropathy should be done as indicated by the history and physical examination. Based on the outcome of this medical evaluation, the patient then should be counseled on treatment options, benefits, and risks. The ultimate goals of treatment must be defined clearly. These goals may be absolute weight loss if obesity is present without other comorbid conditions. If improvement in blood glucose, blood cholesterol, and hypertension are primary goals, then these must be defined appropriately, such as target levels for low-density-lipoprotein cholesterol, glycosylated hemoglobin, or blood pressure. For these patients, weight loss goals may be as little as 5% of starting weight.[61] In contrast, if obesity is causing physical problems such as impaired mobility, osteoarthritis, or sleep apnea, then 10% to 20% of starting weight may be more appropriate. All too often patients expect to lose weight "overnight," only to be disappointed. Thus it is important to set a time course for the plan. A reasonable rate of weight loss is typically about 0.5 kg per week.

NONPHARMACOLOGIC THERAPY

BEHAVIORAL MODIFICATION

Behavior modification is common to almost all weight loss interventions. The primary aim is to help patients choose lifestyles that are conducive to safe and sustained weight loss. Behavioral therapy is based on principles of human learning and therefore attempts to substitute learned undesirable habits with desirable behaviors using a combination of stimulus control and reinforcement. Most such programs use self-monitoring of diet and exercise both to increase patient awareness of behavior and as a tool for the clinician to determine patient compliance as well as patient motivation.[45,63] Behavior is reinforced by techniques including behavioral contracting, social support, relapse prevention, and in some cases booster treatments. Behavioral contracts are written agreements jointly developed by the patient and clinician. Components of these agreements include goals of therapy, methods to achieve these goals, and rewards for achieving these goals successfully. Social support requires the active participation of a close friend or relative who is involved in monitoring compliance and reinforcing behavior. Relapse prevention is geared to identifying high-risk situations for relapse such as social events and training the individual to avoid these circumstances. Eventually, the patient is trained to deal with these situations actively, such as refusing high-fat foods assertively rather than avoiding such social events.

DIET

Numerous diet or nutrition plans exist to aid in weight loss.[64,65] Whichever diet program is selected, it is clear that energy consumption must be less than energy expenditure to achieve weight loss (see Fig. 140–2). The challenge has been to develop a diet plan that leads to compliance by the patient and therefore sustained weight loss. Two broad categories of diet have been used in practice: low calorie and very low calorie. Low-calorie diets allow the consumption of less than 800 kcal/d. Very low-calorie diets generally contain approximately 500–800 kcal/d. These highly restrictive diets often result in early weight loss but have been disappointing in the long term in part because it is difficult for individuals to maintain compliance.[66] Other investigators have proposed total or modified fasts.[57] The obvious problem with total fasts is that both fat and lean body mass are lost. In addition, because of diuresis, significant mineral losses occur. Because of the problem with total fasting, alternate regimens called protein supplemented modified fasts (PSMFs), became popular. With a PSMF, the protein is given in the form of either formula or natural foods such as fish or lean meat. The consensus is that it is dangerous to allow these diets to be continued for longer than 15 weeks at a time.[66] Patients may lose 1.5 to 2.3 kg per week on these diets. All these types of severe calorie-restricted diets need vitamin and mineral supplementation.[67]

A more reasonable goal for individuals is weight reduction of about 0.5 kg per week achieved by a negative calorie balance of approximately 500 kcal/d. This translates into a diet of approximately 20 kcal/kg of desirable body weight for most adults. The dietary regime should be well balanced in fat, carbohydrates, and proteins as well as micronutrients. Generally 0.8 g of protein per kilogram of desirable body weight is recommended, with at most 30% of calories from fat.

SURGERY

Surgery remains the most effective intervention for moderate to severe obesity. Surgical procedures either reduce the absorptive surface of the alimentary tract, resulting in some degree of malabsorption, or reduce the stomach volume. In some cases, a combination of these two approaches is used. The most common procedure performed in the past was some form of intestinal bypass.[68] This type of procedure reduces the surface area available for nutrients and in particular calories to be absorbed, resulting in malabsorption and subsequent weight loss. The early procedures of jejunocolic bypass (anastamosis of jejunum to colon) had serious side effects as well as an unacceptable mortality. Further developments in bypass procedures subsequently led to the use of a safer and more acceptable bypass procedure known as a jejunoileal bypass (jejunum-to-ileum anastamosis).

Jejunoileal bypass was the standard surgical procedure for obesity in the 1970s, until the advent of gastric restriction surgery. The operative risk of jejunoileal procedures was less than 1% and resulted in weight loss of approximately one-third of preoperative weight. Although this procedure did result in a state of malabsorption and loss of ingested calories in the stool, up to 75% of the weight loss observed in these patients could be accounted for by a reduction in caloric ingestion. In addition, animal studies suggest that bacterial overgrowth in the blind loop of the procedure may contribute to the weight loss observed. Unfortunately, the complications of this procedure, which in part may be secondary to this bacterial colonization and overgrowth, resulted in hepatic steatosis, cirrhosis in up to 4% of patients, and in some cases liver failure.[66] Other long-term complications include arthritis, skin lesions, vasculitis, enteritis, electrolyte abnormalities, osteomalacia, renal stones and in some cases renal failure, an increased risk of tuberculosis, and systemic fungal infection.[68] These complications have led to this procedure becoming obsolete.

Gastric bypass is a procedure in which a loop of bowel is attached the stomach in a roux-en-Y method. This procedure ultimately may result in the loss of approximately one-third of body weight. Common complications include gallstone formation, prolonged nausea and vomiting, and ulceration and stenosis at the site of anastamosis.[68] Very rarely, hepatic failure has been reported. Many gastric reduction procedures have been described, including numerous versions of gastroplasty and gastric balloon procedures. All are designed to reduce

TABLE 140–3. Surgical Procedures, Outcomes, and Complications

Procedure	Weight Loss (% of Initial Weight)	Operative Mortality (%)	Complications
Jejunoileal bypass	33	<1	Hepatic steatosis, cirrhosis, bacterial overgrowth, nephrolithiasis, renal failure
Gastric bypass	30–35	<1	Cholelithiasis, prolonged nausea, stomal ulceration and stenosis, anemia
Gastroplasty	20–25	<1	Cholelithiasis, nausea, stomal ulceration and stenosis, weight regain is more common

the volume of the stomach by either surgically reducing the stomach volume or insertion of a silicone balloon into the stomach cavity so that it acts like a bezoar. The most successful of these procedures has been the vertically banded gastroplasty.[68] The complications of this procedure are similar to those seen with gastric bypass. Both gastric bypass and gastroplasty result in maximum weight loss around 18 months postoperatively. However, late weight gain and the need for surgical revision are greater in patients undergoing vertically banded gastroplasty. Recent surgical developments have allowed this procedure to be performed via a laporoscope. Long-term results using this approach are not yet available.

It is clear that great attention needs to be paid to selection of the appropriate patient for surgery and subsequently identifying the correct procedure. The input of an experienced surgeon working with a multidisciplinary team is invaluable (Table 140–3)

PHARMACOLOGIC THERAPY

Strategies for the pharmacologic management of obesity have been focused on modulating central and/or peripheral sites that regulate human energy balance. Figure 140–4 depicts sites of action and Table 140–4 lists the most common classes of agents currently in use or of recent use. Since the 1970s, numerous studies of the effects of central appetite suppressant agents on weight status have been completed.[9,69] The quality and interpretability of some of the data have been questioned.[70] The National Task Force on the Prevention and Treatment of Obesity concluded that short-term anorexic agent use was difficult to justify because of the predictable weight regain that occurs on discontinuation of pharmacotherapy. However, long-term pharmacotherapy may have a place in the treatment of obesity for patients who have no obvious contraindications to available drug therapy.[71] Additionally, the American Association of Clinical Endocrinologists (AACE) and the American College of Endocrinology (ACE) have developed a guideline for multidisciplinary obesity team approach to therapy.[72] Routine implementation awaits the development of medications that are effective and safe with long-term exposure. Recent discovery of cardiac valve disease in relation to serotonergic appetite suppressant use affirms the task force's warning for further study of available therapies prior to widespread implementation of routine obesity pharmacotherapy.[73–75] Bray and Greenway recently completed an extensive review of current and potential drugs for the treatment of obesity.[9] The next sections outline the current status of pharmacologic agents for obesity therapy, focusing on proposed mechanisms, dosing recommendations, potential side effects, and monitoring parameters.

NORADRENERGIC AGENTS

Amphetamines

Appetite suppressant effects of the amphetamines were well recognized in the 1930s. Amphetamines activate central noradrenergic receptor systems as well as dopaminergic pathways, at higher doses, by

TABLE 140–4. Obesity Pharmacotherapeutic Agents

Class	Availability	Daily Dosages (mg)
Noradrenergic Agents		
Methamphetamine HCl (desoxyephedrine HCl)	Rx[a]	5–15
Amphetamine sulfate	Rx[a]	5–30
Dextroamphetamine sulfate (Dexedrine)	Rx[a]	5–30
Amphetamine/dextroamphetamine mixtures (Adderall)	Rx[a]	5–30
Benzphetamine (Didrex)	Rx[a]	25–150
Phendimetrazine (Prelu-2, Bontril, Plegine, X-Trazine)	Rx	70–105
Phentermine (Fastin, Oby-trim, Adipex-P, Ionamin)	Rx	15–37.5
Diethylpropion (Tenuate, Tenuate Dospan)	Rx	75
Mazindol (Mazanor, Sanorex)	Rx	1–3
Phenylpropanolamine (Accutrim, Dexatrim, others)	Removed from market	75
Ephedrine (various)	OTC/unlabeled use	20–60
Serotonergic Agents		
Fenfluramine (Pondamin)	Removed from market	60–120
Dexfenfluramine (Redux)	Removed from market	15–30
Fluoxetine (Prozac)	Rx/unlabeled use	60
Sertraline (Zoloft)	Rx/unlabeled use	200
Noradrenergic/Serotonergic Agent		
Sibutramine (Meridia)	Rx	5–15
Gastrointestinal Lipase inhibitor		
Orlistat (Xenical)	Rx	*360*

[a]High abuse potential, not recommended for routine use.

stimulating neurotransmitter release. Increases in blood pressure and mild bronchodilation are attributed to peripheral α- and β-receptor activation. The central nervous system (CNS) stimulant and addiction potential of amphetamine relative to other compounds has been described as amphetamine > methamphetamine > phentermine > mazindol > diethylpropion.[72] The powerful stimulant and addictive potential of the amphetamines relative to other available agents has resulted in their general avoidance for the treatment of obesity.[72,76]

Phentermine

Phentermine is structurally similar to amphetamine, but it has less severe CNS stimulation and a lower abuse potential. Its mechanism of action is related to enhanced norepinephrine and dopamine neurotransmission. Phentermine is available in both immediate-release and sustained-release formulations. However, the value of sustained-release formulations can be questioned based on the reported phentermine plasma half-life of 12 to 24 hours.[9] A single dose of 30 mg once daily in the morning provides effective appetite suppression throughout the day. Divided doses of 8 mg immediately prior to meals, however, are common. Doses above 30 mg daily do not improve effectiveness.[77] Evening or nighttime dosing should be avoided because of insomnia. Significant increases in blood pressure, palpitations, and arrhythmias can occur with phentermine administration. Use is not advisable in hypertensive patients and those with unstable cardiovascular function. The potential for hypertensive crisis with coadministration of phentermine and monoamine oxidase (MAO) inhibitors is noted in product labeling because of the documented cases of this syndrome seen with coadministration of amphetamine or noradrenergic derivatives and MAO inhibitors.[78] Similar warnings have been noted regarding concomitant use of tricyclic antidepressants, but this is less well documented.[79] With MAO inhibitors, a minimum washout time of 14 days prior to use of any adrenergic agent is suggested to avoid excessive adrenergic stimulation syndromes. Phentermine use is contraindicated in patients who are abusers of substances such as cocaine, phencyclidine, and methamphetamine, again because of the potential for excessive adrenergic stimulation syndromes and abuse potential. Mydriasis from adrenergic stimulation can worsen glaucoma, and patients diagnosed with glaucoma should not receive phentermine. Diabetic patients may experience altered insulin or oral hypoglycemic dosage requirements soon after beginning therapy and prior to any substantial weight loss.

Phentermine is an effective adjunct to diet, exercise, and behavior modification for producing weight loss in excess of that seen with placebo.[9,80] Intermittent phentermine therapy appears to elicit comparable weight loss when compared with continuous use.[81] However, most individuals experience weight regains during therapy and generally always after discontinuing use.[9] Despite its extensive off-label use in combination with the fenfluramine derivatives and the occurrence of cardiac valvulopathy, phentermine currently remains on the market as a short-term pharmacotherapy for obesity.

Mazindol

Although chemically distinct from amphetamines and phentermine, mazindol's tricyclic structure results in amphetamine-like appetite suppression. Direct stimulation of hypothalamic activity and norepinephrine reuptake inhibition are potential mazindol mechanisms.[82] Mazindol undergoes extensive hepatic metabolism, and approximately 50% of an administered dose is recovered in urine, mostly as conjugated metabolites. The pharmacokinetics of mazindol have not been described extensively; however, dosing is based on an elimination half-life of 10 hours.[9] Clinically, the drug is given once daily, 1 to 3 mg, prior to the morning or noon meal. However, some clinicians employ multiple small doses, 1 mg, given just prior to meals. Efficacy trials of single versus multiple daily doses are not available. Dry mouth commonly occurs with mazindol use, and difficulty with urination is possible. Mazindol use results in fewer CNS stimulant complaints than either phentermine or the amphetamines. Additionally, fewer cardiovascular adverse effects have been reported, and thus obese patients with mild to moderate hypertension may be treated with mazindol. Contraindications for use are similar to phentermine and include concurrent MAO inhibitors, glaucoma, symptomatic cardiovascular disease, and stimulant substance abuse. Mazindol has been noted to cause lithium toxicity with concurrent use.[83] Early studies in type 2 diabetic patients treated with mazindol demonstrated no need for changes in oral hypoglycemic therapy.[84] More recently, improved insulin sensitivity with mazindol treatment was documented using euglycemic clamp studies.[85] Caution and close monitoring of insulin or oral hypoglycemic dosage needs are advisable when treating obese diabetic patients with this therapy. Several placebo-controlled trials have demonstrated the effectiveness of mazindol as a short-term therapy for weight reduction.[9]

Diethylpropion

Diethylpropion stimulates norepinephrine release from presynaptic storage granules. Increased adrenergic neurotransmitter concentrations activate hypothalamic centers, which results in decreased appetite and food intake. This drug undergoes extensive first-pass hepatic metabolism. Active metabolites are eliminated renally and account for approximately 70% of administered dose. The elimination half-life of these metabolites is approximately 8 hours.[77] Less than 10% of the parent compound is recovered in urine. No specific dosing recommendations exist for use in patients with renal or hepatic insufficiency. Diethylpropion can be taken in divided daily doses, generally 25 mg three times daily before meals. An extended-release formulation is also employed by some clinicians, usually as 75 mg taken once daily in the morning or midmorning. Both dosing regimens are effective in achieving short-term weight loss in excess of placebo.[9] Complaints of insomnia increase if late afternoon dosing is used. Diethylpropion causes less CNS stimulation than mazindol and generally causes less insomnia than phentermine. Patients with severe hypertension or significant cardiovascular disease should not receive diethylpropion. However, it is one of the safest noradrenergic appetite suppressants, and its use has been recommended in patients with mild to moderate hypertension or angina pectoris.[86] Diabetic patients may experience decreased insulin or oral hypoglycemic dosage requirements soon after beginning therapy and prior to any substantial weight loss. More frequent blood glucose self-monitoring and medical follow-up are warranted when treating diabetic patients with diethylpropion.

Phenylpropanolamine

Although commonly classified as a noradrenergic anorexic, phenylpropanolamine (PPA) is atypical with regard to its mechanism and site of action. PPA racemates, D- and L-norephedrine, have chemical structures quite similar to amphetamine.[9] PPA has been used for many years as a constituent of over-the-counter appetite suppressants and various cough and cold preparations. However, because of persistent case reports of hemorrhagic stroke related to PPA exposure, the

U.S. Food and Drug Administration (FDA) and pharmaceutical manufacturers partnered to complete a case-control study known as the Hemorrhagic Stroke Project (HSP) during the 1990s. The final report of the HSP was submitted to the FDA in May 2000. In October 2000, the Nonprescription Drugs Advisory Committee discussed the HSP report and concluded that PPA is not safe for continued use. The FDA issued a public health warning in early November 2000 requesting that all manufacturers discontinue marketing of PPA-containing products.

A peer-reviewed publication based on the HSP report suggests that PPA in appetite suppressants and possibly cough and cold preparations appears to increase the risk of hemorrhagic stroke in women.[87] No increased risk was noted in men. Based on the accepted background prevalence of stroke and the odds ratios defined by the HSP report, Kernan and colleagues estimate that 1 woman may experience PPA-related stroke for every 107,000 to 3,268,000 women exposed to PPA appetite suppressants.[87] Despite the very low risk of hemorrhagic stroke, the FDA believes that a favorable risk-benefit no longer exists for any PPA-containing products. As such, PPA-containing products have either been reformulated without PPA or removed from the market in the United States.

Ephedrine

Chemically related to PPA (± norephedrine), ephedrine may be a viable obesity pharmacotherapy. It appears to suppress appetite and increase energy expenditure via release of presynaptic norepinephrine and direct stimulation of thermogenic β-adrenergic receptors.[88] The efficiency of ephedrine stimulation is somewhat blunted by physiologic feedback systems involving adenosine and various prostaglandins.[89] This notion has stimulated research to characterize the effect of ephedrine in the presence of adenosine and prostaglandin antagonists such as caffeine and aspirin.[90,91] Ephedrine in combination with caffeine has enhanced appetite suppression and thermogenesis as compared with placebo and other anorectics over time periods of up to 6 months.[69,88,92] Oral doses of 20 mg ephedrine and 200 mg caffeine up to three times daily have been studied.[93,94] The spectrum of side effects with ephedrine and ephedrine-caffeine combinations is similar to that seen with other noradrenergic agents. Side effects are more notable at higher doses and most commonly include tremor, agitation, nervousness, increased sweating, and insomnia; palpitations and tachycardia also have been reported. Patients with diabetes, hypertension, or cardiovascular disease (including arrhythmic conditions) should not self-medicate with ephedrine-containing products without evaluation by a qualified physician. Ephedrine is available both with and without a prescription; neither form is labeled by the FDA for use as an obesity therapy.[95,96]

SEROTONERGIC AGENTS

Serotonin is an important neurotransmitter involved in many human physiologic systems. Sleep-wake cycles, sensitivity to pain, blood pressure, mood, and eating behaviors have links to serotonin activity. Increasing central serotonin levels decreases the amount of food consumed and prolongs the time between food intake.[76] Some serotonergic agents increase central serotonin concentrations via stimulating release of presynaptic stores and/or inhibition of reuptake into storage granules. Additionally, either the parent compound or metabolites of these agents also may stimulate postsynaptic 5-HT receptors directly.[97] Peripheral serotonin effects that have an impact on appetite, such as slowing gastric motility, also have been described.[76] A major distinction between serotonergic and noradrenergic anorexiants is that serotonergic agents lack the central stimulant effects and thus the abuse potential seen with the noradrenergic compounds.[9,98] Conversely, decreased wakefulness, altered sleep patterns, and changes in affect can be seen.

Fenfluramine

Fenfluramine is an orally active racemic mixture (D,L-fenfluramine) that was used extensively as monotherapy for appetite suppression for many years. Fenfluramine increases synaptic serotonin concentration via reuptake inhibition and possibly by increasing serotonin release. An early double-blind, placebo-controlled trial in obese patients demonstrated that fenfluramine 20 mg three times daily had similar efficacy to daily phentermine 30 mg.[99] Average weight loss after 20 weeks of therapy ranged from 7.5 to 10 kg. Both medications were more effective than placebo, which attained 4.4 kg average loss.[99] Additionally, this trial was one of the first to include a treatment arm employing the combination of fenfluramine (30 mg prior to the evening meal) and phentermine (15 mg in the morning). Combination dosages were half that used in the monotherapy arms and achieved average weight loss of 8.5 kg with fewer reported side effects. Subsequently, Weintraub and colleagues completed classic placebo-controlled studies in a small cohort of obese patients that stimulated widespread interest and use of the combination of fenfluramine and phentermine (fen-phen) for weight management.[100–108] The combination provided, in most cases, enhanced anorexia with weight loss in excess of placebo.[9,109] Additionally, it appears that phentermine coadministration decreased some of the anxiety and confusion sometimes associated with fenfluramine.[98] Weight loss with this combination was associated with improvements in blood pressure, lipid profile, and glucose tolerance.[106,107,110] The long-term effectiveness of this combination was never clearly documented, and weight regain, while less than that lost, occurred during the second year of use in many patients.[110,111] Fenfluramine was withdrawn from worldwide markets in 1997 due to a relationship with cardiac valvular insufficiency and valvular structural abnormalities (see "Severe Adverse Effects" below).[73–75,112]

Dexfenfluramine

The D-isomer of fenfluramine was used extensively in Europe prior to its release in the United States in 1996. Dexfenfluramine increased synaptic serotonin concentrations via reuptake inhibition. Additionally, in vitro observations demonstrated that its metabolite, dexnorfenfluramine, directly stimulated 5-HT_{2C} receptors.[97] This compound was the first in the United States to receive labeling for chronic use. Dexfenfluramine was more effective than placebo in promoting weight loss as part of a program in conjunction with diet and exercise.[9,69] Additional effectiveness with the addition of phentermine also was noted with this agent.[113] As a derivative of fenfluramine, it also was removed from worldwide markets because of potential cardiac valve problems (see "Severe Adverse Effects" below).[75,114]

Antidepressants: Selective Serotonin Reuptake Inhibitors

It is interesting to note that some of the serotonergic appetite-suppressing agents were first studied as antidepressants and then noted subsequently to have effects on weight. As a class, the serotonin reuptake inhibitors generally are weight neutral as opposed to other commonly used compounds such as the tricyclic antidepressants.[32,115] The National Task Force on the Prevention and Treatment of Obesity has reviewed multiple randomized, double-blinded, placebo-controlled weight loss clinical trials using fluoxetine and one with sertraline.[71,116] Patients receiving fluoxetine (60 mg/day) demonstrate initial weight loss of up to 2 to 4 kg on average, but weight regain occurs despite continued medication use such that no difference is noted between fluoxetine and placebo over periods of up to 1 year.[117] Similar findings are noted using sertraline (200 mg/day) as an adjunct to help maintain weight lost with a very low calorie diet.[116] A direct relationship exists between amount of weight lost and the sum of fluoxetine and norfluoxetine plasma concentrations. Higher plasma concentrations are associated with greater weight loss.[118] The antidepressant serotonin reuptake inhibitors are not approved by the FDA as weight management agents and are not recommended currently for routine treatment of obesity.[71,72] Some practitioners continue to prescribe these agents for the treatment of obesity "off label" either alone or in combination with phentermine.[119] The safety and efficacy of phentermine-serotonin reuptake inhibitor combinations are currently unclear. A case report of adverse experiences (e.g., impaired mentation, tremor, hyperreflexia, and gastrointestinal symptoms) with unintentional concurrent use of phentermine and fluoxetine reinforces the need for caution by prescribers of unlabeled combination therapy.[120] Serious adverse effects such as primary pulmonary hypertension and cardiac valve abnormalities (see "Severe Adverse Effects" below) in excess of background prevalence have not been reported in relation to selective serotonin reuptake inhibitor (SSRI) use for obesity therapy.

NORADRENERGIC-SEROTONERGIC AGENTS

Sibutramine

An orally active racemic mixture, sibutramine, became available in the United States in early 1998. The parent compound and two active metabolites appear to increase synaptic concentrations of serotonin, norepinephrine (NE), and dopamine via reuptake inhibition. The active metabolites (M_1 and M_2) are more potent than the parent sibutramine. Reuptake inhibition appears to be greatest for NE, followed by serotonin, with dopamine the least inhibited. Sibutramine, M_1, and M_2 do not directly stimulate serotonergic (5-HT_1 or 5-HT_2), noradrenergic (α_1, α_2, β_1, β_2, β_3), or dopamine receptors.[121] It is thought that sibutramine induces weight loss by both decreasing appetite and maintaining or increasing thermogenesis via the combined effects on 5-HT and NE reuptake inhibition.[122] In humans, the degree to which these effects can be attributed to central versus peripheral activity is currently unknown. Sibutramine is subject to hepatic first-pass metabolism via cytochrome P450 3A4.[123] Moderate changes in sibutramine and/or metabolite disposition have been seen with ketoconazole coadminstration.[124] M_1 and M_2 area under the curve increased by 58% and 20%, respectively, with concurrent ketoconazole (200 mg twice daily for 7 days). Smaller changes have been noted with concurrent erythromycin and cimetidine. The active metabolites M_1 and M_2 exhibit elimination half-lives of 14 and 16 hours, respectively.[123,125] Further metabolism of the active metabolites results in conjugates that are eliminated renally. The pharmacokinetics of sibutramine allow for single daily oral dosing.

Sibutramine has been studied in clinical trials in doses from 1 to 30 mg daily and demonstrates a relatively clear dose-response relationship. Weight loss from daily doses of 1 mg is, on average, no different than from placebo. The recommended starting dose is 10 mg daily, with a recommended dose range of 5 to 15 mg daily. Dry mouth, anorexia, insomnia, constipation, appetite increase, dizziness, and nausea were noted two- to threefold more frequently in sibutramine-treated subjects than in placebo-treated subjects.[123,125] Significant increases in both systolic and diastolic blood pressure and pulse rate have been noted with sibutramine use.[123] Baseline blood pressure should be established prior to beginning therapy, and close monitoring is required when using this agent. Sibutramine product labeling indicates that it should not be used in patients with a history of coronary artery disease, stroke, congestive heart failure, or arrhythmias.[125] Like other centrally acting appetite suppressants, sibutramine should not be used in patients receiving MAO inhibitor therapies. Sibutramine is listed as a schedule IV prescription substance despite being noted as having no street value by recreational substance users.[121] Primary pulmonary hypertension has not been reported with sibutramine use. Echocardiographic assessments of a small cohort of patients from clinical trials with approximately 6 months exposure do not demonstrate the cardiac valve problems seen with the fenfluramine derivatives. Based on 12-month clinical trials, weight loss with sibutramine therapy appears to be most significant during the first 6 months of therapy. Twenty-nine percent of placebo-treated patients in these trials attained a 5% reduction in total body weight after 12 months.[125] Using sibutramine at 10–15 mg/day resulted in 56% and 65% of patients, respectively, achieving at least a 5% reduction in total body weight.[125] A 10% reduction in body weight was achieved by 8% of placebo-treated patients, whereas 30% and 39% of those taking sibutramine 10–15 mg/day, respectively, obtained this level of weight reduction. There is, on average, a tendency for weight regain after 6 months of treatment. As with other centrally active appetite suppressants, weight regain occurs with cessation of therapy.[126] Safety and efficacy beyond 1 year of exposure to sibutramine are currently uncertain.

LIPASE INHIBITORS

Orlistat

The percentage of dietary intake as fat has been implicated as a contributing factor in the development of obesity. Fat represents an extremely dense energy source, providing 9 kcal/g as compared with approximately 4 kcal/g from protein or carbohydrate. In humans, most of accumulated body fat excess is derived from dietary sources because of a limited capacity to synthesize fat from carbohydrate. Gastrointestinal (gastric, pancreatic, and carboxylester) lipases are essential in the absorption of the long-chain triglycerides commonly found in Western diets. Additionally, lipase is known to play a role in facilitating gastric emptying and secretion of other pancreaticobiliary substances.[127] Orlistat (Xenical, RO 18-0647) is a synthetic derivative of lipstatin, a natural lipase inhibitor produced by *Streptomyces toxyticini*. Orlistat is minimally absorbed and selectively inhibits gastrointestinal lipases.[128] Lipase inhibition results in decreased formation of free fatty acids from dietary triglyceride. Additionally, lower luminal free fatty acid concentrations result in malabsorption of cholesterol.[70] Orlistat induces weight loss by a persistent lowering of dietary fat absorption. Clinical studies employing orlistat as an adjunct to diet therapy demonstrated dose-dependent reductions in fat absorption. Pharmacodymanic modeling using early clinical trial data demonstrated half-maximal inhibition of fat absorption from orlistat doses of 98 mg/day, with maximal effects at around 400 mg/day.[129] Clinically, as much as a 30% reduction in fat absorption occurs with daily doses of 360 mg.[129,130] No additional decreases in fat absorption occur with doses above 400 mg/day.[129] The drug must be taken with foods that contain fat in order to exert its effect. However, varying either meal content with regard to fat-fiber ratio or timing of drug ingestion relative to meal demonstrated little effect on the inhibition of fat absorption.[131,132]

At least one gastrointestinal complaint (soft stools, abdominal pain/colic, flatulence, fecal urgency, or incontinence) is reported initially in up to 80% of individuals using orlistat.[133,134] These complaints are most common in the first 1 to 2 months of therapy, are mild to moderate in severity, and tend to improve with continued orlistat use. Orlistat in addition to a low-calorie diet over a 1-year time period resulted in a small cohort of obese subjects who maintained a 7% to 9% decrease in body weight as opposed to placebo-treated subjects, who experienced weight regain at 6 to 7 months of therapy.[135] Orlistat-induced malabsorption of fat-soluble vitamins has been documented.[135,136] Therefore, vitamin supplementation should be considered during therapy with this agent. Despite its definite effects on fat absorption and gastrointestinal motility, orlistat does not appear to change the pharmacokinetic or dynamic profiles of numerous other agents. Controlled studies of concurrent administration documenting minimal effects include oral contraceptives, digoxin, glyburide, phenytoin, pravastatin, warfarin, extended-release nifedipine, captopril, atenolol, furosemide, and ethanol.[128]

Results from a series of 1- to 2-year clinical trials indicate that this agent may prove to be an acceptable long-term medication supplement in medically supervised weight loss programs. A 1-year, randomized, double-blind, placebo-controlled trial of orlistat in obese type 2 diabetics was completed.[137] This trial demonstrated that prolonged use of orlistat results in significant sustainable weight loss with improvements in glycemic control and lipid profile. Additionally, a significant number of orlistat-treated diabetics either decreased or discontinued oral sulfonylurea therapy during and throughout the trial. A slowing of progression to the development of type 2 diabetes has been demonstrated by an analysis of data pooled from three randomized, double-blind, placebo-controlled multicenter clinical trials with orlistat.[138] Obese study participants showed a slower rate of progression to impaired glucose tolerance and type 2 diabetes when orlistat was added to conventional weight loss therapy.[138] In a 2-year study, orlistat-treated patients lost significantly more weight than placebo-treated patients after 1 year, and during the second year, orlistat therapy was associated with less weight regain than placebo treatment.[139] Orlistat use in addition to diet significantly promoted weight loss and less weight regain during another 2-year randomized, double-blind, placebo-controlled study.[140] In this study, in addition to weight loss, orlistat use was associated with improvements in lipid profile and a sustained reduction in fasting insulin levels. Finally, a 2-year randomized, double-blind, placebo-controlled multicenter study completed in a primary care setting demonstrated similar outcomes with respect to orlistat utility as a supplement to medically supervised weight loss.[141] Although unanimously recommended for approval by an FDA advisory committee in 1997, the FDA subsequently requested further information regarding the occurrence of breast cancer during clinical trials. An overall breast cancer incidence of 0.6% (nine cases, all female) was noted in the orlistat treatment versus 0.1% (one case, female) with placebo. In retrospect, evidence of malignancy prior to study participation was apparent in eight of the nine orlistat-treated patients. Clarification of this issue resulted in orlistat approval by the FDA in 1998 and its arrival in U.S. markets in 1999.

PEPTIDES

Multiple different endogenous peptides, which play a role in the regulation of food intake, have been identified in animals and humans. Leptin originates in the adipocyte and is proposed to function as a peripheral feedback messenger with respect to fat storage (discussed earlier in the chapter). NPY and galanin are two CNS peptides that appear to similarly stimulate food consumption but have differing effects on preference to carbohydrate or fat as well as substrate metabolism.[142] Currently, NPY and galanin are thought to exert minimal effects on protein intake, but a third, less well described CNS peptide, growth hormone-releasing factor, stimulates protein ingestion. Carbohydrate ingestion and use are related to NPY hypothalamic activity, specifically in the arcuate and medial paraventricular nucleus. Galanin activity, centering in the lateral paraventricular nucleus and medial preoptic areas, increases both carbohydrate and fat intake with preferential effects on fat consumption and utilization.[142] NPY enhances fat synthesis via increased respiratory quotient and use of carbohydrate. Galanin appears to slow energy expenditure. NPY and galanin modulate the release of insulin, corticosterone, and vasopressin, further affecting nutrient intake behaviors and substrate metabolism. NPY is associated with increased levels of insulin, corticosterone, and vasopressin, whereas decreases are seen with galanin.[142] The macronutrient intake, energy use, and endocrine effects of NPY are most consistent with those seen in chronic obesity. Future pharmacotherapies may develop based on knowledge of the effects of these endogenous peptides.

Currently, recombinant leptin has been administered subcutaneously to humans.[143] A phase I tolerability and dose-ranging study demonstrated some initial prospects for exogenous leptin administration. Participants were randomly assigned to receive either leptin or placebo and were given exercise and nutrition counseling. The placebo-controlled study was not designed to demonstrate efficacy, but preliminary data analysis of 165 male and female participants showed that 19% of placebo-treated patients versus 30% to 45% of leptin-treated subjects lost at least 2 kg over 28 days of study. Thirty obese participants remained on the study through 90 days of therapy. Not all the leptin doses studied elicited weight loss. Placebo-treated individuals lost an average of 1.5 kg, and subjects exposed to some of the leptin doses lost 2 to 4 kg. These potentially effective doses are being used in phase II trials involving obese patients with and without type 2 diabetes. Some study participants suffered local injection-site reactions, and systemic antibodies were detected at higher leptin doses in some patients. Second-generation leptin molecules are being developed to reduce injection-site reactions, which potentially will improve tolerability for higher doses.

HERBAL, NATURAL, AND FOOD SUPPLEMENT WEIGHT LOSS THERAPIES

Many individuals choose to undertake weight loss regimens without medical monitoring that incorporate the ingestion of herbal, natural, or food supplement products. It is important to remember that the FDA does not strictly regulate the manufacture and labeling of these products. Table 140–5 lists some of the common constituents found in many of these products.

CHROMIUM

The inclusion of chromium as an effective agent for weight loss is unclear. The hexavalent form of this trace element is thought to be *carcinogenic*, whereas the trivalent form found in human food sources is essentially nontoxic.[144] Chromium is considered an essential nutrient and experimentally in animals is an insulin cofactor active in carbohydrate, protein, and lipid metabolism.[144] In humans,

TABLE 140–5. Weight Loss Agents in Herbal, Natural, and Food Supplements[a]

Herbal/Natural/ Food Supplements	Active Moiety	Proposed Effect
Chromium picolinate	Chromium	Mechanism unclear
Ma huang	Ephedrine derivatives	Noradrenergic
St. John's wort	Hypericin	Serotonergic/MAO inhibition
White willow bark	Salicylate	Inhibit norepinephrine breakdown
Calcium pyruvate	Pyruvate	Mechanism unclear
Guarana extract	Caffeine	Noradrenergic
Various tea extracts	Caffeine	Noradrenergic
Garcinia gambogia extract (citrin)	Hydroxycitric acid	Mechanism unclear
Chitosan	Cationic polysaccharide	Block fat absorption

[a]Safety and efficacy not documented.

insulin resistance has been reported in a few cases of apparent severe chromium deficiency during long-term total parenteral nutrition (see Chapter 137). Currently, there is no reliable means of assessing total body chromium status, making diagnosis of deficiency difficult. The tryptophan metabolite, picolinic acid, forms a complex with trivalent chromium, which improves bioavailability. Food sources with highly available chromium include brewer's yeast, calf liver, American cheese, and wheat germ.[144] A double-blind, placebo-controlled study of chromium picolinate as a supplement to aerobic exercise in the treatment of obesity failed to demonstrate any effectiveness.[145]

MA HUANG

Ma huang is a traditional Chinese medicine manufactured from various plant parts of the *Ephedraceae* species. This species is known to produce L-ephedrine, D-pseudoephedrine, L-norephedrine, D-norpseudoephedrine, L-*N*-methylephedrine, and D-*N*-methylpseudoephedrine.[146] The FDA Center for Food Safety and Applied Nutrition completed an analysis of several products labeled as containing ma huang; ephedrine-type alkaloids were detected in concentrations ranging from 0–56 mg/g.[146] Although it is quite difficult to determine actual exposure to active entities when using ma huang, side effects and cautions would be similar to those listed earlier for ephedrine. Recently, the FDA proposed constraints on allowable ephedrine alkaloid concentrations and combinations with other stimulants such as caffeine in dietary supplements.[147] From 1994 through July 1997, the FDA received over 800 reports of serious adverse events, including seizures, stroke, and death, coincident with ephedrine-containing dietary supplement use. An in-depth review of 140 reports of adverse events related to ephedrine alkaloid-containing dietary supplements demonstrated that approximately half the reports involved cardiovascular symptoms.[148] These preparations probably are best avoided in patients with diabetes, hypertension, and other cardiovascular disease. The problem with many marketed products is the lack of consistency in labeling versus actual product content.

ST. JOHN'S WORT

A perennial flowering plant (*Hypericum perforatum*), St. John's wort has been employed as a medicinal herb for thousands of years. Its use in weight loss and herbal supplements probably is based on the proposed effects of its constituent naphthodianthrones (hypericin and pseudohypericin). These are thought to be inhibitors of MAO and would be expected to increase synaptic concentrations of monoamines such as serotonin and NE. Consistent with these assumptions, *Hypericum* extracts appear to be more effective than placebo in the treatment of depression.[149] However, in vitro studies have not been able to substantiate direct MAO inhibition at physiologic hypericin concentrations, and recognized antidepressant effects may be due to other constituents.[150,151] The risks of concurrent use of *Hypericum* derivatives and other adrenergic and serotonergic compounds have not been characterized. Currently, St. John's wort has not been studied with respect to its role in obesity management, and its safety and efficacy as a treatment modality in the self-management of obesity are unclear.

WHITE WILLOW BARK

White willow bark is a source of salicylate, a prostaglandin inhibitor. Prostaglandin inhibition may enhance adrenergic stimulation via inhibition of NE breakdown (see the earlier discussion of ephedrine).

GUARANA EXTRACT AND VARIOUS TEA EXTRACTS

Guarana and tea are sources of caffeine that have inherent adrenergic properties as well as increasing the effects of stimulant substances such as ephedrine or ephedra alkaloids (see the earlier discussion of ephedrine).

CHITOSAN

Chitosan is a cationic polysaccharide, specifically a partially *N*-deacetylated form of chitin. This nonhydrolyzable fiber exhibits properties similar to cellulose.[152] In vitro and preclinical data has indicated that chitosan may be effective in blocking absorption of fat from the gut. It has been suggested that orally administered chitosan may be an effective weight reduction agent by blocking calories ingested as fat. Chitosan is a major constituent in several heavily advertised weight management food supplements and over-the-counter preparations. However, a small number of properly randomized and blinded or open-label investigations currently demonstrate that orally administered chitosan is not an effective inhibitor of fat absorption in humans.[152–154] Additionally, head-to-head comparisons of chitosan versus orlistat have been completed. These investigations clearly demonstrate that orlistat blocks 30% to 40% of ingested fat versus negligible effects with chitosan.[155,156] While further research may be warranted with respect to the appropriate dose in humans needed to impair fat absorption, current claims of chitosan effectiveness in humans are unsubstantiated.

SEVERE ADVERSE EFFECTS

Severe adverse effects have been reported with almost all the appetite-suppressant agents discussed in this chapter. Because of combination use or multiple use patterns by many patients, it is often difficult to identify direct causal relationships. Therefore, all practitioners dealing with patients who are current users of or have been exposed to anorectic agents should maintain a high index of suspicion for the occurrence of severe adverse effects. Primary pulmonary hypertension and cardiac valvulopathy, discussed next, appear to occur most frequently with the use of fenfluramine derivatives.

PRIMARY PULMONARY HYPERTENSION

Primary pulmonary hypertension (PPH) is a condition in which high pressures of unknown etiology in the pulmonary vasculature result in increased right ventricular afterload. Various causal relationships have been suggested, including recent pregnancy, cocaine use, cirrhosis, genetic susceptibility, oral contraceptive use, and infection with the human immunodeficiency virus. Afflicted individuals have an impaired ability to increase cardiac output in response to exertion and can present with vague complaints of dyspnea, chest pains, and sometimes syncope. Progression of this disorder causes right-sided heart failure and death. About 50% of cases may remit spontaneously. In the unremitting cases, the condition responds poorly to medical management, and patients have a median survival from diagnosis of about 2.5 to 3 years. The estimated annual incidence of this condition is 1 to 2 cases per million population. In Europe during the 1960s, an increase in the incidence of PPH was noted during the same time period that an adrenergically active appetite suppressant, aminorex fumarate, was marketed. A return to the baseline incidence of PPH was observed after aminorex was removed from use. Overall, an increased risk of developing PPH appears possible with use of some of the noradrenergic and serotonergic appetite suppressants, either alone or in combination.[157–160] Specifically, the estimated odds ratio for occurrence of PPH with use of fenfluramine derivatives is stated as about 6 and possibly greater than 20 with use over 3 months.[159,160] The 20-fold increased PPH prevalence is similar to the rate of fatality from penicillin anaphylaxis (10–20/million exposures).[161] To date, PPH has not been identified as a problem with PPA, sibutramine, or the SSRI compounds.

CARDIAC VALVULOPATHY

Cardiac valve disease is known to occur coincident with serotonergic compounds (methysergide and ergotamine) and disease states (carcinoid disease) that result in systemic elevations of serotonin.[162,163] A form of cardiac valvular disease has been recognized coincident with the use of serotonergic appetite suppressants. Clinician investigators described 24 cases of symptomatic valvular heart disease in women, mean age 44 years, with no previous history of cardiac disease and a common association with exposure to the combination of fenfluramine-phentermine (fen-phen).[73] Cardiac ultrasonography demonstrated multivalvular regurgitation and abnormal valve morphology. Eight of the 24 patients demonstrated newly documented pulmonary hypertension with right ventricular systolic pressures ranging from 52 to 93 mm Hg. Mitral valve replacement was required in 5 of the 24 patients. Three of these five were exposed concurrently to SSRI or tricyclic antidepressant compounds. Average exposure to fen-phen was 11 months (range, 1–28 months). Subsequently, a prevalence study using echocardiography was performed in 233 appetite-suppressant-exposed patients and 233 control subjects matched for age, gender, and BMI.[75] A significantly increased prevalence of mostly aortic insufficiency was observed in the exposed patients who had been treated with dexfenfluramine alone, dexfenfluramine-phentermine, or fen-phen for an average of 20.5 months. The investigators found that 1.3% of control subjects versus 22.7% of exposed patients demonstrated mild or greater aortic insufficiency. This study demonstrated a highly significant risk for cardiac valve insufficiency with appetite-suppressant use (odds ratio 22.6; $P < .001$; 95% confidence interval 7.1–114.2). Fewer individuals demonstrated mitral or tricuspid insufficiency than the original case reports. Of note, this study demonstrates that the background prevalence of mild or greater aortic insufficiency in unexposed obese patients is similar to that of the general population under 50 years of age.

Three additional studies have reported risk estimates for this drug-related valvular insufficiency.[164–166] The differing study designs, populations, and duration of exposure can, in part, explain the variability of these risk estimates. Weissman and colleagues studied patients from a prematurely terminated, placebo-controlled dexfenfluramine treatment trial.[165] The average exposure to dexfenfluramine at the time of study termination was 2.5 months. Using cardiac ultrasound, they demonstrated a significantly higher prevalence of aortic insufficiency in those exposed (17%) versus those in the placebo arm (11.8%; $P = 0.03$).[155] A population-based follow-up study with nested case-control analysis by Jick and colleagues evaluated the prevalence of significant valve regurgitation in patients who used fenfluramine or dexfenfluramine for less than 3 months versus 4 or more months.[164] Those with 4 months or more of use demonstrated a significantly greater odds ratio (7.4; $P = 0.01$) for valve insufficiency. Two research groups have estimated the incidence of this drug-related disease by documenting valve disease prior to and after fenfluramine or dexfenfluramine exposure in small numbers of patients.[166,167] They reported a valve insufficiency incidence of 4% to 16.5% with periods of exposure of less than 1 year. Although a relationship between fenfluramine-like drug use and valve insufficiency seems certain, the exact incidence and possible risk factors for developing the problem are not well defined.[168,169] Two echocardiographic follow-up studies of patients approximately 1 year after stopping dexfenfluramine or fenfluramine use both demonstrated no significant progression of valve insufficiency and significant trends for improvement in valve function.[170,171]

Valvular insufficiency is not readily appreciated on physical examination in many patients with appetite-suppressant-related valvular disease but is detectable via cardiac ultrasonography. An understanding of risk factors, etiology, progression, and natural history of this drug-related valve disease is evolving. The U.S. Department of Health and Human Services has issued interim recommendations for health care providers to deal with this valvulopathy. These include antibiotic prophylaxis for some dental and surgical procedures depending on the degree of valve incompetence.[112] Most of the current research regarding this valvulopathy has centered around serotonergic pharmaceuticals. Interestingly, significant aortic insufficiency has been reported in women who have consumed "Chinese herbs" as part of a weight loss routine.[172] However, direct causal relationship with the herbal preparations is unclear because these weight loss routines also included use of fenfluramine and diethylpropion.[172]

SEROTONIN SYNDROME

Concern regarding the potential occurrence of the serotonin syndrome has been heightened with the ever-increasing number of serotonergic agents being employed in the treatment of obesity, depression, and migraine headache. The serotonin syndrome is defined by a spectrum of symptoms that develop coincident with the administration of multiple serotonergic agents.[173] Excess peripheral and central serotonergic stimulation may be involved, leading to a constellation of symptoms.[174] Specific diagnostic criteria include the presence of at least three of the following: fever, shivering, confusion, agitation, tremor, ataxia, hyperreflexia, sweating, or diarrhea. Although the syndrome generally is mild, severe episodes can include seizures, dyspnea, hypotension, hypertension, arrhythmias, renal failure, disseminated intravascular coagulation, and death. The syndrome occurs most commonly in patients consuming combinations of serotonergic agents. The largest number of reported cases center around MAO inhibitors taken concurrently with SSRIs, dextromethorphan, meperidine, and tricyclic antidepressants.[173] Case reports also include combinations of SSRIs with tryptophan, lithium, pentazocine, and dextromethorphan. Sumatriptan, a popular therapy for migraine headache, has been linked to syndrome development in a small number of patients who also were receiving an SSRI.[175] Interestingly, this review compiled a number of cases of SSRI-sumatriptan and MAO inhibitor-sumatriptan use without problems. No information regarding the safety of sumatriptan and noradrenergic or serotonergic obesity therapies was given. The apparent unpredictable nature of combination serotonergic therapy dictates extreme caution in these polypharmacy situations.

MONITORING THE PHARMACEUTICAL CARE PLAN

OUTCOME MEASURES

Specific weight goals should be established that are consistent with medical needs and patient personal desire. For most obese patients, a weight loss goal of 5% to 10% to no more than 30% of initial weight is reasonable. An average rate of weight loss after the first month of therapy is around 1 lb per week. Patients should not be allowed to attain weight less than their estimated ideal weight. Assessment of patient progress should be documented in a health care setting once or twice monthly for 1 to 2 months and then monthly thereafter.[72] Each encounter should document weight, WC, BMI, blood pressure, medical history, and patient assessment of obesity medication tolerability.[72] Chronic use of obesity medications should be consistent with the approved product labeling. Medication therapy should be discontinued after 3 to 4 months if the patient has failed to demonstrate weight loss or maintenance of prior weight. A recent AACE/ACE statement on obesity provides a patient evaluation checklist, a validated survey of general well-being, and sample informed consent that could be used in screening and follow-up of patients receiving obesity pharmacotherapy as part of a weight loss program.[72] The Short Form 36 (SF-36) also has been used as a quality-of-life evaluation tool for obese patients undergoing programmatic weight loss. Quarterly assessments of well-being and quality of life using validated assessment tools can be helpful in objectively quantifying the effectiveness of therapy as well as potential drug-induced side effects (e.g., depression).[72]

Diabetic patients receiving weight loss medication require more intense medical monitoring and self-monitoring of blood glucose. Some centrally acting weight loss agents, such as the serotonergic agents, have direct effects that immediately improve glucose tolerance, even prior to significant weight loss. Insulin therapy therefore may need to be adjusted with the start of obesity medication therapy. Peripherally active agents, such as orlistat, also have been shown to decrease oral hypoglycemic agent requirements in type 2 diabetic patients.[137] However, this effect was noted later in therapy and correlated more directly with weight loss. Some diabetic patients may require daily telephone contact with a health care provider to assist in adjusting their hypoglycemic therapy. Weekly patient visits to a health care setting may be necessary for 1 to 2 months until the effects of diet, exercise, and weight loss medication become more predictable. As frequent as quarterly assessment of hemoglobin A_{1c} may be appropriate in type 2 diabetics who lose weight to aid in adjustment of hypoglycemic therapy. Lipid profiles can normalize or improve with weight loss. Lipid status should be assessed semiannually or annually in patients with hyperlipidemia to determine need for continued hyperlipidemia therapies. Weight loss also can result in normalization of blood pressure in hypertensive obese patients. Assessment of appropriateness of antihypertensive therapy should occur with each follow-up visit.

PHARMACOECONOMIC CONSIDERATIONS

There are few data regarding economic consequences of treating obesity. One study evaluated the savings in prescription costs following a 12-week weight reduction program in 40 type 2 diabetic patients.[176] Patients lost an average of 33.7 lb over the study period. A cost analysis was completed on 32 of 40 patients who were taking antihypertensive and or antidiabetic medications using the out-of-pocket costs for these medications at the beginning of the study and after 1 year. The patients sustained a mean weight loss of 19.8 lb over the next year. The average cost of these prescriptions at the beginning as compared to the 1-year follow-up was $63.30 versus $32.50 per month. The estimated annual average saving in prescription costs per patient was $443. *Money* magazine caught consumer eyes with a 1997 article entitled, "Shrink Your Weight While Keeping Your Wallet Plump."[177] This analysis evaluated out-of-pocket expenses per pound lost for several different diet options, including Weight Watchers, Ultra Slim Fast, Redux (dexfenfluramine), Jenny Craig, and Optifast. Jenny Craig costs included purchase of food products, and Redux and Optifast costs included physician monitoring. Weight Watchers and Ultra Slim fast were lowest at $8 to $9 per pound lost, whereas Jenny Craig and Optifast came in high at $59 and $84, respectively, per pound lost. Redux fell in the middle at $28 per pound lost. Cost of side effects, quality-of-life parameters, and probability of long-term weight loss with the various products/services were not included in this analysis. A more objective assessment of costs related to orlistat use has been published based on data obtained from three peer-reviewed publications.[178] In this report from the United Kingdom, the cost utility of orlistat was estimated at £46,000 (approximately $75,000) per quality adjusted life year (QALY) gained. Sensitivity analysis from this report demonstrated variability in this estimate of £14,000 to £132,000 (approximately $23,000 to $215,200). The authors raised questions about the potential long-term value of pharmacotherapy for obesity.[178]

Finally, Martin and colleagues compared the costs associated with medical and surgical treatment of obesity.[179] Medical therapy groups received diet therapy only (no medications), and cost included weekly clinic visits for behavioral modification. A successful outcome was defined as loss of at least one-third of excess body weight above ideal body weight. They monitored all patients for 2 years and some for as long as 7 years so that long-term weight control could be addressed. As expected, the costs of surgery were much higher than medical therapy over the first 2 years ($24,000 versus $3000). However, when costs were extrapolated out to 6 years, the cost per pound lost for medical therapy exceeded surgical therapy (about $313 versus $261 per pound lost). It is clear from the preceding data that weight loss can be expensive for the consumer. Prospectively designed cost-benefit or cost-effectiveness analyses are needed to determine if costs of weight loss therapy or surgery are balanced by lower costs of hospitalizations for other medical problems associated with obesity or the additional life years gained. Quality-of-life measures also need to be taken into consideration when evaluating these types of data.

EVALUATION OF THERAPEUTIC OUTCOMES

An expert committee of the National Institutes of Health, Heart, Lung, and Blood Institute has completed and extensive summary of clinical guidelines for the assessment and treatment of obesity.[180] This report provides guidance with evidence-based, graded assessment and treatment recommendations from an extensive metaanalysis of the available obesity literature to date. The evaluation and management of a patient with obesity requires careful clinical, biochemical, and, if necessary, psychological evaluation. The evaluation must include an assessment of current medical conditions and medications the patient uses. Clearly, a multidisciplinary team including but not limited to a physician, nutritionist, psychologist, and pharmacist best achieves this. The algorithm in Figure 140–5 shows an approach to determining appropriate types of treatment for the overweight individual. The decision to treat any overweight/obese patient depends on the degree and distribution of obesity present, the motivation of the patient to lose weight, and the potential benefits and risks of weight loss. The initial step in this process should be to verify the presence of clinically significant excess body weight. In the clinical setting, this is done most often by measuring height, weight, and WC of the individual and calculating BMI. If the BMI is greater than 25 kg/m^2 and/or WC is greater than 40 inches for males or 35 inches for females, it is likely that the patient will benefit from weight loss. The next step is to assess whether the patient actually is motivated to lose weight. No matter what the treatment options are, they all require significant effort on the part of the patient to change lifestyle and comply with the management plan. If it is clear the patient is not yet ready to meet these expectations, then early counseling will reduce the chance of frustration for the patient, clinician, and in some cases other family members. This does not exclude the possibility of educating the

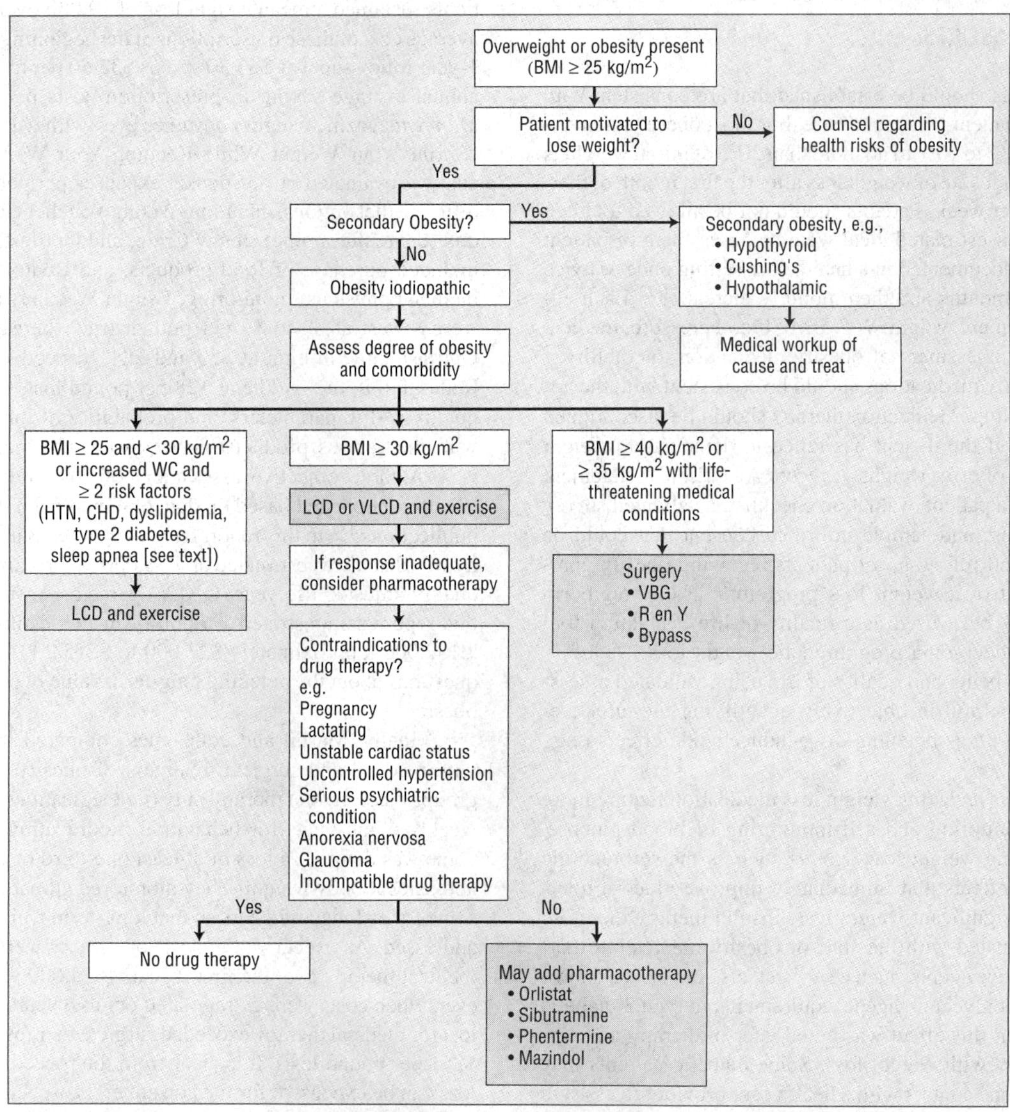

FIGURE 140–5. Pharmacotherapy treatment algorithm. A select population of individuals may benefit from medication therapy as an adjunct to a program of weight loss that includes diet, exercise, and behavioral modification. Increased WC >40 inches for males and >35 inches for females. (BMI = body mass index; CHD = coronary heart disease; LCD = low-calorie diet; VLCD = very-low-calorie diet; VBG = vertically banded gastroplasty; R en Y = Roux-en-Y; WC = waist circumference.)

patient about potential risks of obesity and the benefits of weight loss. This type of basic information in certain cases can lead to a significant change in motivation and desire to lose weight and improved compliance.

Pharmacotherapy may be appropriate for some overweight individuals (e.g., those with a BMI of 30 kg/m^2 or more without weight-related, immediate life-threatening medical conditions). It also should be considered for those with BMI of 27 kg/m^2 or more or an increased WC who have two or more risk factors. From the health care providers' perspective, drug therapy for obesity always should be considered as a supplement to an integrated program of diet, exercise, and behavior modification (including group support). A complete medical and medication history is essential in determining appropriate obesity drug therapy. Consideration must be given to alcohol, nicotine, caffeine, and herbal or food supplement use as well as prescription and nonprescription drugs.

CONCLUSIONS

The prevalence of obesity has increased dramatically in the latter part of this century. Obesity is determined by a combination of genetic and environmental factors. Epidemiologic studies provide evidence for a causative role of environmental factors in the development of obesity in those individuals who are genetically susceptible. Furthermore, there are clear differences in racial susceptibility to obesity and its complications such as diabetes. The precise role of genetic and environmental factors in the development is unknown. It is clear, though, that obesity is a lifelong condition. Currently, orlistat is the only pharmacotherapy available in the United States that has been demonstrated to be effective for up to 2 years in selected patients. Longer-term results will require further research. Weight regain occurs in the majority of individuals regardless of the therapeutic modalities used. Nevertheless, in recent years, increasingly effective treatments have been developed. These agents have augmented the role of lifestyle changes and diet and therefore serve a useful role as adjunct therapies for obesity.

Every patient seeking help for the management of obesity should be evaluated for secondary causes of obesity. Although a secondary cause is rare, it is important to identify and manage. Treatment of obesity needs to be individualized. It is important to consider factors such as patient desires, age, degree and duration of obesity, and the presence or absence of medical conditions both directly related to obesity and those which may have an impact on the therapeutic decisions. Whatever combinations of therapeutic modalities are used, it is clear that management is a lifelong process requiring patient support and careful monitoring for safety and efficacy.

▶ PRINCIPLES OF PHARMACOTHERAPY

- A sufficient degree of obesity (BMI $\geq$ 30 kg/m^2 and/or WC $\geq$ 40 inches for males or 35 inches for females, or BMI of 27–30 kg/m^2 with obesity risk factors) should be present before pharmacotherapy-facilitated weight loss is considered.
- Medication therapy for obesity is appropriate only as an adjunct to a regimen of diet, exercise, and behavioral modification.
- Concurrent use of noradrenergic and serotonergic obesity medications is contraindicated in the presence of MAO inhibitors, and extreme caution is needed with other serotonergic combinations.
- Exposure to some appetite suppressants (fenfluramine derivatives) can result in cardiac valve disease. Valvular insufficiency may improve after stopping exposure to drug.
- Obese individuals with concurrent diseases such as diabetes and hypertension require intensive monitoring when undertaking a weight loss program.
- Some herbal and food supplement diet agents contain sources of pharmacologically active substances that should be used with caution or avoided in obese patients with conditions such as diabetes, hypertension, and significant cardiovascular disease.
- The FDA does not regulate labeling of herbal and food supplement diet agents, and content is not guaranteed.
- There is a high probability of weight regain when obesity pharmacotherapy is discontinued.
- Safe and efficacious long-term obesity pharmacotherapy remains to be demonstrated.

REFERENCES

1. Horm J, Anderson K. Who in America is trying to lose weight? Ann Intern Med 1993;119:672–676.
2. Lovejoy JC, Smith SR, Bray GA, et al. A paradigm of experimentally induced mild hyperthyroidism: Effects on nitrogen balance, body composition, and energy expenditure in healthy young men. J Clin Endocrinol Metab 1997;82:765–770.
3. Williamson DF, Pamuk E, Thun M, et al. Prospective study of intentional weight loss and mortality in never-smoking overweight U.S. white women aged 40–64 years. Am J Epidemiol 1995;141:1128–1141[published erratum appears in Am J Epidemiol 1995;142(3):369].
4. Lissner L, Odell PM, D'Agostino RB, et al. Variability of body weight and health outcomes in the Framingham population. New Engl J Med 1991;324:1839–1844.
5. The painful business of losing weight. The Economist January, 1997; 45–47.
6. Rippe JM. Overweight and health: Communications challenges and opportunities. Am J Clin Nutr 1996;63:470S–473S.
7. Kassirer JP, Angell M. Losing weight: An ill-fated New Year's resolution. New Engl J Med 1998;338:52–54.
8. Stevens J, Cai J, Pamuk ER, et al. The effect of age on the association between body-mass index and mortality. New Engl J Med 1998;338: 1–7.
9. Bray GA, Greenway FL. Current and potential drugs for treatment of obesity. Endocr Rev 1999;20:805–875.
10. Kuczmarski RJ. Prevalence of overweight and weight gain in the United States. Am J Clin Nutr 1992;55:495S–502S.
11. Abraham S, Carroll MD, Najjar MF, Fulwood R. Obese and overweight adults in the United States. Vital Health Stat 1983;11:1–93.
12. McDowell A, Engel A, Massey JT, Maurer K. Plan and operation of the Second National Health and Nutrition Examination Survey, 1976–1980. Vital Health Stat 1981;1:1–144.
13. Metropolitan Life Insurance Company. Metropolitan height and weight tables. Stat Bull Metropol Life Insur Co 1983;64:2–9.
14. Williamson DF. Descriptive epidemiology of body weight and weight change in U.S. adults. Ann Intern Med 1993;119:646–649.
15. Wang ZM, Pierson RN Jr, Heymsfield SB. The five-level model: a new approach to organizing body-composition research. Am J Clin Nutr 1992;56:19–28.
16. Harsha DW, Bray GA. Body composition and childhood obesity. Endocrinol Metab Clin North Am 1996;25:871–885.
17. Bray GA. Topography of body fat. Adv Endocrinol Metab 1994;5: 297–322.
18. Kelley DE, Thaete FL, Troost F, et al. Subdivisions of subcutaneous abdominal adipose tissue and insulin resistance. Am J Physiol Endocrinol Metab 2000;278:E941–E948.

19. Pouliot MC, Despres JP, Lemieux S, et al. Waist circumference and abdominal sagittal diameter: Best simple anthropometric indexes of abdominal visceral adipose tissue accumulation and related cardiovascular risk in men and women. Am J Cardiol 1994;73:460–468.
20. Flier JS, Foster DW. Eating disorders: Obesity, anorexia nervosa, bulimia nervosa. In: Wilson JD, Foster DW, Kronenberg HM, Larsen PR, eds. Williams' Textbook of Endocrinology, 9th ed. Philadelphia, Saunders, 1998:1061–1097.
21. Bray GA. Overweight is risking fate: Definition, classification, prevalence, and risks. Ann NY Acad Sci 1987;499:14–28.
22. Kuczmarski RJ, Flegal KM, Campbell SM, Johnson CL. Increasing prevalence of overweight among U.S. adults: The National Health and Nutrition Examination Surveys, 1960–1991. JAMA 1994;272:205–211.
23. Abraham S, Collins G, Nordsieck M. Relationship of childhood weight status to morbidity in adults. HSMHA Health Rep 1971;86:273–284.
24. Guo SS, Roche AF, Chumlea WC, et al. The predictive value of childhood body mass index values for overweight at age 35 years. Am J Clin Nutr 1994;59:810–819.
25. Sorensen TI, Sonne-Holm S. Risk in childhood of development of severe adult obesity: Retrospective, population-based case-cohort study. Am J Epidemiol 1988;127:104–113.
26. Power C, Lake JK, Cole TJ. Body mass index and height from childhood to adulthood in the 1958 British-born cohort. Am J Clin Nutr 1997;66:1094–1101.
27. Garn SM, Clark DC. Trends in fatness and the origins of obesity Ad Hoc Committee to Review the Ten-State Nutrition Survey. Pediatrics 1976;57:443–456.
28. West DB. Genetics of obesity in humans and animal models. Endocrinol Metab Clin North Am 1996;25:801–813.
29. Hill JO, Peters JC. Environmental contributions to the obesity epidemic. Science 1998;280:1371–1374.
30. Lissner L, Levitsky DA, Strupp BJ, et al. Dietary fat and the regulation of energy intake in human subjects. Am J Clin Nutr 1987;46:886–892.
31. Baez M, Kursar JD, Helton LA, et al. Molecular biology of serotonin receptors. Obes Res 1995;3(Suppl 4):441S–447S.
32. Bloom FE. Neurotransmission and the central nervous system. In: Hardman JG, Gilman AG, Limbird LE, eds. Goodman and Gilman's: Pharmacologic Basis of Therapeutics, 9th ed. New York, McGraw-Hill, 1996:267–293.
33. Caro JF, Sinha MK, Kolaczynski JW, et al. Leptin: the tale of an obesity gene. Diabetes 1996;45:1455–1462.
34. Misra A, Garg A. Leptin, its receptor and obesity. J Invest Med 1996;44:540–548.
35. Makimura H, Mizuno TM, Roberts J, et al. Adrenalectomy reverses obese phenotype and restores hypothalamic melanocortin tone in leptin-deficient *ob/ob* mice. Diabetes 2000;49:1917–1923.
36. Giacobino JP. Role of the β_3-adrenoceptor in the control of leptin expression. Horm Metab Res 1996;28:633–637.
37. Considine RV, Sinha MK, Heiman ML, et al. Serum immunoreactive-leptin concentrations in normal-weight and obese humans. New Engl J Med 1996;334:292–295.
38. Barinaga M. New appetite-boosting peptides found. Science 1998;279:1134.
39. Woods SC, Seeley RJ, Porte DJ, Schwartz MW. Signals that regulate food intake and energy homeostasis. Science 1998;280:1378–1383.
40. DeLany JP, Lovejoy JC. Energy expenditure. Endocrinol Metab Clin North Am 1996;25:(4)831–846.
41. Roberts SB, Savage J, Coward WA, et al. Energy expenditure and intake in infants born to lean and overweight mothers. New Engl J Med 1988;318:461–466.
42. Fogelholm M, Kukkonen-Harjula K. Does physical activity prevent weight gain: A systematic review. Obesity Rev 2000;1:95–111.
43. Larsen PR, Davies TF, Hay ID. The thyroid gland. In: Wilson JD, Foster DW, Kronenberg HM, Larsen PR, eds. Williams' Textbook of Endocrinology, 9th ed. Philadelphia, Saunders, 1998:389–515.
44. Pi-Sunyer FX. Obesity. In: Bennett JC, Plum F, eds. Cecil Textbook of Medicine, 20th ed. Philadelphia, Saunders, 1998:1161–1168.
45. Clark MM, Pera V, Goldstein MG, et al. Counseling strategies for obese patients. Am J Prev Med 1996;12:266–270.
46. Bouchard C. The genetics of obesity. Boca Raton, FL, CRC Press, 1994:
47. Bouchard C, Perusse L, Leblanc C, et al. Inheritance of the amount and distribution of human body fat. Int J Obes 1988;12:205–215.
48. Comuzzie AG, Allison DB. The search for human obesity genes. Science 1998;280:1374–1377.
49. Garrow JS. Energy Balance and Obesity in Man, 2d ed. New York, Elsevier/North Holland Biomedical Press, 1978.
50. Lowell BB, Flier JS. Brown adipose tissue, β_3-adrenergic receptors, and obesity. Annu Rev Med 1997;48:307–316.
51. Vidal-Puig A, Solanes G, Grujic D, et al. UCP3: An uncoupling protein homologue expressed preferentially and abundantly in skeletal muscle and brown adipose tissue. Biochem Biophys Res Commun 1997;235:79–82.
52. Liu YL, Toubro S, Astrup A, Stock MJ. Contribution of β_3-adrenoceptor activation to ephedrine-induced thermogenesis in humans. Int J Obes Relat Metab Disord 1995;19:678–685.
53. Large V, Hellstrom L, Reynisdottir S, et al. Human beta-2 adrenoceptor gene polymorphisms are highly frequent in obesity and associate with altered adipocyte beta-2 adrenoceptor function. J Clin Invest 1997;100:3005–3013.
54. Clement K, Vaisse C, Manning BS, et al. Genetic variation in the beta 3-adrenergic receptor and an increased capacity to gain weight in patients with morbid obesity. New Engl J Med 1995;333:352–354.
55. Hubert HB, Feinleib M, McNamara PM, Castelli WP. Obesity as an independent risk factor for cardiovascular disease: A 26-year follow-up of participants in the Framingham Heart Study. Circulation 1983;67:968–977.
56. Manson JE, Colditz GA, Stampfer MJ, et al. A prospective study of obesity and risk of coronary heart disease in women. New Engl J Med 1990;322:882–889.
57. Garfinkel L. Overweight and cancer. Ann Intern Med 1985;103:1034–1036.
58. Messerli FH. Cardiovascular effects of obesity and hypertension. Lancet 1982;1:1165–1168.
59. Williamson DF, Thompson TJ, Thun M, et al. Intentional weight loss and mortality among overweight individuals with diabetes. Diabetes Care 2000;23:(10)1499–1504.
60. Diamanti-Kandarakis E, Zapanti E. Insulin sensitizers and antiandrogens in the treatment of polycystic ovary syndrome. Ann NY Acad Sci 2000;900:203–212.
61. Barnard RJ, Ugianskis EJ, Martin DA, Inkeles SB. Role of diet and exercise in the management of hyperinsulinemia and associated atherosclerotic risk factors. Am J Cardiol 1992;69:440–444.
62. Sacks FM, Svetkey LP, Vollmer WM, et al. Effects on blood pressure of reduced dietary sodium and the dietary approaches to stop hypertension (DASH) diet. New Engl J Med 2001;344:3–10.
63. Williamson DA, Perrin LA. Behavioral therapy for obesity. Endocrinol Metab Clin North Am 1996;25:943–954.
64. National Institute of Diabetes and Digestive and Kidney Diseases (NIDDK). Health Information, Nutrition and Obesity. Available at *http://www.niddk.nih.gov/health/nutrit/nutrit.htm.* Accessed October 1998.
65. Weight-Control Information Network. Available at *http://www.niddk.nih.gov/health/nutrit/win.htm.* Accessed October 1998.
66. Wadden TA, Stunkard AJ, Brownell KD. Very low calorie diets: Their efficacy, safety, and future. Ann Intern Med 1983;99:675–684.
67. Pi-Sunyer FX. Obesity. In: Shils ME, Olson JA, Shike M, eds. Modern Nutrition in Health and Diesease, 8th ed. Philadelphia, Lea & Febiger, 1994:984–1006.
68. Greenway FL. Surgery for obesity. Endocrinol Metab Clin North Am 1996;25:1005–1027.
69. Cerulli J, Lomaestro BM, Malone M. Update on the pharmacotherapy of obesity. Ann Pharmacother 1998;32:88–102.
70. Drent ML, van der Veen EA. Lipase inhibition: a novel concept in the treatment of obesity. Int J Obes Relat Metab Disord 1993;17:241–244.

71. National Task Force on the Prevention and Treatment of Obesity. Long-term pharmacotherapy in the management of obesity. JAMA 1996;276: 1907–1915.
72. Bray GA. AACE/ACE obesity statement. Endocr Pract 1997;3:163–208.
73. Connolly HM, Crary JL, McGoon MD, et al. Valvular heart disease associated with fenfluramine-phentermine. New Engl J Med 1997;337: 581–588 [published erratum appears in New Engl J Med 1997;337 (24):1783].
74. Graham DJ, Green L. Further cases of valvular heart disease associated with fenfluramine-phentermine. New Engl J Med 1997;337:635.
75. Khan MA, Herzog CA, St. Peter JV, et al. The prevalence of cardiac valvular insufficiency assessed by transthoracic echocardiography in obese patients treated with appetite-suppressant drugs. New Engl J Med 1998;339:713–718.
76. Noach EL. Appetite regulation by serotoninergic mechanisms and effects of D-fenfluramine. Neth J Med 1994;45:123–133.
77. Silverstone T. Appetite suppressants: A review. Drugs 1992;43:820–836.
78. Dawson JK, Earnshaw SM, Graham CS. Dangerous monoamine oxidase inhibitor interactions are still occurring in the 1990s. J Accid Emerg Med 1995;12:49–51.
79. Lasagna L. Safety. In: Lasagna L, ed. Phenylpropanolamine: A review. New York, Wiley, 1988:191–300.
80. Valle-Jones JC, Brodie NH, O'Hara H, et al. A comparative study of phentermine and diethylpropion in the treatment of obese patients in general practice. Pharmatherapeutica 1983;3:300–304.
81. Truant AP, Olon LP, Cobb S. Phentermine resin as an adjunct in medical weight reduction: a controlled, randomized, double-blind prospective study. Curr Ther Res Clin Exp 1972;14:726–738.
82. Angel I. Central receptors and recognition sites mediating the effects of monoamines and anorectic drugs on feeding behavior. Clin Neuropharmacol 1990;13:361–391.
83. Amdisen A. Lithium and drug interactions. Drugs 1982;24:133–139.
84. Sanders M, Breidahl H. The effect of an anorectic agent (Mazindol) on control of obese diabetics. Med J Aust 1976;2:576–577.
85. Nishikawa T, Iizuka T, Omura M, et al. Effect of mazindol on body weight and insulin sensitivity in severely obese patients after a very-low-calorie diet therapy. Endocrinol Jpn 1996;43:671–677.
86. American Medical Association. Drugs Used in Obesity. Chicago: American Medical Association, 1995:2439.
87. Kernan WN, Viscoli CM, Brass LM, et al. Phenylpropanolamine and the risk of hemorrhagic stroke. New Engl J Med 2000;343:1826–1832.
88. Astrup A, Breum L, Toubro S. Pharmacological and clinical studies of ephedrine and other thermogenic agonists. Obes Res 1995;3(Suppl 4): 537S–540S.
89. Dulloo AG. Ephedrine, xanthines and prostaglandin-inhibitors: Actions and interactions in the stimulation of thermogenesis. Int J Obes Relat Metab Disord 1993;17(Suppl 1):S35–S40.
90. Dulloo AG, Seydoux J, Girardier L. Paraxanthine (metabolite of caffeine) mimics caffeine's interaction with sympathetic control of thermogenesis. Am J Physiol 1994;267:E801–E804.
91. Dulloo AG, Seydoux J, Girardier L. Potentiation of the thermogenic antiobesity effects of ephedrine by dietary methylxanthines: Adenosine antagonism or phosphodiesterase inhibition? Metabolism 1992;41: 1233–1241.
92. Breum L, Pedersen JK, Ahlstrom F, Frimodt-Moller J. Comparison of an ephedrine/caffeine combination and dexfenfluramine in the treatment of obesity: A double-blind multicenter trial in general practice. Int J Obes Relat Metab Disord 1994;18:99–103.
93. Astrup A, Breum L, Toubro S, et al. The effect and safety of an ephedrine/caffeine compound compared to ephedrine, caffeine and placebo in obese subjects on an energy restricted diet: A double-blind trial. Int J Obes Relat Metab Disord 1992;16:269–277.
94. Astrup A, Toubro S, Cannon S, et al. Thermogenic synergism between ephedrine and caffeine in healthy volunteers: A double-blind, placebo-controlled study. Metabolism 1991;40:323–329.
95. Williams DM, Self TH. Asthma products. In: Covington TR, Berardi RR, Young LL, eds. Handbook of Nonprescription Drugs, 11th ed. Washington, American Pharmaceutical Association, 1996:157–177.
96. Tietze KJ. Cold, cough, and allergy products. In: Covington TR, Berardi RR, Young LL, eds. Handbook of Nonprescription Drugs, 11th ed. Washington, American Pharmaceutical Association, 1996:133–156.
97. Curzon G, Gibson EL, Oluyomi AO. Appetite suppression by commonly used drugs depends on 5-HT receptors but not on 5-HT availability. Trends Pharmacol Sci 1997;18:21–25.
98. Brauer LH, Johanson CE, Schuster CR, et al. Evaluation of phentermine and fenfluramine, alone and in combination, in normal, healthy volunteers. Neuropsychopharmacology 1996;14:233–241.
99. Weintraub M, Hasday JD, Mushlin AI, Lockwood DH. A double-blind clinical trial in weight control: Use of fenfluramine and phentermine alone and in combination. Arch Intern Med 1984;144:1143–1148.
100. Weintraub M. Long-term weight control: the National Heart, Lung, and Blood Institute funded multimodal intervention study. Clin Pharmacol Ther 1992;51:581–585 [published erratum appears in Clin Pharmacol Ther 1992;52(3):323].
101. Weintraub M, Sundaresan PR, Madan M, et al. Long-term weight control study: I (weeks 0 to 34). The enhancement of behavior modification, caloric restriction, and exercise by fenfluramine plus phentermine versus placebo. Clin Pharmacol Ther 1992;51:586–594.
102. Weintraub M, Sundaresan PR, Schuster B, et al. Long-term weight control study: II (weeks 34 to 104). An open- label study of continuous fenfluramine plus phentermine versus targeted intermittent medication as adjuncts to behavior modification, caloric restriction, and exercise. Clin Pharmacol Ther 1992;51:595–601.
103. Weintraub M, Sundaresan PR, Schuster B, et al. Long-term weight control study: III (weeks 104 to 156). An open- label study of dose adjustment of fenfluramine and phentermine. Clin Pharmacol Ther 1992;51: 602–607.
104. Weintraub M, Sundaresan PR, Schuster B, et al. Long-term weight control study: IV (weeks 156 to 190). The second double-blind phase. Clin Pharmacol Ther 1992;51:608–614.
105. Weintraub M, Sundaresan PR, Schuster B, et al. Long-term weight control study: V (weeks 190 to 210). Follow-up of participants after cessation of medication. Clin Pharmacol Ther 1992;51:615–618.
106. Weintraub M, Sundaresan PR, Cox C. Long-term weight control study: VI. Individual participant response patterns. Clin Pharmacol Ther 1992;51:619–633.
107. Weintraub M, Sundaresan PR, Schuster B. Long-term weight control study: VII (weeks 0 to 210). Serum lipid changes. Clin Pharmacol Ther 1992;51:634–641.
108. Weintraub M. Long-term weight control study: Conclusions. Clin Pharmacol Ther 1992;51:642–646.
109. Tuominen S, Hietola M, Kuusankoski M. Double-blind trial comparing fenfluramine, phentermine and dietary advice on treatment of obesity. Int J Obes 1980;14:138.
110. Hartley GG, Nicol S, Halstenson C, et al. Long-term results from phentermine, fenfluramine, diet, behavior modification, and exercise for treatment of obesity. Obes Res 1997;5:58S.
111. Spitz AF, Schumacher D, Blank RC, et al. Long-term pharmacologic treatment of morbid obesity in a community practice. Endocr Pract 1997;3:(5)269–275.
112. Cardiac valvulopathy associated with exposure to fenfluramine or dexfenfluramine: U.S. Department of Health and Human Services interim public health recommendations, November 1997. Morbid Mortal Week Rep 1997;46:1061–1066.
113. Khan MA, St. Peter JV, Hartley GG, et al. The effect of adding phentermine to weight management therapy in patients with declining response to dexfenfluramine alone. Obes Res 1997;5:22S.
114. Wisenbaugh T, Sinovich V, Dullabh A, Sareli P. Six month pilot study of captopril for mildly symptomatic, severe isolated mitral and isolated aortic regurgitation. J Heart Valve Dis 1994;3:197–204.
115. Fluoxetine (Prozac) and other drugs for treatment of obesity. Med Lett 1994;36:107–108.
116. Wadden TA, Bartlett SJ, Foster GD, et al. Sertraline and relapse prevention training following treatment by very-low-calorie diet: A controlled clinical trial. Obes Res 1995;3:549–557.

117. Goldstein DJ, Rampey AHJ, Enas GG, et al. Fluoxetine: A randomized clinical trial in the treatment of obesity. Int J Obes Relat Metab Disord 1994;18:129–135.
118. Goldstein DJ, Rampey AHJ, Roback PJ, et al. Efficacy and safety of long-term fluoxetine treatment of obesity: Maximizing success. Obes Res 1995;3(Suppl 4):481S–490S.
119. Anchors M. Fluoxetine is a safer alternative to fenfluramine in the medical treatment of obesity. Arch Intern Med 1997;157:1270–1270.
120. Bostwick JM, Brown TM. A toxic reaction from combining fluoxetine and phentermine. J Clin Psychopharmacol 1996;16:189–190.
121. Stock MJ. Sibutramine: A review of the pharmacology of a novel anti-obesity agent. Int J Obes Relat Metab Disord 1997;21(Suppl 1):S25–S29
122. Wales JK. The effect of fenfluramine on weight loss during restricted dietary regimes. Int J Obes 1980;4:127–132.
123. Knoll Pharmaceutical Company. Sibutramine hydrochloride monohydrate (Meridia) product information. Mount Olive, NJ, Knoll Pharmaceutical Company, 1997.
124. Preston PG, Ford MJ, Munro JF, Campbell DB. The variable response to fenfluramine in obesity. Int J Obes 1979;3:359–361.
125. Lean ME. Sibutramine: A review of clinical efficacy. Int J Obes Relat Metab Disord 1997;21(Suppl 1):S30–S36
126. Bray GA, Ryan DH, Gordon D, et al. A double-blind randomized placebo-controlled trial of sibutramine. Obes Res 1996;4:263–270.
127. Schwizer W, Asal K, Kreiss C, et al. Role of lipase in the regulation of upper gastrointestinal function in humans. Am J Physiol 1997;273: 612–620.
128. Guerciolini R. Mode of action of orlistat. Int J Obes Relat Metab Disord 1997;21(Suppl 3):S12–S23.
129. Zhi J, Melia AT, Guerciolini R, et al. Retrospective population-based analysis of the dose-response (fecal fat excretion) relationship of orlistat in normal and obese volunteers. Clin Pharmacol Ther 1994;56:82–85.
130. Hauptman JB, Jeunet FS, Hartmann D. Initial studies in humans with the novel gastrointestinal lipase inhibitor Ro 18-0647 (tetrahydrolipstatin). Am J Clin Nutr 1992;55:309S–313S.
131. Guzelhan C, Odink J, Niestijl Jansen-Zuidema JJ, Hartmann D. Influence of dietary composition on the inhibition of fat absorption by orlistat. J Int Med Res 1994;22:255–265.
132. Hussain Y, Guzelhan C, Odink J, et al. Comparison of the inhibition of dietary fat absorption by full versus divided doses of orlistat. J Clin Pharmacol 1994;34:1121–1125.
133. Tonstad S, Pometta D, Erkelens DW, et al. The effect of the gastrointestinal lipase inhibitor, orlistat, on serum lipids and lipoproteins in patients with primary hyperlipidaemia. Eur J Clin Pharmacol 1994;46:405–410.
134. Drent ML, Larsson I, William-Olsson T, et al. Orlistat (Ro 18-0647), a lipase inhibitor, in the treatment of human obesity: a multiple dose study. Int J Obes Relat Metab Disord 1995;19:221–226.
135. James WP, Avenell A, Broom J, Whitehead J. A one-year trial to assess the value of orlistat in the management of obesity. Int J Obes Relat Metab Disord 1997;21(Suppl 3):S24–S30.
136. Melia AT, Koss-Twardy SG, Zhi J. The effect of orlistat, an inhibitor of dietary fat absorption, on the absorption of vitamins A and E in healthy volunteers. J Clin Pharmacol 1996;36:647–653.
137. Hollander PA, Elbein SC, Hirsch IB, et al. Role of orlistat in the treatment of obese patients with type 2 diabetes: A 1-year randomized, double-blind study. Diabetes Care 1998;21:1288–1294.
138. Heymsfield SB, Segal KR, Hauptman J, et al. Effects of weight loss with orlistat on glucose tolerance and progression to type 2 diabetes in obese adults. Arch Intern Med 2000;160:1321–1326.
139. Rossner S, Sjostrom L, Noack R, et al. Weight loss, weight maintenance, and improved cardiovascular risk factors after 2 years treatment with orlistat for obesity. European Orlistat Obesity Study Group. Obes Res 2000;8:49–61.
140. Davidson MH, Hauptman J, DiGirolamo M, et al. Weight control and risk factor reduction in obese subjects treated for 2 years with orlistat: A randomized, controlled trial (See comments). JAMA 1999;281:235–242 [published erratum appears in JAMA 1999;281(13):1174].
141. Hauptman J, Lucas C, Boldrin MN, et al. Orlistat in the long-term treatment of obesity in primary care settings. Arch Fam Med 2000;9:160–167.
142. Lebowitz NE, Bella JN, Roman MJ, et al. Prevalence and correlates of aortic regurgitation in American Indians. J Am Coll Cardiol 2000;36:461–467.
143. Anonymous. Amgen announces leptin causes weight loss in humans and plans for two phase 2 trials. Available at *http://www.Amgen.com*, 1997.
144. National Research Council. Trace elements. In: Anonymous, ed. Recommended Dietary Allowances, 10th ed. Washington, National Academy Press, 1998:195–246.
145. Trent LK, Thieding-Cancel D. Effects of chromium picolinate on body composition. J Sports Med Phys Fitness 1995;35:273–280.
146. Betz JM, Gay ML, Mossoba MM, et al. Chiral gas chromatographic determination of ephedrine-type alkaloids in dietary supplements containing ma huang. J AOAC Int 1997;80:303–315.
147. FDA proposes constraints on ephedrine dietary supplements. Am J Health Syst Pharm 1997;54:1578
148. Effects of age, duration and treatment of insulin-dependent diabetes mellitus on residual beta-cell function: Observations during eligibility testing for the Diabetes Control and Complications Trial (DCCT). The DCCT Research Group. J Clin Endocrinol Metab 1987;65:30–36.
149. Linde K, Ramirez G, Mulrow CD, et al. St. John's wort for depression: An overview and meta-analysis of randomised clinical trials. Br Med J 1996;313:253–258.
150. Cott JM. In vitro receptor binding and enzyme inhibition by *Hypericum perforatum* extract. Pharmacopsychiatry 1997;30(Suppl 2):108–112.
151. Bladt S, Wagner H. Inhibition of MAO by fractions and constituents of hypericum extract. J Geriatr Psychiatry Neurol 1994;7(Suppl 1): S57–S59.
152. Kanauchi O, Deuchi K, Imasato Y, et al. Mechanism for the inhibition of fat digestion by chitosan and for the synergistic effect of ascorbate. Biosci Biotechnol Biochem 1995;59:786–790.
153. Pittler MH, Abbot NC, Harkness EF, Ernst E. Randomized, double-blind trial of chitosan for body weight reduction. Eur J Clin Nutr 1999;53: 379–381.
154. Stern JS, Gades MD, Halsted CH. Chitosan does not block fat absorption in men fed a high fat diet. Obes Res 2000;8:91S.
155. Guerciolini R, Radu-Radulescu L, Boldrin M, et al. Comparative evaluation of faecal fat excretion induced by orlistat and chitosan. Obes Res 2000;8:43S.
156. Lengsfeld H, Fleury A, Nolte M, et al. Effect of orlistat and chitosan on faecal fat excretion in young healthy volunteers. Obes Res 1999;7:50S.
157. Brenot F, Herve P, Petitpretz P, et al. Primary pulmonary hypertension and fenfluramine use. Br Heart J 1993;70:537–541.
158. Thomas SH, Butt AY, Corris PA, et al. Appetite suppressants and primary pulmonary hypertension in the United Kingdom. Br Heart J 1995;74:660–663.
159. Abenhaim L, Moride Y, Brenot F, et al. Appetite-suppressant drugs and the risk of primary pulmonary hypertension. International Primary Pulmonary Hypertension Study Group. New Engl J Med 1996;335:609–616.
160. McCann UD, Seiden LS, Rubin LJ, Ricaurte GA. Brain serotonin neurotoxicity and primary pulmonary hypertension from fenfluramine and dexfenfluramine: A systematic review of the evidence. JAMA 1997;278:666–672.
161. Chambers HF, Neu HC. Penicillins. In: Mandell GL, Bennett JE, Dolin R, eds. Principles and Practice of Infectious Diseases, 4th ed. New York, Churchill-Livingstone, 1995:233–246.
162. Redfield MM, Nicholson WJ, Edwards WD, Tajik AJ. Valve disease associated with ergot alkaloid use: Echocardiographic and pathologic correlations. Ann Intern Med 1992;117:50–52.
163. Robiolio PA, Rigolin VH, Wilson JS, et al. Carcinoid heart disease: Correlation of high serotonin levels with valvular abnormalities detected by cardiac catheterization and echocardiography. Circulation 1995;92: 790–795.
164. Jick H, Vasilakis C, Weinrauch LA, et al. A population-based study of appetite-suppressant drugs and the risk of cardiac-valve regurgitation. New Engl J Med 1998;339:719–724.

165. Weissman NJ, Tighe JFJ, Gottdiener JS, Gwynne JT. An assessment of heart-valve abnormalities in obese patients taking dexfenfluramine, sustained-release dexfenfluramine, or placebo. Sustained-Release Dexfenfluramine Study Group. New Engl J Med 1998;339:725–732.
166. Wee CC, Phillips RS, Aurigemma G, et al. Risk for valvular heart disease among users of fenfluramine and dexfenfluramine who underwent echocardiography before use of medication. Ann Intern Med 1998;129:(11)870–874.
167. Ryan DH, Bray GA, Helmcke F. et al. Echocardiographic abnormalities in patients treated with fenfluramine (F) or dexfenfluramine (D). Int J Obes 1998;22:-S77.
168. Devereux RB. Appetite suppressants and valvular heart disease. New Engl J Med 1998;339:765–766.
169. Parisi AF. Diet-drug debacle. Ann Intern Med 1998;129:(11)903–905.
170. Khan MA, St.Peter JV, Herzog CA, Vessey JT. Does the severity of appetite suppressant-related aortic valve insufficiency change over time after stopping exposure to drug? Circulation 2000;102:II-369.
171. Gardin JM, Weissman NJ, Leung CY, et al. One year echocardiographic follow-up of patients previously treated with phentermine-fenfluramine or dexfenfluramine. Circulation 2000;102:II–474.
172. Reginster F, Jadoul M, van Ypersele de Strihou C. Chinese herbs nephropathy presentation, natural history and fate after transplantation. Nephrol Dial Transplant 1997;12:81–86.
173. Sporer KA. The serotonin syndrome: Implicated drugs, pathophysiology and management. Drug Saf 1995;13:94–104.
174. Brown TM, Skop BP, Mareth TR. Pathophysiology and management of the serotonin syndrome. Ann Pharmacother 1996;30:527–533.
175. Gardner DM, Lynd LD. Sumatriptan contraindications and the serotonin syndrome. Ann Pharmacother 1998;32:33–38.
176. Collins RW, Anderson JW. Medication cost savings associated with weight loss for obese non-insulin-dependent diabetic men and women. Prevent Med 1995;24:369–374.
177. Shrink your weight while keeping your wallet plump. Money February, 1997; 162–167.
178. Foxcroft DR, Milne R. Orlistat for the treatment of obesity: Rapid review and cost-effectiveness model. Obes Rev 2000;1:121–126.
179. Martin LF, Tan TL, Horn JR, et al. Comparison of the costs associated with medical and surgical treatment of obesity. Surgery 1995;118: 599–606.
180. Clincal guidelines on the identification, evaluation, and treatment of overweight and obesity in adults: The evidence report. National Institutes of Health. Obes Res 1998;6(Suppl 2):51S–209S.

INDEX

Note: Page numbers followed by *f* refer to illustrations; page numbers followed by *t* refer to tables.

E

G

H

L

M

O

Q

S

T

W

X

Y

ISBN 0-07-136361-0
90000
9 780071 363617
DIPIRO/PHARMACOTHERAPY,5E